NELSON Textbook *of* Pediatrics

FOURTEENTH EDITION

RICHARD E. BEHRMAN, M.D.
Managing Director
Center for the Future of Children
David and Lucile Packard Foundation;
Clinical Professor of Pediatrics
Stanford University and UCSF;
Attending Physician
Lucile Salter Packard
Children's Hospital at Stanford
Stanford, California

Associate Editor
ROBERT M. KLIEGMAN, M.D.
Vice Chairman and Associate Director of Pediatrics
Rainbow Babies and Childrens Hospital
Cleveland, Ohio;
Professor of Pediatrics
Case Western Reserve University School of Medicine
Cleveland, Ohio

Senior Editors
WALDO E. NELSON, M.D.
Professor of Pediatrics
Medical College of Pennsylvania and
Temple University School of Medicine;
Attending Physician
St. Christopher's Hospital for Children
Philadelphia, Pennsylvania

VICTOR C. VAUGHAN III, M.D.
Clinical Professor of Pediatrics
Stanford University;
Attending Physician
Lucile Salter Packard
Children's Hospital at Stanford
Stanford, California

W. B. SAUNDERS COMPANY
Harcourt Brace Jovanovich, Inc.

Philadelphia London Toronto Montreal Sydney Tokyo

W. B. SAUNDERS COMPANY
Harcourt Brace Jovanovich, Inc.

The Curtis Center
Independence Square West
Philadelphia, Pennsylvania 19106

Library of Congress Cataloging-in-Publication Data

Nelson textbook of pediatrics / editor, Richard E. Behrman; associate editor, Robert M. Kliegman; senior editors, Waldo E. Nelson, Victor C. Vaughan, III.—14th ed.

p. cm.

Includes bibliographical references and index.

1. Pediatrics. I. Nelson, Waldo E. (Waldo Emerson). II. Behrman, Richard E. III. Kliegman, Robert M. IV. Title: Textbook of pediatrics. [DNLM: 1. Pediatrics. WS 100 N432]

RJ45.N4 1992 618.92—dc20 DNLM/DLC

ISBN 0-7216-2976-8 90-9181

French—Vol. I (*10th Edition*)—Doin Editeurs, S.A., Paris, France

French—Vol. II (*10th Edition*)—Doin Editeurs, S.A., Paris, France

Russian—(*12th Edition*)—Meditsina Publishing House, Moscow, U.S.S.R.

Indonesian—(*12th Edition*)—EGC Medical Publishers, Jakarta, Indonesia

Spanish—(*13th Edition*)—McGraw-Hill Interamericana de Espana, Madrid, Spain

Portuguese—(*13th Edition*)—Editora Guanabara-Koogan S.A., Rio de Janeiro, Brazil

Editor: Lisette Bralow
Designer: Paul Fry
Production Manager: Linda R. Garber
Manuscript Editors: Marjory I. Fraser and Ruth Low
Illustration Coordinator: Walt Verbitski
Indexers: Julie Figures and Angela Holt

Nelson Textbook of Pediatrics ISBN 0-7216-2976-8

Printed in the United States of America.

Last digit is the print number: 9 8 7 6 5 4 3 2 1

This edition is dedicated to Waldo E. Nelson, M.D., whose vision, wisdom, and constructive criticism over the years have contributed so much to the quality of care for children and to this textbook.

CONTRIBUTORS

Taro Akabane, M.D., Ph.D.
Chairman and Professor of Pediatrics, Shinshu University School of Medicine; Attending Physician, Shinshu University Hospital, Japan
CHAPTER 26: ENVIRONMENTAL HEALTH HAZARDS

James E. Arnold, M.D.
Assistant Professor of Otolaryngology–Head and Neck Surgery and Pediatrics, Case Western Reserve University School of Medicine; Director, Pediatric Otolaryngology, Rainbow Babies and Children's Hospital, Cleveland, Ohio
CHAPTER 14: THE RESPIRATORY SYSTEM

Stephen C. Aronoff, M.D.
Associate Professor, Departments of Pediatrics and Microbiology/Immunology, West Virginia University School of Medicine; Chief, Section of Allergy/Immunology/Infectious Diseases, West Virginia University Children's Hospital, Morgantown, West Virginia
CHAPTER 12: INFECTIOUS DISEASES
CHAPTER 26: ENVIRONMENTAL HEALTH HAZARDS

David M. Asher, M.D.
Medical Officer, Laboratory of CNS Studies, National Institute of Neurological Disorders and Stroke, National Institutes of Health, Bethesda; Instructor in Oncology and Pediatrics, Johns Hopkins University School of Medicine; Associate Staff, Johns Hopkins Hospital, Baltimore, Maryland
CHAPTER 12: INFECTIOUS DISEASES

John N. Aucott, M.D.
Assistant Professor, Division of Infectious Diseases, Case Western Reserve University School of Medicine; Divisions of Infectious Diseases and General Internal Medicine, Wade Park Veterans Administration Hospital, Cleveland, Ohio
CHAPTER 12: INFECTIOUS DISEASES

Victor H. Auerbach, Ph.D.
Senior Research Professor in Pediatrics, Temple University School of Medicine; Formerly Director of Laboratories, St. Christopher's Hospital for Children, Philadelphia, Pennsylvania
CHAPTER 8: METABOLIC DISEASES

Robert L. Baehner, M.D.
Chairman, Department of Pediatrics, University of Southern California School of Medicine; Physician-in-Chief, Childrens Hospital Los Angeles, Los Angeles, California
CHAPTER 11: IMMUNITY, ALLERGY, AND DISEASES OF INFLAMMATION

William F. Balistreri, M.D.
Dorothy M. M. Kersten Professor of Pediatrics, University of Cincinnati College of Medicine; Director, Division of Pediatric Gastroenterology and Nutrition, Children's Hospital Medical Center, Cincinnati, Ohio
CHAPTER 13: THE DIGESTIVE SYSTEM

Giulio J. Barbero, M.D.
Professor of Child Health, University of Missouri School of Medicine and University of Missouri Hospital, Columbia, Missouri
CHAPTER 6: GENERAL CONSIDERATIONS IN THE CARE OF SICK CHILDREN

Lewis A. Barness, M.D.
Visiting Professor of Pediatrics, University of Wisconsin and University of Wisconsin Hospital, Madison, Wisconsin; Professor of Pediatrics (on leave), University of South Florida College of Medicine, Tampa, Florida
CHAPTER 4: NUTRITION AND NUTRITIONAL DISORDERS

Richard E. Behrman, M.D.
Managing Director, Center for the Future of Children, David and Lucile Packard Foundation; Clinical Professor of Pediatrics, Stanford University and UCSF; Attending Physician, Lucile Salter Packard Children's Hospital at Stanford, Palo Alto, California
CHAPTER 1: THE FIELD OF PEDIATRICS
CHAPTER 9: THE FETUS AND THE NEONATAL INFANT
CHAPTER 12: INFECTIOUS DISEASES
CHAPTER 13: THE DIGESTIVE SYSTEM
CHAPTER 24: THE BONES AND JOINTS
CHAPTER 25: UNCLASSIFIED DISEASES

Jerry Michael Bergstein, M.D.
Professor, Department of Pediatrics, Indiana University School of Medicine; Director, Section of Nephrology, James Whitcomb Riley Hospital for Children, Indianapolis, Indiana
CHAPTER 18: THE URINARY SYSTEM AND PEDIATRIC GYNECOLOGY

James B. Besunder, D.O.
Assistant Professor of Pediatrics, Case Western Reserve University School of Medicine; Director, Pediatric Critical Care and Pharmacology, MetroHealth Medical Center, Cleveland, Ohio
CHAPTER 12: INFECTIOUS DISEASES

Charles D. Bluestone, M.D.
Professor of Otolaryngology, University of Pittsburgh School of Medicine; Director, Department of Pediatric Otolaryngology, Children's Hospital of Pittsburgh, Pennsylvania
CHAPTER 22: DISORDERS OF THE EYE AND EAR

Thomas F. Boat, M.D.
Professor and Chairman, Department of Pediatrics, University of North Carolina School of Medicine; Chief of Pediatrics, North Carolina Childrens Hospital, Chapel Hill, North Carolina
CHAPTER 14: THE RESPIRATORY SYSTEM

Laurence A. Boxer, M.D.
Professor of Pediatrics, University of Michigan School of Medicine; Director, Pediatric Hematology/Oncology, C. S. Mott Children's Hospital, Ann Arbor, Michigan
CHAPTER 16: DISEASES OF THE BLOOD

Philip A. Brunell, M.S., M.D.
Professor of Pediatrics, University of California, Los Angeles; Associate Director and Head of Infectious Diseases, Department of Pediatrics, Cedars Sinai Medical Center, Los Angeles, California
CHAPTER 12: INFECTIOUS DISEASES

Carrie Byington, M.D.
Resident, Department of Pediatrics, Baylor College of Medicine, Houston, Texas
CHAPTER 12: INFECTIOUS DISEASES

Hugo F. Carvajal, M.D.
Professor of Pediatrics and Surgery and Director, Pediatric Critical Care Unit, Department of Pediatrics, University of Texas Medical School, Houston, Texas
CHAPTER 6: GENERAL CONSIDERATIONS IN THE CARE OF SICK CHILDREN

James D. Cherry, M.D., M.Sc.
Professor of Pediatrics and Chief, Division of Infectious Diseases; Department of Pediatrics, University of California, Los Angeles School of Medicine; Attending Physician, UCLA Medical Center, Los Angeles, California
CHAPTER 12: INFECTIOUS DISEASES

Russell Wallace Chesney, M.D.
Le Bonheur Professor and Chair, Department of Pediatrics, The University of Tennessee, Memphis; Vice President for Academic Affairs, Le Bonheur Children's Medical Center, Memphis, Tennessee
CHAPTER 24: THE BONES AND JOINTS

J. Julian Chisolm, Jr., M.D.
Associate Professor of Pediatrics, Johns Hopkins University School of Medicine; Director, Lead Poisoning Prevention Program, Kennedy Institute for Handicapped Children; Staff Pediatrician, Johns Hopkins Hospital; Senior Staff Pediatrician, Francis Scott Key Medical Center, Baltimore, Maryland
CHAPTER 8: METABOLIC DISEASES
CHAPTER 26: ENVIRONMENTAL HEALTH HAZARDS

Thomas G. Cleary, M.D.
Professor of Pediatrics, University of Texas Medical School at Houston; Attending Physician, Hermann Hospital, L. B. Johnson Hospital, and M. D. Anderson Hospital, Houston, Texas
CHAPTER 12: INFECTIOUS DISEASES

Mary Lou Clements, M.D., M.P.H.
Professor and Head, Division of Vaccine Sciences, Department of International Health, Johns Hopkins University School of Hygiene and Public Health, Baltimore, Maryland
CHAPTER 12: INFECTIOUS DISEASES

David F. Clyde, M.D., Ph.D., D.T.M.&H.
Adjunct Professor, Johns Hopkins University School of Medicine; Research Professor of Medicine, University of Maryland School of Medicine, Baltimore, Maryland
CHAPTER 12: INFECTIOUS DISEASES

Paul M. Coates, Ph.D.
Research Professor of Pediatrics and Biochemistry, University of Pennsylvania School of Medicine; Research Director, Division of Gastroenterology, Nutrition and Lipid–Heart Research Center, The Children's Hospital of Philadelphia, Philadelphia, Pennsylvania
CHAPTER 8: METABOLIC DISEASES

A. W. Conn, M.D., B.Sc.(Med), F.A.C.A., F.R.C.P.(C), F.A.A.P.
Professor Emeritus, Department of Anaesthesia, Faculty of Medicine, University of Toronto; Chief Emeritus of Anaesthesia and Director Emeritus of Pediatric Intensive Care, Hospital for Sick Children, Toronto, Ontario, Canada
CHAPTER 6: GENERAL CONSIDERATIONS IN THE CARE OF SICK CHILDREN

James J. Corrigan, Jr., M.D.
Professor of Pediatrics, Section of Pediatric Hematology/Oncology, Vice Dean for Academic Affairs, Tulane University School of Medicine; Attending Physician, Tulane University Medical Center and Charity Hospital, New Orleans, Louisiana
CHAPTER 16: DISEASES OF THE BLOOD

Jean A. Cortner, M.D.
Professor of Pediatrics, University of Pennsylvania School of Medicine; Director, Lipid–Heart Research Center, The Children's Hospital of Philadelphia, Philadelphia, Pennsylvania
CHAPTER 8: METABOLIC DISEASES

Richard F. Dalton, Jr., M.D.
Associate Professor of Psychiatry and Pediatrics, Division of Child Psychiatry, Tulane University; Director of the Children's Neuropsychiatric Inpatient Unit, Tulane University Hospital, New Orleans, Louisiana
CHAPTER 3: GROWTH AND DEVELOPMENT

Franklin L. DeBusk, M.D.
Professor of Pediatrics, University of Florida College of Medicine; Attending Pediatrician, Shands Hospital, Gainesville, Florida
CHAPTER 25: UNCLASSIFIED DISEASES

Angelo M. DiGeorge, M.D.
Professor of Pediatrics, Temple University School of Medicine; Section of Endocrinology, Diabetes, and Metabolism, St. Christopher's Hospital for Children, Philadelphia, Pennsylvania
CHAPTER 19: THE ENDOCRINE SYSTEM

John J. Downes, M.D.
Professor of Anesthesia and Pediatrics, University of Pennsylvania School of Medicine; Director, Department of Anesthesiology and Critical Care Medicine, The Children's Hospital of Philadelphia, Philadelphia, Pennsylvania
CHAPTER 6: GENERAL CONSIDERATIONS IN THE CARE OF SICK CHILDREN

Nancy B. Esterly, M.D.
Professor of Pediatrics and Dermatology, The Medical College of Wisconsin; Head, Division of Dermatology, Children's Hospital of Wisconsin, Milwaukee, Wisconsin
CHAPTER 23: THE SKIN

Hugh E. Evans, M.D.
Professor of Pediatrics, New Jersey Medical School; Attending Staff, Department of Pediatrics, University Hospital, Newark; Consultant, Department of Pediatrics, St. Joseph's Hospital and Medical Center, Patterson, New Jersey
CHAPTER 12: INFECTIOUS DISEASES

James C. Fallis, M.D., F.R.C.S.(C)
Assistant Professor in Surgery and Pediatrics, University of Toronto; Past Director, Emergency Services, Past Chief, Division of Emergency Pediatrics, and Active Staff, Division of General Surgery, Hospital for Sick Children, Toronto, Ontario, Canada
CHAPTER 13: THE DIGESTIVE SYSTEM

Ralph D. Feigin, M.D.
Distinguished Service Professor and J. S. Abercrombie Professor and Chairman, Department of Pediatrics, Baylor College of Medicine; Physician-in-Chief, Texas Children's Hospital; Physician-in-Chief, Pediatric Services, Ben Taub General Hospital; Chief, Pediatric Services, The Methodist Hospital, Houston, Texas
CHAPTER 12: INFECTIOUS DISEASES

Kathleen M. Finta, M.D. (formerly Antishin)
Postdoctoral Fellow in Pediatric Cardiology, Department of Pediatrics, University of Michigan Medical Center, Ann Arbor, Michigan
CHAPTER 12: INFECTIOUS DISEASES

J. Pérez Fontán, M.D.
Associate Professor of Pediatrics, Yale University School of Medicine; Attending Pediatrician and Associate Director, Pediatric Intensive Care Unit, Yale/New Haven Hospital, New Haven, Connecticut
CHAPTER 14: THE RESPIRATORY SYSTEM

Marc A. Forman, M.D.
Professor of Psychiatry and Pediatrics and Director, Division of Child and Adolescent Psychiatry; Vice-Chairman, Department of Psychiatry and Neurology, Tulane University School of Medicine, New Orleans, Louisiana
CHAPTER 3: GROWTH AND DEVELOPMENT

Norman Fost, M.D., M.P.H.
Professor and Vice Chairman, Department of Pediatrics; Director, Program in Medical Ethics, University of Wisconsin; Attending Physician, University of Wisconsin Hospital, Madison, Wisconsin
CHAPTER 2: ETHICAL AND CULTURAL ISSUES IN PEDIATRICS

Welton M. Gersony, M.D.
Professor of Pediatrics, College of Physicians and Surgeons of Columbia University; Attending Pediatrician and Director, Division of Pediatric Cardiology, Babies Hospital, Columbia-Presbyterian Medical Center, New York, New York
CHAPTER 15: THE CARDIOVASCULAR SYSTEM

Ricardo Gonzalez, M.D.
Professor, Department of Urologic Surgery, and Director of Pediatric Urology, University of Minnesota; Attending Urologist, University of Minnesota Hospital, The Variety Club Childrens Hospital, and Minneapolis Childrens Medical Center, Minneapolis, Minnesota
CHAPTER 18: THE URINARY SYSTEM AND PEDIATRIC GYNECOLOGY

Samuel P. Gotoff, M.D.
Professor and Chairman of Pediatrics, Rush Medical College; Chairman, Department of Pediatrics, Rush–Presbyterian–St. Luke's Medical Center, Chicago, Illinois
CHAPTER 9: THE FETUS AND THE NEONATAL INFANT

N. Thorne Griscom, M.D.
Professor of Radiology, Harvard Medical School; Radiologist, Children's Hospital and Brigham and Women's Hospital, Boston, Massachusetts
CHAPTER 6: GENERAL CONSIDERATIONS IN THE CARE OF SICK CHILDREN

Mark A. Groshek, M.D.
Pediatrician, Kaiser Permanente Arapahoe Medical Center, Littleton, Colorado
CHAPTER 12: INFECTIOUS DISEASES

Gabriel G. Haddad, M.D.
Professor of Pediatrics and Director, Section of Respiratory Medicine, Department of Pediatrics, Yale University School of Medicine; Attending Physician, Yale–New Haven Hospital, New Haven, Connecticut
CHAPTER 14: THE RESPIRATORY SYSTEM
CHAPTER 25: UNCLASSIFIED DISEASES

Robert J. Haggerty, M.D.
Clinical Professor of Pediatrics, Cornell University Medical School; Pediatrician, New York Hospital, New York, New York
CHAPTER 5: PREVENTIVE PEDIATRICS AND EPIDEMIOLOGY

Scott B. Halstead, M.D.
Director, Health Sciences Division, The Rockefeller Foundation, New York, New York
CHAPTER 12: INFECTIOUS DISEASES

J. Richard Hamilton, M.D., F.R.C.P.(C)
Professor and Chairman, Department of Pediatrics, McGill University; Physician-in-Chief, Montreal Childrens Hospital, Montreal, Quebec, Canada
CHAPTER 13: THE DIGESTIVE SYSTEM

Robert H. A. Haslam, M.D., F.R.C.P.(C)

Professor and Chairman, Department of Pediatrics, and Professor of Medicine (Neurology), University of Toronto; Pediatrician-in-Chief, The Hospital for Sick Children, Toronto, Ontario, Canada

CHAPTER 20: THE NERVOUS SYSTEM

John J. Herbst, M.D.

Professor and Chairman, Department of Pediatrics, Louisiana State University at Shreveport; Chief of Staff, Pediatrics, Louisiana State University Medical Center, Shreveport, Louisiana

CHAPTER 13: THE DIGESTIVE SYSTEM

Kurt Hirschhorn, M.D.

Herbert H. Lehman Professor of Pediatrics and Chairman, Jack and Lucy Clark Department of Pediatrics, Mount Sinai School of Medicine; Pediatrician in Chief, Mount Sinai Hospital, New York, New York

CHAPTER 7: PRENATAL DISTURBANCES

Peter R. Holbrook, M.D.

Professor of Anesthesiology and Pediatrics, George Washington University School of Medicine; Chairman, Department of Critical Care Medicine, Children's National Medical Center, Washington, D.C.

CHAPTER 6: GENERAL CONSIDERATIONS IN THE CARE OF SICK CHILDREN

Lewis B. Holmes, M.D.

Professor of Pediatrics, Harvard Medical School; Pediatrician and Chief, Embryology-Teratology Unit, Massachusetts General Hospital, Boston, Massachusetts

CHAPTER 7: PRENATAL DISTURBANCES

Richard Hong, M.D.

Professor of Pediatrics, University of Wisconsin Medical School; Attending Physician, University of Wisconsin Hospital, Madison, Wisconsin

CHAPTER 11: IMMUNITY, ALLERGY, AND DISEASES OF INFLAMMATION

George R. Honig, M.D., Ph.D.

Professor and Head, Department of Pediatrics, University of Illinois College of Medicine, Chicago, Illinois

CHAPTER 16: DISEASES OF THE BLOOD

R. Rodney Howell, M.D.

Professor and Chairman, Department of Pediatrics, University of Miami School of Medicine; Pediatrician-in-Chief, Children's Hospital Center and University of Miami/Jackson Memorial Medical Center, Miami, Florida

CHAPTER 8: METABOLIC DISEASES

George Hug, M.D.

Professor of Pediatrics, University of Cincinnati College of Medicine; Director, Division of Enzymology, and Attending Physician, Children's Hospital Medical Center; Active Staff Member, University of Cincinnati Hospital, Cincinnati, Ohio

CHAPTER 8: METABOLIC DISEASES

David C. Johnsen, D.D.S., M.S.

Professor and Chairperson, Department of Pediatric Dentistry, Case Western Reserve University; University Hospitals of Cleveland, Cleveland, Ohio

CHAPTER 13: THE DIGESTIVE SYSTEM

Richard B. Johnston, Jr., M.D.

William H. Bennett Professor of Pediatrics, University of Pennsylvania School of Medicine; Senior Physician, The Children's Hospital of Philadelphia, Philadelphia, Pennsylvania

CHAPTER 11: IMMUNITY, ALLERGY, AND DISEASES OF INFLAMMATION

Kenneth Lyons Jones, M.D.

Professor of Pediatrics and Vice-Chairman for Education, Department of Pediatrics, University of California, San Diego, La Jolla; Director, California Teratogen Registry, UCSD Medical Center, San Diego, California

CHAPTER 7: PRENATAL DISTURBANCES

Niranjan Kanesa-thasan

Fellow, Department of Pediatrics, Divisions of General Pediatrics and Geographic Medicine, Case Western Reserve University, Cleveland, Ohio

CHAPTER 12: INFECTIOUS DISEASES

Edward L. Kaplan, M.D.

Professor of Pediatrics, School of Medicine, and Adjunct Professor (Epidemiology), School of Public Health, University of Minnesota; Attending Physician, University of Minnesota Hospital and Clinic, Minneapolis, Minnesota

CHAPTER 11: IMMUNITY, ALLERGY, AND DISEASES OF INFLAMMATION

Sheldon L. Kaplan, M.D.

Professor, Department of Pediatrics, Baylor College of Medicine; Chief, Infectious Disease Service, Texas Children's Hospital; Attending Physician, Ben Taub General Hospital, Houston, Texas

CHAPTER 12: INFECTIOUS DISEASES

James W. Kazura, M.D.

Professor of Medicine and Chief, Division of Geographic Medicine, Case Western Reserve University School of Medicine; Physician, University Hospitals of Cleveland, Cleveland, Ohio

CHAPTER 12: INFECTIOUS DISEASES

John A. Kirkpatrick, Jr., M.D.

Professor of Radiology, Harvard Medical School; Radiologist-in-Chief, Children's Hospital, Boston, Massachusetts

CHAPTER 6: GENERAL CONSIDERATIONS IN THE CARE OF SICK CHILDREN

Robert M. Kliegman, M.D.

Vice Chairman and Associate Director of Pediatrics, Rainbow Babies and Childrens Hospital; Professor of Pediatrics, Case Western Reserve University School of Medicine; Cleveland, Ohio

CHAPTER 6: GENERAL CONSIDERATIONS IN THE CARE OF SICK CHILDREN
CHAPTER 9: THE FETUS AND THE NEONATAL INFANT
CHAPTER 12: INFECTIOUS DISEASES
CHAPTER 13: THE DIGESTIVE SYSTEM

Richard D. Krugman, M.D.
Professor of Pediatrics and Acting Dean, University of Colorado School of Medicine; Director, C. Henry Kempe National Center for the Prevention and Treatment of Child Abuse and Neglect, Denver, Colorado
CHAPTER 3: GROWTH AND DEVELOPMENT

Margaret W. Leigh, M.D.
Associate Professor, Department of Pediatrics, University of North Carolina at Chapel Hill School of Medicine; Staff Physician, North Carolina Children's Hospital and University of North Carolina Hospitals, Chapel Hill, North Carolina
CHAPTER 25: UNCLASSIFIED DISEASES

Brigid G. Leventhal, M.D.
Associate Professor of Oncology and Pediatrics, Johns Hopkins University School of Medicine; Director, Clinical Research Administration, Johns Hopkins Oncology Center, Johns Hopkins Hospital, Baltimore, Maryland
CHAPTER 17: NEOPLASMS AND NEOPLASM-LIKE STRUCTURES
CHAPTER 25: UNCLASSIFIED DISEASES

Melvin D. Levine, M.D.
Professor of Pediatrics, University of North Carolina School of Medicine; Director, The Clinical Center for the Study of Development and Learning, University of North Carolina, Chapel Hill, North Carolina
CHAPTER 3: GROWTH AND DEVELOPMENT

Iris F. Litt, M.D.
Professor of Pediatrics, Stanford University School of Medicine; Director, Division of Adolescent Medicine, Department of Pediatrics, Stanford University Hospital and Lucile Salter Packard Children's Hospital at Stanford, Stanford, California
CHAPTER 3: GROWTH AND DEVELOPMENT
CHAPTER 10: SPECIAL HEALTH PROBLEMS DURING ADOLESCENCE

Adel A. F. Mahmoud, M.D.
Professor of Medicine and Molecular Biology and Microbiology, Case Western Reserve University; Physician-in-Chief, Department of Medicine, University Hospitals of Cleveland, Cleveland, Ohio
CHAPTER 12: INFECTIOUS DISEASES

Ameeta B. Martin, M.D.
Fellow, Pediatric Cardiology, Texas Children's Hospital, Baylor College of Medicine, Houston, Texas
CHAPTER 12: INFECTIOUS DISEASES

Lois J. Martyn, M.D.
Associate Professor of Ophthalmology and Associate Professor in Pediatrics, Temple University School of Medicine; Attending Ophthalmologist, St. Christopher's Hospital for Children, Philadelphia, Pennsylvania
CHAPTER 22: DISORDERS OF THE EYE AND EAR

Reuben H. Matalon, M.D., Ph.D.
Professor, Department of Biology, College of Health, Florida International University; Director, Research Institute, and Director of Genetics and Metabolism, Miami Children's Hospital, Miami, Florida; Professor, Department of Nutrition, University of Illinois, Chicago, Illinois
CHAPTER 8: METABOLIC DISEASES

Paul L. McCarthy, M.D.
Professor of Pediatrics, Yale University School of Medicine; Head, Section of General Pediatrics, Yale–New Haven Medical Center, New Haven, Connecticut
CHAPTER 6: GENERAL CONSIDERATIONS IN THE CARE OF SICK CHILDREN

Kenneth McIntosh, M.D.
Professor of Pediatrics, Harvard Medical School; Chief, Division of Infectious Diseases, Children's Hospital, Boston, Massachusetts
CHAPTER 12: INFECTIOUS DISEASES

Rima McLeod, M.D.
Professor of Medicine, Immunology and Microbiology, The University of Illinois at Chicago; Lecturer in Medicine and The Committee on Immunology, The University of Chicago, Pritzker School of Medicine; Attending Physician, Humana Hospital–Michael Reese, Chicago, Illinois
CHAPTER 12: INFECTIOUS DISEASES

Jack H. Medalie, M.D., M.P.H., F.A.A.F.P.
Dorothy Jones Weatherhead Professor of Family Medicine, Professor of Pediatrics, and Professor of Medicine, Case Western Reserve University School of Medicine; Active Staff, University Hospitals of Cleveland and Mount Sinai Medical Center, Cleveland, Ohio
CHAPTER 3: GROWTH AND DEVELOPMENT

Donald N. Medearis, Jr., M.D.
Charles Wilder Professor of Pediatrics, Harvard Medical School; Chief, Children's Service, Massachusetts General Hospital, Boston, Massachusetts
CHAPTER 12: INFECTIOUS DISEASES

Robert B. Mellins, M.D.
Professor of Pediatrics and Director, Pediatric Pulmonary Division, Columbia University College of Physicians and Surgeons; Attending Physician, Babies Hospital/Columbia-Presbyterian Medical Center, New York, New York
CHAPTER 25: UNCLASSIFIED DISEASES

Michael H. Merson, M.D.
Director, Global Programme on AIDS, World Health Organization, Geneva, Switzerland
CHAPTER 12: INFECTIOUS DISEASES

Richard A. Miller, M.D.
Assistant Professor of Medicine, University of Washington School of Medicine; Chief, Infectious Disease Division, Seattle Veterans Administration Medical Center, Seattle, Washington
CHAPTER 12: INFECTIOUS DISEASES

Robert W. Miller, M.D., Dr.P.H.
Clinical Professor of Pediatrics, Georgetown University; Chief, Clinical Epidemiology Branch, National Cancer Institute, Bethesda, Maryland
CHAPTER 26: ENVIRONMENTAL HEALTH HAZARDS

Thomas P. Monath, M.D.
Chief, Virology Division, U.S. Army Medical Research Institute of Infectious Diseases, Fort Detrick, Frederick, Maryland
CHAPTER 12: INFECTIOUS DISEASES

Edward A. Mortimer, Jr., M.D.
Elisabeth Severance Prentiss Professor of Epidemiology and Biostatistics and Professor of Pediatrics, Case Western Reserve University School of Medicine; Active Staff, University Hospitals of Cleveland and Cleveland Metropolitan General Hospital, Cleveland, Ohio
CHAPTER 5: PREVENTIVE PEDIATRICS AND EPIDEMIOLOGY

Hugo W. Moser, M.D.
Professor of Neurology, Johns Hopkins University School of Medicine; Active Staff, Kennedy Institute and Johns Hopkins Hospital (Neurology and Pediatrics), Baltimore, Maryland
CHAPTER 8: METABOLIC DISEASES

Betty A. Muller, M.D.
Associate Professor of Clinical Psychiatry and Training Director for Child Psychiatry, Tulane University School of Medicine, New Orleans, Louisiana
CHAPTER 3: GROWTH AND DEVELOPMENT

John F. Nicholson, M.D.
Associate Professor of Pediatrics and Pathology, College of Physicians and Surgeons, Columbia University; Director, Clinical Chemistry Service, and Associate Attending Pediatrician, The Presbyterian Hospital in the City of New York, New York, New York
CHAPTER 27: LABORATORY MEDICINE AND REFERENCE TABLES

Nadia Nogueira, M.D., Ph.D.
Adjunct Professor, Department of Molecular Parasitology, The Rockefeller University, New York, New York; Senior Associate Medical Director, Berlex Laboratories, Wayne, New Jersey
CHAPTER 12: INFECTIOUS DISEASES

Michael E. Norman, M.D.
Professor and Associate Chairman, Department of Pediatrics, Jefferson Medical College of Thomas Jefferson University, Philadelphia, Pennsylvania; Chairman of Pediatrics, Medical Center of Delaware, and Pediatrician-in-Chief, Alfred I. duPont Institute, Wilmington; Chairman of Pediatrics, Christiana Hospital, Newark, Delaware
CHAPTER 24: THE BONES AND JOINTS

Robert J. Nozza, Ph.D.
Assistant Professor, Otolaryngology, University of Pittsburgh School of Medicine; Director of the Audiology Center, Children's Hospital of Pittsburgh, Pittsburgh, Pennsylvania
CHAPTER 22: DISORDERS OF THE EYE AND EAR

Lee M. Pachter, D.O.
Assistant Professor, Department of Pediatrics, University of Connecticut School of Medicine; Associate Director, Pediatric Inpatient Services, St. Francis Hospital and Medical Center, Hartford, Connecticut
CHAPTER 2: ETHICAL AND CULTURAL ISSUES IN PEDIATRICS

Demosthenes Pappagianis, M.D., Ph.D.
Professor, Department of Medical Microbiology and Immunology, School of Medicine, University of California, Davis, Davis, California
CHAPTER 12: INFECTIOUS DISEASES

James M. Perrin, M.D.
Associate Professor of Pediatrics, Harvard Medical School; Director, Ambulatory Care Programs and General Pediatrics, Children's Service, Massachusetts General Hospital, Boston, Massachusetts
CHAPTER 3: GROWTH AND DEVELOPMENT

Michael A. Pesce, Ph.D.
Associate Professor of Clinical Pathology, Department of Clinical Pathology, Columbia University College of Physicians and Surgeons; Director of the Special Chemistry Laboratory, Columbia-Presbyterian Medical Center, New York, New York
CHAPTER 27: LABORATORY MEDICINE AND REFERENCE TABLES

Carol F. Phillips, M.D.
Professor and Chairman, Department of Pediatrics, University of Vermont College of Medicine; Chief, Pediatric Service, Medical Center Hospital of Vermont, Burlington, Vermont
CHAPTER 12: INFECTIOUS DISEASES
CHAPTER 26: ENVIRONMENTAL HEALTH HAZARDS

Stanley A. Plotkin, M.D.
Professor of Pediatrics and Microbiology, University of Pennsylvania School of Medicine; Professor of Pediatrics, Division of Infectious Diseases and Immunology, Children's Hospital of Philadelphia, Philadelphia, Pennsylvania
CHAPTER 12: INFECTIOUS DISEASES

Dwight A. Powell, M.D.
Associate Professor, Department of Pediatrics, The Ohio State University College of Medicine; Chief, Section of Infectious Diseases, Children's Hospital, Columbus, Ohio
CHAPTER 12: INFECTIOUS DISEASES

Albert W. Pruitt, M.D.
Ellington Charles Hawes Professor and Chairman, Department of Pediatrics, Medical College of Georgia; Chief of Pediatrics, Medical College of Georgia Hospital and Clinics, Augusta, Georgia
CHAPTER 15: THE CARDIOVASCULAR SYSTEM

Russell C. Raphaely, M.D.
Professor of Anesthesia and Pediatrics, School of Medicine, University of Pennsylvania; Director, Division of Critical Care Medicine; Associate Director, Department of Anesthesiology and Critical Care Medicine; and Director, Pediatric Critical Care Complex, The Children's Hospital of Philadelphia, Philadelphia, Pennsylvania
CHAPTER 6: GENERAL CONSIDERATIONS IN THE CARE OF SICK CHILDREN

Michael D. Reed, Pharm.D., F.C.C.P., F.C.P.
Associate Professor of Pediatrics, Case Western Reserve University School of Medicine; Attending Physician, Division of

Pediatric Pharmacology and Critical Care, Rainbow Babies and Children's Hospital, Cleveland, Ohio
CHAPTER 6: GENERAL CONSIDERATIONS IN THE CARE OF SICK CHILDREN

Jack S. Remington, M.D.
Professor of Medicine, Division of Infectious Diseases, Stanford University School of Medicine; Chairman, Department of Immunology and Infectious Diseases, Marcus A. Krupp Research Chair, Research Institute, Palo Alto Medical Foundation, Palo Alto, California
CHAPTER 12: INFECTIOUS DISEASES

Iraj Rezvani, M.D.
Professor of Pediatrics, Temple University School of Medicine; Chief, Section of Endocrine, Diabetes and Metabolism, St. Christopher's Hospital for Children, Philadelphia, Pennsylvania
CHAPTER 8: METABOLIC DISEASES

Luther K. Robinson, M.D.
Assistant Professor of Pediatrics, State University of New York at Buffalo, School of Medicine and Biomedical Sciences; Director of Dysmorphology and Clinical Genetics, The Children's Hospital of Buffalo, Buffalo, New York
CHAPTER 24: THE BONES AND JOINTS

Alan M. Robson, M.D., F.R.C.P.
Professor of Pediatrics, Louisiana State University School of Medicine and Tulane University School of Medicine; Medical Director, Childrens Hospital, New Orleans, Louisiana
CHAPTER 6: GENERAL CONSIDERATIONS IN THE CARE OF SICK CHILDREN

Barry H. Rumack, M.D.
Professor of Pediatrics, University of Colorado School of Medicine; Director, Rocky Mountain Poison and Drug Center; Attending Physician, University of Colorado Health Science Center, Denver General Hospital, and The Children's Hospital, Denver, Colorado
CHAPTER 26: ENVIRONMENTAL HEALTH HAZARDS

Robert A. Salata, M.D.
Assistant Professor of Medicine and International Health, Divisions of Infectious Diseases, Geographic Medicine, and General Medical Sciences, Case Western Reserve University School of Medicine; Attending Physician and Consultant, University Hospitals of Cleveland and the Cleveland Veterans Administration Medical Center; Director, Travelers' Healthcare Center, Cleveland, Ohio
CHAPTER 5: PREVENTIVE PEDIATRICS AND EPIDEMIOLOGY
CHAPTER 12: INFECTIOUS DISEASES

Joseph S. Sanfilippo, M.D.
Professor of Obstetrics and Gynecology, University of Louisville School of Medicine; Chief of Obstetrics and Gynecology, Norton and Kosair Childrens Hospitals, Louisville, Kentucky
CHAPTER 18: THE URINARY SYSTEM AND PEDIATRIC GYNECOLOGY

Harvey B. Sarnat, M.D., F.R.C.P.(C).
Professor of Paediatrics, Pathology, and Clinical Neurosciences, University of Calgary Faculty of Medicine; Attending Physician, Alberta Children's Hospital, Foothills Regional Provincial Hospital, and Calgary General Hospital, Calgary, Alberta, Canada
CHAPTER 21: NEUROMUSCULAR DISORDERS

Jane Green Schaller, M.D.
Professor and Chairman, Department of Pediatrics, Tufts University School of Medicine; Pediatrician-in-Chief, Floating Hospital for Infants and Children and New England Medical Center Hospitals, Boston, Massachusetts
CHAPTER 11: IMMUNITY, ALLERGY, AND DISEASES OF INFLAMMATION

Barton D. Schmitt, M.D.
Professor of Pediatrics, University of Colorado School of Medicine; Director of Consultative Services, The Children's Hospital, Denver, Colorado
CHAPTER 3: GROWTH AND DEVELOPMENT

Gloria L. Sellman, M.D.
Assistant Professor, Department of Anesthesiology, University of North Carolina School of Medicine; Attending Physician, North Carolina Memorial Hospital, Chapel Hill, North Carolina
CHAPTER 6: GENERAL CONSIDERATIONS IN THE CARE OF SICK CHILDREN

Barry Shandling, M.B., Ch.B., F.R.C.S.(Eng.), F.R.C.S.(C), F.A.C.S.
Associate Professor, Department of Surgery, University of Toronto; Senior Staff Surgeon, Hospital for Sick Children; Director, Bowel Clinic, Hugh McMillan Medical Centre; Consultant Surgeon, Sunnybrook Hospital and North York General Hospital, Toronto, Ontario, Canada
CHAPTER 13: THE DIGESTIVE SYSTEM

Jack P. Shonkoff, M.D.
Professor of Pediatrics, University of Massachusetts Medical School; Chief, Division of Developmental and Behavioral Pediatrics, University of Massachusetts Medical Center, Worcester, Massachusetts
CHAPTER 3: GROWTH AND DEVELOPMENT

David O. Sillence, M.B., B.S.(Syd.), M.D.(Melb.), F.R.A.C.P., F.R.C.P.A.
Professor of Medical Genetics, University of Sydney, Sydney; Head, Medical Genetics and Dysmorphology Unit, Children's Hospital, Camperdown, Australia
CHAPTER 24: THE BONES AND JOINTS

Joseph E. Simon, M.S., M.D.
Clinical Assistant Professor of Pediatrics, Medical College of Georgia; Medical Director, Pediatric Emergency Services, Scottish Rite Childrens Medical Center, Atlanta, Georgia
CHAPTER 6: GENERAL CONSIDERATIONS IN THE CARE OF SICK CHILDREN

R. Michael Sly, M.D.
Professor of Pediatrics, The George Washington University School of Medicine and Health Sciences, Chairman of Allergy and Immunology, Children's National Medical Center, Washington, D.C.
CHAPTER 11: IMMUNITY, ALLERGY, AND DISEASES OF INFLAMMATION

Rebecca Snider, M.D.
Dermatology Resident, Medical University of South Carolina, Charleston, South Carolina
CHAPTER 12: INFECTIOUS DISEASES

William T. Speck, M.D.
Gertrude Lee Chandler Tucker Professor and Chairman, Department of Pediatrics, Case Western Reserve University School of Medicine; Director of Pediatric Infectious Diseases, Rainbow Babies and Childrens Hospital, Cleveland, Ohio
CHAPTER 12: INFECTIOUS DISEASES
CHAPTER 26: ENVIRONMENTAL HEALTH HAZARDS

Mark A. Sperling, M.D.
Professor and Chairman, Department of Pediatrics, University of Pittsburgh School of Medicine; Pediatrician-in-Chief, Children's Hospital of Pittsburgh, Pittsburgh, Pennsylvania
CHAPTER 8: METABOLIC DISEASES

Lynn T. Staheli, M.D.
Professor of Orthopedic Surgery, University of Washington; Director, Department of Orthopedics, Children's Hospital and Medical Center, Seattle, Washington
CHAPTER 24: THE BONES AND JOINTS

Charles A. Stanley, M.D.
Professor of Pediatrics, University of Pennsylvania School of Medicine; Senior Endocrinologist, The Children's Hospital of Philadelphia, Philadelphia, Pennsylvania
CHAPTER 8: METABOLIC DISEASES

Robert C. Stern, M.D.
Professor of Pediatrics, Case Western Reserve University School of Medicine; Associate Pediatrician, Rainbow Babies and Childrens Hospital, Cleveland, Ohio
CHAPTER 14: THE RESPIRATORY SYSTEM

James A. Stockman, III, M.D.
Professor and Chairman, Department of Pediatrics, Northwestern University Medical School; Centennial Professor and Chairman of Medicine, Childrens Memorial Hospital, Chicago, Illinois
CHAPTER 16: DISEASES OF THE BLOOD

Marshall L. Stoller, M.D.
Assistant Professor and Director, Urinary Stone Center, Department of Urology, University of California at San Francisco, San Francisco, California
CHAPTER 12: INFECTIOUS DISEASES

Frederick J. Suchy, M.D.
Professor of Pediatrics, Yale University School of Medicine; Chief, Pediatric Gastroenterology/Hepatology Section, Yale–New Haven Hospital; Attending Physician, Yale–New Haven Hospital and Children's Hospital, New Haven, Connecticut
CHAPTER 13: THE DIGESTIVE SYSTEM

Robert W. Sugerman, M.D.
Pediatric Resident, Department of Pediatrics, University of Cincinnati College of Medicine, Cincinnati, Ohio
CHAPTER 12: INFECTIOUS DISEASES

Andrew M. Tershakovec, M.D.
Assistant Professor, Department of Pediatrics, University of Pennsylvania School of Medicine; Assistant Physician, Division of Gastroenterology and Nutrition, The Children's Hospital of Philadelphia, Philadelphia, Pennsylvania
CHAPTER 8: METABOLIC DISEASES

Philip Toltzis, M.D.
Assistant Professor, Department of Pediatrics, Case Western Reserve University School of Medicine; Attending Physician, Pediatric Infectious Diseases, Rainbow Babies and Childrens Hospital, Cleveland, Ohio
CHAPTER 12: INFECTIOUS DISEASES

Victor C. Vaughan III, M.D.
Clinical Professor of Pediatrics, Stanford University School of Medicine; Attending Physician, Lucile Salter Packard Children's Hospital at Stanford, Stanford, California
CHAPTER 3: GROWTH AND DEVELOPMENT

Steven L. Werlin, M.D.
Professor of Pediatrics, Medical College of Wisconsin; Director, Division of Gastroenterology, Department of Pediatrics, Medical College of Wisconsin, Milwaukee, Wisconsin
CHAPTER 13: THE DIGESTIVE SYSTEM

Robert E. Wood, Ph.D., M.D.
Professor of Pediatrics, University of North Carolina School of Medicine; Chief, Pediatric Pulmonary Medicine, University of North Carolina Children's Hospital, Chapel Hill, North Carolina
CHAPTER 14: THE RESPIRATORY SYSTEM

David J. Wyler, M.D.
Professor of Medicine and of Molecular Biology and Microbiology, Tufts University School of Medicine; Physician, New England Medical Center Hospitals; Director, Travelers' Health Service, New England Medical Center, Boston, Massachusetts
CHAPTER 12: INFECTIOUS DISEASES

Michael A. Zasloff, M.D., Ph.D.
Charles E. H. Upham Professor of Pediatrics, University of Pennsylvania School of Medicine; Chief, Division of Human Genetics and Molecular Biology, The Children's Hospital of Philadelphia, Philadelphia, Pennsylvania
CHAPTER 7: PRENATAL DISTURBANCES

PREFACE

The publication of the Fourteenth Edition of *Nelson Textbook of Pediatrics* comes at a time of significant advance in the application of molecular biology, genetics, and cell biology to understanding health and disease in children and to the development of new prevention and treatment modalities. However, it also occurs at a time when the circumstances of many children are desperate in terms of the incidence of preventable deaths and disabilities and the loss of opportunity to fulfill their potential as healthy, productive, and happy adults.

The editors of this textbook continue their commitment to provide a comprehensive, concise, and current one-volume edition, addressing the full range of problems related to the health and welfare of children that are faced by practitioners, house staff, and medical students. We have tried to do this in a manner that encompasses both the science and art of pediatrics.

This edition represents a major revision based on a complete review of the field of pediatrics and includes many new sections and substantial modification and expansion of others, in terms of understanding, diagnosis, and treatment. Practically no area of the book has been left untouched and, we hope, no section unimproved. Although to an affected child and family even the rarest disorder is of vital importance, it is not possible to cover all health problems in the same degree of detail in a general textbook of pediatrics. Therefore, leading articles and subspecialty texts are included in the references and should be consulted when more information is desired. This textbook reflects the hard work, thought, and energy of our contributors to achieve completeness, relevance, and conciseness. We are indebted to their efforts aimed at producing an edition that we hope will continue to be helpful to persons caring for children or to those wishing to know more about them.

Since the last edition, we have lost *one* contributor through death. The participation of Harold Harrison is greatly missed.

In this edition we have had informal assistance from faculty and house staff of the Department of Pediatrics at Stanford and Case Western Reserve Universities. The help of these individuals and the numerous pediatricians elsewhere in the United States and around the world who have taken the time to offer thoughtful suggestions is greatly appreciated.

We especially wish to express our heartfelt thanks to Ann Behrman and Sharon Kliegman for their patience, understanding, and help, without which this textbook would not have been possible.

RICHARD E. BEHRMAN, M.D.
ROBERT M. KLIEGMAN, M.D.

CONTENTS

12

13

15

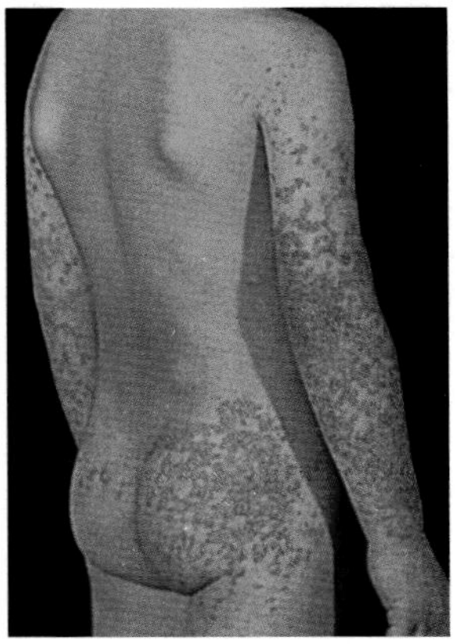

Figure 11–20. Henoch-Schönlein purpura (anaphylactoid purpura). (From Korting GW: Hautkrankheiten bei Kindern und Jugendlichen, 3rd ed. Stuttgart, Germany, FK Schattauer Verlag, 1982.)

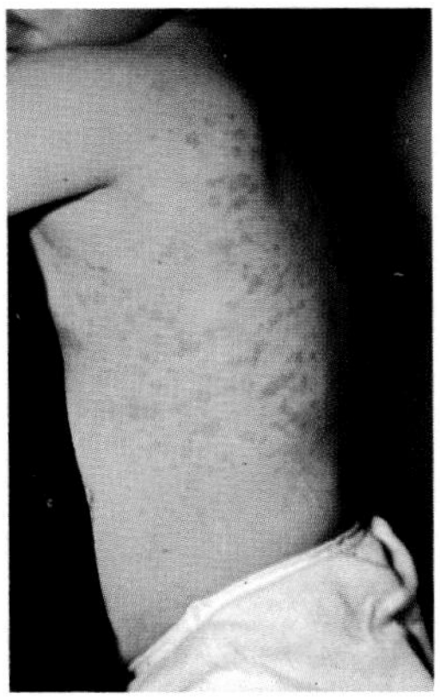

Figure 11–14. Rash of rheumatoid arthritis.

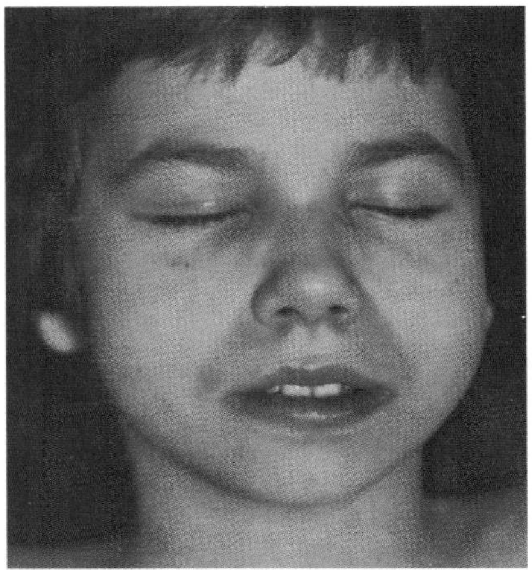

Figure 11–21. The facial rash of dermatomyositis. Note the faint erythema over the bridge of the nose and malar areas and the heliotropic discoloration of the upper eyelids.

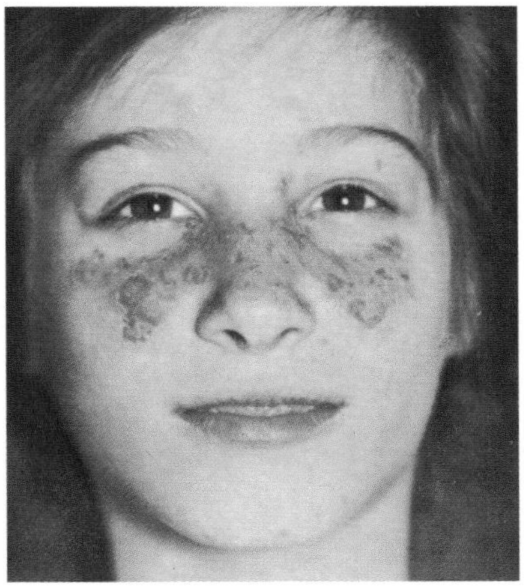

Figure 11–19. The butterfly rash of systemic lupus erythematosus.

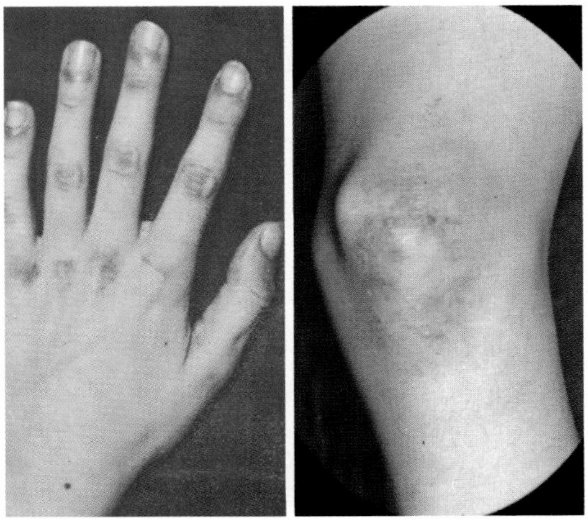

Figure 11–22. Rash of dermatomyositis. Note the skin changes over the knuckles *(left)* and over the knee *(right)*.

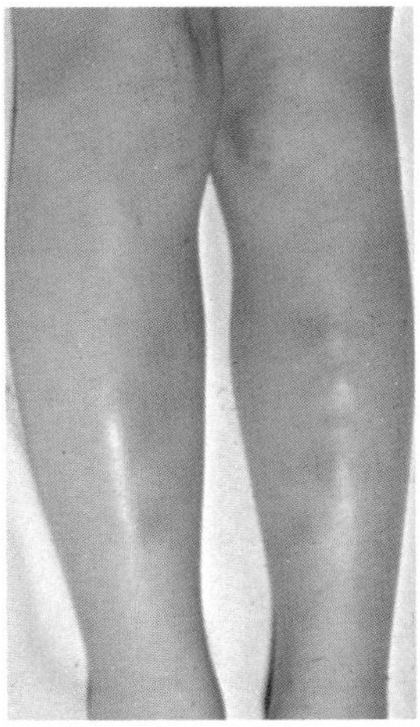

Figure 11–24. Erythema nodosum.

COLOR PLATES

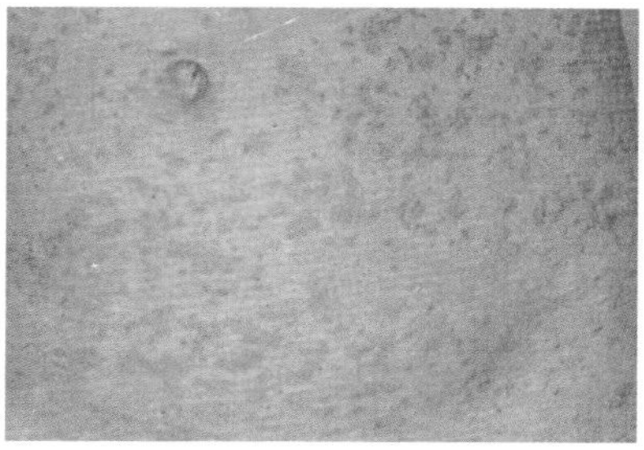

Figure 12–12. Maculopapular rash of measles. (From Korting GW: Hautkrankheiten bei Kindern und Jugendlichen, 3rd ed. Stuttgart, Germany, FK Schattauer Verlag, 1982.)

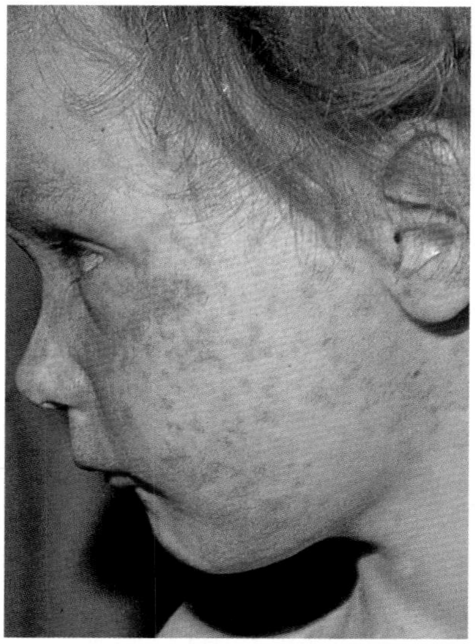

Figure 12–14. Rash of rubella (German measles). (From Korting GW: Hautkrankheiten bei Kindern und Jugendlichen, 3rd ed. Stuttgart, Germany, FK Schattauer Verlag, 1982.)

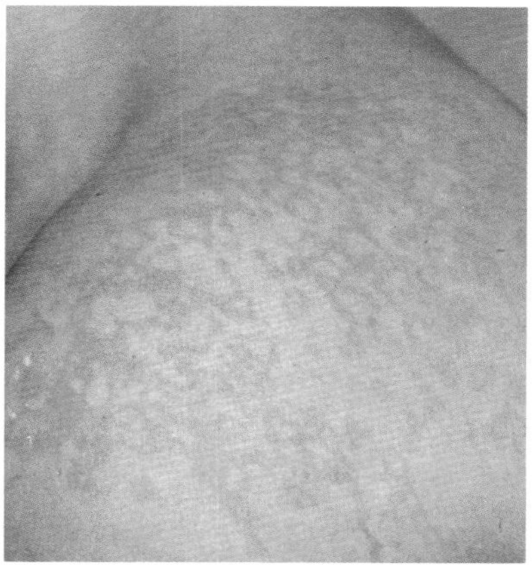

Figure 12–15. Erythema infectiosum. (From Korting GW: Hautkrankheiten bei Kindern und Jugendlichen, 3rd ed. Stuttgart, Germany, FK Schattauer Verlag, 1982.)

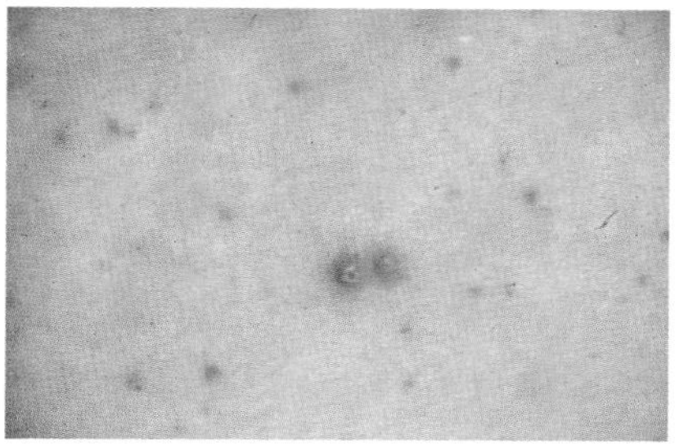

Figure 12–19. Skin lesions of chickenpox. Note the varying stages of development (macules, papules, and vesicles) present at the same time. (Courtesy of PF Lucchesi, M.D.)

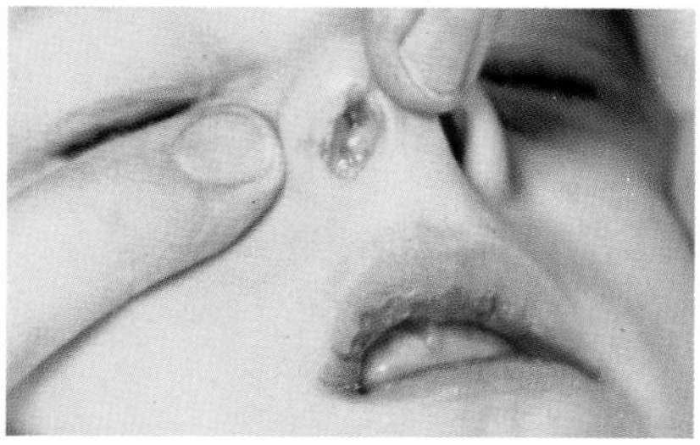

Figure 12–4. Nasal diphtheria. (Courtesy of Robert A Lyon, M.D.)

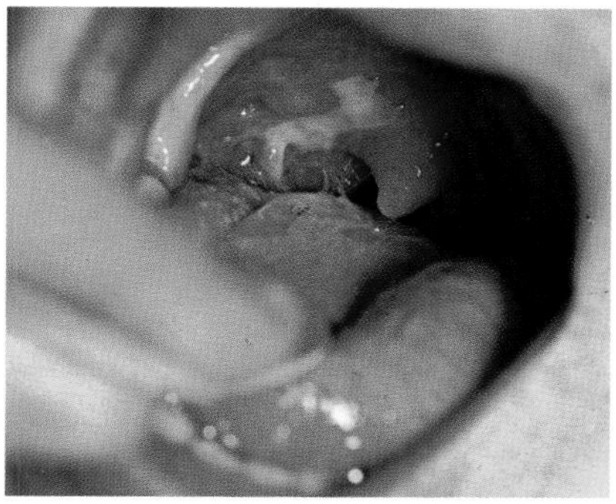

Figure 12–5. Pharyngotonsillar membrane of diphtheria. (Courtesy of Robert A Lyon, M.D.)

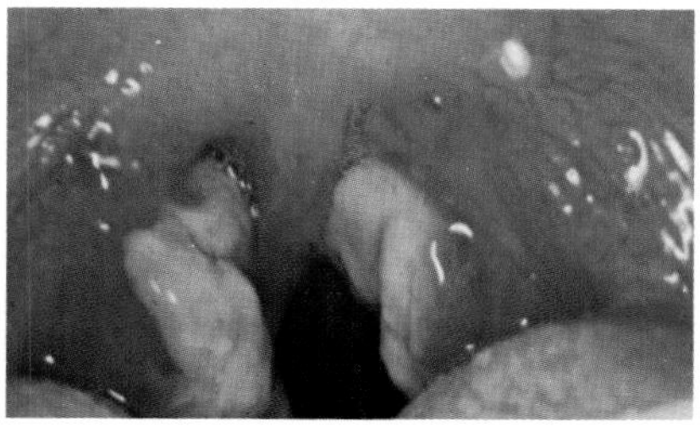

Figure 12–22. Tonsillitis with membrane formation in infectious mononucleosis. (Courtesy of Alex J. Steigman, M.D.)

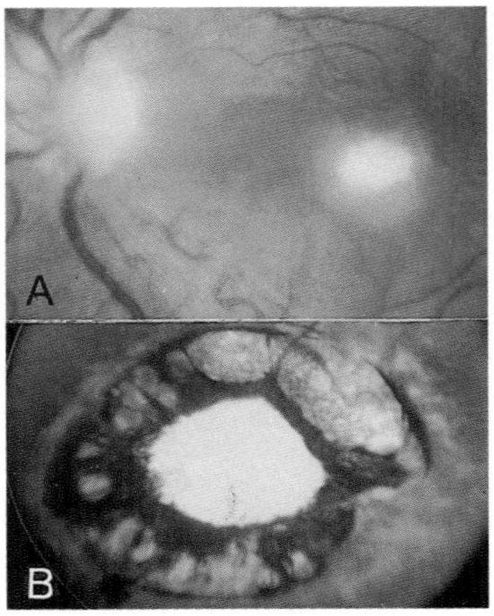

Figure 12–38. Toxoplasmic chorioretinitis. *A*, Active acute lesion by indirect ophthalmoscopy. *B*, Old, quiescent lesion. (*B*, Adapted from Desmonts G, Remington J: Congenital Toxoplasmosis. *In*: Remington J, Klein J [eds]: Infectious Diseases of the Fetus and Newborn Infant, 3rd ed. Philadelphia, WB Saunders, 1991).

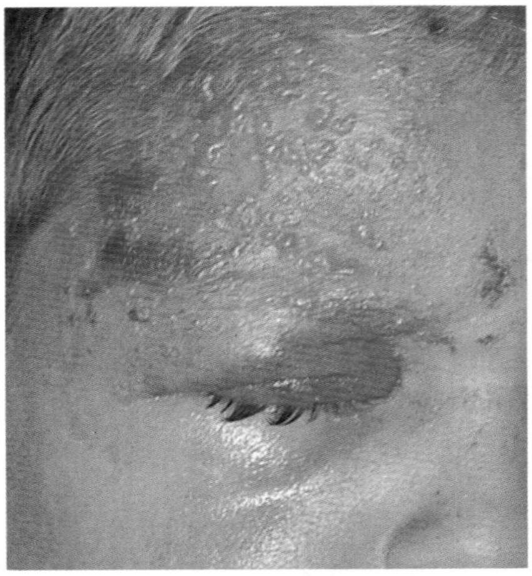

Figure 12–21. Herpes zoster ophthalmicus. (From Korting GW: Hautkrankheiten bei Kindern und Jugendlichen, 3rd ed. Stuttgart, Germany, FK Schattauer Verlag, 1982.)

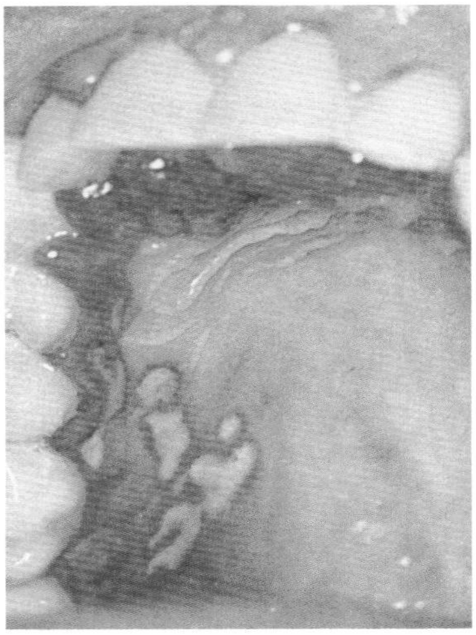

Figure 12–30. Herpangina. (From Korting GW: Hautkrankheiten bei Kindern und Jugendlichen. Stuttgart, Germany, FK Schattauer Verlag, 1969.)

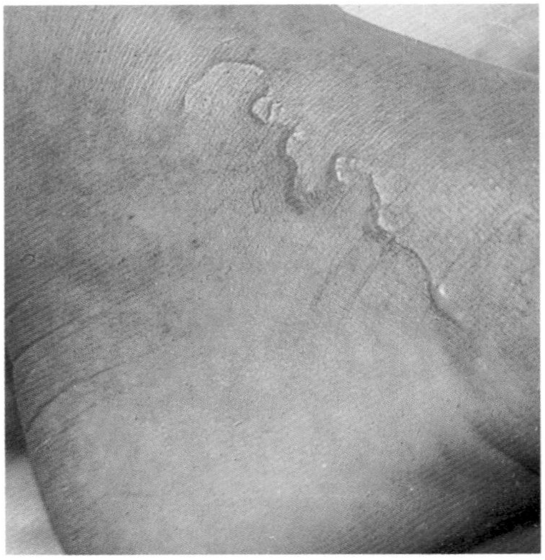

Figure 12–43. Creeping eruption of cutaneous larva migrans. (From Korting GW: Hautkrankheiten bei Kindern und Jugendlichen. Stuttgart, Germany, FK Schattauer Verlag, 1969.)

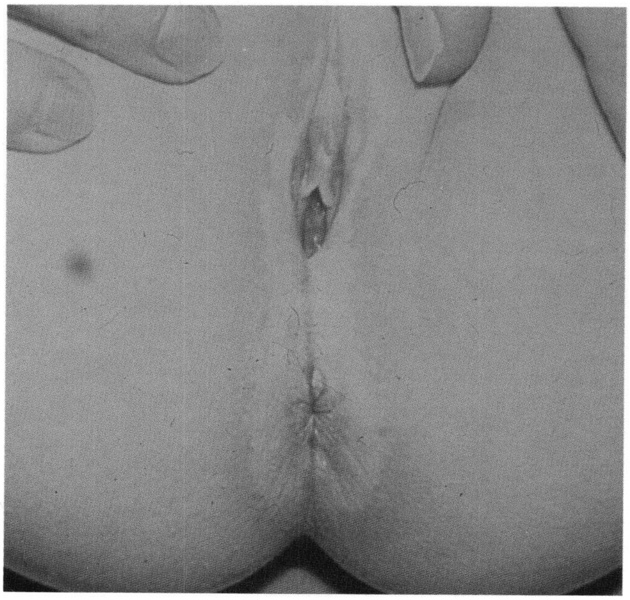
Figure 18–45. Lichen sclerosus.

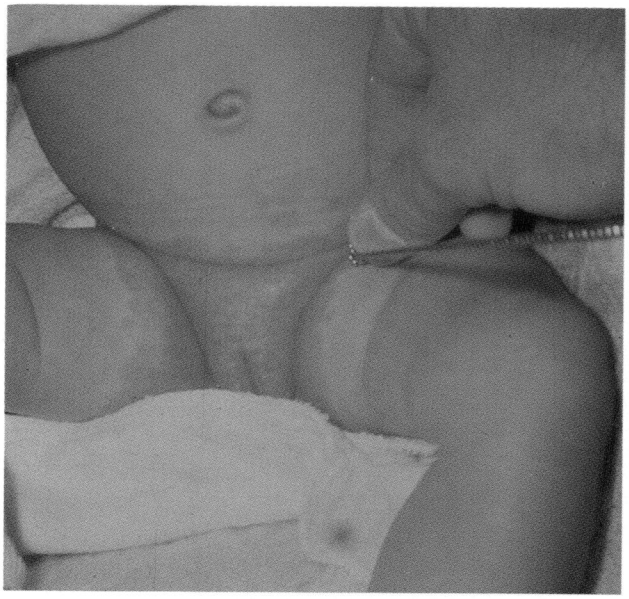
Figure 18–46. Vulvar psoriasis.

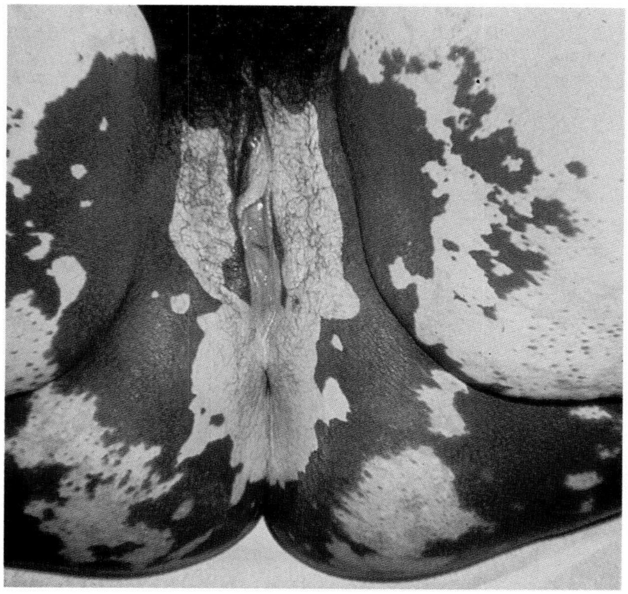
Figure 18–47. Vitiligo.

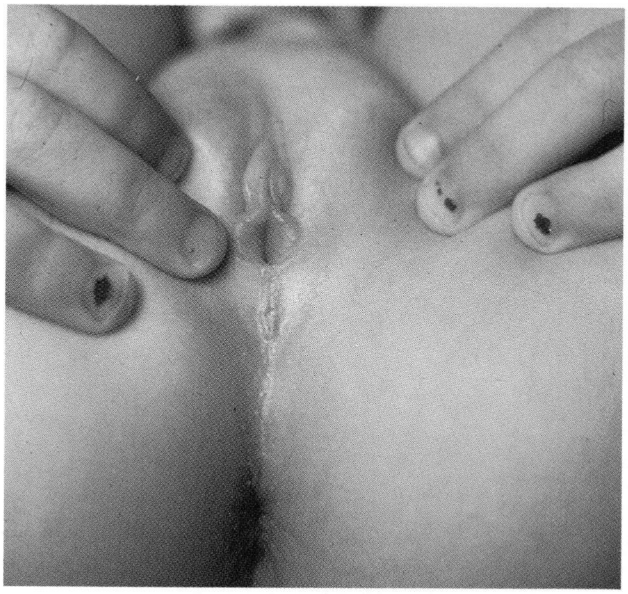
Figure 18–48. Labial adhesions.

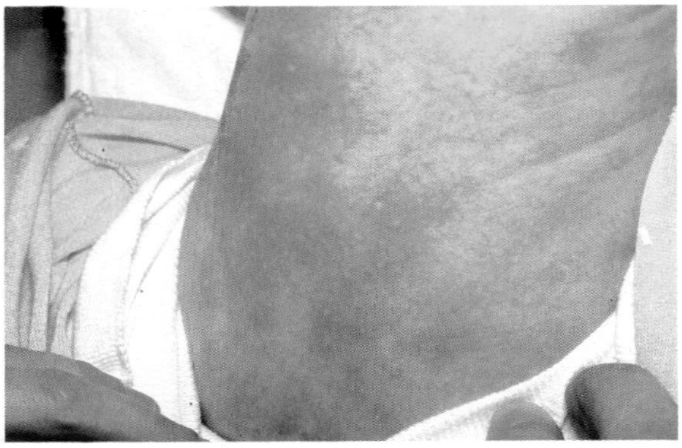

Figure 23–1. Erythema toxicum on the trunk of a newborn infant.

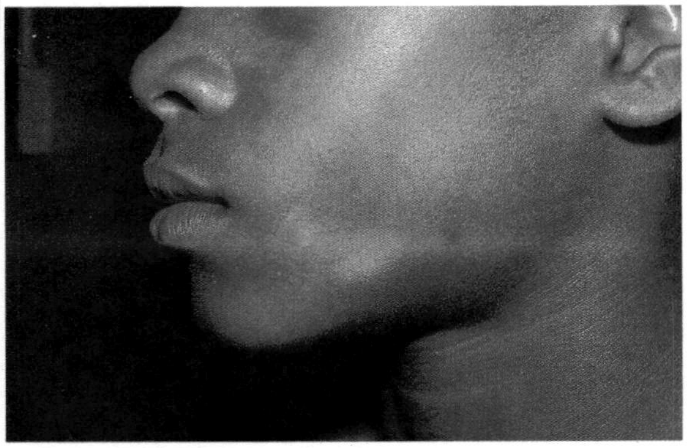

Figure 23–22. Patchy hypopigmented lesions with diffuse borders characteristic of pityriasis alba.

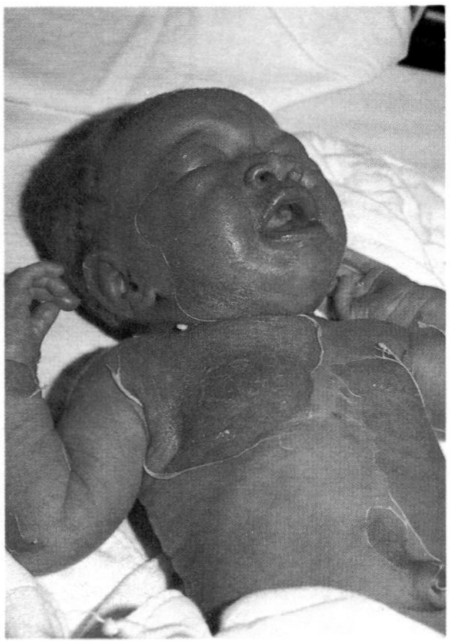

Figure 23–40. Infant with staphylococcal scalded skin syndrome.

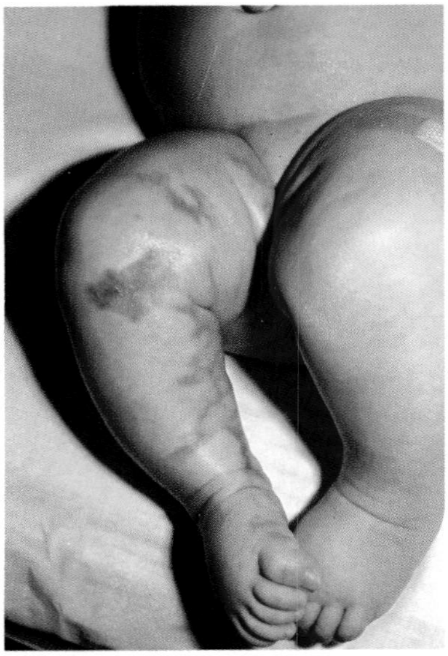

Figure 23–7. Marbled pattern of cutis marmorata telangiectatica congenita on the right leg.

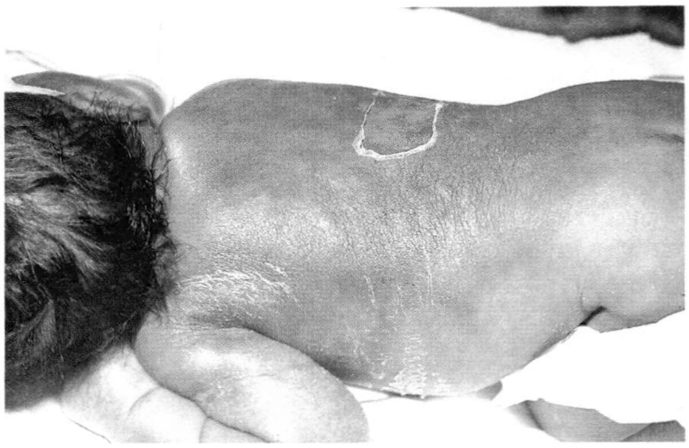

Figure 23–36. Red purple nodular infiltration of skin of back and upper arms due to subcutaneous fat necrosis.

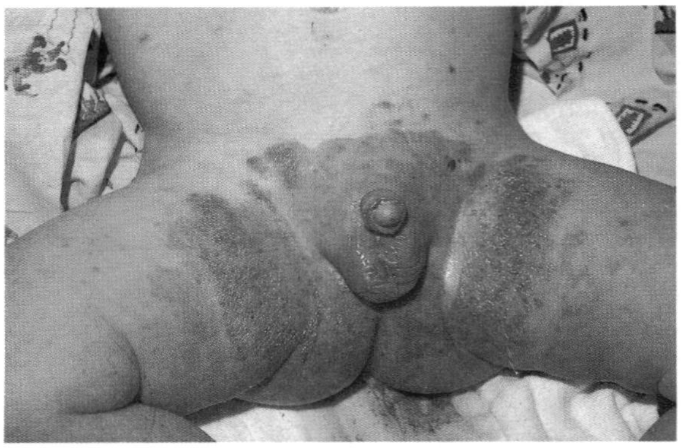

Figure 23–45. Erythematous confluent plaque with satellite pustules due to candidal infection.

1

THE FIELD OF PEDIATRICS

Pediatrics is concerned with the health of infants, children, and youths, their growth and development, and their opportunity to achieve full potential as adults. As physicians who assume a responsibility for children's physical, mental, and emotional progress from conception to maturity, pediatricians must be concerned with social or environmental influences, which have a major impact on the health and well-being of children and their families, as well as with particular organ systems and biologic processes. The young are often among the most vulnerable or disadvantaged in society, and thus their needs require special attention.

SCOPE AND HISTORY OF PEDIATRICS

Over a century ago, pediatrics emerged as a medical specialty in response to an increasing awareness that the health problems of children differ from those of adults and that the child's response to illness and stress varies with age. The emphasis and scope of pediatrics continue to change, but this basic observation remains valid.

The health problems of children vary widely among the nations of the world depending on a number of factors, which are often interrelated. These factors include (1) the prevalence and ecology of infectious agents and their hosts; (2) climate and geography; (3) agricultural resources and practices; (4) educational, economic, social, and cultural considerations; (5) stage of industrialization and urbanization; and (6), in many instances, the gene frequencies for some disorders.

Not only do problems differ in various parts of the world, but priorities do also, because they must reflect local concerns, resources, and needs. The assessment of the state of health of any community must begin with a description of the incidence of illness and must continue with studies that show the changes that occur with time and in response to programs of prevention, case finding, therapy, and adequate surveillance. As contemporary problems in any community yield to study and to improved management, new problems become the foci of the attention and efforts of pediatric clinicians and research workers. Accordingly, with time, there may be major changes in the relative importance of the various causes of childhood morbidity and mortality.

In the late 19th century in the United States, of every 1,000 children born alive 200 might be expected to die before the age of 1 yr of conditions such as dysentery, pneumonia, measles, diphtheria, and whooping cough. The efforts of pediatricians, combined with those of scientists and pioneers in public health, have led to such better understanding of the origin and management of many problems of infants that in the past half century the infant mortality in the United States has fallen from around 75/1,000 live births in 1925 to approximately 9.9 in 1988. Both neonatal (<1 mo) and postneonatal (1–11 mo) mortality have had major reductions. The majority of deaths of infants under 1 yr of age occur within the first 28 days of life, most of these within the first 7 days; moreover, a large proportion of those within the first 7 days occur within the 1st day. However, an increasing number of severely ill infants born at low birthweight survive the neonatal period and die later in infancy from neonatal disease, its sequelae, or its complications. Table 1–1 shows the disproportionately high death rate within the 1st yr, compared with the remainder of childhood.

Postneonatal infant mortality for the United States in 1986 was 3.6/1,000 live births (6.3/1,000 for black infants and 3.1/1,000 for white infants). The leading cause of death in this age group was the sudden infant death syndrome, followed in order by congenital anomalies, perinatal conditions, respiratory system diseases, accidents, and infectious and parasitic diseases. Maternal risk characteristics, such as unmarried status, teenage, high parity, and less than 12 yr of education, are correlated significantly with increased risk of postneonatal mortality and morbidity and low birthweight.

Early in the 20th century, efforts at control of infectious disease began to be complemented by better understanding of nutrition. New and continuing discoveries in these areas led to establishment of well-child clinics. Along with acute infections and the chronic disturbances associated with deficits of calories, vitamins, minerals, or proteins, the acute nutritional and metabolic disturbances that accompany acute diarrhea also received attention.

In the middle years of the 20th century, a profound revolution in child health was brought about by the introduction of antibacterial chemicals and antibiotic agents. With improved control of infectious disease through both prevention and treatment and with other scientific and technical advances, pediatric medicine turned its attention increasingly to conditions affecting relatively small numbers of children. These included both potentially lethal conditions and temporarily or permanently handicapping conditions; among these disorders were leukemia, cystic fibrosis, diseases of the newborn infant, congenital heart disease, mental retardation, genetic defects, rheumatic diseases, renal diseases, and metabolic and endocrine disorders.

More recently, increasing attention has been given to behavioral and social aspects of child health, ranging from a reexamination of child-rearing practices to the creation of major programs aimed at prevention and management of abuse and neglect of infants and children. Developmental psychologists, child psychiatrists, sociologists, anthropologists, ethnologists, and others have brought us new insights into human potential, including new views of the importance of the circumstances surrounding birth and the early hours together of infants and parents (Sec. 3.3, 3.4, and 9.6).

Table 1–2 shows the five leading causes of death in various age groups in 1985 and 1988. Tables 1–3, 1–4, and 5–1 to 5–5 show how certain problems of these children have changed in the United States over a generation. Tables 1–2, 5–4, and 5–5 highlight the impact of violent deaths on mortality in older children, adolescents, and young adults.

Figure 9–1 shows that the nonwhite children of the United States have not fully benefited from the changes in infant mortality in this century owing to a variety of socioeconomic and other disadvantages that have resisted the efforts of many who have struggled to reduce this disparity, including many pediatricians. Similar disparities between races occur in sev-

TABLE 1–1. Death Rates* for All Causes, According to Sex, Race, and Age: United States, Selected Years, 1950–1985†

	1950		1960		1970		1980		1985	
	White	*Black*	*White*	*Black*	*White*	*Black*	*White*	*Black*	*White*	*Black*
Male										
<1 yr	3,401	1,413 (<1 yr and 1–4 yr combined)	2,694	5,307	2,113	4,299	1,230	2,587	1,034	2,135
1–4 yr	136		105	209	84	151	66	111	52	89
5–14 yr	67	95	53	75	48	67	35	47	30	41
15–24 yr	152	290	144	212	171	321	167	209	136	174
Female										
<1 yr	2,567	1,139 (<1 yr and 1–4 yr combined)	2,008	4,162	1,614	3,369	963	2,124	787	1,757
1–4 yr	112		85	173	66	129	49	84	40	70
5–14 yr	45	73	35	54	30	44	23	31	19	28
15–24 yr	72	213	55	108	62	112	56	71	48	60

*Death rates per 100,000 population.
†Adapted from Table 21, Health, United States, 1987. DHHS (PHS) Pub No 88–1232, pp. 56–57. Hyattsville, MD, National Center for Health Statistics, 1988.

eral indices of health, such as rates of diseases of the heart and homicides.

In the United States, existing programs for meeting child health problems are not available to all families in need, with gaps between eligibility for public support and ability to pay costs. Needed services are often either nonexistent or fragmented among programs, agencies, or policies. Programs are often poorly coordinated and the data collection is inadequate. The resources available for maternal and child health care services are also generally inadequate. These findings reflect a need, not just in the United States but in many other parts of the world as well, for continuing re-examination and revision of the system of health care, especially with regard to its impact on the health status of children.

TABLE 1–2. Causes of Death and Age

Rank	Causes	Subrank	Rate
	Under 1 Yr: All Causes*		692† (992.9‡)
1	Perinatal conditions		
	Intrauterine growth retardation/low birthweight	1	
	Respiratory distress syndrome	2	
	Intrauterine hypoxia/birth asphyxia	3	
	Birth trauma	4	
	Others		
2	Congenital anomalies		
3	Sudden infant death syndrome		
4	Pneumonia		
5	Gastrointestinal disorders		
	1–4 Yr: All Causes†		43.3†
1	Injuries		
2	Congenital anomalies		
3	Malignant neoplasms		
4	Homicide		
5	Diseases of the heart‖		
	5–9 Yr: All Causes§		18.5†¶
1	Injuries		
2	Malignant neoplasms		
3	Congenital anomalies		
4	Homicide		
5	Diseases of the heart‖		
	10–14 Yr: All Causes§		18.5†¶
1	Injuries		
2	Malignant neoplasms		
3	Suicide		
4	Homicide		
5	Congenital anomalies		
	15–24 Yr**: All Causes§		52.0†
1	Injuries		
2	Suicide		
3	Homicide		
4	Malignant neoplasms		
5	Diseases of heart‖		

*Adapted from Monthly Vital Statistics Report 37(13):16, 26, 1989. Ranking is for 1988 (Prov.).
†1988 (Prov.) rate per 100,000 population.
‡1988 (Prov.) rate per 100,000 live births.
§Leading causes of death by age, 1985. National Center for Health Statistics.
‖Excludes congenital heart anomalies.
¶Mortality rate per 100,000 population ages 5–14 yr for 1988 (Prov.).
**Ranking is for ages 15–19 in 1985.

These problems are exacerbated by social and demographic changes in the United States. By 1986, 24% (14.8 million) of all children under 18 yr of age were living with one parent, a 15% increase since 1960. Of these one-parent families, 88% consisted of children living with their mother, and black children were three times more likely to be living in a single-parent household than were white children. Furthermore, in 1986, 54% of mothers with children under 6 yr of age and 70% of mothers of children 6–17 yr of age worked full-time or part-time. More than 20% of children under 5 yr whose mothers worked outside the home were in day-care. One in five children were living in poverty (13 million under 18 yr) and a black or Hispanic child was more than three times as likely to be living in poverty as a white child. This increase in childhood poverty in the United States has been accompanied by a large increase in the number of children without adequate health insurance; by 1985, more than 11 million children were completely uninsured.

The aforementioned findings have generated three sets of goals. The 1st set included that all families have access to adequate perinatal, preschool, and family-planning services; that governmental activities be effectively coordinated at national and local levels; that services be so organized that they reach populations at special risk; that there be no insurmountable or inequitable financial barriers to adequate care; that the health care of children have continuity from prenatal through adolescent age periods; and that ultimately every family have access to *all* necessary services, including dental, genetic, and mental health services. A 2nd set of goals addresses the needs for reducing accidents and environmental risks, for meeting nutritional needs, and for health education aimed at fostering health-promoting life styles. A 3rd set of goals covers needs for research in biomedical and behavioral science, in fundamentals of bioscience and human biology, and in the particular problems of mothers and children.

The unfinished business in the quest for physical, mental, and social health in the community is illustrated by the disparities with which deaths due to disease, to accidents, and to violence are distributed between white and nonwhite children. Homicide has become a major cause of adolescent deaths and has increased in rate also among the very young, among whom the increase may in part represent the more

TABLE 1–3. Death Rates* for Diseases of the Heart According to Sex, Race, and Age: United States, Selected Years, 1950–1985†

	1950		1960		1970		1980		1985	
	White	*Black*	*White*	*Black*	*White*	*Black*	*White*	*Black*	*White*	*Black*
Male										
<1 yr	4.1	4.8	6.9	13.9	12.0	33.5	22.5	42.8	23.8	46.7
1–4 yr	1.1		1.0	3.8	1.5	3.9	2.1	6.3	1.7	4.4
5–14 yr	1.7	6.4	1.1	3.0	0.8	1.4	0.9	1.3	0.8	1.5
15–24 yr	5.8	18.0	3.6	8.7	3.0	8.3	2.9	8.3	3.0	7.2
Female										
<1 yr	2.7	3.9	4.3	12.0	7.0	31.3	15.7	43.6	18.3	39.5
1–4 yr	1.1		0.9	2.8	1.2	4.2	2.1	4.4	1.6	5.2
5–14 yr	1.9	8.8	0.9	3.0	0.7	1.8	0.8	1.7	0.9	1.7
15–24 yr	5.3	19.8	2.8	10.0	1.7	6.0	1.7	4.6	1.7	4.6

*Death rates per 100,000 population.
†Adapted from Table 23, Health, United States, 1987. DDHS (PHS) Pub No 88–1232, pp. 60–61. Hyattsville, MD, National Center for Health Statistics, 1988.

accurate identification of child abuse (Sec. 3.51); among adolescents it may reflect unresolved social tensions, the epidemic of substance abuse (especially cocaine and crack), and an unhealthy preoccupation in our society with violence. Some of the issues underlying these problems are discussed in Sec. 2.8, 3.16–3.18, 3.20, 5.5, 10.1, 10.3, and 10.4.

PATTERNS OF HEALTH CARE

In 1987, children (0–21 yr) made up 30.3% (78.4 million) of the population of the United States. The number of births has been increasing since 1976 and is expected to continue to increase at 1–2% annually. There were 3,829,000 live births in 1987. Table 1–5 indicates the distribution of children in the population by age. The population of children less than 5 yr of age increased 11% between 1980 and 1987 and will reach a peak in 1990. The adolescent population (15–19 yr of age) has been decreasing since the 1970s but will reach a crest in 2005, reflecting the peak of younger children. However, the proportion of children is decreasing relative to the adult population.

There were 132 million office visits to physicians by children aged 0–19 yr in 1987. About 50% of these children were examined by pediatricians, with the greatest number of visits being by children under 2 yr (59.3 visits/100 children/yr, under 2 yr) and the least by older children (67 visits/100 children/yr, 10–19 yr). Office visits represent about two thirds of all physician contacts with children. Seven to 10% receive all their care from a physician in an institutional setting (hospital or free-standing clinic). Nonwhite children are four times more likely than are white children to use hospital facilities for their ambulatory care.

Hospitals, particularly in urban areas, are sources of both routine and intensive child care, with medical and surgical services which may range from immunization and developmental counseling to open heart surgery or renal transplantation. Clinical conditions and procedures requiring intensive care are likely to be clustered in university-affiliated centers serving as regional resources. However, it is also important to appreciate that chronic illness and impairments resulting in limitation of usual activities affect about 5% of children but account for 31% of hospital days and for two and one-half times the number of physician contacts as do acute childhood conditions.

PLANNING A SYSTEM OF CARE

Physicians caring for children have been increasingly called upon to advise in the management of disturbed behavior or in relationships between child and parent, child and school, or child and community and are increasingly concerned with problems of mental, social, and societal health. There is also an increasing concern with disparities in how the benefits of what we know about child health reach various groups of children. Just as in many developing countries, so in the United States the health of children lags far behind what it could be if the means and will to apply current knowledge could be brought to bear. The medical problems of the children are often intimately related to problems of mental and social health. The children most at risk are disproportionately represented among ethnic minority groups. Pediatricians have a responsibility to address themselves aggressively to problems such as these.

Linked with these views of the broad scope of pediatric

TABLE 1–4. Death Rates* for Malignant Neoplasms According to Sex, Race, and Age: United States, Selected Years, 1950–1985†

	1950		1960		1970		1980		1985	
	White	*Black*	*White*	*Black*	*White*	*Black*	*White*	*Black*	*White*	*Black*
Male										
<1 yr	9.6	8.2	7.9	6.8	4.3	5.3	3.5	4.5	3.1	2.4
1–4 yr	13.1		13.1	7.9	8.5	7.6	5.4	5.1	4.4	3.3
5–14 yr	7.6	5.8	8.0	4.4	7.0	4.8	5.2	3.7	4.0	3.6
15–24 yr	9.9	7.9	10.3	9.7	10.6	9.4	7.8	8.1	6.5	6.4
Female										
<1 yr	7.8	7.0	6.8	6.7	5.4	3.3	2.7	3.0	3.0	4.3
1–4 yr	11.3		9.7	6.9	6.9	5.7	3.6	3.9	3.5	2.5
5–14 yr	5.3	3.9	6.2	4.8	5.4	4.0	3.7	3.4	3.1	3.0
15–24 yr	7.5	8.8	6.5	6.9	6.2	6.4	4.7	5.7	4.3	4.3

*Death rates per 100,000 population.
†Adapted from Table 25, Health, United States, 1987. DHHS (PHS) Pub No 88–1232, pp. 64–65. Hyattsville, MD, National Center for Health Statistics, 1988.

TABLE 1–5. Distribution of Children by Age in the United States in 1987*

Age (Yr)	% of Total†
<1	1.5
1–5	7.0
6–9	5.4
10–14	6.4
15–17	4.3
18–21	5.7

*From the US Bureau of the Census.
†Total population of children and adults.

concern is the concept that access to at least a basic level of services to promote health and treat illness is a right of every person. The failure of health services and health benefits to reach all who need them has led to re-examination of the design of health care systems in many countries; but unresolved problems remain in most health care systems, such as the maldistribution of physicians, institutional unresponsiveness to the perceived needs of the individual, failure of medical services to be adapted to the need and convenience of the patient, and deficiencies in health education. Efforts to make the delivery of health care more efficient and effective have led imaginative pediatricians to create new categories of health care providers, such as pediatric nurse practitioners, and to participate in new organizations for providing care to children.

New insights into the needs of children have reshaped the child health care system in other ways. Growing understanding of the need of the infant for certain qualities of stimulation and care has led to restudy and revision of the care of the newborn infant (Sec. 3.3, 3.4, and 3.14) and of procedures leading to adoption or to placement with foster families (Sec. 3.16 and 3.17). For handicapped children the massive centralized institutions of past years are being replaced by community-centered arrangements offering a better opportunity for these children to achieve their maximal potential. Pediatricians have been involved in shaping these and other institutions that provide services to children, and their insights and active contributions will continue to be needed.

COSTS OF HEALTH CARE

The growth of high technology, the redesign of health institutions (particularly with respect to the needs for and the uses of personnel), the public's demand for medical services, and the manner in which the costs of health care are paid (by public or private insurance programs based on fee-for-service) have driven the costs of health care in the United States up to a point at which they represent a significant proportion of the gross national product (11.5% in 1988). Efforts to contain these costs have led to revisions of the way in which physicians and hospitals are paid for services. Limits have been set on the fees for some services, capitated prepayment and a variety of managed care systems flourish, a program of reimbursement (diagnosis-related groups [DRGs]) based on the diagnosis rather than on the particular services rendered to the individual patient has been implemented, and a relative value scale for varying rates of payment among different physician services is being implemented. These changes in the system of financing health services raise important ethical issues for pediatricians to address (Sec. 2.8).

EVALUATION OF HEALTH CARE

The shaping of health care systems to meet the needs of children and their families requires accurate statistical data and difficult decisions in the setting of priorities. Along with growing concerns about the design and cost of health care systems and their ability to equitably distribute health services has come more intense preoccupation with the quality of health care and with both its efficiency and its effectiveness. There are large local and regional variations among similar populations of children in the rates of use of procedures and of hospital admissions. These variations require continuing evaluation and explanation in terms of the actual impact of medical and surgical services on health status and the outcome of illness. The need for technology assessment is increasing.

GROWTH OF SPECIALIZATION

The amount of information relevant to child health care is rapidly expanding, and no person can become master of it all. Physicians are increasingly dependent on one another for the highest quality of care for their patients; group practices in pediatrics are on the rise, each member developing some special knowledge and skills. The vast majority of pediatricians are generalists, but as many as 25% claim an "area of special interest."

The growth of specialization within pediatrics has taken a number of different forms: interests in problems of *age groups* of children have created neonatology and adolescent medicine; interests in *organ systems* have created pediatric cardiology, allergy, hematology, nephrology, gastroenterology, pulmonology, endocrinology, and specialization in metabolism and genetics; interests in the *health care system* have created pediatricians devoted to ambulatory care on the one hand or to intensive care on the other; and finally, multidisciplinary subspecialties have grown up around the problems of *handicapped children,* to which pediatrics, neurology, psychiatry, psychology, nursing, physical and occupational therapy, special education, speech therapy, audiology, and nutrition all make essential contributions. This growth of specialization has been most conspicuous in university-affiliated departments of pediatrics and medical centers for children. The development of such areas of special interest among private practitioners is particularly likely among pediatricians who practice in groups.

NEED FOR CONTINUING SELF-EDUCATION

The explosion of information has also created a need for continuing education, which was felt much less keenly in earlier years, when the new information in any field of medicine was easily accessible through a relatively small number of journals, texts, or monographs. Now, relevant information is so widely scattered among the many journals published that elaborate electronic data systems are necessary to make it accessible. New auditory and visual aids to learning abound as well as postgraduate courses through which the participating physician can be brought up to date on various aspects of child health care. The American Board of Pediatrics and the American Academy of Pediatrics have arranged for the close linkage of continuing education of the pediatrician to recertification in pediatrics.

There is no touchstone through which physicians can ensure that the process of their own continuing education will keep them abreast of advancing knowledge in the field, but they must find a way if they are to discharge their responsibility to their patients. An essential element of this process may be for the physician to take an *active* role, such as participating in medical student and resident education. Efforts in continuing self-education will also be fostered, for example, if clinical problems can be made a stimulus for a review of standard literature, alone or in consultation with an appropriate colleague or consultant. This continuing review will do much to identify those inconsistencies or contradictions that will indicate, in the ultimate best interest of the patient, that things are not what they seem or have been said to be. Physicians still learn most from their patients, but this will not be the case if they fall into the easy habit of accepting their patients' problems casually or at face value because they appear to be simple.

The tools that the physician must use in dealing with the problems of children and their families fall into three main categories: *cognitive* (up-to-date factual information regarding diagnostic and therapeutic issues, available on recall or easily found in readily accessible sources); *interpersonal or manual* (e.g., the ability to carry out a productive interview, execute a reliable physical examination, perform a deft venipuncture, or manage cardiac arrest or the resuscitation of a depressed newborn infant); and *attitudinal* (the physician's commitment to fullest possible implementation of knowledge and skills on behalf of children and their families in an atmosphere of empathetic sensitivity and concern). With regard to this last category, it is important that children participate with their families in informed decision-making about their own health care in a manner appropriate to their stage of development and the nature of the particular health problem.

The workaday needs of professional persons for knowledge and skills in care of children vary widely. The primary care physician needs depth in developmental concepts and in the ability to organize an effective system for achieving quality and continuity in assessing and planning for health care during the entire period of growth. There may often be little or no need for immediate recall of esoterica. On the other hand, the consultant or subspecialist not only needs a comfortable grasp of esoterica within his or her field and perhaps within related fields but must be able also to cope with controversial issues, with flexibility that will permit adaptation of a variety of points of view to the best interest of his or her unique patient.

At whatever level of care (primary, secondary, or tertiary), or in whatever role (as student, as pediatric nurse practitioner, as resident pediatrician, as a practitioner of pediatrics or of family medicine, or as a pediatric or other subspecialist), professional persons dealing with children must be able to identify their roles of the moment and their levels of engagement with a child's problem; each must determine whether his or her experience and other resources at hand are adequate to deal with this problem and must be ready to seek other help when they are not. Among the necessary resources will be general textbooks, more detailed monographs in subspecialty areas, selected journals, audiovisual materials, and, above all, colleagues with exceptional or complementary experience and expertise. The intercommunication of all these levels of engagement with medical and health problems of children offers the best hope of bringing us closer to the goal of providing the opportunity for all children to achieve their maximum potential.

RICHARD E. BEHRMAN*

Advance Report of Final Natality Statistics, 1987. Monthly Vital Statistics Report 38(3), Suppl. 1989. Washington, DC, US Department of Health and Human Services. Public Health Service, Centers for Disease Control.

American Medical Association, Department of Data Release Services, Division of Survey and Data Resources: Physician Characteristics and Distribution in the US. 1987 ed. Chicago, IL, 1988.

Annual Summary of Births, Marriages, Divorces, and Deaths: United States, 1988. Monthly Vital Statistics Report 37(13), 1989. Washington, DC, US Department of Health and Human Services. Public Health Service, Centers for Disease Control.

Both DR, Garduque L (eds): Social Policy for Children and Families: Creating an Agenda: A Review of Selective Reports. National Forum on the Future of Children and Families. Institute of Medicine. National Research Council. Washington, DC, National Academy Press, 1989.

Child Health USA, 1989. US Department of Health and Human Services.

Health United States, 1987. US Department of Health and Human Services. Centers for Disease Control. National Center for Health Statistics.† Hyattsville, MD, 1988. DHHS Pub No (PHS) 88–1232.

Kins NMP, Cross AW: Children as decision makers: Guidelines for pediatricians. J Pediatr 115:10, 1989.

Martinez GA, Ryan AS: The pediatric market place. Am J Dis Child 143(8):924, 1988.

Newacheck PW, Starfield B: Morbidity and use of ambulatory services among poor and non-poor children. Am J Public Health 78:927, 1988.

The 1990 Health Objectives for the Nation: A Midcourse Review. Public Health Service, US Department of Health and Human Services. Office of Disease Prevention and Health Promotion, November 1986.

*Modified from the original version of this chapter written by Victor C. Vaughan, III.

†Inquiries regarding the publications of the National Center for Health Statistics (NCHS) can be made to National Center for Health Statistics, Center Building, Room 1–57, 3700 East-West Highway, Hyattsville, MD 20782. Telephone: (301) 436–8500.

2

ETHICAL AND CULTURAL ISSUES IN PEDIATRICS

ETHICS IN PEDIATRIC CARE

Ethical issues permeate all interactions between physicians and patients: How much information should be disclosed? Is this patient consuming an unfair share of the physician's or society's resources? Should clinical decisions be made by the patient, the parent, or the physician? In pediatrics, these familiar dilemmas are compounded by the variable competence of the patient, the sometimes competing interests of parents and children, and the longstanding tradition of treating children more paternalistically than is acceptable for adult patients.

The following sections review the major conceptual principles in medical ethics; identify the central issues in the common clinical/ethical dilemmas involving children; identify areas of apparent consensus; and suggest a procedural approach to ethical decision-making.

2.1 CONCEPTUAL ISSUES

AUTONOMY. This is a central principle in contemporary medical ethics. Its purpose is to allow competent patients to make their own health care decisions, based on their own values. In the United States and many other nations, a competent patient has almost an absolute right to decide what shall be done to his or her own body. This right is not contingent on the patient making rational decisions. Thus, a patient may permissibly refuse life-saving care for religious or other reasons, even though others may believe that he or she is making a foolish or unwise decision. This principle is particularly relevant in adolescence, when a patient's competence begins to resemble that of an adult, but younger children are also sometimes competent to make their own health care decisions.

COMPETENCE. The principle of autonomy is intertwined inextricably with the concept of competence, because only competent patients are granted the right to make their own health care decisions. The most common definition of competence is based on the patient's ability to understand the possible consequences of his or her decision and the available alternatives. Many adolescents meet this standard, creating potential conflicts when they are still under the supervision of their parents.

PATERNALISM. This is defined as interfering with the liberty of another person for his or her own benefit. It is generally considered to be a duty of parents, although this assumption has been questioned, and is morally unjustified with regard to competent patients, with limited exceptions. Physicians have historically believed that they had a right and duty to be paternalistic, based on the claim that their responsibility is *beneficence*—to promote the patient's health, not his or her autonomy. There is general support for the opinion that paternalism is justified at least in circumstances when there is a high probability of serious harm; when interference with the patient's liberty is likely to prevent the harm; and when there is a reasonable likelihood that the patient would want to be treated in this manner or will appreciate it later on. This view of justified paternalism provides the justification for many intrusions done for the benefit of children over their apparent objection, such as surgery for suspected appendicitis or immunizations against serious diseases, but raises questions about the appropriateness of intrusions of uncertain effectiveness if the child objects or of intrusions for the purpose of preventing uncertain or minimal harms.

TRUTH TELLING. The duty to tell the truth is a requisite for any moral community. It has special importance in the physician-patient relationship, in which trust is essential because of unequal power and because of the serious consequences of medical decisions. Failure to respect this principle occurs by active lying, which is wrong under almost all circumstances in the health care setting, or by omission of information. Omissions should not be made for the purpose of deception or of manipulating the patient's response. Some consider that all intentional deceptions are examples of lying, which is only justified under exceptional circumstances.

CONFIDENTIALITY. Patients need to trust their physicians not to disclose private information to others because confidentiality facilitates full disclosure of information relevant for providing effective personal health care, may prevent disorders that threaten others in the community, and possibly reduces the total human and financial cost of illness and related disability through early treatment. There is an implied promise by the physician not to disclose information except with the consent of the patient, or his or her representative, or when required by law. Exceptions to this principle are generally limited to circumstances in which there is a high risk of serious physical harm to others that is most likely to be prevented only by unconsented disclosure (e.g., reporting suspected child abuse on the basis of information obtained from the potential abuser in what was presumed to be a confidential relationship).

CONFLICTS OF INTEREST. Because the child/patient is usually represented by someone else, there is an increased potential for the pediatrician to perceive the best interests of the child differently from the way in which they are appreciated by the parent(s) or guardian(s). In addition, the physician's sense of responsibility for the rest of the family may also result in conflicts between the interests of the family and the interests of the child patient (e.g., see the following section on "Baby Doe").

COMMON CLINICAL ETHICAL DILEMMAS

2.2 WITHHOLDING AND WITHDRAWING LIFE SUPPORT

This is one of the most important ethical dilemmas that physicians have to deal with. In pediatrics, these issues arise most commonly in the newborn period, involving infants with limited prospects for survival without significant lifelong morbidity. These cases, however, are only one part of the general question of the justifications for withholding or withdrawing life support from children with a variety of illnesses from birth through adolescence (see also Sec. 3.59).

There is a strong ethical consensus in the United States that a competent person has an almost absolute right to determine what shall be done with his or her own body. This implies a right to refuse health care, even if the patient has excellent prospects for long-term survival and death is the certain result of refusing treatment. There is a similar tradition in the law. A familiar example is the common occurrence of a Jehovah's Witness refusing a lifesaving blood transfusion; religious justifications are not an essential aspect of this ethical or legal principle. Accordingly, an adolescent patient who is competent in the sense of understanding the consequences of his or her decision, including the prospects for survival and the likely quality of life if treatment is accepted and the certainty of death if treatment is withheld, should play a major role in such decisions. The more problematic cases involve younger adolescents at the boundary of competence and disorders with limited prospects for long-term survival.

Most pediatric patients are clearly not competent to make their own decisions with regard to the termination of care. Although parents have traditionally made such decisions on behalf of their children with little controversy, there has been increased questioning of the limits of such authority. This has occurred primarily in decisions involving handicapped or critically ill newborns—the so-called "Baby Doe" controversy.

"BABY DOE" DILEMMA. This term arose in a 1982 conflict over an infant with Down syndrome and esophageal atresia who was allowed to die at 6 days of age at the parents' request. The case was similar to many others that had occurred during the preceding decade, particularly involving undertreatment of newborns with Down syndrome and spina bifida. Many of these children appeared to have excellent prospects for long, happy lives, suggesting that the decisions were not being made in the interests of the children. Furthermore, in two large surveys, most pediatricians supported parental control of such decisions; some pediatricians stated that they considered their duty was not to serve the interests of their patient but rather to serve the interests of the parents. These problems were compounded by the fact that many decisions were being based on erroneous medical assumptions, including inappropriately pessimistic prognoses.

As a consequence of concern about this issue in the United States, regulations were eventually promulgated under the authority of the child abuse law that prohibited withholding medically beneficial treatment because a child might survive with handicaps, however severe. This rule removed the central reason for discontinuing life-sustaining care from any patient; namely, the likelihood that continued biologic existence would not serve the patient's interests precisely because he or she would be so handicapped as to make the burdens of treatment greater than the benefits. The result of this rule has been an apparent shift from undertreatment to widespread overtreatment of critically ill newborns, defined as life-prolonging treatment that, in the opinion of the physician, does not serve the interests of the child.

The effort to find an acceptable middle ground between undertreatment and overtreatment has led to increasing support for a procedural approach to deciding what is in the interests of the child based on the "Ideal Observer Theory." A decision is morally acceptable if it could be approved of by an ideal ethical observer with five characteristics: (1) *omniscience,* the decision has included all the readily available and relevant facts; (2) *omnipercipience,* the decision has empathically taken into account the feelings of those involved; (3) *disinterest,* the decision is not based on vested interests; (4) *dispassionate,* the decision is not made under conditions in which strong emotions obscure critical thinking; and (5) *consistency,* the hallmark of ethical reasoning, meaning similar cases are decided similarly. Because no person can attain this ideal, a collaborative process is used to approximate these characteristics, such as hospital ethics or infant care review committees. The number of these committees has grown rapidly on a voluntary basis, and this trend has been accompanied by a virtual disappearance of the problems of undertreatment. Such committees play a consultative role in cases in which parents and medical staff cannot agree on the proper course of action.

WITHHOLDING VERSUS WITHDRAWING TREATMENT. It is widely accepted that there is no moral distinction between withholding and withdrawing treatment. Although historically and psychologically physicians and nurses are more reluctant to discontinue a treatment once it has begun, the withdrawal of treatment is more justified for two reasons. First the withdrawal of treatment has the benefit of coming after a clinical trial, resulting in more data regarding the likely outcome than if treatment had been withheld. Good ethics start with good facts, and it is generally preferable to avoid irreversible decisions in the presence of major uncertainty. Second, the traditional prohibition of withdrawing treatment led some physicians to withhold treatment from some infants who had reasonable prospects of benefit, for fear that if the outcome were later shown to be bleak, there would be no recourse other than to keep the patient alive as long as technology would allow; for example, a very small premature infant allowed to die in the delivery room without the benefit of a clinical trial. No physician in the United States has ever been found liable, civilly or criminally, for withholding or withdrawing any life-sustaining treatment from any patient for any reason.

ACTIVE VERSUS PASSIVE EUTHANASIA. As the preceding discussion implies, there has been broad support for passive euthanasia—allowing a patient to die owing to some intrinsic disease or defect. Active euthanasia, in comparison, is considered to be more problematic and generally opposed. The reasons for this are only partly related to concerns for the interests of the patient. If a decision has been made that continued survival is not in the patient's interest, it would seem irrelevant whether he or she died by active or passive means. Indeed, active euthanasia might be preferable because of the opportunity to minimize suffering. The objections are based, in part, on the swiftness and irreversibility of action, precluding the possibility of changing course if it is discovered that the decision was wrong. The greater concern, however, has been for "slippery slope" effects: the claim that lowering the barrier against killing will make it easier for physicians to kill others, that boundaries will become less distinct, and that patients without a clear interest in dying will be harmed. The accounts of the two countries with the greatest experience in active euthanasia, Germany in the 1930s and contemporary Holland, lends some support to this concern.

2.3 SCREENING

Screening is the search for asymptomatic illness in a defined population, which is usually performed for the purpose of treatment but is sometimes done for counselling or research. Several programs, such as screening for inborn errors of metabolism (e.g., phenylketonuria [PKU] and hypothyroidism), are counted among the triumphs of contemporary pediatrics. The success of such programs obscures serious ethical issues that continue to arise in proposals to screen for other conditions, such as human immunodeficiency virus (HIV) infection.

The central ethical principle that should justify screening programs is no different from that which should guide all medical care: *do no harm without compensating benefit and informed consent.* In the context of drugs and devices, the implementation of this principle means that these treatments are not offered or imposed on patients until benefits and risks have been demonstrated, costs have been found to be acceptable, and then only with the informed consent of the patient or his or her representative. In addition, tests that identify candidates for treatment need to have demonstrated sensitivity, specificity, and high predictive value, lest individuals be falsely labeled and subject to possibly toxic treatments or to psychosocial risks. These safeguards have not been systematically applied to screening programs. In the early years of PKU screening, the significance of high blood phenylalanine was not understood, and some infants with benign hyperphenylalaninemia were falsely labeled. Concurrently, the toxic effects of a restricted phenylalanine intake were not fully appreciated, resulting in iatrogenic retardation in some normal children. Similar problems arose in screening premature infants with respiratory distress syndrome for acidosis. For more than a decade, concentrated bicarbonate solutions were given to infants with abnormal laboratory results until careful studies showed the limited benefits and the hazard of intracranial hemorrhage. Other examples include presymptomatic detection of cystic fibrosis, which has not been shown to have health benefits, and fetal monitoring, which has contributed to the rising rate of cesarean sections with little benefit for many infants.

The growing epidemic of acquired immunodeficiency syndrome (AIDS) infection has stimulated interest in screening newborns for HIV infection, particularly in high prevalence areas. Whether such screening will have benefits proportional to the risks remains to be shown. This requires overcoming the obstacles of finding a test that can distinguish infected newborns from those with passive transfer of antibodies; demonstrating health benefits from early intervention; and unavoidably identifying infected mothers, who are subject to stigmatization to a degree that exceeds that of most other laboratory tests.

Screening has become such a ubiquitous and accepted component of the health care of healthy and sick patients that its benefits are often assumed and the risk is rarely assessed. Routine pediatric procedures, such as the annual physical examination, urine cultures, and developmental screening prior to school entry may be examples of common interventions of uncertain benefit and potential risks, organic and psychosocial. Two ethical principles are important in making judgments about screening: new programs should be considered experimental until the risks and benefits are demonstrated; and parents should generally be given the opportunity to exercise informed consent or refusal. Concern is often expressed that seeking informed consent is ethically inappropriate for tests of clear benefit, such as the PKU program in its present form, because refusal would constitute neglect. It is also claimed that such efforts are unduly time consuming. In fact, compliance with PKU testing is higher in some states in the United States without a mandatory program, and one study showed that a reasonable attempt at consent could be done without excessive time or cost.

2.4 ADOLESCENT HEALTH CARE

See also Sec. 10.22.

Many adolescents resemble adults more than they do children in their competence to consent to health care. Competence, however, is not a global quality: A teenager may not be able to support himself or herself, yet may still be competent to consent to health care.

In addition to the role of competence, there are public health reasons for allowing an adolescent to consent to his or her own health care with regard to reproductive decisions and treatment of sexually transmitted diseases, such as the epidemics of teenage pregnancy, with its adverse consequences for the adolescent parent and her offspring, and sexually transmitted diseases, including HIV infection. Strict requirements for parental consent may deter many adolescents from seeking health care, with serious implications for their health and other community interests.

Weighed against these concerns are the legitimate interests of parents in maintaining responsibility and authority for child-rearing, including the opportunity to influence the sexual attitudes and practices of one's children. There is also the claim that public support for access to such treatment, particularly contraception and abortion, implicitly endorses and encourages sexual activity, aggravating rather than ameliorating the problems. Similar concerns underlie the objection to providing sterile needles for intravenous drug abusers, for the purpose of reducing the risk of acquiring hepatitis or HIV. Critics complain that such programs give children the message that illegal drug use is supported by the state as long as it is done safely. The pediatrician's role and behavior in these disputes will be influenced by his or her own moral beliefs, assessments of the competing arguments, and understanding of adolescent psychologic development. The physician needs to consider the possibility that a moralistic position may deter the adolescent from seeking health care or counseling.

2.5 EXPERIMENTATION

Prior to the late 1960s, there were few laws, regulations, or formally articulated principles guiding experimentation on adults or children. Disclosures of egregiously unethical studies led, after a period of debate and analysis, to the formulation of national regulations in the United States.

The central ethical distinction between experimentation and standard clinical practice is the investigator's commitment to future patients, or societal interests, in addition to his or her responsibility for the patient who is the human subject of the investigation. Research is defined in the federal regulations as the "systematic collection of information for the benefit of others." In *therapeutic research,* there is the expectation that the patient/subject may also benefit, but the uncertainty about benefits and risks is typically greater compared with standard treatment. In addition, the need to collect data may be greater than would normally be necessary, thus exposing the patient to more discomfort or risk.

In *nontherapeutic research,* there is usually no expected benefit for the subject, therefore, any risk presents a very high risk/benefit ratio. Some argue that children, along with other nonconsenting subjects, should never be used in nontherapeutic research, because of the violation of Kant's dictum that a person should never be used solely as a means to an end. The more widely held opinion is that children may be exposed to at least *minimal risks,* although the reasons for this exception are disputed. Some argue that children have a duty to contribute to the social welfare, although the federal regulations do not allow competent adults to be used as research subjects without their consent, or that the very low risk is the reason for exclusion of children. The federal regulations define minimal risk as risks "similar to those encountered in the course of a routine office visit." Some interpret this to include procedures similar to those done in routine office visits, but others claim that an invasive procedure such as a liver biopsy may be done if the risks, in the hands of a particular investigator, are empirically no higher than those of a routine office visit or if the procedure is routine for a visit to a specialist.

Innovative therapy is defined as a new and unproven intervention done primarily for the benefit of the patient, with no intent to gather new information. Such innovations may be more hazardous and ethically more problematic than research, in part because they are not subject to peer review and because toxicity is not being systematically assessed. This therapy is also subject to abuse because its definition is a matter of intent, difficult for others to disprove.

As with all medical care, *informed consent* of the patient or his or her representative is at the core of protecting subjects. The standard for consent in the experimentation setting is higher because the risks and benefits are typically less clear, the investigator has a conflict of interest, and historically humans have been subjected to unauthorized risks when strict requirements for consent were not respected. Adolescents who are competent may sometimes consent to be research subjects. It is also generally acknowledged that children should be given the opportunity to *dissent,* particularly for nontherapeutic research when there cannot be a claim that participation is in the child's interest. In the United States national regulations require that reasonable efforts be made to at least inform the child over the age of 7 that participation is not part of his or her care and that, therefore, the child is free to refuse to participate.

In addition to the protection that informed consent is intended to provide, virtually all research in the United States is reviewed by an institutional review board, required by federal regulations for institutions receiving federal research funds. It is uncertain whether such review is legally required for research that is not federally funded or for research in settings that receive no federal funds, such as private clinics. The principles of ethical decision-making that led to the involvement of ethics committees in clinical decisions argue for similar review of research involving children, regardless of the source of funding.

2.6 DEFINITION OF DEATH

There is a general consensus that a patient is legally dead when brain death occurs, which is defined as irreversible cessation of all brain activity, including the brain stem (Sec. 20.56). The method of determining when brain death occurs is a medical question, not generally specified by the law, and it is subject to changing technology and understanding of brain physiology and its assessment. The criteria useful for assessing brain death in adults can be applied to children, down to the age of approximately 1 wk in term infants. Below 1 wk of age these criteria are subject to significant error, and the diagnosis cannot be made with complete confidence.

There is a continuing ethical controversy with regard to the appropriateness of using brain death as the criterion for death of the person. The possibility of retrieving organs from infants with anencephaly has stimulated consideration of relying on absence of the cortex or evidence of death of cortical tissue as the criterion for death. This is based on the claim that all functions that we associate with personhood reside in the cortex.

2.7 MATERNAL-FETAL CONFLICTS

In addition to the continuing debate over abortion in the United States, there is increased discussion about the proper balancing of maternal and fetal interests when a pregnant woman's behavior affects the well-being of the fetus. This is usually not limited to maternal-fetal conflicts of interest, because in virtually all cases the concern is also over the well-being of future infants and children.

The most dramatic of these conflicts arise when a pregnant woman refuses standard, effective treatment essential for the benefit of a fetus/infant who is at high risk of death or serious disability, such as refusal of cesarean section for placenta previa in a voluntary pregnancy near term involving a presumably normal fetus/infant. Courts in the United States have usually decided that a woman can be required to undergo such a procedure when the benefit to the emergent child is clear. A federal court has decided that such an order was inappropriate in a case involving a 26 wk-old-fetus and, by implication, other cases in which the benefit of intervention was in doubt. Pediatricians may be required in such cases prenatally to initiate or support court proceedings in the interests of the future child or to consider postnatal sanctions, including reporting of child abuse or neglect.

Child abuse statutes have also been invoked in attempts to modify the behavior of women who ingest alcohol or illicit drugs during pregnancy and expose their fetus/infants to harm. The pediatrician considering reporting such cases must consider the likelihood of benefit from reporting, the harms to the child as well as to the mother if criminal charges or custody changes are sought, and the possible effects that reporting may have in driving pregnant women away from the health care system, particularly from prenatal care.

2.8 ALLOCATION OF LIMITED HEALTH CARE RESOURCES (DISTRIBUTIVE JUSTICE)

The most serious ethical problem in health care in the United States may be the great inequality in access to care in the population. Large numbers of citizens are affected, and there are serious consequences in terms of death and disability. Approximately 20% of children are estimated to lack access to the health care system, most commonly because they lack private insurance and are not eligible for Medicaid programs (see Chapter 1). The total amounts to more than 10 million children who have a variety of preventable illnesses and disabilities, including prematurity, inadequate immunization, and delayed diagnosis and treatment for conditions commonly detected through routine health supervision. In ethical terms, it is argued that the prevailing system of distribution is unjust because it is chosen and maintained by those who are already well served and generally financially and socially advantaged. Some advocate that health care services are so basic to life, well-being, and equal opportunity that access to a basic level of effective services should be guaranteed to all members of society.

NORMAN FOST

Beauchamp T, Walters L: Contemporary Issues in Bioethics, 3rd ed. Belmont, CA, Wadsworth Pub Co, 1989.
Culver CM, Gert B: The justification of paternalistic behavior. *In:* Philosophy in Medicine: Conceptual and Ethical Issues in Medicine and Psychiatry. New York, Oxford U Pr, 1982.
Fost N: Ethical issues in pediatric AIDS. *In:* Pizzo P, Wilfert C (eds): Pediatric AIDS: The Challenge of HIV Infection in Infants, Children, and Adolescents. Baltimore, Williams & Wilkins, 1990.
Fost N, Cranford R: Hospital ethics committees: Administrative aspects. JAMA 253:2687, 1985.
Gaylin W, Macklin R (eds): Who Speaks for the Child?: The Problems of Proxy Consent. New York, Plenum Press, 1982.
Holder AR: Legal Issues in Pediatric and Adolescent Medicine, 2nd ed. New Haven, Yale Press, 1985.
Levine R: Ethics and Regulation of Clinical Research, 2nd ed. Baltimore, Urban and Schwarzenberg, 1986.
Menzel PT: Strong Medicine: The Ethical Rationing of Health Care. Oxford, New York, 1990.
O'Neill O, Ruddick W: Having Children: Philosophical and Legal Reflections of Parenthood. New York, Oxford U Pr, 1979.
Weir R: Selective Nontreatment of Handicapped Newborns: Moral Dilemmas in Neonatal Medicine. New York, Oxford U Pr, 1984.

2.9 CULTURAL ISSUES IN PEDIATRIC CARE

The physician who takes care of children and families from diverse ethnic backgrounds needs to be aware of the culturally accepted ways in which individuals deal with health, illness, and the health care system. These health beliefs and behaviors constitute a group's way of defining and maintaining health. They include assumptions concerning the cause, identification, classification, and treatment of illness as well as interactions with therapists. How an individual experiences illness is to a great extent culturally determined and has a significant impact on the interaction between the patient and the physician. Knowledge of cultural beliefs about sickness and health may help the physician increase the effectiveness of, and satisfaction with, the clinical encounter. This section discusses these issues and strategies for providing culturally appropriate medical care.

INTRACULTURAL DIVERSITY. Because individuals subscribe to group norms to varying degrees, an individual's health beliefs and behaviors consist of a combination of cultural standards mixed with personal experiences and perceptions. Not all people from a particular cultural heritage think and act in the same manner. More variations in behavior often exist within cultural groups than between groups. The clinician should be aware of possible differences and should attempt to identify individuals for whom specific beliefs may be a barrier to effective health care.

In the multicultural setting, the degree of adherence to cultural standards is related to the individual's level of *acculturation,* the changes in cultural beliefs due to contact with the "mainstream" culture, such as acceptance of the "Western" biomedical culture. The level of acculturation has been positively correlated with (1) length of residency in the host cultural area; (2) second generation or greater in the host cultural area; (3) level and location of formal education; (4) ease with which one speaks the host language; (5) residence outside of an ethnic enclave; (6) less contact with the cultural area of origin; and (7) family composition (with older, more traditional relatives present, cultural transmission increases and acculturation decreases).

The clinician should determine a patient's or parent's level of acculturation by asking questions that pertain to these variables when the social history is being taken. When less acculturated families are identified, the clinician should ask about specific beliefs and practices concerning health care.

CAUSES OF ILLNESS. Different cultural groups may have theories and explanations for *illness causation* that do not fit into the biomedical paradigm. Some cultures believe that health is a product of a state of *natural balance* and that illness and disease result from a disruption of this balance. The Oriental beliefs of *yin* and *yang* and the *humoral* (or hot/cold) theory of illness found in many Latino cultures (which has its historical roots in the Hippocratic belief in the four cardinal humors) are examples of this concept. People in other cultures may consider that illness is a *retribution for sins,* and some distinguish *natural and supernatural* causes of illness. These categorizations often have implications regarding what type of healer to consult for treatment—for example, sometimes patients go to the physician for relief of *symptoms* while they also consult a folk healer for identifying a spiritual or supernatural *cause.* The physician should become familiar with the common beliefs that are held in the cultural groups that he or she serves and should inquire nonjudgmentally about the patient's or parent's thoughts concerning the cause of the illness. If the parent relates beliefs that are inconsistent with the biomedical explanatory model but will have no adverse effect on the outcome of the illness, it is best not to contradict the parent but to offer the biomedical explanation and treatment plan *in addition.* Attempts to change long-held beliefs in a short clinical visit will most likely fail.

Many cultures have strict rules regarding conduct during times when the body is thought to be susceptible to illness. For example, many ethnic groups believe that the postpartum period is a critical time in which the newborn and mother are at risk for disease. For a particular period of time, the mother and child are often kept at home in isolation and may have special dietary restrictions, such as in traditional Haitian and Mexican *(la cuarentena, la dieta)* cultures. Another time of increased susceptibility in many traditional cultures is during menstruation. Appointments for well-child care during these periods may be missed for fear of having the mother or infant go outside of the home.

ILLNESS DEFINITION AND SYMPTOM EXPRESSION. *Folk illnesses* are culturally derived clusters of symptoms that are believed to exist as syndromes by members of an ethnic group. Examples believed to affect infants and children include *empacho* (a gastrointestinal syndrome, found in Mexicans, Puerto Ricans, Central Americans, Filipinos), *caida de mollera* ("fallen fontanelle," found in Mexicans), and *mal (de) ojo* (found in Latin America), *malocchio* (found in Italy) and other "evil-eye" beliefs (found in Europe and the Middle East). Parents may present their child to a pediatrician even when they suspect that the child has a folk illness. The reasons for this vary and include the fear that friends and family might consider the parents negligent if they did not bring their child to the physician. Although they may present for medical care, these parents usually do not express their thoughts about folk etiology to the physician, and a cycle of miscommunication may begin.

Some folk illnesses are cultural explanations for illnesses

that have a pathophysiologic cause and may require biomedical treatment, such as the Mexican folk illness *caida de mollera*, or "fallen fontanelle," which may be a folk description for moderate dehydration. Other syndromes do not fit into a medical disease category, and if the physician diagnoses "nothing wrong" or a self-limiting illness that requires no treatment, it is likely that the patient may seek further care with a folk healer (a culturally sanctioned lay healer who treats folk illness). Often this is appropriate, especially when the physician decides that the illness does not require medical intervention. However, some remedies and treatments that folk healers recommend to patients may have adverse health effects or may interfere with other medications that the patient is taking. For example, harmless treatments for *empacho* (a gastrointestinal syndrome) include herbal teas, dietary restrictions, and going to a folk healer who performs massage and prays. Some healers in the southwestern United States and Mexico, however, have recommended that the child should also drink certain folk remedies *(greta, azarcon,* and *ayalbalde)*, which were found to have a high content of lead oxides, resulting in lead toxicity in many of the children.

Another folk illness, *Mal (de) ojo,* is believed to be an illness of infancy brought on by a spell put on the child by someone who secretly covets him or her. Any person who displays excessive attention or strong glances directed at the child may be thought by the parents to be casting a spell on their child. Pediatricians, who usually enjoy smiling at and praising children, should be aware that their display may be misinterpreted by some parents and grandparents. The physician should know how to allay this concern—for example, in the Puerto Rican culture, saying the words "dios le (la) bendiga" ("God bless him [her]") will dispel concerns of malevolence. The level of acculturation may provide insight into which parents may believe in folk illnesses; another clue may be the display of protective objects, such as charms and amulets, attached to the baby's clothing or worn around chains. The culturally sensitive physician should be aware of the reasons for these protective amulets and should not ask the parent to remove them, especially when the child is ill. If the physician is concerned about injury owing to necklaces or bracelets on an infant, he or she should recommend that the object be safely attached to underclothing instead of being placed on a chain.

CULTURALLY NORMATIVE INTERACTIVE STYLES. Another area in which cross-cultural miscommunication may occur concerns different *interactive styles*. For example, many people display a deferential style when interacting with strangers, elders, and those of higher education and social class. This type of behavior may occur more often in Puerto Ricans (who call it *respeto*), Asians, and Native Americans than in others, although it can be manifest in any individual and stereotyping should be avoided. Part of this behavior style often includes reticence with regard to asking questions of authority figures. The "nod of the head" in response to a physician's comment does not mean necessarily that the patient agrees with or understands the instructions given. An open and sensitive approach on the part of the physician, as well as asking the patient to repeat the instructions, may improve communication. Other cultural groups display a more inquisitive and openly questioning style of interaction. The physician who is unaware of this may mistake it for hostility.

Nonverbal communication is also culturally determined. The maintenance of eye contact with the patient is regarded as exhibiting caring and understanding in some cultures, but in other cultures eye contact may be considered to be a display of challenge or aggression (especially from the opposite sex). The use of physical contact can also be interpreted as showing care in some groups or as culturally inappropriate behavior by others.

Cultures often have strict definitions of what should be discussed with members of the opposite sex, such as traditional Chinese, Italians *(vergogna)*, Mexican-Americans, and Puerto Ricans. For example, a mother who is concerned with masturbatory behavior in her preschool daughter, or an adolescent presenting with penile or vaginal discharge or for contraceptive planning, may, at the sight of a physician of the opposite sex, not reveal the true reason for the visit. Likewise, a mother may feel uncomfortable discussing the foreskin care of her newborn boy. If these concerns exist, the physician may need to elicit help from health care workers of the opposite sex and attempt to involve both parents in the history-taking and treatment plan.

LANGUAGE BARRIERS. Clinicians working in the multicultural setting often find themselves in a situation in which the patient or parents are not sufficiently fluent in the language of the physician to adequately describe medical and health care concerns. The culturally sensitive physician who makes an effort to learn the language of his or her patients will meet with increased acceptance by the patient, but it should be understood that effective communication requires total understanding on the part of both the physician and the patient; therefore, it may be prudent to enlist the services of an interpreter as well. A good interpreter is an individual who, in addition to being fluent in both languages, has a basic knowledge of medical terminology as well as a good understanding of the interactive style and rules of communication in the cultural group being interpreted The sex of the interpreter may have important implications, depending on the topic of discussion. More time will need to be allotted for a patient visit when translation services are needed. When a professional interpreter is not available, certain guidelines are helpful when choosing an interpreter (Table 2–1). When the patient brings an adult friend or family member who is fluent in both languages and accepts the role as interpreter, the clinician should utilize him or her but remember that the individual may not be familiar with medical terms. Also, the "friend" interpreter, by definition, has a tie with the patient and may consciously or unconsciously edit or editorialize the physician's discourse. During critically important discussions, it may be wise to have present a second bilingual "observer," chosen by the physician, to monitor the translation.

CULTURALLY SENSITIVE METHODS TO INCREASE COMPLIANCE. Lack of adherence to therapeutic suggestions is a problem in clinical care. The acknowledgment of culturally mediated health beliefs and behaviors and their incorporation into the medical care plan, when appropriate, may improve compliance. For example, in many cultural groups certain numbers and colors have magical or religious connotations; administering medications on a schedule that incorporates

TABLE 2–1. Guidelines for Choosing an Appropriate Interpreter and Strategies to Increase Effective Communication During Use of an Interpreter

Never use a child to interpret because this may disrupt social roles and put undue stress on the child.
Do not ask a stranger from the waiting room to interpret because of potential confidentiality problems.
It is usually appropriate to use an adult who the patient brings to the visit for this purpose. However, there may be problems of medical terminology, confidentiality, and editorialization.
Always ask the patient if the designated translator is acceptable to him or her.
Maintain visual contact with the patient or parent during translation; you may pick up important nonverbal clues regarding comprehension.
Ask the interpreter to translate as literally as possible.
Use nonlanguage aids (e.g., charts, diagrams) whenever possible.

the beneficial ones, such as red and 3 in traditional gypsy culture, for example, prescribing a pink antibiotic three times a day for otitis media, may be met with more acceptance (than a white antibiotic four times a day). Compliance may also be increased by administering medications with culturally appropriate foods. In addition, identifying patients or parents who utilize nonharmful folk remedies and incorporating these remedies into the medical treatment plan may help increase compliance with prescribed medical therapy.

The care of children and families from different cultural heritages provides the clinician with insights regarding the relationship between biology, culture, and society. Most interventions aimed at increasing the quality of care in these circumstances only require that the physician recognize the need for nonjudgmental inquiry regarding cultural health beliefs and behaviors and remain open-minded and sensitive to the responses obtained.

LEE M. PACHTER

Clark AL (ed): Culture and Childrearing. Philadelphia, FA Davis, 1981.

Harwood A: Ethnicity and clinical care: Selected issues in treating Puerto Rican patients. Hosp Phys 17(9):113, 1981.

Harwood A (ed): Ethnicity and Medical Care. Cambridge, Harvard University Press, 1981.

Kleinman A: Concepts and a model for the comparison of medical systems as cultural systems. Soc Sci Med 12:85, 1978.

Kleinman A: Selected issues in treating the Chinese patient. Hosp Phys 18(7):58, 1982.

Kleinman A, Eisenberg L, Good B: Culture, illness, and care: Clinical lessons from anthropologic and cross-cultural research. Ann Intern Med 88:251, 1978.

Martinez RA (ed): Hispanic Culture and Health Care. St. Louis, CV Mosby, 1978.

Pachter LM, Bernstein B, Osorio A: Clinical implications of a folk illness: Empacho in mainland Puerto Ricans. Med Anthropol 13(4), 1991.

Shields MN: Ethnicity and clinical care: Selected issues in treating gypsy patients. Hosp Phys 17:85, 1981.

Snow LF: Ethnicity and clinical care: American blacks. Hosp Phys 18(3):90, 1982.

Spector RE: Cultural Diversity in Health and Illness. East Norwalk, CT, Appleton-Century-Crofts, 1985.

Trotter RT II: Folk medicine in the Southwest: Myths and medical facts. Postgrad Med 78:167, 1985.

3

GROWTH AND DEVELOPMENT

3.1 INTRODUCTION

The basic science of pediatrics is growth and development. All health personnel having responsibility for the care of children should be familiar with the normal patterns and milestones of development and be able to recognize deviations from the norm as early as possible, so that underlying disorders may be promptly identified and given appropriate attention.

The term *growth and development* refers to the process by which the fertilized ovum becomes an adult person. *Growth* implies principally changes in size of the body as a whole or of its individual parts; *development* embraces other aspects of differentiation of form, including those driven by genetic endowment, but also involves changes of function, including those that are shaped mainly by interactions with the environment, whether these produce structural, emotional, or social changes.

Manifestations of *physical growth and development* range from those at the molecular level, such as the activation of enzymes in the course of differentiation, to the complex interplay of metabolic and physical changes associated with puberty and adolescence.

Neurodevelopmental processes, such as the acquisition of basic gross and fine motor skills, depend to a great extent on maturation of neural structures, but they may be profoundly modified by the environment and by experience.

Cognitive growth and development depends on both genetic and environmental factors. In early infancy this process may be difficult to differentiate from neurologic and behavioral maturation. In later infancy and childhood, cognitive and intellectual functions are increasingly measured by communicative skills and by the ability to handle abstract and symbolic material.

The *psychosocial development* of the child integrates all of the foregoing in a process that incorporates genetic constitution, cognition, and experience into the continuing and ultimate definition of the individual as a unique person and personality.

Genetic factors may set limits to biologic potential, but these are intimately interwoven with the environment. *Physical trauma* may be prenatal or postnatal, nutritional, chemical, residual from infection, or immunologic. *Nutritional* factors may reflect primarily *socioeconomic* realities. *Social and emotional* factors affecting growth potential include the sex of the child, the position of the child in the family, the quality of interaction of the infant or child with siblings, parents, and others, the personal concerns and needs of the parents, and the child-rearing patterns of the parents and of the community. *Cultural considerations* may either limit or expand the range of behavior of children by establishing conventional expectations and may alter the schedule for acquisition of skills, such as sitting or walking, which were once regarded as depending almost entirely on maturation. *Politics* and culture are closely related, inasmuch as the political life of any community provides the arena in which public priorities are set, including those that may have profound effects on children.

The experience of each child is unique, and the patterns of development may be profoundly different for individual children within the broad limits that designate "normality." Patterns of physical growth and development, for example, have such variability that they can often be expressed only in statistical terms.

STATISTICAL PRINCIPLES IN ASSESSMENT OF VARIABILITY IN GROWTH AND DEVELOPMENT

When biologic measurements vary over a range of normal values, the largest number of values found tend to cluster about an *average* or *mean* value. When such data are plotted on a graph, the result is often a close approximation of the theoretical or gaussian bell-shaped curve (Fig. 3–1) that describes the ideal distribution of continuously variable values about a population mean. Statistical treatment of such data may generate a number of useful measurements, the most important of which are the *mean* or *average* value and the *standard deviation (SD) of the mean.*

The *SD* measures the degree of dispersion of observed values around the mean value. In the ideal gaussian distribution the values lying between the points 1 SD below and 1 SD above the mean value will include approximately 68% of all values. The range *mean* ± *2 SD* includes approximately 95% of values distributed about this mean (excluding 2.5% above and 2.5% below the range); the range *mean* ± *3 SD* includes about 99.7% of such values.

In an ideal distribution of random normal values the mean or average value will be the one most commonly found (i.e., the *modal* or *normal* value [*mode* or *norm*]) within the population under study. If, on the other hand, a set of values includes a disproportionately larger number of high values than low, or vice versa, the most common value (the mode or norm) may differ from the average value for the population being investigated. Asymmetric curves are generated, which are said to be *skewed.* Under these circumstances, the *median* or central value (see later) may be more representative of the population. Symmetric curves may show *kurtosis* in accordance with whether they are unusually peaked (leptokurtic) or flattened (platykurtic). (The ideal curve is mesokurtic.) When a *bimodal* curve is found, it may be inferred that not one but two populations are being measured, which have some feature differentiating them from each other.

When quantitative data are arranged in order of ascending or descending magnitude, a value, the *median,* can be found, on either side of which lie half of the observations. In the distribution described by the symmetric ideal curve, the median, the mean, and the mode fall at the same point. Values may also be designated that divide the data into two groups at the first *quartile* point, below which will lie one quarter of the values, at the second quartile point (the median), and at the third quartile point, below which lie three quarters of the observed values. *Percentile (or centile)* points in a distribution of ordered data have similar meaning, one tenth of observations falling below the 10th percentile, three tenths

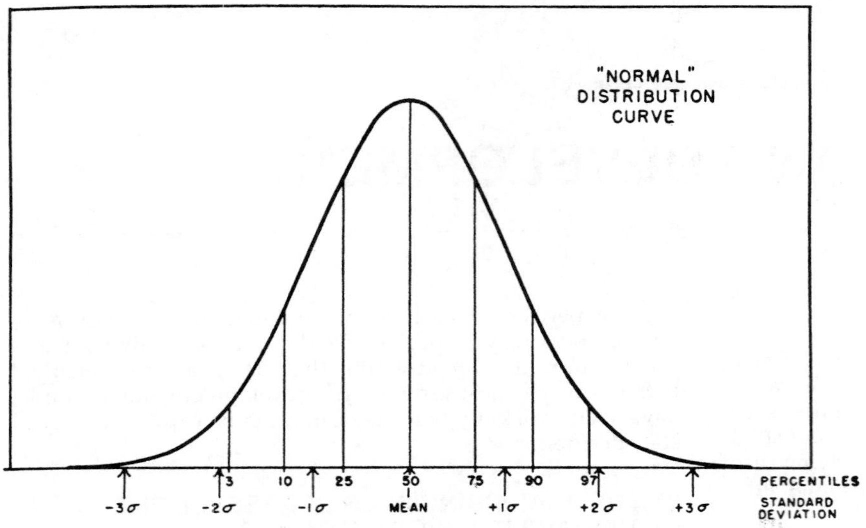

Figure 3–1. "Normal" (gaussian) distribution curve. This curve represents the theoretical distribution of values for many biologic measurements. The percentiles indicate certain positions within this distribution, as do the standard deviations from the mean. (From Nelson WE [ed]: Textbook of Pediatrics, 7th ed. Philadelphia, WB Saunders, 1959, p 18.)

below the 30th percentile, one twentieth (5%) above the 95th percentile, and so on.

Percentile location is commonly used to designate where an individual member of a population stands with respect to the other members. The growth charts commonly used for following the course of physical development of children with age show curves at positions corresponding to distances from average values, either above or below the mean. Approximately 10% of normal persons fall either above the 95th percentile (5%) or below the 5th percentile (5%) for any normally distributed measurement.

When two samples or populations differ with respect to average values for some biologic trait, it is often difficult to evaluate the meaning of this difference unless the distribution or dispersion of values in each sample is known. When the *SDs* of the two samples are known, the *probability* (p) can be calculated that an observed difference between them might have occurred by chance alone, the samples having been drawn from a homogeneous population. When the observed difference is very unlikely to have occurred by chance, it may be inferred that the observed difference is likely to represent a real (and perhaps significant) differential factor between the two groups.

When it seems unlikely (e.g., $p < 0.05$, or < 0.001) that a particular difference would have occurred by chance, this does not prove that the difference is real rather than an artifact. When the likelihood that an observed deviation from a mean value or a difference between two means would be expected by chance less than once in 20 comparisons of random data, the deviation or difference is often said to be "statistically significant." A p value of less than 0.01 or 0.001 will carry more confidence that a deviation or difference is significant or real. The choice of a value of p is arbitrary; if "statistical significance" is defined as p less than 0.05, such "significance" will be found by chance in about 1 in 20 examinations made in a homogeneous population with normally distributed values.

These considerations set the basis for the use of percentile (centile) designations in following the growth and development of children. Examination of their percentile location helps to identify children whose substantial distance from the norm (e.g., above the 95th percentile or below the 5th percentile [in an ideal distribution, beyond 1.645 SD above or below the mean]) suggests that their developmental progress may need careful evaluation before any judgment is made with regard to whether their deviation from the norm represents a variant normal growth pattern or an abnormality.

3.2 FETAL GROWTH AND DEVELOPMENT

Intrauterine life comprises *embryonic* and *fetal* periods. The embryonic period is usually considered to be the first 8 wk of growth, during which the ovum differentiates into an organism with most of the gross anatomic features of the human form. Organogenesis continues beyond 8 wk in some systems, so that some prefer to designate the embryonic period as the 1st trimester of pregnancy, or the first 12 wk. The circulatory system of the fetus, for example, attains its final form between the 8th and 12th wk of gestation. (The details of its structure and the changes that occur with birth are discussed in Chapters 9 and 15.) The period between the 12th and 40th wk of gestation, the fetal period, is marked by rapid growth and elaboration of function. Not until the 24th–26th wk, however, is the fetus generally *viable.*

PHYSICAL DEVELOPMENT. The 1st wk of embryonic life is *germinal;* its chief feature is cellular division. During the 2nd wk, the cell mass differentiates into two layers (ectoderm and entoderm); during the 3rd wk, mesoderm is added. During the 4th wk, the growing organism elaborates the somites and undergoes rapid differentiation between the 4th and 8th wk into an essentially human form. At 8 wk of age, the fetus weighs about 1 g and is about 2.5 cm in length; at 12 wk it weighs about 14 g and is about 7.5 cm long, and at 16 wk it is about 100 g and 17 cm long. By the end of the 1st trimester the sex of the fetus can be distinguished on external examination. During the *2nd trimester of pregnancy* there is rapid acquisition of new functions. By the end of the 2nd trimester (28 wk), the fetus weighs about 1,000 g and is about 35 cm (14 in) in length. During the *3rd trimester* the increase in size of the fetus involves primarily subcutaneous tissue and muscle mass.

Respiratory movements of the fetus occur as early as the 18th wk of gestation, but the level of development of alveolar structures usually does not permit survival until the 24th–26th wk. The development of pulmonary surfactant is underway by 20 wk of gestation but may not be adequate until late in the 3rd trimester (see Sec. 9.32). The tidal flow of amniotic fluid into and out of the developing lung may contribute to pulmonary arborization. Late in pregnancy, when amniotic fluid contains more cells and may contain meconium and other debris, aspiration may deposit these materials into the alveoli, leading to respiratory difficulties following delivery (see Sec. 9.35).

The hemoglobin of the fetus is predominantly fetal in type (Hgb F). At a given oxygen tension, Hgb F carries more oxygen than adult hemoglobin (Hgb A). Hgb A is produced in late fetal life and represents approximately 30% of the hemoglobin in the mature newborn infant (see also Sec. 16.2).

Bile begins to be formed by about 12 wk of gestation and digestive enzymes soon thereafter. Meconium, the distinctive intestinal content of the fetus, is present by 16 wk; it consists of desquamated intestinal cells and fluids, and of squamous cells and lanugo hair from amniotic fluid swallowed by the fetus.

The fetus makes swallowing movements as early as the 14th wk of gestation; at 17 wk the upper lip may protrude on stimulation in the oral area, and by the 20th wk both lips protrude. At 22 wk the lips are pursed on stimulation, and by 26–28 wk the fetus may actively suck in attempting to gain nourishment.

The *placenta* is the chief route of metabolic exchange between the mother and the fetus. Its most urgent function is to provide for gas exchange; for this, adequate perfusion is needed on both the fetal and the maternal side. The placenta elaborates hormones and enzymes that participate in the regulation of pregnancy, and it effects the selective transfer of nutrients and metabolites between the mother and the infant. Maternal hormones and drugs may also be transferred to the infant. Placental permeability is selective even for such closely related substances as the antibodies against viruses and those against bacteria; the former (e.g., immunoglobulin G [IgG]) are more readily transmitted than the latter (e.g., IgM). Much of the transfer of calcium, iron, and IgG to the infant occurs in the last trimester, with the result that the infant born prematurely may have a greater need than the full-term infant for calcium and iron and may be more susceptible to infection (see Sec. 9.58).

NEURODEVELOPMENT. Neurologic activity in the fetus is first manifest by about 8 wk of gestation, when isolated muscular contractions may be seen in response to local stimulation. By 9 wk, contralateral flexion may be followed by ipsilateral flexion, and some spontaneous movements occur. By 9 wk of gestation, the palms and soles have become reflexogenic; by 13–14 wk, graceful flowing movements may be produced by stimulation of all areas except the back, the back of the head, and the vertex. At this time, the movements of the fetus may first be felt by the mother. The grasp reflex is evident by 17 wk and is generally well developed by 27 wk. Weak phonation may occur in the fetus delivered at 22 wk. By 25 wk, the earliest signs of the Moro response can be elicited. In late pregnancy the fetus is capable of *habituation* to certain sensory stimuli; for example, fetal movement and acceleration of the fetal pulse in response to noise transmitted through the mother's abdomen are blunted on repetition of the noise (see *orienting response*, later).

Fetuses differ in levels of activity, and there is evidence that fetal activity may respond to maternal emotions, possibly as a result of placental transfer of epinephrine or other substances. Little is known about how the activity of newborn infants or the quality of the infant's demands during the first few weeks of life may reflect aspects of gestation that are dependent on maternal emotional states. The comfort that some newborn infants receive from rhythmic motion or rhythmic sound may stem from similar sensations imparted by maternal motion, breathing, or heart sounds.

PROBLEMS OF EMBRYONIC AND FETAL LIFE. Mortality during the embryonic period is probably higher than at any other time of life. Causes include abnormalities of genes and chromosomes and alterations in maternal health. These may be interrelated; advanced maternal age, for example, disposes to certain chromosomal abnormalities. Maternal infection or the administration of certain drugs to the mother during the 1st trimester may alter the differentiation of the fetus and may result in congenital anomalies. Intrauterine environmental factors responsible for defects in differentiation exert their effects principally within the 1st trimester (see Sec. 9.9).

Morbidity during the fetal period may result from a variety of intrauterine factors. These include interference with oxygenation secondary to disturbances of the placenta or umbilical cord; infections of bacterial, viral, or protozoan origin; injury by radiation, trauma, or noxious chemicals; immunologic disorders due to maternal immunization and transfer of isoantibodies; and maternal nutritional disturbances.

The effects of *intrauterine malnutrition* on cerebral structure or function in later life are not fully understood. The rate of increase in the number of neurons is high during gestation, and their number probably continues to increase at a decreasing rate until about 18 mo of postnatal age. In this postnatal period there is also an increase in the number and complexity of dendritic connections, in the number of neuroglial cells, in the size of neurons and glial cells, and in myelinization. The effects on the central nervous system of malnutrition that occurs after this time can be much more readily reversed than those that result from undernutrition during periods of rapid cellular proliferation.

3.3 THE NEWBORN INFANT

PHYSICAL DEVELOPMENT. The weight of the newborn infant averages about 3.4 kg (7½ lb); boys are slightly heavier than girls. About 95% of full-term newborn infants weigh between 2.5 and 4.6 kg (5½–10 lb). Length averages about 50 cm (20 in); approximately 95% of infants are within the range of 45–55 cm (18–22 in). Head circumference averages about 35 cm (14 in), ranging from 32.6 to 37.2 cm (5th–95th percentiles).

Body proportions of newborn infants differentiate them sharply from older infants, children, and adults (Fig. 3–2). The head is relatively larger, the face rounder, and the mandible smaller than in older children or adults. The chest tends to be rounded rather than flattened anteroposteriorly; the abdomen is relatively prominent and the extremities relatively short. The midpoint of stature of the newborn infant is near the level of the umbilicus, whereas in the adult it is at the symphysis pubis.

At birth, minor traumatic effects of labor may be apparent, such as edema of the vertex or overriding of cranial bones, and infrequently there may be more severe injuries. There may be other minor anatomic variants of little or no significance. Normal anatomic features differentiating the newborn from the older child include external auditory canals that are relatively short and straight, with thicker eardrums that are placed more obliquely to the canal. The middle ear contains a mucoid substance that may be mistaken for an exudate of infection. The eustachian tube is short and broad. There is usually a single mastoid cell in the antrum; maxillary and ethmoid sinuses are small, and the frontal and sphenoidal ones are undeveloped. The liver and spleen are commonly felt at or just below the costal margins, and the kidneys are often palpable.

The posture of the newborn infant tends to be one of partial flexion, simulating the fetal posture. The latter can often be determined by "folding" the infant into its most comfortable position, in which a more or less ovoid shape is created. Sometimes minor and occasionally major orthopedic abnormalities of the infant reflect the effect of intrauterine posture and pressure on the growing fetus.

PHYSIOLOGY. The prime need of the newborn infant is

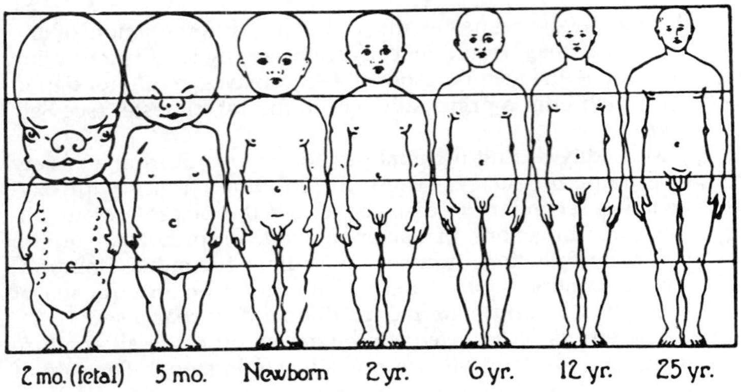

Figure 3–2. Changes in body proportions from the 2nd fetal mo to adulthood. (From Robbins WJ, Brody S, Hogan AG, et al: Growth. New Haven, Yale University Press, 1928. By permission of publisher.)

to establish adequate respirations for the exchange of gases. The rate of established respirations ranges generally from 35–50 breaths/min; brief excursions outside this range are common.

Cardiac adjustments of the neonatal period are often associated with transient murmurs. The heart rate ranges from 120 to 160 beats/min. The heart of the newborn infant seems large in proportion to the thorax when assessed by adult standards.

Activity of newborn infants directed toward meeting nutritional needs includes crying when hungry and a tendency when hungry to turn the head toward and to "root" about for the nipple or another stimulus placed close to the oral area (rooting reflex). Sucking, gagging, and swallowing reflexes are active. The newborn infant is capable of nausea and of vomiting (see also Sec. 9.41).

The infant initially expresses hunger at irregular intervals, but by the end of the 1st wk will usually be reasonably comfortable feeding at intervals ranging from 2 to 5 hr. No schedule of feedings will meet the demands or needs of all infants; if the infant and mother are close to each other during the immediate postnatal period, such as in a rooming-in arrangement, the opportunities for comfortably finding the baby's patterns of sleeping, awakening, and feeding will be as optimal as can be expected.

The first stools are generally passed within 24 hr and consist of meconium. When milk feedings are established, these stools begin to be replaced on the 3rd–4th day by *transitional stools*, which are greenish brown and may contain milk curds. The typical milk stool of the older infant follows after an interval of 3–4 days. The frequency of stools in the newborn infant seems closely related to the frequency of feeding and to the amount of food obtained, averaging 3–5/day by the end of the 1st wk. On any given day during the 1st wk about 1 infant in 50 will have no stool at all; it is not unusual for a healthy infant to have as many as 6–7 stools/day after the 2nd day, particularly if he or she has been breast-fed.

At delivery the body temperatures of mother and infant are virtually the same. The infant's temperature falls quickly but transiently; it is usually restored within 4–8 hr. The caloric requirement of the newborn infant for maintenance of body heat and basal activity is usually about 55 kcal/kg/24 hr. By the end of the 1st week the total caloric needs will be approximately 110 kcal/kg/24 hr, of which 50% supplies basal metabolic needs, 40% is invested in growth and in activity, 5% is needed for the specific dynamic action of protein, and 5% is lost in feces and urine.

In the newborn infant the extracellular fluid compartment may constitute up to 35% of body weight. During the 1st few days of life there is a loss of fluid that, in the absence of unusual oral intake, generally averages about 6% of body weight and may occasionally exceed 10%. When this loss is excessive, there may be dehydration or inanition fever on the 3rd–4th day. After the 1st wk the need for water ranges between 120 and 150 mL/kg/24 hr. About half of this is devoted to formation of urine and the rest to insensible loss by lungs and skin and to other losses. Insensible water loss has a relatively fixed relationship to the calories metabolized by the infant (about 40 mL/100 kcal). Losses in stool are variable, those in sweat minimal.

Because metabolism in newborn infants favors the anaerobic or glycolytic pathway, they are more tolerant of periods of hypoxia than older infants, children, or adults. This tolerance for hypoxia is only relative, however. If oxygenation of the newly born infant is not quickly established, a rapidly progressive metabolic and respiratory acidosis may ensue (due to accumulation of lactic acid and carbon dioxide), and hypoxic tissue injury may occur.

Glomerular filtration rate (GFR) and urine output are low in the 1st days of life but increase rapidly in the 1st 2 wk. The GFR does not approach adult standards until the end of the first year. During the 1st wk proteinuria is common, and the urine may contain an abundance of urates, which may give the diaper a pink stain. Urea clearance is low, and the ability to concentrate urine is limited. Production of ammonium ion also is limited, and phosphate clearance is low. The blood urea nitrogen (BUN) level may rise transiently.

The hemoglobin level of the newborn infant ranges around 17–19 g/dL, and mild reticulocytosis and normoblastemia may be observed for the 1st day or two of life (see Table 16–3). Leukocytes number about 10,000/mm^3 at birth and generally increase in number for the first 24 hr, with a relative neutrophilia. Counts as high as 25,000–35,000 may be encountered. After the 1st wk the total white cell count is likely to be below 14,000, with the characteristic relative lymphocytosis of infancy and early childhood. Stressful situations in the newborn infant, including overwhelming infections, may be associated with little or no leukocytosis and even with leukopenia.

There is little or no transfer of certain clotting factors from mother to infant. Establishment of normal hemostatic mechanisms depends on the acquisition of normal intestinal flora and elaboration of vitamin K (see Sec. 16.71).

Placental transfer of maternal hormones produces temporary changes in the breasts and genitalia of the newborn infant (see Sec. 9.9) and possibly in other tissues as well, and the withdrawal of maternal hormones or other metabolites may contribute to temporary hypofunction of the parathyroid gland. Maternal hyperglycemia may dispose the infant to hyperinsulinemia and hypoglycemia (see Sec. 9.56). Blood levels of sugar and of calcium are normally relatively low in the newborn infant, and further decreases (below about 20 mg/dL of sugar or about 7.5 mg/dL of calcium) may cause convulsions.

The gamma globulin level of the newborn infant (almost entirely maternal IgG) is slightly higher that that of the mother due to an active transport mechanism. The IgG affords protection against many viral and some bacterial diseases. On the other hand, IgM antibodies (which include the natural isohemagglutinins) do not cross the placenta in substantial numbers, nor does IgA or IgE. The IgM fraction of maternal immunoglobulins contains her antibodies against certain antigens of gram-negative enterobacteria; infants denied these are, accordingly, at increased risk of gram-negative bacillary infection. IgM antibodies may be formed by the fetus, however, in reponse to intrauterine infection. An elevated IgE level in the cord blood of the infant indicates an increased risk of allergic disorder following intrauterine sensitization. T lymphocyte functions are somewhat reduced in newborn infants.

The gamma globulin level of the infant falls to a low level by about 3 mo of age as maternal antibody disappears; a rise then occurs, as the infant produces his or her own immunoglobulins, to the levels that characterize older children and adults. Responses to artificial immunizations are relatively sluggish in term newborn infants and markedly so in premature infants. Antibodies of the major blood group system (ABO) usually appear by the 2nd mo of life.

The digestive enzymes are usually adequate for the diet of the newborn infant, although fat is handled somewhat less well than protein or carbohydrate. At the cellular level, however, a number of metabolic deficiencies (or neonatal immaturities) may have important clinical consequences. The red blood cells have relatively low levels of reduced glutathione, which may contribute to increased hemolysis under a variety of circumstances. A deficiency in capacity of the liver to conjugate bilirubin with glucuronic acid leads to hyperbilirubinemia, often with no evidence of hemolysis. A diminished capacity to metabolize certain drugs may place the newborn infant at increased risk when drug therapy is needed.

NEURODEVELOPMENT. Many of the behavioral features and neurologic responses of the newborn infant are described in Sec. 9.3 and 20.1. As indicated there and in Sec. 3.4, these responses depend on the level of maturity of the infant. Beyond the conventional neurologic or reflex behavior of the term newborn infant, however, lies a capacity for interaction with the environment, unappreciated until recently, that gives evidence of a complex neurologic organization.

The quality of the behavior that can be elicited from the newborn infant is highly dependent on the *behavioral state* or the level of arousal of the infant. Six levels of arousal have been defined (Prechtl and Beintema): deep sleep; sleep with rapid eye movement (REM); a drowsy state; a quiet, alert state; an awake and active state; and a state of active, intense crying. It is in the quiet and alert state (state 4) that newborn infants are capable of engaging in the most responsive and complex interactions with the environment. Sleep patterns of newborn infants begin to change as early as the 2nd day from the predominantly REM-type sleep of the older fetus toward the patterns of older infants and children.

Within the first hour or two after normal delivery of an unanesthetized and unsedated infant, the infant commonly spends a good deal of time in state 4. Within the next few days the amount of time spent by the baby in this state amounts to about 10% of the day and then increases with age.

From the moment of birth the infant is able to fixate objects visually and to follow the movements of these objects, and even in the first minutes of life, the term infant, among somewhat similar and rather complex figures, gives preferential attention to figures that resemble the human face. Within the first few days he or she is capable of visually scanning simple geometric figures. During the 1st wk, infants are also able to maintain visual fixations on faces, light, or movement against passive movements of their bodies (doll's eye reflex). Responses are originally partly vestibular but become increasingly oculomotor.

Certain behaviors of infants in response to environmental change have been called the *orienting response.* As a new stimulus is received in the auditory and /or visual or other sensory field, the infant becomes more alert, as shown by a suppression of spontaneous movement, by a likely turning of the head toward the stimulus, and by physiologic changes such as changes in heart rate. Acceleration occurs when a totally unfamiliar or noxious stimulus is received, whereas the heart rate tends to decelerate when the baby orients to a more or less familiar stimulus. When a substantially unchanging new stimulus becomes repetitive, the orienting response rapidly *habituates;* there is less startle reaction or cardiac acceleration, and, as the stimulus becomes familiar, cardiac deceleration may supervene.

Brazelton has brought together a number of observations of neonatal behavior to form a *Neonatal Behavioral Assessment Scale (NBAS)* that may provide a more helpful assessment of the behavior of the newborn infant than a traditional neurologic examination. The scale assesses the behavior of the infant in four dimensions: *interactive* processes (orientation, alertness, consolability, cuddliness); *motor* processes (muscular tone, motor maturity, defensive reactions, hand-to-mouth activity, general activity level, and reflex behavior); *control of physiologic state* (habituation to a bright light, a rattle, a bell, and a pinprick; self-quieting behavior); and *response to stress* (tremulousness, lability of skin color, and startle reaction).

The NBAS has been used to identify deficits in neurobehavioral function, to describe the level and quality of normal behavior, to assess the impact on behavior of injury, drugs, or other interventions, and to attempt to predict future development and function. In this last use, the results of the Brazelton evaluation may give a more accurate prognosis during the first week or two than the Apgar score at 1 and 5 min, and as late as 1 wk after delivery the use of this examination has detected changes in the infant's behavior due to drugs given to the mother (e.g., phenobarbital). The demonstration to parents of some of the items in the scale may foster healthy attachment as they reveal the infant's complexity and early evidence of the infant's personality and individuality (see Temperament, Sec. 3.15).

PSYCHOSOCIAL DEVELOPMENT. The infant is born into a social milieu in which he or she has for some time already been an important participant, as represented in the hopes and fears of the parents and particularly in the mother's experiences during pregnancy. To these earlier experiences are added the events surrounding the mother's labor and the delivery of the child. These experiences have the effect of *bonding* the parents in greater or lesser degree to the child. Bonding consists of those emotional ties and commitments that characterize the relationship between each parent or other participant in this social event and the infant who becomes the central figure. During the next hours, days, weeks, and months the infant reciprocates this bonding with his or her *attachment* to the significant persons in the environment to whom he or she will turn in the future for protection, nurturance, and love. Studies of analogs of bonding and attachment in animals and their newborn, under the designation of *imprinting,* have greatly enriched the study of socialization in human infants.

The equipment that the infant brings to bonding and attachment is striking in its complexity, beginning with the observation that the infant in the first minutes of life responds visually preferentially to figures that resemble the human face. Such behavior may be important in facilitating or eliciting those interactions that lead to the formation of social bonds. For example, the steady gaze of the newborn infant into the mother's eyes is often experienced by her as a powerful stimulus to her emotional attachment. Moreover, newborn infants give attention preferentially to high-pitched or female voices and within the 1st wk of life turn their heads more readily toward the sound of their own mothers' voices than to voices not previously heard, and they are even able to distinguish a familiar sound in the mother's voice. Furthermore, the motor behavior of infants is responsive to the cadences of speech of a person engaging them in a social relationship. This responsiveness to vocal stimulation may have importance for social bonding, and its lack may give a mother her first clue that her infant is abnormal, without either her or her physician knowing at first that the infant is deaf.

The attraction of the newborn infant to the human face may have a basis in some predetermined and poorly understood preprogramming of a genetic nature. The existence of a preregistration of what may be seen is evidenced by the fact that the infant imitatively sticks out the tongue to someone who sticks out a tongue at him or her. Other evidence of intersensory organization in the infant is shown by the fact that the infant will at the moment of birth turn the eyes with more than random likelihood toward a sound heard at one side of the head, perhaps reflexly, but as if knowing that to hear a sound from that source means that there is something there to be seen.

Prenatal and postnatal experiences involve kinesthetic, somesthetic, thermal, olfactory, and proprioceptive stimuli. Reactions to some of these may reflect the intrauterine experience. For example, the baby is exposed in utero to the regular rhythm and rate of the maternal heart beat and respiration, and it has been shown that sounds having the quality, rhythm, and rate of a normal heart beat can sometimes comfort fretful infants. The responsiveness to the maternal voice, referred to earlier, has been shown to have a prenatal component. Infants are capable within the 1st wk of life of differentiating breast pads containing the odor of the milk and breast of their own mothers. Other sensory modalities have been less well studied for their social implications.

The first hour or two after birth, when the infant is in the quiet, alert state, may offer a particularly favorable opportunity for facilitating bonding and attachment. Events at this time may influence not only the quality of the relationship established between mother and infant, but also, to some degree, between the infant and other persons sharing the experience, even if only as onlookers (e.g., as godparents). It is not known whether there exist for bonding and attachment in humans *critical periods* comparable with those used for imprinting in animals. It seems unlikely, given the resilience with which many infants, parents, and families surmount neonatal experiences that might have had devastating effects. On the other hand, for some fragile infants or parents the loss of some opportunities for harmonious interaction may be irretrievable within a few hours or days. These lost opportunities may be in some instances a first step in the development in later life of emotional disorders, child abuse and neglect, or failure to achieve potential levels of intellectual or social development.

Growing appreciation of the importance of childbirth as a social rather than a medical event has led to substantial revision of traditional practices. Mothers and fathers have both become involved in prenatal programs oriented toward education for childbirth and for child rearing. There has been encouragement of family-centered activities for pregnancy and childbirth, of greater restraint in the use of analgesic and anesthetic medication in labor, of breast-feeding, and of rooming-in arrangements in the neonatal period that will optimize the opportunities for newborn infants, their mothers, and their families to get to know each other within the first hours and days of life.

3.4 INFANT BORN PREMATURELY

The fetus born prematurely begins to have a substantial chance of survival at about 26–28 wk of gestation. The physical features of infants between the gestational ages of 26 and 40 wk are described in detail in Sec. 9.17. Their behavioral characteristics also evolve with their increasing gestational age.

NEURODEVELOPMENT. Infants whose birthweights range from 1,000 to 1,500 g tend to be predominantly hypotonic and to lie in a tonic neck attitude, often with little motion of the extremities. Vocalization is weak, as are the grasp and Moro responses. Sucking responses may also be weak, and these infants may show little evidence of hunger on deprivation of food. It is difficult to tell whether they are awake or asleep, although they can be stimulated to greater alertness.

Infants weighing from 1,500 to 2,000 g have good muscle tone when stimulated, a more vigorous grasp, and complete Moro responses. A sleep pattern is easily discernible, and they are able visually to fixate some objects in their environment. The more vigorous of these infants are able to manage breast-feeding.

Infants weighing between 2,000 and 2,500 g at birth generally have the appearance of small full-term infants, from which they cannot usually be differentiated by developmental examination. They have good cry and sustained muscle tone.

Although a moderate-sized premature infant (1,500 g or more) may seem more alert and active by the time he or she reaches the expected date of delivery than a full-term baby born on that day, the actual developmental level reached within a few weeks will generally be lower than that indicated by the chronologic age. The deficit in development tends to correspond to the level of prematurity. These differences generally disappear by the end of the 2nd year of life as long as no complicating factors occur.

PROBLEMS. The premature infant faces difficulties resulting from failure of adequate maturation of enzymatic, respiratory, renal, metabolic, hematologic, and immunologic mechanisms (see Chapter 9). Developmental defects are more common in premature infants than in full-term infants and often include impairments of motor or intellectual function. The latter are commonly due to residual damage resulting from anoxia or infection.

The premature infant is particularly vulnerable to the effects of sensory or social deprivation in the neonatal period due to the restrictions imposed by the necessities of care and by the sometimes prolonged period of relative isolation. Recent studies emphasize the importance of involving the mothers of even the smallest babies in some aspects of their care as early as possible to enhance the opportunities for mutual emotional bonding and attachment (see Sec. 3.3 and 9.6) and to prevent the long-term anxiety that may lead to the *vulnerable child syndrome*.

3.5 THE 1ST YEAR

PHYSICAL DEVELOPMENT. Most full-term infants regain their birthweights by the age of 10 days. The full-term infant generally doubles birthweight by 5 mo and triples it by 1 yr (Table 3–1). The premature infant is likely to gain about 6–7 kg (13–15 lb) in the 1st yr, which is about the average gain for full-term infants. The length of the normal infant increases during the 1st yr by 25–30 cm (10–12 in). An increase in subcutaneous tissue in the early months of life reaches its peak at about 9 mo (see Fig. 3–10).

The anterior fontanel may increase in size after birth but generally diminishes after 6 mo and may become effectively

TABLE 3–1. Formulas for Approximate Average Height and Weight of Normal Infants and Children

Weight	Kilograms	(Pounds)
(a) At birth	3.25	(7)
(b) 3–12 mo	$\frac{\text{age (mo)} + 9}{2}$	(age [mo] + 11)
(c) 1–6 yr	age (yr) × 2 + 8	(age [yr] × 5 + 17)
(d) 7–12 yr	$\frac{\text{age (yr)} \times 7 - 5}{2}$	(age [yr] × 7 + 5)
Height	**Centimeters**	**(Inches)**
(e) At birth	50	(20)
(f) At 1 yr	75	(30)
(g) 2–12 yr	age (yr) × 6 + 77	(age [yr] × 2½ + 30)

closed between 9 and 18 mo. The posterior fontanel is usually closed to palpation by 4 mo.

Head circumference (normally 34–35 cm [13.4–13.8 in] at birth) increases to approximately 44 cm by 6 mo and to 47 cm by 1 yr (Table 3–2). The head circumference is slightly larger than that of the chest at birth, but the two measurements become equal by the end of the first year.

The first deciduous teeth erupt in most children between 5 and 9 mo. The first to appear are the lower central incisors, followed by the upper central and then the upper lateral incisors. The lower lateral incisors, the 1st deciduous molars, cuspids (canines), and 2nd deciduous molars follow in that order. By the age of 1 yr most children have 6–8 teeth. Occasionally an infant has as few as 2 teeth at 1 yr without other evidence of any growth disturbance.

FIRST 3 MONTHS OF LIFE

NEURODEVELOPMENT. The newborn infant prone on a firm surface is able to avoid suffocation by turning the face from side to side; by 4 wk of age the head is lifted above the surface as it is turned. By then a rather symmetric flexed posture has become more relaxed, and the infant is likely to lie, when supine, in a tonic neck posture (head turned to one side with the extremities extended on that side).

When the infant within the first 4–8 wk of life is pulled from a supine to a sitting position, the head lags, and when the infant is in the upright position, head control is absent. By 12 wk there is some control of the head as the infant is drawn to a sitting position, but the head is tilted a little forward on the upright body; irregular head control results in a bobbing motion.

When held in ventral suspension (*Landau response*—the infant is lifted from the prone position by a hand held under the trunk), the newborn infant will be in a posture of flexion of head and extremities around the supporting hand. By 1 mo of age the infant will raise the head momentarily to the plane of the body, and by 2 mo he or she will be able to sustain the head in that plane. By 3 mo the head will be raised above the plane of the body, and the legs will be extended as well.

In the first days of life infants visually fixate best on those objects that are placed close to or moved through their line of vision. Depending on their level of interest, they may maintain fixation with movement of the eyes and head to nearly 90 degrees to either side of the midline. By 2 mo of age a supine infant will be able to follow an object presented 90 degrees from the midline through an arc of 180 degrees.

Reaching and grasping movements evolve out of earlier coordinate but incomplete motions of the arms and hands in response to the sight of objects in motion nearby ("larval reach"). Within 4 wk, some infants will make contact with stationary objects within their reach. Reflex grasp persists until the age of about 8 wk, after which, with growing eye and hand coordination, an active grasp becomes more evident. By 12 wk, the infant attempts to make contact with an offered object and will hold it briefly if appropriate contact is made. The coordination of eye and hand implicit in this activity seems to be facilitated in some measure by the tonic neck attitude.

The infant begins at about 4 wk to make small throaty noises; some vowel sounds are produced at 8 wk, and these are uttered with evident pleasure on social contact by 12 wk.

PSYCHOSOCIAL DEVELOPMENT. With neonatal experiences fostering bonding and attachment, and with continuing social interaction, infants soon show that they differentiate persons and objects in their environment. As early as 2–6 wk of age they can be shown to be more comfortable with familiar persons than with strangers.

Newborn and even prematurely born infants often display fragmentary *smiles,* usually in response to internal stimuli of uncertain nature during REM sleep or moments of drowsiness. A fully developed social smile becomes manifest usually between 3 and 5 wk of age. There is evidence that the smile of the very young infant may be elicited primarily by the infant's discovery that he or she has control over some contingencies in the environment, such as securing care or attention from the mother or another caretaker or recognizing an ability to control the behavior of inanimate objects. The infant who does not have a social smile by the age of 8–12 wk should be regarded as possibly seriously deviant with respect to developmental potential or to quality of environmental experience.

The earliest days and weeks of life find the infant attaining control of reflex and homeostatic mechanisms and entering into interactions with the personal and inanimate environment. Patterns or rhythms of feeding and sleeping have evolved, along with the ability to control his or her own state through self-stimulation, as by finger-sucking or thumb-sucking. A major part of the interaction between the mother and the infant in the first weeks of life is initiated by the infant, not simply as changes of state indicating distress or immediate need but as part of a growing and complex system of signals between the infant and the mother (or other caretaker). Through these communicative exchanges emotional attachments are formed; the infant learns to interpret his or her own internal states and to convey information regarding them, and the mother learns to read and to respond appropriately to the infant's signals with activities that comfort, reassure, or at times make tolerable any appropriate or necessary frustration or postponement of gratification.

There is reason to think that during this period the sense of security of the infant will be optimally fostered when care is given by the mother or mother-figure in a prompt, loving, and confident manner. There is evidence that the *responsive environment* is more crucial to development than attempts on the part of parents or others to initiate care in anticipation of the needs of the infant.

Both consistency and promptness seem important in the responses of the caretakers to the behavior of the infant. In instances of defective mothering the infant's normal or appropriate behavior may not be consistently or reliably rewarded by a reduction of tension, or an effective maternal response may come so late and after so much anxiety or tension that the infant cannot associate any specific action of his or her

TABLE 3–2. Median Head Circumferences of Infants and Children*

Boys					Girls			
Median	Percentiles (5th–95th)	Median	Percentiles (5th–95th)		Median	Percentiles (5th–95th)	Median	Percentiles (5th–95th)
Centimeters		(Inches)		Age	Centimeters		(Inches)	
34.8	32.6–37.2	(13.7)	(12.8–14.7)	Birth	34.3	32.1–35.9	(13.5)	(12.6–14.1)
37.2	34.9–39.6	(14.7)	(13.7–15.6)	1 mo	36.4	34.2–38.3	(14.3)	(13.5–15.1)
40.6	38.4–43.1	(16.0)	(15.1–17.0)	3 mo	39.5	37.3–41.7	(15.6)	(14.7–16.4)
43.8	41.5–46.2	(17.2)	(16.3—18.2)	6 mo	42.4	40.3–44.6	(16.7)	(15.9–17.6)
45.8	43.5–48.1	(18.0)	(17.1–18.9)	9 mo	44.3	42.3–46.4	(17.4)	(16.7–18.3)
47.0	44.8–49.3	(18.5)	(17.6–19.4)	1 yr	45.6	43.5–47.6	(18.0)	(17.1–18.7)
48.4	46.3–50.6	(19.1)	(18.2–19.9)	1.5 yr	47.1	45.0–49.1	(18.5)	(17.7–19.3)
49.2	47.3–51.4	(19.4)	(18.6–20.2)	2 yr	48.1	46.1–50.1	(18.9)	(18.2–19.7)
49.9	48.0–52.2	(19.7)	(18.9–20.6)	2.5 yr	48.8	47.0–50.8	(19.2)	(18.5–20.0)
50.5	48.6–52.8	(19.9)	(19.1–20.8)	3 yr	49.3	47.6–51.4	(19.4)	(18.8–20.2)

Estimating Formula (First Year Only)†	Boys and Girls Combined‡	Centimeters	(Inches)
Normal range of head circumference (5th–95th percentile) = $\left[\frac{\text{Length (cm)}}{2} + 9.5\right] \pm 2.5$	Median head circumference at 4 yr	50.4	(19.8)
	at 5 yr	50.8	(20.0)

*From Health Survey of National Center for Health Statistics, 1976 (see footnote to Table 3–8).
†After Dine et al., 1981.
‡From Studies of Harvard School of Public Health (see text).

own with relief of that tension. Such infants may come to feel that they are unable to affect their environment through their own actions. Long-term retreat, anxiety, or hostility may be the consequence.

3–6 MONTHS

By the age of 3 mo an infant in the prone position on a firm surface is generally able to raise the head and chest with the arms extended. From the same position, by 4 mo he or she is able to raise the head to a vertical axis and turn it easily from side to side. When the infant of 4 mo is pulled from a supine to a sitting position, the head is brought up without lag; in the upright position the head tilts a little forward but is held steady without bobbing. The head can be maintained erect and steady by 5 mo of age. At 5–6 mo of age the infant begins purposefully to roll over, at first from the prone to the supine position and then in the reverse direction.

Between 3 and 4 mo of age the infant gradually abandons the tonic neck attitude as the predominant posture, and the head becomes generally maintained in the midline, with the arms and legs in more or less symmetric positions and the hands often brought together in the midline or at the mouth (*symmetrotonic posture*). In this position the 4- to 6-mo-old infant often develops a bald spot over the occiput.

By 4–5 mo the infant enjoys being supported in an upright posture and becomes increasingly attracted to objects presented on a plane surface. By 6 mo he or she is able to change the orientation of the entire body to reach out toward a desired object.

By 4 mo the infant becomes more adept at making contact with objects brought within reach and often brings them to the midline and to the mouth for visual and oral exploration. At this age the infant is able to grasp an object of moderate size but has only limited interest in a small object, such as a pellet. By 7 mo the pellet is promptly seen and may be vigorously pursued by raking motions of the fingers, but the infant is not apt to be able to pick it up. After 6 mo the functions of the hands involve increasingly the structures on the radial side, the thumb being used in conjunction with the palm. By 6–6½ mo most infants can grasp a large object such as a rattle and transfer it from hand to hand.

With growing skills in manipulation of the arms and hands, infants discover the rest of their body, the face at first and then the head, trunk, lower extremities, and genitalia. Their discovery that the genitalia can be handled with pleasure may engender anxiety in parents.

At 5–6 mo infants can often be pulled from a sitting to a standing position and can support their weight on extended legs. At 6–6½ mo in this same position they often flex the knees momentarily and then return to a standing posture. At this age infants are often able to sit alone, leaning forward on their hands or with slight support of the pelvis; they have not yet developed a lumbar lordosis, and the spine has a gentle kyphotic curve from the cervical region to the sacrum.

PSYCHOSOCIAL DEVELOPMENT. As infants become more intricately related to objects and persons in the environment, their smiles continue as catalysts of social exchange. By 4 mo they begin to laugh aloud at pleasurable social contacts. They may also, on interruption of a pleasant social contact, show displeasure by changes of expression, fussing, or crying. Between 4 and 7 mo of age infants become increasingly responsive to the emotional tone of social contacts, and by 7 mo will respond to changes in the facial expressions of those having close rapport with them. By the end of the 6th mo normal infants have developed clear preferences for social contact with the persons giving them the most care and, particularly when in the mother's arms, begin to show anxiety at the approach of strangers. By contrast, in a setting where they are alone with a stranger, new social contacts may be accepted without protest. Development of separation anxieties and fear of strangers may depend in some measure on the depth to which infants have developed comfortable patterns of communication and emotional exchange with primary caretakers.

6–12 MONTHS

NEURODEVELOPMENT. By 7 mo the infant in the prone position is able to *pivot* in pursuit of an object, but if it is not within reach, he or she may be unable to attain it. By 9–10 mo most infants have learned to *creep* or to *crawl*.

Supine infants are able by 6 mo or so to lift their heads and become increasingly interested in their legs and feet. By 8–9 mo they are able to assume a sitting position without help and are soon able to maintain it with the back straight. They are often able at 8 mo to stand steadily for a short time as long as their hands are held, and by 9 mo may be able to take some steps with both hands held.

Between 6 and 9 mo the *radial-palmar grasp* becomes clearly elaborated into movements involving the thumb and forefinger. The index finger is used to poke at objects by 9 mo, and at this time the thumb and forefinger can be brought into sufficiently accurate apposition to permit a pellet to be picked up with a pincer motion. This movement is apt to be made with the ulnar surface of the hand supported on the same surface on which the pellet lies. By 12 mo, the pincer will be executed without this ulnar support.

Between 6 and 12 mo the infant's behavior becomes more *imitative*. At 6 mo the infant may crudely imitate the tapping of a pencil on a table. At 9 mo the infant can wave bye-bye or bring the hands together imitatively; at 12 mo a child may enter into very simple games with a toy such as a ball.

At 9 mo an infant may be able to release an object on request if the object is grasped as the request is made. By 1 yr most infants extend the object and release it into an offered hand.

COGNITIVE DEVELOPMENT. A significant developmental achievement of the 2nd half of the 1st yr is the infant's discovery of *object permanence*. By 9 mo, if an object that has attracted attention is covered with a cloth before the infant has an opportunity to grasp it, he or she can uncover it and seize it, with apparent knowledge that its being out of sight does not mean that it is not available.

LANGUAGE. The infant is able to make repetitive vowel sounds by 6½ mo and by 8 mo is likely to produce repetitive consonant sounds, such as ba-ba, ma-ma, and da-da, although not necessarily associating these sounds with objects. Children of 8–9 mo become attentive to the sounds of their own names. They may knowingly use a few words besides ma-ma or da-da by the age of 1 yr and may show by their behavior that they know the names of some objects.

PSYCHOSOCIAL DEVELOPMENT. The preference for the mother that was manifested at 6 mo often evolves into separation anxiety between the ages of 6 and 8 mo. About this same time a mother may experience difficulty in putting a baby to sleep who always went willingly before. Sometimes a mother whose child is fretful when she leaves the room can comfort him or her by maintaining vocal contact. Peek-a-boo often becomes a pleasant game about this time and gives the infant an opportunity to test and retest his or her ability to re-create the absent parent. By 9–10 mo infants begin to be less dependent on the physical presence of the mother, partly because with creeping or crawling they are increasingly able to follow her around.

At the end of the 1st yr, with a secure interactive system in place between the infant and the mother and other caretakers, including the father and sometimes siblings, and with the development of locomotion, the infant is ready to choose independent activities and to explore a larger world.

3.6 THE 2ND YEAR

PHYSICAL DEVELOPMENT. During the 2nd yr of life there is a further deceleration in the rate of growth; the average child gains about 2.5 kg (5–6 lb) and about 12 cm (5 in) (Table 3–3). After 10 mo of age there is often a decrease in appetite extending into the 2nd yr. The result is a loss during the 2nd yr of some of the subcutaneous tissue, which reached its maximal development around 9 mo; the plump infant begins to change gradually into the lean and muscular child. With the upright posture, the mild lordosis and protuberant abdomen appear that are characteristic of the 2nd and 3rd yr of life.

The growth of the brain continues its deceleration during the 2nd yr. Head circumference, which increased approximately 12 cm during the 1st yr, increases only 2 cm during the 2nd yr. By the end of the 1st yr the brain has reached approximately two thirds, and at the end of the 2nd yr, four fifths of its adult size. During the 2nd yr 8 more teeth erupt, making a total of 14–16, including the 1st deciduous molars and the cuspids (canines). The order of eruption may be irregular; the cuspids commonly appear after the 1st molars have erupted.

NEURODEVELOPMENT. During the 2nd yr the infant moves from an awkward upright stance in which he or she could walk with support to a high degree of locomotor control. By 12 mo infants are generally able to rise independently and walk a few steps alone. By 15 mo creeping is discarded, and by 18 mo the infant is able to run stiffly. At 18 mo the infant can climb stairs if one hand is held, going up one step at a time; by 20 mo he or she is able to go downstairs, one hand held, and may be able to climb stairs holding onto the stair railing. By 24 mo children normally enter the "runabout" age. They are able to move quickly from a safe environment into danger and need constant surveillance.

The child who at 12 mo was able to release a pellet into the hand of a person requesting it will at 15 mo generally be able to put the pellet into a small bottle. He or she may attempt to remove the pellet from the bottle by inserting a finger and by 18 mo is able to dump it from the bottle.

By 15 mo the child is able to put a 1-in cube on top of another in response to a demonstration; by 18 mo he or she is able to make a tower of four cubes and by 24 mo a tower of seven cubes. Imitative and conceptual behavior continues to evolve, with spontaneous scribbling and imitation of vertical lines at 18 mo; by 24 mo the child imitates circular strokes and can make a horizontal line.

During the 2nd yr children enter a period when they vigorously and imitatively exploit the objects in their environment. They can empty wastebaskets, drawers, and shelves and may try to examine anything within reach. *Household poisons, drugs, and chemicals must be kept in places inaccessible to them.*

COGNITIVE DEVELOPMENT. During the 2nd yr the child develops a sense of self as separate from other persons and recognizes his or her own capacity for taking initiative and making choices in behavior. There is an increasing concern with the expectations of adults, standards of behavior (Kagan), and order in the daily arrangement of things.

LANGUAGE. The child normally has a vocabulary of 10 words by 18 mo. There is wide variation in the times at which words begin to flow readily; it is not unusual for a normal child to have few or no sounds conveying definite meaning until 18 mo or later. Some children in whom development of recognizable speech is delayed have a rich jargon before communicative sounds appear; this jargon often has many of the intonations and punctuations of speech but otherwise conveys no meaning. In normal children in whom speech is delayed to 18–20 mo, rapid acquisition of words and meanings often occurs after this time, with the result that most normal children by their second birthday are able to put three words together.

PSYCHOSOCIAL DEVELOPMENT. During the 2nd yr imitative behavior extends to persons other than the mother, including siblings and playmates. Until the end of the 2nd yr, however, *play* is generally solitary and consists in active manipulation of available objects and sometimes in contests with other children over control or possession of such objects.

By 18–24 mo most children are able to verbalize their toilet needs and can be helped at this time to follow acceptable social patterns in meeting them. Whenever the young child has comfortable and adequate models, toilet training need

TABLE 3–3. Length, Weight, and Head Circumference by Age
Boys and Girls: Birth to 36 Months

	Boys: Percentiles								Girls: Percentiles						
	5th	10th	25th	50th	75th	90th	95th	Measurement	5th	10th	25th	50th	75th	90th	95th
	46.4 (18¼)	47.5 (18¾)	49.0 (19¼)	50.5 (20)	51.8 (20½)	53.5 (21)	54.4 (21½)	Length-mm (in)	45.4 (17¾)	46.5 (18¼)	48.2 (19)	49.9 (19¾)	51.0 (20)	52.0 (20½)	52.9 (20¾)
BIRTH	2.54 (5½)	2.78 (6¼)	3.00 (6½)	3.27 (7¼)	3.64 (8)	3.82 (8½)	4.15 (9¼)	Weight-kg (lb)	2.36 (5¼)	2.58 (5¾)	2.93 (6½)	3.23 (7)	3.52 (7¾)	3.64 (8)	3.81 (8½)
	32.6 (12¾)	33.0 (13)	33.9 (13¼)	34.8 (13¾)	35.6 (14)	36.6 (14½)	37.2 (14¾)	Head C-cm (in)	32.1 (12¾)	32.9 (13)	33.5 (13¼)	34.3 (13½)	34.8 (13¾)	35.5 (14)	35.9 (14¼)
	50.4 (19¾)	51.3 (20¼)	53.0 (20¾)	54.6 (21½)	56.2 (22¼)	57.7 (22¾)	58.6 (23)	Length-cm (in)	49.2 (19¼)	50.2 (19¾)	51.9 (20½)	53.5 (21)	54.9 (21½)	56.1 (22)	56.9 (22½)
1 mo	3.16 (7)	3.43 (7½)	3.82 (8½)	4.29 (9½)	4.75 (10½)	5.14 (11¼)	5.38 (11¾)	Weight-kg (lb)	2.97 (6½)	3.22 (7)	3.59 (8)	3.98 (8¾)	4.36 (9½)	4.65 (10¼)	4.92 (10¾)
	34.9 (13¾)	35.4 (14)	36.2 (14¼)	37.2 (14¾)	38.1 (15)	39.0 (15¼)	39.6 (15½)	Head C-cm (in)	34.2 (13½)	34.8 (13¾)	35.6 (14)	36.4 (14¼)	37.1 (14½)	37.8 (15)	38.3 (15)
	56.7 (22¼)	57.7 (22¾)	59.4 (23½)	61.1 (24)	63.0 (24¾)	64.5 (25½)	65.4 (25¾)	Length-cm (in)	55.4 (21¾)	56.2 (22¼)	57.8 (22¾)	59.5 (23½)	61.2 (24)	62.7 (24¾)	63.4 (25)
3 mo	4.43 (9¾)	4.78 (10½)	5.32 (11¾)	5.98 (13¼)	6.56 (14½)	7.14 (15¾)	7.37 (16¼)	Weight-kg (lb)	4.18 (9¼)	4.47 (9¾)	4.88 (10¾)	5.40 (12)	5.90 (13)	6.39 (14)	6.74 (14¾)
	38.4 (15)	38.9 (15¼)	39.7 (15¾)	40.6 (16)	41.7 (16½)	42.5 (16¾)	43.1 (17)	Head C-cm (in)	37.3 (14¾)	37.8 (15)	38.7 (15¼)	39.5 (15½)	40.4 (16)	41.2 (16¼)	41.7 (16½)
	63.4 (25)	64.4 (25¼)	66.1 (26)	67.8 (26¾)	69.7 (27½)	71.3 (28)	72.3 (28½)	Length-cm (in)	61.8 (24¼)	62.6 (24¾)	64.2 (25¼)	65.9 (26)	67.8 (26¾)	69.4 (27¼)	70.2 (27¾)
6 mo	6.20 (13¾)	6.61 (14½)	7.20 (15¾)	7.85 (17¼)	8.49 (18¾)	9.10 (20)	9.46 (20¾)	Weight-kg (lb)	5.79 (12¾)	6.12 (13½)	6.60 (14½)	7.21 (16)	7.83 (17¼)	8.38 (18½)	8.73 (19¼)
	41.5 (16¼)	42.0 (16½)	42.8 (16¾)	43.8 (17¼)	44.7 (17½)	45.6 (18)	46.2 (18¼)	Head C-cm (in)	40.3 (15¾)	40.9 (16)	41.6 (16½)	42.4 (16¾)	43.3 (17)	44.1 (17¼)	44.6 (17½)
	68.0 (26¾)	69.1 (27¼)	70.6 (27¾)	72.3 (28½)	74.0 (29¼)	75.9 (30)	77.1 (30¼)	Length-cm (in)	66.1 (26)	67.0 (26½)	68.7 (27)	70.4 (27¾)	72.4 (28½)	74.0 (29¼)	75.0 (29½)
9 mo	7.52 (16½)	7.95 (17½)	8.56 (18¾)	9.18 (20¼)	9.88 (21¾)	10.49 (23¼)	10.93 (24)	Weight-kg (lb)	7.00 (15½)	7.34 (16¼)	7.89 (17½)	8.56 (18¾)	9.24 (20¼)	9.83 (21¾)	10.17 (22½)
	43.5 (17¼)	44.0 (17¼)	44.8 (17¾)	45.8 (18)	46.6 (18¼)	47.5 (18¾)	48.1 (19)	Head C-cm (in)	42.3 (16¾)	42.8 (16¾)	43.5 (17¼)	44.3 (17½)	45.1 (17¾)	46.0 (18)	46.4 (18¼)
	71.7 (28¼)	72.8 (28¾)	74.3 (29¼)	76.1 (30)	77.7 (30½)	79.8 (31½)	81.2 (32)	Length-cm (in)	69.8 (27½)	70.8 (27¾)	72.4 (28½)	74.3 (29¼)	76.3 (30)	78.0 (30¾)	79.1 (31¼)
12 mo	8.43 (18½)	8.84 (19½)	9.49 (21)	10.15 (22½)	10.91 (24)	11.54 (25½)	11.99 (26½)	Weight-kg (lb)	7.84 (17¼)	8.19 (18)	8.81 (19½)	9.53 (21)	10.23 (22½)	10.87 (24)	11.24 (24¾)
	44.8 (17¾)	45.3 (17¾)	46.1 (18¼)	47.0 (18½)	47.9 (18¾)	48.8 (19¼)	49.3 (19½)	Head C-cm (in)	43.5 (17¼)	44.1 (17¼)	44.8 (17¾)	45.6 (18)	46.4 (18¼)	47.2 (18½)	47.6 (18¾)
	77.5 (30½)	78.7 (31)	80.5 (31¾)	82.4 (32½)	84.3 (33¼)	86.6 (34)	88.1 (34¾)	Length-cm (in)	76.0 (30)	77.2 (30½)	78.8 (31)	80.9 (31¾)	83.0 (32¾)	85.0 (33½)	86.1 (34)
18 mo	9.59 (21¼)	9.92 (21¾)	10.67 (23½)	11.47 (25¼)	12.31 (27¼)	13.05 (28¾)	13.44 (29½)	Weight-kg (lb)	8.92 (19¾)	9.30 (20½)	10.04 (22¼)	10.82 (23¾)	11.55 (25½)	12.30 (27)	12.76 (28¼)
	46.3 (18¼)	46.7 (18½)	47.4 (18¾)	48.4 (19)	49.3 (19½)	50.1 (19¾)	50.6 (20)	Head C-cm (in)	45.0 (17¾)	45.6 (18)	46.3 (18¼)	47.1 (18½)	47.9 (18¾)	48.6 (19¼)	49.1 (19¼)
	82.3 (32½)	83.5 (32¾)	85.6 (33¾)	87.6 (34½)	89.9 (35½)	92.2 (36¼)	93.8 (37)	Length-cm (in)	81.3 (32)	82.5 (32½)	84.2 (33¼)	86.5 (34)	88.7 (35)	90.8 (35¾)	92.0 (36¼)
24 mo	10.54 (23¼)	10.85 (24)	11.65 (25¾)	12.59 (27¾)	13.44 (29¾)	14.29 (31½)	14.70 (32½)	Weight-kg (lb)	9.87 (21¾)	10.26 (22½)	11.10 (24½)	11.90 (26¼)	12.74 (28)	13.57 (30)	14.08 (31)
	47.3 (18½)	47.7 (18¾)	48.3 (19)	49.2 (19¼)	50.2 (19¾)	51.0 (20)	51.4 (20¼)	Head C-cm (in)	46.1 (18¼)	46.5 (18¼)	47.3 (18½)	48.1 (19)	48.8 (19¼)	49.6 (19½)	50.1 (19¾)
	87.0 (34¼)	88.2 (34¾)	90.1 (35½)	92.3 (36¼)	94.6 (37¼)	97.0 (38¼)	98.7 (38¾)	Length-cm (in)	86.0 (33¾)	87.0 (34¼)	88.9 (35)	91.3 (36)	93.7 (37)	95.6 (37¾)	96.9 (38¼)
30 mo	11.44 (25¼)	11.80 (26)	12.63 (27¾)	13.67 (30¼)	14.51 (32)	15.47 (34)	15.97 (35¼)	Weight-kg (lb)	10.78 (23¾)	11.21 (24¾)	12.11 (26¾)	12.93 (28½)	13.93 (30¾)	14.81 (32¾)	15.35 (33¾)
	48.0 (19)	48.4 (19)	49.1 (19¼)	49.9 (19¾)	51.0 (20)	51.7 (20¼)	52.2 (20½)	Head C-cm (in)	47.0 (18½)	47.3 (18½)	48.0 (19)	48.8 (19¼)	49.4 (19½)	50.3 (19¾)	50.8 (20)
	91.2 (36)	92.4 (36½)	94.2 (37)	96.5 (38)	98.9 (39)	101.4 (40)	103.1 (40½)	Length-cm (in)	90.0 (35½)	91.0 (35¾)	93.1 (36¾)	95.6 (37¾)	98.1 (38½)	100.0 (39¼)	101.5 (40)
36 mo	12.26 (27)	12.69 (28)	13.58 (30)	14.69 (32½)	15.59 (34½)	16.66 (36¾)	17.28 (38)	Weight-kg (lb)	11.60 (25½)	12.07 (26½)	12.99 (28¾)	13.93 (30¾)	15.03 (33¼)	15.97 (35¼)	16.54 (36½)
	48.6 (19¼)	49.0 (19¼)	49.7 (19½)	50.5 (20)	51.5 (20¼)	52.3 (20½)	52.8 (20¾)	Head C-cm (in)	47.6 (18¾)	47.9 (18¾)	48.5 (19)	49.3 (19½)	50.0 (19¾)	50.8 (20)	51.4 (20¼)

These data are those of the National Center for Health Statistics (NCHS), Health Resources Administration, DHEW. They were based on studies of The Fels Research Institute, Yellow Springs, Ohio. Metric data have been smoothed by a least-squares cubic spline technique. For details see Hamill PVV, et al: NCHS Growth Charts, 1976. Monthly Vital Statistics Report 25(3):1, 1976.

not become the focus either of emotion-laden educational activity or of disciplinary concern.

The expectation and requirement that children at this age submit to increasing control of their bodies and of their environment by social and cultural pressures often produce frustration and anger. Temper tantrums, breath-holding spells, and less dramatic outbursts are common. These episodes respond best to management by firm and loving parents who are able to set the necessary limits for the child (see Sec. 3.15 and 3.38).

3.7 PRESCHOOL YEARS

PHYSICAL DEVELOPMENT. During the 3rd, 4th, and 5th yr of life gains in weight and height are relatively steady at approximately 2.0 kg (4.5 lb) and about 6–8 cm (2.5–3.5 in)/yr (Tables 3–4*A* and *B*, and 3–5*A* and *B*; see also Table 3–3). Most children are lean in comparison with their earlier body configuration. The lordosis and protuberant abdomen of late infancy tend to disappear by the 4th yr, as do the pads of fat that earlier camouflaged the normal arches of the feet.

Text continued on page 27

TABLE 3–4*A*. Stature and Weight by Age* Boys: 2 to 18 Years

{ **Stature:** centimeters and (inches)
{ **Weight:** kilograms and (pounds)

Age Years	Boys: Percentiles						
	5th	*10th*	*25th*	*50th*	*75th*	*90th*	*95th*
2.0†	82.5 (32½) 10.49 (23¼)	83.5 (32¾) 10.96 (24¼)	85.3 (33½) 11.55 (25½)	86.8 (34¼) 12.34 (27¼)	89.2 (35) 13.36 (29½)	92.0 (36¼) 14.38 (31¾)	94.4 (37¼) 15.50 (34¼)
2.5†	85.4 (33½) 11.27 (24¾)	86.5 (34) 11.77 (26)	88.5 (34¾) 12.55 (27¾)	90.4 (35½) 13.52 (29¾)	92.9 (36½) 14.61 (32¼)	95.6 (37¾) 15.71 (34¾)	97.8 (38½) 16.61 (36½)
3.0	89.0 (35) 12.05 (26½)	90.3 (35½) 12.58 (27¾)	92.6 (36½) 13.12 (29¾)	94.9 (37¼) 14.62 (32¼)	97.5 (38½) 15.78 (34¾)	100.1 (39½) 16.95 (37¼)	102.0 (40¼) 17.77 (39¼)
3.5	92.5 (36½) 12.84 (28¼)	93.9 (37) 13.41 (29½)	96.4 (38) 14.46 (32)	99.1 (39) 15.68 (34½)	101.7 (40) 16.90 (37¼)	104.3 (41¼) 18.15 (40)	106.1 (41¾) 18.98 (41¾)
4.0	95.8 (37¾) 13.64 (30)	97.3 (38¼) 14.24 (31½)	100.0 (39¼) 15.39 (34)	102.9 (40½) 16.69 (36¾)	105.7 (41½) 17.99 (39¾)	108.2 (42½) 19.32 (42½)	109.9 (43¼) 20.27 (44¾)
4.5	98.9 (39) 14.45 (31¾)	100.6 (39½) 15.10 (33¼)	103.4 (40¾) 16.30 (36)	106.6 (42) 17.69 (39)	109.4 (43) 19.06 (42)	111.9 (44) 20.50 (45¼)	113.5 (44¾) 21.63 (47¾)
5.0	102.0 (40¼) 15.27 (33¾)	103.7 (40¾) 15.96 (35¼)	106.5 (42) 17.22 (38)	109.9 (43¼) 18.67 (41¼)	112.8 (44½) 20.14 (44½)	115.4 (45½) 21.70 (47¾)	117.0 (46) 23.09 (51)
5.5	104.9 (41¼) 16.09 (35½)	106.7 (42) 16.83 (37)	109.6 (43¼) 18.14 (40)	113.1 (44½) 19.67 (43¼)	116.1 (45¾) 21.25 (46¾)	118.7 (46¾) 22.96 (50½)	120.3 (47¼) 24.66 (54¼)
6.0	107.7 (42½) 16.93 (37¼)	109.6 (43¼) 17.72 (39)	112.5 (44¼) 19.07 (42)	116.1 (45¾) 20.69 (45½)	119.2 (47) 22.40 (49½)	121.9 (48) 24.31 (53½)	123.5 (48½) 26.34 (58)
6.5	110.4 (43½) 17.78 (39¼)	112.3 (44¼) 18.62 (41)	115.3 (45½) 20.02 (44¼)	119.0 (46¾) 21.74 (48)	122.2 (48) 23.62 (52)	124.9 (49¼) 25.76 (56¾)	126.6 (49¾) 28.16 (62)
7.0	113.0 (44½) 18.64 (41)	115.0 (45¼) 19.53 (43)	118.0 (46½) 21.00 (46¼)	121.7 (48) 22.85 (50¼)	125.0 (49¼) 24.94 (55)	127.9 (50¼) 27.36 (60¼)	129.7 (51) 30.12 (66½)
7.5	115.6 (45½) 19.52 (43)	117.6 (46¼) 20.45 (45)	120.6 (47½) 22.02 (48½)	124.4 (49) 24.03 (53)	127.8 (50¼) 26.36 (58)	130.8 (51½) 29.11 (64¼)	132.7 (52¼) 32.73 (72¼)
8.0	118.1 (46½) 20.40 (45)	120.2 (47¼) 21.39 (47¼)	123.2 (48½) 22.09 (51)	127.0 (50) 25.30 (55¾)	130.5 (51½) 27.91 (61½)	133.6 (52½) 31.06 (68½)	135.7 (53½) 34.51 (76)
8.5	120.5 (47½) 21.31 (47)	122.7 (48¼) 22.34 (49¼)	125.7 (49½) 24.21 (53¼)	129.6 (51) 26.66 (58¾)	133.2 (52½) 29.61 (65¼)	136.5 (53¾) 33.22 (73¼)	138.8 (54¾) 36.96 (81½)
9.0	122.9 (48½) 22.25 (49)	125.2 (49¼) 23.33 (51½)	128.2 (50½) 25.40 (56)	132.2 (52) 28.13 (62)	136.0 (53½) 31.46 (69¼)	139.4 (55) 35.57 (78½)	141.8 (55¾) 39.58 (87¾)
9.5	125.3 (49¼) 23.25 (51¼)	127.6 (50¼) 24.38 (53¾)	130.8 (51½) 26.88 (58¾)	134.8 (53) 29.73 (65½)	138.8 (54¾) 33.46 (73¾)	142.4 (56) 38.11 (84)	144.9 (57) 42.35 (93¼)
10.0	127.7 (50¼) 24.33 (53¾)	130.1 (51¼) 25.52 (56¼)	133.4 (52½) 28.07 (62)	137.5 (54¼) 31.44 (69¼)	141.6 (55¾) 35.61 (78½)	145.5 (57¼) 40.80 (90)	148.1 (58¼) 45.27 (99¾)
10.5	130.1 (51¼) 25.51 (56¼)	132.6 (52¼) 26.78 (59)	136.0 (53½) 29.59 (65¼)	140.3 (55¼) 33.30 (73½)	144.6 (57) 37.92 (83½)	148.7 (58½) 43.63 (96¼)	151.5 (59¾) 48.31 (106½)
11.0	132.6 (52¼) 26.80 (59)	135.1 (53¼) 28.17 (62)	138.7 (54½) 31.25 (69)	143.33 (56½) 35.30 (77¾)	147.8 (58¼) 40.38 (89)	152.1 (60) 46.57 (102¾)	154.9 (61) 51.47 (113½)
11.5	135.0 (53¼) 28.24 (62¼)	137.7 (54½) 29.72 (65½)	141.5 (55¾) 33.08 (73)	146.4 (57¾) 37.46 (82½)	151.1 (59½) 43.00 (94¾)	155.6 (61¼) 49.61 (109¼)	158.5 (62½) 54.73 (120¾)
12.0	137.6 (54¼) 29.85 (65¾)	140.3 (55¼) 31.46 (69¼)	144.4 (56¾) 35.09 (77¼)	149.7 (59) 39.78 (87¾)	154.6 (60¾) 45.77 (101)	159.4 (62¾) 52.73 (116¼)	162.3 (64) 58.09 (128)
12.5	140.2 (55¼) 31.64 (69¾)	143.0 (56¼) 33.41 (73¾)	147.4 (58) 37.31 (82¼)	153.0 (60¼) 42.27 (93¼)	158.2 (62¼) 48.70 (107¼)	163.2 (64¼) 55.91 (123¼)	166.1 (65½) 61.52 (135¾)
13.0	142.9 (56¼) 33.64 (74¼)	145.8 (57½) 35.60 (78½)	150.5 (59¼) 39.74 (87½)	156.5 (61½) 44.95 (99)	161.8 (63¾) 51.79 (114¼)	167.0 (65¾) 59.12 (130¼)	169.8 (66¾) 65.02 (143¼)
13.5	145.7 (57¼) 35.85 (79)	148.7 (58½) 38.03 (83¾)	153.6 (60½) 42.40 (93½)	159.9 (63) 47.81 (105½)	165.3 (65) 55.02 (121¼)	170.5 (67¼) 62.35 (137½)	173.4 (68¼) 68.51 (151)
14.0	148.8 (58½) 38.22 (84¼)	151.8 (59¾) 40.64 (89½)	156.9 (61¾) 45.21 (99¾)	63.1 (64¼) 50.77 (112)	168.5 (66¼) 58.31 (128½)	173.8 (68½) 65.57 (144½)	176.7 (69½) 72.13 (159)
14.5	152.0 (59¾) 40.66 (89¾)	155.0 (61) 43.34 (95½)	160.1 (63) 48.08 (106)	166.2 (65½) 53.76 (118½)	171.5 (67½) 61.58 (135¾)	176.6 (69½) 68.76 (151½)	179.5 (70½) 75.66 (166¾)
15.0	155.2 (61) 43.11 (95)	158.2 (62¼) 46.06 (101½)	163.3 (64¼) 50.92 (112¼)	169.0 (66½) 56.71 (125)	174.1 (68½) 64.72 (142¾)	178.9 (70½) 71.91 (158½)	181.9 (71½) 79.12 (174½)
15.5	158.3 (62¼) 45.50 (100¼)	161.2 (63½) 48.69 (107¼)	166.2 (65½) 53.64 (118¼)	171.5 (67½) 59.51 (131¼)	176.3 (69½) 67.64 (149)	180.8 (71¼) 74.98 (165¼)	183.9 (72½) 82.45 (181¾)
16.0	161.1 (63½) 47.74 (105¼)	163.9 (64½) 51.16 (112¾)	168.7 (66½) 56.16 (123¾)	173.5 (68¼) 62.10 (137)	178.1 (70) 70.26 (155)	182.4 (71¾) 77.97 (172)	185.4 (73) 85.62 (188¾)
16.5	163.4 (64¼) 49.76 (109¾)	166.1 (65½) 53.39 (117¾)	170.6 (67¼) 58.38 (128¾)	175.2 (69) 64.39 (142)	179.5 (70¾) 72.46 (159¾)	183.6 (72¼) 80.84 (178¼)	186.6 (73½) 88.59 (195¼)
17.0	164.9 (65) 51.50 (113½)	167.7 (66) 55.28 (121¾)	171.9 (67¾) 60.22 (132¾)	176.2 (69¼) 66.31 (146¼)	180.5 (71) 74.17 (163½)	184.4 (72½) 83.58 (184¼)	187.3 (73¾) 91.31 (201¼)
17.5	165.6 (65¼) 52.89 (116½)	168.5 (66¼) 56.78 (125¼)	172.4 (67¾) 61.61 (135¾)	176.7 (69½) 67.78 (149½)	181.0 (71¼) 75.32 (166)	185.0 (72¾) 86.14 (190)	187.6 (73¾) 93.73 (206¾)
18.0	165.7 (65¼) 53.97 (119)	168.7 (66½) 57.89 (127½)	172.3 (67¾) 62.61 (138)	176.8 (69½) 68.88 (151¾)	181.2 (71¼) 76.0 (167¾)	185.3 (73) 88.41 (195)	187.6 (73¾) 95.76 (211)

*Data in Tables 3–4*A* and 3–4*B* are those of the National Center for Health Statistics, Health Resources Administration, DHEW, collected in its Health Examination Surveys. Metric data have been smoothed by the least-squares cubic spline technique. For details see footnote to Table 3–3.

†Stature data for 2.0–3.0 yr include some recumbent length measurements, which make values slightly higher than if all measurements had been of stature.

TABLE 3–4*B*. Stature and Weight by Age* Girls: 2 to 18 Years { **Stature:** centimeters and (inches) **Weight:** kilograms and (pounds)

Age Years	Girls: Percentiles													
	5th		*10th*		*25th*		*50th*		*75th*		*90th*		*95th*	
2.0	81.6	(32¼)	82.1	(32¼)	84.0	(33)	86.8	(34¼)	89.3	(35¼)	92.0	(36¼)	93.6	(36¾)
	9.95	(22)	10.32	(22¾)	10.96	(24¼)	11.80	(26)	12.73	(28)	13.58	(30)	14.15	(31¼)
2.5	84.6	(33¼)	85.3	(33½)	87.3	(34½)	90.0	(35½)	92.5	(36½)	95.0	(37½)	96.6	(38)
	10.80	(23¾)	11.35	(25)	12.11	(26¾)	13.03	(28¾)	14.23	(31¼)	15.16	(33½)	15.76	(34¾)
3.0	88.3	(34¾)	89.3	(35¼)	91.4	(36)	94.1	(37)	96.6	(38)	99.0	(39)	100.6	(39½)
	11.61	(25½)	12.26	(27)	13.11	(29)	14.10	(31)	15.50	(34¼)	16.54	(36½)	17.22	(38)
3.5	91.7	(36)	93.0	(36½)	95.2	(37½)	97.9	(38½)	100.5	(39½)	102.8	(40½)	104.5	(41¼)
	12.37	(27¼)	13.08	(28¾)	14.00	(30¾)	15.07	(33¼)	16.59	(36½)	17.77	(39¼)	18.59	(41)
4.0	95.0	(37½)	96.4	(38)	98.8	(39)	101.6	(40)	104.3	(41)	106.6	(42)	108.3	(42¾)
	13.11	(29)	13.84	(30½)	14.80	(32¾)	15.96	(35¼)	17.56	(38¾)	18.93	(41¾)	19.91	(44)
4.5	98.1	(38½)	99.7	(39¼)	102.2	(40¼)	105.0	(41¼)	107.9	(42½)	110.2	(43½)	112.0	(44)
	13.83	(30½)	14.56	(32)	15.55	(34¼)	16.81	(37)	18.48	(40¾)	20.06	(44¼)	21.24	(46¾)
5.0	101.1	(39¾)	102.7	(40½)	105.4	(41½)	108.4	(42¾)	111.4	(43¾)	113.8	(44¾)	115.6	(45½)
	14.55	(32)	15.26	(33¾)	16.29	(36)	17.66	(39)	19.39	(42¾)	21.23	(46¾)	22.62	(49¾)
5.5	103.9	(41)	105.6	(41½)	108.4	(42¾)	111.6	(44)	114.8	(45¼)	117.4	(46¼)	119.2	(47)
	15.29	(33¾)	15.97	(35¼)	17.05	(37½)	18.56	(41)	20.36	(45)	22.48	(49½)	24.11	(53¼)
6.0	106.6	(42)	108.4	(42¾)	111.3	(43¾)	114.6	(45)	118.1	(46½)	120.8	(47½)	122.7	(48¼)
	16.05	(35½)	16.72	(36¾)	17.86	(39¼)	19.52	(43)	21.44	(47¼)	23.89	(52¾)	25.75	(56¾)
6.5	109.2	(43)	111.0	(43¾)	114.1	(45)	117.6	(46¼)	121.3	(47¾)	124.2	(49)	126.1	(49¾)
	16.85	(37¼)	17.51	(38½)	18.76	(41¼)	20.61	(45½)	22.68	(50)	25.50	(56¼)	27.59	(60¾)
7.0	111.8	(44)	113.6	(44¾)	116.8	(46)	120.6	(47½)	124.4	(49)	127.6	(50¼)	129.5	(51)
	17.71	(39)	18.39	(40½)	19.78	(43½)	21.84	(48¼)	24.16	(53¼)	27.39	(60½)	29.68	(65½)
7.5	114.4	(45)	116.2	(45¾)	119.5	(47)	123.5	(48½)	127.5	(50¼)	130.9	(51½)	132.9	(52¼)
	18.62	(41)	19.37	(42¾)	20.95	(46¼)	23.26	(51¼)	25.90	(57)	29.57	(65¼)	32.07	(70¾)
8.0	116.9	(46)	118.7	(46¾)	122.2	(48)	126.4	(49¾)	130.6	(51½)	134.2	(52¾)	136.2	(53½)
	19.62	(43¼)	20.45	(45)	22.26	(49)	24.84	(54¾)	27.88	(61½)	32.04	(70¾)	34.71	(76½)
8.5	119.5	(47)	121.3	(47¾)	124.9	(49¼)	129.3	(51)	133.6	(52½)	137.4	(54)	139.6	(55)
	20.68	(45½)	21.64	(47¾)	23.70	(52¼)	26.58	(58½)	30.08	(66¼)	34.73	(76½)	37.58	(82¾)
9.0	122.1	(48)	123.9	(48¾)	127.7	(50¼)	132.2	(52)	136.7	(53¾)	140.7	(55½)	142.9	(56¼)
	21.82	(48)	22.92	(50½)	25.27	(55¾)	28.46	(62¾)	32.44	(71½)	37.60	(83)	40.64	(89½)
9.5	124.8	(49¼)	126.6	(49¾)	130.6	(51½)	135.2	(53¼)	139.8	(55)	143.9	(56¾)	146.2	(57½)
	23.05	(50¾)	24.29	(53½)	26.94	(59½)	30.45	(67¼)	34.94	(77)	40.61	(89½)	43.85	(96¾)
10.0	127.5	(50¼)	129.5	(51)	133.6	(52½)	138.3	(54½)	142.9	(56¼)	147.2	(58)	149.5	(58¾)
	24.36	(53¾)	25.76	(56¾)	28.71	(63¼)	32.55	(71¾)	37.53	(82¾)	43.70	(96¼)	47.17	(104)
10.5	130.4	(51¼)	132.5	(52¼)	136.7	(53¾)	141.5	(55¾)	146.1	(57½)	150.4	(59¼)	152.8	(60¼)
	25.75	(56¾)	27.32	(60¼)	30.57	(67½)	34.72	(76½)	40.17	(88½)	46.84	(103¼)	50.57	(111½)
11.0	133.5	(52½)	135.6	(53½)	140.0	(55)	144.8	(57)	149.3	(58¾)	153.7	(60½)	56.2	(61½)
	27.24	(60)	28.97	(63¾)	32.49	(71¾)	36.95	(81½)	42.84	(94½)	49.96	(110¼)	54.00	(119)
11.5	136.6	(53¾)	139.0	(54¾)	143.5	(56½)	148.2	(58¼)	152.6	(60)	156.9	(61¾)	159.5	(62¾)
	28.83	(63½)	30.71	(67¾)	34.48	(76)	39.23	(86½)	45.48	(100¼)	53.03	(117)	57.42	(126½)
12.0	139.8	(55)	142.3	(56)	147.0	(57¾)	151.5	(59¾)	155.8	(61¼)	160.0	(63)	162.7	(64)
	30.52	(67¼)	32.53	(71¼)	36.52	(80½)	41.53	(91½)	48.07	(106)	55.99	(123½)	60.81	(134)
12.5	142.7	(56¼)	145.4	(57¼)	150.1	(59)	154.6	(60¾)	158.8	(62½)	162.9	(64½)	165.6	(65¼)
	32.30	(71¾)	34.42	(76)	38.59	(85)	43.84	(96¾)	50.56	(111½)	58.81	(129¾)	64.12	(141¼)
13.0	145.2	(57¼)	148.0	(58¼)	152.8	(60¼)	157.1	(61¾)	161.3	(63½)	165.3	(65)	168.1	(66¼)
	34.14	(75¼)	36.35	(80¼)	40.55	(89½)	46.10	(101¾)	52.91	(116¾)	61.45	(135½)	67.30	(148¼)
13.5	147.2	(58)	150.0	(59)	154.7	(61)	159.0	(62½)	163.2	(64¼)	167.3	(65¾)	170.0	(67)
	35.98	(79¼)	38.26	(84¼)	42.65	(94)	48.26	(106½)	55.11	(121½)	63.87	(140¾)	70.30	(155)
14.0	148.7	(58½)	151.5	(59¾)	155.9	(61½)	160.4	(63¼)	164.6	(64¾)	168.7	(66½)	171.3	(67½)
	37.76	(83¼)	40.11	(88½)	44.54	(98¼)	50.28	(110¾)	57.09	(125¾)	66.04	(145½)	73.08	(161)
14.5	149.7	(59)	152.5	(60)	158.8	(61¾)	161.2	(63½)	165.6	(65¼)	169.8	(66¾)	172.2	(67¾)
	39.45	(87)	41.83	(92¼)	46.28	(102)	52.10	(114¾)	58.84	(129¾)	67.95	(149¾)	75.59	(166¾)
15.0	150.5	(59¼)	153.2	(60¼)	157.2	(62)	161.8	(63¾)	166.3	(65¼)	170.5	(67¼)	172.8	(68)
	40.99	(90¼)	43.38	(95¾)	47.82	(105½)	53.68	(118¼)	60.32	(133)	69.54	(153¼)	77.78	(171½)
15.5	151.1	(59½)	153.6	(60½)	157.5	(62)	162.1	(63¾)	166.7	(65¾)	170.9	(67¼)	173.1	(68¼)
	42.32	(93¼)	44.72	(98½)	49.10	(108¼)	54.96	(121¼)	61.48	(135½)	70.79	(156)	79.59	(176½)
16.0	151.6	(59¾)	154.1	(60¾)	157.8	(62¼)	162.4	(64)	166.9	(65¾)	171.1	(67¼)	173.3	(68¼)
	43.41	(95¾)	45.78	(101)	50.09	(110½)	55.89	(123¼)	62.29	(137¼)	71.68	(158)	80.99	(178½)
16.5	152.2	(60)	154.6	(60¾)	158.2	(62¼)	162.7	(64)	167.1	(65¾)	171.2	(67½)	173.4	(68¼)
	44.20	(97½)	46.54	(102½)	50.75	(112)	56.44	(124½)	62.75	(138¼)	72.18	(159¼)	81.93	(180½)
17.0	152.7	(60)	155.1	(61)	158.7	(62½)	163.1	(64¼)	167.3	(65¾)	171.2	(67½)	173.5	(68¼)
	44.74	(98¾)	47.04	(103¾)	51.14	(112¾)	56.69	(125)	62.91	(138¾)	72.38	(159½)	82.46	(181¾)
17.5	153.2	(60¼)	155.6	(61¼)	159.1	(62¾)	163.4	(64¼)	167.5	(66)	171.1	(67¼)	173.5	(68¼)
	45.08	(99½)	47.33	(104¼)	51.33	(113¼)	56.71	(125)	62.89	(138¾)	72.37	(159½)	82.62	(182¼)
18.0	153.6	(60½)	156.0	(61½)	159.6	(62¾)	163.7	(64½)	167.6	(66)	171.0	(67¼)	173.6	(68¼)
	45.26	(99¾)	47.47	(104¾)	51.39	(113¼)	56.62	(124¾)	62.78	(138½)	72.25	(159¼)	82.47	(181¾)

*See footnotes to Table 3–4*A*.

TABLE 3–5*A*. Weight by Length*
Boys and Girls Younger Than 4 Years

Recumbent Length	Boys: Weight Percentiles, kg and (lb)							Girls: Weight Percentiles, kg and (lb)						
	5th	*10th*	*25th*	*50th*	*75th*	*90th*	*95th*	*5th*	*10th*	*25th*	*50th*	*75th*	*90th*	*95th*
48–50 cm (19–19¾ in)			2.86 (6¼)	3.15 (7)	3.50 (7¾)					3.02 (6¾)	3.29 (7¼)	3.59 (8)		
50–52 cm (19¾–20½ in)			3.16 (70)	3.48 (7¾)	3.86 (8½)					3.25 (7¼)	3.55 (7¾)	3.89 (8½)		
52–54 cm (20½–21¼ in)			3.52 (7¾)	3.88 (8½)	4.28 (9½)					3.56 (7¾)	3.89 (8½)	4.26 (9½)		
54–56 cm (21¼–22 in)	3.49 (7¼)	3.65 (8)	3.95 (8¾)	4.34 (9½)	4.76 (10½)	5.13 (11¼)	5.33 (11¾)	3.54 (7¾)	3.64 (8)	3.93 (8¾)	4.29 (9½)	4.70 (10¼)	5.02 (11)	5.21 (11½)
56–58 cm (22–22¾ in)	3.90 (8½)	4.09 (9)	4.43 (9¾)	4.84 (10¾)	5.29 (11¾)	5.69 (12½)	5.88 (13)	3.93 (8¾)	4.05 (9)	4.37 (9¾)	4.76 (10½)	5.20 (11½)	5.55 (12¼)	5.77 (12¾)
58–60 cm (22¾–23½ in)	4.37 (9¾)	4.58 (10)	4.94 (11)	5.38 (11¾)	5.84 (12¾)	6.28 (13¾)	6.47 (14¼)	4.38 (9¾)	4.50 (10)	4.85 (10¾)	5.27 (11½)	5.73 (12¾)	6.12 (13½)	6.36 (14)
60–62 cm (23½–24½ in)	4.88 (10¾)	5.10 (11¼)	5.49 (12)	5.94 (13)	6.42 (14¼)	6.88 (15¼)	7.08 (15½)	4.85 (10¾)	4.99 (11)	5.37 (11¾)	5.82 (12¾)	6.30 (14)	6.70 (14¾)	6.95 (15¼)
62–64 cm (24½–25¼ in)	5.43 (12)	5.65 (12½)	6.05 (13¼)	6.52 (14¼)	7.02 (15½)	7.50 (16½)	7.72 (17)	5.35 (11¾)	5.50 (12)	5.91 (13)	6.39 (14)	6.89 (15¼)	7.30 (16)	7.55 (16¾)
64–66 cm (25¼–26 in)	5.99 (13¼)	6.20 (13¾)	6.62 (14½)	7.11 (15¾)	7.63 (16¾)	8.13 (18)	8.36 (8½)	5.87 (13)	6.03 (13¼)	6.47 (14¼)	6.97 (15¼)	7.48 (16½)	7.90 (17½)	8.15 (18)
66–68 cm (26–26¾ in)	6.55 (14½)	6.76 (15)	7.19 (15¾)	7.70 (17)	8.23 (18¼)	8.75 (19¼)	8.99 (19¾)	6.38 (14)	6.56 (14½)	7.02 (15½)	7.55 (16¾)	8.07 (17¾)	8.50 (18¾)	8.75 (19¼)
68–70 cm (26¾–27½ in)	7.10 (15¾)	7.31 (16)	7.75 (17)	8.27 (18¼)	8.82 (19½)	9.35 (20½)	9.62 (21¼)	6.89 (15¼)	7.08 (15½)	7.56 (16¾)	8.11 (17¾)	8.64 (19)	9.08 (20)	9.33 (20½)
70–72 cm (27½–28¼ in)	7.63 (16¾)	7.84 (17¼)	8.28 (18¼)	8.82 (19½)	9.39 (20¾)	9.93 (22)	10.21 (22½)	7.37 (16¼)	7.58 (16¾)	8.08 (17¾)	8.64 (19)	9.18 (20¼)	9.63 (21¼)	9.88 (21¾)
72–74 cm (28¼–29¼ in)	8.13 (18)	8.33 (18¼)	8.78 (19¼)	9.33 (20½)	9.92 (21¾)	10.48 (23)	10.77 (23¾)	7.82 (17¼)	8.05 (17¾)	8.56 (18¾)	9.14 (20¼)	9.68 (21¼)	10.15 (22½)	10.41 (23)
74–76 cm (29¼–30 in)	8.58 (19)	8.78 (19¼)	9.24 (20¼)	9.81 (21¾)	10.43 (23)	10.99 (24¼)	11.29 (25)	8.24 (18¼)	8.49 (18¾)	9.00 (19¾)	9.59 (21¼)	10.14 (22¼)	10.63 (23½)	10.91 (24)
76–78 cm (30–30¾ in)	9.00 (19¾)	9.21 (20¼)	9.68 (21¼)	10.27 (22¾)	10.91 (24)	11.48 (25¼)	11.78 (26)	8.62 (19)	8.90 (19½)	9.42 (20¾)	10.02 (22)	10.57 (23¼)	11.08 (24½)	11.39 (25)
78–80 cm (30¾–31½ in)	9.40 (20¾)	9.62 (21¼)	10.09 (22¼)	10.70 (23½)	11.36 (25)	11.94 (26¼)	12.25 (27)	8.99 (19¾)	9.29 (20½)	9.81 (21¾)	10.41 (23)	10.97 (24¼)	11.51 (25¼)	11.85 (26)
80–82 cm (31½–32¼ in)	9.77 (21½)	10.01 (22)	10.49 (23¼)	11.12 (24½)	11.80 (26)	12.39 (27¼)	12.69 (28)	9.34 (20½)	9.67 (21¼)	10.19 (22½)	10.80 (23¾)	11.37 (25)	11.93 (26¼)	12.29 (27)
82–84 cm (32¼–33 in)	10.14 (22¼)	10.39 (23)	10.88 (24)	11.53 (25½)	12.23 (27)	12.83 (28¼)	13.13 (29)	9.68 (21¼)	10.04 (22¼)	10.57 (23¼)	11.18 (24¾)	11.75 (26)	12.35 (27¼)	12.72 (28)
84–86 cm (33–33¾ in)	10.49 (23¼)	10.76 (23¾)	11.27 (24¾)	11.93 (26¼)	12.65 (28)	13.26 (29¼)	13.56 (30)	10.03 (22)	10.41 (23)	10.94 (24)	11.56 (25½)	12.15 (26¾)	12.76 (28¼)	13.15 (29)
86–88 cm (33¾–34¾ in)	10.85 (24)	11.14 (24½)	11.67 (25¾)	12.34 (27¼)	13.07 (28¾)	13.69 (30¼)	14.00 (30¾)	10.39 (23)	10.78 (23¾)	11.33 (25)	11.95 (26¼)	12.55 (27¾)	13.19 (29)	13.57 (30)
88–90 cm (34¾–35½ in)	11.22 (24¾)	11.53 (25½)	12.08 (26¾)	12.76 (28¼)	13.50 (29¾)	14.13 (31¼)	14.44 (31¾)	10.76 (23¾)	11.17 (24½)	11.74 (26)	12.36 (27¼)	12.98 (28½)	13.63 (30)	14.01 (31)
90–92 cm (35½–36¼ in)	11.60 (25½)	11.94 (26¼)	12.52 (27½)	13.20 (29)	13.94 (30¾)	14.58 (32¼)	14.90 (32¾)	11.16 (24½)	11.58 (25½)	12.17 (26¾)	12.80 (28¼)	13.45 (29¾)	14.10 (31)	14.45 (31¾)
92–94 cm (36¼–37 in)	12.00 (26½)	12.37 (27¼)	12.97 (28½)	13.65 (30)	14.40 (31¾)	15.05 (33¼)	15.39 (34)	11.59 (25½)	12.02 (26½)	12.63 (27¾)	13.27 (29¼)	13.95 (30¾)	14.61 (32¼)	14.92 (33)
94–96 cm (37–37¾ in)	12.42 (27½)	12.81 (28¼)	13.45 (29¾)	14.14 (31¼)	14.88 (32¾)	15.54 (34¼)	15.90 (35)	12.05 (26½)	12.48 (27½)	13.12 (29)	13.77 (30¼)	14.48 (32)	15.14 (33½)	15.42 (34)
96–98 cm (37¾–38½ in)	12.88 (28½)	13.28 (29¼)	13.96 (30¾)	14.66 (32¼)	15.39 (34)	16.06 (35½)	16.43 (36¼)	12.55 (27¾)	12.98 (28½)	13.64 (30)	14.31 (31½)	15.04 (33¼)	15.71 (34¾)	15.99 (35¼)
98–100 cm (38½–39¼ in)	13.37 (29½)	13.78 (30½)	14.50 (32)	15.21 (33½)	15.94 (35¼)	16.62 (36¾)	17.00 (37½)	13.10 (29)	13.51 (29¾)	14.19 (31¼)	14.87 (32¾)	15.63 (34½)	16.32 (36)	16.64 (36¾)
100–102 cm (39¼–49¼ in)	13.90 (30¾)	14.30 (31½)	15.06 (33¼)	15.81 (34¾)	16.54 (36½)	17.22 (38)	17.60 (38¾)	13.68 (30¼)	14.08 (31)	14.77 (32½)	15.46 (34)	16.25 (35¾)	16.96 (37½)	17.39 (38¼)
102–104 cm (49¼–51 in)	14.48 (32)	14.85 (32¾)	15.65 (34½)	16.45 (36¼)	17.18 (37¾)	17.87 (39½)	18.24 (40¼)							

*Data in Tables 3–5*A* and 3–5*B* are those of the National Center for Health Statistics (NCHS), Health Resources Administration, DHEW. Data of Table 3–5*A* are based on studies of the Fels Research Institute, Yellow Springs, OH; those of Table 3–5*B* are based on the Health Examination Surveys of the NCHS. For details see footnote to Table 3–3.

TABLE 3–5*B*. Weight by Stature*
Boys and Girls: Prepubescent

Stature	Boys: Weight Percentiles, kg and (lb)							Girls: Weight Prcentiles, kg and (lb)						
	5th	*10th*	*25th*	*50th*	*75th*	*90th*	*95th*	*5th*	*10th*	*25th*	*50th*	*75th*	*90th*	*95th*
90–92 cm (35½–36¼ in)	11.70 (25¾)	11.97 (26½)	12.59 (27¾)	13.41 (29½)	14.35 (31¾)	15.25 (33½)	15.72 (34¾)	11.45 (25¼)	11.67 (25¾)	12.28 (27)	13.14 (29)	14.11 (31)	14.98 (33)	15.74 (34¾)
92–94 cm (36¼–37 in)	12.07 (26½)	12.36 (27¼)	13.03 (28¾)	13.89 (30½)	14.84 (32¾)	15.87 (35)	16.41 (36¼)	11.86 (26¼)	12.10 (26¾)	12.74 (28)	13.63 (30)	14.63 (32¼)	15.57 (34¼)	16.42 (36¼)
94–96 cm (37–37¾ in)	12.46 (27½)	12.77 (28¼)	13.49 (29¾)	14.38 (31¾)	15.34 (33¾)	16.45 (36¼)	17.06 (37½)	12.26 (27)	12.53 (27½)	13.21 (29)	14.12 (31¼)	15.14 (33½)	16.13 (35½)	17.05 (37½)
96–98 cm (37¾–38½ in)	12.87 (28¼)	13.21 (29)	13.98 (30¾)	14.89 (32¾)	15.87 (35)	17.01 (37½)	17.69 (39)	12.66 (28)	12.97 (28½)	13.70 (30¼)	14.62 (32¼)	15.66 (34½)	16.69 (36¾)	17.65 (39)
98–100 cm (38½–39¼ in)	13.31 (29¼)	13.67 (30¼)	14.48 (32)	15.43 (34)	16.41 (36¼)	17.56 (38¾)	18.29 (40¼)	13.06 (28¾)	13.42 (29½)	14.19 (31¼)	15.13 (33¼)	16.19 (35¾)	17.24 (38)	18.23 (40¼)
100–102 cm (39¼–40¼ in)	13.77 (30¼)	14.15 (31¼)	15.00 (33)	15.98 (35¼)	16.98 (37½)	18.11 (40)	18.89 (41¾)	13.48 (29¾)	13.88 (30½)	14.69 (32½)	15.65 (34½)	16.73 (37)	17.80 (39¼)	18.80 (41½)
102–104 cm (40¼–41 in)	14.25 (31½)	14.65 (32¼)	15.54 (34¼)	16.65 (36½)	17.57 (38¾)	18.67 (41¼)	19.50 (43)	13.91 (30¾)	14.36 (31¾)	15.21 (33½)	16.20 (35¾)	17.28 (38)	18.38 (40½)	19.38 (42¾)
104–106 cm (41–41¾ in)	14.76 (32½)	15.18 (33½)	16.10 (35½)	17.13 (37¾)	18.18 (40)	19.25 (42½)	20.12 (44¼)	14.36 (31¾)	14.85 (32¾)	15.75 (34¾)	16.75 (37)	17.86 (39¼)	18.98 (41¾)	19.98 (44)
106–108 cm (41¾–42½ in)	15.30 (33¾)	15.73 (34¾)	16.68 (36¾)	17.74 (39)	18.82 (41½)	19.86 (43¾)	20.76 (45¾)	14.84 (32¾)	15.37 (34)	16.30 (36)	17.33 (38¼)	18.46 (40¾)	19.62 (43¼)	20.61 (45½)
108–110 cm (42½–43¼ in)	15.85 (35)	16.31 (36)	17.28 (38)	18.37 (40½)	19.49 (43)	20.51 (45¼)	21.45 (47¼)	15.35 (33¾)	15.91 (35)	16.87 (37¼)	17.94 (39½)	19.09 (42)	20.30 (44¾)	21.29 (47)
110–112 cm (43¼–44 in)	16.43 (36¼)	16.91 (37¼)	17.90 (39½)	19.02 (42)	20.18 (44½)	21.22 (46¾)	22.18 (49)	15.90 (35)	16.48 (36¼)	17.47 (38½)	18.56 (41)	19.76 (43½)	21.03 (46¼)	22.03 (48½)
112–114 cm (44–45 in)	17.04 (37½)	17.53 (38¾)	18.54 (40¾)	19.70 (43½)	20.91 (46)	21.98 (48½)	22.98 (50¾)	16.48 (36¼)	17.09 (37¾)	18.08 (39¾)	19.22 (42¼)	20.47 (45¼)	21.81 (48)	22.84 (50¼)
114–116 cm (45–45¾ in)	17.66 (39)	18.18 (40)	19.20 (42¼)	20.39 (45)	21.66 (47¾)	22.82 (50¼)	23.85 (52½)	17.11 (37¾)	17.72 (39)	18.72 (41¼)	19.91 (44)	21.23 (46¾)	22.67 (50)	23.73 (52¼)
116–118 cm (45¾–46½ in)	18.32 (40½)	18.85 (41½)	19.89 (43¾)	21.11 (46½)	22.45 (49½)	23.73 (52¼)	24.80 (54¾)	17.77 (39¼)	18.40 (40½)	19.40 (42¾)	20.64 (45½)	22.04 (48½)	23.60 (52)	24.71 (54½)
118–120 cm (46½–47¼ in)	18.99 (41¾)	19.55 (43)	20.60 (45½)	21.85 (48¼)	23.28 (51¼)	24.73 (54½)	25.83 (57)	18.48 (40¾)	19.11 (42¼)	20.11 (44¼)	21.42 (47¼)	22.92 (50½)	24.62 (54¼)	25.81 (57)
120–122 cm (47¼–48 in)	19.70 (43½)	20.28 (44¾)	21.34 (47)	22.63 (50)	24.15 (53¼)	25.80 (57)	26.96 (59½)	19.22 (42¼)	19.85 (43¾)	20.87 (46)	22.25 (49)	23.88 (52¾)	25.73 (56¾)	27.03 (59½)
122–124 cm (48–48¾ in)	20.43 (45)	21.03 (46¼)	22.11 (48¾)	23.45 (51¾)	25.07 (55¼)	26.96 (59½)	28.18 (62¼)	19.99 (44)	20.64 (45½)	21.68 (47¾)	23.13 (51)	24.91 (55)	26.95 (59½)	28.37 (62½)
124–126 cm (48¾–49½ in)	21.20 (46¾)	21.82 (48)	22.92 (50½)	24.32 (53½)	26.05 (57½)	28.18 (62¼)	29.50 (65)	20.80 (45¾)	21.47 (47¼)	22.54 (49¾)	24.09 (53)	26.05 (57½)	28.27 (62¼)	29.87 (65¾)
126–128 cm (49½–50½ in)	21.99 (48½)	22.64 (50)	23.77 (52½)	25.24 (55¾)	27.10 (59¾)	29.48 (65)	30.92 (68¼)	21.65 (47¾)	22.34 (49¼)	23.47 (51¾)	25.11 (55¼)	27.28 (60¼)	29.71 (65½)	31.51 (69½)
128–130 cm (50½–51¾ in)	22.82 (50¼)	23.50 (51¾)	24.67 (54½)	26.22 (57¾)	28.21 (62¼)	30.86 (68)	32.44 (71½)	22.53 (49¾)	23.25 (51¼)	24.46 (54)	26.22 (57¾)	28.63 (63)	31.28 (69)	33.33 (73½)
130–132 cm (51¼–52 in)	23.69 (52¼)	24.59 (53¾)	25.62 (56½)	27.26 (60)	29.41 (64¾)	32.31 (71¼)	34.07 (75)	23.44 (51¾)	24.22 (53½)	25.52 (56¼)	27.40 (60½)	30.09 (66¼)	32.99 (72¾)	35.33 (78)
132–134 cm (52–53¾ in)	24.59 (54¼)	25.32 (55¾)	26.62 (58¾)	28.38 (62½)	30.68 (67¾)	33.82 (74½)	35.81 (79)	24.38 (53¾)	25.22 (55½)	26.66 (58¾)	28.68 (63¼)	31.68 (69¾)	34.84 (76¾)	37.53 (82¾)
134–136 cm (52¾–53½ in)	25.53 (56¼)	26.30 (58)	27.68 (61)	29.58 (65¼)	32.05 (70¾)	35.40 (78)	37.67 (83)	25.35 (56)	26.28 (58)	27.88 (61½)	30.06 (66¼)	33.41 (73¾)	36.84 (81¼)	39.93 (88)
136–138 cm (53½–54¼ in)	26.51 (58½)	27.32 (60¼)	28.80 (63½)	30.86 (68)	33.51 (74)	37.05 (81¾)	39.65 (87½)	26.34 (58)	27.39 (60½)	29.19 (64¼)	31.54 (69½)	35.29 (77¾)	39.01 (86)	42.54 (93¾)
138–140 cm (54½–55 in)	27.53 (60¾)	28.38 (62½)	29.99 (66)	32.23 (71)	35.08 (77¼)	38.77 (85½)	41.74 (92)							
140–142 cm (55–56 in)	28.59 (63)	29.48 (65)	31.25 (69)	33.70 (74¼)	36.75 (81)	40.55 (89½)	43.97 (97)							
142–144 cm (56–56¾ in)	29.70 (65½)	30.64 (67½)	32.58 (71¾)	35.27 (77¾)	38.54 (85)	42.39 (93½)	46.32 (102)							
144–146 cm (56¾–57½ in)	30.86 (68)	31.85 (70¼)	34.00 (75)	36.95 (81½)	40.45 (89¼)	44.29 (97¾)	48.80 (107½)							

*See footnote to Table 3–5*A*.

By 2½ yr the 20 deciduous teeth have usually erupted. During the rest of the preschool period the face tends to grow proportionately more than the cranial cavity, and the jaw widens preparatory to the eruption of permanent teeth.

NEURODEVELOPMENT. Refinement of motor skills includes alternation of feet in ascending stairs by 3 yr and alternation in descending stairs by 4 yr. By 3 yr most children can stand for a short period on one foot; by 5 yr they are generally able to hop on one foot and soon to skip.

By 3 yr a child may be able to imitate crudely the drawing of a cross. By 4 yr the cross figure may be copied without prior demonstration, by some as a four-element figure. By 4–5 yr the child can make correctly proportionate copies of the figures and for the first time is able to copy figures with slanting lines such as triangles. A diamond-shaped figure may not be accurately and proportionately reproduced until the 6th yr.

By the age of 3 yr the child can respond to the request to draw a person. The first figures consist of a circular head with arms and legs attached as sticks. During the next years the child adds the trunk, two-dimensional extremities and other anatomic detail, clothing, and the like in increased detail and sophistication.

By the age of 6 yr the child begins to develop the ability to translate abstract conceptions into figures and structures (e.g., the sound of T into the letter T, the idea of two into the figure 2).

LANGUAGE. During the 3rd yr the child puts short sentences together to sustain a brief conversation. During the 4th yr longer sentences and conversations are produced, and by the 5th yr language is used in social functions such as role-playing. The rate and quality of growth of language depend heavily on the quantity and quality of the language used within the home.

PSYCHOSOCIAL DEVELOPMENT. By 3 yr most children can state their ages and whether they are boys or girls. With increasing awareness that they are destined to become larger children and adults, children in the later preschool period begin to seek adequate models from whom to learn. The most accessible models are, of course, parents and other members of the immediate family. The child's imperfect perception of the realities of the future often engenders conflicting pressures and anxieties. A child of 4, 5, or 6 yr assumes those habits of thought, feeling, and action that represent his or her growing perception or fantasy of the future. Inside the home the child's fantasies about future roles include playing the part of the parent of the same sex, and there may be increasing curiosity and concern about what the realities of these roles may be.

Outside the home, fantasies and concerns about future roles are likely to be expressed in play. During the 3rd yr of life children move increasingly into play activities in which other children are involved, at first in parallel play (doing the same thing) rather than in reciprocating actions or exchanges. By the end of the 4th year the child is increasingly engaged in activity with other children in which the group begins to enact imaginative roles and activities. This tendency toward role-playing increases during the school years. The interest of children of this age in sex differences, which often appears as questions inside the home, may commonly appear in the form of sex play among children of both sexes, which is to be expected.

Changing patterns of parent-child interaction and of other relationships in and out of the home often leave elements of anxiety, hostility, or aggression in the child's behavior, thoughts, or fantasies. Anxieties may be expressed as nightmares or as fears of separation, death, or bodily injury. Children with serious problems may resume or continue bedwetting or thumb-sucking, show speech or learning difficulties, be unable to enter into a comfortable sharing relationship, or display temper tantrums or other behavior appropriate to earlier years.

3.8 EARLY SCHOOL YEARS

PHYSICAL DEVELOPMENT. The early school years are a period of relatively steady growth ending in a preadolescent growth spurt by about the age of 10 yr in girls and about 12 yr in boys. The average gain in weight during these years is about 3–3.5 kg (7 lb)/yr, and in height about 6 cm (2.5 in)/yr. Growth in head circumference is slowed, the circumference increasing from about 51 cm (20 in) to 53–54 cm (21 in) between the ages of 5 and 12 yr. At the end of this period the brain has reached virtually adult size. The development of the facial bones is active during the school years, particularly with enlargement of the nasal accessory sinuses. The frontal sinus has usually made its appearance by the 7th yr.

The 1st permanent teeth, the 1st molars, most often erupt during the 7th yr of life. With these so-called 6-yr molars in place, the shedding of deciduous teeth begins; it follows approximately the same sequence as occurred in their acquisition. They are replaced at a rate of about four teeth/yr during the next 5 yr. The 2nd permanent molars commonly erupt by the 14th yr; the 3rd molars may not appear until the early 20s.

The school years are a time of vigorous physical activity. The spine becomes straighter, but the child's body is supple, and postures may be assumed that are disturbing to parents and to teachers. Mild degrees of knock-knee or flatfoot, which may have been apparent in the late preschool years, tend to correct themselves during the first year or two of the school years. The motor activities of the earlier years, such as running and climbing, become increasingly directed toward more specialized activities and games requiring particular motor and muscular skills.

Lymphatic tissues are at the peak of their development during these years and generally exceed the amount of such tissue in the normal adult. The abundance of lymphoid tissue during this time of life bears some relationship to the frequency with which tonsillectomy and adenoidectomy are incorrectly recommended. Respiratory infections are common during these years, and the response of the child to infection begins to be more like that of the adult than of the infant or young child. The usual number of respiratory infections during the school years is high; as many as six to seven illnesses/yr are not uncommon.

NEURODEVELOPMENT. The neurodevelopmental features of the school-aged child are discussed in Sec. 3.11.

COGNITIVE DEVELOPMENT. During the school years the child develops an increasing ability to monitor his or her own mental processes. Concepts of conservation of volume and mass against deformities are achieved. In art, the notion of perspective is evolved.

PSYCHOSOCIAL DEVELOPMENT. With the removal of a large portion of the child's life from the home to the school environment, children begin increasingly to live independently and to look outside the home for goals and for standards of behavior. This shifting of interests is often anxiety-provoking for parents, and if earlier problems between parent and child have not been adequately resolved, adjustments to forces outside the home are likely to be difficult.

A major task of the school years is the creation in the child of the senses of duty, of responsibility, and of realistic accomplishment. There is a possibility of great frustration for parents and children when the child's achievement does not measure up to parental hopes. The child who is unable to meet expected standards may learn for the first time the sense of *failure* and may react with anxiety, depression, or hostility. Antisocial behavior may develop through which the child attempts to gain recognition that he or she cannot attain otherwise (see Sec. 3.38).

VICTOR C. VAUGHAN III
IRIS F. LITT

Bower TGR: A Primer of Infant Development. San Francisco, WH Freeman, 1977.
Bower TGR: Human Development. San Francisco, WH Freeman, 1979.
Brazelton TB: Neonatal Behavior Assessment Scale. Clin Dev Med Ser No 50. London, William Heinemann, 1973.
Brazelton TB, Parker WB, Zuckerman B: Importance of assessment of the neonate. Curr Prob Pediatr 7:1, 1976.
Brazelton TB, Vaughan VC III (eds): The Family: Setting Priorities. New York, Science & Medicine Publishing Co, 1979.
Erikson EH: Childhood and Society. New York, WW Norton, 1985
Ginsburg H, Opper S: Piaget's Theory of Intellectual Development. Englewood Cliffs, NJ, Prentice-Hall, 1979.
Kagan J: The Second Year: The Emergence of Self-Awareness. Cambridge, Harvard University Press, 1981.
Klaus MH, Kennell JH: Parent-Infant Bonding, 2nd ed. St. Louis, CV Mosby, 1982.
Prechtl H, Beintema D: The Neurological Examination of the Full Term Newborn Infant. Clin Dev Med Ser No 12. Philadelphia, JB Lippincott, 1975.
Rosenblith JF, Sims-Knight JE: In the Beginning: Development in the First Two Years. Monterey, Brooks/Cole, 1985.
Vaughan VC, Brazelton TB (eds): The Family—Can It Be Saved? Chicago, Year Book Medical Publishers, 1976.
Vaughan VC, Litt IF: Child and Adolescent Development: Clinical Implications. Philadelphia, WB Saunders, 1990.

3.9 ADOLESCENCE

Adolescence begins and progresses across a wide range of chronologic ages and differs between the sexes. Attempts to categorize chronologically the changes of adolescence are therefore fraught with boundary problems. The most important organizing process is the development of sexual maturity. Accordingly, it is reasonable to define *early, middle,* and *late* adolescence in terms of *stages of pubertal development,* since these follow a consistent pattern for individuals regardless of chronologic age. The stages are defined by the development of primary and secondary sex characteristics (pubic hair and breasts in females, genitalia and pubic hair in males); these changes are illustrated in Figures 3–3 and 3–4 and are described later. The *sex maturity ratings* (*SMRs, Tanner stages*) that they generate are defined in Tables 3–6 and 3–7.

Unfortunately, many of the physiologic and other data about adolescence have been derived in accordance with age criteria that limit their potential usefulness. When possible, we will reorganize existing information into the model of stage of physical maturation in order to present a developmentally integrated picture of the adolescent at each stage. Within each stage, physical, psychologic, and social development will be described, with emphasis on those areas of particular interest to health professionals as well as on tools and methods of assessment.

Early adolescence will refer to the first stage of puberty (SMR 2), which normally ranges in age of onset (approximately, mean ± 2 SD [95% confidence limits]) from 10.5 to 14 yr in boys and from 10 to 13 yr in girls, and lasts from 0.5 to 2 yr in boys and from 0.2 to 1.2 yr in girls. *Middle* adolescence (SMR 3 and 4) has an age of onset that normally ranges from 12.5 to 15 yr in boys and from 12 to 14 yr in girls, and lasts from 0.5 to 2 yr in boys and from 0.9 to 3 yr (pubic hair) or 7 yr (breast) in girls. *Late* adolescence (SMR 5) has its onset normally from 14 to 16 yr in boys and from 14 to 17 yr in girls. The end of the changes that define late adolescence determines the status of *young adulthood;* this is generally reached between the ages of 17 and 21 yr.

EARLY ADOLESCENCE

PHYSICAL DEVELOPMENT. The earliest stage of puberty (SMR 2) is initiated by sleep-augmented pulsatile secretion of pituitary gonadotropins and growth hormone. During the early stages of pubertal maturation (corresponding to SMR 1 [late] and 2), gains in weight and height differ little from those achieved in the preceding years, approximating 2.0 kg and 6–8 cm each year, respectively. This apparent continuity with earlier years belies the changes in body composition that occur with the onset of puberty.

In *females,* an increase in body fat content is associated with each successive stage of pubertal development. Subscapular skinfold thickness, a measure of adiposity, increases an average of about a third in the transition from SMR 1 to 2, about a quarter from SMR 2 to 4, and about another 50% from SMR 4 to 5. Between SMR 1 and 5, the total fat content of the female body increases from approximately 8 to about 25%.

Males become more muscular, rather than fatter, during puberty, but there is little increase in muscle tissue between SMR 1 and 2. Body fat content has been shown to decrease in males reaching SMR 2 (genital).

In *females* breast development results from stimulation by ovarian estrogens that are secreted in response to follicle-stimulating hormone (FSH). The predominant effect of FSH is to stimulate growth of the ovaries, beginning during late SMR 1, approximately 1 yr before the stage of breast budding

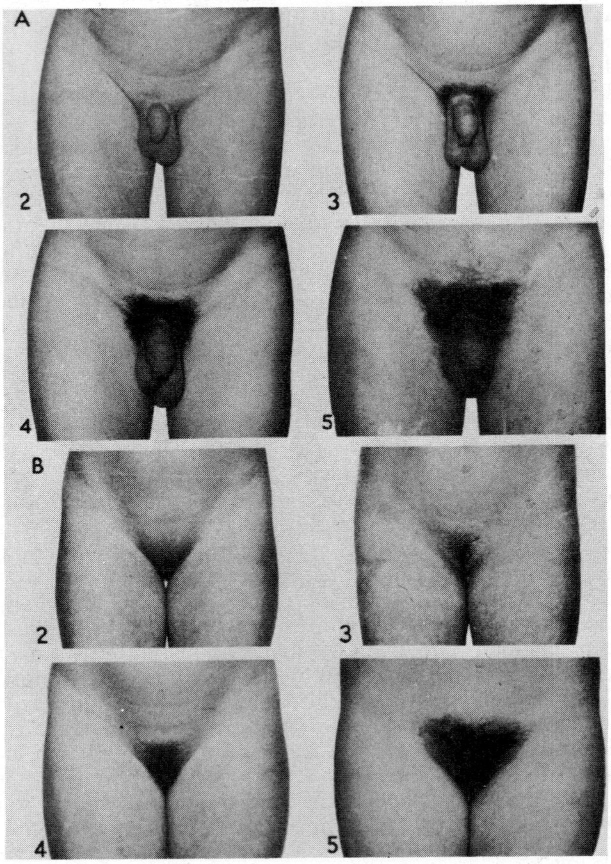

Figure 3–3. Sex maturity ratings of pubic hair changes in adolescent boys and girls. (Courtesy of JM Tanner, M.D., Institute of Child Health, Department of Growth and Development, University of London, London, England.)

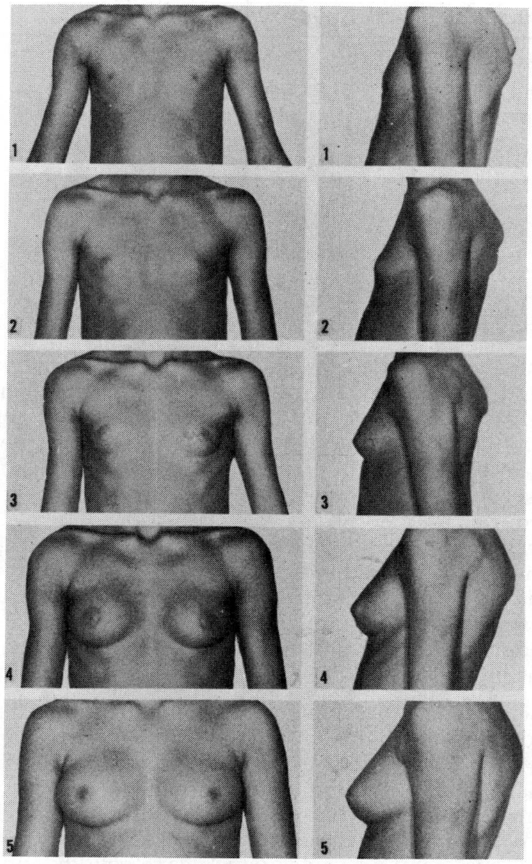

Figure 3–4. Sex maturity ratings of breast changes in adolescent girls. (Courtesy of JM Tanner, M.D., Institute of Child Health, Department of Growth and Development, University of London, London, England.)

(SMR 2). Other effects of ovarian estrogen production include thickening of the vaginal mucosa, increased pigmentation, vascularization, and eroticization of the labia majora, and slight enlargement of the clitoris, as well as enlargement of the uterus, which is at this stage equally divided between corpus and cervix. Endometrial thickening and differentiation begin, as do myometrial increases in the cellular content of actinomysin, creatine kinase (CK), and adenosine triphosphate (ATP), presumably in preparation for menses and childbirth. Increased deposition of glycogen within the cells of the vaginal mucosa is another effect of estrogen; it favors the growth of acid-forming bacteria (Döderlein bacillus) and results in an acid pH as well as increased susceptibility to yeast infections.

TABLE 3–6. Classification of Sex Maturity Stages in Girls*

SMR Stage	Pubic Hair	Breasts
1	Preadolescent	Preadolescent
2	Sparse, lightly pigmented, straight, medial border of labia	Breast and papilla elevated as small mound; areolar diameter increased
3	Darker, beginning to curl, increased amount	Breast and areola enlarged, no contour separation
4	Coarse, curly, abundant but amount less than in adult	Areola and papilla form secondary mound
5	Adult feminine triangle, spread to medial surface of thighs	Mature; nipple projects, areola part of general breast contour

*Adapted from Tanner JM: Growth at Adolescence, 2nd ed. Oxford, Blackwell Scientific Publications, 1962.

In *males* SMR 2 consists of enlargement of the testes owing to an increase in the size of seminiferous tubules and in the number of Leydig and Sertoli cells; secretion of testosterone is responsible for enlargement of the epididymis, seminal vesicles, and prostate. The epididymis grows proportionately less than the testes, coincident with thinning and hypervascularity of the scrotum. The latter assumes the adult configuration, with a narrower proximal portion and the left testis lower than the right. Enlargement of the penis begins shortly thereafter; it remains thinner in proportion to its length until later puberty, when acceleration of the growth of the corpora cavernosa penis over that of the urethra eventually results in the adult width. Some breast development (gynecomastia) occurs also in 30–50% of males during the pubertal period; it is variable in degree (usually mild) and inconsistent in its timing (see later).

In addition to secretion of testosterone in males, increased concentrations of adrenal androgens occur in both sexes and are responsible for initiation of growth of pubic and axillary hair. The consistency and distribution of pubic hair follow a predictable pattern and give a reliable index of pubertal progression in conjunction with breast development in females and development of the genitalia in males. The relationships among these events are diagrammed in Figures 3–5 and 3–6. At SMR 2 pubic hair is fine and silky and appears on the labia at the midline in females and surrounding the base of the penis in males. Another effect of androgen is to increase both the size and secretions of the sebaceous follicles. These effects are the forerunners of acne, which may thus also be considered a secondary sex characteristic (see Sec. 23.32).

Dramatic functional as well as structural changes take place in the genitalia during puberty. Ejaculation, usually initially in response to masturbation, occurs approximately 1 yr following the onset of testicular growth at the time of appearance of pubic hair.

DENTITION. The cuspids (canines) and 1st molars of the primary dentition are shed by early adolescence; the permanent cuspids, 1st and 2nd premolars, and molars erupt during this period. There is close correlation between the time of menarche and the eruption of the 2nd permanent molar ($r = 0.62$).

NEURODEVELOPMENT. Although no gross changes in brain morphology become apparent during adolescence, electroencephalographic studies demonstrate continuing neurodevelopmental maturation; an increase in α_2-wave activity parallels a decrease in θ waves and is most dramatic in girls during *early* adolescence. By early adolescence an individual should manifest a "mature" response on all items of a standardized neurodevelopmental assessment. The last of the items to mature do so by the age of 12 yr; they include the ability to identify correctly stimulated fingers in a finger localization task, to distinguish left and right starting from new bases, such as those in marching commands, and to separate the third and fourth fingers without "overflow" movement to other fingers.

COGNITIVE DEVELOPMENT. Until recently, cognitive development has been described largely in relation to chronologic age. Accordingly, the relationship between stages of pubertal development and cognitive development remains unclear. Since the age of onset of SMR 2 in females spans the ages from 10 to 13 yr (mean ± 2 SD) and that for males is broader (from 10.5 to 14.5 years), it is apparent that in the piagetian sequence (see Sec. 3.31) some children at each age will be at the stage of concrete operations and others will be at the stage of formal operations. At the latter stage, the individual is capable of generating hypotheses to be tested before action is initiated, can think abstractly, can entertain multiple contingencies simultaneously, and can generalize

TABLE 3–7. Classification of Sex Maturity Stages in Boys*

SMR Stage	Pubic Hair	Penis	Testes
1	None	Preadolescent	Preadolescent
2	Scanty, long, slightly pigmented	Slight enlargement	Enlarged scrotum, pink texture altered
3	Darker, starts to curl, small amount	Longer	Larger
4	Resembles adult type, but less in quantity; coarse, curly	Larger; glans and breadth increase in size	Larger, scrotum dark
5	Adult distribution, spread to medial surface of thighs	Adult size	Adult size

*Adapted from Tanner JM: Growth at Adolescence, 2nd ed. Oxford, Blackwell Scientific Publications, 1962.

and consider possible consequences of behavior in a logical manner without actually experiencing them first. Attainment of the level of formal operations has potential implications for health. Inasmuch as health behaviors are influenced by the patient's ability to understand the consequences of a proposed therapy (or the risk of pregnancy, for example), an adolescent may not be in a position to enter into a mature, confidential relationship with a physician until he or she has reached the stage of formal operations. Achievement of this stage is often associated with the development of interests in the occult or in mysticism as well as in religion.

Piagetian theory describes the development of cognition in terms of clear-cut, discrete stages. These changes may be better conceptualized in terms of developmental trends that evolve during childhood and adolescence and that involve more overlap and variation than implied by the discrete stages (Flavell). These trends include

1. *Information-processing capacity.* Adolescents appear superior to younger children in their functional information-processing capacities, but it is not yet known whether this reflects any increase in "hard-wired structural capacity" with age.
2. *Domain-specific knowledge.* As a child ages, he or she accumulates more and more organized knowledge in different specific domains, allowing for problem-solving by memory processes unavailable to the younger child.
3. *Concrete and formal operations.* The younger child's approach is viewed as more "empirico-deductive"; that of the adolescent is more "hypothetico-deductive."
4. *Quantitative thinking.* Adolescents tend to approach problems with a "more quantitative, measurement-oriented set" than younger children as a result of acquisition "of the concept of a unit measure."
5. *"A sense of the game."* With increasing age, children become increasingly interested in thinking as a competitive game and are challenged by it.
6. *Metacognition.* This concept refers to thinking about thinking and is divided by Flavell into metacognitive knowledge and metacognitive experiences. The former "refers to accumulated declarative and procedural knowledge concerning cognitive matters" and the latter refers to affective experiences of the "Eureka!" or, conversely, of the "This doesn't make sense to me" variety. Metacognition develops considerably during adolescence.
7. *Improving existing competencies.* The maturation of competencies once acquired is a continuing process during development. Sex differences appear to emerge during early adolescence with boys performing better in areas of spatial ability and mathematics and girls excelling in verbal ability. Their cause is unclear.

Closely related to cognitive development is the development of moral thought, an area explored by Kohlberg (see Sec. 3.15). At the time of entry into formal operations in the piagetian schema, the individual should be at the postconventional level of moral development in the Kohlberg classification. This level is "characterized by a major thrust toward autonomous moral principles which have validity and application apart from authority of the groups or persons who hold them and apart from the individual's identification with those persons or groups."

PSYCHOSOCIAL DEVELOPMENT. The early adolescent must function in three arenas: the family, peer group, and school. In each arena there exists a complex interplay of determinants of successful function. The major psychosocial developmental task of early adolescence is that of initiating independence from the *family*, and it is at this time that earlier familial homeostasis may be most evidently disrupted. Often at the same time, the onset of pubertal development signals

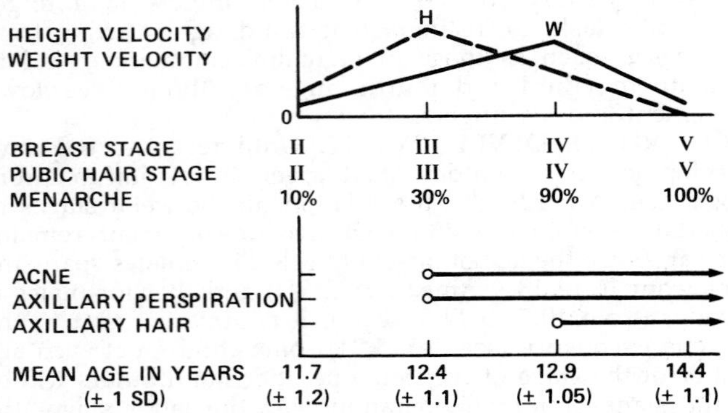

Figure 3–5. Sequence of maturational events in females. (Adapted from Marshall WA, Tanner JM: Variations in pattern of pubertal changes in girls. Arch Dis Child 44:291, 1969.)

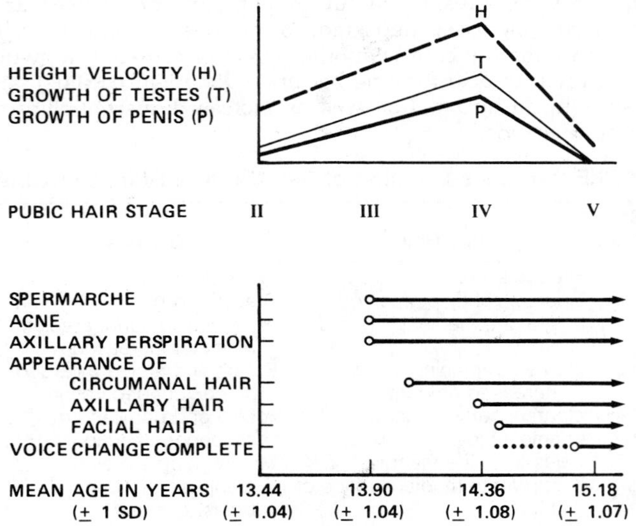

Figure 3–6. Sequence of maturational events in males. (Adapted from Marshall WA, Tanner JM: Arch Dis Child 44:291, 1969.)

a wish for privacy and often for increased distance from a physically affectionate parent of the opposite sex. The adolescent's unspoken wish for limit-setting is in conflict with his or her need for autonomy. Unresolved parental needs are often reawakened by these stresses. As a result, the adolescent tends to turn toward a same-sex peer group.

Friendships at this early adolescent stage of development are typically with members of the same sex and tend to center more on joint activity than on the interaction itself, according to Douvan and Adelson, who describe the friendships of early adolescence as relatively devoid of depth or mutuality. A very high degree of conformity exists in the peer groups of early adolescence, with little difference in this regard between males and females.

Function in the *school* setting at this age is determined by many factors. Synchrony of pubertal development with that of the peer group is particularly important in adjustment. Gross and Duke found that boys who were late maturers performed less well in school and had lower educational expectations and aspirations than early-maturing males. Simmonds and associates found that early-maturing girls in a middle school setting had a poorer self-image and lower grade point averages than their later-maturing peers or those who were still in an elementary school (8th grade or less) setting. The emergence of sex differences in cognition in early adolescence described earlier may contribute to changes in school performance.

MIDDLE ADOLESCENCE

Middle adolescence refers to the period corresponding to SMR 3 and 4. It is the period of the most dramatic growth and change. There is at this time acceleration in weight and linear growth as well as further development of secondary sex characteristics. The height velocity curve peaks, followed in approximately 6 mo by the peak of the weight velocity curve. During this phase the bulk of fat tissue is deposited in females and that of muscle mass in males. In males the peak of grip strength occurs about 14 months after the peak of the height velocity curve.

PHYSICAL DEVELOPMENT. During the *growth* spurt of middle adolescence, females average an increment in height of 8 cm/yr at a mean age of 12 yr; the later growth spurt of males (at a mean age of 14 yr) averages 10 cm/yr. There is an orderly pattern of progression of skeletal growth from the distal to proximal parts of the body, beginning with growth of the feet. This is followed approximately 6 mo later by growth of the calf and then the thigh. A similar pattern occurs in the upper extremity, the resulting disproportionately large hands and feet contributing to the apparent clumsiness of adolescents. The peak acceleration of growth of leg length is followed approximately 4 mo later by that of the chest and hips. Elongation of the trunk and an increase in the anteroposterior diameter of the chest are the last manifestations of the pubertal growth spurt.

Just as sex differences arise in soft tissue growth during middle adolescence, they also occur in patterns of skeletal growth. The greater biachromial width of males is androgen-determined, whereas the wider bitrochanteric diameter that contributes to the adult female contour is estrogen-determined. The longer arms and legs of males, relative to total body length, result from the later onset of their growth spurt compared with females. The carrying angle of the male arm is less than that of the female as a result of differential growth of cartilage of the lateral humeral epicondyle during puberty.

In middle adolescence development of *secondary sex characteristics* involves enlargement of the female breast and areola and, in about 75% of girls (in SMR 4), demarcation of the contours of the breast and areola by an elevation of the latter. Pubic hair darkens, coarsens, curls, and extends proximally and laterally to cover the mons (SMR 3 and 4). In the male, the penis elongates and widens, the testes enlarge, and the scrotum becomes more pigmented.

The most dramatic event of puberty for the female is *menarche;* it occurs at a mean age of 12.5 yr in the United States. Its timing is closely linked to other pubertal events: It occurs at SMR 2 in 10%, SMR 3 in 20%, SMR 4 in 60%, and SMR 5 in 10% of girls. The timing of menarche is closely related to the peak of the weight velocity curve and is determined by a number of factors, the most important of which are undoubtedly genetic. There is a close concordance between a mother's and daughter's ages at menarche and an even closer correlation among those of siblings. Other factors, such as nutritional status, are also important; obese girls have their menarche earlier than those who are lean. Very lean girls, particularly athletes or those with anorexia nervosa, often have a delayed menarche. Any chronic illness that adversely affects nutritional status or tissue oxygenation will also delay pubertal maturation and ultimately the timing of menarche.

Much more variable in timing of appearance is growth of circumanal *hair,* which tends to antedate axillary and facial hair; the latter two appear at about the time pubic hair reaches SMR 4. In males facial hair first appears at the corners of the upper lip and spreads medially. Coincident with the appearance of axillary hair is that of *body odor,* which results from androgenic stimulation of apocrine sweat glands and is often a source of concern to the already self-conscious adolescent.

It is also typically during middle adolescence that many males manifest *gynecomastia,* which may be bilateral or unilateral and can persist up to 18 mo after onset. It usually consists of a round nubbin of tissue, 0.5 to 2 cm in diameter, directly behind the nipple. It may be tender, and although common and nonpathologic, it often causes consternation. Reassurance that this is normal is appropriate even in the absence of inquiry by the patient.

NEURODEVELOPMENT. Neurodevelopmental maturity appears to be reached before or during early adolescence. Although no apparent neurodevelopmental change or growth of the central nervous system occurs during middle adolescence, sleep studies suggest that physiologic changes do occur. As an individual moves from SMR 3 to SMR 4, there is a decrease in sleep latency time and an increase in daytime sleepiness. Parents may misinterpret these normal events as signs of laziness.

COGNITIVE DEVELOPMENT. The trends in cognitive development described in the section on early adolescence continue.

PSYCHOSOCIAL DEVELOPMENT. The contexts of adolescents' behavior in relation to family, school, and peer groups during this middle adolescent stage remain similar to those of early adolescence: School and peer group gain in importance, and sex differences in peer relationships now become apparent. According to Savin-Williams, "the developmental tasks during adolescence for boys are dominated by needs for achievement and independence, best worked through in a group; for girls, developing interpersonal skills and love, which are best achieved in dyadic relationships." Loyalty and commitment and intimacy of shared information are more valued in female than in male friendships.

Puberty may change the *interaction between parents and their offspring.* For example, pubertal males and their mothers interrupt each other more often during than before or after middle adolescence. Puberty in females is associated with more arguments with mothers and distancing from fathers as well as with more rigidity in patterns of interaction within the family. Familial homeostasis tends to be re-established when puberty is completed.

During middle adolescence, *social groups* may extend to include members of the opposite sex, and paired dating may begin. A developmental progression in dating behavior has been described by Schofeld: Stage 1 consists of dating without physical contact; stage 2 of kissing, with touching of clothed breasts; stage 3 of touching of unclothed breasts or genital apposition; stage 4 of sexual intercourse with a single partner; and stage 5 of intercourse with multiple partners. Although there is a great deal of variability among subgroups of adolescents, it appears that the majority of teenagers in the middle adolescent years do not progress to the fourth stage. For those who do, however, the risk of unintended pregnancy and sexually transmitted disease is quite high, making prevention of pregnancy an important health issue in caring for those in this age group (see Chapter 10).

During middle adolescence vocational and educational decisions are often made. As indicated earlier, synchrony with the peer group in timing of physical maturation can influence *school* performance as well as aspirations for educational achievement. The physical effects of pubertal development are incorporated into one's self-image during these years, often with profound consequences. When the increased adiposity of pubertal development is viewed negatively by the young woman, a chain of events culminating in anorexia nervosa may ensue. Asymmetric breast development may cause an adolescent to view herself as abnormal. Poor self-image is a common problem during this time, particularly for females and those with chronic illness. Development of self-image also involves "trying on" or experimenting with different social roles. In the eriksonian categorization of life crises, it is the time for self-definition or development of an identity. It is also the time when sexual identity becomes solidified and a sense of sexual adequacy is developed.

LATE ADOLESCENCE

PHYSICAL DEVELOPMENT. It is during this phase of development that the body approximates its young adult proportions and size. Little additional linear growth is achieved after the growth spurt of middle adolescence. Remaining epiphyses, such as those of the femur, humerus, and sternoclavicular junction, become fused, sometimes as late as the early 20s. Development of secondary sex characteristics is completed (SMR 5) with spread of pubic hair to the medial aspects of the thighs in both sexes, attainment of adult genitalia, full reproductive capacity in the male, and adult breast configuration in the female. In the male, facial hair spreads to the chin, and chest hair appears as the last event in the progression of hair growth. The deepening of the voice is completed as testosterone stimulates growth of the thyroid and cricoid cartilages and of the laryngeal muscles. In the female, the adult relationship of a larger uterine fundus to a smaller cervix is attained.

NEURODEVELOPMENT. Neurophysiologic structures and functions appear to be completely developed by the end of middle adolescence. Although no further developmental processes are known, cognitive, social, and moral development may continue to evolve through the rest of life.

PSYCHOSOCIAL DEVELOPMENT. In late adolescence issues of career decisions are usually firmly and sometimes finally faced, and the rebelliousness of earlier stages, if manifest, is often replaced by a gradual return to the family, albeit on a new footing. Although still often moralistic and absolute in their thinking, adolescents at this stage are often more able to engage in a dialogue with their parents. The ability to engage in an empathetic, intimate relationship with another person begins, supplanting the sometimes exploitative, narcissistic sexual relationships of earlier stages. By the age of 19 years, approximately 60% of females and 80% of males in the United States have had sexual intercourse. Even in same-sex relationships, differences in priorities emerge in late adolescence: loyalty, trust, and support in an emotional crisis become the characteristics most valued in friendships of 17-year-olds, whereas among 13-year-olds the emphasis tends to be on good moral character and "niceness" in friendships.

If the psychosocial crisis of earlier adolescence was, in Erikson's schema, that of identity, then that of late adolescence is the need to develop the capacity for intimacy. Once the individual has a self to give, he or she is capable of giving this self.

IRIS F. LITT
VICTOR C. VAUGHAN III

Bazan MT: Anomalous dental development with medical and genetic implications. Pediatr Ann 14:108, 1985.
Chess S, Thomas A, Cameron M: Sexual attitudes and behavior patterns in a middle-class adolescent population. Am J Orthopsychiatry 4:46, 1976.
Costanzo PR, Shaw ME: Conformity as a function of age level. Child Develop 37:967, 1966.
Diamond R, Carey S, Back KJ: Genetic influences on the development of spatial skills during early adolescence. Cognition 13:167, 1983.
Douvan E, Adelson J: The Adolescent Experience. New York, John Wiley & Sons, 1966.
Flavell J: Cognitive Development, 2nd ed. Englewood Cliffs, NJ, Prentice Hall, 1985.
Gross RT, Duke PM: The effect of early versus late physical maturation on adolescent behavior. Pediatr Clin North Am 27:71, 1980.
Katchadourian HA: Biology of Adolescence. San Francisco, WH Freeman, 1977.
Kohlberg L, Gilligan C: The adolescent as a philosopher: the discovery of the self in a postconventional world. *In:* Kagan J, Coles R (eds): 12 to 16. Early Adolescence. New York, WW Norton, 1972.
Levine MD: Developmental assessment. *In:* Levine MD, Carey W, Crocker A, et al (eds): Developmental-Behavioral Pediatrics. Philadelphia, WB Saunders, 1983.
Peterson AC: Pubertal change and cognition. *In:* Brooks-Gunn J, Peterson AC (eds): Girls at Puberty. New York, Plenum Press, 1983.
Savin-Williams R: Dominance hierarchies in groups of early adolescents. Child Develop 50:923, 1979.
Schofeld M: The Sexual Behavior of Young People. Boston, Little, Brown, 1965.
Simmonds RG, Blyth DA, McKinney KL: The social and psychological effects of puberty on white females. *In:* Brooks-Gunn J, Peterson AC (eds): Girls at Puberty. New York, Plenum Press, 1983.
Steinberg L: Reciprocal relation between parent-child distance and pubertal maturation. Devel Psychol 24:1, 1988.
Tanner JM: Growth at Adolescence, 2nd ed. Oxford, Blackwell Scientific Publications, 1962.

3.10 ASSESSMENT OF GROWTH AND DEVELOPMENT

The accurate assessment of developmental status is critical to health care of the infant, child, or adolescent. Many structural and functional details of growth and development are inconspicuous in the broad patterns of growth outlined earlier but take on significance when they are factors in the evaluation of clinical problems. The physician who monitors the growth and development of the child will need to know or have access to information about the limits of normal variability in these details, not only quantitatively and qualitatively but also with respect to their interrelationships. Appraisal of growth and development is most useful when the data obtained are accurate and usually when they are obtained through *serial measurements* taken over periods of months or years.

ASSESSMENT OF PHYSICAL GROWTH AND DEVELOPMENT

In the infant the most useful routine physical measurements are *head circumference, length,* and *weight.* These are supplemented by observation of the nutritional state, dentition, and size or patency of the fontanels. In older children measurements of stature and weight may be supplemented by measurements of the lengths of body segments (extremities, span, and sitting height). Interpretation of the growth status of adolescents requires, in addition to height and weight, assessment of the *sex maturity rating*, *height velocity*, and *body fat content*. Measurements of skinfold thickness and arm or leg circumference may be useful in the estimation of muscle mass or of body fat content.

Charts depicting patterns of normal growth, with indications of its variability, were developed more than 50 yr ago. Among them were the Harvard and Iowa charts, data for which were derived from white children of predominantly middle class origin, and the Wetzel grid, which drew from a wider assortment of sources. Such charts may not now reflect the characteristics of growth patterns of contemporary ethnic, genetic, or socioeconomic groups. There is evidence that ethnic differences depend primarily on differences in the prevalence of malnutrition and infectious disease in various parts of the world; accordingly, there is no contemporary universal standard.

The National Center for Health Statistics (NCHS) has conducted a large survey of characteristics of the growth of children in the United States, from which the data were developed that are shown in Tables 3–2 to 3–4 and in Figures 3–7 and 3–8. The children studied represented a cross-section of ethnic and economic groups; accordingly, some genetic, ethnic, and socioeconomic differences are imbedded in the data. The data and the derived charts are best regarded, therefore, as *reference standards* rather than as descriptive of any particular group of children. As such standards, they have some justification: (1) they are reasonably up-to-date; (2) they reflect the status of generally well-nourished children whose health has been about as good as is likely to be achieved in an industrially developed country; and (3) they appear to indicate conditions close to asymptotic for the secular trend toward increasing growth in height that has been evident for several centuries.

Tables 3–3 and 3–4 and Figure 3–7*A* and *B* present data on the relationship of distributions of length (or stature) and weight to age. Table 3–5 and Figure 3–8*A* and *B*, on the other hand, present data relating to the distributions of relationships between weight and length (or stature) regardless of age. In conjunction with data relating height to age, the latter data may be particularly informative. For example, children with low heights for age who have acceptable weight for height may have experienced nutritional or growth failure in the past, whereas if both height for age and weight for height are strikingly low, then both past and current nutritional or growth failure may be suspected. In contrast, children with normal height for age who have conspicuously low weight for height are likely to have either relatively acute nutritional or growth problems or variant physiques. Children whose weights are at less than the 5th or over the 95th percentile for their actual heights should be evaluated. A physical assessment in conjunction with a review of the history of illness, dietary habits, family patterns of growth, and the psychosocial circumstances of the family will suggest whether more extensive studies are indicated.

Measurements of weight, height, and head circumference at any given time indicate the status of a child in relation to other children of the same age, but only sequential measurements indicate the quality of the process through which each child is achieving his or her growth potential. A child below the 10th percentile in weight for age may be suspected of being undernourished, but 10% of normal children are below this level. If such children manifest regular sequential growth in height and weight along a percentile curve above the 3rd or 5th percentile, they often are manifesting normal physical growth. On the other hand, children whose height and weight are at higher percentiles for their ages may be found to be significantly below their own ideal levels when sequential measurements are evaluated; alternatively, some obese or ill children may be found to have height or weight above that expected for their age.

The growth curves of each healthy child at or near his or her appropriate percentile point in the normal distribution are so smooth that any substantial perturbation of the growth line is likely to reflect physical illness, nutritional disturbance, or psychosocial difficulties. Early recognition of such disturbances may depend heavily on the care with which regular and accurate measurements are made.

It is useful in assessing children's height to take into account family patterns. Tanner and associates have developed for children between the ages of 2 and 9 yr standards for height that have been appropriately adjusted for parental height. Wingerd and associates also have indicated how an appraisal of the preadolescent child's height can take parental height into account.

Inasmuch as the NCHS data relating height and weight to age represent averages of the population at each age, the data obscure differences that distinguish early- from late-maturing adolescents. For these two groups the curves that relate growth velocity to age are markedly different, and it is unlikely that any adolescent will follow precisely the standard curve. Reliable estimates of growth velocity require accurate measurements at relatively frequent intervals (3–6 mo).

The standard height, weight, and head circumference charts are inappropriate for children with intrinsic growth disorders. Special reference growth charts are available for children who have Down, Turner, and Klinefelter syndromes or classic achondroplasia.

VARIABILITY IN BODY PROPORTIONS

Besides the usual changes in body proportions from fetal to adult life (see Fig. 3–2), there are individual differences that express innate growth potential and environmental influences. These variations in body forms of normal persons may be expressed by differences in *physique*. *Somatotype* connotes loosely the potentialities at the time of birth for the development of a particular physique: ectomorphic, mesomorphic, or endomorphic. The ectomorph is characterized by relative linearity, light bone structure, and small mass with respect to body length. The endomorph is characterized by a relatively stocky build, with large amounts of soft tissue. The physique of the mesomorph is in between and is often relatively muscular. Some functional attributes, including some psychologic ones, may be loosely related to somatotype.

Somatotype may be evident in early childhood or may become clear only with the termination of the growth period. Somatotype does not seem closely related to the ultimate height or weight achieved, but the endomorph appears to mature earlier than the ectomorph. As a result of this early maturation, the endomorphic child may have a tendency to be taller than the ectomorphic one in late childhood, the differences being reduced as the ectomorph completes growth.

Other variations in body proportions depend on the different rates of growth of body parts. The size of the brain and cranial cavity approaches adult levels much more rapidly than the size of the face or the length of the legs. This relative preponderance of growth at the cranial end of the body (with corresponding early elaboration of function) has been termed the cephalocaudad progression.

Alterations in proportionate sizes of trunk, extremities, and head are characteristic of certain growth disturbances and may give insight into the underlying pathophysiologic proc-

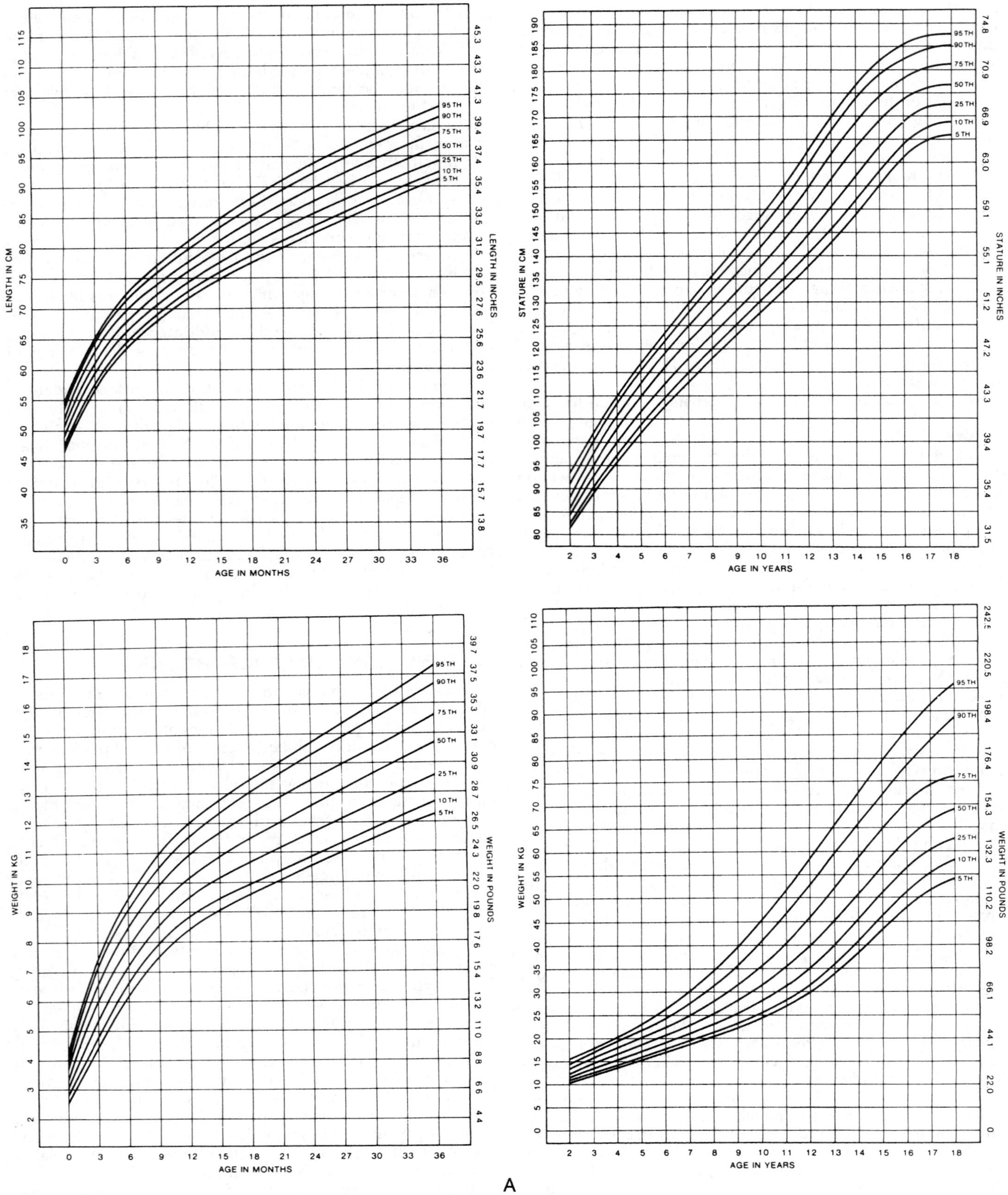

A

Figure 3–7. *A* (*above*) and *B* (*opposite*). Charts for BOYS (*A*) and GIRLS (*B*) of length (or stature) by age (*upper curves*) and weight by age (*lower curves*), each curve corresponding to the indicated percentile level. These charts are based on the data in Tables 3–3 and 3–4. (*A* and *B*, From Hamill PVV, Drizd TA, Johnson CL, et al: Physical growth: National Center for Health Statistics percentiles. Am J Clin Nutr 32:609–610, 1979.)

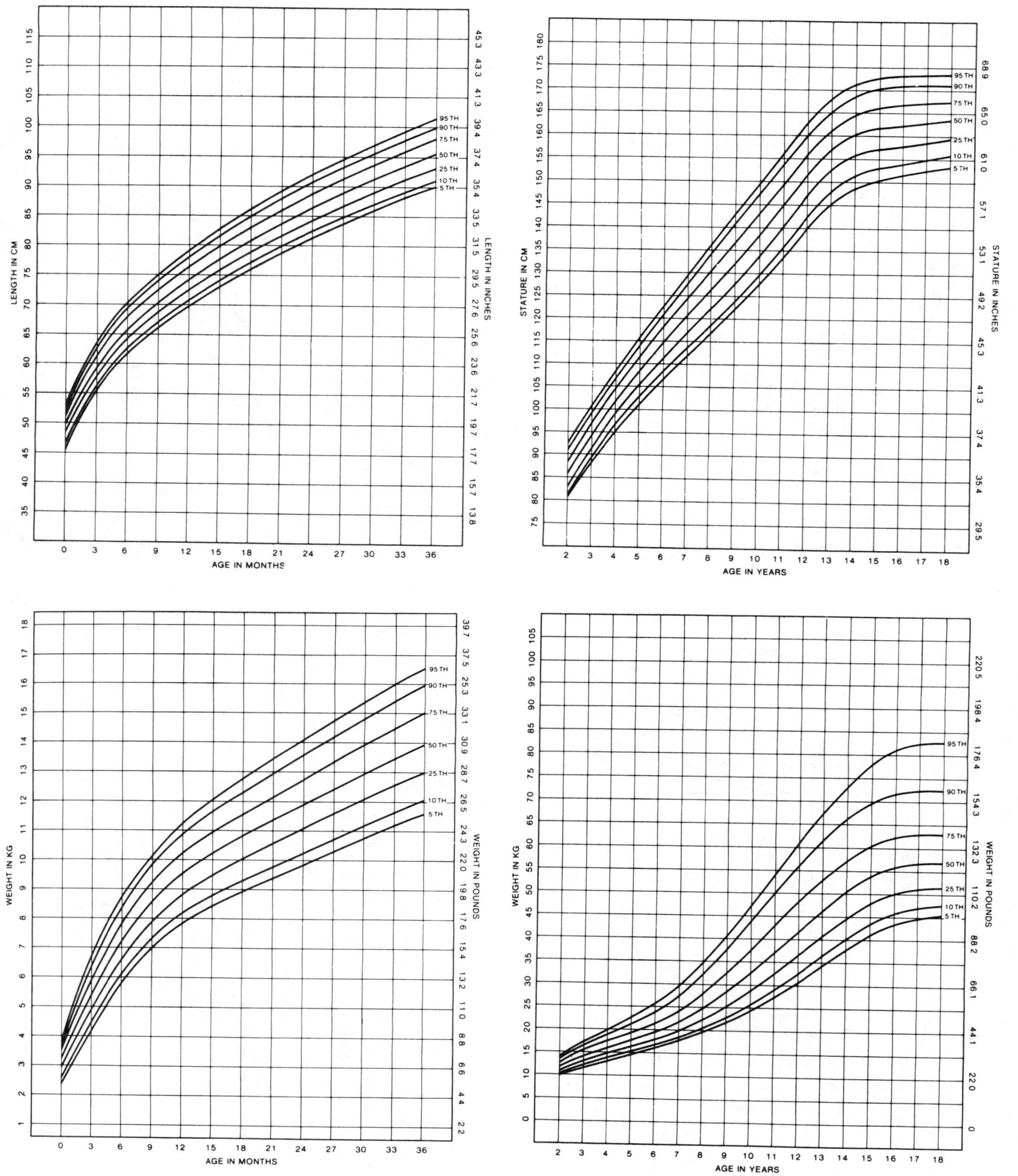

B

Figure 3–7*B*. See legend on opposite page.

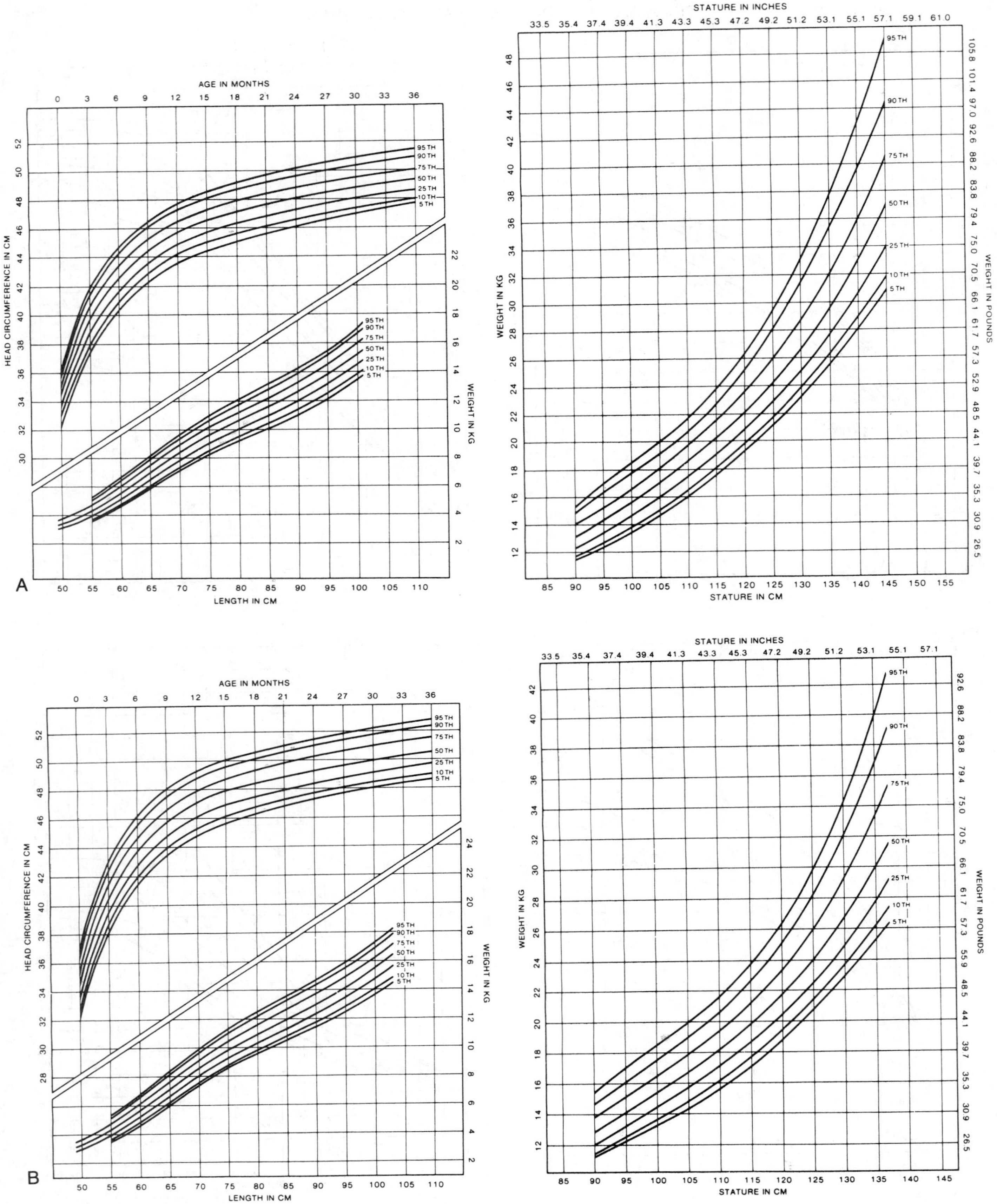

Figure 3–8. Charts for BOYS (Fig. 3–8*A*, above), and for GIRLS (Fig. 3–8*B*, below) of weight by length (or stature), for infants and young children (left) and for older (prepubertal) children (right). *Head circumference by age* is given for infants and young children (upper left). These charts are based on the data in Tables 3–3 and 3–5. (*A* and *B*, From Hamill PVV, Drizd TA, Johnson CL, et al: Physical growth: National Center for Health Statistics percentiles. Am J Clin Nutr 32:614, 1979.)

esses. Helpful measurements include sitting and standing heights, span, body weight, and head circumference. Normally, sitting height represents about 70% of length in the newborn infant, 57% at 3 yr, and about 52% at the time of menarche (SMR [Tanner stage] 3) in girls and at about SMR 4 in boys. There is then a slight increase of 1–2 percentage points because the trunk shows some growth after the limbs have ceased growing.

Figure 3–9 illustrates the proportionate rates of growth for several body systems and shows distinctive variations in patterns of growth, which are often closely correlated with function. Standards for weights of organs at various ages show certain organ-specific patterns; these may be designated as lymphoid, neural, general, and genital. There may be variations within patterns: Whereas the ovary and testis follow the designated genital pattern, the uterus and adrenals are relatively large at birth and show involution in the early weeks of life. The absolute amount of lymphoid tissue in the school-aged child may exceed that in the normal adult; involution is evident at puberty. The weight of the thymus is labile in childhood, decreasing rapidly during illness. It tends to follow the general pattern of growth during the 1st 5 yr of life, with involution occurring at adolescence. The spleen appears to follow the lymphoid pattern and the liver the general one. Skeletal muscle follows the general pattern but is slow to achieve its ultimate mass. Cardiac muscle is initially proportionately large relative to body size, but after the neonatal period it follows the general growth curve.

The proportionate mass of subcutaneous tissue is greatest at about 9 mo; it decreases steadily to about 6 yr, when the increase begins that presages the "fat spurt" of preadolescence, at which time sex differences become apparent (Fig. 3–10). The ratio of total body water to body weight may be a more accurate measurement of body fat than skinfold thickness (SFT), correlating at about 0.62 with SFT. In office practice, however, measurements of triceps and subscapular SFT generally are sufficient and can be referred to standards such as those prepared by Tanner and Whitehouse.

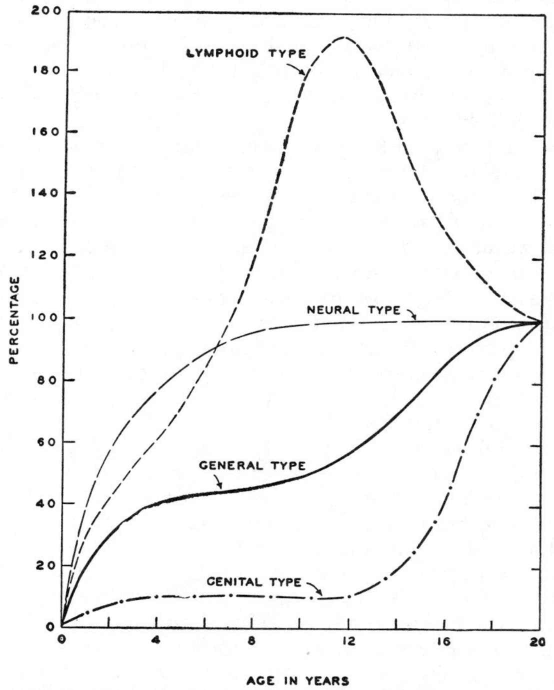

Figure 3–9. Main types of postnatal growth of the various parts and organs of the body. (After Scammon: The measurement of the body in childhood. *In:* Harris B et al [eds]: The Measurement of Man. Minneapolis, University of Minnesota Press, 1930.)

EVALUATION OF OSSEOUS MATURATION

Ossification of the fetal skeleton begins at about the 5th mo of gestation and makes increasing demands on the maternal supply of bone-forming substances. Ossification appears first in the clavicles and membranous bones of the skull and follows rapidly in the long bones and spine. The distal femoral and proximal tibial epiphyses are usually ossified in the normal full-term infant. The fusion of the humeral capitellum with the shaft is said to mark the end of the period of most rapid growth in girls and to predict menarche within 1 year.

A general index of growth status is given by the bone age, as determined from roentgenograms. Bone age is based on (1) the number and size of the epiphyseal centers, (2) the size, shape, density, and sharpness of outline of the ends of bones, and (3) the distance separating the epiphyseal center and the zone of provisional calcification or the degree of fusion between these two elements. Examination of the hand and wrist is useful at all ages; useful information can also be derived from the leg, especially in early infancy.

Tables 3–8 and 3–9 show the expected times of appearance and fusion of the various ossification centers, together with normal variations. Since girls are more advanced than boys in skeletal development at all ages, separate standards are necessary. Variability is less for girls than for boys, especially in later childhood. In boys the standard deviation of bone age in relation to chronologic age is about 2 mo in the 1st yr of life, increasing to 4 mo during the 2nd yr, 6 mo during the 3rd yr, and 10 mo by the 7th yr. Thereafter, for the rest of the growth period, the standard deviation is about 12–15 mo. Larger standard deviations during adolescence reflect the different rates of pubertal maturation; bone age corresponds more closely to sex maturity rating than to chronologic age.

EVALUATION OF DENTAL DEVELOPMENT

See also Chapter 13.

Calcification of teeth begins during approximately the 7th mo of fetal life; it involves deciduous teeth until shortly before term, when calcification begins in those permanent teeth that will be the first to erupt.

Table 3–10 lists the times of eruption of the deciduous and permanent teeth. Delay in eruption of deciduous teeth occurs in children with hypothyroidism and other nutritional and growth disturbances, but the normal variability in dental eruption prevents such a delay from being useful as an indicator of a disorder of growth. In some families the children have conspicuously early or late dentition without other signs of retardation or acceleration of growth.

The first permanent teeth to erupt are the 6-yr molars; they may be mistaken for deciduous teeth. The first permanent molars stabilize the dental arch and have a great deal to do with the ultimate shape of the jaw and the orderly arrangement of teeth. Caries or other defects in them should receive prompt attention; extraction of these teeth should be avoided.

Nutritional disorders, prolonged illness, or use of certain drugs (such as tetracyclines) in infancy or childhood may interfere with the calcification of deciduous and permanent teeth. Such disturbances, if temporary, may leave defects in the enamel ranging from a line of small pits across the tooth to a broader band of hypoplasia. It is possible at times to date a nutritional disturbance by these pits or bands.

The formation of healthy tooth structure is fostered by a diet adequate in protein, calcium, phosphate, and vitamins, especially vitamins C and D, and depends further on an adequate

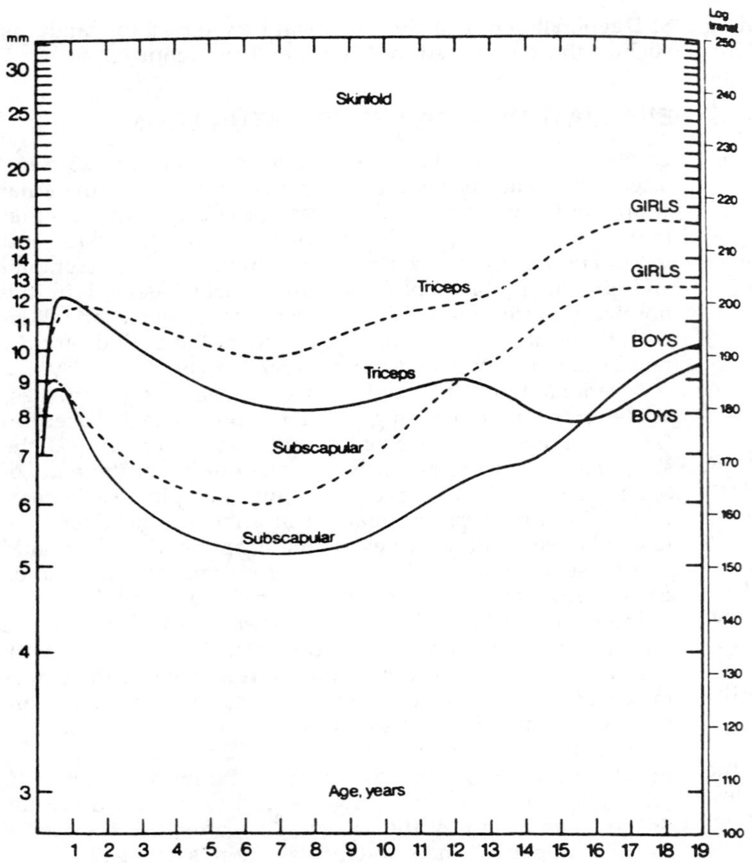

Figure 3–10. Skinfold thickness by age and sex, as measured by Harpenden skinfold calipers over triceps and under scapula. Scale is in millimeters on the left side and logarithmic transformation units on the right side. The lines shown are the 50th percentiles for British children. (Reprinted by permission from Tanner JM: Fetus into Man: Physical Growth from Conception to Maturity. Cambridge, MA, Harvard University Press, 1978.) The data generating these curves are those of Tanner and Whitehouse (1975).

supply of thyroid hormone. Resistance to dental caries is increased when the diet contains optimal amounts of fluoride.

SPECIAL FEATURES OF GROWTH IN THE RESPIRATORY TRACT

The status of the sinuses in the newborn infant is described in Sec. 3.3. The sphenoidal sinuses appear by about the age of 3 yr, and the frontal sinuses between 3 and 7 yr of age. Figure 3–11 shows the changes in respiratory rate that occur with age, with 10th and 90th percentile lines, and also shows how the rates differ for boys and girls and the distinctive changes occurring at adolescence (see also Sec. 12.1–12.3).

SPECIAL FEATURES OF GROWTH IN THE CARDIOVASCULAR SYSTEM

The heart is relatively large at birth, and there is a pubertal growth spurt in heart size that parallels the general growth spurt. As a result, different standards for radiologic interpretation of cardiac diameter in adolescents may be necessary. Figure 3–12 shows how the pulse rate varies with age, and Figures 15–1 to 15–6 show the changes in blood pressure with age. The mean systolic pressure for boys continues to advance with age after that of girls has begun to reach an asymptote. The levels of serum urate increase and those of high-density lipoprotein (HDL) cholesterol decrease with advancing age in male adolescents (see Sec. 8.20).

SPECIAL ASPECTS OF METABOLISM AND NUTRITION

Caloric needs increase with growth in size but maintain a relatively constant relationship to body surface area, which appears to be as closely correlated with the body's mass of metabolically active tissue as any other simple measurement. Measurements of body surface that correspond to given heights and weights are available; estimates can be obtained from nomograms (see Chapter 27). Crude estimates for children of average physique are given by the simple formulas shown in Table 3–11.

When referred to body surface, basal caloric needs appear to be somewhat lower in premature infants than in full-term ones. They increase during the 1st yr of life from about 30 kcal/m^2/hr to about 50 kcal by the 2nd yr, with a subsequent fall to adult levels of 35–40 kcal/m^2/hr. The rate of fall is slowed or may be reversed during the prepubertal or adolescent years by the need for additional energy to support the increase in growth rate that occurs at this time. This increased need for calories is matched by an increased need for other nutritional factors, including iron for both sexes (for muscular development in males and to replace menstrual blood loss in postmenarchal females).

Needs for water and electrolytes remain roughly constant in relation to body surface area through most of the growing period; the inevitable variations in intake are met by the capacity of homeostatic mechanisms to adjust to varying conditions of supply and demand.

Adolescent growth is particularly susceptible to impairment by dietary fads or by behaviors that deprive the youngster of essential calories or other nutritional substances. Drugs also may impair adolescent growth; among these are certain of the stimulants given for attention deficit disorders or learning disabilities (methylphenidate or dextroamphetamines).

A variety of metabolic changes in adolescence are reflected in changes in normal values for levels of serum components. Alkaline phosphatase activity increases during the period of

TABLE 3–8. Time of Appearance in Roentgenograms of Centers of Ossification in Infancy and Childhood

BOYS—Age at Appearance: Mean ± Std. Deviation*	Bones and Epiphyseal Centers	GIRLS—Age at Appearance: Mean ± Std. Deviation*
3 wk	*Humerus*, head	3 wk
	Carpal bones	
2 mo ± 2 mo	Capitate	2 mo ± 2 mo
3 mo ± 2 mo	Hamate	2 mo ± 2 mo
30 mo ± 16 mo	Triangular†	21 mo ± 14 mo
42 mo ± 19 mo	Lunate†	34 mo ± 13 mo
67 mo ± 19 mo	Trapezium†	47 mo ± 14 mo
69 mo ± 15 mo	Trapezoid†	49 mo ± 12 mo
66 mo ± 15 mo	Scaphoid†	51 mo ± 12 mo
No standards available	Pisiform†	no standards available
	Metacarpal bones	
18 mo ± 5 mo	II	12 mo ± 3 mo
20 mo ± 5 mo	III	13 mo ± 3 mo
23 mo ± 6 mo	IV	15 mo ± 4 mo
26 mo ± 7 mo	V	16 mo ± 5 mo
32 mo ± 9 mo	I	18 mo ± 5 mo
	Fingers (epiphyses)	
16 mo ± 4 mo	Proximal phalanx, 3rd finger	10 mo ± 3 mo
16 mo ± 4 mo	Proximal phalanx, 2nd finger	11 mo ± 3 mo
17 mo ± 5 mo	Proximal phalanx, 4th finger	11 mo ± 3 mo
19 mo ± 7 mo	Distal phalanx, 1st finger	12 mo ± 4 mo
21 mo ± 5 mo	Proximal phalanx, 5th finger	14 mo ± 4 mo
24 mo ± 6 mo	Middle phalanx, 3rd finger	15 mo ± 5 mo
24 mo ± 6 mo	Middle phalanx, 4th finger	15 mo ± 5 mo
26 mo ± 6 mo	Middle phalanx, 2nd finger	16 mo ± 5 mo
28 mo ± 6 mo	Distal phalanx, 3rd finger	18 mo ± 4 mo
28 mo ± 6 mo	Distal phalanx, 4th finger	18 mo ± 5 mo
32 mo ± 7 mo	Proximal phalanx, 1st finger	20 mo ± 5 mo
37 mo ± 9 mo	Distal phalanx, 5th finger	23 mo ± 6 mo
37 mo ± 8 mo	Distal phalanx, 2nd finger	23 mo ± 6 mo
39 mo ± 10 mo	Middle phalanx, 5th finger	22 mo ± 7 mo
152 mo ± 18 mo	Sesamoid (adductor pollicis)	121 mo ± 13 mo
	Hip and knee	
Usually present at birth	Femur, distal	Usually present at birth
Usually present at birth	Tibia, proximal	Usually present at birth
4 mo ± 2 mo	Femur, head	4 mo ± 2 mo
46 mo ± 11 mo	Patella	29 mo ± 7 mo
	Foot and ankle‡	

*To nearest month.

†Except for the capitate and hamate bones, the variability of carpal centers is too great to make them very useful clinically.

‡Standards for the foot are available, but normal variation is wide, including some familial variants, so that this area is of little clinical use.

The norms in Tables 3–8 and 3–9 present a composite of published data from the Fels Research Institute, Yellow Springs, Ohio (Pyle SI, Sontag L. Am J Roentgenol Vol. 49, 1943), and unpublished data from the Brush Foundation, Case Western Reserve University, Cleveland, OH, and the Harvard School of Public Health, Boston, MA. Compiled by Lieb, Buehl, and Pyle.

increase in height velocity. Changes in levels of somatomedins, hematocrit, HDL cholesterol, serum iron, and other measurements correlate more closely with sex maturity rating than with chronologic age. An increase in creatinine level is correlated with increasing muscle mass in males.

DEVELOPMENTAL ASPECTS OF DRUG METABOLISM

Changes in metabolic activity with age may significantly alter the child's response to drugs and may require adjustments of dosage. This is particularly evident with respect to administration of drugs to newborn infants (see Sec. 6.55). Some variability in rates of metabolism reflects the rapidity with which the infant or child acquires a normal capacity to metabolize drugs for which the metabolic pathways are at birth incomplete or incompletely activated. Normal activities of glucuronidase, phenylalanine transaminase, and other enzymes may be achieved only after days, weeks, or months, sometimes with clinical consequences.

During puberty changes in body composition, such as increased adipose tissue in females and decreased total body water in both sexes, will affect the patterns of drug distribution. Competition for enzymes that metabolize drugs may result from increased levels of sex steroids as well. In male adolescents high levels of androgens increase the binding

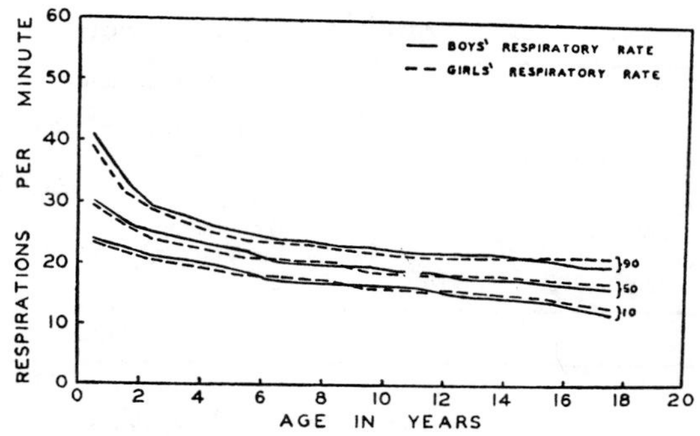

Figure 3–11. Respiratory rates in infants and children.

capacity of the cytochrome P450 system. The rate of elimination of theophylline is more closely related to sex maturity than to age. A similar relationship can be expected for other drugs.

Genetic variability also may determine the rate of metabolism or the pharmacologic effect of some substances. Acetylation, methylation, demethylation, sulfation, and other processes may be involved. For example, the rapidity of acetylation and excretion of such drugs as isoniazid, hydralazine, and some sulfonamides is genetically set by autosomal recessive genes. Persons who are fast acetylators may need larger doses of drugs and respond poorly to them; slow acetylators are at higher risk of toxic effects associated with elevated drug levels.

Other developmental aspects of pharmacology that are not well understood include the paradoxic reactions of some children to some drugs; excitement as a response to phenobarbital and abatement of hyperkinesis with amphetamine are examples. Moreover, children appear to have increased sensitivity or reactivity to the effects of some drugs under other conditions; children with deficiencies of glucose-6-phosphate dehydrogenase (G-6-PD) for example, have generally more severe reactions from ingestion of the offending drugs than do susceptible adults.

TECHNIQUES OF PHYSICAL MEASUREMENTS

Accuracy of measurement is essential to the reliable interpretation of growth data; slight variations in technique may result

TABLE 3–9. Modal Age at Onset and Completion of Fusion in Skeletal Areas in Adolescence

BOYS—Modal Age Between	Area	GIRLS—Modal Age Between
	Elbow	
13.0–13.5 yr	Onset in humerus	11.0–11.5 yr
15.0–15.5	Complete in ulna	12.5–13.0
	Foot and Ankle	
14.0–14.5	Onset in great toe	12.5–13.0
15.5–16	Complete in tibia, fibula	14.0–14.5
	Hand and Wrist	
15.0–15.5	Onset in distal phalanges	13.0–13.5
17.5–18.0	Complete in radius	16.0–16.5
	Knee	
15.0–15.5	Onset in tibial tuberosity	13.5–14.0
17.5–18.0	Complete in fibula	16.0–16.5
	Hip and Pelvis	
15.5–16.0	Onset in greater trochanter	14.0–14.5
after 18.0	Complete in symphysis	17.5–18.0
	Shoulder and Clavicle	
15.5–16.0	Onset in greater tubercle of humerus	14.0–14.5
after 18.0	Complete in clavicle	17.5–18.0

See footnotes to Table 3–8.

TABLE 3–10. Chronology of Human Dentition Primary or Deciduous Teeth*

	Calcification		Eruption		Shedding	
	Begins at	***Complete at***	***Maxillary***	***Mandibular***	***Maxillary***	***Mandibular***
Central incisors	5th fetal mo	18–24 mo	6–8 mo	5–7 mo	7–8 yr	6–7 yr
Lateral incisors	5th fetal mo	18–24 mo	8–11 mo	7–10 mo	8–9 yr	7–8 yr
Cuspids (canines)	6th fetal mo	30–36 mo	16–20 mo	16–20 mo	11–12 yr	9–11 yr
First molars	5th fetal mo	24–30 mo	10–16 mo	10–16 mo	10–11 yr	10–12 yr
Second molars	6th fetal mo	36 mo	20–30 mo	20–30 mo	10–12 yr	11–13 yr

Secondary or Permanent Teeth

	Calcification		Eruption	
	Begins at	***Complete at***	***Maxillary***	***Mandibular***
Central incisors	3–4 mo	9–10 yr	7–8 yr	6–7 yr
Lateral incisors	Max, 10–12 mo Mand, 3–4 mo	10–11 yr	8–9 yr	7–8 yr
Cuspids (canines)	4–5 mo	12–15 yr	11–12 yr	9–11 yr
First premolars (bicuspids)	18–21 mo	12–13 yr	10–11 yr	10–12 yr
Second premolars (bicuspids)	24–30 mo	12–14 yr	10–12 yr	11–13 yr
First molars	Birth	9–10 yr	6–7 yr	6–7 yr
Second molars	30–36 mo	14–16 yr	12–13 yr	12–13 yr
Third molars	Max, 7–9 yr Mand, 8–10 yr	18–25 yr	17–22 yr	17–22 yr

*Adapted from chart prepared by PK Losch, Harvard School of Dental Medicine, who provided the data for this chart.

in significantly large errors in the placement of children according to percentile rank.

HEIGHT. Recumbent length can be more accurately measured than standing height in children under the age of 5 yr; after this time measurement of standing height is generally more convenient. Recumbent length is measured as the child lies on a firm table that has a measuring stick of at least 125 cm or 50 in fastened along one edge. The soles of the feet are held firmly against a fixed upright placed at the zero mark. A movable upright crosses the table above the head and is brought firmly against the vertex. If recumbent length is used after 5 yr of age, the value obtained may be reduced by 1 cm from that for standing height.

Standing height is measured as the child stands erect, with heels, buttocks, upper part of the back, and occiput placed against a vertical upright; the heels should be close together, and the arms should hang naturally at the sides. (The external auditory meatus and the lower border of the orbit should be in a plane parallel with the floor.) A wooden headpiece with two faces at right angles may be placed firmly on the head against a 2-m or 6-ft measuring scale attached to the vertical surface against which the child is positioned.

During adolescence serial measurements of height should be plotted on a *height velocity* chart to document the acceleration of growth that should occur at this time. Moreover, the interpretation of findings should take into account the sex maturity rating of the patient in order to determine whether the velocity curve is consistent with that expected for the developmental stage. Standards have been prepared by Tanner and associates.

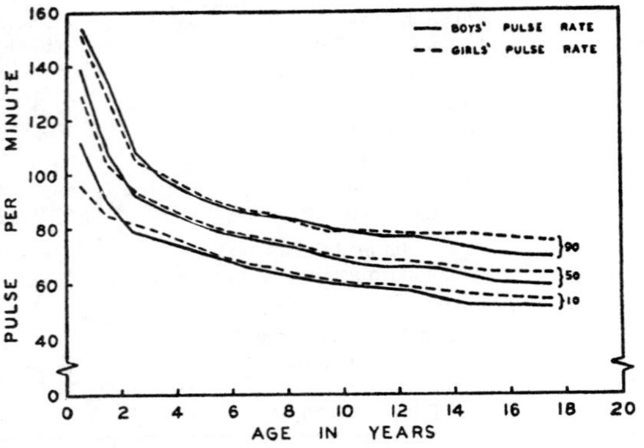

Figure 3–12. Pulse rates in infants and children.

BODY COMPOSITION. Measurement of SFT provides a rough estimate of body composition. Triceps SFT is measured over the posterior surface of the triceps of the left arm by calipers placed at a point halfway between the acromion and the olecranon as the arm hangs vertically in a relaxed fashion at the patient's side. Subscapular SFT is measured below the angle of the left scapula. Values obtained may be converted to estimates of body fat using conversion tables. SFT and arm circumference together give crude information about muscle mass.

SEX MATURITY RATING. Inspection of the patient is generally adequate to establish his or her SMR, which is based on examination of the breasts and pubic hair in girls and on examination of the testes, penis, and pubic hair in boys. Tables 3–6 and 3–7 list the criteria used for determining SMR. Staging of testicular size is aided by use of an orchiometer.

HEAD CIRCUMFERENCE. The head circumference measurement is particularly valuable in infants; it need not be taken routinely after 3 yr of age. The tape is applied firmly over the glabella and supraorbital ridges anteriorly and on that part of the occiput that gives the maximal circumference. Difficulties sometimes arise when the head has an unusual or abnormal shape, as in hydrocephalus. Under these circumstances, serial measurements of the changing size of the head may best be made by positioning the tape over whatever points on the forehead and occiput give the maximal circumference. If cloth tapes are used, they may stretch with aging

TABLE 3–11. Approximation of Surface Area (m^2) to Weight (kg)

Weight Range*	Approximate Surface Area
1–*5* kg	$m^2 = (0.05 \times kg) + 0.05$
6–*10* kg	$m^2 = (0.04 \times kg) + 0.\mathit{10}$
11–*20* kg	$m^2 = (0.03 \times kg) + 0.\mathit{20}$
21–*40* kg	$m^2 = (0.02 \times kg) + 0.\mathit{40}$

*The figures 5, 10, 20, and 40 are given in italics to indicate a simple mnemonic. The formula $m^2 = (0.02 \times kg) + 0.40$ gives reasonable estimates from 21 to 70 kg.

TABLE 3–12. Emerging Patterns of Behavior During the First Year of Life*

	Neonatal Period (First 4 Wk)
Prone:	Lies in flexed attitude; turns head from side to side; head sags on ventral suspension
Supine:	Generally flexed and a little stiff
Visual:	May fixate face or light in line of vision; "doll's-eye" movement of eyes on turning of the body
Reflex:	Moro response active; stepping and placing reflexes; grasp reflex active
Social:	Visual preference for human face
	At 4 Wk
Prone:	Legs more extended; holds chin up; turns head; head lifted momentarily to plane of body on ventral suspension
Supine:	Tonic neck posture predominates; supple and relaxed; head lags on pull to sitting position
Visual:	Watches person; follows moving object
Social:	Body movements in cadence with voice of other in social contact; beginning to smile
	At 8 Wk
Prone:	Raises head slightly farther; head sustained in plane of body on ventral suspension
Supine:	Tonic neck posture predominates; head lags on pull to sitting position
Visual:	Follows moving object 180 degrees
Social:	Smiles on social contact; listens to voice and coos
	At 12 Wk
Prone:	Lifts head and chest, arms extended; head above plane of body on ventral suspension
Supine:	Tonic neck posture predominates; reaches toward and misses objects; waves at toy
Sitting:	Head lag partially compensated on pull to sitting position; early head control with bobbing motion; back rounded
Reflex:	Typical Moro response has not persisted; makes defensive movements or selective withdrawal reactions
Social:	Sustained social contact; listens to music; says "aah, ngah"
	At 16 Wk
Prone:	Lifts head and chest, head in approximately vertical axis; legs extended
Supine:	Symmetric posture predominates, hands in midline; reaches and grasps objects and brings them to mouth
Sitting:	No head lag on pull to sitting position; head steady, tipped forward; enjoys sitting with full truncal support
Standing:	When held erect, pushes with feet
Adaptive:	Sees pellet, but makes no move to it
Social:	Laughs out loud; may show displeasure if social contact is broken; excited at sight of food
	At 28 Wk
Prone:	Rolls over; pivots; crawls or creep-crawls (Knobloch)
Supine:	Lifts head; rolls over; squirming movements
Sitting:	Sits briefly, with support of pelvis; leans forward on hands; back rounded
Standing:	May support most of weight; bounces actively
Adaptive:	Reaches out for and grasps large object; *transfers* objects from hand to hand; grasp uses radial palm; rakes at pellet
Language:	Polysyllabic vowel sounds formed
Social:	Prefers mother; babbles; enjoys mirror; responds to changes in emotional content of social contact
	At 40 Wk
Sitting:	Sits up alone and indefinitely without support, back straight
Standing:	Pulls to standing position; "cruises" or walks holding on to furniture
Motor:	Creeps or crawls
Adaptive:	Grasps objects with *thumb and forefinger;* pokes at things with forefinger; picks up pellet with assisted pincer movement; uncovers hidden toy; attempts to retrieve dropped object; releases object grasped by other person
Language:	Repetitive consonant sounds (mama, dada)
Social:	Responds to sound of name; plays peek-a-boo or pat-a-cake; waves bye-bye
	At 52 Wk (1 Yr)
Motor:	Walks with one hand held (48 wk); rises independently, takes several steps (Knobloch)
Adaptive:	Picks up pellet with unassisted pincer movement of forefinger and thumb; releases object to other person on request or gesture
Language:	A few words besides mama, dada
Social:	Plays simple ball game; makes postural adjustment to dressing

*Data are derived from those of Gesell (as revised by Knobloch), Shirley, Provence, Wolf, Bailey, and others.

and should be checked frequently against wooden or steel standards.

CHEST CIRCUMFERENCE. Measurement is made in mid-respiration at the level of the xiphoid cartilage or substernal notch. Measurement is made in the recumbent position up to the age of 5 yr, and while standing thereafter.

ABDOMINAL CIRCUMFERENCE. This measurement is taken only in patients up to 3 yr old and is of value principally in recognizing and following the course of chronic intestinal disturbances. Measurement is made in the plane of the umbilicus when the infant is recumbent.

3.11 ASSESSMENT OF NEURODEVELOPMENTAL STATUS

See also Sec. 3.2–3.7 and 20.1.

An informal assessment of the neurodevelopmental status of infants and children should be a routine part of each clinical encounter. Only with such an assessment will the physician be adequately sensitive to deviations indicating slight impairment or retardation and only with such knowledge will he be able to inform parents, respond to their questions, or make

TABLE 3–13. Emerging Patterns of Behavior from 1 to 5 Years of Age*

	15 Mo
Motor:	Walks alone; crawls up stairs
Adaptive:	Makes tower of 3 cubes; makes a line with crayon; inserts pellet in bottle
Language:	Jargon; follows simple commands; may name a familiar object (ball)
Social:	Indicates some desires or needs by pointing; hugs parents
	18 Mo
Motor:	Runs stiffly; sits on small chair; walks up stairs with one hand held; explores drawers and waste baskets
Adaptive:	Makes a tower of 4 cubes; imitates scribbling; imitates vertical stroke; dumps pellet from bottle
Language:	10 words (average); names pictures; identifies one or more parts of body
Social:	Feeds self; seeks help when in trouble; may complain when wet or soiled; kisses parent with pucker
	24 Mo
Motor:	Runs well; walks up and down stairs, one step at a time; opens doors; climbs on furniture; jumps
Adaptive:	Tower of 7 cubes (6 at 21 mo); circular scribbling; imitates horizontal stroke; folds paper once imitatively
Language:	Puts 3 words together (subject, verb, object)
Social:	Handles spoon well; often tells immediate experiences; helps to undress; listens to stories with pictures
	30 Mo
Motor:	Goes up stairs alternating feet
Adaptive:	Tower of 9 cubes; makes vertical and horizontal strokes, but generally will not join them to make a cross; imitates circular stroke, forming closed figure
Language:	Refers to self by pronoun "I"; knows full name
Social:	Helps put things away; pretends in play
	36 Mo
Motor:	Rides tricycle; stands momentarily on one foot
Adaptive:	Tower of 10 cubes; imitates construction of "bridge" of 3 cubes; copies a circle; imitates a cross
Language:	Knows age and sex; counts 3 objects correctly; repeats 3 numbers or a sentence of 6 syllables
Social:	Plays simple games (in "parallel" with other children); helps in dressing (unbuttons clothing and puts on shoes); washes hands
	48 Mo
Motor:	Hops on one foot; throws ball overhand; uses scissors to cut out pictures; climbs well
Adaptive:	Copies bridge from model; imitates construction of "gate" of 5 cubes; copies cross and square; draws a man with 2 to 4 parts besides head; names longer of 2 lines
Language:	Counts 4 pennies accurately; tells a story
Social:	Plays with several children with beginning of social interaction and role-playing; goes to toilet alone
	60 Mo
Motor:	Skips
Adaptive:	Draws triangle from copy; names heavier of 2 weights
Language:	Names 4 colors; repeats sentence of 10 syllables; counts 10 pennies correctly
Social:	Dresses and undresses; asks questions about meaning of words; domestic role-playing

*Data are derived from those of Gesell (as revised by Knobloch), Shirley, Provence, Wolf, Bailey, and others. After 5 yr the Stanford-Binet, Wechsler-Bellevue, and other scales offer the most precise estimates of developmental level. In order to have their greatest value, they should be administered only by an experienced and qualified person.

appropriate recommendations for further study. Tables 3–12 and 3–13 list the expected behaviors of infants and children at various ages. In evaluating these behaviors the examiner often uses materials (such as readily available toys or other materials) that have not been standardized but do reveal whether a standardized screening test or a formal psychologic evaluation is indicated. The casual examination should be interpreted with caution, particularly when an infant or child who is irritable, hungry, or ill does not perform at his or her expected level. For such patients a future examination should be scheduled. For the infant born prematurely, the observed developmental level should be adjusted in relation to chronologic age during the 1st 2 yr of life.

PROCEDURE. For the young infant the examination may begin with observation of the infant in the prone and supine positions, note being made of spontaneous behavior and then of the manner in which the infant adjusts to being pulled from a supine to a sitting position and to being held in ventral suspension (*Landau response*). The reaction to moving persons or objects within the visual field or line of sight or within reach can be observed, both for relatively large objects, such as a rattle or stethoscope, and for small objects such as a raisin or pellet. Behavior when standing with support should also be observed.

After 6 mo of age the infant may be given blocks (1-in cubes), and after 12 mo blocks and crayon and paper, for observing the child's ability to imitate or copy patterns of construction with blocks or the drawings of simple figures as demonstrated by the examiner. After 2½ yr the child can be asked to draw a person or geometric figures and to count pennies or raisins.

STANDARDIZED SCREENING TESTS. A number of relatively simple tests permit the physician or his or her assistant to make helpful assessments of the developmental or cognitive levels of older children as a part of normal office practice. Some of these are in the form of questionnaires for parents; others are administered directly, using standardized materials. Such tests include the Quick Test, the Raven Matrices, the Thorpe Developmental Inventory, the Denver Developmental Screening Test (DDST), and the Revised Developmental Screening Inventory (based on Gesell by Knobloch). In using these or other tools to evaluate performance, the tester should become thoroughly familiar with the procedures used, the rules for their administration, and their limitations.

3.12 ASSESSMENT OF PSYCHOSOCIAL DEVELOPMENT

Assessment of psychosocial problems and their management are discussed in Sec. 3.22 and subsequent sections.

VICTOR C. VAUGHAN III
IRIS F. LITT

Bayer LM, Bayley N: Growth Diagnosis. Chicago, University of Chicago Press, 1959.

Bayley N: Bayley Scales of Infant Development. New York, The Psychological Corporation, 1969.

Dine MS, Gartside PS, Glueck CJ, et al: Relationship of head circumference to length in the first 400 days of life: A mnemonic. Pediatrics 67:506, 1981.

Frankenburg WK, Thornton SM, Cohrs ME: Pediatric Developmental Diagnosis. New York, Thieme-Stratton Inc, 1981.

Greulich WW, Pyle SI: Radiographic Atlas of Skeletal Development of the Hand and Wrist, 2nd ed. Stanford, CA, Stanford University Press, 2nd ed., 1959.

Hamill PVV, Drizd TA, Johnson CL, et al: Physical growth: National Center for Health Statistics percentiles. Am J Clin Nutr 32:607, 1979.

Hein K, Dell R, Pesce M, et al: Effects of adolescent development on theophylline half-life. Pediatr Res 19 (Suppl): 173A, 1985.

Iliff A, Lee VA: Pulse rate, respiratory rate, and body temperature of children between two months and eighteen years of age. Child Develop 23:237, 1952.

Knobloch H, Pasamanick B (eds): Gesell and Amatruda's Developmental Diagnosis, 3rd ed. Hagerstown, MD, Harper & Row, 1974.

Knobloch H, Stevens F, Malone AF: Manual of Developmental Diagnosis. Hagerstown, MD, Harper & Row, 1980.

Pyle SI, Reed RB, Stuart HC: Patterns of skeletal development in the hand. Pediatrics 24:886, 1959.

Roche AF, Himes JH: Incremental growth charts. Am J Clin Nutr 33:2041, 1980.

Special Growth Charts (Annotation): Arch Dis Child 63:1179, 1988.

Tanner M, Davies PSW: Clinical longitudinal standards for height and weight velocity of North American children. J Pediatr 107:317, 1985.

Tanner JM, Whitehouse RH: Revised standards for triceps and subscapular skinfolds in British children. Arch Dis Child 50:142, 1975.

Vaughan VC III, Litt IF: Child and Adolescent Development: Clinical Implications. Philadelphia, WB Saunders Co, 1990.

Wingerd J, Solomon IL, Schoen EJ: Parent-specific height standards for preadolescent children of three racial groups, with method for rapid determination. Pediatrics 52:555, 1973.

PSYCHOSOCIAL DIMENSIONS OF PEDIATRICS

3.13 INTRODUCTION

The term *psychosocial* recognizes that the activities, functions, and behaviors of a child include two dimensions: *psychic* or *internal,* which consists of feelings, attitudes, thoughts, fantasies, memory, judgment, values, and self-image; and *social, external,* or *interactional,* encompassing relationships with the environment, people, and circumstances within which the child lives. The psychosocial orientation in no way neglects the biologic or organic aspects of development. Biologic (physiologic or pathologic) facts significant to psychosocial development or disturbances will be identified.

The psychosocial viewpoint considers the child's emotional and social development and its deviations and disturbances in terms of *interaction* between fetus, infant, or child and the environment. For example, to state that an infant's cry indicates hunger is to infer a physiologic or biologic state. The inference seems justified when the cry subsides after feeding. But the process of feeding has had, besides its nutritional significance, emotional and social aspects for both infant and mother. Holding, cuddling, crooning to, or talking to the infant expresses emotional and social states of the mother, and the infant perceives and feels ("ingests") and responds to these aspects of the feeding relationship as surely as to the food itself.

Maturation involves those intrinsic processes that are genetically or otherwise organically programmed; but even maturational features of development depend for their healthy achievement on environmental factors. *Development* refers to the progressive differentiation, refinement, and specialization of the organism and its constituent parts. Development is interactional and depends on both general and specific internal and environmental conditions. The major intrapsychic dimensions of psychosocial development include the *cognitive* and the *affective.* Cognitive processes underlie perceptual reasoning, judgment, and memory—generally, the intellectual features of intrapsychic function. Affective states include anxiety, depression, fear, anger, sadness, joy, elation, jealousy, calmness, and placidity (the dimensions of feeling or emotion).

Most activities of the child integrate both affective and cognitive processes. The risk for most clinicians is that attention to affective distress may be neglected until it is blatant. The affective component in a child's temper tantrum is unmistakable; but a child's poor performance in school may be too easily construed as only a cognitive or perceptual difficulty, with little attention given to strong feelings of guilt, discouragement, fear of failure, and displaced anger. Both acute and chronic illnesses frequently produce in children lassitude and sadness, bordering on depression.

The formation of *conscience* and its exercise are psychic processes with important cognitive and affective features. Anxiety and the desire for approval are early affective precursors. Identifying and remembering approved and disapproved actions and choosing among behavioral alternatives are cognitive aspects of the formation and function of conscience.

3.14 SOME CONCEPTUAL MODELS OF CHILD DEVELOPMENT

No single psychosocial theory adequately accounts for all aspects of the development or behavior of children, whether normal or disturbed. Although each specific theory offers detailed explanations and rationales for a certain perspective from which to evaluate or understand a child, one theoretical view alone cannot account for the multiply variant processes that occur in child development. To fully appreciate the complex process of child development, the physician should be aware of the major contributions from each important theoretical viewpoint. Knowledge of the rudiments of the basics of child development allows the pediatrician to better evaluate the entire child and to offer sound and appropriate advice or recommendations.

The first theoretical model is generally called the *medical* or *physiologic* model. Throughout the 1st 18 yr of life, each person undergoes extensive changes in the nervous, endocrine, cardiovascular, musculoskeletal, gastrointestinal, and other organ systems. The pediatrician should be familiar with the normal development of these different systems and have a keen awareness of abnormal variations. Extensive education focuses on how to handle the abnormal or disease process. Frequently, however, little attention is given to the impact of the disease process on the simultaneously developing emotional, cognitive, and social aspects of the child. This psychosocial dimension should be recognized as an integral part of the medical or physiologic model.

Sigmund Freud postulated the *psychoanalytic model,* in which the child is seen as motivated by basic sexual and aggressive drives and passes through successive, critical stages influenced initially by parents and then by an enlarging group of social experiences. In the first half of the 1st yr of life, the *oral stage,* basic trust is learned as long as both the child's physical apparatus and the environment are intact and supportive. At 2–3 yr of age the child enters the *anal stage* of development, marked by toilet training and the development of competence. The *oedipal stage* occurs at 4–5 yr of age and is marked by the child's competitive relationship with the parent of the same sex for the attention of the parent of the opposite sex. At 5–6 yr of age the child enters the *latency stage* in which aggressive and sexual urges have traditionally been thought to be dormant but actually are not. This is a very active phase in regard to social development, peer orientation, and the learning of the rules and regulations of society. During puberty, *phallic stage,* the adolescent faces physiologic changes, emerging sexuality, and the task of identity formation.

Erikson expanded the psychoanalytic theory beyond the nuclear family and emphasized the *interaction of the person with society.* Rather than focusing on the childhood experience with parents as the main determinant of personality development, Erikson maintained that the personality develops from continual interaction between the person and his or her environment throughout life. Conflicts with the environment are considered inevitable and facilitate a growth process. Erikson proposed that development occurs in eight stages, each one focused on an essential conflict related to that developmental level. For example, the conflict in infancy is whether the infant will learn to trust that the environment will respond to biologic and emotional needs or to mistrust the environmental response. Erikson considered personality development to be a process occurring throughout the life cycle. He stressed the interplay between the person's relative skills and the environment. How a person negotiates each developmental stage is dependent on his or her level of functioning at that time and the environmental response. The resolution of each stage helps to determine the resolution of successive stages. However, changes in the environment or in the person can promote new or different resolutions, resulting in variability in development.

Mahler asserted that the psychologic development of an individual proceeded in a continually unfolding process, with critical stages during the first 3–4 yr of life. Initially, the infant is biologically and psychologically bound to the mother; the infant has difficulty in distinguishing himself or herself from others. As the infant's sensory and motor skills improve, he or she is increasingly capable of greater and newer experiences with the mother and the environment, which foster a greater awareness of being separated from the mother. The more interactions that the infant has with the environment, the more the infant learns how to distinguish himself or herself from others. The infant gradually develops a sense of himself as separate from others, as an individual. The interaction between the mother and the infant determines how secure and successful the infant is in achieving *separation-individuation.* This process of separation-individuation is of fundamental importance in childhood development. Mahler proposed that this process determines further personality development and forms the basis of relationships with others.

In recent years, less emphasis has been placed on motivation of the child by basic sexual and aggressive drives, and more attention has been given to the importance of relationships in the child's development of the sense of identity or of the sense of how to use relationships to mediate basic biologic and emotional needs. In addition, more attention has been focused on the child's temperament and on the basic genetic and biologic capacity (e.g., memory, intelligence, sensory, motor abilities) to perceive and interact with the world.

A more circumscribed, conceptual model is the *cognitive model,* which was primarily proposed by Jean Piaget through his studies of the step-by-step acquisition of knowledge. According to this model, there are several different stages of intellectual development, which are somewhat biologically determined and occur in an epigenetic sequence across all cultures. Initially, the child begins to develop an awareness of self and the world through sensory motor modalities; the infant's perception of the world is based on brief experiences with caregivers and the physical environment. With increasing interactions and experiences, the infant develops a knowledge base on which a primitive structure of the world is formulated. As more information is added through sensory-motor input, the infant's conception of the world expands and changes. Through the processes of assimilation (adding new objects and experiences to the existing knowledge base) and accommodation (modifying the knowledge base as a result of new experiences), the infant (and later the child and adult) develops a more sophisticated and realistic view of himself and the environment. As neurologic competence grows, the infant appreciates more complex relationships and acquires massive amounts of information, which further promote the refinement and maturation of intelligence. After the sensory-motor stage of cognitive development, the child acquires knowledge in more complex interactions and experiences. However, interpretations of the new information remain concrete and egocentric. The world revolves around the toddler, and the toddler personalizes every experience. By the age of 7, 8, or 9, the school-aged child develops an ability to process information in a more factual manner. Increasingly complex relationships between objects and people are appreciated. Multiple dimensions of a single variable are recognized. In the final stage of cognitive development, formal thought operations, the adolescent thinks in abstract ways. Inductive reasoning and "thinking about thinking" become possible. Contrasting views or facts can be thought about, understood, and reconciled.

The *behavioral model* of child development is less concerned with what goes on in the mind or body than with predictable patterns in the child's overt response to external stimuli at different age levels. This model is based on learning theories and emphasizes that most of the behavior of children is learned. Appropriate behavior may be positively reinforced by pleasant, rewarding experiences. Similarly, inappropriate behavior may be diminished or eliminated not by reinforcing it but by ignoring it. Use of this model helps physicians to counsel parents about how to teach children (e.g., to go to bed without undue delay). The model helps parents to see how their own behavior determines the responses of their children. Some parents do not know that unwanted behaviors are just as learned as wanted ones. The child who finds that screaming is the only stimulus that gets a response from mother will use that behavior when the need for mother overrides the consideration that her attention may be aversive. The behavioral model can help plan strategies aimed at changing such specific behaviors as enuresis, avoidance due to phobias, and others.

No single theoretical framework can adequately explain the multiple facets of human behavior and the complex layers of the developmental process. Although cognitive, physical, social, and emotional developments appear to proceed along divergent pathways, they are interdependent and influence each other. Each theory of development describes a particular aspect that contributes to the whole process of forming a complete individual. An integrated view of development in each phase of the individual's growth to adulthood is necessary to understand how to serve and help that individual in times of health and disease.

3.15 PHASES OF DEVELOPMENT

PRENATAL PHASE. As each individual matures from infancy to adulthood, the learning and experiences that occur during previous years of living and past relationships with parents, siblings, and friends greatly contribute to the quality and types of relationships developed with significant other adults. Often, marital or other intimate relationships reflect early, primary relationships. If the parent-child relationship was satisfying or nurturing, the later marital relationship has a better chance of being satisfactory. If the parent-child relationship was deficient in understanding, love, or acceptance, intimate relationships with others are more likely to be perceived as frustrating and lacking in providing support and love.

Couples may unite in part to satisfy unspoken or unrecognized needs in one another. If the couple can successfully meet the needs of each other, the relationship will probably continue to grow. If the decision to have children is predicated primarily on securing love and acceptance from the mate or from the unborn child, the tremendous amount of emotional and physical sacrifice that is inherent in child-rearing may go unrecognized or poorly acknowledged. To provide a child with the optimal growth-promoting environment, the mother and father should each feel fulfilled within themselves. A relative degree of independence and autonomy in each of the parents is an indication of maturity. They can then unite together to share in a mutual endeavor that requires the skills and talents of each to provide for the survival and growth of another human being.

Ideally, potential parents should have some sense that their future relationship with their child will reflect their own early relationships. If there are unresolved issues or bad feelings with one's own parents or early environment, the parents should take time to explore current feelings about those relationships before starting their own family in order to increase the likelihood that the marriage will be sufficiently stable to absorb a major stress such as childbirth. The mother and father may have different expectations and attitudes about the child, which are determined mainly by their own experiences as well as their own religious and sociocultural opinions. Conflicting views about child-rearing are common, and differences should be discussed to avert serious disagreements. The ability to compromise is fundamental for successful marital and parenting relationships.

Once the parents decide to conceive, it is helpful for them to talk about their hopes, expectations, and desires. These discussions can improve a couple's mutual understanding of each other. During the prenatal phase, it is normal for expectant mothers and fathers to have elaborate fantasies about their unborn child. These fantasies may consist of expectations for huge success and also fears of deformity and failure. However, children who are conceived to satisfy unmet emotional needs are at great risk for disappointing their parents or for being seen as failures by their parents.

Previous miscarriages and abortions, even an early pregnancy loss through planned or spontaneous abortion, should be adequately grieved for prior to the new pregnancy. The parents' sense of loss should be acknowledged, and they should be allowed to feel sad and disappointed. A stillbirth can represent a devastating emotional experience for both parents. If desired, parents should be allowed to see or hold the infant and to arrange for funeral or burial services. Supportive counseling should be made available. A physician should meet with the parents several weeks after the loss to assess how they are dealing with their grief. The timing of a subsequent pregnancy should be the parents' decision, but the pediatrician should explain the positive and negative consequences of deciding to delay further pregnancies.

During pregnancy, while the embryologic process is occurring in utero, the expectant mother and father are undergoing major emotional changes. The mother gradually shifts her focus from the external environment to the happenings within her body. More time is spent on taking care of herself, emotionally and physically. More demands are placed on the father to meet the mother's emotional needs. Much thought is given to the expected newborn. Some fathers experience multiple physical discomforts (couvade syndrome) that parallel the mother's complaints. The parents must plan for specific changes in their finances, their physical environment, and their work schedules.

INFANCY. The preconception and prenatal relationship between the parents provides the foundation for the major emotional and physical adjustments that accompany the birth of a baby. For some the early, perinatal interaction between infants and parents may be critical to the development of the permanent emotional bond that exists among them for the rest of their lives. After the birth, both mother and father carefully examine the newborn and begin the process of reconciling previous fantasies with the reality of the new individual.

While the parents are reorganizing their emotional relationship with each other to include the new child, the infant also exerts a powerful influence in redefining this relationship. Infants are biologically programmed to engage in interactions with adults that facilitate needed emotional attachments, which ensure their survival in a state of dependency. At birth, the infant is capable of brief periods of eye contact and sucking at the breast or bottle. Quiet alert states allow the infant and parents time for mutual visual exploration. Various inborn behaviors (crying, sucking, grasping, smiling, and looking) allow continued opportunities for parent-infant interactions. Increased interactions offer greater opportunities for caregivers to provide the appropriate emotional and physical environment in which the infant can thrive.

During early infancy, the interactions between infant and caregivers promote attachment and bonding and set the tone for further developmental gains (see Sec. 3.31). A parent's prompt, reliable, and consistent response to the crying infant and the infant's reciprocal response foster a trusting and nurturing relationship. The infant learns to rely on others to care for him or her in a predictable and satisfying manner, thus leading to the belief that relationships are positive and facilitating appropriate social development. On the other hand, if parents are chronically unresponsive to the infant's needs, the infant's subsequent experience of distress without relief can be destructive to the development of caregiving relationships and further personality growth. Relationships are experienced as antagonistic and unsatisfactory.

The infant's individual temperamental style is important in his or her development. *Temperament* refers to the individual's particular pattern of physiologic organization, probably genetically determined, through which a uniquely personal way of thinking, feeling, and acting is demonstrated. How the infant usually responds to a feeding routine, sleeping schedule, elimination needs, and stressful or comforting situations form the basis of temperament. Temperament later encompasses adaptability, energy expenditure, mood, and focus of attention. Chess and Thomas identified nine specific characteristics that categorize temperamental styles: activity level, rhythmicity, approach/withdrawal, adaptability, threshold, intensity, mood, distractibility, and attention span and persistence. When these characteristics were analyzed in a large sample of normal babies, three major types of temperamental styles were identified. The *difficult child* is described as biologically irregular, predominantly negative in mood, intense in expressiveness, slow to adapt, and withdrawn in new situations. Children with this temperamental style are often difficult to rear, especially in infancy because of such irregularity in biologic rhythms. These children require great patience and tolerance from parents. In contrast is the *easy child,* who is characterized as biologically predictable, positive in mood, mildly or moderately energetic, quickly adaptive, and eager to approach new stimuli. Most parents appreciate the easy child because he or she offers parents early rewards and satisfaction for their caring efforts. The *slow-to-warm-up* child is the third type of temperamental constellation. These children are slowly adaptive, mildly withdrawn in new situations (shy), mildly negative in mood, susceptible to biologic irregularity, and mildly intense in expressiveness.

In their longitudinal study of temperamental styles, Chess and Thomas found that the difficult child had the greatest risk of developing behavior disorders by 5 yr of age. However, the easy child and slow-to-warm-up child are susceptible to future behavior problems if the temperamental style conflicts with the parental style. "Goodness of fit" reflects the ability of an infant and parent to communicate and interact effectively with one another. When there is a conflict of temperaments, the parents must be more flexible in their caregiving responses because the infant has a limited ability to adapt. If the parents are too rigid in their demands and expectations, the infant may become a disappointment to the parents. Feelings of frustration and failure may overshadow the interactions between the parents and the child, inhibiting and distorting normal development.

In the middle of the 1st yr of life, the infant begins to be mobile by crawling or scooting away from the caregiver. For many parents, this is the first tangible sign that the infant is an independent being with an increasing ability to regulate biologic rhythms and communicate needs more directly. When the infant begins to walk and talk, the emerging ability to separate from the parent and to display individuality is established. The infant must become comfortable with an optimal balance of dependence and independence to promote the emerging sense of self. Many parents feel uneasy as the infant struggles to gain increasing control over the environment. Struggles with regard to eating, sleeping, and toileting are extremely common. Most infants fight to get immediate responses to their demands, and temper tantrums are not unusual responses to their frustrated efforts. Parents need to understand such behavior for what it is—the developmental process of learning to deal with frustration. This process begins at birth, but the toddler of 2–3 yr of age is much more aware of desires and has a greater repertoire of behaviors for achieving goals than the infant. At this stage, parents need to establish consistent, predictable, and reasonable rules and expectations and take into account their needs as well as the child's.

PRESCHOOL YEARS. Winnicott's statement about hide-and-go-seek, "It is a joy to be hidden and a disaster not to be found," contains the essence of preschool psychologic development. The game demonstrates the child's struggle to gain independence and autonomy but emphasizes the continued need to be nurtured.

With greatly improved motor skills, the toddler is capable of actively moving away from parents and *pursuing self-interests.* Most preschoolers insist on greater freedom in choosing play activities, food items, and clothes, as well as individual styles for accomplishing tasks. Toddlers appear to have an internal drive or "instinct" to test their new physical and cognitive skills. They actively seek new or challenging situations in an attempt to extract a satisfactory interaction with novel stimuli. Toddlers learn important information about how to approach new objects or situations and incorporate the feedback, whether positive or negative, for future reference. Parents should encourage this independent exploration, allowing themselves to become background figures who are available for support or limited assistance. Parents thus help modulate the child's level of frustration, contributing to the child's burgeoning ability to delay gratification. As the child continues to pursue individual challenges within the environment, a developing sense of competence and mastery contributes to advancing identity and individuality.

During the preschool years, tremendous strides are made in acquiring self-help skills. *Toilet training* is usually introduced at this time by the parents. The onset should coincide with the child's level of development and interest. Children progress to this stage at variable times; some are reliably trained at 2 yr of age, whereas others achieve bowel and bladder control at 3–4 yr of age. Toilet training proceeds more smoothly and quickly if parents remain attentive to the child's cues. If the child requires tangible rewards (candy, toys, and so on) in addition to verbal praise, they should be provided. If the toddler wishes to return to diapers after an initial trial, the parents should be willing to postpone the process until the child is ready to resume training. Occasional accidents are not uncommon for several weeks or months after the major thrust of toilet training has been completed. These accidents should not be handled in a punitive manner. Because toilet training occurs at a time when the preschooler is psychologically struggling with issues of control and autonomy, parents should avoid authority struggles.

Even before toilet training, toddlers openly express interest in body parts and explore their own bodies as well as the bodies of parents and others as a way of defining themselves and their environment. This *self-exploration* continues throughout the preschool years with greater emphasis on body function during toilet training. It is natural for infants and toddlers to experience sensory excitation when touching genital areas. It is similar to the pleasurable response they feel when touching other parts of their bodies. Because of the sensitivity of the genital area, toddlers enjoy sexual arousal. It is not uncommon for males of 10 mo to 1 yr to have erections. During diaper changes and toilet training, most toddlers inquire about the names of their sexual parts. By 2½–3 yr of age, toddlers have achieved a sense of gender identity and an understanding of maleness and femaleness. Expected behavior from the sex type has already been incorporated into the toddler's choice of clothes, games, toys, and other interests and behaviors.

At 4–5 yr of age, the preschooler becomes especially attracted to the parent of the opposite sex. Girls develop an unusual fondness for fathers; boys become unusually interested in their mothers. The same-gender parent becomes an ambivalent object of affection; often the toddler feels direct competition with that parent for the affection and attention of the other parent. Boys make claims of being as strong and as big (if not stronger or bigger) as father, asserting that they can take care of mother and the house without father. Girls become more cuddly and solicitous of father. While feeling ambivalent about and rivalry with the same-gender parent, the preschooler continues to interact with that parent to reinforce and expand the appropriate sex-stereotyped behavior. The same-gender parent continues to serve as a base for nurturance, support, and discipline.

Parents should not be alarmed at the competitiveness that develops during this phase. Both parents should accept this stage as part of the development of the beginnings of heterosexual relationships. Parents need to maintain their relationship with one another, not allowing the child to disrupt their relationship. Each parent should affirm their love for the other while reassuring the child of their love for him or her. Gradually, the preschooler accepts his position within the family structure, enjoying special relationships with mother and father, while the mother and father maintain their special relationship with each other.

Because of the preschooler's advances in independence and self-reliance, *day-care and nursery school* placement are often considered. Many parents place their children at much earlier ages in out-of-home care for financial and career reasons. For many families, day-care offers the best alternative method of child care. Day-care centers can be nurturing, stimulating, and stable. Although children from highly stressed or chaotic families are at greater risk for the development of insecure attachments and behavioral problems, quality day-care facilities can minimize these negative consequences.

Early studies showed that infants and toddlers attending day-care centers were not adversely affected by the experience, particularly with a child-to-caregiver ratio of 4:1 for infants and 6–8:1 for toddlers. Children placed early were found to be as emotionally secure and attached to their parents as children reared at home. Research suggested that day-care children might have more aggressive behavior than others but were more socially assured and independent. It also suggested that day-care offered a stimulating environment, both emotionally and intellectually, for children from disadvantaged or high-risk families and environments. This early research, however, was not well controlled for differences in family backgrounds and values and was primarily based on high-quality day-care centers. More recent studies suggest that children placed in day-care prior to 1 yr of age are at high risk for insecure attachments to parents. These studies have been controlled for various day-care settings, family backgrounds, and socioeconomic and marital situations. Boys were noted to be more vulnerable to the negative effects of day-care, showing greater insecurity regarding parental attachments and more aggressive behavior during the early school years. However, these newer findings also must be cautiously interpreted because the instrument used to measure attachment (Ainsworth Strange Situation) may not be a valid indicator of attachment for children who have experienced repeated and consistent separations from their mothers and fathers. Furthermore, family background variables have not been adequately controlled.

Individual differences in children and families, as well as differences in child-care settings, need to be considered in making recommendations to parents about child care, especially for infants. The pediatrician should explore the parents' expectations and life style and should provide guidelines for optimal child care. If possible, infants should remain within the home. If the mother must return to work prior to the first birthday, the infant should be in the type of care that offers at least a 4:1 child-to-caregiver ratio. Toddlers should be placed in environments that stress nurturance as well as cognitive stimulation. The pediatrician should emphasize that parents need to investigate child-care settings and options thoroughly. Parents need to visit different centers, personally interview the child-care workers, and observe the caregiving staff interacting with children. The more questions they ask, the more information they will have with which to make the right choice for their particular situation. Once placed in day-care, parents should make unannounced visits to determine how the child is adjusting to the situation.

During the toddler years, motor, social, cognitive, and emotional growth progresses. The decision to have another child is sometimes made when the preceding child is 2–3 yr old because of the toddler's greater independence and autonomy. The timing of siblings is not critical; parents should consider their own emotional needs as well as the needs of the family.

The impact of *sibling relationships* in childhood development is extremely variable. Sibling relationships provide the potential for intimacy and competitiveness and the opportunity for children to learn a balance between the two as well as how to tolerate the inherent ambivalence when two such strong emotions coexist. Siblings have strong influences on one another. Older siblings who are aggressive contribute to the development of aggressive behavior in younger siblings. Conversely, friendly, cooperative, and affectionate older siblings promote similar behavior in younger brothers and sisters. The age gap and gender differences between siblings are not consistently related to the development of conflicts. Different parental behavior (especially the mother's) toward siblings does relate to sibling conflict, however. The emotional climate of the family is another important determinant of the development of conflict. Increased stress within the family leads to increased sibling conflict. Maternal sensitivity to the needs of each sibling and the mother's ability to share each sibling's needs with the other is associated with greater friendliness and cooperation between siblings.

Families with chronically ill or handicapped children usually face greater stress. Often marital relationships and the financial status of families are greatly influenced by the presence of a handicapped child. Some studies show that healthy children who have handicapped or ill siblings develop more considerate and kind sibling relationships than would otherwise be the case. Conflicts between healthy and disabled siblings are reportedly more troublesome or difficult for the healthy one. How the healthy child perceives the disabled sibling is partially dependent both on how the disabled sibling treats the healthy one and on the healthy child's relationship with the mother.

As the preschooler becomes more aware of and more comfortable with independence and autonomy, increasing efforts to control the parents are attempted. Toddlers actively test *external limits and controls.* Although this is a healthy process, children need to learn to regulate their demands and wishes to conform to the rules, regulations, and expectations of the family and society. Parents provide the external structure that allows children to mature and develop in a safe, secure environment. *Discipline* is the means by which parents educate and control their children's behavior as part of the training and socializing process. Discipline consists of a complex set of attitudes, behaviors, instructions, and consequences that foster internalization of appropriate ideals, values, and behaviors.

It is important for parents to agree on their values and expectations as well as their styles of discipline. Consistency and predictability are the keys to effective discipline. If parents contradict one another or displace a marital conflict into the arena of discipline, ambiguity and inconsistency result. Of course, this displacement also undermines the disciplining efforts of each of the parents.

The emotional climate in which the child is reared and disciplined is another important factor in the effectiveness of discipline. Children respond best if discipline occurs in the context of a warm, affectionate, accepting relationship. Parents can effectively set limits while being nurturing and sensitive to the needs of the child. Behavioral consequences should be paired with praise and approval for acceptable behavior. Positive reinforcements are extremely effective and powerful in obtaining desired results. Demonstrated approval of desired behavior works to reinforce that behavior; with active efforts to show approval, negative reinforcement may be increasingly unnecessary. Parents act as role models for acceptable and expected behavior. How parents handle their own anger, affection, and anxiety and how they process and act in difficult situations serve to demonstrate the type of behavior they want. Children are quick to imitate and identify with the parents' behavior.

The type of negative consequences that parents employ as discipline is dependent on their family values, social norms, and religious and cultural beliefs, e.g., corporal punishment, verbal reprimands, ignoring certain behaviors, and temporary withdrawal of approval or attention. Whatever the chosen method, to be effective the consequences should occur shortly after the disordered behavior and should be appropriate to the transgression. The shorter the delay between the transgression and the consequence, the greater the chance of preventing its repetition. Consequences also should be of sufficient intensity to create mild to moderate amounts of anxiety in the child. However, the anxiety should not be overwhelming or so extreme that the child is frightened or infuriated.

Physical punishment is a popular method of discipline. However, it is often presented inconsistently, indiscriminately, too frequently, and while the parent is angry. For some children, physical punishment inadvertently promotes aggression, particularly if the parents use it in an aggressive way. Withdrawal of approval, verbal reprimands, physical withdrawal (time-out), and loss of privileges are more effective methods of enforcing rules and regulations while simultaneously helping the child to internalize self-control. When parents utilize nonphysical consequences and then help the child to process the offending incident, greater effectiveness is achieved. For toddlers, short withdrawals of approval, verbal reprimands, and brief time-out periods are effective. Clear and simple reasons for the consequences should be given, and the punishment should not last more than 5–15 min. Lingering feelings of anger and resentment should be resolved so that the parent and child can engage in positive and mutually satisfying interactions after the consequence.

SCHOOL-AGED CHILDREN. The period of development between 6 and 12 yr of age has been traditionally called latency, a time in which *cognitive growth* is emphasized. Children begin to attend daily school where organized and structured learning occurs. New and more diverse expectations are placed on the child to produce in a cognitive, intellectual manner. Schoolwork and school performance offer the opportunity to expand the quest for mastery and competence. Learning new information can be exciting and stimulating for most children. In school, children can develop skills and work habits that promote a sense of competence and industry.

For some, learning during latency can become frustrating and may lead to a sense of failure. If learning problems or intellectual delays are detected early, undue suffering can be averted. Behavioral or emotional problems that interfere with the educational process should be quickly identified so that appropriate interventions can be implemented. With the enactment of Public Law 94–142, each child is guaranteed the right to an educational setting and level of instruction that appropriately address individual learning needs. The law mandates that school systems provide appropriate teaching environments and the necessary adjunctive therapy to facilitate each child's formal education.

School-aged children are engaged in active learning in other arenas besides formal education. The process of *socialization* is greatly accelerated during latency. Because school becomes an environment away from home for a large portion of the day, latency-aged children must learn to function outside the security and safety of the home. School-aged children interact with a wide variety of children and adults. New and more complex rules, regulations, and expectations for behavior are presented and enforced. They become ardent game players. This serves to enhance the process of socialization. Strict game rules are diligently learned, and adherence to the rules is stressed among peers. Transgressions are quickly noted and disavowed by peer disapproval or punishment (exclusion from the game or a peer group). Following the rules of the game provides a forum for learning and following the rules in society. School-aged children develop a code of ethics and a sense of honesty among peers. Lying and cheating are discouraged through negative feedback by peers.

As part of the continued socialization process, children consolidate the development of *conscience formation.* In early childhood, the conscience consists of a primitive internalization of the parents' prohibitions and the modeling of parental behaviors, attitudes, and values. Initially, toddlers vocalize their thinking when facing a "moral" decision; one hears the child say "no" when going close to the stove. Later, children mentally talk to themselves without verbalizing prohibitions. Finally, solutions to the problem of right versus wrong are decided by a series of thoughts. When children enter school, they experience a wider range of prohibited or accepted behaviors. Peers and teachers add additional values to those previously learned from parents and family members.

Several operational models of conscience formation have been developed. The psychoanalytic model contends that the conscience is a function of the superego, which develops from the child's desire to have basic biologic and emotional needs met as well as the environment's response to those needs. The superego incorporates both the ideals and the prohibitions of the parents and society. It governs the child's behavior by leading to positive feelings about the self when "ideal" behavior is achieved and through feelings of guilt when rules are disregarded. Guilt acts as a personal and internal punishment for disregarding the superego's (parents' and society's) prohibitions.

Another popular model of conscience formation has been proposed by Kohlberg. In this conceptualization, an epigenetic development of the conscience occurs in six stages, each successive stage building on the preceding one. The final stages of conscience formation are not attained by everyone. Initially, the primitive conscience is determined by consequences of behavior, both positive and negative. Interactions with others allow the child to learn what behaviors elicit certain responses. Later, the child maintains behavior in accordance with the rules and regulations of others to retain the support and affection of others. The next stage emphasizes the intention of actions rather than the actual outcome. Older children feel guilty when they deliberately break one cup but not so guilty when they accidentally break several cups. After this stage, the child appreciates that "right" behavior is expected. It is the child's obligation or duty to uphold the rules and regulations of society. In the final stages of conscience development, individuals perceive themselves as part of a society in which individual rights and responsibilities must be balanced with the needs and rights of the group. One's sense of justice, morality, and ethics broadens significantly.

Although education and formal learning become the primary objectives of the latency-aged child, *the school environment* offers the child an opportunity to further develop independence and separation from the family. In school, children begin to sense how others perceive them and how they fit into a broader community of people. In this new setting, the child is judged by individual capacities and attributes. Teachers and peers differ in their values. Latency-aged children must learn that others evaluate them differently from family members; unconditional acceptance is not guaranteed. Approval is earned through performance. The sense of self must expand to include a concept of how one relates to others and how one is valued by others.

Latency-aged children spend an increasing amount of time

in *peer interactions*. Not only do these interactions add another dimension to their socialization, they also serve to reinforce or redefine sex-stereotyped behavior. Although gender identity has been established by 2½–3 yr of age, the behaviors that typify the sexes are learned in an ongoing process from toddlerhood through adolescence and adulthood. School-aged children quickly expand their repertoire of feminine or masculine behaviors as new interactions and relationships occur with different adults and peers. Occasionally, peer pressure or school environments restrict the amount of flexibility allowed in the development of gender role behaviors. Cultural, religious, and community values enhance or limit the range of sex role standards.

Prepubertal children have an active interest in sex. Masturbation has been shown to occur in 10% of 7-yr-old boys and 80% of 13-yr-old boys. Kissing the opposite sex occurs quite frequently; over 60% of 10 yr olds and 85% of 12 yr olds have reportedly kissed boyfriends or girlfriends. Most prepubertal children openly express interest in the opposite sex. Group dating commonly begins at 11–13 yr of age. Both boys and girls are acutely aware of their physical differences. Boys compare themselves to other boys, girls compare themselves to other girls, and the sexes compare themselves to one another. A major component of the self-esteem of 10- to 13-yr-old children is determined by their perceptions of their own attractiveness. Great emphasis is placed on physical appearance. It is during latency, however, that children strive to repress and suppress regressive, sexual urges to concentrate on learning and social mastery.

ADOLESCENCE (See also Chapter 10). Between the final stages of childhood and the beginning of adulthood is the period commonly referred to as adolescence. It spans 8–10 yr. Biologic, psychologic, and sociologic maturation, in preparation for independent living, occur. Each of these maturational courses proceeds along different developmental lines, yet each is interdependent on the others. By late adolescence and early adulthood, an integrated series of physical, psychologic, and social developmental steps consolidates identity formation and prepares each individual for intimate relationships.

Sexual maturation is paramount in adolescent development. These changes are described in Sec. 3.9 and Chapter 10. Other physical changes also occur while the marked sexual maturational process unfolds.

The actual onset of adolescence varies among individuals of the same sex as well as between the sexes. Girls commonly enter adolescence 2 yr earlier than boys, and their sexual and physical maturation is usually completed 1½ to 2 yr before that of boys. Studies addressing the effects of early versus late maturation show that adverse sequelae accompany both extremes of timing. Girls who perceive themselves to be average in their development express a more positive self-image. Late developers have a more positive self-image than early developers. Girls are more sensitive to social pressures than boys and seem to be more adversely affected if the pace of their physical development is deviant. In contrast, early-maturing boys seem to fare better than average- or late-maturing boys. Those maturing early are perceived as more popular, athletically skilled, attractive, and capable of leadership. In late adolescence, early-maturing boys display more self-confidence and less dependence. Later maturers show more personal and social problems throughout their adolescent development. In late adolescence, late-maturing boys appear to have negative self-concepts, increased dependency, more feelings of rebelliousness toward parents, and strong feelings of rejection by peers.

Important social, emotional, and psychologic changes occur during adolescence. Most 12 and 13 yr olds enter junior high school, where different academic and social structures exist. Junior high school students are given greater freedom and flexibility. They move from one class to another and interact with a greater variety and number of teachers and students. More emphasis is placed on self-motivation and self-discipline. A greater amount of independent study is expected. These changes become more pronounced in high school, where academic achievement and self-direction are emphasized even more. For many, a decision to pursue formal education beyond the required high school years becomes critical. How an adolescent adjusts to the increased academic demands often determines his or her opportunities and choices for employment.

Controversy exists about whether adolescence is synonymous with conflict and turmoil. Although a major developmental task is the establishment of individual autonomy and independence, most adolescents remain financially and physically dependent on their parents. Traditional psychoanalytic theory has held that this is a period of turmoil marked by a desire for independence, a quest for sexual identity and maturity, and a casting off of parental images and values to solidify one's own personality structure. Turmoil is regarded as an inevitable, necessary part of growth. This view held, furthermore, that if turmoil does not occur, individuals will pay the cost later in inhibition, constriction of personality, or dependency. More recent, well-controlled studies of large groups of boys and girls suggest that less conflict is present. Rutter and associates found in a review of normative studies that most adolescents are not actually critical of their parents, and very few reject them. Parents and adolescents have disagreements, and most adolescents prefer their parents to be less restrictive, but the great majority tend to admire their parents, get along quite well with them, and are generally satisfied and happy at home. Contrary to popular belief, they are more worried about parental disapproval than about the disapproval of friends. Normal adolescents experience the anxiety and depression inherent in growing up, but they do not show signs of major turmoil, confusion, or withdrawal.

Although most adolescents maintain ties and loyalties to their families, *peer relationships* gain increasing importance. More time is spent in peer-related activities than in family activities. Conformity to peer values (e.g., dress style, music) is more important in early adolescence than in later adolescence. Girls seem to invest more time and energy in establishing friendships and usually tolerate more conflicts within those relationships than boys. Girls also seem to have more intimate friendships with a greater sharing of personal thoughts and feelings than boys. For both, characteristics associated with popularity among peers are cheerfulness, friendliness, enjoying jokes, initiating games, and physical attractiveness. Those who tend to be restless, overtalkative, or physically unattractive are more likely to be unpopular.

Heterosexual interests and activities greatly increase throughout this time. Although many prepubescent boys and girls display heterosexual interest and activity, the degree and amount of sexual activity among adolescents is increased. In recent years sexual experience among adolescents has greatly increased. In 1971, 30% of unmarried female teenagers between 15 to 19 yr residing in metropolitan areas had experienced sexual intercourse; this increased to 43% by 1976 and to 50% by 1979. In 1976, the use of birth control measures, especially the pill, was increasing, although more than a third were "unprotected" at the time of their last intercourse. In 1979, contraceptive use continued to increase, but there was also an increase in the use of ineffective measures such as withdrawal, and 13% of unmarried teenage girls had become pregnant. Sorenson found that 59% of American adolescent boys and 45% of adolescent girls had had sexual intercourse. They saw sexual activity in adolescents as occurring in the context of a relationship, as a means of communication, as a part of self-realization, and as an aspect of love. About half of the boys and 62% of the girls (16–19 yr olds) had used contraception during their most recent intercourse. Many adolescents who did not use birth control relied on the possibility of abortion or rearing the baby without getting married.

Cognitively, the *stage of formal thought operations* is achieved during adolescence. Abstract reasoning, the use of logic, and increased sophistication in moral reasoning occur. Adolescents commonly "think about thinking" and play with ideas. Many become preoccupied with ideals or liberal ways of thinking. They frequently discuss and argue with peers and parents about religion, philosophy, politics, sociology, and ethics.

By the end of adolescence, it is expected that the individual will have succeeded in establishing *a stable identity or self-concept*. To this end, the adolescent must integrate all of the physical, cognitive, emotional, and social changes into some sort of meaningful whole. As a teenager progresses through this time frame, an increased awareness of the sense of self as an independent and effective being is realized. Many engage in active exploration of new ideas and behaviors as a method of expanding their sense of self. This exploration and experimentation can result in *risk-taking behavior*, as the adolescent tests the limits of what can and cannot be done and what is and is not desirable as an expression of the self. Most do not endanger themselves. They become more cautious as they mature. By late adolescence, most have formed a coherent sense of identity. Plans and goals for the future are established. Late adolescence can be prolonged for those who decide to further their education and delay their entrance into the work force.

In guiding the adolescent, the physician must take into account the developmental tasks that are inherent during this phase and understand the changing relationships between adolescents and parents and between adolescents and peers. Young adolescents vacillate between attempts at extreme independence and sudden reversions to overt or camouflaged dependence. They actively test new ideas and new relationships and try to negotiate the old relationships with parents to win somewhat new and different terms. One of the most important roles of a physician is to point out to teenagers, and particularly to parents, that they are entering a new phase of their relationship. Both must get used to the idea that they are in a process of psychologically separating from each other. Parental attitudes that are most threatening to the adolescent may be related to either premature total emancipation on the one hand or inappropriately severe restrictions on the other. Parental indifference may also be threatening. Physicians can help parents and teenagers to avoid power struggles in which the loss of trust by the parent or child is a frequent outcome.

Anxiety and depression are to be expected at times, on the part of either the child or the parent, during adolescence. Teens in the United States are under great pressure to succeed both academically and vocationally. They may expect too much of themselves, become discouraged, and give up or strive inordinately hard, paying a high price emotionally, socially, and sometimes medically. *Suicide attempts* reach a peak incidence between 15 and 25 yr of age; the suicide rate in this age group increased by 140% from 1960 to 1981 (see Sec. 3.37). Discussions among teenage peers about coping with stress can be very supportive. Humor is a major coping strategy, the targets of which may be parents, adult-dominated institutions, and the adolescents themselves.

Occasionally, other serious problems occur during adolescence. Eating disorders are occurring at an increasing rate among girls. The physician should be familiar with the signs and symptoms of anorexia nervosa and bulimia (see Sec. 10.14). Physicians must be adequately informed and aware of drug and alcohol use and abuse among teenagers (see Sec. 10.4). Although depression and anxiety are common, physicians should be able to determine whether these states are of sufficient duration and intensity to impair the adolescent's usual level of functioning (see Sec. 3.33). Extreme conflicts between teenagers and parents should alert the physician to the possibility of major difficulties in negotiating this phase of development. Although uncommon in the adolescent population, the development of major thought disorders, manic-depressive illness, and other serious psychiatric disturbances can occur (see Sec. 3.43). The physician who treats adolescents should be aware of some of the indications for these disorders and when appropriate should quickly refer the adolescent and family for appropriate evaluation and treatment.

SOCIAL ISSUES

3.16 ADOPTION

Most adopted children and their families handle this issue with considerable common sense and sensitivity, but some problems of adoption require comment.

Adoptions accomplished through approved agencies are preferred to independent adoptions, since these agencies tend to assess the psychosocial setting of the prospective adoptive family more adequately and perhaps provide better safeguards for the physical condition of the infant. Adoptive placement should be made as soon after birth as possible in order to foster attachment and bonding between infant and adoptive mother (see Sec. 3.3). Adoptions of older children, or across religious and ethnic lines, or by single parents are, in appropriate instances, reasonable alternatives to having adoptable children languish in institutions or temporary foster homes, but adoptions of older children present some increased risks. For example, a family seeking to adopt a 4- to 5-yr-old child with a history of severe emotional deprivation and multiple foster home placements may find that the child has been severely traumatized and will later display major psychologic disturbances, even in the best of adoptive homes.

Adopted children should be told of their adoption as soon as they have achieved reasonably good verbal facility and comprehension, by the age of 3 or at the latest 4 yr. The explanation can be repeated when circumstances are appropriate, such as during a family discussion about the birth of a neighbor's baby, but should not become ritual. Children's books on adoption can be read to young children; later they can read them themselves.

Controversy continues about whether adopted children are at increased risk for development of emotional problems. If they are, it is likely to reflect problems of parental management. Since the adopted child generally arrives in the context of marital infertility, he or she may be treated with considerable overindulgence as a "special child." Adoption need not be perceived by the child as a threat to self-esteem, but in the case of individual and family problems, the child's adoptive status may reinforce otherwise existing doubts about his or her competence and worth. Not infrequently a natural child is born following an adoption to previously "infertile" parents. For the adopted child the event may initiate a competitive struggle requiring both understanding and firmness on the part of the parents.

Occasionally, foster parents wish to adopt a child who has been in their care for a number of years but has not been legally relinquished by the natural parents. Historically, the courts have upheld the claim of biologic parents for the child, even in those instances in which the natural parents abandoned the child and the foster parents had been essentially the child's only longstanding, nurturant, and consistent (psychologic) parents. Such legal decisions reinforced the notion that children were treated as property rather than as people having their own needs and rights. Recent decisions to the contrary, however, show the courts' growing appreciation of the child's need for continuity of care.

In some states, adopted persons who have attained their majority are entitled to have access to their adoption records and to information about their biologic parents. On the whole, this is a commendable development; this right-to-know must be weighed, however, against the rights of biologic parents to privacy if they desire it.

3.17 FOSTER CARE

Placement in foster care is typically provided by local welfare authorities for abandoned, severely neglected, or abused children. For many children, foster care offers a lifesaving environment that gives them the opportunity to be physically replenished, to grow, and to develop innate potential. For others, however, foster care represents yet another episode in a lifelong history of deprivation. The number of infants born to substance-abusing pregnant women has increased significantly, especially to women addicted to cocaine or crack. The toxic effects of these latter drugs on the developing fetal nervous system often make the care of these infants particularly difficult. Their behavior may be erratic, agitated, and unresponsive or inconsolable, and their subsequent development may be delayed or abnormal (see Sec. 9.54).

Unfortunately, we have yet to develop in the United States a comprehensive and well-supervised system of foster care that provides integrated services for children already at risk. Undermanned and underbudgeted departments of public welfare are often unable adequately to prepare, supervise, and support foster parents who may have to deal with difficult, traumatized children. Children are transferred from one foster home to another because foster parents move, the child doesn't "adjust," or unsupervised foster parents are deemed to be inadequate. Some children move in and out of placement according to the whims of natural parents who can neither care for them nor let them go permanently. For some children multiple foster care placements have disastrous effects on their abilities to learn, trust, and relate to others. Such children, already made vulnerable by the circumstances that led to their placement, are placed at further risk by the vagaries of foster care. Serious retardation in reading, antisocial behavior, apathetic states, and defects in socialization have all been compellingly described by Eisenberg as the sequelae of such experiences. This situation will not change until the needs of children receive high priority in social planning and legislation. Only recently have trends in state and federal legislation been aimed at "permanency planning," with the use of adoptive placement or permanent foster care, and with earlier relinquishment or termination of the rights of parents who are unwilling or unable to care for their own children.

3.18 EFFECTS OF A MOBILE SOCIETY

A significant proportion of the population of the United States changes residence each year. The effects of this movement on children and families are frequently overlooked. For children the move is essentially involuntary; they move because a parent has obtained employment elsewhere, because the birth of a sibling has made a larger home desirable, or for other reasons. When such changes in family structure as divorce or death precipitate moves, children face the stresses created by both the precipitating events and moving itself. When parents are sad because of the circumstances surrounding the move, this unhappiness will be transmitted to their children. Children who move lose their old friends, the comfort of a familiar bedroom and house, and their ties to school and community. Not only must they sever old relationships, they are also faced with developing new ones in new neighborhoods and new schools. Because movement upward in social standing often accompanies a geographic move, children may enter neighborhoods with new and different customs and values. And since academic standards and curricula vary from community to community, children who have performed well in one school may find themselves struggling in a new one. Frequent moves during the school years are likely to have adverse consequences on social and academic performance.

Parents should prepare children well in advance of any move and allow them to express any unhappy feelings or misgivings. Parents should acknowledge their own mixed feelings and agree that they will miss their old home while looking forward to a new one. Visits to the new home in advance are often useful preludes to the actual move. Transient periods of regressive behavior may be noted in preschool children after moving, and these should be understood and accepted. Parents should assist the entry of their children into the new community, and exchanges of letters with old friends and visits, whenever possible, should be encouraged.

3.19 SEPARATION AND DEATH

Relatively brief separations of children from their parents, such as vacations, usually produce minor transient effects. But more enduring and frequent separations may cause significant sequelae. The potential impact of each event must be considered in the light of the age and stage of development of the child and the particular relationship with the absent person as well as the nature of the separation. For example, it is more frightening for children to be separated from a parent in a hospital than within the familiar surroundings of home. In a marital separation the child is faced with a relative loss of one parent who may be vilified by the other.

In young children the initial reaction to separation may involve crying, either of a tantrum-like, protesting type or of a quieter, sadder type. After a few hours or a day or so of separation, the child may appear more subdued, withdrawn, and quiet or irritable, fussy, moody, and resistant to authority. Disturbance of appetite may occur, and there may be special difficulties at bedtime, such as reluctance in going to bed and problems in getting to sleep, with a resurgence of old fears, and in younger children perhaps such regressive behavior as bedwetting. Children may repeatedly ask where the absent parent is and when he or she will return home; some children may not refer to parental absence at all. The child may go to the window or door or out into the neighborhood looking for the absent parent; a few may even leave home or their places of temporary placement to try to find where their parents are. This last rather unusual response needs to be considered when a child cannot be found for a while shortly after the separation or departure of a parent.

The child's response to reunion may surprise or alarm the parent who is not prepared. The parent who joyfully returns to the family may be met by wary or cautious children, who, after a brief interchange of affection, may move away from the parent and seem indifferent to his or her return. The interpretation of this response will depend on the child and his or her style; it may indicate anger at being left and wariness that the event will happen again, or, because children tend to personalize, the child may have felt that he or she caused the parent's departure. For instance, if the mother who frequently says, "Stop it, or you'll give me a headache," is hospitalized, the child may unrealistically feel at fault and guilty. As a result of these feelings, children may seem to be more closely attached to the other parent than to the absent one, or even to the grandparent or babysitter who cared for them during their parent's absence. Immediately after the reunion or after a few days, some children, particularly younger ones, may become more clinging and dependent than they were prior to separation, while continuing any regressive behavior that had occurred during separation. Such behavior may engage the returned parent more closely and help to re-establish the bond that the child felt was broken. Usually such reactions are transient; within a week or two the child will have recovered his or her usual behavior and equilibrium. Recurrent separations may tend to make the child more wary and guarded about re-establishing the relationship with the repeatedly absent parent, and these traits may affect other personal relationships. Parents should not try to ameliorate a child's behavior by threatening to leave.

Experiences of loss such as divorce or placement in foster care can give rise to the same kinds of reactions listed earlier, but more intense and possibly more lasting. School-aged children may respond with evident depression, seem indifferent, or be markedly angry. Other children appear to deny or avoid the issue, behaviorally or verbally. Most children may cling to the hope or fantasy that the actual placement or separation is not real. Guilt may be generated by the child's feeling that this loss, separation, or placement represents rejection and perhaps punishment for misbehavior. The child may protect the parents at his or her own expense, believing and asserting that one's own badness caused the parent to depart or to place him or her with relatives or strangers rather than that the parent has been bad or irresponsible. Besides having their own feelings of guilt, children cannot blame their parents because they sense it may be fairly risky. The parent who discovers that the child harbors resentment might punish further for these thoughts or feelings. Children who feel that their misbehavior caused their parents to separate or become divorced have the fantasy that their own trivial or recurrent behavioral patterns have caused their parents to become angry with each other. Some children develop behavioral or psychosomatic symptoms and unwittingly adopt a "sick" role as a strategy for reuniting the parents.

In response to separation and divorce of parents, older children and adolescents commonly show more intense anger. Almost all children cling to the magical belief that their parents will reunite. Wallerstein and Kelly found that 5 yr after the break-up about one third of the children studied were "consciously and intensely unhappy and dissatisfied with their life in the post-divorce family." Another third showed clear evidence of a quite satisfactory adjustment, and the remaining third demonstrated "a mixed picture with good achievement in some areas and faltering achievement in others." After 10 yr 45% were doing well, but 41% were poorly adjusted with academic, social, and emotional problems. As they entered adulthood many were reluctant to form intimate relationships, fearful of repeating their parents' experience. Good adjustment in children after a divorce is related to ongoing involvement with two psychologically healthy parents who minimize conflict and to the support system offered by siblings and other relatives. Joint custody arrangements may reduce ongoing parental conflict, but a study by Steinman revealed that one third of children in joint custody "felt overburdened by the demands and requirements of maintaining a strong presence in 2 homes."

As to the ultimate separation—death of a parent—most preadolescent children do not seem to go through a typical mourning process as psychoanalytically defined. The child's mourning may be masked by behavior not typically seen in adults. Among school-aged to adolescent children who had lost a parent through death, Wolfenstein found that immediately after the loss sad feelings were not markedly evident, nor was there much crying. Children continued in daily activities, the major mechanism in dealing with catastrophe being denial, both overt and unconscious, and maintained by the magical wish and hope for reunion and reappearance. Some children seemed to maintain remarkably good moods; some were more active than usual. Wolfenstein saw these good moods as an effective accompaniment of denial: "If one does not feel bad, then nothing bad has happened." Some children show hostile and angry feelings toward the surviving parent and tend to identify with and idealize the lost parent, sometimes with reunion fantasies accompanying denial. Guilt may be present, reflecting the child's egocentric tendency. Alternatively, some children show considerable sorrow at the time of the parent's death or after a delay when the defense of denial is no longer effective.

Children under the age of 5 yr view death as reversible, possibly with belief in the dead coming back to life and in ghosts. In the next stage, up to 8–9 yr, death is personified, for example as the "grim reaper" who punishes and avenges. Only after this age does the child realistically understand death as a universal and final biologic process.

The physician can help children and surviving caretakers through a period of separation or adjustment to death of parent or sibling, first by helping them recognize that the adults themselves are going through a period of grief and mourning. It is not unhealthy for children to see their surviving or remaining parent mourn the loss of a mate or grieve for a divorced or separated spouse. In the case of a dead parent the child needs the support and reassurance of having the remaining parent or other important caretakers available. Close physical contact and emotional exchange, with verbal explanations and reassurance for those children who can understand, are important aspects of support. Children should not be expected or forced to discuss all their feelings or to put into words their reactions to a parent's death. They should not be expected to interrupt usual social or recreational activities for weeks or months after death of a parent, either out of respect for that parent or in recognition of the remaining parent's sorrow or grief. Continuance of usual activities should not be interpreted by adults or older children as callousness or indifference but rather as the child's way of dealing at his or her stage of development with what is as much a catastrophe for him or her as it is for the adult. Further, the child should not be expected to serve as a primary support to the remaining parent or others in their grief.

In most cases it seems helpful for the child to participate appropriately in the rituals that generally surround the death and burial of a parent. A young child can attend a funeral, viewing, or wake so long as there is no morbid preoccupation or demand that the child remain a long time or be involved in prolonged religious ceremonies. To keep the young child away from some participation in the burial rituals, whatever they are, will be a misguided effort to protect and ultimately will be more confusing and isolating than helpful.

3.20 IMPACT OF TELEVISION

It is estimated that American children watch television for an average of 30–40 hr/wk. This is more time than they spend in school, and for many it is their major scheduled activity. Television places children in passive roles and offers them entertainment generally requiring little engagement or imagination. It entices them away from important activities such as reading, hobbies, physical exercise, and relationships with peers and with other family members.

Educational programs aimed at preschool children through television may enhance cognitive development in reading readiness and acquisition of vocabulary. At best, however, such programs can only supplement rather than substitute for the activities of parents in conveying knowledge, skills, and information, and in motivating learning (see Sec. 3.15). Television may inform older children of current events, politics, history, and science; it more commonly, however, displays scenes of violence that serve as models for aggressive behavior. Exposure to violence in films increases interpersonal aggressiveness among children. Most children may be able to separate themselves from the steady diet of violence they witness on television, but children readily imitate all types of models, and the effects of television violence on children may be considerably more pervasive than we now know. It is certain that some children who are already emotionally disturbed may act out aggressively as the direct result of crime or horror programs and that the action may follow the models presented.

All parents should know what their children are watching on television, should decide whether certain programs are appropriate, and should feel in no way reluctant to meet their own standards in imposing restrictions on the time and content of television viewing.

3.21 ASSESSMENT AND INTERVIEWING

THE CLINICAL INTERVIEW (HISTORY)

The clinical interview is the most common procedure in medicine, but the nature of the process is often poorly defined. The interview is not simply history-taking; still less is it a cross-examination of the patient that attempts to fulfill the requirements of a review of systems. It is basically a working alliance between the patient and the physician, aimed at the orderly exchange of any and all clinically relevant information between them (see also Sec. 6.1). The patient is seeking reassurance or help, and the physician possesses knowledge, skills, and the social sanction to be helpful. *The most useful perspective in which to view the clinical interview is as a major means of engaging the patient in the active management of his or her own care.*

One well-practiced aspect of the clinical interview in most pediatric and general medical settings is the simple collection of those historical medical data that disclose and review the signs and symptoms of a presenting illness, the nature and course of past medical illnesses, the family history, and a review of systems. Other aspects of the patient's life, such as the psychosocial aspects, often get less or scant attention in interviewing. Physicians need to find ways to use clinical interviews to assess the emotional states of their patients, their usual reactions to stress, their levels of self-concept, their systems of values, the natures of their personal relationships, something of their personalities, the quality of their coping abilities, and clues that might point to psychosocial distress or disturbance.

To become an effective interviewer requires motivation, skill, and continuous attentive practice. The skills required develop throughout the course of one's professional life. They are frequently overlooked in medical school, poorly taught, seen as related only to psychiatric patients, or taken for granted once medical school is completed. The development of effective interviewing skills is facilitated when the student has the opportunity to practice with simulated patients, to make and watch recordings of his or her work with simulators or with actual patients, and to have these activities supervised by competent teachers or consultants.

TIME. An interview that attempts comprehensively to explore both psychosocial and biomedical aspects of the condition of a stranger who has just become a new patient needs at least 30–40 min for significant exchange of the most basic relevant information. Physician and patient must have time to become comfortable with each other and to establish the rapport that facilitates the exploration of psychologic and social information. When patient and physician have had an adequate earlier initial interview, and the physician therefore knows some of the major aspects of the patient's psychosocial status, it is possible to focus on particular issues in periods as brief as 10 min, but an initial interview of 10 min is ineffective and it may communicate to the family a lack of respect for the sensitivity and importance of material given such casual attention.

SETTING. Privacy is essential, but unfortunately it is often difficult to maintain in children's hospitals or in busy outpatient clinics. The need for privacy is most likely to be overlooked with children, who are frequently managed with less respect and sensitivity than are given adults. It is difficult to carry on an interview in a relatively unsheltered cubicle in an outpatient department or at bedside, even with curtains drawn to shield the child or family from visual intrusion or distractions. If possible, it is often more productive to seat the hospitalized child in a chair next to the bed rather than to converse with the child while he or she lies in bed. Adverse physical conditions negatively affect the quality and the effectiveness of the clinical interview. Though it may be difficult, it is worth considerable effort to find a private place; in hospitals this may be a treatment room, an empty conference room, or even an unoccupied office or patient's room. Privacy is more easily arranged in the office of the practicing physician, where closed doors and reasonable comfort are ordinarily routine.

GOALS. The most common deficiency within an interview is the failure of the clinician to define clearly the goals of that particular encounter. No single interview can accomplish everything that needs to be done to complete a clinical assessment. *The clinician must set, define, and state priorities.* These will depend on the nature of the patient's condition, whether the interview is an initial visit or a follow-up one, and whether the physician has to elicit sensitive material or to transmit unpleasant or unhappy diagnostic or prognostic information to patient or family. Physicians must become sufficiently familiar with their own styles and learn enough from past experiences to be able to judge accurately what can be accomplished in each interview. For example, if the work of the first interview is to establish a working alliance with a child and family and to identify the primary problems or concerns, then it may be a mistake to attempt a total developmental, family, or school survey on such an occasion.

COMMUNICATION. The major purpose and process of the clinical interview is the exchange of information. When the patients are children, this exchange occurs between parents and physician, between child and parents, and between parents, as well as between child and physician. In any social interaction communication has two major features: one is the *content* or *message;* the other is the *process,* or the manner in which content is exchanged within the relationship. See also Sec. 2.9.

The notion of *content* refers to the literal meaning of the words exchanged between communicating parties; content is the message or the *what* of communication. The notion of *process* refers to the relational or nonverbal aspects of communication. The tone of voice, the rate of speech, the inflection of words and phrases, facial expressions, head movements, hand gestures, and body postures and movement all communicate meaning, often more accurately than the words exchanged. The words usually capture the major conscious attention, but the process may frequently determine the success of the venture. The nonverbal features of communication are continually monitored by each sender and receiver, often preconsciously or subconsciously. The nonverbal expression conveys the cognitive, emotional, social, or global state of the sender with respect to what he or she is saying and indicates to the receiver *how the content is to be interpreted.*

Children attend to and interpret nonverbal communication before they understand the meanings of words. Reciprocal communication of basic feelings and emotions between parent and infant takes place through sounds, gestures, and body contacts long before the infant or the toddler can identify feelings or know what words appropriately express them. Physicians should be aware of how their own facial expressions, tones of voice, or gestures influence children's reactions and determine how messages are interpreted; this knowledge contributes greatly to skill in interviewing. The complementary skill required of the physician is to recognize and correctly interpret the child's emotional state through careful observation of facial expression, tone and inflection of voice, body posture, gestures, and other responses. Children may be unresponsive to questions because they are upset by the loudness of the physician's voice, by the suddenness with which he or she initiates an examination, or even by the closeness of the physician's body. Some children have temperamental characteristics predisposing them to anxiety in new or unfamiliar situations and the physician has the responsibility for recognizing the signs and knowing how anxiety may be dealt with. Many children are frightened of unfamiliar office or hospital settings, of physical pain, of separation, of uncertainty, of persons or figures to whom they may attribute awesome authority and power, and of all else that goes with the word "doctor."

Children need continually to know what is happening and what is going to happen to them in the immediate future. Their anxiety will be significantly reduced when physicians take time to explain what they are doing and what they are going to do, and when they engage the child as an active participant as much as the clinical situation and good judgment will allow. Making life predictable, within the framework of a short or even a 50-min encounter in office or hospital, can have a profound effect on the likelihood of obtaining the cooperation of children.

Some children as young as 3–4 yr and most children by the age of 8 yr can participate verbally as well as physically in their own health care. All too frequently, conversation involves only the clinician and the parent, with the interaction between clinician and child being limited to the physical examination and some pleasantries. Children can and will respond relevantly to seriously posed questions about themselves.

By the age of 13 yr the young person is to be considered the primary informant and should be dealt with directly in his or her own right. If parents are at hand, they may be interviewed with the adolescent or separately, but at this age all explanations of diagnostic and treatment procedures should be directed first to the young person rather than to the parents. This procedure does not imply that the patient has veto power over the recommendations of the physician. The patient is still dependent on his or her parents, and the parents are still the major decision makers. Physical examinations of adolescents should be conducted with their parents not present, unless the patient requests otherwise.

TALKING WITH CHILDREN. Professional conversations with children have certain rules:

1. Don't talk to children in a condescending manner, but as a physician talks with any patient.
2. Don't convey to the child your thought that his or her feelings, concerns, or ideas are "childish."
3. Don't laugh at what a child says unless you are quite sure the child intends to be humorous.
4. Don't try always to be funny or amusing to children. Such efforts are best saved for few occasions only, and for children you know and who know you very well. Children know the difference between doctors and funny people.
5. Never tease a child unless you know him or her *very* well and the child knows that he or she has permission to tease you in return.
6. Initial or casual encounters with young children are often made easier when introduced in a whisper, which young children may find more personal, private, and reassuring than jollity; they commonly whisper in response.
7. When children are old enough, at 4–5 yr, form the habit of discussing with them their symptoms, diagnoses, and treatments in terms they can understand. The use of drawings to illustrate and explain medical problems can be very useful.
8. Never discuss the illness or treatment of a hospitalized child who has acquired receptive language functions in the child's presence unless you are discussing it with him or her as well.
9. When a child fails to cooperate in his or her care in office or hospital, the first assumption should be that negativism or struggling means that he or she is frightened and reacting to fear in a customary personal manner; such behavior is often erroneously perceived as immature and irritating, embarrassing, provocative, or frightening by parents and other adults.

OTHER ASPECTS OF THE INTERVIEW. Certain signs indicate that the progress of an interview or examination should be assessed or reassessed for the effectiveness of communication.

1. When parents do not appear readily reassured by the diagnostic and treatment procedures, look for hidden anxiety from unanswered questions that they may have difficulty recognizing or stating. Latent anger may have the same result. The physician should make it comfortable and easy for parents to ask "stupid" questions or to admit "shameful" thoughts or "ungrateful" or angry feelings.
2. When a child is giving evidence of feeling pain, it is a psychologic impossibility that nothing hurts. When parents scold a child with "That doesn't hurt," they must be helped to understand that pain is a purely subjective experience and needs to be respected. Their acceptance of this may help greatly to clear the air.
3. Parents will sometimes be heard denigrating or shaming a child by using such terms as "baby," which is almost as bad as being intentionally cruel or frightening. Such behavior should be dealt with by the physician promptly and its inappropriateness discussed, with as much empathy for the parents' position as possible. "I can see that it's upsetting to you to have your child behaving this way, but I don't think

that this approach is going to help us. Let's look at it from her (his) point of view . . ."

4. Exhortation and other emotional appeals to reason are frequently used by parents and are among the weakest methods of attempting to alter behavior or attitudes. Again, ". . . Let's look at it from the child's point of view . . ."

5. When only one parent accompanies the child, it is almost always the mother. In many families, including those with working mothers, issues of health care are considered as maternal responsibilities. Physicians should feel increasingly uncomfortable as time passes and they have not yet met the fathers of children for whom they have assumed the responsibility of continuing care. Many fathers will be found eager to see a physician who extends a specific invitation, has clearly stated expectations, and will accommodate his time and schedules.

6. The physician will often, if he or she adequately explores the matter, find that parents have not complied with recommendations made for the care of their children. Compliance is not simply a matter of hearing, understanding, and doing what the doctor says, nor is noncompliance to be explained simply as ignorance, neglect, or a personality clash. The parent who fails to comply with recommendations may do so for a number of reasons, and these must be accurately identified.

Did the parent really understand what was prescribed or recommended? Does noncompliance express the parent's reservations as to the appropriateness of the recommendations or were the recommendations beyond the capacity of these parents to execute them, for technical, emotional, or financial reasons? Had the parents enough opportunity to ask questions and to discuss the details and ramifications of the child's condition and treatment? Is a noncompliant parent being influenced or torn by information or advice contrary to that of the physician, which may come from the other parent, a grandmother, a friend, a newspaper or magazine article, or television programs?

Does the parent or do the parents have personal or marital problems which so upset and distract them that they cannot be effective, or does the child's illness itself have them so emotionally upset that they cannot accept the initiative and responsibility that has been thrust on them? Depressed mothers can be so psychologically depleted as to be unavailable to the child even though they may consciously want or intend to carry out recommendations. Is the parent expressing anger at the physician through noncompliance? Is the parent of an anxious and resistant child unable to execute a prescribed regimen that may be difficult or uncomfortable because he or she fears that the child may become hurt, resentful, or angry if the required firmness is exercised?

OTHER SOURCES FOR ASSESSMENT

INSTITUTIONS OR AGENCIES. Besides the clinical interview, other data can greatly help in psychosocial assessment. Birth records, for example, may help in questions of injury during pregnancy or at birth. Such records are often deficient, but they may provide the only objective view of events of the patient's birth and early days. Other health records, including those from other physicians or agencies who have cared for the patient, may provide essential information concerning acute or chronic illness, show a pattern of unusually frequent visits to the physician's office for relatively minor problems, or reveal an obsessive focus on certain areas of the body.

School reports are important to the psychosocial assessment, especially if they include both an academic assessment and a description of the child's relationships with schoolmates and teachers. Requests for school reports should be made only with the written permission of the child's parents or legal guardians.

Reports from child care agencies may also be helpful, especially in the case of adopted children or children in foster care. Such agencies often have extensive background material and may have reports of earlier psychologic examinations.

PSYCHOLOGIC TESTING. Relatively simple screening tests such as the Peabody Picture Vocabulary Test, the Denver Developmental Screening Test (see Sec. 3.11), the Thorpe Developmental Inventory, and others may be administered by the trained pediatrician or by his or her assistant. They may indicate areas of possible or patent intellectual or perceptual dysfunction that need further study. The major danger of these tests is that they may be relied on too heavily as giving definitive assessments, whereas they should be regarded purely as screening tests.

Some psychologic tests should be administered and interpreted only by or under the supervision of trained psychologists; others can be used by trained school personnel. They are generally of four types. The first type is concerned with *perceptual-motor* integrity. This type is felt to be especially sensitive to "organicity" or to reflect structural or physiologic abnormalities in the central nervous system. The Bender-Gestalt test is probably the best known test in this category. The second category is that of *intelligence* tests such as the Stanford-Binet or the Wechsler Intelligence Scale for Children-Revised (WISC-R). The WISC-R is a 10-category test that gives both verbal and performance IQ scores. The third type of test includes the *achievement* tests that are usually administered in schools. Tests such as the Wide Range Achievement Test (WRAT) report the grade level of achievement in such subject areas as reading, spelling, and mathematics. The fourth type includes the *projective* tests such as the Rorschach test (ink blot) or the Thematic Apperception Test (TAT). These give some indication of the fantasy life of the child as well as the reality testing and personality characteristics. When tests have already been done by the school, the results should be examined before new tests that may prove redundant or unnecessary are requested.

Other assessment instruments include various rating scales, questionnaires, checklists, and specific parent-child interactive measures. For example, the *Achenbach Child Behavior Checklist* provides a profile of the child's behavior problems. Ainsworth and associates have developed a structured mother-child paradigm that assesses attachment and affective and cognitive development in infancy. *The Nursing Child Assessment Feeding and Teaching Scales* (Barnard and Eyres) may be used by pediatricians and nurses to evaluate parent-child interaction according to sensitivity to cues and distress, responsiveness, and whether or not the interaction fosters cognitive growth. The *Child Assessment Schedule* (CAS) developed by Hodges and associates is used in a structured interview setting with the child and correlates with the standard classification system for psychiatric disorders.

The tests to be used should be chosen by the psychologist after the physician and psychologist have discussed the nature of the problem and the reason for consultation. As much as possible, tests should be chosen to assess specific problems rather than as an exhaustive battery, some of which may have only a vague relationship to any clearly defined problems or goals. When the physician is at all uncertain of the nature of the tests or the implications conveyed in their interpretation, a joint meeting should be arranged with the psychologist and parents for an interpretive review; otherwise, costly tests may be ordered, the results of which are never fully exploited.

Occasionally, genetic, endocrine, or neurologic studies will be required to determine whether organic problems may contribute to or be responsible for psychologic disorders.

PSYCHIATRIC CONSULTATION. A psychiatric consultation may be a valuable part of the assessment of children in whom vague or unexplained physical symptoms may have substantial psychogenic determinants; it will often be most acceptable and useful when the child has been hospitalized for study. Other indications include the evaluation of depression in children with major acute or chronic illness, of chronic anxiety problems, of underachievement, and of serious aggressive difficulties. The physician should inform both parent and child of the reasons for the psychiatric consultation, obtain their consent, and prepare them for what to expect.

CORRELATION OF DATA. The physician must avoid early diagnostic closure even when the parents' initial description of their problem gives a reasonably clear idea of what is going on. So long as the physician remains a receptive and perceptive listener, new and important information will emerge, as parents and perhaps patient begin to feel more trusting, and as they are educated by the physician's questions. Furthermore, the weighing of data must be done in the context of the family's sociocultural pattern. It is important that the physician not use his or her personal value system or style of living as a yardstick against which to measure the family's behavior or their success or failure in coping with their life situation. Their own feelings of anger, frustration, anxiety, failure, or depression are more valid indicators of where they need help.

It is important that the principal item of concern be accurately identified. Parents may present as the prime concern, for example, a problem such as bedwetting of many years' duration. Why then have they come for help now? It is important to determine whether there may, in fact, be more important hidden issues the parents do not recognize or acknowledge, or cannot face. By the same token, it must be understood that the parents' assessment of the problem is critical for the child. Sometimes a physician, having collected and assessed appropriate data, can conclude only that a child presented by his or her parents as having a problem is functioning within normal limits. In such a case it must be determined what personal, familial, social, or cultural considerations compel the parents to see the child's behavior as a major problem. It must then be determined what re-education they may need to feel reassured and not be left with the impression that their anxiety has been casually dismissed.

REFERRAL. When problems have not been internalized by the child it may be sufficient simply to counsel the parents or school personnel, or both. If this has been done and a maladaptive child or situation continues to present problems, the child and family will probably require more intensive or extensive help and should be referred to a child psychiatrist or to a psychiatric clinic. It is important that physicians avoid the position that psychiatric referral is a last resort. The need for a psychiatric consultation or referral can perhaps best be expressed in terms of the joint need of the family and physician for help in areas where the psychiatrist has special expertise, with the understanding that the collaboration of physician and family in management of the other health-care needs of the child remains intact.

3.22 PSYCHOSOCIAL PROBLEMS

A psychosocial disorder in a child may become manifest as a disturbance in feelings (e.g., depression, anxiety), in bodily functions (psychosomatic disorders), in behavior (e.g., conduct disturbances, passive-aggressive behavior), or in performance (learning problems). Dysfunction may involve any or all of these areas. Psychosocial problems may be produced by such physical or emotional stresses as birth defects, physical injury, inconsistent and contradictory child-rearing practices, marital conflict, child abuse and neglect, overindulgence, chronic illness, and so on. Particular agents do not, however, produce specific symptoms or disorders; rather, children's psychosocial problems are multifactorial in origin, their expression depending on many variables, including temperament, developmental level, the nature and duration of stress, past experiences, and the coping and adaptive abilities of the family. In general, chronic stresses, or a series of stressful events, are much more difficult for child and family to manage than a single acute stressful episode. Children may react immediately to traumatic events or may keep their feelings dormant until maladaptive reactions become apparent during later periods of vulnerability.

Anticipatory guidance during periods of stress may considerably help children and their families to achieve more positive outcomes. Parents should be encouraged to prepare their children in advance for potentially traumatic events that can be anticipated (e.g., elective surgery, separation, or divorce). Children should be allowed or encouraged to express their feelings of dismay, fear, or anger rather than being told to be a "good girl" or "brave boy."

Infants and toddlers tend to react to stressful situations with impairment of physiologic functions, such as disturbances of feeding and sleep, with relatively global expressions of anger or fear, as in temper tantrums, or with withdrawal and avoidance behavior. School-aged children demonstrate their difficulties through altered interpersonal relationships with peers and family members, through impairment of school performance, by the development of specific psychologic syndromes, such as phobias or psychosomatic disorders, or by "regressing" to earlier, more "childish" modes of functioning.

Parents are frequently concerned whether the particular behaviors of their children are "normal" or whether they represent problems that require intervention. Some "symptomatic" actions of children may be part of normal development. For example, a temper tantrum may express the normal negativism of a toddler; on the other hand, temper tantrums on slight provocation in a 6 yr old may indicate psychosocial disturbance. Whether behavior is judged to be a developmental variation or evidence of a more serious problem depends on the age of the child, on the frequency, intensity, and number of symptoms, and especially on the degree of functional impairment. The decision of parents to seek help is determined, in turn, by the characteristics of their children's behavior, by the amount of distress it causes the children, parents, teachers, and others, and by their past experiences in discussing psychosocial matters with their physicians.

3.23 PSYCHIATRIC CONSIDERATIONS OF CENTRAL NERVOUS SYSTEM INJURY

Psychiatric difficulties may follow infection, injury, or intoxication, or genetic, metabolic, or idiopathic illness involving the central nervous system. These are not to be confused with the manifestations of "minimal cerebral dysfunction" (also known as minimal brain dysfunction, dysfunctional child, attention deficit disorder, or, in behavioral terms, the hyperactive or hyperkinetic child. For the last condition see Sec. 3.39).

Brain injury increases the risk of both intellectual impairment and psychiatric disorder, especially when the injury is severe. Social disinhibition appears to be a specific sequela of brain injury, but no typical psychiatric syndrome is associated. The particular expression of disturbance depends more on the child's developmental level, past history, temperament, and family relationships than on the nature of the insult. Psychosis is not a typical result of brain injury or illness in childhood. Chess has reported an autism-like syndrome in children who have had congenital rubella, but autistic psychosis is probably the result primarily of unspecified genetic, physiologic, and organic factors (see Sec. 3.44).

Psychiatric disorder accompanies or follows brain injury or illness or epilepsy in a significant percentage of affected children. The epidemiologic survey of the Isle of Wight found brain-injured or epileptic children 5–15 yr old to have five times the normal risk of psychiatric disorders. Mentally retarded children also are at increased risk of psychiatric disorders.

Prenatal factors have long been suspected of causing brain damage and psychiatric or behavioral disorders. Prematurity and neonatal complications involving hypoxia have been seen as causing such conditions as hyperactivity, impulsivity, difficulties in socialization, and poor control of emotions, especially anger. On the other hand, Graham's study of 350 children at the age of 3.5 yr who had suffered neonatal asphyxia found no more behavioral or emotional disturbances than were found in a control group matched for social class and family factors.

Children under the age of 3 yr who survive encephalitis or meningitis seem to show more lasting effects on personality and behavior than those who have these illnesses later. The result contradicts the notion that the brain might in the earlier years have greater potential for recovery without significant residual dysfunction.

Children with hydrocephalus and motor deficits have a seven times greater than average incidence of psychiatric disorder. The additional findings of low intelligence, language disorder, or bilaterality of the motor handicap increase the incidence of psychiatric disturbance significantly, but again there is no specificity in the type of disturbance encountered.

When children with brain damage or injury have problems with impulse or anger control, aggressiveness, hyperactivity, or other emotional reactions, these do not differ in quality from those of children with intact nervous systems who have the same disturbances.

The most significant factor in the child's adjustment to a chronic handicapping organic condition is the capacity of his parents to adjust and cope.

In some affected children stimulant drugs improve the ability to perform in school, smooth out emotional reactivity, and facilitate social interactions with peers and adults. Such medication taken for extended periods may produce growth retardation, which must be weighed against possible beneficial effects. Neuroleptics may lessen anxiety and improve emotional control and behavior, but they tend also to produce obtundation and somnolence, which may interfere with learning. In addition, they may have serious side effects (see Sec. 3.48).

Most children with psychologic disturbances related to central nervous system injuries and their families benefit from understanding psychosocial support. A frequently beneficial approach is to help the child to identify his or her ineffective reaction patterns, along with more successful patterns. The approach combines "coaching" and education with an opportunity to discuss depression, isolation, and anger and those feelings of being different, rejected, or exploited that so much affect self-esteem. The parents have their own needs and will need advice, counseling, and emotional support in dealing with their child's emotional and behavioral problems, both in family matters and in his or her life at school and with friends. Fair, firm discipline is always useful. Behavior modification techniques can help children in whom specific target behaviors can be identified; the technique may be used at home or at school. Both aberrant psychosocial behaviors and learning difficulties may respond to these techniques (see Sec. 3.14).

3.24 PSYCHOSOMATIC DISORDERS

Psychologic conflict that significantly alters somatic function is the hallmark of the psychosomatic disorders. Any kind of emotional distress may be associated with any type of psychosomatic disorder in a child or adolescent; particular types of feeling or conflict do not produce specific kinds of psychosomatic illness. There appear to be both innate, constitutional vulnerabilities and environmental factors, neither of which are well understood, that determine why one organ or system becomes dysfunctional rather than another.

Conversion disorder, the loss or alteration of physical functioning without a demonstrable organic illness, is a type of somatoform disorder that usually presents in adolescence or adulthood. However, numerous childhood cases have occurred. Conversion reactions usually start suddenly, can often be traced to a precipitating environmental event, and end abruptly after a period of short duration. Voluntary musculature and organs of special sense are the most frequent target sites for the "hysterical" expressions of psychologic conflict. Such reactions may take many forms, including hysterical blindness, paralysis, diplopia, gait disturbances, and the like. Physical examination often fails to reveal objective abnormalities. Deep tendon reflexes can be elicited in a paralyzed leg, and pupillary responses to light are noted in patients with hysterical blindness. Affected children and their families tend to be rather dramatic and hypochondriacal and often give a past history of previous conversion episodes. The few follow-up studies that do exist suggest that more than one third of children and adolescents who are initially diagnosed with a conversion disorder ultimately are found to have a not readily apparent organic disorder.

Hypochondriasis, preoccupation with the fear of having a serious illness, and *somatization disorder,* the use of multiple somatic complaints as a means of assuaging inner tension, are also somatoform disorders. As with conversion hysteria, these disorders provide alternate routes and mechanisms for the discharge of physiologic and emotional tension. Adolescence and early adulthood are the most common times for the presentation of each, although both can be seen in some anxious, usually dependent, school-aged children who often have an adult role model with a similar symptom picture.

Psychophysiologic disorders have a more insidious onset. Chronic anxiety produces functional abnormalities within the autonomic nervous system that lead to structural changes within organ systems. Eczema, bronchial asthma, ulcerative colitis, and peptic ulcer are considered to be psychophysiologic disorders or at least to have significant psychophysiologic components in some children. Although these children have been reported to be obsessive and inhibited, there is no compelling evidence for specific personality characteristics.

Several general principles guide the management of children with psychosomatic disorders: (1) The symptoms of affected children are not within their conscious control; they are not acting or malingering, and their pain and their problems are real. (2) It is essential for a psychiatric assessment to be arranged early in the management of these disorders; otherwise, after elaborate and expensive tests have been done, the child and family will often be convinced that the patient has a very serious illness for which a "real" cause exists that cannot be found. (3) An explanation of the role of the emotions and the genesis of these disorders must be accepted by the parents before truly effective intervention can be accomplished. (4) Psychotherapy for the child and counseling for the family are often indicated, as well as pediatric management. The psychiatrist and pediatrician must be in close communication with each other in a therapeutic alliance. Modest amounts of minor tranquilizing medication may be a useful adjunct. (5) Child and family should be helped to live as normally as possible to avoid crippling psychologic invalidism. Stress should be placed on early return to school after acute illness, participation in recreational activities, and normal peer interactions. Parents should know that some children unconsciously use their symptoms to maintain dependency, and that firm, gentle insistence on the fullest possible range of activities for the child is indicated. (6) The physician should be alert for indications of psychosomatic or physical illness in parents, with which children may unconsciously identify; successful treatment of parental illness may be necessary to ensure a favorable outcome in the child.

3.25 DISORDERS RELATED TO VEGETATIVE FUNCTIONS

OBESITY. See Sec. 4.20.
ANOREXIA NERVOSA AND BULIMIA. See Sec. 10.14.

3.26 RUMINATION DISORDER

The hallmark of this disorder is a weight loss or failure to gain at the expected level because of repeated regurgitation of food without nausea or associated gastrointestinal illness. This rare disorder occurs more commonly in males and usually appears between 3 and 14 mo of age. It is potentially fatal; some reports indicate that up to one fourth of affected children die. There are psychogenic and self-stimulating ruminators. The former type occurs in infants with otherwise normal development, although there is often a disturbed parent-child relationship. The self-stimulating variety is usually seen in mentally retarded individuals of any age and often occurs even in the presence of nurturing parents.

Behavioral *treatment* is directed toward positively reinforcing correct eating behavior and negatively reinforcing rumination. Adverse conditioning is often used. Parent counseling and family therapy are often necessary to discern underlying conflicts and to help educate the parents about appropriate approaches to be taken toward the child and the problem.

3.27 PICA

This habit disorder involves repeated or chronic ingestion of non-nutrient substances, which may include plaster, charcoal, clay, wool, ashes, paint, and earth. The age of onset is usually 1–2 yr of age but may be earlier. Mental retardation and lack of parental nurturing (psychologic and nutritional) are predisposing factors. Although tasting or mouthing of objects is normal in infants and toddlers, pica after the 2nd yr of life needs investigation. It is often a symptom of family disorganization, poor supervision, and affectional neglect. Pica appears to be more prevalent in the lower socioeconomic classes. Children with pica are at an increased risk for lead poisoning (see Sec. 26.16) and parasitic infections (see Sec. 12.105).

3.28 ENURESIS (Bedwetting)

The involuntary discharge of urine after the age at which bladder control should have been established is one of the most common and perplexing problems brought to the attention of the pediatrician. The prevalence at age 5 yr is 7% for males and 3% for females. At age 10, it is 3% for males and 2% for females, and at age 18, it is 1% for males and extremely rare in females. Twin studies show that there is a marked familial pattern.

CLINICAL MANIFESTATIONS. Bedwetting may be divided into the persistent (or primary) type, in which the child has never been dry at night, and the regressive type, in which a previously continent child begins to wet the bed again. Persistent nocturnal enuresis is often the result of inadequate or inappropriate toilet training. Parents who demand coercively that the child become toilet trained promptly may generate an angry response, the child unconsciously defying them by wetting the bed. On the other hand, parents who are not sufficiently close to the needs of the child to support toilet training may undermine his or her attempts at bladder mastery. Chronic psychologic stress, unrelated to toilet training experiences but occurring during the toddler period, can also impair the child's ability to achieve bladder control.

The regressive type of bedwetting is precipitated by stressful environmental events, such as a move to a new home, marital conflict, birth of a sibling, or death in the family. Such bedwetting is intermittent and transitory; the prognosis is better and management is less difficult than in a child with primary enuresis.

In both types of bedwetting, organic pathology can be found in only a very small number of cases. Physical examination and urinalysis are indicated, but procedures such as urography and cystoscopy are usually not warranted and should not be pursued unless there is some indication of an organic lesion.

TREATMENT. Management of the child with enuresis depends on an understanding of the possible specific causative factors suggested by an adequate psychosocial evaluation and physical examination. For example, a child can be helped to deal with feelings about a younger sibling, or the parent may be helped to establish proper attitudes and climate for a child's success in toilet training. Some general suggestions are as follows: (1) It is important to enlist the cooperation of the child to deal with the problem. Rewarding the child for being dry at night is a useful step. The child or parent can chart the dry nights, and with one or two dry nights, a small reward can be given. More substantial rewards should be given for increasing success. (2) Older children should be expected to launder their own soiled bed clothes and pajamas. (3) Children should be given no liquids after dinner time. (4) The child should void before retiring. (5) Waking the child repeatedly to take him or her to the bathroom is useful in only a few children and may further engender or aggravate anger in child or parent. (6) Punishment or humiliation of the child by parents or others should be strongly discouraged.

The use of conditioning devices (e.g., an alarm that rings when the child wets a special sheet) is usually not necessary and should be reserved for persistent and refractory cases in which the child's self-esteem has been seriously eroded. Consent of the child should be a prerequisite for use of such a device. A positive reinforcement system that charts the child's progress is successful in 80–85% of cases. Conditioning devices have been shown to be successful in well over 90% of cases. Imipramine (Tofranil) administration is generally effective only briefly, and drug tolerance is common. Its use in children with enuresis should be discouraged because of the exacerbation of symptoms after the drug has been discontinued and because of side effects of the medicine.

3.29 ENCOPRESIS

This term refers to the passage of feces into inappropriate places at any age after bowel control should have been established. This predominantly male disorder affects 1% of 5 yr olds. It is more commonly seen in children from low socioeconomic backgrounds. Organic defects are rarely found. Encopresis indicates a more serious emotional disturbance than enuresis.

CLINICAL MANIFESTATIONS. Chronic soiling may persist from infancy onward (primary) or may appear as a regressive (secondary) phenomenon. It is often associated with chronic constipation, fecal impaction, and overflow incontinence and may progress to psychogenic megacolon. This symptom usually represents unconscious anger and defiance in the child, and the parents may respond with retaliatory, punitive measures. School performance and attendance may be affected as the child becomes the target of scorn and derision from schoolmates because of the offensive odor.

TREATMENT. Measures similar to those used for the supportive treatment of enuresis may be useful, but the fixed and disabling nature of the symptom frequently requires psychotherapeutic intervention with the child and family. Treatment of secondary encopresis can be facilitated by the judicious use of mineral oil and a high-fiber diet. Sitting on the toilet 10–15 min after each meal is often necessary. Rewards for compliance should be offered. Power and autonomy struggles should be avoided, if possible, and records of the child's elimination should be kept. Primary encopresis is more difficult to treat. Initially, enemas may be needed to evacuate the colon. However, chronic use of enemas and laxatives should be avoided. The child is encouraged to use the bathroom at specific times and is rewarded accordingly. If the child does not produce a reasonable amount of fecal material, glycerine suppositories may be necessary. A nonhumiliating examination of the child's clothing at the end of the day is necessary. Rewards are offered for nonsoiling, and mild, nonjudgmental consequences are used for soiling.

3.30 SLEEP DISORDERS

These are common in childhood and may be temporary, intermittent, or chronic in nature.

CLINICAL MANIFESTATIONS. A substantial portion of children have struggles around bedtime. Many use a special toy or a nightlight to help them fall asleep. Infants who show difficulty in establishing regular night-time sleep patterns may also show general fussiness and irritability as a temperamental characteristic. Sleep disorders in infancy may be a result of parental anxiety or strife. Older children may experience transient night-time fears (of burglars, noises, thunder and lightning, being kidnapped, and so on) that interfere with sleep. Children may express their fears overtly, or they may disguise them, often by invoking tactics designed to delay bedtime. The fearful child may also seek to sleep in the parents' bedroom or may attempt to come into their bedroom after they are asleep.

Separation anxiety often contributes to this problem. Children may unconsciously and symbolically consider sleep as a time when they are removed from parental love and concern. If there is conflict within the family or if separation or divorce has occurred, such anxiety will be exacerbated. Bedtime fears are often related to normal separations such as occur with the child's first attendance in nursery school or kindergarten. As growing children become more aware of death, they may be unwilling to go to sleep at night for fear that they may die. This fear will be heightened if a family member has recently died. Anxiety related to any other areas of the child's life—family, peers, school performance—may be expressed as a sleep disorder. Depression also causes sleep disturbances.

About 5% of the general population report current problems with *nightmares*. Anxiety dreams occur during REM sleep; the child awakens, becomes lucid quickly, and usually remembers the content of the dream. Nightmares occur more often in girls than boys and usually begin before the age of 10.

Night terrors usually begin in the preschool years and occur with arousal from stage 4 (non-REM) sleep; the child is confused and disoriented, shows signs of intense autonomic activity (labored breathing, dilated pupils, sweating, tachypnea, tachycardia), may complain of peculiar visual phenomena, and appears to be frightened. A period of *somnambulism* (sleepwalking) may occur, during which the child may be at risk for injury. Some minutes may pass before the child seems to be oriented. Usually the child cannot recall the content of the dream causing the night terror. Night terrors are often self-limited and may be related to a specific developmental conflict or to a precipitating traumatic event. The incidence in children is said to be from 1 to 4%, and it is more common in boys than in girls. There is a familial pattern in the development of night terrors, and febrile illness may be a predisposing factor.

TREATMENT. Parental support, reassurance, and encouragement are vital for alleviating sleep disorders. Angry threats and punitive measures should be avoided. Parents should adopt calm, understanding, but firm attitudes. Bedtime should be set for a regular, stated time, variations being kept to a minimum. The parents should discourage the child from sleeping in their room but may temporarily allow a fearful child to sleep in a sibling's room. A nightlight and permission to leave the child's door open are often reassuring. The interval before bedtime should be quiet and restful; stimulating television programs should be avoided. A warm bath, a light snack, and a quiet affectionate moment with parents are conducive to sleep. Some children may become drowsy if they are allowed to read a favorite book for a few minutes after they are settled in bed. Diphenhydramine may serve as a mild sedative.

The treatment of persistent nightmares involves an understanding of the underlying anxiety and the provision of reasonable support for the individual. Night terrors are treated in the same fashion, although the addition of diazepam is beneficial.

For sleep disorders in adolescents, see Sec. 10.13.

3.31 HABIT DISORDERS

Habit disorders include tension-discharging phenomena, such as head banging, body-rocking, thumbsucking, nail biting, hair pulling (trichotillomania), teeth grinding (bruxism), hitting or biting parts of one's own body, body manipulations, repetitive vocalizations, breath-holding, and swallowing air (aerophagia). Tics, which involve the involuntary movement of various muscle groups of the body, are also included. Stuttering is discussed with the habit disorders, although it is not generally regarded as a tension-relieving activity.

All children at various developmental points show repetitive patterns of movement that can be described as habits. Whether they are considered disorders depends on the degree to which they interfere with the child's physical, emotional, or social functioning. Some habit patterns may be learned by imitation of adults. Many begin as a purposeful movement that for some reason becomes repetitive, the habit losing its original significance and becoming a means of discharging tension. For example, a child who has an eye irritation or is attempting not to shed tears might try closing the eyelids several times in rapid succession. This activity may become repetitive and incorporated into the child's behavior as an outlet for tension. Such symptoms are often reinforced by attention from parents or others. Other movements, such as rhythmic head banging and rocking in early life, can persist without parental reinforcement, occurring when the child is put to bed or is alone; these movements seem to provide a kind of sensory solace for the child who is feeling otherwise uncared for or understimulated by human touch or interaction. These movements represent a kind of internal stroking. Such patterns are often seen in the mentally retarded or in children suffering from maternal or emotional deprivation. Equivalent movements are evident in children who twist their hair or touch or play with parts of their bodies in repetitive ways. As involved children become older, they learn to inhibit some of their rhythmic habit patterns, particularly in social situations. The prevalence of habit disorders is not known. The natural course can vary, depending on whether the behavior is part of a chronic problem (e.g., mental retardation) or results from an episodic disorder.

Teeth grinding seems to result from tension originating in unexpressed anger or resentment. It may create problems in dental occlusion. Helping the child to find ways to express resentment may relieve the problem. Bedtime can be made more enjoyable and relaxed by reading or talking with the child, permitting re-experience and review of some of the fears or angers experienced during the day. Praise and other emotional support are useful at these times.

Thumbsucking is normal in early infancy. It makes the older child appear immature and may interfere with normal alignment of the teeth. Like other rhythmic patterns, it can be seen as a way of securing extra self-nurturance. The best strategy for dealing with thumbsucking is to provide the child with evidence of interest in his or her well-being and other forms of satisfaction. Parents should ignore the symptom if possible, while giving attention to more positive aspects of the child's behavior. The child who actively tries to restrain thumbsucking should be given praise and encouragement.

Tics involve repetitive movements of muscle groups and represent discharges of tension originating in emotional and physical states that have no apparent useful function. They may have been initially intentional, sometimes becoming nonintentional very quickly. Parts of the body most frequently involved are the muscles of the face, neck, shoulders, trunk, and hands. There may be lip-smacking and grimacing, tongue-thrusting, eye blinking, throat-clearing, and so on. It is very difficult for a person with a tic to inhibit it. Tics can be distinguished from variants of minor seizures in that the child does not experience a transient loss of consciousness or amnesia. They can be distinguished from dyskinetic movements and dystonias by their discontinuation during sleep and by virtue of the conscious control that can be achieved for short periods of time. Tics usually accompany other psychiatric syndromes or follow encephalitis. In most cases, they seem to have had no physical antecedents and are transient. Undue parental attention can reinforce tics, whereas ignoring them may diminish their occurrence. Electroencephalographic (EEG) findings and cognitive testing do not differentiate patients with tics from controls.

Gilles de la Tourette syndrome, which has a lifetime prevalence rate of 0.5/1,000 individuals, is a rare condition in children. It is characterized by multiple tics, compulsive barking, or shouting obscene words. It is more common in the 1st-degree relatives of patients with Tourette syndrome than in the general population and affects boys 3–4 times more often than girls. Children with Gilles de la Tourette syndrome often suffer from secondary behavioral and emotional disorders. Although the etiology is uncertain, research has shown that drugs that increase dopaminergic action precipitate or worsen tics and Gilles de la Tourette syndrome. Many environmental precipitants have been noted to serve as emotional stressors, which also precipitate or increase tics and Gilles de la Tourette syndrome. Gilles de la Tourette syndrome can be fairly well managed with haloperidol, a dopamine antagonist, and pimozide, a more powerful dopamine antagonist. The disorder usually persists throughout life, but studies have shown a significant diminution in symptoms in half to two thirds of cases 10–15 yr after the initial evaluation and treatment.

Primary *stuttering* usually begins as an atypical development during the learning of speech. It starts gradually, initially with the repetition of consonants, often followed by a repetition of words and phrases. As the child becomes aware of the dysfluency, anxiety and behavioral responses may occur. As the condition becomes fixed, secondary compulsive and repetitive movements of various muscle systems occur as the child attempts to "force" out the words and release the built-up tension. About 5% of children stutter. Most cases resolve spontaneously, although about 20% continue to suffer the disability in adulthood. A strong family incidence has been noted, and the disorder seems to remit more readily in girls than in boys.

The physician can help parents accept the child's early patterns of dysfluent speech; a decreased emphasis on these early patterns portends a better outcome. The child should be made to feel successful and cared for in other ways. If the pattern persists, a speech therapist should be consulted. Approaches to treatment include breath-control exercises and the use of a miniaturized metronome that "paces" the rhythm of speech.

3.32 ANXIETY DISORDERS

Anxiety, fearfulness, and worrying are regularly experienced as part of normal development. When they become disattached from specific situations or events or when they become disabling to the point that they negatively affect social interactions and development, they are pathologic and warrant intervention. Separation anxiety disorder, avoidant disorder, overanxious disorder, obsessive-compulsive disorder, phobias, and post-traumatic stress disorder are all defined by the occurrence of either diffuse or specific anxiety related to predictable situations. The Isle of Wight study reported by Rutter and associates noted the prevalence of anxiety disorders to be 6.8%. About one third of these children were overanxious, and another third had specific fears or phobias that were disabling. Other studies estimate the prevalence of phobias as 7%, of which 2% are clinically disabling.

The antecedents of developmentally normal anxiety initially present at 7–8 mo of age. As infants begin to differentiate from their primary caregivers they often develop wariness and mood changes that previously did not exist when in the company of strangers. This *stranger reaction* is to be differentiated from *stranger anxiety,* which is a more intense discomfort that includes obvious psychologic and physiologic distress. Although stranger reaction is typically seen in early development, stranger anxiety often heralds later problems related to attachment and separation. Preschoolers typically develop specific fears related to the dark, animals, and imaginary situations. Parental reassurance is usually sufficient to help the child through this period. School-aged children slowly give up imaginary fears and replace them with fears of bodily harm as well as with other potentially real worries. Social anxieties often develop during the teenage years.

There are a number of theories about the origin of fears and phobias. The psychoanalytic view postulates that internal conflict that is not expressed leads to the development of neurotic symptoms. Social learning theory proposes that fears and anxieties are learned within the context of the child's environment. Others think that excessive worrying is related to maternal anxiety.

Children with *phobias* are anxious only under specific conditions. They try to avoid specific objects or situations that will automatically lead to anxiety. As with other forms of anxiety, phobias become pathologic when they interfere with social, professional, and interpersonal functioning. The parents of phobic children should remain calm in the face of the child's anxiety or panic. If they become upset, the child will conclude that there is, in fact, something to fear. Behavioral therapy is indicated, including systematic desensitization, the process of exposing the patient to the fear-inducing situation or object. Anxiety is managed through relaxation techniques. A thorough interpretive session with the parents and child designed to convey an understanding of what is happening is important to the development of a trusting therapeutic relationship. Parent training designed to help the family be supportive during stressful periods is also important.

School phobia, a syndrome in which a child will not attend school because of various reasons, occurs in about 1–2% of children. The literature has underscored the hostile-dependent nature of the relationship between mother and child that often contributes to this disorder. Bernstein and Garfinkel have shown that 70% of these children suffer with depression, 60% with an anxiety disorder, and 50% with both depression and anxiety. Management of the disorder involves treatment of the underlying psychiatric problems, family therapy, parent management training, and liaison work with the child's school.

Separation anxiety disorder is characterized by unrealistic and persistent worries of possible harm befalling primary caregivers, reluctance to go to school or to sleep without being near the parents, persistent avoidance of being alone, nightmares involving themes of separation, and numerous somatic symptoms and complaints of subjective distress. These are children who come from the middle to lower socioeconomic classes. Often the first clinical sign of this disorder does not appear until 3rd or 4th grade, typically after the Christmas holidays or after a period in which the child has been absent from school because of an illness. Parents frequently encourage the disability in conscious and unconscious ways.

Children are referred for psychiatric therapy when the usual supportive approaches have failed to return the child to school or to reduce the symptoms. After a thorough assessment, the therapist clearly states to the child the expectations of the family regarding the child's return to school. A program involving the school, the parents, and the child is coordinated by the therapist to minimize the child's use of splitting and manipulation. Parent training as well as family therapy is often necessary to delineate underlying motivations and to teach appropriate ways to help the child fulfill reasonable expectations regarding school attendance. A large percentage of children with separation anxiety disorder develop feelings of panic when they are coerced to separate from their parents. A judicious use of either antidepressant or antianxiety medicines is often necessary to facilitate treatment goals.

Avoidant disorder is characterized by an excessive fear of contact with unfamiliar people that leads to social isolation. These children and adolescents maintain the desire for involvement with family and familiar peers. Some clinicians think that this diagnosis does not really exist but is part of a generalized anxiety picture.

Children who suffer from *overanxious disorder* have unrealistic worries about future events, the appropriateness of past behavior, and concerns about competence. They frequently present with somatic complaints, are markedly self-conscious, need large amounts of reassurance, and have trouble relaxing. Onset may be gradual or sudden. The disorder is usually seen in white children who are the eldest in their families. The families are usually of a higher socioeconomic status than the families of children with other anxiety disorders and are often overconcerned about issues of competence of their own. Boys and girls are equally affected. Overanxious children are more likely than children with separation anxiety to be diagnosed as having a simple phobia or panic disorder as well. Frequently, overanxious disorder does not become manifest until puberty.

Many children present with repetitive thoughts that invade consciousness or repetitive rituals or movements that do not obviously contribute to a high level of adaptation in any given situation (an obsessive-compulsive disorder). In times of stress (e.g., bedtime, preparing for school), some children touch certain objects, verbalize certain words, or wash their hands continually. The most common *obsessions* are concerned with bodily wastes and secretions, the fear that something calamitous will happen, or the need for sameness. The most common *compulsions* are hand-washing, continual checking of locks, and touching. These thoughts and acts occur consciously, often causing great distress in the child. Some children externalize the ritualized behavior, attempting to involve their parents in their compulsions.

These behaviors become part of a disorder when they cause distress, consume time, or interfere with usual occupational or social functioning. The lifetime prevalence rate is about 1%. This disorder may be associated with anorexia nervosa, Gilles de la Tourette syndrome, and epilepsy. Recent positron-emission tomography (PET) studies have demonstrated increased metabolic activity in the frontal lobes and the basal ganglia in affected children. Treatment consists of behavioral therapy and pharmacotherapy. Overexposure of the patient to the situations that lead to the symptoms and anxiety is a major therapeutic technique, used especially for rituals. Clomipramine, fluoxetine, and fluvoxamine have all shown promise in ameliorating obsessive-compulsive symptoms. Because each blocks the neuronal re-uptake of serotonin, some have hypothesized that excessive serotonergic activity may be the basis for the disorder. However, Rapoport cautions that other neurotransmitters, particularly dopamine, are also probably involved.

Post-traumatic stress disorder is characterized by recurrent and intrusive recollections and dreams of noxious events in addition to intermittently intense psychologic and physiologic distress in situations that symbolize the original trauma. Individuals with this disorder typically try to avoid stimuli associated with the original trauma. Although typically described as an adult illness, it occurs in children and adolescents, especially those who have been physically or sexually abused. Studies examining the effects of natural disasters, terrorism, and physical trauma clearly indicate that children are as vulnerable as adults to the psychologic sequelae of perceived trauma. Treatment centers on relaxation therapy, psychotherapy, and pharmacotherapy.

3.33 AFFECTIVE DISORDERS

Major depressive disorder, dysthymic disorder, and bipolar disorder with alternating mania and depression are the three major types of affective disorder seen in children and adolescents. *Major depression* is characterized by dysphoria and an obvious loss of interest and pleasure in usual activities but also includes a significant weight change secondary to decreased or increased food intake, insomnia or hypersomnia, psychomotor agitation or retardation, fatigue or loss of energy almost every day, feelings of worthlessness and excessive guilt, diminished ability to think and concentrate, and recurrent thoughts of death. In addition, the melancholic subtype of depression also includes marked anhedonia and greater feelings of depression in the morning with early morning awakening. *Dysthymic disorder* is a less severe but more protracted syndrome involving depressed mood for at least 1 yr. In addition poor appetite, sleep problems, decreased energy and self-esteem, and feelings of hopelessness are present. *Bipolar disorder* involves both mania and depression. *Mania* is characterized by a persistently elevated, expansive, or irritable mood with grandiosity and inflated self-esteem, decreased need for sleep, increased loquaciousness, flights of ideas, distractibility, and an increase in goal-directed activities.

3.34 MAJOR DEPRESSION

The concept of the existence of depression in children has been controversial. Many have argued that because depression has a component replete with feelings of hopelessness and helplessness about the future, an individual can become depressed only after achieving the ability to string together hypothetical thoughts about the future. Because formal operations, which develop during adolescence, are required for such hypothetical thinking, the preponderant belief has been that depression cannot develop until then. However, researchers have now abundantly shown by using structured interviews and other psychologic scales that prepubertal children do manifest mood disturbance, anhedonia, and vegetative symptoms associated with depression. Although some still argue that children assign different values and importance to questions of mood, thus leading to a number of false-positive responses, it has become fairly well accepted that both prepubertal children and adolescents suffer mood disturbances not unlike those affecting adults.

EPIDEMIOLOGY. The prevalence of depressive disorders in childhood has been estimated to be between 0.15 and 2%. In a population that has clinical problems it has been estimated between 10 and 20%. The prevalence of major depression in prepubertal children has been reported as 1.8% and in adolescents between 3.5 and 5%. Girls report significantly more depressive symptoms than boys.

ETIOLOGY. Although the causes of depression have not been established, there is ample evidence of a genetic basis for major depressive disorders. Twin studies have shown a 76% concordance for depression among monozygotic twins reared together and 67% for monozygotic twins reared apart, compared with 19% for dizygotic twins reared together. Many studies have demonstrated an increased rate of depression (3–6 times greater) in 1st-degree relatives of patients suffering from a major affective disorder; some researchers have theorized that there is a possible X-linked basis for major depression. In attempting to assess exactly what it is that is genetically transmitted, researchers have focused on biogenic amines and neurotransmitters. Because of the low urinary levels of MHPG (3-methoxyhydroxyphenylglycol) and 5-HIAA (5-hydroxyindoleacetic acid) in depressed patients, low functional levels of norepinephrine and serotonin are thought to be important genetic markers. These views are reinforced by the therapeutic responses to antidepressants that block their presynaptic re-uptake. Cognitive theories have attributed the development of depression to feelings of hopelessness and helplessness secondary to an actual loss or the perception of loss by the individual. Learning theory has postulated that depression is learned within the environment because of a lack of reasonable reinforcers.

CLINICAL MANIFESTATIONS. Depressive symptoms vary according to age and developmental level. Spitz described the *anaclitic depression of infancy.* Separation from a primary caregiver after 6–7 mo of age leads to protest (crying, searching, panic-like behavior, and hypermotility of both arms and legs). This is followed by the infant's close scrutiny of each approaching adult, looking for the caregiver. The child turns away from everyone else. The final phase involves apathy in which the infant becomes hypotonic and inactive, exhibiting an obviously sad facial expression. These babies cry silently and stare into space. When picked up, they search again for the familiar face; they cling to the stranger and cry, but are not consoled.

Depressed school-aged children present with a variety of symptoms. Sad facial expressions, easy tears, irritability, withdrawal from usually pleasurable interests, and vegetative symptoms involving eating and sleeping disturbances are common. Half of depressed children also present with obvious anxiety symptoms, and 20–30% have behavioral disturbances. Adolescents typically present with impulsivity, fatigue, depression, and suicidal ideation. Psychotically depressed adolescents frequently present with both hallucinations and delusions, whereas psychotically depressed children usually do not have delusions. Hopelessness is much more frequently seen in depressed adolescents than in children.

The symptoms of a major depressive episode usually develop over a period of days or weeks. Sometimes they may develop suddenly secondary to a severe precipitant. The duration of the symptoms is quite variable. Untreated, symptoms often persist for 6 mo. Sometimes, however, they continue for 2–3 yr before they remit. Although the natural history of major depression has not been fully elucidated, several longitudinal studies clearly show that children and adolescents who are depressed are at risk for the development of later episodes of depression. Children who have depression at age 9 have been shown to have numerous depressive symptoms at 11–13 yr of age. Other studies have shown that within 2 yr of the first depressive episode, 40% of children who have had a major depressive disorder experience a relapse. As many as 20% of teenagers hospitalized because of major depressive disorders develop a manic episode within 3–4 yr of discharge. Three predictors of such an outcome are (1) a depressive symptom cluster characterized by rapid onset, psychomotor retardation, and mood-congruent psychotic features; (2) a family history of either bipolar illness or other affective illness; and (3) induction of hypomania by antidepressant medication.

DIAGNOSIS. Two measures have been developed that are somewhat useful in diagnosing depression: structured interviews or questionnaires and biologic methods that measure physiologic and neuroendocrine dysfunctions. The Children's Depression Inventory, Children's Depression Scale, Depression Self-Rating Scale, and the Center for Epidemiological Studies Depression Scale for Children have all been shown to be useful in diagnosing depression in children and adolescents, although some researchers have questioned the validity of some scales. There are no biologic tests specific for depression. During major depressive episodes some children have been shown to hyposecrete growth hormone in response to insulin-induced hypoglycemia. Some preliminary reports have also suggested that depressed prepubertal children produce higher growth hormone peaks during sleep. Dexamethasone suppression tests have been shown to be inconclusive in children and adolescents, although they show some efficacy in diagnosing depressed adults. Sleep EEG reports in depressed children and adolescents are inconclusive. In short, although psychologic and biologic tests show promise in their ability to differentiate depression from other psychopathologic syndromes as well as from a normal state, additional work is needed in regard to their sensitivity and specificity.

TREATMENT. Major depression in childhood and adolescence is treated with antidepressant medications and various psychologic therapies. Tricyclic antidepressants (imipramine, desipramine) are useful in ameliorating symptoms. It is particularly important that these medicines in children and adolescents be followed by adequate determination of blood levels of the drug; children treated with subtherapeutic levels are much less likely to respond efficaciously than those whose drug levels are in the therapeutic range. The more recently developed serotonin re-uptake blockers (trazodone, fluoxetine) are also efficacious and have perhaps fewer side effects.

Nonpharmacologic treatment, including psychotherapy, is indicated and is especially important for those children who have dual disorders; anxiety disorders and conduct disorders frequently coexist with depression. Play therapies and various talking therapies are important in ameliorating symptoms secondary to these diagnoses in combination with affective disorders.

3.35 DYSTHYMIC DISORDER

In this disorder the dysphoria is generally more intermittent, with periods of normal mood lasting several days to several weeks, than in a major depression. The dysphoria is less intense but more chronic, lasting up to several years.

ETIOLOGY. Although the genetic basis of major affective disorder has been demonstrated, it is questionable whether there is also a genetic basis for dysthymic disorder. Dysthymia may be a partial phenotypic expression of an underlying genetic disorder or a different syndrome altogether that has certain symptom clusters in common with major depression.

Ten per cent of latency-aged children give positive answers to questions pertaining to depression and dysphoria. Other studies have shown a prevalence rate of 3.3% for dysthymia in adolescence.

CLINICAL MANIFESTATIONS. With the exception of hallucinations and delusions, the other symptoms of major depression may be present. Dysthymia frequently is the consequence of pre-existing, chronic disorders such as anorexia nervosa, somatization disorder, or anxiety disorder. Children who have dysthymia have had frequent disruptions of important relationships, often beginning as early as infancy. There is often a history of depressive illness in both parents. Affected children show more general emotional and social maladjustment. They often present the picture of helpless, passive, clinging, dependent, and lonely children. Others relate in a more hardened, aloof, negativistic manner. They are reluctant to invest emotion or trust in relationships and frequently develop rather manipulative or expedient approaches to human affairs. They are less likely than acutely depressed children to show episodes of crying. These children attempt to hide their depressed affect. They frequently experience problems in school achievement and in their relationships with family and peers. They are at risk for the development of conduct disorders or substance abuse. Studies show that untreated dysthymic disorder lasts approximately 3 yr. The recovery rate for dysthymic disorder is significantly worse than that for a major affective disorder. The younger the child when dysthymia emerges, the longer it takes to recover.

TREATMENT. Antidepressant pharmacotherapy may be useful in the treatment of dysthymic patients. It is especially helpful for dysthymic patients who display vegetative symptoms of depression. Because the occurrence of dysthymic disorder predisposes the individual to major depression, therapies necessary in the treatment of major depression are often also indicated for the treatment of dysthymic disorder. However, when the dysthymic symptoms are a secondary reaction to an underlying disorder (anorexia, somatization disorder, substance abuse disorder, physical illness, personality disorder), the issues leading to the underlying disorder should be addressed as well. This often requires a full spectrum of therapies including alliance building and dynamic psychotherapy, family therapy, parent management training, and community liaison work.

3.36 BIPOLAR DISORDER

This illness typically presents in the 2nd or 3rd decade of life, but there are descriptions of cases beginning before puberty. Initially, patients may present with either a depressive episode or mania. During the first few years of the illness, manic episodes are more common than depressive episodes. Many adolescents misdiagnosed as schizophrenic are correctly diagnosed in their adult years as suffering with bipolar illness. Twenty per cent of adolescents presenting with major depressive symptoms have been shown to develop manic episodes later.

Clinical manifestations in adolescents are similar to those in adults. Overactivity, loquaciousness, insomnia, a grandiose sense of self, expansive mood, paranoid delusions, and overspending are all seen in both populations. The earlier the onset of bipolar symptoms, the more susceptible the patient is to later suicide, increased frequency of episodes, and rapid cycling. See also Sec. 10.2.

Lithium carbonate has proved to be very effective in the *treatment* of bipolar illness and manic symptoms. This is administered orally and is followed by blood levels. The ideal therapeutic range for the initial treatment of acute symptoms is 1.0–1.2 mEq/L, and the recommended level for maintenance therapy is 0.5–0.8 mEq/L. During the acute manic phase, neuroleptic medication may also be required because of the psychotic nature of the symptoms. Carbamazepine, a tricyclic compound used as an antiseizure medicine, has also been effective in controlling manic symptoms in adults. Alliance-building psychotherapy and parent work designed to help manage the behavioral sequelae of mania are also important.

3.37 SUICIDE AND ATTEMPTED SUICIDE

See also Chapter 10.3.

Adolescents may turn to suicide as a solution to psychologic and environmental problems. In addition, although few prepubertal children kill themselves, many in this age group also consider suicide as a means of handling problems.

EPIDEMIOLOGY. Nine to 18% of nonpsychiatrically disturbed preadolescents entertain suicidal ideas, whereas 1.5% actually make suicidal threats. The incidence of suicide for children under the age of 15 yr is rising. For boys the suicidal rate tripled from 1950 to 1977, reaching a peak of 1.6/100,000 deaths; the rate declined to 1.1/100,000 by 1979. The rate for girls has steadily increased, and by 1979 it had reached 0.5/100,000, 5 times the incidence since 1950. The number of deaths due to suicide in the 15- to 19-yr age group was 7.64/100,000 or 7.95% of all deaths in this age group.

The individual and family variables associated with suicidal ideation are different from those associated with suicide. Factors influencing suicidal thoughts include depression, preoccupation with death, and general psychopathologic factors. No particular diagnosis has been associated with suicidal threats. However, a wide range of psychosocial variables were found not to be associated with suicidal ideation: age, sex, social status, race, family size, intelligence, academic achievement, impulse control, reality testing, parental separation and divorce, parental medical and psychiatric problems, and drug or alcohol abuse. Variables associated with completed suicides are different. The preponderance of white, older adolescent males among child and adolescent suicide victims readily points to age, sex, and race as important factors.

CLINICAL MANIFESTATIONS. Fifteen to 40% of completed suicides are preceded by other suicide attempts. Depression and general psychopathologic factors are also related to completed suicides. In one third of suicides, a parent, a sibling, or other 1st-degree relative had previously shown overt suicidal behavior. Just as with suicidal ideation, children and adolescents who have killed themselves show an especially prominent preoccupation with death and dying, a wish to die, and feelings of hopelessness or worthlessness prior to the act. In adolescents, the notion of revenge or hostility is particularly prominent, directed either outwardly or against the self; it is present in at least half of those who succeed in killing themselves. Family studies have shown that fathers of suicidal youngsters have been more often noted to be depressed themselves and to have low self-esteem, whereas mothers have experienced greater anxiety or suicidal ideation. Both parents have tended to consume more alcohol than usual. Drug use is a common family problem.

Firearms serve as the major method of death in adolescent suicide. Death from carbon monoxide poisoning and medication overdoses are also prominent. Males are more likely to use violent methods than females. Among preadolescents, jumping from heights is the most common method, followed by self-poisoning, hanging, stabbing, and running into traffic. Episodes of self-poisoning that occur after age 6 yr are less likely to be accidental and should be treated as if the behavior had suicidal potential or as a possible case of child abuse and neglect.

School-aged children in general are surprisingly knowledgeable about the subject of suicide. The major difference between children and adolescents lies in the congruence among knowledge, fantasy, and method. Among adolescents there is a very high correspondence among knowledge about the kinds of acts that will lead to death, fantasies about what will happen to them if they commit one of these acts, and the particular method chosen for suicide. Prepubertal children, on the other hand, show discrepancies between what they know to be a suicidal act and their fantasies of what will kill and what will not. This may, in part, be why so few prepubertal children kill themselves compared with adolescents.

TREATMENT OF THREATS AND ATTEMPTS AT SUICIDE. Threats of suicide should be seen as acts communicating desperation, and all such threats or attempts should be taken seriously. Physicians, parents, and others must scrupulously avoid sarcasm, kidding, daring, or belittling the individual making such threats. If a suicidal threat is labeled "manipulative," power or control becomes a major issue influencing behavior.

The physician assessing suicidal behavior of a child or adolescent should carefully explore, in detail, the child's life during the 48–72 hr prior to either the threat or the suicide attempt. The precipitating events should be identified. The degree of premeditation or impulsivity should be assessed. It is important to understand whether the patient intended to stop or to be discovered and whether the behavior prior to or subsequent to the attempt promoted or impeded the patient's being discovered before or after the attempt. The physician should judge the margin of error allowed by the patient in terms of the method used or proposed, the closeness or remoteness of available help, whether the patient actually called for help after the attempt if it was not immediately discovered, and whether the patient calculated correctly whether the family would return in time to discover the attempt. The most significant factor in assessing intent is the possibility and probability of rescue as foreseen by the child or adolescent.

When the patient is able, the physician should investigate the child's frame of mind, the degree of hopelessness, helplessness, or overwhelming shame or guilt, and the presence or absence of anger (directed toward others or toward the self). The degree of depression should be evaluated carefully in terms of both the seriousness of the attempt and whether or not the patient presents a continuing risk. It is important to determine whether the child acted out a psychotic delusion or paranoid ideation or whether the act was the result of hallucinatory experiences that produce intolerable anxiety or panic. After recovery, it is important to assess the patient's frame of mind, to determine whether the suicide intent persists, and to assess whether there is now a more optimistic sense of being able to solve or to seek help for problems in a more constructive manner.

When suicidal patients have been seen in the physician's office or the emergency room, it is often best to admit them for a day or more to the hospital so that a more adequate evaluation can be made of the patient's frame of mind and of the circumstances of the family or environment. Such admissions usually require 2–3 days, unless medical needs require a longer stay or unless serious psychiatric disorders such as depression or psychosis are found. If social service and psychiatric assessments are adequate and arrangements for appropriate follow-up care can be made, disposition can be made fairly rapidly. The physician must give careful attention to how the family and friends have responded to the patient's act. A hostile and angry family, such as occurs frequently, will necessitate a different disposition or resolution than a family that is supportive, sympathetic, and understanding. The latter supports a decision for the patient to return home. Some families may completely deny the seriousness of the behavior; this can be discouraging and provocative to the patient, whose act has been a desperate attempt to compel a different response. The family members should be helped to examine their roles in the interactions that preceded the attempt, without being made to feel overly guilty.

In planning care of patients after suicidal threats or attempts the physician should consider the following factors:

1. Has the patient been restored physiologically? The patient's state of consciousness, orientation, memory, attention, and concentration should be evaluated. Drugs taken during the suicide attempt may produce an acute brain syndrome or delirium that persists after the coma or stupor phase is no longer present. It is important to determine whether the effects of the drugs have cleared the system.
2. Is the patient less depressed, or is the depression masked? This is difficult to determine quickly and may require a pediatric psychiatric consultation. The family can sometimes help determine if or when the patient seems to be returning to his or her usual self.
3. Does the patient appreciate the seriousness of the act, or does he or she still want to die? Answers to these questions are important in deciding about future psychiatric hospitalization as well as in determining the appropriate time to discharge the patient home.
4. Are the precipitating events or other reasons that provoked the suicidal behavior still actively influential? The answer requires assessment of the family and environment by a health care worker.
5. Have the family, friends, teachers, and other persons significant to the patient responded in a relatively positive manner? It is important to determine whether the parents or other significant adults have recovered from their anger or excessive guilt because the child will need their support after discharge. Have the parents and child been able to identify

for themselves some changes that they can make to improve things at home, school, or in the neighborhood?

6. Does the child show evidence of a future orientation after the return home?

7. Have the child's anger, disappointment, shame, guilt, depression, grief, and other strong feelings moderated to the point at which he or she does not feel at the mercy of impulses and feelings? It is particularly important to assess whether hopelessness and helplessness have declined and whether a sense of control over one's life or one's situation has reappeared.

3.38 DISRUPTIVE BEHAVIORAL DISORDERS

Numerous behaviors considered appropriate at certain developmental levels are obviously pathologic when they present at later ages. Lying, impulsiveness, breath-holding, defiance, and temper tantrums are frequently noted around the ages of 2–4 yr when children begin to need autonomy but do not have the motor and social skills necessary for successful independence. These behaviors are probably the result of frustration and anger.

Breath-holding is not unusual during the first years of life. It is frequently used by infants and toddlers in an attempt to control their environment and their caregivers. Whereas some children hold their breath until they lose consciousness, sometimes leading to a seizure, there is no increased risk of their later developing a seizure disorder. Parents are best advised to ignore the behavior and leave the room in response. Without sufficient reinforcement, the behavior soon disappears.

Defiance, oppositionalism, and *temper tantrums* are often used by children 18 mo to 3 yr of age who feel frustrated by their conflicting desires to be in control of their environment on the one hand, and, on the other, to be taken care of and pampered in a developmentally regressed way. Parental and caregiver response to this behavior is very important. Caregivers who respond to toddler defiance with punitive anger run the risk of reinforcing the defiance and teaching the child that out-of-control emotions are a reasonable response to frustration. In response to tantrums and oppositionalism, parents are advised to acknowledge verbally to the child that the reasons for frustration are understandable but that the particular response is not acceptable. The child should be given time and space to recover. If the child is unable to give up this behavior but instead presents with escalating oppositionalism, parents should nonemotionally place the child on time out or a room restriction until he or she is able to adjust more reasonably.

Children are often frightened by the strength and intensity of their own angry feelings as well as by the intensity of the angry feelings they arouse in their parents. It is therefore of prime importance that parents provide models for control of their own anger and aggressive feelings that they wish their children to follow. Many parents who are horrified at their children's loss of control of anger are unable to see that they have often lost control themselves; they are not, therefore, helping their children to internalize controls. Physicians must learn from the parents how they handle anger before making recommendations about how the child's problems are to be helped. One way to help the toddler develop a sense of autonomy and to feel more in control is to allow the child to have simple choices of activities that the parents can accept. This helps to provide the child with options, thus reducing his or her potential feelings of being powerless, overwhelmed, or engulfed. Such negative, internalized feelings may later have adverse effects on developing interpersonal relationships, intimacy, and personality development.

Lying is often used by 2–4 yr olds as a method of playing with the language. By observing the reactions of parents and caregivers, preschoolers learn cognitively and affectively about expectations for honesty in communication. In another sense, lying is a form of fantasy for children, who describe things as they wish them to be rather than as they are. For instance, a child who has not done something that a parent wanted may say that it has been done to avoid an unpleasant confrontation. The child's sense of time and reason does not permit the realization that this only postpones an even angrier confrontation.

In school-aged children, lying most often represents the child's attempt to avoid the pain of a relative loss of self-esteem. That is, most lying is an effort to cover up something that the child does not want to accept in his or her own behavior. The lie is invented, therefore, to achieve temporary good feeling. Lying can be the result of parental modeling, in which case the child's interpretations of reality are often conflicting, confusing, or unclear. For instance, when mothers and fathers accuse each other frequently of lying, the child may become hopelessly unsure of how the word lying is to be interpreted; moreover, a loyalty conflict is added to the already distorted process of reality testing.

Many adolescents lie because they fear that their parents would disapprove of what they are doing. Chronic lying, however, often occurs in combination with several other antisocial behaviors and is a sign of underlying psychopathology. As with other antisocial behaviors, lying is often used as a method of rebellion.

Regardless of the age or developmental level, when lying becomes a frequent way of managing conflict and anxiety, intervention is warranted. Initially, the parents should confront the child to give a clear message of what is acceptable. Sensitivity and support are necessary for a successful intervention because children and adolescents are so developmentally vulnerable to shame and embarrassment. If the situation cannot be equitably resolved (i.e., parental understanding of the situation and the child's understanding that lying is not a reasonable alternative), professional intervention is indicated.

Almost all children *steal* something at some point in their lives. It becomes a problem when it happens more than once or twice. Some preschoolers and school-aged children steal as a response to a sense of internal loss. They frequently feel neglected and are in fact emotionally deprived. Their stealing is impulsive, but the gratification derived does not satisfy the underlying need. In children and adolescents stealing can sometimes be an expression of anger or revenge for real or imagined frustrations by the parents. In many instances of children's stealing there is a strong wish by the child to be caught. Stealing becomes one way in which the child or adolescent can manipulate and attempt to control interactions with parents. Like lying, stealing can be learned from parents. Parents who boast about outwitting tax laws or exceeding speed limits are implicitly condoning stealing as an acceptable behavior.

It is important for parents to help the child undo the theft by returning the stolen articles or by rendering their equivalent either in money that the child can earn or in services. When it is apparent that children are not able to control temptation, money and valuable objects should not be left where they can reach them, to decrease the chances of stealing. It is also important that the act not be overemphasized, lest the behavior or the response to it becomes so exciting that it is reproduced in future periods of discontent.

Unlike the previous behaviors, *truancy* and *run-away behavior* are never developmentally appropriate. Some children skip school because they are afraid of peers or teachers or because of the sense of humiliation secondary to learning difficulties. Others are truant because of separation anxiety symptoms. Most often, truancy represents disorganization within the home, developing personality problems, or both. Whereas younger children often threaten to run away out of frustration or a desire to get back at parents, children who run away with nowhere to go are almost always expressing a serious underlying problem. During the latency years, the most common causes are related to abuse and neglect within the home. In adolescence, disagreements with the parents, developing personality problems, and abuse and neglect all must be considered as possible precipitants.

Although the interest in fire is ubiquitous in early childhood, unsupervised *fire-setting* is always inappropriate. Early school-aged children tend to set fires because of latent hostility secondary to deprivation within a disorganized and neglectful family. These young children set fires by themselves within their homes. In adolescence, fire-setting is a more delinquent sign. Teenagers usually set fires in small groups, seeking revenge from school and community authorities.

At the very least, fire-setting requires intervention by the parents, but most often also intervention by mental health professionals. A combination of family therapy, alliance-building individual therapy, parent management training, and community involvement is often necessary to effect a reasonable change. The recidivistic young fire-setter is very difficult to manage, however. Many adult arsonists were childhood fire-setters.

Although there is no totally satisfactory theory about the nature and causes of human *aggressive behavior*, the main extant theories are not mutually exclusive. The drive theory proposes that aggressive responses are biologically programmed within the human species. The phenomenologic approach suggests that everyday life is sufficiently depriving and frustrating that aggression is to be expected. Social learning theory proposes that aggression is learned and successively reinforced throughout young childhood and adolescence. In addition, social theorists suggest that modern crowding, the breakdown of commonly shared values, the demise of traditional family patterns of child-rearing in kinship systems, and social alienation both in individuals and in large groups are leading to increased aggression in children, adolescents, and adults. Aggression in childhood has also been correlated with family unemployment, discord, criminality, and psychiatric disorders.

Several factors contribute to aggression. Boys are almost universally reported to be more aggressive than girls. In many animals, administration of male sex hormones to females produces more aggressive behavior. Large children are often more aggressive than smaller ones. More active and intrusive children are perceived as more aggressive. Difficult temperament and later aggressiveness have been shown to be related. Children from larger families are often more aggressive than those from smaller families. Marital discord between parents and aggression within the home certainly contribute to aggression within children.

Clinically, it is important to differentiate the causes and motives for childhood aggression. Many hyperactive, clumsy children are called aggressive because of the accidental results of their behavior. Intentional aggression may be primarily instrumental, to achieve an end, or primarily hostile, to inflict physical or psychologic pain. The relationship between individual aggression and emotional disturbance, school failure, brain damage, overactivity, and character pathology has been recently underscored in several studies. Of particular importance is the relationship between severe reading retardation and the development of symptoms of aggressive conduct disorder, especially in boys. In a review of the Isle of Wight study, Wolff noted that both one third of retarded readers suffered from conduct disorder and one third of children with conduct disorder suffered from reading retardation.

The child of 2–5 yr may show aggressive outbursts ranging from temper tantrums and screaming to hurting others or destroying toys and furniture. This behavior is frequently the product of particular frustrations and the toddler's inability to manage them. In toddlerhood, aggression is usually directed toward parents; during the preschool years, it is more likely to be directed toward siblings or peers. Verbal aggression increases between 2 and 4 yr, and after 3 yr of age, revenge and retaliation become more prominent as determinants of aggression.

Aggressive behavior in boys is relatively consistent from the preschool period through adolescence; a boy with a high level of aggressive behavior from 3 to 6 yr of age has a high probability of carrying this behavior into adolescence. On the other hand, girls under 6 yr who are aggressive toward peers are less likely to demonstrate that behavior at older ages.

Children exposed to aggressive models on television or in play display more aggressive behavior compared with children not exposed to these models. Parents' anger and aggressive or harsh punishment model behavior that children may imitate when they are physically or psychologically hurt.

Passive-aggressive behaviors are common in childhood and adolescence. Prevalence rates of 16–22% have been noted. Children with passive-aggressive behavior express hostility indirectly as procrastination, stubbornness, or resistance. Parents often complain that such children do not hear them and that they fail to respond to repeated requests. Academic underachievement is common. Early histories may reveal excessive negativism during infancy and toddlerhood with feeding disturbances and problems in bladder and bowel training.

Children may unconsciously adopt passive-aggressive strategies for a variety of motives: to gain independence while maintaining dependency; to counter underlying low self-esteem; to maintain control and autonomy when threatened by anxiety; and to get revenge. These children are fearful of direct expression of aggression and hostility. The child-rearing styles of their parents are often intimidating, critical, and inconsistent or, on the other hand, indulgent and permissive. Both children and parents often find it difficult to deal directly with anger.

Parents should be encouraged to handle passive-aggressive behavior by setting firm limits and expectations for the child. Parents and child should reach agreement on what they consider to be the child's important tasks and responsibilities. The most important issues need to be managed first. Age-appropriate assertiveness and independence should be promoted and rewarded. More refractory cases often require psychiatric intervention.

Conduct disorder is a distinct clinical entity manifested by several different antisocial behaviors: stealing, lying, fire-setting, truancy, property destruction, cruelty to animals, rape, use of a weapon while fighting, armed robbery, physical cruelty to others, and repeated attempts to run away from home. A pattern of such behaviors that has existed for at least 6 mo warrants the diagnosis of a conduct disorder. *Oppositional defiant disorder* is defined by less severe behavior than a conduct disorder: temper tantrums, continual arguing, defiance of rules, continual blaming of others, angry and resentful affect, spiteful and vindictive behavior, and frequent use of obscene language.

Many argue that conduct disorder is not a unitary illness but instead contains three different syndromes characterized primarily by *aggression, intermittent antisocial behaviors,* and *delinquency.* The latter two types of behavior are differentiated by the number and frequency of antisocial behaviors committed by the child. Little is known about the antecedents or outcome of patients suffering from each of these subtypes.

The risk factors (from child, parent, and environment) associated with the development of conduct disorders are very similar to those previously mentioned in association with the development of specific antisocial and aggressive behaviors. Specific antisocial symptoms in children have been related to similar behavior in their parents. For example, Robins reported a relationship between truancy and the parents' premature discontinuance of their own education. Aggressive behavior is stable across generations within families. Inconsistent parenting practices as well as overly punitive disciplinary measures have been associated with conduct disordered children. Parents of conduct disordered children are less accepting of their children and show less warmth and support of their children. However, not all children showing antisocial behavior continue that behavior into adulthood. An early age of onset of disordered behavior, an increased number of episodes and varieties of antisocial behaviors, seriousness of the behavior as well as the types of symptoms, parental criminality, and marital discord are associated with continuation of antisocial behavior into the adult years.

Many different approaches have been used in the *treatment* of children and adolescents with aggressive behavior, conduct disorder, and oppositional disorder. Individual therapy focusing on alliance building and conflict resolution is sometimes useful in establishing the basic trust necessary for a positive therapeutic outcome; however, this has not been shown to be especially effective in ameliorating behavioral problems. Group therapy has shown some promise in treating adolescents with behavioral difficulties but has been relatively ineffective with latency-aged children. Training in problem-solving skills involves modeling, role play, and practicing to help children deal more successfully with interpersonal relations and is somewhat effective in modifying maladaptive styles of relating and behaving. The most effective results have been obtained with parent management training in which parents are trained directly to promote prosocial behaviors within the home and to place reasonable limits on unwanted, destructive behaviors. Family therapy designed to improve communication among family members and to elicit underlying conflicts to allow them to be more equitably resolved is also somewhat effective. Pharmacotherapy is, by and large, not indicated for this problem. However, children with underlying biologic vulnerability (intermittent psychotic disorders, attention deficit problems) may benefit from judicious use of appropriate medication. There are no medicines specifically intended for treatment of antisocial behaviors. Although lithium and haloperidol have some usefulness in treatment of aggression, it is not clear whether they are helpful in conduct disordered children or in patients with psychotic and affective symptoms. Physicians are sometimes pressured by caregivers to use both major and minor tranquilizers to help control specific behavior problems. This pressure should be resisted. Some children present with such severe behavioral problems that residential treatment and psychiatric hospitalization are necessary for a successful outcome.

3.39 ATTENTION DEFICIT HYPERACTIVITY DISORDER (ADHD)

See also Sec. 3.55.

This disorder is characterized by poor ability to attend to a task, motoric overactivity, and impulsivity. These children are fidgety, have a difficult time remaining in their seats in school, are easily distracted, have difficulty awaiting their turn (impulsively blurt out answers to questions), have difficulty following instructions and sustaining attention, shift rapidly from one uncompleted activity to another, talk excessively, intrude on others, often seem not to listen to what is being said, lose items regularly, and often engage in physically dangerous activities without considering possible consequences. It is difficult to distinguish adequately between ADHD and conduct disorder, on the one hand, and between ADHD and learning disabilities on the other. Restlessness, inattentiveness, distractibility, and vigilance deficits are commonly seen in conduct disordered children. In several studies learning disabled children could not be differentiated from children with ADHD on the basis of attention or distractibility. Hyperactive behaviors often cannot be shown to be separate from aggressive and antisocial behaviors.

ETIOLOGY. There is no tenable hypothesis of a single neurotransmitter deficit. Dopaminergic, noradrenergic, and serotonergic mechanisms have been postulated, but a unitary biologic model has not been established. Children with ADHD differ from normal children in terms of cognitive style, levels and types of arousal, and response to rewards. Zametkin and Rapoport have demonstrated abnormal PET scans with reduced glucose metabolism in premotor and superior prefrontal cortex in adults having ADHD. These areas involve control of attention and motor activities.

EPIDEMIOLOGY. Some studies differentiate ADHD from both conduct and anxiety disorders because the former overwhelmingly occurs in males and is primarily a disorder of cognitive impairment, in contrast to the other disorders. European and American investigators differ in their estimates of the prevalence of ADHD. The Isle of Wight study found two hyperactive children in a group of over 2,000. Studies in the United States have suggested a prevalence rate of 1.5–4%. The difference underscores the confusion concerning the diagnostic criteria defining the disorder. The syndrome is 4–6 times more likely to occur in males than in females. In about half the cases the age of onset occurs before 4 yr. Central nervous system and neurologic disorders serve as predisposing factors for this syndrome. ADHD, developmental disorders, alcohol abuse, conduct disorder, and antisocial personality disorder have all been shown to be more common in 1st-degree relatives of children with ADHD than in the general population.

CLINICAL MANIFESTATIONS. A description of the problem behaviors in specific situations and environments is elicited. A *history* of aggression and fears, poor relationships with peers, academic difficulty, behavioral problems at school, and reaction to authority define the breadth of the problem and provide useful information about the concurrent presence of conduct disorder, anxiety disorders, and learning disabilities. The history should include events of the birth and delivery, a description of the child's temperament, examples of manifestations of early separation reaction and separation anxiety, a description of the child's behavior between 18 and 30 mo when the child was psychologically separating from the primary caregiver, and the child's activity level between 2 and 5 yr. ADHD is associated with neurologic problems, and some parents of hyperactive children report problems during pregnancy and delivery as well as during infancy. Some children are also described as "colicky," temperamentally difficult, and overactive from a very early age, with sleep and feeding abnormalities. Many parents report excessive temper tantrums and oppositionalism during the preschool years, suggesting a conduct disorder.

The initial identification of many children with this problem commonly occurs when they enter nursery or elementary school. They are often reported as being uncontrollable, refusing to sit still, intruding into the space and activities of other children, being boisterous and inattentive, and refusing to follow instructions. They often provoke others to anger and rarely learn from their mistakes.

During the *examination* of a child who is said to be hyperactive, it is not uncommon for signs and symptoms to be absent. Many hyperactive children are able to suppress characteristic behavior in a structured situation. Although some children have neurologic "soft signs" (mixed hand preference, impaired balance, astereognosis, dysdiadochokinesia), these findings are very inconsistent and do not contribute to the final assessment. Many of these neurologic signs occur in normal children and in various other syndromes.

DIAGNOSIS AND DIFFERENTIAL DIAGNOSES. Laboratory studies do not establish the diagnosis of ADHD. Slow wave activity on electroencephalograms is not relevant unless the child also suffers from a neurologic disorder or epilepsy. It is uncertain whether hyperactive children have significantly lower IQ scores than children appropriately matched for age, school grade level, and socioeconomic status who do not have the syndrome. Some studies have suggested that hyperactive children have higher verbal scores than performance scores on the Wechsler Intelligence Scale for Children-Revised (WISC-R) and lower scores on the Attention-Concentration Subset. Educational levels, as measured on the Peabody Individual Achievement Test and the Wide Range Achievement Test, may be lower than expected for age and IQ, especially for children who also have learning disabilities. Specific tests for learning disabilities (Woodcock Reading Mastery Test, Key Math Diagnostic Test) should be administered to pinpoint areas of difficulty. Projective psychologic tests are not useful in establishing the diagnosis.

Children in whom attention deficit problems are suspected should be evaluated for conduct disorder problems and learning disabilities. Sensory impairment, particularly auditory impairment, should be investigated in children who present with difficulty in concentrating. Petit mal epilepsy should be considered, because it can mimic the concentration and attention problems seen in children with ADHD. Various medications (antipsychotics, anticonvulsants) may cause overactivity and attention problems. Overanxious children and those suffering with dysthymic and depressive disorders also may show increased activity and social disturbances similar to those seen in ADHD. Gilles de la Tourette syndrome may coexist with ADHD.

TREATMENT. Stimulant medications should be used only as a part of an ongoing treatment plan of behavioral and psychosocial therapy involving the child, parents, and school. This approach is most likely to be efficacious.

A program that gives *structure to the child's environment* decreases the effects of the handicap and helps in academic and social learning. Children should have a regular daily routine, which they are expected to follow promptly and for which they are rewarded with praise. Rules should be simple, clear, and as few in number as possible, and should be coupled with firm limits, enforced fairly and sympathetically through restrictions and deprivation for transgressions. Overstimulation and excessive fatigue should be avoided. There should be time for relaxation after play, particularly after vigorous physical activity. The period before bedtime should be quiet, with avoidance of exciting television programs and rough and tumble games. Children with obvious hyperactivity problems should not be taken on long trips in automobiles or on extensive shopping trips. The home should be arranged so that all valuable, dangerous, or breakable objects are out of reach of young hyperactive children. Parents should reward even partially successful efforts to control behavior or to perform academic responsibilities with recognition, affection, and regular praise. More formal operant conditioning techniques that reward the child with stars or tokens contingent on improved behavior are often helpful.

Close communication between the physician and school personnel is essential. Depending on the level of the disability, some children may require special classes in which contingency or operant conditioning is used. Such approaches can be very helpful when carefully planned and implemented. Behavior therapy is a more efficacious treatment than pharmacotherapy for aggression and physical acting-out in children with ADHD. Decisions about medication should be made in consultation with school personnel as well as with parents.

When severe psychosocial difficulties have produced serious family distress or when the child has internalized the obvious disapproval rendered by others so that low self-esteem results, *referral* to a mental health professional is indicated. There is no evidence that psychotherapy is primarily beneficial in ADHD, but individual and family therapy are indicated when hyperactivity is complicated by depression, social withdrawal, conduct disorder, eroded self-esteem, or family conflict.

Several *controversial therapies* are not efficacious. There is no evidence to support the use of dietary management. Megavitamins, restriction of sugar, and supplementary trace minerals are not effective. Although a small percentage of affected children may respond to diets low in food additives or coloring, these treatments are not superior to the more conventional approaches.

Methylphenidate, dextroamphetamine, magnesium pemoline, and various tricyclic antidepressants are efficacious in reducing overactivity, increasing attention span, improving interaction between the child and the mother and between the child and other family members, and improving academic performance. The long-term benefits of these medicines have not yet been established.

Methylphenidate is the most commonly used stimulant; it is efficacious in 75–80% of patients when administered in a dose ranging from 0.3 to 1.0 mg/kg. It generally has an effect for 2–4 hr, although the sustained-release form, available only in 20-mg tablets, lasts considerably longer. Studies of plasma levels suggest that a dose of 0.3 mg/kg helps to improve attention, whereas amelioration of behavioral problems requires 0.7 mg/kg. Methylphenidate should usually be given for at least 2–3 wk so that efficacy can be adequately determined.

Dextroamphetamine is efficacious in approximately 70–75% of patients. Its optimal dose range is 0.2–0.5 mg/kg. It has a longer half-life than methylphenidate, although the therapeutic effect of amphetamine preparations is reported to be no longer than 4 hr. Both dextroamphetamine and methylphenidate should be given about 20–30 min before meals to avoid their deactivation. They should not be given after 4.00 P.M. to avoid insomnia. The response to both medications should be noticeable soon after they are started. Children who do not respond will show little or no change in behavior with increasing doses.

Magnesium pemoline is effective in 65–70% of children. Its effect develops more slowly, and it may take 2–3 wk to fully evaluate its efficacy. An initial dose of 18.75 mg should be given and increased by half a tablet per week as needed (see Table 3–14, max 112.5 mg/24 hr). About 1–2% of children treated with this medicine may show changes in liver function; accordingly, pretreatment studies and monitoring of liver function are required.

Tricyclic antidepressants are efficacious in 60–70% of children. When used for hyperactivity, it is not necessary to determine blood levels in these patients. Many clinicians feel that patients that respond best with a diminution of overactivity are those who also suffer from an underlying dysthymic or depressive disorder. Because of possible side effects, these medications should not be used initially.

Stimulant drugs can cause complications such as increased nervousness and jitteriness. Major short-term side effects include anorexia, upper abdominal pain, and difficulty with sleeping. The abdominal discomfort usually remits spontaneously. Long-term side effects may include increased heart rate and growth suppression. The effects of increased heart rate are not known. Some researchers feel that the decreased growth rate is a short-term problem, but others have reported a drop in height of 2 percentile points in children taking an average of 40 mg/day of a stimulant medicine for 2–4 yr. The growth of children receiving stimulants should be monitored, and drug-free holidays (weekends, holidays, summer vacations) should be employed when practical. Stopping the medication each summer permits the parents and child to reassess the need for continued medication. At the very least, a drug-free period of 2–3 wk/yr should be tried routinely for this purpose. It is difficult to predict which children will respond most favorably to stimulants. The action of these drugs is the same in both hyperactive and nonhyperactive, conduct disordered children. Some studies suggest that children with the poorest levels of concentration respond best to pharmacotherapy. Inattentive behavior not due to anxiety is the most appropriate reason to use stimulant drugs.

PROGNOSIS. Some anecdotal studies propose that hyperactivity continues into adolescence and adulthood and is associated with adult alcoholism, sociopathy, and hysteria. Other studies strongly suggest that hyperactive children do well in adulthood if they are successfully employed. The most consistent, predictive symptom of later psychopathology is the presence of aggression in childhood, a symptom not used to define this syndrome.

3.40 SEXUAL BEHAVIOR AND ITS VARIATIONS

See also Sec. 3.9.

Gender identity refers to the individual's sense of self as a male or a female. *Gender role,* on the other hand, refers to those behaviors within a culture commonly thought to be associated with maleness or femaleness. Thus, one's gender identity is intact when a biologic male identifies himself as a man and a biologic female identifies herself as a woman. If the male performs the sort of behavior associated with being a man within his culture, he is said to fit comfortably within his gender role. However, if a man is uncomfortable with those behaviors identified with men within his culture, the implication is that he has trouble with his gender role. The same is true for women. Of course, as society changes, the issue becomes more complicated. In the past, gender roles were shaped by traditionally defined masculine and feminine roles. As the economics of family life have changed—and both sexes have become potentially self-sufficient economically—gender roles, as they relate to job choices and performance, have changed dramatically or, in some cases, have simply disappeared. Fewer behaviors are specific solely to one gender.

Children identify themselves as boys or girls by about 18 mo of age (i.e., establish a gender identity). Between 18 and 30 mo of age children establish *gender stability,* the concept that boys become men and girls become women. By 30 mo gender constancy, the immutability of one's gender, is firmly established and resistant to change. Although there are numerous theories suggesting which environmental and biologic factors are most important to the establishment of a firm gender identity, at this point we still do not understand, in a way that has treatment implications, which factors are most important in any given child.

Children are naturally curious about their bodies. The 2-yr-old child ought to be taught the proper names for the parts of the body, including the genitals. Parents should react calmly when their children explore and manipulate their own bodies with enjoyment, although open masturbation by older children suggests poor awareness of social reality or lack of parental censorship. Parents should inform their children that *masturbation* is not a social activity and should be limited to the bedroom when the child is alone. An overly excited or overly punitive reaction will only serve to excite the child. It is important for masturbation to be accepted as a normal aspect of the child's sexual life and for guilt to be avoided. By puberty, children should be given explanations of its normality. This can be done in conjunction with explanations of ejaculation, orgasm, and menstruation so that children can understand them, too, as normal bodily functions.

It is quite common for preschool children to hug and kiss each other. More explicit sexual behavior, such as oral contact, attempts at simulated intercourse, or anal stimulation are probably learned through observation or direct involvement with older children or adults. Intervention designed to uncover the source of the child's knowledge and appropriate subsequent action is indicated in these situations.

Especially between the ages of 10 and 12 yr, boys and girls typically explore sexual issues with best friends (same-sex friends) as a means of gathering information. This should not be viewed as a prelude for homosexuality but as a developmental stage in most children. At any age, the compulsive need for sex serves as a defense against underlying dependency, separation, and autonomy issues. It is often during adolescence that the final decision about gender object choice is made. The teenager's actual or perceived sexual experiences and their reinforcements are important in shaping the individual's ultimate sexual choices.

Transsexualism, the conviction by a person biologically of one gender that he or she is a member of the other gender, is the most obvious example of gender identity confusion. Transsexual adolescents feel discomfort and a sense of inappropriateness about their assigned sex. They spend years trying to figure out how to get rid of the primary and secondary sexual characteristics that define them biologically. Gender roles of the opposite biologic sex are usually adopted.

The prevalence of transsexualism is 1/30,000 for males and 1/100,000 for females. Individuals with this disorder usually have a difficult time with social and occupational functioning. Concurrent psychopathology and depression are part of the reason; societal consternation is the other part. The natural history of transsexualism is not well understood. A preponderance of adult transsexuals had gender identity disorders as children and adolescents. Extreme femininity in boys is a predisposing factor. Some say that they remember being confused about gender identity as early as 2 yr of age. Which particular effeminate boys will later show transsexual behavior cannot be accurately predicted.

Treatment of transsexualism has taken two directions. Many transsexual adults have opted for hormonal and surgical therapies to produce primary and secondary sexual characteristics of the gender with which they identify. Follow-up studies consistently show continued distress after these treatments. Long-term dynamic and behavioral therapies also have been tried. Although there are anecdotal reports of successful re-identification with the given biologic sex, without statistical controls it is impossible to know whether this represents a response to therapy or a spontaneous change that would have occurred otherwise. Spontaneous remissions have been shown to occur.

Transvestism, cross-dressing, may occur transiently, in preschool boys who dress up in their mothers' clothing, or it may occur chronically in preschool and school-aged boys who feel genuinely excited when dressed in women's clothing. Cross-dressing in girls is rarely an identified problem. Chronic cross-dressing should be a source of parental concern because it is most often associated with other gender role behaviors typically seen in effeminate boys. When parents approach the physician with concerns of chronic cross-dressing in boys, the physician should investigate other areas of gender identification. Does the child verbalize a preference to be the opposite sex? Does the child deny or disparage his or her own sexual anatomy or assert that opposite anatomic structures will develop? Three to 6% of school-aged boys and 10–12% of school-aged girls often behave like the opposite sex, but fewer than 2% of boys and 2–4% of girls actually wish to be the opposite sex.

3.41 GENDER IDENTITY DISORDER (GID)

Persistent distress about being a particular gender while being preoccupied with cross-gender roles or repudiation of given anatomic genital structures is the hallmark of GID. It encompasses transsexualism, transvestism, and effeminacy in boys. The etiology of GID is similar to that postulated for homosexuality.

CLINICAL MANIFESTATIONS. Many GID children develop the disorder prior to 4 yr of age. They are often ostracized by peers and have a difficult social adjustment, sometimes with subsequent depression. One half or more of the boys develop a homosexual orientation during adolescence and adulthood. Because the social opprobrium is so much greater for effeminate boys than for masculine girls, it is often difficult to identify girls with GID, making it difficult to understand the natural course of the disorder in girls. GID is associated with numerous other childhood and adolescent disorders. Using the Child Behavior Checklist, it has been shown that 84% of feminine boys display behavioral disturbances similar to those seen within a clinic population. Sixty per cent endorsed items related to peer difficulties and met the criteria for the diagnosis of separation anxiety disorder. Others have found that GID is unrelated to ethnic background, religion, or educational level.

TREATMENT. The relationship between GID and separation anxiety disorder and other disturbances supports the importance of dynamic, alliance-building psychotherapy. Children with GID are not a heterogeneous group, however. Other approaches are often employed and have been shown to be helpful. Parenting techniques that specify which behaviors are appropriate and what is expected of the child regarding gender role behaviors have shown promise in managing a significant percentage of children with GID. The physician needs to help the parents control their own frustration and disappointment to minimize judgmental, rejecting behavior. Punishment, castigation, or shaming will not support the child's attempts to struggle with whatever intrapsychic, interpersonal, or cultural conflicts exist. Underlying family conflicts and parent-child conflicts need to be managed therapeutically.

3.42 HOMOSEXUALITY

Homosexuality, the romantic and physical attraction to someone of the same gender, has occurred throughout the ages in 5–10% of men and women. Historically, acceptance of homosexuality has waxed and waned within societies. The view is currently held by some that homosexuality is best regarded as an alternative life style. The American Psychiatric Association no longer lists it among mental disorders.

The *etiology* is uncertain. Many view its development as a normal variant of sexual development; others point to problematic parent-child relationships. It has been postulated that an overly close or poor relationship with either parent may predispose a child to homosexuality. The absence of a father figure or a father who is weak or frightening may prevent a boy from identifying with a male role, thereby engendering an overly close mother-son relationship. Wanting to be like his mother, the boy may develop a feminine identification and later seek love and intimacy with males during adolescence. On the other hand, the absence of a mother figure and an overly close relationship with the father can lead to powerful love feelings that influence the adolescent girl's orientation. Distaste for the mother's role as a dominated or abused housewife, or a father's rejection, can contribute to a homosexual orientation. A strongly eroticized attachment may, through the incest taboo, rule out other male choices. Considering the connection between GID and separation anxiety disorder, some boys may become homosexual because of an overidentification with the mother that serves to minimize anxiety secondary to actual or perceived separation. However, there is no appreciable difference between children of lesbian mothers and the general population in social and emotional adaptation or in gender identification. Others choose homosexuality in adolescence as a response to a fear of women or a fear of their own sexual performance with women.

Biologic etiologies have also been proposed. Focusing on the perceived homology between homosexual behavior in humans and lower animals, researchers have proposed the "dual mating center" theory, stating that there are hypothalamic areas that regulate male and female sexual behavior. It is hypothesized that too little androgen production in males during a critical prenatal period causes the female center to overdevelop; conversely, excessive androgen production in females leads to overdevelopment of the male center. Proponents point to the fact that some homosexual men demonstrate "estrogen feedback responses," in which, because of decreased androgen levels, administration of estrogen causes increased production of luteinizing hormone. Many other investigators dispute this theory because of a lack of consistent findings (e.g., XY males with testicular feminization syndrome do not exhibit this response). There may be multiple possible mechanisms leading to homosexual object choice in adolescence and adulthood.

If a child is found to be engaging in homosexual behavior, parents should not immediately suspect that this means that the child has already made a homosexual object choice. Children explore sexually in the same way they explore other parts of their environment. The first task of the physician or parents is to help the younger child feel safe and less guilty. Parents should avoid suspicious, scolding, threatening, shaming, or guilt-inducing attitudes or behaviors toward the child. The physician can serve as a model for the parent through his or her own calm, sensitive, careful exploration of feelings and behavior with the child. The physician should expect denials on the part of the child and avoidance of and embarrassment with the subject, but discussion will help the child to understand that sexual behavior is comprehensible and that sexual feelings and curiosity are normal. It is important to know whether the child's information and understanding of sexual matters are appropriate to his or her age.

If the same-sex behavior involves another child in the family, he or she should be treated in the same manner. If an older child is the initiator or seducer, he or she should be told clearly and firmly that such behavior will not be tolerated and that he or she will be expected to act with responsibility and control. The older child should talk with a physician or mental health professional, and if concerns about emotional and social adjustment become evident, referral for psychiatric evaluation is indicated. Physicians must not let their own negative feelings aggravate the disgust, anger, or punitive feelings that parents may have for an older child seen as a perpetrator, especially if the older child is not a member of the younger child's family. The physician may need to help parents of exploited children refrain from ill-considered acts of revenge against offenders. If, on the other hand, there has been physical violence or psychologic coercion, both psychiatric and legal interventions are indicated.

Very little can be done to change one's sexual object choice unless that individual wants to change. Even in these cases, significantly fewer than half of those who try are able to change sexual orientation with various behavioral and dynamic therapies. Psychotherapy is more appropriately used for concurrent disorders (separation anxiety disorder, conduct disorder, dysthymic disorder, depression). Families usually need assistance in coping with this knowledge and their attendant anger and disappointment. Children need help in understanding how to cope with the reactions of others.

3.43 PSYCHOSIS IN CHILDHOOD

EARLY ONSET

3.44 INFANTILE AUTISM

This psychosis develops before 30 mo of age. It is characterized by a qualitative impairment in verbal and nonverbal communication, in imaginative activity, and in reciprocal social interactions.

CLINICAL MANIFESTATIONS. Among the most notable symptoms and signs are nondeveloped or poorly developed verbal and nonverbal communication skills, abnormalities in speech patterns, impaired ability to sustain a conversation, abnormal social play, lack of empathy, and an inability to make friends. Stereotypic body movements, a marked need for sameness, very narrow interests, and a preoccupation with parts of the body are also frequent. The autistic child is withdrawn and often spends hours in solitary play. Ritualistic behavior prevails, reflecting the child's need to maintain a consistent, predictable environment. Tantrum-like rages may accompany disruptions of routine. Eye contact is minimal or absent. Visual scanning of hand and finger movements, mouthing of objects, and rubbing of surfaces may indicate a heightened awareness and sensitivity to some stimuli, whereas diminished responses to pain and lack of startle responses to sudden loud noises reflect lowered sensitivity to other stimuli. If speech is present, echolalia, pronomial reversal, nonsense rhyming, and other idiosyncratic language forms may predominate.

IQ by conventional psychologic testing usually falls in the functionally retarded range; however, the deficits in language and socialization make it difficult to obtain an accurate estimate of the autistic child's intellectual potential. Some autistic children perform adequately in nonverbal tests, and those with developed speech may demonstrate adequate intellectual capacity. Occasionally, an autistic child may have an isolated, remarkable talent, analogous to that of the adult autistic savant.

Although first described as a social illness, most research studies have focused on the communicative and cognitive deficits of autism and particularly on the types of cognitive processing deficits most apparent in emotional situations. Deficits in verbal sequencing, abstraction, rote memory, and reciprocal verbal exchange are typical in autistic children.

EPIDEMIOLOGY. The prevalence is generally thought to be 3–4/10,000 children, although a North Dakota study found 21 children among 180,000 who met the criteria for the diagnosis of infantile autism. The disorder is much more common in males than in females (3–4:1). Autism tends to be more common in siblings of autistic children than in the general population. Several systemic, infectious, and neurologic illnesses produce autistic-like symptoms or predispose patients to the development of autistic symptoms. An increased association with seizures also has been noted.

ETIOLOGY. The cause of autism is speculative. Theories have centered on a variety of possibilities, including brain injury, constitutional vulnerability, developmental aphasia, deficits in the reticular activating system, an unfortunate interplay between psychogenic and neurodevelopmental factors, and structural cerebellar changes. Dopamine functioning appears to be normal in autistic children who have not been treated with neuroleptics. Contrary to notions in vogue in the past, autism is not induced by parents.

TREATMENT. Different therapeutic approaches have been advocated to treat and manage autistic children, but success has been limited. Gains in speech acquisition have been reported with behavior therapy utilizing operant conditioning. Destructive behavior and aggression can often be modified by behavior management. Neuroleptics have shown promise in reducing self-injurious behavior, outwardly directed aggression, stereotypic behavior, and social withdrawal. Potent opiate antagonists have recently been shown to alter behavioral problems, withdrawal, and stereotypies. Day treatment models using play, language therapy, and structured interpersonal exercises have also shown promise.

PROGNOSIS. This is guarded. Some children, especially those with speech, may grow up to live marginal, self-sufficient, albeit isolated, lives in the community, but for most, chronic placement in institutions is the ultimate outcome. The relationship between autism and schizophrenia is uncertain. Cases in which autistic children have later developed schizophrenia have been reported but are not common.

3.45 PERVASIVE DEVELOPMENTAL DISORDER

Some children have a qualitative impairment in the development of reciprocal social interaction and verbal and nonverbal communication but do not have the quantity of symptoms necessary for a diagnosis of autism. Though somewhat socially aware, these children appear to others to be peculiar and eccentric. The prevalence is said to be 2.0/10,000 children. In adulthood, these patients are often diagnosed as having a schizoid personality disorder or Asperger syndrome.

LATE ONSET

Psychotic reactions in older children tend more closely to resemble the psychoses of adulthood, and the same diagnostic criteria apply. Affective psychoses have been described earlier.

In *childhood schizophrenia*, prominent symptoms include thought disorder, delusions, and hallucinations. The latter two symptoms, in addition to later onset, higher IQ scores, and fewer perinatal complications, differentiate schizophrenia from autism. As the symptoms imply, schizophrenic children often appear to be chaotic. They may have paranoid delusions, aggressive behavior, hebephrenic silliness, social withdrawal, and alternating moods not apparently related to environmental stimuli, among other possibilities.

The prevalence of adult schizophrenia is 1% of the population. Because the typical age of onset is late adolescence to early adulthood, a very small percentage of preschool and latency-aged children actually show symptoms that meet the criteria for a diagnosis of schizophrenia. The prognosis is poor. The symptoms in childhood that most predict psychotic adult psychopathology are affective blunting and disturbed interpersonal relationships, as opposed to delusions and hallucinations.

A multimodal therapeutic approach is necessary to manage this illness. Parent training is necessary to teach effective techniques to modify the schizophrenic child's behavior to a reasonable extent. Individual therapy designed to build a positive alliance is also very important. Neuroleptic therapy is often effective in managing hallucinations and psychotic delusions. School and community liaison work can establish and maintain a day-to-day schedule for the patient.

3.46 BORDERLINE PERSONALITY DISORDER

The majority of children with late-onset psychosis suffer from this disorder, also called interactive psychosis or symbiotic psychosis. These children present with a marked instability of mood, interpersonal relationships, and sense of self. They make suicidal threats and gestures, often abuse themselves and others physically, and are very impulsive. Behavioral disorders are almost always present, and unpredictability is frequent, as are rage reactions and manipulativeness. They rarely hallucinate, although they may be suspicious and have paranoid-like thinking.

Although underlying biologic vulnerabilities may be present, most of these children experience a great deal of difficulty with attachment and separation issues. Their behavior often seems to be a product of the child's underlying desire to maintain a self-image of being the center of his or her own environment. Rage reactions result when this desire is frustrated. These children require very consistently applied limits in addition to alliance-building dynamic psychotherapy designed to improve object relations.

Most nonorganically induced psychotic reactions and behaviors in children are a product of either autism, pervasive developmental disorder, affective disorder, schizophrenia, or borderline personality disorder. Some children may present with intermittent psychotic-like behavior (withdrawal, hysterical acting-out) in response to a traumatic situation or an ongoing series of psychologic and physical insults. These are either post-traumatic or adjustment reactions.

3.47 PSYCHOLOGIC TREATMENT OF CHILDREN AND ADOLESCENTS

All clinical phenomena relate to a variety of organizational levels: molecular, anatomic, physiologic, intrapsychic, interpersonal, familial, and social. Accordingly, the physician should focus on the patient's discomfort rather than on a categorization of clinical manifestations as either organically or psychologically determined. The psychologic aspects of illness should be evaluated from the outset, and the physician should act as a model for the parents and the child by showing interest in the child's feelings and demonstrating that it is possible and appropriate to communicate discomfort in verbal, symbolic language.

For *the hospitalized child*, potential challenges include coping with separation, adapting to a new environment, adjusting to multiple caregivers, often associating with very sick children, and sometimes experiencing the disorientation of intensive care, anesthesia, and surgery. To help mitigate potential problems, a preadmission visit to the hospital is often important to meet the people who will be offering care and to ask questions about what will happen. For children under 5–6 yr of age, parents should room with the child if feasible. Creative and active recreational or socialization programs, with liberal visiting hours (including visits from siblings), and chances to act out feared procedures in play with dolls or mannequins are all helpful. Sensitive, sympathetic, and accepting attitudes toward the child and parents by the hospital staff are very important. There is often an underlying tension between the hospital caregivers and the parents. Hospital routines and schedules often serve to complicate the relationship between parents and hospital workers. Guilt and anger can result, unnecessarily complicating an already difficult situation.

Ambulatory care in clinics where patients receive discontinuous care from a series of physicians whose intercommunication is often limited may create a problem. Parents often become confused and unable to verbalize major concerns about their children. Recommendations for care may become inappropriate or irrelevant, and compliance with advice or directions becomes poor. At the end of any initial diagnostic or management activity, the physician should habitually inquire whether there are other things parents or children may wish to ask or talk about during this visit. In busy emergency rooms of hospitals and urban centers, conflicting expectations between how the professional staff expects the emergency room to be used and what patients actually need can lead to confusion. When these different expectations are critically examined, ways may be found to deal more effectively with the patterns of use of emergency services.

With *chronically or fatally ill children*, every symptom is experienced by the patient and parent as a threat to physical integrity and life. The more serious the clinical state, the greater the intensity of the emotions aroused. By 9 yr of age, children begin to conceive of death as meaning more than just going away. By adolescence they think of death in philosophic terms much as adults do, albeit with limited experience.

In dealing with chronic illness that shortens life, such as cystic fibrosis, parents need the physician's early support in developing a relatively guilt-free understanding of the disease and how to manage it. They need guidance to help them comfortably answer the child's questions about the disease. The young child will take most cues from the parents. With the older child, and especially the adolescent, parents must be prepared to deal with the anger of the child because of his or her fate. The child needs both the parents' psychologic strengths and resources and the physician's availability and objectivity.

The role of the physician is difficult. He or she must stand for hope and for relief of discomfort, ready to help parents and child avoid emotionally crippling psychologic handicaps. For example, parents must be encouraged to meet their own needs, even when this requires temporary and perhaps recurrent separation from the child; at times this may help the child to learn to tolerate frustration. Parents of critically or fatally ill children may creatively support each other in group meetings under the professional guidance of physicians, psychologists, or social workers.

In *potentially fulminant lethal processes,* the intensity of parental anxiety, guilt, and despair may be greater than it is with more chronic illnesses. With most children over 9–10 yr of age it is most supportive to treat fatal illness factually with the child, so far as diagnosis and prognosis are concerned, but always offering realistic hope. Children do not usually ask the physician if and when they are going to die, though they may reveal their fears to others in the hospital. Young children primarily want to be reassured that their parents will not desert them and that they are loved. A hospital team approach representing medical, nursing, psychologic, and social work disciplines, among others, should provide support. The primary physician needs to stay involved and close to the child and to the clinical situation.

Organ transplants in children have most often involved the kidney. Dialysis may precede renal transplant for varying lengths of time and begins in the hospital, but parents may be expected to learn to carry out this procedure at home. They may be ambivalent about being given control of a life-threatening process. The child receiving dialysis becomes psychologically dependent and often withdrawn. Bone marrow transplants also involve many psychologic considerations, such as donor relationships and the stress of isolation.

Family problems multiply with the question of who will donate an organ. If relatives are available as donors, there may be tension about who should "make the sacrifice." In some cases guilt may be relieved if the physician arbitrarily (but thoughtfully) makes this decision. A medical support team of carefully chosen staff is essential to facilitate decision-making and continuing care. Although there is a high suicide rate among adults on hemodialysis, this procedure appears to be less traumatic in children, probably owing to the child's greater capacities for denial and acceptance of a support system. Adolescents are concerned with distortions of body image, which they cannot always express verbally.

After *the death of a child* the parents will need opportunities to talk out their feelings with the physician, one of whose goals should be to help them avoid psychologically encapsulating the lost child in an unmourned state. Many parents can be helped and comforted by being with and holding the dying infant or child or seeing and touching him or her after death. The physician needs the patience to listen (both to the stated and to the implied questions and misconceptions), to answer questions, and to help families with funeral arrangements (see Sec. 3.59).

3.48 PSYCHOPHARMACOLOGY
(Table 3–14)

Using drugs to modify children's behavior is controversial. Their effects on behavior are influenced by the maturity of the central nervous system, by intrapsychic and psychosocial factors, by the personality or charisma of the physician prescribing them, by the problem itself, and by the milieu (e.g., patient, parents, time of day given).

Neuroleptics are appropriately used for hallucinations, delusions, thought disorders, and severe agitation. They are primarily indicated for children and adolescents suffering with schizophrenic disorders, mood-congruent and mood-incongruent psychotic reactions secondary to major affective disorders, pervasive developmental disorders, autistic patients presenting with stereotypic and withdrawal symptoms and self-abuse, and Gilles de la Tourette syndrome. Some advocate the use of haloperidol for aggressive behavior in children and adolescents, but this usage remains somewhat controversial. Serious question has been raised about the efficacy of neuroleptics in childhood schizophrenia. This class of medicine is inappropriately used for anxiety, conduct disorder without extreme aggression, and attention deficit disorder.

Neuroleptics can be subdivided into low-potency, midpotency, and high-potency types. Chlorpromazine and thioridazine are both low-potency medicines and usually require a higher dose than the other neuroleptics for symptom remission. They are both rather sedative, producing numerous anticholinergic side effects but causing comparatively fewer extrapyramidal symptoms. Mesoridazine, a midpotency medicine, produces more extrapyramidal symptoms than the low-potency drugs. Thiothixene (Navane) and haloperidol (Haldol) are high-potency medicines that produce comparatively the greatest number of extrapyramidal symptoms.

The most worrisome side effect of the neuroleptics is the development of *tardive dyskinesia.* This is characterized by choreoathetoid movements of trunk, limbs, and facial musculature; these movements develop in approximately 20–30% of children treated long-term with neuroleptics. Dyskinesia can occur during the treatment with the drug or after it has been discontinued, in which case it is referred to as withdrawal dyskinesia. This latter type of dyskinesia, whose symptoms can include nausea, vomiting, diaphoresis, ataxia, oral dyskinesia, and various dystonic movements, is reversible in most cases, whereas the dyskinesia developing during drug use improves in only one half to two thirds of appropriately managed cases. The treatment involves decreasing or discontinuing the medication if possible, although it has been noted that increasing the neuroleptic causes a temporary diminution of dyskinetic symptoms. Prophylactic measures involving drug-free holidays and periodic discontinuation of neuroleptics are also advisable to help mitigate the development of tardive dyskinesia.

Extrapyramidal symptoms, a Parkinson-like syndrome (akisthesia, bradykinesis, torticollis, drooling, and involuntary hand movements, among others), develop in at least one fourth of children treated with neuroleptics. The imbalance created by the dopaminergic blocking action of the antipsychotic medication disrupts a needed balance between that system and the cholinergic system within the basal ganglia. The high-potency neuroleptics, which contain few anticholinergic properties, are the most likely to produce extrapyramidal symptoms. This syndrome can be treated by decreasing the neuroleptic or adding an anticholinergic agent (trihexyphenidyl HCl, benztropine mesylate).

Stimulant medications are used to treat the signs and symptoms of attention deficit hyperactivity disorder. Although the mechanism of action is not entirely clear, these medications have been shown to increase children's ability to attend, to improve classroom behavior, and to increase social acceptance in various situations. These stimulants should be used concurrently with individual, family, and community therapy, but often this is not done.

Antidepressants and lithium carbonate are useful in the treatment of patients with affective disorders. Antidepressants generally are effective for depression, whereas lithium has shown efficacy with mania. Bipolar and unipolar adult patients are often treated with long-term pharmacotherapy, and this is becoming more common in childhood and adolescence. Because of the propensity of tricyclic antidepressants to cause heart block, a pretreatment electrocardiogram (ECG) and follow-up ECGs are necessary. Children and adolescents taking tricyclic antidepressants should be followed by serial blood levels until an adequate dose is determined. This usually takes at least a few weeks. A pretreatment lithium evaluation includes thyroid studies and renal function tests. Lithium blood levels should also be determined adequately while the patient is taking the medication.

Other medicines have shown clinical efficacy in pediatric psychiatric patients. *Clonidine* has been partially successful in treating children with attention deficit hyperactivity disorder as well as in those who have a personal history of tics (including Gilles de la Tourette syndrome). *Pimozide* has been shown to reduce vocal and motor tics effectively in both tic disorder and Gilles de la Tourette syndrome. *Carbamazepine*, an antiepileptic medicine, is effective in the treatment of mania and episodic dyscontrol syndrome. β-*Blocking agents* (Nadolol) appear to decrease aggressiveness in the mentally retarded; their use as an antianxiety agent with adults has been well established. *Opiate antagonists* significantly change some behaviors in autistic children and have promise in the treatment of self-injurious behavior in severely and profoundly mentally retarded individuals. *Clomipramine* is efficacious in the treatment of obsessive-compulsive disorder. Seizures have been reported secondary to its use, however.

Because some parents are adamantly opposed to the use of psychotropic medications, the physician contemplating their use must make sure of parental attitudes. If drugs are used, it should be for as short a time as possible. As with any clinical disorder, the physician should avoid using multiple medications and should not shift back and forth from one medication to another when no immediate response occurs. Because psychotropic medications have significant biochemical effects on the developing child, it is important for the physician to give an appropriate explanation to the parents and child about the rationale for medication. Even with thought disorders, in which chemotherapy has a definite place, medication is rarely if ever the sole treatment indicated. The complexity of emotional conditions demands an integrated approach involving various therapies: psychodynamic (individual, family, or group), behavioral, milieu, medication, and the use of resources in the family, school, and community. These factors must be knowledgeably selected, judiciously coordinated, and skillfully applied to ensure that maximal benefit for the child results.

3.49 PSYCHOTHERAPY

When it has been determined that psychopathology exists in a child or within a family that requires intervention, the

TABLE 3–14. Psychopharmacology

Medication Class	Indications	Dosage	Side Effects/Toxicity/Cautions
Antipsychotics	All classes: Severe agitation; childhood and adolescent schizophrenia; emotional lability and aggressiveness; pervasive developmental disorder; mania; stereotypic symptoms of pervasive developmental disorder and autism; self-abuse, pica, and aggressiveness in mental retardation High-potency class: Gilles de la Tourette syndrome; other tic disorders (haloperidol)	Low-potency: 30–150 mg/24 hr in divided doses; available in concentrated form Mid-potency: 10–75 mg/24 hr in divided doses High-potency: 1–6 mg/24 hr in divided doses	All classes: Sedation, weight gain; anticholinergic effects (dry mouth, blurred vision, constipation); hypersensitivity reactions (hepatic, skin); blood dyscrasias; parkinsonism Long-term effects: Risk of tardive dyskinesia and "withdrawal-emergent" syndrome (see text)
Low potency/high dosage: Thioridazine (Mellaril), Chlorpromazine (Thorazine)			
Midpotency/mid-dosage: Mesoridazine (Serentil)			
High potency/low dosage: Trifluoperazine (Stelazine), Thiothixene (Navane), Haloperidol (Haldol)			
Stimulants (6 yr and older)			Insomnia, decreased appetite, possible weight loss; irritability and tearfulness; abdominal pain, headache; elevated systolic blood pressure; development and worsening of tics. A long-term effect may be height and weight reduction (Sec. 3.39). *Pemoline* is associated with hypersensitivity reactions, especially hepatic
Methylphenidate (Ritalin)	Attention deficit disorder	0.3–1.0 mg/kg/24 hr	
Dextroamphetamine (Dexedrine)	Attention deficit disorder	0.2–0.5 mg/kg/24 hr	
Pemoline (Cylert)	Attention deficit disorder	37.5–112.5 mg/24 hr	
Antidepressants			
Desipramine (Norpramin)	Major depressive disorder; separation anxiety; attention deficit disorder unresponsive to stimulants (12 yr and older)	For major depressive disorder and separation anxiety; 2–3 mg/kg/24 hr in divided doses	ECG and blood pressure should be monitored for hypertension, orthostatic hypotension, cardiac arrhythmia, or lengthening of PR or QRS interval (see Sec. 3.34). Monitor plasma levels for therapeutic range
Fluoxetine (Prozac)	Major depressive disorder (12 yr and older)	20–40 mg/24 hr	Agitation, insomnia, appetite and weight loss

pediatrician may develop and implement the therapeutic plan or may refer to a more specialized level of care within the community. The choice of treatment should be left to the consultant, with the referring physician reassuring the family and patient that close communication with the consultant will be maintained. The primary physician should continue to evaluate the child's progress throughout the treatment process and to provide medical care for the patient.

There are many types of individual psychotherapy. Most involve the development of an alliance with the patient that provides an opportunity to look at the problems precipitating therapy. Younger children often express their concerns and developmental issues in play therapy, a specific modality designed to foster symbolic and metaphoric individual expression. Older children and adolescents are more likely to participate in talking during therapy. *Dynamic therapy* is designed to understand the psychologic motivations for the child's problems and to develop a therapeutic process based on that understanding. *Behavior therapy* is used to modify specific behaviors through consistently applied positive and negative reinforcements.

There are several types of *family therapy:* directive, structural, strategic, and object-relations. In each, the therapist works primarily with the family to impart understanding or to help organize change. A particular directive approach, *parent management training,* is very useful in the treatment of conduct disorders. This approach involves training parents to respond in specific and consistent ways to the child's behavior.

Group therapy is especially useful for children suffering from poorly developed social skills. Group therapy for preadolescents tends to emphasize physical and other structured activities through which therapist and children alike can discover how they relate to each other and find ways to change. It is an especially profitable approach for treating the social problems of adolescents.

Barriers to involving the generalist or pediatrician in psychotherapeutic activities with children include a presumed lack of time and lack of adequate conceptual background. Although psychotherapy primarily emphasizes listening and interviewing, two skills important to all fields of medicine, experience is an important and necessary asset for the psychotherapist.

3.50 HOSPITALIZATION

At times hospitalization of the disturbed or emotionally ill child in a general or pediatric hospital is helpful or necessary, and it may serve a number of functions. In children with many psychosomatic disorders or in a suicidal or drugged adolescent, indications may be medical as well as psychiatric. If treatment of a child in a psychiatric hospital is thought necessary, consultation with a child psychiatrist or social agency is essential for decision-making and planning. Admission to residential treatment reflects the family's decompensation as often as the child's.

RICHARD F. DALTON, JR.
MARC A. FORMAN
BETTY A. MULLER

GENERAL

Adams PL, Fras I: Beginning Child Psychiatry. New York, Brunner/Mazel, 1988.
Chess S, Hassibi M: Principles and Practice of Child Psychiatry, 2nd ed. New York, Plenum, 1986.
Erikson E: Childhood and Society, 2nd ed. New York, Norton, 1963.
Flavell JH: The Developmental Psychology of Jean Piaget. Princeton, Van Nostrand, 1963.
Kagan J: The Nature of the Child. New York, Basic Books, 1984.
Rutter M, Herzov L (eds): Child and Adolescent Psychiatry, 2nd ed. Oxford, Blackwell, 1985.

CHILD AND ADOLESCENT DEVELOPMENT

Ainsworth M: Object relations, dependency, and attachment: A theoretical review of the infant-mother relationship. Child Dev 40:969, 1969.
Aronfreed J: Conduct and Conscience: The Socialization of Internalized Control Over Behavior. New York, Academic Press, 1968.
Bakeman R, Brown JV: Early interaction: Consequences for social and mental development at three years. Child Dev 51:437, 1980.
Belsky J: Infant day care and socioemotional development: The United States. J Child Psychol Psychiatry 29:397, 1988.
Belsky J, Rovine M: Non-maternal care in the first year of life and the security of infant-parent attachment. Child Dev 59:157, 1988.
Bloom B: Support for families with unsuccessful pregnancies. Birth Defects 23:45, 1987.
Bowlby J: Attachment. New York, Basic Books, 1969.
Bowlby J: Attachment and Loss, Vol. 2. Separation. New York, Basic Books, 1973.
Carey WB, McDevitt SC: Revision of the infant temperament questionnaire. Pediatrics 61:735, 1978.
Chess S: The plasticity of human development. J Am Acad Child Adol Psychiatry 17:80, 1978.
Clarke ADB, Clarke AM: Constancy and change in the growth of human characteristics. J Child Psychol Psychiatry 25:191, 1984.
Coates S, Person E: Extreme boyhood femininity: Isolated behavior or pervasive disorder? J Am Acad Child Adol Psychiatry 24:702, 1985.
Davis D, Stewart M, Harmon R: Postponing pregnancy after perinatal death: Perspectives on doctor advice. J Am Acad Child Adol Psychiatry 28:481, 1989.
Deur JL: The effects of inconsistent punishment on aggression in children. Dev Psychobiol 2:403, 1970.
Dunn J: Sibling influences on childhood development. J Child Psychol Psychiatry 29:119, 1988.
Fagot B, Leinbach M: Gender identity: Some thoughts on an old concept. J Am Acad Child Adol Psychiatry 24:684, 1985.
Fullard W, McDevitt SC, Carey WB: Assessing temperament in one to three year old children. J Pediatr Psychol 9:205, 1984.
Ginsburg H, Opper S: Piaget's theory of intellectual development, 2nd ed. Englewood Cliffs, NJ, Prentice-Hall, 1979.
Green R: Atypical sex role behavior. *In:* Noshpitz JD (ed): Basic Handbook of Child Psychiatry. New York, Basic Books, 1979.
Green R: Sexual identity of 37 children raised by homosexual and transsexual parents. Am J Psychiatry 135:692, 1978.
Graham M, Thompson S, Estrada M, et al: Factors affecting psychological adjustment to a fetal death. Am J Obstet Gynecol 157:254, 1987.
Gross R, Duke P: The effect of early versus late maturation on adolescent behavior. Pediatr Clin North Am 27:71, 1980.
Hegvik RL, McDevitt SC, Carey WB: The middle childhood temperament questionnaire. J Dev Behav Pediatr 3:197, 1982.
Hodgman C: Current issues in adolescent psychiatry. Hosp Comm Psychiatry 34:514, 1983.
Jones M: Psychological correlates of somatic development. Child Dev 36:899, 1965.
Kagan J: Acquisition and significance of sex typing and sex role identity. *In:* Hoffman ML, Hoffman LW (eds): Review of Child Development Research, Vol. 1. New York, Russell Sage Foundation, 1964.
Kaplan H, Freedman A, Sadock B: Comprehensive Textbook of Psychiatry, Vol. 3. Baltimore, Williams & Wilkins, 1980.
Klaus M, Kennell J: Parent-Infant Bonding, 2nd ed. St. Louis, CV Mosby, 1982.
Kohlberg L: Stages of moral development as the basis for moral education. *In:* Beck C, Sullivan E, Crittendon D (eds): Moral Education. Toronto, University of Toronto Press, 1971.
Landenburger G, Delp K: An approach for supportive care before, during, and after selective abortion. Birth Defects 23:84, 1987.
Mahler M, Pine F, Bergman A: The Psychological Birth of the Human Infant. New York, Basic Books, 1975.
Masterson JF: The psychiatric significance of adolescent turmoil. Am J Psychiatry 124:107, 1968.
McCartney K, Galanopoulos A: Child care and attachment: A new frontier the second time around. Am J Orthopsychiatry 58:16, 1988.
McDevitt SC, Carey WB: The measurement of temperament in 3–7 year old children. J Child Psychol Psychiatry 19:245, 1978.
Money J, Ekhardt AA: Man and Woman, Boy and Girl. Baltimore, Johns Hopkins University Press, 1972.
Ounstead C, Taylor DC (eds): Gender Differences: Their Ontogeny and Significance. Edinburgh, Churchill Livingstone, 1972.
Parke RD: The role of punishment in the socialization process. *In:* Hoppe RA, Milton GA, Simmel EC (eds): Early Experience and the Process of Socialization. New York, Academic Press, 1970.
Rutter M, Chadwick OFD, Yule W: Adolescent turmoil: Fact or fiction? J Child Psychol Psychiatry 17:35, 1976.
Schonfeld W: Adolescent development: Biological, psychological, and sociological determinants. Adol Psychiatry 1:296, 1971.

Schwartz J, Strickland RG, Krolick G: Infant day care: Behavioral effects at preschool age. Dev Psychol 10:502, 1974.
Siegel AE: Working mothers and their children. J Am Acad Child Adol Psychiatry 23:486, 1984.
Smith BM: Competence and socialization. *In:* Clausen JA (ed): Socialization and Society. Boston, Little, Brown, 1968.
Sorensen RC: Adolescent Sexuality in Contemporary America. New York, World Publishing, 1972.
Stierman E: Emotional aspects of perinatal death. Clin Obstet Gynecol 30:352, 1987.
Theut S, Pederson F, Zaslow M, et al: Perinatal loss and parental bereavement. Am J Psychiatry 146:635, 1989.
Thomson E: Early pregnancy loss. Birth Defects 23:37, 1987.
Winnicott D: Playing and Reality. London, Tavistock, 1971.
Zeanah C: Adaptation following perinatal loss: A critical review. J Am Acad Child Adol Psychiatry 28:467, 1989.
Zigler E, Hall N: Day care and its effect on children: An overview for pediatric health professionals. Dev Behav Pediatr 9:38, 1988.
Zelnik M, Kantner JF: Sexual activity, contraceptive use and pregnancy among metropolitan-area teenagers: 1971–1979. Fam Plan Perspect 12:230, 1980.

SOCIAL ISSUES

Abarbanel L: Shared parenting after separation and divorce: A study of joint custody. Am J Orthopsychiatry 49:320, 1979.
Derdeyn AP, Scott E: Joint custody: A critical analysis and appraisal. Am J Orthopsychiatry 54:199, 1984.
Eisenberg L: The sins of the fathers: Urban decay and social pathology. Am J Orthopsychiatry 32:5, 1962.
Fine S: Children in divorce, custody and access situations: The contributions of the mental health professional. J Child Psychol Psychiatry 21:353, 1980.
Gardner R: The Boys' and Girls' Book About Divorce. New York, Science House, 1970.
Goodman JD, Silberstein RM, Mandell W: Adopted children brought to child psychiatric clinics. Arch Gen Psychiatry 9:451, 1963.
Ilfield F, Ilfield H, Alexander JR: Does joint custody work? A first look at outcome data of relitigation. Am J Psychiatry 139:62, 1982.
Keilin WG, Bloom LJ: Child custody evaluations: A survey of experienced professionals. Prof Psychol 17:338, 1986.
Nagy M: The child's meaning of death. *In:* Feifel H (ed): The Meaning of Death. New York, McGraw-Hill, 1959.
Rothenberg MB: The role of television in shaping the attitudes of children. J Am Acad Child Adol Psychiatry 22:86, 1983.
Rutter M, Maughan B, Mortimore P, et al: Fifteen Thousand Hours: Secondary Schools and Their Effects on Children. London, Open Books, 1979.
Steinman S: The experience of children in a joint custody arrangement: A report of a study. Am J Orthopsychiatry 51:403, 1981.
Wallerstein JS: Children of divorce: The psychological tasks of the child. Am J Orthopsychiatry 53:230, 1983.
Wallerstein JS, Blakeslee S: Second Chances: Men, Women and Children a Decade After Divorce. London, Ticknor & Fields, 1989.
Wallerstein JS, Kelly JB: Surviving the Breakup: How Children Actually Cope with Divorce. New York, Basic Books, 1980.
Wolfenstein M: How is mourning possible? *In:* The Psychoanalytic Study of the Child. New York, International Universities Press, 1966.

ASSESSMENT AND INTERVIEWING

Achenbach TM, Edelbrock CS: Manual for Child Behavior Checklist and Revised Child Behavior Profile. Burlington, University of Vermont, Dept of Psychiatry, 1983.
Ainsworth MDS, Bell SM: Attachment, exploration, and separation illustrated by the behavior of one-year-olds in a strange situation. Child Dev 41:49, 1970.
Barnard KE, Eyres SJ (eds): Child Health Assessment, Part 2: The First Year of Life. Publ. No. DHEW HRA 79-25. Washington D.C., US Government Printing Office, 1979.
Cohen DJ: The diagnostic process in child psychiatry. Psychiatr Ann 6:29, 1976.
Conners CK: A teacher rating scale for use in drug studies with children. Am J Psychiatry 126:884, 1969.
Freeman RD: The home visit in child psychiatry: Its usefulness in diagnosis and training. J Am Acad Child Adol Psychiatry 6:276, 1967.
Goodall J: Opening windows into a child's mind. Dev Med Child Neurol 18:173, 1976.
Hodges K, McKnew D, Cytryn L, et al: The Child Assessment Schedule (CAS) diagnostic interview: A report on reliability and validity. J Am Acad Child Adol Psychiatry 21:468, 1982.
Rich J: Interviewing Children and Adolescents. London, Macmillan, 1968.
Simmons JE: Psychiatric Examination of Children, 4th ed. Philadelphia, Lea & Febiger, 1987.
Wood DJ: Talking to young children. Dev Med Child Neurol 24:856, 1982.

PSYCHOSOCIAL DISORDERS

Ablon SL, Mark JE: Sleep disorders. *In:* Noshpitz JD (ed): Basic Handbook of Child Psychiatry. New York, Basic Books, 1979, pp 643–660.
American Psychiatric Association: Diagnostic and Statistical Manual of Mental Disorders III-R. Washington, DC, American Psychiatric Association, 1987.
August GJ, Stewart MA: Familial subtypes of childhood hyperactivity. J Nerv Ment Dis 171:362, 1983.
Bandura A: Aggression: A Social Learning Analysis. Engelwood Cliffs, NJ, Prentice-Hall, 1973.
Beeghly JHL: Anxiety and anxiety disorders in childhood. *In:* Munoz RA (ed): Treating Anxiety Disorders. New Directions for Mental Health Services. San Francisco, Jossey-Bass, 1986.
Berg I: Day wetting in children. J Child Psychol Psychiatry 16:289, 1975.
Bernstein G, Garfinkel B: School phobia: The overlap of affective and anxiety disorders. J Am Acad Child Adol Psychiatry 25:235, 1986.
Bleiberg E, Jackson L, Ross J: Gender identity disorder and object loss. J Am Acad Child Adol Psychiatry 25:58, 1986.
Cantwell D: Depressive disorders in children. Psychiatr Clin North Am 8:779, 1985.
Carlson G, Asarnow J, Orbach I: Developmental aspects of suicidal behavior in children. J Am Acad Child Adol Psychiatry 26:186, 1987.
Chess S: Autism in children with congenital rubella. J Autism Child Schizophrenia 1:33, 1971.
Costello AJ: Assessment and diagnosis of affective disorders in children. J Child Psychol Psychiatry 27:565, 1986.
Earls F: The epidemiology of depression in children and adolescents. Pediatr Ann 13:23, 1984.
Eisenberg L: The epidemiology of suicide in adolescents. Pediatr Ann 13:47, 1984.
Eron L, Walden L, Lefkowitz M: Learning of Aggression in Children. Boston, Little Brown, 1971.
Eth S, Pynoos R: Post-Traumatic Stress Disorder in Children. Washington, DC, APA Press, 1985.
Forman MA: Psychosomatic illness. *In:* Gellis S, Kagan B (eds): Current Pediatric Therapy 12. Philadelphia, WB Saunders, 1986.
Garber J, Kriss M, Koch M, et al: Recurrent depression in adolescents: A follow-up study. J Am Acad Child Adol Psychiatry 27:49, 1988.
Garfinkel BD, Froese A, Hood J: Suicide attempts in children and adolescents. Am J Psychiatry 139:1257, 1982.
Golombok S, Spencer A, Rutter M: Children in lesbian and single-parent households: Psychosexual and psychiatric appraisal. J Child Psychol Psychiatry 24:551, 1983.
Goodyer I: Hysterical conversion reactions in childhood. J Child Psychol Psychiatry 22:179, 1981.
Graham FK, Ernhardt CB, Thurston CB, et al: Development three years after perinatal anoxia and other potentially damaging newborn experiences. Psychol Monographs 76:1, 1962.
Graham P, Rutter M: Organic brain dysfunction and child psychiatric disorder. Br Med J 3:697, 1968.
Greenberg HR, Sarner CA: Trichotillomania: Symptoms and syndrome. Arch Gen Psychiatry 12:482, 1965.
Greenman DA, Gunderson JG, Cane M, et al: An examination of the borderline diagnosis in children. Am J Psychiatry 143:8, 1986.
Gross M, Tofanelli R, Butzinus S, et al: The effect of diets rich in and free from additives on the behavior of children with hyperkinetic and learning disorders. J Am Acad Child Adol Psychiatry 26:53, 1987.
Guilleminault C, Anders TF: Sleep disorders in children. *In:* Schulman I (ed): Advances in Pediatrics, Vol. 22. Chicago, Year Book Medical Publishers, 1976.
Haenlein M, Caul W: Attention deficit disorder with hyperactivity: A specific hypothesis of reward dysfunction. J Am Acad Child Adol Psychiatry 26:356, 1987.
Hansen CR, Cohen D: Multimodality approaches in the treatment of attention deficit disorders. Pediatr Clin North Am 31:499, 1984.
Hawton K: Suicide and Attempted Suicide among Children and Adolescents. Beverly Hills, Sage Publications, 1986.
Hersov L: Emotional disorders. *In:* Rutter M, Hersov L (eds): Child and Adolescent Psychiatry, 2nd ed. Oxford, Blackwell, 1985.
Hetznecker W, Forman MA: Developmental issues and psychosocial problems in children: I. Normal development and minor behavioral problems. II: More serious behavioral and performance disorders. *In:* Smith DWS (ed): Introduction to Clinical Pediatrics, 2nd ed. Philadelphia, WB Saunders, 1977.
Hoare P: The development of psychiatric disorder among schoolchildren with epilepsy. Dev Med Child Neurol 26:3, 1984.
Hoberman H, Garfinkel B: Completed suicide in children and adolescents. J Am Acad Child Adol Psychiatry 27:689, 1988.
Jones P, Berney T: Early onset rapid cycling bipolar affective disorder. J Child Psychol Psychiatry 28:731, 1987.
Kazdin AE: Conduct disorders in childhood and adolescence. Beverly Hills, Sage Publications, 1986.
Kandel DB, Davies M: Epidemiology of depressive mood in adolescents. Arch Gen Psychiatry 39:1205, 1982.
Kashani JH, Husain A, Shekim WO, et al: Current perspectives on childhood depression: An overview. Am J Psychiatry 138:143, 1981.
Kashani JH, McGee RO, Clarkson RE, et al: Depression in a sample of nine-year-old children. Arch Gen Psychiatry 40:1217, 1983.
Keith PR: Night terrors. J Am Acad Child Adol Psychiatry 14:147, 1975.
King AC, Ollendick TH: Gilles de la Tourette disorder: A review. J Clin Child Psychol 13:2, 1984.

Kirkpatrick M, Smith C, Roy R: Lesbian mothers and their children: A comparative study. Am J Orthopsychiatry 51:545, 1981.
Kovacs M, Feinberg TL, Crouse-Novak M, et al: Depressive disorders in childhood: A longitudinal prospective study of characteristics and recovery. Arch Gen Psychiatry 41:229, 1984.
Kovacs M, Feinberg TL, Crouse-Novak MA, et al: Depressive disorders in childhood. II: A longitudinal study of the risk for a subsequent major depression. Arch Gen Psychiatry 41:643, 1984.
Lahey BB, Piacentini JC, McBurnett K, et al: Are attention deficit disorders with and without hyperactivity similar or dissimilar disorders? J Am Acad Child Adol Psychiatry 23:302, 1984.
Lahey BB, Piacentini JC, McBurnett K, et al: Psychopathology in the parents of children with conduct disorder and hyperactivity. J Am Acad Child Adol Psychiatry 27:163, 1988.
Last C, Hersen M, Kazdin A, et al: Comparison of DSM III separation anxiety and overanxious disorders: Demographic characteristics and patterns of comorbidity. J Am Acad Child Adol Psychiatry 26:527, 1987.
Lazare A: Current concepts in psychiatry: Conversion symptoms. N Engl J Med 305:745, 1981.
Lewis DO, Lovely R, Yeager C, et al: Toward a theory of the genesis of violence: a follow-up study of delinquents. J Am Acad Child Adol Psychiatry 28:431, 1989.
Levine MD: Encopresis: Its potentiation, evaluation and alleviation. Pediatr Clin North Am 29:315, 1982.
Marriage K, Fine S, Moretti M, et al: Relationship between depression and conduct disorder in children and adolescents. J Am Acad Child Adol Psychiatry 25:687, 1986.
Mattes J, Gittleman R: Effects of artificial food coloring in children with hyperactive symptoms. Arch Gen Psychiatry 38:714, 1981.
Mattison R, Bagnato S: Empirical measurement of overanxious disorder in boys 8 to 12 years old. J Am Acad Child Adol Psychiatry 26:536, 1987.
Mayes SD, Humphrey F, Handford A, et al: Rumination disorder: Differential diagnosis. J Am Acad Child Adol Psychiatry 27:300, 1980.
McGee R, Williams S: A longitudinal study of depression in nine-year-old children. J Am Acad Child Adol Psychiatry 27:342, 1988.
McGlashan TH: Adolescent versus adult onset mania. Am J Psychiatry 145:221, 1988.
McIntire MS, Angle CR (eds): Suicide Attempts in Children and Adolescents. Hagerstown, MD, Harper and Row, 1980.
Meyer-Bahlburg H: Gender identity disorder of childhood. J Am Acad Child Adol Psychiatry 24:681, 1985.
Mitchell J, McCauley E, Burke P, et al: Phenomenology of depression in children and adolescents. J Am Acad Child Adol Psychiatry 27:12, 1988.
Nunn K: The episodic dyscontrol syndrome in childhood. J Child Psychol Psychiatry 27:439, 1986.
Patterson G, Chamberlain P, Reid J: A comparative evaluation of a parent-training program. Behav Ther 13:638, 1982.
Pfeffer C: Clinical aspects of childhood suicidal behavior. Pediatr Ann 13:56, 1984.
Pfeffer C, Lipkins R, Plutchik R, et al: Normal children at risk for suicidal behavior: A two-year follow-up study. J Am Acad Child Psychiatry 27:34, 1988.
Pfeffer C, Newcorn J, Kaplan G, et al: Suicidal behavior in adolescent psychiatric inpatients. J Am Acad Child Adol Psychiatry 27:357, 1988.
Prior M, Sanson A: Attention deficit disorder with hyperactivity: A critique. J Child Psychol Psychiatry 27:307, 1986.
Prugh DG, Eckhardt DL: Psychophysiological disorders. *In:* Noshpitz JD (ed): Basic Handbook of Child Psychiatry. New York, Basic Books, 1979.
Puig-Antich J: Clinical and treatment aspects of depression in childhood and adolescence. Pediatr Ann 13:37, 1984.
Rapaport JL: Childhood obsessive-compulsive disorder. J Child Psychol Psychiatry 27:289, 1986.
Rapoport J: The neurobiology of obsessive-compulsive disorder. JAMA 260:2888, 1988.
Raskin L, Shaywitz S, Shaywitz B, et al: Neurochemical correlates of attention deficit disorder. Pediatr Clin North Am 31:387, 1984.
Reeves J, Werry J, Elkind G, et al: Attention deficit, conduct, oppositional, and anxiety disorders in children. II: Clinical characteristics. J Am Acad Child Adol Psychiatry 26:144, 1987.
Rey JM, Bashir MR, Schwarz M, et al: Oppositional disorder: Fact or fiction? J Am Acad Child Adol Psychiatry 27:157, 1988.
Rivinius TM, Jamison DL, Graham PG: Childhood organic neurological disease presenting as psychiatric disorder. Arch Dis Child 50:115, 1975.
Robins LN: Deviant Children Grown Up: A Sociological and Psychiatric Study of Sociopathic Personality. Baltimore, Williams & Wilkins, 1966.
Robins LN: Sturdy childhood predictors of adult antisocial behavior: Replications from longitudinal studies. Psychol Med 8:611, 1978.
Rock NL: Conversion reactions in childhood. J Am Acad Child Adol Psychiatry 10:65, 1971.
Rutter M: Relationships between child and adult psychiatric disorders. Acta Psychiatr Scand 48:3, 1972.
Rutter M: Family, area and school influences in the genesis of conduct disorder. *In:* Hersov LA, Berger M, Shaffer D (eds): Aggression and Antisocial Behavior in Childhood and Adolescence. Oxford, Pergamon Press, 1978.
Rutter M: Psychological sequelae of brain damage in children. Am J Psychiatry 138:1533, 1981.
Rutter M, Tizard J, Yule W, et al: Research report: Isle of Wight studies, 1964–1974. Psychol Med 6:313, 1976.
Satin M, Winsberg B, Monetti C, et al: A general population screen for attention deficit disorder with hyperactivity. J Am Acad Child Adolesc Psychiatry 24:756, 1985.
Scott JP: Biology and human aggression. Am J Orthopsychiatry 40:568, 1970.
Shaffer D: Suicide in childhood and early adolescence. J Child Psychol Psychiatry 15:275, 1974.
Shaffer D: Depression, mania and suicidal acts. *In:* Rutter M, Hersov LA (eds): Child and Adolescent Psychiatry, 2nd ed. Oxford, Blackwell, 1985.
Shaffer D, Garland A, Gould M, et al: Preventing teenage suicide: A review. J Am Acad Child Adolesc Psychiatry 27:675, 1988.
Shapiro AK: Gilles de la Tourette Syndrome, 2nd ed. New York, Raven Press, 1988.
Shaywitz S, Shaywitz B: Diagnosis and management of attention deficit disorder: A pediatric perspective. Pediatr Clin North Am 31:429, 1984.
Shekim W, Kashani J, Beck N, et al: The prevalence of attention deficit disorders in a rural midwestern community sample of nine-year-old children. J Am Acad Child Adol Psychiatry 24:765, 1985.
Spitz R: The First Year of Life. New York, International Univ Press, 1965.
Sreenivasan V: Effeminate boys in a child psychiatric clinic: Prevalence and associated factors. J Am Acad Child Adolesc Psychiatry 24:689, 1985.
Stoller RJ: Male childhood transsexualism. J Am Acad Child Adolesc Psychiatry 7:193, 1968.
Strober M, Carlson G: Bipolar illness in adolescents with major depression. Arch Gen Psychiatry 39:549, 1982.
Taylor E: Syndrome of overactivity and attention deficit. *In:* Rutter M, Hersov LA (eds): Child and Adolescent Psychiatry, 2nd ed. Oxford, Blackwell, 1985.
Thomas A, Chess S: Genesis and evolution of behavioral disorders from infancy to early adult life. Am J Psychiatry 141:1, 1984.
Varley C: Diet and the behavior of children with attention deficit disorder. J Am Acad Child Adolesc Psychiatry 23:182, 1984.
Voeller KKS: Right-hemisphere deficit syndrome in children. Am J Psychiatry 143:8, 1986.
Weiss G, Hechtman L: The hyperactive child syndrome. Science 205:1348, 1979.
Wender PH, Wender EH: The Hyperactive Child and The Learning Disabled Child. New York, Crown, 1978.
Werry J, Reeves J, Elkind G, et al: Attention deficit, conduct, oppositional, and anxiety disorders in children. I: A review of research on differentiating characteristics. J Am Acad Child Adolesc Psychiatry 26:133, 1987.
West D: Delinquency. *In:* Rutter M, Hersov LA (eds): Child and Adolescent Psychiatry, 2nd ed. Oxford, Blackwell, 1985.
Whalen C, Henker B: Hyperactivity and the attention deficit disorders: Expanding frontiers. Pediatr Clin North Am 31:397, 1984.
Wolff S: Non-delinquent disturbances of conduct. *In:* Rutter M, Hersov LA (eds): Child and Adolescent Psychiatry, 2nd ed. Oxford, Blackwell, 1985.
Zametkin AJ, Nordahlte A, Gross M, et al: Cerebral glucose metabolism in adults with hyperactivity of childhood origin. N Engl J Med 323(20):1361, 1990.
Zametkin A, Rapoport J: Neurobiology of attention deficit disorder with hyperactivity: Where have we come in 50 years? J Am Acad Child Adolesc Psychiatry 26:676, 1987.
Zucker KJ: Childhood gender disturbance: Diagnostic issues. J Am Acad Child Adolesc Psychiatry 21:274, 1982.

PSYCHOSIS IN CHILDHOOD

Burd L, Kerbeshian J: Psychogenic and neurodevelopmental factors in autism. J Am Acad Child Adolesc Psychiatry 27:252, 1988.
Burd L, Fisher W, Kerbeshian J: Childhood onset pervasive developmental disorder. J Child Psychol Psychiatry 29:155, 1988.
Chess S: Autism in children with congenital rubella. J Aut Child Schiz 1:33, 1971.
Gillberg C: The neurobiology of infantile autism. J Child Psychol Psychiatry 29:257, 1988.
Green WH, Campbell M, Hardesty AS, et al: A comparison of schizophrenic and autistic children. J Am Acad Child Adolesc Psychiatry 23:399, 1984.
Howells JG, Giurguis W: Childhood schizophrenia 20 years later. Arch Gen Psychiatry 41:123, 1984.
Kanner L: Early infantile autism. Am J Orthopsychiatry 19:416, 1949.
Kolvin I: Psychoses in childhood. *In:* Rutter M (ed): Infantile Autism—Concepts, Characteristics and Treatment. London, Churchill Livingstone, 1971.
Mahler MS, Furer M, Settlage CF: Severe emotional disturbances in childhood psychoses. *In:* Arieti S (ed): American Handbook of Psychiatry, Vol. 1. New York, Basic Books, 1959.
Nuechterlein K: Childhood precursors of adult schizophrenia. J Child Psychol Psychiatry 27:133, 1988.
Orntiz EM, Ritvo ER: The syndrome of autism: A critical review. Am J Psychiatry 133:609, 1976.
Petty L, Ornitz E, Michelman EG, et al: Autistic children who become schizophrenic. Arch Gen Psychiatry 41:1229, 1984.
Rutter M: Cognitive deficits in the pathogenesis of autism. J Child Psychol Psychiatry 24:513, 1983.
Snow M, Hertzig M, Shapiro T: Rate of development in young autistic children. J Am Acad Child Adolesc Psychiatry 26:834, 1987.

Tanguay P, Cantor S: Schizophrenia in children. J Am Acad Child Adolesc Psychiatry 25:591, 1986.
Tantam D: Asperger's syndrome. J Child Psychol Psychiatry 29:245, 1988.
Treffert DA: Epidemiology of infantile autism. Arch Gen Psychiatry 22:431, 1970.
Treffert DA: The idiot savant: A review of the syndrome. Am J Psychiatry 145:563, 1988.
Watkins JM, Asarnow RF, Tanguay PE: Symptom development in childhood onset schizophrenia. J Child Psychol Psychiatry 29:865, 1988.
Wolff S, Narayan S, Moyes B: Personality characteristics of parents of autistic children: A controlled study. J Child Psychol Psychiatry 29:143, 1988.

PSYCHOLOGIC TREATMENT OF CHILDREN AND ADOLESCENTS

Adams PL: A Primer of Child Psychotherapy. Boston, Little Brown, 1982.
Bergman T: Children in the Hospital. New York, International Univ Press, 1966.
Bernstein NR, Sanger S, Fras I: The functions of the child psychiatrist in the management of severely burned children. J Am Acad Child Adolesc Psychiatry 8:620, 1969.
Brunnquell D, Hall MD: Issues in the psychological care of pediatric oncology patients. Am J Orthopsychiatry 52:32, 1982.
Camp BW, et al: "Think aloud": a program for developing self-control in young aggressive boys. J Abnorm Child Psychol 5:157, 1977.
Campbell M: Fenfluramine treatment of autism. J Child Psychol Psychiatry 29:1, 1988.
Campbell M, Spencer EK: Psychopharmacology in child and adolescent psychiatry: A review of the past five years. J Am Acad Child Adolesc Psychiatry 27:269, 1988.
Dalton R: Psychiatry on the burn unit. *In:* Salisbury R, Dingeldein P, Newman N (eds): A Guide to Burn Unit Therapies. Boston, Little, Brown, 1984.
Dalton R, Haslett N, Daul G: Alternative therapy with a recalcitrant firesetter. J Am Acad Child Adolesc Psychiatry 25:713, 1986.
Dalton R, Muller B, Forman M: Psychiatric hospitalization of children: An overview. Child Psychiatry Human Dev 19:231, 1989.
Denckla MB, Bemporad JR, Mackay MC: Tics following methylphenidate administration. JAMA 235:1349, 1976.
Douglas JWB: Early hospital admissions and later disturbances of behavior and learning. Dev Med Child Neurol 17:456, 1975.
Douglas VI, Barr RG, Amin K, et al: Dosage effects and individual responsivity to methylphenidate in attention deficit disorder. J Child Psychol Psychiatry 29:453, 1988.
Farber J: Psychopharmacology of self-injurious behavior in the mentally retarded. J Am Acad Child Adolesc Psychiatry 26:296, 1987.
Forman MA, Hetznecker W: The physician and the handicapped child: Dilemmas of care. JAMA 247:3325, 1982.
Freund BL, Siegel K: Problems in transition following bone marrow transplantation: Psychosocial aspects. Am J Orthopsychiatry 56:244, 1986.
Gualtieri CT, Guimond M: Tardive dyskinesia and the behavioral consequences of chronic neuroleptic treatment. Dev Med Child Neurol 23:255, 1981.
Halpern W: The treatment of encopretic children. J Am Acad Child Adolesc Psychiatry 16:478, 1977.
Hansen CR, Cohen D: Multimodality approaches in the treatment of attention deficit disorders. Pediatr Clin North Am 31:499, 1983.
Kalachnik JE, Sprague RL, Sleator EK, et al: Effect of methylphenidate hydrochloride on stature of hyperactive children. Dev. Med Child Neurol 24:586, 1982.
Kornberg MS, Kaplan G: Risk factors and preventive intervention in child psychopathology: A review. J Prev 1:71, 1980.
Lansky SB: Childhood leukemia. J Am Acad Child Adolesc Psychiatry 13:499, 1974.
Minuchin S: Families and Family Therapy. Cambridge, Harvard University Press, 1974.
Newman LE: Treatment for the parents of feminine boys. Am J Psychiatry 133:683, 1976.
Quinton D, Rutter M: Early hospital admissions and later disturbances of behavior: An attempted replication of Douglas' findings. Dev Med Child Neurol 18:447, 1976.
Robinson LH: Psychiatric consultation for physically ill children. Prim Care 3:563, 1976.
Safer DJ, Allen RP, Barr E: Growth rebound after termination of stimulant drugs. J Pediatr 86:113, 1975.
Schacher R, Taylor E, Wieselberg M, et al: Changes in family function and relationships in children who respond to methylphenidate. J Am Acad Child Adolesc Psychiatry 26:728, 1987.
Solnit AJ, Green M: Psychologic considerations in the management of deaths on pediatric hospital services. I: The doctor and the child's family. Pediatrics 24:106, 1959.
Solnit AJ, Stark M: Mourning and the birth of a defective child. Psychoanal Study Child 16:523, 1961.
Spinetta JJ: The dying child's awareness of death. Psychol Bull 81:256, 1974.
Tisza VB, Dorsett P, Morse J: Psychological implications of renal transplantation. J Am Acad Child Adolesc Psychiatry 15:709, 1976.
Van Dongen-Melman JEWM, Sanders-Woudstra JAR: The chronically ill child and his family. *In:* Solnit AJ, Cohen DJ, Schowalter J (eds): Child Psychiatry (Psychiatry, Vol. 6). Philadelphia, JB Lippincott, 1986.
Van Dongen-Melman JEWM, Sanders-Woudstra JAR: The fatally ill child and his family. *In:* Solnit AJ, Cohen DJ, Schowalter J (eds): Child Psychiatry (Psychiatry, Vol. 6). Philadelphia, JB Lippincott, 1986.
Wallinga J: Human ecology: Primary prevention in pediatrics. Am J Orthopsychiatry 52:141, 1982.
Werry JS: An overview of pediatric psychopharmacology. J Am Acad Child Adolesc Psychiatry 21:3, 1982.
Werry JS, Wollersheim JP: Behavior therapy with children. A broad overview. J Am Acad Child Adolesc Psychiatry 6:346, 1967.
Wiener JM: Psychopharmacology in childhood disorders. Psychiatry Clin North Am 7:831, 1984.
Film: You See, I Had a Life. The Eccentric Circle Cinema Workshop, PO Box 1981, Evanston IL, 60204.

The authors wish to acknowledge the contributions of John M. Dunn, William Hetznecker, and Wesley E. Kerschbaum to this section in previous editions.

ABUSE AND NEGLECT OF CHILDREN

Child abuse is any maltreatment of children or adolescents by their parents, guardians, or other caretakers. Physicians must be able to recognize abused children and confirm the diagnosis; recognition is especially important in the first 6 mo of life because if the diagnosis is missed at this age, risk of fatality is high. Physicians have three main responsibilities toward abused children: detection, reporting, and prevention. In all 50 states the laws require physicians to report suspected cases of child abuse or neglect to a local child protective agency; laws protect physicians from liability should their suspicions be unsubstantiated.

3.51 THE SPECTRUM OF CHILD ABUSE AND NEGLECT

The types of child abuse and neglect seen by physicians are approximately 70% physical abuse, 25% sexual abuse, and 5% failure to thrive due to underfeeding. *Physical abuse* or non-accidental trauma inflicted by a caretaker may include bruises, burns, head injuries, fractures, and the like; their severity can range from minor bruises to fatal subdural hematomas. Corporal punishment that causes bruises, draws blood, or leads to an injury that requires medical treatment is outside the range of normal disciplinary action; reckless and dangerous punishment (e.g., kicking a child in the abdomen) is absolutely unacceptable, even if injuries do not occur. *Nutritional neglect* or psychologic underfeeding is the most common cause of underweight in infancy and may account for over half of the cases of failure to thrive. *Sexual abuse* can occur within the family (incest) or by acquaintances or strangers (extrafamilial). It is the most often overlooked type of child abuse.

Intentional drugging or poisoning includes giving children medications that are harmful or are not intended for children, or sharing illegal drugs with them. Cocaine, crack-cocaine, barbiturates, and tranquilizers are the drugs most frequently given. Occasionally, the parent has lethal intent. *Neglect of medical care* recommended for a child with chronic disease may lead to deterioration in the condition and require court-enforced supervision or placement in foster care. Court orders to hospitalize and treat are also needed when an emergency exists for the child that parents will not acknowledge or will not permit to be treated. Accidents to children from *neglect of safety* constitute child neglect if there is gross lack of supervision, especially if the child involved is under 3 yr of age. Rare types of child abuse include hypernatremic dehydration due to water deprivation, hyponatremia from forcing water, hypothermia due to cold water punishment, near drowning following forced immersion, intentional suffocation, deprivational dwarfism, and kwashiorkor due to cult diets.

The term *Munchausen syndrome by proxy* describes cases in which children are victims of illnesses fabricated or induced by parents. The children are usually under 6 yr old and too young to reveal the deception. The induced symptoms and signs lead to unnecessary medical investigations, hospital admissions, and treatment. Occasionally a child dies, as when the parent induces apnea. The involved parent often is a nurse or has an illness with features similar to those being induced in the child. Factitious symptoms often include bleeding from various sites. If specimens are requested, the parent adds his or her own blood to them. Factitious signs include recurrent sepsis (often polymicrobial) from injecting contaminated fluids, chronic diarrhea from laxatives, false renal stones from pebbles, fever from rubbing or heating thermometers, or rashes from rubbing the skin or applying caustic substances. All such cases should be reported to child protective services and the police in order to prevent the child's being taken to a different hospital or a fatal outcome.

Emotional abuse is the frequent rejection, scapegoating, isolation, criticism, or terrorizing of a child by caretakers; severe verbal abuse is usually part of this picture. Emotional abuse is difficult to prove. The diagnostic criteria include psychopathology in the child, as determined by a mental health professional, with persistent refusal by the parents of treatment for the child. Psychologic terrorism (e.g., locking a child in a dark cellar or threats of mutilation) requires automatic reporting. The social and economic costs of emotional abuse are great.

3.52 PHYSICAL ABUSE

EPIDEMIOLOGY. Each year in the United States approximately 1% of children are reported to be abused or neglected. Substantiated new cases of physical abuse are 1,200/million population/yr. About 10% of injuries to children under 5 yr of age seen in hospital emergency rooms are due to abuse. The mortality is about 3% or 4,000 deaths/yr. The ages of victims of physical abuse are estimated to be one third under 1 yr, one third from 1–6 yr of age, and one third over 6 yr. Premature infants are at a 3-fold greater risk of abuse.

ETIOLOGY. The abuser is a related caretaker or a male friend of the mother in 95% of cases, an unrelated babysitter in 4%, and a sibling in 1%. Parents who abuse their children exist in all ethnic, geographic, religious, educational, occupational, and socioeconomic groups. Groups living in poverty may have an increased incidence of child abuse because of the increased number of crises in their lives (e.g., unemployment or overcrowding) and because they have limited access to economic or social resources. An increased incidence of child physical abuse has been noted on military bases. The presence of spouse abuse doubles the likelihood of child abuse. Women are more likely to be the victims of abuse than are men, but this is not usually the case in families in which the fathers are home, unemployed. Many cases involve the concomitant use of drugs and alcohol.

Over 90% of abusing parents have neither psychotic nor criminal personalities; they tend to be lonely, unhappy, angry adults under heavy stress. They injure their children in anger after being provoked by some misbehavior, and often themselves have experienced physical abuse as children. They usually believe that all misbehavior is deliberate and that severe punishment is necessary in teaching children to respect authority. If parents do not fit this description, suspicion of abuse should turn to babysitters and other parties.

The occurrence of physical abuse requires not only the particular parent but also a specific child and occasion. The child often has characteristics that make him or her provocative, such as negativism or a difficult temperament; some of the more offensive misbehaviors are intractable crying, wetting, soiling, and spilling. The occasion initiating the abuse is usually a family crisis; the most common crises include loss of a job or home, marital strife or upheavals, birth of a sibling, or physical exhaustion.

CLINICAL MANIFESTATIONS. Many cases of physical abuse are first suspected because the injury is unexplained. More commonly, an explanation is offered but is implausible. Inconsistencies are common between the history offered of a minor accident and the physical findings of a major injury, or between the history and the child's developmental level. Normal parents usually know to the moment when and where their children were hurt, and bring their children immediately for examination. In the case of abused children, there is often delay in seeking medical help, sometimes for several days.

Bruises, welts, lacerations, and scars identify physical abuse. The most common sites of accidental bruises are over the forehead, anterior tibia, and other bony prominences; however, bruises confined to the buttocks and lower back are almost always related to spanking. Finger and thumb prints may be found on the arms where a child has been forcefully grabbed. A slap leaves a bruise on the cheek with two or three parallel lines running through it. Attempts to silence a screaming child with impatient, forced attempts at feeding may bruise the upper lip and frenulum. Human bite marks are distinctive, paired, crescent-shaped bruises facing each other. When a blunt instrument is used in punishment, a bruise or welt will often resemble it in shape. Loop marks or scars on the skin are secondary to a doubled-over cord or rope. Lash marks are seen after beating with a belt, tree branch, or hard-edged ruler. Choke marks may be seen on the neck, or circumferential marks of ropes tied around the ankles or wrists. Traumatic alopecia may occur when the hair is yanked; the scalp has a normal appearance and the damaged hairs are broken off at varying lengths. A subgaleal hematoma may form under the site. Bruises and scars may be found at various stages of healing. Noninflicted petechiae of the face and shoulders may follow intense retching, coughing, or crying. A mongolian spot may be mistaken for a bruise, but the color of the spot is solely blue-gray without any red hue.

Approximately 10% of cases of physical abuse involve burns. Hot solid burns are easiest to diagnose. The shape of the burn may be pathognomonic as when the child is held against a heating grate or electric hot plate. Cigarette burns produce circular, punched-out lesions of uniform size. These are often found on the hands or feet. By contrast, bullous impetigo is characterized by sores of variable size that grow in number and diameter if untreated.

Hot water burns are the most common type of inflicted burn; blisters are usually present. A dunking burn occurs when a parent holds the thighs against the abdomen and places the buttocks and perineum in scalding water as punishment for enuresis or resistance to toilet training. This results in a circular type of burn restricted to the buttocks. With deeper, forced immersions, the scald extends to a clear-cut water level on the thighs and waist. The hands and feet are spared, which is incompatible with falling into a tub or turning on the hot water while in the bathtub. Forcible immersion of a hand or foot as punishment can be suspected when a burn goes well above the wrist or ankle. Toxic epidermal necrolysis is usually easy to distinguish from scalds.

Subdural hematoma is the most dangerous inflicted injury, often causing death or serious sequelae. More than 95% of serious intracranial injuries during the first year of life are the result of abuse. Affected infants often present with coma, convulsions, apnea, and increased intracranial pressure. Subdural hematomas may be associated with skull fractures secondary to a direct blow to the head, but most cases involve no skull fracture or bruises. These cases are the result of violent, shaking injuries and slamming the head against a mattress or wall. The latter impact may produce devastating contusions of the posterior cortex. Retinal hemorrhages are nearly always present, and there may be grab mark bruises of the upper extremities, shoulders, or chest.

Intra-abdominal injuries are the second most common cause of death in battered children. Affected children may present with recurrent vomiting, abdominal distention, absent bowel sounds, localized tenderness, or shock. Because the abdominal wall is flexible, the force of the blow is usually absorbed by the internal organs and the overlying skin is free of bruises. The most common finding is a ruptured liver or spleen. Much rarer are tears or other injuries of the small intestine at sites of ligamental support such as the duodenum and proximal jejunum. Intramural hematomas at these sites can lead to temporary obstruction. Chylous ascites and pseudocyst of the pancreas have been reported.

LABORATORY DATA. Screening tests for a bleeding diathesis should be obtained if medically indicated or if the parents deny the possibility of inflicted injury and give a history of easy bruisability.

When physical abuse is suspected in a child under 2 yr of age, a roentgenologic bone survey consisting of films of skull, thorax, and long bones should be made; pelvis and spine films may be indicated if any of the preceding films are positive. These films are of great diagnostic value, since the clinical findings of fracture often disappear in 6–7 days even without orthopedic care. For most children 2–4 yr of age, a bone survey is indicated unless the child is verbal, has very minor injuries, or has been in a supervised setting (e.g., preschool). For verbal children (usually over the age of 4 or 5 yr) roentgenograms need be obtained only if there is bone tenderness or a limited range of motion on physical examination. If films of a tender site are initially negative, they should be repeated in 2 wk to detect any calcification of subperiosteal bleeding or nondisplaced epiphyseal separations that may have occurred. Bone trauma is found in 10–20% of physically abused children.

Most inflicted fractures are due to wrenching or pulling injuries that damage the metaphysis, and the classic early finding is a chip fracture in which a corner of the metaphysis of a long bone is torn off, along with the epiphysis and periosteum. Ten to 14 days later calcification of subperiosteal bleeding becomes visible at the periphery. By 4–6 wk after the injury the subperiosteal calcification will be solid and start to smooth out and remodel. Inflicted fractures of the shaft are usually spiral rather than transverse, and spiral fractures of the femur prior to the age of walking are usually inflicted. Fractures of the ribs, scapula, or sternum should arouse suspicion of nonaccidental trauma. Cardiopulmonary resuscitation (CPR) rarely causes rib fractures in children.

DIAGNOSIS. A tentative diagnosis of physical abuse should be made if the medical findings are unexplained or inconsistent with the history offered. Often a child over the age of 3 yr will be able to tell a sensitive and skillful interviewer that a particular adult hurt him or her. Certain bruises, burns, and scars are pathognomonic, and subdural hematomas do not occur spontaneously. Roentgenographic findings of metaphyseal fractures or multiple bony injuries at different stages of healing, implying repeated assaults, are also diagnostic.

Rare bone diseases such as scurvy and syphilis may resemble nonaccidental bone trauma, but the bony changes in these diseases are often symmetric. Children with osteogenesis imperfecta, severe osteomalacia, or sensory deficits (e.g., myelomeningocele or paraplegia) have an increased incidence of pathologic fractures, but not of the metaphysis.

TREATMENT. A child suspected of being abused must be reported to a child protective service (CPS) agency by phone immediately. Reporting the incident should secure evaluation, treatment, follow-up, and access to the Juvenile Court when necessary. The official written medical report is required within 48 hr. In large metropolitan areas, CPS caseworkers are on call 24 hr a day. Children with suspected abuse cannot be legally discharged from the clinic or office without consulting the county CPS agency. The caseworker either will concur with the physician's recommendation that the child can be safely released to the parent, or will come to the hospital and evaluate the family about the safety of the home. The 20% or so of children at risk for serious re-abuse usually can be placed in emergency receiving homes.

At this time, the only patients requiring admission are those with major trauma requiring ongoing medical care, those from an outlying county, or young children in whom the diagnosis is unclear. If in doubt, the physician should err on the side of protecting the child through hospitalization. If parents refuse hospitalization, a police or court order should be obtained.

The parents should be told by the physician when an inflicted injury is suspected, the reasons for this concern, and that the physician is legally obligated to report it. It should be emphasized that this problem is treatable, that a CPS social worker will be involved, and that in family-related abuse the goal is not to punish but to help the parents find better ways of dealing with their child's needs. Siblings should have full examinations within 24 hr of the report of child abuse in the family. Approximately 20% of them will also be found to have signs of physical abuse.

Feeling angry with abusing parents is natural, but expressing the anger damages rapport, making the cooperation of parents less likely. Repeated interrogations, confrontations, and accusations must be avoided. For hospitalized children, the parents should be encouraged to visit their children, and the hospital staff must do their best to be courteous and helpful. The primary physician should see the parents or telephone them daily. An evaluation by hospital social services should be obtained to determine the nature of problems in the family and environment and the safety of the home. A psychiatric evaluation may be appropriate in some instances.

Every hospital caring for children should designate a group of professionals who are responsive to the needs of abused or neglected children and their families. The group should include a pediatric consultant, a hospital social worker, a pediatric nurse, a psychologist or psychiatrist, and a coordinator. There should be clearly defined liaisons with public agencies and the courts, and legal consultants should be available. Within 1 wk of admitting any child for abuse or neglect, evaluations should be completed, and the team should meet with the child's physician and nurse, the child protective service representative, and, as appropriate, the police or any other community agencies involved with the family, to decide on the best immediate and long-range plans.

The pediatrician can coordinate the health care of the abused child, who needs more intensive surveillance and well-child care than the average child. Child welfare agencies are primarily responsible for coordinating and making home visits and for evaluating the therapy of the entire family. Because of the number of difficulties experienced by most abusive families, usually no single agency or discipline can provide all the needed services. Innovative types of therapy that have been successful when designed for individual families include Parent Aides, Homemakers, Parents Anonymous groups, telephone hotlines, environmental crisis therapy, substance abuse treatment, and child-rearing counseling. Traditional psychotherapy is often ineffective.

PREVENTION. Parents at high risk for being unable to love and care for their offspring adequately can be identified early if attention is given to such things as abuse of a previous child, drug addiction or serious psychiatric illness in a new mother, negative parental comments about the newborn infant, lack of evidence of maternal attachment, infrequent visits to a new baby whose discharge is delayed because of prematurity or illness, the spanking of a young infant, or the severe neglect of infant hygiene. Abuse and serious neglect may be prevented when such families receive intensive support with well-baby care, including prenatal classes, contact between mother and baby in the delivery room, rooming-in, increased parental contact with premature infants, extra help with calming the crying infant, more frequent office visits, ongoing counseling regarding discipline and nonphysical response to annoying behaviors, visits of public health nurses, parenting classes, close follow-up of acute illnesses, telephone lifelines, arrangement for day care or preschool, and assistance in family planning.

PROGNOSIS. With comprehensive, intensive treatment of the entire family, 80–90% of families involved in child abuse or neglect can be rehabilitated to provide adequate care for their children. Approximately 10–15% of such families (especially those with substance abuse) can only be stabilized and will require an indefinite continuation of supporting services until their children are old enough to leave home. Termination of parental rights or continued foster placement is required in 2–3% of cases.

Of abused children returned to their parents without any intervention, about 5% will be killed and 25% seriously injured. Children with repeated injuries to the central nervous system may develop mental retardation, organic brain syndrome, seizures, hydrocephalus, or ataxia. Common emotional traits of abused children are fearfulness, aggression, and hyperactivity. Further, untreated families tend to produce children who become the juvenile delinquents and violent members of our society and the next generation of child abusers.

3.53 SEXUAL ABUSE

See also Sec. 3.51.

Three types of sexual abuse are molestation, sexual intercourse, and rape. Child molestation includes touching or fondling the genitals of the child or asking the child to fondle the adult's genitals; forced exposure to sexual acts or pornography is also part of this definition. Sexual intercourse includes vaginal, oral, or rectal penetration (or attempted penetration) on a nonassaultive basis. Without detection and intervention molestation almost always progresses to full sexual intercourse. Less than 10% of sexual abuse is assaultive, forced intercourse (family-related rape).

Sexual mistreatment of children by family members (incest) is the most common type. Sexual abuse by friends and acquaintances of the child or family is the next most common. Least common is sexual abuse by strangers. Intrafamilial sexual abuse is more difficult to manage because the child must be protected from additional abuse at the same time that one tries to preserve the family unit.

EPIDEMIOLOGY. At least 0.2–0.3% of children have been involved in persistent incestuous relationships for an average period of 5 yr. Brief sexual encounters occur more frequently. The victims of incest are 90% female and 10% male. (In cases of third-party molestation in child care centers, which are being recognized with increasing frequency, the sex ratio is more nearly equal.) No age of child is exempt. Approximately one third are younger than 6 yr of age, one third 6–12, and one third 12–18. Incest is often repeated with successive daughters. The offenders are 99% male; females are more often perpetrators in child care settings. The incidence among stepfathers is about 5 times higher than among natural fathers. Incest cuts across socioeconomic lines to a greater degree than physical abuse.

ETIOLOGY. Most incest involves fathers and daughters. Sexual relationships usually begin gradually and without any violence. The father brings to this relationship a need for sexual gratification, and the daughter brings a need for tender affection and nurturance. The father is usually rigid, patriarchal, and emotionally immature. He is unlikely to engage in extramarital relationships, but he may have a tendency toward alcoholism. Mothers are often chronically depressed, unavailable to their husbands because of work or illness, and often themselves the childhood victims of sexual abuse. The child victim tends to be pseudomature and has taken on many of the housekeeping tasks. The families are often closely knit and socially isolated. In cases of violent family-related rape, the father is usually a sociopath, and his sexual abuse extends outside the family circle.

CLINICAL MANIFESTATIONS. A child may disclose an incestuous relationship to her mother and be brought to a physician at that time. If the mother does not believe the child, the child may later tell a girlfriend, friend's mother, or school counselor. Some adolescents will disclose their secret to a physician in a private interview. At other times the physician must elicit the history of incest on suspicion. Medical conditions associated with sexual abuse include genital infections, genital or anal trauma, recurrent urethritis and urinary tract infections, enuresis, encopresis, and inappropriate sexual behavior. In addition, run-away behavior, substance abuse, suicide attempts, and pregnancy may be the first sign that the child has been sexually abused. Because of the secrecy enforced by the abuser, the cause of these findings is often masked or hidden. The main cause of venereal disease in the prepubertal child is sexual transmission from adults.

Investigation of the possibility of incest requires sensitive and thorough history-taking because fewer than half of the victims have any abnormal physical or laboratory findings. A detailed explicit account of sexual experiences by a prepubertal child should be considered hard evidence in these cases. Physical findings are usually absent because of the long delay before the victim feels safe in telling someone about his or her plight. Interviewing should proceed gently and at the child's pace. Pictures or dolls can be used to clarify body parts; the child's vocabulary should be learned from the parent. If a social worker or law enforcement officer has carried out the initial interview, the physician can review this material and may not need to repeat the interview.

Female victims usually prefer that a female physician examine them, but this is not mandatory. An examination of the skin should be carried out for any signs of trauma, especially about the neck and mouth. If present, bite marks can be used to identify the perpetrator. The abdominal examination should assess the possibility of pregnancy. The mouth should be examined for signs of trauma such as redness, abrasions, or purpura. The rectum should be examined for signs of trauma or laxity. The external genitals should be examined for signs of trauma, laxity, or discharge. Most acute genital injuries occur between the 4 and 8 o'clock positions. The labia minora and posterior fourchette are damaged first, followed by tears of the posterior hymenal ring. The hymenal orifice is measured in the horizontal direction while lateral traction is applied to the labia. During the first 5 yr of life, a horizontal diameter >5 mm is abnormal and suspicious for vaginal penetration. From age 5 to 9, an additional 1 mm is allowed per year of age. A diameter >9 mm is considered abnormal for any girl 9 or older who has not yet entered puberty (Tanner stage 2). Magnification using a colposcope or otoscope helps identify past injuries of the hymen (usually hymenal scars). A speculum examination of the vagina is indicated when the victim is postpubertal or when nonmenstrual vaginal bleeding or major trauma of the external genitals is present.

LABORATORY DATA. The amount of laboratory evidence sought depends on the history. Molestation victims usually receive only a vulvar washing for sperm. Sexual intercourse victims should have routine tests for sperm, acid phosphatase, and gonorrhea and *Chlamydia* cultures from all sites. In the vagina, motile sperm can be found for 6 hr and nonmotile for 72 hr or longer. Acid phosphatase is present for 24 hr. Sperm and semen may also be recovered from the mouth and rectum. While the presence of semen substantiates the victim's history, the absence of semen does not contradict the history of vaginal intercourse. Cultures should be taken from the mouth, vagina, and anal canal; occasionally they are positive at sites initially denied by the child because of embarrassment. Fewer than 5% of the victims have positive cultures for gonorrhea. Symptomatic victims should also have tests for syphilis. When epidemiologically indicated, human immunodeficiency virus (HIV) and hepatitis B tests should be performed. Additional materials that may help to identify the perpetrator in third-party cases include pubic hair, scalp hair, fingernail scrapings, blood samples, and sperm. The specimens are usually transferred to the forensic laboratory in sealed, signed, and dated envelopes.

DIAGNOSIS. The diagnosis of child molestation and most instances of sexual intercourse rest on the graphic history offered by the victim. False accusations are rare except in cases involving psychotic patients or in some custody disputes. The physical examination may corroborate a child's history but is not often diagnostic. Abnormal physical findings in a child (e.g., an enlarged hymenal opening or scarred rectum) raise the suspicion of abuse and require a full investigation. Data are only now being gathered on the genital findings of nonabused children, thus caution should be exercised in assigning specificity to a particular physical finding. If sexual intercourse has occurred within the previous 72 hr, laboratory evidence of acid phosphatase or sperm helps to confirm the diagnosis. In rape cases, the diagnosis is readily confirmed by evidence of recent trauma as well as positive laboratory findings. Normal physical and laboratory examinations, however, are compatible with most types of sexual abuse. In one study of 18 victims whose abusers confessed to vaginal penetration, seven children had normal genital examinations.

TREATMENT. Evaluation and management of sexual abuse is similar to but more complex than that of physical abuse. Unlike physical abuse, which is dealt with primarily by the civil court and child protective service agency, *all* sexual abuse is considered a criminal offense and is investigated by the police. All victims of sexual abuse require psychologic support. Often both parents deny the girl's accusation and rebuke or punish her for reporting the incident. Victims of a single nonviolent episode of molestation may need only reassurance and a chance to express their feelings about the event on one or two occasions. Usually they are less distressed by the incident than are their parents. In a single, violent episode of family-related rape the patient is usually in serious emotional distress and requires the services of a child psychiatrist and/or rape victim advocate. Most such patients make a good adjustment after several sessions in age-appropriate psychotherapy. The victims of multiple episodes of sexual abuse almost always need long-term psychotherapy. The victim may be able to return home if the perpetrator is out of the home or has confessed and is in therapy. The child should be placed in foster care if this is his or her desire, if the mother doesn't believe the child's story, if family life is chaotic, or if collection of evidence is not yet complete. Medication to prevent pregnancy may be given to postmenarcheal girls in midcycle, who have experienced vaginal intercourse within the previous 72 hr. Victims are treated with antibiotics to prevent sexually transmitted disease if the perpetrator is known to be infected, the victim has signs of infection, or the likelihood of follow-up is poor (see Sec. 10.17). At a minimum all victims should revisit their physicians within 2 wk to evaluate their psychologic functioning and to assess the services that have been implemented.

Many incest offenders are treatable but success requires a coordinated, multidisciplinary approach. The offending parent requires a psychiatric evaluation, and the spouse should be evaluated by a social worker. Offenders are always investigated by the police, and criminal prosecution commonly occurs. Sentencing is usually deferred if the father becomes honestly involved in therapy. Both parents usually need psychotherapy and marital therapy. The offender in family-related rape cases is usually placed in jail, and criminal prosecution and sentencing do occur. The sociopaths are usually untreatable. Offenders with alcoholism may be helped by Alcoholics Anonymous groups.

PREVENTION. The primary prevention of sexual abuse includes encouraging children to "not keep secrets," "say no," and to "tell someone." Over two hundred books, plays, cartoons, films, and mime shows on sexual abuse are currently available in the United States. Such programs may bring out declarations by children already sexually abused, but whether they will protect others from seductive or predatory adults is not clear. At present, the best protection for children is alert adults who will not leave them in high-risk situations (e.g., day-care centers that prohibit visiting) and who will listen to them and recognize their symptoms of stress. The burden of preventing sexual abuse should be borne by adults, not children.

PROGNOSIS. With intervention most incest victims can lead normal adult lives. Without intervention many of them run away from home and become adolescent prostitutes and drug addicts; those who stay at home manifest depression, suicidal gestures, and conversion reactions; as adults most of them have difficulties with close relationships, may enter abusive relationships with men, and need psychiatric help.

3.54 NONORGANIC FAILURE TO THRIVE (from neglect)

See also Sec. 6.30.

Failure to thrive (FTT) has several causes. Approximately 70% of cases are nonorganic and 30% are organic. The nonorganic group is composed of 50% neglectful or psychologic FTT and 20% accidental, e.g., errors in formula preparation or errors in feeding techniques. Here we will consider neglectful failure to thrive, which rarely occurs after 2 yr of age because older children can obtain food for themselves. Under bizarre circumstances an older child can lose weight or gain poorly because he or she is confined to a room or deliberately starved. The main cause of FTT in infancy is that the infant is not fed enough. The mother may neglect feeding because she is busy with external problems (e.g., overwhelmed with work), preoccupied with inner problems, or doesn't like the infant. Emotional deprivation is inevitably concurrent with nutritional deprivation. Most of the involved mothers feel deprived and unloved themselves; many are acutely or chronically depressed. The infant is usually unplanned and unwanted. Multiple and continuing crises, frequently compounded by the physical absence of the father, may overwhelm the mother, who reacts by neglecting her infant.

CLINICAL MANIFESTATIONS. The dietary history in infants with nutritional neglect is usually not helpful because the parent reports that the baby is receiving adequate calories. In some cases, the mother's report that the infant has vomiting and diarrhea is not confirmed by the baby's hospital course. The parents have not usually sought medical care for their infant, and immunizations are not up-to-date. By contrast, the feeding history is extremely helpful in accidental FTT because the parents are open about their feeding errors and have actively sought medical assistance.

The infant with FTT usually exhibits thin extremities, a narrow face, prominent ribs, and wasted buttocks. Neglect of hygiene is often evidenced by rampant diaper rash, unwashed skin, untreated impetigo, uncut fingernails, or filthy clothing. A flattened occiput points to being left unattended for many hours. Delays in social and speech development are common but are rarely detected before 4 mo of age. Findings include an avoidance of eye contact, an expressionless face, and the absence of a cuddling response. The amount of time the mother spends holding, playing with, and talking to her baby is usually reduced or inappropriate. A rejecting mother will often feed her baby with anger and unnecessary force.

LABORATORY DATA. Investigation of the etiology of failure to thrive is discussed in Sec. 6.30. Extensive laboratory evaluation should usually be delayed until dietary management has been attempted for at least 1 wk and has failed. A skeletal survey is indicated in those infants who have a rejecting parent or evidence of associated physical abuse.

DIAGNOSIS. Most children with FTT should be hospitalized and given unlimited feedings for a minimum of 1 wk of a diet appropriate for age that approaches 150 kcal/kg (ideal weight)/24 hr. The formula should be similar to the one allegedly given at home. Infants with neglectful FTT will gain over 2 oz /24 hr for 1 wk (approximately 1 lb/wk) or have a gain that is strikingly greater than that achieved during a similar time period at home. Most such infants also display a ravenous appetite. If deprivational behaviors are also present, another diagnostic finding is their improvement or resolution in the hospital setting.

TREATMENT. All cases of FTT due to underfeeding from maternal neglect should be reported to a child protective agency. After appropriate hospital management approximately 75% of infants are discharged home with added services for the family, 20% go into temporary foster care while the parents receive therapy, and 5% enter long-term foster care with plans for relinquishment or termination of parental rights. This dispositional decision is based mainly on the potential responsiveness of the mother to treatment. Those infants who are discharged to their natural home require intensive intervention. The parents should be provided with clear, written dietary instructions at discharge and encouraged to hold the infant closely during feedings and to give appropriate stimulation. Many families require homemaker, public health nurse, health visitor, and other types of outreach services. Weekly medical follow-up is needed to monitor progress.

PROGNOSIS. Without detection and intervention a small percentage of infants with nutritional neglect die from starvation. Approximately 5–10% of these infants sustain superimposed physical abuse. Weight loss and understature from malnutrition are reversible, but normal head circumference and brain growth may not be achieved if the infant has had marasmus persisting beyond 6 mo of age. Emotional and educational problems occur in over half of these children.

BARTON D. SCHMITT
RICHARD D. KRUGMAN

PHYSICAL ABUSE

Billmire ME, Myers PA: Serious head injury in infants: accident or abuse? Pediatrics 75:340, 1985.
Bruce DA, Zimmerman RA: Shaken impact syndrome. Pediatr Ann 18(8):482, 1989.
Cupoli JM: Piecing together the pattern of child abuse. Contemp Pediatr 4(12):12, 1987.
Ellerstein NS, Norris KJ: Value of radiologic skeletal survey in assessment of abused children. Pediatrics 74:1075, 1984.
Feldman KW, Schaller RT, Feldman JA, et al: Tap-water scald burns in children. Pediatrics 62:1, 1978.
Kempe CH: The battered child syndrome, JAMA 181:17, 1962.
Kempe CH, Helfer RE (eds): The Battered Child, 3rd ed. Chicago, University of Chicago Press, 1980.
Krugman RD: Fatal child abuse: Analysis of 24 cases. Pediatrician 12:68, 1985.
Schmitt BD: The child with non-accidental trauma. *In:* Kempe CH, Helfer RE (eds): The Battered Child, 4th ed. Chicago, University of Chicago, 1987, pp 178–196.
Shaw A: Are you sure it's child abuse? Contemp Pediatr 3(1):92, 1986.
Wilson EF: Estimation of the age of cutaneous contusions in child abuse. Pediatrics 60:751, 1977.

SEXUAL ABUSE

Cantwell HB: Vaginal inspection as it relates to child sexual abuse in girls under thirteen. Child Abuse Neglect 7:171, 1983.
Emans SJ, Woods ER, Flagg NT, et al: Genital findings in sexually abused symptomatic and asymptomatic girls. Pediatrics 79:778, 1987.
Enos WF, Conrath TB, Byer JC: Forensic evaluation of the sexually abused child. Pediatrics 78:385, 1986.
Heger A, Emans SJ: Introital diameter as the criterion for sexual abuse. Pediatrics 85:222, 1990.
Horowitz DA: Physical examination of sexually abused children and adolescents. Pediatr Rev 9:25, 1987.
Krugman RD: Recognition of sexual abuse in children. Pediatr Rev 8:25, 1986.
Neinstein LS, Goldenring J, Carpenter S: Nonsexual transmission of sexually transmitted diseases: an infrequent occurrence. Pediatrics 74:67, 1984.
Strickland SL: Sexual abuse assessment. Pediatr Ann 18(8):495, 1989.

FAILURE TO THRIVE

Goldbloom RB: Failure to thrive. Pediatr Clin North Am 29:151, 1982.
Neifert MR, Seacat MJ, Jobe WE: Lactation failure due to insufficient glandular development of the breast. Pediatrics 76:823, 1985.
Powell GF, Low JF, Speers MA: Behavior as a diagnostic aid in failure to thrive. J Dev Behav Pediatr 8:18, 1987.
Pugliese MR, Weyman-Daum M, Moses N, et al: Parental health beliefs as a cause of nonorganic failure to thrive. Pediatrics 80:175, 1987.
Rosenn DW, Loeb LS, Jura MB: Differentiation of organic from non-organic failure to thrive in infancy. Pediatrics 66:698, 1980.
Schmitt BD, Mauro RD: Nonorganic failure to thrive: An outpatient approach. Child Abuse Neglect 13:235, 1989.
Sills RH, Sills IN: Don't overlook environmental causes of failure to thrive. Contemp Pediatr 3:25, 1986.

OTHER TYPES OF CHILD MALTREATMENT

Dine MS, McGovern ME: Intentional poisoning of children—an overlooked category of child abuse: Report of seven cases and review of the literature. Pediatrics 70:32, 1982.
Garbarino J: The psychologically battered child: Toward a definition. Pediatr Ann 18(8):502, 1989.
Kessler DB, New MI: Emerging trends in child abuse and neglect. Pediatr Ann 18(8):471, 1989.
Rosen CL, Frost JD, Bricker T, et al: Two siblings with recurrent cardiorespiratory arrest: Münchausen syndrome by proxy or child abuse? Pediatrics 71:715, 1983.
Schmitt BD: Child neglect. *In:* Ellerstein NS (ed): Child Abuse and Neglect: A Medical Reference. New York, John Wiley & Sons, 1981, p 297.
Zitelli BJ, Seltman MF, Shannon RM: Manchausen's syndrome by proxy and its professional participants. Am J Dis Child 141:1099, 1987.

3.55 NEURODEVELOPMENTAL DYSFUNCTION IN THE SCHOOL-AGED CHILD

Neurodevelopmental dysfunctions engender considerable agony for school-aged children who are struggling to feel effective. These so-called low-severity impairments of development are commonly associated with academic underachievement, behavioral difficulties, and problems with social adjustment. It has been estimated that 5–15% of school children harbor these insidious handicaps. The prevalence may be higher if one includes discrete dysfunctions leading to a transient self-limited disorder in learning a particular subject area.

ETIOLOGY

Diverse etiologies underlie the developmental dysfunctions of children. Some reading and spelling disabilities have genetic causes. Studies have suggested causal associations between learning disorders and abnormal chromosome patterns, low-level lead intoxication, recurrent otitis media, meningitis, acquired immune deficiency syndrome (AIDS), intraventricular hemorrhage, serious head trauma, and low birthweight. Poor nutrition and sociocultural deprivation have also been implicated as etiologies, or at least potentiators, of developmental dysfunction. In individual cases, a definite cause usually cannot be ascertained.

CLINICAL MANIFESTATIONS

Children with developmental dysfunctions vary widely with regard to clinical symptoms. Their specific patterns of academic performance and behavior represent final common pathways, the convergence of multiple forces, including interacting cognitive strengths and deficits, environmental or cultural factors, temperament, educational experience, and intrinsic resiliency. Thus, a memory dysfunction will have different manifestations in a child with strong language skills, good attention, and a supportive home environment from those evident in an economically deprived youngster whose memory problems are accompanied by weaknesses of attention and difficulties with language. Consequently, our full understanding of an academically dysfunctional child necessitates a broad view, an important component of which is the description of key areas of developmental function. Eight functions (Table 3–15) are especially germane and are described in more detail.

ATTENTION AND ATTENTION DEFICITS. Dysfunctions of selective attention are probably the most common of the neurodevelopmental dysfunctions affecting children. Although there is considerable variation, most youth with attention deficits have varying degrees of difficulty with sustained, focused concentration. They often show signs of *distractibility,* which may be principally sensory, because they are sidetracked by irrelevant sounds, visual stimuli, or their own tactile explorations. Other children are extremely restless, yearn for stimulation, and often complain of being bored. Still others are predisposed to distraction by association (the free flight of ideas or daydreaming). Their uncontrolled tide of associations prevents them from concentrating on salient material. In addition, many children with attention deficits are socially distractible; they seem unable to focus in the presence of other children.

Impulsivity is commonly encountered in children with attention deficits. An inability to control impulses can lead to behavior problems and to "verbal disinhibition" (inappropriate candor and loquaciousness). Some of these children exhibit cognitive impulsivity; they have trouble planning and organizing tasks prior to engaging in them. Their impulsive approach leads them to work too quickly (and carelessly). Other traits commonly associated with attention deficits include poor self-monitoring (of behavior, social interactions, or academic work), emotional lability, social skill deficits, performance inconsistency, and overactivity and conduct problems. It is important to stress that many children have attention deficits without being overactive and without manifesting any behavior problems. This is particularly true among girls with attention deficits.

There is considerable confusion and disagreement about the appropriate terminology to be applied to children with attentional difficulties. The DSM III-R uses the term ADHD (Attention Deficit Hyperactivity Disorder). Over the years, such terms as attention deficit disorder (ADD), hyperactivity, hyperkinetic impulse disorder, and minimal brain dysfunction have been used. In part, the taxonomic flux stems from the marked heterogeneity of groups of affected children. The traits summarized in Table 3–16 are variably present and are of different degrees of severity from case to case. In addition, children with attention deficits show variable patterns of developmental, academic, or behavioral difficulties. It is likely, therefore, that there are multiple subtypes of attention deficits.

DYSFUNCTIONS OF MEMORY (Table 3–17). As children proceed through school, there is a progressively increasing reliance on memory. Students are expected to be selective, systematic, and strategic in entering skills and data in memory. They must become efficient in their use of both long- and short-term memory to retrieve stored rules, facts, concepts, and procedures. By secondary school, rapid and precise recall is heavily stressed. Not surprisingly, some students experience tremendous frustration when memory dysfunctions prevent them from satisfying academic demands.

There are children who experience difficulty with the initial *registration* of information in short-term memory. They have trouble keeping pace with the information flow in a classroom. In some cases children with attention deficits experience considerable difficulty in being selective, alert, and sufficiently aroused to register salient information in memory. Other students have highly specific registration weaknesses. Some may have trouble with registering visual-spatial data in memory, whereas others may be deficient in the registration of sequences of data or of language. Some children can register data in the short-term memory but cannot do so quickly enough. Others have trouble capturing information that comes in "large chunks"; they simply are unable to assimilate sizable portions of data.

TABLE 3–15. Academically Relevant Neurodevelopmental Functions

Attention	Temporal-sequential ordering
Memory	Neuromotor function
Language	Higher order cognition
Visual-spatial ordering	Social cognition

TABLE 3–16. Common Indicators of Attention Deficit

Weak concentration	Inconsistency
Distractibility	Poor self-monitoring
Insatiability	Poor modulation of activity
Free flight of ideas	Lack of behavioral control
Impulsivity	

TABLE 3–17. Common Memory Dysfunctions

Weak registration in short-term memory (generalized, or specific to visual, verbal, or sequential data)
Active working memory failure
Poor consolidation in long-term memory
Deficient recall

Many children experience problems with *active working memory*. They are ineffective at suspending information in memory temporarily while they are working on it. Normally active working memory enables a student to keep in mind all of the different components of a task, such as a mathematics problem, while completing it. A student with an active memory dysfunction might, for example, carry a number and then forget what it was that she intended to do after she had carried it! Active working memory also enables children to remember the beginning of a paragraph when they arrive at the end of it. Thus, children with active working memory disorders can have trouble performing computations in mathematics and difficulty in remembering and retelling what they have read.

There are other youngsters who have particular problems with *consolidating* information in long-term memory. They are ineffective at filing data for later access. Ordinarily, consolidation in long-term memory is accomplished in one or more of four ways: (1) pairing two bits of information together (such as a combination of letters and the sound it represents); (2) classifying data in categories (e.g., filing all the insects together in memory); (3) linking new information to established rules (so-called rule-based learning); and (4) arranging knowledge in logical chains (such as the months of the year, the alphabet, or the events in a story). Some students struggle unsuccessfully with specific kinds of paired association learning, with categories, with rules, or with chains.

Some children can register and consolidate information in memory but seem to have inordinate difficulty recalling such data when they need it. Their recall may be painfully slow or imprecise. Some of them encounter difficulty with *simultaneous recall;* they have trouble recalling several facts or procedures at once. This can be especially disabling when it comes to writing, a task requiring the simultaneous recall of spelling, punctuation, capitalization, letter formation, ideas, vocabulary, and the directions given for the assignment. Consequently, many children with simultaneous recall problems have their greatest difficulty with written output. When they try to write, they contend with a memory overload, often manifest in illegibility (due to a crowding out of memory for letter formation), poor use of punctuation and capitalization, deficient spelling, and surprisingly primitive ideation. Some of these children also do poorly in mathematics.

LANGUAGE (Table 3–18). Linguistically proficient children have a distinct advantage in school, since much of what is taught is delivered in literate language. All of the basic academic skills are conveyed largely through language. Therefore, it is not surprising that children with language dysfunctions usually have troubled educational careers.

There are many forms of language disorder. Some children have particular problems with *phonology*. They experience unclear reception of English language sounds. They may have trouble discriminating between and forming associations with the sounds of their native language. Commonly, a weak phonologic sense has a negative effect on reading. A student with a poor appreciation of language sounds is likely to form unstable associative linkages between those sounds and visual symbols (i.e., letter combinations). Other common language lesions include difficulty with acquiring vocabulary (either receptive or expressive), problems with syntax (word order), an underdeveloped sense of how language works (weak metalinguistics), and trouble with drawing appropriate inferences from language.

It is common to distinguish between *receptive language dysfunctions* (those affecting understanding) and *expressive language dysfunctions* (those impeding production or communication). Children with primarily receptive language problems may have serious difficulty in following instructions in the classroom, understanding verbal explanations, and interpreting what they have read. Expressive weaknesses include oromotor problems affecting articulation and verbal fluency. In addition, some children display weaknesses of *word retrieval;* despite an adequate vocabulary, they have problems in finding exact words when they need them (as in a class discussion). Still others with expressive impediments have trouble formulating sentences, using grammar effectively, and organizing spoken (and possibly written) narrative. Some children with expressive language problems are hesitant when they speak, so that their verbal communication is unduly laborious. They may become passive, taciturn, and nonelaborative in communication. Some studies have linked expressive language dysfunction to delinquent behavior. This is especially true when an expressive language disorder occurs in a context of environmental deprivation or turmoil.

Language dysfunctions may be subtle and diagnostically elusive. For example, some children with mild language difficulties function reasonably well in school until they are required to master a second language.

Students with strong language function may make use of their linguistic facility to overcome other learning problems. For example, it may be possible to verbalize one's way through a mathematics curriculum, thereby overcoming a tendency to be confused by predominantly nonverbal concepts (such as ratio, equation, and diameter).

VISUAL-SPATIAL ORDERING. Visual perceptual abilities entail the appreciation of spatial attributes. Shape, position, relative size, foreground and background relationships, and form constancy (the notion that a shape retains its identity regardless of its position in space) are among the constituents of visual-spatial ordering. Children with visual-spatial deficiencies may encounter some initial problems with letter recognition. Spelling may emerge as a weakness because these children commonly experience trouble recalling precise visual configurations of words. In general, however, children who are confused about spatial attributes are unlikely to have longstanding or serious academic problems unless their visual-spatial weaknesses are complicated by other developmental dysfunctions. At one time it was thought that visual-spatial dysfunctions were a common cause of chronic reading disabilities; recent research has refuted this opinion.

Children with visual-spatial dysfunctions may be late in discriminating between left and right. They may show signs of fine or gross motor clumsiness because they may be poor

TABLE 3–18. Some Common Language Dysfunctions

Weak phonologic sense—problems in appreciating (and recalling) language sounds
Poorly developed vocabulary—trouble in acquiring or using new words
Confusion over syntax—difficulty in understanding how word *order* affects meaning
Inadequate metalinguistic awareness—inability to reflect on how language works
Trouble with inference drawing—difficulty in supplying missing information while listening
Word retrieval problems—slow or imprecise recall of words during speech
Narrative dysfluency—hesitant, imprecise, or disorganized verbal communication while describing or explaining

at making use of visual-spatial data to program motor responses.

TEMPORAL-SEQUENTIAL ORDERING. Awareness of time and sequence is an important developmental function. Students in school need to be able to manage time, to process and produce multistep explanations and procedures, and to develop memory capacity for extended sequences. The latter includes the preservation of serial order in spelling, in narrative, and in various mathematical algorithms.

Children who have difficulties with temporal-sequential ordering may be delayed in learning to tell time. They may have great difficulty in following multistep commands, performing acts that necessitate a sequence of steps in the proper order, or organizing narrative. Affected children may also have trouble in managing time. They may be frustrated in adhering to schedules, in learning the order of their classes in school, or in meeting deadlines.

NEUROMOTOR FUNCTION. Fine and gross motor skills ordinarily develop rapidly throughout childhood. However, some children experience considerable humiliation related to their insufficiently developed motor abilities. Fine motor skills are especially germane when it comes to writing. Several subtypes of fine motor dysfunction significantly impede the graphomotor fluency of children. Some youngsters exhibit signs of *finger agnosia;* they have trouble localizing their fingers while they write. As a result, they need to keep their eyes very close to the page. Ultimately, their writing becomes agonizingly slow and laborious. Others struggle with fine motor *dyspraxias.* Such students have trouble planning the highly coordinated motor sequences needed for writing. Although they may understand and be able to visualize what it is they need to write, they have difficulty with the sequential facilitation and inhibition of distinct muscle groups in their hands. Some of these students also display oromotor dyspraxias, resulting in speech articulation problems. Some students seem to have *visual-motor memory* weaknesses. They have trouble picturing the configurations of letters and words as they write. Their written output tends to be poorly legible, and their problems with visualization frequently result in poor spelling as well.

Some children harbor underlying *gross motor weaknesses* with or without fine motor problems. They may exhibit generalized gross motor delays or highly specific deficits. Examples of the latter include problems in using visual-spatial information to guide their gross motor actions; these children are inept at catching or throwing a ball because they cannot form accurate judgments about trajectories in space. Others are unable to satisfy the motor praxis demands of certain gross motor activities. It is hard for them to plan complex motor procedures (such as those needed for dancing, gymnastics, and swimming). Still others have poor *body position sense.* They fail to receive or interpret feedback from peripheral joints and muscles. They are likely to be impaired when activities demand balance and the ongoing tracking of body movement.

Children with gross motor problems may suffer a significant loss of self-esteem. They may incur considerable embarrassment in physical education classes. Gross motor weaknesses can lead to social rejection, withdrawal, and generalized feelings of inadequacy.

HIGHER ORDER COGNITION. This function consists of sophisticated thinking skills. Included in this area of development are the formation of concepts, problem-solving skills, critical thinking, brainstorming (and creativity), and metacognition.

Children vary considerably in their capacities to understand the conceptual bases of skills and content areas. Some of them acquire only a *tenuous grasp of concepts.* As students progress through their education, concepts become increasingly abstract and complex. New concepts are likely to contain old concepts. Those youngsters who have chronically tenuous grasps of concepts are likely to underachieve. Some students may have a pervasive weak grasp of concepts, whereas others may have difficulty only with concepts in certain domains (e.g., mathematics, social studies, or science). There are some students who prefer to conceptualize verbally, whereas others are more comfortable in forming concepts without the interposition of language. Many of the best students try to portray their concepts both linguistically and nonverbally.

Problem-solving skills are an important part of mathematics as well as virtually every other subject in school. Children with good problem-solving skills are good strategists. They are excellent at previewing or estimating answers, coming up with multiple alternative techniques to meet challenges, selecting the best techniques, and monitoring what they are doing so that they can deploy alternative strategies as needed. Poor problem-solvers, on the other hand, tend to be rigid or impulsive. They fail to come up with the best strategic approaches. Instead, they become committed irreversibly to a particular technique whether or not it works. They may then encounter significant difficulties in course work requiring methodical strategy deployment and flexible problem-solving.

Brainstorming skill is needed to develop a topic for a report, to think about the best way to undertake a project, and to deal with a variety of other open-ended academic challenges. Some students have real difficulty in generating original ideas. They prefer to be told exactly what to do. They balk at having to choose a topic, deploy imagination, develop an argument, or think freely and independently.

Critical thinking skills represent another higher cognitive ability acquired during childhood. Successful students often demonstrate an ability to evaluate statements, products, and people using objective criteria. They are able to tease out their own personal biases and appreciate the viewpoints of others. They are effective in comparing and contrasting their own values and views with those of an author. They can think and talk about the qualities of a person. They become adept at assembling qualitative criteria to judge the products they see on television or in stores.

Metacognition has received considerable attention in recent years. A child's metacognitive abilities refer to her or his capacity to think about thinking. Children with good metacognition are able to observe themselves thinking or studying. They develop an understanding of thought processes, enabling them to enhance their personal learning strategies and become more efficient students. Those youngsters who lack metacognition tend to perform intellectual tasks the hard way. They are unlikely to appropriate effective techniques to study for a test, to write a report, or to meet other complex academic challenges.

SOCIAL COGNITION. A student's social abilities are stringently tested throughout the school day as well as in the neighborhood after school. There is increasing evidence that social cognition exists as a discrete developmental function. Some children are extremely adept in social abilities, whereas others exhibit debilitating social skill deficits. There are multiple subskills within social cognition. These include an ability to enter smoothly into new relationships, a capacity to time and stage interactions effectively, a sensitivity to social feedback cues, a knowledge of how to resolve social conflict without aggression, a facility with the use of language in social contexts (verbal pragmatics), a pattern of establishing reciprocal (sharing) relationships with others (especially peers), and an inclination to overcome one's innate egocentricity in order to praise or nurture others. In addition to these skills, students need to be conscious of their own "image development" and to be adept at marketing themselves to peers. Regrettably, there are some children who have no idea of how adversely they are affecting others. As a result, they experience agonizing isolation with little or no insight into the reasons for their rejection.

The plight of a socially unskilled child can be tragic. He or she may sustain verbal abuse, bullying, and outright rejection, as well as various subtle forms of repudiation. Such students may seek refuge in the company of younger children, animals, a fantasy world, or adults. Social skill deficits can exert an enduring negative effect on behavioral adjustment, mental health, and, ultimately, success in a career.

ACADEMIC EFFECTS. The neurodevelopmental dysfunctions enumerated earlier are likely to occur in varying clusters within individual children. Combinations of dysfunctions commonly result in academic delays, particularly in the basic skills of reading, spelling, writing, and mathematics, which are reviewed subsequently.

Reading. Reading disabilities may stem from multiple developmental factors (Table 3–19). Most commonly, subtle or blatant language dysfunctions are present in children with significant reading delays. Initially, such children have difficulty in appreciating language sounds (phonology). They may then have debilitating problems forming associations in memory between English language sounds and combinations of letters. This gap results in deficiencies at the level of decoding individual words. An affected child may be slow to acquire a *sight vocabulary* (a repertoire of words he can identify instantly). When decoding skills are delayed or overly laborious, reading comprehension is often seriously compromised.

Students with visual-spatial dysfunctions may have trouble learning to read, but this is a relatively rare cause of reading difficulty. Children with weaknesses of temporal-sequential ordering may experience difficulty in breaking down words into their component sounds (phonemes) and reblending them into correct sequences. Memory difficulties can cause problems with reading recall, with associative memory for sounds and symbols, and with the acquisition of vocabulary. Some youngsters with higher order cognitive deficiencies experience trouble in understanding what they read because they lack a strong grasp of the concepts in a text.

Commonly, children with reading difficulties avoid reading. Thus, it is not unusual for a child whose reading is deficient to superimpose on this problem a lack of reading practice. Consequently, a delay in reading proficiency becomes increasingly pronounced over time.

Spelling. Impairments in spelling ability take various forms, depending in part on the nature of a child's developmental dysfunctions. Those with language disorders may have difficulty in applying a knowledge of phonology to spelling. They may overuse their visual (configurational) sense of words, so that their attempts at spelling are phonetically poor approximations yet visually comparable to the actual word (e.g., faght for fight). Other youngsters seem to have trouble with revisualization or the recall of word configurations. When their phonologic abilities are adequate, their spelling efforts are often phonetically correct but visually far afield (e.g., fite for fight).

Children with certain memory disorders can spell words adequately during a spelling bee or on a spelling list, but they misspell the same words when writing a paragraph. They appear to have a memory problem leading to difficulty in sustaining several different operations simultaneously. As a result, spelling becomes "eclipsed" by other task components.

TABLE 3–19. Types of Reading Problems

Poor decoding—deficient translation of written words into sounds and meanings
Delayed comprehension—inability to understand written sentences and passages
Incomplete recall—defective memory during reading
Deficient summarization—problems in restating what has been read

Some students commit mixed spelling errors, many of which are orthographically illegal (i.e., they deploy letter combinations never found in English). Such children have the worst prognoses with regard to spelling proficiency.

Writing (Table 3–20). Writing is an anathema to many youngsters with learning problems. As children proceed through school, there are growing demands for large amounts of well-organized written output. In many cases, writing is laborious because of an underlying fine motor dysfunction. In such instances, a child's graphomotor fluency fails to keep pace with ideation and language production. Thoughts are literally forgotten or underdeveloped during writing because the mechanical effort is so taxing.

TABLE 3–20. Types of Writing Problems

Graphomotor—problems with the motor fluency needed for writing
Linguistic—difficulty in using language during writing
Mnemonic—poor or slow recall of procedures and facts during writing
Organizational—trouble with arranging ideas appropriately on paper
Attentional—weak focus on detail, poor monitoring of writing quality (careless errors)

Just as students with simultaneous memory deficiencies experience difficulty with spelling in paragraphs, they are also prone to serious problems with writing in general. Their written output is often inconsistent in its legibility, ideation, and use of rules (of punctuation, capitalization, and grammar). Children with sequential ordering problems may have difficulty in organizing their ideas effectively when they write. Those with language disabilities may not be able to use language effectively on paper.

Mathematics. Delays in mathematical ability can be especially refractory to correction. In a recent community study, it was found that no student who was delayed more than 6 mo in mathematics in 6th grade ever caught up. Thus, significant mathematical weaknesses can become virtually insurmountable. Various forms of mathematics disability plague students.

1. Some children experience mathematics failure because of discrete higher order cognitive weaknesses. They cannot grasp arithmetical concepts. Good mathematicians are able to deploy both verbal and nonverbal conceptual abilities to understand such concepts as fractions, percentages, equations, and proportion. Impaired student mathematicians may have serious difficulty in moving back and forth from abstract to concrete thinking. It may also be hard for them to apply concepts effectively in solving word problems or when confronted with practical situations.

2. There are youngsters who show circumscribed memory weaknesses that compromise mathematical ability. Some have trouble in automatizing mathematics facts (such as the multiplication tables). Others have difficulty in recalling appropriate procedural sequences (such as the steps involved in solving a long division problem). Still others harbor weaknesses of active working memory, so that when they focus on one portion of a mathematics problem they are likely to forget other components of the same problem.

3. Some students with language dysfunctions have difficulty in mathematics because they have trouble understanding their teachers' verbal explanations of quantitative concepts and operations. Such students are likely to experience frustration in solving word problems.

4. Many students with attention deficits falter in mathematics classes because they are poor at focusing on fine detail (such as operational signs). Consequently, they commit frequent careless errors.

It is not unusual for individuals with mathematics disabilities to develop superimposed mathematics phobias. Anxiety over mathematics can be especially disheartening and can aggravate an underlying skill delay.

Content Area Subjects. Children with neurodevelopmental dysfunctions may experience difficulty in a wide range of content areas. The sciences may be a special problem, especially because they necessitate the processing of dense verbal material in textbooks and the rapid convergent recall of facts. Social studies courses often entail use of sophisticated language as well as a mastery of verbal abstract concepts (e.g., democracy, liberalism, and taxation with representation). Students with higher cognitive weaknesses may fail to grasp such concepts.

Foreign language learning can be a serious problem for students with language disorders or memory gaps. Some adolescents require foreign language waivers to graduate from high school and enter college.

Many students with attention deficits can succeed only in content areas that they find romantically attractive. They are likely to exhibit poor performance in courses that contain a great deal of not very exciting detail. They may have trouble distinguishing important data from trivia in a text because their selective attention is too diffuse.

Students with organizational problems commonly suffer in content area subjects. They often lack effective learning strategies. Some are too impulsive to make use of techniques to facilitate studying and work output. Others struggle because they are unable to maintain a systematized notebook, keep track of assignments, get to places on time, meet deadlines, find things, organize a locker, and remember what books to take home from school. Many disorganized students also have trouble studying for tests. They seem not to know how and what to study and for how long. They frequently lack self-testing skills.

NONACADEMIC IMPACTS. Neurodevelopmental dysfunctions commonly exert impacts that extend far beyond school. Some nonacademic impacts are closely related to the dysfunctions themselves, whereas other sequelae are secondary to persistent failure and frustration.

Children with attention deficits are particularly prone to experience nonacademic impacts. Their impulsivity and lack of effective self-monitoring may lead to behavioral maladaptation. A child affected by attentional dysfunction may be aggressive or disruptive in the classroom and at home. She or he may have serious difficulty in accepting behavioral limits, assuming responsibilities, and delaying gratification. The child's insatiability may lead to highly provocative behaviors, as she perpetually seeks intense experience (be it ever so negative). These negative behaviors often subvert the function of an entire family.

In some cases, children with neurodevelopmental dysfunctions have excessive performance anxiety or clinical depression. Sadness, self-deprecatory comments, declining self-esteem, chronic fatigue, loss of interests, and even suicidal ideation may ensue. Some children with neurodevelopmental dysfunctions lose motivation. They tend to give up and exhibit "learned helplessness," a sense that they have no personal control over their destinies. Therefore, they feel no need to exert effort. Such feelings ultimately can promote depression, pessimism, and a loss of ambition.

DIAGNOSIS (ASSESSMENT)

A child who is functioning poorly during the school years requires a careful multidisciplinary evaluation. It is unlikely that any one professional can adequately assess the diverse sources and broad effects of underachievement. An optimal evaluation team should consist of a pediatrician, a psychologist or psychiatrist, and a psychoeducational specialist. The latter is a professional (usually a special educator or educational psychologist) who can undertake a detailed analysis of academic skills. Other professionals should become involved as needed in individual cases, such as a speech and language pathologist, an occupational therapist, a neurologist, and a social worker.

Many children undergo evaluations in school. Such assessments are guaranteed in the United States under Public Law 94–142. Multidisciplinary evaluations conducted in schools are usually very helpful, but they are susceptible to biases or conflicts of interest. For example, if a school does not have a language therapist, that school's evaluation team might tend to be reluctant to recommend language therapy. School budgeting constraints may also affect the quality of evaluations and the extent of recommended services. Because of such limitations, there has been a growing demand for independent evaluations, for second opinions outside of the school setting. Many pediatricians become involved in such outside assessments.

The evaluation of a child with suspected neurodevelopmental dysfunctions should include complete physical, neurologic, and sensory examinations. A physician may also perform an extended neurologic and developmental assessment. Available pediatric neurodevelopmental examination instruments that facilitate direct sampling of various neurodevelopmental functions, such as attention, memory, and so on, include the PEET, the PEER, the PEEX, and the PEERAMID. Examinations of this type also include direct behavioral observations as well as assessment of minor neurologic indicators (sometimes called "soft signs"). The latter include various associated movements and other phenomena frequently associated with neurodevelopmental dysfunction (see also Sec. 3.11).

The pediatrician can be helpful in gathering and organizing data relating to a child with neurodevelopmental dysfunctions. He or she can obtain such data through the use of questionnaires completed by the parents, the school, and (if old enough) the child. These questionnaires can provide up-to-date information about behavioral adjustment, patterns of academic performance, and traits associated with specific developmental dysfunctions. Additionally, questionnaires can elicit relevant data concerning the child's health history, family background, and demographic variables relevant to a child's learning difficulty. The ANSER System Questionnaires have been developed for this purpose. There also exist standardized behavioral checklists that can aid in evaluation. Among these are the Yale Child Behavioral Inventory, the Connors Questionnaire (for hyperactivity), and the Achenbach Child Behavioral Checklist.

Commonly, an evaluation includes *intelligence testing*. Although an overall IQ is seldom helpful, it can be useful in relating specific subtest scores to other diagnostic data. Such comparisons can uncover revealing patterns suggestive of specific neurodevelopmental dysfunctions.

Psychoeducational tests yield relevant data, especially when such assessments include careful analyses that pinpoint where breakdowns are occurring in the processes of reading, spelling, writing, and mathematics. The psychoeducational specialist, making use of input from multiple sources, can help the pediatrician formulate specific recommendations for regular and special educational teachers.

A mental health specialist can be valuable in identifying family-based issues that may be complicating or aggravating neurodevelopmental dysfunctions. Specific psychiatric disorders also may be a part of the clinical picture.

TREATMENT

Just as assessment requires a multidisciplinary approach, the management of children with neurodevelopmental dysfunctions often needs to be multimodal. Most children with neurodevelopmental dysfunctions require at least several of the following forms of intervention.

DEMYSTIFICATION. Many children with neurodevelopmental dysfunctions have little or no understanding of the nature or sources of their difficulties. Once an appropriate descriptive assessment has been performed, it is especially important to explain to the child the nature of the dysfunction as well as his or her strengths. This explanation should be provided in nontechnical, optimistic, and nonaccusatory language.

BYPASS STRATEGIES. Numerous techniques can enable a child to circumvent neurodevelopmental dysfunctions. Ordinarily, such bypass strategies are used in the regular classroom, while individual forms of intervention in other settings are aimed at strengthening deficient functions. Examples of bypass strategies include using a calculator while solving mathematical problems, writing essays with a word processor, presenting oral instead of written reports, solving fewer mathematics problems, seating a child with attention deficits closer to the teacher to minimize distraction, offering visually presented demonstration models of correctly solved mathematical problems, and granting permission for a student to take scholastic aptitude tests (SATs) untimed. These bypass strategies do not "cure" neurodevelopmental dysfunctions but minimize their academic and nonacademic impacts.

REMEDIATION OF SKILLS. Tutorial programs are commonly used to bolster deficient academic skills. Reading specialists, mathematics tutors, and other such professionals can make use of diagnostic data to select techniques that make use of a student's neurodevelopmental strengths in an effort to improve decoding skills, writing ability, or mathematical computation. Often remediation takes place in a resource room or learning center at school. To qualify for these services in school, students may need to be labeled or classified as "learning disabled." To be so designated, testing must document a substantial discrepancy between the child's IQ and his or her academic skill. Unfortunately, some needy students with significant neurodevelopmental dysfunctions fail to display such a discrepancy. They commonly "fall between the cracks" and so may require tutoring outside of school.

Remediation need not focus exclusively on specific academic areas. Many students need assistance in acquiring study skills, cognitive strategies, and productive organizational habits.

DEVELOPMENTAL THERAPIES. Considerable controversy exists about the efficacy of treatments to enhance weak developmental functions. It has not been demonstrated convincingly that it is possible to improve substantially a child's fine motor skills, memory, problem-solving proficiency, or temporal-sequential ordering abilities. Nevertheless, some forms of developmental therapy are widely accepted. *Speech and language pathologists* commonly offer intervention for youngsters with various forms of language disability. *Occupational therapists* strive to improve the motor skills of certain students with writing problems or gross motor clumsiness. Recently, there has been considerable interest in *social skills training* that usually takes the form of small group sessions in which school children are helped to become more aware of the dynamics of social interaction. *Cognitive-behavioral therapy* is another recently introduced intervention. In this modality of treatment, children learn about their neurodevelopmental dysfunctions and are given specific exercises aimed at enhancing the weak areas. For example, a child with attention deficits may be taught about her impulsivity and then provided with exercises that encourage reflection, planning, and a less frenetic tempo.

CURRICULUM MODIFICATION. Many children with developmental dysfunctions require alterations in the school curriculum to succeed. This is particularly true as students progress through secondary school. For example, students with memory weaknesses may need to have their courses selected for them so that they do not have an inordinate cumulative memory load in any one semester. The timing of a foreign language, the selection of a mathematics curriculum, and the choice of science courses are critical issues for many of these struggling adolescents.

STRENGTHENING OF STRENGTHS. In all cases children with developmental dysfunctions need to have their affinities, potential, and talents identified clearly and exploited widely. It is as important to strengthen strengths as it is to attempt to remedy deficiencies. Athletic skills, artistic inclinations, creative talents, and mechanical aptitudes are among the potential assets of certain students who are underachieving academically. Parents and school personnel need to create opportunities for such students to build on these proclivities and to achieve respect and praise for their efforts. The strengthening of strengths is essential for sustaining self-esteem and motivation.

INDIVIDUAL AND FAMILY COUNSELING. When learning difficulties are complicated by family problems or identifiable psychiatric disorders, psychotherapy may be indicated. Clinical psychologists or child psychiatrists may offer long- or short-term therapy. Such intervention may involve the child alone or the entire family. It is essential, however, that the therapist have a firm understanding of the nature of a child's neurodevelopmental dysfunctions. Both parents and child can become confused if a psychotherapist attributes a child's learning difficulties exclusively to environmental factors, thus ignoring the potent influence of an underlying language disability, attention deficit, or memory problem. Most families do not require a heavily psychoanalytic or psychodynamic approach, but instead can benefit from a counseling program that offers them practical advice on behavioral management.

ADVOCACY. Children with developmental dysfunctions require informed advocacy. They need to have their rights upheld in school and in the community. A physician can be especially helpful in advocating for a child in school. Some children, for example, are devastated by being held back in a grade, and the likelihood of benefit is minimal. A physician may need to represent the rights of the child in opposing such grade retention as well as other sources of public humiliation. A physician may also need to argue strongly for a child to receive services in school or to benefit from modifications in the curriculum. Physicians can also perform advocacy by becoming vocal citizens of their communities. In serving on a school board, for example, a physician can exert a major influence on local policy and on the allocation of resources to school children with special educational needs.

MEDICATION. Certain psychopharmacologic agents may be especially helpful in lessening the toll of neurodevelopmental dysfunctions. Most commonly, stimulant medications are used in the management of children with attention deficits. They are never a panacea because most youngsters with attention deficits have other associated dysfunctions (such as language disorders, memory problems, motor weaknesses, or social skill deficits). Nevertheless, medications such as methylphenidate, dextroamphetamine, and pemoline can be important adjuncts to treatment because they seem to help youngsters focus more selectively and control their impulsivity. Stimulant medication and its administration is described in more detail elsewhere in Sec. 3.48. When depression or excessive anxiety is a significant component of the clinical picture, antidepressants can be prescribed.

Children receiving medication need regular follow-up visits that include a review of current behavioral checklists, a physical examination, and appropriate modifications of medication dose. Treated children should be given periodic "medication holidays," intervals when they are off the drug so that they can strive to be in control of themselves.

LONGITUDINAL CASE MANAGEMENT. All children with neurodevelopmental dysfunctions can benefit from the support and guidance of a case manager, a professional who can offer advice in a continuing manner and be available to monitor function over the years. The pediatrician may be an ideal professional to assume this responsibility. With time, new questions inevitably emerge as a child's neurodevelopmental dysfunctions evolve and academic expectations undergo progressive changes. Because children with neurodevelopmental dysfunctions represent an extremely heterogeneous group, no two children require the same management plan. Nor is it possible to predict with certainty at age 7 the needs of a youngster when he or she is 14 yr of age. Consequently, affected children and their families require vigilant follow-up and individualized objective advice throughout their academic careers.

MELVIN D. LEVINE

Kavanagh JF, Truss TJ (eds): Learning Disabilities: Proceedings of the National Conference. Parkton, MD, York Press, 1988.

Levine MD: Attention and memory: Progression and variation during the elementary school years. Pediatr Ann 18:366, 1989.

Levine MD, Melmed RD: The unhappy wanderers: Children with attention deficits. Pediatr Clin North Am 29:105, 1982.

Levine MD, et al: The Pediatric Assessment System for Learning Disorders. (Questionnaires and Neurodevelopmental Examinations.) Cambridge, MA, Educators Publishing Service, 1982.

Levine MD: Developmental Variation and Learning Disorders. Cambridge, MA, Educators Publishing Service, 1987.

Levine MD: Keeping a Head in School: A Student's Book About Learning Abilities and Learning Disorders. Cambridge, MA, Educators Publishing Service, 1990.

Luria A: Higher Cortical Function in Man. New York, Basic Books, 1980.

Ross DM, Ross SA: Hyperactivity: Current Issues, Research, and Theory. New York, Wiley Interscience, 1982.

Torgeson JK, Wong BYL (eds): Psychological and Educational Perspectives on Learning Disabilities. Orlando, FL, Academic Press, 1986.

Wallach GP, Butler KG: Language Learning Disabilities in School-Age Children. Baltimore, Williams & Wilkins, 1984.

3.56 CHILDREN WITH SPECIAL HEALTH NEEDS: AN OVERVIEW

Children with special health needs comprise a heterogeneous population that includes youngsters with a wide variety of developmental disabilities and chronic illnesses. In some cases, persistent problems may overlap, such as when a child with bronchopulmonary dysplasia also has delayed development, or when a child with mental retardation develops diabetes mellitus. Other children fit more clearly into one group or another, such as a youngster with cystic fibrosis who has no cognitive or developmental problems, or a physically healthy child with a complex learning disorder. Nevertheless, a core of basic considerations is applicable to most children with special health needs, and these issues are discussed first in this section.

Most children receive the majority of their health care from a single provider and are educated in regular school settings that require no modifications to meet special developmental or health concerns. Children with special health needs, on the other hand, may see a variety of health care specialists (e.g., neurologists, orthopedists, and cardiologists), interact with multiple professionals (e.g., occupational therapists, respiratory therapists, nutritionists, and psychologists), and need major adaptive modifications in their school setting (e.g., barrier-free facilities, special education services, and specialized nursing care).

Some chronic conditions that are determined genetically are wholly preventable through utilization of new measures for determining carrier states prior to conception and through techniques for prenatal diagnosis. Although emerging advances in molecular genetics are likely to diminish further the incidence of inherited disease, the wide range of conditions that lead to special health needs during childhood and the continued lack of understanding of the causes of many of these disorders make it likely that large numbers of youngsters will continue to manifest chronic impairments of health or development.

An appreciation of the multiple levels at which prevention or treatment efforts can be implemented for children with special health needs requires an understanding of the differences inherent among the concepts of disease, disability, and handicap. *Disease* refers to a specific health condition affecting a child, such as arthritis or congenital cytomegalovirus (CMV) infection. *Disability* refers to the functional problem brought about as a result of the symptoms of the disease, such as a poorly functioning knee or a hearing impairment. *Handicap,* on the other hand, refers to the social implications or consequences of having the disease or disability, such as the inability to participate competitively in sports or the social isolation that results from difficulty in communicating orally.

Physicians can play a key role in preventing the occurrence of many special health needs and in diminishing their impact on a child's growth and development. Intervention may be targeted at any level—that of the disease, the disability, or the handicap. For the child with arthritis, efforts are directed both toward reducing joint inflammation and toward removing barriers to participation in age-appropriate physical activities. For the child with congenital CMV and deafness, successful management focuses on both audiologic habilitation and social integration. Both types of children have a chronic health condition, although neither may necessarily be perceived as "chronically ill." The two terms (condition and illness) are used interchangeably in the following sections.

Early detection of persistent conditions, amelioration of the functional consequences of specific disabilities, and prevention of secondary psychosocial handicaps are central to the provision of care for children with special health needs. However, health-care providers occasionally and inappropriately refer to such children by the name of their condition, such as "asthmatics," "sicklers," "leukemics," or "Down's babies." This tendency to characterize children by their disease or disability influences both parental and professional attitudes as well as their assessments of the child's current abilities and their expectations for his or her future. In general, parents and professionals should work together on behalf of a child who has a disease rather than allowing the disease to define the child.

The importance of early intervention programs as a mechanism for decreasing the impact of special health or developmental needs on children and their families is increasingly recognized. Because of their strategic relationship with young children and their parents, physicians have an important responsibility with regard to early identification of children at risk and referral to the appropriate services. This includes the need to maintain accurate and updated information on all available resources within a community to ensure that families have access to a full range of needed services. Programs that incorporate the best practices provide individualized services designed to strengthen the inherent adaptiveness of participating children and families. Furthermore, because the best predictors of the well-being of children with special health needs include factors that relate to family functioning, effective pediatric management should embody a comprehensive approach to the child within the context of the family, addressing the needs of all of its members. This will enhance the prospects for a positive outcome.

Several public programs exist in the United States to help children with chronic health conditions. Title V Services for Children with Special Health Needs in each of the states provide a variety of coordinating and multidisciplinary clinical services for children with many chronic illnesses and developmental disabilities and their families. Public Law 94–142 (1975) mandates an appropriate education in the least restrictive environment for all school-aged children with developmental disabilities. More recently, Public Law 99–457 (1986) lowered the mandated age of eligibility for special educational services to 3 yr and offered incentives to states to establish systems of early intervention programs beginning at birth. Section 504 of the Rehabilitation Act similarly serves to diminish barriers to education programs (and other public services) for children with disabilities.

In summary, children with special health needs and their families are a diverse group who share common experiences. Those who have symptoms of illness for more than 3 mo or who require hospitalization or extensive home- or community-based health services for more than 1 mo in a 12-mo period are said to have a chronic disease. Children with developmental disabilities, on the other hand, have been defined by the federal Developmental Disabilities Assistance and Bill of Rights Act Amendments of 1987 as individuals with impairments in physical or mental abilities that are manifested before 22 yr of age, are likely to persist indefinitely, and result in functional limitations in major life activities. Mental retardation is the prototypic developmental disability; others include cerebral palsy, specific learning disabilities, pervasive developmental disorder, autism, visual or hearing impairments, and disorders of communication. Distinctions between youngsters with mental retardation and those with chronic illness are discussed in the following sections.

JAMES M. PERRIN
JACK P. SHONKOFF

3.57 CHRONIC ILLNESS IN CHILDHOOD

EPIDEMIOLOGY

The epidemiology of chronic illness in childhood differs in important ways from the epidemiology of long-term illness in adults. Adults face a relatively small number of common chronic conditions (e.g., diabetes, osteoarthritis, and coronary artery disease) and few rare diseases. Children, in contrast, face a wide variety of mainly quite rare diseases. Only two groups of chronic conditions in childhood are common: allergic disorders (mainly asthma, eczema, and hayfever) and neurologic disorders (mainly seizure disorders and neuromuscular conditions such as cerebral palsy). Other conditions often thought to be common, such as childhood diabetes, occur only in about 1 in 1,000 children under 16 yr of age, a much lower rate than that seen in adults. Many of the conditions described in this textbook occur with a frequency of much less than 1 in 1,000. Table 3–21 indicates prevalence rates for representative childhood conditions. Given the wide variety of conditions that may affect children, the total number of children with individually very rare conditions is relatively high.

These epidemiologic distinctions have implications for both physicians and families. The adult epidemiologic pattern means that health care providers for adults have frequent daily experience with the common chronic illnesses of adults, remaining current and knowledgeable about such conditions as hypertension. Similarly, an adult who has been newly diagnosed with high blood pressure probably knows something about the disease and has friends or family members with hypertension. The practicing pediatrician, however, may see a new case of a malignancy only once a decade and will make the diagnosis of cystic fibrosis or even diabetes infrequently. A family whose child has been newly diagnosed with a rare condition may never even have heard the name of the disease prior to its onset in their child. These epidemiologic facts mean that child health care providers have a difficult task in identifying children with rare conditions and in staying current with the new technologies applicable to rare diseases. Families typically feel very isolated when a rare disease is detected in their child.

The aggregate number of children with all types of chronic health conditions is high, despite the rarity of individual conditions. At least 10–20% of American and British children have some chronic condition, and some studies indicate that the number may be even higher. This percentage translates into at least 10 million or more children in the United States with some kind of chronic health condition. Most chronic conditions are mild, such as acne, hayfever, or mild congenital deformity causing a small limp. Only about 10% of chronically ill children (1–2 million children) have diseases of such physiologic severity that they interfere with a child's usual daily activities on a regular basis.

The percentage of children with severe long-term illnesses has approximately doubled in the past 2 decades (Fig. 3–13). This change partly reflects major advances in the technology of medical and surgical care. Current estimates are that, even among severely ill children, at least 80% survive to young adulthood, although often with significant long-term morbidity. New technologies will probably improve the longevity of children who today die in the first 2 decades of life and significantly increase the total number of children with chronic

TABLE 3–21. Estimated Prevalence of Representative Childhood Chronic Conditions, Ages 0–20, United States, 1980*

Chronic Conditions	Rates/1,000
Asthma (moderate and severe)	10.00
Congenital heart disease	7.00
Seizure disorder	3.50
Arthritis	2.20
Diabetes mellitus	1.80
Cleft lip/palate	1.50
Down syndrome	1.10
Spina bifida	0.40
Sickle cell anemia	0.28
Cystic fibrosis	0.20
Hemophilia	0.15
Acute lymphocytic leukemia	0.11
Chronic renal failure	0.08
Muscular dystrophy	0.06

*Adapted from Gortmaker SL, Sappenfield W: Chronic childhood disorders: Prevalence and impact. Pediatr Clin North Am 31:3–18, 1984.

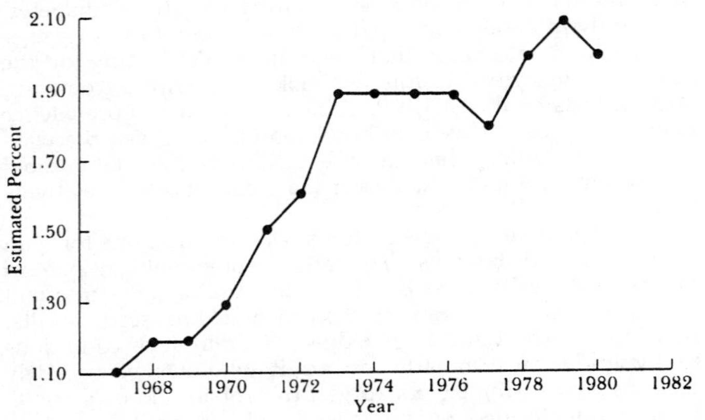

Figure 3–13. Estimated percentage of American children, aged birth through 16 yr, with limitation of activity due to chronic conditions (1967–1980). (From the National Center for Health Statistics, Current Estimates from the National Health Interview Survey, Series 10, Annual Reports 1967–1980.)

conditions. Conditions that may show major changes in incidence, thereby affecting the size of the total population of children with severe illnesses, include AIDS, the aftereffects of fetal substance abuse, and major pulmonary or neurologic disease in children leaving neonatal intensive care units. Alternatively, new genetic techniques allow the prenatal and preconception diagnosis of increasing numbers of health conditions, and genetic counseling and other interventions may diminish the incidence of several diseases.

Severity, a notion simple in concept, is difficult to measure in most chronic illnesses. Few illnesses have a clear biologic marker that is relatively independent of environmental influences and treatment (the factor VIII level in hemophilia is an exception to this rule). Physiologic measures of severity (e.g., asthma rating scales or hemoglobin A_{1C} in diabetes) reflect the interaction of biologic susceptibility, treatment, and other environmental factors. The impact of the condition on the child's functioning with friends or in school or on his or her psychologic status are other aspects of severity. Although this section focuses on health conditions that are relatively severe in physiologic terms, many of the issues discussed affect children with milder conditions. Further, one type of severity (e.g., physiologic) may correlate poorly with others (e.g., psychologic or functional).

ISSUES COMMON TO DIVERSE CHRONIC CONDITIONS

Health care providers typically view each chronic illness as a distinct and separate entity that has its own etiology, natural history, treatment, complications, and physiologic impact. However, families whose children have a variety of long-term illnesses face several issues in common, reflecting chronicity itself rather than aspects of the specific disease (Table 3–22).

First, many chronic childhood illnesses are high-cost health conditions. A small percentage of children with major chronic illnesses utilize a large proportion of the child health dollar; 2–4% of children with severe long-term illnesses account for at least 25% of all child health expenditures. These figures really reflect only what is paid by public or private insurance. Families face many other costs, such as the costs of transportation, long-distance phone calls, and special diets, few of which may be reimbursed. Furthermore, chronic illness in a child makes it more difficult for both parents to work outside the home, thereby diminishing families' financial resources.

TABLE 3–22. Common Issues for Children with Chronic Illnesses and Their Families

Costly treatments	Unpredictability
Burden of care on families	Pain
Multiple providers and treatments	Effects on child's daily life
Rarity and isolation	Stress and psychologic impact

Second, the daily burden of care rests mainly on the families, and that burden can be extensive, as with a family with two teenagers with muscular dystrophy, both wheelchair bound and requiring transportation from place to place, or with a youngster with cystic fibrosis who needs extensive pulmonary care prior to leaving for school each day. These daily burdens greatly extend the work of families.

Third, whereas most children require only a single health care provider for most of their health care and supervision, children with long-term health conditions frequently have multiple providers and multiple treatments. A child with hemophilia may have contact with a hematologist, a pediatrician, a specialized dentist, an orthopedist, a hematology nurse, a physical therapist, a psychologist, and a social worker, among others. The recommendations of any one member of this group may vary from those of another, and families must often choose among conflicting advice. Clinically, there usually are trade-offs among the choices, such as the optimal time to do a surgical procedure or the trade-off between seizure control and alertness. Families need help to make informed decisions.

Fourth, the comparative rarity of most childhood chronic conditions makes families feel isolated. They often wonder why they have been singled out by an unusual condition and feel that no other families have had similar experiences. Several programs in specialty centers (e.g., cystic fibrosis or arthritis centers) and several parent advocacy programs have worked to break this sense of isolation through groups that help parents learn from each other how to raise children with chronic illnesses.

Fifth, many of these conditions are unpredictable in their implications, longevity, complications, and developmental impact on the individual child. The parent whose child has leukemia wonders whether new bleeding signals a relapse that will have a fatal outcome or will be followed by a permanent remission. The parent whose child has mild wheezing at bedtime does not know whether the child will sleep well through the night or awaken severely dyspneic in the middle of the night in need of emergency care. Parents speak frequently of how difficult this unpredictability is for them and how they wish for clear answers to difficult questions, even if the answers may be unfavorable. Many important aspects of chronic disease are unpredictable, both because of great variability in environmental influences and biologic responsiveness to specific conditions and treatments and because little information is available about many rare diseases.

Sixth, many chronic conditions and their treatments cause great pain, far in excess of that faced by other children. Sickle cell anemia, hemophilia, arthritis, and leukemia are all examples of conditions characterized at times by severe pain.

Seventh, chronic illness has a pervasive influence on a child's daily life. Frequent interactions with the medical care system, occasional hospitalizations, and greater dependency on parents and health care providers characterize their experience. A chronic health impairment may create a sense of "differentness," of being unable to do many things that other children can do.

Finally, a chronic illness creates additional stresses and demands on families and on children that apparently healthy children do not face. Perhaps as a result, chronically ill children have about twice the frequency of psychologic or behavioral problems found in healthy controls; children with significant neurologic handicaps or sensory deficits have as much as a 5 times greater risk for these problems. The level of severity correlates poorly with psychologic status. Despite this greater risk of psychologic maladjustment, most children with chronic health conditions are psychologically healthy.

DEVELOPMENTAL ASPECTS OF LONG-TERM ILLNESS

Two issues are central to an understanding of the developmental implications of long-term childhood illness: the development of children's understanding of illness mechanisms and the impact of illness at different stages of child development.

Clinicians working with children who have long-term illnesses should understand the developmental stage of their patients' understanding of illness in order to explain illness and its mechanisms in age-appropriate terms. Because children's understanding follows a typical pattern of growth in cognitive abilities, children need different explanations of their continuing disease as they mature. Young children of preschool or early school age tend to have a concrete and relatively superficial understanding of illness. They view illness as a response to their bad behavior or not following the rules (such as wearing a coat when you go outside in the cold). Children at this age believe that getting well occurs by adhering to another set of rules. By about the 4th–6th grade, children begin to differentiate themselves from external events that may cause illness. For this age group, germ theory seems very important; with the notion that germs cause almost all illnesses, illness can be prevented by avoiding germs, and better results will be gained from taking medicines, which are seen as fighting germs. This notion of germs can cause confusion or isolation for children of this age who have conditions such as leukemia or diabetes. By 8th grade or even later, children begin to understand the physiologic mechanisms for illness, appreciating the many interrelated causes of illness and the several symptoms of illness. At this age children usually begin to understand the interaction of body parts, for example, that lungs and hearts are not only near each other but actually work together to maintain body functions.

Physical illness has different impacts on children based on their stage of development. In infancy, the illness may affect the parameters of growth and development by influencing feeding, sleeping, motor abilities (and therefore exploration of the environment), or sensory functions. Physical deformity or fatigue may affect a child's responsiveness to parents, who may in turn react differently to this child. Frequent hospitalizations may interfere with the normal development of trusting relationships within a family. In later preschool years, when children are developing autonomy, mobility, and self-control, illness may again interfere with these important developmental functions. Early school-aged children may be subject to teasing from classmates; they may need to be absent from school for illness or its treatment and thus miss normal opportunities for early socialization. Middle childhood and adolescence are periods when children expand their areas of competence; responsibility for the care of the child's health condition should shift gradually from the parents to the child. Chronic illness may interfere with this process.

In adolescence, illness may affect the individual's developing independence, greater responsibility for self-care, growing intimacy, and planning for the future. The disease or its treatment may be particularly embarrassing for adolescents and may affect their body image. Adolescence is frequently a time to test the limits of the illness and compliance with recommended therapies. Health conditions that require another person for some care, such as the teenager with cystic fibrosis who needs pulmonary physical therapy before each day of high school, may hinder growth toward independence. Sensitivity to the developmental impact of chronic illness will help clinicians provide their patients with appropriate planning and anticipatory guidance and help children and their families find acceptable ways of fulfilling the normal developmental tasks of childhood and adolescence.

Children should take increasing responsibility for the management of their own health condition commensurate with their level of maturity, developmental stage, and understanding of their illness. Areas of responsibility include monitoring the condition, assessing indicators of change and exacerbation, asking for help, and self-medication (both at home and at school). Families may need help in learning ways to foster responsibility, and children need education and advice in learning how to become independent in appropriate ways.

CHARACTERISTICS OF PROGRAMS AND SERVICES FOR FAMILIES

Changing interests of families and changing notions of the civil rights of people with disabilities have fostered an increasing emphasis on family-centered services for children with chronic conditions. Parents increasingly take responsibility for monitoring and managing the care of their child, and more care is provided in or near the child's home and less in hospitals. Families want most care to be community-based, both in the sense of receiving as many services as close to home as possible and in the sense of integrating their chronically ill child into the usual community activities, not limiting him or her to services provided for children with special health needs. The Iowa model of providing most care for children with malignancies through community-based physicians, with supervision and coordination of specialty care provided at the university health center, illustrates that complex health services can be delivered close to home.

Community-based services also strengthen early socialization of the child, mainly through participation in community services such as day-care, and later social and educational development through participation in regular school programs. Chronic illness accounts for a sizable number of school absences by children. Part of that time away from classes reflects the direct effects of illness, such as increased fatigue or necessary hospitalization; however, some represents the need to travel great distances for treatments that are often available only during regular school hours.

Some children with chronic illnesses, especially those with cognitive impairments, need special education services. However, most children with long-term illnesses have no intrinsic cognitive impairment and should be in regular education programs. They may need specialized health services (e.g., access to medicines or planning for emergencies) in order to participate in school, and children who must miss classes frequently need home-bound and hospital-bound instruction to allow them to keep up with their classmates.

Families whose children have long-term health conditions should have access to a wide range of coordinated and comprehensive services. The specific services needed by any one family may vary considerably from those needed by another and will probably change over time as the child's needs and the family's needs change. The main groups of services that should be available for families include appropriate primary and specialized medical and surgical care; nursing services, especially those that will help to strengthen a family's own skills in caring for their child; preventive and therapeutic mental health services; social services; educational planning; and certain special therapies, such as physical therapy, occupational therapy, or nutritional services. Preventive mental health services help to diminish the risk of psychologic problems related to the chronicity of the child's condition.

Partly because of the emphasis on specialized medical services, children with chronic health conditions lack regular pediatric health supervision more than other children. Chronically ill children have lower rates of immunization and screening for common health problems and often lack anticipatory guidance in key areas of growth and development, such as behavior and discipline in the preschool years, preparation for entry to school, and preparation for adolescence, with developing sexuality, growth of independence, and opportunity for substance abuse. All children need primary care services, and each of these areas has special significance for children who are chronically ill.

Teamwork among the multiple professionals and the family and coordination of care are important to serve families of chronically ill children effectively. For some families, especially in the first months or years after the initial diagnosis of a long-term condition, care coordination by another person is an essential service. Most parents prefer to coordinate the care for their children themselves, especially after they become knowledgeable about their child's condition and its management. Therefore, the education of both parents and child about the disease process, its management, its complications, and its developmental implications is a central part of the therapeutic effort.

PEDIATRIC CARE IN THE COMMUNITY

Community-based pediatricians can help coordinate the medical care needed by chronically ill children and collaborate with those providing other community-based services, such as schools, social agencies, and home health care providers. They must communicate effectively with the specialty consultants who have responsibility for the management of disease-specific aspects of care, such as monitoring complications, recommending specific treatments, providing access to newer technologies, carrying out specialized procedures, and educating families and community care providers about specific disease issues. Lack of clear allocation of responsibilities may lead to limited provision of certain services such as genetic counseling; for example, different members of the health care team may believe that other members are providing genetic information when in fact no one is.

Communication is extremely important for these families. Communication among primary and specialty physicians and among providers of health care and other community services, all involving parents themselves, is essential. The child should also participate in developmentally appropriate ways. Community physicians can help parents gain the information on which to make decisions and facilitate a growing role for the child in decision-making as he or she gets older. Sharing of necessary information so that parents and child can make informed choices can be very time-consuming, especially in situations in which there is much uncertainty.

JAMES M. PERRIN

Hobbs N, Perrin JM, Ireys HT: Chronically Ill Children and Their Families. San Francisco, Jossey-Bass, 1985.

Kisker CT, Strayer F, Wong K, et al: Health outcomes of a community-based therapy program for children with cancer. Pediatrics 66:900, 1980.

Leikin SL: Minors' assent or dissent to medical treatment. J Pediatr 102:169, 1983.

Perrin EC, Gerrity PS: There's a demon in your belly: Children's understanding of illness. Pediatrics 67:841, 1981.

Perrin EC, Gerrity PS: Development of children with chronic illness. Pediatr Clin North Am 31:19, 1984.

Stein REK (ed): Caring for Children with Chronic Illness. New York, Springer, 1989.

Stein REK, Gortmaker SL, Perrin EC, et al: Severity of illness: Issues and concepts. Lancet 2:1506, 1987.

3.58 MENTAL RETARDATION

Mental retardation is a condition of both clinical and social importance. It is characterized by limitations in performance that result from significant impairments in measured intelligence and adaptive behavior. It also confers a social status that can be more handicapping than the specific disability itself. Because the boundaries between "normality" and "retardation" frequently are difficult to delineate, the pediatric identification, evaluation, and care of children with cognitive difficulties and their families require a considerable level of both technical sophistication and interpersonal sensitivity.

Dramatic changes in social and political attitudes toward persons with developmental disabilities during the last 2 decades have revolutionized the pediatric approach to children with mental retardation. Previous practices of withholding lifesaving measures from neonates with congenital abnormalities have been replaced by legally sanctioned treatments for children with profound and irreversible disorders. The practice of almost automatically placing young children with disabilities in residential institutions has been replaced by extensive efforts to develop community-based service systems that coordinate resources for both children and their families. The pediatric responsibility has shifted from helping to "put the child away" to "normalizing" the life of the child and his or her family.

Concurrent with this shift in sociopolitical values, our theoretical and empiric understanding of the phenomenon of mental retardation has also changed. The expanding knowledge base has led to a rejection of the simplistic debate over "organic" versus "environmental" causes of retardation and to a growing recognition of the mutually interactive contributions of both nature and nurture to the development of all children. Consequently, the traditional narrow focus on neuropathology has been expanded to an assessment of the interplay among the biologic factors in the child, the adaptive characteristics of the family, and the social context in which they live.

ETIOLOGY AND PATHOGENESIS. The determinants of competence in any individual are complex and multifactorial. Regardless of his or her level of performance, each child's abilities are influenced by both the integrity and maturational status of the nervous system and by the nature and quality of his or her life experience. Some children sustain significant neurologic insults and develop normal skills. Others manifest severe cognitive impairment despite the absence of recognizable focal neurologic findings or historical evidence of significant risk factors for central nervous system dysfunction. The neurobiologic roots of mental retardation may be found among such diverse factors as structural malformations of the brain, metabolic abnormalities, and CNS deficits related to infection, malnutrition, or hypoxic-ischemic injury. The experiential precursors of retardation may be identified in histories of dysfunctional caregiving related to parental psychopathology, extreme family disorganization, or the stresses of poverty. Children who live in poverty are particularly susceptible to the cumulative burdens of both social stress and the greater biologic vulnerability related to a higher prevalence of such risk factors as perinatal complications and nutritional deficiencies.

Table 3–23 lists the potential contributing factors in the pathogenesis of mental retardation from preconception through the early childhood years. Few of the etiologic factors

TABLE 3–23. Potential Contributing Factors in the Pathogenesis of Mental Retardation

- Preconceptual disorders
  - Single gene abnormalities (e.g., inborn errors of metabolism, neurocutaneous disorders)
  - Chromosomal abnormalities (e.g., X-linked disorders, translocations, fragile-X)
  - Polygenic familial syndromes
- Early embryonic disruptions
  - Chromosomal disorders (e.g., trisomies, mosaics)
  - Infections (e.g., cytomegalovirus, rubella, toxoplasmosis, human immunodeficiency virus)
  - Teratogens (e.g., alcohol, radiation)
  - Placental dysfunction
  - Congenital central nervous system malformations (idiopathic)
- Fetal brain insults
  - Infections (e.g., human immunodeficiency virus, toxoplasmosis, cytomegalovirus, herpes simplex)
  - Toxins (e.g., alcohol, cocaine, lead, maternal phenylketonuria)
  - Placental insufficiency/intrauterine malnutrition
- Perinatal difficulties
  - Extreme prematurity
  - Hypoxic-ischemic injury
  - Intracranial hemorrhage
  - Metabolic disorders (e.g., hypoglycemia, hyperbilirubinemia)
  - Infections (e.g., herpes simplex, bacterial meningitis)
- Postnatal brain insults
  - Infections (e.g., encephalitis, meningitis)
  - Trauma (e.g., severe head injury)
  - Asphyxia (e.g., near drowning, prolonged apnea, suffocation)
  - Metabolic disorders (e.g., hypoglycemia, hypernatremia)
  - Toxins (e.g., lead)
  - Intracranial hemorrhage
  - Malnutrition
- Postnatal experiential disruptions
  - Poverty and family disorganization
  - Dysfunctional infant-caregiver interaction
  - Parental psychopathology
  - Parental substance abuse
- Unknown influences

included in this table, however, provide a complete explanation for the phenomenon of retardation in any single individual. Rather, a developmental disability reflects the complex interplay among multiple risk and protective factors.

EPIDEMIOLOGY. Just under 3% of the general population has an IQ of less than 68 (<2 standard deviations below the mean). It has been estimated that 80–90% of persons with mental retardation function within the mild range, whereas only 5% of the population with mental retardation is severely to profoundly impaired. Table 3–24 summarizes the distinguishing features of different levels of severity of disability. The prevalence of mild retardation varies inversely with socioeconomic status, whereas moderate to severe disability occurs with equal frequency across all income groups. Because a diagnosis of mental retardation relies on an assessment of adaptive behavior and not solely on IQ, the epidemiology varies with the life cycle. The reported incidence of retardation increases initially with age, the numbers rising sharply in the early school years and then declining in late adolescence as individuals with borderline or mild retardation leave the formal education setting and are assimilated into the "normal" adult world. Identification of children with mild retardation in the preschool period is most commonly precipitated by concerns about the development of language.

CLINICAL MANIFESTATIONS. Children with physical findings suggestive of recognizable syndromes that are associated with mental retardation may be identified at birth or during early infancy. Down syndrome and primary microcephaly are examples of such conditions. These disorders, however, represent a small percentage of the population of youngsters with intellectual impairment. The overwhelming majority are identified because of their failure to meet age-appropriate expectations.

Delayed achievement of developmental milestones is the cardinal symptom of mental retardation. Although youngsters with severe impairment show marked delays in psychomotor skills in the first year of life, children with moderate retardation typically exhibit normal motor development and present with delayed speech and language abilities in the toddler years. Mild retardation, on the other hand, may not be suspected until after entry to school, although participation in a nursery school or day-care program can highlight discrepancies in the performance of a preschooler with significantly subaverage abilities.

The natural history of mental retardation is highly variable and dependent on the availability of appropriate educational and therapeutic experiences as well as on neuromaturation and the presence of associated disabilities. Although many youngsters may experience transient "plateau periods" during which measurable progress may be minimal, most individuals with mental retardation acquire new skills and continue to learn throughout their lifetimes. The ability to formulate specific prognoses, except for children who manifest severe to profound retardation, is quite limited, especially during the preschool years. Children with histories that suggest a loss of previously acquired skills represent an important subgroup for whom the diagnosis of a progressive rather than a static neurologic disorder must be investigated. In such cases, developmental deterioration is rarely reversible, yet a precise diagnosis is important for genetic counseling and informed family support.

A thorough pediatric history is essential to identify the relevant contributing factors as well as to document the evolving pattern of the child's developmental skills over time. The product of the history should be a comprehensive inventory of the risk factors (both within the child and within his

TABLE 3–24. Levels of Severity of Mental Retardation

Category	Descriptive Features
Borderline (IQ 68–83)	Strictly speaking, children with IQ scores above 69 do not meet the criteria for mental retardation, but they are vulnerable to educational problems. Many such children are able to function adequately with special help in regular classes. Most achieve independent social and vocational adjustment
Mild (IQ 52–67)	This group includes almost 90% of children formally classified as mentally retarded. Most need at least some special class placement, although mainstreaming should be considered, and some can achieve 4th–6th grade reading levels. Those who have well-developed adaptive skills may be able to function independently as adults
Moderate (IQ 36–51)	Educational goals for children in this group focus primarily on gaining maximal self-care and perhaps some academic skills up to a 2nd grade level. Those who are well adjusted may be able to function semi-independently in supervised living and sheltered workshop settings
Severe (IQ 20–35)	Children in this group can learn minimal self-care and simple conversational skills. They need much supervision throughout their lives
Profound (IQ below 20)	Children in this group require total supervision. Very minimal self-care skills are possible, and few individuals are toilet trained. Language development generally is minimal

or her environment) that increase the likelihood of developmental dysfunction as well as protective factors that may contribute to more adaptive functioning (see Table 3–23). Common protective factors include good physical health, a normal rate of growth, healthy parent-child attachment, and a cohesive family unit within a supportive social network.

A systematic physical examination may reveal findings that help to explain the etiology of the child's disability or that identify particular treatment needs. Table 3–25 lists a number of atypical physical features that have been associated with a higher incidence of mental retardation. In some cases, a particular cluster of phenotypic characteristics may suggest a specific syndrome related to a chromosomal abnormality or known teratogenic effect. It should be emphasized, however, that many of these features are found in children without developmental disabilities, some tend to be familial, and several appear with greater prevalence among specific ethnic groups.

DIAGNOSIS. The primary care pediatrician is strategically situated to identify young children with possible mental retardation through routine developmental surveillance in the context of general pediatric care. Parental report of a child's typical skills and behaviors in conjunction with the use of in-office screening procedures are important complementary sources of information. For young children involved in a program outside of the home (e.g., day-care or preschool), the impressions of the caregiver or teacher are also valuable. Concerns raised by parents, nonparental caregivers, or teachers or by direct observation of the child require systematic investigation. The extent to which a comprehensive developmental assessment can be performed within the primary care setting depends on the expertise of the physician and his or her office staff.

Ultimately, the diagnosis of mental retardation requires confirmation of significantly subaverage general intellectual functioning (i.e., more than 2 standard deviations below the mean for age) in association with deficits in adaptive behavior (e.g., limitations in self-care or social skills) as demonstrated through formal psychologic evaluation. Screening instruments (e.g., the Denver Developmental Screening Test) and nonstandardized developmental scales are unacceptable substitutes for validated and reliable diagnostic measures (e.g., the Bayley Scales of Infant Development, the Stanford-Binet Intelligence Scale, or the Wechsler Scales). After the psychometric diagnosis of mental retardation has been confirmed, a comprehensive medical evaluation is necessary to complete the assessment process.

A range of laboratory studies must be considered in the medical evaluation of a youngster with mental retardation. Table 3–26 lists important studies and the indications for their use.

A comprehensive history, physical examination, and laboratory evaluation often lead to identification of specific factors that contribute to the phenomenon of mental retardation. A thorough diagnostic formulation highlights those contributing factors that are amenable to specific treatments (e.g., hypothyroidism or an excessive lead burden), suggests associated problems that require intervention or continued surveillance (e.g., a seizure disorder or a sensory impairment), and provides a comprehensive data base that can inform ongoing management decisions. More commonly, however, the results of the medical evaluation are nonspecific and inconclusive. In such cases, when there is no evidence of a specific central nervous system insult, a family history of disability, or identifiable environmental problems, the retardation is presumed

TABLE 3–25. Atypical Physical Features that May Be Associated with Increased Incidence of Mental Retardation

Hair	Head
Double whorl	Microcrania
Fine, friable, prematurely gray or white locks	Macrocrania
Sparse or absent hair	
	Hands
Eyes	Short 4th or 5th metacarpals
Microphthalmia	Short, stubby fingers
Hypertelorism	Long, thin tapered fingers
Hypotelorism	Broad thumbs
Upward-and-outward or downward-and-outward slant	Clinodactyly
Inner or outer epicanthal folds	Abnormal dermatoglyphics (e.g., distal triradius)
Coloboma of iris or retina	Transverse palmar crease
Brushfield spots	Abnormal nails
Eccentrically placed pupil	
Nystagmus	Feet
	Short 4th or 5th metatarsals
Ears	Overlap of toes
Low-set pinna	Short, stubby toes
Simple or abnormal helix formation	Broad, large big toes
	Deep crease leading from angle of 1st and 2nd toes
Nose	Abnormal dermatoglyphics
Flattened bridge	
Small size	Genitalia
Upturned nares	Ambiguous genitalia
	Micropenis
Face	Large testicles
Increased length of philtrum	
Hypoplasia of maxilla or mandible	Skin
	Café-au-lait spots
Mouth	Depigmented nevi
Inverted V shape of upper lip	
Wide or high-arched palate	Teeth
	Evidence of abnormal enamelogenesis
	Abnormal odontogenesis

TABLE 3–26. Indications for Laboratory Assessment of the Young Child With Mental Retardation

- Chromosomal karyotype
  - Unusual number or character of atypical physical features
  - History of maternal exposure to a teratogen
  - Major congenital malformations
  - Abnormal genitalia
- Serum amino or organic acids
  - Unexplained seizures in early infancy
  - Failure to thrive
  - Unusual smell of urine or skin
  - Unusually light-colored hair
  - Microcephaly
  - Dermatitis
  - Unexplained acidosis
  - Family history
- Urine mucopolysaccharides
  - Coarse facial features
  - Kyphosis
  - Short extremities
  - Short trunk
  - Hepatosplenomegaly
  - Cloudy corneas
  - Impaired hearing
  - Short stature
  - Stiff joints
- Urine-reducing substances
  - Cataracts
  - Hepatomegaly
  - Seizures
- Plasma ammonia
  - Episodic vomiting and metabolic acidosis
- Urine ketoacids
  - Seizures
  - Short friable hair
- Blood lead
  - History of pica
  - Anemia
- Serum zinc
  - Acrodermatitis
- Serum copper and ceruloplasmin
  - Involuntary movements
  - Cirrhosis
  - Kayser-Fleischer rings
- White blood cell lysosomal enzyme analysis or skin biopsy
  - Loss of motor or cognitive milestones or functions
  - Optic atrophy
  - Retinal degeneration
  - Recurrent cerebellar ataxia
  - Myoclonus
  - Hepatosplenomegaly
  - Coarse loose skin
  - Seizures
  - Enlarged head beginning after 1 yr of age
- Urine vanillylmandelic acid
  - Episodic vomiting
  - Poor suck
  - Symptoms of autonomic dysfunction
- Serum uric acid
  - Self-mutilation
  - Rage attacks
  - Gout
  - Choreoathetosis
- Plasma very long chain fatty acids
  - Atypical phenotypic features
  - Hepatomegaly
  - Early seizures and hypotonia
  - Hearing loss
  - Retinal degeneration
  - Renal cysts
  - Aberrant bone calcification
- Blood lactate and pyruvate
  - Metabolic acidosis
  - Myoclonic seizures
  - Progressive weakness
  - Ataxia
  - Retinal degeneration
  - Ophthalmoplegia
  - Recurrent stroke-like episodes
- Viral titers for congenital infection
  - Sensorineural hearing impairment
  - Neonatal hepatosplenomegaly
  - Neonatal petechial rash
  - Chorioretinitis
  - Microphthalmia
  - Intracranial calcifications
  - Microcephaly
- Electroencephalogram
  - Suspected seizure disorder
  - Severe receptive language impairment
- Cranial computed tomography (CT) or magnetic resonance imaging (MRI)
  - Progressive enlargement of head
  - Tuberous sclerosis
  - Suspected gross malformation of brain
  - Focal seizures
  - Suspected intracranial mass

to be secondary to an unknown congenital influence on the development of the brain.

TREATMENT. Management of a child with mental retardation is multidimensional and highly individualized. Although the potential need for a highly specialized multidisciplinary effort should be considered, not all children with mental retardation are served best by a complex array of services and professionals. Wise decisions about resource needs are most likely when they are informed by the development of an individualized plan whose goals and objectives flow from a careful consideration of the specific risk and protective factors inherent in the child and his or her family.

One of the critical and most demanding roles played by the physician involves the initial synthesis and presentation of diagnostic findings to the family. This process involves a highly sensitive interaction whose details are often remembered and recounted verbatim by parents for many years thereafter. A skilled clinician provides complete and accurate information about what is known about the nature and possible causes of the child's disability, identifies areas of relative competence and adaptive behaviors, provides emotional support, works with the family to define specific goals and objectives and to formulate a strategy for further management, provides sufficient opportunities for parents to identify their own needs for further information, and responds honestly to unanswerable questions. When managed well, the initial informing interview can provide a strong foundation for ongoing parent-professional collaboration.

Specialized educational and therapeutic services are central elements in the multidisciplinary treatment of children with mental retardation. During the adolescent years, issues related to sexuality, vocational training, and community living become more prominent than at earlier stages. The role of the physician necessarily varies with the needs of the child and family. All children must be assured of routine health maintenance services including immunizations, monitoring of growth, and prompt treatment of minor illnesses. Specific medical complications that occur with greater frequency among children with developmental disabilities (e.g., seizure disorders, impairments of vision or hearing, and nutritional problems) require accurate diagnosis and prompt management. Ongoing health surveillance should be guided by knowledge of the relative risks of specific associated disorders (e.g., slowly progressive hearing impairment in children with congenital cytomegalovirus infection or the development of hypothyroidism in youngsters with Down syndrome). Finally, the physician has an important responsibility to ensure the provision of sophisticated genetic counseling whenever the diagnosis of a heritable disorder is considered.

Collaboration between the primary care physician and an early intervention service system is particularly important in the management of children with developmental impairments in the first years of life. Early identification and prompt referral ensure access to individualized therapeutic and educational services for the child in conjunction with flexible support services for the family. Such services are delivered best when they focus on the family as a dynamic system and view child and family adaptation as interdependent and mutually influenced by the environment in which they live. Although significant methodologic limitations compromise the ability to evaluate adequately the full range of effects of early intervention programs on young children with disabilities, a substantial body of research demonstrates the presence of positive short-term benefits on standardized developmental test scores. The effects of early intervention on children's social competence, their long-term efficacy, and the influence of services on family adaptation are largely unknown.

PREVENTION. Although most pathogenetic mechanisms remain unknown, an increasing number of disorders can be detected through prenatal diagnostic studies such as ultrasound, amniocentesis, or chorionic villous biopsy. The provision of complete information and sensitive medical management are therefore essential to ensure informed family decisions about all available prenatal intervention options, including experimental fetal surgeries (such as the placement in utero of an intracranial shunt) and the elective termination of a pregnancy. When specific early treatments are available for infants with metabolic disorders and structural abnormalities, successful prevention requires prompt diagnosis and sophisticated management, such as for phenylketonuria. In contrast, identifiable metabolic disorders for which specific therapies are not yet available, such as the mucopolysaccharidoses, must await further advances in molecular biology before effective prevention efforts can be realized.

The central theme common to all efforts to prevent mental retardation is the promotion of healthy brain development and the provision of a nurturing and growth-promoting environment. Because most of the population of mentally retarded individuals are mildly retarded, and because mild retardation is disproportionately prevalent among lower socioeconomic groups, substantial prevention efforts must focus on the biologic well-being and the early life experiences of children living in poverty. In this regard, prenatal care and family support services represent major prevention strategies.

JACK P. SHONKOFF

Featherstone H: A Difference in the Family. New York, Basic Books, 1980.

Freeman JM (ed): Prenatal and Perinatal Factors Associated with Brain Disorders. NIH Publication No. 85-1149. Washington, DC, US Department of Health and Human Services, 1985.

Gould SJ: The Mismeasure of Man. New York, WW Norton, 1981.

Jones KL: Smith's Recognizable Patterns of Human Malformation. Philadelphia, WB Saunders, 1988.

Meisels SJ, Shonkoff JP (eds): Handbook of Early Childhood Intervention. New York, Cambridge University Press, 1990.

Shonkoff JP: Biological and social factors contributing to mild mental retardation. *In:* Heller K, Holtzman W, Messick S (eds): Placing Children in Special Education: A Strategy for Equity. Washington, DC, National Academy Press, 1982.

Turnbull HR, Turnbull AP: Parents Speak Out—Then and Now, 2nd ed. Columbus, OH, Merrill, 1985.

Zigler E, Balla D (eds): Mental Retardation: The Development-Difference Controversy. Hillsdale, NJ, Lawrence Erlbaum Associates, 1982.

3.59 CARE OF THE CHILD WITH A FATAL ILLNESS

From time to time every physician has the painful duty of caring for a child with a chronic fatal illness. It is then his or her responsibility to help the family cope with their pain and grief in such ways that the experience may become growth-promoting rather than destructive of family integrity or emotional well-being. When physicians accept these goals as realistic and commit professional skills to them, their efforts will help to blunt their own senses of frustration, grief, or professional inadequacy. (See also Sec. 2.1).

CARE OF PARENTS

When the physician is certain that a condition will have a fatal outcome, there should be no equivocation in conveying the diagnosis to the family in a direct and empathetic way. If both parents are available, the fact that their child has an illness from which recovery is not expected should be conveyed to them when they are together. The words chosen and the manner of the physician should be gentle and honest, and he or she should be prepared to meet the parents' anguish or disbelief with answers to their questions and with information as to what measures will be taken to try to forestall what seems to be inevitable (see Sec 2.2).

The place in which this conversation occurs should be apart from the other activities of the hospital or office and should be available for an adequate, uninterrupted time. The privacy of this place and time should be carefully protected. Much of the conversation will not be fully registered or accurately remembered by the parents of the sick child, and the physician should plan another session later in the day or on the next day when the information given can be reviewed and new or recurring questions answered.

Ordinarily the physician should avoid taking the position that nothing can be done but should emphasize the positive steps that the physician and parents together can take to surmount the difficulties ahead. Physicians should generally avoid detailed predictions of the course or duration of the illness, emphasizing that in such situations one generally lives from day to day and that it is usually possible to avoid undue suffering or pain. When the illness may endure for months or years, it may not be inappropriate to hold out hope that medical research may provide methods of control that are not currently available.

Parents are often reluctant to ask whether some other physician or the resources of some other medical center may offer more hope, or whether the diagnosis may be in doubt. They will need help in expressing these concerns and should be encouraged and helped to seek additional medical opinions if they wish. These matters should be discussed in such a way that the family should feel no embarrassment, and they should know that they are causing none. They can be told that medical communication is generally good enough to provide prompt dissemination of any real breakthrough in the management of the otherwise fatal illness of their child. It is also reasonable to advise them that they may do the ill child and the rest of the family a disservice if they dissipate the family's emotional and other resources in a frantic search for something that is not available.

It is natural and inevitable that parents will ask themselves whether the fatal illness of their child was not somehow avoidable. Some will seek causes in inadequate medical care, in incompetent physicians, or in other environmental circumstances; others will assume a burden of guilt at their own failure to recognize the symptoms of illness or to take action quickly enough so that a cure could have been effected. Each of these reactions may be irrational. When these feelings are implicit in questions or responses of parents, the physician should make them explicit, point out the inevitability of such feelings, and, when it can be honestly done, reassure the parents that there are no grounds for their shouldering blame for a situation that no one could say might have been averted. The feeling of guilt or of punishment may be particularly strong in genetic disorders. Here it may be helpful to encourage the family to regard genetic mutations as tragic accidents, almost always beyond the ability of man to avoid.

In the management of the affected child parents should be encouraged to handle the life situation of the child as normally as possible. This may be difficult for guilt-ridden or grieving parents who may think that their usual disciplinary activities may make the child's pain or illness worse. The parents should be encouraged to maintain the child in the normal place in the family hierarchy. Special arrangements, such as the celebration of Christmas in the summertime or public dramatizations of the child's illness, should be discouraged; they may be more anxiety-provoking for the child than fulfilling of any need. As much as possible, the parents should be encouraged to participate in the care of the child in the hospital as long as their responsibilities to other children at home are adequately met. They may also need encouragement to take adequate respite from the care of the ill child.

As the physician follows the evolution of a fatal illness in a child, the manner in which the parents are coping with the situation should be observed. For example, some parents may increasingly turn their attention to other sick children in the hospital. This is a healthy sign if it is not premature; if it comes too early, it may represent the parents' unresolved burden of guilt or their pain in facing the ill child. This turning away to help other children is healthy as long as the parents still have adequate resources and strength for the needs of their own child.

At times the guilt of parents is intensified by a wish that the illness were over or by an unexpected sense of relief or release at the terminal event itself. The considerate and skillful physician will be on the watch for signs of these reactions and find the right words of reassurance or encouragement that such feelings are normal and that the parents have given everything that could have been expected of them in a situation that they have found very trying and toward which they will forever have sensitive and tender feelings.

CARE OF THE CHILD

What to tell the child who has a fatal illness about the future will vary with the condition and circumstances. Most young children do not ask whether they are going to die. They can often be told that they have an illness that may last for some time and has ups and downs, and that it is important for them to get adequate rest and to be active when they feel up to it. Unrealistic reassurances that they look well and are doing fine will be less helpful than the frank recognition of the child's feeling that being ill is no fun and that having it going on so long is discouraging. If the child is in a stage of illness requiring temporary hospitalization, he or she needs reassurance that school and normal activity will begin again as soon as possible. Meanwhile it is supportive, when appropriate, for the child to receive attention from schoolteachers and play therapists in the hospital, who will help blunt the sense of inevitability of worsening illness.

In the case of preadolescent or adolescent children with chronic and fatal illness, the plan for care may often include sharing the diagnosis with the child and examining with parents and child together the implications of diagnosis and prognosis, answering their questions, and laying out with them a program of action and support that will have as its goal keeping the patient as comfortable as possible and forestalling any conclusion to the effort as long as possible. In this atmosphere of frankness, trust, and cooperation, free of secrets or evasions, many families and patients will find an unexpectedly healthy climate for the expression of tenderness and love toward each other, and the physician may find his or her own work easier. As a chronic illness becomes terminal, this climate makes it easier to meet the needs of the patient for a sense of not being abandoned, for assurances of the continuing love and affection of those around, and for reasonably prompt responses to needs for care. The decision as to when or how the diagnosis of a potentially fatal illness is to be shared with the child must have the full understanding, consent, and cooperation of parents, and the parents will need to have given some thought to how the news of the child's illness is to be handled with siblings, relatives, and neighbors.

OTHER RESOURCES

In dealing with the problems of patient and family around a fatal illness, the physician often calls on other professional persons for help. The family minister or other spiritual advisor can be of immense comfort. When family problems can be ameliorated by use of community resources, the help of a social worker may be important. When the family is not intact, owing to the death or previous separation of a parent, the likelihood of emotional difficulties complicating the management of the illness is sufficiently great that social service resources should probably be involved from the time the diagnosis is known.

The fatal chronic illnesses of children tend to cluster around certain diseases, such as leukemia or other malignancy, cystic fibrosis, and metabolic or degenerative disorders (e.g., Tay-Sachs disease). When groups of families who share a common problem can be brought together to discuss aspects of the care of their children under the guidance of a knowledgeable and skillful professional person (physician, social worker, or nurse), they can often help one another in the management of the illness as well as in coping with the feelings that go with the inevitability of ultimate loss.

MANAGEMENT OF PAIN

The prevention or relief of pain in children or adolescents who have terminal illness depends on the sensitivity of the physician or others to the indications given by each patient that he or she is in distress (also see Sec. 6.53). Children, especially very young children, do not always or readily complain vocally of discomfort but may give other signs, such as immobility or a facial expression of depression. It is not sufficient to order medication for the relief of pain to be given on indication or "prn"; such a procedure makes it inevitable that the child will suffer some pain before relief comes. Rather, medication should be given at regular intervals or continuously, in a suitable dosage.

Older children and adolescents can be given some responsibility for and control of their own medication. Apparatus exists that will permit continuous intravenous administration of analgesics at designated rates and doses, with the patient able to increase the dose if necessary by calling on an additional pulse of injection. The interval between such pulses can be controlled. There is no evidence that the administration of opiates in this manner is addictive for children or adolescents who need relief from pain; the total amount of medication required is sometimes less than if it were administered prn.

When chronic discomfort is punctuated by the acute distress of diagnostic or therapeutic intrusions, relief may be obtained for some children by hypnosis, with the use of relaxation imagery.

TERMINAL CARE

In the management of terminal illness physicians should not leave decisions about what is to be done for the child to parents but should give positive advice as to what they plan to do. The physician should be responsive, however, to the suggestions of parents when these represent helpful and realistic appraisals of their children's needs.

When death is imminent, the patient should be kept comfortable and the parents, as much as possible, should be close at hand. The physician should be available both to parents and to the patient. The physician's control of his or her own feelings is important; if the physician's personal distress is allowed to increase the distance from or decrease involvement with the patient, the anger of the child or parents with what may be perceived as abandonment of them may make terminal care much more difficult. The continued interest and concern of the physician are important in preventing the emotional situation from deteriorating at this time.

As the moment of death approaches, the child should be in a room where he or she can be alone with parents or loved ones at the bedside or nearby. The sensitive physician will see that the occasion is accorded appropriate dignity and not rendered more frustrating or agonizing by efforts to prolong vital functions in a climate of fruitless hyperactivity.

When death has occurred, the patient, bed, and room should be made neat, and the paraphernalia of illness removed. If the parents are not at hand, they should be asked to come to the hospital and be informed of the circumstances. Parents should be given the opportunity to be with the child a little while in the relatively peaceful and uncluttered setting that has been created. A brief and tender parting may help the parents in the adjustments they must ultimately make.

After an infant or child has died, the opportunity for groups of parents with similar experiences to share them may be as important and as supportive as before the death of the child, as long as professional guidance is adequate. Members of such groups can help each other with the process of mourning and can foster the reassurance that comes with sharing such common and otherwise frightening experiences as the guilt felt at the sense of relief that the illness is over, or the fear of losing touch with reality that comes with having set a place at the table for the dead child, or with finding oneself listening for or hearing his or her footstep or voice. Regardless of whether such parent programs exist, physicians should plan for a number of visits with the parents in the weeks after a child's death in order to review such matters with them, to answer their continuing questions, and to assess their status.

DEATH OF THE NEWBORN INFANT

The management of the death of the newborn infant serves as a model for the management of the *acute* and often unanticipated death of an infant, child, or adolescent. Acute fatal illnesses have a major cluster in the neonatal period, and neonatal nurseries and intensive care units must be responsive to the needs of parents who have had no preparation for a catastrophic loss. Mother and infant are usually apart at the moment of death. The body of the newborn infant can often be taken to the mother or to both parents at her bedside or at some other point in the hospital where the chance to hold and examine the baby may be the mother's only opportunity to establish for herself the reality of the birth and death of her infant and to adjust toward reality her current or future fantasies as to what the baby might *really* have been like or what might *really* have happened. For the mother of the malformed infant this may be even more important than for the mother of the otherwise intact infant. The defects can be examined by her in reality rather than in fantasy and their implications gently discussed, with the observation perhaps that the baby was in every other way perfectly formed.

Mothers whose infants have died are in critical need of help in mourning; they should be as involved as they may wish or as circumstances permit in decisions occasioned by the death, including such ceremonial leave-taking as funerals or memorial services.

Neonatal intensive care units find it helpful to maintain small discussion groups for mothers who have lost infants, within which, during the first few weeks of mourning, they can share their experiences with others. Such experiences may include the illusion of hearing the baby (even the stillborn infant) cry in the night. Sharing of such normal but distressing experiences may allay anxiety. The quality of professional guidance of such groups is crucial to their success.

Physicians should make sure that parents understand that the mourning process for a dead infant or older child ought to be reasonably complete and a stable state reached before they decide to have another child. This generally requires 9 mo to a year or more. A new infant conceived too soon is likely to be too closely identified with the dead child and to be surrounded by inordinate anxiety or inappropriate expectations.

POST MORTEM EXAMINATION

A request for post mortem examination should be made by the responsible physician who knows the family best, often not the house officer but the attending or referring physician. The need for post mortem examination should be urged as strongly as conviction permits. Parents can be assured that such examinations are always helpful, that information is gathered and saved which may be useful in years to come in solving similar problems of other children or in providing definitive answers to questions of other children in the family or of their relatives or descendants concerning the patient's illness. Later the physician should describe the important and relevant findings of the gross post mortem examination for the parents in simple terms, and they should have a chance to discuss them as freely as they desire.

VICTOR C. VAUGHAN III

Bluebond-Langner M: The Private Worlds of Dying Children. Princeton, NJ, Princeton University Press, 1978.

Davidson GW: Death of the wished-for child: A case study. Death Educ 1:265, 1977.
Howell DA: A child dies. J Pediatr Surg 1:2, 1966.
Kübler-Ross E: On Death and Dying. New York, Macmillan, 1969. (Available also in paperback.)
McGrath PJ, Unruh AM: Pain in Children and Adolescents. Amsterdam, Elsevier, 1987.
Olness K, Gardner GG: Hypnosis and Hypnotherapy with Children. Philadelphia, Grune & Stratton, 1988.
Schulman JL, Kupst MJ: The Child with Cancer: Clinical Approaches to Psychosocial Care—Research in Psychosocial Aspects. Springfield, IL, Charles C Thomas, 1980.

3.60 INTERACTION BETWEEN THE CHILD AND THE FAMILY

Infants are born completely dependent on the people in their surroundings, and their gradual development toward maturity and independence is greatly influenced by the nurturance given them in the early years of life. This nurturance is provided by the infant's primary intimate group, which in most cases is the family.

As in all developmental biologic processes, the earlier that something goes right or wrong, the more widespread are its effects on the whole organism. Thus, the value of a nurturant (in utero) environment during pregnancy and in the first few years of life cannot be overemphasized. Nurturant intrafamily surroundings, together with sufficient stimulation and fostering of development, need to continue throughout later childhood and puberty to produce a healthy functioning teenager and young adult.

There is tremendous variation in the interactions between a child and his or her family. This section deals first with the basic assumptions and tenets that should influence the physician's understanding of and relations with families and then reviews coping processes and the application of the assumptions and tenets to clinical practice.

BASIC ASSUMPTIONS AND TENETS

ASSUMPTIONS. Society and culture influence the infant and child mainly through the intervention and mediation of his or her primary group of relationships. The most intimate of these is the family, which contributes to the child's physical and emotional health as well as to his or her attitudes, beliefs, understanding, and behavior pertaining to health and disease. It follows that the characteristics of the family (i.e., its structure, function, and developmental stage) have a marked influence on all aspects of the child's life. The second assumption accepts the fact that the family is a system of dynamic interrelating people. Whenever one member, for example, a child, becomes seriously ill, it affects each member of the family as well as the family as a whole. Similarly, anything that affects the family as a whole, for example, loss of the home or moving to a different city, affects each member. At all stages of this interaction there is continuous feedback to and from the sick child, and this influences the sick child's reaction. The premise of this *interactive systems model* is that all disease is multifactorial in origin, resulting from the interaction of the factors related to the specific illness, the child, the child's family, and the surrounding environment. Last, except for occasional acute emergencies, the most effective way to diagnose and manage a sick child is by working with, actively involving, and supporting the family of the child.

DEFINITION OF FAMILY. For health care purposes, this definition includes the *biologic* family, those related by blood, marriage, and adoption; the *unit of living or household;* and the *functional* family, that is, the people who are closest to the patient. These might include biologic or fictive kin, friends, or neighbors whom the patient regards as his or her primary social support network. Fictive kin designates friends who can be counted on, have a mutual consensual relationship, live together or near one another, and assume the responsibilities of kin.

FAMILY INFLUENCES ON THE CHILD. The family may be the means by which a disease is transmitted, as may occur genetically (sickle cell), intrauterine (rubella), at birth (herpes), or by infections (enteritis). In addition, family clustering occurs in many disorders whose exact mode of transmission is unknown, for example, atopic dermatitis, allergies, asthma, enuresis, peptic ulcers, obesity, and hypertension. Children's attitudes, beliefs, and behavior related to eating or not eating certain types of food, smoking, drinking alcohol, reaction to pain, or feelings about physicians develop through processes such as imitating, identifying with, role modeling, or learning in response to rewards and punishments.

Family functioning affects children in numerous positive and negative ways. Marital conflict, lack of bonding at birth, pathologic sibling rivalry, abnormal boundaries between generations, parental deprivation, and child abuse are examples of family dysfunction that have deleterious effects on children (discussed in other sections of this chapter). Adults who were severely deprived of love and affection when very young often are unable to maintain intimate relationships and deprive their own children of love. Family support has an important role in helping the child cope with everyday hassles and stresses as well as with chronic health problems.

FAMILY STRUCTURE AND CHARACTERISTICS. Families vary in their composition and stage of development. The *nuclear* family, two parents and children, constituted 80% of American families a few decades ago. Currently, this type of family accounts for fewer than 40% of all families. The nuclear family is suited for differentiation of roles and responsibilities. *Single-parent households,* usually a mother with children, constitute more than 20% of American families. The mother may never have been married, or she may be divorced, separated, or widowed. Because the parent usually has to work full-time, the problem of being the sole income provider as well as fulfilling the roles of mother and father is very difficult for both parent and children. Some studies suggest that many children from single-parent households do not do as well educationally or emotionally as children from households with two parents.

The *three-generation* family can be a nuclear family or a single-parent household with the grandparent(s) of the children. The presence of grandparents is usually a positive feature, whether they live in the same household or in close proximity. They make life easier for the parents, especially in single-parent households; for example, often the mother works while the grandmother does the "mothering." In some cases grandparents are replaced by or complemented by the presence of aunts or parental siblings. This extended kin network may provide a good support system.

Reconstituted families result from remarriage of divorced, separated, or widowed parents. Thus, the children may have to adjust to the biologic offspring of one parent and the step-children of the other and to siblings and step-siblings, and perhaps later, half-siblings. In addition, they often have continuing involvement with the other divorced parent. The potential for problems is increased in such families.

Serial monogamy is the term given to an adult, usually a woman, who in the course of her adult years has a series of husbands or companions. She has a monogamous relationship with each one for a period of time. Children may result from one or more of these relationships. This type of living often is associated with a great deal of social pathology and an increased amount of childhood morbidity and recurrent hospitalizations.

Children sometimes find themselves in other types of living arrangements such as foster homes, orphanages, and, recently, adopted by couples of the same sex.

Each family goes through a developmental process in which a number of distinct sequential stages may be recognized. These begin with the growing stage of family formation, continuing through the expanding stages of child-bearing, child-rearing, and child launching, to the contracting periods of the "empty nest," widowhood, and finally, termination. As the family unit evolves through these stages, the developmental needs of individual members of a family may overlap and complement each other, or may conflict and compete with one another. During each stage, as well as during the transition from one stage to another, certain developmental events occur in most families. Physiologic changes include standing, walking, bowel control, puberty, childbirth, and menopause, and sociocultural transitions include entering preschool or school, graduating from or leaving school, the first date, the first job, leaving home, and so on. In contrast to normal transitions, there are unexpected ones such as an accident, failure at school, robbery, fire, sudden acute illness, diagnosis of serious chronic disease, or a life-threatening episode such as a rape. In each of these stages, there are a number of specific developmental tasks that should be accomplished as they affect family relationships and functioning. If these tasks are not accomplished, the individual and the family are at a disadvantage at subsequent stages.

Although this description is based on the cycle of the nuclear family, other types of families also go through their own life cycle stages. These vary from those of the nuclear family, but they all go through some of the same stages, albeit with a different constellation of family members and with variations depending on the composition of a particular family. For example, the empty nest period may not be experienced at all in an extended family, but the same principles of developmental tasks hold true. These family stages are highly interrelated with the life development of each member of the family, as described in other sections. It is important for physicians to appreciate the effect that different stages of an illness may have on the development of both the individual child and the family.

THE ENVIRONMENT. The physical, economic, and social environment have significant effects on the health of the children and their families. These are discussed in various other sections.

APPLICATIONS AND IMPLICATIONS FOR CLINICAL PRACTICE

STRESS AND COPING. Disruptive stressful life events, such as bereavement, are associated directly or indirectly (through increased susceptibility) with mild to severe physical and mental disorders. The short-term effects of stress are often readily apparent in children; the long-term effects are complex and difficult to establish with certainty.

The process of stress and coping is conceptualized in Figure 3–14. X stands for stressors or activators that arise from an internal or environmental stimulus. Unmet expectations or fear can, on occasion, act as stressors. Some obvious stressors of childhood are hospitalizations, birth of a sibling, parental divorce, parental death, and so on. Reactions (Y) are the biologic reactions (changes in cells, blood glucose, blood pressure) or psychologic responses (anger, hostility) of an individual to a stressor. Consequences (Z) are the sequelae to reactions, such as long-term health changes or positive results such as increased schoolwork productivity. Mediators are the filters and modifiers that act on each stage in the X–Y–Z sequence to produce the individual variations. They may vary from a genetic predisposition or a physical or psychologic setting that can produce or alleviate anxiety to a social situation that can be helpful or destructive. Included in this group of mediators are risk factors for specific diseases, which often are the study objectives of experimental, clinical, or epidemiologic research.

In humans there is tremendous variation in actual and potential stressors, which leads to great variation in reactions and consequences. The same activator may produce variations in reactions depending on the characteristics of the individual (age, sex, temperament, genetic factors) and family involved as well as on the mediating factors. The importance of social support in helping the child deal with stressors cannot be overemphasized. As children and families traverse their life cycle stages their reactions and coping abilities also change, based on their developing maturity and experience in dealing with various types of stressors. The basic methods and strategies of dealing with stressors remain the same, but the ability to use them changes with the development of the individual and the family.

The sick child's ability to cope with the stress of illness depends in large measure on the loving presence of the child's parents and the empathetic understanding of the health care team (see Sec. 3.59). From the family's point of view, there are three basic coping strategies following the initial shock stage: (1) seeking information and understanding of the stressor, such as the meaning of the diagnosis of diabetes; (2) mobilizing the family by improving communication between family members when there is a need to restructure the family's functioning, trying to take an optimistic view of the situation, mobilizing the family's resources, and developing new skills; and (3) seeking social support from others.

COPING WITH NORMAL TRANSITIONS. These are usually adequately dealt with by individuals and families even though some transitions, such as adolescence, are more difficult for some families to deal with. Occasionally the reaction to a normal transition that occurs out of its time sequence, for example, puberty at an early age, or a parent dying when children are younger than 12 yr of age, is similar to an unexpected transition and may lead to a crisis situation.

COPING WITH ACUTE ILLNESS AND CRISIS. An acute

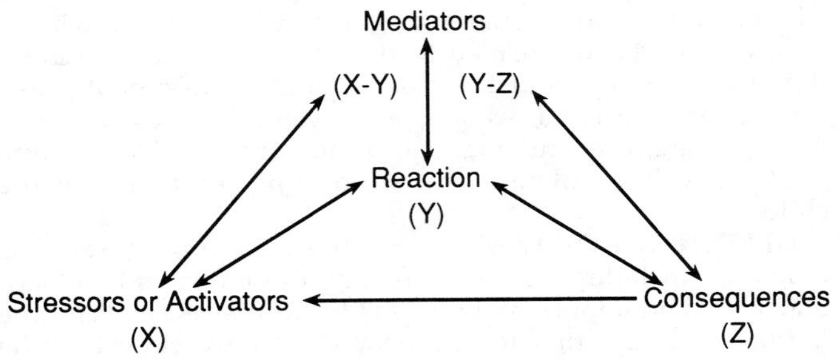

Figure 3–14. A framework for interactions between the individual and the environment.

severe illness, accident, or fatality to a child can create a crisis situation for the entire family, an event in which the individual's or family's coping abilities are inadequate to meet the demands of the situation. An average family's reaction to crisis can be divided into four related and overlapping phases.

1. The phase of shock, denial, and bewilderment. Activities are carried out automatically, and explanations by physicians and others are not absorbed unless they are repeated and reinforced.
2. A period of changing emotions such as anxiety, resentment, and blame (toward the sick child, another member of the family, or the physician), depression, apathy, and guilt. Daily activities are carried on automatically at a minimal level. At this stage a person's defenses are weakened, and most people are more open to suggestions, changes, and other forms of assistance.
3. Gradual acknowledgment and acceptance, which leads to the 4th stage.
4. Reorganization of the family system in an attempt to adjust to the new situation and to continue functioning. This *family reorganization* can result in: (1) Re-establishment of the family's precrisis state of functioning. Following bereavement, this usually occurs within 1 yr but may take as long as 3 yr; (2) beneficial changes and improved family functioning; (3) a reduced level of functioning that may show itself in development of various illnesses in several individuals, such as asthma, arthritis, ulcerative colitis, recurrent infections; or (4) rapid or gradual entry into a state of disorganization or disintegration that leads to parental separation or divorce.

COPING WITH CHRONIC ILLNESS

See Sec. 3.57.

THE HIDDEN PATIENT. Whenever a family has a child with a serious illness, the burden of caretaking usually falls primarily on one person—usually the mother. If this person does not receive adequate support from the rest of the family as well as from outside resources, during the course of time she or he is very likely to develop an illness or disease. Physicians should be aware of these hidden patients.

Occasionally, the whole family becomes dysfunctional with the possibility of numerous members showing signs of illness. Another and perhaps more common occurrence in the dysfunctional family is the maintenance of homeostasis at the expense of one child who becomes the family "scapegoat." This child may manifest abnormal behaviors at home or at school or may begin to develop various illnesses.

THE EFFECT OF ILLNESS IN FAMILIES ON CHILDREN. There are many instances when the sick child is a symptom or the result of family pathology. Parents or families with severe conflicts in or between them may achieve a type of equilibrium by projecting their hostilities onto one of their children (scapegoating). For example, when adolescents and their parents have severe conflicts, some sort of equilibrium may be maintained by scapegoating a younger defenseless sibling.

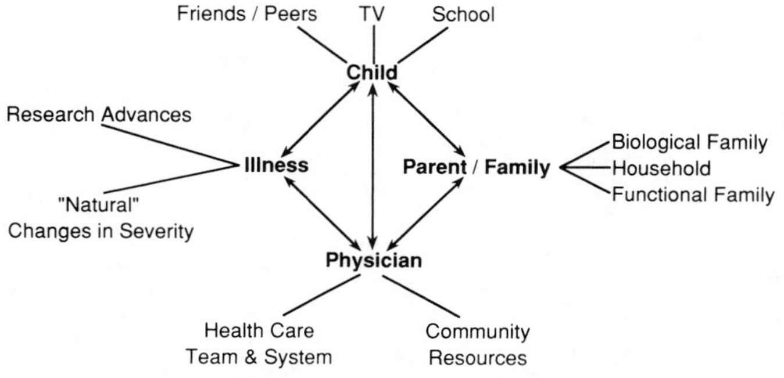

Figure 3–15. The extended therapeutic quadrate.

In addition, serious illness of parents or loss of a family member may have untoward effects on children. Depression of one parent may produce increased morbidity and visits to physicians in children during and after the depression. Acute life-threatening illness in one member of a family may increase the number of contacts for serious complaints in the unaffected members of families who have inadequate coping resources. There is an increased number of physician contacts for all types of morbidity in children of families with unsatisfactory or disturbed relationships compared to those with satisfactory ones. Weissman et al found that the children of parents of whom one had a history of major depression showed significant differences in the following respects: They reached a number of developmental landmarks significantly later than normal (sitting with assistance, urinary and bowel control); had more injuries, accidents, and seizures; showed more school learning and attention problems despite having no difference in IQ levels; and exhibited higher rates of depression, anxiety, and suicidal gestures.

Children growing up in families in which one or more adult is an alcoholic suffer many short- and long-term effects. Approximately 50% of alcoholic families exhibit definite inherited tendencies. Alcoholic families also tend to react in patterned and even predictable ways when one member becomes alcoholic. Some of the problems that occur in children of alcoholics at a higher incidence than others in the population include fetal alcohol syndrome, child and sexual abuse, behavior problems, school problems, chemical dependency, depression, and suicide attempts. The family dynamics of alcoholics often produce patterns of behavior in children, such as the family hero (the successful child), the scapegoat who often acts out his or her anger with aggression and defiance, the lost child who is withdrawn and isolated but not a troublemaker, and the family mascot, who provides the comic relief but in reality is a very anxious and often hyperactive child. These children and the whole family can be helped to overcome their problems if they receive appropriate and sufficient assistance, including family therapy, Alcoholics Anonymous, Alanon, Alateen, and other self-help groups.

THERAPEUTIC PROCESS. In every encounter with a child patient, the physician deals with the child, the illness, the child's family, and the physician's own attitudes and knowledge (Fig. 3–15). The child is affected by the illness, by his or her family, and by the influence of television, school, and friends. The behavior of the parents is the product of their experiences from their families of orientation, friends, and neighbors, economic status, and social network. Similarly, the physician has his or her own background of experiences in addition to those of the current health care system and community resources, which impinge on his or her diagnostic and therapeutic decisions. These influences play important roles in every physician-patient encounter. Pediatricians should supplement the recent advances made in disease processes with a family orientation when dealing with sick children, especially those with chronic diseases.

JACK H. MEDALIE

Elliott GR, Eisdorfer C (eds): Stress and Human Health: A Study by the Institute of Medicine/National Academy of Sciences. New York, Springer-Verlag, 1982.
Griner ME, Griner PF: Alcoholism and the family. *In:* Barnes HN, Aronson MD, Delbanco TL (eds): Alcoholism: A Guide for the Primary Care Physician. New York, Springer-Verlag, 1987, pp 159–166.
Hamburg BA: Chronic illness. *In:* Levine MD, Carey WB, Crocker AC, et al (eds): Developmental Behavioral Pediatrics. Philadelphia, WB Saunders, 1983, pp 455–463.
Hamburg BA, Killilea A: Relation of social support, stress, illness and use of

health services. *In:* Healthy People Report, Institute of Medicine. Washington, National Academy of Sciences Press, 1979, pp 253–276.

Klaus MH, Kennell JH: Maternal–Infant Bonding. St. Louis, CV Mosby, 1976.

Osterweis M, Solomon F, Green M (eds): Bereavement: Reactions, Consequences and Care. Washington, National Academy of Sciences Press, 1984.

Patterson JM: Chronic illness in children and the impact on families. *In:* Chilman CS, Nunnally EW, Cox FM (eds): Chronic Illness and Disability. Newbury Park, CA, Sage, 1988, pp 69–107.

Patterson JM, McCubbin HI: Chronic illness: Family stress and coping. *In:* Figley CR, McCubbin HI (eds): Stress and the Family, Vol. 2: Coping With Catastrophe. New York, Brunner/Mazel, 1983, pp 21–36.

Rolland JS: A conceptual model of chronic and life-threatening illness and its impact on families. *In:* Chilman CS, Nunnally EW, Cox FM (eds): Chronic Illness and Disability. London, Sage, 1988, pp 17–68.

Weissman MM, John K, Merikangas KR, et al: Depressed parents and their children. Am J Dis Child 140:801, 1986.

Whitt JK: Children's adaptation to chronic illness and handicapping conditions. *In:* Eisenberg MC, Sutkin LC, Jansen MA (eds): Chronic Illness and Disability Through the Life Span. New York, Springer-Verlag, 1984, pp 69–102.

4

NUTRITION AND NUTRITIONAL DISORDERS

NUTRITIONAL REQUIREMENTS

Individual nutritional requirements vary with genetic and metabolic differences. For infants and children, however, the basic goals are satisfactory growth and the avoidance of deficiency states. Good nutrition helps to prevent acute and chronic illness and to develop physical and mental potential; it should also provide reserves for stress.

The Food and Nutrition Board (NAS-NRC, 1989) has identified appropriate dietary allowances for a number of substances that prevent deficiency states in most persons (Table 4–1). Because some essential substances remain unidentifiable, a varied diet may be the only prudent way of providing them after early infancy. Only human milk appears to supply all essentials for a prolonged time. Although some essential foods should be included in the daily diet, others are stored by the body and may be supplied periodically.

Although any diet producing good nutrition varies considerably, mild excesses of nutrients or calories may be as undesirable as mild deficiencies. Because dietary influence on aspects of the aging process, for example, atherosclerosis and longevity, remains incompletely understood, avoidance of excessive caloric and fat intake appears to be wise at all ages.

4.1 WATER

Water (Sec. 6.3) is essential for existence; a lack of it results in death in a matter of days. The water content of infants is relatively higher (70–75% of the body weight) than that of adults (60–65%). Although fluids provide the principal source of water, some water is obtained from the oxidation of foods (mixed diets yield about 12 g H_2O/100 kcal) and body tissues.

Human needs for water are related to caloric consumption, to insensible loss, and to the specific gravity of the urine. The infant must consume much larger amounts of water per unit of body weight compared with the adult, but when calculated per unit of caloric intake, the amounts required are almost identical (Tables 4–2 and 4–3). The daily consumption of fluid by the healthy infant is equivalent to 10–15% of body weight, compared with 2–4% in the adult. The usual food of infants and children is high in water content; most of the solid food in the child's diet contains 60–70% water, and many of the fruits and vegetables contain 90%.

Water is absorbed throughout the intestinal tract. The quantity of water in the interstitial compartment is readily changed to maintain homeostatic balance between the intracellular and vascular compartments. The interchange of water among these compartments depends on their respective protein and electrolyte concentrations. Depending on the rate of growth, about 0.5–3% of the fluid intake will be retained. Retention of water is in the range of 9–13 mL/24 hr for the "male reference infant" in the first year of life.

Water balance depends on variables such as fluid intake, protein and mineral content of diet, solute load presented for renal excretion, metabolic and respiratory rates, and body temperature. Water requirements for low-birthweight infants are estimated at 85–170 mL/kg/24 hr. Fecal losses are small (3–10% of intake). Evaporation from lungs and skin accounts for 40–50% of intake (sometimes more) and renal excretion for 40–50% or more. The kidney preserves the fluid and electrolyte equilibrium of the body by varying the osmolar content and volume of urine. Urine usually has a greater osmotic pressure (300–1,000 mOsm/L) than the internal environment (293 mOsm/L); maximum normal urinary concentration is approximately 600–700 mOsm/L.

4.2 CALORIES

The unit of heat in metabolism is the large calorie or kilocalorie (1 Cal = 1 kcal); it is used to refer to the energy content of food. A kilocalorie is defined as the amount of heat necessary to raise the temperature of 1 kg of water from 14.5 to 15.5° C. The production of heat varies in the oxidation of different foods, so that measuring the amount of oxygen consumed or measuring the end products of oxidation, carbon dioxide, and water approximates the values obtained by direct calorimetry.

Energy needs of children at different ages and under various conditions (Fig. 4–1) vary greatly. The approximate average expenditures of energy by the child 6–12 yr of age are basal metabolism, 50%; growth, 12%; physical activity, 25%; and fecal loss, about 8%, mainly as unabsorbed fat.

Basal metabolism is measured at room temperature (20° C) 10–14 hr after a meal, with the patient physically and emotionally quiet. For each centigrade degree of fever, basal metabolism increases approximately 10%. The basal requirement in infants is about 55 kcal/kg/24 hr; it decreases to 25–30 kcal/kg/24 hr at maturity. The term *specific dynamic action* (SDA) refers to the increase in metabolism over the basal rate by the ingestion and assimilation of food. Protein digestion may increase metabolism as much as 30% above the basal level, except when it is being deposited in tissues, whereas fat and carbohydrate, which have a "sparing" effect on the specific dynamic action of protein and upon each other, cause increases of only 4 and 6%, respectively. In infants, about 7–8% of the total caloric intake goes to SDA, whereas in older children on an ordinary mixed diet it is unlikely to constitute more than about 5% of total intake. The estimated energy necessary to build body tissue *(growth)* is the difference between the calories ingested and those expended for other purposes. The average requirement for *physical activity* is 15–25 kcal/kg/24 hr, with peak utilizations as high as 50–80 kcal/kg/24 hr for short periods. The amount of energy-producing

TABLE 4–1. Food and Nutrition Board, National Academy of Sciences—National Research Council Recommended Dietary Allowances (Revised 1989)*†

							Fat-Soluble Vitamins			Water-Soluble Vitamins								Minerals						
Category	Age (yr) or Condition	Weight‡ (kg)	Weight‡ (lb)	Height‡ (cm)	Height‡ (in)	Protein (g)	Vitamin A (μg RE)§	Vitamin D (μg)‖	Vitamin E (mg α-TE)¶	Vitamin K (μg)	Vitamin C (mg)	Thiamin (mg)	Riboflavin (mg)	Niacin (mg NE)**	Vitamin B_6 (mg)	Folate (μg)	Vitamin B_{12} (μg)	Calcium (mg)	Phosphorus (mg)	Magnesium (mg)	Iron (mg)	Zinc (mg)	Iodine (μg)	Selenium (μg)
Infants	0.0–0.5	6	13	60	24	13	375	7.5	3	5	30	0.3	0.4	5	0.3	25	0.3	400	300	40	6	5	40	10
	0.5–1.0	9	20	71	28	14	375	10	4	10	35	0.4	0.5	6	0.6	35	0.5	600	500	60	10	5	50	15
Children	1–3	13	29	90	35	16	400	10	6	15	40	0.7	0.8	9	1.0	50	0.7	800	800	80	10	10	70	20
	4–6	20	44	112	44	24	500	10	7	20	45	0.9	1.1	12	1.1	75	1.0	800	800	120	10	10	90	20
	7–10	28	62	132	52	28	700	10	7	30	45	1.0	1.2	13	1.4	100	1.4	800	800	170	10	10	120	30
Males	11–14	45	99	157	62	45	1,000	10	10	45	50	1.3	1.5	17	1.7	150	2.0	1,200	1,200	270	12	15	150	40
	15–18	66	145	176	69	59	1,000	10	10	65	60	1.5	1.8	20	2.0	200	2.0	1,200	1,200	400	12	15	150	50
	19–24	72	160	177	70	58	1,000	10	10	70	60	1.5	1.7	19	2.0	200	2.0	1,200	1,200	350	10	15	150	70
	25–50	79	174	176	70	63	1,000	5	10	80	60	1.5	1.7	19	2.0	200	2.0	800	800	350	10	15	150	70
	51+	77	170	173	68	63	1,000	5	10	80	60	1.2	1.4	15	2.0	200	2.0	800	800	350	10	15	150	70
Females	11–14	46	101	157	62	46	800	10	8	45	50	1.1	1.3	15	1.4	150	2.0	1,200	1,200	280	15	12	150	45
	15–18	55	120	163	64	44	800	10	8	55	60	1.1	1.3	15	1.5	180	2.0	1,200	1,200	300	15	12	150	50
	19–24	58	128	164	65	46	800	10	8	60	60	1.1	1.3	15	1.6	180	2.0	1,200	1,200	280	15	12	150	55
	25–50	63	138	163	64	50	800	5	8	65	60	1.1	1.3	15	1.6	180	2.0	800	800	280	15	12	150	55
	51+	65	143	160	63	50	800	5	8	65	60	1.0	1.2	13	1.6	180	2.0	800	800	280	10	12	150	55
Pregnant						60	800	10	10	65	70	1.5	1.6	17	2.2	400	2.2	1,200	1,200	320	30	15	175	65
Lactating	1st 6 months					65	1,300	10	12	65	95	1.6	1.8	20	2.1	280	2.6	1,200	1,200	355	15	19	200	75
	2nd 6 months					62	1,200	10	11	65	90	1.6	1.7	20	2.1	260	2.6	1,200	1,200	340	15	16	200	75

*The allowances, expressed as average daily intakes over time, are intended to provide for individual variations among most normal persons as they live in the United States under usual environmental stresses. Diets should be based on a variety of common foods in order to provide other nutrients for which human requirements have been less well defined. See text for detailed discussion of allowances and of nutrients not tabulated.

†Designed for the maintenance of good nutrition of practically all healthy people in the United States.

‡Weights and heights of Reference Adults are actual medians for the population in the United States of the designated age, as reported by NHANES II. The median weights and heights of those under 19 years of age were taken from Hamill H, et al: Physical Growth: National Center for Health Statistics Percentiles. The use of these figures does not imply that the height-to-weight ratios are ideal.

§Retinol equivalents. 1 retinol equivalent (RE) = 1 μg retinol or 6 μg β-carotene. See text for calculation of vitamin A activity of diets as retinol equivalents.

‖As cholecalciferol. 10 μg cholecalciferol = 400 IU of vitamin D.

¶α-Tocopherol equivalents. 1 mg *d*-α tocopherol = 1 mg α-TE. See text for variation in allowances and calculation of vitamin E activity of the diet as α-tocopherol equivalent.

**1 NE (niacin equivalent) is equal to 1 mg of niacin or 60 mg of dietary tryptophan.

TABLE 4–2. Water Requirements

Urine Specific Gravity	Infant—3 kg 300 Calories* Intake			Adult—70 kg 3,000 Calories* Intake		
	Water Intake			*Water Intake*		
	mL	*g/100 kcal*	*g/kg*	*mL*	*g/100 kcal*	*g/kg*
1.005	650	217	220	6300	210	90
1.015	339	113	116	3180	106	45
1.020	300	100	100	2790	93	40
1.030	264	88	91	2430	81	35

*In this sense Calorie = large calorie = 1 kcal = 1 Cal (see text).

food lost in the stools, except when absorption is impaired, is not more than 10% of the intake.

Although caloric requirements can best be predicted from the surface area rather than from age or weight, the final criteria for evaluating the child's needs depend on the growth pattern, the sense of well-being, and satiety. The daily requirement is approximately 80–120 kcal/kg for the first year of life, with subsequent decreases of about 10 kcal/kg for each succeeding 3-yr period. Periods of rapid growth and development near puberty require increased caloric consumption. The distribution of calories in human milk, in most formulas, and in a well-balanced diet is similar. Approximately 9–15% of the calories are derived from protein, 45–55% are derived from carbohydrate, and 35–45% are derived from fat.

Each gram of ingested protein or carbohydrate provides 4 kcal. One gram of short-chain fatty acids provides 5.3 kcal; 1 g of medium-chain fatty acid gives 8.3 kcal; and 1 g of long-chain fatty acids provides 9 kcal. A continued caloric intake greater or less than the body expenditure will increase or decrease body fat. In general, a consistent caloric imbalance of 500 kcal/24 hr changes body weight by about 450 g (1 lb)/wk.

4.3 PROTEINS

Protein constitutes about 20% of adult body weight. Its amino acids are essential nutrients in forming cell protoplasm. The kind, number, and arangement of amino acids in a protein molecule determine its characteristics. Twenty-four amino acids have been identified; nine were found to be essential for infants (threonine, valine, leucine, isoleucine, lysine, tryptophan, phenylalanine, methionine, and histidine). Arginine, cystine, and taurine are essential for low-birthweight infants. Nonessential amino acids can be synthesized and need not be supplied in the diet. New tissue cannot be formed without all of the essential amino acids simultaneously present in the diet; the absence or deficiency of only one essential amino acid results in a negative nitrogen balance.

TABLE 4–3. Range of Average Water Requirements of Children at Different Ages Under Ordinary Conditions

Age	Average Body Weight (kg)	Total Water in 24 hr (mL)	Water per kg Body Weight in 24 hr (mL)
3 days	3.0	250–300	80–100
10 days	3.2	400–500	125–150
3 mo	5.4	750–850	140–160
6 mo	7.3	950–1100	130–155
9 mo	8.6	1,100–1,250	125–145
1 yr	9.5	1,150–1.300	120–135
2 yr	11.8	1,350–1,500	115–125
4 yr	16.2	1,600–1,800	100–110
6 yr	20.0	1,800–2,000	90–100
10 yr	28.7	2,000–2,500	70–85
14 yr	45.0	2,200–2,700	50–60
18 yr	54.0	2,200–2,700	40–50

Proteins are broken down in the digestive process to oligopeptides and α-amino acids. The hydrochloric acid of the stomach provides the optimal pH for peptide cleavage by pepsin. Chymosin changes casein of milk to paracasein, which pepsin hydrolyzes along with other proteins. The various proteases show preference for splitting specific peptide linkages; some cleave linkages in the interior of the peptide chain, and others act at more terminal junctures. In the alkaline medium of the intestine, trypsin, chymotrypsin, and carboxypeptidase from the pancreas hydrolyze these proteins and peptones to peptides and to some amino acids; other peptidases from the intestinal juices carry digestion to the amino acid stage.

Minute amounts of certain proteins may be absorbed unchanged, as shown by immunologic reactions, but the hydrolytic products, the amino acids, and some peptides are normally absorbed through the intestinal mucosa. Large oligopeptides may be absorbed in the first few months of life or after episodes of gastroenteritis. The amino acids are carried to the liver by the portal circulation, and from there they are distributed to other tissues. Amino acids are reconstituted to functional human proteins (e.g., albumin, hemoglobin, hormones). Excess amino acids undergo deamination, and the nitrogenous portions are converted to urea in the liver and excreted by the kidneys. The carbon from amino acids is oxidized much like that of carbohydrate or fat; some amino acids are glycogenic; others are ketogenic. Proteins cannot be effectively stored. In protein depletion states, proteins from muscle may be broken down to supply amino acids for more essential sites, such as brain and enzymes.

Aberrations in the metabolism of protein and the amino acids constitute a significant portion of the disease entities known as inborn errors of metabolism (see Chapter 8).

Protein requirements at various ages are listed in Table 4–1. "Biologic value" of proteins indicates effectiveness of utilization; proteins of high biologic value have the quantity and distribution of essential amino acids appropriate for resynthesis of body tissues and provide little waste, as determined by nitrogen balance studies (Table 4–4). Abundant protein is available for children in the United States, but the supply in many countries is limited.

4.4 CARBOHYDRATES

Carbohydrates, while supplying the necessary bulk of the diet, also supply most of the body's energy needs. In its

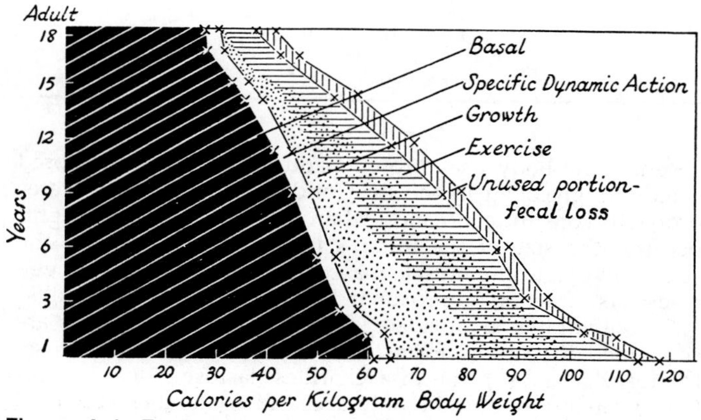

Figure 4–1. Total daily expenditure of calories with approximate distribution among individual factors in relation to age and weight. (Calorie = large calorie = 1 kcal = 1 Cal).

TABLE 4–4. Functions, Effects of Deficiency and Excess, Requirements, and Sources of Water, Proteins, Carbohydrates, and Fats

Foodstuffs	Functions	Effects of Deficiency	Effects of Excess	Requirements	Sources
Water	Structure of cells; solvent for cellular changes; medium for ions; transport of nutrients and waste products; regulation of body temperature	Thirst, dryness of tongue, dehydration, anhydremia, high sp. gr. of urine, loss of kidney function (acidosis, oliguria, uremia, death)	Abdominal discomfort, headache, cramps (water without salt), intoxication, convulsions, edema, and circulatory failure	See Tables 4–2 and 4–3 Related to calories consumed; greater in hot weather	Water as such All foods
Proteins	Supply amino acids for growth and repair of tissue cells; sols for osmotic equilibrium; ions in acid-base balance. With prosthetic groups to form hemoglobin, nucleoproteins, glycoprotein, and lipoproteins. Enzymes, hormones, cellular respiratory substance, antibodies. Protective structures (nails and hair). Source of energy	Lassitude, abdominal enlargement, edema; depletion of plasma proteins, negative nitrogen balance (no clinical syndrome due to lack of specific amino acid); kwashiorkor (protein malnutrition); marasmus (protein-calorie malnutrition)	Prolonged high protein intake probably not harmful. Important in certain anomalies involving amino acid and protein metabolism	See Table 4–1	Milk, eggs, meat, fish, poultry, cheese, soybeans, peas, beans, cereals, nuts, lentils
Carbohydrates	Readily available source of energy, antiketogenic, structure of cells, antibodies, source of stored calories (glycogen and fat), conversion to fat, resynthesis of amino acids, roughage	Ketosis if intake is less than 15% of calories or in starvation; underweight if total calories are low	Overweight if total calories are high. Various syndromes due to inborn errors of sugar metabolism	To supply 25–55% of calories	Milk, cereals, fruits, sucrose, syrups, starches, vegetables
Fats	Concentrated source of energy; physical protection for vessels, nerves, organs; insulation against changes in temperature; structure of body tissues, cell membranes, and nuclei; vehicle for absorption of vitamins (A, D, E, and K); appetite appeal; aids satiety (delays emptying time of stomach); avoids necessity of ingestion of large bulk of foods; spares protein, vitamin A, and thiamine; supplies linoleic acid	Lack of satiety (craving for fat); underweight; skin changes with intakes very low in linoleic acid	Overweight; abdominal symptoms in familial hyperlipidemia; high cholesterol intakes may be harmful to selected populations	Minimal not known; 1–2% of calories as linoleic acid	Milk, butter, egg yolk, lard, bacon, meat, fish, cheese, nuts, vegetable oils Breast milk usually supplies 4–5% of calories as linoleic acid; vegetable oils vary greatly, safflower, corn, soy, and others being especially rich

absence, the body uses proteins and fats for energy. Stored chiefly as glycogen in the liver and muscles, carbohydrates probably constitute no more than 1% of the body weight. Because the size of the infant's liver is 10% of that of the adult's liver and the muscle mass is 2%, the infant's glycogen reserve is a fraction (approximately 3.5%) of that of the adult's.

Carbohydrates are oxidized as glucose (dextrose) but are consumed in various forms: the monosaccharides (glucose, fructose, galactose), the disaccharides (lactose, sucrose, maltose, isomaltose), and the polysaccharides (starches, dextrins, glycogen, gums, cellulose). Pentoses are poorly absorbed.

Through a series of enzymatic and chemical reactions in the digestive tract, complex carbohydrates are split into simpler structures. Salivary and pancreatic amylases are principally involved in the breakdown of starch to oligosaccharides (dextrins) and disaccharides (primarily maltose). Intestinal amylase may be decreased during the first 4 mo of life. The disaccharides are absorbed intact into the intestinal brush border cells, where the various disaccharidases in the membrane fraction of the microvilli complete the hydrolysis to the monosaccharides: 1 molecule of maltose to 2 molecules of glucose; sucrose to glucose and fructose; lactose to glucose and galactose. The monosaccharides are absored rapidly; glucose and galactose are actively taken up against concentration gradients, whereas fructose absorption is passive. During absorption, phosphoric acid "carrier" radicals combine with hexose sugars in the intestinal mucosa for transport across the cell membrane. Sodium must be present for absorption to continue when the intraintestinal sugar concentration is low. These hexose-phosphates separate again into their component parts, permiting the sugar to diffuse into the portal bloodstream.

Some glucose may be oxidized directly, such as in the brain and heart. Most of the absorbed sugar is converted to glycogen in the liver, although glycogenesis also occurs in other tissues. Up to 15% of the weight of the liver and 3% of the muscle may be glycogen; small amounts are also found in practically all other organs. Glycogenolysis in the liver yields glucose as the chief product, whereas glycogen breakdown in the muscle yields lactic acid. The overall oxidation of glucose has two phases, the anaerobic (glycolysis) and the aerobic (tricarboxylic acid cycle). In the former, glucose is broken down to pyruvic acid; in the aerobic cycle pyruvic acid is completely oxidized to carbon dioxide and water. Insulin and the pituitary and adrenal hormones are involved in these processes, and nicotinic acid, thiamine, riboflavin, and pantothenic acid take part in the enzymatic reactions. Carbohydrate that is not oxidized or stored as glycogen is converted to fat.

The principal carbohydrate metabolic disorders are diabetes mellitus, glycogen storage disease, galactosemia, fructose intolerance, and glucose intolerance; deficiencies of sugar-splitting enzymes in the intestines (lactase, sucrase, maltase) are associated with diarrhea and malabsorption resulting from the osmotic effect of the unabsorbed sugar and from fermentation of the carbohydrate by intestinal bacteria.

4.5 FATS

Fats or their metabolic products form an integral part of cellular membranes and are efficient stores of energy. They impart palatability to food and serve as vehicles for fat-soluble vitamins A, D, E, and K. Approximately 98% of natural fats are triglycerides, three fatty acids combined with glycerol. The remaining 2% include free fatty acids, monoglycerides, diglycerides, cholesterol, and phospholipids (including lecithin, cephalin, sphingomyelin, and cerebrosides).

Naturally occurring fats contain straight-chain fatty acids, both saturated and unsaturated, varying in length from 4 to 24 carbon atoms. The degree of absorption generally varies with the melting point, the degree of unsaturation, and the positions of the fatty acids on the glycerol molecule.

Ingested triglycerides are partially hydrolyzed by lingual lipase and emulsified in the stomach. In the duodenum, pancreatic lipase hydrolyzes the triglycerides to monoglycerides and fatty acids; intraluminal solubility is enhanced greatly by the presence of bile salts. The remaining unsplit diglycerides and triglycerides are insoluble even in the presence of bile salts. Low-birthweight infants have decreased amounts of bile and decreased absorption of fat.

Long-chain fatty acids and monoglycerides (those with more than 10 carbon atoms) are presumably absorbed into the mucosal cell by diffusion. Transport across the cell involves re-esterification of these fatty acids and monoglycerides to triglycerides, which are then "coated" with lipoprotein to form the chylomicron, in which the fat is transported in the lymph system to the venous circulation via the thoracic duct. Transport proteins include very-low-density (VLDL), low-density (LDL), and high-density (HDL) lipoproteins synthesized in the liver.

Short- and medium-chain triglycerides are handled differently; they are readily hydrolyzed by pancreatic lipase to free fatty acids which are transported through the cell. Even when intraluminal hydrolysis is inadequate because of deficiency of pancreatic lipase or of bile salts, these fats will be absorbed and hydrolyzed to free fatty acids within the cell by mucosal lipase. With neither esterification to triglycerides nor subsequent chylomicron formation, these free fatty acids directly enter the intestinal veins and pass to the liver via the portal system. This alternate pathway for short- and medium-chain triglycerides is utilized in nutritional formulations for children with severe absorptive problems.

ESSENTIAL FATTY ACIDS. Humans do not synthesize linoleic acid (an ^{18}C atom chain with 2 double bonds, one in the ω-6 position) or linolenic acid (18 carbons with 3 double bonds, the last in the ω-3 position). Both must be supplied in the diet. Linoleic acid is the precursor of arachidonic acid, the prostaglandins, and the leukotrienes. Linolenic acid modulates the rate of production of arachidonic acid metabolites and forms longer chain unsaturated fatty acids, which may be essential for central nervous system structure and function. Unsaturated fatty acids are necessary for growth, skin and hair integrity, regulation of cholesterol metabolism, lipotropic activity, decreased platelet adhesiveness, and reproduction. Diets containing less than 1–2% of the calories as linoleic acid require greater caloric consumption for comparable growth. In children with essential fatty acid deficiency, serum levels of trienoic acid increase relative to tetraenoic acids. Excess unsaturated acids increase peroxidation and may cause membrane destruction. Rapidly growing young infants maintained on diets very low in linoleic acid develop intertrigo and dryness, thickening, and desquamation of the skin.

The relation of dietary fat intake to intimal fat streaking in the major arterial vessels in early life and atheromatous changes in adults remains to be clarified (see Sec. 8.28–8.33).

4.6 MINERALS

The physiologic roles and dietary sources of the principal minerals with nutritional significance are summarized in Table 4–5. Requirements are shown in Table 4–1, except for several of the trace elements.

The ash content of the fetus is about 3% of the body weight at birth. It increases continuously throughout childhood. Adult ash content is 4.35% of body weight; 83% is in the skeleton and 10% is in the muscle. For each gram of protein retained, 0.3 g of mineral mattter is deposited. The principal cations are calcium, magnesium, potassium, and sodium; the comparable anions are phosphorus, sulfur, and chloride. Iron, iodine, and cobalt appear in important organic complexes. The trace elements fluorine, copper, zinc, chromuim, and manganese have known metabolic roles; selenium, silicon, boron, nickel, aluminum, arsenic, bromine, molybdenum, and strontium are present in the diet and in the body.

4.7 VITAMINS

The word "vitamin" refers to organic compounds required in minute amounts to catalyze cellular metabolism essential for growth or maintenance of the organism. Vitamin requirements for infants and children are listed in Table 4–1. For vitamin functions and disorders, see Table 4–6 and Sec. 4.21–4.33.

MISCELLANEOUS FACTORS

FIBER. The quantity of indigestible vegetable fiber in acceptable diets may be as much as 170–300 mg/kg/24 hr. Most children who receive well-balanced diets obtain sufficient

TABLE 4–5. Physiology and Sources of Nutritionally Important Minerals

Mineral	Function and Metabolism	Effects of Deficiency	Effects of Excess	Sources
Calcium	Structure of bone and teeth, muscle contraction, nerve irritability, coagulation of blood, cardiac action, production of milk Absorbed from upper small intestine: aided by vitamin D, ascorbic acid, lactose, acid reaction; hindered by excesses of dietary oxalic acid, phytic acid, fat, fiber, phosphate. Deposited in bone trabeculae and maintained in dynamic equilibrium with body tissue through action of parathyroid hormone and thyrocalcitonin About 70% excreted in feces, 10% in urine; 15–25% retained, depending on growth rate. Serum level 9–11 mg/dL, 60% ionized	Poor mineralization of bones and teeth; osteomalacia; osteoporosis; tetany; rickets; impairment of growth	Unknown (dietary) Heart block and renal stones (parenteral)	Milk, cheese, green leafy vegetables, canned salmon, clams, oysters
Chloride	Osmotic pressure; acid-base balance; HCl in gastric juice Readily absorbed; about 92% of intake is excreted, mainly in the urine, some in feces and sweat; comprises about ⅔ of the blood plasma anions; blood serum level, 99–106 mEq/L; in intracellular and extracellular fluids; parallels sodium intake and output	Hypochloremic alkalosis may occur with prolonged vomiting or excessive sweating, with parenteral administration of glucose without saline, with excessive ACTH therapy, and with congenital alkalosis	Unknown	Table salt, meat, milk, eggs
Chromium	Glycemia regulation and insulin metabolism	Diabetes in animals	None known	Yeast
Cobalt	Component of vitamin B_{12} (cobalamin) molecule and of erythropoietin Not utilized for synthesis of cobalamin by humans; readily absorbed and excreted	None known ? Hypothyroidism	Cardiomyopathy; medicinally it may be goitrogenic or may produce cardiomyopathy	Widely distributed
Copper	Essential for production of red blood cells; catalyst in hemoglobin formation; absorption of iron. Associated with activities of tyrosinase, catalase, uricase, cytochrome C oxidase, δ-aminolevulinic acid dehydrase, lysyl oxidase. Absorbed with sulfur-rich proteins; transported in plasma bound to plasma proteins and in ceruloplasmin; present in erythrocytes in a labile form and the more stable hemocuprein; highest concentration in liver and central nervous system (cerebrocuprein); excreted mainly via the intestinal wall and bile; deranged metabolism in Wilson disease (hepatolenticular degeneration), and Menkes syndrome	May be cause of refractory anemia, osteoporosis, neutropenia, depigmentation and ataxia Increased serum cholesterol	? Cirrhosis	Liver, oysters, meats, fish, whole grains, nuts, legumes
Fluorine	Tooth and bone structure Retained when intake is above 0.6 mg/day; excreted in urine and sweat; deposited in bones as fluorapatite (dynamic equilibrium)	Tendency to dental caries	Fluorosis: mottling of teeth with intake of more than 4–8 mg/24 hr	Water, sea foods, plant and animal foods (dependent on content in soil and water)
Iodine	Constituent of thyroxine (T_4) and triiodothyronine (T_3) Readily absorbed from intestine; circulates as inorganic and organic iodide; selectively concentrated about 25:1 in the thyroid gland, quickly iodized and incorporated into a complex known as thyroglobulin; proteolytic enzymes release thyroxine and triiodothyronine into the blood. Excretion mainly in urine. Antithyroid compounds interfere with iodine metabolism: goitrins and brassicae; certain drugs	Simple goiter, endemic cretinism	Not harmful (less than 1 mg/24 hr); medicinally may cause goiter	Iodized salt, sea food, food grown in nongoitrous areas

Table continued on opposite page

TABLE 4–5. Physiology and Sources of Nutritionally Important Minerals *Continued*

Mineral	Function and Metabolism	Effects of Deficiency	Effects of Excess	Sources
Iron	Structure of hemoglobin and myoglobin for O_2 and CO_2 transport; oxidative enzymes; cytochrome C and catalase Absorbed in ferrous form according to body need, aided by gastric juice and ascorbic acid; hindered by fiber, phytic acid, steatorrhea Transported in plasma in ferric state bound to transferrin (a β-globulin); stored in liver, spleen, bone marrow, and kidney as ferritin and hemosiderin; carefully conserved and reused; minimal losses in urine and sweat; about 90% of intake excreted in the stool	Anemia: hypochromic, microcytic, growth failure, hyperactivity (?)	Hemosiderosis in Bantu people of Africa due to low phosphorus and high iron contents of diet Poisoning by medicinal iron	Liver, meat, egg yolk, green vegetables, whole grains, legumes, nuts
Magnesium	Structure of bones and teeth; activation of enzymes in carbohydrate metabolism; muscle and nerve irritability, important intracellular cation, essential to metabolic processes Principal cation of soft tissue; absorption from small intestine varies with intake; some urinary excretion, but excellent renal conservation; antagonist to calcium action	Occurs in malabsorption and deficiency states; may be expressed clinically as tetany; associated frequently with hypocalcemia, hypokalemia	None (dietary); toxicity from intravenous medication	Cereals, legumes, nuts, meat, milk
Manganese	Enzyme activation, especially superoxide dismutase; normal bone structure, carbohydrate metabolism Poor absorption from intestine; transported in plasma; particularly high turnover rate in mitochondria; excretion mainly via the intestine in bile; competes with iron	Not known	Non (dietary); toxicity from chronic inhalation (encephalopathy)	Legumes, nuts, whole grain cereals, green leafy vegetables
Molybdenum	Component of enzymes: xanthine oxidase for conversion to uric acid and mobilization of ferritin iron in liver, liver aldehyde oxidase Readily absorbed from intestine; excreted chiefly in urine, some in bile	Not observed in humans	Not established	Legumes, grains, dark green leafy vegetables, animal organs
Phosphorus	Constituent of bones and teeth; structure of nucleus and cytoplasm of all cells; acid-base balance; key position in energy transformations and transmission of nerve impulses; metabolism of carbohydrate, protein, and fat About 70% of intake absorbed as free phosphates from intestine; vitamin D and parathormone implicated in intestinal absorption and kidney retention; excreted in urine and feces; occurs in blood as phospholipids, organic esters, and inorganic phosphates; inorganic phosphates in blood serum of infants and children, 4–7 mg/dL; ratio of inorganic to organic phosphates in whole blood is about 1:20	Rickets may develop in rapidly growing, very low-birthweight babies with low intakes of both P and Ca; muscle weakness	Possibility of tetany during recovery from rickets or in newborn on formula with low Ca:P (1:1) ratio	Milk, milk products, egg yolk, fresh foods, legumes, nuts, whole grains
Potassium	Muscle contraction; nerve impulse conduction; intracellular osmotic pressure and fluid balance; heart rhythm Primarily intracellular; absorption via intestine; excretion 80% in urine—some in sweat and feces; about 8% retained by growing child; blood serum level 4.0–5.6 mEq/L	In starvation or in such pathologic conditions as diarrhea, diabetic acidosis, ACTH excess: muscle weakness, anorexia, nausea, abdominal distention, nervous irritability, drowsiness, confusion, tachycardia; deficiency exaggerates effects of sodium	Heart block at serum levels of 10 mEq/L; important in Addison disease, renal failure, or administration of K-containing salts	All foods
Selenium	Cofactor for glutathione peroxidase in tissue respiration	Muscle diseases in animals. Kashan cardiomyopathy, arthritis (?)	Toxicity observed in animals	Vegetables, meats

Table continued on following page

TABLE 4–5. Physiology and Sources of Nutritionally Important Minerals *Continued*

Mineral	Function and Metabolism	Effects of Deficiency	Effects of Excess	Sources
Sodium	Osmotic pressure; acid-base balance; water balance; muscle and nerve irritability Readily absorbed from intestine; excreted chiefly in urine (98%); parallels choride intake; renal excretion controlled by adrenal cortical hormone; extracellular cation, but small amount in muscle and cartilage; blood serum level, 135–145 mEq/L	Nausea; diarrhea, muscle cramps, dehydration, hypotension	Edema if inadequate excretion or excessive parenteral fluids	Table salt, flesh foods, milk, eggs, sodium compounds as baking soda and powder, glutamate, seasonings, and preservatives
Sulfur	Constituent of all cellular protein; cocarboxylase; melanin; mucopolysaccharides of mucous secretions, vitreous humor, synovial fluid, connective tissues, cartilage, heparin, insulin; metabolism of nerve tissue; detoxification mechanisms; tissue metabolism as SH group in coenzyme A, cystathionine, and glutathione Only sources utilized are cystine and methionine; inorganic forms unavailable to body; excreted as inorganic sulfate or ethereal sulfate via urine and bile	Not known; growth failure from protein deficiency may be due in part to deficiency of sulfur-containing amino acids	Not harmful; excreted in urine as sulfates	Protein foods contain about 1%
Zinc	Constituent of several enzymes: carbonic anhydrase (in erythrocytes) essential for CO_2 exchange; carboxypeptidase of intestine for hydrolysis of protein; dehydrogenase of liver Found in liver and organs, muscles, bones, red and white blood cells; higher tissue concentration in young subjects; excreted chiefly from intestine, competes with copper	Dwarfism, iron deficiency anemia, hepatosplenomegaly, hyperpigmentation and hypogonadism, acrodermatitis enteropathica, depression of immunocompetence, poor wound healing	Gastrointestinal upsets (from galvanized iron cooking utensils); copper deficiency; decreased high-density lopoprotein	Meat, grain, nuts, cheese

amounts of fiber. Highly refined foods contain little fiber and may be associated with increased incidence of constipation, appendicitis, diverticulitis, and other intestinal disorders. High-fiber intake may result in decreased absorption of cholesterol as well as zinc and other essential nutrients.

DIGESTIBILITY. The relative amount of a given nutrient available for assimilation is high in most of the common food classes: carbohydrate, 97%; fat, 95%; protein, 92%. Cooking is a factor in digestibility. For example, the boiling of milk reduces the size of the curd and renders it more digestible; on the other hand, heating destroys activity of vitamin C.

SATIETY. The ingestion of a meal should provide a sense of well-being. Whole milk, cream, eggs, and fatty foods have high satiety values; sugar increases the flow of gastric juice and delays emptying of the stomach, thus increasing satiety. Bread and potatoes have relatively low satiety values, as do lean meat, fish, vegetables, and many fruits.

AVAILABILITY. Poverty, ignorance, and lack of practical education in buying and preparing food are the main causes of malnutrition in children. Diets of lower-income families are often deficient in milk, fruits, fresh vegetables, and meats. A suggested method for planning low-cost meals is to divide the money available for food into fifths: one fifth each for vegetables and fruits; for milk and cheese; for meats, fish, and eggs; for bread and cereals; and for fats, sugar, and other food adjuncts.

Geographic location may influence the availability of foods and the development of deficiency disorders, especially among low socioeconomic populations; for example, the relation of dental caries to lack of fluoride in communal water supplies.

BACTERIAL SYNTHESIS OF VITAMINS. Certain vitamins are synthesized in the human gastrointestinal tract; however, the extent to which they can meet the body's needs is uncertain. Once the bacterial flora of the intestinal tract have been established, vitamin K is produced and is available to the body. Pantothenic acid and biotin, essential to human metabolism, can be supplied by bacterial synthesis alone. Thiamine, riboflavin, niacin, vitamin B_6, vitamin B_{12}, and folic acid are synthesized in some species, but synthesis is limited or does not exist in humans. The kind of food or the nature of intestinal flora may affect vitamin production or availability. For instance, 3% of the population in Kobe, Japan, harbored intestinal bacteria that split thiamine; evidence of beriberi appeared in these persons.

ANTIMICROBIAL FACTORS. Administration of antimicrobial agents may affect nutritional status. Appetite is sometimes impaired or bacterial flora producing vitamin K are sufficiently altered to precipitate borderline deficiency. Several antibiotics are known to produce steatorrhea. Orally administered broad-spectrum antibiotics decrease nitrogen balance. Isoniazid combines with pyridoxal phosphate and may produce symptoms of vitamin B_6 deficiency. Antimicrobial compounds may be transmitted in breast milk or in foods from animals that are fed these compounds.

ENDOCRINE FACTORS. Antithyroid substances that increase the requirement for iodine (goitrogens) have been found in turnips, rutabagas, cabbage, soybeans, cobalt-containing foods, food additives, and medications. Administering adenocorticotropic hormone (ACTH) or corticosteroids necessitates an increase in protein and calcium and a decrease in sodium intake. Transient hypoparathyroidism with tetany has been observed in the neonatal period after excessive intake of vitamin D or of phosphates.

RADIOACTIVITY. Apparently, little danger results from ^{14}C because of its low activity. ^{131}I is removed from milk by aeration or storage. ^{137}Cs, which may be found in meat and milk products, can be counteracted by a high potassium intake or by acetazolamide. Only 10% of ^{90}St ingested by the cow is found in cow's milk.

EMOTIONAL FACTORS. Along with increased knowledge of the significance of various nutrients, excessive parental and

TABLE 4–6. Physical and Metabolic Properties and Food Sources of the Vitamins

Name and Synonyms	Characteristics	Biochemical Action	Effects of Deficiency	Effects of Excess	Sources
Vitamin A: Retinol (vitamin A_1) is an alcohol of high molecular weight *Provitamin A:* The plant pigments, α-, β-, and γ-carotenes and cryptoxanthin	Fat-soluble; heat-stable; destroyed by oxidation, drying; bile necessary for absorption; stored in liver; protected by vitamin E	Component of retinal pigments, rhodopsin and iodopsin, for vision in dim light; bone and tooth development; formation and maturation of epithelia	Nyctalopia, photophobia, xerophthalmia, conjunctivitis, keratomalacia leading to blindness; faulty epiphyseal bone formation; defective tooth enamel; keratinization of mucous membranes and skin; retarded growth	Excessive carotene intake may produce carotenemia with xanthosis cutis. Individual variation in sensitivity includes anorexia, slow growth, drying and cracking of skin, enlargement of liver and spleen, swelling and pain of long bones, bone fragility, increased intracranial pressure	Liver, fish-liver oils, whole milk, milk fat products, egg yolk, fortified margarines. Carotenoids from plants—green vegetables, yellow fruits and vegetables
Vitamin B Complex: *Thiamine:* Vitamin B_1; antiberiberi vitamin; aneurin	Water- and alcohol-soluble; fat-insoluble; stable in slightly acid solution; labile to heat, alkali, sulfites	Component of thiamine pyrophosphate carboxylases, which act in various oxidative decarboxylations, including that of pyruvic acid	Beriberi—fatigue, irritability, anorexia, constipation, headache, insomnia, tachycardia, polyneuritis, cardiac failure, edema; elevated pyruvic acid in the blood Wernicke encephalopathy—mental confusion, ataxia	None from oral intake	Liver, meat, especially pork, milk, whole grain or enriched cereals, wheat germ, legumes, nuts
Riboflavin: Vitamin B_2	Sparingly soluble in water; sensitive to light and alkali; stable to heat, oxidation, acid	Constituent of flavoprotein enzymes important in hydrogen transfer reactions; amino acid, fatty acid, and carbohydrate metabolism and cellular respiration. Retinal pigment for light adaptation	Ariboflavinosis; photophobia, blurred vision, burning and itching of eyes, corneal vascularization, poor growth	Not harmful	Milk, cheese, liver and other organs, meat, eggs, fish, green leafy vegetables, whole or enriched grains
Niacin: Nicotinamide; nicotinic acid; antipellagra vitamin	Water- and alcohol-soluble; stable to acid, alkali, light, heat, oxidation	Constituent of coenzymes I and II, cofactors in a number of dehydrogenase systems	Pellagra; multiple B-vitamin deficiency syndrome	Nicotinic acid (not the amide) is vasodilator; skin flushing and itching, may induce hepatopathy	Meat, fish, poultry, liver, whole grain and enriched cereals, green vegetables, peanuts
Folacin: Group of related compounds containing pteridine ring, para-amino benzoic acid, and glutamic acid. Pteroylglutamic acid (PGA)	Slightly soluble in water; labile to heat, light, acid	Concerned with formation and metabolism of one-carbon units; participates in synthesis of purines, pyrimidines, nucleoproteins, and methyl groups	Megaloblastic anemia (infancy, pregnancy); usually is secondary to malabsorption disease	Unknown	Liver, green vegetables, nuts, cereals, cheese
Vitamin B_6: 3 active forms: pyridoxine, pyridoxal, pyridoxamine	Water-soluble; destroyed by ultraviolet light and by heat	Constituent of coenzymes for decarboxylation, transamination, transsulfuration; fatty acid metabolism	Irritability, convulsions, hypochromic anemia; peripheral neuritis in patients receiving isoniazid; oxaluria (Sec. 8.8)	Sensory neuropathy	Meat, liver, kidney, whole grains, peanuts, soybeans
Cobalamin: Vitamin B_{12}	Slightly soluble in water; stable to heat in neutral solution; labile in acid or alkaline ones; destroyed by light Castle intrinsic factor of the stomach required for absorption	Transfer of one-carbon units in purine and labile-methyl group metabolism; essential for maturation of red blood cells in bone marrow; metabolism of nervous tissue; adenosylcobalamin is the coenzyme for methylmalonyl CoA mutase	Juvenile pernicious anemia, due to defect in absorption rather than to dietary lack; also secondary to gastrectomy, celiac disease, inflammatory lesions of small bowel, long-term drug therapy (PAS, neomycin); methylmalonic aciduria; homocystinuria	Unknown	Muscle and organ meats, fish, eggs, milk, cheese
Biotin	Crystallized from yeast; soluble in water	Coenzyme of all 4 carboxylases; involved in CO_2 transfer	Dermatitis, seborrhea; inactivated by avidin in raw egg white	None known	Yeast, animal products; synthesized in intestine

Table continued on following page

TABLE 4–6. Physical and Metabolic Properties and Food Sources of the Vitamins *Continued*

Name and Synonyms	Characteristics	Biochemical Action	Effects of Deficiency	Effects of Excess	Sources
Vitamin C: *Ascorbic acid:* Vitamin C; antiscorbutic vitamin	Water-soluible; easily oxidized, accelerated by heat, light, alkali, oxidative enzymes, traces of copper or iron	Integrity and maintenance of intercellular material in all tissues; facilitates absorption of iron and conversion of folic acid to folinic acid; metabolism of tyrosine and phenylalanine, contributes to activity of succinic dehydrogenase and serum phosphatase in infants, not in adults	Scurvy and poor wound healing	Oxaluria (see also Sec. 8.8 and discussions of hyperoxaluria oxalosis)	Citrus fruits, tomatoes, berries, cantaloupe, cabbage, green vegetables. Cooking has destructive effect
Vitamin D: Group of sterols having similar physiologic activity. D_2-calciferol is activated ergosterol. D_2 is activated 7-dehydrocholesterol	Fat-soluble; stable to heat, acid, alkali, and oxidation; bile necessary for absorption	Regulates absorption and deposition of calcium and phosphorus, presumably by affecting permeability of intestinal membrane; regulates level of serum alkaline phosphatase, which is believed to be concerned with calcium phosphate deposition in bones and teeth	Rickets (high serum phosphatase level appears before bone deformities); infantile tetany, poor growth, osteomalacia	Wide variation in tolerance; in general over 500 μg/24 hr toxic when continued for weeks; prolonged administration of 45 μg/24 hr may be toxic (Sec. 4.31); manifestations are nausea, diarrhea, weight loss, polyuria, nocturia, calcification of soft tissues, including heart, renal tubules, blood vessels, bronchi, stomach	Vitamin D–fortified milk and margarine, fish-liver oils, exposure to sunlight or other ultraviolet sources
Vitamin E: Group of related chemical compounds—tocopherols—with similar biologic activities	Fat-soluble; unstable to ultraviolet light, alkali; readily oxidized by oxygen, iron, rancid fats. Antioxidant; bile necessary for absorption	Minimizes oxidation of carotene, vitamin A, and linoleic acid in the intestine	Requirements related to polyunsaturated fat intake; red blood cell hemolysis in premature infants, loss of neural integrity	Unknown	Germ oils of various seeds, green leafy vegetables, nuts, legumes
Vitamin K: Group of naphthoquinones with similar biologic activities; K_1 is phytoquinone	Natural compounds are fat-soluble; water-soluble products have been developed (menadione). Stable to heat and reducing agents; labile to oxidizing agents, strong acids, alkali, light; bile salts necessary for intestinal absorption of fat-soluble forms	Prothrombin formation, coagulation factors II, VII, IX, X and osteocalcin are K-dependent	Hemorrhagic manifestations; bone metabolism	Not established; medicinally may produce hyperbilirubinemia in premature infants	Green leafy vegetables, pork liver. Widely distributed

professional concern has developed with regard to the food that the individual infant or child eats. The mother, developing a sense of fear or guilt about her child's eating habits, may create a battle of wits between her and her child that may have far-reaching effects. For example, misdirected efforts to control obesity and hypercholesterolemia have led to severe malnutrition in young children.

4.8 EVALUATION OF DIET

See Tables 4–7 and 27–9 and 27–10.

The recall interview for determining children's food habits is usually satisfactory, but for a more accurate accounting the mother should observe and record the actual food intake and convert to "servings" appropriate to the child's age (see Table 4–7). It is important to include items that may not be consumed daily.

The dietary guide according to food groups provides flexibility. A food intake record can indicate possible nutritional imbalances. An excessive intake of foods of one group may result in a high caloric level producing an overweight child while at the same time leading to a dangerously low intake of some essential nutrients, such as the overconsumption of milk and the underconsumption of meat and eggs, the resultant danger of which is iron deficiency anemia. When key foods, such as milk, eggs, and citrus fruits, are eliminated for personal or medical reasons, the deficiencies may be compensated for by judicious substitutions. A list of the principal food groups' nutrients follows:

Milk: high-quality protein, calcium, and phosphorus; riboflavin; vitamin A; vitamin D (if fortified)
Meat and eggs: high-quality protein, iron, B vitamins; vitamin A from liver and eggs
Fruits and vegetables: vitamin C; provitamin A from green and yellow ones; trace elements; fiber

TABLE 4–7. Recommended Food Intake for Good Nutrition According to Food Groups and the Average Size of Servings at Different Age Levels*

Food Group	Servings/Day	Average Size of Servings					
		1 Yr	***2–3 Yr***	***4–5 Yr***	***6–9 Yr***	***10–12 Yr***	***13–15 Yr***
Meat and cheese (1.5 oz cheese = 1 C† milk)	4	½ C†	½–¾ C	½–¾ C	½–1 C	½–1 C	½–1 C
Meat group (protein foods)	3 or more						
Egg		1	1	1	1	1	1 or more
Lean meat, fish, poultry (liver once a week)		2 Tbsp‡	2 Tbsp	4 Tbsp	2–3 oz (4–6 Tbsp)	3–4 oz	4 oz or more
Peanut butter			1 Tbsp	2 Tbsp	2–3 Tbsp	3 Tbsp	3 Tbsp
Fruits and vegetables							
Vitamin C source (citrus fruits, berries, tomato, cabbage, cantaloupe)	At least 4, including: 1 or more (twice as much tomato as citrus)	⅓ C (citrus)	½ C	½ C	1 medium orange	1 medium orange	1 medium orange
Vitamin A source (green or yellow fruits and vegetables)	1 or more	2 Tbsp	3 Tbsp	4 Tbsp (¼ C)	¼ C	⅓ C	½ C
Other vegetables (potato and legumes, etc.) *or*	2	2 Tbsp	3 Tbsp	4 Tbsp	⅓ C	½ C	¾ C
Other fruits (apple, banana, etc.)		¼ C	⅓ C	½ C	1 medium	1 medium	1 medium
Cereals (whole-grain or enriched)	At least 4						
Bread		½ slice	1 slice	1½ slices	1–2 slices	2 slices	2 slices
Ready-to-eat cereals		½ oz	¾ oz	1 oz	1 oz	1 oz	1 oz
Cooked cereals (including macaroni, spaghetti, rice, etc.)		¼ C	⅓ C	½ C	½ C	¾ C	1 C or more
Fats and carbohydrates	To meet caloric needs						
Butter, margarine, mayonnaise, oils: 1 Tbsp = 100 Calories (kcal)		1 Tbsp	1 Tbsp	1 Tbsp	2 Tbsp	2 Tbsp	2–4 Tbsp
Desserts and sweets: 100-Calorie portions as follows: ⅓ C pudding or ice cream, 2 3″ cookies, 1 oz cake, 1⅓ oz pie, 2 tbsp jelly, jam, honey, sugar		1 portion	1½ portions	1½ portions	3 portions	3 portions	3–6 portions

*Modified with Mildred J. Bennett, Ph.D., from "Four Food Groups of the Daily Food Guide," Institute of Home Economics, U.S.D.A., and Publication No. 30, Children's Bureau of the United States Department of Health, Education, and Welfare.

†C = 1 cup or 8 oz or 240 mL.

‡Tbsp = Tablespoon (1 Tbsp = 15 mL = ½ oz).

Cereals: less expensive and supplementary amounts of protein, minerals, fiber, B vitamins

Suspected dietary insufficiencies may be corroborated by appropriate laboratory tests and clinical evaluation. When malnutrition, either as dietary deficiency or excess, or failure to thrive exists despite an apparently satisfactory food intake, the infant or child's family relationships must be evaluated, not only for organic causes but especially for psychosocial ones (see Sec. 3.22).

(References follow next section.)

4.9 FEEDING OF INFANTS

Successful infant feeding requires cooperation between the mother and her baby, beginning with the initial feeding experience and continuing throughout the child's period of dependency. Promptly establishing comfortable, satisfying feeding practices contributes greatly to the infant's and mother's emotional well-being (see Sec 9.6). Feeding time should be pleasurable for both mother and child. Because maternal feelings are readily transmitted to the baby and largely determine the emotional setting in which feeding takes place, tense, anxious, irritable, easily upset, or emotionally labile mothers are more likely to experience a difficult feeding relationship, but they frequently become more comfortable and confident with appropriate guidance and support from an empathetic and experienced relative, friend, or physician.

As soon after birth as an infant can safely tolerate enteral nutrition, as judged by normal activity, alertness, suck, and cry, feedings should be initiated to maintain normal metabolism and growth during the transition from fetal to extrauterine life, to promote maternal-infant bonding and to decrease the risks of hypoglycemia, hyperkalemia, hyperbilirubinemia, and azotemia. Mistakes are made by feeding the infant too much or too little. Inadequate fluid intake, particularly in hot weather, may result in "dehydration fever." Most infants may start feeding by 6 hr of life. When any question about the tolerance of feeding arises because of physical or neurologic status, feeding should be withheld and parenteral fluids should be substituted. The schedule of initial feeding in a hospital is less important than the principle of the unhurried beginning and patient assistance and support for the mother.

Mothers who wish to initiate breast-feeding in the delivery room and continue on a demand basis thereafter should be supported. However, when rooming-in is unavailable or not desired and demand feeding is impractical, the infant can be taken to the mother for the first feeding at 10.00 A.M. or 6.00 P.M., whichever is nearer the end of a 6-hr postpartum rest. Subsequent formula or breast-feedings are given every 3–4 hr/day and night by the mother. Artificially fed infants should receive sterile water for the first feeding, because regurgitation and aspiration of this liquid are less likely to cause significant irritation of the respiratory tract.

The feeding of infants requires practical interpretation of specific nutritional needs and of the widely varying limits of the normal baby's appetite and behavior regarding food. The time that it takes the infant's stomach to empty may vary from 1 to 4 hr or more; thus, considerable difference in the infant's desire for food is expected at different times of the day. Ideally, the feeding schedule should be based on this reasonable "self-regulation." Variation in the time between feedings and in the amount taken per feeding is to be expected in the first few weeks during the establishment of the self-regulation plan. By the end of the first month more than 90% of infants will have established a suitable and reasonably regular schedule.

Most healthy, bottle-fed infants will want 6–9 feedings/24 hr by the end of the first week of life. Some will take enough at one feeding to satisfy themselves for approximately 4 hr; others who are smaller or whose gastric emptying time is more rapid will want milk about every 2–3 hr; breast-fed infants often prefer shorter intervals. Most term infants will rapidly increase their intake from 30 mL to 80–90 mL every 3–4 hr at 4–5 days of life. Feeding should be considered as having progressed satisfactorily if the infant is no longer losing weight by 5–7 days and is gaining weight by 12–14 days. Some infants will not awaken for a middle-of-the-night feeding after 3–6 wk of age; some may never want it. Many will not want a late evening feeding between 4 and 8 mo of age and will be satisfied with 3 meals/day by 9–12 mo. However, individual feeding needs are quite variable, and one infant should not be expected to fit the pattern of another infant.

It is important to appreciate that infants cry for other reasons besides hunger, and *they need not be fed every time they cry;* some infants are placid, some are unusually active, and some are irritable. Sick infants are often uninterested in food. Infants who awaken and cry consistently at short intervals may not be receiving enough milk at each feeding or may have discomfort from some cause other than hunger, such as too much clothing; colic; soiled, wet, or uncomfortable diapers and clothing; swallowed air ("gas"); uncomfortably hot or cold environment; or illness. Some infants cry to gain sufficient or additional attention, whereas others deprived of adequate mothering become indifferent. Some infants simply need to be held. Those who stop crying when they are picked up or held do not usually need food, but those who continue to cry when held and when food is offered should be carefully evaluated for other causes of distress. The habit of offering frequent, small feedings or of holding and feeding to pacify all crying should not be cultivated.

However, the advantages in satisfying the infant's true hunger needs as they are expressed are several: physiologic requirements are met promptly; the infant does not learn to associate prolonged crying and discomfort with feeding; and the infant is less likely to develop poor eating practices such as gulping the feedings or taking small amounts too frequently. Infants soon establish a regular schedule that permits the family to resume normal function. If this does not occur, individual feedings or the whole day's schedule can be moved ahead or delayed sufficiently to avoid conflicts with necessary family activities.

Some mothers will not understand the goals of infant "self-regulation"; some will misinterpret the physician's instructions; and others may be unable to adjust themselves to the regimen of the infant. *The orderly, overanxious, and compulsive parent may do better with a more specific outline for the infant's activities.*

The postpartum period is often a time of great anxiety and insecurity for the first-time mother, who may be temporarily overwhelmed by the responsibilities of motherhood. The hospital setting and the attitude of the hospital personnel should be comforting and supporting while the mother finds and develops confidence in her maternal abilities. *Time should be set aside to consider the questions of inexperienced or uncertain mothers at the hospital or in the home.* Fathers and other household members should be included by physicians in these anticipatory guidance sessions. Knowing the personalities and expectations of both parents is invaluable in helping to avert physical and psychologic problems centered on feeding. Parental misconceptions and confusion about the dietary and satiety needs of infants and children are often the bases for abnormal parent-child relations that can be avoided by appropriate counseling.

4.10 BREAST-FEEDING

Breast-feeding continues to have practical and psychologic advantages that should be considered when the mother selects the method for feeding. Human milk is the most appropriate of all available milks for the human infant because it is uniquely adapted to his or her needs.

ADVANTAGES. *Breast milk is the natural food for full-term infants during the first months of life.* It is always readily available at the proper temperature and needs no time for preparation. The milk is fresh and free of contaminating bacteria, which reduces the chances of gastrointestinal disturbances. Although little if any difference exists in mortality rates in formula-fed and breast-fed infants receiving good care, among the lower socioeconomic groups and those living in unsanitary conditions, the breast-fed infant is more likely to survive.

Allergy and intolerance to cow's milk create significant disturbances and feeding difficulties that are not seen in breast-fed infants. The symptoms include diarrhea, intestinal bleeding, and occult melena. "Spitting up", colic, and atopic eczema are less common in infants receiving human milk (see also Sec. 14.71).

Human milk contains bacterial and viral antibodies, including relatively high concentrations of secretory IgA antibodies, which prevent micro-organisms from adhering to the intestinal mucosa. Breast-fed infants of mothers with high antipoliomyelitis titers are relatively resistant to infection by the attenuated live poliomyelitis vaccine viruses, an effect that may be pronounced in the neonatal period but does not seem to interfere with active immunization at 2, 4, and 6 mo of age. Growth of the mumps, influenza, vaccinia, and Japanese B encephalitis viruses can be inhibited by substances in human milk. These ingested antibodies from human colostrum and milk may provide local gastrointestinal immunity against organisms entering the body via this route.

Macrophages normally present in human colostrum and milk may be able to synthesize complement, lysozyme, and lactoferrin. Breast milk is also a source of lactoferrin, the iron-binding whey protein that is normally about one third saturated with iron, which has an inhibitory effect on the growth of *Escherichia coli* in the intestine. The stool of the breast-fed infant has a pH lower than that of the infant fed cow's milk. The intestinal flora of infants fed human milk may protect them against infections caused by some species of *E. coli*. Bile salt–stimulated lipase kills *Giardia lamblia* and *Entamoeba histolytica*.

Milk from the mother whose diet is sufficient and properly balanced will supply the necessary nutrients, except, perhaps, fluoride and, after several months, vitamin D (Sec. 4.29). Iron stores are sufficient for the first 6–9 mo in term infants. Human milk iron is well absorbed by the infant; breast-fed infants may not require supplemental iron during the first year, but their diets should be supplemented after 6 mo of age by the addition of cereal and meat or by administration of one of the ferrous iron preparations. Human milk contains sufficient vitamin C for the infant's needs, provided the mother's intake is adequate.

The psychologic advantages of breast-feeding for both mother and infant are well recognized, and successful breast-feeding is a satisfying experience for both. The mother is personally involved in the nurturing of her baby, gaining both a feeling of being essential and a sense of accomplishment. The infant is provided with a close and comfortable physical relationship with the mother. Breast-feeding offers increased opportunity for close sensual contact between the mother and the infant (see Sec. 9.6).

The mother who is unable or does not wish to nurse her infant, however, need have no less sense of accomplishment or of affection for her baby. The quality of attachment and mothering and the degree of security and affection provided can be identical.

CONTRAINDICATIONS. For the average, healthy, full-term infant there are no disadvantages to breast-feeding, provided that the mother's milk supply is ample and that her diet contains sufficient amounts of protein and vitamins. Infrequently, allergens to which the infant is sensitized may be conveyed in the milk. In such cases, an attempt should be made to find the specific allergen and to remove it from the mother's diet; its presence rarely is a valid reason for weaning the baby.

From the mother's standpoint there are few contraindications to breast-feeding. Markedly inverted nipples may be troublesome. Fissuring or cracking of the nipples can usually be avoided if engorgement is prevented. Mastitis may be alleviated by continued and frequent nursing on the affected breast to keep it from becoming engorged, local heat applications, and antibiotics. Acute infection in the mother may contraindicate breast-feeding if the infant does not have the same infection; otherwise there is no need to stop nursing unless the condition of either necessitates it. When the infant is unaffected and the mother's condition permits, the breast may be emptied and the milk given to the infant. Septicemia, nephritis, eclampsia, profuse hemorrhage, active tuberculosis, typhoid fever, and malaria are permanent contraindications to nursing, as are chronic poor nutrition, substance abuse, debility, severe neuroses, and postpartum psychoses.

The resumption of menstruation should not deter continued nursing, although temporary behavior changes of mother or baby may call for reassurance. Pregnancy does not necessitate immediate cessation of nursing, but the combined demands of supplying milk to the infant and nutrients to the fetus are formidable and require special attention to maternal nutrition.

Prematurely born infants weighing 2,000 g (4½ lb) or more usually thrive on breast milk. Infants of lesser birthweights, however, may have such rapid rates of growth that human milk alone may not supply sufficient essential nutrients for normal growth (see Sec. 9.17). Low-birthweight infants too weak to suck or those tiring before ingesting an adequate volume may be given human milk by gavage. Many such infants have thrived.

The low vitamin K content of human milk may contribute to hemorrhagic disease of the newborn. *Administration of 1 mg of vitamin K_1 parenterally at birth is recommended for all infants, especially for those who will be breast-fed.*

Unconjugated hyperbilirubinemia in breast-fed infants is discussed in Sec. 9.44.

Hemolytic disease of the newborn (erythroblastosis fetalis) is not a contraindication to breast-feeding if the infant's general condition warrants it, because antibodies in the mother's milk are inactivated in the intestinal tract and do not contribute to further hemolysis of the infant's blood cells.

PREPARATION OF THE PROSPECTIVE MOTHER. Most women are physically capable of breast-feeding, provided they receive sufficient encouragement and are protected from discouraging experiences and comments while the secretion of breast milk is becoming established. The physician interested in aiding the prospective mother to breast-feed should discuss its advantages during the midtrimester of pregnancy or whenever the mother begins planning for her baby. Many mothers ambivalent toward breast-feeding will be able to nurse successfully if they are reassured and supported. If the mother rejects the suggestion that she should nurse her infant, overpersuasion may be detrimental to mother-infant relationships.

Physical factors conducive to a good breast-feeding experience include establishing and maintaining a state of good health, proper balance of rest and exercise, freedom from worry, early and sufficient treatment of any intercurrrent disease, and adequate nutrition.

Retracted nipples usually benefit from daily manual breast-pump traction during the latter weeks of prregnancy; truly inverted nipples may be helped by the use of milk cups, starting as early as the 3rd mo of pregnancy.

The mother may be confidently told that she need not gain or lose weight if her diet is adequate. She should be reassured that breast tone will be preserved by the use of a properly fitted brassiere to support the breasts, especially before delivery and during the nursing period. During the latter part of pregnancy, the mother gains weight and stores fat, which is utilized in lactation. Nutritional requirements for lactation are listed in Table 4–1.

ESTABLISHING AND MAINTAINING THE MILK SUPPLY

The most satisfactory stimulus to the secretion of human milk is regular and complete emptying of the breasts; milk production is reduced when the secreted milk is not drained. Once lactation is well established, mothers are capable of producing more milk than their infants need. There are many reasons for incomplete nursing, but the principal ones are unsupportive hospital practices, weakness of the infant, and failure to initiate the natural hunger cycle. Efforts should be directed toward the early establishment of normal, vigorous nursing by letting the infant empty the breast frequently during the time when only colostrum is being formed. The infant should be allowed to nurse when hungry, whether or not there appears to be any milk.

Breast-feeding should be begun as soon after delivery as the condition of the mother and of the baby permits, preferably within several hours. Infants who cannot be fed on demand should be brought to the mother for feeding about every 3 hr during the day and every 4 hr during the night. Many infants are hungry within 2 hr of a satisfying nursing episode, and about 75% of the breast's milk has been replenished by this time.

Appropriate care for tender or sore nipples should be instituted before severe pain from abrasions and cracking develops. Exposing the nipples to air; applying pure lanolin; avoiding soap, alcohol, and tincture of benzoin; frequently changing disposable nursing pads lining the brassiere cups; nursing more frequently; manually expressing milk; nursing in different positions; and keeping the breast dry between feedings are recommended. When the tenderness causes the mother apprehension the *milk-ejection reflex* may be delayed, leading to frustration in the infant and to increasingly vigorous nursing, which further injures the nipple and areolar area. Occasionally, nipple shields may be helpful.

The first 2 wk of the neonatal period are crucial for establishing breast-feeding. Lactogenic hormones are ineffective in stimulating human breast secretion. Daily weight gains are overly emphasized, and early supplemental bottle feedings given to achieve this goal compromise attempts at breast-feeding. The infant usually finds that it is easier to get milk from a bottle than from a breast and becomes satiated. The difference between breast and bottle nipples may also confuse the infant, leading to disruption of the feeding pattern or to injury of the mother's nipples.

On the day that the mother is discharged from the hospital lactation may not be well established, and the excitement of going home may impede an initially successful nursing experience there. A wise physician anticipates this experience and discusses it with the mother. In some cases, providing her with enough isocaloric formula for 1–2 complementary feedings may prevent discouragement that might prejudice further nursing.

PSYCHOLOGIC FACTORS. No factor is more important than a happy, relaxed state of mind. Worry and unhappiness are the most effective means for decreasing or abolishing breast secretions.

Mothers may worry that their infants are abnormal when they cry, are drowsy, sneeze, or regurgitate milk. Mothers are upset by any suggestion that their milk may be lacking in quantity or quality. They may be disturbed at the scanty supply of colostrum, at tenderness of the nipples, and at the fullness of the breast on the 4th or 5th day. Many mothers do not feel comfortable when trying to nurse in an open ward or with another person in the room. Mothers may worry about what is going on at home while they are in the hospital or about what is going to happen when they arrive home. An alert physician recognizes and appreciates these worries, particularly if the baby is a first born, and by tactful reassurance and explanation can help prevent or minimize worry, thus contributing to successful breast-feeding.

FATIGUE. Avoiding fatigue is important, but the mother should exercise sufficiently to promote her sense of physical well-being.

HYGIENE. Once a day the breasts should be washed. If soap is drying to the nipple and areolar area, it should be discontinued. The nipple area should be kept dry. *Boric acid must not be used.* Care should be taken to prevent irritation and infection of the nipples caused by prolonged initial nursing, maceration from wetness of the nipple, or rubbing of clothing.

Some mothers may be more comfortable if they wear a properly fitted brassiere day and night. Plastic liners should be removed. An absorbent pad (commercially available) or a clean cloth or handkerchief may be placed inside the brassiere to absorb any milk that leaks out.

DIET. The diet should contain enough calories to compensate for those secreted in the milk as well as for those required to produce it. The nursing mother needs a varied diet, sufficient to maintain her weight and high in fluid, vitamins, and minerals. She should avoid weight-reducing diets. Milk is important but should not replace other essential foods. If the mother is allergic to or dislikes milk, 1 g of calcium may be added to her daily diet. The fluid intake should approximate 3 quarts daily; urinary output is a good measure of the adequacy of fluid in the daily diet.

The idea that substances such as milk, beer, oatmeal, and tea are galactogenic is mistaken. Singular foods in the mother's diet seldom disturb the breast-fed infant. Occasionally, however, eating certain berries, tomatoes, onions, members of the cabbage family, chocolate, spices, and condiments may cause gastric distress or loose stools in the infant. No food need be withheld from the mother unless it causes distress to the infant. Whenever possible, nursing mothers should not take drugs because many preparations are harmful to the neonate and many have not been evaluated (see Table 9–5). Antithyroid medications, lithium, anticancer agents, isoniazid, and phenindione are contraindicated. Temporary cessation of nursing is recommended if the mother requires diagnostic radiopharmaceuticals, chloramphenicol, metronidazole, sulfonamides, or anthroquinone-derivative laxatives. Lactating women should not eat sport fish from waters contaminated with polychlorinated biphenyls (PCBs). It is better to control maternal constipation by inclusion in her diet of raw and cooked fruits and vegetables, whole wheat bread, and an adequate amount of water than by use of laxatives. Smoking cigarettes and drinking alcoholic beverages should be discouraged. Substances such as arsenicals, barbiturates, bromides, iodides, lead, mercurials, salicylates, opium, atropine, most antimicrobial agents, and cascara may be transmitted through the milk and exert an effect on the infant.

TECHNIQUE OF BREAST-FEEDING

The technical aspects of breast-feeding require careful consideration. Breast-feeding sometimes becomes impossible simply because the attending physician fails to recognize that the difficulties are in the feeding technique.

At feeding time the infant should be hungry, dry, neither too cold nor too warm, and held in a comfortable, semisitting position for his or her enjoyment and for ease of eructation without vomiting. The mother, too, must be comfortable and completely at ease. When she is able to be out of bed, a moderately low chair with an armrest is preferable, and a low stool is advantageous for resting her foot and raising her knee on the nursing side. The baby is supported comfortably with the face held close to the mother's breast by one arm and hand while the other hand supports the breast so that the nipple is easily accessible to the infant's mouth and yet does not obstruct the infant's nasal breathing. The baby's lips should be expected to engage considerable areola as well as nipple.

Success in infant feeding depends greatly on the adjustments made during the first few days of life. Difficulties often result from attempts to adapt the infant to a nursing procedure rather than designing a procedure that satisfies the infant's natural desires. Rigidly adhering to clock schedules and the "assembly line" manner in which babies are handled in many nurseries may make adjustment at home more difficult. Most problems can be avoided by conforming to the infant's spontaneous pattern. If the infant is breast-fed when he or she normally cries in hunger and feeding ends when the baby's appetite is satisfied, the fundamental requirements are met.

At birth the normal infant is equipped with several reflexes, or behavior patterns, that facilitate breast-feeding. These reflexes are concerned with obtaining food—rooting, sucking, swallowing, and satiety reflexes. The *rooting reflex* is the first to come into play. When infants smell milk they move their heads around, attempting to find its source. If their cheek is touched by a smooth object (the mother's breast), they will turn toward that object, opening their mouths in anticipation of grasping the nipple (rooting with their mouths for the nipple).

The infant's rooting reflex brings the entire areolar area into the mouth; the contact of the nipple against the palate and posterior tongue elicits sucking or "milking," and the buccal fat pads help to keep the nipple in place. This *sucking reflex* is a process of squeezing the sinuses of the areola rather than simply suction on the nipple. The infant's sucking results in afferent impulses to the mother's hypothalamus and then to both anterior and posterior pituitary. Prolactin from the anterior pituitary stimulates milk secretion in the cuboidal cells in the acini or alveoli of the breast. Finally, milk in the infant's mouth triggers the *swallowing reflex*. In contrast, bottle-feeding requires the infant to compress the nipple to avoid choking.

Mothers should know that if the infant is not hungry, he or she will not search for the nipple or suck. Infants are usually sleepy for several days and most, initially, are not avid suckers. On the 3rd day, when there has been some weight loss, mothers become anxious about infants who seem uninterested in nursing. It reassures them to learn that most healthy babies "wake up" and become good nursers on the 4th day. Infants whose mothers received obstetric sedation during labor suck at lower rates and pressures and consume less milk than comparable infants of mothers given no sedation.

Some infants will empty a breast in 5 min; others nurse more leisurely for 20 min. Most of the milk is obtained early in the feeding: 50% in the first 2 min and 80–90% in the first 4 min. The infant should be permitted to suck until satisfied unless the mother has sore nipples. If the infant does not "unlatch" from the breast, a finger inserted into the corner of the infant's mouth decreases suction and facilitates removal. The infant should not be pulled from the breast. Waking a sleepy infant to nurse by slapping feet, pinching, or shaking is usually unsuccessful.

At the end of the nursing period the infant should be held erect over the mother's shoulder or on her lap with or without gently rubbing or patting the back to assist in expelling swallowed air; often this "burping" procedure is necessary one or more times during the feeding as well as 5–10 min after the infant has been put into the crib. It is an essential procedure during the early months but should not be overdone. When nursing is completed, the infant should be placed in the crib on the abdomen or on the right side to facilitate emptying of the stomach into the intestines and to reduce the chances of regurgitation or aspiration.

ONE OR BOTH BREASTS PER FEEDING. The infant should empty at least one breast at each feeding; otherwise it will not be stimulated to refill. Both breasts should be used at each feeding in the early weeks to encourage maximal production of milk. After the milk supply has been established, the breasts may be alternated at successive feedings, and the infant will usually be satisfied with the amount obtained from one. If the secretion of milk becomes too great, both breasts may again be offered at each feeding and incompletely emptied with the intent of securing a partial decrease in lactation.

DETERMINING ADEQUACY OF MILK SUPPLY. If the infant is satisfied after each nursing period, sleeps 2–4 hr, and gains weight adequately, the milk supply is sufficient. Infants who are "light sleepers" require a lot of body contact with the mother during the first months. Mothers of these wakeful and alert infants should not be thought to have a poor milk supply. However, if the infant nurses avidly and completely empties both breasts but appears unsatisfied afterwards, does not go to sleep, or sleeps fitfully and awakens after 1–2 hr, and fails to gain weight satisfactorily, the milk supply is probably inadequate. The program of La Leche League,* which establishes close relationships between successful nursing mothers and mothers needing assistance, is often helpful in such circumstances.

The "let-down" or *milk-ejection reflex* in the mother is an important sign of successful nursing. Sucking or psychologic stimuli associated with nursing lead to secretion of oxytocin by the posterior pituitary. As a result, the myoepithelial cells surrounding the alveoli deep in the breast contract, squeezing milk into the larger ducts, where it is more easily available to the sucking infant. When this reflex functions well, milk flows from the opposite breast as the infant begins to nurse. This reflex is frequently absent or erratic during periods of pain, fatigue, or emotional distress, and its malfunction is thought to be responsible for milk retention in women unsuccessful in breast feeding.

In general, a mother's weighing her infant before and after nursing is neither necessary nor desirable in judging milk supply adequacy. The amount of milk an infant takes at a time is usually unimportant (the amount ingested at each feeding ranges from one to several ounces throughout a 24-hr period), and the results obtained are readily misinterpreted. Small gains may worry the mother and in turn may diminish her milk supply. She may give the infant a bottle to reassure herself that the infant is getting enough to eat. The better result with the "test bottle" may be so discouraging that subsequent breast-feeding becomes impossible, even when she has an adequate supply of milk. Before assuming that the mother produces insufficient milk, three possibilities should be excluded: (1) errors in feeding technique responsible for the infant's inadequate progress; (2) remediable maternal factors related to diet, rest, or emotional distress; or (3) physical disturbances in the infant that interfere with eating or with gain in weight. Infrequently infants who seem to be nursing well may not thrive because of insufficiency of milk; increased frequency of feeding may be indicated. Nursing more than every 2 hr, however, may inhibit prolactin secretion of the anterior pituitary, decreasing production; this is usually corrected by delaying feedings to 2½-hr intervals. Other aids include stimulation of prolactin secretion by administering small doses of chlorpromazine for a few days or by devices such as the Lact-aid, which supplement the infant's intake.

MANUAL EXPRESSION OF BREAST MILK. This is achieved by two movements. First, the whole breast is compressed between the hands, starting at the base and continuing toward the areola. Firm pressure maintained throughout the movement, which is repeated several times, impels milk to the lacteal sinuses. The second movement empties the sinuses: the breast is supported with one hand while the tissue just behind the areola is compressed repeatedly between the thumb and first finger of the other hand. The force is directed backward toward the center of the breast rather than toward the nipple. The fingers remain in this initial position, and the skin over the breast tissue is never rubbed. The procedure should not be painful, even if the nipples are sore and cracked.

MECHANICAL EXPRESSION OF BREAST MILK. Hand pumps are often ineffectual and may increase the irritation and pain in congested breast and nipple tissues. Many mothers prefer electric breast pumps.

SUPPLEMENTARY FEEDINGS. An occasional replacement feeding, after the first 6 wk when nursing has been adequately established, permits the mother greater freedom in her activities. For the normal, healthy infant who is getting insufficient breast milk, artificial feeding may be offered either immediately after or in place of one or more breast-feedings. An attempt should first be made to increase the supply of breast milk. Any of the milk formulas described in Sec. 4.11 may be offered to the infant in sufficiently satisfying amounts. If formula is to be given after the infant has completed a breast-feeding, the warmed bottle should be available so it

---

*La Leche League International, 9616 Minneapolis Avenue, Franklin Park, Illinois 60131, has many local affiliates composed of successfully nursing mothers willing to assist other mothers desiring to nurse.

can be offered immediately after the infant has been burped. The holes in the nipples should not be so large that the infant gets this portion of food without any effort, or the infant will quickly abandon any efforts to suck adequately at the mother's breast.

WEANING. Most infants gradually reduce the volume and frequency of their demand for breast-feedings at 6–12 mo of age, and they become accustomed to increasing amounts of solid foods and liquids by bottle and cup. As they demand less breast milk, the mother's supply gradually diminishes, causing the mother no discomfort from engorgement. Weaning should be initiated by substituting formula or cow's milk by bottle or cup for part of a breast-feeding, and subsequently for all of a breast-feeding. Over several days, one of the breast-feedings is replaced and then subsequently another, and so on, until the infant is weaned completely. Occasionally, the infant takes the cup as readily as the bottle, avoiding the intermediate transfer from bottle to cup. These changes should be made gradually for they should provide a pleasant experience, not a conflict, for the mother and infant. Praise, loving attention, and cuddling are vital to successful weaning.

When cessation of nursing is necessary at an earlier age because of maternal illness or prolonged illness or death of the infant, a tight breast binder may be used and ice bags may be applied for a few days to decrease milk production. Restriction of the mother's fluid intake is also helpful. Hormones, such as small doses of estrogen for 1–2 days, also may help decrease milk production at the termination of nursing.

4.11 FORMULA FEEDING

Whole cow's milk or its modified form is the basis for most formulas, although other milks and milk substitutes are available for infants who cannot tolerate it. Sterilization and refrigeration of the formula greatly reduce morbidity and mortality from gastrointestinal infections. Milk processing (ranging from simple home boiling to commercial pasteurization, homogenization, and evaporation) alters the casein so that small and readily digestible curds form in the stomach, eliminating the principal cause for indigestibility of cow's milk protein.

Although breast-feeding is considered superior to formula feeding for normal infants, many infants receive formula from birth. Changing social and cultural patterns may encourage formula feeding. Because they are employed outside the home, many mothers are reluctant to nurse their infants. Others believe that nursing will limit their activities. Some refuse to nurse because they fear failure at nursing. Others regard weight gain and loss of breast tone as unattractive, and some consider breast-feeding as socially unacceptable. Whatever the reasons, the present popularity of artificial feeding could not have been reached without prior improvements in the safety and quality of the substitute milks.

Objective nutritional studies of growing infants (e.g., rate of growth in weight and length, normality of various constituents in blood, performance in metabolic studies, body composition) show relatively small differences between infants fed human milk and those fed cow's milk. Although such techniques may not record small but important variations, these investigations attest to the normal infant's ability to thrive by making satisfactory physiologic adjustments to wide ranges of ingested protein, fat, carbohydrate, and minerals.

Conventional formulas of whole and evaporated cow's milk provide approximately 3–4 g of protein/kg/24 hr ("high-protein" intake largely exceeding the basic need), whereas breast milk and many commercially prepared feedings simulating the composition of breast milk supply 1.5–2.5 g/kg/24 hr ("low-protein" intake supplying a smaller degree of excess).

Fomon has calculated the rate of increase in total body protein mass in the "male reference" term infant to average approximately 3.5 g/24 hr in the first 4 mo of life. Assuming 0.5 g/24 hr nitrogen loss from the skin, total protein need is estimated to be about 4 g/24 hr during the first 4 mo and slightly less during the remainder of the first year.

Commercial formulas are modified from a cow's milk base, and their protein and ash levels are reduced nearer to those of human milk, thus decreasing osmolality and renal excretory load. The saturated fat of cow's milk is replaced with some unsaturated vegetable fatty acids, and vitamins are added. The concentration of lactose is lower in cow's milk than in human milk. Some formulas include higher lactoproteins and lower casein, such as in breast milk. Low-birthweight infants in particular may benefit from the increased cystine of lactoproteins. Until more information is available, breast-feeding for all infants appears prudent, but if this is impossible, then a formula as compositionally close to breast milk as possible is desirable.

TECHNIQUE OF ARTIFICIAL FEEDING

The setting should be similar to that for breast-feeding, with the mother and infant in a comfortable position, unhurried, and free from distractions. The infant should be hungry, fully awake, warm, and dry and be held as though being breast-fed. The bottle should be held so that milk, not air, channels through the nipple. Bottle propping, even with a "safe" holder, should be avoided, because it not only deprives the infant of the physical contact, comfort, and security of being held but may also be dangerous to small infants, who may aspirate if unattended. Otitis media is more common in infants fed with the propped bottle.

The bottle of milk is customarily warmed to body temperature, although no harmful effects have been demonstrated from feedings at room temperature or cooler. The temperature may be tested by dropping milk onto the wrist. The nipple holes should be of the size so that milk will drop slowly.

Especially during the first 6–7 mo of life, the eructation of air swallowed during feeding is important for avoiding regurgitation and abdominal discomfort. This technique is similar to that described after breast-feeding. A few infants relieve themselves best after being replaced in the crib. All infants will, at times, regurgitate or "spit up" a small amount of milk after feeding, a fact that the mother should know. Spitting up occurs more often in the artificially fed than in the breast-fed infant.

A feeding may last from 5 to 25 min, depending on the vigor and the age of the infant. Because the appetite varies from one feeding to another, each bottle should contain more than the average amount taken per feeding. In no case should the infant be urged to take more than desired, and excess milk should be discarded.

COMPARISON OF HUMAN MILK AND COW'S MILK

Average values for the various constitutents of human milk and whole fresh cow's milk are listed in Table 4–8. Both differ during the various stages of lactation and among individuals, although the differences in human milk from women with adequate diets are insignificant. Milk late in pregnancy and early after birth contains more protein, calcium, and other minerals than later during lactation.

COLOSTRUM. The secretion of the breasts during the latter part of pregnancy and for the 2–4 days after delivery is

TABLE 4–8. Approximate Composition of Colostrum, Human Milk, and Cow's Milk*

Constituent (g/100 g)	Human Milk	Human Colostrum	Cow's Milk
Water	88	87	88
Protein	0.9	2.7	3.3
Casein	0.4	1.2	2.7
Lactalbumin	0.4		0.4
Lactoglobulin	0.2	1.5	0.2
Fat	3.8	2.9	3.8
% polyunsaturated	8.0	7.0	2.0
Lactose	7.0	5.3	4.8
Ash	0.2	0.5	0.8
Calcium (mg/100g)	34	30	117
Phosphorus (mg/100g)	15	15	92
Sodium (mEq/L)	7	48	22
Potassium (mEq/L)	13	74	35
Chloride (mEq/L)	11	80	29
Magnesium (mg/100 g)	4	4	12
Sulfur (mg/100 g)	14	22	30
Chromium (μg/L)			10
Manganese (μg/L)	10	tr	30
Copper (μg/L)	400	600	300
Zinc (mg/L)	4	6	4
Iodine (μg/L)	30	120	47
Selenium (μg/L)	30		30
Iron (mg/L)	0.5	0.1	0.5
Amino acids (mg/100 mL)			
Histidine	22		95
Leucine	68		228
Isoleucine	100		350
Lysine	73		277
Methionine	25		88
Phenylalanine	48		172
Threonine	50		164
Tryptophan	18		49
Valine	70		245
Arginine	45		129
Alanine	35		75
Aspartic acid	116		166
Cystine	22		32
Glutamic acid	230		680
Glycine	0		11
Proline	80		250
Serine	69		160
Tyrosine	61		179
Vitamin			
Vitamin A (IU)	1,898		1,025
Thiamine (μg)	160		440
Riboflavin (μg)	360		1,750
Niacin (μg)	1,470		940
Pyridoxine (μg)	100		640
Pantothenate (mg)	2		3
Folcin (μg)	52		55
B_{12} (μg)	0.3		4
Vitamin C (mg)	43		11
Vitamin D (IU)	22		14
Vitamin E (mg)	2		0.4
Vitamin K (μg)	15		60

*Collated largely from Fomon SJ: Infant Nutrition, 2nd ed. Philadelphia, WB Saunders, 1974, pp. 360 ff; Macy IG, Kelly HJ, Sloan RE: The Composition of Milks. NAS-NRC Publ. 254, 1953.

called "colostrum." It has a deep lemon yellow color, its reaction is alkaline, and its specific gravity is 1.040–1.060, in contrast to the average specific gravity of 1.030 for mature breast milk. The total amount of colostrum secreted daily is 10–40 mL. Human or cow colostrum contains several times the protein of mature breast milk, more minerals, but less carbohydrate and fat. Human colostrum also contains some unique immunologic factors. After the first few days of lactation, colostrum is replaced by secretion of a transitional form of milk that gradually assumes the characteristics of mature breast milk by the 3rd or 4th wk.

WATER. The relative amounts of water and solids in human and cow's milks are about the same.

CALORIES. The energy value of each milk may vary slightly and is approximately 20 kcal/oz or 0.67 kcal/mL.

PROTEIN. There are quantitative differences between the proteins of the two milks. Human milk contains only 1–1.5% protein compared with approximately 3.3% in cow's milk. The increased protein of cow's milk results almost entirely from its 6-fold higher content of casein. Human milk protein consists of approximately 70% whey proteins, largely lactalbumins and lactoglobulins, and 30% casein; the cow's milk ratio is reversed to 18:82.

CARBOHYDRATE. Human milk contains 6.5–7%, and cow's milk contains about 4.5% lactose. About 10% of the carbohydrate in human milk consists of polysaccharides and glycoproteins.

FAT. The fat content of milks is about 3.5%. In human milk fat content varies somewhat with maternal diet; during a single nursing it is higher in the latter portion of the feeding, which may help satiate the infant at the conclusion of nursing.

The milks of different breeds of cattle vary in fat content. Most market milk in urban areas, however, is pooled, and the fat content is adjusted to a standard level, generally from 3.25–4%.

Qualitative differences exist in the fats of human milk and cow's milk. The fats of each consist principally of the triglycerides olein, palmitin, and stearin, but human milk contains twice as much of the more absorbable olein. The volatile fatty acids (butyric, capric, caproic, and caprylic) comprise only about 1.3% of human milk fat but about 9% of cow's milk fat. The small amount of linoleic acid in cow's milk is usually sufficient to prevent deficiency. The premature or debilitated infant may have steatorrhea after ingesting cow's milk fat. For such infants it is wise to substitute a more readily assimilated vegetable fat or human milk.

MINERALS. Cow's milk contains much more of all the minerals except iron and copper than human milk; total mineral content of cow's milk is 0.7–0.75%; that of human milk is 0.15–0.25%. Cow's milk contains inadequate iron; breast-milk iron, although low, may be sufficient for the infant because it is better absorbed, and during the first 4 mo or so of life iron stored during fetal life compensates for the milk's deficiency. Although the need for calcium and phosphorus is great during periods of rapid growth, adequate balances are maintained on breast milk despite its low content of these minerals.

VITAMINS. The vitamin content of each milk varies with the maternal intake, although each has large amounts of vitamin A. Cow's milk is low in vitamins C and D. Breast milk usually contains adequate vitamin C, if the mother eats appropriate foods, and adequate vitamin D unless she is insufficiently exposed to sunlight or is darkly pigmented. Cow's milk contains more thiamine and riboflavin than human milk and about an equal amount of niacin. Both types of milk seem to contain adequate amounts of vitamin A and the B-complex vitamins for the nutritional needs of infants in the first months of life.

BACTERIAL CONTENT. Although human milk is essentially uncontaminated by bacteria, pathogenic organisms in significant numbers may enter the milk from mastitis. Tubercle and typhoid bacilli and herpes, hepatitis B, rubella, mumps, human immunodeficiency virus (HIV), and cytomegaloviruses may be found at times in the milk of women infected with these organisms. Cow's milk is regularly contaminated, but in most cases by bacteria that are not harmful to humans. Milk, however, is a good culture medium for pathogenic bacteria, and many infections are milk-borne, including streptococcal diseases; diphtheria; typhoid fever; salmonellosis; tuberculosis; and brucellosis. Furthermore, certain bacteria that may not affect older children or adults may cause diarrhea in infants. In most cities pasteurization of all marketed whole milk is required. In addition, terminal sterilization or boiling the milk immediately before mixing the infant's formula is advisable.

DIGESTIBILITY. The stomach empties more rapidly after human milk than after whole cow's milk; however, no appreciable difference in gastrointestinal passage time exists between human milk and processed milk formulas during the first 45 days of life. The curd of cow's milk is reduced in size by boiling; it is made considerably less tough and much smaller by the heating required in evaporation, by the addiiton of acid or alkali, and by homogenization. In contrast, the curd of breast milk is fine and flocculent and readily broken down in the stomach. The fat of cow's milk is less readily digested than that of breast milk.

MILK USED IN FORMULAS

RAW MILK. This is not advised for infant feeding; it forms large curds in the stomach, is slowly digested, and is easily contaminated with pathogenic organisms. Its sale is forbidden in most urban communities in the United States.

PASTEURIZED MILK. Pasteurization destroys pathogenic bacteria and modifies casein so that smaller, less tough curds are produced in the stomach. Raw milk is pasteurized by holding heated milk at a specified temperature for a specified length of time, such as at 63°C (145°F) for 30 min or, more commonly, at 72°C (161°F) for 15 sec, then rapidly cooling it to 65°C (148°F) or lower (60°C [140°F]). Standards for the bacterial content of pasteurized milk vary in different cities and countries, tolerable counts ranging as high as 50,000 nonpathogenic bacteria/mL; average counts in many cities, however, are as low as 5,000–10,000. Pasteurized milk should be boiled when used for infant feeding. If it is allowed to stand in the refrigerator for as long as 48 hr, its bacterial count may increase significantly.

HOMOGENIZED MILK. During the process of homogenization, the fat globules are broken into minute particles and remain dispersed. The principal advantage of homogenized milk is the smaller, less tough curd produced in the stomach.

EVAPORATED MILK. This milk has many advantages, including almost universal availability. The unopened can will keep for months without refrigeration. The casein curd produced in the stomach is softer and smaller than that of boiled whole milk; homogenization of the fat also contributes to smaller curd formation. The lactalbumin appears to be less allergenic than that of fresh milk. The sugar is unchanged. When necessary, evaporated milk can be fed in higher concentrations than whole milk formulas. The standard can contains 13 fluid oz* (384 mL). Each fluid oz equals about 44 kcal; in practice the value is generally considered to be 40 kcal. Vitamin D is usually added in the processing so that each reconstituted quart contains 10 μg.

PREPARED MILKS. Many commercially prepared modified milks requiring only the addition of water in a 1:1 proportion are used widely in infant feeding (Tables 4–9 and 4–10). Most are derived from cow's milk, and many are available in both liquid and powder forms. The composition of the majority simulates breast milk in various ways. All are fortified with vitamin D; many contain other vitamins, and some have added iron.

These milks are nutritionally adequate for normal infants, simple to prepare, and convenient to use. They cost more than evaporated milk–water formulas.

Other prepared milks that may have virtue for special circumstances are now available. Those with very low electrolyte content (mineral content similar to that in human milk) may be helpful for infants having congestive heart failure, nephrogenic diabetes insipidus, or marginal renal function.

*One fluid oz is equivalent to approximately 29.57 mL.

TABLE 4–9. Natural Milks, Prepared Milks, and Milk Substitutes Used in Infant Feeding

	Normal Dilution (kcal/oz)*	Approximate Percentage Composition in Normal Dilution (g/100 mL)					Approximate Electrolyte Composition in Normal Dilution (Milliequivalents/Liter)			Milligrams/Liter		
		Protein	*Carbohydrate*	*Fat*	*PUFA*	*Minerals*	*Na*	*K*	*Cl*	*Ca*	*P*	*Fe*
Human milk, mature, average	22	1.1	7.0	3.8	—	0.21	7	14	12	340	150	1.5
Cow's milk, market, average	20	3.3	4.8	3.7	—	0.72	25	35	29	1,170	920	1.0
Cow's milk, evaporated	22	3.8	5.4	4.0	—	0.80	28	39	32	1,300	1,100	1.0
Prepared formulas, cow's milk based												
Aptamil Milupa	20	1.5	7.2	3.6	0.43	0.30	7.8	21.2	11.2	580	350	8.0
Bebelac No. 1, Lijemph	—	1.8	8.6	3.0	—	0.40	—	—	—	950	540	0.4
Dumex Baby Food, Dumex	22	2.0	7.3	3.2	—	0.42	9.0	15.0	13.0	594	396	7.9
Dutch Baby Food, Friesland	20	1.9	6.6	3.0	0.33	—	5.8	13.7	11.5	408	274	0.4
Enfamil, Mead Johnson	20	1.5	6.9	3.8	0.67	0.30	9.0	18.0	12.0	460	320	1.0
Frisolac, Friesland	20	1.4	7.4	3.4	0.60	—	5.5	12.8	10.3	455	274	0.4
Gerber Baby Formula	20	1.4	6.9	3.5	—	0.22	9.1	14.0	12.6	480	370	11.5
Good Start, Carnation	20	1.6	7.4	3.4	0.30	0.19	7.0	16.5	11.3	430	240	10.0
Lactalac V, Friesland	20	3.5	4.9	3.7	0.10	—	23.0	45.0	32.1	1,340	1145	0.1
Lactogen, Nestle	20	1.9	7.1	3.1	0.40	0.41	11.7	21.0	17.7	670	520	8.0
Lactogen FP, Nestle	20	3.1	7.5	2.7	0.35	0.69	20.0	35.0	29.2	1,110	860	12.0
Mamex, Dumex	22	1.6	7.3	3.5	—	0.26	6.0	14.0	10.0	500	333	7.7
Nan, Nestle	20	1.6	7.4	3.4	0.44	0.30	7.4	19.2	14.4	530	300	8.0
Nativa, Nestle	20	1.8	6.9	3.6	0.36	0.31	9.1	16.7	11.0	580	380	8.0
Nutricia	20	1.8	7.1	3.4	0.28	0.23	8.3	17.2	12.0	600	370	8.0
Perlargon, Nestle	20	1.9	7.7	3.1	0.39	0.43	12.6	22.3	18.3	690	540	8.0
Similac, Ross (also 13, 24, 27 kcal/oz)	20	1.5	7.2	3.6	0.87	0.23	8.3	18.7	12.9	510	390	12.0
Similac PM 60/40, Ross	20	1.5	6.9	3.8	1.2	0.22	7.0	15.0	11.0	380	190	1.5
Similac with Whey + Iron, Ross	20	1.5	7.2	3.6	1.4	0.34	10.0	19.0	12.0	400	300	12.0
SMA, Wyeth (also 13, 24, 27 kcal/oz)	20	1.5	7.2	3.6	0.35	0.25	6.5	14.0	11.0	443	290	12.7
Soy Based												
Alsoy, Nestlē	20	1.9	7.4	3.3	0.8	0.35	10.0	20.5	13.8	600	430	8.0
Isomil (soy), Ross	20	1.8	6.8	3.7	1.4	—	13.0	18.0	15.0	700	500	12.0
Nursoy (soy), Wyeth	20	2.1	6.9	3.6	0.34	0.35	8.7	18.9	10.6	634	443	12.7
ProSobee (soy), Mead Johnson	20	2.0	6.9	3.6	0.67	0.4	13.0	20.0	16.0	630	500	12.7
Soyalac (soy), Loma Linda	20	2.1	6.8	3.7	1.9	0.4	13.0	20.0	13.0	635	370	1.3

Table continued on opposite page

TABLE 4–9. Natural Milks, Prepared Milks, and Milk Substitutes Used in Infant Feeding *Continued*

	Normal Dilution (kcal/oz)	Approximate Percentage Composition in Normal Dilution (g/100 mL)				Approximate Electrolyte Composition in Normal Dilution (Milliequivalents/Liter)			Milligrams/Liter	
		Protein	*Carbohydrate*	*Fat*	*Notes*	*Osm*	*Na*	*K*	*Ca*	*P*
Specialty Products										
Advance, Ross	16	2.0	5.5	2.7	—	200	8	20	510	390
Alfare, Nestlé	20	2.2	7.0	3.3	—	—	17	21	540	340
Alimentum, Ross	20	1.9	6.9	3.8	2	370	13	20	710	510
Attain, Sherwood	30	4.0	12.0	4.0	—	300	30	30	625	625
Compleat, Sandoz	32	4.3	12.8	4.3	—	405	56	22	670	1,300
Comply, Sherwood	45	6.0	18.0	6.0	—	410	48	47	1,000	1,000
Criticare HC, Mead Johnson	32	3.8	22.0	0.5	2	650	27	34	530	530
Electrodialyzed Whey, Wyeth	100 g	3.5	56.0	3.0	—	—	15	43	700	419
Enfamil Human Milk Fortifier, Mead Johnson	14	0.7	2.7	0.04	—	—	7	15	60	3
Enrich, Ross	33	4.0	16.2	3.7		480	37	43	720	720
Ensure, Ross	32	3.7	14.5	3.7		470	37	40	530	530
Ensure HN	32	4.4	14.1	3.5		470	40	40	750	750
Ensure Plus	45	5.5	20.0	5.3		690	50	54	700	700
Ensure Plus HN	45	6.3	20.0	5.0		650	51	47	1,050	1,050
Entera, Fresenius	32	4.0	14.6	3.6		420	35	34	800	640
Entralife, Corpak	30	3.5	13.6	3.5		300	26	25	500	500
Entralife HN30	4.2	13.3	3.4			300	40	32	800	800
Good Nature, Carnation	20	2.0	8.8	2.6		—	11.3	22.5	900	600
Isocal, Mead Johnson	32	3.4	13.3	4.4		300	23	34	630	530
Isocal HCN	60	7.5	20.0	10.2		690	35	43	1,000	1,000
Isocal HN	32	4.4	12.4	4.4		300	41	41	850	850
Jevity, Ross	32	4.4	15.2	3.7		310	40	40	912	759
Magnacal, Sherwood	60	7.0	25.0	8.0		590	43	32	1,000	1,000
Meritine, Sandoz	30	5.8	11.0	3.2		505	38	41	1,200	1,200
Newtrition, Knight	32	3.6	41.0	4.0		450	26	26	600	600
Newtrition Isotonic	32	3.6	14.8	3.6		300	26	26	600	600
Newtrition Isofiber	36	5.0	16.0	3.7		310	36	32	847	847
Nutrapak, Corpak	32	3.7	14.5	3.7		450	37	40	530	530
Nutren 1.0, Clintec	30	4.0	12.7	3.8		340	22	32	500	500
Nutren 1.5	45	6.0	17.0	6.7		600	33	48	750	750
Nutren 2.0	60	8.0	19.6	10.6		800	43	64	1,000	1,000
Nutramigen, Mead Johnson	20	2.2	8.8	2.6	2	—	14	18	630	420
Osmolite, Ross	32	3.7	14.5	3.8		300	28	26	530	530
Pediasure, Ross	30	3.0	11.0	4.9		325	16	33	970	800
Peptamen, Clinitec	30	4.0	12.7	3.9	1	260	22	32	600	500
Pepti 2000, Sherwood	30	4.0	19.0	1.0	1	490	30	30	725	625
Portagen, Mead Johnson	20	2.4	8.0	3.2		220	16	22	635	470
Pregestimil PO, Mead Johnson	20	1.9	6.9	3.6	2	—	14	19	630	420
Profiber, Sherwood	30	4.0	13.2	4.0		300	32	32	667	667
Pulmocare, Ross	45	6.0	10.5	9.2		490	57	49	1,050	1,050
RCF, Ross	40	2.0	0	3.6		74	13	19	700	500
Resource, Sandoz	32	3.7	14.5	3.7		430	30	30	550	550
Resource Plus	38	5.5	20.0	5.3		600	39	45	630	630
S14, Wyeth	20	1.1	7.1	3.7		280	7	12	420	320
S-29, Wyeth	20	1.7	10.1	2.3		360	0.4	8	140	170
S-44, Wyeth	20	1.7	10.1	2.3		360	0.4	8	140	170
Sustacal, Mead Johnson	30	6.1	14.0	2.3		620	41	54	1,010	930
Sustacal, fiber	32	4.6	14.0	3.5		480	31	36	845	704
Sustacal HC	45	6.1	19.0	5.8		650	36	38	850	850
Tolerex, Norwich	30	2.1	22.6	0.15	3	550	20	30	550	550
Traumacal, Mead Johnson	45	8.3	14.3	6.8		490	51	36	750	750
Vital HN, Ross	30	4.1	18.0	1.1	4.5	500	20	34	670	670
Vitaneed, Sherwood	30	4.0	12.8	4.0		300	30	32	670	670
Vivonex, Norwich	30	3.8	20.6	0.3	3	630	20	20	500	500

(1) Hydrolyzed whey, (2) Hydrolyzed casein, (3) Amino acids, (4) Partially hydrolyzed whey, (5) and others.

Other specialty formulas are available from various manufacturers, low or free of carbohydrate, protein, sodium, phenylalanine, branched chain amino acids, histidine, homocystine, lysine, tyrosine, and methionine.

Table continued on following page

TABLE 4–9. Natural Milks, Prepared Milks, and Milk Substitutes Used in Infant Feeding *Continued*

	Normal Dilution (kcal/oz)*	Approximate Percentage Composition in Normal Dilution (g/100 mL)					Approximate Electrolyte Composition in Normal Dilution (Milliequivalents/Liter)			Milligrams/Liter		
		Protein	Carbohydrate	Fat	PUFA	Minerals	*Na*	*K*	*Cl*	*Ca*	*P*	*Fe*
Formulas for low-birthweight infants												
Alprem, Nestlê	21	2.0	8.0	3.4	0.31	0.31	10	18.5	11.3	550	300	8
Enfamil, Premature Formula, Mead Johnson	24	2.4	8.9	4.1	0.8	0.5	14	23	19.4	950	480	1.3
Similac 24 LBW, Ross	24	2.2	8.5	4.5	0.6	0.5	13	31	23	730	560	3
Similac Special Care, Ross	24	2.2	8.6	4.4	0.6	0.5	15	27	19	1,440	720	1.5
SMA Preemie, Wyeth	24	2.0	8.6	4.4	0.4	0.4	13.9	19	15	750	400	3

Table continued on opposite page

A low sodium milk, containing about 1 mEq of sodium per reconstituted quart, is commercially available for managing infants having congestive heart failure but should be used with caution. Milks prepared from hydrolysed whey or casein may be useful for infants having malabsorption or milk allergy. Special formulas with specific amino acid elimination are useful for infants and children having inborn metabolic errors.

CONDENSED MILK. About 45% cane sugar has been added in sweetened condensed milk, making the carbohydrate content approximately 60% in the evaporated form before dilution. The usual dilutions (1:10–14) are disproportionately high in sugar and low in fat and protein. Although readily digestible, it has no use in infant feeding for more than short periods when a high-calorie diet is desired.

DRIED WHOLE MILK. The fat content of fluid milk is adjusted to 3.5%, and the milk is rapidly evaporated to powder form by spray-, freeze-, or roller-drying. Reconstituted dried milk has most of the advantages of evaporated milk but does not keep well when exposed to air.

DRIED SKIM MILK. Both nonfat skim milk (fat content 0.5%) and half-skim milk (fat content 1.5%) are available for infants with fat intolerance or for children consuming diets with lowered fat content. Skim milk should not be used in the first year of life. Its high protein and mineral content in proportion to calories may cause severe dehydration. Many of these products do not contain added vitamin D.

ACID AND FERMENTED MILK. So-called acid milks are prepared by adding acid to previously boiled and cooled cow's milk formulas, or these milks are fermented by adding lactic acid–producing organisms. These milks require less hydrochloric acid for gastric digestion. The casein is altered so that smaller, less tough curds form in the stomach. Acidified milks are now rarely used in infant feedings, because they are likely to cause acidosis.

GOAT'S MILK. In many countries goat's milk is used extensively for infant feeding; in the United States its use is limited to managing cow's milk allergies.

Although similar in composition to cow's milk, goat's milk contains less sodium, more potassium and chloride, and more linoleic and arachidonic acids. Its fat may be more digestible and its curd tension lower than that found in cow's milk. It is low in vitamin D, iron, and folic acid; infants fed exclusively on goat's milk are susceptible to megaloblastic anemia due to folate deficiency. Because the goat is especially susceptible to brucellosis, its milk should be boiled before use. It is commercially available in evaporated and powdered forms.

MILK PROTEIN. Powdered protein is used chiefly for increasing protein content of some formulas fed to premature or debilitated infants or to infants with diarrhea. Because of the increased metabolic products and the easy conversion from a balanced to an unbalanced diet, such products should be used carefully and for short durations.

MILK SUBSTITUTES AND HYPOALLERGENIC MILKS. A number of milks and milk substitutes are available for infants allergic to cow's milk. These include evaporated goat's milk, a preparation in which nutrient nitrogen is supplied as an amino acid mixture (casein or whey hydrolysate), and nonmilk foods in which the protein is derived from soybeans. All appear to be nutritionally satisfactory and have a place in the management of infants who cannot tolerate cow's milk; those not containing lactose are useful for infants with galactosemia. Powdered casein (Casec) and medium-chain triglycerides (MCT oil) are available for special purposes.

FILLED AND IMITATION MILKS. Imitation milk products and nondairy "white" beverages in which vegetable fat is substituted for cow (butter) fat are being tested for use in countries where milk and other high-quality protein sources are in short supply. Many of these products lack the full nutritional benefits of fluid milk; they are not intended as formula for infants or as a substitute for breast milk. When they are used for older children, the physician should be aware of the composition and limitations of the product.

ELEMENTAL DIETARY SUBSTITUTES FOR MILK. A number of specialty products have been developed to meet complicated dietary and nutritional problems in children and adults with malabsorption due to primary disease or extensive surgical resection of the small bowel. These include diets prepared with known quantities of purified chemical elements (free glucose, amino acids, and essential fatty acids). All are low residue, chemically defined, and nutritionally adequate, at least for short-term use. They have been most useful in treating severely ill infants with intractable diarrhea, in reducing stooling or "resting" the colon in inflammatory bowel disease, in making maximum use of short bowel segments after surgery, and in maintaining very ill patients in positive nitrogen balance while decreasing the bulk and bacterial content of the colon prior to and after major bowel surgery (see Table 4–9).

MILK FORMULAS

The formulas combine milk, sugar, and water, and some modification for a more desirable, smaller curd formation. They should contain about 20 kcal/oz.

CALORIC REQUIREMENTS (Sec. 4.2). The average caloric requirements of full-term infants are about 45–55 kcal/lb or 80–120 kcal/kg during the first few months of life and about 45 kcal/lb or 100 kcal/kg by 1 yr of age; individual variations are significant, and for many infants intakes of this order exceed caloric need.

FLUID REQUIREMENTS (see Table 4–3). Fluid requirements are high during infancy. During the first 6 mo of life they range from 2 to 3 oz/lb/24 hr, or 130 to 190 mL/kg/24 hr and may increase during hot weather. As a rule, the infant regulates his or her own fluid intake, provided adequate amounts are offered. Most of the fluid required is in the formula, but some is supplied in orange juice and other foods and by water between feedings.

NUMBER OF FEEDINGS DAILY. The number of feedings required per day decreases throughout the first year; by 1 yr of age most infants are satisfied with 3 meals/day (Table 4–

TABLE 4–9. Natural Milks, Prepared Milks, and Milk Substitutes Used in Infant Feeding *Continued*

Carbohydrate Supplements	kcal/g	kcal/mL
LC, Corpak	—	2.5
Moducal, Mead Johnson	3.8	—
Nutrisource, Sandoz	—	3.2
PC, Corpak	4.0	—
Pollycose, Ross	3.8	2.0
Sumacal, Sherwood	3.8	—
Fat Supplements	**kcal/g**	**kcal/mL**
Liposyn, Abbott 10%	1.1	1.1
Liposyn, Abbott 20%	2.0	2.0
Intralipid, Cutter 10%	1.1	1.1
Intralipid, Cutter 20%	2.0	2.0
MCT Oil, Mead Johnson	7.7	7.1
MCT Supplement, Corpak	6.1	—
Microlipid, Sherwood	4.5	2.2
Nutrisource LCT, Sandoz	2.2	0.5
Nutrisource MCT	2.0	0.5
Protein Supplements	**kcal/g**	**kcal/mL**
Casec, Mead Johnson	3.7	—
Pro-Mix, Corpak	3.4	—
Pro-Mod, Ross	4.2	—
Propac, Sherwood	4.0	—
Nutrisource Prot, Sandoz	4.0	—

*Kcal = kilocalories = Cal.

11). The interval between feedings differs considerably among infants but, in general, ranges from 3–5 hr during the first year of life, averaging 4 hr for full-term, healthy infants. Small or weak infants may prefer feedings at 2- to 3-hr intervals. For the first month or two, feedings are taken throughout the 24-hr period, but thereafter, as the quantity of milk consumed at each feeding increases and the infant adjusts his or her demand to the family pattern of daytime activity, the infant usually sleeps for longer periods at night. As the infant develops psychologically and the loving relationship between the parent and infant evolves, demand feeding should gradually progress to a feeding regimen that accounts for the needs of both the infant and the parents.

QUANTITY OF FORMULA. Although the quantity taken at a feeding varies with different infants of the same age and with the same infant at different feedings, it is important to know the average amounts taken at various ages.

Each infant must be primarily responsible for determining the quantity of intake (Table 4–12). Rarely will an infant want to take more than 7–8 oz of milk at one feeding, if caloric and nutritional needs are adequately supplemented by other foods. The relative requirement for milk is somewhat less in the first 2 wk than in the succeeding 5–6 mo. After this time milk, although still of great value, has diminishing importance in meeting total nutritional requirements.

TABLE 4–10. Recommended Ranges of Nutrient Levels in Infant Formulas*

Nutrient (per 100 kcal)	Adequate	Not to Exceed
Protein (g)	1.8†	4.5
Fat (g)	3.3 (30% of Cal)	6 (54% of Cal)
Including essential fatty acid (linoleate) (mg)	300 (2.7% of Cal)	
Vitamins		
A (IU)	250 (75 μg)‡	750 (225 μg)‡
D (μg) cholecalciferol)§	1	2.5
K (μg)	4	—
E (tocopherol equivalents)‖	0.5 (at least 0.5/g linoleic acid)	
C (ascorbic acid) (mg)	8	—
B_1 (thiamine) (μg)	40	—
B_2 (riboflavin) (μg)	60	—
B_6 (pyridoxine) (μg)	20 μg/g protein	—
B_{12} (μg)	0.15	
Niacin (μg)	250 (or 0.8 niacin equivalent)	—
Folic acid (μg)	4	—
Pantothenic acid (μg)	300	—
Biotin (μg)	1.5	—
Choline (mg)	7¶	—
Inositol (mg)	4¶	—
Minerals**		
Calcium (mg)	60‡‡	—
Phosphorus (mg)	30‡‡	—
Magnesium (mg)	6	—
Iron (mg)	0.15	2.5‡‡
Iodine (μg)	5	25
Zinc (mg)	0.5	—
Copper (μg)	60	—
Manganese (μg)	5	100
Selenium (μg)	3	—
Sodium (mg)	20 (5.8 mEq/L)	60 (17.5 mEq/L)
Potassium (mg)	80 (13.7 mEq/L)	200 (34.3 mEq/L)
Chloride (mg)	55 (10.4 mEq/L)	150 (28.3 mEq/L)

*AAP Committee on Nutrition, 1976 Recommendations with 1982 Modifications.

†Nutritionally equivalent to casein. For use of other proteins refer to the Commentary on Breast Feeding and Infant Formulas, including Proposed Standards for Formulas. Pediatrics 57:278, 1976.

‡Retinol equivalents.

§1 μg cholecalciferol = 40 IU vitamin D.

‖1.49 IU = 1 mg *d*-α-tocopherol equivalent. The β and γ isomers have less activity.

¶Average present in milk-based formulas; should be included in this amount in other formulas.

**Formula should be made with water low in fluoride and in all cases contain less than 45 μg/100 kcal. For explanation see Statement on Fluoride Supplementation: Revised Dosage Schedule. Pediatrics 63:150, 1979.

††Calcium to phosphorus ratio should not be less than 1.1 or more than 2.

‡‡Prudence indicates there should be an upper limit for iron. If formula is labeled " infant formula with iron," it must not contain less than 1 mg/100 kcal.

TABLE 4–11. Average Number of Feedings per 24 Hours

Age	Average No. of Feedings in 24 Hours
Birth–1 wk	6–10
1 wk–1 mo	6–8
1–3 mo	5–6
3–7 mo	4–5
4–9 mo	3–4
8–12 mo	3

It is rarely necessary to use more than 1 can (13 fluid oz) of evaporated milk or 1 quart of whole milk/day. By the time the infant is taking these quantities, other foods will be added to the diet in increasing amounts. Ingesting more milk has no advantage, but the disadvantage is that other essential foods may be displaced. Some of the milk may be incorporated in the cereal and in the preparation of foods such as custards, soups, and sauces.

During the first few months the high quantity of protein and minerals in undiluted cow's milk makes such unmodified milk unsuitable for most infants. Diluting the milk supplies free water, and adding carbohydrate increases the caloric content (Table 4–13).

Whereas lactose is the milk sugar of most mammals, it is expensive and other carbohydrates are usually used in home-prepared formulas. Cane sugar, dextrin-maltose preparations, or other easily digestible sugars can be added. Ingested lactose produces a lower pH in the intestine than formulas containing other sugars. The acid pH improves calcium absorption.

Representative evaporated or whole milk formulas for the first 10 days of life are given in Table 4–14. These formulas are satisfactory for an initial prescription. Subsequent adjustments of milk and water should be made in accordance with the infant's satiety and the growth curve.

PREPARATION OF FORMULA. Several more bottles than the number required for feedings are needed for holding water and orange juice. Bottles should be made of heat-resistant glass; they should be smooth inside; and they should be marked in ounces or milliliters. A wide-mouthed bottle is preferable because it is cleaned more easily, and those with an adequate cover for the nipple are preferable if the baby is to be fed away from home. There should be several more nipples than the number required for feedings. Alternatively, disposable bottles are now widely used in some communities. Other useful utensils include a graduate made of heat-resistant glass and marked in ounces or milliliters, a saucepan for heating and mixing the formula, a container for nipples, a glass funnel if narrow-mouthed bottles are used, a large kettle or special bottle sterilizer, a measuring spoon, a can opener, a knife, a standard tablespoon, and a strainer.

All utensils required for the mixing and storing of the formula should be sterilized by boiling for 5–10 min. The rubber nipples and caps should not be boiled more than 5 min. After each feeding the bottle and nipple should be flushed thoroughly, and the bottle should be filled with water until washed with water and a detergent.

The hands should be scrubbed thoroughly, and the sterilized bottles and utensils should be arranged on a clean table. If whole milk is used, the bottle is shaken so that its contents are mixed, and the top is washed with hot water before the cap is removed. The water for the formula (it is necessary to allow for a slight loss in boiling) is brought to the boiling point in a saucepan; the amount of whole milk is added; and the mixture is boiled for 5 min. Constant stirring is necessary. The sugar is added while the milk is still warm.

TABLE 4–12. Average Quantity of Feedings

Age	Average Quantity Taken in Individual Feedings
1st and 2nd wk	2–3 oz (60–90 mL)
3 wk–2 mo	4–5 oz (120–150 mL)
2–3 mo	5–6 oz (150–180 mL)
3–4 mo	6–7 oz (180–210 mL)
5–12 mo	7–8 oz (210–240 mL)

TABLE 4–13. Household Measures of Some Commonly Used Sugars*

	Tablespoonfuls per Ounce
Lactose	3
Sucrose (cane)	2
Dextrin-maltose preparations:	
Mead's Dextri-Maltose	4
Karo	2
Cartose	2
Dexin	6
Polycose fluid	2

*Caloric value of each is 120 Calories per ounce, except Dexin, 115, and polycose, 60.

If evaporated milk is used, the top of the can is washed with soap and hot water and rinsed with hot water; two holes are punctured in it. The water for the formula is boiled for 5 min, and the evaporated milk and sugar are added to it. No further boiling is necessary.

The freshly prepared and sterile formula is poured in appropriate amounts into sterilized nursing bottles. The bottles are capped by aseptic technique and stored in the refrigerator until time for the feedings.

TERMINAL HEATING. This method is most commonly used today; it has practical advantages and does not require presterilization of bottles or utensils. The formula is poured into clean nursing bottles, and the nipples are applied. The nipples are then covered loosely with glass, metal, or paper caps and the bottles are placed in a rack in a container tall enough to prevent the bottles from touching the lid. The container is filled with water to about the midpoint of the bottles, covered, and placed over a moderate flame. The water is allowed to boil gently for 25 min. The bottles are then removed with tongs and placed in a container of cold water for 10 min. The caps are then tightened, and the bottles are stored in a refrigerator. Bottles containing formula should not be warmed in a microwave oven, because uneven heating may cause the formula to burn the infant.

4.12 OTHER FOODS

VITAMINS. Most marketed whole and artificial milks are fortified with 10 μg of vitamin D per reconstituted quart, and

TABLE 4–14. Representative Formulas*

	1–3 Days	Cal	4–10 Days	Cal	10 Days	Cal
Evaporated milk	6 oz	240	7 oz	280	13 oz	520
Sugar	1 tbsp	60	1 tbsp	60	3 tbsp	180
Water	14 oz	___	14 oz	___	17 oz	___
	20 oz	300	21 oz	340	30 oz	700
Cal/oz		14		16		22
Cal/100 mL		47		56		70
Whole milk	12 oz	240	14 oz	280	26 oz	520
Sugar	1 tbsp	60	1 tbsp	60	3 tbsp	180
Water	8 oz		7 oz		6 oz	
	20 oz	300	21 oz	340	32 oz	700

*Total volume is divided into six bottles, and the total intake is regulated by the infant.

commercially prepared milks vary in the content of other vitamins. Therefore, knowing the vitamin content of the milk is essential before prescribing additional vitamins for the bottle-fed baby.

Orange and other citrus fruit juices are natural sources of *vitamin C*, but because many young infants do not seem to tolerate them in amounts large enough to supply an adequate vitamin intake, it is preferable to give 50 mg of ascorbic acid. When at least 2 oz of fresh, frozen, or canned orange juice (or equivalent amounts of other sources of vitamin C) is taken daily, the ascorbic acid may be discontinued.

Vitamin D should be started early in the neonatal period with a daily intake of approximately 10 μg only if the infant is taking a formula that does not contain vitamin D or is receiving an insufficient volume of milk to meet the daily requirement. Low-birthweight infants require supplementation (Sec. 9.17). Vitamin D supplement is not necessary during the first few months of breast-feeding of white infants but may be for black infants and those not exposed to adequate sunlight. Concentrates in water-miscible vehicles are desirable to avoid aspiration of oil.

IRON. Foods rich in iron are less available in the diet of poor families. The most effective way to prevent iron deficiency is to provide iron supplementation in the form of an iron-fortified milk formula or medicinal iron (2 mg/kg up to a total of 15 mg/24 hr) beginning at 6 wk of age. It is doubtful whether iron-supplemented cereals provide sufficient supplementation for infants with reduced iron stores.

"SOLID" FOODS. The caloric contents of the various prepared baby foods differ widely (see Table 27–10). Egg yolk, cereals with added milk, meats, and puddings have greater caloric density than milk, whereas vegetables and fruits have an energy value similar to or lower than milk. Without appropriate advice, many mothers do not know how to select foods for their infants. Among their errors is the tendency to select foods with high caloric values that result in obesity. The inclusion of solid foods to the diet before 4–6 mo of age does not contribute significantly to the health of the normal infant.

Any new food should be initially offered once a day in small amounts (1–2 teaspoonfuls). Any small spoon that easily fits the baby's mouth may be used. New foods are generally best accepted if fairly thin or dilute. Food is frequently pushed out by the tongue rather than back because the baby cannot yet swallow efficiently. This should be mentioned to the mother, who might otherwise interpret the "spitting out" of new foods as dislike. It is usually wise to offer the same food daily until the baby becomes accustomed to it and not to introduce new foods more often than every 1–2 wk.

The feeding at which these foods are offered is not particularly important. They should be given when the baby's hunger is no longer satisfied by milk alone and when they fit into the daily schedule. There is no reason for persisting with or forcing a particular food that is definitely disliked. The family's dislikes and prejudices for particular foods are contagious and should not be displayed before the infant. The physician should avoid prescribing a definite amount of a given food lest the mother interpret the suggestion too literally. *Many infants are overfed by overzealous parents who mistake acceptance of food for appetite.* The infant's appetite is the best index of the proper amount, and respect for the infant's wishes will avoid many problems.

Cereal. The various precooked cereals on the market provide in a convenient form a variety of grains excellent for infants. Most contain iron and factors of the vitamin B complex.

Fruits. Strained or puréed cooked fruits furnish minerals and some water-soluble vitamins and usually have a mildly laxative effect. Raw ripe mashed banana is readily digested and enjoyed by most infants. Many infants who are slow in accepting new foods seem to prefer fruits.

Vegetables. Vegetables are moderately good sources of iron and other minerals and of the B complex vitamins. They should be freshly cooked and strained or commercially prepared. Vegetables are usually added to the infant's diet by about 7 mo of age.

Meats, Eggs, and Starchy Foods. Eggs and starchy foods are usually introduced during the second 6 mo of life, although some physicians offer egg yolk at an earlier age. The yolk of the egg is used initially and is preferably hard-cooked. As with all new foods, a small amount is offered at first, with gradual increases up to a whole yolk 1–3 times a week. Egg white should be introduced with equal caution to minimize any possible allergic manifestations.

Potatoes, rice, spaghetti, bread, and similar starchy foods have principally a caloric value. As a rule, they are not included in the infant's diet until the more essential foods mentioned earlier are being taken regularly. Zwieback, toast, or graham crackers may be offered to the infant when he or she shows an interest in "gumming" on coarser foods (usually 6–8 mo of age). It is with such foods that infants learn to chew and to feed themselves.

Meat is an excellent source of protein as well as of iron and vitamins. Ground fresh beef or liver or the strained canned meats may be used initially by about 6 mo of age. Meats may be more readily accepted when mixed with another food.

The commercial soups and meat and vegetable mixtures are relatively high in carbohydrate and are not considered optimal sources of iron or protein. Many home-prepared soups are bulky out of proportion to their food value, and much of the vitamin content is lost by overcooking.

Desserts. Puddings, junkets, and custard are good foods for older infants, particularly if they temporarily prefer milk in that form. If, however, such foods are given as a bribe or reward or only after other foods have been finished, poor eating habits are likely to be established. Sweet foods should be offered as casually as the rest of the meal and at any place in the meal that the child desires.

SALT INTAKE. To increase their palatability, particularly for the parent, excessive salt used to be added to baby foods. This practice has been discontinued. The significance of large intakes of sodium, which are in the ranges seen in populations with a high incidence of hypertension, is not clear, but the possibility that they might contribute to the development of hypertension later in life cannot be ignored.

FOOD ADDITIVES. Naturally occurring chemicals and food additives, particularly the artificial flavors and colors, have been implicated in health problems. It has been estimated that more than 3,000 flavors are currently being used, and few children are spared exposure to them in their daily diet. Artificial flavors and colors have been associated with respiratory allergic disorders, with urticaria and angioedema, with lesions of the tongue and buccal mucosa, with digestive disturbances, with arthralgia and hydrarthroses, and with headache and behavioral disturbances, including hyperkinesis in childhood.

4.13 FIRST-YEAR FEEDING PROBLEMS

UNDERFEEDING. Underfeeding is suggested by restlessness and crying and by failure to gain weight adequately, despite complete emptying of the breast or bottle. Underfeeding may also result from the infant's failure to take a sufficient quantity of food even when offered. In these cases the frequency of feedings, the mechanics of feeding, the size of the holes in the nipple, the adequacy of eructation of air, the possibility of abnormal mother-infant "bonding," and possible systemic disease in the baby should be investigated (Sec. 6.1). The extent and duration of underfeeding determine the clinical manifestations. Constipation, failure to sleep, irritability, and excessive crying are to be expected. There may be poor gain in weight or an actual loss. In the latter case the skin becomes dry and wrinkled, subcutaneous tissue disappears, and the infant assumes the appearance of an "old man." Deficiencies of vitamins A, B, C, and D and of iron and protein may be responsible for characteristic clinical manifestations.

Treatment consists of increasing the fluid and caloric intake, correcting deficiencies in vitamin and mineral intake, and instructing the mother in the art of infant feeding. If some underlying systemic disease or psychologic problem is responsible, specific management of these disorders is necessary.

OVERFEEDING. Overfeeding may be quantitative or qualitative. Regurgitation and vomiting are frequent symptoms of overfeeding. As a rule, infants can be depended on not to take excessive quantities, but occasionally an infant who has postprandial discomfort from eating too much may nonetheless gain weight excessively. Diets too high in fat delay gastric emptying, cause distention and abdominal discomfort, and may cause excessive gain in weight. Diets too high in carbohydrate are likely to cause undue fermentation in the intestine, resulting in distention and flatulence and in too rapid gain in weight. Such diets may be deficient in essential protein, vitamins, and minerals. Formulas too high in caloric content in the first 1–2 wk of life are likely to result in loose or diarrheal stools. Obesity is undesirable at any time in life; often the excessively fed infant becomes the obese child and adult.

REGURGITATION AND VOMITING. The return of small amounts of swallowed food during or shortly after eating is called "regurgitation" or "spitting up." More complete emptying of the stomach, especially occuring some time after feeding, is called "vomiting." Within limits, regurgitation is a natural occurrence, especially during the first 6 mo or so of life. It can be reduced to a negligible amount, however, by adequate eructation of swallowed air during and after eating, by gentle handling, by avoiding emotional conflicts, and by placing the infant on the right side for a nap immediately after eating. The head should not be lower than the rest of the body during the rest period, because gastroesophageal reflux is common during the first 4–6 mo.

Vomiting, one of the most common symptoms in infancy, may be associated with a variety of disturbances, both trivial and serious. It should be distinguished from rumination; its cause should always be investigated (Sec. 13.13, 13.14, and 13.16).

LOOSE OR DIARRHEAL STOOLS. Acute infectious diarrhea and chronic diarrheal conditions are discussed in Sec. 12.10 and 13.59–13.61; only mild disturbances of dietary origin are considered here.

The stool of the breast-fed infant is naturally softer than that of the infant fed cow's milk. From about the 4th to the 6th day of life the stools go through a transitional stage in which they are rather loose and greenish yellow and contain mucus; within a few days the typical "milk stool" appears. Subsequently, the use of laxatives or the ingestion of certain foods by the mother may be temporarily responsible for an infant's loose stools. Excessive intake of breast milk may also increase the frequency and the water content of the stool. Actual diarrhea in a breast-fed infant is unusual and should be considered infectious until proved otherwise.

Although the stools of artifically fed infants tend to be firmer than those of breast-fed infants, loose stools may result from artificial feeding. In the first 2 wk or so of life, overfeeding is likely to cause loose, frequent stools. Later, formulas too concentrated or too high in sugar content, especially in lactose, may produce loose, frequent stools. Many temporary diarrhea disturbances in artifically fed infants result from food contaminations that would not disturb an older child and are not serious enough to cause prolonged difficulty for the infant. The ease with which artificially fed infants acquire diarrheal disturbances and their potential seriousness are strong arguments for extreme care in providing food free of pathogenic bacteria.

Mild diarrheal disturbances due to overfeeding respond quickly to temporary decrease or cessation of feeding. Withholding all solid food and one or several milk feedings, substituting boiled water or a balanced electrolyte solution, is usually all that is required.

CONSTIPATION (Sec. 13.14). Constipation is practically unknown in breast-fed infants receiving an adequate amount of milk and is rare in artificially fed infants receiving an adequate diet. The nature of the stool, not its frequency, is the mark of constipation. Although most infants have one or more stools daily, an infant will occasionally have a stool of normal consistency only at intervals of 36–48 hr. Whenever constipation or obstipation is present from birth or shortly thereafter, a rectal examination should be performed. Tight or spastic anal sphincters may be responsible occasionally for obstipation, and correction usually follows finger dilatation. Anal fissures or cracks may also cause constipation. If irritation is alleviated, healing usually occurs quickly. Aganglionic megacolon may be manifested by constipation in early infancy; the absence of stool in the rectum on digital examination suggests this possibility.

Constipation in the artificially fed infant may be caused by an insufficient amount of food or fluid. In other cases it may result from diets too high in fat or protein or deficient in bulk. Simply increasing the amount of fluid or sugar in the formula may be corrective in the first few months of life. After this age, better results are obtained by adding or increasing the amounts of cereal, vegetables, and fruits. Prune juice (½–1 oz) may be given as a temporary measure, but it is better to add foods with some bulk. Enemas and suppositories should never be more than temporary measures. Milk of magnesia may be given in doses of 1–2 teaspoonfuls but should be reserved for unresponsive or severe constipation.

COLIC. The term "colic" describes a frequent symptom complex of paroxysmal abdominal pain, presumably of intestinal origin, and of severe crying. It occurs usually in infants under 3 mo of age.

The clinical pattern is characteristic: the attack usually begins suddenly; the cry is loud and more or less continuous; so-called paroxysms may persist for several hours; the face may be flushed, or there may be circumoral pallor; the abdomen is distended and tense; the legs are drawn up on the abdomen, though they may be momentarily extended; the feet are often cold; the hands are clenched. The attack may terminate only when the infant is completely exhausted, but often there is apparent relief with the passage of feces or flatus.

Certain infants seem to be peculiarly susceptible to colic. The cause of recurrent attacks is usually not apparent, although they may be associated with hunger and with swallowed air that has passed into the intestine. Overfeeding may also cause discomfort and distention. Certain foods, especially those of high carbohydrate content, may be responsible for excessive fermentation in the intestines, but a change in diet only occasionally prevents further colic attacks. Crying from intestinal discomfort is seen in infants with intestinal allergy, but colic is not limited to this group. Intestinal obstruction or peritoneal infection may mimic an attack of colic. Recurrent attacks commonly occur late in the afternoon or evening, suggesting that events in the household routine may possibly cause them. Worry, fear, anger, or excitement may cause vomiting in an older child and may cause colic in an infant. No single factor consistently accounts for colic, nor does any treatment consistently provide satisfactory relief. Careful physical examination is important to eliminate the possibility of intussusception, strangulated hernia, hair in eye, otitis, pyelonephritis, or other disorders.

Holding the baby upright or permitting the baby to lie prone across the lap or on a hot water bottle or heating pad helps occasionally. Passage of flatus or fecal material spontaneously or with expulsion of a suppository or enema sometimes affords relief. Carminatives before feedings are ineffective in preventing the attacks. Sedation is occasionally indicated for a prolonged attack and is sometimes given to the parent or child for a period of time if other measures fail. Temporary hospitalization of the infant, often without more than a change in the infant's feeding routine and providing a period of rest for the mother, may help in extreme cases. Prevention of attacks should be sought by improving feeding techniques, including burping, providing a stable emotional environment, identifying possibly allergenic foods in the infant's or nursing mother's diet, and avoiding underfeeding or overfeeding. Colic rarely persists after 3 mo of age. A supportive, sympathetic physician is important in successfully resolving the problem.

4.14 FEEDING DURING THE SECOND YEAR OF LIFE

Most infants naturally adapt themselves to a schedule of three meals a day by about the end of the 1st yr of life. Although considerable latitude in the diet of each infant should be permitted to allow for personal idiosyncrasies and family habits, the mother should be given an outline of the daily basic dietary needs (see Table 4–7).

REDUCED CALORIC INTAKE. Toward the end of the 1st yr of life and during the 2nd yr, because of the constantly decelerating rate of growth, there is a gradual reduction in the infant's caloric intake per unit of body weight. In addition, it is not unusual to have temporary periods of lack of interest in certain foods or even in food in general. Failure to recognize these features, especially the decreasing caloric needs, results in attempts to force feed. The child naturally rebels and feeding problems ensue. Because preventing problems is more effective than correcting them, the changing pattern of the infant's food habits during the 2nd yr of life should be explained to the mother before it appears.

SELF-SELECTION OF DIET. Children's strong likes or dislikes of particular foods should be respected whenever possible and practicable. Spinach is an example of a nonessential food whose virtues have been overemphasized. When consistently rejected foods include basic staples such as milk and eggs, food allergy should be considered.

Children, including infants, tend to select diets which, over several days, assume a balanced nature. Thus, the child may be permitted a wide choice of foods, as long as he or she eats adequately over the longer period. Normally, the child determines the quantity to be eaten of a given food and of the entire meal. At this age eating habits may be strongly influenced by older children in the family, particularly in respect to food likes and dislikes. Eating patterns and habits developed in the first 2 yr of life usually persist for several years.

SELF-FEEDING BY INFANTS. Before 1 yr of age the infant should be permitted to participate in the act of feeding. By approximately 6 mo the infant can hold a bottle; within another 2–3 mo, a cup. Zwieback, graham crackers, or other hand-held foods can be introduced by the age of 7–8 mo. A spoon may be used as soon as it can be held and directed to the mouth, possibly by 10–12 mo of age. Mothers often inhibit this learning process because they object to its messiness.

Acquiring the ability to feed oneself is an important step in developing self-reliance and responsibility. By the end of the second year of life, infants should be largely responsible for feeding themselves.

Permitting infants and children to go to sleep while sucking intermittently from a bottle of formula, whole milk sweetened fruit juice, or water should be discouraged. Pedodontists emphasize the correlation between this habit and enamel erosion in deciduous teeth, calling it the "baby bottle syndrome."

Although nutritional requirements per unit of body weight constantly decrease with increasing age (110 kcal/kg in infancy; 50 kcal/kg at 15 yr), the need for calories as well as for protein, vitamins, and minerals is relatively greater in children than it is in adults.

DAILY BASIC DIET. Parents should be given a daily basic diet for the child from which the family menu can be prepared. Daily selection from each of the food groups provides a balanced diet with sufficient macronutrients and micronutrients. The quantity of intake after the basic requirements have been met can be determined usually by the healthy growing child. The child's history of dietary habits is essential for evaluating the nutritive intake, but such histories are often unreliable unless an accurate dietary diary is kept for several days. From such information, correcting the diet may be more effective. The recommended daily dietary intake is shown in Table 4–7.

The older child should learn the content of a basic diet and its importance to proper growth and good health, but this information should never be presented as a threat to enforce rigid feeding practices.

EATING HABITS. Eating habits formed in the first year or two of life distinctly affect those of the subsequent years. Feeding difficulties between the ages of 2 and 5 yr frequently result from excessive parental insistence on eating and subsequent anxiety when the child does not conform to some arbitrary standard. The child's negative reactions naturally result from undue mealtime stress, and correction requires improvement in parent-child relations. Other factors that disturb eating are too much confusion at mealtime, insufficient time for eating, either on the part of the adult or of the child, food dislikes of other members of the family, and poorly prepared and unattractively served food. A comfortable chair of proper height with a foot-rest is important for a child's ease at the table. Mealtimes should be happy and the conversation should be on subjects of interest to the entire family. The child's appetite should be respected; if his or her desire for food at times is below average, there should be no persuasion to eat more. Adults should realize that eating habits are taught better by example than by formal explanation.

SNACKS BETWEEN MEALS. During the second year and even for several years thereafter, orange juice or other fruit juice or fruit, together with a cracker, may be given in either or both of the between-meal periods. Snacks served in nursery schools and kindergartens should be nutritious. Older children should avoid between-meal snacking if it reduces their appetite for the next meal. After-school snacks, especially of fruit, should be encouraged if they produce greater enthusiasm and energy for play and do not reduce the appetite for the evening meal.

VEGETARIAN DIET

All-vegetable diets supply all necessary nutrients when vegetables are selected from different classes. Vegetables are high in fiber content, vitamins, and minerals. Vegetarians usually have faster gastrointestinal transit time, bulkier stools, and low serum cholesterol levels and are said to have less diverticulitis and appendicitis than meat eaters. Those who consume eggs are ovovegetarians. Those who consume milk are lactovegetarians. Those who consume neither are vegans. Vegans may develop vitamin B_{12} deficiency and, because of high-fiber intake, may develop trace mineral deficiency. Nursing vegan mothers must be given added vitamin B_{12} to prevent methylmalonic acidemia in their infants. Vegetarian infants may not grow as rapidly as omnivores in the first 2 yr.

DIET FOR ATHLETIC ACTIVITIES

Adequate caloric intake is necessary for growth and activity. A varied diet supplies all necessary nutrients. Special food supplements are unnecessary and may be harmful. Water intake should be scheduled regularly before and during athletic events.

American Society for Parenteral and Enteral Nutrition, Inc.: Product Resource Manual, 2nd ed, 1982.
Bahna SL, Heiner DC: Cow's milk allergy. Adv Pediatr 25:1, 1978.
Barr RG, Kramer MS, Pless B, et al: Feeding and temperament as determinants of early infant crying/fussing behavior. Pediatrics 84:514, 1989.
Chesney RW: Requirements and upper limits of vitamin D intake in the term neonate, infant, and older child. J Pediatr 116:159, 1990.
Committee on Nutrition, AAP: Pediatric Nutrition Handbook, 2nd ed, 1985.
Committee on Nutrition, AAP: On the feeding of supplemental foods to infants. Pediatrics 65:1178, 1980.
Committee on Nutrition, AAP: Toward a prudent diet for children. Pediatrics 71:78, 1983.
Cunningham AS: Morbidity in breast-fed and artificially fed infants. J Pediatr 90:726, 1977.
Fomon, SJ: Infant Nutrition, 2nd ed. Philadelphia, WB Saunders, 1974.
Food and Nutrition Board: Recommended Dietary Allowances, 9th ed. National Academy of Sciences, 1980.
Gaull GE: Taurine in pediatric nutrition: Review and update. Pediatrics 83:433, 1989.
Goldfarb J, Tibbetts E: Breast-feeding Handbook. Hillside, NJ, Enslow Publ, 1980.
Goldman AS, Pong AJH, Goldblum RM: Host defenses: Development and maternal contributions. Adv Pediatr 33:71, 1985.
La Leche League International: The Womanly Art of Breast Feeding. Franklin Park, IL, La Leche League International, 1976.
Lebenthal E (ed): Textbook of Gastroenterology and Nutrition in Infants, 2nd ed. New York, Raven Press, 1989.
Lockitch G, Jacobson B, Quigley G, et al: Selenium deficiency in low birthweight neonates: An unrecognized problem. J Pediatr 114:865, 1989.
Lothe L, Lindberg T: Cow's milk whey protein elicits symptoms of infantile colic in colicky-formula-fed infants: A double blind crossover study. Pediatrics 83:262, 1989.
Macy IG, Kelly HJ, Sloan RE: The composition of milks: A compilation of the comparative composition and properties of human, cow and goat milk, colostrum and transitional milk. Washington, DC, Pub No 254, National Academy of Science–National Research Council, 1953.
Reeves JD, Vichinsky E, Addiego J, et al: Iron deficiency in health and disease. Adv Pediatr 30:281, 1983.
Reina D: Infant nutrition. Clin Perinatol 2:373, 1975.
Sampson HA: Infantile colic and food allergy? Fact or fiction. J Pediatr 115:583, 1989.

NUTRITIONAL DISORDERS

4.15 MALNUTRITION

Worldwide, malnutrition is one of the leading causes of morbidity and mortality in childhood (Sec. 5.4).

Malnutrition may be due to improper or inadequate food intake or may result from inadequate absorption of food. Insufficient food supply, poor dietary habits, food faddism, and emotional factors may limit intake. Certain metabolic abnormalities may also cause malnutrition. Requirements for essential nutrients may be increased during stress and disease and during the administration of antibiotics or of catabolic or anabolic drugs. Malnutrition may be acute or chronic, reversible or irreversible.

Precise evaluation of nutritional status is difficult. Severe disturbances are readily apparent, but mild disturbances may be overlooked, even after careful physical and laboratory examinations. The diagnosis of malnutrition rests on an accurate dietary history; on evaluation of present deviations from average height, weight, head circumference, and past rates of growth; on comparative measurements of midarm circumference and skinfold thickness; and on chemical and other tests. Decreased skinfold thickness suggests protein-calorie malnutrition; excessive thickness indicates obesity. Muscle mass is calculated by subtracting skinfold measurements from arm circumference. For older children and adults midarm muscle circumference (cm) = arm circumference (cm) − (skinfold thickness [cm] × 3.14). Lean body mass can be estimated from 24-hr creatinine excretion. Deficiencies of some nutrients may be revealed by finding low blood levels of them or their metabolites, by observing biochemical or clinical effects of administration of the nutrients or their products, or by giving the patient substantial amounts of appropriate nutrients and noting the rate at which they are excreted. Protein reserves are assessed from serum albumin and rapid turnover proteins. The levels of rapid turnover proteins, transthyretin with a half-life of 12 hours, pre-albumin with a half-life of 1.9 days, and transferrin with a half-life of 8 days, decrease due to inadequate visceral protein synthesis or depletion of protein stores. Serum levels of essential amino acids may be lower than those of nonessential amino acids. Excretion of hydroxyproline is decreased and of 3-methylhistidine increased, and hair is easily plucked out in the severely malnourished child.

The most acute nutritional disturbances are those which involve water and electrolytes, especially sodium, potassium, chloride, and hydrogen ions (see Chapter 6). Chronic malnutrition usually involves deficits of more than a single nutrient. Immunologic insufficiency is common in malnutrition and is demonstrated by total lymphocyte counts less than $1,500/mm^3$ and anergy to skin test antigens, such as streptokinase-streptodornase, *Candida*, mumps, or tuberculin in exposed persons (Sec. 11.22 and 13.53).

4.16 MARASMUS

(Infantile Atrophy, Inanition, Athrepsia)

Severe malnutrition in infants is common in areas with insufficient food, inadequate knowledge of feeding techniques, or poor hygiene. The synonyms of marasmus listed earlier apply to patterns of clinical illness emphasizing one or more features of protein and calorie deficiency.

ETIOLOGY. The clinical picture of marasmus originates from an inadequate caloric intake due to insufficient diet, to improper feeding habits such as those of disturbed parent-child relations, or to metabolic abnormalities or congenital malformations. Severe impairment of any body system may result in malnutrition.

CLINICAL MANIFESTATIONS. Initially, there is failure

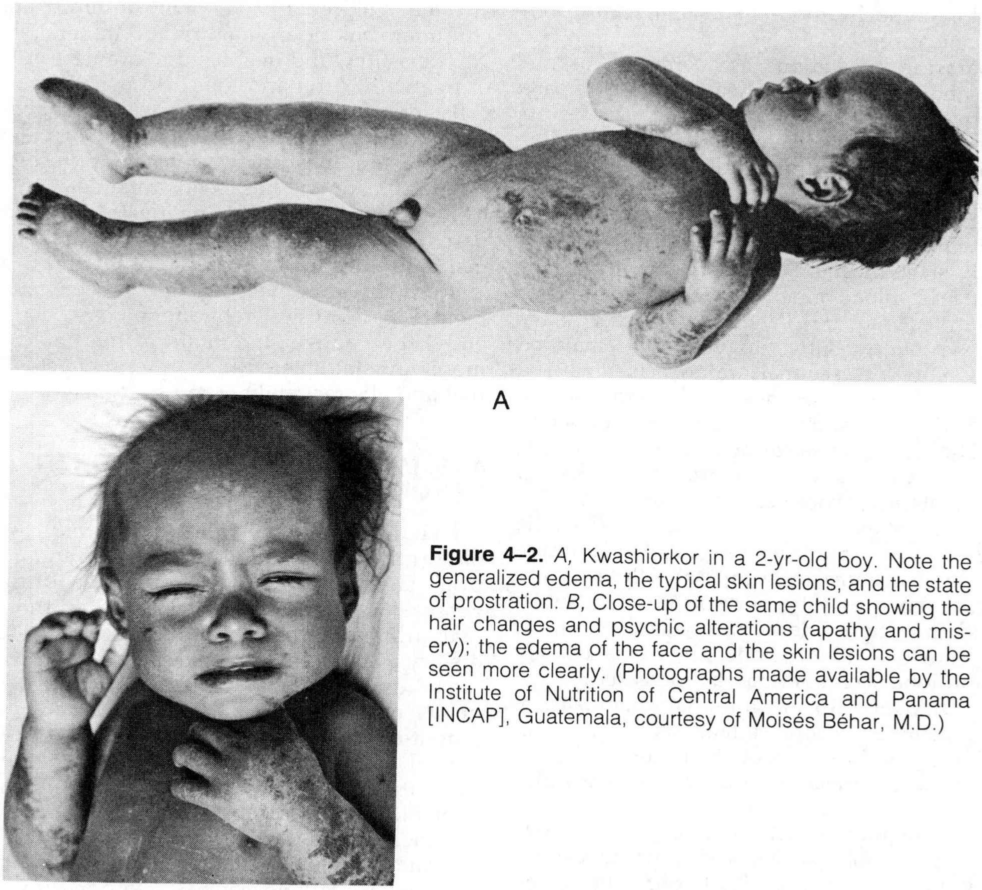

A

B

Figure 4–2. *A*, Kwashiorkor in a 2-yr-old boy. Note the generalized edema, the typical skin lesions, and the state of prostration. *B*, Close-up of the same child showing the hair changes and psychic alterations (apathy and misery); the edema of the face and the skin lesions can be seen more clearly. (Photographs made available by the Institute of Nutrition of Central America and Panama [INCAP], Guatemala, courtesy of Moisés Béhar, M.D.)

to gain weight, followed by loss of weight until emaciation results, with loss of turgor in skin that becomes wrinkled and loose as subcutaneous fat disappears. Because fat is lost last from the sucking pads of the cheeks, the infant's face may retain a relatively normal appearance for some time before becoming shrunken and wizened. The abdomen may be distended or flat, and the intestinal pattern may be readily visible. Atrophy of muscle occurs, with resultant hypotonia. Edema may be present.

The temperature is usually subnormal, the pulse may be slow, and the basal metabolic rate tends to be reduced. At first the infant may be fretful but later becomes listless, and the appetite diminishes. The infant is usually constipated, but the so-called starvation type of diarrhea may appear, with frequent, small stools containing mucus.

4.17 PROTEIN MALNUTRITION
(Protein-Calorie Malnutrition [PCM], Kwashiorkor)

Because they are growing, children must consume enough nitrogenous food to maintain a positive nitrogen balance, whereas adults need only maintain nitrogen equilibrium.

ETIOLOGY. Although deficiencies of calories and other nutrients complicate the clinical and chemical patterns, the principal symptoms of protein malnutrition are due to insufficient intake of protein of good biologic value. There may also be impaired absorption of protein, such as in chronic diarrheal states, abnormal losses of protein in proteinuria (nephrosis), infection, hemorrhage or burns, and failure of protein synthesis, such as in chronic liver disease.

Kwashiorkor is a clinical syndrome that results from a severe deficiency of protein and an inadequate caloric intake. It is the most serious and prevalent form of malnutrition in the world today, especially in industrially underdeveloped areas.

Kwashiorkor means "deposed child," that is, the child no longer suckled; it may become evident from early infancy to about 5 yr of age, usually after weaning from the breast. Although gains in height and weight are accelerated with treatment, these measurements never equal those of consistently well-nourished children.

CLINICAL MANIFESTATIONS (Fig. 4–2). Early clinical evidence of protein malnutrition is vague but does include lethargy, apathy, or irritability. When well advanced, it results in inadequate growth, lack of stamina, loss of muscular tissue, increased susceptibility to infections, and edema. Secondary immunodeficiency is one of the most serious and constant manifestations. For example, measles, a relatively benign disease of the well nourished, can be devastating and fatal in malnourished children. The child may develop anorexia, flabbiness of subcutaneous tissues, and loss of muscle tone. The liver may enlarge early or late; fatty infiltration is common. Edema usually develops early; failure to gain weight may be masked by edema, which is often present in internal organs before it can be recognized in the face and limbs. Renal plasma flow, glomerular filtration rate, and renal tubular function are decreased. The heart may be small in the early stages of the disease but is usually enlarged later.

Dermatitis is common. Darkening of the skin appears in irritated areas but not in those exposed to sunlight, a contrast to the situation in pellagra (Sec. 4.25). Dyspigmentation may occur in these areas after desquamation or may be generalized. The hair is often sparse and thin and loses its elasticity. In dark-haired children, dyspigmentation may result in streaky red or gray hair color (hypochromotrichia). Hair texture becomes coarse in chronic disease.

Infections and parasitic infestations are common, as are anorexia, vomiting, and continued diarrhea. The muscles are weak, thin, and atrophic, but occasionally there may be an excess of subcutaneous fat. Mental changes, especially irritability and apathy, are common. Stupor, coma, and death may follow.

LABORATORY DATA. Decrease in the concentration of serum albumin is the most characteristic change. Ketonuria is common in the early stage of inanition but frequently disappears in the later stages. Blood glucose values are low, but glucose tolerance curves may be diabetic in type. Urinary excretion of hydroxyproline relative to creatinine may be decreased. Plasma values of essential amino acids may be decreased relative to nonessential ones, and there may be increased aminoaciduria. Potassium and magnesium deficiencies are frequent. The serum cholesterol level is low, but it returns to normal after a few days of treatment. The serum values of amylase, esterase, cholinesterase, transaminase, lipase, and alkaline phosphatase are decreased. There is diminished activity of the pancreatic enzymes and of xanthine oxidase, but these values return to normal shortly after the onset of treatment. Anemia may be normocytic, microcytic, or macrocytic. Other nutritional deficiencies, as of vitamins and minerals, are usually evident. Bone growth is usually delayed. Growth hormone secretion may be increased.

DIFFERENTIAL DIAGNOSIS. Differential diagnosis of protein deprivation includes chronic infections, diseases in which there is an excessive loss of protein through urine or stools, and conditions with a metabolic inability to synthesize protein.

PREVENTION. This requires a diet containing an adequate quantity of protein of good biologic quality. Because kwashiorkor has not only a serious and often fatal course but often permanent and devastating aftereffects in recovered children and their offspring, adequate dietary instruction and food distribution are urgently needed in endemic areas.

TREATMENT. Immediate management of any acute problems such as those of severe diarrhea, renal failure, and shock (Sec. 6.35) and, ultimately, the replacement of missing nutrients is essential. Moderate or severe dehydration, manifest or suspected infection, eye signs of severe vitamin A deficiency, severe anemia, hypoglycemia, continuing or recurrent diarrhea, skin and mucous membrane lesions, anorexia, and hypothermia all must be treated. For mild to moderate dehydration fluids are administered orally or by nasogastric tube (Sec. 6.17). A breast-fed infant should be nursed as often as he or she wants. For severe dehydration, intravenous fluids are necessary (Sec. 6.18). If intravenous fluids cannot be given, a rapid intraosseous (marrow) or intraperitoneal infusion of 70 mL/kg of half-strength Ringer lactate solution may be lifesaving. Effective antibiotics should be given parenterally for 5–10 days.

When dehydration is corrected, oral feeding starts with small, frequent feeds of dilute milk; strength and volume are gradually increased and frequency decreased over the next 5 days. By day 6–8, the child should receive 150 mL/kg/day in 6 feeds. Cow's milk, or yogurt for the lactose-intolerant, should be made with 50 g sugar/L. Special feeds are available from UNICEF. In the recovery period, high-energy feeds made with milk, oil, and sugar are needed. Skim milk, casein hydrolysates, or synthetic amino acid mixtures may be used to supplement the basic fluid and nutritional regimen.

When high-calorie and high-protein diets are given too early and rapidly, the liver may become enlarged, the abdomen becomes markedly distended, and the child improves more slowly. Vegetable fat is better absorbed than cow's milk fat. Impaired glucose tolerance may be improved in some affected children by the daily administration of 250 μg of chromium chloride. Vitamins and minerals, especially vitamin A, potassium, and magnesium, are necessary from the outset of treatment. Iron and folic acid usually correct the anemia.

Bacterial infections must be treated concomitantly with the dietary therapy, whereas treatment of parasitic infestations, if not severe, may be postponed until recovery is under way.

After treatment has been initiated, the patient may lose weight for a few weeks, owing to loss of apparent or inapparent edema. Serum and intestinal enzymes return to normal, and intestinal absorption of fat and protein improves.

If growth and development has been extensively impaired, mental and physical retardation may be permanent. Apparently, the younger the infant at the time of deprivation, the more devastating are the long-term effects. Deficits in perceptual and abstract abilities are especially long-lasting.

4.18 MALNUTRITION IN CHILDREN BEYOND INFANCY

ETIOLOGY. Malnutrition in children may be a continuation of an undernourished state begun in infancy, or it may arise from factors that become operative during childhood. In general, the causes are the same as those responsible for malnutrition in infants. The problem may be complex. Poor dietary habits may be associated with a generally poor hygienic situation, with chronic disease, with finicky eating habits of other members of the family, or with disturbed parent-child relations (Sec. 6.30).

Poor eating habits in children under the age of 5 or 6 yr can often be traced directly to parental factors, of which overconcern about the quantity or quality of the diet is a common one. In children of all ages, insufficient sleep and too much emotional excitement, such as that associated with the movies and television, are important factors. School-aged children often develop irregular or inappropriate eating habits, especially at breakfast and lunch, because sufficient time is not allotted or because the meals may be inadequate. Some children as young as 5–8 yr eat little because of fear of obesity. These children respond readily to dietary advice and explanation, in contrast to children who have anorexia nervosa. Eating between meals, especially of items such as candy and snack foods, usually reduces the mealtime appetite.

CLINICAL MANIFESTATIONS. Malnutrition does not invariably result in underweight. Fatigue, lassitude, restlessness, and irritability are frequent manifestations. Restlessness and overactivity are frequently misinterpreted by parents as evidences of lack of fatigue. Anorexia, easily induced digestive disturbances, and constipation are common complaints, and even in older children the starvation type of mucoid diarrheal stool may be observed. Malnourished children often have a limited span of attention and do poorly in school. They have increased susceptibility to infections. Muscular development is inadequate, and the flabby muscles result in a posture of fatigue, with rounded shoulders, flat chest, and protuberant abdomen. Such children often look tired; the face is pale, the complexion is "muddy," and the eyes lack luster. Hypochromic anemia is common. In protracted cases there may be delayed epiphyseal development, irregularities in dentition, and delayed puberty.

Evaluation should always include a careful history of dietary habits, psychosocial maladjustments, physical hygiene, and illness; a thorough physical examination; and appropriate laboratory examinations.

TREATMENT. There is a great need for individualized treatment aimed at correcting underlying psychologic and physical disturbances. An adequate diet (Sec. 4.14) should be outlined; vitamin concentrates may be added and continued for a time after the dietary intake has become adequate. When anorexia is a problem, the essential items of the diet should be provided in as concentrated a form as possible, and the fat content should be low. Between-meal snacks need not be prohibited if they do not interfere with the appetite for the next meal; milk or candy should not be given at such times; fruit or fruit juices are appropriate. Re-educating the entire family about eating habits may be necessary (Sec. 3.60).

Cupoli JM, Hallock JA, Barness LA: Failure to thrive. Current Probl Pediatr No. 11, Sept, 1980.
Graham GG, Lembeke J, Lancho E, et al: Quality protein maize: Digestibility and utilization by recovering malnourished infants. Pediatrics 83:416, 1989.
Hegsted DM: Protein-calorie malnutrition. Am Scientist 66:61, 1978.
Katz M, Stiehm ER: Host defense in malnutrition. Pediatrics 59:490, 1977.
Robinson H, Picou D: A comparison of fasting plasma insulin and growth hormone concentrations in marasmic, kwashiorkor, marasmic-kwashiorkor and underweight children. Pediatr Res 11:637, 1977.
Sleisenger MH, Kim YS: Protein digestion and absorption. N Engl J Med 300:659, 1979.
Zain BK, Haquani AH, Quereshi N, et al: Studies on the significance of hair root protein and DNA in protein calorie malnutrition. Am J Clin Nutr 30:1094, 1977.

4.19 PROTEIN EXCESS

Excessive protein intake, especially in the absence of sufficient water, may lead to signs of dehydration—protein fever. Signs of protein excess are rare, but premature infants fed a high-protein diet may have an increased morbidity. Marasmic infants fed high-protein diets during the recovery phase may develop hyperammonemia; protein intoxication has also been noted in children with other liver disease. Some weight reducing diets with high-protein content may be responsible for protein intoxication.

Barness LA, Omans WB, Rose CS, et al: Progress of premature infants fed a formula containing demineralized whey. Pediatrics 32:52, 1963.

4.20 OBESITY

No exact line separates good nutrition and overnutrition; practically, the diagnosis is made from the child's appearance rather than from an arbitrary weight excess. Stocky children may have relatively large skeletal frames and more than the average amount of muscular tissue so that their weight and height as well as their "bigness" exceed those of the average child of their age, but they should not be considered obese. Obesity or overnutrition is a generalized, excessive accumulation of fat in subcutaneous and other tissues that can be quantitated by measuring skinfold thickness with calipers.

ETIOLOGY. Obesity is usually due to an excessive intake of food. Appetite may be influenced by a variety of factors that include psychologic disturbances; hypothalamic, pituitary, or other brain lesions; and hyperinsulinism. Genetic predisposition to obesity occurs in certain animals and may occur in humans. In a study of adults, obesity was found to be seven times more common in the lowest than in the highest socioeconomic class. Lack of activity may be responsible for obesity even though intake of food may not be unusual. Illnesses that keep a child in bed for prolonged periods may also result in obesity. Some inherited syndromes such as the Laurence-Moon-Biedl, Prader-Willi, and Cushing usually include obesity, on either an endocrine or inactivity basis.

Obesity may result from increases in numbers or in size of fat cells, adipocytes. Adipocytes appear to increase in number when caloric intake is increased, especially in the gestational months and during the first year of life. This stimulus to increase in number continues, although at a reduced rate, throughout puberty, so that during periods of adolescent weight reduction, the size but not the number of adipocytes decreases.

The obese may become resistant to insulin, resulting in an increase in levels of circulating insulin. Insulin decreases lipolysis and increases fat synthesis and uptake. The obese respond to a carbohydrate meal with increased insulin and a decreased utilization of free fatty acids. During weight reduction regimens, the obese deliver less food to their cells than the lean, owing to decreased mobilization of free fatty acids. In starvation after obesity, fat is mobilized as serum insulin decreases. Protein conservation is facilitated as the brain utilizes ketones for energy. During starvation, serum alanine levels decrease and glycine levels rise.

Purified sugars as well as high-protein diet may cause greater secretion of insulin than do complex carbohydrates.

The chronic and uncritical offering of a bottle as a method of dealing with a fretful or crying infant may establish a habit that leads the infant to expect or seek food whenever experiencing frustration. If obesity is initiated early, it is likely to persist. Similarly, the uncritical early introduction of high-calorie solid foods may lead to rapid weight gain and to obesity.

CLINICAL MANIFESTATIONS. Obesity may become evident at any age, but it appears most frequently in the first year of life, at 5–6 yr of age, and during adolescence. The child whose obesity is due to excessively high caloric intake is usually not only heavier than others in his or her cohort but also taller, and bone age is advanced. The facial features often appear disproportionately fine. The adiposity in the mammary regions of boys is often suggestive of breast development and therefore an embarrassing feature. The abdomen tends to be pendulous, and white or purple striae are often present. The external genitalia of boys appear disproportionately small but actually are most often of average size; the penis is often imbedded in the pubic fat. Puberty may occur early, with the result that the ultimate height of the obese may be less than that of their slower maturing peers. The development of the external genitalia is normal in the majority of girls, and menarche is usually not delayed. The obesity of the extremities is usually greater in the upper arm and thigh and is sometimes limited to them. The hands may be relatively small and the fingers tapering. Genu valgum is common.

Psychologic disturbances are common in obese children. Even in the apparently well-adjusted child adequate psychologic evaluation often discloses significant underlying emotional problems. These may have initially contributed to the causes of obesity and usually are an additive factor in its maintenance.

PREVENTION AND TREATMENT. Because obesity may be self-perpetuating for psychologic or physiologic reasons, children of obese parents or those with obese siblings should be encouraged to adhere to a systematic program of energetic exercise and a balanced low-calorie diet. Idealized weight is desirable not only for esthetic reasons but also to prevent complications of obesity such as diabetes, shortness of breath, and early death. Untreated overweight infants frequently remain overweight as adults. Treatment of the obese child usually fails unless the child is motivated to lose weight. Feeding the infant on demand shortly after birth, providing food only at signs of hunger in the first year, avoiding cueing by showing attractive foods or regimenting feeding times by the clock, and by teaching the child to eat only when hungry may effectively prevent overeating and obesity. Modifying behavior to include increased activity is helpful.

In planning a diet, the basic nutritional needs must be met. All the essential dietary needs may be included in an 1,100- to 1,300-calorie diet for children 10–14 yr of age for several months (Table 4–15). Some children avoid excessive eating

TABLE 4–15. 1,100–1,300 Calorie Diet

Breakfast
½ cup orange juice
¾ cup ready-to-eat cereal
6 oz 1% milk
1 tsp sugar
Lunch
2 oz turkey or lean meat
½ cup noodles or bread
½ cup carrots
1 tsp margarine
1 cup 1% milk
Dinner
2 oz lean ground beef
1 oz cheese
½ tomato
1 cup 1% milk
2 taco slices, taco sauce
1 nectarine
Lettuce
Snack
6 Saltines
1 apple

Total "exchanges": 3 fruit, 2 vegetables, 4 starch, 2¾ milk, 3 medium-fat meat, 2 low-fat meat, 2 fat. Try to incorporate egg, high-fiber sources (e.g., beans, some combination foods).

after they have been allowed to return to a free choice of diet. The diet should contain as much bulk as possible. At times greater cooperation is secured if small portions of the diet are permitted between meals, especially in the afternoon. If there is doubt that the daily vitamin intake is adequate, vitamin concentrates may be prescribed. Vitamin D should be included, as for all growing children. Rapid decreases in weight should not be attempted, and medical supervision should be maintained. During the growing years, maintenance of weight while the child increases in height is often a sufficient goal. At best there is a limited place for drug therapy. Psychologic support is often an essential element in management, and both dietary and psychologic treatment should involve the entire family.

The *pickwickian syndrome* (for the fat boy, Joe, in Dickens' *Pickwick Papers*) is a rare complication of extreme exogenous obesity, in which there is severe cardiorespiratory distress. The extreme obesity causes alveolar hypoventilation, with a decrease in pulmonary, tidal, and expiratory reserve volumes. The manifestations include polycythemia, hypoxemia, cyanosis, cardiac enlargement, congestive cardiac failure, and somnolence. High concentrations of oxygen may be dangerous in treating the cyanosis because respiration may depend solely on the stimulatory effect of hypoxia. Weight reduction is extremely important and should be accomplished as rapidly as feasible.

American Academy of Pediatrics Committee on Nutrition: Obesity in infancy and childhood. Pediatrics 68:880, 1981.

Bistrian BR, Blackburn GL, Stanbury JB: Metabolic aspects of a protein-sparing modified fast in the dietary management of Prader-Willi obesity. N Engl J Med 296:774, 1977.

Mossberg H: 40-year follow-up of overweight children. Lancet II:491, 1989.

VITAMINS

Vitamins are essential nutrients that must be supplied exogenously. Functions of vitamins are summarized in Table 4–6, and recommended daily allowances in Table 4–1. Toxicity is seen more commonly with excesses of the fat-soluble vitamins A and D than with the water-soluble vitamins. The vitamin-dependent states are summarized in Table 4–16.

4.21 VITAMIN A DEFICIENCY

The term vitamin A is a generic label for all β-ionone derivatives other than provitamin A carotenoids. Retinol signifies vitamin A alcohol retinyl ester, vitamin A ester; retinal, vitamin A aldehyde; and retinoic acid, vitamin A acid.

"Provitamin A carotenoids" is the generic term for all carotenoids that have the biologic activity of β-carotene. They

TABLE 4–16. Vitamin Dependency States

Vitamin	Disease	Untreated State	Daily Dosage
A	Darier	Hyperkeratosis follicularis	7,500 μg
B_1	Leigh—pyruvic-lactic acidosis	Ataxia, retardation	600 mg
	Thiamine responsive anemia	Megaloblastic anemia	20 mg
	Maple syrup urine disease	Hypotonia, seizures	10 mg
Riboflavin	Pyruvate kinase deficiency	Hemolysis	10 mg
	Glutaric acidemia (II)	Hypoglycemia	100–300 mg
Niacin	Hartnup	Ataxia, eczema	200 mg
B_6	Cystathioninuria	No symptoms	200 mg
	Homocystinuria	Retardation	200 mg
	B_6-anemia	Hypochromic microcytic anemia	10 mg
	B_6-seizures	Seizures	25 mg
	Xanthurenic aciduria	Retardation	10 mg
	Gyrate atrophy of choroid	Blindness	100 mg
	Oxaluria	Oxalate crystals	100 mg
Folic acid	Formiminotransferase deficiency	Retardation	5 mg
	Folate reductase deficiency	Megaloblastic anemia	5 mg
	Homocystinuria	Retardation	10 mg
B_{12}	Methylmalonic acidemia	Retardation	1 mg
Biotin	Propionic acidemia	Retardation	10 mg
	β-Methylcrotonyl glycinuria	Coma	10 mg
	Biotinidase deficiency	Seizures	5–20 mg
	Holocarboxylase deficiency	Hypotonia	10 mg
C	Chédiak-Higashi	Infections	50 mg
D	Dependency	Rickets	100 μg
	Familial hypophosphatemia	Rickets	2,500 μg

or their derivatives with vitamin A activity are required in the diets of infants and children.

β-Carotene is partly absorbed by the intestinal lymphatics; the remainder is cleaved into two molecules of retinol. Dietary retinyl ester is hydrolyzed to retinol in the intestine. Retinol is esterified inside the mucosal cell with palmitic acid and is stored in the liver as retinyl palmitate; this in turn is hydrolyzed to free retinol for transport to its site of action. Zinc is required for this mobilization. Normal plasma values of retinol in infants are 20–50 μg/dL; in children and adults, 30–225 μg/dL.

Heavy ingestion of carotenoids may result in large amounts of carotene in the blood and in yellow discoloration of the skin but not of the sclera. This disorder, carotenemia, is especially likely to occur in children with liver disease, diabetes mellitus, or hypothyroidism and in those who have congenital absence of enzymes that convert provitamin A carotenoids.

ETIOLOGY. The liver at birth has a low vitamin A content that is rapidly augmented because colostrum and breast milk furnish large amounts of the vitamin. Breast milk and whole cow's milk are satisfactory sources of vitamin A. Other foods (vegetables, fruits, eggs, butter, liver) or vitamin supplements also provide vitamin A. Loss of it in cooking, canning, and freezing of foodstuffs is small; oxidizing agents, however, destroy it.

The risk of vitamin A deficiency is small in healthy children with balanced diets. Deficient diets commonly cause disease by 2–3 yr of age. Vitamin A deficiency also results from inadequate intestinal absorption, such as, for example, with chronic intestinal disorders, celiac disease, hepatic and pancreatic diseases, iron deficiency anemia, chronic infectious diseases, or chronic ingestion of mineral oil. Low intake of dietary fat results in low vitamin A absorption. Vitamin A excretion is increased in cancer, urinary tract disease, and chronic infectious diseases. Low protein intake results in deficient carrier protein and in decreases in plasma concentration of vitamin A.

PATHOLOGY. The human retina contains two distinct photoreceptor systems: the rods are sensitive to light of low intensity, the cones to colors and to light of high intensity. Retinal is the prosthetic group of the photosensitive pigment in both rods and cones. The major difference between the visual pigments in rods (rhodopsin) and in cones (iodopsin) is the nature of the protein bound to retinal. All-*trans* retinal isomerizes in the dark to 11-*cis* form. This combines with opsin to form rhodopsin. Energy from light quanta reconverts 11-*cis* retinal back to the all-*trans* form; this energy exchange, transmitted via the optic nerves to the brain, results in visual sensation. β-Carotene has been effective in ameliorating photosensitivity in patients with erythropoietic protoporphyria. It has also been suggested that retinitis pigmentosa may be related to a defect in retinol-binding protein.

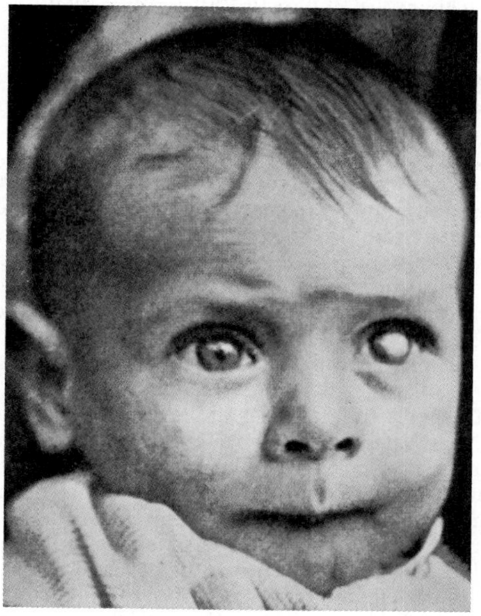

Figure 4–3. Recovery from xerophthalmia, showing permanent eye lesion. (From Bloch CE: Blindness and other diseases arising from deficient nutrition [lack of fat-soluble A factor]. Am J Dis Child 27:139, 1924.)

Vitamin A is apparently necessary for membrane stability. Both excess and deficiency of vitamin A lead to rupture of lysosomal membranes with release of hydrolases.

The vitamin plays a role in keratinization, cornification, bone metabolism, placental development, growth, spermatogenesis, and mucus formation. Characteristic changes in epithelium include proliferation of basal cells, hyperkeratosis, and the formation of stratified, cornified, squamous epithelium. Epithelial changes in the respiratory system may result in bronchiolar obstruction. Squamous metaplasia of the renal pelves, ureters, urinary bladder, enamel organs, and pancreatic and salivary ducts may lead to an increase in infections in these areas.

CLINICAL MANIFESTATIONS. Ocular lesions develop insidiously. Initially, the posterior segment of the eye is affected, with impairment of dark adaptation resulting in night blindness. Later, drying of the conjunctiva (xerosis conjunctivae) and of the cornea (xerosis corneae) is followed by wrinkling and cloudiness of the cornea (keratomalacia) (Fig. 4–3). Dry, silver-gray plaques may appear on the bulbar conjunctiva (Bitot spots), with follicular hyperkeratosis and photophobia.

Vitamin A deficiency may result in retardation of mental and physical growth and in apathy. Anemia with or without hepatosplenomegaly is usually present.

The skin is dry and scaly, and at times follicular hyperkeratosis may be found on the shoulders, buttocks, and extensor surfaces of the extremities. The vaginal epithelium may become cornified, and epithelial metaplasia of the urinary tract may contribute to pyuria and hematuria. Increased intracranial pressure with wide separation of cranial bones at the sutures may occur. Hydrocephalus, with or without paralyses of the cranial nerves, is an infrequent manifestation.

DIAGNOSIS. Dark adaptation tests may be helpful. Xerosis conjunctivae can be detected by biomicroscopic examination of the conjunctiva. Examination of the scrapings from the eye and vagina is recommended as a diagnostic aid. The plasma carotene concentration falls quickly, but that of vitamin A decreases more slowly. A standard absorption test for vitamin A is available. Low absorption curves are obtained in children with cystic fibrosis, celiac disease, obliteration of the bile ducts, and cretinism (Sec. 13.49).

PREVENTION. Infants should receive at least 500 μg daily; older children and adults, 600–1500 μg of vitamin A or carotene. The average diets of infants and children in this country supply enough vitamin A to prevent symptoms of deficiency.

For therapeutic reasons low-fat diets should be supplemented with vitamin A. In disorders with poor absorption of fat or increased excretion of vitamin A, water-miscible preparations should be administered in amounts several times the usual daily requirement. Premature infants, who absorb fats and vitamin A less efficiently than do full-term infants, should also receive water-miscible preparations. In areas of the world where vitamin A deficiency occurs, 30,000 μg of vitamin A should be given orally in a water-miscible base 4 times yearly;

the same dose should be given postpartum to the mothers of breast-fed infants in these regions.

TREATMENT. In cases of latent vitamin A deficiency, a daily supplement of 1,500 μg of vitamin A is sufficient. For xerophthalmia, 1,500 μg/kg/24 hr is given orally for 5 days and then continued with intramuscular injection of 7,500 μg of vitamin A in oil daily until recovery occurs.

HYPERVITAMINOSIS A. Acute hypervitaminosis A may occur in infants after ingesting 100,000 μg or more. The symptoms are nausea, vomiting, drowsiness, and bulging of the fontanel. Diplopia, papilledema, cranial nerve palsies, and other symptoms suggestive of brain tumor (*pseudotumor cerebri*) may also occur.

Chronic hypervitaminosis A appears after ingestion of excessive doses for several weeks or months. The child has anorexia, pruritus, and a lack of weight gain. There is increased irritability, limitation of motion, and tender swelling of the bones. Alopecia, seborrheic cutaneous lesions, fissuring of the corners of the mouth, increased intracranial pressure, and hepatomegaly may develop. Craniotabes and desquamation of the palms and soles are common. Roentgenograms reveal hyperostosis affecting several long bones; it is most notable at the middle of the shafts (Fig. 4–4).

Severe congenital malformations may occur in infants of mothers consuming large amounts of oral retinoids used in treating acne.

A history of excessive ingestion of vitamin A helps to differentiate it from cortical hyperostosis (Sec. 24.55). Besides a history of excess, the serum vitamin A level is elevated and hypercalcemia or liver cirrhosis occurs occasionally.

Fisher KD, Carr CJ, Huff JE, et al: Dark adaptation and night vision. Fed Proc 29:1605, 1970.
Goodman DS: Vitamin A metabolism. Fed Proc 39:2716, 1980.
Leung AKC: Carotenemia. Adv Pediatr 34:223, 1987.
Mahoney CP, Margolis T, Knauss TA, et al: Chronic vitamin A intoxication in infants fed chicken liver. Pediatrics 65:893, 1980.

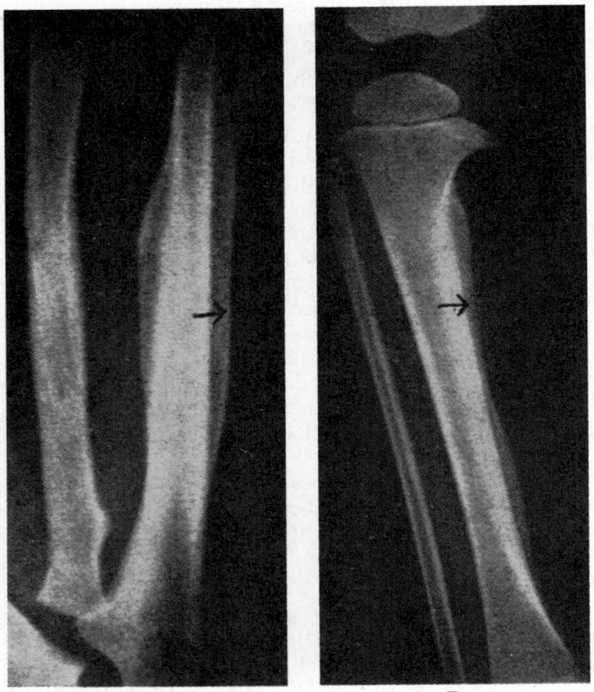

A B

Figure 4–4. Hyperostosis of the ulna and the tibia in an infant 21 mo of age, resulting from vitamin A poisoning. *A*, Long, wavy cortical hyperostosis of the ulna. *B*, Long, wavy cortical hyperostosis of the right tibia; striking absence of metaphyseal changes. (From Caffey J: Pediatric X-ray Diagnosis, 5th ed. Chicago, Year Book, 1967, p 994.)

McLaren DS, Shirajain E, Tchallian M, et al: Xerophthalmia in Jordan. Am J Clin Nutr 17:117, 1965.
Moon RC: Comparative aspects of carotenoids and retinoids as chemopreventive agents for cancer. J Nutr 119:127, 1989.
Peck GL: Prolonged remissions of cystic and conglobate acne with 13-*cis*-retinoic acid. N Engl J Med 300:299, 1979.

4.22 VITAMIN B COMPLEX DEFICIENCY

Vitamin B complex includes several factors whose chemical composition and function vary widely (see Table 4–6). All are important constituents of enzyme systems. Because many of these enzymes are closely related functionally, lack of a single factor can interrupt an entire chain of chemical processes, producing diverse clinical manifestations.

Diets deficient in any one factor of the B complex are frequently poor sources of other B vitamins. Because manifestations of several B deficiencies can usually be found in the same patient, it is generally practical to treat the patient with the entire B complex.

Factors such as pantothenic acid, choline, and inositol are important for the normal functioning of the human organism, but at present no specific deficiency syndromes can be ascribed to their lack in the diets of children.

4.23 THIAMINE DEFICIENCY

(Beriberi)

ETIOLOGY. Vitamin B_1 (thiamine) is water-soluble and, as thiamine pyrophosphate or cocarboxylase, functions as a coenzyme in carbohydrate metabolism. Thiamine is required for the synthesis of acetylcholine, and deficiency results in impaired nerve conduction. It is the coenzyme in transketolation and in decarboxylation of α-keto acids. Transketolase participates in the hexose monophosphate shunt that generates nicotinamide adenine dinucleotide phosphate (NADPH) and pentose.

Breast milk or cow's milk, vegetables, cereals, fruits, and eggs are sources of thiamine. Infants whose source of food is the milk of thiamine-deficient mothers may develop beriberi. Older children whose diet contains good sources of thiamine such as meats and legumes do not require thiamine supplements.

Thiamine is easily destroyed by heat in neutral or alkaline media and is readily extracted from foodstuffs by cooking water. An enzyme factor destructive to thiamine is present in some fish. Because the covering of grains of cereals contains most of the vitamin, polishing reduces its availability.

Thiamine absorption decreases with gastrointestinal or liver disease. Requirements increase with fever, surgery, or stress. Thiamine dependency has been described in a child with megaloblastic anemia and in an infant with otherwise typical maple syrup urine disease. The urine of children with *Leigh encephalomyelopathy* and of their parents inhibits the formation of thiamine pyrophosphate. Large doses of thiamine improve some of the physical abnormalities associated with the disease.

PATHOLOGY. In fatal cases of beriberi, lesions are located principally in the heart, peripheral nerves, subcutaneous tissue, and serous cavities. The heart is dilated, and fatty degeneration of the myocardium is common. Generalized edema or edema of the legs, serous effusions, and venous engorgement may be present. The peripheral nerves undergo varying degrees of degeneration of myelin and axon cylinders, with wallerian degeneration, beginning in the distal locations. The nerves of the lower extremities are affected first. Lesions in the brain include vascular dilatation and hemorrhage.

CLINICAL MANIFESTATIONS. Early manifestations of deficiency include fatigue, apathy, irritability, depression, drowsiness, poor mental concentration, anorexia, nausea, and abdominal discomfort. Signs of progression include peripheral neuritis with tingling, burning, and paresthesias of the toes and feet; decreased tendon reflexes; loss of vibration sense; tenderness and cramping of leg muscles; congestive heart failure; and psychic disturbances. There may be ptosis of the eyelids and atrophy of the optic nerve. Hoarseness due to paralysis of the laryngeal nerve is a characteristic sign. Muscle atrophy and tenderness of nerve trunks are followed by ataxia, loss of coordination, and loss of deep sensation. Paralytic symptoms are more common in adults than in children. Later, signs of increased intracranial pressure, meningismus, and coma occur.

In *dry* beriberi the child may appear plump but is pale, flabby, listless, and dyspneic; the heart rate is rapid and the liver enlarged. In *wet* beriberi the child is undernourished, pale, and edematous and has dyspnea, vomiting, and tachycardia. The skin appears waxy. The urine may contain albumin and casts.

The cardiac signs at first are slight cyanosis and dyspnea. Tachycardia, enlargement of the liver, loss of consciousness, and convulsions may develop rapidly. The heart is enlarged, especially to the right. The electrocardiogram shows increased Q-T interval, inversion of T waves, and low voltage, changes that rapidly revert to normal with treatment. Cardiac failure may lead to death in either chronic or acute beriberi.

Wernicke Encephalopathy. This is characterized by irritability, somnolence, and ocular signs, and less commonly by mental confusion and ataxias, infrequently occurring in malnourished infants and children. Malignancy, infection, gastrointestinal disorders, and prematurity have been associated findings in these patients.

DIAGNOSIS. Since the early symptoms are encountered in many types of nutritional disturbances besides thiamine deficiency, demonstrations of lowered red blood cell transketolase and high blood or urinary glyoxylate values have been proposed as diagnostic tests. Excretion after an oral loading dose of thiamine or its metabolites, thiazole or pyrimidine, may help to identify the deficiency state. Clinical response to administration of thiamine remains the best test for thiamine deficiency.

PREVENTION. A maternal diet containing sufficient amounts of thiamine prevents this deficiency in breast-fed infants (see Table 4–1). Thiamine requirements increase with a high-carbohydrate content of the diet.

TREATMENT. If beriberi occurs in a breast-fed infant, both the mother and child should be treated with thiamine. The daily dose for adults is 50 mg and for children 10 mg or more. Oral administration is effective unless gastrointestinal disturbances prevent absorption. Thiamine should be given intramuscularly or intravenously to children with cardiac failure. Such treatment is followed by dramatic improvement, although complete cure requires several weeks. The heart is not permanently damaged. Because patients with beriberi often have other B complex deficiencies, all other vitamins of the B complex should be administered, in addition to large doses of thiamine chloride.

4.24 RIBOFLAVIN DEFICIENCY
(Ariboflavinosis)

Riboflavin deficiency without deficiencies of other members of the B complex is rare. Riboflavin, a yellow, fluorescent, water-soluble substance, is stable to heat and acids but is destroyed by light and alkalis. The coenzymes flavin mononucleotide (FMN) and flavin adenine dinucleotide (FAD) are synthesized from riboflavin, forming the prosthetic groups of several enzymes important in electron transport. Riboflavin is essential for growth and tissue respiration; it may have a role in light adaptation and is required for conversion of pyridoxine to pyridoxal phosphate. Large amounts of riboflavin occur in liver, kidney, brewer's yeast, milk, cheese, eggs, and leafy vegetables; cow's milk contains about five times as much riboflavin as human milk.

Riboflavin deficiency is usually caused by inadequate intake. Faulty absorption may contribute in patients with biliary atresia or hepatitis or in those receiving probenecid, phenothiazine, or oral contraceptives. Phototherapy destroys riboflavin.

CLINICAL MANIFESTATIONS. Evidences of riboflavin deficiency include cheilosis (perlèche), glossitis, keratitis, conjunctivitis, photophobia, lacrimation, marked corneal vascularization, and seborrheic dermatitis. Cheilosis begins with pallor at the angles of the mouth, followed by thinning and maceration of the epithelium. Superficial fissures often covered by yellow crusts develop in the angles of the mouth and extend radially into the skin for distances of 1–2 cm. Epidemics of cheilosis occur in institutions and in families whose diet is inadequate. With glossitis the tongue is smooth, and loss of papillary structure occurs. A normocytic, normochromic anemia with bone marrow hypoplasia is common.

DIAGNOSIS. Urinary excretion of riboflavin below 30 μg/24 hr is abnormally low. Levels of erythrocyte glutathionine reductase, a flavoprotein requiring FAD, may reflect the stores of riboflavin. A patient with hemolysis owing to pyruvate kinase deficiency and reduced erythrocyte glutathionine reductase had both enzyme activities restored to normal on administration of riboflavin.

PREVENTION. Recommended daily allowances are presented in Table 4–1. Riboflavin deficiency is usually prevented by a diet that contains adequate amounts of milk, eggs, leafy vegetables, and lean meats.

TREATMENT. Treatment consists in the oral administration of 3–10 mg of riboflavin daily. If no response occurs within a few days, intramuscular injections of 2 mg of riboflavin in saline solution may be made three times daily. The child should also be given a well-balanced diet and, at least temporarily, more than the usual requirements of the B complex.

4.25 NIACIN DEFICIENCY
(Pellagra)

ETIOLOGY. Pellagra (*pellis*, skin; *agra*, rough), a deficiency disease caused mainly by a lack of niacin (nicotinic acid), affects all tissues of the body. Niacin forms part of two enzymes important in electron transfer and glycolysis: nicotinamide adenine dinucleotide (NAD) and nicotinamide adenine dinucleotide phosphate (NADP). Although dietary tryptophan can partially substitute for niacin, other sources of niacin are necessary. Liver, lean pork, salmon, poultry, and red meat are good sources, but most cereals contain only small amounts of it. Pellagra occurs chiefly in countries where corn (maize), a poor source of tryptophan, is a basic foodstuff. Milk and eggs, which contain little niacin, are good pellagra-preventive foods because of their high content of tryptophan. Because niacin is a stable compound, there are only small losses in cooking.

PATHOLOGY. Histologically, edema and degeneration of the superficial collagen of the dermis occur. The papillary vessels are engorged, and there is perivascular lymphocytic infiltration in the dermis. The epidermis is hyperkeratotic and later becomes atrophic.

Changes comparable with those in the skin are present in the tongue, buccal mucous membranes, and vagina. These changes may be associated with secondary infection and ulceration. The walls of the colon are thickened and inflamed with patches of pseudomembrane; later the mucosa atrophies. Changes in the nervous system occur relatively late in the disease and consist of patchy areas of demyelinization and degeneration of ganglion cells; demyelinization in the spinal cord may involve the posterior and lateral columns.

CLINICAL MANIFESTATIONS. The early symptoms of pellagra are vague. Anorexia, lassitude, weakness, burning sensations, numbness, and dizziness may be prodromal symptoms. After a long period of niacin deficiency the characteristic symptoms appear. The classic triad consists of dermatitis, diarrhea, and dementia. Manifestations in children who have parasites or chronic disorders may be especially severe.

The most characteristic manifestations are the cutaneous ones, which may develop suddenly or insidiously and may be elicited by irritants, particularly by intense sunlight. They first appear as symmetric erythema of the exposed surfaces that may resemble sunburn and in mild cases may escape recognition. The lesions are usually sharply demarcated from the healthy skin around them, and their distribution may change frequently. The lesions on the hands sometimes have the appearance of a glove (pellagrous glove) (Fig. 4–5), and similar demarcations are occasionally seen on the foot and leg (pellagrous boot) or around the neck (Casal necklace). In some cases vesicles and bullae develop (wet type), or there may be suppuration beneath the scaly, crusted epidermis; in others the swelling disappears after a short time and desquamation begins. The healed parts of the skin may remain pigmented.

The cutaneous lesions are sometimes preceded by stomatitis, glossitis, vomiting, or diarrhea. Swelling and redness of the tip of the tongue and its lateral margins may be followed by intense redness of the entire tongue and of the papillae and even ulceration.

Nervous symptoms include depression, disorientation, insomnia, and delirium.

The classic symptoms of pellagra are usually not well developed in infants and children. Anorexia, irritability, anxiety, and apathy are common in "pellagra families." They may also have sore tongues and lips, and the skin is usually dry and scaly. Diarrhea and constipation may alternate and a moderate secondary anemia may occur. Children who have pellagra often have evidence of other nutritional deficiency diseases.

DIAGNOSIS. Diagnosis is usually made from the physical signs of glossitis, gastrointestinal symptoms, and a symmetric dermatitis. Rapid clinical response to niacin is an important confirming test. *N*-methylnicotinamide, a normal metabolite of niacin, is almost undetectable in urine during niacin deficiency.

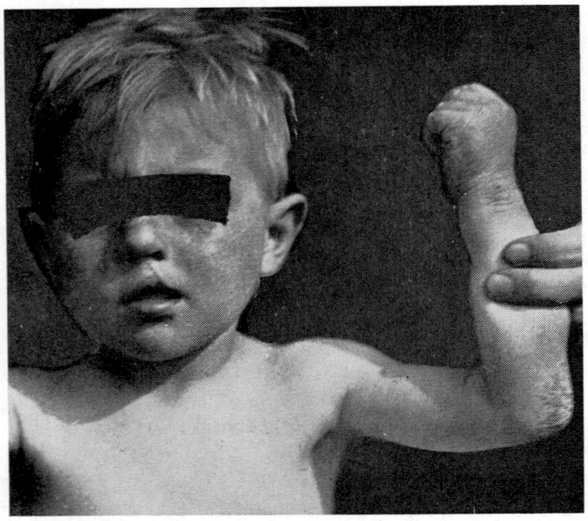

Figure 4–5. Pellagra in a boy 3 yr of age, showing lesions on the hand and elbow and an early lesion over the nose and malar eminences.

PREVENTION. A well-balanced diet containing meat, vegetables, eggs, and milk meets the recommended daily allowances (see Table 4–1), thus supplements of niacin are necessary only in breast-fed infants whose mothers have pellagra or in children on restricted diets.

TREATMENT. Children respond rapidly to antipellagral therapy. A liberal and well-balanced diet should be supplemented with 50–300 mg/day of niacin; 100 mg may be given intravenously in severe cases or in cases of poor intestinal absorption. Administering large doses of niacin is often followed within a half hour by a sensation of increased local heat and flushing and burning of the skin, unpleasant effects that are not produced by niacinamide. But large doses of niacin may cause cholestatic jaundice or hepatotoxicity.

The diet should be supplemented with other vitamins, especially with other members of the B complex. Sun exposure should be avoided during the active phase; the skin lesions may be covered with soothing applications. A blood transfusion may be helpful when there is severe anemia; less severe hypochromic anemia should be treated with iron. The diet of the cured pellagrin should be supervised continuously to prevent recurrence.

THIAMINE DEFICIENCY

Borgna-Pignatti C, Marradi P, Pinelli L, et al: Thiamine-responsive anemia in DIDMOAD syndrome. J Pediatr 114:405, 1989.

Brin M: Erythrocyte as a biopsy tissue for functional evaluation of thiamin adequacy. JAMA 187:762, 1964.

McCandless DW, Schenker S: Neurologic disorders of thiamine deficiency. Nutr Rev 27:213, 1969.

Pihko H, Soarinen U, Paetau A: Wernicke encephalopathy: A preventable cause of death: Report of 2 children with malignant disease. Pediatr Neurol 5:237, 1989.

Vrochota K, Oberg CN, Harris KN: Beriberi in a southeast Asian adolescent. Am J Dis Child 143:270, 1989.

RIBOFLAVIN DEFICIENCY

Rillotson JA, Baker EM: An enzymatic measurement of the riboflavin status in man. Am J Clin Nutr 25:425, 1972.

Rivlin RS: Hormones, drugs and riboflavin. Nutr Rev 37:241, 1979.

Staal GEJ, Van Berkel TJC, Nijessen JG, et al: Normalization of red blood cell pyruvate kinase in pyruvate kinase deficiency by riboflavin treatment. Clin Chim Acta 60:323, 1975.

NIACIN DEFICIENCY

Darby WJ, McNutt KW, Todhunter EN: Niacin. Nutr Rev 33:289, 1975.

4.26 PYRIDOXINE (VITAMIN B_6) DEFICIENCY

Vitamin B_6 includes pyridoxal, pyridoxine, and pyridoxamine. These are converted to pyridoxal-5-phosphate (or pyridoxamine-5-phosphate), which acts as a coenzyme in decarboxylation and transamination of amino acids, such as in the decarboxylation of 5-hydroxytryptophan in the formation of serotonin, and in the metabolism of glycogen and fatty acids. Vitamin B_6 is also essential for the breakdown of kynurenine. When this does not occur, xanthurenic acid appears in the urine. Adequate functioning of the nervous system depends on pyridoxine, deficiency of which leads to seizures and to peripheral neuropathy. Pyridoxal phosphate is the coenzyme for both glutamic decarboxylase and γ-aminobutyric acid transaminase; each is necessary for normal brain metabolism. It participates in active transport of amino acids across cell membranes, chelates metals, and participates in the synthesis of arachidonic acid from linoleic acid. If it is lacking, glycine metabolism may lead to oxaluria. It is excreted largely as 4-pyridoxic acid.

ETIOLOGY. Pyridoxine is adequately available in human

and cow's milk and in cereals, but prolonged heat processing of the latter two destroys it. Diseases with malabsorption, such as celiac syndrome, may contribute to vitamin B_6 deficiency.

There are several types of *vitamin B_6 dependency syndromes*, presumably the result of errors in enzyme structure or function, in which the patient responds to very large amounts of pyridoxine. These syndromes include B_6-dependent convulsions, a B_6-responsive anemia, xanthurenic aciduria, cystathioninuria, and homocystinuria.

Pyridoxine antagonists, such as isonicotinic acid hydrazide (isoniazid) used in the treatment of tuberculosis, increase the requirements for pyridoxine, as do pregnancy and drugs such as penicillamine, hydralazine, and the oral progesterone-estrogen contraceptives.

CLINICAL MANIFESTATIONS. Deficiency symptoms are not as common in children as in adults. Four clinical disturbances caused by vitamin B_6 deficiency have been described in humans: convulsions in infants, peripheral neuritis, dermatitis, and anemia.

Infants fed a formula deficient in vitamin B_6 for 1–6 mo exhibit irritability and generalized seizures. Gastrointestinal distress and an aggravated startle response are common.

Peripheral neuropathy may occur during treatment of tuberculosis with isonicotinic acid hydrazide. The neuropathy responds to administration of pyridoxine or to a decrease in the dose of the drug. Administration of isonicotinic acid may also be followed by manifestations of pellagra.

Skin lesions include cheilosis, glossitis, and seborrhea around the eyes, nose, and mouth. Microcytic anemia, oxaluria, oxalic acid bladder stones, hyperglycinemia, lymphopenia, decreased antibody formation, and infections also occur.

Convulsions from B_6 dependency may occur several hours to as long as 6 mo after birth. Seizures are typically myoclonic with hypsarrhythmic patterns on the electroencephalogram. In several cases the mother had received large doses of pyridoxine during pregnancy for control of emesis.

In *B_6-dependent anemia* the red blood cells are microcytic and hypochromic. There are increased serum iron concentrations, saturation of iron-binding protein, hemosiderin deposits in bone marrow and liver, and failure of iron utilization for hemoglobin synthesis.

Xanthurenic aciduria following tryptophan load tests is an apparently benign occurrence in some families. Xanthurenic acid excretion becomes normal following large doses of vitamin B_6. *Cystathioninuria* is similarly not accompanied by any clear clinical disturbance. Cystathioninase is vitamin B_6 dependent (Sec. 8.5).

In some patients with *homocystinuria*, serum levels of homocysteine will fall following B_6 administration. Cystathionine synthetase is B_6 dependent (Sec. 8.5).

LABORATORY DATA. Anemia is not common in affected infants. After administration of 100 mg/kg of tryptophan, large amounts of xanthurenic acid will be found in the urine of patients with pyridoxine deficiency; in normal persons none is detected. The result of this test may be normal in patients with "pyridoxine dependency."

DIAGNOSIS. Infants with seizures should be suspected of having vitamin B_6 deficiency or dependency. If more common causes of infantile seizures, such as hypocalcemia, hypoglycemia, and infection, can be eliminated, 100 mg of pyridoxine should be injected. If the seizure stops, B_6 deficiency should be suspected, and a tryptophan loading test is indicated. Similarly, in older children with seizure disorders, 100 mg of pyridoxine may be injected intramuscularly while the electroencephalogram (EEG) is being recorded; a favorable response of the EEG suggests pyridoxine deficiency.

Erythrocyte glutamic pyruvic transaminase is reduced in pyridoxine deficiency; its concentration may be used as an indicator of vitamin B_6 status.

PREVENTION. Balanced diets usually contain enough pyridoxine so that deficiency is rare. Children receiving high-protein diets should have vitamin B_6 added. Infants whose mothers have received large doses of pyridoxine during pregnancy are at increased risk of seizures due to pyridoxine dependency. Any child receiving a pyridoxine antagonist such as isoniazid should be carefully observed for neurologic manifestations. If these develop, either pyridoxine should be administered or the dose of the antagonist decreased. Daily intake of 0.3–0.5 mg of pyridoxine in the infant, 0.5–1.5 mg in the child, or 1.5–2.0 mg in the adult prevents deficiency states.

TREATMENT. For convulsions possibly due to pyridoxine deficiency, 100 mg of the vitamin should be given intramuscularly. One dose should suffice if the diet is adequate. For "pyridoxine-dependent" children, 2–10 mg intramuscularly or 10–100 mg orally may be necessary daily.

TOXICITY. Excessive intake may cause sensory neuropathy.

Cinnamon AD, Beaton JR: Biochemical assessment of vitamin B_6 status in man. Am J Clin Nutr 26:96, 1970.

Frimpter GW, Andelman RJ, George WF: Vitamin B_6-dependency syndromes. Am J Clin Nutr 22:794, 1959.

Hansson O, Hagberg B: Effect of pyridoxine treatment in children with epilepsy. Acta Soc Med Upsal 73:35, 1968.

Schaumburg H, Kaplan J, Windebank, A, et al: Sensory neuropathy from pyridoxine abuse. N Engl J Med 309:445, 1983.

Scriver CR: Vitamin B_6 deficiency and dependency in man. Am J Dis Child 113:109, 1967.

4.27 BIOTIN

Biotin deficiency is rare. It is found in those consuming the biotin antagonist, avidin, found in raw egg white. Many microorganisms produce biotin.

ETIOLOGY. Biotin is discussed in Sec. 8.7. Avidin ingestion causes symptoms of deficiency. Deficiencies have appeared in those receiving all their nutrition parenterally and occasionally in infants whose mothers are deficient in biotin.

CLINICAL MANIFESTATIONS. Brawny dermatitis, somnolence, hallucinations, and hyperesthesia with accumulation of organic acids are common. Other neurologic signs and defective immunity may occur.

DIAGNOSIS. Elevated organic aciduria, particularly propionic and hydroxy–short chain acids, with response to clinical and biochemical abnormalities following treatment, suggests biotin deficiency.

PREVENTION AND TREATMENT. Parenteral solutions should contain biotin. Deficient patients respond to oral administration of 10 mg.

VITAMIN B_{12} (see Sec. 16.10).

4.28 VITAMIN C (ASCORBIC ACID)

(Scurvy)

Ascorbic acid is essential for the formation of normal collagen; the defects in collagen structure arising from deficiency of the vitamin produce many of the metabolic and clinical manifestations of scurvy. Alterations in collagen formation are partly due to failure to incorporate hydroxyproline and proline.

Vitamin C is a potent reducing agent that is easily oxidized and destroyed by heating. The adrenals and lenses have particularly high contents of vitamin C.

Ascorbic acid functions in a number of enzymatic activities (Table 4–6 and Sec. 8.3). Transient tyrosinemia in the neonatal period, relatively common among low-birthweight infants and occasionally seen in full-term ones fed high-protein diets, is corrected by administering ascorbic acid (Sec. 9.17).

Ascorbic acid deficiency may also be a factor in some cases of megaloblastic anemia by interfering in the conversion of folic acid or other conjugates (Table 4–6 and Sec. 16.10).

ETIOLOGY. The infant is born with adequate stores of vitamin C if the mother's intake has been adequate; the vitamin C content of cord blood plasma is 2–4 times greater than that of maternal plasma. Under these circumstances breast milk contains about 4–7 mg/dL of ascorbic acid and is an adequate source of vitamin C. Deficiency of vitamin C in the mother's diet may result in scurvy in her breast-fed infant. Infants fed with formula must receive vitamin C supplements; such supplements will provide additional protection for the breast-fed infant.

The need for vitamin C is increased by febrile illnesses, particularly infectious and diarrheal diseases, and by iron deficiency, cold exposure, protein depletion, or smoking.

PATHOLOGY. During vitamin C deficiency formation of collagen and of chondroitin sulfate is impaired. The tendencies to hemorrhage, defective tooth dentin, and loosening of the teeth are caused by deficient collagen. Because osteoblasts no longer form their normal intercellular substance (osteoid), endochondral bone formation ceases. The bony trabeculae that have been formed become brittle and fracture easily. The periosteum becomes loosened, and subperiosteal hemorrhages occur, especially at the ends of the femur and tibia. In severe scurvy there may be degeneration in skeletal muscles, cardiac hypertrophy, bone marrow depression, and adrenal atrophy.

CLINICAL MANIFESTATIONS. Scurvy may occur at any age but is rare in the newborn infant. The majority of cases occur in infants 6–24 mo of age. Clinical manifestations require time to develop; after a variable period of vitamin C depletion, vague symptoms of irritability, tachypnea, digestive disturbances, and loss of appetite appear. The irritability becomes progressively greater, and there is evidence of general tenderness, especially noticeable in the legs when the infant is picked up or when the diaper is changed. The pain results in pseudoparalysis, and the legs assume the typical "frog position" (Fig. 4–6), in which the hips and knees are semiflexed with the feet rotated outward. Edematous swelling along the shafts of the legs may be present, and in some cases a subperiosteal hemorrhage can be palpated at the end of the femur. The facial expression is apprehensive. Changes in the gums, most noticeable when the teeth are erupted, are characterized by bluish purple, spongy swellings of the mucous membrane, usually over the upper incisors. There may be a "rosary" at the costochondral junctions and a depression of the sternum. The angulation of the "scorbutic beads" is usually sharper than that of the rachitic rosary, because it is produced by a subluxation of the sternal plate at the costochondral junction (see Fig. 4–6) rather than by widening of the softened epiphyses as occurs in rickets (Sec. 4.29).

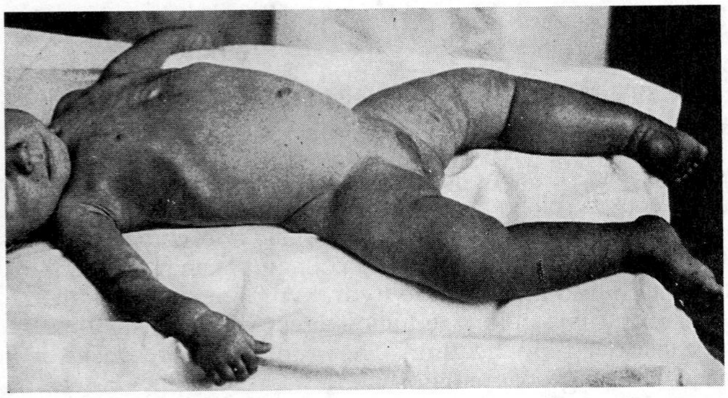

Figure 4–6. Scorbutic rosary, depression of sternum, and the so-called frog position.

Petechial hemorrhages may occur in the skin and mucous membranes. Hematuria, melena, and orbital or subdural hemorrhages may be found. Low-grade fever is usually present. Anemia may reflect inability to utilize iron or impaired folic acid metabolism (Sec. 16.10). Wound healing is delayed, and apparently healed wounds may break down. Swollen joints and follicular hyperkeratosis may develop, as well as the "sicca" syndrome of Sjögren, which is usually associated with collagen disorders and includes xerostomia, keratoconjunctivitis sicca, and enlargement of the salivary glands (Sec. 11.72).

ROENTGENOGRAPHIC MANIFESTATIONS. The diagnosis of scurvy is usually based on roentgenographic changes in the long bones, especially at their distal ends. Changes are greatest, as a rule, in the area of the knee. In the early stages the appearance resembles that of simple atrophy of bone. The trabeculae of the shaft cannot be discerned, and the bone assumes a "ground-glass" appearance. The cortex is reduced to "pencil-point thinness," and the epiphyseal ends are sharply outlined. The white line of Fraenkel, which represents the zone of well calcified cartilage, can be clearly discerned as an irregular but thickened white line at the metaphysis. The epiphyseal centers of ossification also have a ground-glass appearance and are surrounded by a white ring (Fig. 4–7).

At this stage, scurvy cannot be diagnosed with certainty from the roentgenogram unless the zone of rarefaction under the white line at the metaphysis becomes apparent. The zone of rarefaction is a linear break in the bone proximal and parallel to the white line. Often it does not traverse the shaft in its entire width and may be seen only in its lateral parts as a triangular defect (see Fig. 4–7*B*). A spur, as a lateral prolongation of the white line, may be present. Epiphyseal separation may occur along the line of destruction, with linear displacement or compression of the epiphysis against the shaft. Subperiosteal hemorrhages are not visible roentgenographically in active scurvy. During healing, however, the elevated periosteum becomes calcified, and the affected bone assumes a dumbbell or club shape.

DIAGNOSIS. Diagnosis is based mainly on the characteristic clinical picture, the roentgenographic apearance of the long bones, and history of poor intake of vitamin C. Occasionally, a mother may have been boiling the infant's fruit juices.

Laboratory tests for scurvy are unsatisfactory. A fasting vitamin C level of the blood plasma of over 0.6 mg/dL aids in the exclusion of scurvy, but a lower vitamin C level does not prove its presence. Evidence of vitamin C deficiency is better furnished by the ascorbic acid concentration in the white cell—platelet layer (buffy layer) of centrifuged oxalated blood. A level of zero in this layer indicates latent scurvy, even in the absence of clinical signs of deficiency. The saturation of the tissues with vitamin C can be estimated from the amount of urinary excretion of the vitamin after a test dose of ascorbic acid. During the 3–5 hr after parenteral administration of the test dose, 80% of it can be found in the urine of normal children. A generalized, nonspecific aminoaciduria occurs in scurvy, while blood values of amino acids remain normal. After a tyrosine load the scorbutic infant excretes metabolites similar to those of the premature infant. Prothrombin time may be greatly increased.

DIFFERENTIAL DIAGNOSIS. The tenderness of the limbs and the pain elicited by movement have often led to a false diagnosis of arthritis or acrodynia. The patient's age aids in differentiating scurvy from rheumatic fever, because rheumatic fever is rare in children under 2 yr of age. Suppurative arthritis and osteomyelitis should be considered in the differ-

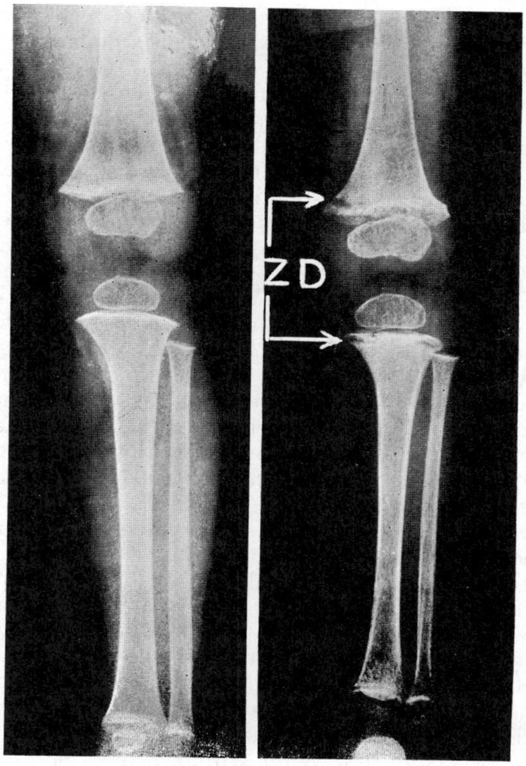

A B

Figure 4–7. Roentgenograms of a leg. *A*, Early scurvy: "white line" is visible on the ends of the shafts of the tibia and fibula; rings around the epiphyses of the femur and tibia. *B*, More advanced scorbutic changes; zones of destruction (ZD) in the femur and tibia.

ential diagnosis. The pseudoparalysis of syphilis occurs usually at an earlier age than does that of scurvy and is often accompanied by other signs of syphilis; a roentgenogram may aid in the diagnosis. Poliomyelitis causes a true flaccid paralysis, and, in infants, the exquisite tenderness present in the limbs in scurvy is absent. Henoch-Schönlein purpura, thrombocytopenic purpura, leukemia, meningitis, or nephritis may be suspected.

PROGNOSIS. With proper treatment recovery occurs rapidly in infants, but the swelling of subperiosteal hemorrhge may require months to disappear. Body growth usually is quickly resumed.

PREVENTION. Scurvy is prevented by a diet adequate in vitamin C; citrus fruits and juices are excellent sources. Formula-fed infants should receive 35 mg of ascorbic acid daily. Lactating mothers should take 100 mg; 45–60 mg/day is needed by children or adults (see Table 4–1).

TREATMENT. The administration of 3–4 oz of orange juice or tomato juice daily will quickly produce healing, but ascorbic acid is preferable. The daily therapeutic dose is 100–200 mg or more, orally or parenterally.

Irwin MI, Hutchins BK: A conspectus of research on vitamin C requirements in man. J Nutr 106:823, 1976.

Levine M: New concepts in the biology and biochemistry of ascorbic acid. N Engl J Med 314:892, 1986.

4.29 RICKETS OF VITAMIN D DEFICIENCY*

Rickets is the term signifying a failure in mineralization of growing bone or osteoid tissue. The characteristic early changes are seen roentgenographically at the ends of long bones; evidence of demineralization also exists in the shafts. Subsequently, if healing is not initiated, clinical manifestations appear (see later). Failure of mature bone to mineralize is called osteomalacia.

ETIOLOGY. During the first third of this century, the predominant cause of rickets was nutritional deficiency of vitamin D due either to inadequate direct exposure to ultraviolet rays in sunlight (296–310 nm; these rays do not pass through ordinary window glass) or to inadequate intake of vitamin D, or both. Vitamin D deficiency rickets has been almost eliminated among infants and children in the industrialized countries by prophylactic means. Deficiency may occur in unsupplemented dark-skinned infants or in breast-fed infants of mothers unexposed to sunlight.

Currently in industrialized countries, it appears that conditions besides inadequate nutritional prophylaxis with vitamin D collectively produce most of the observed rachitic lesions (Sec. 24.59–24.65). These conditions include clinical entities that interfere with the metabolic conversion and activation of vitamin D, such as hepatic and renal lesions, or that disrupt calcium and phosphorus homeostasis in other ways.

Two forms of vitamin D are of practical importance. Vitamin D_2, or calciferol, available as irradiated ergosterol, largely replaced the fish liver oils (cod and percomorph) as a source of dietary and therapeutic vitamin D. Vitamin D_3, now available synthetically, is naturally present in human skin in the provitamin stage as 7-dehydrocholesterol. It is activated photochemically to cholecalciferol and transferred to the liver. Each of these irradiated sterols is hydroxylated in the liver to 25-OH-cholecalciferol and, subsequently, in the renal cortical cells to 1,25-dihydroxycholecalciferol, an end product considered a hormone. Its antirachitic functions include facilitation of intestinal absorption of calcium and phosphorus and of reabsorption of phosphorus in the kidney and a direct effect on mineral metabolism of bone (deposition and reabsorption). In conjunction with parathormone and calcitonin, it has a major role in homeostasis of calcium and phosphorus in the body's fluids and tissues.

The diet of infants may contain only small amounts of vitamin D; cow's milk contains only 0.1–1 μg/quart.† Cereals, vegetables, and fruits contain only negligible amounts. Egg yolk contains 3–10 μg/g. Most marketed cow's milk is fortified with 10 μg of vitamin D per quart, and most commercially prepared milks for infant formulas are also fortified.

Besides lack of dietary vitamin D and the skin's lack of exposure to ultraviolet irradiation, several factors may predispose to vitamin D deficiency. Rickets or epiphyseal dysplasia is particularly likely to develop during rapid growth, such as in low-birthweight infants and in adolescents. Black children are singularly susceptible to rickets, owing to either the pigmentation of their skin or inadequate penetration of sunlight.

Children with disorders of absorption, such as celiac disease, steatorrhea, pancreatitis, or cystic fibrosis, may acquire rickets because of deficient absorption of vitamin D and calcium or of both. Anticonvulsant therapy, such as for example with the phenytoins or with phenobarbital, may interfere in the metabolism of vitamin D; rickets has been seen with some frequency in institutionalized children receiving such therapy who also have inadequate exposure to sunlight (Sec. 24.63). Glucocorticoids appear to be antagonistic to vitamin D in calcium transport.

PATHOLOGY. New bone formation is initiated by the

*For a review of the rachitic lesions reference should be made to Table 4–5 and Sec. 6.6 and 6.10 for calcium and phosphorus metabolism; Sec. 4.29 and 6.28 for hypocalcemic tetany; Sec. 19.16 for parathormone, vitamin D, and calcitonin activities; and to Table 4–6 and Sec. 24.59–24.65 for additional discussion of vitamin D metabolism and its activities.

†1μg = 40 IU.

osteoblast, which is responsible for matrix deposition and its subsequent mineralization. Osteoblasts secrete collagen, and changes in polysaccharides, phospholipids, alkaline phosphatase, and pyrophosphatase follow until mineralization occurs in the presence of adequate calcium and phosphorus. Resorption of bone occurs when osteoclasts secrete enzymes on the bone surface, dissolving and removing matrix and mineral. Osteocytes covered by bone both resorb and redeposit bone. Factors affecting bone growth are poorly understood, but phosphorus, calcium, fluoride, and growth hormone all have some influence.

In rickets defective growth of bone results from retardation or suppression of normal growth of epiphyseal cartilage and of normal calcification. These changes depend on a deficiency in serum of calcium and phosphorus salts for mineralization. Cartilage cells fail to complete their normal cycle of proliferation and degeneration, and subsequent failure of capillary penetration occurs in a patchy manner. The result is a frayed, irregular epiphyseal line at the end of the shaft. Failure of osseous and cartilaginous matrix to mineralize in the zone of preparatory calcification, followed by deposition of newly formed uncalcified osteoid results in a wide, irregular, frayed zone of nonrigid tissue (the rachitic metaphysis) (Fig. 4–8). This zone, responsible for many of the skeletal deformities, becomes compressed and bulges laterally, producing flaring of the ends of the bones and the rachitic rosary (Figs. 4–9 and 4–10).

Mineralization is also lacking in subperiosteal bone; preexisting cortical bone is resorbed in a normal manner but is replaced by osteoid tissues over the entire shaft, which fails to mineralize. If this process continues, the shaft loses its rigidity, and the resultant softened and rarified cortical bone is readily distorted by stress; deformities and fractures result (Fig. 4–10).

Healing Rickets. With healing, degeneration of cartilage cells occurs along the metaphyseal-diaphyseal border, capillary penetration of the resultant spaces is resumed, and calcification takes place in the zone of preparatory calcification. This calcification, occurring approximately at the line at which normal calcification would have occurred had the rachitic process not supervened, produces a line clearly demonstrable in roentgenograms (Figs. 4–11*A* and *B*). As healing progresses, the osteoid tissue between this line of preparatory calcification and the diaphysis also becomes mineralized (see Fig. 4–8). Osteoid tissue in the cortex and about the trabeculae in the shaft rapidly becomes mineralized. Months or years may be required to repair the deformities, and in extreme cases complete repair may be impossible.

Chemical Pathology. In healthy infants the inorganic serum phosphorus concentration is 4.5–6.5 mg/dL, whereas in rachitic infants it is usually reduced to 1.5–3.5 mg/dL. The serum calcium level is usually normal, but under certain conditions it too is reduced, and tetany may develop.

Vitamin D deficient rickets can be assumed to be the body's attempt to maintain normal serum calcium levels, presumably because calcium is necessary for normal function of nerve, muscle, and endocrine glands and for intercellular bridging. In the absence of vitamin D, less calcium is absorbed from the intestine. With slightly lowered serum calcium, parathormone is secreted, leading to mobilization of calcium and phosphorus from the bone. The serum calcium concentration is thus maintained, but secondary effects occur, including the changes of rickets in bone, the lowered serum phosphorus concentration (because parathormone decreases phosphorus reabsorption in the kidney), and elevated serum phosphatase (due to increased osteoblastic activity).

The alkaline phosphatase of serum, which in normal children is less than 200 IU/dL, is elevated in mild rickets to more than 500 IU/dL. As rickets heals, the phosphatase value returns slowly to the normal range. Serum alkaline phosphatase may be normal in infants with rickets who are protein or zinc depleted.

Calcium and phosphorus homeostasis depends on the intestinal absorption of dietary calcium and phosphorus. Maximum calcium absorption occurs in humans when the ratio of calcium to phosphorus in the diet is about 2:1; increase in phosphate decreases absorption of calcium. Acidity of intestinal contents increases absorption of calcium. An increase in calcium absorption also occurs when lactose is the dietary sugar. Chelating agents such as ethylenediaminetetra-acetic acid (EDTA) or the phytates of cereals may decrease calcium absorption, and dietary iron may decrease absorption of phosphate. High dietary levels of stearic and palmitic acids, which are poorly absorbed, also decrease calcium absorption.

Calcium absorption is facilitated by 1,25-dihydroxycholecalciferol or similar hydroxylated forms of vitamin D. Calcium deficiency alone rarely leads to the failure of calcification as seen in rickets and osteomalacia; it results in a diminished amount of bone.

Vitamin D deficiency is also accompanied by generalized aminoaciduria, a decrease of citrate in bone and its increased urinary excretion, decreased ability of the kidneys to make an acid urine, phosphaturia, and, occasionally, mellituria. The parathyroid glands hypertrophy in rickets, and urinary cyclic adenosine monophosphate (AMP) is increased.

CLINICAL MANIFESTATIONS. Osseous changes of rickets can be recognized after several months of vitamin D deficiency. In breast-fed infants whose mothers have osteomalacia, rickets may develop within 2 mo. Florid rickets appears toward the end of the 1st and during the 2nd yr of life. Later in childhood manifest vitamin D deficient rickets is rare.

One of the early signs of rickets, craniotabes, is due to thinning of the outer table of the skull and detected by pressing firmly over the occiput or posterior parietal bones. A ping-pong ball sensation will be felt. Craniotabes near the suture lines is a normal variant. Low-birthweight infants are particularly susceptible to the early development of rickets and to craniotabes. Palpable enlargement of the costochondral junctions (the "rachitic rosary") (see Fig. 4–9) and thickening of the wrists and ankles (see Fig. 4–11) are other early evidences of osseous changes. Increased sweating, particularly around the head, may also be present.

Advanced Rickets. Signs of advanced rickets are easily recognized.

HEAD. Craniotabes may disappear before the end of the 1st yr, although the rachitic process continues. The softness of the skull may result in flattening and, at times, permanent asymmetry of the head. The anterior fontanel is larger than normal; its closure may be delayed until after the 2nd yr of life. The central parts of the parietal and frontal bones are often thickened, forming prominences or bosses, which give the head a box-like appearance (caput quadratum). The head may be larger than normal and may remain so throughout life. Eruption of the temporary teeth may be delayed, and there may be defects of the enamel and extensive caries. The permanent teeth that are calcifying may also be affected; the permanent incisors, canines, and first molars usually show enamel defects.

THORAX. Enlargement of the costochondral junctions may become prominent; the beading of the ribs is not only palpable but also visible (see Fig. 4–9). The sides of the thorax become flattened, and the longitudinal grooves develop posterior to the rosary. The sternum with its adjacent cartilage appears to be projected forward, producing the so-called pigeon breast deformity. Along the lower border of the chest develops a horizontal depression, Harrison groove (Fig. 4–12), which corresponds with the costal insertions of the diaphragm.

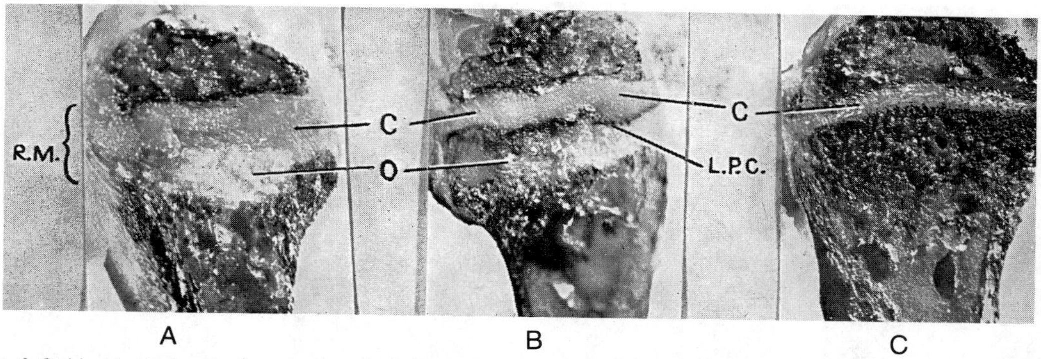

Figure 4–8. Line tests in rats (proximal end of the tibia) (calcified tissue stained with silver appears black). *A*, Active rickets. The light broad zone between the epiphysis and the shaft represents the rachitic metaphysis (R.M.). (C = cartilage; O = osteoid). *B*, Healing rickets. The line of preparatory calcification (L.P.C.) between the zone of cartilage (C) and the osteoid (O). *C*, Healed rickets. Cartilaginous disk (C) between the epiphysis and the normal shaft.

There may be a variety of other thoracic deformities, including those of the shoulder girdle.

Spinal column. Slight to moderate degrees of lateral curvature (scoliosis) are common, and a kyphosis may appear in the dorsolumbar region of rachitic children when sitting. Lordosis of the lumbar region may be seen in the erect position.

Pelvis. In children with lordosis there is frequently a concomitant deformity of the pelvis, which is also retarded in growth. The pelvic entrance is narrowed by a forward projection of the promontory; the exit, by a forward displacement of the caudal part of the sacrum and the coccyx. In the female these changes, if they become permanent, add to the hazards of childbirth and may necessitate cesarean section.

Extremities. As the rachitic process continues, the epiphyseal enlargement at the wrists and ankles becomes more noticeable. The enlarged epiphyses can be seen (see Fig. 4–11) or palpated but are not distinct in roentgenograms because they consist of cartilage and uncalcified osteoid tissue. Bending of the softened shafts of the femur, tibia, and fibula results in bowlegs or knock-knees; the femur and the tibia may also acquire an anterior convexity. Coxa vara is sometimes the result of rickets. Greenstick fractures occur in the long bones; often there are no clinical symptoms.

Deformities of the spine, pelvis, and legs result in reduced stature, rachitic dwarfism.

Ligaments. Relaxation of ligaments helps to produce deformities and partly accounts for knock-knees, overextension of the knee joints, weak ankles, kyphosis, and scoliosis.

Muscles. The muscles are poorly developed and lack tone. As a result, children with moderately severe rickets are late in standing and walking. The common condition of potbelly (see Figs. 4–10 and 4–12) depends to a large extent on weakness of the abdominal muscles; weakness of the gastric and intestinal walls may contribute.

DIAGNOSIS. The diagnosis of rickets is based on a history of inadequate intake of vitamin D and on clinical observation; it is confirmed chemically and by roentgenographic examination. The serum calcium level may be normal or low, the serum phosphorus level is below 4 mg/dL, and the serum alkaline phosphatase is elevated. Urinary cyclic AMP is elevated, and serum 25-hydroxycholecalciferol is decreased.

Roentgenographic Changes (see Fig. 4–11). **Active rickets.** A roentgenogram of the wrist is best for early diagnosis, because characteristic changes of the ulna and radius occur at an early stage. The distal ends appear widened, concave (cupping), and frayed, in contrast to the normally sharply demarcated and slightly convex ends. The distance from the

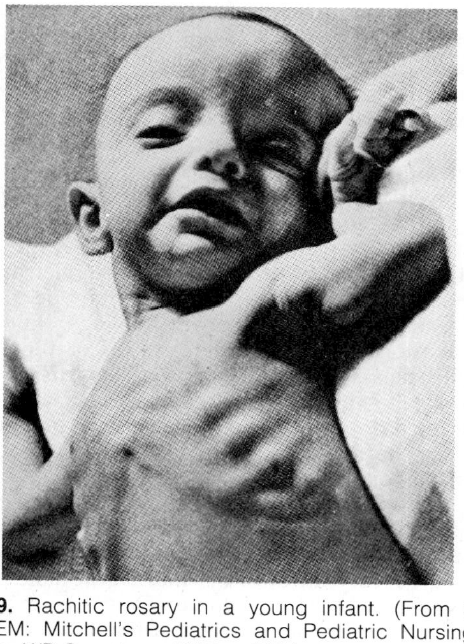

Figure 4–9. Rachitic rosary in a young infant. (From Lyons RA, Wallinger EM: Mitchell's Pediatrics and Pediatric Nursing, 3rd ed. Philadelphia, WB Saunders, 1950, p 267.)

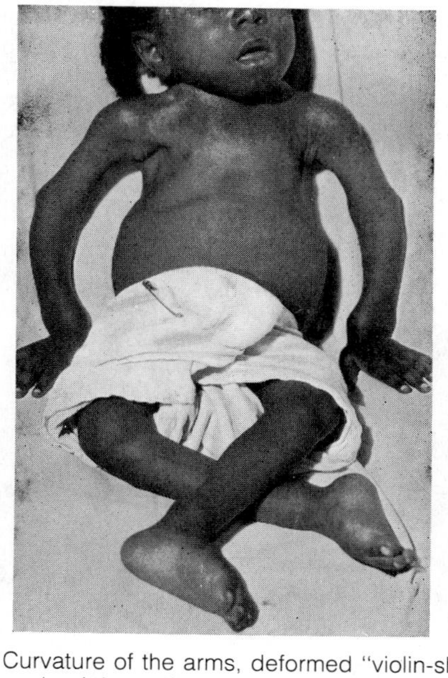

Figure 4–10. Curvature of the arms, deformed "violin-shaped" chest, potbelly, enlarged epiphyses in a child with rickets, 3 yr of age.

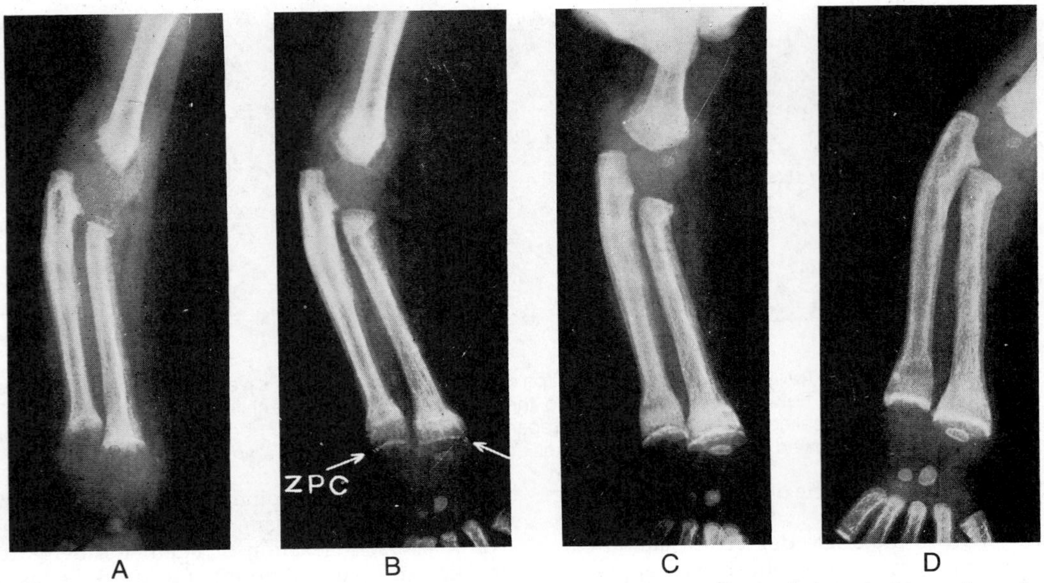

Figure 4–11. *A*, Active rickets; cupping and fraying of the distal ends of the radius and ulna; double contour along the lateral outline of the radius (periosteal osteoid). The two dense zones in the shaft of the ulna are calluses of greenstick fractures. *B*, Healing rickets after 12 days of treatment with vitamin D. Zones of preparatory calcification (ZPC); above them in the rachitic metaphyses there is beginning calcification. *C*, Healing rickets after 18 days of treatment. The zones of preparatory calcification are well defined, and the rachitic metaphyses appear well calcified. The epiphysis of the radius has become visible. *D*, Healing rickets after 29 days of treatment. Zones of preparatory calcification, rachitic metaphyses, and shafts have become united.

distal ends of the ulna and radius to the metacarpal bones is increased because the large rachitic metaphysis, which is not calcified, does not appear on the roentgenogram. The density of the shafts is decreased, but the trabeculae are unusually prominent.

HEALING RICKETS (see Fig. 4–11). Initial healing is indicated by the appearance of the line of preparatory calcification. This line is separated from the distal end of the shaft by a zone of decreased calcification, the zone of the osteoid tissue. As healing progresses and the osteoid tissue becomes calcified, the shaft "grows" toward the line of preparatory calcification until it becomes united with it.

DIFFERENTIAL DIAGNOSIS. Nonrachitic craniotabes, at times present in the immediate postnatal period, tends to disappear before rachitic softening of the skull would become manifest (2nd–4th mo of life). Craniotabes also occurs in hydrocephalus and osteogenesis imperfecta, but it is not difficult to differentiate these conditions from rickets.

Enlargement of the costochondral junctions occurs in rickets, scurvy, and chondrodystrophy. The enlargements in rickets are rounded knobs, but in scurvy a ledge-like depression with the chondral or sternal portion is displaced below the osseous ribs. In chondrodystrophy there may be irregular, concave outlines of the distal ends of the bones, but no roentgenographic evidence of fraying. Other epiphyseal lesions that may require differentiation include congenital epiphyseal dysplasia, cytomegalic inclusion disease, syphilis, rubella, and copper deficiency. It is sometimes difficult to distinguish rachitic deformities of the chest from congenital ones. Bowlegs can be the result of rickets but may be a familial characteristic. Vitamin D resistant rickets and other metabolic disturbances with osseous lesions resembling rickets must also be differentiated (Sec. 24.59).

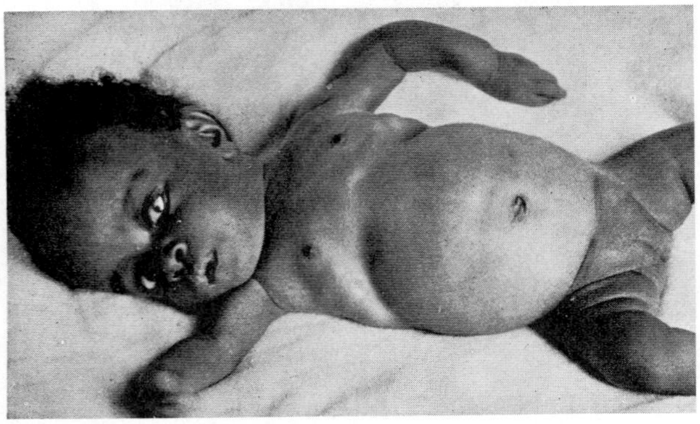

Figure 4–12. Deformities in rickets, showing the curvature of the limbs, potbelly, and Harrison groove.

COMPLICATIONS. Respiratory infections such as bronchitis and bronchopneumonia are common in rachitic infants, and pulmonary atelectasis is frequently associated with severe deformities of the chest. Anemia due to iron deficiency or accompanying infections often develops in severe rickets.

PROGNOSIS. If sufficient amounts of vitamin D are administered, healing begins within a few days and progresses slowly until the normal bony structure is restored. In many instances, the enlargement of the epiphyses of the long bones, including the ribs, and the deformities of the skull disappear only after months or years of treatment. Even rather severe bowing of the legs may disappear within several years without osteotomies. In advanced cases there may be permanent osseous alterations in the form of bowlegs, knock-knees, curvature of the upper arms, deformities of the chest and spine, rachitic pelvis and coxa vara, and dwarfism.

Rickets in itself is not a fatal disease, but complications and intercurrent infections such as pneumonia, tuberculosis, and enteritis are more likely to cause death in rachitic children than in normal children.

PREVENTION. Rickets can be prevented by exposure to ultraviolet light or by oral administration of vitamin D. Sunlight, as a prophylactic agent, may be effective in the temperate zones only during the summer months in haze-free areas.

The daily requirement of vitamin D is 10 μg or 400 IU. Much of the whole milk available in urban areas and evaporated milk are fortified with vitamin D concentrate so that

1 quart of fresh, whole milk or a can of evaporated milk contains this amount. Prematurely born infants or breast-fed infants whose mothers are not exposed to adequate sunlight should receive supplemental vitamin D daily.

Vitamin D should also be administered to pregnant and lactating mothers.

TREATMENT. Natural and artificial light are effective therapeutically, but oral administration of vitamin D is preferred. The daily administration of 50–150 μg of vitamin D_3 or 0.5–2 μg of 1,25-dihydroxycholecalciferol will produce healing demonstrable on roentgenograms within 2–4 wk except in the unusual cases of vitamin D refractory rickets.

Administering 15,000 μg of vitamin D in a single dose without further therapy for several months may be advantageous. More rapid healing will follow, possibly with earlier differential diagnosis from genetic vitamin D-resistant rickets and less dependence on parents for daily administration of the vitamin. If no healing occurs, the rickets is probably resistant to vitamin D (Sec. 24.61). After healing is complete, the dose of vitamin D should be lowered to 10 μg/day.

Rasmussen H: Cell communication, calcium ion, and cyclic adenosine monophosphate. Science 170:404, 1970.

Reichel H, Koeffler HP, Norman AW: The role of the vitamin D endocrine system in health and disease. N Engl J Med 320:980, 1989.

Root AW, Harrison HE: Recent advances in calcium metabolism. I. Mechanisms of calcium homeostasis. II. Disorders of calcium homeostasis. J Pediatr 88:1, 177, 1976.

Yetgin S, Ozsoylu S, Raucan S, et al: Vitamin D-deficiency rickets and myelofibrosis. J Pediatr 114:213, 1989.

4.30 TETANY OF VITAMIN D DEFICIENCY
(Infantile Tetany)

See also Sec. 6.27.

Tetany due to deficiency of vitamin D occasionally accompanies rickets. Relatively common in former times, this type of tetany is rare today owing to the widespread prophylactic use of vitamin D. Occasionally, tetany is associated with celiac disease, probably as a result of deficient absorption of both vitamin D and calcium. Tetany of vitamin D deficiency occurs most frequently between the ages of 4 mo and 3 yr.

CHEMICAL PATHOLOGY. When the serum calcium concentration falls below 7–7.5 mg/dL, muscular irritability occurs, apparently owing to the loss of the inhibitory control that serum ionized calcium exerts on the neuromuscular junctions. It remains unclear why serum calcium is occasionally decreased in association with rickets; failure of the parathyroids to compensate for the low serum calcium level may be a factor.

CLINICAL MANIFESTATIONS. The symptoms and signs of tetany are manifested, and rickets usually occurs concurrently. Vitamin D deficient tetany may exist in either a latent or a clinically manifest stage.

Latent Tetany. Symptoms are not evident, but they can be elicited by means of the Chvostek, Trousseau, and Erb procedures. The serum calcium level is less than 7–7.5 mg/dL.

Manifest Tetany. Spontaneous clinical manifestations include carpopedal spasm, laryngospasm, and convulsions. The serum calcium level is often well under 7 mg/dL.

DIAGNOSIS. The diagnosis is based on the combined presence of rickets, low serum calcium level, and symptoms of tetany. The serum phosphorus level is usually low; the serum alkaline phosphatase level is increased. In the differential diagnosis causes of tetany such as hypoparathyroidism, hypomagnesemia, and ingestion of phenothiazine must be eliminated.

PROGNOSIS. The prognosis is good unless treatment is delayed. Death rarely occurs, though it may result from laryngospasm and possibly from cardiac dilatation, so-called cardiac tetany.

PREVENTION. Prophylactic treatment is identical to that for rickets (Sec. 4.29).

TREATMENT. Active treatment raises the serum calcium above the tetany level. This level may be attained by administration of calcium chloride in 1–2% solution in milk. For the first 1–2 days, 4–6 g/day may be given in 1-g doses, the initial dose being 2–3 g; smaller doses of 1–3 g/day should then be continued for 1–2 wk. Calcium chloride in more concentrated solution may cause severe gastric ulceration, and large doses may cause acidosis. Calcium lactate may be added to milk in doses of 10–12 g/day for 10 days. When oral medication is impractical, calcium gluconate (5–10 mL of a 10% solution) can be administered intravenously but not subcutaneously or intramuscularly owing to the dangers of local necrosis.

Oxygen inhalation is indicated during convulsive seizures. When intravenously administered calcium gluconate does not quickly control the attacks, sodium phenobarbital may be given intramuscularly. Prolonged attacks of laryngospasm are usually controlled by sedation and by administering calcium salts. Intubation is only occasionally necessary. After the acute manifestations have been controlled, vitamin D in daily doses of 50–100 μg should be started and the oral administration of calcium continued (see earlier). When the rickets is healed, the dose of vitamin D should be decreased to the usual prophylactic one.

Fraser D, Kook SW, Scriver CR: Hyperparathyroidism as the cause of hyperaminoaciduria and phosphaturia in human vitamin D deficiency. Pediatr Res 1:425, 1967.

4.31 HYPERVITAMINOSIS D

Ingesting excessive amounts of vitamin D results in signs and symptoms similar to those of idiopathic hypercalcemia (Sec. 24.68), which may be due to hypersensitivity to vitamin D. Symptoms develop after 1–3 mo of large intakes of vitamin D; they include hypotonia, anorexia, irritability, constipation, polydipsia, polyuria, and pallor. Hypercalcemia and hypercalciuria are notable. Evidence of dehydration is usually present. Aortic valvular stenosis, vomiting, hypertension, retinopathy, and clouding of the cornea and conjunctiva may occur.

The urine may show proteinuria. With continued excessive intake, renal damage and metastatic calcification occur. Roentgenograms of the long bones reveal metastatic calcification and generalized osteoporosis.

Excessive intake of vitamin D may result from inadvertently substituting its concentrated form for one more dilute, from the parents' increasing their child's prescribed dose, and from inadequately controlling dosages for children receiving large amounts of vitamin D for chronic hyperphosphatemic states (Sec. 24.69).

DIFFERENTIAL DIAGNOSIS. Metastatic calcification occurs in chronic nephritis, hyperparathyroidism, and idiopathic hypercalcemia. The latter two are accompanied by hypercalcemia.

PREVENTION. Prevention requires careful evaluation of vitamin D dosage.

TREATMENT. This includes discontinuing vitamin D intake and decreasing intake of calcium. For severely involved infants, aluminum hydroxide by mouth, cortisone, or sodium versenate may be used.

Forbes GB, Cafarelli C, Manning J: Vitamin D and infantile hypercalcemia. Pediatrics 42:203, 1968.

4.32 VITAMIN E DEFICIENCY

The effects of vitamin E deficiency vary in different animal species. Vitamin E (α-tocopherol) is a fat-soluble antioxidant that may be involved in nucleic acid metabolism, but its precise biochemical action is unclear. Vitamin E is present in many foods (see Table 4–6).

Deficiency may occur in malabsorption states such as cystic fibrosis and acanthocytosis. Diets high in unsaturated fatty acid increase the vitamin E requirement in premature infants who absorb vitamin E poorly. Excess iron administration exaggerates signs of vitamin E deficiency.

Some patients deficient in vitamin E have creatinuria, ceroid deposition in smooth muscle, focal necrosis of striated muscle, and muscle weakness. Some improvement may occur after administration of vitamin E. Vitamin E deficiency has been suggested as a causative factor in the anemia of kwashiorkor. Premature infants may have low serum levels of tocopherol, with development of a hemolytic anemia at 6–10 wk of age, correctable by administration of vitamin E. The role of vitamin E in retinopathy of prematurity is discussed in Sec. 9.17 and 22.13. Patients with malabsorption and vitamin E deficiency due to biliary atresia develop a degenerative neurologic syndrome.

In deficiency states, platelet adhesiveness increases, as do blood platelet levels. Treatment of hemolysis in glucose-6-phosphate dehydrogenase (G-6-PD) deficiency, of sickle cell anemia, of leg cramps, or of coronary artery disease represents unsubstantiated use of vitamin E.

DIAGNOSIS. If vitamin E has recently been administered, 3 days should elapse before determination of blood levels, because oral vitamin E may circulate for 1–2 days.

PREVENTION. Minimal daily requirements of vitamin E are not known; 0.7 mg/g of unsaturated fat in the diet appears adequate. Children with deficient fat absorption should take more. Premature infants may be given 15–25 IU/24 hr. Large oral or parenteral doses of vitamin E may prevent permanent neurologic abnormalities in children with biliary atresia or abetalipoproteinemia.

Gross S: Hemolytic anemia in premature infants: Relationship to vitamin E, selenium, glutathione peroxidase, and erythrocyte lipids. Semin Hematol 13:187, 1976.

Sokol RJ: Vitamin E and neurologic deficits. Adv Pediatr 37:119, 1990.

4.33 VITAMIN K DEFICIENCY

Vitamin K is a naphthoquinone that participates in oxidative phosphorylation. Its absence or its failure to be absorbed from the intestinal tract results in hypoprothrombinemia and decreased hepatic synthesis of proconvertin. Prothrombin (factor II) and proconvertin (Factor VII) are important to the 2nd stage of coagulation (Sec. 16.63). The 2nd stage of coagulation is studied by the 1-stage prothrombin time (Quick). Administering vitamin K to the newborn infant increases concentrations of prothrombin, proconvertin, plasma thromboplastin component (factor IX, PTC), and Stuart-Prower factor (factor X). Four vitamin K-dependent proteins contain γ-carboxyglutamate. All require calcium for activity. Factors C and S are anticoagulants. Factors Z and M stimulate platelet activity. Vitamin K-dependent calcium binding proteins such as osteocalcin promote phospholipid interactions in coagulation and in calcium metabolism.

SOURCES OF VITAMIN K. Naturally occurring vitamin K is fat soluble; it is found in high concentrations of hog's liver, soybeans, and alfalfa and in smaller amounts in some vegetables, such as spinach, tomatoes, and kale. The natural vitamin (2-methyl-3-phytyl-1,4-naphthoquinone) has been labeled vitamin K_1 to distinguish it from synthetic naphthoquinones with vitamin K activity.

Many bacteria, including normal intestinal flora, are capable of synthesizing quinones with vitamin K activity. Suppression of intestinal bacteria by various antibiotics may be responsible for vitamin K deficiency, which results in diminution of prothrombin. Irradiated foods have produced vitamin K deficiency in animals. Cow's milk has more vitamin K than human milk.

CLINICAL MANIFESTATIONS. Deficiency of vitamin K or hypoprothrombinemia should be considered in all patients with a hemorrhagic disturbance. The incidence of hemorrhagic disease of the newborn (Sec. 9.49) has been sharply decreased by the prophylactic administration of vitamin K. In childhood, the deficiency is usually due to factors affecting absorption or utilization of fat or to factors limiting its synthesis in the intestine, such as prolonged use of antibiotics. Diarrhea in infants, particularly breast-fed ones, may cause vitamin K deficiency. Diseases of the liver may lead to hypoprothrombinemia, which usually does not respond to administration of vitamin K.

Hypoprothrombinemia may also result from administering certain drugs. Dicumarol (or bishydroxycoumarin), obtained from spoiled sweet clover, is used specifically for the production of hypoprothrombinemia in the prevention and treatment of venous thrombosis. Dicumarol is thought to prevent the liver from utilizing vitamin K without exerting an effect on prothrombin. Blood prothrombin is continually destroyed in the body; since dicumarol prevents its replacement, a fall in prothrombin occurs. If a dangerously low-level results, massive doses of vitamin K_1 may be necessary to restore prothrombin, and whole blood transfusions may also be necessary.

Salicylic acid, a degradation product of dicumarol, produces hypoprothrombinemia by similar action. The fall in prothrombin resulting from salicylates, however, is mild compared with that of dicumarol. The hemorrhagic manifestations in acute rheumtic fever may be due in some cases to large doses of salicylates; vitamin K is effective in neutralizing this action. Its use in children receiving large doses of salicylates would appear justified.

TREATMENT. Oral administration of vitamin K may correct mild prothrombin deficiency. One to 2 mg/day for an infant will usually suffice. If prothrombin deficiency is severe and hemorrhagic manifestations have appeared, 5 mg/day of vitamin K_1 should be given parenterally. Large doses of synthetic vitamin K analogs, but not of vitamin K_1, may result in hyperbilirubinemia and kernicterus in the G-6-PD–deficient newborn and in the premature infant. In hypoprothrombinemia owing to liver damage, vitamin K_1 may be given, but whole blood is usually also necessary.

LEWIS A. BARNESS

Corrigan JJ: The vitamin K dependent proteins. Adv Pediatr 28:57,1981.

Peters C, Casella JF, Marlar RA, et al: Homozygous protein C deficiency. Pediatrics 81:272, 1988.

5

PREVENTIVE PEDIATRICS AND EPIDEMIOLOGY

Remarkable improvements in child health, not only in mortality but also in acute and chronic morbidity, have occurred in the United States and other developed nations since the turn of this century. Most of the increase in years of expected life since 1900 in the United States is attributable to enhanced survival in infancy and childhood (Table 5–1). Although exact data are not available for many disorders, it is clear that acute morbidity, particularly from infectious disease, and to a considerable extent chronic morbidity have also declined. Examination of Table 5–1 indicates that for the first 40 yr of the 20th century the average annual increase in life expectancy was 0.39 yr compared with 0.26 yr for the next 47 yr. The decline before the 1940s cannot be attributed to the advances in pharmacologic and surgical therapies that have developed since World War II; instead, this early decline must be explained mainly by social and economic changes plus public health measures, including preventive pediatrics.

The importance of preventive pediatrics is more evident now than it was 50 yr ago for several reasons. First, therapeutic medicine and surgery have their limitations, often producing new problems (e.g., the enhanced survival of handicapped children) and consuming a high proportion of money for health care. Second, modern epidemiology has clarified the etiology and pathogenesis of many disorders that affect adults, including the recognition that they often originate in infancy and childhood. Third, new disorders, such as acquired immunodeficiency syndrome (AIDS), and old problems that have increased in frequency, including drug abuse and adolescent pregnancy, require vigorous programs for prevention.

Preventive pediatrics consists of efforts to avert rather than to cure disease and disability. It includes primary prevention, which is directed at avoiding disorders before they begin, such as by tetanus immunization or by chlorination of water supplies; secondary prevention, the recognizing and eliminating of the precursors of disease, such as screening programs for elevated blood levels and the Papanicolaou (Pap) smear, and also by efforts to identify and reverse disease in its early stages, such as a screening program for scoliosis in adolescents; and tertiary prevention, the measures for ameliorating or halting the disabilities arising from established disease, such as physiotherapy to prevent contractures in patients with chronic neurologic disorders. Most successful primary preventive measures require understanding the cause, the pathogenesis, and the natural history of disease. For secondary or tertiary prevention, however, determining the cause is not essential. Many preventive measures, such as tetanus immunization, are effective only for the individual recipient; others are applied to the entire community (e.g., water fluoridation). Some primary prevention measures that are directed at the individual recipient also benefit others; vaccination against measles and poliomyelitis is an example.

Significant changes have occurred in child health in the United States during the 20th century as a result of primary preventive medicine. Table 5–2 shows that in 1987, infant mortality was 1/16 that for 1900 and 1/3 that for 1950. A preliminary estimate for 1990 indicates that infant mortality had fallen to 9.1/1,000. Table 5–2 indicates that more than half of this decrease is due to the control of infections in infants; 20% is attributable to a decline in mortality due to perinatal causes. Because of the striking diminution in deaths due to infection and perinatal causes, other conditions now loom proportionately larger in importance. For example, although deaths due to congenital anomalies declined more than 50% between 1900 and 1987, approximately 20% of deaths in infants in 1987 were due to birth defects compared with only 3% in 1900. Similarly, despite the fact that the sudden infant death syndrome has not increased in frequency over the years, it is now estimated to be responsible for 1/7 of all infant deaths. Table 5–3 indicates that in 1900 almost 2% of all children 1–4 yr old died annually and that four of five deaths in this age group were caused by infection. By 1987, overall mortality in this age group was reduced by 97%, primarily owing to the reduction of death due to infection. Neoplasms, congenital anomalies, and violence *in toto* caused less than 5% of deaths in this age group in 1900 compared with 63% in 1987 and are, therefore, proportionately more important now despite an actual decrease in the rate of each.

The United States, however, has not been as successful in reducing its infant mortality rate as have several other countries; 21 other nations have lower infant mortality rates. An

TABLE 5–1. Life Expectancy at Birth, Selected Years, 1900–1987*

Year	Life Expectancy	Year	Life Expectancy
1900	47.3	1950	68.2
1910	50.0	1960	69.7
1920	54.1	1970	70.9
1930	59.7	1980	73.7
1940	62.9	1987	75.0

*Published March 20, 1990.

TABLE 5–2. Infant Mortality Rates, 1900, 1950, and 1987, for All Causes and Certain Conditions*†

Causes	1900	1950	1987
All	162.9	33.0	10.2
Infection	85.9	5.4	0.5
Enteric	42.1	1.4	<0.1
Anomalies	4.7	4.5	2.1
Perinatal	35.9	19.4	4.8
Sudden infant death syndrome‡	—	—	1.4
Accidents and violence	1.3	1.1	0.3
All others	34.2	2.6	1.1

*Deaths per 1,000.
†Published March 20, 1990.
‡Data not available until 1979.

TABLE 5–3. US Mortality Rates, Children 1–4 Years of Age, 1900, 1950, and 1987, for All Causes and Certain Conditions*†

Causes	1900	1950	1987
All	1,980	141	51.6
Infection	1,566	51	5.3
Respiratory	479	21	1.5
Neoplasms	8	13	3.8
Anomalies	9	11	6.4
Accidents, violence	74	37	22.6
All others	323	29	16.5

*Deaths per 100,000/yr.
†Published March 20, 1990.

explanation for part of this disparity lies in the high infant mortality rate for black infants in the United States, who constitute approximately 17% of all live births. The birth rate among blacks is almost 50% greater than that for whites, and the infant mortality rate is more than twice as high. For all major causes of death, the rates in blacks exceed those for whites in the United States; the major contributors among these causes are prematurity and various perinatal conditions.

The reductions in childhood mortality are attributable partly to medical advances (e.g., immunization, anti-infective drugs, and various other diagnostic and therapeutic developments) and partly to certain public health measures (e.g., filtration and chlorination of public water supplies, hygienic food handling [especially of milk], mosquito control, and isolation of infected persons). The indirect effects of social, economic, and educational advances have also played a role, although their benefits have not affected all population groups equally. However, many of the salutary changes in childhood mortality cannot be fully explained; for example, the annual crude mortality rates from measles declined 98% from 1900 to 1955 before the introduction of measles vaccine.

As a consequence of the decline in mortality, substantial changes in emphases in pediatric practice have occurred. Except for accident prevention and the development of effective methods for preventing prematurity, there is little further that can be done to reduce mortality in infancy and childhood, which may be approaching an irreducible minimum. Thus, increasing emphasis is placed on maintaining and enhancing the quality of the child's life and on ensuring that each child reaches adult life as physically, intellectually, and emotionally healthy as possible. Activities such as anticipatory guidance, developmental counseling, assisting families with children's school-related problems, sexual counseling, secondary prevention by screening for incipient disease, and attempting to ameliorate the precursors of adult disease have become integral parts of pediatric practice.

In addition, three increasingly prevalent and interrelated problems that endanger the lives and future well-being of the young currently demand urgent attention. These problems include substance abuse, adolescent pregnancy, and AIDS. The problems of alcohol and drug use by adolescents and even younger children, particularly in (but not limited to) inner cities and among minorities, are increasingly widespread. The implications of all of these problems, and of related violence, for maturing, education, and the ultimate future of the individual are enormous. Substance abuse is discouragingly difficult to ameliorate in the adult; successful intervention and prevention in the young are even harder to achieve (Sec. 10.4). Although the teenage birth rate is less than that in the early 1970s, possibly because of the abortion, it has not changed subsequently (Sec. 10.15). There were 310,000 births to females less than 19 yr old in 1987. More than 70% of the mothers were unmarried. The effects of the teenage pregnancy on the mother and her education and on the infant are well known. AIDS in children is usually acquired from an infected mother at birth (Sec. 12.82). As of 1988, more than 1,300 children with AIDS had been identified; this total does not include asymptomatic human immunodeficiency virus (HIV)-infected children. In 1988 among the 31,001 new cases of AIDS reported in the United States, 678 (2.2%) were children and adolescents less than 20 yr of age. Two thirds of these were less than 10 yr old, in most of whom the infection was maternally derived and, in the remainder, acquired from transfusions or blood products. However, more than one fifth were 10 to 19 yr old, many of whom were infected from sexual or drug-related sources. Thus, prevention of AIDS in young children must be addressed through the control of risk factors in the child-bearing population, including adolescents with risk-taking behaviors, who may jeopardize themselves as well as future offspring (Sec. 10.17). Deaths in children with AIDS in 1988 totalled 360.

5.1 PRIMARY PREVENTION

Primary prevention occurs both within the community and in the pediatrician's office.

COMMUNITY PRIMARY PREVENTION. Several measures preventing disease at the community level have had enormous effects on childhood morbidity and mortality in the United States: sewage disposal and water sanitation, improved housing, hygienic control of food, including pasteurization of milk, iodination of salt, and control of arthropod vectors of disease (e.g., mosquito control by swamp drainage in malarial areas). In areas of the world where these measures are still incompletely adopted, the spectrum of childhood mortality resembles that of the United States in 1900.

Many other public health programs of proven merit have not been universally adopted, even in the United States.

Fluoridation of public water supplies is efficacious in reducing dental caries. Its safety and high benefit-to-cost ratio are well established. However, fluoridated water is currently available to only about one third of all infants and children in the United States, because they live either in areas without communal water supplies or in communities where fluoridation, although feasible, has not been instituted for social, political, or economic reasons. Community fluoridation programs should be supported. In unfluoridated areas, school programs should be established to provide fluoride tablets or rinses as alternative approaches. Additional measures include fluoride supplements from birth.

Pasteurization of milk prevents outbreaks of diarrheal disease caused by contaminating pathogenic bacteria. However, the recent interest in the United States in "natural foods" has led to the increased consumption of raw milk under the fallacious assumption that it is nutritionally superior to pasteurized milk. Consequently, local outbreaks of diarrheal disease, which include fatalities, have occurred owing to the presence of strains of *Salmonella, Brucella, Campylobacter,* and other gram-negative bacilli transmitted by milk. Pediatricians should educate parents and local authorities concerning the risks of raw milk (whether certified or not).

External causes of death, including accidents, poisonings, homicides, and suicides (Sec. 6.31), currently account for half of all deaths in individuals from 1 to 24 yr of age. Table 5–4 shows the changes that occurred between 1950 and 1987 in overall mortality and that were due to external causes for

TABLE 5–4. Death Rates* for All Causes and Certain External Causes, 1987, and Percentage Change Since 1950, by Age Groups

Causes	1–4 Yr	5–14 Yr	15–24 Yr
All	51.6 (−63)	25.6 (−58)	99.4 (−22)
All external	22.5 (−49)	14.2 (−39)	75.8 (+10)
Accidents	20.2 (−45)	12.3 (−46)	48.9 (−11)
Automobile	6.8 (−41)	7.0 (−20)	37.8 (+10)
Homicide	2.3 (−66)	1.2 (+500)	14.0 (+41)
Suicide	—	0.7 (+40)	12.9 (+87)

*Deaths per 100,000.

specific age groups. Death rates from all causes decreased by more than 50% between 1 and 14 yr but by only about one fifth between the ages of 15 and 24 yr. Death from external causes between 1 and 14 yr decreased, but at a lower rate, and proportionately now account for about half of all deaths in this age group. In addition, although overall death rates between 15 and 24 yr decreased by more than one fifth, deaths due to external causes actually increased by 10%. Deaths from accidents in this age group decreased even though automobile-related deaths increased. Most of the increase in deaths due to external causes is due to higher rates of homicide and suicide in this older age group. Currently 76% of deaths in persons 15–24 yr of age are due to external causes; half of these are related to automobile accidents and one fourth are caused by homicide and suicide. In relation to overall death rates, male mortality exceeds that of females in all age groups, and rates for blacks are at least 50% greater throughout childhood and adolescence, mainly as a result of external causes. In terms of morbidity, injuries and poisoning accounted for one seventh of all postneonatal hospital admissions for individuals less than 15 yr of age in 1986, ranking only behind respiratory disorders, and accounted for about one eighth of all hospital days for this age group.

Of concern and not entirely explicable is that the downward trends in mortality in persons 1–25 yr of age, evident for many decades, appear to have reversed between 1983 and 1988 in some segments of this population, compared with infant mortality, which has declined slowly but steadily in all groups. In 1988, death rates in ages 15–24 for white and black women increased 8% and 20%, respectively, from their nadirs in 1983 and 1985. For black females aged 5 to 14 yr, there has been a 27% increase since 1983. For black men aged 15–24, there has been a 31% increase in mortality between 1983 and 1988, and white men have shown a 5% increase. For other age groups of both sexes and both races less than 25 yr old, continuing declines in mortality have been observed. Although exact data are not yet available, it is likely that the increases in mortality in persons aged 15–24 are related mainly to drugs and violence. The remarkable increase for black females aged 5–14 yr has not yet been explained.

Accident prevention in young children is difficult because of the diversity of childhood injuries (see also Sec. 6.31). Three approaches to primary prevention have been used:

1. Public health education, such as encouraging "childproofing" of the home.
2. Changes in children's environment, either mandated by law or voluntarily built in by manufacturers, such as flame-resistant fabrics, childproof containers, paint of minimal lead content, window guards for apartment buildings, safe spacing of crib rails, and others. As of 1985, all but one state in the United States had passed an infant car seat law. These measures have been much more effective than public education.
3. One-on-one parent education by the child's physician.

To provide effective parental guidance, the physician should know the household risk factors and the propensities of children at various ages for different types of accidents (Sec. 6.37, 6.38, and 10.1). Areas that are particularly important are the medicine cabinet; places where toxic household chemicals, such as solvents and furniture polish, are stored; the stove; matches; electrical wires and devices; and sharp objects, such as glassware and knives. Outside the home, the automobile and unprotected bodies of water endanger toddlers.

Widome has suggested that our efforts to prevent accidents to the young need to be directed somewhat differently. Rather than focusing excessively on the host, both in assigning responsibility for various preventive measures to parents or to children and adolescents whose judgments are immature and in placing blame after the fact (poor judgment), more attention should be given to the agents of injury and the environment in which injuries occur. Thus, reducing injury requires greater emphasis on effective public health measures, such as with the infectious disease model. If we relied on personal use of insect sprays rather than on widespread mosquito control by draining swamps and other public health measures, malaria would be a "usual childhood disease." Driver training does not reduce accidents; it is a convenience for parents and a route to a driver's license rather than an effective preventive measure. Instead, measures such as better highways, safer vehicles, raising the permissible driving age, reduced speed limits with strict enforcement, and control of alcohol use by the young may be much more effective. Safer all-terrain vehicles, banning of recreational trampolines, and some approach to reducing the availability of guns are methods of controlling agents of injury. Similarly, to encourage teenagers to refuse to take drugs and to maintain sexual abstinence cannot be expected to exert much impact on two major problems of the young.

For the pediatrician to concentrate more on the agent and the environment and less on the individual host requires active participation in the public health decision-making process at various levels, both as an individual and through organizations and agencies concerned with child health. The effectiveness of the influence of pediatric health care professionals in developing and implementing school immunization laws, car seat regulations, restrictions on raw milk, and other salutary measures is only one example of how the host, the agent, and the environment can be modified through public health efforts.

Poisoning became proportionately more important as a child health problem as others were ameliorated during the first 70 yr of this century. In 1900, the death rate attributed to accidental poisoning was 5-fold that of 1970 but accounted for only 0.4% of all deaths compared with 1.8% in 1970. From 1970 to 1985 children's death rates from poisoning have further declined by 72%, no doubt due mainly to the activities of poison control centers, safety caps on medicine bottles, and the like (Sec. 26.4). Pediatricians should work for primary prevention of poisoning not only from their offices but also in the community by supporting efforts at educating parents, childproofing containers, properly storing and disposing of toxic substances, and establishing poison control centers.

Homicides accounted for 4.5% and 14% of deaths in 5–14 and 15–24 yr olds, respectively, in 1987 (see Table 5–4). Homicide rates for young black males during the last 15 yr have been greater than those for other groups; in 1985 for white males the homicide rate was 7.3/100,000 and the rate for black males aged 15–19 was 46.4/100,000. More than 75% of these deaths were caused by firearms and were usually unrelated to criminal activities. The amount of permanent disability occurring to survivors of gunshot wounds can only be speculated. *Suicide* rates in persons aged 15–19 yr increased more than 40% between 1976 and 1985; rates are higher for males, particularly white males. Sixty per cent are carried out with firearms. The causes of homicide and suicide (Sec. 10.3) are undoubtedly numerous and include complex social and economic factors. Pediatricians should warn parents of the dangers of firearms and should participate in developing a public solution.

Adolescent Pregnancy. A problem involving all aspects of prevention is sexuality and consequent pregnancy in adolescents (Sec. 10.15). Teenage pregnancy causes major social, psychologic, educational, and financial burdens for the young parent(s). The infant of a teenage mother is at enhanced risk physically and developmentally, although, after adjustment for socioeconomic status and prenatal care, the only immediate consequences attributable to maternal youth are increases in pre-eclampsia and in low-birthweight infants. From 1970 to 1983 rates of live births to teenage females decreased slightly but absolute numbers of births to teenagers did not, because of increases in the adolescent population. Since 1983, rates have remained steady except for girls less than 15 yr in whom they have increased. In 1987, live births occurred to 10,311 girls less than 15 yr of age; induced abortions were performed on almost 14,000 others. At current rates, 1 of 70 girls becomes pregnant between her 10th and 15th birthdays, and 1 in 160 girls delivers a live baby in this interval. Similarly, 1 in 2.4 females becomes pregnant between her 15th and 20th birthdays; 1 in 4 females has a liveborn child. Rates in nonwhites are more than double those in whites.

The multiple and complex reasons for teenage pregnancies make control difficult to achieve; not all conceptions are accidental. Although precise data are not available, teenage sexual activity and pregnancy affect all population groups, but pregnancy occurs more frequently in lower socioeconomic groups.

The optimal solution to the problem would be the reduction or avoidance of sexual activity during adolescence. Because educational and motivational programs have had very limited success, most efforts should be directed at encouraging and facilitating use of contraceptives by sexually active teenagers (Sec. 10.16). The key factors in successful programs directed are outreach, nonjudgmental counseling to reduce ambivalent feelings about pregnancy and contraceptives, making contraceptives readily available, and linking services with school health programs. For pregnant teenagers, counseling about reproductive options and encouraging regular prenatal care are important, as are helping to develop plans for care of the infant, continuing the mother's education, and preventing further pregnancies until maturity.

Substance abuse is discussed in Sec. 10.4.

PRIMARY PREVENTION IN THE PEDIATRICIAN'S OFFICE. The purposes of routine child health care are to foster the normal development of the child from infancy to adulthood and to help ensure that each child achieves his or her full physical, intellectual, and emotional adult potential. In infancy, interaction between the pediatrician and the child is mediated mainly by the parents; in later childhood and adolescence, a direct relationship between the physician and the child increasingly develops. Children's regularly scheduled health maintenance checkups should be evaluative and preventive. Evaluations include the usual interval history and inquiries into any perceived problem, assessment of growth and development by history and examination, and screening for various abnormalities or their precursors. Preventive management includes efforts to correct or ameliorate any abnormalities; specific preventive measures, such as immunization; and anticipatory guidance. The following general recommendations derived from the American Academy of Pediatrics comprise general guidelines for the care of normal infants and children; the needs of individual children and their families may require modification. For example, an experienced family with a third child may require fewer visits than new anxious parents whose prior pregnancy terminated in death due to prematurity.

Prenatal Period. It is desirable, particularly with first pregnancies, for the parents to talk with their pediatrician sometime during the 3rd trimester about any of their problems or concerns. At this time they can review the pediatrician's role in the subsequent care of the child, which includes care in the newborn nursery, the proposed schedule of visits, and planned immunizations. Financial arrangements may also be discussed. Other topics might include desirability of breastfeeding, the advantages and disadvantages of circumcision, the living arrangements for the baby, and what help may be available at home during the first few weeks after birth. The pediatrician should also help to instill confidence in the parents by pointing out that there is no single correct method of caring for the baby and that, for the most part, their own instincts in dealing with the infant from one day to another should be followed.

Newborn Care. See also Sec. 9.4–9.6. Every infant should receive prophylaxis for ophthalmia neonatorum and a single intramuscular dose of a vitamin K preparation (0.1–0.2 mg of menadione sodium bisulfite or 0.5 mg of vitamin K_1). A test for phenylketonuria (PKU) should be done, and T_4 should be measured. Ten to 15 mL of cord blood should be collected at birth and saved in the refrigerator for 7 days for typing, Coombs testing, and other tests if needed.

Just before discharge from the hospital, it is important to sit down with the parents to review care at home, to reassure the parents that they have a normal infant, and, particularly, to encourage them to enjoy their baby. The parents also should be assured of the availability of the pediatrician by telephone. A telephone conversation with the parents is desirable after the baby has been home for 1–2 wk.

Follow-up. The optimal time for the first routine follow-up visit depends on the status of the infant and the experience of the parents. An office visit at 3–4 wk after birth ensures that feeding is going well, provides answers to questions that have arisen, identifies and solves minor problems, and reassures the parents. Schedules for evaluation and preventive measures at specific ages are given in Table 5–5*A* and *B*.

Routine Immunization. The schedule for immunization is that recommended for routine protection of children by the Committee on Infectious Diseases of the American Academy of Pediatrics and the Advisory Committee on Immunization Practices (ACIP), United States (US) Public Health Service. Pediatricians should understand the benefits and risks of children's vaccines and should adequately inform parents about them. Untoward events following immunization must be reported to the US Department of Health and Human Services.

DIPHTHERIA AND TETANUS TOXOIDS AND PERTUSSIS (DTP) VACCINE. Immunization is usually started at 8 wk of age; two additional doses are given at 2-mo intervals. A 4th dose is given at approximately 15–18 mo of age, and a 5th dose is given at the time of school entry. DTP is not given after the 7th birthday. Instead, tetanus and diphtheria toxoids (Td) for adult use, combined Td, containing a smaller amount of diphtheria toxoid are recommended at 10-yr intervals. DTP and Td should be given intramuscularly, preferably in the anterolateral thigh in young infants and either in the thigh or deltoid in older children. Although the first three doses of DTP may be given at 1-mo intervals with the initial dose at 4 wk of age if widespread pertussis is occurring, the 2-mo interval avoids unnecessary expense and inconvenience to parents.

There are three contraindications to administering DTP:

(1) an acute febrile illness, because confusion may result as to the cause of subsequent symptoms (a minor respiratory infection is not a contraindication); (2) an evolving or suspected neurologic illness (for the same reason); and (3) a severe reaction to a prior dose of DTP.

DTP immunization of infants with underlying neurologic disorders, real or suspected, presents a special problem. Because DTP may precipitate or unmask manifestations of pre-existing neurologic problems and because temporal coincidence may result in confusion about causation, delaying initiation of DTP in such an infant for a few months until the situation is resolved is recommended. Detailed recommendations for immunizing these infants, published by the American Academy of Pediatrics and the US Public Health Services, should be consulted.

Reactions that follow DTP injection may be of three varieties. The first is minor, including local swelling and tenderness at the site of injection, slight fever, and irritability. A fever of greater than 40.5° C (105° F) is a contraindication to further doses of DTP. Second, reactions that are upsetting but without demonstrated sequelae include excessive somnolence beyond that attributable to a visit to a pediatrician and disruption of daily schedule, protracted inconsolable crying that may last 4 hr or more, and an unusual shock-like syndrome that also may last for hours. The pathogenesis of these reactions is unknown. The shock-like syndrome is a contraindication to further injections of DTP. The degrees of excessive somnolence or inconsolable crying sufficient to warrant discontinuation of DTP are matters of judgment. Third, neurologic reactions within 3 days of DTP that contraindicate further doses including occasional convulsions and, fortunately only rarely, manifestations of acute encephalopathy. The vast majority of, if not all, cases of acute encephalopathy following pertussis vaccine represent the precipitation of inevitable symptoms of previously existing but as yet unrecognized central nervous system disorders. Most experts agree that the often-quoted incidence of one case of permanent brain damage for every 310,000 doses of pertussis vaccine is a substantial overestimate; if it ever occurs, the rate is too low to be measurable. Because most of the reactivity of DTP is due to the pertussis component, the occurrence of one of these reactions does not contraindicate the continuation of immunization against diphtheria and tetanus using diphtheria and tetanus toxoids (DT) for pediatric use. Although local and febrile reactions to this preparation may occur, they are less severe than those to DTP and, except for extraordinarily rare anaphylactic reactions to tetanus toxoid, are not dangerous. Because no firm evidence exists that decreasing the dose of DTP significantly reduces the reactivity of the pertussis component, and because administering partial doses of DTP needs to be continued until the full 12 units of pertussis vaccine (1.5 mL) are given, such divided doses are not warranted.

Poliovirus Vaccines. Two types of vaccine are licensed in the United States: OPV, a live, attenuated trivalent poliovirus vaccine (Sabin), and IPV, an inactivated (killed) trivalent poliovirus vaccine (Salk). A full course of either vaccine protects the recipient against paralytic poliomyelitis almost without exception. Because rare cases of paralytic poliomyelitis occur in recipients of OPV or in their close contacts, some have advocated returning to IPV for routine immunization of children. Epidemiologic support for this recommendation comes from Sweden and other countries in which eradication of poliomyelitis has been achieved by IPV alone. The current IPV preparation, more potent than the earlier product, is presently being field tested in the United States. However, immunization advisory groups in the United States have continued to recommend OPV for routine immunization of children because of the virtual eradication of poliomyelitis from the United States by OPV and because of the belief that circulation of wild virus in the community is controlled better by the greater intestinal immunity afforded by OPV.

The first dose of OPV should be given at approximately 2 mo of age and the second dose should be given 2 mo later. Ninety-five per cent of recipients are protected against all three strains of poliomyelitis by this regimen. In communities close to areas of high endemicity of poliomyelitis, such as the southwestern United States, a third dose at 6 mo of age is recommended. An additional dose is given to all children at approximately 15–18 mo of age and another dose should be given prior to school entry. An interval of at least 2 mo between doses of OPV is required because intestinal carriage of vaccine virus may persist for up to 6 wk with consequent viral interference. The doses administered at 15–18 mo and prior to school entry are considered as "fillers" rather than as boosters in case one of the original doses did not "take." The same schedule is recommended for IPV.

OPV should not be given to individuals proven or suspected to be immunocompromised, including those with congenital and acquired immunodeficiencies and those whose immune mechanisms are impaired by therapy. OPV also should not be given to household contacts of immunocompromised individuals or to subsequent siblings of a child with congenital immunodeficiency until the younger child is shown to be normal. In circumstances in which OPV is contraindicated, IPV should be given at 2, 4, and 6 mo of age and 6–12 mo after the 3rd dose for primary immunization.

Unimmunized parents of infants scheduled for poliomyelitis immunization represent a special problem owing to their risk, albeit remote, of acquiring paralytic poliomyelitis from the vaccinated infant. In this situation, two courses of action are acceptable. The first is administering OPV to the infant, regardless of the immune status of household contacts, which is the usual practice in the United States. The second is to give three consecutive monthly doses of IPV to the adult household contacts, administering the initial dose of OPV to the infant at the time of the third dose of IPV to the contacts. If the adult household contacts have been partially immunized with OPV or IPV, they should be given OPV or IPV, respectively, at the same time that the initial dose of OPV is administered to the infant. Adults and children traveling to areas where poliomyelitis is endemic should be fully immunized with poliovirus vaccine (Sec. 5.6).

Measles-Mumps-Rubella (MMR) Vaccine, Combined. Routine immunization with these live, attenuated viruses, combined in a single preparation (MMR), should be initiated at 15 mo of age; since 1989, a second dose of MMR has been recommended by the American Academy of Pediatrics and the US Public Health Service. The reason for this second dose is that reported cases of measles, which declined to a low of 1,500 in 1983 following widespread use of measles vaccine, steadily rose to 16,000 with 45 deaths in 1989, with peak incidence rates in unvaccinated preschool children and previously vaccinated teenagers. The reasons for this recrudescence are numerous, the most important of which is unacceptably low rates of immunization of preschool children who are unaffected by school entrance laws. Other factors include vaccine failures secondary to persistence of transplacental antibody into the second year of life, simultaneous use of immune serum globulin, improper handling of vaccines (particularly the less stable preparation used prior to 1979), and, probably, waning immunity. For the second dose, MMR, rather than monovalent measles vaccine, is recommended to provide enhanced protection against rubella and mumps as well. Approximately 10% of women of childbearing age remain serosusceptible to rubella and about half of the few cases reported annually occur in individuals older than 14 yr, probably because of primary vaccine failure or lack of immu-

TABLE 5–5*A*. Evaluation at Specific Ages*

Procedure	Months							Years									
	2	4	6	9	12	15	18	2	3	4	5	6	8	10	12	14	16
Interview																	
Family history	+											+					+
Pregnancy and delivery	+																
Neontal course	+																
Other past history	+																
Development evaluation (see Sec. 3.11)	+	+	+	+	+	+	+	+	+	+	+	+	+	+	+	+	+
Body systems (for special attention)																	
Hearing, vision	+	+	+	+	+		+	+	+	+	+	+	+	+	+	+	+
Gastrointestinal (defecation, etc.)	+			+				+	+	+	+	+	+	+	+	+	+
Urinary	+							+									
Dental care									+	+	+	+	+	+	+	+	+
Drugs, alcohol, tobacco															+	+	+
Pica					+	+	+	+	+	+							
Sexual behavior														+	+	+	+
Physical examination																	
Height and weight	+	+	+	+	+	+	+	+	+	+	+	+	+	+	+	+	+
Head circumference	+	+	+	+	+												
Blood pressure									+	+	+	+	+	+	+	+	+
Vision																	
Fixes eyes	+																
Red reflex	+																
Fundus			+						+								
Strabismus			+														
Snellen chart									+		+			+			
Hearing																	
Gross	+			+													
Audiometer											+	+		+			
Speech					+			+	+								
Hip dislocation	+	+	+														
Gait						+	+	+									
Scoliosis													+	+	+	+	+
Pubertal development														+	+	+	+
Laboratory																	
Hgb or Hct				+				+					+				+
Urinalysis			+					+					+				+
Urine culture (girls)					+						+			+		+	
Tuberculin					+				+			+	+	+	+	+	+

**Note:* Interval history and dietary and sleep patterns should be included in each routine visit and are not listed on the table. Items not previously performed, as with an older child who is a new patient, should be carried out at the initial visit.

nization. Waning immunity following rubella vaccine does not appear to be a problem nor has there been an increase in incidence in recent years, compared with measles. However, although most cases of mumps represent failure to vaccinate, there is a suggestion of waning immunity following immunization with this vaccine.

Contraindications to MMR are pregnancy, immunodeficiency, therapeutic immunosuppression, or an acute febrile illness. Although no deleterious effects on the fetus have occurred when the vaccine is given in the 1st trimester, not giving MMR to pregnant women is prudent. Additionally, women of childbearing age given MMR should be warned to avoid pregnancy for the next 3 mo. As with any live virus vaccine, immunocompromised individuals should not be immunized. Immunization of individuals receiving immunosuppressive therapy should be delayed until at least 3 mo after the discontinuation of therapy. The measles and mumps vaccines are grown in chick-embryo cell culture. Because allergic reactions to these vaccines have been reported in at least five children with prior anaphylaxis from egg ingestion, such children should not receive either vaccine. Other types of egg allergy are not contraindications. Compared with OPV, transmission of measles, mumps, or rubella vaccine virus to susceptible contacts has not occurred. Therefore, the presence of a pregnant or immunocompromised household contact does not contraindicate immunization with MMR.

Adverse reactions to MMR attributable to the measles component include transient rashes and fever up to 39.4° C (103° F) occurring in a few individuals at 6–11 days after immunization. If subacute sclerosing panencephalitis (SSPE) occurs after measles vaccine, which is doubtful, it does so at a much lower rate than that following natural measles. Additionally, because of the rubella component, transient arthralgia, rarely arthritis, and paresthetic pains may occur in 1–2% of children and a higher percentage of adults, especially females, 2–8 wk after immunization; this is less common than after natural rubella. Recurrent or permanent arthritis may follow rubella vaccine, especially in adult females, in association with persistence of vaccine virus; this observation requires confirmation. Recognizable reactions to the mumps component have not occurred.

***Haemophilus influenzae* b (Hib) Vaccine.** In 1987 the first conjugated Hib vaccine (PRP-D) was licensed for use in 18-mo-old children and replaced the former unconjugated PRP preparations that were T cell independent and, therefore, ineffective in children less than 2 yr of age. More recently,

TABLE 5–5*B*. Preventive Measures at Specific Ages

Procedure	Months							Years									
	2	4	6	9	12	15	18	2	3	4	5	6	8	10	12	14	16
Immunizations																	
DTP	+	+	+			+*					+†						
Td																+	
OPV	+	+	±	(optional)		+*	+				+						
MMR										(+)‡					(+)§		
Haemophilus influenzae type b	+	+	+			+											
Influenza viral (high risk only)					+			Annually hereafter									
Pneumococcal (high risk only)								+									
Counseling (for special attention)																	
Diet	+	+	+	+	+	+	+	+	+					+	+	+	
Sleep	+	+	+		+		+	+	+			+		+	+	+	
Toilet training						+	+	+									
Accidents (see Sec. 6.31)																	
Day care									+								
School problems											+	+	+	+	+	+	+
Puberty and sexuality														+	+	+	+
Substance abuse													+	+	+	+	+

*The fourth dose of DTP and the third dose of OPV may be given simultaneously with the MMR at 15 mo, or DTP and OPV may be deferred until 18 mo.
†Immunization should be on entry to school at 4–6 years.
‡AAP recommends second dose of MMR at 5 yr of age.
§United States Public Health Service recommends 2nd dose of MMR at 12 yr of age.

studies of newer conjugated PRP vaccines have demonstrated efficacy when administered at 2 mo of age, and the first of these (HbOC) was licensed for such use in 1990. It is therefore now recommended that PRP vaccine (HbOC) be given in three doses at 2, 4, and 6 mo of age simultaneously with DTP and OPV but at a different site. A 4th dose is advised at 15 mo of age. For infants who did not receive the first three doses, two doses are recommended between 7 and 11 mo with a 3rd dose at 15 mo. For children 12 to 15 mo of age who have received no previous Hib vaccine, two doses are recommended with at least 2 mo between injections. A single dose of a conjugated vaccine is recommended for those older than 15 mo. The second licensed conjugated vaccine (PRP-OMP) is also recommended for initial immunization at 2–6 mo. Initially, 2 doses are administered at 2 mo intervals and a 3rd dose given at 12 mo of age. Initial administration after 6 mo is similar to that of HbOC. Although only a conjugated vaccine licensed for use less than 15 mo of age should be used prior to that age, any of the conjugated preparations is satisfactory for use at 15 mo of age and older. There is no interference among DTP, OPV, MMR, and these Hib vaccines. Because these recommendations, as well as those for other vaccines, may change over time, the recommendations of the American Academy of Pediatrics and the U.S. Public Health Service should be consulted.

Delayed Immunization. Infants more than 2 mo but less than 14 mo of age without any immunization should be started on the same sequence of immunizations and intervals, except for Hib vaccine (see earlier), between doses as those recommended for young infants. Infants and children who previously received one or more doses of any vaccine at intervals longer than those routinely recommended do not require initiation of the series; completion of full immunization, counting the original doses, should be undertaken.

Children 14 mo to 7 yr of age who have received no immunizations should receive DTP, OPV, and a tuberculin test at the first visit. Hib vaccine should be given as noted earlier. To provide prompt protection against measles, MMR should be given 1 mo later, followed by DTP and OPV after an additional month. Approximately 2 mo after the second DTP and OPV (4 mo after the initial doses), the third dose of DTP and, in poliomyelitis-endemic areas, the third dose of OPV should be given. DTP and OPV should be repeated approximately 1 yr later. For a child more than 4 yr of age at completion of this regimen, further immunization before school entry is unnecessary; otherwise DTP and OPV should be given again between 5 and 7 yr of age. All children should receive a dose of Td in early adolescence.

When immunization is delayed, questions arise about simultaneously administering multiple antigens, such as DTP, OPV, Hib, and MMR at the initial visit. There is no interference between DTP and OPV (or IPV). Although one study suggested that DTP and MMR given at the same time resulted in reduced seroconversion rates for measles, others have shown no difference. MMR and the "filler" dose of OPV are effective when given simultaneously in the 2nd year; whether giving MMR and the first dose of OPV at this time compromises immune response is unknown. If there is any interference with immunogenicity of one or another of these vaccines when given simultaneously, it is almost certainly slight and is outweighed by the advantage of ensuring that they have been given. Therefore, when such an older unimmunized child is seen in whom the adequacy of followup is doubtful, the simultaneous administration of DTP, OPV and MMR is reasonable. An interval of at least 1 mo should always be allowed between doses of the same or different vaccines (2 mo between doses of OPV) when they are not given simultaneously.

Special Vaccines. Annual immunization against *viral influenza* diseases is inappropriate for normal children but *should* be given to children at high risk from infections of the lower respiratory tract. Examples include children susceptible to pulmonary infections, such as those with congenital or acquired heart disease (e.g., left to right shunts); children with disorders that compromise pulmonary function, including cystic fibrosis, severe asthma, neuromuscular and orthopedic conditions that distort or weaken the thoracic cage, and pulmonary dysplasia as a consequence of the neonatal respiratory distress syndrome; children with chronic azotemic renal disease or the nephrotic syndrome; children with diabetes mellitus; and children with chronic severe anemia, such as thalassemia or sickle cell anemia. Immunodeficient and immunocompromised children may also benefit. Because the constituents of influenza vaccine must be changed annually owing to shifts in prevalent influenza viruses, annual recommendations of the US Public Health Service, published in the *Morbidity and Mortality Weekly Report*, should be consulted for doses and schedules.

The 23-valent *pneumococcal vaccine* presently licensed in the United States is not recommended for routine use in children. As with other polysaccharide vaccines, its efficacy is minimal in children under 2 yr of age. Experience with children having sickle cell anemia indicates that the vaccine is useful in children older than 2 yr who have functional or anatomic asplenia. The dose is 0.5 mL intramuscularly or subcutaneously; because antibodies persist and because reactivity is high even as long as 4 yr after the initial dose, reimmunization with pneumococcal vaccine is currently not indicated. The vaccine is probably ineffective in preventing otitis media.

Screening and Immunization for Viral Hepatitis. All newborn infants should be immunized with hepatitis B vaccine. All pregnant women should be screened for hepatitis B carriage and, if the result is positive, their infants should receive hepatitis immune globulin (HBIG) in addition to active immunization (see Sec. 9.62 and 12.79). Passive immunization with immune serum globulin should be given to all infants and children exposed to hepatitis A; there is no vaccine (see Sec. 12.79).

Miscellaneous Vaccines. The indications for the occasional use of other vaccines, such as meningococcal polysaccharide vaccine and typhoid vaccine, are discussed under those disease sections and in Sec. 5.6. Mixed respiratory vaccines and autogenous respiratory vaccines, oral or injected, are ineffective. Smallpox vaccine is not indicated for children under any circumstances.

Tuberculin Test. This should be performed early in the 2nd year of life. It may be given before or, for convenience, at the time when MMR is administered. Subsequent tuberculin testing is advisable before school entry and in early adolescence, but the physician should deviate from this schedule when circumstances, such as the local prevalence of tuberculosis, dictate.

OTHER PRIMARY PREVENTIONS. In 1987 there were 2,123,000 deaths in the United States. Arteriosclerotic heart disease and stroke accounted for almost 43% and cancer for 22% of these deaths. Because there is evidence that the factors responsible for *degenerative vascular disease* commence in childhood and that they may be somewhat controllable, considerable interest has developed in screening children for risk factors for premature degenerative cardiovascular disease and in attempting to change these risks. Risk factors include hyperlipidemia (Sec. 8.22), obesity (Sec. 4.20), hypertension (Sec. 15.81), smoking (Sec. 10.10), and, perhaps, sedentary habits. Although there are uncertainties about the role of these risk factors, their interactions, and the effects of intervention in the young, it seems prudent to discourage obesity and the initiation of smoking and to monitor blood pressure of all children. Children whose parent or grandparent had early coronary artery disease are at highest risk and, therefore, should be screened for hyperlipidemia after 2 yr of age.

Reducing the likelihood of *cancer* in later life by childhood intervention is an even more difficult problem. Age-adjusted cancer mortality rates increased 11% between 1940 and 1987; this was almost entirely due to the more than 5-fold increase in mortality from respiratory cancer, which is attributable mainly to cigarettes. Thus, preventing the initiation of smoking would produce enormous benefits. Other personal activities, including dietary habits, are variably associated epidemiologically with excessive rates of cancer at certain anatomic sites. For example, an apparent relationship between meat ingestion and bowel cancer suggests that perhaps a high-fiber diet may reduce the risk of intestinal cancer; these data have led some authorities to encourage changes in children's diets, although definitive information is not available. The effects of environmental pollution are even more uncertain. Although occupational exposure to some substances, such as arsenic, asbestos, and vinyl chloride, is known to be responsible for certain tumors (Sec. 17.1 and 26.17), the effect of general environmental pollution on cancer incidence or mortality is yet unclear. This uncertainty may be due to the long latent period between the exposure and the appearance of neoplasia and to the fact that the dramatic increase in exposure to chemicals began only 2–3 decades ago.

5.2 SECONDARY AND TERTIARY PREVENTION

Many facets of routine pediatric care (see Table 5–5*A* and *B*) represent *secondary preventive efforts*. The family history, monitoring of development, sensory evaluation, blood pressure screen programs, and the like are designed to identify the susceptibilities to, or antecedents of, later disease and thus are secondary preventive measures. Others include screening for tuberculosis, urinary tract infections, proteinuria, scoliosis, and early signs of congenital hip dysplasia. Care for the common, acute childhood illnesses also largely represents secondary prevention in that treatment for such illnesses in many cases prevents sequelae that would occur in very few. For example, streptococcal pharyngitis is treated to prevent rheumatic fever and suppurative complications, such as peritonsillar abscesses. Furthermore, acute bacterial otitis media will subside spontaneously in up to 95% of cases; the major benefit of antimicrobial therapy is the prevention of mastoiditis or chronic perforation of the ear drum (Sec. 22.22).

Similarly, a great deal of care for chronic illness and disability in childhood represents *tertiary prevention* (Sec. 3.57). Examples include many facets of care for children with cystic fibrosis, orthopedic measures for cerebral palsy and neural tube defects, antistreptococcal prophylaxis for those having had rheumatic fever, and physiotherapy for children with rheumatoid arthritis. The pediatrician is additionally responsible for providing continuous support to the family while ameliorating as much as possible the social, psychologic, and financial effects of chronic illness on the child and other family members. Because such children often require the attention of subspecialists and various services, such as physiotherapy, occupational therapy, and nutritional counseling, the pediatrician must coordinate these activities while providing regular child health care and treatment of intercurrent illness. The pediatrician should ensure that care proffered or recommended by other providers, including subspecialists and nonmedical health care professionals, is considered comprehensively, with respect to all aspects of the child and the family and to the probabilities that diagnostic and therapeutic benefits will outweigh the risks, untoward effects, and costs.

5.3 EPIDEMIOLOGY IN PEDIATRICS

Epidemiology is the scientific study of factors influencing health, disease, and the control of disease in populations rather than in individuals. Historically, epidemiology began with the search for clues to the causation of disease; more recently it has been used in assessing preventive and therapeutic measures and in evaluating health services, including costs.

Physicians are constantly applying *clinical epidemiology* as a science of probabilities in making decisions. For example, whether to obtain a throat culture from a child with fever and an injected pharynx is a decision involving an assessment of the likelihood that group A streptococci will be recovered from the culture, which depends on a wide spectrum of variables, including the age of the child, the season of the year, existing disease patterns in the community, the clinical features of the child's illness, and the chance of the child's developing rheumatic fever if streptococcal pharyngitis is not recognized and treated because the throat was not cultured. These variables consist of a series of probabilities established by observations of large groups of children (with and without streptococcal pharyngitis) and by the physician's own experiences. These probabilities cannot always be precisely quantitated and are subject to judgment; nonetheless, they are useful in clinical decision-making.

Much of this clinical epidemiology is intuitive or informal and is not recognized as such by the physician; an example is the influence of knowing "what's going around" the community at the moment, such as "the flu" or parainfluenza infections associated with croup. The recognition that a school has an excess of cases of streptococcal pharyngitis or that a child attending day-care developed *Haemophilus influenzae* meningitis is important mini-epidemiology. Knowledge of current community epidemiology is often invaluable and extends beyond infectious disease epidemiology. For example, impressions about substance abuse in a local secondary school may provide clues about the appearance of behavioral changes in an adolescent. It is also important to have general knowledge of community problems that may influence the well-being of children and adolescents, ranging from "gangs" or rates of teenage pregnancy to the closing of a factory that may have economic implications.

Such informal or intuitive epidemiology should be combined with more formal clinical epidemiologic information in the management of health and disease in children. Formal epidemiology, derived from the medical literature, guides the physician in the use of diagnostic measures, assessing the risks and benefits of therapy, and estimating a prognosis. Recommendations of public health advisory committees, such as those of the American Academy of Pediatrics, are usually based on studies that are published in the medical literature. Information intended to influence patient management is provided by other sources as well, including reports at meetings, colleagues, pharmaceutical manufacturers, and, sometimes, the media; this information varies in validity. Accordingly, in order to provide optimum care, the physician should be able to assess the soundness of the evidence that he or she should adopt a new modality of care and the methods by which that evidence was obtained, which is often epidemiologic.

There are three types of epidemiologic studies. *Descriptive epidemiology* records the incidence and prevalence of death, disability, and disease of various types and causes. National, state, county, city, and local health departments and other agencies in the United States tabulate current information about health and disease. The National Center for Health Statistics and the Centers for Disease Control publish detailed morbidity and mortality data for the entire United States, for individual states, and, to a limited extent, for counties and metropolitan areas. *Causative (analytic) epidemiology* searches for clues to the causes of disease based on the fact that disease does not occur randomly in the population. Differences exist between those who incur a disease and those who do not, which may be due to inherent characteristics of the individuals themselves or to the experiences of the individual. A given characteristic is said to be "associated" with a disease when it is found more often in those with the illness than in those without it. *Experimental epidemiology* uses clinical trials to compare responses to different therapies in groups of subjects.

There are three subtypes of causative epidemiology studies: cross-sectional, prospective, and retrospective. *Cross-sectional studies* are usually surveys that determine differences in prevalences of disease among various segments of the population at a particular time. A *prospective study* identifies a cohort of individuals who exhibit a particular characteristic, such as hypertension or exposure to an environmental pollutant, and follows them over time for the development of disease; a comparable cohort of persons without hypertension or exposure would also be similarly followed over time for the development of disease. The major advantage of such studies is that the actual rate of disease attributable to the factor in question can be determined because the numbers of those at risk, those not at risk, and those who develop disease in both groups are available. Disadvantages are that the investigator must suspect in advance which factor is associated with the disease, an unrecognized causative factor may exist but not be considered, and the disease must be reasonably frequent, because the cohorts of exposed and unexposed persons would otherwise be of unwieldy size. Sometimes conducting a prospective study by retrospection is possible by identifying cohorts of exposed and unexposed persons from prior records; an example is the study of gynecologic abnormalities in female offspring of women who did or did not receive diethylstilbestrol (DES) during their pregnancies.

Retrospective (case-control) epidemiologic studies start with disease and search for previous differences in exposure or other characteristics between groups of affected and nonaffected persons. This type of study is useful particularly in two situations: first, when few or no clues to causation exist; and second, when the causative agent is strongly suspected but the disorders in question are so rare that prospective studies are not feasible logistically and economically. An example of the first type is a study of Reye syndrome in which parents of patients and controls were asked about possible exposures to different types of medications and to various environmental substances; a strong association between salicylate use and subsequent Reye syndrome was observed.

Retrospective studies have certain disadvantages. The **absolute risk** of disease after exposure (the number of cases per 100,000 exposed persons) cannot be determined because the denominator of exposed individuals is unavailable. Only an estimate of **relative risk** (ratio or disease frequencies in exposed and unexposed persons) can be obtained. There is also considerable potential for bias in the selection of controls and in the differences of recall that exist between patients and controls.

Causative epidemiologic studies are frequently criticized because association does not prove causation. This is true; however, the strength of the association (i.e., the magnitude of the difference between cases and controls) and the lack of a plausible alternative for explaining the difference may be such that association is tantamount to causation even though the specific etiologic mechanism is unknown. Causation studies often require a judgmental decision, such as with aspirin and Reye syndrome.

In *experimental epidemiology* or a *clinical trial,* the effect of a new preventive or therapeutic measure is compared with another form of treatment or to no treatment by randomly assigning comparable patients to each measure. Groups of patients are usually necessary for comparison purposes because the outcomes of most diseases are variable, which prevents drawing conclusions from only one or several individuals. Randomization within certain subgroups, such as by age or sex, is sometimes desirable and is called stratified randomization. In a double-blind study, both the experimenters and the subjects are unaware of treatment assignment. In a single-blind study, the experimenters but not the patients are aware of treatment assignment. In a triple-blind study, not only the experimenters and patients but also those conducting the analyses are unaware of treatment assignment.

In comparative epidemiologic studies (causative and experimental epidemiology), there is always potential for three types of **bias:** selection, confounding, and observational. Selection bias is an inherent difference between the study and control groups that might influence the results. For example, in a clinical trial of a new drug or a new surgical procedure, if the control group is more seriously ill than the study group, the benefits might be mistakenly attributed to the new measure. Alternatively, if the study group consisted of more severe cases, a beneficial effect of the new treatment might be obscured. Selection bias may occur in causative epidemiology if the control group differs, in addition to the factor in question, in some other inherent characteristic or exposure related to the outcome. An example is the reported association between coffee consumption and cancer of the pancreas. Coffee consumption by patients and controls hospitalized with other diseases was determined by interview. Patients with alcohol- and tobacco-related diseases were excluded from the control group; however, because alcohol and tobacco use are associated with coffee consumption, it is possible that persons who drink little or no coffee were overly represented in the control group. The association may therefore be spurious.

Confounding bias occurs when another factor linked to the disease or to the issue in question is also associated with the characteristic being studied. For example, one might conclude that chronic tonsillitis occurred more frequently in a suburban community than in the inner city because of the greater number of tonsillectomies performed in the suburbs. However, this conclusion is unjustified, because affluence is associated both with an increased tonsillectomy rate and with living in a suburb. Confounding bias may also occur in clinical trials when there are differences in management of the groups being compared other than the therapeutic modality being evaluated. For example, if antibiotic A is being compared with antibiotic B in the treatment of otitis media, but myringotomy is also performed on those who receive antibiotic A, apparent superiority of antibiotic A over antibiotic B cannot be attributed to antibiotic A, because benefit may well have been due to the myringotomy, which is then said to be a confounder.

Observational bias occurs either when the study or the control group is observed more intensively that the other group, when there is greater interest in recalling previous events by patients than by controls, or when there is a placebo effect. An example of observational bias due to the placebo effect is a study of a cold vaccine conducted on the University of Minnesota students before World War II. Students reporting undue susceptibility to colds received a vaccine and during the subsequent year noted a 70% reduction in colds. However, unknown to the students, about half of them received a saline placebo, and those students in this group experienced the same reduction.

Pediatricians are exposed constantly to new information intended to modify the way in which they practice medicine, and they have a responsibility to evaluate such information critically, using their basic medical knowledge and their knowledge of study design and analysis. They should examine the studies' methods, particularly for the possibility of bias. Because degrees of bias are inescapable in almost all studies, it is important to make a judgment based on medical knowledge about whether the bias is sufficient to negate the conclusions. If the results seem valid, pediatricians should then decide whether these results apply to their patient population and whether they should alter their own medical practices.

BIOSTATISTICS. This method is used in clinical epidemiology to determine the likelihood that an observed difference between the groups studied is explained by chance. A *p value* of less than 0.05, for example, indicates that the probability that the difference between the groups due to chance is less than 5%; one is 95% certain that the difference is not due to chance. Three corollaries of this approach should be kept in mind. First, a p value indicates only the probability of a true difference, but this does not mean that the true difference is exactly that which has been observed; it may turn out to be more or less if the study populations were expanded to include infinite numbers of subjects. *Confidence limits* are frequently provided to indicate the range of probabilities created by the use of a finite number of subjects. For example, a causative epidemiologic study might find that, compared with no exposure, exposure to a given chemical increases the likelihood of developing a particular cancer 12-fold (a relative risk of 12). But if the study was based on only 20 patients with the tumor, it would be reported as a relative risk of 12 (95% confidence interval 7.3–18.5), meaning that one can be 95% confident that exposure to the chemical increases the risk of that cancer between 7-fold and 18-fold. If the lower limit of the 95% confidence interval is less than 0, the significance is less than 5%.

Second, a p value of 0.05 means that one *expects* a difference as large as that observed to occur once in 20 times owing to chance. Thus, if statistical tests are made of 100 variables in a study, one should not be surprised to find that five tests produced p values of 0.05; indeed one of them should reach the 0.01 level. For example, in repeatedly flipping a coin, the probability that heads will appear five times in a row is 0.03125 ($p < 0.04$). This also means that, if one flips a coin in repeated series of five tosses, all heads should occur once in every 32 series of five flips.

The third corollary is that biostatistical significance tests are not a substitute for critically assessing the study methods combined with medical judgment, which includes assessing the importance of the health problem in question.

There are many statistical tests, with each or several being applicable to special situations. Most commonly used are tests for differences between proportions, such as the percentage of patients cured with one drug compared with those cured with another (e.g., the chi-square test). For comparisons of means, Student's t-test is used. Reference texts should be consulted for further explanation of these and other methods of statistical and epidemiologic analysis.

GENERAL

Fulginiti VA, Bartlett VE, Book LS, et al: Pediatric patient education: Challenge for the '80s. Pediatrics 74(Suppl):913, 1984.

Roghmann KJ, Hoekelman RA, McInerny TK: The changing pattern of primary pediatric care: Update for one community. Pediatrics 73:363, 1984.

MORBIDITY AND MORTALITY

Centers for Disease Control: Summary of notifiable diseases, United States, 1988. MMWR 37(54), 1989.

National Center for Health Statistics: Advance Report of Final Mortality Statistics, 1987: Monthly Vital Statistics Report, Vol 38, no 5 suppl. Hyattsville, MD, Public Health Service, 1989.
National Center for Health Statistics (D Graham): Detailed diagnoses and procedures for patients discharged from short-stay hospitals, United States, 1986. Vital Health Statistics. Series 13, No 95. DHHS Pub No (PHS) 88–1756. Public Health Service. Washington, US Government Printing Office, 1988.
National Center for Health Statistics and its predecessors: Vital Statistics of the United States, 1900–1985.
US Bureau of the Census: Historical Statistics of the United States: Colonial Times to 1970, Bicentennial ed, Part 2. Washington, DC, 1975.
Wegman ME: Special article. Annual summary of vital statistics—1988. Pediatrics 84:943, 1989.

PUBLIC HEALTH MEASURES

Centers for Disease Control: AIDS and human immunodeficiency virus infection in the United States: 1988 update. MMWR 38(Suppl 5–4):1, 1989.
Horowitz AM, Thomas HB (eds): Promoting the use of fluorides in communities: Past accomplishments and future perspectives. A symposium. Presented at the annual session of the American Association for Dental Research, March 20, 1980, Los Angeles. J Public Health Dent 40:211, 1980.
Jones RB, Mormann DN, Durtsche TB: Commentary: Fluoridation referendum in LaCrosse, Wisconsin: Contributing factors to success. Am J Public Health 79:1405, 1989.

ACCIDENTS, VIOLENCE, AND SUBSTANCE ABUSE

Boyce WE, Sprunger LW, Sobolewski S, et al: Epidemiology of injuries in a large urban school district. Pediatrics 74:342, 1984.
Centers for Disease Control: Playground-related injuries in preschool-aged children—United States, 1983–1987. MMWR 37:629, 1988.
Centers for Disease Control: Temporal patterns of motor-vehicle-related fatalities associated with young drinking drivers—United States, 1983. MMWR 33:699, 1984.
Centers for Disease Control: Violent deaths among persons 15–25 years of age—United States, 1970–1978. MMWR 32:453, 1983.
Chafee-Bahamon C, Lovejoy FH Jr: Effectiveness of a regional poison center in reducing excess emergency room visits for children's poisonings. Pediatrics 72:164, 1983.
Chandler JK, Tingle AJ, Petty RE: Persistent rubella infection with chronic arthritis in children. N Engl J Med 313:1117, 1985.
Committee on Accident and Poison Prevention, American Academy of Pediatrics: Automatic passenger protection systems. Pediatrics 74:146, 1984.
Committee on Accident and Poison Prevention, American Academy of Pediatrics: Skateboard injuries. Pediatrics 83:1070, 1989.
Decker MD, Dewey MJ, Hutcheson RH Jr, et al: The use and efficacy of child restraint devices. JAMA 252:2571, 1984.
Dolan MA, Knapp JF, Andres J: Three-wheel and four-wheel all-terrain vehicle injuries in children. Pediatrics 84:694, 1989.
O'Malley PM, Bachman JG, Johnston LD: Period, age and cohort effects on substance use by young Americans: A decade of change, 1976–86. Am J Public Health 78:1315, 1989.
Sudak HS, Ford AB, Rushforth NB: Suicide in the Young. Boston, MA, John Wright-PSG Inc, 1984.
Torg J, Das M: Trampoline-related quadriplegia: Review of the literature and reflections on the American Academy of Pediatrics' position statement. Pediatrics 74:804, 1984.
Westman JS, Morrow G III: Moped injuries in children. Pediatrics 74:820, 1984.
Widome MD: Commentary: On the relevance of poor judgment. Pediatrics 84:724, 1989.

ADOLESCENT PREGNANCY

National Center for Health Statistics: Advance Report of Final Natality Statistics, 1987. Monthly Vital Statistics Report, Vol 38, No 3(Suppl). Hyattsville, MD, Public Health Service, 1989.
National Center for Health Statistics: Annual Summary of Births, Marriages, Divorces and Deaths: United States, 1988: Monthly Vital Statistics Report, Vol 37, No 13. Hyattsville, MD, Public Health Service, 1989.

ROUTINE CHILD HEALTH MAINTENANCE

Casto DT, Brunell PA: Safe handling of vaccines. Pediatrics 87:108, 1991.
Centers for Disease Control: National Childhood Vaccine Injury Act: Requirements for permanent vaccination records and for reporting of selected events after vaccination. MMWR 37:197, 1988.
Cody CL, Baraff LJ, Cherry JD, et al: Nature and rates of adverse reactions associated with DTP and DT immunizations in infants and children. Pediatrics 68:650, 1981.
Committee on Practice and Ambulatory Medicine, American Academy of Pediatrics: Recommendations for Preventive Pediatric Care. Elk Grove Village, IL, American Academy of Pediatrics, 1987.
Committee on Psychosocial Aspects of Child and Family Health, American Academy of Pediatrics: The prenatal visit. Pediatrics 73:561, 1984.
Current status of Haemophilus influenza type b vaccines. Pediatrics (Suppl)85 (Part 2):631, 1990.
Miller DL, Ross EM, Alderslade R, et al: Pertussis immunisation and serious acute neurological illness in children. Br Med J 282:1595, 1981.
Plotkin SA, Mortimer EA Jr: Vaccines. Philadelphia, WB Saunders, 1988.
Recommendation of the Immunization Practices Advisory Committee (ACIP): Diphtheria, tetanus, and pertussis: Guidelines for vaccine prophylaxis and other preventive measures. MMWR 34:405, 1985.
Report of the Committee on Infectious Diseases, 20th ed. Elk Grove Village, IL, American Academy of Pediatrics, 1988.

PREVENTION OF DISEASE IN LATER LIFE

American Heart Association. Inter-Society Commission for Heart Disease Resources: Special report: Optimal resources for primary prevention of atherosclerotic diseases. Circulation 70:153A, 1984.
Committee on Nutrition, American Academy of Pediatrics: Toward a prudent diet for children. Pediatrics 71:78, 1983.

EPIDEMIOLOGY

Diehl HS, Baker AB, Cowan DW: Cold vaccines. JAMA 111:1168, 1938.
Fletcher RH, Fletcher SW, Wagner EH: Clinical Epidemiology: The Essentials, 2nd ed. Baltimore, Williams & Wilkins, 1982.
Friedman GD: Primer of Epidemiology, 2nd ed. New York, McGraw-Hill, 1980.
Goldbloom R: Science and empiricism in pediatrics. Pediatrics 73:693, 1984.
Halpin TJ, Holtzhauer FJ, Campbell RJ, et al: Reye's syndrome and medication use. JAMA 248:687, 1982.
Haynes RB: How to read clinical journals. II: To learn about a diagnostic test. Can Med Assoc J 124:703, 1981.
Hennekens CH, Buring JE, Mayrent SL: Epidemiology in Medicine. Boston, Little, Brown, 1987.
MacMahon B, Yen S, Trichopoulos D, et al: Coffee and cancer of the pancreas. N Engl J Med 304:630, 1981.
Mausner JS, Kramer S: Epidemiology: An Introductory Text. Philadelphia, WB Saunders, 1985.
Sackett DL: How to read clinical journals. I: Why to read them and how to start reading them critically. Can Med Assoc J 124:555, 1981.
Sackett DL: How to read clinical journals. V: To distinguish useful from useless or even harmful therapy. Can Med Assoc J 124:1156, 1981.
Trout KS: How to read clinical journals. IV: To determine etiology or causation. Can Med Assoc J 124:985, 1981.
Tugwell PX: How to read clinical journals. III: To learn the clinical course and prognosis of disease. Can Med Assoc J 124:869, 1981.

5.4 CHILD HEALTH IN THE DEVELOPING WORLD

The health status of most children in the world is pathetically different from that in developed countries, such as the United States. In the developing world 15% or more of children born each year die before they reach 5 yr of age compared with 1.3% of such children in the United States. In 1987 in five countries (Afghanistan, Mali, Mozambique, Angola, and Sierra Leone) the mortality rate under 5 yr of age exceeded 27%, a rate half again higher than that of the United States in 1900. These enormous differences exist for many reasons, the most important of which are social, political, and economic, and access to the beneficial effects of modern medical science depends to a great extent on solutions to these underlying problems.

Immediate contributing medical causes of childhood death and morbidity in developing countries are the high prevalence of infants born at low birthweight, of children with inadequate nutrition, and of infants and children with serious infectious diseases, especially diarrhea, respiratory infections, and parasitic infestations (Sec. 12.105). For 1987, it is estimated that there were 137 million births worldwide; of these, 119 million (87%) occurred in the developing world. Of the 14.7 million under-5-yr deaths in 1987, 14.3 million (97%) occurred in the developing world. Approximately 3.5 million (24%) of these deaths were attributed to four vaccine-preventable diseases (measles, pertussis, poliomyelitis, and neonatal tetanus). Thirty to 50% of deaths were attributable to diarrhea and malnutrition, and the remainder were attributable to respiratory disease and other causes.

Vital statistics on health in the developing world are imprecise and vary from one country to another. Furthermore, their interpretation is confounded by the interaction of malnutrition with infection, especially the debilitating cycle of diarrhea and malnutrition. For example, measles is clearly associated with higher mortality in young children of borderline nutritional status who experience enteritis shortly before or during measles. Conversely, episodes of enteritis soon after recovery from measles are more likely to be fatal. Moreover, measles may itself exacerbate chronic diarrheal states.

Comparison of patterns of childhood mortality in currently developing countries with those that existed at the turn of the 20th century in the now-developed countries suggests certain similarities and differences. For example, in 1900 more than 60% of childhood deaths in the United States were attributed to infection, as they are in developing countries today. However, children in the developing world at present probably suffer somewhat more from malnutrition and have more parasitic diseases. It is also important to note that the decline in such mortality in the developed countries began before the application of preventive and therapeutic medical measures, such as immunizations and antimicrobial agents, suggesting that other factors, known and unknown, had major roles in reducing childhood mortality.

Because of interactions among low birthweight, malnutrition, and infections, there is a need to address these problems concurrently. Furthermore, because the severity of these problems parallels that of social, economic, educational, and political problems and because these problems are sometimes complicated by unanticipated natural disasters, nonmedical problems should be addressed concomitantly with direct medical intervention to achieve optimum results.

LOW BIRTHWEIGHT (See also Sec. 9.7). About 27 million of the 137 million infants born annually worldwide weigh less than 2,500 g; increased mortality rates in surviving infants continue throughout the first few years of life, in part because low-birthweight infants are more likely to become malnourished children. In countries with infant mortality rates exceeding 100/1,000 live births in 1987, the proportion of low-birthweight infants (< 2,500 g) averaged 2½ times that in developed countries; in some countries, it is up to 5-fold greater. These low-birthweight infants are two to three times as likely to die in infancy as are those of normal weight.

Three factors amenable to intervention contribute to low birthweight: (1) maternal malnutrition, which may date back to childhood as well as result from inadequate food during pregnancy (food supplements for such pregnant women are associated with higher birthweights of their infants); (2) maternal infection, such as tuberculosis, malaria, and other parasitic diseases (this is mediated through aggravation of nutritional deficits as well as having an independent effect); and (3) short intervals between pregnancies. Encouragement of breast-feeding, which interferes with conception, and family planning can reduce this problem.

CHILDHOOD MALNUTRITION (Sec. 4.15). Inadequate nutrition is often preceded by low birthweight; these small infants are 3–4 times more likely to become malnourished children than infants of normal weight. Malnutrition in childhood is aggravated further by diarrhea and other infections. Countries with the highest infant mortality rates also have the highest death rates for children 1–4 yr old. In these countries, the average caloric intake is 30% less than in countries with the lowest mortality; in many countries, the caloric deficits are greater, and within each of these countries there are populations with even greater deficits.

Morley thinks that the most important cause of childhood malnutrition is infection, including repeated diarrhea, parasitic diseases, measles, pertussis, and tuberculosis. These infections, whether acute or chronic, induce anorexia and divert nutrient energy from growth and development. He also points out that diets based mainly on grain (e.g., gruel and pap) have such a low-calorie content that the sheer bulk required for normal energy and growth requirements exceeds the ingestion capacity of many small children. This problem is uncommon in developed countries where high-calorie fats and oils constitute a larger part of children's diets. Furthermore, in some cases, caloric intake is adequate, but there is deficient protein consumption (Sec. 4.17). Lastly, Morley cites inadequate knowledge of elementary diet requirements as a major cause of malnutrition. In deprived areas, mothers also often do not recognize that their children are malnourished, because they look no different from other children whom they see.

These factors, in combination with each other and often with low birthweight, constitute a debilitating complex of causation that is not easily overcome. Mortality is high, and in survivors growth is stunted, and psychologic and emotional development is impaired. Furthermore, the malnourished child has little energy available for the usual childhood activities that contribute to normal development; the daily caloric expenditure of malnourished African children in play is approximately 40% that of their European counterparts. Amelioration of childhood malnutrition in the developing world requires attracting the attention of affected populations, especially the mothers, to the problem and educating them about its solutions. Morley advocates providing a simple chart for the mother as well as for health care workers that graphically indicates growth in height and weight and development. If the mothers are literate, messages about family planning, immunizations, available resources for health care, and other information may be included with the chart.

DIARRHEA AND OTHER ENTERIC DISEASES. The United Nations International Children's Emergency Fund (UNICEF) and the World Health Organization (WHO) estimate that worldwide one child dies of diarrhea every 6 sec. Rates of enteric infection and consequent mortality are related closely to the lack of sanitary water supplies and to improper food handling. Safe public water is available to few in the developing world; refrigeration, food inspection, and other measures for control of enteric disease are usually lacking. For economic, political, logistic, and other reasons, these deficits are unlikely to be corrected in the near future. However, two interventions useful in ameliorating this illness are breast-feeding and oral rehydration therapy (ORT).

Unfortunately, about 25 yr ago a trend away from breast-feeding and toward bottle feeding began in the developed world. Bottle feeding requires safe water, sterilization, and refrigeration, resources that are often unavailable. Furthermore, powdered milk is costly and, therefore, may be overdiluted to save money. Illiterate parents also may make errors in preparing formula. The result is often contaminated formula, improperly diluted, leading to diarrhea and malnutrition. Recognizing that the widespread use of artificial infant feeding contributes significantly to morbidity and mortality from diarrhea in developing countries, WHO, UNICEF, and various governments instituted measures to encourage breast-feeding and discourage artificial feeding. In 1981, the WHO issued stringent guidelines (a Code) to limit the marketing of artificial milk substitutes by prohibiting or restricting various advertising and promotional practices. Governments were also urged to vigorously encourage breast-feeding. Where these recommendations have been observed, sharp reductions in morbidity and mortality from infant diarrhea have occurred.

ORT is based on the observation that diarrheal dehydration rarely occurs if the affected infants can drink and retain adequate fluid containing small amounts of electrolyte and carbohydrate (Sec. 6.17 and 6.18). WHO and UNICEF, as well as certain countries, distribute 300 million individual ORT packets each year containing 3.5 g of NaCl, 2.5 g of $NaHCO_3$, 1.5 g of KCl, and 20 g glucose in dried form, to be dissolved in 1 liter of water. More than 90% of diarrheal episodes in children can be treated with ORT. In some communities in which ORT has been used, childhood mortality from diarrhea has been reduced by 50–60%. However, there are 1 billion or more episodes of childhood diarrhea worldwide with more than 5 million deaths from dehydration each year. The number of ORT packets produced annually is insufficient; many children reside in areas that are too remote for supplies to be available; and a high proportion of community health workers are not trained in its use. In some countries, indigenous health care workers and mothers are trained to substitute ingredients that are readily available locally for those in the packet. For example, in Bangladesh, mothers are instructed to mix a three-finger pinch of salt and a fistful of molasses in a "seer" (approximately 1 quart) of water; analyses of the electrolyte content of these mixtures indicate that a safe and effective solution almost always results. Worldwide approximately 25% of diarrhea episodes in children less than 5 yr old are treated with ORT (Fig. 5–1).

IMMUNIZATION-PREVENTABLE DISEASES. Since 1977, WHO and UNICEF have conducted vigorous efforts (the Expanded Program on Immunization [EPI]) to make immunization against six illnesses available to all children in the developing world. These diseases are diphtheria, pertussis, tetanus, measles, poliomyelitis, and tuberculosis, which are estimated to kill one child every 6 sec and to disable another child every 6 sec (Fig. 5–2). As of 1983, WHO estimated that immunization was unavailable to 80% of the more than 100 million children born annually in the developing world. The major problems in achieving a goal of universal immunization are societal and organizational.

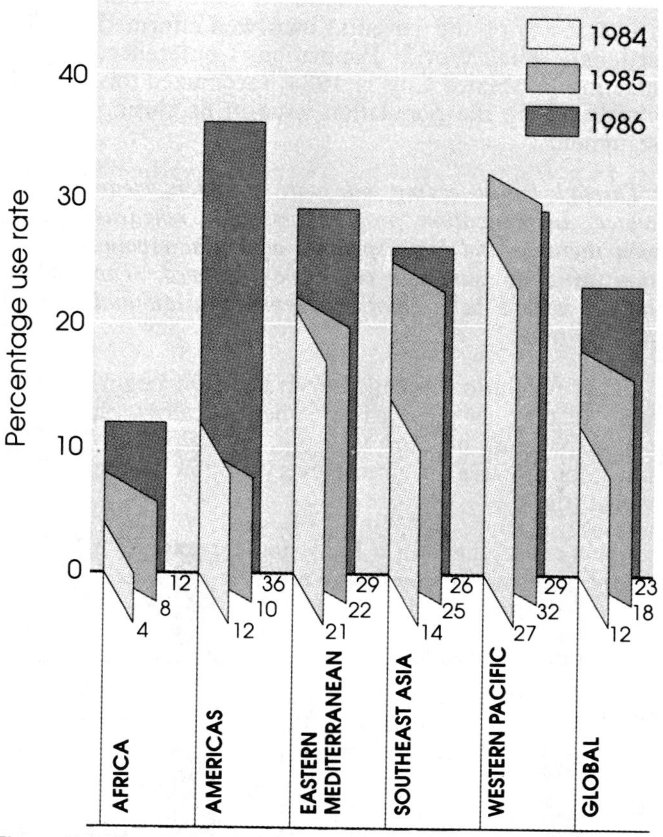

Figure 5–1. Percentage of diarrhea episodes in children under 5 yr of age being treated with ORT, 1984–1986. (Reproduced from State of the World's Children, 1989 [UNICEF] with permission.)

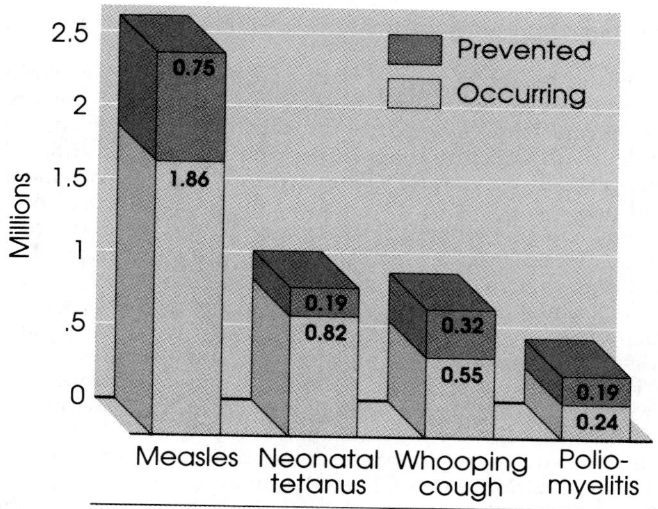

Figure 5–2. Estimated deaths and prevented deaths from vaccine-preventable diseases, in the developing world in 1988. (Reproduced from State of the World's Children, 1989 [UNICEF] with permission.)

The EPI plan was for WHO and UNICEF to encourage and assist individual countries in developing their own EPIs. Although many countries have done so and indeed are beginning to keep records of the incidence of these diseases and the numbers of children immunized, major problems in implementation have occurred. Senior- and middle-level managers have been trained by EPI, but the subsequent recruitment, training, and supervision of the thousands of field workers who are ultimately responsible for the delivery of these vaccines to children have been impeded by the lack of governmental commitment and delegation of authority, insufficient financial resources, and increasing ineffectiveness in the quality of training as it passed from one level to the next. There are also major logistic problems in reaching children who live in poverty in cities and who live in remote areas.

Achieving compliance with the full immunization series is also extremely difficult: parents may not understand the importance, they may have other pressing responsibilities, and access to the field health center, although short in miles, may be limited owing to the absence of roads, vehicles, and other methods of transportation.

There are also technical problems, particularly in remote areas. Maintenance of the "cold chain" necessary for vaccine preservation may not be possible because of the absence of electricity. Attempts are being made to develop new methods of refrigeration and new methods for determining whether a vaccine has been inactivated by breaks in the cold chain. There are also problems with sterilization; disposable syringes and needles are too expensive and impractical for many areas. An additional problem is that several vaccines require multiple doses; efforts are being made to provide slow- or intermittent-release preparations that will require fewer or single doses. Nonetheless, despite all these problems, at present two thirds of infants in developing countries receive bacille Calmette-Guerin (BCG), 3 DTP, 3 OPV, and measles vaccine. Currently, immunization is unavailable to only 20% of the world's children. Unfortunately, only 25% of mothers receive tetanus toxoid.

The health problems of children in the developing world require that immunization be combined with other primary health care services, including prenatal care, family planning for mothers, efforts to control enteric diseases, and nutritional services. These services depend on community involvement and interest, which in turn depend on social, political, economic, and geographic considerations. Furthermore, the customs, mores, attitudes, and priorities as well as the political and organizational situations in developing countries usually differ from those in the developed world, as well as from each other. Sensitivity to these differences is critical to successful implementation of preventive health measures.

Finally, effects of the outcome of a particular preventive program on other problems should be considered. A reduction of infant mortality by immunization and ORT in a community with inadequate nutritional resources to feed increased numbers of children requires family planning, greater food production, and other changes in order to achieve real benefits from the increased survival.

Additionally, many serious problems remain and new ones, such as AIDS, have occurred (Sec. 12.82). Maternal mortality remains high (½ million deaths annually, of which about 40% are due to illegal abortion), and adequate family planning is unavailable to most women. In developing nations there has also been a decline in spending for social, educational, and health efforts since 1980, in part owing to weakening of economic growth.

EDWARD A. MORTIMER, JR

Abed FH: Household teaching of ORT in rural Bangladesh: Case study. Assignment Children (UNICEF) 61/62:249, 1983.

Kerr RA: Fifteen years of African drought. Science 227:1453, 1985.

McKeown T: The Role of Medicine: Dream, Mirage or Nemesis? Princeton, NJ, Princeton University Press, 1979.

Morley D: Growth monitoring. *In:* State of the World's Children 1984. New York, Oxford University Press, 1983, p 77.

UNICEF: State of the World's Children 1989. New York, Oxford University Press, 1989.

WHO/UNICEF. The management of diarrhea and use of oral rehydration therapy: A joint WHO/UNICEF statement. Assignment Children 61/62:77, 1983.

5.5 CHILDREN AT SPECIAL RISK

In this section, the health issues faced by some of the most socioculturally disadvantaged children in the United States are discussed: native Americans, migrants, immigrants, homeless children and runaways, and children in foster care. The biologic causes of special risk are covered elsewhere. Both groups of causes often overlap.

Most children in the United States today grow up loved and supported, although many have problems that disturb their parents and blight their future. However, for a small but significant number of children, their circumstances are so dismal that one wonders how many survive. Examples of children with even more dismal futures than these also exist elsewhere in the world, such as children growing up in the midst of the Israel-Palestine conflict, or in Northern Ireland, Eritrea, Uganda, Soweto, or Beirut. Many of the children growing up in these environments will be damaged and their futures will be compromised, unless effective interventions are mounted. However, in all of these situations, a few children are so resilient that they survive and actually thrive. Werner has characterized these children as "vulnerable but invincible." The fact that a few defy the odds does not absolve society from attempting to help the majority of those who do not, although these resilient ones can teach us what it takes to survive.

The majority of children at special risk need a nurturant environment but have had their futures compromised by actions or policies arising from their environment: their families, schools, communities, and nation. The challenge is to improve the environment of children at risk so that most can achieve their full potential. Many of the problems of these children are due to multiple causes, and many of these causes are similar, whether the end result is homeless children, runaways, children in foster care, or other disadvantaged groups. From a preventive point of view, the most effective approach involves alleviation of poverty, poor housing, and lack of jobs. From a medical point of view, optimal care of these children requires specially organized programs, multidiscipline teams, and special financing.

NATIVE AMERICANS, INCLUDING ALASKAN ESKIMOS AND ALEUTS

Children of native Americans have higher than average rates of many physical and psychologic disorders. They are one group in the United States for whom a separately organized health service has long been in place, the Indian Health Service. There are approximately 1.3 million Indian and Alaskan native Americans, 44% of whom are under 20 yr of age, a much higher proportion of children than for the remainder of the United States. Both the unemployment and poverty levels of native Americans are twice those of the national average, and far fewer native Americans graduate from high school or go on to college (Fig. 5–3).

The rate of *low birthweight* is less than the national average (especially for babies of younger mothers), 6% compared with 6.8% for the United States as a whole, and less than half that of blacks; and the *neonatal mortality* rate is only 0.6 times the national average, whereas the *postneonatal mortality* rate is 1.4 times the average in the United States (Fig. 5–4). Deaths during the 1st yr of life from sudden infant death syndrome and pneumonia and influenza are higher than the average in the United States, whereas deaths from congenital anomalies, respiratory distress syndrome, and disorders relating to short gestation and low birthweight are all lower. These deviations from the usual higher rates of low birthweight and resultant neonatal deaths found in other poverty groups are poorly understood. It is doubtful whether it results from good prenatal care alone, although prenatal care is readily available and accepted on many reservations. It probably arises from

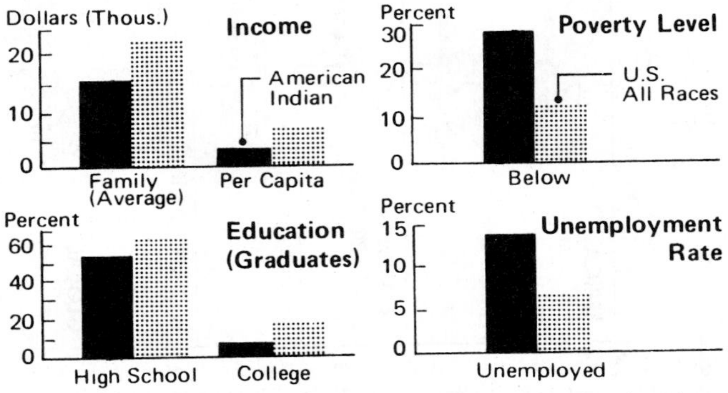

Figure 5–3. Social and economic characteristics of native Americans and all races in the United States.

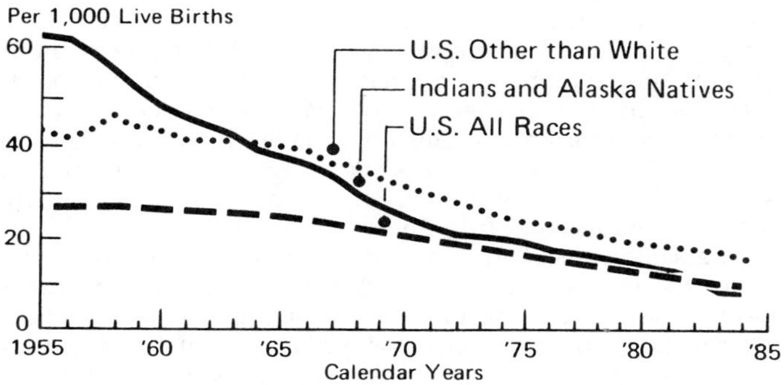

Figure 5–4. Infant mortality rate of native Americans, all races in the United States, and other nonwhites.

certain biologic factors as well. Because many more adult native Americans have adult onset diabetes mellitus, it is interesting to speculate that natural selection has increased the number of women with higher risk of adult onset diabetes, but also with lower risk of low-birthweight infants, due to the fact that prediabetic women bear larger infants.

After the newborn period, *accidental deaths* are the most common cause of death in all childhood populations (with the exception that in New York City in 1988, AIDS was the most common cause of death in children from 1–4 yr of age). But accidental death among native Americans occurs at twice the rate for other United States populations, whereas deaths from congenital malformations and malignant neoplasms are lower. During adolescence and young adulthood, *suicide* and *homicide* are the second and third causes of death in this population and also occur at about twice the rates of the rest of the population.

Recurrent otitis media is an especially frequent problem among native American children. As many as three quarters of these children have recurrent otitis media and high rates of hearing loss. This results in learning problems for many children. Other infectious disorders, such as tuberculosis and gastroenteritis, which were so much more common among native Americans in the past, now occur at about the national average.

Psychosocial problems are more prevalent in these populations than in the general population: depression, alcoholism, drug abuse, out-of-wedlock teenage pregnancy, school failure and dropout, and child abuse and neglect. The reasons for these differences are not clear, but the cultural disruption of native American populations is probably, in part, responsible.

INDIAN HEALTH SERVICE. Since 1954, the Indian Health Service has been the responsibility of the Public Health Service; and since the 1975 Indian Self-Determination Act, tribes have been given the option of managing Indian health services in their communities. Thus today the Indian Health Service is managed through local administrative units, and some tribes contract outside of the Indian Health Service for health care. A great deal of emphasis is on adult services: treatment for alcoholism, nutrition and dietetic counseling, and public health nursing services. In addition to programs on Indian reservations, there are currently more than 40 urban programs for native Americans, with an emphasis on increasing access of this population to existing health services, providing special social services, and developing self-help groups. In an effort to accommodate traditional Western medical, psychologic, and social services to the native American cultures, such programs increasingly include the "Talking Circle," the "Sweat Lodge," and other interventions based on native American culture. The efficacy of any of these programs, especially those to prevent and treat the sociopsychologic problems peculiar to native Americans, has not been assessed.

The United States has played a long and ambivalent role in dealing with its native American population. Health services have been among its more socially responsible activities, and today there is increased recognition of the need to maintain cultural sensitivity and to utilize traditional healing models, while at the same time bringing the benefits of modern medicine and social services to this group at special risk.

CHILDREN OF MIGRANT FARM WORKERS

Despite increased mechanization of farms, there are still more than 1 million migratory farm workers and their families in the United States. The eastern stream of workers winters primarily in Florida, while the western stream comes from Texas and the border states, as well as from Mexico. Many children travel with their parents in the migrant streams. The circumstances of migrants often include poor housing, frequent moves, and a socioeconomic system controlled by a crew boss who arranges the jobs, provides transportation, and often, together with the farm owners, provides food, alcohol, and drugs under a "company store" system that leaves the migrant family with little money, or even in debt at the end of the year. Children often go without schooling because of the moves, and medical care is usually limited.

The medical problems of children of migrant farm workers are similar to those of children of homeless families: increased frequency of infections, trauma, poor nutrition, poor dental care, and developmental delays. In the experience of the program at the University of Rochester, there were fewer than expected congenital malformations seen. One reason given by mothers was that children with these problems were left behind because they were too sick to travel.

In 1964, the Public Health Service initiated a special program to provide funds for local groups to organize medical care for migrant families. This program has continued to grow. In addition, many migrant health projects, which were staffed initially by part-time providers and were open for only part of the year, have been transformed into community health care centers that provide services not only for migrants but also for other residents in the area. However, health services for migrant farm workers often need to be organized separately from existing primary care programs because the families are migratory. Special record-keeping systems that link the health care provided during winter months in the south with the care provided during the migratory season in the north are difficult to maintain in ordinary group practices or individual physicians' offices. Outreach programs that take medical care to the often remote farm sites are necessary, and specially organized Head Start, early education, and remedial education programs should also be provided. Similar to other groups discussed in this section, children of migrant farm workers require health care that is more extensive than physicians' services; and this sort of health care often requires separate organizations to deliver it.

CHILDREN OF IMMIGRANTS

The United States has always been a country of immigrants, and in the last 10 yr immigration has once again increased, especially from Southeast Asia, South America, and the Soviet Union. Families of different origins obviously bring different health problems and different cultural backgrounds, which influence health practices and use of medical care and need to be understood to provide good services. Children from Southeast Asia and South America have growth patterns that are generally below the norms established for children of Western European origin, and high rates of hepatitis, parasitic diseases, and nutritional deficiencies are prevalent, as well as high degrees of psychosocial stress. The high prevalence of hepatitis among women from Southeast Asia makes use of hepatitis B vaccine necessary for newborns in this group. While special health care programs have been developed for many of these children (e.g., children of immigrant migrant workers), children of immigrant families have usually been more readily incorporated into traditional medical practice in the United States than some of the other groups of children at special risk.

HOMELESS CHILDREN

Estimates are that in the late 1980s as many as 3 million people were homeless in the United States, and the estimated number of children among the homeless ranged between 220,000 and 750,000. The population of homeless children has been increasing as a consequence of more families with children living in poverty, fewer available affordable dwellings for these families, decreasing public assistance programs for the non-elderly poor, and the rising prevalence of substance abuse.

Homeless children have an increased frequency of illness, including intestinal infections, anemia, neurologic disorders, seizures, mental illness, and dental problems, as well as increased frequency of trauma and substance abuse. Homeless children are admitted to hospitals at a much higher rate than the national average, and the likelihood of their being victims of abuse and neglect is much higher. In one study, 50% of such children were found to have psychosocial problems, such as developmental delays, severe depression, or learning disorders.

Because families tend to break apart under the strain of poverty and homelessness, many homeless children end up in foster care. And even if their families remain intact, frequent moves make it very difficult for them to receive continuity of medical care. Even in the United Kingdom, which offers the easiest access to primary care of all Western democracies, studies have shown that homeless persons rarely have a family physician, and therefore special programs generally need to be developed to provide health services for this population. Mobile vans, with a team consisting of a physician, nurse, social worker, and welfare worker, have been shown to provide effective comprehensive care, ensure delivery of immunizations, link the children to school health services, and bring the children and their families into a stable relation with the traditional medical system. A special record-keeping system is necessary to enhance continuity and to provide a record of care once the family has moved to a permanent location. Because of the high frequency of developmental delays in this group, linkage of preschool homeless children to Head Start programs is an especially important service. Medical and social services for the parents of homeless children are also essential for preservation of those families.

The basic problem of homeless families cannot, of course, be solved by physicians. Provision of adequate housing, job retraining for the parents, and mental health and social services are necessary to prevent homelessness from occurring. But physicians can play an important role in motivating society to adopt the social policies that will prevent homelessness from occurring by pointing out the likelihood that these homeless children will become burdens both to themselves and to society if their special health needs are not met.

RUNAWAY YOUTH

It is estimated that in the United States more than 1 million young people 10–17 yr of age run away from home each year; some are clearly forced to leave by their families. The usual definition of a runaway is a youth under 18 yr of age who is gone for at least one night from his or her home without parental permission. Most runaways leave home only once, stay overnight with friends, and have no contact with the police or other agencies. This group is no different from their "healthy" peers in psychologic status. A smaller but unknown number become multiple or permanent "runners" and are significantly different from the one-time "runners."

The same constellation of causes common to many of the other special-risk groups is characteristic of permanent runaways. These causes include environmental problems (family dysfunction, abuse, poverty), as well as personal problems of the young person (poor impulse control, psychopathology, or school failure). The reason why one child enters the group of runaways while another child enters foster care, the juvenile justice system, or mental health systems is not clear.

The minority of runaway youths who become homeless street people have a high frequency of problem behaviors. Three quarters engage in some type of criminal activity and half engage in prostitution as a means of support. A majority of permanent runaways have serious mental problems; more than one third are the product of families who engage in repeated physical and sexual abuse. These children also have a high frequency of medical problems, including traditional infections, hepatitis, sexually transmitted diseases, and drug abuse. Although runaways usually distrust most social agencies, they will come to and use medical services. Thus, medical care may become the point of re-entry into mainstream society, and to needed services.

Services for the permanent runaways need to be comprehensive and should include social, psychiatric, foster home, drug detoxification, as well as more traditional medical services. The only approach that has been successful has been long-term team efforts by people who develop the trust of runaway youths and then can help them to work out a better solution to their problems than by running away, drug use, and prostitution.

Although there may be significant legal considerations involved in the treatment of homeless minor adolescents, most states, through their "good Samaritan" acts and definitions of "emancipated minors," authorize treatment of homeless youths. Physician liability is based on the usual malpractice standards. Legal barriers should not be used as an excuse to refuse medical care to runaway youths.

The Runaway Youth Act, Title III of the Juvenile Justice and Delinquency Prevention Act of 1974 (Public Law 93-414), and its amended version (Public Law 95-509) have supported shelters and provide a toll-free 24-hour telephone number (1-800-621-4000) for youth who wish to contact their parents or request help after having run away.

Parents who seek a physician's advice about a runaway child should be asked about the child's past history of running away, the presence of family dysfunction, and personal aspects of the child's development. If the youth contacts the physician, he or she should be examined and the youth's health status should be assessed, as well as his or her willingness to return home. If it is not feasible for the youth to return home, foster care, a group home, or an independent living arrangement should be sought by referral to a social worker or a social agency.

FOSTER CHILDREN

Most children placed in foster care have a higher than average number of health problems, as well as social problems. The frequency of placement of children in foster care is greater among most of the populations of children at special risk and children from broken families and single-parent families than in the general population. Although extended families (especially grandparents) are frequently the initial source of continuing care, their abilities to cope are often overtaxed and their wards end up receiving foster care from strangers. Innovative preventive programs such as *Homebuilders,* which has been successful in reducing family break-up, are not feasible for families with drug addiction, HIV infection, or child abuse, nor for migrant or native American families.

Although the number of children in foster care decreased in the first half of the last decade, due to the Adoption Assistance and Child Welfare Act of 1980 (Public Law 96-272), faster adoption procedures, and limits to the amount of time that children were allowed to stay in foster care, the total number has been increasing in recent years due primarily to an influx of infants and adolescents. The total number of children in foster care dropped from over 300,000 to about 275,000 by 1985. But by 1988, the number had risen to 340,000 nationally. Substance abuse and poverty have contributed significantly to this trend. Public Law 96-272 offers financial incentives to help states prevent foster care placement by encouraging either early reunification of foster care children with their parents or adoption.

Infants who have a positive test result for HIV infection and children whose mothers are substance abusers present special problems. They are especially difficult to place in foster care or adoption and often cannot be returned to their biologic homes. Parental drug abuse is a factor in 35–40% of all foster care placements and is increasing. It contributes significantly to child abuse, both physical and sexual, and to neglect and abandonment of children.

Adolescents have always been difficult to place for adoption, and most who are in foster care have such severe emotional and physical problems that adoption is impossible. They often end up permanently in foster care, revolving in and out of different foster homes. More than 80% have experienced sexual or physical abuse, or neglect. There is need to prepare adolescents in foster care for independent living when they reach maturity. The Federal Foster Care Independent Living Initiative (Section 477, Title IV E of the SSA) of 1980 permits payment for such discharge planning, without which many of these youths would end up chronically on welfare.

General considerations concerning foster care and adoption are discussed in Sec. 3.16 and 3.17, but children at special risk present the social service and medical systems with especially difficult problems. Every child entering foster care should have a complete health assessment and provision of a medical record. However, it is difficult to provide standard health care to many of these children because frequent moves from one foster home to another obstruct continuity of medical care. Successful medical care programs usually involve special organizations to provide continuity of care. One of the most effective of these is the Chesapeake Health Plan in Baltimore, a prepaid group practice affiliated with Johns Hopkins University, which contracts with the state of Maryland to provide continuity of health care to all the foster children in their system, wherever their families move.

Foster children are also more likely to have chronic health problems, especially psychoeducational ones. They are often depressed and insecure, and they may have lifelong difficulty in developing intimate relationships. These complex sociomedical problems are another reason why there is a need for specially organized health care programs for children in foster care. Because most foster children are eligible for Medicaid, it is also important to enroll them in this source of funding.

CHILDREN IN POVERTY

Poverty and economic loss diminish the capacity of parents to be supportive, consistent, and involved with their children. Clinicians need to be especially alert to the development and behavior of children whose parents have lost their jobs or who live in permanent poverty. Fathers who become unemployed frequently develop psychosomatic symptoms, and their children often develop similar symptoms. Young children who grew up in the Great Depression and whose parents were subject to acute poverty suffered more than older children, especially if the older ones were able to take on responsibilities for helping the family economically. Such responsibilities during adolescence seem to give purpose and direction to an adolescent's life. But the younger children, faced with parental depression, and unable to do anything to help, suffered a higher frequency of illness and a diminished capacity to lead productive lives even as adults. Children who are poor have higher than average rates of death and illness from almost all causes (exceptions being suicide and motor vehicle accidents, which are most common among white, nonpoor children) (Table 5–6).

Although physicians cannot cure poverty, they have an obligation to ask parents about their economic resources, adverse changes in their financial situation, and the family's attempts to cope. Encouraging concrete methods of coping, suggesting ways to reduce stressful social circumstances while increasing social networks that are supportive, and referring patients and their families to appropriate welfare, job training, and family agencies can significantly improve the health and functioning of children at risk when their families live in poverty. In many cases special services, especially social services, need to be added to the traditional medical services, and outreach is required to find and encourage parents to use health services and bring their children into the health care system.

Poverty among children in the United States has increased during the last 20 yr (Fig. 5–5). One in five children lives in poverty, a higher percentage than in any other developed country. Many factors associated with poverty are responsible for the illnesses seen in these children—crowding, poor hygiene and health care, poor diet, environmental pollution, poor education, and stress. The basic support for poor families in the United States comes from the Aid to Families with Dependent Children program (AFDC). Support for these families is the foundation on which specially organized health care programs for children at special risk must be built. Unfortunately, AFDC has not kept up with inflation, has been subject to fraud, and varies greatly from one state to another.

TABLE 5–6. Morbidity Associated with Low Income Status*

Increased frequency of:
Low birthweight
Cytomegalic inclusion disease
Iron deficiency anemia
Lead poisoning
Poor vision
Hearing disorders
Psychologic problems
More disability days:
More hospital days/yr
Longer average length of stay in hospitals
Lower survival when ill with leukemia
More likely to be unable to attend regular school because of a chronic condition

*From Starfield B: Family income, ill health, and medical care of U.S. children. J Publ Health Policy 3:244–259, 1982.

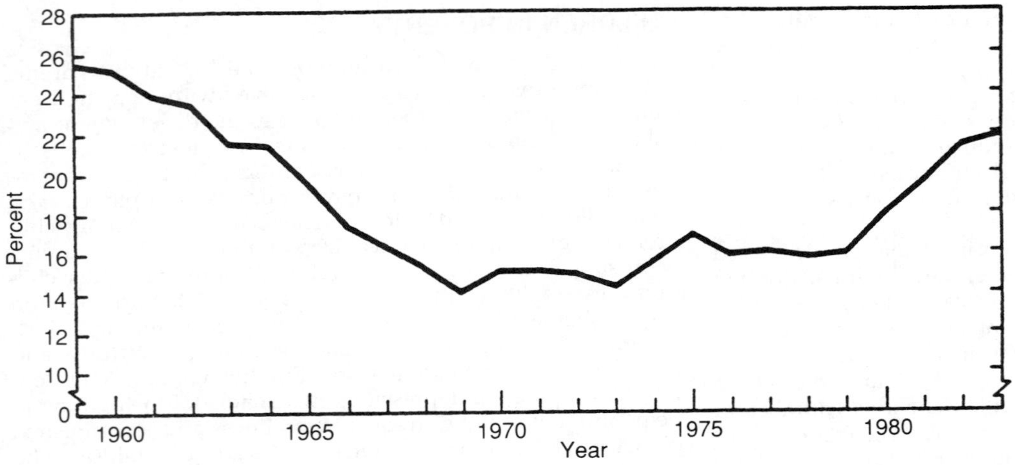

Figure 5–5. Poverty rate among children in the United States, aged 0–17 yr from 1960 to 1983. (From the Congressional Budget Office.)

INHERENT STRENGTHS IN VULNERABLE CHILDREN AND INTERVENTIONS

By 20–30 yr of age, many children who were at special risk will have made moderate successes of their lives. Furstenberg's study of teenage mothers and Werner's study of children in Kauai, most of whom were born prematurely or in poverty, demonstrate that by this age the majority in each study had defied the odds and made the transition to stable marriages and jobs and were accepted by their communities as responsible citizens.

Certain biologic characteristics are associated with success over the long term, such as being born with an accepting temperament. Avoidance of additional social risks is even more important. Premature infants or preadolescent boys with conduct disorders and poor reading skills, who must also face a broken family, poverty, frequent moves, and family violence, are at much greater risk than children with only one of these handicaps. But perhaps most important are the protective buffers that have been found to enhance children's resilience, because these can be added by an effective care system. Children generally do better if they can gain social support, either from family members or from a nonjudgmental adult outside the family, especially an older mentor or peer. Providers of medical services should develop ways to "prescribe" supportive "other" persons for children who are at risk and isolated. Promotion of self-esteem and self-efficacy seems to be a very central factor in protecting against risks. It is essential to promote competence in some area of these children's lives.

Providers of medical services need the patience to work over a long time frame and the willingness to accept limited improvement. In addition, prediction of the consequences of risk is never 100% accurate. Health professionals as well as families should have hope. However, the confidence that even without aid, many such children will achieve a good outcome by age 30 does not justify ignoring or withholding services from them in early life. It should teach us how to focus our resources on those most in need and provide a basis for hope in individual cases.

Programs that seem to work for high-risk children have a similar group of characteristics. A *team* is needed, because it is rare for one individual to be able to provide the multiple services needed for high-risk children. At the same time, successful programs are characterized by at least *one caring person* who can make personal contact with these children and their families. Most successful programs are relatively *small* (or are large programs divided up into small units) and nonbureaucratic but are *intensive, comprehensive,* and *flexible.* They work not only with the individual but also with the *family, school, community,* and even at broader societal levels. In addition, generally the *earlier* the programs are started, in terms of the age of children involved, the better is the chance of success. It is also important for services to be continued over a long period.

ROBERT J. HAGGERTY

GENERAL

Committee on Economic Development: Children in Need: Investment Strategies for the Educationally Disadvantaged. Washington, DC, Committee on Economic Development, 1987.

Macchiarola FJ, Gardner A: Caring for America's children. Proc Acad Political Science 37:1, 1989.

US House of Representatives, Select Committee on Children, Youth and Families: Report of the Select Committee on Children, Youth and Families: U.S. Children and Their Families: Current Conditions and Recent Trends. Washington, DC, US Government Printing Office, 1989.

Weissberg RP, Caplan MZ, Siva PJ: A conceptual framework for establishing school-based social competence promotion programs. *In:* Bond LA, Compas BE (eds): Primary Prevention and Promotion in the Schools. Newbury Park, CA, Sage, 1989, pp 255–296.

Werner EE: Vulnerable but Invincible: A Longitudinal Study of Resilient Children and Youth. New York, McGraw-Hill, 1982.

Werner EE, Smith RS: Against the Odds: A Longitudinal Study of High-Risk Children from Birth to Adulthood. Ithaca, NY, Cornell University Press (in press)

Wilson WJ: The Truly Disadvantaged: The Inner City, the Underclass and Public Policy. Chicago, Chicago University Press, 1987.

Zuckerman B, Weitzman M, Alpert JJ (eds): Children at risk: Current social and medical challenges. Pediatr Clin North Am 35:1169, 1988.

NATIVE AMERICAN, ALASKAN ESKIMO, AND ALEUT CHILDREN

McShane DA, Plas JM: Otitis media and psychoeducation difficulties and American Indians: A review and a suggestion. Preventive Psychiatry 1(3):277, 1982.

US Congress Office of Technology Assessment: Mental Health Status of American and Alaskan Native Youth. Part I: Historical Interest, Specific Problems, and Future Challenges; Part II: Current Systems, Typical Forms of Intervention and New Service Models. Washington DC, 1990.

US Department of Health and Human Services, Public Health Service, Indian Health Service, Office of Planning, Evaluation and Legislation, Division of Program Statistics: Trends in Indian Health, 1989. Washington, DC, 1989.

HOMELESS CHILDREN

Alperstein G, Rappaport C, Flanigan JM: Health problems of homeless children in New York City. Am J Public Health 78:1232, 1988.

American Academy of Pediatrics: Report of the Committee on Community Health Services: Health needs of homeless children. Pediatrics 82:938, 1988.

CHILDREN OF MIGRANT FARM WORKERS

Chi PSK: Medical utilization patterns of migrant farmworkers in Wayne County, New York. Public Health Reports 100:480, 1985.

Haggerty RJ: The migrant health project: Care or conflict? *In:* Haggerty RJ, Roghmann KJ, Pless IB (eds): Child Health and the Community. New York, John Wiley, 1975, pp 265–273.

RUNAWAY YOUTH

US Department of Health and Human Services: Runaway and Homeless Youth: National Program Inspection, Office of Inspector General, Region X, 1983.

CHILDREN OF IMMIGRANTS

Baldwin LM, Sutherland S: Growth patterns of first generation Southeast Asian infants. Am J Dis Child 142:526, 1988.

FOSTER CHILDREN

Committee on Early Childhood: Adoption and dependent care: Report: Health care of foster children. Pediatrics 79:644, 1989.

Health guidelines for the attendance in daycare and foster care settings of children infected with human immunodeficiency virus. Pediatrics 79:466, 1987.

Schor EL: Foster care. Pediatr Rev 10:209, 1989.

CHILDREN IN POVERTY

Five million children: A statistical profile of our poorest young citizens. New York, National Center for Children in Poverty, 1990.

5.6 HEALTH ADVICE FOR TRAVELING CHILDREN

Each year, more than 8 million United States citizens travel to developing countries and over 1 million visit malaria-endemic areas. Many of these travelers are children. This major increase in international travel, as well as the resurgence of malaria and other infectious diseases worldwide, brings the issues regarding prevention and management of health problems in travelers into the office of every physician caring for children. However, many physicians trained in industrialized countries are unfamiliar with the health hazards and rapidly changing information and requirements related to travel. Furthermore, the risks, needs, and requirements for children who are traveling (particularly those less than 2 yr of age) may sometimes differ from those of adults. The purpose of this section is to provide updated information on pretravel health advice and immunization for traveling children.

GENERAL RECOMMENDATIONS

Parents of traveling children should seek medical consultation well in advance of their departure in order to obtain a realistic assessment of risks, for immunization and chemoprophylactic measures, and for advice on dealing with disease if it occurs. For traveling small children, particularly infants, additional concerns relate to inadequate primary immunizations, lack of demonstrated efficacy and safety of many vaccines in infants, excretion of prophylactic drugs in breast milk, and increased morbidity and possible mortality associated with some diseases acquired abroad.

General advice to parents should first include a discussion of *eating and drinking habits,* because most travel-related health problems occur through the ingestion of contaminated food or water. Consultation should then focus on the common *problems related to travel,* including jet lag, altitude sickness, environmental exposures, the hazards of insects as vectors of many infections (e.g., malaria, yellow fever, dengue, filariasis, trypanosomiasis, onchocerciasis), and the means to avoid these vectors. Travelers to remote areas should be warned about venomous animals, rabies (predominantly transmitted by domestic dogs and cats), and exposure to rodents (because of plague), as well as the hazards of swimming in fresh water (schistosomiasis, noncholera vibrios, or leptospirosis). Most of the illnesses that develop in traveling children are related to behaviors that can be modified with proper advice and supervision by parents.

With AIDS becoming more prevalent abroad, the hazards of casual sexual encounters for adolescents as well as of needle and blood and blood product exposure should be emphasized. Blood sources in developing countries currently must be suspect. Children should have their blood typed before departure so that transfusions from family members or travel companions with similar blood types are possible in dire emergencies. Several agencies can provide emergency evacuation to industrialized countries if the situation dictates. HIV is not transmitted through casual contacts, sources of food or water, contact with inanimate objects, mosquitoes, or other insect vectors.

Children with pre-existing medical problems are traveling more extensively and are in greatest need of consultation prior to departure. Conditions on which travel has the greatest impact include chronic cardiopulmonary disease, diabetes, allergies, and gastrointestinal problems, especially diarrhea (malabsorption or inflammatory bowel disease). Special arrangements should be made for patients with bleeding disorders, those on anticoagulation therapy, and those who require hemodialysis.

Children with medical conditions should take with them a brief medical summary. For children requiring care by specialists, an international directory for that specialty can be consulted. In addition, a directory of physicians worldwide who speak English and who have met certain qualifications is available from the International Association for Medical Assistance to Travelers (736 Center St., Lewiston, NY 14092; telephone: [716] 754-4883). If medical care is needed urgently when abroad, sources of information include the American embassy or consulate, hotel managers, travel agents catering to foreign tourists, and missionary hospitals. Parents should be counseled, however, to take a sufficient supply of prescription medications for their children and to ensure that bottles are clearly identified. A travel health kit consisting of prescription medications and nonprescription items is also often useful. Travelers also need to ascertain whether their health insurance will cover medical care abroad.

IMMUNIZATIONS (See also Sec. 5.1)

General Considerations

Immunization is only one feature of a comprehensive disease prevention program for traveling children (Table 5–7). No vaccine is completely safe or effective; benefits and risks must be considered for all immunobiologic agents. One of the most important issues related to vaccinations of traveling children is a modification in the immunization schedule for the unvaccinated or inadequately vaccinated child, especially those less than 2 yr of age. The routine childhood immunizations (i.e., measles, mumps, rubella, *Haemophilus influenzae* type B conjugate vaccines, diphtheria, tetanus, and pertussis) are most frequently affected and involve alterations in both the minimum age for immunization and the minimum interval between doses (Table 5–8). Issues related to the minimum age at administration also arise for those immunizations that are considered solely because of specific travel-related needs (e.g., cholera, hepatitis B, Japanese encephalitis [JE], meningococcal, rabies, typhoid, and yellow fever vaccines and immune globulin).

Parents should allow 4–6 wk before departure for optimal administration of vaccines to their children, because some

TABLE 5–7. Immunization for Traveling Children

Live Attenuated Virus Vaccines*	Inactivated Vaccines	Toxoids	Immunoglobulins
Measles†	Cholera‡	Diphtheria§	Immune globulin
Mumps†	HbCV	Tetanus§	Rabies immune globulin
Rubella†	IPV		
OPV	Hepatitis B		
Yellow fever‡	Japanese encephalitis‖		
	Meningococcal		
	Pertussis§		
	Plague		
	Rabies		
	Typhoid¶		

*Generally contraindicated in immunodeficient children. An exception is measles vaccination, which is recommended for both asymptomatic and symptomatic HIV-infected children. Live vaccines should be given simultaneously or at least 30 days apart. Live, attenuated immunizations should not be coadministered with immune globulin (OPV and yellow fever are exceptions); administer these vaccines at least 3 mo after immune globulin use. Immune globulin should be administered no sooner than 2–4 wk after a live virus vaccine is given.

†Administered together as MMR or separately.

‡May be required for entry into certain countries.

§Administered together as DTP or DT.

‖Not available in the United States. May be obtained in endemic areas for high-risk individuals.

¶A new licensed oral live attenuated typhoid vaccine (Vivotif, Ty21a) can be given to immunocompetent children >6 yr of age.

HbCV = *Haemophilus influenzae* type B conjugate vaccine; IPV = injectable polio vaccine (enhanced); OPV = oral polio vaccine.

immunizations require multiple doses for full protection and some immunobiologic agents are incompatible with others. In general, inactivated vaccines can be given simultaneously, although both local and systemic adverse reactions may be cumulative. Live attenuated viral vaccines should always be administered together (see Table 5–7); if not administered concurrently, live vaccines should be given at least 30 days apart whenever possible. Inactivated and live vaccines can be given together at any time. The notable exception is yellow fever and cholera vaccines, which should not be given simultaneously or within 3 wk of each other, because the antibody response to both vaccines may be decreased. Because immune globulin can interfere with the replication of live attenuated viruses, live vaccines should not be given within 6 wk and preferably should be delayed until 3 mo after use of immune globulin. Immune globulin should be administered no sooner than at least 2 wk and preferably 4 wk after a live virus vaccine is given. Vaccine products produced in eggs may contain an allergenic substance that cause hypersensitivity responses, including anaphylaxis in persons with known egg sensitivity. Screening by history of ability to eat eggs without adverse effect is a reasonable way to identify those at allergic risk from receiving yellow fever, measles, mumps, rubella, or influenza vaccines.

TABLE 5–8. Modification of Routine Immunization Schedules for Traveling Children

Vaccine	Modified Schedule
MMR	Children younger than 6 mo of age should not be vaccinated because of maternal antibodies. Children aged 6–12 mo should receive one dose of measles vaccine before departure and revaccination with MMR at 15 mo of age or at 12 mo if remaining in a high-risk area. If the child is 12–14 mo of age, MMR should be given and revaccination should be considered when the child starts school. Older children who were previously immunized with measles vaccine before 1980 should be revaccinated.
OPV	Children should receive at least three doses at intervals of 6 wk when time permits. When traveling infants are less than 6 wk old, an initial dose should be given and 3 additional doses at 6,10, and 14 wk should be administered if remaining in the endemic areas. Children traveling to endemic areas who have received a first or second dose of the primary series should receive their second/third doses 4 wk after their prior dose. Children who have received less than the primary series and who remain in endemic areas should complete the primary series within the endemic area with doses at 4-wk intervals.
HbCV	See Sec. 5.1 and Table 5–5*B*.
DTP	Young infants should receive three doses, the first no sooner than 6 wk and the next two doses at intervals of no less than 4 wk. Children less than 7 yr old who have received fewer than three doses and who will remain in endemic areas should complete their remaining doses at 4-wk intervals.

DTP = diphtheria and tetanus toxoids and pertussis vaccine; HbCV = *Haemophilus influenzae* type B conjugated vaccine; MMR = measles, mumps, rubella; OPV = oral polio vaccine.

Rapid viral replication after administration of live vaccines occurs in *immunodeficient hosts*. These patients include those with lymphoreticular malignancy, generalized malignancies, or AIDS, or those receiving corticosteroids, cytotoxic agents, or radiation. In general, live virus vaccines are contraindicated in these individuals. An exception is measles vaccine, which is recommended for both asymptomatic and symptomatic HIV-infected children because of severe, life-threatening measles infection found in children with AIDS. Although children with symptomatic HIV infection should not receive yellow fever vaccine, asymptomatic HIV-infected children may be vaccinated if the risk from yellow fever remains significant (see later). These immunocompromising conditions may also reduce immunologic responses to inactivated vaccines and toxoids; inactivated vaccines and toxoids are not contraindicated in immunodeficient children.

Routine Childhood Vaccines and Toxoids

DIPHTHERIA, TETANUS, AND PERTUSSIS. Tetanus is a ubiquitous problem, is a major cause of worldwide neonatal mortality, and is most prevalent in tropical countries. Diphtheria is also endemic in many developing countries. Pertussis is common in the Third World as well as in some industrialized nations where pertussis immunization is not practiced as widely as in the United States. Guidelines for optimum protection against these three infections in the first year of life are presented in Sec. 5.1. The immunization schedule for DTP should be modified for young infants and inadequately or unimmunized children according to the guidelines in Table 5–8. For children less than 7 yr of age with a contraindication to pertussis vaccine, DT should be used. Partially immunized infants for whom further doses of pertussis vaccine are contraindicated should have DT substituted for each of the remaining scheduled DTP doses.

POLIO VACCINE. In most developed nations, the risk of poliomyelitis is usually no different from that seen in the United States. On the other hand, most developing countries are still endemic for poliomyelitis. Children traveling to such countries are at increased risk for developing poliomyelitis and adequate immunization must be undertaken.

In the United States, a primary series of OPV should be given to individuals less than 18 yr of age (see Sec. 5.1). In cases in which this standard immunization schedule cannot be followed, then the age of vaccination can be lowered and the interval between doses can be shortened (see Table 5–8).

Although not considered the vaccine of choice for children, enhanced potency IPV may be indicated for children who are immunocompromised or who are in close contact with immunocompromised individuals. The primary series of enhanced IPV is begun ideally at 8 wk of age with an interval of 8 wk between the 1st two doses and a 12-mo interval between the 2nd and 3rd doses. When necessary, immunization can be started as early as 6 wk of age with a 4-wk interval between the 1st and 2nd doses and between the 2nd and 3rd doses and a 4th dose administered 6 mo later.

MEASLES, MUMPS, AND RUBELLA VACCINES. Measles is endemic in many developing countries as well as in some industrialized nations. Individuals traveling abroad should be immune to measles. Measles vaccine, preferably in combination with mumps and rubella vaccines, should be given to all children at 15 mo of age and older, unless there is a contraindication (Sec. 5.1). The age of vaccination should be lowered for children traveling to endemic areas according to the schedule in Table 5–8.

In the United States, measles vaccine failures have been observed increasingly in children immunized before 1980. These children should be revaccinated, particularly before travel outside the United States.

***HAEMOPHILUS INFLUENZAE* TYPE B CONJUGATE VACCINE.** Severe *H. influenzae* type B infection is most common in children 6 mo to 1 yr in age, but one third of cases of invasive infection are found in children 18 mo of age and older. The risk of developing serious *H. influenzae* infection when traveling outside the United States may be comparable with that found in the United States. See Sec 5.1 for the immunization schedule of conjugated Hib. Unimmunized children up to 23 mo of age should be vaccinated (Sec. 5.1). Children who previously received the polysaccharide vaccine should be revaccinated with *H. influenzae* type B conjugate vaccine.

Special Vaccines for Travel

YELLOW FEVER. Yellow fever is a mosquito-borne viral illness resembling other hemorrhagic fevers but with more prominent liver involvement (Sec. 12.84). Yellow fever exists in jungle areas of South America and Africa. In South America, sporadic infection is found in forestry, agricultural, and other occupationally exposed workers. In Africa, the virus is transmitted to young children in the moist savanna zones of West Africa during the rainy season.

Yellow fever vaccine is a live, attenuated vaccine developed in chick embryos and is extremely safe and effective. Yellow fever vaccination is required by law by some countries for travelers arriving from endemic areas. Some African countries require evidence of vaccination from all entering travelers. The most recent recommendations can be obtained by contacting state or local health departments or the Division of Vector-Borne Viral Diseases, Centers for Disease Control (CDC), telephone no. (303) 221-6400.

Most countries accept a medical waiver for children who are too young to be vaccinated (< 4 mo of age) and for individuals with a contraindication to vaccination, such as immunodeficiency. Children with asymptomatic HIV infection may be vaccinated if exposure to the yellow fever virus cannot be avoided.

The vaccine, made from the attenuated 17D strain, is given as a single 0.5-mL dose. Long-lived, perhaps lifetime immunity develops; however, international travel certificates require proof of immunization within 10 yr. Cholera vaccine given 3 wk before or simultaneously with yellow fever vaccine reduces but does not prevent an antibody response to yellow fever immunization (see earlier).

CHOLERA VACCINE. Cholera is an acute noninflammatory diarrheal illness caused by *Vibrio cholera* O group 1 acquired through the ingestion of contaminated food or water (Sec. 12.31). In children less than 2 yr of age, cholera is frequently a mild disease. Although there has been continued spread since the 7th worldwide pandemic of cholera of 1961, travelers rarely contract cholera. There were only 10 cases of cholera reported to the CDC between 1961 and 1982; no childhood cases were reported. Two of five internationally acquired cases in 1986 were in children.

Although cholera vaccination can reduce the rate of illness by 50%, it provides only short-term protection. Vaccine efficacy is low particularly in children less than 5 yr of age. WHO and the CDC do not recommend cholera vaccination for international travel. However, a few countries still require evidence of vaccination for travelers entering from endemic areas. In that case, a single dose of 0.2 mL (subcutaneously or intramuscularly) is sufficient to satisfy this requirement. Because cholera vaccination is not recommended for children less than 6 mo of age, a medical waiver should be given before departure.

TYPHOID VACCINE. *Salmonella typhi* infection, or typhoid fever, is not uncommon in young children (Sec. 12.29). American international travelers are at risk of contracting typoid especially in the Indian subcontinent and western South America. Typhoid vaccination is recommended when a person travels to an endemic area and when exposure to contaminated food and water is likely. The heat-phenol-inactivated vaccine (60–80% efficacy), available in the United States, has been widely used for many years. Children 6 mo of age and older who are traveling to a typhoid endemic area should be considered for vaccination with 0.25 mL subcutaneously of the heat-phenol-inactivated vaccine (0.5 mL if older than 10 yr) on two occasions, separated by 4 wk or more. A local reaction to the heat-phenol typhoid vaccination is common and may be associated with fever, headache, and malaise. Hyperpyrexia in reaction to the heat-phenol-inactivated preparation can be severe in young children, and febrile seizures may occur. Acetominophen can be administered as may be done with DTP vaccination.

A newly licensed oral live-attenuated vaccine (Vivotif, manufactured from the Ty21a strain of *S. typhi*) has undergone field trials among Egyptian and Chilean school children with an estimated efficacy of 67% for at least 4 yr. Because of the lack of efficacy data in children less than 5 yr of age, Ty21a vaccine is not recommended for children less than 6 yr old. It is also not recommended for immunocompromised children; the inactivated vaccine should be used for these children.

MENINGOCOCCAL VACCINE. Meningococcal meningitis is a worldwide disease (Sec. 12.23); epidemic disease has been reported in India, Nepal, Saudi Arabia, and sub-Saharan Africa. Cases in American travelers in such areas are infrequent; however, prolonged contact with the local population could increase the risk of infection and makes vaccination a reasonable precaution. Saudi Arabia requires evidence of meningococcal vaccination for travel to parts of that country. Serogroup A is the most common cause of epidemics outside the United States, but serogroup C and, rarely, serogroup B have been associated with epidemics.

Only one vaccine is available in the United States, the quadrivalent A/C/Y/W-135 vaccine. This vaccine is effective against serogroup A in infants less than 3 mo of age and may be only partially effective in children 3 to 11 mo old. Children less than 2 yr of age are not protected against serogroup C. A dose of 0.5 mL is given subcutaneously. Children vaccinated before 4 yr of age should be revaccinated after 2 or 3 yr if they remain in an endemic area.

IMMUNOGLOBULIN FOR HEPATITIS A. This is recommended for children traveling to developing countries if their travel is done on the usual tourist routes, if they will be eating or drinking water in areas of questionable sanitation, or if they will have contact with local children in settings of poor sanitation. Immunoglobulin is also recommended for children residing in developing countries. Clinical hepatitis may not be symptomatic in young children (< 5 yr of age); infected children can, however, transmit infection to older children and adults, in whom it is usually symptomatic (Sec. 12.79). Immunoglobulin should be given at 0.02 mL/kg for a visit of 3 mo or less and 0.06 mL/kg every 5 mo for longer travel. Immunoglobulin produced in developing countries may not meet the same standards for purity set in developed countries.

HEPATITIS B VACCINE. Hepatitis B is highly endemic in eastern and southeastern Asia, sub-Saharan Africa, and the Pacific Basin. Infants and children traveling to such areas may be at risk if they are exposed directly to blood from the local population. Cases in which disease transmission can occur include receipt of blood transfusions not screened for HBsAg, exposure to unsterilized needles, or close contact with local children who have open skin lesions. Exposure to hepatitis B is more likely if the child is living for prolonged periods in the endemic areas. Vaccination for hepatitis B is recommended for children staying in an endemic area for 6 mo or longer or who may have the aforementioned exposures. The recombinant hepatitis B vaccine is given in three doses of 0.5 mL each (2nd dose 1 mo after the 1st and the 3rd dose 5 mo after the 2nd dose). Optimally, vaccination should begin at least 6 mo before departure; some protection occurs by one or two doses.

RABIES VACCINE. The risk of rabies is currently the highest in countries where rabies in dogs is uncontrolled, including Columbia, Ecuador, El Salvador, Guatemala, India, Mexico, Nepal, Philippines, Thailand, and Vietnam. Rabies is also endemic in most other countries of Africa, Asia, and Central and South America. Pre-exposure prophylaxis is given to individuals at risk as three 1-mL doses on days 7 and 28. Postexposure prophylaxis is given as five 1-mL doses on days 0, 3, 7, 14, and 28 if unimmunized and in two doses of 1 mL on days 0 and 3, if previously vaccinated. Intramuscular administration is the preferred route for postexposure and pre-exposure immunization in the setting of travel. Rabies immune globulin is also indicated after exposure in unvaccinated children (20 IU/kg), with one half of the dose infiltrated into the wound, when possible, and the other given intramuscularly (Sec. 12.81).

JAPANESE ENCEPHALITIS (JE) VACCINE. JE vaccine is not currently available in the United States, but it can be obtained abroad in endemic areas. Worldwide, JE is the leading cause of viral encephalitis and occurs in the People's Republic of China, India, Bangladesh, Nepal, Sri Lanka, Hong Kong, Korea, Japan, Taiwan, Philippines, eastern Russia, and Southeast Asia. In endemic areas, the age-specific incidence is highest in young children. The risk for travelers is associated with the extent of exposure to the mosquito vectors. Since 1981, six cases of JE have been seen among adult expatriate Americans. Fortunately, most cases are asymptomatic, but mortality rates of 50% or significant neurologic sequelae in one third of survivors have been seen in symptomatic cases. An inactivated vaccine purified from infected suckling mouse brain has been well tolerated and widely used in Asia with an efficacy of greater than 95%. The CDC recommends immunization for travelers with a high risk of exposure to the mosquito vectors and who will stay for several weeks or more in rural endemic areas during transmission season. JE vaccine is available in Japan and Korea and at individual clinics in other Asian countries.

TRAVELERS' DIARRHEA

Travelers' diarrhea, characterized by a 2-fold or greater increase in the frequency of unformed bowel movements, has been observed in up to 40% of all travelers overseas. A large number of infectious agents (bacteria, viruses, and parasites) have been associated with travelers' diarrhea; enterotoxic *Escherichia coli* is the most frequent cause. The most important risk factor for travelers' diarrhea is the country of destination. High-risk areas (attack rates of 25–50%) are developing countries of Latin America, Africa, the Middle East, and Asia. Intermediate risk occurs in the Mediterranean, China, and Israel, whereas low-risk areas include North America, Northern Europe, Australia, and New Zealand.

Careful selection and preparation of food and water can reduce the risk of developing travelers' diarrhea. Breastfeeding is the best alternative for young infants. Great care should be taken in the preparation of formula and selection of pasteurized dairy products for non–breast-fed infants. Carbonated and boiled water is safest. Uncooked vegetables and undercooked meat and fish should be avoided. Fruits should be peeled by parents.

There are few data on the use of antidiarrheal drugs in children. Chemoprophylactic agents have been discouraged in children because potential adverse effects greatly outweigh any prophylactic benefit. Antimicrobial therapy for travelers' diarrhea in infants and young children should generally be administered in consultation with a physician. This is true particularly if the illness is severe or there is associated high fever or the stools are bloody. If empiric antimicrobial agents are administered by parents in cases of mild illness, trimethoprim (4 mg/kg) and sulfamethoxazole (20 mg/kg) twice a day for 3 days may be effective for infants (2 mo of age or greater) and older children. Furazolidone (5 mg/kg/day in four divided doses) should also be considered, given its efficacy against both bacterial pathogens and *Giardia lamblia*. Antimotility agents like diphenoxylate HCl (Lomotil) should be avoided; mortality and morbidity from infection caused by *Salmonella* and *Shigella* are higher with diphenoxylate HCl therapy.

Dehydration is the greatest threat presented by a diarrheal illness in a small child. Education of parents regarding the symptoms and signs of dehydration is necessary. Parents should carry with them either prepackaged oral rehydration solutions recommended by the WHO or a recipe for a home formula if their children develop an acute, dehydrating diarrheal illness.

MALARIA CHEMOPROPHYLAXIS

Malaria, a mosquito-borne infection, is the leading parasitic cause of death worldwide (Sec. 12.109). Of the four *Plasmodium* species that infect humans, *P. falciparum* causes the

TABLE 5–9. Drugs Used in Chemoprophylaxis and Presumptive Treatment of Malaria in Children

	Drug	Pediatric Dosage
Areas of chloroquine-**sensitive** *Plasmodium falciparum*	Chloroquine phosphate*	5 mg/kg base (8.3 mg/kg of salt) once per wk, up to maximum adult dose of 300 mg base
Areas of chloroquine-**resistant** *P. falciparum*	Chloroquine phosphate*	5 mg/kg base (8.3 mg/kg of salt) once per wk, up to maximum adult dose of 300 mg base
	PLUS Proguanil† (East Africa)	<2 yr: 50 mg qd 2–6 yr: 100 mg qd 7–10 yr: 150 mg qd >10 yr: 200 mg qd
	PLUS Pyrimethamine-sulfadoxine‡	2–11 mo: ¼ tablet 1–3 yr: ½ tablet 4–8 yr: 1 tablet 9–14 yr: 2 tablets >14 yr: 3 tablets Take single dose of the aforementioned for self-treatment of febrile illness when medical care is not immediately available.
	OR Mefloquine§	15–19 kg: ¼ tab/wk (62.5 mg/wk) 20–30 kg: ½ tab/wk (125 mg/wk) 31–45 kg: ¾ tab/wk (187.5 mg/wk) >45 kg: 1 tab/wk (250 mg/wk)
Prevention of relapses	Primaquine phosphate‖	0.3 mg/kg base (0.5 mg/kg of salt) orally, once a day for 14 days, or 0.9 mg/kg base (1.5 mg/kg of salt) orally, once a wk for 8 wk

*If chloroquine phosphate is not available, hydroxychloroquine sulfate is as effective; 400 mg of hydroxychloroquine sulfate is equivalent to 500 mg of chloroquine phosphate.

†Proguanil (Paludrine-Ayerst, Canada, ICI) is not available in the United States.

‡Recommended for travel to sub-Saharan Africa, the Indian subcontinent, South America (except the Amazon basin), Oceania, Hainan Island, and the southern provinces of China. Pyrimethamine-sulfadoxine (Fansidar) is contraindicated in patients with a history of sulfonamide intolerance, in pregnancy at term, and in infants less than 2 mo old.

§Mefloquine is not recommended for children less than 15 kg.

‖Primaquine is only recommended to prevent relapse of *P. vivax* and *P. ovale* infection. Primaquine phosphate can cause hemolytic anemia, especially in patients with glucose-6-phosphate dehydrogenase (G-6-PD) deficiency. This deficiency is most common in blacks, Orientals, and Mediterranean people. Children should be screened for G-6-PD deficiency before treatment.

greatest morbidity and mortality. In the United States, a growing number of malaria cases is being reported annually in travelers and immigrants. In 1986, 1,123 cases of malaria were reported in the United States. Between 1975 and 1983, *P. falciparum* infections acquired by American citizens traveling to east Africa increased 21-fold. Given this major resurgence of malaria, physicians in developed countries will be increasingly required to give advice on the prevention, as well as the diagnosis and treatment, of malaria.

Malaria transmission occurs primarily between dusk and dawn, and parents should be advised of the importance of *measures to reduce mosquito contact* during these times. Measures to avoid the insect vector, including the use of appropriate clothing, netting, and insect repellents, are extremely important and should be emphasized. Insect repellent should be purchased before departure. The most effective repellents contain *N,N*-diethyl-meta-toluamide (DEET). The higher the concentration of DEET, the longer it lasts as a repellent. Toxic encephalopathy, however, has occurred in children exposed to DEET. Frequent application of products containing high concentrations of DEET should be avoided in children.

Prophylactic medication has also been shown to be extremely effective. Unfortunately, only 28% of the 410 American citizens with *P. falciparum* malaria acquired in Africa between 1980 and 1984 were using a recommended drug for prophylaxis. One survey of 4,042 returning American travelers to Africa and Haiti demonstrated that 58% of these individuals did not take recommended prophylactic agents regularly. Travelers are more likely to use prophylactic antimalarial drugs if appropriate recommendations and education are provided to them by physicians before their departure. However, in one survey, only 14% of persons who sought medical advice obtained correct information regarding malaria prevention and prophylaxis.

Resistance of *P. falciparum* to the 1st-line chemoprophylactic agent, chloroquine, is rapidly increasing worldwide. Because of this growing problem of resistance, 2nd-line agents are increasingly utilized. In the United States, pyrimethamine-sulfadoxine (Fansidar) was given concurrently to travelers visiting areas of chloroquine-resistant *P. falciparum* malaria between 1982 and 1985. During that period, however, numerous cases of severe cutaneous reactions and seven deaths were reported in individuals taking long-term prophylaxis. As a result, the recommendations for malaria prophylaxis have changed several times during the last few years.

Several factors are important in choosing appropriate chemoprophylactic regimens for malaria. The travel itinerary should be reviewed thoroughly in relation to information regarding areas of risk within a particular country. The risk for acquiring chloroquine-resistant *P. falciparum* should also be determined. Finally, allergic or other known adverse reactions to antimalarial agents should be considered, as well as the availability of medical care during travel.

Chloroquine is still the mainstay of chemoprophylaxis for children traveling to most malaria-endemic areas (Table 5–9). *P. vivax, P. ovale,* and *P. malariae* and the other species infecting humans remain chloroquine-sensitive. In areas where *P. falciparum* is developing resistance to chloroquine, sensitive strains coexist. In one study, decreased parasitemia and milder illness were also seen in individuals who took chloroquine but still developed chloroquine-resistant falciparum malaria. Malaria chemoprophylaxis should begin 1–2 wk before departure to ensure adequate serum levels and to screen for adverse effects. Chloroquine should be also continued for 4 to 6 wk after leaving an endemic area. Chloroquine is manufactured in the United States only in tablet form and tastes quite bitter. Pediatric doses should be carefully calculated per unit body weight because of the risk of severe toxicity. Pharmacists can pulverize tablets and prepare gelatin capsules. Alternatively, mixing pulverized doses in food or drink may facilitate compliance in children. Chloroquine suspension is also widely available overseas.

Parents of children traveling to areas where chloroquine-resistant malaria exists should be warned about the possibility of acquiring resistant malaria, and they should be supplied with **pyrimethamine-sulfadoxine** (Fansidar) for presumptive treatment if a febrile illness develops (see Table 5–9). After giving presumptive treatment with pyrimethamine-sulfadoxine, the parents should seek medical care for the child as soon as possible.

Proguanil, which is currently not available in the United States, is recommended by some authorities for prophylaxis against chloroquine-resistant *P. falciparum* in East Africa. Limited data with this dihydrofolate reductase inhibitor suggest that this drug is not effective in Thailand, the Amazon Basin, Papua New Guinea, and possibly West Africa. Proguanil (see Table 5–9) should be used in combination with weekly chloroquine phosphate.

Mefloquine is highly effective against chloroquine- and pyrimethamine-sufadoxine–resistant *P. falciparum*. This drug has been approved by the Food and Drug Administration in the United States. In preliminary studies of Peace Corps workers, mefloquine is 67% more effective than chloroquine in malaria endemic areas where chloroquine-resistant *P. falciparum* exists. This drug should not be used in children who weigh less than 15 kg because of insufficient efficacy and tolerance data.

Doxycycline has been recommended for travelers to areas of multidrug-resistant *P. falciparum* (Thailand, Burma, Kampuchea, the Amazon Basin) and for travelers allergic to sulfa drugs. This drug is contraindicated in children less than 8 yr of age. Parents should be discouraged from taking a child on a trip if there will be evening or night-time exposure in rural areas of countries with chloroquine- (or multidrug-) resistant *P. falciparum* or if the child is allergic to sulfa drugs or is too young to take sulfa drugs.

Primaquine is given to prevent relapses of malaria seen in *P. vivax* or *P. ovale* infection. Prophylaxis is generally indicated for children who have prolonged exposure in malaria-endemic areas (see Table 5–9). Primaquine can cause severe hemolysis in individuals deficient in glucose-6-phosphate dehydrogenase (G-6-PD). Testing for G-6-PD deficiency should be performed in children before administration of primaquine.

Small amounts of antimalarial drugs, including chloroquine and sulfa compounds, are secreted into breast milk of lactating women. The amounts of transferred drug are not considered to be harmful or sufficient to provide adequate prophylaxis against malaria.

Lastly, because of changes in the risk of developing malaria, resistance patterns, and recommendations for prophylaxis and treatment, physicians should contact the Centers for Disease Control, Division of Parasitic Diseases, at telephone no. (404) 639–1610 to obtain the most recent information.

ROBERT A. SALATA

Hill DR, Pearson RD: Health advice for international travel. Ann Intern Med 108:839, 1988.

Nahlen BL, Parsonnet J, Preblud SR, et al: International travel and the child younger than two years. II: Recommendations for prevention of travelers' diarrhea and malaria chemoprophylaxis. Pediatr Infect Dis 8:735, 1989.

Preblud SR, Tsai TF, Brink EW, et al: International travel and the child younger than two years. I: Recommendations for immunization. Pediatr Infect Dis 8:416, 1989.

Salata RA, Olds GR: Infectious diseases in travelers and immigrants. *In:* Warren KS, Mahmoud AAF (eds): Tropical and Geographical Medicine. 2nd ed. New York, McGraw-Hill, 1990, pp 228–242.

US Department of Health and Human Services, Public Health Services, Centers for Disease Control: Health Information for International Travel. Health and Human Services Publication, 1991.

6

GENERAL CONSIDERATIONS IN THE CARE OF SICK CHILDREN

6.1 CLINICAL EVALUATION OF THE WELL AND SICK CHILD: OBSERVATION, HISTORY, AND PHYSICAL EXAMINATION

The most powerful diagnostic maneuver available to the pediatrician is the clinical evaluation: the process of observing the child, taking a history, and performing the physical examination. In order for the pediatrician to maximize the benefit of the clinical evaluation, some of the complexities of this process must be appreciated.

UNIQUE CHARACTER OF THE PEDIATRIC CLINICAL EVALUATION. This evaluation involves the physician, the parent(s), and the child. Historical information is often taken from the parents, and it is not until the child reaches later developmental stages that he or she can contribute information about symptoms more actively. These considerations change the manner in which the pediatrician gathers data about symptoms. Rather than asking, for example, if the child has abdominal pain, the physician asks questions that focus on the manner in which abdominal pain would present to an observer. Thus, questions about loss of appetite, sudden episodes of crying and drawing the legs up in a fetal position, or the child's crying when the parent has placed pressure on the abdomen are appropriate. The 24-mo-old child with a sore throat often does not complain of this, but rather is observed by the parents to have more difficulty handling oral secretions, refuses solids, and has a foul breath odor. Questions are tailored to elicit this information.

As the child becomes older, he or she may begin to add historical information that expresses symptoms in unique ways. At times the information provided by the child suggests the diagnosis precisely, but, at other times, the child's information may reflect a less developed sense of cause-effect relationships and be at variance with the data provided by the parents. Thus, the 4-yr-old child with a urinary tract infection may be observed by the parent to be holding his or her abdomen and to have a subtle change in the frequency of urination. The child, on the other hand, may perceive that his or her abdominal complaints are related to a specific food that was ingested just prior to the onset of symptoms. In this instance, the pediatrician may conclude that the parent's history suggests the correct diagnosis (a urinary tract infection) by eliciting further information about, for example, discomfort when urinating.

PARENTS AND CHILD AS PARTICIPANTS IN THE CLINICAL EVALUATION. It is often left to the judgment of parents whether clinical symptoms should be brought to the attention of a physician. Moreover, children's interpretation of symptoms is intimately related to their developmental stage; this also influences the manner in which they transmit clinical information to the physician. Both parents and children must believe that the pediatrician is interested in their concerns, and that interactions with the pediatrician provide them support and enhance the acuity of their clinical perceptions. This process occurs at both well and sick child visits. At well child visits the parent or child might describe a specific behavior or symptom. The pediatrician demonstrates concern by listening attentively and by asking follow-up questions demonstrating that the behavior or symptom has been understood. These follow-up questions provide an opportunity for the parent or child to explore their own interpretation of these behaviors or symptoms, to explore what emotional response they have had, and to learn from the interpretation provided by the physician. For example, parents reporting that their 9-mo-old child cries when being put to bed and has difficulty falling asleep is an opportunity for the pediatrician to explore their interpretations of this behavior, to discuss their response to it, and to discuss the developmental dimensions of individuation. Based on this discussion and a more precise appreciation of the meaning of that behavior, strategies can evolve as an appropriate response to that behavior.

The same interaction and education process occur during sick child visits. Upper respiratory symptoms may concern parents. The pediatrician's discussing the predominance of nasal breathing in younger children, the more prominent symptoms that arise from nasal stuffiness because of this, and the absence of other evidence of serious pulmonary involvement such as tachypnea enhance parents' abilities to interpret respiratory symptoms during subsequent upper respiratory infections. Similarly, the pediatrician can explain cause-effect relationships between infection and symptoms to the older child. Such encounters, during both well and ill child visits, serve to enhance the confidence of parents and children in their role as participants in the clinical evaluation. Studies have demonstrated the ability of parents to evaluate clinical data reliably and the ability of children, when given developmentally appropriate information, to improve their understanding of clinical causality.

DEVELOPMENTAL DIMENSIONS. The data generated from observation, history (see earlier), and physical examination are greatly influenced by the child's developmental stage. A portion of the observational assessment of a child focuses on signs related to specific organ systems that are intimately related to age. The child of 1 mo has a more rapid respiratory rate (30 breaths/min) than the 3-yr-old child. The infant's respiratory rate is more sensitive to other influences, such as gastric pressure on the diaphragm caused by the recent ingestion of a meal, than that of the older child. Other portions of observational assessment focus on data that are indicators of the child's overall state of well-being or functional status, such as how the child responds visually to the environment. The pediatrician should not only be aware that visual responses undergo developmental change, but of the manner in which stimuli should be presented to elicit the child's optimal visual response at different developmental stages. The 1-mo-old infant, for example, is more near-sighted and tends to focus on objects held within 1 to 2 ft of the face; objects presented in the peripheral fields of vision may be ignored. The ability of the young infant to maintain attention on a visual stimulus is less developed than in the older child. Thus, the pediatrician must be aware of the developmental dimensions of observing children in order to gather and interpret clinical information accurately.

The data generated during the physical examination are also closely linked to the child's stage of development. Specific findings may be normal in one age group and abnormal in another. For example, the 1-mo-old child normally has a rooting reflex, which facilitates suckling. On the other hand, a rooting reflex found in a 2-yr-old child indicates central nervous system abnormalities. Not only do specific findings differ in different age groups, but the manner in which physical examination findings are elicited varies from one developmental stage to another. The 8-mo-old child, for example, is beginning to develop a sense of individuality and is aware of strangers and frightened by separation. To elicit accurate physical examination data, the child should remain cooperative and not resist the examination, especially during auscultation of the chest and heart. Based on an appreciation of the developmental stage of an 8-mo-old, the examiner should allow the child to remain close to the parent and make his or her approach as unobtrusively as possible. Factors that would lessen the strangeness of a situation, such as the warmth of the room, the stethoscope, and the examiner's voice, help facilitate data gathering. The older child is usually more comfortable with strangers and in separating from the parents and hence, after initial assurances, the physical examination may be done on the examination table.

The pediatric clinical evaluation is a complex situation because of the manner in which information flows among the participants, and because of the influence of developmental trends on gathering and interpreting the observation, history, and physical examination data.

GUIDELINES FOR EVALUATION. During the clinical encounter it is often difficult to separate each component of the evaluation. As the physician is taking a history from the parent, he or she is observing the child and observing the interaction with the parent; as the physician performs the physical examination, he or she is evaluating the child's global responses to the specific maneuver being performed. Nevertheless, certain guidelines can be followed during each part of the evaluation.

Observation is best done with the younger child in a comfortable position, usually on the parent's lap. Upset and anxiety on the parent's part are easily transmitted to the child, thus the parent and child must be placed at ease with a greeting and reassuring words. The tone of the examiner's voice is important and should convey a willingness to listen and a sensitivity to concerns being expressed. The manner in which the examiner is oriented to the parent and child is also important: if the examiner sits in one corner and regards only the notation page, a sense of unwillingness to communicate is conveyed. Sitting close to the parents and child and facing them directly is more effective. The examiner should observe the manner in which the parent and child are interacting—how are the parents responding to the child's needs and, in turn, how is the child responding to the parents? The pediatrician can modulate the stimuli in this situation to gather important observation information. The child may initially be clinging to the parent, so the pediatrician should interact with the child, offer the child an object, or attempt some separation of the child and parent to observe the child's response.

The history is best taken with the child in a comfortable position. If the child is quiet and comfortable, the parent can focus better on specific questions. Physicians vary in their amount of note taking during the history. Some prefer to write the history directly to progress notes; others note only key words and, at the end of the examination, transfer the information to the medical record. Whichever technique is used, it is critical that the physician remain responsive to the information being presented. If highly sensitive information is being conveyed and the parent or child is responding emotionally, the physician must convey empathetic understanding. This is impossible, however, if note taking continues without interruption. Additionally, note taking during this critical moment can interfere with important observations about the parent and child and their interaction.

The precision and clarity with which parents and children describe symptoms vary. Ongoing interaction with the family over a period of time enables the pediatrician to learn how clinical information is perceived and transmitted within each family. If, for example, the parents perceive the child as vulnerable, minor symptoms may be overemphasized; the pediatrician can adjust the assessments accordingly.

The portions of the physical examination that require optimal cooperation are completed initially—the blood pressure measurement, pulmonary and cardiac examinations, and evaluations of the eyes and central nervous system. The younger child may be held by the parent or seated on the parent's lap for these parts of the examination. The older child can be seated on the examination table. The pattern and rate of respirations is evaluated initially. Is there tachypnea? Is there increased work of breathing, as manifested by subcostal, intercostal, and/or supraclavicular retractions? Is there an expiratory grunt indicating that the child is expiring against a closed glottis to keep the small airways open longer? What are the colors of the skin, nails, and mucous membranes? After these assessments have been made, the physician may proceed to palpation, percussion (if indicated), and auscultation. It is not uncommon for the younger child to cry as the stethoscope is placed on the chest, but this can usually be overcome by patience and by increasing the child's comfort, such as offering the infant a bottle. The same sequence may be followed for the cardiac examination. The ophthalmologic examination requires that the child be quietly wakeful; ophthalmoscopy can be done with the child in the parent's lap or as the child is being carried over the parent's shoulder. Sometimes the other parent can provide visual stimuli; the retina can be seen more easily as the child focuses on such stimuli. Many portions of the neurologic examination, such as the eliciting of reflexes, also require cooperation and a state of quiet wakefulness. In the older child this can be accomplished with the child on the examination table but it is usually more helpful for the younger child to remain on the parent's lap.

After these portions of the examination the examiner proceeds to the parts of the examination that are usually more bothersome to the child. The abdominal examination requires that the child be on the examination table. It is helpful to have the parent hold a younger patient's hand and speak reassuringly. Thus, the child does not tense the abdominal musculature unnecessarily, which might occur during crying. After the abdominal examination, the pulses may be palpated, the genitalia examined, and the hips and extremities evaluated for clinical abnormalities. It is at this time that the examiner proceeds to the most intrusive portions of the examination, the evaluation of the ear canals and tympanic membranes and the examination of the oropharynx. During the ear examination, the parent may hold the child's head to minimize movement against the otoscope. The examiner should recognize that the ear canals are highly sensitive, and the speculum should be introduced gently. The free hand of the examiner can be used to put gentle traction on the pinna to straighten the canal. A portion of the hand holding the otoscope, usually the 5th finger, should rest against the head so that the otoscope moves with the head. At times, depending on the level of cooperation, the ears may be examined with the child in the parent's lap and the head resting against the parent's shoulder. The oropharyngeal examination is performed last and the tongue blade is introduced gently.

The sequence of performing those portions of the physical examination that require inspection, palpation, percussion, and auscultation (pulmonary, cardiac, and abdominal) varies according to organ system. The most bothersome maneuvers are performed last. For example, during the cardiac examination, inspection can be followed by palpation and percussion and then by auscultation. For the abdominal examination, inspection should be followed by auscultation before percussion and palpation are completed.

With appropriate sensitivity to the child and the parent, an appreciation of the child's developmental stage, and concern for minimizing the discomfort of an examination, the pediatrician can almost always obtain accurate clinical information and not cause undue upset to the child.

WELL CHILD EVALUATION. The broad principles outlined earlier also apply to the clinical evaluation during the well child examination. Well child visits are recommended prenatally, in the newborn period, at 2 wk, 2, 4, 6, 9, 12, 15, 18, and 24 mo, annually between 3 and 6 yr, and every 2 yr thereafter (see Table 5–5). For children with chronic or intercurrent problems, this sequence can vary. Certain considerations should be addressed at each visit.

Open-Ended Questions. The physician should ask general questions that allow the parent or child to voice concerns that might not be raised if questions were too specific. Open-ended questions such as "How are you?" or "How is the baby?" transmit an interest in the general well-being of the child and family, as do the behavioral clues that were outlined previously. When such open-ended questions are asked, it is important that the physician explore the leads provided by the parents or child; ending the interaction prematurely, without appropriate follow-up questions, is frustrating to the parents and child and sends a mixed message about the physician's interest and concern.

Development. Each well child visit should determine the child's developmental achievements, such as by the widely used Denver Developmental Screening Test. Questions in the gross motor, person-social, language, and fine motor-adaptive realms can be presented and scored. Previous scores serve as a reference point for future visits; the rate of change in specific dimensions, such as language, can be more easily appreciated. As the child matures beyond 5 and 6 yr of age, questions that focus on school performance and talented accomplishments can be substituted for the Denver test. Reviewing developmental milestones provides the parents with a sense of satisfaction in their child's progress and reinforces the efforts they are making to nurture and teach their children. Reviewing the older child's accomplishments is an important demonstration of support for these activities.

Feeding and Diet. Many changes occur in the dietary intake of those in the pediatric age group, and these should be reviewed with the parents and children. During the first 12 mo of life, for example, breast milk or infant formula is the major source of calories and nutrients. The introduction of infant cereals (strained, then junior) and finally table foods, the change from formula to milk, and the use of vitamins and fluoride are issues of daily concern for parents. In the older child the intake of excessive salt, carbohydrates, or cholesterol can affect health adversely. If the rationale underlying the introduction of certain foods and dietary changes is discussed with parents and children, they can more easily play an active role in and feel comfortable with this process.

Accident Prevention. At each well child care visit accident prevention should be reviewed. Potential hazards around the home are emphasized, as well as the importance of car safety measures. Syrup of ipecac is provided at the 6-mo visit and the phone number of the local Poison Control Center should be given to the parents. In order for the parents and older children to participate more fully in this process, the developmental aspect of accident prevention should be stressed. For example, the child's ability to crawl and to grasp and place objects in the mouth make the issue of poison prevention especially critical when these developmental milestones have been reached. The necessity for having ipecac in the house and for "accident-proofing" the home then becomes clearer.

Growth. At each well child visit the height, weight, and head circumference are measured. These are plotted on standard graphs, such as those provided by the National Center for Health Statistics (see Sec. 3.10). It is important to review growth parameters with parents and children, because these are objective indicators of the child's progress. If abnormalities in the rate of growth are noted, the clinical evaluation can focus on possible causes. When interpreting these data the pediatrician must focus on what is normal for this child, given the family background. Growth charts rely on normative data from populations with selected growth characteristics; thus, if both parents are slightly below the 3rd percentile for height, this normative data requires appropriate interpretation to allay undue concern in regard to this child's growth.

Family and Social Relations. To grow and develop normally, children rely on the support and nurturance provided by their family and the social environment (see Sec. 3.1). They are sensitive to disturbances in these supports, which can lead to nonoptimal growth, altered development, and adverse behavioral changes. The pediatrician should assess these supports by observation and asking questions. Observations can include the hygiene of the child and the child's general level of interest and response to people. How do the parents respond to the child's needs? What is the tone of parents' voices as they discuss the child? In what terms do the parents describe the child? If the child begins crying or is disruptive, how do the parents respond? Do the parents face the young child or do they show disinterest or lack of concern? Does the child appear depressed or inappropriately anxious? Specific questions from the pediatrician may elucidate other stresses or strengths in the environment. Is there an extended network of friends and family that provides support to the children and parents? Is the family under significant stress, such as through illness or loss of a job? The pediatrician's willingness to gather information about these issues and to address them demonstrates a realistic attitude toward what constitutes health or dysfunction for the child and family.

A particular challenge to all who care for children is represented by the special needs of children who live in impoverished environments (see Sec. 5.5). Empathizing with the difficulties of raising children in these circumstances and recognizing the obstacles that such children often face in realizing their potential are major concerns of pediatric care. Demonstrating a willingness to assist parents and children in resolving some of these adversities can provide them with a sense of hope and optimism about the future.

Anticipatory Guidance. Based on a developmental orientation, the physician should be aware of issues that might present problems or questions for the parents or child between the current and next visits. For example, the rate of growth of the 24 mo old lessens as compared with that of previous months, and this results in a diminished appetite. Rather than have the parents be unnecessarily concerned about this, it is prudent to preview the child's rate of growth in the next 6 mo and to discuss its impact on food intake. The developmental achievements the parents might expect over the next several months and the type of activities that facilitate these developments can also be discussed. For example, the 12 mo old's ability to grasp and bring objects to the mouth make finger foods an option for the child at this age. In addition, this ability points out the necessity of removing small objects (e.g., peanuts) from the environment to minimize choking and aspiration hazards. The anticipatory guidance that is provided should also review issues in daily caretaking, such as hygiene and sleep patterns. Again, every effort should be made to integrate these caretaking issues into a wider developmental perspective.

Other Concerns. At the initial well child visit, data should be entered into the medical record about the family medical history and the prenatal and perinatal history. At each well child visit, the physician should record and provide a record of immunizations to parents. Notes should be made about any intercurrent illnesses, such as otitis media or bronchitis. At each well child visit, a review of systems is carried out to ascertain whether there have been any symptoms related to specific organ systems, such as the gastrointestinal or neurologic. Finally, a flow sheet of laboratory screening tests, such as hemoglobin level, should be updated.

After the aforementioned considerations have been addressed and the physical examination completed, the pediatrician should summarize the child's health status. The parents should be complimented on their strengths as caregivers and the child complimented about his or her achievements and progress. It is also important to recognize problems and to express a willingness to work on these along with the family. The pediatrician's availability, if problems arise before the next visit, should be stressed. In this way the parents and child are reassured about the pediatrician's involvement in ongoing care. Parents and children should again be given an opportunity to ask questions or raise concerns about any aspect of the well child visit.

SICK CHILD EVALUATION. Many of the approaches presented for the well child evaluation are also applicable to the sick child evaluation. There are a number of reasons for a sick child visit but most visits are made because of acute intercurrent infections, and often the child is febrile. This discussion focuses on this type of illness, but the principles outlined are relevant to most sick child visits.

When evaluating an acutely ill, febrile child, the pediatrician must be aware of statistics about the occurrence of serious illness, because one of the major goals of the sick child visit is to identify the seriously ill child who requires the most vigorous therapeutic intervention. The risk among children with acute febrile illnesses for serious illnesses and the cause of the serious illness vary, depending on the child's age. In the first 3 mo of life, because of an immature immunologic system, the infant is more susceptible to sepsis and meningitis caused by group B streptococcus and gram-negative organisms. Additionally, urinary tract infections are seen more commonly in male infants; these infants more often have an underlying anatomic abnormality of the urinary tract than older children with urinary tract infections. As the infant matures beyond 3 mo, the bacterial pathogens that usually cause sepsis and meningitis are *Haemophilus influenzae* type b and *Streptococcus pneumoniae*. Urinary tract infections are seen more commonly in females than males. As the child matures, immunity is developed to the bacterial pathogens common during the 1st 3 to 4 yr of life. At this time, *Neisseria meningitidis* becomes the leading cause of bacterial meningitis. In children older than 36 mo, pharyngitis caused by group A streptococcus is a common bacterial infection. *Mycoplasma pneumoniae* assumes increasing importance as a cause for pulmonary infiltrates in children beyond 5 yr of age. The diagnosis of serious illnesses documented in 996 children in the first 3 yr of life who presented consecutively with fever and acute illnesses are shown in Table 6–1. These children were seen in a university hospital and in private practices.

Identifying the acutely ill child with a serious illness is accomplished by careful observation, history, physical examination, appreciation of age and temperature as risk factors, and the judicious use of screening laboratory tests. Based on these data, the physician can make informed decisions about the need for more definitive laboratory tests (e.g., urine culture), therapy, and the advisability of hospital admission.

Observation is a key factor in the evaluation of children with acute problems for the possibility of a serious illness. The child should be observed for specific evidence of a serious illness, such as grunting, which might indicate pneumonia or sepsis, or a bulging fontanelle, which might indicate bacterial meningitis. *Most observational data that the pediatrician gathers during an acute illness should focus, however, on assessing the child's response to stimuli.* How does the child's crying respond to parents' comforting? If the child is sleeping, how quickly does the child awaken with a stimulus? Does the child smile when the examiner interacts with the child? As noted previously, assessing responses to stimuli—and often providing those stimuli—requires a knowledge of normal responses for different age groups, the manner in which those normal responses are elicited, and to what degree a response might be impaired.

Sometimes the manner in which the child responds to stimuli is readily apparent—for example, the child vocalizes and smiles as the examiner enters the room. At other times, more effort and more stimuli are needed to cause the child to act in a more normal manner. Often, the fussing, irritable child begins to look around and focus on the examiner when held and walked by the parent. This normal visual behavior is an important indicator of well-being. Thus, during observation, the pediatrician must be both clinically and developmentally oriented.

Six observation items and their scales (the Acute Illness Observation Scales) that have reliably and validly identified serious illness in febrile children are shown in Figure 6–1. The normal point is scored as 1, moderate impairment as 3, and severe impairment as 5. The best possible score is 6 items $\times$ 1 = 6; the worst score is 6 items $\times$ 5 = 30. The chance of serious illness is 1–2% if the total score is $\leq$10; if the score is

TABLE 6–1. Diagnosis of Serious Illnesses During 996 Episodes of Acute Infectious Illness in Febrile Children Younger Than 36 Mo*

Diagnosis	Cases No.	Cases %
Bacterial meningitis	9	0.9
Aseptic meningitis	12	1.2
Pneumonia	30	3.0
Bacteremia	10	1.0
Focal soft-tissue infection	10	1.0
Urinary tract infection	8	0.8
Bacterial diarrhea	1	0.1
Abnormal electrolytes, abnormal blood gases	9	0.9
Total	89	8.9

*From McCarthy PL: Acute infectious illness in children. Comp Ther 14:51, 1988.

>10, the risk of serious illness increases at least tenfold. It is not clear whether these scales can be used in the first 2–3 mo of life, because infants may not have developed the skills required to score some of these items.

The complex nature of history taking has been outlined previously. Parents must transmit how a younger child has been "feeling." In addition, they should also provide information on specific symptoms, such as bloody diarrhea or cyanosis when coughing. The older child's perception of his or her symptoms may reflect a less developmentally mature understanding of the cause of the illness. The examiner pursues the historical information provided by the parents or child to define the symptoms precisely. For example, if the complaint is blood in the stool, additional questions can be asked about other evidence of bowel inflammation, such as watery stools, mucus in the stools, or increased frequency of stooling. On the other hand, if the historical information indicates crying with defecation and streaks of blood on the outer portion of a hard stool, without other changes in the character or frequency of the stool, a diagnosis of a rectal fissure is tenable.

Questions should focus on those entities that are seen most commonly in acute childhood illnesses. The more serious diagnoses are outlined in Table 6–1. Because most acute illnesses in children are caused by minor viral infections, specific questions about the epidemiology of the illness can provide important insights. Are there other children in the family with similar symptoms? Has the child had other illness exposures? Finally, it is important to be aware of any underlying chronic problems that might predispose the child to recurring infections and/or a serious acute illness; for example, the child with IgA deficiency may have a propensity to recurring upper respiratory tract infections and to pneumonia.

The approach to the physical examination has been discussed. The examiner should be aware of the illnesses that might be present in the acutely ill febrile child and seek evidence of those illnesses by examination. The child with pneumonia might have a severe cough, grunting, nasal flaring, tachypnea, subcostal retractions, and abnormal findings on auscultation; the child with meningitis might be more irritable when held by the parent (holding a child places increased traction on the meninges and results in "paradoxic" irritability), might have nuchal rigidity, and might manifest Kernig and Brudzinski signs. A careful evaluation of the skin and extremities might yield evidence of soft tissue infection, such as buccal cellulitis or septic arthritis.

The sensitivity of clinical evaluation is approximately 90% for serious illness. Each component of the clinical evaluation is as effective as the others in identifying serious illness, and careful data gathering is necessary by observation, history, and physical examination. Other data, however, should be sought to improve this sensitivity level. In the child with an acute febrile illness, the other important supplemental data are age, temperature, and screening laboratory tests. Febrile children in the first 3 mo of life have yet to achieve immunologic maturity, and therefore are more susceptible to severe infections and to infections by unusual organisms. Thus, the febrile infant is at greater risk for serious illness than the child

6 OBSERVATION ITEMS AND THEIR SCALES

(PLEASE CHECK BOXES THAT DESCRIBE YOUR CHILD'S APPEARANCE AND BEHAVIOR)

OBSERVATION ITEM	NORMAL	MODERATE IMPAIRMENT	SEVERE IMPAIRMENT
1. **QUALITY OF CRY**	STRONG WITH NORMAL TONE ☐ *OR* CONTENT AND NOT CRYING ☐	WHIMPERING ☐ *OR* SOBBING ☐	WEAK ☐ *OR* MOANING ☐ *OR* HIGH PITCHED ☐
2. **REACTION TO PARENT STIMULATION** (Effect on crying when held, patted on back, jiggled on lap, or carried)	CRIES BRIEFLY, THEN STOPS ☐ *OR* CONTENT AND NOT CRYING ☐	CRIES OFF AND ON ☐	CONTINUAL CRY ☐ *OR* HARDLY RESPONDS ☐
3. **STATE VARIATION** (Going from awake to asleep or asleep to awake)	IF AWAKE, THEN STAYS AWAKE ☐ *OR* IF ASLEEP AND STIMULATED, THEN WAKES UP QUICKLY ☐	EYES CLOSE BRIEFLY, THEN AWAKENS ☐ *OR* AWAKENS WITH PROLONGED STIMULATION ☐	WILL NOT ROUSE ☐ *OR* FALLS TO SLEEP ☐
4. **COLOR**	PINK ☐	PALE HANDS, FEET ☐ *OR* ACROCYANOSIS (BLUE HANDS AND FEET) ☐	PALE ☐ *OR* BLUE ☐ *OR* ASHEN (GRAY) ☐ *OR* MOTTLED ☐
5. **HYDRATION** (Moisture in skin, eyes, mouth)	SKIN NORMAL *AND* EYES, MOUTH MOIST ☐	SKIN, EYES NORMAL *AND* MOUTH SLIGHTLY DRY ☐	SKIN DOUGHY OR TENTED *AND* EYES MAY BE SUNKEN *AND* DRY EYES AND MOUTH ☐
6. **RESPONSE TO SOCIAL OVERTURES** (Being held, kissed, hugged, touched, talked to, comforted)	SMILES ☐ *OR* ALERTS ☐ (2 months or less)	BRIEF SMILE ☐ *OR* ALERTS BRIEFLY ☐ (2 months or less)	NO SMILE, FACE ANXIOUS ☐ *OR* DULL, EXPRESSIONLESS ☐ *OR* NO ALERTING ☐ (2 months or less)

Figure 6–1. Clinical evaluation of the well and sick child. (From McCarthy PL, Sharpe MR, Spiesel SZ, et al: Observation scales to identify serious illness in febrile children. Pediatrics 70:802, 1982. Reproduced by permission of Pediatrics.)

beyond 3 mo of age (see Sec. 12.1–12.4). In febrile children of any age, the higher the fever the greater the risk for selected illnesses. The risk of bacteremia increases as the degree of fever increases; at ≥40° C the risk is 7%. The limit of physiologic thermoregulation is 41.1° C; fevers in this range and higher indicate not only bacteremia but also possible central nervous system infection.

Screening laboratory tests can be helpful in identifying the febrile child at increased risk for common serious illnesses (see Fig. 6–1). For example, a white blood cell count (WBC) ≥15,000/μL and/or erythrocyte sedimentation rate (ESR) ≥30 mm/hr in children younger than 24 mo with a temperature ≥40° C places those children at five times the risk of bacteremia (15% versus 3%) compared to children in whom the WBC is <15,000/μL and the ESR is <30 mm/hr. A similar association with bacteremia has been found with a WBC ≥15,000/μL, a polymorphonuclear neutrophil count >10,000/μL, and a band count ≥500/μL. The risk of any serious illness in all febrile children is approximately twice as great if the WBC is ≥15,000/μL and/or the ESR ≥30 mm/hr than if neither of these elevations were present.

Diagnostic Approach. See also Sec. 12.3.

If the febrile child is older than 3 mo, appears well, the history or physical examination does not suggest a serious illness, and no age or temperature risk factors are present, the child may be followed expectantly. If otitis media is present, it should be treated. This profile applies to most children with acute infectious illnesses. If, on the other hand, the child appears ill or the history or physical examination suggests a serious illness, definitive laboratory tests appropriate for those findings are indicated (e.g., a chest roentgenogram for a child with grunting). The area of greatest controversy is the necessity of performing laboratory studies on the febrile child who appears well and has no abnormalities on history and physical examination to suggest serious illness but who is less than 3 mo of age or whose temperature is ≥40° C. Most would agree that a sepsis work-up is indicated in the febrile child <3 mo (see Sec. 9.60).

If the physician feels comfortable in following the child in whom no specific diagnosis has been established on an outpatient basis, a follow-up examination often provides a diagnosis. During the initial visit, or from one visit to the next during the acute illness, the change in symptoms or in the physical examination over time may provide important diagnostic clues. For the child in whom a diagnosis has already been established and hospitalization is not required, follow-up by phone or an office visit should be used to monitor the course of the illness and further educate and support the parents.

PAUL L. McCARTHY

American Academy of Pediatrics: Guidelines for Health Supervision. Elk Grove Village, IL, American Academy of Pediatrics Press, 1985.

Green M: Pediatric interview and history. *In* Haggerty R, Green M (eds): Ambulatory Pediatrics, 4th ed. Philadelphia, WB Saunders, 1990.

McCarthy PL, et al: Mother's clinical judgment: A randomized trial of the Acute Illness Observation Scales. J Pediatr (in press).

Roberts KB (ed): The Febrile Infant and Occult Bacteremia. The Nineteenth Ross Round Table on Critical Approaches to Common Pediatric Problems. Columbus, OH, Ross Laboratories, 1988.

6.2 PATHOPHYSIOLOGY OF BODY FLUIDS

There are three components when considering the physiology of body fluids:

1. *The total amounts of water and solutes in the body as a whole.* These result from carefully regulated balances between intake and output. Many controlling mechanisms, especially for substances having physiologic significance, are extremely complex. Those especially important to the clinician are discussed in some detail.
2. *The distribution of water and solutes in the various compartments of the body.* This is critically important with considerable energy being required to maintain steady-state equilibrium for most substances.
3. *The concentration of the solutes within each compartment.* This depends on the relative amounts of both solute and solvent (water) in that compartment. Thus, concentration can be changed by altering the content of either or both.

Regulatory mechanisms appear to be designed to prevent the large changes in solute concentrations that can lead to profound functional alterations. Generally the rate and percentage of change in concentration of the various solutes are more physiologically and clinically significant than absolute change. For example, an alteration of 3 mEq/L from normal in the extracellular fluid concentration of potassium represents a change of approximately 70% and may result in profound physiologic effects, but an alteration of 3 mEq/L in the extracellular fluid sodium concentration represents a change of only 2%, is well tolerated, and is of little clinical significance.

Changes in volume are relatively well tolerated, although percentage and rate of change are again more critical than absolute change. Thus, the loss of 100 mL of blood in a few minutes produces a negligible disturbance in an adolescent but results in shock in a newborn infant; extended over several days, the same hemorrhage in the infant could be fairly well tolerated.

6.3 WATER

TOTAL BODY WATER

Water constitutes 78% of body weight at birth but drops to the adult level of approximately 60% by 1 yr of age (Fig. 6–2). A close linear relationship exists between total body water (TBW) and body weight (wt), described by the equation TBW (L) = 0.611 wt (kg) + 0.251. Thus, estimates of TBW can be approximated from body weight alone. However, since fat is low in water content, TBW represents a smaller percentage of body weight in an obese than in a normal person. Because mature females have a higher body fat content than do mature males, their TBW is 55% of their body weight compared with 60% of the males'. A more exact estimate of TBW can be obtained from lean body mass (LBM) in which the relationship is TBW (L) = 0.72 LBM (kg).

FLUID COMPARTMENTS. Body water consists of intracellular and extracellular components (Fig. 6–3). In the fetus, *extracellular fluid* (ECF) volume is larger than the intracellular space, but the ratio of extracellular water to intracellular water falls to the adult level by 9 mo of postnatal life (see Fig. 6–2). This relative loss of extracellular fluid results from the increasing growth of cellular tissue and the decreasing rate of growth of collagen relative to muscle during the early months of life. Thereafter, extracellular fluid bears a fairly straight-line relation to weight (ECF = 0.239 wt [kg] + 0.325) and to total body water in normal infants and children. Under conditions of normal hydration in the older child (see Fig. 6–3), it constitutes 20–25% of body weight and is composed of plasma

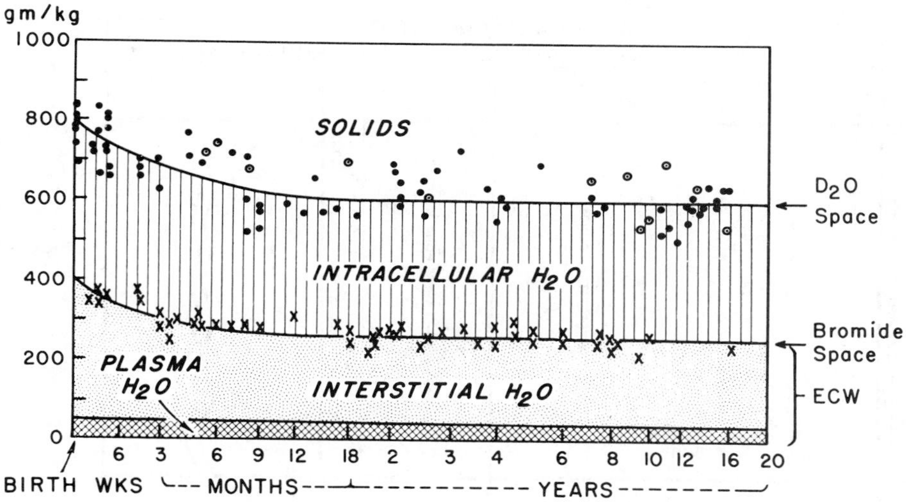

Figure 6–2. Body content and distribution of water at various ages. Deuterium oxide (D_2O) space represents total body water. (ECW = extracellular water.) (From Talbot NB, Richie RH, Crawford JD: Metabolic Homeostasis. Boston, Harvard University Press, 1959, p 3. Reprinted by permission.)

water (5% of body weight), interstitial water (15% of body weight), and transcellular water (1–3% of body weight).

The *transcellular water* compartment is composed primarily of gastrointestinal secretions plus cerebrospinal, intraocular, pleural, peritoneal, and synovial fluids. Transcellular fluid is usually considered a specialized fraction of extracellular fluid, although it is probably more accurate to consider the fluid in the gastrointestinal tract as extracorporeal. The volume of the transcellular compartment varies greatly, depending on the absorptive and secretory activities of the intestine; during the fasting state it represents about 1–3% of body weight.

Intracellular fluid (ICF) volume, the difference between total body water and extracellular water, approximates 30–40% of body weight. Although frequently considered a homogeneous phase, intracellular fluid represents the sum of fluids from cells in different locations with varying functions and differing intracellular compositions.

REGULATION OF BODY WATER

The plasma osmolality, the concentration of solute particles in plasma, remains almost constant at 285–295 mOsm/kg H_2O regardless of day-to-day fluctuations in solute and water intake. This is largely a result of precise control of the amount of water in the body through a finely regulated feedback system involving osmoreceptors and volume receptors, the hypothalamus, the posterior pituitary, and the collecting ducts of the nephrons. To maintain a constant state, the amount of body water derived from intake and from oxidation of carbohydrate, fat, and protein of both exogenous and endogenous origin must equal losses from the kidneys, lungs, skin, and gastrointestinal tract. Water balance is controlled by regulating both intake and excretion, the latter being the more important regulatory mechanism.

INTAKE. Intake of water is normally stimulated by a sensation of *thirst;* this mechanism is a major defense against fluid depletion and hypertonicity. Thirst, regulated by a center in the midhypothalamus, occurs either when plasma osmolality increases by as little as 1–2% or when the volume of body fluids is reduced 10% or more, as occurs with hemorrhage or sodium depletion. The changes in osmolality are monitored by osmoreceptors (see later) located in the hypothalamus and possibly in the pancreas and hepatic portal vein. The mechanisms by which volume depletion induces thirst are less well understood, but it may be monitored by baroreceptors in the atria and elsewhere in the vascular bed. Considerable circumstantial evidence suggests that elevated plasma levels of angiotensin II stimulate drinking and may mediate thirst in hypovolemic and hypotensive states. The kidney may also be involved in regulating water intake, possibly through the renin-angiotensin system.

In clinical situations, when conflicting stimuli such as hypotonicity and decreased intravascular volume occur together, the volume signal is dominant and thirst causes increased water intake, restoring volume at the expense of tonicity.

The thirst mechanism and the release of antidiuretic hormone (ADH) may be interrelated. However, at least some of the thirst centers are separated functionally and physically from those involved in release of ADH.

Disorders of the thirst mechanism may be seen in psychologic disorders associated with diseases of the central nervous system, in potassium deficiency, and in malnutrition. These may lead to increased drinking, even though the content of body water is greater than usual and osmolality decreased.

ABSORPTION. Ingested water is absorbed in the gastrointestinal tract by passive diffusion in response to active transport of solute from intestinal lumen to interstitial fluid and plasma. The active transport of sodium is the chief process responsible for generating the osmotic gradient leading to water movement. Any inhibition of sodium transport or failure of reabsorption of solute, as in disaccharidase deficiency, can lead to the presence of large volumes of unabsorbed intestinal water, resulting in diarrhea.

EXCRETION. Loss of water occurs from the lungs, skin, gastrointestinal tract, and kidneys. The losses from the lungs and skin are evaporative and, in conjunction with that part of the urine volume necessary to excrete its solute load, are referred to as *obligatory losses*. These losses represent the minimum volume of fluid a person must ingest every day to maintain fluid balance.

Water excretion is regulated by varying the rate of urine flow. A fall in plasma osmolality, indicating relative excess of water, is corrected by the excretion of an increased volume of dilute urine which has an osmolality below that of plasma. This loss of free water restores plasma osmolality to normal. Conversely, when plasma osmolality rises above normal, the volume of urine falls and its osmolality rises above that of plasma. This regulation of urine volume and concentration depends principally on the neurohypophyseal-renal axis, the effector of which is ADH. However, because urine volume can be reduced to only that necessary to excrete the solute load, it is influenced by diet. Other factors that influence urine flow include glomerular filtration rate (GFR), the state of the renal tubular epithelium, and plasma concentrations of adrenal steroids.

Unlike the excretion of water by the kidneys, which responds to the content of water in the body, evaporative water

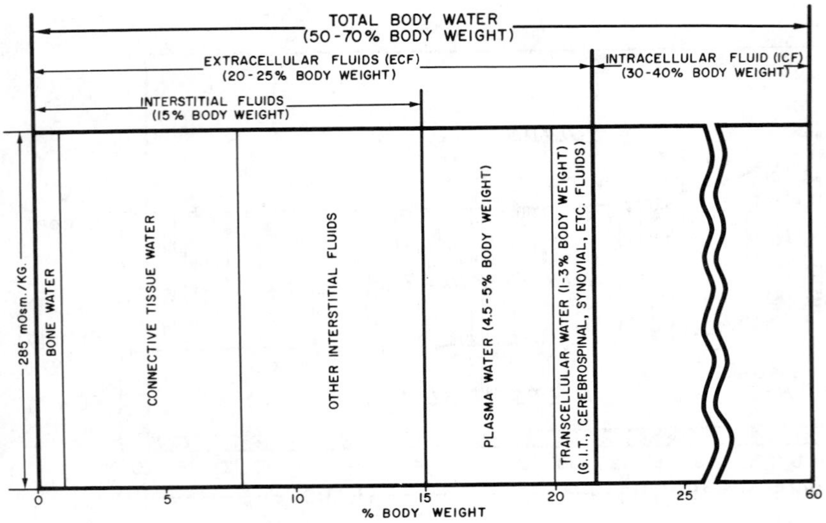

Figure 6–3. The distribution of water in the body of the older child (G.I.T. = gastrointestinal tract.)

losses are regulated by factors generally independent of body water. They are proportionate to the surface area of the body and are influenced by body and environmental temperatures, by the rate of respiration, and by the partial pressure of water vapor in the environment. Thus, evaporative water losses cannot be used to regulate water losses that occur because of changes in the body's water content. The rate of sweating varies with the body temperature and is controlled in part by the autonomic nervous system. It may be reduced in heat stress, by *severe* deficits in volume of body fluids or by concentration of electrolytes, but still does not represent a major mechanism for regulating body water.

Antidiuretic Hormone (ADH). Human ADH (arginine vasopressin), a cyclic octapeptide, is synthesized in the supraoptic nuclei. This neurosecretory substance is transported down axons that descend through the infundibular stem to be stored in the terminal arborizations in the pars nervosa of the posterior pituitary. Release of ADH into the bloodstream occurs by exocytosis in response to stimuli from the hypothalamus. Depletion of ADH in the posterior pituitary occurs in animals deprived of water; storage occurs when water loads are administered (see also Sec. 19.4).

Secretion of ADH is regulated by the effective osmotic pressure of the extracellular fluid—that is, that produced by solutes (primarily sodium and chloride) that do not readily penetrate cell membranes. This regulation is monitored by vesicles in the supraoptic nuclei that act as osmoreceptors: they swell when the osmolality of extracellular fluid is less than that of the intracellular fluid and shrink when the osmolality of extracellular fluid exceeds that of the intracellular fluid. Thus, administering urea, which readily diffuses across cell membranes to increase the osmolality of both extracellular and intracellular fluids, produces little shift of water between cells and interstitial fluid and does not evoke consistent antidiuresis. On the other hand, intravenous hypertonic saline solution evokes intense antidiuresis; the sodium remains predominantly in the extracellular fluid, increasing its osmolality in relation to that of intracellular fluid. Conversely, administering water inhibits the release of ADH.

Normally, the threshold for release of ADH is 280 mOsm/kg H_2O. Release of vasopressin may be initiated or inhibited with changes in plasma osmolality of as little as 1–2%. Response is graded, permitting the urine volume and the osmolality of extracellular fluid to be continuously regulated, thus preventing the fluctuations in osmolality that would occur as a consequence of normal variations in intake of fluid and solutes. Levels of ADH also increase significantly after 8% or greater dehydration, the rise being exponential with more marked dehydration.

The primary action of ADH is to increase the permeability of the renal collecting ducts to water. Under conditions of antidiuresis, the interstitium of the renal medulla has an osmolality of up to 1,200 mOsm/kg H_2O at the level of the papilla. This level of osmolality is achieved by the actions of the countercurrent multiplier (loops of Henle) and the exchange (medullary vasa recta blood vessels) systems. In the presence of ADH, luminal urine entering the collecting duct has an osmolality of about 285 mOsm/kg H_2O and becomes progressively more concentrated along the course of the collecting duct as water diffuses out of the urine into the hypertonic medullary interstitium by passive osmotic diffusion. By the time the urine enters the calyces, it has achieved the same concentration as the fluid in the hypertonic medullary papillae. If ADH is absent, continued reabsorption of sodium in the distal tubule and collecting duct leads to further dilution of the urine. Because, in the absence of ADH, these segments of the nephron are impermeable to water, diffusion into the hypertonic medulla does not occur and dilute urine is formed.

Influence of Disease States. Interruption of the supraoptic hypophyseal system causes diabetes insipidus. A failure of the renal collecting ducts to respond to ADH results in nephrogenic diabetes insipidus. Both are accompanied by an inability to concentrate the urine. Release of ADH may be stimulated or inhibited by emotional factors. Stressful stimuli such as pain or the mass discharge of peripheral receptors resulting from trauma, burns, or surgery increase ADH output and are important considerations in fluid therapy. Nicotine, prostaglandins, and cholinergic and β-adrenergic drugs are potent stimulators of ADH output. Demerol, morphine, and barbiturates are probably antidiuretic in this way, although their reduction of GFR may contribute to their reduction of urine flow. Alcohol is a potent inhibitor of ADH release with a consistent dose-response relation. Diphenylhydantoin and possibly glucocorticoids also inhibit ADH release. Anesthesia reduces urinary flow, probably by altering renal hemodynamics. The presence of nonabsorbable, osmotically active solutes in the renal tubular lumen (e.g., glucose in diabetes mellitus) reduces the amount of water that can diffuse into the hypertonic medulla, thus limiting the ability of ADH to conserve water.

MECHANISMS FOR DISTRIBUTING FLUID WITHIN THE BODY

The distribution of water between intracellular and extracellular spaces is determined by physical factors. *Intracellular volume* is maintained relatively constant by osmotic forces operating across cell membranes freely permeable to water. The maintenance of these forces depends on active transport of potassium into and sodium out of cells by energy-requiring processes. No evidence exists for active transport or secretion of water per se. A rise in extracellular osmolality (e.g., with a sodium load) results in a decrease in cell water. Conversely, water intoxication decreases extracellular osmolality and leads to an increase in cell volume. Disturbances in cellular function may also result in an increase in the fluid content of cells.

The volume of fluid in the *intravascular space* (plasma water) is maintained in a steady state by a balance between filtration and oncotic forces at the capillary level. Oncotic pressure (colloid osmotic pressure) represents only a small fraction of total osmotic pressure,* but its osmotic pressure is exerted by molecules, primarily albumin, which do not readily pass through the capillary pores. Thus, colloid osmotic pressure produces an effective osmotic gradient across capillary walls. At the arteriolar end of the capillaries the dominant effect of intracapillary hydrostatic pressure results in a net loss of plasma ultrafiltrate. Normally, at the venous end of the capillary, oncotic pressure causes the net return of a somewhat smaller amount of fluid and electrolytes, with the difference being returned to the vascular space through the lymphatic system.

Decreases in protein concentration (as in the nephrotic syndrome) lead to reductions in plasma volume and equivalent increases in *interstitial volume.* These changes may compromise the intravascular volume enough to reduce the GFR and blood flow to other vital organs but, because the volume of plasma is only one third that of interstitial fluid, plasma volume reduction by shifting of water into the interstitial space may not be observed clinically as *edema.* An increase in capillary permeability to protein, as in angioneurotic edema, produces a rise in protein concentration of the interstitial fluid. This rise reduces oncotic pressure, causing a net shift of fluid, which increases interstitial volume. The increase may be localized, appearing as a wheal or urticaria, or may be generalized. Interstitial fluid volume may also be increased by an increase in the hydrostatic pressure at the venous end of the capillary, as occurs with increased venous pressure associated with heart failure or with retention of sodium and resultant hypervolemia in glomerulonephritis.

The *transcellular fluid* space may increase markedly in inflammatory bowel disease (e.g., eosinophilic gastroenteropathy), in early severe diarrhea, or in ileus with multiple fluid levels.

OSMOLALITY OF BODY FLUIDS

Individual solute concentrations in the extracellular and intracellular fluids vary (Fig. 6–4). However, the osmolality in each compartment is comparable (see Fig. 6–3); the chemical activity of water (i.e., the tendency of molecules to escape to another compartment) is the same in each compartment. Nevertheless, the water content of the different body fluids does differ considerably, and variations from normal in these values can be clinically significant. For example, when serum solids such as the proteins and lipids are elevated, as may occur in diabetic ketosis with hyperlipemia, the water content in the serum is markedly decreased (when expressed per liter of serum) because of volume displacement of water by lipids. Because electrolytes are dissolved in the aqueous phase of serum, electrolyte concentrations such as that of sodium determined by flame photometry and expressed as milliequivalents per liter of serum appear decreased even though the concentration per liter of serum water is normal. Treatment of such *pseudohyponatremia* is unnecessary and may be detrimental to the patient. Its occurrence can be recognized by measuring serum osmolality by freezing point depression. This measures solute concentration of the water fraction of serum and more accurately reflects sodium concentration in the serum water. The problem of pseudohyponatremia is avoided by methods measuring sodium concentration with ion-specific electrodes.

*The principal colloids in the plasma are the plasma proteins, which exert an osmotic pressure of approximately 28 mm Hg compared with the 5,100 mm Hg exerted by the plasma's crystalloidal solutes. However, the capillary walls are very permeable to the crystalloidal solutes, which therefore exert no osmotic force across the capillary walls. Albumin, the most abundant plasma protein and the one having the lowest molecular weight, is the principal solute responsible for colloid osmotic pressure and for regulating net water movement across capillary walls.

6.4 SODIUM

BODY CONTENT OF SODIUM

Sodium, the bulk cation of the extracellular fluid, is the principal osmotically active solute responsible for the maintenance of intravascular and interstitial volumes. The quantity of sodium in the body approximates 58 mEq/kg, more than 30% of which is either nonexchangeable or only slowly exchangeable. Of total body sodium, 6.5 mEq/kg (11.2% of total) is present in the plasma sodium pool, 16.8 mEq/kg (29%) in the interstitial lymph fluid, and 1.4 mEq/kg (2.4%) in the intracellular fluid. About 25 mEq/kg (43.1%) is present in bone, but only one third of the sodium in bone is exchangeable. Dense connective tissue and cartilage sodium is 11.7%.

The *exchangeable sodium content of the fetus* averages approximately 85 mEq/kg compared with the adult value of 40 mEq/kg because the fetus has relatively large amounts of cartilage, connective tissue, and extracellular fluid (all of which contain considerable amounts of sodium) and a relatively small mass of muscle cells (which have a low sodium content).

REGULATION OF SODIUM

INTAKE. The amount of sodium in the body is determined by the balance between intake and excretion. When compared with the thirst mechanism for water, the regulatory mechanism of sodium *intake* is poorly developed but may respond to large changes; for example, salt craving may occur in some patients with salt-wasting syndromes. However, sodium intake normally depends on cultural customs. In the United States the average adult usually takes in about 170 mEq/day, equivalent to 10 g of salt. Children take in less, proportionate to their smaller food intake. However, infants generally have a relatively high sodium intake because of the high sodium content of cow's milk.

ABSORPTION. Occurring throughout the gastrointestinal tract, minimally in the stomach and maximally in the jejunum, absorption probably takes place by way of a sodium-potassium–activated adenosine triphosphatase (ATPase) system, a transport mechanism augmented by aldosterone or desoxycorticosterone acetate (DCA).

EXCRETION. This occurs in the urine, sweat, and feces, with the kidney the principal organ for the facultative regulation of sodium output. Normally, the concentration of sodium in sweat ranges from 5 to 40 mEq/L. Higher values are seen in cystic fibrosis and Addison disease and lower

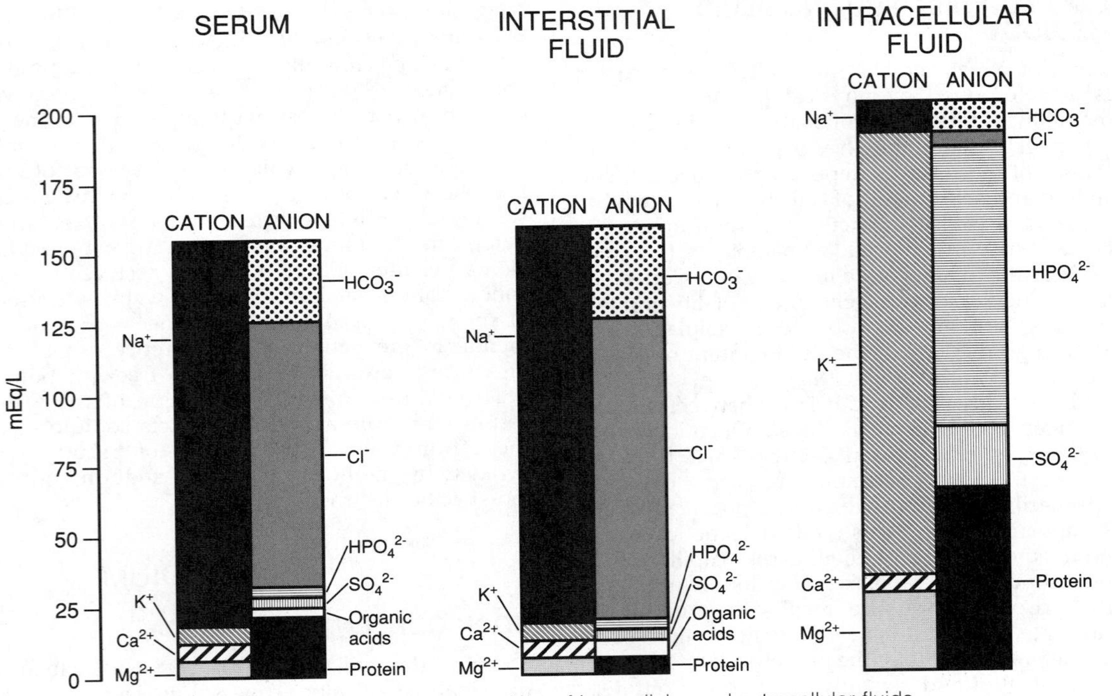

Figure 6–4. Differences in composition of intracellular and extracellular fluids.

values in sodium depletion and hyperaldosteronism, but there is little evidence that changes in the level of sodium in sweat are part of the excretory mechanism for regulating the sodium content of the body. In the absence of diarrhea, fecal concentrations of sodium are low.

RENAL REGULATION OF SODIUM EXCRETION. This depends on a balance between glomerular and tubular functions. Normally, the amount of sodium filtered daily by the kidneys is more than 100 times that ingested and more than five times the total amount of sodium in the body. However, less than 1% of the filtered sodium is excreted in the urine; the remaining 99% is reabsorbed along the length of the renal tubule.

Under normal conditions changes in glomerular filtration rate (GFR) do not affect sodium homeostasis; changes in the filtered load of sodium produced by alterations in GFR are compensated for by appropriate changes in tubular reabsorption of sodium. Moreover, sodium balance can be achieved even when sodium intake varies and GFR remains stable. However, the reduction in GFR that occurs with severe depletion of the volume of extracellular fluid and the increase that accompanies volume expansion may facilitate sodium regulation. Even then it has been shown that experimentally induced changes in GFR, over a wide range, are accompanied by proportional changes in sodium reabsorption in the proximal tubule. Such glomerular-tubular balance reduces changes in the delivery of sodium to more distal segments of the nephron, even when the filtered load of sodium alters markedly, and presumably acts as a protective mechanism.

Approximately two thirds of the filtered sodium is reabsorbed by the *proximal convoluted tubule.* With contraction of extracellular fluid volume this fraction increases; with volume expansion, it decreases. The percentages of filtered sodium and water reabsorbed in the proximal tubule are proportional, so that the fluid remaining at the end of the proximal convoluted tubule has a sodium concentration comparable to that in the blood. Net movement of sodium out of the proximal tubule represents the balance between sodium reabsorbed from the luminal fluid and that returned through intercellular spaces. Because such a high flux of sodium enters the epithelial cells across the luminal membranes, the sodium flux is unlikely to occur by purely passive mechanisms. Reabsorbed sodium is actively transported out of the cells across their basolateral membranes, producing an osmotic gradient that causes the movement of an equivalent amount of water. The resulting hydrostatic force in the intercellular spaces and interstitial fluid, as well as the exertion of oncotic pressure by the plasma protein in the peritubular capillary, is responsible for returning the reabsorbed sodium and water into the vascular space. The balance between glomerular filtration rate and reabsorption of fluid from the proximal tubule (glomerulotubular balance) may be modulated through changes in the protein concentration in the blood at the level of the glomerular and peritubular capillaries.

Sodium reabsorption in the proximal tubules may be regulated by altering the amount of sodium returned to the lumen through the intercellular spaces and tight junctions. It may also be controlled by a natriuretic hormone secreted from the midbrain or hypothalamic region. Although considerable indirect evidence supports this hypothesis, such a hormone has yet to be isolated.

Significant sodium reabsorption occurs in the *loop of Henle* and is central to the countercurrent multiplier system essential for water balance and the concentration of urine (see earlier). Water reabsorption occurs in the descending limb of the loop of Henle, sodium reabsorption in the ascending limb. Sodium transport at this site may be secondary to the active transport of chloride rather than primary as it is at most other sites. Although the loop of Henle is important in the overall control of sodium reabsorption, no precise regulating mechanism has yet been delineated, nor has a maximal rate for sodium transport at this site been demonstrated. When the load of sodium delivered to the loop is increased, by changes either in GFR or in sodium reabsorption in the proximal tubule, most of the excess load is reabsorbed in the loop, providing a further protective mechanism and limiting the magnitude of changes of sodium delivery to the distal convoluted tubule.

The fine regulation of sodium balance probably occurs

throughout the distal nephron in both the *distal convoluted tubules* and the *collecting ducts.* Sodium reabsorption at these sites is stimulated by aldosterone, whose secretion is governed by the renin-angiotensin system, by some aspect of potassium balance (Fig. 6–5), and by a tropic hormone. The stimulus for release of renin may be a decrease in renal perfusion pressure or a change in sodium concentration (or delivery) in the distal tubule at the level of the macula densa; either system provides a servomechanism to prevent excessive changes in sodium balance. Throughout the distal tubule and collecting duct, sodium is reabsorbed against a large concentration gradient from lumen to plasma. However, in comparison with the proximal convoluted tubule and the loop of Henle, the total capacity for sodium reabsorption is more limited. Thus, if the load of sodium reaching the distal tubule increases significantly, reabsorption does not increase proportionately and the added load is excreted in the urine.

Additional mechanisms may be responsible for the renal regulation of sodium. Cortical nephrons, which have short loops of Henle, may be sodium-losing nephrons and the juxtamedullary nephrons with long loops of Henle may be sodium-retaining nephrons. Sodium balance could be accomplished by altering the proportion of renal blood flow directed to these two populations of nephrons. Such a regulatory mechanism could be intrarenal and respond to local release of renin.

Granules in the cardiac atria contain peptides that are released into the circulation with volume loading. One of the most potent of these is a 24-amino acid peptide referred to as atriopeptin III, which causes marked dilatation of blood vessels and induces a diuresis and natriuresis of an order of magnitude greater than that produced by diuretics. These peptides may represent one of the major regulators of sodium balance, probably exerting their influence through selective modulation of vascular tone.

In health, less than 1% of filtered sodium is normally excreted in the urine. However, to maintain sodium balance, this figure may increase to 10% or higher with a high sodium intake and can decrease to very low levels in response to reduced dietary sodium. Thus, there is considerable flexibility, which prevents a significantly positive or negative sodium balance when dietary sodium intake fluctuates. However, it takes about 3 days for a new steady state to be achieved after dietary intake of sodium has been markedly altered.

DISTRIBUTION OF BODY SODIUM

Although cell membranes are relatively permeable to it, sodium is predominantly extracellular in distribution. Intracellular concentrations are maintained at levels of approximately 10 mEq/L and extracellular concentrations at approximately 140 mEq/L. The low intracellular concentration is achieved by active extrusion of sodium from cells by the sodium-potassium–activated and magnesium-activated ATPase systems. No other cation can replace sodium stimulation of ATPase, but potassium can be replaced by ammonium, rubidium, cesium, and lithium. Calcium inhibits ATPase, as do ouabain and related cardiac glycosides.

Although intracellular concentrations of sodium are low and represent a small part of total body sodium, they may be critical in modifying certain intracellular enzyme activities. Thus, intracellular sodium content is usually relatively constant, and changes in total body sodium reflect mostly changes in extracellular sodium. However, redistribution of sodium between the intracellular and extracellular compartments may occur in the absence of significant changes in total body sodium. Such a change may be observed in the severely ill patient, in whom it usually is referred to as the "sick cell syndrome."

Because of the Donnan distribution of anionic proteins, the concentration of sodium in interstitial fluid is approximately 97% that of the serum sodium value; changes in concentration of sodium in the serum are reflected by proportional changes in the concentration of sodium in the interstitial fluid. Concentrations of sodium in transcellular fluids vary considerably because such fluids are not in simple diffusion equilibrium with plasma (Table 6–2). Unexpected changes in composition of these fluids may occur and may necessitate the changing of therapeutic regimens designed to replace their abnormal loss.

INFLUENCE OF DISEASE STATES

In many disease states the body loses its ability to regulate sodium normally. Such abnormalities usually result in changes in volume rather than in changes in sodium concentration. Retention of sodium is typically compensated for by a retention of an equivalent amount of water, so that edema develops. Sodium concentration remains in, or near, the normal range. Excessive losses of sodium may cause hypo-

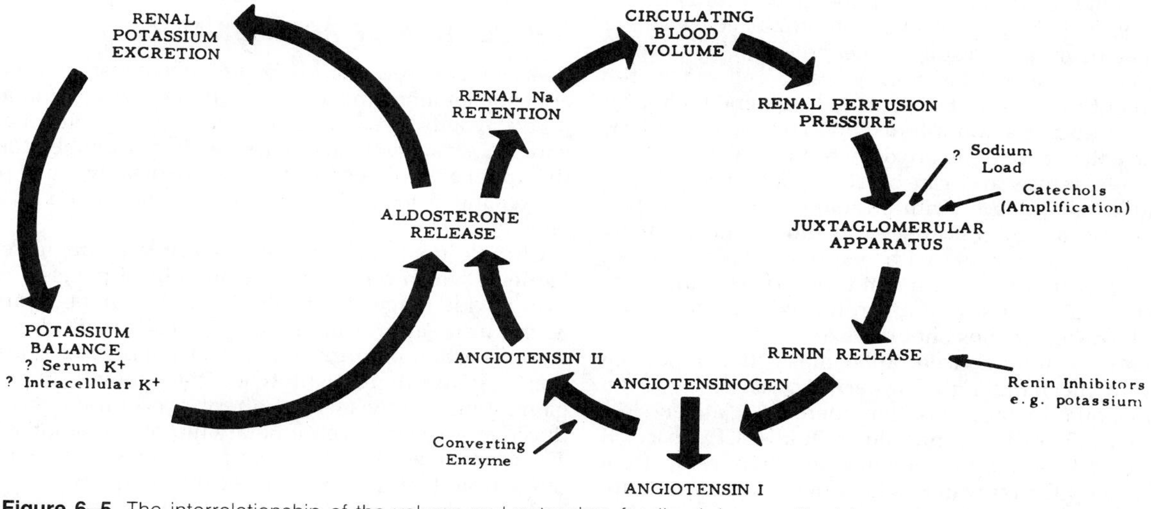

Figure 6–5. The interrelationship of the volume and potassium feedback loops with aldosterone secretion. Integration of signals from each loop determines the level of aldosterone secretion. (From Williams GH, Dluhy RG: Aldosterone biosynthesis: Interrelationship of regulating factors. Am J Med 53:595, 1972.)

TABLE 6–2. Sodium, Potassium, and Chloride Concentrations in Transcellular Fluids*

Fluid	Concentration (mEq/L)†		
	Sodium	*Potassium*	*Chloride*
Saliva	33.1 ± 13.4	19.5 ± 3.4	33.9 ± 10.2
Gastric juice	60.4 (9–116)	9.2 (0.5–32.5)	84.0 (7.8–154.5)
Ileal fluid	129.4 (105.4–143.7)	11.2 (5.9–29.3)	116.2 (90–136.4)
Cecal fluid	52.5	7.9	42.5
Pancreatic juice	141.1 (113–153)	4.6 (2.6–7.4)	76.6 (54.1–95.2)
Bile	148.9 (131–164)	4.98 (2.6–12)	100.6 (89–117.6)
Cerebrospinal fluid	140.0 (130–150)	3.3 (2.7–3.9)	126.8 (115.5–132.4)
Aqueous humor (rabbits)	143.0 (141.7–145.0)	4.7	107.9 (106.2–109.5)
Sweat	See Table 6–8		

*From Edelman IS, Liebman J: Anatomy of body water and electrolytes. Am J Med 27:256, 1959.
†Range in parentheses.

natremia, but they are often paralleled by comparable losses of water, thus resulting in volume contraction with little change in sodium concentration.

Patients with *chronic renal disease* can usually modify their rate of sodium excretion, but both the upper and lower limits of sodium tolerance are characteristically limited. Some renal diseases, especially those affecting the tubules, are associated with a limited renal ability to conserve sodium. In such patients the unnecessary restriction of sodium results in volume contraction and a further reduction in renal function. Conversely, exceeding the upper limit for sodium tolerance produces positive sodium balance and edema, a condition most often seen in patients with glomerular diseases. However, patients with chronic renal disease frequently do not develop positive sodium balance until their GFR falls to levels below 5 and 10% of normal or unless they have a nephrotic syndrome. Positive sodium balance may also be found in association with acute decreases in GFR such as that seen in acute glomerulonephritis and may also result from a decrease in the oncotic pressure of plasma (e.g., with the nephrotic syndrome), from a decrease in effective arterial volume (e.g., with congestive heart failure), or from the administration or increased secretion of steroids with mineralocorticoid effects.

In *diabetes mellitus* the high level of osmotically active solute in the tubular urine is a result of the presence of glucose, which retards passive reabsorption of water and causes the limiting gradient for sodium transport to be attained inappropriately, thus reducing sodium transport. This osmotic effect, exerted principally beyond the proximal tubule, produces both natriuresis and diuresis and can cause negative sodium balance. Negative salt balance (with an inappropriate elevation of sodium in the urine) is also seen in those with Addison disease and in some patients with neurologic lesions. More commonly, it results from extrarenal losses of sodium, such as those that occur with severe or protracted diarrhea when urine sodium concentrations should be low.

Alterations in sodium concentration most often reflect an abnormality in the handling of water. *Hyponatremia* (serum sodium <135 mEq/L) indicates that there is relatively less sodium than water in the extracellular fluid (ECF) space. It can be caused by ECF sodium depletion but often results from expansion of the ECF by water, which may arise from inappropriate reduction of water loss—for example, with the inappropriate ADH syndrome, or from excessive water administration (Sec. 6.25). In diabetes mellitus, hyperglycemia increases ECF osmotic pressure and draws water out of cells, causing a decrease in the sodium concentration of 1.6 mEq/L for each 100 mg/dL increase in glucose. Mild degrees of hyponatremia result in remarkably few symptoms. With more severe decreases in sodium concentration the presenting symptom typically is confusion. When serum sodium concentrations fall to 120 mEq/L or less, they should be treated promptly, because convulsions may occur as the osmotically induced movement of water into cerebral cells causes them to swell and produce seizures.

Hypernatremia (serum sodium >150 mEq/L) occurs when the amount of sodium in the ECF is increased in relation to the amount of water in this space. The content of sodium in the ECF may be increased but can be normal or even decreased if there have been major losses of water. Thus, as with hyponatremia, hypernatremia can result from derangements of sodium or water balance either alone or in combination. Examples include the following: (1) sodium retention resulting from excess sodium administration either as saline or as salt tablets or with accidental substitution of salt for sugar in infant formulas; and (2) negative water balance resulting from inadequate replacement of either excessive losses (e.g., patients with central or nephrogenic diabetes insipidus) or normal losses (e.g., a comatose patient) (see Sec. 6.26).

6.5 POTASSIUM

BODY CONTENT OF POTASSIUM

The body content of potassium, the major intracellular cation, correlates well with lean body mass. Because potassium is predominantly intracellular, the change in body potassium content that occurs with growth is an excellent index of cellular mass at different ages. In the adult, potassium approximates 53 mEq/kg body weight, 95% of which is exchangeable. Intracellular potassium amounts to 48 mEq/kg (89.6%); extracellular (plasma [0.4%], interstitial lymph [1.0%], dense connective tissue and cartilage [0.4%], and bone [7.6%]) amounts to only 5.5 mEq/kg (9.4%), of which 4 mEq/kg is in bone.

Intracellular concentrations of potassium approximate 150 mEq/L of cell water. Most is unbound and osmotically active, but sequestration by active transport in subcellular particles, such as mitochondria, is likely. Extracellular concentrations of potassium are maintained normally at 4–5 mEq/L.

REGULATION OF POTASSIUM

Potassium is present in remarkably constant quantities in almost all animal and vegetable tissues. A daily intake of 1–2 mEq/kg body weight is recommended, but intakes vary widely. Absorption of potassium is reasonably complete in the upper gastrointestinal tract. More distally, body potassium is exchanged for sodium present in the lumen of the lower bowel.

Chronic potassium balance is primarily regulated by the kidneys, which can adjust the amount of potassium excreted over a wide range. Normally, the rate of potassium excretion in the urine approximates 10–15% of that filtered. With the administration of large amounts of potassium, urinary excretion may be more than twice the amount filtered at the glomerulus. Conversely, urinary concentrations can be reduced to very low levels if potassium conservation is required. Thus, in the adult, rates of urinary potassium excretion may range from less than 5 mEq to 1,000 mEq/day.

Potassium is freely filtered in the glomerulus. Its concentration along the length of the proximal convoluted tubule is similar to that of plasma, indicating that reabsorption of potassium in this segment of the nephron is proportionate to that of water, with 60% or more of the filtered potassium being absorbed. Concentrations of potassium are increased in the loop of Henle. However, by the time tubular fluid reaches the early distal convoluted tubule, its potassium concentration is below that of plasma, so that the amount of potassium delivered to more distal segments of the nephron is less than 10% of the filtered load. Under states of maximal potassium conservation, continued reabsorption occurs in the distal tubule; when dietary intake is normal or when excretion is increased for other reasons, secretion of potassium takes place in the distal tubule and possibly in the collecting duct. Most of the potassium in the final urine probably results from tubular secretion rather than glomerular filtration.

The mechanisms responsible for the control of net secretion of potassium in the distal nephron are extremely complex and not fully understood. Potassium transfer across the luminal membrane is passive and depends on electrical and chemical gradients as well as on the membrane's potassium permeability. The electrical gradient generated by reabsorption of sodium from the fluid in the distal tubule represents a major driving force for this potassium secretion. The rate of potassium secretion, however, is always less than that of sodium reabsorption. Moreover, the variable ratio of the two rates indicates that the processes are not tightly coupled. Furthermore, the hydrogen ion is also excreted into the distal tubule in exchange for sodium, and renal production of ammonia, a regulatory system for acid-base balance, is also intimately related to potassium homeostasis. These observations may explain the interrelation of hydrogen ion and potassium excretion and account for the effects of acid-base balance on urinary losses of potassium. For example, kaliuresis and hypokalemia frequently occur with systemic alkalosis.

The concentration gradient for potassium between the distal tubular fluid and the distal tubular cells also modifies the addition of potassium to the fluid in the distal nephron. This process may be regulated in large part by modulation of intracellular concentrations of potassium through the active transport of potassium at the contraluminal cell membrane. Such a scheme could account for the observation that potassium excretion frequently cannot be correlated with serum potassium levels but may be better correlated with intracellular concentrations of the cation. An increased flow rate of distal tubule fluid increases the concentration gradient as well as the rate of loss of potassium in the urine.

Active transport of potassium may also occur at the luminal membrane, from the tubular fluid back into the cells. It has been proposed that this process could represent the final regulating mechanism. In summary, factors affecting distal nephron potassium secretion include mineralocorticoid activity, dietary potassium, acid-base status, distal tubular flow rate, and sodium delivery to the distal tubule.

Aldosterone plays a major role in potassium regulation in the kidney as well as in other tissues. Injected intravenously into a patient with Addison disease, it reduces urinary excretion of sodium and increases that of potassium. It acts at the distal tubule by altering permeability of the luminal membrane to sodium, thus allowing increased exchange between luminal sodium and intracellular potassium. Aldosterone secretion appears to be affected by both sodium and potassium balance (see Fig. 6–5).

Potassium is also lost in the feces and the sweat. The exchange of plasma potassium for sodium present in the colonic contents contributes to sodium conservation and permits the colon to participate in potassium homeostasis. However, even under conditions of chronic potassium loading, fecal potassium constitutes only a small percentage of the total amount of potassium excreted. The human colon responds to mineralocorticoids by decreasing sodium and increasing the potassium content of the stool. Glucocorticoids have a similar effect.

The potassium content of sweat, normally 10–25 mEq/L, is increased by mineralocorticoids and may be elevated in aldosteronism as well as in cystic fibrosis. Losses of potassium by this route, however, usually are insignificant, even in disease states.

Acute potassium loads require well-developed extrarenal mechanisms to prevent severe hyperkalemia and to avoid potassium toxicity. In the first 4–6 hr following a potassium load, only half of the potassium is excreted by the kidneys. Some is secreted into the intestinal tract. More than 40%, however, is translocated into cells, primarily in the liver and muscle. This process is an important protective mechanism and is regulated by both insulin and epinephrine, which enhance potassium uptake. The catecholamine effect appears to be mediated through β-receptors. Stimulation of α-adrenergic receptors impairs extrarenal disposal of an acute potassium load. Aldosterone plays a key role in the extrarenal handling of potassium. Its primary site of action may be the gastrointestinal tract, although it also affects muscle transport of potassium. Glucocorticoids may also be important in extrarenal potassium homeostasis. Glucagon infusion causes a transient hyperkalemia, but its role in potassium regulation is not clear.

Acid-base balance affects intracellular shifts of potassium. Systemic acidosis results in movement of potassium out of cells; alkalosis produces the opposite effect. For every 0.1 unit change in blood pH, the plasma potassium concentration changes 0.3–1.3 mEq/L in the opposite direction. The changes depend on numerous factors; for example, the increase in serum potassium accompanying respiratory acidosis is much less than that with metabolic acidosis.

POTASSIUM DEPLETION. Abnormally low amounts of total body potassium occur in various disease states, such as muscular dystrophy, which are characterized by a decrease in muscle mass. These disorders are not necessarily accompanied by *hypokalemia.* A low serum potassium level may result from a prolonged decreased intake, from increased renal excretion, or from increased extrarenal losses. Renal losses may be increased by the use of diuretics including osmotic diuretics and carbonic anhydrase inhibitors; by tubular defects such as renal tubular acidosis; by acid-base disturbances; in endocrinopathies such as Cushing syndrome, primary aldosteronism, and thyrotoxicosis; in diabetic ketoacidosis; in Bartter syndrome; and in magnesium deficiency. Extrarenal losses may occur from the bowel (e.g., with diarrhea, chronic catharsis, frequent enemas, protracted vomiting, biliary drainage, or enterocutaneous fistulas), or from the skin if there is profuse sweating. Movement of potassium into cells during correction of a metabolic acidosis, for example, may also result in hypokalemia, as may *familial hypokalemic periodic paralysis,* a rare disorder in which episodes of paralysis are usually accompanied by an abrupt and marked hypokalemia caused by movement of potassium into an extravascular body compartment (see Sec. 21.22).

External losses of potassium result in a shift of potassium from the intracellular to the extracellular fluid. Intracellular potassium is replaced in part by sodium, hydrogen ions, and dibasic amino acids. If these changes become severe, intracellular acidosis in the renal tubular cells may result in excessive exchange of intracellular hydrogen for sodium in the distal tubular fluid leading to aciduria, with the increased urinary excretion of ammonia and to systemic alkalosis.

The relation of extracellular to intracellular potassium concentration is vital to cell function. Membrane depolarization, the process responsible for initiating muscle contraction, requires the abrupt influx of sodium into cells and a comparable efflux of potassium out of them. The process is reversed with repolarization. With hypokalemia the ratio of intracellular to extracellular potassium concentrations is increased. The transmembrane electrical potential gradient increases so that a wider differential between the resting and excitation potentials exists, which interferes with impulse formation, propagation, and muscle contraction. Thus, hypokalemia produces functional alterations in skeletal muscle, in smooth muscle, and in the heart. Although it is impossible to predict the degree of potassium loss from the body accurately by measuring serum potassium, a 1-mEq/L decrease in serum potassium concentration secondary to potassium loss generally corresponds to a loss of approximately 5–10% of body potassium. Many patients tolerate this degree of loss without symptoms. Rate of change in potassium levels as well as magnitude of losses probably affects severity of symptoms. Weakness is an early manifestation typically noted first in limb muscles before trunk and respiratory muscles. Areflexia, paralysis, and death from respiratory muscle failure can develop. Paralytic ileus and gastric dilation reflect smooth muscle dysfunction. Electrocardiographic abnormalities, especially a lowered T-wave voltage and the appearance of a U wave, are characteristic. In the kidney, potassium deficiency results in vacuolar changes in the tubular epithelium. If sustained for a long time, it leads to nephrosclerosis and interstitial fibrosis, pathologic lesions indistinguishable from those of chronic pyelonephritis. The kidney has a reduced ability to concentrate or dilute the urine, with polyuria and polydipsia developing. An increase in bicarbonate reabsorption and hydrogen ion secretion results in systemic alkalosis. When the source of potassium loss is not apparent, measuring urinary potassium may help. A urine concentration of 15 mEq/L or less indicates renal conservation of potassium and suggests that the loss occurred from a nonrenal source.

INCREASES IN BODY POTASSIUM. Increases comparable in magnitude to the deficits discussed have not been described; they probably would be lethal. Indeed, *hyperkalemia* with serum potassium levels of 5.5 mEq/L or greater may result from surprisingly small increases in total body potassium. Because the kidney has a large capacity to excrete excess potassium and to prevent hyperkalemia, this electrolyte abnormality is most often seen when renal excretory mechanisms are impaired. Thus, it may occur in acute or chronic renal failure, in adrenal insufficiency, in hyporeninemic hypoaldosteronism, and with the use of potassium-sparing diuretics. Acute increases in potassium intake may also result in hyperkalemia, although it is typically transient in duration. Sources of such potassium include the use of potassium salts of penicillin (1.7 mEq/1 million units) and of salt substitutes by patients on a salt-restricted diet. Acute tissue breakdown, such as from trauma, major surgery, or burns, can also release sufficient potassium into the extracellular fluid to cause hyperkalemia. Finally, transcellular redistribution of potassium may cause an elevated serum potassium level seen typically in metabolic acidosis. It may also occur shortly before death or in severely ill patients. Certain drugs may increase the serum potassium level by similar mechanisms. Succinylcholine inhibits membrane repolarization, which requires cellular uptake of potassium. Severe digitalis overdose may cause severe hyperkalemia, presumably by inhibiting sodium-potassium exchange by cell membranes. Because intracellular levels of potassium are 30 times as high as those in the extracellular fluid, lysis of red cells during the collection or handling of a blood sample or release of potassium from platelets during clotting may result in pseudohyperkalemia, in which apparent elevations of serum potassium levels are recorded by the laboratory.

The major consequences of hyperkalemia are a result of its neuromuscular effects. It reduces transmembrane potential toward threshold levels and therefore results in delayed depolarization, faster repolarization, and a slowing of conduction velocity. Paresthesias are followed by weakness and eventually by flaccid paralysis if treatment is not instituted. The heart is particularly vulnerable to hyperkalemia. The electrocardiogram typically shows peaking of the T waves. Lengthening of the P-R interval and widening of the QRS complex develop later and are particularly ominous, because they often herald the development of ventricular fibrillation. Because the sequence of cardiotoxic events often progresses rapidly, hyperkalemia should be treated as a medical emergency (Sec. 6.26).

6.6 CALCIUM

BODY CALCIUM

See also Sec. 4.6, 6.27, and 24.58.

At all ages 99% of the body's calcium is in bone. Because the bones of infants are less densely mineralized than are those of adults, the body contents of calcium in infants and adults are significantly different, i.e., about 400 and 950 mEq/kg of body weight, respectively.

In health the extracellular pool of calcium remains remarkably constant despite fairly free exchange with the enormous reservoir in bone. The calcium concentration in serum is also maintained within narrow limits, averaging 2.5 mM/L (10 mg/dL). Approximately 40% is protein-bound, with the remaining 60% being ultrafilterable. One gram of albumin binds 0.8 mg of calcium, whereas 1 g of globulins binds only 0.16 mg. Thus, 80–90% of the bound calcium is bound to albumin, so that decreases in serum albumin concentration result in decreases in total serum calcium levels. Of the ultrafilterable calcium, 14% is complexed with anions such as phosphate and citrate and the remaining 46% (1.2 mM/L, or 4.8 mg/dL) is present as free ionic calcium. The ionized calcium is of greatest physiologic importance. Changes in hydrogen ion activity in the plasma modify the percentage of calcium that is ionized; for example, a change of 1.0 pH unit alters the concentration of ionized calcium by 10%. Acidosis increases and alkalosis decreases the proportion ionized. Although ionized calcium concentrations can be measured, a useful approximation can be estimated for clinical purposes from the aforementioned information if the patient's acid-base status is known, and from the assumption that each 1-g/dL decrease in serum albumin concentration decreases bound and therefore total serum calcium by 1 mg/dL.

REGULATION

Body calcium content is regulated primarily through the gastrointestinal tract. The recommended daily dietary intake is 360 mg in the first 6 mo of life, 540 mg in the second 6 mo, 800 mg from ages 1–10 yr, and 1,200 mg from ages 11–18. Dairy products constitute the most important single source. Dietary calcium is absorbed along the small intestine, primarily in the duodenum and early jejunum by a process enhanced by 1,25-dihydroxy vitamin D_3. It is proposed that hypocalcemia stimulates release of parathyroid hormone (PTH), which in turn increases the renal conversion of 25-hydroxy vitamin D_3 to its 1,25-derivative.

The efficiency of intestinal absorption of dietary calcium is increased on a low calcium intake, in the growing child, in pregnancy, and during depletion of body calcium stores. The mechanisms responsible for this adaptation are unknown. Administering vitamin D and PTH also increases calcium absorption, the latter probably by its effect on vitamin D metabolism. Increases in absorption leading to hypercalcemia occur in sarcoidosis, carcinomatosis, and multiple myeloma.

Decreased absorption of calcium results from the presence in the gastrointestinal tract of phytate, oxalate, and citrate (all of which complex the dietary calcium); from increased gastric motility; from reduction of bowel length; and from protein depletion, which may cause a deficiency of the calcium-binding protein in the intestinal mucosa. Some calcium is secreted into the intestinal lumen by the bowel, but this process probably does not represent a regulatory mechanism.

EXCRETION. Plasma non–protein-bound calcium (ultrafilterable calcium) is filtered at the glomerulus. Normally, about 99% of this filtered calcium is reabsorbed by the tubules, ionized calcium being transported more easily than the complexed form. Reabsorption occurs throughout the nephron. That which occurs in the proximal tubule (50–55%) and loop of Henle (20–30%) appears to parallel sodium reabsorption; factors influencing transport of one of these cations also affect the other. Calcium transport in the distal convoluted tubule (10–15%) and the collecting duct (2–8%) is independent of sodium transport; these sites probably represent the mechanisms that are specifically calciuric. Calcium reabsorption is stimulated specifically by 1,25-dihydroxy vitamin D_3 and inhibited by thyrocalcitonin. Parathyroid hormone increases reabsorption of calcium by the renal tubules, but this effect may be masked by the concomitant hypercalcemia and resultant increase in the glomerular filtered load of calcium seen in hyperparathyroidism. Urinary excretion of calcium is also increased by many nonspecific mechanisms. These include expansion of extracellular fluid volume; the administration of osmotic diuretics, furosemide, thiazides, growth hormone, thyroid hormone, or glucagon; metabolic acidosis; prolonged fasting; and an increase in the serum phosphate level.

There is a diurnal variation in the excretion of calcium, which peaks at the middle of the day. Alterations in dietary calcium result in only small changes in urinary excretion of calcium, probably reflecting adaptive changes in intestinal absorption of calcium. Physical inactivity is associated with increased urinary excretion of calcium and, if prolonged, may result in formation of renal stones.

INFLUENCE OF DISEASE STATES. The amount of ionized calcium is physiologically important in determining the significance of changes in plasma calcium concentration. Because some calcium is bound to protein, especially albumin, total calcium levels vary directly with the level of serum albumin. However, with hypoalbuminemia, a low total calcium level in the serum is rarely associated with symptoms or signs of hypocalcemia because the level of serum ionized calcium remains normal.

The balance between deposition and mobilization of calcium in bone largely determines the concentration of ionized calcium in the blood. PTH and 1,25-dihydroxy vitamin D_3 promote increased calcium resorption from bone and elevate the serum calcium. Thyrocalcitonin has the opposite effects. Plasma pH modifies concentrations of plasma-ionized calcium, as do the amounts of calcium absorbed from the renal tubular fluid and from the bowel, but to a lesser extent. In addition, the serum concentrations of sodium and potassium may play some role in the balance between deposition and mobilization of bone calcium; thus, treating hypernatremia with fluids low in potassium content may result in hypocalcemia.

Symptomatic *hypocalcemia* caused by a low concentration of ionized calcium results from vitamin D deficiency, which in turn is caused by nutritional deficiency, malabsorption, or abnormal metabolism of vitamin D. Hypocalcemia may also be a result of hypoparathyroidism or pseudohypoparathyroidism, hyperphosphatemia, magnesium deficiency, and acute pancreatitis. Because acidosis increases and alkalosis decreases the proportion of calcium that is ionized, symptomatic hypocalcemia may be seen during rapid correction or overcorrection of acidosis or with alkalosis.

The neonate is particularly susceptible to hypocalcemia in association with hypoparathyroidism, abnormal vitamin D metabolism, a low calcium intake, or a high phosphate intake (Sec. 6.10, 6.28, 9.54, and 19.17). Bone mineralization is frequently inadequate in very low birthweight infants during the neonatal period, increasing the incidence of radiologic rickets and fractures. These lesions most likely result from an inadequate intake of calcium and phosphorus at the time of rapid postnatal growth and may not respond to vitamin D metabolites.

Causes of *hypercalcemia* include primary or tertiary hyperparathyroidism, hyperthyroidism, vitamin D intoxication, immobilization, malignancies (especially those which metastasize to bone), use of thiazide diuretics, milk-alkali syndrome, and sarcoidosis. An idiopathic form may occur in infancy associated with typical "elfin" facies and supravalvular aortic stenosis; this syndrome may be caused by hypersensitivity to vitamin D. If their dietary intake of phosphorus is inadequate, low-birthweight infants may develop hypercalcemia as a result of resorption of both phosphorus and calcium from bone.

Calcium loading increases renal excretion of sodium and potassium and profoundly reduces the ability to concentrate the urine, an effect that may explain the polyuria and polydipsia seen clinically in patients with hypercalcemia resulting from hypervitaminosis D. Concentrated calcium solutions should always be administered cautiously, using electrocardiographic monitoring whenever possible to minimize cardiac arrhythmias (Sec. 15.62).

6.7 MAGNESIUM

Magnesium, the fourth most abundant cation in the body, plays a major role in cellular enzymatic activity, especially glycolysis and the stimulation of the ATPases.

TOTAL BODY MAGNESIUM

Total body magnesium amounts to approximately 22 mEq/kg in the infant. It increases in adults to 28 mEq/kg. Sixty per cent of body magnesium is in bone, of which about one third is freely exchangeable. Most of the remaining 40% is intracellular; more than 50% is in muscle and much of the remainder in liver. Only 20–30% of the intracellular magnesium is exchangeable, the remainder being bound to proteins, RNA, and ATP.

Extracellular magnesium accounts for only 1% of body magnesium. Although freely exchangeable with the large exchangeable pools in bone and cells, extracellular concentrations are maintained at low levels within a relatively narrow normal range. Serum magnesium normally ranges from 1.5–1.8 mEq/L, although wider normal ranges have been reported. Approximately 80% is ultrafilterable; this consists of 55% ionized and 25% complexed. The remaining 20% is protein-bound.

REGULATION

INTAKE. The intake of magnesium in children ranges from 10 to 25 mEq/day, depending on age; the highest intakes are required during periods of rapid growth. Green vegetables and many other foods contain high concentrations of magnesium; the intake of most individuals exceeds the minimum requirement of 3.6 mg/kg/day (12 mg of magnesium is equivalent to 1 mEq or 0.5 mM). Absorption of dietary magnesium occurs primarily in the upper gastrointestinal tract by mechanisms that are not fully delineated. Vitamin D, PTH, and increased sodium absorption enhance magnesium absorption;

calcium, phosphorus, and increased intestinal motility decrease it. Absorption is far from complete; an amount of magnesium equal to about two thirds the intake is present in the feces. A small proportion of this magnesium is secreted by the bowel.

MAINTENANCE OF BALANCE. Maintenance of balance depends primarily on urinary excretion. Normally, less than 5% of the filtered load of magnesium appears in the urine. Twenty to 30% is reabsorbed in the proximal tubule and most of the remainder in the loop of Henle, especially the thick ascending limb. Regulation of magnesium absorption is incompletely understood. Under various conditions magnesium reabsorption parallels that of calcium and sodium. There is competition between magnesium and calcium for transport. Urinary excretion of magnesium usually amounts to about one third of intake. It is increased by expansion of extracellular fluid volume; by osmotic, thiazide, mercurial, and loop diuretics; by glucagon; and by calcium loading. Conversely, volume contraction, magnesium deficiency, thyrocalcitonin, and PTH increase the renal reabsorption of magnesium.

The maintenance of magnesium balance and serum magnesium concentrations, however, requires a complex interaction of both renal and nonrenal factors. For example, a low-magnesium diet results in reduced urinary magnesium. This reduction may be the consequence of modest reductions in the serum concentration of magnesium, which have been shown to increase the release of PTH. In turn, PTH release decreases urinary loss of magnesium and also causes the release of both magnesium and calcium into the extracellular fluid, with increased concentrations of both cations. Tubular reabsorption of filtered magnesium can be almost complete. However, the gastrointestinal tract continues to secrete small amounts of magnesium, and depletion may result.

INFLUENCE OF DISEASE STATES. The concentration of magnesium in serum depends not only on intake and output but also on mobilization of magnesium from both bone and soft tissue. It is not always a reliable indicator of magnesium balance but may remain normal, even with marked *magnesium depletion*. Thus, in severe nutritional deficiency states such as kwashiorkor, serum levels of magnesium may be normal even though the content of magnesium in the muscle is decreased. Conversely, reduced levels may be seen in the absence of appreciable losses.

Hypomagnesemia occurs in various clinical states, including malabsorption syndromes, hypoparathyroidism, diuretic therapy, hypercalcemia, renal tubular acidosis, primary aldosteronism, alcoholism, and prolonged intravenous fluid therapy with magnesium-free fluids. At special risk are infants who undergo surgery and receive such fluids for protracted periods of time. Infants with either early or late neonatal tetany often also have hypomagnesemia (Sec. 6.28, 9.54, and 19.17). When associated with early neonatal tetany, it tends to be mild and transient and may not require treatment with magnesium. In late neonatal tetany, hypocalcemia may fail to respond to treatment until magnesium levels have been returned to normal.

The symptoms of hypomagnesemia are primarily those of increased neuromuscular irritability and include tetany, severe seizures, and tremors. Personality changes, nausea, anorexia, abnormal cardiac rhythms, and electrocardiographic changes may also be seen. Symptoms do not always correlate with serum magnesium levels, perhaps because serum levels do not always reflect the body content of magnesium, a predominantly intracellular cation. Alternatively, the symptoms of hypomagnesemia may be minor compared with the symptoms of the primary disease causing the magnesium depletion. A third possibility is that symptoms may reflect whether hypomagnesemia is complicated by hypocalcemia. Severe hypomagnesemia interferes with the release of PTH and induces skeletal resistance to the action of PTH. Thus, hypomagnesemia and hypocalcemia often coexist.

Hypermagnesemia, or an increase in body magnesium, rarely occurs in the absence of decreased renal function. Normally, the kidney prevents elevations of serum magnesium to dangerous levels even when large magnesium loads are administered. However, hypermagnesemia with serum levels exceeding 5 mEq/L can occur. The usual sources of a magnesium load include magnesium-containing laxatives, enemas, and intravenous fluids. Severe hypermagnesemia may be seen in neonates born of mothers who were treated with intramuscular injections of magnesium sulfate for the hypertension of pre-eclampsia. Neonates born prematurely with asphyxia and/or hypotonia are at special risk, although it remains to be determined whether the elevated magnesium is the cause or consequence of these abnormalities. Serum magnesium levels tend to spontaneously return to normal within 72 hr. There is also an increased incidence of hypermagnesemia in patients with Addison disease. Symptoms of hypermagnesemia occur when levels exceed 5 mg/dL. Hyporeflexia antedates respiratory depression, drowsiness, and coma. They are rapidly reversed by intravenous administration of calcium. Coma and death usually occur when the serum magnesium level increases above 15 mg/dL.

6.8 HYDROGEN ION
(Acid-Base Balance)

TERMINOLOGY

Acid-base balance has been complicated historically by a confusion of terminologies. The current approach emphasizes the *hydrogen ion*—or proton—which is a hydrogen atom with its neutralizing electron removed. *pH* is the negative logarithm of the concentration of free hydrogen ions. An *acid* is a proton (hydrogen ion) donor. Hydrochloric, sulfuric, phosphoric, and carbonic acids are conventional acids, each dissociating to liberate protons. A strong acid is one that is highly dissociated and, therefore, presents a high concentration of hydrogen ions; a weak acid is one that is poorly dissociated. A *base* is a hydrogen ion acceptor. Thus, bases bind free hydrogen ions, reducing their concentration. Examples include hydroxyl ions, ammonia, and the anions of weak acids. A *buffer* is defined as a substance that reduces the change in free hydrogen ion concentration of a solution on the addition of an acid or base. The presence of a buffer in a solution increases the amount of acid or alkali that must be added to cause a change in pH. The addition of a strong acid to any of these buffer systems results in the production of a neutral salt and a weak acid. By generating a poorly dissociated acid, the buffer significantly reduces the increment in free hydrogen ion concentration when the reaction is compared to one that is not buffered. *Aprotes* are either cations such as sodium, potassium, calcium, and magnesium that carry one or more positive charges, depending on valence, or anions such as chloride and sulfate that carry negative charges. Because aprotes can neither donate nor accept protons, they are not acids, bases, or buffers.

REGULATING MECHANISMS

The number of potential hydrogen ions in the body is huge. Most are buffered and, therefore, are not in free form. At the usual pH of 7.4 the concentration of free hydrogen ions in the blood is only 0.0000398 mEq/L or 3.98×10^{-8} Eq/L (often expressed as 40 nEq/L):

$$pH = -\log(H^+) = -\log(3.98 \times 10^{-8}) = -(0.60 - 8.0) = 7.4$$

Normally, the hydrogen ion concentrations of body fluids are maintained in relatively narrow ranges by the presence of buffers. Buffers represent the first line of defense against changes in pH, but they cannot maintain acid-base balance. Because, in the presence of disease states or abrupt alteration of hydrogen ion production, buffer systems may not be able to maintain a normal pH for a prolonged period, their action needs to be supplemented by compensatory and corrective physiologic changes in the lungs and the kidneys.

Compensation of a primary acid-base disorder is a slower process than buffering, but it is more effective in returning pH to normal. In a primary metabolic disorder the respiratory system provides the compensating mechanism; the kidneys compensate in a primary respiratory disorder. Compensation reduces pH changes but must be followed by *correction,* which returns all acid-base measurements to normal. This occurs when the primary disorder is cured. The kidneys correct a metabolic disorder, the lungs a respiratory one. Although discussed separately, the buffering, pulmonary, and renal systems are interdependent and act in concert with one another.

BUFFER SYSTEMS. The principal buffer in the extracellular fluid is the bicarbonate-carbonic acid system; intracellular buffers include various proteins and organic phosphates. In the urine, phosphate in its mono- and dihydrogen forms is the major buffer. Only the extracellular fluid buffer mechanisms are considered in detail.

Hydrogen ions, when added to the plasma, are buffered in large part by bicarbonate with the generation of a neutral salt and carbonic acid:

$$HA + NaHCO_3 \rightarrow NaA + H_2CO_3$$

Carbonic acid is a weak acid with a relatively low solubility coefficient and is in equilibrium with dissolved carbon dioxide, as follows:

$$[H^+] \cdot [HCO_3^-] \rightleftharpoons H_2CO_3 \rightleftharpoons CO_2 + H_2O$$

The addition of hydrogen ions drives this equation to the right, generating CO_2 and H_2O. Thus, despite the addition of hydrogen ions, the buffering mechanisms result in relatively little change in free hydrogen ion concentration and in pH. However, buffering is accomplished at the expense of a decrease in bicarbonate concentration (this decrease has been referred to as representing *base deficit*) and an increase in carbon dioxide (P_{CO_2}) levels. The Henderson-Hasselbalch equation indicates that these changes must result in some change in pH:

$$pH = pK + \log \frac{\text{base}}{\text{acid}}$$

In the bicarbonate–carbonic acid system, pK (a constant derived from the dissociation of the acid-base pair) is 6.1. Thus,

$$pH = 6.1 + \log \frac{\text{bicarbonate}}{\text{carbonic acid}}$$

Because carbonic acid is in equilibrium with dissolved carbon dioxide, measurement of the partial pressure of carbon dioxide (P_{CO_2}) can be used as a clinical estimate of carbonic acid concentration. By decreasing bicarbonate concentration and increasing P_{CO_2}, the addition of hydrogen ion to the plasma still results in some decrease in pH despite the presence of buffers. However, the changes are of lesser magnitude than would occur in the absence of the buffering mechanism.

PULMONARY MECHANISMS. The aforementioned equation indicates that pH depends not on absolute levels of bicarbonate and carbonic acid (P_{CO_2}) but on the *ratio* of the two concentrations. A decrease or increase in concentration of bicarbonate does not modify pH if the P_{CO_2} is lowered or increased in proportion. Thus, by altering the rate at which carbon dioxide is excreted, the lungs can regulate P_{CO_2} and modify pH. Although enormous quantities of carbon dioxide are produced from normal metabolic activity (Table 6–3), little change in pH results because of the unique properties of the bicarbonate–carbonic acid buffer system and a highly developed respiratory control mechanism. An increased respiratory rate, stimulated by increased levels of carbon dioxide, increases the excretion of carbon dioxide, decreases P_{CO_2}, and thus increases pH. Conversely, a decreased respiratory rate results in an increase in P_{CO_2} and a decrease in pH.

Even though the lungs can modify pH by changing P_{CO_2} and altering the ratio of carbonic acid to bicarbonate, this process cannot cause any loss (or gain) in hydrogen ions. The lungs are incapable of regenerating bicarbonate to replace that lost when hydrogen ion was buffered. The generation of new bicarbonate and, when required, the excretion of bicarbonate are the responsibilities of the kidneys.

RENAL MECHANISMS. The excretion of excess hydrogen ions, with generation of new bicarbonate or the excretion of bicarbonate, occurs by regulation of two basic steps. First, reclamation of nearly all the filtered bicarbonate occurs in the proximal tubule. No net hydrogen ion excretion results but, in the adult, this process is responsible for reclaiming up to 5,000 mEq of bicarbonate, which is filtered through the glomeruli each day. If this bicarbonate were not reclaimed, its loss would be equivalent to the retention of an equal amount of hydrogen ions, which would result in severe systemic acidosis. Second, generation of new bicarbonate occurs in more distal segments of the nephron and results in the net secretion of hydrogen ions needed to maintain hydrogen ion balance under most circumstances.

The mechanisms for both these steps are highly developed, energy-requiring, active transport processes, in contrast to the pulmonary excretion of carbon dioxide, which results from simple, passive diffusion. Both steps require the generation of hydrogen ions by the same basic reaction. Figure 6–6 shows that the proximal renal tubular cells, under the influence of carbonic anhydrase, hydrolyze carbon dioxide to carbonic acid. This carbonic acid is then dissociated into hydrogen ion and bicarbonate. The hydrogen ions are transported into the proximal tubule and exchanged for filtered sodium, which is reabsorbed into the peritubular capillaries with the bicarbonate generated from the formation of hydrogen ion. In the lumen of the proximal tubule the hydrogen ion combines with filtered bicarbonate to form carbon dioxide and water. These mechanisms ensure that virtually no bicarbonate passes to more distal segments of the nephron and that an amount of sodium bicarbonate equal to the amount filtered is returned to the peritubular capillaries.

Hydrogen ions are generated in the distal tubular cells by the same process as that described for the proximal tubular cells. They are also excreted into the lumen in exchange for sodium, probably by an active process. The transport of

TABLE 6–3. Approximate Order of Magnitude of Certain Factors in Hydrogen Ion Metabolism

Factor	Value†
Total CO_2 turnover	24,000 mM/24 hr
Total hydrogen ion turnover	69 mEq/24 hr
Total buffer in body	2,100 mEq
Total hydrogen ion in buffer (maximum capacity)	700 mEq
Total hydrogen ion in buffer (normal amount)	105 mEq
Total free hydrogen ion in body fluids	0.0021 mEq

*From Elkinton JR: Hydrogen ion turnover in health and in renal disease. Ann Intern Med 57:660, 1962.

†For an average man with a body surface area of 1.73 m^2.

hydrogen ions at this site appears to be gradient-limited, with the distal tubule able to generate a gradient for free hydrogen ion from tubular lumen to tubular cell of up to 1,000:1. Transport is thus facilitated by the presence of buffers in the tubular fluid that decrease the concentration of free hydrogen ion and permit increased movement of hydrogen ion from cells into the tubular fluid. The principal buffers at this site are phosphate and ammonia.

Under most conditions large amounts of *phosphate* are present in the distal tubular fluid. In the presence of a high concentration of free hydrogen ions, the phosphate is converted from a monohydrogen to a dihydrogen form (see Fig. 6–6), reducing the concentration of free hydrogen ion in the tubular fluid. The amount of hydrogen ion excreted in the urine in this form can be measured by determining the amount of alkali required to bring the urine to a neutral pH and is termed *titratable acidity*.

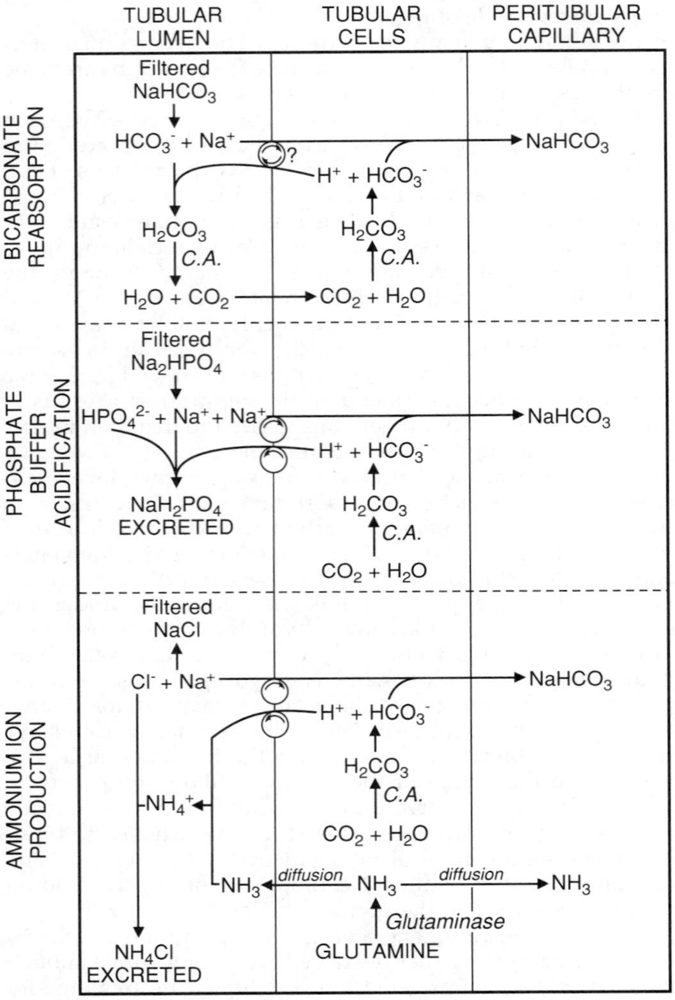

SIGNIFIES ACTIVE TRANSPORT

C.A. = CARBONIC ANHYDRASE

Figure 6–6. The renal mechanisms involved in acid-base homeostasis. Bicarbonate reabsorption normally occurs in the proximal tubule, where the presence of carbonic anhydrase on the luminal brush border facilitates the conversion of bicarbonate to carbon dioxide and water. This mechanism does not effect any net excretion of hydrogen ion from the body but results in the reclamation of bicarbonate in an amount equal to that lost from the plasma into the glomerular filtrate. Incomplete reabsorption of bicarbonate in the proximal tubule results in bicarbonate entering the distal nephron, where it decreases the amount of hydrogen ion available for producing ammonium and titrating phosphate to sodium dihydrogen phosphate, thus reducing net acid excretion. It is still uncertain whether the movement of sodium and hydrogen ions across the luminal border of the proximal tubular cell occurs by an active linked-transport mechanism.

Ammonia, a hydrogen ion acceptor, is synthesized in tubular cells from the deamidation and deamination of glutamine in the presence of glutaminase; this reaction is stimulated by systemic acidosis. Ammonia diffuses through the lipid membrane of the cells into the tubular fluid, where it reacts with hydrogen ion to form ammonium ion, NH_4^+. This charged cation cannot readily diffuse back from luminal fluid.

These two processes, by reducing free hydrogen ion concentration in the tubular fluid, enable an increased rate of transport of hydrogen ions into the distal renal tubule fluid and allow the generation of new bicarbonate, which can enter the plasma and replenish depleted levels of plasma bicarbonate (see Fig. 6–6).

The absolute net rate of excretion of hydrogen ions by the kidney is calculated as the sum of the excretion rates in the urine of titratable acid and ammonium ion minus urine bicarbonate. Living on an average mixed diet, an adult in the United States must excrete about 70 mEq of hydrogen ions each day to maintain balance. Approximately one third is excreted as titratable acid, the remaining two thirds as ammonium.

A number of factors cause an increase in the rate of hydrogen ion secretion in the proximal tubules and lead to increased bicarbonate reabsorption with consequent elevation of the serum bicarbonate level. These include elevation of plasma P_{CO_2}, hypokalemia, reduction in effective arterial blood volume (e.g., after vomiting or hemorrhage), and administration of mineralocorticoids. Conversely, hydrogen ion secretion, and thus bicarbonate reabsorption, is decreased by a decreased plasma P_{CO_2}, by expansion of extracellular fluid volume, by inhibition of carbonic anhydrase (e.g., by drugs such as acetazolamide), and by mineralocorticoid deficiency. Reduction in the plasma bicarbonate level may occur in these situations. Similarly, disease states such as cystinosis or heavy metal poisoning associated with structural or functional damage to the proximal tubule may limit bicarbonate reabsorption at this site and result in systemic acidosis. The distal acidification mechanisms may be impaired by intrinsic defects in the tubule, which cause primary distal renal tubular acidosis, or by various insults such as nephrocalcinosis, vitamin D intoxication, or amphotericin B administration, which produce secondary forms of distal renal tubular acidosis.

USUAL ACID-BASE BALANCE

Most mixed diets produce a net amount of hydrogen ions; true vegetarians ingest a neutral ash diet. Protein is the largest source of hydrogen ions; its metabolism accounts for approximately 65% of the total, generated primarily from the oxidation of sulfur-containing amino acids to yield sulfuric acid and from the oxidation and hydrolysis of phosphoproteins to yield phosphoric acid. The remainder of the hydrogen ions comes from the incomplete catabolism of carbohydrates, fats, and organic acids such as pyruvic, lactic, acetoacetic, and citric acids. Complete oxidation of these compounds does not produce excess hydrogen ions, because water and carbon dioxide are the final reaction products; incomplete metabolism results in the formation of organic acids and adds hydrogen ions. Thus, milk and meat diets generate about 70 mEq of hydrogen ions/day in the adult and require the kidney to excrete an equal amount daily to maintain a normal blood pH of 7.35–7.45. The infant and child must excrete proportionally similar amounts of hydrogen ion. In consequence the daily turnover of hydrogen ions is large, amounting to more than

50% of the hydrogen ions usually present in the body buffers and 10% of the maximum storage capacity of the buffers (see Table 6–3). This hydrogen ion is initially buffered by the intra- and extracellular fluid buffers, and then there is respiratory compensation before the kidneys excrete the hydrogen ion to maintain balance.

DISTURBANCES OF ACID-BASE BALANCE

Systemic acidosis or alkalosis may result from either primary metabolic or respiratory abnormalities. Recovery is unlikely to occur if the blood pH falls below 6.80 or increases above 7.80.

METABOLIC ACIDOSIS. Systemic acidosis may result from increased production or inadequate excretion of hydrogen ions or from excessive loss of bicarbonate in the urine or stools. Rapid expansion of the extracellular fluid space by a bicarbonate-free solution may also produce metabolic acidosis by diluting the bicarbonate in the extracellular fluid. The hydrogen ion load is buffered initially by bicarbonate in the extracellular fluid and by intracellular buffers such as hemoglobin and phosphate. Bone may be a further source of buffer. The serum bicarbonate level and pH fall (but to a lesser extent than if no buffering mechanism were available) and P_{CO_2} rises. The resulting systemic acidosis and increased P_{CO_2} stimulate the respiratory center (and possibly peripheral chemoreceptors in the carotid artery and aorta) to increase the respiratory rate, thereby increasing the rate of excretion of carbon dioxide. Plasma P_{CO_2} and carbonic acid levels fall, partially or almost totally correcting the acidosis but at the expense of lowering both plasma bicarbonate and P_{CO_2}. Thus, blood pH is decreased but rarely drops as low as might be predicted from the low level of plasma bicarbonate.

The acidosis also stimulates the kidney to increase ammonia production and hydrogen ion excretion into the urine. As a result, there is an increased generation of new bicarbonate, returning the plasma bicarbonate level to normal if the primary disease process has been alleviated. In turn, the respiratory rate subsequently decreases, with the P_{CO_2} returning to normal. At this point the patient's acid-base status has returned to the normal state that existed before the hydrogen ion load was administered.

The clinical picture of metabolic acidosis is usually dominated by its underlying cause and by the deep, rapid respirations *(Kussmaul breathing)* needed for respiratory compensation. However, severe acidosis itself may cause a decrease in peripheral vascular resistance and cardiac ventricular function, resulting in hypotension, pulmonary edema, and tissue hypoxia. The laboratory findings are decreased serum pH, as well as decreased bicarbonate level and P_{CO_2}. For every 1 mEq/L fall from normal in the plasma bicarbonate level, arterial P_{CO_2} should decrease 1.0–1.5 mm Hg. If this does not occur, a mixed disturbance should be suspected (see below). When the acidosis is a result of bicarbonate loss, the anion gap is normal and hyperchloremia is present. An increased anion gap usually signifies the increased production of hydrogen ion or its decreased excretion. A more detailed discussion of anion gap is presented in Sec. 6.9.

Renal Causes. Renal causes of metabolic acidosis are numerous. Diseases involving the proximal tubules may limit the ability of this segment of the nephron to secrete hydrogen ions and cause incomplete bicarbonate reabsorption. Increased amounts of bicarbonate are presented to the distal tubular fluid, resulting in the proximal form of *renal tubular acidosis.* In distal renal tubular acidosis the distal tubule cannot maintain a normal hydrogen ion gradient so that urine pH remains relatively alkaline, rarely falling below 5.5. A reduction of titratable acid, decreased secretion of hydrogen ion, and systemic acidosis result. With *chronic renal insufficiency,* acidification mechanisms work normally or at supranormal rates. However, the reduced tubular mass limits the ability of the kidney to generate sufficient ammonia and thus to excrete adequate amounts of hydrogen ions. A *low GFR,* such as in the newborn, also limits the renal capacity to excrete hydrogen ion. In addition, the filtered load of phosphate is reduced, the bulk being reabsorbed in the proximal tubule; little is left for buffering of added hydrogen ion in the distal tubule. Hydrogen ion transport is thus reduced by rapid attainment of a maximal concentration gradient in the absence of buffer. Rarely, *reduction in ammonia synthesis,* as in the cerebro-oculorenal syndrome of Lowe, limits the ability to excrete hydrogen ions.

Other Causes. Metabolic acidosis may also develop in *diabetic ketoacidosis* from incomplete metabolism of body lipids and catabolism of body protein, accompanied by the production of large amounts of acetoacetic, β-hydroxybutyric, phosphoric, and sulfuric acids. In *salicylism,* metabolic acidosis results not only from hydrogen ion derived from salicylic acid but also from the uncoupling of oxidative phosphorylation by salicylate. In severe *diarrhea* the increased losses of bicarbonate in diarrheal fluid and, possibly, the formation of organic acids from incomplete breakdown of carbohydrate in the stools result in metabolic acidosis. *Hyperalimentation, lactic acidosis, starvation,* and *poisoning with either methyl alcohol or ethylene glycol* cause systemic acidosis by increased production of various strong acids. Metabolic acidosis is seen also in certain *inherited aminoacidurias* (e.g., methylmalonicaciduria), in hypoxemia, and in shock.

METABOLIC ALKALOSIS. This may result from three basic mechanisms: (1) excessive loss of hydrogen ion, as in prolonged gastric aspiration or persistent vomiting associated with pyloric stenosis; (2) increased addition of bicarbonate to the extracellular fluid, which may result from excessive administration by the parenteral route or by oral intake, as in the milk-alkali syndrome, or from increased renal reabsorption of bicarbonate caused by profound potassium depletion, primary hyperaldosteronism, Cushing syndrome, Bartter syndrome, or excessive intake of licorice; and (3) contraction of the extracellular fluid volume, which increases bicarbonate concentration in this fluid space and increases bicarbonate reclamation in the renal tubule.

The buffer systems minimize pH change, but both the plasma bicarbonate level and pH are increased. Respiration may be depressed with some increase in plasma P_{CO_2}, but this response is limited by increasing hypoxia so that respiratory compensation is always incomplete and never restores pH to normal. The renal threshold for bicarbonate is exceeded, and bicarbonate appears in the urine, which may have a pH as high as 8.5–9.0. However, factors such as volume depletion and hypokalemia often coexist and they, along with the increased P_{CO_2} itself, tend to increase renal reabsorption of bicarbonate, maintaining the metabolic alkalosis. Metabolic alkalosis may be refractory to treatment in the presence of either hypokalemia or depletion of extracellular fluid volume and often can only be treated after these deficiencies have been corrected.

The diagnosis of metabolic alkalosis should be considered in any patient with an appropriate history; there are no pathognomonic signs of this electrolyte disturbance. Patients may have cramps or feel weak and may have the signs of tetany if ionized calcium has been reduced by the alkalosis.

Characteristically, pH, plasma bicarbonate level, and P_{CO_2} of arterial blood are elevated. Hypochloremia and hypokalemia are usually present, the latter principally resulting from increased urinary losses of potassium. Classically, the urine pH is alkaline, but in the presence of severe depletion of potassium, the urinary potassium level is low and paradoxic aciduria is present. In those patients with volume depletion who are responsive to sodium chloride, urine chloride concentrations should be less than 10 mEq/L. In contrast, patients who have metabolic alkalosis resulting from excessive mineralocorticoid activity or potassium depletion have a urine chloride level exceeding 20 mEq/L and are resistant to sodium chloride treatment.

RESPIRATORY ACIDOSIS. This disturbance results from inadequate pulmonary excretion of carbon dioxide in the presence of normal production of this gas. It may be seen acutely in neuromuscular disorders such as brain stem injury, Guillain-Barré syndrome, or sedative overdose; in airway obstruction such as that caused by a foreign body, severe bronchospasm, or laryngeal edema; in vascular diseases such as massive pulmonary embolism; and in other conditions such as pneumothorax, pulmonary edema, or severe pneumonia. Chronic respiratory acidosis may accompany the pickwickian syndrome, poliomyelitis, chronic obstructive airway disease, kyphoscoliosis, or chronic administration of sedatives.

In health, increased production of CO_2 stimulates its increased respiratory excretion so that a normal P_{CO_2} is maintained and acid-base status remains normal. In any of the disease states causing respiratory acidosis, the level of P_{CO_2} increases until it is elevated sufficiently to cause pulmonary excretion of carbon dioxide equal to its production. Although a new steady state is reached, the increase in P_{CO_2} (hypercapnia) causes a systemic acidosis by increasing serum concentrations of carbonic acid and, therefore, of hydrogen ions.

Because CO_2 is a major component of the principal buffer system of the extracellular fluid, the rise in P_{CO_2} must be buffered initially by the nonbicarbonate buffers—that is, the proteins in the extracellular fluid and phosphate, hemoglobin, other proteins, and lactate in the cells. The acidosis and increased P_{CO_2} stimulate the kidney to increase hydrogen ion excretion as ammonium and titratable acid and to generate and reabsorb more bicarbonate; thus, plasma bicarbonate levels may be increased somewhat above normal. At this stage the increase in the plasma bicarbonate level compensates for the primary increase in P_{CO_2} so that pH returns toward normal and the respiratory acidosis has been "compensated" by renal mechanisms. The only way to *correct* the abnormality is to reverse the primary disorder.

Causes of acute respiratory acidosis are often associated with hypoxemia, which usually dominates the clinical picture, along with the signs of respiratory distress. Hypercapnia results in vasodilatation, increases cerebral blood flow, and may be responsible for the headaches and raised intracranial pressure sometimes found in these patients. Severe hypercapnia may be a cerebral depressant; arterial pH is low, P_{CO_2} elevated, and plasma bicarbonate level elevated moderately.

RESPIRATORY ALKALOSIS. Excessive pulmonary losses of carbon dioxide in the presence of normal production results in a fall in P_{CO_2} and respiratory alkalosis. It may be observed with hyperventilation of psychogenic origin, with overventilation from mechanically assisted ventilation, and in the early stages of salicylate overdosage as a result of stimulation of the respiratory center by salicylate or of increased sensitivity of the respiratory center to P_{CO_2}.

Plasma P_{CO_2} falls and pH rises. A rapid buffering of this pH change occurs, with hydrogen ions released from body buffers to decrease plasma bicarbonate. Approximately 99% of this hydrogen ion is released from intracellular buffers and the remaining 1% from extracellular buffers. The renal excretion of bicarbonate, slowly increasing by mechanisms that are incompletely understood, reduces plasma bicarbonate levels and compensates for the excessive loss of carbon dioxide, returning pH toward normal. However, correction cannot occur until the causative disorder has been removed.

The clinical picture usually is that of the underlying disease process. However, acute hypercapnia may result in neuromuscular irritability and paresthesias in the extremities and perioraly, because of a decrease in the concentration of ionized calcium. Arterial pH is elevated, P_{CO_2} and plasma bicarbonate level decreased. Despite systemic alkalosis the urine usually remains acid.

MIXED DISORDERS. Under certain circumstances, mixed disturbances may occur in which more than a single primary cause is responsible for the abnormal acid-base balance. For example, in respiratory distress syndrome metabolic and respiratory acidoses often coexist. The respiratory disease prevents the compensatory fall in P_{CO_2}, and the metabolic component limits the ability to increase the plasma bicarbonate level, which would normally buffer a respiratory acidosis. In such a situation the decrease in pH is often profound, of greater magnitude than that seen when only a single disturbance exists.

Other types of mixed disturbances may be seen. Patients with congestive heart failure and chronic respiratory acidosis may develop a component of metabolic alkalosis if they use diuretics excessively. The plasma bicarbonate level and pH are higher than in a simple chronic respiratory acidosis. Indeed, pH may be normal or even slightly elevated. Patients with hepatic failure may have both a metabolic acidosis and a respiratory alkalosis. The plasma bicarbonate level and P_{CO_2} may be lower than expected with a simple disorder, whereas pH may be little changed from normal. Respiratory and metabolic alkaloses may also coexist under some circumstances.

CLINICAL ASSESSMENT OF ACID-BASE DISORDERS

For clinical purposes acid-base status is determined from serum pH, P_{CO_2}, and bicarbonate levels. This approach has replaced measuring base excess or deficit and estimating buffer base as the sum of concentrations of the buffer anions of whole blood—that is, bicarbonate, plasma proteins, and hemoglobin. Base excess was measured by titration of whole blood with a strong acid to pH 7.40 at a P_{CO_2} of 40 mm Hg at 37° C and base deficit was measured by titrating with base. Values were expressed as mEq/L.

MEASUREMENTS. Blood pH can be measured accurately with small blood samples; normal values are from 7.35 to 7.45. The concentration of carbonic acid (H_2CO_3) in biologic fluids is quantitatively negligible compared with dissolved carbon dioxide. The latter is measured as the partial pressure of carbon dioxide (P_{CO_2}) in a gas phase in equilibrium with the biologic fluid; the normal value approximates 40 mm Hg.

The concentration of bicarbonate ion in plasma can be measured directly, but the precision of this determination is not required for clinical purposes. It is customary to determine total carbon dioxide concentration of the serum as an estimate of bicarbonate level. This value is 1–2 mEq/L higher than that of true bicarbonate. It is obtained either by titration or by generation of carbon dioxide from serum with a strong acid. The carbon dioxide is derived principally from bicarbonate but also from dissolved carbon dioxide, carbonic acid, carbonate ion, and carbamino compounds. The normal value is 25–28 millimoles (mM)/L, except in the 1st yr of life, when values are 20–23 mM/L, probably because of the low renal threshold for bicarbonate.

If only two of these values are known, the third can be derived from one of the nomograms developed for this purpose (Fig. 6–7) or can be calculated by one of the several

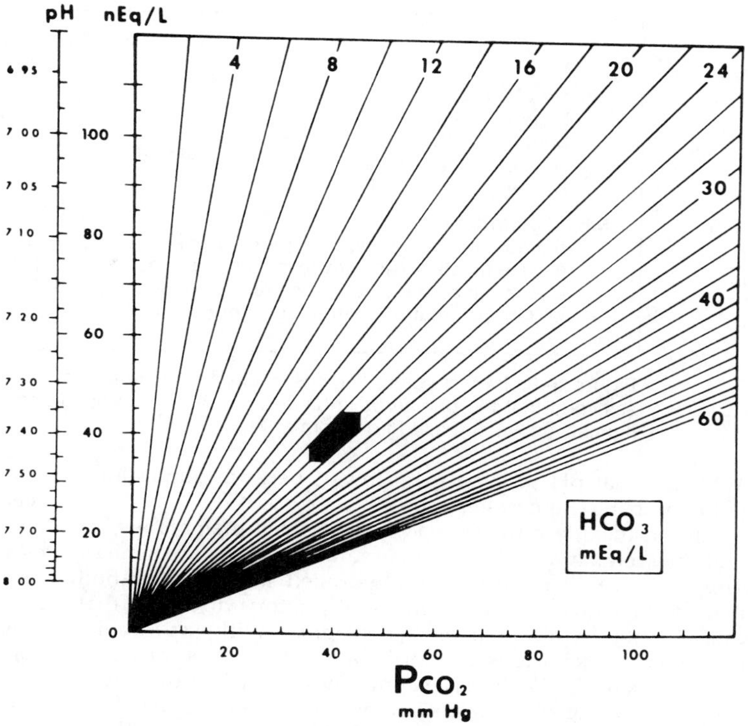

Figure 6–7. A nomogram permitting estimation of pH, Pco_2, or serum bicarbonate levels when only two of these measurements have been determined in the laboratory. The shaded area in the center of the plot represents the normal values. (From Cohen JJ: A new acid-base nomogram featuring hydrogen ion concentration. Henderson revisited. Ann Intern Med 66:159, 1967.)

methods based on the Henderson-Hasselbalch equation.* If all three measurements have been made, the same formulas can be used to check the validity of the values.

INTERPRETATION. It is relatively easy to diagnose a simple acid-base disorder correctly, given blood pH, Pco_2, and bicarbonate levels and using an acid-base nomogram such as that shown in Figure 6–8 or the summary of laboratory findings shown in Figure 6–9. Diagnosing a mixed disorder, however, is more difficult. In simple disorders Pco_2 and bicarbonate levels always change in the same direction. If any patient's values do not show this relationship, a mixed disorder should be considered. Similarly, results that plot outside any of the shaded areas shown in Figure 6–8 indicate a 95% chance of a mixed disorder, which can be diagnosed from the clinical setting, as discussed, and from the information presented in Figure 6–9.

There are significant arteriovenous differences in acid-base values. In patients with normal cardiac output, central venous pH is lower than arterial by an average of 0.03 unit, with the venous Pco_2 being higher by about 6 mm Hg. These differences increase with moderate heart failure and are substantial with severe circulatory failure (pH difference averages 0.1 unit; Pco_2 differences average 24 mm Hg). Large arteriovenous differences (up to 0.35 pH unit and up to 56 mm Hg for Pco_2) occur in patients during cardiac arrest with mechanical maintenance of ventilation and during cardiorespiratory arrest after sodium bicarbonate administration. Thus, arterial and central venous blood samples are required to assess acid-base status optimally in patients with critical hemodynamic compromise. Arterial samples provide information about pulmonary gas exchange and central venous samples provide more accurate information on the acid-base status of tissues during conditions of severe hypoperfusion.

INTRACELLULAR pH

Normal intracellular pH has been estimated to be 6.8; values as low as 6.0 have been obtained using microelectrodes.

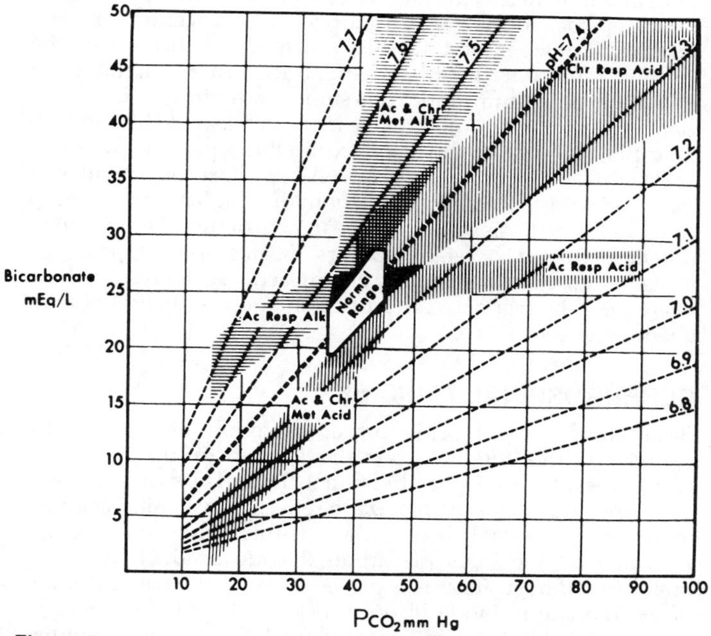

Figure 6–8. Determining simple acid-base disorders from measurements of pH, Pco_2, and serum bicarbonate. (Ac = acute; Acid = acidosis; Alk = alkalosis; Chr = chronic; Met = metabolic; Resp = respiratory.) (From Arbus GS: An in vivo acid-base nomogram for clinical use. Can Med Assoc J 109:291, 1973.)

---

*Pco_2 may be estimated from the equation

$$Pco_2 = \frac{[H^+] \times [\text{total } CO_2 \text{ content in mEq/L}]}{25}$$

$[H^+]$, expressed as nanoequivalents per liter (nEq/L), can easily be estimated from serum pH. At a pH of 7.40, $[H^+]$ is approximately 40 nEq/L (see Regulating Mechanisms). Each decrease in pH of 0.01 unit is associated with an increased $[H^+]$ of 1 nEq/L. Conversely, each increase in pH of 0.01 unit is associated with a decreased $[H^+]$ of 1 nEq/L. Thus, $[H^+]$ at a pH of 7.30 is 50 nEq/L and at 7.45 is 35 nEq/L. The maximum error in Pco_2 calculated by this simple formula is 7% for pH values from 7.10–7.50 and even less in the pH range of 7.28–7.45. (See N Engl J Med 272:1067, 1965.)

	PH	PCO_2	BICARBONATE
Simple disorders			
Metabolic acidosis	↓	↓	
Metabolic alkalosis	↑	↑	↑
Respiratory acidosis	↓	↑	↑
Respiratory alkalosis	↑	↓	↓
Mixed disorders			
Metabolic acidosis with respiratory acidosis	↓ ↓	↑ ,N, ↓	↑ ,N, ↓
Metabolic alkalosis with respiratory acidosis	↑ ,N, ↓	↑	↑
Metabolic acidosis with respiratory alkalosis	↑ ,N, ↓	↓	↓
Metabolic alkalosis with respiratory alkalosis	↑ ↑	↑ ,N, ↓	↑ ,N, ↓

Figure 6–9. Typical serum findings in clinical disturbances of acid-base balance. In the simple disorders it has been assumed that the primary acid-base disturbance has been compensated (see text for details). (↑ = increased from normal; ↓ = decreased from normal; N = normal.)

Mitochondrial pH may be even lower, because intracellular pH is probably inhomogeneous.

Carbon dioxide diffuses readily across cell membranes, so that intracellular and extracellular values for P_{CO_2} are similar. Thus, intracellular changes in hydrogen ion concentration may occur as a result of primary respiratory disorders that cause either hypocapnia or hypercapnia. With *hypo*capnia, intracellular alkalosis is proportional to the degree of extracellular alkalosis. With *hyper*capnia, however, because intracellular bicarbonate concentrations cannot be adjusted as rapidly as those in the extracellular fluid, intracellular acidosis may be proportionally greater than that seen in the extracellular fluid. In contrast to the situation in respiratory acidosis, intracellular pH may be maintained in the face of severe metabolic acidosis until extracellular pH drops below 7.0.

The effects of extracellular acidosis and alkalosis on cellular functions are not fully understood. A low pH produces a slight change in the Donnan distribution across the capillary membrane; therefore, some decrease in oncotic pressure results in a reduced plasma volume. Low pH also seems to reduce myocardial contractility and impair catecholamine action, and it increases the likelihood of arrhythmia, particularly with hypoxia. Moreover, if hydrogen ion concentration rises rapidly, it may inhibit further transport of the ion in the kidney. Metabolic disturbances also lead to an alteration in exchange of sodium and potassium for hydrogen ion; deficiency of potassium may result in a decrease in the intracellular pH at the same time that extracellular pH is elevated.

Changes in intracellular pH probably affect the activities of many enzymes. Decrease in carbohydrate tolerance has been observed in acidosis, and increase in neuromuscular irritability (latent or manifest tetany) occurs in alkalosis. Hypocapnia leads to an increase in the blood lactic acid level, with a decrease in bicarbonate concentration and production of metabolic acidosis.

CEREBROSPINAL FLUID pH

Bicarbonate–carbonic acid represents virtually all the buffering capacity in this fluid. Carbon dioxide can diffuse freely between the blood and cerebrospinal fluid. Thus, increases or decreases in P_{CO_2} in the blood are reflected by similar changes in the cerebrospinal fluid, although this latter value is also modified by the rates of carbon dioxide production in the brain. In contrast, increases or decreases in the concentration of bicarbonate in blood lead only slowly to small changes in the bicarbonate level in cerebrospinal fluid. Consequently, the concentration of hydrogen ion in the cerebrospinal fluid does not change instantaneously with changes in extracellular pH; the pHs of these fluids may differ significantly at times, especially if active respiratory compensation of a metabolic acidosis or alkalosis has occurred. Particular problems may be seen if a compensated metabolic acidosis is corrected too quickly. Correction results in an increase in both P_{CO_2} and bicarbonate levels in the extracellular fluid, but only the P_{CO_2} rises in the cerebrospinal fluid. The pH of the extracellular fluid returns to normal, but that of the cerebrospinal fluid falls even further. Thus, continuing neurologic symptoms and abnormalities in respiration may result.

6.9 CHLORIDE

Chloride is the major anion of extracellular fluid. Total body chloride amounts to 33 mEq/kg. Most of it is in the extracellular (plasma chloride, 13.6%; interstitial lymph, 37.3%; dense connective tissue and cartilage, 17%; bone, 15.2%) and transcellular (4.5%) fluids, with small quantities present intracellularly (12.4%). Exchangeable chloride remains relatively constant per unit of body weight at different ages.

The intake and output of chloride parallel those of sodium. Its transport is largely passive and travels down an electrochemical gradient created in part by sodium transport. However, chloride transport at several sites, including the thick ascending limb of the loop of Henle, may be active. The potency of furosemide as a diuretic may be a result of the specific inhibition of this mechanism.

Under most clinical circumstances alterations in chloride concentration in the blood parallel those of sodium. Thus, hypo- and hyperchloremia are usually associated with comparable degrees of hypo- and hypernatremia, respectively, and are seen most often with dehydration secondary to diarrhea. Occasionally, however, changes in chloride concentration are not accompanied by equivalent changes in sodium concentration.

Chloride is not directly involved in regulating the concentration of free hydrogen ion. Nevertheless, as metabolic adjustments within the kidney are made and plasma levels of bicarbonate change secondary to secretion of hydrogen ions, reciprocal changes in the plasma concentration of chloride generally occur. Thus, *hypochloremia* is typically seen in metabolic alkalosis. It occurs also when chloride is lost from the body in excess of sodium losses. Examples include loss from the bowel with vomiting or gastric drainage or in chloride diarrhea, a rare congenital disorder in which there is a defect in bowel transport of chloride. Urinary losses of chloride may exceed those of sodium during the correction of metabolic acidosis and in potassium deficiency. Indeed, with potassium deficiency, both potassium and chloride must be given before the potassium deficits can be corrected. Similarly, administering chloride is necessary to correct most cases of metabolic alkalosis irrespective of whether it is associated with potassium deficiency. In patients with metabolic alkalosis, using either potassium or sodium chloride, as appropriate, results in the prompt excretion of bicarbonate into the urine and correction of the alkalosis. Hypochloremia also results from a protracted inadequate intake of chloride. Thus, infants fed a chloride-deficient milk formula for several months developed chronic depletion of body chloride, severe hypochloremia (serum sodium levels usually remained normal), severe hypokalemic metabolic alkalosis, loss of appetite, failure to thrive, muscle weakness, and lethargy. Although adding chloride to the diet quickly reverses the electrolyte abnormalities, long-term sequelae may develop, including disturbed behavioral patterns.

Hyperchloremia may result when chloride is conserved by the kidney in excess of sodium and potassium. It occurs when alkaline urine is formed during the renal correction of alkalosis. An increased fractional reabsorption of chloride in the renal proximal tubule in distal renal tubular acidosis also results in hyperchloremia. Early amino acid solutions used in parenteral alimentation contained excessive amounts of chloride, and their administration resulted in hyperchloremic acidosis. Substituting acetate has largely solved this problem.

Measurements of the serum chloride level are necessary to determine a patient's *anion gap.* The concentration of the most abundant serum cation (sodium) is greater than the sum of the two most abundant serum anions (chloride and bicarbonate). The difference, referred to as the anion gap, is normally about 12 mEq/L (range 8–16 mEq/L). It results from the effect of the combined concentrations of the unmeasured anions such as phosphate, sulfate, proteins, and organic acids, which exceed those of the unmeasured cations, primarily potassium, calcium, and magnesium. Calculating the anion gap permits the detection of an abnormal concentration of an unmeasured anion or cation. An increased anion gap in renal failure is a result of increased concentrations of phosphate and sulfate; in diabetic ketoacidosis, to β-hydroxybutyrate and acetoacetate; in lactic acidosis, to lactate; in hyperglycemic nonketotic coma, to unidentified organic acids; and in disorders of amino acid metabolism, to various organic acids. Increased anion gap also follows the administration of large amounts of penicillin. After ethylene glycol ingestion, it is caused by glycolate production; after methanol ingestion, by formate production; and after salicylate poisoning, by the salicylate anion and various organic anions secondary to the uncoupling of oxidative phosphorylation.

A decreased anion gap occurs less frequently. It may be found in nephrotic syndrome, in which it is caused by a decreased serum concentration of albumin, which is anionic at pH 7.4; after lithium ingestion, lithium being an unmeasured cation; and in multiple myeloma, because of the presence of cationic proteins.

6.10 PHOSPHORUS

Confusion may exist in understanding the physiology of phosphorus, because the terms "phosphorus" and "phosphate" have frequently and erroneously been used interchangeably. Measurements of "phosphate" in biologic samples are usually performed as and expressed in terms of total elemental phosphorus concentration. Because the atomic weight of phosphorus is 30.98, a concentration of 3.1 mg/dL (31 mg/L) of phosphorus is equivalent to 1 mM phosphorus/L. Most of the measured plasma phosphorus exists as both monovalent and divalent orthophosphate and thus behaves as though it has a valence of 1.8 at pH 7.40. Consequently, at pH 7.40, 1 mM of phosphate is equivalent to 1.8 mEq of phosphate (mM × valence = mEq).

BODY PHOSPHORUS

Infants retain phosphorus avidly. A 3-kg infant may retain 40–80 mg/day, which is more than 50% of usual intake. Consequently, total body phosphorus per unit of fat-free body weight (FFBW) increases throughout childhood; it doubles from birth to adulthood, at which time its value is approximately 12 g/kg FFBW. This doubling is primarily the result of an increase in skeletal phosphorus content; more than 80% of body phosphorus is in bone, and the remainder is distributed throughout all soft tissues.

In plasma, two thirds of phosphorus is present as phospholipids (Table 6–4). These compounds are insoluble in acid and are not measured in routine "plasma phosphorus" determinations. The measured portion of plasma phosphorus is acid-soluble and is composed of inorganic phosphorus, primarily orthophosphate, 10% of which is bound to protein. The remaining 90% is ultrafilterable, 5% of which is complexed as calcium, magnesium, and sodium phosphates and 85% of which is present as "free phosphate." Of the latter, 80% is the divalent anion (HPO_4^{2-}) and 20% the monovalent anion ($H_2PO_4^-$). Concentrations of phosphorus are low in interstitial fluids, but this fluid is not a simple ultrafiltrate of plasma. Each organ may have an interstitial fluid composition to meet its own needs.

Cellular phosphorus is present in cell membranes and subcellular organelles as organic phosphoglycerides and sphingolipids. Acid-soluble moieties of intracellular phosphorus include ATP and other nucleotides, various glucose-phosphate compounds, creatinine phosphate, and a small amount of cytosolic inorganic phosphate. Thus, intracellular phosphate plays an essential role in forming and releasing energy, as well as in intracellular enzyme activity. Inorganic phosphorus is the principal urinary buffer and plays a critical function in the regulation of free hydrogen ions (see earlier).

The principal sources of *dietary phosphorus* are milk, milk products, and meat. The recommended daily intake is 880 mg/day for ages 1–10 yr and 1,200 mg for older children. Breast-fed infants ingest 25–30 mg of phosphorus/kg/24 hr. Up to two thirds of the dietary phosphate is absorbed from the bowel, primarily in the jejunum. This absorption is stimulated by vitamin D and its metabolites as well as by parathyroid hormone (PTH); it is decreased by thyrocalcitonin, by the presence in the bowel of binders such as aluminum hydroxide and carbonate and, at least in animals, by a high dietary calcium intake.

Even though phosphate is actively transported across the bowel wall, it is the kidney that plays a major role in regulating body phosphate. Renal handling of phosphate consists of glomerular filtration with facultative reabsorption by the tu-

TABLE 6–4. Major Components of Plasma Phosphorus

	Total Plasma Phosphorus			3.9 mM/L
	Acid-insoluble		2.6 mM/L	
	Organic (phospholipids)			
	Acid-soluble		1.3 mM/L	
	Organic (esters)	0.1 mM/L		
	Inorganic	1.2 mM/L		
A*	Pyrophosphate (0.003 mM/L)			
A*	Orthophosphate (1.2 mM/L)			
A*	—10% Protein bound (0.12 mM/L)			
A*, B†	—5% Complexed (0.07 mM/L)			
A*, B†	—85% "Free"‡ (1.01 mM/L)			

*A, measured as plasma phosphorus.
†B, ultrafilterable phosphorus.
‡At pH 7.4: 17% as $H_2PO_4^-$ (0.20 mM/L), 68% as HPO_4^{2-} (0.81 mM/L).

bule. Ultrafilterable phosphate is freely filtered at the glomerulus with an average of 90% of this filtered load normally being reabsorbed. Sixty to 70% of the reabsorption occurs in the proximal tubule and the remainder in more distal segments. Under certain circumstances phosphate may also be secreted by the distal tubules. Although a maximal rate for tubular reabsorption of phosphate (Tm phosphate) exists, it varies with filtration rate and is not attained under normal circumstances. Urinary excretion of phosphate shows a circadian rhythm—lowest in the morning and highest in early evening.

Tubular reabsorption of phosphate is regulated by *PTH,* the effects of which are mediated by the adenylate cyclase system. This hormone reduces tubular reabsorption of phosphorus and is associated with phosphaturia. Conversely, large doses of vitamin D stimulate reabsorption of phosphate in the proximal tubule, as does growth hormone. Under many circumstances renal tubular transport of phosphate parallels that of sodium. Thus, expansion of extracellular fluid results in phosphaturia, as does the administration of diuretics, especially those that inhibit carbonic anhydrase. Phosphate transport is also linked to that of glucose and to changes in pH; therefore, hyperglycemia results in phosphaturia and reduced Tm for phosphorus. Similarly, conditions that result in an alkaline urine also decrease reabsorption of phosphate.

REGULATION OF PLASMA PHOSPHATE

In addition to the factors already discussed, plasma phosphate concentration is affected by the continuous exchange of phosphate between the large stores in bone and those in the extracellular fluid. Net reabsorption of phosphate from bone is promoted by 1,25-dihydroxyvitamin D_3 and PTH but is opposed by thyrocalcitonin. Phosphate is also readily transported across all cell membranes. Administering glucose or insulin decreases plasma phosphate concentration, probably because of an intracellular flux of phosphate secondary to the phosphorylation of glucose. Hyperventilation, alkalosis, and administration of epinephrine also decrease plasma phosphate concentration. Marked, acute increases in plasma phosphate concentration result in hypocalcemia. Changes in calcium concentration, however, do not necessarily reciprocally alter plasma phosphate concentration.

Plasma phosphorus concentrations are high during infancy and childhood. Values at birth range from 1.4 to 2.8 mM/L and increase progressively in the 1st week of life to 2.0–3.3 mM/L before declining slowly during childhood. Levels fall to those of the adult (1.0–1.3 mM/L) on completion of growth. Premature infants also have high plasma phosphorus values of 2.5–3.0 mM/L, provided their intake of phosphorus is adequate.

Hyperphosphatemia is characteristic of hypoparathyroidism but rarely occurs in the absence of renal insufficiency. Although small changes in GFR have little effect on phosphate excretion in health, *reduction in GFR* to below 25% leads to an elevation of the serum inorganic phosphate level and to reciprocal changes in the serum calcium level, resulting in secondary hyperparathyroidism. This process begins with small decreases in GFR but usually does not clinically appear until GFR has fallen to low levels. *In the young infant* GFR is low in relation to active cell mass and the dietary phosphorus intake is high; consequently, the serum inorganic phosphorus level is high. Hence, reduction in GFR or relative hypoparathyroidism in infants rapidly leads to very high serum values of phosphate, with consequent depression of calcium concentration and latent or manifest tetany (Sec. 6.27, 6.28, 9.54, and 19.17). Hyperphosphatemia may also result from the excessive administration of phosphate by the oral or intravenous routes or as phosphate-containing enemas. Using cytotoxic drugs to treat malignancies, especially lymphomas or leukemias, results in cytolysis, with hyperphosphatemia caused by release of phosphate into the circulation. The major clinical consequences of hyperphosphatemia are symptoms of the resulting hypocalcemia.

Hypophosphatemia may result from phosphate deficiency in association with, for example, starvation, protein-calorie malnutrition, and malabsorption syndromes. It may result from intracellular shifts of phosphate such as those that occur with respiratory or metabolic acidosis, during the treatment of diabetic ketoacidosis (typically during the first 24 hr), and following the administration of corticosteroids. Increased urinary losses of phosphate may be sufficiently severe to reduce plasma concentration; this reduction is observed in primary and tertiary hyperparathyroidism, in renal tubular defects, after ECF volume expansion, or after administration of diuretics. Often a combination of pathophysiologic mechanisms is responsible for the hypophosphatemia. Examples include vitamin D-deficient (Sec. 4.29) and vitamin D–resistant rickets (Sec. 24.59). The very low birthweight infant requires a high phosphorus intake at the time of rapid postnatal growth. Inadequate intake results in phosphorus depletion and hypophosphatemia. In addition, bone demineralization, hypercalcemia, and calciuria may occur, probably as a result of mobilization of phosphorus and calcium from the bone.

In most instances, hypophosphatemia is mild or moderate in degree and is asymptomatic. Occasionally, plasma phosphate concentration may fall to very low levels (0.3 mM/L; 1.0 mg/dL or less). Such low levels have been observed with the *prolonged use of intravenous alimentation without phosphate supplements* and may result in a very severe, well-defined syndrome. Red cell concentrations of 2,3-diphosphoglycerate and ATP are decreased. The resulting decrease in release of oxygen by the red cells produces tissue anoxia. Increased hemolysis may also occur, as may leukocyte and platelet dysfunction. Some patients display the symptoms of a metabolic encephalopathy, including irritability, paresthesias, confusion, seizures, and coma, and some may develop abnormalities in the electroencephalogram. Hypercalcemia, thought to be a result of increased release of calcium from bone, rhabdomyolysis, cardiomyopathy, and possibly hepatocellular dysfunction have also been reported. Renal tubular defects may occur, and the kidney's ability to excrete hydrogen ions is impaired. Promptly recognizing and treating this syndrome, preferably by orally administering phosphate salts, is beneficial, but permanent defects may result. Thus, prevention of severe hypophosphatemia should always be the goal.

Ad Hoc Committee on Acid-Base Terminology: Report. Ann NY Acad Sci 133:25, 1966.

Adrogué HJ, Rashad N, Gorin AB, et al: Assessing acid-base status in circulatory failure. N Engl J Med 320:1312, 1989.

Bronner F, Coburn JW (eds): Disorders of Mineral Metabolism. Vol. II: Calcium Physiology. Vol. III: Pathophysiology of Calcium, Phosphorus and Magnesium. New York, Academic Press, 1981.

Chan JCM, Gill JR, Jr (eds): Kidney Electrolyte Disorders. New York, Churchill Livingstone, 1990.

Cooke RE (ed): The Biologic Basis of Pediatric Practice. New York, McGraw-Hill, 1968.

Emmett M, Narins RG: Clinical use of the anion gap. Medicine 56:38, 1977.

Hellerstein S, Duggan E, Merveille O, et al: Follow-up studies on children with severe dietary chloride deficiency during infancy. Pediatrics 75:1, 1985.

Hicks JM, Boeckx RL (eds): Pediatric Clinical Chemistry. Philadelphia, WB Saunders, 1984.

Klahr S (ed): The Kidney and Body Fluids in Health and Disease, 2nd ed. New York, Plenum Press, 1984.

Needleman P, Adams SP, Cole BR, et al: Atriopeptins as cardiac hormones. Hypertension 7:469, 1985.

Plum F, Price RW: Acid-base balance of cisternal and lumbar cerebrospinal fluid in hospital patients. N Engl J Med 289:1346, 1973.

Schrier RW (ed): Renal and Electrolyte Disorders, 2nd ed. Boston, Little, Brown & Co, 1980.

6.11 PARENTERAL FLUID THERAPY

Infants and young children are especially susceptible to the consequences of illnesses that affect fluid balance. The infant's usual daily turnover of water is equal to almost 25% of total body water, compared with 6% in the adult. Thus, the effects of any disease that reduces fluid intake (e.g., vomiting) or increases fluid losses (e.g., diarrhea) appear much more rapidly in the infant than in the adult. Diarrhea remains a scourge in developing countries and a problem in developed countries. For example, in the United States, it is responsible for about 400 deaths/yr in the 1st year of life and for about 200,000 hospital admissions/yr in the 1st 5 yr of childhood.

DETERMINATION OF REQUIREMENTS. Fluid therapy is considered in three phases. *Maintenance therapy* is designed to replace ongoing normal and abnormal losses of fluids and electrolytes. The purpose is to maintain patients in normal balance and to prevent deficits from developing. *Deficit therapy* is designed to replace losses of fluids and electrolytes resulting from an illness before the patient was brought for medical care. Its goal is to return volume and composition to normal. *Supplemental therapy* is used in certain diseases that require specific fluids and electrolytes in addition to those for repair of deficits and maintenance.

Total fluid and electrolyte needs are calculated as the sum of these individual phases of treatment. For example, after uncomplicated surgery a patient may only require normal maintenance—the replacement of the usual losses of fluids and electrolytes that occur through the lungs and as urine, sweat, and feces. A postoperative patient with gastric drainage requires maintenance therapy to replace both the normal losses and the increased losses of water and electrolytes in the gastric fluid. A dehydrated patient with severe diarrhea requires deficit therapy to replace the losses resulting from the diarrhea and maintenance therapy to replace normal losses as well as the continuing abnormal stool losses for as long as the diarrhea persists. A patient with severe salicylate intoxication requires replacement of deficits that occurred prior to hospital admission; replacement of usual losses as well as the increased losses caused by hyperventilation and fever; and supplemental treatment in which alkalinization of the urine and induction of diuresis are frequently employed to increase salicylate excretion in the urine.

Each of these phases of fluid therapy is considered separately. *As with potentially lethal drugs, amounts of fluids and electrolytes should preferably be calculated independently by at least two people, and the results should be reconciled before administration is begun.*

MONITORING OF PATIENT. Regardless of the accuracy of planning a therapeutic regimen, a patient's response is not always predictable. Consequently, frequent assessment is required so that appropriate modifications of therapy can be instituted promptly, if needed. Typically, such monitoring consists of frequent physical examinations to determine changes in body weight and frequent review of intake and output charts. These clinical determinations may need to be supplemented by repeated laboratory determinations. Serial measurements of levels of serum electrolytes, blood urea nitrogen, and serum creatinine, and blood counts may be essential; the interval between determinations depends on the patient's clinical status.

6.12 MAINTENANCE THERAPY

6.13 REPLACEMENT OF NORMAL LOSSES

A healthy person deprived of a normal oral intake continues to lose basal amounts of fluids and electrolytes from the body as urine, sweat, and feces and has additional losses of water from the lungs as evaporation in exhaled air. Water and electrolytes are required to replace these obligatory losses, or deficits result. Protein and calories are also required, but complete parenteral replacement is difficult and is not essential unless oral intake is restricted for a week or longer.

Two methods for calculating normal maintenance requirements are presented. Because the amount and type of these losses may be modified by disease states, the influences of diseases on maintenance requirements are discussed after normal maintenance needs have been analyzed.

Calculation of Normal Maintenance Therapy

BASIC METHOD. Fluid and electrolyte requirements for purposes of maintenance are directly related to metabolic rate. An increase in metabolic rate requires an increase in catabolism of metabolic fuels and has three effects: (1) it increases the rate of endogenous water production from the oxidation of carbohydrate, fats, and protein; (2) it increases urinary solute excretion, which in turn increases obligatory urine flow rates and urinary water losses; and (3) it increases heat production, which increases water loss as sweat and water loss through respiration. Similarly, the turnover rates of electrolytes are related to water loss and to metabolic rate. Therefore, if a patient's caloric expenditure can be estimated, his or her maintenance requirements of fluids and electrolytes can be calculated because the amounts of water, sodium, and potassium required for every 100 kcal metabolized are well established.

Calculation of Caloric Expenditure. Metabolic rate depends on age, body weight, degree of activity, and body temperature. *Basal metabolic rate* can be obtained from Table 6–5, which depicts the values by sex at various body weights. The basal values must *be adjusted for the patient's activity, body temperature, and any pathologic state* to estimate caloric expenditure. Adjustments for activity are made from observing the patient. No increments are needed for patients in coma or under anesthesia. Usual activity in bed rarely increases basal expenditure by more than 30%. Caloric expenditure is increased by fever (12%/°C rise in body temperature) and by hypermetabolic states such as salicylism and hyperthyroidism (25–75%). It is decreased by hypothermia (12%/°C fall in body temperature) and by hypometabolic states such as hypothyroidism (10–25%).

These calculations permit a good estimate of caloric expenditure in all but the very young infant and the obese subject. In the neonate, activity during the first 3–5 days of life is low; total caloric expenditure does not usually exceed 50 kcal/kg of body weight/day; this figure should be used to calculate maintenance requirements during this period. In obese infants and children, "ideal" weight (50th percentile for age and height) should be used to calculate basal metabolic rate.

Translation of Caloric Expenditure to Water and Electrolyte Requirements. Table 6–6 depicts the usual losses of water and electrolytes from lungs, skin, stool, and urine in relationship to caloric expenditure. For every 100 kcal metabolized the patient requires a total of approximately 125 mL of water, 3.2 mEq of sodium, and 2.4 mEq of potassium to replace normal losses. However, maintenance requirements for water have to be reduced by 10–15 mL/100 kcal metabolized to allow for the release of an equivalent volume of water during oxidation of endogenous and exogenous carbohydrate, fat, and protein. Thus, water requirements for normal maintenance therapy are estimated at 115 mL for every 100 kcal metabolized; the equivalent values for sodium and potassium

TABLE 6–5. Standard Basal Caloric Output

Weight (kg)	Output (kcal/24 hr) Male	Male and Female	Female
3		140	
5		270	
7		400	
9		500	
11		600	
13		650	
15		710	
17		780	
19		830	
21		880	
25	1,020		960
29	1,120		1,040
33	1,210		1,120
37	1,300		1,190
41	1,350		1,260
45	1,410		1,320
49	1,470		1,380
53	1,530		1,440
57	1,590		1,500
61	1,640		1,560

Increments or decrements:
1. Add or subtract 12% of above for each degree C (8% for each degree F) above or below rectal temperature of 37.8° C (100° F).
2. Add 0 to 30% increments for activity.

can be rounded off to 3 mEq and 2.5 mEq, respectively. Bottle-fed infants require a higher fluid intake of 140 mL/100 kcal of food, because their milk diet has a high protein content, which increases the solute load to be excreted by the kidneys and, thus, the obligatory renal water loss.

These recommendations assume that the kidney can adjust rates of urine flow and electrolyte excretion over wide ranges. The maintenance requirements calculated here do not require maximal renal concentration or dilution of urine or exceed the solute load that can be excreted by the kidney or its ability to conserve electrolytes. The designated requirements thus provide some latitude in the amounts of fluids and electrolytes that can be administered safely. With renal damage, or in other disease states, this is frequently not the case, and maintenance requirements must be modified precisely, as outlined later.

ALTERNATIVE METHOD. Several alternate methods have been developed to estimate caloric expenditure and to calculate fluid and electrolyte requirements. They are derived from the principles outlined previously but do not require the availability of reference tables. More simple to use, they relate maintenance requirements to either body weight or body surface.

One such method for estimating caloric expenditure is shown in Table 6–7. The values are for the average hospitalized patient and allow for usual activity in bed. Although values for caloric expenditure are slightly higher than those

TABLE 6–6. Water and Electrolyte Losses/100 kcal Metabolized Under Normal Conditions and in Disease States

Route of Loss	Usual Loss H_2O (mL)	Usual Loss Na (mEq)	Usual Loss K (mEq)	Range Observed in Disease States H_2O (mL)	Na (mEq)	K (mEq)
Evaporative						
Lungs	15	0	0	10–60	0	0
Skin	40	0.1	0.2	20–100	0.1–3.0	0.2–1.5
Stool	5	0.1	0.2	0–50	0.1–4.0	0.2–3.0
Urine	65	3.0	2.0	0–400	0–30.0	0–30.0
Total	125	3.2	2.4			

TABLE 6–7. Simplified Alternative Method for Calculating Caloric Expenditure from Body Weight

Body Weight (kg)	Caloric Expenditure/Day
Up to 10	100 kcal/kg
11–20	1,000 kcal + 50 kcal/kg for each kg above 10 kg
Above 20	1,500 kcal + 20 kcal/kg for each kg above 20 kg

used in the basic system, the derived values for maintenance requirements are identical, because it is recommended that for every 100 kcal expended only 100 mL of fluid should be administered (compared with 115 mL with the basic system); this solution should contain 25 mEq/L of sodium, 20 mEq/L of potassium, and 5% dextrose. Commercially prepared solutions with this composition are available (see Table 27–8) that also provide magnesium (3 mEq/L), phosphate (3 mEq/L), and either lactate or acetate (23 mEq/L).

COMPARISON OF METHODS. Maintenance requirements calculated by the alternative method are virtually identical to those calculated by the basic method. For example, for an afebrile, previously healthy male child weighing 45 kg, basic caloric expenditure obtained from Table 6–5 would be 1,410 kcal. Allowing a 20% increment for physical activity, the estimated caloric expenditure would be 1,692 kcal. Daily water requirements would be 16.92 × 115 = 1,946 mL; sodium requirements, 16.92 × 3 = 51 mEq (equivalent to 26 mEq/L of administered solution); and potassium requirements, 16.92 × 2.5 = 42 mEq (or 21 mEq/L of administered solution). The administered fluid should contain 5% dextrose. Using the alternative system (see Table 6–7) caloric expenditure would be estimated as 2,000 kcal, which would indicate the need to administer 2,000 mL of the maintenance solution containing 5% dextrose, 25 mEq/L of sodium, and 20 mEq/L of potassium.

6.14 MODIFICATION OF MAINTENANCE REQUIREMENTS BY DISEASE STATES

Disease states may result in either markedly increased or decreased losses of water and/or electrolytes (see Table 6–6). Maintenance therapy must be adjusted appropriately to maintain a patient's fluid and electrolyte balance.

DECREASED REQUIREMENTS. In *anuria* or extreme oliguria, urine output may be negligible, often less than 10 mL/100 kcal, compared with a normal 65 mL. Only stool and evaporative water losses occur. The rate of fluid administered must be reduced accordingly and rarely exceeds 45 mL for each 100 kcal. It is preferable to underestimate rather than to overestimate fluid requirements in such cases, because it is easier to administer additional fluids later if needed than to remove excess fluid administered inappropriately. Administration of electrolytes should also be reduced in anuric patients. In the absence of complications such as diarrhea, sodium and potassium losses through the sweat and stools are usually negligible, and no electrolytes may be required for maintenance in these patients.

In some patients, particularly those with *meningitis*, excessive or inappropriate release of antidiuretic hormone may occur. The rate of flow of urine is markedly reduced, and fluid intake should be reduced to reflect these decreased losses. *Patients in highly humidified atmospheres* (e.g., incubators or croup tents) also have reduced fluid requirements, because the high humidity may reduce evaporative losses of water by 20–50%. In *congestive heart failure* restriction of sodium and water intake is indicated when planning parenteral as well as oral intake.

INCREASED REQUIREMENTS. The amount and nature

of abnormally increased losses of fluids and electrolytes depend on the underlying disease process and the site of loss. Considerable variation exists in the composition of abnormal *gastrointestinal losses* from patient to patient and from time to time in the same patient. An estimate of the composition of the more common fluid losses can be based on Table 6–8. These losses should be replaced as nearly as possible, volume for volume and milliequivalent for milliequivalent as they occur to prevent physiologic readjustment that may further deplete the body of water and electrolytes. If such estimates are too imprecise, the electrolyte concentrations in the fluid being lost should be measured to determine the exact replacement needs.

In general, losses in gastric or intestinal drainage can be replaced satisfactorily by isotonic or somewhat hypotonic solutions that contain more chloride than sodium for gastric replacement and more sodium than chloride for intestinal replacement. Although gastric fluid contains relatively little potassium, the alkalosis that develops from the loss of significant quantities of hydrogen ion in the gastric juice usually results in increased urinary potassium loss; therefore, replacement fluid for a patient with gastric drainage should contain 10–20 mEq of potassium/L (provided renal function is well maintained).

Increased losses of sodium chloride in *sweat* usually are of little significance except in adrenal insufficiency and cystic fibrosis; heat stress should be avoided in such patients. In *hyperventilation* and *heat stress*, evaporative losses of water may increase as much as 90 and 120 mL/100 kcal, respectively.

When *renal* concentrating and diluting ability is lost, as in chronic renal disease, water requirements may rise to 150 mL/100 kcal and, as in diabetes insipidus of nephrogenic or hypothalamic origin, to as high as 400 mL/100 kcal.

Under most circumstances fluid losses are replaced volume for volume and electrolyte losses milliequivalent for milliequivalent, but sometimes this is inappropriate. For example, the increased urine output seen in the diuretic phase of acute tubular necrosis may eliminate fluid retained during the oliguric phase of the disease. All these increased losses are not replaced, because such therapy would only perpetuate the presence of edema. Sodium and water losses can be replaced rapidly. Potassium losses are replaced over a more protracted period of time, especially if administered parenterally.

THIRD SPACING. Less easily recognized but equally important losses are those that may result from sequestration of fluid in a body space. For example, a patient with paralytic ileus may have pooling of fluid in the gastrointestinal tract. Even though total body fluid and electrolyte content may not be changed, this pooled fluid may not be in equilibrium with the vascular compartment and may cause a functional deficit.

TABLE 6–8. Composition of External Abnormal Losses

Fluid	Electrolyte (mEq/L)			Protein (g/dL)
	Sodium	*Potassium*	*Chloride*	
Gastric	20–80	5–20	100–150	—
Pancreatic	120–140	5–15	90–120	—
Small intestine	100–140	5–15	90–130	—
Bile	120–140	5–15	80–120	—
Ileostomy	45–135	3–15	20–115	—
Diarrheal	10–90	10–80	10–110	—
Sweat:*				
Normal	10–30	3–10	10–35	—
Cystic fibrosis	50–130	5–25	50–110	—
Burns	140	5	110	3–5

*Sweat sodium concentrations progressively increase with increasing sweat flow rates.

ADMINISTRATION OF MAINTENANCE REQUIREMENTS

Losses should be replaced by mouth, if possible, or else by the intravenous route. Using subcutaneous injections of fluids is not recommended because of variable rates of absorption and other complications. However, if technical or other difficulties dictate that therapy be given by this route, glucose in water or in very dilute electrolyte solution should not be given because diffusion of sodium chloride into such an extravascular pool and the subsequent loss of fluid from the extracellular fluid may reduce plasma volume acutely and precipitate shock.

Replacing large quantities of fluid precisely may be difficult. In such instances, thirst, changes in body weight, and urinary output are usually more reliable indicators of the patient's needs than are the physician's estimates. Such patients should be re-evaluated every 8 hr, or more frequently.

Caloric Intake

In a patient receiving maintenance fluids parenterally, matching caloric expenditure with adequate caloric intake is difficult and, fortunately, is unnecessary if maintenance therapy is needed for only short periods. However, administering maintenance electrolytes in a 5% dextrose solution is desirable as a routine measure to provide approximately 20% of the calories metabolized, to produce a decreased catabolism of endogenous protein and a decreased solute load to be excreted by the kidney, and to reduce the risk of hypoglycemia in the young infant. Concentrations of dextrose above 5% are not recommended, because when they are administered at infusion rates sufficient to meet water requirements, they frequently result in hyperglycemia. The consequent loss of dextrose in the urine may actually increase water requirements through an osmotic diuretic effect. At slower infusion rates, such as those used in the anuric patient or in the neonate, higher concentrations of dextrose may be used, but they increase the risk of intravenous thrombosis and infection.

Intravenous Alimentation

The foregoing regimens for replacing and maintaining fluid and electrolytes are calorically inadequate and cannot sustain growth. They are suitable, therefore, for short periods only. In some infants and children, especially newborns undergoing major surgery and children with protracted diarrhea, parenteral nutrition for prolonged periods is necessary. Regimens developed to meet this need may effectively maintain positive nitrogen balance and growth for periods of 60 days or longer.

The standard infusate is prepared from a crystalline amino acid solution and contains 20% glucose and various electrolytes (Table 6–9). A multiple vitamin preparation is added to the solution, avoiding excess amounts of vitamin E; zinc, copper, chromium, and manganese are added in recommended trace amounts. The solution is infused into a central vein by means of a constant speed infusion pump through a catheter tunneled subcutaneously to reduce the risk of infection. Infused at rates of up to 135 mL/kg/24 hr, this solution provides approximately 120 cal/kg/24 hr and meets protein requirements estimated to be in the range of 2.0–3.0 g/kg/24 hr. Lipids may be given daily, but the more cost-effective intravenous transfusion of 20 mL/kg of lipids (containing linolenic and linoleic acids) every 10 days provides adequate amounts of essential fatty acids.

In patients in whom it is impossible to use a central venous catheter and in neonates, parenteral nutrition may be given by peripheral vein. The glucose concentration in these infusates should be reduced to 10%. To compensate partially for

TABLE 6–9. Composition of Typical Infusate Used in Intravenous Alimentation

Constituent	Concentration (Per L)	Approximate Infusion Rate (Per kg/day)*
Amino acids (g)†	16	2.2
Glucose (g)	200	27
Sodium (mEq)‡	32	4.3
Potassium (mEq)‡	30	4.1
Chloride (mEq)‡	30	4.1
Acetate (mEq)	32	4.1
Calcium (mEq)§	9	1.2
Magnesium (mEq)	8	1.1
Sulfate (mEq)	8	1.1
Phosphate (mM)	10	1.4
Total calories (kcal)	864	117
Osmolality (mOsm)	1,462	209
pH	6.4	

*Based on an infusion rate of 135 mL/kg/day.
†Derived from crystalline amino acid preparations such as FreAmine III or Trophamine (McGaw) Neoaminosol (Abbott Laboratories), or Travasol (Baxter Laboratories).
‡May be adjusted to meet individual patient's needs.
§Some sources recommend a higher calcium concentration.

the reduced caloric content of this infusate, the amino acid content is increased to 30 g/L if an older child is to be treated. Because neonates do not tolerate this solution well, they should receive a solution containing the lower amino acid and glucose content even though it provides only 464 cal/L. The neonates should, however, receive lipids daily (see Sec. 9.17).

Complications of intravenous alimentation are common. They include sepsis; severe hyperglycemia, especially in the early stages of treatment of low-birthweight infants; profound hypophosphatemia, which can be life-threatening and can occur most often in the first week of the parenteral nutrition of malnourished patients; hyperammonemia, typically seen in small infants with bowel disease; severe metabolic acidosis; and other disturbances in electrolyte concentrations. To minimize complications, inserting catheters and changing lines should be performed only by persons trained in these techniques; the patient's clinical status and state of hydration should be monitored closely; urines should be regularly checked for glucosuria, especially in the first week of treatment; and serum electrolyte, phosphate, glucose, urea nitrogen, and hemoglobin levels should be measured before treatment is started and at weekly intervals thereafter. Serum calcium, ammonia, and albumin levels should be measured at less frequent intervals. Checking liver function and certain trace metal or vitamin levels may also be necessary if these studies are indicated on clinical grounds.

6.15 DEFICIT THERAPY

Deficits in body water and electrolytes may result from reduced intake with continuing normal losses, from excessive losses occurring with or without usual intake, or from a combination of these mechanisms. The *absolute deficits* of water and electrolytes observed in dehydration produced by different disease states are estimated in Table 6–10, which provides some representative values and illustrates the similarity in the magnitudes of deficits irrespective of the precipitating condition. This similarity is not surprising, because deficits reflect not only the results of direct losses but also the physiologic readjustments by the patient. As a consequence, *patients with deficits resulting from many different causes can be treated successfully in a similar manner.* In most instances, management is

TABLE 6–10. Estimated Deficits of Water and Electrolytes in Infants with Moderately Severe Dehydration*

Condition	H_2O (mL)	Na (mEq)	K (mEq)†	Cl (mEq)
Fasting and thirsting	100–120	5–7	1–2	4–6
Diarrhea				
Isonatremic	100–120	8–10	8–10	8–10
Hypernatremic	100–120	2–4	0–4	−2–−6‡
Hyponatremic	100–120	10–12	8–10	10–12
Pyloric stenosis	100–120	8–10	10–12	10–12
Diabetic acidosis	100–120	8–10	5–7	6–8

*Per kg of body weight.
†Converted for breakdown of tissue cells: −1 g N = 3 mEq of K.
‡Negative balance of chloride indicates an excess at the beginning of therapy.

dictated more by the severity and type of deficit than by its underlying cause. The *severity of the clinical disturbances* typically depends on the magnitude of the deficit in relation to body reserves and on the rate at which the deficit developed. The *type of deficit* depends on the relationship between the magnitude of loss of water and that of electrolytes, principally sodium.

SEVERITY OF DEFICIT

The magnitude or severity of a deficit can be gauged from change in body weight. Any loss of body weight in excess of 1%/day represents loss of body water. In young infants a weight loss of up to 5% (50 mL/kg) is considered mild, 5–10% moderate, and 10–15% severe dehydration, the last of which is frequently associated with peripheral circulatory failure. Deficits in excess of 15% of body weight are rarely compatible with life. Any percentage loss of body weight is equivalent to a disproportionately greater percentage loss of body water. Thus, a 15% loss of body weight (150 mL/kg) is equivalent to an approximately 25% loss of body water.

In older children and adults total body water and extracellular fluid volume each represents a smaller percentage of body weight than in the infant. In these patients, any given percentage loss of body weight resulting from fluid and electrolyte deficits indicates more severe depletion than in infants. Thus, comparable figures for severity of the deficit in older patients are 3% (mild), 6% (moderate), and 9% (severe).

The rapidity with which a deficit develops is also important. A 10% weight loss occurring over 24 hr in an infant is severe. The same weight loss developing over several days is better tolerated, and its effects typically are only moderately severe.

6.16 TYPES OF DEHYDRATION

The serum sodium level in dehydrated patients may be normal, low, or high, depending on the relative losses of water and electrolytes. Dehydration is classified on this basis, being termed *isonatremic* when serum sodium levels are 130–150 mEq/L, *hyponatremic* when serum sodium levels are less than 130 mEq/L, and *hypernatremic* when serum sodium levels are above 150 mEq/L. Because plasma osmolality in large part reflects sodium concentrations, these forms of dehydration are usually *isotonic*, *hypotonic*, and *hypertonic*, respectively. Changes in tonicity do not always correspond to changes in sodium concentration, however, so the two sets of terms cannot be used interchangeably. For example, in diabetic ketoacidosis or in uremia, serum sodium concentration may be low, but the plasma is hypertonic as a result of elevated plasma levels of glucose or urea, respectively.

Classifying dehydration into these three types, based on sodium concentrations, is of practical importance. Each form is associated with different relative losses of fluid from intracellular (ICF) and extracellular (ECF) compartments. In *isona-*

tremic dehydration the fluid and electrolyte losses are in proportion to one another; the extracellular fluid remains isotonic. Because there is no osmotic gradient across cell walls, intracellular fluid volume remains virtually constant; the majority of fluid loss is borne by the extracellular compartment. In *hyponatremic* dehydration the hypotonicity of the extracellular fluid results in an osmotically induced movement of fluid from the extracellular compartment into cells, resulting in even further depletion of extracellular fluid and some increases in intracellular fluid. Conversely, in *hypernatremic* dehydration, the increase in osmolality of the extracellular fluid results in movement of fluid out of the cells so that the intracellular fluid volume is depleted; depletion of extracellular fluid is less than expected. This analysis assumes that the plasma does not contain pathologic concentrations of other molecules that are osmotically effective across cell walls. As a consequence of these differences, the three forms of dehydration are characterized by variations in clinical presentation and in physical findings, each requiring appropriate modification in therapeutic approach.

6.17 ESTIMATION OF MAGNITUDE AND TYPE OF DEFICIT

This assessment should consist of a detailed history and a thorough physical examination, often augmented by appropriate laboratory studies.

HISTORY. Some important aspects are shown in Table 6–11. If a patient's preillness weight is known, the change from this value provides an accurate estimate of the magnitude of fluid losses. Without such information, a detailed estimate of losses and the exact quantities and composition of the infant's feedings prior to being seen may permit a less exact assessment of the magnitude of the deficit and also indicate the type of dehydration. It is important to remember that body composition of dehydrated patients is influenced not only by losses but also by *concomitant intake.* Historical information about intake is always more accurate than that obtained from estimating losses. The severity and type of dehydration are the result of the sum of intake and losses of both water and electrolytes. For example, a patient with severe diarrhea, losing fluid with a sodium concentration as low as 40 mEq/L, may continue to drink tap water containing virtually no sodium. Water losses are partially compensated for by the water intake but sodium losses are not replaced. Thus, despite the primary loss of excessive quantities of hyponatremic fluid (diarrhea), this patient may still present with hyponatremia. Conversely, the same patient treated with homemade electrolyte mixtures given by mouth may be hypernatremic, especially if the solution has been prepared with excessive amounts of salt or sodium bicarbonate, an all too common problem that has frequently been observed to result in severe hypernatremia.

TABLE 6–11. Historical Data Required in Estimating Magnitude and Types of Deficit and in Planning Deficit Therapy

- Intake (during period of illness)
  - Quantity and how given
  - Type: water, electrolyte, protein, drugs
- Output (during period of illness)
  - Quantity
  - Type: urine, vomiting, diarrhea, sweat, drainage
- Balance
  - Weight change
- General medical
  - Age
  - Cardiovascular, respiratory, renal, or central nervous system disease

The time and frequency of recent urinations, whether excessive or suppressed, may provide some appreciation of the severity of dehydration or indicate its cause. Urine output characteristically is decreased with dehydration, except in some low-birthweight infants. Continued frequent and excessive urination with dehydration suggests diabetes mellitus, diabetes insipidus, or nephrogenic diabetes insipidus. Output of usual amounts of urine without increased intake of water, in association with physical signs of dehydration, indicates a loss in the ability of the kidneys to conserve water and suggests renal disease.

PHYSICAL EXAMINATION. Table 6–12 details the physical findings associated with dehydration of different degrees of severity. In general, these findings occur irrespective of the etiology of the volume of depletion. Table 6–13 summarizes how different types of dehydration modify the physical signs.

Most infants and children appear ill when dehydrated. Mild dehydration may result only in thirst with no abnormal findings on physical examination. When fluid deficits reach 50 mL/kg, tachycardia usually develops, although it may also be a manifestation of fever or infection. With increasing degrees of dehydration the eyes may appear sunken and the skin around them dark. Intraocular pressure, elicited by lightly pressing on the closed eyes, is low. The mucous membranes of the mouth are usually dry, but prolonged mouth breathing or the tachypnea of acidosis may cause dry mucous membranes in the absence of dehydration. Tissue elasticity, sometimes referred to erroneously as turgor, may be reduced. Normally, when the skin and subcutaneous tissue are pinched between the thumb and 1st finger and then released, they return to position immediately. Delay in return (*tenting*) indicates dehydration. Skin and subcutaneous tissue must be tested together, or laxity of the skin may be misinterpreted as dehydration. Skin over the abdominal and chest walls and of the thigh should be tested. Testing over the abdomen alone may miss the sign if abdominal distention is present. Skin elasticity may remain relatively normal in the dehydrated, well-nourished child and decreased in the undernourished subject and, thus, is not an infallible sign. Depression of the anterior fontanel in the infant is apparent when fluid losses exceed 50 mL/kg but can be a misleading sign unless the state of the fontanel was known prior to the dehydration.

Signs of circulatory failure appear with increasing degrees of dehydration. The skin is cool and appears mottled. There may be postural hypotension. Shock manifested by tachycardia, a thin, thready pulse, cyanosis, and low blood pressure may supervene with severe dehydration. A fall in central blood pressure of 20 mm Hg or more usually indicates the loss of 150 mL/kg. Blood pressure is frequently hard to determine, but a useful estimate of systolic pressure only can often be obtained by palpation. The Doppler technique may enable an accurate measurement of blood pressure. The state of the peripheral circulation can be assessed by the warmth and color of the skin and by the rapidity of filling of the cutaneous capillary bed after pressure over the ear lobe, the nail bed, and the dorsum of the hand or the foot. However, peripheral circulation can be affected by local factors such as ambient temperature, and care must be taken when evaluating these signs. Attempts have been made to quantitate losses based on changes in capillary refill time. This is determined by pinching the abdominal skin or by blanching the ball of the patient's thumb or great toe with pressure, and either estimating or timing the number of seconds it takes for blood to reappear in the tissue. A refill time of less than 2 sec indicates a loss of less than 50 mL fluid/kg; a 2- to 3-sec refill time occurs with losses of 50 to 90 mL/kg; refill times in excess of 3 sec are associated with losses of 100 mL/kg or more and with the presence of or potential for shock.

TABLE 6–12. Clinical Assessment of Severity of Dehydration

Signs and Symptoms	Mild Dehydration	Moderate Dehydration	Severe Dehydration
General appearance and condition:			
Infants and young children	Thirsty; alert; restless	Thirsty; restless or lethargic but irritable to touch or drowsy	Drowsy; limp, cold, sweaty, cyanotic extremities; may be comatose
Older children and adults	Thirsty; alert; restless	Thirsty; alert; postural hypotension	Usually conscious; apprehensive; cold, sweaty, cyanotic extremities; wrinkled skin of fingers and toes; muscle cramps
Radial pulse	Normal rate and strength	Rapid and weak	Rapid, feeble, sometimes impalpable
Respiration	Normal	Deep, may be rapid	Deep and rapid
Anterior fontanel	Normal	Sunken	Very sunken
Systolic blood pressure	Normal	Normal or low	Less than 90 mm Hg, may be unrecordable
Skin elasticity	Pinch retracts immediately	Pinch retracts slowly	Pinch retracts very slowly (>2 sec)
Eyes	Normal	Sunken (detectable)	Grossly sunken
Tears	Present	Absent	Absent
Mucous membranes	Moist	Dry	Very dry
Urine flow	Normal	Reduced amount and dark	None passed for several hours; empty bladder
Body weight loss (%)	4–5	6–9	10 or more
Estimated fluid deficit (mL/kg)	40–50	60–90	100–110

Modified from World Health Organization guide.

Physical examination may also help determine the type of dehydration (see Table 6–14). Patients with hyponatremic dehydration have relatively greater losses of fluid from the extracellular fluid compartment and are more likely to develop shock; conversely, evidence of depletion of intracellular fluid may be apparent in patients with hypernatremic dehydration and may be reflected by a doughy or putty-like consistency of the skin and subcutaneous tissue on palpation, a marked loss of intraocular pressure, or a small, shriveled tongue. These signs rarely occur unless fluid deficits exceed 100 mL/kg. Less severe losses are usually characterized by a poor ability to focus attention, a lethargic state with increased irritability to external stimuli, and increased muscle tone with hyper-reflexia.

Some disease states result in specific losses. For example, severe diarrhea is associated with marked losses of bicarbonate resulting in systemic acidosis. In pyloric stenosis, major losses of hydrogen and chloride cause a hypochloremic alkalosis. Chronic diarrhea may result in hypomagnesemia from continuing losses of magnesium. The findings on physical examination that may indicate such deficits are summarized in Table 6–14. Such signs are not infallible or uniform. For example, the characteristic signs of metabolic acidosis (relatively slow, regular breathing with increased depth and a prolonged expiratory phase, referred to as *Kussmaul breathing*) may be less marked in the presence of severe circulatory insufficiency. The compensatory diminution in breathing associated with alkalosis, although usually absent in adults, may be seen in infants with pyloric stenosis. Deficiencies of potassium, calcium, or magnesium may exist without obvious physical findings. Hypokalemia may not always be present, even when the cells are depleted of potassium, so that such deficits may have to be inferred from history alone.

LABORATORY DATA. Admission laboratory values are helpful in characterizing the type of deficit and in planning therapy. None is so essential, however, that adequate therapy cannot be initiated without it. Serial laboratory determinations are of greater importance. They permit the assessment of the results of treating deficits and guide subsequent maintenance therapy.

Hemoconcentration (increase in *hemoglobin, hematocrit,* and *plasma proteins*) may indicate the severity of dehydration.

TABLE 6–13. Effects of Type of Dehydration on Physical Signs

Parameter	Isonatremic Dehydration (Proportionate Loss of Water and Sodium)	Hyponatremic Dehydration (Loss of Sodium in Excess of Water)	Hypernatremic Dehydration (Loss of Water in Excess of Sodium)
ECF volume*	Markedly decreased	Severely decreased	Decreased
ICF volume*	Maintained	Increased	Decreased
Physical signs			
Skin			
Color†	Gray	Gray	Gray
Temperature	Cold	Cold	Cold or hot
Turgor‡	Poor	Very poor	Fair
Feel	Dry	Clammy	Thickened, doughy
Mucous membranes	Dry	Slightly moist	Parched§
Eyeball	Sunken and soft	Sunken and soft	Sunken
Fontanel	Sunken	Sunken	Sunken
Psyche	Lethargic	Coma	Hyperirritable
Pulse†	Rapid	Rapid	Moderately rapid
Blood pressure†	Low	Very low	Moderately low

*ECF, extracellular fluid; ICF, intracellular fluid.
†Signs of shock rather than of dehydration itself.
‡Reflects magnitude of fluid loss from ECF.
§Tongue often has shriveled appearance because of loss of cellular fluid.

TABLE 6–14. Physical Signs of Variations in Concentration of Specific Ions

Ion	Concentration	Condition	Sign(s)
Hydrogen	Increased	Acidosis (metabolic)	Respiration: increased depth and rate
Hydrogen	Decreased	Alkalosis (metabolic)	Respiration: decreased depth and rate; latent or manifest tetany
Potassium	Decreased	Hypopotassemia	Heart: fast or slow, poor quality to heart sounds; skeletal muscle: weakness or paralysis, diminished reflexes; smooth muscle: abdominal distention, ileus
Potassium	Increased	Hyperpotassemia	Heart: slow or fast, poor quality to heart sounds; skeletal muscle: fibrillation, paralysis
Calcium	Decreased	Hypocalcemia	Latent tetany (Sec. 6.27); manifest tetany (Sec. 6.28)
Calcium	Increased	Hypercalcemia	Gastrointestinal: fecal masses; hypotonia
Magnesium	Decreased	Hypomagnesemia	Latent or manifest tetany; muscular twitching
Magnesium	Increased	Hypermagnesemia	Decreased deep tendon reflexes; central nervous system depression

However, with pre-existing anemia, both hemoglobin and hematocrit may be normal even with severe dehydration. Similarly, the measurement of plasma proteins may have limited usefulness at the beginning of therapy, especially in the malnourished patient. Despite such limitations, these measurements, when correlated with physical findings, may be useful in planning therapy. Repeat measurements help assess effectiveness of treatment.

Dehydration may result in a decrease in GFR so that both *blood urea nitrogen* and *creatinine* levels increase, the former often being raised more than the latter. Azotemia may also result from intrinsic renal disease, however. Measuring urine concentration can help separate these two entities; *urinalysis* showing a specific gravity of less than 1.020 with dehydration indicates a defect in urinary concentrating mechanisms and suggests intrinsic renal disease. With dehydration there may be mild to moderate proteinuria and the urine may contain hyaline and granular casts, white blood cells and, occasionally, red blood cells. Such findings do not necessarily indicate intrinsic renal disease, but urinalysis should be repeated after recovery from the dehydration. Serial measurements of urinary output and specific gravity are of value in evaluating the effectiveness of therapy and in guiding it.

Serum or *plasma electrolyte values* are especially useful. Serum sodium concentration reflects the relative losses of water and electrolytes. *Total body sodium is typically depleted in all patients with dehydration, even in those with hypernatremia.* Serum potassium concentrations at the beginning of therapy are of limited value, because they do not help determine body content of this cation. Values may be elevated because of anoxia, diminished renal function, or acidosis, even when significant cellular deficits exist. Serial electrocardiograms may provide clues to disturbances of intracellular potassium and calcium. *Serum bicarbonate* concentrations help define whether the patient has acidemia or alkalemia. Values may have to be supplemented by determining blood pH and P_{CO_2}. These determinations are particularly valuable as guides to the severity of metabolic disorders or of respiratory disorders, such as occur in patients receiving assisted or artificial respiration. Measuring *serum chloride* concentration permits calculation of the anion gap (see Sec. 6.9). Normally, the difference between the sum of measured cations (sodium and potassium) and that of measured anions (chloride and bicarbonate) is 15 ± 5 mEq/L. This value is increased in renal disease, as a result of retention of phosphate, sulfate, and other unmeasured anions, as well as in ketosis and lactic acidosis. The difference may also indicate the possibility of laboratory error in electrolyte determinations.

6.18 PRINCIPLES OF THERAPY

In some dehydrated patients, such as those in shock, administering fluids must be treated as a medical emergency. A complete evaluation of the patient can be undertaken after fluid therapy has begun and the patient's condition has been stabilized. However, most errors in fluid management occur in the initial stages of rehydration. When possible, it is preferable not to administer fluids until the patient's state of hydration has been assessed clinically and the type and amounts of fluids to be given for initial rehydration have been carefully determined. When planning this therapy for the dehydrated patient, the important considerations are the magnitude of the sodium and water deficits, the qualitative changes in body composition that have resulted from relative losses of electrolytes in relation to water, and the status of both potassium and hydrogen ion balances. *Similar basic therapeutic approaches with only minor modification may be used for patients having dehydration resulting from widely differing etiologies.*

Oral rehydration may be appropriate in patients with mild or moderate dehydration. Amounts of fluid and electrolytes adequate to correct the deficits can often be administered by mouth to such patients (see Sec. 6.20). Parenteral administration is required for patients with more severe dehydration, for those who are vomiting, or for those having profound ongoing losses; for example, it is recommended for any patient with diarrhea of amounts greater than 100 mL/kg/hr. The intravenous route is preferred for the parenteral replacement of deficits, although replacement fluids have been given by the intraperitoneal and subcutaneous routes.

Parenteral rehydration therapy has three phases. *Initial therapy* consists of rapid re-expansion of extracellular fluid volume and is designed to improve circulatory dynamics and renal function which are of primary importance in the morbidity and mortality of dehydration. *Subsequent therapy* is aimed at replacing the remaining intracellular and extracellular deficits of water and electrolytes but at a slower rate, with sodium replacement preceding potassium replacement. The *final phase* consists of the return of the patient's normal nutritional state and usually begins when the patient is able to return to oral feedings.

INITIAL THERAPY. This phase is designed to treat or prevent shock by rapidly expanding the volume of extracellular fluid, especially the plasma. Ideally, the entire fluid used for initially treating dehydration should remain in the vascular space. Whole blood, however, is not the treatment of choice. Delays during typing and cross-matching the blood may occur, and thrombosis accompanying the administration of blood in the dehydrated patient is a risk. Similarly, the risk of hepatitis makes the use of pooled plasma undesirable. Instead, an electrolyte solution with a sodium concentration similar to that of blood is recommended. Glucose should be included in this fluid, because the sick infant is susceptible to hypoglycemia. Suitable preparations that fulfill these criteria are commercially available (see Table 27–8). Isotonic saline (0.9%; sodium and chloride both 154 mEq/L) containing glucose, 5 g/dL, is one especially useful alternative in dehydrated patients with metabolic alkalosis (e.g., from pyloric stenosis).

Using this solution in a patient with acidosis is less optimal, because it does not correct the acidosis unless renal perfusion is increased, thus permitting increased excretion of hydrogen ions by the kidneys. Indeed, saline administration can aggravate the acidosis by further diluting the plasma bicarbonate. In an acidotic patient a solution containing some bicarbonate or a bicarbonate precursor is preferred—for example, adding 28 mL of 7.5% sodium bicarbonate solution to 750 mL of 0.9% sodium chloride solution and increasing the final volume to 1 L with 5% dextrose in water. This solution contains 140 mEq of sodium, 115 mEq of chloride, and 25 mEq of bicarbonate/L. Similar commercial solutions containing lactate or acetate instead of bicarbonate are available but have the disadvantage that the bicarbonate precursor may not be readily metabolized to bicarbonate in severely dehydrated patients with impaired circulation; thus, therapy with these solutions may aggravate the existing acidosis.

The solution chosen for the initial phase of therapy can be started immediately even though serum electrolyte values are not known. The volume given should equal 20–30 mL/kg and be administered as rapidly as possible if there are signs of shock, or within 1 hr in less severely ill patients. If clinical signs of shock persist, a second and, rarely, a third infusion of 20–30 mL/kg may be necessary to restore circulation. Ordinarily, however, normal circulation is restored by the time 20 mL/kg has been administered, at which point the laboratory findings are usually available and one can proceed more slowly with logically planned subsequent therapy. If large volumes of fluid are administered, monitoring central venous pressure is desirable to minimize the danger of volume overload.

This therapy is equally appropriate in hypo-, iso-, and hypernatremic dehydration; the administered fluid tends to return the serum sodium level toward normal in most cases. In some patients with hypernatremic dehydration, the serum sodium level may increase even further on administering isotonic saline solution, the mechanism for which is unclear. However, this increase is usually 5 mEq/L or less and does not appear to affect the clinical course adversely.

Potassium should not be administered at this stage of therapy unless the patient is severely hypokalemic. It should be given only after establishing that the kidneys are functioning.

Occasionally, the therapy outlined is inadequate to reverse shock, and blood (10 mL/kg) or some other plasma volume expander is required.

SUBSEQUENT THERAPY. Once circulation has been restored, therapy during the remainder of the first 24 hr is aimed both at completely correcting the remaining sodium and water deficits and at replacing ongoing abnormal and normal obligatory losses. Replacement of potassium losses may be started but is not essential. Frequently, it is not attempted until after the first 24 hr. The exception is the presence of proven hypokalemia or a situation known to be associated with severe losses of potassium. Examples include the hypochloremic alkalosis of pyloric stenosis, prolonged diarrhea, or diabetes acidosis, when potassium may be administered even when pretreatment serum levels are normal or only mildly reduced. Even in such patients, however, potassium should not be administered until urine flow has been established.

By the time this phase of therapy is reached, the patient's serum electrolytes should be known and, as discussed next, therapy can be modified, depending on the presenting serum sodium level.

Isonatremic Dehydration. In this disorder there are not only external losses of sodium from the extracellular fluid but also movement of sodium from extracellular into intracellular fluid to compensate for intracellular potassium losses. Therefore, administering sodium in an amount equal to the loss from the extracellular fluid would be excessive and would result in an increase in the patient's total body sodium; the increment of sodium in the intracellular fluid would later return to the extracellular fluid when potassium was administered, resulting in expansion of the latter compartment. To avoid this, only two thirds of the approximate losses of sodium and water from the extracellular fluid is replaced during the first 24 hr of treatment.

For example, in a patient with severe isonatremic dehydration and a 15% loss of body weight, the calculated fluid deficit would be 150 mL/kg (15% of body weight) and the sodium deficit 21 mEq/kg (assuming a serum sodium concentration of 140 mEq/L). In the first 24 hr only 100 mg/kg of water and 14 mEq/kg of sodium should be administered. Of this, 20–30 mL/kg of fluid and 3–4 mEq/kg of sodium (possibly more if the patient did not respond to this treatment) would be administered in the first 2–3 hr as initial therapy to expand the extracellular fluid. The remaining 70–80 mL/kg of water and 10–11 mEq/kg of sodium would then be given during the ensuing 21–22 hr. The fluid used for this phase of therapy would be similar to that used in the first 2–3 hr (i.e., 0.9% saline or its equivalent), and treatment is aimed at replacing the bulk of the deficits of water and sodium.

In addition to replacing deficits, total fluid and electrolyte administration during this and subsequent phases of treatment must include replacement for both ongoing normal losses and any continuing abnormal losses such as those from diarrhea, intestinal suction, and so forth (see Sec. 6.14). They are added to those needed to correct initial deficits, and thus an estimate of total requirements for the first 24 hr of treatment can be obtained.

After the first 24 hr, the objective is to achieve complete replacement of sodium and water losses and to start replacing potassium losses. The sodium and water requirements at this point can be estimated by adding 25% to estimated normal maintenance requirements and by adding requirements for any ongoing abnormal losses. Potassium losses in dehydration may equal sodium losses, but potassium is lost almost exclusively from the intracellular fluid and has to be replaced by administration into the extracellular compartment. If potassium were replaced at a rate comparable to that used to replace sodium, severe hyperkalemia would almost certainly result. Thus, potassium losses are usually replaced over a 3- to 4-day period. Potassium should also not be administered if the serum potassium is elevated or until it is established that the kidneys are functioning. Moreover, in the presence of severe acidosis, it should be administered cautiously. Except under unusual circumstances, the concentration of potassium in the administered fluid should not exceed 40 mEq/L, and the rate of potassium administration should not exceed 3 mEq/kg/24 hr.

Hyponatremic Dehydration. This condition results from relatively greater losses of sodium than of water. The extra sodium loss can be calculated from the formula

$$\text{Sodium deficit [mEq]} = (135 - S_{Na}) \times \text{total body water [in L]}$$

where S_{Na} represents the measured serum sodium concentration and 135 is the low-normal value for serum sodium. Because the patient is dehydrated, total body water should be estimated at 50–55% of admission weight rather than as the usual value of 60%. Even though sodium is principally an extracellular cation, total body water is used for calculating sodium deficit. This allows for repletion of sodium lost from the extracellular fluid, for any expansion of the extracellular fluid that occurs with repletion, and for repletion of sodium lost from other pools of exchangeable sodium, such as that in bone.

Treatment of hyponatremic dehydration is similar to isonatremic dehydration, except that when calculating sodium administration, the extra losses of that ion should be taken into account. Administering the extra amounts of sodium needed to replace the additional losses can be spread over several days so that gradual correction of the hyponatremia is accomplished as volume is expanded. Sodium concentrations should not be abruptly elevated by administering hypertonic saline solutions unless symptoms of water intoxication, such as convulsions, are present. Symptoms rarely occur unless serum sodium levels fall below 120 mEq/L, and they are usually rapidly controlled by intravenous administration of a 3% solution of sodium chloride at a rate of 1 mL/min to a maximum of 12 mL/kg of body weight. More details are presented in Sec. 6.26. *Hypotonic solutions should be avoided, especially in the initial phase of treatment, because of the risk of inducing symptomatic hyponatremia.*

Hypernatremic Dehydration. This presents one of the more difficult problems in fluid therapy because severe hyperosmolality may result in cerebral damage, with widespread cerebral hemorrhages and thromboses or subdural effusions. This cerebral injury may result in permanent neurologic deficit. Even in the absence of such obvious pathologic lesions, seizures are common in patients with severe hypernatremia. The diagnosis of cerebral injury secondary to hypernatremia is assisted by finding an elevated protein level in the cerebrospinal fluid.

Frequently, seizures occur during treatment as the serum sodium is returning to normal. They may result from an increase in the sodium content of cerebral cells during the period of dehydration, which in turn results in an excessive movement of water into these cells during rehydration before excess sodium is extruded. Although the mechanism by which this water movement results in seizures is uncertain, the incidence may be reduced by correcting hypernatremia slowly over a period of days. Therefore, therapy is adjusted to return serum sodium levels toward normal by not more than 10 mEq/L/24 hr.

The sodium deficit in hypernatremic dehydration is relatively small and the extracellular fluid volume relatively well maintained so that the amounts of both sodium and water to be administered in this phase of therapy are reduced, compared with those in hypo- or isonatremic dehydration. A suitable regimen is to administer 60–75 mL/kg/24 hr of a 5% dextrose solution containing 25 mEq/L of sodium as a combination of the bicarbonate and chloride.

Amounts of maintenance fluid and sodium should be reduced by about 25% during this phase because the hypernatremic patient has high levels of antidiuretic hormone (ADH), resulting in a low volume of urine. Replacement of ongoing abnormal losses does not require modification.

If seizures do occur, they may often be controlled by intravenous administration of 3–5 mL/kg of a 3% sodium chloride solution or by administering hypertonic mannitol.

Treatment of hypernatremic dehydration with large amounts of water, with or without salt, frequently results in expansion of the extracellular fluid volume before there is any notable excretion of chloride or correction of the acidosis. As a consequence, edema and cardiac failure may develop, necessitating digitalization. Hypocalcemia is also seen occasionally during treatment of hypernatremic dehydration; it may be prevented by administering appropriate amounts of potassium. Once developed, it may require intravenous administration of calcium. Another complication is renal tubular injury with azotemia and loss of concentrating ability, which may necessitate modification of the therapeutic regimen.

Although hypernatremic dehydration can be successfully treated, management is difficult and seizures frequently occur, even with the best-designed regimens. Treatment of such seizures is detailed in Sec. 6.20. It is better to emphasize prevention, because this particularly dangerous form of dehydration is frequently iatrogenic in etiology.

CORRECTION OF NUTRITIONAL DEFICIENCIES. Although parenteral fluid therapy results in a caloric intake inadequate to meet the patient's needs, the inadequate calories are rarely a cause for concern because of the short periods of time usually involved. When the patient can return to a normal diet, any deficits in body fat and protein are soon corrected.

If parenteral fluid therapy is required for prolonged periods (e.g., when patients are unable to eat or when they develop severe diarrhea as oral feeding is restarted), increased caloric and nutritional intake may be required to prevent the development of serious malnourishment. This intake is best given by the intravenous alimentation technique (Sec. 6.14).

ASSESSMENT OF RESPONSE. Many factors modify the amounts and types of fluids to be administered. Thus, it is vitally important that the clinician monitor the response to therapy, which should include frequent clinical observation emphasizing the child's cry, degree of activity, skin turgor, and blood pressure. In addition, frequent measurements of body weight and careful charting of intake and output, by recording stool and urine volumes separately, is valuable in assessing response to therapy. Under certain circumstances, serially measuring serum and urine electrolyte levels, osmolality, and central venous pressure, as well as monitoring the electrocardiogram, may also be required. In the severely ill child, recording these serial determinations on a carefully maintained flow sheet and using them as a guide for adjusting therapy may be lifesaving. Unpredicted responses to therapy are not uncommon; hence, monitoring should be meticulous and, when indicated, appropriate modifications of the regimens should be instituted promptly.

SIMPLIFIED METHODS TO CALCULATE REQUIREMENTS

These alternative methods are based on the principles outlined previously and estimate deficit and maintenance needs together. They are implemented once initial therapy for treating or preventing shock (see Sec. 6.18) has been completed.

One method in widespread use expresses fluid and electrolyte requirements per unit of body surface—the *meter-squared system* (Table 6–15). In health, the kidneys have the ability to regulate water and electrolyte balances over wide ranges of intakes. As shown in the table, various disease states may reduce the maximum (ceiling) or increase the minimum (floor) amounts of water or electrolytes that can be tolerated. However, the average dehydrated child with functioning kidneys still has relatively large ranges of tolerance. If water and electrolytes are provided in adequate quantities within the limits of tolerance, the patients cure themselves with renal function providing final regulation.

According to the meter-squared system, normal maintenance of water and electrolytes in older infants and children is provided by 1,500 mL/m^2/24 hr of a solution containing 5% dextrose, 25 mEq/L of sodium, and 20 mEq/L of potassium. This rate of administration may be increased 2- or 3-fold in dehydration or reduced in overhydration. With experience the clinician can determine fluid and electrolyte requirements using these guidelines and need not go through the several stages of calculations presented earlier. The important exceptions to this generalization are found in patients with marked renal insufficiency, craniopharyngioma, adrenal insufficiency, or other defects in the homeostatic mechanisms responsible for regulating water and sodium metabolism. In such patients severe impairment of renal or other regulatory mechanisms

TABLE 6–15. Principles of Meter-Squared System for Determining Fluid and Electrolyte Therapy

Substance	Range of Tolerance (in Health)	Ceiling Lowered	Floor Raised
Water	1–13 L/m²/24 hr (1–5 in 1st wk of life)	General anesthesia; morphine and related drugs; "nephritis;" hypothalamic lesions; circulatory failure; neonatal period	Diabetes insipidus; nephrogenic diabetes insipidus; cellular potassium deficiency; sodium intoxication
Sodium	5–250 mEq/m²/24 hr	Zero potassium intake; hypoalbuminemia; cardiac failure; severe stress; corticosteroid therapy; Cushing syndrome; renal disease	Hypoadrenocorticism; abnormal loss of gastrointestinal fluids; extensive burns; renal tubular disease (diuretic therapy)
Potassium	10–250 mEq/m²/24 hr	Marked dehydration; circulatory failure; low sodium intake; reduced glomerular filtration rate; hypoadrenocorticism; congenital adrenal hyperplasia	Diarrhea; gastrointestinal drainage; high sodium intake; corticosteroid therapy
Phosphorus	0–4,000 mg/m²/24 hr (expressed as phosphorus)	Normal newborn; reduced glomerular filtration rate; hypoparathyroidism; pseudohypoparathyroidism; circulatory failure	Vitamin D intoxication; hyperparathyroidism
Chloride	0–250 mEq/m²/24 hr		
Bicarbonate	5–250 mEq/m²/24 hr		
Glucose	50–300 g/m²/24 hr		

markedly limits the ranges of tolerance and requires that each component of fluid and electrolyte therapy be carefully calculated for the individual on a daily or even more frequent basis.

6.19 THERAPY IN SPECIFIC DISEASE STATES

6.20 DIARRHEA

See Sec. 12.10 and 13.14.

ACUTE DIARRHEA. Diarrhea continues to be a serious problem in many areas of the world. It results in large losses of both water and electrolytes, especially sodium and potassium (see Table 6–10), and frequently is complicated by severe systemic acidosis.

In approximately 70% of patients, the losses of water and sodium are proportionate, with *isonatremic dehydration* developing. *Hyponatremic dehydration* is seen in approximately 10% of all patients with diarrhea. It occurs when large amounts of electrolytes, especially sodium, are lost in the stool out of proportion to fluid losses. Thus, it is seen more frequently with bacillary dysentery or cholera. In these diseases, as opposed to diarrhea caused by rotavirus, to other nonspecific (presumably viral) infections, and to many noninfectious causes, the concentration of sodium in the stool rises with increasing volume of stool. Hyponatremia may be accentuated or produced if, during the period of diarrhea, a considerable oral intake consisting of low-electrolyte or electrolyte-free fluids is administered.

Disproportionately large net losses of water compared to electrolytes result in *hypernatremic dehydration,* which is seen in approximately 20% of patients with diarrhea and may result during the course of diarrhea from oral administration of homemade electrolyte solutions with too high concentrations of salt. It may also occur in young infants with diarrhea if their renal ability to conserve water is limited, especially if the renal solute load is increased by feeding boiled skim milk. Such factors may be potentiated by fever, high environmental temperatures, or hyperventilation, each of which increases evaporative water loss significantly.

Using intravenous fluids for treating dehydration from severe diarrhea is discussed in Sec. 6.18. An important development is the demonstration that dehydration from diarrhea of any etiology can be treated effectively, in a wide range of age groups, using a simple glucose-electrolyte solution given by mouth. Such oral rehydration is used in many countries and significantly reduces the mortality rate from acute diarrhea and lessens diarrhea-associated malnutrition. Patients in shock, those with severe dehydration or with uncontrollable vomiting, those with amounts of diarrhea exceeding 100 mL/kg/hr, those unable to drink because of extreme fatigue, stupor, or coma, or those with other serious complications such as severe gastric distention require intravenous therapy. However, oral rehydration can be attempted in the remainder, provided adequate supervision is available.

The composition of the oral rehydration solution (ORS) recommended by the Diarrhea Disease Control Program of the World Health Organization is shown in Table 6–16. The ingredients should be available in powder form in preweighed packages. Using teaspoons or other household items for measuring the amount of the solutes is inaccurate and is not recommended. In the United States, a suitable preparation is available commercially (*Hydra-Lyte*). Alternatively, an ORS with similar composition can be prepared from readily available solutions as follows: NaCl (0.9% saline solution) 390 mL; glucose (5% in water) 400 mL; KCl (2 mEq/mL) 10 mL; $NaHCO_3$ (1 mEq/mL) 30 mL; water to 1 L. Glucose is the preferred sugar for use in ORS, because its high concentration facilitates the transport of sodium across the bowel wall. Sucrose can be substituted but has a slightly lower success rate, possibly because it has to be hydrolyzed before being absorbed as glucose. The concentration of sucrose in g/L

TABLE 6–16. Comparison of Composition of Oral Solutions (mM/L)

Component	WHO (ORS)*	Traditional Solution†	Reformulated Solution†‡
Sodium	90	30	50
Potassium	20	25	25
Chloride	80	25	45
Bicarbonate	30	36	30
Glucose	111	28§	28§

*World Health Organization oral rehydration solution composed of (g/L water): NaCl, 3.5; $NaHCO_3$, 2.5; KCl, 1.5; glucose 20.0.

†Bicarbonate usually present as a precursor, such as citrate. Also contains (mEq/L): Ca, 4; Mg, 4; SO_4, 4; PO_4, 5.

‡Lytren (Mead Johnson). Other solutions are similar except for sodium and chloride concentrations which range from 45 to 75 mEq/L.

§Additional sugars provided as corn syrup to total carbohydrate content of 77 g/L.

should be twice that of glucose to obtain the same osmolarity. Solutions containing rice-syrup solids may also be effective.

As a guideline for oral rehydration, 50 mL/kg of the ORS should be given within 4 hr to patients with mild dehydration and 100 mL/kg over 6 hr to those with moderate dehydration. The amounts and rates should be increased if the patient continues to have diarrhea or if rehydration does not appear complete; they should be decreased if the patient appears fully hydrated earlier than expected or develops periorbital edema. Breast-feeding should be allowed ad libitum after treatment has been started in infants who are breast-fed; in other patients, plain water should be offered. Vomiting may occur during the first 2 hr of administration of ORS but does not prevent successful oral rehydration. To reduce vomiting, the ORS should be given slowly, in small amounts, at short intervals. If sustained severe vomiting occurs, intravenous therapy should be used. The patient's progress should be assessed frequently, and changes in body weight monitored, if possible, to determine the degree of rehydration.

When rehydration is complete, maintenance therapy can be started. Patients with mild diarrhea can be treated at home. Using 100 mL ORS/kg/24 hr until diarrhea stops is recommended. Breast-feeding or supplemental water intake should be maintained. Those patients with more severe diarrhea require continued supervision. The volume of ORS ingested should equal the volume of stool losses. If stool volume cannot be measured, an intake of 10–15 mL ORS/kg/hr is appropriate.

This regimen has not been universally accepted. The sodium concentration of ORS (90 mM/L) is three times that of fluids (such as *Pedialyte* or *Lytren;* see Tables 6–16 and 27–8) that have traditionally been recommended for oral therapy in patients with diarrhea. These low-sodium solutions were advocated because hypernatremia was seen frequently in the United States when oral electrolyte solutions with sodium concentrations of 50 mEq/L or more were used to treat infantile diarrhea. In contrast, extensive use of ORS in many developing countries has documented hypernatremia to be a rare complication, probably because ORS has been used primarily for rehydration (the major previous role for oral therapy was to prevent dehydration or for maintenance), because large amounts of water are ingested in addition to ORS, and because ORS has been administered under close supervision by trained personnel. Oral rehydration has been found effective in treating acute diarrheal illnesses in well-nourished children in developed countries. Hypernatremia did not occur even when solutions containing sodium 90 mEq/L were used. Several commercially available electrolyte solutions for oral use have been reformulated with a sodium concentration increased to 50 mEq/L or higher (Table 6–16).

Occasionally, an infant receiving 2–3 L/day of carbohydrate and electrolyte mixtures by mouth may have an apparently related increase in the volume of stools, but such instances are sufficiently rare that they do not contraindicate an initial trial of oral therapy.

It has been traditional to omit oral feedings initially when treating infants having more severe diarrhea. However, even during acute diarrhea, the small intestine can absorb various nutrients and may absorb up to 60% of the food eaten. Because better weight gain has been documented in infants given a liberal dietary intake during diarrhea when compared to others on a more restricted intake, because fasting has been shown to further reduce the ability of the small intestine to absorb nutrients, and because no physiologic basis exists for giving the bowel a "rest" during acute diarrhea, regimens in developing countries for treating acute diarrhea have encouraged continuing the oral intake of nutrients. This approach may cause, in a minority of subjects, an increase in the volume of stool resulting in continuing large losses of fluid and electrolytes (see Table 6–6), which must be replaced and may require instituting or extending parenteral therapy for several days. Despite this occasional complication, studies have shown that rehydration occurs as rapidly with oral as with parenteral therapy in most patients.

Typically, frequency and volume of stools lessen within 48 hr in fasted patients treated with intravenous therapy. When stooling subsides, oral feeding of one of the carbohydrate and electrolyte mixtures may be initiated, providing gastric distention and vomiting are absent. As soon as oral feeding is tolerated without exacerbating the diarrhea, the caloric intake may be increased gradually by substituting mixtures that also contain fat and protein until the usual dietary intake is attained, which usually occurs within 7–8 days. Prematurely administering large quantities of calories in the form of milk may exacerbate diarrhea. In the young infant with a family history of allergy, a hypoallergenic feeding mixture is recommended for the recovery phase, because permeability of the gastrointestinal tract to whole protein may be increased during this time. The routine use of lactose-free formulas in children with diarrhea does not lessen recovery time.

In addition to replacing the deficits of water and electrolytes, efforts should be made to obtain an etiologic diagnosis so that specific antimicrobial therapy may be given if indicated. Antibiotics are required in cases in which the diarrhea results from cholera, shigella, amebic dysentery, or acute giardiasis. Such treatment does not modify fluid therapy. Drugs such as opiates, which inhibit peristaltic activity of the bowel, or absorbents such as kaolin or pectin have relatively little or no effect on the course of infantile diarrhea and are not recommended.

DIARRHEA IN CHRONICALLY MALNOURISHED CHILDREN. Severe malnutrition complicated by diarrheal dehydration is common in tropical and subtropical countries and occurs occasionally in the temperate zones. Therapy should be adapted to meet the specific disturbances in body composition characteristic of the dehydrated *and* malnourished infant, in whom there appears to be an overexpansion of the intracellular space, accompanied by extracellular and presumably intracellular hypo-osmolality. Serum sodium, potassium, and magnesium levels tend to be low, and tetany may occasionally result from magnesium deficiency. Serum protein levels are frequently below 3.6 g/dL. The sodium content of muscle is high; potassium and magnesium contents are low. The electrocardiogram frequently shows tachycardia, low amplitude, and flat or inverted T waves. Cardiac reserve seems lowered and heart failure is a common complication.

Despite clinical signs of dehydration and reduced body water, urinary osmolality may be low in the chronically malnourished child. This defect in renal concentration may result from the relative absence of urea to contribute to a hypertonic fluid in the renal papillae, a defect associated with a low dietary protein intake and resulting in a failure of tubular conservation of water. However, the GFR is low, resulting in a smaller loss of water than would otherwise be expected, and renal concentrating ability returns after several days of high-protein feedings.

Survival of the malnourished infant with diarrhea is limited by caloric deficit to a greater extent than by water and electrolyte deficit. Reparative calories can be given by slow drip through an indwelling nasogastric tube while electrolytes and water are given parenterally. If appetite is poor and vomiting and gastric distention are absent, feeding is begun early (30–40 cal/kg/24 hr), given by slow intragastric drip. Increases to 50–100 cal/kg/24 hr and 1–2 g of protein/kg/24 hr are made in a few days. Ad lib intake should be permitted in the succeeding weeks, up to 250–300 cal/kg/24 hr, and should include an adequate supply of iron and copper.

Initial parenteral therapy is designed to improve the circulation and to expand extracellular volume. The repair solutions recommended resemble those of hyponatremic dehydration. If edema is present, the quantity of fluid and rate of administration should be reduced from recommended levels to avoid pulmonary edema. Blood should be given if the patient is in shock, severely ill, or anemic. Potassium salts can be given early if urine output is good. Controlled trials suggest that survival can be improved by the intramuscular injection of 1.0–1.5 mL of a 50% solution of magnesium sulfate (4.0 mEq/mL) every 12 hr for 1–3 days. Clinical and electrocardiographic improvement may be more rapid with magnesium therapy, and seizures occurring during recovery from diarrhea complicating severe malnutrition may respond to magnesium.

CHRONIC DIARRHEA. Parenteral alimentation (Sec. 6.14) may be required when diarrhea is severe and prolonged. Occasionally, this therapy must be supplemented by full oral feedings during chronic diarrhea, especially in severe malnutrition. Cow's milk protein allergy or specific disaccharidase deficiencies should be suspected in infants having persistent diarrhea. Acquired disaccharidase deficiency (especially for lactose) may develop as a complication of many chronic disorders of the gastrointestinal or other systems. Hypoallergenic feeding mixtures containing monosaccharides as the sole carbohydrate should be administered until the diarrhea ceases and nutrition improves. Specific tests of carbohydrate (disaccharide) splitting and absorption and of milk protein sensitivity can then be carried out but can be potentially dangerous, sometimes resulting in severe diarrhea with marked fluid and electrolyte losses.

CONGENITAL ALKALOSIS OF GASTROINTESTINAL ORIGIN. Rarely, chronic diarrhea may result from a congenital defect in the transport of chloride in both the small and large bowel. The watery stools of such patients have a high content of chloride and alkalosis results from the ensuing volume depletion. Potassium is lost in the stools and in the urine, the latter losses being a consequence of the alkalosis. Treatment of fluid and electrolyte deficits is similar to that for pyloric stenosis. Long-term therapy must provide an adequate dietary intake of potassium and chloride. A rare, acute, chloride-losing diarrhea may also occur.

6.21 PYLORIC STENOSIS

This condition exemplifies the correction of deficits associated with alkalosis. The therapy differs little from that for other causes of dehydration, except that potassium replacement should begin early, as soon as the child has urinated, and relatively more sodium and potassium should be given as the chloride salt than is usual in treating dehydration, partly because of the larger deficit of chloride seen in pyloric stenosis and partly because this results in some correction of the alkalosis as volume is expanded. Correction of the hypochloremia and alkalosis by administering ammonium chloride without correcting the potassium deficit is not recommended because it results in continued dysfunction of renal tubular and other cells.

Severe depletion of intracellular potassium results in increased exchange of hydrogen ion for sodium in the distal tubules of the kidney. Thus, the paradoxic presence of an acid urine with systemic alkalosis should be interpreted as signifying a marked potassium deficit and a need to increase the amount of potassium used for repletion.

It is not uncommon for deficits to be replaced and serum levels of electrolytes returned to normal within 12 hr. However, except in the mildly ill infant without signs of dehydration, it is preferable to delay surgery for at least 36–48 hr to achieve optimal readjustment of body functions. During this preparation period adequate fluid therapy prevents dehydration, and the stomach may be decompressed by gentle suction (Sec. 6.5 and 13.27).

6.22 FASTING AND THIRSTING

Parenteral fluid therapy is usually required in initially treating the infant or child who has taken little or no water and food for 1–5 days. Such infants are deficient not only in water, which has evaporated from the lungs and skin, but also in electrolytes, particularly sodium and chloride, which have been excreted in the urine (see Table 6–10). Administering electrolyte-free solutions under such circumstances leads only to an increase in urine volume, with possible increased losses of electrolytes, and may actually increase the dehydration. If fasting and thirsting continue beyond 4–5 days, urinary output falls to such low levels there is no significant continued loss of electrolytes. Further severe deficiency of water alone occurs because of evaporative losses and results in hypernatremia.

Therapy is begun with an isonatremic solution to produce rapid and safe expansion of extracellular volume and to improve renal function. Subsequent therapy is described in Sec. 6.18. Because relatively smaller extracellular reservoirs exist as age increases, children and adults should be given approximately one fourth to one third less water and sodium per kilogram than infants for a given degree of clinical dehydration. Potassium deficits are relatively the same in infants, children, and adults. Water, carbohydrate, and electrolytes may be administered to the mildly ill patient by mouth. Infants, however, often vomit when they are dehydrated, and for this reason initial therapy is usually given parenterally.

For a detailed discussion of the fluid therapy of children with diabetic ketoacidosis and burns, see Sec. 8.53 and Sec. 6.37, respectively.

6.23 SALICYLATE POISONING

The treatment of salicylate intoxication exemplifies the importance of supplemental therapy in which water and electrolytes are given above the usual needs, even in the absence of specific deficits, to facilitate excretion of the drug (see also Sec. 26.6).

Initially, high blood concentrations of salicylate sensitize the respiratory center to carbon dioxide. The resultant hyperventilation, with its characteristic marked prolongation of the expiratory phase of respiration, leads to increased evaporative losses of water and to respiratory alkalosis, for which the kidneys compensate by excreting large amounts of sodium and potassium bicarbonate. In addition, toxic levels of salicylate uncouple oxidative phosphorylation and may reduce hepatic glycogen, usually resulting in ketonemia and ketonuria. Hyperglycemia and glycosuria are common; hypoglycemia may be seen occasionally.

The loss of sodium and potassium in excess of chloride and the accumulation of acetoacetic and β-hydroxybutyric acids eventually produce severe metabolic acidosis, which is aggravated by the release of two moles of free hydrogen ion from each mole of aspirin absorbed and hydrolyzed. Thus, a dose of salicylate of 200 mg/kg adds an acute hydrogen ion load of 2 mEq/kg. Transition from respiratory alkalosis to a mixed disturbance of acid-base balance with severe metabolic acidosis complicated by respiratory alkalosis may be relatively rapid; therefore, therapy must be followed by periodic monitoring of the serum carbon dioxide content and the pH of the blood and urine.

Except in poisoning resulting from repeated therapeutic administration of salicylates, the significance of an isolated blood salicylate level depends in part on the interval between the time the drug was ingested and the time the blood sample was obtained; a level of 35 mg/dL 36 hr after an acute ingestion or after the start of aspirin therapy may be more significant than a level of 60 mg/dL 2 hr after acute ingestion when peak levels may be expected. Figure 6–10 can help determine the severity of an acute overdose, given the serum salicylate level and the time since ingestion.

In chronic ingestion it should be remembered that even though a salicylate level of 35 mg/dL may be required to obtain therapeutic benefits in older children, fatal cases of salicylism have occurred in infants with lower blood levels; the need for active treatment depends only in part on blood levels of salicylate and on whether the overdose is acute or chronic. Clinical factors are equally important. Coma, convulsions, marked hyperventilation, oliguria, respiratory depression, severe azotemia, or marked reduction in the plasma level of bicarbonate or P_{CO_2} indicates the need for active therapeutic intervention.

Treatment is designed to prevent further absorption of salicylate, to correct deficits and replace ongoing losses of fluids and electrolytes (which are increased above normal), and to reduce tissue levels of salicylate by facilitating excretion of the drug.

The efficacy of attempting to empty the gastrointestinal tract of salicylate is controversial. However, in the absence of central nervous system depression, gastric emptying can be attempted for up to 10 hr following ingestion of the salicylate. Syrup of ipecac (dose in children over 1 yr of age: 1 tbsp [15 mL] repeated after 20 min if vomiting does not occur) is probably still the most effective emetic, and a slurry of activated charcoal can be given later in an attempt to prevent further absorption of any remaining salicylate from the bowel.

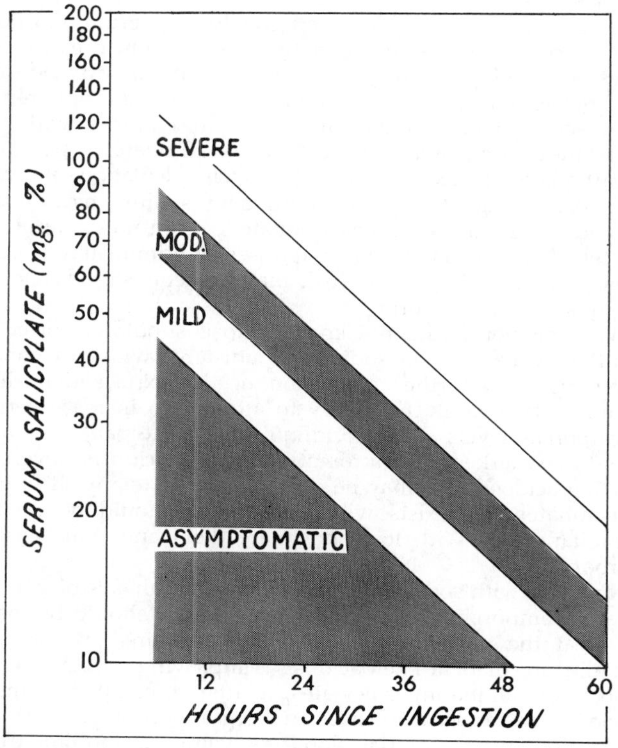

Figure 6–10. Nomogram relating serum salicylate concentration and expected severity of intoxication at varying intervals following the ingestion of a single dose of salicylate. (From Done AK: Salicylate intoxication: Significance of measurements of salicylate in blood in cases of acute ingestion. Pediatrics 26:800, 1960. Copyright 1960. Reproduced by permission of Pediatrics.)

If the patient is in shock, an isonatremic solution is indicated to expand plasma volume; otherwise, a hyponatremic solution can be used to replace fluid and electrolyte deficits.

The amount of fluid required ranges in individual patients from 2,000 to 5,500 mL/m²/24 hr. This fluid should contain sodium, 40–50 mEq/L, some of which should be sodium bicarbonate and, if there is adequate renal function, potassium, to 40 mEq/L. Oral potassium salts may be used to supplement the intravenous therapy. Administering carbohydrate appears to improve prognosis; intravenous fluids should contain at least 5% glucose.

Treatment is designed to replace maintenance losses of fluids and electrolytes, which may be twice normal because of increased evaporative losses, to replace deficits, and to maintain a diuresis to facilitate excretion of salicylate. A urine volume of at least 2,000 mL/m²/24 hr with a specific gravity of less than 1.010 is a reasonable goal. The early administration of sodium bicarbonate to maintain an alkaline urine (pH higher than 7.5) facilitates excretion of salicylate by reducing its back-diffusion in ionized form from tubular urine through the lipid membranes of the renal tubular cells; the clearance of salicylate with a urine pH greater than 8.0 is 20 times that at a urine pH of 6.0. The dose of bicarbonate necessary to alkalinize the urine is approximately 2 mEq/kg, given over 1 hr. An additional 2 mEq/kg of sodium bicarbonate should be given if the urine pH does not reach 7.0. The urinary pH should then be checked every 30 min. If the pH falls below 7.0, additional sodium bicarbonate should be given with appropriate amounts of potassium to avoid renal tubular potassium depletion and paradoxic aciduria.

Acetazolamide (5 mg/kg repeated 2 or 3 times in 24 hr) also increases salicylate excretion; this therapy has not received general acceptance because of reported complications, including seizures, and an increased mortality in experimental animals. Peritoneal dialysis or hemodialysis should be considered for severely ill patients as a means for removing additional amounts of salicylate loosely bound to plasma proteins. Such patients include those with blood levels of salicylate above 100 mg/dL, those with an elevated P_{CO_2}, those with severe acidosis, or those who have failed to respond adequately to alkalinization. The efficiency of dialysis is increased by the addition of albumin to the dialysis fluid. Exchange transfusion is a relatively inefficient means of removing salicylate in the critically ill patient. If done, heparinized blood should be used because of the often lethal exacerbation of acidosis if citrated blood is used.

Vitamin K_1 oxide (Konakion) should be given intramuscularly to offset possible prothrombin deficiency.

6.24 ELECTROLYTE DISTURBANCES ASSOCIATED WITH CENTRAL NERVOUS SYSTEM DISORDERS

Diseases of the central nervous system are frequently associated with disturbances in sodium concentration. Three types of changes have been described:

1. Patients with diverse lesions, such as surgical or traumatic damage to the brain, encephalitis, bulbar poliomyelitis, cerebrovascular accidents, tumors of the 4th ventricle, and subdural hematomas, may lose large amounts of sodium in the urine. Dehydration, hypotension, and azotemia result unless large amounts of salt are administered and the intake of water is limited.

2. Patients with tuberculous meningitis who are severely ill and comatose are frequently hyponatremic but exhibit no symptoms that can be attributed to hyponatremia. This situation may be analogous to the asymptomatic hyponatremia of severe malnutrition or pulmonary disease. Relatively large

amounts of salt may be lost in the urine when attempts are made to correct the hyponatremia by salt loading. Careful clinical and laboratory observations are essential to ensure that salt depletion and water intoxication do not occur. Potassium should be administered in amounts at least 50% greater than with usual maintenance therapy.

3. Patients with acute infections of the central nervous system occasionally have symptoms of acute water intoxication, with a rapid fall in the serum sodium level. These patients retain an excessive amount of water and have increased thirst. Convulsions are severe and resistant to drug therapy but respond to the intravenous administration of hypertonic saline solution and subsequent restriction of fluid.

These disorders may result from lesions involving the thirst center, osmoreceptors, or supraopticohypophyseal tract, from inappropriate secretion of ADH, or from other lesions.

Convulsions or other symptoms from cerebral edema may respond to hypertonic mannitol solution, although care in its administration should be taken in patients with impaired renal function.

6.25 PREOPERATIVE, INTRAOPERATIVE, AND POSTOPERATIVE FLUIDS

See Sec. 6.48–6.52.

Preoperatively preparing a patient having no pre-existing deficit or in whom the deficit has been repaired consists mainly of supplying carbohydrate to ensure adequate storage of glycogen in the liver. Usual maintenance requirements of water and electrolytes are appropriate. Young infants who are not vomiting should receive carbohydrate and sodium chloride mixtures by mouth until 3 hr before operation. Such fluids are readily absorbed from the gastrointestinal tract and do not produce aspiration pneumonitis if vomited and aspirated.

Preoperatively preparing the newborn involves certain unique hazards. Deficits of water and electrolytes from vomiting or from stasis caused by intestinal obstruction should be replaced before operating. If aspiration pneumonitis is suspected, it should be treated with antibiotics. Nasogastric suction may be inadequate. If so, *gastrostomy* should be performed to aid in decompression and in postoperative feeding. In intestinal obstruction conjugated bilirubin may be deglucuronidated by intestinal enzymes; an enterohepatic circulation of unconjugated bilirubin can then lead to high serum levels and kernicterus. Hypoprothrombinemia should be prevented by administering 1 mg of vitamin K_1 oxide.

The most common error in administering parenteral fluid during and after surgery is overadministration, particularly of dextrose in water. Table 6–17 lists maintenance water requirements during surgery. Additional amounts of blood, plasma, saline, or other volume expander must be given if blood loss or tissue trauma is significant. The magnitude of such losses is best judged by the experienced surgeon as he or she operates.

Under most circumstances no potassium should be administered during this time, because extensive tissue trauma or anoxia may result in the release of large amounts of intracellular potassium with the potential of causing hyperkalemia. Moreover, if shock occurs, it may be complicated by acute renal failure, making treatment of the hyperkalemia more difficult.

Postoperatively, intake should be limited for 24 hr. Thereafter, usual maintenance therapy is gradually resumed. The water intake should not exceed 85 mL/100 kcal metabolized because of antidiuresis resulting from trauma or circulatory readjustment unless renal ability to concentrate the urine is limited (e.g., in sickle cell anemia). If the intake of water is not limited, whether given parenterally or by mouth, water intoxication may result. Maintenance sodium intake should also be low because of the low caloric expenditure during anesthesia and postoperatively.

Some postoperative children have elevated blood ADH levels but not the inappropriate ADH syndrome. Rather, the ADH release is an appropriate response to very severe fluid restriction with resultant volume contraction.

6.26 ISOLATED DISTURBANCES IN CONCENTRATIONS OF ELECTROLYTES

ACIDOSIS. *Respiratory acidosis,* in which the pH may be markedly lowered, primarily as a result of retention of carbon dioxide, may be seen with severe respiratory insufficiency, with respiratory distress syndrome in the newborn infant, and in patients receiving assisted ventilation for any reason. Mild metabolic acidosis may also exist because hypoxia leads to the accumulation of lactic and other organic acids in the extracellular fluid. Measurements of blood pH and gases should guide correction of acidosis. The appropriate treatment is to improve ventilation by assisting respiration rather than by administering sodium bicarbonate, which may produce hyperosmolality and cardiac failure.

Metabolic acidosis, resulting, for example, from renal tubular acidosis or from accumulation of organic acids, may require the administration of alkali, especially if symptoms are evident. In lactic acidosis, in glycogen disorders, or in circulatory insufficiency and hypoxia, sodium lactate may not be adequately metabolized; in these situations sodium bicarbonate is the preferred agent. The usual initial dose is 1–2 mEq/kg. However, a more precise estimate of the dosage required is given by the general formula

$$(C_d - C_a) \times f_d \times \text{body weight [in kg]} = \text{mEq required}$$

where C_d and C_a represent, respectively, the serum bicarbonate concentration desired and the one actually present, expressed as mEq/L; and f_d represents that fraction of the total body weight in which the administered material is apparently (not actually) distributed (the value for f_d varies with the substance administered). The f_d for bicarbonate or potential bicarbonate approximates 0.5–0.6. Such calculations indicate that 0.5 mL/kg of a molar solution of sodium bicarbonate would raise the serum bicarbonate concentration approximately 1 mEq/L. However, responses to administered bicarbonate vary widely, because it may be sequestered in bone or muscle or lost in urine.

With glomerular insufficiency, acidosis should be corrected cautiously, because the sodium administered with bicarbonate may result in further expansion of the extracellular fluid volume. It is rarely necessary to attempt to increase serum bicarbonate levels above 15 mEq/L unless the patient continues to be markedly symptomatic from the acidosis. Overcorrecting acidosis also may be complicated by tetany. If hyperphosphatemia coexists with acidosis, it should be treated simultaneously with low-phosphate diets and oral calcium carbonate.

Treating with sodium bicarbonate should always be considered a temporizing measure; every attempt should be made to treat the underlying cause, such as using glucose and insulin in diabetic ketoacidosis, improving circulation in shock, or eliminating salicylates, methanol, or other toxins.

Severe metabolic acidosis is an integral part of *cardiovascular shock.* Relying on arterial blood gas values to monitor treatment in patients in shock and receiving mechanical ventilation is misleading. There is an exaggerated difference between arterial and central venous values for pH and P_{CO_2} in this situation, necessitating additional sampling of venous blood through a central venous line (see Sec. 6.34).

TABLE 6–17. Approximate Requirements of Water Without Electrolytes During Operation*

Weight (kg)	Basal (kcal/24 hr)	Evap. Water, mL/hr (90 mL/100 kcal/24 hr)†	Urine Water, mL/hr (30 mL/100 kcal/24 hr)‡	Total (mL/hr)§
3	150	6	2	8
5	270	10	3	13
7	410	15	5	20
10	550	21	7	28
20	850	32	10	42
30	1,100	41	14	55
40	1,300	49	16	65

*From Harned HS Jr, Cooke RE: Surg Gynecol Obstet 104:543, 1957. By permission of Surgery, Gynecology & Obstetrics.
†This value is assumed to be high because of possible sweating and hyperventilation.
‡This value is assumed to be low because of probable antidiuresis.
§This does not include abnormal losses of fluid (hemorrhage, wound edema, suction) that must be replaced by appropriate electrolyte-containing fluids.

ALKALOSIS. Normally, the kidney has an enormous capacity to excrete bicarbonate, and increased amounts of blood bicarbonate are promptly excreted. However, under certain circumstances, *metabolic alkalosis* may develop and be maintained. Typically, it is caused by the administration of excess amounts of alkali, by the loss of hydrogen ion, or by volume contraction with disproportionate losses of chloride. Severe hypokalemia can result in alkalosis, too, or may perpetuate it.

The plasma bicarbonate level is elevated and respiratory compensation results in hypoventilation and an increase in P_{CO_2}. Rarely, respiration may be so depressed in infants with severe hypochloremic alkalosis that blood oxygenation is diminished. Severe alkalotic tetany may also occur. In such instances, administering ammonium chloride may effect symptomatic improvement; the dose may be calculated from the general formula presented above, with the probable f_d being 0.2–0.3. Such therapy only relieves symptoms and should not be used in place of correcting the contracted volume of body fluids or administering potassium chloride to repair intracellular deficits.

Metabolic alkalosis associated with volume contraction responds to measures designed to expand volume and replace the chloride and potassium deficits. It occurs in patients with acid-base disorders caused by vomiting, gastric suction, congenital chloride diarrhea, dietary chloride deficiency, or administration of diuretics. Their urinary chloride concentration is low (10 mM/L or less). A minority of patients are "chloride-resistant," with urinary chloride concentrations of 15 mM/L or greater because of hyperadrenalism, Bartter syndrome, severe potassium depletion, or licorice ingestion. Potassium repletion, using potassium chloride and not potassium phosphate, as well as specific therapy directed to the underlying condition, is indicated.

Respiratory alkalosis occurs in salicylate intoxication, in various central nervous system diseases such as trauma, infection, or tumors, with anxiety or fever, and in congestive heart failure, hepatic insufficiency, and gram-negative septicemia. Treatment should be directed at removing the underlying cause, although measures designed to return the P_{CO_2} to normal may be indicated. Acidifying agents such as ammonium chloride are not indicated.

HYPONATREMIA. The serum sodium level is most commonly reduced as a result of either sodium depletion or water "intoxication" or a combination of both (Table 6–18). A low serum sodium level, thought to be a result of redistribution of total body sodium, may also occur in association with severe illnesses or in the terminally ill patient. In addition, *apparent* hyponatremia may be observed as an artifact, such as in diabetic ketoacidosis when the water content of plasma is reduced by the presence of increased quantities of lipids. This error is avoided by laboratory methods that determine sodium activity rather than concentration.

Patients with a serum sodium below 120 mEq/L are usually symptomatic (e.g., convulsions, shock); those with lesser degrees of hyponatremia are frequently asymptomatic. Treatment of *asymptomatic hyponatremia* depends on its cause. With water overload, fluid restriction is the appropriate measure; the serum sodium level may return rapidly to normal if there is good renal function but may take several days or weeks with the inappropriate ADH syndrome. When sodium deficits are present, adding extra salt to the diet or increasing the

TABLE 6–18. Clinical States Complicated by Hyponatremia

- Expansion of extracellular space by water
  - Excessive intake
    - Parenteral fluid therapy—glucose in water
    - Oral (with diminished output)
    - Tap water enemas
    - Allergy to cow's milk (very rare)
  - Diminished output (usual intake)
    - Renal
      - Intrinsic: nephritis, nephrotic syndrome, tubular necrosis, prematurity
      - Extrinsic
        - Excess of antidiuretic hormone: acute and chronic central nervous system disease, vasopressin therapy, surgery, pulmonary disease
        - Circulatory: heart failure, cardiovascular surgery, malnutrition
    - Skin: premature infant in very humid environment
- Deficiency of extracellular sodium
  - Inadequate intake
    - Low-salt diet
    - Parenteral therapy with glucose in water
  - Excessive losses
    - Gastrointestinal: vomiting, salivary, gastric, biliary, pancreatic drainage, diarrhea, resin therapy, tap water enemas (especially in megacolon)
    - Genitourinary
      - Intrinsic renal disease: chronic nephritis, acute tubular necrosis (recovery phase), nephrotic syndrome (diuresis)
      - Extrinsic influences: diuretics, acetazolamide, hypoadrenalism, central nervous system disease (rare), expanded volume (Pitressin, excessive water therapy)
    - Skin
      - Normal sweat
      - Abnormal sweat: cystic fibrosis, adrenal insufficiency
      - Burn therapy with silver nitrate (hypochloremia)
    - Cerebrospinal fluid
      - Draining myelomeningocele
      - Arachnoureterostomy
      - Continuous drainage of cerebrospinal fluid (e.g., in lead encephalopathy)
    - Parenteral: thoracentesis, paracentesis, burns
  - Redistribution
    - Severe malnutrition
    - Potassium deficiency
    - Trauma

sodium concentration of parenterally administered fluid often corrects the deficit. Measuring urine sodium concentration helps determine the cause of hyponatremia. Typically, with sodium depletion, urine sodium concentration is 10 mEq/L or less, although such low values are also found in nephrotic syndrome, congestive heart failure, or hepatic failure. Expansion of the extracellular fluid with water or renal tubular injury results in a higher urinary sodium concentration (around 50 mEq/L). The wrong treatment does not correct the defect and may be detrimental. For example, administering sodium to a patient with hyponatremia resulting from water excess, such as that seen with the chronic edema of heart failure, nephrotic syndrome, or cirrhosis, may result only in further expanding the extracellular fluid without correcting the serum sodium level.

Treatment of *symptomatic hyponatremia* consists of administering a hypertonic saline solution, calculated according to the formula in the preceding section on acidosis, with C representing serum sodium rather than bicarbonate. Because there is osmotic equilibrium between cells and extracellular water, changes in osmolality are distributed over total body water so that the value for f_d should be 0.6–0.7. A dose of 12 mL/kg of body weight of 3% sodium chloride solution (6 mEq sodium/kg) usually raises the serum sodium level by approximately 10 mEq/L. Correction of hyponatremia may be associated with myelinolysis in the central nervous system. Therefore, the initial rapid therapeutic increase in the serum sodium level should only be to a value of about 125 mEq/L. Subsequent elevation of the sodium concentration should be effected in small increments (5–10 mEq/L) over 1–4 hr. Hypernatremia should be avoided.

HYPERNATREMIA. This may result from faulty preparation of infant formulas: using condensed instead of evaporated milk or using heaped or packed instead of level measures of milk powder. These errors increase the solute load to be excreted by the kidney relative to the amount of water provided and may result in an osmotic diuresis and negative water balance. The accidental ingestion of excessive amounts of sodium chloride (*salt poisoning*) may also result in hypernatremia with serious residuals. The accidental substitution of salt for cane sugar in private homes and institutions occurs with sufficient frequency to justify the routine use of liquid sugars in infant feeding. The excessive intake of sodium is accompanied by increases in total body sodium and in the volume of extracellular water. Severe acidosis results from a shift of organic acids and free hydrogen ions to extracellular fluid. With shift of water from brain cells distention of cerebral vessels occurs, leading to subdural, subarachnoid, and intracerebral hemorrhage. The complications and residuals of salt poisoning are similar to, but may be more severe than, those seen with hypernatremic dehydration.

Hypernatremia is still associated with a high mortality rate, especially if the serum sodium concentration exceeds 158 mEq/L. Treatment is directed toward the rapid removal of excess sodium from the body. Intravenous fluids should consist of glucose in water, potassium acetate, and calcium, as needed. *Intermittent peritoneal dialysis* with glucose solutions can remove large quantities of sodium, correcting the hyperosmolality without the danger of pulmonary edema and heart failure. Approximately 45 mL/kg of a commercial dialysis solution containing 4.25% glucose can be injected intraperitoneally for severe hypernatremia (serum sodium concentration more than 200 mEq/L) and withdrawn 1 hr later. As the concentration of sodium in the serum falls, subsequent dialysis may be carried out using a solution with 1.5% glucose so as not to remove too much water and dehydrate the patient. Exchange transfusion is not a substitute for dialysis, because enormous quantities of blood would be required to effect a change in osmolality of total body water. Phenobarbital should be administered to prevent or control seizures. Digitalization may be necessary to counteract heart failure.

The treatment of hypernatremic dehydration is discussed in Sec. 6.18.

HYPOKALEMIA. Disturbances in the potassium concentration occurring without changes in volume of body fluids have been described in primary hyperaldosteronism and in Bartter syndrome. Large amounts of potassium are lost in the urine, resulting in low serum potassium and high serum bicarbonate concentrations. In congenital alkalosis of gastrointestinal origin, large amounts of potassium and chloride are lost in the stools. Using thiazide and loop diuretics (e.g., ethacrynic acid and furosemide) causes kaliuresis and natriuresis; prolonged use may result in significant potassium loss and hypokalemia.

Severe hypokalemia may result in weakness of skeletal muscles, decreased peristalsis, ileus, and an inability of the kidney to concentrate urine. Prolonged hypokalemia results in characteristic pathologic changes in the kidney and a decrease in function, which may persist even after potassium repletion.

Treatment consists of administration of large amounts of potassium (usually up to 3 mEq/kg/24 hr); in Bartter syndrome up to 10 mEq/kg may have to be given orally.

HYPERKALEMIA. Marked elevation of the serum potassium level results in ventricular fibrillation and death. Levels above 6.5 mEq/L should be treated promptly. The possibility of orally or parenterally administering excessive amounts of potassium should be considered and all potassium intake discontinued. The rapid intravenous administration of sodium bicarbonate (up to 2 mEq/kg over a 5- to 10-min period) or glucose and insulin (0.5 g of glucose/kg with 0.3 unit crystalline insulin/g of glucose, given over a 2-hr period) results in the intracellular movement of potassium and lowers the serum potassium level. Intravenous calcium gluconate (up to 0.5 mL of a 10% solution/kg given over 2–4 min) counters the cardiac toxicity of potassium, but the ECG should be monitored while it is being administered. None of these measures removes significant quantities of potassium from the patient; they are temporizing measures until negative potassium balance is established by the use of ion exchange resins (Kayexalate, 1 g/kg/24 hr, in divided oral doses twice daily or as a retention enema), by hemodialysis, or by peritoneal dialysis.

HYPOCALCEMIA AND HYPERCALCEMIA. These are discussed in Sec. 4.30, 6.27, 6.28, 9.54, and 19.17.

HYPOMAGNESEMIA. The importance of magnesium in intravenous therapy is reviewed in Sec. 6.7 and 6.29. The only definitive symptom complex associated with hypomagnesemia (serum magnesium level less than 1.3 mEq/L) is that of latent or manifest tetany. Convulsions, muscular twitching, disorientation, athetoid movements, carpopedal spasm, and hyper-reactivity to mechanical and auditory stimulation have been observed. Lowered serum concentrations and whole body deficits of magnesium are found in chronic diarrhea or vomiting, sprue, celiac disease, prolonged parenteral fluid therapy, and hyperaldosteronism. Low serum magnesium levels have been observed in infantile tetany, presumably on the basis of transient hypoparathyroidism. The intramuscular injection of 0.1 mL of a 24% solution of $MgSO_4 \cdot 7H_2O$ (0.2 mEq/kg) repeated every 6 hr for three or four doses produces symptomatic and biochemical improvement. Adding 3 mEq/L of magnesium to maintenance fluids for patients requiring long-term therapy may decrease the chance of serious deficiency (see Sec. 9.54).

HYPERMAGNESEMIA. Levels of serum magnesium higher than 10 mEq/L are accompanied by drowsiness and, occasionally, coma. Such levels rarely occur in the absence of renal failure. Deep tendon reflexes may also be abolished, and respiratory depression may occur at higher concentrations. Disturbances in atrioventricular and intraventricular conduction may be detected at levels of 5 mEq/L. Acute renal failure and Addison disease are accompanied by significantly elevated serum magnesium levels. Iatrogenic poisoning can result from using magnesium in treating hypertension or toxemia of pregnancy; deaths have been reported from using magnesium sulfate enemas in megacolon and from orally administering it for purging.

Intravenously administering calcium gluconate rapidly reverses the depressant effects of hypermagnesemia as well as the associated cardiac abnormalities.

PARENTERAL SOLUTIONS

Table 7–8 lists some solutions commercially available for use in fluid therapy. The many carbohydrate and electrolyte mixtures available permit great flexibility and individualization of therapy.

Ayus JC, Krothapali RK, Arieff A: Changing concepts in treatment of severe symptomatic hyponatremia. Am J Med 78:897, 1985.
Bezerra JA, Duncan B, Udall J: Dietary management of acute diarrhea: Fast or feed. Int Pediatr 5:30, 1990.
Darrow DC, Pratt EL: Fluid therapy: Relation to tissue composition and expenditure of water and electrolyte. JAMA 154:365, 1950.
Feliciano DV, Telander RL: Total parenteral nutrition in infants and children. Mayo Clin Proc 51:647, 1976.
Fomon SJ (ed): Infant Nutrition, 2nd ed. Philadelphia, WB Saunders, 1974.
Ichikawa I (ed): Pediatric Textbook of Fluids and Electrolytes. Baltimore, Williams & Wilkins, 1990.
Levine MM, Pizarro D: Advances in therapy of diarrheal dehydration: Oral rehydration. Adv Pediatr 31:207, 1984.
Lipschitz CH, Carrazza F: Effect of formula carbohydrate concentration on tolerance and macronutrient absorption in infants with severe chronic diarrhea. J Pediatr 117:378, 1990.
MacKenzie A, Barnes G, Shann F: Clinical signs of dehydration in children. Lancet 2:605, 1989.
Nalin DR, Levine MM, Mata L, et al: Oral rehydration and maintenance of children with rotavirus and bacterial diarrheas. Bull WHO 57:453, 1979.
Pizarro D, Posada G, Sandi L, et al: Rice-based oral electrolyte solutions for the management of infantile diarrhea. N Engl J Med 324:517, 1991.
Segar WE: Parenteral Fluid Therapy. Current Problems in Pediatrics. Chicago, Year Book Medical Publishers, 1972.
Snyder JD: Use and misuse of oral therapy for diarrhea: Comparison of US practices with American Academy of Pediatrics recommendations. Pediatrics 87:28, 1991.
Weil WB: A unified guide to parenteral fluid therapy. J Pediatr 75:1, 1969.
WHO Treatment and prevention of dehydration in diarrheal diseases. Guide for use of primary health care personnel. Scientific Publication No. 336, 1977.
Wu PYK (ed): Fluid balance in the newborn infant. Clin Perinatol 9:645, 1982.

6.27 TETANY

TETANY. Tetany, the state of hyperexcitability of the central and peripheral nervous systems, results from abnormal concentrations of ions in the fluid bathing nerve cells. These abnormalities may be decreases of H^+ (alkalosis), of Ca^{2+}, or of Mg^{2+}. Decrease of H^+ may precipitate tetany when concentrations of Ca^{2+} or Mg^{2+} may otherwise lie above the threshold for manifest tetany. A decrease of K^+ can prevent tetany despite low Ca^{2+} concentrations, but a rising K^+ can precipitate tetany in a patient with low Ca^{2+}. Hypomagnesemic tetany, on the other hand, can occur despite reduction of K^+ concentration. Thus, a range of ionic concentrations exists at which tetany can be either latent or manifest.

The serum calcium level, as usually measured, includes both ionized calcium (Ca^{2+}) and undissociated calcium proteinate; albumin is the chief serum protein to form a complex with calcium. Ca^{2+} can be measured, but the procedure is unavailable in most clinical laboratories. At normal concentrations of serum albumin about 40–50% of the total calcium is ionized—that is, 4.0–5.2 mg/dL. When the serum albumin level is reduced, total serum calcium is decreased without a decrease in CA^{2+}; a rule of thumb states that with each decrease of 1 g/dL of albumin, a decrease of 0.8 mg/dL of calcium results. A nephrotic child with a serum albumin level of 1 g/dL might, therefore, be expected to have a total serum calcium concentration of 7.5–8.0 mg/dL without reduction of Ca^{2+}.

At physiologic concentrations of H^+ and K^+, tetany may develop at Ca^{2+} concentrations of less than 3.0 mg/dL and is almost always manifest at Ca^{2+} concentrations less than 2.5 mg/dL. At normal concentrations of serum albumin, these levels correspond to total serum calcium concentrations of approximately 7 mg/dL and 5 mg/dL, respectively.

The normal level of magnesium in serum ranges from 1.6 to 2.6 mg/dL, of which about 75% is Mg^{2+}. Total serum magnesium reduced to less than 1.0 mg/dL may be associated with hyperexcitability of the nervous system.

MANIFEST TETANY. The classic signs of peripheral hyperexcitability of motor nerves are spasms of the muscles of the wrists and ankles (carpopedal spasm) and of the vocal cords (laryngospasm). In *carpopedal spasm* the wrists are flexed, the fingers extended, the thumbs adducted over the palms, and the feet extended and adducted. These muscular spasms can be quite painful. *Laryngospasm* causes inspiratory obstruction accompanied by a high-pitched inspiratory crow; apnea may result. The sensory manifestations are paresthesias, particularly numbness and tingling of the hands and feet. Motor excitability of the central nervous system may be manifested by often brief but recurrent convulsions, which are usually generalized but may be localized to one side of the body. Between seizures the patient may be apparently conscious, but after a prolonged series of convulsions a postictal state may result. In young infants convulsions are frequently the only evidence of the nervous system's hyperexcitability.

LATENT TETANY. This is the condition in which ischemia or mechanical or electrical stimulation of motor nerves is required to produce the motor response characteristic of tetany. Carpopedal spasm may be induced in latent tetany through the production of ischemia of the motor nerves by reducing the arterial blood supply with a tourniquet *(Trousseau sign)*; a blood pressure cuff on the arm is inflated above the systolic blood pressure for 3 min. Motor nerve impulses can be elicited by mechanical tapping, but under normal physiologic conditions this is not possible. The facial nerve can be stimulated by tapping anterior to the external auditory meatus. Contraction of the orbicularis oris occurs with a twitch of the upper lip or entire mouth *(Chvostek sign)*. The peroneal nerve can be stimulated by tapping the place where it passes over the head of the fibula; a positive *peroneal sign* is dorsiflexion and abduction of the foot.

The motor nerves can also be stimulated electrically. *Erb sign* is a positive response of motor nerves to electrical stimulation by galvanic currents of amperage less than that required for their stimulation under normal physiologic conditions.

Another manifestation of reduced Ca^{2+} concentrations is a prolonged Q-T interval for a given heart rate on the electrocardiogram.

ALKALOTIC TETANY. This is very rare in infants and young children. Tetany can be induced through spontaneous overventilation, producing respiratory alkalosis; such hyperventilation is most often of psychogenic origin. The treatment of alkalotic tetany resulting from spontaneous hyperventilation is to have the patient rebreathe into a bag or balloon to increase P_{CO_2}. In patients with low Ca^{2+} concentrations tetany may be precipitated by overventilation or by a metabolic alkalosis following administration of sodium bicarbonate, but the metabolic alkalosis resulting from loss of gastric juice caused by pyloric obstruction is rarely associated with tetany. Alkalotic tetany has occurred in patients with renal disease who have been protected by concurrent metabolic acidosis from the consequences of low Ca^{2+} concentration; correcting the acidosis has caused tetany and convulsions.

6.28 HYPOCALCEMIC TETANY

DISORDERS OF PARATHYROID FUNCTION. The most common disorder of parathyroid function is transient physiologic hypoparathyroidism of the newborn infant, sometimes referred to as *neonatal hypocalcemia*. Clinically, these infants can be separated into two groups, one group with hypocalcemia during the first 36 hr of life, usually before achieving a significant oral intake of milk, and a second group with hypocalcemia resulting from high phosphate load, which develops only after receiving cow's milk for a number of days. The onset of symptoms in the second group occurs most commonly during the 1st 5–10 days of life; clinical manifestations have occasionally appeared as late as 6 wk of age. Both forms presumably result from physiologically inactive parathyroid glands that fail to respond normally to low Ca^{2+} concentrations. Serum calcium values correlate directly with gestational age, and less mature infants have a greater chance of developing hypocalcemia.

In addition to a relative lack of parathyroid hormone output in the newborn period, a partial refractoriness of the target cells to parathyroid hormone may exist. Moreover, excessive secretion of thyrocalcitonin may be a major contributing factor in persistent hypocalcemia of premature infants, particularly those stressed by anoxia. The low-birthweight infant whose mother has had an inadequate intake of vitamin D and little exposure to sunshine also has a low plasma concentration of 25-hydroxy vitamin D_3, the deficiency of which is associated with relative refractoriness to parathyroid hormone.

The relative hypoparathyroidism of the newborn has been attributed to the increased serum calcium level of the fetus, which reflects a calcium gradient across the placenta. In addition, this inhibition of the fetal parathyroids by calcium ion may be augmented by mild maternal hyperparathyroidism. Physiologic hyperparathyroidism, indicated by increased parathyroid hormone levels found during pregnancy, may occur more intensely in diabetic women. Occasional cases of infant transient hypoparathyroidism have been associated with maternal clinical hyperparathyroidism.

Early Hypocalcemia. The infants at greatest risk are low-birthweight infants, especially those with intrauterine growth retardation, infants born of diabetic mothers, and infants who have been subjected to prolonged, difficult deliveries (see Sec. 9.54). Calcium intake may also be decreased because of the infant's small size or illness, and endogenous phosphate may be increased from catabolism. The incidence of hypocalcemia in prematurely born infants is extremely high, particularly in those with respiratory distress and those who have received intravenous sodium bicarbonate. Evaluating the role of hypocalcemia in the morbidity and mortality of such infants is difficult. Although hypocalcemia should be suspected as a possible cause of convulsions, it can be diagnosed only by determining serum calcium concentrations.

Asymptomatic hypocalcemia of premature infants usually resolves spontaneously. However, when possible, oral calcium gluconate should be given, because it usually obviates the subsequent need for intravenous therapy and its attendant complications.

Treatment requires the intravenous injection of 10% calcium gluconate in a dose of about 2 mL/kg (18 mg Ca/kg), which must be given slowly, while monitoring the cardiac rate for bradycardia; blood containing excessive calcium concentration that reaches the right auricle may inhibit the rhythmic electrical activity of the sinus node, causing cardiac arrest. Tissue necrosis and calcification may occur if this solution extravasates or is given intramuscularly. The intravenous dose of calcium gluconate can be repeated at 6- to 8-hr intervals until calcium homeostasis becomes stable, or the calcium gluconate (75 mg elemental Ca/kg/24 hr) can be added to a constant intravenous infusion. Administering either 1,25-dihydroxy vitamin D_3 or 25-hydroxy vitamin D_3 in the 1st day of life to prematurely born infants at risk for hypocalcemia has successfully prevented or reduced the severity and duration of hypocalcemia, but neither is recommended for routine prevention. If hypomagnesemia is present, it usually requires treatment before hypocalcemia responds to therapy. Calcium gluconate or calcium lactate also may be added to the feeding (see later) at the same time. There may be a gradual return to normal calcium levels after 1–3 days. Oral calcium should be continued for about 1 wk.

Late Hypocalcemia. Following the feeding of high phosphate milk, tetany can occur in both full-term and prematurely born infants and in infants whose clinical histories have been benign. The intake of a high-phosphate food (cow's milk) in relatively large volume leads to an elevated serum phosphate level because of relatively high tubular reabsorption of phosphate and the physiologically low GFR of the newborn. The elevated serum phosphate level depresses the serum calcium level through deposition of calcium phosphate in bone, and possibly in other tissues. The normal physiologic response would be an increased output of parathyroid hormone, which would increase both the solubilization of bone mineral and urine phosphate. This would restore the normal serum levels of both calcium and phosphate. If the infant's parathyroid glands are not yet able to respond with such an increase of parathyroid hormone, the level of serum calcium progressively falls and symptomatic hypocalcemia may result.

Clinical Manifestations. The most important presentation of hypocalcemia in infants is convulsions; carpopedal spasm is not usually seen and, because the Chvostek sign is common in newborn infants, it cannot be interpreted as a sign of tetany. Laryngospasm with cyanosis and apneic episodes may occur. Irritability, muscular twitchings, jitteriness, and tremors are frequent clinical manifestations in the newborn. In addition to the characteristic signs from increased excitability of the nervous system, the nonspecific symptoms clinically suggestive of sepsis may also occur, such as poor feeding, vomiting, and lethargy rather than irritability. Serum calcium determinations and other diagnostic studies should be made in infants suspected of having sepsis. Bradycardia with heart block is rarely noted. A prolonged Q-T interval on the electrocardiogram suggests hypocalcemia. A serum calcium concentration below 7 mg/dL establishes the diagnosis; one below 7.5 mg/dL is suggestive. The serum phosphate level is increased, sometimes to 10–12 mg/dL. The blood urea nitrogen level is not elevated, distinguishing this condition from the hyperphosphatemia of severe renal dysfunction. Normal newborns fed cow's milk have serum phosphate concentrations of 6–8 mg/dL; normal premature infants may have concentrations even higher. Hypomagnesemia may also be present.

A favorable response to administering calcium is insufficient in itself to make the diagnosis, because calcium may act nonspecifically during seizures. Furthermore, symptoms such as irritability and tremors may subside spontaneously, and convulsions resulting from cerebral edema, anoxia, or injury may not be repeated during the neonatal period. Examination of the spinal fluid is indicated because of the possibility of a convulsion caused by infection or hemorrhage in the central nervous system.

Treatment. Initial treatment of the convulsing infant is intravenous injection of 10% calcium gluconate, 2 mL/kg, with the precautions given previously. The response may be dramatic. After this, specific treatment aims at reducing the serum phosphate level in late hypocalcemia. Because human milk is low in phosphorus, breast-fed infants rarely, if ever, develop hypocalcemia. "Humanized" infant foods prepared from dialyzed whey of cow's milk are considerably higher in phosphate than is human milk. Phosphate absorption from food can be suppressed, however, by adding to the formula a great excess of calcium, which precipitates as calcium phosphate in the lumen of the gut (e.g., adding calcium lactate or gluconate to the milk feeding to achieve a calcium to phosphorus ratio of 4:1). Calcium lactate powder is preferred, and its addition to milk produces no significant gastrointestinal disturbances. Because calcium lactate is 13% calcium, 770 mg of this salt provides 100 mg of calcium; calcium gluconate is 9% calcium, so that 1,100 mg of it provides 100 mg of calcium. A soluble preparation of calcium gluconate (syrup of Neo-Calglucon), containing 92 mg Ca/tsp, is a less desirable method of adding calcium, because the required amounts have caused diarrhea. Calcium chloride may cause gastric irritation and hyperchloremic acidosis. Because the salt must dissolve in the milk, calcium lactate tablets should not be used, because compressed tablets are insoluble even if fragmented. A sample calculation follows.

An infant taking a volume of prepared infant feeding estimated to contain 300 mg of P and 450 mg of Ca can achieve a 4:1 ratio of Ca to P by adding 750 mg of calcium, for a total calcium intake of 1,200 mg. This requires the addition of 6 g of calcium lactate powder to the total feeding, or 1 g/feeding given every 4 hr.

As treatment decreases the serum phosphorus level, the serum calcium level returns to normal, possibly even rising to hypercalcemic levels. At this point, the calcium supplement is reduced in steps, not stopped abruptly, because the serum phosphorus level may rise precipitously and the calcium concentration fall again to tetanic levels. In most infants restoration of normal calcium homeostasis and presumably normal parathyroid responsiveness occurs in 1–2 wk.

Occasionally, a more prolonged calcium supplementation period is needed, in which case the treatment must be individualized by serial measurements of calcium and phosphate concentrations. If the infant responds poorly to treatment, the calculations should be checked to determine if sufficient calcium is being added, and the feeding should be examined to see if the calcium lactate or gluconate has been dissolving completely. If no errors are found and the therapeutic response is inadequate, the diagnosis of congenital hypoparathyroidism should be entertained or, in older infants, vitamin D deficiency or an absorptive or metabolic abnormality of vitamin D.

The *prognosis* of early hypocalcemia with seizures depends on the primary disease; infants with late tetany have an excellent prognosis.

CONGENITAL ABSENCE OF THE PARATHYROIDS. This can occur in association with aplasia of the thymus *(DiGeorge syndrome)*, in combination with abnormalities of the great vessels of the heart, or as an isolated parathyroid aplasia (Sec. 19.17). Such patients present the same symptoms as those in infants with transient physiologic hypoparathyroidism but respond incompletely to the simple treatment outlined previously and have relapsing hypocalcemia, which requires more definitive treatment. In total parathyroid deficiency, substituting pharmacologic amounts of vitamin D, vitamin D metabolites, or vitamin D analogs for parathyroid hormone is required. Dihydrotachysterol is preferable; at pharmacologic doses, it is more potent than vitamin D in correcting hypocalcemia. Because it is also more rapidly inactivated in the body, it is not stored as is vitamin D and is not as cumulatively toxic. In the young infant 0.05–0.1 mg of dihydrotachysterol should be given daily and the dose adjusted by determining serum calcium concentrations, which should be returned to levels of about 9–10 mg/dL. The highly active vitamin D metabolite, 1,25-dihydroxy vitamin D_3, is now available and in doses of 0.25–0.5 μg/24 hr is effective in treating hypoparathyroidism. As the child grows, the dosage of either steroid must be increased, as indicated by serum calcium concentrations. Hypoparathyroidism in older children is discussed in Sec. 19.16.

HYPOCALCEMIA AND TETANY CAUSED BY VITAMIN D DEFICIENCY OR ABNORMALITIES OF VITAMIN D METABOLISM. The onset of vitamin D deficiency tetany usually occurs at 3–6 mo of age, because depletion of the infant's vitamin D stores requires this amount of time. However, an infant born of a vitamin D–deficient mother may develop hypocalcemia from vitamin D deficiency within the first week of life. Tetany and nutritional vitamin D deficiency are now rare, but the latter occasionally develops in a breast-fed infant whose mother, unaware of human milk's vitamin D deficiency, does not provide supplementary vitamin D (see Sec. 4.30).

Hypocalcemia may also be a result of failure of normal metabolism of vitamin D, which undergoes two hydroxylation steps, first in the liver and second in the kidney, before becoming the metabolically active 1,25-dehydroxy vitamin D_3. Infants with liver disease, such as neonatal hepatitis, cytomegalic inclusion disease, or atresia of the bile ducts, may show manifestations of vitamin D deficiency with hypocalcemia because of failure of the liver to metabolize vitamin D. In atresia of the bile ducts, malabsorption of vitamin D may complicate the problem. In the genetic defect of vitamin D metabolism called vitamin D–dependent (pseudodeficient) rickets, the probable failure of the 1-hydroxylation step in the kidney affects infants who may also present with hypocalcemia. Vitamin D deficiency can also result from steatorrhea caused by pancreatic lipase deficiency or by intrinsic intestinal mucosal disorders. In addition, rickets and osteomalacia are associated with the treatment of convulsive disorders by large doses of combined anticonvulsant drugs, principally phenobarbital, diphenylhydantoin, and primidone, which alter the liver's metabolism of vitamin D. Diphenylhydantoin also inhibits intestinal transport of calcium, and patients may present with hypocalcemia as well as skeletal changes (see Sec. 24.63).

Initially, patients with tetany resulting from vitamin D deficiency or failure of normal metabolism of vitamin D can be symptomatically relieved by intravenous injection of 10 mL of 10% calcium gluconate, with the usual precautionary monitoring of heart rate to prevent a too rapid injection. The definitive treatment is a highly concentrated vitamin D preparation, which should be given in amounts adequate to achieve a rapid physiologic effect (e.g., vitamin D, 600,000 units, in a single dose) or divided into several doses over a 24-hr period. The common solution of vitamin D in propylene glycol (Drisdol), 10,000 units/g, is unsuitable for this type of therapy, because the large volume of propylene glycol is depressant. An alternative therapy is 10,000 units of vitamin D daily for 3 wk. These large doses of vitamin D given orally are effective in true vitamin D deficiency. If there is impaired vitamin D absorption or a defect in the metabolism of vitamin D, larger doses may be required. The active vitamin D metabolites, 25-hydroxy vitamin D_3 and 1,25-dihydroxy vitamin D_3, are available for treatment. The hypocalcemia of hepatic disorders or of vitamin D–dependent rickets responds to large doses of vitamin D, but more precise treatment with 25-hydroxy vitamin D_3 or 1,25-dihydroxy vitamin D_3 is possible. Treatment must be individualized and patients closely monitored to avoid vitamin D intoxication (see also Sec. 4.31).

6.29 HYPOMAGNESEMIC TETANY

Hypomagnesemia has reportedly caused tetany associated with either low or normal serum calcium concentrations. In transient physiologic hypoparathyroidism of the newborn, low serum magnesium concentrations may accompany the hyperphosphatemia and hypocalcemia. This hypomagnesemia usually responds to treatment directed at reducing the serum phosphate concentration. Occasionally, newborn infants with hypomagnesemia require specific magnesium therapy, which can be injected intramuscularly with 0.2 mL/kg of a 50% solution of $MgSO_4 \cdot 7H_2O$ (25% solution of $MgSO_4$). This treatment raises serum Mg concentrations into the normal range within an hour and should maintain adequate concentrations for several hours. Often, no further therapy is needed. The mechanism of this transient hypomagnesemia is not understood. Hypomagnesemic tetany and convulsions seen beyond the newborn period may result from congenital disorders of magnesium transport, causing either failure of absorption of dietary magnesium or failure of tubular reabsorption of magnesium with excessive urinary loss. In Bartter syndrome, hypomagnesemia, hypokalemia, and tetany can occur secondary to a renal tubular dysfunction. Intestinal malabsorption of magnesium also results from acquired intestinal injury such as inflammatory bowel disease or resection of small intestine. Renal loss of magnesium may be secondary to nephropathy caused by aminoglycosides or *cis*-platinum. Magnesium depletion, whatever the pathogenesis, can be associated with hypocalcemia, because magnesium is needed for both secretion of parathyroid hormone and responsiveness of target tissues to the hormone. Treatment requires magnesium administered either intramuscularly (see earlier), intravenously, 2–10 mL/kg of 1% magnesium sulfate solution by slow infusion, or orally in the form of magnesium salts, such as the chloride or gluconate (see also Sec. 6.7).

ALAN M. ROBSON

Bakwin H: Tetany in newborn infants. Am J Dis Child 54:1211, 1937.

Booth BE, Johanson A: Hypomagnesemia due to renal tubular defect in reabsorption of magnesium. J Pediatr 84:350, 1974.

Broner CW, Stidham GL, Westenkirchner DF, et al: A prospective, randomized, double blind comparison of calcium chloride and calcium gluconate therapies for hypocalcemia in critically ill children. J Pediatr 117:986, 1990.

Brown DR, Steranka BH, Taylor FH: Treatment of early-onset neonatal hypocalcemia. Am J Dis Child 135:24, 1981.

Callenbach JC, Sheehan MB, Anderson SJ, et al: Etiologic factors in rickets of very low-birth-weight infants. J Pediatr 98:800, 1981.

Changaris DG, Purohit DM, Balentine JD, et al: Brain calcification in severely stressed neonates receiving parenteral calcium. J Pediatr 104:941, 1984.

Colletti RP, Pan MW, Smith EWP, et al: Detection of hypocalcemia in susceptible neonates. The Q-oTc interval. N Engl J Med 290:931, 1974.

Gardner LI: Tetany and parathyroid hyperplasia in the newborn infant. Influence of dietary phosphate load. Pediatrics 9:534, 1962.

Harrison HE, Harrison HC: Disorders of Calcium and Phosphate Metabolism in Childhood and Adolescence. Philadelphia, WB Saunders, 1979.

Harrison HE, Lifshitz F, Blizzard RM: Comparison between crystalline dihydrotachysterol and calciferol in patients requiring pharmacologic vitamin D therapy. N Engl J Med 276:894, 1967.

Paunier L, Radde IC, Kooh SW, et al: Primary hypomagnesemia with secondary hypocalcemia in an infant. Pediatrics 41:385, 1968.

Richens A, Rowe DJF: Disturbance of calcium metabolism by anticonvulsant drugs. Br Med J 4:73, 1970.

Tsang RC, Light IJ, Sutherland JM, et al: Possible pathogenetic factors in neonatal hypocalcemia of prematurity. J Pediatr 82:423, 1973.

6.30 FAILURE TO THRIVE

Failure to thrive identifies infants and children who, without superficially evident cause, fail to gain weight and often lose weight. This problem occurs most often in infants but also is observed later in childhood. It can occur commonly among institutionalized children, especially those who are mentally retarded.

ETIOLOGY. Failure to thrive usually results from psychosocial circumstances, not always immediately apparent, that adversely affect the child's intake, absorption, or utilization of food. Emotional deprivation and neglect or abuse (Sec. 3.51), including the withholding of food, are commonly associated with this condition. An increased incidence of failure to thrive, accompanied by malabsorption, has been reported among children with autism and adults who later develop schizophrenia. Sometimes the physical or emotional deprivation of the child is related to a physical handicap, such as cerebral palsy or cleft palate, or to difficult behavior resulting from temperament or hyperactivity. The syndrome may also result from rare organic abnormalities as well as from easily discoverable diseases in which growth failure occurs. For many children who experience a period of failure to thrive with no ascertainable organic or environmental cause, retrospective analysis indicates the likelihood of psychosocial origin. Table 6–19 lists some of the psychosocial and organic conditions associated with failure to thrive.

CLINICAL MANIFESTATIONS. Failure to gain weight or to grow at the expected rate may be the only sign. More characteristically, this is accompanied by signs of developmental retardation and of physical and emotional deprivation, such as apathy, poor hygiene, intense eye contact with people, and withdrawing behavior, and disorders of oral intake, which may be manifested as anorexia, voracious appetite, or pica. Vomiting, regurgitation, diarrhea, and general neuromuscular spasticity or hypotonia may be concurrent.

DIAGNOSIS AND DIFFERENTIAL DIAGNOSIS. The diagnosis of failure to thrive is complex, because of the many factors that affect a child's growth. History may provide clarification of whether inadequate intake, increased losses from vomiting or diarrhea, or disturbed food utilization is the mechanism leading to the growth failure. Frequently, the mechanism is unclear, but information gathered from other observers and through repeated interviews may reveal unsuspected adverse factors in the child's environment.

Constructing and studying both a growth chart and a developmental flow sheet may identify when the child began failing to thrive and may help uncover the environmental or physical factors responsible (Sec. 3.10). If growth parallels the normal growth pattern but is below the expected level (e.g., usually below the 5th percentile), constitutional short stature, and endocrine, genetic, and other systemic disorders should be considered. A physical examination that reveals no abnormality except for growth and development is usually compatible with an environmental cause, although some organic etiologies may show no gross physical findings.

Hospitalizing the child provides an opportunity for quantitating factors governing the net caloric intake (food intake, vomiting, stools) and for observing the child's interactions—especially during feeding and play—with parents, health personnel, and other children. Hospitalization frequently leads to dramatic improvement in weight gain and in social responses and thus provides evidence that environmental

TABLE 6–19. Some Causes of Failure to Thrive and Screening Tests

Cause	Screening Tests
Environmental and psychosocial	
Inadequate caloric intake	History; observation in hospital
Emotional deprivation and disruptions	History; observation in hospital
Rumination; chronic diarrhea, gastroesophageal reflux	History; observation in hospital
Anorexia nervosa and bulimia	History; examination
Secondary to impact of organic disease	History and observation
Organic	
Central nervous system abnormalities, infection	Neurodevelopmental assessment; transillumination of skull; brain scan
Gastrointestinal system	
Malabsorption, cystic fibrosis, inflammatory bowel disease, parasites, aganglionic megacolon; liver disease; gastroesophageal reflux	Examination of stools: stool fat, sweat test, stool ova and parasites; liver function tests; barium swallow, sedimentation rate
Partial cleft palate	Physical examination; observation of feeding
Chronic heart failure	Physical examination; chest roentgenography; echocardiography
Endocrine disorders	Growth chart; thyroid function; blood tests; bone age
Pulmonary disease	
Bronchopulmonary dysplasia; bronchiectasis	Physical examination; chest roentgenography; tuberculin test, pulmonary function tests
Renal disease	Urinalysis; blood urea nitrogen; ultrasound; urinary amino acid screen; urine pH
Anomalies; infection; renal failure; renal tubular disorder	
Chromosomal disorders	Chromosomal analysis; identification of peculiar facies or multisystem defects
Turner syndrome	
Other metabolic or inborn errors	Urine amino acid screen
Chronic infection	Tuberculin test; appropriate laboratory identification of infectious agent
Tuberculosis, mycotic, congenital	
Chronic inflammation	Physical examination; sedimentation rate
Juvenile rheumatoid arthritis	
Immunodeficiency disease	History of rash and diarrhea; thymus size; tonsil size; skin tests; complete blood count
DiGeorge syndrome; combined immunodeficiency	
AIDS or AIDS-related complex	HIV test
Malignancies (kidney, adrenal, brain)	Roentgenography of abdomen, chest; ultrasonography; brain scan
Congenital syndromes caused by alcohol, Dilantin, drugs, infection	Physical examination

factors are causative, eliminating the need for searching further for underlying organic disease.

If the history or physical examination suggests disturbance in any organ system, appropriate diagnostic study is warranted, beginning with screening tests (e.g., routine blood count, sweat test, and urinalysis) and proceeding further only if these are positive. Extensive study to rule out underlying organic lesions is justified only if the initial data base has failed to provide clues pointing to a specific environmental or organic etiology; failure of a favorable response to hospitalization should also be demonstrated.

Children chronically deprived of food may have stools consistent with malabsorption when an adequate dietary intake is initiated. They gain weight, however, and resume a normal stool pattern after some weeks or months.

PREVENTION. Failure to thrive arising from psychosocial factors is exceedingly difficult to prevent, because it frequently results from complex social or familial disruptions and intense stress. Preventive counseling involves the identification of families with a new infant having significant current life stresses, of problems during the pregnancy and perinatal period, and of poor relationships between parent and infant in the postnatal period. The family relationships may be characterized by violence and hostility, and members may have limited support systems. The involvement of a supporting network of community volunteers may facilitate the growth of parental capability and self-esteem.

TREATMENT. For necessary evaluation, a temporary change of environment, such as the hospital, may relieve transient tension among family members. Aggressive intervention with hospitalization is often vital to promote improved growth and development. When hospitalization is coupled with counseling and support from a physician, social worker, and family service agency, as appropriate, the family may be able to make adjustments needed to ensure adequate care of the child when he or she returns home. Temporary or permanent placement in a foster home may be necessary in some cases. Identified organic disease should be appropriately treated.

PROGNOSIS. It is difficult to generalize about the prognosis of nonorganic failure to thrive because of the many variables involved for each patient. Children involved in a significant crisis affecting the family over a limited period may eventually achieve adequate physical growth and development. However, studies have shown that some may later exhibit neurotic or antisocial traits, reading problems, and poor verbal development. In some patients, inadequate rate of growth and development continues for a protracted time. A number of children with failure to thrive are also abused, and some may even die under suspicious circumstances (see Sec. 3.52). The personality of the child, the degree of deprivation, and the nature of the environmental experiences are all important variables in the ultimate outcome of this disturbance.

GIULIO J. BARBERO

Barbero GJ, Shaheen E: Environmental failure to thrive: A clinical view. J Pediatr 59:73, 1967.
Berwick D, Levy J, Kleinerman R: Failure to thrive: Diagnostic yield of hospitalization. Arch Dis Child 57:347, 1982.
Drotar D (ed): New Directions in Failure to Thrive. New York, Plenum Press, 1984.
Drotar D, Eckeole D: The family environment in non-organic failure to thrive: A controlled study. J Pediatr Psychol 14:245, 1989.
Fryer GE: The efficacy of hospitalization of non-organic failure-to-thrive children: A meta-analysis. Child Abuse Negl 12:375, 1988.
Powell GF, Low JF, Speers MA: Behavior as a diagnostic aid in failure-to-thrive. Dev Behav Pediatr 8:18, 1987.

6.31 ACCIDENTAL INJURY AND EMERGENCY MEDICAL SERVICES FOR CHILDREN

Accidents are a major cause of morbidity and mortality in children. Of children 1–14 yr of age, accidents cause more deaths annually in the United States than the next six most prevalent causes combined, resulting in about four times more deaths than those from cancer, the second highest cause. In total, 8,500 children younger than 14 yr of age die and 100,000 suffer permanent disability each year as a result of accidental injury. One in five children requires care in an emergency room each year for an accidental injury. The emergency medical services (EMS) systems in this country that were developed to respond to the needs of accident victims, as well as to the needs of the victims of acute life-threatening illnesses, have until recently largely ignored the special needs of the pediatric patient. However, the advent of pediatric emergency medicine as a separate specialty within pediatrics has heightened awareness of the special emergency medical needs of infants, children, and adolescents. Accordingly, the concept of an EMS-C (Emergency Medical Services for Children) system, or a "system within a system" is evolving and, in many areas of the country, is being implemented.

ACCIDENTAL INJURY

EPIDEMIOLOGY. Most accidental injuries and deaths of children occur on the streets, at home, in school, and on the farm.

The Road. Motor vehicle accident (MVA) deaths are the leading cause of death for individuals 1–25 yr of age. MVA deaths among teenagers have a higher incidence in rural compared to urban communities. Persons under the age of 20 yr account for 10% of the drivers but 18% of the automobile fatalities. Teenagers drive 20% of their total driving hours after dark but experience 50% of their traffic fatalities during these hours. Alcohol is a factor in 50% of MVAs involving teenagers. One in 50 teenagers is injured in a car accident every year.

Infants are another particularly vulnerable group, having an alarming occupant death rate of 9.1/100,000/yr. The body of an 8-kg, 6-mo-old infant attains a force equivalent to almost 350 kg during a collision at 30 mph, the equivalent of a fall from a 3rd-story window. The lap-carried infant in the front seat is at great risk because he or she can be subjected to both a direct blow against the dashboard in front and a crush injury from the adult following behind. The adult usually survives.

Motorcycles, motor scooters, motorbikes, and mopeds are increasingly used for transportation because of their low initial cost and relative fuel economy, and many riders of these vehicles are adolescents. The number of motorcycles in the United States contributes disproportionately to the number of accidental deaths. In 1988 there were 75 fatalities/100,000 registered motorcycles, over three times the rate for other registered motor vehicles. The death rate for all motor vehicles was 2.46 deaths/100,000,000 mi, but 41 deaths/100,000,000 motorcycle mi. In 1988 motorcycles accounted for 3% of the registered motor vehicles and 7% of motor vehicle fatalities.

Bicycle accidents result in significant mortality (600 deaths in 1988 in the United States); they cause many injuries and are the most common cause of product-related injury. One in 80 children 6–12 yr old requires hospital care for a bicycle injury each year. Of pediatric patients hospitalized after bicycle accidents in one study, 67% had craniocerebral trauma, 18% had upper limb fractures, and 7% had lower limb fractures.

Most bicycle-related injuries to infants occur when they are carried as passengers. Their feet and legs can get caught in the wheel of the bicycle where spokes can cause a laceration and where the infant's extremity can be squeezed between the wheel and frame of the bicycle, resulting in crush and shearing injuries.

Most fatal bicycle accidents involve a motor vehicle, and the injury leading to death is usually craniocerebral trauma (80%). The type of accident causing the greatest proportion of deaths (24.6%) is the motor vehicle overtaking the bicyclist from the rear.

Children under 13 yr old account for 10% of bicycle traffic but 28% of bicycle injuries. One study showed that in 38% of accidents motorists received traffic citations, with failure to yield the right of way as the most common charge. Bicyclists were in violation of traffic laws in 70% of accidents; most of them were guilty of wrong-way riding (riding facing traffic), failure to yield the right of way, and turning violations. Young children may be unable to process their perceptions of road situations quickly enough to ride safely in traffic.

Pedestrian motor vehicle accidents involving children and young adults under the age of 24 yr account for nearly 60% of all pedestrian fatalities (over 3,000 in 1986). Most commonly injured is the 3- to 7-yr-old age group, followed by the 18- to 19-yr-old age group. As in most other types of accidents, boys outnumber girls. Four out of every 1,000 7 yr olds are struck by cars each year. Usually, children are unsupervised by adults at the time of the accident, and often dart out into the street. Frequently, prior to an accident, a child is hidden from the driver by parked cars, bushes, or other roadside objects.

Home. The home is frequently the site of fatal and nonfatal accidents, and children in the 2- to 3-yr-old age group are most commonly involved. Many types of accidents occur in the home, with the most common accidents involving falls down stairs and against low furniture or objects, such as coffee tables and fireplace hearths. One in 40 children 0–5 yr of age requires hospital care for a fall-related injury each year. The number of steps or height of the fall are generally of lesser importance than the surface impacted when determining the severity of injury. One in three infants using an infant walker suffers an accidental injury; 8,600 of these require hospital care, and 54% are secondary to falls down stairs. Nevertheless, 1,000,000 walkers are sold each year despite research indicating that they actually delay walking. Injuries caused by toys are also common, accounting for 131,000 emergency room visits in 1987.

One study found 13 significant child safety violations in the average household. The most common were stairway hazards, windows in poor repair, water temperature higher than 120° F, accessible medications, and crib slats more than 2⅜ in apart. See Sec. 6.36 and Sec. 6.37 for discussion of burns, drowning, and near-drowning, respectively.

School. Between the ages of 5 and 18 yr, children spend up to 20% of their waking hours in school. For children in the primary grades, physical education and unorganized activities have the highest accident rates. For older children, accidents most commonly occur in physical education activities, the school building in general, interscholastic sports, and shops and laboratories. Overall, injuries occur at a rate of 49 injuries/1,000 students—severe injuries, amputations, 3rd-degree burns, concussions, crush injuries, fractures, and multiple injuries occur at a rate of about 9 injuries/1,000 students. Adolescent males suffer 30% of all injuries.

Playground equipment is frequently the source of product-related injury. Approximately 118,000 children annually have accidents related to playground equipment, resulting in injuries severe enough to require an emergency room visit. Most of these injuries relate to falls from the equipment, and approximately 50% of these falls result in injuries to the head and neck. The surface over which the playground equipment is installed may be a critical factor; often this surface is concrete or asphalt rather than an energy-absorbing material, such as loose sand, wood chips, or foam mats. A fall from a height of 1 ft onto concrete or asphalt can create forces sufficient to cause death if the child lands directly on his or her head. A fall from 3 ft onto packed dirt can also lead to death. Falls onto energy-absorbing material, however, can be tolerated from a much greater height.

The older the children, the more likely they are to be injured in physical education activities. Although these injuries are usually relatively minor, they are frequent—almost 4 injuries/100 participants a year—and cause the loss of slightly more than 1 school day/injury.

The injury rate in interscholastic sports is higher in each succeeding school level. It is highest for boys in high school football (2.3 accidents/100,000 student days) and highest for girls in high school basketball (0.23 accident/100,000 student days). Wrestling, hockey, gymnastics, and skating also have high accidental injury rates. In one study, over 50% of high school hockey players experienced significant facial trauma. One in 14 teenagers requires hospital care for a sports-related injury each year, and two thirds of these injuries occur during practice rather than during competition. Over 10% of all sports injuries occur as a result of rule violations; 25% occur as a result of returning to competition after inadequate rehabilitation.

The Farm. Accidental farm injuries in children account for 300 deaths and over 20,000 significant injuries each year in the United States. Corn augers, tractors, power takeoff units, and gravity boxes are the most commonly involved types of farm equipment. A concentration of injuries during planting and harvest times suggests a relationship between periods of increased use of farm equipment and of decreased supervision of children.

PREVENTION. Studies about the causes and prevention of accidental injury have been hampered by the term "accident," which implies an event that is unpredictable and unavoidable. Research is beginning, however, to define effective strategies for the prevention of accidental injury in childhood. These can be categorized into "active" and "passive," depending on the level of ongoing participation of the child and/or parent in the process. For example, an active strategy for the prevention of drowning in a home swimming pool would be enrollment of child and parent in a water safety course when the child reaches 18 mo of age. A passive strategy would be a community ordinance requiring that pools be fenced *on all four sides,* with automatically locking gates. In the case of teenagers involved in MVAs, an active strategy would be requiring drivers' education courses in school and a passive strategy would be to raise the drinking age from 18 to 21 yr. Research has clearly demonstrated that passive strategies are more effective than active strategies in the prevention of childhood injuries. Table 6–20 lists common childhood injuries and strategies for their prevention.

Another area of accidental injury research that has yet to produce feasible preventive strategies is the effect of the child's psychosocial make-up on accidental injury risk. Surprisingly, although children with aggressive behavior characteristics have an increased incidence of accidental injury, the correlation is lower than might be suspected. On the other hand, social stress factors such as those listed in Table 6–21 appear to play a very significant role in accidental injury risk. Developmental factors have long been known to be significant in accidental injury risk. Research in this area indicates that the concept of the "accident-prone child," based on personality traits, is being replaced by the concept of "accident-prone periods" during childhood. Age, developmental stage, and social stress factors act in conjunction to create an ever-changing group of accident-prone children.

Finally, although accidental injury is the greatest risk to a child's health, one study revealed that only 4% of the time spent during an average pediatric office visit is devoted to anticipatory guidance in accidental injury prevention, but at least one study has shown that the most effective counselor is a family's personal physician.

6.32 EMERGENCY MEDICAL SERVICES FOR CHILDREN

When a child is injured or experiences a medical emergency, the resources available to deal with that problem are known as the Emergency Medical Services (EMS) system; the EMS components for children are known as the EMS-C system. Children account for 21 million emergency room visits annually, but the significant role of emergency care in the overall health and well-being of children is not fully appreciated. It is of even greater significance that more than 80% of pediatric mortality results from EMS-related conditions—conditions that activate hospital and prehospital emergency medical services.

The components of an EMS-C system are listed in Table 6–22. Through retrospective analysis, one study has documented the potential of such a system for preventing pediatric trauma mortality. Another study has documented improved survival of ill and injured children cared for within an optimally designed EMS-C system.

PREHOSPITAL CARE

EPIDEMIOLOGY. Although the pediatric population accounts for 30% of the total population, only 10% of ambulance EMS calls involve pediatric patients. Furthermore, only 8% of all pediatric calls are of a life-threatening nature, and less than 1% of all pediatric calls require emergency medical technicians (EMTs) to use their cardiopulmonary resuscitation (CPR) skills. Infants and adolescents constitute disproportionately high percentages of all pediatric EMS calls. Trauma accounts for 54% of all pediatric calls. The most frequently occurring medical conditions are seizures, respiratory distress, and ingestion of poisonous substances.

Few studies have evaluated the quality and effect of pediatric prehospital care on final outcome. Several studies have shown a dismal success rate for pediatric prehospital CPR. This lack of success, however, may be a function of the causes of pediatric prehospital cardiopulmonary arrest rather than of the skills of the resuscitators. Most causes of pediatric prehospital cardiopulmonary arrest (Table 6–23), such as sudden infant death syndrome and drowning, represent unwitnessed arrests—arrests for which bystander CPR is delayed several minutes or much longer. Success rates for these resuscitations would be expected to be low in comparison with adult cardiac arrests, which are more frequently witnessed.

Accordingly, the rates of success for prehospital pediatric CPR vary from 0 to 7%, compared to 20% for adult prehospital CPR. In three series no infant under 15 mo of age survived a prehospital arrest. In one series the effectiveness of basic life support (ventilation and compressions) was compared with that of advanced life support (intubation and drugs), and was found to be the same. Consequently, improved training of

TABLE 6–20. Accidental Injury Prevention Strategies

Mechanism and Age Affected (yr)	Active Strategies	Passive (One-Time) Strategies
Motor vehicle accident (MVAs)*	Lower driving speed;† lap or shoulder belt (parents must act as role models)	Use air bag, automatic seat belts; redesign automobiles and roadways
0–5 (40 lb)	Use properly installed infant safety seat†, ‡ or convertible safety seat†	
2–8 (30–60 lb)	Use booster seat, † child safety lock	
8–16		Ban sale of some all-terrain vehicles, regulate design and advertising of others
16 and up	Raise drinking age†§; use extended provisional driver's license with insurance incentives for compliance (example: invalid after 10 P.M.);† SADD: Students Against Drunk Driving program	
Pedestrian motor vehicle accidents	Wear clothing reflector; teach "left-right-left," road avoidance instruction beginning at age of 2 yr; walk facing traffic	Fence playground, install speed bumps, sidewalks; decrease number of intersections with right turn on red; change parallel parking to 20-degree angle parking; raise the legal driving age; use properly designed infant/child carriers
Bicycles, motorcycles, mopeds, snowmobiles	Wear helmet,† "reflectorized" clothing, protective clothing, bicycle safety education; avoid use of headphones while riding, ride with traffic	Ride proper-sized bicycle with good pedal brakes
Falls		
0–4	Use nonaccordion stairway gate, seat belt in shopping cart, carpeted stairway	Ban sales of infant walkers, remove low, sharp-edged furniture Install window guards above first floor‖
1–10	Modify playground surface and equipment	
11 and over	Restrict use of trampolines to organized gymnastics	
Skateboards	Wear helmets, knee/elbow padding, mouth guard	Pass laws restricting areas of use
Sports-related injuries	Encourage proper conditioning and rehabilitation, use of suitable equipment, competition commensurate with level of skill, aggressive enforcement of game rules	Eliminate field hazards
Firearms	Remove guns from homes with children; lock guns and ammunition in separate places; pass laws making adults responsible for accidents involving children†	Pass handgun control legislation; regulate design and sale of nonpowder firearms
Farm equipment	Include farm safety in rural school curriculum	Incorporate child safety features into farm equipment design; pass laws restricting children's participation in farm work
Burns		
0–5	Carry out fire prevention inspections, have fire escape plan ready; use caution with hot drinks and when preparing hot foods	Install smoke detectors;¶ use flame-resistant children's clothing; reduce home hot water temperature to ≤120° F; install floor furnace guards; require automatic sprinklers in new construction; put plastic covers on extension cord plugs; advocate greater restrictions on sale of firecrackers
Drowning**		
0–5	Promote water safety education; *never* leave infants or children alone in a bathtub; use a certified life preserver *only* as a flotation device	Restrict diving boards to *carefully* supervised pools;†† use fencing with automatic gates around pools on all four sides; install sonar pool alarms
15–21	Install tamper-proof pool covers; teach the dangers of hyperventilation before diving	
Poisoning	Advocate poison prevention education; install cabinet locks; use safety caps on medication bottles	Add bitter additives to potential poisons

*Driver's education is not listed because of equivocal results. Although providing clear benefits, these classes may indirectly increase teenaged MVAs by increasing the number of teenaged drivers.

†Laws, to the extent enforced, may effectively move these to passive strategies.

‡Decrease mortality by 90% and serious injury by 80%.

§Can decrease teenaged MVA deaths by 31%.

‖Laws requiring guards on apartment windows have been very effective.

¶Batteries must be checked regularly.

**Swimming instruction is not listed because it is not a viable strategy for children under 5 yr of age, but teaching water safety may be of benefit under 5 yr.

††Availability of insurance may be a mechanism for "enforcing" this strategy.

TABLE 6–21. Social Stress Factors Correlated with Accidental Injury Risk

Maternal factors
Single
Unemployed
Ill
Pregnant
Drug- and/or alcohol-dependent
Limited education
Life events
Death in the family or of a close friend
Birth of a sibling
Move to a new residence
Change in parental employment
Marriage of a parent

EMTs probably cannot improve the success rate of resuscitation of pediatric patients who have a prehospital arrest. Enhanced pediatric prehospital care for conditions other than cardiopulmonary arrest, however, could improve outcome. In a study of 100 consecutive pediatric trauma deaths, 19 of 53 patients judged to have been potentially salvageable were found to have had significantly deficient prehospital care.

ASSESSMENT AND MANAGEMENT. Because rapid transport to a hospital is critical. The focus of the EMT's work is on the vital physiologic functions of ventilation and circulation, with minimal regard for underlying diagnosis. Assessment of an adult's vital signs and cardiac rhythm (rhythm strip) are key to the EMT's evaluation of an adult patient's vital functions, but these parameters are less useful for pediatric patients. The rhythm strip is not of much use except in the arrest situation. Vital signs in children in the field are difficult to assess and vary greatly with the child's age, temperature, and anxiety level. Taking the blood pressure, in particular, requires special cuff sizes that are frequently unavailable. Furthermore, children maintain blood pressure in the face of considerable volume loss far better than adult patients, making this parameter even less useful when assessing circulation in children.

Table 6–24 describes the basic primary survey (rapid assessment of vital functions) of a child in the prehospital setting.

Airway. Airway assessment is similar to that of the adult—breath sounds provide the key. If an obstruction is indicated by wheezing, stridor, or diminished breath sounds, despite vigorous respiratory efforts, the basic decision the EMT must make is whether to use the hands-off or hands-on approach. Unlike the situation with an adult, which is almost always an

TABLE 6–22. Components of an Emergency Medical Services for Children (EMS-C) System

Parent education: It is the responsibility of primary care physicians to educate parents about when and how to access the EMS-C system. All parents should also know basic CPR, a subject easily incorporated into prenatal classes.

Office preparedness for pediatric emergencies: Minimal pediatric resuscitation equipment should be available in the office of every physician who evaluates children. Surveys of office preparedness for pediatric emergencies have been published along with equipment recommendations.

911: A community emergency communications system should be in place. Dispatchers should be trained to incorporate into their dispatch decision-making considerations such as level of the pediatric training of and the pediatric equipment carried by various rescue units. Distance to a pediatric regional center should be considered in choosing the mode of transportation to be dispatched to the scene.

EMT (emergency medical technician) training in pediatrics: EMTs need special training and periodic recertification in pediatric prehospital care. Their training should emphasize rapid assessment techniques, management of the pediatric airway, pediatric CPR, and maintenance of body temperature of small infants. (See section on Pediatric Prehospital Care.)

Rescue squad equipment for pediatric emergency care: Minimal essential equipment includes pediatric resuscitation masks, endotracheal tubes, suction catheters, and laryngoscope blades; drugs in pediatric concentrations; pediatric cervical collars and traction splints; pediatric blood pressure cuffs; and newborn resuscitation equipment, including bulb syringe and warming packs.

Pediatric medical supervision (control) of prehospital care personnel: Physicians providing radio guidance to EMTs in the field need to be both knowledgeable in pediatric emergency care and familiar with field conditions and the pediatric care capabilities of the region's EMTs. Regionally developed pediatric prehospital care protocols should guide physicians' orders to EMTs. Such protocols guarantee consistency and serve as a basis for training and quality assurance evaluation.

Early warning devices: Any child with a chronic medical condition should wear a Med-Alert bracelet, shoe tag, or similar device that will alert EMS personnel to the underlying medical condition.

Field triage: Local protocols need to define a mechanism for grading the severity of a pediatric emergency to determine the appropriate choice of receiving facility. The pediatric trauma score is an example of pediatric trauma grading system that may be useful for this purpose.

Categorization of receiving facilities: The pediatric emergency care capabilities of local and regional medical centers must be clearly defined. This enables EMTs and medical supervisors to choose an appropriate receiving facility on the basis of a field triage evaluation system. Local categorization of receiving facilities should be done in a manner that encourages development of an appropriate number of facilities within each category. In some regions this has taken the form of designating levels I and II pediatric trauma centers. In the Los Angeles area, for example, the concept of EDAPs (Emergency Departments Approved for Children) and PCCCs (Pediatric Critical Care Centers) has evolved to meet the need for categorization and definition of institutional capabilities.

Interhospital pediatric transport system: The American Academy of Pediatrics has developed guidelines for pediatric transport systems.

Transfer agreements: Any hospital that lacks comprehensive pediatric emergency care and critical care capabilities should have a transfer agreement with a level I pediatric center. This agreement should guarantee the prompt acceptance of any pediatric patient subject only to the availability of resources at the receiving hospital and the availability of an appropriate means of transport.

Data gathering/quality assurance/education: No system is complete without an objective means of evaluating the quality of care it provides to the region's children. Scoring systems are available to allow comparison of regional results to national standards. For example, the Modified Injury Severity Score is available to assess pediatric trauma care. Other scores have been developed for children requiring pediatric intensive care. The information generated from these data should be used to refine the system through education as well as other means that encourage compliance with the effective components of the system.

TABLE 6–23. Causes of Prehospital Pediatric Cardiopulmonary Arrests*

Cause	Cases	
	No/Total	%
SIDS	38/119	32
Drowning	26/119	22
Unknown	17/119	14
Respiratory	11/119	9
Chronic illness	10/119	8
Other	17/119	14

*From Eisenberg M, Bergner L, Hallstrom A: Epidemiology of cardiac arrest and resuscitation in children. Ann Emerg Med 12:672, 1983.

immediate hands-on approach, the child with airway obstruction is often best managed with minimal or no intervention. It is difficult for the EMT to become accustomed to this difference. When apnea, gasping, or cyanosis dictates the need for aggressive airway management, the skills needed are not difficult for most EMTs to carry out and are similar to those used on the adult patient. Manual airway opening maneuvers (e.g., jaw thrust, chin lift, suction) are more consistently effective on the pediatric patient. Oral airways are usually not needed and risk inducing gagging and vomiting if used indiscriminately. Airway devices used on adult patients, such as the esophageal obturator airway and needle cricothyroidotomy, should not be used in the field setting on pediatric patients. Endotracheal intubation of children is essential if prolonged positive-pressure ventilation (PPV) is anticipated, or if a route is needed for the administration of resuscitation drugs. EMTs can learn this procedure and maintain their skill with a high degree of proficiency.

Breathing. Breathing is assessed by the child's work of breathing, color and, to a lesser extent, respiratory rate. In the future, field use of pulse oximetry may aid considerably in making this assessment. Oxygen should be offered to any pediatric patient in distress, even if color appears adequate, because cyanosis is a later indicator of hypoxia in pediatric patients. If the oxygen mask causes agitation and increases work of breathing, however, it should be withheld. Apnea, gasping, and cyanosis, despite high-concentration oxygen therapy, are the indicators for supporting ventilation with PPV. This is initially performed with bag-valve-mask (BVM) ventilation, a key skill for the EMT to master. Performed properly, this can overcome airway obstruction, ventilate the apneic patient, partially correct the acidosis of the child in circulatory failure, and even lower increased intracranial pressure. The most common mistake is underventilation with the BVM because of the perception that the child's small lung volume predisposes to a high risk of pneumothorax during PPV; as a result, too little volume is delivered. Training EMTs to gauge their success at BVM by constantly monitoring chest rise can overcome this frequent error.

Circulation. Circulation is assessed by the strength of peripheral pulses, temperature and color of the extremities and, less importantly, by heart rate and blood pressure. Accurate assessment of circulation in a child lying by the side of the road in a cold, dark environment is extremely difficult and frequently inaccurate. Rapid transport takes priority in this situation.

Although establishment of an IV line prior to transport is commonly regarded as an essential step in advanced life support, its advisability has been challenged by many pediatric emergency medicine specialists. Two studies have shown that establishing IV access requires 8 min in a pediatric patient in the field. In urban settings this is usually longer than transport time to the receiving hospital. Although success rates as high as 66% have been reported, these decline with decreasing age to less than 30% for infants under 1 yr old. In the arrest situation, IV access attempts are successful less than 50% of the time and are almost never successful in children younger than 6 yr. Another argument against establishing IV access in the pediatric patient in arrest is that, unlike the adult patient, the most important drugs to be administered in this situation can all be delivered through the endotracheal tube. Finally, pediatric pneumatic antishock garments (PASG) have been developed for children in shock and, although their efficacy remains to be proven, they may be an alternative to IV therapy in the field.

Another method for obtaining circulatory access in the prehospital setting is the placement of an intraosseous needle (Fig. 6–11). Used selectively, this technique may overcome the problems of delay and high failure rate associated with placing an IV line.

Disability. Disability in regard to central nervous system (CNS) function is assessed using the Modified Glasgow Coma Scale (MGCS), pupillary responses, and fontanel tension. The MGCS (Table 6–25) is a quantification of a child's responses to verbal and painful stimuli. The actual determination of a number using the MGCS is less important (and often unrealistic in the field setting) than making and recording observations of the child's responses to specific verbal and painful stimuli.

LOAD-AND-GO VERSUS STABILIZATION. One of the most critical judgments an EMT makes is when to load the patient and depart for the hospital. Arguments for spending less time at the scene of an accident or injury (and therefore using fewer stabilizing maneuvers on pediatric patients than on adult patients) include the following: (1) the difficulty of successfully achieving IV access at the scene; (2) better physiologic compensation of the pediatric patient; (3) increased risk of hypothermia from prolonged field treatment; (4) data showing no difference in survival from prehospital arrest when basic rather than advanced life support techniques are used; and (5) greater risk that certain procedures performed on a pediatric patient may actually precipitate clinical deteri-

TABLE 6–24. Prehospital Primary Survey (ABCDs)

Airway	Breath sounds
Breathing	Work of breathing; color; respiratory rate
Circulation	Strength of peripheral pulses; color and temperature of extremities; heart rate; blood pressure
Disability	Modified Glasgow Coma Scale (see Table 6–25); pupillary responses; fontanel tension

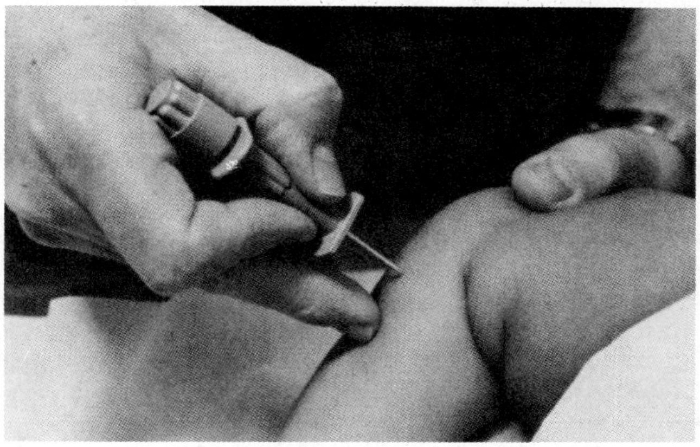

Figure 6–11. Intraosseous infusion.

TABLE 6–25. Modified Glasgow Coma Scale

Score	>1 Yr	<1 Yr	
	Eyes Opening		
4	Spontaneously	Spontaneously	
3	To verbal command	To shout	
2	To pain	To pain	
1	No response	No response	
	Best Motor Response		
Score	**>1 Yr**	**<1 Yr**	
6	Obeys	Spontaneous	
5	Localizes pain	Localizes pain	
4	Flexion-withdrawal	Flexion-withdrawal	
3	Flexion-abnormal (decorticate rigidity)	Flexion-abnormal (decerebrate rigidity)	
2	Extension (decerebrate rigidity)	Extension (decerebrate rigidity)	
1	No response	No response	
	Best Verbal Response		
Score	**>5 Yr**	**2–5 Yr**	**0–23 Mo**
5	Oriented and converses	Appropriate words and phrases	Smiles, coos appropriately
4	Disoriented and converses	Inappropriate words	Cries, consolable
3	Inappropriate words	Persistent cries or screams	Persistent inappropriate crying or screaming
2	Incomprehensible sounds	Grunts	Grunts, agitated or restless
1	No response	No response	No response

oration (e.g., increased agitation of the child in respiratory distress). The average time spent at the scene in two studies was 18 min for pediatric patients compared with 26 min for adults. This suggests that EMTs do recognize the advantage of a load-and-go approach for children as opposed to adults. Conversely, one argument supporting greater efforts at stabilization at the scene is the longer transport times for systems in which EMTs are permitted to bypass local hospitals in favor of going to a regional pediatric medical center.

HOSPITAL-BASED PEDIATRIC EMERGENCY CARE

EPIDEMIOLOGY. Pediatric patients account for 26% of all emergency room visits, but they account for less than 5% of hospital admissions from emergency rooms and only 2.5% of all cases of arrest managed in general emergency rooms. (A general emergency medicine physician therefore, can manage 40 adult CPRs for every pediatric patient resuscitated.)

Infants and toddlers from families of (low) socioeconomic groups IV and V (Hollingshead's classification) comprise a disproportionate percentage of pediatric emergency room visits. Ten per cent of pediatric emergency room visits are judged by the treating physician to be emergent, 60% are judged urgent, and 30% nonurgent. Factors that reduce the number of nonurgent pediatric emergency room visits include availability of a regular primary health care provider, availability of telephone advice, and membership in a prepaid health plan. Contrary to common belief, the availability of transportation and parental hours of employment do not substantially influence the decision to use an emergency room.

Urgent medical visits occur with twice the frequency of urgent surgical visits. Fever, respiratory distress, and gastrointestinal complaints account for most urgent medical visits; minor trauma accounts for most urgent surgical visits. Actual medical and surgical emergencies account for 6 and 4% of pediatric emergency room visits, respectively. The typical medical emergency is an infant with meningitis, respiratory failure, or severe dehydration. The typical surgical emergency is a school-aged child with appendicitis or injuries sustained in a pedestrian motor vehicle accident.

Sixty-two per cent of pediatric emergency room visits occur between 4 P.M. and midnight. Major and minor trauma occur with increased frequency in the spring and summer; urgent and emergent medical conditions predominate in the fall and winter. Visits to a pediatric emergency room at a pediatric medical center account for only 10% of all emergency room visits by pediatric patients, and the remaining 90% are managed in general emergency rooms.

Many factors contribute to the unique medical environment of the emergency room. The most important is that the number of patients and the gravity of their condition in the emergency room at any given time are uncontrollable (and unpredictable). This not only influences the orientation and style of emergency medical care, but can also affect the quality of that medical care. The uncontrollable nature of patient flow places a premium on efficiency. The emergency room physician's role, therefore, has traditionally been to triage and stabilize. Complete evaluation and definitive care are left to primary physicians and subspecialists, freeing the emergency room physician for the next influx of patients. The quality of care provided is heavily dependent on the degree to which the hospital's medical staff supports the emergency room. The medical staff must accept responsibility for close follow-up of patients triaged by the emergency room physician as sufficiently stable to be discharged. In the case of a critically ill patient whose condition has been stabilized by the emergency room physician, the medical staff must promptly assume responsibility for definitive care. The community's primary care pediatricians and other pediatric subspecialists should assist in the development of policies and procedures for dealing with children in the emergency room, in quality assurance evaluation of pediatric emergency care, and in the formulation of a systems perspective to guarantee maximal community response to a child with an emergency medical problem.

DIAGNOSIS AND TREATMENT. Because the role of the emergency room is identification and treatment of emergency conditions, diagnostic accuracy must be extremely high. Therefore, the most useful laboratory tests are those with very high predictive values. (The predictive value of a test is the frequency with which a positive result is diagnostic of a given disease entity or a negative result rules out a given disease entity. A test's predictive value is derived from its sensitivity and specificity and from the incidence of the disease entity in question.) Tests possessing only moderate predictive values delay decision-making, compromising an emergency room's efficiency. Consequently, a major thrust of emergency medicine research has been to refine the indications for selecting laboratory tests in the emergency room setting. The results of much of this research have been to downgrade the usefulness of extensive laboratory evaluation in the emergency room setting and to reaffirm the value of experienced clinical skills and judgment in identifying emergency conditions in pediatric patients.

The treatment objectives of the emergency department, in addition to minimizing mortality and long-term morbidity, include pain control and limiting the need for inpatient care. Pain and discomfort can be managed with various agents and modalities, many of which are listed in Table 6–26 (see Sec. 6.54). The use of physical restraints should be a last resort. The need for hospitalization is minimized through the use of

TABLE 6–26. Pain Control Measures in Pediatric Emergency Medicine

Psychologic	
	Reassurance
	Suggestion
	Hypnosis
Oral	
	Chloral hydrate
	Midazolam
Inhalation	
	Nitrous oxide
Intramuscular	
	Meperidine, promethazine, chlorpromazine (used in combination)
Intravenous	
	Meperidine and a benzodiazepine
	Fentanyl
Topical	
	TEC (tetracaine, epinephrine, cocaine)
	4% lidocaine
Local	
	Lidocaine with bicarbonate
Regional	
	Bier block

holding areas, parenteral antibiotics with long half-lives, and close follow-up provided by the child's primary care physician.

For more specific discussions of the assessment and management of pediatric emergency medical conditions, see the relevant sections in this text. The approach to the major trauma victim is discussed here in detail.

MAJOR TRAUMA MANAGEMENT IN THE EMERGENCY DEPARTMENT

Blunt trauma accounts for 88% of pediatric trauma, compared to 60% for the general population. Blunt trauma is associated with a higher incidence of occult injury and a lesser need for acute surgical intervention compared to penetrating injury. Two thirds of pediatric major trauma victims have an isolated head injury. Another 15% have a major head injury as part of their constellation of injuries.

ASSESSMENT AND MANAGEMENT. The pediatric major trauma victim is best managed by direct transfer to a pediatric trauma center staffed by a well-organized team of physicians that is led by a pediatric surgeon with special expertise in pediatric trauma. This team should have a prompt response time, appropriate in-house radiologic, operating room, laboratory, and intensive care unit (ICU) support, and a system of compiling, reviewing, and reporting its results to a National or Regional Trauma Registry. Validated scoring systems are available to allow comparison of a center's results with regional or national standards.

The overall approach to the pediatric trauma victim is the same as that for the adult trauma victim: cervical spine stabilization, assessment of airway, breathing, circulation, and disability (ABCD), and secondary survey. Within each category, however, are important differences (see also Sec. 6.33).

Cervical Spine Stabilization. The first step is stabilization of the child's cervical spine with towel rolls or foam blocks taped to a spine board. The cervical spine is immobilized in the neutral position when the ear aligns to the shoulder. In younger children this requires placing a folded towel under the shoulders to prevent the child's large occiput from causing cervical spine flexion. A cervical collar alone is insufficient for pediatric cervical spine control. Most pediatric cervical spine injuries are high in the cervical spine—an area not well immobilized by cervical collars, particularly if not of proper size. Immobilization should only be removed in the emergency department if cervical spine injury is ruled out both radiologically and clinically. Up to 50% of small children with cervical spine injuries have a normal lateral neck roentgenogram. Many of these suffer from the SCIWRA syndrome—spinal cord injury without radiographic abnormality. Computed tomography (CT), magnetic resonance imaging (MRI), or carefully performed flexion-extension roentgenograms may be necessary to rule out cervical cord or cervical spine injury.

Airway. The airway is assessed with breath sounds. If the airway cannot be maintained by suction or manual maneuvers, or if positive pressure ventilation (PPV) is needed, intubation under direct visualization is the preferred technique for airway management. Blind nasotracheal intubation is ineffective in children. Establishing an oral airway risks vomiting and aspiration. One exception to this is the child with massive facial trauma who may need temporary airway management with a needle cricothyroidotomy. The difficulty with oral intubation in the pediatric multiple trauma victim is not the technical challenge of the procedure itself, but the risk of exacerbating increased intracranial pressure secondary to hypoxia, hypercapnia, or gagging. This is most successfully avoided using a drug sequence prior to intubation that includes a paralyzing agent and a sedative. In addition, lidocaine 1 mg/kg may both depress intracranial pressure waves and decrease the risk of gagging.

Breathing. Breathing in the pediatric major trauma victim is most commonly compromised by pulmonary contusions or a distended stomach that is impeding diaphragmatic movement. All these children should be treated with high-concentration oxygen and a nasogastric tube (or an oronasogastric tube if a basilar skull fracture is suspected based on serous drainage from the nose or midfacial fracture.) Because the pediatric rib cage is so pliable, rib fractures, hemothoraces, and pneumothoraces occur less commonly than in adults. When a pneumothorax does occur, however, it has more devastating consequences because of the child's mobile mediastinum. The great vessels become obstructed, resulting in shock and hypoxia. The diagnosis is based on auscultatory findings and, if time permits, on a chest roentgenogram. Tracheal deviation and neck vein distention are not useful signs of a pneumothorax in a pediatric patient. The treatment is needle thoracostomy followed by tube thoracostomy. Indications that breathing must be supported with PPV in the pediatric major trauma victim include hypoxia, hypercarbia, unacceptable work of breathing in the presence of shock, and the need to hyperventilate to decrease intracranial pressure.

Circulation. Circulation is initially assessed using the heart rate and signs of peripheral perfusion. The blood pressure should be taken but interpreted cautiously. Pediatric patients may maintain a normal blood pressure in the presence of up to 25% blood volume loss. Obvious external hemorrhage, which may in itself be sufficient in a child to produce shock, should be tamponaded with direct pressure. Two large-bore peripheral IV lines should be started with an isotonic solution and run slowly if the child is well perfused to avoid exacerbating any increased intracranial pressure. If shock is present, however, successive 20-mL/kg boluses should be promptly administered pending the availability of blood and while monitoring for the development of shock lung syndrome. For shock unresponsive to fluid boluses, intra-abdominal bleeding and mediastinal injuries should be considered early during the secondary survey.

Disability. Disability is the catchword for CNS status. Isolated CNS injury accounts for over 60% of pediatric trauma mortality and is a complicating factor in an additional 15% of trauma deaths. Disability is assessed using the child's mental status, pupils, peripheral tone and, in the case of the infant, the fontanel. Any alteration in consciousness demands an emergency CT scan. When mental status is profoundly affected (MGCS $\leq$ 8), intubation with appropriate pharmacologic support and hyperventilation is indicated. If there are lateralizing neurologic findings that persist or progress despite hyperventilation, the use of IV mannitol and/or emergency burr holes may be warranted. Shock must be aggressively treated with fluid when increased intracranial pressure is also suspected. Although the fluid therapy may exacerbate the increased intracranial pressure, the lack of perfusion to the brain represents an even greater threat.

Secondary Survey. After the ABCDs have been stabilized the child is fully exposed and examined from head to toe, being careful to avoid hypothermia in the process. Special attention should be directed to the abdomen, a vulnerable area in children because the abdominal viscera are close to the surface and are less well protected by the rib cage and abdominal musculature. Distention, tenderness, bruising, or a suspicious mechanism of injury in the unconscious victim, without any abdominal findings, should raise the suspicion of intra-abdominal injury. If the child is stable, a contrast abdominal CT that does not delay monitoring and therapy of the child's CNS injuries may help define intra-abdominal pathology with a high degree of reliability and safety. This CT scan should include the lower chest to screen for occult pulmonary injury. If the child is unstable, peritoneal lavage is the most appropriate diagnostic procedure. Other important components of the secondary survey include a careful HEENT examination, auscultation of heart sounds and over all body cavities, bony palpation, and a rectal examination. Laboratory studies that can aid in the assessment include a complete blood count (CBC), determination of amylase and liver enzyme levels, and a urinalysis. The urine sample should be obtained with an indwelling Foley catheter to monitor urine output if shock is present or if mannitol is used. Finally, the child who is conscious during this intense evaluation must be comforted in an age-appropriate fashion to minimize the long-term psychologic effects of the child's accident and subsequent treatment.

PROGNOSIS. The prognosis for the major trauma victim who reaches the hospital alive and receives timely and expert acute and rehabilitative care is excellent. Over 95% of these children are left with minimal or no residual disabilities. Even children who have been comatose for more than 24 hr have, in most series, a greater than 50% chance of a reasonable recovery.

JOSEPH E. SIMON

GENERAL REFERENCES

American Medical Association Commission on Emergency Medical Services: Pediatric emergencies. Pediatrics 85:879, 1990.
McIntire MS (ed): American Academy of Pediatrics, Committee on Accident and Poison Prevention: Injury Control for Children and Youth. Elk Grove Village, IL, American Academy of Pediatrics Press, 1987.
Munoz E: Economic costs of trauma. United States, 1982. J Trauma 24:237, 1984.
National Safety Council: Accident Facts, 1989. Chicago, National Safety Council, 1989.
Rivara FP, Kamitsuka MD, Quan L: Injuries to children younger than one year of age. Pediatrics 81:93, 1988.
Runyan CW, Gerken EA: Epidemiology and prevention of adolescent injury. JAMA 266:2273, 1989.

ROAD AND FARM INJURIES

Automobiles: Drivers and Passengers

Agran PF, Dunkle DE, Winn DG: Effects of legislation on motor vehicle injuries to children. Am J Dis Child 141:959, 1987.
Bull MJ, Strup KB, Gerhart S: Misuse of car safety seats. Pediatrics 81:98, 1988.
Decker MD, Dewey MJ, Hutcheson RH, et al: The use and efficacy of child restraint devices. The Tennessee experience, 1982 and 1983. JAMA 252:2571, 1984.
Mohan D, Schneider LW: An evaluation of adult clasping strength for restraining lap-held infants. Hum Factors 21:635, 1979.
Robertson LS: Crash involvement of teenaged drivers when driver education is eliminated from high school. Am J Public Health 70:599, 1980.
Scherz R: Restraint systems for the prevention of injury to children in automobile accidents. Am J Public Health 66:451, 1976.

All-Terrain Vehicles

American Academy of Pediatrics, Committee on Accident and Poison Prevention: Policy statement: All-terrain vehicles: two-, three-, and four-wheeled unlicensed motorized vehicles. Pediatrics 79:306, 1987.
Stevens WS, Rodgers BM, Newman BM: Pediatric trauma associated with all-terrain vehicles. J Pediatr 109:25, 1986.

Motorcycles

Robertson LS: An instance of effective legal regulation: Motorcycle helmet and daytime headlamp laws. Law Soc Rev 10:467, 1976.
Watson GS, Zador PL, Wilks A: A repeal of helmet use laws and increased motorcyclist mortality in the United States, 1975–1978. Am J Public Health 70:579, 1980.

Bicycles

Cross K, Fisher G: A Study of Bicycle/Motor Vehicle Accidents: Identification of Problem Types and Countermeasure Approaches, Vol I. Santa Barbara, CA, Anacapa Sciences, Inc, 1977.
Thompson RS, Rivara FP, Thompson DC: A case-control study of the effectiveness of bicycle safety helmets. N Engl J Med 320:1361, 1989.

Farm Equipment

Salmi LR, Weiss HB, Peterson PL, et al: Fatal farm injuries among young children. Pediatrics 83:267, 1989.
Swanson JA, Sachs MI, Dahlgren KA, et al: Accidental farm injuries in children. Am J Dis Child 141:1276, 1987.

Pedestrians

Sandels S: Young children in traffic. Br J Educ Psychol 40:111, 1970.

HOME AND SCHOOL INJURIES

Boyce WT, Sprunger LW, Sobolewska S, et al: The epidemiology of injuries in large, urban school districts. Pediatrics 79:342, 1984.
Goldberg B, Rosenthal PP, Robertson LS, et al: Injuries in youth football. Pediatrics 81:255, 1988.
Joffe M, Ludwig S: Stairway injuries in children. Pediatrics 82:457, 1988.
Miller JL, Shermeta DW: Falls in urban children. Am J Dis Child 141:1271, 1987.
Reichelderfer TE, Overback A, Greensher J: Unsafe playground. Pediatrics 56:526, 1979.

Accident-Prone Child

Beautrais AL, Fergusson DM, Shannon FT: Life events and childhood morbidity: A prospective study. Pediatrics 70:935, 1982.
Bijur P, Golding J, Haslum M, et al: Behavioral predictors of injury in school-age children. Am J Dis Child 142:1307, 1988.
Boyce WT, Sobolewski S: Recurrent injuries in schoolchildren. Am J Dis Child 143:338, 1989.
Larson CP, Pless IB: Risk factors for injury in a 3-year-old birth cohort. Am J Dis Child 142:1052, 1988.
Padilla ER, Rohsenow DJ, Bergman AB: Predicting accident frequency in children. Pediatrics 58:223, 1976.
Schor EL: Unintentional injuries. Patterns within families. Am J Dis Child 141:1280, 1987.

Reducing Injury

American Academy of Pediatrics, Committee on Accident and Poison Prevention: The Injury Prevention Program. Elk Grove Village, IL, American Academy of Pediatrics Press, 1989.
Haddon W: Energy damage and the ten countermeasure strategies. J Trauma 13:21, 1973.
Phillips WR, Little TL: Continuity of care and poisoning prevention education. Patient Counseling Health Information 170:73, 1980.
Schaplowsky A: Community injury control—a management approach. Am J Public Health 53:252, 1973.
Schlesinger ER, Dickenson DG, Westag J, et al: Study of health education in accident prevention. Am J Dis Child 111:490, 1966.

EMERGENCY MEDICAL SERVICES FOR CHILDREN

General References

Alterra M, Bellet J, Scott H: Preparedness for pediatric emergencies encountered in the practitioner's office. Pediatrics 85:710, 1990.
American Academy of Pediatrics, Committee of Hospital Care: Guidelines for air and ground transportation of pediatric patients. Pediatrics 78:943, 1986.
Pollock M, Alexander S, Clarke N, et al: Evaluation of Oregon pediatric critical care outcome by hospital resource level. Presented at the National Conference on Pediatric Trauma, Boston, Sept 1987.
Simon JE, Smookler S, Guy B: A regionalized approach to pediatric emergency care. Pediatr Clin North Am 28:677, 1981.
Tendler C, Grossman S, Tenenbaum J: Medication dosages during pediatric emergencies: A simple and comprehensive guide. Pediatrics 84:731, 1989.

Prehospital Care

Applebaum D: Advanced prehospital care for pediatric emergencies. Ann Emerg Med 14:656, 1985.
Holbrook P: Prehospital care of critically ill children. Crit Care Med 8:537, 1980.
Ramenotsky M, Luterman A, Curreir PW: EMS for pediatrics: Optimum treatment or unnecessary delay? J Pediatr Surg 18:498, 1983.
Siedel JS, Hornbein M, Yoshuyama K: Emergency medical services and the pediatric patient: Are the needs being met? Pediatrics 73:769, 1984.
Simon JE, Goldberg AT: Prehospital Pediatric Life Support. St. Louis, CV Mosby, 1989.
Tsai A, Kallsen G: Epidemiology of pediatric prehospital care. Ann Emerg Med 16:284, 1987.

Hospital Care

Billmire D, Neale H, Gregory R: Use of IV fentanyl in outpatient treatment of pediatric facial trauma. J Trauma 26:1079, 1985.
Bonadio W, Wagner V: Efficacy of TAC topical anesthetic for repair of pediatric lacerations. Am J Dis Child 142:203, 1988.
Chessare J: Utilization of emergency services among patients of a pediatric group practice. Pediatr Emerg Care 2:27, 1986.
Dagan R, Phillip M, Watember M: Outpatient treatment of serious community-acquired pediatric infections using once-daily intramuscular ceftriaxone. Pediatr Infect Dis 6:1080, 1987.
Fifield G, Magnuson C, Carr WP: Pediatric emergency care in a metropolitan area. J Emerg Med 1:495, 1984.
Halperin R, Meyers A, Alpert J: Utilization of pediatric emergency services. Pediatr Clin North Am 26:747, 1979.
Hiker TL: Nonemergency visits to a pediatric emergency department. Journal of the American College of Emergency Physicians 7:3, 1978.
Li M, Baker MD, Ropp LS: Pediatric emergency medicine. Pediatrics 84:336, 1989.
Losek J, Walsh-Kelly C, Glaeser P: Pediatric emergency departments. Pediatr Emerg Care 2:215, 1986.
Pryor G, Kilpatrick W, Opp D: Local anesthesia in minor lacerations: Topical TAC versus lidocaine infiltration. Ann Emerg Med 9:568, 1980.
Rosenstein BJ, Baker D: Pediatric outpatient intravenous rehydration. Am J Emerg Med 5:183, 1987.
Wilbert C, Davis AT, Herman JJ: Short-term holding room treatment of asthmatic children. J Pediatr 106:707, 1985.

THE CHILD WITH MAJOR INJURY

Buntain WL, Gould HR, Maull KI: Predictability of splenic damage by computerized tomography. J Trauma 28:24, 1988.
Buntain WL, Lynch FP, Ramenofsky ML: Management of the acutely injured child. Adv Trauma 2:43, 1987.
Haller JA, Shorter N, Miller D, et al: Organization and function of a regional pediatric trauma center: Does a system of management improve outcome? J Trauma 23:691, 1983.
Holmes MJ, Reyes HM: A critical review of urban pediatric trauma. J Trauma 24:253, 1984.
Karp MP, Cooney DR, Berger PE: The role of computerized tomography in the evaluation of blunt abdominal trauma in children. J Pediatr Surg 16:316, 1981.
Mayer T, Matlok ME, Johnson DG, et al: The modified injury severity scale in pediatric multiple trauma patients. J Pediatr Surg 15:719, 1980.
Miller JL, Little AG, Shermeta DW: Thoracic trauma in children. Pediatrics 74:813, 1984.
Pang D, Wilberger JE: Spinal cord injury without radiographic abnormalities in children. J Neurosurg 57:114, 1982.
Ramenofsky M, Luterman A, Quindlen E: Maximum survival in pediatric trauma: The ideal system. J Trauma 24:818, 1984.
Rothenberg S, Moore E, Marx J: Selective management of blunt trauma in children—the triage role of peritoneal lavage. J Trauma 27:1101, 1987.
Velecek FT, Weiss A, DiMaio D: Traumatic death in children. J Pediatr Surg 12:375, 1977.

REFERENCES FOR PARENTS

American Academy of Pediatrics, 141 Northwest Point Road, PO Box 927, Elk Grove Village, IL, 60007.
Child Restraint Systems for Your Automobile. United States Department of Transportation, National Highway Traffic Safety Administration, Washington, DC, 20590.
Don't Risk Your Child's Life! Physicians for Automotive Safety, PO Box 930, Armonk, NY, 10504.

6.33 PEDIATRIC CRITICAL CARE

The child who has life-threatening or potentially disabling illness or injury and who requires immediate treatment is, fortunately, rare. Critical care pediatrics is the subspecialty devoted to the care of these children and encompasses resuscitation from life-threatening events, transportation (see Sec. 6.32), and intensive care. It is not restricted by organ system, discipline, or the presence of a medical or surgical condition. Ideally, the primary caregiver, who knows the child, the family, and the pre-existing diseases, and the critical care physician should work closely together until evolution of the acute process is complete.

RECOGNITION OF THE CRITICALLY ILL CHILD. There are certain clinical manifestations of critical illness, some relatively subtle, which must be recognized immediately if a child is to have maximal likelihood of recovery. Although some of these findings may be found in disease states that are not critical illnesses, the clinician should respond to these "red flags" rather than to assume that the patient is not seriously ill. See also Sec. 6.1.

Signs and symptoms of critical illness referable to the central nervous system (CNS) include alterations in levels of consciousness and musculoskeletal positioning. Changes in the level of consciousness can be produced by the involvement of large amounts of cortical brain tissue, such as in patients with intoxication, hypoxia, or other global conditions, or by more discrete lesions in the reticular activating system (RAS), such as hemorrhage into the brain stem or compression of the RAS during herniation. The alteration may be in the direction of increased consciousness (e.g., cocaine intoxication) or decreased consciousness (e.g., the obtundation induced by shock). An alteration of level of consciousness should always be presumed to be caused by a critical illness.

Alarming musculoskeletal changes include posturing and flaccidity. Posturing is found when there is unopposed or incompletely opposed contraction of muscle groups. This signifies injury or illness in the CNS and is always of concern. Flaccidity is caused by impairment of the neuromuscular axis at some point from the cortex to the muscle unit. Because neuromuscular degeneration is exceptional in children, the presence of flaccidity is of great significance.

A major cardiovascular sign of critical illness is poor perfusion of the capillary beds. Three beds are readily assessed by the clinician and should be evaluated initially in screening for severe illness: the CNS, where hypoperfusion is manifested by depressed levels of consciousness; the renal capillary bed, where poor perfusion decreases urine output; and the skin, which shows poor capillary refill (longer than 3 sec) if poor perfusion is present.

Cyanosis (a blue coloring of the skin), which is usually caused by the circulation of deoxygenated hemoglobin in the arterial system, is only apparent when there is circulation of at least 50 g/L of deoxygenated hemoglobin. Thus, significant desaturation may exist without cyanosis or, in the anemic patient, cyanosis may not even be evident. The absence of cyanosis is not a reliable predictor of good oxygen saturation.

Clinical manifestations of respiratory insufficiency include noisy, difficult breathing, retractions, flaring, and tachypnea (see Sec. 14.17). Because of the broad range of normal respiratory rates found at different ages in children, it is easy to overlook significant tachypnea. In addition, the pattern of respiration may indicate severe disease. Seesaw respirations (abdominal protrusion with inhalation) indicate poor pulmonary or chest wall compliance. Irregular respirations with periodic deep sighs may indicate CNS dysfunction. Similarly, an increasing-decreasing depth of respiration, often followed by apnea (Cheyne-Stokes breathing) and by rapid, deep breathing (central hyperventilation) are found in brain herniation syndromes (see Sec. 20.57). Grunting, or forced exhalation against a transiently closed glottis, is also associated with significant respiratory dysfunction. It is important to identify this sign and determine its cause.

Metabolic collapse is heralded by changes in the vital signs. Tachypnea (and, more importantly, hyperpnea) is an early finding in the various metabolic acidosis syndromes, such as diabetic ketoacidosis. Tachycardia is usual. In addition, poor perfusion and a depressed level of consciousness are typical.

CARDIOPULMONARY RESUSCITATION (CPR). This is the sequence of events undertaken in an attempt to reverse life-threatening cardiopulmonary insufficiency immediately. Because the urgency of the situation demands action, resuscitation sequences have been codified into plans of action that are simple, largely rote, and easily communicated to all who might need to resuscitate a patient. Resuscitation of the traumatized child (Sec. 6.32) does not differ in principle from resuscitation of other children. Several different sequences are recognized depending on the age, location, and presentation of the patient. All resuscitation protocols involve mastery of psychomotor skills and require practice. Courses in CPR are available from a number of organizations.

The primary target organ for any resuscitation attempt is the brain. The greatest threats to the child's brain are hypoxia (lack of oxygen) and ischemia (lack of flow). Frequently, these two cannot be separated. Establishment of an adequate airway, supporting breathing, addressing the circulation of the patient, the ABCDs of resuscitation, are fundamental to the provision of sufficient oxygen and the maintenance of adequate blood flow. In addition, the integrity of the spinal column must be protected.

Airway control is essential for resuscitation and should be the first priority. A patent airway is demonstrated by smooth, quiet air flow in and out of the patient and a rising and falling of the chest with ventilation. Manual establishment of the airway begins by placing the patient in the supine position, gently extending the occiput, and flexing the cervical spine on the thoracic spine. This may be done by inserting a hand under the child's neck and lifting upward, which result in straightening the airway into the "sniffing position" (Fig. 6–12). Lifting the mandible from the angle of the jaw also may be of benefit. If the child is apneic, two quick breaths are given. If this does not produce chest expansion or, if the child is breathing but air flow is not smooth, a second attempt can be made to position the child, as just described. If this fails, airway obstruction resulting from the presence of a foreign body should be considered. Chest thrusts, abdominal thrusts, and back blows are all successful in dislodging foreign bodies. After one or more of these maneuvers the child is repositioned into the sniffing position and air flow is reassessed. If air flow is still compromised, there are two options. The first involves upper airway visualization, removal of any foreign body, and insertion of an endotracheal tube, if necessary (Fig. 6–13). There should be consideration of whether the child has a full stomach and compression of the esophagus and appropriate muscle relaxation drugs provided, as necessary. In prolonged respiratory or circulatory arrest, intubation of the trachea is important to provide high oxygen concentrations, reduce aspiration risks, and maintain the airway. Alternatively, the upper airway may be bypassed by a cricothyrotomy, but this is a very difficult technique in a small child.

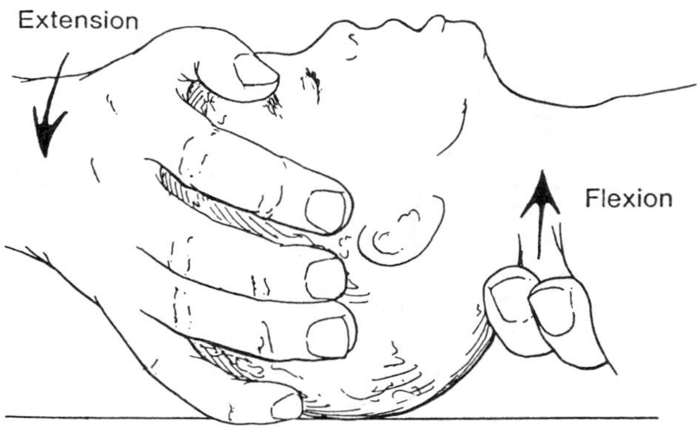

Figure 6–12. "Sniffing position." (From American Academy of Pediatrics/American College of Emergency Medicine: Advanced Pediatric Life Support. Elk Grove Village, IL, American Academy of Pediatrics Press, 1989, p 4. Copyright 1989. Reproduced by permission.)

Once airway control has been achieved, breathing is initiated, if necessary. Mouth-to-mouth ventilation can always be done, but breathing for the patient with a bag-valve-mask combination is preferable because of the higher level of oxygen that can be administered. Whichever technique is used, it is essential for the child's chest to rise with inflation. No other means of assessing breathing is more important than the rise and fall of the chest.

Circulation should be addressed only after a patent airway and breathing are ensured. The presence of pulses is sought in the femoral, brachial, carotid, or cardiac apical regions. If absent, closed-chest cardiac massage is begun. Thumb, two-finger, one-hand, or two-hand compression may be used, depending on the size of the child. Although it remains controversial as to whether the heart or the entire chest is being compressed in the adult during CPR, evidence has shown that it is direct force on the heart that moves the blood forward during pediatric CPR. Thus, the chest should be compressed enough to promote emptying of the heart. Pulses should be palpated by an assistant. If the patient has inadequate pulses, measures for improving the circulation are carried out next. Active bleeding should be stopped and intravenous or intramedullary fluids (see Fig. 6–11) of sufficient amount to restore blood volume should be administered immediately (see later, Circulatory Collapse).

Selected cardiovascular drugs, indications, and dosages are listed in Tables 6–27, 6–28, and 6–29. In addition, sodium bicarbonate (1–2 mEq/kg) is indicated for correction of documented metabolic acidosis; other indications for the use of bicarbonate in CPR have not been established. Calcium therapy is indicated for patients with documented hypocalcemia.

While the ABCDs are being pursued, close attention should be paid to preservation of the integrity of the cervical spine (Sec. 6.32).

PROGNOSIS. The prognosis after CPR correlates with the procedures needed to restore the patient. If establishment of the airway was all that was necessary, and the patient experienced no circulatory or CNS embarrassment, the prognosis is good. If respiratory arrest has occurred but not circulatory embarrassment, the prognosis is also good, and the underlying disease determines the outcome. Circulatory arrest, however, carries a grim prognosis unless reversed very quickly. Primary dysrhythmias are uncommon in children and circulatory embarrassment is usually the result of respiratory, CNS, or metabolic disease. Under these conditions, circulation failure frequently occurs after a long period of pansystemic dysfunction; circulatory resuscitation may be difficult and the added insult of hypoxia and ischemia caused by the circulatory arrest may prove lethal. If the traumatized patient has not experienced circulatory collapse, the outcome

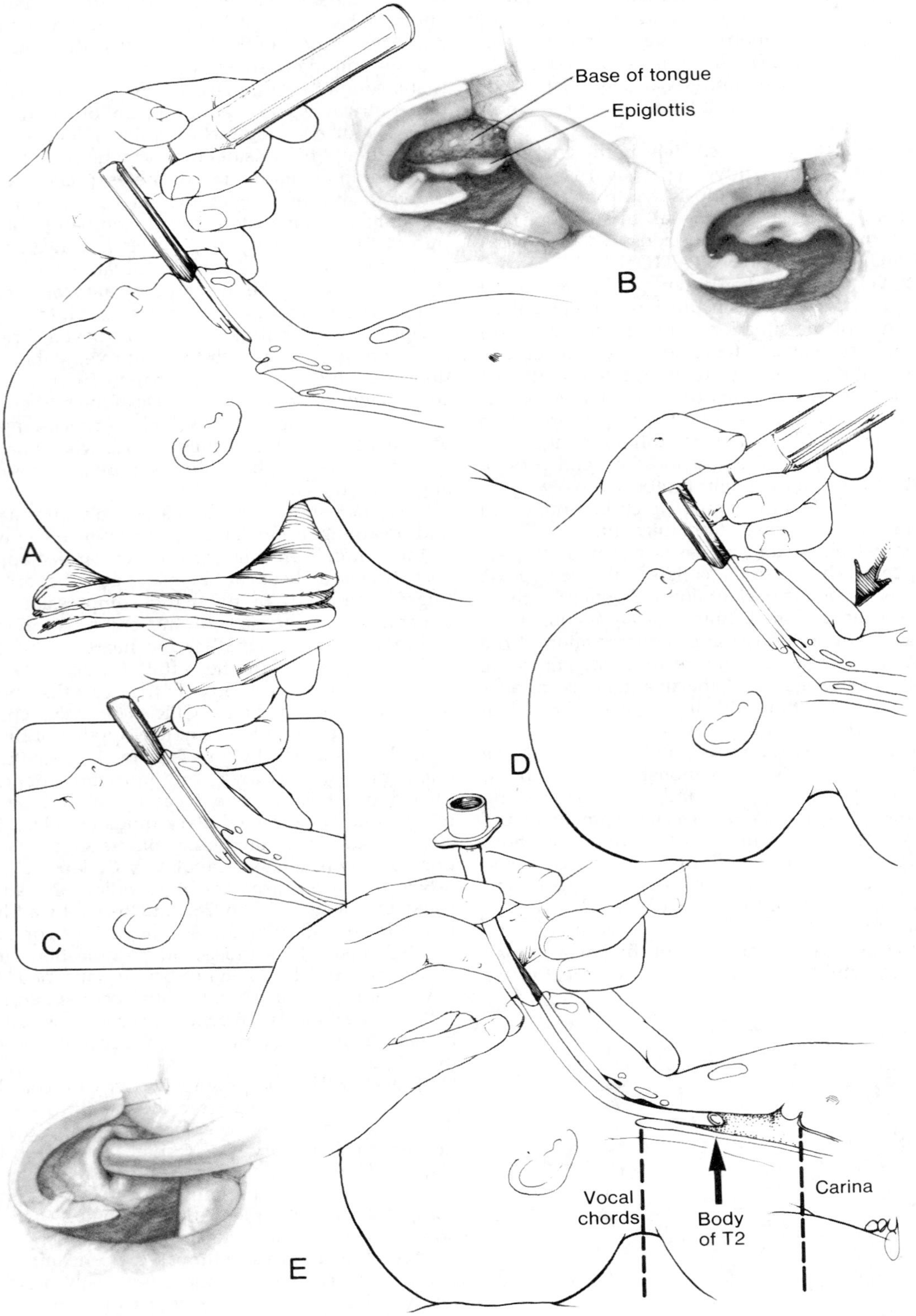

Figure 6–13. Intubation technique. (From Fleisher G, Ludwig S: Textbook of Pediatric Emergency Medicine. Baltimore, Williams & Wilkins, 1983, p 1250.)

TABLE 6–27. Cardiovascular Agents and Procedures Affecting Heart Rate

Indication	Agent	Dose	Comment
Cardiac arrest	Epinephrine	10 μg/kg	Cardiac and vascular stimulation, ET*
Fibrillation	Defibrillation	2 watt-sec/kg	Double intensity if unsuccessful
Bradycardia	Atropine	0.01–0.03 mg/kg	Vagolytic, ET
	Isoproterenol	0.1 μg/min	Vasodilator
Supraventricular tachycardia	Cardioversion†	0.5–1 watt-sec/kg	Double intensity if unsuccessful
Ventricular tachycardia	Cardioversion†	0.5–1 watt-sec/kg	Double intensity if unsuccessful
	Lidocaine	1 mg/kg bolus	ET
	Bretylium	5 mg/kg bolus	
	Phenytoin	15 mg/kg	Give 1 mg/kg/min

*ET may be administered through an endotracheal tube.
†If the patient is in cardiovascular collapse, cardioversion is indicated. For further details on dysrhythmia therapy see Chapter 15.

is determined by the underlying injuries. Cardiac arrest in the trauma patient, however, regardless of underlying injury, carries a grave prognosis. Because of the poor prognosis after circulatory arrest in children, there has been a growing concern about how long to persist with resuscitative efforts. In the absence of hypothermia or other confounding variables, the persistence of efforts beyond two administrations of appropriate medications without improvement is usually unwarranted.

American Academy of Pediatrics, American College of Emergency Physicians: Advanced Pediatric Life Support. Elk Grove Village, IL, American Academy of Pediatrics Press, 1989.
American Heart Association: Standards for CPR and ECC. JAMA 255:2954, 1986.
Schleien CL, Berkowitz ID, Traystman R, et al: Controversial issues in cardiopulmonary resuscitation. Anesthesiology 71:133, 1989.

6.34 INTENSIVE CARE OF THE CHILD

Intensive care of the child has two broad components in addition to treatment of the underlying disease: support of vital organs and monitoring for early detection of potentially life-threatening or disabling conditions.

ORGAN SYSTEM SUPPORT. Supportive care for the brain is still based on limited information. Adequate oxygenation of the blood and blood flow to the brain are essential. Thus, correction of airway abnormalities, establishment of sufficient breathing function, and provision of adequate circulation are fundamental. Other therapies (e.g., hyperventilation) must not compromise oxygenation and blood flow to the brain.

Increased intracranial pressure (ICP) is a common result of injury to the brain. If it is high enough to compromise blood flow to the CNS, it adds hypoxic and ischemic injury to the underlying problem and may decrease the likelihood of return of function. However, it has now been recognized that increased ICP is more frequently a marker of the severity of the underlying injury than a primary, treatable problem. Treatment of severely increased ICP in patients with head trauma and hypoxia and ischemia has not resulted in an improved outcome. The successful treatment of moderate increases in ICP may improve outcome in head trauma patients, but no improvement has been noted by treating increased ICP in hypoxic and ischemic patients. In the absence of treatment aimed at the underlying disease, treatment of increased ICP alone may not be indicated.

Treatment of increased ICP is based on the hypothesis that the intracranial contents within the rigid, bony skull take up too much space. These contents consist of brain tissue, brain water, blood, and cerebrospinal fluid (CSF). The goal of treatment is to reduce the volume of one or more of the intracranial contents. Immediate reduction of pressure is achieved by raising the patient's head above the heart and maintaining the head in the midline, thus promoting drainage of blood out of the skull. Hyperventilation is the next quickest method of reducing an increased ICP by decreasing blood volume, secondary to a reduction in blood flow. The patient may be hyperventilated manually by bag and mask or tube or may be mechanically ventilated. A Pa_{CO_2} of 25 mm Hg is the usual target for reducing ICP without severely reducing cerebral blood flow; additional reductions in ICP can be achieved if a lower Pa_{CO_2} is selected but blood flow may decrease further.

Removal of CSF by ventricular puncture may also be lifesaving but usually requires special skills (see Sec. 20.1).

Increased ICP also may be reduced by administering osmotic agents intravenously. By establishing a gradient between the blood and brain, water can be drawn into the circulation and excreted by the kidneys. Mannitol in a dose of 0.25–1.0 g/kg is the usual agent given. Diuretics such as furosemide also promote water loss, although not selectively from the CNS. Carbonic anhydrase inhibitors such as Diamox reduce the production of CSF and promote diuresis, but they do not work quickly enough to be acutely effective.

Intravenous lidocaine (1 mg/kg) also lowers an increased ICP, as do barbiturates. Barbiturates reduce blood flow and cerebral metabolic rate and function—the patient is anesthetized. Corticosteroids reduce the swelling caused by many CNS tumors, although they are not clearly effective for other causes of increased ICP.

There are many complications of the use of aggressive therapy aimed at decreasing an increased ICP. Hyperventilation depresses cardiac output if it is too vigorous. Diuretics may cause dehydration and electrolyte imbalance. Barbiturates depress the CNS (thus interfering with the clinical examination) and the circulation if given in large doses.

TABLE 6–28. Cardiovascular Agents Affecting Contractility

Agent	Dose	Comment
Dobutamine	3–20 μg/kg/min	Preferable in chronic heart failure states
Dopamine	3–20 μg/kg/min	Selective renal/splanchnic vasodilator
Epinephrine	0.1–3 μg/kg/min	Intense vasoconstriction at higher doses
Isoproterenol	0.1–3 μg/kg/min	Risk of subendocardial ischemia, dysrhythmias; risk of vasodilatation

TABLE 6–29. Cardiovascular Agents Affecting Afterload

Agent	Dose	Comment
Nitroprusside	0.5–10 μg/kg/min	Cyanide toxicity risk with prolonged administration
Nitroglycerin	0.5–10 μg/kg/min	
Isoproterenol	0.1–3 μg/kg/min	Tachycardia, increased myocardial oxygen demands

Other than ensuring adequate oxygenation and ventilation, control of increased ICP (if indicated), and control of seizures, effective supportive therapy for the brain is limited at present. Indeed, it is still not clear whether blood flow should be enhanced or curtailed to a damaged area of the brain.

Life support of the *cardiovascular system* is highly developed. Multiple agents are available for control of different types of dysrhythmias (see Chapter 15), and there are many agents available to aid poor cardiac and vascular function (Tables 6–27, 6–28, and 6–29). Cardiac output is determined by preload, heart rate, contractility, and afterload; preload may be altered with fluid infusion and the other variables by pharmacologic agents. Rarely, mechanical devices such as ventricular aortic balloon counterpulsation, military antishock trousers (MAST), abdominal compression, or cardiopulmonary bypass are necessary to support the circulation.

Supportive therapy is available for nearly all components of *respiratory tract function* (see Sec. 14.2). Airway failure is acutely addressed by the aforementioned emergency procedures. For most children beyond the neonatal age group a nasotracheal airway is more stable and thus preferable. The greater skill required for insertion, the side effect of an increased chance of sinus infection, and the possibility of nasal injury are usually outweighed by the greater stability achieved. Tracheostomy is the procedure of choice if airway support is expected for more than 45–60 days. All airway bypass techniques increase the risk of pulmonary atelectasis, infection, and aspiration. Recurrent chest roentgenograms, strict asepsis, and surveillance cultures may prevent or allow early discovery of these complications. Although subclinical aspiration is common, most critical care pediatricians nourish intubated patients enterally, if gastrointestinal function is normal.

Disorders that result in inadequate gas exchange require respiratory support. Supplemental oxygen, pressure applied to the airway (continuous positive airway pressure [CPAP] using a face mask or endotracheal tube), and mechanical ventilation with or without positive end-expiratory pressure (PEEP) are routinely used. Supplemental oxygen and additional airway pressure (CPAP, PEEP) support oxygenation and increases in minute ventilation aid carbon dioxide removal.

Mechanical ventilators may be classified as positive or negative pressure, depending on the pressure applied to the airway. Positive-pressure machines may be further subclassified on the basis of the normal mechanism used to stop the flow of gases. Time-cycled, volume-cycled, or pressure-cycled machines stop flow when a preset time, volume, or pressure has been reached, respectively. All machines allow for discontinuing a breath when a given pressure has been reached, so a time-cycled machine can be pressure-limited.

Usually, a child is mechanically ventilated by selecting a tidal volume (usually 15 mL/kg body weight) at a rate that mimics that of the normal child, and the effectiveness of ventilation is assessed by measuring arterial blood gases (see Sec. 14.14). When mechanical problems (e.g., air leak around a tracheostomy) preclude effective delivery of the necessary tidal volume or when there is special concern about generated pressures, pressure-limited ventilation may be necessary.

Negative-pressure ventilators do not usually allow the fine tuning necessary for titrated support of the patient, and are rarely used in critical care units. Similarly, the use of high-frequency ventilators is rarely indicated. When mechanical ventilation fails to achieve adequate gas exchange, extracorporeal membrane oxygenation (ECMO) may be considered (see Sec. 9.36).

Support of *acute liver failure* (e.g., fulminant hepatitis, certain intoxications, Reye syndrome) is rarely necessary in pediatrics. Careful attention to intravascular fluid balance (often decreased, despite total body fluid overload), reduction of ammonia precursors (e.g., by restriction of dietary protein, elimination of blood in the gastrointestinal tract), and sterilization of the distal bowel (e.g., by eliminating nitrogen-fixing bacteria) are standard support measures (see Sec. 13.99). Also see Sec. 6.43 and 13.84.

Renal function can be supported by the use of various techniques. Uncomplicated renal failure is not a common cause of admission to the intensive care unit (ICU). Renal failure commonly accompanies other organ system failure in the ICU, however, and successful management of potassium, fluid, and acid overload by dialysis (vascular or peritoneal) or continuous arteriovenous hemofiltration (CAVH) or venovenous hemofiltration (CVVH), with or without dialysis, may be lifesaving (see Sec. 18.35).

Skin failure (e.g., burns, scalded skin syndrome, epidermolysis bullosa, hypersensitivity reactions, or graft-versus-host disease) is also life-threatening. Meticulous attention to fluid shifts, intravascular volume changes, asepsis, and nutrition are essential to preserve life (see Sec. 6.15 and 6.37).

American Academy of Pediatrics, American College of Emergency Physicians: Advanced Pediatric Life Support. Elk Grove Village, IL, American Academy of Pediatrics Press, 1989.

Mickell JJ, Ward JD: Monitoring and management of increased intracranial pressure. *In:* Pollack JM, Myer EC (eds): Neurologic Emergencies in Infancy and Childhood, 2nd ed. New York, Raven Press, 1990.

Shoemaker WC, Ayres S, Grenvik A, et al: Textbook of Critical Care, 2nd ed. Philadelphia, WB Saunders, 1989.

MONITORING. Monitoring the critically ill patient to assess current status and anticipate problems is essential to pediatric critical care. These techniques allow collection of information that would not otherwise be available. A given technique should be employed when the benefit of the information gained outweighs the risk to the patient.

Monitoring of the CNS is done clinically by assessments of cognition, consciousness, motor capabilities, posturing, and reflexes (both cranial nerve and peripheral). Special attention is paid to focality. A commonly used screening system is the MGCS (see Table 6–25). Initially designed to predict outcome in head trauma patients 6 hr after injury, it is commonly used in the ICU to assess a patient's overall neurologic status.

Intracranial pressure may be measured with various invasive devices. All present a small risk of infection at the insertion site. Intraventricular catheters offer a monitoring and therapeutic option (drainage of ventricular fluid) if the ventricles have not collapsed. Noninvasive techniques such as measurement of the anterior fontanel pressure have not proven reliable.

Measurements of cerebral blood flow and other parameters of brain metabolism have been made but are currently investigative techniques.

Continual or intermittent measurement of electroencephalographic (EEG) discharge is helpful in patients who are at risk for convulsions or who are undergoing brain depressant therapy with agents such as barbiturates.

Electrocardiographic and respiratory rate monitoring are universal in ICUs and alarms, hard-copy triggers, and dysrhythmia detection and analysis programs are available. The relative infrequency of dysrhythmias in children limits the usefulness of these latter techniques.

Arterial waveforms can be assessed by intra-arterial monitoring. Such waveform analysis may provide information on the intravascular volume status of the patient and may suggest an arterial runoff lesion (e.g., arteriovenous shunts). Arterial lines allow ready access to arterial blood for gas analysis and blood samples, obviating the need for painful arterial or venous punctures (see Sec. 14.14).

Oxygenation may be measured transcutaneously, but this technique is being replaced by measurement of the light absorbance of oxygenated and deoxygenated hemoglobin (pulse oximetry). All noninvasive blood gas techniques must be calibrated against a blood sample but, once calibrated, offer continuous read-outs.

Carbon dioxide tensions in the blood may be measured directly by blood gas analysis. In addition, end-tidal CO_2 ($ETCO_2$), carbon dioxide measured at the end of an exhaled breath, correlates well with arterial PCO_2 in patients with good ventilation-perfusion matching. Changes in $ETCO_2$ may provide an early warning of acute cardiopulmonary changes.

Invasive continuous oxygen saturation and pH catheters are available, but the small size of the pediatric vessels limits their use. Analysis of the partial pressure of oxygen in capillary blood is a poor substitute for arterial blood analysis, although the pH and partial pressure of carbon dioxide from capillary samples may be comparable with those from arterial samples in young infants.

Central venous pressure (CVP) may be measured directly with a catheter. CVP correlation with left ventricular end-diastolic pressure (LVEDP) is unreliable, and central venous blood gases do not reflect true mixed venous (i.e., pulmonary artery) gases. The central venous catheter is most frequently used as a large-bore access to the central circulation.

Right ventricular pressure and pulmonary artery pressure (PAP) may be measured directly with a pulmonary artery catheter. In addition, the pulmonary artery occlusion (wedge) pressure is an approximation of the LVEDP. The LVEDP is related to left ventricular end-diastolic filling volume (LVEDV), so wedge pressure is an approximation of the volume status of the systemic side of the circulation. PAP may be calculated by echocardiography if Doppler technology is added, as may the LVEDV.

Pulmonary artery gas concentrations may only be measured by direct catheterization. Cardiac output may be determined by various techniques. Pulmonary artery catheterization allows cardiac output calculation by measuring indicator (dye or thermal) dilution across the heart. Echocardiographically determined cardiac output is increasingly being used.

6.35 PATTERNS OF PRESENTATION IN CRITICAL CARE

COMA. Coma is always an emergency. It may be caused by diffuse injury to the cerebral cortex or by discrete injury to the reticular activating system. Coma itself is not life-threatening, but is a marker of severe disease affecting the CNS. When a patient presents in coma, primary attention should be directed to determining the presence of other threats to the patient's life (e.g., airway obstruction, apnea, shock, dysrhythmias). Once these have been considered, attention can be given to the CNS. The differential diagnosis of coma involves many factors and is discussed in more detail in Sec. 20.55.

HERNIATION. Herniation of portions of the brain through passages with rigid margins can lead to compression and infarction of brain tissue (see Sec. 20.57). One or more of the following components of the neurologic examination are found to be abnormal during herniation states: level of consciousness (usually depressed), pupils (may be pinpoint and minimally reactive, midposition and nonreactive, or unilaterally or bilaterally dilated and fixed), ocular movements (inability to move one or both eyes laterally or upward), respirations (may be shallow and rapid, Cheyne-Stokes type [see earlier], rapid and deep, irregular, or absent), and gross movements (unilateral or bilateral paresis, plegia, hypertonicity, decerebrate or decorticate posturing). If any of these findings are noted, especially in combination, consideration should be given to measures to reduce intracranial pressure. Immediate and continuing neurologic evaluation is essential.

STATUS EPILEPTICUS. Status epilepticus, or continual, repetitive convulsions without intervening return of consciousness, is a frequently encountered emergency (Sec. 20.23). Continuous seizures may damage neuronal structures and should be terminated. The use of barbiturates, benzodiazapines, and other drugs to stop seizures may make the patient apneic, and thus dependent on respiratory life support. However, this possibility should not deter the clinician from treating seizures aggressively, because respiratory life support is usually easily instituted and is well tolerated by the child. Because the cause of many seizures is self-limited, the period of respiratory life support required may be short.

Although grand mal status is readily recognized, less dramatic variations may occur; staring, coma, paralysis, or tonic deviations of portions of the body may indicate seizures. If in doubt, a trial of an anticonvulsant may be indicated.

CIRCULATORY COLLAPSE (SHOCK). This may be the result of failure of the heart as a pump (cardiogenic shock), vascular obstruction (obstructive shock), the loss of effective blood volume (hypovolemic shock), or a maldistribution of the blood flow (distributive shock). This latter type is most frequently a result of sepsis (septic shock). Shock results from both the effects of the underlying illness and the body's response to the insult.

Shock is a clinical syndrome consisting of poor perfusion (see earlier) and signs of toxicity such as tachycardia, tachypnea, acidosis and, especially in older children, perspiration, cold, clammy skin, and a sense of doom. Hypotension is usually a late finding. Signs of infection (hyperthermia or hypothermia, increased or decreased white blood cell count) are also found in septic shock; some septic shock patients have warm, dry skin.

For cardiogenic shock, augmentation of cardiac muscle performance by direct stimulation and reduction in afterload with vasodilators may improve performance (see Tables 6–27, 6–28, and 6–29). Dysrhythmias require additional support.

Hypovolemic syndromes are reversed by the administration of fluids and by the restoration of an effective circulating blood volume. The choice of fluid is less important than the provision of enough fluid to restore the volume. Patients should be given boluses of 10 mL/kg of a colloid-containing solution or 20 mL/kg of crystalloid solution as quickly as possible. Vital signs and perfusion are then reassessed and the bolus is given again, as necessary. This process is repeated until the patient responds or there are objective signs of intravascular hypervolemia.

Sepsis is treated with careful selection of appropriate antibiotics for the putative infection. Collections of pus, which may serve as a nidus for continuing infection, should also be evacuated. Cardiovascular support agents are usually required.

Early, aggressive treatment of shock with fluids, appropriate antibiotics, cardiovascular support medications, and support of organ system dysfunction can lead to reversal of the shock process and recovery. More severe cases may develop a *multiple organ failure syndrome* (MOFS), an ill-defined but malignant, progressive deterioration of body functions that frequently follows sepsis or other pansystemic insults. *Adult respiratory distress syndrome* (ARDS) is the pulmonary component of MOFS. ARDS is pathologically similar to infantile respiratory distress syndrome and represents damage to the terminal alveolar capillary unit, resulting in accumulation of fluid, electrolytes, and protein in the interstitium of the lung. Ventilation-perfusion abnormalities follow and cause hypoxia. See Sec. 14.79. The development of MOFS is ominous. Mortality in patients who develop ARDS is approximately 60%, although only a few deaths are a result of lung disease; the remainder succumb to other organ system dysfunction.

Upper airway failure results from obstruction, which may occur above the glottis (usually bacterial supraglottitis, rarely diphtheria), at the glottis (usually a foreign body, but also various congenital and acquired lesions), or below the glottis (usually viral laryngotracheobronchitis, but now also bacterial tracheitis; Sec. 14.44). The patient presents with noisy breathing and varying degrees of decreased air movement. Gasping is an ominous sign. Treatment of airway failure involves removal of the offending agent or bypassing the airway, as outlined previously (see also Sec. 14.17).

Lower airway failure is usually caused by asthma (see Sec. 11.41), or bronchiolitis (see Sec. 14.54). The clinical presentation is of wheezing and respiratory distress. Blood gas abnormalities, especially carbon dioxide retention, are common. Respiratory failure is present when the P_{CO_2} stays above 55 mm Hg (see Sec. 14.17). The treatment of status asthmaticus (asthma unresponsive to initial therapy) consists of the administration of oxygen to correct hypoxia, fluids to correct dehydration, and β_2-sympathomimetics and theophylline to break bronchospasm (see Sec. 14.41). Sympathomimetics may be administered by the inhalation route if sufficient air is being moved by the patient to deliver the medication to the distal airways. In asthmatic patients in the ICU this is frequently not the case, and parenteral sympathomimetics must be used. Continuous infusions may be necessary. Corticosteroids and inhalation of atropine are recommended, and treatment of infection is an important adjunct. Mechanical ventilation is rarely necessary but, when used, differs from conventional ventilation. Because of delayed emptying of the lungs, very low ventilator rates with long expiratory times are used.

METABOLIC COLLAPSE. This may be caused by various insults, such as intoxications (e.g., ethanol, methanol, ethylene glycol, carbon monoxide, salicylate), diabetic ketoacidosis, liver or kidney failure, tissue infarction (e.g., dead bowel), or an inborn error of metabolism. The usual presentation is one of alterations in vital signs (e.g., tachypnea, hyperpnea, tachycardia, altered mentation). Treatment consists of correction of the acidosis with alkali (sodium bicarbonate, 1–2 mEq/kg) while searching for the cause.

The poisoned child presents with one or more of the following symptoms: CNS hyperactivity (agitation, seizures) or hypoactivity (obtundation or coma), which may be caused by many agents, including those causing hypoxia; metabolic acidosis, especially in patients with an increased anion gap; cardiac dysrhythmias (especially tricyclic antidepressants); and gastrointestinal irritation (nausea, vomiting, cramps, diarrhea, or burns of lips, mouth, and esophagus from ingestion of a caustic substance). Treatment is aimed at support of vital functions while a precise diagnosis is made (see Sec. 26.4). With such an approach fatalities resulting from such ingestion are rare in patients who arrive to the ICU alive.

PETER R. HOLBROOK

Holbrook P: Issues in Airway Management. Crit Care Clin 4:789, 1988.

Plum F, Posner JB: Diagnosis of Stupor and Coma. Philadelphia, FA Davis, 1980.

Zaritsky A, Eisenberg MG: Ontogenetic considerations in the pharmacotherapy of shock. *In:* Chernow B, Shoemaker WC (eds): Critical Care: State of the Art, Vol. 7. Fullerton, CA, Society of Critical Care Medicine Press, 1986.

Zimmerman JJ, Dietrich KA: Current perspectives on septic shock. Pediatr Clin North Am 34:131, 1987.

6.36 DROWNING AND NEAR-DROWNING

Drowning is death from suffocation by submersion in water; severe asphyxia results from respiratory obstruction, with or without the aspiration of water. Death may be immediate or may follow unsuccessful resuscitation. Successful resuscitation, termed *near-drowning,* is the complete or temporary survival following a submersion incident. The victim may later die (termed *near-drowning with delayed death*) or may recover completely or partially. Fortunately, for each near-drowned child who later dies, there are four who survive, and most (92%) make a complete recovery.

Most drownings are accidental: infants drown in bathtubs; inadequately attended toddlers drown in swimming pools; small children fall into ponds, streams, and flooded excavations; accomplished swimmers overestimate their endurance; occupants of pleasure boats fall overboard without life jackets; and the incautious of all ages plunge through thin ice.

INCIDENCE. Annually, approximately 140,000 people die worldwide from drowning. In the United States, there are about 7,000 deaths/yr, with a higher proportion of males than females and of nonwhites than whites. Over half the victims are children, adolescents, and young adults (younger than 25 yr old), and nearly half of these drownings occur in creeks, rivers, and other bodies of water.

The highest incidence (in those younger than 25 yr) occcurs in the 1- to 4-yr age group, and the bathtub is the site in almost 20% of cases. Bathtub drownings most often occur to children unsupervised at the time of the accident and, particularly, to those 10- to 12-mo old who are the youngest or next to youngest members of larger families. Swimming pools are the site of the highest death rates for children 1–3 yr old, and in about three fourths of the drownings, the children were unsupervised in a pool having no fence around it. The incidence of drownings and near-drownings could be decreased, especially in this group, if all swimming pools were required to be enclosed on all four sides by a fence with a self-latching gate. In addition, parents need to be taught that young children should never swim or bathe unsupervised.

PATHOPHYSIOLOGY. Drowning is characterized by increasing hypoxemia affecting all organs and tissues, the severity of which is determined by the *duration of submersion,* the presence of *pulmonary aspiration,* and by the *individual's responses.*

The duration of submersion is critical because arterial oxygen tension falls exponentially during asphyxia. The maximum submersion period before irreversible damage occurs is uncertain, although it is probably usually 3–5 min. However, cases have been reported of prolonged submersion (10–40 min) with complete recovery, especially of children in cold water who developed acute hypothermia. Although full recovery is rare after more than 20 min submersion, resuscitation should always be attempted.

Pulmonary aspiration, which occurs in 80–90% of all cases, may have profound effects. The near-drowned patient's subsequent course depends on the nature, composition, and amount of aspirate, which includes such variables as sea water or fresh water, cold water or warm water, pathogenic bacteria or fungi, toxic chemicals, mud and vegetable matter, and gastric contents. Aspirated sea water produces hypoxia by mechanisms that differ from those of fresh water. Because sea water is hypertonic (approximately 3% saline), body fluid is initially drawn into the alveoli, producing hypoxia. In contrast, aspirated hypotonic fresh water alters the surface tension properties of pulmonary surfactant, resulting in unstable alveoli, which become atelectatic, thus producing intrapulmonary shunting and hypoxemia. In both types, pulmonary insufficiency with intrapulmonary shunting and ventilation-perfusion mismatching occurs, lung compliance decreases, dead space to tidal volume ratio increases, and airway resistance increases.

Of greater immediate consequence is systemic absorption of the aspirated water and its temperature and volume. In drowning animals, aspirated cold fresh water is rapidly absorbed and can produce significant "core" cooling (including cerebral hypothermia) prior to circulatory arrest. This process, "acute submersion hypothermia," may delay the onset of irreversible damage, making complete recovery possible despite prolonged submersion. Aspirated cold sea water is less likely to be rapidly absorbed and cause such profound central cooling, although the lung may function as a heat exchanger. Alternatively, humans who hyperventilate when submerged in icy water may have massive absorption and movement of cold water into their circulation; they may drown immediately from severe intravascular hemolysis with hyperkalemic circulatory arrest or from acute core hypothermia with unconsciousness or ventricular fibrillation. More commonly, aspiration of smaller volumes occurs and may produce mild hemolysis with hematuria and possible renal failure.

The volume of fresh water aspirated during a brief period of submerged respiration can exceed 100 mL/kg body weight, and Swann showed that the blood volume could increase up to 10 times in dogs submerged for 2–3 min.

The water load may be exacerbated by administering large volumes of fluid during resuscitation, producing excessive third-space fluid and late complications. Regardless of large fluid shifts during drowning, no clinically significant electrolyte changes are present within 15 min of successful resuscitation.

The acute aspiration of as little as 2.2 mL/kg of water produces a profound decrease in arterial oxygen tension and, after aspiration of 11 mL/kg of fresh water or sea water, the Pa_{O_2} consistently drops to values of 30–40 mm Hg and remains depressed for at least 72 hr in survivors. In the recovery phase, there may be hypoxia during room air breathing that was not evident during oxygen breathing, suggesting persistent areas of ventilation-perfusion mismatching. The Pa_{CO_2} initially increases following aspiration in experimental animals but rapidly returns to normal as hyperventilation supervenes; measurements of Pa_{CO_2} in human near-drowning victims are variable. Carbon dioxide levels may be elevated by hypoventilation but rapidly return to normal with increased spontaneous or mechanical ventilation, indicating no barrier to the elimination of carbon dioxide. In the late recovery period, pulmonary function returns to normal and lung sequelae are rare.

Pulmonary damage may be exacerbated by inhaled irritating chemicals, virulent microorganisms, and mud or other vegetative material. In addition, near-drowned victims may swallow large volumes of fluid, develop gastric distention, and then regurgitate, which accounts for the water often seen issuing from the mouth after rescue. Stomach contents are aspirated in nearly 25% of cases, especially during cardiopulmonary resuscitation (CPR).

Aspiration does not occur in about 10% of drownings and 12% of near-drownings. These drowning victims die acutely from breath-holding, laryngospasm, or cardiac arrhythmias. Near-drowning victims who do not aspirate develop severe hypoxia and hypercarbia, but if rescued and given artificial ventilation prior to circulatory arrest, they usually recover completely.

All body organ systems are affected by progressive hypoxemia and hypercarbia. However, the primary responses of the central nervous and cardiovascular systems while the victim is submerged are of greatest importance. Initially, panic and anxiety with breath-holding occur, followed by swallowing and loss of consciousness. Subjective sensations are rarely reported because of retrograde amnesia in severe cases. Later, involuntary respiration usually occurs, followed by apnea from medullary depression. In animals, initially there is tachycardia followed after a minute or so by extreme hypertension (presumably the result of endogenous catecholamine release) with reflex bradycardia. Increasing cardiac irregularities follow, and within 3–5 min the circulation suddenly fails, secondary to myocardial hypoxia (producing "pulselessness"). The heart continues to beat briefly, but effective perfusion is absent, and successful resuscitation rapidly becomes impossible. In humans, without significant core hypothermia, a similar narrow margin exists between the onset of pulselessness and the inability to resuscitate. With cardiac arrest, total ischemia-anoxia supervenes and multiple organ failure results.

PATHOLOGY. Post mortem changes after drowning are nonspecific. Cutis anserina (goose flesh), water wrinkling of the skin of the hands and feet, pale or sanguineous water foam from the nose and mouth, and vomitus and aquatic debris in the respiratory tract are common. The lungs may be irregularly congested and hyperinflated. Inhaled water interacts with mucus present in small airways to produce copious amounts of froth, which obstruct the exit of alveolar air. Microscopic sections show varying degrees of alveolar distention, edematous protein precipitate, infiltrates, and focal intralveolar hemorrhage. In forensic medicine, the findings of diatoms, flagellates, or algae in the lung establish death by drowning.

The whole brain of drowning victims always looks swollen, but in delayed death after near-drowning its microscopic appearance varies with the degree of anoxia and duration of survival. With early death, edema and anoxic perivascular hemorrhages may be the only changes. In late death from near-drowning with prolonged and severe hypoxia, the changes may progress to cystic degeneration of the basal ganglia or midbrain. The heart usually appears normal, but some left ventricular dilation may occur. The liver, spleen, and kidneys appear congested, and the stomach may contain swallowed fluid.

CLINICAL MANIFESTATIONS. Clinical death at the time of rescue does not always signify biologic death, especially in hypothermic children. Because such patients may have a good prognosis, substantial efforts to resuscitate are justified, despite the difficulties of restarting a cold, anoxic heart. After successful resuscitation, cardiac irregularities and low output are rare, unless severe hypoxia and metabolic acidosis persist as a result of prolonged submersion. Pulmonary edema frequently occurs in the immediate postresuscitation period secondary to increased capillary permeability from anoxia, massive fluid overload, or myocardial failure. Severe pulmonary infection associated with aspiration is a common complication requiring vigorous respiratory care. Later, CNS dysfunction may become obvious as the result of cerebral hypoxia, ischemia, or both. Cerebral edema rarely develops; brain perfusion and cellular integrity may be further compromised by intracranial hypertension.

The ambient water temperature may play an important role in the clinical course of a marine accident victim, especially at the extremes of temperature. Studies of unprotected subjects exposed to cold water have shown the relentless development of immersion hypothermia, starting with surface cooling and leading to death from hypothermia and/or drowning. Investigations of animal drowning in cold fresh water have shown that massive aspiration can cause immediate core cooling, termed "acute submersion hypothermia." This latter mechanism can prevent brain damage despite prolonged submersion in cold water, and this argues for initiating and continuing resuscitation in such cases. At the other extreme, the increasing use of hot tubs and Jacuzzis has resulted in infants and toddlers drowning in hot water. Reported cases suggest that the submersion time resulting in irreversible brain damage in these children is much reduced from the generally accepted 3- to 5-min period in warm water. Near-drowning victims may also develop massive gram-negative pneumonia from aspiration of warm water.

TREATMENT. Following rescue, and unless contraindicated, immediate resuscitation at the scene is recommended for all children. Delay in treatment should be avoided, even though usually the duration of submersion is uncertain, the water temperature is unknown, the clinical-biologic state is equivocal, and accurate predictors of the victim's future course are nonexistent. Occasional unexpected recovery occurs and there is, therefore, an ethical obligation to initiate resuscitative measures. Decisions regarding the continuation of treatment should be made subsequently in the intensive care unit (Sec. 6.33 and 6.34).

Therefore, if the patient is apneic, mouth-to-mouth ventilation should begin at once and be replaced as soon as possible with positive-pressure ventilation. Closed-chest massage should be added to ventilatory support if effective circulation is not present. CPR should be maintained continuously during transport to the hospital (see Sec. 6.32). If the patient was diving into water, near-drowning may be complicated by injury to the head or cervical spine, and care must be taken to maintain the neck in a neutral position. In the emergency room, routine resuscitative measures usually include intravenous administration of sodium bicarbonate, because severe metabolic acidosis is common. Measurement of core temperature and assessment for neurologic classification (Table 6–30) are valuable for prognostic purposes.

All patients with a history of significant submersion, even though asymptomatic, should be admitted to the hospital and observed for at least 24 hr, because of the risk of pulmonary insufficiency, infection, and neurologic depression.

Subsequent respiratory and circulatory support should be appropriate to the patient's condition. If the patient is alert and ventilating adequately to clear carbon dioxide, CPAP may be applied to the airway using a tight-fitting mask to increase functional residual capacity and to prevent alveoli from collapsing. A nasogastric tube should be inserted and the face observed for pressure points. CPAP should be titrated to the level at which the least intrapulmonary shunt occurs without harmful effects on cardiovascular function. If hypovolemia is present, CPAP, particularly at high levels, may decrease cardiac output and increase the need for circulatory support. Withdrawal from CPAP should be in decremental steps; sudden discontinuation of CPAP or of routine suctioning may result in significant deterioration of oxygenation. If the patient cannot maintain a normal $Paco_2$, if respirations are labored, or if the Pao_2 does not significantly improve, the trachea should be intubated and intermittent mandatory ventilation (IMV) should be provided at the rate determined by the arterial pH and Pco_2. If hypotension or low output exists or recurs, the use of inotropes and volume expanders is indicated (Sec. 6.35).

If the patient is comatose, additional intensive care measures are required (Sec. 6.34). Intubation is necessary to protect the airway and to provide ventilatory support as indicated by the arterial blood gases. Maintaining a $Paco_2$ of less than 30 mm Hg and a Pao_2 of greater than 55 mm Hg may diminish the development of cerebral edema. The patient's inability to maintain an adequate arterial oxygen tension at inspired oxygen concentrations of less than 40% necessitates aggressive ventilatory therapy, which may include mechanical ventilation with PEEP and respiratory paralysis.

Nebulized isoproterenol, racemic epinephrine, or intravenous aminophylline may be useful if bronchospasm is present. Occasionally, diuretics may also be beneficial in mobilizing interstitial pulmonary edema, but they must be used cautiously in the hypovolemic patient. Inotropic agents and plasma in large amounts may be necessary to maintain perfusion. Bronchoscopy is indicated only if food or solid material has been aspirated. Decompressing gastric dilatation with a nasogastric tube decreases the risk of regurgitation and aspiration and also may improve ventilation by decreasing intra-abdominal pressure. Prophylactic use of corticosteroids or antibiotics is not recommended.

Only after the circulation has remained stable for several hours following resuscitation should diuretics be given. Usually, maintenance fluid is decreased for several days. However, with sea water aspiration, large amounts of protein may be lost through the lungs, and colloid replacement may be indicated. Pulmonary edema after aspirating fresh or sea water may cause the loss of large volumes of fluid into the lung, which requires circulatory replacement. Pulmonary edema may also occur secondary to congestive heart failure and require fluid and pharmacologic management (see Sec. 15.73 and 14.78), as well as PEEP. Significant electrolyte imbalances, coagulopathy, or anemia should be appropriately diagnosed and corrected.

Near-drowning may precipitate multiple organ system failure. Therefore, appropriate cardiopulmonary, renal, and central nervous system monitoring is required. The initial chest roentgenogram may be relatively clear even in the presence of extreme hypoxia, particularly after aspiration of fresh water. Atelectasis, shock lung (see Sec. 6.35 and 14.79), pneumothorax (see Sec. 14.91), and pneumomediastinum (see Sec. 14.92) may occur. Associated injuries, such as those of the spinal cord and intracranial bleeding, should also be ruled out.

Intracranial pressure monitoring and treatment with hyperventilation, muscle relaxants, diuretics, mannitol infusion, hypothermia, and barbiturates have been used to prevent subsequent anoxic and ischemic injury to the brain. The risks and benefits of these therapies are controversial and they should not be used routinely.

PROGNOSIS. The mortality rate for children admitted to the hospital following a near-drowning incident approximates 20%; most deaths occur in the first few days from cardiopulmonary failure. Among the survivors, the most serious sequela is neurologic damage, the reported incidence of which ranges from 0 to 21%. Although no prospective studies on the subject exist, retrospective studies suggest that those who are awake at the scene of rescue, or unconscious at the scene but fully awake on arrival at the emergency room (even after CPR), did not suffer serious neurologic sequelae (see Table 6–30). The results seem similar for patients with a blunted level of consciousness (e.g., lethargic, semicomatose, agitated, confused, or combative on arrival at the hospital). In these groups, treatment consisted of cardiopulmonary support without aggressive cerebral resuscitation. In contrast, patients comatose on arrival at the hospital who required appropriate cardiopulmonary support were found to have nearly a 50% survival rate without brain damage, whether treated with only mild hyperventilation and steroids or with aggressive hyperventilation, fluid restriction, hyperoxia, steroids, muscle paralysis, and barbiturate coma. Aggressive treatment may decrease morbidity and mortality in those with decorticate or decerebrate signs but, in general, severe anoxic injury occurs in the flaccid comatose patient, in those submerged for more

TABLE 6–30. Fresh Water Drowning and Near-Drowning (1970–1982), Hospital for Sick Children, Toronto

Neurologic Category	Total No. of Cases	Results: *Dead*	*Abnormal CNS*	*Normal*
A (Awake)	56	0	0	56 (100%)
B (Blunted)	19	1 (5.5%)	0	18 (94.5%)
C (Comatose)	65	25 (38.5%)	9 (13.8%)	31 (47.7%)
Total no. of cases	140	26 (18.6%)	9 (6.4%)	105 (75%)

than 6 min in warm water, in those requiring cardiopulmonary resuscitation in the emergency room, or in those needing continual mechanical ventilation. Rarely, following cold water drowning, hypothermic children who appeared clinically dead have recovered completely.

A. W. CONN

Biggart MJ, Bohn DJ: Effect of hypothermia and cardiac arrest on outcome of near drowning accidents in children. J Pediatr 117:179, 1990.
Conn AW, Barker GA: Fresh water drowning and near-drowning. Can Anaesth Soc J 31:S38, 1984.
Conn AW, Bunegin L, Gelineau J, et al: Acute submersion hypothermia in dogs. *In:* Laursen GA, Pozos RS, Hendel FG (eds): Human Performance in the Cold. Bethesda, MD, Undersea Medical Society, 1986.
Conn AW, Montes JE, Barker GA, et al: Cerebral salvage in near-drowning following neurological classification by triage. Can Anaesth Soc J 27:201, 1980.
Golden FStC, Rivers JF: The immersion incident. Anaesthesia 30:364, 1975.
Modell JH, Graves SA, Kuck EJ: Near-drowning: Correlation of level of consciousness and survival. Can Anaesth Soc J 27:211, 1980.
Peterson B: Morbidity of childhood near-drowning. Pediatrics 29:364, 1977.
Swann HG, Spafford NR: Body salt and water changes during fresh and sea water drowning. Tex Rep Biol Med 9:356, 1981.

6.37 BURN INJURIES

Burns are a result of the effects of thermal injury on skin and other tissues. Human skin can tolerate temperatures up to 42–44° C (107–111° F) for relatively long periods, but temperatures above this level produce a logarithmic increase in tissue destruction. The degree of tissue damage correlates with both the temperature and duration of exposure to the heat source. The skin of newborns and infants is more susceptible to tissue damage than that of older children or adults. At relatively low temperatures (lower than 45° C) the resulting changes are reversible but, when the temperature exceeds 45° C (113° F), protein denaturation exceeds the capability for cellular repair. Clinically, burns are classified as 1st, 2nd, 3rd, or 4th degree, according to the depth of tissue injured.

In 1st-degree burns, such as sunburn, only the epithelium is involved. These are characterized solely by pain and redness. The injured cells peel away within a few days, leaving a totally healed base without scarring.

In 2nd-degree burns the epithelium and part of the corium are destroyed, but dermal appendages from which re-epithelialization may occur are spared. Depending on the extent of vertical damage, 2nd-degree burns are best subclassified as superficial or deep partial-thickness burns. Unless optimal conditions for preservation of dermal elements and epidermal appendages are present, deep partial-thickness burns may convert to full-thickness necrosis.

In 3rd-degree burns the entire thickness of the dermis is destroyed, and healing can only occur by the ingrowth of epithelium from the margins of the wound or by grafting of skin from nonburned areas of the body.

In 4th-degree burns the injury extends to subjacent tissues such as subcutaneous fat, fascia, muscle, or bone. Closure of such wounds may necessitate, in addition to grafting, local or regional flaps for definitive coverage.

Burns are also classified according to the extent of the injury as mild (less than 10%), moderate (10–30%), or severe (greater than 30%). Morbidity and mortality increase with increasing extent and depth of the burn. In children, hospitalization is usually recommended for burns exceeding 10% of the body surface or whenever the injury involves the face, hands, feet, and/or genitalia.

INCIDENCE. Approximately 2 million patients receive medical attention, 100,000 are hospitalized, and 7,800 die each year in the United States because of burn injuries. Fires produce the 2nd highest death rate worldwide and the highest among industrialized nations. Burns are the 2nd leading cause of nonvehicular accidental deaths; 30% of these deaths occur in children under 15 yr old. Among children aged 1–4 yr burns are the leading cause of accidental death in the home, secondary only to vehicular injuries. Among children 5–14 yr, burns are the 3rd leading cause of accidental deaths.

ETIOLOGY. The young, the elderly, and the socioeconomically disadvantaged are at increased risk for burn injuries. Almost all burns in children occur in the home during waking hours. The major vectors of heat energy are hot liquids and solids, flammable fabrics, volatile flammable liquids, and domestic dwellings. Combustible materials are most commonly ignited by matches, poorly guarded space heaters, kitchen ranges, or water heaters. Scalds are the leading cause of burn injuries during the first 3 yr of life and are usually limited to small areas of the body. Chemical burns are rare and usually benign, except for those involving the esophagus (see Sec. 26.10). Burns resulting from the ignition of combustible materials are most common in older children and the resultant injuries are usually extensive and life-threatening.

PREVENTION. Preventing burn injuries requires educating the public about potential risks and ways to avoid them, regulating product safety, and attenuating the vectors of heat energy and their ignitors through technologic advances. Common strategies to prevent burns by controlling the source and expenditure of energy are outlined in Table 6–31. Physicians have a major responsibility for educating parents and for encouraging appropriate legislative controls. For example, physicians strongly supported the passage of federal regulation regarding the flammability of childrens' sleepwear, which considerably reduced the hazard of burn injury from flammable garments. Similar efforts are being made to regulate the maximum temperature of home water heaters and the ignition and burning power of cigarettes and matches.

PATHOPHYSIOLOGY. Hemodynamic, autonomic, cardiopulmonary, renal, and metabolic disturbances develop rapidly following severe burns. Within seconds of injury cardiac output decreases, presumably because of exaggerated reflex responses and decreased venous return. Myocardial contractility is not affected at this time. A plasma factor that depresses myocardial contractility has been isolated from severely burned animals and humans during the latter stages of shock, but its significance remains poorly understood.

Soon after injury the permeability of the entire vascular tree increases; this is accompanied by the loss of water, electrolytes, and proteins from the vascular compartment into the interstitium of injured and noninjured tissues. Animal studies

TABLE 6–31. Prevention of Burn Injuries

General Principles	Examples of Application to Burns
Prevent marshaling of latent energy	Do not store gasoline in the home
Reduce the amount of marshaled energy	Reduce temperature of bath or shower water
Modify the rate at which energy can propagate	Use flame-retardant fabrics
Separate the energy from the susceptible structure in time or space	Locate water heaters away from flammable liquids
Separate by interposition of a barrier	Use safeguards for space heaters
Strengthen the structure that might be damaged by energy	Apply more stringent building and fireproofing codes
Detect the danger and counter its rapid continuation and extension	Use fire alarms, sprinkler systems, fire extinguishers

suggest that in the injured skin this effect is maximal 30 min after the burn, but capillary integrity is not restored until 8–12 hr after injury. In noninjured tissues only mild and transient leaks occur, even when the total burn extends to 40% of the body surface.

Within minutes following a substantial burn the renal plasma flow and GFR decrease. Oliguria develops and tubular function is at least transiently compromised. Increased secretion of antidiuretic hormone and aldosterone further contributes to reduced urine formation; tubular reabsorption of sodium is stimulated, excretion of potassium is enhanced, and the urine is maximally concentrated. This antidiuresis is most prominent during the 1st 12–24 hr after the burn, but it may persist for several days.

Destruction of red blood cells in the period immediately after a burn seldom exceeds 10% of circulating erythrocytes. Additional losses may occur, however, in the ensuing days, as partly damaged cells are lysed and blood is lost from granulation tissues. Thus, anemia is likely to develop within 4–7 days of major burn injuries.

TREATMENT

Emergency Management of Severe Burns. It is imperative that care be administered in an orderly fashion (Table 6–32). First, the adequacy of the airway should be established, especially in a child with facial burns or one who has inhaled smoke. A rapid assessment is then made that includes the following: (1) inspection of the wounds; (2) assessment of the cardiorespiratory status; and (3) evaluation of previously unrecognized injuries. An intravenous infusion is started to expand the blood volume. Lactated Ringer's solution, isotonic saline, or plasma may be infused at a rate of 20 mL/kg/hr until more accurate estimates of fluid requirements have been made.

The stomach is emptied with a nasogastric tube to prevent gastric dilatation, vomiting, or aspiration of stomach contents. A urinary catheter is then inserted so that output can be monitored.

Because the quantities of fluids and medications to be administered depend on the size of the patient and the extent of injury, the weight and length of the patient should be measured carefully and the areas of total body surface and burned surface should be estimated. Weight is measured before dressings, bedclothes, or restraints are applied. The wounds are cleansed and debrided, their depth assessed, and the extent of 2nd- and 3rd-degree burns estimated by using body surface charts corrected for age (Fig. 6–14). The wounds should then be covered with dressings saturated with an antimicrobial agent. In addition, circumferential 3rd-degree burns should be identified and escharotomies performed to prevent the ischemia of distal limbs and respiratory embarrassment from chest wall involvement.

If there are no injuries to the central nervous system, sedatives may be given, preferably by the intravenous route. Respiratory depressants should be avoided.

For analgesia, morphine (0.05–0.1 mg/kg of body weight may be given; however, once the wounds are dressed, Valium (5 mg/m^2 of body surface/dose/6–8 hr) is usually sufficient to control pain and anxiety.

Tetanus toxoid and parenteral benzathine penicillin are indicated for prophylaxis against tetanus and β-hemolytic streptococcal infections, respectively. Passive protection with tetanus immunoglobulin (TIG) is indicated only when the patient has received one or no previous injection of tetanus toxoid. The recommended dose for TIG is 250–500 units intramuscularly.

Fluid, Electrolyte, and Colloid Therapy During the 1st 24 Hr. The primary goal of fluid resuscitation during the first 24 hr after the burn is restoration of the patient's volume and electrolyte homeostasis while simultaneously minimizing the degree of organ dysfunction and edema formation. This is achieved by replacing antecedent and concurrent deficits of fluid, electrolytes, and proteins. In addition, therapy should anticipate and replace maintenance fluid and electrolyte requirements before significant deficits develop.

The specific aims of fluid management are to attain and maintain a normal or near-normal state of hydration in all body fluid compartments; to correct acid-base imbalance; and to restore cardiovascular, pulmonary, and renal hemodynamics. Restoration and maintenance of perfusion pressures should lead to maximal oxygenation of injured and noninjured tissues, which promotes spontaneous healing, prevents wound conversion, minimizes bacterial colonization, and prepares the injured areas for early grafting.

Rehydration should be accomplished without overloading the circulation, preferably over a period of 24 hr. Attempts to replace deficits over a shorter period are usually fraught with multiple complications, including excessive edema formation, and should be discouraged. Restoration of fluid and electrolyte homeostasis and organ function, however, does not imply a return to normal of all physiologic variables. Oliguria, for example, may persist for 48 to 72 hr or even longer after the burn because of excessive secretion of antidiuretic hormone (ADH). Cardiac output, generally low during the first 24 hr despite aggressive resuscitation, may increase beyond preburn levels after the first 24 hr and a state of hypercatabolism may persist for several days after the burn. Thus, the physician's expectations should take into consideration not only the physiologic make-up of the child, which differs significantly from that of the adult, but also the specific responses of various organs to the burn injury.

During the immediate postburn period, errors in fluid therapy may have grave consequences. Underhydration can

TABLE 6–32. Priorities of Medical Procedures in the Emergency Phase of Burn Injuries

Procedure	Indication	Comment
Establish an adequate airway	Burns of the face Laryngeal edema Smoke inhalation	Avoid emergency tracheostomy
Examine for trauma to head, skeleton, or nervous system	Explosions	Remove clothing; radiologic examination helpful
Begin intravenous infusion	To prevent intravascular dehydration	Use isotonic fluids
Empty stomach through a nasogastric tube	To prevent gastric dilatation, vomiting, or aspiration	Antacids may be helpful
Insert an indwelling urinary catheter	To monitor hourly urine output	Use a closed drainage system
Examine the burn wound	To estimate depth and extent	Use burn charts corrected for age
Clean, debride, and dress the burn area	To minimize microbial colonization	Use topical antimicrobial therapy
Administer medications	To treat infections; to prevent tetanus; for sedation	Use intravenous route for sedation
Begin fluid, electrolyte, and protein replacement	To correct antecedent deficits and concurrent losses	Use appropriate formula to estimate requirements

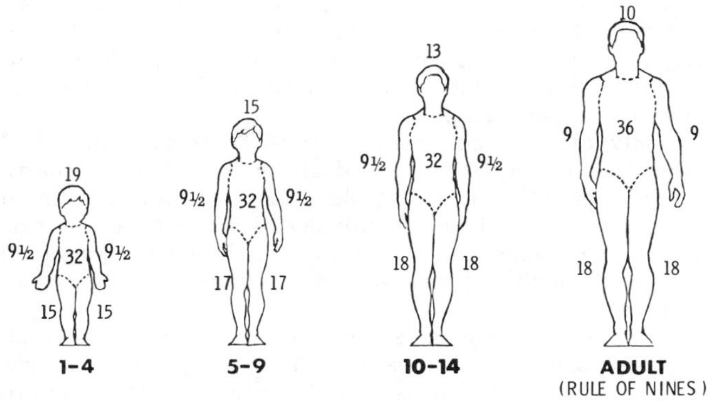

Figure 6–14. Burn assessment chart. Numbers under the figures indicate age; the others indicate the percentage of body surface. (Body proportions modified from Lund CL, Brower NC: The estimation of areas of burns. Surg Gynecol Obstet 79:352, 1944.)

prolong the state of shock, worsen metabolic acidosis, and induce organ dysfunction; overhydration fosters edema formation and pulmonary congestion. Accurate prediction of fluid requirements is especially difficult, because most formulas for the fluid therapy of burn victims were designed for adults. These formulas are based only on body weight and on the percentage of body surface burned, and make no separate allowances for maintenance fluids and the fluid needed to replace burn-related losses; consequently, they tend to underhydrate small children and to overestimate the fluid requirements of the large or obese child. Similar errors can also be committed at the extremes of burn size. Because of these and other reasons, the use of a "single-figure" formula, such as the Parkland or the modified Brooke formula, is not recommended for hydration of burned children.

Compared to adults, children, and particularly infants, have high rates of heat exchange relative to their size and weight, high rates of water exchange in relation to total body water, and significant differences in muscle water and electrolyte composition. Children also require relatively larger volumes of urine for excretion of waste products and insensible water losses, when expressed in terms of body weight, are significantly greater than those in adults. Therefore, calculating fluid and electrolyte requirements on the basis of body surface area offers greater accuracy, consistency, and simplicity.

When these concepts are applied to managing the burned child, the quantity of fluids to administer during the 1st 24 hr after the burn can be estimated as follows:

2,000 mL/m^2 of body surface/24 hr
plus
5,000 mL/m^2 of body surface *burned*/24 hr

Half of this amount should be administered during the 1st 8 hr and the other half during the subsequent 16 hr. No ceiling for burn size is used. Fluid received prior to arrival at a center for definitive care should be reviewed and appropriate adjustments made.

For example, a 4-yr-old boy having a body surface area of 0.68 m^2 sustained 3rd-degree burns to approximately 40% of his body surface. Despite having received 200 mL of lactated Ringer solution during the 1st hr, after the injury he appeared dehydrated on admission.

1. Fluids received during the initial evaluation period (lactated Ringer, saline, or plasma) need not be included in the calculation of requirements for the 1st 24 hr. These fluids may be given at a rate of approximately 20 mL/kg/hr for 1–2 hr.
2. Calculation of 1st 24 hr requirements:

2,000 mL/m^2 of body surface/24 hr

The boy's body surface area is 0.68 m^2, so

$$2{,}000 \times 0.68 = 1{,}360 \text{ mL/24 hr}$$

plus

5,000 mL/m^2 of body surface burned/24 hr

In this case the body surface burned is 40% of body surface. Therefore,

$$5{,}000 \times 0.68 \times 0.4 = 1{,}360 \text{ mL/24 hr}$$

The total requirement for the 1st 24 hr (maintenance plus burn replacement) is

$$1{,}360 \text{ mL} + 1{,}360 \text{ mL} = 2{,}720 \text{ mL}$$

3. Half of the estimated amount (2,720 mL) is given during the 1st 8 hr and half during the subsequent 16 hr:

Thus, in this example the rate of fluid administration during the 1st 8 hr is 170 mL/hr (8 hr × 170 mL/hr = 1,360 mL), and 85 mL/hr (8 hr × 85 mL/hr = 680 mL) during the 2nd and 3rd 8 hour periods for a total of 2720 mL for the first 24 hr.

Although this method offers definite advantages in children, it still provides only reasonable estimates of the quantities of fluid needed for the first 24 hr. Successful fluid resuscitation of the burned child requires not only the use of an appropriate formula but also a clear understanding of the fluid therapy *program* as a whole, which includes the following:

1. Burn charts, properly corrected for age, to assess the extent of the injury (see Fig. 6–14)
2. Careful measurement of height and weight to estimate surface area from standard nomograms (see Figs. 27–1 and 27–2)
3. Accurate prediction of fluid requirements using the surface area formula
4. An appropriate hydrating solution
5. Well-defined guidelines to monitor the state of hydration

Choice of Hydrating Solutions. The composition of fluids to be used for resuscitation is controversial. Over the years, various solutions such as plasma and saline, dextrose, lactated Ringer, and hypertonic saline have been proposed. The major issue is whether the initial use of crystalloid or colloid-containing solutions improves the outcome of severe burns. Although this question remains unanswered, evidence now suggests that leakage of albumin from the intravascular to the interstitial spaces is a short-lived phenomenon, lasting 8–12 hr, and of significance only for the 1st 6 hr after the burn; that the addition of albumin to resuscitation fluids reduces fluid requirements and consequently edema formation; that the addition of 12.5 g of albumin/L of fluid given during the 1st 24 hr prevents the development of hypoalbuminemia and its consequences; and that isotonic solutions containing 130–135 mEq/L of sodium and 20–30 mEq/L of bicarbonate or lactate maintain serum osmolality and electrolytes within normal limits, and promptly correct any underlying metabolic acidosis. Thus, for resuscitation of the burned child, an isotonic salt solution containing albumin, lactate or bicarbonate, and adequate quantities of carbohydrate (e.g., 5% glucose) are recommended to provide a protein-sparing effect. Such solutions can be prepared by adding 12.5 g of human serum albumin (50 mL of 25% solution) to 950 mL of lactated Ringer in 5% dextrose. The final composition of the mixture is as follows: sodium, 132 mEq/L; chloride, 109 mEq/L; lactate, 28 mEq/L; potassium, 4 mEq/L; glucose, 47.5 g/L; and albumin, 12.5 g/L.

For infants less than 1 yr of age the concentration of sodium in the hydrating fluids should be decreased to avoid hypernatremia. Thus, this recommended mixture includes 930 mL of 5% dextrose in 0.3% sodium chloride solution with 20 mL of sodium bicarbonate (1 mEq/mL) and 50 mL of 25% human serum albumin. The final composition of this mixture is as follows: sodium, 77 mEq/L; chloride, 57 mEq/L; bicarbonate, 20 mEq/L; glucose, 46.5 g/L; and albumin, 12.5 mg/L.

Potassium is not added to IV fluids during the first 24 hr, because large amounts of this ion are released from injured cells into the extracellular compartment. Acidosis and renal failure may also result in dangerous hyperkalemia. After the 1st day, depending on the blood urea nitrogen level, urine output, and condition of the patient, 20–30 mEq of potassium in its phosphate form may be added to each liter of intravenous fluid.

A major advantage of using a composite solution is that fluids, electrolytes, and albumin can be simultaneously replaced in quantities that approximate those of the patient's losses. The rate of infusion, then, is the only adjustment needed, and the total volume needed for resuscitation can be prepared in advance. This method also avoids so-called "piggybacks," and permits a more accurate control of fluid intake.

No fluids other than ice chips should be given orally for the first 24 hr; during this time, absorption of fluid and electrolytes from the gastrointestinal tract is unpredictable and paralytic ileus and vomiting may develop. Similarly, the routine use of antacids to retard the development of stress ulcers is not recommended.

Monitoring Hydration Therapy. No one criterion suffices to guide the adjustment of fluid therapy. Because renal function and ADH secretion in burned patients are modified by factors other than blood volume, urine output may not accurately reflect the state of hydration. Significant oliguria, however, does not occur unless there is renal damage or severe dehydration. The urine output varies considerably from hour to hour but, when averaged at 4- to 8-hr intervals, 30 mL/hr/m^2 of body surface is the usual rate of urine production during the 1st 24 hr. Attempts to increase urine output beyond these limits usually cause increased peripheral and/or pulmonary edema. The state of hydration is better judged by frequent periodic assessment of many variables, such as sensorium, pulse, blood pressure, venous capillary filling, body weight, hematocrit, blood urea nitrogen, and serum and urine electrolytes and osmolality. Trends rather than individual measurements should be followed. Invasive techniques for measuring hemodynamic variables (e.g., cardiac output, pulmonary capillary wedge pressure, central venous pressure) are seldom necessary.

Fluid, Electrolyte, and Protein Replacement During the 2nd and Subsequent Days. After the 1st 24 hr, and once capillary permeability has been restored, fluid and electrolyte losses occur primarily in the form of burn exudate and evaporation through denuded skin. Fluid requirements usually average three fourths of the 1st day's allowance and may be estimated as follows:

1,500 mL/m^2 of body surface/24 hr
plus
3,750 mL/m^2 of body surface *burned*/24 hr

Because water loss by evaporation is electrolyte-free, sodium requirements after the 1st 48 hr are markedly curtailed and, in children, can be satisfied by administering oral or IV solutions with a sodium concentration of 50 mEq/L. Infants less than 1 yr of age require lower concentrations of sodium, usually in the range of 35–40 mEq/L.

In the absence of renal functional impairment, potassium requirements after the 1st day may be satisfied by administering solutions with concentrations of 30–40 mEq/L. Potassium phosphate instead of potassium chloride is preferred, because it allows the preparation of a more physiologic fluid mixture (sodium to chloride ratio of 3:2) while simultaneously replacing exaggerated phosphate losses.

Usually, the transition from IV to oral fluids is accomplished during the 2nd postburn day. Beginning at 24 hr postburn, homogenized milk or a suitable enteral formula is offered hourly. The IV fluid rate is adjusted downward as the oral intake is increased so that the hourly fluid intake is maintained constant. A small soft diet is usually tolerated by the 2nd or 3rd day.

Maximum weight gain (edema) is usually attained within 2–3 days postinjury. Thereafter a daily reduction in weight should follow (diuretic phase) until the 13th to 14th postburn day, at which time the patient's "preburn weight" is usually attained.

During the next several days (subacute phase) the child is supported medically to facilitate the healing of 2nd-degree burns and the autografting of 3rd-degree burns. Management includes daily irrigation and debridement of the wounds with antiseptic solutions, topical antimicrobial therapy, splinting of affected parts, and other indicated surgical procedures. Body weight, serum electrolyte, and plasma protein levels, colloid osmotic pressure, hematocrit, and hemoglobin should be monitored to detect any developing fluid or electrolyte disturbance, hypoalbuminemia, or anemia. Serum albumin levels should be maintained above 2 g/dL and oncotic pressure above 15 mm Hg to prevent edema and contraction of the intravascular volume. This may be accomplished by infusing human serum albumin as a 5% solution over 3–6 hr. The usual quantity of human serum albumin needed to maintain the recommended serum level varies from 100–150 mg/m^2 of burned body surface/wk, in 3 divided doses. An equivalent amount of plasma can be used instead, but the risk of hepatitis and/or transfusion reactions should be considered.

Blood lost as a direct result of the injury or from complications needs to be replaced during the 2nd–5th day after the burn, depending on its severity. Except for the patient with active bleeding or severe concomitant hypoproteinemia, transfusions of packed red blood cells are safer than whole blood and are better tolerated. In most cases, packed cells in the amount of 10 mg/kg, given over a 3- to 4-hr period, are sufficient. Although transfusions may be needed at intervals of 3–4 days, quantities of blood in excess of 15 mL/kg should not be given within a 24-hr period unless the patient is actively bleeding. Transfusing packed cells in larger quantities frequently results in cardiopulmonary congestion and/or dangerous hypertension.

Caloric Requirements. Hypermetabolism, increased glucose requirement, and severe protein and fat wasting are characteristic of the response to major trauma and infection. In no disease state is this response as great as it is following thermal injury. The resting metabolic rate increases in a curvilinear fashion with increasing burn size, from near-normal for burns less than 10% total body surface to 1.5 times normal for 25% total body surface burns to a maximum of twice normal for burns in excess of 40% total body surface area.

The precise energy requirements needed to reach weight and nitrogen balance have been calculated in adults from linear regressive analysis of weight change versus predicted dietary intake. This has been found to be approximately 25 kcal/kg plus 40 kcal/% body surface area burned/24 hr. For children, maintenance caloric requirements should be estimated on the basis of 1,800 kcal/m^2 of body surface/day, and the calories required for the burn itself should be estimated on the basis of 2,200 kcal/m^2 of body surface burned/day. Hildreth and Carvajal found that only 3 of 45 severely burned children with an average caloric intake equal to or in excess of that recommended by this formula lost weight; the others either gained or maintained their weight and clinically appeared well nourished.

In children, the increased caloric demands are usually met by oral feedings of milk or a lactose-free formula, plus a well-balanced diet containing 15% protein calories, 40% fat calories, and 45% carbohydrate calories. Most patients tolerate hourly feedings well and welcome oral fluid administration. In some cases, however, continuous nasogastric tube feeding may be preferable to promote normal sleeping habits.

Lactose intolerance may lead to diarrhea severe enough to limit enteral alimentation. The use of lactose-free formulas from the onset or soon after the diagnosis of disaccharidase deficiency, if suspected, frequently decreases or completely eliminates diarrhea.

COMPLICATIONS. A number of complications may ensue following burn injuries.

Cardiac Dysfunction. With appropriate fluid therapy, cardiac output usually returns to normal in 24–48 hr. The cause of persistent cardiac dysfunction in burns is unknown but may involve a circulating substance, presumably of pancreatic origin, with a molecular weight of less than 1,000, which has been reported in severely burned patients and those having septic shock. This myocardial depressant factor (MDF) decreases myocardial contractility and reduces cardiac output. Burned children are prone to congestive failure and pulmonary edema during septic shock and to renal failure. Treatment may require digitalis, diuretic agents (e.g., furosemide) and, in extreme cases, phlebotomy or peritoneal dialysis may be necessary. The development of overt congestive failure in burned children and septic patients can be prevented by cautious hydration or by maintaining patients in a slightly underhydrated state.

Respiratory Problems. These are common, particularly with smoke inhalation or facial burns (Sec. 14.70). Phillips and Cope found that pulmonary lesions contributed to or were directly responsible for 80% of burn deaths. The most common respiratory problems are pulmonary edema, tracheobronchitis, bronchopneumonia, and the alveolar-capillary block syndrome (also called ARDS, the adult respiratory distress syndrome). In addition, poisoning by inhalation of toxic gases, such as carbon monoxide, may occur in burns.

Severe Oliguria. During the immediate postburn period severe oliguria is usually the result of ADH secretion and a reduction in the glomerular filtration rate, but the possibility of renal damage should continue to be considered until normal renal function has been demonstrated. For example, in the presence of oliguria, the inability to concentrate the urine or conserve sodium may indicate renal dysfunction.

Renal Failure. In burns renal failure may be transient, associated with acute hypovolemia or shock, or persistent. With persistent azotemia the patient may be oliguric. The prognosis for oliguric azotemia is extremely poor, but with adequate supportive therapy recovery is still possible. Recognizing nonoliguric renal failure is important, because an adequate urine output may mask a relatively fixed urine volume; water and sodium retention, hypervolemia, and congestive heart failure may then develop. If, on the other hand, the condition is promptly recognized, appropriate restrictions of water, salt, and protein intake usually sustain relatively normal fluid balance and allow for recovery of renal function. When renal failure (particularly of the oliguric type) complicates burns, peritoneal dialysis or hemodialysis is often required.

Sepsis. This is the leading cause of death in burned children. In addition to the loss of the protective skin barrier, additional defects in host resistance such as deficiencies in thymus-dependent lymphocytes, phagocytic function, complement, and macrophage activation may predispose the patient to infection for some weeks. Serum levels of immunoglobulins fall in the 1st week because of loss of plasma into the interstitium, but antibody formation is spared. The infecting organisms vary with exposure, but the principal pathogens are *Staphylococcus aureus* and gram-negative bacteria such as *Pseudomonas aeruginosa*. The main portals of entry are the wound, respiratory tract, urinary tract, intravenous catheters, and possibly gastrointestinal tract. Successful treatment depends on early diagnosis and prompt institution of parenteral antibiotic therapy. No clinical signs are pathognomonic of sepsis. The diagnosis must be suspected when there is wound infection, hyperthermia or hypothermia, tachypnea, gastrointestinal symptoms, thrombocytopenia, a sudden change in sensorium, oliguria, or arterial hypertension.

With such findings, blood and other appropriate cultures are obtained and antibiotic therapy is begun. The bacteriologic history of the patient should be reviewed to choose the most appropriate antibiotic, but usually a combination of tobramycin and a penicillinase-resistant penicillin (e.g., oxacillin, dicloxacillin, methicillin) is adequate. Both drugs must be administered in maximal therapeutic doses (see Table 27–11) and continued for a minimum of 10 days. Whenever possible therapy should be adjusted on the basis of in vitro antibiotic sensitivity tests, serum antibiotic levels, and assessment of the minimal inhibitory concentrations of the antibiotics in use.

The condition of septic burned children is unstable and vascular collapse may lead to death within a few hours. Fluctuating body temperature, profuse sweating, anxiety, clouded sensorium, and changes in vital signs, especially blood pressure, and urine output should be considered incipient manifestations of septic shock (see Sec. 6.35 and 12.14).

Endotoxemia. This usually has a number of untoward effects on renal, respiratory, and cardiovascular function. Fluid management should therefore be conservative: a reasonable objective is to maintain the blood pressure just above shock levels and to be satisfied with minimal urine production. Isotonic fluids containing albumin may be used initially, but, as soon as the colloid osmotic pressure and arterial blood pressure have stabilized, lower concentrations of sodium solutions without albumin should be administered. The cautious use of vasoactive drugs (e.g., isoproterenol, dopamine, dobutamine) and digitalis is recommended to maintain blood pressure and to avoid administering excessive quantities of fluids.

REHABILITATION. Because the physical and psychologic effects of burns are potentially crippling, a vigorous rehabilitation program should be instituted as soon as possible to counter these effects. Residual deformities or loss of function may greatly impair the child's body image and self-esteem, and prolonged hospitalization may lead to a dependency reaction that extends beyond the period of confinement. The child or parents may harbor guilt feelings about the injury. In the parent, such feelings tend to interfere with the ability to cope with the illness of the child; confronting these issues early (by the child and family) may ameliorate this problem. The services of a mental health professional and social worker may be required. Psychologic support should be closely coordinated with other essential rehabilitative measures, including physical therapy, play therapy, and continuation of schoolwork.

Plans should be made to return the child to as normal a home life as possible. The parents and child should be instructed in home care procedures, such as the application of wound dressing, splints, and pressure dressings, and physical therapy. Such measures are particularly important in reducing hypertrophic scars. The child should return to school and other social activities as soon as feasible. Generally, this should be within the 1st week after the end of hospitalization.

The continuing rehabilitation of the burned child involves the cooperative efforts of the family physician, physical therapist, mental health professional, and reconstructive surgeon. Their involvement should be planned so that they interfere minimally with the child's schoolwork and other normal social activities.

HUGO F. CARVAJAL

Baxter CR, Moncrief JA, Prager MH, et al: A circulating myocardial depressant factor in burn shock. *In:* Matter P, Barclay TL, Kowicfova S (eds): Research in Burns. Transactions of the Third International Congress on Research in Burns, Prague. Berne, Switzerland, Hans Huber Publishers, 1971.
Berman W Jr, Goldman AS, Reichelderfer T, et al: Childhood burn injuries and deaths. Pediatrics 51:1069, 1973.
Bernstein NR: Emotional Care of the Facially Burned and Disfigured. Boston, Little, Brown, & Co, 1976.
Carvajal HF: A physiologic approach to fluid therapy in severely burned children. Surg Gynecol Obstet 150:379, 1980.
Carvajal HF: Controversies in fluid resuscitation and their impact on pediatric populations. *In:* Carvajal HF, Parks DH (eds): Burns in Children. Pediatric Burn Management. Chicago, Year Book Medical Publishers, 1988, pp 51–77.
Carvajal HF: Resuscitation of the burned child. *In:* Carvajal HF, Parks DH (eds): Burns in Children. Pediatric Burn Management. Chicago, Year Book Medical Publishers, 1988, pp 78–98.
Carvajal HF, Feinstein R, Traber DL, et al: An objective method for early diagnosis of gram-negative septicemia in burned children. J Trauma 21:221, 1981.
Clark AM: Burns in childhood. World J Surg 2:175, 1978.
Durtschi MB, Kohler TR, Finley A, et al: Burn injury in infants and young children. Surg Gynecol Obstet 150:651, 1980.
Granger ND, Gabel JC, Drake RE, et al: Physiologic basis for the clinical use of albumin solutions. Surg Gynecol Obstet 146:97, 1978.
Gump FE, Kinney JM: Energy balance and weight loss in burned patients. Arch Surg 103:442, 1971.
Hildreth M, Carvajal HF: Caloric requirements in burned children: A simple formula to estimate daily caloric requirements. J Burn Care Rehabil 3:78, 1982.
Holleman JH, Gable JC, Hardy JD: Pulmonary effects of intravenous fluid therapy and burn resuscitation. Surg Gynecol Obstet 149:161, 1978.
Janzekovic Z: The burn wound from a surgical point of view. J Trauma 15:42, 1975.
Larson DL: Burns in childhood: Invited commentary. World J Surg 2:181, 1978.
Larson DL, Abston S, Willis B, et al: Contracture and scar formation in the burn patient. Clin Plast Surg 1:653, 1974.
Moncrief JA: Burns. N Engl J Med 288:444, 1973.
Pruitt BA Jr: Advances in fluid therapy and the early care of the burn patient. World J Surg 2:139, 1978.
Stoll AM, Chianta MA: Heat transfer through fabrics as related to thermal injury. Trans NY Acad Sci 33:649, 1971.

6.38 TRANSPLANTATION MEDICINE

Organ and tissue transplantation are important therapies for pediatric end-stage organ failure. Transplantation of bone marrow for aplastic anemia and leukemia and of kidney, liver, and heart for end-stage organ disease are standard therapies if a suitable donor is available. Transplantation is also useful in correcting inborn errors of metabolism, even without end-stage organ failure. Furthermore, bone marrow and hepatic transplantation have been used as adjuvants or cures for benign tumors or various systemic or localized malignancies (Tables 6–33 and 6–34).

Organ transplantation has many potential complications associated with the risks of graft rejection, graft-versus-host disease, nonspecific effects of immunosuppressive drugs, and specific nonimmune toxicities of these immunosuppressive agents. The risks of chronic immunosuppressive therapy include infection with opportunistic microorganisms (see Sec. 12.13) and the delayed onset of a new malignancy. In addition, the original disease may recur in the transplanted organ, with varying effects on graft survival. Nonetheless, organ transplantation has many advantages and decreases the morbidity and mortality of end-stage organ failure in most children.

6.39 TRANSPLANTATION IMMUNOLOGY

Donor tissues from genetically disparate people are recognized as foreign (nonself) and rejected by the recipient's immune system. The recipient's recognition of alloantigens of the major histocompatibility complex (MHC) initiates graft rejection by host T lymphocytes. The human MHC, called the human leukocyte antigen (HLA) complex, is encoded on the short arm of chromosome 6, representing 2% of the chromosome's DNA. Included in this complex are the class I molecules (HLA-A, HLA-B, HLA-C) and the class II molecules (HLA-DP, HLA-DQ, HLA-DR), which determine antigen recognition by T lymphocytes. Class I molecules are constitutively present on all nucleated cells, whereas class II molecules are expressed constitutively on a few cells, including macrophages, monocytes, dendritic cells, and B lymphocytes. Class II antigen expression may be induced on other cells (e.g., T lymphocytes, pancreatic β cells, endothelial cells, renal tubular cells) by γ-interferon and other agents. See also Sec. 11.50.

Class I and II gene-encoded cell surface antigens are codominantly expressed and are inherited in a mendelian pattern, with haplotype linkage of HLA-A, HLA-B, HLA-C, and HLA-

TABLE 6–33. Diseases Treated by Bone Marrow Transplantation

Bone marrow failure: Anemia
Aplastic anemia (severe)
Osteopetrosis
β-Thalassemia
Kostmann agranulocytosis
Erythrophagocytic lymphohistiocytosis
Fanconi anemia
Diamond-Blackfan anemia
Paroxysmal nocturnal hemoglobinuria
Radiation injury
Malignancy*
Acute lymphoblastic leukemia (multiple relapses)
Acute myelogenous leukemia (1st remission)
Non-Hodgkin lymphoma (relapsing)
Hodgkin disease (relapsing)
Ewing sarcoma
Neuroblastoma
Wilms tumor
Myeloproliferative disease
Chronic myeloid leukemia
Immunodeficiency disease or syndrome
Adenosine deaminase deficiency
Severe combined immunodeficiency disease
Wiskott-Aldrich syndrome
Chédiak-Higashi disease
Leukocyte adhesion deficiency
Reticular dysgenesis
Chronic granulomatous disease
Cartilage hair hypoplasia
AIDS (?)
Metabolic disease
Hurler syndrome
Other mucopolysaccharidoses
Metachromatic leukodystrophy
Gaucher disease

*Includes allogeneic, autologous (with ex vivo treatment of remission marrow to remove residual cancer), or syngeneic (from an identical twin).

TABLE 6–34. Diseases Treated by Liver Transplantation

- Acute liver failure
  - Hepatitis B virus
  - Non-A–non-B hepatitis (C virus)
  - Acetaminophen or other drug- or toxin-induced severe hepatotoxicity
  - Neonatal hepatitis
  - Neonatal iron storage disease
  - Liver allograft rejection
- Biliary tract
  - Biliary atresia
  - Cystic fibrosis
  - Primary biliary cirrhosis
  - Sclerosing cholangitis
  - Familial cholestasis (Byler disease)
  - Alagille syndrome
  - Biliary hypoplasia
- End-stage liver disease
  - Cirrhosis
  - Budd-Chiari syndrome
  - Congenital hepatic fibrosis
  - Chronic active hepatitis
  - Portal vein thrombophlebitis (varices)
- Malignancy
  - Nonmetastatic primary hepatic tumor
- Metabolic disease
  - Oxalosis (with renal transplant)
  - Wilson disease
  - α_1-Antitrypsin deficiency
  - Homozygous familial hypercholesterolemia
  - Tyrosinemia
  - Galactosemia
  - Types I and IV glycogen storage disease
  - Crigler-Najjar syndrome
  - Urea cycle enzyme deficiency
  - Protein C deficiency
  - Hemophilia A and B
  - Sea-blue histiocyte syndrome
  - Protoporphyria

DR antigens within the maternal and paternal chromosomes. There are approximately 24 HLA-A, 51 HLA-B, 11 HLA-C, 20 HLA-DR, 9 HLA-DQ, and 6 HLA-DP alleles responsible for an equal number of cell surface antigens and thus for an extensive number of genetic combinations. The ability to match haplotypes between donor and recipient is closest among immediate family members and is most remote for nonrelated donors who have the large possibility of multiple allelic combinations. The chance of histoidentity among unrelated individuals is 1 in 10,000.

HLA matching is important for related living donor tissue, but may be less significant for cadaveric allograft survival. Because the HLA-DR antigens are the strongest transplantation antigens (followed by HLA-B, HLA-A, and HLA-C), many renal transplant centers match specifically for HLA-DR antigens, hoping to include other HLA group matches in the process. The advent of pregraft blood transfusions and/or the use of cyclosporine has greatly increased the survival of such cadaveric grafts. Nonetheless, close matching (one or both haplotypes) is beneficial in bone marrow transplantation from related or unrelated living donors to reduce the risk of rejection and graft-versus-host disease. Although the HLA system probably represents the MHC, other tissue antigenic groups (minor histocompatibility antigens) may result in graft rejection or graft-versus-host disease (GVHD). The donor and recipient should be matched for ABO blood group antigens for renal but not necessarily bone marrow transplantation.

ALLOGRAFT REJECTION. The physiologic function of MHC molecules is to present foreign antigens to T lymphocytes. During graft rejection, the MHC molecules of the donor tissue serve as both the presenting and the foreign antigen. The afferent limb of graft rejection involves antigen recognition of class I and II antigens by host T lymphocytes following presentation by host antigen-presenting cells (Fig. 6–15). Antigenic determinants on the surface of the intrinsic cell of the graft (e.g., hepatocyte), graft vascular endothelium, or donor "passenger" leukocytes may sensitize the host immune system. Donor cells with dendritic cell morphology constitutively express class I and II MHC antigens, are antigen-presenting cells, migrate from the donor tissue to host lymphoid tissue, and may be one critical component of host sensitization. Subsequent lymphocyte activation (CD4, CD8) by cytokines (interferon, interleukins) results in antibody production and cellular cytotoxicity in the efferent arc of graft rejection (see Fig. 6–15).

Mechanisms for allograft rejection include delayed-type hypersensitivity reactions, infiltration of activated macrophages, and collaboration of the CD4 (helper-inducer cell) and CD8 (cytotoxic-suppressor cell) subsets of T lymphocytes (see Fig. 6–15). CD4 cells responding to class II MHC antigens may initiate the rejection process and release cytokines, whereas CD8 cells propagate and amplify graft rejection. Cell products such as interleukin 2 function as mediators to amplify the immunologic cascade by activating lymphocytes.

GRAFT-VERSUS-HOST DISEASE (GVHD) (see Sec. 11.21). Engraftment by donor lymphocytes in an immunologically compromised host (congenital, radiation, or chemotherapy-induced immune defects) results in donor T cell activation against host MHC antigens, predominantly in the skin, gastrointestinal tract, and liver. GVHD is seen in 30–70% of patients following allogeneic bone marrow transplant and develops in 20–50% of HLA-identical marrow transplants from siblings.

Acute GVHD. This develops 7–14 days after transplantation but, by definition, not later than 100 days. Manifestations are divided into four clinical grades. Grade 1 demonstrates a maculopapular sunburn-like rash involving less than 50% of the body, serum bilirubin levels of 2–3 mg/dL, and no diarrhea or change in overall activity. Grade 2 demonstrates the rash involving 50–100% of the skin, bilirubin levels of 3–6 mg/dL, diarrhea (500–1,500 mL/24 hr) in adolescents and adults, and a mild reduction in activity. Grade 3 demonstrates the generalized erythrodermic rash, bilirubin levels of 6–15 mg/dL, diarrhea of more than 1,500 mL/24 hr, persistent fever higher than 38.5° C, and moderate to marked reduction in activity. Grade 4 demonstrates a toxic, epidermal necrolysis–like erythroderma with bullae and generalized desquamation, bilirubin levels higher than 15 mg/dL, diarrhea of more than 1,500 mL/24 hr, extreme toxicity, fever, and reduction of activity. Eosinophilia, lymphocytosis, protein-losing enteropathy, bone marrow aplasia (neutropenia, thrombocytopenia, anemia), peripheral edema, and secondary infections may ensue. Some GVHD may be beneficial in patients with prior malignancy, because graft versus cancer-directed T lymphocyte activity may improve the outcome related to the primary malignancy by destroying residual tumor cells.

Chronic GVHD. This develops more than 100 days after bone marrow transplantation and resembles a multisystem autoimmune process manifesting as Sjögren (Sicca) syndrome, eosinophilic fasciitis, systemic lupus erythematosus, scleroderma, lichen planus, primary biliary cirrhosis, and polyclonal hypergammaglobulinemia. Recurrent infections (sepsis, sinusitis, pneumonia) with encapsulated bacteria and interstitial pneumonia are common in patients with chronic GVHD. Prophylaxis with trimethoprim-sulfamethoxazole reduces the incidence of interstitial pneumonia. Risks for chronic GVHD include increasing age, prior acute GVHD, and buffy coat transfusions.

Treatment of GVHD is difficult and includes prednisone, cyclosporine, or antithymocyte globulin. Prevention of GVHD

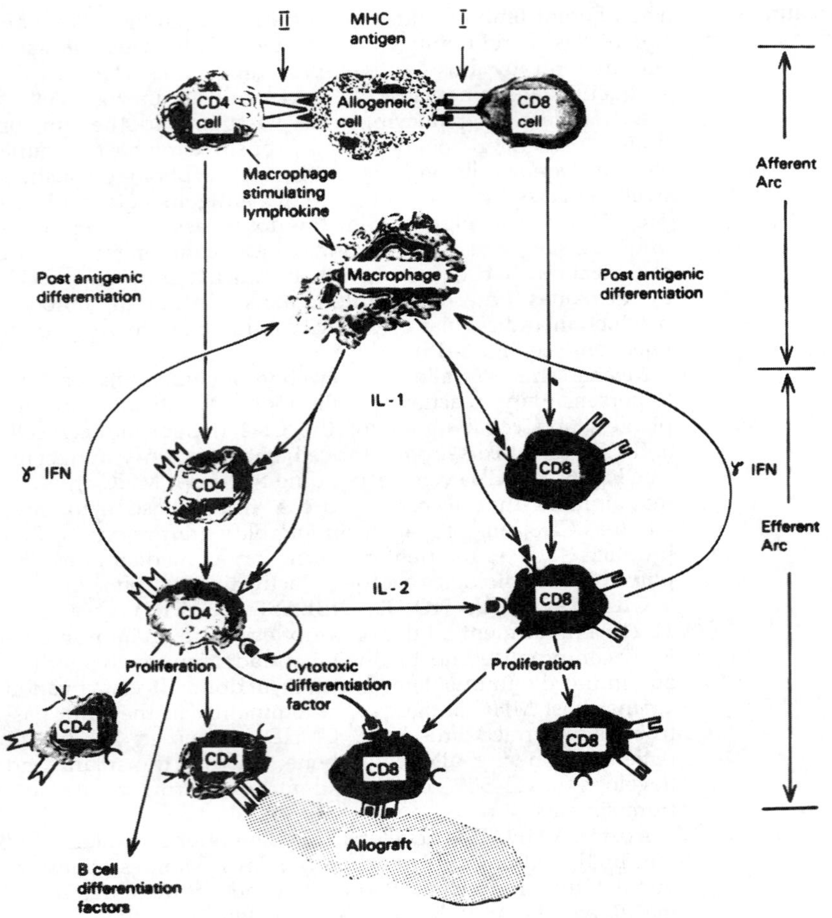

Figure 6–15. Scheme of allograft rejection response, involving antigen-induced interactions between macrophages. CD4+ and CD8+ lymphocytes and their humoral products are critical for the completion of the rejection response. (From Tilney N, Kupiec-Weglinski J: Immunobiology of acute allograft rejection. *In:* Brent L, Sells R [eds]: Organ Transplantation. London, Baillière Tindall, 1989.)

is most important and includes in vivo prophylaxis with methotrexate, cyclophosphamide, cyclosporine, prednisone, antithymocyte globulin, or various combinations of these agents immediately following transplantation. In vitro techniques include donor marrow T cell depletion with monoclonal antibodies or other methods to separate T lymphocytes. In vitro T cell depletion of donor marrow may increase the risk of graft rejection and leukemic recurrence.

6.40 PRINCIPLES OF IMMUNOSUPPRESSION

Immunosuppressant agents are needed to prevent and treat allograft rejection and GVHD. Because differences in major or minor histocompatibility antigens induce recipient T lymphocyte activation with subsequent donor allograft rejection, immunosuppression is needed in all tissue transplantation, except that from identical twins. Immunosuppression for solid organ transplants is lifelong, whereas that for bone marrow transplantation may be needed for 6–12 mo. Newer, more potent immunosuppressant agents permit tissue transplantation to occur across greater degrees of mismatched HLA antigens. The ideal immunosuppressive agent inhibits the lymphocyte subsets that mediate allograft rejection without altering immunity against infection, autoimmune processes, or malignancy. Furthermore, the idiosyncratic drug reactions associated with the specific immunosuppressant agent should be minor and distinguishable from those of organ rejection.

CORTICOSTEROIDS. Prednisone, usually in combination with another immunosuppressive agent, is frequently used to prevent or treat allograft rejection. Corticosteroids may interfere with T lymphocyte proliferation by directly blocking activation of the genes for interleukins 1 and 6. Because interleukin 2 (IL 2) secretion depends, in part, on IL 1 and IL 6 release, steroids indirectly block IL 2 action. Corticosteroids also produce a more rapid anti-inflammatory response by inducing the production of lipocortin, an inhibitor of phospholipase A_2, thus reducing the synthesis of inflammatory prostaglandins. Corticosteroids may also lyse small populations of activated lymphocytes and reduce the migration of monocytes to sites of inflammation.

Nonspecific and pronounced immunosuppressant effects of corticosteroids place the patient at risk for serious opportunistic infections, such as viral (varicella-zoster), bacterial *(Mycobacterium tuberculosis)*, fungal *(Candida albicans)*, or protozoal *(Pneumocystis carinii)* infection (see Sec. 12.13). Other long-term complications include growth failure, cushingoid appearance, hypertension, cataracts, gastrointestinal bleeding, pancreatitis, psychosis, hyperglycemia, osteoporosis, aseptic necrosis of the femoral head, and suppression of the pituitary adrenal axis.

AZATHIOPRINE. This imidazole derivative of 6-mercaptopurine blocks DNA synthesis by inhibiting purine synthesis, and is useful for preventing the primary immune response but not for reversal of allograft rejection. Azathioprine and 6-mercaptopurine inhibit T cell activation and decrease the number of migrating mononuclear cells. Toxic effects include myelosuppression (neutropenia), secondary infections, megaloblastic anemia, hepatic veno-occlusive disease, hepatitis, pancreatitis, and secondary malignancies (e.g., lymphoma, squamous cell carcinoma).

CYCLOSPORINE. This lipophilic (hydrophobic), cyclic, 11-

amino acid peptide is a potent and specific immunosuppressive agent that selectively inhibits the translation of IL 2 mRNA and thus IL 2 synthesis by helper T cells. Cyclosporine may also inhibit IL 1, IL 3, and γ-interferon synthesis. In the absence of IL 2, T cell activation is attenuated. Cyclosporine has no myelosuppressive activity nor is it an anti-inflammatory agent, but it has been very successful in preventing tissue rejection. Because of these beneficial properties and its potent immunosuppressive action, cyclosporine has greatly advanced the field of tissue transplantation.

Cyclosporine is metabolized by the hepatic cytochrome P-450 enzyme system and can be involved in a number of drug interactions. Cyclosporine levels increase in the presence of ketoconazole, erythromycin, methylprednisolone, warfarin, verapamil, ethanol, imipenem-cilastatin, metoclopramide, and fluconazole; cyclosporine levels decrease in the presence of phenytoin, phenobarbital, carbamazepine, valproate, nafcillin, and rifampin.

Cyclosporine has significant nonimmunosuppressant toxic effects, including neurotoxicity (tremors, paresthesias, headache, confusion, somnolence, seizures, coma), hypertrichosis, gingival hyperplasia, anorexia, nausea, vomiting, hepatotoxicity (cholestasis, cholelithiasis, hemorrhagic necrosis), endocrinopathies (ketosis, hyperprolactinemia, hypotestosteronemia, gynecomastia, impaired spermatogenesis), metabolic disorders (hypomagnesemia, hyperuricemia, hyperglycemia, hyperkalemia, hypocholesterolemia), vascular derangements (hypertension, increased sympathetic nervous system activation, vasculitic-hemolytic uremic syndrome–like illness, atherogenesis), and nephrotoxicity. Renal toxicity is a significant limitation of cyclosporine use and is manifested as an increased creatinine level, oliguria, hypertension, fluid retention, vasoconstriction of the afferent glomerular arteriole, reduced glomerular filtration rate, renal tubular damage, and hemolytic uremic syndrome–like lesions. Chronic nephrotoxicity (interstitial fibrosis, tubular atrophy) may require a reduction of the cyclosporine dose or change to other immunosuppressant drugs, such as azathioprine. Renal biopsy may be needed to differentiate nephrotoxicity from other causes of renal impairment (rejection, acute tubular necrosis, infection). Nephrotoxicity may be exacerbated by aminoglycosides, amphotericin B, acyclovir, digoxin, furosemide, indomethacin, or trimethoprim. It may be reduced by careful monitoring of blood cyclosporine levels and use for as short a period as possible. The therapeutic window for trough cyclosporine levels is not well defined; the therapeutic ranges vary with assay technique, which may be highly sensitive or may detect metabolites in addition to the active compound. Cyclosporine is frequently used in combination with prednisone and/or azathioprine to reduce its dose in an attempt to avoid its potential serious side effects.

FK506. This experimental macrolide immunosuppressive drug produced by the fungus *Streptomyces tsukubaensis,* is chemically distinct from cyclosporine but has similar effects on the immune system. Rapamycin is structurally similar to FK506 and also has immunosuppressive properties. FK506 has a low incidence of post-transplant hypertension, hirsutism, and gingival hyperplasia but is associated with hypocholesterolemia, nephrotoxicity, and neurotoxicity. Preliminary trials suggest that FK506 is a potent agent that may have fewer serious side effects than cyclosporine. More experience in pediatric transplantation patients is needed to determine the usefulness of this new drug.

ANTITHYMOCYTE GLOBULIN. Heterologous antilymphocyte globulins produced by immunization of horses or rabbits against human peripheral blood or splenic cells has been used to prevent and treat transplant rejection in combination with other agents. Side effects of antilymphocyte globulin include a 1st-dose flu-like illness caused by lymphocytolysis and cytokine release (fever, chills, myalgia) and, later, development of serum sickness (or, rarely, anaphylaxis). The potent immunosuppressant T cell–depleting effects increase the risk for opportunistic infections.

OKT3. Mouse monoclonal antibodies directed against T lymphocytes are effective in reversing graft rejection. OKT3, an IgG antibody, is directed against the T3 (CD3) surface glycoprotein complex on mature post-thymic T cells. OKT3 produces T lymphocyte elimination by the hepatic and splenic reticuloendothelial system. Binding of OKT3 to the lymphocyte also prevents T cell activation.

OKT3 can induce recipient anti-OKT3 antibodies, thus reducing the effectiveness of this immunosuppressant agent with time. Concomitant use of immunosuppressant drugs reduces the 1st-treatment incidence of antibody formation to 30%. Failure of retreatment with OKT3 is associated with high-titer (1:1,000) antibodies against OKT3. Antibody titers can be determined prior to each treatment with OKT3.

Adverse effects of OKT3 include a 1st-dose (occasionally 2nd or 3rd) syndrome of fever, chills, dyspnea, wheezing, chest tightness, nausea, vomiting, and diarrhea, which may begin 45 min after the dose and last several hours. This flu-like lymphocytolytic reaction is caused by released cytokines, but it may be partly attenuated by pretreatment with methylprednisone and simultaneous administration of intravenous hydrocortisone with oral diphenhydramine and acetaminophen. Other complications include pulmonary edema in fluid-overloaded patients, aseptic meningitis, and an increased risk for opportunistic infections.

6.41 ORGAN DONATION

Inadequate referral of suitable donors, rather than a lack of potential donors, is the rate-limiting factor in the treatment of the many patients on waiting lists for tissue transplantation. To increase the referral of appropriate donors, regional organ procurement agencies have been established to coordinate and provide education for health professionals and the public, organ retrieval, tissue preservation, and transportation, and medical-legal services. The North American Transplant Coordinating Organization and the United Network of Organ Sharing are two computerized registries used to match donors and recipients.

A suitable donor must be declared brain-dead following a well-defined life-threatening event (e.g., drowning, cerebral trauma, brain tumor, asphyxia, intracranial hemorrhage). Care of the prospective donor includes optimal management of respiration, blood pressure, and renal perfusion and prevention of nosocomial infection. Neurogenic or hypovolemic shock should be treated with fluid resuscitation, but α-adrenergic vasoconstrictor agents should be avoided to prevent ischemic organ injury. The Pa_{O_2} should be maintained between 70 and 100 mm Hg and the pH kept between 7.35 and 7.45. Diuresis should be maintained with fluid therapy and careful attention directed to patients with excessive urine output caused by central diabetes insipidus, which is treatable with volume replacement and controlled intravenous infusions of vasopressin.

Prior to transplantation, the donor organ is preserved at 4° C for varying periods of cold ischemia time. This time can be extended for some allografts following perfusion or storage with the University of Wisconsin solution, which contains compounds to reduce cold-induced cell swelling and ischemia-induced loss of intracellular metabolites. These compounds include lactobionic acid, glutathione, adenosine, hydroxyethyl starch, raffinose, magnesium, insulin, dexamethasone, and phosphate. Preservation times are 48–72 hr for renal, 10–48 hr for liver, 4 hr for lungs, and 5 hr for heart allografts.

Living relatives may donate renal and partial (reduced size) lung, pancreas, or hepatic allografts. Living, related organ donation has psychologic and medical implications for the donor and recipient. The benefits of living, related donor organ transplantation include better assessment of the donor's health status; improved histocompatibility with a lower risk of rejection, less frequent graft injury secondary to hypotension or cold preservation, and no underlying or secondary medical conditions associated with brain death; nonemergent planning of the operative procedures; and time to initiate immunosuppression in the recipient or to administer donor-specific transfusions in some renal transplant recipients.

6.42 BONE MARROW TRANSPLANTATION

Transplantation of bone marrow may be autologous (reinfusion of patients previously stored marrow), syngeneic (from an identical twin), or allogeneic (from a sibling or, less often, from an unrelated donor). Allogeneic donors are most frequently used. Indications for bone marrow transplantation primarily include bone marrow failure (severe aplastic anemia), malignancy, and immunodeficiency syndromes, but an increasing number of other disorders are being treated with bone marrow transplantation (see Table 6–33). Bone marrow transplantation differs from solid organ transplantation because the donor tissue contains viable lymphocytes able to react to host antigens, which results in acute or chronic GVHD (see Sec. 6.39 and 11.21). Furthermore, except for patients with aplastic anemia who have identical twins, or those with primary T cell immunodeficiency, other patients undergoing allogeneic transplantation require pretreatment conditioning with high-dose myeloablative chemotherapy (e.g., with busulfan, cytosine arabinoside, or cyclophosphamide) or fractionated total body irradiation to prevent graft rejection. Conditioning regimens make room in the host marrow space for the new marrow, provide immunosuppression and, in the case of prior malignancy, attempt to eradicate residual malignant cells. Post-transplant immunosuppression is then usually needed to prevent GVHD.

HLA typing identifies HLA-identical antigens and the mixed lymphocyte culture confirms antigenic identity between host and recipient. Without an identical match there is a high risk for rejection and GVHD. Although most donors are HLA-identical siblings, the advent of new, potent immunosuppressive regimens has permitted transplantation from HLA-nonidentical (one haplotype mismatch) related donors or HLA-identical nonrelated donors. These alternative donors increase the donor pool and possibility of bone marrow transplantation, but such transplantation is associated with an increased risk for GVHD, delayed or failed (rejected) marrow engraftment, and infections. T cell–depleted marrow may reduce the incidence of GVHD but increase the risk of recurrent malignancy.

Engraftment in recipients of HLA-identical marrow can occur as early as 2 wk in patients with severe combined immunodeficiency disease, as determined by normal B and T lymphocyte function. The period of immunodeficiency is usually more prolonged in other patients (9–12 mo) and is extended by the presence of GVHD. Immunologic reconstitution following nonidentical or nonrelated matches may only be partially achieved or take longer than that for HLA-identical sibling transplants. Hematopoietic reconstitution (erythrocyte, myeloid, and megakaryocyte engraftment) occurs in the 2nd–3rd week; myeloid production may be augmented by recombinant human granulocyte-macrophage (GM-CSF) colony-stimulating factor. Prior to bone marrow engraftment, patients frequently need erythrocyte and platelet transfusions. In the absence of severe GVHD, cyclosporine is discontinued after 6 mo in patients with prior leukemia and after 12 mo in patients with aplastic anemia.

Complications of bone marrow transplantation include opportunistic infections (Sec 12.13), acute and chronic GVHD, toxicity related to conditioning (idiopathic interstitial pneumonia, cardiac toxicity, delayed gonadal or thyroid dysfunction, hepatic veno-occlusive disease, cataracts), graft rejection, recurrent malignancy, induced secondary malignancy (Epstein-Barr virus–positive non-Hodgkin B cell lymphoma, leukemia, solid organs), hemolytic uremic syndrome, thrombotic thrombocytopenia, transfer of IgE-mediated hypersensitivity, avascular necrosis of bone (hip>knee>ankle>shoulder), diffuse alveolar hemorrhage, and obstructive lung disease (preparative conditioning or GVHD). The incidence or severity of complications may be reduced by using fractionated total body irradiation, administering prophylactic antimicrobial agents (acyclovir for herpes simplex, intravenous immunoglobulin for cytomegalovirus [CMV], trimethoprim-sulfamethoxazole for *Pneumocystis carinii*), avoiding CMV-seropositive blood products in CMV-seronegative recipients, using cyclosporine to prevent GVHD, and avoiding prior sensitizing blood transfusions in patients with aplastic anemia to ensure engraftment. Secondary malignancy (lymphoma) may be managed by reducing the dose of immunosuppressive agents and/or chemotherapy.

The prognosis for graft survival in patients treated with HLA-identical allogeneic bone marrow transplantation for severe aplastic anemia is excellent. Untransfused patients have a long-term survival of 80% versus 65–75% for previously transfused patients. The success rate in HLA-identical marrow transplantation in patients with severe combined immunodeficiency disease is 60–65% (35–40% if HLA-mismatched marrow is used). The long-term prognosis in patients with lymphoma or leukemia depends on the patient's age (younger than 20 yr is optimal) and the timing of transplantation (1st remission is optimal in acute myelogenous leukemia, AML). Recurrent malignancy, occurring in 20–60% of patients, is the major morbidity. Children with acute lymphocytic leukemia (ALL) with standard risk factors should be treated with chemotherapy, because the prognosis is excellent; bone marrow transplantation should be reserved for the 2nd remission (see Sec. 17.5).

AUTOLOGOUS BONE MARROW TRANSPLANTATION. This has been employed in patients with various lymphoproliferative malignancies and solid tumors following ablative high-dose cancer chemotherapy or total body irradiation. In cancer patients without bone marrow involvement, the bone marrow is removed and cryopreserved prior to ablative cancer chemotherapy. If there is bone marrow involvement, the marrow is removed during remission and may undergo further purging ex vivo to remove residual malignant cells. The use of monoclonal antibodies directed against the tumor is the most common method for removing residual cancer cells.

Autologous bone marrow transplantation has few direct complications, because there are no risks for rejection or GVHD. If too few stem cells are returned, however, graft failure may ensue. Recurrent malignancy is the most troublesome problem, either at the original site (neuroblastoma) or in the bone marrow (ALL). There may be a higher malignancy recurrence rate with autologous transplantation compared with allogeneic marrows, because the former is not subject to GVHD and, therefore, there are no donor-induced activated lymphocytes against the recipient's (host) antigens on the malignant cells. Prognosis is related to the original tumor type (poorest for glioma, neuroblastoma; best for ALL, lymphoma), with disease-free survival rates ranging from 10–60%.

6.43 LIVER TRANSPLANTATION

Orthotopic liver transplantation is an accepted therapy for acute or chronic end-stage liver disease, various metabolic disorders, primary hepatic malignancy, irreparable structural lesions, and other serious hepatic conditions (see Table 6–34). Biliary atresia is the most common pediatric indication, followed by acute fulminant hepatitis, α_1-antitrypsin deficiency, intrahepatic cholestasis, and other inborn errors of metabolism.

Contraindications to liver transplantation include extrahepatic primary or metastatic malignancy, acceptable alternative therapy, irreversible nonhepatic infection, disease that would be expected to recur (carrying chronic hepatitis B is not an absolute contraindication), severe pulmonary arteriovenous shunting with hypoxia, poor social support, and significant disease or impairment in extrahepatic organs.

Allocation of the donor allograft depends on similar ABO blood groups, distance from the center (0–50 mi optimal; >2,500 mi least desirable), and the severity of the patient's status. The highest priority is given to patients with acute fulminant hepatic failure (including liver transplant graft failure), followed by those requiring intensive care treatment for liver disease, by hospitalized patients, and by those living at home. Patients with refractory ascites, variceal hemorrhage, recurrent cholangitis, and failure to thrive are also given higher priority. Currently, there is no HLA matching performed for liver transplantation. An ABO mismatch between an O donor and an A, B, or AB recipient may produce hemolysis for 4–6 wk of mild to moderate significance.

The operative procedure may be complicated by coagulopathy, previous portal hypertension with extensive portosystemic collateral vessels, scarring from a previous Kasai procedure, and difficulties in dissection and isolation of the common bile duct, suprahepatic vena cava, intrahepatic vena cava, portal vein, and hepatic artery. The total recipient operation may take 6–24 hr (usually 8–10 hr) and requires meticulous vascular and bile duct anastomoses and large volumes of blood replacement.

Immediate postoperative complications include graft failure (technically suboptimal operation, unrecognized donor liver disease, graft ischemia, accelerated rejection), vascular thrombosis (portal or hepatic vein, hepatic artery) and subsequent ischemic injury to the liver and bile duct with an increased risk of infectious *(Candida)* peritonitis, other fungal and bacterial infections, hypertension (treated with captopril, labetalol, nitroprusside, propranolol, or hydralazine), coagulopathy (not treated too aggressively in order to avoid vascular thrombosis), oliguria lasting 24–48 hr, post-transplant metabolic alkalosis, right-sided atelectasis, phrenic nerve plalsy, pleural effusion, and delayed recovery from anesthesia. Bacterial infection can be prevented by the postoperative administration of ampicillin and cefotaxime, and acyclovir can be given to prevent herpes simplex infection.

Graft function is monitored by determination of serial serum liver enzyme and bilirubin levels, coagulation times, and bile flow through the biliary drain, Doppler assessment of vascular sites, and liver biopsy, if needed. Serum glutamate dehydrogenase (GLDH), a mitochondrial enzyme, is a sensitive marker for hepatic ischemia. Routine liver transaminase levels peak at 48 hr post-transplantation and subsequently decline in healthy allografts. Coagulation status, the blood glucose level, arterial pH, and mental status should return to near-normal by 24–48 hr.

Complications occurring after the immediate postoperative period include hypertension, abdominal bleeding, opportunistic infection, seizures, encephalopathy, benign isolated elevations of serum alkaline phosphatase levels, episodes of endotoxemia, vascular thrombosis, ascites, cholangitis caused by bile duct stricture, vanishing bile duct syndrome secondary to prior ischemia, CMV infection, aplastic anemia caused by non-A, non B-hepatitis, recurrence of native disease (cancer, hepatitis B or C, Budd-Chiari syndrome), delayed onset lymphoma, and rejection. Secondary lymphoma can be managed by reducing the dose of immunosuppressive agents, which must be balanced against the risk of allograft rejection.

Immunosuppression is begun perioperatively and usually includes cyclosporine, methylprednisolone, and azathioprine. Rejection occurs in as many as 75% of patients and is treated with increasing doses of methylprednisolone and the addition of OKT3. The 1st episode of rejection usually occurs within the 1st 3 wk; rejection episodes are unusual after 3 mo post-transplantation. Rejection affects the bile ducts and vascular endothelium and is manifested by elevated levels of liver enzymes such as γ-glutamyltranspeptidase (GGTP) and alkaline phosphatase, a rising direct bilirubinemia, fever, tachypnea, hepatic tenderness, a sepsis-like appearance, percutaneous biopsy evidence of activated lymphocyte infiltration in the portal areas, inflammation of the vascular endothelium (endothelialitis), and injury to the interlobular bile ducts.

The prognosis for pediatric liver transplant recipients is usually excellent once the problems of the operative and immediate post-transplant periods have been resolved. The graft survival rate approaches 60–80% in experienced centers. New advances such as split liver ex vivo reduction hepatectomy of cadaver donor organs and reduced-size hepatic left lateral lobe transplantation from related living donors should increase the availability of allografts for the many patients on waiting lists.

6.44 RENAL TRANSPLANTATION

The management of end-stage renal disease (ESRD) includes dialysis and/or renal transplantation. Patient survival, quality of life, growth and development, success in school and employment, and cost effectiveness are superior following transplantation, which is the preferred choice of therapy for ESRD. The causes of ESRD include reflux nephropathy, obstructive nephropathy, renal dysplasia, acquired chronic glomerulonephritis and, rarely, primary oxalosis, cystinosis, Wilms' tumor, or juvenile-onset diabetes mellitus (more common in adults). Contraindications to renal transplantation include active systemic infection, intravenous drug use, systemic malignancy, and irreversible brain or other organ injury. The risk of recurrence of the original renal disease in the allograft is not a contraindication to transplantation. The incidence and significance of recurrent disease on graft survival vary with the primary process: focal segmental glomerulosclerosis, membranoproliferative glomerulonephritis, hemolytic uremic syndrome, dense deposit disease, and primary oxalosis (without liver transplant) have a moderate-to-high recurrence rate with subsequent severe impairment of the allograft; IgA nephropathy, membranous nephropathy, and Henoch-Schönlein purpura have a moderate recurrence rate with minor graft impairment; hereditary nephritis, systemic lupus erythematosus, Wegener granulomatosis, polyarteritis nodosa, diabetes mellitus, and cystinosis have a low-to-rare risk of recurrence.

The transplanted kidney may come from a related living donor (older than 18 yr), an unrelated living donor (rarely), or a cadaveric donor (more often). Preoperative evaluation for living donor transplantation includes a donor-recipient cross-match of the donor's lymphocytes against those of the recipient to identify preformed cytotoxic antibodies. A negative cross-match is a prerequisite for living donor and cadaveric transplantation. Preformed cytotoxic antibodies cause an acute humoral vasculitis-like rejection directed against ABO or HLA antigens. Chronic humoral rejection also causes graft failure. Humoral rejection is difficult to manage (compared with T lymphocyte–directed rejection) and is refractory to antirejection therapy.

Graft survival is optimal when an identical twin is the donor (full HLA match), followed by a parent or sibling (single or full haplotype identity) and then closely by cadaveric transplantation. Donors should not possess blood group A or B if the recipient does not possess the same blood group. Ideally, cadaveric donors should have the fewest mismatched HLA antigens with the recipient. Nonetheless, HLA matching is not always possible, and this is not an absolute contraindication for transplantation.

The transplant procedure is not technically difficult. The recipient's native kidneys are usually left in place, except in the presence of intractable nephrotic syndrome, malignancy, severe hypertension, or refractory infection. In infants weighing less than 20 kg the donor kidney is placed in the intraperitoneal space, the renal artery is anastomosed to the aorta, the renal vein is connected to the vena cava, and the ureter is reimplanted using a posterior Leadbetter-Politano procedure (similar to that used for vesicoureteral reflux). In larger children the iliac vessels are used for vascular anastomoses and the kidney is placed in the extraperitoneal iliac fossa. Immediately prior to revascularization of the allograft, the systemic arterial and venous pressures are elevated with fluid therapy, and furosemide (Lasix) or mannitol is administered, as is methylprednisolone. Infants who receive an adult kidney may have massive fluid and electrolyte losses (e.g., calcium, phosphorus, magnesium, sodium, bicarbonate) and require careful fluid replacement. Oliguria may be managed with colloid or crystalloid fluid therapy (raising the central venous pressure to 10–15 cm Hg) and with diuretics (furosemide, bumetanide).

Immunosuppression for prevention of rejection includes a combination of prednisone, azathioprine, and cyclosporine. Rejection is treated with a higher dose of intravenous methylprednisolone and with OKT3. Rejection may be immediate, recurrent, or occur as long as 3–4 yr post-transplantation. It is manifested as fever, anorexia, malaise, hypertension, oliguria, abdominal pain, allograft swelling and tenderness, increase in blood urea nitrogen and serum creatinine or phosphorus levels, decreased GFR, and biopsy evidence of rejection. Late-onset problems include hypertension caused by cyclosporine, native disease, renal artery stenosis, thromboembolism, erythrocytosis, osteonecrosis, and complicated pregnancies.

The 5-yr graft survival has improved with the advent of new immunosuppressant regimens and antirejection therapy, and now approaches 70%. Related living donor allografts have a better long-term survival than cadaveric transplanted kidneys. Children transplanted at 10–15 yr of age (70–80%) have a better graft prognosis than those younger than 2 yr of age (40–60%). Patient survival (not allograft) is nonetheless good (85–90%), and for most the quality of life is greatly improved following renal transplantation.

6.45 HEART TRANSPLANTATION

Orthotopic cardiac transplantation is an acceptable treatment for intractable, irreversible heart disease. Indications for cardiac transplantation in infants include hypoplastic left heart syndrome and other complex congenital heart lesions, cardiomyopathy, and cardiac allograft rejection; in older children indications include cardiomyopathy (including doxorubicin-induced cardiomyopathy), myocarditis, cardiac allograft rejection, complex congenital heart disease, extensive myocardial nonmalignant tumors, and coronary artery disease.

Contraindications include the presence of uncontrolled infections, active malignancy, active peptic ulcer disease, poorly controlled diabetes mellitus, a positive lymphocyte cross-match (indicative of preformed cytotoxic antibodies), ABO incompatibility, and elevated pulmonary vascular resistance (such patients may be candidates for combined heart-lung transplantation). Pulmonary vascular resistance of 6–8 Woods units is not necessarily an absolute contraindication. HLA matching is usually not done because of urgency of organ procurement, transportation, and transplantation.

The operative procedure is performed while the patient is on cardiopulmonary bypass. The recipient's atria and great arteries distal to the semilunar valves are left in place for anastomosis to the allograft. The atrial anastomoses create two large atria and two foci of electrical discharge, often resulting in two distinct P waves.

Immediate postoperative complications include bradycardia (titrated with isoproterenol and an atrial pacemaker) and poor cardiac output (treated with dopamine, dobutamine, nitroprusside). Later complications include opportunistic infections (see Sec. 12.13), hypertension (cyclosporine, plus other factors), lymphoproliferative disease (Epstein-Barr virus), and graft coronary atherosclerosis (noted in 30–50% of patients), and possibly associated with repeated rejection, hyperlipidemia, hypertension, and CMV infection. Allograft rejection occurs in the 1st 6 mo after transplantation and is manifested as fever, fatigue, heart failure, cardiomegaly, atrial arrhythmias or heart block, reduced ECG voltage, and transcatheter endomyocardial biotome biopsy evidence of rejection. Tissue histology in rejection is graded as mild (sparse perivascular or endocardial mononuclear cell infiltration, no myocyte necrosis), moderate (increased cell infiltration, patchy myocyte necrosis), or severe (florid interstitial mononuclear and neutrophilic infiltration, hemorrhage, and myocyte necrosis). Noninvasive methods such as Doppler or two-dimensional echocardiography and radionuclide angiography to evaluate ventricular function, coupled with the physical examination and ECG evidence, may reduce the need for repeated biopsies. Rejection may be prevented by chronic immunosuppression, including the use of cyclosporine, prednisone, and azathioprine; acute rejection is treated with intravenous pulse methylprednisolone and OKT3. Young infants may have a lower incidence of rejection.

The 5-yr survival rate approaches 60–70%. The 3-yr survival rate in infants approaches 80%. Atherosclerosis, lymphoproliferative disease, opportunistic infection, and chronic graft rejection are important causes of morbidity and mortality. Adults treated with OKT3 may have an increased incidence of lymphoproliferative disorders.

6.46 LUNG AND HEART-LUNG TRANSPLANTATION

There is limited experience with lung, partial lung, or combined heart-lung transplantation on children. Indications for *lung transplantation* include pulmonary fibrosis (single lung), primary pulmonary hypertension, congenital heart disease with hypoplastic pulmonary arteries, and cystic fibrosis (double lung) without cor pulmonale. Indications for *combined heart-lung transplantation* include chronic pulmonary disease, elevated pulmonary vascular resistance, and cor pulmonale (cystic fibrosis, bronchiectasis, emphysema), Eisenmenger syndrome, and possibly primary pulmonary hypertension. In some heart-lung transplantation procedures the recipient's heart is removed and transplanted to another recipient.

Complications include opportunistic infections (see Sec. 12.13), particularly CMV pneumonia, tracheal or bronchial dehiscence, bronchial stenosis, severe pleural hemorrhage (especially in patients with previous chest surgery), and bronchiolitis obliterans (possibly a form of chronic rejection).

Acute lung rejection is manifested as fever, cough, rales, new infiltrates on chest roentgenogram, hypoxia, respiratory failure, and transbronchial biopsy evidence of lymphocyte infiltration of the perivascular space. Acute rejection is managed with pulse intravenous methylprednisolone and OKT3. Chronic immunosuppression requires combinations of cyclosporine, prednisone, and azathioprine. Acute cardiac allograft rejection is discussed in Sec. 6.45.

In experienced centers patient survival approaches 70–75% at 2 yr post-transplantation.

6.47 PANCREATIC TRANSPLANTATION

Insulin-dependent patients with diabetes mellitus who develop end-stage renal disease (see Sec. 6.44) are candidates for combined renal and pancreatic transplantation. The risks of pancreatic transplantation and chronic immunosuppression are too great, balanced against the alternate therapy of the judicious use of multiple insulin injections, to justify isolated pancreatic transplantation. Pancreatic transplantation might also be indicated for those diabetics who eventually develop severe retinopathy or nephropathy. Unfortunately, it remains difficult to predict who may develop these severe diabetic vascular complications (see Sec. 8.53).

The cadaveric whole pancreatic allograft is drained directly into the recipient's bladder to avoid autodigestion by pancreatic enzymes. In combined renal and pancreatic transplants rejection is manifested by a deterioration in renal function; pancreatic rejection is manifested as a decline of the urine amylase levels.

Long-term pancreatic allograft survival currently approaches 50–60%. Pancreatic transplantation usually produces euglycemia, with the occasional need for exogenous insulin. Nonetheless, because of the risks of rejection and chronic immunosuppression, pancreatic transplantation should be reserved for those adolescents or adults with ESRD who require a simultaneous (or have had a prior) renal transplant.

ROBERT M. KLIEGMAN

GENERAL TRANSPLANTATION

Bach FH, Sachs DH: Transplantation immunology. N Engl J Med 317:489, 1987.
Bennett WM, Porter GA: Cyclosporine-associated hypertension. Am J Med 85:131, 1988.
Brayman KL, Vianello A, Morel P, et al: The organ donor. Crit Care Clin 6:84, 1990.
Carpenter CB: Immunosuppression in organ transplantation. N Engl J Med 322:1224, 1990.
Hong R: Transplantation immunity: Basic principles and future projections. Adv Pediatr 37:285, 1990.
House RM, Thompson TL II: Psychiatric aspects of organ transplantation. JAMA 260:535, 1988.
Kahan BD: Cyclosporine. N Engl J Med 321:1725, 1989.
Krensky AM, Weiss A, Crabtree G, et al: T-lymphocyte–antigen interactions in transplant rejection. N Engl J Med 322:510, 1990.
MacLeod AM, Catto GRD: Cancer after transplantation: The risks are small. Br Med J 297:4, 1988.
MacLeod AM, Thomson AW: FK 506: An immunosuppressant for the 1990s? Lancet 337:25, 1991.
Odom NJ: Organ donation. Br Med J 300:1571, 1990.
Reznik VM, Jones KL, Durham BL, et al: Changes in facial appearance during cyclosporin treatment. Lancet 1:1405, 1987.
Sands M, Brown RB: Interactions of cyclosporine with antimicrobial agents. Rev Infect Dis 11:691, 1989.
Scherrer U, Vissing SF, Morgan BJ, et al: Cyclosporine-induced sympathetic activation and hypertension after heart transplantation. N Engl J Med 323:693, 1990.
Starzl TE, Fung J, Jordan M, et al: Kidney transplantation under FK506. JAMA 264:63, 1990.
Wallwork J: Organs for transplantation: Improvements needed in supply and use. Br Med J 299:1291, 1989.

BONE MARROW TRANSPLANTATION

Brandt SJ, Peters WP, Atwater SK, et al: Effect of recombinant human granulocyte-macrophage colony-stimulating factor on hematopoietic reconstitution after high-dose chemotherapy and autologous bone marrow transplantation. N Engl J Med 318:869, 1988.
Cheson BD, Lacerna L, Leyland-Jones B, et al: Autologous bone marrow transplantation: Current status and future directions. Ann Intern Med 110:51, 1989.
Fischer A, Griscelli C, Friedrich W, et al: Bone-marrow transplantation for immunodeficiencies and osteopetrosis: European survey, 1968–1985. Lancet 2:1080, 1986.
Fischer A, Landais P, Friedrich W, et al: European experience of bone-marrow transplantation for severe combined immunodeficiency. Lancet 336:850, 1990.
Krivit W, Whitley CB: Bone marrow transplantation for genetic diseases. N Engl J Med 316:1085, 1987.
Lucarelli G, Galimberti M, Polchi P, et al: Bone marrow transplantation in patients with thalassemia. N Engl J Med 322:417, 1990.
Nisbet NW: Bone marrow transplantation in precocious osteopetrosis. Br Med J 294:463, 1987.
Rollins BJ: Hepatic veno-occlusive disease. Am J Med 81:297, 1986.
Sanders JE, Whitehead J, Storb R, et al: Bone marrow transplantation experience for children with aplastic anemia. Pediatrics 77:179, 1986.
Witherspoon RP, Fisher LD, Schoch G, et al: Secondary cancers after bone marrow transplantation for leukemia or aplastic anemia. N Engl J Med 321:784, 1989.

RENAL TRANSPLANTATION

Frey DJ, Matas AJ: Renal transplantation. Crit Care Clin 6:899, 1990.
Kalia A, Brouhard BH, Travis LB, et al: Renal transplantation in the infant and young child. Am J Dis Child 142:47, 1988.
Moran M, Mozes MF, Maddux MS, et al: Prevention of acute graft rejection by the prostaglandin E_1 analogue misoprostol in renal-transplant recipients treated with cyclosporine and prednisone. N Engl J Med 322:1183, 1990.
Ortho Multicenter Transplant Study Group: A randomized clinical trial of OKT3 monoclonal antibody for acute rejection of cadaveric renal transplants. N Engl J Med 313:337, 1985.
Read AE, Wiesner RH, LaBrecque DR, et al: Hepatic veno-occlusive disease associated with renal transplantation and azathioprine therapy. Ann Intern Med 104:651, 1986.
Reinhart JB, Kemph JP: Renal transplantation for children: Another view. JAMA 260:3327, 1988.
Sheldon CA, McLorie GA, Churchill BM: Renal transplantation in children. Pediatr Clin North Am 34:1209, 1987.
Snydman DR, Werner BG, Heinze-Lacey B, et al: Use of cytomegalovirus immune globulin to prevent cytomegalovirus disease in renal-transplant recipients. N Engl J Med 317:1049, 1987.
Taube DH, Neild GH, Williams DG, et al: Differentiation between allograft rejection and cyclosporin nephrotoxicity in renal-transplant recipients. Lancet 2:171, 1985.
Trompeter RS: Renal transplantation. Arch Dis Child 65:143, 1990.
Trompeter RS, Bewick M, Haycock GB, et al: Renal transplantation in very young children. Lancet i:373, 1983.

LIVER TRANSPLANTATION

Chapman RW, Forman D, Peto R, et al: Liver transplantation for acute hepatic failure? Lancet 335:32, 1990.
Esquivel CO, Koneru B, Karrer F, et al: Liver transplantation before 1 year of age. J Pediatr 110:545, 1987.
Fishbein MH, Whittington PF: Update on pediatric liver transplantation in the treatment of end-stage liver disease. Int Pediatr 5:9, 1990.
Shaw BW, Wood RP, Kaufman SS, et al: Liver transplantation therapy for children: Part 1. J Pediatr Gastroenterol Nutr 7:157, 1988.
Shaw BW, Wood RP, Kaufman SS, et al: Liver transplantation therapy for children: Part 2. J Pediatr Gastroenterol Nutr 7:797, 1988.
Starzl TE, Demetris AJ, van Thiel D: Liver transplantation (first of two parts). N Engl J Med 321:1014, 1989.
Starzl TE, Demetris AJ, van Thiel D: Liver transplantation (second of two parts). N Engl J Med 321:1092, 1989.
Strong RW, Lynch SV, Ong TH, et al: Successful liver transplantation from a living donor to her son. N Engl J Med 322:1505, 1990.

Whitington PF, Balistreri WF: Liver transplantation in pediatrics: Indications, contraindications, and pretransplant management. J Pediatr 118:169, 1991.

HEART TRANSPLANTATION

Addonizio LJ, Rose EA: Cardiac transplantation in children and adolescents. J Pediatr 111:1034, 1987.
Boucek MM, Kanakriyeh MS, Mathis CM, et al: Cardiac transplantation in infancy: Donors and recipients. J Pediatr 116:171, 1990.
Fricker FJ, Griffith BP, Hardesty RL, et al: Experience with heart transplantation in children. Pediatrics 79:138, 1987.
Gersony WM: Cardiac transplantation in infants and children. J Pediatr 116:266, 1990.
Green M, Wald ER, Fricker FJ, et al: Infections in pediatric orthotopic heart transplant recipients. Pediatr Infect Dis J 8:87, 1989.
Pahl E, Fricker J, Armitage J, et al: Coronary arteriosclerosis in pediatric heart transplant survivors: Limitation of long-term survival. J Pediatr 116:177, 1990.
Reid CJ, Yacoub MH: Determinants of left ventricular function one year after cardiac transplantation. Br Heart J 59:397, 1988.
Swinnen LJ, Costanzo-Norden MR, Fisher SG, et al: Increased incidence of lymphoproliferative disorder after immunosuppression with monoclonal antibody OKT3 in cardiac transplant recipients. N Engl J Med 323:1723, 1990.

LUNG TRANSPLANTATION

Grossman RF, Frost A, Zamel N, et al: Results of single-lung transplantation for bilateral pulmonary fibrosis. N Engl J Med 322:727, 1990.
Kirklin JK: Heart-lung transplantation. Am J Med 85:3, 1988.
Scott J, Higenbottam T, Hutter J, et al: Heart-lung transplantation for cystic fibrosis. Lancet ii:192, 1988.
Theodore J, Lewiston N: Lung transplantation comes of age. N Engl J Med 322:772, 1990.
Toronto Lung Transplant Group: Unilateral lung transplantation for pulmonary fibrosis. N Engl J Med 314:1140, 1986.
Toronto Lung Transplant Group: Experience with single-lung transplantation for pulmonary fibrosis. JAMA 259:2258, 1988.

PANCREATIC TRANSPLANTATION

Allen D, MacDonald M: Pancreas and islet cell transplantation for type I diabetes mellitus: Does it have a role for children? Adv Pediatr 37:391, 1990.
Bilous RW, Mauer SM, Sutherland DER, et al: The effects of pancreas transplantation on the glomerular structure of renal allografts in patients with insulin-dependent diabetes. N Engl J Med 321:80, 1989.
Skolnick A: Advances in islet cell transplantation: Is science closer to a diabetes cure? JAMA 264:427, 1990.
Tattersall R: Is pancreas transplantation for insulin-dependent diabetics worthwhile? N Engl J Med 321:112, 1989.
Transplantation or insulin. Lancet 335:1271, 1990.

6.48 PREANESTHETIC AND POSTANESTHETIC CARE

Safe and effective anesthesia for infants and children requires a thorough comprehension of the basic principles of modern anesthetic practice and of pediatric physiology and pharmacology. The anesthesiologist must understand the following: (1) the ways in which pediatric patients differ from adults in anatomy, physiology, and response to drugs; (2) the emotional reactions to anesthesia and surgery by various pediatric age groups; and (3) the physical status of the patient, the nature of the surgical lesion, and the operation to be performed. These factors enable the anesthesiologist to make an appropriate preoperative evaluation, to produce the desired degree of preanesthetic sedation, to select the least hazardous anesthetic agents and techniques that produce satisfactory operating conditions, to determine the appropriate modes for monitoring various vital functions, and to provide for maintenance of an adequate alveolar ventilation and circulating blood volume as well as fluid, electrolyte, and acid-base equilibrium.

6.49 PREANESTHETIC EVALUATION

A careful history enables the anesthesiologist to plan more effectively the management of anesthesia and the postanesthetic period. It should include specific information about the following:

The child's previous anesthetic and surgical procedures
Family history of major anesthetic complications
History of apnea, breathing irregularities, or cyanosis (especially in infants under age 6 mo)
Recent upper respiratory tract infection
Exposure to exanthems
Previous laryngotracheitis (croup)
History of allergies, drug hypersensitivities, asthma, or wheezing during respiratory infections
Abnormal weight loss
Exercise tolerance
Bleeding tendencies
Blood transfusion reactions
Current medications
Prior administration of corticosteroids
Emotional reactions of the child to the proposed operation
When and what the child last ate (especially in emergency procedures)

Other considerations are also important. A history of frequent croup requires special airway management during anesthesia. A familial history of abnormal response to muscle relaxants might indicate a genetically abnormal pseudocholinesterase, which the anesthesiologist must consider when selecting a muscle relaxant. Infants and children receiving cortisone, antiepileptic or sedative drugs, or certain antibiotics may have altered responses to anesthetic and adjuvant agents. Finally, a patient with a full stomach risks aspiration during induction of anesthesia.

Following inhalation anesthesia, infants less than 6 mo of age born at a gestational age less than 36 wk may be prone to periodic breathing, with an increased risk of postoperative apnea, arterial oxyhemoglobin desaturation, bradycardia, and cardiac arrest. The mechanisms by which anesthetics affect the control of breathing in infants remain unclear. These infants are at even greater risk if they have a history of apneic or cyanotic episodes and if their postconceptual age is less than 1 yr. Regional or spinal anesthesia has limited application in infants and each presents its own side effects, including postanesthetic apnea. Intravenous caffeine given at the induction of anesthesia may be effective in preventing apnea in some, but not all, infants. Because of these considerations, as well as the occasional unexplained postanesthetic apnea in a young infant born at term, delaying *purely elective* operations is recommended until after a postconceptual age of 55–60 wk in former preterm infants and 44 wk in infants born at term.

With the increased survival of severely premature infants (<1,500 g birthweight) and their propensity to develop inguinal hernias, the risk of early operation must be weighed against the risks of delaying the hernia repair. This delay leads to the possibility of developing an incarcerated or strangulated hernia and acute intestinal obstruction requiring an emergency herniorrhaphy at a time when the infant may be in less than optimal condition. If proceeding with the operation is decided, the infant should be observed with ECG and respiratory monitoring in the recovery room for at least 2 hr. If the infant also presents with one or more of the high risk factors associated with postanesthetic apnea with bradycardia cited earlier, in-hospital monitoring with close nursing surveillance for 24–48 hr is usually indicated.

The physical examination of any infant or child considered for anesthesia and operation should emphasize the heart, lungs, and upper airways. The presence of heart murmurs, rales in the chest, or wheezing requires careful cardiac or pulmonary evaluation before proceeding. Small, narrow nares filled with secretions, loose teeth, tonsils and adenoids large enough to cause mouth-breathing, or a small, underdeveloped mandible with a protruding maxilla may contribute to upper airway obstruction after sedation or induction of anesthesia. Tracheal intubation may be difficult if the larynx lies cephalad and anterior to its normal position, as in the Pierre-Robin anomalad or Treacher-Collins syndrome.

Laboratory tests desirable before anesthesia include determination of hemoglobin or hematocrit, white cell count, and urinalysis. In patients with serious systemic disease or those about to undergo extensive surgery, a preoperative roentgenogram of the chest and measurement of arterial pH, Pa_{O_2} and Pa_{CO_2}, and of serum electrolyte, blood glucose, or urea nitrogen levels, may be indicated. For healthy infants and children undergoing elective superficial operations, many pediatric anesthesiologists require only a hemoglobin determination to ensure adequate blood oxygen transport ability.

6.50 PREANESTHETIC PREPARATION AND SEDATION

Children are frightened on leaving the security and familiarity of home, especially those 1–4 yr of age, who are unable to understand the purpose of hospitalization. Terrifying experiences during induction of anesthesia or in the immediate postoperative period can produce disabling psychologic changes such as night terrors, enuresis, and temper tantrums. Certain steps can minimize the psychologic trauma. For the child over 3 yr of age, parents should explain the purpose of the proposed operation in simple terms, telling of the probable sequence of events and discomfort involved. Parents should be encouraged to display confidence and cheerfulness; their tension and anxiety are readily transmitted to the child. The anesthesiologist should visit the child prior to operation, in the presence of the parents if possible, so that the child regards the anesthesiologist as a sympathetic, caring friend. Preanesthetic sedation, when used, should permit the child to be transported to the operating room lightly asleep, allow induction of anesthesia without awakening, and provide some analgesia during postanesthetic recovery.

Improvements in pediatric anesthesia over the past 25 yr permit children with no organic disturbances or some mild to moderate abnormalities to be admitted to a surgical facility, undergo general anesthesia and superficial, noncomplex operative procedures, recover, and return home on the same day. The requirements for safe "day surgery" include a history and physical examination, basic laboratory studies, and a visit with the anesthesiologist, preferably within 30 days prior to operation as well as a brief preanesthetic review by the anesthesiologist on the day of operation; and an extended recovery period to ensure that the child has voided, is not vomiting, and has adequate relief of pain.

Elective anesthesia and operation in the healthy infant less than 6 mo of age carries an increased risk of certain serious, even potentially lethal, complications. Infants, in contrast to older children and adults, experience more rapid uptake from the lungs and require higher blood levels to achieve effective anesthesia with halothane (Fluothane), the most widely used volatile anesthetic agent. Severe systemic arterial hypotension at an effective anesthetic dose occurs more frequently in the infant, indicating a narrow margin of safety. Unexplained apneic episodes in apparently recovered infants may occur after anesthesia, resulting in severe brain damage and death if undetected. Hemoglobin concentration may be at its nadir and limit oxygen content reserves in the blood. Delayed or partial recovery from muscle relaxants may also occur during this period, especially if the infant's body temperature falls below 36° C (96.8° F). All these complications are rare, yet are more likely to occur in the infant born preterm who is less than 44 wk postconception. Appropriate use of halothane, isoflurane (Forane), muscle relaxants, and oxygen provides safe, reliable anesthesia in infants; however, extending postanesthetic observation and maintaining body temperature helps ensure the safety of anesthesia in this age group.

A wide variety of drugs are used for preanesthetic sedation. Table 6–35 lists appropriate oral and intramuscular drugs and dosages for various age groups. Atropine provides more effective abolition of vagal reflexes than does scopolamine and, therefore, is preferred in infants under 1 yr of age, in whom vagal reflexes tend to be more active. In children over 1 yr of age a small-volume oral preanesthetic sedation in a fruit-flavored syrup containing meperidine, diazepam, and atropine given 2 hr prior to anesthetic induction is safe and effective. Painful intramuscular injections of preanesthetic sedatives are indicated only rarely, and an equivalent sedative and analgesic effect can be achieved with the use of an appropriate inpatient oral regimen (see Table 6–35). Postoperative analgesia can be ensured initially by regional anesthetic block with a long-acting agent, such as bupivacaine, or by the intravenous injection of a short-acting narcotic in an analgesic dose, such as fentanyl (1–2 μg/kg), prior to termination of anesthesia.

Although the child's stomach should be free of solids prior to anesthesia, it is important not to interrupt fluid intake longer than necessary. No milk or solids should be given less than 12 hr prior to anesthesia. Clear liquids with glucose should be given up to 4 hr prior to inducing anesthesia in infants and children. Because this preoperative oral fluid regimen may not prevent mild dehydration, intravenous isotonic electrolyte solution with glucose is warranted for all but the shortest minor procedures (see Sec. 6.25).

Before proceeding with an operation the anesthesiologist should correct dehydration, decrease excessive fever, correct acidosis, and restore a depleted blood volume.

The febrile, dehydrated child who requires emergency surgery, such as appendectomy, should receive at least partial rehydration rapidly, along with correction of any concomitant metabolic acidosis by intravenous sodium bicarbonate (2–3 mEq/kg). General endotracheal anesthesia with neuromuscular blockade and controlled ventilation followed by surface cooling with water mattresses on the anterior and posterior body surfaces can then be instituted. Cooling should be continued until the colonic or esophageal temperature is under 38° C (100.4° F).

Newborn infants who require immediate surgery and who have made little or no recovery from birth asphyxia or who have a body temperature below 35° C (95° F) require oxygen, intravenous infusion of sodium bicarbonate (1–3 mEq/kg) over 30–60 min, and elevation of body temperature toward 37° C

TABLE 6–35. Oral Preanesthetic Medication

Drug	Dosage (mg/kg)
Atropine	0.02
Meperidine	1.5 (outpatient)*
	3.0 (inpatient)
Diazepam	0.15 (outpatient)
Pentobarbital	4.0 (inpatient)

*Outpatient: meperidine-diazepam-atropine; inpatient: meperidine-pentobarbital-atropine. This can be prepared in a fruit-flavored syrup in fixed concentrations so that it can be prescribed in mL/kg (e.g., 0.25 mL/kg).

(98.6° F). Analyzing blood for pH, $Paco_2$, Pao_2, sodium, potassium, ionized calcium, glucose, osmolality, and hematocrit is essential to initial monitoring and to evaluate the patient's ventilation and metabolic status.

6.51 INTRAOPERATIVE MANAGEMENT

Infants and children of all ages, including the smallest preterm infant, should receive anesthesia for operative procedures, unless the patient is in such a compromised cardiopulmonary condition that the agents are likely to cause cardiac arrest. Local and regional anesthesia can be used to supplement the use of more potent narcotic and inhalation agents in some severely ill infants. Blocking the stress of pain perception has beneficial effects on the newborn's and young infant's metabolic stability by attenuating the stress response, which is characterized by excessive catecholamine release, hyperglycemia, and protein catabolism.

All the common inhalation agents have been used in children, but during the past 25 yr halothane, isoflurane, and nitrous oxide with neuromuscular blockage have replaced flammable agents such as cyclopropane and diethyl ether. For induction, most anesthesiologists prefer gravity flow of nitrous oxide and halothane over the face, with application of a face mask only after the child has lost consciousness. Intravenous induction, using a No. 25–27 gauge scalp vein needle, may be achieved rapidly with intravenous thiopental (3–4 mg/kg); ketamine can also be used for intravenous induction in infants and young children, but is contraindicated in older children and adolescents because of the frequency of postanesthetic hallucinations in this age group. In equipotent dosage isoflurane causes less arterial hypotension, fewer cardiac dysrhythmias, and greater skeletal muscle relaxation than halothane. Regional anesthesia has become more widely applied as a supplement to inhalation anesthesia and as the primary form of anesthesia in infants over the past decade. Infants and children are at no greater risk than adults for adverse drug reactions or accidental overdosage, provided the total drug dose and route of administration are appropriate for the patient's size and physical status.

Experience has shown that nondepolarizing muscle relaxants (metubine, *d*-tubocurarine, pancuronium, and the shorter acting atracurium and vecuronium) can be used with effectiveness and safety, even in the newborn infant. Tracheal intubation and controlled ventilation provide optimal gas exchange, and neostigmine preceded by atropine restores neuromuscular transmission at the conclusion of anesthesia.

Tracheal intubation is indicated in the following: (1) operations of the head and neck; (2) intrathoracic, intraperitoneal, and intracranial procedures; (3) operations in the prone position; (4) most procedures in infants under 1 yr of age; and (5) virtually all emergency procedures, because there is uncertainty about the contents of the stomach. Ventilation should be controlled manually or mechanically in all intrathoracic and intraperitoneal operations and in patients lying in the prone position.

During anesthesia, monitoring of heart tones with a precordial stethoscope, a continuous electrocardiogram (lead 2), continuous measurement of rectal temperature with a thermistor probe, and assessment of arterial pressure by the Riva-Rocci or ultrasonic Doppler method are mandatory for all age groups. For children in poor physical condition or those undergoing extensive surgery, inserting a plastic cannula into an artery for continuous direct measurement of arterial pressure and for blood sampling is usually indicated.

Pulse oximetry and expired carbon dioxide analysis are also basic monitoring techniques that should be used. The pulse oximeter accurately and precisely measures arterial oxygen saturation (Sao_2), even when mean systemic arterial pressures are as low as 30 mm Hg; skin pigmentation does not affect its reading. The unheated sensor can be attached to an infant's finger, hand, or foot for many hours without replacement and remains accurate without harming the infant's skin. Continuously measuring end-tidal expired carbon dioxide concentration by infrared or mass spectrometry and pulse oximetry can noninvasively provide important information about the child's gas exchange. Mass spectrometry semicontinuously assesses inspired and end-tidal carbon dioxide, oxygen, nitrous oxide, and volatile anesthetics such as halothane, enhancing both the efficacy and safety of anesthesia. National anesthesia machine standards call for a device to measure continuously the inspired oxygen concentration and for safety devices that preclude the delivery of a hypoxic gas mixture to the patient.

Shock from hypovolemia may occur suddenly, and cardiac arrest ensue (see Sec. 6.35). Being aware of the infant's approximate blood volume (80–90 mL/kg in the newborn, 75 mL/kg in the older infant) and immediately replacing losses exceeding 10–15% of that volume can prevent hypovolemic shock. Blood for rapid infusion should be warmed to 37° C immediately before use because rapid infusion of cold blood may produce cardiac arrest. When the anticipated losses exceed one third of the patient's estimated blood volume, CPD (citrate-phosphate-dextrose) blood less than 10 days old should be used because older blood becomes extremely acidotic (pH 6.5–6.7) and depleted of clotting factors. Serial arterial pH, Pco_2, and electrolyte determinations can detect the acidosis, hypocalcemia, and hyperkalemia that may be associated with rapid, massive blood replacement. Selecting the appropriate blood products and balanced electrolyte solutions often permits the restoration of intravascular volume without using whole blood.

Continuous monitoring of body temperature is essential during general anesthesia. In air-conditioned operating rooms inadvertent hypothermia (colonic temperature under 35° C, 95° F) develops frequently in small infants undergoing laparatomy or thoracotomy and is associated with ventilatory depression, peripheral vasoconstriction, and a moderate metabolic acidosis in the immediate postanesthetic period. Overhead radiant heaters, circulating warm water mattresses, heated humidification of inspired gases, and wrapping the head and extremities with cotton or other heat-retaining, nonabrasive materials can minimize this thermal stress. *Malignant hyperpyrexia* (MH), the abrupt and unexplained rise in body temperature above 41° C (105.8° F) during or following (immediately or after several hours) inhalation anesthesia or administration of succinylcholine, occurs in children over 1 yr of age and in young adults. Typically, there is also tachypnea, tachycardia, and hypertension. The overall mortality rate approaches 75% unless detected at the outset and treated. Successful management demands immediate recognition of a rapid rise in temperature, cessation of anesthesia, and hyperventilation with oxygen. Treatment also includes packing the patient in ice, ice-water gastric lavage, rapid infusion of intravenous fluids at 5–10 times the maintenance rate until adequate urine output is established, and intravenous administration of sodium bicarbonate (4–7 mEq/kg) and dantrolene (1 mg/kg, to a total of 10 mg/kg). The patient at risk of MH by prior personal or family history requires consultation with an anesthesiologist well in advance of the day of operation. Preparation for such patients involves purging of the anesthesia machine with oxygen for 12 hr, selecting the anesthetic agents and adjuvant drugs least likely to trigger MH, and often providing prophylactic therapy with dantrolene (see also Sec. 21.23).

6.52 POSTANESTHETIC RECOVERY

Recovery room facilities and nursing must be available to provide constant surveillance of airway patency, adequate ventilation, and circulatory stability. Infants less than 6 mo of age should remain in the recovery room for at least 2 hr to ensure full recovery of respiratory control, neuromuscular function, and upper airway reflexes. Common sequelae of general anesthesia in infants and children include postanesthetic excitement, vomiting, and pain. Postanesthetic excitement occurs most frequently in patients who have undergone painful procedures involving the head and neck and the abdomen; intravenous narcotics in an appropriate dose are most effective in managing this complication. Vomiting occurs commonly following myringotomy, tonsillectomy, procedures on the eyes, and intra-abdominal operations. It can sometimes be relieved with intravenous droperidol, a benzodiazepine, diazepam, or phenothiazine in small doses. For control of severe pain, such as that associated with extensive orthopedic procedures, morphine (0.05–0.10 mg/kg by slow intravenous injection) should provide relief for at least 3 hr. Malignant hyperpyrexia may also occur in the immediate postanesthetic period; therefore, initial measurement of body temperature and repeated monitoring of heart rate and, if tachycardia occurs, rectal temperature, remains important.

Patients with upper airway anomalies, operations in the pharynx or upper airway, or a history of upper airway obstruction during sleep require exceptionally careful and longer observation. They may develop lethal airway obstruction when sedated and should be observed in an intensive care unit for 24 hr.

Following tracheal intubation, patients between 6 mo and 6 yr of age may develop subglottic edema, especially if they have a history of croup or recent upper respiratory tract infection, which can often be relieved by inhaling aerosolized racemic epinephrine (0.2%) in addition to supportive measures, including receiving humidified oxygen and intravenous fluids. Intravenous corticosteroids may have some beneficial effect. Rarely, orotracheal intubation followed by nasotracheal intubation or tracheostomy is required for 2–5 days to guarantee an adequate airway.

6.53 PAIN MANAGEMENT

Over the past decade, dramatic improvement has occurred in the development and availability of safe and effective techniques for the management of pain in infants and children from all causes, including postoperative pain (see also Sec. 6.54). No child should suffer acute or chronic intense pain without therapy to ameliorate the pain and lessen the accompanying fear and anxiety. One of the newer techniques applicable to children is continuous epidural anesthesia with a long-acting analgesic. Some currently used agents and procedures include the following: (1) bupivacaine mixed with morphine or fentanyl; (2) patient-controlled infusion pumps for intravenous narcotic administration on demand, with a "lockout" timing mechanism to prevent excessive dosage; (3) continuous intravenous narcotic infusion to maintain a constant analgesic plasma concentration; (4) combinations of antidepressant and analgesic medications for chronic and terminal pain management; and (5) the use of relaxation therapy and self-hypnosis. Effective implementation of these and other methods usually requires a multidisciplinary team dedicated to pain management in children. Emergency department physicians can also play an important role in alleviating pain by using appropriate local and field blocks supplemented by low intravenous doses of short-acting narcotics. The efficacy and safety of nitrous oxide analgesia (up to 50% inspired concentration in oxygen) remain to be proven in prospective, large-scale studies of pediatric emergency department patients with pain.

JOHN J. DOWNES
RUSSELL C. RAPHAELY

GENERAL REFERENCES

Gregory GA (ed): Pediatric Anesthesia, Vols. 1 and 2, 2nd ed. New York, Churchill-Livingstone, 1989.
Motoyama E, Davis P (eds): Smith's Anesthesia for Infants and Children, 5th ed. St. Louis, CV Mosby, 1990.
Ryan JF, Todres ID, Cote CJ, et al (eds): A Practice of Anesthesia for Infants and Children. New York, Grune & Stratton, 1986.

GENERAL ANESTHESIA AND SEDATION

Anand KJS, Sippell WG, Aynsley-Green A: Randomized trial of fentanyl anesthesia in preterm babies undergoing surgery. Effects on the stress response. Lancet 1:243, 1987.
Brustowicz RM, Nelson DA, Betts EK, et al: Efficacy of oral premedication for pediatric outpatient surgery. Anesthesiology 60:475, 1984.
Keenan RL, Boyan CP: Cardiac arrest due to anesthesia. A study of incidence and causes. JAMA 253:2373, 1985.
Nicolson SC, Betts EK, Jobes DR, et al: Comparison of oral and intramuscular preanesthetic medication for pediatric inpatient surgery. Anesthesiology 71:8, 1989.

POSTOPERATIVE APNEA

Kurth CD, Spitzer AR, Broennle AM, et al: Post-operative apnea in preterm infants. Anesthesiology 66:483, 1987.
LeBard SE, Kurth CD, Spitzer AR, et al: Preventing postoperative apnea by neuromodulator antagonists. Anesthesiology 71:A1026, 1989.
Welborn LG, DeSoto H, Hannallah RS, et al: The use of caffeine in the control of post-anesthetic apnea in former preterm infants. Anesthesiology 68:796, 1988.

REGIONAL ANESTHESIA

Dalens B: Regional anesthesia in children. Anesth Analg 68:654, 1989.

PAIN MANAGEMENT

McGrath PJ, Unruh AM: Pain In Children and Adolescents. New York, Elsevier, 1987.
Tyler DC, Krane EJ: Post-operative pain management in children. Anesthesiol Clin North Am 7:155, 1989.

6.54 PAIN MANAGEMENT IN CHILDREN

The management of pain in the pediatric patient has lagged markedly behind that in the adult resulting, in large part, from misconceptions regarding the existence of the pain sensation and its tolerance in children. Additionally, the difficulty in assessing pain in preverbal or cognitively immature individuals, coupled with the ill-founded notion that infants and children exhibit a greater sensitivity to pain medication, have further hampered the rational management of pain syndromes in children.

MISCONCEPTIONS OF PAIN. Pain is a subjective experience comprised of both sensory and emotional components. The intensity of the pain experience and the mechanisms for coping with it, therefore, vary among individuals for any given injury. The inability of the pediatric patient, however, to communicate his or her pain experience clearly has led to accumulation of complex societal beliefs and medical misjudgments that have resulted in the undertreatment of their pain. Some misconceptions about pain in children include the following: (1) children have a higher tolerance to pain; (2) pain perception in children is decreased because of biologic immaturity; (3) children have little or no memory of a painful experience; (4) children are more sensitive to the side effects of analgesics; and (5) children are at special risk for addiction to narcotics. There is no evidence to substantiate these beliefs.

PATHOPHYSIOLOGY. Neurologic immaturity does not render the preterm and term neonate incapable of painful sensation and memory. The neurosensory pathways necessary for nociceptive transmission are anatomically and functionally intact in the newborn infant. Anatomic studies show that peripheral innervation and central nervous system connections at the spinal cord dorsal horn cell level exist early in fetal development. Spinal nerve tracts for pain transmission are myelinated by mid- to late gestation and the basic nerve pathways necessary for completing synaptic pain transmission to the level of the neocortex are intact and completely myelinated by the 3rd trimester of gestation. In addition, nociceptive transmitters (substance P) and pain modulator substances (endogenous opioids) function in the fetus, and concentrations of these neuropeptides are significantly increased in the perinatal period.

In the neonate, as in the adult, unmyelinated C fibers transmit nociceptive information peripherally. Nerve pulse transmission in incompletely myelinated A-δ fibers is delayed, not blocked, until myelination has been completed postnatally. The shorter distances necessary for impulse travel offset any delay in conduction velocity. Therefore, lack of well-developed inhibitory control in the newborn may result in exaggerated, hyperalgesic responses to afferent stimuli until postnatal maturation occurs.

Furthermore, evaluation of the neonate undergoing painful procedures (e.g., heel lance, circumcision) without anesthesia indicates a pattern of autonomic response to pain manifested by increases in blood pressure, heart rate, pulmonary vascular resistance, intracranial pressure, palmar sweat, and by a decrease in the transcutaneous partial pressure of oxygen. Behavior responses are diffuse and exaggerated but purposeful, and are characterized by prolonged withdrawal, particularly in the preterm neonate, correlating with increased neuropeptide concentrations at available receptor sites spread diffusely over the cerebral cortex. Pain from such procedures elicits individualized behavioral responses, with some infants actually decreasing activity during painful stimulation. Behavioral changes persist after the pain is over, suggesting memory. Newborns also demonstrate hormonal responses to the pain of surgery with the release of catecholamines, corticosteroids, glucagon, and growth hormone, with simultaneous suppression of insulin release. These metabolic alterations result in marked hyperglycemia, persisting in the postoperative period, and a prolonged state of catabolism leading to the breakdown of protein substrate. Endocrine responses to the stress of various types of surgical pain can be attenuated or blocked by the use of potent inhaled anesthesia or fentanyl anesthesia, respectively. A lack of attenuation of the neuroendocrine stress response correlates with intraoperative instability and increased postoperative metabolic and circulatory complications, as compared to the course of infants receiving fentanyl anesthesia. Therefore, there may be a benefit from the attenuation of the hormonal response to the stress of surgical pain in children.

CLINICAL MANIFESTATIONS AND ASSESSMENTS. The assessment of pain in the infant is necessarily indirect and includes the observation of cry, facial expression, autonomic responses, and behavior or motor activity. Facial expression is the most consistently valid indicator of pain in infants. As infants become older anticipatory behavior also occurs, manifest by posturing and protective limb movement. Preschool children, aged 3–7 yr, have a limited cognitive ability to qualify or quantify their pain. Ladder or linear analog scales using photographed facial expression, serial line-drawn faces, or color schemes may be useful for validating the discomfort of preschool children. Self-reporting methods using numerical rating scales for pain intensity have proven particularly useful for school-aged children and correlate well with simultaneous parent ratings. The psychologic and emotional aspects of the adolescent pain experience are more likely to be factored into self-reporting of their pain. Because behavior is more restrained, and in the absence of a validated pain assessment tool specific to the adolescent's needs, reliance on a more comprehensive self-reporting instrument, such as the McGill Pain Questionnaire, may be helpful. Regardless of age, time must be provided for instruction and practice using self-reporting instruments. Pain assessment should be performed regularly and frequently, and is facilitated by the patients' better understanding of their pain and the reasons it exists.

TREATMENT. The first step in a comprehensive pain management program is the evaluation of each patient's individual needs with the help of a team of pediatric medical and psychosocial specialists, when possible. There should be age-appropriate education and discussion regarding the proposed care plan or any planned procedure, including introducing the patient and family to caregivers, offering hands-on play with benign medical equipment, and encouraging practice sessions with dolls. These techniques may help reveal some of the patient's fears that would otherwise not be easily expressed. By permitting patient participation and incorporating patient preferences in the treatment plan, insofar as possible, patient confidence and cooperation can be improved at almost any age.

The mainstay of the pharmacologic treatment of severe acute or chronic pain is systemic opioid medication. Other analgesic medications given systemically or locally (local anesthetics) can act to provide synergism with opioids or can eliminate the need for systemic opioids (Table 6–36).

Whenever feasible, a child should be offered an appropriate analgesic by a noninvasive route, orally or through an existing intravenous line. It is important to realize that administering intramuscular injections to children reporting pain sends them the message that, to achieve pain relief, more pain must be administered. This is a concept that, even if understood, rarely meets with patient acceptance and inevitably leads to the open denial of active pain by fearful children.

Postoperative Pain. Pain control in the perioperative period should be a continuum, beginning with preoperative teaching and medication and followed by intraoperative analgesia with a regional block or systemic drug, either or both of which can be continued throughout the postoperative period. In the absence of a regional block (Sec. 6.53), most postoperative pain can be treated effectively by oral preparations of opioids or by their intravenous administration with intermittent or continuous infusion. Continuous infusion is helpful in maintaining uniform plasma drug levels and permits constancy of pain relief, unlike the cycles of alternating pain and analgesia that result from intermittent parenteral administration. The side effects of opioid use can be limited by combination therapy with acetaminophen or nonsteroidal anti-inflammatory drugs (NSAID). Moderate to mild postoperative pain may be well controlled with nonopioid analgesics alone but, unlike opioids, nonopioids have ceiling effects for analgesia, and increasing doses may lead to a higher incidence of side effects without improved analgesia. Also, the practice of prn dosing results in inadequate pain relief and is not recommended.

TABLE 6–36. Recommended Schedules and Dosages of Analgesic Medication in Infants and Older Children

Medication	Dosing Schedule		Comments
	Infants <3 mo	*Children >3 mo*	
Morphine	IV: bolus—0.1 mg/kg q3–4 hr; loading—0.05 mg/kg; then infusion—0.01–0.015 mg/kg/hr	Oral: 0.3–0.6 mg/kg q8–12 hr; IV: bolus—0.1 mg/kg q1–2 hr; infusion—0.04–0.06 μg/kg/hr	MS-Contin Apnea monitoring <3 mo or at risk; bolus over 20 min; beware of hypotension and bronchospasm; naloxone reversal (10 μg/kg) available at all times
		Subcutaneous: bolus—0.1–0.15 mg/kg q3–4 hr; infusion—0.05–0.06 mg/kg/hr	>20 mo, syringe pump
Fentanyl	IV: bolus—0.5–2 μg/kg q1–2 hr; loading—1–2 μg/kg; then infusion—1–5 μg/kg/hr	IV: bolus—0.5–2 μg/kg q2–3 hr; increments—0.5 μg/kg q1–2 min; loading—1–2 μg/kg; then infusion—1–5 μg/kg/hr	Intubation or apnea monitoring in infants <3 mo or at risk; beware chest wall rigidity and bradycardia; naloxone standby
Alfentanil		IV increments: 1–2 μg/kg q2–3 min	Potent, ultrashort-acting opioid
Methadone		Oral: 0.1 mg/kg q4 hr × 3; then q6–8 hr IV, bolus: 0.1 mg/kg q2 hr × 2, then 0.04–0.09 mg/kg q4–8 hr	Full analgesia and toxicity may not be evident until plasma steady state, 3–5 days
Codeine		Oral: 0.5–1 mg/kg q4 hr	Gastric irritation
Tylenol	Oral: 10–15 mg/kg; R*-15–20 mg/kg	Oral: 10–15 mg/kg R-15–25 mg/kg	Prolonged plasma half-life in neonates; acute hepatotoxicity with excess dosing
Ibuprofen		Oral: 4–10 mg/kg q6–8 hr	Children >2 yr old; can cause gastritis; risk of nephrotoxicity and hepatoxicity with prolonged use
Naprosyn		Oral: 5–7 mg/kg q8–12 hr	
Tolectin		Oral: 5–7 mg/kg q6–8 hr	
Ketorolac		IM: 1.5 mg/kg q12 hr (60 mg max dose)	New NSAID: pain relief comparable to morphine. Less risk of gastritis and bleeding than other NSAID. Can inhibit platelet function. Soon available IV.
Amitriptyline		Oral: 0.5–1.5 mg/kg q HS†	Neuropathic pain; 3–5 days therapy required for pain reduction
Midazolam		Oral: 0.03 mg/kg q4–5 min	Potent benzodiazepine; 4-hr half-life; airway resuscitation equipment

*R = rectal
†HS = at bedtime

Morphine and fentanyl can be safely administered to children of 3 mo and older for postoperative pain control. This age group has the same ability as adults for drug clearance and comparable susceptibility to the respiratory side effects of opioids. On the other hand, drug clearance in neonates is highly variable. Therefore, infants younger than 3 mo old may safely receive opioid analgesia but must be monitored for apnea until 24 hr after their last dose. This age group, especially preterm infants and those at risk because of underlying disease (e.g., cystic fibrosis), should be intensively observed with immediate access to airway resuscitation available. These patients are at higher risk for apnea after general anesthesia and should be monitored appropriately.

Older children benefit greatly from the use of a pre-programmed computerized pump device for the self-administration of intravenous opioids. This method—patient-controlled analgesia (PCA)—has the advantages of timely drug administration for the maintenance of adequate analgesia, patient participation in self-care, and demonstrated safety in those aged 8–18 yr. It is strongly favored by both patient and caregivers. Younger patients may also be acceptable candidates for PCA, but those of all ages must be selected individually according to manual dexterity and conceptual understanding.

Cancer and Other Pain Syndromes. Patients with cancer suffer pain from the disease process, chemotherapy side effects, and repeated diagnostic and therapeutic procedures. It is imperative to establish the precise etiology of all pain to rule out unexpected complications of the underlying disease process. In addition to oral and intravenous opioids, alternative methods of drug administration are sometimes necessary because of patient tolerance, such as when mucositis or nausea preclude the administration of oral medication, or when intravenous access is limited. Options include the following: intermittent, continuous, or PCA subcutaneous infusion of morphine or methadone; transdermal or nasal fentanyl; or an opioid agent administered by indwelling epidural or intrathecal catheter. Corticosteroid therapy is also important in the relief of pain resulting from widespread tumor invasion of bone or of the central and peripheral nervous systems, resulting in nerve compression or elevated intracranial pressure.

Adjuvant therapies for potentiating or replacing opioid analgesia (in the case of non–cancer-related pain) include the use of NSAIDs, tricyclic antidepressants, anxiolytic agents, and transcutaneous electrical nerve stimulation (TENS). For example, the most effective pharmacologic therapy for the relief of the neuropathic pain from nerve injury is low-dose tricyclic medication. The pain of sickle cell disease or juvenile rheumatoid arthritis is best treated on a chronic basis by acetaminophen (Tylenol) or NSAIDs. Occasionally, however, as in acute vaso-occlusive crisis of sickle cell disease, opioid therapy is indicated. In such a case, morphine is the parenteral agent of choice. Generally, meperidine is not recommended because its long-acting metabolite, normeperidine, has poor analgesic properties and is associated with central nervous system excitement and seizures. Also, prolonged administration of normeperidine leads to its accumulation and carries a significant incidence of dysphoria and other toxic effects, particularly in patients with renal dysfunction.

Procedural Pain. Children with chronic illnesses often report that procedural pain related to bone marrow aspirations, lumbar punctures, and intrathecal chemotherapy is their greatest source of anxiety and pain in the hospital setting. Yet these procedures, as well as burn dressing changes and debridements and various intensive care and emergency room procedures, are widely performed without the benefit of a sedative, analgesic, or other coping strategy. Hypnosis and other cognitive-behavioral techniques can be extremely important adjuncts to pain management in this setting and emphasize patient participation. Children report that the single most helpful factor in coping with any pain experience is for their parent(s) to be present.

Effective topical local anesthetic preparations are available to anesthetize a skin area planned for a procedure. A small amount of sodium bicarbonate added to a local anesthetic solution can minimize the pain of subcutaneous infiltration prior to line placement or suturing. Fixed combinations of three or more systemic analgesics and tranquilizers are no longer considered safe; they are associated with significantly higher complication rates than more individualized schedules using one or two short-acting medications. By effectively combining the preceding methods the vast majority of procedures can be performed efficiently without prolonged medication effects, and with a significant reduction in the painful distress otherwise suffered by these patients.

With the assistance of a pediatric anesthesiologist in a well-equipped treatment room or in the operating suite, monitored care with profound sedation and analgesia using ultra–short-acting agents or general anesthesia can also be provided. The patient has almost complete or total amnesia of the experience and is pain-free when emerging from the sedation. Physicians regularly managing procedures of very brief duration should be well acquainted with the pharmacologic and clinical effects of these potent drugs, such as midazolam and alfentanil or fentanyl, and should rely on the anesthesiologist for instruction until they are more experienced. A qualified assistant to the physician should be dedicated to monitoring the patient closely during and after the procedure. Early detection of hypoventilation or airway obstruction is possible with vigilant observation and oxygen saturation monitoring by pulse oximetry. Equipment for airway management and resuscitation should be immediately available at all times.

GLORIA L. SELLMAN

Anand KJS, Hichey PR: Pain and its effects in the human neonate and fetus. N Engl J Med 317:1321, 1987.

Anand KJS, Sippell WG, Aynsley-Green A: Randomized trial of fentanyl anaesthesia in preterm babies undergoing surgery: Effects on the stress response. Lancet 1:243, 1987.

Berde C, Sethna NF, Masek B, et al: Pediatric pain clinics: Recommendations for their development. Pediatrician 16:94, 1989.

Berde CB, Fischel N, Filardi JP: Caudal epidural morphine analgesia for an infant with advanced neuroblastoma: Report of a case. Pain 36:219, 1989.

Beyer JE, DeGood DE, Ashley LC, et al: Patterns of postoperative analgesic use with adults and children following cardiac surgery. Pain 17:71, 1983.

Halperin DL, Koren G, Attias D, et al: Topical skin anesthesia for venous subcutaneous drug reservoir and lumbar punctures in children. Pediatrics 84:281, 1989.

Hertzka RE, Fisher DM, Gauntlett IS, et al: Are infants sensitive to respiratory depression from fentanyl? Anesthesiology 67:A512, 1987.

Lynn AM, Slattery JT: Morphine pharmacokinetics in early infancy. Anesthesiology 66:136, 1987.

Mather L, Mackie J: The incidence of postoperative pain in children. Pain 15:271, 1983.

McGrath PJ, Unruh AM: Pain in Children and Adolescents. New York, Elsevier, 1987.

Miser AW, Davis DM, Hughes CS, et al: Continuous subcutaneous infusion of morphine in children with cancer. Am J Dis Child 137:383, 1983.

Schechter NL, ed: Acute pain in children. Pediatr Clin North Am 36:781, 1989.

Truog R, Anand KJS: Management of pain in the postoperative neonate. Clin Perinatol 16:61, 1989.

Webb CJ, Stergios DA, Rodgers BM: Patient-controlled analgesia as postoperative pain treatment for children. J Pediatr Nurs 4:162, 1989.

6.55 PRINCIPLES OF DRUG THERAPY

Clinical pharmacology is concerned with the clinical application of a drug's pharmacokinetic and pharmacodynamic profile to optimize drug therapy. *Pharmacokinetics* is the quantitative evaluation of each component of a compound's disposition—that is, the processes of absorption, distribution, metabolism, and excretion. The ability to estimate a drug's pharmacokinetic parameters accurately depends on the ability to determine the concentration of that drug in a specific body fluid (e.g., blood, cerebrospinal fluid, urine, joint fluid). A drug concentration in a specific body fluid is, in theory, a reflection of the drug concentration in tissue, and thus reflects its concentration at its site of action, the receptor. A drug's concentration in blood (or other body fluid), however, is not necessarily equal to the drug's concentration in tissue or at its cellular receptor site. In pediatric practice, it is important to appreciate the factors involved in determining drug concentrations in body fluids, including physical access of that body fluid, available volume that can be safely removed, and the sensitivity and specificity of available laboratory methodology. Biologic fluid sampling in pediatrics is challenging because of the limited volume of biologic fluid present in the patient and the desirability for noninvasive sampling.

Pharmacodynamics is the study of the biochemical and physiologic effects of drugs—that is, their mechanism(s) of action. The pharmacologic or toxicologic effects of most drugs are a result of their interaction with macromolecular components of cells or receptors. Rational prescribing of drugs depends on a fundamental understanding of a drug's pharmacokinetic and pharmacodynamic profile. Understanding the effect of age is essential to understanding pediatric drug therapy, because age is one of the most important variables that influences the processes responsible for a drug's disposition and action in children. Designing an optimal pharmacologic therapy involves integrating an understanding of the pharmacokinetics and pharmacodynamics of a drug with the patient variables of disease and age.

INFLUENCE OF AGE ON DRUG THERAPY

Drug Absorption (see also Sec. 13.26)

Drugs administered extravascularly must cross many physiologic membranes before entering the systemic circulation and being distributed to their site of action.

GASTROINTESTINAL ABSORPTION. Although certain xenobiotics and nutrients are absorbed by active transport or facilitated diffusion, most drugs are absorbed from the gastrointestinal tract by passive diffusion. A number of important patient variables can affect the rate and extent of a drug's gastrointestinal absorption, including pH-dependent diffusion, the presence, absence, and/or type of gastric contents, gastric emptying time, and gastrointestinal motility. These physiologic processes reflect a clear but highly variable dependence on a patient's age. Patient and chemical factors that affect drug absorption are shown in Table 6–37.

Gastric pH. At birth this approaches neutrality, but within hours rapidly falls to between 1.5 and 3.0. Postnatally, gastric acid secretion displays a biphasic pattern: the highest gastric

TABLE 6–37. Factors Influencing Drug Absorption

Physicochemical factors
Molecular weight
Degree of ionization under physiologic conditions
Product formulation characteristics
Disintegration and dissolution rates for solid dosages
Drug-release characteristics for time-release preparations
Cosolutes and complex formation
Patient factors
Surface area available for absorption
Gastric and duodenal pH
Gastric emptying time
Bile salt pool size
Bacterial colonization of the gastrointestinal tract
Presence and extent of underlying diseases
Presence or absence of metabolic pathways or enzymes necessary for biotransformation

acid concentrations occur within the 1st 10 days of life and the lowest between 10 and 30 days of life. Corrected for body weight, the secretion of gastric acid approaches the lower limit of adult values by 3 mo of age. The ability to secrete pepsin and intrinsic factor appears to parallel that of gastric acid. Depending on a drug's pK_a, these differences in rate and amount of gastric acid can influence a drug's rate and/or extent of gastrointestinal absorption by influencing the amount of drug present in the ionized or nonionized form. Decreased ionization favors absorption.

Gastric Emptying Time and Intestinal Motility. Most orally administered drugs are absorbed from the small intestine, so the rate of gastric emptying is an important determinant of the rate and possibly overall extent of a drug's absorption. The gastric emptying rate during the neonatal period varies greatly. It is characterized by irregular and unpredictable peristaltic activity, and it is prolonged relative to that in the adult. The rate of gastric emptying is directly related to gestational and postnatal age, and is influenced by the type of feeding (solid or liquid). Gastric emptying time approaches adult values within the 1st 6–8 mo of life.

Similarly, small intestinal motility in the perinatal period is highly variable and is influenced by the presence or absence of food. Contractions of the duodenum in term neonates occur at rates similar to those observed in fasting adults, although the number of contractions/burst is lower. In addition, fasting or interdigestive motor activity is also shorter in children. These physiologic perturbations may influence the time course and extent of drug absorption from the gastrointestinal tract.

Pancreatic Enzyme Activity. The activity of pancreatic enzymes is decreased at birth, and it is lower in premature than in full-term neonates. Lipase activity is present by 34–36 wk gestation and increases 5-fold during the 1st week and 20-fold during the first 9 mo of postnatal life. In contrast, amylase activity can be detected as early as the 22nd wk of gestation but remains low even after birth (approximating 10% of adult values). There is decreased duodenal amylase activity in both fasting and fed infants during the 1st year of life. Trypsin secretion and response to pancreatin and secretin administration are blunted in term infants, but develop during the 1st year of life. Thus, any drug that requires cleavage from its salt by pancreatic enzymes prior to absorption (e.g., chloramphenicol palmitate) may demonstrate highly variable bioavailability during the 1st 1–3 mo of life.

Other Processes. The development of other physiologic processes also may influence the gastrointestinal absorption of drugs and other compounds. Bile salt metabolism during the first few months of life is affected by a progressive maturation of gallbladder emptying, intestinal motility and absorption, and hepatic uptake. Also, colonization of the gastrointestinal tract by bacterial flora, a process that influences the metabolism of bile salts and drugs and intestinal motility, varies with respect to age, type of delivery, type of feeding, and concurrent drug therapy. The gastrointestinal tract of a full-term, formula-fed, vaginally delivered infant is colonized with anaerobic bacteria by 4–6 days of postnatal life. The metabolic ability and activity of gastrointestinal bacterial microflora vary greatly. There are differences in the ability of gastrointestinal microflora to metabolize specific substrates among infants, children, and adults. In healthy subjects, complete metabolic activity of gastrointestinal bacterial flora approaches adult values for bile acids and neutral sterols by the age of 4 yr, but the effect of these maturational changes in intestinal flora on drug metabolism is uncertain. For example, although children are colonized with intestinal bacteria able to metabolize digoxin by the age of 2 yr, the ability to inactivate the drug develops only gradually, and the metabolic pattern observed in adults is not achieved until adolescence. This finding suggests, at least for digoxin, that intestinal colonization by digoxin-reducing organisms in children approaches adult values. Such variation clearly influences a drug's absorption profile, which can directly influence a patient's clinical response.

ALTERNATIVE ROUTES OF DRUG ABSORPTION. The primary means of extravascular drug administration in infants and children, other than the oral route, is the intramuscular route. Similar physiologic and physicochemical factors that affect the rate and extent of drug absorption in the gastrointestinal tract also influence the absorption of drugs from injection sites and through the skin (see Table 6–37). Drugs administered intramuscularly should be water-soluble at physiologic pH to prevent precipitation and the resultant decreased, delayed, or erratic absorption from the injection site. Lipid solubility of a drug favors diffusion into the capillaries. Blood flow to and from the injection site should be adequate to ensure absorption into the systemic circulation. This physiologic requirement may be compromised in seriously ill infants and children with poor peripheral perfusion resulting from low cardiac output and respiratory disease.

The skin is another important but often overlooked organ for the absorption of various therapeutic agents and environmental chemicals. This is exemplified by the many toxic effects noted in newborn infants exposed to hexachlorophene, aniline-containing disinfectant solutions, and hydrocortisone. The percutaneous absorption of a compound is directly related to the degree of skin hydration and inversely related to the thickness of the stratum corneum. The full-term newborn's integument is a more effective functional barrier than the skin of a premature infant. More importantly, however, the ratio of the newborn's skin surface area to body weight is approximately three times greater than that of an adult. Therefore, the amount of drug absorbed into the systemic circulation (bioavailability) for an identical percutaneous dose of a drug is approximately three times greater in an infant than in an adult. These characteristics of skin make topical creams and patch formulations of drugs important means of drug delivery in infants with adequate perfusion.

Thus, the effects of maturational changes on the bioavailability of a drug are unpredictable. A prolonged gastric emptying time and irregular intestinal peristaltic activity can lead to erratic rates of drug absorption, reducing the amount of drug absorbed and/or blunting or delaying the peak serum concentration. Reducing the rate and/or amount of total drug absorbed into the body can be therapeutically important, whereas blunting or delaying a drug's peak concentration may be of only minor clinical significance. The extent to which maturational changes influence gastrointestinal drug absorption also depend on the specific drug formulation administered. Solid dosage forms (e.g., tablets, capsules) must dissolve into solution before the drug can cross cell membranes. Most drugs administered to infants and young children are available in a liquid formulation, some as a suspension.

Drug Distribution

Understanding a drug's distribution characteristics in the body is paramount when selecting the dose to be administered. Although a drug's distribution volume (apparent volume of distribution, V_d) does not denote any real physiologic volume, an estimate of this pharmacokinetic parameter provides insight into the total amount of drug present in the body relative to its concentration in blood. Knowledge of a drug's V_d is important when designing an optimal drug dosage regimen to attain a selected target concentration. The value of the V_d for a number of drugs differs markedly in newborns, infants, and children as compared to adults. These differences are a result of many important age-dependent variables, including the composition and size of body water compartments, protein binding characteristics, and hemodynamic factors, including cardiac output, regional blood flow, and membrane permeability. The absolute amounts and distribution of body water and fat depend on a child's age and are well characterized (see Sec. 6.3). Changes in body water compartment sizes and water distribution account for the differences observed in the V_d in infants and children (see Fig. 6–2).

The extent to which a drug is bound to circulating plasma proteins directly influences the distribution characteristics of the drug. Only the free, unbound drug can be distributed from the vascular space into other body fluids and tissues, where it binds to its receptor and stimulates a response. Drug binding to plasma proteins depends on a number of age-related variables, including the absolute amount of proteins available, their respective number of available binding sites, the affinity constant of the drug for the protein, the influence of pathophysiologic conditions, and/or the presence of endogenous substances, which may compete for protein binding (e.g., protein displacement interactions). These and other clinically important variables can affect drug protein binding relative to age. The extent to which a drug is bound to protein markedly influences its V_d and body clearance (Cl).

Albumin, α_1-acid glycoprotein (orosomucoid), and lipoproteins are the most important circulating proteins responsible for drug binding in plasma. Basic drugs bind mainly to albumin, α_1-acid glycoprotein, and lipoprotein, whereas acidic and neutral compounds bind primarily to albumin. Serum albumin and total protein concentrations are decreased during infancy, approaching adult values by the age of 10–12 mo. A similar pattern of maturation is observed with α_1-acid glycoprotein; concentrations appear to be approximately 3-fold lower in neonatal plasma compared to those in maternal plasma, achieving values comparable to those of adults by 12 mo of age.

Because the free (unbound) drug can diffuse from the vascular compartment into tissues and bind to its receptor, the developmental perturbations described earlier are of utmost importance when designing optimal dosage regimens. Significantly greater concentrations of free drug in cord blood than in adult plasma has been described for many drugs. Decreased binding of drugs to α_1-acid glycoprotein has also been observed. These differences in the degree of drug protein binding in neonates and young infants may alter therapeutic drug concentrations compared to those in adults.

In addition to drugs, several endogenous substances present in human plasma may bind to plasma proteins and compete for available drug binding sites. During the neonatal period, free fatty acids, bilirubin, and 2-hydroxybenzoylglycine compete for albumin binding sites and influence the resultant balance between free and bound drug concentrations. 2-Hydroxybenzoylglycine is a strong competitor for albumin binding sites in newborn infants and, combined with other endogenous substrates, is a particularly important determinant of drug protein-binding differences between infants and adults.

Bilirubin is noncovalently bound to albumin; the binding affinity of bilirubin for albumin is independent of gestational age at birth and is much lower for the newborn infant than the adult, but by the age of 5 mo it approaches the adult value. This compromised binding affinity of bilirubin for albumin in neonates is a contributing factor in their susceptibility to the development of kernicterus. Clinically significant protein binding displacement reactions occur only when a drug is 80–90% protein-bound, the drug's body clearance (Cl) is limited, and its apparent V_d is small, usually <0.15 L/kg. It is prudent to assess a drug's potential for displacement of bilirubin from protein binding sites prior to its administration to premature and newborn infants.

Knowledge of a drug's V_d relative to body weight (i.e., 1/kg) permits rapid calculation of the dose necessary to achieve a specific target concentration (see later, Volume of Distribution). Imbalances between bound and free drug concentration caused by changes in protein binding or displacement interaction can influence the intensity of pharmacologic effect and the rate of drug removal from the body (i.e., free drug is metabolized and/or excreted from the body).

Drug Metabolism

The moment a drug molecule is present within the body, the process of its removal from the body begins. The overall rate of drug removal is described by the pharmacokinetic parameter clearance (Cl), or body Cl. A drug's body Cl is the summation of all clearance mechansims involved in removing that compound from the body (see later, Clearance).

The primary organ for drug metabolism is the liver, although the kidney, intestine, lung, adrenal, and skin can also biotransform certain compounds. For most drugs (e.g., lipophilic weak acids or weak bases), biotransformation to more polar, water-soluble compounds facilitates their elimination from the body through the bile, kidney, or lung. Although the biotransformation of most drugs results in pharmacologically weaker or inactive compounds, parent compounds may be transformed into active metabolites or intermediates (e.g., theophylline to caffeine, procainamide to *N*-acetylprocainamide, or carbamazepine to 10,11-carbamazepine epoxide). Conversely, pharmacologically inactive parent compounds or prodrugs may be converted to an active moiety (e.g., chloramphenicol succinate to active chloramphenicol base, cefuroxime axetil to active cefuroxime) prior to subsequent biotransformation and body elimination.

Drug metabolism within the hepatocyte involves two primary enzymatic processes: phase I, or nonsynthetic, and phase II, or synthetic reactions. Phase I reactions include oxidation, reduction, hydrolysis, and hydroxylation reactions, whereas phase II reactions primarily involve conjugation with glycine, glucuronide, or sulfate. Most drug-metabolizing enzymes are located in the smooth endoplasmic reticulum of cells that are recovered as the microsomal fraction on homogenation. Of these mixed function oxidase systems, the cytochrome P-450 system has been studied in greatest detail. In addition, the extent of fetal hepatic drug metabolism may be influenced by hepatocyte concentrations of ligandin. Ligandin, or Y protein, is a basic protein responsible for substrate uptake by metabolizing cells. Ligandin binds bilirubin and organic anions, including drugs. Although concentrations of ligandin at birth are low, values comparable to those in adults have been observed in the 1st 5–10 days of postnatal life.

At birth, the concentration of drug-oxidizing enzymes in fetal liver (corrected for liver weight) is similar to that in adult liver. The activity of these oxidizing enzyme systems is reduced, however, which is reflected by a prolonged body elimination for drugs that depend on oxidation pathways in newborns (e.g., phenytoin, diazepam). Postnatally, the hepatic cytochrome P-450 mono-oxygenase system appears to mature rapidly; metabolic activity similar to or in excess of the adult value is achieved by approximately 6 mo of age.

In contrast to mono-oxygenase activity, other phase I enzyme systems have been studied in less detail. Alcohol dehydrogenase activity is detectable by the age of 2 mo at levels lower than or equal to 3–4% of adult activity. The activity of certain hydrolytic enzymes, including blood esterases, is also reduced during the neonatal period, and appears to account for the highly erratic and variable rates of hydrolysis observed in the conversion of chloramphenicol succinate to the active chloramphenicol base. Blood esterases are also important for the metabolic clearance of cocaine; the reduced activity of these plasma esterases in the newborn may account for the delay often observed in the onset of clinical signs and symptoms of cocaine relative to the infant's time of delivery.

Phase II enzymatic reactions are primarily responsible for the synthesis of more water-soluble compounds, augmenting their renal or biliary elimination. These phase II reactions are also catalyzed by the hepatic microsomal enzyme systems located on the smooth endoplasmic reticulum. Glucuronidation is the most common conjugation reaction because of the relative availability of UDP glucuronic acid (see Sec. 9.44) and the variety of functional groups with which it can combine.

In addition to an altered activity of phase I and II hepatic metabolic pathways, the hepatic metabolism of certain drugs is different in neonates as compared to older children and adults. The *N*-methylation of *theophylline* to caffeine occurs in preterm and full-term infants, whereas adults primarily *N*-demethylate and *C*-oxidate theophylline to monomethylxanthenes and methyluric acid. Caffeine is rarely measured in the serum of older infants, children, or adults because *N*-methylation represents only a minor pathway in these individuals and their renal function is active enough to excrete the parent compound effectively (theophylline), and any metabolite (caffeine) that may be formed. The caffeine that accumulates because of the reduced renal excretion of aminophylline or theophylline administration in young infants most likely acts additively or synergistically with theophylline, both therapeutically and in the development of adverse affects. A metabolic pattern for theophylline degradation and excretion similar to that of adults is observed by approximately 7–9 mo of age. Similarly, age-related differences in the biotransformation of acetaminophen occur.

Numerous attempts have been made to stimulate or induce the activity of phase I and II enzyme systems by either maternal or fetal administration of known enzyme inducers, such as phenobarbital. To date, however, only limited experience is available with such pharmacologic maneuvers, and the erratic and unpredictable nature of enzyme induction raises questions about the overall therapeutic value of this approach.

Understanding the sequence of maturation of processes of drug metabolism is important when developing dosage recommendations for drugs that undergo extensive hepatic metabolism. An example of the consequences of failing to appreciate these processes is the tragedy that occurred following the administration of usual doses of chloramphenicol (e.g., 100+ mg/kg/24 hr) to premature and newborn infants (fatal grey baby syndrome) and the resultant beneficial use of this compound in the same patient population when the dose was appropriately adjusted (e.g., 15–50 mg/kg/24 hr) to compensate for the decreased hepatic ability for glucuronidation. Chloramphenicol glucuronide is the primary metabolite of chloramphenicol, which is then excreted through the kidneys.

Drug Excretion

The amount of drug that is filtered by the glomerulus/unit of time depends on the functional ability of the glomerulus, on the integrity of renal blood flow, and on the extent of drug-protein binding (see also Sec. 18.2). The amount of drug filtered is inversely related to the degree of protein binding. Only the free drug is filtered by the glomerulus and excreted. Although highly variable, renal blood flow averages 12 mL/min at birth, approaching the adult value by approximately 5–12 mo of age. The glomerular filtration rate is approximately 2–4 mL/min in full-term infants, increases to approximately 8–20 mL/min by 2–3 days of life, and approaches the adult value by approximately 3–5 mo of age. Before 34 wk of gestation, glomerular filtration is markedly reduced and increases slowly.

PHARMACOKINETICS

Basic Concepts

Pharmacokinetics is the mathematical expression of the time course of drug movement in the body. It is clinically useful only when integrated with the drug's pharmacodynamic characteristics. Because the pharmacologic effects of most drugs are reversible, the time of onset, intensity, and duration of effect of a drug are proportional to the amount of drug in the body at any point in time. Pharmacokinetic-based methods can be used to predict drug concentration at any time after a dose is administered and can facilitate calculation of a drug dose to achieve a desired concentration. The recognition that a drug's pharmacologic and/or toxicologic effects correlate best with its concentration in a biologic fluid (e.g., blood) rather than the absolute dose administered is the foundation of applied clinical pharmacokinetics.

The biodisposition of most drugs used clinically is best described using the principles of linear or first-order pharmacokinetics—that is, the serum concentration or, more appropriately, the amount of drug in the body is directly proportional to the dose administered. For example, if the dose of a drug that follows linear pharmacokinetics is doubled, its resultant concentration in blood (at steady state) also doubles. This characteristic of proportionality, combined with appropriate patient monitoring, is often used clinically to make adjustments in drug dosing (see later, Individualization of Drug Therapy). In contrast, some drugs such as phenytoin, salicylate, and alcohol exhibit saturation kinetics; their elimination pathways become "saturated" and the resultant drug concentration in the blood changes disproportionately to the dose administered. Under usual clinical conditions these drugs exhibit linear (first-order) elimination characteristics at low doses (i.e., low serum concentrations) but, as the amount of drug in the body increases with increasing dose, their elimination pathways become saturated. Such drugs are often referred to as drugs that follow the principles of zero-order or Michaelis-Mentin kinetics. The principles of elimination half-life ($t^{1/2}$) and clearance (Cl) do not apply to drugs that exhibit zero-order kinetics.

DRUG ABSORPTION AND BIOAVAILABILITY. To be effective, a drug must be absorbed from its site of administration into the systemic circulation, from where it is distributed to its site of action and eliminated from the body. Bioavailability is a measure of the amount of drug absorbed into the systemic circulation over a finite period. With few exceptions (e.g., prodrugs), a drug administered intravenously is 100% bioavailable. A drug's bioavailability is most often described as a fraction of the amount absorbed following extravascular drug administration relative to intravenous (IV) drug administration. Drugs administered as prodrug formulations require cleavage of the parent compound from their ester salt-liberating active drug. For example, chloramphenicol succinate and palmitate are inactive prodrug formulations of the antibiotic chloramphenicol that are administered intravenously and orally, respectively. Both require cleavage of the ester salt from the parent compound to liberate (release) antibacterially active chloramphenicol; the succinate ester is hydrolyzed after IV administration in blood by nonspecific plasma and hepatic esterases, whereas the palmitate ester is cleaved from the parent drug by pancreatic enzymes in the duodenum after oral administration.

A drug's absorption profile is a composite that depends on both the bioavailability and the rate of absorption into the systemic circulation. A drug's rate and extent of absorption are influenced by a number of physicochemical and patient-related factors, some of which are outlined in Table 6–37. These variables and others (e.g., concurrent drug therapy) may interfere with a drug's rate of absorption but not affect its bioavailability. For example, the presence of food in the stomach and duodenum can decrease the rate but generally does not affect the overall extent of absorption of many orally administered drugs. The clinical relevance of this interaction depends on whether the drug's efficacy is related to its peak serum concentration (i.e., decreased rate would blunt the peak concentration) or the total amount of drug in the body. Appreciating a drug's rate of absorption can be important in anticipating the onset of toxicologic symptoms in cases of drug overdose. In contrast, a disease or a drug interaction that results in a decrease in drug bioavailability would be expected to influence a patient's response to therapy.

VOLUME OF DISTRIBUTION. The V_d refers to the hypothetical volume of body fluid in which a drug is distributed; it is a proportionality constant that relates the amount of drug in the body to its serum concentration. The apparent V_d is expressed by the equation $V_d = D/C_p$, where D is the dose of the drug administered and C_p is the peak concentration of drug following administration of the dose D. The V_d may be used to calculate the initial or loading dose (LD) of a drug needed to achieve a desired serum concentration (C_p). If a desired C_p is selected and an age-appropriate "average" V_d is known or obtained from the literature, a dose necessary to obtain that concentration can be easily calculated:

$$LD = C_p \times V_d \times \text{patient's body weight}$$

where C_p is in mg/L, V_d is in L/kg, and the patient's body weight is in kg. Furthermore, it is apparent from this relationship that drug elimination from the body, or drug clearance, does not influence the initial or loading dose of a drug. For example, although a drug may be eliminated from the body only through the kidneys, the initial dose is the same for patients with normal renal function as for those with compromised or no renal function. The 1st dose of drug achieves an equilibrium concentration between body fluids and tissues while undergoing metabolism and elimination. Subsequent doses must account for drug elimination from the body to maintain a desired serum concentration without drug accumulation.

ELIMINATION HALF-LIFE. A drug's elimination half-life (t½) is the time required for any given concentration in blood (or other biologic fluid) to decrease to half of the initial value—that is, the time required for half the amount of drug present in the fluid to be cleared. The t½ can be determined as $t½ = 0.693/k_d$, where k_d is equal to the slope of the terminal portion of the natural log of the linear serum concentration versus time curve. The t½ depends on both the drug's Cl and V_d. A more useful formula for t½, which reflects these important relationships, would be $t½ = (0.693V_d)/Cl$. Thus, a change in t½ does not necessarily reflect a change in body elimination (i.e., Cl) of a drug. Despite this important distinction, the t½ is often used clinically to adjust dosing intervals, primarily because it can easily be calculated. A drug's t½ is also used to determine the time necessary to achieve a steady-state concentration—that is, the point at which the amount of drug administered (dose) is equivalent to the amount of drug cleared from the body (Fig. 6–16). After three half-lives, 87.5% of a drug's steady-state concentration is achieved, after four half-lives it is 93.8%, and after five half-lives it is 100%. When integrated with a target concentration strategy, a drug's t½ is often used to determine a drug's dosage interval.

CLEARANCE. Clearance (Cl) is the pharmacokinetic parameter that estimates the theoretical volume from which a drug is removed/unit of time. A drug's body clearance reflects the amount of drug removed or eliminated from the body/unit of time, whereas renal Cl reflects the amount of drug cleared by the kidneys/unit of time. Total body Cl is the summation of all Cl mechanisms for a given drug (e.g., Cl renal, Cl hepatic, Cl lung). The body Cl can be calculated as $Cl = (0.693V_d)/t½$. Knowledge of a drug's Cl is fundamental when determining the need for a drug and how often its dose

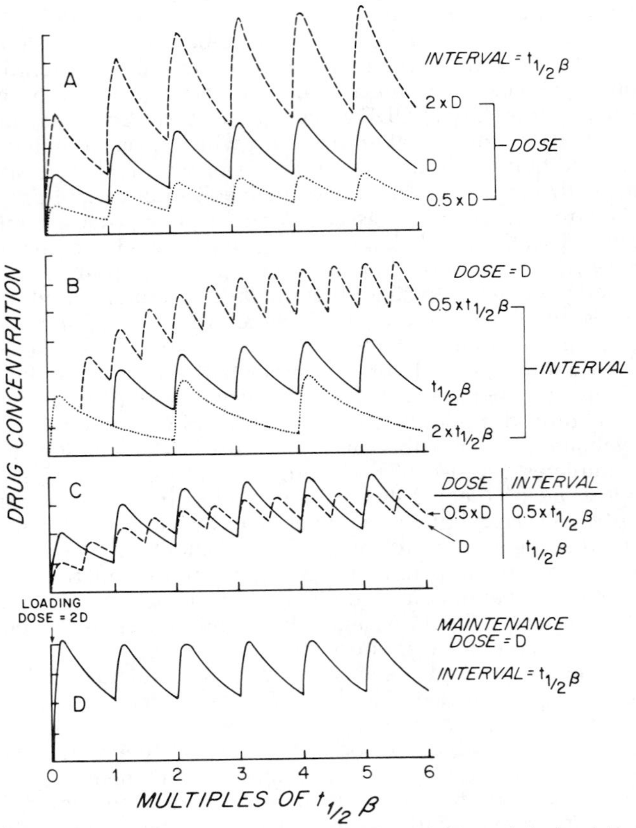

Figure 6–16. The influence of differing drug dose and dosing interval on drug concentrations following repeated dose administration. *A*, Varying the dose while maintaining the dosing interval constant; *B*, Varying the dosing interval while maintaining the dose constant; *C*, Decreasing both the dose and the dosing interval by one half reduces the amount of fluctuation but maintains the mean steady-state drug concentration unchanged; *D*, Administration of an appropriate loading dose eliminates the delay in achieving steady state. (Adapted from Greenblatt DJ, Koch-Weser J: Clinical pharmacokinetics. Part II. N Engl J Med 293:967, 1975. Reprinted with permission from the New England Journal of Medicine.)

must be repeated to maintain a given serum concentration. It is the most important pharmacokinetic parameter for determining the steady-state drug concentration for a given dose rate. Changes in organ function responsible for the removal of a drug from the body are reflected as a change in the drug Cl. A drug's body Cl is influenced by the integrity of blood flow and by the functional ability of the organ(s) involved in removing the drug from the body.

INDIVIDUALIZATION OF DRUG DOSE. The clinical response to an average or usual recommended dose of drug can vary considerably, even when the dose is administered relative to a patient's body weight, surface area, and stage of maturation. This variation is a result of interindividual differences in drug pharmacokinetics and pharmacodynamics and a number of biologic variables, including genetic differences in metabolism and concurrent pathophysiology. Individual variability with respect to drug efficacy and possibly toxicity frequently necessitates the adjustment of dosage regimens for specific patients, especially when prescribing drugs with a low therapeutic index. For some drugs, including dopamine, nitroprusside, and furosemide, the drug dose may be adjusted according to the patient's immediate and readily quantifiable clinical response. For other drugs, dosage adjustments may be guided more appropriately by combining clinical response with measuring the concentration of drug in plasma or serum. Such an approach to therapy is often referred to as a target concentration strategy, where a drug's pharmacologic or toxicologic response can be directly related to a specific serum concentration range.

Reported therapeutic concentration ranges for drugs (Table 6–38) are usually determined from studies of only a limited number of patients, mostly adults, and these therapeutic ranges represent an average mean value, and therefore 49% of the population is encompassed within the two standard deviations that surround this mean value. Thus, the clinical monitoring of serum drug concentrations serves only as a guide to pharmacologic intervention and dose adjustment. Serum drug concentration values must be interpreted individually for individual patients. For example, one patient may have a complete clinical response when the serum concentration of drug X is within the "low" portion of the therapeutic range or window. Conversely, the next patient, with the same disease of similar severity requiring the same drug X, may require a serum drug concentration above or below the reported therapeutic concentration range to achieve the same degree of positive therapeutic response. Toxicity, however, may limit how much above the therapeutic range the serum drug concentration may safely be raised. Therefore, therapeutic ranges for serum drug concentrations serve only as guidelines for therapy. Drug efficacy must be assessed by clinical response.

TABLE 6–38. Therapeutic Serum Drug Concentration Ranges for Selected Drugs*

Drug	Usual Therapeutic Range
Amikacin	25–35 μg/mL (peak) <10 μg/mL (trough)
Carbamazepine	6–12 μg/mL
Chloramphenicol	25–30 peak 5–10 trough
Digoxin	0.9–2 ng/mL
Ethosuximide	40–100 μg/mL
Gentamicin, tobramycin, netilmicin	5–10 μg/mL (peak) <2 μg/mL (trough)
Lidocaine	1.5–5 μg/mL
Lithium	0.6–1.4 mEq/L
Phenobarbital	15–40 μg/mL
Phenytoin	10–20 μg/mL
Primidone	5–12 μg/mL
Procainamide	10–30 μg/mL
Quinidine	2–6 μg/mL
Theophylline	10–20 μg/mL
Valproic acid	50–100 μg/mL
Vancomycin	30–40 μg/mL peak 5–10 μg/mL trough

*Usual therapeutic range shown (see text). Consult a clinical pharmacy/clinical pharmacology service for assistance in the interpretation and appropriate time to obtain a blood sample relative to the specific agent and route of drug administration.

Serum drug concentration-time values or profiles may also be compared to previously determined patient-specific values or literature reports to assess patient compliance with a prescribed drug regimen. More commonly, the determination of a drug concentration in biologic fluid helps to achieve an optimal therapeutic regimen while reducing the likelihood of drug toxicity. Finally, the determination of a drug concentration in a biologic fluid provides a means to assess the influences, if any, of disease process or drug interaction on a drug's disposition profile.

Therapeutic drug monitoring is not appropriate, necessary, or practical for all drugs. Drugs with well-defined and easily recognizable and monitored pharmacodynamic effects do not warrant routine monitoring (e.g., diuresis with diuretics, lowering of blood pressure by an antihypertensive). For therapeutic drug monitoring to be of clinical value, a clear concentration-response or -toxicity relationship should be identifiable. Patient age and the extent or severity of disease can influence the relationships among drug concentration, efficacy, and toxicity.

A number of variables should be considered when designing strategies to monitor therapy using serum drug concentration. When measuring a drug's concentration in blood the pharmacokinetic characteristics of that drug must be remembered, so that blood samples can be obtained at appropriate times in relation to administration of the drug. This permits proper interpretation of drug concentrations and therapeutic effects and helps avoid serious therapeutic errors. Peak drug concentrations in blood usually do not refer to the highest concentration achieved in blood with that drug but usually to the postdistribution peak drug concentration. Thus, a lag time often exists between the time of drug administration and the time that is recommended to obtain the "peak" blood sample. Also, most clinical determinations of drug concentrations in biologic fluids routinely measure (report) the total drug concentration in that fluid (i.e., free drug concentration plus concentration of drug bound to protein equals total drug concentration). This approach assumes a constant ratio of free to bound drug at various concentrations and differing pathophysiologic conditions, which may not always be true, and caution must be exercised in its extrapolation. For example, clinically important imbalances between free and total drug concentrations have been observed with the drug phenytoin in critically ill trauma patients and in patients with severe renal disease. As a result, many laboratories are now beginning to report both free *and* total serum concentrations of drugs or have these results available on request. Despite these differences, it is generally unusual for an imbalance in this ratio to be clinically significant, except for those drugs whose protein binding, under normal circumstances, is greater than 90%.

ADDITIONAL CONSIDERATIONS

METHOD OF DRUG ADMINISTRATION. Although it is often assumed that drugs administered intravenously are administered rapidly and completely, this is not always true, especially in pediatrics. The length of time necessary to infuse the total dose of an intravenously administered drug depends on a number of factors, including the flow rate of the IV fluid, the dead space of the system into which the drug is injected, and the total volume in which the drug is diluted. Because most standard IV fluid delivery systems, including their tubing, are designed for adult use, they contain a large volume/unit of length. This introduces a relatively large dead space factor, which causes substantial infusion delays when operated at the slow flow rates necessary for infants and children. For example, a dose of ceftazidime placed in a volume chamber of an IV system and administered at a flow rate of 25 mL/hr does not begin to infuse into the infant or small child until 1 hr after dosing, and may take up to 3 hr to infuse 90% of the dose. Such a slow infusion rate may profoundly affect the serum concentration and the therapeutic efficacy of the drug. Several steps can be taken to minimize problems with IV drug administration to small infants and children. These include the following: standardization and documentation of the total administration time; documentation of the volume and content of the solution used to "flush" an IV dose; standardization of specific infusion techniques (i.e., infusion duration, volumes) for drugs with a narrow therapeutic index; standardization of dilution and infusion volumes for drugs given by intermittent IV injection; avoidance of attaching lines for drug infusion to a central hub with other solutions infused concurrently at widely disparate rates; preferential use of large-gauge cannula; maintenance of the recommended solution at a specific height for use with a gravity-based controller; and the use of low-volume tubing and the most distal sites for access of the drug into an existing IV line.

DRUG-DRUG INTERACTIONS. When two or more drugs are administered to the same patient, the pharmacokinetic and pharmacodynamic properties of each agent may be modified by their combined interaction. Drugs may interact by a number of different mechanisms; these may be classified on a pharmaceutic, pharmacokinetic, and/or pharmacodynamic basis. These interactions may result in unpredictable clinical effects or toxicologic responses. Pharmaceutic interactions include those resulting in drug inactivation when compounds are mixed together physically prior to patient administration, as in syringes, infusion tubing, or parenteral fluid preparations. The inactivation of aminoglycosides by certain β-lactam antibiotics when these drugs are mixed together in the same IV solution represents a common, clinically relevant example of this type of interaction.

Pharmacokinetic interactions can occur when the disposition characteristics of one compound (e.g., absorption, distribution, metabolism, and/or excretion) are influenced by those of another. This type of interaction may involve one or more aspects of a drug's pharmacokinetic profile. For example, one drug may reduce the rate but not the overall extent of absorption, or a compound may displace a drug from its protein binding sites while concomitantly retarding its elimination from the body.

Finally, drugs may interact pharmacodynamically—that is, compete for the same receptor or physiologic system—thus altering a patient's response to drug therapy. The number of known, clinically important drug interactions, combined with the ever-increasing number of available pharmacologic agents, emphasizes the need to make a critical assessment of the possibility or presence of drug-drug interactions in any patient receiving multiple drugs.

DRUGS IN HUMAN MILK. Almost all drugs administered to lactating women are secreted to some extent into their milk and may be ingested by the nursing infant. In general, drug use should be as minimal as possible during lactation; a few drugs have been reported to affect the nursing infant adversely (see Sec. 9.6). Obviously, it is not possible nor desirable for lactating women to stop taking needed medications. If a question exists about the amount of drug a breast-feeding infant may be receiving and/or possible drug effects on the infant, a sample of the mother's milk should be analyzed.

PRESCRIBING MEDICATIONS. Factors such as taste, smell, color, consistency, and cost affect the degree to which patients comply with their therapeutic drug regimen. Prescribing generically equivalent medications can sometimes reduce the cost of a drug for a patient—if the generic brand affords equivalent bioavailability, bioeffectiveness, and patient acceptability. Complete bioequivalence data are not available for all drugs and, when in doubt, the prescribing physician should consult with the pharmacist.

A prescription issued by the prescribing physician should always direct the dispensing of just enough drug to treat the patient, leaving only a small amount of drug left over after the prescribed course of therapy has been completed. This small residual leaves some drug available for when doses are spilled or lost. Parents should be instructed to discard all remaining doses of a prescribed medication after the course of therapy to protect against accidental poisoning or improper self-medication at a later date. Patient instruction on the prescription should state the specific number of doses the patient should receive each day and the total duration of therapy (number of days of therapy). The number of times the prescribing physician allows the prescription to be refilled should be noted on the prescription label; if no refills are to be permitted, this should also be specified.

COMPLIANCE WITH THE PRESCRIBED REGIMEN. Little is known about the many factors that determine the degree of compliance with a physician's instructions, but it is clear that many patients frequently do not take medication consistently or in the manner intended or prescribed. Moreover, patients frequently take medications not recommended or prescribed by their physician. A child's compliance with a prescribed therapeutic regimen is usually only as good as that of the parents. Compliance can often be maximized by carefully educating the family about the nature of the child's illness, the action of the medications prescribed, and the importance of following the instructions precisely. Often, if the instructions are written down clearly and in detail for the family, and if the regimen results in minimal interference with the daily living schedule (particularly parental sleeping habits), compliance with the therapeutic regimen may be improved.

MICHAEL D. REED

Besunder JB, Reed MD, Blumer JL: Principles of drug biodisposition in the neonate: A critical evaluation of the pharmacokinetic-pharmacodynamic interface. Clin Pharmacokinet 14:189 (Part I); 14:261 (Part II), 1988.

Gal P: Therapeutic drug monitoring in neonates: Problems and issues. Drug Intell Clin Pharmacol 22:317, 1988.

Gilman JT: Therapeutic drug monitoring in the neonate and pediatric age group. Problems and clinical pharmacokinetic implications. Clin Pharmacokinet 19:1, 1990.

Greenblatt DJ, Koch-Weser J: Clinical pharmacokinetics. N Engl J Med 293:702 (Part I); 293:964 (Part II), 1975.

Holford NHG, Sheiner LB: Kinetics of pharmacologic response. Pharmacacol Ther 16:143, 1982.

Kearns GL, Reed MD: Clinical pharmacokinetics in infants and children. A reappraisal. Clin Pharmacokinet 17 (Suppl 1):29, 1989.

Kenakin T: Drugs and receptors. An overview of the current state of knowledge. Drugs 40:666, 1990.

Lee EJD, Williams KM, Chirality LS: Clinical pharmacokinetic and pharmacodynamic considerations. Clin Pharmacokinet 18:339, 1990.

Oosterhuis B, Van Boxtel CJ: Kinetics of drug effects in man. Ther Drug Monitor 10:121, 1988.

6.56 IMAGING PROCEDURES FOR CHILDREN

There has been a revolution in diagnostic imaging in the last 15 years; ultrasonography (US), computed tomography (CT), magnetic resonance imaging (MRI), and new nuclear medicine techniques have become available. Furthermore, various interventional radiologic techniques are now widely used. In the recent past pediatric diagnostic imaging primarily depended on radiography and occasionally fluoroscopy, sometimes facilitated by introducing contrast materials. The new techniques now account for over half of the expenditure in time and money. Formerly, diagnostic imaging relied heavily on displacement of structures and other indirect evidence. Now, US, CT, and MRI can often reveal the pathology directly. Diagnostic precision has greatly increased, and the necessity for and number of exploratory operations has declined steeply. This change has been particularly marked in prenatal diagnosis because of the use of ultrasonography.

These developments make it important to frame the diagnostic question as precisely as possible based on detailed knowledge of the child's condition, because an exact answer is often possible. Furthermore, the newer examinations are seldom stereotyped. There are only a few ways of radiographing the chest, but many more ways to employ ultrasonographic, computed tomographic, and magnetic resonance imaging, depending on the particular problem of the patient. It is also critical to intelligently choose among the use of these new procedures; MRI is useful in the examination of the mediastinum, for example, but CT is better for demonstrating the adjacent lungs. Diagnostic procedures need to be preceded by thought and consultation.

This rich diagnostic armamentarium has also brought problems. There is a tendency to substitute an imaging procedure for a careful history and thorough physical examination. Many new procedures are expensive, and require preparation of the patient (e.g., fluid restriction and sedation). In addition, interventional procedures are associated with various complications. Finally, there is a tendency to ignore cost (in dollars, time, inconvenience, pain, complications, radiation) in the often vain hope that the diagnostic benefits outweigh these disadvantages.

CONVENTIONAL RADIOLOGY. This term refers to almost all radiology as it was practiced in 1970. Excluded are nuclear medicine, US, CT, MRI, and interventional radiology. Conventional radiology shows anatomy by a radiographic projection. The x-ray beam passes through the object to be studied, and every structure in its path contributes to the final shadow. Conventional studies are quicker and less expensive than the newer techniques and are less physician-intensive. Their judicious use often makes more sophisticated examinations unnecessary.

Most conventional studies are plain films that involve no fluoroscopy, tomography, or contrast material. Right angle and oblique views allow anatomic relationships to be determined. The position of the patient (upright, supine, prone, decubitus) can be critical; thoughtful radiologists frequently use gravity to characterize gas or liquid, particularly when both are contained in the same anatomic space. The physiologic state at the moment of radiography is important, particularly the degree of inspiration at which the heart and lungs are depicted. The development of high-quality portable equipment has made it possible to have frequent bedside examinations, especially in intensive care units. Radiographic exposure factors are so low for chest films in neonatal intensive care units and collimation so satisfactory that the radiation hazard to bystanders is almost nonexistent.

Plain Films. These remain the dominant technique for examining the extremities for trauma. Chest films are still unrivalled in depicting diseases of the lungs simply and rapidly; pneumonia, atelectasis, and their variations seldom require any further delineation. Neonatal pulmonary disease requires repeated radiography of the chest, usually supine anteroposterior (AP) views; these are obtained to show the position of catheters and changes in the pulmonary process itself. In the abdomen, suspicion of intestinal obstruction or appendicitis indicates the need for recumbent and upright anteroposterior films. There are many other indications for plain radiography, but most are well known and are discussed elsewhere in this text.

Fluoroscopy. This is the observation of dynamic roentgenographic images on a fluorescent screen. It is used less frequently than in the past, but fluoroscopy of the chest is still an excellent way to detect a bronchial foreign body by differential ventilation. It often helps characterize a difficult or uncertain pulmonary abnormality, because the fluoroscopist can ascertain the most informative obliquity and obtain a radiograph in that projection. Intraoperative fluoroscopy often guides the correction of orthopedic deformities.

Contrast Examinations. Contrast examinations of the gastrointestinal tract are also used somewhat less frequently than formerly, largely because of the availability of endoscopy and body section imaging. The contrast material is usually barium sulfate, which is highly opaque and chemically inert; special situations require the use of water-soluble contrast material. Among the conditions well revealed by upper gastrointestinal series and barium enemas are malrotation, Crohn disease, ulcerative colitis, and Hirschsprung disease. Pyloric stenosis is convincingly shown by a barium study, although ultrasonography is now an acceptable diagnostic alternative in many cases. Intussusception is usually diagnosed with barium or air by enema. Reduction may be achieved with a positive-contrast substance (e.g., barium or water-soluble material) or air. Water-soluble contrast enemas are often useful to alleviate meconium ileus.

Intravascular Injection of Contrast Material. This can be used to examine the heart (angiocardiography), the brain (cerebral arteriography), the vessels themselves, or the urinary tract (intravenous urography). The increasing sophistication and lack of side effects of echocardiography have made angiocardiography less indispensable in diagnosing congenital heart disease than it was a decade ago. Its most common use now is to refine diagnoses already reached by echocardiography. Magnetic resonance imaging and computed tomography have largely replaced cerebral and peripheral arteriography. The indications for cranial angiography in children are currently limited to the following: (1) arteriovenous malformation or its suspicion; (2) arteritis or stroke; and (3) the need to characterize an unusual tumor, especially in regard to meningeal arterial blood supply. In the rest of the body, arteriography is limited almost entirely to malformations and diseases of the vessels themselves, whereas formerly it was used to reveal tumors and other processes by vascular displacement. Because of the availability of ultrasonography and the advent of radionuclide scintigraphy, intravenous urography is less frequently performed than a few years ago, although it is still useful for evaluating renal structure and function. Intravenous urography to show abdominal masses has been largely replaced by CT, MRI, and US.

Voiding Cystourethrography. This method (VCUG) is the most common examination involving direct introduction of contrast material into a child's urinary tract. Using fluoroscopy the examination readily shows valves, ureteroceles, diverticula, reflux, and other abnormalities of the bladder and urethra. The current approach to a 1st urinary tract infection in an infant or young child is to search for reflux using VCUG; radionuclide voiding cystography is a reasonable alternative. If reflux is found excretory urography is usually required, although renal scintigraphy shows function and anatomy with reasonable precision. If no reflux has been found the kidneys should be evaluated with ultrasonography. After a 1st infection in later childhood, ultrasonography alone usually suffices.

Conventional Tomography. This procedure, as opposed to CT, is also now less frequently employed than previously. It is used to show contrast material within poorly functioning kidneys and to characterize bony lesions. The plane of its images is usually parallel to the long axis of the body or of the extremity, whereas CT yields cross-sectional images.

The performance of these conventional examinations has changed only moderately, but systems of recording, transmitting, and storing the results of these and other examinations are changing rapidly. Digital techniques are being used to manipulate the contrast and brightness of computed tomographic and magnetic resonance images and to record them; they are also beginning to be used for plain films. Digitizing an image allows its transmission over telephone lines or by satellite to a remote location and permits its storage on a disk. Immediate transmission of digitized images to intensive care units is already available. These digital approaches may eventually permit the storage of radiographic film to be abandoned altogether. Disk storage and instantaneous retrieval are also available for voice reports that have not yet been transcribed.

ULTRASONOGRAPHY. Pediatric ultrasonography is now part of the diagnostic evaluation of many hospitalized and ambulatory children. The transducer translates the reflection of sound waves from interfaces in tissues into cross-sectional images of normal and pathologic anatomy. Bone and gas are obstacles to sound waves. Sufficient high-frequency sound cannot penetrate into or beyond them to produce a useful image, but there are several windows around and through these barriers, so that pediatric ultrasonography can evaluate a child from head to toe.

The anterior fontanel serves as an ultrasonic window to the brain of the neonate. Premature infants can be examined for intracranial hemorrhage, the infant having a myelomeningocele for ventricular dilatation, the dysmorphic infant for the presence of intracranial anomalies, and the infant with a large head for ventricular dilatation and extra-axial fluid. The eye can also be scanned at any age, but most pediatric eye diseases are best evaluated with a combination of ophthalmoscopy, CT, and MRI.

The soft tissues of the neck and face, the thyroid, and the arteries and veins of the neck are uncommon sites of pathology in children. In children who are suspected of having cervical adenitis, ultrasonography can confirm the diagnosis, reveal suppuration, and guide the needle aspiration of pus. In the chest, empyema can be localized if the collection of fluid is peripheral and thus visible between the ribs.

Cardiac ultrasonography has replaced angiocardiography in many cases, and has allowed the angiographic investigation to be more focused in others. Intraesophageal probes with the transducers placed directly adjacent to the heart produce images of the highest resolution.

Every solid organ in the abdomen is ultrasonographically accessible. Not only is the gross anatomy displayed but, in some cases, histologic changes in an organ cause recognizable parenchymal patterns. For example, a child with sickle cell anemia may have cholelithiasis, obstruction of intrahepatic ducts by a stone in the common bile duct, splenic infarction with deposition of hemosiderin, and parenchymal changes in the kidneys caused by sickling of erythrocytes in the medullae; all of these are detectable by careful ultrasonography. Although gas in the intestinal tract is a hindrance, intestinal dilatation with fluid and thickening of the bowel wall are both recognizable. Some gastrointestinal conditions usefully displayed by ultrasonography are pyloric stenosis, intussusception, and appendicitis.

The urinary tract is the most frequently scanned system in the abdomen for the following reasons: (1) congenital anomalies often affect the kidneys, ureters, and bladder; (2) masses in children are usually renal or perirenal; (3) infection of the urinary tract is common in infancy and childhood; and (4) urine, like any liquid, serves as a useful acoustic window.

Pelvic ultrasonography is used to evaluate anomalies of the gynecologic tract, masses in the ovaries or uterus, and changes caused by abnormal hormonal stimulation. Scanning of the scrotum is an ideal technique for evaluating swelling or a mass. An ultrasonographic search for an undescended testis is sometimes successful.

Ultrasonography has replaced radiography in the diagnosis of congenital dysplasia of the hip in neonates. Although bone is a barrier to ultrasound, the cartilage, muscles, and other soft tissues around the joint are not. The bones themselves are defined by their abrupt reflection of sound; thus, the entire outline of the hip can be displayed. Because ultrasonography is a presentation in real time, the effect of motion or stress on the hip can be shown.

Doppler ultrasonography provides some physiologic information along with the anatomic findings. Pulsed Doppler and color Doppler techniques reveal the direction of flow in vessels. With manipulation and quantification of the image, the arterial waveform can be integrated and the volume of blood flow calculated if the cross-sectional area of the vessel is measurable. Venous occlusion can also be shown.

Prenatal ultrasonography has had an enormous impact on evaluation of the fetus. Growth and development can be assessed throughout pregnancy, and congenital disorders can also be detected. This permits prompt evaluation and therapy after delivery and opens the door to the possibility of intrauterine treatment.

COMPUTED TOMOGRAPHY. CT is digitized cross-sectional radiographic imaging. The roentgenographic tube and detectors are on opposite sides of the patient. The image is obtained by rapid bursts of x-rays during one revolution of both the tube and detectors. The computer forms a cross-sectional image of the patient from the enormous quantity of information generated. Each cross-sectional image takes a finite amount of time, often 2 sec; motion during this interval degrades the image. For children below the age of 4 yr, sedation is usually required. CT is excellent for detecting fine differences in roentgenographic absorption (density). The images can be "enhanced" with intravenous injection of contrast material; enhanced images reveal the opacified vessels and extracellular spaces, distinguish among structures, and allow deductions to be made about vascularity. Computed tomographic images can be reconstructed in three dimensions, which is particularly useful in cases of complex hip disease and in planning reconstructive craniofacial surgery. CT easily distinguishes cerebrospinal fluid from the brain itself, and is therefore well suited to the study of hydrocephalus. It is more useful than MRI for the evaluation of recent trauma to the head and brain because of its relative simplicity and its ability to demonstrate acute hemorrhage and bony abnormalities. It is less suitable for distinguishing white from gray matter and for detecting demyelination; if tumor or demyelinating illness is the primary consideration, MRI should be employed.

CT is the preferred examination for the detection of pulmonary metastases, bronchiectasis, and subtle interstitial disorders. It is less satisfactory than MRI in showing the precise extent of a mediastinal mass. It is usually the only imaging procedure required in abdominal trauma—it reveals hepatic, splenic, renal, and pancreatic injuries well and is reasonably satisfactory at detecting intestinal injury. CT has replaced lymphangiography in the search for retroperitoneal adenopathy in lymphoma and testicular tumors and readily shows primary retroperitoneal malignancies, such as Wilms tumor and neuroblastoma. Among its orthopedic applications are the display of tarsal coalitions, the precise measurement of femoral anteversion, and the demonstration of the satisfactory reduction of dislocated hips through a cast. Tumorous destruction of cortical bone is more easily detected by CT than by MRI, although the latter shows soft tissue extensions and marrow replacement better.

NUCLEAR MEDICINE. Nuclear medicine imaging, also known as radionuclide scintigraphy, relies on external detection of the distribution of radiopharmaceuticals in the body using special imaging devices (gamma cameras and computer systems) that produce static or dynamic images. These images provide unique information; they are often functional complements to strictly anatomic modalities. Single-photon emission computed tomography (SPECT) produces three-dimensional images and improved definition of lesions. Radiation exposures in nuclear medicine are generally in the lower range of those produced by other radiologic procedures.

Radionuclide angiocardiography consists of rapid imaging of the heart and great vessels after IV injection of ^{99m}Tc-pertechnetate. It permits detection and quantitation of left-to-right shunts and measurement of right and left ventricular ejection fractions. The gated blood pool scan, using labeled red blood cells, allows evaluation of global and regional ventricular contractility and of ejection fractions, as well as measurement of regurgitant fractions. Other agents such as ^{201}Tl permit the visualization of regional myocardial perfusion.

^{67}Ga–citrate and ^{111}In–labeled white blood cells can be used to detect hidden sites of infection. ^{67}Ga–citrate helps in the localization of osteomyelitis when the conventional bone scan is negative or equivocal.

Planar brain imaging with tracers that do not cross the blood-brain barrier (^{99m}Tc-pertechnetate or -diethylenetriamine penta-acetic acid [DTPA]) is now performed less frequently because of the higher resolution of CT and MRI. These tracers can be used to confirm the diagnosis of brain death. Some radiopharmaceuticals are distributed according to regional cerebral blood flow and permit three-dimensional imaging of the brain with SPECT and PET (positron emission tomography). Because of this new technology, the use of radionuclide imaging of the brain is likely to increase in the next few years. Cerebral hypometabolism at the site of an epileptogenic focus has been shown using ^{18}F–fluorodioxyglucose. SPECT and PET may eventually be used to localize the focus in patients with inconclusive clinical and electrophysiologic findings or in patients with seizures who are candidates for surgery.

Skeletal scintigraphy greatly facilitates the evaluation of sports-related bone injuries. SPECT of the spine, for example, has greatly improved the localization of stress injury of the pars interarticularis in athletes. Magnification scintigraphy has been used successfully to diagnose vascular disorders of the hip and as an intraoperative guide in the resection of osteoid osteomas.

Renal scintigraphy using agents that are cleared rapidly by the kidneys (e.g., ^{99m}Tc–DTPA) may be helpful in evaluating patients with obstructive uropathy preoperatively and postoperatively and in reassessing newborn infants carrying the prenatal diagnosis of obstructive uropathy. Dynamic renal scintigraphy is also valuable in the evaluation of transplanted kidneys. Cortical scintigraphy with ^{99m}Tc-dimercaptosuccinic acid (DMSA) reveals the distribution of functioning renal cortex in reflux nephropathy and renal hypertension. Radionuclide cystography is well established for diagnosing and following vesicoureteral reflux.

Scrotal scintigraphy evaluates testicular perfusion and is indicated in boys with acute testicular pain to differentiate surgical from nonsurgical conditions.

Ventilation and perfusion scans of the lungs with ^{133}Xe help evaluate regional abnormalities of lung function, such as in cystic fibrosis, airway obstruction, aspiration, bronchopulmonary dysplasia, pectus excavatum, and bronchiectasis. Perfusion scintigraphy using ^{99m}Tc–macroaggregated albumin shows regional pulmonary blood flow when pulmonary embolism is suspected and after pulmonary angioplasty.

Hepatobiliary scintigraphy helps distinguish biliary atresia from neonatal hepatitis. This technique is also useful in evaluating right upper quadrant pain in adolescents without demonstrable biliary calculi (acalculous cholecystitis), as well as after hepatic transplantation. A site of bleeding in the abdomen may be found by ^{99m}Tc-pertechnetate, which localizes in functioning ectopic gastric mucosa, as in a Meckel diverticulum.

The use of ^{99m}Tc–labeled red blood cells permits imaging of the extravasation of blood itself. Nonabsorbable radiopharmaceuticals such as ^{99m}Tc–sulfur colloid can be used to evaluate gastroesophageal reflux, gastric emptying, and aspiration.

MAGNETIC RESONANCE IMAGING. MRI generates signals according to nuclear characteristics and yields images reflecting magnetic differences in body tissues rather than differences in x-ray absorption or acoustic reflection. The images are readily presented in the sagittal, coronal, and axial planes. MRI is an excellent procedure for imaging fat, marrow, white and gray matter, cerebrospinal fluid, vessels, ligaments and tendons, muscle, and solid abdominal viscera, but it is insensitive to calcium and cortical bone. Gadolinium DTPA, an IV contrast material for MRI, has a distribution similar to that of the IV iodinated contrast material used in CT.

Approximately 70% of MRI of children is presently used for imaging the central nervous system. MRI is particularly valuable for displaying brain tumors and demyelinating disorders, but is less satisfactory in acute head trauma. It is the procedure of choice for evaluating the spinal cord and canal.

Indications for MRI outside the central nervous system include congenital heart disease, abnormalities of the great vessels, hilar and mediastinal adenopathy, and masses involving the pleura, chest wall, and mediastinum. Hepatic masses, hemosiderosis, neuroblastoma, and pelvic tumors are well shown by MRI, but CT is preferable for renal masses. In the musculoskeletal system, tumors of the soft tissues and bones, abnormalities of the joints, slipped capital femoral epiphyses, aseptic necrosis, vascular anomalies, and growth plate injuries are well shown by MRI.

INTERVENTIONAL RADIOLOGY. Image-guided therapeutic procedures allow treatment of certain pediatric illnesses with less morbidity than alternative surgical procedures. Vascular interventional procedures include embolization, percutaneous transluminal angioplasty, thrombolysis, and retrieval of foreign bodies. Embolization has been used to treat vascular malformations. Selective embolization of hemangioendotheliomas of the liver is used to control congestive heart failure. Embolization alleviates discomfort and bleeding in patients with angiomyolipomas of the kidney and may control hemoptysis in patients with cystic fibrosis. Percutaneous transluminal angioplasty may be the treatment of choice in renal vascular hypertension caused by renal artery stenosis. Stenoses of vascular access shunts and of vessels serving transplanted organs caused by thrombosis have been successfully treated with this technique. Localized thrombolysis with uro-

TABLE 6–39. Range of Radiation Doses Received in Various Medical and Nonmedical Activities

Type of Radiation	Dose (Rad, Rem; Very Approximate)*	Length of Exposure	Where Received
Medical			
Chest film, newborn	0.004	Msec	Skin entrance dose; exit dose lower
CT, contiguous slices, child	2–5	Sec	Scanned volume
Lateral of lumbosacral spine, adult	0.5	Sec	Skin entrance dose; exit dose much lower
Cardiac catheterization	10–100	Hr	Skin entrance dose; exit dose much lower
Curative radiotherapy	7,000	Wk	Tumor and adjacent structures
Nonmedical			
Natural background at sea level	0.08	Yr	Whole body
Some professional jet pilots and flight crews, from cosmic rays	1	Yr	Whole body
Residents of certain areas of India with radioactive soil	3	Yr	Whole body
Radiation workers, current permitted dose	5	Permitted/yr	Radiation badge (usually worn on neck)
Dose at which half of population dies, nuclear warfare	450	Min	Whole body

*To convert to grays, divide by 100.

kinase, streptokinase, or tissue-specific plasminogen delivered directly into the clot through a vein or artery may be more effective and entail less bleeding than when those agents are used systemically.

Most nonvascular interventional procedures are percutaneous aspirations and drainages of abscesses, biopsies of tumors, and placements of nephrostomy tubes. These techniques can be guided by fluoroscopy, ultrasonography, computed tomography, or magnetic resonance imaging. Ultrasonography and fluoroscopy are usually preferable, because the real-time nature of the imaging allows for accurate placement of the needle or catheter. Percutaneous drainage of abscesses with catheters is often successful; a similar technique may be used to drain noninfected spaces, such as obstructed renal pelves, pancreatic pseudocysts, and obstructed bile ducts. Gastrostomy and gastroenterostomy can also be performed successfully using percutaneous methods.

OTHER PROCEDURES. Some imaging procedures are now of limited usefulness such as skull films to diagnose calcifications or increased intracranial pressure or intravenous urography to diagnose renal tumors. New diagnostic studies are adopted more rapidly than obsolescent ones are abandoned or appropriately held in reserve, for occasional judicious application. Also, some imaging procedures are sometimes overused. The usefulness of medical procedures depends on the particular circumstances of the case, many of which are extrinsic to the procedure itself. An imaging study justified in one instance might not be warranted in another.

The revolution in diagnostic imaging has brought benefits and problems. The major advantage is a striking improvement in diagnostic precision. The major problem is the increased need to consider the costs and benefits before requesting a diagnostic study. The greatest difficulty in imaging is now not with the procedure, though the hazards of radiation can not be ignored (Table 6–39), but with its ill-considered use.

These new procedures compound the problem of deciding what diagnostic approach is most appropriate under the circumstances. Thinking in terms of costs and benefits (Table 6–40) makes this principle easy to state, although difficult to apply. Few costs and benefits can be expressed numerically, as is the situation with other medical technologies. Nevertheless, decisions must be made. The need for technology assessment is particularly urgent in pediatric radiology.

TABLE 6–40. Costs and Benefits of Imaging Procedures*

Costs	Benefits
Pain, discomfort	Longer life
Time, disruption of personal life (for both child and parents)	Healthier life
Anxiety aroused by the procedure and its results	Reassurance
Hazards of the use of instrumentation, sedation, contrast material, radiation	
Consequences of false-positives (for example, unnecessary surgery)	
Consequences of false-negatives (for example, abandonment of needed therapy)	
Expense of the procedure to parents or others	

*None of the following are necessarily beneficial: a positive examination; greater diagnostic precision; a change in therapy.

JOHN A. KIRKPATRICK JR.
N. THORNE GRISCOM

Adler DD, Blane CE, Coran AG, et al: Splenic trauma in the pediatric patient: The integrated roles of ultrasonography and computed tomography. Pediatrics 78:576, 1986.
Cleveland RH, Foglia RP: CT in the evaluation of pleural versus pulmonary disease in children. Pediatr Radiol 18:14, 1988.
Davis PC, Hoffman JC Jr, Ball TI, et al: Spinal abnormalities in pediatric patients: MR imaging findings compared with clinical, myelographic, and surgical findings. Radiology 166:679, 1988.
Diament MJ, Bird CR, Stanley P: Outpatient performance of invasive radiologic procedures in pediatric patients. Radiology 166:401, 1988.
Dickinson DF, Wilson N, Partridge JB: Digital subtraction angiography in infants and children with congenital heart disease. Br Heart J 51:485, 1984.
Eisenberg JM, Schwartz JS, McCaslin FC, et al: Substituting diagnostic services: New tests only partly replace older ones. JAMA 262:1196, 1989.
Gu L, Alton DJ, Daneman A: Intussusception reduction in children by rectal insufflation of air. AJR 150:1345, 1988.
Hayden CK, Swischuk LE (eds): Pediatric Ultrasonography. Baltimore, Williams & Wilkins, 1987.
Kirks DR: Practical Pediatric Imaging. Boston, Little, Brown & Co, 1984.
Lebowitz RL, Mandell J: Urinary tract infection in children: Putting radiology in its place. Radiology 165:1, 1987.
Leung MP, Mok CK, Lau KC, et al: The role of cross-sectional echocardiography and pulsed Doppler ultrasound in the management of neonates in whom congenital heart disease is suspected. Br Heart J 56:73, 1986.
Radkowski MA, Naidich TP, Tomita T, et al: Neonatal brain tumors: CT and MRI findings. J Comput Assist Tomogr 12:10, 1988.
Sweet EM: The impact of new imaging systems on pediatric radiology. Clin Radiol 34:361, 1983.

7

PRENATAL DISTURBANCES

PRENATAL FACTORS IN DISEASES OF CHILDREN

7.1 MOLECULAR GENETICS

There has been a growing appreciation of the importance of genetic factors in human disease. At the same time, revolutionary developments have occurred in the basic science of genetics. Major efforts have focused on the application of molecular genetics to an understanding of heritable disease, and extraordinary progress has been made to use these advances in the practice of medicine. The approach to diagnosis, genetic counseling, and screening of individuals at risk for genetic disease have been revolutionized by the application of molecular genetics.

The scope of molecular genetics extends from the structure of genes to the functioning of their products in a cell. This field is dominated by powerful and rapidly changing technology involving the manipulation of DNA, RNA, and protein, resulting in a constant interchange between new insights in basic science and application to medical problems. A fundamental goal of molecular genetics is to identify a heritable disease at the level of the affected gene and to chemically define the precise mutation. Once the mutation has been identified, efforts are made to understand what impact it has on the functioning of the cell, on the tissue and organ, and on the organism. The mutation is traced from DNA to the corresponding RNA copies from the gene, to the protein translated from the RNA. Studies at this level of the effects of mutations generally provide novel insights into the biologic design of the normal cellular constituents.

With knowledge of the nature of mutations available at the DNA level, diagnosis of a mutation is aimed at direct examination of an individual's DNA. Diagnosis can now be achieved by examination of the DNA from a single cell, and almost any cell from an individual can suffice. Although our diagnostic possibilities still exceed our therapeutic capabilities, molecular genetics promises the treatment of disease through direct correction of a mutation at the DNA level. In some cases, a gene can be corrected in a somatic cell by replacement with a normal or modified gene and, in a few examples, similar replacement of a gene into the germ line of an animal has been accomplished.

One portion of this section reviews certain essential facts that provide an understanding of how our genetic equipment is organized; another section discusses applications that have an impact on the study of human disease. There are numerous excellent texts that provide a clear and reasonably up-to-date review of the general field of molecular genetics, and the reader is advised to refer to them for a deeper appreciation of the subject matter addressed in this section.

HUMAN GENOME. Each human somatic cell contains two copies of the entire human genome, amounting to 6 billion base pairs (bp) of DNA. DNA is a double-stranded helix, each "step" of the helix comprising a base from one strand bonded to that from the other (a base pair). DNA is portioned into 23 large fragments, each contained in a specific autosomal chromosome or the X or Y chromosome. Between 10,000 and 50,000 genes are encoded in human DNA, a number similar to what characterizes most mammals. In any one type of cell, it is estimated that about 10,000 genes operate to maintain the viability and specialized functions of the cell. The genes within a cell are expressed at widely varying levels. Some genes are responsible for the specialized function of a cell, like the globin genes of a red blood cell, and most cells have no more than ten or so of these genes. Other genes are considered to have a "housekeeping" value and consist of genes (the products of which are common to most cells) that are needed for the maintenance of basic cellular functioning. A major question of modern molecular biology is to explain why certain genes, such as globin in a red blood cell or myosin in the muscle cell, are capable of extraordinary activity in some cells but remain silent in others. In general, expression of large amounts of a particular gene in a specialized cell results from heightened activity of that gene, rather than from an increase in the number of copies of a gene in a particular cell.

We do not know why genes are located at particular sites in the genome or why they are present on a particular chromosome. Frequently, however, highly related genes are clustered in a particular region of a chromosome. A well-studied example are the genes for β-globin on chromosome 11. At this location we find a cluster of six related globin genes. In the case of this globin cluster, one gene is turned on in red blood cells during embryonic life, another gene is turned on during the neonatal period, whereas the β-globin gene is turned on at approximately 6 months of life and remains active into adulthood. It is believed that precise developmental regulation of the genes within the globin family depends partly on their physical proximity to each other within the cluster.

Many proteins consist of different component proteins, which together are needed for complete function. Generally, the genes encoding these component proteins are located on different chromosomes. A well-studied example is the genes for the α- and β-globin, the proteins that assemble into the tetrameric hemoglobin molecule. The genes for α-globin are on chromosome 16, whereas the gene for the β chain is on chromosome 11. The cell carefully regulates the expression of these physically unconnected genes.

It is surprising, but only a small fraction of the DNA that makes up the human genome appears to be represented by genes, perhaps only about 10% of the total. Most of the human genome consists of DNA sequences without any clear function. This large fraction of DNA consists of sequences that are present in many copies in the genome, from a few thousand to up to a million, depending on the specific sequence. In some cases, the particular repeated sequences lie tandemly on a site on a specific chromosome. Other classes of repeated sequences are scattered in an almost random fashion through the genome. As an example, consider the **Alu** sequence. The Alu sequence consists of about 300 base pairs of DNA and is present in about 500,000 copies in humans, all scattered about. These sequences can be found in DNA between genes and, in some cases, within the bodies of genes. Because no obvious function has emerged as yet for most of these highly repeated DNA sequences, they have been considered by some investigators to be **junk**; however, we presume that, in time, functions will be described.

Almost, but not all, DNA in a human cell is contained in the nucleus. Some genes are also found in the mitochondria. These organelles, which serve energy-producing needs of cells, contain their own genome. The mitochondrial genome consists of a circular double-stranded molecule containing about 16,000 base pairs of DNA, which has been completely sequenced. Each mitochondrion may harbor several copies each of this circular DNA molecule and, during mitochondrial division, the mitochondrial genome is replicated. A cell may contain different mitochondria with distinctly different genomes. What is remarkable about the mitochondrion is that it is built up from proteins that are encoded on its own genome as well as proteins that are encoded on genes contained in the cell nucleus. Proteins that are encoded in the mitochondrial genome appear to be synthesized within the mitochondrion, whereas those encoded in the nucleus are made in the cell's cytoplasm and transported into the mitochondrion. The design principle on which the mitochondrion is built has an impact on the patterns of inheritance that are observed for mitochondrial characteristics. On fertilization, the sperm does not carry mitochondria into the oocyte. The fertilized egg, therefore, only receives mitochondria from the maternal gamete. Thus, genes expressed on the mitochondrial genome are inherited maternally and, as a consequence, diseases resulting from mutations of mitochondrial genes exhibit a maternal inheritance pattern.

STRUCTURE OF GENES. A gene is a functional unit of DNA from which RNA is copied *(transcribed)*. Most genes implicated in human disease express a class of RNA that is translated by cellular machinery into protein (messenger RNA [mRNA]). The size of a gene is usually proportional to the protein product that is ultimately to be made. Genes range in length from between several hundred base pairs and almost 1 million base pairs of DNA. A specialized nuclear enzyme, *RNA polymerase*, recognizes the beginning or start sequence of a gene, attaches to the double-stranded DNA, and proceeds to copy one strand of the gene's DNA sequence into a single strand of RNA as it travels along the length of the gene. At a certain point along the length of the gene, the enzyme recognizes another punctuation signal and falls off the gene, releasing the RNA strand. The RNA strand is then *processed*. The processing reactions involve additions of certain nucleic acids at both ends and splicing of certain internal sequences. These processing reactions are necessary for the RNA to be transported from the nucleus to the cytoplasm and to be used effectively by the protein synthetic machinery of the cytoplasm, which must translate this RNA into protein.

The most striking processing reaction involves the splicing out of stretches of the RNA, each splicing event taking place at a very precise point in the precursor. In some cases, the total length of RNA removed exceeds the final length of the matured product. Because of this process, matured RNA differs in sequence from the original DNA template. RNA sequences that are retained are called **exons** of a gene, and those that are excised are called **introns**.

The cellular equipment that splices the RNA precursor accurately is complex and consists of many proteins and small RNA species that are, for the most part, only vaguely characterized. The basic principle underlying splicing is that nuclear splicing machinery somehow recognizes proper splice junctions, cleaves the RNA precisely at these junctions, and rejoins the pieces. The excised piece is destroyed in the nucleus and appears to serve no further function in most cases.

Splicing is a very complicated process, fraught with possible opportunities for errors to occur. Mutations have been identified, for example, that prevent normal splicing by altering critical sequences around the splice junction.

Why are most eukaryotic genes designed in this manner? No clear answer is yet available. However, this splicing mechanism permits a cell to produce different RNA molecules from a single gene by splicing the initial RNA differently. For example, in a muscle cell the initial tropomyosin RNA transcript is spliced into as many as ten different alternative patterns. Each alternatively spliced RNA actually yields a distinctly different final protein product. From a single gene a family of different proteins, corresponding to RNAs alternatively spliced, can be expressed. This design permits different proteins to be expressed from a single gene. An RNA may be spliced in one way in one cell and in another way in a different cell type, permitting some degree of tissue specificity over the nature of the product expressed from a gene. Splicing permits another level of control and compresses the amount of DNA that we must harbor in our genome.

What causes a particular gene to be expressed in a given cell, and how is the activity of that gene regulated? We know that certain controls exist that can activate a particular battery of genes in a cell (e.g., the genes activated in response to a hormone). Other specialized controls are necessary for activating genes expressing an abundant product in a specific tissue. Another level of control exists to turn on genes at specific times in development. Many of these controls appear to lie on very small DNA sequences residing in the general neighborhood of the gene, consisting of DNA sequences of about 10 to 20 base pairs in length. They are commonly found at the front end of the gene (5′-end) outside the DNA sequence itself that is copied into RNA. The essential control elements of a gene comprise a *promoter* and, in almost every gene, such a group of essential control sequences have been identified. Specific proteins bind to these control sequences and make the gene more accessible to productive transcription by RNA polymerase. The precise mechanism by which proteins accomplish this is not known, but it is thought that they permit RNA polymerase to gain access more easily than when they are absent. For example, it appears that steroid hormone-responsive genes are activated by specific proteins that bind to DNA sequences around responsive genes when associated with a specific hormone.

The control elements that are needed for tissue specific activation are called *enhancers*. These enhancers appear to be special sequences that interact with proteins present only in cells of a specific tissue. The presence of this sequence in the vicinity of a gene may be sufficient to lead to its expression in a tissue-specific fashion.

If DNA were fully extended, the total length of the DNA contained in the nucleus of a cell would stretch to about 1 m. Because DNA is condensed into a considerably smaller volume, it is obvious that DNA must be packaged. Packaging is complicated by the requirement that genes and other sequences must be accessed. In addition, our DNA must be replicated during cellular division. Extensive studies have demonstrated that our nuclear DNA is packaged with a set of five proteins, *histones*, into a DNA-protein assembly called *chromatin*. The histones themselves organize to form spherical particles around which about 200 base pairs of DNA are draped. These "beads on a string" are coiled coaxially to form thicker ropes, which are then draped on proteins that comprise the scaffolding of the chromosomes. It is generally believed that when a gene is active the chromatin assembly containing the gene is less condensed, or more "open" and, at certain sequences, histones may be replaced by specialized proteins.

After a gene sequence has been copied to an RNA, and that RNA has subsequently matured, the RNA is transported to the cytoplasm of a cell. In the cytoplasm, the RNA is translated by the ribosome and associated enzymes into a nascent protein. In some cases, the protein remains in the cytoplasm where it will ultimately function (e.g., glycolytic enzymes). In other cases, the messenger RNA (mRNA) directs its protein product into the internal membrane system of a cell, the endoplasmic reticulum, and the newly made protein is shuttled through the internal membrane compartments of a cell. It can be directed from the endoplasmic reticulum to membrane compartments, such as the Golgi network, where chemical modifications, such as the addition of carbohydrate, occur. Proteins are subsequently delivered into intracellular vesicles, such as lysozomes, or secreted constitutively from the cell, or delivered to any of the membranes of the cell, such as the plasma membrane. In some cases, proteins synthesized in the cytoplasm are transported into membrane-enclosed organelles, such as the mitochondrion, the peroxisome, or the nucleus. The precise nature of the signals that specify the particular intracellular compartment a protein will ultimately find itself is the subject of intense investigation.

NATURE OF MUTATIONS. Human genetics deal with the variations between humans. These variations are reflections of differences that exist at the DNA level. Variations that have an impact on the functioning of a gene are usually referred to as *mutations*. Other variations that do not have an impact on the health or functioning of an organism are called *polymorphisms*. Mutations may arise in somatic cells as well as in our germ cells. But only those DNA changes that are present in the germ line will be heritable.

Mutations result from a change of a single base pair of DNA, the loss or addition of DNA, and rearrangements. A mutation in which a base is changed within an exon, resulting in change of a corresponding amino acid in the protein, is called a *missense mutation*. Such a mutation may result in a dramatic loss of function or may only mildly affect the protein. In some cases, a single base change can add a new punctuation signal to an RNA molecule, commanding the ribosome to terminate translation *(nonsense mutation)*, and would yield either a shortened protein or, more generally, no protein at all. A gene can be profoundly altered by the deletion or addition of DNA, depending on the extent. Similarly, a gene can be disrupted by *translocation*, an event that joins a segment of DNA on one chromosome with a segment normally located on another chromosome, resulting in an aberrant fusion product.

Mutations also can affect the functioning of a gene by altering the splicing efficiency of the RNA transcribed from the gene. A mutation might lie in an intron and lead to reduced amounts of normally spliced RNA. The classic examples of mutations of this type include several forms of β-thalassemia.

Mutations can profoundly disturb a cell by altering the normal regulated function of a gene, rather than through disturbing the quality of the actual protein. An example is the expression of the *myc* gene, a growth promoting nuclear protein whose gene is translocated into the neighborhood of immunoglobulin heavy chain genes in certain lymphoid tumors. The *myc* gene, which is normally regulated when present in its usual chromosomal setting, is activated when it is translocated beside the immunoglobulin gene, normally active in the plasma cell. The activation of the *myc* gene in this cell, in an unregulated fashion, results in unrestrained growth and a malignant phenotype.

Rearrangements in the human genome occur naturally between generations. In meiosis, it has been observed for many years that *crossing-over* occurs, a process by which paternal and maternal chromosomes undergo reciprocal translocations in which DNA is broken and rejoined. Approximately 30 to 40 discrete and presumably random events take place during meiosis (one to two cross-overs per chromosome). The crossing-over mechanism appears to be exquisitely precise. Exchange of DNA even occurs between portions of the short arm of Y and X chromosomes, the so-called pseudoautosomal regions of the sex chromosomes. Translocations of this type result in the exchange of segments of DNA between the parental pairs of chromosomes. In addition, mutations occur in the germ line. These mutations, if transmitted in a gametic cell, represent potential mechanisms for the origin of inherited disease or variation.

Translocations also take place in somatic cells. The most well understood are the rearrangements that occur in lymphoid cells. These rearrangements are required for the formation of functional immunoglobulin in B cells and antigen-recognizing receptors on the T cell. Large segments of DNA, which code for the variable and the constant regions of either immunoglobulin or the T cell receptor, are physically joined at a specific stage in the development of an immunocompetent lymphocyte. The rearrangements take place during lymphoid cell lineage in humans and result in the extensive diversity of the genes for immunoglobulin and T cell receptors. It is as a result of this post germ line DNA rearrangement that no two individuals, not even identical twins, are really identical, because mature lymphocytes from each will have undergone random DNA rearrangements at these loci.

During the last decade, as human genes have been cloned and sequenced, and variations in particular sequences compared between individuals, certain striking patterns have emerged that characterize DNA variations in humans. We have learned that segments of a gene that play a critical functional role, at any level of the pathway of expression of that gene into a functional product, will exhibit very little variation between individuals. In contrast, segments of our genome that seem to be less "important" (e.g., regions of DNA between genes) exhibit extensive variation between individuals. Indeed, if these less important areas are examined at the level of nucleic acid sequence, the variation in a specific segment of DNA (e.g., an intron in a globin gene) may amount to a different base in every several hundred. As a result of this pattern of variation, a gene and all of the associated sequences that are critical for function may be considered as an "island" lying in a sea of highly variable DNA. The sequences surrounding this "gene island" can exhibit significant sequence difference when these segments, which tolerate variation, are compared between individuals from different pedigrees, while the genes themselves are strikingly similar. We sometimes say that the polymorphic framework that surrounds a gene, and a particular framework, is called a *haplotype*. The variations that characterize the DNA in which the gene is embedded can be used to identify the particular chromosome from an individual and (if the sequence of the framework is known in sufficient detail and number) would provide a **fingerprint**, enabling us to distinguish the particular chromosomal region within a population. If a mutation were to arise in the gene of one individual, that mutation could be followed directly (or by tracking the variations in the neighborhood of the gene that distinguish that individual's chromosomes). This linkage concept underlies much of the diagnostic methodology of molecular genetics in use today.

This picture of the genome as consisting of islands of conserved genes embedded in a framework, that tolerates considerably more variation, also helps us to understand the patterns of variation that are observed across evolution. As we compare specific genes between mammals, for example, less variation is noted in the sequences of the genes than in the surrounding genetic environment. When segments of DNA between species are compared by sequence, segments that are conserved in sequence across many species generally mark the presence of genes.

TECHNOLOGY OF MOLECULAR GENETICS. Molecular genetics, as a field, is driven to a large degree by technology, and novel methods are introduced almost monthly that improve and significantly modify experimental approaches to the study of gene structure and function. Both DNA and RNA can be sequenced directly. DNA can be cloned, meaning that a DNA sequence can be amplified to yield unlimited amounts. The procedure involves the insertion of a specific DNA sequence into a *vector* (e.g., a virus or antibiotic-resistant plasmid) that can be propagated indefinitely in bacteria. By simple procedures, the vector, containing an inserted DNA sequence, can be purified and the inserted DNA sequence can be cleaved out. RNA can be transcribed into DNA enzymatically and can be cloned and sequenced. Small amounts of DNA (< 100 base pairs) can be synthesized efficiently by purely chemical methods. DNA can be manipulated through the use of a variety of enzymes purified from natural sources. Duplex DNA segments can be ligated to each other enzymatically. DNA and RNA can be chemically tagged with radioactive or fluorescent markers. Enzymes (e.g., restriction nucleases, isolated from a variety of microorganisms) cleave specific DNA sequences (between four and eight nucleotides in length) and are used to fragment DNA at specific sites. These tools and others provide an extraordinary ability to manipulate and characterize nucleic acids.

In addition, specific DNA sequences can be detected with high specificity. All methods of detection rely on the double-stranded design of DNA. A single-stranded DNA sequence of sufficient length (a *probe*), corresponding to a segment of DNA in the human genome, will find its complementary sequence when exposed to a preparation of human DNA that has been "melted" into single strands. By several different methods, the formation of such a duplex between a probe and any DNA preparation to which it has been *hybridized* can be readily detected.

Molecular hybridization is used in procedures such as Southern blotting and in situ hybridization. In **in situ hybridization**, a chromosome spread is prepared in the same manner as one would prepare a karyotype (Sec. 7.11). A DNA sequence, corresponding to a sequence within the human genome, is applied to the chromosome spread after the DNA strands have been separated (or denatured). After a period of time the probe will hybridize to its complementary sequence at a precise location on a specific chromosome. The method of detecting the location of the probe varies. If the probe is made radioactive, an emulsion is laid over the slide and the probe is detected by generation of silver grains overlying the location. Fluorescent-tagged probes have been used more frequently, and their location can be determined by observation of the karyotype under a fluorescent microscope. The precise chromosomal locus can be determined by comparison with karyotypic landmarks. Another technique utilizing molecular hybridization is called **Southern blotting**. In this procedure, DNA is fragmented with a specific restriction nuclease, which is generally chosen empirically. The digestion of DNA with a specific restriction endonuclease permits a preparation of DNA to be fragmented into discrete pieces at cleavage sites dependent on the particular sequence recognized by the nuclease utilized. Thus, the DNA from every cell is fragmented in the same way, and a uniform population of fragments is generated. In the classic procedure, the fragments are separated on the basis of size by electrophoresis in agarose: they are denatured and then transferred (with their position preserved) onto a plastic sheet. The sheet bearing the fragments is exposed to a probe, and the position on the sheet bearing the complement is detected. This procedure tells us the presence of and the size of the fragment bearing the sequence of interest.

RNA can be studied by a similar method called **Northern blotting**. In this procedure RNA is isolated, analyzed by electrophoresis in agarose, and transferred to a nitrocellulose membrane. The presence of a specific RNA, and its size, is detected by hybridization of the sheet with a probe complementary to the expected RNA sequence.

Southern blotting, along with application of sets of restriction enzymes, permits one to examine the nucleic acid sequence around a gene. Thus, if a sequence necessary for the cutting of a restriction enzyme is missing, that fragment will not be present. A fragment of a different size will result. These differences are called *restriction fragment length polymorphisms* (RFLPs).

Another technique called *polymerase chain reaction* (PCR) has become increasingly important to molecular genetics. This method permits one to enzymatically amplify a DNA sequence, using short synthetic DNA probes. If a sequence is known, by use of two oligonucleotides, one can specifically amplify the DNA sequence bracketed by the probes. From the DNA contained in a single cell, enough DNA corresponding to a specific sequence can be generated to sequence, to probe by hybridization, or to clone. This method permits direct examination of mutations and can be applied to situations in which very limited DNA is available. In practice, the procedure is used to amplify a segment of DNA to be examined. The presence of the mutation is then detected by hybridization methodology or by direct sequencing. In hybridization techniques, the geneticist determines whether or not a probe corresponding to the exact, normal sequence hybridizes to the amplified sequence under conditions in which a perfect match can be distinguished from one that is not perfect.

The power of DNA methodology is that mutations can be studied in essentially every cell. Other very powerful techniques have an impact, not so much on diagnosis, but on the search for genes. When a mutation is identified, the dilemma is to prove that the mutation is a gene and is not a polymorphism (e.g., that a particular nucleic acid variation observed in an individual is not simply a polymorphism). It is possible to express genes in several systems. A gene can be transcribed directly in RNA and can be translated into protein. The gene can be transferred into a living eukaryotic cell, and expression of the gene is examined. The gene can be redesigned and expressed in bacterial or yeast cells and protein products produced in large quantity. In some cases, it is possible to transfer DNA back into the germ line of an animal (e.g., the mouse) and to explore its expression and its effect on development. In the most perfect case, the gene can be returned back to a cell bearing a mutant phenotype and the genetic disease can be corrected.

Perhaps the most important point in this section is that in the past we diagnosed a disease by looking for a specific enzymatic defect or for the presence of an abnormal protein. In the present setting, once a disease is suspected or a carrier suspected, we can make a diagnosis by examination of the individual's DNA. The gene encoding a liver-specific enzyme or red blood cell's protein can be examined in any available cell from that individual and from every member of the kindred. Any tissue with chemically intact DNA can be studied. With the advent of PCR, it is now possible to perform this study on a single cell's worth of DNA and it need not even be physically intact. The DNA from a single cell of a human blastomere can be defined genetically, or the DNA can be obtained from a single sperm cell or from a few nucleated cells present in a drop of blood.

HUMAN LINKAGE MAP. The chromosomal location of about a thousand human genes is known. In many cases, the precise location on a chromosome, as well as the relative position between individual genes on the same chromosome are known. This body of data comprises the *human linkage map*. In some cases, positional information about DNA sequences is available for which there is no known function. These sequences have been mapped to precise locations and help to orient us in a particular region of a chromosome, providing us with further guideposts for mapping.

There are several approaches to mapping genes and other DNA sequences to specific chromosomes. In the classic approach, genes located on the X chromosome were identified on the basis of sex-linked patterns of inheritance (Sec. 7.6–7.7). Other disorders were mapped by virtue of the association of a disease with a visible chromosomal alteration, either a translocation or a deletion (Sec. 7.20–7.21). It was assumed that segments deleted or disrupted when chromosomes break and rejoin represented the positions of the genes lost or altered and that they were responsible for the disease. By this association, the gene responsible for retinoblastoma was localized to chromosome 13 and that of Wilms' tumor was localized to chromosome 11. The precise location of the gene for Duchenne muscular dystrophy (DMD) on the X chromosome was identified by the finding of a deletion encompassing a large enough segment of the X chromosome to be visible by routine cytogenetics.

Another powerful technique for the mapping of genes was the use of human rodent somatic cell hybrids. By this method, cells of a human and rodent are fused in tissue cultures. Through repeated cell cycle passage, human chromosomes are randomly lost, resulting in a variety of hybrid cells containing one or several human chromosomes. Because the chromosomes of humans and rodents are very distinguishable by karyotype analysis, the human chromosomes persisting in the hybrid can be readily identified. By analyzing each of the cell lines for the presence of specific human enzymes or other biochemical markers, it has been possible to assign the genes expressing specific proteins to individual human chromosomes.

The introduction of molecular genetic techniques has dramatically expanded our ability to localize genes to specific chromosome loci. As mentioned earlier in this section, through application of in situ hybridization, a DNA probe can be physically mapped directly, providing the most powerful and direct approach to this problem.

To construct detailed linkage maps, which relate genes too closely spaced to be visualized as physically distinct on microscopic examination of chromosomes (this amounts to around 1 million base pairs of DNA), Southern hybridization and related methods are utilized. In this approach, DNA is fragmented, as described previously, into large pieces using restriction endonucleases. To determine if two genes (or DNA sequences) are chromosomal neighbors, one experimentally asks whether or not they lie on the same DNA fragment generated by a restriction nuclease. In addition, once a single gene (or sequence) has been mapped, one can *walk* around the chromosomal region, by cloning segments of DNA that are contiguous with the DNA sequence of interest. By this route, detailed "maps" of many chromosomal loci are assembled and this body of information grows daily.

FINDING A "DISEASE" GENE. The power of modern molecular genetic methodologies is best appreciated in the approach taken to define a gene by "reverse" rather than "forward" or classic genetic methods. When molecular genetics is applied to the study of the cause of disease by the "classic" or "forward" approach, the pathophysiology of a disease is determined to a degree or detail that includes our identification of the specific protein that is defective, and we begin a search for the mutation at the genetic level. The protein is purified, and the chemical sequence of that purified protein is determined. A comparison between that sequence and the normal sequence determines the nature of the amino acid error. This was the way that the molecular basis of sickle cell anemia was determined, now known to result from a valine to glutamic acid substitution in position 6 of β-globin. In the molecular genetic era, the mRNA for β-globin was isolated, cloned, and sequenced; the gene was subsequently sequenced; and the nature of the mutation was determined at the RNA and DNA level. A similar pathway of discovery characterized the elucidation of the defect in Tay-Sachs disease. After discovering that this degenerative disease of the nervous system resulted from expression of a defective enzyme, *hexosaminidase A*, the enzyme was purified. The protein was partially sequenced, and the corresponding mRNA for the enzyme was cloned and sequenced. Molecular genetic methods revealed heterogeneity to the disease. Those of Ashkenazi Jewish origin exhibited the disease as a result of a frameshift mutation in the coding portion of the hexosaminidase A gene, whereas those from other ethnic backgrounds (e.g., French Canadian kindred) seemed to be missing a segment of the gene.

By the "reverse" genetic approach, it is possible to identify the cause of disease through purely genetic techniques. The defective protein and the biologic processes underlying the disease are studied *after* the gene has been identified by direct genetic analysis. This approach is exemplified by the discovery of the gene that is defective in DMD. It was known for many years that DMD was an X-linked disorder and, although pathophysiology was unclear, the defect was profoundly expressed in muscle tissue. After the discovery of a visible deletion on the X-chromosome associated with DMD in a single individual, the chromosomal neighborhood was identified. By use of several techniques, DNA probes were isolated from human DNA, which mapped to the region identified by the deletion. These probes provided a powerful tool. The probes were used to identify genes in the suspected locus that encoded proteins that were expressed in muscle. After one gene was identified successfully, it was later shown that the product of that gene was absent from muscle of many patients with DMD. The protein, **dystrophin**, was shown to be very large in size and appeared to be associated with certain membrane functions involved in coupling of electrical activity and muscle contractions. At the present time, considerable effort is directed to understanding how defects in dystrophin function results in DMD (Sec. 21.11).

Another example of this "reverse" genetic approach coupled with a linkage approach is the identification of a strong candidate for the gene responsible for cystic fibrosis (CF). Unlike the situation with DMD, no patient has been identified with a visible deletion. Although it was known that the disease was associated with a gene on chromosome 7, the precise location of the gene was not evident. To find this gene required precise mapping of the suspicious region of chromosome 7, narrowing down the neighborhood through careful linkage studies at the molecular genetic level by analysis of many different pedigrees. As the region around chromosome 7 linked to CF narrowed, potential candidate genes were surveyed in the region, using probes to determine if any genes were present that expressed RNA in tissues affected in CF, exocrine tissues. One such candidate gene was identified. After cloning of the RNA product of that gene from the tissues of those with CF and those without, it fortunately appeared that a three-nucleotide deletion occurred in the deduced gene product in about 70% of the common Caucasian stock. From the nucleic acid sequence of the putative CF gene product, it was possible to "translate" a protein on paper from the genetic code. The protein sequence deduced appeared to be novel but resembled a group of proteins that were implicated in multidrug resistance, proteins that pump out many different classes of drugs that permeate our cells. Although the biochemical basis of CF is unknown, it appeared that epithelial cells from the respiratory mucosa exhibited a defect in the transport of chloride resulting from aberrant chloride channels. How this putative gene product, deduced by pure linkage assignment, explains the abnormal chloride transport data is not yet clear. Furthermore, individuals with CF do not seem to lack this gene product, which is the case of those with DMD. To be completely certain that a gene such as that described for CF is correctly assigned, the molecular geneticist must prove that the mutation inactivates the gene. To do this, the gene must be introduced into a cell exhibiting a defective phenotype and must be corrected. Introduction of the "defective" gene should not correct the defect. Until this is accomplished, assignment of a gene by linkage remains circumstantial.

Huntington chorea is an example of a disease in which localization of the gene to a large neighborhood has been accomplished by extensive linkage studies. At this time, however, attempts to identify a precise gene on the short arm of chromosome 4 have failed. Thus, although we know where the gene is located, reverse genetics has not yielded any clue with regard to the nature of the defective gene or the pathophysiology of Huntington chorea.

The power of reverse genetics is that it relies on molecular biologic techniques almost exclusively for gene assignment, and these methods can be applied to almost any genetic disorder. Furthermore, in the process of identification of a disease gene, probes are accumulated that can be used to trace chromosomes bearing the responsible mutation throughout a pedigree. This may lead to the progressive refinement of diagnostic tools available for both carrier detection and prenatal diagnosis.

DIAGNOSIS

The most striking advantage of the diagnosis of genetic disease through the molecular genetic approach is that a gene can be identified through examination of the DNA from almost any cell of a patient. The cell can be obtained at any time in the life of the individual. Frequently, whole blood is used as a source of DNA, coming from the nucleated cells present in the circulation. Alternatively, buccal epithelial cells, cells shed from the urinary tract, and even a single sperm can serve as a source for DNA to be examined. In prenatal diagnosis, chorionic villus sampling can be used, or amniocytes can be obtained from amniocentesis. Rare fetal cells in the maternal circulation also can be isolated, providing a noninvasive access to fetal DNA. In combination with in vitro fertilization, a cell can be dissected from the cultured human embryo (without apparent harm!) and used for diagnosis before implantation.

Diagnosis of a genetic disorder can be accomplished by either the direct approach or the indirect approach. In the direct approach, we examine a gene for mutations associated with a disease; in the indirect approach, generally applied before a gene has been characterized, we follow a "disease" gene by its linkage with defined sequences that are inherited with high probability. In general, the direct examination of a gene provides a diagnosis with absolute certainty and represents an essential goal in the advancement of the diagnostic arm of molecular genetics.

If a disease is associated with a single mutation, we can readily determine whether an individual carries the mutant gene. Thus, the diagnosis of sickle cell anemia or the determination of a carrier state involves positive identification of the specific mutation within the β-globin gene (Sec. 16.19). This is accomplished by the application of PCR methodology or by hybridization with DNA, with short DNA probes specific for either normal or mutant DNA sequences, permitting direct examination of the presence of a specific sequence at the DNA level associated with expression of the mutant protein.

In diseases such as DMD or factor VIII deficiency, in which numerous mutations within the corresponding genes have been identified to result in a disease with a common phenotype, the gene is examined for mutations that are observed with highest frequency. If no previously recognized mutation can be localized, the gene itself can be sequenced directly (in some cases, a major research effort), and variations from normal, which appear to be linked to the disease phenotype, can be deduced directly. As data accumulate defining the mutations within a gene responsible for specific diseases, our ability to identify a mutation within a gene directly increases, and catalogues of such data grow more detailed continually at an extraordinary pace.

In many diseases, however, the responsible defective gene has not been identified. Prenatal diagnosis and carrier status must be determined through linkage analysis. An attempt is made to identify DNA sequences that are inherited with the disease phenotype and serve to *mark* the chromosome that has been implicated in carrying the defective allele. In general, these linked sequences lie physically close to the gene and are part of the framework referred to earlier (Nature of Mutations), representing the somewhat polymorphic DNA in which genes are embedded. Molecular genetic methods are used to try to distinguish the DNA neighborhood of the defective gene from the DNA neighborhood or framework surrounding a gene unaffected in a kindred. As stated earlier, sufficient polymorphisms exist in DNA in which our genes are embedded to distinguish nonidentical chromosomal segments (e.g., alleles deriving from either parent). In practice, considerable effort at an investigational level is mounted to determine highly polymorphic DNA sequences that are linked through patterns of inheritance with a disease. When an individual case is presented for diagnosis, the molecular geneticist must first attempt to *fingerprint* the chromosome associated with the disease gene in the pedigree. If the disorder is recessive, both chromosomal neighborhoods harboring the defective gene must be fingerprinted. The fingerprint amounts to a collection of polymorphic sequences that can distinguish a particular chromosomal framework from another. In the case of a recessive disorder, the chromosomes bearing the defective gene must first be identified by examination of the DNA of the affected child. Then, a determination is made with regard to which of the two maternal and paternal chromosomes is associated with the defective gene. If an unaffected sibling is present, that individual should not have inherited the same set of alleles as that of the affected individual and provides a control for the molecular genetic analysis. Prenatal diagnosis involves a search for the presence of the set of maternal and paternal chromosomes bearing mutations. If only one is inherited, the patient is a *heterozygote* or *carrier*. If neither chromosome is inherited, the patient will not have inherited the defective gene. Carrier detection within the extended family is based on the same general principle, that involving a tracking of the affected chromosome on which the disease gene is linked.

Prenatal diagnosis or carrier detection through linkage analysis requires an analysis of the DNA of an affected individual. This provides a method of fingerprinting the chromosomes bearing the mutation; DNA from both parents permits the characterization of the chromosome that carries the unaffected gene and, ideally, DNA of a sibling of the proband who is unaffected provides a "proof" that the chromosomal linkage is correct. The larger the pedigree and the more discriminating the sequence differences characterizing the chromosomal neighborhood in which the gene is embedded, the more accurate will be the diagnosis. It must be appreciated, however, that diagnosis by linkage analysis can never offer 100% certainty about the inheritance of a defective gene. Because, by this method, we do not actually examine the defective gene, but only track it by association of its immediate chromosomal neighborhood, linkage is never perfect. Significant uncertainty results from a probability that the gene will be separated from the linked DNA sequences during meiosis, and this probability increases as the distance between these linked sequences and the gene increases. In general, however, once the chromosomal neighborhood of a gene has been established, major efforts are directed to characterization of the defective gene itself. If this is accomplished, the diagnosis can be made by direct examination of a gene for the presence of associated mutations.

Molecular genetic diagnosis can be performed on any cell from an individual. Therefore, diseases expressed in highly specialized tissues (e.g., the liver), appearing late in development, can be determined through direct examination of a gene examined from almost any cell of an individual. When a defective gene responsible for human disease is identified, and the mutations associated with it are characterized, it will be possible to screen populations for the presence of these mutations. Ethical and societal pressures frequently determine how we apply these techniques in practice (Sec. 2.3).

THERAPY

In addition to providing powerful techniques for the prevention and diagnosis of genetic disease, molecular genetics has an extraordinary potential for therapeutic intervention. First, genes encoding human proteins that are defective can be synthesized by application of recombinant DNA technology (genetic engineering). In this approach, a human gene, encoding a critical protein, is redesigned to be efficiently expressed in a bacterial cell. The product is made in industrial quantities. By this method, human insulin and growth hormone were made available. Any disorder in which the administration of a human protein to an individual can be corrective or of benefit is amenable to therapeutic intervention by this route.

Molecular genetics can also be used to attempt to correct a disease by introducing a normal gene into some somatic cells of the individual or into the embryo, with subsequent transfer through growth throughout the cells and tissues of the organism, including the germ cells. In somatic cell genetic correction (or *gene therapy*), DNA bearing a functional gene must be introduced into a cell and the cell must be replaced into the individual. Introduction may occur by several possible routes, including the use of certain viruses that permit high-efficiency integration of DNA carried into cells. Alternatively, one proposal is to introduce DNA directly into humans by the use of a virus that is trophic for a particular tissue and would, thus, deliver the gene to the correct location. In this approach, the physiology of the correction must make sense. To correct sickle cell anemia, hematologic precursors would be removed from marrow, a normal gene would be introduced, and the modified cells would be returned to the individual. That gene must produce enough β-globin per cell to effectively correct the disease and must produce it in a regulated fashion so as not to interfere with the normal hematologic development of a hematopoietic cell. Interference with red blood cell production might eliminate the stem cell. Certain central nervous system disorders would require the introduction of a gene into the central nervous system to produce high levels of a protein within the confines of the blood-brain barrier. Once again, it is critical to introduce such a gene in a fashion permitting normal regulation and minimum disturbance of normal cell function and development. Treatment of diabetes mellitus presents another interesting example for potential gene therapy. It has been suggested that the insulin gene be introduced into certain cells, such as endothelium, and, in this way, implant a permanent source of an insulin-expressing cell. This approach makes little meaningful sense, physiologically, unless the expression of insulin can be tightly regulated.

At the present stage of technology, it is not possible to control the precise chromosomal location of a gene that is introduced into a patient's cells. Thus, although with understanding of the design of a specific gene, including DNA sequences that are necessary for modulation of its activity, it becomes theoretically possible to transfer an intact, functional gene into a cell and then reintroduce the cell back into the individual, there are major concerns about the potential untoward effects on a patient. The extraneous piece of DNA may have a mutagenic effect. Genes may be disrupted at the site of insertion of this "foreign" DNA sequence. Damage may occur in the course of manipulation of the cells leading to cell death or development of a malignant phenotype. The inserted gene may be lost from the engineered cell after several cell divisions, either physically or functionally.

These uncertainties surrounding gene introduction into humans are of profound concern when we consider the introduction of genes into the embryo. At present, genetic manipulation of mammalian embryos is being actively studied in rodents and animals of commercial value. Several avenues of genetic manipulation have been used successfully. In one approach, DNA is introduced into the fertilized zygote, often into the male pronucleus. Every cell of the resulting individual will carry the introduced DNA sequence. In a second procedure, DNA is introduced into an embryonic blastula-stage cell, propagated in culture, and the cell is then physically reintroduced into a blastocyst-stage embryo. The engineered animal will develop as a mosaic: some cells derive from the manipulated embryonic cell bearing the introduced DNA, with others deriving from original embryonic cells. As applied to the embryo, the gene must be introduced with all essential regulatory elements needed for both correct tissue expression as well as developmental expression. This has already been accomplished in several cases in mice. However, it should be appreciated that by using such methods as are proposed to correct genetic disorders, in part related to the inability to precisely target the chromosomal location of the introduced gene, mutations have resulted from direct disruption of essential genes. There may also be other effects on the embryo, not yet known, that will appear during development as a result of genetic manipulation. For human therapy, these long-term consequences are very important.

Scientific uncertainties related to limitations of our current techniques of introducing DNA into an embryo may be resolved in the future. More recent work suggests that it may be possible to precisely direct foreign DNA into a particular chromosomal site in such a way as to "splice" in a correct DNA sequence and replace the mutation. This technique, called *homologous recombination*, has been used successfully in bacteria and yeast and has also been used to a very limited extent in the cells of mice and humans. It is not beyond the realm of possibility that in the future, an oocyte, taken from a female carrying a mutation in one gene, would be fertilized in vitro; the fertilized ovum would be cultured to the four-cell stage; and a cell would be removed for PCR diagnosis for the presence of that gene. If present, DNA bearing the correct sequence would be introduced in such a way as to correct the defective sequence. Similarly, in the future, there is the possibility that not only will genes be corrected, but new genes might also be introduced that are not part of our evolutionary array to confer viral resistance or help us detoxify certain environmental agents. The ethical and policy issues that have already been raised with regard to current genetic engineering will also become more pressing with future advances.

MICHAEL A. ZASLOFF

Alberts B, Bray D, Lewis J, et al: Molecular Biology of the Cell, 2nd ed. New York, Garland Publishing, 1989.

Collins FS, Gelehrter TD: Principles of Medical Genetics. Baltimore, Williams & Wilkins, 1990.

Kerem B-S, Rommens JM, Buchanan JA, et al: Identification of the cystic fibrosis gene: Genetic analysis. Science 245:1073, 1989.

Koenig M, Hoffman EP, Bertelson CJ, et al: Complete cloning of the Duchenne muscular dystrophy (DMD) cDNA and preliminary genomic organization of the DMD gene in normal and affected individuals. Cell 50:509, 1987.

Lewin B: Genes IV. New York, Oxford UP, 1990.

MacDonald ME, Haines JL, Zimmer M, et al: Recombination events suggest potential sites for the Huntington's disease gene. Neuron 3:183, 1989.

McKusick VA: Mendelian Inheritance in Man: Catalogs of Autosomal Dominant, Autosomal Recessive, and X-linked Phenotypes, 8th ed. Baltimore, The Johns Hopkins University Press, 1988.

Neufeld EF: Natural history and inherited disorders of a lysosomal enzyme β-hexosaminidase. J Biol Chem 264:10927, 1989.

Riordan JR, Rommens JM, Kerem B-S, et al: Identification of the cystic fibrosis gene: Cloning and characterization of complementary DNA. Science 245:1066, 1989.

Rommens JM, Iannuzzi MC, Kerem B-S, et al: Identification of the cystic fibrosis gene: Chromosome walking and jumping. Science 245:1059, 1989.

Rossiter BJF, Caskey CT: Molecular scanning methods of mutation detection. J Biol Chem 265:12753, 1990.

7.2 GENETIC ABNORMALITIES

Genetic abnormalities are a common cause of disease, handicap, and death among infants and children. Genetic disease accounts for the primary diagnosis of 11–16% of patients admitted to the pediatric units of teaching hospitals. One per cent of newborn infants have a hereditary malformation, and an additional 0.5% have an inborn error of metabolism or an abnormality of the sex chromosomes that causes no physical abnormalities and that can be detected only by specific laboratory tests.

The types of biochemical abnormalities that have been identified as causes of genetic disease include: substitution of a single amino acid (e.g., sickle cell disease, Sec. 16.19) or synthesis of extra amino acid residues (e.g., hemoglobin Constant Spring) in a protein molecule; deficient activity of an enzyme located normally in the lysosomes, mitochondria, or extracellular space (e.g., phenylketonuria due to deficiency of dihydropteridine reductase, Sec. 8.2, and Ehler-Danlos syndrome, type VII due to deficiency of procollagen peptidase, Sec. 23.18); lack of production of a specific protein or protein sugar complex (e.g., macular corneal dystrophy due to failure to synthesize keratan sulfate proteoglycan); or defective biosynthesis (e.g., of the C_1 esterase inhibitor in hereditary angioneurotic edema).

Many genes have been localized to specific chromosomes (Table 7–1). Molecular biology technology now makes gene mapping possible so that gene deletions and point mutations due to the loss or the substitution of a few base pairs can be identified (Sec. 7.1). New methods for staining human chromosomes and identifying subtle duplications and deficiencies of chromosomal material have also enlarged the understanding of human chromosomal abnormalities.

A more complete understanding of the basic defect in many of the genetic diseases has altered current clinical classifications. For example, homocystinuria, once considered a single disease, has been shown to be the manifestation of several different metabolic abnormalities. The lethal type of osteogenesis imperfecta, once considered a single disorder, has been shown to be caused by several different alterations of the collagen gene, including internal deletions in the gene's structure, its failure to properly form the collagen triple helix, and failure to secrete the precursors of collagen from cells. Furthermore, although lethal osteogenesis imperfecta was once considered to be due to an autosomal recessive gene, spontaneous and presumably autosomal dominant mutations are now known to be the basis for most affected infants. The study of common genetic disorders has shown that for some, like cystic fibrosis and phenylketonuria (PKU), most affected individuals have the same mutation, whereas others, like hemophilia, are due to many different mutations. The identification of genetic markers, called restriction length polymorphisms, that are close to mutant genes is making it possible to trace mutant genes in diseases, such as Huntington disease, through successive generations (Sec. 7.1).

Four categories of genetic defects have been identified in humans: the single mutant gene, abnormalities of the chromosomes, multifactorial inheritance, and cytoplasmic or mitochondrial inheritance. Other genetic abnormalities have been postulated but not proved, for example, delayed mutation expressed in response to environmental factors, or from a deletion in a chromosome that accentuates the effect of an adjacent gene or permits the expression of the effect of a mutant recessive gene on the homologous chromosome.

When clinically appraising and managing the child with an inherited disorder, three phases are critical: (1) recognizing that the condition is inherited, (2) identifying the pattern of inheritance, and (3) clarifying the clinical nature of the disorder, which includes understanding the risk of the disease's occurrence in siblings or other members of the family. Recognition that a condition is hereditary may be difficult when the patient has no affected relatives. The physician should be familiar with the different types of genetic diseases and be able to identify their patterns of inheritance using appropriate references such as *Mendelian Inheritance in Man* by McKusick, which lists conditions caused by single mutant genes. No catalog is available for disorders attributed to multifactorial inheritance; their recognition depends on the physician's knowledge of these disorders. For chromosomal abnormalities there is a laboratory test for providing visible evidence of the underlying genetic disorder (Sec. 7.13).

7.3 SINGLE MUTANT GENES

Each single mutant gene exhibits one of the four patterns of mendelian inheritance: autosomal recessive, autosomal dominant, X-linked recessive, and X-linked dominant. This method of grouping genetic diseases is often helpful in understanding the clinical presentation of a disorder. Concepts such as the basic structure of the DNA molecule and the transmission of genetic information, initially to messenger RNA and then to the formation of a specific polypeptide, help in understanding the basis of diseases such as the various

TABLE 7–1. Partial List of Cloned Genes Responsible for Known Hereditary Disorders and Examples of Gross Alterations and Point Mutations in Selected Disorders*

Genes	Chromosome	Disorder	Gross Gene Alterations	Point Mutations (PM)
Antithrombin III	1q	Antithrombin III deficiency	del	
Fucosidase	1p	Fucosidosis		
Protein 4.1	1p	Elliptocytosis-1	del	
Glycocerebrosidase	1q	Gaucher's disease		PM
Uroporphyrinogen decarboxylase	1p	Porphyria cutanea tarda		
Medium-chain acyl-CoA dehydrogenase	1p	Medium-chain acyl-CoA dehydrogenase deficiency		
α-Spectrin	1q	Elliptocytosis-2, spherocytosis		
Carbamylphosphate synthetase deficiency	2p	Carbamylphosphate synthetase deficiency		
Apolipoprotein B	2p	Hypobetalipoproteinemia, premature atherosclerosis?		PM
α_1(III)-Procollagen	2p	Ehlers–Danlos syndrome type IV		
Protein C	2	Thrombophilia due to protein C deficiency		
β-Propionyl-CoA carboxylase	3q	Propionic acidemia type II		
Transferrin	3q	Atransferrinemia		
Fibrinogen α, β, and γ	4q	Dysfibrinogenemias		
β-Hexosaminidase	5q	Sandhoff's disease		
Factor XIII	6p	Factor XIII deficiency		
Steroid 21-hydroxylase	6p	Congenital adrenal hyperplasia	del	
Complement factor 2	6p	C2 deficiency		
Complement factor 4	6p	C4 deficiency	del	
Plasminogen	6q	Thrombophilia due to plasminogen variant		
Argininosuccinate lyase	7q	Argininosuccinic aciduria		
β-Glucuronidase	7q	Mucopolysaccharidosis VII		
α_2(1)-Procollagen	7q	Osteogenesis imperfecta, Ehlers–Danlos syndrome type VII A2	del	PM
Plasminogen activator	8p	Thrombophilia due to plasminogen activator deficiency		
Carbonic anhydrase	8q	Renal tubular acidosis with osteopetrosis		
Thyroglobulin	8q	Hereditary congenital hypothyroidism		
Argininosuccinate synthetase	9q	Citrullinemia		
Fructose-1-phosphate aldolase	9q	Fructose intolerance		
Ornithine aminotransferase	10q	Gyrate atrophy		PM
Steroid 17-hydroxylase/17,20-lyase	10	Congenital adrenal hyperplasia		
Insulin	11p	Diabetes mellitus due to abnormal insulins		PM
β-Globin	11p	Sickle cell anemia, β-thalassemia		PM
γ-Globin	11p	Hereditary persistence of fetal hemoglobin	del	PM
Parathyroid hormone	11p	Familial hypoparathyroidism (one form)		
Catalase	11p	Acatalasemia		
Apolipoprotein A1, C3, and A4	11q	Premature coronary artery disease	inv	
Muscle glycogen phosphorylase	11q	McArdle's disease		
Porphobilinogen deaminase	11q	Acute intermittent porphyria		

Table continued on following page

disorders of hemoglobin structure in which the primary abnormalities include amino acid substitutions and deletions, elongated globin chains, and fused or "hybrid" globin chains. Other concepts explaining the mechanisms for the occurrence of genetic abnormalities that are apparent in the study of microorganisms, such as defective function of repressor genes and regulator genes, may also be applicable to understanding human genetic diseases (Sec. 7.1).

In discussing single mutant genes a number of special terms are used. The 23 chromosomes in the sperm combine with the 23 chromosomes in the egg to form a *zygote* with 23 *pairs* of chromosomes. The *gene locus* is the particular location of a specific gene in a specific chromosome. Recent studies show that the coding portions of a gene are interrupted by *intervening sequences* of DNA of variable lengths (Sec. 7.1). These intervening sequences, *introns*, are not represented in the mature messenger RNA that corresponds to the gene. Errors in splicing out the introns are the basis for the most common types of β-thalassemia. Each gene has an analog with a similar location in the homologous (other of a pair) chromosome; the identical pair of loci are called *homologous loci*. The genes at the homologous loci are called *alleles*. Allelic genes are analogous (i.e., affect the nature of the same characteristic) but are often not identical; extensive variation may be observed in many of the different types of serum proteins among people of the same as well as different races. Because of the genetic variation that exists at many gene loci, it is arbitrary to consider some genes as mutant; usually the distinction is that the mutant gene has a major, harmful effect. When a person has a mutant gene at a locus in one chromosome but not at the homologous locus of the other, the person is *heterozygous* for that mutant gene. If the mutant gene does not affect the heterozygous individual, it is called a *recessive gene*. If the mutant gene has an effect in the heterozygous state, it is a *dominant gene*. A person having the same mutant gene at both homologous loci is *homozygous* for that gene. Autosomal recessive genes manifest their clinical effect only in the *homozygote*. The distinctions between recessive and dominant genes become arbitrary when identifying the heterozygote by biochemical testing or when the heterozygote only mildly expresses the disorder. Furthermore, molecular genetic studies have demonstrated that many persons consid-

TABLE 7–1. Partial List of Cloned Genes Responsible for Known Hereditary Disorders and Examples of Gross Alterations and Point Mutations in Selected Disorders* *Continued*

Genes	Chromosome	Disorder	Gross Gene Alterations	Point Mutations (PM)
Pyruvate carboxylase	11q	Pyruvate carboxylase deficiency		
von Willebrand factor	12p	von Willebrand's disease	del	
Triosephosphate isomerase	12p	Triosephosphate isomerase deficiency		
Phenylalanine hydroxylase	12q	Phenylketonuria		PM
Retinoblastoma gene	13q	Retinoblastoma	del	
Factor VII	13q	Factor VII deficiency		
Factor X	13q	Factor X deficiency		
α-Propionyl-CoA carboxylase	13	Propionic acidemia type I		
α-Antitrypsin	14	α_1-Antitrypsin deficiency		PM
Liver phosphorylase	14	Hers' disease (glycogen storage disease VI)		
α_1-Hexosaminidase	15q	Tay–Sachs disease	del	PM
P-450 side-chain cleavage enzyme/20,22-desmolase	15	Lipid adrenal hyperplasia		
α-Globin	16p	α-Thalassemia	del	PM
Tyrosine aminotransferase	16q	Tyrosinemia type II		
Lecithin–cholesterol acyltransferase	16q	Lecithin–cholesterol acyltransferase deficiency		
Growth hormone	17q	Isolated familial growth hormone deficiency	del	
α_1(1)-Procollagen	17q	Osteogenesis imperfecta, Ehlers–Danlos syndrome type VII A1	del	PM
Complement factor 3	19p	C3 deficiency		
Apolipoprotein E, C2, and C1	19q	Dyslipoproteinemia		
Low-density-lipoprotein receptor	19q	Familial hypercholesterolemia	del	PM
Adenosine deaminase	20q	Severe combined immunodeficiency due to adenosine deaminase deficiency		
Cystathionine β-synthase	21q	Homocystinuria		
Steroid sulfatase	Xp	X-linked ichthyosis	del	
Ornithine transcarbamylase	Xp	Ornithine transcarbamylase deficiency	del	PM
Chronic granulomatous disease gene	Xp	Chronic granulomatous disease		
Gene for Duchenne's muscular dystrophy	Xp	Duchenne's muscular dystrophy	del	
α-Galactosidase	Xq	Fabry's disease		
Phosphoglycerate kinase	Xq	Phosphoglycerate kinase deficiency		
Hypoxanthine guanine phosphoribosyltransferase	Xq	Lesch–Nyhan syndrome	del	
Factor IX	Xq	Hemophilia B	del	PM
Factor VIII	Xq	Hemophilia A	del ins	PM
Green/red cone pigment	Xq	Color blindness	del	
Glucose-6-phosphate dehydrogenase	Xq	Glucose-6-phosphate dehydrogenase deficiency		

*From Antonarakis SE: Diagnosis of genetic disorders at the DNA level. Reprinted with permission from *The New England Journal of Medicine* 320:153, 1980.
del = deletion; inv = inversion; ins = insertion.

ered homozygous for the same autosomal recessive gene actually have two different mutations (Sec. 7.1).

Each mendelian pattern of inheritance has characteristics that may be useful in establishing a diagnosis or in planning family studies that may be important for a clear explanation to the parents of an affected child.

7.4 AUTOSOMAL RECESSIVE INHERITANCE

The pedigree illustrating this pattern of inheritance (Fig. 7–1) shows the following characteristics: the child of two heterozygous parents has a 25% chance of being homozygous (i.e., a 1 chance in 2 of inheriting the mutant gene from each parent: $1/2 \times 1/2 = 1/4$); males and females are affected with equal frequency; the affected individuals are almost always born in only one generation of a family; the children of the affected (homozygous) person are all heterozygotes; the children of a homozygote can be affected only if the spouse is a heterozygote, which is a rare event because of the low incidence of most adverse recessive genes in the general population.

If the frequency of an autosomal recessive disease is known, the frequency of the heterozygote or carrier state can be calculated from the Hardy-Weinberg formula: $p^2 + 2pq + q^2 = 1$, in which p is the frequency of one of a pair of alleles and q is the frequency of the other. For example, if the frequency of cystic fibrosis among white Americans is 1 in 2,500 (p^2), then the frequency of the heterozygote (2 pq) can be calculated: if $p^2 = 1/2500$, then $p = 1/50$ and $q = 49/50$; $2pq = 2 \times 1/50 \times 49/50$ or approximately 1/25 (or 3.92%).

Every human probably has several rare, harmful, recessive genes. Because these mutant genes are frequently not identifiable by laboratory tests, the heterozygous adult usually learns about his or her harmful recessive genes after the birth of a homozygous (and therefore affected) child. Related parents are much more likely to be heterozygous for the same harmful recessive genes because they have a common ancestor. Consanguineous matings are rare in the United States and in many other countries. Therefore, few genetic studies have been carried out to establish the overall risk for healthy but related parents. Based on the information available, the risk for parents who are first cousins of having a newborn child with a birth defect is about double the 2–3% risk faced by healthy, unrelated parents.

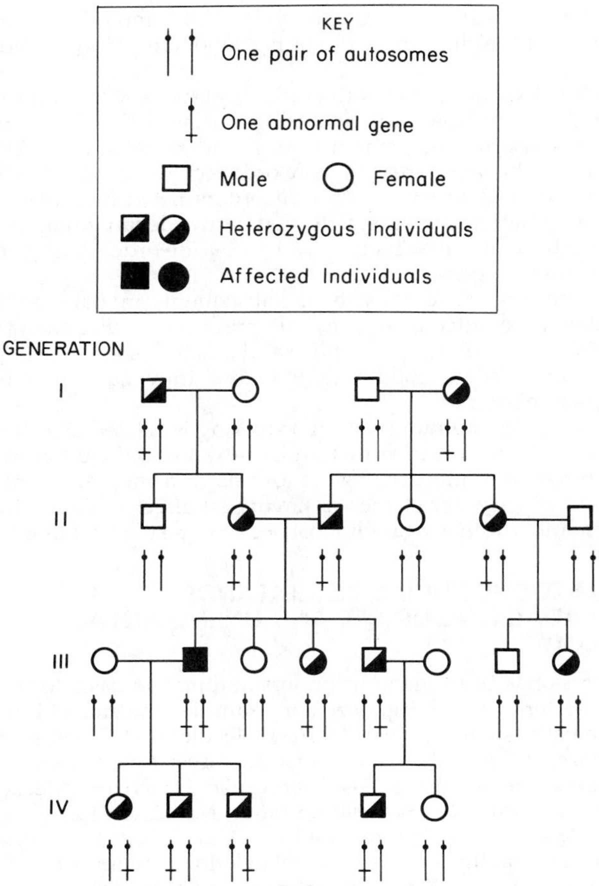

Figure 7–1. Autosomal recessive inheritance.

7.5 AUTOSOMAL DOMINANT INHERITANCE

The pedigree in Figure 7–2 shows that both males and females are affected, that transmission occurs from one parent to child and that the responsible mutant gene can arise by spontaneous mutation. The risk is 50% that an offspring of the affected person will inherit the chromosome that contains the mutant gene.

7.6 X-LINKED RECESSIVE INHERITANCE

The pedigree in Figure 7–3 shows that only males are clinically affected; that affected males are related through carrier females; that all daughters of affected males are carriers of the mutant gene; and that affected males do not have affected sons but may have affected grandsons born to carrier females. The female carrier has a 50% chance of giving her chromosome that bears the mutant gene to each of her children. In other words, each daughter of a carrier has a 50% chance of being a carrier, and each son has a 50% chance of inheriting the mutant gene and having the disease that it causes. Therefore, in each pregnancy the female carrier has a 25% chance of having an affected son.

Initially, both X chromosomes of a female zygote are active. Random inactivation of portions of one X in each cell occurs early in fetal development. The inactivated X, which replicates later than the active X, is the sex chromatin mass or Barr body, which may be observed in the nucleus of a cell near the nuclear membrane. This random inactivation, also called *lyonization*, protects the carrier female from the effect of the X-linked recessive mutant gene because there is as much

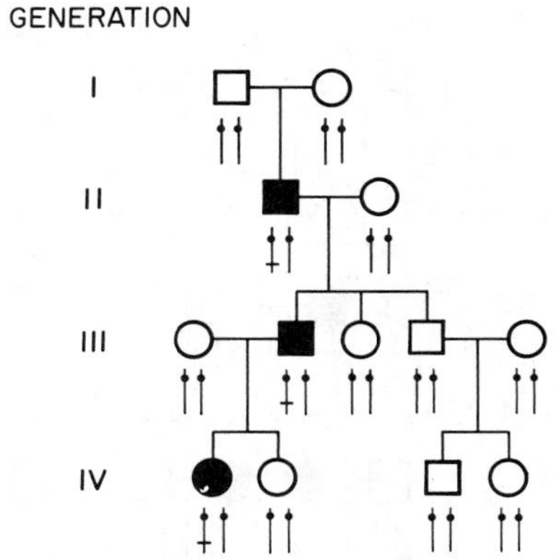

Figure 7–2. Autosomal dominant inheritance. (See Figure 7–1 for key.)

chance that the X chromosome that carries the mutant gene will be inactivated as that the other X chromosome will. Therefore, the carrier expresses the effect of the mutant gene in an average of 50% of her cells. For this reason the female carrier of classic hemophilia will have a reduced level of factor VIII activity but a level not nearly as low as that in her affected son or brother.

7.7 X-LINKED DOMINANT INHERITANCE

Very few X-linked dominant genes have been identified in humans. Two examples are vitamin D-resistant rickets and the Melnick-Needles syndrome of multiple malformations. The pedigree in Figure 7–4 shows the essential characteristics: both males and females are affected, but males are often more severely affected; the disorder is transmitted from generation to generation; all daughters of an affected father will be affected, but none of his sons.

7.8 MULTIFACTORIAL INHERITANCE

The term multifactorial inheritance refers to the process in which a disease or abnormality is the result of the additive effect of one or more abnormal genes and environmental factors (Sec. 7.1). These disorders include some of the most

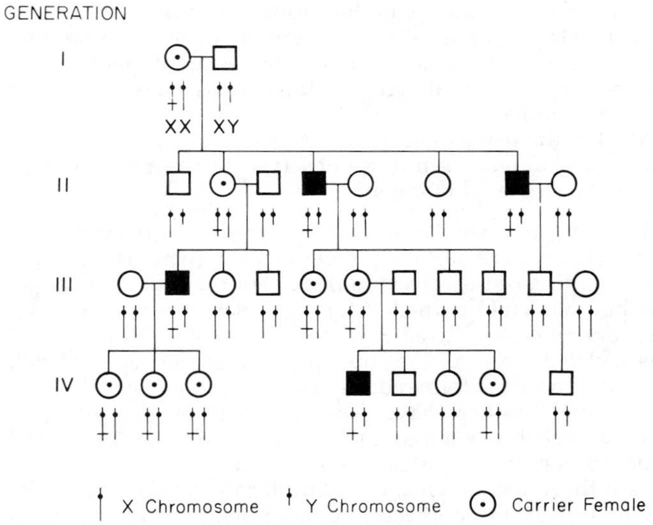

Figure 7–3. X-linked recessive inheritance. (See Figure 7–1 for key.)

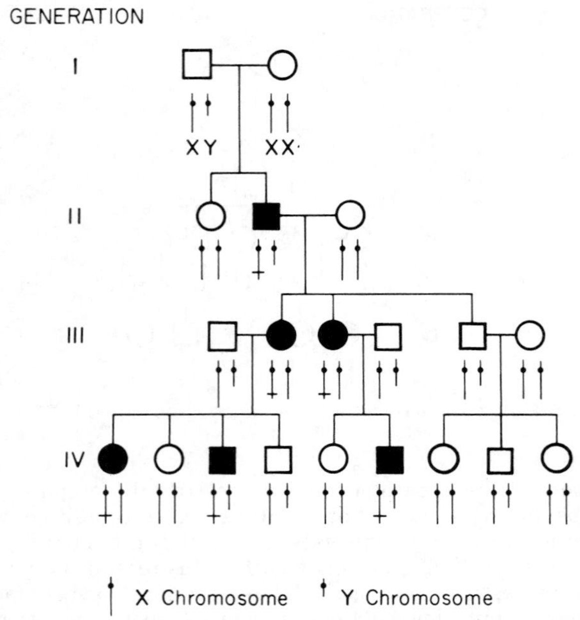

Figure 7–4. X-linked dominant inheritance. (See Figure 7–1 for key.)

common malformations as well as medical conditions such as allergic disorders, schizophrenia, and some types of hyperlipidemia (Table 7–2 and Sec. 8.22). The number of genes involved is unknown. Some investigators have postulated that the genes involved are "minor genes," which individually are not harmful but whose cumulative effect is harmful; others postulate that genes that exert a major effect are also involved. Few of the environmental factors have been identified in humans, but studies of conditions caused by multifactorial inheritance in animals emphasize their relevance. Some of the environmental factors identified in humans include seasonal variation in the occurrence of the disorder, increased frequency in families living in poor socioeconomic conditions, and associations with an altered uterine environment (see Table 7–13). Considerable data must be available on many affected persons and their families before the disease or malformation can be attributed to multifactorial inheritance. This term should not be used simply because the reason for familial occurrence is poorly understood.

Some of the features of multifactorial inheritance are similar to mendelian inheritance of single mutant genes, for example, the incidence of specific conditions varies according to racial background; this racial predisposition persists after migration to other countries.

Most of the features of multifactorial inheritance, however, are quite different from those observed in mendelian inheritance of a single mutant gene:

1. There is a similar rate of recurrence (usually 2–10%; Table 7–2) among all first-degree relatives (parents, siblings, and offspring of the affected infant). For example, if a couple has had one child with cleft lip and palate, the risk that the next one will be affected is approximately 4%; if one parent has a cleft lip and palate, the chance that the 1st child will have the same malformation is also approximately 4%.
2. Some disorders have a sex predilection. For example, pyloric stenosis is more common in males, whereas congenital dislocation of hips is more common in females.
3. If there is an altered sex ratio, the affected person of the sex less likely to be affected is more likely to have affected children. For example, a woman who had pyloric stenosis as an infant has a 25% chance of having a child similarly affected; the risk for the children of the father who had pyloric stenosis is only 4%.
4. The likelihood that both of identical twins will be affected with the same malformation is less than 100% but much greater than the chance that both nonidentical twins will be affected. The frequency of concordance for identical twins ranges from 21 to 63% for the disorders listed in Table 7–2. This distribution contrasts with that of mendelian inheritance, in which identical twins always share a disorder owing to a single mutant gene.
5. The risk of recurrence in subsequent pregnancies depends on the outcome in previous pregnancies. For example, the risk of recurrence for cleft lip and palate is 4% for a couple with one affected child, but 9% after they have had two affected children.
6. The risk of abnormality in offspring is related directly to the severity of the malformation. For example, the infant who has congenital intestinal aganglionosis of a long segment of bowel has a greater chance of having an affected sibling than the infant who has aganglionosis of only a small segment.

7.9 MITOCHONDRIAL INHERITANCE, GONADAL MOSAICISM, AND UNIPARENTAL DISOMY

Progress has been made in understanding the basis for unusual patterns of inheritance. For example, the mitochondria contains a small circular DNA molecule that is only 16.5 kilobases (kb) long (by contrast the dystrophin gene that contains the abnormalities that cause DMD and Beckers' muscular dystrophy is 2,000 kb long). Mitochondrial myopathies (e.g., Kearns-Sayre syndrome) and Leber hereditary optic neuropathy are caused by deletions in mitochondrial DNA (see Sec. 21.25). The affected male cannot have any affected sons or daughters, whereas the affected woman can have affected sons and daughters. Furthermore, females with gonadal mosaicism have mutations in only some of their eggs; the female is not shown to be a carrier but has more than one affected son, a phenomenon observed in DMD and in X-linked hemophilia. Last, in uniparental disomy the child inherits both chromosomes in one pair from one parent and does not have a chromosome from that pair from the other parent.

7.10 GENERAL CLINICAL PRINCIPLES IN GENETIC DISORDERS

NEGATIVE FAMILY HISTORY. A child with a genetic disease or malformation is usually the only known affected member of his or her family. This reflects the fact that the rates of recurrence are very low for common abnormalities of the chromosomes and for conditions attributed to multifactorial inheritance. For example, the recurrence risk for Down syndrome associated with 21-trisomy is 1%; for conditions attributed to multifactorial inheritance it varies from 2 to 10% (see Table 7–2). The recurrence risk for disorders with a mendelian pattern of inheritance is much higher (e.g., 25% for autosomal recessive disorders), but in small families it is more likely that an autosomal recessive disorder will affect only 1 of 3 or 4 children rather than 2. In the case of autosomal dominant disorders, the child may be affected by a spontaneous genetic mutation rather than by inheriting the mutant gene from an affected parent. Generally speaking, a negative family history may be misleading.

ENVIRONMENTAL FACTORS. Since the family history is usually negative for the disorder under consideration, the

TABLE 7–2. Genetic Disorders Attributed to Multifactorial Inheritance

Abnormality	Race	Prevalence in General Population (%)	Risk of Recurrence Among Family Members of an Affected Individual (%)		
			Siblings	Offspring	Identical Twin
Malformations					
Cardiac defects					
Ventricular septal defect		0.23	4.4	3.7	
Atrial septal defect		0.1 (1/1,000)	3.3	3.5 (parents)	
Patent ductus arteriosus		0.05	1.4	2.8	
Tetralogy of Fallot		0.03	1.1	1.6	
Cleft lip and palate	Whites	0.13 (1/750)	3.9	3.5	31
	Blacks	0.04			
	Navajos	0.2			
	Japanese	0.16			
Cleft palate	Whites	0.05 (1/2,000)	3.0	6.2	40
	Blacks	0.04			
	Navajos	0.03			
Club foot (talipes equinovarus)		0.01	2.9		33
Dislocation of hip, congenital		0.07 (1/1,400)	4.3		35
Hirschsprung disease		0.02 (1/5,000)	3.8*		
			12.5†		
Hypospadias	Whites	0.8 (1/120)	7.0	6.0	
	Blacks	0.2 (1/500)			
Legg-Perthes disease		0.07 (Canada)	3.7*		
			4.3†		
Meningomyelocele, anencephaly, encephalocele	Whites	0.3 (1/330) (London)	4.4	3.0	21
		0.14 (1/700) (Boston)	2		
	Jews	0.08			
	Blacks	0.07			
	Puerto Ricans	0.2			
Pyloric stenosis		0.2 (1/500) (London)	3.2*	25.4‡	22
			6.5†	4.2§	
Other Diseases					
Ankylosing spondylitis			7.0*		
			2.0†		
Atopic disease		2–3	5.8		24
Psoriasis		1–2	7.8		63
Schizophrenia		1–3	6–12	10	40

*If brother affected.
†If sister affected.
‡If mother affected.
§If father affected.

parents often blame themselves and look for environmental factors that might have been the cause. The physician should anticipate their feelings of guilt and should carefully discuss the events, including medications taken, to which congenital disorders may be attributed inappropriately by parents.

GENETIC HETEROGENEITY. A single clinical manifestation may have more than one cause. An elevation in serum phenylalanine may be associated with classic phenylketonuria (either the absence or deficiency of phenylalanine hydroxylase); absence or deficiency of the enzyme pteridin reductase; or deficient biopterin synthesis. Arachnodactyly may be an isolated characteristic of a tall, thin person, or it may be a feature of a number of genetic disorders, including Marfan syndrome and contractural arachnodactyly.

PLEIOTROPISM. Some genetic disorders have many different features, all of which are the pleiotropic effect of a single mutant gene. For example, in classic galactosemia, cataracts, hepatomegaly, malabsorption, neonatal sepsis, and mental deficiency are all related to deficiency of the transferase enzyme, which is the primary effect of the underlying autosomal recessive mutant gene. In neurofibromatosis, café-au-lait spots, subcutaneous nodules, solid tumors, scoliosis, and mental deficiency are caused by a single autosomal dominant gene.

VARIABLE EXPRESSION. Publications often present the extreme manifestations of a clinical disorder but rarely describe its milder forms. The clinician must appreciate that 2 or 3 café-au-lait spots may be either innocent birth marks or the earliest signs of neurofibromatosis in which additional features may become manifest at an older age. This diagnostic dilemma can be resolved only by a careful diagnostic evaluation and sometimes long-term follow-up. In the case of hereditary disorders without progressive changes, such as the Treacher Collins syndrome (mandibulofacial dysostosis), the affected child may have microtia, severe hearing loss, colobomas of the lower eyelids, and marked maxillary hypoplasia, whereas the affected parent may have only mild hearing loss, a downward slant of the palpebral fissures, and a decreased number of lashes on the lower eyelid.

NOT EVERYTHING FAMILIAL IS GENETIC. Environmental factors, such as infection and teratogens (see Table 7–15), may simulate genetic conditions; occasionally two or more children of healthy parents may be affected.

ESTABLISHING THE PATTERN OF INHERITANCE REQUIRES EXTENSIVE DATA. Data from a small number of families cannot establish a pattern of inheritance. For example, when a presumed genetic disorder has occurred in a son and daughter of healthy parents, it is often concluded that each child is homozygous for an autosomal recessive mutant gene. However, a familial chromosomal abnormality and multifactorial inheritance could also cause the same pattern. Similarly, the pattern of occurrence in families with a disorder due to multifactorial inheritance may simulate mendelian inheritance; for example, the parent and child with a cleft lip and palate mimic autosomal dominant inheritance. With the rate of recurrence among parents and siblings only 4% for Caucasians, almost all children with cleft lip and palate are the only affected members of their families. Data on hundreds of families were needed to establish multifactorial inheritance as the basis for the disorder and to exclude the possibility of mendelian inheritance.

LEWIS B. HOLMES

Antonarakis SE: Diagnosis of genetic disorders at the DNA level. N Engl J Med 320:153, 1989.
Fraser FC: The multifactorial/threshold concept: Uses and misuses. Teratology 14:267, 1976.
Hall JG, Powers EK, McIlvaine RT, et al: The frequency and financial burden of genetic disease in a pediatric hospital. Am J Med Genet 1:417, 1978.
Hoffman EP, Kunkel LM: Dystrophin abnormalities in Duchenne/Becker muscular dystrophy. Neuron 2:1019, 1987.
Kazazian HH Jr, Boehm CD: Molecular basis and prenatal diagnosis of β-thalassemia. Blood 72:1107, 1988.
Kerem B-S, Rommems JM, Buchanan JA, et al: Identification of the cystic fibrosis gene: genetic analysis. Science 245:1073, 1989.
McKusick VA: Mapping and sequencing the human genome. N Engl J Med 320:910, 1989.
Schmickel RD: Contiguous gene syndromes: A component of recognizable syndromes. J Pediatr 109:231, 1986.
Scriver CR, Claw CL: Phenylketonuria: Epitome of human biochemical genetics. N Engl J Med 303:1336, 1394, 1980.
Singh G, Lott MT, Wallace DC: A mitochondrial DNA mutation and a cause of Leber's hereditary optic neuropathy. N Engl J Med 320:1300, 1989.
Spence JE, Perciaccante RG, Greig GM, et al: Uniparental disomy or a mechanism for human genetic disease. Am J Hum Genet 42:217, 1988.
Woo SLC: Molecular basis and population genetics of phenylketonuria. Biochemistry 28:1, 1989.

GENERAL

McKusick V: Mendelian Inheritance in Man: Catalogs of Autosomal Dominant, Autosomal Recessive and X-Linked Phenotypes, 8th ed. Baltimore, Johns Hopkins University Press, 1988.
Vogel F, Motulsky AG: Human Genetics: Problems and Approaches. New York, Springer-Verlag, 1979.
Watson JD, Tooze J, Kurtz DT: Recombinant DNA: A Short Course. New York, Scientific American Books, WH Freeman, 1983.

7.11 CHROMOSOMES AND THEIR ABNORMALITIES

Scientific and technologic advances permitted Hsu and Levan in 1952 to observe accurately human chromosomes and Tjio and Levan in 1956 to discover that the correct systemic chromosome number in humans is 46. In 1959 Lejeune observed that patients with Down syndrome have 47 chromosomes, including an extra chromosome 21 (21-trisomy). These seminal observations were rapidly followed by the discovery of other trisomies in congenital malformation syndromes, abnormalities in the number of sex chromosomes in Klinefelter and Turner syndromes, and the first detection of chromosomal mosaics and abnormalities of chromosome structure. Cytogenetic abnormalities are now recognized as important etiologic factors in human disease. During the ensuing 30 years, laboratory procedures were developed to identify precisely the individual chromosomes (and chromosomal segments), enabling the interpretation of complex chromosomal rearrangements as well as minor morphologic variations. These techniques have led to more accurate clinical diagnosis as well as to more precise genetic counseling.

Because chromosome studies are complicated and expensive, candidates for these procedures must be carefully identified. The most important clinical indications are congenital malformations, especially if more than one system is involved, and mental retardation of unknown origin. Some of the more common features of children with chromosome abnormalities are odd facies, abnormal ears, heart and kidney malformations, abnormal hands and feet, simian creases, a single crease on the 5th finger, and low birthweight. It has been estimated that about 1 in 150 newborn infants has a chromosomal abnormality. Table 7–3 lists the incidence of various chromosomal abnormalities in liveborn infants.

In addition, the fact that 50–60% of the products of early spontaneous abortion have a chromosomal abnormality suggests that at least 10% of human conceptions have a karyotypic abnormality. At 16–18 wk of gestation, the incidence of chromosomal abnormalities as detected by amniocentesis is greater than in liveborn infants, suggesting the loss of additional cytogenetically unbalanced fetuses in mid- and late pregnancy. Approximately 90% of karyotypically abnormal conceptions do not survive pregnancy. Of the chromosomal abnormalities observed in liveborn infants, about half involve the autosomes and half the sex chromosomes. Chromosomal abnormalities are associated with approximately 50% of cases of primary amenorrhea, 10% of male sterility, and 20% of mental retardation, and are found in most neoplastic cells. Their discoverable frequency should increase as more accurate methods for detection of minor structural alterations become available.

METHODOLOGY

CELL CULTURE. The small lymphocyte, which is readily stimulated to divide with the plant mitogen phytohemagglutinin (PHA), is commonly used for chromosome investigation. The dividing cells are arrested in metaphase and the chromosomes are dispersed and air dried.

Cultures of fibroblasts may be necessary for studies of mosaicism and biochemical defects. For diagnosing blood dyscrasias, bone marrow preparations are best, but chromo-

TABLE 7–3. Incidence of Chromosomal Abnormalities Among Liveborn Infants

Down syndrome (21-trisomy)	1/800
18-trisomy syndrome	1/8,000
13-trisomy syndrome	1/20,000
Turner syndrome (females)	1/10,000
Klinefelter syndrome (males)	1/1,000
Poly-X anomalies (females)	1/1,000
XYY karyotype (males)	1/1,000
Balanced structural rearrangement	1/520
Unbalanced structural rearrangement	1/1,700
Fragile X (males)	1/2,000
(females)	1/1,000
Total	1/150

somes of peripheral blood myelocytes can be used. The methodology for culturing amniotic fluid cells is similar to that for fibroblasts. Cytogenetic analysis is complete in 2–3 wk.

A much more rapid method for fetal chromosome analysis, chorionic villus biopsy, consists of obtaining a small sample of chorionic villi by ultrasonically guided transcervical suction biopsy followed by directly observing chromosomes in the sample or in cells cultured from the sample. The procedure is performed at 8–11 weeks of gestation, and results are generally available before the end of the 1st trimester.

Chromosome staining methods have been replaced mainly by the development of techniques that can yield characteristic patterns of alternating light and dark (or bright and dull) bands for each chromosome. These bands appear to be associated with the composition of base pairs forming the DNA, as well as the distribution of the various histone and nonhistone proteins along the length of the chromosome (Sec. 7.1). Staining with quinacrine derivatives or similar compounds, followed by microscopic investigation using an ultraviolet light source, produces fluorescent bands called *Q bands*, while corresponding *G bands* are produced by a modified Giemsa staining procedure. Another method, using Giemsa or acridine orange, produces staining intensities opposite to Q and G bands, which are called reverse or *R bands*. All qualified cytogenetic laboratories now use at least one of these banding methods to assure a reliable diagnosis. Other procedures available in more advanced laboratories include C-banding to stain constitutive heterochromatin found near the centromere of each chromosome; a *C-band* stain (G-11) specific for No. 9; NOR, using ammoniacal silver to stain the nucleolar organizing regions of satellited chromosomes; and SCE, a procedure that reveals exchanges between sister chromatids.

An important newer development consists of examining chromosomes during late prophase, at which time they are much less contracted than at metaphase when they are commonly examined. This procedure allows the analysis of 600–1,400 bands as opposed to the usual 200–400, permitting the discovery of very small deletions and duplications.

KARYOTYPING. Chromosomal DNA replicates during the S stage of interphase, but the double-structured nature of the chromosomes becomes clearly visible only at the beginning of mitosis; each chromosome consists of two identical long thin strands called sister chromatids, which coil progressively tighter, giving the appearance of short, thick arms held together by the centromere. At metaphase, when they are at their shortest length, the chromosomes are photographed and arranged in pairs. This systematized arrangement from a single cell is referred to as a karyotype. Only "banded" karyotypes are acceptable for diagnoses, and most laboratories study 10–40 metaphase karyotypes per subject. If mosaicism is suspected, more cells, as well as cells of other tissues, should be analyzed. When finer details are required, prophase or prometaphase chromosomes are examined because they are longer and show more bands.

7.12 NORMAL KARYOTYPE

The diploid number of human chromosomes is 46, consisting of 23 pairs; 23 is the haploid number found in the gametes. At metaphase each chromosome, consisting of 2 chromatids, has a characteristic morphology determined by the position of the centromere, or primary constriction, which delineates the long and short arms (Fig. 7–5*A*). Examples of the three normal characteristic shapes are Nos. 1, 3, and 16 *(metacentric)*, Nos. 4 and 5 *(submetacentric)*, and Nos. 21 and 22 *(acrocentric)*. The short arms of all acrocentric chromosomes except the Y have a secondary constriction and satellite. Following the accurate identification of each chromosome, accomplished on the basis of size, morphology, and banding pattern, a number system was agreed upon (Fig. 7–6).

A few morphologic variants have been observed in the normal karyotype with conventional stains. Best known are elongation of the paracentromeric region in the long arm of Nos. 1, 9, and 16, extended or deleted short arms or enlarged satellites of acrocentric chromosomes, and a secondary constriction on the short arm of No. 17 (Fig. 7–7; see also Fig. 7–5*B*). The Y chromosome may also vary in length and shape. Although the banding patterns are constant for each chromosome, normal variants have been revealed by fluorescent stains, for example, variation in intensity of fluorescent bands near the centromeres of chromosomes 3 and 4 and satellites on the acrocentric chromosomes (see Fig. 7–7). The variation in length of the Y chromosome is the result of extension or loss of the brilliant Q band, which appears to have no effect on the phenotype. Morphologic variants were first observed in abnormal subjects and were thought to be associated with disease, but it soon became apparent that they were inherited in mendelian fashion, and some occur in sufficiently high frequencies to be considered polymorphisms ("normal variants"). Therefore, they are useful genetic markers and also help to localize genes to specific chromosomes.

Cell-to-cell variation in chromosome number has been found in older people. A tendency exists for women aged 55 yr and older to lose an X chromosome and for men over 65 yr of age to lose a Y chromosome.

Another category of variation is the presence or absence of fragile sites. Whereas most of these are not associated with specific syndromes, the presence of such a site near the end

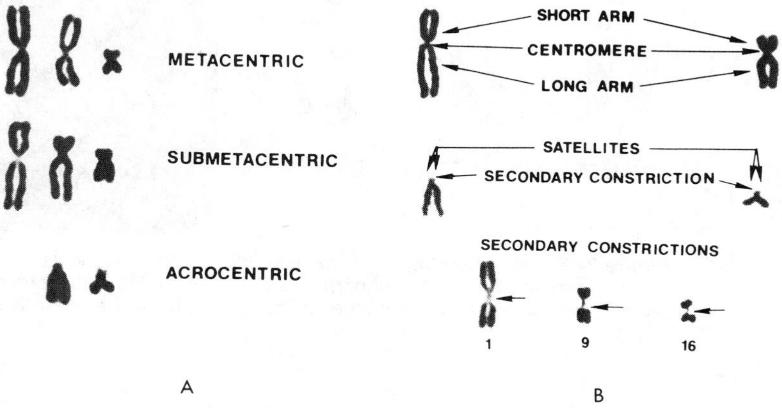

Figure 7–5. *A*, Centromere position determining the three types of chromosomes seen in the normal human karyotype—metacentric, submetacentric, and acrocentric. *B*, Morphologic landmarks useful in chromosome identification.

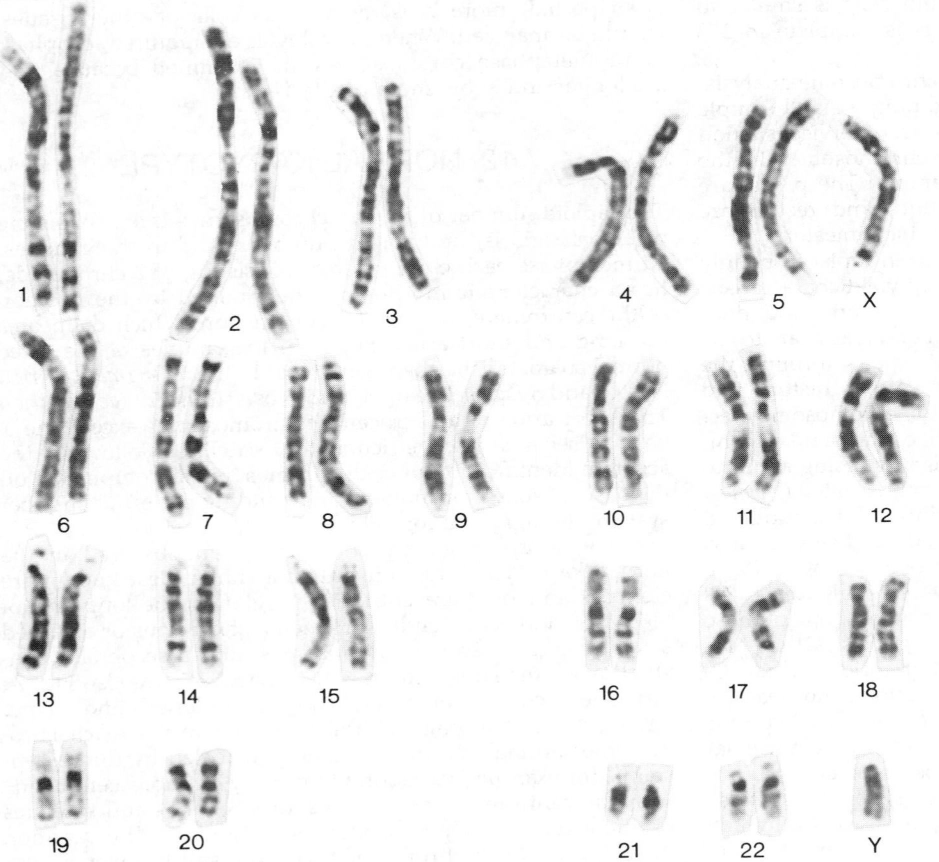

Figure 7–6. Karyotype of normal male with chromosomes in late prophase. The chromosomes are longer and a greater number of bands are seen than when chromosomes are photographed at metaphase.

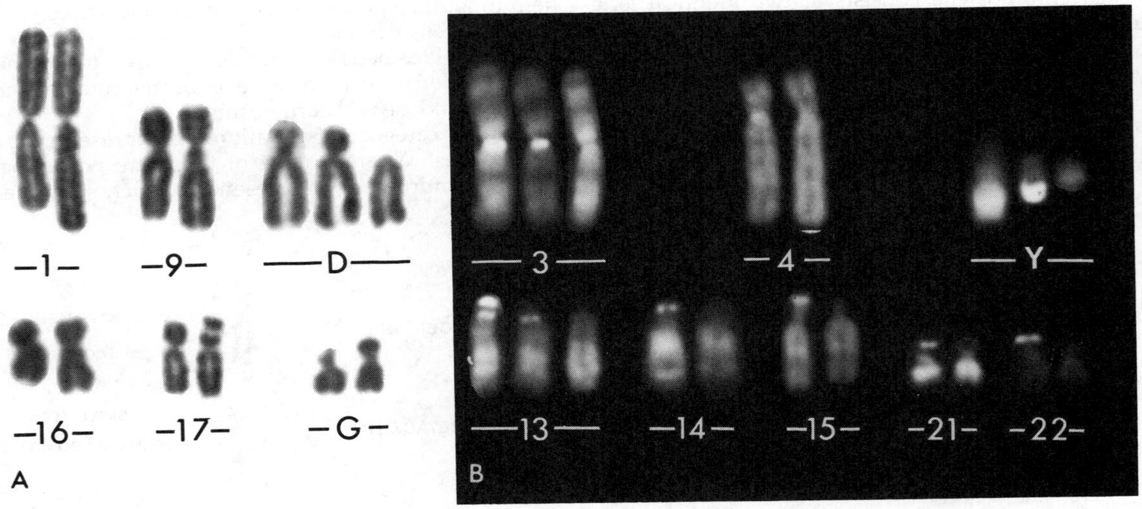

Figure 7–7. Some morphologic variants found in normal subjects. *A*, Chromosomes stained with aceto-orcein. The left-hand chromosome of each pair or triad is a usual or "nonmarker" chromosome. *B*, Chromosomes stained with quinacrine dihydrochloride showing differences in intensity of fluorescent bands among homologues.

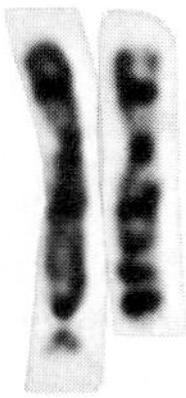

Figure 7–8. X chromosomes with the one on the left showing a fragile site near the lower end of the long arm (fra(X) (q28)).

of the long arm of the X chromosome (Fig. 7–8) is associated with mental retardation (Sec. 7.30).

7.13 ABNORMAL KARYOTYPES

NUMERIC ABNORMALITIES. Chromosomal aberrations are divided into numeric and structural types. A cell with the exact multiple of the haploid number (e.g., 46, 69, 92) is referred to as *euploid*. Euploid cells with more than the normal *diploid* number of 46 chromosomes are called *polyploid*. Cells deviating from one of the euploid numbers are called *aneuploid*.

The most common type of aneuploidy is *trisomy*, that is, 3 homologous chromosomes instead of the pair normally present. Lack of a chromosome is called *monosomy* (for the affected pair). Aneuploid individuals may be trisomic for more than one pair of chromosomes or may even combine trisomy and monosomy. During meiosis, synapsis occurs between each chromosome and its homologue; after separation each proceeds to an opposite pole of the dividing cell. Failure of synapsis or failure to separate *(nondisjunction)* interferes with orderly segregation and may result in aneuploidy (Fig. 7–9).

Nondisjunction occurring during mitotic division results in *mosaicism*, that is, the presence of more than one population of cells with differing chromosome numbers in the same individual (Fig. 7–10). The older the mother, the greater is the likelihood of nondisjunction and trisomy. Monosomy may result from chromosome loss or *anaphase lag*, that is, failure of a chromosome to reach either pole during anaphase, which also results in mosaicism (see Fig. 7–10). The timing of mitotic nondisjunction in embryonic development may result in mosaicism with two or three different populations of cells present (Fig. 7–11).

Pure polyploidy is lethal in humans, but individuals with mosaicism have been known to survive. *Triploidy* (3 haploid sets, totaling 69 chromosomes) has been found most frequently among abortuses and stillbirths. It arises by fertilization of the ovum by two spermatozoa or by the union of a haploid with a diploid gamete. Tetraploid cells have been found in aborted material, in persons with malignant disease, and, rarely, in dysmorphic infants. *Tetraploidy* occurs occasionally in cultured cells, particularly amniotic fluid cells, and increases during culture.

STRUCTURAL ABERRATIONS. These abnormalities result from chromosome breaks and rearrangements. *Deletion syndromes*, such as cri-du-chat (5p −), may result from a simple deletion or from the inheritance of a deleted translocation chromosome. Interstitial deletions result from the loss of a segment within the chromosome arm (Fig. 7–12).

All structural defects require at least two chromosomal breaks followed by reunion of the broken ends. *Translocations*, which may be inherited or arise de novo, are most common. *Reciprocal translocations* result from the exchange of segments between 2 nonhomologous chromosomes (see Fig. 7–12). Carriers of reciprocal translocations are usually phenotypically normal since they have a full complement of genes. Children of such "translocation carriers" will be abnormal if they

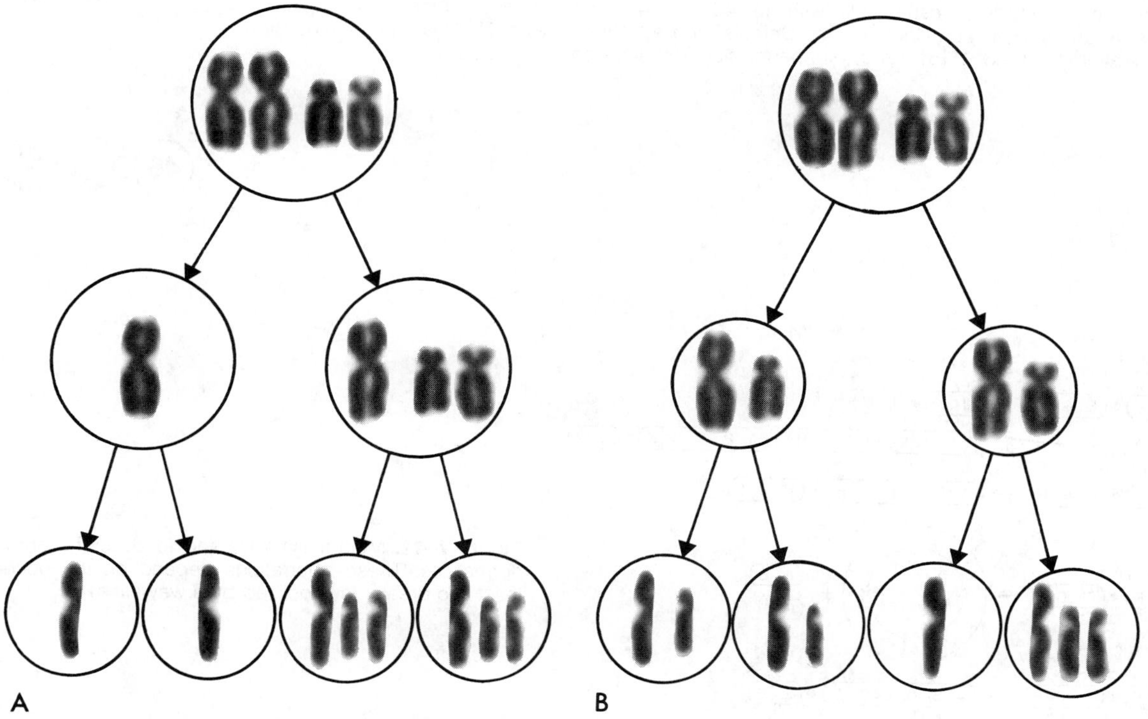

Figure 7–9. Nondisjunction during meiosis illustrated with two pairs of chromosomes. *A*, First division nondisjunction with failure of smaller homologues to separate gives rise to gametes with no small chromosome or with an extra one. *B*, Second division nondisjunction following division of centromere. Two newly formed chromosomes fail to separate in cell on the right.

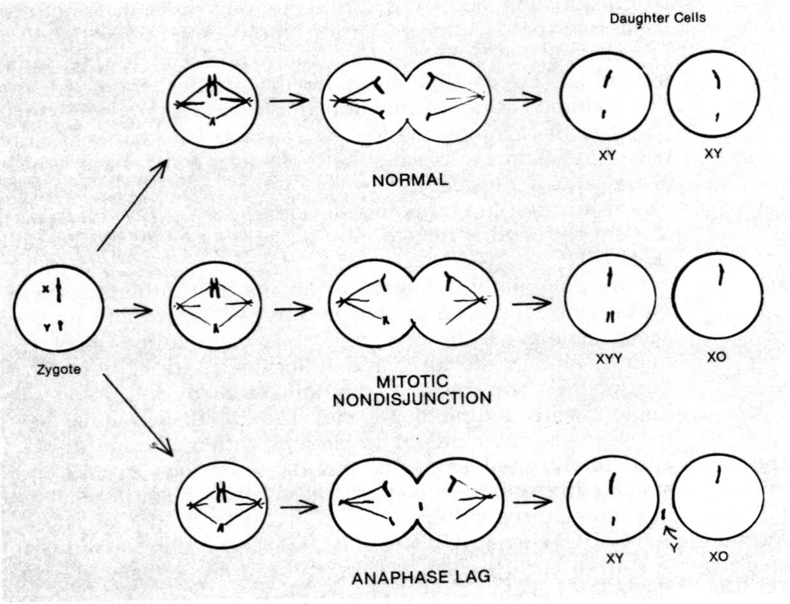

Figure 7–10. The formation of mosaicism. The X and Y chromosomes are used to illustrate two common errors leading to chromosomally abnormal cell populations. In normal mitosis *(top)* duplicated chromosomes separate and become incorporated into daughter cells. If one replicated chromosome fails to separate, mitotic nondisjunction occurs *(middle)*. Occasionally, normal separation occurs, but one member fails to migrate. This is known as anaphase lag *(bottom)*. (From Wisniewski LP, Hirschhorn K: A Guide to Human Chromosome Defects, 2nd ed. White Plains, NY, March of Dimes Birth Defects Foundation, BD:OAS, 16[6], 1980, with permission from the copyright holder.)

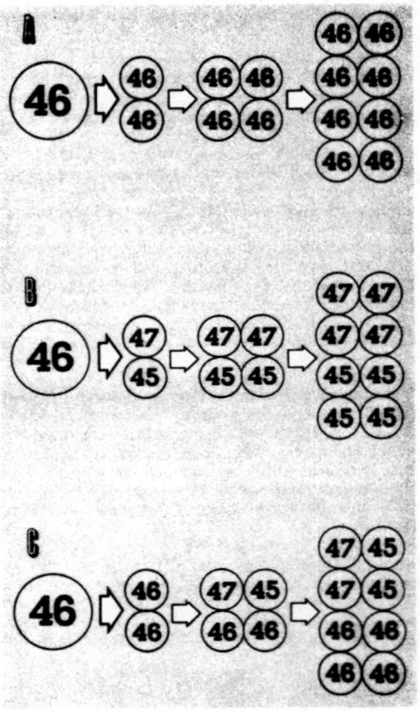

Figure 7–11. Relationship of the timing of mitotic nondisjunction to the proportion of abnormal cells in a mosaic embryo. *A,* Normal mitosis; all resulting cells contain 46 chromosomes. *B,* Error occurring during the first mitosis after conception; two types of cells subsequently compose the developing embryo (half containing 47 chromosomes, half containing 45). *C,* An error occurs after some growth has been achieved; three different cell populations result (cells with 45, 46, and 47 chromosomes). (From Wisniewski LP, Hirschhorn K: A Guide to Human Chromosome Defects, 2nd ed. White Plains, NY, March of Dimes Birth Defects Foundation, BD:OAS, 16[6], 1980, with permission from the copyright holder.)

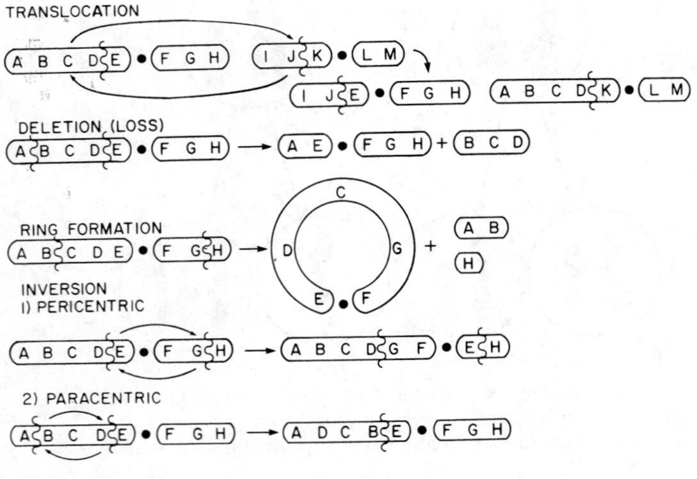

Figure 7–12. Mechanisms leading to structural chromosome abnormalities. These aberrations depend on the occurrence of at least two breaks (symbolized by a *wavy line*).

receive only 1 of the 2 translocation chromosomes and thus become affected by duplication-deficiency syndromes (Fig. 7–13). Depending on the amount of material duplicated or deficient, the aberration is referred to as *partial trisomy* or *partial monosomy*. A special type of translocation, the *centric fusion* or *Robertsonian translocation*, involves acrocentric chromosomes in which the breaks occur adjacent to the centromeres of "recipient" and "donor" chromosomes. The centromere of the donor chromosome and the short arms of both chromosomes are usually lost. Centric fusion commonly involves No. 14 and No. 21 and therefore may result in Down syndrome (Fig. 7–14). Since the short arms of acrocentric chromosomes appear to be genetically inactive, the loss of material in such translocations has no apparent phenotypic effect on carriers.

Ring chromosomes are formed when both tips of a chromosome are broken and the ends of the centric fragment rejoin forming a chromosome with a deletion of both arms (see Fig. 7–12). This unstable closed structure leads to difficulties in mitosis. *Inversions* (see Fig. 7–12) of two types may result when the segment between two breaks in a single chromosome is inverted and the order of the genes reversed. Because an inversion may cause difficulty in synapsis, it may increase the risk of nondisjunction.

During meiosis, crossing over of genes between chromatids of homologous chromosomes is a normal phenomenon readily proved by the recombination or separation of genes originally linked on the same chromosome. Exchanges between chromatids may also occur during mitosis and may involve the chromatids of two homologous or nonhomologous chromosomes. Since at metaphase the sister chromatids have not yet separated, such exchanges result in *quadriradial* configurations that resemble crossroads. It is more difficult to prove the existence of *sister chromatid exchanges* (SCE) in mitotic cells because replicated chromatids carry identical genes and no unusual configurations are formed. This can be done with staining techniques. The various types of chromatid exchanges are found in breakage syndromes (Sec. 7.22) and in cells exposed to mutagenic agents.

NOMENCLATURE

The nomenclature for describing a karyotype has been standardized to avoid confusion. First, the total number of chromosomes, and second, the sex chromosome complement are recorded; then any aberration is described. The short arm is referred to as *p* and the long arm as *q*. Any addition or loss of chromosomal material is denoted by a plus (+) or minus (−) sign placed before the chromosome number if a whole chromosome is involved and after a symbol if any increase or decrease in length is involved. Chromosomes involved in a translocation are written in brackets preceded by a *t*; for example, t(14q21q) describes the translocation most frequently found in Down syndrome. (Most children with Down syndrome, however, have three No. 21 chromosomes, the extra denoted as +21.)

The regions within the chromosomes are now also delineated by their characteristic bands. Each chromosome arm is divided and subdivided into regions so that the breakpoints in chromosomal rearrangements can be identified and the aberration described with some accuracy. This nomenclature is complicated, and the clinician dealing with chromosomal disorders will often need to consult a cytogeneticist.

DERMATOGLYPHICS

Before the advent of human cytogenetics, the analysis of hand and footprints was used as one criterion for diagnosing Down syndrome. The subsequent development of techniques for chromosomal analysis has decreased their relative importance in the clinical assessment of patients suspected of having a chromosomal abnormality.

Dermatoglyphics refers to configurations formed by the dermal ridges, not by the flexion creases. The most important landmarks are the patterns on the distal phalanges of the digits, the position of the triradius in the axis of the palm, and the pattern in the hallucal area of the soles. The size of a pattern is determined by counting the number of dermal

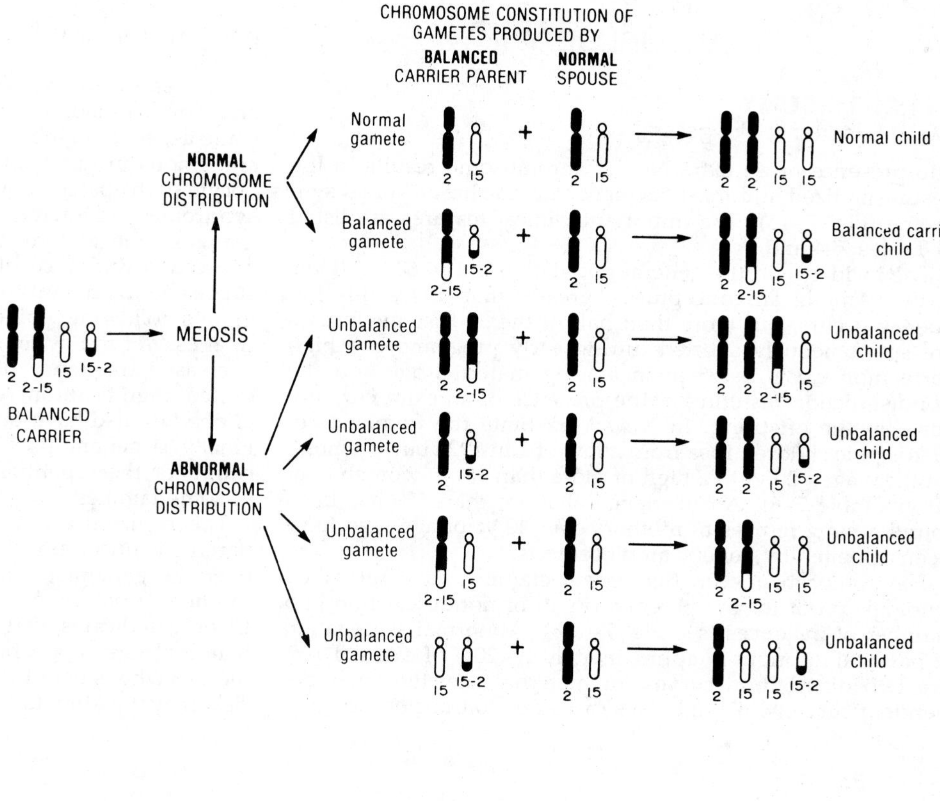

Figure 7–13. The inheritance of a 2/15 translocation. (From Wisniewski LP, Hirschhorn K: A Guide to Human Chromosome Defects, 2nd ed. White Plains, NY, March of Dimes Birth Defects Foundation, BD:OAS, 16[6], 1980, with permission from the copyright holder.)

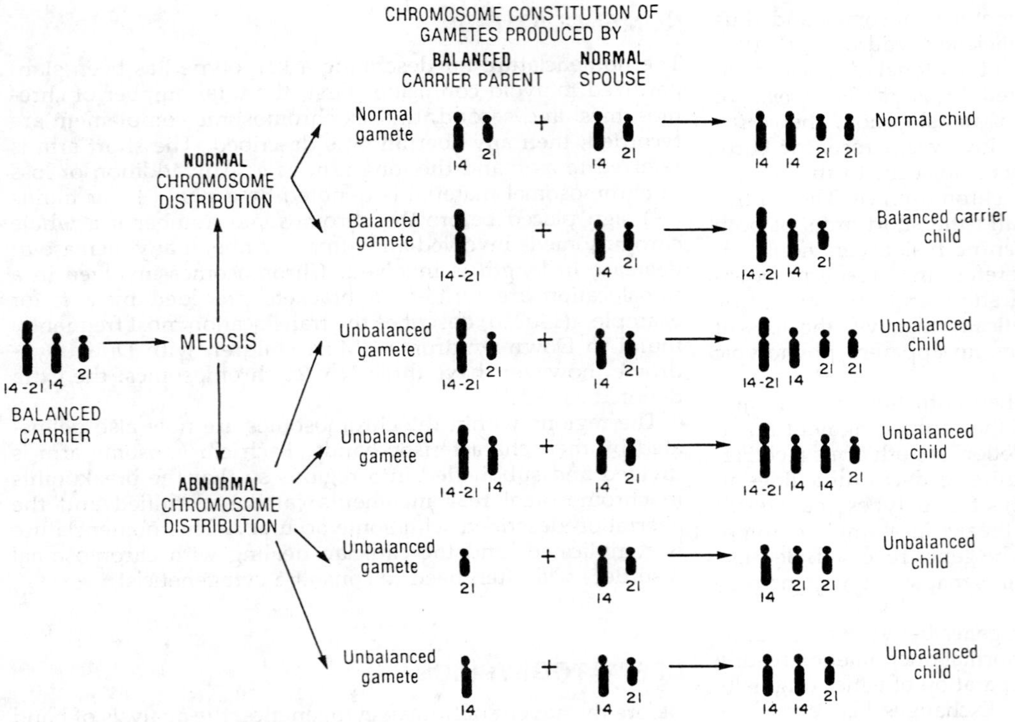

Figure 7–14. The inheritance of a 14/21 centric fusion. Although this translocation can also result in abnormalities of chromosome 14 and monosomy 21, conceptions with these defects rarely, if ever, survive. (From Wisniewski LP, Hirschhorn K: A Guide to Human Chromosome Defects, 2nd ed. White Plains, NY, March of Dimes Birth Defects Foundation, BD:OAS, 16[6], 1980, with permission from the copyright holder.)

ridges between the center or core of the pattern and the triradius that determines its periphery. Whorls usually have the highest ridge counts while an arch has a count of 0 because it has no triradius. Digital pattern size is important in certain syndromes.

There is a strong correlation between dermatoglyphics and chromosomes. Characteristic dermal patterns are established for 13-, 18-, and 21-trisomies and in 18 and G deletion syndromes. They are described under the respective syndromes.

CLINICAL ABNORMALITIES OF THE AUTOSOMES

ANEUPLOIDY

7.14 21-TRISOMY
(Down Syndrome; Mongolism)

The presence of an extra No. 21 chromosome results in the best recognized and most frequent human chromosomal syndrome (Fig. 7–15). The important clinical features are listed in Tables 7–4 and 7–5.

The incidence in the general population is 1 in 600–800 live births. Among all conceptuses, greater than twice this frequency occurs, but more than half of the 21-trisomic fetuses are spontaneously aborted during early pregnancy. A high correlation exists between increasing maternal age and the nondisjunction resulting in the presence of an extra chromosome in the offspring. In New York State the frequency of 21-trisomic children rose from a low of 1 in 1925 births among mothers aged 20 yr to a high of more than 1% in women over 40 yr (Table 7–6). An incidence of more than 5% has been found among fetuses of mothers over 40 yr of age who have been screened by genetic amniocentesis.

Heteromorphisms on fluorescent staining have furnished cytologic proof for the parental origin of nondisjunction in a number of instances (see Fig. 7–15*B*). Abnormal segregation is paternal in origin in approximately 10–20% of cases. There are two distribution curves for maternal age: the age-independent curve, which includes cases due to translocation and probably paternal nondisjunction, and the age-dependent curve.

The reason for the correlation between late maternal age and nondisjunction is unknown. It is thought to be due to some aspect of aging of the oocyte, which lives in suspended animation during meiotic division from late fetal life until that oocyte participates in ovulation. The incidences of both Down syndrome and maternal exposure to diagnostic roentgenograms of the abdomen correlate with maternal age. Virus-induced disturbance of chromosomal segregation has been suggested to account for the clustering of births of 21-trisomic infants following epidemics of infectious hepatitis. "Overripeness" of the ovum due to delayed fertilization because of decreased frequency of coitus with age has also been suggested. Significant increases in the frequency of thyroid autoantibodies also have been observed in patients and mothers. Finally, a genetic predisposition to nondisjunction could account for the repetition of 21-trisomy and other aneuploidy in some families.

The recurrence risk of trisomy to chromosomally normal parents is uncertain. Estimates range from no increase in risk over the general population to a 50-fold increase in young mothers. Analysis of data using only chromosomally proven trisomy indicates that the risk of recurrence, regardless of maternal age, appears to be about the same as that for a mother who is over the age of 45 yr (i.e., 1/80). This increased risk may be due to undetected mosaicism in a parent or

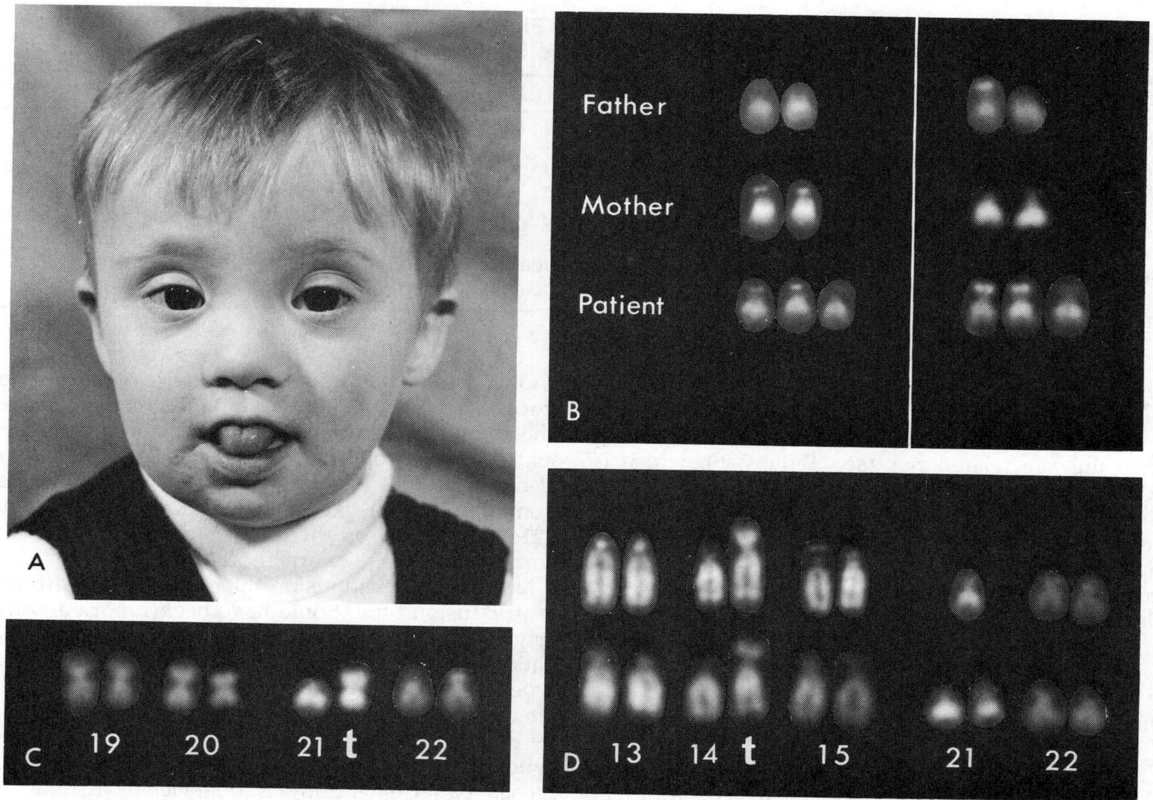

Figure 7–15. Partial karyotypes from patients with Down syndrome. *A,* Patient with trisomy 21. *B,* Chromosomes 21 from 2 patients and their parents. *Left*: 2 of a patient's chromosomes with brightly fluorescent satellites were transmitted by the mother. *Right*: 2 chromosomes with bright satellites resulted from paternal nondisjunction at second meiotic division. *C,* 21q21q translocation. *D,* 14q21q translocation in a mother *(above)* and her affected child *(below)*.

TABLE 7–4. Major Clinical Features of the Three Most Common Autosomal Trisomic Syndromes

Characteristic Features	21-Trisomy	18-Trisomy	13-Trisomy
General	Mental retardation; hypotonia	Mental retardation; hypertonia; failure to thrive; preponderance of females; low birthweight	Mental retardation; failure to thrive; capillary hemangiomas; increased nuclear projections in neutrophils; persistent fetal hemoglobin; seizures; apneic episodes
Craniofacies	Flat occiput; oblique palpebral fissures; epicanthic folds; speckled irides (Brushfield spots); protruding tongue; prominent, malformed ears; flat nasal bridge	Prominent occiput; small features; micrognathia; low-set, malformed ears	Microcephaly; cleft lip ± palate; midline scalp defects; microphthalmia; colobomata; low-set malformed ears; apparent deafness
Thorax	Congenital heart disease, mainly septal defects, especially of the endocardial cushion	Congenital heart disease, mainly VSD* and PDA†; short sternum; diaphragmatic hernia	Congenital heart disease, mainly septal defects, PDA
Abdomen and pelvis	Decreased acetabular and iliac angles; small penis; cryptorchidism	Horseshoe kidney; small pelvis; cryptorchidism; limited hip abduction; inguinal or umbilical hernia	Polycystic kidneys; bicornuate uterus; cryptorchidism
Hands and feet	Simian crease; short, broad hands; hypoplasia of middle phalanx of 5th finger; gap between 1st and 2nd toes	Flexion deformity of fingers; short, dorsiflexed big toes; rockerbottom feet or equinovarus; phocomelia (rare)	Polydactyly; hyperconvex or hypoplastic fingernails; simian crease
Other features observed with significant frequency	High-arched palate; strabismus; broad, short neck; small teeth; furrowed tongue; intestinal atresia; imperforate anus; Hirschsprung disease	Cleft lip ± palate; ocular anomalies; simian crease; hypoplasia of fingernails; widely spaced nipples; webbed neck; single umbilical artery; tracheoesophageal fistula	Flexion deformity of fingers; single umbilical artery; shallow supraorbital ridges; micrognathia; retroflexible thumb; rockerbottom feet; omphalocele

*VSD = ventricular septal defect.
†PDA = patent ductus arteriosus.

TABLE 7–5. Important Dermatoglyphic Patterns and Flexion Creases Found in the Three Common Autosomal Trisomic Syndromes

Areas	21-Trisomy	18-Trisomy	13-Trisomy
Digits	Ulnar loops on most fingers; radial loops on fingers 4 and 5	Arches on fingers and toes	—
Palms	Distal axial triradius or large *atd* angle	—	Distal axial triradius or large *atd* angle
Soles	Arch tibial or small loop distal in hallucal area	—	Arch fibular or arch fibular-S in hallucal area
Flexion creases	Simian crease; single crease on finger 5	Single crease on finger 5 or on all fingers	Simian crease

repeated exposure to the same environmental insult. In pregnancies subsequent to the birth of a 21-trisomic infant, the risk of recurrence can generally be estimated for counseling as 1% above the age related risk (see Table 7–6), which is significant only for women under 37 yr.

TRANSLOCATION DOWN SYNDROME. "Regular" trisomy comprises some 95% of cases of Down syndrome. Approximately 1% of cases are mosaic (this estimate is minimum because some mosaics probably remain undetected, particularly among phenotypically normal parents of trisomic offspring); the remainder are the result of translocation.

The majority of translocations giving rise to the Down syndrome consist of centric fusions between No. 21 and chromosomes 13, 14, or 15; approximately half of these are inherited. The vast majority are t(14q21q) (see Fig. 7–15) and a few are t(15q21q). The rarity of t(13q21q) probably accounts for the absence of 13-trisomy syndrome, which would be expected to occur among the offspring of phenotypically normal carriers of the 13q21q translocation. Carrier mothers produce three types of viable offspring: normal phenotype and karyotype, phenotypically normal translocation carrier, and the translocation 21-trisomy (Fig. 7–16). Theoretically, these three types of offspring should occur with equal frequency, but only 10% have been abnormal, probably because of an increased lethality to the unbalanced zygote or fetus. The expected frequency of one third affected has been observed, however, among fetuses studied early in gestation. Carrier fathers rarely have affected offspring, although they do produce both normals and carriers.

TABLE 7–6. Estimated Rates of Down Syndrome (New York State Study)*

Maternal Age in Years†	Estimated Rate	Maternal Age in Years†	Estimated Rate
20	1/1,925	35	1/365
21	1/1,695	36	1/285
22	1/1,540	37	1/225
23	1/1,410	38	1/175
24	1/1,300	39	1/140
25	1/1,205	40	1/110
26	1/1,125	41	1/85
27	1/1,050	42	1/67
28	1/990	43	1/53
29	1/935	44	1/41
30	1/885	45	1/32
31	1/825	46	1/25
32	1/725	47	1/20
33	1/590	48	1/16
34	1/465	49	1/12

*Adapted from Hook EB and Chambers GM: Estimated rates of Down syndrome in live births by one year maternal age intervals of mothers aged 20–49 . . . . *In*: Bergsma D and Lowry RB (eds): Numerical Taxonomy of Birth Defects and Polygenic Disorders. New York, Alan R. Liss for the National Foundation-March of Dimes, BD:OAS XIII(3A):126, 1977

†Age at last birthday at delivery.

Only 5% of cases of translocation Down syndrome involving chromosomes 21 or 22 are inherited from a carrier parent. The small metacentric translocation chromosome may represent centric fusion of chromosomes 21 and 22 or of two No. 21 chromosomes (see Fig. 7–15*C* and *D*). All viable offspring from a t(21q21q) carrier would have Down syndrome. A t(21q22q) carrier, on the other hand, can produce carrier and normal as well as abnormal offspring.

Not all translocations producing Down syndrome are of the centric fusion type. Some have been reported with increased length of the long arm of one chromosome No. 21. Other patients with Down syndrome and apparently normal karyotypes may have a hidden translocation (i.e., part of No. 21 attached to a larger chromosome), which can be demonstrated by banding techniques. However, most children with Down syndrome and apparently normal karyotypes probably have mosaic patterns with low frequencies of trisomic cells.

The frequency of acute leukemia among individuals with Down syndrome is higher than in the general population; the majority are of the lymphoblastic type. The Philadelphia (Ph^1) chromosome found in patients with chronic myelogenous leukemia involves No. 22, in which the distal portion of the long arm has been reciprocally translocated to the long arm of chromosome 9.

A number of biochemical alterations have been reported in patients with Down syndrome, but most have not been consistent enough to provide useful genetic information. Several gene loci have been assigned to chromosome 21. Studies of two of these, the genes for the soluble form of the *superoxide dismutase* (SOD_s) and for the interferon receptor have revealed a dose relation proportional to the number of No. 21 chromosomes in a cell. The level of SOD_s in cells from patients with 21-trisomy has been shown to be approximately 1.5 times normal.

7.15 18-TRISOMY SYNDROME

This is the second most common autosomal aberration, originally referred to as the E-trisomy syndrome until improved techniques permitted distinction between chromosomes 17 and 18. Small, delicate facial features serve to distinguish children with 18-trisomy from other trisomics (Fig. 7–17). The principal clinical characteristics are listed in Tables 7–4 and 7–5.

Incidence is about 1 in 8,000 births. Affected infants are usually born after term, but the birth weight is low. The sex ratio is 1 male to 4 females. Almost all have a cardiac malformation, a major factor in the characteristically early demise, most frequently within the first 3 mo of life. Exceptional long-lived patients have been reported, the oldest being 15 yr of age. As with 21-trisomy, advanced maternal age is etiologically important.

TRANSLOCATIONS OF CHROMOSOME 18. These, although rare, have given rise to partial 18-trisomy syndromes,

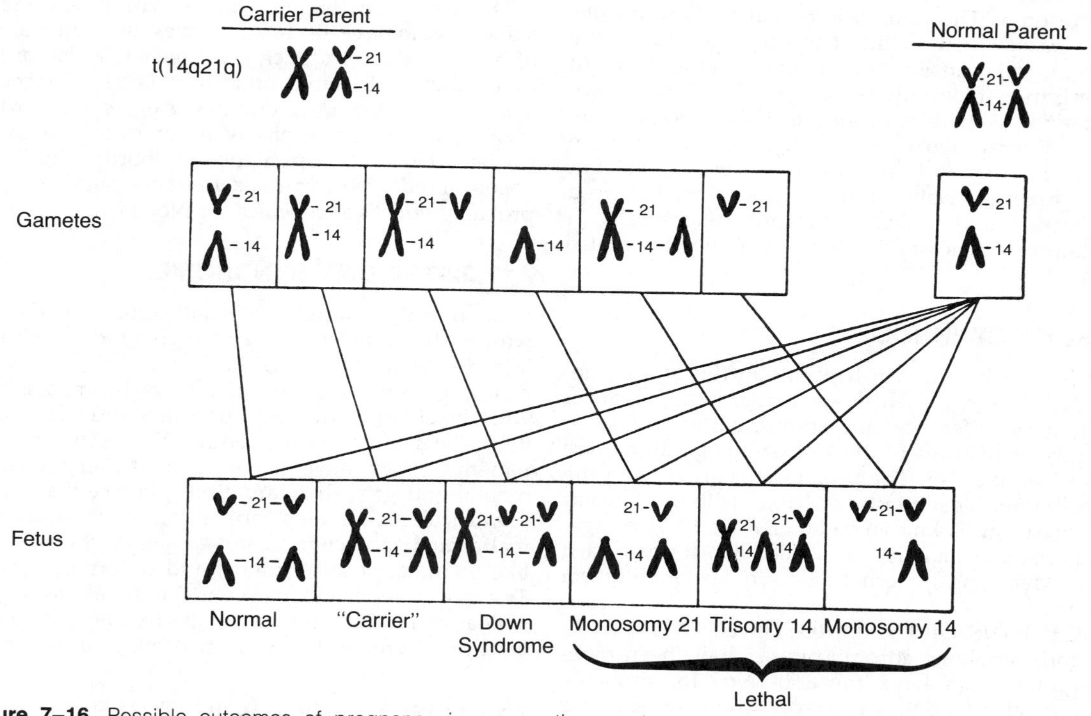

Figure 7–16. Possible outcomes of pregnancy in segregation products of a balanced carrier of a Robertsonian translocation.

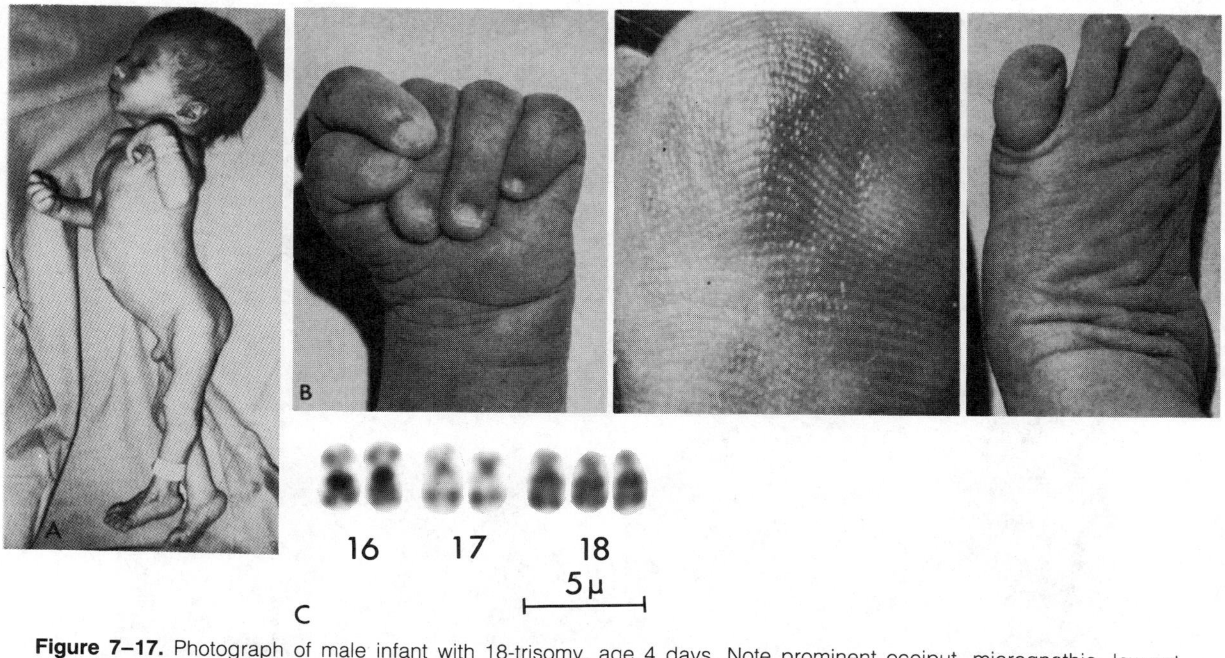

Figure 7–17. Photograph of male infant with 18-trisomy, age 4 days, Note prominent occiput, micrognathia, low-set ears, short sternum, narrow pelvis, prominent calcaneus, and flexion abnormalities of the fingers. (Courtesy of Robert E. Carrel.) *B,* Several of the common anomalies in the 18-trisomy syndrome, including the unusual position of the fingers with hypoplasia of 5th fingernail; the simple arch pattern of the fingers; and the dorsiflexed hallux with hypoplasia of toenails. (From Smith DW: Autosomal abnormalities. Am J Obstet Gynecol 90:1055, 1964.) *C,* Partial karyotype of 18-trisomy prepared with modified Giemsa stain.

that is, only part of one No. 18 chromosome is duplicated either by elongation of its long arm or by translocation to another chromosome. The diagnosis of partial trisomy has generally been based on the clinical picture, because in the absence of reciprocal translocation in one parent it is not possible to confirm cytologically the origin of the extra chromosomal material. As with translocation Down syndrome, offspring of six different chromosomal types can result from segregation of the chromosomes of a carrier parent, but probably only three are viable: normal karyotype, balanced translocation carrier, and partial 18-trisomy, theoretically in equal proportions. Mosaics and double trisomics have also been reported.

7.16 13-TRISOMY SYNDROME

Chromosome No. 13 is found in triplicate in this syndrome. Trisomies for No. 14 and 15, which are similar in appearance, can be identified by differences in banding patterns (Fig. 7–18). The phenotypic features of the 13-trisomy syndrome are listed in Tables 7–4 and 7–5. The prognosis is grave as in the 18-trisomy syndrome. Most infants affected die in the 1st year of life, but at least one is known to be alive at 10 yr of age. The incidence is approximately 1 in 20,000 live births and it increases with advancing maternal age. No sex predilection has been observed.

TRANSLOCATIONS OF CHROMOSOMES 13, 14, AND 15. Translocations involving chromosome 13 have been more frequently reported than have those of No. 18, probably because of the greater tendency of acrocentric chromosomes to break and rearrange and the ease of identification due to chromosome length. Most are formed by centric fusion, but some consist of two chromosomes attached in tandem to form a very long acrocentric chromosome. The pattern of inheritance is similar to that of other Robertsonian translocations discussed earlier.

There are many large pedigrees with phenotypically normal subjects who have 45 chromosomes, including a centric fusion of No. 13 or 14, but such a carrier has a risk of less than 1% of producing trisomic offspring; larger chromosomes with symmetric arm lengths tend to segregate in an orderly fashion, giving rise to karyotypically normal individuals or balanced carriers. However, spontaneous abortion and infertility are encountered with increased frequency and the abortuses are probably effective trisomics for No. 14.

7.17 22-TRISOMY SYNDROME

Patients with an additional small acrocentric chromosome but without the clinical signs of Down syndrome were originally interpreted as having 22-trisomy, XYY, or partial trisomy resulting from deletions of larger chromosomes. However, with the aid of marker chromosomes and fluorescent banding, it has been possible to identify 22-trisomy in some of these patients. They have a clinical syndrome characterized by mental and growth retardation; microcephaly; micrognathia; preauricular skin tags, appendages, or sinuses; low-set or malformed ears; cleft palate; congenital heart disease; finger-like or malopposed thumbs; and deformed lower limbs. 22-Trisomy is seen less frequently than 21-trisomy despite the similarity in size and shape of the chromosomes, probably because of greater loss of 22-trisomics during pregnancy.

7.18 TRISOMY INVOLVING OTHER AUTOSOMES

Accurate identification of chromosomes has led to the description of new autosomal trisomy syndromes due to 8-trisomy

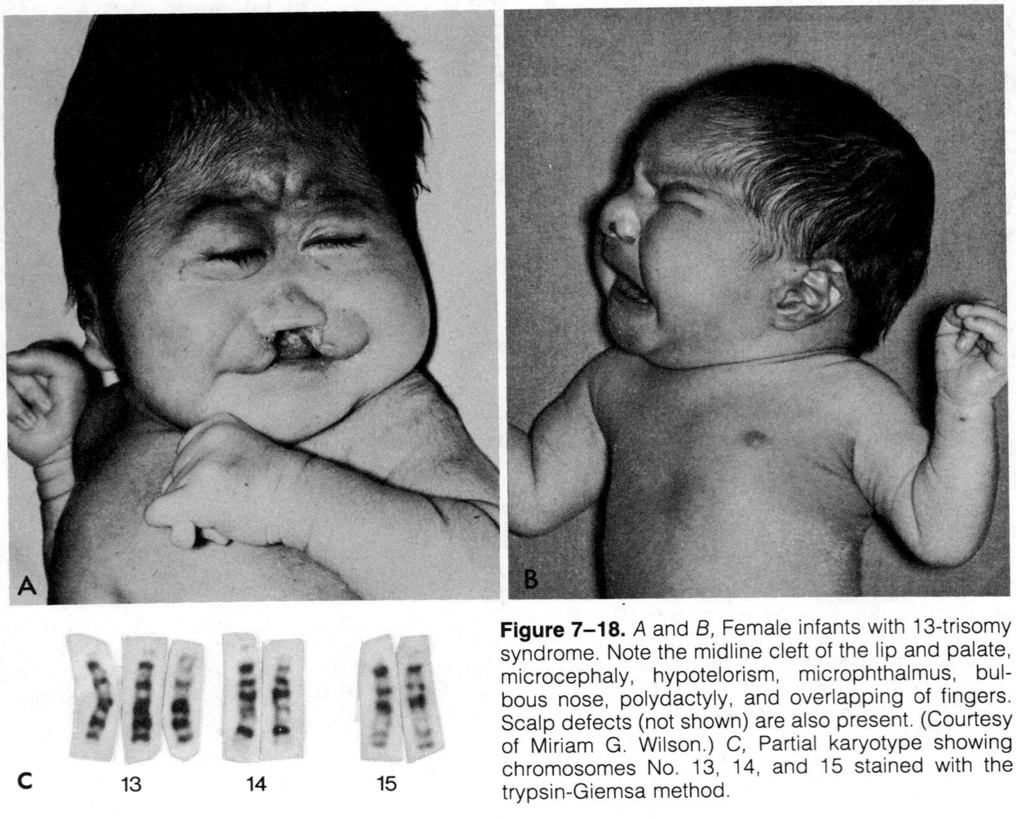

Figure 7–18. *A* and *B*, Female infants with 13-trisomy syndrome. Note the midline cleft of the lip and palate, microcephaly, hypotelorism, microphthalmus, bulbous nose, polydactyly, and overlapping of fingers. Scalp defects (not shown) are also present. (Courtesy of Miriam G. Wilson.) *C*, Partial karyotype showing chromosomes No. 13, 14, and 15 stained with the trypsin-Giemsa method.

TABLE 7–7. Major Clinical Features of the 8-Trisomy and 9-Trisomy Syndromes

Feature	8-Trisomy	9-Trisomy
General	Mental retardation, short stature, decreased weight, vertebral anomalies	Mental retardation
Craniofacies	Dysmorphic skull, prominent forehead, dysplastic ears, strabismus, plump nose with broad base, low-set ears, everted lower lip, high palate, cleft soft palate, micrognathia	Microcephaly, abnormal cranial sutures, prominent forehead, deep-set eyes, protuberant ears, prominent nose, fishmouth, micrognathia
Thorax	Congenital heart disease	Congenital heart disease
Abdomen and pelvis	Urinary tract anomaly, narrow pelvis	Urinary tract anomaly
Limbs	Patellar dysplasia, limited joint mobility, deep flexion creases on palms and soles	Congenital hip/knee dislocation, clinodactyly, digital hypoplasia, nail hypoplasia, syndactyly, simian palmar creases, absent B and C palmar digital triradii

and 9-trisomy (Table 7–7). Full (i.e., not in mosaic association with a chromosomally normal cell line) trisomies for other chromosomes have also been reported, but documentation is lacking. Trisomy for virtually every autosome has been documented in the products of early spontaneous abortion; most full trisomies are probably lethal. Partial trisomy (duplication or duplication-deficiency state) for almost all the autosomes produced by segregation of a translocation or inversion has been described, as has partial trisomy for an unattached segment of an autosome.

7.19 AUTOSOMAL MONOSOMY

Several cases of monosomy involving chromosome 21 or 22 have been reported, but few have been adequately documented as complete monosomy. Syndromes produced by deletion (partial monosomy) of part of the long arm of chromosome 21 or 22 have been well documented, as have deletions of parts of other chromosomes (Table 7–8).

STRUCTURAL ABERRATIONS

7.20 TRANSLOCATIONS

These are the most common structural aberrations. Exchange of segments between two nonhomologous chromosomes is known as a *reciprocal* or *balanced translocation*. Although early reports of translocations suggested the presence of *simple translocations* (i.e., a segment of one chromosome broken off and attached to the unbroken end of the recipient chromosome), no convincing evidence exists for the occurrence of simple translocations in humans.

In phenotypically normal individuals translocations are assumed to be *reciprocal* and *balanced* because the loss or gain of chromatin material usually results in an abnormal phenotype. An exception is the balanced (Robertsonian, Sec. 7.13) translocation discussed earlier. Unbalanced karyotypes associated with *duplication-deficiency syndromes* are found among the offspring of carriers of balanced translocations (see Fig. 7–13).

Except for translocation resulting in well-known clinical syndromes, it is difficult and often impossible, even with the aid of banding patterns, to identify with certainty the origin of excess chromosomal material in the absence of a reciprocal translocation in a parent. Another exception is the translocation of a large segment of the X chromosome that can be positively identified by the X chromatin or thymidine-labeling pattern. When a parent is a translocation carrier, the origin of the extra (trisomic) or missing (monosomic) chromosomal material can be accurately determined, and the delineation of new clinical syndromes becomes possible. Banding techniques can identify small duplications and deletions in karyotypes that were thought to be normal with conventional stains.

Syndromes have been described as the result of partial trisomy (duplication) for chromosomes 1q, 2p, 2q, 3p, 3q, 4p, 4q, 5p, 6q, 7q, 9p, 9q, 10q, 12p, 14q, 18q, and 22q. The best known and most frequently documented partial trisomy is the 9p-trisomy syndrome (Fig. 7–19). Translocation of the short arm of chromosome 9 to a variety of autosomes has been reported, and many kindreds have been described in which reciprocal translocations are carried by many members and transmitted through several generations. Characteristic features include mental retardation, microcephaly, hypertelorism, oblique palpebral fissures, enophthalmos, bulbous nose, downward slanting mouth, low-set protruding ears, and single palmar crease.

The most commonly observed reciprocal translocation occurs between the long arms of 11 and 22 (Fig. 7–20). A number of the offspring of balanced carriers of this translocation (t[11;22]) have 47 chromosomes, the extra one consisting of a part of both chromosomes 11 and 22. These infants show microcephaly, a wide face with a short flat nose, a prominent philtrum, microretrognathia, cleft palate, low set abnormal ears with preauricular pits and tags, a micropenis, heart defects, renal anomalies, anal anomalies, and dislocated hips. They, therefore, share abnormalities with children with 22-trisomy and those with partial trisomy of the long arm of No. 11. The phenotypic results of translocations depend on the parts of the chromosomes involved, so that new syndromes are constantly being described.

Although all chromosomes are subject to breaks that result in structural aberrations, the chromosomes most frequently involved in translocations appear to be the acrocentrics of chromosomes 13, 14, 15, 21, and 22, probably because of their close association as nucleolar organizers—that is, the stalks of the satellites have the capacity to organize diffuse nucleolar material into one or more compact bodies during interphase. These translocations and their modes of transmission have been discussed in the respective sections under *Aneuploidy*.

7.21 DELETIONS

Chromosomal deletions are associated with several clinical syndromes. Some lead to a less severely affected phenotype than do trisomies. Clinical features of the more common deletions are listed in Table 7–8.

CHROMOSOMES 4 AND 5 (4p- AND 5p- SYNDROMES). The cri du chat syndrome (5p-) (Fig. 7–21*A*) is so named because the cry of affected infants resembles that of a kitten and is characterized by high-pitched, tense phonation. This distinguishing trait probably accounts for the apparently greater frequency of 5p- compared to other deletions. How-

TABLE 7–8. Important Clinical Features

Feature	4p−	5p−	9q−	11p−
General	LBW, severe MR, delayed ossification	LBW, MR, cat-like cry	MR	MR, growth retardation
Craniofacies	Microcephaly, hypertelorism, epicanthus, ptosis, colobomata, beaked nose, short broad philtrum, cleft palate, micrognathia, simple ears	Microcephaly, round face, hypertelorism, epicanthus, antimongoloid palpebral fissure, micrognathia, low-set malformed ears, preauricular tags	Trigonocephaly, upward slanting palpebral fissures, epicanthal folds, depressed nasal bridge, anteverted nares, long philtrum, low-set ears, high palate, micrognathia, short and webbed neck	Aniridia
Thorax		CHD (occasional)	Widely spaced nipples, cardiac murmur	
Pelvis and abdomen	Inguinal hernia, sacral dimples, hypospadias, cryptorchidism	Inguinal hernia, diastasis recti, small iliac wings		Wilms tumor, gonadoblastoma, ambiguous genitalia in males
Hands and feet		Short metacarpals or metatarsals, partial syndactyly, pes planus, simian crease	Long fingers, square nails	

CHD = congenital heart disease; LBW = low birthweight; MR = mental retardation; TRC = total ridge count.

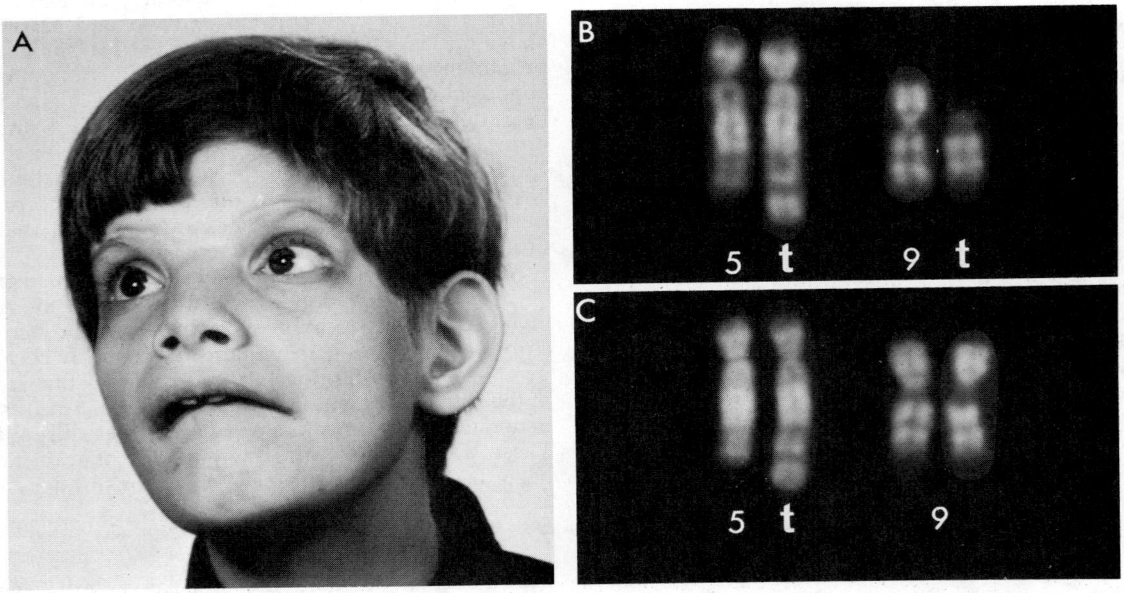

Figure 7–19. *A,* Patient with 9p-trisomy syndrome showing some of the characteristic features: hypertelorism, bulbous nose, downward slanting mouth, low-set protruding ears. *B,* Balanced t(5q/9p) translocation carried by mother. *C,* Unbalanced translocation resulting in 9p-trisomy syndrome in above patient. (t = translocation chromosome.)

of the Deletion Syndromes

13q−	18p−	18q−	21q−	22q−
LBW, severe MR, failure to thrive	LBW, variable MR, short stature, Turner syndrome-like stigmata	LBW, severe MR, seizures, hypotonia	MR, hypertonia, skeletal malformations, growth retardation	MR, hypotonia
Microcephaly; trigonocephaly; flat, wide nasal bridge; hypertelorism; ptosis, epicanthus, microphthalmia, colobomata; retinoblastoma; micrognathia	Hypertelorism, epicanthus, flat nasal bridge, micrognathia, low-set, large floppy ears	Microcephaly, ophthalmologic defects, carp-shaped mouth, apparently protruding mandible, atretic ear canals	Microcephaly, downward-slanting palpebral fissures, high palate, large or low-set ears, prominent nasal bridge, micrognathia	Microcephaly, high palate, large or low-set ears, epicanthal folds, ptosis of eyelids, bifid uvula
CHD		CHD (occasional), supernumerary ribs		
Hip dysplasia, cryptorchidism		Small penis, cryptorchidism, hypoplastic genitalia in females	Pyloric stenosis, inguinal hernia, hypospadias, cryptorchidism	
Hypoplastic or absent thumbs, clinodactyly of 5th fingers, syndactyly of toes	Stubby hands with high-set thumbs, partial webbing of toes, large digital patterns with high TRC	Long, tapering fingers; abnormal implantation of toes; large digital patterns with high TRC	Nail anomalies	Syndactyly of toes, clinodactyly

ever, the typical cry tends to disappear in late infancy, and a similar cry has been noted occasionally in other retarded infants. Most cases arise sporadically, but reciprocal translocation is sometimes present in a parent. Ring chromosomes with loss of material from both ends may produce the same syndrome.

Patients with a deletion of chromosome 4 (see Fig. 7–21*B*) are much more severely malformed and retarded and do not have the typical cry. The clinical signs are listed in Table 7–8.

CHROMOSOME 9 (9p-SYNDROME). A small number of infants have been described with deletion of the short arm of chromosome 9 (see Table 7–8).

CHROMOSOME 11 (11p-SYNDROME). Deletion in the short arm of chromosome 11, always including band 11p13, results in aniridia and is frequently associated with Wilms' tumor. Additional abnormalities include mental and growth retardation, ambiguous genitalia in the male patients, and gonadoblastoma in some of the patients. Most cases occur de novo but familial chromosomal rearrangements are occasionally responsible (see Table 7–8).

CHROMOSOME 13 (13q- SYNDROME). A deletion of the long arm of chromosome 13, including band 13q14, is associated with retinoblastoma (Sec. 17.21). Other clinical findings depend on the amount of the chromosome deleted. These are listed in Table 7–8.

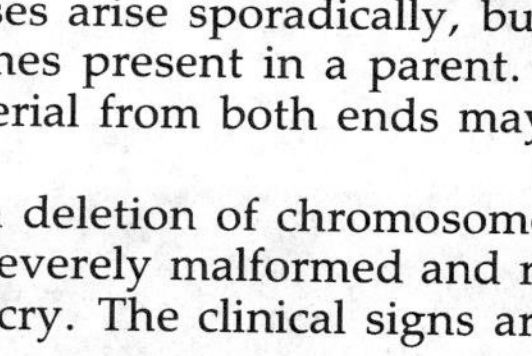

t11 t12

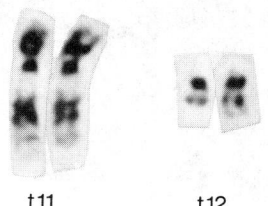

Figure 7–20. Translocation between the long arms of chromosomes 11 and 22 (t(11; 22) (q23; q11)).

CHROMOSOME 18 (18p- AND 18q- SYNDROMES). Deletions of chromosome 18 take 3 forms: loss of the entire short arm, 18p-; loss of part of the long arm, 18q-; and deletions of both ends to form a ring, r(18). Patients with 18p- are phenotypically extremely variable. A few are severely affected, with arrhinencephaly, cyclopia, or cleft lip and palate, but most have only minor malformations and are only moderately retarded (Fig. 7–22; see also Table 7–8). Turner syndrome is often suspected. On the other hand, children with 18q- are severely retarded and have more characteristic malformations (Fig. 7–23). Children with a ring chromosome 18 have phenotypic features of both short and long arm deletions since the ends of both arms of the chromosome are lost during ring formation.

A number of characteristics are common to the three types of deletion. Prognosis for survival seems to be good. IgA deficiency has been noted in some patients. Large dermal patterns are present on the digits, mainly whorls, giving a very high total ridge count similar to that seen in the Turner syndrome. This is in sharp contrast to 18-trisomy syndrome, in which the presence of arches results in a very low ridge count.

CHROMOSOMES 19, 20, 21, AND 22. Deficiencies in these chromosomes have resulted mainly in formation of ring chromosomes. Loss of material from the long arm has occurred in some subjects, but deletions compatible with life may often be too small to identify unless a ring is formed. *Aberrations* in chromosomes 19 and 20 were first reported only in studies of aborted material and patients with blood dyscrasias, but a few patients with severe mental retardation have now been described; others with deletions in only some of their cells (mosaics) appear to be phenotypically normal.

Because many more cases have been described with *deletions* of chromosomes 21 and 22, two syndromes have emerged, one attributed to 21q- and the other to 22q-. The phenotypic features of these syndromes, some of which are shared by both, are enumerated in Table 7–8. Because some of the clinical signs of chromosome 21 deletions are variations of

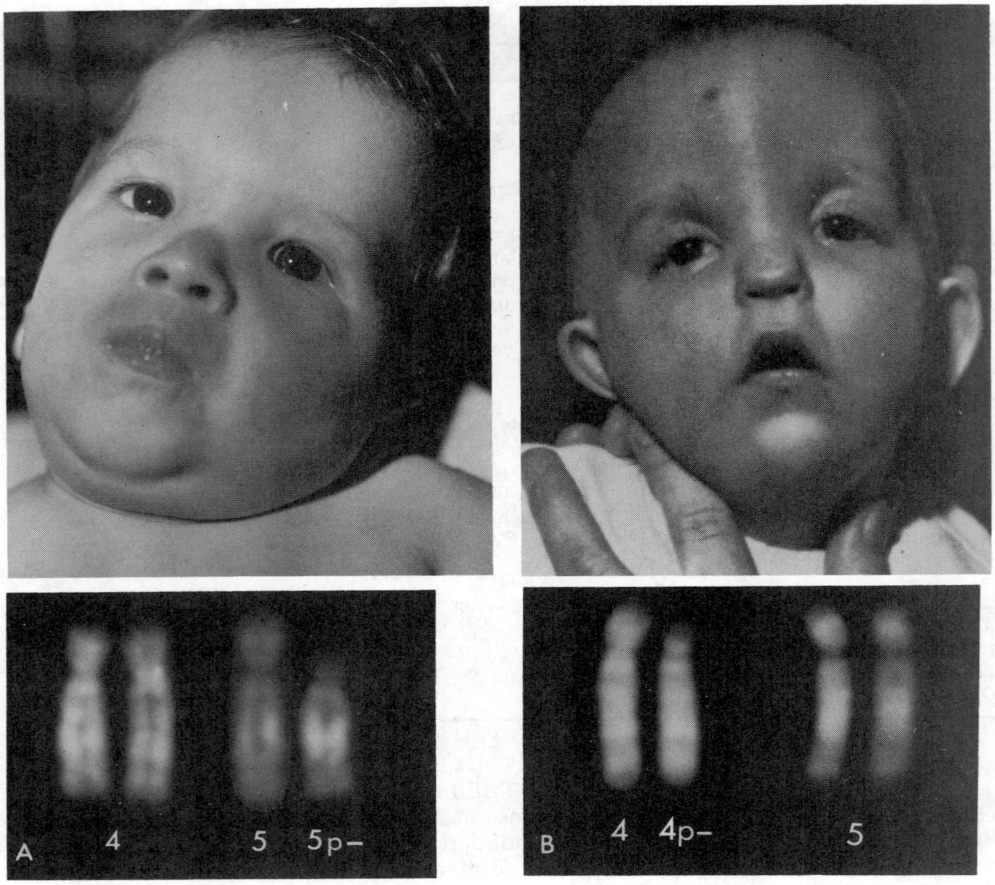

Figure 7–21. Patients with partial deletion of short arm chromosomes No. 4 and 5. *A,* An 8-mo-old boy with cri du chat syndrome and deletion of part of the short arm of one chromosome No. 5 (5p −). *B,* 1-yr-old boy with partial deletion of the short arm of one chromosome No. 4. (Courtesy of W. R. Breg.)

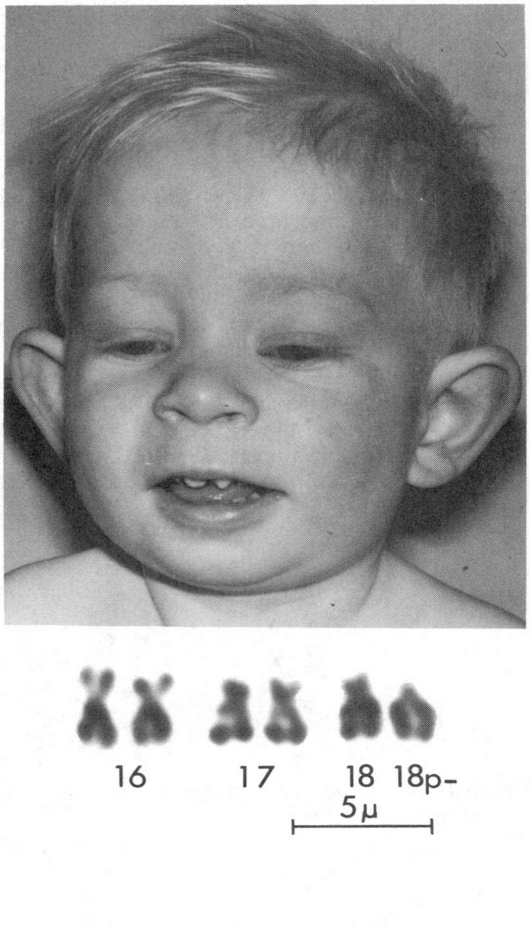

Figure 7–22. Patient with 18 short arm deletion, 18p −.

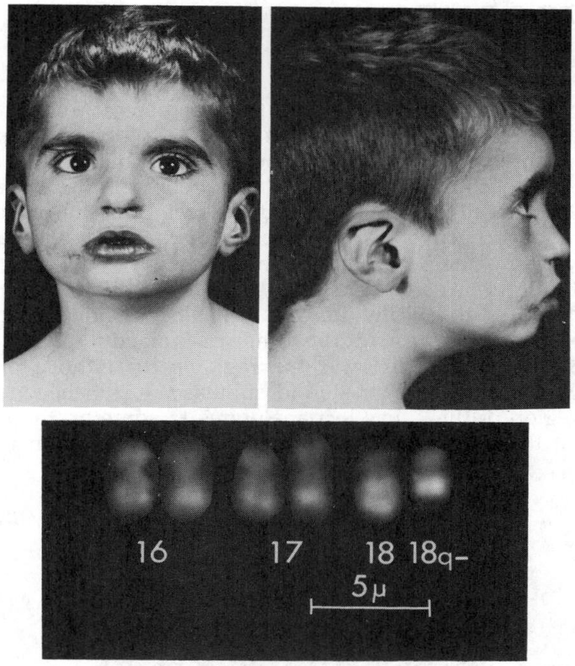

Figure 7–23. Patient with partial deletion of long arm of chromosome No. 18. (Courtesy of P. S. Gerald and W. Wertelecki.) Partial karyotype showing 18q−, stained with quinacrine dihydrochloride.

those of the Down syndrome, this syndrome has also been referred to as "antimongolism."

7.22 BREAKAGE SYNDROMES

Chromosomal breakage, structural rearrangements, and aneuploidy have been reported as inconsistent findings during viral diseases, such as measles, chickenpox, and infectious hepatitis. Specific rearrangements have been described in a number of neoplastic diseases, primarily leukemias and lymphomas. These include the following translocations with their associated conditions: acute myelogenous leukemia, t(8; 21); chronic myelogenous leukemia, t(9; 22) (Philadelphia chromosome); acute promyelocytic leukemia, t(15; 17); acute monocytic leukemia, t(11; 19); Burkitt lymphoma, t(8; 14), t(8; 22), and t(2; 8). In Burkitt lymphoma the break point in the long arm of chromosome 8, common to the three observed translocations, occurs at the site of the oncogene c-*myc*, whereas the break points in chromosomes 14, 22, and 2 occur at the sites of the genes for immunoglobulin (14: heavy chains; 22: λ light chains; 2: κ light chains). It is probable that these rearrangements put the oncogene under the regulation of the immunoglobulin genes, causing inappropriate activity of factors leading to abnormal growth of the cells. It is likely that other translocations will be shown to work in an analogous fashion.

There is a group of autosomal recessive diseases with high frequencies of chromosome breaks and rearrangements, together with an increased risk of leukemia and other malignancies: Bloom syndrome (congenital telangiectatic erythema with dwarfism, Sec. 23.15), constitutional aplastic pancytopenia (Fanconi anemia, Sec. 16.34), ataxia-telangiectasia (Louis-Bar syndrome, Sec. 11.19 and 20.45), and xeroderma pigmentosum (Sec. 23.10).

In addition to breaks and gaps, the characteristic chromosomal aberration of Bloom syndrome is the quadriradial, formed by the exchange of chromatid segments, usually between two chromosomes of the No. 6–12 and No. 19–20 groups. In almost all cases the breaks occur at corresponding sites in homologous chromosomes (Fig. 7–24). The number of sister chromatid exchanges is much higher in cultured cells from affected children than in cells from homozygous normals or heterozygotes for the Bloom syndrome allele.

In the Fanconi pancytopenia syndrome, endoreduplication and a variety of gaps, breaks, and rearrangements involving nonhomologues as well as homologues have been observed. The number of sister chromatid exchanges per cell is lower than that found in the cells of normal subjects. Chromosomal studies of the Louis-Bar syndrome have revealed an increase in gaps and breaks, an increase in rearrangements such as dicentrics and abnormal monocentrics, and the presence of distinct, stable cell subpopulations (clones) with translocations involving particularly chromosome 14.

Chromosomal gaps, breaks, and rearrangements have not been seen in xeroderma pigmentosum, but chromosomally abnormal clones have been observed in cultured skin fibroblasts from affected patients. An increased number of ultraviolet light-induced chromosome breaks and sister chromatid exchanges occur in cultured lymphocytes.

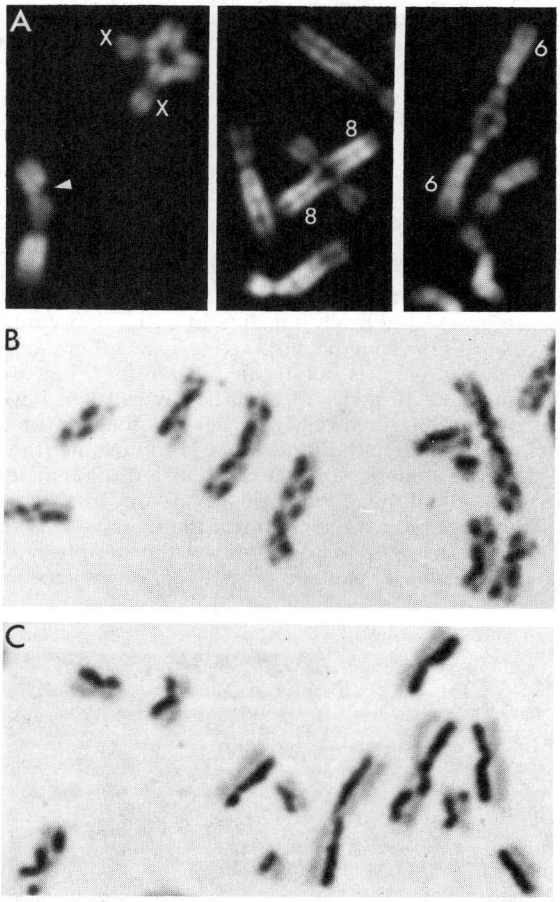

Figure 7–24. Partial spreads showing chromosome aberrations in cells from patient with Bloom syndrome, compared with a normal subject. *A*, Fluorescent-stained spreads with quadriradial figures formed by homologous chromosomes, typical of this syndrome. *B*, Harlequin effect resulting from high frequency of sister chromatid exchanges (SCE) in cells of patient with Bloom syndrome, treated with 5-bromodeoxyuridine (BrdU). *C*, Low rate of sister chromatid exchanges in cells of normal subject.

7.23 SEX CHROMOSOMES

The normal sex chromosome complement in the female is XX and in the male XY. The following sections deal with departures from that norm. In the Q-banded karyotype, the Y is ordinarily the most brightly fluorescent chromosome. The brightly fluorescent segment of the long arm may be greatly extended or completely deleted (see Fig. 7–7*B*) without producing any discernible phenotypic effect. The only clinically relevant gene loci known to occupy the Y chromosome are those involving male sex determination; they are found in the pale-fluorescing region of the short arm.

7.24 SEX CHROMATIN

Tests for sex chromatin most often utilize cells scraped from the buccal mucosa, the *buccal smear*. Other tissues used include vaginal epithelial cells, hair root sheath cells, and cells from amniotic fluid. Because of limitations described earlier, X- and Y-chromatin determinations should not be relied on for the definitive diagnosis of an abnormal sex chromosome constitution. However, such determinations may be useful, along with chromosomal analysis by banding techniques, in genetic studies and in identification of structural rearrangements of the sex chromosomes.

X-CHROMATIN

Because females have two X chromosomes, they have two alleles for each X-linked gene; the male, with a single X, is therefore hemizygous for each X-linked allele. The lack of quantitative differences between the two sexes in the products of X-linked genes suggests *dosage compensation*. Lyon provided evidence that one of the two X chromosomes in the cells of females becomes genetically inactive in early embryonic life. In each cell of a normal female the active X, whether paternally or maternally derived, is determined at random, but, once it is determined, all progeny of a particular cell will have the same active X. Thus each cell, whether in a male or a female, contains only one genetically active X chromosome (the *Lyon hypothesis*). The genetic consequence is that all females are mosaic for any heterozygous alleles located in the X chromosome. The cytologic manifestation of the inactive X is the *X-chromatin mass* or *"Barr body,"* found at the periphery of the resting or interphase nucleus (Fig. 7–25*A*). In a cell all X chromosomes in excess of one are inactive and form X-chromatin masses. By counting the number of X-chromatin masses (in at least 100 cells), it is possible to obtain an index of the number of X chromosomes present in the cells of a subject (i.e., one more than the number of X-chromatin masses per cell). Because cell survival requires the presence of one entire active X chromosome, any X with a deletion always forms the X-chromatin mass.

Although it is generally stated that one X chromosome in a female cell is genetically inactive, it has been shown that the tip of the short arm of the otherwise inactive X remains genetically active. The loci in this region include those for the Xg blood group and for steroid sulfatase. It is believed that this region of the X has loci analogous to some on the short arm of the Y chromosome and that these regions on the X

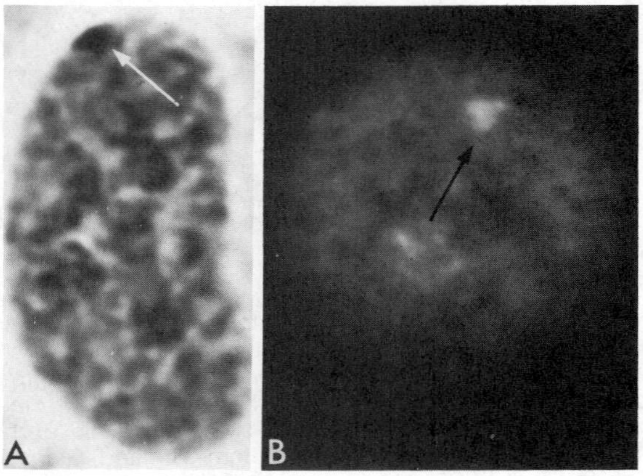

Figure 7–25. Sex chromatin bodies in interphase nuclei. *A*, X-chromatin mass (Barr body) seen at the periphery of the nucleus. *B*, Bright fluorescent Y-chromatin mass in the nucleus of a normal male.

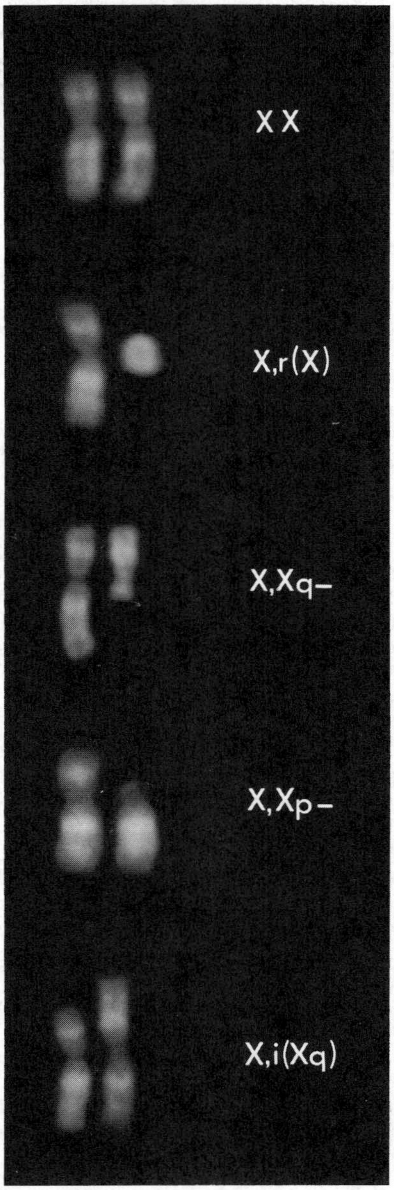

Figure 7–26. Structural aberrations of the X chromosome. Normal X chromosome on the left of each pair. On the right, from top to bottom: normal X, ring X, deletion of long arm, deletion of short arm, long arm isochromosome. All are X chromatin-positive.

and the Y associate during meiosis, thus allowing for exchange of genetic material. The area on the Y may include genes for masculinization which, if translocated to the X, could result in an XX male in the next generation (Sec. 7.29).

X-CHROMATIN IN TURNER SYNDROME. Determining X-chromatin is a valuable diagnostic and screening technique only if its limitations are kept in mind. Some Turner syndrome patients who are X-chromatin-positive have two X chromosomes, one of which is structurally altered (Fig. 7–26). If X-chromatin determination were the sole cytologic basis for diagnosing Turner syndrome, then the presence of an X-chromatin mass would erroneously exclude the diagnosis. Almost 40% of patients having Turner syndrome are X-chromatin-positive.

Y-CHROMATIN

Q-banding has led to a second type of chromatin determination. In the interphase nucleus the Y chromosome remains tightly condensed and appears as a small, brilliantly fluorescent mass of chromatin (see Fig. 7–25*B*). The number of Y-chromatin masses in a nucleus bears a 1:1 relation to the number of Y chromosomes present. However, the Y-chromatin test also has limitations. Some acrocentric chromosomes bear fluorescent satellites that are large and brilliant enough to resemble a Y-chromatin body in an interphase nucleus. Moreover, if all or most of the brilliantly fluorescent segment of the Y chromosome has been deleted, a Y-chromatin mass will not be detected.

ABNORMALITIES OF THE SEX CHROMOSOMES

These make up about half of all chromosomal abnormalities encountered in newborn infants (see Table 7–3). Their consequences may be varied, but almost all have some effect on gonadal function.

7.25 TURNER SYNDROME

See Sec. 19.23 for clinical features.

Turner syndrome is defined as the spectrum of phenotypic features resulting from complete or partial monosomy of the *short arm* of the X chromosome. The most frequent abnormality, accounting for about 55% of cases, is complete monosomy-X, with a karyotype 45,X. Its frequency is approximately 1 in 10,000 live female births, but this figure represents only a small proportion of conceptuses with a 45,X karyotype, at least 95% of which are estimated to be spontaneously aborted. The 45,X karyotype is one of the most common chromosomal aberrations found among the products of spontaneous abortion and is the only well documented chromosomal monosomy in humans. Turner syndrome may result from a number of abnormalities of the X chromosome other than 45,X (Table 7–9 and Fig. 7–26). The most frequently encountered structural aberration is the isochromosome of the long arm designated i(Xq). A metacentric X resembling the i(Xq) may be formed by a translocation following breaks in the paracentromeric regions of the short arms of two X chromosomes to form a dicentric. Simple deletion of the short arm of an X[del (Xp)] also produces Turner syndrome. However, patients with deletion of part or most of the long arm, while manifesting gonadal dysgenesis and its phenotypic results, do not have the other somatic features of Turner syndrome.

The most important characteristic features of Turner syndrome are short stature, gonadal dysgenesis with "streak" gonads, and primary amenorrhea. Although mental retardation has not ordinarily been considered a feature of Turner syndrome, one review noted its presence in 18% of patients. In the absence of mental retardation, an abnormality in spatial perception has been reported in some cases. The characteristic dermatoglyphic feature is the large size of dermal patterns on the digits (high ridge count).

A mosaic karyotype is common in Turner syndrome; 45,X/46,XX is most frequent. In general, the presence of a 46,XX cell line in addition to the 45,X line mitigates the effects of X-monosomy. Secondary sex development, menses, and even fertility have been reported in patients with 45,X/46,XX mosaicism. Fertility has also been described in a few cases of nonmosaic 45,X Turner syndrome. One form of mosaicism, 45,X/46,XY (mixed gonadal dysgenesis, Sec. 19.23), predisposes the patient to gonadal neoplasia and is an indication for surgical removal of the gonads. A buccal smear for X-chromatin is misleading in 45,X/46,XY mosaicism because it does not reflect the presence of the XY cell line. Chromosomal analysis is needed in all patients suspected of Turner syndrome.

Unlike autosomal trisomy and 47,XXY Klinefelter syndrome, Turner syndrome is not associated with advanced maternal age, suggesting that the underlying mechanism can involve the loss of either a paternal or a maternal sex chromosome. In 75% of testable cases of 45,X Turner syndrome, the *paternal* X or Y is absent. The frequency of mosaic karyotypes implicates a postfertilization error in cell division as the cause of many cases. Once parents have had a child with Turner syndrome, their risk for producing a second affected infant is *not* increased.

TABLE 7–9. Abnormalities of the Sex Chromosomes

	% of Cases	Population Frequency
Turner syndrome		1/10,000 females
45,X	57	
Mosaics 45,X/46,XX;45,X/47,XXX, etc.	12	
Mosaics 45,X/46,XY	4	
46,X,i (Xq) including mosaics	17	
46,X,del (Xq) including mosaics	1	
Other [del (Xp), r(X), mosaics]	9	
	100	
Klinefelter syndrome		1/1,000 males
47,XXY	82	
48,XXXY	3	
49,XXXXY	<1	
Mosaics	8	
Other (XXYY, XXXYY)	6	
	100	
Poly-X females		1/1,000 females
47,XXX	98+	
48,XXXX	Rare	
49,XXXXX	Rare	
Mosaics	Rare	
	100	
Fragile X [fra(X)(q28)]		1/2,000 males 1/1,000 females
Y-polysomy		1/1,000 males
47,XYY	98+	
Other (XXYY,XXXYY)	Rare	
	100	

7.26 KLINEFELTER SYNDROME

See Sec. 19.30 for clinical features.

Klinefelter syndrome is defined as the spectrum of phenotypic features resulting from a sex chromosome complement that includes two or more X chromosomes and one or more Y chromosomes. The 47,XXY Klinefelter syndrome occurs in approximately 1 per 1,000 liveborn males but very rarely among spontaneous abortuses. The syndrome with karyotypes other than 47,XXY is rare. The somatic features are few and nonspecific. It is not often detected in the prepubertal male unless found in an X-chromatin screening program of a population, such as the males in an institution for the mentally abnormal. One helpful diagnostic feature is the presence of small patterns on the digits with a low ridge count. Klinefelter syndrome is associated with advanced maternal age.

Klinefelter syndrome is not a serious pediatric problem because, aside from infertility, most affected males lead normal lives; they are not identified until they are examined more closely because of the infertility and are found to have small testes and azoospermia.

Somatic abnormalities are more common in the Klinefelter syndrome when it is caused by chromosomal abnormalities other than 47,XXY. A direct correlation is apparent between the increased likelihood and severity of mental retardation and increasing number of X chromosomes. A specific identifiable phenotype has been attributed to the 49,XXXXY karyotype (Table 7–10).

7.27 47,XXX FEMALE

The 47,XXX karyotype occurs with the same frequency among females as does 47,XXY among males (1/1,000). There is no characteristic phenotype, and affected females are usually identified by chance, through X-chromatin screening programs, newborn surveys, or amniocentesis ordered for other reasons; or they may be identified when an unrelated chromosomal abnormality is discovered in a child or other relative of a proband in a family study. They usually have normal gonadal function and are fertile, but they may have offspring with an abnormal sex chromosome complement. 47,XXX females may also have an increased frequency of delayed motor and speech development, mild intellectual deficit, and disturbed interpersonal relationships. More than three X chromosomes have been found in females, the largest number being five X. As in males, mental retardation or psychiatric abnormality appears to increase in females with increasing numbers of X chromosomes.

TABLE 7–10. Phenotypic Features of the 49,XXXXY Male

Feature	Frequency (%)
Skeletal abnormalities (radioulnar synostosis; coxa valga; rib anomalies; abnormal ossification centers in hands; fusion of vertebral arches; pseudoepiphyses in hands and feet; absent radial heads; short, bowed radius and ulna)	70
Genital anomalies	
Hypoplastic scrotum	70
Cryptorchidism	30
Small penis	85
Small testicles	80
Decreased or female distribution of pubic hair	40
Mental retardation	100
Facial features	
Upward slanting palpebral fissures	75
Epicanthal folds	80
Strabismus	57
Hypertelorism	87
Malformed ears	73
Broad nasal bridge	86
Depressed nasal bridge	68
Short neck	70
Increased frequency of digital arch patterns	

7.28 XYY MALE

A stigma has become attached to the 47,XYY sex chromosome complement because of studies, carried out in a prison population, reporting an association with aggressive antisocial behavior. The other feature claimed to be characteristic of XYY males is tall stature. Another study, although finding an elevated crime rate, did not relate the criminal behavior to aggression. Difficult ethical problems are raised by such studies. Among children, the XYY karyotype has occasionally been found in those referred for chromosomal analyses because of difficult personality problems in school. The frequency of XYY has been estimated from newborn surveys as 1 in 1,000 live births.

7.29 ATYPICAL SEX CHROMOSOME KARYOTYPES

46,XX in Phenotypic Males

A 46,XX karyotype has been reported in phenotypic males with characteristics resembling those of Klinefelter syndrome. Their internal and external genitalia are male. Most affected males are discovered at or after puberty because of sterility or failure of development of secondary sex characteristics (Sec. 3.9).

The occurrence of an XX sex chromosome constitution in a phenotypic male is contrary to the concept that a Y chromosome is necessary for male sex determination and differentiation. Possible explanations for the phenomenon include (1) undetected 46,XX/46,XY chimerism or 46,XX/47,XXY mosaicism, (2) translocation of the male sex-determining segment of the Y to the X chromosome or to an autosome, and (3) a mutant gene or genes. Available evidence suggests that the second explanation is likely in most cases, although the first explanation cannot be completely ruled out. The translocation of the male-determining segment of the Y to the X could produce an apparently XX male by the inactivated X-chromatin mechanism. The occurrence in the same family of an XX male and an XX true hermaphrodite is consistent with the suggestion of a mutant gene that may produce sex reversal in the 46,XX person.

46,XY in a Phenotypic Female

See also Sec. 19.34.

The XY sex chromosome constitution exerts an effect on the early embryo to cause the gonads and the internal and external genitalia to differentiate into the definitive genital apparatus of the male; otherwise the embryo will differentiate as a female. The influence of the XY chromosome constitution is not completely understood but is mediated through induction of testicular differentiation. Testicular Leydig cells then secrete testosterone, which is converted peripherally to dihydrotestosterone. Target cells must have the capacity to respond to testosterone and dihydrotestosterone. If any of these steps fails, then masculinization of the embryo will not occur and the infant may have a female genital phenotype. Female phenotype may be seen in a 46,XY infant as the result of (1) complete insensitivity of target tissue to androgen (testicular feminization), (2) testicular unresponsiveness to luteinizing hormone (LH) and human chorionic gonadotropin (hCG) (Leydig cell aplasia), (3) a severe defect in the biosynthesis of testosterone, and (4) the syndrome of XY pure gonadal dysgenesis (Swyer syndrome).

7.30 FRAGILE X SYNDROME

"Heritable fragile sites" form another category of clinically significant chromosome breaks. These sites, reported to exist on several chromosomes, manifest themselves as spontaneous breaks inherited in a mendelian fashion whose appearance may be enhanced by the use of special tissue culture media or specific pretreatments of the cells. The most important of such fragile sites occurs on the long arm of the X chromosome (band q27-28) (see Fig. 7–8) and is associated with a syndrome of mental retardation, with or without macro-orchidism in males. The "fragile-X syndrome" may account for up to 30% of X-linked mental retardation in males and perhaps 10% of all mild mental retardation in females (heterozygotes). The assessment of the mentally retarded male is incomplete without testicular measurement and chromosome study for this X chromosome marker.

SPONTANEOUS ABORTIONS

More than 20%, and perhaps as many as 50%, of all conceptuses are spontaneously aborted, at least half because of chromosomal aberrations, the most common being aneuploidy. Loss of a sex chromosome has been found most frequently. Chromosomal banding techniques have resulted in the identification of trisomies for all chromosomes except No. 1. Trisomy 16 is the most common, followed by trisomies of the small and large acrocentrics with the notable exception of No. 13. Autosomal monosomies have not been found, probably owing to their lethality before implantation. Another relatively common finding in abortuses is polyploidy, usually triploidy (69 chromosomes), a condition resulting either from fertilization of an ovum by two sperm (dispermy) or from retention of the second polar body. No evidence exists of an association of polyploidy or other types of aberrations with birth control pills. In about 5 to 10% of couples who have had two or more spontaneous abortions, one or the other parent carries a balanced translocation. Such couples deserve cytogenetic study, because they are also at risk for producing chromosomally abnormal offspring.

7.31 GENETIC COUNSELING IN CHROMOSOMAL DISORDERS

See Sec. 7.33.

KURT HIRSCHHORN

Bergsma D (ed): Birth Defects Compendium, 2nd ed. New York, AR Liss, 1979.
Boué A, Boué J, Gropp A: Cytogenetics of pregnancy wastage. Adv Human Genet 14:1, 1985.
deGrouchy J, Turleau C: Clinical Atlas of Human Chromosomes, 2nd ed. New York, John Wiley & Sons, 1984.
Hamerton JL: Human Cytogenetics, Vols I and II. New York, Academic Press, 1971.
LeBeau MM, Rowley JD: Chromosomal abnormalities in leukemia and lymphoma. Adv Hum Genet 15:1, 1985.
Paris Conference (1971): Standardization in Human Cytogenetics. Birth Defects—Original Article Series. Vol 8. New York, The National Foundation—March of Dimes, 1971.
Paris Conference (1971) Suppl (1975): Standardization in Human Cytogenetics. Birth Defects—Original Article Series. Vol II. New York, The National Foundation—March of Dimes, Suppl 1975.
Simpson JL: Disorders of Sexual Differentiation: Etiology and Clinical Delineation. New York, Academic Press, 1977.
Thompson MW: Thompson & Thompson Genetics in Medicine, 4th ed. Philadelphia, WB Saunders, 1986.
Turner G, Jacobs P: Marker (X)-linked mental retardation. Adv Human Genet 13:83, 1983.

PATIENT EDUCATION

Smith DW, Wilson AA: The Child with Down's Syndrome (Mongolism). Philadelphia, WB Saunders, 1973.
Wisniewski LP, Hirschhorn K: A Guide to Human Chromosome Defects, 2nd ed. Birth Defects: Original Article Series Vol 16(6), New York, March of Dimes Birth Defects Foundation, 1980.

Acknowledgments. Acknowledgment is made to Sophie Paciuc, Elizabeth Byrnes, and Paula R. Martens for the preparation of karyotypes. I am grateful to Drs. Maimon M. Cohen and Henry N. Nadler for permission to use portions of their chapter from the thirteenth edition.

7.32 CONGENITAL MALFORMATIONS

About 2% of newborn infants have a major malformation. The incidence is as high as 5% if one includes malformations detected later in childhood, such as abnormalities of the heart, kidneys, lungs, and spine. Malformations are more common among spontaneous abortuses; many of these are severe and may cause abortion. About 9% of perinatal deaths are due to malformations. Treatment of malformations is one of the common reasons children are hospitalized.

A simple and arbitrary terminology has evolved for describing malformations. A *major malformation* is a structural abnormality that has serious medical, surgical, or cosmetic consequences. A *minor anomaly* and a *normal variation* have no serious consequences and are arbitrarily differentiated: a minor anomaly occurs in 4% or less of children of the same race, whereas a normal variation occurs more commonly in children of the same racial group. For example, the incidence of features such as simian crease, clinodactyly of the 5th finger, extra nipples, Brushfield spots, and sacral dimple varies with race (Table 7–11).

A *syndrome* refers to a recognized pattern of malformations considered to have a single and specific cause, such as the Holt-Oram syndrome, an autosomal dominant disorder with malformations of the heart and upper extremities. *Association* is used to indicate a non-random cluster of malformations for which no specific etiology has been identified, such as the VATER association of *v*ertebral, *a*nal, *t*racheo*e*sophageal, *ra*dial upper limb, and *r*enal anomalies. A *morphogenic complex* (or sequence or developmental field defect) comprises a primary malformation and its derived structural changes (e.g., Pierre Robin syndrome of cleft palate, glossoptosis, and micrognathia) but does not specify a cause.

ETIOLOGY. In a prospective study of 69,227 newborn

TABLE 7–11. Incidence of Minor Anomalies and Normal Variations in Newborn Infants*

Physical Feature	White Infants (%) (No. = 3989)	Black Infants (%) (No. = 827)
Third sagittal fontanel	3.1	9.8
Epicanthal folds, bilateral	1.4	1.0
Brushfield spots, bilateral	7.2	0.2
Preauricular sinus, left or right	0.8	5.3
Extra nipple, left or right	0.5	4.6
Umbilical hernia	0.7	6.1
Sacral dimple	4.8	0.6
Clinodactyly of both 5th fingers	5.2	4.5
Simian crease, both hands	0.7	0.5
Syndactyly of toes 2 and 3, left or right	1.7	2.3

*From Holmes LB: The Malformed Newborn—Practical Perspectives. Boston, Developmental Disabilities Council, 1976.

infants 1,549 major malformations (2.2%) occurred, 51% of which were attributed to genetic abnormalities; 0.2% of the infants had malformations attributed to chromosomal abnormalities, 0.07% to single mutant genes, 0.5% to multifactorial inheritance, and 0.3% to uncertain patterns of inheritance. The number of chromosomal abnormalities is less than the 0.6% incidence of all types of chromosomal abnormalities in newborn infants because many of the common disorders, such as 47,XXY, 47,XYY, and 47,XXX, have no detectable physical characteristics in the newborn infant. Teratogens and other environmental factors were identified as causes of malformations in 48/69,227 of the infants or 3.2% of all malformations, an incidence lower than many clinicians expect. Teratogens include drugs and maternal conditions such as diabetes mellitus; other environmental factors include amniotic constrictive bands, vascular abnormalities, and oligohydramnios. Vascular abnormalities, including absence of arteries, an abnormal persistence of embryonic vessels, and occlusion of vessels, have been shown to be associated with some types of bowel atresia, hydranencephaly, absence of the pectoralis major muscle (Poland anomaly), and absence of long bones. Twinning is associated with a higher incidence of malformations than that in singletons; the acardiac infant syndrome occurs only in monozygous twins.

The causes of 43% of the 1,549 major malformations were not detected. Malformations of unknown cause include imperforate anus, gastroschisis, Goldenhar syndrome, omphalocele, cloacal exstrophy, and diaphragmatic hernia through the foramen of Bochdalek.

UNDERLYING MECHANISMS. The understanding of malformations has been derived principally from the study of animals. Basic abnormalities identified include (1) abnormal cell shape; (2) abnormalities of the collagens or of the proteoglycans, major constituents of the extracellular matrix; (3) errors in circulation during fetal development; and (4) lack of appropriate death of cells during morphogenesis. An example of abnormal cell shape is the defect in the Bergmann glial cells that normally provide the latticework for migration of neuronal cells. When they are defective because of the autosomal recessive gene *weaver* in the mouse, hypoplasia of the cerebellum results. Several types of Ehlers-Danlos syndrome have been identified by clinical and genetic studies in humans, some of which have been shown to be due to different defects in collagen metabolism. For example, in type VI the collagen is deficient in hydroxylysine because of a deficiency of lysyl hydroxylase; in type VII there is an inability to convert procollagen to collagen; in type IV there is a lack of type III collagen.

The malformation *hemifacial microsomia* can be caused by a failure of the vascular supply to be transferred from the stapedial artery to the external carotid artery, a switchover that normally occurs during the 6th and 7th wk of gestation in humans. *Synostosis of bones* can be due to a lack of appropriate death of cells between the developing long bones in a limb. *Cleft palate* reflects a failure of the palate shelves to meet and fuse, a process in which death of cells in the epithelium must precede the fusion of the underlying palatal mesenchyme.

CLINICAL EVALUATION. Any child with a major or with multiple minor malformations deserves diagnostic evaluation. This includes a history of defects in other family members and of any untoward events during the pregnancy as well as a thorough physical examination. In the examination, objective measurements should be used when a physical feature seems too long, short, narrow or wide. Many normal standards are included in Smith's *Recognizable Patterns of Human Malformation*. Chromosomal analysis by banding techniques should be obtained when there are multiple malformations, especially if the infant is mentally retarded, is stillborn, or dies soon after birth (Sec. 7.11). For such studies on a deceased infant, cells obtained from biopsies of skin, gonad, thymus, or spleen grown in tissue culture are preferable to those obtained from a blood sample taken when the infant is moribund. The likelihood of finding a chromosomal abnormality in infants in the aforementioned categories is only 10–20%. Screening for metabolic diseases is also warranted in malformed infants. Glutaric aciduria type II has been observed in some malformed infants, especially in association with genitourinary abnormalities.

The same clinical signs or malformations may be caused by a variety of genetic accidents. For example, the split-hand/split-foot syndrome, an unusual malformation in which there is a cleft in the middle of the hand, foot, or both, may be due to lack of development of the middle digits and metatarsals and metacarpals. The same deformity occurs in focal dermal hypoplasia, a multiple malformation syndrome, and in the autosomal dominant disorder in which the deformities are limited to the limbs.

Coco R, Penchaszadeh VB: Cytogenetic findings in 200 children with mental retardation and multiple congenital anomalies of unknown cause. Am J Med Genet 12:155, 1982.

Gorlin RJ, Pindborg JJ, Cohen MM Jr: Syndromes of the Head and Neck, 2nd ed. New York, McGraw-Hill, 1976.

Hootnick DR, Levinsohn EM, Randall PA, et al: Vascular dysgenesis associated with skeletal dysplasia of the lower limb. J Bone Joint Surg 62A:1123, 1980.

Jones KL: Smith's Recognizable Patterns of Human Malformation, 4th ed. Philadelphia, WB Saunders, 1988.

Leppig KA, Werler MM, Cann CI, et al: Predictive value of minor anomalies. I: Association with major malformations. J Pediatrics 110:531, 1987.

Machin GA: Chromosome abnormality and perinatal death. Lancet 1:549, 1974.

Mueller RF, Sybert VP, Johnson J: Evaluation of a protocol for post-mortem examination of stillbirths. N Engl J Med 309:586, 1983.

Nelson K, Holmes LB: Malformations due to presumed spontaneous mutations in newborn infants. N Engl J Med 320:19, 1989.

Poswillo D: The pathogenesis of the first and second branchial arch syndrome. Oral Surg 35:302, 1973.

Sweetman L, Nyhan WL, Tranner DA, et al: Glutaric acidemia type II. J Pediatr 96:1020, 1980.

Van Allen MI, Hoyme HE, Jones KL: Vascular pathogenesis of limb defects. I:Radial artery anatomy in radial aplasia. J Pediatr 101:832, 1982.

Warkany J: Congenital Malformations. Chicago, Year Book Medical Publishers, 1971.

Winter RM, Knowles SAS, Bieber FR, et al: The malformed fetus and stillbirth: A Diagnostic Approach. New York, John Wiley & Sons, 1988.

7.33 GENETIC COUNSELING

Genetic counseling is a communication process dealing with the human problems associated with the occurrence or risk of occurrence of a genetic disorder in a family. Many are unaware of their risks, whereas some request genetic information and counseling. The latter most commonly are couples whose first child has just been born with a birth defect or medical problem. Older couples are also frequently concerned about genetic risks and wish to learn about prenatal diagnosis. Others seek information before marriage or before having children because of medical problems of their relatives. The physician should recognize which birth defects and medical problems are hereditary and offer genetic information to all families, not just to those who request it. Genetic counseling becomes more complex when detection of carriers is possible or when the relevance of prenatal diagnosis must be explained.

PRINCIPLES OF GENETIC COUNSELING

The first step in genetic counseling is to make certain that the diagnosis is correct. The physician must, for example, distinguish isolated cleft lip and palate (multifactorial inheritance) from cleft lip and palate with lip pits (autosomal dominant); distinguish Duchenne muscular dystrophy (X-linked recessive) from the Becker type of muscular dystrophy (X-linked recessive), the latter being much less severe; distinguish the perinatal type of infantile polycystic kidney disease (autosomal recessive) from unilateral multicystic kidney (nonhereditary).

With diagnosis established, the steps in the counseling process follow:

1. Have both parents present for the discussion (a teenager in the family should be offered the opportunity of a separate discussion).

2. Discuss the medical consequences of the defect; if relevant, the variability of associated features that might develop in future years should be explained.

3. Review the family history of each parent and identify any unrecognized genetic risks.

4. Review the interpretations the family has made or which have been offered by others to explain the condition under discussion.

5. Describe the genetic basis for the problem, using *visual aids* (pictures demonstrating phenotypic or other features of the problem, pictures of chromosomes, diagrams of patterns of inheritance) as much as possible.

6. Explain the genetic risks in terms the family can understand.

7. Outline the options available, such as having no children, having children and accepting the risks, adopting a child if possible, artificial insemination (this option is particularly pertinent in the case of all autosomal recessive disorders and serious paternal autosomal dominant disorders); note whether prenatal diagnosis is possible.

8. Provide the persons counseled with a summary of the issues discussed and, if possible, meet with them again to help them decide the option most appropriate for them.

9. Stay in contact with families previously counseled to provide new information that may become available, such as new methods for carrier detection in a parent or for prenatal diagnosis.

Parents often first become aware of their genetic risks after the birth of a child having a birth defect. Coping with this knowledge usually includes periods of denial, anger, and depression before it is assimilated and accepted. Each family's situation is different and their reaction to counseling unique. A frequent problem for families is conceptualizing the genetic abnormality, such as a single mutant gene, an abnormal chromosome, or, in the case of multifactorial inheritance, the interaction of several genes and environmental factors. In the case of chromosomal abnormalities, it may be advantageous to show the abnormal karyotype compared with a normal one (Sec. 7.31). Another problem is the fact that most infants and children with a genetic disorder are the first affected member of the family. Parents may assume a problem cannot be hereditary if no other relatives are affected. It is helpful for the counselor to discuss in detail how healthy parents with no affected relatives can have a child with a hereditary disorder.

GENETIC COUNSELING WHEN DETECTION OF CARRIERS IS POSSIBLE

Genetic counseling is simplified, more specific, and probably more effective when the carrier state for the genetic abnormality in question can be identified by laboratory tests. Those at risk can be identified, and their relatives who were tested and found not to be carriers can be reassured. The concept of genetic risk is more concrete when an individual has a venipuncture and can be shown the test results in comparison with the normal. Carrier detection is possible for some biochemical disorders, for certain abnormalities of the chromosomes, and through DNA analysis techniques, such as gene mapping and the identification of a restriction length polymorphism that is closely linked to a mutant gene.

BIOCHEMICAL DISORDERS. Persons heterozygous for some autosomal recessive inborn errors of metabolism and abnormalities of hemoglobin can be identified. These inborn errors include abnormalities such as hemoglobins S and C, thalassemia, Tay-Sachs disease, and α_1-antitrypsin deficiency. If the assay is appropriate for screening large numbers of individuals, testing high-risk populations may be conducted. This type of testing has been used to screen Jews of Eastern European origin for Tay-Sachs disease, persons of Mediterranean ancestry for thalassemia, and blacks for hemoglobins S and C. Screening for genetic diseases may have untoward psychologic effects by focusing on a racial or ethnic group.

Progress in DNA analysis has greatly improved the ability to identify female carriers of the two most common X-linked recessive disorders, DMD, and hemophilia A (Sec. 7.1 and 16.64). DMD in affected males is associated with deletions in the large dystrophin gene in 73% of cases and is due to point mutations in the remainder. Prenatal diagnosis is highly reliable for almost any female in the family of an affected male, although the carrier status cannot always be determined. DNA markers are available that flank the DMD gene, as well as intragenic probes. Errors due to crossing over usually have a frequency of less than 4%.

Experience in DNA studies of families with males with the X-linked hemophilia A has shown that about half of the affected males are sporadic (i.e., affected as the result of a new genetic mutation). The high mutation rate for the factor VIII gene also makes carrier detection more difficult. Carrier diagnosis is best when the mutation itself can be detected directly by intragenic probes.

CHROMOSOMAL TRANSLOCATIONS. When a child is abnormal because of an excess or deficiency of chromosomal material, the parents should be studied to identify whether or not either is the carrier of a balanced translocation. A carrier parent can then be counseled as to his or her risk of having children with an unbalanced translocation, and other blood relatives may be tested to determine whether they, too, are carriers. Related chromosomal abnormalities of the fetus of the carrier of a balanced translocation may be identified through culture of fetal cells obtained by amniocentesis.

GENETIC COUNSELING WHEN PRENATAL DIAGNOSIS IS POSSIBLE

Many couples seek genetic counseling to learn more about prenatal diagnosis. The most common indications for prenatal diagnosis are advanced maternal age (see Table 7–6) and a previous child with either Down syndrome or anencephaly-meningomyelocele.

In general, prenatal diagnosis by amniocentesis is recommended for all women over 35 yr of age, because their risk of having a child with any type of chromosomal abnormality is at least 1%. There has been a steady decline during the last 30 yr in the percentage of infants with Down syndrome born to women over 35 yr of age. Thus 80% of the infants with Down syndrome are now born to women under 35 yr of age, because this group is not routinely offered prenatal diagnosis as an option. Further, in about 1 of 5 cases, the extra No. 21 chromosome is derived from the father (Sec. 7.14).

Couples at risk for having children with metabolic diseases and hemoglobinopathies are a less common indication for prenatal diagnosis. Diagnostic testing of DNA from tissue removed by chorionic villus sampling (CVS) should be done by those laboratories experienced in conducting such assays.

Prenatal diagnosis by *amniocentesis* is usually undertaken at

15–16 wk of gestation, when the uterus extends high enough out of the pelvis to facilitate the procedure, although early amniocentesis at 12–13 wk of gestation is now available at many medical centers. Ultrasound is used to locate the placenta and to determine whether there is more than one fetus; the incidence of twin pregnancy is about 1 in 80. Using aseptic technique and local anesthesia, a 22-gauge spinal needle with trocar in place is inserted through the abdomen at the most favorable site, as indicated by the ultrasonogram, and is advanced into the amniotic cavity. The trocar is removed and the first 2 mL of fluid is discarded to minimize the risk of contamination of the sample with cells from the mother's skin; then 10–30 mL of amniotic fluid is withdrawn into a second syringe, sealed in the syringe, and taken directly to the laboratory. (A small amount of fluid is withdrawn in early amniocentesis.) The specimen is tested for the presence of fetal blood and centrifuged to separate the fluid from the cells; the cells are then placed in tissue culture medium under sterile conditions in an incubator.

Fetal loss from amniocentesis is less than 0.5%. Three per cent of women have transient cramps and leakage of amniotic fluid. Occasionally, the amniocentesis must be repeated, either because no amniotic fluid was obtained with the first amniocentesis or because there was insufficient growth of cells.

Results can be provided within 14–21 days of the amniocentesis. If the tests show that the fetus is abnormal and the parents elect to have the fetus aborted, most obstetricians prefer to terminate the pregnancy before 20 wk of gestation, although up to 24 wk is permissible by law in the United States.

Prenatal diagnosis based on CVS is performed at 9–11 wk of pregnancy. The tissue is obtained by inserting a sampling device either through the cervix and up into the fetal placenta or transabdominally with needle insertion similar to amniocentesis. The tissue obtained can be used for direct DNA analysis or for cell culture. The risk of fetal loss after CVS is about the same as for amniocentesis, although there is an additional chance of 1% that tissue mosaicism will be found that can be resolved by subsequent amniocentesis.

Tissues and Technical Procedures Used in Prenatal Diagnosis

CELLS IN THE AMNIOTIC FLUID. The cells obtained by amniocentesis can be used for chromosomal analysis, biochemical assay, or DNA analysis. Two to 3 wk are needed for the cells to multiply and reach a number adequate for testing; it is more difficult to obtain good metaphase preparations from amniotic fluid cells than from peripheral lymphocytes. Chromosomal abnormalities such as polyploidy and mosaicism with both normal and abnormal cell lines are also more common in amniotic fluid cells obtained at 14–16 wk of gestation than in cells of infants at birth.

AMNIOTIC FLUID

α-Fetoprotein (AFP). The level of this constituent of amniotic fluid, which is synthesized by the fetal liver, gastrointestinal tract, and yolk sac, is increased whenever transudation across a thin membrane occurs, such as in anencephaly, meningomyelocele, encephalocele, and omphalocele. The most common use of measuring AFP is to evaluate subsequent pregnancies of couples who have had a child with anencephaly, meningomyelocele, or encephalocele; omphalocele is usually not hereditary. Increased AFP levels have also been used to identify the **Meckel syndrome** (an autosomal recessive disorder that includes encephalocele, polycystic kidneys, polydactyly, cleft lip and palate, and anomalies of the genitals and eyes) and congenital nephrosis (a rare autosomal recessive disorder).

The level of AFP is highest between 14 and 18 wk of gestation and falls steadily after that; it is important to obtain an estimate of gestational age by ultrasonography before amniocentesis. The concentration of AFP may be increased by the presence of fetal blood, fetal spontaneous abortion, fetal death, Rh sensitization, congenital nephrosis, and the presence of intestinal atresia. The measurement of acetylcholinesterase in amniotic fluid is helpful in confirming the presence of a neural tube defect and in eliminating false-positive elevations of AFP. The AFP level is often normal if a neural tube defect, such as meningocele or encephalocele, is covered by skin.

Routine prenatal screening of pregnant women by measuring the level of AFP in serum by radioimmunoassay is effective in identifying 80–90% of fetuses with anencephaly and meningomyelocele. This test is performed at 16–18 wk of pregnancy. If the serum AFP is 2.0 times the median value, the fetus is examined by ultrasound and amniocentesis. In addition to detecting neural tube defects, serum AFP screening will also identify the presence of other malformations such as omphalocele, growth retardation, and twinning.

Low levels of maternal serum AFP occur in about 20% of fetuses with 21-trisomy and 18-trisomy. Expanding serum AFP screening to include estriol and hCG may detect 60% of affected fetuses, but this expanded screening is still being developed.

ULTRASOUND. Ultrasound is used primarily to determine gestational age, to localize the placenta, to rule out multiple pregnancies, and to diagnose congenital malformations (Sec. 6.56 and 9.9).

PERCUTANEOUS UMBILICAL CORD BLOOD SAMPLING (PUBS). This technique is being used to obtain a blood sample, primarily for chromosome studies, at about 20 wk of gestation after fetal abnormalities have been identified by prenatal ultrasound.

FETOSCOPY. Direct inspection of the fetus is possible, but the risk to the fetus is about 5%. It has been used for obtaining skin biopsies and liver biopsies. A difficulty with this technique is the small area that can be seen at one time. Improvements in ultrasound and PUBS techniques have almost eliminated the use of fetoscopy.

RADIOGRAPHY. Roentgenograms of the fetus may be helpful when the fetus is at risk for a severe deficiency of the long bones, such as in thrombocytopenia with radial aplasia, and to identify vertebral malformations, as in the Jarcho-Levin syndrome. However, this technique is being replaced by ultrasound.

GENETIC COUNSELING

Lippman-Hand A, Fraser FC: Genetic counseling, provisions and reception of information. Am J Med Genet 3:113, 1979.

Reif M, Baitsch H: Psychological issues in genetic counseling. Hum Genet 70:193, 1985.

Wertz DC, Fletcher JC: Attitudes of genetic counselors: a multinational survey. Am J Hum Genet 42:592, 1988.

Zare N, Sorenson JR, Heeren T: Sex of provider as a variable in effective genetic counseling. Soc Sci Med 19:671, 1984.

CARRIER DETECTION

Koenig M, Hoffman EP, Bertelson CJ, et al: Complete cloning of the Duchenne muscular dystrophy (DMD) cDNA and preliminary genomic organization of the DMD in normal and affected individuals. Cell 50:509, 1987.

Schwaab R, Oldenburg J, Higuchi M, et al: Hemophilia A: carrier detection by DNA analysis. Blut 57:85, 1988.

PRENATAL DIAGNOSIS

Benacerraf BR, Pober BR, Sanders SP: Accuracy of fetal echocardiography. Radiology 165:847, 1987.

Canick JA: Screening for Down syndrome using maternal serum alpha-fetoprotein, unconjugated estriol, and HCG. J Clin Immunoassay 13:36, 1990.

Juberg RC, Mowney PN: Origin of nondisjunction in trisomy 21 syndrome. Am J Med Genet 16:111, 1983.
Kazazian HH Jr, Boehm CD: Molecular basis and prenatal diagnosis of β-thalassemia. Blood 72:1107, 1988.
Landegren U, Kaiser R, Caskey CT, et al: DNA diagnostics: Molecular techniques and automation. Science 242:229, 1988.
Manchester DK, Pretorius DH, Avery C, et al: Accuracy of ultrasound diagnoses in pregnancies complicated by suspected fetal anomalies. Prenat Diagn 8:109, 1988.
Palomaki GE: Collaborative study of Down syndrome screening using maternal serum alpha-fetoproteins and maternal age. Lancet ii:1460, 1986.
Rhoads GG, Jackson LG, Schlesselman SE, et al: The safety and efficacy of chorionic villus sampling for early prenatal diagnosis of cytogenetic abnormalities. N Engl J Med 320:609, 1989.

7.34 TERATOGENS

When an infant or child is malformed or mentally retarded, the parents often wrongly blame themselves and attribute the child's problems to events that occurred during pregnancy. Because infections occur and several drugs are often taken during many pregnancies, the pediatrician must evaluate the presumed viral infections and the drugs ingested to help parents understand their child's birth defect. The causes of approximately 40% of congenital malformations are unknown. While only a relatively few agents teratogenic in humans are

TABLE 7–12. Teratogenic Agents in Humans

Teratogen	Phenotypic Effect	Period of Greatest Sensitivity	Likelihood of Harmful Effect
Drugs Taken by Pregnant Mother			
Aminopterin or amethopterin (folic acid antagonist)	Hydrocephalus, craniosynostosis, shortened limbs, absent digits, mental deficiency	?	?
Angiotensin-converting enzyme (ACE) inhibitor	Renal tubular dysplasia, oligohydramnios, skull hypoplasia	2nd and 3rd trimester	?
Carbamazepine	Craniofacial abnormalities, growth retardation	?	?
Cocaine	Prematurity, perinatal morbidity, abruptio placentae	?	?
Diethylstilbestrol	Carcinoma and adenosis of vagina in exposed females; genitourinary anomalies in exposed males	1st 2 months	>50% of females 25% of males
Iodides and propylthiouracil	Goiter, fetal hypothyroidism	?	?
Isotretinoin	Brain malformations, microtia, thymic hypoplasia, coronatruncal heart defects	1st trimester	>20-fold increase
Phenytoin	Heart defects, nail hypoplasia, growth retardation	1st trimester	3-fold increase
Progestogens contaminated with testosterone	Masculinization of female fetus	?	?
Tetracyclines	Enamel dysplasia	2nd and 3rd trimester	?
Thalidomide	Phocomelia, anomalies of ears, teeth, eyes, and intestine	Days 34–50 (menstrual age)	>20-fold increase
Valproic acid	Spina bifida, facial anomalies, developmental delay	First trimester	>20-fold increase
Warfarin (vitamin K antagonist)	Hypoplasia of nose, shortened digits, stippled epiphyses, mental deficiency in some	Weeks 7–12 (menstrual age)	?
Maternal Conditions			
Chronic, severe alcoholism	Growth retardation, mental deficiency, microcephaly, heart defects, flexion contractures	?	30–50%
Diabetes mellitus	Heart defects; all types of birth defects; sacral agenesis; anencephaly and spina bifida	1st trimester	3-fold increase
Lupus erythematosus	Congenital heart block	?	?
Phenylketonuria	Microcephaly, mental deficiency, heart defects	?	?
Smoking cigarettes	Decrease in birthweight; abnormal placentation	?	?
Smoking marijuana	Decrease in birthweight	?	?
Trace Metals			
Lead	Decrease in intelligence	?	?
Mercury	Microcephaly, spasticity, mental deficiency	?	?
Intrauterine Infections			
Cytomegalovirus	Microcephaly, mental deficiency	1st trimester	?
Rubella	Heart defects, microcephaly, cataracts, deafness, mental deficiency	1st trimester	15–40%
Toxoplasmosis	Macrocephaly or microcephaly, microphthalmia, mental deficiency	1st trimester	?
Varicella	Skin scars, hypoplasia of limbs, microphthalmia, cataracts, mental deficiency	?	?
Parvovirus	Hemolytic anemia, stillbirth	?	1%
Uterine Factors			
Septate uterus	Positional deformities	Throughout	?
Severe oligohydramnios	Lung hypoplasia, deformities caused by pressure from surrounding structures	Throughout	100%

recognized (Table 7–12), additional agents, such as valproic acid (used to treat or prevent convulsions) and isotretinoin (used to treat severe cystic acne), continue to be identified.

Several generalizations can be made about teratogens. None is harmful to every exposed fetus; some drugs (e.g., phenytoins) and maternal conditions (e.g., diabetes mellitus) may cause only a 2- to 3-fold increase in the overall incidence of malformations. Because the increase caused by a teratogen may be relatively small, harmful effects may be difficult to demonstrate. In general, exposure during the 1st trimester of pregnancy is probably the most harmful. The exact age of the fetus when a particular drug is most harmful has been established only for thalidomide (days 34–50). Even less information is available on the effects of exposure during the 2nd and 3rd trimesters.

If a child has multiple structural malformations, such as polydactyly, cleft palate, meningomyelocele, or absence of a long bone, it is inappropriate to consider intrauterine infections as a possible cause. It is true that rubella infection in utero causes cardiac anomalies, but its other effects, such as microcephaly, cataracts, and deafness, are the results of infection of the tissues concerned, not structural malformations. Likewise, congenital toxoplasmosis may cause hydrocephalus, and intrauterine infection with cytomegalovirus may cause cerebral cysts. However, none of these intrauterine infections causes multiple major and minor *structural* malformations, as can be caused by chromosomal abnormalities, single mutant genes, and teratogenic drugs.

The mechanism of action is known or postulated for very few teratogens. Warfarin, an anticoagulant because it is a vitamin K antagonist, prevents carboxylation of gamma-carboxyglutamic acid (GLA) that are components of osteocalcin and other vitamin K-dependent bone proteins. The teratogenic effect on developing cartilage, especially nasal cartilage, appears to be avoided if the pregnant woman's treatment between weeks 6 to 12 of gestation is switched from warfarin to heparin. Hypothyroidism in the fetus may be caused by maternal ingestion of an excessive amount of iodides or of propylthiouracil; each interferes with the conversion of inorganic to organic iodides. Phenytoin may be teratogenic because of the accumulation of a metabolite due to deficiency of epoxide hydrolase.

Recognition of teratogens offers the opportunity for prevention of related birth defects. For example, if a pregnant woman is informed of the potentially harmful effects of alcohol on her unborn infant, she may be motivated to control this problem during pregnancy. The woman with insulin-dependent diabetes mellitus may decrease significantly her risk for having a child with birth defects by achieving good control of her disease before conception.

Physicians are often asked about the risks of exposure in utero to drugs that have not been proved to be teratogenic. These include caffeine, diazepam, lysergic acid (LSD), marijuana, heroin, blighted potatoes, aspirin, and phenothiazine derivatives, such as Bendectin. Current references should be consulted before drawing conclusions.

Genetic factors play a role in determining teratogenicity that may represent multifactorial inheritance in which the inherited factor is susceptibility to a teratogenic environmental factor. Variation in susceptibility to teratogens is apparent not only between different species of animals but also within species (e.g., different genetic strains of rats show different degrees of susceptibility to cortisone as a teratogenic agent that induces cleft palate in the rat fetus). The parents of a child with anticonvulsant-induced malformations have an increased risk of a subsequent child developing this drug-induced embryopathy in comparison with parents whose exposed children are not malformed. This increased risk may reflect a genetic difference in metabolizing the anticonvulsant.

Other conditions are also teratogenic, such as oligohydramnios, and uterine constraint. Oligohydramnios may result from bilateral renal agenesis, severe polycystic kidney disease, chronic leakage of amniotic fluid, and extrauterine pregnancy. Its consequences are lung hypoplasia, club foot deformity, a flattened face, and amnion nodosum.

Ardinger HH, Atkin JF, Blackston RD, et al: Verification of the fetal valproate syndrome phenotype. Am J Med Genet 29:171, 1988.
Bellinger D, Leviton A, Waternaux C, et al: Longitudinal analyses of prenatal and postnatal lead exposure and early cognitive development. N Engl J Med 316:1037, 1987.
Dunn PM: Congenital postural deformities. Br Med Bull 32:71, 1976.
Heinonen OP, Slone D, Shapiro S: Birth Defects and Drugs in Pregnancy. Littleton, MA, Publishing Science Groups, 1976.
Jones KJ, Lacro RV, Johnson KA, et al: Pattern of malformations in the children of women treated with carbamazepine during pregnancy. N Engl J Med 320:1661, 1989.
Lammer EJ, Chen CT, Hoar RM, et al: Retinoic acid embryopathy. N Engl J Med 313:837, 1985.
Litsey SE, Noonan JA, O'Connor WN, et al: Maternal connective tissue disease and congenital heart block. N Engl J Med 312:98, 1985.
Newman CGH: Teratogen update: Clinical aspects of thalidomide embryopathy—a continuing preoccupation. Teratology 32:133, 1985.
Pauli RM, Lian JB, Mosher DF, et al: Association of congenital deficiency of multiple vitamin K-dependent coagulation factors and the phenotype of the warfarin embryopathy: Clues to the mechanism of teratogenicity of coumarin derivatives. Am J Hum Genet 41:566, 1987.
Shepard TH: Catalog of Teratogenic Agents, 6th ed. Baltimore, The Johns Hopkins University Press, 1989.
Stickler SM, Dansky LV, Miller MA, et al: Genetic predisposition to phenytoin-induced birth defects. Lancet ii:746, 1985.
Streissguth AP, Barr HM, Sampson DD, et al: Attention, distraction and reaction time at age 7 years and prenatal alcohol exposure. Neurobehavioral Toxicology and Teratology 8:717, 1986.
Zuckerman B, Frank DA, Hingson R, et al: Effects of maternal marijuana and cocaine use on fetal growth. N Engl J Med 320:762, 1989.

7.35 RADIATION

Accidental exposure of pregnant women to radiation is a common cause for anxiety among women, their families, and their physicians, usually about whether the fetus will have birth defects or genetic abnormalities. It is unlikely that exposure to either diagnostic or therapeutic radiation will cause gene mutations; no increase in genetic abnormalities has been identified in the offspring exposed as unborn fetuses to the atomic bomb explosions in Japan in 1945.

A more realistic concern is whether the exposed human fetus will show birth defects or a higher incidence of malignancy. The recommended occupational limit of maternal exposure to radiation from all sources is 500 millirads (mrad) for the entire 40 wk of a pregnancy. Estimates of the gonadal exposure for the mother and the whole body exposure of the fetus from several common roentgenographic examinations are shown in Table 7–13. The limited data on human fetuses

TABLE 7–13. Radiation Exposure of the Fetus*

Type of Study	Millirad†
Roentgenogram of:	
Chest	1
Thoracic spine	11
Abdomen	221
Pelvis	210
Hips	124
Roentgenographic contrast studies	
Upper gastrointestinal series	171
Barium enema	903
Cholangiogram	78
Intravenous pyelogram	588

*From US DHEW: Gonad Doses and Genetically Significant Dose from Diagnostic Radiology; US, 1964 and 1970. Washington, DC,US Government Printing Office, 1976.

†Due to variation in techniques these estimates may be exceeded.

show that large doses of radiation (10,000–30,000 millirads) are harmful to the central nervous system.

Therapeutic abortion is often recommended when exposure exceeds 10,000 mrad. It is more likely that a human fetus will be exposed to 1,000–3,000 mrad, an amount not shown to cause malformations. There is controversy with regard to whether this level of exposure is associated with an increased risk of developing cancer or leukemia. (See also Sec. 6.56 and Sec. 26.1).

LEWIS B. HOLMES

Brent RL: Radiation teratogenesis. Teratology 21:281, 1980.
The Effects on Populations of Exposure to Low Levels of Ionizing Radiation (BEIR Report). Washington DC, National Academy of Sciences. National Research Council, November, 1972.
Griem ML, Meier P, Dobben GD: Analysis of the morbidity and mortality of children irradiated in fetal life. Radiology 88:347, 1967.
US Department of Health, Education, and Welfare: Gonad Doses and Genetically Significant Dose from Diagnostic Radiology: US., 1964 and 1970. Washington, DC, US Government Printing Office, 1976.
Webster EW: On the question of cancer induction by small X-ray doses. Am J Roentgenol 137:647, 1981.
Yamazaki NJ: A review of the literature on the radiation dosage required to cause manifest central nervous system disturbances from in utero and postnatal exposure. Pediatrics 37:877, 1966.

7.36 DYSMORPHOLOGY—THE APPROACH TO STRUCTURAL DEFECTS OF PRENATAL ONSET

The field of dysmorphology has expanded dramatically as the number of recognizable patterns of malformation has more than tripled during the last 20 yr; new insights have been gained into the pathogenesis of various structural defects, the potential prenatal effect of various drugs, chemicals, and environmental agents has been better appreciated, and the number of defects in which prenatal detection is possible has increased. Because of their vast number, a listing of all known recognizable patterns of malformation will not be presented. Rather, this section provides an approach to the child with the prenatal onset of structural defects. The approach is predicated upon the concept that the nature of the structural defects represents a clue to the time of onset, mechanism of injury, and possible etiology of the problem, all of which determine the necessary evaluation. This permits a systematic narrowing of the diagnostic possibilities so that other sections of this textbook or one of the basic compendiums on dysmorphology may be used to make a specific diagnosis.

Structural defects of prenatal onset can be separated into those that represent a *single primary defect* in development and those that represent a multiple malformation syndrome. In most cases, the defect involves only a single structure, the child being otherwise completely normal. The seven most common single primary defects in development are congenital hip dislocation (Sec. 24.8), talipes equinovarus (Sec. 24.2), cleft lip with or without cleft palate (Sec. 13.5), cleft palate alone (Sec. 13.5), cardiac septal defects (Sec. 15.30), pyloric stenosis (Sec. 13.27), and defects in neural tube closure (Sec. 20.2–20.5). For most, the etiology is unknown, and counseling as to recurrence risk is difficult. However, most single primary defects are explained on the basis of multifactorial inheritance (Sec. 7.8), which carries a recurrence risk of between 2% and 5% for the next child of unaffected parents with one affected child.

The extent to which multifactorial inheritance contributes to the etiology of some of the less common single defects in development is unclear. The fact that single primary defects are etiologically heterogeneous implies that some have an environmental etiology and others result from dominantly or recessively inherited single altered genes. Craniosynostosis (Sec. 20.16) secondary to in utero constraint is an example of the former, whereas postaxial polydactyly (Sec. 24.23) illustrates the latter. Before multifactorial risk figures are used for counseling when a single primary defect is recognized, references should be consulted to determine whether other risk figures are available.

In contrast to the concept of the single primary defect in development, the designation *multiple malformation syndrome* is used when several observed structural defects all have the same known or presumed etiology. The defects usually include a number of anatomically unrelated errors in morphogenesis. Multiple malformation syndromes are caused by chromosomal abnormalities, by teratogens, and by single gene defects inherited in mendelian patterns. Risks of recurrence range from 0 in cases that represent fresh gene mutations or are caused by teratogens to 100% in the case of a child with the Down syndrome in which the mother is a balanced 21/21 translocation carrier (Sec. 7.14).

SINGLE PRIMARY DEFECTS IN DEVELOPMENT. These defects are subcategorized according to the nature of the error in morphogenesis that has produced the observed structural defect: malformation, deformation, or disruption of developing structure. A *malformation* is a primary structural defect arising from a localized error in morphogenesis. A *deformation* is an alteration in shape or structure of a part that has differentiated normally. The term *disruption* is used for a structural defect resulting from destruction of a previously normally formed part. Of the deformations noted at birth, 90% correct spontaneously; of those that do not, most can be corrected with early postural intervention. If correction of malformations or disruptions is at all possible, surgery is virtually always required.

Malformations. Most children with a localized malformation such as cardiac septal defect or pyloric stenosis are otherwise completely normal. After surgical correction, prognosis is excellent. When neither dominant nor recessive inheritance is established, multifactorial recurrence risk factors (2–5%) apply to unaffected parents.

Deformations. Most deformations involve the musculoskeletal system and are probably caused by intrauterine molding. The pressure producing such molding may be intrinsic, due to neuromuscular imbalance within the fetus, or may be extrinsic, secondary to fetal crowding. In either case, the impaired ability of the fetus to kick results in decreased fetal movement, an important factor in development of the normal musculoskeletal system, particularly with respect to normal joint development. In addition, marked positional deformation of any body part can occur when the fetus is unable to change position and thus alter the direction along which potentially deforming forces are being directed.

Intrinsically derived positional deformation of prenatal onset occurs in disorders involving muscle degeneration, such as the Steinert myotonic dystrophy syndrome, and disorders involving motor neurons, such as Werdnig-Hoffmann disease (Sec. 21.36). Early defects in development of the central nervous system are more common causes of positional deformations and should be seriously considered whenever a structural defect is thought to be intrinsically derived.

Fetal crowding, the common cause of an extrinsically derived deformation of prenatal onset, is usually due to a decreased volume of amniotic fluid, a situation that occurs normally during the later weeks of gestation when the fetus is undergoing extremely rapid growth. However, it also occurs abnormally with diminished fetal urinary output and chronic leakage of amniotic fluid.

Other extrinsic factors associated with the development of deformations include breech presentation and the shape of the amniotic cavity. When a fetus is in the breech position, the legs may be trapped between the body and the uterine wall. In that position, the fetus is unable to kick optimally, resulting in a 10-fold increase in the incidence of deformations. The shape of the amniotic cavity, which has profound influence on the shape of the fetus that lies within it, is influenced by many factors, including uterine shape; volume of amniotic fluid; size and shape of the fetus; presence of more than one fetus; site of placental implantation; presence of uterine tumors; shape of the abdominal cavity, which is influenced by the pelvis, sacral promontory, and neighboring abdominal organs; and tightness of abdominal musculature.

Various forms of talipes and congenital hip dislocation are the most frequently observed congenital postural deformities. Most children with these deformations are otherwise completely normal, and their prognosis is excellent. Correction usually occurs spontaneously. However, recognizing that a structural defect represents a deformation does not always imply "normal" fetal crowding and should lead to careful consideration of other etiologic possibilities that might have far greater significance to the child. For example, because decreased fetal movement can be secondary to serious neurologic abnormalities, multiple joint contractures should alert the physician to the possibility of a malformation in central nervous system development. Although congenital hip dislocations and talipes have a 2–5% recurrence risk, most deformations are the result of physiologic crowding and have a lower recurrence risk. Deformations that are due to pathologic crowding (e.g., uterine tumors or malformation) have a much higher recurrence risk unless the factors leading to crowding are altered prior to subsequent pregnancies. Deformations that are the result of an underlying malformation (e.g., renal agenesis) have a recurrence risk similar to that of the underlying malformation.

DISRUPTION. These defects occur when there is destruction of a previously normally formed part. At least two basic mechanisms are known to produce disruption. One involves entanglement followed by the tearing apart or amputation of a normally developed structure, usually a digit, arm, or leg, by strands of amnion floating within amniotic fluid (i.e., amniotic bands) (Sec. 24.23). The second involves the interruption of blood supply to a developing part leading to infarction, necrosis, and/or resorption of structures distal to the insult. If interruption of blood supply occurs early in gestation, the disruptive defect that is seen at term usually involves atresia or absence of a particular part. If the infarction occurs later, necrosis is more likely to be present. Examples of disruptive single primary defects for which infarctive mechanisms have been implicated include nonduodenal intestinal atresia, gastroschisis (Sec. 13.28), and porencephaly (Sec. 20.11). The extent to which disruption of a developing structure plays a role in dysmorphogenesis is unknown.

Genetic factors play a minor role in the pathogenesis of disruptions; most are sporadic events in otherwise normal families. The prognosis for a disruptive defect is determined entirely by the extent and location of the tissue loss. Thus a child with a limb amputation has an excellent prognosis for normal function, whereas a child with porencephaly does not.

Sequence. The pattern of multiple anomalies that occurs when a single primary defect in early morphogenesis produces multiple abnormalities through a cascading process of secondary and tertiary errors in morphogenesis is called a sequence. When evaluating a child with multiple anomalies, the physician must differentiate between multiple anomalies secondary to a single localized error in morphogenesis (a sequence) and a multiple malformation syndrome. In the former recurrence risk counseling for the multiple anomalies depends entirely on the recurrence risk for the single localized malformation.

The words malformation, deformation, and disruption sequence are used to describe only the initiating error in morphogenesis of a sequence if it is known. For example, the Robin malformation sequence (Sec. 13.5) is a pattern of multiple anomalies, all of which are produced by a single prenatal onset defect in development, mandibular hypoplasia. Because the tongue is relatively small for the oral cavity, it drops back (glossoptosis), blocking closure of the posterior palatal shelves and causing a U-shaped cleft palate. Recognizing that all of the observed defects are due to a single localized error permits recurrence risk counseling based on the single defect.

The patient shown in Figure 7–27 has bathrocephaly, torticollis, facial asymmetry, a dislocated hip, and valgus anomalies of both feet resulting from compression of developing fetal parts. This pattern is the *breech deformation sequence.* Intrauterine crowding occurred because the large-sized infant was delivered from a breech position to a small, primigravida mother; recurrence risk is therefore negligible. Recognizing the deformational nature of the abnormalities is helpful with respect to prognosis. All of the problems should resolve spontaneously or with postural therapy.

In the *amniotic band disruption sequence* all of the craniofacial and limb defects are secondary to constrictions caused by entanglement in multiple fibrous strands of amnion extending from the placental insertion of the umbilical cord to the surface of the amnion-denuded chorion or floating freely within the chorionic sac (Fig. 7–28). These strands of amnion, which result from disruption of the normally formed membrane, can cause secondary defects through several mechanisms. Malformations occur if a strand of amnion interferes with the normal sequence of development; for example, a strand of amnion may interrupt fusion of the facial processes so that a cleft lip results. Disruptions occur secondary to tearing apart of structures that have previously developed normally; for example, an amniotic band might cleave areas in the developing craniofacies along lines not conforming to the normal planes of facial closure.

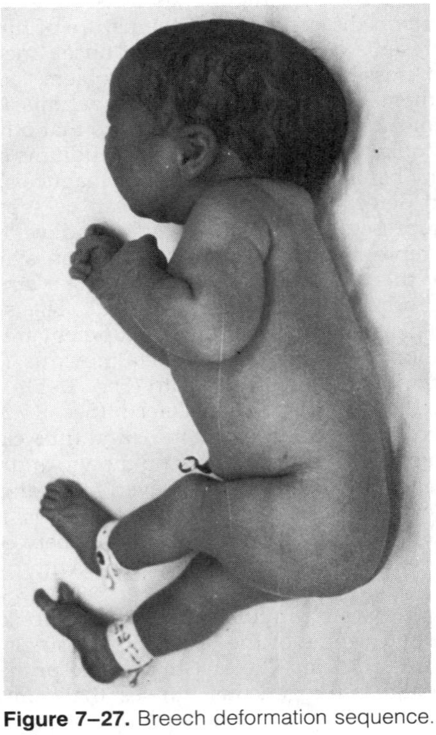

Figure 7–27. Breech deformation sequence.

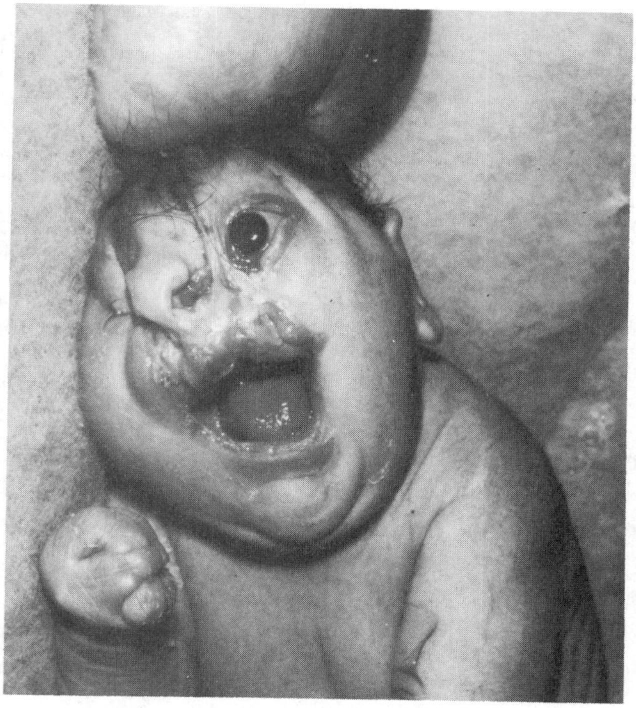

Figure 7–28. Amniotic band disruption sequence.

Deformations due to fetal compression occur secondary to oligohydramnios or tethering of a fetal part. The former may result from rupture of both amnion and chorion, leading to chronic leakage of amniotic fluid. Tethering occurs when the fetus or one of its parts becomes immobilized by the constraining effect of an amniotic band so that it is unable to change positions and thus alter the direction along which potentially deforming forces are being directed. The recurrence risk is based upon the recurrence risk for amnion rupture; unaffected parents have not been reported to have given birth to more than one child affected with this disorder.

MULTIPLE MALFORMATION SYNDROMES. This category includes patients in whom one or more developmental anomalies of two or more systems have occurred, all of which are thought to be due to common etiology. Other than Down syndrome, with an incidence of 1:660, and XXY syndromes (1:500 males), none of these disorders occurs more frequently than 1 in 3,000 live births.

Multiple malformation syndromes may be caused by chromosomal and genetic abnormalities and by teratogens. A number of these are associated with chromosome abnormalities (Sec. 7.11).

Disorders due to single mutant genes (dominant or X-linked in males) or to pairs of mutant genes (autosomal recessive) also cause a number of recognizable multiple malformation syndromes of prenatal onset. Their correct diagnosis depends on clinical recognitions, since in most cases there is no laboratory test to confirm the diagnosis. A family history of a similarly affected individual is extremely helpful. However, in many patients with multiple malformation syndromes of genetic etiology, the occurrence is sporadic and thus represents fresh gene mutations. In such situations, all family members are normal, and the diagnosis depends entirely on the evaluation of the patient's phenotype.

Disorders caused by teratogens include multiple malformation syndromes due to the effect of specific infections or of pharmacologic or chemical agents with which the embryo or fetus has come into contact during gestation. These conditions may be prevented before conception, particularly in the case of drugs and chemicals if the mother is aware that the agent in question can affect her baby. It is difficult, on the other hand, for a pregnant woman to avoid contact with all infectious agents.

A careful history of drug intake (Sec. 9.12) and chemical exposure (Sec. 26.17) should be obtained from the parents of all children with multiple malformation syndromes, especially when the etiology of the disorder is unknown. *A Catalog of Teratogenic Agents* by T. H. Shepard is an excellent reference for determining whether the agent the mother has been exposed to is a known teratogen.

Specific and easily distinguishable phenotypes do not exist for each of the infectious diseases which are commonly associated with altered fetal development, but intrauterine infection can frequently be suspected if there is an overall pattern of malformation (Sec. 9.73). Any patient should be suspected of having had an intrauterine infection if he or she is small for gestational age, developmentally delayed, or affected by microcephaly or hydrocephalus, ocular defects including microphthalmia, chorioretinitis, cataracts, or glaucoma, and hepatosplenomegaly and thrombocytopenia. Intrauterine infections have a wide spectrum of clinical manifestations from the severely affected newborn infant with multiple malformations to the child with no malformations who first manifests learning disabilities at school age.

There are also some well-recognized multiple malformation syndromes in which virtually all cases have been sporadic in otherwise normal families and the etiology is unknown. The *Cornelia de Lange syndrome*, the *Williams syndrome*, the *Prader-Willi syndrome*, and the *Rubinstein-Taybi syndrome* are the most common disorders in this category. Each occurs with a frequency greater than 1 per 10,000. Despite the lack of knowledge of etiology, experience with many children with each of these disorders has provided a vast amount of information that can be extremely helpful to parents in understanding their child's behavior and to educators in planning an appropriate curriculum. For example, a specific behavioral phenotype has been delineated for the de Lange syndrome; the parents' awareness that the child's aberrant behavior is "normal" for the de Lange syndrome rather than "their fault" can be extremely helpful in relieving their anxiety and guilt. For Williams syndrome, a characteristic psychologic profile that indicates delayed motor and perceptual development with relatively good verbal performance and sociability has been demonstrated. This knowledge of a child's particular strengths and weaknesses may allow educators to develop a curriculum that will give affected children a better chance to reach their potential.

Finally, there are certain nonrandom associations of malformations for which it has not been determined whether the pattern is a sequence or a syndrome. These are designated associations. One important clinical example is the VATER association, which includes *v*ertebral defects, *a*nal atresia, *t*racheo*e*sophageal fistula with atresia, *r*adial upper limb hypoplasia, and *r*enal defects. Single umbilical artery and cardiac and genital anomalies also occur in this association. These defects are likely to occur together in almost any combination of two or more and usually represent a sporadic occurrence in an otherwise normal family.

The ultimate goal in evaluating a child with structural defects is making a specific overall diagnosis. When this is achieved, appropriate recurrence risk counseling for the parents, accurate prognostication about the child's future development, and an appropriate plan to help the child reach his or her potential usually are possible. When an overall diagnosis is lacking, the most that can be expected is a better understanding of the nature and onset of the problem, which often may be helpful to parents and to others dealing with the child.

KENNETH LYONS JONES

Bennett FC, Vanderveer B, Sells CJ: The Williams elfin facies syndrome: A psychological profile. Clin Res 25:170a, 1970.

Dunn PM: Congenital postural deformities. Br Med Bull 32:71, 1976.

Gorlin RJ, Cohen MM Jr, Pinburg JJ: Syndromes of the Head and Neck, 2nd ed. New York, McGraw-Hill, 1975.

Higginbottom MC, Jones KL, Hall BD, et al: The amniotic band disruption complex. Timing of amniotic rupture and variable spectra of consequent defects. J Pediatr 95:544, 1979.

Hobbins JC, Romero R, Grannum P, et al: Antenatal diagnosis of renal anomalies with ultrasound.

Johnson HG, Ekman P, Frieseu W, et al: A behavioral phenotype in the deLange syndrome. Pediatr Res 10:843, 1976.

Kalter H, Warkany J: Congenital malformation, etiologic factors and their role in prevention. N Engl J Med 308:424, 1983.

Kazazian HH Jr: The nature of mutation. Hosp Pract, Feb, 1985, p 55.

McKusick VA: Mendelian Inheritance in Man. Catalog of Autosomal Dominant, Autosomal Recessive and X-linked Phenotypes. 8th ed. Baltimore, The Johns Hopkins University Press, 1988.

Shepard TH: A Catalog of Teratogenic Agents, 5th ed. Baltimore, The Johns Hopkins University Press, 1986.

Jones KL: Smith's Recognizable Patterns of Human Malformation, 4th ed. Philadelphia, WB Saunders, 1988.

8

METABOLIC DISEASES

8.1 INTRODUCTION

Many disorders originate in mutational events that alter the genetic constitution of an individual, disrupting normal function. Hundreds of human hereditary biochemical disorders, termed "inborn errors of metabolism" by Garrod at the turn of the century, have been discovered, and they are continually being discovered.

Now modern biochemical genetics can describe how genetic information is translated into the synthesis of proteins having specific metabolic or structural properties (see Sec. 7.1). An inherited mutational event can result in the alteration of either primary protein structure or the amount of the specific protein being synthesized. In either case, the functional ability of the protein, whether it is an enzyme, receptor, transport vehicle, membrane pump, or structural element, may be relatively or seriously compromised.

If the process affected by an inborn error of metabolism is essential for well-being and if the degree of alteration is sufficient to affect the system, clinical consequences may result. Some genetic changes are clinically inconsequential and are responsible only for the many polymorphic differences that set individuals apart. Others produce changes that express themselves only under conditions that may not be encountered during the lifetime of an individual. Still others, however, produce a disease state, which may range from very mild to lethal. Most inborn errors of metabolism exhibiting clinical consequences manifest themselves (or can be detected) in the newborn period or shortly thereafter. It is also now possible to screen and detect many of these disorders in utero (see Sec. 9.13).

Children with inborn errors of metabolism may present with one or more of a large variety of signs and symptoms (Table 8–1). These may include metabolic acidosis (Table 8–2), persistent vomiting, failure to thrive, developmental abnormalities, elevated blood or urine levels of a particular metabolite, for example, an amino acid or ammonia, a peculiar odor (Table 8–3), or physical changes such as hepatomegaly. Diagnosis is facilitated by considering those presenting in the neonatal period separately from children presenting later in life.

TABLE 8–1. Some Clinical Findings Often Associated with Inborn Errors of Metabolism

Symptoms or Signs	Examples of Associated Diseases
Neurologic abnormalities	Almost all categories
Metabolic acidosis and ketosis	All organic acidemias
Poor feeding, persistent vomiting, and failure to thrive	Organic acidemias, urea cycle defects, PKU, galactosemia, adrenal insufficiency
Liver disease	Tyrosinemia, glycogen storage, galactosemia, Wilson disease, hereditary fructose intolerance, α_1-antitrypsin deficiency, hemochromatosis, lipidoses
Miscellaneous	
Clinical: dislocated lenses, renal stones, thrombosis, deafness, microcephaly, cataracts, hematuria, self-mutilation, abnormal urine odor (see Table 8–3) or color, coarse facies, persistent eczema, abnormal hair	
Laboratory: osteoporosis, rickets, hypoglycemia, unexplained jaundice, abnormal liver function	

NEONATAL PERIOD. Inborn errors of metabolism causing *clinical manifestations* in the neonatal period are usually severe and are often lethal if proper therapy is not promptly initiated. Clinical findings are usually nonspecific and similar to those seen in infants with generalized infections. An inborn error of metabolism should be considered in the differential diagnosis of a severely ill neonatal infant, and special studies should be undertaken if the index of suspicion is high (Fig. 8–1).

Neonatal infants with metabolic disorders are usually normal at birth; however, signs and symptoms such as lethargy, poor feeding, convulsions, and vomiting may develop as early as a few hours after birth. A history of clinical deterioration in a previously normal neonate should suggest an inborn error of metabolism. This clinical course contrasts with many other genetic disorders or perinatal insults, which cause abnormalities from the time of birth. Occasionally, vomiting may be severe enough to suggest the diagnosis of pyloric stenosis, which is usually not present, although it has simultaneously occurred in such infants. Lethargy, poor feeding, convulsions, and coma may also be seen in infants with hypoglycemia (see Sec. 9.57) or hypocalcemia (see Sec. 6.28). Response to intravenous injection of glucose or calcium usually establishes these diagnoses. Since most inborn errors of metabolism are inherited as autosomal recessive traits, a history of consanguinity and/or death in the neonatal period in the immediate family should increase suspicion of this diagnosis. Physical examination usually reveals nonspecific findings, with most signs related to the central nervous system. Hepatomegaly, however, is a common finding in a variety of inborn errors of metabolism. Occasionally, an unusual odor may offer an invaluable aid to the diagnosis (see Table 8–3). A physician caring for a sick infant should smell the patient and his or her excretions; patients with maple syrup urine disease have the unmistakable odor of maple syrup in their urine and their bodies.

Diagnosis usually requires a variety of specific *laboratory studies*. Measuring serum concentrations of ammonia, bicarbonate, and pH is often very helpful in differentiating major causes of metabolic disorders (see Fig. 8–1). Elevation of blood ammonia is usually due to defects in urea cycle enzymes. These infants with elevated blood ammonia levels commonly have normal serum pH and bicarbonate, and without measurement of blood ammonia they may remain undiagnosed and succumb to their disease. Elevation of serum ammonia,

TABLE 8–2. Inborn Errors of Metabolism That May Have Metabolic Acidosis as a Major Component

Disease	Major Metabolites (Acids)
Aminoacidopathies	
Maple syrup urine disease	α-Ketoisocaproic, α-keto-β-methylvaleric, α-ketoisovaleric, indoleacetic, ketones*
Isovaleric acidemia	Isovaleric, *N*-isovalerylglycine, β-hydroxyisovaleric, ketones*
3-Methylcrotonylglycinuria	3-Methylcrotonylglycine, β-hydroxyisovaleric, 2-oxoglutaric, ketones*
3-Hydroxy-3-methylglutaric aciduria	3-Hydroxyisovaleric, 3-methylglutaric, 3-methylglutaconic, 3-hydroxy-3-methylglutaric
α-Methylacetoacetic aciduria	α-Methyl-β-hydroxybutyric, α-methylacetoacetic, ketones*
Propionic acidemia	Propionic, propionylglycine, β-hydroxypropionate, methylcitric, ketones*
Methylmalonic acidemia	Methylmalonic, ketones*
Pyroglutamic acidemia	Pyroglutamic (5-oxoproline)
α-Ketoadipic aciduria	α-Ketoadipic, α-hydroxyadipic, α-aminoadipic,1,2-butenedicarboxylic
Glutaric acidemia	Glutaric, lactic, isobutyric, isovaleric, α-methylbutyric
Multiple carboxylase deficiency	α- and β-Hydroxybutyric, 3-hydroxyisovaleric, propionic, 3-methylcrotonylglycine, lactic ketones*
Hawkinsinuria	4-Hydroxycyclohexylacetic, hawkinsin
Organic Acidemias	
Multiple acyl-CoA dehydrogenase deficiency (glutaric acidemia type II)	2-Ethylmalonic, adipic, glutaric, C8 and C10 dicarboxylic, ω-hydroxy acids, glutaric hexanoylglycine, ketones*
Ethylmalonic aciduria	2-Ethylmalonic, adipic
γ-Hydroxybutyric aciduria	γ-Hydroxybutyric
Defects in Carbohydrate Metabolism	
Diabetes mellitus	Lactic, ketones*
Fructose-1,6-diphosphatase deficiency	Lactic, pyruvic, ketones*
Succinyl-CoA transferase deficiency	Ketones*
Glycogen storage disease, type I	Lactic, pyruvic, ketones*
Pyruvate carboxylase deficiency	Lactic, pyruvic
Pyruvate dehydrogenase complex deficiency	Lactic, pyruvic

*Acetoacetic and β-hydroxybutyric.

Diagnosis of the diseases listed among the aminoacidopathies can be made through detection of the corresponding metabolite in urine by various techniques such as column or gas or high-pressure liquid chromatography or by measuring enzyme activity in cultures of skin fibroblasts. Of the carbohydrate defects, only succinyl-CoA transferase deficiency can be detected in fibroblasts. Deficiency of fructose-1,6-diphosphatase can be demonstrated in white cells. Glycogen storage type I and pyruvate carboxylase defects must be detected in liver biopsies. In addition to the above, acidosis has been reported in a patient with acute tyrosinemia and in patients with oxalosis and renal tubular acidosis, in whom persistent acidosis is due primarily to a renal defect rather than being a direct effect of the metabolic error.

however, has also been observed in some infants with certain organic acidemias. These infants are severely acidotic because of accumulation of organic acids in body fluids.

When blood ammonia, pH, and bicarbonate are normal, other aminoacidopathies such as hyperglycinemia and galactosemia should be considered; galactosemic infants may also manifest cataracts, hepatomegaly, ascites, and jaundice.

Most inborn errors of metabolism presenting in the neonatal period are lethal if specific *therapy* is not initiated immediately. Specific diagnosis, even in an infant in whom death seems inevitable, is of great importance for genetic counseling of the family (see Sec. 7.33). Therefore, every effort should be made to determine the diagnosis while the infant is alive; postmortem examination is usually not helpful.

CHILDREN AFTER THE NEONATAL PERIOD. Most inborn errors of metabolism that cause symptoms in the first few days of life exhibit milder variant forms that have a more insidious onset. These forms may escape detection during the neonatal period, and the diagnosis may be delayed for months or even years. The early clinical manifestations in children with these forms are commonly nonspecific and may be attributed to perinatal insults.

TABLE 8–3. Inborn Errors of Amino Acid Metabolism Associated with Abnormal Odor

Inborn Error of Metabolism	Urine Odor
Glutaric acidemia (type II)	Sweaty feet
Hawkinsinuria	Swimming pool
Isovaleric acidemia	Sweaty feet
Maple syrup urine disease	Maple syrup
Methionine malabsorption	Cabbage
β-Methylcrotonylglycinuria	Tomcat urine
Oasthouse urine disease	Hop-like
Phenylketonuria	Mousy or musty
Trimethylaminuria	Rotting fish
Tyrosinemia	Rancid, fishy, or cabbage-like

Clinical manifestations such as mental retardation, motor deficits, and convulsions are the most constant findings in some of these children. There may be an episodic or intermittent pattern with episodes of acute clinical manifestations separated by periods of seemingly disease-free states. The episodes are usually triggered by a stress or a nonspecific insult such as an infection. The child may die during one of these acute attacks. An inborn error of metabolism should be considered in any child with one or more of the following manifestations: (1) unexplained mental retardation, developmental delay, motor deficits, or convulsions; (2) unusual odor, particularly during an acute illness; (3) intermittent episodes of unexplained vomiting, acidosis, mental deterioration, or coma; (4) hepatomegaly; or (5) renal stones.

Inborn errors of metabolism of a given pedigree run true to type. Thus, although symptomatology may vary among siblings, usually if one child in a family has the form of maple syrup urine disease manifested during the neonatal period, the next affected sibling will have the same defect, not the variant that occurs only intermittently later in childhood.

IRAJ REZVANI
VICTOR H. AUERBACH

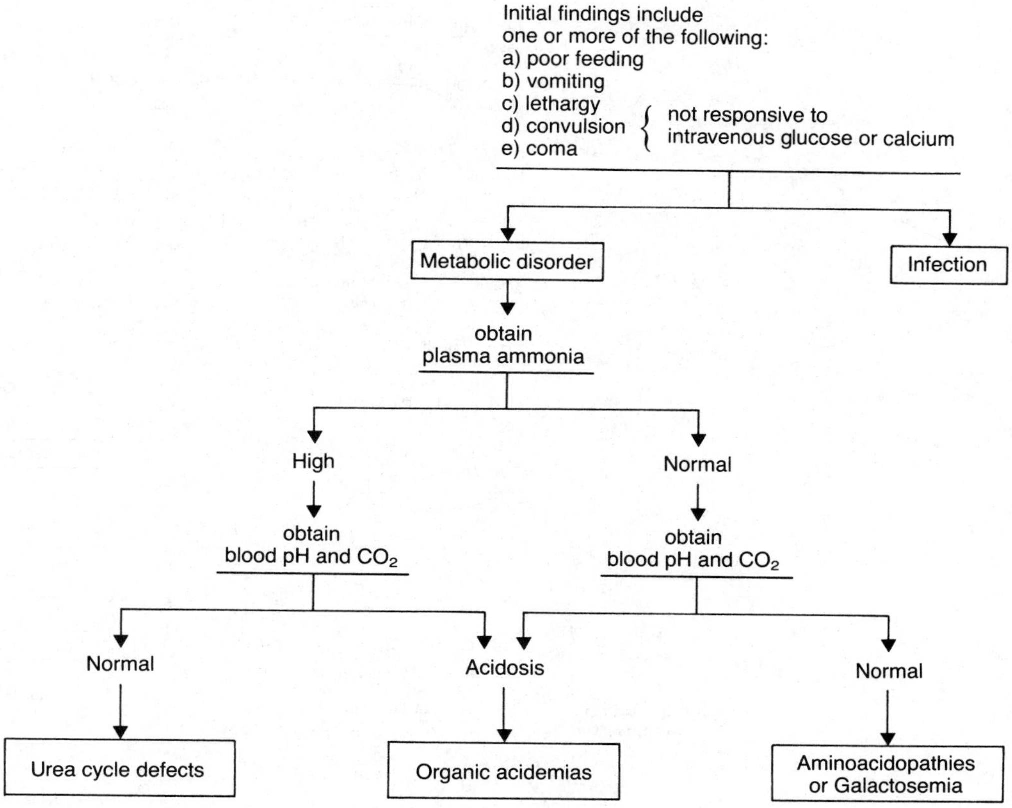

Figure 8–1. Clinical approach to a newborn infant with a suspected metabolic disorder. This schema is a guide to the elucidation of some of the metabolic disorders in newborn infants. Although some exceptions to this schema exist, it is appropriate for most cases.

DEFECTS IN METABOLISM OF AMINO ACIDS

8.2 PHENYLALANINE

Phenylalanine is an essential amino acid. Dietary phenylalanine not utilized for protein synthesis is normally degraded via the tyrosine pathway (Fig. 8–2). Deficiency of the enzyme phenylalanine hydroxylase or of its cofactor tetrahydrobiopterin causes accumulation of phenylalanine in body fluids. Several clinically and biochemically distinct forms of hyperphenylalaninemia exist.

CLASSIC PHENYLKETONURIA (PKU). This form of the disorder is caused by the complete or near-complete deficiency of phenylalanine hydroxylase. Excess phenylalanine is transaminated to phenylpyruvic acid or decarboxylated to phenylethylamine (see Fig. 8–2). These and subsequent metabolites, along with excess phenylalanine, disrupt normal metabolism and cause brain damage.

Clinical Manifestations. The affected infant is normal at birth. Mental retardation may develop gradually and may not be evident for a few months. It has been estimated that an untreated infant loses about 50 points in IQ by the end of the 1st yr of life. Mental retardation is usually severe, and most patients require institutional care. Vomiting, sometimes severe enough to be misdiagnosed as pyloric stenosis, may be an early symptom. Older untreated children become hyperactive with purposeless movements, rhythmic rocking, and athetosis.

On physical examination these infants are blonder than unaffected siblings; they have fair skin and blue eyes. Some may have a seborrheic or eczematoid skin rash, which is usually mild and disappears as the child grows older. These children have an unpleasant odor of phenylacetic acid, which has been described as musty, mousey, or wolf-like. There are no consistent findings on neurologic examination. However, most infants are hypertonic with hyperactive deep tendon reflexes. About one fourth of children have seizures, and more than 50% have electroencephalographic (EEG) abnormalities. Microcephaly, prominent maxilla with widely spaced teeth, enamel hypoplasia, and growth retardation are other common findings in untreated children. The clinical manifestations of classic PKU are rarely seen in those countries in which neonatal screening programs for the detection of PKU are in effect.

Diagnosis. Infants with PKU are clinically normal at birth, and tests of their urine for phenylpyruvic acid may be negative in the first few days of life; accordingly, the diagnosis depends on measuring blood levels of phenylalanine. The bacterial inhibition assay method of Guthrie is widely used in the newborn period to screen for PKU. This test requires a few drops of capillary blood, which are placed on a filter paper and mailed to the laboratory for assay. Blood phenylalanine in affected infants may rise to levels necessary to render the Guthrie test positive as early as 4 hr after birth in the absence of any protein feeding. It is recommended, however, that the blood for screening be obtained after 72 hr of life and preferably after feeding proteins in order to reduce the possibility of false-negative results. When this test indicates an elevated level of phenylalanine, the phenylalanine and tyrosine concentrations of the plasma should be measured. The criteria for diagnosis of classic PKU are: (1) a plasma phenylalanine level above 20 mg/dL (1.2 mM); (2) a normal plasma tyrosine level; (3) increased urinary levels of metabolites of phenylalanine (phenylpyruvic and o-hydroxyphenylacetic acids); and (4) a normal concentration of the cofactor tetrahydrobiopterin.

Treatment. The goal of therapy is to reduce phenylalanine

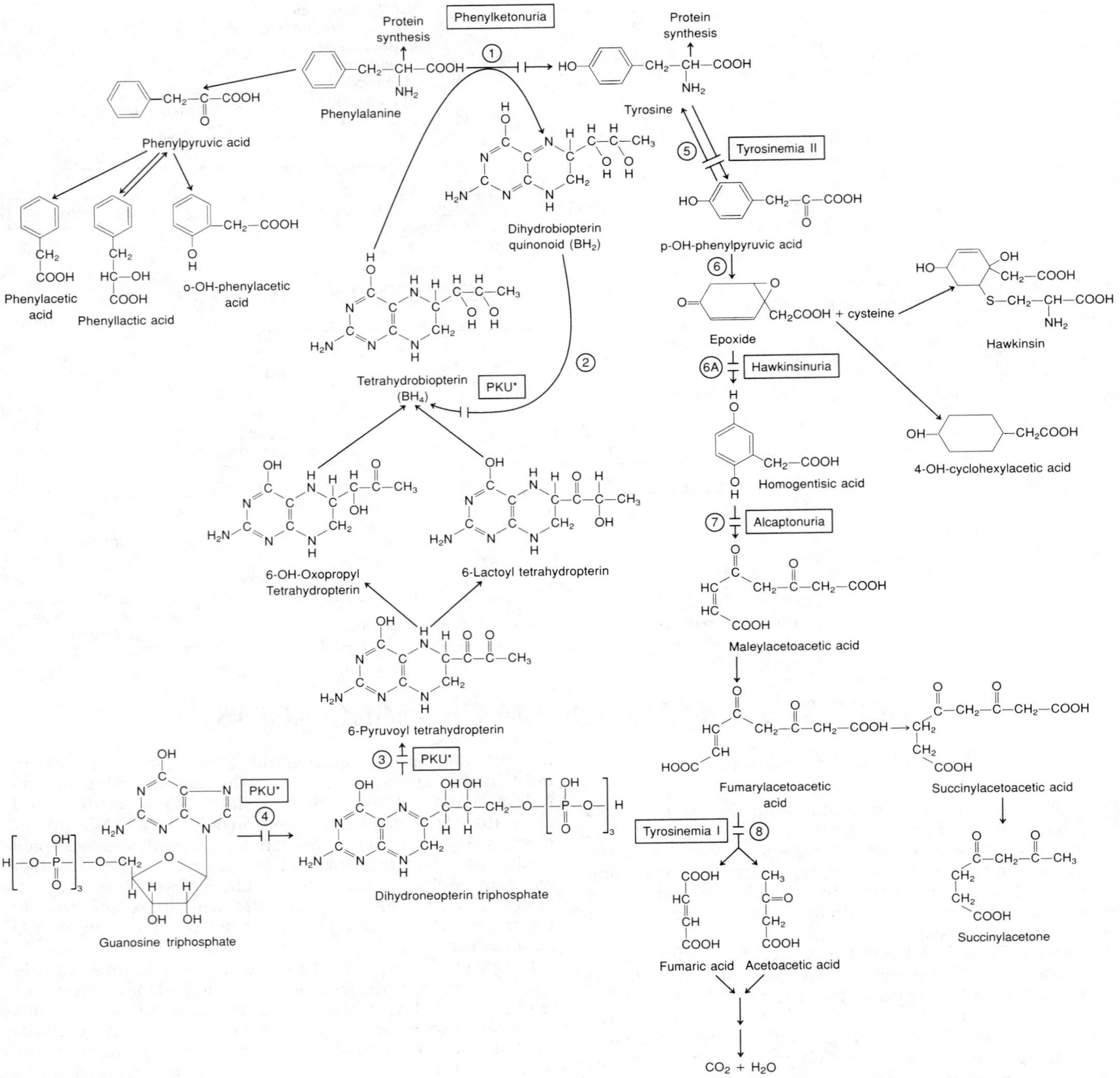

Figure 8–2. Pathways of phenylalanine and tyrosine metabolism. Inborn errors are depicted as bars crossing the reaction arrow(s). PKU* refers to defects of BH_4 metabolism that affect the phenylalanine, tyrosine, and tryptophan hydroxylases. See Figures 8–3 and 8–5. **Enzymes**: (1) phenylalanine hydroxylase; (2) dihydropteridine reductase; (3) 6-pyruvoyltetrahydropterin synthase; (4) guanosine triphosphate (GTP) cyclohydrolase; (5) tyrosine aminotransferase (6 + 6A)-p-OH-phenylpyruvic acid oxidase; (6) intramolecular rearrangement; (7) homogentisic acid oxidase; (8) fumarylacetoacetate hydrolyase.

and its metabolites in body fluids in order to prevent or minimize brain damage. This can be achieved by instituting a diet low in phenylalanine; formulas low in this essential amino acid are now available commercially.* Administration of the low-phenylalanine diet requires close nutritional supervision and frequent monitoring of the serum concentration of phenylalanine. The optimal serum level to be maintained probably lies between 3 mg/dL (0.18 mM) and 15 mg/dL (0.9 mM). Because phenylalanine is not synthesized in the body, "overtreatment," particularly in rapidly growing infants, may lead to phenylalanine deficiency, manifested by lethargy, anorexia, anemia, rashes, diarrhea, and even death; moreover, tyrosine becomes an essential amino acid in this disorder

*Dietary management with this milk substitute is described in "Phenylketonuria—Low Phenylalanine Dietary Management with Lofenalac", a pamphlet available from Mead Johnson Laboratories, Evansville, Indiana 47721.

and its adequate intake must be ensured. Dietary treatment should be started as soon after birth as the diagnosis is established.

The duration of diet therapy is controversial. Although rigid diet control may be relaxed after 6 yr of age, some form of restriction in dietary phenylalanine may be necessary indefinitely. Dietary management is almost inevitably complicated by emotional problems resulting from dietary restriction and the abnormal eating habits imposed upon child and family. Therefore, parents and children need continuous skillful and empathetic support and guidance.

Pregnancy in Mothers with PKU. Pregnant women with PKU who are not on a low-phenylalanine diet have a higher risk of spontaneous abortion than the general population. Infants born to such mothers are often mentally retarded and may have microcephaly and/or a congenital heart anomaly. These complications seem to be related to high levels of blood phenylalanine. Prospective mothers who have PKU should be started on a low-phenylalanine diet before conception, and every effort should be made to keep blood phenylalanine levels below 10 mg/dL throughout pregnancy.

HYPERPHENYLALANINEMIA DUE TO DEFICIENCY OF COFACTOR TETRAHYDROBIOPTERIN (BH_4). In about 2% of infants with hyperphenylalaninemia, the defect resides in one of the enzymes necessary for production or recycling of BH_4. Historically, these infants were diagnosed as having PKU, but they deteriorated neurologically despite adequate control of serum phenylalanine; BH_4 was then shown to be a cofactor for tyrosine and tryptophan hydroxylases, which are essential for biosynthesis of the neurotransmitters dopamine (see Fig. 8–3) and serotonin (see Fig. 8–5). Today, patients with BH_4 deficiency are diagnosed very early in life because all patients with hyperphenylalaninemia are tested for the possibility of this cofactor deficiency.

BH_4 is synthesized from guanosine triphosphate and is oxidized to quinonoid dihydrobiopterin (BH_2) during the hydroxylation of phenylalanine by phenylalanine hydroxylase. The quinonoid dihydrobiopterin is reduced by the enzyme dihydropteridine reductase to regenerate BH_4 (see Fig. 8–2). Three enzyme deficiencies leading to defective BH_4 formation have been described. More than half of the reported patients have had a deficiency of 6-pyruvoyltetrahydropterin synthase (6-PTS). Four patients with a deficiency of guanosine triphosphate cyclohydrolase have been reported. The remaining patients have had a deficiency of dihydropteridine reductase.

The *clinical manifestations* of these disorders are similar and are usually indistinguishable from those of classic PKU. These patients are identified during screening programs for PKU because of evidence of hyperphenylalaninemia, but neurologic manifestations such as loss of head control, hypertonia, drooling, swallowing difficulties, and myoclonic seizures develop after 3 mo of age despite adequate dietary therapy. Plasma phenylalanine levels may be as high as those in classic PKU or in the range of benign (persistent) hyperphenyalaninemia (<1.0 mM).

Diagnosis of BH_4 deficiency and the responsible enzyme defect may be established by performing one of the following tests:

1. Measurement of neopterin (oxidative product of dihydroneopterin triphosphate) and biopterin (oxidative product of dihydro- and tetrahydrobiopterin) in body fluids, especially urine. In patients with 6-pyruvoyltetrahydropterin synthase deficiency, there is a marked elevation of neopterin and a concomitant decrease in biopterin excretion (neopterin-biopterin ratio is high). In patients with GTP cyclohydrolase deficiency, urinary excretion of both neopterin and biopterin is very low, and in patients with dihydropteridine reductase deficiency, neopterin is normal, but biopterin is very high (neopterin-biopterin ratio is low). Excretion of biopterin increases in this enzyme deficiency because the quinonoid dihydrobiopterin cannot be recycled into BH_4.

2. BH_4 loading test. An oral or intravenous (more reliable if feasible) dose of BH_4 (2–10 mg/kg) normalizes plasma phenylalanine in patients with BH_4 deficiency within 4–6 hr. This test should be done while the child is receiving normal amounts of phenylalanine in the diet. Some patients with dihydropteridine reductase deficiency may not respond to this loading test.

3. Enzyme assay. The activity of dihydropteridine reductase can be measured in many tissues including liver, leukocytes, red blood cells, and cultured fibroblasts. 6-Pyruvoyltetrahydropterin synthase can be measured in liver, kidney, and red blood cells. GTP cyclohydrolase can be measured in liver and in phytohemagglutinin-stimulated lymphocytes (the enzyme activity is normally very low in unstimulated lymphocytes). Measurement of the last two enzymes is technically difficult, and assays are not readily available.

Treatment. The long-term efficacy of various therapies is unknown. The various treatment methods include the following:

1. Low-phenylalanine diet. Although phenylalanine does not prevent neurologic damage, such a diet in conjunction with the following therapies is recommended for at least the first 2 yr of life. High levels of phenylalanine inhibit synthesis of neurotransmitters.

2. Neurotransmitter precursors. Administration of L-dopa and 5-hydroxytryptophan seems to be the most effective treatment and may prevent neurologic damage if started early in life. Therefore, *all patients with PKU and hyperphenylalaninemia should be tested for BH_4 deficiency as early as possible*. Treatment started after 6 mo of age, although resulting in some improvement, has not reversed existing neurologic damage.

3. BH_4 replacement. Oral administration of the cofactor in small daily doses normalizes serum levels of phenylalanine. This compound, unless given at high doses (20–40 mg/kg/24 hr), does not readily cross the blood-brain barrier, and neurologic damage may continue to progress.

BENIGN HYPERPHENYLALANINEMIA. Infants with hyperphenylalaninemia are occasionally identified whose blood levels of phenylalanine are only slightly elevated; these concentrations are not enough (less than 20 mg/dL or 1.2 mM) to result in the excretion of phenylpyruvic acid. Like infants with classic PKU, these patients presumably have a deficiency of the phenylalanine hydroxylase enzyme but with some residual enzyme activity; measured activity has ranged from 1–35% of normal, in contrast to the nondetectable enzyme activity found in classic PKU. These infants have been detected by screening tests in the neonatal period; they are asymptomatic and may develop normally without special dietary treatment. They should, however, be tested for the presence of the cofactor tetrahydrobiopterin, and if it is deficient they should be treated accordingly (see earlier).

For infants who have serum phenylalanine concentrations in the range of 10–20 mg/dL, with normal tyrosine values and no PKU, a simple reduction of dietary protein intake may be sufficient to control serum concentrations of phenylalanine; if this is not effective, specific restriction of dietary phenylalanine is indicated. All infants who are not treated with dietary restriction should be systematically monitored with repeated determinations of plasma phenylalanine and developmental evaluations to establish the safety of continuing partial treatment or nontreatment. Periodic challenges with natural protein may be helpful in determining the need for continuing dietary restriction.

TRANSIENT HYPERPHENYLALANINEMIA. Moderately elevated levels of phenylalanine occur in transient tyrosinemia of the newborn infant (see Sec. 8.3). When the infant's ability to oxidize tyrosine matures, the elevated levels of tyrosine and phenylalanine return to normal.

Absence of or delayed maturation of phenylalanine transaminase can also produce hyperphenylalaninemia if the patient is fed milk with a high protein content. Such infants cannot produce much phenylpyruvic acid even when their blood levels of phenylalanine approach 30 mg/dL; they have normal blood levels when fed milk products having the protein content of human milk.

GENETICS AND PREVALENCE. All defects causing persistent hyperphenylalaninemia and PKU are inherited as autosomal recessives. They have a collective prevalence of 1:10,000 to 1:20,000 live births, with classic PKU being the most common and GTP cyclohydrolase the rarest. The gene for phenylalanine hydroxylase is located on the long arm of chromosome 12. Prenatal diagnosis and carrier detection are possible using specific genetic probes in cells obtained from chorionic villus biopsy.

8.3 TYROSINE

Tyrosine, obtained from ingested protein and synthesized endogenously from phenylalanine, is used for protein synthesis and is a precursor of dopamine, norepinephrine, epinephrine, melanin, and thyroxine. Excess tyrosine is metabolized to carbon dioxide and water (see Fig. 8–2). At least two distinct clinical entities are associated with a persistent increase in plasma concentrations of tyrosine, but only in tyrosinemia type II are signs and symptoms attributed to high levels of tyrosine in body fluids. In hereditary tyrosinemia type I the causal relationship with increased tyrosine levels remains unclear. There are also patients who present varied clinical findings and tyrosinemia but do not fit into any specific category, and a transient form of tyrosinemia is seen in newborn infants.

TYROSINEMIA TYPE I (Tyrosinosis, Hereditary Tyrosinemia, Hepatorenal Tyrosinemia). In this condition, caused by a deficiency of the enzyme fumarylacetoacetate hydrolyase, a moderate elevation of serum tyrosine is associated with severe involvement of the liver, kidney, and central nervous system. These findings are thought to be due to an accumulation of intermediate metabolites of tyrosine in the body, especially succinylacetone. Decreased activities of 4-hydroxyphenylpyruvic acid oxidase and maleylacetoacetate hydroxylase observed in this condition are presumed to be secondary phenomena (see Fig. 8–2).

Clinical Manifestations. There are two main forms of the disease: the neonatal or acute form, which comprises most reported cases, and the chronic or latent form. Intermediate forms also occur. Acute and chronic forms have been observed within the same family.

Infants having the *acute form* become symptomatic within the first 6 mo of life. Failure to thrive, developmental delay, irritability, vomiting, diarrhea, and fever are among the early manifestations. Hepatomegaly, jaundice, hypoglycemia, and bleeding tendencies as manifested by melena, hematuria, and ecchymosis are common findings. A cabbage-like odor of some infants is related to metabolites of methionine. Death from hepatic failure usually occurs before the 2nd yr of life.

In the *chronic form,* clinical manifestations may not appear until after the 1st yr of age. Failure to thrive, developmental delay, progressive cirrhosis, renal tubular dysfunction (Fanconi syndrome), and vitamin D–resistant rickets are characteristic. Episodes of acute polyneuropathy resembling acute porphyria have been observed in about 40% of affected infants. These episodes are characterized by severe pains in the legs (occasionally in the abdomen), hypertonia, vomiting, paralytic ileus, and occasionally self-mutilation. Elevation of urinary δ-aminolevulinic acid (presumably due to inhibition of δ-aminolevulinic hydratase by succinylacetone) has been observed in these patients, but the relationship of this abnormality to the polyneuropathic crises is unclear because the urinary excretion of δ-aminolevulinic acid remains elevated between the attacks. Death usually occurs by 10 yr of age from liver failure or hepatoma.

Laboratory findings include normocytic anemia and marked elevations of serum bilirubin (both conjugated and unconjugated), serum transaminases, and α-fetoprotein. An increase in serum levels of α-fetoprotein has been observed in the cord blood of affected infants indicating intrauterine liver damage. Plasma levels of tyrosine and other amino acids, especially methionine, are moderately increased. Generalized aminoaciduria occurs. Urinary excretion of δ-aminolevulinic acid may be increased. The presence of succinylacetoacetate and succinylacetone in serum and urine is diagnostic (see Fig. 8–2). Liver histology is usually compatible with chronic active hepatitis and nonspecific cirrhosis. Hyperplasia of pancreatic islet cells is also a common finding.

This condition should be differentiated from other causes of hepatitis and hepatic failure in infants including galactosemia, hereditary fructose intolerance, and giant cell hepatitis. *Diagnosis* is established by measurement of fumarylacetoacetate hydrolyase activity in liver biopsy specimens or fibroblast cultured cells. The degree of residual enzyme activity dictates the severity of the disease.

Treatment. A diet low in tyrosine, phenylalanine, and methionine may result in some clinical improvement in some patients. However, in most patients the progression of the disease cannot be halted by diet alone. Liver transplantation may be the only effective treatment for patients who do not respond to diet therapy.

Tyrosinemia type I is an autosomal recessive trait. Most reported patients have a French-Canadian ancestry. The prevalence of the condition is estimated to be 1 in 12,000 in the French-Canadian population of Quebec. Prenatal diagnosis has been achieved by measurement of succinylacetone in amniotic fluid and by the enzyme assay in chorionic villus biopsy.

TYROSINEMIA TYPE II (Richner-Hanhart Syndrome, Oculocutaneous Tyrosinemia). This rare autosomal recessive disorder results in mental retardation, palmar and plantar punctate hyperkeratosis, and herpetiform corneal ulcers. Corneal lesions usually occur during the first few months of life and are presumed to be due to tyrosine deposition; skin lesions may develop later in life. Mental retardation is usually mild to moderate and may be associated with self-mutilation.

Significant hypertyrosinemia (20–50 mg/dL) and tyrosinuria are present. The condition is due to the deficiency of the cytosolic fraction of hepatic tyrosine amino transferase (tyrosine transaminase). In contrast to tyrosinemia type I, liver and kidney functions, as well as serum concentrations of other amino acids, are normal.

Treatment with a diet low in tyrosine and phenylalanine has not only corrected the chemical abnormalities but has also resulted in dramatic healing of the skin and eye lesions. Mental retardation may be prevented by early dietary restriction of tyrosine. The gene for tyrosine aminotransferase is located on the long arm of chromosome 16.

TRANSIENT TYROSINEMIA OF THE NEWBORN. In 0.5–10% of newborn infants, plasma tyrosine may rise to as high as 60 mg/dL during the first 2 wk of life. Most affected infants are premature and are receiving high-protein diets. Lethargy, poor feeding, and decreased motor activity occur in some of them, but most are asymptomatic and come to medical attention because of a high blood phenylalanine level, rendering the Guthrie test for PKU screening positive. Tyrosinemia usually resolves spontaneously during the 1st mo of life. The condition is presumably due to delayed maturation of *p*-hydroxyphenylpyruvic acid oxidase. The condition is often corrected promptly by reducing the amount of protein in the diet (to 2–3 g/kg/24 hr) and by administering vitamin C (200–400 mg/24 hr). Mild intellectual deficits have been reported in some full-term infants with this disorder. Since vitamin C is necessary for optimal functioning of the oxidase, it is not surprising that tyrosinemia occurs in patients with scurvy.

HAWKINSINURIA. This rare condition (named after the first affected family) is due to a deficiency of one of the components of the 4-hydroxyphenylpyruvic acid oxidase enzyme complex. This enzyme oxidizes 4-hydroxyphenylpyruvic acid to form an epoxide intermediate first; the epoxide metabolite undergoes a rearrangement to form the final product, homogentisic acid (see Fig. 8–2). A block in the rearrangement step leads to an accumulation of the epoxide intermediate, which either is reduced to form 4-hydroxycyclohexylacetic acid (4-HCAA) or reacts with glutathione (or cysteine) to form the unusual organic acid 2-L-cysteine-S-yl-1-4 dihydroxycyclohex-5-en-1-yl-acetic acid (hawkinsin).

Individuals with this disorder become symptomatic only during infancy. The symptoms usually appear after weaning from breast-feeding with the introduction of a high-protein diet. Severe metabolic acidosis, ketosis, failure to thrive, mild hepatomegaly, and an unusual odor (like that of a swimming pool) are common findings. These infants respond well to a diet low in both phenylalanine and tyrosine, and their clinical manifestations resolve spontaneously by 1 yr of age. Adults with this condition are usually asymptomatic despite metabolic abnormalities. Mental development is usually normal.

Affected children and adults excrete 4-hydroxyphenylpyruvic acid and 4-hydroxyphenylacetic acid as well as the two very unusual organic acids 4-HCAA and hawkinsin in their urine.

Treatment consists of a low-protein diet (such as breast milk) or a diet low in phenylalanine and tyrosine. Large doses of vitamin C (up to 1,000 mg/24 hr) are also recommended. No therapy is needed after 1 yr of age. The condition is inherited as an autosomal dominant trait, and all affected patients reported to date have been presumed to be heterozygous for the trait.

ALBINISM. This condition is due to defects in the biosynthesis and distribution of melanin. Melanin is synthesized by melanocytes from tyrosine in a membrane-bound intracellular organelle called the melanosome. The first two steps in the conversion of tyrosine to dopa and dopaquinone are catalyzed by the same enzyme, tyrosinase (Fig. 8–3). Dopaquinone either reacts with cysteine to make pheomelanine, a yellow-red pigment, or undergoes several nonenzymatic steps to form eumelanine, which is brown-black. Genes involved in the biosynthesis and distribution of melanin have not yet been elucidated. As a result, no unified classification for albinism has been developed. Several forms that are presently segregated on the basis of clinical and ethnic differences may prove to be either the allelic forms of one gene or heterozygotic compounds of two different genes. In this section only the major forms are discussed. Albinism (all types) has a worldwide prevalence of 1 in 20,000.

Clinical manifestations common in almost all forms of albinism include depigmentation of skin, iris, and retina. Nystagmus, strabismus, photophobia, decreased visual acuity, and the presence of red reflex are common eye findings. Binocular vision is absent because of a decussation defect in which all optic nerve fibers from one eye completely cross to the other

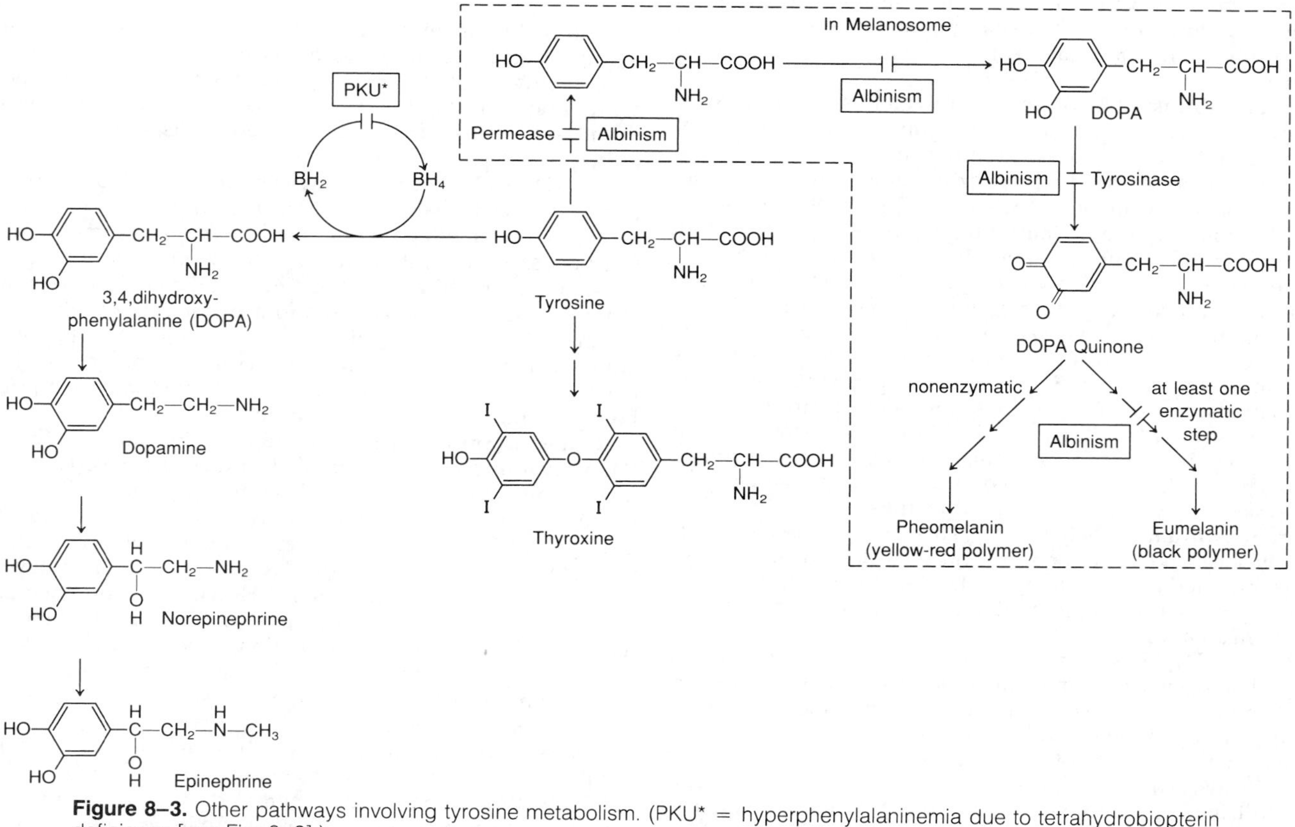

Figure 8–3. Other pathways involving tyrosine metabolism. (PKU* = hyperphenylalaninemia due to tetrahydrobiopterin deficiency [see Fig. 8–2].)

side at the chiasma. Blindness and skin cancer are the two major late sequelae of albinism in its severe forms.

Three major forms can be identified on the basis of clinical manifestations and genetic transmission: oculocutaneous albinism (generalized albinism), which is inherited as an autosomal recessive trait (except for a rare type that is dominantly inherited); ocular albinism, which is inherited as an X-linked or autosomal recessive trait; and partial albinism (piebaldism), which is inherited as an autosomal dominant trait.

Oculocutaneous Albinism. There are at least 10 different variants reported. The most common form is *tyrosinase-positive albinism*. In this condition, some pigment is formed when a plucked hair bulb is incubated with tyrosine. The nature of the defect is not known. However, the cause is expected to be a block in eumelanine synthesis distal to dopaquinone.

Tyrosinase-negative albinism is the second most common and the most severe form of oculocutaneous albinism. In these patients the enzymatic defect resides in the first step of melanin synthesis, and no pigment is made.

Chédiak-Higashi syndrome is a tyrosinase-positive form of partial albinism in which there are abnormal granules in leukocytes and other cells and a susceptibility to infection (see Sec. 16.59). Patients who survive childhood may develop a terminal lymphofollicular malignancy. These patients have reduced numbers of melanosomes, which are abnormally large (macromelanosomes).

Hermansky-Pudlak syndrome is a tyrosinase-positive generalized albinism associated with platelet dysfunction owing to the absence of platelet-dense bodies and an accumulation of ceroids in tissues. The degree of albinism is variable in these patients. This is the third most common cause of albinism and is most prevalent in Puerto Rico. Bleeding tendencies and a prolonged bleeding time are seen in all patients. Ceroid storage disease manifested as restricted fibrotic lung disease and renal failure occurs during the 4th–5th decades of life.

Other types of oculocutaneous albinism include platinum albinism, yellow-mutant albinism, minimal pigment albinism, brown albinism, refous albinism, and autosomal dominant albinism.

Ocular Albinism. In these patients albinism is limited to the eyes (iridis and retina). Nystagmus, decreased visual acuity, and photophobia are common findings in all forms. Skin and hair color are within normal limits but are usually lighter than those in nonaffected siblings. Eyes are usually pale blue to light green. Hair bulb tyrosinase is positive in all cases. Four forms of this condition have been identified, differentiated by their mode of inheritance and additional associated anomalies. Ocular albinism of *Nettleship-Falls* and ocular albinism with *sensorineural deafness* are inherited as X-linked traits. In these forms only the hemizygote male has the complete syndrome. Some abnormal pigmentation of the eye may also be seen in heterozygote female carriers. *Autosomal recessive ocular albinism* is the third type of ocular albinism; it has manifestations similar to those of the X-linked form. The fourth form of the condition is *autosomal dominant ocular albinism*, with lentigines and deafness.

Partial Albinism (Piebaldism). This disorder is characterized by localized areas of skin and hair devoid of pigment and is inherited as a dominant trait. In some instances a white forelock or patch of depigmented hair elsewhere may be the sole manifestation.

ALCAPTONURIA. This autosomal recessive disorder is due to a deficiency of homogentisic acid oxidase, which causes large amounts of homogentisic acid to accumulate in the body and then to be excreted in the urine (see Fig. 8–2).

Clinical manifestations of alcaptonuria consist of ochronosis and arthritis. These findings may not become evident until midadult life. The only sign of the disorder in the pediatric age group is a darkening of the urine to almost a black color on standing. This is caused by oxidation and polymerization of the homogentisic acid and is enhanced with an alkaline pH. Therefore, an acid urine may not become dark even after many hours of standing. This is one of the reasons why darkening of the urine may never be noted in an affected person, and the diagnosis may be delayed until adulthood, when arthritis or ochronosis occurs. **Ochronosis**, a term used to describe the darkening of tissue, is due to a slow accumulation of the black polymer of homogentisic acid in cartilage and other mesenchymal tissues. It is manifested clinically as dark, blackened spots in the sclera or as diffuse blackish pigmentation of the conjunctiva, cornea, and ear cartilage. Arthritis is the only disabling effect of this condition, which occurs in almost all affected subjects with advancing age. It involves the large joints (spine, hip, and knee) and is usually more severe in men. The arthritis has the clinical characteristics of rheumatoid arthritis, but the radiologic findings are typical of osteoarthritis. Degenerative changes in the lumbar spine are quite characteristic with narrowing of the joint spaces and fusion of the vertebral bodies. The pathogenesis of arthritic changes remains unclear. High incidences of heart disease (mitral and aortic valvulitis, calcification of the heart valves, and myocardial infarction) have also been noted.

The *diagnosis* is confirmed by measurement of homogentisic acid in urine. Affected subjects may excrete as much as 4–8 g of this compound daily. Homogentisic acid is a strong reducing agent that produces a positive reaction with Fehling or Benedict reagent (but not with glucose oxidase). The dark urine of phenol poisoning and that associated with melanotic tumors do not have these reducing properties. The enzyme is expressed only in the liver and kidneys.

There is no effective *treatment* for this disorder.

8.4 METHIONINE

The normal pathway for catabolism of methionine, an essential amino acid, produces *S*-adenosylmethionine, which serves as a methyl group donor for methylation of a variety of compounds in the body, and cysteine, which is formed through a series of reactions called trans-sulfuration (Fig. 8–4).

HOMOCYSTINURIA (Homocystinemia). Most homocysteine, an intermediate compound of methionine degradation, is normally remethylated to methionine. This methionine-sparing reaction is catalyzed by the enzyme methionine synthase, which requires a metabolite of folic acid (5-methyltetrahydrofolate) as a substrate and a metabolite of vitamin B_{12} (methylcobalamin) as a cofactor (see Fig. 8–4). Homocysteine (and its dimer homocystine) ordinarily is not detectable in plasma or urine. Three major forms of homocystinemia and homocystinuria have been identified.

Homocystinuria Due to Cystathionine Synthase Deficiency (Homocystinuria Type I, Classic Homocystinuria). This is the most common inborn error of methionine metabolism. The prevalence of this autosomal recessive condition is estimated at 1 in 200,000 live births. The gene for cystathionine synthase is located on the long arm of chromosome 21. Heterozygote carriers are usually asymptomatic. However, thromboembolic disease has been shown to be more common in these individuals than in the normal population. About 40% of affected patients respond to high doses of vitamin B_6 and usually have milder clinical manifestations than those who are unresponsive to vitamin B_6 therapy.

Infants with this disorder are normal at birth. *Clinical manifestations* during infancy are nonspecific and may include failure to thrive and developmental delay. The diagnosis is usually made after 3 yr of age, when subluxation of the ocular

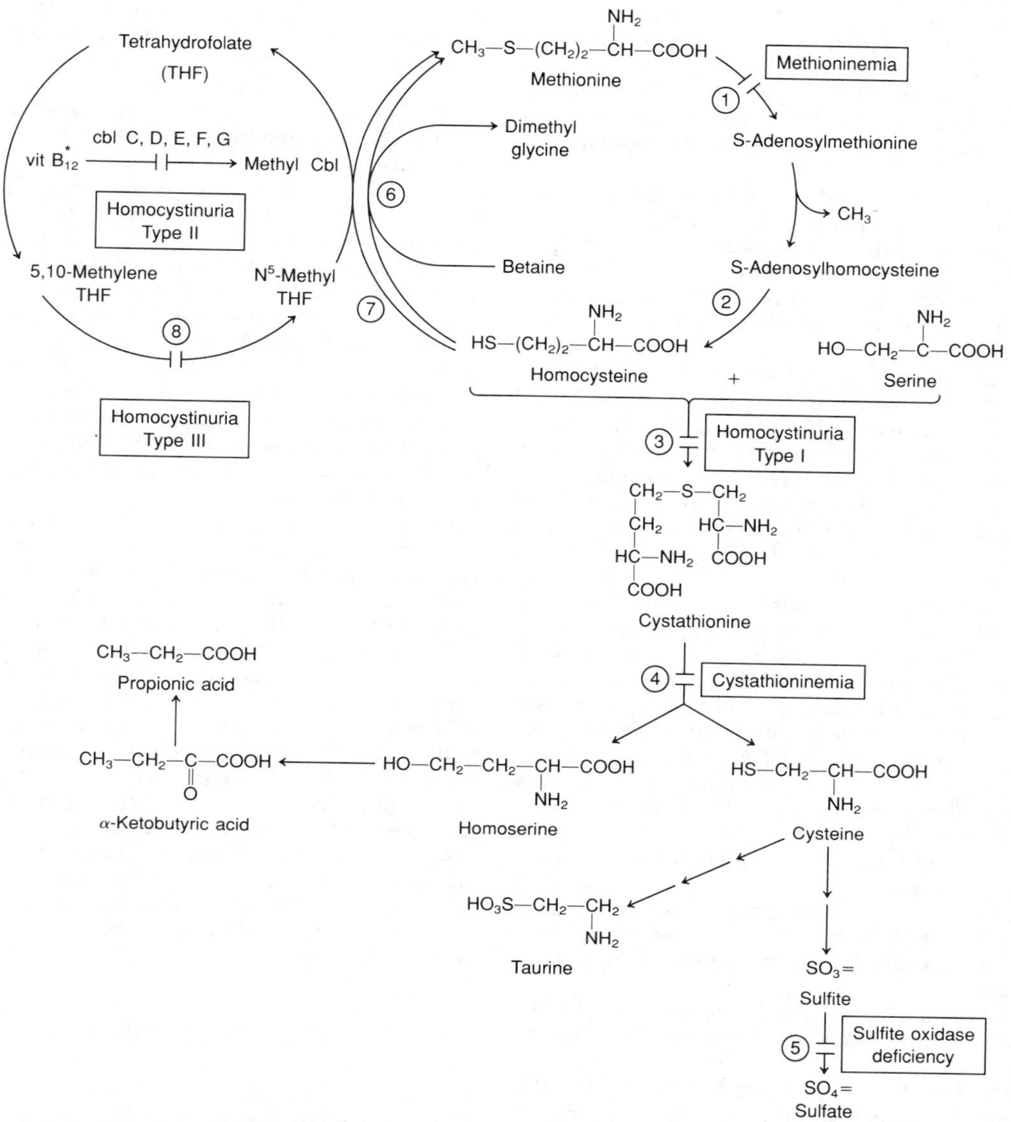

Figure 8–4. Pathways in the metabolism of the sulfur-containing amino acids. **Enzymes**: (1) methionine adenosyltransferase; (2) adenosylhomocysteine hydrolase; (3) cystathionine synthase; (4) cystathionase; (5) sulfite oxidase; (6) betaine homocysteine methyltransferase; (7) methionine synthase; (8) methylene tetrahydrofolate reductase.
*See Figure 8–6 for details of vitamin B_{12} metabolism.

lens (ectopia lentis) occurs. This causes severe myopia and iridodonesis (quivering of the iris). Astigmatism, glaucoma, staphyloma, cataracts, retinal detachment, and optic atrophy may develop later in life. Progressive mental retardation is common. Normal intelligence, however, has been reported in some patients. Psychiatric disorders have been observed in more than 50% of affected patients. Convulsions occur in about 20% of patients. Affected individuals with homocystinuria manifest skeletal abnormalities resembling those of Marfan syndrome (see Sec. 24.56); they are usually tall and thin with elongated limbs and arachnodactyly. Scoliosis, pectus excavatum or carinum, genu valgum, pes cavus, high arched palate, and crowding of the teeth are commonly seen. These children usually have fair complexions, blue eyes, and a peculiar malar flush. Generalized osteoporosis is the main roentgenographic finding. Thromboembolic episodes involving both large and small vessels, especially those of the brain, are common and may occur at any age. Optic atrophy, paralysis, seizure disorders, cor pulmonale, and severe hypertension (due to renal infarcts) are among the serious consequences of thromboembolism, which is due to changes in the vascular walls and increased platelet adhesiveness secondary to elevated homocystine levels. The risk of thromboembolism increases following surgical procedures.

Elevations of both methionine and homocystine (or homocysteine) in body fluids are the diagnostic *laboratory findings*. Freshly voided urine should be tested for homocystine, since this compound is unstable and may disappear as the urine is stored. Cystine is low or absent in plasma. The *diagnosis* may be established by assay of the enzyme in liver biopsy specimens, cultured fibroblasts, or phytohemagglutinin-stimulated lymphocytes. Prenatal diagnosis is feasible by performing an enzyme assay of cultured amniotic cells or chorionic villi.

Treatment with high doses of vitamin B_6 (200–1,000 mg/24 hr) causes dramatic improvement in patients who are responsive to this therapy, but some patients may not respond because of folate depletion; therefore, a patient should not be considered unresponsive to vitamin B_6 until folic acid (1–5 mg/24 hr) has been added to the treatment regimen. Restriction of methionine intake in conjunction with cysteine supplementation is recommended for all patients regardless of their response to vitamin B_6. Betaine (trimethylglycine, 6–9 g/24 hr), which also serves as a methyl group donor, lowers homocysteine levels in body fluids by remethylating homocysteine to methionine. This treatment has produced clinical improvement in patients who are unresponsive to vitamin B_6 therapy.

Homocystinuria Due to Defects in Methylcobalamin Formation (Homocystinuria Type II). Methylcobalamin is the cofactor for the enzyme methionine synthase, which catalyzes remethylation of homocysteine to methionine. There are at least five distinct defects in the intracellular metabolism of cobalamin that may interfere with the formation of methylcobalamin. These are designated as *cbl* C, *cbl* D, *cbl* E, *cbl* G, and *cbl* F (see Figs. 8–4 and 8–6). However, the exact nature of these defects is unknown. Patients with *cbl* C, *cbl* D, and *cbl* F defects have methylmalonic aciduria in addition to homocystinuria because formation of both adenosylcobalamin and methylcobalamin is impaired (see Sec. 8.7). Patients with *cbl* E and *cbl* G defects are unable to form methylcobalamin and develop homocystinuria without methylmalonic aciduria (see Fig. 8–6); only a few patients with these two defects have been reported.

The *clinical manifestations* are similar in patients with all of these defects. Vomiting, poor feeding, lethargy, hypotonia, and developmental delay may occur in the first few months of life. However, one patient with *cbl* G defect was not symptomatic (except for mild developmental delay) until she was 21 yr old, when she developed difficulty in walking and numbness of the hands. *Laboratory studies* reveal megaloblastic anemia, homocystinuria, and hypomethioninemia. The presence of hypomethioninemia and megalobastic anemia differentiates these defects from homocystinuria due to either cystathionine synthase deficiency or methylene tetrahydrofolate reductase deficiency.

Diagnosis is established by proper complementation studies performed in cultured fibroblasts. Prenatal diagnosis has been accomplished by performing complementation studies in amniotic cell cultures.

Treatment with vitamin B_{12} (1–2 mg/24 hr) has been effective in correcting clinical and biochemical findings in these patients.

Homocystinuria Due to Deficiency of Methylene Tetrahydrofolate Reductase (Homocystinuria Type III). This enzyme reduces 5–10 methylene tetrahydrofolate to form 5-methyltetrahydrofolate, which provides the methyl group needed for remethylation of homocysteine to methionine (see Fig. 8–4). The majority of reported patients with this disorder have been female. The condition is transmitted as an autosomal recessive trait.

The severity of the enzyme defect and of the *clinical manifestations* varies considerably in different families. Complete absence of enzyme activity results in neonatal apneic episodes and myoclonic seizures that may lead rapidly to coma and death. Partial deficiency may result in a more chronic clinical picture manifested by mental retardation, convulsions, microcephaly, and spasticity. One 15-yr-old patient developed schizophrenia and mental deterioration at 11 yr of age.

Laboratory studies reveal moderate homocystinemia and homocystinuria. The methionine concentration is low or low normal. This finding differentiates this condition from classic homocystinuria due to cystathionine synthase deficiency. Absence of megaloblastic anemia distinguishes this condition from homocystinuria due to methylcobalamin formation (see earlier). Thromboembolism of vessels has also been observed in these patients. *Diagnosis* may be confirmed by the enzyme assay in liver biopsy specimens, cultured fibroblasts, and leukocytes.

Treatment with a combination of folic acid, vitamin B_6 and vitamin B_{12}, methionine supplementation, and betaine has produced dramatic responses in some patients.

HYPERMETHIONINEMIA. Increased concentration of plasma methionine occurs in liver disease, tyrosinemia type I, and homocystinuria type I. Hypermethioninemia has also been found in premature and some full-term infants on high-protein diets, in whom it may represent delayed maturation of the enzyme methionine adenosyltransferase; lowering the protein intake usually resolves the abnormality. Hypermethioninemia due to the deficiency of hepatic methionine adenosyltransferase has also been reported. These children were diagnosed in the neonatal period during screening for homocystinuria and have remained asymptomatic for at least 13 yr.

CYSTATHIONINEMIA. Cystathionine, an intermediate metabolite of methionine degradation, is normally cleaved by cystathionase to cysteine and homoserine (see Fig. 8–4). This enzyme requires vitamin B_6 as a cofactor. Cystathionase is not present in normal fetal and newborn liver, and thus cysteine becomes an essential amino acid during the newborn period, particularly in the premature infant.

Cystathioninuria occurs in patients with vitamin B_6 or B_{12} deficiency, liver disease (particularly when the liver damage is secondary to galactosemia), thyrotoxicosis, hepatoblastoma, neuroblastoma, ganglioblastoma, or defects in remethylation of homocysteine (homocystinuria types II and III).

Cystathionase deficiency results in massive cystathioninuria and mild to moderate cystathioninemia; cystathionine is not normally detectable in blood. Deficiency of this enzyme is inherited as an autosomal recessive trait. Affected subjects with a wide variety of clinical manifestations have been reported. Lack of a consistent clinical picture and the presence of cystathioninuria in a number of normal persons suggest that cystathionase deficiency perhaps is of no clinical significance. A majority of reported cases are responsive to oral administration of large doses of vitamin B_6 (100 mg or more/24 hr). Once cystathioninuria is discovered in a patient, vitamin B_6 treatment seems indicated, but its beneficial effect has not been established.

8.5 CYSTEINE/CYSTINE

Cysteine is a sulfur-containing nonessential amino acid that is synthesized from methionine (see Fig. 8–4). In the presence of oxygen, two molecules of cysteine are oxidized to form cystine. The most common disorders of cysteine/cystine metabolism, cystinuria (see Sec. 18.48) and cystinosis (see Sec. 24.72), are discussed elsewhere.

SULFITE OXIDASE DEFICIENCY (Molybdenum Cofactor Deficiency). As the last step in cysteine metabolism, sulfite is oxidized to sulfate by sulfite oxidase, and the sulfate is excreted in the urine. This enzyme requires a molybdenum-containing compound named molybdenum cofactor. This cofactor is also necessary for the function of two other enzymes in humans, xanthine dehydrogenase (which oxidizes xanthine and hypoxanthine to uric acid) and aldehyde oxidase. Most patients who were originally diagnosed as having sulfite oxidase deficiency have proved to have molybdenum cofactor deficiency. The condition is inherited as an autosomal recessive trait.

Both deficiencies produce identical *clinical manifestations.* Refusal to feed, vomiting, seizures (tonic, clonic, and myoclonic), and severe mental retardation may develop within a few weeks after birth. Bilateral dislocation of ocular lenses is a common finding in patients who survive the neonatal period.

These children excrete large amounts of sulfite, thiosulfate, *S*-sulfocysteine, xanthine, and hypoxanthine in their urine.

Urinary and serum levels of uric acid and urinary concentration of sulfate are diminished. The urine can be screened for the presence of sulfite by a commercially available strip test (Macherey-Nagel strip). Fresh urine should be used for screening purposes and for quantitative measurements of sulfite, since oxidation at room temperature may produce false-negative results.

Diagnosis is confirmed by measurement of sulfite oxidase and molybdenum cofactor in fibroblasts and liver biopsies, respectively. Prenatal diagnosis is possible by performing an assay of sulfite oxidase activity in cultured amniotic cells or in samples of chorionic villi.

No effective treatment is available, and most children die during the first 2 yr of life.

8.6 TRYPTOPHAN

Tryptophan is an essential amino acid and a precursor for nicotinic acid and serotonin (Fig. 8–5). Presumed deficiencies of a variety of different enzymes involved in tryptophan metabolism have been reported in isolated cases, but in none of these cases has the enzyme deficiency been documented by direct assay of the enzyme activity. Moreover, because of the paucity of reported patients, the relationship between the symptoms and the putative enzyme deficiency has remained uncertain. Therefore, only disorders of tryptophan metabolism that have been well documented are discussed in this section. The most common disorder involving tryptophan metabolism is Hartnup disorder.

HARTNUP DISORDER. In this autosomal recessive disorder, named after the first reported family, there is a single defect in the transport of monoamino-monocarboxylic amino acids (neutral amino acids) by the intestinal mucosa and renal tubules.

Data from routine urine screening of newborn infants have revealed that most children with Hartnup defect remain asymptomatic. The major *clinical manifestation* in the rare symptomatic patient is cutaneous photosensitivity. The skin becomes rough and red after moderate exposure to the sun, and with greater exposure a pellagra-like rash may develop. The rash may be pruritic, and a chronic eczema may appear. The skin changes have been reported in affected infants as young as 10 days of age. Some patients may have intermittent ataxia with or without the skin rash. Mental deficiency, perhaps an incidental finding in the original kindred, has not been observed in other cases. Episodic psychologic changes such as irritability, emotional instability, and suicidal tendencies have been observed; these changes are usually associated with bouts of ataxia.

Identification of asymptomatic children with Hartnup defect suggests that it can be a benign disorder. The clinical polymorphism may be related to the severity of the defect, especially in the intestinal mucosa. Patients with a severe defect may develop marked amino acid deficiency following minor stress such as diarrhea or a low-protein diet and may then become symptomatic. This theory also explains the episodic nature of the symptoms and the long intervals of spontaneous remission in patients with Hartnup disorder. Hartnup defect, with an overall prevalence of 1 in 24,000 (range 1 in 18,000–42,000) ranks among the most common amino acid disorders in man. The molecular nature of the defect has not yet been elucidated. Pregnancy in women with Hartnup disorder has not produced any ill effects in either mother or fetus.

The main *laboratory finding* is aminoaciduria, which is restricted to neutral amino acids (alanine, serine, threonine,

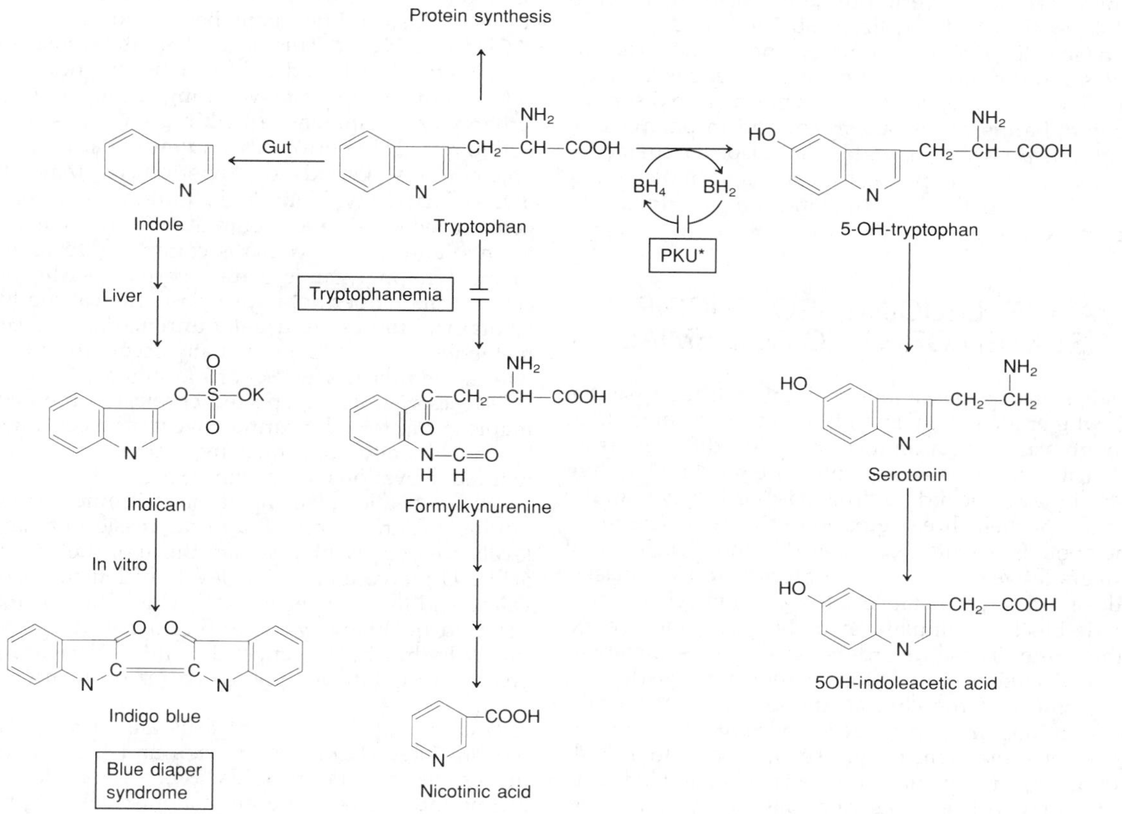

Figure 8–5. Pathways in the metabolism of tryptophan. *Hyperphenylalaninemia due to tetrahydrobiopterin deficiency (see Fig. 8–2).

valine, leucine, isoleucine, phenylalanine, tyrosine, tryptophan, and histidine). Urinary excretion of proline, hydroxyproline, and arginine remains normal. This is an important diagnostic finding that differentiates Hartnup disorder from other causes of generalized aminoaciduria such as Fanconi syndrome. Plasma concentrations of neutral amino acids are usually within normal limits. This seemingly unexpected finding is due to absorption of the amino acids as dipeptides because the transport system for small peptides remains intact in Hartnup disorder. The indole derivatives (especially indican) are usually excreted in large amounts in this disorder owing to bacterial breakdown of unabsorbed tryptophan in the intestines.

Treatment with nicotinic acid or nicotinamide (50–300 g/24 hr) and a high-protein diet have resulted in a favorable response in symptomatic patients.

SEROTONIN DEFICIENCY. The first step in serotonin synthesis is the hydroxylation of tryptophan by tryptophan hydroxylase. This enzyme requires tetrahydrobiopterin as a cofactor. Defects in biopterin metabolism (see Sec. 8.2) cause a deficiency of serotonin in addition to phenylketonuria. This fact explains why treatment of patients with PKU due to biopterin defects with the usual low-phenylalanine diet alone does not prevent neurologic manifestations.

TRYPTOPHANEMIA. Some children with mental and physical retardation, ataxia, and photosensitive pellagra-like skin rash have been reported who were found to have mild elevations in plasma concentrations of tryptophan and tryptophanuria. A block in the conversion of tryptophan to formyl kynurenine is postulated as the cause on the basis of decreased urinary kynurenine after an oral tryptophan load. No direct enzyme assay has been performed on these patients.

INDICANURIA (Tryptophan Malabsorption). This condition occurs when tryptophan, poorly absorbed from the gastrointestinal tract, is converted there by bacterial action to indole. Indole is absorbed, oxidized, sulfated, and excreted as an indican (see Fig. 8–5). Indicanuria is commonly observed whenever stasis in the bowels occurs, such as in constipation or in the *blind loop syndrome*; it also occurs in Hartnup disorder, in which tryptophan is poorly absorbed, and in phenylketonuria. The *blue diaper syndrome*, a familial disorder characterized by hypercalcemia, nephrocalcinosis, and indicanuria, derives its name from the fact that indican is oxidized to indigo blue on exposure to air.

8.7 VALINE, LEUCINE, ISOLEUCINE, AND RELATED ORGANIC ACIDEMIAS

The early steps in the degradation of these three essential amino acids, the branched-chain amino acids, are similar (Fig. 8–6). Although valine transaminase may be different from leucine-isoleucine transaminase, only one enzyme system (branched-chain α-ketoacid dehydrogenase) is involved in the decarboxylation of their three ketoacid derivatives. The intermediate metabolites are all organic acids, and deficiency of any of the degradative enzymes, except for the transaminases, causes acidosis; in such instances, the organic acids before the enzymatic block accumulate in body fluids and are excreted in the urine. These disorders cause severe metabolic acidosis, which usually occurs during the first few days of life. Although most of the clinical findings are nonspecific, some manifestations may provide important clues to the nature of the enzyme deficiency. An approach to infants suspected of having an organic acidemia is presented in Figure 8–7. Definitive diagnosis is usually established by identifying and measuring specific organic acids in body fluids, especially urine, and by the enzyme assay.

Organic acidemias are not limited to defects in the catabolic pathways of branched-chain amino acids. Disorders causing accumulation of other organic acids include those derived from lysine (see Sec. 8.13), those associated with lactic acid (see Sec. 8.36), and dicarboxylic acidemia associated with defective fatty acid degradation (see Sec. 8.15).

DEFICIENCY OF BRANCHED-CHAIN AMINOTRANSFERASE. Only one Japanese girl with hypervalinemia and two siblings from France with hyperleucine-isoleucinemia have been reported. The symptoms were nonspecific (failure to thrive, seizures, mental deficiency). The infant with hypervalinemia had only increased concentrations of valine in blood and urine with normal levels of leucine and isoleucine. Impaired transamination of valine was demonstrated in leukocytes. The siblings with hyperleucine-isoleucinemia had elevated plasma concentrations of leucine, isoleucine, and proline with normal levels of valine. Assay of leukocytes revealed no abnormalities of branched-chain ketoacid dehydrogenase or of valine aminotransferase, but there was a 50% reduction in leucine and isoleucine aminotransferase. The urine of these infants neither contained branched-chain ketoacids nor had the odor of maple syrup.

The presence of hypervalinemia and hyperleucine-isoleucinemia as separate entities suggests that there may be more than one aminotransferase for these amino acids.

MAPLE SYRUP URINE DISEASE (MSUD). Decarboxylation of leucine, isoleucine, and valine is accomplished by a complex enzyme system (branched-chain α-ketoacid dehydrogenase) using thiamine pyrophosphate as a coenzyme. This mitochondrial enzyme consists of four subunits: $E_{1\alpha}$, $E_{1\beta}$, E_2, and E_3. The E_3 subunit is shared with two other dehydrogenases in the body, namely, pyruvate dehydrogenase and α-ketoglutarate dehydrogenase. Deficiency of this enzyme system causes MSUD (see Fig. 8–6), named after the sweet odor of maple syrup found in body fluids, especially urine. Several forms of this condition have been reported.

Classic MSUD. This form has the most severe *clinical manifestations*. Affected infants who are normal at birth develop poor feeding and vomiting during the 1st wk of life; lethargy and coma ensue within a few days. Physical examination reveals hypertonicity and muscular rigidity with severe opisthotonos. Periods of hypertonicity may alternate with bouts of flaccidity. Neurologic findings are often mistaken for generalized sepsis and meningitis. Convulsions occur in most infants, and hypoglycemia is common. However, in contrast to most hypoglycemic states, correcting the blood glucose concentration does not improve the clinical condition. Routine laboratory studies are usually unremarkable except for severe metabolic acidosis. Death usually occurs in untreated patients within the first few weeks or months of life.

Diagnosis is often suspected because of the peculiar odor of maple syrup found in urine, sweat, and cerumen (see Fig. 8–7). It is usually confirmed by amino acid analysis showing marked elevations in plasma levels of leucine, isoleucine, valine, and alloisoleucine (a stereoisomer of isoleucine not normally found in blood) and depression of alanine. Leucine levels are usually higher than those of the other three amino acids. Urine contains high levels of leucine, isoleucine, and valine and their respective ketoacids. These ketoacids may be detected qualitatively by adding a few drops of 2,4-dinitrophenylhydrazine reagent (0.1% in 0.1 N HCl) to the urine; a yellow precipitate of diphenylhydrazine is formed in a positive test.

Treatment of the acute state is aimed at quick removal of the branched-chain amino acids and their metabolites from the tissues and body fluids. Since renal clearance of these compounds is poor, hydration alone does not produce a rapid improvement. Peritoneal dialysis is the most effective mode of therapy and should be promptly instituted; significant

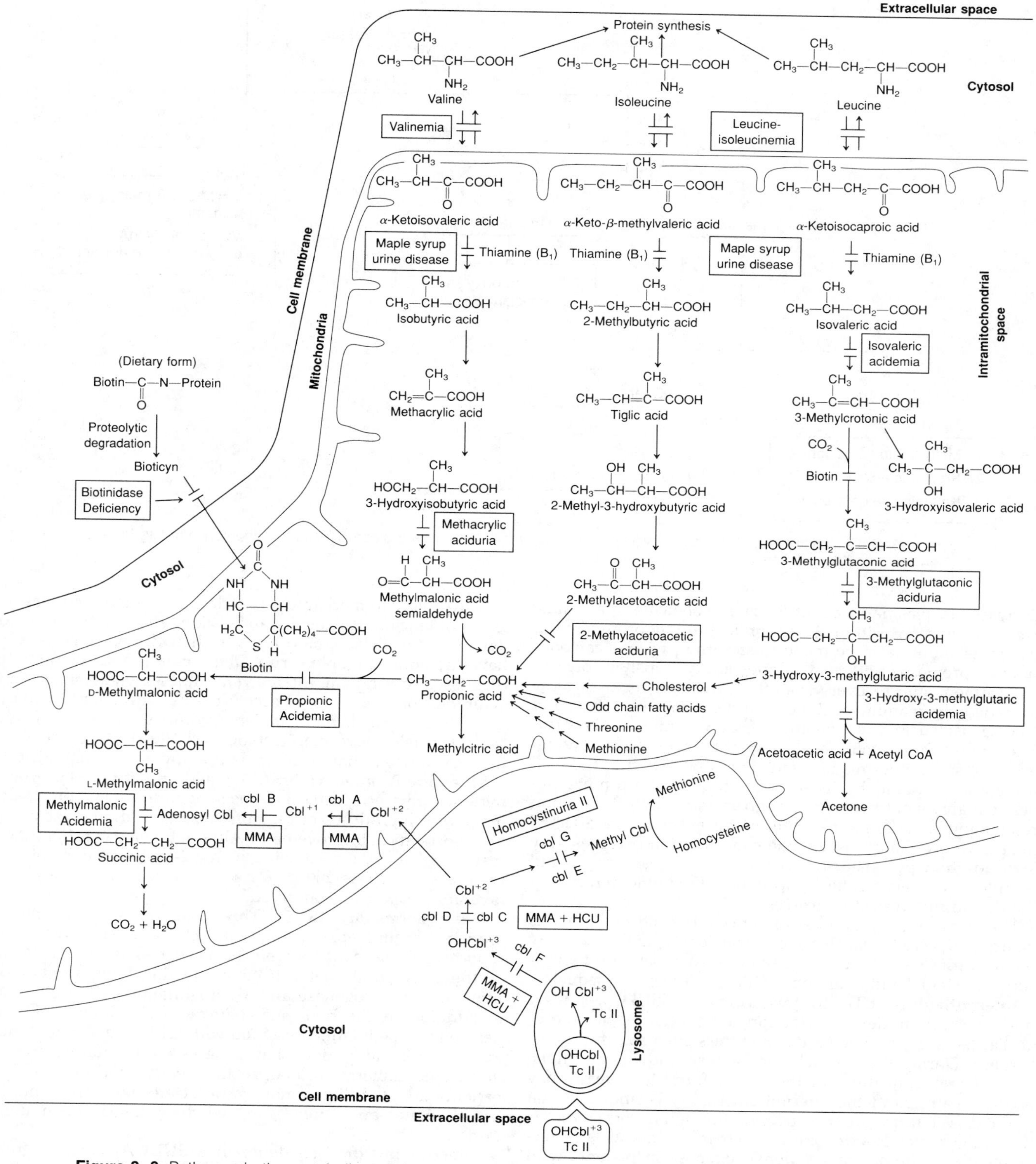

Figure 8–6. Pathways in the metabolism of the branched-chain amino acids, biotin, and vitamin B_{12} (cobalamin). Many of the intermediates (the organic acids) are metabolized via their coenzyme A (CoA) derivatives. For the sake of simplicity, this is not indicated in most of the cases. (MMA = methylmalonic acidemia; HCU = homocystinuria; Cbl = cobalamin; OHCbl = hydroxycobalamin; cbl = defect in metabolism of cobalamin; Tc = transcobalamin.)

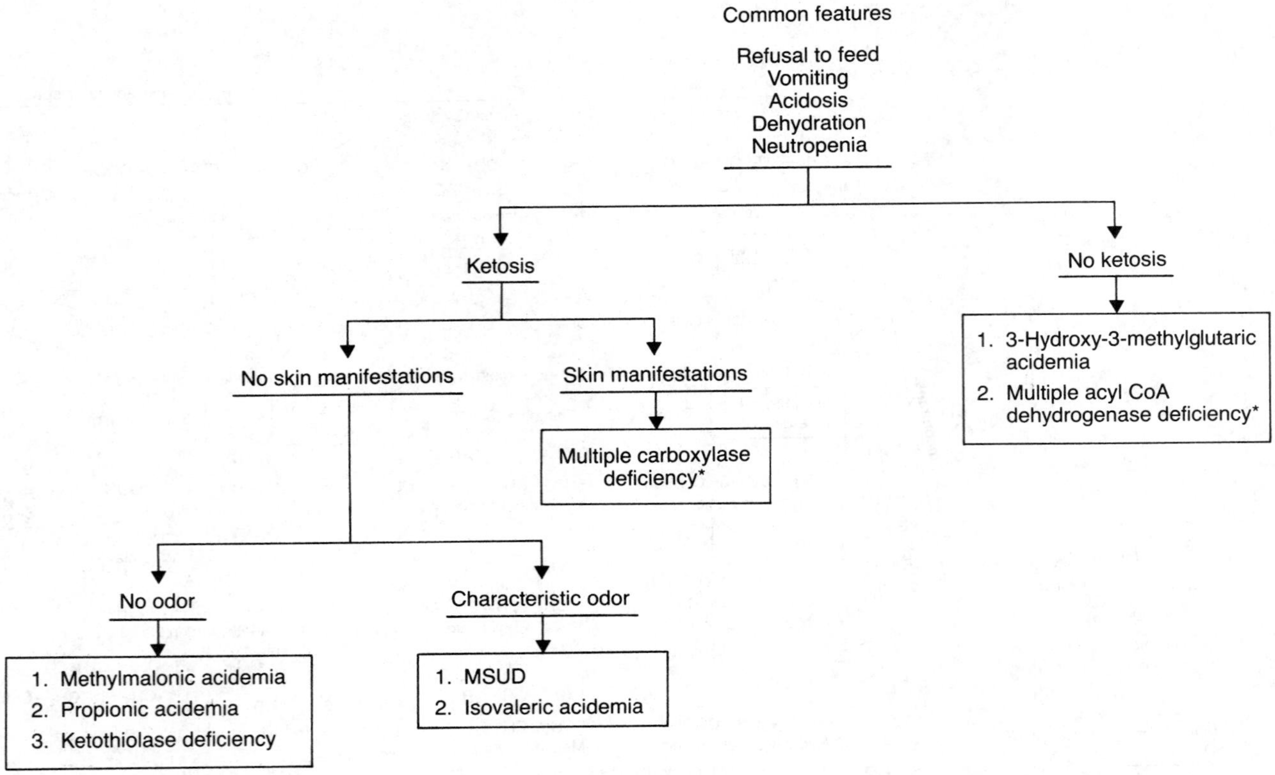

Figure 8–7. Clinical approach to infants with organic acidemia. Asterisks indicate disorders in which patients have a characteristic odor (see text).

decreases in plasma levels of leucine, isoleucine, and valine are usually seen within 24 hr of institution of treatment. Attempts should also be made to stop the patient's catabolic state by providing sufficient calories intravenously or orally.

Treatment after recovery from the acute state requires a low branched-chain amino acid diet. Synthetic formulas devoid of leucine, isoleucine, and valine are now commercially available.* Since these amino acids cannot be synthesized endogenously, small amounts of them should be added to the diet; the amount should be titrated carefully by performing frequent analyses of the plasma amino acids. A clinical condition resembling acrodermatitis enteropathica occurs in affected infants whose plasma isoleucine concentration becomes very low; addition of isoleucine to the diet causes a rapid and complete recovery. Patients with MSUD should remain on the diet for the rest of their lives.

The long-term *prognosis* of affected children remains guarded. Severe ketoacidosis, cerebral edema, and death may occur during any stressful situation such as infection or surgery. Mental and neurologic deficits are common sequelae.

Intermittent MSUD. In this form of MSUD seemingly normal children develop vomiting, odor of maple syrup, ataxia, lethargy, and coma during stress such as infection or surgery. During these attacks, laboratory findings are indistinguishable from those of the classic form, and death may occur. Treatment of the intermittent variety is similar to that of the classic form. After recovery, although a normal diet is tolerated, a diet low in branched-chain amino acids is recommended. The activity of dehydrogenase in patients with the intermittent form is higher than that in the classic form and may reach 8–16% of the normal activity.

Mild (Intermediate) MSUD. In this form affected children develop milder disease after the neonatal period. They are usually mildly to moderately retarded, have increased plasma levels of leucine, isoleucine, and valine, and excrete ketoacid derivatives of these amino acids in their urine. They usually have the odor of maple syrup. These children are commonly diagnosed during an intercurrent illness when signs and symptoms of classic MSUD occur. The dehydrogenase activity is 2–8% of normal. Since patients with thiamine-responsive MSUD usually have manifestations similar to those seen in the mild form, a trial of thiamine therapy is recommended.

Thiamine-Responsive MSUD. Children with mild or intermittent forms of MSUD have been reported in whom treatment with high doses of thiamine results in dramatic clinical and biochemical improvement. Although some children have responded to treatment with 10 mg/24 hr thiamine, others require as much as 200 mg/24 hr for at least 3 wk before a favorable response is observed.

Other Forms of MSUD. Three patients with combined branched-chain ketoaciduria and lactic acidosis have been reported. These patients were believed to have a deficiency of the E_3 subunit that caused a functional impairment of pyruvate dehydrogenase and α-ketoglutarate dehydrogenase in addition to the branched-chain ketoacid dehydrogenase deficiency. The infants presented with acidosis and hypotonia in the neonatal period that progressed to ataxia, severe neurologic impairment, and death in early childhood. These patients excreted large amounts of lactate, pyruvate, and α-ketoglutarate, and three branched-chain ketoacids in their urine.

Genetics and the Prevalence of MSUD. All forms of this disorder are inherited as an autosomal recessive trait. The deficiency of different subunits of the enzyme may account for the wide clinical and biochemical variability seen in different affected families. Patients with the classic form may have $E_{1\alpha}$, $E_{1\beta}$, or E_2 subunit deficiency. The gene for $E_{1\alpha}$ is mapped to chromosome 19 and that of E_2 to chromosome 1. Patients

*MSUD Formula, Mead Johnson Laboratories, Evansville, Indiana.

with the mild and intermittent forms may also be "double heterozygotes" with two different mutant alleles. The enzyme activity can be measured in leukocytes and fibroblasts, making it possible to diagnose heterozygotes and affected fetuses. The incidence in the United States is about 1 in 200,000; however, the classic form of the disease is more common among Mennonites.

ISOVALERIC ACIDEMIA. This rare condition is due to the deficiency of isovaleryl CoA dehydrogenase, which catalyzes the conversion of isovaleric acid to 3-methylcrotonic acid in the leucine degradative pathway (see Fig. 8–6). Isovaleric acidemia is inherited as an autosomal recessive trait. The gene frequency in the general population is not known.

Clinical manifestations in the acute form include vomiting and severe acidosis in the first few days of life. Lethargy, convulsions, and coma ensue, and death may occur if proper therapy is not initiated. The vomiting may be severe enough to suggest pyloric stenosis. The characteristic odor of "sweaty feet" may be present (see Fig. 8–7). A milder form of the disease also exists in which the first clinical manifestation (vomiting, lethargy, acidosis, or coma) may not appear until the infant is a few months or a few years old (chronic intermittent form).

Laboratory findings reveal severe ketoacidosis, neutropenia, thrombocytopenia, and occasionally pancytopenia. Hypocalcemia and moderate to severe hyperammonemia may be present in some patients. Increases in plasma ammonia may suggest a defect in the urea cycle. However, in the latter conditions the infant is not acidotic. Hyperglycemia may be present in some patients.

Diagnosis is established by demonstrating marked elevations of isovaleric acid and its metabolites (isovalerylglycine, 3-hydroxyisovaleric acid) in body fluids, especially urine. Isovaleric acid is volatile and may disappear from the urine if the specimen is not handled properly; however, isovalerylglycine is a stable compound that is more reliable for diagnostic purposes. Measuring the enzyme in cultured skin fibroblasts confirms the diagnosis. Intrauterine diagnosis has been accomplished by measuring isovalerylglycine in amniotic fluid.

Treatment of the acute attack is aimed at hydration, correction of metabolic acidosis (by infusing sodium bicarbonate), and removal of the excess isovaleric acid. Since isovalerylglycine has a high urinary clearance, administration of glycine (250 mg/kg/24 hr) is recommended to enhance formation of isovalerylglycine. Carnitine (100 mg/kg/24 hr) also increases removal of isovaleric acid by forming isovalerylcarnitine, which is excreted in the urine. Adequate calories should be provided orally or intravenously to minimize the catabolic state. In patients with significant hyperammonemia (blood ammonia >200 μM) measures that reduce blood ammonia should be employed (Sec. 8.11). Exchange transfusion and peritoneal dialysis may be needed if the above measures fail to induce significant clinical and biochemical improvement. Patients should be kept on a low-protein diet (1.0–1.5 g/kg/24 hr) and should be given glycine and carnitine supplements after recovery from the acute attack. Normal development can be achieved with early and proper treatment.

MULTIPLE CARBOXYLASE DEFICIENCY (Defects in Utilization of Biotin). Biotin is a water-soluble vitamin that acts as a cofactor for all carboxylases in the body: pyruvate carboxylase, acetyl CoA carboxylase, propionyl CoA carboxylase, and 3-methylcrotonyl CoA carboxylase. The latter two of these carboxylases are involved in the metabolic pathways of leucine, isoleucine, and valine (see Fig. 8–6).

Dietary biotin is bound to protein (carboxylases); free biotin is generated in the intestine by the action of digestive enzymes and perhaps biotinidase. The latter enzyme, which is found in serum and most tissues in the body, is also essential for the recycling of biotin in the body by releasing it from a carboxylase (see Fig. 8–6). Free biotin must form a covalent peptide bond with the apoprotein of the above carboxylases in order to render them active. This binding is catalyzed by holocarboxylase synthetase. Deficiencies in this enzyme or in biotinidase result in malfunction of all the carboxylases and in organic acidemia.

Holocarboxylase Synthetase Deficiency (Multiple Carboxylase Deficiency—Infantile or Early Form). Infants with this rare autosomal recessive disorder become symptomatic in the first few weeks of life with breathing difficulties (tachypnea, apnea), hypotonia, seizures, vomiting, and failure to thrive. The urine may have a peculiar odor, which is described as similar to tomcat urine. The clinical finding that may differentiate this disorder from other organic acidemias, especially propionic acidemia, is the skin manifestations, which include generalized erythematous rash with exfoliation and alopecia totalis (see Fig. 8–7).

Laboratory findings include metabolic acidosis, ketosis, and the presence of organic acids such as lactic acid, propionic acid, 3-methylcrotonic acid, 3-methylcrotonylglycine, and 3-hydroxyisovaleric acid in body fluids. Significant hyperammonemia has occurred in some patients. These infants may also have an immunodeficiency manifested by a decrease in the number of T cells.

Treatment with biotin (10 mg/24 hr) results in a dramatic response. Prenatal diagnosis has been accomplished by means of an assay of enzyme activity in cultured amniotic cells and by measurement of intermediate metabolites (3-hydroxyisovalerate and methylcitrate) in amniotic fluid. Prenatal treatment of the mother with biotin has produced normal offspring in two women in whom prenatal diagnosis of holocarboxylase synthetase deficiency was made.

Biotinidase Deficiency (Multiple Carboxylase Deficiency—Juvenile or Late Form). The absence of biotinidase results in biotin deficiency. The prevalence of this autosomal recessive trait is estimated at 1 in 60,000.

Infants with this deficiency may develop clinical manifestations similar to those seen in infants with holocarboxylase synthetase deficiency, but, unlike the latter, symptoms may appear later when the child is several months or several years old. The delay is presumably due to the presence of sufficient free biotin derived from the mother or the diet. Atopic or seborrheic dermatitis, alopecia, ataxia, myoclonic seizures, hypotonia, developmental delay, hearing loss, and immunodeficiency may occur. Measurement of biotinidase in 100 Japanese children with intractable seborrheic dermatitis revealed two children with partial (15–30% activity) deficiency of the enzyme; these children were otherwise asymptomatic, and their dermatitis resolved with biotin therapy. Patients with partial deficiency of the enzyme have been identified on neonatal screening and in family members of these infants. Symptoms of biotinidase deficiency were observed in a few of these individuals. Episodes of metabolic acidosis may also occur.

Laboratory findings and the pattern of organic acids in body fluids resemble those associated with holocarboxylase synthetase deficiency (see earlier). *Diagnosis* can be established by measurement of the enzyme activity in the serum. A simplified method of neonatal screening for biotinidase deficiency is now available that requires a small amount of blood spotted on a filter paper.

These children respond dramatically to administration of free biotin (10 mg/24 hr).

Multiple Carboxylase Deficiency Due to Dietary Biotin Deficiency. Acquired deficiency of biotin may occur in infants receiving total parenteral nutrition without added biotin, in patients receiving prolonged anticonvulsant drugs, or in children with short gut syndrome or chronic diarrhea who are receiving formulas low in biotin. Excessive ingestion of raw eggs may also cause biotin deficiency because the protein avidin in egg white binds biotin and makes it unavailable for absorption. Infants with biotin deficiency develop dermatitis, alopecia, and moniliasis.

3-METHYLGLUTACONIC ACIDURIA. Clinical manifestations have ranged from mild motor and speech retardation to severe neurologic deficits with self-mutilation. Patients excrete large amounts of 3-methylglutaconic acid, an intermediate metabolite in the catabolism of leucine, in their urine. It is not clear whether the metabolic defect is the cause of the clinical manifestations.

β-KETOTHIOLASE DEFICIENCY (2-Methylacetoacetyl CoA Thiolase Deficiency). 2-Methylacetoacetyl CoA thiolase is one of the three existing ketothiolases in the body. This enzyme cleaves 2-methylacetoacetyl CoA to acetyl CoA and propionyl CoA (see Fig. 8–6). Although deficiencies of the other β-ketothiolases have also been reported (in a total of three patients), the term β-ketothiolase deficiency is traditionally reserved for patients with 2-methylacetoacetyl CoA thiolase deficiency. Fourteen patients with this deficiency have been reported. This condition is inherited as an autosomal recessive trait and may be more prevalent than has been appreciated.

The *clinical manifestations* are quite variable, ranging from an asymptomatic course in an adult to severe episodes of acidosis starting in the 1st yr of life. These children have intermittent episodes of severe acidosis, ketosis, and moderate to severe hyperammonemia that may lead to coma and death. These episodes usually occur following an intercurrent infection and respond quickly to intravenous fluids and bicarbonate therapy. The child may be completely asymptomatic between episodes and may tolerate a normal protein diet well. Mental development is normal in most children. The episodes may be misdiagnosed as salicylate poisoning because of the similarity of clinical findings and the interference of elevated blood levels of acetoacetate with the colorimetric assay for salicylate. In an unreported case of our own, the diagnosis was not made until the child was 3½ yr of age when a third episode of severe acidosis occurred following an upper respiratory infection. The second episode at 14 mo of age was diagnosed as salicylate ingestion. The child had normal development.

Laboratory findings during the acute attack include acidosis, ketosis, and hyperammonemia. The urine contains large amounts of 2-methylacetoacetate, 2-methyl-3-hydroxybutyrate, and tiglylglycine. Hyperglycinemia may also be present. The clinical and biochemical findings should be differentiated from those seen with propionic and methylmalonic acidemias (see later). *Diagnosis* may be established by assay of the enzyme in cultured fibroblasts.

Treatment of acute episodes includes hydration and infusion of bicarbonate to correct the acidosis; a 10% glucose solution with the appropriate electrolytes and intravenous lipids may be used to minimize the catabolic state. Hyperammonemia should be treated promptly (see Sec. 8.11). Peritoneal dialysis may be required if the above measures do not produce significant clinical improvement. Restriction of protein intake (1–2 g/kg/24 hr) is recommended for long-term therapy. L-Carnitine (50–100 mg/kg/24 hr) may be used to prevent possible secondary carnitine deficiency.

3-HYDROXY-3-METHYLGLUTARIC (HMG) ACIDEMIA. This rare condition (a total of 19 patients have been reported) is due to a deficiency of hydroxymethylglutaryl (HMG) CoA lyase (see Fig. 8–6). About 60% of these patients become symptomatic between 3 and 11 mo of age, whereas 30% develop symptoms in the first few days of life. One child remained asymptomatic until 2 yr of age. Episodes of vomiting, severe hypoglycemia, hypotonia, acidosis, and dehydration may rapidly lead to lethargy, ataxia, and coma. These episodes often occur during an intercurrent infection. Hepatomegaly is a common physical finding.

Laboratory studies reveal hypoglycemia, moderate to severe hyperammonemia, acidosis, and abnormal liver function test results. There is no ketosis (see Fig. 8–7) because 3-hydroxy-3-methylglutaric acid cannot be converted to acetoacetic acid and β-hydroxybutyric acid. 3-Hydroxy-3-methylglutaryl CoA is also an obligatory intermediate metabolite in the formation of ketone bodies from any other source. Urinary excretion of 3-hydroxy-3-methylglutaric acid and other proximal intermediate metabolites of leucine catabolism (3-methylglutaconic acid and 3-hydroxyisovaleric acid) is markedly increased. This condition should be differentiated from medium-chain acyl CoA dehydrogenase (MCAD) deficiency. The urinary metabolites described earlier are characteristic of 3-hydroxy-3-methylglutaric acidemia and are not found in MCAD deficiency. *Diagnosis* may be confirmed by enzyme assay in cultured fibroblasts, leukocytes, or liver specimens. Prenatal diagnosis has been accomplished by means of an assay of the enzyme in a biopsy specimen of the chorionic villi.

Treatment of acute episodes includes hydration, infusion of glucose to control hypoglycemia, and administration of bicarbonate to correct acidosis. Hyperammonemia should be treated promptly (see Sec. 8.11). Exchange transfusion and peritoneal dialysis may be required in patients with severe hyperammonemia. Restriction of protein and fat intake is recommended for long-term management of these patients. L-Carnitine (50–100 mg/kg/24 hr) may be used to prevent secondary carnitine deficiency. Prolonged fasting should be avoided. There may be some risk in performing immunization of these children because one child has died following immunization.

PROPIONIC ACIDEMIA (Propionyl CoA Carboxylase Deficiency). Propionic acid is an intermediate metabolite of isoleucine, valine, threonine, methionine, odd-chain fatty acids, and cholesterol catabolism. It is normally carboxylated to methylmalonic acid by the mitochondrial enzyme propionyl CoA carboxylase, which requires biotin as a cofactor (see Fig. 8–6). The enzyme is composed of two nonidentical subunits, α and β. Biotin is bound to the α subunit.

The prevalence of propionic acidemia, inherited as an autosomal recessive trait, is not known. The gene for the α subunit is located on chromosome 13 and that of the β subunit is mapped to the long arm of chromosome 3.

Clinical manifestations are nonspecific. The majority of patients develop symptoms in the first few weeks of life. Poor feeding, vomiting, hypotonia, lethargy, dehydration, and clinical signs of acidosis progress rapidly to coma and death. Seizures occur in about 30% of affected infants. If an infant survives the first attack, similar episodes may occur during an intercurrent infection, constipation, or following ingestion of a high-protein diet. Less frequently, the infant may come to medical attention later in life because of mental retardation without acute attacks of ketosis. Some affected children may have episodes of unexplained severe ketoacidosis separated by periods of seemingly normal health. The severity of clinical manifestations may also be variable within a family; in one kindred, a brother was diagnosed at 5 yr of age, whereas his 13-yr-old sister, with the same level of enzyme deficiency, was asymptomatic. The reason for this polymorphism remains unclear.

Laboratory studies during the acute attack reveal severe metabolic acidosis with a large anion gap, ketosis, neutropenia, thrombocytopenia, and hypoglycemia. Moderate to severe hyperammonemia is commonly seen in these infants. Plasma concentration of ammonia usually correlates with the severity of the disease. Measurement of plasma ammonia is especially helpful in planning therapeutic strategy during episodes of exacerbation in a patient whose diagnosis has been established previously. Hyperglycinemia is common in patients with propionic acidemia. Elevations in plasma and urinary levels of glycine have also been observed in patients with methylmalonic acidemia, isovaleric acidemia, and β-ketothiolase deficiency. These disorders formerly were collectively referred to as **ketotic hyperglycinemia** before the specific enzyme deficiencies were elucidated. The reason for hyperglycinemia in these disorders remains unclear. Concentrations of propionic acid and methylcitric acid (presumably made by the condensation of propionyl CoA with oxaloacetic acid) are markedly elevated in the plasma and urine of infants with propionic acidemia. Measurement of methylcitric acid is especially helpful in making the diagnosis because, unlike propionic acid, which is volatile, methylcitric acid is a stable compound and does not disappear from the specimen during shipping and handling. 3-Hydroxypropionic acid, propionylglycine, and other intermediate metabolites of isoleucine catabolism such as tiglic acid, tiglylglycine, and 2-methyloacetoacetic acid are also found in urine.

The *diagnosis* of propionic acidemia should be differentiated from multiple carboxylase deficiency (see earlier description and Fig. 8–7). Patients with propionic acidemia responsive to biotin in earlier reports were later found to have multiple carboxylase deficiency. The latter infants may have skin manifestations and excrete large amounts of lactic acid, 3-methylcrotonic acid, and 3-hydroxyisovaleric acid in addition to propionic acid. The presence of hyperammonemia may suggest a genetic defect in the urea cycle enzymes. However, infants with defects in the urea cycle are usually not acidotic (see Fig. 8–1). Hyperammonemia is believed to be due to inhibition of carbamylphosphate synthetase (CPS I) by the organic acid. Definitive diagnosis of propionic acidemia can be established by measuring the appropriate enzyme activity in leukocytes or cultured fibroblasts.

Prenatal diagnosis has been accomplished by measuring the enzyme activity in cultured amniotic cells and in samples of uncultured chorionic villi.

Treatment of acute attacks includes rehydration, correction of acidosis, and prevention of the catabolic state by provision of adequate calories through parenteral hyperalimentation. Minimal amounts of protein (0.25 g/kg/24 hr), preferably a protein deficient in propionate precursor, should be provided in the hyperalimentation fluid very early in the course of treatment. To control the possible production of propionic acid by intestinal bacteria, sterilization of the intestinal tract flora by antibiotics (e.g., oral neomycin) should be promptly initiated. Constipation should also be treated. Patients with propionic acidemia may develop carnitine deficiency, presumably as a result of urinary loss of propionylcarnitine formed from the accumulated organic acid. Administration of L-carnitine (50–100 mg/kg/24 hr) normalizes fatty acid oxidation and improves acidosis. In patients with concomitant hyperammonemia measures to reduce blood ammonia should be employed (see Sec. 8.11). Very ill patients with severe acidosis and hyperammonemia require peritoneal dialysis or hemodialysis to remove ammonia and other toxic compounds (Sec. 8.11). Although infants with true propionic acidemia are rarely responsive to biotin, this compound should be administered (10 mg/24 hr) to all infants during the initial attack and should be continued until a definitive diagnosis is established.

Long-term treatment consists of a low-protein diet (1.0–1.5 g/kg/24 hr) and administration of L-carnitine (50–100 mg/kg/24 hr). Synthetic proteins deficient in propionate precursors* (isoleucine, valine, methionine, and threonine) may be used to increase the amount of dietary protein (to 1.5–2.0g/kg/24hr) while causing minimal change in propionate production. However, excessive supplementation with these proteins may cause a deficiency of the essential amino acids. To avoid this problem, natural proteins should comprise most of the dietary protein (50–75%). Some patients may require chronic alkaline therapy to correct low-grade chronic acidosis. The concentration of ammonia in blood usually normalizes between attacks, and chronic treatment of hyperammonemia is rarely needed. Stressful situations that may trigger acute attacks (e.g., infections) should be treated promptly and aggressively. Close monitoring of blood pH, amino acids, urinary content of propionate and its metabolites, and growth parameters is necessary to ensure the proper balance of the diet and the success of therapy.

Long-term *prognosis* is guarded. Death may occur during an acute attack. Normal psychomotor development is possible, but most children manifest some degree of permanent neurodevelopmental deficit despite adequate therapy.

METHYLMALONIC ACIDEMIA. Methylmalonic acid, a structural isomer of succinic acid, is normally derived from propionic acid as part of the catabolic pathways of isoleucine, valine, threonine, methionine, cholesterol, and odd-chain fatty acids. Two enzymes are involved in the conversion of D-methylmalonic acid to succinic acid, methylmalonyl CoA racemase (which forms the L-isomer) and methylmalonyl CoA mutase (which converts the L-methylmalonic acid to succinic acid) (see Fig. 8–6). The latter enzyme requires adenosylcobalamin, a metabolite of vitamin B_{12}, as a coenzyme. Deficiency of either the mutase or its coenzyme causes an accumulation of methylmalonic acid and its precursors in body fluids. Deficiency of the racemase has not yet been conclusively identified.

At least two forms of mutase apoenzyme deficiency have been identified. These are designated *mut*^{0}, meaning no enzyme activity, and *mut*$^-$, indicating partial deficiency of the mutase activity. About half of the reported patients with methylmalonic acidemia have a deficiency of the mutase apoenzyme (*mut*^{0} or *mut*$^-$). These patients are not responsive to vitamin B_{12} therapy. In the remaining patients with methylmalonic acidemia, the defect resides in the formation of adenosylcobalamin.

Defects in Metabolism of Vitamin B_{12} (Cobalamin). Dietary vitamin B_{12} requires intrinsic factor, a glycoprotein secreted by the gastric parietal cells, for absorption in the terminal ileum. It is transported in the blood by three carrier proteins, transcobalamin I, II, and III. The complex of transcobalamin II-cobalamin (TcII-Cbl) is recognized by a specific receptor on the cell membrane and enters the cell by endocytosis (see Fig. 8–6). The TcII-Cbl complex is hydrolyzed in the lysosome, and free cobalamin is released into the cytosol. The cobalt of the molecule is reduced in the cytosol from three valences (cob(III)alamin) to two (cob(II)alamin) before it enters the mitochondria, where further reduction to cob(I)alamin occurs. The latter compound reacts with adenosine to form adenosyl cobalamin (coenzyme for methylmalonyl CoA mutase). The free cobalamin in the cytosol may also undergo a series of poorly understood enzymatic steps to form methylcobalamin (coenzyme for methionine synthase, which catalyzes the remethylation of homocysteine to methionine, see Fig. 8–4).

At least seven different defects in the intracellular metabolism of cobalamin have been identified. These are designated *cbl* A through G (*cbl* stands for a defect in any step of cobalamin metabolism). *cbl* A is due to a deficiency of mitochondrial cobalamin reductase; *cbl* B is caused by a deficiency of adenosylcobalamin transferase. Both cause methylmalonic acidemia only. The precise enzymatic deficiencies in the remaining defects are not known. In patients with *cbl* C, *cbl* D, and *cbl* F defects, synthesis of both adenosylcobalamin and methylcobalamin is impaired, causing homocystinuria in addition to methylmalonic acidemia. Defects E and G involve

* Milupa OS1. Milupa Corporation, Darien, CT.

only the synthesis of methylcobalamin, resulting in homocystinuria without methylmalonic acidemia. All of the above defects including apoenzyme deficiency (mut^0 and mut$^-$) are inherited as autosomal recessive traits and have an overall prevalence of about 1 in 48,000.

Clinical manifestations of patients with *mut*^{0} and *mut*$^-$ and *cbl* A and *cbl* B are similar to those of patients with propionic acidemia (see earlier). However, fulminating neonatal forms causing severe ketosis, acidosis, hyperammonemia, neutropenia, coma, and death are more common in patients with methylmalonic acidemia than in patients with propionic acidemia. If the infant survives the first attack, similar exacerbations may occur during an intercurrent infection or following ingestion of a high-protein diet. The condition may present later in life with failure to thrive, hypotonia, and developmental delay. Some infants with methylmalonic acidemia have characteristic facial features with a triangular mouth and high forehead (Fig. 8–8). Patients with severe clinical manifestations in the first few days of life tend to have mutase deficiency (*mut*^{0} or *mut*$^-$). However, there are wide variations in the clinical presentation regardless of the nature of the enzyme deficiency. Asymptomatic patients with mutase apoenzyme deficiency have been identified through screening of newborn infants. These patients tolerate a normal protein intake and accumulate high levels of methylmalonate in their body fluids.

Laboratory findings include ketosis, acidosis, anemia, neutropenia, thrombocytopenia, hyperglycinemia, hyperammonemia, hypoglycemia, and the presence of large quantities of methylmalonic acid in body fluids (see Fig. 8–7). Propionic acid and its metabolites 3-hydroxypropionate and methylcitrate are also found in urine. Hyperammonemia may suggest the presence of genetic defects in the urea cycle enzymes. However, patients with defects in urea cycle enzymes are not acidotic (see Fig. 8–1). The increase in ammonia in patients with methylmalonic acidemia is believed to be due to inhibition of CPS I by the organic acid.

Diagnosis can be confirmed by measuring mutase activity and by performing complementation studies in cultured fibroblasts. Prenatal diagnosis has been accomplished by performing an assay of the mutase enzyme activity in cultured amniotic cells.

Treatment of acute attacks is similar to that of attacks in patients with propionic acidemia (see earlier) except that large doses (1–2 mg/24 hr) of vitamin B_{12} are used instead of biotin. Long-term treatment consists of a low-protein diet (1.0–1.5 g/kg/24 hr) and administration of L-carnitine (50–100 mg/kg/24 hr) and vitamin B_{12} (1 mg/24 hr for only those patients with defects in vitamin B_{12} metabolism). The protein composition of the diet is similar to that prescribed for patients with propionic acidemia. Chronic alkaline therapy is usually required to correct low-grade chronic acidosis. Blood levels of ammonia usually normalize between the attacks, and chronic treatment of hyperammonemia is rarely needed. Stressful situations that may trigger acute attacks (such as infection) should be treated promptly. Close monitoring of blood pH, amino acid levels, urinary content of methylmalonate, and growth parameters is necessary to ensure proper balance in the diet and the success of therapy.

Prognosis depends largely on the type of enzymatic defect that is present. Patients with mutase apoenzyme deficiency (*mut*^{0}, *mut*$^-$) have a worse prognosis. Unexplained infarcts of brain and renal dysfunction have been observed in some of these patients.

COMBINED METHYLMALONIC ACIDURIA AND HOMOCYSTINURIA (*cbl* C, *cbl* D, AND *cbl* F Defects). Fewer than two dozen patients with methylmalonic acidemia and homocystinuria due to *cbl* C, *cbl* D, and *cbl* F defects (see Figs. 8–4 and 8–6) have been reported. The majority of the patients had the *cbl* C defect; only two brothers with *cbl* D and two patients with *cbl* F defects have been identified.

Neurologic findings were prominent in patients with *cbl* C and *cbl* D defects. Most of these patients came to medical attention in the first 2 mo of life because of failure to thrive, lethargy, poor feeding, mental retardation, and seizures. However, late-onset defects with sudden development of dementia and myelopathy have been reported. Megaloblastic anemia was a common finding in patients with *cbl* C defect. Mild to moderate increases in concentrations of methylmalonic acid and homocysteine were found in body fluids. Neither hyperammonemia nor hyperglycinemia has been observed in these patients. Both reported patients with *cbl* F defect were females in whom poor feeding, growth and developmental delay, and persistent stomatitis became manifest in the first 3 wk of life. The first patient did not have megaloblastic anemia and homocystinuria, but both these signs were present in the second infant. Moderate methylmalonic acidemia was present in both infants. Patients with *cbl* E and *cbl* G defects do not have methylmalonic acidemia and are discussed further in the section on homocystinuria (see Sec. 8.41).

Experience with *treatment* of patients with *cbl* C, *cbl* D, and *cbl* F defects is very limited. Large doses of vitamin B_{12} (1–2 mg/24 hr) in conjunction with betaine (6–9 g/24 hr) seem to produce biochemical improvement with little clinical effect. Unexplained severe hemolytic anemia and congestive heart failure have been major complications in patients with *cbl* C defect.

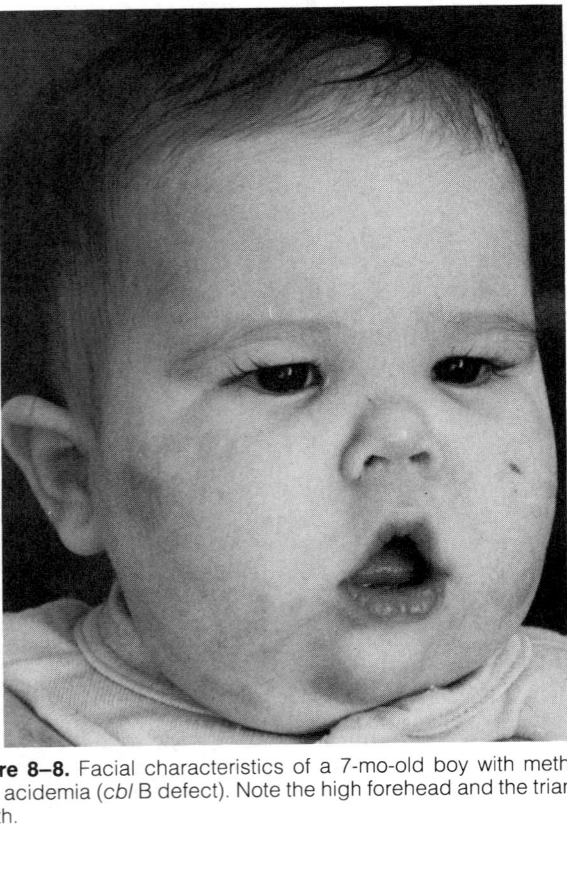

Figure 8–8. Facial characteristics of a 7-mo-old boy with methylmalonic acidemia (*cbl* B defect). Note the high forehead and the triangular mouth.

8.8 GLYCINE

Glycine is a nonessential amino acid synthesized mainly from serine and threonine. The main catabolic pathway requires the complex glycine cleavage enzyme system to cleave the first carbon of glycine and convert it to carbon dioxide. The second carbon is transferred to tetrahydrofolate (THF) to form hydroxymethyltetrahydrofolate, which may either react with another mole of glycine to form serine (Fig. 8–9) or form methyltetrahydrofolate, which serves as a methyl group donor for many reactions in the body (see Fig. 8–4).

HYPERGLYCINEMIA. Elevated levels of glycine in body fluids occur in patients having a number of inborn errors of metabolism, including propionic acidemia, methylmalonic acidemia, isovaleric acidemia, and β-ketothiolase deficiency. These disorders have been collectively referred to as *ketotic hyperglycinemia* because episodes of severe acidosis and ketosis occur. The pathogenesis of hyperglycinemia in these disorders is not fully understood, but inhibition of the glycine cleavage enzyme system by the various organic acids has been shown to occur in some of the affected patients. The term nonketotic hyperglycinemia is reserved for the clinical condition caused by the genetic deficiency of the glycine cleavage enzyme system (see Fig. 8–9). In this condition hyperglycinemia is present without ketosis.

Nonketotic Hyperglycinemia. The majority of patients with this disorder become ill during the first few days of life. The *clinical manifestations* of poor feeding, failure to suck, and lethargy may progress rapidly to a deep coma, apnea, and death. Convulsions, especially myoclonic seizures, and hiccups are common. This disorder is usually fatal; current therapeutic measures may produce only transient improvement. The rare infant who survives this state will have severe mental retardation, repeated myoclonic seizures, and microcephaly. Milder forms of the condition have also been reported; mental retardation, convulsions, and spasticity are

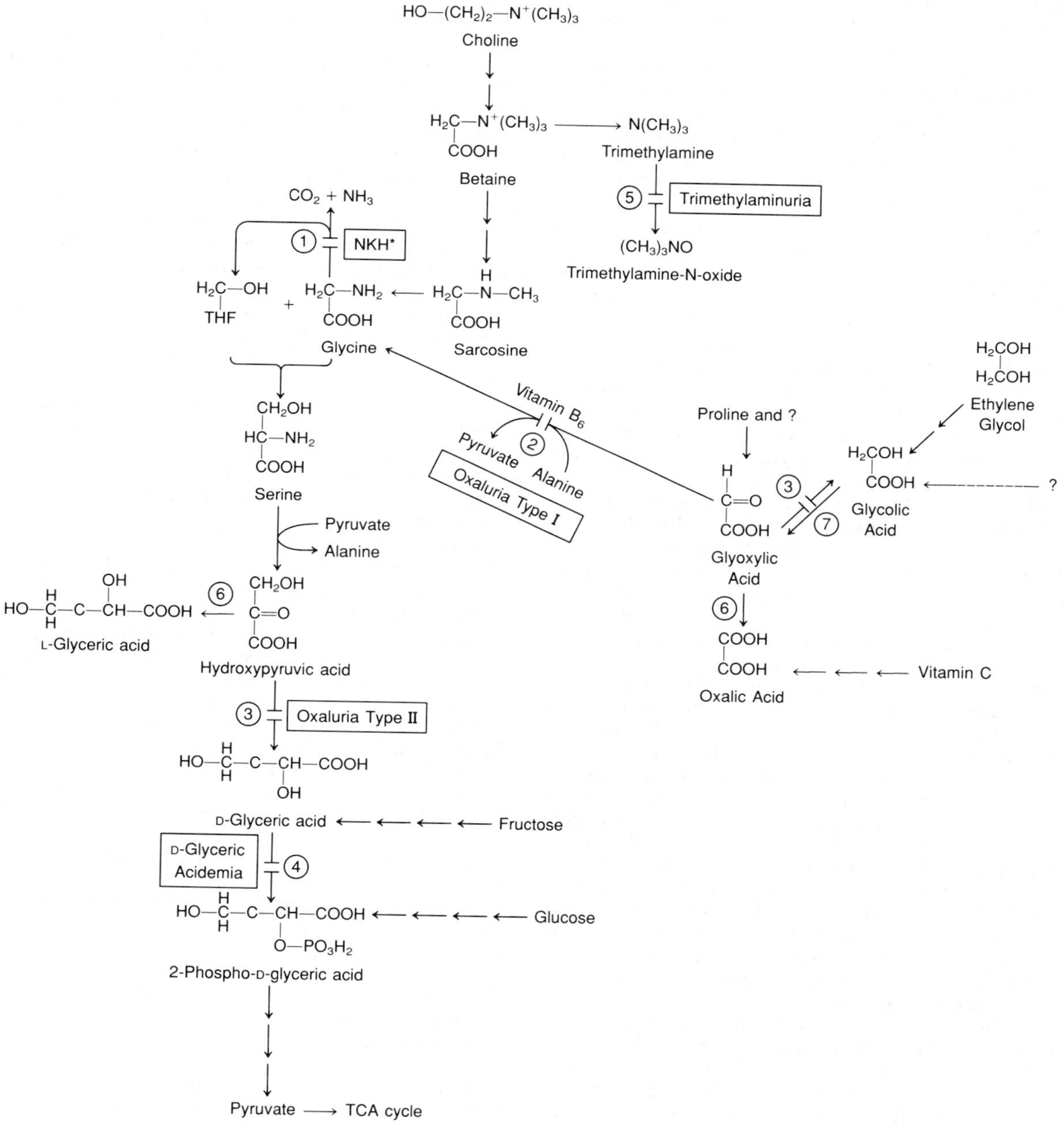

Figure 8–9. Pathways in metabolism of glycine and glyoxylic acid. **Enzymes**: (1) glycine cleavage enzyme; (2) alanine: glyoxylate aminotransferase; (3) D-glyceric acid dehydrogenase; (4) glycerate kinase; (5) trimethylamine oxidase; (6) lactate dehydrogenase; (7) glycolate oxidase. (NKH* = nonketotic hyperglycinemia; THF = tetrahydrofolate.)

frequent findings in these patients. Heterogeneity in clinical severity of the disease has also been observed within a given family.

Laboratory findings reveal moderate to severe hyperglycinemia and hyperglycinuria, and an increased glycine concentration in the spinal fluid. The high ratio of glycine concentration in the spinal fluid to that in blood has been used to differentiate nonketotic hyperglycinemia from other hyperglycinemic states. Plasma serine levels are usually low. Serum pH is usually normal. Organic acidemias that cause hyperglycinemia (propionic and methylmalonic acidemias) should be ruled out by proper urinary assays. Diagnosis of nonketotic hyperglycinemia may be suggested in infants who are receiving the anticonvulsant drug valproic acid because this medication is known to cause moderate increases in blood and urinary glycine concentrations. Repeat assays after removal of the drug should establish the diagnosis. The rare condition D-glyceric acidemia, which may cause hyperglycinemia, should also be ruled out (see later).

No effective *treatment* is known. Exchange transfusion, dietary restriction of glycine, and administration of sodium benzoate or folate have not altered the neurologic outcome. Drugs that counteract the effect of glycine on the neuronal cells, such as strychnine and diazepam, have been used; beneficial effects have been observed in some patients with the mild form of the condition.

Nonketotic hyperglycinemia appears to be inherited as an autosomal recessive trait and is more common in Finland than in any other part of the world. The enzyme system may be assayed in specimens obtained from liver or brain. Prenatal diagnosis has been accomplished by performing an assay of enzyme activity in biopsy specimens of chorionic villi.

SARCOSINEMIA. Increased concentrations of sarcosine (*N*-methylglycine) have been observed in both blood and urine, but no consistent clinical picture can be attributed to this metabolic defect. This is probably a recessively inherited inborn error involving sarcosine dehydrogenase, the enzyme that converts sarcosine to glycine (see Fig. 8–9).

D-GLYCERIC ACIDEMIA. D-Glyceric acid is an intermediate metabolite of serine and fructose metabolism (see Fig. 8–9). At least two forms of this rare condition have been identified. In one form (seen in three patients) clinical manifestations of severe encephalopathy (hypotonia, seizures, and mental and motor deficits) and the laboratory findings of hyperglycinemia and hyperglycinuria were suggestive of nonketotic hyperglycinemia. However, these patients excreted large quantities of D-glyceric acid (this compound is not normally detectable in urine). Enzyme studies indicated a deficiency of glycerate kinase in one patient and decreased activity of D-glyceric dehydrogenase in another.

In the other form, the major findings were persistent metabolic acidosis and developmental delay. This infant excreted large amounts of D-glyceric acid without hyperglycinemia. The enzyme defect in this patient was not identified.

TRIMETHYLAMINURIA. Trimethylamine is normally produced in the intestine from the breakdown of dietary choline and trimethylamine oxide by bacteria. Eggs and liver are the main sources of choline, and fish is the major source of trimethylamine oxide. Trimethylamine thus produced is absorbed and oxidized in the liver by trimethylamine oxidase to trimethylamine oxide, which is odorless, and is excreted in the urine. Deficiency of this enzyme results in massive excretion of trimethylamine in urine. Several asymptomatic patients with trimethylaminuria have been reported; there is a foul body odor that resembles that of a rotten fish. Restriction of fish, eggs, liver, and other sources of choline (such as nuts and grains) in the diet significantly reduces the odor.

HYPEROXALURIA AND OXALOSIS. Normally, oxalic acid is derived mostly from the oxidation of glyoxylic acid and, to a lesser degree, from oxidation of ascorbic acid (see Fig. 8–9). Glyoxylic acid is formed from the oxidation of glycolic acid in the peroxisomes. However, the source of glycolic acid remains unclear. Foods containing oxalic acid, such as spinach and rhubarb, are the main exogenous sources of this compound. Oxalic acid cannot be further metabolized in man and is excreted in the urine as oxalates. Calcium oxalate is relatively insoluble in water and precipitates in tissues (kidney and joints) if its concentration increases in the body.

Secondary hyperoxaluria has been observed in pyridoxine deficiency (cofactor for alanine-glyoxylate aminotransferase, see Fig. 8–9), following ingestion of ethylene glycol or high doses of vitamin C, after administration of the anesthetic agent methoxyflurane (which oxidizes directly to oxalic acid), and in patients with inflammatory bowel disease or extensive resection of bowel **(enteric hyperoxaluria)**. Acute, fatal hyperoxaluria may develop after ingestion of plants with a high oxalic acid content such as sorrel. Intentional ingestion of oxalic acid was a common suicidal agent at the turn of the century when oxalic acid was easily accessible as a common household cleaning agent. Precipitation of calcium oxalate in tissues causes hypocalcemia, liver necrosis, renal failure, cardiac arrythmia, and death. The lethal dose of oxalic acid is estimated to be between 5 and 30 g.

Primary hyperoxaluria is a rare genetic disorder in which large numbers of oxalates accumulate in the body. Two types of primary hyperoxaluria have been identified. The term **oxalosis** refers to deposition of calcium oxalate in parenchymal tissue.

Primary Hyperoxaluria Type I. This rare condition is the most common form of primary hyperoxaluria. It is due to a deficiency of the peroxisomal enzyme alanine-glyoxylate aminotransferase, which requires pyridoxine (vitamin B_6) as its cofactor. In the absence of this enzyme, glyoxylic acid, which cannot be converted to glycine, is transferred to the cytosol, where it is oxidized to oxalic acid (see Fig. 8–9). It is inherited as an autosomal recessive trait.

There is wide variation in the age of presentation. The majority of patients become symptomatic before 5 yr of age. In about 10% of cases symptoms develop before 1 yr of age (neonatal oxaluria). The initial *clinical manifestations* are related to renal stones and nephrocalcinosis. Renal colic and asymptomatic hematuria lead to a gradual deterioration of renal function, manifestated by growth retardation and uremia. Most patients die before 20 yr of age from renal failure. Acute arthritis is a rare manifestation and may be misdiagnosed as gout, since uric acid is usually elevated in patients with type I hyperoxaluria. Late forms of the disease presenting during adulthood have also been reported.

A marked increase in urinary excretion of oxalate (normal excretion 10–50 mg/24 hr) is the most important *laboratory finding*. The presence of oxalate crystals in urinary sediment is rarely helpful for diagnosis because such crystals are often seen in normal individuals. Unlike the situation with hyperoxaluria type II, urinary excretion of glycolic acid and glyoxylic acid is increased in patients with type I hyperoxaluria. Diagnosis can be confirmed by performing an assay of the enzyme in liver specimens.

Treatment has been largely unsuccessful. In some patients administration of large doses of pyridoxine reduces urinary excretion of oxalate. Renal transplantation in patients with renal failure has not improved the outcome in most cases because oxalosis has recurred in the transplanted kidney. Combined liver and kidney transplants have resulted in a significant decrease in plasma and urinary oxalate in a few patients and this may be the most effective treatment of this disorder to date.

Primary Hyperoxaluria Type II. This disorder, which has

been described in only four patients from two pedigrees, is due to the deficiency of D-glyceric acid dehydrogenase (see Fig. 8–9). In the absence of this enzyme, hydroxypyruvate (the ketoacid of serine) is reduced to L-glyceric acid by lactic dehydrogenase. The reason for increased oxalate production in this disorder is not clear. Clinically, these patients are indistinguishable from those with hyperoxaluria type I. Renal stones presenting with renal colic and hematuria may develop before age 2 yr. However, renal failure has not been observed in patients with type II oxaluria; the urine contains large amounts of L-glyceric acid in addition to high levels of oxalate (L-glyceric acid is not normally present in urine). Urinary excretion of glycolic acid and glyoxylic acid is not increased. The presence of L-glyceric acid without increased levels of glycolic and glyoxylic acids in urine differentiates this type from type I hyperoxaluria. A similar disease has been recently described in cats.

8.9 PROLINE AND HYDROXYPROLINE

Proline and hydroxyproline are found in high concentrations in collagen. Neither of these amino acids is normally found in urine in the free form except in early infancy. Excretion of "bound" hydroxyproline (dipeptides and tripeptides containing hydroxyproline) reflects collagen turnover and is increased in disorders of accelerated collagen turnover, such as rickets or hyperparathyroidism.

HYPERPROLINEMIA. Two types of this rare autosomal recessive condition have been described. *Type I hyperprolinemia* is due to a deficiency of proline oxidase (dehydrogenase), and *type II* is due to a defect in Δ'-pyrroline-5-carboxylic acid dehydrogenase enzyme (Fig. 8–10). Neither type causes any specific clinical manifestation. Increased blood concentrations of proline (more pronounced in type II) and prolinuria are found in both types. Hydroxyproline and glycine are also excreted in abnormal amounts in the urine because of the saturation of the common tubular reabsorption mechanism by the massive prolinuria. The presence of Δ'-pyrroline-5-carboxylic acid in plasma and urine differentiates type II from type I. No treatment is recommended for the affected individuals.

HYPERHYDROXYPROLINEMIA. This rare autosomal recessive condition is presumably due to a deficiency of hydroxyproline oxidase (see Fig. 8–10). Patients with this disorder are usually asymptomatic. A marked increase in blood concentration of hydroxyproline is diagnostic. These patients also excrete large quantities of proline and glycine in their urine. No treatment is recommended.

PROLIDASE DEFICIENCY. During collagen degradation imidodipeptides (such as glycylproline) are released and are normally cleaved by tissue prolidase. This enzyme requires manganese for its proper activity. Deficiency of prolidase, which is inherited as an autosomal recessive trait, results in the accumulation of imidodipeptides in body fluids. The gene for prolidase has been mapped to chromosome 19.

The *clinical manifestations* of this rare condition (only 28 patients are known) and the age of onset are quite variable. Skin lesions (recurrent ulcers, fine purpuric rash, crusting erythematous dermatitis), mental and motor deficits, susceptibility to infections, and joint laxity are major findings. Some patients have characteristic craniofacial features with ptosis, ocular proptosis, and prominent cranial sutures. Asymptomatic cases have also been reported. A marked increase in urinary excretion of imidodipeptides is diagnostic. Enzyme assay may be performed in erythrocytes or cultured skin fibroblasts.

Oral supplementation with proline, ascorbic acid, and manganese and the topical use of proline and glycine result in an improvement in leg ulcers.

FAMILIAL IMINOGLYCINURIA. This asymptomatic defect in renal tubular reabsorption of proline is inherited as an autosomal recessive trait. Since proline, hydroxyproline, and glycine are all transported by a common mechanism, patients with familial iminoglycinuria also excrete proline and hydroxyproline in abnormal amounts. The serum concentrations of these amino acids are normal. Many persons so affected also have impaired intestinal transport of proline, and a few may be coincidentally mentally retarded. In a screening program, iminoglycinuria was found in 1 in 15,000 infants. Iminoglycinuria is also seen in patients with hyperprolinemia, hyperhydroxyprolinemia, and Fanconi syndrome.

8.10 GLUTAMIC ACID

Glutathione (γ-glutamylcysteinylglycine) is the major product of glutamic acid in the body. This ubiquitous tripeptide is synthesized and degraded through a complex cycle called the γ-glutamyl cycle (Fig. 8–11). Because of its free sulfhydryl (−SH) group and its abundance in the cell, glutathione protects other sulfhydryl-containing compounds (such as en-

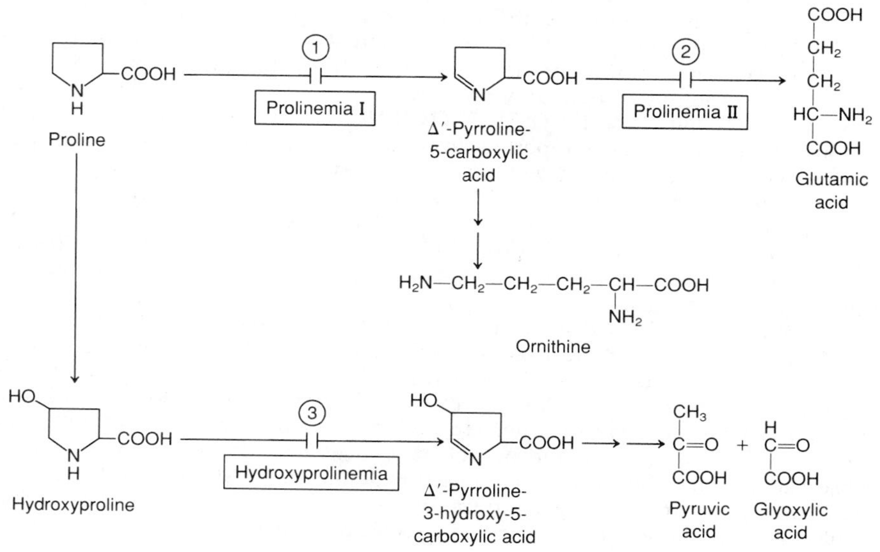

Figure 8–10. Pathways in the metabolism of the imino acids. **Enzymes**: (1) proline oxidase; (2) Δ¹-Pyrroline-5-carboxylic acid dehydrogenase; (3) hydroxyproline oxidase.

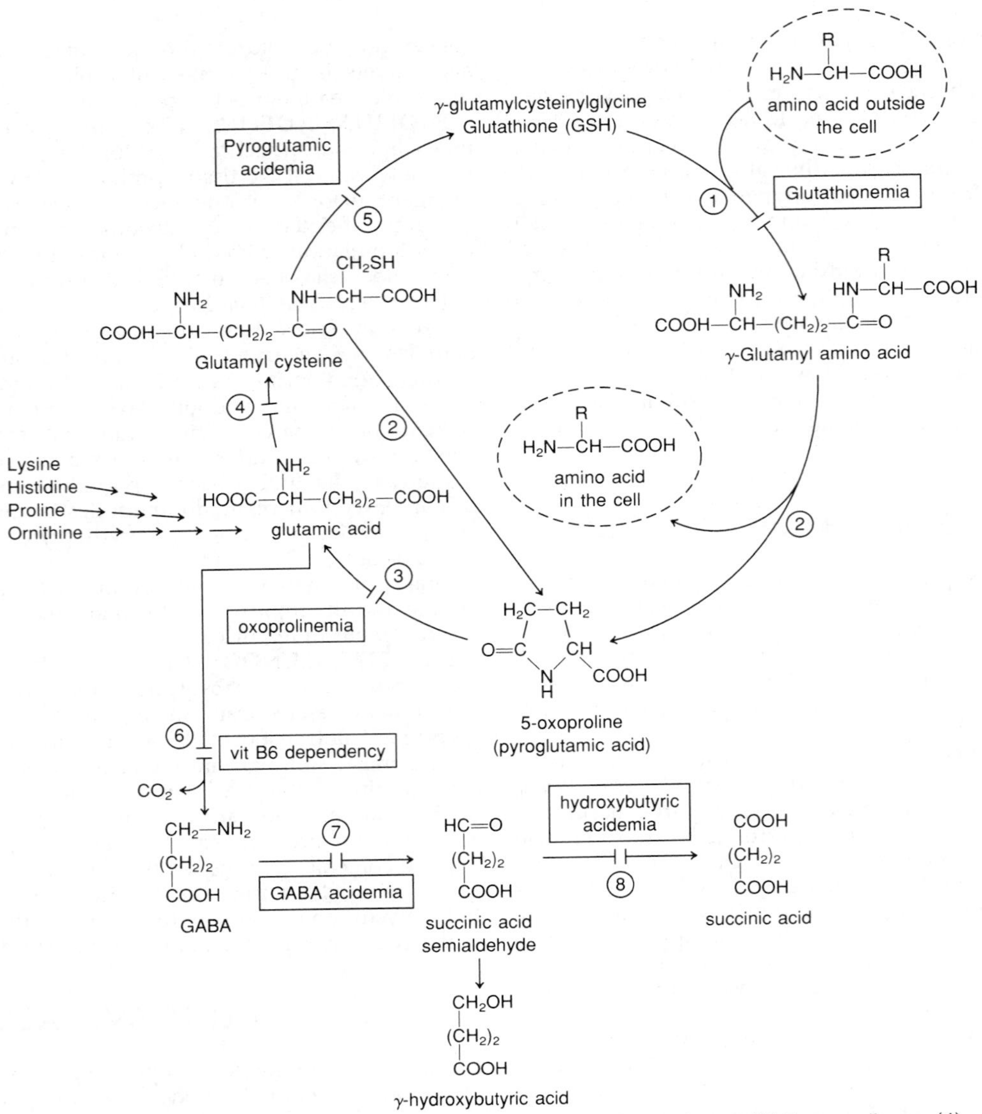

Figure 8–11. Enzymes: (1) γ glutamyl transpeptidase; (2) γ glutamyl cyclotransferase; (3) 5-oxoprolinase; (4) γ glutamylcysteine synthetase; (5) glutathione synthetase; (6) glutamic acid decarboxylase; (7) GABA transaminase; (8) succinic semialdehyde dehydrogenase.

zymes and coenzyme A) from oxidation. It is also involved in the detoxification of peroxides, including hydrogen peroxide, and in keeping the cell content in a reduced state. Glutathione may also participate in amino acid transport across the cell membrane through the γ-glutamyl cycle.

GLUTATHIONE SYNTHETASE DEFICIENCY. Two forms of this condition have been reported. In the *severe form*, which is due to generalized deficiency of the enzyme, severe acidosis and 5-oxoprolinuria are the rule. In the *mild form*, in which the enzyme deficiency is limited to red blood cells only, neither 5-oxoprolinuria nor acidosis has been observed. In both forms, patients have hemolytic anemia secondary to glutathione deficiency.

Glutathione Synthetase Deficiency, Severe Form (Pyroglutamic Acidemia, 5-Oxoprolinuria). Chronic metabolic acidosis and mild to moderate hemolytic anemia, which become manifest in the first few days of life, are cardinal findings in this rare autosomal recessive disorder (16 patients had been reported as of 1988). Mental and neurologic deficits have been observed in some affected children. Life-threatening metabolic acidosis may occur following a surgical procedure or intercurrent infection. These patients excrete massive amounts (up to 40 g/24 hr) of 5-oxoproline (pyroglutamic acid) in urine. High concentrations of this compound are also found in blood. The glutathione content of erythrocytes is markedly decreased. Increased synthesis of 5-oxoproline in this disorder is believed to be due to the conversion of γ-glutamylcysteine to 5-oxoproline by the enzyme γ-glutamyl cyclotransferase (see Fig. 8–11). γ-Glutamylcysteine production increases greatly because the inhibitory effect of glutathione on the γ-glutamylcysteine synthetase enzyme is removed. A deficiency of glutathione synthetase has been demonstrated in a variety of cells. *Treatment* is mainly directed toward correcting the acidosis, avoiding drugs and oxidants that may cause hemolysis, and preventing stressful states.

Glutathione Synthetase Deficiency, Mild Form. These patients have mild hemolytic anemia and jaundice without 5-oxoprolinuria and acidosis. The enzyme deficiency is limited to the red blood cells.

5-OXOPROLINASE DEFICIENCY. No clear clinical picture has yet been established because only three patients with this disorder have been reported. Two brothers had enterocolitis and renal stones. The other patient had only a low IQ. These findings may be unrelated to the enzyme deficiency. Patients excrete moderate quantities of 5-oxoproline in the urine but, unlike patients with glutathione synthetase deficiency, they are neither acidotic nor have hemolytic anemia. Glutathione and glutamate deficiencies do not occur in this disorder mainly because glutamic acid is produced from other sources in the body (see Fig. 8–11).

γ-GLUTAMYLCYSTEINE SYNTHETASE DEFICIENCY. Chronic hemolytic anemia, peripheral neuropathy, progressive spinocerebellar degeneration, and generalized aminoacidemia have been reported in two siblings who had very low erythrocytic glutathione levels and a marked deficiency of γ-glutamylcysteine synthetase. Inability to synthesize γ-glutamyl compounds results in impairment of amino acid transport in renal tubules and aminoaciduria (see Fig. 8–11).

GLUTATHIONEMIA (γ-Glutamyl Transpeptidase Deficiency). Mental retardation and severe behavioral problems are the major clinical manifestations of this rare disorder. Patients have glutathionemia, glutathionuria, and deficient activity of γ-glutamyl transpeptidase in leukocytes and cultured fibroblasts.

INBORN ERRORS OF METABOLISM OF γ-AMINOBUTYRIC ACID (GABA). GABA is synthesized mostly from glutamic acid and, to a lesser degree, from ornithine (see Fig. 8–11). GABA is most abundant in the brain and functions as an inhibitory factor for neurotransmitters.

Vitamin B_6 (Pyridoxine) Dependency. This autosomal recessive condition is due to a deficiency of glutamic acid decarboxylase activity in the brain, which results in decreased production of GABA. This enzyme requires vitamin B_6 as a cofactor (see Fig. 8–11). Diagnosis of pyridoxine dependency should be considered in infants in whom seizures in early life are poorly controlled with conventional anticonvulsant therapy but in whom administration of large doses (10–100 mg/kg) of vitamin B_6 results in dramatic improvement of both seizure activity and EEG abnormalities. Since this defect cannot be detected in fibroblasts, the diagnosis is usually made on the basis of a clinical response to vitamin B_6. Decreased activity of glutamic acid decarboxylase, reversible by the addition of pyridoxine, has been demonstrated in renal tissue but not in the brain. These children require high daily doses of vitamin B_6 indefinitely.

γ-Aminobutyric Acidemia (GABA Transaminase Deficiency). This condition is manifest as severe psychomotor retardation, hypotonia, and accelerated linear growth. There is a marked elevation of GABA and β-alanine in cerebrospinal fluid and blood (see Fig. 8–11). Increased linear growth occurs, possibly as a result of hypersecretion of growth hormone induced by GABA. GABA transaminase deficiency has been demonstrated in liver biopsy and lymphocytes. Treatment with high doses of vitamin B_6 is ineffective.

γ-Hydroxybutyric Acidemia. A defect in succinic semialdehyde dehydrogenase, inherited as an autosomal recessive disorder, leads to increased production of γ-hydroxybutyric acid, a normal minor metabolite of GABA, which is abundant in the brain (see Fig. 8–11). Ataxia, hypotonia, and neurologic deficits are the main clinical manifestations, which may occur in early infancy. Ataxia improves with advancement of age. Large amounts of γ-hydroxybutyrate and moderate quantities of succinic semialdehyde are found in the urine. Elevated levels of γ-hydroxybutyrate are also detected in the blood and cerebrospinal fluid. These levels may become normal with advancing age. The enzyme deficiency has been demonstrated in lymphocyte lysates. No effective treatment is yet available.

8.11 UREA CYCLE AND HYPERAMMONEMIA

Catabolism of amino acids results in the production of free ammonia, which is highly toxic to the central nervous system. Ammonia is detoxified to urea through a series of reactions known as the Krebs-Henseleit or urea cycle (Fig. 8–12). Five enzymes are required for the synthesis of urea: carbamylphosphate synthetase (CPS), ornithine transcarbamylase (OTC), argininosuccinate synthetase (AS), argininosuccinate lyase (AL), and arginase. A sixth enzyme, *N*-acetylglutamate synthetase, is also required for synthesis of *N*-acetylglutamate, which is an activator of the CPS enzyme. Individual deficiencies of these enzymes have been observed, and with an overall prevalence of 1 in 30,000 live births, they are the most common genetic causes of hyperammonemia in infants.

GENETIC CAUSES OF HYPERAMMONEMIA. In addition to genetic defects of the urea cycle enzymes, a marked increase in plasma level of ammonia is also observed in other inborn errors of metabolism (Table 8–4). In this section only defects of urea cycle enzymes and transient hyperammonemia of the newborn are discussed.

CLINICAL MANIFESTATIONS OF HYPERAMMONEMIA. In the *neonatal period*, symptoms and signs are mostly related to brain dysfunction and are similar regardless of the cause of the hyperammonemia. In general, the affected infant is normal at birth but becomes symptomatic after a few days of protein feeding. Refusal to eat, vomiting, tachypnea, and lethargy quickly progress to a deep coma. Convulsions are common. Physical examination may reveal hepatomegaly in addition to the neurologic signs of deep coma. In *infants and older children*, acute hyperammonemia is manifested by vomiting and neurologic abnormalities such as ataxia, mental confusion, agitation, irritability, and combativeness. These manifestations may alternate with periods of lethargy and somnolence that may progress to coma.

Routine *laboratory studies* show no specific findings when hyperammonemia is due to defects of the urea cycle enzymes. Blood urea nitrogen is usually very low. In infants with organic acidemias, hyperammonemia is commonly associated with severe acidosis. Newborn infants with hyperammonemia are often misdiagnosed as having a generalized infection, and they may succumb to the disease without a correct diagnosis. Autopsy is usually unremarkable. It is therefore imperative to measure plasma ammonia levels in any ill infant whose clinical manifestations cannot be explained by an obvious infection.

DIAGNOSIS. The main criterion for diagnosis is hyperammonemia. The plasma ammonia concentration in the ill infant is usually above 200 μM (normal values <35 μM). An approach to the differential diagnosis of hyperammonemia in the newborn infant is illustrated in Figure 8–13. Patients with a deficiency of carbamylphosphate synthetase or of ornithine transcarbamylase have no specific abnormalities of plasma amino acids except for increased levels of glutamine, aspartic acid, and alanine secondary to hyperammonemia. A marked increase in urinary orotic acid in patients with ornithine transcarbamylase deficiency differentiates this defect from carbamylphosphate synthetase deficiency. Patients with a deficiency of argininosuccinic acid synthetase, argininosuccinic acid lyase, or arginase have a marked increase in the plasma level of citrulline, argininosuccinic acid, or arginine, respectively. Differentiation between the carbamylphosphate synthetase deficiency and the *N*-acetylglutamate synthetase deficiency may require an assay of the respective enzymes. Clinical improvement occurring after oral administration of carbamylglutamate, however, may suggest *N*-acetylglutamate synthetase deficiency.

TREATMENT OF ACUTE HYPERAMMONEMIA. Acute hyperammonemia should be treated promptly and vigorously. The goal of therapy is to remove ammonia from the body and provide adequate calories and essential amino acids to halt further breakdown of endogenous proteins (Table 8–5). Adequate calories, fluid, and electrolytes should be provided

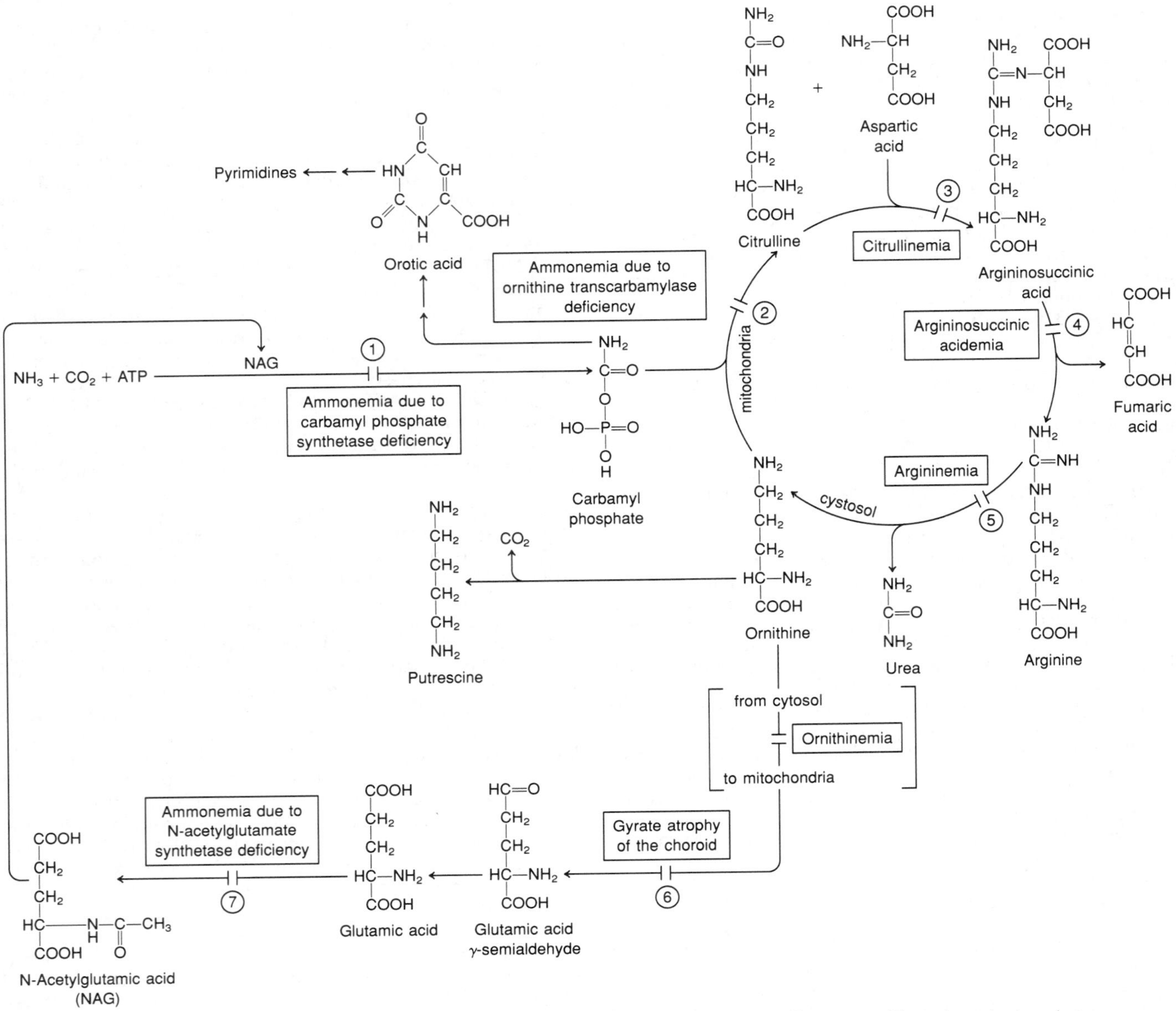

Figure 8–12. Pathways in the metabolism of ammonia and in the urea cycle. **Enzymes**: (1) carbamyl phosphate synthetase (CPS); (2) ornithine transcarbamylase (OTC); (3) argininosuccinic acid synthetase; (4) argininosuccinic acid lyase; (5) arginase; (6) ornithine 5-aminotransferase; (7) *N*-acetylglutamate synthetase.

intravenously. Lipids for intravenous use (1 g/kg/24 hr) provide an effective source of calories. Minimal amounts of protein (0.25 g/kg/24 hr), preferably in the form of essential amino acids, should be added to the intravenous fluid to prevent a catabolic state. To supply these essential amino acids without increasing the nitrogen load, ketoacid analogs of essential amino acids have been used by some, but the beneficial effects of these compounds have not been proved clinically. Oral feeding with a low-protein formula (0.5–1.0 g/kg/24 hr) through a nasogastric tube should be started as soon as sufficient improvement in the clinical condition permits it.

Since ammonia is poorly cleared by the kidneys, its removal from the body must be expedited by formation of compounds with a high renal clearance. Sodium benzoate forms hippuric acid with endogenous glycine; hippurate is cleared from the kidney at 5 times the glomerular filtration rate. Each mole of benzoate removes 1 mole of ammonia as glycine. Phenylacetate conjugates with glutamine to form phenylacetylglutamine, which is readily excreted in the urine. One mole of phenylacetate removes 2 moles of ammonia as glutamine from the body.

Arginine administration is effective in the treatment of hyperammonemia that is due to defects of the urea cycle (except in patients with arginase deficiency) because it supplies the urea cycle with ornithine and *N*-acetylglumate (see Fig. 8–12). In patients with citrullinemia, 1 mole of arginine reacts with 1 mole of ammonia (as carbamylphosphate) to form citrulline. In patients with argininosuccinic acidemia, 2 moles of ammonia (as carbamylphosphate and aspartate) form argininosuccinic acid with arginine through the urea cycle. Citrulline and argininosuccinic acid are far less toxic and more readily excreted by the kidneys than ammonia. In patients with CPS or ornithine transcarbamylase (OTC) deficiency, arginine administration is indicated because arginine becomes an essential amino acid in these disorders. Patients with OTC deficiency benefit from citrulline supplementation (200 mg/kg/24 hr) because 1 mole of citrulline can accept 1 mole of

TABLE 8–4. Inborn Errors of Metabolism Causing Hyperammonemia

Deficiencies of the urea cycle enzymes (Sec. 8.11)
- Carbamyl phosphate synthetase (CPS)
- *N*-acetylglutamate synthetase
- Ornithine transcarbamylase (OTC)
- Argininosuccinate synthetase (AS)
- Argininosuccinate lyase (AL)
- Arginase

Organic acidemias (Sec. 8.7)
- Propionic acidemia
- Methylmalonic acidemia
- Isovaleric acidemia
- Ketothiolase deficiency
- Multiple carboxylase deficiency
- Fatty acid acyl CoA dehydrogenase deficiency (glutaric acidemia type II)
- 3-Hydroxy-3-methylglutaric acidemia

Lysinuric protein intolerance (Sec. 8.13)

Hyperornithinemia-hyperammonemia-homocitrullinemia syndrome (Sec. 8.11)

Periodic hyperlysinuria with hyperammonemia (?) (Sec. 8.13)

Transient hyperammonemia of the newborn (Sec. 8.11)

ammonia (as aspartic acid) to form arginine. In patients whose hyperammonemia is secondary to organic acidemias, treatment with arginine is not indicated because no beneficial effect from such therapy can be expected. However, in a newborn infant with a first attack of hyperammonemia, arginine should be used until the diagnosis is established.

Benzoate, phenylacetate, and arginine may be administered together for maximal therapeutic effect. A priming dose of these compounds is followed by continuous infusion until recovery from the acute state occurs (see Table 8–5). It should be noted that both benzoate and phenylacetate are supplied as concentrated solutions and should be properly diluted (1–2% solution) for intravenous use. The recommended therapeutic doses of both compounds deliver a substantial amount of sodium to the patient that should be calculated as part of the daily sodium requirement. Benzoate and phenylacetate should be used with caution in newborn infants with hyperbilirubinemia because they may potentiate the risk of hyperbilirubinemia by displacing bilirubin from albumin. In infants at risk, it is advisable to reduce bilirubin to a safe level by exchange transfusion before administering benzoate or phenylacetate.

If the foregoing therapies fail to produce any appreciable change in the blood ammonia level within a few hours, hemodialysis or peritoneal dialysis should be used. Exchange transfusion has little effect on reducing total body ammonia. It should be used only if dialysis cannot be employed promptly or when the patient is a newborn infant with hyperbilirubinemia (see earlier). Hemodialysis, although the most effective measure for removal of ammonia, is technically difficult to perform and may not be readily available in all centers. Peritoneal dialysis, therefore, is the most practical and expeditious method for treatment of patients with severe hyperammonemia; there is usually a dramatic decrease in the plasma ammonia level within a few hours of dialysis, and in most patients the plasma ammonia returns to normal within 48 hr of initiation of peritoneal dialysis. In a patient whose hyperammonemia is due to an organic acidemia, peritoneal dialysis effectively removes both the offending organic acid and ammonia from the body.

To curtail the possible production of ammonia by intestinal bacteria, oral administration of neomycin and lactulose through a nasogastric tube should be initiated very early in the course of therapy. There may be considerable lag between the normalization of ammonia and an improvement in the neurologic status of the patient. Several days may be needed before the infant becomes fully alert.

Long-Term Therapy. Once the infant is alert, therapy should be tailored to the underlying cause of the hyperammonemia. In general, all patients require some degree of protein restriction (1–2 g/kg/24 hr) regardless of the enzymatic defect. In patients with defects in the urea cycle, chronic administration of benzoate (250–500 mg/kg/24 hr), phenylacetate (250–500 mg/kg/24 hr), and arginine (200–400 mg/kg/24 hr), or citrulline in patients with OTC deficiency (200–400 mg/kg/24 hr), is effective in maintaining blood ammonia levels within the normal range. Phenylacetate may not be accepted by the patient and family because of its offensive odor. Carnitine supplementation has also been recommended for treatment of these patients because benzoate and phenylacetate may cause carnitine depletion, but the clinical benefits of this compound remain to be proved. Catabolic states triggering hyperammonemia should be avoided.

CARBAMYLPHOSPHATE SYNTHETASE (CPS) AND *N*-ACETYLGLUTAMATE SYNTHETASE DEFICIENCIES. Deficiencies of these two enzymes produce similar *clinical and biochemical manifestations*. Affected infants usually become symptomatic in the first few days of life with refusal to eat, vomiting, lethargy, convulsions, and coma. Late forms of the CPS deficiency, characterized by mental retardation with episodes of vomiting and lethargy, have also been reported.

Laboratory findings reveal hyperammonemia without an increase in any specific amino acids in plasma; marked elevations in plasma concentrations of glutamine and alanine seen in these patients are secondary to hyperammonemia. Urinary orotic acid is usually low or may be absent (see Fig. 8–13).

Treatment of patients with CPS deficiency is similar to that outlined above for hyperammonemia. The single reported case of *N*-acetylglutamate synthetase deficiency was shown to benefit from oral administration of carbamylglutamate. It is, therefore, important to differentiate between these two enzyme deficiencies by assay of the enzyme activities in biopsies obtained from the liver.

CPS deficiency is inherited as an autosomal recessive trait; the enzyme is normally present in liver and intestine. The gene is mapped to the short arm of chromosome 2.

TABLE 8–5. Treatment of Acute Hyperammonemia in an Infant

1. Provide adequate calories, fluid, and electrolytes intravenously (10% glucose and intravenous lipids 1 g/kg/24 hr). Add minimal amounts of protein as a mixture of essential amino acids (0.25 g/kg/24 hr) during the first 24 hr of therapy.
2. Give priming doses of the following compounds:

Sodium benzoate 250 mg/kg* Sodium phenylacetate 250 mg/kg* Arginine hydrochloride 200–800 mg/kg† as a 10% solution	To be added to 20 mL/kg of 10% glucose and infused within 1–2 hr

3. Continue infusion of sodium benzoate* (250–500 mg/kg/24 hr), sodium phenylacetate* (250–500 mg/kg/24 hr), and arginine (200–800 mg/kg/24 hr†) following the above priming doses. These compounds should be added to the daily intravenous fluid.
4. Initiate peritoneal dialysis or hemodialysis if above treatment fails to produce an appreciable decrease in plasma ammonia.

*These compounds are usually prepared as a 5–10% solution for intravenous use. Sodium from these drugs should be included as part of the daily sodium requirement.

†The higher dose is recommended in the treatment of patients with citrullinemia and argininosuccinic aciduria. Arginine is not recommended in patients with arginase deficiency and in those whose hyperammonemia is secondary to organic acidemias.

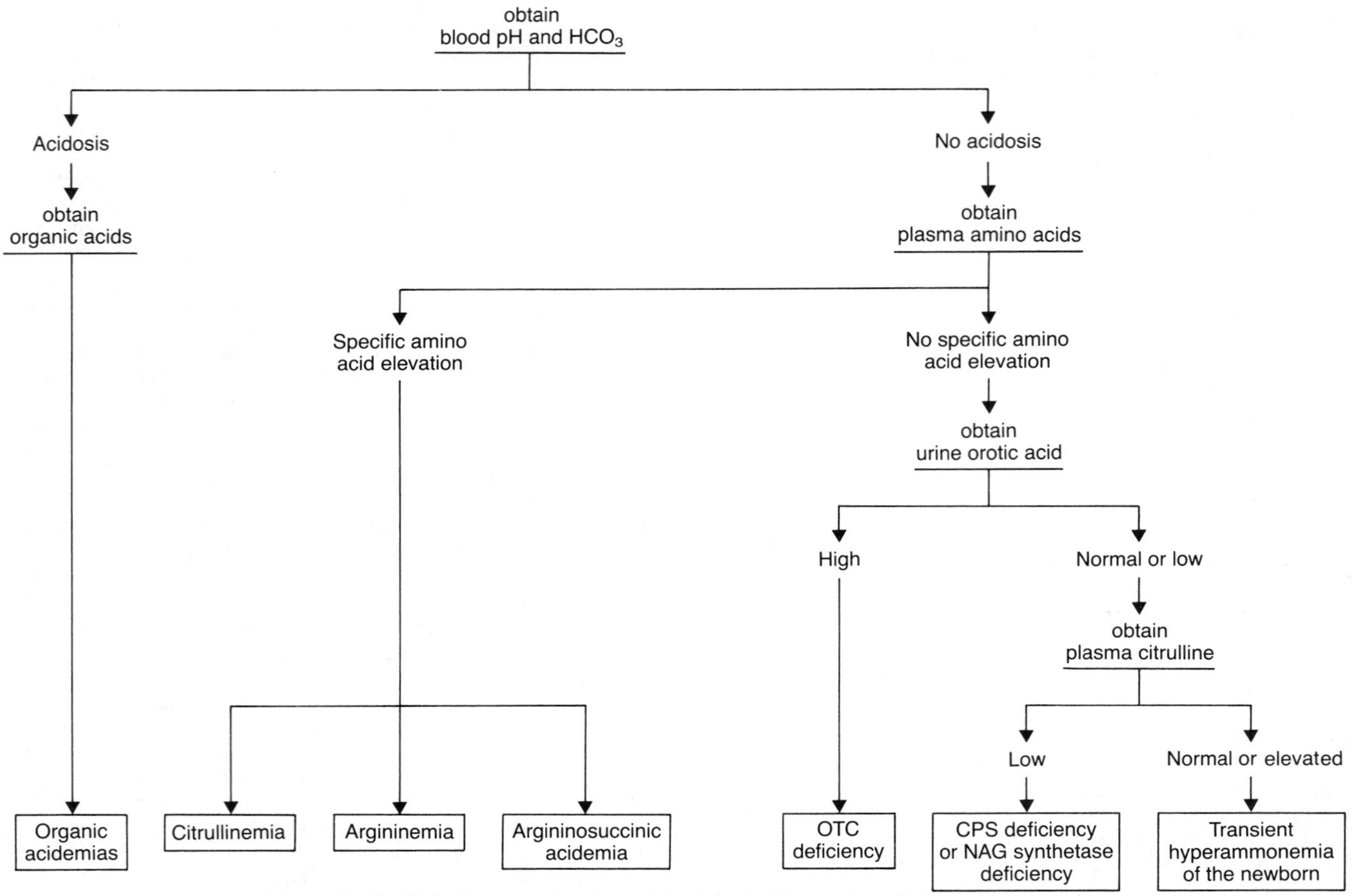

Figure 8–13. Clinical approach to a newborn infant with symptomatic hyperammonemia.

N-acetylglutamate synthetase has been assayed only in liver specimens obtained at biopsy.

ORNITHINE TRANSCARBAMYLASE (OTC) DEFICIENCY. In this X-linked dominant disorder the hemizygote males are more severely affected than heterozygote females. The latter may have either mild disease or no clinical manifestations. This is probably the most common of all the urea cycle disorders.

Clinical manifestations in a male newborn infant are those of severe hyperammonemia. Milder forms of the condition are commonly seen in heterozygote females and in some affected males. These forms characteristically have episodic manifestations. Episodes of hyperammonemia (manifested by vomiting and neurologic abnormalities such as ataxia, mental confusion, agitation, and combativeness) are separated by periods of wellness. Onset may occur in early infancy or early childhood. These episodes usually occur following a high-protein diet or during a situation of stress or infection. Hyperammonemic coma and death may occur during one of these attacks. Some affected children have been diagnosed as having recurrent Reye syndrome. Mental development may proceed normally. However, mild to moderate mental retardation is common.

The major *laboratory finding* during the acute attack is hyperammonemia without an increase in any specific amino acid in the blood. As with CPS deficiency, elevation of the plasma concentrations of glutamine and alanine are secondary to hyperammonemia. A marked increase in the urinary excretion of orotic acid differentiates this condition from CPS deficiency (see Fig. 8–13). Orotates may precipitate in urine as gravel or stones. In the mild form, these laboratory abnormalities may revert to normal between attacks. This form should be differentiated from all the episodic conditions of childhood and from poisoning. In particular, lysinuric protein intolerance (Sec. 8.13) mimics the clinical and biochemical characteristics of OTC deficiency. Increased urinary excretion of lysine, ornithine, and arginine and elevated blood concentrations of citrulline, which are salient features of lysinuric protein intolerance, are not seen in patients with OTC deficiency.

The *diagnosis* may be confirmed by performing an assay of enzyme activity that is normally present only in liver. Perinatal diagnosis has been achieved by means of fetal liver biopsy and, more recently, by studying the characteristic DNA polymorphism in chorionic villus samples. Asymptomatic heterozygous female carriers may be identified by using an oral protein load, which increases plasma ammonia and urinary orotic acid levels. A marked increase in urinary excretion of orotidine following an allopurinol loading test has also been used to detect obligate female carriers. Asymptomatic female carriers have mild cerebral dysfunction compared with their unaffected siblings.

Treatment is similar to that given for CPS deficiency except that citrulline may be used in place of arginine.

ARGININOSUCCINIC ACID SYNTHETASE DEFICIENCY (Citrullinemia). Citrullinemia is inherited as an autosomal recessive trait. The gene is located on the long arm of chromosome 9. The severity of the abnormality of the mutant genes inherited from each parent is different in a given patient, indicating that most affected patients are "double or compound" heterozygotes. This disorder shows considerable clinical and biochemical heterogeneity.

The spectrum of *clinical manifestations* ranges from severe forms to asymptomatic ones. The signs and symptoms in the neonatal form are identical to those seen in the severe forms of CPS and OTC deficiencies (see earlier). Mild forms may have a gradual onset with failure to thrive, frequent vomiting, developmental delay, and dry, brittle hair or, like mild forms of OTC deficiency, may appear episodically (see earlier). In some patients symptoms may not appear until 20 yr of age.

Laboratory findings are similar to those found in patients with OTC deficiency except that the plasma citrulline concentration is markedly elevated in patients with citrullinemia (see Fig. 8–13). Urinary secretion of orotic acid is moderately increased in patients with citrullinemia, and crystalluria due to precipitation of orotates may also occur. Patients with argininosuccinic aciduria also show some increase in the plasma concentration of citrulline in addition to elevated levels of argininosuccinic acid. The *diagnosis* is confirmed by performing an assay of the enzyme activity that is normally present in cultured fibroblasts. Prenatal diagnosis is based on an assay of the enzyme activity in cultured amniotic cells.

Treatment is similar to that for other urea cycle disorders (see earlier). Although *prognosis* is very poor for symptomatic neonates, patients with the mild disease usually do well on a protein-restricted diet. Mild to moderate mental deficiency is a common sequela even in a well-treated patient.

ARGININOSUCCINATE LYASE DEFICIENCY (Argininosuccinic Aciduria). This deficiency is inherited as an autosomal recessive trait with a prevalence of about 1 in 70,000 live births. The gene is located on chromosome 7.

The severity of the *clinical and biochemical manifestations* varies considerably. In the neonatal form severe hyperammonemia develops in the first few days of life, and mortality is usually high. In the subacute or late form the major finding is mental retardation, which is associated with episodic vomiting, failure to thrive, and hepatomegaly. Abnormalities of the hair (characterized by dryness and brittleness) are of special diagnostic value. Microscopically, the hair appears similar to that seen in patients with trichorrhexis nodosa. Less severe hair abnormalities are also seen in patients with citrullinemia.

Laboratory findings reveal hyperammonemia, moderate elevation in liver enzymes, nonspecific increases in plasma levels of glutamine and alanine, moderate increase in plasma levels of citrulline (less than that seen in citrullinemia), and marked increase in plasma levels of argininosuccinic acid. In most amino acid analyzers, argininosuccinic acid appears within the isoleucine or methionine region, which may cause confusion in the diagnosis. Argininosuccinic acid can also be found in large amounts in urine and spinal fluid. The levels in the spinal fluid are usually higher than those in plasma. The enzyme is normally present in erythrocytes, liver, and cultured fibroblasts. Prenatal diagnosis is based on measuring the enzyme activity in cultured amniotic cells. Argininosuccinic acid is also elevated in the amniotic fluid of affected fetuses.

Treatment is similar to that described for citrullinemia.

ARGINASE DEFICIENCY (Hyperargininemia). This defect is inherited as an autosomal recessive trait. There are two genetically distinct arginases in humans. One is cystosolic and is expressed in liver and erythrocytes, and the other is found in the renal mitochondria. The cytosolic enzyme, which is the one deficient in patients with arginase deficiency, is mapped to the long arm of chromosome 6.

The *clinical manifestations* of this rare condition are quite different from those of other urea cycle enzyme defects. The onset is insidious; the infant usually remains asymptomatic in the first few months or sometimes years of life. A progressive spastic diplegia with scissoring of the lower extremities, choreoathetotic movements, and loss of developmental milestones in a previously normal infant may suggest a degenerative disease of the central nervous system. Mental retardation is progressive; seizures are common, and episodes of severe hyperammonemia are not usually seen in this disorder. Hepatomegaly may be present.

Laboratory findings reveal marked elevation of arginine in plasma and cerebrospinal fluid (see Fig. 8–13). Urinary orotic acid is moderately increased. Plasma ammonia levels may be normal or mildly elevated. Urinary excretion of arginine, lysine, cystine, and ornithine is increased, which may suggest a diagnosis of cystinuria. Therefore, determination of plasma amino acid is important in any child with increased urinary excretion of these dibasic amino acids. The guanidino compounds (guanidinoacetic acid and guanidinobutyric acid) are also markedly increased in the urine. The *diagnosis* is confirmed by assaying arginase activity in erythrocytes. Prenatal diagnosis has not yet been achieved.

Treatment consists of a low-protein diet devoid of arginine. Administration of a synthetic protein made of essential amino acids usually results in a dramatic decrease in plasma arginine concentration and an improvement in neurologic abnormalities. The composition of the diet and the daily intake of protein should be monitored by frequent plasma amino acid determinations. Sodium benzoate (250–375 mg/kg/24 hr) is also effective in controlling hyperammonemia.

TRANSIENT HYPERAMMONEMIA OF THE NEWBORN. Although the plasma levels of ammonia in normal full-term infants are within the normal limits of those seen in older children, a majority of premature infants with low-birth-weights have a *mild transient hyperammonemia* (40–50 μM), which lasts for about 6–8 wk. These infants are asymptomatic, and follow-up studies up to 18 mo of age have not revealed any significant neurologic deficits.

Severe transient hyperammonemia has been observed in newborn infants. The majority of affected infants have been premature and have had mild respiratory distress syndrome. Hyperammonemic coma may develop within 2–3 days of life, and the infant may succumb to the disease if treatment is not started immediately. Laboratory studies reveal marked hyperammonemia (plasma ammonia as high as 4,000 μM), with moderate increases in plasma levels of glutamine and alanine. Plasma concentrations of urea cycle intermediate amino acids are usually normal except for citrulline, which may be moderately elevated. The cause of the disorder is unknown. Urea cycle enzyme activities are normal. Treatment of hyperammonemia should be initiated promptly and continued vigorously. Recovery without sequelae is common, and hyperammonemia does not recur even with a normal protein diet.

ORNITHINE. Ornithine is one of the intermediate metabolites of the urea cycle that is not incorporated into natural proteins. Rather, it is generated in the cytosol from arginine and must be transported into the mitochondria, where it is used as a substrate for the enzyme OTC to form citrulline. Excess ornithine is catabolized by two enzymes, ornithine 5-aminotransferase, which is a mitochondrial enzyme and converts ornithine to a proline precursor, and ornithine decarboxylase, which resides in the cytosol and converts ornithine to putrescine (see Fig. 8–12). Two genetic disorders result in hyperornithinemia: gyrate atrophy of the retina and ammonemia-hyperornithinemia-homocitrullinemia syndrome.

Gyrate Atrophy of the Retina and Choroid. This is an autosomal recessively inherited disorder due to the deficiency of the enzyme ornithine 5-aminotransferase. About half of the reported cases are from Finland. Clinical manifestations are limited to the eyes and include night blindness, myopia, loss of peripheral vision, and posterior subcapsular cataracts. These eye changes start between 5 and 10 yr of age and progress to complete blindness by the 4th decade of life. Atrophic lesions in the retina resemble cerebral gyri. These patients usually have normal intelligence. There is a 10- to 20-fold increase in plasma levels of ornithine. There is no occurrence of hyperammonemia and no increase in any other amino acids. Some patients respond to high doses of pyridoxine (500–1,000 mg/24 hr) and low dietary arginine.

Hyperammonemia-Hyperornithinemia-Homocitrullinemia Syndrome (HHH Syndrome). In this rare autosomal recessively inherited disorder the defect is in the transport system of ornithine from the cytosol into the mitochondria, causing an accumulation of ornithine in the cytosol and a deficiency of ornithine inside the mitochondria. The former causes hyperornithinemia and the latter results in disruption of the urea cycle and hyperammonemia. Homocitrulline is formed from the reaction of mitochondrial carbamylphosphate with lysine, which occurs because of the intramitochondrial deficiency of ornithine. Acute episodes of hyperammonemia in early infancy may result in coma. Failure to thrive, mental retardation, and seizures are common findings between the attacks. The onset may be delayed until adulthood in some affected patients. No ocular lesions have been observed in these patients. Marked increases in plasma levels of ornithine and homocitrulline are usually diagnostic. Restriction of protein intake improves hyperammonemia. Ornithine supplementation may produce clinical improvement in some patients.

8.12 HISTIDINE

Histidine is an essential amino acid only during infancy. Its synthetic pathway in older children and adults is poorly understood. Histidine is degraded through the urocanic acid pathway to glutamic acid (Fig. 8–14).

HISTIDINEMIA. This disorder is due to a deficiency of histidase, which normally converts histidine to urocanic acid (see Fig. 8–14). The disorder is inherited as an autosomal recessive trait; its overall prevalence is estimated at 1 in 10,000 worldwide.

Clinical manifestations include impaired speech, growth retardation, or mental retardation. However, the relationship of these findings to histidinemia remains unclear; routine amino acid screening has uncovered a significant number of asymptomatic subjects with histidinemia.

Laboratory studies reveal marked increases in plasma and cerebrospinal fluid concentrations of histidine. There is also an unexplained elevation in the blood level of alanine. Urine contains large amounts of histidine and its transaminated product imidazolepyruvate. The latter compound, like phenylpyruvate, reacts with ferric chloride to produce an intense blue-green color. The *diagnosis* of histidinemia may be confirmed by assay of histidase in liver or skin. Prenatal diagnosis has not yet been achieved because histidase is not present in amniotic cells.

Treatment with a diet low in histidine has produced excellent biochemical control. However, no clinical improvement in symptomatic patients has been observed. Unlike phenylketonuria, maternal histidinemia does not cause any ill effect in the offspring.

UROCANIC ACIDURIA. This disorder is characterized by mental and growth retardation and massive urocanic aciduria (see Fig. 8–14). Urocanase deficiency has been shown in liver biopsies of three of the four reported children. However, the relation of this enzyme deficiency to the clinical findings may be coincidental because normal infants with urocanic aciduria have been identified through routine urine screening of newborns.

HISTIDINURIA. The urinary excretion of histidine normally increases in pregnant women. Histidinuria also occurs as an overflow phenomenon in patients with histidinemia. Isolated histidinuria without histidinemia due to defective

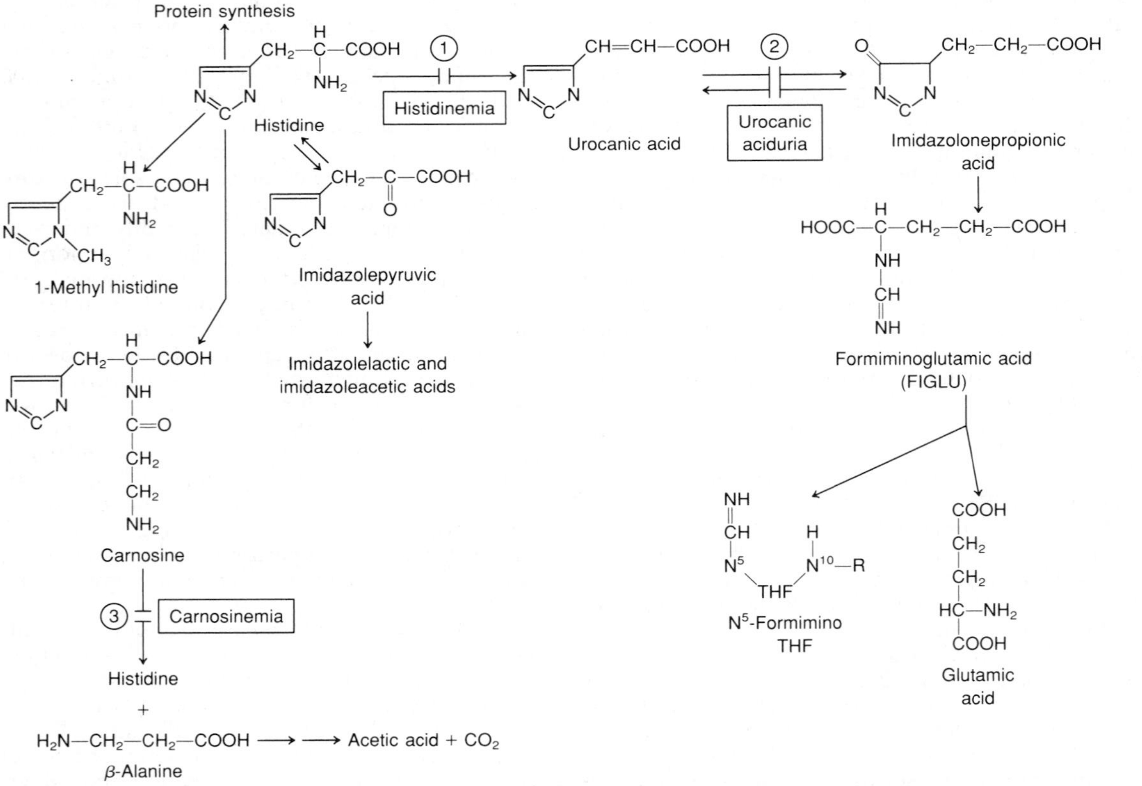

Figure 8–14. Pathways in the metabolism of histidine. (THF = tetrahydrofolic acid.) **Enzymes**: (1) histidase; (2) urocanase; (3) carnosinase.

renal tubular reabsorption may occur in children whose parents and siblings have been shown to be heterozygotic for the defect.

8.13 LYSINE

Lysine is an essential dibasic amino acid with a unique catabolic pathway, which starts with its condensation with α-ketoglutaric acid to form saccharopine rather than with its transamination. Saccharopine is then broken down to acetoacetic acid through a series of reactions (Fig. 8–15). The first two enzymes involved in the catabolic pathway of lysine, α-ketoglutarate reductase and saccharopine dehydrogenase, are very likely part of a one-protein complex controlled by a single gene. In a minor pathway for the catabolism of lysine, transamination is the first step and pipecolic acid is formed (see Fig. 8–15). This pathway is most active in the brain.

HYPERLYSINEMIA. Marked elevations of plasma lysine may occur as persistent or periodic disorders; the latter is also associated with hyperammonemia.

Persistent Hyperlysinemia. This rare, presumably autosomal recessive disorder is due to a deficiency of the putative enzyme complex lysine ketoglutarate reductase/saccharopine dehydrogenase system.

Clinical manifestations range from severe mental and physical retardation, joint laxity, and convulsions to perfectly normal children (who were identified through routine screening). Hyperlysinemia is not generally believed to be the cause of clinical manifestations in symptomatic patients.

Laboratory findings reveal hyperlysinemia, saccharopinemia, lysinuria, and saccharopinuria (saccharopine is not normally detected in blood or urine) in the majority of the patients. Affected persons with hyperlysinemia but without saccharopinemia have also been reported. In addition, homocitrulline and homoarginine are found in body fluids (see Fig. 8–15). Combined deficiencies of the enzymes lysine ketoglutarate reductase and saccharopine dehydrogenase have been found in all patients having these measurements except one who had a complete deficiency of saccharopine dehydrogenase with a mild decrease in lysine ketoglutarate reductase activity.

Hyperlysinemia/saccharopinemia is an example of a double

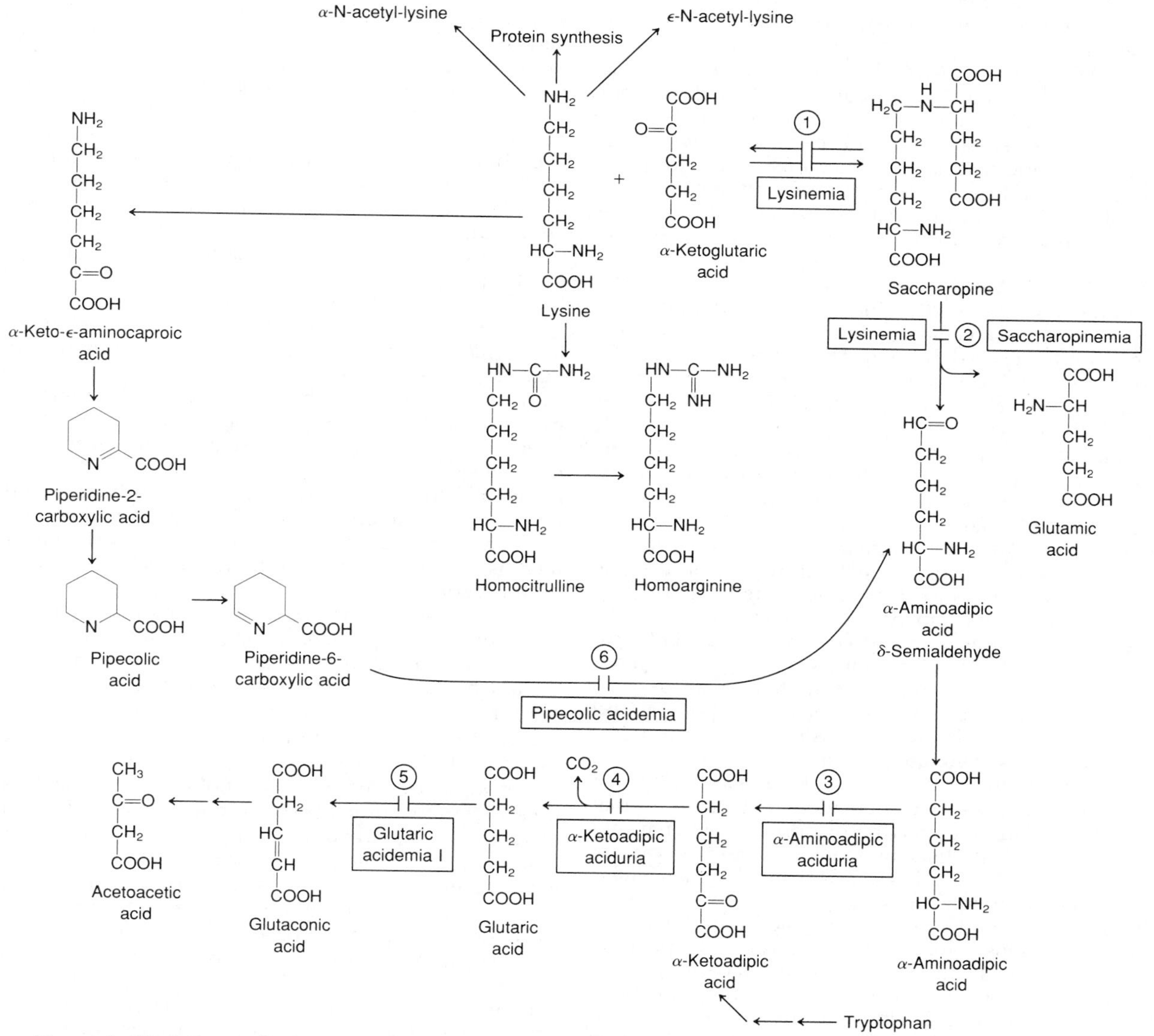

Figure 8–15. Pathways in the metabolism of lysine. **Enzymes**: (1) lysine ketoglutarate reductase; (2) saccharopine dehydrogenase; (3) α-aminoadipic acid transferase; (4) α-ketoadipic acid dehydrogenase; (5) glutaryl CoA dehydrogenase; (6) α-aminoadipic semialdehyde oxidase.

deficiency of two sequential enzymes. Another example is the enzyme deficiency causing orotic aciduria (see Sec. 8.47).

The need for treatment of patients with hyperlysinemia is controversial.

Periodic Hyperlysinemia with Hyperammonemia. Patients with this disorder have episodes of hyperammonemia and hyperlysinemia that may start in the newborn period. They are triggered by a diet high in lysine or in protein. A low-protein diet normalizes plasma concentrations of lysine and ammonia. Patients may have increased levels of plasma arginine or citrulline during the attacks. Enzymes of the urea cycle were within normal limits in patients in the original reports, but subsequently deficiency of the enzyme argininosuccinic synthetase was reported. The basic defect in these patients is obscure but may be a deficiency of one of the urea cycle enzymes because plasma lysine is elevated in some patients with deficiencies of the urea cycle enzymes.

α-AMINOADIPIC ACIDEMIA. Normal children and children with multiple bony anomalies and learning disabilities who excrete large amounts of α-aminoadipic acid have been reported. No relationship could be established between the clinical abnormalities and the biochemical defect. Since lysine loads increased the α-aminoadipic acid excretion, the block is presumed to be an inability to convert α-aminoadipic to α-ketoadipic acid.

α-KETOADIPIC ACIDEMIA. Neonatal seizures, ichthyosis, mild metabolic acidosis, and subsequent marked retardation are associated with elevated α-ketoadipic acid levels in plasma and urine. A defect in the decarboxylation of α-ketoadipic to glutaric acid has been demonstrated. However, the same biochemical defects have been found in a clinically normal sibling of an affected patient, raising doubts about any relationship between the metabolic defect and the mental retardation.

GLUTARIC ACIDURIA TYPE I. Glutaric acid is an intermediate in the degradation of lysine (see Fig. 8–15), hydroxylysine, and tryptophan. Glutaric aciduria type I, an autosomal recessive disorder caused by a deficiency of glutaryl CoA dehydrogenase, should be differentiated from glutaric aciduria type II, a distinct clinical and biochemical disorder caused by deficiencies of acyl CoA dehydrogenases (see Sec. 8.15). The incidence of the disorder is not known, but it may be more common than has been realized. The disease may be more prevalent in Sweden and among the Pennsylvania Amish in the United States.

Clinical Manifestations. Affected patients with glutaric aciduria type I may develop normally up to 2 yr of life. The hallmark of the disease is a progressive dystonia and dyskinesia (choreoathetoic movements). Symptoms of hypotonia, choreoathetosis, seizures, generalized rigidity, opisthotonos, and dystonia may occur suddenly following a minor infection. In other patients, these signs and symptoms may develop gradually during the first few years of life. Hypotonia and choreoathetosis may gradually progress into rigidity and dystonia. Acute episodes of vomiting, ketosis, seizures, and coma with hepatomegaly, hyperammonemia, ketosis, and elevation of serum transaminases, a combination of symptoms that resembles Reye syndrome, may occur during an intercurrent infection or stress. Death usually occurs in the first decade of life during one of these episodes. The intellectual abilities may remain relatively intact in some patients.

Laboratory Findings. During acute episodes mild to moderate metabolic acidosis and ketosis may occur. Hypoglycemia, hyperammonemia, and elevation of serum transaminases have been seen in some patients. High concentrations of glutaric acid are usually found in urine and blood. 3-Hydroxyglutaric acid may also be present in the urine. This finding differentiated glutaric aciduria type I from type II. In glutaric aciduria type II, 2-hydroxyglutaric rather than 3-hydroxyglutaric acid is elevated. Plasma amino acid concentrations are usually within normal limits. Laboratory findings may be unremarkable between attacks. Severely affected children without glutaric aciduria also have been reported. Therefore, in any child with progressive dystonia and dyskinesia, activity of the enzyme glutaryl CoA dehydrogenase should be measured in leukocytes or cultured fibroblasts.

Treatment. A low-protein diet (especially a diet restricted in lysine and tryptophan) and high doses (200–300 mg/24 hr) of riboflavin (the coenzyme for glutaryl CoA dehydrogenase) and carnitine (50–100 mg/kg/24 hr) have resulted in a dramatic decrease in the levels of glutaric acid in body fluids, but the clinical effect has been variable. The addition of a GABA analog (baclofen) and valproic acid to the therapeutic regimen has produced clinical improvement in some affected children.

PIPECOLATEMIA (Pipecolic Acidemia). Pipecolic acid is one of the intermediate metabolites of the minor pathway of lysine catabolism (see Fig. 8–15). It is oxidized to α-aminoadipic acid within the peroxisomes. Therefore, pipecolic acidemia is a common finding in patients with generalized peroxisomal defects including Zellweger syndrome (see Sec. 8.16), neonatal adrenoleukodystrophy (see Sec. 8.16), and infantile Refsum disease (see Sec. 8.16). Previous reported patients with isolated pipecolatemia who all had severe neurologic deficits and hepatomegaly most probably had unrecognized forms of Zellweger syndrome or neonatal adrenoleukodystrophy. The existence of pipecolatemia as a distinct clinical disorder remains doubtful at this time. Pipecolic acidemia is also found in patients with persistent hyperlysinemia.

LYSINURIC PROTEIN INTOLERANCE (Familial Protein Intolerance). This rare autosomal recessive disorder is due to a defect in the transport of lysine, ornithine, and arginine in both kidney and intestine. Unlike patients with cystinuria, urinary excretion of cystine is not increased in these patients. Most reported cases are from Finland, where the prevalence has been estimated to be 1 in 60,000.

Clinical manifestations include refusal to eat, failure to thrive, hypotonia, and repeated episodes of vomiting and diarrhea that may appear anytime after birth. Breast-fed infants may thrive well as long as they are not receiving supplemental protein, perhaps because of the low protein content of human milk. Severe episodes of hyperammonemia leading to coma may develop after ingestion of a high-protein diet. Mild to moderate hepatosplenomegaly, sparse, brittle hair, and osteoporosis are common physical findings in patients in whom the condition has remained undiagnosed. Mental development is usually normal, but moderate mental retardation has been observed in about 20% of patients.

Laboratory studies may reveal hyperammonemia, which develops only after protein feeding. Fasting blood ammonia is usually normal. Urinary orotic acid is elevated, even in patients who are receiving protein-restricted diets. Plasma concentrations of lysine, arginine, and ornithine are usually mildly decreased, but urinary levels of these amino acids, especially lysine, are greatly increased. The exact mechanism producing hyperammonemia is not clear. All enzymes of the urea cycle are normal. Hyperammonemia is thought to be related to a disturbance of the urea cycle secondary to a deficiency of arginine and ornithine. However, in patients with cystinuria, who also have defects in the transport of lysine, arginine, and ornithine in both intestine and kidney, hyperammonemia is not observed. Plasma concentrations of alanine, glutamine, serine, glycine, and citrulline are usually increased. These abnormalities may be secondary to hyperammonemia and are not specific to this disorder.

Mild anemia and increased serum levels of ferritin, lactic dehydrogenase (LDH), and thyroxine-binding globulin also have been observed in these patients. This condition should be differentiated from hyperammonemia due to urea cycle defects (see Sec. 8.11), especially the female heterozygote with OTC deficiency. Increased urinary excretion of lysine, ornithine, and arginine and elevated blood levels of citrulline are not seen in patients with OTC deficiency.

Treatment with a low-protein diet (1.0–1.5 g/kg/24 hr), supplemented with citrulline (1–4 mmol/kg/24 hr), has produced biochemical and clinical improvement. Episodes of hyperammonemia should be treated promptly (see Sec. 8.11). Supplementation with lysine is not useful because it is poorly absorbed and tends to produce diarrhea and abdominal pain.

A potential fatal complication in survivors is interstitial pneumonia of unknown etiology. Pathologic examination of the lungs has revealed alveolar proteinosis. One patient so far has responded to treatment with prednisone.

IRAJ REZVANI
VICTOR AUERBACH

Arn PH, Hauser ER, Thomas GH, et al: Hyperammonemia in women with a mutation at the ornithine carbamyltransferase locus. N Engl J Med 322:1652, 1990.

Azen CG, Koch R, Gross-Friedman E, et al: Intellectual development in 12-year-old children treated for phenylketonuria. Am J Dis Child 145:35, 1991.

Blau N: Inborn errors of pterin metabolism. Annu Rev Nutr 8:185, 1988.

Danpure CJ: Recent advances in the understanding, diagnosis and treatment of primary hyperoxaluria type 1. J Inherited Metab Dis 12:210, 1989.

Danpure CJ, Jennings PR, Mistry J, et al: Enzymological characterization of a feline anlogue of primary hyperoxaluria type 2: A model for the human disease. J Inherited Metab Dis 12:403, 1989.

Dhondt JL: Tetrahydrobiopterin deficiencies: Preliminary analysis from an international survey. J Pediatr 104:501, 1984.

Finkelstein JE, Hauser ER, Leonard CO, et al: Late onset ornithine transcarbamylase deficiency in male patients. J Pediatr 117:897, 1990.

Hauser ER, Finkelstein JE, Valle D, et al: Allopurinol-induced orotidinuria. N Engl J Med 322:1641, 1990.

Hayasaka K, Tada K, Fueki N, et al: Prenatal diagnosis of nonketotic hyperglycinemia: Enzymatic analysis of the glycine cleavage system in chorionic villi. J Pediatr 116:444, 1990.

Hereditary tyrosinemia (Editorial). Lancet 1:1500, 1990.

Holtzman NA, Kronmal RA, Van Doorninck W, et al: Effects of age at loss of dietary control on intellectual performance and behavior of children with phenylketonuria. N Engl J Med 314:593, 1986.

Koletzko B, Bachmann C, Wendel U: Antibiotic therapy for improvement of metabolic control in methylmalonic aciduria. J Pediatr 117:99, 1990.

Levy HL: Phenylketonuria—1986. Pediatr Rev 7:269, 1986.

Mahoney MJ, Bick D: Recent advances in the inherited methymalonic acidemias. Acta Paediatr Scand 76:689, 1987.

McKusick V: Mendelian Inheritance in Man, 9th ed. Baltimore, The Johns Hopkins University Press, 1990.

Michalski AJ, Berry GT, Segal S: Holocarboxylase synthetase deficiency: Nine year follow-up of a patient on chronic biotin therapy and a review of the literature. J Inherited Metab Dis 123:312, 1989.

Mudd SH, Skovby F, Levy HL, et al: The natural history of homocystinuria due to cystathionine B-synthetase deficiency. Am J Hum Genet 37:1, 1985.

Nyhan WL: Abnormalities in amino acid metabolism in clinical medicine. Norwalk, CT, Appleton-Century Crofts, 1984.

Nyhan WL, Sakati NO: Diagnostic recognition of genetic disease. Philadelphia, Lea & Febiger, 1987.

Riviello J, Rezvani I, DiGeorge A: Cerebral edema in patients with maple syrup urine disease. J Pediatr (in press).

Scriver CR, Beaudet AL, Sly WS, et al: The Metabolic Basis of Inherited Disease, 6th ed. New York, McGraw-Hill, 1989.

Secor-McVoy JR, Levy HL, Lawler M, et al: Partial biotinidase deficiency: Clinical and biochemical features. J Pediatr 116:78, 1990.

Spritz RA, Strunk KM, Giebel LB, et al: Detection of mutations in the tyrosinase gene in a patient with type IA oculocutaneous albinism. N Engl J Med 322:1724, 1990.

Wold B, Heard GS: Screening for biotinidase deficiency in newborns: Worldwide experience. Pediatrics 85:512, 1990.

8.14 ASPARTIC ACID (CANAVAN DISEASE)

N-Acetylaspartic acid is a derivative of aspartic acid that is synthesized in the brain and is found in a high concentration similar to that of glutamic acid. Its function is unknown, but excessive amounts of *N*-acetylaspartic acid in urine and a deficiency of the enzyme that cleaves the *N*-acetyl group from *N*-acetylaspartic acid are associated with Canavan disease.

CANAVAN DISEASE (see also Sec. 20.58). Canavan disease is an autosomal recessive disorder characterized by spongy degeneration of the white matter of the brain leading to a severe form of leukodystrophy. It is more prevalent in individuals of Ashkenazi Jewish descent than in other ethnic groups.

Etiology and Pathology. The basic defect is a deficiency of the enzyme aspartoacylase, which leads to the accumulation of *N*-acetylaspartic acid in brain, especially in white matter, and massive urinary excretion of this compound. Excessive amounts of *N*-acetylaspartic acid are also present in the blood and cerebrospinal fluid. There is striking vacuolization and astrocytic swelling in white matter. Electron microscopy reveals distorted mitochondria. As the disease progresses, the ventricles tend to enlarge, leading to brain atrophy.

Clinical Manifestations. The severity of Canavan disease comprises a wide spectrum of manifestations. In general, infants appear normal at birth and may not manifest symptoms of the disease until 3–6 mo of age, when they develop progressive macrocephaly, severe hypotonia, and persistent head lag. As the infant grows older, delayed milestones become evident. These children are usually hyperreflexic and hypotonic, although joint stiffness may be encountered because of disuse. Seizures and optic atrophy develop as they grow older. Feeding difficulties, poor weight gain, and gastroesophageal reflux occur in the 1st yr of life; swallowing deteriorates during the 2nd and 3rd yr of life, and nasogastric feeding or permanent gastrostomy may be required. Most patients die in the 1st decade of life; however, with improved nursing care they may survive through the second decade.

Diagnosis. Computed tomography (CT) scans and magnetic resonance imaging (MRI) suggest diffuse white matter degeneration, primarily in the cerebral hemispheres with less involvement in the cerebellum and brain stem. Repeated evaluations may be required. The differential diagnosis of Canavan disease should include Alexander disease, which is another leukodystrophy with macrocephaly. Progression is usually slow in Alexander disease, and hypotonia is not as pronounced as it is in Canavan disease. Brain biopsy shows spongy degeneration of the myelin fibers, astrocytic swelling, and elongated mitochondria. The diagnosis may also be established by finding elevated amounts of *N*-acetylaspartic acid in the urine and a deficiency of aspartoacylase in cultured skin fibroblasts. Levels of *N*-acetylaspartic acid in normal urine are only trace amounts (less than 10 μmol/mmol creatinine), whereas in patients with Canavan disease they are in the range of 3,000 ± 1,800 μmol/mmol creatinine. High levels of *N*-acetylaspartic acid in plasma, cerebrospinal fluid (CSF), and brain tissue can also be detected. The activity of aspartoacylase in the fibroblasts of obligate carriers is about half or less of the activity found in normal individuals. Prenatal diagnosis can also be established by using samples of cultured chorionic villi and amniotic cells and by monitoring the amniotic fluid for elevated levels of *N*-acetylaspartic acid.

Treatment and Prevention. No specific treatment is available. Feeding problems and seizures should be treated on an individual basis. Genetic counseling, carrier testing, and prenatal diagnosis are the only methods of prevention.

REUBEN H. MATALON

Adachi M, Schneck L, Cazara J, et al: Spongy degeneration of the central nervous system (van Bogaert and Bertrand type; Canavan's disease). Human Pathol 4:331, 1973.

Matalon R, Kaul RK, Casanova J, et al: Aspartoacylase deficiency: The enzyme defect in Canavan disease. J Inher Met Dis 12:329, 1989.

Matalon R, Michals K, Sebasta D, et al: Aspartoacylase deficiency and N-acetylaspartic aciduria in patients with Canavan disease. Am J Med Genet 29:463, 1988.

DEFECTS IN METABOLISM OF LIPIDS

8.15 DISORDERS OF FATTY ACID OXIDATION

Infants and children with genetic defects in fatty acid oxidation most commonly present either with episodes of coma and hypoglycemia that are induced by fasting or with chronic, progressive muscle weakness and cardiomyopathy. These clinical manifestations reflect the importance of fatty acids as a major fuel for mitochondrial oxidative phosphorylation in the fasted state and in the aerobic metabolism and functioning of heart and skeletal muscle. These defects are inherited in autosomal recessive fashion.

Recognizing the defects in fatty acid oxidation clinically is often difficult because the only specific clue to the diagnosis may be the finding of inappropriately low levels of urinary ketones in a patient who has hypoglycemia. Similarly, defects in ketone utilization may be overlooked because ketosis is an expected finding with fasting hypoglycemia. In addition, because these disorders are often completely silent until a patient fasts for too long a period, attacks of illness may seem mysterious and can easily be mistaken for an acquired disease or misdiagnosed as Reye syndrome or sudden infant death syndrome.

The steps involved in mitochondrial oxidation of a typical long-chain fatty acid are outlined in Figure 8–16. The fatty acid is first activated to its coenzyme-A ester in the cytosol and then shuttled across the inner mitochondrial membrane in a cycle that requires carnitine. Within the mitochondrial matrix, successive turns of the four-step β-oxidation cycle produce $FADH_2$ and NADH, which in turn yield adenosine triphosphate (ATP) through the electron-transport chain and degrade the fatty acid to acetyl-CoA. In most organs, acetyl-CoA is then further oxidized by the tricarboxylic acid cycle. In the liver and kidney, acetyl-CoA is used largely to synthesize the ketones, β-hydroxybutyrate and acetoacetate, which are then released as fuels for the brain and other tissues.

DEFECTS IN THE INTRAMITOCHONDRIAL OXIDATION PATHWAY

These are a closely related group of disorders that involve single-enzyme defects either in one of the β-oxidation steps for fatty acids or in the pathway that transfers electrons from $FADH_2$ to the electron-transport chain. Except for the severe infantile form of electron transfer flavoprotein (ETF) and electron transfer flavoprotein dehydrogenase (ETF-DH) deficiencies, patients with these disorders appear to be healthy until an excessive period of fasting stress triggers an episode of illness. In some of the disorders, there are no signs of impaired muscle function; in others, evidence of muscle involvement may be prominent, especially during attacks of illness, with severe cardiomyopathy and skeletal muscle weakness. Laboratory features of these disorders include "hypoketotic hypoglycemia," elevated urinary levels of dicarboxylic and other organic acids during illnesses, and secondary carnitine deficiency.

MEDIUM-CHAIN ACYL-CoA DEHYDROGENASE (MCAD) DEFICIENCY. Deficiency of medium-chain acyl-CoA dehydrogenase activity is the most common fatty acid oxidation defect.

Clinical Manifestations. Patients with this defect appear to be perfectly normal until stressed by a period of 12–16 hr of fasting. The first episode of illness usually occurs between 6 mo and 2 yr of age. Episodes of illness are often life-threatening, and up to 25% of patients may die during the first attack. Clinical features include vomiting, lethargy progressing rapidly to coma, and occasionally seizures. The liver size may be normal or slightly enlarged.

Laboratory Findings. These include hypoglycemia with inappropriately low urinary and plasma ketone levels ("hypoketotic hypoglycemia"), mild acidemia, and elevations of plasma urea, ammonia, uric acid, transaminases, and prothrombin and partial thromboplastin times. Liver biopsies at times of acute illness show increased neutral lipid deposits in either a micro- or macrovesicular pattern. Urinary organic acid quantitation at times of illness or fasting stress shows low levels of ketones together with elevated levels of medium-chain dicarboxylic acids derived from microsomal ω-oxidation of fatty acids. In common with patients with all of the other intramitochondrial matrix fatty acid oxidation defects and some defects in amino acid oxidation, these patients have secondary carnitine deficiency. Plasma and tissue total carnitine levels are reduced to about 25% of normal, and the fraction of plasma total carnitine that is esterified is increased. The mechanism of this secondary carnitine deficiency is not known. *Diagnosis* can be made by demonstrating the presence of octanoyl-carnitine or of glycine conjugates of hexanoic and phenylpropionic acid in urine or by demonstrating deficient enzyme activity in cultured fibroblasts or leukocytes.

Treatment. Acute illnesses should be promptly treated with intravenous fluids containing 10% dextrose in order to suppress lipolysis as rapidly as possible. Chronic therapy consists of instituting minor adjustments in diet to ensure that patients never fast for more than 10–12 hr. Some investigators think that dietary fat restriction or carnitine therapy is also helpful.

Prognosis. Patients with MCAD deficiency do not have muscle weakness or cardiomyopathy and appear to have an excellent long-term prognosis.

LONG-CHAIN ACYL-COA DEHYDROGENASE (LCAD) DEFICIENCY. In general, this disorder is similar to, but more severe than, MCAD deficiency. The 14 affected patients identified to date have usually presented with attacks of fasting-induced coma and hypoglycemia early in the 1st yr of life. At the time of illness they also often have evidence of muscle weakness and hypertrophic cardiomyopathy. Some have persistent skeletal muscle weakness, resembling a mild form of muscular dystrophy. Physical and laboratory findings during the acute illness are similar to those seen in patients with MCAD deficiency, with mild hepatomegaly, hypoketotic hypoglycemia, and abnormal liver function test results. These patients also have a secondary carnitine deficiency. Urinary organic acid profiles taken at the time of illness show inappropriately low ketone levels and elevations of medium-chain dicarboxylic acids. The specific diagnosis can be made only by assay of enzyme activity in cultured fibroblasts or leukocytes. Treatment is similar to that given for MCAD deficiency except that continuous nasogastric feeding has been necessary in some patients who were severely ill at the time of diagnosis.

SHORT-CHAIN ACYL-COA DEHYDROGENASE (SCAD) DEFICIENCY. There is some uncertainty about the clinical features of this disorder, since only three cases have been reported. One patient presented with symptoms resembling those of MCAD deficiency, whereas another presented with chronic acidosis, failure to thrive, developmental delay, and muscle weakness. The urinary organic acid profile shows elevations of ethylmalonic acid as well as medium-chain dicarboxylic acids. These patients also have secondary carnitine deficiency. Specific diagnosis requires an assay of enzyme activity in leukocytes or cultured fibroblasts. Treatment appears to be the same as that for MCAD deficiency: avoidance of fasting stress by dietary therapy.

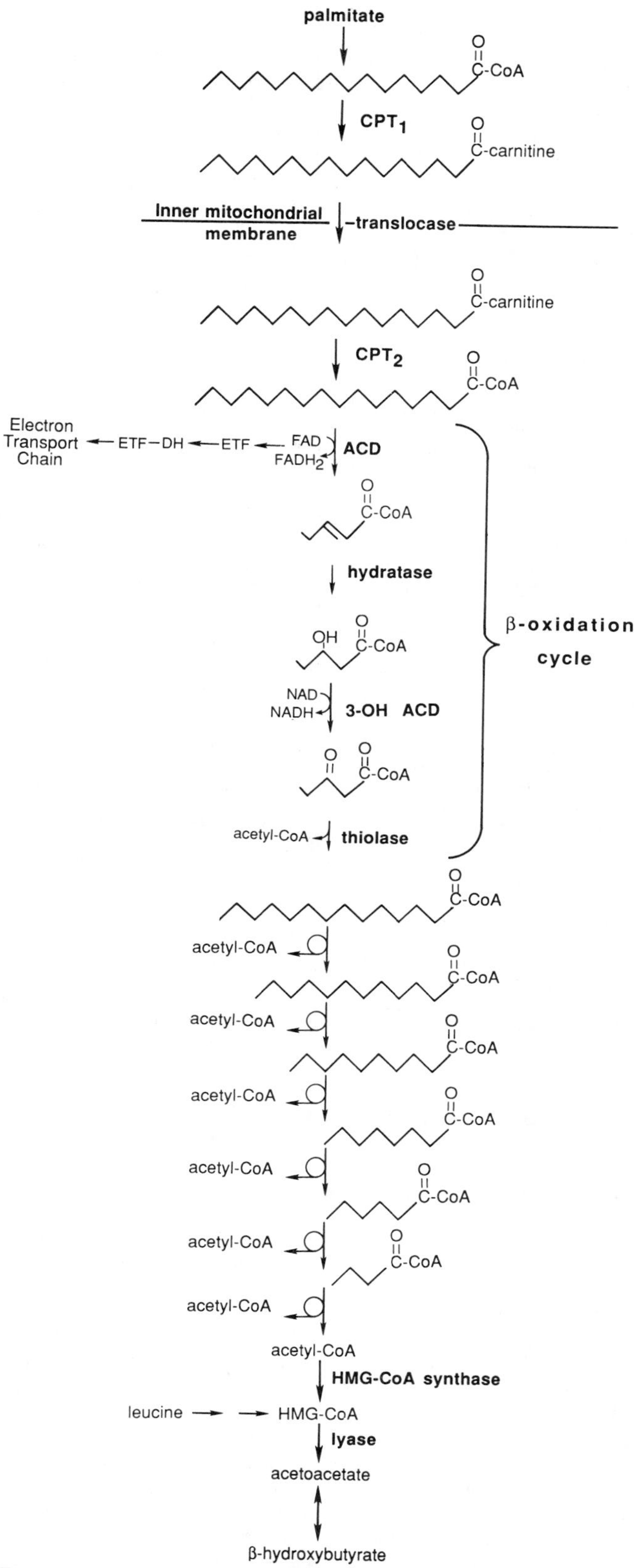

Figure 8–16. Pathway of mitochondrial oxidation of a typical long-chain fatty acid. Enzyme steps include the carnitine palmityltransferases (CPT) 1 and 2, carnitine translocase, acyl-CoA dehydrogenase (ACD), enoyl-CoA hydratase, 3-hydroxy acyl-CoA dehydrogenase (3-OH ACD), β-ketothiolase, electron transfer flavoprotein (ETF), ETF-dehydrogenase (ETF-DH), β-hydroxy-β-methylglutaryl-CoA (HMG-CoA) synthase, and HMG-CoA lyase.

LONG-CHAIN 3-HYDROXYACYL-COA DEHYDROGENASE (3-OH ACD) DEFICIENCY. Only two children with this disorder have been identified. One had symptoms similar to those of LCAD deficiency with episodes of fasting hypoglycemia, coma, and weakness. The second presented with hepatomegaly and progressive liver failure leading to death before 1 yr of age. The urinary organic acid profile shows increased levels of 3-hydroxydicarboxylic acids as well as the increased levels of medium-chain saturated dicarboxylic acids seen in the other β-oxidation enzyme defects. Secondary carnitine deficiency is also noted. Treatment with diet to avoid periods of fasting, together with the use of medium-chain triglyceride (MCT) oil as a source of fat that bypasses the enzyme block, was successful in the one surviving patient with this defect.

ELECTRON-TRANSFER FLAVOPROTEIN (ETF) AND ELECTRON-TRANSFER FLAVOPROTEIN DEHYDROGENASE (ETF-DH) DEFICIENCIES (MULTIPLE ACYL-CoA DEHYDROGENATION DEFECTS [MADD], GLUTARIC ACIDURIA TYPE II). These two enzymes transfer electrons into the electron-transport chain complex from the dehydrogenation steps catalyzed by the three acyl-CoA dehydrogenases of fatty acid oxidation as well as three other dehydrogenases involved in the oxidation of branched-chain amino acids and glutaric acid. Deficiency of these enzymes produces a disorder that combines the features of a defect in fatty acid oxidation with those of a defect in amino acid oxidation such as isovaleric acidemia. Complete absence of the activity of either ETF or ETF-DH causes severe illness in the newborn period characterized by acidosis, hypoglycemia, coma, and hypotonia. Some of these infants have also had congenital abnormalities with mild facial dysmorphia and polycystic kidneys. Most severely affected patients have died within a few weeks of birth. The urinary organic acid profile is distinctive, showing evidence of blocks in fatty acid oxidation (dicarboxylic acids, ethylmalonic acid), lysine (glutaric acid), and the branched-chain amino acids (glycine conjugates of isovaleric, isobutyric, and α-methylbutyric acids).

Partial deficiency of ETF activity produces a milder disease that presents in a manner similar to MCAD or LCAD deficiency with episodes of hypoglycemia, vomiting, coma, and muscle weakness triggered by fasting stress. The urinary organic acid profile reveals elevations of dicarboxylic and ethylmalonic acids. Patients with either the mild or severe form of these enzyme deficiencies have secondary carnitine deficiency. Therapy for patients with the mild form of deficiency simply requires altering the diet to avoid fasting stresses. A few patients with the mild form of MADD have shown improvement with riboflavin treatment, suggesting that these individuals may have an underlying defect in the metabolism of FAD, the cofactor for ETF and the acyl-CoA dehydrogenase enzymes.

DEFECTS IN TRANSPORTATION OF FATTY ACIDS INTO MITOCHONDRIA

Three defects in the carnitine-dependent cycle that transports long-chain fatty acids into the mitochondria have been described. Unlike the β-oxidation defects described earlier, patients with these disorders do not have dicarboxylic aciduria (see Sec. 8.39).

PLASMA MEMBRANE CARNITINE TRANSPORT DEFECT (Primary Carnitine Deficiency). The most common clinical presentation of this disorder is a relentlessly progressive cardiomyopathy and skeletal muscle weakness that begins at 2–4 yr of age. A smaller number of patients present with episodes of fasting hypoketotic hypoglycemia during the 1st yr of life before they develop myopathy. The underlying defect involves the plasma membrane carnitine transport system that is normally present in heart, muscle, and kidney and serves to maintain intracellular carnitine levels 20–50 times greater than plasma concentrations. Patients with this defect cannot maintain adequate carnitine levels in muscle tissue for fatty acid oxidation and also have severe renal wastage of carnitine. Plasma and tissue carnitine levels are reduced to 1–2% of normal.

In marked contrast to patients with secondary carnitine deficiency (see Sec. 8.39), in whom carnitine therapy does not correct the metabolic defect, these patients respond dramatically to high doses of oral carnitine, regaining strength and cardiac function to nearly normal within a few months of starting therapy. Muscle carnitine levels remain very low during therapy, suggesting that carnitine does not become a rate-limiting factor in fatty acid oxidation until the tissue levels are less than 5–10% of normal. The disorder can be strongly suspected from the extreme severity of the tissue carnitine deficiency and confirmed by studies of carnitine transport in cultured fibroblasts.

CARNITINE PALMITYLTRANSFERASE (CPT) DEFICIENCY ("LIVER" FORM). The two patients who had this disorder presented with episodes of fasting hypoketotic hypoglycemia during the 1st yr of life. No evidence of muscle weakness or cardiomyopathy was found. Unlike patients with β-oxidation enzyme defects, these patients had normal plasma and tissue carnitine levels and no dicarboxylic aciduria or other abnormalities in their urinary organic acid profiles. Simple avoidance of prolonged fasting was successful in managing these patients. The underlying defect involved a form of the CPT-1 enzyme, which is expressed in liver but not in muscle tissue. The defect can be demonstrated in cultured fibroblasts.

CARNITINE PALMITYLTRANSFERASE (CPT) DEFICIENCY ("MUSCLE" FORM). Patients with this disorder present with exercise-induced episodes of aching muscle pain, rhabdomyolysis, and myoglobinuria. The first episode usually does not occur until late childhood or adolesence. The myoglobinuria is frequently severe enough to cause acute renal failure. During attacks, plasma levels of creatine kinase are elevated to 5,000–10,000 U or more. Fasting or cold stress seems to aggravate attacks. Although ketogenesis is impaired in some of these patients, none have presented with hypoketotic, hypoglycemic coma. Muscle biopsy shows increased deposition of neural fat. The underlying defect involves a deficiency of carnitine palmityltransferase activity, probably of the CPT-2 enzyme, which may be present in all tissues. The diagnosis is made by assaying enzyme activity in muscle tissue. Levels of carnitine and urinary excretion of organic acids are normal. Long-term treatment consists primarily of avoiding fasting or excessively strenuous and prolonged exercise.

DEFECTS IN KETONE SYNTHESIS

β-HYDROXY-β-METHYLGLUTARYL-CoA(HMG-CoA) LYASE DEFICIENCY. See Sec. 8.7.

DEFECTS IN KETONE UTILIZATION

The ketones, β-hydroxybutyrate and acetoacetate, which are end products of hepatic fatty acid oxidation, serve as important metabolic fuels, particularly for the brain, during the late stages of fasting. Two defects in ketone utilization by extrahepatic tissues that present with episodes of "hyperketotic" hypoglycemia have been identified.

SUCCINYL-CoA–ACETOACETYL-CoA TRANSFERASE DEFICIENCY. One patient with this defect has been described. He presented with recurrent episodes of severe ketoacidosis beginning in the newborn period and expired at 6 mo of age. Treatment of acute episodes required infusion of glucose and large amounts of bicarbonate for 3–4 days. The defect is located in the enzyme step that initiates the oxidation of acetoacetate in peripheral tissues by transferring coenzyme A from succinyl-CoA to form acetoacetyl-CoA. Deficient enzyme activity occurs in brain, muscle, and fibroblasts.

β-KETOTHIOLASE DEFICIENCY. See Sec. 8.7.

CHARLES A. STANLEY

GENERAL

Roe CR, Coates PM: Acyl-CoA dehydrogenase deficiencies. *In*: Scriver DR, Beaudet AL, Sly WS, et al (eds): The Metabolic Basis of Inherited Disease, 6th ed. New York, McGraw Hill, 1989, p 889.

Stanley CA: New genetic defects in mitochondrial fatty acid oxidation and carnitine deficiency. Adv Pediatr 34:59, 1987.

SPECIFIC

Coates PM, Hale DE, et al: Genetic deficiency of short-chain acyl-coenzyme A dehydrogenase in cultured fibroblasts from a patient with muscle carnitine deficiency and severe skeletal muscle weakness. J Clin Invest 81:171, 1988.

Demaugre F, Bonnefort JP, et al: Hepatic and muscular presentation of carnitine palmitoyl transferase deficiency: Two distinct entities. Pediatr Res 24:308, 1988.

Frerman FE, Goodman SL: Deficiency of electron transfer flavoprotein: Ubiquinone oxidoreductase in glutaric acidemia type II fibroblasts. Proc Natl Acad Sci 82:4517, 1985.

Gregersen N, Wintzensen H, Kolvraa S, et al: C6–C10-Dicarboxylic aciduria: Investigation of a patient with riboflavin responsive multiple acyl-CoA dehydrogenation defects. Pediatr Res 16:861, 1983.

Hale DE, Batshaw ML, et al: Long-chain acyl coenzyme A dehydrogenase deficiency. Pediatr Res 19:459, 1985.

Leonard JV, Middleton B, et al: Acetoacetyl CoA thiolase deficiency presenting as ketotic hypoglycemia. Pediatr Res 21:211, 1987.

Robinson BH, Oei J, et al: Hydroxymethylglutaryl CoA lyase deficiency: Features resembling Reye syndrome. Neurology 30:714, 1980.

Stanley CA, Hale DE, et al: Medium-chain acyl-CoA dehydrogenase deficiency in children with non-ketotic hypoglycemia and low carnitine levels. Pediatr Res 17:877, 1983.

Tildon JT, Cornblath M: Succinyl-CoA: 3-ketoacid CoA transferase deficiency: A cause for ketoacidosis in infancy. J Clin Invest 51:493, 1972.

Treem WR, Stanley CA, et al: Primary carnitine deficiency due to a failure of carnitine transport in kidney, muscle, and fibroblasts. N Engl J Med 319:1331, 1988.

8.16 DISORDERS OF VERY LONG CHAIN FATTY ACIDS

PEROXISOMAL DISORDERS

The peroxisomal diseases represent a group of genetically determined disorders in which the major cause of pathology is either the failure to form or maintain the peroxisome or a defect in the function of a single enzyme that normally is located in this organelle. These disorders cause serious disability in childhood and occur more frequently and present a wider range of phenotype than has been recognized in the past.

ETIOLOGY. Table 8–6 shows the current classification of the peroxisomal disorders. The group 1 disorders involve the failure to form normal peroxisomes, and they are therefore referred to as disorders of peroxisome biogenesis. Peroxisomes normally are present in all cells other than mature erythrocytes. The peroxisome is a subcellular organelle surrounded by a single membrane; at least 40 enzymes have been localized to the peroxisome. Some of these enzymes are involved in the production and decomposition of hydrogen peroxide. Other enzymes are concerned with lipid and amino acid metabolism. Most peroxisomal enzymes are first synthesized in their mature form in free polyribosomes and then

TABLE 8–6. Classification of Peroxisomal Disorders

Group 1	Group 2	Group 3
Peroxisomes reduced or absent; multiple enzyme defects	Peroxisome normal; single enzyme defect	Peroxisomes present, but structure abnormal; more than one defective enzyme
Zellweger syndrome Neonatal adrenoleukodystrophy Infantile Refsum disease	X-linked adrenoleukodystrophy Acatalasemia Hyperoxaluria type 1 3-oxoacyl-CoA thiolase deficiency "pseudo-Zellweger syndrome" Acyl-CoA oxidase deficiency Bifunctional enzyme deficiency	Rhizomelic chondrodysplasia punctata Zellweger-like syndrome

enter the cytoplasm and are targeted to the peroxisome. It appears that malfunction of the enzyme import mechanisms is the key abnormality in the disorders of peroxisome biogenesis. In the group 2 disorders, peroxisome structure is normal, and there is dysfunction of a single peroxisomal enzyme. The mechanisms of the group 3 disorders are complex and poorly understood.

EPIDEMIOLOGY. Except for X-linked adrenoleukodystrophy, all the peroxisomal disorders listed in Table 8–6 are inherited as autosomal recessive traits. Their combined incidence is estimated to be between 1 in 25,000 and 1 in 50,000. All races are affected.

PATHOLOGY. Absence or reduction in the number of peroxisomes is the pathognomonic feature of disorders of peroxisome biogenesis. In most of these disorders there are membranous sacs that contain peroxisomal integral membrane proteins but lack the normal complement of matrix proteins; these are referred to as peroxisome "ghosts." Pathologic changes are observed in many organs. These include profound and characteristic defects in neuronal migration; micronodular cirrhosis of the liver; renal cysts; chondrodysplasia punctata; corneal clouding, congenital cataracts, glaucoma, and retinopathy; congenital heart disease; and dysmorphic features.

PATHOGENESIS. It is likely that all pathologic changes are secondary to the peroxisome defect. Multiple peroxisomal enzymes fail to function in the group 1 disorders. Table 8–7 lists the defective reactions that are clinically significant. The enzymes that are diminished or absent are synthesized normally but are degraded abnormally fast, presumably because they are unprotected outside of the peroxisome. It is not clear how the defective peroxisome functions lead to the widespread pathologic manifestations.

The mechanisms that control the import of peroxisomal enzymes are incompletely understood, but certain of the enzymes have been shown to have specific sequences that are required for appropriate targeting. Complementation studies have subdivided the disorders of biogenesis into six separate groups. It is likely that each of these groups represents a distinct genotype, and this suggests that the import of peroxisomal enzymes is controlled by at least six separate mechanisms.

CLINICAL MANIFESTATIONS (Disorders of Peroxisome Biogenesis [Group 1]). The three group 1 disorders represent a spectrum of severity. The Zellweger cerebrohepatorenal syndrome is the most severe, infantile Refsum disease the least severe, and neonatal adrenoleukodystrophy intermediate in severity. These distinctions are not definitive. Complementation studies have shown that all three phenotypes are found within a single large complementation group, and the Zellweger phenotype is represented in four of the small complementation groups. However, it seems wisest to retain the current designations until the biochemical basis of the various genotypes is defined.

Newborn infants with *Zellweger syndrome* show striking and consistent abnormalities that are easily recognized. Of central diagnostic importance are the typical facial appearance (high forehead, unslanting palpebral fissures, hypoplastic supraorbital ridges, and epicanthal folds [Fig. 8–17]), severe weakness and hypotonia, neonatal seizures, and eye abnormalities (cataracts, glaucoma, corneal clouding, Brushfield spots, pigmentary retinopathy, and optic nerve dysplasia). Because of the hypotonia and "mongoloid" appearance, Down syndrome is sometimes suspected in these infants. Infants with Zellweger syndrome rarely live more than a few months. More than 90% show postnatal growth failure. Table 8–8 lists the main clinical abnormalities.

Patients with *neonatal adrenoleukodystrophy* show fewer and occasionally no dysmorphic features. Neonatal seizures occur frequently. Some degree of psychomotor development is present, but function remains in the severely or profoundly retarded range and may regress after 3–5 yr of age, probably owing to a progressive leukodystrophy. Several patients are now in a stable, albeit severely handicapped, state in their midteens. Enlarged liver and impaired liver function, pigmentary degeneration of the retina, and severely impaired hearing are almost always present. Adrenocortical function is usually impaired, but overt Addison disease is rare. Chondrodysplasia punctata and renal cysts are absent.

Infants with Refsum disease have survived to the 2nd decade or longer. They are able to walk, although gait may be ataxic and broad-based. Cognitive function is in the severely retarded range. All have sensorineural hearing loss and pigmentary degeneration of the retina. They have moderately dysmorphic features that may include epicanthal folds, flat bridge of the nose, and low-set ears. Early hypotonia and enlarged liver with impaired function are common. Levels of plasma cholesterol and high- and low-density lipoprotein are often moderately reduced. Chondrodysplasia punctata and renal cortical cysts are absent. Postmortem study has been performed in only one child with infantile Refsum disease, who died at 12 yr of age. This revealed micronodular liver cirrhosis and small hypoplastic adrenals. The brain showed no malformations except for severe hypoplasia of the cerebel-

TABLE 8–7. Abnormal Laboratory Findings Common to Disorders of Peroxisome Biogenesis

Peroxisomes absent or reduced in number
Catalase in cytosol
Deficient synthesis and reduced tissue levels of plasmalogens
Defective oxidation and abnormal accumulation of very long chain fatty acids
Deficient oxidation and age-dependent accumulation of phytanic acid
Defects in certain steps of bile acid formation and accumulation of bile acid intermediates
Defects in oxidation and accumulation of L-pipecolic acid
Increased urinary excretion of dicarboxylic acids

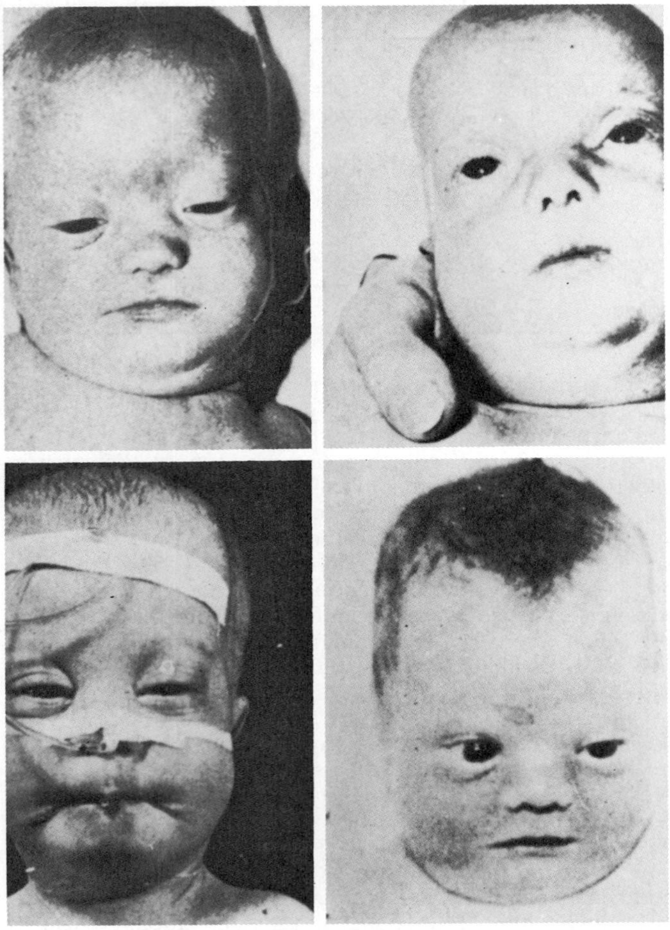

Figure 8–17. Four patients with the Zellweger cerebrohepatorenal syndrome. Note the high forehead, epicanthal folds, and hypoplasia of supraorbital ridges and midface. (Courtesy of Hans Zellweger, M.D. Used by permission.)

lar granule layer and ectopic locations of the Purkinje cells in the molecular layer. Although initial reports indicated a preponderance of males, the mode of inheritance is probably autosomal recessive.

The designation of *hyperpipecolic acidemia* was applied to four patients subsequently shown to have diminished or absent peroxisomes, but because of the resemblance of this condition to the Zellweger syndrome or neonatal adrenoleukodystrophy, this disorder is no longer classified as a separate phenotype.

Structurally Abnormal Peroxisomes and Defective Enzymes (Group 3). *Rhizomelic chondrodysplasia punctata (RCDP)* is characterized by the presence of stippled foci of calcification within the hyaline cartilage and is associated with dwarfing, cataracts (72%), and multiple malformations due to contractures. Vertebral bodies have a coronal cleft filled by cartilage that is a result of an embryonic arrest. Disproportionate short stature affects the proximal parts of the extremities (Fig. 8–18*A*). Radiologic abnormalities consist of shortening of the proximal limb bones, metaphyseal cupping, and disturbed ossification (see Fig. 8–18*B*). Height, weight, and head circumference are below the 3rd percentile, and the children are severely retarded mentally. Skin changes such as those observed in ichthyosiform erythroderma are present in about 25% of patients.

Isolated Enzyme Defects of Peroxisomal Fatty Acid Oxidation (Group 2). These rare disorders include oxidase deficiency (pseudoneonatal adrenoleukodystrophy), 3-oxoacyl-CoA thiolase deficiency (pseudo-Zellweger syndrome), and bifunctional enzyme deficiency. Clinically, they resemble the disorders of peroxisome biogenesis and can be distinguished only through laboratory studies.

LABORATORY FINDINGS. The *group 1 disorders* display a spectrum of biochemical abnormalities that are secondary to the defect in peroxisome structure (Table 8–9). The pathognomonic feature is the diminished number or absence of peroxisomes combined with defective function of multiple peroxisomal enzymes.

In the *group 2 disorders* there is a defect in a single peroxisomal enzyme: lignoceroyl-CoA ligase in X-linked adrenoleukodystrophy; alanine:glyoxylate aminotransferase in hyperoxaluria type 1; catalase in acatalasemia; and acyl-CoA oxidase, bifunctional enzyme, or 3-oxoacyl-CoA thiolase, respectively, in the three recently described disorders in which a single peroxisomal β-oxidation enzyme fails to function. "Classic" or "adult" Refsum disease, previously classified as a peroxisomal disorder, is a defective mitochondrial enzyme disorder (phytanic acid oxidase) and is no longer included in the peroxisome disease category.

The *group 3 disorder (RCDP)* shows three biochemical abnormalities: (1) impaired capacity to oxidize phytanic acid, (2) impaired capacity to synthesize plasmalogens, and (3) failure to process the peroxisomal thiolase enzyme so that it is present in the precursor rather than the mature form. These three defects are also a feature of the group 1 disorders. RCDP differs from them in that the peroxisome structure is intact, and the oxidation of very long chain fatty acids and pipecolic acid is unimpaired.

The *Zellweger-like syndrome,* represented by a single case, has physical findings that resemble those of the Zellweger

TABLE 8–8. Main Clinical Abnormalities in Zellweger Syndrome*

	Cases in Which Information About the Feature Was Available		Cases in Which the Feature Was Present	
Abnormal Feature	***No.***	**%**	***No.***	**%**
High forehead	60	53	58	97
Flat occiput	16	14	13	81
Large fontanelle(s), wide sutures	57	50	55	96
Shallow orbital ridges	33	29	33	100
Low/broad nasal bridge	23	20	23	100
Epicanthus	36	32	33	92
High arched palate	37	32	35	95
External ear deformity	40	35	39	97
Micrognathia	18	16	18	100
Redundant skin fold of neck	13	11	13	100
Brushfield spots	6	5	5	83
Cataract/cloudy cornea	35	31	30	86
Glaucoma	12	11	7	58
Abnormal retinal pigmentation	15	13	6	40
Optic disk pallor	23	20	17	74
Severe hypotonia	95	83	94	99
Abnormal Moro response	26	23	26	100
Hyporeflexia or areflexia	57	50	56	98
Poor sucking	77	68	74	96
Gavage feeding	26	23	26	100
Epileptic seizures	61	54	56	92
Psychomotor retardation	45	39	45	100
Impaired hearing	21	18	9	40
Nystagmus	37	32	30	81

*From Heymans HSA: Cerebro-hepato-renal (Zellweger) syndrome. Clinical and biochemical consequences of peroxisomal dysfunctions. Thesis, University of Amsterdam, 1984.

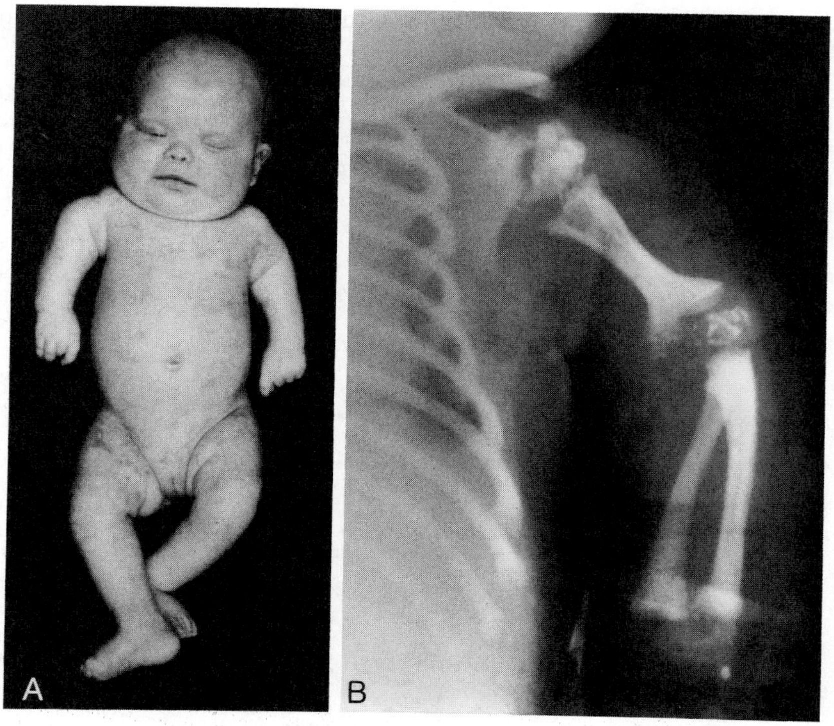

Figure 8–18. *A*, A newborn infant with RCDP. Note the severe shortening of the proximal limbs, the depressed bridge of the nose, hypertelorism, and widespread scaling skin lesions. *B*, Note the marked shortening of the humerus and epiphyseal stippling at the shoulder and the elbow joints. (Courtesy of John P. Dorst, M.D., Johns Hopkins Hospital.)

syndrome and multiple peroxisomal enzyme deficiencies; liver peroxisomes have a normal structure.

DIAGNOSIS. There now are several noninvasive laboratory tests that permit precise and early diagnosis of peroxisomal disorders (see Table 8–9). For the clinician the main decision is when to order these tests. The main challenge in group 1 disorders is to differentiate them from the large variety of other conditions that can cause hypotonia, seizures, failure to thrive, or dysmorphic features. Experienced clinicians can readily recognize classic Zellweger syndrome by its clinical manifestations. However, group 1 patients often do not show the full clinical spectrum of disease and may be identifiable only by laboratory assays. Clinical features that may serve as indications for these diagnostic assays include: severe psychomotor retardation; weakness and hypotonia; dysmorphic features; neonatal seizures; retinopathy, glaucoma, or cataracts; hearing deficits; enlarged liver and impaired liver function; and chondrodysplasia punctata. The combined presence of one or more of these abnormalities increases the likelihood of this diagnosis.

Patients with the isolated defects of peroxisomal fatty acid oxidation (group 2) resemble those with group 1 disorders and can be detected by demonstrating abnormally high levels of very long chain fatty acids.

Patients with RCDP must be distinguished from patients with other causes of chondrodysplasia punctata. In addition to warfarin embryopathy and the Zellweger syndrome, these disorders include the milder autosomal dominant form of chondrodysplasia punctata *(Conradi-Hünermann syndrome)* that is characterized by longer survival, absence of severe limb shortening, and usually intact intellect, an X-linked dominant form, and an X-linked recessive form associated with a deletion of the terminal portion of the short arm of the X chromosome. RCDP is suspected clinically because of the shortness of limbs, psychomotor retardation, and ichthyosis. The most decisive laboratory test is the demonstration of abnormally low plasmalogen levels in red blood cells and an impaired capacity to synthesize plasmalogens in cultured skin fibroblasts. These biochemical defects are not present in other types of chondrodysplasia punctata.

COMPLICATIONS. Patients with the Zellweger cerebrohepatorenal syndrome have multiple disabilities involving muscle tone, swallowing, cardiac abnormalities, liver disease, and seizures. These are treated symptomatically, but the prognosis is poor, and most patients succumb during the first few months of life.

PREVENTION. See later section Genetic Counseling.

TREATMENT. Because of the multiplicity and severity of deficits, only supportive and symptomatic care is recommended for patients with the classic Zellweger syndrome. For patients with the somewhat milder variants, considerable success has been achieved with multidisciplinary early intervention, including physical and occupational therapy, hearing aids, alternative communication, nutrition, and support for the parents. Although most patients continue to function in the profoundly or severely retarded range, some make significant gains in self-help skills, and several now are in stable condition in their teens or even early twenties. Specific experimental therapies include the oral administration of plasmalogens in the form of batyl alcohol 5–10 mg/kg/24 hr in 3–5 divided doses and restricted phytanic acid intake. It is not known whether these nutritional measures are of benefit.

GENETIC COUNSELING. All of the peroxisomal disorders can be diagnosed prenatally. Except for hyperoxaluria type 1, all can be identified prenatally in the 1st or 2nd trimester. The tests used are similar to those described for postnatal diagnosis (see Table 8–9) and utilize chorionic villus samples or amniocytes. More than 300 pregnancies have been monitored, and more than 60 affected fetuses have been identified so far without diagnostic error. Because of the 25% recurrence risk, couples who have previously had an affected child must be advised about the availability of prenatal diagnosis. Except for X-linked adrenoleukodystrophy, there are no techniques for the identification of heterozygotes.

Brul S, Westerveld A, Strijland A, et al: Genetic heterogeneity in the cerebro-hepato-renal (Zellweger) syndrome and other inherited disorders with a generalized impairment of peroxisomal functions: A study using complementation analysis. J Clin Invest 81:1710, 1988.

Budden SS, Kennaway NG, Buist NRM, et al: Dysmorphic syndrome with

TABLE 8–9. Peroxisomal Disorders: Biochemical Diagnostic Assays

Disease	Assay	Findings
Disorders of peroxisome biogenesis: Zellweger syndrome, neonatal adrenoleukodystrophy, infantile Refsum disease, hyperpipecolic acidemia	Plasma:	VLCFAs* Pipecolic acid Phytanic acid Bile acids
	RBCs†:	Plasmalogens
	Fibroblasts:	Plasmalogen synthesis Catalase subcellular localization
X-linked ALD‡ hemizygote	Plasma/RBCs:	VLCFAs
	Fibroblasts:	VLCFAs
X-linked ALD heterozygotes	Plasma:	VLCFAs
	Fibroblasts:	VLCFAs
	DNA probe	
Rhizomelic chondrodysplasia punctata	Plasma:	Phytanic acid
	RBCs:	Plasmalogens
	Fibroblasts:	Plasmalogen synthesis Phytanic acid oxidation
Isolated defects of VLCFA degradation	Plasma:	VLCFAs
	Fibroblasts:	VLCFAs VLCFA oxidation Immunoblot of peroxisomal fatty acid oxidation enzymes
Hyperoxaluria, type 1	Urine:	Organic acids
	Liver:	Alanine: Glyoxalate amino transferase in percutaneous liver biopsy
Acatalasemia	RBCs:	Catalase

*VLCFAs = very long chain fatty acids.
†RBCs = red blood cells.
‡ALD = adrenoleukodystrophy.

phytanic acid oxidase deficiency, abnormal very long chain fatty acids, and pipecolic acidemia: Studies in four children. J Pediatr 108:33, 1986.
Danpure CJ, Jennings PR, Watts RW: Enzymological diagnosis of primary hyperoxaluria type 1 by measurement of hepatic alanine:glyoxylate aminotransferase activity. Lancet 1:289, 1987.
Hoefler G, Hoefler S, Watkins PA, et al: Biochemical abnormalities in rhizomelic chondrodysplasia punctata. J Pediatr 112:726, 1988.
Kelley RJ, Datta NS, Dobyns WB, et al: Neonatal adrenoleukodystrophy: New cases, biochemical studies and differentiation from Zellweger and related peroxisomal polydystrophy syndromes. Am J Med Genet 23:869, 1986.
Lazarow PB, Fujiki Y: Biogenesis of peroxisomes. Annu Rev Cell Biol 1:489, 1985.
Moser AE, Singh I, Brown FR III, et al: The cerebro-hepato-renal (Zellweger) syndrome: Increased levels and impaired degradation of very long chain fatty acids and their use in prenatal diagnosis. N Engl J Med 310:1141, 1984.
Moser HW: Peroxisomal diseases. *In*: LA Barnes (ed): Advances in Pediatrics, Vol. 36. Chicago, Year Book Medical Publishers, 1989, pp 1–38.
Schutgens RBH, Heymans HSA, Van Den Ende A, et al: Peroxisomal disorders: A newly recognized group of genetic diseases. Eur J Pediatr 114:430, 1986.

8.17 Adrenoleukodystrophy (X-linked)

X-linked adrenoleukodystrophy (ALD) is a genetically determined disorder associated with the accumulation of saturated very long chain fatty acids and a progressive dysfunction of the adrenal cortex and nervous system white matter.

ETIOLOGY. The key biochemical abnormality is the tissue accumulation of saturated very long chain fatty acids. These are unbranched with a carbon chain length of 24 or more. Excess hexasanoic acid (C26:0) is the most striking and characteristic feature. This accumulation of fatty acids is due to a genetically determined deficient capacity to degrade them, a function that is normally carried out in the peroxisome. The defect probably involves the enzyme lignoceroyl-CoA ligase, a peroxisomal enzyme that catalyzes the formation of the coenzyme-A derivatives of very long chain fatty acids. The adrenoleukodystrophy gene has been mapped to chromosome Xq28, the terminal segment of the long arm of the X chromosome.

EPIDEMIOLOGY. X linkage has been confirmed by analysis of more than 500 kindreds. All races are affected. Minimum incidence is 1 in 100,000, and this figure is probably an underestimate because of a failure to diagnose the disorder. The various phenotypes often occur in members of the same kindred.

PATHOLOGY. Characteristic lamellar cytoplasmic inclusions can be demonstrated with the electron microscope in adrenocortical cells, testicular Leydig cells, and nervous system macrophages. These inclusions probably consist of cholesterol esterified with very long chain fatty acids. They are most prominent in cells of the zona fasciculata of the adrenal cortex, which at first are distended with lipid and later atrophy.

The nervous system of patients with childhood ALD shows acute and relatively symmetric demyelinative lesions that involve the parieto-occipital regions most severely. In addition to the myelin breakdown, there is perivascular infiltration of lymphocytes resembling that seen in multiple sclerosis. Most other tissues are intact. Peroxisomes are normal in number and structure.

PATHOGENESIS. The adrenal dysfunction is probably a direct consequence of the accumulation of very long chain fatty acids. The cells in the zona fasciculata are distended with abnormal lipids. Cholesterol esterified with very long chain fatty acids is relatively resistant to ACTH-stimulated cholesterol ester hydrolases, and this limits the capacity to convert cholesterol to endocrinologically active steroids. In addition, C26:0 excess increases the viscosity of the plasma membrane, and this in turn may interfere with receptor and other cellular functions.

There is no correlation between the severity of the nervous system lesions and the biochemical defect or between the degree of adrenal involvement and that of nervous system involvement. One third or more of patients with adrenoleukodystrophy are free of nervous system involvement or develop a milder disability in adulthood. Thus, nervous system involvement depends on some factor or factors in addition to the very long chain fatty acid excess. These factors may involve autoimmune reactions that are triggered in some way by the very long chain fatty acid excess.

CLINICAL MANIFESTATIONS. There are seven relatively distinct phenotypes, three of which present in childhood with symptoms and signs. In all of the phenotypes development is usually normal during the first 3–4 yr.

In the *childhood cerebral* form of ALD, symptoms are first noted most commonly between the ages of 4 and 8 yr, 2 yr at the earliest. The most common initial manifestations are hyperactivity, which is often mistaken for an attention deficit disorder, and worsening school performance in a child who had previously been a good student. Auditory discrimination is often impaired although tone perception is preserved. This may be evidenced by difficulty in using the telephone and greatly impaired performance on intelligence tests in items that are presented verbally. Spatial orientation is often impaired. Other initial symptoms are disturbances of vision, ataxia, poor handwriting, seizures, and strabismus. Visual disturbances often are due to involvement of the cerebral cortex, which leads to variable and seemingly inconsistent visual capacity. Seizures occur in more than one third of the patients and may represent the first manifestation of the disease. Some patients present with increased intracranial pressure or with unilateral mass lesions. Impaired cortisol response to ACTH stimulation is present in 85% of patients, and mild hyperpigmentation is often noted. However, in most patients with this phenotype adrenal dysfunction is recognized only after the condition is diagnosed because of the cerebral symptoms. Cerebral childhood adrenoleukodystrophy tends to progress rapidly with increasing spasticity and paralysis, visual and hearing loss, and loss of ability to speak or swallow. The mean interval between the first neurologic symptom and an apparently vegetative state is 1.9 ± 2 yr. Patients may continue in this apparently vegetative state for 10 or more yr.

Adolescent ALD designates patients who develop neurologic symptoms between the ages of 10 and 21 yr. The manifestations resemble those of childhood cerebral ALD except that progression is slower.

Adrenomyeloneuropathy first becomes manifest in late adolescence or adulthood as a progressive paraparesis due to long-tract degeneration in the spinal cord. Approximately one third of the patients also have involvement of the cerebral white matter.

The "Addison only" phenotype is an important and underdiagnosed condition. Studies in developed countries, where tuberculosis is no longer a common cause, suggest that as many as 50% of male patients with Addison disease have the biochemical defect of ALD. Many of these patients have intact neurologic systems, whereas others have subtle neurologic signs. Many develop adrenomyeloneuropathy in adulthood.

The term presymptomatic ALD is applied to boys up to 10 yr old who have the biochemical defect of ALD but are free of neurologic or endocrine disturbances. Boys in this category who are 10 yr or older are referred to as asymptomatic. A few persons with the biochemical defect of ALD who are relatives of clinically affected patients with ALD have remained asymptomatic even in the 6th or 7th decade.

Approximately 10–15% of female heterozygotes develop a syndrome that resembles adrenomyeloneuropathy but is milder and of later onset. Adrenal insufficiency is very rare.

LABORATORY FINDINGS. Very Long Chain Fatty Acids. The most specific and important laboratory finding is the demonstration of abnormally high levels of very long chain fatty acids in plasma, red blood cells, or cultured skin fibroblasts. The test should be performed in a laboratory that has experience with this specialized procedure. Positive results are obtained in all male patients with X-linked ALD and in approximately 85% of female carriers of X-linked ALD.

Computed Tomography and Magnetic Resonance Imaging. Patients with childhood cerebral or adolescent ALD show cerebral white matter lesions that are characteristic with respect to location and attenuation patterns on CT or MRI. In 80% of patients the lesions are symmetric and involve the periventricular white matter in the posterior parietal and occipital lobes. Noncontrast CT scans show bilateral hypodensities in this location. The second characteristic, observed following intravenous injection of contrast material, is the demonstration of a garland of accumulated contrast material adjacent and anterior to the posterior hypodense lesions (Fig. 8–19*A*). This zone corresponds to the zones of intense perivascular lymphocytic infiltration where the blood-brain barrier breaks down. In 12% of patients the initial lesions are frontal. Unilateral lesions that produce a mass effect suggestive of a brain tumor may occur. MRI provides a clearer delineation of normal and abnormal white matter than CT and may demonstrate abnormalities missed by CT (see Fig. 8–19*B*).

Impaired Adrenal Function. More than 85% of patients with the childhood form of ALD have elevated levels of ACTH in plasma and a subnormal rise of cortisol levels in plasma following intravenous injection of 250 μg of $ACTH_{1-24}$ (Cortrosyn).

DIAGNOSIS AND DIFFERENTIAL DIAGNOSIS. The earliest manifestations of childhood cerebral ALD are difficult to distinguish from the much more common attention deficit disorders or learning disabilities. Rapid progression, signs of dementia, or difficulty in auditory discrimination suggests ALD. Even in early stages CT or MRI may show strikingly abnormal changes. Other leukodystrophies or multiple sclerosis may, however, mimic these radiographic findings. Definitive diagnosis depends on demonstration of very long chain fatty acid excess, which occurs only in X-linked ALD and the peroxisomal disorders. The latter may be distinguished from X-linked ALD by their clinical presentation during the neonatal period.

Cerebral forms of ALD may present with increased intracranial pressure and unilateral mass lesions. These have been misdiagnosed as gliomas even after brain biopsy, and several patients have received radiotherapy before the correct diagnosis was made. Measurement of very long chain fatty acids in plasma or brain biopsy specimens is the most reliable differential test.

Adolescent or adult cerebral ALD can be confused with psychiatric disorders, epilepsy, or dementing disorders. The first clue to the diagnosis of ALD may be the demonstration of white matter lesions by CT or MRI; assays of very long chain fatty acids should be confirmatory.

ALD cannot be distinguished clinically from other forms of Addison disease, and it is recommended that assays of very long chain fatty acid levels be performed in all male patients with Addison disease. ALD patients almost never have antibodies to adrenal tissue in their plasma.

COMPLICATIONS. An avoidable complication is the occurrence of adrenal insufficiency. The most difficult problems are those related to bed rest, contracture, coma, and swallowing disturbances. Other complications involve behavioral disturbances and injuries associated with defects of spatial orientation, impaired vision and hearing, and seizures.

TREATMENT. Steroid replacement for adrenal insufficiency or adrenocortical hypofunction is effective (see Sec. 19.21). Adrenal function should be tested periodically at minimum intervals of 1 yr.

The progressive behavioral and neurologic disturbances associated with the childhood form of ALD are extremely difficult for the family to cope with. ALD patients require the establishment of a comprehensive management program and partnership between the family, physician, visiting nursing staff, school authorities, and counselors. In addition, parent support groups are often helpful.* Communication with school authorities is important because under the provisions of Public Law 94–142 children with ALD qualify for special services as "other health impaired" or "multihandicapped." Depending on the rate of progression of the disease, special needs might range from relatively low level resource services within a regular school program to home- and hospital-based teaching programs for children who are not mobile.

Management challenges vary with the stage of the illness. The early stages are characterized by subtle changes in affect, behavior, and attention span. Counseling and communication with school authorities are of prime importance. Changes in the sleep-wake cycle can be benefited by the judicious use at night of sedatives such as chloral hydrate (10–50 mg/kg), pentobarbital (5 mg/kg), or diphenhydramine (2–3 mg/kg).

As the leukodystrophy progresses, the modulation of muscle tone and support of bulbar muscular function are major concerns. Baclofen in gradually increasing doses (5 mg twice a day to 25 mg 4 times a day) is the most effective pharmacologic agent for the treatment of acute episodic painful muscle spasms. Other agents may also be used, care being taken to monitor the occurrence of side effects and drug

*United Leukodystrophy Foundation, 2304 Highland Drive, Sycamore, IL 60178.

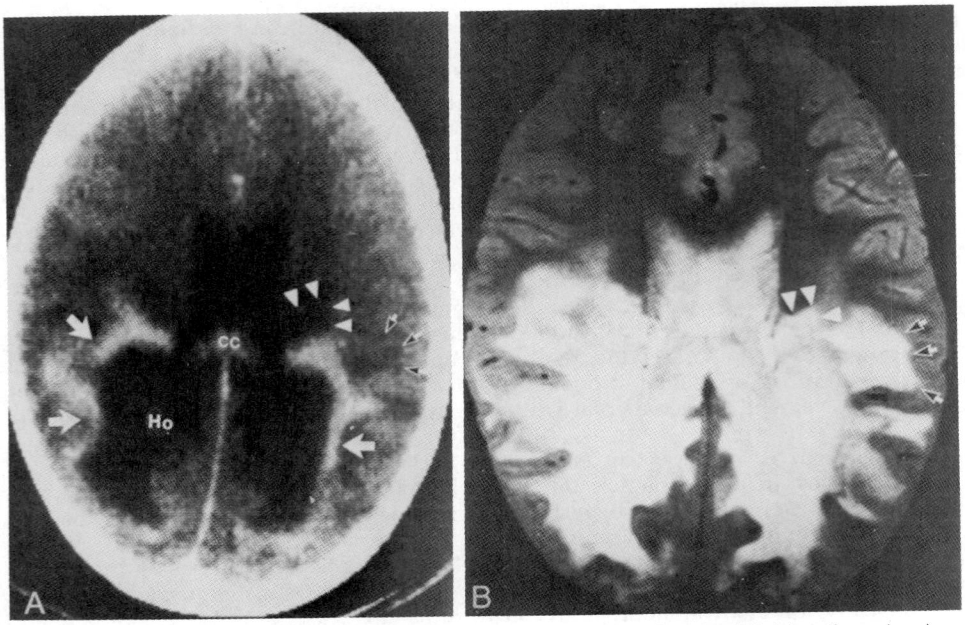

Figure 8–19. *A*, Contrast-enhanced CT abnormalities in ALD with typical parieto-occipital location, showing symmetric bilateral hypodense inactive zones (Ho). The enhancing active periphery zone of hypodensity is demarcated by *arrows*. Compare the anterior zone of hypodensity *(arrowheads)* with the MRI. (CC = corpus callosum.) (From Kumar et al, 1987—with permission.) *B*, An MRI of the same patient and area shown by CT scanning. MRI-T_2-weighted image shows a high-intensity signal of the abnormally bright parieto-occipital white matter. Subcortical involvement is better identified on MRI. Separation of active zones may be better appreciated by CT scanning, because both inactive and active zones are seen at high-signal areas on MRI. However, it is assumed that such major distinctions afforded by CT will also be demonstrable when IV enhancement (paramagnetic enhancement) becomes readily available. Note the hypodense involvement of CT scanning *(arrowheads* and *arrows)* in *A* compared with the well-resolved lesions on MRI in *B*. (From Kumar et al: Adrenoleukodystrophy: Correlating MR Imaging with CT. Radiology 165:497–504, 1987.)

interactions. As the leukodystrophy progresses, bulbar muscular control is lost. Although initially this can be managed by changing the diet to soft and pureed foods, most patients eventually require a nasogastric tube or a surgical procedure such as gastrostomy or lateral esophagostomy. At least one third of patients have focal or generalized seizures, which usually respond readily to standard anticonvulsant medications.

Treatment with oral administration of glyceryl trierucate and glyceryl trioleate oils combined with dietary restriction of very long chain fatty acids to prevent or ameliorate neurologic disability is now being evaluated in an international trial. It is possible to normalize very long chain fatty acid levels within 4 wk by specific dietary therapy. This approach is without significant risk and has a rational justification. Bone marrow transplantation is an experimental procedure for patients who have very early neurologic involvement and for whom a matched donor is available.

GENETIC COUNSELING AND PREVENTION. The very long chain fatty acid assay can identify 85% of female carriers, and the accuracy of carrier identification can be increased by use of the DXS-52 DNA probe. Prenatal diagnosis of affected male fetuses can be achieved by measurement of very long chain fatty acid levels in cultured amniocytes or chorionic villus cells. Whenever a new patient with X-linked ALD is identified, a detailed pedigree should be constructed, and efforts should be made to identify all at-risk female carriers and affected males. These investigations should be accompanied by careful and sympathetic attention to social, emotional, and ethical issues during counseling.

HUGO W. MOSER

Aubourg P, Blanche S, Jambaqué I, et al: Reversal of early neurologic and neuroradiologic manifestations of X-linked adrenoleukodystrophy by bone marrow transplantation. N Engl J Med 332:1860, 1990.
Aubourg PR, Sack GH Jr, Meyers DA, et al: Linkage of adrenoleukodystrophy to a polymorphic DNA probe. Ann Neurol 21:349, 1987.
Kumar AJ, Rosenbaum AE, Naidu S, et al: Role of magnetic resonance imaging in adrenoleukodystrophy. Radiology 165:497, 1987.
Lazo O, Contreras M, Hashmi M, et al: Peroxisomal lignoceroyl-CoA ligase deficiency in childhood adrenoleukodystrophy and adrenomyeloneuropathy. Proc Natl Acad Sci USA 85:7647, 1988.
Moser HW, Moser AB, Singh I, et al: Adrenoleukodystrophy: Survey of 303 cases: Biochemistry, diagnosis and therapy. Ann Neurol 16:628, 1984.
Moser HW, Moser AB, Trojak JE, et al: Identification of female carriers of adrenoleukodystrophy. J Pediatr 103:54, 1983.
Rizzo WB, Leshner RT, Odone A, et al: Dietary erucic acid therapy for X-linked adrenoleukodystrophy. Neurology 39:1415, 1989.
Wanders RJA, Van Roermund CWT, Van Wijland MJA, et al: Direct demonstration that the deficient oxidation of very long chain fatty acids in X-linked adrenoleukodystrophy is due to an impaired ability of peroxisomes to activate very long chain fatty acids. Biochem Biophys Res Commun 153:618, 1988.

8.18 LIPID STORAGE DISORDERS
(Lipidoses)

The lipidoses are lysosomal lipid storage diseases, each caused by deficiency of a specific hydrolase. The lipid material stored within the lysosomes, usually a glycosphingolipid, leads to the pathophysiology characteristic of the specific lipid storage disease. For example, if the sphingolipid is stored only in the peripheral tissues, sparing the central nervous system (CNS), then hepatosplenomegaly may be noted and the disease suspected, as in Gaucher disease. On the other hand, if the glycosphingolipid is stored in the CNS only and not in peripheral tissues, there is no hepatosplenomegaly, and the storage disease may not be suspected, as in Tay-Sachs disease. When the CNS is involved, mental retardation and neurologic deterioration are major components of the storage disease. In lipidoses in which storage material accumulates in the periphery and in the CNS, mental retardation together with hepatosplenomegaly is characteristic of the disease, as in Niemann-Pick disease.

The *sphingolipids*, which are components of the cell membrane, are found in every cell of the body. Their basic structure is identical, and all sphingolipids are based on sphingosine (Fig. 8–20). The structure of sphingosine is achieved by the condensation of the amino acid serine with palmitic acid. This compound combines the C_{18} nonpolar region of palmitate and the polar region of serine, which contains an amino group and two hydroxyl groups. Another fatty acid is added to sphingosine through the amino group of serine, forming ceramide. The first hydroxyl group (C_1) of ceramide can become a recipient to sugars, for example, ceramide-glucose, which is also called glucocerebroside. Ceramide-galactose is another ceramide-monohexoside, also known as galactocerebroside. Phosphocholine may substitute for the sugars, forming sphingomyelin. More than one sugar can be added to ceramide, and branches of sialic acid (neuraminic acid [NANA]) may be added, resulting in a rather complex compound (see Fig. 8–20). When neuraminic acid is added to the sphingolipid, the resulting compound is called a ganglioside. Despite their complexity, such membrane-associated compounds have similar building blocks and must be degraded or recycled by lysosomal enzymes. A general outline of the stepwise degradation of sphingolipids is shown in Figure 8–21 and 8–22. A defect in any step results in a lysosomal storage disease. The storage of a specific compound in a specific tissue depends on the distribution of that compound in the body.

GM_1 GANGLIOSIDOSIS. This is a group of lysosomal disorders with variable clinical findings. GM_1 ganglioside is a monosialoganglioside found in normal cerebral gray and white matter and in peripheral tissues. There are two major forms of GM_1 gangliosidosis, infantile (type 1) and juvenile (type 2). There is also an adult form, type 3 (see Sec. 20.59).

Etiology. The biochemical defect of both forms of GM_1 gangliosidosis is a deficiency of the lysosomal enzyme β-galactosidase, which hydrolyzes the terminal galactose from GM_1 ganglioside (see Fig. 8–22). The diagnosis is confirmed by demonstrating deficiency of β-galactosidase in white blood cells or cultured skin fibroblasts.

Clinical Manifestations (see also Sec 20.59). The *infantile form* of GM_1 gangliosidosis may be noted at birth by the presence of hepatosplenomegaly, edema of the extremities, and rashes that cannot be explained by the usual newborn skin eruptions. Psychomotor retardation soon becomes evident. A cherry-red spot in the macula is present in 50% of the patients. Umbilical and inguinal hernias with edema of

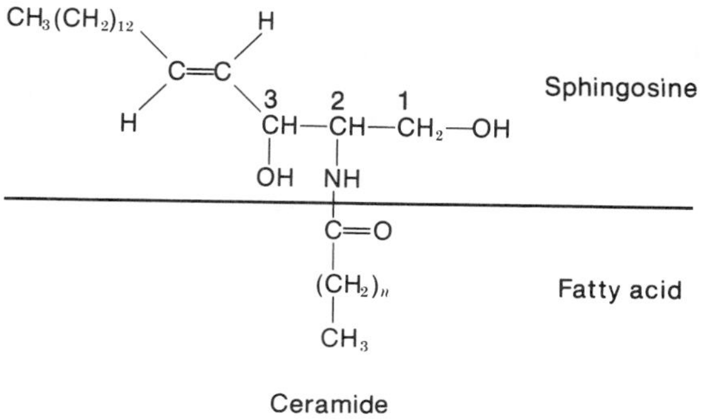

Figure 8–20. Basic structure of sphingolipids. All additions to ceramide are made through the hydroxyl group of carbon atom 1: Glycosphingolipids = ceramide plus one or more sugars attached to C-1. Gangliosides = glycosphingolipids plus one or more sialic acid residues. Sphingomyelin = ceramide plus phosphorylcholine attached to C-1.

the scrotum are usually present at birth (Fig. 8–23). Because of the coarse facial features and macroglossia these children may be suspected of having Hurler disease. Enlargement of the heart and signs of ventricular hypertrophy occur in most patients with GM_1 gangliosidosis. Lumbar kyphosis and some stiffening of the joints are also characteristic of GM_1 gangliosidosis as well as of Hurler disease. However, rapid mental deterioration, macular cherry-red spot, and early onset of seizures are more characteristic of GM_1 gangliosidosis. The patient becomes dysphagic, deaf, and blind, and death occurs at 3–4 yr of age.

Radiologic changes are those of *dysostosis multiplex*. Vertebral changes occur with anterior beaking, the sella turcica is large, and the calvarium may be thickened. Although these changes are similar to those seen in the mucopolysaccharidoses, they are less severe. CT scans and MRI of the brain show ventricular dilatation and generalized brain atrophy.

Late-onset GM_1 gangliosidosis is clinically distinct. The age of onset varies, and such patients may present with ataxia, dysarthria, and cerebral palsy-like spasticity. Deterioration is slow, and patients may survive through the 4th decade of life. These patients lack visceral involvement, do not have coarse facial features, and do not have dysostosis multiplex.

Biochemical and Pathologic Findings. There are foam cells in bone marrow aspirates and in histologic preparations of tissues such as the lungs and liver. GM_1 ganglioside accumulates in the brain and peripheral tissues. In addition, keratan sulfate, a mucopolysaccharide, accumulates in liver and is excreted in the urine of patients with GM_1 gangliosidosis.

Diagnosis. GM_1 gangliosidosis is suspected clinically by developmental delay, coarse facial features, enlarged tongue, hepatosplenomegaly, and a cherry-red spot of the macula. Hurler disease, I-cell disease, and Niemann-Pick disease should be considered. Radiologic evaluation should rule out Niemann-Pick disease because it is the only one of these conditions that does not show dysostosis multiplex. Urinary mucopolysaccharides that include excessive keratan sulfate are characteristic of GM_1 gangliosidosis. The diagnosis is confirmed by enzymatic assay of white blood cells or cultured skin fibroblasts showing a deficiency of β-galactosidase. Prenatal diagnosis can be accomplished by assaying amniocytes or chorionic villi for β-galactosidase.

Genetics and Treatment. GM_1 gangliosidosis is inherited as an autosomal recessive trait. Carriers can be detected using white blood cells or cultured skin fibroblasts to assay for β-galactosidase. There is no specific treatment for either form of GM_1 gangliosidosis other than symptomatic care.

TAY-SACHS (GM_2 GANGLIOSIDOSIS I). Because this lysosomal storage disease primarily involves the central nervous system, no evidence of peripheral storage is evident on physical examination. Tay-Sachs disease is the most devastating of the lipid storage diseases and occurs frequently among individuals of Ashkenazi Jewish descent.

Etiology. The basic defect is a deficiency of the heat-labile lysosomal enzyme β-hexosaminidase A; two isoenzymes, A and B, are responsible for the total activity. Two polypeptide chains, α and β, are required for the formation of β-hexosaminidase A and B. Isoenzyme A is formed with α and β chains, whereas isoenzyme B is composed of β chains only. Therefore, a defect in the α chain results in deficient activity in β-hexosaminidase A, as occurs in both forms of Tay-Sachs disease. Several mutations at the gene locus affecting the production of the α chain of β-hexosaminidase have been identified. A defect in the β chain affects the activity of both isoenzymes A and B, thus causing a deficiency of the total activity of β-hexosaminidase (see later discussion of Sandhoff Disease). The enzyme β-hexosaminidase A requires for its hydrolytic activity an activator that binds to the enzyme and

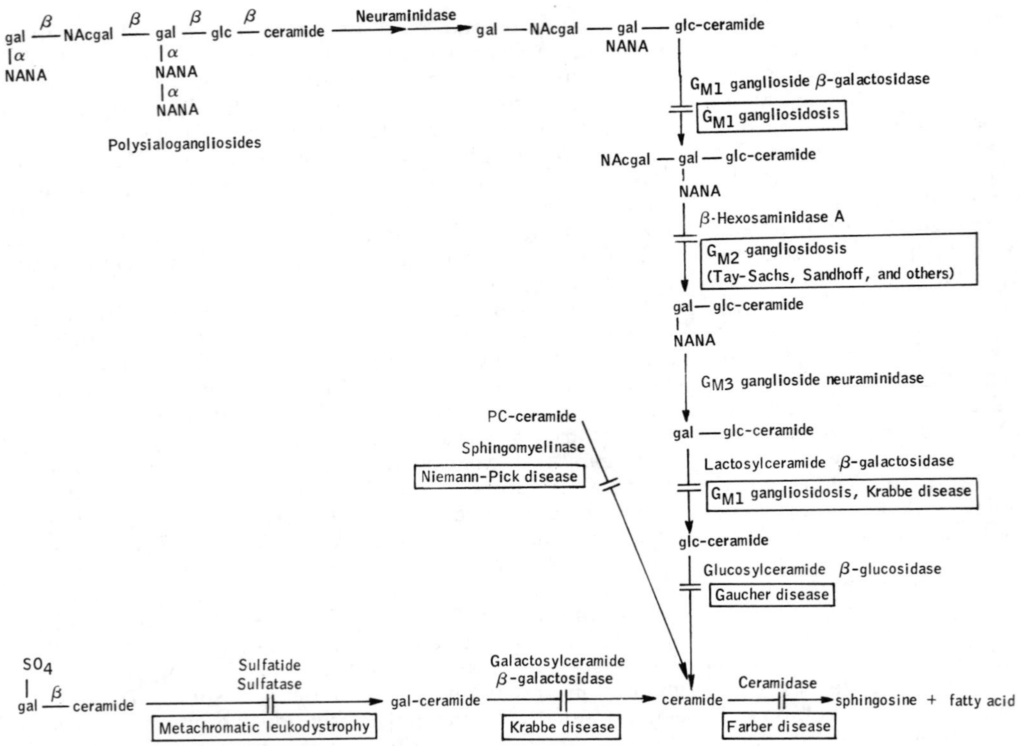

Figure 8–21. Pathways in the metabolism of sphingolipids found in nervous tissues. The name of the enzyme catalyzing each reaction is given with the name of the substrate acted on. Inborn errors are depicted as bars crossing the reaction arrows, and the name of the associated defect or defects is given within the nearest box. The gangliosides are named according to the nomenclature of Svennerholm. Anomeric configurations are given only at the largest starting compound. (gal = galactose; glc = glucose; NAcgal = *N*-acetyl-galactosamine; NANA = *N*-acetyl-neuraminic acid; PC = phosphorylcholine.)

to the natural substrate GM_2 ganglioside. Very rarely, patients with Tay-Sachs disease may have normal activity of β-hexosaminidase A when it is assayed in a test tube. In such cases the disease is caused by *activator deficiency*, and an assay for the activator should be performed.

Clinical Manifestations. Infants develop normally until about 5 mo of age. Usually decreased eye contact and focusing are noted first, along with an exaggerated startle response to noise, **hyperacusis**. By the end of the 1st yr an infant with Tay-Sachs disease becomes severely hypotonic. Physical examination is often characterized by severe hypotonia, blindness, and hyperacusis. Funduscopic examination of the eye may reveal a cherry-red spot of the macula. Such infants assume a frog-like position and interact very little with their surroundings. The head size may enlarge more than 50%, but this enlargement is not associated with hydrocephalus. Sei-

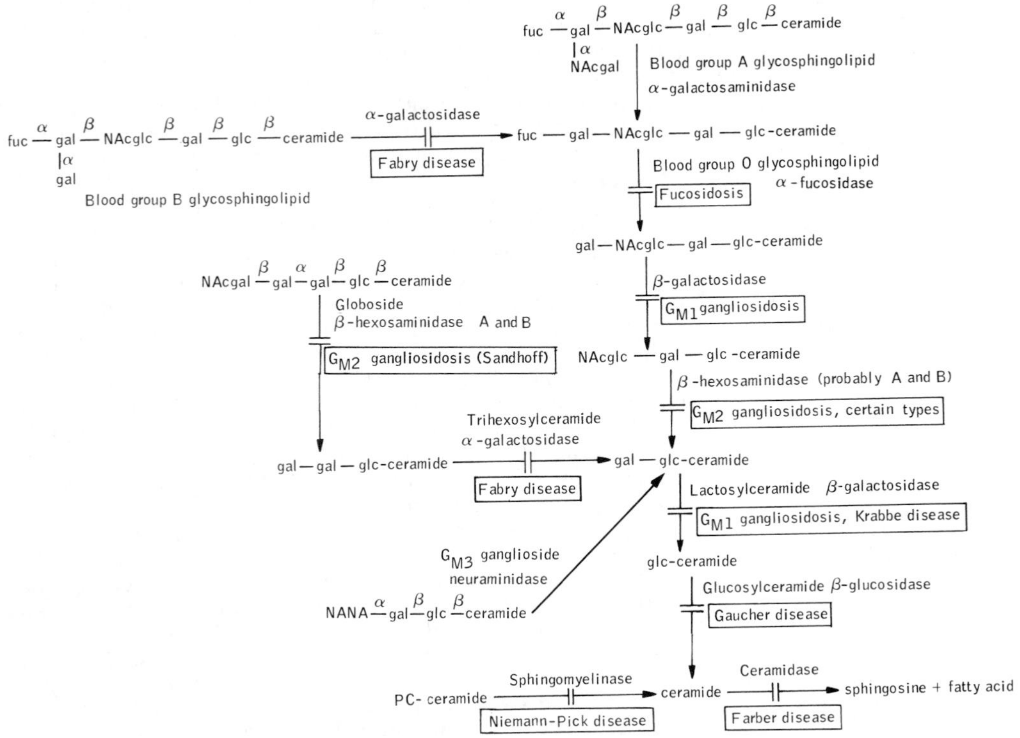

Figure 8–22. Pathways in the degradation of sphingolipids found in visceral organs and red or white blood cells. See also the legend for Figure 8–21. (fuc = fucose; NAcglc = *N*-acetylglucosamine.)

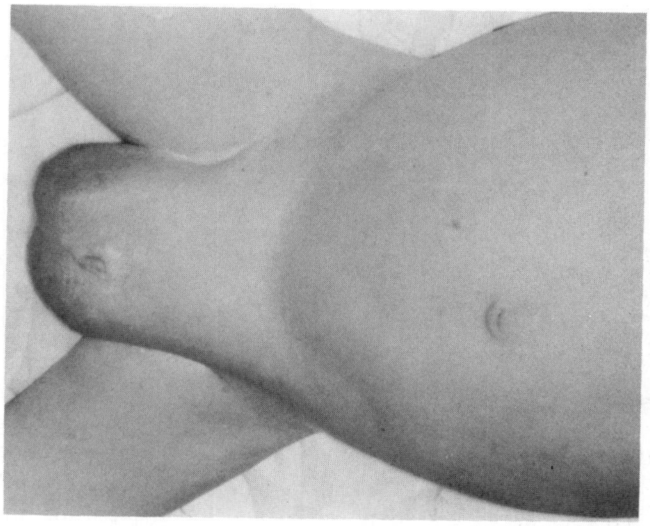

Figure 8–23. Bilateral inguinal hernias, with scrotal edema, in a baby with the infantile form of GM_1 gangliosidosis.

zures may complicate the disease in the 2nd yr of life, and death usually occurs between the 2nd and 4th yr of age.

Late-onset or juvenile Tay-Sachs disease (GM_2 gangliosidosis III) is a variant of Tay-Sachs disease. Onset may occur as early as 2 yr of life but can also occur in the 2nd or 3rd (adult GM_2 gangliosidosis) decade of life (see Sec. 20.59). Mental retardation is not associated in the early phase of this condition, and the major manifestations are those of ataxia, choreoathetosis, and dysarthria. Blindness and spasticity may occur prior to death. Juvenile Tay-Sachs disease is not associated with cherry-red spot of the macula, and there is no organomegaly. Tay-Sachs disease is not associated with bony changes. CT scan and MRI of the brain reveal enlarged ventricles and brain atrophy with gray matter degeneration.

Diagnosis. Tay-Sachs disease is usually suspected in a severely retarded infant with a cherry-red spot of the macula and lack of visceral storage. Several sphingolipidoses are associated with cherry-red spot, but only patients with Tay-Sachs disease lack hepatosplenomegaly (Table 8–10). The juvenile form of Tay-Sachs disease should be suspected in a child whose ataxia and dysarthria become progressive. The assay for β-hexosaminidase A is diagnostic and can be carried out on plasma, cultured skin fibroblasts, or white blood cells. Carriers for Tay-Sachs disease and juvenile Tay-Sachs disease can be detected by performing an assay for the specific activity of hexosaminidase A.

Genetics and Prevention. There is considerable heterogeneity at the gene level, and the major group of mutations responsible for Tay-Sachs disease in the Jewish population is different from that in non-Jewish people. The mutation for the infantile form of Tay-Sachs disease is different from that for the juvenile form.

Both forms of Tay-Sachs disease are inherited as autosomal recessive traits, and both are more frequent among Ashkenazi Jews. The frequency of Tay-Sachs disease is 1 in 3,500–4,000 births, making the carrier rate among Ashkenazi Jews 1 in 30. This high frequency and the availability of carrier testing have led to mass carrier blood screening for β-hexosaminidase A. Carrier testing, counseling, and prenatal diagnosis have markedly decreased the frequency of Tay-Sachs disease among Jewish couples.

Treatment. There is no treatment for either form of Tay-Sachs disease.

SANDHOFF DISEASE (GM_2 Gangliosidosis II). This autosomal recessive disease is associated with total β-hexosaminidase deficiency because both A and B isoenzymes are deficient. *Clinical manifestations* vary but usually mimic those of Tay-Sachs disease in its infantile form. However, Sandhoff disease is associated with hepatosplenomegaly, indicating peripheral storage of GM_2 ganglioside, an *N*-acetylglucosamine containing oligosaccharide. Foam cells are found in bone marrow aspirates. The cherry-red spot of the macula is also seen in Sandhoff disease. A juvenile form of Sandhoff disease presents in the latter half of the 1st decade of life with ataxia, dysarthria, and mental deterioration. No visceral enlargement or macular cherry-red spot is associated with this form of the disease. There is no preponderance of Sandhoff disease among Ashkenazi Jews.

TABLE 8–10. Lipidoses Associated with Cherry-Red Spot of the Macula

Disease	Enzyme Defect	Visceral Involvement
Tay-Sachs	β-Hexosaminidase A	No organomegaly
Sandhoff	β-Hexosaminidase A and B	Hepatosplenomegaly
Niemann-Pick	Sphingomyelinase	Hepatosplenomegaly
GM_1 gangliosidosis	β-Galactosidase	Hepatosplenomegaly
Mucolipidosis 1	Sialidase (neuraminidase)	Hepatosplenomegaly

The *basic defect* is an abnormal β chain in β-hexosaminidase that affects both the A and B isoenzymes. *Diagnosis* of Sandhoff disease is achieved by demonstrating a total deficiency of β-hexosaminidase on assay of plasma white blood cells or cultured fibroblasts.

NIEMANN-PICK DISEASE (Type A). This is an autosomal recessive disorder of sphingomyelin and cholesterol storage within the lysosomes. Niemann-Pick disease is found more frequently among Jewish individuals of Ashkenazi descent.

Etiology. There are increased levels of sphingomyelin and cholesterol in bone marrow cells, liver, spleen, and brain. The enzyme defect is sphingomyelinase deficiency (see Figs. 8–21 and 8–22). Failure to cleave phosphocholine from sphingomyelin results in the storage of sphingomyelin. Storage of cholesterol is not well understood, but there seems to be a close relationship between the metabolism of sphingomyelin and that of cholesterol.

Clinical Manifestations. These begin at 3–4 mo of age with feeding difficulties and failure to thrive. Neurologic deterioration may not be overt because these children are able to sit, stand, and learn other skills, although their development is globally delayed. Physical examination is characterized by hepatosplenomegaly. The liver may be enlarged earlier than the spleen. Bone marrow aspirates show characteristic foam cells containing sphingomyelin and cholesterol. As the disease progresses, children with Niemann-Pick disease begin to look more severely malnourished and have protruding abdomens. Mental retardation becomes more pronounced as new skills are not achieved and existing skills regress. Muscle strength diminishes, and the children become hypotonic. Hearing and vision deteriorate, and blindness occurs in the advanced stages of the disease. Hypoacusis is present. A cherry-red spot on the macula is seen in 50% of cases. Death occurs before the 4th yr of life.

Major bony abnormalities are not associated with Niemann-Pick disease, although some widening of the medullary cavity and thinning of the cortex are observed. CT scan and MRI of the brain show gray matter degeneration, demyelination, and cerebellar atrophy.

Late-onset variants of Niemann-Pick disease are associated with dystonic movements, athetosis, and seizures. Hepatosplenomegaly and sphingomyelinase deficiency are diagnostic.

Diagnosis. Hepatosplenomegaly, mental retardation, foam cells in bone marrow or peripheral blood smears, and a cherry-red spot suggest the diagnosis. Sphingomyelinase deficiency in white blood cells, cultured skin fibroblasts, or other tissues is diagnostic. Carrier detection and prenatal diagnosis are available using a sphingomyelinase assay. Recently, the gene for sphingomyelinase was cloned, which should facilitate further understanding of the various mutations leading to the different clinical forms of Niemann-Pick disease.

Treatment. There is no therapy.

Niemann-Pick Disease (Type B). This is a benign form of sphingomyelinase deficiency that is associated with hepatosplenomegaly and the presence of foam cells in the bone marrow but minor or no neurologic involvement. This disease has an autosomal recessive mode of inheritance but is not associated with any particular ethnic group. It is compatible with a normal life span.

Niemann-Pick Disease (Types C and D). These two autosomal recessive disorders are *not associated with sphingomyelinase deficiency*, although the enzyme activity may be reduced. Hepatosplenomegaly exists, and foam cells are present in the bone marrow. Type C is associated with normal development until the age of 2–3 yr, when extrapyramidal symptoms develop. Type D is similar to type C but is found more frequently in Nova Scotia.

The enzyme defect in these disorders is not known but seems to be associated with cholesterol rather than sphingomyelin metabolism. Diagnosis of Niemann-Pick disease type C or D is based on the morphology of foam cells in the bone marrow aspirate in a patient with splenomegaly and normal sphingomyelinase activity.

GAUCHER DISEASE. In this disorder glucosylceramide (glucocerebroside) is stored in the reticuloendothelial system. The classic form of Gaucher disease, sometimes referred to as the chronic or adult form, is common among Ashkenazi Jews and does not involve the central nervous system. There is an infantile form that is neuropathic and also a juvenile form that is associated with late-onset neurologic deterioration.

Etiology. The enzyme defect is deficiency of beta-glucosidase. Enzyme determination can be performed on white blood cells or cultured skin fibroblasts.

Clinical Manifestations. The chronic form of Gaucher disease is characterized by reticuloendothelial system involvement resulting in splenomegaly. Splenomegaly is usually the first clinical sign of Gaucher disease, but symptoms of hypersplenism and bone marrow failure may occur as early as birth and as late as 80 yr of age. Splenomegaly can be striking, and the spleen may occupy a major portion of the abdomen. In the Ashkenazi Jewish population Gaucher disease may not be identified until the 2nd or 3rd decade of life. The storage of glucocerebroside in the spleen and bone marrow leads to anemia, leukopenia, and thrombocytopenia. In rare cases, thrombocytopenia leads to bleeding. Involvement of the liver is minimal, although moderate hepatomegaly may be encountered. Bone marrow aspirates and cells from the spleen show the characteristic Gaucher cells engorged with glucocerebroside (Fig. 8–24). Radiologic changes include the Erlenmeyer flask shape of the long bones, especially the distal femora.

Diagnosis. Splenomegaly with mild anemia that is unexplained should lead to suspicion of Gaucher disease. Bone marrow aspirates showing Gaucher cells strengthen the suspicion. Gaucher disease is confirmed by the demonstration of a deficiency of β-glucosidase.

Genetics. Gaucher disease is inherited as an autosomal recessive disease. It is very common among Ashkenazi Jews, with a frequency as high as 1 in 500 births, which exceeds the frequency of Tay-Sachs disease. Carrier testing and prenatal diagnosis are possible.

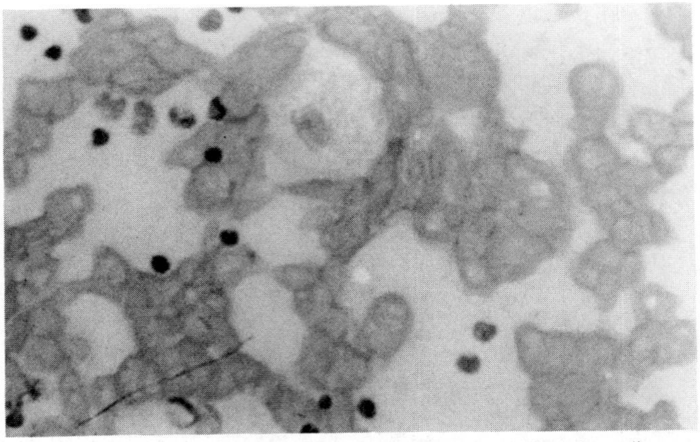

Figure 8–24. Cells from a spleen of a patient with Gaucher disease. A characteristic spleen cell is shown engorged with glucocerebroside.

Treatment. Splenectomy alleviates hypersplenism, improves the blood count, and causes remission for years. Other forms of therapy that are currently under evaluation include repeated injections of the enzyme glucocerebrosidase (β-glucosidase) and bone marrow transplantation.

Infantile Gaucher Disease. This form of the disease involves the central nervous system. The disease may present with splenomegaly, strabismus, trismus, and dorsiflexion of the head. Seizures are common, and such children usually die around 3–4 yr of age. The diagnosis is made by demonstrating a deficiency of glucocerebrosidase in the tissues.

Juvenile Gaucher Disease. This form of disease has variable age of onset, with neurologic signs occurring in the 1st or 2nd decade of life. Neurologic symptoms include ataxia, peripheral neuropathy, myoclonus, ophthalmoplegia, and dementia. The diagnosis is made by documenting a deficiency of glucocerebrosidase (β-glucosidase). This autosomal recessive disorder is panethnic in distribution.

FABRY DISEASE. This X-linked recessive sphingolipid storage disease results from a deficiency of the enzyme α-galactosidase. Glycosphingolipid with two and three sugar residues with α-galactosyl at the terminal end is deposited and cannot be degraded (see Fig. 8–22).

Clinical Manifestations. Symptoms usually occur in adolescent males and include pain crises of the extremities caused by deposition of sphingolipids in the vascular endothelium supplying the peripheral nerves. Skin eruptions around the naval and over the buttocks and angiokeratomas (tiny dark purple-blue telangiectasias) are characteristic of Fabry disease. Hypohydrosis and corneal lenticular opacities may also be seen early in the course of the disease.

As males with Fabry disease get older, the deposition of sphingolipids in the vascular system increases, leading to cardiac manifestations such as mitral insufficiency, conduction defects, ischemic heart attacks, and thromboses. Fabry disease is not associated with mental retardation. Kidney involvement begins with proteinuria and ends with kidney failure. Corneal changes are the most frequent complication found in female heterozygotes.

Diagnosis. Fabry disease should be considered in a male with pain crises of the extremities, angiokeratomas, proteinuria, and signs of kidney malfunction. A kidney biopsy will show lipid accumulation in epithelial and endothelial cells of the glomeruli and tubules. Confirmation is achieved by documenting α-galactosidase deficiency in white blood cells or cultured skin fibroblasts. Enzymatic tests in females at risk of being carriers of Fabry disease are difficult to perform, but the gene for α-galactosidase has been cloned, and molecular methods can now be used for carrier testing. Prenatal diagnosis can be done using an α-galactosidase assay on amniocytes or chorionic villi.

Treatment. Pain crises should be treated symptomatically. Renal failure may require renal transplantation.

SCHINDLER DISEASE (α-*N*-Acetylgalactosaminidase Deficiency). This is a newly described autosomal recessive neurodegenerative disorder. Glycolipid with α-*N*-acetylgalactosamine accumulates in brain throughout the cortex, leading to axonal degeneration; other tissues may also contain this lipid. The enzyme defect is α-*N*-acetylgalactosaminidase deficiency, a lysosomal enzyme. This disease should not be confused with α-*N*-acetylglucosaminidase deficiency (Sanfilippo syndrome type B).

These children appear normal until about 1 yr of age. Developmental regression starts in the 2nd yr of life, followed by cortical blindness, myoclonic seizures, spasticity, decerebrate rigidity, and profound retardation. Demonstration of α-*N*-acetylgalactosaminidase deficiency in white blood cells or cultured skin fibroblasts confirms the diagnosis.

METACHROMATIC LEUKODYSTROPHY (MLD). This autosomal recessive disorder is caused by a deficiency of arylsulfatase A, which is required for the hydrolysis of sulfated glycosphingolipid. Therefore, sulfatide is stored within lysosomes, especially those of white matter, since sulfatide is a component of myelin. In the infantile, juvenile, and adult forms, the enzyme is defective; however, in the disease form in which the activator protein (SAP-1) is defective, arylsulfatase A is intact, but sulfatide nevertheless cannot be cleaved.

Clinical Manifestations. Metachromatic leukodystrophy represents a spectrum of clinical severity and has variable ages of onset. The *late infantile* form of MLD is the most severe and also the most common. It usually becomes manifest between 12 and 18 mo of life with irritability, inability to walk, and hyperextension of the knee causing genu recurvatum. Deep tendon reflexes are diminished or absent. Muscle wasting, weakness, and hypotonia become gradually evident, and these children eventually become bedridden. Nystagmus, myoclonic seizures, optic atrophy, and quadriparesis are features of the end stage of the disease. Patients with the *late infantile form* usually die in the 1st decade of life. The *juvenile form* of MLD has a slower course, and its onset may occur as late as 20 yr of age. The disease presents with ataxia, mental deterioration, and emotional difficulties. The *adult form* is similar to the juvenile form in its clinical manifestations except that emotional difficulties and psychosis are more prominent and the age of onset is usually after the 2nd or 3rd decade of life. Dementia, seizures, diminished reflexes, and optic atrophy are features of the juvenile and adult forms of MLD. An additional form of MLD is caused by a *deficiency of a sphingolipid activator protein* (SAP-1), a protein required for the formation of substrate-enzyme complex. In this disorder arylsulfatase activity is normal when assayed in the test tube, so an assay for the activator protein is required for the diagnosis.

Pathophysiologic and Pathologic Findings. The undegraded sulfatide is stored primarily in white matter. Therefore, no visceral or bone marrow involvement is encountered. White matter from the brain of patients with MLD undergoes demyelination with deposition of many metachromatic bodies, which stain strongly positive with periodic acid-Schiff (PAS) and Alcian blue. Oligodendroglial cells are markedly reduced in number. Neuronal inclusions are also seen in nerve cells of the midbrain, pons, medulla, retina, and spinal cord, and demyelination occurs in the peripheral nervous system. Biopsies of sural nerve stained with acid cresyl violet show many brown metachromatic deposits containing granules, which accumulate in the perinuclear cytoplasm of Schwann cells and in perivascular histiocytes. All involved areas show a loss of oligodendroglial elements. In patients with MLD excessive amounts of sulfatide are excreted in urine.

Diagnosis. The clinical features of leukodystrophy along with decreased nerve conduction velocities, increased cerebrospinal fluid protein, metachromatic deposits in biopsied segments of sural nerve, and metachromatic granules in urinary sediment suggest MLD. The juvenile and adult forms are more difficult to suspect. In none of the forms of MLD is peripheral storage encountered. Brain CT scan or MRI shows attenuation of white matter. Confirmation of the diagnosis is based on enzymatic studies on leukocytes or on cultured skin fibroblasts, indicating a deficiency of arylsulfatase A activity. Enzymatic studies do not differentiate the various forms of MLD. Measurement of the ability of cultured fibroblasts to metabolize radioactive sulfatide in the culture medium sometimes is required to establish the diagnosis of MLD.

Sphingolipid activator protein–deficient patients can be diagnosed by measuring the concentration of SAP-1 using specific antibodies to leukocytes and cultured skin fibroblasts. A low level of cross-reacting material is found. Carrier detection and prenatal diagnosis can be attained using the specific enzyme assay of arylsulfatase A or an assay for SAP-1. Some carriers of MLD have arylsulfatase A levels near those found in affected children. Therefore, parents of affected children should be checked for their carrier status before prenatal testing is undertaken to avoid abortion of a nonaffected but low-activity child.

Treatment. There is no treatment for any form of MLD—only supportive care can be given. Attempts have been made to treat young patients with MLD with bone marrow transplantation. Although normal enzyme levels can be achieved in peripheral blood, no clear evidence indicates that the treatment decreases the neurologic deterioration.

Prognosis. Patients with the late infantile form usually live 2–4 yr after diagnosis, and those with the juvenile form live 4–6 yr. Some children with the adult form have lived to the 5th decade.

Multiple Sulfatase Deficiency. This is another autosomal recessive disease with deficiencies of arylsulfatases A, B, and C. Sulfatides, mucopolysaccharides, steroid sulfates, and gangliosides accumulate in the cerebral cortex and visceral tissues. The neurologic picture is similar to that of late infantile MLD, but the bony involvement may suggest a mucopolysaccharidosis. Severe ichthyosis occurs in many patients with multiple sulfatase deficiency. Examination of urine for mucopolysaccharides is positive. There is a striking abnormality of granulation in the leukocytes. Carrier testing and prenatal diagnosis can be performed. There is no specific treatment for multiple sulfatase deficiency other than supportive care.

KRABBE DISEASE. Krabbe disease, or globoid cell leukodystrophy, is a progressive cerebral degenerative disease affecting the white matter primarily. There is storage of ceramide galactose within lysosomes, leading to degeneration of the white matter. A high incidence of disease occurs in persons of Scandinavian descent. Inheritance is autosomal recessive. The name globoid cell comes from the globular distended multinucleated bodies found in the basal ganglia, pontine nuclei, and cerebellar white matter.

Clinical Manifestations. Onset of Krabbe disease may occur very early in life in the *infantile form*, usually around 3 mo of age. These infants are irritable, develop seizures, and are hypertonic. Optic atrophy is evident in the 1st yr of life, and mental development is severely impaired. As the disease progresses, these infants develop opisthotonos and usually die before 3 yr of age. Patients with the *late infantile form* of Krabbe disease become symptomatic after the 2nd yr of life. The clinical course is similar to that of the infantile form but much slower.

Pathophysiologic and Pathologic Findings. The white matter contains large numbers of globoid histiocytes in areas of demyelination. These cells cluster around blood vessels; they have a lacy, pink cytoplasm (on hematoxylin-eosin stain) and prominent staining of intracellular material on PAS stain. The pathologic abnormalities are almost entirely restricted to the white matter. There may, however, be some damage to the cortical gray matter, but the intense intraneuronal deposition usually observed in other cerebral lipidoses is lacking. Visceral organs are usually not involved because of their paucity of galactosylceramide lipids.

Galactosylceramide accumulation is the result of a deficiency of the lysosomal enzyme that cleaves galactosylceramide. This is a specific β-*galactosidase* referred to as *galactocerebrosidase* or galactosylceramide-β-galactosidase. The deficiency can be documented in leukocytes or cultured skin fibroblasts. As a result of this deficiency, galactosylceramide concentration in the brain of patients with Krabbe disease may be 100 times the normal level.

Diagnosis. Diagnosis of Krabbe disease should be suspected in any patient with white matter disease; attenuation of white matter can be found by MRI or CT scan of the brain. Nerve conduction is reduced, and protein is elevated in the CSF (100–500 mg/dL). Elevation of protein in the cerebrospinal fluid is also found in MLD. A definite diagnosis can be made following the demonstration of galactosylceramide-β-galactosidase deficiency in white blood cells or cultured skin fibroblasts. Carriers have lower than normal levels of galactocerebrosidase activity in white blood cells or cultured skin fibroblasts. Prenatal diagnosis can be performed by measuring this activity in chorionic villi or cultured amniocytes.

Treatment. There is no specific therapy for Krabbe disease.

BATTEN DISEASE. The neuronal storage diseases in this heterogeneous group are sometimes given different labels based on the age of onset: Spielmeyer-Vogt, Jansky-Bielschowsky, and Kufs or amaurotic familial idiocy. Because the storage material, a fluorescent lipopigment, is referred to as lipofuscin, this group of disorders is sometimes called *lipofuscinosis*.

Clinical Manifestations. In the early form of Batten disease *(late infantile)* a child may develop normally until the age of 2–5 yr. Onset may begin with visual disturbances, intellectual retardation, ataxic gait, or seizures. Patchy macular degeneration and retinitis pigmentosa are also features, especially in the late-onset forms. The *juvenile form* begins at the end of the 1st decade or in the early teens. Visual disturbances may be the first symptom noted. Handwriting becomes unintelligible, and school performance declines. The *adult form* presents in the 2nd decade of life with signs of ataxia, dementia, and choreoathetosis.

Pathologic and Pathophysiologic Findings. There is loss of neuronal perikarya, and neurons contain granules that stain for ceroid and lipofuscin. The neurons also contain cytoplasmic inclusions that resemble fingerprints called *curvilinear bodies*. These inclusions also are found in circulating lymphocytes. The exact biochemical defect is unknown, although *dolichol*, a long-chain lipid containing repeating units of five carbon groups, is excreted in excessive amounts in the urine of many, but not all, patients with Batten disease.

Diagnosis. Young patients with retinitis pigmentosa or other retinal changes, ataxia, or myoclonic seizures should be suspected of having Batten disease. Increased amounts of dolichol in the urine and curvilinear bodies in lymphocytes are diagnostic. Skin, conjunctival, or rectal biopsy may be needed to show lipofuscin storage. No carrier detection is available for this autosomal recessive trait because no enzyme defect has been identified.

Treatment. No treatment is available except control of seizures and symptomatic supportive measures.

FARBER DISEASE. This autosomal recessive disease is a result of lysosomal storage of ceramide in various tissues, especially joints.

Clinical Manifestations. Symptoms can begin as early as in the 1st yr of life with painful joint swelling and nodule formation (Fig. 8–25). Sometimes rheumatoid arthritis is suspected in these patients. As the disease progresses these children fail to thrive. Nodule or granulomatous formation affects the vocal cords and leads to hoarseness and breathing difficulties. Children with Farber disease may die from recurrent pneumonias in their teens.

Pathologic and Pathophysiologic Findings. The nodules over the joints are granulomas made of foam cells containing ceramide, the lipid backbone of glycolipids. The kidneys, liver, lungs, and lymph nodes contain an excess of ceramide ranging from 10- to 60-fold. A deficiency of ceramidase leads to a failure to cleave the amino-linked fatty acid attached to sphingosine.

Diagnosis. The diagnosis should be suspected in patients who have nodule formation over the joints but no findings of rheumatoid arthritis. In such patients ceramidase activity should be assayed in cultured skin fibroblasts or white blood cells. Carrier detection is based upon the finding of a lower than normal ceramidase activity. Prenatal diagnosis depends on the presence of ceramidase levels in cultured chorionic villi or amniocytes.

Treatment. There is no specific therapy.

WOLMAN DISEASE. This autosomal recessive lysosomal storage disease of cholesteryl esters is caused by a deficiency of a lysosomal lipase, *acid lipase*. Cholesterol and cholesteryl esters are stored in histiocytic foam cells of visceral organs. The disease is associated with failure to thrive, relentless vomiting, abdominal distention, and hepatosplenomegaly. Calcification of the adrenals is pathognomonic. Usually the disease occurs in the first few weeks of life, and death occurs within 6 mo owing to cachexia and peripheral edema. Diagnosis and carrier identification are based on measuring decreased acid lipase activity in white blood cells or cultured skin fibroblasts. Prenatal diagnosis depends on measuring decreased enzyme levels in cultured chorionic villi or amniocytes. There is a milder form of this acid lipase cholesteryl storage disease that is compatible with long life. There is no specific treatment for Wolman disease.

FUCOSIDOSIS. This is an autosomal recessive lysosomal

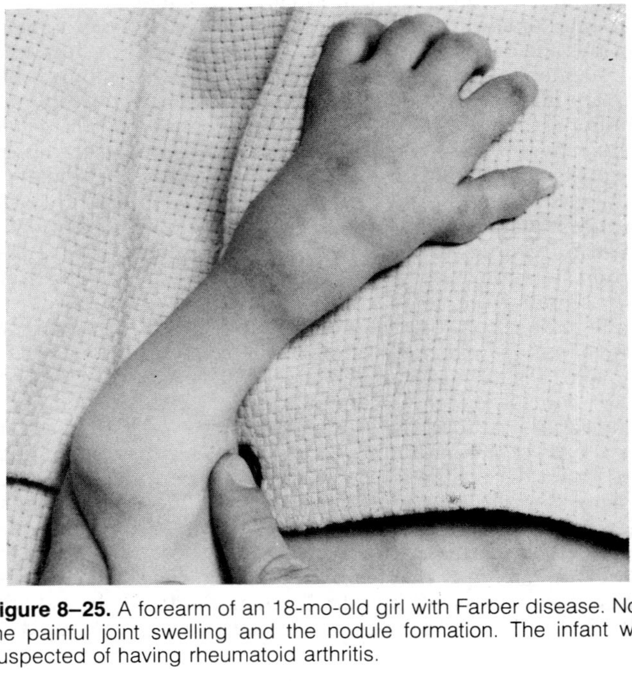

Figure 8–25. A forearm of an 18-mo-old girl with Farber disease. Note the painful joint swelling and the nodule formation. The infant was suspected of having rheumatoid arthritis.

storage disease of fucose-containing glycosphingolipids and glycoproteins.

Pathologic and Pathophysiologic Findings. Lysosomal storage material is found in the liver, brain, and other organs. The hepatocytes and Kupffer cells contain multilamellar structures rich in glycosphingolipid and glycoprotein. The cells in the central nervous system also store this material, and as the disease progresses the features of leukodystrophy become more evident. α-Fucosidase, the enzyme that is deficient in fucosidosis, can be measured in white blood cells, plasma, and cultured skin fibroblasts.

Clinical Manifestations. Children have psychomotor retardation, seizures, hepatosplenomegaly, frontal bossing, coarse facial features, and macroglossia reminiscent of the mucopolysaccharidoses. As they grow older these children develop contractures of the joints and lumbar kyphosis. A *juvenile form* is associated with milder mental involvement and skin lesions over the abdomen and angiokeratomas, similar to those seen in Fabry disease. Fucosidosis is associated with roentgenographic findings of dysostosis multiplex. An MRI or CT scan of the head may suggest the existence of white matter degeneration. Although the radiologic findings of fucosidosis are similar to those of the mucopolysaccharidoses, an enzymatic determination is required to differentiate the former from the latter.

Diagnosis. Visceral storage disease is suggested by hepatosplenomegaly, coarse facial features, and frontal bossing. Urine does not contain mucopolysaccharides but does contain fucose-rich oligosaccharides. In the infantile form, sweat chloride levels are elevated. The diagnosis is confirmed by the demonstration of α-fucosidase deficiency in white blood cells or cultured skin fibroblasts. Carrier detection and prenatal diagnosis can be achieved by performing assays for α-fucosidase. Some ethnic groups, such as Italians and Spanish-Americans, have a high incidence of fucosidosis.

Treatment. There is no specific therapy.

Barranger JA, Ginns EL: Glucosylceramide lipidoses: Gaucher disease. *In*: Scriver CR, Beaudet AL, Sly WS, et al (eds): The Metabolic Basis of Inherited Disease, 6th ed. New York, McGraw Hill, 1989, p 1677.

Barranger JA, Murray GJ, Ginns EI: Genetic heterogeneity of Gaucher's disease. *In*: Barranger JA, Brady RO (eds): Molecular Basis of Lysosomal Storage Disorders. New York, Academic Press, 1984, p 311.

Beaudet AL, Thomas GH: Acid lipase deficiency: Wolman disease and cholesteryl ester storage disease. *In*: Scriver CR, Beaudet AL, Sly WS, et al (eds): The Metabolic Basis of Inherited Disease, 6th ed. New York, McGraw Hill, 1989, p 1623.

Desnick RJ, Bishop DF: Fabry disease: α-galactosidase deficiency; Schindler disease: α-*N*-acetylgalactosaminidase deficiency. *In*: Scriver CW, Beaudet AL, Sly WS, et al (eds): The Metabolic Basis of Inherited Disease, 6th ed. New York, McGraw Hill, 1989, p 1751.

Fujibayashi S, Inui K, Wenger DA: Activator protein deficient metachromatic leukodystrophy: Diagnosis in leukocytes using immunologic methods. J Pediatr 104:739, 1984.

Inui K, Emmett M, Wenger DA: Immunological evidence for a deficiency of an activator protein for sulfatide sulfatase in a variant form of metachromatic leukodystrophy. Proc Natl Acad Sci USA 80:3074, 1983.

Johnson WG: The clinical spectrum of hexosaminidase deficiency diseases. Neurology 31:1453, 1981.

Kolodny EH: Metachromatic leukodystrophy and multiple sulfatase deficiency: Sulfatide lipidosis. *In*: Scriver CW, Beaudet AL, Sly WS, et al (eds): The Metabolic Basis of Inherited Disease, 6th ed. New York, McGraw Hill, 1989, p 1721.

Kolodny EH, Ullman MD, Mankin HJ, et al: Phenotypic manifestations of Gaucher disease: Clinical features in 48 biochemically verified type 1 patients and comments on type 2 patients. Progr Clin Biol Res 95:33, 1982.

Matthew SW, Callahan WJ: Sphingomyelin-cholesterol lipidoses: The Niemann-Pick group of diseases. *In*: Scriver CW, Beaudet AL, Sly WS, et al (eds): The Metabolic Basis of Inherited Disease, 6th ed. New York, McGraw Hill, 1989, p 1655.

Moser HW, Moser AB, Winston CW, et al: Ceramidase deficiency: Farber lipogranulomatosis. *In*: Scriver CR, Beaudet AL, Sly WS, et al (eds): The Metabolic Basis of Inherited Disease, 6th ed. New York, McGraw Hill, 1989, p 1645.

Moser HW, Moser AE, Trojak JE, et al: Identification of female carriers of adrenoleukodystrophy. J Pediatr 103:54, 1983.

O'Brien JS: β-Galactosidase deficiency (GM_1 gangliosidosis, galactosialidosis and Morquio syndrome type 8); Ganglioside sialidase deficiency (mucolipidosis IV). *In*: Scriver CW, Beaudet AL, Sly WS, et al (eds): The Metabolic Basis of Inherited Disease, 6th ed. New York, McGraw Hill, 1989, p 1787.

Polten A, Fluharty AL, Fluharty CB, et al: Molecular bases of different forms of metachromatic leukodystrophy. N Engl J Med 324:18, 1991.

Sandhoff K, Conzelmann E, Neufeld EF, et al: The GM_2 gangliosidoses. *In*: Scriver CW, Beaudet AL, Sly WS, et al (eds): The Metabolic Basis of Inherited Disease, 6th ed. New York, McGraw Hill, 1989, p 1807.

Suzuki K, Suzuki Y: Galactosylceramide lipidosis: Globoid cell leukodystrophy (Krabbe disease). *In*: Scriver CW, Beaudet AL, Sly WS, et al (eds): The Metabolic Basis of Inherited Disease, 6th ed. New York, McGraw Hill, 1989, p 1699.

Zimran A, Gross E, West C, et al: Prediction of Gaucher's disease by identification at DNA level. Lancet 2:349, 1989.

8.19 MUCOLIPIDOSES

Patients with mucolipidoses exhibit clinical features of both lipidoses and mucopolysaccharidoses (see Sec. 8.43). Despite their name, there is little evidence of true storage of lipids or mucopolysaccharides in the organs of affected patients. Technically, fucosidosis, GM_1 gangliosidosis, and multiple sulfatase deficiency are mucolipidoses because there is evidence of storage both of lipids (as glycosphingolipids) and of glycosaminoglycans in various organs. All of the mucolipidoses are inherited as autosomal recessive traits. There is no specific treatment for these disorders.

Mucolipidosis (ML-I), lipomucopolysaccharidosis, or sialidosis type 2 (infantile onset) produces symptoms in the 1st yr of life. There are Hurler-like features, with dysostosis multiplex, moderate mental retardation, visceromegaly, corneal clouding, cherry-red spot, seizures, vacuolated lymphocytes, and coarse fibroblast inclusions, but no mucopolysacchariduria. Some of these children may appear relatively normal at birth, but all patients develop progressive severe clinical manifestations. There is also a congenital type 2 form characterized by hydrops fetalis and neonatal ascites, hepatosplenomegaly, stippling of the epiphyses, periosteal cloaking, and stillbirth or death during infancy. These patients have an isolated neuraminidase deficiency. There is, in addition, a "juvenile" type 2 form of sialidosis (ML-1), sometimes designated *galactosialidosis*, which is characterized by primary β-galactosialidase deficiency as well as neuraminidase deficiency. In these patients clinical manifestations may begin at any time from infancy to adulthood. In early infancy there may be a phenotype similar to that of GM_1 gangliosidosis with edema, ascites, skeletal dysplasia, and cherry-red spot. Later, the main features are dysostosis multiplex, visceromegaly, mental retardation, dysmorphism, corneal clouding, progressive neurologic deterioration, and bilateral cherry-red spots. The storage compounds in this disorder are predominantly sialylated oligosaccharides similar to those excreted by children with other types of sialidoses.

Sialidosis type 1 is distinguished from type 2 by the cherry-red spot–myoclonus phenotype and the absence of somatic features such as coarse facies and dysostosis multiplex. The age of onset is variable, but usually the disorder occurs in the 2nd decade of life.

Sialidosis types 1 and 2 result from inherited deficiencies of neuraminidase, of which there are at least two forms. Sialic acid terminal oligosaccharides and sialylglycopeptides are excreted in large amounts in the urine. Kupffer cells and hepatocytes are vacuolated, and sural nerve biopsy reveals metachromatic myelin degeneration. These patients are deficient in glycoprotein sialidase activity. Ganglioside sialidase is normal. Diagnosis is based on measurement of neuraminidase activity in fibroblasts or white blood cells. Carriers can be identified, and prenatal diagnosis can be made using cultured amniotic cells.

ML-II or **I-cell** disease is manifest within the first few months of life. The clinical pattern somewhat resembles Hurler syndrome and GM_1 gangliosidosis (type 1). Affected patients may have congenital dislocation of the hips, inguinal hernias, hypertrophy of the gums, restriction of motion in the shoulders, generalized hypotonia, thick and tight skin, and hepatomegaly. The coarse facial features become more conspicuous with age. Progressive psychomotor retardation occurs as well. Characteristic bone changes related to severe dysostosis multiplex occur, leading to a cloaking of the appearance of long tubular bones, to shortening of vertebral bodies, and to other significant changes in the pelvis, hands, ribs, and skull. Death from pneumonia or congestive heart failure usually occurs at 2–8 yr of age.

Urinary mucopolysaccharides are normal, but sialyloligosaccharides are elevated. Fibroblast cultures reveal characteristic inclusions, which initially set this disease apart from the mucopolysaccharidoses. Enzyme studies show greatly increased lysosomal enzymes in serum, whereas values in leukocytes are near the normal range. Activities of almost all lysosomal enzymes are deficient in cultured skin fibroblasts, whereas the culture medium has an excess of these enzymes compared with those of control fibroblast lines. Normally, the targeting of lysosomal enzymes to lysosomes is mediated by receptors that bind mannose-6-phosphate recognition markers on the enzymes. The marker is synthesized in a two-step reaction in the Golgi complex. UDP-*N*-acetylglucosamine: lysosomal enzyme *N*-acetylglucosaminyl-1-phosphotransferase, the enzyme catalyzing the first step in this process, is defective in ML-II and ML-III. Thus, newly formed lysosomal enzymes cannot be phosphorylated. In the absence of these phosphate groups, which serve as part of a recognition marker, the newly synthesized enzymes do not get into the lysosomes but are excreted from the cell. This specific phosphotransferase activity can be measured in fibroblast cultures, providing a specific diagnostic test for patient and carrier identification and for prenatal diagnosis.

ML-III or pseudo-Hurler polydystrophy is a milder form of ML-II. After possibly delayed early psychomotor development, affected 3- to 4-yr-old children may present with progressive joint stiffness, short stature, mild dysostosis multiplex, mild gingival hyperplasia, and normal urinary mucopolysaccharide levels. Corneal clouding or nystagmus may be present. The IQ may range from normal to as low as 50. The prognosis is unknown; some patients have attained the 3rd decade of life. Orthopedic treatment may be indicated in some cases. As in I-cell disease, serum lysosomal enzymes are elevated, and cultured skin fibroblasts reveal characteristic inclusions and decreased activities for many lysosomal enzymes. Measurement of UDP-*N*-acetylglucosamine-1-phosphotransferase activity using exogenous substrate shows more residual activity than in ML-II. Prenatal diagnosis is possible through examination of cultured amniotic fluid cells.

ML-IV is a recently described mucolipidosis. Most cases reported so far have occurred in children of Ashkenazi Jewish descent. Usually, soon after birth affected children present with bilateral corneal opacities and strabismus. Retinal degeneration may also occur. After 6 mo hypotonia and psychomotor retardation become more evident. Surviving patients are usually retarded to about the 1-yr level. There is no skeletal dysplasia or excess excretion of mucopolysaccharides in the urine. There are grossly abnormal storage bodies in the cells of the liver, brain, conjunctiva, and fibroblasts. The prognosis is uncertain. One patient has reached 24 yr of age. Treatment to correct the corneal opacities may improve the vision, but no other treatment is available.

Diagnosis is based on examining fibroblast cultures for the characteristic lamellated multivesicular membrane bodies. Patients have been found to have a partial deficiency of ganglioside sialidase activity. Although some obligate heterozygotes have less than normal activity, it has still not been proved whether or not this is the primary defect. Prenatal diagnosis is made by examining cultured amniotic fluid cells for the characteristic storage bodies.

REUBEN H. MATALON

Banerjee A, Burg J, Conzelmann E, et al: Enzyme-linked immunosorbent assay for the ganglioside G_{M2}-activator protein. Hoppe-Seyler's Z Physiol Chem 365:347, 1984.

Crandall BF, Philippart M, Brown WJ, et al: Mucolipidosis IV. Am J Med Genet 12:301, 1982.

Gillow JE, Lowden JA, Gaskin MB, et al: Congenital ascites as a presenting sign of lysosomal storage disease. J Pediatr 104:225, 1984.

Lowden JA, O'Brien JS: Sialidosis: A review of human sialidase deficiency. Am J Hum Genet 31:1, 1979.

O'Reilly RJ, Brochstein J, Dinsmore R, et al: Marrow transplantation for congenital disorders. Semin Hematol 21:188, 1984.

Poenaru L, Kaplan L, Dumez J, et al: Evaluation of possible first trimester prenatal diagnosis in lysosomal diseases by trophoblast biopsy. Pediatr Res 18:1032, 1984.

Reitman ML, Varki A, Kornfeld S: Fibroblasts from patients with I-cell disease and pseudo-Hurler polydystrophy are deficient in uridine 5'-diphosphate-N-acetylglucosamine: glycoprotein N-acetylglucosaminylphosphotransferase activity. J Clin Invest 67:1574, 1981.

Scriver CR, Beaudet AL, Sly WS, et al: The Metabolic Basis of Inherited Disease, 6th ed. New York, McGraw-Hill, 1989.

8.20 DISORDERS OF LIPOPROTEIN METABOLISM AND TRANSPORT

The Framingham study and other similar studies have demonstrated that the higher the plasma cholesterol level, the greater the risk of myocardial infarction secondary to the premature development of atherosclerosis. In 1984, the Lipid Research Clinics Coronary Primary Prevention Trial showed that for every 1% drop in plasma cholesterol obtained by cholestyramine therapy in adult males, there was a 2% reduction in the incidence of myocardial infarction. These and other studies suggest that children at risk for developing premature atherosclerosis in adulthood because they have inherited one or more genes for hypercholesterolemia should be identified early in life in order to try to reduce the associated risk of premature heart disease. They also suggest the need to intervene to lower even moderately raised cholesterol levels. Hypertriglyceridemia, although generally considered to be a less significant risk factor than hypercholesterolemia, is also known to be associated with the early development of atherosclerosis. This section focuses on the metabolism and transport of cholesterol and triglycerides; "normal" plasma levels of these lipids; the risk of moderate plasma cholesterol elevations; strategies for screening and intervention; primary (i.e., genetic) and secondary defects of lipoprotein metabolism that can result in abnormal lipid levels in children; and the diagnosis and management of pediatric patients with these disorders. Finally, disorders associated with low circulating levels of lipoproteins are discussed.

8.21 Plasma Lipoprotein Metabolism and Transport

Cholesterol and triglycerides are transported in the circulation in macromolecular complexes termed lipoproteins; the protein components of the complexes are called apolipoproteins. Dietary lipoproteins (chylomicrons) are formed in and secreted by the small intestine; other lipoproteins (e.g., very low density lipoproteins, VLDL) are synthesized in the liver. Still others (high-density lipoproteins, HDL) reach their mature form in the circulation after exchanging components with other circulating lipoproteins or with tissues.

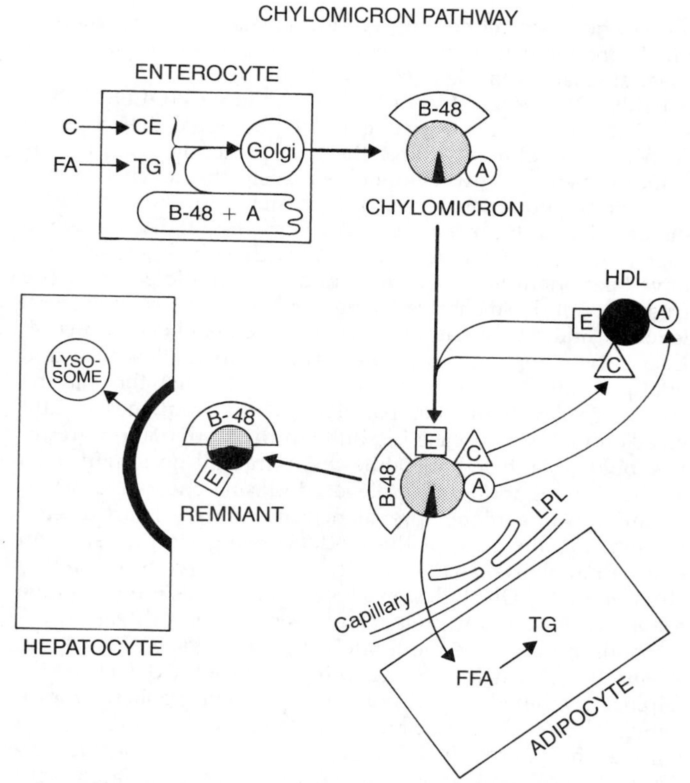

Figure 8–26. Pathway of chylomicron metabolism in human plasma. Fatty acids (FA) and cholesterol (C) are esterified in the intestinal mucosa to form triglycerides (TG) and cholesteryl esters (CE), respectively. They combine with apoA and apoB-48 to form chylomicrons, which are secreted into the circulation: TG *(shaded area)* and CE *(black area)*. Chylomicrons undergo lipolysis in the capillary endothelium near adipose tissue and muscle tissue, losing TG via lipoprotein lipase (LPL), gaining apoE from HDL, and losing apoA and apoC to HDL. The resultant chylomicron remnants are taken up by hepatic apoE receptors for degradation by lysosomes. (Adapted from Havel RJ: Approach to the patient with hyperlipidemia. Med Clin North Am 66:319, 1982.)

TRANSPORT OF EXOGENOUS (DIETARY) LIPIDS (Fig. 8–26). After ingestion of a fat-containing meal and hydrolysis by intestinal and pancreatic lipases, free fatty acids and cholesterol are re-esterified in the intestinal epithelium to form triglycerides and cholesteryl esters, respectively. These lipids are then packaged together with phospholipids, free cholesterol, and at least two apolipoproteins (apoA-I and apoB-48) to form chylomicrons. The chylomicrons are then secreted into the intestinal lymph and pass through the thoracic duct into the peripheral circulation. In the circulation, chylomicrons acquire additional apolipoproteins, mainly apoE and several forms of apoC. Triglycerides, which constitute most of the chylomicron mass, are immediately hydrolyzed by lipoprotein lipase at the capillary endothelium. The free fatty acid products of this hydrolysis are transferred primarily to adipose tissue for storage as triglycerides or to muscle tissue for β-oxidation. The lipoprotein particles, now smaller and more dense because they have lost most of their triglyceride content, are called chylomicron remnants. They have retained virtually all of their cholesteryl ester content and transferred some of their apolipoproteins (apoC and apoA-I) primarily to HDL. They also have become enriched with respect to their apoB-48 and apoE content. These remnants are recognized, bound, and internalized in part through hepatic membrane receptors specific for the apoE on the particles. By this mechanism, dietary cholesterol is delivered to the liver, where it plays a role in the regulation of hepatic cholesterol metabolism. Under normal circumstances, chylomicrons and their remnants are very short-lived in the circulation; following a 12-hr fast, there are normally no lipoproteins of dietary origin remaining in the plasma.

TRANSPORT OF ENDOGENOUS LIPIDS FROM THE LIVER (Fig. 8–27). The liver secretes the class of lipoproteins called VLDL, which contain free and esterified cholesterol, triglycerides, phospholipids, and a characteristic set of apolipoproteins, notably apoB-100, apoC, and apoE. Like chylomicrons, VLDL exchange apolipoproteins with other circulating particles and deliver triglycerides to adipose tissue through lipoprotein lipase. In the process, they become smaller and more dense and are termed VLDL remnants or intermediate-density lipoproteins. Some of these remnant particles are taken up through hepatic cell membrane receptors, and some undergo conversion to low-density lipoproteins (LDL); this latter process involves removal of the remaining triglycerides and all apolipoproteins except apoB-100 and results in a particle that is almost entirely made up of cholesteryl esters and apoB-100. A specific LDL receptor is present on most cell membranes that recognizes, binds, and

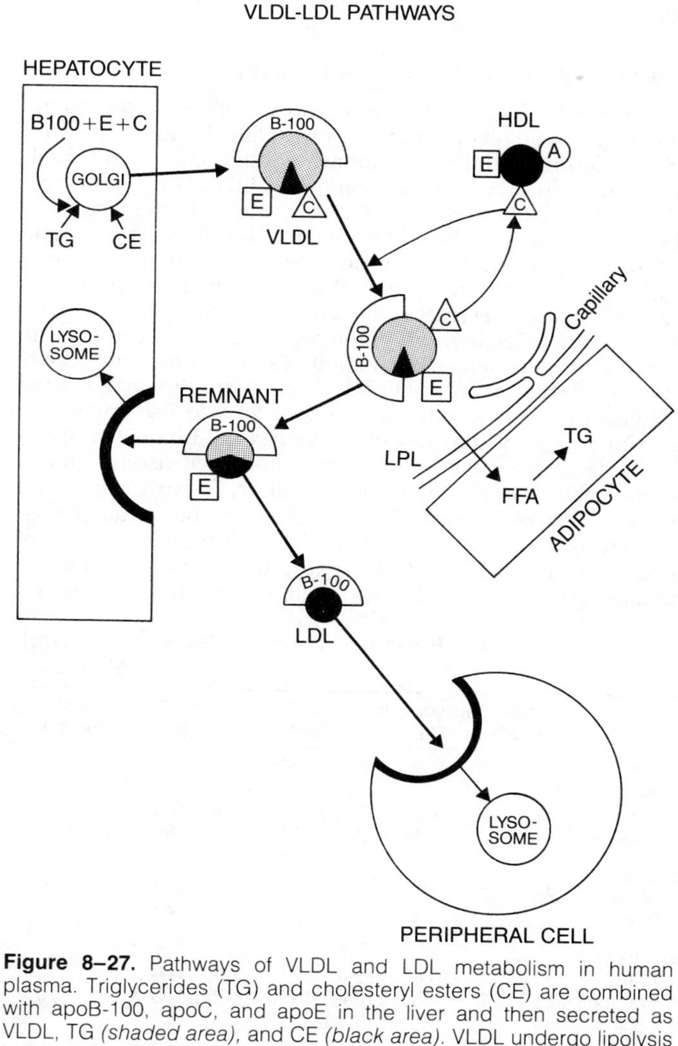

Figure 8–27. Pathways of VLDL and LDL metabolism in human plasma. Triglycerides (TG) and cholesteryl esters (CE) are combined with apoB-100, apoC, and apoE in the liver and then secreted as VLDL, TG *(shaded area)*, and CE *(black area)*. VLDL undergo lipolysis in the capillary endothelium near adipose tissue and muscle tissue, losing TG via lipoprotein lipase (LPL). The resulting VLDL remnants are either converted to low-density lipoproteins (LDL) for transport to peripheral cells via LDL receptor-mediated uptake or are taken up by hepatic receptors. (FFA = free fatty acids.) (Adapted from Havel RJ: Approach to the patient with hyperlipidemia. Med Clin North Am 66:319, 1982.)

internalizes LDL. By this mechanism, LDL particles can deliver cholesterol to extrahepatic tissues to serve their requirements for membrane synthesis; in addition, tissues involved in steroid hormone synthesis can meet their cholesterol needs by receptor-mediated uptake of LDL. LDL particles can circulate in the plasma for several days.

HDL AND REVERSE CHOLESTEROL TRANSPORT. In contrast to chylomicrons and VLDL, which are secreted into the circulation as mature particles, HDL are secreted from the liver and small intestine as nascent discoidal particles composed primarily of phospholipids and proteins (apoE and apoA). The particles accept cholesterol from VLDL and LDL as well as from tissues; this cholesterol is esterified through the lecithin-cholesterol acyltransferase reaction. Part of the cholesteryl ester is stored in the core of HDL, making it a spherical particle, and part of it is transferred back to VLDL and LDL. LDL and remnants of VLDL metabolism can be taken up by the liver, providing a method of return of tissue-derived cholesterol to the liver (reverse cholesterol transport). HDL itself can also be metabolized by the liver, providing another possible vehicle for the return of tissue-derived cholesterol to the liver. The liver can then excrete cholesterol in bile.

Plasma Lipid and Lipoprotein Levels

NORMAL. Table 8–11 shows normal plasma cholesterol and triglyceride levels from birth through the first 2 decades of life. During the first few months of life, cholesterol levels increase, largely because of changes in LDL. During the next 15–20 yr, in both males and females, there is little change in the total cholesterol level; the mean value fluctuates around 150–165 mg/dL. Mean LDL cholesterol levels remain slightly under 100 mg/dL in both males and females during this period. HDL cholesterol levels are comparable in males and females early in life; they remain essentially constant in females but decline markedly in males during the 2nd decade to a level that is maintained through adulthood. Plasma triglyceride levels, on the other hand, tend to rise transiently in both males and females in the 1st yr, fall to a mean of 50–60 mg/dL in the ensuing few years, and then rise to a mean of approximately 75 mg/dL by age 20 yr. In early adulthood there is a marked rise in plasma cholesterol that is due almost exclusively to an increase in LDL cholesterol. The rate of increase during the next 30 yr is greater in males than in females. When coupled with their lower HDL cholesterol levels and their higher triglyceride levels, this puts men at much greater risk than women for atherosclerotic heart disease, at least up to the age of 50–60 yr.

RISK OF MODERATELY ELEVATED CHOLESTEROL LEVELS. In the past, it was generally accepted that children with cholesterol levels above the 95th percentile were hypercholesterolemic. Now evidence suggests that even children with more moderately raised cholesterol levels may be at increased risk for premature coronary heart disease when they grow older. Changes consistent with early atherosclerosis have been identified in young children and adolescents. The frequency of these changes correlates with plasma cholesterol levels. Children's cholesterol levels have also been shown to track along percentiles as they grow into adolescence and young adulthood and to correlate well with the plasma cholesterol levels of their parents and the frequency of atherosclerotic heart disease in adults in their population group. It should be noted that, while there are still no longitudinal studies linking moderately elevated plasma cholesterol levels in children to a higher prevalence of coronary heart disease in later life, the bulk of the evidence suggests that such an association exists. As a result, there is a consensus that children with LDL cholesterol levels above the 75th percentile are at greater risk for premature coronary heart disease.

Children may have moderately raised cholesterol levels for a variety of reasons. Some primary genetic defects (e.g., familial combined hyperlipidemia and hyperapobetalipoproteinemia) may be associated with only mild elevations of plasma cholesterol. In addition, common polymorphic variants of apoE and apoB are known to be associated with moderate elevations of plasma LDL cholesterol. Furthermore, there are secondary causes of hyperlipoproteinemia (e.g., other disease states) that need to be considered. Finally, inappropriate dietary habits, by themselves or by interacting with any of the above factors, can contribute to moderately raised cholesterol levels.

SCREENING FOR HYPERCHOLESTEROLEMIA. Children over the age of 2 yr with a family history of hyperlipidemia or early atherosclerotic heart disease should undergo routine screening for hyperlipidemia. However, this screening rationale may miss more than half of the children with elevated plasma cholesterol. Electively screening all children older than the age of 2 yr for elevated cholesterol levels as part of regular well-child care may be a more prudent approach. Initial screening tests that are positive (see later)

TABLE 8–11. Plasma Cholesterol and Triglyceride Levels in Childhood and Adolescence: Means and Percentiles

	Total Triglyceride (mg/dL)					Total Cholesterol (mg/dL)					LDL Cholesterol (mg/dL)					HDL Cholesterol (mg/dL)*				
	5th	*Mean*	*75th*	*90th*	*95th*	*5th*	*Mean*	*75th*	*90th*	*95th*	*5th*	*Mean*	*75th*	*90th*	*95th*	*5th*	*10th*	*25th*	*Mean*	*95th*
Cord	14	34	—	—	84	42	68	—	—	103	17	29	—	—	50	13	—	—	35	60
1–4 yr																				
Male	29	56	68	85	99	114	155	170	190	203	—	—	—	—	—	—	—	—	—	—
Female	34	64	74	95	112	112	156	173	188	200	—	—	—	—	—	—	—	—	—	—
5–9 yr																				
Male	28	52	58	70	85	125	155	168	183	189	63	93	103	117	129	38	42	49	56	74
Female	32	64	74	103	126	131	164	176	190	197	68	100	115	125	140	36	38	47	53	73
10–14 yr																				
Male	33	63	74	94	111	124	160	173	188	202	64	97	109	122	132	37	40	46	55	74
Female	39	72	85	104	120	125	160	171	191	205	68	97	110	126	136	37	40	45	52	70
15–19 yr																				
Male	38	78	88	125	143	118	153	168	183	191	62	94	109	123	130	30	34	39	46	63
Female	36	73	85	112	126	118	159	176	198	207	59	96	111	129	137	35	38	43	52	74

*Note that different percentiles are listed for HDL cholesterol.

Data for cord blood from Strong W: Atherosclerosis: Its pediatric roots. *In*: Kaplan N, Stamler J (eds): Prevention of Coronary Heart Disease. Philadelphia, WB Saunders, 1983. Data for children 1–4 yr from Tables 6, 7, 20, and 21, and all other data from Tables 24, 25, 32, 33, 36, and 37 in Lipid Research Clinics Population Studies Data Book, Vol. 1, The prevalence study. NIH Publication No. 80–1527. Washington, DC, National Institutes of Health, 1980.

should be repeated and verified in a certified laboratory before any intervention is undertaken.

Determination of total cholesterol in a nonfasting, capillary blood sample is the most easily available and efficient initial screening test for hypercholesterolemia. (As it becomes more available, measurement of apoB may be a more effective initial test. Persons with high levels of apoB are at increased risk for atherosclerotic disease; they may have normal total cholesterol levels and thus be missed by screening for elevated total cholesterol only.) Those with a total cholesterol level above the 75th percentile (approximately 176 mg/dL) and without a secondary cause for hyperlipidemia (see Sec. 8.32) should have a venous blood sample drawn for evaluation of total cholesterol, HDL cholesterol, and triglycerides after a 12-hr fast. LDL cholesterol can then be estimated using the following equation:

$$\text{LDL cholesterol} = \text{total cholesterol} - [\text{HDL cholesterol} + (\text{total triglycerides}/5)]$$

Triglycerides must be less than 400 mg/dL to derive an accurate estimate of LDL cholesterol with this method.

A significant number of children have an elevated total cholesterol level because they have a high HDL cholesterol level. These children are thought to be protected from premature atherosclerotic disease. In children with LDL cholesterol levels above the 75th percentile, however, repeat evaluation should be undertaken prior to beginning dietary modification. Owing to sample variability, both biologic and laboratory, in plasma cholesterol levels, it is recommended that levels be measured in two fasting venous samples obtained over the span of a few weeks and the two levels averaged. If the average LDL cholesterol level is above the 75th percentile, dietary modification is recommended. Children in whom only one measurement is above the 75th percentile (and the average value is less than the 75th percentile) should be re-evaluated in 1 yr. Because some forms of familial hyperlipidemia may not be expressed until the child is older, children with normal plasma cholesterol levels and a family history consistent with a familial form of hyperlipidemia should be re-evaluated 5 and 10 yr after the initial evaluation.

Good standards for the 75th percentile of LDL cholesterol in 2- to 4-yr-old children do not exist. Thus, it may be best to re-evaluate 2- to 4-yr-old children with moderately elevated LDL cholesterol levels (e.g., significantly greater than the mean but less than the 95th percentile) at 5 yr of age before considering dietary modification (see Sec. 8.22).

Children with triglyceride levels above the 95th percentile also should be evaluated further. Although elevated triglyceride levels per se do not represent an independent risk factor for premature cardiovascular disease, levels above the 95th percentile can be a marker for some patients with genetic forms of hyperlipidemia, even with a normal total cholesterol level.

8.22 Dietary Management of Hyperlipidemias

For hyperlipidemic children over the age of 2 yr, dietary modification is the best initial intervention. Dietary intake should provide 30% of total calories as fat (equally distributed among saturated, monounsaturated, and polyunsaturated fats) and no more than 100 mg cholesterol/1,000 calories (maximum total 300 mg)/24 hr. This is referred to as the **prudent diet**. It is recommended that this diet be adopted by all family members above the age of 2 yr to encourage optimal compliance.

This dietary modification program and similar ones are effective and safe in the treatment of hyperlipidemia in adults. Several investigators have demonstrated similar effectiveness and safety in children over the age of 2 yr. A large multicenter trial confirming the safety and efficacy of such a program in children is ongoing. It must be emphasized that these recommendations are meant only for children over the age of 2 yr. Children under the age of 2 placed on a similar or more restrictive diet and older children placed on more restrictive diets by well-meaning caregivers have shown poor growth. Proper supervision to ensure the appropriateness of any dietary modification in children should be undertaken. Because most pediatricians are unable to provide detailed guidance for such dietary modifications, referral to a trained pediatric dietitian is usually indicated. Prior to undertaking a screening program, the physician should ensure the availability of such referral for his or her patients. Considering the limited number of properly trained pediatric dietitians, development of programs to provide this guidance and service to pediatricians and the community is necessary before widespread screening can be undertaken.

It is important that a child with a positive result on a screening test not assume the role of or be labeled a chronically ill child. Intervention programs need to emphasize that a moderately raised LDL cholesterol level is a risk factor, not a disease, and should stress the positive aspects of appropriate life style modification. At the same time, some children and families may have difficulty in accepting the recommendations of a dietary modification program owing to the perceived amorphous nature of the risk of moderately raised plasma cholesterol levels. Modification programs need to take into account these and other special needs of the growing child.

Those children who follow the recommendations of the intervention program but do not respond appropriately by demonstrating a lower LDL cholesterol level should be re-evaluated for familial forms of hyperlipidemia or more obscure causes of secondary hyperlipidemia. For example, persons with familial combined hyperlipidemia may demonstrate further elevations in dietary lipids even when following a dietary modification program.

PRIMARY GENETIC DEFECTS

One third of patients who have suffered their first myocardial infarction before the age of 50 yr (in men) or 60 yr (in women) have hyperlipoproteinemia, and about half of these patients have a dominantly inherited disorder of lipoprotein metabolism. During a recent 2-yr period, the Lipid-Heart Research Center at The Children's Hospital of Philadelphia diagnosed a dominantly inherited disorder of lipoprotein metabolism in 75% of children found to have hyperlipidemia and a strongly positive history for premature coronary artery disease: 21% had familial hypercholesterolemia (FH); 67% had familial combined hyperlipidemia (FCHL); 11% had hyperapobetalipoproteinemia; and 1% had familial hypertriglyceridemia (FHTG).

8.23 Familial Hypercholesterolemia (FH)

HETEROZYGOUS FH. This dominantly inherited disease affecting lipoprotein metabolism (and hence plasma lipid levels) has a prevalence of at least 1 in 500 in the population and is a common form of inherited hyperlipidemia recognized in childhood. FH results from defects of the LDL receptor, and there are at least 20 separate allelic mutations in the gene for the LDL receptor that impair the receptor-mediated uptake of LDL from the circulation (see Fig. 8–27). Most patients with FH are heterozygous for one of these alleles, and hence half of their receptors are normal and half are defective, resulting in marked elevation of the plasma LDL cholesterol level from birth.

Clinical Manifestations. The most important problem is premature coronary atherosclerosis that typically does not develop until the 3rd or 4th decade. The peak incidence of myocardial infarction in affected men occurs in the 4th–5th decades; by 60 yr of age, 85% have had a myocardial infarction. In women, the mean age of onset is about 10 yr later. Most adult patients present with a strong family history of premature coronary artery disease and tendon xanthomas (nodular swellings involving the Achilles and other tendons due to cholesteryl ester deposition in macrophages), as well as deposits in the soft tissue of the eyelid (xanthelasmas) and in the cornea (arcus corneae). Except for tendon xanthomas, which are occasionally found in affected teenagers, these signs are rarely present in pediatric patients with heterozygous FH. Owing to its rarity in healthy children, therefore, Achilles tendinitis in a teenager should suggest the diagnosis of FH.

Diagnosis. Diagnosis of FH is supported by a strong family history of early myocardial infarctions, tendon xanthomas, and total plasma cholesterol levels greater than 300 mg/dL in affected adults. Affected children usually have total cholesterol levels above 250 mg/dL, with LDL cholesterol above 200 mg/dL.

Treatment. Weight control has relatively little impact on the plasma cholesterol level in patients with heterozygous FH. The prudent diet is recommended for FH patients and may produce a significant reduction (by as much as 15%) in LDL cholesterol, but diet alone will rarely return the LDL cholesterol level to normal. Consequently, cholestyramine or colestipol resin is recommended to further reduce LDL cholesterol in children 6 yr of age or older. These nonabsorbable drugs interrupt the enterohepatic cycle through the binding of bile acids in the intestine; they have the additional benefit of inducing LDL receptors in the liver. Most children tolerate this medication quite well; the side effects of constipation and abdominal discomfort usually can be managed effectively. Both drugs may interfere with the absorption of fat-soluble vitamins; supplements may be required, and assessment of plasma vitamin A levels and prothrombin time may be indicated. Cholestyramine is available in 9-g packets (equivalent to 4 g of active drug). The dose of drug varies with age and with the severity of hypercholesterolemia, ranging from as little as 1/2 packet (2 g of active drug) twice a day before meals to as much as 2–3 packets (16–24 g) twice a day. Up to 3 packets (24 g) twice a day is usually well tolerated by teenagers and may reduce LDL cholesterol by 50–100 mg/dL. Colestipol is available in 5-g packets, all of which is active drug; dosage (in terms of packets) is similar to that for cholestyramine. If LDL cholesterol persists above the 95th percentile, nicotinic acid, which is the next drug of choice in adults, should be considered. Sometimes, however, the side effects of nicotinic acid (e.g., flushing, gastrointestinal upset, hepatic toxicity) preclude its effective use in children. Lovastatin and other HMG-CoA reductase inhibitors that have been successfully used in adults have not been approved for use in patients younger than 19 yr of age.

HOMOZYGOUS FH. A rare patient (about 1 in a million) with severe FH is either homozygous for one abnormal allele or is a compound heterozygote for two alleles that impair LDL-receptor function. Homozygotes have plasma cholesterol levels of 600 mg/dL or higher from birth. They have unique planar cutaneous xanthomas over the knees, elbows, and buttocks, which are often evident at birth and almost always appear by 6 yr of age. Tendon xanthomas, xanthelasmas, and arcus corneae are virtually always present. Coronary atherosclerosis frequently has its onset before 10 yr of age; most patients die of complications from myocardial infarction before 30 yr of age.

Drugs and diet do not have a major impact on the clinical outcome of persons with homozygous FH. Consequently, regular plasmapheresis and aggressive therapies, such as ileal bypass surgery and portacaval shunt, have been attempted with some success. Another promising therapy is LDL-apheresis, the specific removal of LDL by plasmapheresis through affinity columns. Liver transplantation has been successful in a few cases.

8.24 Familial Combined Hyperlipidemia (FCHL)

This familial, multiple lipoprotein type of hyperlipoproteinemia is the most frequent inherited disorder of lipoprotein metabolism in adults (1–2/100) and is associated with a high risk of myocardial infarction (10% of first episodes). In this dominantly inherited disease, approximately one third of the hyperlipidemic family members have hypertriglyceridemia, one third have hypercholesterolemia, and one third have elevations of both cholesterol and triglycerides. The lipid elevations tend to be modest, often fluctuating between the 90th and 95th percentiles. In addition, the lipoprotein abnormalities can change from time to time in the same affected individual. This disorder is not usually associated with tendon xanthomas, but obesity, hyperinsulinism, and glucose intolerance are frequently found in adults. Although adults who inherit this gene have hyperlipoproteinemia, affected children may not manifest significant hypercholesterolemia or hypertriglyceridemia until the 2nd or 3rd decade owing to gradual gene expression. The reasons for the varied expression of hyperlipidemia are unclear, but the disease is known to be associated with overproduction of VLDL.

In families with FCHL identified through an affected child, half of the siblings younger than 20 yr of age have hyperlipidemia; this proportion is compatible with full gene penetrance. At least 0.5% of all children have hyperlipidemia due to FCHL.

The risk of premature heart disease is considerable despite the fact that lipid levels may be only moderately elevated. Children in these families, therefore, should be identified, and dietary intervention should be aimed at controlling the hypercholesterolemia (using the prudent diet), with or without controlled carbohydrate intake to reduce hypertriglyceridemia. However, the response to diet is variable, and an occasional patient will experience an increase in plasma cholesterol or triglycerides despite documented compliance with the diet. If the hypercholesterolemia cannot be controlled by dietary modification alone, these patients should be treated with resin as are patients with FH.

8.25 Hyperapobetalipoproteinemia

In this condition the plasma apoB level is significantly increased, but the plasma cholesterol and triglyceride levels are within normal limits, although they are usually above mean values. When this condition occurs in a family with a positive family history of premature coronary artery disease, it is probably a variant of FCHL and should be evaluated and managed in a similar fashion. Unfortunately, measurement of plasma apoB levels is not routinely available.

8.26 Familial Dysbetalipoproteinemia

This rare condition, also known as type 3 hyperlipoproteinemia, is characterized by abnormal plasma lipoproteins designated β-VLDL or "floating β-lipoproteins."

CLINICAL MANIFESTATIONS. The presence of planar xanthomas along the palmar creases of the hands (xanthoma striata palmaris) is virtually diagnostic. Other clinical features include tuberoeruptive xanthomas of the trunk, tuberous xanthomas over the elbows and knees, and tendinous xanthomas. Coronary artery disease and peripheral vascular disease are common.

ETIOLOGY. The specific genetic abnormality is a mutation that alters the structure of apoE, decreasing the binding of apoE-containing lipoproteins to the liver receptor (see Figs. 8–26 and 8–27) and thereby retarding the uptake of chylomicron and VLDL remnants. There are three common alleles at the apoE gene locus, resulting in six phenotypes of apoE that can be distinguished by isoelectric focusing of VLDL proteins. One of these phenotypes, designated apoE 2/2, occurs in about 1% of the population, but more than 90% of patients with familial dysbetalipoproteinemia have this phenotype. Since familial dysbetalipoproteinemia is quite rare (less than 1/10,000 adults), the majority of individuals with apoE 2/2 appear to tolerate this clearance disorder well. If they overproduce chylomicrons (e.g., because of dietary indiscretion) or VLDL (e.g., because of a gene for another familial hyperlipidemia), their clinical disease may be fully expressed.

DIAGNOSIS. Diagnosis can be made on the basis of clinical manifestations or by demonstrating abnormal lipoproteins by electrophoresis. The abnormal chemical composition of the particles also can be demonstrated. The cholesterol content of VLDL in these patients is high; the ratio of their VLDL cholesterol to total triglycerides is greater than 0.3. ApoE phenotyping is not generally available but can be performed in specialized laboratories.

TREATMENT. Familial dysbetalipoproteinemia, unlike the other inherited hyperlipidemias, is often exquisitely sensitive to dietary intervention. Weight loss to a level appropriate for height, coupled with institution of the prudent diet, often causes the lipid levels to return to normal. There is little experience with drug treatment of this disorder in children, but adults with familial dysbetalipoproteinemia whose lipid elevations fail to respond to dietary intervention have been treated with fibric acid derivatives.

8.27 Sitosterolemia

(Phytosterolemia)

This rare inherited disorder is characterized by increased plasma levels of cholesterol and plant sterols. Patients may present in childhood with severe hypercholesterolemia associated with tendon and tuberous xanthomas, and the disease may therefore be confused with homozygous FH. However, by contrast, the hypercholesterolemia associated with sitosterolemia is very responsive to the prudent diet and bile acid–binding resins. The basic defect is unknown, but both excessive intestinal plant sterol absorption and impaired sterol excretion in bile have been implicated. It has been hypothesized that the increased absorption of plant sterols and cholesterol is a compensating response to a deficiency of the rate-limiting enzyme in cholesterol biosynthesis, HMG-CoA reductase.

8.28 Familial (Endogenous) Hypertriglyceridemia

This disorder occurs with a frequency of 2–3/1,000 adults but has a considerably lower risk of premature atherosclerosis than either FH or FCHL. It can be diagnosed only by family studies, which commonly show elevation of the fasting plasma triglyceride level in the range of 200–500 mg/dL, no association with hyperchylomicronemia, and a dominant mode of inheritance. There are families with endogenous hypertriglyceridemia in which some members have, in addition, hyperchylomicronemia (see Sec. 8.29). Only 10–20% of children in families with familial hypertriglyceridemia have elevated triglyceride levels before the age of 25, whereas 50% of adults (i.e., those who have inherited the gene) are affected with hypertriglyceridemia. Obesity, insulin resistance, hyperinsulinemia, glucose intolerance, and hyperuricemia are often associated findings. Although the precise metabolic defect is unknown, some patients have overproduction of VLDL triglycerides, whereas others have reduced clearance of VLDL.

Children older than 2 yr can usually be managed by means of weight control and use of the prudent diet. Occasionally, further modification of the carbohydrate-fat ratio may be required. The risk-benefit ratio does not ordinarily justify drug intervention.

8.29 Endogenous and Exogenous Hypertriglyceridemia

Patients with this rare disorder (<1 in 5,000), also known as type 5 hyperlipoproteinemia, have marked elevations of both chylomicron and VLDL triglycerides. Clinical findings include eruptive xanthomas, lipemia retinalis, pancreatitis, and abnormal glucose tolerance associated with hyperinsulinism. The disorder is usually not expressed in childhood, but several families have been found in which the unidentified defect or defects are expressed early in life. Treatment consists primarily of weight control and dietary modification. Carbohydrate restriction may also be required to reduce endogenous overproduction of VLDL triglycerides. Patients should avoid alcohol and restrict fat intake. Aggressive dietary measures should be tried before drug therapy is considered to reduce the VLDL triglyceride level.

8.30 Exogenous Hypertriglyceridemia

(Hyperchylomicronemia)

LIPOPROTEIN LIPASE (LPL) DEFICIENCY. This is an extremely rare (<1 in 100,000) autosomal recessive disorder. Although demonstrable shortly after birth, the massive elevation of plasma triglycerides (1,000–4,000 mg/dL) is clinically silent and is often not discovered until the patient's blood is sampled for another reason; the chylomicronemia is striking. *Clinical manifestations* include eruptive xanthomas over the trunk, lipemia retinalis, mild hepatosplenomegaly, and recurrent bouts of pancreatitis. The hyperchylomicronemia results from a failure of hydrolysis of chylomicrons due to genetic deficiency of lipoprotein lipase on the endothelial surface of the capillaries. The *diagnosis* of LPL deficiency is made by measuring the enzyme activity in plasma after administration of heparin (postheparin lipolytic activity).

Although patients with this disorder are not at increased risk for early development of atherosclerosis, recurrent bouts of pancreatitis can be life-threatening. *Treatment* of these disorders is aimed at keeping the diet low enough in long-chain fatty acids to keep the patient asymptomatic and free of recurrent bouts of pain. Using medium-chain triglyceride (MCT) oil in food preparation serves both to make the diet more palatable and to provide sufficient calories for growth. MCT are absorbed directly into the portal vein and transported to the liver without requiring chylomicron formation and transport through the systemic circulation. None of the presently available hypolipidemic drugs has any sustained effect.

ApoC-II DEFICIENCY. The clinical and laboratory manifestations of genetic deficiency of apoC-II, a cofactor for LPL, are similar to those of LPL deficiency. The diagnosis of this autosomal recessive disorder is made by isoelectric focusing of VLDL proteins.

8.31 Familial Hyperalphalipoproteinemia

Unlike elevation of other lipoproteins, elevation of plasma HDL cholesterol has a protective effect against the development of atherosclerotic heart disease, presumably because of its role in reverse cholesterol transport. The inherited elevation of HDL cholesterol has been described as a longevity syndrome in families that appear to be at a lower than normal risk for the development of premature atherosclerosis. Therefore, HDL cholesterol levels should be measured in children with moderate hypercholesterolemia. Those with hyperalphalipoproteinemia have HDL cholesterol levels at the upper end of the normal distribution, and their LDL cholesterol levels are often within normal limits.

8.32 SECONDARY HYPERLIPIDEMIAS

Much of the hypertriglyceridemia and, to a smaller extent, hypercholesterolemia seen in clinical practice is secondary to exogenous factors or underlying clinical disorders. Obesity, for example, is probably the major cause of mild elevations of plasma triglycerides, and the hypertriglyceridemia is frequently normalized following a return to desirable weight. Weight loss also reduces cholesterol levels in overweight individuals.

Pediatric conditions associated with hypercholesterolemia include hypothyroidism, nephrotic syndrome, congenital biliary atresia and other causes of cholestasis, anorexia nervosa, systemic lupus erythematosus, and the use of steroids. Secondary causes of hypertriglyceridemia include diabetes mellitus, renal disease, hypothyroidism, and occasionally other endocrine and metabolic disorders such as type I glycogen storage disease.

Excessive alcohol intake is a well-known cause of hypertriglyceridemia in adults and should be considered in teenagers. Oral contraceptives generally increase triglyceride levels, with varying effects on LDL and HDL cholesterol levels. Other drugs that raise triglyceride levels are isotretinoin, thiazide diuretics, and some β-adrenergic blocking agents.

Treatment of the underlying condition or removal of the offending drug is usually the first management approach to the patient with secondary hyperlipidemia. If the elevated lipid level persists, however, consideration must be given to the possibility that the patient has an underlying primary form of hyperlipoproteinemia, and therapy appropriate to the particular disease should be initiated.

HYPOLIPOPROTEINEMIAS

8.33 HDL Deficiency States

Low levels of HDL cholesterol (hypoalphalipoproteinemia) are associated with an increased risk of atherosclerosis, whereas high levels appear to be protective. Most patients with extremely low levels of HDL cholesterol (<10 mg/dL plasma) have an inherited HDL deficiency state such as Tangier disease.

Homozygotes for *Tangier disease* have HDL particles that are structurally abnormal and are present in markedly reduced concentrations. Associated lipoprotein abnormalities include extremely low apoA-I and low apoA-II levels, low to normal LDL cholesterol levels, and high plasma triglyceride levels. The major clinical manifestations, some of which can be detected in childhood, result from deposition of cholesteryl esters in a number of tissues: enlarged yellowish tonsils, splenomegaly, peripheral neuropathy, hepatomegaly, lymphadenopathy, and diffuse corneal infiltration. Heterozygotes have approximately 50% of normal levels of HDL cholesterol, apoA-I, and apoA-II but none of the clinical manifestations noted above. Coronary artery disease, however, is common in both homozygotes and heterozygotes for Tangier disease, but only after 40 yr of age. The precise molecular defect is unknown, but abnormalities in apoA-I synthesis and metabolism have been identified.

Other rare inherited HDL deficiency states have been described (apoA-I and apoC-III deficiency, HDL deficiency with planar xanthomas, fish-eye disease) that share some of the features of Tangier disease. There is no specific treatment for these disorders, but a diet restricted in fat is recommended.

In view of the numerous observations that HDL cholesterol levels tend to be low in patients with premature coronary artery disease, attempts have been made to identify other inherited causes of reduced HDL. Families have been described with low (50% of normal) HDL cholesterol levels apparently segregating in an autosomal dominant fashion and associated with premature vascular disease. There have been few systematic clinical studies of *familial hypoalphalipoproteinemia*, and it is not known whether therapies that act on HDL levels in the general population (i.e., exercise, moderate alcohol intake) will influence HDL cholesterol levels in this group of patients.

8.34 Abetalipoproteinemia and Hypobetalipoproteinemia

Abetalipoproteinemia is a rare autosomal recessive disease characterized in childhood by fat malabsorption and diarrhea, retinitis pigmentosa, cerebellar ataxia, and acanthocytosis (also see Sec. 13.64). All forms of apoB are absent from plasma; thus, homozygotes have no detectable chylomicrons, VLDL, or LDL, and their plasma cholesterol and triglyceride levels are extremely low (usually less than 30 mg/dL). Heterozygotes have no known clinical or biochemical abnormalities. The underlying defect in abetalipoproteinemia is unknown but probably involves the abnormal synthesis or secretion of apoB-containing lipoproteins. The clinical manifestations are directly referable to the failure of transport of lipids and lipid-soluble vitamins. Treatment is symptomatic. Large doses of vitamin E may retard the progress of neurologic and retinal degeneration; water-soluble vitamin A and vitamin K may alleviate symptoms of night blindness and coagulopathy, respectively. Restriction of dietary long-chain fat may lessen the diarrhea. MCT oil may help maintain caloric balance.

Hypobetalipoproteinemia is distinguished from abetalipoproteinemia by its autosomal dominant inheritance. Homozygotes are clinically similar to patients with abetalipoproteinemia. Heterozygotes have low plasma cholesterol and low-to-normal triglyceride levels but are otherwise usually asymptomatic.

8.35 Lecithin: Cholesterol Acyltransferase (LCAT) Deficiency

Deficiency of this plasma enzyme is associated with markedly reduced levels of cholesteryl esters in lipoproteins. It results in alterations of virtually all of the plasma lipoproteins: HDL and LDL cholesterol levels are low; triglycerides are generally high; and lipoproteins have abnormal electrophoretic mobility. LCAT deficiency may present early in childhood with corneal opacities, anemia, and proteinuria; sea-blue histiocytes in bone marrow and spleen are reported. This extremely rare disorder (probably less than 1 in 1 million) can be diagnosed by measuring LCAT activity in plasma. There is no specific treatment. Dietary management includes stringent fat restriction.

JEAN A. CORTNER
PAUL M. COATES
ANDREW M. TERSHAKOVEC

American Academy of Pediatrics, Committee on Nutrition: Indications for cholesterol testing in children. Pediatrics 83:141, 1989.
Belamarich PF, Deckelbaum RJ, Starc TJ, et al: Response to diet and cholestyramine in a patient with sitosterolemia. Pediatrics 86:977, 1990.
Breslow JL: Genetic basis of lipoprotein disorders. J Clin Invest 84:373, 1989.
Brunzell JD: Familial lipoprotein lipase deficiency and other causes of the chylomicronemia syndrome. *In*: Scriver CR, Beaudet AL, Sly WS, et al (eds): The Metabolic Basis of Inherited Disease, 6th ed. New York, McGraw-Hill, 1989, p 1165.
Brunzell JD, Schrott HG, Motulsky AG, et al: Myocardial infarction in the familial forms of hypertriglyceridemia. Metabolism 25:313, 1984.
Cortner JA, Coates PM, Gallagher PR: Prevalence and expression of familial combined hyperlipidemia in childhood. J Pediatr 116:514, 1990.
Dennison BA, Kikuchi DA, Srinavasan SR, et al: Parental history of cardiovascular disease as an indication for screening for lipoprotein abnormalities in children. J Pediatr 115:186, 1989.
The Framingham Study: An Epidemiologic Investigation of Cardiovascular Disease. NIH Publication No. 76-1083. Washington DC, National Institutes of Health, 1976.
Frerichs RR, Srinavasan SR, Webber LS, et al: Serum cholesterol and triglyceride levels in 3,446 children from a biracial community. The Bogalusa heart study. Circulation 54:302, 1976.
Goldstein JL, Brown MS: Familial hypercholesterolemia. *In*: Scriver CR, Beaudet AL, Sly WS, et al (eds): The Metabolic Basis of Inherited Disease, 6th ed. New York, McGraw-Hill, 1989, p 1215.
Granot E, Deckelbaum RJ: Hypocholesterolemia in childhood. J Pediatr 115:171, 1989.
Grundy SM: Hypertriglyceridemia: Mechanisms, clinical significance, and treatment. Med Clin North Am 66:519, 1982.
Grundy SM, Chait A, Brunzell JD: Familial combined hyperlipidemia workshop. Arteriosclerosis 7:203, 1987.
Havel RJ: Approach to the patient with hyperlipidemia. Med Clin North Am 66:319, 1982.
Lauer RM, Clarke WR: Use of cholesterol measurements in childhood for the prediction of adult hypercholesterolemia. JAMA 264:3034, 1990.
Lipid Research Clinics Population Studies Data Book. Vol. 1; The Prevalence Study. NIH Publication No. 80-1527. Washington DC, National Institutes of Health, 1980.
Lipid Research Clinics Program: The Lipid Research Clinics Coronary Primary Prevention Trial results. I and II. JAMA 251:351, 365, 1984.
Mahley RW, Rall SC: Type III hyperlipoproteinemia. *In*: Scriver CR, Beaudet AL, Sly WS, et al (eds): The Metabolic Basis of Inherited Disease, 6th ed. New York, McGraw-Hill, 1989, p 1195.
National Institutes of Health Consensus Development Conference: Lowering blood cholesterol to prevent heart disease. JAMA 253:2080, 1985.
Newman WP, Freedman DS, Voors AW, et al: Relation of serum lipoprotein levels and systolic blood pressure to early atherosclerosis: The Bogalusa heart study. N Engl J Med 314:138, 1986.
Schaefer EJ: Clinical, biochemical, and genetic features in familial disorders of high density lipoprotein deficiency. Arteriosclerosis 4:303, 1984.
Weidman W, Kwiterovich PO, Jesse MJ, et al: AHA Committee Report: Diet in the healthy child. Circulation 67:1411a, 1983.

DEFECTS IN METABOLISM OF CARBOHYDRATES

8.36 INTESTINAL DEFECTS OF CARBOHYDRATE METABOLISM

Nutritional carbohydrates in man's diet include starch (the glucose polymers from plants) and glycogen (from animals), the disaccharides lactose and sucrose, and the monosaccharides glucose, galactose, and fructose (see Sec. 4.4).

Sucrase-Isomaltase Deficiency

See Sec. 13.63.

Lactose Intolerance

See Sec. 13.63.

Glucose-Galactose Malabsorption

See Sec. 13.64.

8.37 DEFECTS IN INTERMEDIARY CARBOHYDRATE METABOLISM

The intracellular conversion of glucose, fructose, and galactose proceeds as shown schematically in Figures 8–28, 8–29, and 8–30.

The demonstration of defective enzyme activity must serve as the basis of diagnosis and therapy in inborn errors of metabolism. However, an enzymatic defect affecting one tissue may not be demonstrable in another tissue for several reasons:

1. The defective enzyme may normally be absent as is glucose-6-phosphatase from muscle. Therefore, the deficiency of this enzyme in liver, kidney, and intestine of glycogen storage disease type I (GSD I) does not affect the skeletal muscle.

2. An enzymatic activity may reflect different enzyme proteins in different tissues. This is the case for glycogen synthetase, phosphorylase, or phosphorylase kinase. Thus, the deficiency of these enzymes in the livers of patients with GSD 0, GSD VI, or GSD IX does not affect their activity in skeletal muscle.

3. There may not have been the opportunity to measure a defective activity in more than one tissue of the patient. Galactokinase deficiency of erythrocytes is likely to affect the liver. However, galactokinase has not been assayed in hepatic tissue of a patient with the defect of this enzyme in erythrocytes.

4. An enzyme may not be effective in vivo although the usual assay indicates in vitro activity. For example, GSD Ia has clinical and biochemical manifestations similar to those of GSD Ib. Glucose-6-phosphatase activity measured in frozen liver homogenates is deficient in GSD Ia but normal in GSD Ib. Hepatocytes of GSD Ib have a defect in the transport of glucose-6-phosphate to glucose-6-phosphatase across the microsomal membranes that normally separate substrate from enzyme in intact liver cells. In vivo, the result of the transport defect is similar to that of the outright defect of the enzyme. However, in hypotonic homogenates of frozen liver tissue, normal intracellular topography is destroyed, and membrane barriers are broken down. Substrate added to GSD Ib homogenate can reach the enzyme, although the transport system is defective. Therefore, in GSD Ib, glucose-6-phosphatase is demonstrable in vitro but remains separated from its substrate in vivo.

5. An apparent enzymatic deficiency revealed by tissue analysis may be an artifact of suboptimal tissue handling. For example, liver phosphorylase activity is low or not demonstrable in autopsy liver, and it is altered nonpredictably in hepatic biopsy specimens unless they are frozen at once after removal from the body.

8.38 DEFECTS WITHOUT LACTIC ACIDOSIS OR ABNORMAL GLYCOGEN STORAGE

Defects in Galactose Metabolism

See Figure 8–28.

GALACTOSEMIA: DEFICIENCY OF GALACTOKINASE. This disorder is characterized by galactosemia, galactosuria, and cataracts without mental deficiency or aminoaciduria.

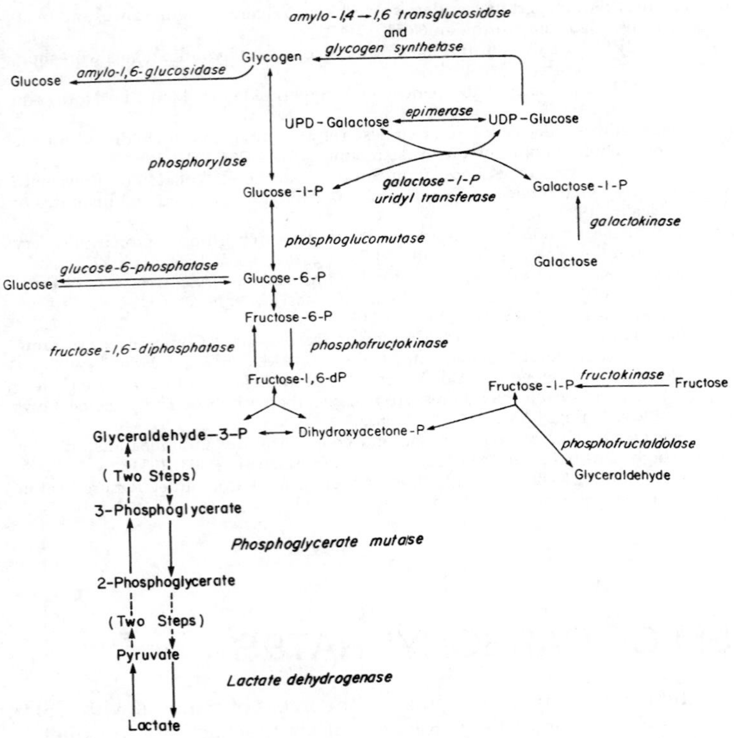

Figure 8–28. Pathway of cytoplasmic glycogen synthesis and degradation.

Cataracts begin to form after birth when the diet contains galactose derived from the lactose in milk. By the time the diagnosis is made, elimination of dietary galactose may come too late to reverse cataract formation, although younger siblings of the patient may be helped and should be tested at birth.

Galactokinase catalyzes the initial phosphorylation of galactose. If its activity is deficient, the ingestion of galactose leads to increased concentration of galactose in blood and in urine, where it can be found as a reducing substance that is not glucose. Urine specimens tested for galactose should be collected following ingestion of a galactose-containing formula. If an affected infant is receiving a diet without galactose such as glucose water prior to the urine collection, galactose may be absent from the urine and the diagnosis will be missed.

Postnatal institution of a galactose-free diet should prevent cataract formation. Since the children are otherwise normal, the prognosis can be good.

Definitive diagnosis is made by showing that erythrocytes are deficient in galactokinase activity, but the defect is assumed to involve the liver. Some galactose is converted into galactitol, which may be responsible for the cataract formation. Erythrocytic galactokinase activity in affected patients is below the limits of measurement; heterozygous parents and siblings have intermediate activity values. Inheritance is autosomal recessive. The incidence of the condition is about 1 in 40,000.

GALACTOSEMIA: DEFICIENCY OF GALACTOSE-1-PHOSPHATE URIDYL TRANSFERASE. "Classic" galactosemia is a serious disease with early onset of symptoms; the incidence is 1 in 50,000. The newborn infant normally receives up to 20% of caloric intake as lactose, which consists of

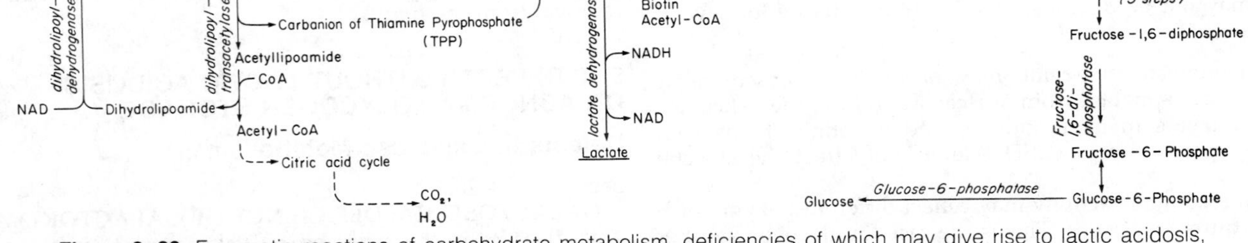

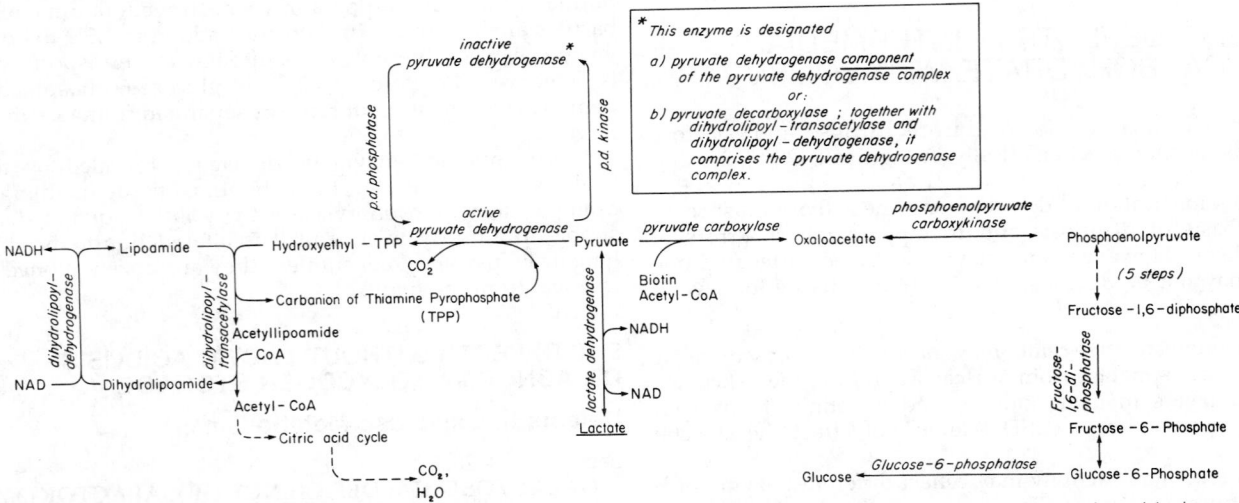

Figure 8–29. Enzymatic reactions of carbohydrate metabolism, deficiencies of which may give rise to lactic acidosis, pyruvate elevations, or hypoglycemia.

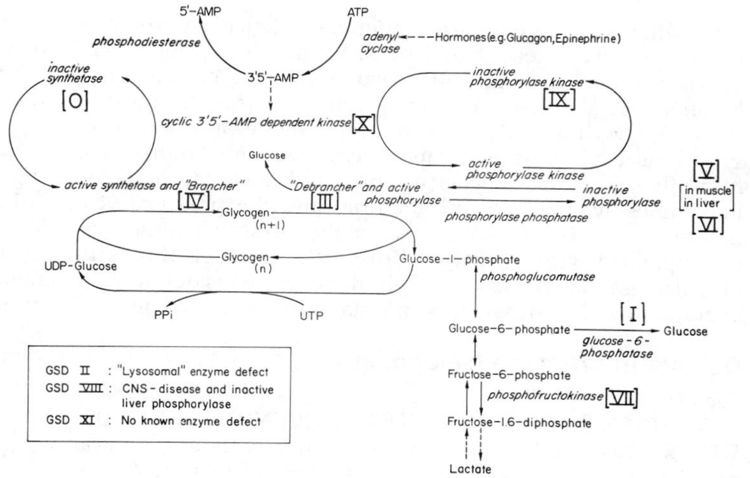

Figure 8–30. Pathway of phosphorylase activation and anaerobic glycolysis. Bracketed numbers refer to the type of glycogenosis in which the activity of the enzyme next to the number is defective. The various types are listed in Table 8–12.

glucose and galactose. Without the transferase the infant is unable to metabolize galactose-1-phosphate, whose accumulation results in injury to parenchymal cells of the kidney, liver, and brain. This injury may begin prenatally in the affected fetus by transplacental galactose derived from the diet of the heterozygous mother, who may metabolize dietary galactose with reduced efficiency.

The diagnosis of uridyl transferase deficiency should be considered in newborn infants or older infants or children with any of the following *clinical manifestations*: jaundice, hepatomegaly, vomiting, hypoglycemia, convulsions, lethargy, irritability, feeding difficulties, poor weight gain, aminoaciduria, cataracts, hepatic cirrhosis, ascites, splenomegaly, or mental retardation. When the diagnosis is not made at birth, damage to the liver (cirrhosis) and brain (mental retardation) becomes increasingly severe and irreversible. Therefore, galactosemia should be considered for the newborn or young infant who is not thriving or who has any of the above findings.

Since galactose is injurious to persons with galactosemia, diagnostic tests dependent on administering galactose orally or intravenously cannot be used. Galactose administration results in high concentrations of intracellular galactose-1-phosphate, which can function as a competitive inhibitor of phosphoglucomutase. This inhibition transiently impairs the conversion of glycogen to glucose and produces hypoglycemia. Galactose-1-phosphate is responsible for hepatotoxicity and mental retardation, but galactitol causes cataracts. Deficiency of either galactokinase or uridyl transferase produces elevations of galactitol.

Light and electron microscopy of hepatic tissue reveals fatty infiltration, the formation of pseudoacini, and eventual macronodular cirrhosis. These changes are consistent with a metabolic disease, but do not indicate the precise enzymatic defect.

The preliminary *diagnosis* of galactosemia is made by demonstrating a reducing substance in several urine specimens collected while the patient is receiving human or cow's milk or another formula containing lactose. The reducing substance found in urine by Clinitest can be identified by chromatography or by an enzymatic test specific for galactose. Clinistix or Testape urine tests are negative because these test materials rely on the action of glucose oxidase, which is specific for glucose and nonreactive with galactose. Deficient activity of galactose-1-phosphate uridyl transferase is demonstrable in hemolysates of erythrocytes, which also exhibit increased concentrations of galactose-1-phosphate. Heterogeneity of the defective enzyme can be shown by electrophoretic techniques using hemolysates. In the complete absence of uridyl transferase activity, very small amounts of galactose may still be metabolized by alternate pathways that are of no clinical significance in most patients.

Primary or secondary amenorrhea was reported in 12 of 18 galactosemic women with transferase deficiency who had laboratory evidence of hypergonadotropic hypogonadism. This condition may result from ovarian toxicity due to galactose and its metabolites, in particular, galactose-1-phosphate, which in patients with galactosemia is present in concentrations toxic to the brain, liver, and kidney. A similar effect is not apparent on the male gonads. This interpretation is consistent with the report of reduced oocytes in offspring of pregnant rats on a high-galactose diet and also with the report that risk factors for ovarian cancer may include increased dietary galactose and decreased transferase activity. We have one adult female patient who has no demonstrable transferase activity; she never adhered to a galactose-free diet because, inexplicably, no clinical symptoms resulted from dietary indiscretion. She is, however, our one patient with primary amenorrhea and hypergonadotropic hypogonadism. She does not show clinical signs of kidney or liver disease and is of moderate intelligence.

The term galactosemia, though adequate for the deficiencies of both galactokinase and uridyl transferase, generally designates the latter for historical reasons.

An occasional infant with galactosemia may tolerate an unexpectedly large amount of food containing lactose, but this is rare. Usually galactose must be excluded from the diet early in life to avoid severe cirrhosis of the liver, mental retardation, cataracts, and recurrent hypoglycemia. With good dietary control the prognosis is generally good.

DEFICIENCY OF URIDYL DIPHOSPHOGALACTOSE-4-EPIMERASE. There are two forms of this defect. Depending on the tissue distribution, the condition can be either completely asymptomatic or clinically identical to that of the classic form of galactosemia in which there is a deficiency of transferase activity.

In the benign form the defect is an incidental finding in an otherwise healthy individual without clinical manifestations. The liver is not enlarged, nor are there cataracts or abnormal neurologic findings. Growth and development are normal on an unrestricted normal diet. Patients may be discovered during a newborn screening examination to have an increased concentration of erythrocyte galactose-1-phosphate; galactokinase and uridyl transferase activity is normal. Inheritance is autosomal recessive. The epimerase deficiency affects leukocytes, lymphocytes, and erythrocytes, but its normal activity in tissues other than blood cells may explain the normal tolerance for galactose and the absence of clinical symptoms. No treatment is required.

In patients with generalized epimerase deficiency, the epimerase activity is less than 10% of normal in fibroblasts, in addition to decreased activity in leukocytes and erythrocytes. Parents have about 50% of normal activity in their fibroblasts, consistent with an autosomal recessive mode of inheritance. The clinical manifestations and course are indistinguishable from those of classic galactosemia and include cataracts, hepatomegaly, jaundice, proteinuria, and the presence of a non-glucose-reducing substance in the urine. Treatment is accomplished with a galactose-free diet. Although this form of galactosemia is very rare, it must be considered in a symptomatic patient who has normal transferase activity.

Defects in Fructose Metabolism

See also Sec. 8.39.

DEFICIENCY OF FRUCTOKINASE (BENIGN FRUCTOSURIA). This condition is not associated with any clinical manifestations. It is an accidental finding usually made because the asymptomatic patient's urine contains a reducing substance. No treatment is necessary. Inheritance is autosomal recessive with an incidence of 1 in 120,000.

Fructokinase deficiency is present in liver, intestine, and kidney. Ingested fructose is not metabolized. Its level is increased in the blood, and it is excreted in urine, there being practically no renal threshold for fructose. Positive Clinitest tests and negative Clinistix tests reveal the urinary-reducing substance to be something other than glucose. It can be identified as fructose by chromatography.

DEFICIENCY OF 1-PHOSPHOFRUCTALDOLASE (Hereditary Fructose Intolerance). This severe disease of infants appears with the ingestion of fructose-containing food. Either fructose or sucrose (table sugar), the disaccharide of glucose and fructose, may be added as a sweetener to baby foods or formulas. Symptoms may occur quite early in life, soon after birth if foods or formulas containing sucrose or fructose are then introduced into the diet. Early *clinical manifestations* may resemble those of galactosemia and include jaundice, hepatomegaly, vomiting, lethargy, irritability, and convulsions. A urinary-reducing substance that is not glucose can be identified as fructose by chromatography.

The deficiency of 1-phosphofructaldolase is practically complete in the liver. Fructose-1-phosphate accumulates in hepatocytes and acts as a competitive inhibitor for phosphorylase in concentrations similar to those of intracellular glucose-1-phosphate. The resulting transient inhibition of the conversion of glycogen to glucose leads to severe hypoglycemia. Some affected children show reduced hepatic conversion of fructose-1,6-diphosphate into the respective trioses in addition to that of fructose-1-phosphate. The concentration of fructose-1-phosphate may be reduced in body tissues by dietary elimination of fructose. However, fructose-1,6-diphosphate is an obligatory metabolite of glycolysis and gluconeogenesis and cannot be eliminated from the body by dietary means.

The severe reduction in the conversion of fructose-1,6-diphosphate in some children may result in *progressive liver disease* despite a fructose-free diet in patients who appear clinically well except for hepatomegaly and elevated levels of serum transaminases. Successive liver biopsies show increasing fatty infiltration and fibrosis, with focal cytoplasmic dissolution, and abnormal appearance of glycogen and mitochondria, and unusual plate-like and needle-like crystals in hepatocytes. The prognosis of fructose intolerance must be guarded in some patients, even with good dietary control. Without such control, the disease can result in death during infancy or early childhood. Some infants with hereditary fructose intolerance show fewer and relatively milder symptoms.

Fructose tolerance tests are contraindicated because they may be followed by hypoglycemia, shock, and death.

Treatment requires completely eliminating fructose from the diet. This may be difficult because fructose is a widely used additive, found even in some aspirin preparations. Inheritance is autosomal recessive, and the incidence (including a mild form in adults) is about 1 in 40,000.

DEFICIENT MUSCLE PHOSPHOGLYCERATE MUTASE. This deficiency has occurred in an otherwise healthy adult exhibiting myoglobinuria and cramps after exercise. The patient was unable to increase blood lactic acid concentration after ischemic exercise, and a muscle biopsy showed normal glycogen concentration and enzyme activities except for low phosphoglycerate mutase activity due to the presence of small normal amounts of B (brain type) isozyme and absence of the M (muscle type) isozyme.

DEFICIENT MUSCLE TYPE LACTATE DEHYDROGENASE. The inability to synthesize the M unit of lactate dehydrogenase (LDH) is inherited as an autosomal recessive disorder and resides on chromosome 11. Affected patients still possess the ability to make the H unit of the enzyme.

The main complaints are fatigue and myoglobinuria after strenuous exercise. There is slightly below normal activity of erythrocyte LDH with a disproportionately high ratio of creatine kinase to LDH activity. Ischemic work results in venous lactate below that of control subjects and venous pyruvate concentration is at least twice that of normal controls. Patients with deficient M type lactate dehydrogenase can convert muscle glycogen to pyruvate, which is then released into the bloodstream rather than converted to lactate.

8.39 DEFECTS IN INTERMEDIARY CARBOHYDRATE METABOLISM ASSOCIATED WITH LACTIC ACIDOSIS

The defects in carbohydrate metabolism associated with lactic acidosis are discussed later; Figure 8–29 depicts the relevant metabolic pathways.

The normal lactic acid blood concentration is less than 18 mg/dL or 2 mM. Hyperlactic acidemia unrelated to an enzymatic defect occurs in hypoxemia. In this case the serum pyruvic acid concentration may remain normal (<1.0 mg/dL), whereas it is usually increased when hyperlactic acidemia results from an enzymatic defect. It is useful, therefore, to measure lactic and pyruvic acid in the same blood specimen and on multiple blood specimens obtained when the patient is symptomatic because dramatic and ultimately fatal hyperlactic acidemia may be intermittent. Thiamine (vitamin B_1) deficiency (as in alcoholism) also can be associated with life-threatening lactic acidosis that is correctable by thiamine administration. Thiamine participates in the pyruvate dehydrogenase reaction (see Fig. 8–29); this participation and lack of thiamine toxicity are the basis of thiamine treatment that is sometimes used for intractable lactic acidosis.

Deep sighing respirations of the Kussmaul variety should suggest acute metabolic acidosis from hyperlactic acidemia (see Sec. 6.8). If not corrected, the acidosis can lead to coma, respiratory failure, cardiovascular collapse, renal insufficiency, and death (see Sec. 6.8).

Hyperlactic acidemia occurs with those defects of carbohydrate metabolism that interfere with the conversion of pyruvate to glucose via the pathway of gluconeogenesis or to CO_2 and water via the mitochondrial enzymes of the citric acid cycle. The concentration of blood lactic acid should be determined in infants and children with unexplained acidosis, especially if the anion gap (see Sec. 6.8) in blood is greater than 16 mM.

DEFICIENCY OF GLUCOSE-6-PHOSPHATASE. GSD I is

the only one of the 12 types of glycogenosis associated with significant lactic acidosis. In most patients the resultant recurrent metabolic acidosis is of minor clinical importance, but in some children it is a life-threatening condition. GSD I is discussed further in Sec. 8.40.

DEFICIENCY OF FRUCTOSE-1,6-DIPHOSPHATASE. These infants are symptom free as long as their diet is limited to human milk. If they receive formulas or food containing fructose or sucrose, they develop intermittent attacks of hypoglycemia, shock, coma, convulsions, and a metabolic acidosis due to hyperlacticacidemia. In symptom-free intervals, physical examination may be normal except for hepatomegaly. If untreated, the disease can lead to psychomotor retardation or death. Inheritance is autosomal recessive.

Fructose-1,6-diphosphatase is one of the four key enzymes of gluconeogenesis. Its activity is markedly reduced or undetectable in hepatic biopsy specimens that show fatty infiltration and reduced glycogen concentration. Other enzymes of fructose metabolism, gluconeogenesis, or glycogen degradation are normal. After glucagon administration, the normal rise in blood glucose concentration may not occur or is abolished after a few hours of fasting. These observations are consistent with reduced stores of liver glycogen. Biochemical analysis of hepatic biopsy tissue indicates that less than 1.5% of wet liver weight may be glycogen (normal: 2–6%).

Administering galactose produces a normal increase in concentration of blood glucose that is not observed after administering fructose, glycerol, or alanine. The latter substances may produce acute hypoglycemia and lactic acidosis; tolerance tests using them should be avoided. Fasting for more than 10 hr may cause hypoglycemia and lactic acidosis. The clinical presentation may resemble "ketotic hypoglycemia" (see Sec. 8.59). Untreated fructose-1,6-diphosphatase deficiency is a serious disease with a poor prognosis. Growth and development are normal if the diet is kept free of fructose, sucrose, and sorbitol and is reasonably restricted in fat and protein.

DEFICIENCY OF PYRUVATE DECARBOXYLASE. This enzyme has also been designated the pyruvate dehydrogenase component or the first enzyme (E_1) of the pyruvate dehydrogenase complex. Its activity was undetected in a 1.3-kg newborn boy of 35-wk gestation who had tachypnea and neurologic signs and died at 6 mo of age despite attempts at dietary control. Plasma concentrations of pyruvate and lactate were high. In contrast, a 9-yr-old boy had 20% of normal enzyme activity in cultured skin fibroblasts and white blood cells. He suffered intermittent episodes of cerebellar dysfunction and choreoathetoid movement, which began at 16 mo of age, occurred from 2 to 6 times a year, lasted a few hours to over 1 wk, and seemed to be triggered by febrile illnesses or other stresses. The episodes ranged in severity from generalized clumsiness to severe ataxia so incapacitating that locomotion was possible only by crawling. Serum concentrations of pyruvate, lactate, and alanine were moderately elevated during attacks but normal between them, as was clinical appearance. Intelligence was normal. Dexamethasone relieved attacks but did not correct the blood chemical abnormalities.

DEFICIENCY OF DIHYDROLIPOYL TRANSACETYLASE. This enzyme is designated the second enzyme (E_2) in the pyruvate dehydrogenase complex, and the only reported patient who might have had this defect was a 9-yr-old boy with profound motor and mental retardation. Blood concentrations of pyruvate and lactate were normal when the patient was fasting but rose to twice the level of controls by 2 hr after a normal meal. A diet high in carbohydrates but not fat (65% and 15%, respectively) precipitated severe lactic acidosis. Dietary thiamine had no effect. Two sisters of the patient had died with severe lactic acidosis; their brains were severely deficient in myelin, but there were no signs of active demyelination. The boy's cultured skin fibroblasts had reduced activity of the pyruvate dehydrogenase complex; activity of the pyruvate decarboxylase was normal. Since the α-ketoglutarate dehydrogenase complex was not defective and since there is evidence that this complex includes an enzyme similar if not identical to E_3 of the pyruvate dehydrogenase complex, it can be inferred that E_2 may have been defective.

DEFICIENCY OF DIHYDROLIPOYL DEHYDROGENASE. The *clinical manifestations* of a deficiency of this third enzyme (E_3) of the pyruvate dehydrogenase complex are severe and include lethargy, hypertonia, irritability, optic atrophy, hyperactive reflexes with muscular hypotonia, lower extremity spasticity, irregular respirations, and laryngeal stridor. Persistent lactic acidosis was not corrected by a diet high in thiamine or fat. Episodes of hypoglycemia may be relieved by alanine. There has been a history of consanguinity.

Laboratory findings include elevations of blood concentrations of pyruvate, lactase, and α-ketoglutarate. Liver function tests may be normal. Dihydrolipoyl dehydrogenase activity in tissues may be as low as 5% of normal. Activities of the pyruvate dehydrogenase complex (but not E_1) and the α-ketoglutarate dehydrogenase complex in liver, muscle, brain, kidney, and skin fibroblasts have also been decreased.

Pathology of the brain in one infant revealed cavitation and lack of myelination in the basal ganglia, thalamus, and brain stem resembling Leigh syndrome.

DEFICIENCY OF PYRUVATE CARBOXYLASE. *Clinical manifestations* of this deficiency have varied from hypoglycemia in infancy to absence of clinical signs and symptoms during the 1st yr of life. Usually psychomotor retardation becomes evident in the 1st yr and may be severe and progressive, culminating in death. Clinical findings have included vomiting, irritability, lethargy, progressive motor and mental retardation, hypotonia, hyporeflexia, abnormal eye movements, optic atrophy, ataxia, and convulsions. There may be a history of psychomotor retardation and death of siblings whose clinical or pathologic findings suggested Leigh syndrome or who were undiagnosed.

Laboratory findings are characterized by elevated concentrations of blood lactate, pyruvate, and alanine. Cerebrospinal fluid protein may be elevated. In one patient, although liver size was normal, glycogen in liver and muscle was increased; there was a normal increase of blood glucose concentration following glucagon administration.

Diagnosis is based upon demonstration of a pyruvate carboxylase deficiency in the liver; a partial defect has been reported in one of two liver pyruvate carboxylases. Activities of the three other gluconeogenic enzymes have been normal.

Treatment with thiamine has prevented episodes of acute metabolic acidosis and controlled the biochemical defect in some patients but has not affected the clinical outcome. Therapy with biotin and lipoic acid is ineffective.

DEFICIENCY OF PYRUVATE CARBOXYLASE SECONDARY TO DEFICIENCY OF HOLOCARBOXYLASE SYNTHETASE OR BIOTINIDASE. See also Sec. 8.7.

Deficiency of either of these enzymes of biotin metabolism results in a secondary deficiency of pyruvate carboxylase (and other biotin-requiring carboxylases and metabolic reactions) and in the symptoms associated with the respective deficiencies as well as in skin rash, lactic acidosis, and alopecia. The course of biotinidase deficiency can be protracted, with intermittent exacerbation of chronic lactic acidosis, failure to thrive, and hypotonia leading to spasticity, lethargy, coma, and death. Initial symptoms of this kind in one of our patients with biotinidase deficiency were reversed by oral biotin, 10 mg/24 hr. In a subsequent sibling the diagnosis was apparent by the finding of less than 5% normal biotinidase activity in serum of cord blood. Biotin therapy prevented the development of discernible symptoms. Because of this curative effect of biotin in an otherwise fatal condition, we believe that in children with compatible symptomatology, especially children with lactic acidosis and/or unexplained skin rash, an assay of serum biotinidase should be done despite the fact that the disease may be rare. The disease can be thought of as biotin dependency. Biotin therapy must be maintained indefinitely.

CARNITINE DEFICIENCY STATES (see also Sec. 8.15.) These states may present with recurrent attacks of severe metabolic acidosis (lactic and pyruvic acidemia), hypoglycemia, and hepatomegaly. Cardiomegaly may be present. Untreated, the patient may die during an attack or develop persistent psychomotor retardation, but correction of acidosis and intravenous glucose may terminate the crisis, usually within 12–24 hr. Carnitine concentration may be reduced in serum, liver, muscle, and/or heart. Administration of L-carnitine, the naturally occurring isomer, benefits some but not all patients. Administration of DL-carnitine is without benefit and may be harmful.

L-Carnitine is synthesized in the liver from lysine in four enzymatic steps. The first three steps can also be executed in muscle and heart. The resulting carnitine precursor is transported through blood to the liver, where the synthesis is completed. The finished L-carnitine is returned into cells of muscle and heart. At the outer side of the inner membrane of the mitochondria, the enzyme carnitine palmitoyl transferase I (CPT I) forms fatty acid–carnitine esters. These esters are transferred into the mitochondria, where CPT II cleaves the esters, freeing fatty acid for energy production by β oxidation. Carnitine exits from the mitochondria to begin the next cycle of fatty acid transfer. Carnitine is indispensable in the transport of fatty acids from the cytoplasm into the mitochondria. A newborn girl with CPT II deficiency demonstrated in heart, liver, muscle, and fibroblasts died at age 5 days of encephalocardiomyopathy, hepatomegaly, hypoglycemia, carnitine deficiency, and acidosis. She had appeared normal for the first 2 days of life, probably living off her tissue glycogen stores. However, entry of fatty acids into mitochondria was impaired and energy production could not be sustained once glycogen was depleted. An infant boy with CPT II deficiency demonstrated in fibroblasts appeared healthy until 3 mo of age when he had an episode of lethargy, seizures, hypoglycemia, and respiratory arrest from which he recovered. He died suddenly at age 17 mo.

Carnitine deficiency states can exist either as primary carnitine deficiency, which is the result of a defect within the metabolism of carnitine itself, or as secondary carnitine deficiency, which is acquired as the result of some other condition. In primary carnitine deficiency the concentration of carnitine in serum and tissues such as liver, muscle, or heart is usually markedly reduced. Carnitine deficiency can occur with CPT II deficiency, in which acylcarnitine ester is formed normally by CPT I but then is not cleaved by the defective CPT II and is excreted with the loss of the carnitine moiety (see Sec. 8.15).

In secondary carnitine deficiency the concentration of carnitine is reduced in serum and/or tissues because of a carnitine loss that may be associated with many different conditions. These conditions are separable into two groups: (1) those with increased loss or decreased intake of carnitine; and (2) those with an accumulation of carnitine esters that are excreted in the urine, draining the body of carnitine. Group 1 includes renal Fanconi syndrome, type XI glycogenosis, cystinosis, Lowe syndrome, suboptimal diet, and renal dialysis. Group 2 includes defects in β oxidation of fatty acids, various types of organic acidemia, and treatment with anticonvulsant drugs, for example, valproic acid, which is excreted in urine as valproylcarnitine ester.

The main danger posed by primary and secondary carnitine deficiencies is the threat to the transfer of fatty acids into the mitochondria and therefore to β oxidation and energy production. The extent to which this threat can be alleviated by carnitine treatment depends on the defective site and mechanism underlying the carnitine reduction. To date, side effects of carnitine treatment are rare and are limited to diarrhea and a fishy body odor. Therefore, after reduced carnitine has been found in serum and/or tissue biopsies, one may consider treatment of children with primary as well as secondary carnitine deficiency with oral L-carnitine in divided doses of up to 200 mg/kg/24 hr.

DEFICIENCY OF PYRUVATE DEHYDROGENASE PHOSPHATASE. This deficiency has been found in a newborn boy who had a metabolic acidosis with high serum concentrations of lactate (up to 7 times normal), pyruvate (2 times normal), and free fatty acids (3 times normal). There was no hypoglycemia or hepatomegaly. The acidosis improved when the intake of glucose was increased and that of fat decreased. Periods of clinical stability and moderate hyperlactic acidemia were interrupted every few days by episodes of severe lactic acidosis. Neurologic damage was evident, with lethargy, convulsions, hypotonia, and irritability. The patient died at 6 mo of age.

The pyruvate dehydrogenase component E_1 of the pyruvate dehydrogenase complex exists in both active and inactive forms. E_1 is inactivated when it is phosphorylated by pyruvate dehydrogenase kinase in the presence of ATP. E_1 is stimulated by calcium. Pyruvate dehydrogenase phosphatase activity was reported deficient in liver and muscle but not in the brain of this child based on the observation that the addition of calcium to a homogenate of liver increased the activity of pyruvate decarboxylase in the patient by 4% and in a control by 50%. Deficiency of this activating phosphatase has been reported in another 7-mo-old boy in whom brain autopsy findings were consistent with Leigh syndrome.

CONGENITAL IDIOPATHIC LACTIC ACIDOSIS. This diagnosis should be considered when there is labored respiration in infancy associated with metabolic acidosis from hyperlactic acidemia. Liver and spleen may be enlarged. Convulsions, hypoglycemia, psychomotor retardation, and neurologic damage usually lead to death in infancy despite dietary administration of thiamine, biotin, steroids, lipoic acid, and other agents. Long-term survival in a few instances is possible.

There are increased serum concentrations of pyruvate, lactate, and alanine, as well as of other amino acids. Cerebral autopsy findings may show severe spongy degeneration and lack of myelination, or there may be only moderate or mild abnormalities.

A variety of deficiencies in enzymatic activities, including those reported above, may lead to lactic acidosis. In patients who have not been examined in a systematic way, excluding the defects described above, the diagnosis of congenital idiopathic lactic acidosis should probably not be made.

LEIGH SUBACUTE NECROTIZING ENCEPHALOPATHY (SNE). This condition is characterized by seizures, psychomotor retardation, optic atrophy, hypotonia, vomiting, abnormal movements, lethargy, and lactic acidosis (also see Sec. 20.58). It is difficult to distinguish this syndrome reliably from many of the enzymatic deficiencies that are associated with lactic acidosis. Gliosis, cavitation, and capillary proliferation in the brain stem, basal ganglia, and thalamus, which are critical criteria for a pathologic diagnosis, may be visible on CT scan. Similar lesions viewed as characteristic have been encountered in patients shown to have pyruvate carboxylase deficiency, or, in one case, defective pyruvate decarboxylase activity in skin fibroblasts. Another boy shown to have SNE by brain autopsy also had a deficiency of pyruvate dehydrogenase phosphatase. The assessment of patients presenting symptoms and signs consistent with Leigh syndrome must include assays of enzymatic activities that result in lactic acidosis. These activities were normal in a 22-mo-old boy who had the cerebral findings of Leigh syndrome associated with increased concentration of endorphin and norepinephrine in CSF and of enkephalins in cerebral cortex.

Thiamine is transiently effective in some patients with Leigh syndrome but not in others. Its use was suggested by the report that extracts of blood, cerebrospinal fluid, and urine of patients with SNE inhibited thiamine pyrophosphate–adenosine triphosphate phosphoryl transferase. Thiamine in pharmacologic doses might have overridden this inhibitor, which has also been found in the urine of as many as 10% of clinically normal persons.

Attempts to correct hyperlactic acidemia with dichloroacetate, which inhibits the inactivating kinase for pyruvate dehydrogenase (E_1; see Fig. 8.29), thereby maintaining dehydrogenase (E_1) activity, have been ineffective in a child with fatal lactic acidosis of unknown cause.

Acute, life-threatening hyperlactic acidemia can be corrected by the intravenous infusion of *tris-hydroxymethyl aminomethane* (THAM), which avoids the sodium overload of sodium bicarbonate administration. This treatment does not alter the poor prognosis for the majority of conditions that are associated with increased concentrations of lactic and pyruvic acid.

8.40 GLYCOGEN STORAGE DISEASES

These diseases are the result of metabolic errors leading to abnormal concentrations or structure of glycogen. The glycogen storage diseases (GSD) or glycogenosis can be classified according to the identified enzymatic defects or sometimes by the distinctive clinical features (Table 8–12). The separation of a new type of GSD is useful to the clinician if the clinical or biochemical characteristics are sufficiently distinctive to permit their recognition in future patients. Figure 8–30 depicts the relevant metabolic pathways.

DEFICIENCY OF GLYCOGEN SYNTHETASE (GSD 0). Early morning convulsions associated with hypoglycemia are typical symptoms of this condition. There is an associated hyperketonemia. Hypoglycemia appears during periods without food and is not responsive to glucagon administration. After administration of glucose the blood glucose level remains elevated for longer than usual. The diagnosis should be made expeditiously, since hypoglycemic episodes and mental retardation can be avoided if the patient is given frequent meals rich in protein. The clinical picture is similar to that of ketotic hypoglycemia (see Sec. 8.59), and patients with the latter diagnosis may benefit from an assay of hepatic glycogen synthetase. Persistent hyperglycemia and an increase in serum lactate concentration after administration of glucose should reveal those with a possible deficiency of glycogen synthetase.

Glycogen synthetase activity is deficient in liver but normal in muscle and in white and red blood cells. Glycogen concentration is low (less than 2%) but not absent in liver and normal in muscle. Differential involvement of tissues reflects the fact that different isozymes of glycogen synthetase exist for various tissues. The activation system for glycogen synthetase is normal.

DEFICIENCY OF GLUCOSE-6-PHOSPHATASE (GSD Ia). In GSD Ia, glucose-6-phosphatase activity is defective, and glycogen concentration is increased in liver, kidney, and intestine. *Clinical manifestations* are summarized in Table 8–12. Mild hypotonia is sometimes also reported in GSD Ia, but the disease does not have a primary effect on muscle, since muscle does not normally contain glucose-6-phosphatase. Marked hypoglycemia may be well tolerated; patients with blood glucose levels as low as 10 mg/dL may display normal behavior. Hyperlipidemia and hyperuric acidemia are marked. In adults the latter produces gout, which must be appropriately treated. There is a secondary impairment of platelet function, which may make bleeding a problem when biopsies are done. Young children with GSD Ia have impressive hepatomegaly, but liver involvement may be easily overlooked in the affected adult. In patients with GSD Ia, the kidneys are moderately but consistently enlarged on roentgenographic examination, which helps to differentiate GSD Ia from GSD III, in which renal size is normal.

Administering galactose or fructose does not produce an elevation of blood glucose concentration; tolerance tests with these sugars should not be done because they can lead to severe acidosis. Administration of fructose, but not of galactose, is followed by increased concentrations of serum insulin. Intravenous administration of glucagon is not followed by a normal rise in blood glucose, regardless of how recently the patient may have eaten. The glucagon tolerance test can, therefore, differentiate between GSD Ia and GSD III; in the latter the concentration of blood glucose will increase if glucagon is given 2 hr after a meal. Subcutaneous administration of epinephrine has no advantage over the glucagon tolerance test and may produce unpleasant side effects.

Acute lactic acidosis may be a recurrent and life-threatening problem. Portacaval shunt has been advocated for its prevention or control, but no patients have benefited from the operation, which has been complicated by closure of the anastomosis and by development of cirrhosis or encephalopathy. Patients in whom this condition is difficult to control can be managed successfully with continuous night-time feedings by nasopharyngeal or gastrostomy tube. Therapeutic success also has been reported with repeated daily drinking of a solution of uncooked cornstarch. With such dietary regimens, children grow satisfactorily, hepatomegaly recedes, and hypoglycemia and lactic acidosis become manageable. However, when the gastric tube feedings are discontinued, the pretreatment tolerance of hypoglycemia may have been lost. Disease-related post-treatment hypoglycemia may result in convulsions. Frequent meals have effects similar to those of gastric tube feedings and may suffice for clinical control. As patients grow older, their metabolic problems become less severe and are more easily manageable. Neither phenobarbital nor phenytoin corrects the biochemical or clinical abnormalities in patients with glycogenoses.

In GSD Ia, hepatocytes contain many lipid droplets ranging in size from smaller than mitochondria to several times that of the nucleus, and the nuclei themselves frequently contain glycogen. Nuclear glycogenosis can also occur in GSD III, in diabetes mellitus, and in Wilson disease. Patients with GSD Ia have an increased incidence of hepatoma. Abdominal examination by ultrasound or CT scan every 6–12 mo may be indicated. Prenatal diagnosis using amniotic fluid cells is not feasible since glucose-6-phosphatase is not normally present in cultured skin fibroblasts; nor can the enzyme be demonstrated in normal white cells.

GSD Ib (Pseudo–GSD I). Clinically, GSD Ib is indistinguishable from GSD Ia except that children with GSD Ib seem to have an increased incidence of neutropenia. Hepatic glycogen concentration is increased but glucose-6-phosphatase activity is normal in hypotonic homogenates made of frozen liver tissue. The activity is decreased, however, in isotonic homogenates made from fresh liver tissue, which is consistent with a defect in GSD Ib of enzymes that transport glucose-6-phosphate across microsomal membranes. Further evidence that this variant of GSD I is associated with an intracellular transport defect is the finding that when fresh liver homogenates from affected patients are treated with deoxycholate, the activity of glucose-6-phosphatase is normal; deoxycholate is known to break up microsomal membranes.

TABLE 8–12. Features of the Glycogen Storage Diseases, Types 0–XI (GSD 0–XI)

Type, Enzyme Affected	Tissue Distribution of Excessive Glycogen and Enzyme Deficiency	Clinical Symptoms and Signs	Comments *Alternate Names*
GSD 0 Glycogen synthetase	Liver but not muscle (other tissues not analyzed); glycogen depletion in liver; hepatic glycogen synthetase less than 2% of normal, but some hepatic glycogen (1%) demonstrable	Fasting hypoglycemia; prolonged hyperglycemia after a meal or glucose administration; mental retardation follows hypoglycemic convulsions—when these are avoided by frequent protein-rich meals, psychomotor development can be normal	*Aglycogenosis*; defect convincingly demonstrated in two unrelated families; early diagnosis and dietary treatment important for prevention of retardation; some children with "ketotic hypoglycemia" may have GSD 0
GSD Ia Glucose-6-phosphatase	Liver, kidney, intestine; frequent intranuclear glycogen seen in these organs not diagnostic; continuous night-time feeding by tube and pump may alleviate clinical symptoms; portacaval shunt risky and clinically disappointing; treatment with phenytoin or phenobarbital ineffective	Enlarged liver and kidneys; "doll face," stunted growth, normal mental development; tendency to hypoglycemia, lactic acidosis, hyperlipidemia, hyperuric acidemia, gout, bleeding; IV* galactose or fructose not converted to glucose (caution: these tests may precipitate acidosis); abortive or no rise in blood glucose after SC† epinephrine or IV glucagon; normal urinary catecholamines; prognosis fair to good	*Von Gierke disease, hepatorenal glycogenosis*; no involvement of skeletal or cardiac muscle, or of leukocytes or cultured skin fibroblasts (glucose-6-phosphatase not normally present in these tissues)
GSD Ib In vitro activity of glucose-6-phosphatase is normal, but translocase is deficient	Activity of glucose-6-phosphatase is normal in frozen liver homogenate but is not demonstrable in isotonic homogenate of fresh liver tissue that has never been frozen	Symptoms are as those of GSD Ia; in addition, frequent neutropenia	Transport defect for glucose-6-phosphate at microsomal membrane
GSD Ic In vitro activity of glucose-6-phosphatase can be demonstrated	Activity of glucose-6-phosphatase is normal in frozen liver homogenate but is deficient in isotonic homogenate of fresh liver tissue that has never been frozen	The patient, an 11-yr-old girl, had hepatomegaly, brittle diabetes, frequent hypoglycemia	Transport defect for inorganic phosphate at microsomal membrane
GSD IIa, b Lysosomal acid α-glucosidase (deficient activity of acid α-1,4- and of α-1,6-glucosidase; the latter could be considered "lysosomal glycogen debrancher")	In the fatal, infantile, classic form (GSD IIa), glycogen concentration excessive in all organs examined; acid α-glucosidase deficiency was generalized in one patient; in others *normal* renal acid α-glucosidase; amniotic *fluid* (in contrast to cultured amniotic fluid cells) contains acid α-glucosidase activity even if the fetus has the disease	Clinically normal at birth, though minimal cardiomegaly, abnormal ECG‡, increased tissue glycogen, abnormal lysosomes in liver and skin, and acid α-glucosidase deficiency demonstrable at birth. Within a few months, marked hypotonia, severe cardiomegaly, moderate hepatomegaly; normal mental development; death usually in infancy (GSD IIa). Cases with involvement of muscle and liver but without cardiomegaly described in children and adults (GSD IIb). Normal blood glucose response to glucagon; normal urinary catecholamines	*Pompe disease, generalized glycogenosis, cardiac glycogenosis;* prenatal diagnosis *within* a few days after amniocentesis by the electron microscopic demonstration of abnormal lysosomes in *uncultured* amniotic fluid cells; for prenatal diagnosis by enzyme analysis, *cultured* amniotic fluid cells required, which also show the abnormal lysosomes GSD IIa: *infantile fatal form* GSD IIb: *late juvenile-adult form*
GSD III Amylo-1,6-glucosidase, "debrancher enzyme"	Liver, muscle, heart, etc., in various combinations; designated types IIIA through D; cultured amniotic fluid cells have diagnostic biochemical abnormality	Moderate to marked hepatomegaly; none to moderate hypotonia; none to moderate cardiomegaly, ECG rarely abnormal; no acidosis, hypoglycemia, or hyperlipemia; glucagon produces a normal rise in blood glucose after a meal but not after fasting; normal mental development; failure of liver or heart rare; normal urinary catecholamines; prognosis fair to good	*Limited dextrinosis, debrancher glycogenosis, Cori disease, Forbes disease*; prenatal diagnosis by enzyme assay of cultured amniotic fluid cells feasible but perhaps unnecessary, owing to the usual benign course
GSD IV Amylo-1,4→1,6-transglucosidase, "brancher enzyme"	Generalized (?); low to normal levels of abnormally structured glycogen (amylopectin-like molecules with fewer branch points than normal in animal glycogen)	Hepatosplenomegaly, ascites, cirrhosis, liver failure; normal mental development; death in early childhood	*Amylopectinosis, brancher glycogenosis, Andersen disease*; prenatal diagnosis of this incurable disease may be feasible and indicated by enzyme analysis of cultured amniotic fluid cells.
GSD V Muscle phosphorylase deficiency (congenital absence of skeletal muscle phosphorylase; phosphorylase-activating system intact)	Skeletal muscle; liver and myometrium normal	Temporary weakness and cramping of skeletal muscle after exercise; no rise in blood lactate during ischemic exercise; symptoms like those of type VII glycogenosis; normal mental development and urinary catecholamines; myoglobinuria in later life; fair to good prognosis	*McArdle syndrome;* liver and smooth muscle phosphorylase not affected; cardiac muscle phosphorylase not examined; prenatal diagnosis not feasible, does not seem indicated

TABLE 8–12. Features of the Glycogen Storage Diseases, Types 0–XI (GSD 0–XI) *Continued*

Type, Enzyme Affected	Tissue Distribution of Excessive Glycogen and Enzyme Deficiency	Clinical Symptoms and Signs	Comments *Alternate Names*
GSD VI Liver phosphorylase deficiency (phosphorylase-activating system intact)	Liver; skeletal muscle normal; leukocytes unsatisfactory for diagnosis	Marked hepatomegaly, no splenomegaly; no hypoglycemia, acidosis, or hyperlipemia; no rise of blood glucose after SC epinephrine or IV glucagon; normal mental development; normal urinary catecholamines; good prognosis	Lack of glucagon-induced hyperglycemia distinguishes GSD VI from GSD IX; the latter shows a normal glucagon response; prenatal diagnosis not feasible, may not be indicated
GSD VII Phosphofructokinase	Skeletal muscle, erythrocytes (in initial report; other tissues not examined); not known whether cultured amniotic fluid cells are affected, but prenatal diagnosis not indicated	Temporary weakness and cramping of skeletal muscle after exercise; no rise in blood lactate during ischemic exercise; normal mental development; symptoms identical to those of type V glycogenosis; good prognosis	Reduction of phosphofructokinase activity severe in skeletal muscle, mild in erythrocytes, not established in other tissues; incapacity may be minimal
GSD VIII No enzymatic deficiency yet demonstrated; total liver phosphorylase normal but most is in inactive form (liver phosphorylase activity reduced because control lost over extent of phosphorylase activation)	Liver, brain; skeletal muscle normal; cerebral glycogen increased; electron microscopy shows some cerebral glycogen in the form of α-particles within axon cylinders and synapses	Hepatomegaly; truncal ataxia, nystagmus, "dancing eyes" may be present; neurologic deterioration progressing to hypertonia, spasticity, decerebration, and death; urinary epinephrine and norepinephrine are increased during acute phase of disease, not in stationary end phase	Predominant clinical problem of the three patients with this presumptive diagnosis was progressive degenerative disease of brain
GSD IX a, b, c Liver phosphorylase kinase deficiency (total phosphorylase content normal but in inactive form, owing to the lack of phosphorylase kinase)	Liver; muscle tissue normal biochemically (in IXa and IXb) and microscopically; diagnosis not possible by using leukocytes; D-thyroxine–induced liver phosphorylase kinase activity in one patient, but not in two others of a different family	Marked hepatomegaly, no splenomegaly; no hypoglycemia or acidosis; normal urinary catecholamines; normal rise in blood glucose after IV glucagon or SC epinephrine; prognosis good; treatment may not be necessary ("benign hepatomegaly" may disappear in early adulthood)	Liver phosphorylase can be activated in vitro by addition of exogenous kinase to the homogenate; not the human counterpart of muscle phosphorylase kinase deficiency in mice; normal glucagon response is a distinguishing feature vs GSD VI; GSD IXa, autosomal recessive; GSD IXb, X-linked recessive; prenatal diagnosis not demonstrated
GSD X Loss of activity of cyclic 3′5′-AMP–dependent kinase in muscle and presumably liver (total phosphorylase content of liver and skeletal muscle normal, but the enzyme completely deactivated in both organs; phosphorylase kinase activity 50% of normal, possibly owing to the loss of 3′5′-AMP–dependent kinase activity)	Liver and muscle (other organs not tested); identical biochemical findings were made in two muscle biopsy specimens taken 6 yr apart	Marked hepatomegaly; patient otherwise clinically healthy initially, but 6 yr after diagnosis mild recurrent muscle pain; no cardiomegaly or hypoglycemia; no rise in blood glucose after IV glucagon; the only individual known to have this condition not incapacitated at 12 yr of age	In vitro activation of the patient's phosphorylase occurs (1) under assay conditions not requiring 3′5′-AMP–dependent kinase, or (2) after the patient's muscle homogenate has been fortified with phosphorylase kinase–deficient mouse muscle that supplied 3′5′-AMP–dependent kinase; postulated defect restricted to the activity of the cyclic 3′5′-AMP–dependent kinase that phosphorylates phosphorylase kinase, other cyclic 3′5′-AMP–dependent phosphorylations being intact
GSD XI All enzymatic activities measured to date are normal (adenyl cyclase, 3′5′-AMP–dependent kinase, phosphorylase kinase, phosphorylase, debrancher, brancher, glucose-6-phosphatase)	Liver, or liver and kidney	Tendency for acidosis; markedly stunted growth; vitamin D–resistant rickets (which can be cured with high doses of vitamin D and oral supplementation of phosphate); hyperlipidemia, generalized aminoaciduria, galactosuria, glucosuria, phosphaturia; normal renal size; no rise in blood glucose after IV glucagon or SC epinephrine; urinary excretion of cyclic 3′5′-AMP increases markedly after administration of glucagon	Muscle usually not affected; GSD XI may include patients with glycogenoses with different enzymatic defects; patients exhibit noncystinotic Fanconi syndrome associated with secondary (acquired) carnitine deficiency

*IV = intravenous administration of.
†SC = subcutaneous administration of.
‡ECG = electrocardiogram.

Phosphatase activity is normal in isotonic homogenate of fresh GSD Ib liver when it is assayed with mannose-6-phosphate, which does not require the translocase system to cross microsomal membranes.

GSD Ic. Transport of glucose-6-phosphate into microsomes (which is defective in GSD Ib) is normally associated with transport of inorganic phosphates in the opposite direction. A deficiency in this phosphate transfer has been described in an 11-yr-old girl with insulin-dependent diabetes (GSD Ic). Liver glycogen concentration was 9.4%, but since the patient had frequent hypoglycemic attacks, the increased glycogen concentration could have resulted from therapeutic glucose administration. The patient's clinical picture appeared to be similar to that of Mauriac syndrome in diabetic children (see Sec. 8.53).

DEFICIENCY OF LYSOSOMAL ACID α-GLUCOSIDASE (GSD II). This disease, whose clinical manifestations are summarized in Table 8–12, occurs in at least two varieties, one affecting infants (GSD IIa), the other affecting older children and adults (GSD IIb). Both varieties have not occurred in members of the same family. Fibroblast studies indicate that in a patient with GSD IIa, the lysosomal acid α-glucosidase is structurally altered, whereas in a patient with GSD IIb, the amount of the enzyme is reduced. Abnormal lysosomes are the morphologic hallmark of GSD II, although we have seen, on rare occasions, similar intracellular vacuoles in liver and muscle of patients with GSD III or GSD IV. The gene for acid α-glucosidase is localized on chromosome 17.

GSD IIa. This is the classic form of generalized glycogenosis and is always fatal, usually within 2 yr after birth. Affected children appear clinically healthy at birth with normal muscle tone and liver size. Heart size and electrocardiographic results are marginally abnormal. However, after a few weeks or months at home, the infant becomes completely flaccid. Sucking becomes weak, respirations shallow, and the cardiac silhouette huge. The liver is typically only moderately enlarged. The patients are alert and normally intelligent. The mouth is kept open and the tongue thrust forward, perhaps more because of air hunger than macroglossia; the resulting facial expression is characteristic. Aspiration pneumonia leads to chronic pulmonary infiltrates, and bronchial compression by the large heart leads to atelectasis. Death is due to failure of respiratory muscles. There is hardly any other condition in which such extreme cardiomegaly and muscular weakness occur in an infant who appears normal at birth. Blood glucose concentrations are normal, as are tolerance tests with glucagon and other carbohydrate test substances.

GSD II is the only lysosomal disease among the glycogenoses; the other types of GSD are associated with defects of enzymes located in the cytoplasm. The deficient acid α-glucosidase is a glycogen-degrading enzyme associated with the lysosomal fraction of tissue homogenates. Fusion of a primary lysosome with an autophagic vacuole normally creates a secondary lysosome. If the primary lysosome is deficient in a lysosomal enzyme (such as α-glucosidase), then the secondary lysosome may become engorged with the material (such as glycogen) that should have been degraded by the defective enzyme. Besides deficiencies of enzymes, other errors in lysosomal mechanisms may be present, such as membrane defects. In GSD IIa the deficiency of lysosomal acid α-glucosidase produces intracellular vesicles (so-called abnormal lysosomes) engorged with glycogen (Fig. 8–31) in cells of liver, muscle, heart and most other tissues of the body. Deficient acid α-glucosidase activity is also associated with the formation of glycogen-filled "abnormal lysosomes" in the cells of placenta and skin of children with I-cell disease (mucolipidosis type II, ML II; see Sec. 8.19).

Increased glycogen concentrations are found in many tissues of affected children. The deficiency of the lysosomal enzyme for glycogen degradation explains the membrane-bound accumulations of glycogen in lysosomes, but it does not explain the excessive accumulation of glycogen in the cytoplasm of heart and muscle cells. This cytoplasmic glycogen accumulates despite the fact that it is probably in contact with the normal glycolytic enzymes of cytoplasm, none of which are known to be defective in GSD II.

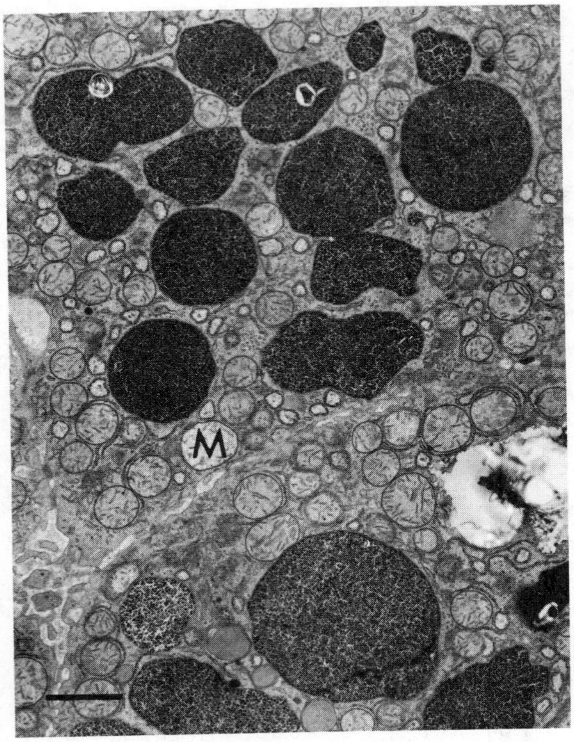

Figure 8–31. Liver autopsy specimen of GSD IIa. "Abnormal lysosomes" with lysosomal glycogen (tightly packed black particles) are ubiquitous, but cytoplasmic glycogen is missing. The absence of cytoplasmic glycogen indicates that this specimen was obtained after starvation or epinephrine treatment, or autopsy. (M = mitochondria.) (Bar: 2 μm.)

The excessive tissue glycogen as such may not be a cause of death; for example, we found the same 7-fold increase in muscle glycogen in a clinically healthy girl at birth and 2 yr later in her tissue obtained post mortem. Glucagon and epinephrine can mobilize cytoplasmic liver glycogen to produce a rise in blood glucose concentrations, but they cannot produce this effect if cytoplasmic liver glycogen is depleted. The lysosomal glycogen can be mobilized from the hepatocytes by administering purified glycogen-degrading enzymes of fungal origin, resulting in the disappearance of the abnormal lysosomes. To a lesser extent, this effect occurs with administered enzymes prepared from human liver or placenta. However, in all these treatment attempts, the normalization of the hepatic ultrastructure is not clinically beneficial for the patient. Bone marrow transplantation in a boy with GSD IIa resulted in engraftment of blood cell lines, but the patient died of GSD IIa 5 mo after the procedure.

The prenatal diagnosis of GSD IIa can be made by electron microscopic examination of cells obtained by chorionic villus biopsy or at amniocentesis (see later).

GSD IIb. Weakness of skeletal muscle begins later in life than in those with GSD IIa. In some the disease is compatible with a normal life span, though it may demand a sedentary life style. In other patients, death from respiratory failure can occur during the 3rd or 4th decade. Cardiomegaly is absent, and the electrocardiogram is normal. The diagnosis is based on electron microscopic examination of skin biopsy showing abnormal lysosomes packed with glycogen particles.

Some cases cannot be explained on the basis of defective activity of lysosomal acid α-glucosidase. For example, a patient who died of unrelated hypertension at 24 yr of age had a deficiency of acid α-glucosidase consistent with GSD IIa. Glycogen concentration was increased in all tissues except heart, though cardiac α-glucosidase activity was deficient. Heart muscle appeared normal on light microscopy; electron microscopy revealed occasional abnormal lysosomes but no excess of glycogen in cytoplasm.

DEFICIENCY OF "DEBRANCHER" ACTIVITY (GSD III). Clinical manifestations are summarized in Table 8–12. In GSD III, hepatomegaly can be as impressive as in GSD I. When generalized, this disorder also affects muscle and heart, but either organ may be clinically involved to a varying degree. Some patients resemble children with muscular dystrophy. Electrocardiographic abnormalities and moderate cardiomegaly are usually found; the size of the kidneys is normal. Patients with GSD III restricted to the liver usually do well. Hypoglycemia is rare and does not present a clinical problem. There may be recurrent pneumonia, but the long-term prognosis is usually good. The serum concentrations of uric acid, lactate, ketones, and lipids are normal. Blood glucose concentration increases if glucagon is given 2 hr after a meal in patients with GSD III but not in those with GSD I, whereas blood glucose levels remain flat in both glycogenoses when glucagon is administered after overnight fasting. These clinical and laboratory findings distinguish GSD III from GSD I.

For "debranching" of the glycogen molecule, two enzymatic reactions need to occur in sequence after phosphorylase activity has reduced the outer chains of the glycogen molecule to within 4 glucose units of the 1,6 branch point. The first reaction is that of a transferase that transfers 3 glucose units of the branched outer chain onto the straight outer chain. The glucose molecule at the branch point becomes exposed and accessible to the subsequent action of α-1,6-glucosidase, which removes it. Both the transferase and the α-1,6-glucosidase activities are deficient in the livers of patients with GSD III. In some patients the activity of transferase in muscle may be low, whereas that of α-1,6-glucosidase remains normal. The overall effect in either liver or muscle is a loss of debrancher activity. Both enzymatic activities may be retained in muscle, the defect being limited to the liver.

Frequently GSD III is a generalized disease, and glycogen concentrations are found to be increased and debranching activity deficient in every (examined) tissue. In generalized GSD III, the concentration of glycogen in muscle may reach the same levels as in GSD II, although patients with the former may be symptom free and those with the latter are markedly hypotonic. In GSD III, starvation induces the degradation of glycogen to within 4 units of the branch point. Glycogen with such short outer chains is called a limit dextrin; hence *limit dextrinosis* is an alternative designation for GSD III. Light microscopic appearance of liver in GSD III is similar to that of GSD I except that GSD III exhibits formation of fibrous septa, more extensive nuclear glycogenosis, and a paucity of intracellular lipid droplets. Hepatic cirrhosis does not usually develop in GSD III; the fibrous septa usually remain stable.

DEFICIENCY OF "BRANCHER" ACTIVITY (GSD IV). This defect is characterized clinically by hepatomegaly and splenomegaly. Progressive portal fibrosis leads to hepatic cirrhosis, ascites, and death in childhood from liver failure. Treatment with corticosteroids may induce temporary remission. Affected children are candidates for liver transplantation; this has been successful in several patients who had the procedure.

Hepatic symptoms are associated with reduced rather than increased concentrations of tissue glycogen. The glycogen resembles amylopectin, since it has fewer than the normal number of branch points. This may be the consequence of deficiency of branching enzyme, though one would expect a defect of this enzyme to result in the synthesis of amylose, the glucose polymer with no branch points. The cirrhosis may be the result of the amylopectin-like glycogen, since this glucose polymer is not normally present even transiently in the liver. The limit dextrin of GSD III may not have this effect because it is a transient form normally encountered during synthesis and degradation of glycogen.

DEFICIENCY OF MUSCLE PHOSPHORYLASE (GSD V) (McArdle Syndrome). This disorder has a wide clinical spectrum, varying from almost no symptoms to recurrent myoglobinuria, attacks of rhabdomyolysis, and unremitting muscle pain. The muscular pains and cramps after exercise that characterize GSD V can be differentiated from muscle cramps related to more common causes by the ischemic exercise test.

The test requires inflation of a blood pressure cuff on the upper arm to above the arterial pressure. The patient is then asked to squeeze a rubber ball with the hand of the same arm about once every second. The healthy person will easily squeeze 70–110 times, with some discomfort but without cramping of the muscle or residual symptoms after deflation of the blood pressure cuff. In the patient with GSD V, muscle cramps may limit the squeeze to 20–30 movements. When the cuff is released, the cramps persist, with the hand in a tetanic position (wrist bent, fingers extended) that cannot be corrected by the patient or by the examiner. After several minutes there is gradual release of the cramp, but pain may persist for 24–48 hr. In the healthy person, blood samples taken from the antecubital vein of the ischemic arm during exercise show a rise in serum lactate, a rise that does not occur in patients with GSD V because of their inability to produce lactate from glycogen. The diagnosis of GSD V also has been made using magnetic resonance spectroscopy by measuring pH, ATP, and phosphocreatine concentration following both aerobic and ischemic exercise. A clinical picture consistent with McArdle syndrome, including recurrent rhabdomylosis, has also occurred in patients with carnitine palmityl transferase deficiency.

Skeletal muscle is without phosphorylase activity. The activity in liver and smooth muscle is normal. The system of phosphorylase activation is intact; patients may have 3 times the normal activity of muscle phosphorylase kinase. Glycogen concentration is increased in muscle but usually not above 4%. Histologically, much of the excessive glycogen is deposited in the cytoplasm beneath the sarcolemma. In patients with phosphorylase deficiency, the energy for muscle contraction can still be provided by glucose entering the myocyte, which may suffice for energy requirements at rest when there are no symptoms. Peak demands for energy, however, which ordinarily are met by supplemental breakdown of muscle glycogen, cannot be satisfied in GSD V because of the phosphorylase defect. The result is pain and cramping during and after exercise, with little or no production of lactic acid. Ischemic exercise tests worsen the situation by interrupting the normal supply of oxygen and glucose.

Treatment with a high-protein diet has been reported.

DEFICIENCY OF LIVER PHOSPHORYLASE (GSD VI). In GSD VI, hepatomegaly may be massive. Otherwise, the affected children are without symptoms and lead normal lives, though there may be some elevation of serum lipids and transaminases (see Table 8–12). Most patients do not have hypoglycemia. The blood glucose concentration does not increase after glucagon administration; this finding can be used to separate GSD VI from GSD IX, in which glucagon tolerance curves are normal. Separation from GSD I also can be made on clinical evidence. The hepatomegaly may recede as the children grow older. Some patients with GSD VI have subtle and unexplained cardiomyopathy.

The low activity of the hepatic phosphorylase system is consistent with but not diagnostic of GSD VI, since low activity may result from a number of defects within the phosphorylase activation system. The diagnosis rests on demonstration of a deficiency in the liver phosphorylase enzyme itself. Leukocyte phosphorylase may also be affected but cannot be relied upon for diagnosis. By light microscopy, formation of fibrous septa is seen in portal areas of the liver. Whether this change remains stationary or progresses to cirrhosis in adulthood is unknown. Phosphorylase activity, glycogen concentration, and histologic appearance are normal in muscle.

DEFICIENCY OF PHOSPHOFRUCTOKINASE (GSD VII). The symptoms of GSD VII resemble those of GSD V, but the muscle pain and cramping after exercise may be somewhat less severe. The disease has been tolerated by a young man who plays tennis for pleasure.

Phosphofructokinase is deficient in skeletal muscle but not in the liver; it is only partially defective in erythrocytes. Since this key glycolytic enzyme affects the use of both glycogen and glucose in muscle, it is surprising that the deficiency may cause fewer symptoms than a deficiency in phosphorylase, which affects only the utilization of glycogen. The concentration of glycogen in muscle is moderately elevated, and its distribution is subsarcolemmal, like that observed in GSD V and GSD X.

PROGRESSIVE BRAIN DISEASE AND DEACTIVATED LIVER PHOSPHORYLASE WITHOUT DEMONSTRATED ENZYME DEFECT (GSD VIII). Hepatomegaly was apparent soon after birth in one of the four patients in whom the disease has been described. However, the *clinical manifestations*, which are unique for GSD VIII among the glycogenoses and are present in all four patients, are related primarily to the central nervous system (see Table 8–12). The infant may develop nystagmus and rolling of the eyes, ataxia, and truncal tremor. The patient becomes hypotonic and then spastic; spasticity may become severe. Gradually the patient loses rapport with the environment, becomes unresponsive and bedridden, develops swallowing difficulties, and may die of aspiration pneumonia. Urinary excretion of epinephrine and norepinephrine may be increased. The glucagon tolerance test is normal.

Glycogen concentration was increased in hepatic and cerebral biopsies; in muscle, it may be normal or increased. In all patients, electron microscopy of cerebral biopsies revealed increased amounts of glycogen in the form of α particles that are about 10 times wider than the β particles usually found in brain. Liver phosphorylase activity may be low. Cerebral enzymes have not been assayed. The low activity of the hepatic phosphorylase system does not reflect a deficiency of phosphorylase enzyme or of any other enzyme in the hepatic system of phosphorylase activation. This is demonstrated by the normal glucagon tolerance curve and also by the fact that in vivo the phosphorylase activity increases to normal within 2 min after the administration of glucagon or epinephrine to the patient. The low phosphorylase activity observed in a liver specimen obtained before glucagon administration could be increased to normal in vitro by the patient's own liver homogenate. Accordingly, the affected child appears to suffer from impaired control of phosphorylase activation.

Since hepatic phosphorylase activity and liver glycogen concentration are as a rule found to be low in normal autopsy specimens, these findings do not reflect what they might have been in biopsies and illustrate why biopsy tissues must be optimally handled prior to assay.

DEFICIENCY OF LIVER PHOSPHORYLASE KINASE (GSD IX). This defect occurs in three forms that differ in their pattern of inheritance and tissue distribution. GSD IXa follows an autosomal recessive pattern of inheritance, and GSD IXb is sex-linked recessive. Otherwise, these two forms are indistinguishable. Skeletal muscle is not affected and is normal biochemically (see Table 8–12) and morphologically. In GSD IXc, with autosomal recessive inheritance, the phosphorylase kinase activity of liver and muscle is deficient. Hepatomegaly is massive in early life but recedes as the children grow older; it may disappear completely in teenagers or adults, though the liver can remain somewhat large. Transaminases are minimally elevated. GSD IX can be classified as a benign hepatomegaly except in patients who also have defective debrancher activity. Glucagon produces a normal rise in blood glucose concentration that serves to distinguish it from GSD VI, in which the glucagon tolerance curve remains flat. Affected children require no treatment, except perhaps in rare instances of combined deficiencies.

The concentration of liver glycogen is increased and phosphorylase activity is low, as is the case in GSD VI. In GSD IX, however, the low activity of phosphorylase results from a deficiency in phosphorylase kinase. Other enzymes of the activating system, including phosphorylase, are normal. Cultured skin fibroblasts and leukocytes have been reported to be affected but are undependable for diagnosis. The defect persists in adulthood, as demonstrated by rebiopsy of the original patient 25 yr later. In the liver, glycogen remained elevated at 11%, phosphorylase kinase activity was still less than 10% of normal, and some fibrous septa were present.

DEFICIENCY OF CYCLIC 3′5′-AMP-DEPENDENT KINASE (GSD X). The patient with this condition had marked hepatomegaly at 6 yr of age, when the clinical picture was indistinguishable from that of GSD IX except that the blood sugar curve remained flat after intravenous administration of glucagon (see Table 8–12). She had no skeletal muscular symptoms at this time, but 6 yr later she complained of muscular pain, cramping after exercise, and a minimal degree of persistent muscular weakness. The ischemic exercise test was normal, and hepatomegaly was persistent. The patient is doing well without specific therapy.

Liver glycogen concentration was high, and hepatic phosphorylase activity was low. Concentration of glycogen in muscle was increased to 2–4%. Light and electron microscopy showed increased glycogen deposition in liver and skeletal muscle cells. Muscle phosphorylase was present only in the inactive form, whereas normally 60–80% of total phosphorylase is in the active form. GSD X reflects a deficiency in activity of cyclic 3′5′-AMP-dependent kinase. The complete inactivation of muscle phosphorylase in GSD X is clinically well tolerated, whereas the complete lack of muscle phosphorylase in GSD V is characterized by cramps and pains. This difference may be due to the ability of inactive phosphorylase b to degrade glycogen in the presence of adenylic acid (5′-AMP), which is normally found in muscle tissue.

HEPATIC GLYCOGENOSIS WITH STUNTED GROWTH (GSD XI). This disorder is characterized by a greatly enlarged liver and markedly stunted growth (see Table 8–12). Serum transaminase and lipid levels may be elevated. Affected children develop severe hypophosphatemic rickets early in life unless they receive oral phosphate supplementation. Orally administering phosphate alone to the extent necessary for correction of the hypophosphatemia may heal the florid rickets, but adequate growth is not attained through this regimen. The marked rachitic bone changes are due to Fanconi syndrome characterized by urinary loss of phosphate, amino acids, glucose, and galactose that can occur in these children. Administering arginine raises the level of growth hormone in serum. After puberty the hepatomegaly may recede (although hepatic glycogen concentration remains increased) and the growth rate may increase (although the ultimate body height remains far below normal). However, after puberty the serum phosphate concentration remains normal without supplementation with phosphate.

Glycogen concentration is markedly increased in liver and kidney but normal in muscle. All measured hepatic glycolytic enzyme activities are normal. Administering glucagon does not increase the blood glucose concentration but does increase urinary excretion of cyclic AMP that is usually induced by glucagon administration. Glucose concentration decreases after the oral administration of 1.75 g/kg of galactose, an amount that normally is followed by a significant increase in blood glucose. Conversely, oral administration of an equivalent amount of fructose is followed by the normal increase in blood glucose concentration. On the basis of these findings, it is reasonable to postulate that patients with GSD XI have a functional deficiency of hepatic phosphoglucomutase despite the fact that the activity of this enzyme is normal in vitro when measured in hypotonic homogenates of frozen liver biopsy specimens.

Prenatal Diagnosis of GSD

The glycogenoses generally follow an autosomal recessive pattern of inheritance except for GSD IXb, in which inheritance is sex-linked recessive. They should be detectable in the fetus through assay of cultured amniotic fluid cells when these cells normally produce the particular enzyme under study. This criterion is not fulfilled for GSD I because glucose-6-phosphate is not found in normal cultured amniotic fluid cells. GSD I, GSD III, GSD VI, GSD IX, and GSD X may not be candidates for prenatal diagnosis because most of the affected children with these conditions lead near-normal lives. In GSD IIa and GSD IV, on the other hand, antenatal diagnosis has been made through assay of cultured amniotic fluid cells. Acid α-glucosidase activity has been present in all amniotic fluid specimens tested, even in GSD IIa. Several weeks may be needed to culture the amniotic fluid cells. Prenatal diagnosis of GSD IIa is feasible within 3 days after amniocentesis through electron microscopic examination of uncultured amniotic fluid cells, which show abnormal intracellular lysosomes that are not present in heterozygous or normal fetuses. These cellular inclusions are also seen by electron microscopy of chorionic villus biopsy specimens in fetal GSD IIa.

DEFICIENCY OF XYLULOSE DEHYDROGENASE
(Essential Benign Pentosuria)

This benign condition is characterized by a reducing substance in the urine of an otherwise healthy individual. Care should be taken not to mistake the reducing substance for glucose. The pentose in the urine reacts with Clinitest but not with glucose oxidase test papers such as Testape or Clinistix dipsticks.

L-Xylulose dehydrogenase converts L-xylulose (which can arise from D-glucuronate) to xylitol. Xylitol is converted to D-xylulose, which becomes D-xylulose-5-phosphate and enters the pentose phosphate shunt. Deficiency of this enzyme leads to increased concentration of L-xylulose in blood and urine. This rare defect is most common in Jews. No therapy is required.

Pentosuria can be observed in normal individuals if the dietary pentose intake is increased, as with the excessive ingestion of fruit containing pentose. Under these circumstances there may be urinary excretion of xylose and arabinose up to 200 mg/24 hr in normal individuals.

DEFICIENCY OF ACID α-MANNOSIDASE
(Mannosidosis)

The appearance of the patient with mannosidosis is similar to that of a patient with Hurler syndrome (see Sec 8.43). The liver and spleen are enlarged in this lysosomal disease; the lymphocytes contain vacuoles. Skeletal roentgenograms reveal structural abnormalities (dysostosis multiplex). Infections are frequent, especially of the middle ear and lungs. There may be corneal or lenticular opacities and psychomotor retardation is usually present. No treatment is available.

Acid α-mannosidase activity is deficient in body fluids and tissues. Mannose-containing macromolecules are stored in the abnormal liver lysosomes, which resemble those characteristic of Hurler syndrome. Mannosidosis exists in heterogeneous forms.

DEFICIENCY OF ACID α-FUCOSIDASE
(Fucosidosis)

See Sec. 8.18.

8.41 DIAGNOSTIC PROCEDURES IN DEFECTS OF METABOLISM OF CARBOHYDRATES

A history of the patient and family, clinical presentation, and findings of the physical examination are indispensable for the diagnosis of metabolic defects in children. A limited number of clinical test procedures, including analyses of blood and urine for constituents unusual in kind or amount, tolerance tests with glucagon, exercise tests, and so on, provide a preliminary assessment (see Table 8–12). Differential diagnosis is helped by gas chromatographic and mass spectroscopic (GC/MS) analysis of urine for organic acid patterns and excretion of unusual metabolites. The ultimate diagnosis depends on the biochemical analysis of tissues, which provides the basis of treatment.

Organ Biopsy and the Handling of Tissue Specimens Obtained at Biopsy or Autopsy

Biopsy should be performed of the organ system that exhibits clinical involvement. For example, hepatomegaly and hypotonia require open liver and abdominal wall biopsies. Needle biopsies of liver and muscle are alternative procedures, but the retrieved tissue is frequently inadequate in quantity or quality, for example, amounts are from 10 to 30 mg, and muscle contraction bands are unavoidable. Success with diagnostic tissue analysis often depends on having a biochemist experienced with the analysis present during the biopsy procedure in order to ensure that an appropriate specimen is obtained and then maintained in optimal condition. For example, assays of the cascade for phosphorylase activation and deactivation require that a small part of a few milligrams of fresh biopsy tissue be separated into fixative for electron microscopy and that most of the specimen be frozen in liquid nitrogen within seconds of the biopsy. Details of the biochemical analysis are decided after electron microscopic evaluation, which may indicate the area of metabolic impairment that should be scrutinized biochemically. Aberrations of mitochondrial ultrastructure are meaningful only in optimally prepared specimens, and the details of this preparation must be known. Measurements of enzymatic activity are informative provided the handling of the specimen has been controlled. Other details of patient management must also be monitored. If the patient receives substantial amounts of glucose infusion before and during the biopsy, increased liver glycogen is consistent with but not diagnostic of hepatic glycogenosis. The principal risks in the diagnosis of metabolic disease can be eliminated if the patient rather than the biopsy specimen is sent to a center with the resources and commitment to optimal study of metabolic disease. If transfer of the patient is not feasible, the cooperating biochemical laboratory should be contacted before the biopsy to discuss the details of the procedure and to provide a clinical summary of the patient, without which a meaningful biochemical analysis cannot be done.

Although analysis of white blood cells is valuable in selected instances, such as the determination of the carrier state of GSD IIa, examination of blood cells is usually only complementary to analysis of tissues of solid organs. Fibroblast cultures of skin biopsy specimens are of limited reliability.

8.42 THERAPY OF DEFECTS IN METABOLISM OF CARBOHYDRATES

For many of these conditions no treatment is effective; for others, none is necessary. The clinician's role may be limited to supportive care or to genetic counseling (see Sec. 7.33).

In a few conditions dietary regimens may offer some help; for some they are lifesaving (galactosemia, fructose intolerance, etc.). Life-threatening symptoms of biotinidase or holocarboxylase synthetase deficiency can be reversed by taking daily large doses of biotin that must be given indefinitely. Future therapies depend upon research to find ways of replacing specific enzymes, adding pharmacologic doses of cofactors (vitamins, etc.) to the diet, or compensating for the enzymatic defect with hormones or drugs.

Enzyme replacement has been carried out by transplanting normal kidneys into patients with Fabry disease (see Sec. 8.18) and by bone marrow transplantation into patients with a variety of lysosomal diseases such as Hunter or Hurler disease (see Sec. 8.43) or with GSD IIa. In Fabry disease, the transplanted normal kidney may provide a "filter" for circulating trihexoside with enough α-galactosidase to initiate its degradation. Bone marrow transplantation may be effective in children with some lysosomal disease, in particular in various types of mucopolysaccharidoses (see Sec. 8.43). Bone marrow transplantation or enzyme infusion has to date not benefited clinically the several patients with GSD II in whom it was tried.

GEORGE HUG

Barranger JA, Brady RO (eds): The Molecular Basis of Lysosomal Storage Disorders. New York, Academic Press, 1984.
Beratis NG, LaBadie GU, Hirschhorn K: Characterization of the molecular defect in infantile and adult acid α-glucosidase deficiency fibroblasts. J Clin Invest 62:1264, 1978.
Brandt NJ, Terenius L, Jacobsen BB, et al: Hyper-endorphin syndrome in a child with necrotizing encephalomyelopathy. N Engl J Med 303:914, 1980.
Brown WJ, Farquhar MG: The mannose-6-phosphate receptor for lysosomal enzymes is concentrated in cis Golgi cisternae. Cell 36:295, 1984.
Chen VT, Mattison DR, Feigenbaum L, et al: Reduction in oocyte number following prenatal exposure to a diet high in galactose. Science 214:1145, 1981.
Chen Y-T, Cornblath M, Sidbury JB: Cornstarch therapy in type I glycogen storage disease. N Engl J Med 310:171, 1984.
Cramer DW, Willett WC, Bell DA, et al: Galactose consumption and metabolism in relation to the risk of ovarian cancer. Lancet II: 66, 1989.
Demaugre F, Bonnefonte J-P, Colonna M, et al: Infantile form of carnitine palmitoyl transferase II deficiency with hepatomuscular symptoms and sudden death. J Clin Invest 87:859, 1991.
DeVivo DC, Haymond MW, Obert KA, et al: Defective activation of the pyruvate dehydrogenase complex in subacute necrotizing encephalomyelopathy (Leigh disease). Ann Neurol 6:483, 1979.
Durand P, Borrone C, Gatti R: On genetic variants in fucosidosis. J Pediatr 89:688, 1976.
Farrell DF, Clark AF, Scott CR, et al: Absence of pyruvate decarboxylase activity in man: A cause of congenital lactic acidosis. Science 187:1082, 1975.
Garibaldi LR, Canini S, Suporti-Furga A, et al: Galactosemia caused by generalized uridine disphosphate galactose-4-epimerase deficiency. J Pediatr 103:927, 1983.
Gitzelmann R, Steinmann B, Mitchell B, et al: Uridine diphosphate galactose 4'-epimerase deficiency. IV. Report of eight cases in three families. Helv Paediatr Acta 31:441, 1976.
Greene HL, Slonim AE, O'Neill JA, et al: Continuous nocturnal intragastric feeding for management of type I glycogen storage disease. N Engl J Med 294:423, 1976.
Gröbe H, von Bassewitz DB, Dominick HC, et al: Subacute necrotizing encephalomyelopathy: Clinical, ultrastructural, biochemical and therapeutic studies in an infant. Acta Paediatr Scand 64:755, 1975.
Harris RE, Hannon D, Vogler C, et al: Bone marrow transplantation in type IIa glycogen storage disease. Birth Defects, Original Article Series 22:119, 1986.
Hofnaegel D, Worster-Hill D, Child EL: Ovarian failure in galactosaemia. Lancet 2:1197, 1979.
Hug G, Chuck G, Walling L, et al: Liver phosphorylase deficiency in glycogenosis type VI: Documentation by biochemical analysis of hepatic biopsy specimens. J Lab Clin Med 84:26, 1974.
Hug G, Schubert WK, Chuck G: Phosphorylase kinase of the liver: Deficiency in a girl with increased hepatic glycogen. Science 153:1534, 1966.
Hug G, Soukup S, Ryan M, Chuck G: Rapid prenatal diagnosis of glycogen storage disease type II by electron microscopy of uncultured amniotic-fluid cells. N Engl J Med 310:1018, 1984.
Hug G, Chuck G, Chen Y-T, et al: Chorionic villus ultrastructure in type II glycogen storage disease (Pompe's disease). N Engl J Med 324:342, 1991.
Hug G, Soukup S, Berry H, and Bove K: Carnitine palmitoyl transferase (CPT): Deficiency of CPT II but not of CPT I with reduced total and free carnitine but increased acylcarnitine. Pediatr Res 25:115A, 1989.
Kornfeld M, LeBaron M: Glycogenosis type VIII. J Neuropathol Exp Neurol 43:568, 1984.
Lerner A, Iancu TC, Bashan N, et al: A new variant of glycogen storage disease type IXc. Am J Dis Chil 136:407, 1982.
McAdams AJ, Hug G, Bove KE: Glycogen storage disease: Type I to X: Criteria for morphologic diagnosis. Hum Pathol 5:463, 1974.
Mehler M, DMauro S: Late-onset acid maltase deficiency. Arch Neurol 33:692, 1976.
Reitman ML, Varki A, Kornfield S: Fibroblasts from patients with I-cell disease and pseudo-Hurler polydystrophy are deficient in UDP-N-acetylglucosamine: glycoprotein *N*-acetylglucosaminylphosphotransferase activity. J Clin Invest 67:1574, 1981.
Robinson BH, Taylor J, Sherwood WG: Deficiency of dihydrolipoyl dehydrogenase: A cause of congenital lactic acidosis. Pediatr Res 11:1198, 1977.
Saul R, Ghidoni JJ, Molyneux RJ, et al: Castanospermine inhibits α-glucosidase activities and alters glycogen distribution in animals. Proc Natl Acad Sci 82:93, 1985.
Slonim AE, Goans PJ: Myopathy in McArdle's syndrome: Improvement with a high-protein diet. N Engl J Med 312:355, 1985.
Towfighi J, Yoss BS, Wasiewski WW, et al: Cerebral glycogenosis, alpha particle type: Morphologic and biochemical observations in an infant. Hum Pathol 20:1210, 1989.
Treem WR, Stanley CA, Fingeold DN, et al: Primary carnitine deficiency due to a failure of carnitine transport in kidney, muscle, and fibroblasts. N Engl J Med 319:1331, 1989.

8.43 DISORDERS OF MUCOPOLYSACCHARIDE METABOLISM

The mucopolysaccharidoses are a group of inherited disorders caused by incomplete degradation and storage of acid mucopolysaccharides (glycosaminoglycans). The clinical manifestations result from the accumulation of mucopolysaccharides in various organs. Specific degradative lysosomal enzyme deficiencies have been identified for all the mucopolysaccharidoses.

The mucopolysaccharides are polyanionic polymers, most of which contain alternating carbohydrate residues of *N*-acetylhexosamine and uronic acid. Although the acid mucopolysaccharides are closely related as a group, individual compounds differ in their distribution in body tissues. Dermatan sulfate, heparan sulfate, and keratan sulfate are the major mucopolysaccharides involved in the pathogenesis of the mucopolysaccharidoses. The structural differences of the mucopolysaccharides explain the need for various lysosomal enzymes required for their degradation.

Since the mucopolysaccharides are major components of

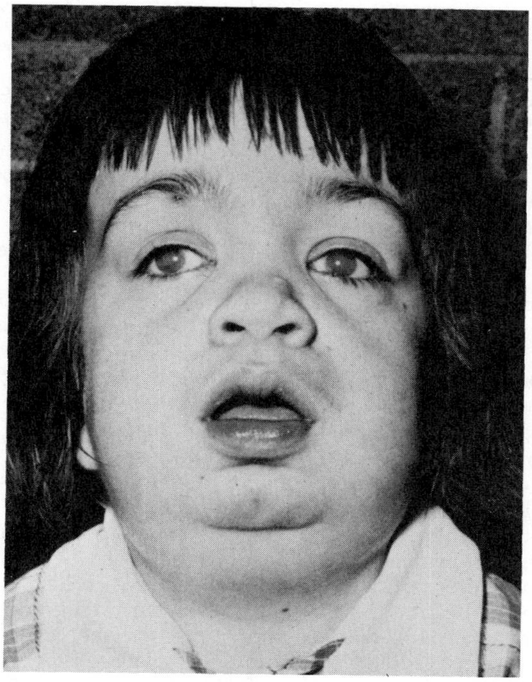

Figure 8–32. Typical appearance of a patient with Hurler syndrome.

the intercellular substance of connective tissue, bony changes are characteristic of the mucopolysaccharidoses. The skeletal deformities seen in roentgenograms are referred to as **dysostosis multiplex**. The central nervous system also may be affected, leading to progressive mental retardation. In addition, the cardiovascular system, liver, spleen, tendons, joints, and skin may be involved. The degree of disability and overall prognosis in each of the mucopolysaccharidoses are determined by the extent of the physical and mental involvement.

The mucopolysaccharidoses follow an autosomal recessive mode of inheritance, with the exception of Hunter syndrome, which is inherited as an X-linked recessive trait. They are suspected on the basis of clinical and radiologic manifestations, and the diagnosis is confirmed by the finding of increased urinary excretion of mucopolysaccharides and deficiency of a specific enzyme.

HURLER SYNDROME (MPS IH). This syndrome is the most severe of the mucopolysaccharidoses. Its relentless progression usually results in death by the early teenage years.

Etiology and Pathology. The basic defect in Hurler disease is a deficiency of α-L-iduronidase, which leads to accumulation of the dermatan and heparan sulfates in tissues and their urinary excretion. Almost every tissue in the body is affected, with widespread occurrence of vacuolated, or "gargoyle," cells, which contain lysosomes engorged with mucopolysaccharide. In the brain, lipid storage also occurs with the mucopolysaccharide accumulation. There is unusual hyalinization of collagen and separation of the collagen bundles. These changes lead to joint deformities and stiffness, thickened meninges, hydrocephalus, peripheral nerve compression, and a tendency to develop hernias. As the disease progresses, narrowing of the coronary arteries, thickening of the cardiac valves and endocardium, and stiffening of the myocardium may lead to congestive heart failure. The constricted thorax contributes to the clinical deterioration of these patients.

Clinical Manifestations. Infants with Hurler syndrome appear normal at birth, and during the 1st year of life only slight developmental delays are noted. Physical examination, however, reveals hepatosplenomegaly, exaggerated kyphosis, persistent nasal discharge, and noisy breathing. The facial features become progressively coarser after the 1st yr of life (Fig. 8–32). The head is large and dolichocephalic, with frontal bossing and prominent sagittal and metopic sutures. The bridge of the nose is depressed, and the nose is broad and flat. Clouding of the corneas becomes evident at about 1 yr of age. Umbilical and inguinal hernias are common. Children afflicted with this disease regress developmentally, and mental retardation becomes obvious. The downhill course continues rapidly after the 2nd or 3rd yr of life. These children become immobile, their joints become progressively stiff and contracted, and they usually die by their early teens.

Roentgenographic Changes. Roentgenograms of patients with Hurler syndrome reveal dysostosis multiplex, which includes a large dolichocephalic skull and thickened calvarium. There may be hyperostosis of the cranium, and the sella turcica may be boot- or J-shaped. The medial third of the clavicle is thickened. The vertebral bodies are ovoid in the lower thorax and upper lumbar regions. They develop beak-like projections on their lower anterior margins, while their upper portions remain hypoplastic (Fig. 8–33). This results in the gibbus deformity commonly seen in these patients. The ribs are spatulated or oar-shaped, and the pelvis shows flaring of the iliac bones, with shallow acetabulae. Roentgenograms of the hips show progressive coxa valga deformity, sometimes resembling the findings of aseptic necrosis. Roentgenograms of the hands show tapering of the terminal phalanges and widening at the distal ends and tapering at the proximal ends of the metacarpals. The 5th metacarpal is the first to show these changes (Fig. 8–34). In the long bones, particularly those of the upper extremities, irregular widenings associated with areas of cortical thinning and expansion of the medullary

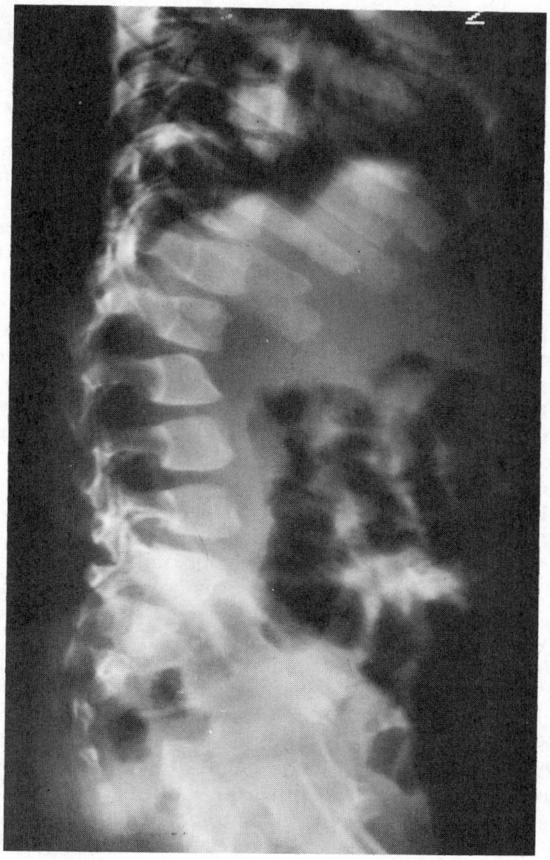

Figure 8–33. Lateral spine roentgenogram of a patient with Hurler syndrome.

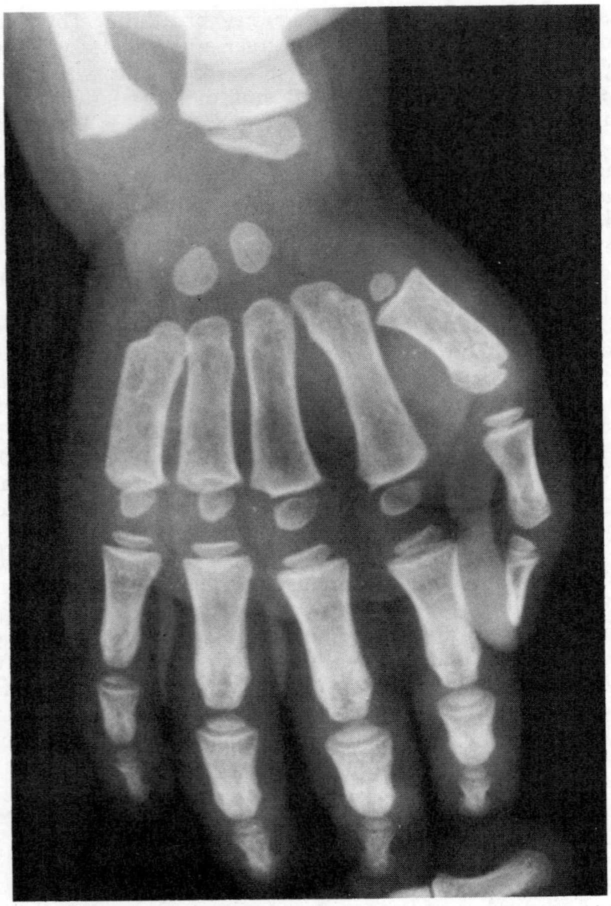

Figure 8–34. Roentgenogram of the hand of a patient with Hurler syndrome.

cavity are seen. Occasionally, there may be cortical thickening. The radius curves toward the ulna, and the articular surfaces of the radius and the ulna face one another, forming a V (see Fig. 8–34). The humerus may be angulated, and the glenoid fossa, like the acetabulum, may be shallow. Severe growth retardation is common in these children.

Diagnosis. The diagnosis of Hurler syndrome is suggested by the presence of the relevant clinical and roentgenographic findings. Urinary excretion of dermatan and heparan sulfates provides further support. Although there are helpful screening methods for quantifying the mucopolysaccharides in the urine, definitive diagnosis requires detection of α-L-iduronidase deficiency in white blood cells, serum, or cultured skin fibroblasts.

SCHEIE SYNDROME (MPS IS). This syndrome is the mildest of the mucopolysaccharidoses. It is a distinct clinical and genetic entity; the enzyme deficiency, α-L-iduronidase, is the same as in Hurler syndrome but is specific for dermatan sulfate, which accumulates in tissues and is excreted in excessive amounts in urine.

Clinical Manifestations. Patients with this disease have normal intelligence, mild facial coarsening with striking prognathism, joint stiffness typified by claw hands, and carpal tunnel syndrome. Corneal clouding is a constant feature that leads to loss of visual acuity. Aortic regurgitation is common. The clinical features do not appear until after 5 yr of age, and the disease is compatible with close-to-normal life expectancy. The patient with Scheie syndrome reaches normal height.

Roentgenographic Changes. Findings on roentgenography include mild dysostosis multiplex, without the vertebral changes or the gibbus deformity seen in Hurler disease. There is coxa valga and slight radial and ulnar obliquity with V formation of their articular surfaces.

Diagnosis. Early clinical diagnosis is more difficult in Scheie than in Hurler syndrome because the somatic changes are mild and mental retardation is not present. Detection of urinary dermatan sulfate is helpful, but the diagnosis is confirmed by demonstrating a deficiency of α-L-iduronidase in white blood cells or in cultured skin fibroblasts.

HURLER-SCHEIE SYNDROME (MPS IH/IS). Few reports exist of patients with this syndrome.

Etiology. The basic defect is α-L-iduronidase deficiency specific for dermatan sulfate, which is excreted in urine and stored in the liver, spleen, and other tissues. It has been suggested that the Hurler-Scheie syndrome is a genetic compound of two recessive genes, analogous to hemoglobin SC disease, but recent work indicates it is best explained as an allelic mutation of the iduronidase gene.

Clinical Manifestations. Patients develop mild coarseness of facial features, corneal clouding, shortness of stature, joint contractures, hepatosplenomegaly, hernias, and cardiac valvular lesions, primarily mitral insufficiency (Fig. 8–35). Mental development is normal. The clinical features, which usually develop in the first 2 yr of life and in early childhood, are often mistaken for manifestations of a variety of skeletal defects causing growth retardation. The disease is compatible with long life.

Roentgenographic Features. Roentgenograms of patients with this syndrome reveal severe dysostosis multiplex with findings identical to those seen in Hurler syndrome, except that there is no gibbus.

Diagnosis. Diagnosis is based upon the findings of dermatan sulfate in the urine and α-L-iduronidase deficiency. The clinical pattern of onset of joint involvement and the severity of skeletal deformities distinguish Hurler-Scheie from Scheie disease.

HUNTER SYNDROME (MPS II). This syndrome is the only X-linked disorder among the mucopolysaccharidoses. It is milder than Hurler syndrome with respect to the skeletal and mental defects, although the mucopolysaccharides, dermatan and heparan sulfate, stored in tissues and excreted in

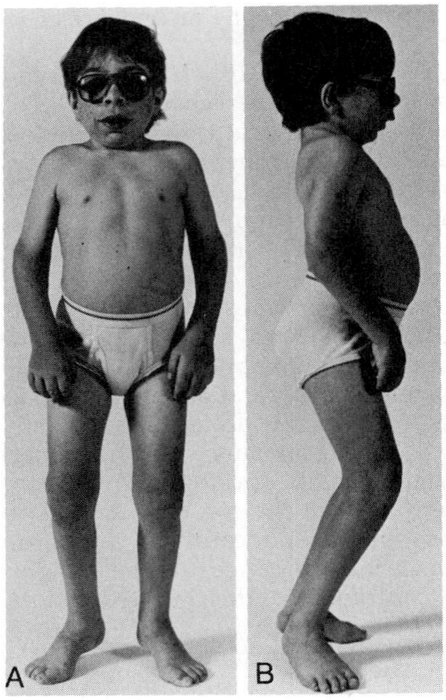

Figure 8–35. A patient with Hurler-Scheie syndrome with normal intelligence. Note the joint stiffness of all extremities.

the urine are similar in the two diseases. The enzyme deficient in tissues is iduronosulfate sulfatase, but there is a considerable phenotypic heterogeneity; there is no biochemical or enzymatic difference between the severe form of the disease, designated *type A*, and the mild disease, *type B*.

Type A. This is the "classic" form of Hunter syndrome. Coarseness of facial features, short stature, joint stiffness, hepatosplenomegaly, and hernias are common clinical manifestations. Mental retardation is severe. Progression of the disease process is slower and the dysostosis multiplex is milder than in Hurler syndrome. Corneal clouding is usually absent, but hearing loss is very common. Skin changes also are frequent, including small raised papules over the skin of the shoulders, the scapulas, and the lower back. Cardiac involvement often occurs. Patients usually do not have gibbus deformity, although mild kyphosis may be present in some. Life expectancy for these patients usually extends into the late teens or early 20s.

Type B. This syndrome is a milder disease than *type A*, even though the enzyme deficiency and urinary mucopolysaccharides are the same. Retardation is usually lacking or very minimal. The physical features are similar to, but milder than, those in type A, and patients have a longer life expectancy. Airway obstruction caused by mucopolysaccharide accumulation in the trachea and bronchi is a complicating feature of type B.

Diagnosis. The physical features, dysostosis multiplex, and dermatan and heparan sulfaturia suggest either Hurler or Hunter syndrome, but sex-linked inheritance is specific to the latter. Enzyme studies showing iduronosulfate sulfatase deficiency in serum, white blood cells, or cultured fibroblasts confirm the diagnosis of Hunter syndrome. Other sulfatases should be examined, since multiple sulfatase deficiency can be confused with Hunter syndrome.

SANFILIPPO SYNDROME (MPS III). This syndrome is a distinct entity and is based on clinical findings and excessive urinary excretion of exclusively heparan sulfate. The coarse facial appearance and skeletal involvement are milder than those seen in the Hurler and Hunter syndromes. There are four enzymatic variants, distinct deficiencies all leading to the same phenotype and mucopolysacchariduria. Heparan sulfate is stored in tissues, and its accumulation is responsible for the neuronal damage and atrophy underlying the profound mental retardation associated with the disease.

Clinical Manifestations. The clinical features of the Sanfilippo syndrome in early life are not very striking. Affected children have delayed developmental milestones and are usually very hyperactive. By the end of the 1st decade there is rapid neurologic deterioration; their gait becomes unsteady, and they become bedridden. Most of the children die in their middle teens. Mental retardation, some joint stiffening, hepatosplenomegaly, hernias, and dysostosis multiplex are common, but dwarfism and corneal clouding are rare.

Patients manifest dysostosis multiplex typical of the mucopolysaccharidoses. The large bones are not as severely involved; the obliquity of the radius and ulna and the tapering of the proximal ends of the metacarpals are very mild.

Diagnosis. Sanfilippo syndrome should be considered in the presence of heparan sulfaturia, hepatosplenomegaly, mental retardation, and dysostosis multiplex. Screening tests for urinary mucopolysaccharides usually give positive results but not as consistently as in the Hurler or Hunter syndrome. The different enzymatic variants can be confirmed by specific enzyme assays provided by special laboratories.

Sanfilippo A Syndrome (MPS III A). Sulfamidase is deficient in this disease, which can be assayed using cultured skin fibroblasts or peripheral blood leukocytes.

Sanfilippo B Syndrome (MPS III B). This form is characterized by α-*N*-acetylhexosaminidase deficiency, which can be assayed on serum, white blood cells, or cultured skin fibroblasts.

Sanfilippo C Syndrome (MPS III C). This syndrome is caused by a deficiency of acetyl CoA:α-glucosaminide *N*-acetyltransferase. The assay requires cultured fibroblasts or white blood cells.

Sanfilippo D Syndrome (MPS III D). This deficiency of *N*-acetylglucosamine-6-sulfatase is specific for heparan sulfate. The enzyme is assayed using a substrate prepared from heparin.

MORQUIO SYNDROME (MPS IV). This disorder is characterized by keratan sulfaturia and skeletal dysplasia. Keratan sulfate is stored in tissues together with chondroitin-6-sulfate. The keratan sulfaturia may decrease with age, but it is always above the normal range. There are two enzyme defects that lead to identical phenotypes in this syndrome.

Clinical Manifestations. The syndrome is associated with severe somatic manifestations and lack of mental involvement. At birth it may not be recognized. Joint laxity and shortness of stature first appear at about 1 yr of age. Skeletal abnormalities include flat vertebrae (platyspondyly universalis), short neck, genu valgum, flat feet, large and unstable knee joints, large elbow joints, and large wrists with ulnar deviation. The platyspondyly leads to short trunk and short stature. The odontoid process is underdeveloped; early on, this may cause atlantoaxial subluxation or translocation, with spinal cord compression. Corneal clouding also may be apparent at an early age. There is midface hypoplasia with a depressed nasal bridge and protrusion of the mandible, which give these patients a permanent grin. Hepatosplenomegaly is not as pronounced as in the other mucopolysaccharidoses, but it is usually present. Cardiac manifestations are secondary to respiratory failure caused by kyphoscoliosis and restricted chest movements, although aortic regurgitation may complicate the Morquio syndrome. Teeth are severely affected and have very thin enamel. Hearing loss may result from recurrent otitis media. Variation in the clinical manifestations is common, and very mild cases may be encountered. Patients usually die in their 3rd or 4th decade of life from cor pulmonale caused by the severe abnormalities of the chest and spine.

Roentgenographic Changes. In the 1st yr of life, roentgenograms may reveal only mild changes in patients with Morquio syndrome. The vertebral bodies show height loss and anterior tongue-like projections. At 2 yr the platyspondyly becomes evident. The hypoplasia of the odontoid process can be clearly seen in tomographic studies. The skull and sella turcica are mildly involved. The long bones are shortened, and the metaphyses appear irregular. There is progressive distortion of the epiphyseal metaphyseal plates. The pelvis shows wide acetabulae with progressive subluxation or dislocation of the femoral heads. The metacarpal bones are short and wide with conical tapering of their proximal ends. The distal ends of the radius and ulna face one another, similar to the obliquity seen in other mucopolysaccharidoses. These changes, especially the coxa valga and the changes in the wrists and lumbar spine, should differentiate Morquio syndrome from other skeletal dysplasias.

Diagnosis. The spondyloepiphyseal dysplasias (see Sec. 24.29) may mimic the signs of Morquio syndrome both clinically and roentgenographically. Screening tests for acid mucopolysaccharides in the urine of these patients can be negative; therefore, quantitative rather than qualitative isolation methods are preferred. The urinary finding of keratan sulfaturia, moreover, is also found in the Kneist syndrome. Therefore, enzyme determinations are essential for differentiating Morquio syndrome from other conditions. There are two enzyme deficiencies:

Morquio Syndrome, Type A (MPS IV A). This syndrome is caused by a deficiency of *N*-acetylgalactosamine-6-sulfate sulfatase, an enzyme that also degrades galactose-6-sulfate.

MORQUIO SYNDROME, TYPE B (MPS IV B). In this syndrome β-galactosidase is deficient. An important clinical difference between the two syndromes is the lack of enamel hypoplasia in type B. In other respects, including roentgenograms of the spine, the two forms may be indistinguishable. Morquio syndrome type B should not be confused with GM_1 gangliosidosis, which also is associated with β-galactosidase deficiency but resembles Hurler syndrome clinically.

KERATAN AND HEPARAN SULFATURIA (MPS VIII). A single case of this unusual form of mucopolysacchariduria has been described. The patient was a boy who was noted to have developmental delay at 18 mo of age. At 2½ yr he was severely retarded, bedridden, and blind. He had scaphocephaly and mild pectus excavatum but no organomegaly; corneal clouding was not noted. Roentgenographic studies showed dysostosis multiplex without the platyspondyly seen in Morquio syndrome.

Urinary studies showed excessive excretion of both keratan and heparan sulfates. Enzymatic assays revealed normal activity for both of the known Morquio enzyme defects. *N*-acetylglucosamine-6-sulfate sulfatase specific for a substrate prepared from keratan sulfate was deficient. This enzyme defect is different from that of Sanfilippo D, in which *N*-acetylglucosamine-6-sulfate sulfatase deficiency is specific for heparan sulfate only.

MAROTEAUX-LAMY SYNDROME (MPS VI). The Maroteaux-Lamy syndrome resembles Hurler disease clinically but does not involve mental retardation. There are two clinical types: the severe form is designated *type A*, and the milder form, with less pronounced skeletal deformities, is designated *type B*.

Clinical Manifestations. Coarse facial features are typical of this syndrome. The head is enlarged, and the neck and trunk are short. The chest shows pectus carinatum deformity. Claw hands and other joint contractures are common. The abdomen protrudes owing to hepatosplenomegaly (Fig. 8–36). Umbilical hernias and corneal opacities are frequent. Mental ability is usually not impaired, although hydrocephalus and increased intracranial pressure are sometimes associated with Maroteaux-Lamy disease. Cardiac involvement includes mitral insufficiency and aortic regurgitation. The roentgenographic findings are those of dysostosis multiplex seen in Hurler syndrome.

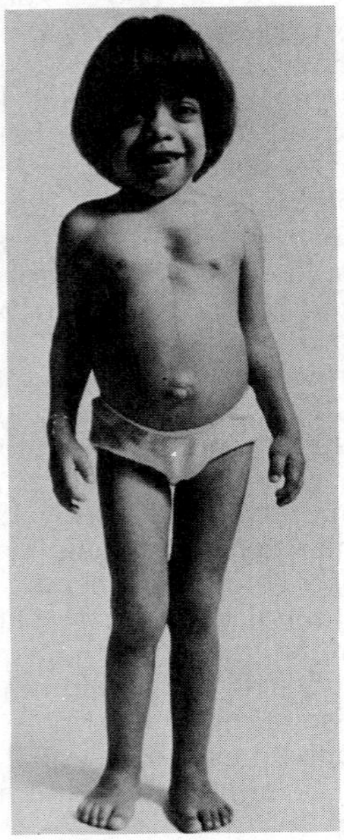

Figure 8–36. A patient with Maroteaux-Lamy syndrome with normal intelligence. The elbows, wrists, and fingers show typical joint stiffness. The abdomen is protuberant with umbilical hernia.

Diagnosis. The elevated urinary mucopolysaccharide in Maroteaux-Lamy syndrome is almost exclusively dermatan sulfate, and *N*-acetylglucosamine-4-sulfate sulfatase (arylsulfatase B) is the deficient enzyme. Types A and B have the same mucopolysacchariduria and the same enzyme deficiency. The findings of somatic changes resembling those of Hurler syndrome, normal mental development, and dermatan sulfaturia suggest either Maroteaux-Lamy or Hurler-Scheie syndrome. Deficiency of arylsulfatase B in white blood cells or cultured fibroblasts confirms the diagnosis of Maroteaux-Lamy syndrome.

β-GLUCURONIDASE DEFICIENCY (MPS VII). Patients with this disease have clinical and skeletal features of mucopolysaccharidoses with hepatosplenomegaly, umbilical hernia, thoracolumbar gibbus, and mental retardation. Variations in the phenotypic expression of this enzyme defect have been reported; some patients have a clinical course similar to that of Hurler disease, whereas others have had no mental retardation and a very mild course. The roentgenographic changes are those of dysostosis multiplex. The severity of the bony changes may vary but at times they are indistinguishable from those seen in Hurler disease.

The biochemical findings are characterized by the mucopolysacchariduria of chondroitin 4/6 sulfate. The definitive diagnosis is made by establishing β-glucuronidase deficiency in white blood cells or in cultured skin fibroblasts.

DIFFERENTIAL DIAGNOSIS OF THE MUCOPOLYSACCHARIDOSES

Diseases with dysostosis multiplex and physical features of the mucopolysaccharidoses are summarized in Table 8–13.

Multiple sulfatase deficiency (see Sec. 8.18) may mimic the mucopolysaccharidoses in its clinical manifestations, roentgenographic findings, and the presence of mucopolysacchariduria. The mental and neurologic deterioration is usually more rapid than that seen in the Hurler or Hunter disease and often resembles metachromatic leukodystrophy. Severe ichthyosis, a constant feature, and hepatomegaly should raise the suspicion of multiple sulfatase deficiency in a patient suspected of having a mucopolysaccharidosis. Urinary screening for mucopolysaccharides and sulfatides is usually positive.

GM_1 gangliosidosis (generalized gangliosidosis) (see Sec. 8.18) shares the clinical features of lipid and mucopolysaccharide storage diseases. Clinically, patients with the infantile severe form of generalized gangliosidosis are mentally retarded and hypotonic and have hepatosplenomegaly. In more than 50% there is a macular cherry-red spot.

Mannosidosis (see Sec. 8.40) is characterized by psychomotor retardation, hearing loss, coarse features with Hurler-like facial appearance, hepatosplenomegaly, muscular hypotonia, and mild dysostosis multiplex. There is no mucopolysacchariduria, but mannose-rich oligosaccharide is found in the urine.

Patients with *fucosidosis* (see Sec. 8.18) show coarse facial features, hepatosplenomegaly, severe psychomotor retardation, and dysostosis multiplex. There is no mucopolysacchariduria, and fucose-containing oligosaccharide is stored in tissues and excreted in urine.

Aspartylglucosaminuria (AGU) has frequently been confused with the Hurler or Hunter syndrome. Children with this disease appear normal at birth but progressively develop coarse facies with broad nose, depressed nasal bridge, thick lips, and anteverted nostrils. Other features include short neck, cranial asymmetry, scoliosis, hepatosplenomegaly, and urinary excretion of aspartylglucosamine.

TABLE 8–13. Diseases to be Considered in the Differential Diagnosis of the Mucopolysaccharidoses

Syndrome	Biochemical Findings	Enzyme Deficiency	Genetics
GM_1 gangliosidosis	GM_1 stored in tissues. "Keratan sulfate–like" glycoprotein stored in tissue and excreted in urine	β-Galactosidase	Autosomal recessive
Mannosidosis	Mannose-containing glycopeptides excreted in urine and stored in tissues	α-Mannosidase	Autosomal recessive
Fucosidosis	Fucose-containing oligosaccharides and glycopeptides stored in tissues and excreted in urine	α-Fucosidase	Autosomal recessive
Aspartylglucosaminuria	Aspartylglucosamine in urine and tissues	Aspartylglucosaminidase	Autosomal recessive
Mucolipidosis I	Sialic acid–containing oligosaccharides excreted in urine and stored in tissues	α-Sialidase	Autosomal recessive
Mucolipidosis II I-cell disease	Very high levels of acid hydrolases, e.g., β-hexosaminidase in urine and serum. Very low levels of the same enzymes in cultured fibroblasts	UDP-*N*-Acetylglucosamine: *N*-acetylglucosamine-1-phosphotransferase	Autosomal recessive
Mucolipidosis III	Same as mucolipidosis II	Same as in mucolipidosis II	Autosomal recessive
Mucolipidosis IV	No consistent findings	Sialidase in some cases	Autosomal recessive
Multiple sulfatase deficiency	Heparan sulfate and sulfatides in urine and tissues	Arylsulfatases A, B, and C, sulfamidase, iduronosulfatase	Autosomal recessive
Kneist syndrome	Keratan sulfaturia	None known	Autosomal dominant
Spondyloepiphyseal dysplasias	No consistent biochemical findings	None known	Several forms: autosomal dominant, recessive, and X-linked

The *mucolipidoses* must also be distinguished from the mucopolysaccharidoses. Patients with mucolipidosis I (see Sec. 8.19) share many clinical and roentgenographic features with the Hurler syndrome, including the skeletal deformities. However, a macular cherry-red spot is frequently a characteristic feature of this disorder. Neurologic deterioration is progressive and is often associated with myoclonic seizures, muscle atrophy, choreoathetotic movements, and nystagmus. Urinary mucopolysaccharides are normal, and sialic acid-bound oligosaccharides are excreted in increased quantities.

Mucolipidosis II: I-Cell Disease (see Sec. 8.19) is often confused with Hurler or Hunter syndrome. I-cell disease is distinguished from the Hurler syndrome by its characteristic rapid psychomotor retardation and early death. Gingival hyperplasia is characteristic in early life. The thorax is small, and cardiac valvular disease is frequent. Corneal clouding is not a feature. Periosteal bone formation is observed in the long bones during the first 6 mo of life, and there is no mucopolysacchariduria.

Mucolipidosis III (see Sec. 8.19), a milder form of mucolipidosis II, is characterized by mild mental retardation and joint stiffness; the skeletal defects are not as pronounced as in I-cell disease. The diagnosis depends on findings of coarse facial features, lack of mucopolysacchariduria, elevated hydrolases in serum and urine, and depressed levels of these enzymes in cultured fibroblasts.

Mucolipidosis IV (see Sec. 8.19) is characterized by corneal clouding and mental retardation without mucopolysacchariduria.

The *spondyloepiphyseal dysplasias* (see Sec. 24.29) are commonly confused with the mucopolysaccharidoses, particularly with the Morquio syndrome. These diseases lack mucopolysacchariduria.

The *Kneist syndrome* (see Sec. 24.29) may be recognized at birth and usually is confused with Morquio syndrome. Full expression of the syndrome becomes obvious after the 1st yr of life and includes short trunk and limbs, large head with depressed nasal bridge, stiffness of fingers and other joints, short neck, bell-shaped chest, tibial bowing, cleft palate, retinal detachment, deafness, and hernias. Later in life exaggerated lordosis and kyphoscoliosis become apparent. Radiographic findings include generalized osteoporosis with poor modeling. The Kneist syndrome is characterized by keratan sulfaturia, which may also occur with the Morquio syndrome. The specific enzyme defects, for example, *N*-acetylgalactosamine-6-sulfate sulfatase or β-galactosidase, which are characteristic of Morquio syndrome, are normal in the Kneist syndrome.

Prenatal diagnosis and carrier detection are available for all the mucopolysaccharidoses.

REUBEN H. MATALON

Dorfman A, Matalon R: The mucopolysaccharidoses (a review). Proc Natl Acad Sci USA 73:630, 1976.

Matalon R: Mucopolysaccharidoses. *In*: Gershwin ME, Robbins DL (eds): Musculoskeletal Diseases of Children. New York, Grune & Stratton, 1983.

McKusick VA, Neufeld EF: The mucopolysaccharide storage diseases. *In*: Stanbury JB, Wyngaarden JB, Fredrickson DS, et al (eds): The Metabolic Basis of Inherited Disease, 5th ed. New York, McGraw-Hill, 1983.

DEFECTS IN METABOLISM OF PURINES AND PYRIMIDINES

Purines and pyrimidines are heterocyclic nitrogen-containing compounds. Combinations of purines and pyrimidines with ribose or deoxyribose and with phosphate create nucleotides. Combined with ribose and phosphate (hence, ribonucleotide), purines and pyrimidines form the elements of ribonucleic acid (RNA); combined with deoxyribose and phosphate (deoxyribonucleotides), they form deoxyribonucleic acid (DNA). The ability to synthesize the purine ring de novo is virtually universal among living organisms. The final product of purine metabolism in man is uric acid.

Other than uric acid, the purine bases recognized to have clinical importance are adenine and guanine. The important pyrimidines are thymine, cytosine, and uracil. The importance of nucleotides as components of DNA rests on the genetic function of this material. RNA is of central importance in the regulation of protein synthesis and as a component of such important energy-producing compounds and nucleotide cofactors as ATP, UDPG, NAD, NADP, and others.

8.44 DISORDERS OF PURINE METABOLISM

GOUT. The hallmark of gout is the elevation of serum uric acid concentration. This disease primarily affects adults and rarely occurs in children except those with type I glycogen storage disease (GSD I), in whom hyperuricemia routinely occurs and gouty arthritis and tophi appear in adolescence (see Sec. 8.40). When hyperuricemia and gout occur in childhood, they are almost always secondary to another disorder.

Elevations of uric acid concentration in serum can result from several general metabolic disturbances. Certain patients have an abnormally active production de novo of uric acid; others have reduction in the renal clearance of uric acid; and some represent combinations of these two major factors.

At least 95% of cases of gouty arthritis are seen in postpubertal males. In a very small group of patients the activity of the enzyme hypoxanthine guanine phosphoribosyl transferase (Fig. 8–37) is reduced to only a few per cent of normal (a total deficiency leads to the Lesch-Nyhan syndrome). In another group of patients overproduction of uric acid and hyperuricemia can be traced to an abnormally high activity of the enzyme phosphoribosylpyrophosphate (PRPP) synthetase (Fig. 8–38). In both of these situations, the increased availability of PRPP leads to an increase in the endogenous production of uric acid. Both enzymes are genetically transmitted as X-linked recessives. The increased availability of PRPP is the mechanism that also leads to hyperuricemia in type I glycogen storage disease; some of the reduction in uric acid clearance that occurs in GSD I may also be due to hyperlactic acidemia, which reduces the renal clearance of uric acid.

Whether or not a patient with elevated levels of uric acid in serum develops gouty arthritis largely depends on the severity and duration of hyperuricemia.

LESCH-NYHAN SYNDROME. Boys with this syndrome are usually normal at birth. The first abnormality consistently noted is a delay in motor development in the first few months of life. Later, extrapyramidal choreoathetoid movements appear, and hyperreflexia, ankle clonus, and spasticity of the legs develop. The most striking clinical abnormality is the dramatic, compulsive self-destructive behavior usually observed. Older children begin to bite and chew their fingers, lips, and buccal mucosa, leading to mutilation. It is not the result of inability to feel pain but of a compulsive urge that appears so irresistible that it is necessary to restrain the patients. Gouty tophi and gouty arthritis are also sometimes seen in older children with the Lesch-Nyhan syndrome. Tophi result from the accumulation of sodium urate crystals in subcutaneous and other tissues; they occur over the extensor surfaces of the elbows, knees, fingers, and toes.

In the Lesch-Nyhan syndrome, serum uric acid concentrations are commonly in the range seen in the adult with gout (10–12 mg/dL); there are marked increases in the production of uric acid and in its urinary excretion. There is an almost total absence of hypoxanthine guanine phosphoribosyltransferase activity in many tissues, including erythrocytes and fibroblasts. This enzyme is important to the "purine salvage" pathway, through which hypoxanthine and xanthine can be converted to nucleotides, inosinic acid, and guanylic acid (see Fig. 8–37). When this enzymatic pathway is not operative, PRPP synthetase activity increases and PRPP accumulates within the cell, giving rise to accelerated purine production de novo and to excesses of uric acid. The salvage pathway may be important in the synthesis of nucleotides within the brain; when this pathway is inactive, the brain may be unable to synthesize required nucleotides.

This syndrome is transmitted as an X-linked condition. Fibroblasts cultured from biopsies of skin of mothers of patients with Lesch-Nyhan syndrome consist of two cell populations, one normal and one deficient in the crucial enzyme, lending support to the Lyon hypothesis (see Sec. 7.24).

The gene for hypoxanthine-guanine phosphoryltransferase has been cloned; the introduction of this gene into patients with Lesch-Nyhan syndrome is currently being considered as an experimental, potentially curative treatment.

OTHER ABNORMALITIES OF URIC ACID METABOLISM. Hyperuricemia is commonly encountered in situations of a marked increase in cell number and cell destruction, as in myeloproliferative disease. The excessive amount of uric acid results from an increased intensity of degradation of nucleotides to purine end products (uric acid). In the treatment of acute leukemia or lymphoma masses, the sudden lysis of cells may provoke hyperuricemia and hyperuricosuria with clinical consequences (see Sec. 17.3).

Hyperuricemia may occur in any condition in which renal clearance is reduced. When the serum concentrations of β-hydroxybutyrate and acetoacetate are increased, as in starvation and diabetic ketoacidosis, there are elevations of serum uric acid concentrations related to reduction in renal clearance. Commonly used drugs, such as salicylates, in low doses may reduce renal clearance and produce hyperuricemia. Patients with Down syndrome regularly display modest hyperuricemia. All of these variables must be weighed in the interpretation of serum uric acid concentrations in children.

Hypouricemia due to an increase in renal clearance of uric acid occurs in proximal renal tubular diseases (e.g., Fanconi syndrome). In a clinically normal patient, hypouricemia has been caused by an isolated defect of renal tubular reabsorption of uric acid; the same situation exists in Dalmatian dogs. Hypouricemia is also a prominent feature of xanthinuria and nucleoside phosphorylase deficiency (see later).

Treatment of Hyperuricemia. Several approaches are used. Avoidance of foods high in purines (such as sweetbreads) is of modest benefit. Probenecid is effective in increasing uric acid clearance and may be used to treat hyperuricemia in patients with normal renal function. Allopurinol, an inhibitor of xanthine oxidase, is also widely used. In persons with no known enzymatic defect in purine biosynthesis, this drug

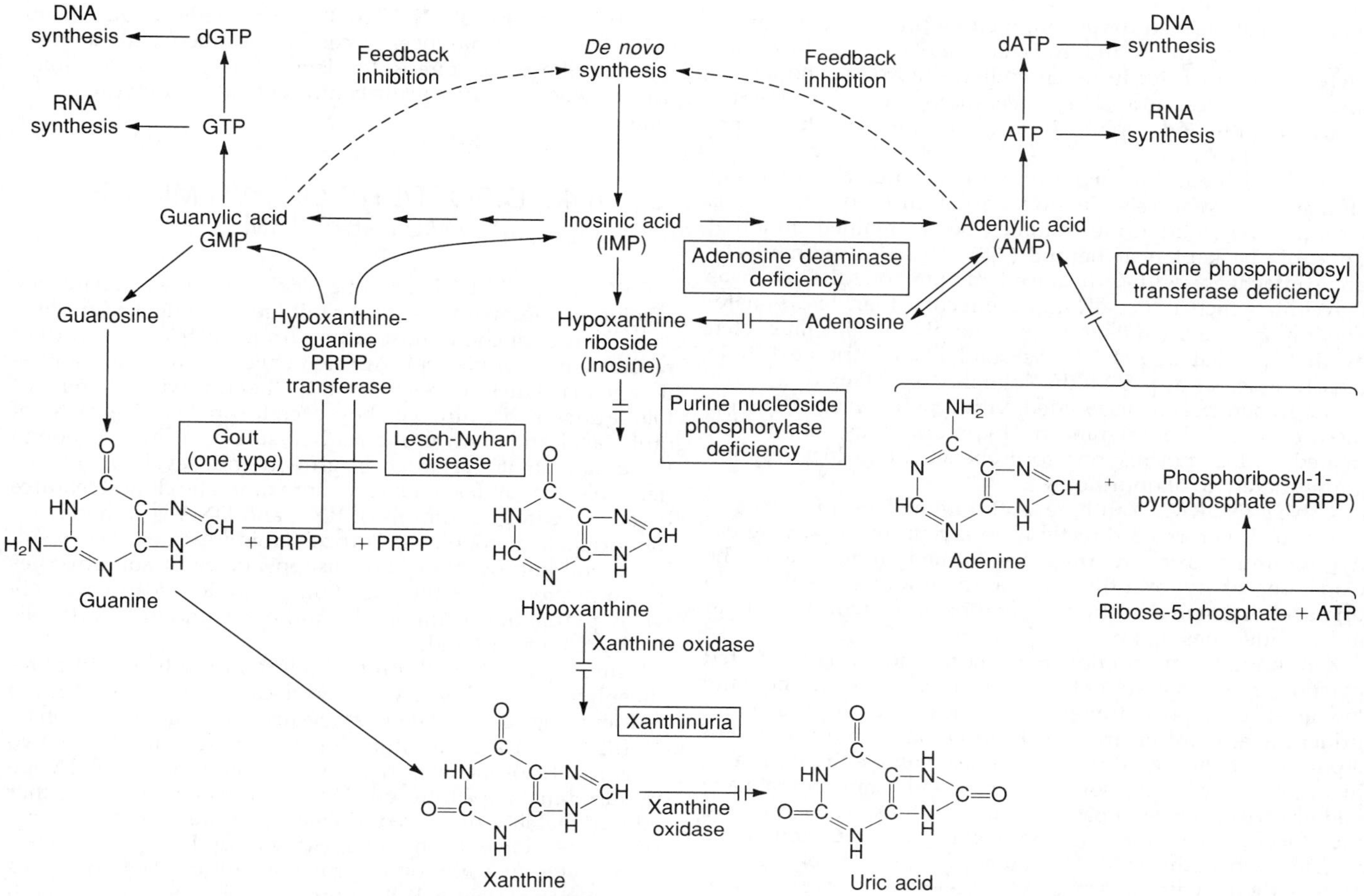

Figure 8–37. Pathways in purine metabolism and salvage.

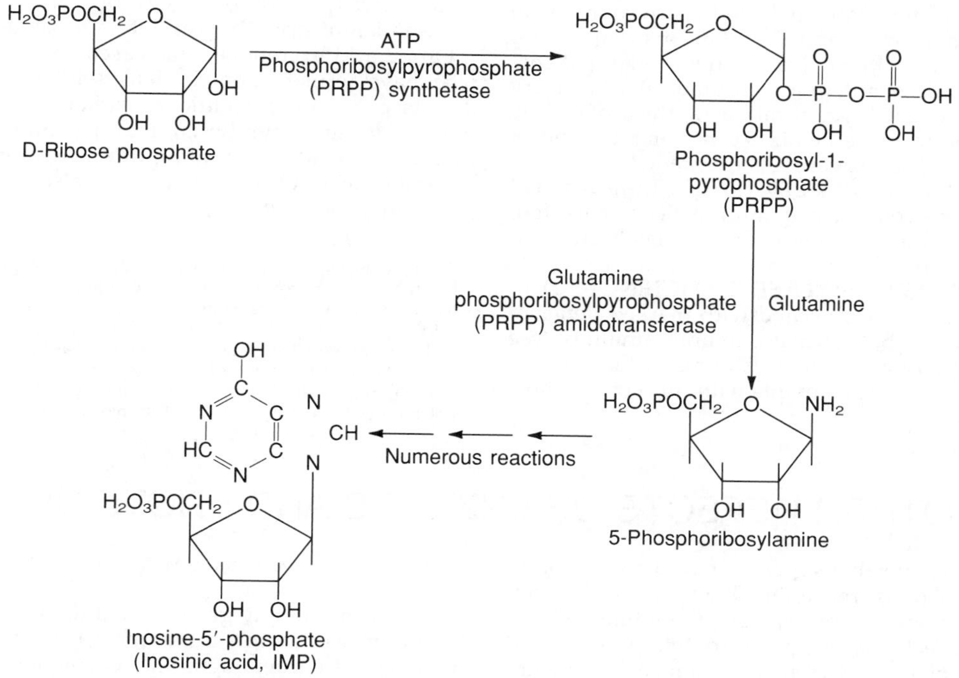

Figure 8–38. Early steps in the biosynthesis of the purine ring.

reduces total purine production, increases the excretion of the oxypurines (xanthine and hypoxanthine), and reduces the excretion of uric acid. In Lesch-Nyhan syndrome, allopurinol treatment reduces uric acid concentrations (and ameliorates gouty arthritis and tophi); there is no effect on the severe neurologic problems.

For any patient with hyperuricosuria, whether as a result of increased synthesis de novo or of drug therapy, it is essential that high urine volumes be maintained and that urine pH be kept near neutral (7.0). This can ordinarily be done effectively with a balanced mixture of salts, such as Polycitra, which is usually more effective than bicarbonate. The importance of adjusting the urine pH to 7.0 is illustrated by the fact that at pH 5.0 the solubility of uric acid is 15 mg/dL, whereas at pH 7.0 the solubility is 200 mg/dL.

The hyperuricemia associated with type I glycogen storage disease, like other significant hyperuricemias, should be treated; it does not respond to probenecid but does respond appropriately to allopurinol.

XANTHINURIA. Xanthine is the immediate precursor of uric acid. It is formed directly from certain purines, whereas hypoxanthine is an intermediary formed from others. The oxidations of hypoxanthine to xanthine and of xanthine to uric acid are mediated by xanthine oxidase, which is found in liver and intestinal mucosa (see Fig. 8–37).

Xanthinuria is uncommon. Serum uric acid levels in affected persons are virtually undetectable (0.1–0.8 mg/dL). There are low levels of hypoxanthine and uric acid in both plasma and urine; the amount of uric acid in urine falls almost to 0 with a purine-free diet. Xanthine is even less soluble than uric acid in urine; accordingly, some patients with xanthinuria have had *urinary calculi* composed of pure xanthine. The stones are radiolucent, except that slight radiopacity was reported in one instance when the stone contained 5% calcium phosphate. Some patients with muscular pain after exertion were shown to have deposits of xanthine crystals in muscles. Jejunal biopsies of affected patients show no activity of xanthine oxidase toward xanthine and only about 5% of normal activity toward hypoxanthine. (Xanthine stones have also been reported as a rare consequence of allopurinol administration.) The enzymes xanthine oxidase and sulfite oxidase require molybdenum as a cofactor. Patients have been recognized to have **molybdenum deficiency** and simultaneous deficiencies of xanthine oxidase and sulfite oxidase activities. All patients with xanthinuria should maintain a high fluid intake, dietary restriction of purines, and alkalinization of the urine. The solubility of xanthine in urine at pH 5.0 is 5 mg/dL, and at pH 7.0 it is 13 mg/dL. The prognosis is excellent.

ADENOSINE DEAMINASE DEFICIENCY. In nearly half of patients with severe combined immunodeficiency (SCID), a deficiency of adenosine deaminase activity has been demonstrated (see Sec. 11.16).

NUCLEOSIDE PHOSPHORYLASE DEFICIENCY. Deficiencies of this enzyme are associated with marked deficiencies of cellular immunity but normal humoral immunity (see Sec. 11.12). Central nervous system dysfunction has been a prominent clinical feature in six infants with nucleoside phosphorylase deficiency.

ADENINE PHOSPHORIBOSYLTRANSFERASE DEFICIENCY. A boy has been recently described with adenine phosphoribosyltransferase deficiency. The prominent clinical feature was urinary calculi composed of 2,8-dihydroxyadenine.

8.45 DISORDERS OF PYRIMIDINE METABOLISM

OROTIC ACIDURIA. Orotic acid is an intermediate metabolite in the synthesis of pyrimidines. Orotic aciduria is a rare disorder of children, resulting from a block in the further metabolism of orotic acid. Affected children have megaloblastic anemia that is unresponsive to therapy with vitamin C, folic acid, or vitamin B_{12}; they excrete up to 1.5 g/24 hr of orotic acid and form orotic acid crystals in urine. Although these patients are retarded in growth and development, the hematologic manifestations are more dramatic clinical features because vigorous synthesis of RNA and DNA is so necessary for normal hematopoiesis. Corticosteroid treatment may result in general improvement, but disappearance of abnormalities in the marrow or of the excretion of orotic acid occurs only when pyrimidine compounds found beyond the metabolic block are administered.

In most patients with orotic aciduria, orotidylic acid pyrophosphorylase and orotidylic acid decarboxylase activities are deficient (Fig. 8–39). The enzyme uridine 5′-monophosphate (UMP) synthase is a bifunctional enzyme with these two activities. In orotic aciduria, normal amounts of mRNA are produced that appear to code for a mutant enzyme with either reduced stability or altered kinetic properties. These enzyme deficiencies have been demonstrated in liver, leukocytes, erythrocytes, and fibroblasts grown in culture. Heterozygotes have approximately half the normal level of activities of both enzymes.

The administration of pyrimidine derivatives lowers the urinary excretion of orotic acid. This effect indicates that enzymes in the pathway leading to orotic acid synthesis are under feedback inhibition control. The hematologic response is due directly to the provision for DNA and RNA synthesis of essential material that cannot be made de novo.

Orotic acid excretion is increased in the urine of children who have primary genetic defects in the urea cycle. These defects result from additional carbamyl phosphate (usually utilized in urea synthesis) that is shunted into de novo pyrimidine synthesis, leading to an apparent overproduction of orotic acid. Orotic aciduria is also seen in nucleoside phosphorylase deficiency.

Willis R, Jolly DJ, Miller AD, et al: Partial phenotypic correction of human Lesch-Nyhan (hypoxanthine-guanine phosphoribosyltransferase-deficient) lymphoblasts with a transmissible retroviral vector. J Biol Chem 259:7842, 1984.

Winkler JK, Suttle DP: Analysis of UMP synthase gene and mRNA structure in hereditary orotic aciduria fibroblasts. Am J Hum Genet 43:86, 1988.

Zegers BJ, Stoop JW: Therapy in adenosine deaminase and purine nucleoside phosphorylase deficient patients. Clin Biochem 16:43, 1983.

OTHER DEFECTS OF ENZYMES AND PROTEINS

Some inborn errors of metabolism cannot be assigned naturally to systems, such as those involved in amino acid, carbohydrate, lipid, pigment, purine, or pyrimidine metabolism. These other defects involving the soluble proteins and formed elements of blood and certain proteins and enzymes of other organs or tissues will be discussed in the following sections.

The absence of any given protein in a specific individual or the presence of a protein that migrates abnormally by electrophoretic and chromatographic techniques is prima facie evi-

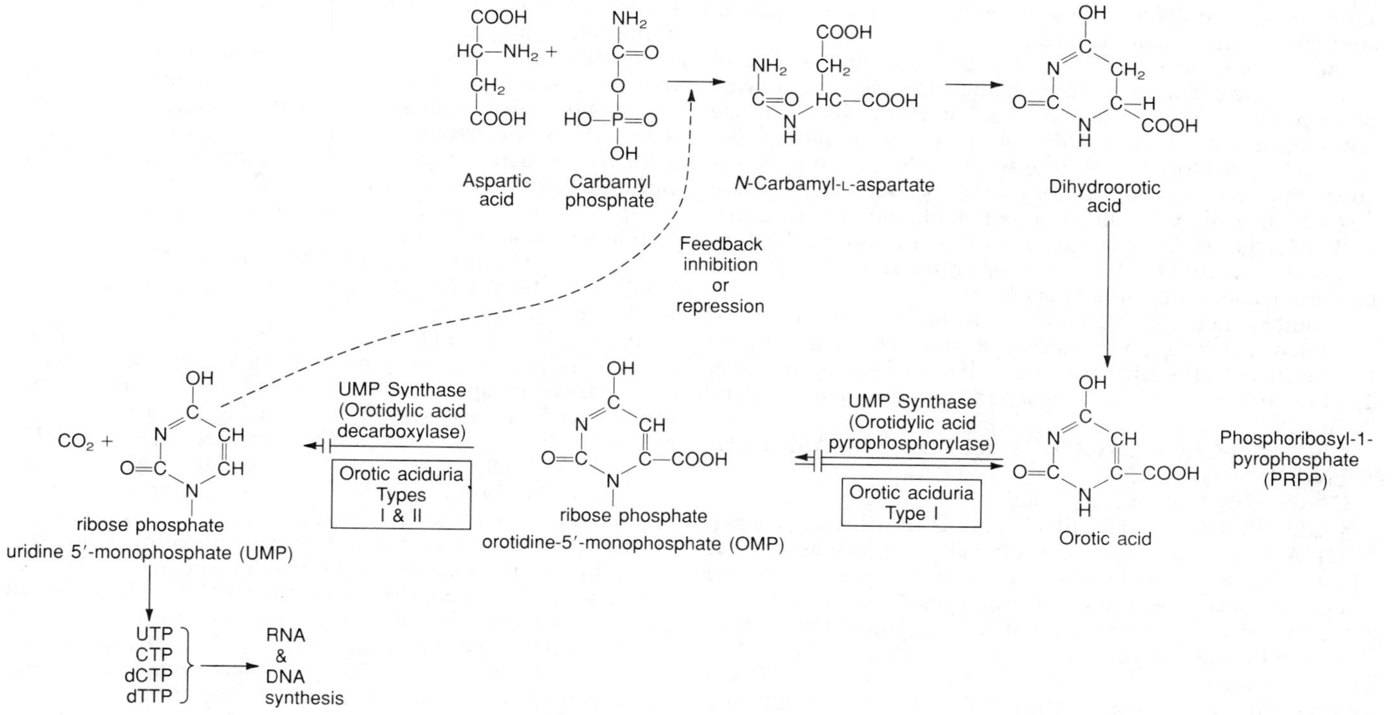

Figure 8–39. Pathways in pyrimidine biosynthesis.

dence of the existence of an inborn error of metabolism. Also, immunologic recognition systems depend upon the presence of a variety of cell-surface macromolecules under genetic control, for example, HLA, and the association of various markers with different diseases. Further, a large array of receptor proteins are found in and on cells that mediate hormonal action. Inborn errors of such protein moieties also occur.

8.46 DEFECTS IN PLASMA PROTEINS

ANALBUMINEMIA. Plasma albumin maintains the oncotic pressure of blood and serves as a vehicle for the transport of many normal blood constituents. Analbuminemia is a very rare, recessively inherited trait. Homozygotes have strikingly few symptoms that can be attributed to the lack of albumin. Some heterozygotes have intermediate levels of albumin. Usually no treatment is necessary. The lack of symptoms in analbuminemia may be the result of lifelong compensations in fluid dynamics that patients with such disorders as nephrosis or protein-losing enteropathy are unable to make.

HAPTOGLOBIN DEFICIENCY. Haptoglobin is an α_2-globulin that binds proteins. There are numerous phenotypic variations (polymorphisms) in the types of haptoglobins among normal persons, which are under genetic control. With severe hemolytic anemia, haptoglobin levels may be greatly decreased or absent. Healthy persons have been found who have no demonstrable circulating haptoglobin without apparent ill effect.

ABETALIPOPROTEINEMIA. See Sec. 8.34.

ANALPHALIPOPROTEINEMIA (TANGIER DISEASE). See Sec. 8.33.

ABSENCE OF TRANSFERRIN. Transferrin, or siderophilin (a β_2-globulin), is a plasma protein that has a prominent role in the transport of iron. Eighteen or more polymorphisms have been identified. The only recorded instance of a congenital absence of transferrin at birth involved a physically retarded girl with hepatomegaly, splenomegaly, and anemia sufficiently severe to require multiple transfusions. The anemia did not respond to any treatment. Iron was absorbed from the intestinal tract and transported to the tissues. Erythrocytes were hypochromic, and the marrow contained many immature erythroblasts. Liver biopsy revealed cirrhosis and siderosis. Antibodies to transferrin developed after multiple transfusions. Sudden death at 7 yr of age was attributed to hemosiderosis. Both parents had lower than normal amounts of transferrin, suggesting autosomal recessive transmission.

C1 ESTERASE INHIBITOR. See Sec. 11.25.

COMPLEMENT DEFICIENCIES. See Sec. 11.24–11.26.

α-ANTITRYPSIN PROTEIN DEFICIENCY. See Sec. 13.93.

TRANSCOBALAMIN II DEFICIENCY. Two different serum proteins bind vitamin B_{12}. One of these, transcobalamin I (an α-globulin), has been reported deficient in two siblings without clinical or hematologic sequelae. Deficiency of the other protein, transcobalamin II (a β-globulin), believed to be the primary B_{12} transport protein, was associated with severe megaloblastic anemia and neurologic manifestations in several infants. Partial deficiency in both parents indicated autosomal recessive inheritance. No abnormalities were found in reactions involving the coenzyme forms of vitamin B_{12}, homocysteine methyltransferase and methylmalonyl CoA mutase (see Sec. 8.7). Treatment consists of parenteral administration of large doses of vitamin B_{12}. Prenatal diagnosis using cultured amniocytes is possible.

8.47 DEFECTS IN PLASMA ENZYMES

PSEUDOCHOLINESTERASE. Pseudocholinesterase is found in plasma, liver, and neural tissue; its physiologic function is poorly understood.

Numerous presumably allelic forms of the altered enzyme are known, in some of which enzyme activity is reduced or absent. Homozygotes for each form and mixed heterozygotes are known. About 1 in 25 persons is heterozygous for one or another of these defects. Among whites heterozygote males are more common than females.

The one person in 3,000 who is homozygous for one of these genes is ordinarily asymptomatic. However, the enzyme participates in the destruction of a commonly used muscle relaxant, succinylcholine. Normally this drug is rapidly destroyed by pseudocholinesterase and therefore has a transient effect. Persons homoyzgous for mutant pseudocholinesterase degrade the drug very slowly or not at all, and apnea results, lasting for hours. Artificial respiration with endotracheal intubation is required. The period of apnea can be shortened by transfusion with normal plasma.

Another genetic alteration of pseudocholinesterase has been described that leads to increased enzyme activity and hence to resistance to the pharmacologic effects of succinylcholine. The human gene has been cloned and mapped to chromosome 3q21–q26.

LECITHIN-CHOLESTEROL ACYLTRANSFERASE DEFICIENCY. See Sec. 8.35.

CARNOSINASE DEFICIENCY. See Sec. 8.12.

γ-GLUTAMYL TRANSPEPTIDASE DEFICIENCY (see Fig. 8–11). A moderately retarded adult male with increased levels of glutathione in blood and urine has been shown to have a deficiency of serum γ-glutamyl transpeptidase, which catalyzes the first step in the degradation of glutathione. There was no other abnormality in amino acid excretion. This serum enzyme produced in the liver appears to be under different genetic control from that synthesized in the renal tubule and intestine.

HYPOPHOSPHATASIA. A variety of genetic abnormalities of alkaline phosphatase have been described that lead to a clinical spectrum of bony disorders, sometimes associated with a grave and fatal disorder in infancy (see Sec. 24.67).

ELEVATED ALKALINE PHOSPHATASE. Elevated serum alkaline phosphatase concentrations (2–10 times normal) usually indicate either liver or bone disease. However, increases (2–4 times normal) also occur in otherwise normal families owing to a genetic alteration, transmitted as an autosomal dominant trait.

8.48 DEFECTS OF PROTEINS IN OTHER TISSUES

MENKES KINKY HAIR SYNDROME. See Sec. 20.66.

MOLYBDENUM COFACTOR DEFICIENCY. Sulfite oxidase deficiency (see Sec. 8.5) and xanthinuria (see Sec. 8.44) have been associated with ocular abnormalities (dislocated lenses, Brushfield spots, and nystagmus), neurologic findings (tonic-clonic seizures), and mental retardation. The defect is an inability to form the molybdenum-containing cofactor whose presence is required for the activity of sulfite oxidase, xanthine dehydrogenase, and aldehyde oxidase. Treatment consists of restricting sulfur-containing amino acids and administering allopurinol.

MYOGLOBIN. Myoglobin, a heme protein found in muscle, is responsible for the intracellular transport of oxygen. Two variants of myoglobin have been identified, and the changes in amino acid sequence producing myoglobinopathies are analogous to the changes responsible for the hemoglobinopathies. Patients have been heterozygous for the normal and for the aberrant molecules. Neuromuscular diseases have not been found in these families.

Autosomal dominant myoglobinuria has been reported in three sucessive generations. Myoglobinuria was precipitated by prolonged exercise, fever, viral illnesses, and alcohol use. There was mild weakness, increased creatine kinase, and enlarged calf muscles. Acute renal failure and death occurred in one such patient.

Myoglobinuria may also occur in a number of disorders of muscle metabolism such as deficient phosphorylase activity (Sec. 8.40), deficient phosphofructokinase activity (Sec. 8.40), deficient phosphoglycerate mutase activity (Sec. 8.38), deficient lactate dehydrogenase activity (Sec. 8.38), and absent carnitine palmityl transferase activity (Sec. 8.15).

X-LINKED ICHTHYOSIS. See Sec. 23.17 for discussion of steroid sulfatase deficiency.

XERODERMA PIGMENTOSUM. See Sec. 23.15.

DYNEIN ARM DEFICIENCY. The absence of this specific ATPase is discussed in Sec. 14.53.

RECEPTOR PROTEINS. Most if not all communications between cells within the same organ or across organ systems are mediated by specific proteins found on the surface of the cell receiving the message. An increasing number of inborn errors involving receptor proteins have been described. The receptor for LDL is an example (see Sec. 8.25). Another example is the absence of functional receptor for the hormone vitamin D_3, which leads to vitamin D–dependent rickets type II (see Sec. 24.62). One form of diabetes mellitus is due to a defect in the specific receptor for insulin (see Sec. 8.53).

PANCREATIC ENZYME DEFICIENCIES. A number of patients have been described in whom malabsorption appears to result from a specific defect involving a pancreatic enzyme or proenzyme (see Sec. 13.75). They have none of the pulmonary or electrolyte abnormalities of cystic fibrosis.

A syndrome with inability to produce trypsin, lipase, and amylase in conjunction with hematologic evidence of bone marrow dysfunction has also been described (see Sec. 13.75).

Lipase Deficiency. Congenital absence of active pancreatic lipase leads to malabsorption of lipids and fatty (and sometimes malodorous) stools. It appears to be inherited in an autosomal recessive fashion. Treatment with pancreatin is effective.

Trypsinogen Deficiency. Severe malnutrition, growth failure, and hypoproteinemic edema resembling kwashiorkor are associated with lack of the ability to synthesize pancreatic trypsinogen. As a result, chymotrypsin and carboxypeptidase activities are also low because these enzymes need to be formed from the corresponding proenzymes by trypsin activity. Treatment with a protein hydrolysate diet and exogenous pancreatic enzymes is recommended. Human trypsin-1 gene has been assigned to chromosome 7q22–7qter.

Amylase Deficiency. Less-defined deficiencies of pancreatic amylase activity have been described in at least two children with malabsorption who did not have cystic fibrosis. One of the children also had reduced trypsin activity.

INTESTINAL ENTEROKINASE DEFICIENCY. Enterokinase, an enzyme secreted by the small intestine, initiates the reactions for the conversion of the pancreatic proenzymes to their active forms. Both the clinical findings in and recommended treatment for deficient enterokinase activity in children are identical to those described above for trypsinogen deficiency. Many if not all of the cases originally described as trypsinogen deficiency may be instances of enterokinase deficiency, with the lack of trypsin activity secondary to inability to form trypsin from trypsinogen. Almost all of the infants presented at birth with failure to thrive and diarrhea. Hypoproteinemia and edema are present in 50% of patients.

COLLAGEN METABOLISM. Collagen refers to a group of fibrous proteins that hold the body together and constitute about one fourth of its total protein. Collagens are the major structural proteins of skin, tendons, cartilage, and bone. Collagen contains large amounts of glycine, hydroxylysine, and hydroxyproline. Although the primary structure of the various collagens is under genetic control, the formation of collagen from procollagen and post-translation hydroxylation of lysine and proline, as well as the addition of various carbohydrate side chains, is controlled by a number of specific enzymes. A growing number of disorders involve collagen metabolism at one stage or another; among these are the numerous variants of both osteogenesis imperfecta (see Sec. 24.51) and Ehlers-Danlos syndrome (see Sec. 23.18), and Marfan syndrome (see Sec. 24.57).

MYOADENYLATE DEAMINASE DEFICIENCY. Patients with muscle cramps, easy fatigability, and muscle pain upon exercise who lack adenylate deaminase in striated muscle have been described. Symptoms may first occur at any time from infancy to adulthood. The enzyme normally converts AMP to IMP (inosine-monophosphate) with the liberation of ammonia. The IMP formed is then normally recycled back to AMP. In the absence of AMP deaminase activity this cycle is broken, and nucleotides are lost from the muscle cell, leading to impaired activity. No blood ammonia is produced upon ischemic forearm exercise, which distinguishes these patients from those with either McArdle disease (see Sec. 8.40) or deficient muscle phosphoglycerate mutase or muscle lactic acid dehydrogenase (see Sec. 8.40) who cannot produce lactic acid upon ischemic forearm exercise. Deficiency of myoadenylate deaminase may be the most common metabolic myopathy.

MITOCHONDRIAL MYOPATHIES. See also Sec. 21.25. Many patients with muscle weakness and lactic acidosis brought on by mild exercise do not have any of the disorders described either in Sec. 8.40 or immediately above. Land and colleagues have prepared a very useful resumé of the defects that exist in mitochondrial myopathies: (1) defects in substrate utilization, as in carnitine deficiency, carnitine palmityl transferase deficiency, and defects in various components of the pyruvate dehydrogenase complex; (2) defects in coupling of mitochondrial respiration to phosphorylation, as in Luft disease and mitochondrial ATPase deficiency; and (3) deficiencies of components of the mitochondrial respiratory chain, such as nonheme iron, protein, cytochrome oxidase, cytochrome b deficiency, and NADH-CoQ reductase. The range of clinical manifestations, even within a given biochemical variant, is wide. Some patients go for many years without any signs or symptoms, others become sick at an early age, and still others have been described with a form that is rapidly fatal in the neonatal period. The patients with mitochondrial myopathies may have partial or complete deficiencies limited to muscle or deficiencies with wide tissue distribution.

ACATALASIA. Catalase is found in most tissues, including the erythrocytes. Persons with a decrease of catalase activity in all tissues, to less than 1% of normal, can be detected through the demonstration that blood placed in contact with hydrogen peroxide turns brown and does not produce the oxygen bubbles usually seen. The disorder is heterogeneous; some instances appear to be mutations of the controller gene. In all instances the mode of inheritance is autosomal recessive; the heterozygote can be detected by quantitative catalase assays. Of the two main types, the Japanese variants have oral gangrene **(Takahara disease)**, whereas the Swiss variants are asymptomatic. A genetic strain of mice with acatalasia is known; catalase encapsulated in semipermeable membranes has been used successfully in their treatment.

STORAGE OF GLUTAMYL RIBOSE-5-PHOSPHATE. A mentally and physically retarded boy with seizures and progressive neurologic deterioration who died of renal failure at 8 yr of age had glutamyl ribose-5-phosphate stored in brain and kidney lysosomes. This compound is normally part of the linkage between histones and poly(ADP-ribose) and is thought to accumulate because of an X-linked deficiency of the enzyme ADP-ribose protein hydrolase.

ASPARTYLGLYCOSAMINURIA. The compound 2-acetamido-1 (β-L-aspartamido)-1,2-dideoxyglucose (AADG) is a substituted hexose that forms one of the linkage points between the carbohydrate moiety and the amino acid groups of many glycoproteins. Large quantities of urinary AADG (as well as other compounds containing AADG) have been found in some patients with mental retardation, petit mal seizures, or manic-depressive psychosis. Other patients have had vacuolated lymphocytes, facial and osseous features similar to those of the mucopolysaccharidoses, hepatomegaly, and lenticular opacities. The defect is in the lack of the enzyme, normally demonstrable in seminal fluid, that hydrolyzes AADG to glucosamine and aspartic acid. The lysosomal enzyme is deficient in liver, brain, and spleen. The structural gene for aspartylglucosaminidase has been assigned to chromosome 4q21–4qter.

ACID PHOSPHATASE DEFICIENCIES. Two groups of patients have been reported with either decreased or absent activity of lysosomal acid phosphatase. Patients with partial activity of this phospholipid-degrading enzyme have a clinical picture characterized by intermittent vomiting, hypotonia, lethargy, opisthotonos, terminal bleeding, and death within the 1st yr of life. Patients with total deficiency exhibit the same symptoms and die in infancy. Some investigators doubt the existence of this disorder. The enzyme involved is distinct from the normal acid phosphatase found in semen or elaborated by prostatic carcinoma.

TRUE CHOLINESTERASE. True cholinesterase, an enzyme essential for neural and muscular function, is also found in erythrocytes, where its function is unknown. There are no clinical manifestations associated with decreased erythrocyte cholinesterase activities.

R. RODNEY HOWELL

Frater-Shroder M: Genetic patterns of transcobalamin II and the relationships with congenital defects. Molec Cell Biochem 56:5, 1983.

Gregersen N: Fatty acyl-CoA dehydrogenase deficiency: Enzyme measurement and studies on alteration metabolism. J Inher Metab Dis 7(Suppl 1):28, 1984.

Land JM, Morgan-Hughes JA, Clark JB: Mitochondrial myopathy: Biochemical studies revealing a deficiency of NADH-cytochrome B reductase activity. J Neurol Sci 50 (1):13, 1981.

McKusick VA: Mendelian Inheritance in Man. Catalogs of Autosomal Dominant, Autosomal Recessive and X-Linked Phenotypes, 8th ed. Baltimore, Johns Hopkins, 1988.

Murray JC, Demopulos CM, Lawn RM, et al: Molecular genetics of human serum albumin; restriction enzyme fragment length polymorphisms and analbuminemia. Proc Natl Acad Sci 80:5951, 1983.

Pike JW, Dokoh S, Haussler MR, et al: Vitamin D_3-resistant fibroblasts have immunoassayable 1,25-dihydroxyvitamin D_3-receptors. Science 224:879, 1984.

Prockop DJ, Kivirikko KI: Heritable diseases of collagen. N Engl J Med 311:376, 1984.

Prody CA, Zevin-Sonkin D, Gnatt A, et al: Isolation and characterization of full length cDNA clones coding for cholinesterase from fetal human tissues. Proc Natl Acad Sci 84:3555, 1987.

Rhead WJ, Amendt BA, Fritchman KS, et al: Dicarboxylic aciduria: Deficient [1-14C] octanoate oxidation and medium-chain acyl-CoA dehydrogenase in fibroblasts. Science 221:73, 1983.

Roesel RA, Bowyer F, Blankenship PR, et al: Combined xanthine and sulfite oxidase defect due to a deficiency of molybdenum cofactor. J Inher Metab Dis 9:343, 1986.

Williams JC, Butler IT, Rosenberg HS, et al: Progressive neurologic deterioration and renal failure due to storage of glutamyl-ribose-5-phosphate. N Engl J Med 311:152, 1984.

DEFECTS IN HEME PIGMENT METABOLISM

This section describes defects of iron and heme pigments. The defects involving melanin and bilirubin are discussed elsewhere (see Sec. 8.3, 9.44, and 13.87).

8.49 THE PORPHYRIAS

This group of syndromes is characterized biochemically by errors in pyrrole metabolism and clinically by photodermatitis and visceral and neuropsychiatric complaints. Incidence is estimated to be 1 in 30,000 in the general population. Table 8–14 classifies the heritable forms according to the organ system in which the error in metabolism is localized: *erythropoietic* and *hepatic* forms are recognized. In some of the heritable forms onset of symptoms occurs during childhood, while in others onset does not occur until after puberty. Acquired or toxic porphyrias may occur at any time during life. Most of the porphyrias have a dominant mode of inheritance. Family studies and close surveillance through adolescence to identify cases in the latent stage are essential because most deaths occur during the late adolescent and early adult years and are attributable to delays in diagnosis that may lead to inappropriate and harmful therapy. Porphyrins should be determined in both urine and stool in all members; in cases of photosensitivity, measurements of erythrocyte protoporphyrin are also necessary. With early diagnosis, proper fluid and dietary therapy, and avoidance of contraindicated drugs, the prognosis for survival and symptomatic relief during acute visceral attacks is good. Enzyme diagnosis using blood, leukocytes, or skin is possible in most of the heritable forms of porphyria.

RELATION OF ABNORMAL HEME BIOSYNTHESIS TO DISEASE STATES. Heme is the prosthetic group of hemoglobin, myoglobin, catalase, peroxidase, and the cytochromes (including P450). Synthesis of heme is regulated by negative feedback control. It is formed via the metabolic pathway shown in Figure 8–40, which is common to all mammalian cells, each cell synthesizing its own heme for the formation of its own particular hemoproteins. The initial step, formation of δ-aminolevulinic acid (ALA),* is mediated by ALA synthase (see Fig. 8–40). This mitochondrial enzyme is inducible, and its availability is rate-limiting for the entire process.

Four basic porphyrin isomers are known and are designated as types I, II, III, and IV. Mammalian hemoproteins only contain type III porphyrin isomers. Protoporphyrin (PROTO) 9 is a type III isomer. Infinitesimal quantities of type I isomers are formed as byproducts of heme synthesis.

The basic genetic defects in the dominantly inherited forms of *hepatic porphyria* associated with neurovisceral manifestations are partial deficiencies (approximately 50%) of porphobilinogen deaminase in *acute intermittent porphyria* (AIP), coproporphyrinogen oxidase in *hereditary coproporphyria* (HCP), and *protoporphyrinogen oxidase* in *porphyria variegata* (PV). These deficiencies are found in all latent cases, but alone they are not associated with neurovisceral attacks. Table 8–14 shows characteristic pyrrole excretion patterns during exacerbation of symptoms in the various porphyrias. In AIP, HCP, and PV

*See Table 8–14 for key to abbreviations used in this section.

TABLE 8–14. Classification of Heritable Porphyrias

Classification	Deficient Enzyme	Inheritance	Age at Clinical Onset	Principal Symptomatology	Increased Erythrocyte Porphyrins*	Excess Excretion of ALA, PBG, Porphyrins*	
						Urine	*Stool*
Erythropoietic Porphyrias							
Congential erythropoietic porphyria (CEP)	Uroporphyrinogen III cosynthase	Autosomal recessive	Early infancy	Photosensitivity	URO COPRO‡	URO‡ COPRO‡	COPRO‡
Erythropoietic protoprophyria (EP)	Ferrochelatase	Autosomal dominant	Early childhood	Photosensitivity	PROTO	Absent	PROTO
Hepatic Porphyrias							
ALA dehydratase deficiency porphyria (ALADP)	ALA dehydratase¶	Autosomal recessive	Childhood	Neurovisceral	PROTO	ALA	—
Acute intermittent porphyria (AIP)	PBG deaminase	Autosomal dominant	Puberty§	Neurovisceral	Absent	ALA, PBG‖	—
Hereditary coproporphyria (HCP)	Coproporphyrinogen oxidase	Autosomal dominant	Childhood	Neurovisceral ± photosensitivity	Absent	ALA, PBG‖, COPRO	COPRO
Porphyria variegata (PV)	Protoporphyrinogen oxidase	Autosomal dominant	Puberty§	Neurovisceral ± photosensitivity	Absent	ALA, PBG‖, COPRO	COPRO, PROTO
Porphyria cutanea tarda (PCT)	Uroporphyrinogen decarboxylase	Variable†	Adult	Photosensitivity	Absent	URO 7-carboxylate porphyrin	ISOCOPRO
Hepatoerythropoietic porphyria (HEP)	Uroporphyrinogen decarboxylase	Autosomal recessive	Early infancy	Photosensitivity ± neurovisceral	PROTO	URO 7-carboxylate porphyrin	ISOCOPRO

*Only major diagnostic findings are listed.
†Autosomal dominant inheritance has been documented in some families but not in others.
‡Type I isomers.
§Occasional clinical onset before puberty.
‖In AIP, HIP, and PV urinary changes may be minimal or absent during remission of neurovisceral symptoms.
¶Also called porphobilinogen synthase.
ALA = δ aminolevulinic acid; PBG = porphobilinogen; URO = uroporphyrin; COPRO = coproporphyrin; ISOCOPRO = isocoporphyrin; PROTO = protoporphyrin.

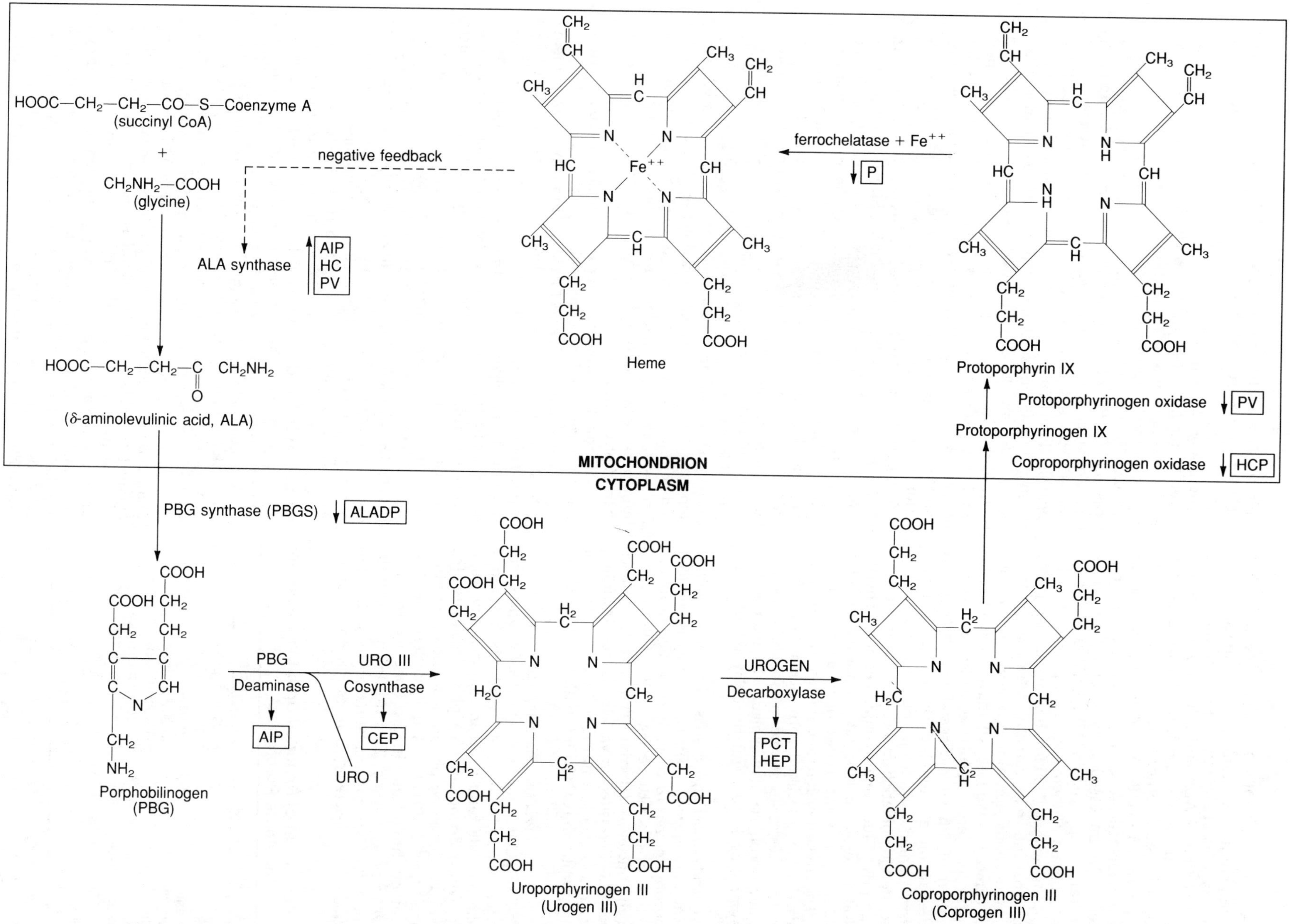

Figure 8–40. Intracellular organization of biosynthesis of heme. The initial and final steps in heme synthesis occur within the mitochondria. ALA is released in the cytoplasm. The metabolites formed in the cytoplasm are those found in the plasma and urine. ALA synthase is the rate-limiting enzyme. Only the fully reduced porphyrin intermediates Urogen III and coproporphyrinogen (Coprogen) III are utilized for heme formation. These colorless, unstable substances do not exhibit fluorescence. Oxidation stabilizes porphyrin molecules and renders them fluorescent. Those portions of Urogen and Coprogen not utilized for heme synthesis are oxidized to UROs I and III and COPROs I and III, and it is in this form that these porphyrins are usually detected in the tissues and excreta. PBG and ALA are also colorless and do not fluoresce; they are measured by chemical methods. Lead (Pb) inhibits PBGS and ferrochelatase (see Chapter 26).

excretion of ALA, PBG, and COPRO in urine may be normal or slightly elevated during remission of symptoms. About 90% of AIP heterozygotes are symptom free and may never show increased excretion of ALA and PBG in urine. Nevertheless, they are thought to be at risk for clinical attacks if exposed to certain drugs and other factors known to exacerbate hepatic porphyrias. Table 8–15 contains a partial list of porphyria-inducing substances. Clinical expression is uniformly associated with increased activity of hepatic ALA synthase, which can be induced in AIP, HCT, and PV by steroid hormones, certain of their metabolites, drugs (particularly those requiring hepatic P450 for their metabolism), and inadequate nutritional intake of carbohydrates and protein. With regard to endogenous steroid metabolism, the majority of patients with clinically manifest AIP have shown a 50% reduction in hepatic 5-α steroid reductase, which favors compensatory formation of 5-β steroid metabolites. Many 5-β steroid metabolites are more potent inducers of ALA synthase than their corresponding 5-α epimers. The same subtle alteration in hepatic steroid metabolism has also been demonstrated in HCP and PV. Glucuronide conjugates of porphyrin-inducing drugs and steroid metabolites do not induce ALA synthase, emphasizing the importance of maintaining good liver function. The hypertension and tachycardia seen in neurovisceral attacks are associated with increased levels of catecholamines. The roles of sex steroid metabolites as potent inducers of hepatic porphyria may explain why the onset of neurovisceral symptoms is so regularly delayed until after puberty.

There are two *erythropoietic porphyrias*. The basic genetic defect in *congenital erythropoietic porphyria* (CEP) is reduced activity of uroporphyrinogen III cosynthase, which results in excessive formation of URO I (see Fig. 8–40). URO I accumulates within the nuclei of defective erythroblasts, diffuses into the circulation, is deposited in various tissues, including teeth and bone, and is excreted in the urine as a mixture of URO I and coproporphyrin (COPRO) I, with URO I predominant.

Erythropoietic protoporphyria is characterized by excessive amounts of free PROTO 9 in marrow reticulocytes and circulating erythrocytes, in which it has a short half-life and readily diffuses into plasma, skin, and liver. In iron deficiency and lead poisoning, which do not involve photosensitivity, the metalloporphyrin zinc protoporphyrin is found in erythrocytes rather than "free" PROTO 9. Activity of ferrochelatase is diminished in erythroid cells in the bone marrow and possibly in liver in *protoporphyria*. This results in substantial accumulation of PROTO 9 in circulating erythrocytes and liver. Excess PROTO 9 is excreted in feces but not in urine.

TABLE 8–15. Partial List of Reported Drug Experience In the Acute Porphyrias*

Unsafe	Safe
Antipyrine	Acetaminophen
Barbiturates	Aspirin
Diphenylhydantoin	Atropine
Griseofulvin	Chloral hydrate
Meprobamate	Glucocorticoids
Primadone	Narcotic analgesics
Sulfonamide antibiotics	Penicillin and derivatives
Synthetic estrogens, progestins	Phenothiazines
Trimethadione	Succinylcholine
Valproic acid	Tetracycline

*For a more complete listing and discussion of unsafe, potentially unsafe, probably safe, and safe drugs for patients with AIP, HCP, and PV see the following reference: Kappas A, Sassa S, Galbraith RA, et al: The porphyrias. *In:* Scriver CR, Beaudet AL, Sly WS, et al (eds): The Metabolic Basis of Inherited Disease, 6th ed. New York, McGraw-Hill, 1989, p 1327.

Gallstones are fairly common. Hepatic disease is uncommon but may be severe and has been associated with a fatal outcome.

The urinary excretion of PBG and ALA does not normally exceed 3 mg/day. The qualitative Hoesch test for PBG (see later) is positive only with a pathologic excess of PBG. Porphyrins normally appear in the excreta in very small amounts: fecal COPRO and PROTO should not exceed 100 μg/g of dry feces/day; COPRO appears in urine at a rate of 2.2 μg/kg (1 μg/lb) of body weight/day. Infections and accelerated erythropoiesis cause a 2- to 3-fold increase in urinary COPRO; hepatitis (infectious and toxic), a 10- to 40-fold increase in urinary COPRO; and lead intoxication, a 10- to 40-fold increase in both ALA and COPRO in urine. Porphyria may cause up to 1,000-fold increases in pyrrole excretion. In acquired porphyria COPRO always exceeds URO in urine, but in the heritable forms the quantity of URO in urine usually exceeds that of COPRO if both are present. Increased fecal porphyrins virtually always indicate a heritable form of porphyria.

RELATION OF METABOLIC ERRORS TO CLINICAL MANIFESTATIONS. Photosensitizing Effects of Porphyrins. Some but not all the skin lesions of both erythropoietic and certain hepatic porphyrias are due to the photosensitizing effect of URO. Erythema, edema, and vesiculation of the exposed skin result when persons with increased uroporphyrinemia are irradiated with a combination of near-ultraviolet (400 nm) and infrared (2,600 nm) monochromatic lights. Protoporphyria is apparently unique among photosensitive dermatitides in that very brief exposure to sunlight can quickly cause intense pain and sensation of heat in the exposed skin. Repeated exposures to near-ultraviolet light lead to urticarial and chronic eczematoid lesions. All the heme precursors (see Fig. 8–40) have been injected into both healthy and porphyric human subjects without demonstrable adverse effect other than photosensitization.

Toxic and Experimental Hepatic Porphyria. Some drugs and chemicals used experimentally to produce hepatic porphyria (see Table 8–15) affect P450, an inducible hemoprotein with short biologic half-life and rapid turnover rate. Phenobarbital, for example, increases the requirement for P450; on the other hand, allylisopropylacetamide increases its destruction. Such findings suggest that patients with heritable hepatic forms of porphyria (AIP, HCP, PV) may not be able to adjust the metabolism of P450 to the effects of the drugs, insecticides, other chemicals, and nutritional and hormonal factors.

DIAGNOSIS AND MANAGEMENT OF THE PORPHYRIAS. Clinical Manifestations. Though the porphyrias are generally genetically determined and the basic metabolic errors are present from birth, clinical symptoms in patients with AIP and PV are rare before puberty in the hepatic forms. Three groups of clinical manifestations are recognized: cutaneous, visceral, and neuropsychiatric. Their onset is insidious, but once they occur, the complaints tend to run an undulating course throughout the remainder of the patient's life. The principal clinical syndromes and patterns of pyrrole excretion encountered in the porphyrias are summarized in Table 8–14.

Acute exacerbations of *dermal lesions* occur with exposure to sunlight. Visceral and neurologic complaints, which almost invariably occur together, may be precipitated by infection, menstruation, pregnancy, alcohol, barbiturates, and other agents (see Table 8–15). The skin lesions are bothersome and may be disfiguring, but the acute visceral and neurologic problems threaten life. The relative frequencies of various abnormal clinical findings encountered during an acute attack are shown in Figures 8–41 and 8–42; none are pathognomonic. Early diagnosis depends upon recognizing the sequence in which the clinical manifestations appear, intensify, and abate, and upon demonstrating excess pyrroles in the excreta. Colicky abdominal pain and varied neuropsychiatric symptoms

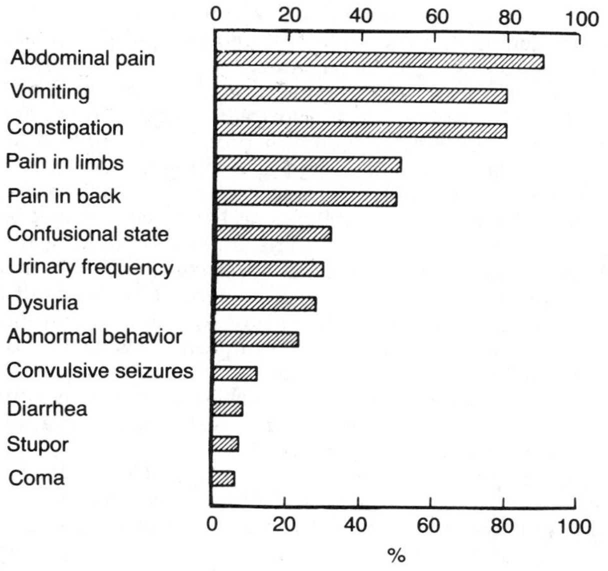

Figure 8–41. The acute attack of porphyria—relative frequency of symptoms. (Adapted from Eales L: Porphyria as seen in Cape Town, a survey of 250 patients and some recent studies. S Afr J Lab Clin Med 9:151, 1963.)

are the usual presenting complaints. Enzymatic assays must substantiate the diagnosis but unfortunately are not widely available.

Colicky abdominal pain, the initial symptom of an acute attack in most patients, is most frequently in the epigastrium or right iliac fossa but may be located anywhere in the abdomen or pelvis. There is considerable variation in its intensity; the pain tends to worsen in an undulating manner over a period of days. Severe colic may persist for hours, often causing the patient to writhe about or assume bizarre positions in bed. Vomiting and constipation develop shortly in all but the mildest attacks. Examination of the abdomen and pelvis reveals minimal signs, which seem insignificant compared with the patient's pain. Diffuse abdominal tenderness is usually present, but does not localize; rigidity and muscle spasm are rare. Leukocytosis and fever are often present. The acute visceral pain of porphyria has been confused with virtually every acute surgical condition of the abdomen, various painful gynecologic disorders, and "hysteria." In the absence of other features and objective findings characteristic of these other conditions, the presence of tachycardia and hypertension makes porphyria a likely diagnosis.

Pain, weakness, and paresthesia in back and limb muscles uncommonly occur as presenting complaints in the absence of abdominal pain. *Personality changes* are observed in most patients suffering from visceral attacks, but they are rarely the predominating features. Patients are variously described as depressed, nervous, hysterical, lachrymose, or "peculiar." These traits wax and wane with the severity of the pain. In severe colic, mental confusion, hallucinations, and disorientation are often present.

After the patient with acute intermittent porphyria or porphyria variegata has had an exacerbation characterized by abdominal pain, vomiting, constipation, tachycardia, and, in more severe cases, hypertension, the end of the attack may often be heralded by the return of blood pressure, pulse, and weight to normal.

The urine is usually colorless at first, although PBG is always present in high concentration and is diagnostic. If the attack progresses, and especially if barbiturates are given, the urine usually becomes red, increasing motor restlessness is noted, and neurologic manifestations, rarely present initially, soon appear. These neurologic manifestations take the form of unpredictable, spotty weakness or paralysis, with diminished or absent tendon reflexes, and pain and tenderness in the involved muscle groups. These signs are attributable to patchy demyelination of peripheral nerves. Muscle paralysis is an ominous sign. Ill-advised abdominal or pelvic surgery may be quickly followed by catastrophic paralysis and coma. Weakness and paralysis may persist for months after the other features of an acute attack have subsided. Death, when it occurs, usually results from quadriparesis or respiratory failure.

A profound disturbance in water and electrolyte homeostasis occurs with severe attacks of porphyria. The serum is hypotonic, with reduced concentrations of sodium and chloride (see Fig. 8–42). The urine is hypertonic, in part because of excessive loss of sodium, which is attributed to inappropriate secretion of antidiuretic hormone. The severity of neurologic injury may be related to the degree of hyponatremia. Hypocalcemia and hypomagnesemia may occur with or without tetany.

Burgundy red urine in the porphyric patient, due to the presence of URO, is a constant finding in patients with congenital erythropoietic porphyria and a frequent finding in patients with cutaneous manifestations of hepatic porphyria.

A variety of *dermal lesions* occur in porphyria. Exposure to sunlight produces vesicles, bullae, and edema on the exposed skin. These photosensitive lesions are prone to secondary infection and heal slowly, with chronic scars which become hyperpigmented. In some patients such lesions may also follow minor mechanical trauma and exposure to indoor sources of ultraviolet light. Macules, papules, eczematous plaques, and urticaria are also seen.

Nearly all patients with cutaneous forms of hepatic porphyria eventually have hypertrichosis and a violaceous hue to their skin. These changes develop insidiously over the years and are most prominent on the exposed parts of the body.

Differential Diagnosis. Porphyria must be included in the differential diagnosis of essential hypertension, hyperthyroidism, painful gynecologic disorders, "hysteria," psychosis, all surgical conditions of the abdomen, lead poisoning, and

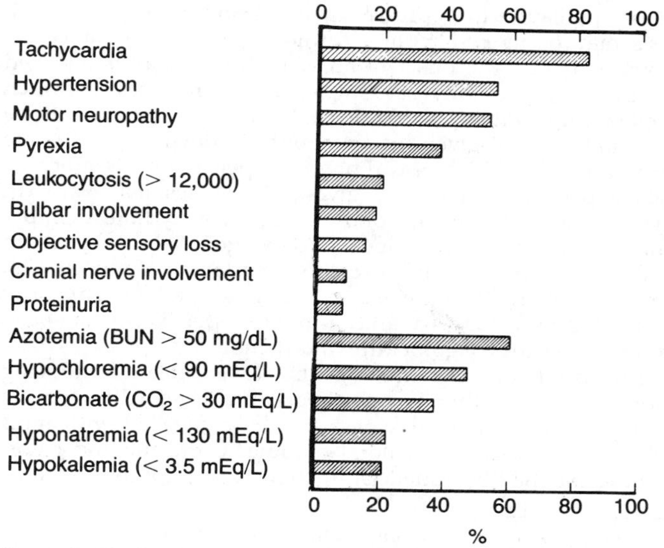

Figure 8–42. The acute attack of porphyria—relative frequency of signs and pertinent laboratory findings. (Adapted from Eales L: Porphyria as seen in Cape Town, a survey of 250 patients and some recent studies. S Afr J Lab Clin Med 9:151, 1963.)

hereditary tyrosinemia. Whenever a diagnosis of such surgical conditions as ulcer, gallbladder disease, or appendicitis cannot be made with confidence, a Hoesch test for PBG should be done prior to surgical exploration. Cutaneous porphyria should be included in the differential diagnosis of photosensitive dermatitides.

Laboratory Diagnosis. Accurate diagnosis requires examination of both urine and feces. PROTO is increased in erythrocytes in erythropoietic protoporphyria (EP), ALAD dehydratase deficiency porphyria (ALADP), and hepatoerythropoietic porphyria (HEP) (see Table 8–14). The excreta of patients and their relatives must be examined to establish the type of pedigree and to identify latent cases. When possible, enzymatic diagnosis should be carried out in all family members. In the hepatic porphyrias, pyrrole excretion patterns may vary according to the presence or absence of visceral symptoms. Porphyrin excretion may be increased 1,000-fold or more over the normal values. The red color imparted to urine by URO must be distinguished from that due to urates, bile, anthrocyanin (from beets), melanin, eosin, hemoglobin, or myoglobin.

The Hoesch test for PBG is simple, specific, and virtually always positive in acute visceral attacks. The test can be performed at the bedside as follows:

To 1 mL of Hoesch reagent (2 g of *p*-dimethylaminobenzaldehyde in 100 mL of 6 N hydrochloric acid) add 1–2 drops of *freshly voided* urine. An instantaneous cherry-red color at the top of the solution, which spreads throughout the solution on brief agitation, is specific for abnormally high amounts of porphobilinogen (PBG). False-positive results due to urobilinogen do not occur. Hoesch reagent is stable for 9 mo.

Newer simplified methods for measuring porphyrins in blood (primarily PROTO) should facilitate the clinical diagnosis of protoporphyria and possibly of other porphyrias associated with photosensitive dermatitis.

Treatment. Management of the neurovisceral attacks characteristic of AIP, HCP, PV, and probably ALADP is basically identical. Disturbances in water and electrolyte homeostasis are not usually seen in mild attacks, but they should be anticipated and the patient treated expectantly. When profound disturbances are present, restricting water and carefully replacing the sodium deficit may result in dramatic clinical improvement. Blood gases should be routinely monitored. Poor ventilation in depressed patients and respiratory paralysis may occur and require cardiopulmonary assistance. In some patients, the onset of an acute attack may be aborted by increasing carbohydrate intake. In severe cases, in which oral administration is not feasible, the patient should be hospitalized and given intravenous 10% dextrose to provide a minimum of 300 g of carbohydrate per 24 hr. As much as 500 g per 24 hr has been given. Responses may vary. In patients who do not respond to high-carbohydrate therapy, intravenous hematin* appears to be generally effective in reducing ALA and PBG excretion, curtailing acute attacks, and possibly reducing the severity of neuropathies. This drug is limited in availability and, although effective, it has been associated with coagulopathy and hemolysis.

Because many chemical agents are capable of inducing porphyria, drug therapy must be approached with extreme caution. Pain and restlessness can be controlled with morphine, diazepam, and chloral hydrate. Cortisone and chlorpromazine may be beneficial in some cases, without obvious effect in others, and deleterious in a few. Adequate caloric and nitrogen intakes should be restored as rapidly as possible.

Successful long-term management requires careful control of infections and absolute avoidance of alcohol and of the drugs listed in Table 8–15. A calorically adequate diet high in carbohydrate content, adequate in protein, and low in fat is beneficial. Many patients fear precipitating colicky episodes and indulge in food fads. In some women, attacks are clearly related to the menstrual cycle; some have been treated with ovulatory suppressants, androgens, and even oophorectomy, with apparent beneficial results. Oral contraceptives in the lowest effective dosage have been beneficial in some but not all cases of acute intermittent porphyria; they are contraindicated in pedigrees with dermal symptoms. Using the long-acting agonist of luteinizing hormone–releasing hormone may prevent cyclic attacks of AIP associated with the menstrual cycle. Persons with latent or manifest hepatic porphyria should wear "Medic Alert" bracelets.

Management of the dermal lesions of CEP, EP, HCP, porphyria cutanea tarda (PCT), and HEP requires avoidance of sunlight, trauma to the skin, and infections. Strict avoidance of alcohol and other precipitating factors is generally recommended. Oral administration of β-carotene to achieve a serum β-carotene level of 600–800 μg/dL is generally effective in improving dermal lesions. This serum level can usually be achieved with oral doses of 100–180 mg of β-carotene daily. Long-term oral administration of activated charcoal also has been associated with promising results. In patients with PCT, excessive stores of iron often occur and are best managed by phlebotomy.

Infants of mothers with hepatic porphyria may have increased pyrrole excretion during the neonatal period; this *passive porphyria* is not associated with any symptoms. The infant's excretion of pyrroles soon returns to normal.

Acquired Hepatic Porphyria

The acquired forms of hepatic porphyria are clinically indistinguishable from the hereditary cutaneous syndromes (see Table 8–14). Visceral manifestations are minimal or absent, and dermal features are usually less severe in the acquired disease, often being limited to hyperpigmentation and hypertrichosis. Acquired porphyria may occur as a rare complication of chronic alcoholism, cirrhosis, tumors involving the liver, and such systemic diseases as Hodgkin disease, disseminated lupus, and leukemia. Red urine due to the presence of URO is usually the clue leading to diagnosis.

Variants of Genetic Porphyria

Congenital erythropoietic porphyria is one of the rarest inborn errors of metabolism. Vastly increased amounts of URO I are found in bone marrow, circulating erythrocytes, plasma, urine, and feces. Lesser amounts of COPRO I are also found in the excreta. The excretion of other pyrroles is normal. The accumulation of URO I in the tissues (including the teeth) and the associated hemolytic anemia account for all the clinical manifestations of this disease. The photodermatitis of this disease is devastating, often causing severe permanent disfigurement. The excretion of urine that is burgundy red as passed, or becomes so upon exposure to light, begins at birth or shortly thereafter and continues for life.

Erythropoietic protoporphyria begins during childhood and continues through adult life. Symptoms that occur are pain, sensation of heat, and, following exposure to sunlight, two types of skin lesions, (1) an urticarial response that resolves without chronic dermal changes and (2) erythema and edema followed by an eczematous eruption on the exposed parts.

*Hemin for injection (Panhematin) is licensed and available on request from Abbott Laboratories, but it should be used only by physicians who are experienced in treating porphyria and practicing in hospitals where the necessary diagnostic and monitoring techniques are available.

This eczematous eruption is chronic rather than recurrent and leaves considerable scarring. These patients also have dull, opaque fingernails without lunulae. Increased amounts of PROTO 9 are always found in erythrocytes, and usually in feces.

Though the major symptoms are due to photosensitivity, a more important prognostic factor may be slowly progressive liver disease, culminating in cirrhosis and hepatic failure. Iron deficiency and other conditions stimulating erythropoiesis should be prevented, good nutrition maintained, hepatic function monitored, and hepatotoxic chemicals avoided.

Among the hepatic porphyrias the visceral, neurologic, and dermal manifestations and the pattern of pyrrole excretion are usually constant within a given pedigree. However, one pedigree varies considerably from another. Of these, *acute intermittent porphyria* and *porphyria variegata* are the most common. In kindreds with acute intermittent porphyria, visceral and neurologic attacks are most frequent and severe in females of childbearing age. In such kindreds, acute attacks often occur without obvious precipitating factors. The occurrence of visceral attacks before puberty is rare. The disorder has an autosomal dominant mode of transmission.

In kindreds with porphyria variegata, symptoms are most common between puberty and the 5th decade of life. Skin lesions are relatively more common in males, and acute visceral attacks are more frequent in females. Barbiturates often precipitate severe acute visceral attacks. There is an autosomal dominant mode of transmission; 50% of adult members of an affected family have a constant increase in excretion of porphyrins in the feces whether or not symptoms occur.

Hereditary coproporphyria is transmitted as an autosomal dominant disorder. Clinically, it resembles acute intermittent porphyria, except that symptoms may begin during childhood. They may be chronic "nervousness" and other psychiatric complaints, with or without recurrent abdominal pain. The unique biochemical feature of this disease is increased fecal excretion of COPRO III. Urinary COPRO III may or may not be increased. In the majority of cases severe visceral attacks are provoked by barbiturates and possibly by other anticonvulsant and tranquilizing drugs. Photosensitivity has been described in 30% of cases.

Patients with PCT can be divided into three groups: (1) those with sporadic disease, (2) patients with evidence of autosomal dominant inheritance, and (3) patients with disease due to exposure to halogenated aromatic hydrocarbons. In familial cases the defect is partial deficiency of uroporphyrinogen decarboxylase in liver, erythrocytes, and possibly in other tissues. The disease may be clinically manifest during childhood. Offending environmental agents must be identified and removed in chemically induced cases of PCT.

A dual form of acute porphyria (Chester porphyria) has been identified in a large family in which a dual enzyme deficiency occurred with reduced activity of both porphobilinogen deaminase, as in AIP, and protoporphyrinogen oxidase, as in PV. Two rare forms of porphyria with autosomal recessive modes of transmission also have been identified. ALADP resembles AIP clinically. HEP probably results from a homozygous defect in uroporphyrinogen decarboxylase activity. This disorder is clinically indistinguishable from CEP and is characterized by excessive synthesis of URO in both liver and bone marrow. Activated charcoal therapy, which has been reported to be effective in patients with CEP, may also prove effective in those with HEP.

8.50 HEREDITARY METHEMOGLOBINEMIAS

The iron of both oxygenated and deoxygenated hemoglobin is normally in the ferrous state, which is essential for its oxygen-transporting function. Oxidation of hemoglobin iron to the ferric state yields methemoglobin, which is nonfunctional and imparts a chocolate hue to the blood; in sufficient concentration it causes cyanosis. The blood of healthy persons contains methemoglobin, but the intraerythrocytic methemoglobin-reducing system maintains its concentration at less than 2% of the total hemoglobin. "Normal" methemoglobin has a characteristic spectral absorption band at 632 nm, which is abolished by treating the blood sample with cyanide. This test is specific for assaying methemoglobin produced by exposure to certain chemicals such as aniline dyes but yields erroneous results when hemoglobin M type pigments are present. Hemoglobin electrophoresis after oxidation with potassium ferricyanide is needed to identify the M hemoglobins. Among familial methemoglobinemias both recessive and dominant patterns of inheritance are recognized; each form involves a distinct metabolic error.

HEREDITARY METHEMOGLOBINEMIA WITH DEFICIENCY OF NADH CYTOCHROME b5 REDUCTASE. There are four types of enzymopenic hereditary methemoglobinemias due to deficiency of cytochrome b5 reductase. All have a recessive mode of inheritance. In type I, the most frequent of these rare disorders, the deficiency of cytochrome b5 reductase is limited to erythrocytes, and cyanosis is the only consequence. Type II is a much more severe and lethal disorder, occurring in about 10–15% of patients with hereditary methemoglobinemia. In this disorder the deficiency of cytochrome b5 reductase is generalized to all tissues. In addition to methemoglobinemia there is a progressive neurologic disorder appearing before 1 yr of age and associated with severe mental retardation, microcephaly, retarded growth, attacks of bilateral athetoid movements, strabismus, opisthotonos, and generalized hypertonia. In type III (hematopoietic cytochrome b5 reductase deficiency), the deficiency is demonstrable in erythrocytes, platelets, lymphocytes, and granulocytes. Clinically, cyanosis is the only manifestation. Type IV, although not clearly defined, appears to involve a lesser deficiency of erythrocyte cytochrome b5 and is associated with chronic cyanosis.

Clinically, cyanosis may vary in intensity with season and diet. The time of onset of cyanosis also varies; in some patients it appears at birth, in others as late as adolescence. Despite the fact that up to 50% of the total circulating hemoglobin may be in the form of nonfunctional methemoglobin, little or no cardiorespiratory distress occurs except on exertion. These comments apply to types I, III, and IV but not to type II, in which neurologic dysfunction, mental retardation, and early death occur in addition to the cyanosis.

Daily oral *treatment* with ascorbic acid (200–500 mg in divided doses) gradually reduces the quantity of methemoglobin to about 10% of the total pigment and alleviates the cyanosis as long as therapy is continued. Chronic high doses of ascorbic acid have been associated with hyperoxaluria and renal stone formation. Methylene blue given intravenously (1–2 mg/kg) promptly eliminates both methemoglobin and cyanosis, and this effect can be maintained by the daily oral administration of methylene blue (3–5 mg/kg).

HEREDITARY METHEMOGLOBINEMIA ASSOCIATED WITH ABNORMAL METHEMOGLOBINS (Hemoglobin M Diseases). The dominantly transmitted forms of methemoglobinemia are collectively known as the hemoglobin M diseases. After all the hemoglobin pigment in a blood sample is oxidized to methemoglobin by treatment with potassium ferricyanide, the abnormal methemoglin M type pigments can be separated from normal methemoglobin by means of starch gel electrophoresis. The several hemoglobin M pigments have substitutions of abnormal amino acid residues in the globin chains. Dissimilar substitutions have been found in different pedigrees. This situation is analogous to that of other hemoglobinopathies (hemoglobin S, hemoglobin C, and others).

Among the several hemoglobin M pedigrees examined, five different hemoglobin M pigments have been identified: HbM_B (abnormal α chain), HbM_S (abnormal β chain), HbM_{M-1} (abnormal β chain), HbM_{M-2}, and HbM_1 (abnormal α chain). Four of the five M hemoglobins result from the substitution of tyrosine for either the proximal or distal histidine residues in close proximity to the prosthetic heme group. It is likely that this substitution stabilizes the iron atom in the oxidized state as methemoglobin. This makes this form of methemoglobin resistant to reduction by both enzymes and reducing agents and so may explain the variable response of patients to ascorbic acid and methylene blue as well as the abnormal spectral properties and differing responses to cyanide treatment of the various hemoglobin M pigments. The entity previously described as "congenital sulfhemoglobinemia" may fall within the hemoglobin M disease group.

Clinically, methemoglobinemia of the hemoglobin M type should be suspected when family studies suggest an autosomal dominant pattern of inheritance and when the blood of the cyanotic patient does not show the absorption band at 632 nm, which is characteristic of normal methemoglobin. The patient's methemoglobin may or may not react with cyanide to yield a normal cyanomethemoglobin absorption curve. This finding varies with the pedigree. In these diseases the quantity of methemoglobin does not exceed 25% of the total hemoglobin; the cyanosis, although persistent from early infancy, is not associated with any disability. There may be a compensatory polycythemia. Affected members of some pedigrees do not respond to ascorbic acid or methylene blue (hemoglobin M_B and hemoglobin M_{M-1}). Fortunately, alleviation of cyanosis is not essential in the hemoglobin M diseases.

8.51 HEMOCHROMATOSIS

The term hemochromatosis refers to impairment of the structure and function of organs (primarily liver, pancreas, heart, gonads, skin, and joints) due to excessive storage of iron, mainly as hemosiderin in the parenchymal cells. *Idiopathic hemochromatosis* has an autosomal recessive mode of inheritance, with full clinical disease limited largely to adult males. The nature of the metabolic defect is unknown. Untreated cases eventually exhibit the classic triad of hepatic cirrhosis, slate or bronze pigmentation of the skin, and diabetes mellitus. Demonstration of massive iron overload distributed in parenchymal rather than in reticuloendothelial cells through elevated serum iron, saturated iron-binding capacity, highly elevated serum ferritin, and needle biopsy of the liver establishes the diagnosis. All siblings of index cases should have HLA typing and the above blood studies to identify heterozygotes and homozygotes in the latent stage, since early detection improves prognosis. Alcohol and excessive iron intake should be avoided. Excess iron stores are removed preferably by repeated phlebotomy.

A number of chronic anemias requiring repeated transfusions are associated with *secondary hemochromatosis.* In such cases chelation therapy with deferoxamine in conjunction with other measures to minimize iron intake is beneficial.

J. JULIAN CHISOLM, JR.

Anderson KE, Spitz IM, Sassa S, et al: Prevention of cyclical attacks of acute intermittent porphyria with a long-acting agonist of luteininizing hormone–releasing hormone. N Engl J Med 311:643, 1984.

Becker DM, Kramer S: The neurological manifestations of porphyria: A review. Medicine 56:411, 1977.

Bloomer JR, Phillips MJ, Davidson DL, et al: Hepatic disease in erythropoietic protoporphyria. Am J Med 58:869, 1975.

Bothwell TH, Charlton RW, Motulsky AG: Hemochromatosis. *In:* Scriver CR, Beaudet AL, Sly WS, et al (eds): The Metabolic Basis of Inherited Disease, 6th ed. New York, McGraw-Hill, 1989, p 1433.

Fujita H, Sassa S, Lundgren J, et al: Enzymatic defect in a child with hereditary hepatic porphyria due to homozygous delta-aminolevulinic acid dehydratase deficiency: Immunochemical studies. Pediatrics 80:880, 1987.

Hellman ES, Tschudy DP, Bartter FC: Abnormal electrolyte and water metabolism in acute intermittent porphyria. Am J Med 32:734, 1962.

Jaffe ER, Hultquist DE: Cytochrome b5 reductase deficiency and enzymopenic hereditary methemoglobinemia. *In:* Scriver CR, Beaudet AL, Sly WS, et al (eds): The Metabolic Basis of Inherited Disease, 6th ed. New York, McGraw-Hill, 1989, p 2267.

Kappas A, Sassa S, Galbraith RA, et al: The porphyrias. *In:* Scriver CR, Beaudet AL, Sly WS, et al (eds): The Metabolic Basis of Inherited Disease, 6th ed. New York, McGraw-Hill, 1989, p 1305.

Lamon J, With TK, Redeker AG: The Hoesch test: Bedside screening for urinary porphobilinogen in patients with suspected porphyria. Clin Chem 20:1438, 1974.

Lamon JM, Frykholm BC, Hess RA, et al: Hematin therapy for acute porphyria. Medicine 58:252, 1979.

McColl KE, Moore MR, Thompson GG, et al: Chester porphyria: Biochemical studies of a new form of acute porphyria. Lancet 2:796, 1985.

Mathews-Roth MM, Pathak MA, Fitzpatrick TB, et al: Beta-carotene therapy for erythropoietic protoporphyria and other photosensitivity diseases. Arch Dermatol 113:1229, 1977.

Pimstone NR, Gandhi SN, Mukerji SK: Therapeutic efficacy of oral charcoal in congenital erythropoietic porphyria. N Engl J Med 316:390, 1987.

Sassa S, Solish G, Levere RD, et al: Studies in porphyria, IV. Expression of the gene defect of acute intermittent porphyria in cultured human skin fibroblasts and amniotic cells: Prenatal diagnosis of the porphyric trait. J Exp Med 142:722, 1975.

Toback AC, Sassa S, Poh-Fitzpatrick MB, et al: Hepatoerythropoietic porphyria: Clinical, biochemical and enzymatic studies in a three generation family lineage. N Engl J Med 316:645, 1987.

Tschudy DP, Valsamis M, Magnussen CR: Acute intermittent porphyria: Clinical and selected research aspects. Ann Intern Med 81:851, 1975.

Weatherall DJ, Clegg JB, Higgs DR, et al: The hemoglobinopathies. *In:* Scriver CR, Beaudet AL, Sly WS, et al (eds): The Metabolic Basis of Inherited Disease, 6th ed. New York, McGraw-Hill, 1989, p 2304.

DIABETES MELLITUS

Diabetes mellitus is a syndrome of disturbed energy homeostasis caused by a deficiency of insulin or of its action and resulting in abnormal metabolism of carbohydrate, protein, and fat. It is the most common endocrine-metabolic disorder of childhood and adolescence with important consequences on physical and emotional development. Individuals affected by insulin-dependent diabetes confront serious burdens that include an absolute daily requirement for exogenous insulin, the need to monitor their own metabolic control, and the need to pay constant attention to dietary intake. Morbidity and mortality stem from metabolic derangements and from long-term complications that affect small and large vessels and result in retinopathy, nephropathy, neuropathy, ischemic heart disease, and arterial obstruction with gangrene of the extremities. The acute clinical manifestations can be fully understood in the context of current knowledge about the secretion and action of insulin; genetic and other etiologic considerations point to autoimmune mechanisms as factors in the genesis of type I diabetes, and there is an emerging consensus that the long-term complications are related to metabolic disturbances. These considerations form the basis of therapeutic approaches to this disease.

8.52 CLASSIFICATION

Diabetes mellitus is not a single entity but rather a heterogeneous group of disorders in which there are distinct genetic patterns as well as other etiologic and pathophysiologic mechanisms that lead to impairment of glucose tolerance. The National Diabetes Data Group has proposed a classification of diabetes and other categories of glucose intolerance based on contemporary knowledge. This classification has been endorsed and accepted by various diabetes associations throughout the world as well as by pediatric investigators (Table 8–16). Three major forms of diabetes and several forms of carbohydrate intolerance have been identified.

TYPE I DIABETES (Juvenile-Onset Diabetes). This condition is characterized by severe insulinopenia and dependence on exogenous insulin to prevent ketosis and to preserve life; it is therefore also termed insulin-dependent diabetes mellitus (IDDM). The natural history of this disease indicates that there are preketotic, noninsulin-dependent phases both before and after the initial diagnosis. Although the onset occurs predominantly in childhood, it may come at any age. Hence, such terms as juvenile diabetes, ketosis-prone diabetes, and brittle diabetes should be abandoned in favor of type I diabetes or IDDM. Type I diabetes is clearly distinct by virtue of its association with certain histocompatibility antigens (HLA), the presence of circulating antibodies to cytoplasmic and cell-surface components of islet cells, antibodies to insulin in the absence of prior exposure to exogenous injection of insulin, lymphocytic infiltration of islets early in the disease, and other autoimmune diseases. With few exceptions, diabetes in children is insulin dependent and fits the type I category.

TYPE II DIABETES. Persons in this subclass (formerly known as adult-onset diabetes, maturity-onset diabetes [MOD], or stable diabetes) are not insulin dependent and only infrequently develop ketosis; some may, however, need insulin for correction of symptomatic hyperglycemia, and ketosis may develop in some during severe infections or other stress.

Serum concentration of insulin may be normal or moderately depressed; it is generally less when compared to that in controls matched for weight, age, and stage of puberty. In the majority of instances, the onset of noninsulin-dependent diabetes mellitus occurs after age 40, but it may occur at any age. It is rare in childhood and adolescence, when it may become manifest as abnormal glucose tolerance, usually in obese individuals. There appears to be adequate secretion of insulin, but there is also resistance to it, and in some individuals it may represent slowly evolving type I diabetes mellitus. As an initial approach, weight reduction is indicated in children who are obese. Abnormal carbohydrate tolerance may also occur in children who have a strong family history of type II diabetes in a pattern suggestive of dominant inheritance; this pattern of diabetes has been termed MODY (maturity-onset diabetes of the young), and it may require treatment with insulin. Most important, in this type of diabetes there is no association with HLAs, autoimmunity, and/or islet cell antibodies.

SECONDARY DIABETES. This subclass contains a variety of types of diabetes, for some of which the etiologic relationship is known. Examples include diabetes secondary to exocrine pancreatic diseases, such as cystic fibrosis; endocrine diseases other than pancreatic diseases (e.g., Cushing syndrome); and ingestion of certain drugs or poisons (e.g., the rodenticide Vacor). Certain genetic syndromes, including those with abnormalities of the insulin receptor, also are included in this category. There are no associations with HLAs, autoimmunity, or islet cell antibodies among the entities in this subdivision.

For all types of diabetes, many believe that the criterion of a fasting blood glucose level in excess of 140 mg/dL is too stringent because normal children do not exceed a fasting blood glucose value of 120 mg/dL.

8.53 TYPE I DIABETES MELLITUS

(Insulin-Dependent Diabetes [IDD]; Juvenile-Onset Diabetes)

EPIDEMIOLOGY. Surveys in the United States indicate that the prevalence of diabetes among school-age children is about 1.9 in 1,000. The frequency, however, is highly correlated with increasing age; available data indicate a range of 1 in 1,430 children at 5 yr of age to 1 in 360 children at 16 yr. Data on prevalence and incidence in relation to racial or ethnic backgrounds indicate a range of nearly 30 new cases annually in 100,000 population in Finland to 0.8 in 100,000 in Japan (Fig. 8–43). Among American blacks the occurrence of insulin-dependent diabetes has been reported to be only 20–30% of that seen in American whites, although it may be as high as two thirds. These observations have implications for genetic counseling (see later). The annual incidence in the United States is about 12–15 new cases per 100,000 of the childhood population (see Fig. 8–43). Males and females are almost equally affected; there is no apparent correlation with socioeconomic status. Peaks of presentation occur in two age groups: at 5–7 yr of age and at the time of puberty. The first peak corresponds to the time of increased exposure to infectious agents coincident with the beginning of school; the latter to the pubertal growth spurt induced by gonadal steroids and increased pubertal growth hormone secretion, which antag-

TABLE 8–16. Summary of Classification of Diabetes Mellitus in Children and Adolescents*

Classification	Criteria
Diabetes mellitus	
1. Insulin-dependent (IDDM, type I)	Typical manifestations: glucosuria, ketonuria, random plasma glucose (PG) >200 mg/dL
2. Noninsulin-dependent (NIDDM, type II)	FPG >140 mg/dL and 2-hr value >200 mg/dL during OGTT on more than one occasion and in absence of precipitating factors
3. Other types	Type I or II criteria in association with certain genetic syndromes (including cystic fibrosis), other disorders, and drugs (see text)
Impaired glucose tolerance (IGT)	FPG <140 mg/dL with 2-hr value >140 mg/dL during OGTT
Gestational diabetes (GDM)	Two or more of following abnormalities during OGTT: FPG >105 mg/dL; 1 hr, >190 mg/dL; 2-hr, >165 mg/dL; 3 hr, >145 mg/dL
Statistical risk classes	
1. Previous abnormality of glucose tolerance	Normal OGTT following a previous abnormal one, spontaneous hyperglycemia or gestational diabetes
2. Potential abnormality of glucose tolerance	Genetic propensity (e.g., identical nondiabetic twin of a diabetic sibling); islet cell antibodies

*Proposed by National Diabetes Data Group (Diabetes 28:1039, 1979) and endorsed by various diabetes associations worldwide.
PG = plasma glucose; FPG = fasting plasma glucose; OGTT = oral glucose tolerance test.

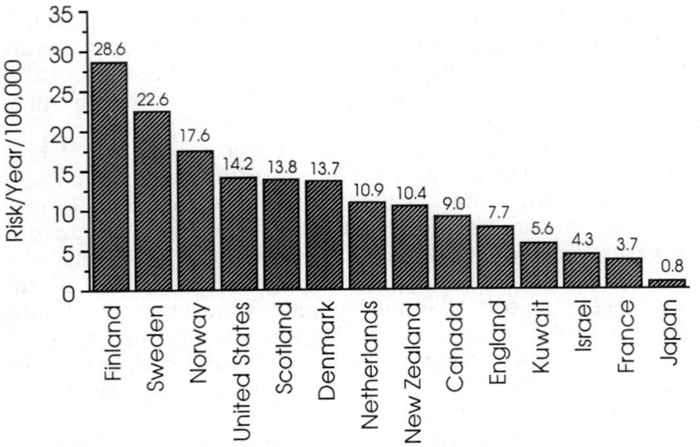

Figure 8–43. Incidence of insulin-dependent diabetes mellitus by country. (Adapted from LaPorte R, et al: Preventing insulin dependent diabetes mellitus: The environmental challenge. Br Med J 295:479, 1987.)

onize insulin action, and to the emotional stresses accompanying puberty. These possible cause-and-effect relationships remain to be proved. The prevalence and incidence of insulin-dependent diabetes in childhood in the United States and elsewhere may reflect the distribution of susceptibility genes encoded on the DQ β chain of the HLA system.

Seasonal and long-term cyclic variations occur in the incidence of insulin-dependent diabetes mellitus. Newly recognized cases appear with greater frequency in the autumn and winter months in the Northern and Southern Hemispheres. Seasonal variations are most apparent in the adolescent years. Attempts to link a pattern of long-term cyclicity with the incidence of mumps or other viral infections when allowance was made for a 4-yr time lag have not been successful. There is, however, a definite increased incidence of diabetes in children with congenital rubella. These associations with viral infections suggest a potential role for viruses as direct or indirect triggering mechanisms in the etiology of diabetes.

ETIOLOGY AND PATHOGENESIS. The basic cause of the initial clinical findings in this predominant form of diabetes in childhood is the sharply diminished secretion of insulin. Although basal insulin concentrations in plasma may be normal in newly diagnosed patients, insulin production in response to a variety of potent secretagogues is blunted and usually disappears over a period of months to years, rarely exceeding 5 yr. In certain individuals considered at high risk for the development of type I diabetes, such as the nonaffected identical twin of a diabetic, a progressive decline in insulin-secreting capacity has been noted for months to years before the clinical appearance of symptomatic diabetes, which usually becomes manifest when insulin-secreting reserve is 20% or less of normal (Fig. 8–44).

The mechanisms that lead to failure of pancreatic β-cell function increasingly point to the possibility of autoimmune destruction of pancreatic islets in predisposed individuals. Type I diabetes has long been known to have an increased prevalence among persons with such disorders as Addison disease, Hashimoto thyroiditis, and pernicious anemia, in which autoimmune mechanisms are known to be pathogenic. These conditions, as well as insulin-dependent type I diabetes mellitus, also are known to be associated with an increased frequency of certain HLAs, in particular HLA-B8, -DR3, -BW15, and -DR4. Located on chromosome 6, the HLA system is the major histocompatibility complex, consisting of a cluster of genes that code transplantation antigens and play a central role in immune responses.

Increased susceptibility to a number of diseases has been related to one or more of the identified HLA antigens. Inheritance of HLA-D3 or -D4 antigens appears to confer a 2- to 3-fold increased risk for developing type I diabetes. When both D3 and D4 are inherited, the relative risk for developing diabetes is increased by 7- to 10-fold. A rare genetic type of properdin factor B (BfF1) that is closely linked to the HLA system on chromosome 6 is found in more than 20% of type I diabetics but in less than 2% of healthy subjects; thus there is a relative risk factor of 15 for those who inherit this genetic marker. Certain blood groups have also been associated with an increased risk of diabetes. Application of newer molecular genetic techniques through analysis of DNA polymorphisms after digestion by specific restriction endonucleases has revealed further heterogeneity in the HLA-D region among individuals with and without diabetes despite the possession in both of the DR3 or DR4 markers, suggesting a yet to be defined "susceptibility" locus within these markers.

There is now considerable evidence that at least one major susceptibility locus may reside in the DQ β_1 gene. The homozygous absence of aspartic acid at position 57 of the HLA-DQ β chain (nonAsp/nonAsp) confers an approximately 100-fold relative risk for developing type I diabetes. Those who are heterozygous with a single aspartic acid at position 57 (nonAsp/Asp) are less likely to develop diabetes but are more susceptible than individuals who contain aspartic acid on both DQ β chains, that is, homozygous Asp/Asp. Indeed, the incidence of type I diabetes mellitus in any given population appears to be proportional to the gene frequency of nonAsp alleles in that population.

These observations provide a rational framework for the long-recognized association of type I diabetes with genetic factors on the bases of the increased incidence in some families, of the concordance rates in monozygotic twins, and of ethnic and racial differences in prevalence. For example, type I diabetes among American blacks is associated with the same HLA genes as it is in American whites. From multiple family pedigrees and HLA typing data it has been determined that if a sibling shares both HLA-D haplotypes with an index case, the risk for that individual is 12–20%; for a sibling sharing one haplotype, the risk for developing IDDM is 5–7%; and with no haplotypes in common, the risk is only 1–2%. HLA typing is not recommended, however, for genetic counseling because no intervention is possible to prevent IDDM at this time. In general, for purposes of genetic counseling, it can be safely assumed that in whites, the overall recurrence risks to siblings are approximately 6% if the proband is under 10 yr of age and 3% if he or she is older at the time of diagnosis. The risk to offspring is 2–5%, with the higher risk in the offspring of a diabetic father. In American blacks, these risks are only one half to two thirds those in whites.

Factors other than pure inheritance must also be involved in evoking clinical diabetes. For example, HLA-D3 or -D4 is found in approximately 50% of the general population and (nonAsp/nonAsp) in approximately 20% of white nondiabetics in the United States, yet the risk for IDDM in these subjects is only one tenth that in an HLA-identical sibling of an index case with IDDM possessing these markers. Even siblings sharing only one haplotype have a 6- to 10-fold greater risk of developing IDDM compared with the normal population. In addition, about 10% of patients with IDDM do not possess either HLA-D3 or -D4, although almost all white diabetics lack at least one aspartic acid at position 57 of the DQ β chain. Most compelling is the fact that the concordance rate among identical twins of whom one has insulin-dependent diabetes is only 30–50%, suggesting the participation of environmental triggering factors or other genetic factors such as the postnatal selection of certain autoreactive T cell clones

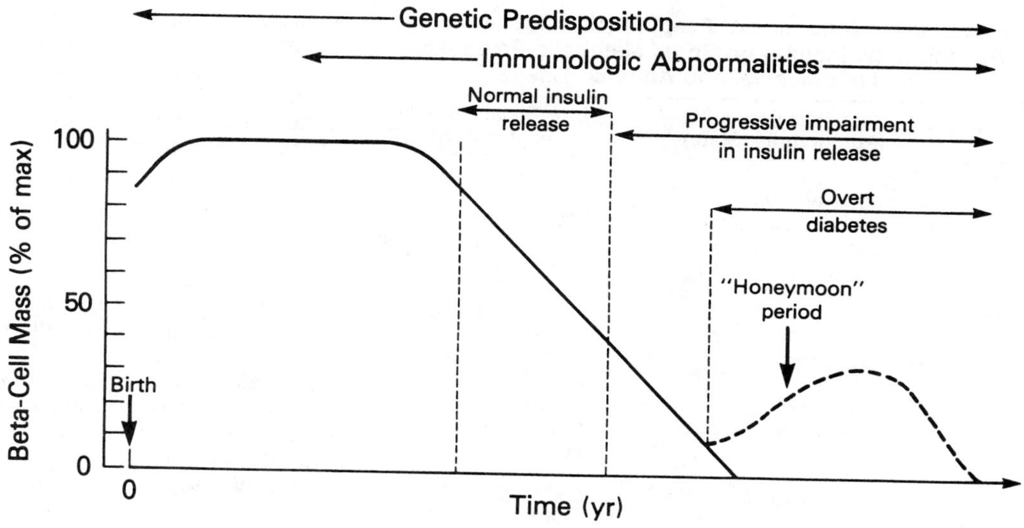

Figure 8–44. Proposed scheme of natural history of β cell defect. (Adapted from Sperling MA [ed]: Physician's Guide to Insulin-Dependent [Type 1] Diabetes Mellitus: Diagnosis and Treatment. Copyright (1988) by the American Diabetes Association. Reprinted with permission.)

Timing of trigger in relation to immunologic abnormalities is unknown. Note that overt diabetes is not apparent until insulin secretory reserves are <10–20% of normal.

that bear receptors recognizing "self." This postnatal process occurs within the thymus and implies that identical twins are not identical with respect to the T cell receptor repertoire they possess.

Triggering factors might include viral infections. In animals, a number of viruses can cause a diabetic syndrome, the appearance and severity of which depend on the genetic strain and immune competence of the species of animal tested. In man, epidemics of mumps, rubella, and coxsackievirus infections have been associated with subsequent increases in the incidence of type I diabetes; the acute onset of diabetes mellitus, presumably induced by coxsackievirus B4, has been described. The viruses may act by directly destroying β cells, by persisting in pancreatic β cells as slow viral infections, or by triggering a widespread immune response to several endocrine tissues. The virus may induce initial β cell damage that results in the presentation of previously masked or altered antigenic determinants. It is also possible that the virus shares some antigenic determinants with those present on β cells, so that antibodies formed in response to the virus may interact with these shared determinants of β cells resulting in their destruction, an example of molecular mimicry. Antecedent stress and exposure to certain chemical toxins have been implicated in the development of IDDM. Histologic examination of pancreas from patients with IDDM who die from incidental causes has revealed lymphocytic infiltration around the islets of Langerhans. Later, the islets become progressively hyalinized and scarred, a process suggesting an ongoing inflammatory response, possibly autoimmune in nature.

Considerable evidence now supports an autoimmune basis for the development of type I diabetes. Some 80–90% of newly diagnosed patients with IDDM have islet cell antibodies (ICA) directed at cell surface or cytoplasmic determinants in their islet cells; the prevalence of these antibodies decreases with the duration of established disease. In contrast, after pancreatic transplantation, ICA may reappear in patients whose sera had become negative for ICA prior to transplantation. Taken together, these findings suggest that ICA disappear as the antigens in the form of pancreatic islets are destroyed and reappear when fresh antigen (transplanted islets) is presented. Studies in identical twins and in family pedigrees demonstrate that the existence of ICA may precede by months to years the appearance of symptomatic IDDM. In vitro, ICA may impair insulin secretion in response to secretagogues and can be shown to be cytotoxic to islet cells, especially in the presence of complement or T cells from patients with type I diabetes. There is also some evidence of abnormal T cell function with an alteration in the ratio of suppressor to killer T cells at the onset of the disease. These findings suggest that type I diabetes, like other autoimmune diseases such as Hashimoto thyroiditis, is a disease of "autoaggression," in which autoantibodies, in cooperation with complement, T cells, or other factors, induce destruction of the insulin-producing islet cells. Thus, inheritance of certain genes intimately associated with the HLA system on chromosome 6 appears to confer a predisposition toward autoimmune disease, including diabetes, when triggered by an appropriate stimulus such as a virus. Although it is understood that some insulin-dependent diabetic patients have none of the frequently associated HLAs, the evidence in favor of an immune basis of islet cell destruction is sufficiently compelling to have fostered several studies of different immunosuppressive agents in the treatment of newly diagnosed diabetics. These immunosuppressive agents must be considered as experimental and should not be viewed as established or recommended therapy. Figure 8–44 summarizes current concepts of the etiology of type I diabetes as an autoimmune disease, the tendency toward which is inherited through the HLA system and in which autoimmune destruction of β cells is triggered by an as yet unidentified agent. The slope of decline in insulin varies, and the point at which clinical features appear corresponds to approximately an 80% destruction of the insulin secretory reserve. This process may take months to years, usually in adolescent and older patients, and weeks in the very young patient. Higher titers of spontaneous autoinsulin antibodies and islet cell antibodies are characteristic of the more active islet cell destruction typically seen in the younger patient and may prove useful in predicting evolving diabetes, though no presently available marker or test can accurately predict the development of type I diabetes mellitus.

PATHOPHYSIOLOGY. The progressive destruction of β cells leads to a progressive deficiency of insulin, a major anabolic hormone. Its normal secretion in response to feeding is exquisitely modulated by the interplay of neural, hormonal, and substrate-related mechanisms to permit controlled disposition of ingested foodstuff as energy for immediate or future use; mobilization of energy during the fasted state

TABLE 8–17. Influence of Feeding (High Insulin) or of Fasting (Low Insulin) on Some Metabolic Processes in Liver, Muscle, and Adipose Tissue*

	High Plasma Insulin (Postprandial State)	Low Plasma Insulin (Fasted State)
Liver:	Glucose uptake Glycogen synthesis Absence of gluconeogenesis Lipogenesis Absence of ketogenesis	Glucose production Glycogenolysis Gluconeogenesis Absence of lipogenesis Ketogenesis
Muscle:	Glucose uptake	Absence of glucose uptake
	Glucose oxidation	Fatty acid and ketone oxidation
	Glycogen synthesis	Glycogenolysis
	Protein synthesis	Proteolysis and amino acid release
Adipose tissue:	Glucose uptake	Absence of glucose uptake
	Lipid synthesis	Lipolysis and fatty acid release
	Triglyceride uptake	Absence of triglyceride uptake

*Insulin is considered to be the major factor governing these metabolic processes. Diabetes mellitus may be viewed as a permanent low-insulin state that, untreated, results in exaggerated fasting.

depends on low plasma levels of insulin. Thus, in normal metabolism there are regular swings between the postprandial, high-insulin anabolic state and the fasted, low-insulin catabolic state that affect three major tissues: liver, muscle, and adipose tissue (Table 8–17). Type I diabetes mellitus, as it evolves, becomes a permanent low-insulin catabolic state in which feeding does not reverse but rather exaggerates these catabolic processes. It is important to emphasize that liver is more sensitive than muscle or fat to a given concentration of insulin—that is, endogenous glucose production from the liver through glycogenolysis and gluconeogenesis can be restrained at insulin concentrations that do not fully augment glucose utilization by peripheral tissues. Consequently, with progressive failure of insulin secretion, the initial manifestation is postprandial hyperglycemia; fasting hyperglycemia indicates excessive endogenous glucose production and is a late manifestation reflecting severe insulin deficiency.

Although insulin deficiency is the primary defect, several secondary changes that involve the stress hormones (epinephrine, cortisol, growth hormone, and glucagon) accelerate and exaggerate the rate and magnitude of metabolic decompensation. Increased plasma concentrations of these counterregulatory hormones magnify metabolic derangements by further impairing insulin secretion (epinephrine), by antagonizing its action (epinephrine, cortisol, growth hormone), and by promoting glycogenolysis, gluconeogenesis, lipolysis, and ketogenesis (glucagon, epinephrine, growth hormone, and cortisol) while decreasing glucose utilization and glucose clearance (epinephrine, growth hormone, cortisol). With progressive insulin deficiency, excessive glucose production and impairment of its utilization result in hyperglycemia with glucosuria when the renal threshold of approximately 180 mg/dL is exceeded. The resultant osmotic diuresis produces polyuria, urinary losses of electrolytes, dehydration, and compensatory polydipsia. These evolving manifestations, especially dehydration, represent physiologic stress, resulting in hypersecretion of epinephrine, glucagon, cortisol, and growth hormone that amplifies and perpetuates the metabolic derangements and accelerates metabolic decompensation. The acute stress of trauma or infection may likewise accelerate metabolic decompensation to ketoacidosis in evolving or established diabetes. Hyperosmolality, commonly encountered as a result of progressive hyperglycemia, contributes to the symptomatology, especially to cerebral obtundation in diabetic ketoacidosis. Serum osmolality (in mOsm/kg) can be estimated by the following formula:

$$[\text{serum Na}^+ \text{ (mEq/L)} + \text{K}^+ \text{ (mEq/L)}] \times 2 + \frac{\text{glucose (mg/dL)}}{18} + \frac{\text{BUN (mg/dL)}}{3}$$

Consideration of serum osmolality has important implications in the therapy of diabetic ketoacidosis.

The combination of insulin deficiency and elevated plasma values of the counterregulatory hormones is also responsible for accelerated lipolysis and impaired lipid synthesis, with resulting increased plasma concentrations of total lipids, cholesterol, triglycerides, and free fatty acids. The hormonal interplay of insulin deficiency and glucagon excess shunts the free fatty acids into ketone body formation; the rate of formation of these ketone bodies, principally β-hydroxybutyrate and acetoacetate, exceeds the capacity for their peripheral utilization and renal excretion. Accumulation of these ketoacids results in metabolic acidosis and in compensatory rapid deep breathing in an attempt to excrete excess CO_2 **(Kussmaul respirations)**. Acetone, formed by nonenzymatic conversion of acetoacetate, is responsible for the characteristic fruity odor of the breath. Ketones are excreted in the urine in association with cations and thus further increase losses of water and electrolytes (Table 8–18). With progressive dehydration, acidosis, hyperosmolality, and diminished cerebral oxygen utilization, consciousness becomes impaired, and the patient ultimately becomes comatose. Thus, insulin deficiency produces a profound catabolic state—an exaggerated state of starvation—in which all of the initial clinical features can be explained on the basis of known alterations in intermediary metabolism mediated by insulin deficiency in combination with counterregulatory hormone excess. Because the counterregulatory hormonal changes are secondary, the severity and duration of the symptoms reflect the extent of the primary insulinopenia.

CLINICAL MANIFESTATIONS. The classic presentation of diabetes in children is a history of polyuria, polydipsia, polyphagia, and weight loss. Duration of these symptoms varies but is often less than 1 mo. A clue to the existence of polyuria may be the onset of enuresis in a previously toilet-trained child. An insidious onset characterized by lethargy, weakness, and weight loss is also quite common. The loss of weight in spite of an increased dietary intake is readily explicable by the following illustration: The average healthy 10-yr-old child has a daily caloric intake of 2,000 or more calories, of which approximately 50% are derived from carbohydrate. With the development of diabetes, daily losses of water and glucose may be as much as 5 L and 250 g,

TABLE 8–18. Fluid and Electrolyte Maintenance Requirements and Estimated Losses in Diabetic Ketoacidosis

	Approximate Daily Maintenance Requirements*	Approximate Accumulated Losses†
Water	1500 mL/m²	100 mL/kg (range 60–100 mL/kg)
Sodium	45 mEq/m²	6 mEq/kg (range 5–13 mEq/kg)
Potassium	35 mEq/m²	5 mEq/kg (range 4–6 mEq/kg)
Chloride	30 mEq/m²	4 mEq/kg (range 3–9 mEq/kg)
Phosphate	10 mEq/m²	3 mEq/kg (range 2–5 mEq/kg)

*Maintenance is expressed in surface area to permit uniformity because fluid requirements change as weight increases. See also Sec. 6.12.

†Losses are expressed per unit of body weight since the losses remain relatively constant in relation to total body weight.

respectively. This represents 1,000 calories lost in the urine or 50% of average daily caloric intake. Therefore, despite the child's compensatory increased intake of food and water, the calories cannot be utilized, excessive caloric losses continue, and increasing catabolism and weight loss ensue.

Pyogenic skin infections and monilial vaginitis in teenage girls are occasionally present at the time of diagnosis of diabetes. They are rarely the sole clinical manifestations of diabetes in children, and a careful history will invariably reveal the coexistence of polyuria and polydipsia.

Ketoacidosis is responsible for the initial presentation of many (approximately 25%) diabetic children. The early manifestations may be relatively mild and consist of vomiting, polyuria, and dehydration. In more prolonged and severe cases, Kussmaul respirations are present, and there is an odor of acetone on the breath. Abdominal pain or rigidity may be present and may mimic appendicitis or pancreatitis. Cerebral obtundation and ultimately coma ensue. Laboratory findings include glucosuria, ketonuria, hyperglycemia, ketonemia, and metabolic acidosis. Leukocytosis is common, and nonspecific serum amylase may be elevated; serum lipase is usually not elevated. In those with abdominal pain, it should not be assumed that these findings are evidence of a surgical emergency before a period of appropriate fluid, electrolyte, and insulin therapy has been tried to correct dehydration and acidosis; the abdominal manifestations frequently disappear after several hours of such treatment.

DIAGNOSIS. Children in whom the diagnosis of diabetes mellitus must be considered may, for practical purposes, be divided into three general categories: (1) those who have a history suggestive of diabetes, especially polyuria with polydipsia and failure to gain weight or a loss of weight in spite of a voracious appetite; (2) those who have a transient or persistent glucosuria; and (3) those who have clinical manifestations of metabolic acidosis with or without stupor or coma. In all instances the diagnosis of diabetes mellitus is dependent on the demonstration of hyperglycemia in association with glucosuria with or without ketonuria. When classic symptoms of polyuria and polydipsia are associated with hyperglycemia and glucosuria, the glucose tolerance test is not needed to support the diagnosis.

Renal glucosuria may be an isolated congenital disorder or a manifestation of the Fanconi syndrome and other renal tubular disorders due to severe heavy metal intoxication, ingestion of certain drugs (e.g., outdated tetracycline), or inborn errors of metabolism (cystinosis). When vomiting, diarrhea, or inadequate intake of food is a complicating factor in any of these conditions, starvation ketosis may ensue, simulating diabetic ketoacidosis. The absence of hyperglycemia eliminates the possibility of diabetes. It is also important to recognize that not all urinary sugar is glucose, and infrequently galactosemia, pentosuria, and the fructosurias will require consideration as diagnostic possibilities.

The discovery of glucosuria, with or without a mild degree of hyperglycemia, during a hospital admission for trauma or infection or even during the associated emotional upheaval may, but usually does not, herald the existence of diabetes; in most of these instances the glucosuria remits during recovery. Because this circumstance may indicate a limited capacity for insulin secretion, which is unmasked by elevated plasma concentrations of stress hormones, these patients should be rechecked at a later date for the possibility of hyperglycemia or clinical features of diabetes mellitus. In these circumstances, a glucose tolerance test may be useful to establish a diagnosis; glucose tolerance testing should be performed several weeks after recovery from the acute illness using a glucose loading dose adjusted for weight. Evidence indicates that the test is most likely to be abnormal in patients with HLA-DR3 and -DR4 and those in whom islet cell antibodies or insulin autoantibodies are detected.

Screening procedures, such as postprandial determinations of blood glucose or oral glucose tolerance tests, have yielded low detection rates in children, even among those considered at risk, such as siblings of diabetic children. Accordingly, such screening procedures are not recommended in children.

Diabetic ketoacidosis must be differentiated from acidosis and/or coma due to other causes; these causes include hypoglycemia, uremia, gastroenteritis with metabolic acidosis, lactic acidosis, salicylate intoxication, encephalitis, and other intracranial lesions. Diabetic ketoacidosis exists when there is hyperglycemia (glucose greater than 300 mg/dL), ketonemia (ketones strongly positive at greater than 1:2 dilution of serum), acidosis (pH less than 7.30 and bicarbonate less than 15 mEq/L), glucosuria, and ketonuria in addition to the clinical features described. Precipitating factors, even for the initial presentation, include stress such as trauma, infection, vomiting, and psychologic disturbances. Recurrent episodes of ketoacidosis in established diabetics often represent deliberate errors in recommended insulin dosage or unusual stress responses that indicate psychologic disturbances and, at times, pleas to be removed from a home environment perceived to be stressful or intolerable. Diabetic ketoacidosis also should be distinguished from nonketotic hyperosmolar coma.

Nonketotic hyperosmolar coma is a syndrome characterized by severe hyperglycemia (blood glucose greater than 600 mg/dL); absence of or only very slight ketosis; nonketotic acidosis; severe dehydration; depressed sensorium or frank coma; and various neurologic signs that may include grand mal seizures, hyperthermia, hemiparesis, and positive Babinski signs. Respirations are usually shallow, but coexistent metabolic (lactic) acidosis may be manifested by Kussmaul breathing. Serum osmolarity is commonly 350 mOsm/kg or higher. This condition usually occurs in middle-aged or elderly individuals who have "mild" diabetes; among them mortality rates have been as high as 40–70%, possibly in part because of delays in recognition and in institution of appropriate therapy. In children this condition is infrequent; among reported cases there has been a high incidence of pre-existing neurologic damage. Profound hyperglycemia may develop over a period of days, and initially the obligatory osmotic polyuria and dehydration may be partially compensated by increasing fluid intake. With progression of disease, thirst becomes impaired, possibly because of alteration of the hypothalamic thirst center by hyperosmolarity and possibly in some instances because of a pre-existing defect in the hypothalamic osmoregulating mechanism.

The low production of ketones is attributed mainly to the hyperosmolarity, which in vitro blunts the lipolytic effect of epinephrine and the antilipolytic effect of insulin; blunting of lipolysis by the therapeutic use of β-adrenergic blockers may contribute to the syndrome. Depression of consciousness is closely correlated with the degree of hyperosmolarity in this condition as well as in diabetic ketoacidosis; hemoconcentration may also predispose to cerebral arterial and venous thromboses.

Treatment of nonketotic hyperosmolar coma is directed at repletion of the vascular volume deficit and correction of the hyperosmolar state (also see later under management of ketoacidosis). One half isotonic saline (0.45% NaCl) is administered at a rate estimated to replace 50% of the volume deficit in the first 12 hr, and the remainder is administered during the ensuing 24 hr. When the blood glucose concentration approaches 300 mg/dL, the hydrating fluid should be changed to 5% dextrose in 0.2 normal (N) saline. Approximately 20 mEq/L of potassium chloride should be added to each of these fluids to prevent hypokalemia. Serum potassium and plasma glucose concentrations should be monitored at 2-hr intervals for the first 12 hr and at 4-hr intervals for the next 24 hr to permit appropriate adjustments of administered potassium and insulin.

Insulin can be given by continuous intravenous infusion beginning with the second hour of fluid therapy. Because blood glucose may decrease dramatically with fluid therapy alone, the intravenous loading dose should be 0.05 U/kg of regular (fast-acting) insulin followed by 0.05 U/kg/hr of the same insulin, rather than 0.1 U/kg/hr as advocated for patients with diabetic ketoacidosis. During the recovery period, therapy with insulin and diet and monitoring of the patient should be the same as those described for patients recovering from diabetic ketoacidosis (see Table 8–18 and related text).

TREATMENT. The management of insulin-dependent diabetes mellitus may be divided into three phases depending on the initial presentation: that of ketoacidosis; the postacidotic or transition period for establishment of metabolic control; and the continuing phase of guidance of the diabetic child and his or her family. Each of these phases has separate goals, although in practice they merge into a continuum. For purposes of management, the transition period corresponds to patients presenting with polyuria, polydipsia, and weight loss but without biochemical decompensation to ketoacidosis.

Ketoacidosis. The immediate aims of therapy are expansion of intravascular volume, correction of deficits in fluids, electrolytes, and acid-base status, and initiation of insulin therapy to correct intermediary metabolism. Treatment should be instituted as soon as the clinical diagnosis is confirmed by the presence of hyperglycemia and ketonemia. Determinations of blood pH and electrolytes should also be obtained; an electrocardiogram (ECG) is useful to provide a rapid reference for the existence of hyperkalemia. If sepsis is suspected as a possible precipitating factor, a blood culture should be obtained and the urine examined for the presence of bacteria and leukocytes. A flow sheet to record chronologically the rate and composition of fluid input, urine output, amount of insulin administered, and the acid-base and electrolyte values of the blood is most useful. Catheterization of the bladder is not routinely recommended in children; bag collection or condom drainage permits an assessment of urinary output, but catheterization may be indicated in comatose patients.

FLUID AND ELECTROLYTE THERAPY (Table 8–19). The expansion of reduced intravascular volume and correction of depleted fluid and electrolyte stores are most important in the treatment of diabetic ketoacidosis (DKA). It must be stressed, however, that exogenous insulin is essential to arrest further metabolic decompensation and restore intermediary metabolism.

Dehydration is commonly on the order of 10%; initial fluid therapy can be based on this estimate, with subsequent adjustments related to clinical and laboratory data. The initial hydrating fluid should be isotonic saline (0.9%). Because of the hyperglycemia, hyperosmolarity is universal in DKA; thus, even 0.9% saline is hypotonic relative to the patient's serum osmolality. A gradual decline in osmolality is desirable because too rapid a decline has been implicated in the development of cerebral edema, one of the major complications of diabetic therapy in children. For the same reason, the rate of fluid replacement is adjusted to provide only 50–60% of the calculated deficit within the initial 12 hr; the remaining 40–50% is administered during the next 24 hr. Also, administration of glucose (5% solution in 0.2 N saline) is initiated when the blood glucose concentration approaches 300 mg/dL in order to limit the decline of serum osmolality and reduce the risk of developing cerebral edema (see below and Table 8–19).

Administration of potassium (K^+) should be started early. Total body potassium may be considerably depleted during acidosis, even when the serum potassium concentration is normal or elevated. Whereas potassium moves from intracellular to extracellular sites during acidosis, the reverse occurs during correction of acidosis, particularly when exogenous insulin and glucose are available in the circulation. This shift of potassium back to the intracellular compartment may result in life-threatening hypokalemia. Hence, after the initial fluid replacement of approximately 20 mL/kg of isotonic saline (0.9%) has been provided, potassium should be added to subsequent infusates if urinary output is adequate; serum potassium concentration should then be monitored periodically. An ECG provides a rapid assessment of serum potassium concentration; T waves are peaked in hyperkalemia and are low and associated with U waves in hypokalemia (see Sec. 6.5). Because the total potassium deficit cannot be replaced within the initial 24 hr of treatment, potassium supplementation should be continued as long as fluids are administered intravenously (see Table 8–19).

It is almost inevitable that the patient will receive an excess of chloride, which may aggravate acidosis. The extent of acidosis, however, can be reduced by substitution of phosphate, which is also significantly depleted in DKA. Moreover, phosphate in conjunction with glycolysis is essential for the formation of 2,3-diphosphoglycerate (2,3-DPG), which governs the oxygen dissociation curve. During deficiency of 2,3-DPG, the oxygen dissociation curve is shifted to the left, that is, more oxygen is retained by hemoglobin and less is available to the tissues, a situation that predisposes to lactic acidosis. Acidosis per se tends to shift the oxygen dissociation curve toward the right (Bohr effect) and thus partially "compensates" for 2,3-DPG deficiency. As acidosis resulting from the accumulation of ketones is corrected by the provision of insulin, with or without administration of bicarbonate, the effects of 2,3-DPG deficiency may no longer be "compensated," and the release of oxygen to tissues may again be impaired. Exogenous phosphate, by contributing to the formation of 2,3-DPG, permits the oxygen dissociation curve to shift to the right and thus facilitates release of oxygen to tissues and aids in the correction of acidosis. Furthermore, resistance to insulin action is associated with hypophosphatemia. Hence, we recommend the administration of potassium phosphate as outlined in Table 8–19. Since excessive use of phosphate may result in hypocalcemia, serum calcium should be measured periodically. Symptomatic hypocalcemia should be corrected with calcium gluconate.

ALKALI THERAPY. With provision of fluids, electrolytes, glucose, and insulin, metabolic acidosis is usually corrected through the interruption of ketogenesis, the metabolism of ketones to bicarbonate, and the generation of bicarbonate by the distal renal tubule. Concerns about the therapeutic administration of bicarbonate center on four issues: (1) alkalosis, by shifting the oxygen dissociation curve to the left, may diminish the release of oxygen to tissues and hence predispose to lactic acidosis; (2) alkalosis accelerates the entry of potassium into cells and hence may produce hypokalemia; (3) provision of bicarbonate according to the calculated base deficit overcorrects and may result in alkalosis; and (4) perhaps most important, bicarbonate may lead to a worsening of cerebral acidosis while the plasma pH is being restored to normal because HCO_3^- combines with H^+ and dissociates to CO_2 and H_2O. Whereas bicarbonate passes the blood-brain barrier slowly, CO_2 diffuses freely, thereby exacerbating cerebral acidosis and possibly cerebral depression. On the other hand, severe acidosis, with a blood pH of 7.1 or less, diminishes respiratory minute volume, may produce hypotension by means of peripheral vasodilation, impairs myocardial function, and may be a factor in insulin resistance. For these reasons, administration of bicarbonate is recommended only when the pH is 7.2 or below (see Table 8–19). At pH 7.1–7.2, 40 mEq of HCO_3^-/m^2, and below pH 7.1, 80 mEq of HCO_3^-/m^2, should be infused over a period of 2 hr; acid-base status should then be re-evaluated prior to continuing further alkali therapy. Bicarbonate should not be given by bolus infusion because it may precipitate cardiac arrhythmias.

TABLE 8–19. Fluid and Electrolyte Therapy for Diabetic Ketoacidosis

Recommendations for replacement of fluid losses and for maintenance of a 30-kg (surface area 1.0 m^2) child with assumed 10% dehydration. Duration of treatment: 36 hours.

REPLACEMENT FLUIDS	Approximate Accumulated Losses with 10% Dehydration	Approximate Requirements for Maintenance (36 hr)	Approximate Totals for Replacement and Maintenance (36 hr)
Water (mL)	3,000	2,250	5,500
Sodium (mEq)	180	65	250
Potassium (mEq)	150	50	200
Chloride (mEq)	120	45	165
Phosphate (mEq)	90	15	100

REPLACEMENT SCHEDULE (continuous intravenous infusion)

Approximate Duration	Fluid (Composition)	Sodium (mEq)	Potassium (mEq)	Chloride (mEq)	Phosphate (mEq)
Hour 1	500 mL of 0.9% NaCl (isotonic saline)	75	—	75	—
Hour 2	500 mL of 0.45% NaCl (0.5 isotonic saline) plus 20 mEq of KCl	35	20	55	—
Hr 3 to 12 (200 mL/hr for 10 hr)	2,000 ml of 0.45% NaCl with 30 mEq/L of potassium phosphate	150	60	150	40
Subtotal initial 12 hr	3,000 mL	260	80	280	40
Next 24 hr 100 mL/hr	5% glucose in 0.2% NaCl with 40 mEq/L of potassium phosphate	75	100	75	60
Total over 36 hours	5,400 mL	335	180	355	100

Note: All replacement values should be halved if dehydration is estimated to be 5%. Maintenance requirements remain the same.

ADDITIONAL GUIDELINES

A **diabetic flow sheet** with laboratory data appropriately recorded must be maintained in the patient's chart.

Insulin therapy by continuous low-dose intravenous method: Priming dose—bolus injection of 0.1 U/kg of regular insulin IV followed immediately by continuous IV infusion of 0.1 U/kg/hr of regular insulin beginning with 2nd hr.

Directions for making insulin infusion: Add 50 U of regular insulin to 500 mL of isotonic saline. Flush 50 mL through the tubing to saturate insulin-binding sites. For 30-kg patient, infuse at rate of 30 mL/hr. When the blood glucose concentration approaches 300 mg/dL, continue the insulin infusion at a reduced rate, or add glucose to the infusate until acidosis is resolved, then start insulin therapy by subcutaneous injections of 0.2–0.4 U/kg of insulin at intervals of 6 hr.

Bicarbonate therapy: For pH >7.20, no therapy necessary. For pH 7.10–7.20, 40 mEq/m^2 of bicarbonate over 2 hr; then re-evaluate. For pH <7.10, 80 mEq/m^2 of bicarbonate over 2 hr; then re-evaluate. New diabetics, <2 yr of age, with diabetic ketoacidosis and 10% dehydration, or any diabetic with pH <7.00, should be managed in an intensive care unit or equivalent setting.

The major life-threatening complication in children treated for DKA is *cerebral edema*. Clinically, cerebral edema develops several hours after the institution of therapy, when clinical and biochemical indices may suggest improvement. The manifestations are those of raised intracranial pressure and include headache, alteration and deterioration in alertness and conscious state, "delirious outbursts," bradycardia, vomiting, diminished responsiveness to painful stimuli, and diminished reflexes. There may be a change in pupillary responsiveness with unequal pupils or fixed dilated pupils. Polyuria, secondary to development of diabetes insipidus, may be erroneously attributed to osmotic diuresis secondary to hyperglycemia, although diabetes mellitus and diabetes insipidus coexist. Prompt recognition of the condition as it evolves, and prompt therapy with mannitol and hyperventilation can be lifesaving. Increasingly, evidence points to the conclusion that subclinical cerebral edema occurs in the majority of patients treated with fluids and insulin for DKA and that in only a minority does it become clinically manifest as a medical emergency.

The evidence that a majority of patients treated for DKA develop subclinical cerebral edema includes increasing cerebrospinal fluid pressure documented by continuous intrathecal monitoring during therapy of DKA in adults and evidence from sequential computed tomography of the head that ventricular size is narrower, compatible with brain swelling, during therapy, than several days after recovery from DKA. Excessive use of fluids, excessive use of bicarbonate, compensatory responses to intracellular acidosis through the NA^+/H^+ exchanger, and large doses of insulin during treatment have all been implicated. The reason that a majority have subclinical brain swelling, whereas only a minority (1–2%) manifest clinically apparent cerebral edema, may be related to the intracranial pressure-volume curve, which shows a steep exponential rise in intracranial pressure beyond a critical volume of cerebral mass.

For these reasons, it is prudent to anticipate clinical cerebral edema in all children treated for DKA by limiting the rate of fluid administration to 4.0 L/m^2/24 hr or less, avoiding the excessive use of bicarbonate as outlined above, and being alert to the clinical manifestations of raised intracranial pressure. Once raised intracranial pressure has become clinically manifest, reduction of the rate of fluid administration, use of mannitol at 10–20 g/m^2 intravenously, repeated at 2- to 4-hr intervals, and hyperventilation are warranted. Preliminary retrospective evidence suggests that these measures, instituted promptly, are lifesaving and may avoid neurologic sequelae.

INSULIN THERAPY. The continuous low-dose intravenous infusion method, in which a priming dose of 0.1 U/kg of regular insulin is followed by a constant infusion of 0.1 U/kg/hr, is outlined in Table 8–19. This method is effective, simple, and physiologically sound and has gained wide acceptance as the preferred method for administering insulin during DKA. It provides a constant steady concentration of insulin in plasma that approximates the peak attained in normal individuals during an oral glucose tolerance test. Presumably, the same steady concentration is attained at the cellular level and permits a steady metabolic response without the fluctuations that must occur with intermittent injections of insulin. Concern that the insulin may adhere to glass and tubing has proved to be unfounded, and effective delivery of insulin can be provided without the use of albumin or gelatin added to the infusate. Moreover, insulin infusion can be provided by gravity drip without the use of a special pump, although such a pump is helpful. A separate infusion set for insulin connected to the infusion line used for fluid and electrolyte therapy is recommended so that adjustments in the dosage of each can be made independently. After the amount of insulin for the initial 6–8 hr has been calculated, this quantity is added to a 250- or 500-mL bottle of 0.9% saline (see Table 8–19 for specific instructions).

When the blood glucose concentration approaches 300 mg/dL, the ongoing potassium requirement is added to 5% glucose in 0.2 N saline, and the rate of insulin infusion may sometimes be reduced to 0.05 U/kg/hr providing that the acidosis is being corrected. The rate of insulin infusion should, however, be periodically adjusted according to the patient's recovery from acidosis and the blood glucose response of each individual.

In treating DKA, it is commonly observed that the blood glucose concentration corrects more quickly than the pH or plasma bicarbonate. Insulin must be provided by infusion or subcutaneous injection as long as acidosis persists even if the glucose concentration is approaching 300 mg/dL. It may be necessary to add glucose to the infusate while continuing insulin infusion at a rate of 0.05–0.1 U/kg/hr until the acidosis is corrected. If acidosis persists despite these measures, a cause such as gram-negative sepsis should be considered.

When the acidosis has been corrected, the continuous infusion may be discontinued and insulin given immediately by subcutaneous injection at a dose of 0.2–0.4 U/kg every 6–8 hr while maintaining the glucose infusion until the child can fully tolerate food. Subcutaneous injections of regular insulin at doses of 0.2–0.4 U/kg every 6–8 hr before meals should be continued for a full 24-hr day after the child is eating. The blood glucose level should be monitored before and 2 hr after each meal, adjusting the insulin dose to maintain the blood glucose concentration in the range of 80–180 mg/dL. The total dose of regular insulin used in this representative day serves as a guide for subsequent insulin treatment with a combination of intermediate- and short-acting insulin as described below.

Insulin treatment during DKA can also be administered by repeated intramuscular or subcutaneous bolus injections; a portion of the dose is also usually injected intravenously. One such regimen based on body weight is outlined in Table 8–20; if plasma ketones are only moderately elevated, the recommended doses may be half of those listed. Administrations of insulin as the fast-acting form are repeated every 2–4 hr, and blood glucose values and acid-base status are monitored as they are during the continuous intravenous insulin approach. When the blood glucose concentration has fallen to approximately 300 mg/dL, subsequent insulin therapy at a dose of 0.2–0.4 U/kg may be given subcutaneously every 6–8 hr while maintaining an infusion of 5% glucose in 0.2 N saline with potassium added (see Table 8–19) until the acidosis is resolved and the child can tolerate solid foods. Sips of clear liquid, broth, or carbonated beverages may be given during this interval. Subcutanous injections of regular insulin at doses of 0.2–0.4 U/kg every 6–8 hr before meals are continued for a full 24-hr day after the child is eating, when the switch to combined intermediate- and short-acting insulins is made as described. Intermediate-acting insulin can usually be begun within 36 hr after commencing therapy for ketoacidosis.

Ketonemia and **ketonuria** may persist despite clinical improvement. The nitroprusside reaction that is routinely used to measure "ketones" reacts with acetoacetate and weakly with acetone but not with β-hydroxybutyrate. The usual ratio of β-hydroxybutyrate to acetoacetate is approximately 3:1, but it is commonly as much as 8:1 or more in patients with DKA. With correction of acidosis, β-hydroxybutyrate dissociates to acetoacetate, which is identified by the nitroprusside reaction. Hence, persistence of ketonuria for a day or more may not reliably reflect the clinical improvement and should not be interpreted as a poor therapeutic response.

Postacidotic Phase or Transition Period for Establishment of Metabolic Control. Diabetic ketoacidosis is usually corrected within 36–48 hr by the foregoing therapeutic regimen. At this time food and fluids are usually tolerated orally, and insulin can be given by subcutaneous injection. The child who presents with classic symptoms and documented hyperglycemia in the absence of clinical dehydration and ketoacidosis can be considered as requiring treatment at this transition stage. For such children, subcutaneous injections of fast-acting insulin are begun at doses of 0.1–0.25 U/kg every 6–8 hr before meals with simultaneous monitoring of the blood glucose concentration and adjustment of the insulin dose for 1–2 days. The initial dose of insulin is lower because these children generally have a lower blood glucose concentration and are more sensitive to insulin than are those presenting in DKA. One to two days of fast-acting insulin therapy are needed to estimate the total daily insulin requirement as a guide to the subsequent use of combined intermediate- and short-acting forms.

The aims of therapy during the transitional period are to treat any recognized precipitating cause of DKA such as infection; to stabilize the patient's metabolic control by adjusting the insulin dosage; to institute an appropriate nutritional pattern for the child; and to educate the parents and patient in the principles of diabetic management. These principles include techniques of insulin injection, monitoring of blood and urine glucose levels, monitoring of a urinary ketone spill, understanding the nutritional requirements, recognition of hypoglycemia (insulin shock) and its management, and ability to make adjustments in insulin dosage during minor illnesses and for regularly planned exercise. This education is best carried out by coordinating the participation of the physician, dietitian, and nurse educator, who have special training in diabetes. For newly diagnosed patients, this phase commonly lasts 5–10 days; less time may be required for the stabilization and re-education of previously diagnosed patients. Ongoing education and adjustment of insulin dosage are continued after discharge from the hospital through patient visits and inquiries by telephone; during this phase, gradual reductions in insulin dosage are frequently required, and the patient should be so advised (see later section on Residual β Cell Function). The details and rationale for insulin and dietary therapy as well as other aspects of long-term management are provided in the following section on insulin regimens.

The immediate goals in the management of children with type I diabetes are to provide adequate nutrition and exogenous insulin in a manner that prevents polydipsia and polyuria, including nocturia, avoids ketoacidosis and severe hypoglycemia, and permits normal growth and development with an active life pattern. These goals are achievable by most patients and their parents if they come to understand the principles of the pathophysiology and management of this disease. Ongoing supervision by the physician is essential and should be provided in a manner that avoids undue anxiety and psychologic dependence on the part of the child or parents or a sense of guilt on the part of the parents.

Evidence is emerging that the long-term complications of diabetes are related to the degree of metabolic control that is achieved. Therefore, one should aim for a metabolism that is as nearly normal as possible. Achievement of a completely normal metabolism, however, is not possible with the standard pattern of treatment that consists of one to two daily injections of insulin and attention to nutritional intake and exercise. In highly motivated adolescents, however, near-normal metabolism can now be achieved in one of two ways: (1) Monitoring of blood glucose values at home with the

TABLE 8–20. Intermittent Insulin Regimen for Diabetic Ketoacidosis

Blood Glucose	Total Insulin Dose	Intravenous Dose	Intramuscular or Subcutaneous Dose	Frequency
>600 mg/dL	1 U/kg	0.5 U/kg	0.5 U/kg	Every 2–4 hr
300–600 mg/dL	0.5 U/kg	0.25 U/kg	0.25 U/kg	Every 2–4 hr
These doses may be halved if serum ketones are only modestly elevated.				

When blood glucose approaches 300 mg/dL, the intravenous infusion for fluid and electrolyte replacement should contain 5% glucose (see Table 8–19 for rate of administration). Continue subcutaneous injections of insulin at 0.2–0.4 U/kg every 6 hr and monitor blood glucose concentration at the same time. If blood glucose concentration rises, increase the next insulin dose by 50%; if glucose concentration falls, decrease the next insulin dose by 50%. Continue this insulin regimen for 24 hr after oral intake of fluid and food is established. See text for subsequent management.

appropriate adjustment of insulin dosage 2–3 times a day and paying close attention to nutritional intake can be effective; (2) continuous subcutaneous insulin infusion by means of a pump worn externally that can be programmed to provide a basal rate of delivery with meal-related increments is also an effective means for highly selected patients. For the majority of pediatric patients, however, these newer approaches are not available or applicable, and routine management rests on three pillars: the provision of insulin and guidance with respect to its dosage, attention to nutritional intake, and exercise.

Insulin Regimens. The diurnal pattern of insulin concentration in the plasma of normal persons is characterized by a basal level on which are superimposed secretory episodes that coincide with intake of food. Each rise in plasma insulin concentration during feeding is synchronous with and proportional to the rise in blood glucose. Plasma insulin concentrations, however, do not reflect total insulin secretion. Because insulin is secreted into the portal circulation, its first target organ is the liver, the key organ governing the initial disposal of a glucose load (see Table 8–17).

Currently *available forms of insulin and their durations of action* are listed in Tables 8–21 and 8–22. They are classified as short-acting, intermediate-acting, and long-acting types; each is available in a concentration of 100 U/mL (U-100); higher concentrations are available for the unusual patient who has high resistance to insulin. Appropriate dilutions can be prepared for younger patients requiring low doses. Refinements in manufacture are now responsible for forms of insulin that have distinctly less contamination than formerly by such other pancreatic hormones as proinsulin, glucagon, pancreatic polypeptide, and somatostatin. Antibodies to these and other contaminants have been demonstrated in the sera of insulin-treated diabetics. It is unclear whether the new and more highly purified insulins facilitate metabolic control, but they probably do result in fewer local and systemic allergic reactions, including lipoatrophy and lipohypertrophy. The currently available insulins are extracted from beef and pork pancreas and are marketed separately or as a mixture of the two forms of insulin. Human insulin, synthesized in bacteria via recombinant DNA technology (synthetic) or by chemical modification of pork insulin (semisynthetic), is also routinely available for therapy. Human insulin may be less allergenic and less likely to induce antibody formation, but the limited data available do not indicate any significant advantages over highly purified pork insulin.

Because exogenous insulins are injected subcutaneously rather than directly into the portal vein, their rate of absorption may be variable, and because the dose injected is determined empirically, it lacks the precision of endogenously secreted insulin. Therefore, a single injection of intermediate-acting insulin cannot duplicate the pattern of normal insulin secretion, and periods of excessive plasma insulin that may produce hypoglycemia and/or periods of inadequate insulin that permit hyperglycemia are virtually inevitable. Even with injections of regular fast-acting insulin prior to each meal, normalization of blood glucose values is not entirely achieved, although the degree of control is clearly improved. Hence, the regimen of insulin administration selected for the diabetic child must represent a compromise designed to achieve as nearly normal an intermediary metabolism as possible that will permit normal growth and development and avoid frequent hypoglycemic reactions and the consequence of unrestrained hyperglycemia.

At the onset of diabetes, or after recovery from ketoacidosis, the total daily dose of insulin is about 0.5–1.0 U/kg. The actual total daily requirement of insulin is estimated from the representative 24-hr period when regular insulin only was administered before each meal during the transition phase after resolution of ketoacidosis or during the initial management of less severely affected patients as outlined earlier. Long-acting insulins are not often used in children. In most instances, one of the intermediate insulins is employed, but, because of its delayed action, a fast-acting (regular) insulin is usually combined with it. With the single-daily dose combined regimen, approximately two thirds of the total dose is an

TABLE 8–21. Common Types of Available Insulin

Product	Form	Strength
Rapid-Acting*		
Humulin R (Regular)[a]	Human	U-100
Regular Iletin I[a]	Mixed beef and pork	U-100
Regular Iletin II[a]	Pork	U-100, U-500
Regular Iletin II[a]	Beef	U-100
Semilente Iletin I[a]	Mixed beef and pork	U-100
Regular Purified Insulin[b]	Pork	U-100
Semitard Insulin Zinc Susp.[b]	Pork	U-100
Actrapid Regular Insulin[b]	Pork or human	U-100
Velosulin Regular[c]	Pork	U-100
Intermediate-Acting†		
Lente Iletin I[a]	Mixed beef and pork	U-100
Lente Iletin II[a]	Pork or beef	U-100
Humulin N (NPH)[a]	Human	U-100
NPH Iletin I[a]	Mixed beef and pork	U-100
NPH Iletin II[a]	Pork or beef	U-100
Lentard Insulin Zinc Susp.[b]	Mixed beef and pork	U-100
Lente Purified[b]	Beef	U-100
Monotard Insulin Zinc Susp.[b]	Pork or human	U-100
NPH (Isophane) Purified[b]	Beef	U-100
Protaphane (NPH) Insulin[b]	Pork	U-100
Insulatard NPH[c]	Pork	U-100
Mixtard NPH + Regular Insulin[c]	Pork	U-100
Long-Acting‡		
Protamine Zinc Iletin I[a]	Mixed beef and pork	U-100
Protamine Zinc Iletin II[a]	Pork or beef	U-100
Ultralente Iletin I[a]	Mixed beef and pork	U-100
Ultratard Zinc Susp.[b]	Beef	U-100

[a]Lilly.
[b]Squibb-Novo.
[c]Nordisk.
*Onset ½–1 hr, peak effect 2–4 hr, duration 6–8 hr.
†Onset 1–2 hr, peak effect 4–12 hr, duration 24 hr.
‡Onset 4–8 hr, peak effect 14–20 hr, duration 24–36 hr.
Onset and duration can vary from person to person.

TABLE 8–22. Insulins by Relative Comparative Action Curves

Insulin	Onset (hr)	Peak (hr)	Usual Effective Duration (hr)	Usual Maximal Duration (hr)
Animal				
Regular	0.5–2.0	3–4	4–6	6–8
NPH	4–6	8–14	16–20	20–24
Lente	4–6	8–14	16–20	20–24
Ultralente	8–14	Minimal	24–36	24–36
Human				
Regular	0.5–1.0	2–3	3–6	4–6
NPH	2–4	4–10	10–16	14–18
Lente	3–4	4–12	12–18	16–20
Ultralente	6–10	?	18–20	20–30

intermediate-acting insulin (e.g., NPH, lente), and the remainder is regular insulin; the injection is given 30 min before breakfast. The two insulins should always be drawn into the syringe in the same sequence (regular first) so that the residual insulin in the "dead space" is always the same type; thus, greater stability of the patient can be assured once a therapeutic dose is established. Disposable syringes with fine needles, minimal dead space, and easy-to-read calibration for use with U-100 insulin are available. For small children syringes calibrated to a maximum of 50 units are also available; in some European countries diluted insulins are marketed.

In order to avoid hypoglycemia, the single-daily dose regimen combining intermediate- and short-acting insulin is initially calculated on the basis of two thirds of the total daily dose, or approximately 0.5 U/kg. Step increases or decreases of 10–15% can then be made daily during the initial phase in the hospital until the desired degree of control is achieved. The initial phase of recovery of metabolic equilibrium is characterized by a period of replenishment of body stores of glycogen, protein, and fat that were depleted during the evolution of diabetes. Hence, insulin requirements for the first few days may on occasion be found to be even greater than 1 U/kg/24 hr. Adjustments in the dose of insulin are made in relation to the pattern of blood glucose values monitored before each meal and/or of the excretion of glucose. If the predominant hyperglycemia or glucosuria occurs in late morning, then the quick-acting form of insulin is increased by 10–15%. If the predominant hyperglycemia or glucosuria occurs in late afternoon or evening, then the intermediate-acting insulin is increased by 10–15%. Should hypoglycemic reactions occur in midmorning to noon, the quick-acting form of insulin is reduced by 10–15%, and, if hypoglycemia occurs in late afternoon or evening, the intermediate-acting insulin is decreased by 10–15%. In anticipation of increased exercise at home, the daily dose of insulin should be decreased by 10% at the time of discharge from the initial hospitalization.

Although many children can be managed with a single daily injection of insulin, *two daily injections* are now routinely recommended (Fig. 8–45). When there is persistent nocturia associated with excessive fasting hyperglycemia and morning glucosuria in response to a single daily injection of insulin, consideration should be given to dividing the total daily dose into two injections. In this plan two thirds of the daily total dose is given before breakfast and one third before the evening meal; each injection consists of intermediate- and short-acting insulins in proportions of 2–3:1. For example, assuming a total daily dose of 1 U/kg for a 30-kg child, 14 units of NPH or lente combined with 6 units of regular insulin would be given before breakfast, and 6 units of NPH or lente with 4 units of regular insulin would be given before the evening meal. As with the single-daily dose regimen, stepwise increases or decreases, each consisting of 10–15%, should be made to minimize hypoglycemic reactions and undue hyperglycemia (see earlier paragraph for guidelines).

Two daily injections of insulin are especially applicable for infants and children under 5 yr of age, in whom intake of food and extent of activity are not always predictable, and for adolescents, especially during the pubertal growth spurt. Two daily injections tend to result in smoother metabolic control with fewer hypoglycemic reactions and less uncontrolled hyperglycemia. This approach is more effective also when the evening meal is the major one (see later section under Nutritional Management). With an explanation of the rationale, adherence to this twice-daily regimen by patients and parents is usually good, and twice-daily insulin is now considered standard therapy. When compliance is not good, which occurs particularly in adolescents, one injection is preferable to none, since there is evidence that two daily injections may not always result in better metabolic control than one daily injection. The physician should in all instances attempt to determine the regimen that will be in the best interest of the patient. For children who insist on only one daily injection of insulin, the daily dose is adjusted according to carefully kept records of blood or urinary glucose values until the best possible degree of metabolic control is achieved. In this way, confidence in the patient-family-physician relationship is maintained, and a sense of guilt in the patient or family is avoided.

The *technique of injection of insulin* should be taught to the parents and to the patient when he or she is ready for it. Injections are given subcutaneously, rotating sites on arms, thighs, buttocks, and abdomen in a regular sequence. An appropriate rotation helps to ensure adequate absorption of

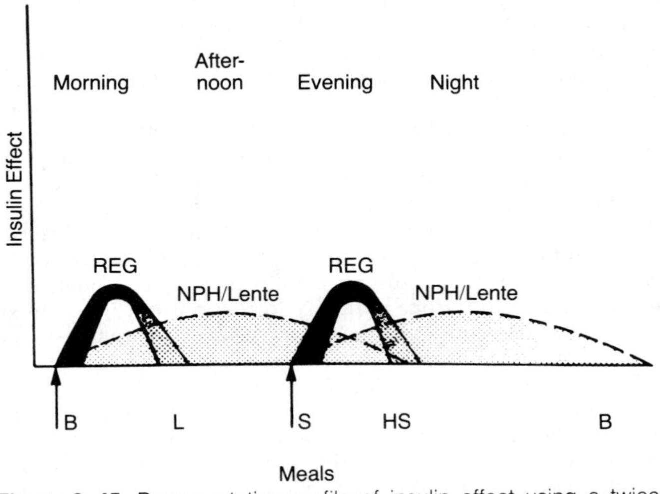

Figure 8–45. Representative profile of insulin effect using a twice-daily injection regimen that combines intermediate-acting insulin (NPH or Lente) with regular (short-acting) insulin (REG). (From Sperling MA: Outpatient management of diabetes mellitus. Pediatr Clin North Am 34:919, 1987.)

insulin, prevent fibrosis, and minimize lipodystrophic changes. With this rotation and the availability of the purer, single-peak insulins, lipoatrophy and lipohypertrophy are quite unusual. Younger children may find injections in the abdominal wall difficult or painful. Depending on their physical and psychologic maturity, children over the age of 10–12 yr should be encouraged to administer their own insulin and to monitor their own responses to it. The assumption of responsibility for self-monitoring will be a gradual process in which the parents and child all participate. Once the child has assumed total responsibility, the parents must resist a tendency toward overprotection. Guidelines for adjusting the dose of insulin based on blood or urinary glucose profiles have been outlined earlier, and those for adjusting the dose of insulin with exercise, illness, and "brittle" diabetes are provided in greater detail in the following section. It should be stressed, however, that the adolescent growth spurt is regularly associated with an increase in insulin requirements, which usually become lower when puberty is completed.

Hypersensitivity to insulin is uncommon in children. Local skin reactions are characterized by erythema or urticaria, with burning, itching, and tenderness within hours or sooner after an injection. These reactions usually resolve spontaneously over a period of days but may require a change from mixed beef-pork to pure pork or human insulin, or from NPH to lente insulin because of allergy to protamine in the former; antihistamines may be used if necessary. Generalized reactions with severe urticaria or angioedema are extremely rare and may also resolve spontaneously, but a change in the type of insulin is usually indicated, for example, from a mixed beef-pork preparation to a pure pork or human preparation. Desensitization may also be necessary, as may a course of systemic corticosteroid therapy for 1–2 wk. Rarely, insulin resistance develops in response to a local tissue enzyme that destroys injected insulin. Some of these patients have benefited from the addition of a protease enzyme inhibitor to the insulin solution; others have required chronic intravenous infusion and are best managed in a hospital with a specialized diabetes unit.

After several months of insulin therapy, nearly all patients will have acquired *antibodies to insulin*. In the majority, these do not interfere with the metabolic response. They may, however, promote instability by creating a reservoir of insulin that may be released at unpredictable times. Rarely, children with antibodies develop true resistance to insulin and require more than 2 units of insulin/kg/24 hr. A change to a preparation of pure pork, pure beef, or human insulin usually resolves this problem; in some instances a period of corticosteroid therapy or a course of desensitization may be necessary. Antibodies causing allergy are usually of the IgE class; IgA and IgM antibodies may be responsible for resistance to insulin.

Nutritional Management. Because the word diet may connote restriction and denial and impose a source of anxiety and/or rebellion on the part of parent or patient, its use should be avoided. Instructional discussion can be provided under such terms as nutritional requirements and meal plans. Actually, there are no special nutritional requirements for the diabetic child other than those for optimal growth and development. However, because the capacity to secrete insulin in response to the intake of food is negligible in the diabetic child, and because the dose of insulin is predicated on caloric intake, regularity of the eating pattern for the determined insulin regimen becomes paramount. In outlining nutritional requirements for the child on the basis of age, sex, weight, and activity, food preferences including any based on cultural and ethnic background should be considered. Although general guidelines are usually applicable, individualization for each child should be programmed.

Total recommended *caloric intake* is based on size or surface area and can be obtained from standard tables. The caloric mixture should consist of approximately 55% carbohydrate, 30% fat, and 15% protein. In general, we recommend that approximately 70% of the carbohydrate content be derived from complex carbohydrates such as starch and that intake of sucrose and highly refined sugars be avoided. Complex carbohydrates require prolonged digestion and absorption so that plasma glucose rises slowly, whereas glucose in refined sugars including those in carbonated beverages is rapidly absorbed and may cause wide swings in the metabolic pattern; carbonated beverages should therefore be of the sugar-free variety. In the United States the ban on saccharin as an artificial sweetener has been removed pending further evidence of its toxic or teratogenic effect. Although in children there is concern about the potential cumulative effect, available data do not support an association of moderate amounts with bladder cancer. Other non-nutritive sweeteners such as aspartame are used in a variety of products. Sorbitol and xylitol should not be used as artificial sweeteners; they are products of the polyol pathway and are implicated in some of the complications of diabetes.

Diets with a *high fiber content* are useful in improving control of blood glucose in diabetic subjects. Inclusion of about 50 g/24 hr of fiber from foods such as vegetables, especially legumes, whole-meal bread, bran cereals, and fruits in the diet of adult diabetics, has led to significant reductions in the concentration not only of blood glucose but also of total and LDL cholesterol. In addition, small amounts of sucrose consumed with fiber-rich foods such as whole-meal bread may have no more glycemic effect than their low-fiber, sugar-free equivalents. The concept of biologic equivalence or a "glycemic index" of foods is currently under investigation. When completed, these studies may provide a listing of foods with more predictable and desirable effects on blood glucose and serum lipid patterns for patients with diabetes.

The *intake of fat* is adjusted so that the polyunsaturated/saturated (P/S) ratio is increased to about 1.2:1.0, in contrast to the estimated American average of 0.3:1.0. Dietary fats derived from animal sources are therefore reduced and are replaced by polyunsaturated fats from vegetable sources. Substituting margarine for butter, vegetable oil for animal oils in cooking, and lean cuts of meat, poultry, and fish for fatty meats such as bacon is advisable. The intake of cholesterol is also reduced by these measures and by limiting the number of egg yolks consumed. There is ample evidence that these simple measures reduce serum LDL cholesterol, a predisposing factor to atherosclerotic disease.

The total daily caloric intake may be divided to provide 20% at breakfast, 20% at lunch, and 30% at dinner, leaving 10% for each of the midmorning, midafternoon, and evening snacks, if they are desired. In older children, the midmorning snack may be omitted and its caloric equivalent added to the lunch. Special brochures and pamphlets describing the exchanges and sample meal plans for children are usually available from regional diabetes associations; their use should be encouraged as part of the educational process. Meal plans are often based on groups of food exchanges; within each of the exchange lists of foods that are principal sources of carbohydrates, proteins, and fats, respectively, there is a wide variety of foods that can be substituted or exchanged. For practical purposes there are few restrictions, so that each child can select a diet based on personal taste or preferences with the help of the physician and/or dietitian. Emphasis should be placed on regularity of food intake and on constancy of carbohydrate intake. Occasional excesses for birthdays and other parties are permissible and are tolerated in order not to foster rebellion and stealth in obtaining desired food. Similarly, cakes, doughnuts, and even candies are permissible on special occasions as long as the food exchange value and carbohydrate content are adjusted in the meal plan. Adjustments in meal planning must be made for anticipated vigorous exercise (see later section, Exercise). Above all, adjustments must constantly be made to meet the needs as well as the desires of each child.

Monitoring. Success in the daily management of the diabetic child can be measured to a considerable extent by the competence acquired by the family, and subsequently by the child, in *assuming responsibility* for daily "diabetic care." Their initial and ongoing instruction in conjunction with their supervised experience can lead to a sense of confidence in making intermittent adjustments in insulin dosage for dietary deviations, unusual physical activity, and even, for some, minor intercurrent illnesses as well as for otherwise unexplained repeated hypoglycemic reactions and excessive glucosuria. Within limits, such acceptance of responsibility should make them independent of the physician for their ordinary care. Independence is good provided that the physician maintains ongoing interested supervision and shared responsibility with the family and with the child.

Self-monitoring is essential to such a plan and necessitates a regimen that includes measurements of blood or urinary glucose and, at times, of ketones, and the keeping of a standardized record of these results and of the corresponding data of dietary deviations, unusual physical activity, hypoglycemic reactions, intercurrent illness, the daily dose of insulin, and other items of possible relevance. Many of these records may be patently unreliable for a number of reasons. There may be self-delusion, reliance on memory with charting just prior to the visit to the physician, attempts to please the physician and avoid rebuke, as well as reluctance to perform some aspects of the blood or urinary tests. In spite of these problems, asking patients to keep records is justified. Initially, following dismissal from the hospital, the parent or patient is apt to be particularly attentive to a prescribed regimen. It is after some months of satisfactory experience that parents or patients tend to become less attentive to detail. When the physician apparently accepts the contrived report, the parent or child may come to find increasing reasons for noncompliance. When the physician mistrusts the report, he may think it justifiable to make evaluations of his own selection (see later). Should his data be counter to those in the parent's or child's report, he can then attempt to clarify the situation with them in such a manner as not to undermine their mutual confidence. Such situations test the physician's skill in the management of patients with persistent but not confining illness.

The *daily tests for glucosuria* are appropriately scheduled to be performed just prior to each of the three major meals and at the time of the evening snack. This timing is designed to secure an estimate of the effect of the prescribed insulin 3–4 hr after each meal. The preciseness of this estimate is increased if the child voids approximately 30 min before the test voiding; the initial specimen is discarded. When reliable measurements consistently indicate 2% or more glucose in the urine for a given portion of the day, the appropriate dose of the short- or intermediate-acting insulin should be increased by 10–15%. Conversely, when urine is consistently free of glucose for any portion of the day, the insulin dose may need to be reduced by 10–15% if hypoglycemic reactions ensue or if the blood glucose concentration, as determined by the glucose oxidase strip, is 60 mg/dL or less. In the absence of symptomatic hypoglycemia or of documented low blood glucose concentrations, absence of glucosuria does not warrant a reduction in insulin dosage; such patients are manifesting desirable metabolic control. Consistent patterns of excessive glucosuria at fixed times in the morning or afternoon are indications for appropriate increases in the morning or evening doses and at times for a change to another type of insulin. When more precise adjustments are deemed necessary, the physician may request a fractional 24-hr collection of urine. The urine should be collected in three fractions: 8.00 A.M. to 2.00 P.M.; 2.00 P.M. to 8.00 P.M.; and 8.00 P.M. to 8.00 A.M. Assessment of volume and semiquantitative or quantitave glucose values in each sample permits a rational basis for adjusting the respective doses of the rapid- and intermediate-acting insulins.

Short-term (daily) blood glucose monitoring has been markedly enhanced by the availability of strips impregnated with glucose oxidase that permit blood glucose measurement from a drop of blood. The blood glucose concentration can be approximated directly by comparison to a color scale or accurately by a portable calibrated reflectance meter. A small spring-loaded device that automates capillary blood-letting in a relatively painless fashion is also commercially available. Parents and patients should be taught to use these devices and to measure blood glucose 3–4 times daily; before breakfast, lunch, and supper and before retiring at night. Initially, in the hospital, the blood glucose measurement should also be performed at 3.00–4.00 A.M. to exclude inappropriate nocturnal hypoglycemia and to avoid the Somogyi phenomenon (see later). Ideally, the blood glucose concentration should range from approximately 80 mg/dL in the fasting state to 140 mg/dL after meals. In practice, however, a range of 60–240 mg/dL is acceptable. Blood glucose measurements that are consistently at or outside these limits, in the absence of an identifiable cause such as exercise or dietary indiscretion, are an indication for a change in the insulin dose. For example, if the fasting blood glucose is high, the evening dose of intermediate-acting insulin is increased by 10–15%; if the noon glucose level exceeds set limits, the morning regular insulin is increased by 10–15%; if the presupper glucose is high, the morning intermediate-acting insulin is increased by 10–15%; and if the prebedtime glucose measurement is high, the evening dose of regular insulin is increased by 10–15%. Similarly, reductions in insulin type and dose should be made if the corresponding blood glucose measurements are consistently below desirable limits.

Daily blood glucose measurements should be continued after discharge from the hospital as long as they are acceptable to the patient. Practical considerations require a reduction in the frequency of blood glucose monitoring at home; few children tolerate capillary blood-letting 4 times daily for prolonged periods. Consequently, after the initial stabilization period of several weeks, when the routine of insulin administration and meal plan has been established, some suggest that home blood glucose monitoring be performed only 2 days per week, varying the days each week to allow a representative profile in time. Monitoring of urine glucose spill is performed on those days when blood glucose measurements are omitted. However, blood glucose measurement should be performed if there are symptoms suggestive of hypoglycemia or if urine glucose spill persists at 2% or greater. In highly motivated adolescents and young adults who become sufficiently knowledgeable about managing their diabetes, self-monitoring of blood glucose levels before and 2 hr after meals, in conjunction with multiple daily injections of insulin, adjusted as necessary, can maintain near-normal glycemia for prolonged periods.

A reliable index of long-term glycemic control is provided by measurement of *glycosylated hemoglobin.* Glycohemoglobin (HbA_{1c}) represents the fraction of hemoglobin to which glucose has been nonenzymatically attached in the bloodstream. The formation of HbA_{1c} is a slow reaction that is dependent on the prevailing concentration of blood glucose; it continues irreversibly throughout the red blood cell's life span of approximately 120 days. The higher the blood glucose concentration and the longer the red blood cell's exposure to it, the higher the fraction of HbA_{1c}, which is expressed as a percentage of total hemoglobin. Since a blood sample at any given time contains a mixture of red blood cells of varying ages, exposed for varying times to varying blood glucose concentrations, an HbA_{1c} measurement reflects the average blood glucose concentration during the preceding 2–3 mo. When measured by standardized methods to remove labile forms, the fraction of HbA_{1c} is not influenced by an isolated episode of hyperglycemia. Consequently, as an index of long-term glycemic control, a measurement of HbA_{1c} is superior to measurements of glycosuria or a single blood glucose determination. Periodic measurements of HbA_{1c} may also help to resolve questions relating the degree of metabolic control to the subsequent development of complications. Although values of HbA_{1c} may vary according to the method used for measurement, in normal individuals the HbA_{1c} fraction is usually less than 7%; in diabetics, values of 6–9% represent very good metabolic control, values of 9–12% fair control, and values above 12% poor control.

Exercise. Exercise is an integral component of growth and development. No form of exercise, including competitive sports of any kind, should be forbidden to the diabetic child, who should not be made to feel different or restricted. Examples of athletes with diabetes who have excelled in national or international sports are not rare. A major complication of exercise in diabetic patients is the presence of a hypoglycemic reaction during or within hours after exercise. If hypoglycemia does not occur with exercise, adjustments in diet or insulin are not necessary, and glucoregulation is likely to be improved through the increased utilization of glucose by muscles. The major contributing factor to hypoglycemia with exercise is an increased rate of absorption of insulin from its injection site. Regular exercise also improves glucoregulation by increasing insulin receptors. In patients who are in poor metabolic control, vigorous exercise may precipitate ketoacidosis because of the exercise-induced increase in the counterregulatory hormones.

In anticipation of vigorous exercise, one additional carbohydrate exchange may be taken prior to the exercise, and glucose in the form of orange juice, carbonated beverage, or candy should be available during and after exercise. With experience and trial and error, each child and parent, guided by the physician, should develop an appropriate regimen for regularly planned exercise that is frequently associated with hypoglycemia; in such instances, the preceding dose of insulin may be reduced by about 10–15% on the day of the scheduled exercise. Prolonged exercise such as long-distance running may require reduction of as much as 50% or more of the usual insulin dose.

Levels of Treatment. The intensity of treatment required for patients with diabetes mellitus must reflect mutually desirable goals negotiated between the physician and the patient and family. These goals may change depending on the age of the patient, his physical and emotional maturity, understanding, commitment, financial means available to the family, and their health beliefs as well as those of the physician. Goals that are not mutually acceptable are doomed to failure. Minimal levels of treatment are preferable to recurrent hospitalization for diabetic ketoacidosis; intensive therapy carries a significant risk for recurrent hypoglycemia, although it may reduce the risk of microvascular complications. The biochemical and clinical characteristics of minimal, average, and intensive treatment are summarized in Table 8–23.

Residual β Cell Function (Honeymoon Period). After the initial stabilization period some 75% of newly diagnosed diabetic children require progressive reductions in the daily dose of insulin from approximately 1 U/kg to 0.5 U/kg or less. Recurrent hypoglycemia is the manifestation that prompts a

TABLE 8–23. Levels of Treatment: Biochemical and Clinical Characteristics

Minimal	
	HbA_{1c} 11.0–13.0% and GHb 13.0–15.0%
	Many SMBG values of ≥300 mg/dL
	Almost constantly positive urine glucose tests
	Intermittent spontaneous ketonuria
Average	
	HbA_{1c} 8.0–9.0% and GHb 10.0–11.0%
	Premeal SMBG 160–200 mg/dL
	Intermittent positive urine glucose
	Rare ketonuria
Intensive	
	HbA_{1c} 6.0–7.0% and GHb 7.0–9.0%
	Premeal SMBG 70–120 mg/dL; postmeal SMBG <180 mg/dL
	Essentially no positive urine glucose or ketones

SMBG = self-monitored blood glucose; HbA_{1c} = glycohemoglobin; GHb = glycosylated hemoglobin.

reduction in the insulin dose. A minority of children can even maintain normoglycemia for a time without any administered insulin; this complete remission occurs in less than 5% of diabetics, but even in these patients glucose tolerance tests demonstrate abnormal carbohydrate metabolism. The duration of this "honeymoon" phase is variable; it commonly lasts several weeks or months but may last as long as 1–2 yr. Recent investigations clearly demonstrate that residual insulin secretion, measured as C-peptide, is present during this remission period and to some extent in virtually all diabetic children in the initial year of their disease; in approximately 20% there is some C-peptide response even after 5 yr. Stable, well-controlled subjects have higher C-peptide secretion than nonstable subjects, and the required dose of insulin is inversely correlated to the basal or stimulated C-peptide response.

It is not completely clear why this residual insulin secretion is inadequate to prevent the evolution of diabetes including ketoacidosis, but the reasons presumably relate to stress-provoked secretion of catecholamines that inhibit still further the insulin secretory capacity of the pancreatic β cells. In any event, the clinical remission phase is limited; with isolated exceptions, insulin-dependent diabetes inevitably recurs. Although opinion varies, insulin treatment should be maintained unless a daily dose of 0.1 U/kg still causes hypoglycemia, in which case insulin treatment should be discontinued and the patient periodically tested for the re-emergence of glycosuria. The physician may decide to discontinue insulin treatment completely if it appears to be in the patient's best interests during this period. The patient and family, however, should not be led to believe that the disease is "cured" and should continue to examine the child's urine for glucose.

Hypoglycemic Reactions (Insulin Shock). Virtually all diabetic children experience a hypoglycemic reaction at some time during the course of their disease. Hypoglycemia occurs suddenly or over a span of minutes, in contrast to diabetic ketoacidosis, which develops over hours or days. The symptoms and signs are those due to an outpouring of catecholamines, which include pallor, sweating, apprehension, trembling, and tachycardia, and those due to cerebral glucopenia, which include hunger, drowsiness, mental confusion, seizures, and coma. Mood and personality changes plus some abnormal physical patterns may be characteristic for an individual and provide an early clue to the more pronounced reaction. There is some evidence that these symptoms may occur with a sudden drop in blood glucose to levels that do not meet the criteria for hypoglycemia (< 60 mg/dL) in healthy subjects.

The occurrence of hypoglycemia in a diabetic child indicates too much insulin relative to food intake and energy expenditure. Common causes include the evolution of the honeymoon phase (see earlier) after the initial diagnosis, deliberate or accidental errors in insulin dosage, inadequate caloric intake, and strenuous and sustained physical activity in the absence of increased caloric intake.

The most important factors in the management of hypoglycemia are an understanding by the patient and family of the symptoms and signs of the reaction, especially of the patient's individual pattern, and avoidance of known precipitating factors. For management of the acute episode a carbohydrate-containing snack or drink such as orange juice or a sugar-containing carbonated beverage or candy (equivalent to 5–10 g of glucose) should be taken. Patients, parents, and teachers should also be instructed in the administration of glucagon; 0.5 mg given intramuscularly is particularly useful when the patient is losing consciousness or is vomiting. If exercise has been the precipitating factor, the patient should be instructed to take additional calories prior to exercise as a preventive measure. If hypoglycemic episodes persist subsequently under similar circumstances, a reduction in the morning and evening dose of insulin by 10–15% for that day is indicated. The avoidance of severe hypoglycemic episodes should be a major objective of treatment; they have been implicated in ultimately provoking epileptic seizures, and there is an increased frequency of abnormal EEG changes in diabetics.

The Somogyi Phenomenon, the Dawn Phenomenon, and "Brittle Diabetes." Hypoglycemic episodes, which may be mild and manifest as late nocturnal or early morning sweating, night terrors, and headaches alternating rapidly (within 4–5 hr) with ketosis, hyperglycemia, ketonuria, and excessive glucosuria, should suggest the possibility of the **Somogyi phenomenon**. This syndrome has been suitably described as "hypoglycemia begetting hyperglycemia" and is believed to be due to an outpouring of counterregulatory hormones in response to insulin-induced hypoglycemia. The coexistence of this brittle form of diabetes with daily doses of more than 2 U/kg of insulin suggests the presence of this phenomenon and the need to reduce the dose of insulin. The term brittle diabetes implies that control of blood glucose fluctuates widely and rapidly despite frequent adjustments of the dose of insulin.

The Somogyi phenomenon should be distinguished from the **dawn phenomenon** in which early morning elevations of blood glucose concentration occur between 5.00 and 9.00 A.M. without preceding hypoglycemia. The dawn phenomenon is a normal event and occurs even in patients treated by continuous subcutaneous infusion of insulin unless the rate of insulin infusion is increased in the early morning hours. The dawn phenomenon reflects the waning effects of biologically available insulin, probably as a consequence of increased clearance of insulin and nocturnal surges of growth hormone that antagonize insulin's metabolic effects; the normal early morning rise in cortisol is not responsible for this phenomenon. Together, the Somogyi and dawn phenomena are the most common causes of instability or "brittleness" in diabetic children. To distinguish between the dawn and Somogyi phenomena, blood glucose concentrations should be measured at 3.00 A.M., 4.00 A.M., and 7.00 A.M. If blood glucose concentrations are over 80 mg/dL in the first two samples and markedly higher in the last, then the dawn phenomenon is likely; an increase in the evening dose of intermediate insulin of 10–15% may be helpful. It may also be helpful to delay the evening dose of intermediate-acting insulin by 2–3 hr so that its delayed peak effect coincides with the anticipated timing of the dawn phenomenon, and excessive increases of blood glucose are avoided or blunted. On the other hand, if the 3.00 A.M. or 4.00 A.M. blood glucose measurement is 60 mg/dL or less followed by rebound hyperglycemia at 7.00 A.M., the Somogyi phenomenon is likely; a reduction of the evening intermediate-acting insulin of 10–15%, or a delay in its injection until approximately 9.00 P.M., is indicated (Fig. 8–46).

In other patients with brittle diabetes better control is often achieved by instituting a change from one to two daily injections of insulin or by a change from beef-pork mixtures to pure pork or human insulin, which may circumvent problems with antibodies that bind insulin. Attention should also be directed to psychologic problems within or outside of the home that may be the bases for deliberate errors in insulin or nutritional intake.

Psychologic Aspects. Diabetes in a child affects the life style and interpersonal relationships of the entire family. Feelings of anxiety and guilt are common in parents. Similar feelings, coupled with denial and rejection, are equally common in children, particularly during the rebellious teenage years. No specific personality disorder or psychopathology is characteristic of diabetes; similar feelings are observed in families with other chronic disorders.

In children with diabetes these feelings find expression in nonadherence to instructions regarding nutritional and insulin therapy and in noncompliance with self-monitoring. Deliberate overdosage with insulin, resulting in hypoglycemia, or omission of insulin, often in association with excesses in nutritional intake, resulting in ketoacidosis, may be pleas for psychologic help or manipulative events to escape an environment perceived as undesirable or intolerable; occasionally they may be manifestations of suidical intent. Frequent admissions to the hospital for ketoacidosis or hypoglycemia should arouse a suspicion of underlying emotional conflict. Overprotection on the part of parents is common and often is not in the best interests of the patient. Feelings of being different or of being alone are common and may be justified in view of the restrictive schedules imposed by testing of urine and blood, administration of insulin, and nutritional limitations. Furthermore, publicity about the likelihood of developing complications and the decreased life span in patients with type I diabetes fosters anxiety. Unfortunately, misinformation abounds about the risks of development of diabetes in siblings or in offspring and of pregnancy in young diabetic women. Even appropriate information often causes further anxiety.

Many, but not all, of these problems can be averted through continued empathic counseling based on correct information

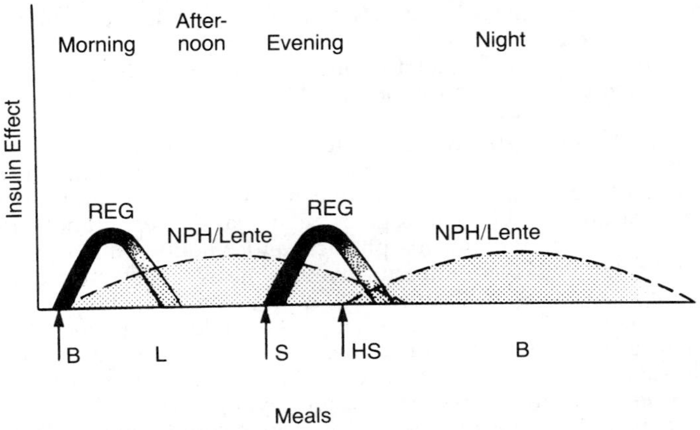

Figure 8–46. Three-dose insulin regimen intended to reduce the likelihood of the Somogyi or the dawn phenomenon. The morning dose comprises a combined short- and intermediate-acting insulin of about one half to two third of the total daily dose. The short-acting dose before supper covers the anticipated glycemic elevation with dinner. The intermediate-acting insulin is delayed till bedtime so that the peak effect is delayed. (From Schade DS, Santiago JV, Skyler JS, et al: Intensive Insulin Therapy, Excerpta Medica, 1983, USA.)

and attempts to build attitudes of normality in the patient as a productive and potentially reproductive member of society. Recognizing the potential impact of these problems, peer discussion groups have been organized in many locales; feelings of isolation and frustration tend to be lessened by the sharing of common problems. Summer camps for diabetic children afford an excellent opportunity for learning and sharing under expert supervision. Education about the pathophysiology of diabetes, insulin dose, technique of administration, nutrition, exercise, and hypoglycemic reactions can be reinforced by medical and paramedical personnel. The presence of numerous peers with similar problems offers new insights to the diabetic child.

The physician managing a child or adolescent with diabetes should be aware of his pivotal role as counselor and advisor and should anticipate the common emotional problems of his patient. When emotional problems are clearly responsible for poor compliance with the medical regimen, referral for psychologic help may be indicated. Such help is often available in pediatric centers, where psychologists form part of the management team for diabetic children.

Management During Infections. Systemic and local infections are no more common in diabetic children than in nondiabetic ones. During intercurrent illnesses, either infectious or traumatic, diabetic children nearly always require additional insulin, especially during prolonged serious episodes that necessitate inactivity. In the latter situations, when glucosuria is excessive, a good working rule is to add 10–20% of the total daily dose as regular (short-acting) insulin prior to each meal. Subsequent increases or decreases should then be based on careful monitoring of urinary and blood glucose values.

Patients who are vomiting should, nevertheless, take some insulin; approximately 50% of the daily dose is a general rule, followed by careful monitoring of urinary or blood glucose and subsequent adjustments of the dose of insulin as indicated. If vomiting continues and the patient cannot tolerate clear liquids, admission to the hospital and consideration of intravenous therapy with glucose, electrolytes, and insulin are warranted.

Management During Surgery. The objectives of management are prevention of hypoglycemia during anesthesia, of severe loss of fluids, and of diabetic acidosis. The regimens described below are generally applicable, but vigilance and individual adjustments for each patient are necessary to achieve these goals.

When surgery is elective, the patient should be admitted to the hospital 24 hr prior to surgery; during this time the usual nutritional requirements and insulin dose are provided. Supplemental regular insulin may be given to achieve better control of blood glucose when the need is demonstrated. On the morning of surgery an infusion of 5% glucose in 0.45% saline solution plus 20 mEq/L of potassium chloride is begun; initially 1 unit of regular insulin is added to the infusate for each 4 g of administered glucose. The rate of infusion should provide maintenance fluid requirements plus estimated losses during surgery. The blood glucose concentration should be monitored at periodic intervals before, during, and after surgery; concentrations of approximately 120–150 mg/dL should be the goal; this can be achieved by varying the rate of infusion of the glucose and electrolyte mixture or the amount of insulin added. This regimen may be discontinued when the patient is awake and capable of taking food and fluid orally. Prior to reinstitution of the patient's usual diet, regular insulin may be administered at a dose of 0.25 U/kg at 6-hr intervals; appropriate adjustments in the dose are based on blood or urinary concentrations of glucose.

An equally effective plan that is particularly useful for surgery of short duration is as follows: On the morning of surgery half of the usual morning dose of insulin is administered subcutaneously, and intravenous infusion of the electrolyte and glucose solution described in the preceding paragraph but minus the insulin is initiated. After surgery, regular insulin in a dose of 0.25 U/kg is administered subcutaneously; subsequent doses at 6-hr intervals are adjusted on the basis of blood glucose concentrations until the patient is ready for his or her usual dietary pattern.

For emergency surgery an intravenous infusion is initiated that provides 5–10% glucose in 0.45% saline solution, 20 mEq of potassium chloride, and 1 unit of regular insulin for each 2–4 g of glucose. Blood glucose concentration should be maintained at approximately 120–150 mg/dL. When possible, rehydration and metabolic balance should precede the surgery. After surgery the regimen described earlier can be instituted.

For minor surgery under local anesthesia the usual insulin and dietary regimens can be maintained. If extensive vomiting occurs, the losses can usually be compensated with glucose solution administered intravenously.

NEUROVASCULAR AND OTHER COMPLICATIONS: RELATION TO GLYCEMIC CONTROL. The increasingly prolonged survival of the diabetic child is associated with an increasing prevalence of complications that affect the microcirculation of the eye (retinopathy), the kidney (nephropathy), the nerves (neuropathy), the large vessels (atherosclerosis), and the lens (cataracts). Retinopathy is present in 45–60% of insulin-dependent diabetics after 20 yr of known disease and in 20% after 10 yr; lens opacities are present in at least 5% of those under 19 yr of age. Diabetic nephropathy is also common; it is present in about 40% of patients after 25 yr of insulin-dependent diabetes whose onset occurred in childhood; this complication may account for about 50% of deaths in long-term insulin-dependent diabetics.

There is an emerging consensus that clinical experience and experimental data strongly suggest an association between glycemic control and the later development of complications. It is not known, however, if this relationship is directly proportional to the degree of hyperglycemia, or if there is a set point of average glycemia above which complications develop exponentially or below which complications may be avoided. In addition, studies implicate possible biochemical pathways that may be responsible for these complications. For example, the process of glycosylation of erythrocytic hemoglobin, which is directly proportional to the blood glucose concentration, also involves other serum and tissue proteins; it has been implicated in basement membrane thickening in the glomeruli. There is evidence that activation of the polyol pathway and disturbances in myoinositol metabolism are related, respectively, to cataracts and to neuropathy. In humans, typical lesions of diabetic nephropathy develop in normal kidneys within several years after they have been transplanted to diabetics with chronic renal failure. By contrast, the early histologic changes of diabetic nephropathy regress when kidneys of a diabetic are transplanted to a nondiabetic recipient with chronic renal failure. Similarly, renal lesions that mimic those of human diabetes develop in animals rendered diabetic, and these changes tend to regress following cure of the diabetes by islet transplantation. Therefore, it appears that the diabetic environment and not the genetic background predisposes to these renal changes. Genetic factors clearly play a role, however, since only 30–40% of patients affected by type I diabetes mellitus eventually develop end-stage renal disease, and only 50% develop proliferative retinopathy.

Other complications described in diabetic children include dwarfism associated with a glycogen-laden enlarged liver **(Mauriac syndrome)**, osteopenia, and a syndrome of limited joint mobility associated with tight, waxy skin, growth impairment, and maturational delay. The Mauriac syndrome is clearly related to underinsulinization; it is now rare because of the availability of the longer-acting insulins. The syndrome of limited joint mobility is frequently associated with the early development of diabetic microvascular complications, such as retinopathy and nephropathy, which may appear before 18 yr of age. None of these complications has been demonstrated in a nondiabetic identical twin, even after 20 yr of recognized diabetes in his or her insulin-dependent twin. As indicated, genetic predisposition to the development of diabetic vascular complications does, however, play a role.

Despite the hard evidence in experimental animals and suggestive evidence in humans with diabetes, the possible relationship of the degree of glycemic control to these complications in humans remains moot because none of the available modes of routine treatment has resulted in sufficiently normal metabolic control to provide an adequate study group. Nevertheless, the persuasive evidence in favor of a relationship, together with improved methods of monitoring glycemic control and of insulin delivery, forms the basis of a multicenter trial examining the relationship between metabolic control and development of complications. Consequently, as long as reduction of these late complications remains a possibility, physicians have the responsibility of maintaining metabolism that is as near normal as is compatible with the physical and psychologic limits of each diabetic child. Despite the potential for development of complications, survival for 40 yr and more is feasible; the goal should be to make these years increasingly free of debilitating diabetic-related disease.

PROGNOSIS. Type I diabetes mellitus is not a benign disease. In one study on the long-term outcome of 45 children under 12 yr of age at the time of diagnosis, there were several deaths within 10–25 yr of diagnosis: three were directly attributable to diabetes, and two were due to suicide; three patients attempted suicide unsuccessfully. Visual, renal, neuropathic, and other complications were relatively frequent. Furthermore, although diabetic children eventually attain a height within the normal adult range, puberty may be delayed, and the final height may be less than the genetic potential. From studies in identical twins it is apparent that, despite apparently satisfactory control, the diabetic twin manifests delayed puberty and a substantial reduction in height, with a mean difference of 5 cm, when onset of disease occurs before puberty. These observations indicate that in the past, conventional criteria for judging control were inadequate and that adequate control of insulin-dependent diabetes was almost never achieved by routine methods.

The introduction of portable devices that can be programmed to provide continuous subcutaneous infusion of insulin with meal-related pulses is one approach to the resolution of these long-term problems. In selected individuals, nearly normal patterns of blood glucose and other indices of metabolic control including HbA_{1c} have been maintained for several years. This approach, however, should be reserved for highly motivated persons who are committed to rigorous self-monitoring of blood glucose and are alert to the potential complications, such as mechanical failure of the infusion device, causing hyperglycemia or hypoglycemia, and infections at the site of needle implantation.

8.54 IMPAIRED GLUCOSE TOLERANCE AND TYPE II NONINSULIN-DEPENDENT DIABETES

In the classification of diabetes mellitus and other clinical impairments of glucose tolerance proposed by the National Diabetes Data Group (see Table 8–16) the term impaired glucose tolerance is used to characterize individuals who have a plasma glucose concentration in excess of 140 mg/dL 2 hr after initiation of the standard oral glucose tolerance test but do not have symptoms of diabetes or fasting hyperglycemia. The indication for an oral glucose tolerance test may be the discovery of isolated or intermittent glucosuria or the occurrence of hyperglycemia during a stressful illness or during corticosteroid therapy. Individuals considered at risk for abnormal glucose metabolism may also need to be tested; these include obese children, those who have symptoms suggestive of reactive postprandial hypoglycemia, and close relatives of known diabetics. An oral glucose tolerance test is not indicated in a child who has characteristic diabetic symptoms and a random blood glucose value in excess of 200 mg/dL.

The term impaired glucose tolerance is suggested as a replacement for such terms as asymptomatic diabetes, chemical diabetes, subclinical diabetes, borderline diabetes, or latent diabetes in order to avoid the stigma associated with the term diabetes mellitus, which may influence the choice of vocation, eligibility for health or life insurance, and self-image. Furthermore, although impaired glucose tolerance represents a biochemical intermediate between normal glucose metabolism and that of diabetes, experience has shown that few children with impaired glucose tolerance go on to develop diabetes; estimates range from 0–10%. There is disagreement about whether the degree of glucose intolerance is useful as a prognostic index of the likelihood of progression, but there is evidence that among the few who do progress, the insulin response during glucose tolerance testing is severely impaired; islet cell or insulin autoantibodies as well as the HLA-DR3 or -DR4 haplotype are commonly found in those who go on to diabetes. In the majority of children with impaired glucose tolerance, particularly the obese, insulin responses during oral glucose tolerance tests are higher than the mean for age-adjusted but not weight-adjusted controls; these individuals have some resistance to the effects of insulin rather than a total inability to secrete it.

In normal children the glucose response during an oral glucose tolerance test is similar at all ages. In contrast, plasma insulin responses during the test increase progressively within the age span of about 3–15 yr and are significantly higher during puberty, so that interpretation of these responses requires comparison with age- and puberty-adjusted criteria.

The performance of the glucose tolerance test should be standardized according to currently accepted criteria. These include at least 3 days of a well-balanced diet containing approximately 50% of calories from carbohydrates; fasting from midnight until the time of the test in the morning; and a dose of glucose for the test of 1.75 g/kg but not more than 75 g. Plasma samples are obtained prior to ingestion of the glucose and at 1, 2, and 3 hr thereafter. The arbitrarily designated response to the test that identifies "impaired glucose tolerance" is a fasting plasma glucose value of less than 140 mg/dL and a value at 2 hr of more than 140 mg/dL. Determination of serum insulin responses during the glucose tolerance test is not a prerequisite for reaching a diagnosis; the magnitude of the response, however, may have prognostic value.

In children with impaired glucose tolerance but without fasting hyperglycemia, repeated oral glucose tolerance tests are not recommended. Investigations in such children indicate that the degree of impaired glucose tolerance tends to remain stable or may actually improve over a period of years, except in patients with markedly subnormal insulin responses. Consequently, apart from reduction in weight for the obese child, no therapy is indicated. In particular, the use of oral hypoglycemic agents should be restricted to investigational studies. If fasting hyperglycemia or characteristic symptoms of diabetes develop, the affected children will have the characteristics of noninsulin-dependent diabetes (type II), previously known as adult-onset diabetes (see Table 8–16 and the brief description in text under Classification). Such children may require insulin for control of hyperglycemia, although they generally do not develop ketosis in the absence of exogenous insulin therapy and hence, by definition, are not insulin dependent.

8.55 DISEASES ASSOCIATED WITH DIABETES

CYSTIC FIBROSIS (see Sec. 14.89). Because of improvements in the medical care of children with cystic fibrosis, many survive to the late teen and early adult years. In addition to the primary insufficiency of pancreatic exocrine function, there is an increasing incidence of pancreatic endocrine dysfunction manifested as glucose intolerance that progresses occasionally to overt diabetes mellitus. When hyperglycemia develops, the accompanying metabolic derangements are usually mild, and, if insulin therapy becomes necessary, relatively low doses usually suffice for adequate management. Ketoacidosis is uncommon but may occur with progressive deterioration of islet cell function. Treatment with insulin is the same as that outlined for type I diabetes, but dietary management may be limited by the constraints of the primary disturbance.

AUTOIMMUNE DISEASES. *Chronic lymphocytic thyroiditis* (Hashimoto thyroiditis) is frequently associated with type I diabetes in children. As many as 1 in 5 insulin-dependent diabetics may have thyroid antibodies in their serum; the prevalence is 2–20 times greater than that observed in control populations. Only a small proportion of these diabetics, however, develop clinical hypothyroidism; the interval between diagnosis of diabetes and development of thyroid disease averages about 5 yr. Periodic palpation of the thyroid gland is indicated in all diabetic children; if the gland feels firm or enlarged, serum measurements of thyroid antibodies and thyroid-stimulating hormone (TSH) should be obtained. A TSH level of greater than 10 μU/mL indicates existing or incipient thyroid dysfunction that warrants replacement with thyroid hormone. Deceleration in the rate of growth may also be due to thyroid failure and is in itself a reason for securing serum measurements of thyroxine and TSH concentrations.

When diabetes and thyroid disease coexist, the possibility of *adrenal insufficiency* should also be considered. It may be heralded by decreasing insulin requirements, increasing pigmentation of the skin and buccal mucosa, salt craving, weakness, asthenia, postural hypotension, or even frank addisonian crisis as evidence of primary adrenal failure. This syndrome is most unusual in the 1st decade of life, but it may become apparent in the 2nd decade or later.

Circulating *antibodies to gastric parietal cells* and to intrinsic factor are 2–3 times more common in patients with type I diabetes than in control subjects. There are good correlations of antibodies to gastric parietal cells with **atrophic gastritis** and of antibodies to intrinsic factor with **malabsorption of vitamin B_{12}**. Although the possibility of **megaloblastic anemia** should be considered in children with type I diabetes, its occurrence is rare.

A variant of the *multiple endocrine deficiency syndrome* (see Sec. 19.17) is characterized by type I diabetes, idiopathic intestinal mucosal atrophy with associated inflammation and severe malabsorption, IgA deficiency, and circulating antibodies to multiple endocrine organs including the thyroid, adrenal, pancreas, parathyroid, and gonads. In addition, nondiabetic family members have an increased frequency of vitiligo, Graves disease, and multiple sclerosis, low complement levels, and a high frequency of antibodies to endocrine tissues. Type I diabetes may itself be an autoimmune disease.

8.56 ACANTHOSIS NIGRICANS WITH INSULIN RESISTANCE TYPE A. This syndrome is characterized by acanthosis nigricans, especially of the axillae and neck, variable degrees of glucose intolerance, including symptomatic diabetes, hirsutism, accelerated growth suggestive of gigantism, and marked endogenous hyperinsulinemia with severe resistance to exogenous insulin. The syndrome occurs predominantly in black females who commonly present during adolescence for evaluation of menstrual irregularities; many are obese and have laboratory findings suggestive of the polycystic ovary syndrome. The carbohydrate intolerance, hyperinsulinemia, and resistance to exogenous insulin result from a congenitally reduced number of insulin receptors, alteration of their molecular structure, or inability to transduce the insulin signal owing to defects in the receptor's tyrosine kinase activity. Weight reduction may ameliorate the carbohydrate intolerance, but exogenous insulin is usually not helpful.

8.57 GENETIC SYNDROMES ASSOCIATED WITH DIABETES MELLITUS

A number of rare genetic syndromes associated with insulin-dependent diabetes mellitus or with carbohydrate intolerance have been described. These syndromes represent a broad spectrum of diseases ranging from premature cellular aging, as in the **Werner** and **Cockayne** syndromes (see Sec. 23.15), to excessive obesity associated with hyperinsulinism, resistance to insulin action, and carbohydrate intolerance, as in the **Prader-Willi syndrome** (see Sec. 19.30). Some of these syndromes are characterized by primary disturbances in the insulin receptor or in antibodies to the insulin receptor without any impairment in insulin secretion. Although rare, these syndromes provide unique models with which to study the multiple causes of disturbed carbohydrate metabolism from defective insulin secretion or from defective insulin action at the cell receptor or postreceptor step.

8.58 TRANSIENT DIABETES MELLITUS OF THE NEWBORN

Onset of persistent insulin-dependent diabetes before the age of 6 mo is very unusual. The syndrome of transient diabetes mellitus in the newborn infant has its onset in the first weeks of life and persists only several weeks to months before resolving spontaneously. It occurs most often in infants who are small for gestational age and is characterized by hyperglycemia and pronounced glycosuria resulting in severe dehydration and at times metabolic acidosis but with only minimal or no ketonemia or ketonuria. Insulin responses to glucose or tolbutamide are low to absent; basal plasma insulin concentrations, however, are normal. After spontaneous recovery, the insulin responses to these same stimuli are brisk and normal. Occurrence of the syndrome in consecutive siblings has been reported. Permanent diabetes is not known to have developed in any affected infant who has recovered from the transient syndrome. This syndrome should be distinguished from severe hyperglycemia that may occur in hypertonic dehydration (see Sec. 6.16); this occurs usually in infants past the newborn period, who respond promptly to rehydration and have a minimal requirement for insulin.

Administration of insulin is mandatory during the active phase of this syndrome. Intermediate-acting insulin, 1–2 U/kg/24 hr given in two divided doses, usually results in dramatic improvement and accelerated growth and gain in weight. Attempts at gradually reducing the dose of insulin may be made as soon as recurrent hypoglycemia becomes manifest or after 2 mo of age. The parents should be assured of the transient nature of the disease and the excellent prognosis. Rarely, **pancreatic agenesis** may be associated with early but permanent diabetes mellitus as well as malabsorption.

MARK A. SPERLING

EPIDEMIOLOGY, ETIOLOGY, PATHOPHYSIOLOGY, AND CLASSIFICATION

Dotta F, Eisenbarth GS: Type I diabetes mellitus: A predictable autoimmune disease with interindividual variation in the rate of β-cell destruction. Clin Immunol Immunopathol 50:S85, 1989.
Eisenbarth GS: Genes, generator of diversity, glycoconjugates, and autoimmune β-cell insufficiency in type I diabetes. Diabetes 36:355, 1987.
Eisenbarth GS: Type I diabetes mellitus: A chronic autoimmune disease. N Engl J Med 314:1360, 1986.
Karam JH, Lewitt PE, Young CW, et al: Insulinopenic diabetes after rodenticide (Vacor) ingestion: A unique model of acquired diabetes in man. Diabetes 29:971, 1980.
LaPorte RE, Dorman JS, Orchard TJ, et al: Preventing insulin dependent diabetes mellitus: The environmental challenge. Br Med J 295:479, 1987.
Maclaren NK: How, when and why to predict IDDM. Diabetes 37:1591, 1988.
National Diabetes Data Group: Classification and diagnosis of diabetes mellitus and other categories of glucose intolerance. Diabetes 28:1039, 1979.
Neufeld M, MacLaren NK, Riley NF, et al: Islet cell and other organ-specific antibodies in US Caucasians and blacks with insulin-dependent diabetes mellitus. Diabetes 29:589, 1980.
Regional variation in diabetes mellitus prevalence—U.S., 1988 and 1989. MMWR 39:805, 1990.
Riley WJ, Winter WE, Maclaren NK: Identification of insulin-dependent diabetes mellitus before the onset of clinical symptoms. J Pediatr 112:314, 1988.
Rosenbloom AL, Kohrman A, Sperling M: Classification and diagnosis of diabetes mellitus in children and adolescents. J Pediatr 98:320, 1981.
Sperling MA (ed): Physician's Guide to Insulin-Dependent (Type I) Diabetes Mellitus: Diagnosis and Treatment. Alexandria, VA, American Diabetes Association, 1988.

GENETICS

Lernmark A: Molecular biology of type I (insulin-dependent) diabetes mellitus. Diabetologia 28:195, 1985.
Morel PA, Dorman JS, Todd JA, et al: Aspartic acid at position 57 of the HLA-DQ β chain protects against type I diabetes: A family study. Proc Natl Acad Sci USA 85:8111, 1988.
Pyke DA: Diabetes: The genetic connections. Diabetologia 17:333, 1979.
Rotter JL, Hodge SE: Racial differences in juvenile-type diabetes are consistent with more than one mode of inheritance. Diabetes 29:115, 1980.
Rotter JL, Rimoin DL: The genetics of diabetes. Hosp Pract May:79, 1987.
Trucco M, Dorman JS: Immunogenetics of insulin-dependent diabetes mellitus in humans. Crit Rev Immunol 9:201, 1989.
Warram JH, Krolewski AS, Gottlieb MS, et al: Differences in risk of insulin-dependent diabetes in offspring of diabetic mothers and diabetic fathers. N Engl J Med 311:149, 1984.
Wassmuth R, Lernmark A: The genetics of susceptibility to diabetes. Clin Immunol Immunopathol 53:358, 1989.

DIABETIC KETOACIDOSIS

Adrogue HJ, Wilson H, Boyd AE III, et al: Plasma acid-base patterns in diabetic ketoacidosis. N Engl J Med 307:1603, 1982.
Arieff AI: Pathogenesis of lactic acidosis. Diabetes Metab Rev 5:637, 1989.
Duck SC, Wyatt DT: Factors associated with brain herniation in the treatment of diabetic ketoacidosis. J Pediatr 113:10, 1988.
Foster DW, McGarry JD: The metabolic derangements and treatment of diabetic ketoacidosis. N Engl J Med 309:159, 1983.
Harris GD, Fiordalisi I, Finberg L: Safe management of diabetic ketoacidemia. J Pediatr 113:65, 1988.
Keller U, Berger W: Prevention of hypophosphatemia by phosphate infusion during treatment of diabetic ketoacidosis and hyperosmolar coma. Diabetes 29:87, 1980.
Krane EJ, Rockoff MA, Wallman JK, et al: Subclinical brain swelling in children during treatment of diabetric ketoacidosis. N Engl J Med 312:1147, 1985.
Matz R. Cerebral edema in diabetic ketoacidosis. Lancet 2:689, 1987.
Riley LJ, Cooper M, Narins RG: Alkali therapy of diabetic ketoacidosis: Biochemical, physiologic, and clinical perspectives. Diabetes Metab Rev 5:627, 1989.
Rosenbloom AL: Intracerebral crisis during treatment of diabetic ketoacidosis. Diabetes Care 13:22, 1990.
Sperling MA: Diabetic ketoacidosis. Pediatr Clin North Am 31:591, 1984.
Van der Meulen JA, Klip A, Grinstein S: Possible mechanism for cerebral edema in diabetic ketoacidosis. Lancet 2:306, 1987.
Winter RJ, Harris CJ, Phillips LS, et al: Diabetic ketoacidosis: Induction of hypocalcemia and hypomagnesemia by phosphate therapy. Am J Med 67:897, 1979.

MANAGEMENT OF TYPE I DIABETES IN CHILDREN

Arky RA: Nutritional therapy for the child and adolescent with type I diabetes mellitus. Pediatr Clin North Am 31:711, 1984.
Bolli GB, Gerich JE: The "dawn phenomenon"—a common occurrence in both non-insulin and insulin-dependent diabetes mellitus. N Engl J Med 310:746, 1984.
Bolli GB, Gottesman IS, Campbell PJ, et al: Glucose counterregulation and waning of insulin in the Somogyi phenomenon (posthypoglycemic hyperglycemia). N Engl J Med 311:1214, 1984.
Cerreto MC, Travis LB: Implications of psychological and family factors in the treatment of diabetes. Pediatr Clin North Am 31:689, 1984.
Goldstein DE: Understanding GHb assays: A guided tour for clinicians. Clin Diabetes 4:7, 1986.
Ingersoll GM, Orr DP, Herrold AJ, et al: Cognitive maturity and self-management among adolescents with insulin-dependent diabetes mellitus. Clin Lab Observ 108:620, 1986.
Kovacs M, Feinberg TL, Paulauskas S, et al: Initial coping responses and psychosocial characteristics of children with insulin-dependent diabetes mellitus. J Pediatr 106:827, 1985.
Menon RK, Sperling MA: Childhood diabetes. Med Clin North Am 72:1565, 1988.
Saggese G, Federico G, Bertelloni S, et al: Hypomagnesemia and parathyroid hormone—vitamin D endocrine system in children with insulin dependent diabetes mellitus: Effects of magnesium administration. J Pediatr 118:220, 1991.
Sperling MA: Insulin biosynthesis and C-peptide. Am J Dis Child 134:1119, 1980.
Stein R, Goldberg N, Kalman F, et al: Exercise and the patient with type I diabetes mellitus. Pediatr Clin North Am 31:665, 1984.
Tamborlane WV, Press CM: Insulin infusion pump treatment of type I diabetes. Pediatr Clin North Am 31:721, 1984.
Wilson DM, Luetscher JA: Plasma prorenin activity and complications in children with insulin dependent diabetes mellitus. N Engl J Med 323:1101, 1990.
Witters LA, Ohman JL, Weir GC, et al: Insulin antibodies in the pathogenesis of insulin allergy and resistance. Am J Med 63:703, 1977.
Zinman B: The physiologic replacement of insulin. N Engl J Med 321:363, 1989.

LONG-TERM OUTCOME OF CHILDHOOD DIABETES: RELATION OF CONTROL TO DEVELOPMENT OF COMPLICATIONS

Abouna GM, Kremer GD, Daddah SK, et al: Reversal of diabetic nephropathy in human cadaveric kidneys after transplantation into non-diabetic recipients. Lancet 2:1274, 1983.
Beyer MM: Diabetic nephropathy. Pediatr Clin North Am 31:635, 1984.
Browning and diabetic complications. Lancet 1:1192, 1986.
Diabetes Control and Complications Trial: Are continuing studies of metabolic control and microvascular complications in insulin-dependent diabetes mellitus justified? N Engl J Med 318:246, 1988.
Diabetic skin, joints and eyes—how are they related? Lancet 2:313, 1987.
Gabbay KH: The sorbitol pathway and complications of diabetes. N Engl J Med 288:831, 1983.
Hostetter TH: Diabetic nephropathy. N Engl J Med 312:642, 1985.
Kirschenbaum DM: Glycosylation of proteins: Its implications in diabetic control and complications. Pediatr Clin North Am 31:611, 1984.
Leslie ND, Sperling MA: Relation of metabolic control to complications in diabetes mellitus. J Pediatr 108:491, 1986.
Rosenbloom AL: Skeletal and joint manifestations of childhood diabetes. Pediatr Clin North Am 31:569, 1984.
Skyler JS: Complications of diabetes mellitus: Relationship to metabolic dysfunction. Diabetes Care 2:499, 1979.
Steffes MW, Sutherland DER, Goetz FC, et al: Study of kidney and muscle biopsy specimens from identical twins discordant for type I diabetes mellitus. N Engl J Med 312:1282, 1985.
White NW, Waltman SR, Krupin T, et al: Reversal of neuropathic and gastrointestinal complications related to diabetes mellitus in adolescents with improved metabolic control. J Pediatr 99:41, 1981.
Winegrad AI: Does a common mechanism induce the diverse complications of diabetes? Diabetes 36:396, 1987.

DISEASES AND SYNDROMES ASSOCIATED WITH DIABETES

Didmoad (Wolfram) syndrome. Lancet 1:1075, 1986.
Flier JS, Kahn CR, Roth J: Receptors, antireceptor antibodies and mechanisms of insulin resistance. N Engl J Med 300:413, 1979.
Lippe BM, Sperling MA, Dooley RR: Pancreatic alpha and beta cell functions in cystic fibrosis. J Pediatr 90:751, 1977.
Low L, Chernausek SD, Sperling MA: Acromegaloid patients with type-A insulin resistance: Parallel defects in insulin and insulin-like growth factor-I receptors and biological responses in cultured fibroblasts. J Clin Endocrinol Metab 69:329, 1989.

National Diabetes Data Group: Classification and diagnosis of diabetes mellitus and other categories of glucose intolerance. Diabetes 28:1039, 1979.
Sullivan MM, Denning CR: Diabetic microangiopathy in patients with cystic fibrosis. Pediatrics 84:642, 1989.
Winter WE, Maclaren NK, Riley WJ, et al: Congenital pancreatic hypoplasia: A syndrome of exocrine and endocrine pancreatic insufficiency. J Pediatr 109:465, 1986.
Winter WE, Maclaren NK, Riley WJ, et al: Maturity-onset diabetes of youth in black Americans. N Engl J Med 316:285, 1987.

TRANSIENT DIABETES OF THE NEWBORN

Blethen SL, White NH, Santiago JV, et al: Plasma somatomedins, endogenous insulin secretion, and growth in transient neonatal diabetes mellitus. J Clin Endocrinol Metab 52:144, 1981.
Pagliara AS, Karl IE, Kipnis DB: Transient neonatal diabetes: Delayed maturation of the pancreatic beta cell. J Pediatr 82:97, 1973.
Schiff D, Colle E, Stern L: Metabolic and growth patterns in transient neonatal diabetes. N Engl J Med 287:119, 1972.

8.59 HYPOGLYCEMIA

Glucose plays a central role in mammalian fuel economy and is a source of energy storage in the form of glycogen, fat, and protein (see Sec. 8.37–8.40). Glucose is an immediate source of energy because it provides 38 moles of ATP/mole of glucose oxidized. It is important for cerebral energy metabolism in that it usually is the preferred substrate whose utilization accounts for nearly all of the O_2 consumption in brain (see later). Cerebral glucose uptake occurs through a carrier-mediated, facilitated diffusion process that is dependent on blood glucose concentration. Neither glucose entry into brain cells nor its subsequent metabolism is dependent on insulin. To maintain the blood glucose concentration and prevent it from precipitously falling to levels that impair brain function, an elaborate regulatory system has evolved.

The defense against hypoglycemia is integrated by the autonomic nervous system and by hormones that act in concert to enhance glucose production through enzymatic modulation of glycogenolysis and gluconeogenesis while simultaneously limiting peripheral glucose utilization. In this context, hypoglycemia represents a defect in one or several of the complex interactions that normally integrate glucose homeostasis during feeding and fasting. This process is particularly important for neonates, in whom there is an abrupt transition from intrauterine life, characterized by dependence on transplacental glucose supply, to extrauterine life, characterized ultimately by the autonomous ability to maintain precise glucose balance. Since prematurity or placental factors may limit tissue nutrient deposits, and genetic abnormalities in enzymes or hormones may become evident in the neonate, hypoglycemia is an important cause of neonatal morbidity.

DEFINITION. In neonates, there is not always an obvious correlation between blood glucose concentration and the classic clinical manifestations of hypoglycemia. The absence of symptoms does not indicate that glucose concentration is normal and has not fallen below some optimal level for maintaining brain metabolism. In addition, there is evidence that hypoxemia and ischemia potentiate the role of hypoglycemia in causing brain damage that may permanently impair neurologic development. Consequently, the lower limit of accepted normality of the blood glucose level in newborn infants with associated illness that already impairs cerebral metabolism has not been determined (see Sec. 9.57). Out of concern for possible neurologic, intellectual, or psychologic sequelae in later life, many authorities now urge that in neonates any value of blood glucose below 40 mg/dL (2.2 mM) be viewed with suspicion and vigorously treated. This is particularly applicable after the initial 2–3 hr of life, when glucose normally has reached its nadir; subsequently, blood glucose levels begin to rise and achieve values of 50 mg/dL (2.8 mM) or higher after 12–24 hr. In older infants and children, a blood glucose concentration of less than 40 mg/dL (10–15% higher for serum or plasma) represents significant hypoglycemia.

SIGNIFICANCE AND SEQUELAE. Metabolism by the adult brain accounts for some 80% of total basal glucose turnover. Studies of in vivo cerebral metabolism indicate that the brain in infants and children can utilize glucose at a rate in excess of 4–5 mg/100 g of brain weight/min. Thus, the brain of a full-term neonate, weighing about 420 g in a 3.5-kg infant, would require glucose at a rate of approximately 20 mg/min, representing glucose production of some 5–7 mg/kg body weight/min. Measurements of the endogenous glucose production rate in infants and children, using stable isotopes, demonstrate values of 5–8 mg/kg/min. Thus, most of the endogenous glucose production in infants and young children can be accounted for by brain metabolism. Furthermore, there is a correlation between glucose production and estimated brain weight at all ages. The correlation between glucose production and body weight demonstrates a marked change in slope beyond 40 kg of body weight, corresponding to the time when brain growth is completed. Since the brain grows most rapidly during the 1st yr of life and since the larger proportion of glucose turnover is utilized for brain metabolism, sustained or repetitive hypoglycemia in infants and children has a major impact on retarding brain development and function. In the rapidly growing brain, glucose may also be a source of membrane lipids and protein synthesis, that is, structural proteins and myelination that are important for normal brain maturation. Under conditions of severe and sustained hypoglycemia, these cerebral structural substrates may be broken down to a variety of energy-usable intermediates such as lactate, pyruvate, amino acids, and ketoacids, which can support brain metabolism at the expense of brain growth. The capacity of the newborn brain to take up and oxidize ketone bodies is about 5-fold greater than that in the adult brain. However, the liver's capacity to produce ketone bodies may be limited in the newborn period, especially in the presence of hyperinsulinemia, which acutely inhibits hepatic glucose output, lipolysis, and ketogenesis, thereby depriving the brain of alternate fuel sources. The deprivation of the brain's major energy source during hypoglycemia and the limited availability of alternate fuel sources during hyperinsulinemia have predictable consequences on brain metabolism and growth: decreased brain oxygen consumption, increased breakdown of endogenous structural components to release amino acids and free fatty acid, and destruction of functional membrane integrity. All of these factors may combine and lead to permanent impairment of brain growth and function. The potentiating effects of hypoxia may exacerbate brain damage, or indeed be responsible for it, when blood glucose values are not in the classic hypoglycemic range.

The major long-term sequelae of severe, prolonged hypoglycemia are neurologic damage resulting in mental retardation, recurrent seizure activity, or both. Subtle effects on personality are also possible but have not been clearly defined. Permanent neurologic sequelae are present in more than half of patients with severe recurrent hypoglycemia under the age of 6 mo, the period of most rapid brain growth. In the long term, these sequelae are reflected in pathologic changes characterized by atrophic gyri, reduced myelination in cerebral white matter, and atrophy in the cerebral cortex. As indicated, these neurologic sequelae are more likely to occur when alternative fuel sources are limited, as occurs with hyperinsulinemia, when the episodes of hypoglycemia are repetitive or prolonged, or when they are compounded by hypoxia. There is no precise knowledge relating the duration or severity of hypoglycemia to subsequent neurologic development in children in a predictable manner. Although less common, hypoglycemia in older children may also produce long-term neurologic defects.

SUBSTRATE, ENZYME, AND HORMONAL INTEGRATION OF GLUCOSE HOMEOSTASIS

IN THE NEWBORN (see also Sec. 9.57). Under nonstressed conditions fetal glucose is derived virtually entirely from the mother through placental transfer. Therefore, fetal glucose concentration usually reflects maternal glucose levels. Catecholamine release, which occurs with fetal stress such as hypoxia, mobilizes fetal glucose and free fatty acids through β-adrenergic mechanisms, reflecting the existence of functionally linked β-adrenergic receptors in fetal liver and adipose tissues. In high doses, catecholamines can exert appropriate modulation of fetal pancreatic hormone secretion by inhibiting insulin and stimulating glucagon release.

The acute interruption of maternal glucose transfer to the fetus at delivery imposes an immediate need to mobilize endogenous glucose. Three related events facilitate this transition: changes in hormones, changes in their receptors, and changes in key enzyme activity. In all mammalian species, there is a 3–5-fold abrupt increase in glucagon concentration within minutes to hours of birth. Insulin, on the other hand, usually falls initially and remains in the basal range for several days without demonstrating the usual brisk response to physiologic stimuli such as glucose. A dramatic surge in spontaneous catecholamine secretion also is characteristic of several mammalian species. These changes in epinephrine, glucagon, and insulin may be interrelated because epinephrine is capable of stimulating glucagon and suppressing insulin release. In addition, epinephrine can augment growth hormone secretion by α-adrenergic mechanisms, and growth hormone levels are considerably elevated at birth. Acting in unison, these hormonal changes at birth mobilize glucose via glycogenolysis and gluconeogenesis, activate lipolysis, and promote ketogenesis. As a result of this process, plasma glucose concentration stabilizes after a transient decrease immediately after birth, liver glycogen stores become rapidly depleted within hours of birth, and gluconeogenesis from alanine, a major gluconeogenic amino acid, can account for approximately 10% of glucose turnover in the human newborn infant by several hours of age. Free fatty acid concentrations also rise sharply in concert with the surges in glucagon and epinephrine and are followed by rises in ketone bodies. In this way, glucose is spared for brain utilization while free fatty acids and ketones provide alternative fuel sources for muscle as well as essential gluconeogenic factors such as acetyl-CoA and NADH from hepatic fatty acid oxidation, which is required to drive gluconeogenesis.

In the early postnatal period, responses of the endocrine pancreas favor glucagon secretion at the relative expense of insulin secretion so that blood glucose concentration can be maintained. These adaptive changes in hormone secretion are paralleled by similarly striking adaptive changes in hormone receptors. The surge in epinephrine and glucagon secretion and their coupling to appropriate receptors augment glucose production and lipolysis. Key enzymes involved in glucose production also change dramatically in the perinatal period. Thus, there is a rapid fall in glycogen synthase activity and a sharp rise in phosphorylase after delivery. Similarly, the rate-limiting enzyme for gluconeogenesis, phosphoenolpyruvate carboxykinase (PEPCK), rises dramatically after birth, activated in part by the surge in glucagon and the fall in insulin. This framework permits an interpretation of the normal mechanisms underlying the transition from intrauterine dependence on maternal glucose to extrauterine autonomy of newborn glucose metabolism. This framework can also explain several causes of neonatal hypoglycemia based on inappropriate changes in hormone secretion, unavailability of adequate reserves of substrates in the form of hepatic glycogen, muscle as a source of amino acids for gluconeogenesis, and lipid stores for the release of fatty acids. In addition, appropriate activities of key enzymes governing glucose homeostasis as outlined in Figure 8–29 are required.

IN OLDER INFANTS AND CHILDREN. Hypoglycemia in older infants and children is analogous to that of adults, in whom glucose homeostasis is maintained by glycogenolysis in the immediate postfeeding period and by gluconeogenesis several hours after meals. The liver of a 10-kg child contains 20–25 g of glycogen, which is sufficient to meet glucose requirements of 4–6 mg/kg/min for only 6–12 hr. Beyond this period, hepatic gluconeogenesis must be activated. Both glycogenolysis and gluconeogenesis depend upon the metabolic pathway summarized in Figure 8–29. Defects in gluconeogenesis may not become manifest in infants until the practice of frequent feeding at 3- to 4-hr intervals ceases and infants sleep through the night, a situation usually present by 3–6 mo of age. The source of gluconeogenic precursors is derived primarily from muscle protein. The muscle bulk of infants and small children is substantially smaller relative to body mass than that in adults, whereas glucose requirements per unit of body mass are greater in children, so the ability to compensate for glucose deprivation by gluconeogenesis is more limited in infants and children, as is the ability to withstand fasting for prolonged periods. The ability of muscle to generate alanine, the principal gluconeogenic amino acid, may also be limited, particularly in children with inborn errors of amino acid metabolism. Thus, in young children, the blood glucose level falls after 24 hr of fasting, insulin concentrations fall appropriately to levels of less than 5–10 μU/mL, lipolysis and ketogenesis are activated, and ketones may appear in the urine.

The switch from glycogen synthesis during and immediately after meals to glycogen breakdown and later gluconeogenesis is governed by hormones, of which insulin is of central importance (see Sec. 8.40). Plasma insulin concentrations increase to peak levels of 50–100 μU/mL after meals, which serves to lower blood glucose through the activation of glycogen synthesis, enhancement of peripheral glucose uptake, and inhibition of gluconeogenesis. In addition, lipogenesis is stimulated, whereas lipolysis and ketogenesis are curtailed. During fasting, plasma insulin concentrations fall to 5–10 μU/mL, and, together with other hormonal changes, this fall results in activation of gluconeogenic pathways (see Fig. 8–29). Fasting glucose concentrations are maintained through the activation of glycogenolysis and gluconeogenesis, inhibition of glycogen synthesis, and activation of lipolysis and ketogenesis. It should be emphasized that a plasma insulin concentration of greater than 10 μU/mL, in association with a blood glucose concentration of 40 mg/dL (2.2 mM) or less, is clearly abnormal, indicating a hyperinsulinemic state and failure of the mechanisms that normally result in suppression of insulin secretion during fasting or hypoglycemia.

The hypoglycemic effects of insulin are opposed by the actions of several hormones whose concentration in plasma increases as blood glucose falls. These counterregulatory hormones are glucagon, growth hormone, cortisol, and epinephrine. Acting in concert, they increase blood glucose concentration by activating glycogenolytic and gluconeogenic enzymes (glucagon and epinephrine); inducing gluconeogenic enzymes (glucagon and cortisol); inhibiting glucose uptake by muscle (epinephrine, growth hormone, cortisol); mobilizing amino acids from muscle for gluconeogenesis (cortisol); activating lipolysis providing glycerol for gluconeogenesis and fatty acids for ketogenesis (epinephrine, cortisol, growth hormone, glucagon); and inhibiting insulin release and promotion of growth hormone and glucagon secretion (epinephrine).

Congenital or acquired deficiencies in these hormones may therefore result in hypoglycemia, which will occur when endogenous glucose production cannot be mobilized to meet energy needs in the postabsorptive state, that is 8–12 hr after meals or during fasting. Concurrent deficiency of several hormones such as occurs in hypopituitarism may result in hypoglycemia that is more severe or appears earlier than that seen with isolated hormone deficiencies.

CLINICAL MANIFESTATIONS OF HYPOGLYCEMIA

See also Sec. 9.57.

Clinical features generally fall into two categories. The first includes symptoms associated with the activation of the autonomic nervous system and epinephrine release, usually associated with a rapid decline in blood glucose (Table 8–24). The second category includes symptoms due to decreased cerebral glucose utilization, usually associated with a slow decline in blood glucose or prolonged hypoglycemia (see Table 8–24). Although these classic symptoms occur in older children, the symptoms of hypoglycemia in infants may be more subtle and include cyanosis, apnea, hypothermia, hypotonia, poor feeding, lethargy, and seizures. Some of these symptoms may be so mild that they are missed clinically. Occasionally hypoglycemia may be asymptomatic in the immediate newborn period. In childhood, hypoglycemia may present as behavior problems, inattention, ravenous appetite, or seizures. It may be misdiagnosed as epilepsy, inebriation, personality disorders, hysteria, and retardation. A blood glucose determination should always be performed in sick neonates, who should be vigorously treated if concentrations are below 40 mg/dL (2.2 mM). At any pediatric age level, hypoglycemia should always be considered a cause of an initial episode of convulsions or a sudden deterioration in psychobehavioral functioning.

TABLE 8–24. Manifestations of Hypoglycemia in Childhood

Features Associated with Activation of Autonomic Nervous System and Epinephrine Release*	Features Associated with Cerebral Glucopenia
Anxiety†	Headache†
Perspiration†	Mental confusion†
Palpitation (tachycardia)†	Visual disturbances (↓ acuity, diplopia)†
Pallor	Organic personality changes†
Tremulousness	Inability to concentrate†
Weakness	Dysarthria
Hunger	Staring
Nausea	Seizures
Emesis	Ataxia, incoordination
Angina (with normal coronary arteries)	Somnolence, lethargy
	Coma
	Stroke, hemiplegia, aphasia
	Paresthesias
	Dizziness
	Amnesia
	Decerebrate or decorticate posture

*Some of these features will be attenuated if the patient is receiving β-adrenergic blocking agents.
†Common.

CLASSIFICATION OF HYPOGLYCEMIA IN INFANTS AND CHILDREN

The classification outlined in Table 8–25 is based on knowledge of the control of glucose homeostasis in infants and children discussed earlier.

NEONATAL. Transient. SMALL-FOR-GESTATIONAL AGE AND PREMATURE INFANTS (see Sec. 9.57). The overall incidence of symptomatic hypoglycemia in newborns varies between 1.3 and 3.0/1,000 live births. This incidence is increased several-fold in certain high-risk neonatal groups (see Table 8–25). The premature, small-for-gestational-age (SGA) infant is especially vulnerable to developing hypoglycemia. The factors responsible for the high frequency of hypoglycemia in this group as well as in other groups outlined in Table 8–25 are related to the inadequate stores of liver glycogen, muscle protein, and body fat needed to sustain the substrates required to meet energy needs. These infants are small by virtue of prematurity or impaired placental transfer of nutrients. In addition, their enzyme systems for gluconeogenesis may not be fully developed.

In contrast to deficiency of substrates and enzymes, the hormonal system appears to be functioning normally at birth in most neonates. Thus, the newborn surge in glucagon secretion occurs normally, low plasma insulin concentrations are usually documented, and plasma concentrations of cortisol and growth hormone are usually normal. Despite the hypoglycemia, plasma concentrations of alanine, lactate, and pyruvate are higher, implying their diminished rate of utilization as substrates for gluconeogenesis. Infusion of alanine elicits further glucagon secretion but causes no significant rise in glucose. During the initial 24 hr of life, plasma concentrations of acetoacetate and β-hydroxybutyrate are lower in SGA infants than in full-term infants, implying diminished lipid stores, diminished fatty acid mobilization, and/or impaired ketogenesis. Diminished lipid stores are most likely, since triglyceride feeding of newborns results in a rise in the plasma levels of glucose, free fatty acids (FFA), and ketones.

The role of FFA and their oxidation in stimulating neonatal gluconeogenesis is essential. The provision of FFA as triglyceride feedings together with gluconeogenic precursors may prevent the hypoglycemia that usually ensues after fasting. For these and other reasons, the practice of delaying feeding of newborns for 12–24 hr has been abandoned, and milk feedings are introduced early (within 4–6 hr) after delivery. In the hospital setting, when feeding is precluded by virtue of respiratory distress or when feedings alone cannot maintain blood glucose concentrations above 40 mg/dL (2.2 mM), intravenous glucose at a rate that supplies approximately 4–8 mg/kg/min should be begun. Infants usually can maintain their blood glucose level spontaneously after 3–5 days of life.

INFANTS BORN TO DIABETIC MOTHERS (see Sec. 9.56). Of the transient hyperinsulinemic states, infants born to diabetic mothers are most common. Gestational diabetes affects some 2% of pregnant women, and approximately 1 in 1,000 pregnant women has insulin-dependent diabetes. At birth, infants born to these mothers may be large and plethoric, and their body stores of glycogen, protein, and fat are replete. Thus, in contrast to the transient hypoglycemia of the SGA infant whose body size and tissue nutrient content reflect diminished placental transfer, infants born to diabetic mothers are examples of nutrient surfeit and represent the opposite extreme of the spectrum.

Hypoglycemia in infants of diabetic mothers is related

TABLE 8–25. Classification of Hypoglycemia in Infants and Children*

Neonatal—Transient Hypoglycemia
- Associated with inadequate substrate or enzyme function
  - Prematurity
  - Small for gestational age
  - Smaller of twins
  - Infants with severe respiratory distress
  - Infant of toxemic mother
- Associated with hyperinsulinemia
  - Infants of diabetic mothers
  - Infants with erythroblastosis fetalis

Neonatal—Infantile or Childhood Persistent Hypoglycemia
- Hyperinsulinemic states
  - Nesidioblastosis
  - β cell hyperplasia
  - β cell adenoma
  - Beckwith-Wiedemann syndrome
  - Leucine sensitivity
  - Falciparum malaria
- Hormone deficiency
  - Panhypopituitarism
  - Isolated growth hormone deficiency
  - ACTH deficiency
  - Addison disease
  - Glucagon deficiency
  - Epinephrine deficiency
- Substrate limited
  - Ketotic hypoglycemia
  - Branched-chain ketonuria (maple syrup urine disease)
- Glycogen storage disease
  - Glucose-6-phosphatase deficiency
  - Amylo-1, 6-glucosidase deficiency
  - Liver phosphorylase deficiency
  - Glycogen synthetase deficiency
- Disorders of gluconeogenesis
  - Acute alcohol intoxication
  - Hyperglycinemia, carnitine deficiency
  - Salicylate intoxication
  - Fructose-1, 6-diphosphatase deficiency
  - Pyruvate carboxylase deficiency
  - Phosphoenolpyruvate carboxykinase (PEPCK deficiency)
  - IGFII—Insulin-like growth factor II
  - IDDM—Insulin-dependent diabetes mellitus
- Other enzyme defects
  - Galactosemia: galactose-1-phosphate uridyl transferase deficiency
  - Fructose intolerance: fructose-1-phosphate aldolase deficiency
- Disorders of fat (alternate fuel) metabolism
  - Primary carnitine deficiency
  - Secondary carnitine deficiency
  - Carnitine palmitoyl transferase deficiency
  - Long-, medium-, short-chain fatty acid acyl-CoA dehydrogenase deficiency

Other Etiologies
- Poisoning—drugs
  - Salicylates
  - Alcohol
  - Oral hypoglycemic agents
  - Insulin
  - Propranolol
  - Pentamidine
  - Quinine
  - Disopyramide
  - Ackee fruit (unripe)–hypoglycin
  - Vacor (rat poison)
- Liver disease
  - Reye syndrome
  - Hepatitis
  - Cirrhosis
  - Hepatoma
- Amino acid and organic acid disorders
  - Maple syrup urine disease
  - Propionic acidemia
  - Methylmalonic acidemia
  - Tyrosinosis
  - Glutaric aciduria
  - 3-Hydroxy-3-methylglutaric aciduria
- Systemic disorders
  - Sepsis
  - Carcinoma/sarcoma (secreting IGFII)
  - Heart failure
  - Malnutrition
  - Malabsorption
  - Anti-insulin receptor antibodies
  - Anti-insulin antibodies
  - Neonatal hyperviscosity
  - Renal failure
  - Diarrhea
  - Burns
  - Shock
  - Postsurgical
  - Pseudohypoglycemia (leukocytosis, polycythemia)
  - Excessive insulin therapy of IDDM

*From Sperling M, Chernausek S: Nelson's Essentials of Pediatrics. Philadelphia, W. B. Saunders, 1990.

mostly to hyperinsulinemia and partly to diminished glucagon secretion. Hypertrophy and hyperplasia of their islets have been documented, as has their brisk, biphasic, and typically adult insulin response to glucose; this insulin response is absent in normal infants. Infants born to diabetic mothers also have a subnormal surge in plasma glucagon immediately after birth, subnormal glucagon secretion in response to stimuli, and, initially, excessive sympathetic activity that may lead to adrenomedullary exhaustion because urinary excretion of epinephrine is diminished. Thus, despite their abundance of tissue stores of available substrate, the normal plasma hormonal pattern of low insulin, high glucagon, and catecholamines is reversed, and their endogenous glucose production is significantly inhibited compared to that in normal infants, thus predisposing to hypoglycemia.

Infants born with *erythroblastosis fetalis* also have hyperinsulinemia and share many physical features, such as large body size, with infants born to diabetic mothers. The cause of the hyperinsulinemia in infants with erythroblastosis is not entirely clear but may be related to compensatory hypersecretion as a result of the hemolysis that provides increased glutathione, which splits the disulfide bonds of insulin.

Mothers whose diabetes has been well controlled during pregnancy generally have babies near normal size who are less likely to develop neonatal hypoglycemia and other complications formerly considered typical of such infants. Nevertheless, treatment of infants born to mothers with diabetes commonly requires provision of intravenous glucose for several days until the hyperinsulinemia abates. In supplying glucose to these infants, it is important to avoid hyperglycemia that evokes prompt insulin release, which may result in rebound hypoglycemia. Usually glucose should be provided at rates of 4–8 mg/kg/min, but the appropriate dose for each patient should be individually adjusted. During labor and delivery, maternal hyperglycemia should be avoided because it results in fetal hyperglycemia, which predisposes to hypoglycemia when the glucose supply is interrupted at birth. Hypoglycemia persisting or occurring after 1 wk of life requires an evaluation for the causes listed in Table 8–25.

HYPOGLYCEMIA IN INFANTS AND CHILDREN. Hyperinsulinemia. Most children with hyperinsulinemia causing hypoglycemia present in infancy. Like infants born to diabetic mothers, they may be macrosomic at birth, reflecting the anabolic effects of insulin in utero. There is, however, no history and no biochemical evidence of maternal diabetes. The onset is from 0.1 to 18 mo. Insulin concentrations are inappropriately elevated at the time of documented hypoglycemia. Thus, when blood glucose concentration is less than 40 mg/dL (2.2 mM), plasma insulin concentration should be less than 5 and no higher than 10 μU/mL. In affected infants, however, plasma insulin concentrations at the time of hypoglycemia are commonly greater than 10 μU/mL. The insulin (μU/mL)-glucose (mg/mL) ratio is 0.4 or above, and plasma ketones and FFA levels are low during hyperinsulinemia. Macrosomic infants may present with hypoglycemia from the first days of life. Infants with lesser degrees of hyperinsulinemia, however, may manifest hypoglycemia after the first few weeks to months, when the frequency of feedings has been decreased to permit the infant to sleep through the night and hyperinsulinemia prevents the mobilization of endogenous glucose. Increasing demands for feeding, wilting spells, jitteriness, and frank seizures are the most common presenting features. Additional clues include the rapid development of fasting hypoglycemia, the need for high rates of exogenous glucose infusion to prevent hypoglycemia, absence of ketonemia or acidosis, and elevated C peptide or proinsulin levels at the time of hypoglycemia. The latter insulin-related products are absent in factitious hypoglycemia from exogenous administration of insulin. Provocative tests with tolbutamide or leucine are not necessary in infants; hypoglycemia is invariably provoked by withholding feedings for several hours, permitting simultaneous measurement of glucose, insulin, ketones, and FFA in the same sample at the time of clinically manifest hypoglycemia. The glycemic response to glucagon at the time of hypoglycemia reveals a brisk rise in glucose of at least 40 mg/dL and implies that glucose mobilization has been restrained by insulin and that glycogenolytic mechanisms are intact (Table 8–26).

Once organic endogenous hyperinsulinism has been established through concurrent measurement of glucose and insulin, the *differential diagnosis* should include **nesidioblastosis, β cell hyperplasia,** and **β cell adenoma**. These three entities cannot be distinguished by the plasma levels of insulin alone. Although they represent diffuse or localized abnormalities in the pancreas, each is characterized by autonomous insulin secretion that is not appropriately reduced when blood glucose declines spontaneously or in response to provocative maneuvers such as fasting. Celiac angiography, which reportedly has a success rate of 60–75% in localizing pancreatic endocrine tumors (adenoma or carcinoma) in adults, has shown only limited success in infants, in whom the nodules may be small and obscured by the normal rich vascular supply. The chances of detecting a tumor "blush" during arteriography must therefore be balanced by the potential risk of causing vascular trauma in infants under 2 yr. When present, however, a tumor blush may be helpful in localizing the tumor prior to surgery. Computed tomography, high-resolution ultrasonography, and MRI may be helpful in localizing a pancreatic adenoma, but most patients have hyperplasia rather than a discreet tumor. The term **islet cell dysmaturation syndrome** has been used to encompass the spectrum of localized or diffuse (nesidioblastosis) disease, and

TABLE 8–26. Analysis of Blood Sample Before and 30 Min After Glucagon*

Substrates	Hormones
Glucose	Insulin
Free fatty acids	Cortisol
Ketones	Growth hormone
Lactate	T_4, TSH†
Uric acid	

*Glucagon 30 μg/kg IV or IM.
†Measure once only before or after glucagon administration.

islet cell histology is highly variable. Rather than a histologically distinct syndrome, the lesions of nesidioblastosis may represent a developmental variant that is present in some normal infants who have hypoglycemia. Islet cell dysmaturity syndrome may produce hyperinsulinism because of an associated deficiency or dysregulation by δ cells, which normally produce somatostatin, a paracrine inhibitor of β insulin-secreting cells.

Because the definitive diagnosis can only be made by histologic examination of removed pancreatic tissue, surgical exploration is usually undertaken in severely affected neonates who are unresponsive to glucose and somatostatin therapy. Near-total resection of 85–90% of the pancreas is recommended. Intraoperative ultrasonography may identify a small unpalpable adenoma, permitting local resection. Further resection of the remaining pancreas may occasionally be necessary if hypoglycemia recurs and cannot be controlled by medical measures, such as the use of somatostatin or diazoxide with cortisone. Surgery should be performed by experienced pediatric surgeons in medical centers equipped to provide the necessary preoperative and postoperative care, diagnostic evaluation, and management.

When the diagnosis is established before 3 mo of life, surgery is usually needed. Frequent feedings coupled with pharmacologic agents such as somatostatin or diazoxide may not consistently maintain blood glucose concentrations or adequately inhibit insulin release. If hypoglycemia first becomes manifest between 3 and 6 mo of life or later, a therapeutic trial using medical approaches with somatostatin, diazoxide, steroids, and frequent feedings can be attempted for up to 2–4 wk. Failure to maintain euglycemia without undesirable side effects from the drugs prompts the need for surgery. Some success in suppressing insulin release and correcting hypoglycemia in patients with nesidioblastosis has been reported with the use of the long-acting somatostatin analog (see later section on treatment). Most cases of neonatal nesidioblastosis are sporadic; familial forms appear to be inherited in an autosomal recessive manner. Also, hyperinsulinism, usually transient (weeks-months), may occur in asphyxiated or small-for-dates infants in whom hypoglycemia usually is attributed to asphyxia-induced catecholamine secretion that depletes glycogen stores.

Hypoglycemia associated with hyperinsulinemia is also seen in approximately 50% of patients with the **Beckwith-Wiedemann syndrome** (see Sec. 9.57). This syndrome is characterized by macrosomia, microcephaly, macroglossia, visceromegaly, and omphalocele. Distinctive lateral ear lobe fissures are present. Diffuse islet cell hyperplasia and nesidioblastosis both occur in those infants with hypoglycemia. The diagnostic and therapeutic approaches are, therefore, the same as those discussed above, although microcephaly and retarded brain development may occur independently of hypoglycemia. In addition, patients with the Beckwith-Wiedemann syndrome have a predilection for the eventual development of tumors, including Wilms tumor, hepatoblastoma, and retinoblastoma.

Leucine-sensitive hypoglycemia is not being diagnosed as often as it was in previous years. Originally it was considered to occur in a subclass of children with "idiopathic hypoglycemia," in whom protein feeding, specifically leucine, triggered hypoglycemic attacks. Leucine-sensitive hypoglycemia is associated with excessive insulin secretion following leucine administration; and β cell hyperplasia, adenoma, and nesidioblastosis may also demonstrate hyperinsulinemia in response to leucine, tolbutamide, and other provocative tests. Because nesidioblastosis may not be diagnosed by a routine histologic examination of islets without employing insulin-specific staining techniques, including immunofluorescent techniques for islet hormones, many of the cases previously diagnosed as leucine-sensitive might now be categorized as nesidioblastosis. Occasionally the diagnosis remains in doubt because histologic examination of pancreatic tissue is not undertaken owing to a satisfactory response to a low-leucine diet and diazoxide with or without additional glucocorticoids. In such cases, a functional hyperinsulinemia with leucine sensitivity serves as a descriptive term for patients who eventually outgrow their propensity for hypoglycemia at 5–7 yr of age. Nevertheless, in view of the similarity of excessive insulin response and documented islet cell hyperplasia in previous patients, it is likely that leucine-sensitive hypoglycemia is a variant of the islet cell dysmaturity syndrome.

After the first 12 mo of life, hyperinsulinemic states are uncommon until islet cell adenomas again reappear after several years of age. Hyperinsulinemia due to **islet cell adenoma** should be considered in any child 5 yr or older presenting with hypoglycemia. The diagnostic approach is outlined in Table 8–26. Fasting for 24–36 hr usually provokes hypoglycemia; coexisting hyperinsulinemia confirms the diagnosis, providing that factitious administration of insulin by the parents, a form of *Munchausen syndrome by proxy*, has been excluded. Occasionally, provocative tests may be required. Exogenously administered insulin can be distinguished from endogenous insulin by simultaneous measurement of C-peptide concentration. If C-peptide levels are elevated, endogenous insulin secretion is responsible for the hypoglycemia; if C-peptide levels are low but insulin values are high, exogenous insulin has been administered, perhaps as a form of child abuse. Islet cell adenomas at this age are treated by surgical excision; familial multiple endocrine adenomatosis type I (Wermer syndrome) or type II should be considered in the differential diagnosis. Antibodies to insulin or the insulin receptor (insulinomimetic action) are also rarely associated with hypoglycemia.

Endocrine Deficiency. Hypoglycemia associated with endocrine deficiency is usually due to adrenal insufficiency with or without associated growth hormone deficiency (see Sec. 19.21 and 19.22). In patients with panhypopituitarism, isolated ACTH or growth hormone deficiency, or combined ACTH deficiency plus growth hormone deficiency, the incidence of hypoglycemia is as high as 20%. In the newborn period, hypoglycemia may be the presenting feature of hypopituitarism; in males, a microphallus may provide a clue to a coexistent deficiency of gonadotropin. Newborns with hypopituitarism often have a form of "hepatitis" and the syndrome of **septo-optic dysplasia**. When adrenal disease is severe, as in congenital adrenal hyperplasia due to cortisol synthetic enzyme defects, adrenal hemorrhage, or congenital absence of the adrenals, disturbances in serum electrolytes with hyponatremia and hyperkalemia or ambiguous genitalia may provide diagnostic clues (Sec. 19.21). In older children, failure of growth should suggest growth hormone deficiency. Hyperpigmentation may provide the clue to Addison disease with increased ACTH levels or adrenal unresponsiveness to ACTH due to a defect in the adrenal receptor for ACTH. The frequent association of Addison disease in childhood with hypoparathyroidism (hypocalcemia), chronic mucocutaneous moniliasis, and other endocrinopathies should be considered. Adrenoleukodystrophy should also be considered in the differential diagnosis of primary Addison disease in older children (see Sec. 8.17).

The etiology of hypoglycemia in cortisol–growth hormone deficiency may be due to decreased gluconeogenic enzymes with cortisol deficiency, increased glucose utilization due to lack of the antagonistic effects of growth hormone on insulin action, or failure to supply endogenous gluconeogenic substrate in the form of alanine and lactate with compensatory breakdown of fat and generation of ketones. Thus, deficiency of these hormones results in reduced gluconeogenic substrate, which resembles the syndrome of ketotic hypoglycemia (see later). Investigation of a child with hypoglycemia, therefore, requires exclusion of ACTH-cortisol or growth hormone deficiency, and if diagnosed, its appropriate replacement with cortisol or growth hormone (see Sec. 19.2).

Epinephrine deficiency could theoretically be responsible for hypoglycemia. Urinary excretion of epinephrine has been diminished in some patients with spontaneous or insulin-induced hypoglycemia in whom absence of pallor and tachycardia was also noted, suggesting that failure of catecholamine release, due to a defect anywhere along the hypothalamic-autonomic-adrenomedullary axis, might be responsible for the hypoglycemia. However, this possibility has been challenged owing to the rarity of hypoglycemia in patients with bilateral adrenalectomy providing they receive adequate glucocorticoid replacement and because diminished epinephrine excretion is found in normal patients with repeated insulin-induced hypoglycemia. In addition, many of the patients described as having hypoglycemia with failure of epinephrine excretion fit the criteria for ketotic hypoglycemia.

Glucagon deficiency in infants or children may rarely be associated with hypoglycemia.

Substrate Limited. KETOTIC HYPOGLYCEMIA. This is the most common form of childhood hypoglycemia. Usually this condition presents between the ages of 18 mo and 5 yr and remits spontaneously by the age of 8–9 yr. Hypoglycemic episodes typically occur during periods of intercurrent illness when food intake is limited. The classic history is of a child who eats poorly or completely avoids the evening meal, is difficult to arouse from sleep the following morning, and may have a seizure or be comatose by midmorning. Another common presentation occurs when parents sleep late and the affected child is unable to eat breakfast, thus prolonging the overnight fast. The possibility of the child ingesting alcoholic drinks must also be considered if there was a preceding evening party.

At the time of documented hypoglycemia, there is associated ketonuria and ketonemia, and plasma insulin concentrations are appropriately low, 5–10 μU/mL, thus excluding hyperinsulinemia. A ketogenic provocative diet, formerly used as a diagnostic test, is not essential to establish the diagnosis because fasting alone will provoke a hypoglycemic episode with ketonemia and ketonuria within 12–18 hr in susceptible individuals. Normal children of similar age can withstand fasting without developing hypoglycemia during the same time period, although even normal children may develop these features by 36 hr of fasting. Thus, the provocative nature of a ketogenic diet appears to be more dependent on its hypocaloric nature than its fat content; its use as a diagnostic tool has been largely replaced by complete caloric restriction.

Children with ketotic hypoglycemia have plasma alanine concentrations that are markedly reduced in the basal state after an overnight fast and decline even further with prolonged fasting. Alanine is the only amino acid that is significantly lower in these children, and infusions of alanine (250 mg/kg body weight) produce a rapid rise in plasma glucose without causing significant changes in blood lactate or pyruvate level, indicating that the entire gluconeogenic pathway from the level of pyruvate is intact but that there is a deficiency of substrate. There is also a normal glycemic response to infusion of fructose and glycerol. Plasma glycerol levels are normal in these children in both the fed and fasted states. Glycogenolytic pathways are also intact because glucagon induces a normal glycemic response in affected children during the fed state. The metabolic response to infusion of β-hydroxybutyrate does not differ from that in normal children. Finally, the levels of hormones that counter hypoglycemia are appropriately elevated, whereas insulin is appropriately low.

Alanine is quantitatively the major gluconeogenic amino acid precursor whose formation and release from muscle during periods of caloric restriction are enhanced by the presence of a glucose-alanine cycle and by de novo formation from other substrates within muscle, principally branched-chain amino acid catabolism. Thus, the release of alanine (and glutamine) for gluconeogenesis exceeds the content of these amino acids in muscle tissue protein.

The *etiology* of ketotic hypoglycemia, which is characterized by hypoalaninemia, may be a defect in any of the complex steps involved in protein catabolism, oxidative deamination of amino acids, transamination, alanine synthesis, or alanine efflux from muscle. Children with ketotic hypoglycemia frequently are smaller than age-matched controls and often have a history of transient neonatal hypoglycemia. Thus, any decrease in muscle mass may compromise the supply of gluconeogenic substrate at a time when glucose demands per unit of body weight are already relatively high, thus predisposing to the rapid development of hypoglycemia, with ketosis representing the attempt to switch to an alternative fuel supply. Children with ketotic hypoglycemia may represent the low end of the spectrum of children's capacity to tolerate fasting. Similar relative intolerance to fasting is present in normal children, who cannot maintain blood glucose after 30–36 hr of fasting, compared with the adult's capacity for prolonged fasting. Although the defect may be present at birth, it may not become manifest until the child is stressed by more prolonged periods of caloric restriction. Moreover, the spontaneous remission observed in children at age 8–9 yr might be explained by the increase in muscle bulk with its resultant increase in supply of endogenous substrate and the relative decrease in glucose requirement per unit of body mass with increasing age. There is also some evidence to support the contention that impaired epinephrine secretion due to immaturity of autonomic innervation contributes to ketotic hypoglycemia.

In anticipation of spontaneous resolution of this syndrome, *treatment* of ketotic hypoglycemia consists of frequent feedings of a high-protein, high-carbohydrate diet. During intercurrent illnesses, parents should test the child's urine for the presence of ketones, the appearance of which precedes hypoglycemia by several hours. In the presence of ketonuria, liquids of high carbohydrate content should be offered to the child. If these cannot be tolerated, the child should be offered a short course of steroids or admitted to the hospital for intravenous glucose administration.

Branched-Chain Ketonuria (Maple Syrup Urine Disease) (see also Sec. 8.7). The hypoglycemic episodes had previously been attributed to high levels of leucine, but evidence now indicates that interference with the production of alanine and its availability as a gluconeogenic substrate during caloric deprivation is responsible for hypoglycemia.

Glycogen Storage Disease. See Sec. 8.40. Glycogen storage diseases associated with hypoglycemia are summarized in the following sections.

Glucose-6-Phosphatase Deficiency (Type I Glycogen Storage Disease) (see also Sec. 8.40). Typically affected children display a remarkable tolerance to their chronic hypoglycemia; blood glucose values in the range of 20–50 mg/dL (1.1–2.7 mM) are not associated with the classic symptoms of hypoglycemia, possibly reflecting the adaptation of the central nervous system to ketone bodies as an alternative fuel.

Affected untreated children manifest growth failure, mental retardation, and a shortened life span unless they are treated. Continuous intragastric feeding or total parenteral nutrition improves the metabolic and clinical findings by reducing the frequency and severity of hypoglycemia, thereby avoiding the secondary hormonal changes that appear to be responsible for the metabolic derangements. Continuous intragastric feeding at night, combined with frequent daytime feedings, produces equally effective amelioration of the biochemical disturbances and avoids the inconvenience of 24-hr continuous gastric feeding and the problems associated with long-term parenteral nutrition. The daytime feedings are given every 3–4 hr: 60–70% of the calories as carbohydrate low in fructose and galactose, 12–15% of the calories as protein, and 15–25% of the calories as fat. At night, a small nasogastric tube is passed by the patient (or a parent, for younger children), and approximately one third of the daily caloric requirements is continuously infused over 8–12 hr using a small continuous infusion pump. One commercially available formula for nocturnal infusion contains 89% of the calories as glucose and glucose oligosaccharides, 1.8% as safflower oil, and 9.2% as crystalline amino acids.* Corn starch nocturnal therapy also has been used successfully, and liver transplantation offers promise of long-term cure.

Amylo-1.6-Glucosidase Deficiency (Debrancher Enzyme Deficiency; Type III Glycogen Storage Disease). See Sec. 8.40.

Liver Phosphorylase Deficiency (Type VI Glycogen Storage Disease). See also Sec. 8.40. Normal liver phosphorylase activity involves a complex cascade of events that degrades liver glycogen both before and after the debranching step. Consequently, low hepatic phosphorylase activity may result from a defect in any of the steps of activation, and a variety of defects have been described. Hepatomegaly, excessive deposition of glycogen in liver, growth retardation, and occasional symptomatic hypoglycemia occur. A diet high in protein and reduced in carbohydrate usually prevents hypoglycemia.

Glycogen Synthetase Deficiency (see also Sec. 8.40). The inability to synthesize glycogen is an extremely rare occurrence. There is fasting hypoglycemia and hyperketonemia, but hyperglycemia occurs with glucosuria after meals. During fasting hypoglycemia, levels of the counterregulatory hormones, including catecholamines, are appropriately elevated or normal, and insulin levels are appropriately low. Gluconeogenic capacity appears to be intact. The liver is not enlarged. Glycogen synthetase activity is markedly reduced in the liver but is normal in muscle. Protein-rich feedings at frequent intervals result in dramatic clinical improvement, including growth velocity. This condition mimics the syndrome of ketotic hypoglycemia and should be considered in the differential diagnosis of that syndrome.

Disorders of Gluconeogenesis. Acute Alcohol Intoxication. The liver metabolizes alcohol as a preferred fuel, and generation of reducing equivalents during the oxidation of ethanol alters the NADH-NAD ratio, which is essential for certain gluconeogenic steps. As a result, gluconeogenesis is impaired, and hypoglycemia may ensue if glycogen stores are depleted by starvation or by pre-existing abnormalities in glycogen metabolism. In toddlers who have been unfed for some time, even the consumption of small quantities of alcohol can precipitate these events. The hypoglycemia responds promptly to intravenous glucose, which should always be given to a child who presents initially with coma or seizure, after taking a blood sample to determine glucose concentration. A careful history allows the diagnosis to be made and may avoid needless and expensive hospitalization and investigation.

Defects in Fatty Acid Oxidation (see also Sec. 8.15). The important role of fatty acid oxidation in maintaining gluconeogenesis is underscored by examples of congenital or drug-induced defects in fatty acid metabolism that may be associated with fasting hypoglycemia.

Various congenital enzymatic deficiencies causing defective

*Vivonex, Eaton Laboratories.

carnitine or fatty acid metabolism also occur. A severe form of fasting hypoglycemia with hepatomegaly, cardiomyopathy, and hypotonia occurs with long- and medium-chain fatty acid coenzyme-A dehydrogenase deficiency. Plasma carnitine levels are low, ketones are not present in urine, but dicarboxylic aciduria is present. Clinically, patients with acyl **CoA dehydrogenase deficiency** present with a Reye-like syndrome, recurrent episodes of severe fasting hypoglycemic coma, and cardiorespiratory arrest (SIDS-like events). Severe hypoglycemia and metabolic acidosis without ketosis also occur in patients with multiple acyl CoA dehydrogenase disorders. Hypotonia, seizures, and acrid odor are other clinical clues. Survival depends on whether the defects are severe or mild; diagnosis is established from studies of enzyme activity in liver biopsy tissue or in cultured fibroblasts from affected patients.

Interference with fatty acid metabolism also underlies the fasting hypoglycemia associated with Jamaican vomiting sickness, with atractyloside, and with the drug valproate. In **Jamaican vomiting sickness**, the unripe ackee fruit contains a water-soluble toxin, hypoglycin, which produces vomiting, CNS depression, and severe hypoglycemia. The hypoglycemic activity of hypoglycin derives from its inhibition of gluconeogenesis secondary to its interference with the acyl CoA and carnitine metabolism essential for the oxidation of long-chain fatty acids. The disease is almost totally confined to Jamaica, where ackee forms a staple of the diet for the poor. The ripe ackee fruit no longer contains this toxic principle. **Atractyloside** is a reagent that inhibits oxidative phosphorylation in mitochondria by preventing the translocation of adenine nucleotides, such as ATP, across the mitochondrial membrane. Atractyloside is a perhydrophenanthrenic glycoside derived from *Atractylis gummifera*. This plant is found in the Mediterranean basin; ingestion of this "thistle" is associated with hypoglycemia and a syndrome similar to Jamaican vomiting sickness. More commonly, the drug **valproate,** now used for the treatment of epilepsy, is associated with side effects, predominantly in young infants, which include a Reye-like syndrome, low serum carnitine levels, and the potential for fasting hypoglycemia. In all of these conditions hypoglycemia *is not associated with ketonuria.*

SALICYLATE INTOXICATION (see also Sec. 26.6). Both hyperglycemia and hypoglycemia occur in children with salicylate intoxication. Accelerated utilization of glucose, due to augmentation of insulin secretion by salicylates, and possible interference with gluconeogenesis may contribute to hypoglycemia. Infants are more susceptible than older children. Monitoring of blood glucose levels with appropriate glucose infusion in the event of hypoglycemia should form part of the therapeutic approach to salicylate intoxication in childhood. Ketosis may occur.

FRUCTOSE-1,6-DIPHOSPHATASE DEFICIENCY (see Sec. 8.39). A deficiency of this enzyme results in a block of gluconeogenesis from all possible precursors below the level of fructose-1,6-diphosphate. Infusion of these gluconeogenic precursors results in lactic acidosis without a rise in glucose, and acute hypoglycemia may be provoked by inhibition of glycogenolysis. Normally, however, glycogenolysis remains intact, and glucagon elicits a normal glycemic response in the fed but not in the fasted state. Accordingly, affected individuals have

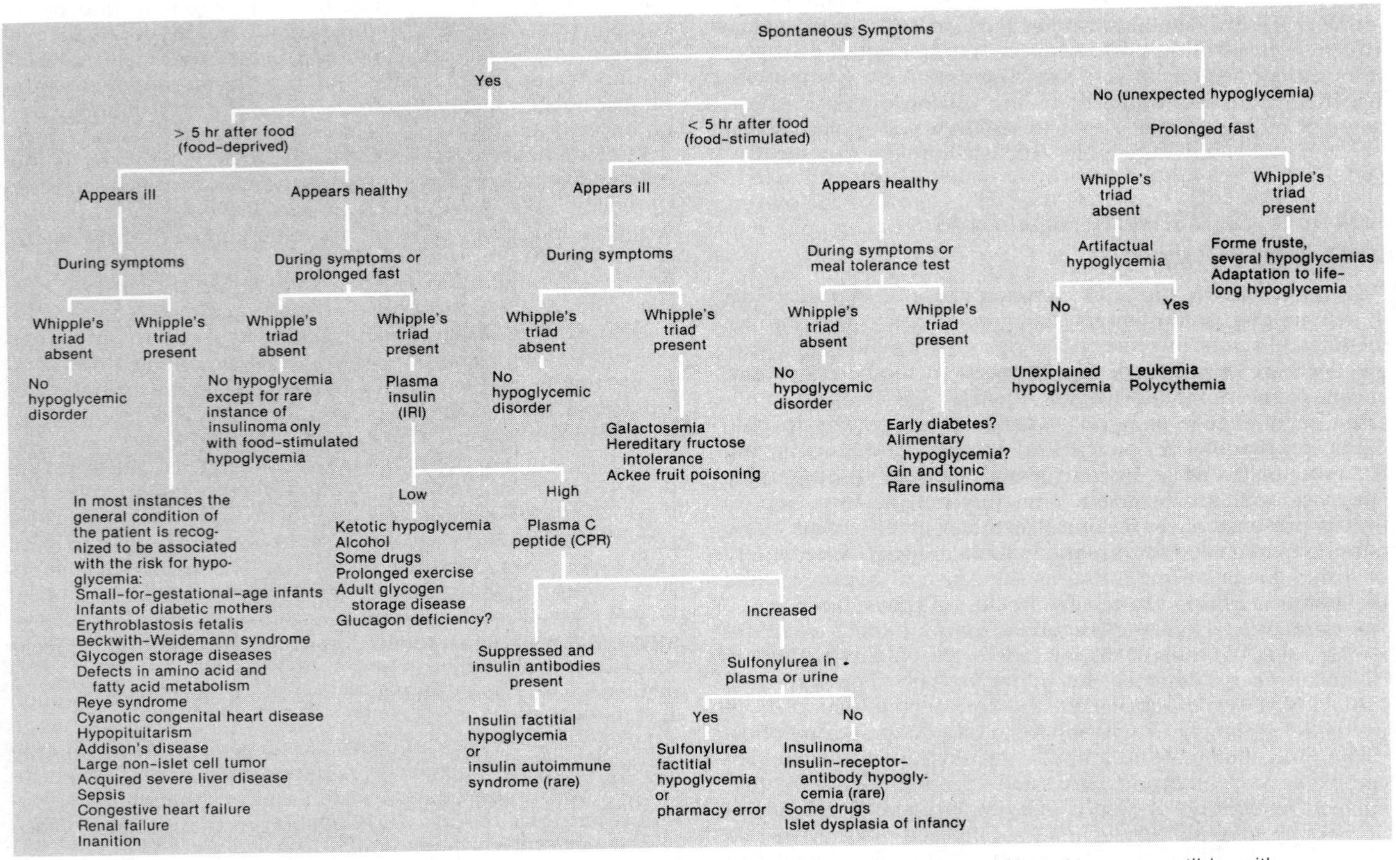

Figure 8–47. Evaluation of hypoglycemic disorders. The Whipple triad includes manifestations compatible with hypoglycemia, low blood glucose levels, and improvement after glucose administration restores blood glucose to normal levels. (From Service FJ: Hypoglycemic disorders. *In*: Wyngaarden JB, Smith LH Jr [eds]: Cecil Textbook of Medicine, 18th ed. Philadelphia, WB Saunders, 1988, p 1383.)

TABLE 8–27. Clinical Manifestations and Differential Diagnosis in Childhood Hypoglycemia

Condition	Hypoglycemia	Urinary Ketones (K) or Reducing* Sugar(s)	Hepatomegaly	Serum		Effect of 24- to 36-hr Fast on Plasma					Glycemic Response to Glucagon		Glycemic Response to Infusion of	
				Lipids	*Uric Acid*	*Glucose*	*Insulin*	*Ketones*	*Alanine*	*Lactate*	*Fed*	*Fasted*	*Alanine*	*Glycerol*
Normal	0	0	0	Normal	Normal	↓	↓	↑	↓	Normal	↑	↓	↑	↑
Hyperinsulinemia	Recurrent severe	0	0	Normal or ↑	Normal	⇊	⇈	⇊	Normal	Normal	↑	↑	↑	↑
Ketotic hypoglycemia	Severe with missed meals	Ketonuria + + +	0	Normal	Normal	⇊	↓	⇈	⇊	Normal	↑	⇊	↑	↑
Hypopituitarism	Moderate with missed meals	Ketonuria + +	0	Normal	Normal	⇊	↓	⇈	⇊	Normal	↑	⇊	↑	↑
Adrenal insufficiency	Severe with missed meals	Ketonuria + +	0	Normal	Normal	⇊	↓	⇈	⇊	Normal	↑	⇊	↑	↑
Enzyme deficiencies														
Glucose-6-phosphatase	Severe–constant	Ketonuria + + +	+ + +	⇈	⇈	⇊	↓	⇈	⇈	⇈	0	0–⇊	0	0
Debrancher	Moderate with fasting	Ketonuria + +	+ +	Normal	Normal	⇊	↓	⇈	⇊	Normal	↑	0–⇊	↑	↑
Phosphorylase	Mild-moderate	Ketonuria + +	+	Normal	Normal	↓	↓	⇈	⇊	Normal	0–↑	0–⇊	↑	↑
Fructose-1, 6-diphosphatase	Severe with fasting	Ketonuria + + +	+ + +	⇈	⇈	⇊	↓	⇈	⇈	⇈	↑	0–⇊	↓	↓
Galactosemia	After milk or milk products	0 Ketones;(s) +	+ + +	Normal	Normal	↓	↓	↑	↓	Normal	↑	0–⇊	↑	↑
Fructose intolerance	After fructose	0 Ketones;(s) +	+ + +	Normal	Normal	↓	↓	↑	↓	Normal	↑	0–⇊	↑	↑

0 = absence.
↑ or ↓ indicates respectively small increase or decrease.
⇈ or ⇊ indicates respectively large increase or decrease.
Details of each condition are discussed in text.

hypoglycemia only during caloric deprivation as in fasting or during intercurrent illness. While glycogen stores remain normal, hypoglycemia does not develop. In affected families there may be a history of siblings with known hepatomegaly who died in infancy with unexplained metabolic acidosis.

Clinical features simulate those of type I glycogen storage disease. However, hepatomegaly in individuals with fructose-1,6-diphosphatase deficiency is due to lipid storage rather than glycogen storage. Lactic acidosis, ketosis, hyperlipidemia, and hyperuricemia occur; their pathogenesis is related to the severity and duration of hypoglycemia and the resultant low levels of insulin and high levels of counterregulatory hormones. Therapy of these infants, consisting of a diet high in carbohydrates (56%, excluding fructose, which cannot be utilized), low in protein (12%), and normal in fat composition (32%), has permitted normal growth and development. Continuous nocturnal provision of calories through the intragastric infusion system described above for type I glycogen storage disease is also applicable to children with fructose-1,6-diphosphatase deficiency. During intercurrent illnesses with vomiting, intravenous glucose infusion is necessary to prevent severe hypoglycemia.

Pyruvate Carboxylase Deficiency (see Sec. 8.39). This is predominantly a disease of the central nervous system characterized by a subacute necrotizing encephalomyelopathy and high levels of blood lactate and pyruvate. Hypoglycemia is not a prominent feature of this syndrome, presumably because gluconeogenesis from precursors other than alanine remains intact because these precursors bypass the pyruvate carboxylase step. The utilization of alanine as well as lactate through pyruvate cannot proceed, however, so that these substrates accumulate in blood, and modest hypoglycemia may result during fasting. Affected patients have usually died from progressive central nervous system disease.

Phosphoenol Pyruvate Carboxykinase (PEPCK) Deficiency. Deficiency of this rate-limiting enzyme, which occupies a key step in gluconeogenesis, is associated with severe fasting hypoglycemia and variable onset after birth. Hypoglycemia may occur within 24 hr after birth, and defective gluconeogenesis from alanine can be documented in vivo. At post mortem, liver, kidney, and myocardium demonstrate fatty infiltration, and atrophy of the optic nerve and visual cortex may occur. Although total hepatic PEPCK activity may be normal, the extramitochondrial (cytosolic) fraction is absent, in contrast to the normal situation, in which one third of enzyme activity is in cytosol. This cytosolic fraction is believed to be physiologically important for gluconeogenesis. Extensive fatty deposition in liver, kidney, and other tissues also occurs in PEPCK deficiency. Hypoglycemia may be profound. Lactate and pyruvate levels in plasma have been normal, but a mild metabolic acidosis may be present. The fatty infiltration of various organs is due to increased formation of acetyl CoA, which becomes available for fatty acid synthesis. Diagnosis of this rare entity can be made with certainty only through appropriate enzymatic determinations in liver biopsy material. Avoidance of periods of fasting through frequent feedings rich in carbohydrate should be helpful because glycogen synthesis and breakdown are intact.

Other Enzyme Defects. GALACTOSEMIA (Galactose-1-Phosphate Uridyl Transferase Deficiency) (see Sec. 8.38).

FRUCTOSE INTOLERANCE. (Fructose-1-Phosphate Aldolase Deficiency). See Sec. 8.38. Acute hypoglycemia is due to the inhibition by fructose-1-phosphate of glycogenolysis via the phosphorylase system and of gluconeogenesis at the level of fructose-1,6-diphosphate aldolase. Affected individuals usually learn spontaneously to eliminate fructose from their diet.

DIAGNOSTIC EVALUATION

Table 8–27 lists the pertinent clinical and biochemical findings in the common childhood disorders associated with hypoglycemia. A careful and detailed history is essential in every suspected or documented case of hypoglycemia (Fig. 8–47). Specific points to be noted include age of onset, temporal relation to meals or caloric deprivation, and a family history of prior infants known to have hypoglycemia or to have unexplained infant deaths. In the 1st wk of life the majority of infants have the transient form of neonatal hypoglycemia as a result of either prematurity/intrauterine growth retardation or by virtue of being born to diabetic mothers. In the absence of a history of maternal diabetes, the characteristic large plethoric appearance of an "infant of a diabetic mother" should arouse suspicion of the islet cell dysmaturation syndrome; plasma insulin concentrations above 10–15 μU/mL in the presence of documented hypoglycemia confirm this diagnosis. The presence of hepatomegaly should arouse suspicion of an enzyme deficiency; if nonglucose-reducing sugar is present in the urine, galactosemia is most likely. In males, the presence of a microphallus suggests the possibility of hypopituitarism, which may be also associated with a hepatic jaundice in both sexes.

Past the newborn period clues to the cause of persistent or recurrent hypoglycemia can be obtained through a careful history, physical examination (see Fig. 8–47), and initial laboratory findings (see Table 8–26), which permit a systematic approach using selective and appropriate investigations. The temporal relation of the hypoglycemia to food intake may suggest that the defect is one of gluconeogenesis if symptoms occur 6 hr or more after meals. If hypoglycemia occurs shortly after meals, leucine sensitivity, galactosemia, or fructose intolerance is most likely, and the presence of reducing substances in the urine will rapidly distinguish these possibilities. The presence of hepatomegaly suggests one of the enzyme deficiencies in glycogen synthesis or breakdown or of gluconeogenesis, as outlined in Table 8–27. The absence of ketonemia or ketonuria at the time of initial presentation strongly suggests hyperinsulinemia or a defect in fatty acid oxidation. In all other causes of hypoglycemia, with the exception of galactosemia and fructose intolerance, ketonemia and ketonuria are present at the time of fasting hypoglycemia. At the time of the hypoglycemia, serum should be obtained for determination of hormones and substrates, followed by repeated measurement after an intramuscular or intravenous injection of glucagon as outlined in Table 8–26. Interpretation of the findings is summarized in Table 8–28. Hypoglycemia with ketonuria in children between the ages of 18 mo and 5 yr is most likely to be ketotic hypoglycemia, especially if hepatomegaly is absent. The ingestion of a toxin, including alcohol or salicylate, can usually be excluded rapidly by the history.

When the history is suggestive but acute symptoms are not present, a 24- to 36-hr fast can usually provoke hypoglycemia and resolve the question of hyperinsulinemia or other conditions (see Table 8–28). Since adrenal insufficiency may mimic ketotic hypoglycemia, plasma cortisol levels should be determined at the time of documented hypoglycemia; increased buccal or skin pigmentation may provide the clue to primary adrenal insufficiency with elevated ACTH (melanocyte stimulating hormone, MSH) activity. Short stature or a decrease in the growth rate may provide the clue to pituitary insufficiency involving growth hormone as well as ACTH. Tests of pituitary-adrenal function such as the arginine-insulin stimulation test for growth hormone and cortisol release may be necessary.

In the presence of hepatomegaly and hypoglycemia, a presumptive diagnosis of the enzyme defect can often be made through the clinical manifestations, presence of hyperlipidemia, acidosis, hyperuricemia, response to glucagon in the fed and fasted states, and the response to infusion of various appropriate precursors (see Tables 8–26 and 8–27). These clinical findings and investigative approaches are summarized in Table 8–27. Definitive diagnosis of the glycogen storage disease may require an open liver biopsy (see Sec. 8.40). Occasional patients with all the manifestations of glycogen storage disease are found to have normal enzyme

TABLE 8–28. Diagnosis of Acute Hypoglycemia in Infants and Children

Acute Symptoms Present	History Suggestive: Acute Symptoms Not Present
1. Obtain blood sample before and 30 min after glucagon administration	1. Careful history for relation of symptoms to time and type of food intake, bearing in mind age of patient (see Table 8–25). Exclude possibility of alcohol or drug ingestion. Assess possibility of insulin injection, salt craving, growth velocity, intracranial pathology
2. Obtain urine as soon as possible. Examine for ketones; if not present and hypoglycemia confirmed, suspect hyperinsulinemia or carnitine deficiency; if present, suspect ketotic, hormone deficiency, inborn error of glycogen metabolism, or gluconeogenesis	2. Careful examination for hepatomegaly (glycogen storage disease; defect in gluconeogenesis); pigmentation (adrenal failure); stature and neurologic status (pituitary disease)
3. Measure glucose in the original blood sample. If hypoglycemia is confirmed, proceed with substrate-hormone measurement as in Table 8–26	3. Admit to hospital for provocative testing: a. 24-hr fast under careful observation; when symptoms provoked proceed with steps 1–4 as when acute symptoms present b. Pituitary-adrenal function using arginine-insulin stimulation test if indicated
4. If glycemic increment after glucagon exceeds 40 mg/dL above basal, suspect hyperinsulinemia	4. Liver biopsy for histology and enzyme determination if indicated
5. If insulin level at time of confirmed hypoglycemia is greater than 10 μU/mL, suspect endogenous hyperinsulinemia; if greater than 100 μU/mL, suspect factitious hyperinsulinemia (exogenous insulin injection). Admit to hospital for provocative testing	5. Oral glucose tolerance test (1.75 g/kg; max 75 g) if reactive hypoglycemia suspected in an adolescent
6. If cortisol less than 10 μg/dL and/or growth hormone less than 5 ng/mL, suspect adrenal insufficiency and/or pituitary disease. Admit to hospital for provocative testing	

THERAPEUTIC CONSIDERATIONS

The prevention of hypoglycemia and its resultant effects on CNS development is very important in the newborn period. For neonates with hyperinsulinemia not associated with maternal diabetes, subtotal pancreatectomy may be needed, unless hypoglycemia can be readily controlled with somatostatin analogs or diazoxide. The therapeutic approach to specific causes is discussed with the description of each condition. As knowledge and understanding of glucose homeostasis have increased, fewer children are labeled as having idiopathic hypoglycemia, and precise rational therapy is possible more often.

Treatment of acute neonatal or infant hypoglycemia includes intravenous administration of 2 mL/kg of $D_{10}W$, followed by a continuous infusion of glucose at 6–8 mg/kg/min, adjusting the rate to maintain blood glucose levels in the normal range.

The management of persistent neonatal or infantile hypoglycemia includes increasing the rate of intravenous glucose infusion to 8–15 mg/kg/min. This may require a central venous catheter to administer a hypertonic, 15–20% glucose solution. In addition, intramuscular hydrocortisone, 5 mg/kg/24 hr given every 8 hr, or oral prednisone, 1–2 mg/kg/24 hr given every 6–12 hr, and intramuscular growth hormone, 1 U/24 hr, may be added if hypoglycemia is unresponsive to intravenous glucose.

Oral diazoxide, 10–25 mg/kg/24 hr given every 6 hr, may reverse hyperinsulinemic hypoglycemia but also produces hirsutism, edema, nausea, hyperuricemia, electrolyte disturbances, advanced bone age, IgG deficiency, and, rarely, hypertension with prolonged use. A long-acting somatostatin analog (octreotide, formerly SMS 201-995) has been effective in controlling hyperinsulinemic hypoglycemia in a small number of patients with islet cell dysmaturity syndrome and islet cell adenoma. Octreotide is administered subcutaneously every 6–12 hr in doses of 20–50 μg in neonates and young infants. Potential but unusual complications include poor growth due to inhibition of growth hormone release, pain at the injection site, vomiting, diarrhea, and hepatic dysfunction (hepatitis, cholelithiasis). Octreotide is usually employed as a temporizing agent for various periods prior to subtotal pancreatectomy for nesidioblastosis. It may be particularly useful for the treatment of refractory hypoglycemia despite subtotal pancreatectomy. Total pancreatectomy is not optimal therapy owing to the risks of surgery, permanent diabetes mellitus, and exocrine pancreatic insufficiency.

MARK A. SPERLING

Antunes JD, Geffner ME, Lippe BM, et al: Childhood hypoglycemia: Differentiating hyperinsulinemic from nonhyperinsulinemic causes. J Pediatr 116:105, 1990.

Aynsley-Green A, Polak JM, Bloom SR, et al: Nesidioblastosis of the pancreas: Definition of the syndrome and the management of the severe neonatal hyperinsulinaemic hypoglycemia. Arch Dis Child 56:496, 1981.

Bennish M, Kalam Azad A, Rahman O, et al: Hypoglycemia during diarrhea in childhood. Prevalence, pathophysiology and outcome. N Engl J Med 322:1357, 1990.

Bergada I, Suissa S, Dufresne J, et al: Severe hypoglycemia in IDDM children. Diabetes Care 12:239, 1989.

Bhowmick SK, Lewandowski C: Prolonged hyperinsulinism and hypoglycemia in an asphyxiated, small for gestation infant. Clin Pediatr 28:575, 1990.

Burchell A, Bell JE, Busuttil A: Hepatic microsomal glucose-6-phosphatase system and sudden infant death syndrome. Lancet 2:291, 1989.

Chaussain JL: Glycemic response to 24 hour fast in normal children and children with ketotic hypoglycemia. J Pediatr 82:438, 1973.

Chaussin JL, Georges P, Olive G, et al: Glycemic response to 24-hour fast in normal children and children with ketotic hypoglycemia: II. Hormonal and metabolic changes. J Pediatr 85:776, 1974.

Corkey BE, Hale DE, Glennon MC, et al: Relationship between unusual hepatic acyl coenzyme A profiles and the pathogenesis of Reye syndrome. J Clin Invest 82:782, 1988.

Cornblath M, Schwartz R: Disorders of Carbohydrate Metabolism in Infancy. Philadelphia, WB Saunders, 1976.

Cross NCP, DeFranchis R, Sebastio G, et al: Molecular analysis of aldolase B genes in hereditary fructose tolerance. Lancet 1:306, 1990.

Cryer PE: Glucose counterregulation in man. Diabetes 30:261, 1981.

DeClue TJ, Malone JI, Bercu BB: Linear growth during long-term treatment with somatostatin analog (sins 201–995) for persistent hyperinsulinemic hypoglycemia of infancy. J Pediatr 116:747, 1990.

Fischer KF, Lees JA, Newman JH: Hypoglycemia in hospitalized patients: Causes and outcomes. N Engl J Med 315:1245, 1986.

Fraker DL, Norton JA: Localization on resection of insulinomas and gastrinomas. JAMA 259:3601, 1988.

Hanse IL, Levy MM, Kerr DS: The 2-deoxyglucose test as a supplement to fasting for detection of childhood hypoglycemia. Pediatr Res 18:490, 1977.

Haymond MW: Hypoglycemia in infants and children. Endocrinol Metab Clin North Am 18:211, 1989.

Haymond MW, Ben-Galim E, Strobel KE: Glucose and alanine metabolism in children with maple syrup urine disease. J Clin Invest 62:398, 1978.

Jackson JA, Hahn HB Jr, Oltorf CE, et al: Long-term treatment of refractory neonatal hypoglycemia with long-acting somatostatin analog. J Pediatr 111:548, 1987.

Katz MD, Restad BI: Octreotide, a new somatostatin analogue. Clin Pharmacol 8:255, 1989.

Koh TH, Aynsley-Green A, Tarbit M, et al: Neural dysfunction during hypoglycemia. Arch Dis Child 63:1353, 1988.

Martin LW, Ryckman FC, Sheldon CA: Experience with 95 percent pancreatectomy and splenic salvage for neonatal nesidioblastosis. Ann Surg 200:355, 1984.

Mayefsky JH, Sarnaik AP, Postellon DC: Factitious hypoglycemia. Pediatrics 69:804, 1982.

Mock DM, Perman JA, Thaler JJ, et al: Chronic fructose intoxication after infancy in children with hereditary fructose intolerance: A cause of growth retardation. N Engl J Med 309:764, 1983.

Pagliara AS, Karl IE, Haymond M, et al: Hypoglycemia in infancy and childhood. J Pediatr 82:365 (part 1) and 558 (part 2), 1973.

Palardy J, Havrankova J, Lepage R, et al: Blood glucose measurements during symptomatic episodes in patients with suspected postprandial hypoglycemia. N Engl J Med 321:1421, 1989.

Phillip M, Bashan N, Smith CPA, et al: An algorithmic approach to diagnosis of hypoglycemia. J Pediatr 110:387, 1987.

Rahier J: Relevance of endocrine pancreas nesidioblastosis to hyperinsulinemic hypoglycemia. Diabetes Care 12:164, 1989.

Schwartz SS, Rich BH, Lucky AW et al: Familial nesidioblastosis: Severe neonatal hypoglycemia in two families. J Pediatr 95:44, 1979.

Schwenk WF, Haymond MW: Optimal rate of enteral glucose administration in children with glycogen storage disease type I. N Engl J Med 314:682, 1986.

Settergren G, Lingblad BS, Persson B: Cerebral blood flow and exchange of oxygen, glucose, ketone bodies, lactate, pyruvate and amino acids in infants. Acta Paediatr Scand 65:343, 1976.

Sperling MA, Ganguli S, Leslie N, et al: Fetal-perinatal catecholamine secretion: Role in perinatal glucose homeostasis. Am J Physiol 247:E69, 1984.

Stanley CA, Baker L: Hyperinsulinism in infants and children: Diagnosis and therapy. Adv Pediatrics 23:315, 1976.

Vidnes J, Oyasaeter S: Glucagon deficiency causing severe neonatal hypoglycemia in a patient with normal insulin secretion. Pediatr Res 11:943, 1977.

Volpe JJ: Hypoglycemia and brain injury. *In*: Volpe JJ (ed): Neurology of the Newborn. Philadelphia, WB Saunders, 1987, pp 364–385.

Ware AJ, Burton WC, McGarry JD, et al: Systemic carnitine deficiency: Report of a fatal case with multisystemic manifestations. J Pediatr 93:959, 1978.

White NJ, Marsh K, Turner RC, et al: Hypoglycemia in African children with severe malaria. Lancet 1:708, 1987.

9

THE FETUS AND THE NEONATAL INFANT

Although the "neonatal period" defines the first 4 wk of life after birth, both fetal and neonatal life form a continuum during which human growth and development are affected by genetic and by intrauterine and extrauterine environmental factors. For example, maternal toxemia may decrease the rate of fetal growth and cause an increased incidence of neonatal hypoglycemia. Social, economic, and cultural influences also affect this continuum. Low economic status is frequently associated with prematurity, which is correlated with high rates of morbidity and mortality, not only in the neonatal period but also throughout infancy. In the United States, the significantly higher black neonatal and infant mortality rate over that of white infants (Fig. 9–1) reflects cultural and socioeconomic factors. Although social influences, such as physician shortages in poor underserved areas, affect the availability of medical care to those most needing it, the failure of many mothers in these areas to use available prenatal and preventive medical care effectively also contributes to fetal and infant morbidity and mortality. Their failure results in part from inadequate public health education, from lack of money to pay for the care, and from limited access to health facilities and providers. Social factors leading to unwed pregnancies and cultural practices, such as the use of illicit drugs, also increase the incidence of fetal and neonatal disease.

Neonatal mortality has progressively decreased (Fig. 9–1); it is highest during the first 24 hr of life, when it accounts for about 65% of deaths under 1 yr of age. Further reduction of mortality and related morbidity depends primarily on preventing the birth of low-birthweight infants, prenatal diagnosis, and early treatment of diseases that result from factors acting during gestation and at delivery (Table 9–1). *Perinatal mortality* designates fetal and neonatal deaths influenced by prenatal conditions and circumstances surrounding delivery. It is often defined as deaths of fetuses and infants from the 20th wk of gestational life through the 28th day after birth.

In the United States each year there are approximately 6,000,000 pregnancies, 3,700,000 live births, and 40,000 infant deaths within the first 12 mo of life. Twelve per cent of births are to women between 15 and 19 years, and 25% are to unmarried women. Fetal deaths are associated with intrauterine growth retardation and conditions such as placental insufficiency that predispose the fetus to asphyxia. Neonatal deaths are due to diseases associated with low birthweight and to lethal congenital anomalies (see Table 9–1).

Infant mortality rates (deaths occurring from birth–12 mo/1,000 live births) vary by country; in 1987 they were lowest in Japan (5.0/1,000 births) and Scandinavia (5.8–8.4/1,000); moderate in the United States (10.1/1,000); and highest in developing countries (30–150/1,000). Although socioeconomic, cultural, and perhaps geographic factors influence perinatal mortality, preventive variables such as health education, prenatal care, nutrition, social support, risk identification, and obstetric care can effectively reduce perinatal mortality. The number of low-birthweight (LBW) infants is a major determinant of both the neonatal mortality rate and, together with lethal congenital anomalies (e.g., cardiac, central nervous system, and respiratory), infant mortality rate and contributes significantly to childhood morbidity. The LBW

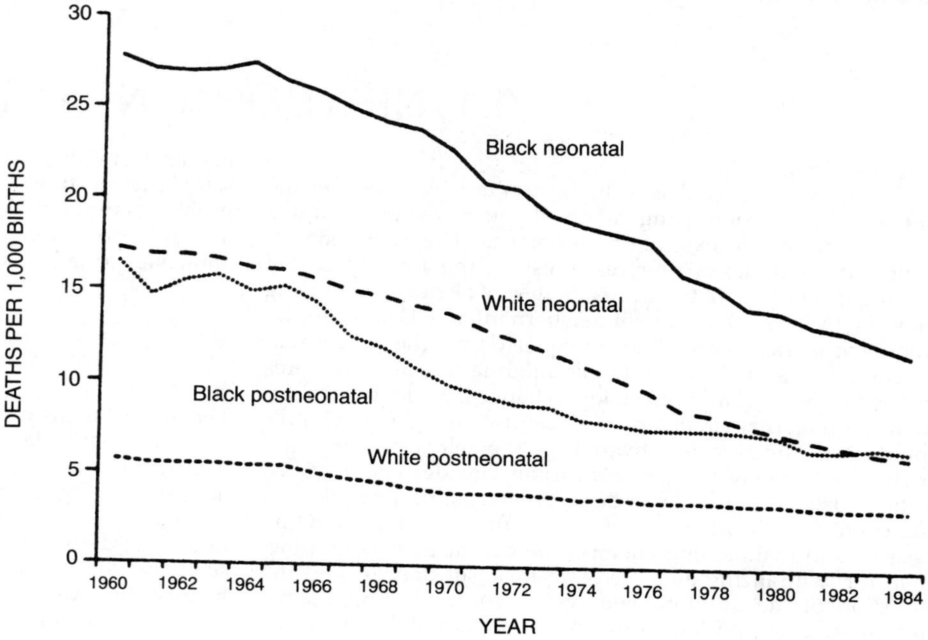

Figure 9–1. Neonatal and postnatal mortality rates among singletons by race and year: USA 1960–1984. (From MMWR 36:1, 1987.)

TABLE 9–1. Major Causes of Perinatal Mortality

Fetal	Preterm	Full-Term
Placental insufficiency Intrauterine infection Severe congenital malformations Umbilical cord accident Abruptio placentae Hydrops fetalis	Respiratory distress syndrome, Bronchopulmonary dysplasia Severe immaturity Intraventricular hemorrhage Congenital anomalies Infection Necrotizing enterocolitis	Congenital abnormalities Birth asphyxia, trauma Infection Meconium aspiration pneumonia Persistent fetal circulation

rate is directly related to the variance of infant mortality rates among different countries. In the United States the low-birthweight rate has declined minimally in the past 15 yr and has not followed the declining mortality rates.

The *low-birthweight rate* (infants weighing 2,500 g or less at birth each year) in recent years has been 6.7–6.9%, and the very low birthweight (VLBW) rate (infants weighing 1,500 g or less at birth) has been 1.1–1.2% of all births. The LBW and VLBW rates and the infant mortality rates are 2 times higher in black infants than in whites. Despite advances in perinatal care, these data suggest a major need for preventive programs.

Although 99% of births occur in hospitals, only 75% of pregnant women receive prenatal care in the 1st trimester. Many women who receive inadequate prenatal care are at risk for perinatal complications. Barriers to prenatal care include absent or insufficient money or insurance to pay for care, poor coordination of services, and inadequate effective education about the importance of prenatal care. Successful and adequate provision of high-quality prenatal and perinatal care requires competent health care professionals and coordination of services among physicians' offices, clinics, community hospitals, special regionalized programs for high-risk mothers and infants, and tertiary care centers. Regional perinatal programs should provide continuing education and consultation in both the community and the referral center and transportation for pregnant women and newborn infants to appropriate hospitals; they should also include a regional hospital with facilities, equipment, and personnel for obstetric and neonatal intensive care.

Fetal deaths slightly exceed neonatal deaths in their contribution to perinatal mortality. The obstetrician has a central role in reducing perinatal mortality and morbidity. Recently, intrapartum fetal deaths have declined more than antepartum fetal deaths, which may reflect an increase in the use of fetal monitoring during labor and a more liberal use of cesarean section for fetal distress and other obstetric complications. It also emphasizes the need for the ability to predict the maturity and functional reserve of the fetus prior to labor. In order to identify as early as possible those fetuses and infants at greatest risk, the obstetrician and pediatrician must effectively interact to anticipate perinatal problems and to take prompt preventive and therapeutic measures.

Along with the need to lower perinatal mortality rates is the need to reduce the incidence of handicaps among high-risk infants. Because both mortality and permanent neurologic sequelae are largely caused by the same or similar disturbances, research and public health measures directed at reducing perinatal mortality should also reduce the conditions contributing to the incidence of handicaps. For example, reducing the high incidence of mental retardation among infants whose births required vigorous and prolonged resuscitation mandates the early diagnosis of fetal asphyxia, appropriate obstetric management, and optimal resuscitation. However, some injury may be unavoidable; retinal damage may occur among those who had prolonged exposure to high concentrations of oxygen in the immediate postnatal period during which attempts were made to reduce the risk of hypoxic brain damage.

Centers for Disease Control: Contribution of birth defects to infant mortality. United States, 1986. MMWR 38:633, 1989.

Committee to Study the Prevention of Low Birthweight: The Prevention of Low Birthweight. Division of Health Promotion and Disease Prevention. Institute of Medicine, National Academy of Sciences. Washington, DC, National Academy Press, 1985.

Gould JB, Le Roy S: Socioeconomic status and low birth weight: A racial comparison. Pediatrics 82:896, 1988.

Hogue C, Yip R: Preterm delivery: Can we lower the black infant's first hurdle? JAMA 262:548, 1989.

Kliegman R, Rottman C, Behrman R: Strategies for the prevention of low birthweight. Am J Obstet Gynecol 162:1073, 1990.

Lubchenco LO, Butterfield J, Delaney-Black V, et al: Outcome of very-low-birth-weight infants: Does antepartum versus neonatal referral have a better impact on mortality, morbidity, or long-term outcome? Am J Obstet Gynecol 160:539, 1989.

Wegman ME: Annual summary of vital statistics—1989. Pediatrics 86:825, 1990.

9.1 NEWBORN INFANT

See also Chapter 3.

The neonatal period is a highly vulnerable time for the infant, who is completing many of the physiologic adjustments required for extrauterine existence. The high neonatal morbidity and mortality rates attest to the fragility of life during this period; in the United States, of all deaths occurring in the 1st yr, two-thirds are of newborn infants. Deaths during the 1st yr mark an annual rate unequaled until the 7th decade.

The infant's intrauterine to extrauterine transition requires many biochemical and physiologic changes. No longer dependent on maternal circulation via the placenta, the newborn's pulmonary function is activated for the self-sufficient respiratory exchange of oxygen and carbon dioxide. The newborn infant also becomes dependent upon gastrointestinal tract function for absorbing food, renal function for excreting wastes and maintaining chemical homeostasis, hepatic function for neutralizing and excreting toxic substances, and the function of the immunologic system for protecting against infection. Unsupported by the maternal placental system, the neonatal cardiovascular and endocrine systems also adapt for self-sufficient functioning. Many of the newborn's special problems are related to poor adaptation following birth due to asphyxia, premature birth, life-threatening congenital anomalies, or adverse effects of delivery.

9.2 HISTORY IN NEONATAL PEDIATRICS

The neonatal history should (1) identify disabling diseases that are amendable by prompt preventive action or treatment (e.g., asphyxia); (2) anticipate conditions that may be of later importance (e.g., gonococcal conjunctivitis); and (3) uncover possible causative factors that may explain pathologic conditions regardless of their immediate or future significance (e.g., screening for inborn errors of metabolism). The perinatal history should include demographic and social data (socioeconomic status, age, race), past medical illnesses in the child and family (cardiopulmonary disorders, infectious diseases, genetic disorders, diabetes mellitus), prior maternal reproductive problems (stillbirth, prematurity, blood group sensitization), events occurring in the present pregnancy (vaginal bleeding, medications, acute illness, duration of rupture of membranes), and a description of the labor (duration, fetal presentation, fetal distress, fever) and delivery (cesarean section, anesthesia or sedation, use of forceps, Apgar score, need for resuscitation).

9.3 PHYSICAL EXAMINATION OF THE NEWBORN INFANT

Many physical and behavioral characteristics of the normal newborn infant are described in Sec. 3.3–3.4, which should be reviewed before reading this section.

The initial examination of the newborn infant should be performed as soon as possible after delivery to detect abnormalities and to establish a baseline for subsequent examinations. For high-risk deliveries this examination should take place in the delivery room and focus on congenital anomalies and pathophysiologic problems that may interfere with a normal cardiopulmonary and metabolic adaptation to extrauterine life. Following a stable delivery room course, a second and more detailed examination should be performed within 24 hr of birth. In healthy infants the mother should be present during this examination; even minor, seemingly insignificant anatomic variations should be explained, since she may become disturbed at her or other relatives' later discovery of them, or she may think the physician is not giving them adequate consideration. However, explaining any problem has the potential for unduly alarming otherwise unworried parents unless it is carefully and skillfully done. No infant should be discharged from the hospital without a final examination, since certain abnormalities, particularly heart murmurs, often appear or disappear in the immediate neonatal period, or there may be evidence of disease that has just been acquired. Pulse, respiratory rate, temperature, weight, length, head circumference, and dimensions of any visible or palpable structural abnormality should be recorded.

Examining the newborn requires patience, gentleness, and procedural flexibility. Thus, if the infant is quiet and relaxed at the beginning of the examination, palpation of the abdomen or auscultation of the heart should be performed first before other, more disturbing manipulations are done.

GENERAL APPEARANCE. Physical activity may be absent during the relaxation of normal sleep or decreased by the effects of illness or drugs; the infant may be either lying with extremities motionless, to conserve energy for the effort of difficult breathing, or vigorously crying with accompanying activity of arms and legs. Both active and passive muscle tone and any unusual posture should be recorded. Coarse, tremulous movements with ankle or jaw myoclonus are more common and less significant in newborn infants than at any other age. Such movements tend to occur when the infant is active, whereas convulsive twitching usually occurs in a quiet state. Edema may produce a superficial appearance of good nutrition. Pitting after applied pressure may or may not be present, but the skin of the fingers and toes will lack the normal fine wrinkles when puffed with fluid. Edema of the eyelids commonly results from irritation caused by administration of silver nitrate. Generalized edema may occur with prematurity, hypoproteinemia secondary to severe erythroblastosis fetalis, nonimmune hydrops, congenital nephrosis, Hurler syndrome, or unknown cause. Localized edema suggests a congenital malformation of the lymphatic system; when confined to one or more extremities of a female infant, it may be the presenting sign of Turner syndrome (Sec. 7.25 and 19.34).

SKIN. Vasomotor instability and peripheral circulatory sluggishness are revealed by deep redness or purple lividity in the crying infant, whose color may darken profoundly with closure of the glottis preceding a vigorous cry, and by harmless cyanosis (acrocyanosis) of the hands and feet, especially when these are cool. Mottling, another example of general circulatory instability, may be associated with serious illness or related to a transient fluctuation in skin temperature. An extraordinary division of the body from forehead to pubis into red and pale halves is **harlequin color change**, a transient and harmless condition. Significant *cyanosis* may be masked by the pallor of circulatory failure or anemia; alternatively, the relatively high hemoglobin content of the first few days and the thin skin may combine to produce an appearance of cyanosis at a higher PaO_2 than in older children. Localized cyanosis is differentiated from ecchymosis by the momentary blanching pallor that occurs following pressure. The same maneuver also helps in demonstrating *icterus*, possibly significant but unnoticed if the skin is suffused with blood. *Pallor* may represent asphyxia, anemia, shock, or edema. Early recognition of anemia may lead to a diagnosis of erythroblastosis fetalis, of subcapsular hematoma of the liver or spleen, subdural hemorrhage, or fetal-maternal or twin-twin transfusion. Without being anemic, postmature infants tend to have paler skin than do term or premature infants. The ruddy-red appearance of *plethora* is seen with polycythemia.

The vernix and common transitory macular capillary hemangiomas of the eyelids and neck are described in Chapter 23. Slate blue, well-demarcated areas of pigmentation are seen over the buttocks, back, and sometimes other parts of the body in more than 50% of black infants and occasionally in white ones. These have no known anthropologic significance despite their name, **mongolian spots**; they tend to disappear within the first year. The vernix, skin, and especially the cord may be stained a brownish yellow if the amniotic fluid has been colored by passage of meconium during or before birth, often because of intrauterine anoxia.

The skin of the premature infant is thin and delicate and tends to be deep red; in extremely premature infants, the skin appears almost gelatinous and bleeds and bruises easily. Fine, soft, immature hair—**lanugo hair**—frequently covers the scalp and brow and may also cover the face in the premature infant. Lanugo hair has usually been lost or replaced by vellus hair in the term infant. Tufts of hair over the lumbosacral spines suggest an underlying abnormality such as an occult spina bifida, sinus tract, or tumor. The nails are rudimentary in the very premature infant, but they may protrude beyond the fingertips in infants born past term. Post-term infants may have a peeling, parchment-like skin (Fig. 9–2), a severe degree of which suggests ichthyosis congenita (Sec. 23.16).

Many neonates develop small, white, occasionally vesiculopustular papules on an erythematous base 1–3 days after birth. This benign rash, *erythema toxicum*, persists for as long as 1 wk, contains eosinophils, and is usually distributed on the face, trunk, and extremities (Sec. 23.4). *Pustular melanosis*, a benign lesion seen predominantly in black neonates, contains neutrophils and is present at birth as a vesiculopustular eruption around the chin, neck, back, extremities, and palms or soles; it lasts 2–3 days. Both lesions need to be distinguished from more dangerous vesicular eruptions such as herpes simplex (Sec. 9.71) and staphylococcal disease of the skin (Sec. 12.19).

Amniotic bands may disrupt the skin, extremities (amputation, ring constriction, syndactyly), face (clefts), or trunk (abdominal or thoracic wall defects). Their etiology is uncertain but may be related to amniotic membrane rupture or vascular compromise with fibrous band formation. Excessive

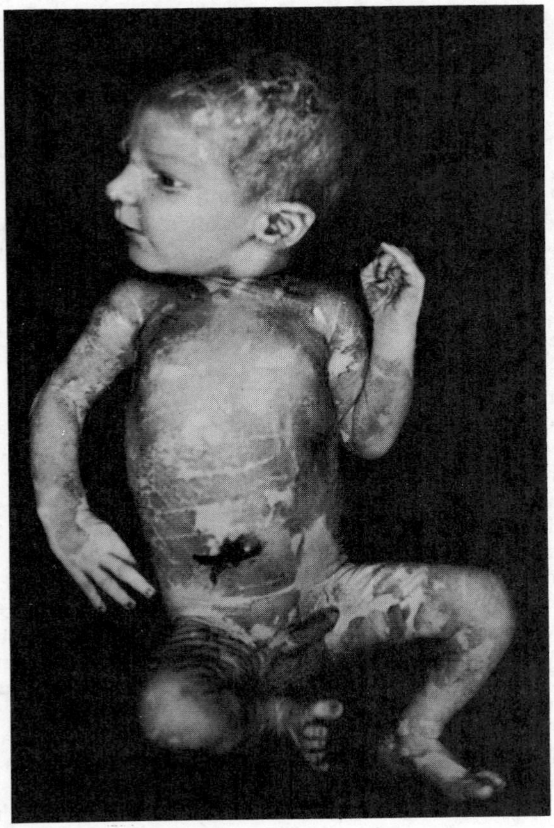

Figure 9–2. Infant with intrauterine growth retardation due to placental insufficiency. Note the long, thin appearance with peeling parchment-like dry skin, alert expression, meconium staining of the skin and long nails. (From Clifford S: Advances in Pediatrics, Vol 9. Chicago, Year Book Medical Publishers, 1962.)

skin fragility and extensibility with joint hypermobility suggest Ehlers-Danlos syndrome, Marfan syndrome, congenital contractural arachnodactyly, or other disorders of collagen synthesis.

SKULL. The skull may be molded, particularly if the infant is the firstborn and if the head has been engaged for a considerable time. The parietal bones tend to override the occipital and frontal bones. The head of an infant born by cesarean section or from a breech presentation is characterized by its roundness. The suture lines and the size and tension of the anterior and posterior fontanels should be determined digitally. Great variation in the size of the fontanels exists at birth; if small, the anterior fontanel usually tends to enlarge during the first few months of life. Persistence of excessively large anterior (normal: 20 ± 10 mm) and posterior fontanels has been associated with several disorders (Table 9–2). Soft areas **(craniotabes)** are occasionally found in the parietal bones at the vertex near the sagittal suture; they are more common in premature infants and in infants who have been exposed to uterine compression. Although usually insignificant, their possible pathologic cause should be investigated if they persist. Soft areas in the occipital region suggest the irregular calcification and wormian bone formation associated with osteogenesis imperfecta, cleidocranial dysostosis, lacunar skull, cretinism, and occasionally Down syndrome. Transillumination of the abnormal skull in a dark room or examination by ultrasound or computed tomography (CT) scan will rule out hydranencephaly or porencephaly (Sec. 20.11). An excessively large head (megalencephaly) suggests hydrocephaly, storage disease, achondroplasia, cerebral gigantism, neurocutaneous syndromes, or inborn errors of metabolism,

TABLE 9–2. Disorders Associated With a Large Anterior Fontanel

Achondroplasia	Osteogenesis imperfecta
Apert's syndrome	Prematurity
Athyrotic hypothyroidism	Pyknodysostosis
Cleidocranial dysostosis	Rubella syndrome
Hallermann-Streiff syndrome	Russell-Silver syndrome
Hydrocephaly	13-, 18-, 21-Trisomies
Hypophosphatasia	Vitamin D deficiency rickets
Intrauterine growth retardation	

or it may be familial. The skull of the premature infant may suggest hydrocephaly because of the relatively larger brain growth compared to that of other organs.

FACE. The general appearance should be noted with regard to dysmorphic features, such as epicanthal folds, widely spaced eyes, microphthalmia, long philtrum, and lowset ears, often associated with congenital syndromes. The face may be asymmetric from a 7th nerve palsy, from hypoplasia of the depressor muscle at the angle of the mouth, or from an abnormal fetal posture (Sec. 7.36); when the jaw has been held against a shoulder or an extremity during the intrauterine period, the mandible may deviate strikingly from the midline. Symmetric facial palsy suggests absence or hypoplasia of the 7th nerve nucleus (Moebius syndrome).

EYES. The eyes often open spontaneously if the infant is held up and tipped gently forward and backward. This maneuver, a result of labyrinthine and neck reflexes, is more successful for inspecting the eyes than forcing the lids apart. *Conjunctival and retinal hemorrhages* are not by themselves seriously significant. The pupillary reflexes are present after 28 wk of gestation. The iris should be inspected for colobomata and heterochromia. A cornea greater than 1 cm in diameter in a term infant suggests congenital glaucoma and requires prompt ophthalmologic consultation. The presence of bilateral *red reflexes* suggests the absence of cataracts or of intraocular pathology (Sec. 22.11–22.15). Leukocoria (white pupillary reflex) suggests cataracts, tumor, chorioretinitis, retinopathy of prematurity, or a persistent hyperplastic primary vitreous and warrants an ophthalmologic consultation.

EARS. Deformities of the pinnae are occasionally seen. Unilateral or bilateral preauricular skin tags occur frequently; if pedunculated, they can be ligated tightly at the base, and dry gangrene and slough will result. The tympanic membrane, easily seen otoscopically through the short, straight external auditory canal, normally appears dull gray.

NOSE. The nose may be slightly obstructed by mucus accumulated in the narrow nostrils.

MOUTH. The normal mouth rarely shows precocious dentition, with natal or neonatal *teeth* in the lower incisor position or aberrantly placed; these teeth are shed before the deciduous ones erupt. Alternatively, neonatal teeth occur in Ellis–van Creveld, Hallermann-Streiff, or other syndromes. Extraction is usually not indicated. Premature eruption of deciduous teeth is even more unusual. The **soft** and **hard palate** should be inspected for a complete or submucosal cleft and the contour noted if the arch is excessively high or the uvula bifid. On the hard palate on either side of the raphe may be temporary accumulations of epithelial cells called **Epstein pearls**. Retention cysts of similar appearance may also be seen on the gums. Both disappear spontaneously, usually within a few weeks of birth. Clusters of small white or yellow follicles or ulcers on an erythematous base may be found on the anterior tonsillar pillars, most frequently on the 2nd–3rd day of life. Of unknown cause, they clear without treatment in 2–4 days.

There is no active salivation. The **tongue** appears relatively large; the **frenulum** may be short, but rarely, if ever, is this a reason for cutting it. Occasionally, the sublingual mucous membrane forms a prominent fold. The **cheeks** have a fullness on both the buccal and the external aspects due to the accumulation of fat making up the **sucking pads**. These pads, as well as the labial tubercle on the upper lip, disappear when suckling ceases. A marble-sized buccal mass is usually due to fat necrosis.

The **throat** of the newborn infant is hard to see because of the arch of the palate; however, it should be clearly viewed because it is easily possible to miss posterior palatal or uvular clefts. The tonsils are small.

NECK. The neck appears relatively short. Abnormalities are not common; they include goiter, cystic hygroma, branchial cleft rests, and lesions of the sternocleidomastoid muscle that are presumably traumatic or are due to fixed positioning in utero that produces either a hematoma or fibrosis, respectively (Sec. 24.22). Redundant skin or webbing in a female infant suggests Turner syndrome (Sec. 7.25). Both clavicles should be palpated for fractures.

LUNGS. Much can be learned by observating breathing. Variations in rate and rhythm are characteristic, fluctuating according to physical activity, state of wakefulness, or presence of crying. Because fluctuations are rapid, the respiratory rate should be counted for a full minute with the infant in the resting state, preferably asleep. Under these circumstances the usual rates for normal term infants are 30–40/min; for premature infants they are higher and fluctuate more widely. Rates consistently over 60/min during periods of regular breathing usually indicate cardiac or pulmonary disease. The premature infant may breathe with a Cheyne-Stokes rhythm, known as periodic respiration, or with complete irregularity. Periodic respiration is rare in the first 24 hr of life. Irregular gasping, sometimes accompanied by spasmodic movements of the mouth and chin, strongly indicates serious impairment of respiratory centers.

The breathing of newborn infants is almost entirely diaphragmatic, so that during inspiration the soft front of the thorax usually is drawn inward while the abdomen protrudes. If the baby is quiet, relaxed, and of good color, this "paradoxic movement" does not necessarily signify insufficient ventilation. On the other hand, labored respiration is important evidence of respiratory distress syndrome, pneumonia, anomalies, or mechanical disturbance of the lungs. A weak groaning, whining cry, or **grunting** during expiration signifies a potentially serious cardiopulmonary disease. Flaring of the alae nasi and retractions of the intercostal muscles and sternum are common signs of pulmonary pathology.

Normally, the breath sounds are bronchovesicular. Suspected pulmonary pathology due to diminished breath sounds, rales, or percussion dullness should always be followed up with a chest roentgenogram.

HEART. The size is difficult to estimate owing to normal variations in the size and shape of the chest. The location of the heart should be determined to detect dextrocardia. There may be transitory murmurs. Congenital heart disease may not initially produce the murmur that will be present later; only a 1:12 chance exists that a murmur heard at birth represents congenital heart disease. Evaluating the heart by roentgenography, echocardiography, and electrocardiography is essential when the possibility of significant lesions exists. The pulse may vary normally from 90/min in relaxed sleep to 180/min during activity. The still higher rate of supraventricular tachycardia may be counted better on an electrocardiogram than by ear. Premature infants, whose resting heart rate is usually 140–150/min, may have a sudden onset of **sinus bradycardia. Pulses** should be palpated in the upper and lower extremities to detect coarctation of the aorta on both admission and discharge from the nursery.

Blood pressure measurements may be a valuable diagnostic aid (Sec. 15.1). The *auscultatory method* is often satisfactory, provided the stethoscope head is small enough. The *Doppler method,* using a transducer in the cuff, transmits and receives ultrasound waves. By detecting movements of the arterial wall, it more accurately measures systolic and diastolic pressures. The *oscillometric method* is currently the easiest and most accurate noninvasive method available. Other methods include the *palpatory method,* in which the systolic blood pressure is understood to be the point at which the pulse distal to the cuff becomes palpable during deflation, and the *flush method,* in which the extremity is first compressed, rendering the area below the cuff relatively bloodless, and then, while deflating the cuff, the mean pressure is recorded at the point where flushing appears in the arm or hand below the cuff. Each of these methods is disadvantageous in that the pulse pressure is not obtained and the reading lies between the systolic and diastolic pressures obtained by the auscultatory method. Continuous or intermittent direct measurement of blood pressure using an umbilical artery catheter may be indicated in special circumstances for infants who are under close observation in an intensive care unit (Fig. 9–3).

ABDOMEN. The liver is usually palpable, sometimes as much as 2 cm below the rib margin. Less commonly, the spleen tip may be felt. The approximate size and location of each kidney can usually be determined on deep palpation. At no other period of life does the amount of air in the gastrointestinal tract vary so greatly, nor is it usually so great under normal circumstances. Gas should normally be present in the rectum on roentgenogram by 24 hr of age. The abdominal wall is normally weak (especially in premature infants), and **diastasis recti** and umbilical hernias are common, particularly among black infants.

Unusual masses should be investigated immediately by ultrasonography. Cystic abdominal masses include hydronephrosis, multicystic-dysplastic kidneys, adrenal hemorrhage, hydrometrocolpos, intestinal duplication, and choledochal, ovarian, omental, or pancreatic cysts. Solid masses include neuroblastoma, Wilms tumor, hepatoblastoma, and teratoma. A solid flank mass may be due to renal vein thrombosis, which becomes manifest with hematuria, hypertension, and thrombocytopenia. Renal vein thrombosis in infants is associated with polycythemia, dehydration, diabetic mothers, asphyxia, sepsis, and coagulopathies such as antithrombin III or protein C deficiencies.

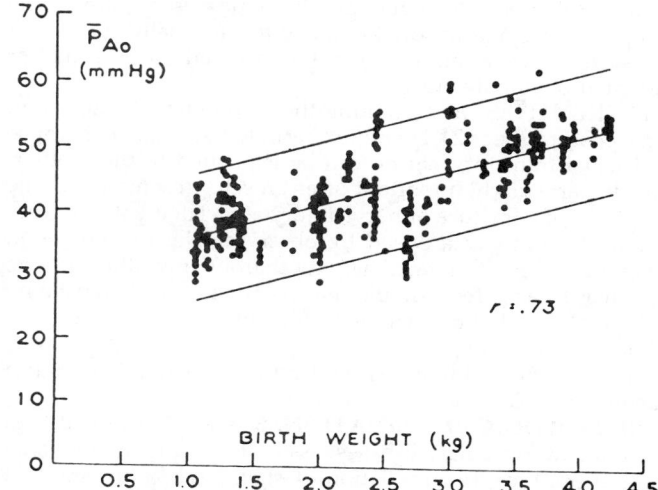

Figure 9–3. Linear regression and 95% confidence limits of mean aortic blood pressure in infants between 2 and 12 hr of age. (From Kitterman JA, Phibbs RH, Tooley WH: Aortic blood pressure in normal newborn infants during the first 12 hours of life. Pediatrics 44:959, 1969. Copyright 1969. Reproduced by permission of Pediatrics.)

Abdominal distention at or shortly after birth suggests either obstruction or perforation of the gastrointestinal tract, often due to meconium ileus; later distention suggests lower bowel obstruction, sepsis, or peritonitis. A scaphoid abdomen in the newborn suggests diaphragmatic hernia. **Abdominal wall defects** produce an omphalocele (Sec. 9.53) when they occur through the umbilicus and a gastroschisis (Sec. 13.26) when they occur lateral to the midline. Omphaloceles are associated with other anomalies and syndromes such as Beckwith-Wiedemann syndrome, conjoined twins, 18-trisomy, meningomyelocele, and imperforate anus. **Omphalitis** is an acute inflammation of the periumbilical tissue that may extend into the portal vein, producing acute pyophlebitis and later chronic portal hypertension.

GENITALIA. The **genitalia** and **mammary glands** normally respond to transplacentally obtained maternal hormones to produce enlargement and secretion of the breasts in both sexes and prominence of the female genitalia, often with considerable nonpurulent discharge. These transitory manifestations require observation but no interference.

Imperforate hymen may result in **hydrometrocolpos** and a lower abdominal mass. The normal scrotum is relatively large; its size may be increased by the trauma of breech delivery or by a **transitory hydrocele**, which is distinguished from a hernia by palpation and transillumination. The testes should be in the scrotum or palpable in the canals. The male black infant usually has dark pigmentation of the scrotum before the rest of the skin assumes its permanent color.

The **prepuce** of the newborn infant is normally tight and adherent. Severe hypospadias or epispadias should always lead one to suspect either the presence of abnormal sex chromosomes (Sec. 7.23) or that the infant is actually a masculinized female with an enlarged clitoris, because this may be the first evidence of the adrenogenital syndrome (Sec. 19.23). Erection of the penis is common and has no significance. Urine is usually passed during or immediately after birth; a period without voiding may normally follow. However, about 95% of preterm and term infants void within 24 hr.

ANUS. Some passage of **meconium** usually occurs within the first 12 hr after birth; 99% of term infants and 95% of premature infants pass meconium within 48 hr of birth. **Imperforate anus** is not always visible and may require evidence obtained by the gentle insertion of the little finger or a rectal tube. Roentgenographic study is required. The dimple or irregularity of skinfold often normally present in the sacrococcygeal midline may be mistaken for an actual or potential pilonidal sinus.

EXTREMITIES. In examining the extremities the effects of fetal posture (Sec. 24.1) should be noted so that their cause and usual transitory nature can be explained to the mother. This is particularly important after breech presentations. The suspicion of a fracture or nerve injury associated with delivery is more commonly aroused by observing the extremities in spontaneous or stimulated activity than by any other means. The hands and feet should be examined for polydactyly, syndactyly, and abnormal dermatoglyphic patterns such as a simian crease.

The hips of all infants should be examined to rule out a congenital dislocation (Sec. 24.8).

NEUROLOGIC EXAMINATION. See Sec. 3.3 and 20.1. In utero neuromuscular diseases associated with limited fetal motion produce a constellation of signs and symptoms that are independent of the specific disease. Severe positional deformation and contractures produce arthrogryposis. Other manifestations of fetal neuromuscular disease include breech presentation, failure to breath at birth, pulmonary hypoplasia, dislocated hips, undescended testes, thin ribs, and club foot.

ORDINARY CARE OF THE NEWBORN INFANT

The basic requirements of the newborn infant are immediate assistance at birth when needed, primarily to *establish respiration;* and subsequent assistance in obtaining *adequate nutrition,* in maintaining a *normal body temperature,* and in *avoiding contact with infection.* The environment meeting these requirements should also provide constant care by a nursing and medical staff alert to any signs of specific illness and should keep to a minimum the time the mother and infant are separated. The care of full-term and premature infants differs only in the degree of emphasis placed on each of these requirements. Problems to be anticipated after the delivery of a normal fetus include hypoventilation-apnea, hemorrhage, hypoxia, bradycardia, hypothermia, hypoglycemia, hypovolemia, hypotension, and unexpected anomalies.

9.4 ROUTINE DELIVERY ROOM CARE

The low-risk infant should be placed head downward immediately after delivery in order to clear the mouth, pharynx, and nose of fluid, mucus, blood, and amniotic debris by gravity; gentle suction with a bulb syringe or soft rubber catheter may also be helpful in removing this material. Wiping the palate and pharynx with gauze may lead to abrasions and the development of thrush, pterygoid ulcers (Bednar aphthae), or, rarely, tooth bud infection with maxillary osteomyelitis and retrobulbar abscess formation. If infants appear to be in satisfactory condition, they may be given to their mothers for immediate bonding and nursing. If there is any concern about respiratory distress, they should be placed under a warmer, with the head dependent.

The **Apgar score** is a practical method of systematically assessing the newborn infant immediately after birth to help identify infants requiring resuscitation for hypoxic acidosis (Table 9–3). A low score does not necessarily signify fetal hypoxia-acidosis; additional factors may reduce the score (Table 9–4). The Apgar score also does not predict neonatal mortality or subsequent cerebral palsy. Indeed, the score is normal in most patients who subsequently develop cerebral palsy, and the incidence of cerebral palsy is very low among infants with Apgar scores of 0–3 at 5 min. The 1-min Apgar score signals the need for immediate resuscitation, and the 5-, 10-, 15-, and 20-min scores indicate the probability of sucessfully resuscitating the infant. Apgar scores of 0–3 at 20 min predict high mortality and morbidity.

Infants with a prolapsed cord or delayed delivery and evidence of intrauterine asphyxia should receive prompt resuscitation and close observation subsequently (Sec. 9.29). The stomachs of infants delivered by cesarean section may contain more fluid than those of infants delivered vaginally. Their stomachs should be emptied by gastric tube to prevent aspiration of gastric contents.

MAINTENANCE OF BODY HEAT. Relative to body weight, the body surface of the newborn infant is approximately 3 times that of the adult, and in low birthweight infants the insulating layer of subcutaneous fat is thinner. The estimated rate of heat loss in the newborn is approximately 4 times that of an adult. Under the usual delivery room conditions (20–25° C), an infant's skin temperature falls approximately 0.3° C/min, and the deep body temperature approximately 0.1° C/min during the period immediately after delivery, resulting usually in a cumulative loss of 2–3° C in deep body temperature (corresponding to a heat loss of approximately 200 kcal/kg). The heat loss occurs by *convection* of heat energy to the cooler surrounding air, by *conduction* of heat to colder materials on which the infant is resting, by

TABLE 9–3. Apgar Evaluation of the Newborn Infant*

Sign	0	1	2
Heart rate	Absent	Below 100	Over 100
Respiratory effort	Absent	Slow, irregular	Good, crying
Muscle tone	Limp	Some flexion of extremities	Active motion
Response to catheter in nostril (tested after oropharynx is clear)	No response	Grimace	Cough or sneeze
Color	Blue, pale	Body pink, extremities blue	Completely pink

*Modified from Apgar V: Res Anesth Analg *32*:260, 1953.

Sixty sec after the complete birth of the infant (disregarding the cord and placenta) the 5 objective signs above are evaluated, and each is given a score of 0, 1, or 2. A total score of 10 indicates an infant in the best possible condition. An infant with a score of 0–3 requires immediate resuscitation.

heat *radiation* from the infant to other nearby solid objects, and by *evaporation* from moist skin and lungs (a function of alveolar ventilation).

Term infants exposed to cold after birth may develop metabolic acidosis, hypoxemia, and hypoglycemia, and increased renal excretion of water and solutes owing to their efforts to compensate for heat loss. They augment heat production by increasing the metabolic rate and oxygen consumption and by releasing norepinephrine, which results in nonshivering thermogenesis through oxidation of fat, particularly of brown fat. In addition, muscular activity may increase. Hypoglycemic or hypoxic infants cannot increase their oxygen consumption when exposed to a cold environment, and their central temperature decreases. After labor and vaginal delivery, many newborn infants have a mild to moderate metabolic acidosis for which they may compensate by hyperventilating, which is more difficult for depressed infants and infants exposed to cold stress in the delivery room. Therefore, it is desirable to ensure that the infant is dried and either wrapped in blankets or placed under a warmer while having skin to skin contact with the mother. Since carrying out resuscitative measures on a covered infant or one enclosed in an incubator is difficult, a radiant heat source should be used to receive the baby immediately.

ANTISEPTIC SKIN AND CORD CARE. To reduce the incidence of skin and periumbilical infections (omphalitis), the entire skin and cord should be cleansed in the delivery room or upon admission to the nursery with sterile cotton soaked in warm water or a mild soap solution. The infant may be rinsed with water at body temperature if care is taken to avoid chilling. The baby is then dried and wrapped in sterile blankets and taken to the nursery. To lessen the chance of carrying pathogenic organisms into the nursery, the outer blanket can be discarded at the nursery door. To reduce colonization with *Staphylococcus aureus* and other pathogenic bacteria the umbilical cord is treated daily with triple dye, a bacteriocidal agent. Alternatively, chlorhexidine washing or, on rare occasions during *S. aureus* epidemics, a single hexachlorophene bath may be employed. Repeated total body exposure to hexachlorophene may be neurotoxic, particularly in low-birthweight infants, and is not recommended. Nursery personnel should use chlorhexidine or iodophor-containing antiseptic soaps for routine handwashing before caring for each infant. Rigidly enforcing hand-to-elbow washing for 2 min in the initial wash and 15–30 sec in the second wash is recommended for staff and visitors entering the nursery. Shorter but equally thorough washes between handling infants also should be required.

TABLE 9–4. Factors Affecting the Apgar Score

False-Positive (No Fetal Acidosis or Hypoxia; Low Apgar)	False-Negative (Acidosis; Normal Apgar)
Immaturity	Maternal acidosis
Analgesics, narcotics, sedatives	High fetal catecholamine levels
Magnesium sulfate	Some full-term infants
Acute cerebral trauma	
Precipitous delivery	
Congenital myopathy	
Congenital neuropathy	
Spinal cord trauma	
CNS anomaly	
Lung anomaly (diaphragmatic hernia)	
Airway obstruction (choanal atresia)	
Congenital pneumonia	
Prior episodes of fetal asphyxia (recovered)	

Regardless of the etiology, a low Apgar score due to fetal asphyxia, immaturity, central nervous system depression, or airway obstruction identifies an infant needing immediate resuscitation.

OTHER MEASURES. The **eyes** of all infants must be protected against gonorrheal infection by instilling 1% *silver nitrate* drops, the best-proved therapy; erythromycin drops are an alternative measure that is also effective against chlamydial conjunctivitis. This procedure may be delayed during the initial short alert period following birth to promote bonding, but once applied, drops should not be rinsed out. Also see Sec. 9.61.

Although hemorrhage in the newborn infant can be due to factors other than *vitamin K deficiency*, an intramuscular injection of 1 mg of water-soluble vitamin K_1 (phytonadione) is recommended for all infants immediately after birth to prevent hemorrhagic disease of the newborn (Sec. 9.49). Higher-dose, repeated administration of oral vitamin K may also be useful, but this treatment is not yet established. Larger intravenous doses predispose to the development of hyperbilirubinemia and kernicterus and should be avoided. Administration of vitamin K to the mother during labor is not recommended owing to unpredictable placental transfer.

Neonatal screening is available for various genetic, metabolic, hematologic, and endocrine diseases. Common screening tests performed on cord or infant heel puncture blood samples include those for hypothyroidism, sickle cell anemia, phenylketonuria, homocystinuria, galactosemia, maple syrup urine disease, and other organic or amino acidopathies. Screening may be cost-effective when timely identification and prompt therapy lessen the morbidity of a disease.

9.5 NURSERY CARE

Non–high-risk infants may be taken after the delivery room examination to the "regular" newborn nursery or placed in the mother's room if the hospital has a rooming-in arrangement.

The bassinet, preferably of clear plastic to allow for easy visibility and care, should be cleaned frequently. All professional care should be given in the bassinet, including the physical examination, clothing changes, temperature-taking, skin cleansing, and other procedures that, if performed elsewhere, would establish a common contact point and possibly provide a channel for cross infection. The clothing and bedding should be minimal, only those needed for the infant's comfort; the nursery temperature should be kept at approximately 24° C (75° F). The infant's temperature should be taken once by rectum and thereafter in the axilla; although the interval between temperature taking depends on many circumstances, it need not be shorter than 4 hr during the first 2–3 days and 8 hr thereafter. Axillary temperatures of 36.0–37.0° C (96.5–98.5° F) are within normal limits. Weighing at birth and daily thereafter is sufficient.

Vernix is spontaneously shed within 2–3 days, much of it adhering to the clothing, which should be completely changed daily. The diaper should be checked before and after feeding and when the baby cries; it should be changed when wet or soiled. Meconium or feces should be cleansed from the buttocks with sterile cotton moistened with sterile water. The foreskin of the male infant should not be retracted.

9.6 PARENT-INFANT BONDING

See also Sec. 3.3.

Normal infant development depends partly on a series of affectionate responses exchanged between a mother and her newborn infant, binding them together psychologically and physiologically. This bonding is facilitated and reinforced by the emotional support of a loving husband and family. The attachment process may be important in enabling some mothers to provide loving care during the neonatal period and subsequently during childhood. It is initiated before birth with the planning and confirmation of the pregnancy and with the growing acceptance of the fetus as an individual. After delivery and during the ensuing weeks, visual and physical contact between mother and baby triggers a variety of mutually rewarding and pleasurable interactions such as the mother's touching the infant's extremities and face with her fingertips and encompassing and gently massaging the infant's trunk with her hands. Touching the infant's cheek elicits responsive turning toward the mother's face or toward the breast with nuzzling and licking of the nipple, a powerful stimulus for prolactin secretion. The infant's initial quiet alert state provides the opportunity for eye-to-eye contact, which is particularly important in stimulating the loving and possessive feelings of many parents for their babies. The infant's crying elicits the maternal response of touching the infant and speaking in a soft, soothing, higher-toned voice. Initial contact between mother and infant should take place in the delivery room, and opportunities for extended intimate contact should be provided within the first hours after birth. Delayed or abnormal maternal-infant bonding, occurring because of prematurity, infant or maternal illness, birth defects, or family stress, may harm infant development and maternal caretaking ability. Hospital routines should be designed to encourage parent-infant contact.

NURSERIES AND BREAST-FEEDING. See Sec. 4.10 and 4.11 for full discussions of breast- and formula feeding, respectively. Many hospital practices contribute to difficulties in breast-feeding by enforcing 4-hr feeding schedules, limiting nursing time, using only one breast at a feeding, washing nipples with substances other than water, delaying the first feeding, providing formula supplements, and using heavy intrapartum sedation.

Hospital practices that encourage successful breast-feeding include immediate postpartum mother-infant contact with suckling, rooming-in, demand feeding, inclusion of fathers in prenatal breast-feeding education, and support from experienced women. Nursing at least 5 min at each breast is reasonable and allows the baby to obtain most of the available breast contents and to provide effective stimulation for increasing milk supply. Nursing episodes should then be extended according to the comfort and desire of the mother and infant. A confident and relaxed mother, supported by an encouraging home and hospital environment, is likely to nurse well (See Sec. 9.6).

DRUGS AND BREAST-FEEDING. Maternal medications may affect the production and safety of breast milk (Table 9–5). Most commonly used medications, such as antihypertensive agents, are safe, but each should be investigated if used

TABLE 9–5. Drugs and Breast-Feeding

Contraindicated	Avoid or Give with Great Caution	Probably Safe But Give with Caution
Antineoplastic agents	Anthroquinones (laxatives)	Anesthetics
Amphetamines	Aspirin (salicylates)	Acetaminophen
Bromocriptine	Atropine	Aldomet
Clemastine	Birth control pills	Antibiotics (not tetracycline)
Cimetidine	Bromides	Antithyroid (not methimazole)
Chloramphenicol	Calciferol	Antiepileptics
Cocaine	Cascara	Antihistamines*
Cyclophosphamide	Danthron	Antihypertensive/cardiovascular
Cyclosporine	Dihydrotachysterol	Bishydroxycoumarin
Diethylstilbestrol	Estrogens	Chlorpromazine*
Doxorubicin	Ethanol	Codeine*
Ergots	Metoclopramide	Digoxin
Gold salts	Metronidazole	Dilantin
Heroin	Narcotics	Diuretics
Immunosuppressants	Phenobarbital*	Furosemide
Iodides	Primidone	Haloperidol*
Lithium	Psychotropic drugs	Hydralazine
Meprobamate	Reserpine	Indomethacin
Methimazole	Salicylazosulfapyridine (sulfasalazine)	Methadone*
Methylamphetamine		Muscle relaxants
Nicotine (smoking)		Prednisone
Phencyclidine (PCP)		Propranolol
Phenindione		Propylthiouracil
Radiopharmaceuticals		Sedatives*
Tetracycline		Theophylline
Thiouracil		Vitamins
		Warfarin

*Watch for sedation.

during breast-feeding. Maternal sedatives may result in the infant's sedation. Maternal drugs that are weak acids, composed of large molecules, plasma bound, or poorly absorbed from the maternal or neonatal intestine are less likely to affect the neonate. When fresh breast milk is fed by tube or bottle, bacteriologic evaluation of stored milk should be performed within 24 hr.

Catlin EA, Carpenter MW, Brann BS IV, et al: The Apgar score revisited: Influence of gestational age. J Pediatr 109:865, 1986.
Committee on Fetus and Newborn: Use and abuse of the Apgar score. Pediatrics 78:1148, 1986.
Frigoletto F, Little G: Guidelines for Perinatal Care, 2nd ed. Am Acad Pediatr. Elk Grove Village, Il, 1988.
Goldfarb J, Tibbetts E: Breast Feeding Handbook: A Practical Reference for Physicians, Nurses, and Other Health Professionals. Hillside, New Jersey, Enslow Publ., 1980.
Klaus M, Kennel J: Parent-Infant Bonding, 2nd ed. St. Louis, CV Mosby, 1982.
Lawrence R: Breast Feeding: A Guide for the Medical Profession, 2nd ed. St. Louis, CV Mosby, 1985.
Lawrence R: Breastfeeding and medical disease. Med Clin North Am 73:583, 1989.

9.7 HIGH-RISK PREGNANCIES

Pregnancies in which factors exist that increase the likelihood of abortion, fetal death, premature delivery, intrauterine growth retardation, fetal or neonatal disease, congenital malformations, mental retardation, or other handicaps are called high-risk pregnancies (Table 9–6; see also Sec. 9.14). Some factors, such as ingestion of a teratogenic drug in the 1st trimester, are causally related to the risk; others, such as hydramnios, are associations that alert the physician to the existence of the risk or risks. Based on their history, 10–20% of pregnant patients can be identified as "high risk"; less than half of all perinatal mortality and morbidity is associated with these pregnancies. Although assessing antepartum risk is important to reducing perinatal mortality and morbidity, some women become high risk only during labor and delivery; therefore, careful monitoring is critical throughout the intrapartum course.

Identifying high-risk pregnancies is important not only because it is the first step toward prevention but also because therapeutic steps may often be taken to reduce the risks to the fetus or neonate if the physician knows of the potential for difficulty. Good prenatal care reduces the incidence of low birthweight infants.

TABLE 9–6. Factors Associated With High-Risk Pregnancy

Economic	**Reproductive**
Poverty	Prior cesarean section
Unemployment	Prior infertility
Uninsured, underinsured health insurance	Prolonged gestation
Poor access to prenatal care	Prolonged labor
Cultural-Behavioral	Prior infant with cerebral palsy, mental retardation, birth trauma, congenital anomalies
Low educational status	Abnormal lie (breech)
Poor health care attitudes	Multiple gestation
No care or inadequate prenatal care	Premature rupture of membranes
Cigarette, alcohol, drug abuse	Infections (systemic, amniotic, extra-amniotic, cervical)
Age less than 16 or over 35 yr	Pre-eclampsia or eclampsia
Unmarried	Uterine bleeding (abruptio placentae, placenta previa)
Short interpregnancy interval	Parity (0 or more than 5)
Lack of support group (husband, family, church)	Uterine or cervical anomalies
Stress (physical, psychologic)	Fetal disease
Black race	Abnormal fetal growth
Biologic-Genetic	Idiopathic premature labor
Previous low-birthweight infant	Iatrogenic prematurity
Low maternal weight at her birth	**Medical**
Low weight for height	Diabetes mellitus
Poor weight gain during pregnancy	Hypertension
Short stature	Congenital heart disease
Poor nutrition	Autoimmune disease
Inbreeding (autosomal recessive?)	Sickle cell anemia
Intergenerational effects	TORCH infection
Hereditary diseases (inborn error of metabolism)	Intercurrent surgery or trauma
	Sexually transmitted diseases

GENETIC FACTORS. The occurrence of chromosomal abnormalities, congenital anomalies, inborn errors of metabolism, mental retardation, or any familial disease in blood relatives increases the risk of the same condition in the infant. Because many parents recognize only obvious clinical manifestations of genetically determined diseases, specific inquiry should be made about any disease affecting one or more blood relative(s).

MATERNAL FACTORS. The lowest neonatal mortality rate occurs in infants of mothers 20–30 yr of age. Both teenage pregnancies and those among women over 35 yr of age, particularly primiparous women, carry an increased risk for intrauterine growth retardation, fetal distress, and intrauterine death.

Maternal illness (Table 9–7); multiple pregnancies, particularly those involving monochorionic twinning; infections (Table 9–8), and certain drugs (Sec. 9.12) increase the risk for the fetus.

Polyhydramnios and *oligohydramnios* indicate high-risk pregnancies. Although there is a rapid turnover rate, during normal pregnancy the amniotic fluid volume gradually increases at a rate of less than 10 mL/day until about the 34th wk of pregnancy, after which it slowly diminishes. The volumes vary widely in normal pregnancy; term volume may be 500–2000 mL. A volume estimated at greater than 2,000 mL in the 3rd trimester constitutes polyhydramnios, and a volume estimated at less than 500 mL indicates oligohydramnios.

Acute polyhydramnios is rare and is usually associated with premature labor and delivery before 28 wk. Chronic polyhydramnios is commonly diagnosed in the 3rd trimester by the discrepancy between uterine size and gestational age; occasionally it goes undiagnosed until the patient has a dysfunctional labor or an abnormally large amount of amniotic fluid is noted during delivery. Polyhydramnios is associated with neuromuscular dysfunction or obstruction of the gastrointestinal tract that interferes with reabsorption of amniotic fluid swallowed by the fetus (Table 9–9). Increased fetal urination or edema formation is also associated with excessive amniotic fluid volume. Ultrasound demonstrates the increased amniotic fluid surrounding the fetus and also detects associated fetal anomalies, hydrops, pleural effusions, or ascites.

Oligohydramnios is associated with congenital anomalies, intrauterine growth retardation, severe renal anomalies, and drugs that interfere with fetal urination (see Table 9–9). This becomes most evident after 20 wk of gestation, when fetal urination is the major source of amniotic fluid. Oligohydramnios causes fetal compression deformations such as club foot and pulmonary hypoplasia and umbilical cord compression

TABLE 9–7. Maternal Disease Affecting the Fetus or Neonate

Disorder	Effects	Mechanism
Cholestasis	Preterm delivery	Unknown
Cyanotic heart disease	Intrauterine growth retardation	Low fetal oxygen delivery
Diabetes mellitus		
Mild	Large for gestational age, hypoglycemia	Fetal hyperglycemia—produces hyperinsulinemia; insulin promotes growth
Severe	Growth retardation	Vascular disease, placental insufficiency
Drug addiction	Intrauterine growth retardation, neonatal withdrawal	Direct drug effect, plus poor diet
Endemic goiter	Hypothyroidism	Iodine deficiency
Graves' disease	Transient neonatal thyrotoxicosis	Placental immunoglobin Passage of LATS and LATS-protector
Herpes gestationis	Bullous rash	Unknown
Hyperparathyroidism	Neonatal hypocalcemia	Maternal calcium crosses to fetus and suppresses fetal parathyroid gland
Hypertension	Intrauterine growth retardation, intrauterine fetal demise	Placental insufficiency, fetal hypoxia
Idiopathic thrombocytopenic purpura	Thrombocytopenia	Nonspecific platelet antibodies cross placenta
Isoimmune neutropenia or thrombocytopenia	Neutropenia or thrombocytopenia	Specific antifetal neutrophil or platelet antibody crosses placenta following sensitization of mother
Malignant melanoma	Placental or fetal tumor	Metastasis
Myasthenia gravis	Transient neonatal myasthenia	Immunoglobin to acetylcholine receptor crosses placenta
Myotonic dystrophy	Neonatal myotonic dystrophy, congenital contractures, respiratory insufficiency	Unknown
Obesity	Macrosomia, hypoglycemia	Unknown
Phenylketonuria	Microcephaly, retardation	Elevated fetal phenylalanine levels
Pre-eclampsia, eclampsia	Intrauterine growth retardation, thrombocytopenia, neutropenia, fetal demise	Uteroplacental insufficiency, fetal hypoxia, vasoconstriction
Renal transplant	Intrauterine growth retardation	Uteroplacental insufficiency
Rhesus or other blood group sensitization	Fetal anemia, hypoalbuminemia, hydrops, neonatal jaundice	Antibody crosses placenta directed to fetal cells with antigen
Sickle cell anemia	Preterm birth, intrauterine growth retardation	Maternal sickling producing fetal hypoxia
Systemic lupus erythematosus	Congenital heart block, rash, anemia, thrombocytopenia, neutropenia	Antibody directed to fetal heart, red and white blood cells and platelets

TABLE 9–8. Maternal Infections Affecting the Fetus or Newborn

Infection	Mode of Transmission	Outcome
Bacteria		
Group B streptococcus	Ascending, cervical	Sepsis, pneumonia
Escherichia coli	Ascending, cervical	Sepsis, pneumonia
Listeria monocytogenes	Transplacental	Sepsis, pneumonia
Ureaplasma urealyticum	Ascending, cervical	Pneumonia, meningitis
Mycoplasma hominis	Ascending, cervical	Pneumonia
Chlamydia trachomatis	Vaginal passage	Conjunctivitis, pneumonia
Syphilis	Transplacental	Congenital syphilis
Borrelia burgdorferi	Transplacental	Prematurity, fetal demise
Neisseria gonorrhoeae	Vaginal passage	Ophthalmia (conjunctivitis)
Mycobacteria tuberculosis	Transplacental	Prematurity, fetal demise
Virus		
Rubella	Transplacental	Congenital rubella
Cytomegalovirus	Transplacental, breast milk (rare)	Congenital CMV, or asymptomatic
Human immunodeficiency virus	Transplacental, vaginal passage, breast milk (rare)	Congenital AIDS
Hepatitis B	Vaginal passage, transplacental, breast milk (rare)	Neonatal hepatitis, chronic HBsAg carrier
Herpes simplex II	Transplacental	Congenital HSV
	Vaginal passage, ascending	Neonatal encephalitis, disseminated viremia
Varicella-zoster	Transplacental, early	Congenital anomalies
	Transplacental, late	Neonatal varicella
Parvovirus	Transplacental	Fetal anemia, hydrops
Coxsackie virus B	Fecal-oral	Myocarditis, meningitis, hepatitis
Poliomyelitis	Transplacental	Congenital poliomyelitis
Epstein Barr	Transplacental	Anomalies (?)
Rubeola	Transplacental	Abortion, fetal measles
Parasites		
Toxoplasmosis	Transplacental	Congenital toxoplasmosis or asymptomatic
Malaria	Transplacental	Abortion, prematurity
Trypanosomiasis	Transplacental	Congenital Chagas' disease
Fungi		
Candida	Ascending, cervical	Sepsis, pneumonia, rash

Table 9–9. Conditions Associated With Disorders of Amniotic Fluid Volume

Oligohydramnios	Polyhydramnios
Intrauterine growth retardation Fetal anomalies Twin-twin transfusion (donor) Amniotic fluid leak Renal agenesis (Potter syndrome) Urethral atresia Prune-belly syndrome Pulmonary hypoplasia Amnion nodosum Indomethacin Angiotensin-converting enzyme (ACE) inhibitors Intestinal pseudo-obstruction	*Congenital anomalies:* Anencephaly, hydrocephaly, tracheoesophageal fistula, duodenal atresia, spina bifida, cleft lip or palate, cystic adenomatoid lung malformation, diaphragmatic hernia *Syndromes:* Achondroplasia, Klippel-Feil, 18-, 21-trisomy, TORCH, hydrops fetalis, multiple congenital anomalad *Other:* Diabetes mellitus, twin-twin transfusion (recipient), fetal anemia, fetal heart failure, polyuric renal disease, neuromuscular diseases, idiopathic

during labor and deliver, which may be alleviated by saline amino-infusion. Ultrasonography may reveal small (1–2 cm) pockets of fluid in addition to the associated growth retardation or anomalies.

Obstetric conditions are understandably important because fetuses weighing more than 2,500 g make up a very high proportion of total fetal deaths, and neonatal mortality is greatest during the first 24 hr after delivery. A pregnancy should be considered high risk when the uterus is inappropriately large or small. A uterus large for the estimated stage of gestation suggests the presence of multiple fetuses, hydramnios, or an excessively large infant; an inappropriately small one suggests oligohydramnios or retardation of intrauterine growth. Rupture of membranes earlier than 24 hr before delivery carries a risk of fetal infection. Prolonged and difficult labors increase the risks of mechanical and hypoxic damage. The risk of neonatal death in uncomplicated labors lasting 24 hr or less is approximately 0.3%; it increases 6-fold in labors lasting over 24 hr and 20-fold (to 6%) in those over 30 hr. A tumultuous short labor, with a precipitate delivery, increases the risk of birth asphyxia and intracranial hemorrhage. Placental separation at any time prior to delivery and abnormal implantation or compression of the cord increase the possibility of brain damage due to fetal anoxia; brown or muddy amniotic fluid suggests that meconium has been passed during an episode of fetal anoxia.

Although the safety of any type of delivery depends on the skill of the obstetrician, additional hazards accompany particular methods and also result from the circumstances that dictated them. Neonatal deaths following deliveries by mid and high forceps, breech extraction, and version are likely to be related to traumatic intracranial injury.

Infants born by *cesarean section* present problems possibly related to the unfavorable obstetric circumstance that necessitated the operation or to prolonged maternal anesthesia. In normal term pregnancies, when there is no indication of fetal distress, delivery through the abdomen carries a greater risk than delivery through the birth canal. However, controversy exists regarding the safest type of delivery for the nondistressed viable immature fetus, especially in a breech presentation; cesarean section may involve less risk than the "stress" of labor and the potentially anoxic effects of uterine contractions during vaginal delivery. A small percentage of mature infants delivered by cesarean section have some degree of respiratory difficulty for 1–2 days. Although transient tachypnea is the most frequently associated problem, hyaline membrane disease may develop, particularly in infants born to diabetic mothers or following asphyxia.

Anesthesia and analgesia affect the fetus as well as the mother; mild maternal hypoxemia due to hypoventilation or hypotension due to epidural anesthesia may result in severe fetal hypoxia and shock. Skilled use of medication avoids severe fetal narcosis while securing the benefits of gentle and unhurried delivery. Even skilled administration often results in a mildly depressed infant whose crying and breathing may be delayed 1–2 min and who may be somewhat inactive for several hours. When anesthesia and analgesia are carelessly used or when their milder effects are added to already unfavorable fetal circumstances such as prematurity, anoxia, or trauma, the result may be catastrophic.

Bargs V, Benacerraf B, Frigoletto F: Second trimester oligohydramnios: A predictor of poor fetal outcome. Obstet Gynecol 64:608, 1984.
Berkowitz R: High Risk Pregnancy—1980. Clin Perinatol 7:Entire issue, 1980.
Blair E, Stanley FJ: Intrapartum asphyxia: A rare cause of cerebral palsy. J Pediatr 112:515, 1988.
Cyr RM, Usher RH, McLean FH: Changing patterns of birth asphyxia and trauma over 20 years. Am J Obstet Gynecol 148:490, 1984.
Diamond MP, Salyer SL, Vaughn WK, et al: Reassessment of White's classification and Pedersen's prognostically bad signs of diabetic pregnancies in insulin-dependent diabetic pregnancies. Am J Obstet Gynecol 156:599, 1987.
Hill LM, Guzick D, Belfar HL, et al: A combined historic sonographic score for the detection of intrauterine growth retardation. Obstet Gynecol 73:291, 1988.
Niswander K, Elbourne D, Redman C, et al: Adverse outcome of pregnancy and the quality of obstetrical care. Lancet 2:827, 1984.
Zuspan F: Preeclampsia-eclampsia. *In:* Fanaroff A, Martin R (eds): Behrman's Neonatal-Perinatal Medicine. St Louis, CV Mosby, 1983.

9.8 THE FETUS

Fetal life begins with the completion of organogenesis at about the 12th wk of gestation. Genetic and environmental influences may affect the embryo and fetus at any time during development; the fetal genome itself plays a role in development and fetal survival. Gene mutations and environmental factors may influence selection and expression of genes.

The mother's health and state of nutrition may affect ovulation, the viability of the ovum and the zygote, and the availability of an adequate site for implantation; women who suffer from malnutrition or debilitating illness have diminished fertility and often diminished frequency of menstruation. Exposure of the embryo or fetus to drugs, chemicals, infectious disease, or other noxious influences may result in structural malformations or aberrant fetal growth. The general health and nutrition of the mother, and possibly her emotional health during pregnancy, also affect the fetus; the infants of malnourished mothers may weigh less and be slightly shorter at birth than those of mothers with adequate nutrition. Illness of the mother may result in miscarriage, fetal death, fetal growth retardation, or premature delivery.

The major emphases in fetal medicine are (1) assessing fetal growth and maturity; (2) evaluating fetal well-being or distress; (3) assessing the effects of maternal disease on the fetus; (4) evaluating the fetal effects of drugs administered to the mother; and (5) identifying and treating fetal disease or anomalies. Increasing knowledge of fetal physiology has paved the way for effective fetal therapy, intervention during fetal distress, and improved adaptation of the newborn infant, particularly of the premature one, to extrauterine life. Some aspects of human fetal growth and development are summarized in Sec. 3.2.

9.9 FETAL GROWTH AND MATURITY

Fetal growth is usually assessed by ultrasonography as early as the 12th wk, but the assessment is more likely to be required between 18 and 20 wk. Serial determinations of the biparietal diameter are most helpful; head-to-abdomen circumference ratios may also be useful. Femoral length and total intrauterine volume measurements are occasionally indicated. An estimate of gestational age by dating of the last menstrual period should also be obtained. Two patterns of fetal growth retardation have been identified: continuous fetal growth 2 standard deviations below the mean for gestational age and a normal fetal growth curve that abruptly slows or flattens later in gestation (Fig. 9–4).

Fetal maturity is usually estimated by determining the amniotic fluid surfactant content (Sec. 9.13 and 9.32). Determination of the extent of calcification by ultrasound (placental maturity index), detection of the first audible fetal heart tones (16–18 wk), and observation of the initial fetal movements (18–20 wk) may also aid in evaluating the maturity of the fetus.

9.10 FETAL DISTRESS

Fetal compromise occurs during the antepartum or intrapartum period. Antepartum fetal distress becomes manifest as intrauterine growth retardation, fetal hypoxia, increased vascular resistance in fetal blood vessels, and, when severe, mixed respiratory and metabolic (lactic) acidosis. The predominant cause of antepartum fetal distress is uteroplacental insufficiency. The antepartum signs of fetal distress (hypoxia-acidosis) do not always produce obvious alterations of fetal heart rate patterns. The signs of early fetal compromise may be assessed with percutaneous umbilical venous blood sampling to detect hypoxia and acidosis (Fig. 9–5, Table 9–10) and with Doppler ultrasound to detect a reduced, absent, or reversed diastolic blood flow wave-form velocity in the fetal aorta or umbilical artery (see Table 9–10).

The *nonstress test (NST)* monitors the presence of fetal heart rate accelerations that follow fetal movement. A reactive (normal) NST result demonstrates fetal heart rate accelerations of at least 15 beats/min lasting 15 sec. A nonreactive NST result suggests fetal compromise and requires further assessment with a *contraction stress test* (CST) or the *biophysical profile* (BPP). A CST observes the fetal heart rate response to spontaneous, nipple-, or oxytocin-stimulated uterine contractions. Fetal compromise is suggested when 3 contractions in 10 min are followed by late decelerations. CST is contraindicated in women in preterm labor and in those with multiple gestations, an incompetent cervix, polyhydramnios, or placenta previa. The goals of fetal monitoring are to prevent intrauterine fetal demise and hypoxic brain injury. Although the CST and NST have low false-negative rates, both have high false-positive rates. Additional methods of assessing fetal well-being have been combined into the biophysical profile to improve the accurate and safe identification of fetal compromise. (The fetus is given a score for breathing movements, body movements, reactive heart rate, and amniotic fluid volume.) Indications for BPP include intrauterine growth retardation, postdate gestation, maternal diabetes mellitus, rhesus-sensitized pregnancy, previous history of stillbirths, and maternal hypertension.

Fetal distress during labor may be detected by monitoring fetal heart rate, uterine pressure, and fetal scalp blood pH (Fig. 9–6).

Continuous fetal heart rate monitoring detects abnormal cardiac patterns by instruments that compute the beat-to-beat fetal heart rate from a fetal electrocardiographic signal. Signals are derived from an electrode attached to the fetal presenting part; from an ultrasonic transducer placed on the maternal abdominal wall to detect continuous ultrasonic waves reflected from the contractions of the heart; or from a phonotransducer placed on the mother's abdomen. Uterine contractions are simultaneously recorded from an amniotic fluid catheter and pressure transducer or from a tocotransducer applied to the maternal abdominal wall overlying the uterus.

Fetal heart rate patterns show various characteristics, some of which suggest fetal distress. Baseline fetal heart rate is the average rate between uterine contractions, which gradually decreases from about 155 beats/min in early pregnancy to about 135 beats/min at term; the normal range at term is 120–160 beats/min. **Tachycardia** (over 160 beats/min) is associated with early fetal hypoxia, maternal fever, maternal hyperthyroidism, maternal β-sympathomimetic or atropine therapy, fetal anemia, and some fetal arrhythmias. The latter do not generally occur with congenital heart disease and tend to resolve spontaneously at birth. **Fetal bradycardia** (less than 120 beats/min) occurs with fetal hypoxia, the placental transfer of local anesthetic agents and β-adrenergic blocking agents, and, occasionally, heart block with or without congenital heart disease.

Normally, the baseline fetal heart rate is variable, with long-term changes of 3–6 cycles/min as well as short-term beat-to-beat variation. This variability may be decreased or lost with fetal hypoxemia or the placental transfer of drugs such as atropine, diazepam, promethazine, magnesium sulfate, and most sedative and narcotic agents. Prematurity, sleep state, and fetal tachycardia may also diminish beat-to-beat variability.

Periodic accelerations or decelerations of fetal heart rate in response to uterine contractions may also be monitored (see Fig. 9–6). **Early deceleration** (type I dips), associated with head compression, is a repetitive pattern of slowing, synchronous with and proportional to, the amplitude of the uterine contraction. **Variable deceleration** (associated with cord compression) is characterized by variable shape, abrupt onset and occurrence with consecutive contractions, and return to baseline at or after the conclusion of the contraction. **Late deceleration** (type II dips), associated with fetal hypoxemia, occurs repetitively after a uterine contraction is well established, is proportional to its amplitude, and persists into the interval following contractions. The late deceleration pattern is usually associated with maternal hypotension or excessive uterine activity but may be a response to any maternal, placental, umbilical cord, or fetal factor that limits effective oxygenation of the fetus. Reflex late decelerations with normal beat-to-beat variability are associated with chronic compensated fetal hypoxia and occur during uterine contractions that temporarily impede oxygen transport to the heart. Nonreflex late decelerations are more ominous and indicate severe hypoxic depression of myocardial function. The latter, together with decreased beat-to-beat variability or spontaneous decelerations in the absence of uterine contractions, either warrants further assessment by fetal blood sampling or is an indication for delivery.

Fetal scalp blood sampling during labor through a slightly dilated cervix may aid in confirming fetal distress suspected on the basis of variations in fetal heart rate or the presence of meconium in the amniotic fluid. The proper use of this technique may result in earlier delivery of depressed infants who thus have a better chance of successful resuscitation, increased survival, and less morbidity. Alternatively, when continuous fetal heart rate monitoring or general clinical evaluation suggests that a fetus is at risk, a normal fetal scalp blood sample may help to avert obstetric intervention.

Women who are reasonably comfortable and pain-relieved during labor and delivery usually exhibit an early mild respiratory alkalosis due to hyperventilation and, just before

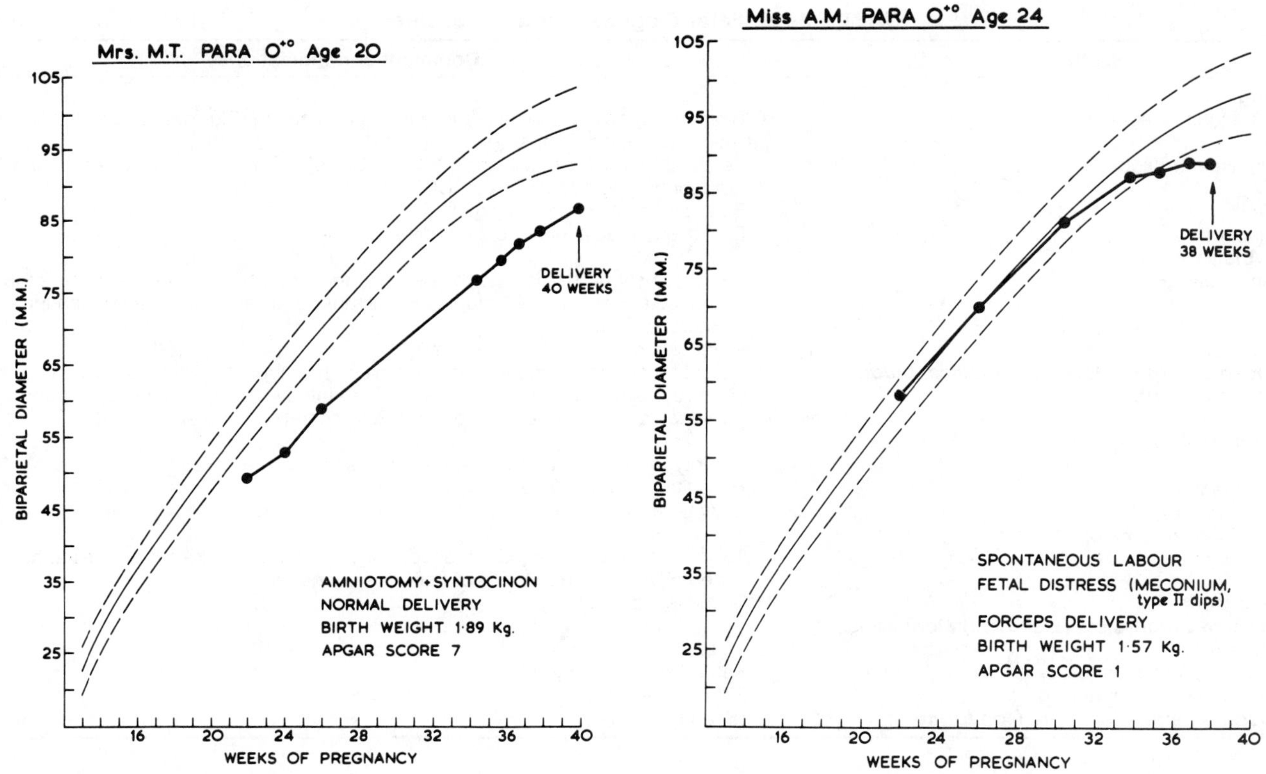

Figure 9–4. *A,* Example of "low profile" growth retardation pattern. Uneventful pregnancy and labor. Baby cried at 1 min and did not develop hypoglycemia. Birth weight was below the 5th percentile weight for gestational age. *B,* Example of "late flattening" growth retardation pattern. Typical history of preeclampsia, intrapartum fetal distress, low Apgar score, and postnatal hypoglycemia. Birth weight was below the 5th percentile weight for gestational age. (From Campbell S: Clin Obstet Gynecol 1:41, 1974.)

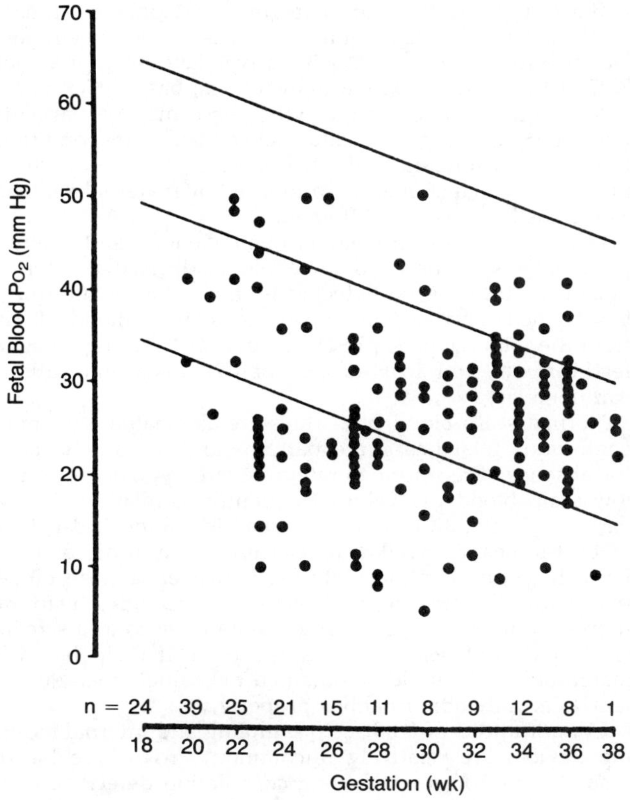

Figure 9–5. Reference range for fetal Po_2 in the umbilical vein between 18–38 wk of gestational age. Note the normal decline of venous Po_2 as gestational age advances. *Circles* depict fetuses with IUGR. (To convert mm Hg to kPa, multiply by 0.133) (From Soothill P: Clin Perinatol 16:755, 1989.)

TABLE 9–10. Fetal Diagnosis and Assessment

Method	Comment and Indications
Imaging	
Ultrasound (real-time)	Biometry (growth), anomaly (morphology) detection. Biophysical profile. Amniotic fluid volume, hydrops
Ultrasound (Doppler)	Velocimetry (blood flow velocity). Detection of increased vascular resistance secondary to fetal hypoxia, IUGR*
Embryoscopy	Early diagnosis of limb anomaly
Fetoscopy	Detection of facial, limb, cutaneous anomalies
Fluid Analysis	
Amniocentesis	Fetal maturity (L/S ratio), karyotype (cytogenetics), biochemical enzyme analysis, molecular genetic DNA diagnosis, bilirubin or α-fetoprotein determination. Bacterial culture
Fetal urine	Prognosis of obstructive uropathy?
Cordocentesis (percutaneous umbilical blood sampling [PUBS])	Detection of anemia, hemoglobinopathies, thrombocytopenia, acidosis, hypoxia, polycythemia, IgM antibody response to infection. Rapid karyotyping and molecular DNA genetic diagnosis. Fetal therapy (see Table 9–14)
Fetal Tissue Analysis	
Chorionic villus biopsy	Karyotype, molecular DNA genetic analysis, enzyme assays
Skin biopsy	Hereditary skin disease
Liver biopsy	Enzyme assay
Maternal Serum α-Fetoprotein	
Elevated	Twins, neural tube defects (anencephaly, spina bifida), intestinal atresia, hepatitis, nephrosis, fetal demise, incorrect gestational age
Reduced	Trisomies, aneuploidy
Antepartum Biophysical (Electrical) Monitoring	
Nonstress test	Fetal distress; hypoxia
Contraction stress test	Fetal distress; hypoxia
Vibroacoustic stimulation	Fetal distress; hypoxia
Intrapartum Fetal Heart Rate Monitoring	(See Fig. 9–7)

*IUGR = intrauterine growth retardation.

delivery, a mild metabolic acidosis due to a lactic acid accumulation that occurs toward the end of labor. However, pain or stress may produce severe hyperventilation, which markedly reduces maternal and subsequent fetal P_{CO_2}; such a reduction may mask fetal acidosis. Fetal scalp blood pH and P_{CO_2} levels fall between values measured in the umbilical vein and artery, in most instances giving a reasonable estimate of systemic fetal acid-base values. Fetal scalp blood pH in normal labor decreases from about 7.33 early in labor to approximately 7.25 at the time of vaginal delivery; the base deficit is about 4–6 mEq/L. Changes in the buffer base may be particularly helpful in assessing fetal status, since they correspond to fetal lactic acid accumulation and do not occur as rapidly as changes in fetal P_{CO_2}, which may be influenced by maternal ventilation as well as by placental diffusion.

Fetal hypoxia and circulatory insufficiency result in a mixed placental respiratory and metabolic acidosis that often, but not invariably, can be detected by the determination of pH, base deficit, and carbon dioxide tension in blood obtained from the fetal scalp. A pH of less than 7.25 strongly suggests fetal distress, and a pH of less than 7.20 is an indication for early delivery.

Normal scalp blood pH values are associated with normal continuous fetal heart rate patterns and accurately indicate the absence of recent moderate to severe hypoxia. In contrast, low scalp blood pH values frequently correlate with severe variable deceleration or late deceleration alone and with loss of beat-to-beat variability or baseline tachycardia associated with these deceleration patterns. However, a wide range of pH is found with these patterns. Accordingly, heart rate–uterine contraction monitoring should be used as a screening technique, and acid-base analysis of fetal scalp blood and maternal blood should be obtained to evaluate many types of fetal heart rate abnormalities properly.

Complications of fetal scalp sampling and internal monitoring devices are relatively uncommon but include bleeding (usually due to an underlying coagulation defect), puncture of the fontanel, and scalp abscesses with or without adjacent osteomyelitis. Abscesses may be due to *Staphylococcus aureus* or gram-negative rods; more often they are sterile.

9.11 MATERNAL DISEASE AND THE FETUS

INFECTIOUS DISEASES (see Table 9–8). Almost any maternal infection with severe systemic manifestations may result in miscarriage, stillbirth, or premature labor. Whether these results are due to infection of the fetus or are secondary to stress is not always clear. Maternal hyperthermia during infections may be associated with an increased incidence of congenital anomalies. Regardless of the severity of the maternal infection, certain agents frequently infect the fetus, with serious sequelae. Such fetuses are frequently small for gestational age. Some infections, such as rubella, may also produce congenital malformations if they occur during the period of organogenesis.

NONINFECTIOUS DISEASES (see Table 9–7). *Maternal diabetes* may result in organomegaly, hypertrophy and hyperplasia of the β cells of the fetal pancreas, and metabolic derangements in the neonate (Sec. 9.56). A high incidence of intrauterine death exists after the 36th wk of gestation in unmonitored and poorly controlled mothers. *Toxemia* of pregnancy, chronic hypertension, and renal disease result in small fetal size for gestational age, prematurity, and intrauterine death, all probably due to diminished uteroplacental perfusion. Uncontrolled maternal *hypothyroidism* or *hyperthyroidism* is responsible for relative infertility, a tendency to abort, premature labor, and fetal death. Maternal *immunologic diseases,* such as idiopathic thrombocytopenic purpura, systemic lupus, myasthenia gravis, and Graves disease, all of which are mediated by IgG autoantibodies that cross the placenta, frequently result in a transient illness in the newborn. Untreated maternal *phenylketonuria* results in miscarriage, congenital malformations, and injury to the brain of the nonphenylketonuric fetus.

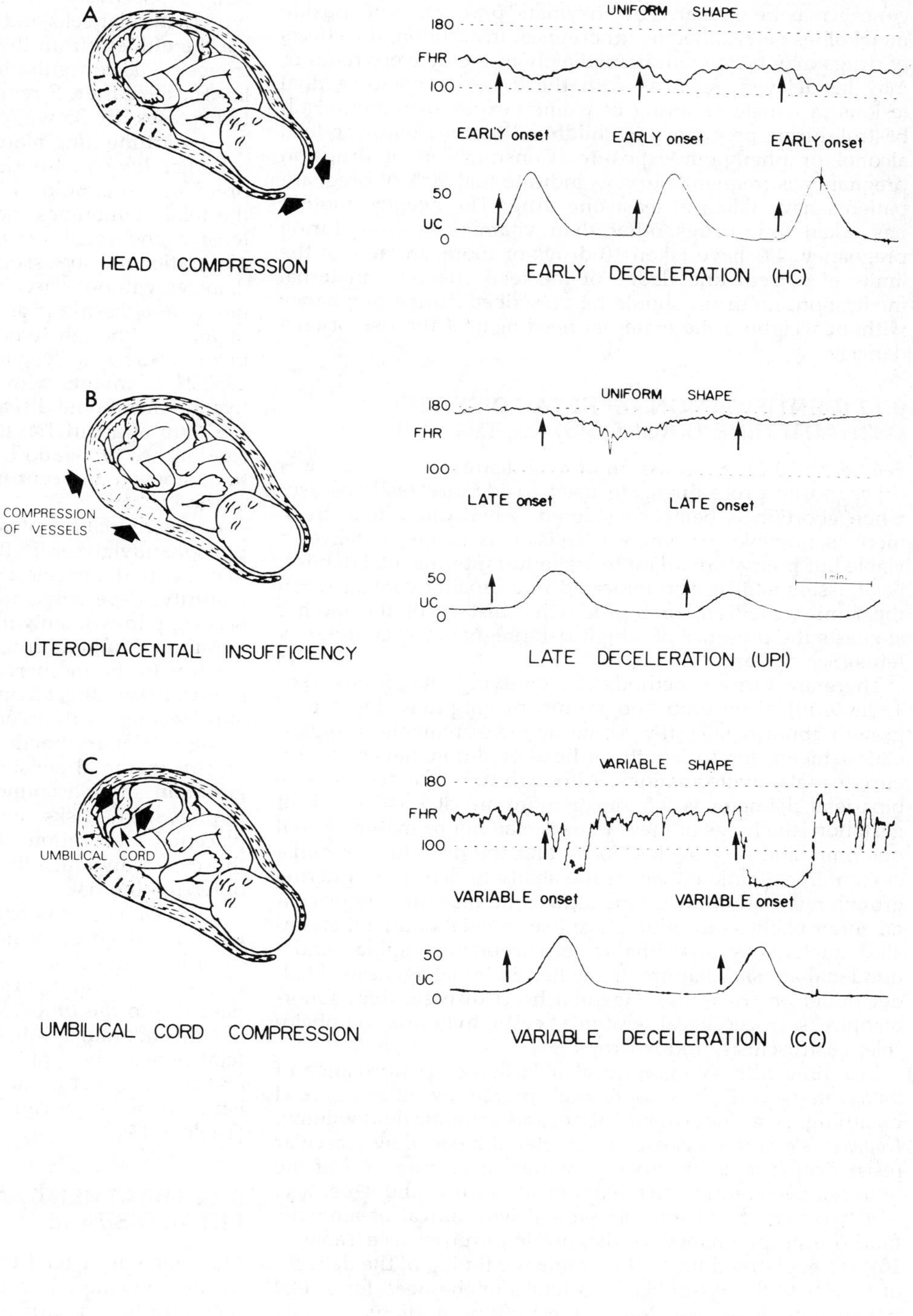

Figure 9–6. Patterns of periodic fetal heart rate decelerations. Tracing in *A* shows early deceleration that occurs during the peak of uterine contractions and is due to pressure on the fetal head; *B*, Late deceleration due to uteroplacental insufficiency; and *C*, Variable deceleration due to umbilical cord compression. *Arrows* denote time relation between the onset of FHR changes and uterine contractions. (From Hon EH: An Atlas of Fetal Heart Rate Patterns. New Haven, CT, Harty Press, Inc, 1968.)

9.12 MATERNAL MEDICATION AND THE FETUS

The effects of drugs taken by the mother vary considerably, especially in relation to the time in pregnancy when they are taken. Miscarriage or congenital malformations result from maternal ingestion of teratogenic drugs during the period of organogenesis. Maternal medications taken later, particularly during the last few weeks of gestation or during labor, tend to affect the function of specific organs or enzyme systems, adversely affecting the neonate rather than the fetus (Tables 9–11 and 9–12). Individual genetic make-up may determine susceptibility to some drugs. For example, phenytoin teratogenesis may be mediated by enzymatic production of epoxide metabolites determined by inheritance. In addition, the effects of drugs may be evident immediately in the delivery room or may be delayed, such as with the development of genital lesions in female offspring of women exposed to diethylstilbestrol during pregnancy or childhood tumors following fetal alcohol or phenytoin exposure. Consumption of drugs in pregnancy is frequent; surveys indicate that 90% of pregnant patients have taken at least one drug. The average mother has taken four drugs other than vitamins or iron during pregnancy; 4% have taken 10 drugs or more. In view of the limits of current knowledge of the fetal effects of maternal medication, no drugs should be prescribed during pregnancy without weighing the maternal need against the risk of fetal damage.

9.13 IDENTIFICATION OF FETAL DISEASE (INTRAUTERINE DIAGNOSIS) (see Table 9–10)

See Sec. 9.10 for a discussion of fetal distress.

Diagnostic procedures are used to identify fetal diseases when abortion is being considered, when direct fetal treatment is possible, or when a decision is made to deliver a viable but premature infant to avoid intrauterine fetal demise. Fetal assessment is also indicated in a broader context when the family, medical, or reproductive history of the mother suggests the presence of a high-risk pregnancy or a high-risk fetus (Sec. 9.7 and 9.15).

There are various methods of identifying fetal disease (see Table 9–10). Fetal ultrasonographic imaging may detect fetal growth abnormalities (by biometric measurements of biparietal diameter, femur length, or head or abdominal circumference) or fetal malformations. Although 95% of fetuses whose biparietal diameter is 9.5 cm or more are at least 37 wk of gestation, the lungs of these fetuses may not be mature. Serial determination of growth velocity and the head-to-abdominal circumference ratio enhances the ability to detect intrauterine growth retardation. Real-time ultrasound may identify placental abnormalities (abruptio placentae, previa) and fetal anomalies such as hydrocephalus, anencephalus, spina bifida, duodenal atresia, diaphragmatic hernia, renal agenesis, bladder outlet obstruction, congenital heart disease, limb abnormalities, sacrococcygeal teratoma, cystic hygroma, omphalocele, gastroschisis, and hydrops.

Real-time ultrasonography also facilitates performance of *cordocentesis* and the biophysical profile by imaging fetal breathing, body movements, tone, and amniotic fluid volume. *Doppler velocimetry* assesses fetal arterial blood flow (vascular resistance) (Sec. 9.10). Roentgenographic examination of the fetus has been replaced by real-time ultrasound and fetoscopy.

Amniocentesis, the transabdominal withdrawal of amniotic fluid during pregnancy for diagnostic purposes (see Table 9–10), is frequently done to determine the timing of the delivery of fetuses with erythroblastosis fetalis or the need for a fetal transfusion. It is also done for genetic indications, usually between the 16th and 18th gestational weeks. The amniotic fluid may be directly analyzed for amino acids, enzymes, hormones, and abnormal metabolic products; and amniotic fluid cells may be cultivated to permit detailed cytologic analysis for the prenatal detection of chromosomal abnormalities and DNA-gene or enzymatic analysis for the detection of inborn metabolic errors. Analysis of amniotic fluid may also help in identifying neural tube defects (elevation of α-fetoprotein), adrenogenital syndrome (elevation of 17-ketosteroids and pregnanetriol), and thyroid dysfunction.

The best available chemical indices of fetal maturity are provided by determinations of amniotic fluid creatinine and lecithin, which reflect the maturity of the fetal kidney and lung, respectively. Lecithin (L) is produced in the lung by type II alveolar cells and eventually reaches the amniotic fluid via the effluent from the trachea. Until the middle of the 3rd trimester, its concentration nearly equals that of sphingomyelin (S); thereafter, S remains constant in amniotic fluid while L increases. By 35 wk, on the average, the L/S ratio is about 2:1, indicating lung maturity.

Earlier lung maturation may occur when there is severe premature separation of the placenta, premature rupture of the fetal membranes, narcotic addiction, or maternal hypertensive and renal vascular disease. A delay in pulmonary maturation may be associated with hydrops fetalis or maternal diabetes without vascular disease. The likelihood of hyaline membrane disease is greatly reduced with L/S ratios of 1 to 2 or more, although hypoxia, acidosis, and hypothermia may increase the risk despite this "mature" L/S ratio. However, 20–25% of infants with L/S ratios less than 2:1 do not have hyaline membrane disease. Maternal and fetal blood have an L/S ratio of about 1:4; thus, contamination will not alter the significance of a ratio of 2:1 or more. Meconium contamination, storage, and centrifugation all may reduce the reliability of the L/S ratio.

A determination of saturated phosphatidylcholine (L) or phosphatidylglycerol (PG) concentrations in amniotic fluid may be more specific and sensitive predictors of pulmonary maturity, especially in high-risk pregnancies such as those occurring in women with diabetes.

Although amniocentesis can be carried out with little discomfort to the mother, there is, even in experienced hands, a small risk of direct damage to the fetus, of placental puncture and bleeding with secondary damage to the fetus, of stimulating uterine contraction and premature labor, of amnionitis, and of maternal sensitization to fetal blood. The earlier in gestation amniotic puncture is done, the greater the risk to the fetus. The risks can be reduced by using ultrasound for placental localization. The procedure should be limited to those cases in which the potential benefits of the findings will outweigh the risk.

Cordocentesis, or percutaneous umbilical blood sampling, is used to diagnose fetal hematologic abnormalities, genetic disorders, infections, and fetal hypoxia (see Table 9–10). Under direct ultrasonographic visualization, a long needle is passed into the umbilical vein at its entrance to the placenta or fetal abdominal wall. Blood may be withdrawn to determine fetal hemoglobin, platelet concentration, lymphocyte DNA, or Pa_{O_2}, pH, P_{CO_2}, and lactate levels. Transfusion or administration of drugs can be given through the umbilical vein (Table 9–13).

9.14 TREATMENT AND PREVENTION OF FETAL DISEASE

Management of fetal diseases continues to depend on coordinated advances in accuracy of diagnosis; understanding of fetal nutrition, pharmacology, immunology, and pathophysiology; availability of antimicrobial and antiviral drugs; and

TABLE 9–11. Agents Acting on Pregnant Women That May Adversely Affect the Fetus

Drug	Effect on Fetus	Dependability of Evidence
Accutane (isotretinoin)	Facial-ear anomalies, heart disease	Conclusive
Alcohol	Congenital anomalies, IUGR*	Conclusive
Aminopterin	Abortion, malformations	Conclusive
Amphetamines	Congenital heart disease, IUGR	Suggestive
Angiotensin converting enzyme inhibitors (ACE)	Renal failure, oligohydramnios	Suggestive
Azathioprine	Abortion	Suggestive
Busulfan (Myleran)	Stunted growth, corneal opacities, cleft palate, hypoplasia of ovaries, thyroid, and parathyroids	Doubtful
Caffeine	Spontaneous abortion, stillbirth, anomalies, or premature birth	Doubtful
Cocaine/crack	Abnormal brain development, microcephaly, LBW, IUGR, anomalies	Conclusive
Chloroquine	Deafness	Suggestive
Cigarette smoking	Low birthweight for gestational age	Conclusive
Cyclophosphamide	Multiple malformations	Suggestive
Dicumarol	Fetal bleeding and death, hypoplastic nasal structures	Conclusive
Lithium	Ebstein anomaly	Suggestive
Meclizine (Bonine)	Congenital malformations	Doubtful
Mepivacaine	Bradycardia, death	Conclusive
6-Mercaptopurine	Abortion	Suggestive
Methimazole	Goiter	Conclusive
Methyl mercury	Minamata disease, microcephaly, deaf, blind, mental retardation	Conclusive
Methyltestosterone	Masculinization of female fetus	Conclusive
17-α-ethinyl-19-nortestosterone (Norlutin)	Masculinization of female fetus	Conclusive
Penicillamine	Cutis laxa syndrome	Suggestive
Phenytoin (Dilantin)	Congenital anomalies, IUGR, tumor	Conclusive
Progesterone	Masculinization of female fetus	Suggestive
Propranolol	Hypoglycemia, bradycardia, respiratory depression	Suggestive
Propylthiouracil	Goiter	Conclusive
Quinine	Abortion, thrombocytopenia, deafness	Suggestive
Radioactive iodine (^{131}I)	Destruction of fetal thyroid	Conclusive
17-α-ethinyl testosterone (Progestoral)	Masculinization of female fetus	Conclusive
Stilbestrol (diethylstilbestrol [DES])	Vaginal adenocarcinoma in adolescence	Conclusive
Streptomycin	Deafness	Suggestive
Sympathomimetic (tocolytic) agents	Tachycardia, heart failure	Suggestive
Tetracycline	Retarded skeletal growth	Suggestive
	Pigmentation of teeth, hypoplasia of enamel	Conclusive
	Cataract, limb malformations	Doubtful
Thalidomide	Phocomelia, other malformations	Conclusive
Trimethadione and paramethadione	Abortion, multiple malformations, mental retardation	Conclusive
Valproate	Spina bifida	Conclusive
Vitamin D	Supravalvular aortic stenosis, hypercalcemia	Doubtful

*IUGR = intrauterine growth retardation.

TABLE 9–12. Agents Acting on Pregnant Women That May Adversely Affect the Newborn Infant

Anesthetic agents (volatile)—central nervous system depression
Adrenal corticosteroids—adrenocortical failure (rare)
Ammonium chloride—acidosis (clinically inapparent)
Aspirin—neonatal bleeding, prolonged gestation
Bromides—rash, CNS depression
Captopril—cardiovascular instability, transient renal failure
Caudal anesthesia with mepivacaine (accidental introduction of anesthetic into scalp of baby)—bradypnea, apnea, bradycardia, convulsions
CNS depressants (narcotics, barbiturates, tranquilizers) during labor—central nervous system depression
Cephalothin—positive direct Coombs test reaction
Cocaine/crack—microcephaly, growth retardation, behavioral disturbances, anomalies
Coumarin derivatives—high perinatal mortality, anomalies
Dilantin—bleeding diathesis (vitamin K deficiency)
Hexamethonium bromide—paralytic ileus
Intravenous fluids during labor (e.g., salt-free solutions—electrolyte disturbances, hyponatremia, hypoglycemia)
Iodides—neonatal goiter
Isoxsuprine—ileus, hypocalcemia, hypoglycemia, hypotension
Magnesium sulfate—respiratory depression, meconium plug, hypotonia
Morphine and its derivatives (addiction)—withdrawal symptoms (poor feeding, vomiting, diarrhea, restlessness, yawning and stretching, dyspnea and cyanosis, fever and sweating, pallor, tremors, convulsions)
Naphthalene—hemolytic anemia (in glucose-6-phosphate dehydrogenase [G-6-PD]–deficient infants)
Nitrofurantoin—hemolytic anemia (in G-6-PD–deficient infants)
Oxytocin—hyperbilirubinemia, hyponatremia
Phenobarbital—bleeding diathesis (vitamin K deficiency)
Primaquine—hemolytic anemia (in G-6-PD–deficient infants)
Propranolol—hypoglycemia, bradycardia, apnea
Reserpine—drowsiness, nasal congestion, poor temperature stability
Sulfonamides (long-acting)—interfere with protein binding of bilirubin; kernicterus at low levels of serum bilirubin
Sulfonylurea—refractory hypoglycemia
Thiazides—neonatal thrombocytopenia (rare)
Vitamin K (excessive amounts)—hyperbilirubinemia

TABLE 9–13. Fetal Therapy

Disorder	Treatment
Hematology	
Anemia with hydrops (erythroblastosis fetalis)	Umbilical vein packed red blood cell transfusion, intraperitoneal transfusion
Thrombocytopenia	
Isoimmune	Umbilical vein platelet transfusion, intravenous immunoglobulin
Autoimmune (ITP)	Maternal steroids, intravenous immunoglobulin, fetal platelet transfusion
Metabolic-Endocrine	
Maternal PKU	Phenylalanine restriction
Fetal galactosemia	Galactose-free diet
Multiple carboxylase deficiency	Biotin
Methylmalonic acidemia	Vitamin B_{12}
21-Hydroxylase deficiency	Dexamethasone
Hypothyroidism	Thyroid hormone (?)
Maternal diabetes mellitus	Tight insulin control
Fetal Distress	
Hypoxia	Maternal oxygen, position
Intrauterine growth retardation	Maternal oxygen, position
Oligohydramnios, premature rupture of membranes with variable deceleration	Amnioinfusion
Supraventricular tachycardia	Maternal digoxin, procainamide, quinidine, propranolol, verapamil
Lupus anticoagulant	Maternal aspirin
Pre-eclampsia	Maternal aspirin
Premature labor	Sympathomimetics, indomethacin, magnesium sulfate
Respiratory	
Pulmonary immaturity	Dexamethasone
Congenital Anomalies	
Neural tube defects	Folate, vitamins (prevention)
Diaphragmatic hernia	Surgery (?)
Hydrocephalus	Ventricular shunt (unproved)
Hydronephrosis (bladder obstruction)	Vesicostomy tube (unproved)
Infectious Disease	
Group B streptococcus	Ampicillin
Chorioamnionitis	Erythromycin (?)
Toxoplasmosis	Spiramycin, pyrimethamine, sulfonamide, and folinic acid
Syphilis	Penicillin
Tuberculosis	Antituberculosis drugs
Lyme disease	Penicillin, ceftriaxone
Parvovirus	Intrauterine red blood cell transfusion
Chlamydia trachomatis	Erythromycin
Other	
Nonimmune hydrops (anemia)	Intrauterine red blood cell transfusion
Narcotic abstinence (withdrawal)	Maternal low-dose methadone
Intraventricular hemorrhage	Vitamin K (?)

(?) Denotes possible but not proved efficacy.

therapeutic procedures. Progress in providing specific treatments for accurately diagnosed diseases has improved with the advent of real-time ultrasonography and cordocentesis (see Table 9–13).

Fetal syphilis is most always present with untreated maternal disease and can be specifically and safely treated (Sec. 12.50). Fetal mortality and prematurity associated with maternal bacterial urinary tract infections can be reduced with appropriate antibiotic treatment of the mother. Immunization has effectively reduced fetal mortality and morbidity from rubella (Sec. 9.73 and 12.65).

The incidence of sensitization of Rh negative women by Rh positive fetuses has been reduced by the prophylactic administration of Rh(D) immunoglobulin to mothers early in pregnancy and after each delivery or abortion, thus reducing the frequency of hemolytic disease in their subsequent offspring. Fetal erythroblastosis (Sec. 9.47) may now be accurately diagnosed by amniotic fluid analysis and treated with intrauterine intraperitoneal or intravenous transfusions of packed Rh negative blood cells to maintain the fetus until it is mature enough to have a reasonable chance of survival.

Fetal hypoxia or distress may now be diagnosed with moderate success (Sec. 9.10). Treatment, however, remains limited to supplying the mother with high concentrations of oxygen, positioning the uterus to avoid vascular compression, and initiating operative delivery before severe fetal injury occurs.

Pharmacologic approaches to fetal immaturity (e.g., administration of steroids to the mother to accelerate fetal lung maturation and to decrease the incidence of respiratory distress syndrome [Sec. 9.32] in prematurely delivered infants) are promising. Inhibiting labor with β-sympathomimetic tocolytic agents is successful in some patients with premature labor. Treatment of definitively diagnosed fetal genetic disease or congenital anomalies consists of parental counseling or abortion; rarely, high-dose vitamin therapy for a responsive inborn error of metabolism (e.g., biotin-dependent disorders) or fetal transfusion (with red blood cells or platelets) may be indicated. The nature of the defect and its consequences as well as the ethical implications for the fetus and the parents must be considered.

Anonymous: Are ACE inhibitors safe in pregnancy? Lancet 2:482, 1989.
Anonymous: Lupus nephritis and pregnancy. Lancet 2:82, 1989.
Frantz T, Lindback T, Skjaeraasen J, et al: Phospholipids in amniotic fluid. II. Lecithin fatty acid patterns related to gestation, maternal disease and fetal outcome. Acta Obstet Gynecol Scand 54:33, 1975.
Fuchs F: Prevention of premature birth. Clin Perinatol 7:3, 1980.
Golbus M, Loughman W, Epstein C, et al: Prenatal genetic diagnosis in 3,000 amniocenteses. N Engl J Med 300:157, 1979.
Goodlin R (ed): Fetal monitoring. Semin Perinatol 5, 1981.
Lombardi SJ, Rosemond R, Ball R, et al: Umbilical artery velocimetry as a

predictor of adverse outcome in pregnancies complicated by oligohydramnios. Obstet Gynecol 74:338, 1989.
Manning F, Morrison I, Lange I, et al: Antepartum determination of fetal health. Composite biophysical profile scoring. Clin Perinatol 9:285, 1982.
Members of the Joint Study Group on Fetal Abnormalities: Recognition and management of fetal abnormalities. Arch Dis Child 64:971, 1989.
Milunsky A, Jick SS, Bruell CL, et al: Predictive values, relative risks, and overall benefits of high and low maternal serum alpha-fetoprotein screening in singleton pregnancies: New epidemiologic data. Am J Obstet Gynecol 161:291, 1989.
Morrow R, Ritchie K: Doppler ultrasound fetal velocimetry and its role in obstetrics. Clin Perinatol 16:771, 1989.
Newton E: The fetus as a patient. Med Clin North Am 73:517, 1989.
Olson EB, Jr, Harline JV, Schneider JM, et al: The use of amniotic bubble stability, L/S ratio, and creatinine concentration in the assessment of fetal maturity. Am J Obstet Gynecol 122:755, 1975.
Pleet H, Graham J, Smith D: Central nervous system and facial defects associated with maternal hyperthermia at 4–14 wk gestation. Pediatrics 67:785, 1981.
Porreco R, Young P, Cousins L, et al: Reproductive outcome following amniocentesis for genetic indications. Am J Obstet Gynecol 143:653, 1982.
Pringle K: Fetal diagnosis and fetal surgery. Clin Perinatol 16:13, 1989.
Reece EA, Copel JA, Scioscia AL, et al: Diagnostic fetal umbilical blood sampling in the management of isoimmunization. Am J Obstet Gynecol 159:1057, 1988.
Report of the International Fetal Surgery Registry: Catheter shunts for fetal hydronephrosis and hydrocephalus. N Engl J Med 315:366, 1986.
Schiff E, Peleg E, Goldenberg M, et al: The use of aspirin to prevent pregnancy-induced hypertension and lower the ratio of thromboxane A_2 to prostacyclin in relatively high risk pregnancies. N Engl J Med 321:351, 1989.
Soothill PW, Nicolaides KH, Campbell S: Prenatal asphyxia, hyperlacticaemia, hypoglycemia, and erythroblastosis in growth-retarded fetuses. Br Med J 294:1051, 1987.
Tejani N, Maran LI, Bhakthavathsalan A, et al: Correlation of fetal heart rate-uterine contraction patterns with fetal scalp blood pH. Obstet Gynecol 46:392, 1975.
Tyrrell S, Obaid AH, Lilford RJ: Umbilical artery Doppler velocimetry as a predictor of fetal hypoxia and acidosis at birth. Obstet Gynecol 74:332, 1989.
Weiner CP, Williamson RA: Evaluation of severe growth retardation using cordocentesis-hematologic and metabolic alterations by etiology. Obstet Gynecol 73:225, 1989.

9.15 HIGH-RISK INFANT

Infants particularly at risk during the neonatal period should be identified as early as possible in order to decrease neonatal morbidity and mortality (see also Sec. 9.7). The term *high-risk* infant designates infants who should be under close observation by experienced physicians and nurses. Approximately 9% of all births require special or neonatal intensive care. Usually needed for only a few days, such observations may last from a few hours to several weeks. Some institutions find it advantageous to provide a special or transitional care nursery for high-risk infants, often within the labor and delivery suite. This facility should be equipped and staffed similarly to a neonatal intensive care area, where well but high-risk term infants can be observed and cared for immediately after birth without being separated from their mothers. Infants in the high-risk category are listed in Table 9–14.

Examination of a fresh *placenta, cord,* and *membranes* may alert the physician to a newborn infant at high risk. Fetal blood loss may be indicated by placental pallor, **retroplacental hematoma**, and tears of a velamentous cord or of chorionic blood vessels supplying succenturiate lobes. **Placental edema** and subsequent deficiency of immunoglobulin G in the newborn may be associated with feto-fetal transfusion syndrome, hydrops fetalis, congenital nephrosis, or hepatic disease. **Amnion nodosum** (granules on the amnion) and **oligohydramnios** are associated with pulmonary hypoplasia and renal agenesis, and small whitish **nodules** on the cord suggest a candidal infection. **Short cords** occur with chromosome abnormalities and omphalocele. **Chorioangiomas** are associated with prematurity, abruptio, polyhydramnios, and intrauterine growth retardation. **Meconium staining** suggests asphyxia and the risk of pneumonia, and opacity of the fetal placental surface suggests infection. **Single umbilical arteries** are associated with an increased incidence of congenital abnormalities.

Many high-risk infants are born prematurely, are breech deliveries, have low weight for gestational age, have significant perinatal asphyxia, or are born with life-threatening congenital anomalies without exhibiting previously identified risk factors. Generally speaking, for any given duration of gestation, the lower the birth weight, the higher the neonatal mortality, and, for any given weight, the shorter the gestational duration, the higher the neonatal mortality (Fig. 9–7). The highest risk of neonatal mortality occurs among infants who weigh less than 1,000 g at birth and whose gestation was less than 30 wk. The lowest risk of neonatal mortality occurs among infants with birthweights of 3,000–4,000 g whose gestational age was 38–42 wk. As birthweight increases from 500 to 3,000 g, a logarithmic decrease in neonatal mortality occurs; for every week increase in gestational age from the 25th to 37th wk, the neonatal mortality rate decreases by approximately one half. Nevertheless, approximately 40% of all *perinatal deaths* occur after 37 wk of gestation in infants weighing 2,500 g or more; many of these deaths occur in the period immediately before birth and are more readily preventable than those of smaller and more immature infants. In addition, neonatal mortality rates rise sharply for infants weighing over 4,000 g at birth and for those whose gestational period is 42 wk or longer. Since neonatal mortality largely depends on birth weight and gestational age, Figure 9–7 helps to identify high-risk infants quickly. However, this analysis is based on total live births and therefore describes the mortality risk only *at birth*. Because most neonatal mortality occurs within the first hours and days after birth, the outlook improves dramatically with increasing postnatal survival.

Behrman RE: Prevention of low birthweight: A pediatric perspective. J Pediatr 107:842, 1985.
Bjerkedahl T, Bakketeig L, Lehmann EH: Percentiles of birth weights of single live births at different gestational periods. Acta Pediatr Scand 62:449, 1973.
Hobel C: Better perinatal health: U.S.A. Lancet 1:31, 1980.
Saigal S, Rosenbaum P, Hattersley B, et al: Decreased disability rate among 3-year-old survivors weighing 501 to 1000 grams at birth and born to residents of a geographically defined region from 1981 to 1984 compared with 1977 to 1980. J Pediatr 114:839, 1989.
Tanner JM, Lejarraga H, Turner G: Within-family standards for birth weight. Lancet 2:193, 1972.
Wariyar U, Richmond S, Hey E: Pregnancy outcome at 24–31 weeks' gestation: Mortality. Arch Dis Child 64:670, 1989.
Wariyar U, Richmond S, Hey E: Pregnancy outcome at 24–31 weeks' gestation: Neonatal survivors. Arch Dis Child 64:678, 1989.
Whitby C, DeCates C, Robertson N: Infants weighing 1.8–2.5 kg: Should they be cared for in neonatal units or postnatal wards? Lancet 1:322, 1982.

9.16 MULTIPLE PREGNANCIES

INCIDENCE. The reported incidence of twins is highest among blacks and East Indians, followed by North European whites, and is lowest among the Oriental races. Specific rates include: Belgium, 1:56, American blacks, 1:70; Italy, 1:86; American whites, 1:88; Greece, 1:130; Japan, 1:150; China, 1:300. Differences in the incidence of twins mainly involve fraternal (polyovular) dizygotic twins. Triplets are estimated to occur in 1 of 86^2 pregnancies and quadruplets in 1 of 86^3 pregnancies in the United States. The incidence of monozygotic twins is unaffected by racial or familial factors (3–

TABLE 9–14. High-Risk Infants

Demographic Social Factors
- Maternal age < 16 or > 40 yr
- Illicit drug, alcohol, cigarette use
- Poverty
- Unmarried
- Emotional or physical stress

Past Medical History
- Diabetes mellitus
- Hypertension
- Asymptomatic bactiuria
- Rheumatologic illness (SLE)*
- Chronic medication (see Table 9–12)

Prior Pregnancy
- Intrauterine fetal demise
- Neonatal death
- Prematurity
- Intrauterine growth retardation
- Congenital malformation
- Incompetent cervix
- Blood group sensitization, neonatal jaundice
- Neonatal thrombocytopenia
- Hydrops
- Inborn errors of metabolism

Present Pregnancy
- Vaginal bleeding (abruptio placentae, placenta previa)
- Sexually transmitted diseases (colonization: herpes simplex, group B streptococcus)
- Multiple gestation
- Pre-eclampsia
- Premature rupture of membranes
- Short interpregnancy time
- Poly-oligohydramnios
- Acute medical or surgical illness
- Inadequate prenatal care

Labor and Delivery
- Premature labor (< 37 wk)
- Postdates (> 42 wk)
- Fetal distress
- Immature L/S ratio: absent phosphatidylglycerol
- Breech presentation
- Meconium-stained fluid
- Nuchal cord
- Cesarean section
- Forceps delivery
- Apgar score < 4 at 1 min

Neonate
- Birthweight < 2,500 or > 4,000 g
- Birth before 37 or after 42 wk of gestation
- SGA†, LGA growth status‡
- Tachypnea, cyanosis
- Congenital malformation
- Pallor, plethora, petechiae

*SLE = Systemic lupus erythematosus.
†SGA = Small for gestational age.
‡LGA = Large for gestational age.

5:1,000). The incidence of twins detected by ultrasonography at 12 wk of gestation (3–5%) is much higher than that occurring later in pregnancy; the vanishing twin syndrome results in a singleton fetus.

ETIOLOGY. The occurrence of monovular twins appears to be independent of genetic influences. Polyovular pregnancies are more frequent beyond the second pregnancy, in older women, and in families with a history of polyovular twins. They may result from simultaneous maturation of multiple ovarian follicles, but follicles containing two ova have been described as a genetic trait leading to twin pregnancies. Twin-prone women have higher levels of gonadotropins. Polyovular pregnancies occur in many women treated for infertility with clomiphene, in vitro fertilization, or gonadotropins.

Conjoined twins (Siamese twins) probably result from relatively late monovular separation, as does the presence of two separate embryos in one amniotic sac. The latter condition has a high fatality rate due to obstruction of the circulation secondary to intertwining of the umbilical cords. The prognosis for conjoined twins depends on the possibility of surgical separation.

Superfecundation, the fertilization of an ovum by an insemination that takes place after one ovum has already been fertilized, and *superfetation,* the fertilization and subsequent development of an ovum when a fetus is already present in the uterus, have been proposed as uncommon explanations for differences in size and appearance of certain twins at birth.

The *prenatal diagnoses of twins* is suggested by a uterine size that is greater than that expected for gestational age and elevated maternal serum α-fetoprotein or human chorionic gonadotropin level and is confirmed by ultrasound. Ninety per cent of twins are detected prior to delivery.

MONOZYGOTIC VERSUS DIZYGOTIC TWINS. Identifying twins as monozygotic or dizygotic (monovular or polyovular) is important because studying monozygotic twins is useful in determining the relative influence of heredity and environment on human development and disease. Twins not of the same sex are dizygotic. In twins of the same sex, zygosity should be determined and recorded at birth through careful examination of the placenta or later through comparison of physical characteristics, detailed blood typing, DNA fingerprinting, or tissue typing.

Examination of the Placenta. If the placentas are separate, they are always dichorionic, but the twins are not necessarily

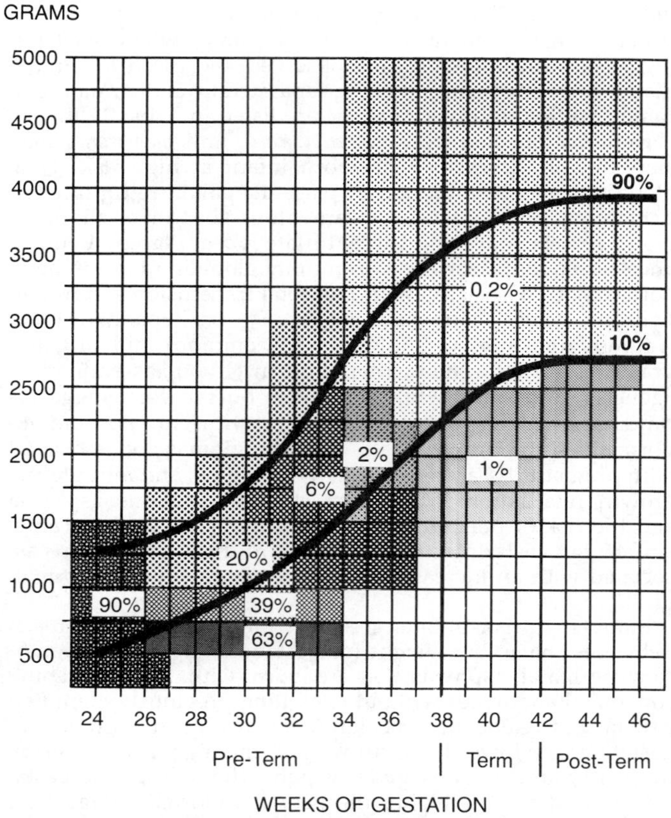

Figure 9–7. Neonatal mortality risk based on actual data from 14,413 live births at the University of Colorado Health Sciences Center from 1974 to 1980. (From Koops B, Morgan L, Battaglia F: J Pediatr 101:969, 1982.)

dizygotic, since initiation of monovular twinning at the first cell division or during the morula state may result in two amnions, two chorions, and even two placentas. One third of monozygotic twins are dichorionic and diamniotic.

An apparently single placenta may be present with either monovular or polyovular twins. Yet inspecting the polyovular placenta usually reveals a separate chorion for each fetus that crosses the placenta between the attachments of the cords and two amnions. Separate or fused dichorionic placentas may be disproportionate in size. The fetus attached to the smaller placenta or portion of placenta is usually smaller than its twin or is malformed. Monochorionic twins may be presumed to be monovular. They are usually diamnionic, and, almost invariably, the placenta is a single mass.

Problems of the twin gestation include polyhydramnios, hyperemesis gravidarum, pre-eclampsia, prolonged rupture of membranes, vasa previa, velamentous insertion of the umbilical cord, and premature labor. Compared with the first-born twin, the second or B twin is at increased risk for respiratory distress syndrome and asphyxia. Twins are at risk for intrauterine growth retardation, twin-twin transfusion, and congenital anomalies that occur predominantly in monozygotic twins. Anomalies are due to uterine compression deformations from crowding (hip dislocation); vascular communication with embolization (ileal atresia, porencephaly) or without embolization (acardiac twin); and unknown factors that cause twinning (conjoined twins, anencephaly, meningomyelocele).

Placental vascular anastomoses occur with high frequency only in monochorionic twins. In monochorionic placentas, the fetal vasculature is usually joined, sometimes in a very complex manner. The vascular anastomoses in monochorionic placentas may be artery-to-artery, vein-to-vein, or artery-to-vein. They are usually well enough balanced so that neither twin suffers. Artery-to-artery communications cross over placental veins, and when anastomoses are present, blood can readily be stroked from one fetal vascular bed to the other. Vein-to-vein communications are similarly recognized and are less common. A combination of artery-to-artery and vein-to-vein anastomoses is associated with *acardiac fetus*. In rare cases one umbilical cord may arise from the other after leaving the placenta. In such cases the twin attached to the secondary cord is usually malformed or dies in utero. Table 9–15 lists the more frequent changes associated with a large uncompensated arteriovenous shunt from the placenta of one twin to that of the other; twins of widely discrepant size are usually monochorionic.

In the **fetal transfusion syndrome**, an artery from one twin delivers blood that is drained into the vein of the other. The latter becomes plethoric and large while the former is anemic and small. By definition, there is a 5 g/dL hemoglobin and 20% body weight difference in this syndrome. Maternal hydramnios in a twin pregnancy suggests the fetal transfusion syndrome. Anticipating this possibility by preparing to transfuse the donor twin or to bleed the recipient twin may be lifesaving. Death of the donor twin in utero may result in generalized fibrin thrombi in the smaller arterioles of the recipient twin, possibly as the result of transfusion of thromboplastin-rich blood from the macerating donor fetus. The surviving twin may develop disseminated intravascular coagulation.

Postnatal Identification. *Physical criteria* for determining monovular twins are as follows: (1) Both must be of the same sex; (2) their features, including ears and teeth, must be obviously alike (but they need not resemble one another more than the lateral halves of one individual); (3) their hair must be identical in color, texture, natural curl, and distribution; (4) their eyes must be of the same color and shade; (5) their skin must be of the same texture and color (nevi may be differently apportioned and distributed); (6) their hands and feet must be of the same conformation and of similar size; and (7) their anthropometric values must show close agreement.

PROGNOSIS. Most twins are born prematurely, and maternal complications of pregnancy are more common than with single pregnancies. Although there is a significant increase in perinatal mortality among monochorionic twins, there is no significant difference between the neonatal mortality rates of twin and single births in comparable weight groups. Yet, since most twins are premature by weight, their overall mortality is higher than that of single births. The perinatal mortality of twins is about 4 times that of singletons. Monoamniotic twins have an increased likelihood of entangling their cords, which may lead to asphyxia. If one of the fetuses is macerated, the live twin is usually delivered first. Theoretically, the second twin is more subject to anoxia than the first because the placenta may separate after the birth of the first twin and before the birth of the second. In addition, the delivery of the second twin may be difficult because it may be in an abnormal presentation (breech, entangled), uterine tone may be decreased, or the cervix may begin to close following the first twin's birth. A growth-retarded twin is at high risk for hypoglycemia. Notable differences in size at birth of monovular twins usually disappear by the time the infants are 6 mo of age. The mortality for multiple gestations with 4–5 fetuses is excessively high for each fetus. Because of this poor prognosis, selective fetal reduction to 2–3 fetuses has been proposed. For ethical reasons this procedure remains controversial.

TREATMENT. Prenatal diagnosis enables the obstetrician and the pediatrician to anticipate the birth of infants who are at high risk because of twinning. Close observation is indicated during labor and in the immediate neonatal period so that prompt treatment of asphyxia or fetal transfusion syndrome can be initiated. The decision to perform an immediate blood transfusion in a severely anemic "donor twin" or to perform a partial exchange transfusion of a "recipient twin" must be based on clinical judgment.

Rausen AR, Seki M, Strauss L: Twin transfusion syndrome: A review of 19 cases studied at our institution. J Pediatr 66:613, 1973.

Soma H, Yoshida K, Tada M, et al: Fetal abnormalities associated with twin placentation. Teratology 12:211, 1975.

Wenstrom K, Gall S: Incidence, morbidity, and mortality and diagnoses of twin gestations. Clin Perinatol 15:1, 1988.

9.17 PREMATURITY AND INTRAUTERINE GROWTH RETARDATION

DEFINITIONS. Liveborn* infants delivered before 37 wk from the first day of the last menstrual period are termed *premature* by the World Health Organization. "Premature" is also often used to denote immaturity. More recently, infants of extremely low birthweight, i.e., less than 750 g, have been referred to as immature neonates. Historically, prematurity was defined by a birthweight of 2,500 g or less, but today infants who weigh 2,500 g or less at birth, "low-birthweight (LBW) infants," are considered to be premature with a shortened gestational period, to be intrauterine growth retarded for their gestational age (also referred to as small for gesta-

*Live birth is defined by the World Health Assembly (1950) as "the complete expulsion or extraction from its mother of a product of conception . . . which, after such separation, breathes or shows any other evidence of life such as beating of the heart, pulsation of the umbilical cord, or definite movement of the voluntary muscles, whether or not the umbilical cord has been cut or the placenta is attached." This definition is approved by the American Public Health Association.

TABLE 9–15. Characteristic Changes in Monochorionic Twins With Uncompensated Placental Arteriovenous Shunts

Twin on Arterial Side—Donor	Twin on Venous Side—Recipient
Oligohydramnios	Polyhydramnios
Small premature	Large premature
Malnourished	Well nourished
Pale	Plethoric
Anemic	Polycythemic
Hypovolemia	Hypervolemic
Hypoglycemia	Cardiac failure
Microcardia	Cardiac hypertrophy
Glomeruli small or normal	Glomeruli large
Arterioles thin-walled	Arterioles thick-walled

tional age [SGA]), or both. Prematurity and *intrauterine growth retardation* (IUGR) are associated with increased neonatal morbidity and mortality. Ideally, the definitions of low birthweight for individual populations should be based on data that are as genetically and environmentally homogeneous as possible. Figure 9–7 presents variations in neonatal mortality based on birthweight with respect to gestational age.

INCIDENCE. During 1985, 6.7% of live births in the United States weighed less than 2,500 g; the rate for blacks (12.4%) was more than twice that for whites (5.6%). The LBW rate has declined only 14% since 1970 compared with a 50% decline in the infant mortality rate. Approximately 30% of LBW infants in the United States have IUGR and are born after 37 wk. At LBW rates greater than 10%, the contribution of IUGR increases and that of prematurity decreases. In developing countries approximately 70% of LBW infants are IUGR. Infants with IUGR have a greater morbidity and mortality than appropriately grown gestational age–matched infants.

THE VERY LOW BIRTHWEIGHT (VLBW) INFANT. VLBW infants weigh less than 1,500 g and are predominantly premature. In the United States in 1985 the VLBW rate was 1.1%: 2.6% among blacks and 0.9% among whites. The VLBW rate is an accurate predictor of the infant mortality rate. VLBW infants account for about 50% of neonatal deaths; their survival is directly related to birthweight, with approximately 20% of those between 500 and 600 g surviving and 85–90% of those between 1,250 and 1,500 g. In the decade of the 80s, the VLBW rate declined minimally in whites and increased in blacks. Perinatal care has improved the rate of survival of LBW infants without yielding a significant overall increase in the rate of serious handicapping conditions. However, compared with term infants, VLBW neonates have a higher incidence of rehospitalization during the 1st yr of life for sequelae of prematurity, infections, and psychosocial disorders (see later discussion in this section on prognosis).

FACTORS RELATED TO PREMATURE BIRTH AND LOW BIRTHWEIGHT. It is difficult to separate completely factors associated with prematurity from those associated with IUGR. (See also Sec. 9.7, 9.11, and 9.12.) A strong positive correlation exists between both premature birth and IUGR and low socioeconomic status. In families of low socioeconomic status there are relatively high incidences of maternal undernutrition, anemia, and illness; inadequate prenatal care; drug addiction; obstetric complications; and maternal histories of reproductive inefficiency (relative infertility, abortions, stillbirths, premature or low birthweight infants). Other associated factors such as single parent families, teenage pregnancies, close spacing of pregnancies, and mothers who have borne more than 4 previous children are also encountered more frequently. Systematic differences in fetal growth have also been described in association with maternal size, birth order, sibling weight, social class, maternal smoking habit, and other factors. The degree to which the variance in birthweights among various populations is due to environmental (extrafetal) rather than to genetic differences in growth potential is difficult to determine.

The *premature birth* of infants whose LBW is appropriate for their preterm gestational age is generally associated with medical conditions in which there is inability of the uterus to retain the fetus, interference with the course of the pregnancy, premature separation of the placenta, or a stimulus to effective uterine contractions prior to term (Table 9–16). *IUGR* is associated with medical conditions that interfere with the circulation and efficiency of the placenta, with the development or growth of the fetus, or with the general health and nutrition of the mother (Table 9–17). Many factors are common to both prematurely born and low-birthweight infants with IUGR.

TABLE 9–16. Identifiable Causes of Preterm Birth

Fetal
- Fetal distress
- Multiple gestation
- Erythroblastosis
- Nonimmune hydrops

Placental
- Placenta previa
- Abruptio placentae

Uterine
- Bicornate uterus
- Incompetent cervix (premature dilation)

Maternal
- Pre-eclampsia
- Chronic medical illness (e.g., cyanotic heart disease, renal disease)
- Infection (e.g., *Listeria monocytogenes*, group B streptococcus, urinary tract infection, chorioamnionitis)
- Drug abuse (e.g., cocaine)

Other
- Premature rupture of membranes
- Polyhydramnios
- Iatrogenic

TABLE 9–17. Factors Often Associated With Intrauterine Growth Retardation

Fetal
- Chromosomal disorders (e.g., autosomal trisomies)
- Chronic fetal infections (e.g., cytomegalic inclusion disease, congenital rubella, syphilis)
- Congenital anomalies
- Radiation injury
- Multiple gestation
- Pancreatic aplasia

Placental
- Decreased placental weight or cellularity or both
- Decreased in surface area
- Villous placentitis (bacterial, viral, parasitic)
- Infarction
- Tumor (chorioangioma, hydatidiform mole)
- Placental separation
- Twin transfusion syndrome (parabiotic syndrome)

Maternal
- Toxemia
- Hypertensive or renal disease or both
- Hypoxemia (high altitude, cyanotic cardiac or pulmonary disease)
- Malnutrition or chronic illness
- Sickle cell anemia
- Drugs (narcotics, alcohol, cigarettes, antimetabolites)

ASSESSMENT OF GESTATIONAL AGE AT BIRTH. Compared with the premature infant of appropriate weight, the infant with retarded intrauterine growth has a reduced birthweight and may appear to have a *disproportionately larger head relative to body size;* infants in both groups lack subcutaneous fat. In some infants (e.g., those with nonbacterial infections or chromosomal anomalies), birthweight and brain growth are severely affected; this is referred to as symmetric growth retardation. In general, neurologic maturity (e.g., nerve conduction velocity) correlates with gestational age despite reduced fetal weight.

Physical signs may be useful in estimating gestational age at birth. Commonly used, the Dubowitz scoring system is accurate to ±2 wk (Figs. 9–8, 9–9, and 9–10). An infant should be presumed to be at high risk of mortality or morbidity if a discrepancy exists between the estimation of gestational age by physical examination, the mother's estimated date of last menstrual period, and fetal ultrasonic evaluation.

SPECTRUM OF DISEASE IN LOW-BIRTHWEIGHT INFANTS. Immaturity tends to increase the severity but reduce the distinctiveness of the clinical manifestations of most neonatal diseases. The principal causes of death among LBW infants are hyaline membrane disease (respiratory distress syndrome), intraventricular hemorrhage, septicemia, asphyxia, birth injuries (principally cerebral), and malformations; prematurity itself should not be considered a cause of death in an infant born alive. The major causes of death at term are asphyxia, infection, anomalies, and aspiration pneumonia (see Table 9–1).

	SCORE				
	0	1	2	3	4
EXTERNAL SIGN					
Edema	Obvious edema of hands and feet; pitting over tibia	No obvious edema of hands and feet; pitting over tibia	No edema		
Skin texture	Very thin, gelatinous	Thin and smooth	Smooth; medium thickness; rash or superficial peeling	Slight thickening; superficial cracking and peeling, especially on hands and feet	Thick and parchmentlike; superficial or deep cracking
Skin color (infant not crying)	Dark red	Uniformly pink	Pale pink; variable over body	Pale; only pink over ears, lips, palms, or soles	
Skin opacity (trunk)	Numerous veins and venules clearly seen, especially over abdomen	Veins and tributaries seen	A few large vessels clearly seen over abdomen	A few large vessels seen indistinctly over abdomen	No blood vessels seen
Lanugo (over back)	No lanugo	Abundant; long and thick over whole back	Hair thinning, especially over lower back	Small amount of lanugo and bald areas	At least half of back devoid of lanugo
Plantar creases	No skin creases	Faint red marks over anterior half of sole	Definite red marks over more than anterior half; indentations over less than anterior third	Indentations over more than anterior third	Definite deep indentations over more than anterior third
Nipple formation	Nipple barely visible; no areola	Nipple well defined; areola smooth and flat; diameter <0.75 cm	Areola stippled, edge not raised; diameter <0.75 cm	Areola stippled, edge raised; diameter >0.75 cm	
Breast size	No breast tissue palpable	Breast tissue on one or both sides <0.5 cm diameter	Breast tissue both sides; one or both 0.5 to 1.0 cm	Breast tissue both sides; one or both >1 cm	
Ear form	Pinna flat and shapeless, little or no incurving of edge	Incurving of part of edge of pinna	Partial incurving whole of upper pinna	Well-defined incurving whole of upper pinna	
Ear firmness	Pinna soft, easily folded, no recoil	Pinna soft, easily folded, slow recoil	Cartilage to edge of pinna, but soft in places, ready recoil	Pinna firm, cartilage to edge; instant recoil	
Genitalia Male	Neither testis in scrotum	At least one testis high in scrotum	At least one testis down in scrotum		
Female (with hips half abducted)	Labia majora widely separated; labia minora protruding	Labia majora almost cover labia minora	Labia majora completely cover labia minora		

Figure 9–8. External characteristics of the Dubowitz examination. Physical criteria are recorded and a final score is obtained following the addition of each category's score. (From Dubowitz L, Dubowitz V: Gestational Age of the Newborn. Reading, MA, Addison-Wesley, 1977.)

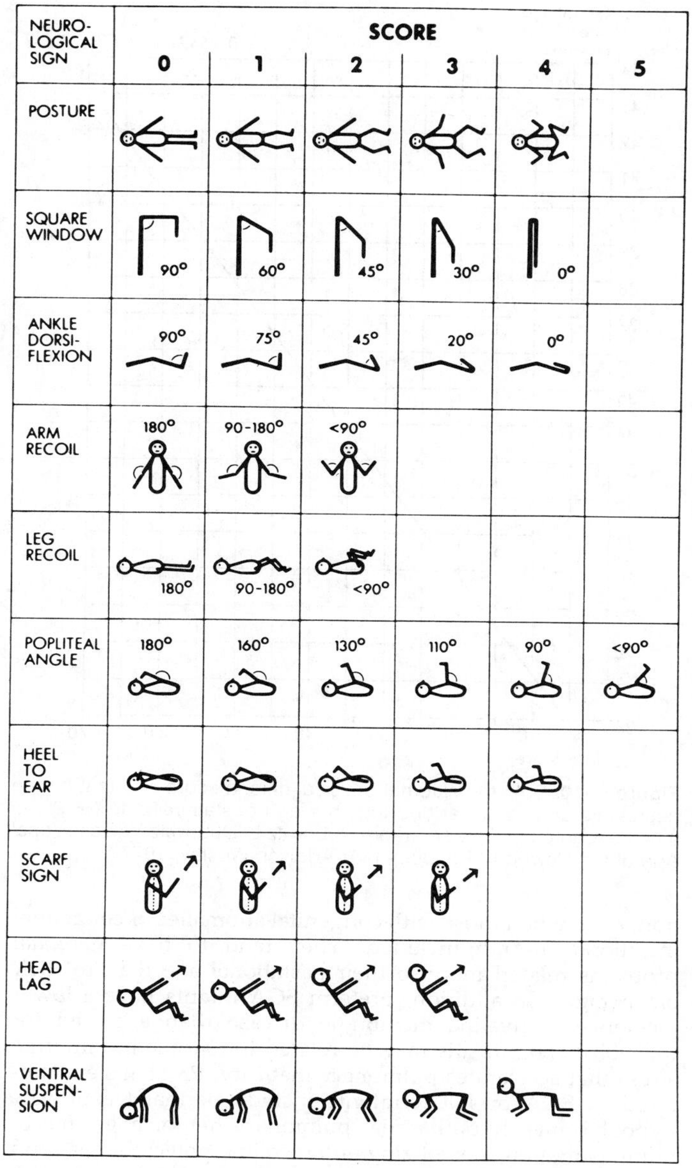

Figure 9–9. Neurologic characteristics of the Dubowitz examination. Neurologic criteria are recorded and added to a final score as performed for the physical assessment. (From Dubowitz L, Dubowitz V: Gestational Age of the Newborn. Reading, MA, Addison-Wesley, 1977.)

Although there is substantial overlap, the incidence of certain neonatal risks varies with birthweight, gestational age, and birthweight for gestational age. Problems of major clinical significance associated with *premature birth* include respiratory distress (hyaline membrane disease, pulmonary hemorrhage, aspiration syndrome, congenital pneumonia, pneumothorax, bronchopulmonary dysplasia), recurrent apnea, hypoglycemia, hypocalcemia, hyperbilirubinemia, anemia, edema, dehydration, cerebral anoxia, circulatory instability, hypothermia, bacterial sepsis, necrotizing enterocolitis, and disseminated intravascular coagulopathy. In addition, preterm infants frequently have weak or uncoordinated ability to feed, prolonged failure to gain weight, and late metabolic acidosis.

Infants *with IUGR (SGA)* are a very heterogeneous popula-

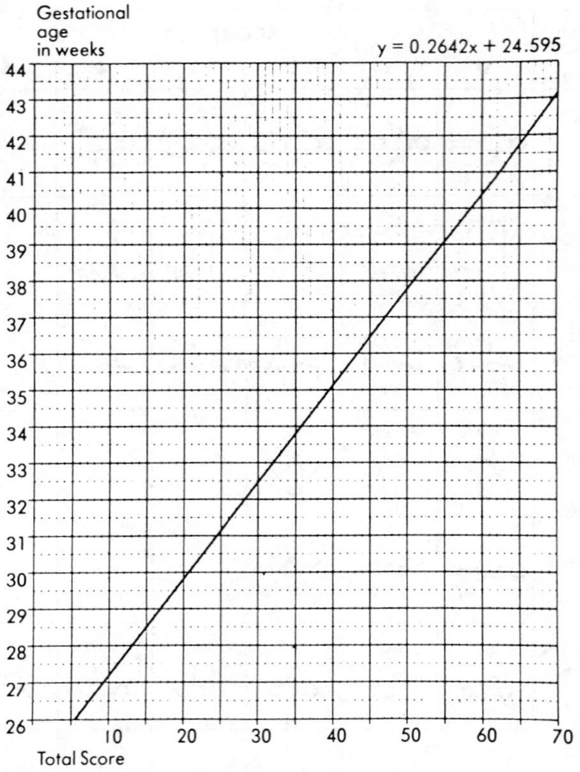

Figure 9–10. Both the external physical criteria score and that for the neurologic criteria are added together and gestational age (± 2 wk) may be read off this graph. (From Dubowitz L, Dubowitz V: Gestational Age of the Newborn. Reading, MA, Addison-Wesley, 1977.)

tion, even when those with congenital anomalies or congenital infections are not included. They tend to have neonatal problems related more to their gestational age than to their birthweight. In addition, preterm SGA infants have a lower incidence of hyaline membrane disease than expected for their birthweight; this may be related to chronic intrauterine stress that accelerates pulmonary maturity. Problems encountered in SGA or IUGR infants include perinatal asphyxia, hypoglycemia, hypothermia, pulmonary hemorrhage, meconium aspiration, necrotizing enterocolitis, polycythemia, and illnesses related to congenital anomalies, syndromes, or infections. The prognosis for these infants depends on the etiology of their growth retardation and on the acute management of these potentially lethal neonatal problems. Head circumference less than the 10th percentile at birth and abnormal neurologic examination in the newborn period are associated with poor growth, later microcephaly, and neurologic deficit.

Hemorrhage (Sec 9.22, 9.23, 9.49, and 16.62), whether associated with trauma, asphyxia, infection, or defect of clotting mechanism, is frequent and often severe in low-birthweight infants. Subcutaneous ecchymoses and subependymal and intraventricular hemorrhage are frequent. Increased capillary fragility, vulnerable arterial and venous capillary networks in friable periventricular germinal tissue, hypernatremia, and increased vascular pressures may be contributing causes. Sudden shock and collapse during the first few days of life are often due to massive **intraventricular hemorrhage** (Sec. 9.22 and 9.23), which occurs predominantly in very small premature infants. It is uncommon in infants who weigh more than 2,000 g at birth or are of more than 34 wk gestational age. Less severe degrees of intraventricular hemorrhage may be associated with lethargy, seizures, apnea, and an acute decline of the hematocrit. Small intraventricular or subependymal hemorrhage may go undetected. Pulmonary hemorrhage has a similar pattern of increased incidence and high mortality in preterm infants, especially those who are SGA.

Hyaline membrane disease (respiratory distress syndrome) occurs most frequently, and mortality is highest, in infants of shortest gestation, and the incidence and mortality fall progressively with increasing gestational age. It is rare in mature infants born at or near term, except in those delivered by cesarean section or born to diabetic mothers (Sec. 9.32).

Congenital malformations (Sec. 7.32) occur with a greater frequency in infants of low birthweight than in all live births. There is a higher malformation rate both in preterm infants and in full-term SGA infants; those with the slowest intrauterine growth rates have the highest incidence of malformations. Breech presentation is common. The incidence of ventricular septal defect is much higher in infants of birthweight less than 2,500 g and gestational age less than 34 wk than among larger or older infants. Infants with chromosome anomalies (e.g., 21-trisomy, 18-trisomy) and those with congenital rubella infection have a high incidence of congenital heart disease and tend to be SGA. Infants with meconium ileus, intestinal obstruction, gastroschisis, and omphalocele are often born prematurely, especially if hydramnios is present.

Patent ductus arteriosus in LBW infants is discussed in Sec. 9.32 and 15.39.

Hypoglycemia may occur in 15% of premature and up to 67% of infants with IUGR (Fig. 9–11). Early feeding and intravenous glucose have reduced its incidence to less than 5% (see Sec. 8.59, 9.56, and 9.57.)

Hyperglycemia is a common problem in extremely premature infants receiving excessive intravenous glucose infusions (over 10 mg/kg/min).

Recurrent apnea (Sec. 9.31), the cessation of breathing for more than 20 sec or long enough to produce cyanosis or bradycardia, has a very high incidence in infants under 1,500 g or under 32 wk gestational age (Table 9–18).

Necrotizing enterocolitis (Sec. 9.43) occurs most commonly in infants of LBW. The highest incidence is among babies weighing less than 1,500 g, but it may also occur in term or normal weight infants.

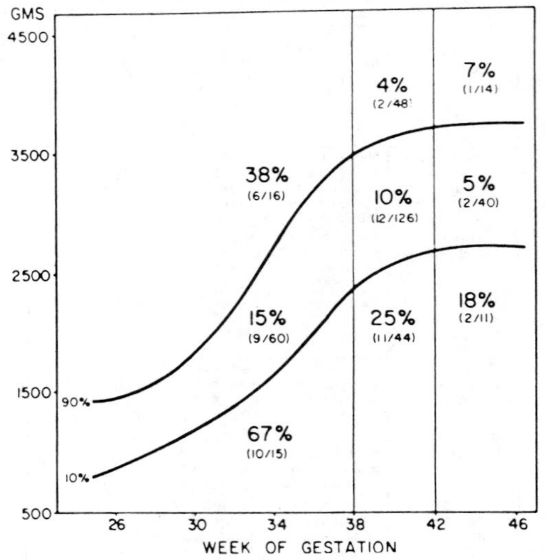

Figure 9–11. Incidence of hypoglycemia by birth weight, gestational age, and intrauterine growth. (From Lubchenco LO [ed]: Incidence of hypoglycemia in newborn infants classified by birth weight and gestational age. Pediatrics 47:832, 1971. Copyright 1971. Reproduced by permission of Pediatrics.)

TABLE 9–18. Potential Causes of Neonatal Apnea and Bradycardia

CNS	IVH, drugs, seizures, hypoxic injury
Respiratory	Pneumonia, obstructive airway lesions, atelectasis, extreme prematurity (< 1,000 g), laryngeal reflex, phrenic nerve paralysis, severe hyaline membrane distress, pneumothorax
Infectious	Sepsis, necrotizing enterocolitis, meningitis (bacterial, fungal, viral)
Gastrointestinal	Oral feeding, bowel movement, gastroesophageal reflux, esophagitis, intestinal perforation
Metabolic	↓ Glucose, ↓ calcium, ↓ Po_2, ↓ ↑ sodium, ↑ ammonia, ↑ organic acids, ↑ ambient temperature, hypothermia
Cardiovascular	Hypotension, hypertension, heart failure, anemia, hypovolemia, vagal tone
Idiopathic	Immaturity of respiratory center, sleep state, upper airway collapse

Retinopathy of prematurity (retrolental fibroplasia) is a disease of the immature, incompletely vascularized retina that occurs in premature infants treated with oxygen at concentrations above ambient air levels (Sec. 22.13). The increased arterial oxygen tensions that result may lead to blindness. The eyes of premature infants exposed to oxygen should be examined at 1 mo of age, after recovery from the illness requiring oxygen therapy, before discharge, and at 3 mo after discharge; cryosurgery has been proposed for severe retinal detachment. The practice of administering oxygen only in the amounts and for the duration of time absolutely necessary for relieving respiratory distress, apnea, hypoxemia, or cyanosis, along with the frequent monitoring of arterial oxygen tensions, has reduced the incidence of this disease and the retinal detachment and scarring that may result from it. The exact level or duration of elevated arterial Po_2 that results in injury is unknown but arterial oxygen tensions should be kept between 55 and 70 mm Hg (7.7–9.8 kPa). Immaturity is an important contributing factor and may rarely be the only identifiable cause. Hypercarbia is another risk factor. Ambient light may also be a factor. The risk of hypoxic brain injury from too little oxygen must be balanced against the risk of blindness from too much oxygen. The prophylactic administration of vitamin E may ameliorate the incidence in some infants; however, its use has also been associated with an increased incidence of sepsis, necrotizing enterocolitis, and other serious systemic toxic effects.

Kernicterus (Sec. 9.44, 9.45) associated with hyperbilirubinemia occurs in 2–20% of autopsies of premature infants. High incidences are probably the result of inappropriate treatment, such as the administration of large amounts of vitamin K analogs to mothers in labor or to newborn infants and the use of sulfisoxazole as chemoprophylaxis. Very low birthweight infants are at increased risk, particularly if they have meningitis; in these immature infants bilirubin levels as low as 10 mg/dL may be dangerous.

Immaturity of anatomic structure or physiologic and biochemical functions is an index of the relative inability of the preterm infant to survive. Deficiencies in these functions affect the infant's ability to withstand demands that do not exist in the protective intrauterine environment, such as control of body heat, pulmonary function, nutrition, disposal of metabolic waste, immunologic function, and detoxification and excretion of toxic substances. The immature infant's respiratory function is limited by the underventilation of perfused alveoli and insufficient surface-active lipid surfactant to prevent collapse of alveoli. Underdeveloped airways and pulmonary tissue and persistence of fluid in the lung result in increased resistance to air flow. The ability to minimize heat loss in response to cold stress is proportional to body size. Decreased stores of hepatic and myocardial glycogen compromise the immature infant's ability to withstand a moderate degree of asphyxia. Renal blood flow, glomerular filtration, and tubular functions are decreased. The cardiopulmonary circulation is transitional between that of a fetus and that of an adult; increased shunting through the ductus arteriosus and foramen ovale may occur in response to stress, hypoxia, or polycythemia and result in circulatory insufficiency or underperfusion of vital organs.

NURSERY CARE. At birth the measures needed for clearing the airway, initiating breathing, caring for the cord and eyes, and administering vitamin K are the same in immature infants as in those of normal weight and maturity (Sec. 9.4). Special care is required to maintain a patent airway and avoid potential aspiration of gastric contents. Additional considerations are (1) need for incubator care and heart rate and respiration monitoring, (2) need for increased oxygen, and (3) need for special attention to the details of feeding. Safeguards against infection can never be relaxed. Everyone involved must be aware that routine procedures that disturb these infants may result in hypoxia. Finally, the need for regular and active participation by the parents in the infant's care in the nursery, the need to instruct the mother in the at-home care of the infant, and the question of prognosis for later growth and development require special consideration. There can be significant untoward effects on the development of a normal mother-infant relationship as a consequence of separation during the neonatal period; these effects may contribute to subsequent behavioral and physical abnormalities, for example, failure to thrive and deprivation syndromes, child neglect, and abuse (Sec. 3.51).

Incubator Care. Modern incubators conserve body heat through provision of a warm atmospheric environment and standard conditions of humidity. They also may provide a regulated oxygen supply and reduced atmospheric contamination if they are scrupulously cleaned. The survival of LBW and sick infants is greater when they are cared for at or near their *neutral thermal environment*. This is a set of thermal conditions, including air and radiating surface temperatures, relative humidity, and air flow, at which heat production (measured as oxygen consumption) is minimal and the infant's core temperature is within the normal range. It is a function of the size and postnatal age of infants; larger, older infants require lower environmental temperatures than smaller, younger infants. The optimal incubator temperature for minimal heat loss and oxygen consumption for the unclothed infant is that which will maintain the infant's core temperature at 36.5–37.0° C. This depends on an infant's size and maturity; the smaller and more immature the infant, the higher the environmental temperature required. A plexiglass heat shield or head caps and body clothing may be required when incubator care alone is insufficient to keep a small premature infant warm.

Maintaining a relative *humidity* of 40–60% aids in stabilizing body temperature by reducing heat loss at lower environmental temperatures; by preventing drying and irritation of the lining of respiratory passages, especially during the administration of oxygen and following or during endotracheal or nasotracheal intubation; and by thinning viscid secretions and reducing insensible water loss from the lungs.

Administering *oxygen* to reduce the risk of injury from hypoxia and circulatory insufficiency must be balanced against the risks of hyperoxia to the eyes (retinopathy of prematurity) and oxygen injury to the lungs. When possible, oxygen should be administered by a head hood, continuous positive airway pressure apparatus, or endotracheal tube to maintain stable and safe inspired oxygen concentration. Although the presence of cyanosis, tachypnea, and apnea are definite clinical indications whose treatment should include only the amount of oxygen needed to eliminate these signs, the potential harm resulting from hypoxia or hyperoxia cannot be minimized without monitoring the oxygen tension (Po_2)of arterial blood and, based on laboratory analysis, continuously readjusting the concentration of oxygen administered. The development of the transcutaneous oxygen electrode and pulse oximetry for routine clinical management of these infants has significantly improved the effectiveness of oxygen monitoring. Capillary blood gases are inadequate for estimating arterial oxygen levels.

If an incubator is not available, the general conditions of temperature and humidity control outlined above can be attained by making intelligent use of radiant warmers, blankets, heating lamps, heating pads, and warm water bottles, and by controlling the temperature and humidity of the room. It may be necessary to administer oxygen temporarily by face mask or through an intubation tube.

The infant should be removed from the incubator only when the gradual change to the atmosphere of the nursery does not result in a significant change in the infant's temperature, color, activity, or vital signs.

Feeding. The method of feeding each LBW infant should be individualized. It is important to avoid fatigue and the aspiration of food by regurgitation or by the feeding process. No feeding method will avoid these problems unless the person feeding the infant has been well trained in the method. Oral feedings (nipple) should not be initiated or should be discontinued in infants with respiratory distress, hypoxia, circulatory insufficiency, excessive secretions, gagging, sepsis, central nervous system depression, immaturity, or signs of serious illness. These infants will require parenteral or gavage feedings to supply calories, fluid, and electrolytes.

Large premature infants can often be fed by bottle or at the breast. Since the effort of sucking is usually the limiting factor, breast-feeding is less likely to succeed until the infant matures. Bottle-feeding of expressed breast milk may be a temporary alternative. In *bottle-feeding,* effort may be reduced by use of special small, soft nipples with large holes. The process of oral alimentation requires, in addition to a strong suck, the coordination of swallowing, epiglottal and uvular closure of the larynx and nasal passages, and normal esophageal motility, a synchronized process that is usually absent prior to 34 wk gestation.

Smaller or less vigorous infants should be fed by *gavage:* A soft plastic tube of No. 5 French external and approximately 0.05 cm internal diameters with a rounded atraumatic tip and two holes on alternate sides is preferable. The tube is passed through the nose until approximately 2.5 cm (1 in) of the lower end is in the stomach. The free end of the tube is then placed under water. If bubbles appear with each expiration, the catheter is in the trachea and must be reinserted into the proper position. The free end of the tube has an adapter into which the tip of a syringe is fitted, and the measured amount of feeding is allowed to flow in slowly by gravity. Such tubes may be left in place for 3–7 days before being replaced by a similar tube through the alternate nostril. Occasionally an infant has enough local irritation from an indwelling tube that he or she may gag or troublesome secretions may gather around it in the nasopharynx. In such cases a catheter may be passed through the mouth by a skilled person and removed at the end of each feeding. Change to bottle- or breast-feeding may be instituted gradually as soon as the infant displays general vigor adequate for oral feeding without fatigue.

Continuous nasogastric and nasojejunal feedings have also been used successfully in LBW infants who are unable to ingest adequate calories by bottle or gavage owing to poor suck, uncoordinated swallowing, and delayed gastric emptying. Intestinal perforation has occurred during nasojejunal feedings.

Gastrostomy feeding is contraindicated in premature infants because of an associated increase in mortality, except as an adjunct to the surgical management of specific gastrointestinal conditions. Partial or total *intravenous alimentation* for premature infants should not be used routinely as a substitute for oral or gavage feedings but only for situations in which the latter are contraindicated by the infant's condition.

Initiation of Feeding. The main principle in the feeding of premature infants is to proceed cautiously and gradually. Careful early feeding of glucose or formula tends to reduce the risk of hypoglycemia, dehydration, and hyperbilirubinemia without the additional risk of aspiration, provided the presence of respiratory distress or other disorders does not present an indication for withholding oral feedings and administering electrolytes, fluids, and calories intravenously.

If the infant is well, is making sucking movements, and is in no distress, oral feeding may be attempted, although most infants weighing less than 1,500 g require tube feeding because they are unable to coordinate breathing, sucking, and swallowing. For infants under 1,000 g, the initial feeding could be 1 mL of either 5% dextrose or 10 cal/oz of premature formula. If this is successful, the next feedings are offered every 2 hr, and the strength of the formula is increased from 10 to 15 to 20 cal/oz. Thereafter, milk volume increments of 1 mL are initiated after 12 successful feedings at the previous volume. The daily milk volume increment should not exceed 20 mL/kg/24 hr. Once a volume of 150 mL/kg/24 hr has been achieved, the caloric content may be increased to 24 or 27 kcal/oz. With high-caloric density, the infant is at risk for dehydration, edema, lactose intolerance, diarrhea, flatus, and delayed gastric emptying with emesis. The feeding protocol for the premature infant weighing over 1,500 g is initiated with increases of milk concentration starting with 4 mL for 3 feeds given every 3 hr until the concentration has increased from 10 to 20 cal/oz. Thereafter, total daily formula volume increments should not exceed 20 mL/kg/24 hr. The expected weight increments for premature infants of various birth-weights are projected from Figure 9–12. Infants with IUGR may not demonstrate the initial weight loss noted in the premature infant.

Regurgitation, vomiting, abdominal distention, or residuals from prior feedings in the early stages of the feeding schedule should arouse suspicion of sepsis, necrotizing entercolitis, or intestinal obstruction; these are indications to drop back in

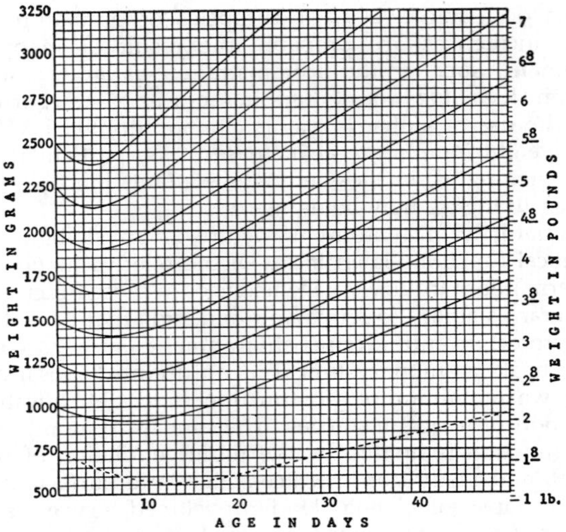

Figure 9–12. Grid for recording weights of premature infants. The average weight increments are indicated on the basis of weight at birth. (From Dancis J, et al: J Pediatr 33:570, 1948.)

the schedule and increase subsequent feedings slowly or to change to intravenous alimentation and to evaluate for more serious problems. Weight gain may not be achieved for 10–12 days, and a daily intake of 130–150 mL/kg or higher may be necessary for some infants. Alternatively, in vigorous infants whose feeding schedule is advanced successfully in calories or volume, weight gain may appear within a few days.

When tube feeding is used, the contents of the stomach should be aspirated before each feeding. If only air or small amounts of mucus are obtained, the feeding is given as planned. If greater than 10% of the previous feeding is obtained, it is advisable to reduce the amount of the feeding and to proceed more gradually with subsequent increases.

The digestive enzyme systems of infants greater than 28 wk gestation are mature enough to permit adequate digestion and absorption of protein and carbohydrate. Fat is less well absorbed owing primarily to inadequate amounts of bile salt; unsaturated fats and the fat of human milk are absorbed better than those of cow's milk. Weight gain of infants weighing under 2,000 g at birth should be adequate when human milk or "humanized" milk (40% casein and 60% whey) with a protein intake of 2.25–2.75 g/kg/24 hr is fed. These two alternatives should provide all amino acids essential for premature infants, including tyrosine, cystine, and histidine. Higher protein intakes may be well tolerated and are generally safe, especially for older, rapidly growing infants. However, protein intakes as high as 4.5 g/kg/24 hr may be hazardous: although linear growth may be promoted, high-protein formulas may cause abnormal plasma aminograms; elevations in blood urea nitrogen, ammonia, and sodium concentrations; metabolic acidosis (cow's milk formulas); and untoward effects on neurologic development. Furthermore, the high protein and mineral contents of balanced cow's milk formulas of high caloric content constitute a large solute load for the kidney, a fact important in maintaining water balance, especially in the infant with diarrhea or fever.

Breast milk may not always be optimal for infants under 1,000 g, since these infants require more calcium, phosphorus, sodium, and protein than is present in pooled, banked breast milk. Premature breast milk obtained from the infant's mother may be more appropriate; specialized premature formulas may also be used.

Although formula in amounts necessary for adequate growth probably contains sufficient amounts of all vitamins, the volume of milk sufficient to satisfy requirements may not be ingested for several weeks. Therefore, LBW infants should be given supplemental vitamins. Since requirements for these infants have not been precisely established, the recommended daily allowances for term infants should be given (see Chapter 4). Furthermore, these infants may have a special need for certain vitamins. Intermediary metabolism of phenylalanine and tyrosine depends, in part, upon vitamin C. Decreased fat absorption with increased fecal fat loss may be associated with decreased absorption of *vitamin D*, other fat-soluble vitamins, and calcium in premature infants. VLBW infants are particularly prone to develop rickets, but their total intake of vitamin D should not exceed 1,500 IU/24 hr. *Folic acid* is essential for the formation of DNA and production of new cells; serum and erythrocyte levels decrease in preterm infants during the first few weeks of life and remain low for 2–3 mo. Therefore, supplementation is recommended, though it does not result in improved growth or increased hemoglobin concentration. Deficiency of vitamin E is associated with increased hemolysis and, if severe, with anemia in premature infants. Vitamin E functions as an antioxidant to prevent peroxidation of polyunsaturated fatty acids in red blood cell membranes; its need may increase because of the increased membrane content of these fatty acids. Vitamin K deficiency is discussed in Sec. 4.33.

In the LBW infant, physiologic anemia due to postnatal suppression of erythropoiesis is exacerbated by smaller fetal iron stores and greater expansion of blood volume resulting from a more rapid growth compared with that of the term infant; therefore, the anemia develops earlier and reaches a lower ultimate level. Fetal or neonatal blood loss accentuates this problem. Iron stores, even in the VLBW neonate, are usually adequate until the infant's birthweight has doubled. In addition, iron supplementation during the period when these infants are at risk for vitamin E deficiency (less than 34 wk postconception age) may enhance hemolysis and reduce vitamin E absorption. Therefore, vitamin E supplementation may be discontinued once the birthweight doubles, at which time iron supplementation (2 mg/kg/24 hr) should be started.

The properly fed premature infant may have from 1–6 daily stools of semisolid consistency; a sudden increase in their number, the appearance of occult or gross blood, or a change to a watery consistency is more reason for concern than any arbitrarily stated frequency.

The premature infant should not vomit or regurgitate. He or she should be satisfied and relaxed after a feeding but may normally show the activity of hunger shortly before the next one.

FLUID REQUIREMENTS. These vary according to gestational age, environmental conditions, and disease states. Assuming minimal water losses in stool of infants not receiving oral fluids, their water needs are equal to insensible water loss, renal solute excretion, and any unusual ongoing losses. Insensible water loss is indirectly related to gestational age; the very immature preterm infant (<1,000 g) may require as much as 2–3 mL/kg/hr, partly because of thin skin, lack of subcutaneous tissue, and a large exposed surface area. Insensible water loss is increased under radiant warmers, during phototherapy, and in the febrile infant. It is diminished when the infant is clothed, is covered by a plexiglass inner heat shield, breathes humidified air, or approaches term. Larger premature infants (2,000–2,500 g) nursed in an incubator may have an insensible water loss of approximately 0.6–0.7 mL/kg/hr.

Fluids also need to be administered to permit excretion of the urinary solute load, e.g., urea, electrolytes, phosphate. The amount varies with dietary intake and the anabolic or catabolic state of nutrition. High-solute load formulas, high protein intake, and catabolism increase the end products that require urinary excretion and thus increase the requirement for water. Renal solute loads may vary between 7.5 and 30 mOsm/kg. Newborn infants, especially those of very low birthweight, also are less able to concentrate urine, thus their fluid intake required to excrete solutes increases.

Water intake in term infants is usually begun at 60–70 mL/kg on day 1 and increased to 100–120 mL/kg by day 2–3. Smaller, more premature infants may need to be started with 70–100 mL/kg on day 1 and advanced to 150 mL/kg or more by day 3–4. Fluid volumes should be titrated individually, although it is unusual to exceed 150 mL/kg/24 hr. Daily weights, urine output and specific gravity, and serum urea nitrogen with electrolytes should be monitored carefully to detect abnormal states of hydration, since clinical observations and physical examinations are poor indicators of the state of hydration of premature infants. Conditions that increase fluid losses, such as glycosuria, the polyuric phase of acute tubular necrosis, and diarrhea, may place additional strain on kidneys that have not yet developed their maximum capacity to conserve water and electrolytes, the results of which may be severe dehydration. Alternatively, fluid overload may lead to edema, congestive heart failure, and a patent ductus arteriosus.

TOTAL PARENTERAL NUTRITION. When oral feeding is impossible for prolonged periods of time, total intravenous alimentation may provide sufficient fluid, calories, amino acids, electrolytes, and vitamins to sustain growth of LBW infants. This technique has been lifesaving for infants who have had intractable diarrheal syndromes or extensive resection of bowel. Infusions may be administered through an indwelling central vein catheter or through a peripheral vein.

The goal of parenteral alimentation is to deliver enough nonprotein calories to allow the infant to use most of the protein for growth. The infusate should contain synthetic amino acids of 2.5 g/dL and hypertonic glucose in the range of 10–25 g/dL in addition to appropriate quantities of electrolytes, trace minerals, and vitamins. The initial daily infusion should deliver 10–15 g/kg/24 hr of glucose and increase gradually to 25–30 g/kg/24 hr when glucose alone is used to meet the full requirements of 100–120 nonprotein kcal/kg/24 hr. If a peripheral vein is used, it is advisable to keep the glucose concentration below 12.5 g/dL. Intravenous fat emulsions such as Intralipid (1.1–2.2 kcal/mL) may be used to provide calories without an appreciable osmotic load, thereby decreasing the need for infusion of the higher concentrations of glucose by central or peripheral vein and usually preventing the development of essential fatty acid deficiency. Electrolytes, trace minerals, and vitamin additives are included in amounts approximating established intravenous maintenance requirements. The content of each day's infusate should be determined after carefully assessing the infant's clinical and biochemical status. Slow and continuous infusion is advisable. A well-trained pharmacist using a laminar flow hood should mix all solutions.

After a caloric intake of greater than 100 kcal/kg/24 hr is established by total parenteral intravenous nutrition, LBW infants can be expected to gain about 15 g/kg/24 hr, with positive nitrogen balances of 150–200 mg/kg/24 hr, if there are no multiple operative procedures, episodes of sepsis, or other severe stress. This goal usually can be achieved and the catabolic tendency during the 1st wk of life reversed with subsequent weight gains by peripheral vein infusions of 2.5 g/kg/24 hr of an amino acid mixture, 10 g/dL of glucose, and 2–3 g/kg/24 hr of Intralipid.

The complications of intravenous alimentation are related to both the catheter and the metabolism of the infusate. **Sepsis** is the most important problem of central vein infusions and can be minimized only by meticulous catheter care and aseptic preparation of the infusate. *Staphylococcus aureus*, *Staphylococcus epidermidis*, and *Candida albicans* are the common infecting organisms. Treatment includes appropriate antibiotics. If an infection persists, the line must be removed. Thrombosis, extravasation of fluid, and accidental dislodgment of catheters have also occurred. Sepsis is rarely attributable to peripheral vein infusions, but phlebitis, cutaneous sloughs, and superficial infection occasionally occur. The **metabolic complications** include hyperglycemia from the high glucose concentration of the infusate, which may lead to an osmotic diuresis and dehydration; azotemia; hypoglycemia from a sudden accidental cessation of the infusate; hyperlipidemia and possibly hypoxemia from intravenous lipid infusions; and hyperammonemia, which may be due to high levels of certain amino acids. Cholestatic jaundice has also been noted. Hyperchloremic acidosis occurs in infants receiving synthetic amino acids unless there is an appropriate balance between cationic and anionic amino acids and salts. Abnormal elevations of blood amino acid levels are an additional potential hazard. If intravenous fat emulsions are not used, essential fatty acid deficiency may also occur. When the infusion is given through a peripheral vein, the osmolality of the solution may limit the length of time an infusion site can be used while, at the same time, it may require greater volumes of fluid than can be tolerated. Continuous chemical and physiologic monitoring of infants receiving intravenous alimentation is indicated because of the frequency and seriousness of complications.

Intravenous Supplementation of Tolerated Oral Feedings. A combination of intravenous and gavage alimentation is the usual method of feeding preterm infants. Once the infant is stable (2nd–3rd day of life), small nasogastric milk feedings are supplemented with peripheral alimentation solutions. Initiation of enteric feeding is possible in the presence of an endotracheal tube and an umbilical artery catheter. Glucose, amino acid mixtures, and lipid emulsions may be infused into peripheral veins when sufficient calories cannot be provided to LBW infants by oral feeding alone. Some infants weighing less than 1,500 g may regain their birthweight sooner and have fewer apneic episodes with a supplemental infusion containing sources of nitrogen. Increases in weight, length, and head circumference approaching those expected in utero have been achieved with mixtures of amino acids, glucose, and Intralipid. Although the complications of both techniques may occur, the combination of nutrient delivery methods allows smaller volumes of enteral feedings, thus decreasing the risk of aspiration. Provision of enteral calories reduces the incidence of cholestatic jaundice and rickets of prematurity.

PREVENTION OF INFECTION. Premature infants have an increased susceptibility to infection, which requires nursery personnel to wash rigorously hand to elbow before and after handling the infant, take measures to reduce contamination of food and objects coming in contact with the infant, prevent air contamination, avoid overcrowding, and limit direct and indirect contacts with themselves and other infants. No one with an infection should be permitted into the nursery. However, the risks of infection must be balanced against the disadvantages of limiting the infant's contacts with the family, which may be detrimental to the infant's ultimate development; early and frequent participation by parents in the nursery care of their infant does not significantly increase the risk when preventive precautions are maintained. Prophylactic administration of gamma globulin to premature infants may be beneficial in preventing bacterial infections.

Preventing transmission of infection from infant to infant is difficult because often neither term nor premature newborn infants manifest clear clinical evidence of an infection early in its course. When epidemics occur within a nursery, cohort nursing and isolation rooms should be employed in addition to routine antiseptic care.

The most important factor in the successful care of premature infants is the skill, experience, and number of the nursing staff. It is the responsibility of the physician to insist on an optimal amount of expert nursing.

IMMATURITY OF DRUG METABOLISM. Renal clearances for almost all substances excreted in the urine are diminished in newborn infants, but more so in premature ones. Intervals between doses may, therefore, need to be extended when administering drugs excreted chiefly by the kidney. Serum creatinine levels may help determine the appropriate dosage. For instance, highly satisfactory levels of penicillin, gentamicin, and kanamycin are maintained on doses given at 12-hr intervals. Drugs detoxified in the liver or requiring chemical conjugation before renal excretion should also be given with caution and in doses smaller than usual. When possible, blood levels should be obtained for potentially toxic drugs, especially if renal or hepatic dysfunction is present. Decisions about the choice and dose of antibacterial agents and route of administration should be made on an individual basis rather than routinely, owing to the dangers of (1) development of infections with organisms resistant to antibacterial agents, (2) destruction or inhibition of intestinal bacteria that manufacture significant amounts of essential vitamins (e.g., vitamin K and thiamine), and (3) harmful interference in important metabolic processes.

Many drugs apparently safe for adults on the basis of toxicity studies may be harmful to newborn infants, especially premature ones. Oxygen and a number of drugs have proved toxic to premature infants in amounts not harmful to term infants (Table 9–19). Thus, administering any drug, particularly in large doses, without pharmacologic testing in premature infants, should be carefully undertaken after weighing risk against benefit.

PROGNOSIS. There is now a 95% or greater chance of survival for infants born weighing between 1,501 and 2,500 g, but those weighing less still have a significantly higher mortality (Fig. 9–13; see also Fig. 9–7). Intensive care has extended the period during which a VLBW infant is likely to die from complications of perinatal disease, such as bronchopulmonary dysplasia, necrotizing enterocolitis, or secondary infection (Table 9–20). The mortality rate of LBW infants who survive to be discharged from the hospital is higher than that of term infants during the first 2 yr of life. Because many of these deaths are attributable to infection, they are at least theoretically preventable. There is also an increased incidence of failure to thrive, sudden infant death syndrome, child abuse, and inadequate maternal-infant bonding among premature infants. Biologic risks from poor cardiorespiratory regulation due to immaturity or to complications of underlying perinatal disease and social risks associated with poverty also contribute to the high mortality and morbidity of these infants. Congenital anatomic anomalies are present in approximately 3–7% of LBW infants.

In the absence of congenital abnormalities, central nervous system injury, VLBW or marked IUGR, physical growth of LBW infants tends to approximate that of term infants during the 2nd yr; this occurs earlier in premature infants of larger birth size. VLBW infants may not catch up, especially if they have severe chronic illness, insufficient nutritional intake, or an inadequate caretaking environment. Premature birth in itself may prejudice later development. In general, the greater the immaturity and the lower the birthweight, the greater the likelihood of intellectual and neurologic deficit (see Fig. 9–13). Small head circumference at birth may be similarly related to poor neurobehavioral prognosis. The incidence of neurologic and developmental handicap in VLBW infants ranges from 10 to 20%, including cerebral palsy (3–6%), moderate to severe hearing and visual defects (1–4%), and learning difficulties (20%). Mean global IQ is 90–97, and 76% have normal school performance. Many surviving LBW infants have hypotonia prior to 8 mo corrected age, which improves by the time they are 8 mo–1 yr old. This transient hypotonia is not a poor prognostic sign.

Mothers of low socioeconomic status are more apt to have LBW babies who tend to develop less well than do those in better postneonatal environments. Major neurologic defects were found to be uncommon in a prospective study of full-term small-for-dates (IUGR) infants, although compared with appropriate-for-gestation term infants, they had an increased incidence of minimal cerebral dysfunction (hyperactivity, short attention span, learning difficulties), electroencephalographic abnormalities, and speech defects.

DISCHARGE FROM HOSPITAL. Before discharge, a premature infant should be taking all nutrition by nipple, either bottle or breast. Growth should be occurring at steady increments of approximately 10–30 g/day. Temperature should be stabilized in an open crib. There should have been no recent apnea or bradycardia, and parenteral drug administration should have been discontinued. Stable infants recovering from bronchopulmonary dysplasia may be discharged on oxygen given by nasal cannula as long as careful follow-up is arranged with frequent pulse oximetry monitoring and outpatient visits. Infants previously treated with oxygen should have an eye examination to determine the presence, stage, or absence of retinopathy of prematurity, while all LBW infants should have a hearing test, and those who had indwelling umbilical arterial catheters should have their blood pressure measured to check for renal vascular hypertension. A hemoglobin level or hematocrit should be determined to evaluate possible anemia. If all major medical problems have resolved and the home setting is adequate, premature infants may then be discharged when their weight approaches 1,900–2,100 g; close follow-up and easy access to health care providers are essential for early discharge protocols. Alternatively, if the medical or social environment is not ideal, high-risk neonates transported to neonatal intensive care units whose major illness has resolved may be returned to their hospital of birth for an additional period of hospitalization. Standard vaccinations with full doses should commence after discharge.

HOME CARE. While the infant is in the hospital the mother should be instructed in how to care for the baby after discharge. This program should include at least one visit to her home by someone capable of evaluating domestic arrangements and advising about any needed improvements.

TABLE 9–19. Adverse Reactions to Drugs Administered to Premature Infants

Drug	Reaction
Sulfisoxazole	Kernicterus
Chloramphenicol	Gray baby—shock, bone marrow suppression
Vitamin K analogs	Jaundice
Novobiocin	Jaundice
Hexachlorophene	Encephalopathy
Benzyl alcohol	Acidosis, collapse, intraventricular bleeding
Intravenous vitamin E	Ascites, shock
Phenolic detergents	Jaundice
$NaHCO_3$	Intraventricular hemorrhage
Amphotericin	Anuric renal failure
Reserpine	Nasal stuffiness
Indomethacin	Oliguria, hyponatremia
Tetracycline	Enamel hypoplasia
Tolazoline	Hypotension, gastrointestinal bleeding
Calcium salts	Subcutaneous necrosis
Aminoglycosides	Deafness, renal toxicity
Enteric gentamicin	Resistant bacteria
Prostaglandins	Seizures, diarrhea, apnea
Phenobarbital	Altered state, drowsiness
Morphine	Hypotension, urine retention, withdrawal
Pancuronium/vecuronium	Edema, hypovolemia, hypotension, tachycardia
Iodine antiseptics	Hypothyroidism
Fentanyl	Seizures, chest wall rigidity, withdrawal
Dexamethasone	Gastrointestinal bleeding, hypertension, infection, hyperglycemia
Lasix	Deafness, hyponatremia, hypokalemia, hypochloremia, nephrocalcinosis, biliary stones
Heparin	Bleeding, intraventricular hemorrhage, thrombocytopenia

9.18 POST-TERM INFANTS

Post-term infants are those born after 42 wk of gestation, calculated from the mother's last menstrual period, regardless of weight at birth. This designation is often used synonymously with the term "postmature" for infants whose gestation exceeds the normal 280 days by 7 days or more. Approximately 25% of all pregnancies end on or after the 287th day of gestation, 12% on or after the 294th day, and 5% on or after the 301st day. The cause of post-term birth or postmaturity is unknown. Large size of the infant correlates poorly

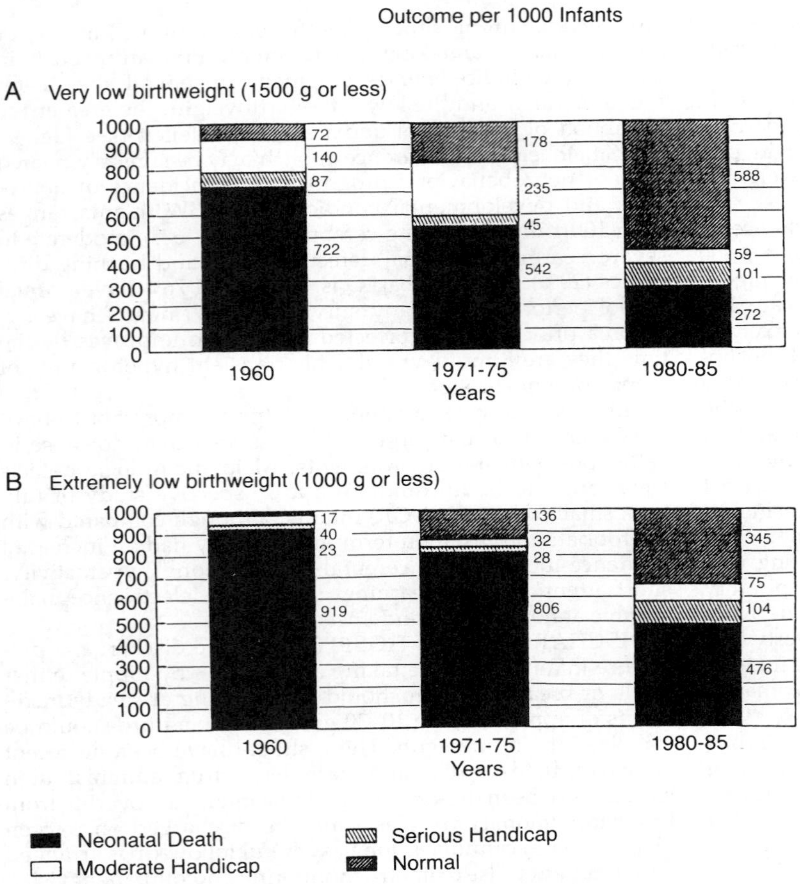

Figure 9–13. *A*, Outcome for VLBW infants born in level III hospitals 1960–1985. *B*, Outcome for extremely low birthweight (ELBW) infants born in level III hospitals 1960–1985. (Adapted from Ehrehaft P, et al. Reprinted with permission from The American College of Obstetricians and Gynecologists [Obstetrics and Gynecology 74:528, 1989].)

with late delivery but does correlate with large size of either parent, multigravidity, or a prediabetic or diabetic state in the mother.

CLINICAL MANIFESTATIONS. Post-term infants may be clinically indistinguishable from term infants, but some have received the designation postmature because their appearance and behavior suggest those of an infant 1–3 wk of age. These post-term, postmature infants are often of increased birthweight and characterized by the absence of lanugo, decreased or absent vernix caseosa, long nails, abundant scalp hair, white parchment-like or desquamating skin, and increased alertness. If *placental insufficiency* occurs, the amniotic fluid and fetus may be meconium stained, and abnormal fetal heart rates may be observed; the infant may have growth retardation. Although this syndrome is frequently confused with postmaturity, *only about 20% of infants with placental insufficiency syndrome are post-term*. The majority of those affected are term and preterm infants, particularly those small for gestational age who are the infants of toxemic mothers, older primigravidas, and women with chronic hypertension. The placentas are often small or poorly attached. This syndrome has been postulated to result from degenerative changes in the placenta that progressively reduce oxygen and nourishment to the fetus.

Those infants born post-term in association with presumed placental insufficiency may have a variety of physical signs: desquamation, long nails, abundant hair, pale skin, alert faces, and loose skin, especially around the thighs and buttocks, giving them the appearance of having recently lost weight; meconium-stained nails, skin, vernix, umbilical cord, and placental membranes (see Fig. 9–2).

PROGNOSIS. When delivery is delayed 3 wk or more beyond term, there is a significant increase in mortality, which in some series has approximated 3 times that of a control group of infants born at term. Mortality has been lowered markedly through improved obstetric management.

TREATMENT. Careful obstetric monitoring, including nonstress testing, biophysical profile, or Doppler velocimetry usually provides a rational basis for choosing a course of nonintervention, induction of labor, or cesarean section. Cesarean section may be indicated in older primigravidas who

TABLE 9–20. Sequelae of Low-Birthweight Infants

Immediate	Late
Hypoxia, ischemia	Mental retardation, spastic diplegia, microcephaly, seizures, poor school performance
Intraventricular hemorrhage	Mental retardation, spasticity, seizures, hydrocephalus
Sensorineural injury	Hearing, visual impairment, retinopathy of prematurity, strabismus, myopia
Respiratory failure	Bronchopulmonary dysplasia, cor pulmonale, bronchospasm, malnutrition, subglottic stenosis, iatrogenic cleft palate, recurrent pneumonia
Necrotizing enterocolitis	Short bowel syndrome, malabsorption, malnutrition, infectious diarrhea
Cholestatic liver disease	Cirrhosis, hepatic failure, carcinoma, malnutrition
Nutrient deficiency	Osteopenia, fractures, anemia, vitamin E, growth failure
Social stress	Child abuse or neglect, failure to thrive, divorce
Other	Sudden infant death syndrome, infections, inguinal hernia, cutaneous scars (chest tube, PDA ligation, IV infiltration), gastroesophageal reflux, hypertension, craniosynostosis, cholelithiasis, urolithiasis, cutaneous hemangiomas

go more than 2–4 wk beyond term, particularly if there is evidence of fetal distress. Meconium aspiration pneumonia or hypoxic encephalopathy are treated symptomatically.

9.19 LARGE FOR GESTATIONAL AGE (LGA)

See also Sec. 9.56.

Neonatal mortality rates decrease with increasing birth weight until approximately 4,000 g, after which mortality increases. These oversized infants are usually born at term, but preterm infants with weights high for gestational age also have a significantly higher mortality than infants of the same size born at term; maternal diabetes and obesity are predisposing factors. Infants who are very large, regardless of their gestational age, have a higher incidence of birth injuries, such as cervical and brachial plexus injuries, phrenic nerve damage with paralysis of the diaphragm, fractured clavicles, cephalhematomas, subdural hematomas, and ecchymoses of the head and face. The incidence of congenital anomalies, particularly congenital heart disease, is also higher than in term infants of normal weight. Intellectual and developmental retardation is statistically more common in high-birthweight term and preterm infants than in babies of appropriate weight for gestational age.

INFANT TRANSPORT

With the advent of regionalized care of high-risk neonates, increasing numbers of sick infants are being transported to neonatal intensive care units in hospitals at which they were not born. Ideally, high-risk mothers should be transported to and delivered at centers where these specialized units are located. Neonatal transport should include consultation about the infant's problem and care before transport, ease of access to the transport team, and transport and stabilization by the team before moving the infant. Securing an airway, providing oxygen, assisting with infant ventilation, providing antimicrobial therapy, maintaining the circulation, providing a warmed environment, and placing intravenous or arterial lines or chest tubes should all be initiated, if indicated, prior to transport. Infant and maternal records, laboratory reports, and a tube of clotted maternal blood should also be provided. Before departing, the mother should be briefly reassured and allowed to see the stabilized infant, if practical; the father should follow the transport vehicle to the unit. The transport officer or nurse should also call ahead to inform the receiving unit about the nature of the patient's illness.

The transport vehicle should be equipped with appropriate medicines, fluids, oxygen tanks, catheters, chest tubes, endotracheal tubes, laryngoscopes, and an infant warming device. It should be well illuminated and have ample room for emergency procedures and monitoring equipment. With efficient transport and appropriately educated nursing and medical staff at the referring hospitals, the mortality of "outborn" neonates should be no higher than that of those born within the tertiary care center.

American Academy of Pediatrics: Hospital Care of Newborn Infants. Evanston IL, The Academy, 1988.

Anderson T, Muttart C, Bieber M, et al: A controlled trial of glucose versus glucose and amino acids in premature infants. J Pediatr 94:947, 1979.

Anonymous: Breast not necessarily the best. Lancet 1:624, 1988.

Bell E, Warburton D, Stonestreet B, et al: Effect of fluid administration on the development of symptomatic patent ductus arteriosus and congestive heart failure in premature infants. N Engl J Med 302:598, 1980.

Committee on Nutrition: Nutritional needs of low-birth-weight infants. Pediatrics 75:977, 1985.

Cross KW, Hey EN, Kennard DL, et al: Lack of temperature control in infants with abnormalities of the CNS. Arch Dis Child 46:437, 1971.

Du JN, Oliver TK Jr: The baby in the delivery room; a suitable microenvironment. JAMA 207:636, 1967.

Dunn L, Hulman S, Weiner J, et al: Beneficial effects of early hypocaloric enteral feeding on neonatal gastrointestinal function: Preliminary report of a randomized trial. J Pediatr 112:622, 1988.

Ehrenhaft PM, Wagner JL, Herdman RC: Changing prognosis for very low birth weight infants. Obstet Gynecol 74:528, 1989.

Ehrenkranz R: Mineral needs of the very low birthweight infant. Semin Perinatol 13:142, 1989.

Gaudy GM, Adamsons K, Cunningham N, et al: Thermal environment and acid base homeostasis in human infants during the first hours of life. J Clin Invest 43:751, 1964.

Gaull GE, Rassin DK, Raiha NCR, et al: Milk protein quantity and quality in low-birth-weight infants. III: Effects on sulfur amino acids in plasma and urine. J Pediatr 90:348, 1977.

Georgieff MK, Weiner S: Nutritional assessment of the neonate. Clin Perinatol 13:73, 1986.

Hack M, Fanaroff A: How small is too small? Considerations in evaluating the outcome of the tiny infant. Clin Perinatol 15:773, 1988.

Heird WC, Hay W, Helms RA, et al: Pediatric parenteral amino acid mixture in low birth weight infants. Pediatrics 81:41, 1988.

Hittner HM, Rudolph AJ, Kretzer FL: Suppression of severe retinopathy of prematurity with vitamin E supplementation. Ophthalmology 91:1512, 1984.

Johnson L, Bowen FW, Abbasi S, et al: Relationship of prolonged pharmacologic serum levels of vitamin E to incidence of sepsis and necrotizing enterocolitis in infants with birth weight 1500 grams or less. Pediatrics 75:619, 1985.

Kashyap S, Schulze KF, Forsyth M, et al: Growth, nutrient retention, and metabolic response in low birth weight infants fed varying intakes of protein and energy. J Pediatr 113:713, 1988.

Kinsey VE, Arnold HJ, Kalina RE, et al: PaO_2 levels and retrolental fibroplasia: A report of the cooperative study. Pediatrics 60:655, 1977.

Kliegman R, King K: Intrauterine growth retardation: Determinants of aberrant fetal growth. *In:* Fanaroff AA, Martin RJ (eds): Behrman's Neonatal Perinatal Medicine. St Louis, CV Mosby, 1987.

Lebenthal E, Leung Y: Feeding the premature and compromised infant: Gastrointestinal considerations. Pediatr Clin North Am 35:215, 1988.

Philips JB, Dickman HM, Resnick MB, et al: Characteristics, mortality and outcome of higher-birth weight infants who require intensive care. Am J Obstet Gynecol 149:875, 1984.

Roy R, Sinclair J: Hydration of the low birth weight infant. Clin Perinatol 2:393, 1975.

Saigal S, Rosenbaum P, Hattersley B, et al: Decreased disability rate among 3-year-old survivors weighing 501 to 1000 grams at birth and born to residents of a geographically defined region from 1981 to 1984 compared with 1977 to 1980. J Pediatr 114:839, 1989.

Sauer P, Visser M: The neutral temperature of very low birth weight infants. Pediatrics 74:788, 1984.

Schanler R: Human milk for preterm infants: Nutritional and immune factors. Semin Perinatol 13:69, 1989.

Shapiro S, McCormick MC, Starfield BH, et al: Relevance of correlates of infant deaths for significant morbidity at 1 year of age. Am J Obstet Gynecol 136:363, 1980.

Shapiro S, McCormick MC, Starfield BH, et al: Changes in morbidity associated with decreases in neonatal mortality. Pediatrics 72:408, 1983.

The Prevention of Low Birthweight. Report of the Committee to Study the Prevention of Low Birthweight. Division of Health Promotion and Disease Prevention. Institute of Medicine. Washington, DC, National Academy of Sciences, National Academy Press, 1985.

Tiffany FM, Dabiri CM, Hallock N, et al: Developmental effects of prolonged pregnancy and postmaturity syndrome. J Pediatr 90:836, 1977.

DISEASES OF THE NEWBORN INFANT: PREMATURE AND FULL-TERM

The infant's physician should appreciate the wide variety of disorders that may originate in utero, during birth, or in the immediate postnatal period, and the need to distinguish them according to their time of onset, etiology, and place of origin. The disorders may represent genetic mutations, chromosomal aberrations, or acquired diseases and injuries.

9.20 CLINICAL MANIFESTATIONS OF DISEASE DURING THE NEONATAL PERIOD

Recognizing disease in the newborn infant depends on knowledge about the disorder and evaluation of a limited number of relatively nonspecific clinical signs and symptoms.

Central cyanosis usually indicates respiratory insufficiency, which may be due to pulmonary conditions or may be secondary to central nervous system depression due to drugs, intracranial hemorrhage, or anoxia (Table 9–21). If it is caused by the former, respirations tend to be rapid and may be accompanied by retraction of the thoracic cage. If it is due to the latter, respirations tend to be irregular and weak and are often slow. Cyanosis persisting for several days, unaccompanied by obvious signs of respiratory difficulty, suggests cyanotic congenital heart disease or methemoglobinemia. Cyanosis resulting from congenital heart disease may, however, be difficult to distinguish clinically from cyanosis caused by respiratory disease. Episodes of cyanosis also may be the presenting sign of hypoglycemia, bacteremia, meningitis, shock, or persistent fetal circulation. Peripheral acrocyanosis is common and usually does not warrant concern.

Pallor, in addition to anemia or acute hemorrhage, should suggest hypoxia, hypoglycemia, sepsis, shock, or adrenal failure.

Convulsions (Sec. 20.17) usually point to a disorder of the central nervous system and suggest hypoxic-ischemic encephalopathy resulting from asphyxia, intracranial hemorrhage, cerebral anomaly, subdural effusion, meningitis, hypocalcemia, hypoglycemia, infarction, and rarely, pyridoxine dependency, hyponatremia, hypernatremia, inborn errors of metabolism, drug withdrawal, or familial seizures. Seizures beginning in the delivery room or shortly thereafter may be due to unintentional injection of maternal local anesthetic into the fetus. Convulsions may also result from administration of large amounts of hypotonic fluids to the mother shortly before and during delivery, leading to subsequent hyponatremia and water intoxication in the infant.

Convulsions (epileptic seizures) should be distinguished from the jitteriness that may be present in normal newborns, in infants of diabetic mothers, in those who experienced birth asphyxia or drug withdrawal, and in polycythemic neonates. Jitteriness resembling simple tremors may be stopped by holding the infant's extremity; it often depends on sensory stimuli and is not associated with abnormal eye movements. Seizures in premature infants are often subtle and associated with abnormal eye or facial movements; the motor component is often that of tonic extension of the limbs, neck, and trunk. Term infants may have focal or multifocal, clonic or myoclonic movements but may also manifest more subtle seizure activity. *Apnea* may be the first manifestation of seizure activity, particularly in a premature infant.

Following severe birth asphyxia infants may have *motor automatisms* characterized by oral-buccal-lingual movements, rotary limb activities (rowing, pedaling, swimming), tonic posturing, or myoclonus. These motor seizures are not usually accompanied by time-synchronized electroencephographic (EEG) discharges, may not signify cortical epileptic activity, respond poorly to anticonvulsant therapy, and are associated with a poor prognosis. Such automatisms may represent cortical depression that produces a brain stem release phenomenon or subcortical seizures.

Lethargy may be a manifestation of infection, asphyxia, hypoglycemia, sedation from maternal analgesia or anesthesia, cerebral defect, and, indeed, of almost any severe disease including inborn errors of metabolism. Lethargy appearing after the 2nd day should, in particular, suggest infection.

TABLE 9–21. Differential Diagnosis of Neonatal Cyanosis

System/Disease	Mechanism
Pulmonary	
Respiratory distress syndrome	Surfactant deficiency
Sepsis, pneumonia	Inflammation, pulmonary hypertension
Meconium aspiration pneumonia	Mechanical obstruction, inflammation, pulmonary hypertension
Persistent fetal circulation	Pulmonary hypertension
Diaphragmatic hernia	Pulmonary hypoplasia, pulmonary hypertension
Transient tachypnea	Retained lung fluid
Cardiovascular	
Cyanotic heart disease with decreased pulmonary blood flow	Right to left shunt as in pulmonary atresia, tetralogy of Fallot
Cyanotic heart disease with increased pulmonary blood flow	Right to left shunt as in d-transposition, truncus arteriosus
Cyanotic heart disease with congestive heart failure	Right to left shunt with pulmonary edema and poor cardiac output as in hypoplastic left heart and coarctation of aorta
Heart failure alone	Pulmonary edema and poor cardiac contractility as in sepsis, myocarditis, supraventricular tachycardia, or complete heart block. High-output failure as in patent ductus arteriosus or vein of Galen or other arteriovenous malformation
Central Nervous System	
Maternal sedative drugs	Hypoventilation, apnea
Asphyxia	CNS depression
Intracranial hemorrhage	CNS depression, seizure
Neuromuscular disease	Phrenic nerve palsy; hypotonia, hypoventilation, pulmonary hypoplasia
Hematologic	
Acute blood loss	Shock
Chronic blood loss	Congestive heart failure
Polycythemia	Pulmonary hypertension
Methemoglobinemia	Low affinity hemoglobin or red blood cell enzyme defect
Metabolic	
Hypoglycemia	CNS depression, congestive heart failure
Adrenogenital syndrome	Shock (salt-losing)

Irritability may be a sign of discomfort accompanying intraabdominal conditions, meningeal irritation, drug withdrawal, infections, congenital glaucoma, or any condition producing pain. As in later infancy, the eardrums should always be examined as a possible source of pain.

Hyperactivity, especially of the premature infant, may be a sign of hypoxia, pneumothorax, emphysema, hypoglycemia, hypocalcemia, central nervous system damage, drug withdrawal, thyrotoxicosis, or discomfort due to a cold environment.

Failure to feed well is seen in most sick newborn infants and should always occasion a careful search for infection, central or peripheral nervous system disorder, and other abnormal conditions.

Fever may be the result of too high an environmental temperature due to weather, overheated nurseries or incubators, or too many clothes or bedclothes. It is also seen in "dehydration fever" of newborn infants. If these causes of fever can be eliminated, then serious infection (pneumonia, bacteremia, viremia, meningitis) must be considered, although such infections often occur without provoking a febrile response in newborn infants (see Sec. 9.60). An unexplained *fall in body temperature* may accompany infection or other serious disturbances of the circulation or central nervous system. A sudden servo-controlled increase in incubator temperature to maintain body temperature is often associated with sepsis.

Periods of *apnea*, particularly in the premature infant, may be associated with a variety of disturbances (see Table 9–19). When apneas recur or when the intervals are longer than 20 sec or are associated with cyanosis or bradycardia, they warrant an immediate diagnostic evaluation.

Jaundice during the first 24 hr of life should be considered to be due to erythroblastosis fetalis until proved otherwise. Septicemia (especially in the low-birthweight infant), cytomegalic inclusion disease, the congenital rubella syndrome, and toxoplasmosis should also be considered, especially if there is an increase in plasma direct-reacting bilirubin.

Jaundice after the first 24 hr may be "physiologic" or may be due to septicemia, hemolytic anemia, galactosemia, hepatitis, congenital atresia of the bile ducts, inspissated bile syndrome following erythroblastosis fetalis, syphilis, herpes simplex, or congenital infections (see Sec. 9.44–9.45).

Vomiting during the 1st day of life suggests obstruction in the upper digestive tract or increased intracranial pressure. Roentgenographic studies are indicated when obstruction is suspected. Vomiting also may be a nonspecific symptom of an illness such as septicemia. It is a common manifestation of overfeeding or inexperienced feeding technique, pyloric stenosis, milk allergy, duodenal ulcer, stress ulcer, or adrenal insufficiency. Infants placed in body casts for orthopedic treatment often vomit transiently. Vomitus containing dark blood is usually a sign of life-threatening illness; the benign possibility of swallowed maternal blood should also be considered. Bile-stained vomitus strongly suggests obstruction below the ampulla of Vater.

Diarrhea may be a symptom of overfeeding (especially high–caloric density formula), acute gastroenteritis, malabsorption, or a nonspecific symptom of infection. It may be seen in conditions accompanied by compromised circulation of part of the intestinal or genital tract, such as mesenteric thrombosis, necrotizing enterocolitis, strangulated hernia, intussusception, and torsion of the ovary or testis.

Abdominal distention, usually a sign of intestinal obstruction or an intra-abdominal mass, may also be seen in infants with enteritis, necrotizing enterocolitis, ileus accompanying sepsis, respiratory distress, or hypokalemia.

Failure to move an extremity (pseudoparalysis) or part of it suggests fracture, dislocation, or nerve injury. It is also seen in osteomyelitis and other infections that cause pain on movement of the affected part.

CONGENITAL ANOMALIES

Congenital anomalies are a major cause of stillbirths and neonatal deaths but are perhaps even more important as causes of physical defects and metabolic disorders. (Anomalies are discussed in general in Chapter 7 and specifically in the chapters on the various systems of the body. For congenital mental defects, see Chapter 3; for congenital metabolic and chemical disorders, see Chapter 8; and for immunologic deficiency disorders, see Chapter 11.) Early recognition of anomalies is important for planning care; for some, such as tracheoesophageal fistula, diaphragmatic hernia, choanal atresia, and intestinal obstruction, immediate medical and surgical therapy is essential for survival (Table 9–22). Parents are likely to have anxiety and guilt upon learning of the existence of a congenital anomaly and require sensitive counseling.

9.21 BIRTH INJURY

The term *birth injury* is used to denote avoidable and unavoidable mechanical and anoxic trauma incurred by the infant during labor and delivery. These injuries may result from inappropriate or deficient medical skill or attention, or they may occur, despite skilled and competent obstetric care, independently of any acts or omissions. In order to avoid later misunderstandings, recriminations, or parental guilt, it is important to counsel parents who have a child with a residuum from birth trauma or anoxia about this broad use of the term "birth injury." The definition does not include injury from amniocentesis, intrauterine transfusion, scalp vein sampling, or resuscitation procedures, all of which are discussed elsewhere.

The incidence of birth injuries has been estimated at 2–7/1,000 live births. Predisposing factors include macrosomia, prematurity, cephalopelvic disproportion, dystocia, pro-

TABLE 9–22. Common Life-Threatening Congenital Anomalies

Name	Manifestations
Choanal atresia	Respiratory distress in delivery room, apnea, unable to pass nasogastric tube through nares. Suspect CHARGE syndrome
Pierre Robin syndrome	Migrognathia, cleft palate, airway obstruction
Diaphragmatic hernia	Scaphoid abdomen, bowel sounds present in chest, respiratory distress
Tracheoesophageal fistula	Polyhydramnios, aspiration pneumonia, excessive salivation, unable to place nasogastric tube in stomach. Suspect VATER syndrome
Intestinal obstruction: volvulous, duodenal atresia, ileal atresia	Polyhydramnios, bile-stained emesis, abdominal distention. Suspect 21-trisomy, cystic fibrosis, cocaine
Gastroschisis, omphalocele	Polyhydramnios, intestinal obstruction
Renal agenesis, Potter syndrome	Oligohydramnios, anuria, pulmonary hypoplasia, pneumothorax
Neural tube defects: anencephalus, meningomyelocele	Polydramnios, elevated α-fetoprotein, decreased fetal activity
Ductal dependent congenital heart disease	Cyanosis, hypotension, murmur

longed labor, and breech presentation. Overall, 5–8/100,000 infants die of birth trauma, and 25/100,000 die of anoxic injuries; such injuries represent 2–3% of infant deaths. Even transient injuries readily apparent to the parents result in anxiety and questioning that require supportive and informative counseling. Some injuries may be latent initially but later result in severe illness or sequelae.

9.22 CRANIAL INJURIES

Caput succedaneum is a diffuse, sometimes ecchymotic, edematous swelling of the soft tissues of the scalp involving the portion presenting during vertex delivery. It may extend across the midline and across suture lines. The edema disappears within the first few days of life. Analogous swelling, discoloration, and distortion of the face are seen in face presentations. No specific treatment is needed, but if there are extensive ecchymoses, early phototherapy for hyperbilirubinemia may be indicated. *Molding* of the head and overriding of the parietal bones are frequently associated with caput succedaneum and become more evident after the caput has receded but disappear during the first weeks of life. Rarely, a hemorrhagic caput may result in shock and require blood transfusion.

Erythema, abrasions, ecchymoses and *subcutaneous fat necrosis* of facial or scalp soft tissues may be seen after forceps deliveries. Their location depends on the area of application of the forceps. Ecchymoses may be seen after manipulative deliveries and occasionally in premature infants for no discernible reason.

Subconjunctival and retinal hemorrhages are frequent, and *petechiae* of the skin of the head and neck are common. All are probably secondary to a sudden increase in intrathoracic pressure during passage of the chest through the birth canal. Parents should be assured that they are temporary and the result of *normal* hazards of delivery.

Cephalohematoma (Fig. 9–14) is a subperiosteal hemorrhage, hence always limited to the surface of 1 cranial bone. There is no discoloration of the overlying scalp, and swelling is usually not visible until several hours after birth, since subperiosteal bleeding is a slow process. An underlying skull fracture, usually linear and not depressed, is occasionally associated with cephalohematoma. Cranial meningocele may be differentiated from cephalohematoma by pulsation, increased pressure on crying, and the roentgenographic evidence of bony defect. Most cephalohematomas are resorbed within 2 wk–3 mo, depending on their size. They may begin to calcify by the end of the 2nd wk. A sensation of central depression suggesting underlying fracture or bony defect is usually encountered on palpation of the organized rim of a cephalohematoma. A few remain for years as bony protuberances and are detectable roentgenographically as widening of the diploic space; cyst-like defects may persist for months or years. Despite these residuals, cephalohematomas require no treatment, although phototherapy may be necessary to ameliorate hyperbilirubinemia. Incision and drainage are contraindicated because of the risk of introducing infection in a benign condition. A massive cephalohematoma may rarely result in blood loss severe enough to require transfusion. It may also be associated with a skull fracture, coagulopathy, and intracranial hemorrhage.

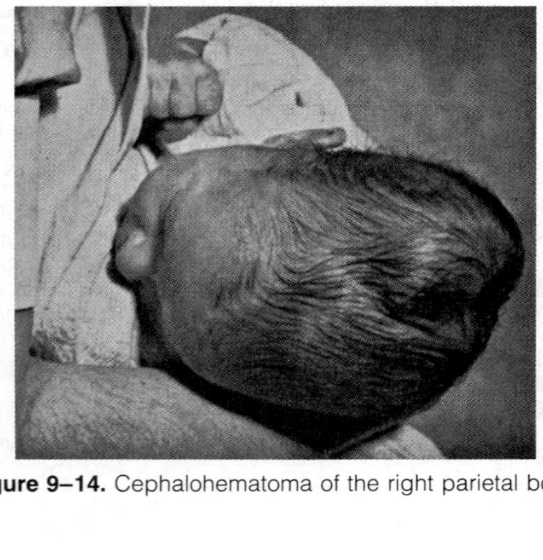

Figure 9–14. Cephalohematoma of the right parietal bone.

Fractures of the skull may occur as a result of pressure from forceps or from the maternal symphysis pubis, sacral promontory, or ischial spines. Linear fractures, the most common, cause no symptoms and require no treatment. Depressed fractures are usually indentations of the calvarium similar to a dent in a ping-pong ball; usually they are a complication of forceps delivery. The infant may be asymptomatic unless there is associated intracranial injury; it is advisable to elevate such depressions to prevent cortical injury from sustained pressure. Fracture of the occipital bone with separation of the basal and squamous portions almost invariably causes fatal hemorrhage owing to disruption of the underlying sinuses. It may result during breech deliveries from traction on the hyperextended spine of the infant with the head fixed in the maternal pelvis.

9.23 INTRACRANIAL (INTRAVENTRICULAR) HEMORRHAGE

ETIOLOGY AND EPIDEMIOLOGY. Intracranial hemorrhage may result from trauma or asphyxia and, rarely, from a primary hemorrhagic disturbance or congenital vascular anomaly. Traumatic epidural, subdural, or subarachnoid hemorrhage is especially likely when the fetal head is large in proportion to the size of the mother's pelvic outlet; when for other reasons the labor is prolonged; when there are breech or precipitate deliveries; or when there is injudicious mechanical interference with delivery. Massive subdural hemorrhages, often associated with tears in the tentorium cerebelli or, less frequently, in the falx cerebri, are rare but are encountered more often in full-term than in premature infants. Primary hemorrhagic disturbances and vascular malformations are rare and usually give rise to subarachnoid or intracerebral hemorrhage. Intracranial bleeding may be associated with disseminated intravascular coagulopathy or idiopathic thrombocytopenia. Intracranial hemorrhages often involve the ventricles **(intraventricular hemorrhage)** of premature infants delivered spontaneously without apparent trauma.

PATHOGENESIS OF INTRAVENTRICULAR HEMORRHAGE (IVH). IVH in the premature infant occurs in the gelatinous subependymal germinal matrix. This periventricular area is the site of embryonal neurons and fetal glial cells, which migrate to the cortex. Immature blood vessels in this highly vascular area may be subjected to various forces that, together with poor tissue vascular support, predispose the premature infant to IVH. By term, the germinal matrix has become attenuated and the tissue's vascular support has strengthened. *Predisposing factors or events* for IVH include prematurity, respiratory distress syndrome, hypoxic ischemic or hypotensive injury, reperfusion of damaged vessels, increased or decreased cerebral blood flow, reduced vascular integrity, increased venous pressure, pneumothorax, hypervolemia, and hypertension. These factors result in rupture of the germinal matrix blood vessels. Similar injurious factors (hypoxic-ischemic-hypotensive) may produce cortical intraparenchymal echodensities (IPE) due to hemorrhagic infarction and *periventricular leukomalacia* (PVL). PVL with or without severe IVH results in necrosis of the periventricular white matter and damage to the corticospinal fibers in the internal capsule.

CLINICAL MANIFESTATIONS. The incidence of IVH increases with decreasing birth weight: 60–70% of 500- to 750-g infants and 10–20% of 1,000- to 1,500-g infants. IVH is rarely present at birth; however, 80–90% of cases occur between birth and the 3rd day of life. Twenty to 40% of cases progress during the 1st wk of life. Delayed hemorrhage may occur in 10–15% of patients after the 1st wk of life. New-onset IVH is rare after the 1st mo of life regardless of birth weight. The most common symptoms are diminished or absent Moro reflex, poor muscle tone, lethargy, apnea, and somnolence. In premature infants with intraventricular hemorrhage there is often a precipitous deterioration on the 2nd or 3rd day of life. Periods of apnea, pallor, or cyanosis, failure to suck well, abnormal eye signs, a high-pitched shrill cry, muscular twitchings, convulsions, decreased muscle tone, paralyses, metabolic acidosis, shock and a decreased hematocrit or its failure to increase after transfusion may be the first indications. The fontanel *may* be tense and bulging. Severe neurologic depression progresses to coma after more severe intraventricular hemorrhages, with associated hemorrhage in the cerebral cortex and ventricular dilation. In a small percentage of cases there may be no clinical manifestations.

PVL is usually asymptomatic until the neurologic sequelae of white matter necrosis becomes manifest in later infancy as spastic diplegia. As a result of nonhemorrhagic ischemic injury, PVL often coexists with IVH. PVL may be present at birth but usually occurs later as an early echo-dense phase (3–10 days of life) followed by the typical echo-lucent (cystic) phase (14–20 days of life).

DIAGNOSIS. Intracranial hemorrhage is diagnosed on the basis of the history, clinical manifestations, and knowledge of the birth weight-specific risks of the type of hemorrhage. The diagnosis of *subdural hemorrhage* in a LGA term infant with cephalopelvic disproportion may be delayed 1 mo until the chronic subdural fluid volume expands, producing megalocephaly, frontal bossing, bulging fontanel, seizures, and anemia. Alternatively, the well neonate with a seizure of short duration may have a benign *subarachnoid hemorrhage*.

Although preterm infants with IVH manifest rapid shock, mottling, anemia, coma, or a bulging fontanel, many signs of IVH are nonspecific or absent. Therefore, it is recommended that the premature infant be evaluated with real-time *cerebral ultrasonography* through the anterior fontanel to detect IVH. Infants weighing under 1,000 g are at high risk for IVH and should be examined within the first 3–5 days of life and again the following week. The ultrasound examination will also detect the precystic and cystic symmetric lesions of PVL and the asymmetric intraparenchymal echogenic lesions of cortical hemorrhagic infarction. Furthermore, the delayed development of cortical atrophy, or porencephaly, and the severity, progression, or regression of posthemorrhagic hydrocephalus can be determined with ultrasonography.

Four levels of increasing severity of IVH are defined by ultrasound for LBW infants: grade I is bleeding confined to the germinal matrix-subependymal region or to less than 10% of the ventricle; grade II is intraventricular bleeding with 10–50% filling of the ventricle; grade III is more than 50% involvement with dilated ventricles; grade IV includes grade III, with corticoperiventricular intraparenchymal lesions that are not necessarily a direct extension of the IVH. Seventy-five per cent of infants with IVH are grade I–II. Severe IVH is independently associated with immaturity and the severity of respiratory distress syndrome (RDS). Immature infants without RDS are at risk for IVH, whereas infants with severe RDS are at greater risk than those with mild or no RDS at the same gestational age.

CT scan is indicated for term infants in whom the diagnosis is suspected, since ultrasound may not reveal intraparenchymal hemorrhage. Lumbar puncture is indicated in the presence of signs of increased intracranial pressure or deteriorating clinical condition to identify gross subarachnoid hemorrhage or to rule out the possibility of bacterial meningitis; the cerebrospinal fluid usually has elevated protein levels with many red blood cells. Not infrequently there is hypoglycorrhachia and a mild lymphocytosis. Since a small amount of bleeding into the cerebrospinal fluid often occurs in the course of normal and even cesarean deliveries, small numbers of red blood cells or slight xanthochromia in subarachnoid fluid does not necessarily indicate significant intracranial hemorrhage. Conversely, the subarachnoid fluid may be absolutely clear in the presence of severe subdural or intracerebral hemorrhage when there is no communication with the subarachnoid space.

PROGNOSIS. Patients with massive hemorrhage associated with tears of the tentorium or falx cerebri rapidly deteriorate and may die after birth. In utero hemorrhage associated with maternal idiopathic or fetal alloimmune thrombocytopenia may occur as severe cerebral hemorrhage or a porencephalic cyst after resolution of a fetal cortical hemorrhage.

Most infants with IVH and acute ventricular distention do not develop *posthemorrhagic hydrocephalus*. Ten to 15% of LBW neonates with IVH have hydrocephalus, which initially may be present without clinical signs such as enlarging head circumference, apnea, bradycardia, lethargy, bulging fontanel, or widely split sutures. In infants who develop symptomatic hydrocephalus, clinical signs may be delayed 2–4 wk despite progressive ventricular distention and compression (thinning) of the cerebral cortex. Posthemorrhagic hydrocephalus is arrested or regresses in 65% of affected infants.

Progressive hydrocephalus requiring ventricular-peritoneal shunting, gestational age of less than 30 wk, prolonged mechanical ventilation ($>$ 28 days), intraparenchymal hemorrhage, and extensive PVL are associated with a poor prognosis. Because PVL and intraparenchymal bleeding represent hypoxic ischemic injury, they are independent risk factors for spastic diplegia and other motor deficits. IVH with intraparenchymal echo-densities greater than 1 cm are associated with a high mortality and a high incidence of motor and cognitive deficits. Grades I–II IVH may be due to factors other than severe hypoxia-ischemia and in such a case it has a lower risk of long-term neurologic sequelae if it is unassociated with PVL or intraparenchymal hemorrhage.

PREVENTION. The incidence of traumatic intracranial hemorrhage may be reduced by judicious management of cephalopelvic disproportion and operative (forceps, cesarean section) delivery. Fetal or neonatal hemorrhage due to maternal idiopathic thrombocytopenic purpura (ITP) or alloimmune thrombocytopenia may be prevented by maternal treatment with steroids, intravenous immunoglobulin, or fetal platelet transfusion. The incidence of IVH may possibly be reduced by neonatal administration of ethamsylate (which decreases bleeding time and limits capillary bleeding), indomethacin, and vitamin E. Wide fluctuations of blood pressure should be avoided.

TREATMENT. IVH associated with hypoxic-ischemic encephalopathy is frequently associated with multiple organ system dysfunction. Seizures are treated with anticonvulsant drugs, anemia-shock requires transfusion with packed red blood cells or fresh frozen plasma, and acidosis is treated with judicious and slow administration of 1–2 mEq/kg sodium bicarbonate. Serial lumbar punctures have no role during the acute hemorrhage; however, repeated lumbar punctures may reduce the symptoms or progression of posthemorrhagic hydrocephalus. Neurosurgical placement of an external ventriculostomy catheter may be needed in the early stage of uncontrolled symptomatic hydrocephalus. After the protein content of the ventricular fluid declines, a permanent ventricular-peritoneal shunt is put in place.

Symptomatic subdural hemorrhage in large term infants should be treated by removing the subdural fluid collection by means of a spinal needle placed through the lateral margin of the anterior fontanel. In addition to birth trauma, child abuse should also be suspected in all infants with subdural effusions.

9.24 SPINE AND SPINAL CORD

Strong traction exerted when the spine is hyperextended or when the direction of pull is lateral, or forceful longitudinal traction on the trunk while the head is still firmly engaged in the pelvis, especially when combined with flexion and torsion of the vertical axis, may produce fracture and separation of the vertebrae. Such injuries, rarely diagnosed clinically, are most likely to occur when difficulty is encountered in delivering the shoulders in cephalic presentations and the head in breech presentations. The injury occurs most commonly at the level of the 7th cervical and 1st thoracic vertebrae. Transection of the cord may occur with or without vertebral fractures, but hemorrhage and edema may produce neurologic signs that are indistinguishable from those of transection except that they are not permanent. There is complete paralysis of voluntary motion below the level of injury, although the persistence of a withdrawal reflex mediated through spinal centers distal to the area of injury is frequently misinterpreted as representing voluntary motion. If the injury is severe, the infant, who from birth may be in poor condition due to respiratory depression, shock, or hypothermia, may deteriorate rapidly to death within several hours before neurologic signs are obvious. Alternatively, the course may be protracted with symptoms and signs appearing at birth or later in the 1st wk; immobility, flaccidity, and associated brachial plexus injuries may not be recognized for several days. Constipation may also be present. Some infants survive for prolonged periods, their initial flaccidity, immobility, and areflexia being replaced after several weeks or months by rigid flexion of extremities, increased muscle tone, and spasms.

The differential diagnosis includes amyotonia congenita and myelodysplasia associated with spina bifida occulta. Treatment of the survivors is supportive, and they often remain permanently injured. When there is compression from a fracture or dislocation, the prognosis is related to the time elapsing before the compression is removed.

9.25 PERIPHERAL NERVE INJURIES

BRACHIAL PALSY. Injury to the brachial plexus may cause paralysis of the upper arm with or without paralysis of the forearm or hand or, more commonly, paralysis of the entire arm. These injuries occur when lateral traction is exerted on the head and neck during delivery of the shoulder in a vertex presentation, when the arms are extended over the head in a breech presentation, or when there is excessive traction on the shoulders.

In **Erb-Duchenne paralysis** the injury is limited to the 5th and 6th cervical nerves. The infant loses the power to abduct the arm from the shoulder, to rotate the arm externally, and to supinate the forearm. The characteristic position consists of adduction and internal rotation of the arm with pronation of the forearm. The power of extension of the forearm is retained, but the biceps reflex is absent; the Moro reflex is absent on the affected side (Fig. 9–15). There may be some sensory impairment on the outer aspect of the arm. The power in the forearm and the hand grasp are preserved unless the lower part of the plexus is also injured; the presence of the hand grasp is a favorable prognostic sign. When the injury includes the phrenic nerve, alteration of the diaphragmatic excursion may be observed fluoroscopically.

Klumpke paralysis is a rarer form of brachial palsy; injury to the 7th and 8th cervical nerves and the 1st thoracic nerve produces a paralyzed hand, and ipsilateral ptosis and miosis if the sympathetic fibers of the 1st thoracic root are also injured.

The mild cases may not be detected immediately after birth. Differentiation must be made from cerebral injury; from fracture, dislocation, or epiphyseal separation of the humerus; and from fracture of the clavicle. Magnetic resonance imaging (MRI) or CT myelography will demonstrate nerve root rupture or avulsion.

The *prognosis* depends on whether the nerve was merely injured or was lacerated. If the paralysis was due to edema and hemorrhage about the nerve fibers, there should be a return of function within a few months; if due to laceration, permanent damage may result. The involvement of the deltoid is usually the most serious problem and may result in a shoulder drop secondary to muscular atrophy. In general, paralysis of the upper arm has a better prognosis than paralysis of the lower arm.

Treatment consists of partial immobilization and appropriate positioning to prevent development of contractures. In upper arm paralysis, the arm should be abducted 90 degrees, with external rotation at the shoulder and with full supination of the forearm and slight extension at the wrist with the palm turned toward the face. This may be done with a brace or splint during the first 1–2 wk. Immobilization should be intermittent through the day while the infant is asleep and between feedings. In lower arm or hand paralysis, the wrist should be splinted in a neutral position and padding placed in the fist. When the entire arm is paralyzed, the same treatment principles should be followed. Gentle massage and range of motion exercises may be started by 7–10 days of age. Infants should be followed closely with active and passive corrective exercises. If the paralysis persists without improvement for 3–6 mo, neuroplasty, neurolysis, end-to-end anastomosis, or nerve grafting offer hope for partial recovery.

PHRENIC NERVE PARALYSIS. Phrenic nerve injury with diaphragmatic paralysis must be considered when cyanosis and irregular and labored respirations develop. Such injuries, usually unilateral, are associated with ipsilateral upper brachial palsy. Because breathing is thoracic in type, the abdomen does not bulge with inspiration. Breath sounds are diminished on the affected side. The thrust of the diaphragm, which often may be felt just under the costal margin on the normal side, is absent on the affected side. The *diagnosis* is established by ultrasonography or fluoroscopic examination, which reveals the elevation of the diaphragm on the paralyzed side and seesaw movements of the two sides of the diaphragm during respiration.

There is no specific *treatment*; the infant should be placed on the involved side and given oxygen if necessary. Initially, intravenous feedings may be needed; later, progressive gavage or oral feedings may be started depending on the infant's condition. Pulmonary infections are a serious complication. Recovery usually occurs spontaneously by 1–3 mo; rarely, surgical plication of the diaphragm may be indicated.

FACIAL NERVE PALSY. Usually, facial palsy is a peripheral paralysis that results from pressure over the facial nerve in utero, from efforts during labor, or from forceps during delivery. Rarely nonobstetric, it may result from nuclear agenesis of the facial nerve. Peripheral paralysis is flaccid and, when complete, involves the entire side of the face, including the forehead. When the infant cries, there is move-

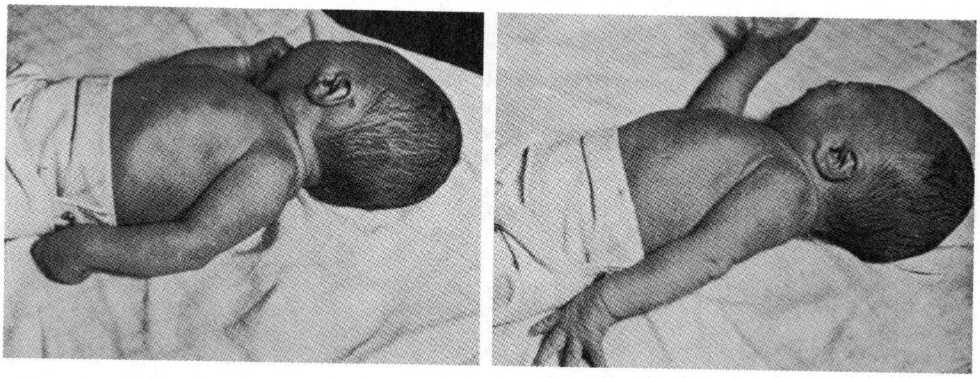

Figure 9–15. Brachial palsy of the left arm (asymmetric Moro reflex).

ment on only the nonparalyzed side of the face, and the mouth is drawn to that side. On the affected side the forehead is smooth, the eye cannot be closed, the nasolabial fold is absent, and the corner of the mouth droops. The forehead will wrinkle on the affected side with central paralysis, since only the lower two thirds of the face is involved. Usually there are also other manifestations of intracranial injury, most commonly a 6th nerve palsy. The *prognosis* depends upon whether the nerve was injured by pressure or whether the nerve fibers were torn. Improvement occurs within a few weeks in the former instance. Care of the exposed eye is essential. Neuroplasty may be indicated when the paralysis is persistent. Facial palsy may be confused with the absence of the depressor muscles of the mouth, which is a benign problem.

Other peripheral nerves are seldom injured in utero or at birth except when they are involved in fractures or hemorrhages.

9.26 VISCERA

The **liver** is the only internal organ other than the brain that is injured with any frequency during birth. The damage usually results from pressure on the liver during delivery of the head in breech presentations. Large infant size, intrauterine asphyxia, coagulation disorders, extreme prematurity, and hepatomegaly are contributing factors. Incorrect cardiac massage is a less frequent cause. The liver is ruptured when there is formation of a subcapsular hematoma, which may tamponade further bleeding. The infant usually appears normal for the first 1–3 days. Nonspecific signs related to loss of blood into the hematoma may appear early and include poor feeding, listlessness, pallor, jaundice, tachypnea, and tachycardia. A mass may be palpable in the right upper quadrant; the abdomen may appear blue. The hematoma may be large enough to cause anemia. Shock and death may occur if the hematoma breaks through the capsule into the peritoneal cavity, reducing pressure and allowing fresh hemorrhage. Early suspicion by means of ultrasonography diagnosis and prompt supportive therapy can decrease the mortality of this disorder. Surgical repair of a laceration may be required.

Rupture of the spleen may occur alone or in association with rupture of the liver. The causes, complications, treatment, and prevention are similar.

Although **adrenal hemorrhage** occurs with some frequency, especially after breech delivery, its cause is undetermined; it may be due to trauma, anoxia, or severe stress, as in overwhelming infections. Calcified central hematomas of the adrenal have been identified roentgenographically or at autopsy in older infants and children, suggesting that not all adrenal hemorrhages are immediately fatal. In severe cases the diagnosis is usually made at post mortem examination. The symptoms are profound shock and cyanosis. There may be a mass in the flank with overlying skin discoloration; jaundice may also develop. If adrenal hemorrhage is suspected, abdominal ultrasonography may be helpful, and treatment for acute adrenal failure may be indicated (Sec. 19.21).

INJURY OF THE STERNOCLEIDOMASTOID

See Torticollis, Sec. 24.22.

9.27 FRACTURES

CLAVICLE. This bone is fractured during labor and delivery more frequently than any other bone; it is particularly vulnerable when there is difficulty in delivery of the shoulder in vertex presentations and of the extended arms in breech deliveries. The infant characteristically does not move the arm freely on the affected side; crepitus and bony irregularity may be palpated, and occasionally discoloration is visible over the fracture site. The Moro reflex is absent on the affected side, and there is spasm of the sternocleidomastoid muscle with obliteration of the supraclavicular depression at the site of the fracture. In greenstick fractures there may be no limitation of movement, and the Moro reflex may be present. Fracture of the humerus or brachial palsy may also be responsible for limitation of movement of an arm and absence of a Moro reflex on the affected side. The *prognosis* is excellent. *Treatment*, if any, consists of immobilization of the arm and shoulder on the affected side. A remarkable degree of callus develops at the site within a week and may be the first evidence of the fracture.

EXTREMITIES

In fractures of the long bones spontaneous movement of the extremity is usually absent. The Moro reflex is also absent from the involved extremity. There may be associated nerve involvement. Satisfactory results of treatment for a fractured humerus are obtained with 2–4 wk of immobilization during which the arm is strapped to the chest, a triangular splint and a Velpeau bandage are applied, or a cast is applied. For fracture of the femur, good results are obtained with traction-suspension of both lower extremities, even if the fracture is unilateral; the legs, immobilized in a spica cast, are attached to an overhead frame. Splints are effective for treatment of fractures of the forearm or leg. Healing is usually accompanied by excess callus formation. The *prognosis* is excellent for fractures of the extremities. Fractures in preterm infants are related to osteopenia (Sec. 9.54).

Dislocations and **epiphyseal separations** rarely result from birth trauma. The upper femoral epiphysis may be separated by forcible manipulation of the infant's leg as, for example, in breech extraction or after version. There is swelling, slight shortening, limitation of active motion, painful passive motion, and external rotation of the leg. The diagnosis is established roentgenographically. The prognosis is good for the milder injuries, but coxa vara frequently results from extensive displacement.

NOSE. The most prevalent injury of the nose is a dislocation of the cartilaginous portion of the septum from the vomerine groove and the columella. The infant may have difficulty in nursing and some impairment in nasal respiration. On physical examination, the nares appear asymmetric and the nose flattened. An oral airway rarely is needed, and surgical consultation should be obtained for definitive treatment.

9.28 HYPOXIA-ISCHEMIA
(Asphyxia)

Anoxia is a term used to indicate the consequences of a complete lack of oxygen owing to a number of primary causes. *Hypoxia* refers to an arterial concentration of oxygen that is less than normal, and *ischemia* refers to blood flow to cells or organs that is insufficient to maintain their normal function. *Hypoxic-ischemic encephalopathy* is an important cause of permanent damage to central nervous system cells, which may result in neonatal death or which may be manifest later as cerebral palsy or mental deficiency. Its prevention and treatment are those of the basic conditions that cause it; death and disability may sometimes be prevented through symptomatic treatment with oxygen or artificial respiration and the correction of associated multisystem dysfunction (Table 9–23).

ETIOLOGY. Fetal hypoxia may result from (1) inadequate oxygenation of maternal blood as a result of hypoventilation during anesthesia, cardiac failure, or carbon monoxide poisoning; (2) low maternal blood pressure as a result of the hypotension that may complicate spinal anesthesia or that may result from compression of the vena cava and aorta by the gravid uterus; (3) inadequate relaxation of the uterus to permit placental filling as a result of uterine tetany caused by excessive administration of oxytocin; (4) premature separation of the placenta; (5) impedance to the circulation of blood through the umbilical cord as a result of compression or knotting of the cord; (6) uterine vessel vasoconstriction by cocaine; and (7) placental insufficiency from numerous causes, including toxemia and postmaturity.

Placental insufficiency often remains undetected on clinical assessment. Chronically hypoxic fetuses may develop intrauterine growth retardation without traditional signs of fetal distress (e.g., bradycardia). Doppler umbilical wave-form velocimetry (demonstrating increased fetal vascular resistance)

TABLE 9–23. Effects of Asphyxia

System	Effect
Central nervous system	Hypoxic-ischemic encephalopathy, infarction, intracranial hemorrhage, seizures, cerebral edema, hypotonia, hypertonia
Cardiovascular	Myocardial ischemia, poor contractility, cardiac stun, tricuspid insufficiency, hypotension
Pulmonary	Persistent fetal circulation, pulmonary hemorrhage, respiratory distress syndrome
Renal	Acute tubular or cortical necrosis
Adrenal	Adrenal hemorrhage
Gastrointestinal	Perforation, ulceration, necrosis
Metabolic	Inappropriate secretion of ADH, hyponatremia, hypoglycemia, hypocalcemia, myoglobinuria
Integument	Subcutaneous fat necrosis
Hematology	Disseminated intravascular coagulation

and cordocentesis (demonstrating fetal hypoxia, see Fig. 9–5) identify the chronically hypoxic infant. Uterine contractions further reduce umbilical oxygenation, depressing the fetal cardiovascular and central nervous systems and resulting in low Apgar scores and postnatal hypoxia in the delivery room.

After birth, hypoxia may result from (1) anemia severe enough to lower the oxygen content of the blood to a critical level due to severe hemorrhage or hemolytic disease; (2) shock severe enough to interfere with the transport of oxygen to vital cells from adrenal hemorrhage, intraventricular hemorrhage, overwhelming infection, or massive blood loss; (3) a deficit in arterial oxygen saturation resulting from failure to breathe adequately postnatally due to a cerebral defect, narcosis, or injury; and (4) failure of oxygenation of an adequate amount of blood resulting from severe forms of cyanotic congenital heart disease or deficient pulmonary function.

PATHOPHYSIOLOGY AND PATHOLOGY. Within minutes of the onset of total fetal hypoxia bradycardia, hypotension, decreased cardiac output, and severe metabolic as well as respiratory acidosis occur. The initial circulatory response of the fetus is increased shunting through the ductus venosus, ductus arteriosus, and foramen ovale with transient maintenance of perfusion of the brain, heart, and adrenals in preference to the lungs (due to pulmonary vasoconstriction), liver, kidneys, and intestine.

The pathology of hypoxia-ischemia is dependent upon the affected organ and the severity of the insult. Early congestion, fluid leak from increased capillary permeability, and endothelial cell swelling may then lead to signs of coagulation necrosis and cell death. Congestion and petechiae are seen in the pericardium, pleura, thymus, heart, adrenals, and meninges. Prolonged intrauterine hypoxia may result in PVL and pulmonary arteriole smooth muscle hyperplasia, which predisposes the infant to pulmonary hypertension (Sec. 9.36). If fetal distress produces gasping, amniotic fluid contents (meconium, squames, lanuga hair) are aspirated into the trachea or lungs.

The combination of chronic fetal hypoxia and acute hypoxic-ischemic injury after birth results in gestational age–specific neuropathology. Term infants demonstrate neuronal necrosis of the cortex (later cortical atrophy) and parasagittal ischemic injury. Preterm infants demonstrate PVL (later spastic diplegia), status marmoratus of the basal ganglia, and IVH. Term more often than preterm infants demonstrate focal or multifocal cortical infarcts that produce focal seizures and hemiplegia. Infarctions are best visualized with CT scanning or MRI. In addition to focal lesions, CT scanning may demonstrate diffuse decreases of tissue attenuation. Cerebral edema with resultant increased intracranial pressure occurs in infants who have severe hypoxic-ischemic encephalopathy.

CLINICAL MANIFESTATIONS. The signs of hypoxia in the *fetus* are usually noted a few minutes to a few days before delivery. IUGR with increased vascular resistance may be the first indication of fetal hypoxia. The fetal heart rate slows, and the beat-to-beat variability declines. Continuous heart rate recording may reveal a variable or late (type II dips) deceleration pattern (see Fig. 9–6), and scalp blood analysis may show a pH less than 7.20. The acidosis is made up of varying degrees of metabolic or respiratory components. Particularly in the infant near term, these signs should lead to the administration of high concentrations of oxygen to the mother and immediate delivery to avoid fetal death or central nervous system damage.

At *delivery* the presence of yellow, meconium-stained amniotic fluid is evidence that there has been fetal distress. At birth these infants are frequently depressed and fail to breathe spontaneously. During the ensuing hours they may remain hypotonic or change from hypotonia to extreme hypertonia, or their tone may appear normal (Table 9–24). Pallor, cyanosis,

TABLE 9–24. Hypoxic-Ischemic Encephalopathy in Term Infants*

Signs	Stage I	Stage 2	Stage 3
Level of consciousness	Hyperalert	Lethargic	Stuporous, coma
Muscle tone	Normal	Hypotonic	Flaccid
Posture	Normal	Flexion	Decerebrate
Tendon reflexes/clonus	Hyperactive	Hyperactive	Absent
Myoclonus	Present	Present	Absent
Moro reflex	Strong	Weak	Absent
Pupils	Mydriasis	Miosis	Unequal, poor light reflex
Seizures	None	Common	Decerebration
Electroencephalographic	Normal	Low voltage changing to seizure activity	Burst suppression to isoelectric
Duration	< 24 hr if progresses, otherwise may remain normal	24 hr to 14 days	Days to weeks
Outcome	Good	Variable	Death, severe deficits

*Modified from Sarnat H, Sarnat M: Neonatal encephalopathy following fetal distress: A clinical and electroencephalographic study. Arch Neurol 33:696, 1976. Copyright 1976, American Medical Association.

apnea, slow heart rate, and unresponsiveness to stimulation also are signs of hypoxic-ischemic encephalopathy. Cerebral edema may develop during the next 24 hr and result in profound brain stem depression. During this time seizure activity may occur that may be severe and refractory to the usual doses of anticonvulsants. Although most often a result of the hypoxic-ischemic encephalopathy, seizures in asphyxiated newborns may also be due to hypocalcemia and hypoglycemia.

In addition to central nervous system dysfunction, congestive heart failure and cardiogenic shock, persistent pulmonary hypertension (persistent fetal circulation), respiratory distress syndrome, gastrointestinal perforation, hematuria, and acute tubular necrosis are also associated with perinatal asphyxia (see Table 9–23).

After delivery hypoxia is due to respiratory failure and circulatory insufficiency (Sec. 9.29 and 9.32).

PROGNOSIS. The outcome of perinatal asphyxia depends on whether its metabolic and cardiopulmonary complications (hypoxia, hypoglycemia, shock) can be treated, the infant's gestational age (outcome is poorest if infant is preterm), and the severity of the hypoxic-ischemic encephalopathy. Severe encephalopathy, characterized by flaccid coma, apnea, absent oculocephalic reflexes, refractory seizures, and a marked decrease of cortical attenuation on CT, is associated with a poor prognosis. A low Apgar score at 20 min, absence of spontaneous respirations, and persistence of abnormal neurologic signs at 2 wk of age also predict death or severe cognitive and motor deficits.

Brain death following neonatal hypoxic-ischemic encephalopathy is diagnosed by the clinical findings of coma that is unresponsive to pain, auditory, or visual stimulation; apnea with P_{CO_2} rising from 40 to over 60 mm Hg (5.3–7.9 kPa); and absent brain stem reflexes (pupil, oculocephalic, oculovestibular, corneal, gag, sucking). These must occur in the absence of hypothermia, hypotension, and elevated levels of depressant drugs (e.g., phenobarbital). The absence of cerebral blood flow on radionuclide scan and electrical activity on EEG (electrocerebral silence)is inconsistently observed in clinically brain dead neonatal infants. Persistence of the clinical criteria for 2 days in term and 3 days in preterm infants predicts brain death in most asphyxiated newborns. Nonetheless, there is no universal agreement about the definition of neonatal brain death. Consideration of withdrawal of life support should include discussions with the family, the health care team, and, if there is disagreement, an ethics committee. The best interest of the infant involves judgments about the benefits and harm of continuing therapy and of avoiding continuing futile therapy.

9.29 PEDIATRIC EMERGENCIES IN THE DELIVERY ROOM

The most common and important emergency related to the newborn infant in the delivery room is the failure to initiate and maintain respirations. Less frequent, but of major importance, are shock, severe anemia (Sec. 9.21–9.23 and 9.46), plethora (Sec. 9.48), convulsions (Sec. 20.17), and management of life-threatening congenital malformations (Sec. 7.32).

RESPIRATORY DISTRESS AND FAILURE. Disorders of respiration in the newborn infant can be categorized as either *central nervous system failure*, representing depression or failure of the respiratory center, or *peripheral respiratory difficulty*, indicating interference with the alveolar exchange of oxygen and carbon dioxide. Cyanosis occurs in both groups (see Table 9–21). The respiratory problems encountered in the delivery room are most frequently those of airway obstruction and of depression of the central nervous system with the absence of adequate respiratory effort.

Respiratory distress in the presence of good respiratory effort should lead to an immediate consideration of peripheral causes; *it is an indication for a roentgenographic examination of the chest*, if this is at all possible.

If respiratory movements are made with the mouth closed but the infant fails to move air in and out of the lungs, bilateral **choanal atresia** (Sec. 14.20) or other obstruction of the upper respiratory tract should be suspected. The mouth should be opened, and the mouth and posterior pharynx cleared of secretions by gentle suction. An oropharyngeal airway should be inserted and the source of the obstruction sought immediately. If effective respiratory flow is not produced by opening the infant's mouth and clearing the airway, laryngoscopy is indicated. With obstructive malformations of the epiglottis, larynx, or trachea, an endotracheal tube should be inserted; prolonged endotracheal intubation or tracheostomy may be required. Respiratory failure due to depression or injury of the central nervous system may require continuous artificial ventilation with a face mask and bag or through an endotracheal tube.

Hypoplasia of the mandible (Pierre Robin syndrome) (Sec. 13.5) with posterior displacement of the tongue may result in symptoms similar to those of choanal atresia, which may be temporarily relieved by pulling the tongue forward. A scaphoid abdomen suggests a **diaphragmatic hernia** or **eventration**, as does asymmetry of contour or movement of the chest or shift of the apical impulse of the heart; these latter manifestations are also compatible with tension pneumothorax.

Causes of peripheral respiratory difficulty are discussed in Sec. 9.30–9.40.

FAILURE TO INITIATE OR SUSTAIN RESPIRATION. This usually originates in the central nervous system owing to asphyxia; immaturity in itself is seldom a causative factor except in infants weighing less than 1,000 g. Intrapulmonary problems, such as the pulmonary hypoplasia associated with Potter syndrome and severe organized intrauterine pneumonia, may at times result in poorly sustained ventilation. The lungs in these infants are very noncompliant, and efforts to begin respirations may be inadequate to start sufficient ventilation.

Narcosis results from heavy doses of morphine, Demerol, barbiturates, reserpine, or tranquilizers administered to the mother shortly before delivery or from maternal anesthesia, given during the second stage of labor. The infant is cyanotic at birth and slow to cry or breathe; when respiration is established, it is extremely slow.

Narcosis should be avoided by using appropriate analgesic and anesthetic practices. Treatment includes initial physical stimulation and securing a patent airway. If effective ventilation is not initiated, artificial breathing with a mask and bag must be instituted. At the same time, if depression is due to morphine or its derivatives, Narcan (naloxone hydrochloride), 0.01 mg/kg, should be given by intravenous, subcutaneous, intratracheal, or intramuscular routes. Ventilation is essential prior to and during the administration of this antidote. If depression is due to other anesthetics or analgesics, artificial respiration should be continued until the infant is able to sustain ventilation. Central nervous system stimulant drugs should not be used because they are ineffective and may be harmful.

Prenatal or **perinatal hypoxia** of whatever cause, if sufficiently severe, will produce brain stem depression and secondary apnea, which is unresponsive to sensory stimulation. Death due to apnea may be prevented by resuscitation, provided the basic cause of the hypoxia can be eliminated within a reasonable time while artificial respiration, if necessary, is being carried out. External cardiac massage, correction of acidosis, and circulatory support with drugs may be important adjuncts to ventilation. Hypothermia as a means of temporarily reducing metabolic needs for oxygen during the period of hypoxia is contraindicated.

Intracranial hemorrhage and **trauma** are discussed in Sec. 9.22 and 9.23. **Central nervous system anomalies** are rarely responsible for respiratory failure.

RESUSCITATION. The *goals* of neonatal resuscitation are to prevent the morbidity and mortality associated with hypoxic-ischemic tissue (brain, heart, kidney) injury and to reestablish adequate spontaneous respiration and cardiac output. High-risk situations should be anticipated by the history of the pregnancy, labor, and delivery and by identification of the signs of fetal distress. Although the Apgar score is helpful in evaluating patients in need of attention, infants who are born limp, cyanotic, apneic, or pulseless require immediate resuscitation prior to assignment of the 1-min Apgar score. Rapid and appropriate resuscitative efforts improve the likelihood of preventing brain damage and achieving a successful outcome.

Immediately after birth an asphyxiated neonatal infant should be placed under a radiant heater (to avoid hypothermia), dried, positioned head down and slightly extended, the airway cleared by suctioning, and gentle tactile stimulation provided (slapping the foot, rubbing the back). Simultaneously, the infant's color, heart rate, and respiratory effort should be assessed.

The steps in neonatal resuscitation follow the ABCs: **A**, anticipate and establish a patent *a*irway by suctioning and, if necessary, performing endotracheal intubation; **B**, initiate *b*reathing using tactile stimulation or positive pressure ventilation with a bag and mask or through an endotracheal tube; **C**, maintain the *c*irculation with chest compression and medications, if needed.

If there are no respirations or if the heart rate is below 100/min, *positive pressure ventilation* with 100% oxygen is given through a tightly fitted face mask and bag for 15–30 sec. Although the first breath may require pressures as low as 15–20 cm H_2O, pressures as high as 30–40 cm H_2O may be needed. Subsequent breaths are given at a rate of 40/min, with pressures of 15–20 cm H_2O. Noncompliant stiff lungs due to hyaline membrane disease, congenital pneumonia, or meconium aspiration need higher pressures (20–40 cm H_2O). Successful ventilation is determined by good chest rise, symmetric breath sounds, improved pink color, heart rate greater than 100/min, spontaneous respirations, and improved tone.

If there is a history of maternal analgesic narcotic drug administration, *Narcan* (naloxone, 0.01 mg/kg, given through the subcutaneous, intramuscular, intravenous, or intratracheal route) is given while adequate ventilation is maintained. Breathing for the depressed infant should be maintained until a response to Narcan is noted. Continuous observation of the infant is important because repeated doses of Narcan may be needed.

If the heart rate does not improve after 15–30 sec with bag and mask (or endotracheal) ventilation and remains below 60/min or if the rate is less than 80/min and not rising, ventilation is continued and *chest compression* with two fingers is initiated over the lower third of the sternum at a rate of 120/min. Bradycardia in neonatal infants is usually due to hypoxia resulting from respiratory arrest and often responds to ventilation with 100% oxygen. Persistent bradycardia despite ventilation with 100% oxygen suggests more severe cardiac compromise or inadequate ventilation techniques. Poor response to ventilation may be due to a loosely fitted mask, poor positioning of the airway, intraesophageal intubation, airway obstruction, insufficient pressure, pleural effusions, pneumothorax, excessive air in the stomach, asystole, hypovolemia, diaphragmatic hernia, or prolonged intrauterine asphyxia.

Endotracheal intubation should be performed by an experienced person in any infant who does not respond to initial bag and mask ventilation or who was born apneic, pulseless, cyanotic, and limp with signs of fetal distress.

Medications should be administered when the heart rate is less than 80/min following 30 sec of combined ventilation and chest compressions or during asystole. Usually the umbilical vein can be readily cannulated and should be used for immediate administration of medications, glucose, and volume expanders during neonatal resuscitation. Epinephrine (0.1–0.3 mL/kg of a 1:10,000 solution, intravenous or intratracheal) is given for asystole or for failure to respond to 30 sec of combined resuscitation. The dose may be repeated every 5 min. Ten to 20 mL/kg of volume expanders (normal saline, blood, 5% albumin, Ringer lactate) should be given for hypovolemia, pallor, electrical-mechanical dissociation (weak pulses with normal heart rate), history of blood loss, suspicion of septic shock, hypotension, or poor response to resuscitation. Sodium bicarbonate (1–2 mEq/kg, 0.5 mEq/mL of a 4.2% solution) should be given slowly (1 mEq/kg/min) if there is a documented metabolic acidosis. Sodium bicarbonate should be given after effective ventilation has been established because such therapy may increase blood CO_2, producing a respiratory acidosis. Restoration of oxygenation and tissue perfusion is the main treatment for the metabolic acidosis associated with asphyxia.

Severe asphyxia also may depress myocardial function, causing cardiogenic shock despite recovery of heart and respiratory rates. Dopamine or dobutamine administered as a continuous infusion (5–20 μg/kg/min) and volume expanders should be started after the initial resuscitation effort to improve cardiac output in an infant with poor peripheral perfusion, weak pulses, hypotension, tachycardia, and poor urine output. Epinephrine (0.1 μg/kg/min) may be indicated for infants in severe shock who do not respond to dopamine or dobutamine.

Less severe degrees of asphyxia can usually be managed by brief periods of bag and mask ventilation of 100% oxygen. Chest compression and medications are not needed for most neonates who have mild to moderate birth depression. Regardless of the severity of asphyxia or the response to resuscitation, asphyxiated infants should be monitored closely for signs of multiorgan hypoxic-ischemic tissue injury (see Table 9–24).

SHOCK. Circulatory insufficiency may present at birth as a result of internal hemorrhage; fetal bleeding during gestation, labor, or delivery (e.g., fetofetal or fetomaternal transfusion syndrome); bleeding from the fetal circulation secondary to a placental tear during amniocentesis; excessive bleeding from a severed or torn umbilical cord; or severe hemolytic anemia. Clinical manifestations include signs of respiratory distress; cyanosis; pallor; flaccidity; cold, mottled skin; tachycardia or bradycardia; hepatosplenomegaly; and, rarely, convulsions. **Edema** and hepatosplenomegaly also may suggest hydrops fetalis or congestive heart failure without shock. Shock from overwhelming infection may also be present after birth.

Supportive treatment with type O, Rh negative blood, plasma, or electrolyte solutions is indicated for hypovolemia. Oxygen should be administered and metabolic acidosis corrected with sodium bicarbonate. β-Sympathomimetic agents such as dopamine or dobutamine may be needed to support cardiac output and blood pressure. The diagnosis and treatment of erythroblastosis fetalis are discussed in Sec. 9.47. If infection is present, appropriate antibiotics must be started as soon as possible.

After supportive measures have stabilized the infant's condition, a specific diagnosis should be established and appropriate continuing treatment instituted.

American Heart Association: Textbook of Neonatal Resuscitation. 1987.

Aylward GP, Pfeiffer SI, Wright A, et al: Outcome studies of low birth weight infants published in the last decade: A meta analysis. J Pediatr 115:515, 1989.

Bada HS, Green RS, Pourcyrous M, et al: Indomethacin reduces the risks of severe intraventricular hemorrhage. J Pediatr 115:631, 1989.

Blair E, Stanley FJ: Intrapartum asphyxia: A rare cause of cerebral palsy. J Pediatr 112:515, 1988.

Catlin EA, Carpenter MW, Brann BS IV, et al: The Apgar score revisited: Influence of gestational age. J Pediatr 109:865, 1986.

Calciolari G, Perlman J, Volpe J: Seizures in the neonatal intensive care unit of the 1980s: Types, etiologies, timing. Clin Pediatr 27:119, 1988.

Chevalier RL, Campbell, F, Brenbridge AG: Prognostic factors in neonatal acute renal failure. Pediatrics 74:265, 1984.

Committee on Fetus and Newborn: Use and abuse of the Apgar score. Pediatrics 78:1148, 1986.

Connell J, Oozer R, DeVries L, et al: Clinical and EEG response to anticonvulsants in neonatal seizures. Arch Dis Child 64:459, 1989.

de Vries LS, Regev R, Dubowitz LMS et al: Perinatal risk factors for the development of extensive cystic leukomalacia. Am J Dis Child 142:732, 1988.

Dykes FD, Dunbar B, Lazzara A, et al: Posthemorrhage hydrocephalus in high-risk preterm infants. Natural history, management, and long-term outcome. J Pediatr 114:611, 1989.

Ergander U, Eriksson M, Zetteretrom R: Severe neonatal asphyxia. Acta Paediatr Scand 72:321, 1983.

Finer NN, Robertson CM, Peters RN, et al: Factors affecting outcome in hypoxic ischemic encephalopathy in term infants. Am J Dis Child 137:21, 1983.

French CE, Waldstern G: Subcapsular hemorrhage of the liver in the newborn. Pediatrics 69:204, 1982.

Graham M, Trounce JQ, Levene MI, et al: Prediction of cerebral palsy in very low birth weight infants: Prospective ultrasound study. Lancet 2:593, 1987.

Gregory G: Resuscitation of the newborn. Anesthesiology 43:225, 1975.

Hall D: Birth asphyxia and cerebral palsy. Br Med J 299:279, 1989.

Hayden CK, Shattuck KE, Richardson CJ, et al: Subependymal germinal matrix hemorrhage in full-term neonates. Pediatrics 75:714, 1985.

Hill A, Volpe J: Perinatal asphyxia. Clinical aspects. Clin Perinatol 16:435, 1989.

Kreusser KL, Tarby TJ, Kovmar E, et al: Serial lumbar punctures for at least temporary amelioration of neonatal posthemorrhagic hydrocephalus. Pediatrics 75:719, 1985.

Lees M, King D: Cyanosis in the newborn. Pediatr Rev 9:36, 1987.

Mangurten HH: Birth injuries. *In* Fanaroff A, Martin R (eds): Behrman's Neonatal-Perinatal Medicine. St Louis, CV Mosby, 1987.

Marrin M, Paes BA: Birth asphyxia: Does the Apgar score have diagnostic value? Obstet Gynecol 72:120, 1988.

McDonald MM, Koops, BL, Johnson ML, et al: Timing and antecedents of intracranial hemorrhage in the newborn. Pediatrics 74:32, 1984.

Mulligan J, Painter M, O'Donoghue P, et al: Neonatal asphyxia. II: Neonatal mortality and long term sequelae. J Pediatr 96:903, 1980.

Perlman JM, Tack ED, Martin T, et al: Acute systemic organ injury in term infants after asphyxia. Am J Dis Child 143:617, 1989.

Ruth VJ, Raivio KO: Perinatal brain damage: Predictive value of metabolic acidosis and the Apgar score. Br Med J 297:24, 1988.

Sarnat HB, Sarnat MS: Neonatal encephalopathy following fetal distress. A clinical and electroencephalographic study. Arch Neurol 33:696, 1976.

Silverman SH, Liebow SG: Dislocation of the triangular cartilage of the nasal septum. J Pediatr 87:456, 1975.

Tzipora D, Skidmore MB, Fong KW, et al: Incidence, severity, and timing of subependymal and intraventricular hemorrhages in preterm infants born in a perinatal unit as detected by serial real-time ultrasound. Pediatrics 71:541, 1983.

Vohr BR, Garcia-Coll C, Mayfield S, et al: Neurologic and developmental status related to the evolution of visual-motor abnormalities from birth to 2 years of age in preterm infants with intraventricular hemorrhage. J Pediatr 115:296, 1989.

Volpe J: Intraventricular hemorrhage and brain injury in the premature infant. Neuropathology and pathogenesis. Clin Perinatol 16:361, 1989.

Volpe JJ: Neonatal seizures: Current concepts and revised classification. Pediatrics 84:422, 1989.

Zelson C, Lee SJ, Pearl M: The incidence of skull fractures underlying cephalhematomas in newborn infants. J Pediatr 85:371, 1974.

DISTURBANCES OF ORGAN SYSTEMS

RESPIRATORY TRACT

Disturbances of respiration in the immediate postnatal period may have originated in utero, in the delivery room, or in the nursery. A wide variety of pathologic lesions may be responsible for one or more of the signs of respiratory distress (see Tables 9–21 and 9–22); cyanosis is common and, if respiratory embarrassment is severe, pallor may also be present. It is occasionally very difficult to distinguish cardiovascular from respiratory disturbances on the basis of clinical signs alone. Signs of respiratory distress in the newborn infant may suggest hyaline membrane disease (respiratory distress syndrome), aspiration syndrome, pneumonia, sepsis, congenital heart disease, congestive heart failure, choanal atresia, hypoglycemia, hypoplasia of the mandible with posterior displacement of the tongue, macroglossia, malformation of the epiglottis, malformation or injury of the larynx, cysts or neoplasms of the larynx or chest, pneumothorax, lobar emphysema, pulmonary agenesis or hypoplasia, congenital pulmonary lymphangiectasis, Wilson-Mikity syndrome, tracheoesophageal fistula, avulsion of the phrenic nerve, hernia or eventration of the diaphragm, intracranial lesions, neuromuscular disorders, and metabolic disturbances. *Any sign of postnatal respiratory distress is an indication for a roentgenogram of the chest.*

9.30 TRANSITION TO PULMONARY RESPIRATION

The establishment of adequate lung function at birth is related to gestational age or maturity. Fluid filling the fetal lung must be removed, gas-containing functional residual capacity (FRC) established and maintained, and a ventilation-perfusion relationship developed that will provide optimal exchange of oxygen and carbon dioxide between alveoli and blood (Sec. 14.3, 14.6, 14.14).

THE FIRST BREATH. During vaginal delivery intermittent compression of the thorax facilitates removal of lung fluid. Surfactant in the fluid enhances aeration of the gas-free lung by reducing surface tension, thereby lowering the pressure required to open alveoli. Nevertheless, the pressures required to inflate the airless lung are higher than those needed at any other period of life; they range from 10–50 cm of H_2O for 0.5- to 1.0-sec intervals compared with about 4 cm for normal breathing in term infants and adults. Most infants require the lower range of opening pressures. Higher pressures necessary to initiate respiration are required to overcome the opposing forces of surface tension (particularly in small airways) and the viscosity of liquid remaining in the airways, as well as to introduce about 50 mL of air into the lungs, 20–30 mL of which remains after the first breath to establish the FRC. Most of the liquid in the lung is removed by the pulmonary circulation, which increases many fold at birth because all of the right ventricular output perfuses the pulmonary vascular bed. The remainder of the fluid is removed by the pulmonary lymphatics, expelled by the infant, swallowed, or aspirated from the oropharynx; removal may be impaired following cesarean section or neonatal sedation.

The stimuli responsible for the first breath are multiple, and their relative importance is uncertain. They include a fall in Po_2 and pH and a rise in Pco_2 due to the interruption of the placental circulation, a redistribution of cardiac output after the umbilical cord is clamped, a decrease in body temperature, and a variety of tactile stimuli.

Compared with the term infant, the LBW infant who has a very compliant chest wall may be at a disadvantage in accomplishing the first breath. The FRC is least in the most immature infants, reflecting the presence of atelectasis. Abnormalities in the ventilation-perfusion ratio are greater and persist for longer periods of time, as does gas trapping. There may be a low Pao_2 (50–60 mm Hg; 6.6–7.9 kPa) and elevated $Paco_2$, reflecting atelectasis, intrapulmonary shunting, and hypoventilation. The smallest immature infants have the most profound disturbances, which may resemble respiratory distress syndrome.

BREATHING PATTERNS IN NEWBORNS. During sleep in the first months of life, normal full-term infants may have infrequent episodes when regular breathing is interrupted with short pauses. This **periodic breathing** pattern, shifting from a regular rhythmicity to cyclic brief episodes of intermittent apnea, is more common in the premature infant, who may have apneic pauses of 5–10 sec followed by a burst of rapid respirations at a rate of 50–60/min for 10–15 sec. There is rarely an associated change in color or heart rate, and it often stops without apparent reason. Periodic breathing persists intermittently usually until premature infants are about 36 wk of gestational age. If the infant is hypoxic, an increase in inspired oxygen concentration will often convert periodic to regular breathing. Transfusion of packed red blood cells or external physical stimulation may also reduce the number of apneic episodes. There is no prognostic significance to periodic breathing, a normal characteristic of neonatal respiration.

9.31 APNEA

Periodic breathing must be distinguished from prolonged apneic pauses, since the latter are associated with serious illnesses. Apnea is due to many primary diseases that affect the neonate (see Table 9–18). Such disorders produce direct depression of the central nervous system's control of respiration (e.g., hypoglycemia, meningitis, drugs, hemorrhage), disturbances of oxygen delivery by perfusion (shock, sepsis, anemia), or ventilation defects (pneumonia, hyaline membrane disease, persistence of fetal circulation).

Idiopathic apnea of prematurity occurs in the absence of identifiable predisposing diseases and may be due to upper airway obstruction (pharyngeal instability, neck flexion, nasal occlusion) characterized by absent air flow but persistent chest wall movement. Pharyngeal collapse may follow negative airway pressures generated during inspiration, or it may result from incoordination of the tongue and other upper airway muscles involved in maintaining airway patency. Apnea of prematurity may also be due to a decrease of *gestational age dependent reduced* central nervous system stimulus to the respiratory muscles characterized by simultaneous absent air flow and chest wall movement. This immaturity of the brain stem respiratory centers is manifest by an attenuated response to carbon dioxide and a paradoxical response to hypoxia, resulting in apnea rather than hyperventilation. The most common pattern of idiopathic apnea among preterm neonates has a mixed etiology, with obstructive apnea preceding (usually) or following central apnea. Short apneas are usually central, whereas apneas of 15 sec or more are often mixed.

Apnea is sleep state dependent; the frequency increases during active (REM) sleep. Paradoxical chest wall movement (inspiratory abdominal expansion and inward chest wall movement) is common during active sleep and may cause a fall in Pao_2 due to ventilation-perfusion defects. Furthermore, increased negative pressure during paradoxical breathing and inhibition of pharyngeal muscle tone during active sleep may contribute to upper airway collapse and obstructive apnea.

CLINICAL MANIFESTATIONS. The incidence of idiopathic apnea of prematurity varies inversely with gestational age. In preterm infants it is rare on the 1st day of life; apnea immediately after birth signifies another illness. The onset of idiopathic apnea occurs on the 2nd–7th day of life. The sudden onset of apnea in a previously well neonate after the 2nd wk of life is a critical event that warrants immediate investigation. In preterm infants serious apnea is defined as cessation of breathing for longer than 10–15 sec. The incidence of associated bradycardia increases with the length of the preceding apnea and correlates with the severity of hypoxia. Short apneas (10 sec) are rarely associated with bradycardia, whereas longer apneas (> 20 sec) have a higher incidence of bradycardia. Bradycardia is associated with apnea in more than 95% of cases; vagal responses and, rarely, heart block are causes of bradycardia without apnea.

TREATMENT. Infants at risk for apnea should be monitored with apnea monitors. Gentle *cutaneous stimulation* is often adequate therapy for the neonatal infant having mild and intermittent episodes. Infants having recurrent and prolonged apnea require immediate *bag and mask ventilation*. *Oxygen* should be administered to treat hypoxia. Apnea of prematurity not due to a precipitating identifiable cause should be treated with *theophylline*. Methylxanthines enhance ventilation through a central mechanism or by improving diaphragmatic strength. Loading doses of 5 mg/kg should be followed by doses of 1–2 mg/kg given every 8–12 hr using oral or intravenous routes. These doses should be monitored by observation of vital signs, clinical response, and serum drug levels (therapeutic levels: theophylline, 5–10 μg/mL; caffeine, 8–20 μg/mL). *Transfusion of packed red blood cells also* may reduce the incidence of idiopathic apnea among anemic infants.

Nasal continuous positive airway pressure (CPAP, 3–5 cm H_2O) is effective therapy for mixed or obstructive apneas. CPAP may splint the upper airway, preventing obstruction. When apnea is due to a precipitating illness, airway stability and oxygenation must be maintained in addition to the therapy of the underlying disease.

PROGNOSIS. Unless severe, recurrent, and refractory to therapy, apnea of prematurity does not alter the infant's prognosis. Associated problems of intraventricular hemorrhage, bronchopulmonary dysplasia, and retinopathy of prematurity are critical in determining the prognosis of apneic infants. Apnea of prematurity usually resolves by 36 wk postconceptional age (gestational age at birth plus postnatal age) and does not predict future episodes of sudden infant death syndrome.

Aranda J, Turmen T: Methylxanthines in apnea of prematurity. Clin Perinatol 6:87, 1979.
Gerhardt T, Bancalari E: Apnea of prematurity. 1: Lung function and regulation of breathing. Pediatrics 74:58, 1984.
Gerhardt T, Bancalari E: Apnea of prematurity. 2: Respiratory reflexes. Pediatrics 74:63, 1984.
Kattwinkel J: Neonatal apnea: Pathogenesis and therapy. J Pediatr 90:342, 1977.
Martin RJ, Miller MJ, Carlo WA: Pathogenesis of apnea in preterm infants. J Pediatr 109:733, 1986.
Miller, MJ, Carlo WA, Martin RJ: Continuous positive airway pressure selectively reduces obstructive apnea in preterm infants. J Pediatr 106:91, 1985.
Southall, Richards JM, Rhoden KJ: Prolonged apnea and cardiac arrhythmias in infants discharged from neonatal intensive care units: Failure to predict an increased risk for SIDS. Pediatrics 70:844, 1982.

9.32 HYALINE MEMBRANE DISEASE (HMD)
(Respiratory Distress Syndrome, [RDS])

INCIDENCE. This condition is a major cause of death in the newborn period. An estimated 50% of all neonatal deaths result from hyaline membrane disease or its complications. The precise incidence is difficult to determine because of differing diagnostic criteria.

Hyaline membrane disease occurs primarily in premature infants; incidence is inversely proportional to the gestational age and birthweight. It occurs in 60–80% of infants less than 28 wk of gestational age, in 15–30% of those between 32 and 36 wk, in about 5% beyond 37 wk, and rarely at term. An increased frequency is associated with infants of diabetic mothers, delivery before 37 wk gestation, multiple pregnancies, cesarean section delivery, precipitous delivery, asphyxia, cold stress, and a history of prior affected infants.

ETIOLOGY AND PATHOPHYSIOLOGY. The failure to develop a functional residual capacity (FRC) and the tendency of affected lungs to become atelectatic correlate with high surface tensions and the absence of surfactant. The major constituents of surfactant are dipalmitylphosphatidylcholine (lecithin), phosphatidylglycerol, apoproteins (surfactant proteins: SP–A, B, C), and cholesterol. With progressive gestational age increasing amounts of phospholipids are synthesized and stored in type II alveolar cells. These active agents are released into the alveoli, reducing the surface tension and helping to maintain alveolar stability by preventing the collapse of small air spaces at end-expiration. However, the amounts produced or released may be insufficient to meet postnatal demands because of immaturity. Surfactant is present in high concentrations in fetal lung homogenates by 20 wk of gestation but does not reach the surface of the lung until later. It appears in the amniotic fluid between 28 and 32 wk. Mature levels of pulmonary surfactant are usually present after 35 wk.

Surfactant synthesis depends in part on normal pH, temperature, and perfusion. Asphyxia, hypoxemia, and pulmonary ischemia, particularly in association with hypovolemia, hypotension, and cold stress, may suppress surfactant synthesis. The epithelial lining of the lung may also be injured by high oxygen concentrations and the effects of respirator management, resulting in further reduction in surfactant.

Alveolar atelectasis, hyaline membrane formation, and interstitial edema make the lungs less compliant, requiring greater pressure to expand the small alveoli and airways. In these infants, the lower chest wall is pulled in as the diaphragm descends and the intrathoracic pressure becomes negative, thus limiting the amount of intrathoracic pressure that can be produced; the result is a tendency to atelectasis. The highly compliant chest wall of the preterm infant offers less resistance than that of the mature infant against the natural tendency of the lungs to collapse. Thus, at end-expiration, the volume of the thorax and lungs tends to approach the residual volume, leading to atelectasis.

Deficient synthesis or release of surfactant, together with small respiratory units and compliant chest wall, produces atelectasis, resulting in perfused but not ventilated alveoli, which causes hypoxia. Decreased lung compliance, small tidal volumes, increased physiologic dead space, increased work of breathing, and insufficient alveolar ventilation eventually results in hypercarbia. The combination of hypercarbia, hypoxia, and acidosis produces pulmonary arterial vasoconstriction with increased right to left shunting through the foramen ovale, ductus arteriosus, and within the lung itself. Pulmonary blood flow is reduced, and ischemic injury to the cells producing surfactant and to the vascular bed results in an effusion of proteinaceous material into the alveolar spaces (Fig. 9–16).

PATHOLOGY. The lungs appear deep purplish red and are liver-like in consistency. Microscopically, there is extensive atelectasis with engorgement of the interalveolar capillaries and lymphatics. A number of the alveolar ducts, alveoli, and respiratory bronchioles are lined with acidophilic, homogeneous, or granular membranes. Amniotic debris, intra-alveolar hemorrhage, and interstitial emphysema are additional but inconstant findings; interstitial emphysema may be marked when an infant has been ventilated with positive end-expiratory pressure. The characteristic hyaline membranes are rarely seen in infants dying earlier than 6–8 hr after birth.

CLINICAL MANIFESTATIONS. Signs of hyaline membrane disease usually appear within minutes of birth, although they may not be recognized for several hours until rapid, shallow respirations have increased to 60 or more/min. The late onset of tachypnea should suggest other conditions. Some patients require resuscitation at birth because of intrapartum asphyxia or initial severe respiratory distress (when birthweight is less than 1,000 g). Characteristically, tachypnea, prominent (often audible) grunting, intercostal and subcostal retractions, nasal flaring, and duskiness are seen. There is increasing cyanosis, which is often relatively unresponsive to oxygen administration. Breath sounds may be normal or diminished with a harsh tubular quality, and, on deep inspiration, fine rales may be heard, especially over the lung bases posteriorly. The natural course is characterized by progressive worsening of signs of air hunger and dyspnea. If inadequately treated, blood pressure and body temperature may fall; fatigue, cyanosis, and pallor increase, and grunting decreases or disappears as the condition worsens. Apnea and irregular respirations occur as infants tire and are ominous signs requiring immediate intervention. There may also be a mixed respiratory-metabolic acidosis, edema, ileus, and oliguria. Signs of asphyxia secondary to apnea or partial respiratory failure occur when there is rapid progression of the disease. The condition may progress to death in severely affected infants, but in milder cases the symptoms and signs may reach a peak within 3 days, after which gradual improvement sets in. Improvement is often heralded by a spontaneous diuresis and the ability to oxygenate the infant with lower inspired oxygen levels. Death is rare on the 1st day of illness, usually occurs between day 2 and 7, and is associated with alveolar air leaks (interstitial emphysema, pneumothorax), or intraventricular hemorrhage. Mortality may be delayed weeks or months if bronchopulmonary dysplasia (BPD) develops in mechanically ventilated infants with severe hyaline membrane disease.

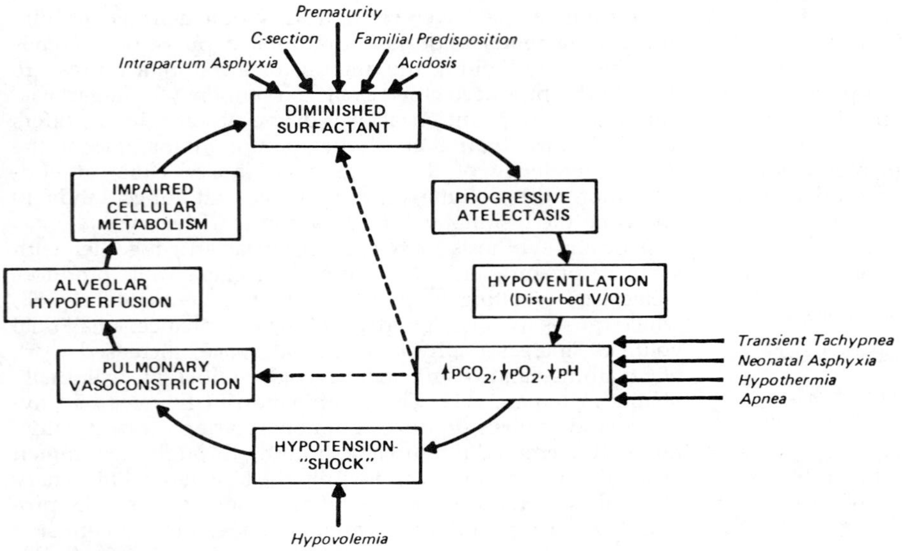

Figure 9–16. Contributing factors in the pathogenesis of hyaline membrane disease. Potential "vicious circle" perpetuating hypoxia and pulmonary insufficiency. (From Farrell P, Zachman R. *In*: Quilligan EJ, Kretchmer N [eds]: Fetal and Maternal Medicine. © 1980. Reprinted by permission of John Wiley & Sons, Inc.)

DIAGNOSIS. The clinical course, roentgenogram of the chest, and blood gas and acid-base values help to establish the clinical diagnosis. Roentgenographically, the lungs may have a characteristic but not pathognomonic appearance, which includes a fine reticular granularity of the parenchyma and air bronchograms that are often more prominent early in the left lower lobe because of the superimposition of the cardiac shadow (Fig. 9–17). Occasionally, the initial roentgenogram is normal, only to develop the typical pattern at 6–12 hr. There may be considerable variation among films, depending on the phase of respiration and the use of CPAP, often resulting in poor correlation between the roentgenograms and clinical course. The laboratory findings are characterized initially by hypoxemia and later by progressive hypoxemia, hypercarbia, and variable metabolic acidosis.

In the *differential diagnosis,* group B streptococcal sepsis may be indistinguishable from hyaline membrane disease. In pneumonia presenting at birth, the chest roentgenogram may be identical to that for hyaline membrane disease; gram-positive cocci in the gastric or tracheal aspirates and buffy coat smear, a positive test of urine for streptococcal antigen, and the presence of marked neutropenia may suggest this diagnosis. Cyanotic heart disease (e.g., total anomalous pulmonary venous return), persistent fetal circulation, aspiration syndromes, spontaneous pneumothorax, pleural effusions, diaphragmatic eventration, and congenital anomalies such as cystic adenomatoid malformation, pulmonary lymphangiectasia, diaphagmatic hernia, or lobar emphysema must be considered and require roentgenographic evaluation. Transient tachypnea may be distinguished by its short and mild clinical course.

PREVENTION. Most important are the prevention of prematurity, including avoidance of unnecessary or poorly timed cesarean section, appropriate management of the high-risk pregnancy and labor, and the prediction and possible in utero treatment of pulmonary immaturity (Sec. 9.14). In timing cesarean section or inducing labor, estimation of the fetal head circumference by ultrasound and determination of the lecithin concentration in the amniotic fluid by the lecithin to sphingomyelin (L/S) ratio decrease the likelihood of delivering a premature infant. Intrauterine antenatal and intrapartum monitoring may similarly decrease the risk of fetal asphyxia, which is associated with an increased incidence and severity of hyaline membrane disease.

The administration of a synthetic corticosteroid to women who do not have toxemia, diabetes, or renal disease 48–72 hr before delivery of fetuses at 32 wk or less of gestation significantly reduces the incidence and mortality from hyaline membrane disease. It may thus be appropriate to administer 1–2 doses of betamethasone intramuscularly to pregnant women whose lecithin in amniotic fluid indicates fetal lung immaturity and who are likely to deliver in 48–72 hr or whose labor can be delayed 48 hr or more.

Administration of one dose of surfactant into the trachea of premature infants immediately after birth or during the first 24 hr of life may not reduce the mortality from hyaline membrane disease or the incidence of BPD but does transiently improve pulmonary function.

TREATMENT. The basic defect requiring treatment is inadequate pulmonary exchange of oxygen and carbon dioxide; metabolic acidosis and circulatory insufficiency are secondary manifestations. Early supportive care of the low birthweight infant, especially in the treatment of acidosis, hypoxia, hypotension, and hypothermia, appears to lessen the severity of hyaline membrane disease. Therapy requires careful and frequent monitoring of heart and respiratory rates, arterial P_{O_2}, P_{CO_2}, pH, bicarbonate, electrolytes, blood glucose, hematocrit, blood pressure, and temperature. Umbilical artery catheterization is frequently necessary. Since most cases of hyaline membrane disease are self-limiting, the goal of treatment is to minimize abnormal physiologic variations and superimposed iatrogenic problems. The management of these infants is best carried out in a specially staffed and equipped hospital unit, the neonatal intensive care nursery.

The general principles for supportive care of any LBW infant should be adhered to, including gentle handling and minimal disturbance consistent with management. To avoid chilling and to minimize oxygen consumption, infants should be placed in an Isolette and core temperature maintained between 36.5 and 37° C (Sec. 9.17). Calories and fluids should be provided intravenously. For the first 24 hr, 10% glucose and water should be infused through a peripheral vein at a rate of 65–75 mL/kg/24 hr. Subsequently, electrolytes should be added and fluid volumes increased gradually to 120–150 mL/kg/24 hr (Sec. 9.17). Excessive fluids contribute to the development of a patent ductus arteriosus (PDA).

Warm humidified oxygen should be provided at a concentration sufficient initially to keep arterial levels between 55 and 70 mm Hg with stable vital signs to maintain normal tissue oxygenation while minimizing the risk of oxygen toxicity. If the arterial oxygen tension cannot be maintained above 50 mm Hg (6.7 kPa) at inspired oxygen concentrations of 70%, applying *continuous positive airway pressure* (CPAP) at a pressure of 6–10 cm of H_2O by nasal prongs is indicated, which usually produces a sharp rise in arterial oxygen tension. Although the course may be protracted, the amount of pressure required usually decreases abruptly at about 72 hr of age, and the infant can be weaned from CPAP shortly thereafter. If an infant on CPAP cannot maintain an arterial oxygen tension above 50 mm Hg while breathing 100% oxygen, assisted ventilation is required.

Infants with severe hyaline membrane disease or those who develop complications resulting in persistent apnea require *assisted mechanical ventilation*. Reasonable indications for its use are (1) arterial blood pH of less than 7.20; (2) arterial blood P_{CO_2} of 60 mm Hg (7.9 kPa) or more; (3) arterial blood P_{O_2} of 50 mm Hg (6.7 kPa) or less at oxygen concentrations of 70–100%; or (4) persistent apnea. Assisted ventilation by constant positive-pressure with variable volume or a constant volume with a variable pressure **respirator** with a nasotracheal tube in place is widely used.

The goals of mechanical ventilation are to improve oxygenation and carbon dioxide elimination without causing excessive pulmonary barotrauma or oxygen toxicity. Acceptable ranges of blood gas values, balancing the risks of hypoxia and acidosis against those of mechanical ventilation, are Pa_{O_2} of 55–70 mm Hg (7.3–9.3 kPa); P_{CO_2} of 35–55 mm Hg (4.6–7.3 kPa); and pH of 7.25–7.45. During mechanical ventilation oxygenation is improved by increasing the Fi_{O_2} or the mean airway pressure. The latter can be increased by increasing the peak inspiratory pressure, gas flow, inspiratory to expiratory ratio, or positive end-expiratory pressure (PEEP). Excessive PEEP may cause a pneumothorax or impede venous return, reducing cardiac output despite improvement of Pa_{O_2} and thus decreasing oxygen delivery. PEEPs of 4–6 cm H_2O are usually safe and effective. Carbon dioxide elimination is achieved by increasing the peak inspiratory pressure (tidal volume) or the rate of the ventilator.

The rate ranges of conventional ventilators are 10–60 breaths/min; of high-frequency jet ventilation (HFJV), 150–600/min; and of oscillators, 300–1,800/min. HFJV and oscillators may improve carbon dioxide elimination, lower mean airway pressure, and occasionally improve oxygenation in patients not responding to conventional ventilators who have hyaline membrane disease, interstitial emphysema, multiple pneumothoraces, or meconium aspiration pneumonia. HFJV may cause necrotizing tracheal damage, especially in the presence of hypotension or poor humidification; and oscillator therapy has been associated with an increased risk of air leaks, interventricular hemorrhage, and periventricular leukomalacia. Both methods may cause gas trapping. Complications of endotracheal intubation (plugging of tube, extubation, subglottic granuloma, and stenosis) and mechanical ventilation (pneumothorax, interstitial emphysema, reduced

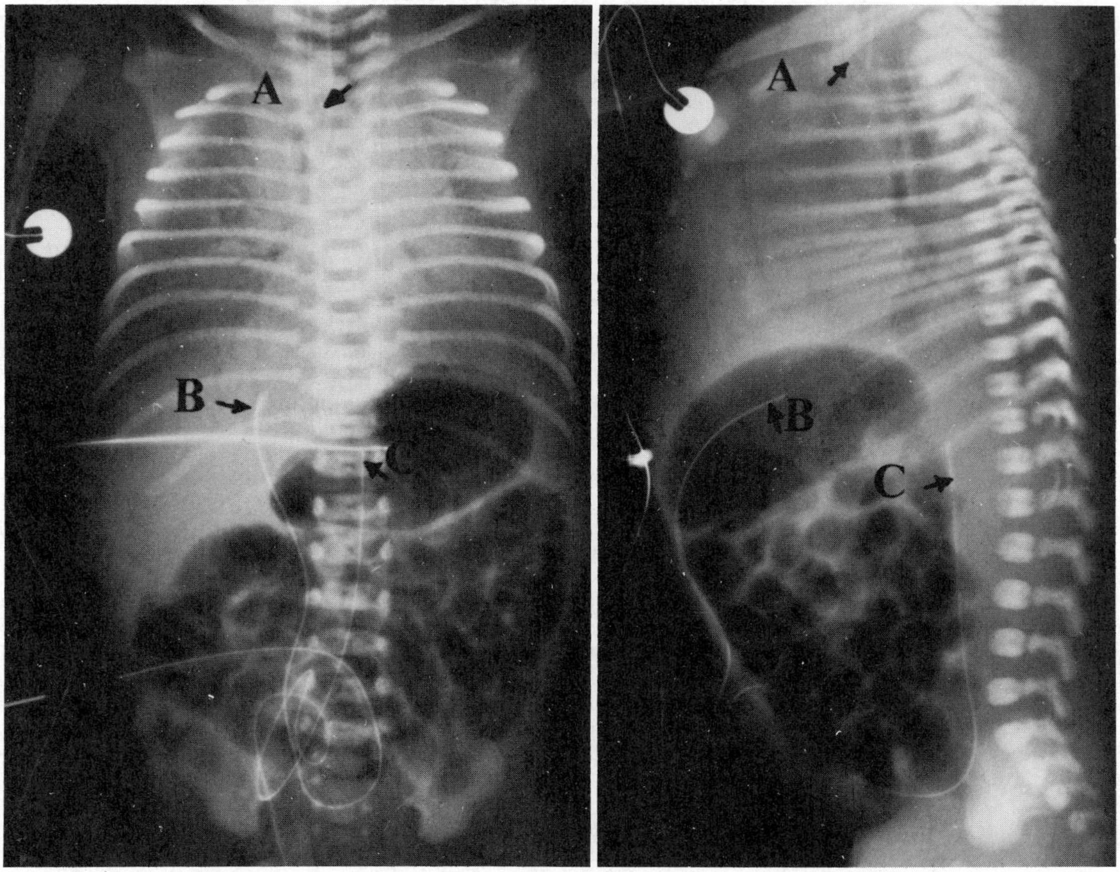

Figure 9–17. Infant with hyaline membrane disease. Note the granular lungs, air bronchogram, and air-filled esophagus. Anteroposterior *(A)* and lateral *(B)* roentgenograms are needed to distinguish umbilical artery from vein catheter and to determine appropriate level of insertion. The lateral view clearly identifies that the catheter has been inserted into an umbilical vein and is lying in the portal system of the liver. *A*, Endotracheal tube; *B*, umbilical venous catheter at the junction of the umbilical vein, ductus venosus, and portal vein; *C*, umbilical artery catheter passed up the aorta to T-12. (Courtesy of Walter E. Berdon, Babies Hospital, New York City.)

cardiac output) may be minimized by the interventions of specially trained physicians, nurses, and respiratory therapists in neonatal intensive care units.

Multidose endotracheal instillation of human amniotic fluid or bovine or artificial *surfactant* to LBW infants requiring 40% oxygen for the treatment of hyaline membrane disease has shown promise. Calf lung surfactant extract (CLSE) is an organic solvent of minced calf lung supplemented with dipalmitoylphosphatidylcholine (DPPC), palmitic acid, and tripalmitin. Artificial lung expanding compound (ALEC) contains DPPC and phosphatidylglycerol (in a ratio of 7:3); other preparations contain nonionic detergents and surfactant phospholipids. The short-term effects of surfactant replacement or "rescue" therapy include improved alveolar-arterial oxygen gradients, reduced mean airway pressure, reduced support from mechanical ventilation, increased pulmonary compliance, decreased incidence of pneumothorax, and improvement of the appearance of the chest roentgenogram. Single-dose surfactant has only a transient beneficial effect, and the incidence of bronchopulmonary dysplasia or death is not reduced. Multiple-dose surfactant given repeatedly may improve the prognosis of hyaline membrane disease.

Although controlled studies have not shown a decrease in mortality as a result of **correcting the acidosis** associated with hyaline membrane disease, the severity of the disease seems to be lessened, and the risks of pulmonary vasoconstriction, ventilation-perfusion abnormalities, untoward shunting through the foramen ovale or ductus arteriosus, hypotension, and arrhythmias are probably diminished. These risks are increased when acidosis is coupled with hypoxia.

Respiratory acidosis may require short-term or prolonged assisted ventilation. In severe respiratory acidosis and hypoxia, treatment with sodium bicarbonate may exacerbate hypercarbia.

Metabolic acidosis in hyaline membrane disease may be a result of perinatal asphyxia and hypotension and is often encountered when an infant has required resuscitation (Sec. 9.29). Sodium bicarbonate, 1–2 mEq/kg, may be administered for treatment over a 10- to 15-min period through a peripheral vein with the acid-base determination repeated within 30 min, or it may be administered over several hours. More often, sodium bicarbonate is administered rapidly on an emergency basis through an umbilical venous catheter. Alkali therapy may result in skin sloughs due to infiltration, increased serum osmolarity, hypernatremia, hypocalcemia, hypokalemia, and liver injury when concentrated solutions are administered rapidly through an umbilical vein.

Monitoring of *aortic blood pressure* through an umbilical arterial catheter or by oscillometric technique may be useful in managing the shock-like state that may occur during the 1st hour or so after premature birth of an infant who has been asphyxiated or who has developed respiratory distress (see Fig. 9–3). Radiopaque catheters should always be used and their position checked roentgenographically after insertion (see Fig. 9–17). The tip of an umbilical artery catheter should lie just above the bifurcation of the aorta (L3–L5) or above the celiac axis (T6–T10). Placement and supervision should be done by skilled and experienced personnel. Catheters should be removed as soon as there is no indication for their continued use, that is, when Pa_{O_2} is stable and the Fi_{O_2} is less than 40%.

Periodic monitoring of arterial oxygen and carbon dioxide tension and of pH is an important part of the management; if assisted ventilation is being used, it is essential. Blood should be obtained from the umbilical or peripheral artery. Temporal artery lines are contraindicated because of cerebral emboli. Tissue P_{O_2} may also be estimated continuously from transcutaneous electrodes or pulse oximetry (oxygen saturation). Capillary blood samples are of limited value for determining P_{O_2} but may be useful for evaluating P_{CO_2} and pH.

Owing to the difficulty of distinguishing some group B streptococcal or other infections from hyaline membrane disease, routinely administering antibacterial agents is indicated until the results of blood cultures are available. Penicillin or ampicillin with kanamycin or gentamicin is suggested, depending on the recent pattern of bacterial sensitivities in the hospital where the infant is being treated (Sec. 9.59 and 9.60).

COMPLICATIONS OF HYALINE MEMBRANE DISEASE AND INTENSIVE CARE. The most serious complications of **tracheal intubation** are asphyxia from obstruction of the tube, cardiac arrest during intubation or suctioning, and the subsequent development of subglottic stenosis. Other complications include bleeding from trauma during intubation, posterior pharyngeal pseudodiverticula, difficult extubation requiring tracheostomy, ulceration of the nares due to pressure from the tube, permanent narrowing of the nostril from tissue damage and scarring from irritation or infection around the tube, erosion of the palate, avulsion of a vocal cord, laryngeal ulcer, papilloma of a vocal cord, and persistent hoarseness, stridor, or edema of the larynx.

Measures to reduce the incidence of these complications include skillfully observing the infant; using polyvinyl endotracheal tubes that do not contain tin, which is toxic to cells; using a tube of the smallest practicable size to reduce local ischemia and pressure necrosis; avoiding frequent changes of the tube; avoiding motion of the tube in situ; avoiding too frequent or vigorous suctioning; and avoiding infection through meticulous cleanliness and frequent sterilization of all apparatus attached to or passed through the tube. The personnel inserting and caring for the endotracheal tube should be experienced and skilled.

The risks of **umbilical arterial catheterization** include vascular embolization, thrombosis, spasm, and perforation, ischemic or chemical necrosis of abdominal viscera; infection; accidental hemorrhage; and impaired circulation to a leg with subsequent gangrene. Although at necropsy the reported incidence of thrombotic complications varies from 1 to 23%, aortography has demonstrated that clots form in or about the tips of 95% of catheters placed in an umbilical artery. Aortic ultrasound can also be used to investigate the presence of thrombosis. The risk of a serious clinical complication resulting from umbilical catheterization is probably between 2 and 5%.

Transient blanching of the leg may occur during catheterization of the umbilical artery. It is usually due to reflex arterial spasm, the incidence of which is lessened by using the smallest available catheters, particularly in very small infants. The catheter should be removed immediately; catheterization of the other artery may then be attempted. Persistent spasm after removal of the catheter may be relieved by warming the opposite leg. Blood sampling from a radial artery may similarly result in spasm or thrombosis, and the same treatment is indicated. Intermittent severe spasm or unrelieved spasm may respond to the cautious local infusion of tolazoline (Priscoline), 1–2 mg injected intra-arterially over 5 min. Accidentally lodging the catheter in a smaller artery, either blocking it completely or causing unrecognized local vascular spasm, may result in gangrene of the organ or area supplied by the vessel. To prevent this complication, the catheter should be removed promptly if blood cannot be obtained through it.

Serious hemorrhage on removal of the catheter is rare. Thrombi may form in the artery or in the catheter; their incidence is lowered by using a smooth-tipped catheter with a hole only at its end, by rinsing the catheter with a small amount of saline solution containing heparin or by continuously infusing a solution containing 1–10 unit/mL of heparin. The risks of thrombus formation with potential vascular occlusion can also be reduced by removing the catheter when there are early signs of thrombosis, such as narrowing of pulse pressure and disappearance of the dicrotic notch. Some prefer to use the umbilical artery for blood sampling only, leaving the catheter filled with heparinized saline between samplings. Renovascular hypertension may occur days to weeks following umbilical arterial catheterization in a small number of neonates.

Umbilical vein catheterization is associated with many of the same risks as artery catheterization. In addition, there is an association with subsequent liver cirrhosis from portal vein thrombosis.

The toxicity to the retina from elevated concentrations of oxygen administered for prolonged periods has been amply demonstrated (Sec. 9.17).

Oxygen is toxic to the lung, particularly if administered by means of a positive-pressure respirator, resulting in **bronchopulmonary dysplasia** (BPD) (see also Sec. 9.38). Instead of showing improvement on the 3rd–4th day, consistent with the natural course in survivors, some infants who have been on prolonged intermittent positive-pressure breathing using increased concentrations of oxygen roentgenographically show a worsening of their pulmonary condition (Fig. 9–18*A*). Respiratory distress persists and is characterized by hypoxia, hypercarbia, oxygen dependency, and the development of right-sided heart failure. The chest roentgenogram is described as gradually changing from a picture of almost complete opacification with air bronchogram and interstitial emphysema to one of small, round, lucent areas alternating with areas of irregular density resembling a sponge (Fig. 9–18*B*). In the histologic picture at this stage (10–20 days after beginning oxygen therapy) there is less evidence of hyaline membrane formation, progressive alveolar coalescence with atelectasis of surrounding alveoli, interstitial edema, coarse focal thickening of the basement membrane, and widespread bronchial and bronchiolar mucosal metaplasia and hyperplasia. This corresponds with a severe maldistribution of ventilation. Most surviving neonates with persistent roentgenographic changes recover by 6–12 mo, but some require prolonged hospitalization and may have respiratory symptoms persisting through infancy. Right-sided heart failure and viral necrotizing bronchiolitis are major causes of death. Pathology reveals cardiac enlargement and pulmonary changes consisting of focal areas of emphysematous alveoli with hypertrophy of the peribronchial smooth muscle of the tributary bronchioles, some perimucosal fibrosis and widespread metaplasia of the bronchiolar mucosa, thickening of basement membranes, and separation of the capillaries from the alveolar epithelial cells.

Infants at risk for BPD have severe respiratory distress requiring prolonged periods of mechanical ventilation and oxygen therapy. Additional associations include the presence of pulmonary interstitial emphysema, lower gestational age, male sex, low P_{CO_2} at 48 hr, patent ductus arteriosus, high peak inspiratory pressure, increased airway resistance in the 1st wk of life, pulmonary infection with *Ureaplasma urealyticum,* and possibly a family history of asthma. Some VLBW infants without hyaline membrane disease who require me-

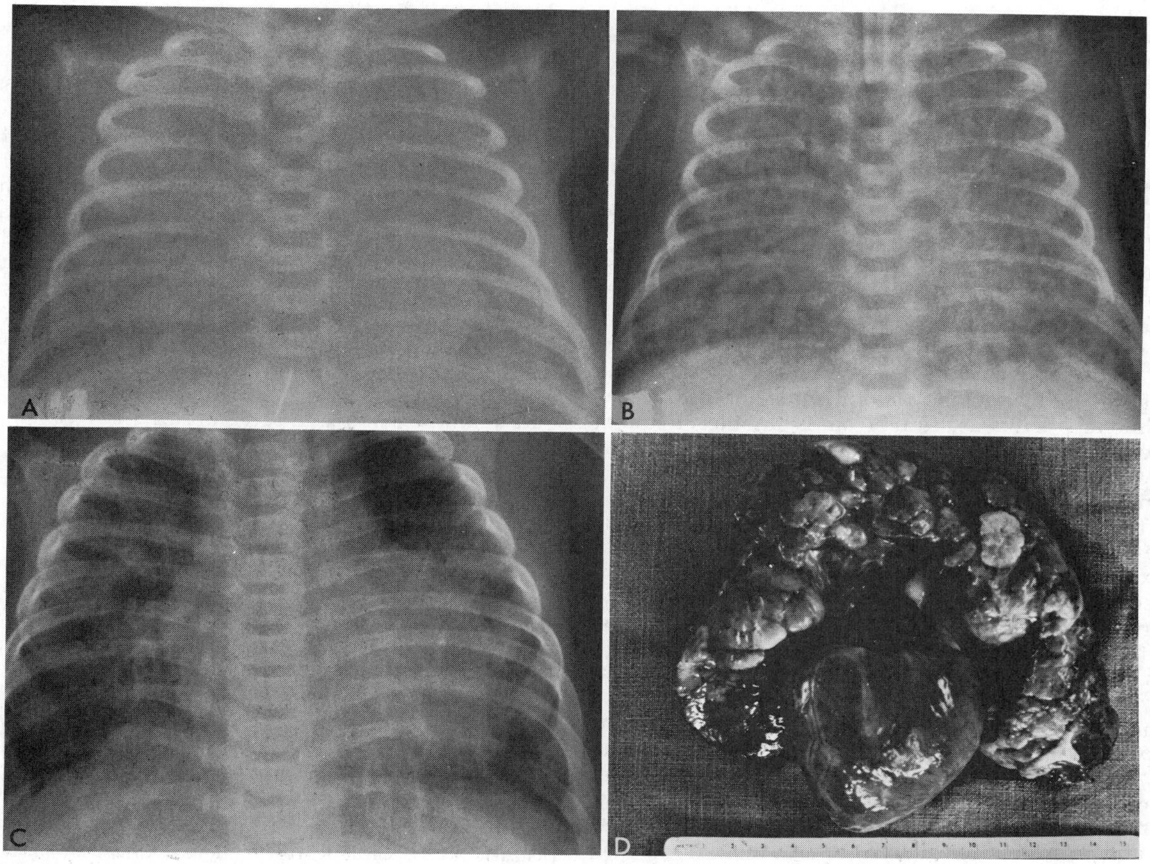

Figure 9–18. Pulmonary changes in infants who were treated in the immediate postnatal period for the clinical syndrome of hyaline membrane disease with prolonged, intermittent positive-pressure breathing with air containing 80 to 100% oxygen. *A,* A 5-day-old infant with nearly complete opacification of lungs. *B,* A 13-day-old infant with "bubbly lungs" simulating the roentgenographic appearance of the Wilson-Mikity syndrome. *C,* A 7-mo-old infant with irregular, dense strands in both lungs, hyperinflation, and cardiomegaly suggestive of BPD. *D,* Large right ventricle and cobbly irregularly aerated lung of an infant who died at 11 mo of age. This infant also had a patent ductus arteriosus. (From Northway WH Jr, Rosan RC, Porter DY: N Engl J Med 276:357, 1967. Reprinted with permission from The New England Journal of Medicine.)

chanical ventilation for apnea develop chronic lung disease that does not follow the classic pattern for BPD. Neonates who remain oxygen dependent and have the chronic chest roentgenographic changes described earlier by 28 days of life are considered to have BPD.

Severe BPD requires continued mechanical ventilation until weaning from the respirator becomes possible. Acceptable blood gas concentrations for a patient with BPD include P_{CO_2} of 50–70 mm Hg (6.7–9.3 kPa) (if pH > 7.30) and Pa_{O_2} of 55–60 mm Hg (7.3–8.0 kPa) with oxygen saturation of 90–95%. Lower levels of Pa_{O_2} may exacerbate pulmonary hypertension and produce cor pulmonale. Airway obstruction in BPD may be due to mucus and edema production, bronchospasm, and collapse of acquired tracheomalacia. These events may contribute to "blue spells." Alternatively, blue spells may be due to acute cor pulmonale or myocardial ischemia.

Treatment of BPD includes use of bronchodilators such as aerosolized β_2-adrenergic agents and theophylline, diuretics, fluid restriction, treatment of infections (*U. urealyticum*, respiratory syncytial virus), high–caloric density formula, CPAP for tracheomalacia, and dexamethasone. Dexamethasone, 0.5 mg/kg/24 hr given in two doses intravenously, is initiated after 2–6 wk of chronic lung disease. This dose is continued for 3 days and then is reduced to 0.3 mg/kg/24 hr for an additional 3 days. Thereafter, the dose is reduced by 10% every 3 days until it reaches 0.1 mg/kg/24 hr. This final dose is given every other day for 1 wk and then is discontinued. The use of steroids has improved the ability to wean patients from ventilators but increases the risk of hypertension and infection. Older infants may respond to vasodilator therapy with reduced pulmonary vascular resistance.

Complications of BPD include growth failure, transient psychomotor retardation, and parental stress, as well as such sequelae of therapy as nephrolithiasis (due to diuretics and total intravenous alimentation), osteopenia, and subglottic stenosis, which may require tracheotomy or an anterior cricoid split procedure to relieve upper airway obstruction.

Patients with BPD often go home on oxygen, diuretics, and bronchodilator therapy. The long-term *prognosis* is good for infants who have been weaned off oxygen prior to discharge from the intensive care unit. Prolonged ventilation, interventricular hemorrhage, pulmonary hypertension, cor pulmonale, and oxygen dependence beyond 1 yr of life are poor prognostic signs. Airway obstruction and hyperactivity and hyperinflation may be demonstrated in some adolescents.

Extrapulmonary extravasation of air is another frequent complication of the management of hyaline membrane disease (Sec. 9.37).

There may be clinically significant shunting through a **patent ductus arteriosus** (PDA) in some neonates with hyaline membrane disease, the delayed closure being due to associated hypoxia, acidosis, increased pulmonary pressure secondary to vasoconstriction, systemic hypotension, immaturity, and local release of prostaglandins, which dilate the ductus. This shunting may be bidirectional or right to left through the ductus arteriosus. As hyaline membrane disease resolves, pulmonary vascular resistance decreases, and there may be left to right shunting leading to left ventricular volume overload and pulmonary edema. The manifestations of PDA may include (1) persistent apnea for unexplained reasons in an infant recovering from hyaline membrane disease; (2) an active heaving precordium, bounding peripheral pulses, wide pulse pressure, and a systolic or to-and-fro murmur; (3) carbon dioxide retention; (4) increasing oxygen dependency; (5) roentgenographic evidence of cardiomegaly and increased pulmonary vascular markings; and (6) hepatomegaly. The diagnosis is confirmed by echocardiographic visualization of a patent ductus arteriosus with Doppler flow evidence of left to right shunting. Most infants respond to general supportive measures including diuretics and fluid restriction. In selected patients in whom spontaneous closure does not occur but in whom there is progressive deterioration despite supportive and cardiotonic treatment, indomethacin, 0.2 mg/kg at 12- to 24-hr intervals for 48 hr, may induce pharmacologic closure by inhibiting prostaglandin synthesis. An alternative protocol is 0.1 mg/kg/24 hr for 6 days; repeated courses of both protocols may be needed. Contraindications to indomethacin include thrombocytopenia (< 50,000/mm³), bleeding disorders, and elevated plasma creatinine level (> 1.8 mg/dL; 159 μmol/L). Indications for surgical closure are failure to close the ductus following indomethacin therapy with persistent heart failure and ventilator dependence.

Anemia secondary to frequent withdrawal of blood samples may also occur as a complication of intensive care. The cumulative amount of blood withdrawn should be carefully recorded. Some of its replacement by transfusion may be indicated if more than 10–15% of estimated total blood volume is removed or if there is a significant decrease in the hematocrit. Oxygen-dependent infants should have their hematocrit maintained close to 40%.

PROGNOSIS. Early provision of intensive observation and care to high-risk newborn infants can significantly reduce morbidity and mortality due to hyaline membrane disease and other acute neonatal illnesses. However, good results depend on the availability of experienced and skilled personnel, specially designed and organized regional hospital units, proper equipment, and lack of complications such as sever fetal or birth asphyxia, intracranial hemorrhage, or irremediable congenital malformation.

Overall mortality for low birthweight infants referred to intensive care centers is steadily declining; about 65% of those under 1,000 g survive, and the mortality progressively decreases at higher weights, with over 95% of sick infants weighing more than 2,500 g surviving. Although 85–90% of all infants surviving hyaline membrane disease after requiring ventilatory support with respirators are normal, the outlook is much better for those weighing above 1,500 g; about 80% of those under 1,500 g have no neurologic or mental sequelae. The long-term prognosis for normal pulmonary function in most infants surviving hyaline membrane disease is excellent.

Avery ME: The argument for prenatal administration of dexamethasone to prevent respiratory distress syndrome. J Pediatr 104:240, 1984.
Behrman RE: The use of acid-base measurements in clinical evaluation and treatment of the sick neonate. J Pediatr 74:632, 1969.
Carlo W, Martin R: Principles of neonatal assisted ventilation. Pediatr Clin North Am 33:221, 1986.
Coates AL, Desmond K, Willis D, et al: Oxygen therapy and long-term pulmonary outcome of respiratory distress syndrome in newborns. Am J Dis Child 136:892, 1982.
Cummings JJ, D'Uegenio DB, Gross SJ: A controlled trial of dexamethasone in preterm infants at high risk for bronchopulmonary dysplasia. N Engl J Med 320:1055, 1989.
Fiascone J, Rhodes T, Grondgeorge S, et al: Bronchopulmonary dysplasia. A review for pediatricians. Curr Probl Pediatr 29:171, 1989.
Gluck L, Kulovich M: Lecithin-sphingomyelin ratios in amniotic fluid in normal and abnormal pregnancy. Am J Obstet Gynecol 115:539, 1973.
Green TP, Thompson TR, Johnson DE, et al: Diuresis and pulmonary function in premature infants with respiratory distress syndrome. J Pediatr 103:618, 1983.
Gregory G, Kitterman J, Phibbs R, et al: Treatment of the idiopathic respiratory distress syndrome with continuous positive airway pressure. N Engl J Med 284:1333, 1971.
Heldt GP, Mellroy MB, Hansen TN, et al: Exercise performance of survivors of hyaline membrane disease. J Pediatr 96:995, 1980.
Holtzman RG, Hageman JR, Yogev R: Role of *Ureaplasma urealyticum* in bronchopulmonary dysplasia. J Pediatr 114:1061, 1989.
Hyde I, English RE, Williams JD: The changing pattern of chronic lung disease of prematurity. Arch Dis Child 64:448, 1989.
Ingram D, Pendergrass E, Bromberger P, et al: Group B streptococcal disease. Am J Dis Child 134:754, 1980.
Jacob J, Edwards D, Gluck L: Early onset sepsis and pneumonia observed as respiratory distress syndrome. Am J Dis Child 134:766, 1980.

Kraybill EN, Runyan DK, Bose CL, et al: Risk factors for chronic lung disease in infants with birth weights of 751 to 1000 grams. J Pediatr 115:115, 1989.
Merritt TA, Hallman M: Surfactant replacement. A new era with many challenges for neonatal medicine. Am J Dis Child 142:1333, 1988.
Milner AD, Hoskyns EW: High frequency positive pressure ventilation in neonates. Arch Dis Child 64:1, 1989.
Northway WH, Rosan RC, Porter DB: Pulmonary disease following respiratory therapy. N Engl J Med 276:357, 1967.
Northway WH Jr, Moss RB, Carlisle KB, et al: Late pulmonary sequelae of bronchopulmonary dysplasia. N Engl J Med 323:1793, 1990.
Robert MF, Neff RK, Hubbell JP, et al: Association between maternal diabetes and the respiratory distress syndrome in the newborn. N Engl J Med 294:357, 1976.
Shapiro D, Notter R: Controversies regarding surfactant replacement therapy. Clin Perinatol 15:891, 1988.
Shelly S, Kovacevic M, Paciga J, et al: Sequential changes of surfactant phosphatidylcholine in hyaline membrane disease of the newborn. N Engl J Med 300:112, 1979.
Stahlman M: Newborn intensive care: success or failure. J Pediatr 105:162, 1984.
Stahlman M, Hedvail G, Lindstrom D, et al: Role of hyaline membrane disease in production of later childhood lung abnormalities. Pediatrics 69:572, 1982.
Stocker JT, Madewell JE: Persistent interstitial pulmonary emphysema: Another complication of the respiratory distress syndrome. Pediatrics 59:847, 1977.
The HIFI Study Group: High-frequency oscillatory ventilation compared with conventional mechanical ventilation in the treatment of respiratory failure in preterm infants. N Engl J Med 320:88, 1989.
Thibeault DW, Emmanoulides GC, Nelson RJ, et al: Patent ductus arteriosus complicating the respiratory distress syndrome in preterm infants. J Pediatr 86:120, 1975.

9.33 TRANSIENT TACHYPNEA OF THE NEWBORN

Transient tachypnea, occasionally called **respiratory distress syndrome type II,** usually follows uneventful normal preterm or term vaginal delivery or cesarean delivery. It may be characterized only by the early onset of tachypnea, sometimes with retractions, or expiratory grunting and, occasionally, cyanosis that is relieved by minimal oxygen. Patients usually recover rapidly within 3 days, although they may rarely appear severely ill and have a more protracted course. The lungs are usually clear without rales or rhonchi, and the chest roentgenogram shows prominent pulmonary vascular markings, fluid lines in the fissures, overaeration, flat diaphragms, and, occasionally, pleural fluid. Hypoxemia, hypercapnia, and acidosis are uncommon. Distinguishing the disease from hyaline membrane disease may be very difficult; the distinctive features of transient tachypnea are the infant's sudden recovery and the absence of a roentgenographic reticulogranular pattern on air bronchography. The syndrome is believed to be secondary to slow absorption of fetal lung fluid resulting in decreased pulmonary compliance and tidal volume and increased dead space.

Avery ME, Gatewood OB, Brumley G: Transient tachypnea of newborn. Possible delayed reabsorption of fluid at birth. Am J Dis Child 111:380, 1966.
Gross TL, Sokol RJ, Kwong MS, et al: Transient tachypnea of the newborn: The relationship to preterm delivery and significant neonatal morbidity. Am J Obstet Gynecol 146:236, 1983.
Sundell H, Garrott J, Blankenship WJ, et al: Studies on infants with type II respiratory distress syndrome. J Pediatr 78:754, 1971.

9.34 ASPIRATION OF FOREIGN MATERIAL
(Fetal Aspiration Syndrome; Aspiration Pneumonia)

During prolonged labors and difficult deliveries, infants often initiate vigorous respiratory movements in utero because of interference with the supply of oxygen through the placenta. Under such circumstances the infant may aspirate amniotic fluid containing vernix caseosa, epithelial cells, meconium, or material from the birth canal, which may block the smallest airways and interfere with alveolar exchange of oxygen and carbon dioxide. Pathogenic bacteria accompany the aspirated material, and pneumonia may ensue, but even in the noninfected cases respiratory distress accompanied by roentgenographic evidences of aspiration is seen (Fig. 9–19).

Pulmonary aspiration of foreign material may also occur in the newborn infant because of tracheoesophageal fistula, esophageal and duodenal obstructions, gastroesophageal reflux, improper feeding practices, and administration of depressant medicines.

The contents of the stomach should be aspirated through a soft rubber catheter just before operation or other procedures that require anesthesia or significantly disturb an infant. Once aspiration has occurred, treatment consists of general and respiratory support and treatment of pneumonia (Sec. 9.60 and 9.65).

Goodwin SR, Graves SA, Haberkern CM: Aspiration in intubated premature infants. Pediatrics 75:85, 1985.

9.35 MECONIUM ASPIRATION

Meconium-stained amniotic fluid is seen in 5–15% of births, but this syndrome usually occurs in term or post-term infants. Usually, but not invariably, fetal distress and hypoxia occur with passage of meconium into the amniotic fluid. These infants are meconium stained and may be depressed and require resuscitation at birth.

CLINICAL MANIFESTATIONS. Either in utero or more often with the first breath, thick meconium is aspirated into the lungs. The resulting small airway obstruction may produce respiratory distress within the first hours with tachypnea, retraction, grunting, and cyanosis in severely affected infants. Partial obstruction of some airways may lead to pneumothorax, pneumomediastinum, or both. Prompt treatment may

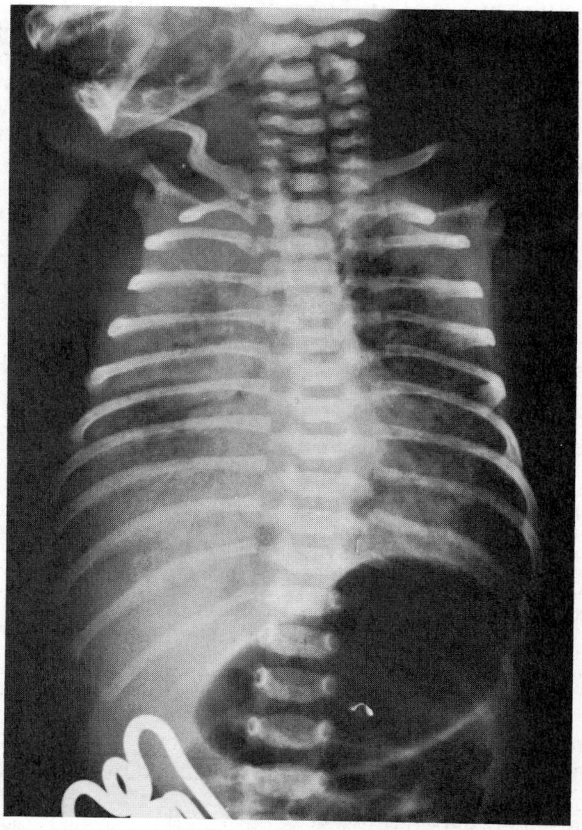

Figure 9–19. Fetal aspiration syndrome (aspiration pneumonia). Note the coarsely granular pattern with irregular aeration typical of fetal distress from aspiration of material, such as vernix caseosa, epithelial cells, and meconium contained in amniotic fluid.

delay the onset of respiratory distress, which may consist only of tachypnea without retractions. Overdistention of the chest may be prominent. The condition usually improves within 48 hr, but when its course requires assisted ventilation, it may be severe and its potential for mortality high. Tachypnea may persist for many days or even several weeks. The typical chest roentgenogram is characterized by patchy infiltrates, coarse streaking of both lung fields, increased anteroposterior diameter, and flattening of the diaphragm. A normal chest roentgenogram in an infant with severe hypoxia and no cardiac malformation suggests the diagnosis of persistent fetal circulation. Arterial Po_2 may be low in either disease, and if hypoxia has occurred, metabolic acidosis is usually present.

PREVENTION. The risk of meconium aspiration may be decreased by paying careful attention to fetal distress and initiating prompt delivery in the presence of fetal acidosis, late decelerations, or poor beat-to-beat variability. DeLee suctioning of the oropharynx after the head is delivered reduces the incidence of meconium aspiration.

TREATMENT. In the absence of fetal distress, a vigorous infant (Apgar score of 8 or more) can be born through thin meconium and may not require treatment. Depressed infants (those with hypotonia, bradycardia, or apnea) and those delivered through thick particulate (pea-soup) meconium-stained fluid should undergo endotracheal intubation, and suction should be applied directly to the endotracheal tube to remove meconium from the airway. The risks of laryngoscopy with endotracheal intubation (bradycardia, laryngospasm, hypoxia, posterior pharyngeal laceration with pseudodiverticulum formation) are less than the risks of meconium aspiration syndrome.

Treatment of meconium aspiration pneumonia includes supportive care and standard management for respiratory distress. The oxygenation benefit of PEEP must be weighed against the risk of pneumothorax. Severe meconium aspiration resembles persistent fetal circulation and requires similar treatment. Patients who are refractory to mechanical ventilation may benefit from extracorporeal membrane oxygenation (ECMO) (see Sec. 9.36).

PROGNOSIS. The mortality of meconium-stained infants is considerably higher than that of nonstained infants, and meconium aspiration accounts for a significant proportion of neonatal deaths. Residual lung problems are rare but include symptomatic cough, wheezing, and persistent hyperinflation for 5–10 yr. Ultimate prognosis depends on the extent of central nervous system injury from asphyxia and the presence of associated problems such as persistence of the fetal circulation.

American Heart Association: Textbook of Neonatal Resuscitation. 1987.
Anonymous: Lung function in children after neonatal meconium aspiration. Lancet 2:317, 1988.
Cunningham A, Lawson E, Martin R, et al: Tracheal suction and meconium: A proposed standard of care. J Pediatr 116:153, 1990.
Gregory GA, Gooding CA, Phibbs RH, et al: Meconium aspiration infants; a prospective study. J Pediatr 85:848, 1974.
Linder N, Aranda JV, Tsur M, et al: Need for endotracheal intubation and suction in meconium-stained neonates. J Pediatr 112:613, 1988.
Murphy JD, Vawter GF, Reid LM: Pulmonary vascular disease in fetal meconium aspiration. J Pediatr 104:758, 1984.
Sunno C, Kosasa TS, Hale RW: Meconium aspiration syndrome without evidence of fetal distress in early labor before elective cesarean delivery. Obstet Gynecol 73:707, 1989.

9.36 PERSISTENT FETAL CIRCULATION (PFC)

(Primary Pulmonary Hypertension of the Neonate: [PPHN])

PFC occurs in term and post-term infants following birth asphyxia, meconium aspiration pneumonia, group B streptococcal sepsis, hyaline membrane disease, hypoglycemia, polycythemia, and pulmonary hypoplasia due to diaphragmatic hernia, amniotic fluid leak, oligohydramnios, or pleural effusions. PFC is often idiopathic.

PATHOPHYSIOLOGY. Persistence of the fetal circulatory pattern of right to left shunting through the patent ductus arteriosus and foramen ovale after birth is due to an excessively high pulmonary vascular resistance. Fetal pulmonary vascular resistance is usually elevated relative to fetal systemic or postnatal pulmonary pressure. This fetal state permits shunting of oxygenated umbilical venous blood to the left atrium (and brain) through the foramen ovale and bypasses the lungs through the ductus arteriosus to the descending aorta. After birth, pulmonary vascular resistance normally declines rapidly as a consequence of vasodilation due to gas filling the lungs, a rise in postnatal Pao_2, a reduction in Pco_2, increased pH, and release of vasoactive substances. Increased neonatal pulmonary vascular resistance may be (1) maladaptive (e.g., not demonstrating normal vasodilation in response to increased oxygen and other changes after birth); (2) the result of increased pulmonary artery medial muscle thickness and extension of smooth muscle layers into the usually nonmuscular, more peripheral pulmonary arterioles in response to chronic fetal hypoxia; (3) due to alveolar capillary dysplasia or pulmonary hypoplasia (diaphragmatic hernia, Potter syndrome); and (4) obstructive due to polycythemia. Apart from the etiology profound hypoxia and normal or elevated Pco_2 are present.

CLINICAL MANIFESTATIONS. Infants become ill in the delivery room or within the first 12 hr of life. PFC due to polycythemia, idiopathic causes, hypoglycemia, or asphyxia may result in severe cyanosis with tachypnea, although initially there may be minimal signs of respiratory distress. Infants who have PFC associated with meconium aspiration, group B streptococcal pneumonia, diaphragmatic hernia, or pulmonary hypoplasia usually have cyanosis, grunting, flaring, retractions, tachycardia, and shock. Multiorgan involvement may be present (see Table 9–23). Myocardial ischemia, papillary muscle dysfunction with mitral and tricuspid regurgitation, and cardiac stun produce cardiogenic shock with decreased pulmonary blood flow, tissue perfusion, and oxygen delivery.

DIAGNOSIS. PFC should be suspected in all term infants with cyanosis with or without fetal distress, intrauterine growth retardation, meconium-stained amniotic fluid, hypoglycemia, polycythemia, diaphragmatic hernia, pleural effusions, and birth asphyxia. Hypoxia is universal and is unresponsive to 100% oxygen given by oxygen hood but may respond transiently to hyperoxic hyperventilation administered after endotracheal intubation or application of a bag and mask. A Pao_2 gradient between a preductal (right radial artery) and a postductal (umbilical artery) site of blood sampling greater than 20 mm Hg suggests right to left shunting through the ductus arteriosus and PFC. Real-time echocardiography combined with Doppler flow studies demonstrate right to left shunting across a patent foramen ovale and a ductus arteriosus. Deviation of the intra-atrial septum into the left atrium is seen in severe PFC. M-mode echocardiography demonstrates an elevated right ventricular pre-ejection period to right ventricular ejection time ratio (RVPEP/RVET > 0.50) because of longer pre-ejection and shorter ejection times due to increased pulmonary hypertension. Tricuspid or mitral insufficiency may be noted on auscultation as a holosystolic murmur and visualized ultrasonographically together with poor contractility when PFC is associated with myocardial ischemia. The second heart sound is accentuated and is not split. In asphyxia-associated and idiopathic PFC the chest roentgenogram is normal, whereas in PFC associated with pneumonia and diaphragmatic hernia it shows the specific lesions of parenchymal opacification and bowel in the chest, respectively. The *differential diagnosis* of PFC includes cyanotic heart disease (especially total anomalous pulmonary venous return) and the associated etiologic entities that predispose to PFC (e.g., hypoglycemia, polycythemia, sepsis).

TREATMENT. Therapy is directed toward correcting any predisposing disease (hypoglycemia, polycythemia) and improving poor tissue oxygenation. The response to therapy is often unpredictable, transient, and complicated by adverse effects of drugs or mechanical ventilation. Initial management includes oxygen administration and correction of acidosis, hypotension, and hypercarbia. Persistent hypoxia should be managed with intubation and mechanical ventilation.

One approach to treatment of severe PFC consists of instituting mechanical ventilation without pancuronium paralysis; ventilator settings are selected to achieve a Pa_{O_2} of 50–70 mm Hg (6.7–9.3 kPa) and a P_{CO_2} of 50–55 mm Hg (6.6–7.3 kPa). Tolazoline (1 mg/kg), a nonselective α–adrenergic antagonist, is used as an adjunct to vasodilate the pulmonary arterial system but also results in systemic hypotension, which is treated with volume expansion and dopamine. In another approach to treating severe PFC, hyperventilation is used to reduce pulmonary vasoconstriction by lowering P_{CO_2} (20–25 mm Hg) (2.7–3.3 kPa) and increasing pH (7.50–7.60). This requires high peak inspiratory pressures and rapid respiratory rates, often necessitating the use of pancuronium paralysis to control ventilation in order to achieve a Pa_{O_2} of between 90 and 100 mm Hg (12.0–13.3 kPa). Complications of hyperventilation include hyperinflation with reduced carbon dioxide elimination, reduced cardiac output, barotrauma, pneumothorax, decreased cerebral blood flow, increased fluid requirements, and edema resulting from pancuronium paralysis. Alkalination with sodium bicarbonate also has been used to elevate the plasma pH to induce pulmonary arterial vasodilation. Both methods of mechanical ventilation may be successful, and specific indications for one or the other have not been defined. Patients not responding to conventional ventilation may later respond to hyperventilation. Cardiogenic shock should be treated with inotropic agents such as dopamine and dobutamine.

Extracorporeal Membrane Oxygenation (ECMO). In 5–10% of patients with PFC there is a poor response to 100% oxygen, mechanical ventilation, and drugs. In such patients, the alveolar-arterial oxygen gradient or the oxygenation index, OI,

$$(\text{mean airway pressure} \times Fi_{O_2} \times 100) \div \text{Postductal } Pa_{O_2}$$

has been used to predict a greater than 80% mortality. AaD_{O_2} gradients of greater than 620 for 8–12 hr and an OI of more than 40 predict a high mortality and are indications for ECMO. ECMO has also been used to treat carefully selected severely ill infants who have hyaline membrane disease, meconium aspiration pneumonia, or group B streptococcal sepsis. ECMO is indicated in hypoxic patients with diaphragmatic hernia, especially when the ventilation index (rate × mean airway pressure) exceeds 1,000 and the P_{CO_2} exceeds 40 mm Hg.

ECMO is a form of cardiopulmonary bypass that augments systemic perfusion and provides gas exchange. Most experience has been with veno-arterial bypass, which requires placement of large catheters in the right internal jugular vein and carotid artery and necessitates carotid artery ligation. Veno-venous bypass avoids this ligation and provides gas exchange but does not support cardiac output. Blood is initially pumped through the ECMO circuit at a rate that approximates 80% of the estimated cardiac output of 150–200 mL/kg/min. Venous return passes through a membrane oxygenator, is warmed, and returns into the aortic arch. Venous oxygen saturations are used to monitor tissue oxygen delivery and subsequent extraction. The rate of ECMO flow is adjusted to achieve satisfactory venous oxygen saturation (>65%) and cardiovascular stability. When an infant is started on ECMO the existing ventilator support is weaned to room air at a low rate and pressure to reduce the risk of oxygen toxicity and barotrauma, thus permitting time for the lungs to rest and heal.

Because ECMO requires complete heparinization to prevent clotting in the circuit, patients with or at risk for IVH (weight < 2 kg, age < 35 wk gestation) are not candidates for this therapy. In addition, infants for whom ECMO is being considered should have reversible lung disease, no signs of systemic bleeding, and an absence of severe asphyxia or lethal malformations, and they should have been ventilated for less than 7–10 days. Complications of ECMO include thromboembolism, air embolization, bleeding, stroke, seizures, atelectasis, cholestatic jaundice, thrombocytopenia, neutropenia, hemolysis, infectious complications of blood transfusions, edema formation, and systemic hypertension.

PROGNOSIS. The outcome for infants with PFC is related to the associated hypoxic-ischemic encephalopathy and the ability to reduce pulmonary vascular resistance. The long-term prognosis for infants with PFC who survive after treatment with hyperventilation is comparable to that for infants who have underlying illnesses of equivalent severity (e.g., birth asphyxia, hypoglycemia, or polycythemia). The outcome for infants who have PFC treated with ECMO is also favorable; 85–90% survive, and 70–75% of survivors appear normal at 1 yr of age. Infants who have diaphragmatic hernia associated with severe PFC do poorly if the pre- and post-surgery P_{CO_2} exceeds 40 mm Hg despite mechanical ventilation. Such patients may respond to ECMO; rarely, it is not possible to wean them from bypass, or they expire after ECMO has been discontinued.

Anonymous: Persistent fetal circulation and extracorporeal membrane oxygenation. Lancet 2:1289, 1988.
Bohn D, Tamura M, Perrin D, et al: Ventilatory predictors of pulmonary hypoplasia in congenital diaphragmatic hernia, confirmed by morphologic assessment. J Pediatr 111:423, 1987.
Carlo WA, Beoglos A, Chatburn RL, et al: High-frequency jet ventilation in neonatal pulmonary hypertension. Am J Dis Child 143:233, 1989.
Fox W, Duara S: Persistent pulmonary hypertension in the neonate: Diagnosis and management. J Pediatr 103:505, 1983.
Gersony W: Neonatal pulmonary hypertension: Pathophysiology, classification and etiology. Clin Perinatol 11:517, 1984.
Hammerman C, Yousefzadeh D, Choi Bui K: Persistent pulmonary hypertension of the newborn. Managing the unmanageable. Clin Perinatol 16:137, 1989.
Wung J-T, James S, Kilchevsky E, et al: Management of infants with severe respiratory failure and persistence of the fetal circulation, without hyperventilation. Pediatrics 76:488, 1985.

9.37 EXTRAPULMONARY EXTRAVASATION OF AIR

(Pneumothorax, Pneumomediastinum, and Pulmonary Interstitial Emphysema)

Asymptomatic pneumothorax, usually unilateral, is estimated to occur in 1–2% of all newborn infants; symptomatic pneumothorax and pneumomediastinum are less common. Pneumothorax is more common in males than in females and in term and post-term infants than in premature ones. The incidence is increased among infants with lung disease, such as meconium aspiration and hyaline membrane disease; in those who have had vigorous resuscitation or are receiving assisted ventilation, especially if high inspiratory pressure or a continuous elevation of end-expiratory pressure is used; and in infants with urinary tract anomalies.

ETIOLOGY AND PATHOPHYSIOLOGY. The most common cause of pneumothorax is overinflation resulting in alveolar rupture. It may be "spontaneous" or idiopathic or secondary to underlying pulmonary disease, such as lobar emphysema or rupture of a congenital or pneumonic cyst; to trauma; or to a "ball-valve" type of bronchial or bronchiolar obstruction resulting from aspiration. Air leaks occur during the first 24–36 hr in infants with meconium aspiration, pneumonia, and hyaline membrane disease when lung compliance is reduced and later during the recovery phase of hyaline membrane disease if inspiratory pressure and PEEP are not reduced simultaneously with improved respiratory function.

Pneumothorax associated with pulmonary hypoplasia is common, occurs in the first day of life, and is due to reduced alveolar surface area and poorly compliant lungs. It is associated with disorders of decreased amniotic fluid volume (Potter syndrome: renal agenesis, renal dysplasia, chronic amniotic fluid leak), decreased fetal breathing movement (oligohydramnios, neuromuscular disease), pulmonary space-occupying lesions (diaphragmatic hernia, pleural effusion, chylothorax), and thoracic abnormalities (asphyxiating thoracic dystrophies).

Air from a ruptured alveolus escapes into the interstitial spaces of the lung, where it may cause *interstitial emphysema* or may dissect along the peribronchial and perivascular connective tissue sheaths to the root of the lung. If the volume of escaped air is great enough, it may follow the vascular sheaths to cause mediastinal emphysema or a rupture with subsequent pneumomediastinum, pneumothorax, and subcutaneous emphysema. Rarely, increased mediastinal pressure may compress pulmonary veins at the hilum, interfering with venous return to the heart and cardiac output. On occasion, air may embolize into the ciruclation, producing cutaneous blanching, air in intravascular catheters, an air-filled heart on chest roentgenograms, and death.

Tension pneumothorax occurs if an accumulation of air within the pleural space is sufficient to elevate intrapleural pressure above atmospheric pressure. A unilateral tension pneumothorax results in impaired ventilation not only in the collapsed lung but also in the normal lung by a mediastinal shift to the other side. Compression of the vena cava and torsion of the great vessels may interfere with venous return.

CLINICAL MANIFESTATIONS. The physical findings of *asymptomatic pneumothorax* are hyper-resonance and diminished breath sounds over the involved side of the chest with or without tachypnea.

Symptomatic pneumothorax is characterized by respiratory distress, which varies from only an increased respiratory rate to severe dyspnea, tachypnea, and cyanosis. Irritability and restlessness or apnea may be the earliest signs. The onset may be sudden or gradual; an infant may rapidly become critically ill. The chest may appear asymmetric with increased anteroposterior diameter and bulging of the intercostal spaces on the affected side, and there may be hyper-resonance and diminished or absent breath sounds. The heart is displaced toward the unaffected side, and the diaphragm is displaced downward, as is the liver with right-sided pneumothorax. Since both sides are affected in approximately 10% of patients, symmetry of findings does not rule out pneumothorax. In tension pneumothorax there may be signs of shock, and the apex of the heart is pushed away from the affected side.

Pneumomediastinum occurs in at least 25% of patients with pneumothorax and is usually asymptomatic. The degree of respiratory distress depends on the amount of trapped air. If it is great, there is bulging of the midthoracic area, the neck veins are distended, and the blood pressure is low. The last two findings are the result of blockage of the circulation by compression of the systemic and pulmonary veins. Although few clinical signs may exist, subcutaneous emphysema in the newborn infant is almost pathognomonic of pneumomediastinum.

Pulmonary interstitial emphysema (PIE) may precede the development of a pneumothorax or may occur independently, resulting in increasing respiratory distress due to decreased compliance, hypercarbia, and hypoxia. The latter is due to an increased alveolar-arterial oxygen gradient and intrapulmonary shunting. Progressive enlargement of blebs or air may result in cystic dilatations and respiratory deterioration resembling pneumothorax. In severe cases PIE precedes the development of bronchopulmonary dysplasia (BPD). Avoidance of high inspiratory or mean ventilatory pressures may prevent the development of PIE. Treatment may include bronchoscopy if there is evidence of mucus plugging, selective intubation of the uninvolved bronchus, oxygen, general respiratory care, and high-frequency jet ventilation.

DIAGNOSIS. Pneumothorax and pneumomediastinum should be suspected in any newborn infant who shows signs of respiratory distress or who displays restlessness or irritability, or has a sudden change in condition. The diagnosis is established roentgenographically with the edge of the collapsed lung standing out in relief against the pneumothorax (see Fig. 13–18), and in pneumomediastinum with hyperlucency around the heart border and between the sternum and the heart border (Fig. 9–20). Transillumination of the thorax is often helpful in the emergency diagnosis of pneumothorax; the affected side transmits excessive light. Associated renal anomalies are identified by ultrasonography. Pulmonary hypoplasia is suggested by signs of uterine compression (extremity contractures), small thorax on chest roentgenogram, severe hypoxia with hypercarbia, and signs of the primary disease (hypotonia, diaphragmatic hernia, Potter syndrome).

Pneumopericardium may be asymptomatic, requiring only general supportive treatment, but usually presents as sudden shock with tachycardia, muffled heart sounds, and poor pulses suggesting tamponade, which requires prompt evacuation of entrapped air. **Pneumoperitoneum** from air dissecting through the diaphragmatic apertures may also be confused with perforation of an abdominal organ.

TREATMENT. Without a continued air leak, asymptomatic and mildly symptomatic small pneumothoraces require only close observation. Frequent small feedings may prevent gastric dilatation and minimize crying, which can further compromise ventilation and worsen the pneumothorax. Breathing 100% oxygen accelerates the resorption of free pleural air into the blood by reducing the nitrogen tension in blood, producing a resultant nitrogen pressure gradient from the trapped air into the blood, but the benefit must be weighed against the risks of oxygen toxicity. With severe respiratory or circulatory embarrassment, emergency needle aspiration is indicated. If there is adequate time, a chest tube should be inserted and attached to underwaterseal drainage. Severe localized interstitial emphysema may respond to selective bronchial intubation. Judicious use of Pavulon in infants fighting the ventilator may reduce the incidence of pneumothorax.

Gonzalez F, Harris T, Black P, et al: Decreased gas flow through pneumothoraces in neonates receiving high-frequency jet versus conventional ventilation. J Pediatr 110:464, 1987.

Hall RT, Rhodes PG: Pneumothorax and pneumomediastinum in infants with idiopathic respiratory distress syndrome receiving CPAP. Pediatrics 55:493, 1975.

Primhak RA: Factors associated with pulmonary air leak in premature infants receiving mechanical ventilation. J Pediatr 102:764, 1983.

Ryan CA, Barrington KJ, Phillips HJ, et al: Contralateral pneumothoraces in the newborn: Incidence and predisposing factors. Pediatrics 79:417, 1987.

9.38 INTERSTITIAL PULMONARY FIBROSIS
(Wilson-Mikity Syndrome; Bronchopulmonary Dysplasia; Pulmonary Insufficiency of the Premature)

See also Sec. 9.32 for discussion of bronchopulmonary dysplasia.

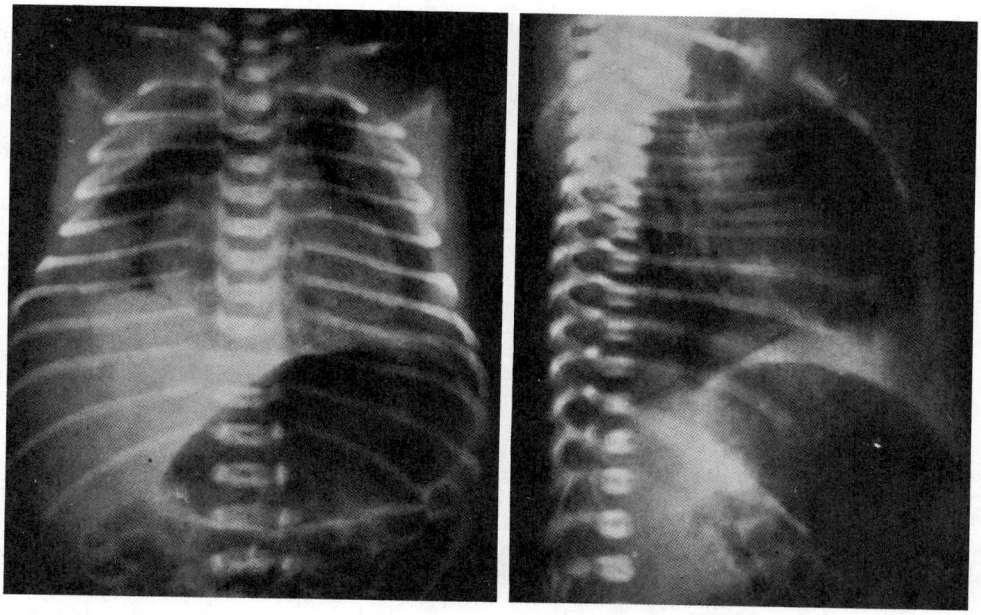

Figure 9–20. Pneumomediastinum in a newborn infant. Anteroposterior view demonstrates compression of lungs and the lateral view shows bulging of the sternum, each resulting from distention of the mediastinum by trapped air.

Wilson and Mikity described a pulmonary syndrome of premature infants, usually of less than 32 wk of gestation and birthweights below 1,500 g, and without a history of hyaline membrane disease; it was characterized by insidious onset of dyspnea, tachypnea, retractions, and cyanosis during the 1st mo of life. Rare cases have been reported in full-term infants, usually those having a history of meconium aspiration or oxygen administration. Viral infections also have been implicated.

Several variations on the clinical presentation have been described with similar roentgenographic findings. Some infants have respiratory distress at birth that is occasionally severe, resembles hyaline membrane disease, and requires oxygen; these may be cases of bronchopulmonary dysplasia. Others show a more gradual development of dyspnea and cyanosis. Others have no early respiratory symptoms or history of exposure to oxygen, and the onset of symptoms occurs at several weeks of life.

Cough, wheezing, and rales may develop, but fever occurs only with concomitant infection. There may be collapse of a lobe or lung; other complications are right-sided heart failure, osteoporosis, and rib fractures. The symptoms usually increase over 2–6 wk with increasing oxygen dependency persisting for several months, followed by gradual resolution or progressive respiratory and cardiac failure. Infants who recover from the severe form may have an increased number of lower respiratory tract infections in the 1st yr of life. The most characteristic features of this syndrome are roentgenographic. Early, they include bilateral coarse reticular streaky infiltrates and, often, overexpansion of the lungs with small areas of emphysema that develop into multicystic lesions. Subsequently, the cysts enlarge and coalesce to give a hyperlucent, bubbly appearance (see Fig. 9–18*B*). The roentgenograms tend to clear gradually over months to several years. The roentgenographic changes in Wilson-Mikity syndrome may be indistinguishable from those of bronchopulmonary dysplasia.

The syndrome must be differentiated from pneumonia due to cytomegalovirus, *Pneumocystis carinii, Ureaplasma urealyticum*, or chlamydia pneumonia, and from cystic fibrosis. *Chronic pulmonary insufficiency of prematurity* is initially different from bronchopulmonary dysplasia. Usually a VLBW infant without respiratory distress syndrome develops severe apnea on day 2–5. Atelectasis and a reduced functional residual capacity follow requiring treatment with CPAP or mechanical ventilation. With prolonged ventilation, a picture of bronchopulmonary dysplasia intervenes.

Treatment consists of supportive measures: oxygen for cyanosis, bronchodilators, diuretics for cardiac failure, acid-base correction, and assisted ventilation when indicated. A trial of erythromycin may be indicated to treat *Chlamydia* or *Ureaplasma* pneumonia.

Abman SH, Wolfe RR, Accurso FJ, et al: Pulmonary vascular response to oxygen in infants with severe bronchopulmonary dysplasia. Pediatrics 75:80, 1985.

Albersheim SG, Solimano AJ, Sharma AK, et al: Randomized, double-blind, controlled trial of long-term diuretic therapy for bronchopulmonary dysplasia. J Pediatr 115:615, 1989.

Hudak BB, Allen MC, Hudal ML, et al: Home oxygen therapy for chronic lung disease in extremely low-birth-weight infants. Am J Dis Child 143:357, 1989.

Toce SS, Farrell PM, Leavitt LA, et al: Clinical and roentgenographic scoring systems for assessing bronchopulmonary dysplasia. Am J Dis Child 138:581, 1984.

Wilson MG, Mikity VG: A new form of respiratory distress in premature infants. Am J Dis Child 99:489, 1960.

LOBAR EMPHYSEMA

See Sec. 14.76.

9.39 LUNG CYSTS

Most lung cysts observed during the neonatal period are acquired as the result of rupture of alveoli by overinflation or infection, often staphylococcal. Congenital cysts are rare; they may be solitary or multiple, air- or fluid-filled, and are believed to result as a developmental anomaly of the bronchial buds (Sec. 14.39). Infants with congenital or acquired cysts may be asymptomatic or may present either with tachypnea and dyspnea at birth or at any time thereafter or with recurrent or persistent pneumonia. Air-filled cysts on the surface of the lung, whatever their origin, sometimes rupture and cause pneumothorax. This is particularly true of multicystic disease. Since most cystic areas discovered only on roentgenographic examination will disappear spontaneously, treatment, which is surgical removal, should be reserved for those cysts causing severe respiratory distress.

9.40 PULMONARY HEMORRHAGE

Massive pulmonary hemorrhage is present in 15% of neonates who come to autopsy in the first 2 wk of life. The reported incidence at autopsy varies from 1–4/1,000 live births. About three fourths of the patients weigh less than 2,500 g at birth.

Most infants in whom pulmonary hemorrhage is demonstrated at autopsy have had symptoms of respiratory distress that are indistinguishable from those of hyaline membrane disease. The onset may occur at birth or may be delayed several days. One fourth to one half of affected infants cough up or regurgitate material containing old or fresh blood from the nose, mouth, or endotracheal tube. Roentgenographic findings are varied and nonspecific, ranging from minor streaking or patchy infiltrates to massive consolidation.

The cause of massive pulmonary hemorrhage is usually not identified; the incidence is increased in association with acute pulmonary infection, severe asphyxia, hyaline membrane disease, assisted ventilation, congenital heart disease, erythroblastosis fetalis, hemorrhagic disease of the newborn, kernicterus, inborn errors of ammonia metabolism, and cold injury. Although in the majority of instances bleeding into other organs is observed at autopsy, bleeding other than through the nostrils and mouth and intraventricular bleeding are relatively rare during life and should suggest the possibility of an additional bleeding diathesis such as disseminated intravascular coagulation (Sec. 16.75). Bleeding is predominantly alveolar in about two thirds of cases and interstitial in the rest. In some infants the pulmonary hemorrhage represents hemorrhagic pulmonary edema due to severe left-sided heart failure resulting from hypoxia.

The little information available that describes the prognosis of infants who bleed through the mouth or nostrils suggests that it is extremely poor. Death occurs in the first 48 hr of life in two thirds of the infants who come to autopsy. Treatment includes blood replacement, positive end-expiratory pressure, and epinephrine aerosols.

Cole VA, Norman ICS, Reynolds EOR, et al: Pathogenesis of hemorrhagic pulmonary edema and massive pulmonary hemorrhage in the newborn. Pediatrics 51:175, 1973.

Trompeter R, Yu VYH, Aynsley-Green A, et al: Massive pulmonary haemorrhage in the newborn. Arch Dis Child 51:123, 1975.

CONGENITAL PULMONARY LYMPHANGIECTASIA

See Sec. 14.41.

CHYLOTHORAX

See Sec. 14.95.

9.41 DIGESTIVE SYSTEM

VOMITING. Infants may vomit mucus, often blood-streaked, in the first few hours after birth. This vomiting rarely persists after the first few feedings; it may be due to irritation of the gastric mucosa by material swallowed during delivery. If the vomiting is protracted, gastric lavage with physiologic saline solution may relieve it.

Vomiting is a relatively frequent symptom during the neonatal period. In the majority of instances it is simply regurgitation from overfeeding or from failure to permit the infant to eructate swallowed air. (See Sec. 13.14 for discussion of gastric emptying and gastroesophageal reflux.) When vomiting occurs shortly after birth and is persistent, the possibilities of intestinal obstruction and increased intracranial pressure must be considered. A history of maternal hydramnios suggests upper intestinal atresia.

Bile-stained emesis suggests intestinal obstruction beyond the duodenum, but it may also be idiopathic. Abdominal roentgenograms (kidney-ureter-bladder [KUB] and cross-table lateral views) should be performed in neonates with persistent emesis and in all infants with bile-stained emesis to detect air-fluid levels, distended bowel loops, characteristic patterns of obstruction (double bubble: duodenal atresia), and pneumoperitoneum (intestinal perforation).

Obstructive lesions of the digestive tract occur most frequently in the esophagus and intestines (see Chapter 13). Vomiting from esophageal obstruction occurs with the first feeding. The diagnosis of **esophageal atresia** can be suspected if there is unusual drooling from the mouth and if resistance is encountered in the attempt to pass a catheter into the stomach. Diagnosis should be made before the infant chokes on oral feedings and risks aspiration pneumonia. Infantile **achalasia** (cardiospasm), a rare cause of vomiting in the newborn infant, is demonstrable roentgenographically by obstruction at the cardiac end of the esophagus, without organic stenosis. Regurgitation of feedings owing to continuous relaxation of the esophageal-gastric sphincter, **chalasia**, is a cause of vomiting, which can be controlled by keeping the infant in a semi-upright position.

Vomiting due to *obstruction of the small intestine* usually begins on the 1st day of life and is frequent, persistent, usually nonprojectile, copious, and, unless the obstruction is above the ampulla of Vater, bile-stained; it is associated with abdominal distention, visible deep peristaltic waves, and reduced or absent bowel movements. **Malrotation** with obstruction from midgut volvulus is an acute emergency that must be considered. Upright roentgenographic films of the abdomen will show the distribution of air in the intestine and often aid in locating the site of the obstruction; malrotation may be identified by contrast studies. Normally, air can be demonstrated roentgenographically in the jejunum by 15–60 min, in the ileum by 2–3 hr, and in the colon by 3 hr after birth. Absence of rectal gas at 24 hr is abnormal. Persistent vomiting may occur with congenital **hernia of the diaphragm** (Sec. 13.103). The vomiting of **pyloric stenosis** may begin any time after birth but does not assume its characteristic pattern before the 2nd–3rd wk. Vomiting may occur with many other disturbances that do not obstruct the digestive tract, such as celiac disease, milk allergy, adrenal hyperplasia of the salt-losing variety, galactosemia, hyperammonemias, increased intracranial pressure, septicemia, meningitis, and urinary tract infections.

THRUSH (ORAL CANDIDOSIS). Thrush of the mouth occurs in healthy infants; later, it is rare except in debilitated infants, in those receiving antibiotic or immunosuppressive therapy, and those with acquired immunodeficiency syndrome (AIDS). Infants with AIDS also manifest failure to thrive, psychomotor retardation, hepatosplenomegaly, diarrhea, lymphadenopathy, and hypergammaglobulinemia (see Sec. 12.82).

Transmission of the infection from maternal vaginal moniliasis to the infant's oral mucosa is the primary means of infection in healthy newborns. Secondary cases develop in the hospital nursery, presumably owing to contact with infected infants and contaminated supplies or caretakers.

Oral thrush in an otherwise healthy infant is usually a self-limited infection, but treatment is advised, especially in the presence of candidal diaper rash (Sec. 9.75).

DIARRHEA. See Sec. 6.20, 9.59, 12.10, 12.27, 13.14, and 13.59–13.61.

CONSTIPATION. More than 90% of full-term newborn infants pass meconium within the first 24 hr, and most of the remainder do so within 36 hr; the possibility of intestinal obstruction should be considered in any infant who does not. Intestinal atresia or stenosis, congenital aganglionic megacolon, milk bolus obstruction, meconium ileus, or meconium plugs may present as constipation. Constipation not present from birth but appearing during the 1st mo of life suggests congenital aganglionic megacolon, cretinism, or anal stenosis. It must be kept in mind that infrequent bowel movements do not necessarily mean constipation. A breast-fed infant usually has frequent bowel movements, whereas a formula-fed infant may have 1–2 movements a day or every other day.

MECONIUM PLUGS. Lower colonic or anorectal plugs (Fig. 9–21) with a lower than normal water content may cause intestinal obstruction. Rarely, a firm mass of meconium may form elsewhere in the intestine and cause intrauterine intestinal obstruction and meconium peritonitis unrelated to cystic fibrosis. Anorectal plugs may also cause intestinal ulceration and perforation. Meconium plugs are associated with small left colon syndrome in the infant of a diabetic mother, cystic fibrosis, rectal aganglionosis, maternal drug abuse, and magnesium sulfate therapy for pre-eclampsia. The plug may be evacuated by irrigating it with isotonic sodium chloride solution. Enemas with the iodinated contrast medium *Gastrografin* usually cause passage of the plug, presumably because the high osmolarity (1,900 mOsm/L) of the medium draws fluid rapidly into the intestinal lumen and loosens inspissated material. Since this rapid loss of fluid into the bowel may result in acute dehydration and shock, it is advisable to dilute the contrast material with an equal amount of water, to correct any existing dehydration and to provide intravenous fluids during and for several hours after the procedure. *After removal of a meconium plug the infant should be observed closely for the possible presence of congenital aganglionic megacolon.*

9.42 MECONIUM ILEUS IN CYSTIC FIBROSIS

In the newborn infant impaction of meconium causes intestinal obstructions often associated with cystic fibrosis. The absence of pancreatic enzymes limits normal digestive activities in the intestine, and meconium is left in a viscid, mucilaginous state. It clings to the intestinal wall and is moved with difficulty. The inspissated and impacted meconium fills the intestinal canal but is most concentrated in the lower ileum.

Clinically, the pattern is that of congenital intestinal obstruction with or without intestinal perforation. Abdominal distention is prominent, and persistent vomiting soon occurs. Infrequently one or more inspissated meconium stools may be passed shortly after birth.

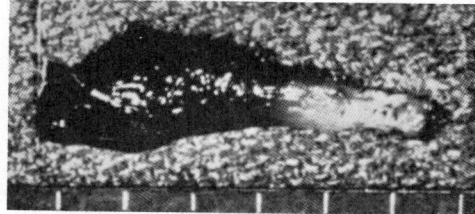

Figure 9–21. Anorectal plug, from child who had not passed meconium for 2 days after birth, is indistinguishable from normal plug. Pale end was adjacent to the anus. (From Emery JL: Arch Dis Child 32:17, 1957.)

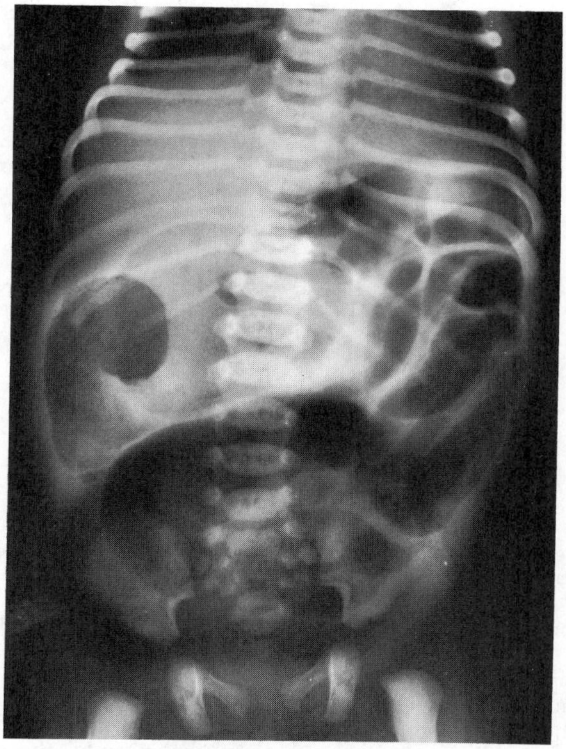

Figure 9–22. Meconium ileus. Impacted meconium with small amounts of air interspersed throughout it in loops of intestine on the right side of abdomen; intestinal loops above this impaction are greatly distended.

The differential diagnosis involves other causes of intestinal obstruction; an exact diagnosis cannot be made except at laparotomy. A presumptive diagnosis can be made on the basis of a history of cystic fibrosis in a sibling, by palpation of doughy or cord-like masses of intestines through the abdominal wall, and by the roentgenographic appearance. Roentgenographically, in contrast to the generally evenly distended intestinal loops above an atresia, the loops may vary in width and are not as evenly filled with gas. At points of heaviest meconium concentration the infiltrated gas may create a bubbly granular appearance (Figs. 9–22 and 9–23). A negative sweat test in the neonatal period may not rule out cystic fibrosis.

The case fatality rate is high, but a number of infants have survived the neonatal period; their subsequent prognosis depends on the basic disturbance, cystic fibrosis (Sec. 14.89).

Treatment is high Gastrografin enemas as described under Meconium Plugs in the previous section. If they are unsuccessful or if there is reason to suspect a perforation of the bowel wall, laparotomy is performed and the ileum opened at the point of greatest diameter of the impaction. Approximately 50% of infants have associated intestinal atresia, stenosis, or volvulus that does not respond to contrast enema and requires surgery. The inspissated meconium is removed by gentle and patient irrigation with warm isotonic sodium chloride or Mucomyst (acetylcysteine) solution introduced through a fine catheter, which may be passed between the impaction and the bowel wall.

MECONIUM PERITONITIS. Perforation of the intestine may occur in utero or shortly after birth. Either the tear may be sealed by natural processes relatively quickly with only a small amount of meconium escaping, or the meconial contents may largely be emptied into the peritoneal cavity. Such

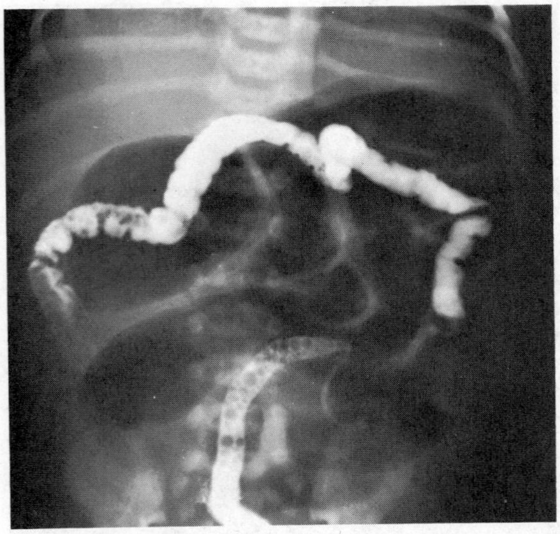

Figure 9–23. Meconium ileus. The colon, outlined by contrast material, is small because meconium has not reached it.

perforations occur most often as a complication of meconium ileus in infants with cystic fibrosis, but occasionally the perforation is due to a meconium plug or intestinal obstruction of another cause.

When the intestinal perforation is spontaneously sealed and only a small amount of meconium has escaped, the event may never be detected, except when some of the meconial particles become calcified and are later fortuitously discovered on roentgenograms of the abdomen. Alternatively, the clinical picture may be dominated by the signs of intestinal obstruction or peritonitis. Characteristically, there is abdominal distention, vomiting, and absence of stools. Treatment consists primarily of elimination of the intestinal obstruction and drainage of the peritoneal cavity.

9.43 NEONATAL NECROTIZING ENTEROCOLITIS (NEC)

This serious disease of the newborn is of unknown etiology and is characterized by varying degrees of mucosal or transmural necrosis of the intestine. No particular race or sex is unduly susceptible to the disease. Incidence ranges from 1 to 5% of admissions to neonatal intensive care units. Since the very small, ill preterm infant is particularly susceptible to NEC, a rising incidence in recent years may reflect improved survival of this high-risk group of patients. The disease does occur occasionally in term infants.

PATHOLOGY AND PATHOGENESIS. Many factors may contribute to the development of a necrotic segment of intestine, the gas accumulation in the submucosa of the bowel wall, and progression of the necrosis leading to perforation, sepsis, and death. The distal ileum and proximal colon are involved most frequently. A variety of factors such as polycythemia, hypertonic milk or medicines, or too rapid feeding protocols may contribute to mucosal injury and subsequent infection leading to bowel necrosis. NEC occurs in premature infants without stress, particularly during epidemics. The clustering of cases suggests a primary role for an infectious agent; *Clostridium difficile, C. perfringens, Escherichia coli, Staphylococcus epidermidis,* and rotavirus have commonly been recovered from cultures.

CLINICAL MANIFESTATIONS. Onset usually occurs in the first 2 wk but can be as late as 2 mo of age in VLBW infants. Meconium is passed normally, and the first signs are abdominal distention with gastric retention. Obvious bloody stools are seen in 25% of patients. The onset is often insidious, and sepsis may be suspected before an intestinal lesion is noted. There is a wide spectrum of illness from mild with only guaiac-positive stools to severe with peritonitis, bowel perforation, shock, and death. Progression may be rapid, but it is unusual for the disease to progress from mild to severe after 72 hr.

DIAGNOSIS. A very high index of suspicion in managing infants at risk is essential. Plain abdominal roentgenograms may demonstrate pneumatosis intestinalis, a finding that is diagnostic of NEC in the newborn infant; 50–75% of patients have pneumatosis when treatment is started. Portal vein gas is a sign of severe disease, and pneumoperitoneum indicates a perforation.

The differential diagnosis of NEC includes specific infections (systemic or intestinal), obstruction, and volvulus. Cultures and roentgenograms may be diagnostic. Gastrografin enema may demonstrate pneumatosis intestinalis, and hepatic ultrasound may detect portal venous gas despite normal abdominal roentgenograms.

TREATMENT. Intensive therapy is advisable for suspected as well as diagnosed cases. Cessation of feeding, nasogastric decompression, and intravenous fluids with careful attention to acid-base and electrolyte balance are very important. Once cultures are taken of blood, stool, and cerebrospinal fluid, systemic antibiotics (antipseudomonas penicillin and an aminoglycoside) should be started. When present, umbilical catheters should be removed, and ventilation should be assisted if distention is contributing to hypoxia and hypercapnia. If hypotension develops, resuscitation with blood, plasma, or crystalloid is essential.

The patient's course should be monitored by frequent cross-table lateral abdominal roentgenograms in search of perforation and by hematocrit, platelet, electrolyte, and acid-base determinations. Gown and glove isolation and grouping infants at similar increased risk into cohorts separate from other infants should be instituted to contain an epidemic.

A surgeon should be consulted early in the course of treatment. Evidence of perforation is usually an indication for resection of necrotic bowel. Pneumoperitoneum and brown-colored paracentesis fluid suggest perforation. Failure to respond to medical management, a single fixed bowel loop, erythema of the abdominal wall, or a mass are additional indications for exploratory laparotomy, resection of necrotic bowel, and external ostomy diversion. Peritoneal drainage may be helpful for the patient in extremis with peritonitis who is unable to withstand bowel resection.

PROGNOSIS. Medical management fails in about 20% of patients in whom there is pneumatosis intestinalis at diagnosis; of these, at least 25% die. Strictures develop at the site of the necrotizing lesion in about 10% of patients. Resection of the stricture is curative. Complications of NEC following massive intestinal resection include short bowel syndrome (malabsorption, growth failure, malnutrition), complications of total parenteral alimentation due to central venous catheters (sepsis, thrombosis), and cholestatic jaundice that may progress to cirrhosis.

Kliegman R, Walsh M: Neonatal necrotizing enterocolitis. Pathogenesis, classification and spectrum of illness. Curr Prob Pediatr 27:215, 1987.

Kosloske A: Pathogenesis and prevention of necrotizing enterocolitis: A hypothesis based on personal observation and a review of the literature. Pediatrics 74:1086, 1984.

9.44 JAUNDICE AND HYPERBILIRUBINEMIA IN THE NEWBORN

Jaundice is observed during the 1st wk of life in approximately 60% of term infants and 80% of preterm infants. The color usually results from the accumulation in the skin of unconjugated, nonpolar, lipid-soluble bilirubin pigment (indirect-reacting) formed from hemoglobin by the action of heme oxygenase, biliverdin reductase, and nonenzymatic reducing agents in the reticuloendothelial cells; it may also be due in part to the deposition of the pigment after it has been converted in the liver cell microsome by the enzyme uridine diphosphoglucuronic acid (UDPGA) glucuronyl transferase to the polar, water-soluble ester glucuronide of bilirubin (direct-reacting). The unconjugated form is neurotoxic for infants at certain concentrations and under various conditions. Conjugated bilirubin is not neurotoxic but indicates a potentially serious disorder. Mild elevations of bilirubin may have antioxidant properties.

ETIOLOGY. The newborn infant's metabolism of bilirubin is in transition from the fetal stage, during which the placenta is the principal route of elimination of the lipid-soluble bilirubin, to the adult stage, during which the water-soluble conjugated form is excreted from the hepatic cell into the biliary system and then into the gastrointestinal tract. Unconjugated hyperbilirubinemia may be caused or increased by any factor that (1) increases the load of bilirubin to be metabolized by the liver (hemolytic anemias, shortened red cell life owing to immaturity or to transfused cells, increased enterohepatic circulation, infection); (2) may damage or reduce the activity of the transferase enzyme (hypoxia, infection, possibly hypothermia and thyroid deficiency); (3) may compete for or block the transferase enzyme (drugs and other substances requiring glucuronic acid conjugation for excretion); or (4) leads to an absence of or decreased amounts of the enzyme or to reduction of bilirubin uptake by the liver cell (genetic defect, prematurity). The risk of toxic effects from elevated levels of unconjugated bilirubin in the serum is increased by factors that reduce the retention of bilirubin in the circulation (hypoproteinemia, displacement of bilirubin from its binding sites on albumin by competitive binding of drugs such as sulfisoxazole, moxalactam, acidosis, increased free fatty acid concentration secondary to hypoglycemia, starvation, or hypothermia), or by factors that increase the permeability of the blood-brain barrier or nerve cell membranes to bilirubin or the susceptibility of brain cells to its toxicity such as asphyxia, prematurity, hyperosmolality, and infection. Early feeding decreases and dehydration increases the serum levels of bilirubin. Meconium has 1 mg bilirubin/dL and may contribute to jaundice by the enterohepatic circulation following deconjugation by glucuronidase. Drugs such as oxytocin and chemicals employed in the nursery such as phenolic detergents may also produce unconjugated hyperbilirubinemia.

CLINICAL MANIFESTATIONS. Jaundice may be present at birth or may appear at any time during the neonatal period, depending on the condition responsible for it. *Its intensity bears no clinically dependable relation to the degree of hyperbilirubinemia,* particularly in infants receiving phototherapy (Sec. 9.45). Therefore, bilirubin determinations should be done on all jaundiced infants. Jaundice resulting from deposition of indirect bilirubin in the skin tends to appear bright yellow or orange; jaundice of the obstructive type (direct bilirubin), a greenish or muddy yellow. This difference is usually apparent only in severe jaundice. The infant may be lethargic and feed poorly. Signs of kernicterus rarely appear on the first day of jaundice (Sec. 9.45).

DIFFERENTIAL DIAGNOSIS. Jaundice, consisting of indirect or direct bilirubin, that is present at birth or appears within the first 24 hr of life may be due to erythroblastosis fetalis, concealed hemorrhage, sepsis, cytomegalic inclusion disease, rubella, or congenital toxoplasmosis. Jaundice in infants who have received intrauterine transfusions may be characterized by an unusually high proportion of direct-reacting bilirubin. Jaundice that first appears on the 2nd or 3rd day is usually "physiologic" but may represent a more severe form called *hyperbilirubinemia of the newborn.* Familial nonhemolytic icterus (Crigler-Najjar syndrome) is seen initially on the 2nd or 3rd day. *Jaundice appearing after the 3rd day and within the 1st wk should suggest septicemia;* it may be due to other infections, notably syphilis, toxoplasmosis, and cytomegalic inclusion disease. Jaundice secondary to extensive ecchymosis or hematoma may occur during the 1st day or later, especially in premature infants. Polycythemia may lead to early jaundice.

Jaundice that is noted initially after the 1st wk of life suggests breast milk jaundice, septicemia, congenital atresia of the bile ducts, hepatitis, rubella, herpetic hepatitis, galactosemia, congenital hemolytic anemia (spherocytosis), or possibly the crises of other hemolytic anemias (such as pyruvate kinase and other glycolytic enzyme deficiencies or hereditary nonspherocytic anemia), or hemolytic anemia due to drugs (as in congenital deficiencies of the enzymes glucose-6-phosphate dehydrogenase, glutathione synthetase, reductase, or peroxidase).

Persistent jaundice during the 1st mo of life suggests the so-called inspissated bile syndrome (which may follow hemolytic disease of the newborn), hyperalimentation-associated cholestasis, hepatitis, cytomegalic inclusion disease, syphilis, toxoplasmosis, familial nonhemolytic icterus, congenital atresia of the bile ducts, or galactosemia. Rarely, physiologic jaundice may be prolonged for several weeks, as in infants with hypothyroidism or pyloric stenosis.

Regardless of the gestational age or time of appearance of jaundice, significant hyperbilirubinemia requires a complete diagnostic evaluation, which should include the determination of the direct and indirect bilirubin fractions, hemoglobin, reticulocyte count, blood type, Coombs test, and an examination of the peripheral blood smear (Table 9–25). Indirect-reacting bilirubinemia, reticulocytosis, and a smear demonstrating evidence of red blood cell destruction suggest hemolysis; in the absence of blood group incompatibility, nonimmunologically induced hemolysis should be considered. If there is direct-reacting hyperbilirubinemia, hepatitis, cholestasis, inborn errors of metabolism, cystic fibrosis, and sepsis are diagnostic possibilities. If the reticulocyte count, Coombs test, and direct bilirubin are normal, physiologic or pathologic indirect hyperbilirubinemia may be present.

PHYSIOLOGIC JAUNDICE (ICTERUS NEONATORUM). Under normal circumstances, the level of indirect-reacting bilirubin in umbilical cord serum is 1–3 mg/dL (17.1–51 μmol/L) and rises at a rate of less than 5 mg/dL/24 hr; thus, jaundice becomes visible on the 2nd–3rd day, usually peaking between the 2nd and 4th days at 5–6 mg/dL and decreasing to below 2 mg/dL between the 5th and 7th days of life. Jaundice associated with these changes is designated "physiologic" and is believed to be the result of increased bilirubin production following breakdown of fetal red blood cells combined with transient limitation in the conjugation of bilirubin by the liver.

Overall, 6–7% of **full-term infants** have indirect bilirubin levels of greater than 12.9 mg/dL and less than 3% have levels greater than 15 mg/dL. Risk factors for indirect hyperbilirubinemia include maternal diabetes, race (Chinese, Japanese, Korean, and American Indian), prematurity, drugs (vitamin K_3, novobiocin), altitude, polycythemia, male sex, 21-trisomy, cutaneous bruising, cephalohematoma, oxytocin induction, breast-feeding, weight loss (dehydration or caloric deprivation), delayed stooling, and a sibling who had physiologic jaundice. Infants without these variables rarely develop indirect bilirubin levels above 12 mg/dL, whereas infants with multiple risks are more likely to have higher bilirubin levels. Indirect bilirubin levels in full-term infants decline to adult

TABLE 9–25. Diagnostic Features of the Various Types of Neonatal Jaundice*

Diagnosis	Nature of Van den Bergh Reaction	Jaundice		Peak Bilirubin Conc.		Bilirubin Rate of Accumulation (mg/dL/day)	Remarks
		Appears	*Disappears*	*mg/dL*	*Age in Days*		
1. "Physiologic jaundice":							1. Usually relates to degree of maturity
Full-term	Indirect	2–3 days	4–5 days	10–12	2–3	< 5	
Premature	Indirect	3–4 days	7–9 days	15	6–8	< 5	
2. Hyperbilirubinemia due to metabolic factors, etc							2. Metabolic factors: hypoxia, respiratory distress, lack of carbohydrate Hormonal influences: cretinism, hormones Genetic factors: Crigler-Najjar syndrome, transient familial hyperbilirubinemia Drugs: vitamin K, novobiocin
Full-term	Indirect	2–3 days	Variable	> 12	1st wk	< 5	
Premature	Indirect	3–4 days	Variable	> 15	1st wk	< 5	
3. Hemolytic states and hematoma	Indirect	May appear in 1st 24 hr	Variable	Unlimited	Variable	Usually > 5	3. Erythroblastosis: Rh, ABO. Congenital hemolytic states: spherocytic, nonspherocytic. Infantile pyknocytosis. Drugs: vitamin K. Enclosed hemorrhage—hematoma
4. Mixed hemolytic and hepatotoxic factors	Indirect and direct	May appear in 1st 24 hr	Variable	Unlimited	Variable	Usually > 5	4. Infection: bacterial sepsis, pyelonephritis, hepatitis, toxoplasmosis, cytomegalic inclusion disease, rubella Drugs: vitamin K
5. Hepatocellular damage	Indirect and direct	Usually 2–3 days	Variable	Unlimited	Variable	Variable can be > 5	5. Biliary atresia; galactosemia; hepatitis and infection as in (4)

*From Brown AK: Pediatr Clin North Am 9:589, 1962.

levels (1 mg/dL) by 10–14 days of life. *Persistent indirect hyperbilirubinemia* beyond 2 wk suggests hemolysis, hereditary glucuronyl transferase deficiency, breast milk jaundice, hypothyroidism, or intestinal obstruction. Jaundice associated with pyloric stenosis may be due to caloric deprivation, deficiency of hepatic UDP-glucuronyl transferase, or ileus-induced increased enterohepatic circulation of bilirubin.

Among **premature infants** the rise in serum bilirubin tends to be the same or a little slower than that in term infants but is of longer duration, which generally results in higher levels, the peak being reached between the 4th and 7th days; the pattern depends upon the time required for the preterm infant to achieve mature mechanisms for the metabolism and excretion of bilirubin. Usually, peak levels of 8–12 mg/dL (136–205 μmol/L) are not reached until the 5th–7th day, and jaundice is infrequently observed after the 10th day.

The diagnosis of physiologic jaundice in term or preterm infants can be established only by excluding known causes of jaundice on the basis of the history and clinical and laboratory findings (Table 9–25). In general, a search to determine the cause of jaundice should be made if (1) it appears in the first 24 hr of life; (2) serum bilirubin is rising at a rate greater than 5 mg/dL/24 hr; (3) serum bilirubin is greater than 12 mg/dL in full-term (especially in the absence of risk factors) or 14 mg/dL in preterm infants; (4) jaundice persists after the 1st wk of life; or (5) direct-reacting bilirubin is greater than 1 mg/dL at any time.

PATHOLOGIC HYPERBILIRUBINEMIA. Jaundice and its underlying hyperbilirubinemia are considered pathologic if their time of appearance, duration, or pattern of serially determined serum bilirubin concentrations varies significantly from that of physiologic jaundice; or if the course is compatible with physiologic jaundice but other reasons exist to suspect that the infant is at special risk from the neurotoxicity of unconjugated bilirubin. It may not be possible to determine precisely the etiology for an abnormal elevation of unconjugated bilirubin. Many of these infants have associated risk factors such as Oriental race, prematurity, breast-feeding, or weight loss; hence the terms **exaggerated physiologic jaundice** and **hyperbilirubinemia of the newborn** are used for those infants whose primary problem is probably a deficiency or inactivity of bilirubin glucuronyl transferase rather than an excessive load of bilirubin for excretion.

The *significance* of hyperbilirubinemia lies in the high incidence of kernicterus associated with serum bilirubin levels over 20 mg/dL (342 μmol/L) in term infants. The correlation between serum bilirubin levels and kernicterus or milder forms of brain injury in infants with erythroblastosis fetalis probably holds for all newborn infants who develop bilirubin concentrations beyond the physiologic range for their weight and gestational age, independent of the etiology of the jaundice. LBW infants develop kernicterus at lower levels (10–12 mg/dL: 171–205 μmol/L) in association with asphyxia, respiratory distress syndrome, hypoglycemia, acidosis, sepsis, intraventricular hemorrhage, and meningitis. Sulfisoxazole also increases susceptibility to kernicterus at relatively low levels (12–15 mg/dL) of serum bilirubin.

JAUNDICE ASSOCIATED WITH BREAST-FEEDING. An estimated 1 of 200 breast-fed term infants develops significant elevations in unconjugated bilirubin between the 4th and 7th days of life, reaching maximum concentrations as high as 10–27 mg/dL (171–462 μmol/L) during the 3rd wk. If breast-feeding is continued, the hyperbilirubinemia gradually decreases and then may persist for 3–10 wk at lower levels. If nursing is discontinued, the serum bilirubin level falls rapidly, usually reaching normal levels within a few days. Cessation of breast-feeding for 2–4 days and substitution of formula for breast milk results in a rapid decline in serum bilirubin, after which nursing can be resumed without a return of the hyperbilirubinemia to its previously high levels. These infants have no other sign of illness, and kernicterus has not been reported. The milk of some of these mothers contains 5-βpregnane-3α, 20-β-diol or nonesterified long-chain fatty acids, which competitively inhibit glucuronyl transferase conjugating activity. In others, the milk contains a glucuronidase that may be responsible for jaundice.

This syndrome must be distinguished from an early onset accentuated unconjugated hyperbilirubinemia in the 1st wk of life, when breast-fed infants have higher bilirubin levels than formula-fed infants (Fig. 9–24). This observation may be due to decreased milk intake with dehydration or reduced caloric intake. Giving supplements of glucose water to breast-fed infants is associated with higher bilirubin levels owing in part to reduced intake of the higher caloric density breast milk. Frequent breast feedings (> 10/24 hr), rooming-in with night feedings, and discouraging 5% dextrose or water supplementation may reduce the incidence of early breast milk jaundice.

Transient Familial Neonatal Hyperbilirubinemia. Severe unconjugated hyperbilirubinemia leading to kernicterus may occur rarely in the first 2 days of life because of a glucuronyl transferase-inhibiting factor present in the serum of mother and infant.

NEONATAL HEPATITIS. See Sec. 13.83 and 13.84.

CONGENITAL ATRESIA OF THE BILE DUCTS. See Sec. 13.84.

INSPISSATED BILE SYNDROME. See Late Complications in Sec. 9.47.

9.45 KERNICTERUS

Kernicterus is a neurologic syndrome resulting from the deposition of unconjugated bilirubin in brain cells. The risk in infants with erythroblastosis fetalis is directly related to serum bilirubin levels, and it is probably similar for infants with hyperbilirubinemia of whatever cause. Lipid-soluble indirect bilirubin may cross the blood-brain barrier and enter the brain by diffusion if the bilirubin-binding capacity of albumin and other plasma proteins is exceeded and plasma free bilirubin levels increase. Alternatively, bilirubin may enter the brain following damage to the blood-brain barrier by asphyxia or hyperosmolality.

The precise blood level above which indirect-reacting bilirubin or free bilirubin will be toxic for an individual infant is unpredictable, but kernicterus is rare in term infants with serum levels under 20 mg/dL (342 μmol/L). The duration of exposure necessary to produce toxic effects is also unknown. There is some evidence that motor disturbances in later childhood are more common among newborn infants whose total serum bilirubin rises above 15 mg/dL. *The less mature the infant, the greater the susceptibility to kernicterus.* Factors that potentiate the movement of bilirubin into brain cells and its adverse effects on them are discussed in Sec. 9.44. In exceptional circumstances kernicterus in VLBW infants with serum bilirubin concentrations as low as 8–12 mg/dL (137–205 μmol/L) has been associated with an apparently cumulative effect of a number of these factors.

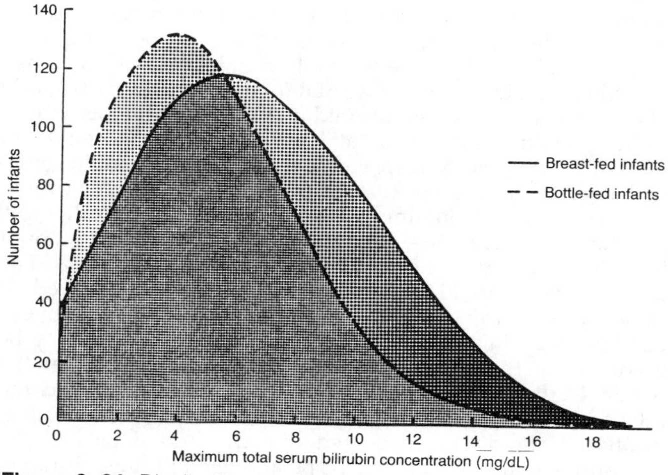

Figure 9–24. Distribution of maximum bilirubin levels during the 1st wk of life in breast-fed and formula-fed white infants >2,500 g. (From Maisels J, Gifford K: Pediatrics 78:837, 1986. Copyright 1986. Reproduced by permission of Pediatrics.)

CLINICAL MANIFESTATIONS. Signs and symptoms of kernicterus usually appear 2–5 days after birth in term infants and as late as the 7th day in premature ones, but hyperbilirubinemia may lead to the syndrome at any time during the neonatal period. The early signs may be subtle and indistinguishable from those of sepsis, asphyxia, hypoglycemia, intracranial hemorrhage, and other acute systemic illnesses in the neonatal infant. Lethargy, poor feeding, and loss of the Moro reflex are common initial signs. Subsequently, the infant may appear gravely ill and prostrated with diminished tendon reflexes and respiratory distress. Opisthotonos, with bulging fontanel, twitching of face or limbs, and a shrill high-pitched cry may follow. In advanced cases convulsions and spasm occur, with the infant stiffly extending his or her arms in inward rotation with fists clenched. Rigidity is rare at this late stage.

Many infants who progress to these severe neurologic signs die; the survivors are usually seriously damaged but may appear to recover and for 2–3 mo manifest few abnormalities. Later in the 1st yr of life opisthotonos, muscular rigidity, irregular movements, and convulsions tend to recur. In the 2nd yr opisthotonos and seizures abate but irregular, involuntary movements, muscular rigidity, or, in some infants, hypotonia increase steadily. By 3 yr of age the complete neurologic syndrome is often apparent, consisting of bilateral choreoathetosis with involuntary muscle spasm, extrapyramidal signs, seizures, mental deficiency, dysarthric speech, high-frequency hearing loss, squints, and defective upward movement of the eyes. Pyramidal signs, hypotonia, and ataxia occur in a few infants. In mildly affected infants the syndrome may be characterized only by mild to moderate neuromuscular incoordination, partial deafness, or "minimal brain dysfunction," occurring singly or in combination; these problems may be inapparent until the child enters school.

PATHOLOGY. The surface of the brain is usually pale yellow. On cutting, certain regions are characteristically stained yellow by unconjugated bilirubin, particularly the corpus subthalamicum, hippocampus and adjacent olfactory areas, striate bodies, thalamus, globus pallidus, putamen, inferior clivus, cerebellar nuclei, and cranial nerve nuclei. Nonpigmented areas may also be damaged. Loss of neurons, reactive gliosis, and atrophy of involved fiber systems are found in late disease. The pattern of injury has been related to the development of oxidative enzyme systems in various regions of the brain and overlaps with that found in hypoxic brain damage. Evidence favors the hypothesis that bilirubin interferes with oxygen utilization by cerebral tissue, possibly by injuring the cell membrane; antecedent hypoxic injury increases the susceptibility of brain cells to injury. Gross bilirubin staining without hyperbilirubinemia or the specific microscopic changes of kernicterus may not be the same entity.

INCIDENCE AND PROGNOSIS. Using pathologic criteria one third of infants with untreated hemolytic disease and bilirubin levels in excess of 20 mg/dL (342 μmol/L) will develop kernicterus. The incidence at autopsy in hyperbilirubinemic premature infants is 2–16% and is related to the risk factors discussed in Sec. 9.44. Reliable estimates of the frequency of the clinical syndrome are not available because of the wide spectrum of manifestations. Overt neurologic signs have a grave prognosis; 75% or more of such infants die, and 80% of affected survivors have bilateral choreoathetosis with involuntary muscle spasm. Mental retardation, deafness, and spastic quadriplegia are common. Infants at risk should have screening hearing tests.

TREATMENT OF HYPERBILIRUBINEMIA. Regardless of etiology, the goal of therapy is to prevent the concentration of indirect-reacting bilirubin in the blood from reaching levels at which neurotoxicity may occur; it is recommended that exchange transfusion or phototherapy be used to keep the maximum total serum bilirubin below the levels indicated in Table 9–26. The risk of injury to the central nervous system from bilirubin must be balanced against the risk inherent in the treatment for each infant. The criteria for initiating phototherapy are not generally agreed on. Since phototherapy may require 12–24 hr to have a measurable effect, it must be started at bilirubin levels below those indicated in Table 9–26. When identified, the underlying cause of the icterus should be treated, for example, antibiotics for septicemia. Physiologic factors that increase the risk of neurologic damage should also be treated (e.g., correction of acidosis).

Exchange Transfusion. This widely accepted treatment should be repeated as frequently as necessary to keep indirect bilirubin levels in the serum under 20 mg/dL (342 μmol/L) in full-term infants. (See Exchange Transfusion in Sec. 9.47.) A variety of factors may alter this criterion in either direction in an individual patient. Appearance of clinical signs suggesting kernicterus is an indication for exchange transfusion at any level of serum bilirubin. A healthy full-term infant with physiologic or breast milk jaundice may tolerate a concentration slightly higher than 20 mg/dL with no apparent ill effect, whereas a sick premature infant may develop kernicterus at a significantly lower level. A level approaching that considered critical for the individual infant may be an indication for exchange transfusion during the 1st day or two of life when a further rise is anticipated but not on the 4th day in term infants or on the 7th day in premature infants, when an imminent fall may be anticipated as the hepatic conjugating mechanism becomes more effective.

Phototherapy. Clinical jaundice and indirect hyperbilirubinemia are reduced on exposure to a high intensity of light in the visible spectrum. Bilirubin absorbs light maximally in the blue range (from 420 to 470 nm). Nonetheless, broad-spectrum white, blue, special narrow spectrum (super) blue, and green lights have been effective in reducing bilirubin levels. Although blue light provides the appropriate wavelengths for photoactivation of free bilirubin, green light may effect photoreactions of albumin-bound bilirubin. Bilirubin in the skin absorbs light energy, which by photoisomerization converts the toxic native unconjugated 4Z,15Z-bilirubin into the unconjugated configurational isomer, 4Z,15E-bilirubin. The latter is the product of a reversible reaction and is excreted in the bile without the need for conjugation. Phototherapy also converts native bilirubin, by an irreversible reaction, to the structural isomer lumirubin, which is excreted by the kidney in the unconjugated state.

TABLE 9–26. Guidelines for Maximal Permissible Total Serum Bilirubin Concentrations (mg/dL)*†

Birthweight Category (g)‡	Uncomplicated Course	Complicated Course§
Less than 1,250	13‖	10
1,250–1,499	15	13
1,500–1,999	17	15
2,000–2,499	18	17
2,500 and up	20	18

*Direct-reacting bilirubin concentrations are not subtracted unless they amount to more than 50% of the total serum bilirubin concentration. This table is applicable during the first 28 days of life.

†From Gartner LM. *In*: Behrman RE (ed): Neonatal-Perinatal Medicine. St. Louis, CV Mosby, 1977.

‡Equivalent gestational age categories may be used in lieu of birth weight for small for gestational age (SGA) infants.

§Complications include perinatal asphyxia and acidosis, postnatal hypoxia and acidosis, significant and persistent hypothermia, hypoalbuminemia, meningitis, and other significant infections, hemolysis, hypoglycemia, and signs of clinical or CNS deterioration.

‖To convert mg/dL to μmol/L, multiply by 17.1.

The use of phototherapy with fluorescent light bulbs has decreased the need for exchange transfusion in LBW infants without hemolytic disease and in LBW infants with hemolysis as well as for repeated exchange transfusion of infants with hemolytic disease. However, when there are indications for exchange transfusion, phototherapy should not be used as a substitute.

Phototherapy is indicated only after the presence of pathologic hyperbilirubinemia has been established. The basic cause(s) of the jaundice should be treated concomitantly. Phototherapy may be initiated at a bilirubin level of 16–18 mg/dL (273–307 μmol/L) in the full-term infant with physiologic jaundice. It is usually begun at bilirubin levels that are 50–75% of the exchange transfusion level in preterm infants. Prophylactic phototherapy in VLBW infants may prevent hyperbilirubinemia and may reduce the incidence of exchange transfusions.

Normal infants receiving phototherapy for 1–3 days have peak serum bilirubin concentrations about one half those of untreated infants. In premature infants without significant hemolysis serum bilirubin usually declines 1–3 mg/dL after 12–24 hr of exposure, and peak levels attained may be decreased by 3–6 mg/dL. The therapeutic effect depends on the light energy emitted in the effective range of wavelengths, the distance between the lights and the infant, and the amount of skin exposed, as well as on the rate of hemolysis and in vivo metabolism and excretion of bilirubin. It is not known whether phototherapy prevents kernicterus or milder forms of brain injury associated with bilirubin toxicity. Available commercial phototherapy units vary considerably in the spectral output and intensity of radiation emitted; therefore, the dose can be accurately measured only at the skin surface. Dark skin does not reduce the efficacy of phototherapy.

Phototherapy is applied continuously, and the infant is turned frequently for maximal skin exposure. It should be discontinued as soon as the indirect bilirubin concentration has been reduced to levels considered safe in view of the infant's age and condition. Serum bilirubin levels and hematocrits should be monitored every 4–8 hr in infants with hemolytic disease or those with bilirubin levels near the range considered toxic for the individual infant. Others, particularly older infants, may be monitored at 12–24 hr intervals. Monitoring should continue for at least 24 hr after cessation of phototherapy, since unexpected rises of serum bilirubin sometimes occur and require further treatment. Skin color cannot be relied on for evaluating the effectiveness of phototherapy; the skin of babies exposed to light may appear almost without jaundice in the presence of marked hyperbilirubinemia. The infant's eyes should be closed and adequately covered to prevent exposure to light (excessive pressure from an eye bandage may injure the closed eyes, or the corneas may be excoriated if the infant can open his or her eyes under the bandage). Body temperature should be monitored, and the infant should be shielded from bulb breakage. If feasible, irradiance should be measured directly, and details of the exposure should be recorded (type and age of bulbs, duration of exposure, distance from light source to infant, and so forth). *In the infant with hemolytic disease, care must be taken not to overlook developing anemia, which may require transfusion.*

Complications of phototherapy include loose stools, rashes, overheating and dehydration (increased insensible water loss, diarrhea), chilling from exposure of the infant, and "bronze baby syndrome." Phototherapy is contraindicated in the presence of porphyria. Eye injury or nasal occlusion from the bandages is uncommon.

The term **bronze baby syndrome** refers to a dark, grayish brown discoloration of the skin sometimes noted in infants undergoing phototherapy. Almost all infants observed with this syndrome have had a mixed type of hyperbilirubinemia with significant elevation of direct-reacting bilirubin and often with other evidence of obstructive liver disease. The discoloration may last for many months.

Wide clinical experience suggests that long-term adverse biologic effects of phototherapy are absent, minimal, or unrecognized. However, those employing phototherapy should remain alert to these possibilities and avoid its unnecessary use, since untoward effects on DNA have been demonstrated in vitro.

Phenobarbital. Phenobarbital enhances the conjugation and excretion of bilirubin. Its administration will limit the development of physiologic jaundice in the newborn infant when administered to mothers in a dose of 90 mg/24 hr prior to delivery or to infants at birth in a dose of 10 mg/kg/24 hr. However, because its effect on bilirubin metabolism is usually not manifest until after several days of administration, because it is less effective than phototherapy in lowering serum bilirubin concentrations, and because it may have an untoward sedative effect and does not add to the response to phototherapy, phenobarbital is not routinely recommended for treating jaundice in the neonatal infant.

Tin (Sn)-protoporphyrin administration has also been proposed for the reduction of bilirubin levels. It may inhibit the conversion of biliverdin to bilirubin by heme oxygenase. Although bilirubin levels may decline, the effect is no greater than that achieved with phototherapy. Complications include transient erythemia if the infant is receiving phototherapy. More data are needed about its efficacy and toxicity before Sn-protoporphyrin can be recommended as therapy for hyperbilirubinemia.

Broderson R: Bilirubin transport in the newborn infant, reviewed with relationship to kernicterus. J Pediatr 96:349, 1980.
Cashore W, Stern L: The management of hyperbilirubinemia. Clin Perinatol 11:339, 1984.
Ennever JF, Knox I, Speck WT: Differences in bilirubin isomer composition in infants treated with green and white light phototherapy. J Pediatr 109:119, 1986.
Fetus and Newborn Committee, Canadian Paediatric Society: Use of phototherapy for neonatal hyperbilirubinemia. Can Med Assoc J 134:1237, 1986.
Gollan, JL, Knapp AB: Bilirubin metabolism and congenital jaundice. Hosp Prac 20:83, 1985.
Gourley GR, Arend RA: Beta-glucuronidase and hyperbilirubinaemia in breast-fed and formula-fed babies. Lancet 2:644, 1986.
Kivlahan C, James EJP: The natural history of neonatal jaundice. Pediatrics 74:364, 1984.
Lewis HM, Campbell RHA, Gambleton G: Use or abuse of phototherapy for physiological jaundice of newborn infants. Lancet 2:408, 1982.
Maisels M: Light versus tin? Pediatrics 81:882, 1988.
Maisels M, Gifford K, Antle C, et al: Jaundice in the healthy newborn infant: A new approach to an old problem. Pediatrics 81:505, 1988.
Maisels MJ, Gifford K: Normal serum bilirubin levels in the newborn and the effect of breast-feeding. Pediatrics 78:837, 1986.
National Institute of Child Health and Human Development: Randomized, controlled trial of phototherapy for neonatal hyperbilirubinemia. Pediatrics (Suppl)75:385, 1985.
Nwaesei CG, Aerde JV, Boyden M, et al: Changes in auditory brainstem responses in hyperbilirubinemic infants before and after exchange transfusion. Pediatrics 74:800, 1984.
Roth P, Polin R: Controversial topics in kernicterus. Clin Perinatol 15:965, 1988.
Scheidt PC, Mellito ED, Hardy JB, et al: Toxicity to bilirubin in neonates: Infant development during the first year in relation to maximum neonatal serum bilirubin concentration. J Pediatr 92:292, 1977.
Turkel S, Guttenberg M, Moynes D, et al: Lack of identifiable risk factors for kernicterus. Pediatrics 66:502, 1980.
Turkel S, Miller CA, Guttenberg M, et al: A clinical pathologic reappraisal of kernicterus. Pediatrics 69:267, 1982.

THE BLOOD

9.46 ANEMIA IN THE NEWBORN INFANT

Fetal hemoglobin increases with advancing gestational age: at term, cord blood hemoglobin is 16.8 g/dL (14–20 g/dL); hemoglobin levels in VLBW infants are 1–2 g/dL below those at term (Fig. 9–25). Determinations of less than the normal range for birthweight and postnatal age are defined as anemia (see Tables 27–2 and 16–2). A "physiologic" decrease in hemoglobin content is noticed at 8–12 wk in term infants (hemoglobin 11 g/dL) and at about 6 wk in premature infants (7–10 g/dL).

Anemia at birth is manifest by pallor, congestive heart failure, or shock (Fig. 9–26). It is usually caused by hemolytic disease of the newborn but may also be the result of tearing or cutting of the umbilical cord during delivery, abnormal cord insertions, communicating placental vessels, placenta previa or abruptio, nuchal cord, incision into the placenta, internal hemorrhage (liver, spleen, or intracranial), α-thalassemia, congenital parvovirus infection or hypoplastic anemias, and twin-twin transfusion in monozygotic twins with arteriovenous placental connections (Sec. 9.16).

Transplacental hemorrhage, with bleeding from the fetal into the maternal circulation, is probably more common than is generally recognized and, unless severe, is usually not sufficient to cause clinically apparent anemia at birth. The cause of transplacental hemorrhage is not clear, but its occurrence has been proved by demonstrating significant amounts of fetal hemoglobin and red blood cells in the maternal blood on the day of delivery by the Kleihaur-Betke test.

Acute blood loss usually results in severe distress at birth, initially with a normal hemoglobin level, no hepatosplenomegaly, and early onset of shock. In contrast, chronic blood loss in utero produces marked pallor, less distress, low hemoglobin level with microcytic indices, and, if severe, congestive heart failure.

Anemia appearing in the first few days after birth is also most frequently the result of hemolytic disease of the newborn. Other causes are hemorrhagic disease of the newborn, bleeding from an improperly tied or clamped umbilical cord, large cephalohematoma, intracranial hemorrhage, or subcapsular bleeding from rupture of the liver, spleen, adrenals, or kidneys. Rapid decreases in hemoglobin or hematocrit values

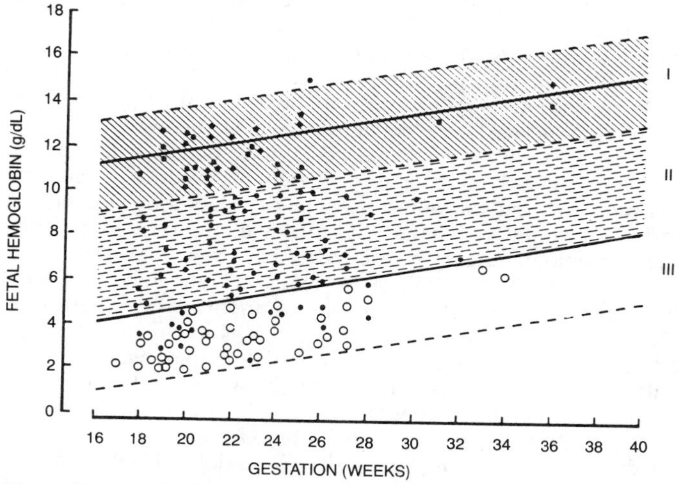

Figure 9–25. Range (mean and 95% confidence limits) of fetal hemoglobin concentration from 16–40 wk of gestational age from normal (zone I) fetuses obtained by cordocentesis. (●) depicts maternal red blood cell isoimmunization, (○) are hemoglobin levels in fetus with ultrasonographic evidence of hydrops (zone III). (From Soothill P: Clin Perinatol 16:755, 1989.)

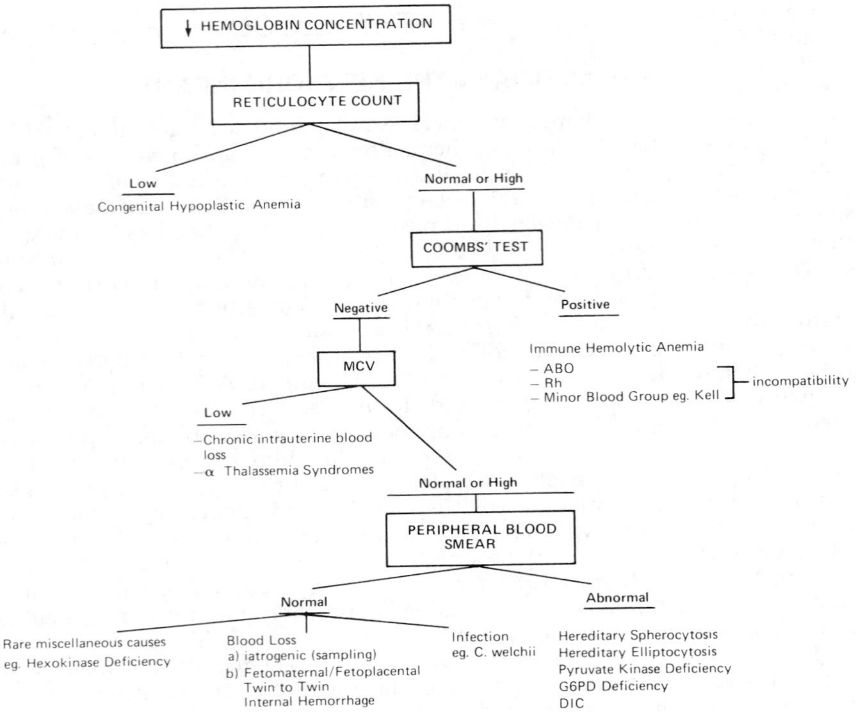

Figure 9–26. Diagnostic approach to anemia in the newborn infant. (From Blanchette V, Zipursky A: Clin Perinatol 11:489, 1984.)

during the first few days of life may be the initial clue to these conditions.

Later in the neonatal period delayed anemia from hemolytic disease of the newborn, with or without exchange transfusion or phototherapy, may be seen. Vitamin K (as Synkayvite) in large doses may cause anemia in premature infants, which is characterized by inclusion bodies (Heinz bodies) in the erythrocytes. Congenital hemolytic anemia (spherocytosis) occasionally appears during the 1st mo of life, and hereditary nonspherocytic hemolytic anemia has been described during the neonatal period secondary to deficiency of such enzymes as G-6-PD and pyruvate kinase. Bleeding from hemangiomas of the upper gastrointestinal tract or from ulcers caused by aberrant gastric mucosa in a Meckel diverticulum or duplication is a rare source of anemia in the newborn. Repeated blood sampling of infants requiring frequent monitoring of blood gases and chemistries may also produce anemia. Deficiency of minerals such as copper may cause anemia in infants on total parenteral nutrition.

Anemia of prematurity occurs in LBW infants 1–3 mo after birth, is associated with hemoglobin levels below 7–10 g/dL, and presents with clinical manifestations such as apnea, poor weight gain, pallor, decreased activity, tachypnea, tachycardia, and feeding problems. Repeated phlebotomy for blood tests, shortened red blood cell survival, rapid growth, and the physiologic effects of the transition from fetal (low PaO_2 and hemoglobin saturation) to neonatal life (high PaO_2 and hemoglobin saturation) contribute to anemia of prematurity. The oxygen available to neonatal tissue is lower than that in adults, but the neonate's erythropoietin response is attenuated for the degree of anemia, resulting in low hemoglobin levels with reticulocytopenia.

Treatment of neonatal anemia by blood transfusion depends on the severity of symptoms, the hemoglobin level, and the presence of co-morbid diseases (bronchopulmonary dysplasia, hyaline membrane disease) that interfere with oxygen delivery. Treatment with blood should be balanced by concern about transfusion-acquired infection (CMV, HIV, hepatitis B and C). The risk of CMV infection can be almost eliminated by the use of CMV antibody–negative blood, while that for HIV and hepatitis B and C viruses is reduced but not eliminated by antibody screening of donated blood.

An asymptomatic full-term infant with a hemoglobin level of 10 g/dL may be observed, whereas the symptomatic neonate born following an abruptio placentae or with severe hemolytic disease of the newborn warrants immediate transfusion. The preterm infant who has repeated episodes of apnea and bradycardia despite theophylline therapy and a hemoglobin level of less than 10 g/dL may benefit from red blood cell transfusion. In addition, infants with hyaline membrane disease or severe bronchopulmonary dysplasia may need hemoglobin levels of 14 g/dL to improve oxygen delivery. Packed red blood cell transfusion (10–15 mL/kg) is given at a rate of 2–3 ml/kg/hr to raise the hemoglobin concentration; 2 mL/kg raises the hemoglobin level 0.5–1 g/dL. Hemorrhage should be treated with whole blood if available; alternatively, fluid resuscitation is initiated and followed by packed red blood cell transfusion.

9.47 HEMOLYTIC DISEASE OF THE NEWBORN
(Erythroblastosis Fetalis)

Erythroblastosis fetalis results from the transplacental passage of maternal antibody active against red blood cell antigens of the infant, leading to an increased rate of red cell destruction. It continues to be an important cause of anemia and jaundice in newborn infants despite the development of a method of prevention of maternal isoimmunization by Rh antigens. Although more than 60 different red blood cell antigens capable of eliciting an antibody response in a suitable recipient have been identified, significant disease is associated primarily with the D antigen of the Rh group and with incompatibility of ABO factors. Rarely, hemolytic disease may be caused by C or E antigens or by other red blood cell antigens, such as C^w, C^x, D^u, K(Kell), M, Duffy, S, and Kidd. Anti-Lewis antibodies do not cause disease.

Hemolytic Disease of the Newborn Due to Rh Incompatibility

The Rh antigenic determinants are genetically transmitted from each parent and determine the Rh type and direct the production of a number of blood group factors (C, c, D, d, E, and e). Each factor can elicit a specific antibody response under suitable conditions; 90% are due to D antigen, the remaining to C or E.

PATHOGENESIS. Isoimmune hemolytic disease from D antigen is approximately three times more frequent in whites than in blacks. When Rh positive blood is infused into an Rh negative woman through error or when small quantities (usually more than 1 mL) of Rh positive fetal blood containing D antigen inherited from an Rh positive father enter the maternal circulation during pregnancy, with spontaneous or induced abortion, or at delivery, antibody formation against D may be induced in the unsensitized Rh negative recipient mother. Once immunization has occurred, considerably smaller doses of antigen can stimulate an increase in antibody titer. Initially, a rise of antibody in the 19S gamma globulin fraction occurs, which later is replaced by 7S (IgG) antibody; the latter readily crosses the placenta, causing hemolytic manifestations.

Hemolytic disease rarely occurs during a first pregnancy, since transfusions of Rh positive fetal blood into an Rh negative mother tend to occur near the time of delivery, too late for the mother to become sensitized and transmit antibody to the infant before delivery. The fact that 55% of Rh positive fathers are heterozygous (D/d) and may have Rh negative offspring and that only 50% of pregnancies have fetal-to-maternal transfusions reduces the chance of sensitization, as does small family size, in which the opportunities for its occurrence are fewer. Finally, the capacity of Rh negative women to form antibodies is variable, some producing low titers even after adequate antigenic challenge. Thus, the overall incidence of isoimmunization of Rh negative mothers at risk is low, with antibody to D detected in less than 10% of those studied, even after five or more pregnancies; only about 5% ever have babies having hemolytic disease.

When mother and fetus are also incompatible with respect to groups A or B, the mother is partially protected against sensitization by the rapid removal of Rh positive cells from her circulation by her anti-A or anti-B, which are IgM antibodies and do not cross the placenta. Once the mother has been sensitized, the infant is likely to have hemolytic disease. There is a tendency for the severity of Rh illness to worsen with successive pregnancies. The possibility that the first affected infant after sensitization may represent the end of the mother's child-bearing potential for Rh positive infants argues urgently for the prevention of sensitization when this is possible. Such prevention consists of injection into the mother of anti-D gamma globulin (RhoGAM) immediately following the delivery of each Rh positive infant (see below).

CLINICAL MANIFESTATIONS. A wide spectrum of hemolytic disease occurs in affected infants born to sensitized mothers, depending on the nature of the individual immune response. The severity of the disease may range from only laboratory evidence of mild hemolysis (15% of cases) to severe anemia with compensatory hyperplasia of erythropoietic tissue, leading to massive enlargement of the liver and spleen. When the compensatory capacity of the hematopoietic system is exceeded, profound anemia results in pallor, signs of cardiac decompensation (cardiomegaly, respiratory distress), massive anasarca, and circulatory collapse. This clinical picture, termed **hydrops fetalis**, frequently results in death in utero or shortly after birth; it may also occur from other nonimmune causes (Table 9–27). The severity of hydrops is related to the level of anemia and the degree of reduction in serum albumin (oncotic pressure), which is due in part to hepatic dysfunction. Failure to initiate spontaneous effective ventilation owing to pulmonary edema or bilateral pleural effusions results in birth asphyxia; following successful resuscitation, severe respiratory distress may ensue. Petechiae, purpura, and thrombocytopenia may also be present in severe cases, reflecting decreased platelet production or the presence of concurrent disseminated intravascular coagulation.

TABLE 9–27. Etiologies of Hydrops Fetalis

Hematologic	Rh and other blood group incompatibilities, thalassemia, twin-twin transfusion, fetomaternal hemorrhage
Infectious	Parvovirus, syphilis, cytomegalovirus, toxoplasmosis, Chagas' disease, leptospirosis
Cardiovascular	Supraventricular tachycardia, heart failure, arteriovenous malformation, umbilical vein thrombosis, congenital heart block, severe congenital heart disease, rhabdomyoma
Pulmonary	Cystic adenomatoid malformation, diaphragmatic hernia, lymphangiectasia, hypoplasia
Tumorous	Congenital neuroblastoma, placental chorioangioma
Hepatic	Hepatitis, fibrosis, cirrhosis
Renal	Nephrosis, prune-belly syndrome, urethral valves
Gastrointestinal	Atresias, volvulus, chylous ascites, cystic fibrosis
Metabolic	Gaucher disease, maternal diabetes mellitus, achondroplasia, other macromolecule storage diseases
Malformation Syndromes	Arthrogryposis, thanatophoric dwarf, Noonan syndrome, Meckel syndrome, amniotic bands
Chromosomal Syndromes	XO, 13-, 18-, 21-triploidy
Idiopathic	

Jaundice is usually absent at birth because of placental clearance of lipid-soluble unconjugated bilirubin, but in severe cases bilirubin pigments stain the amniotic fluid, cord, and vernix caseosa yellow. Icterus is generally evident on the 1st day of life because the infant's bilirubin-conjugating and excretory systems are unable to cope with the load resulting from massive hemolysis. Indirect-reacting bilirubin therefore accumulates postnatally and may rapidly reach extremely high levels, which represent a significant risk of bilirubin encephalopathy. There may be a greater risk of developing kernicterus from hemolytic disease than from comparable nonhemolytic hyperbilirubinemia, although the risk in an individual patient may be a function only of the severity of illness (anoxia, acidosis, and so on). Hypoglycemia occurs frequently in infants with severe isoimmune hemolytic disease and may be related to hyperinsulinism and hypertrophy of the pancreatic islet cells in these infants.

Infants born after intrauterine transfusion for prenatally diagnosed erythroblastosis are generally severely affected, since the indications for the transfusion are evidence of already severe disease in utero (e.g., hydrops, fetal anemia). Such infants usually have very high (but extremely variable) cord levels of bilirubin, which reflects the severity of hemolysis and its effects on hepatic function. Anemia from continuing hemolysis may be masked by the prior intrauterine transfusion, and the clinical manifestations of erythroblastosis may be superimposed upon various degrees of immaturity due to spontaneous or induced premature delivery.

LABORATORY DATA. Prior to treatment, the direct Coombs test is usually positive. Anemia is usual. The cord blood hemoglobin varies, usually proportionally to the severity of the disease; with hydrops fetalis it may be as low as 3–4 g/dL (30–40 g/L). Alternatively, despite hemolysis, it may be within the normal range owing to compensatory bone marrow and extramedullary hematopoiesis. The blood smear usually shows polychromasia and a marked increase in nucleated red blood cells. The reticulocyte count is increased. The white blood cell count is usually normal but may be elevated, and there may be thrombocytopenia in severe cases. The cord bilirubin is usually between 3 and 5 mg/dL (51–86 μmol/L); only rarely is there a substantial elevation of direct-reacting (conjugated) bilirubin. The indirect-reacting bilirubin rises rapidly to high levels in the first 6 hr of life.

After intrauterine transfusions the cord blood may show a normal hemoglobin concentration, negative direct Coombs test, predominantly type O Rh negative adult red cells, and a relatively normal smear. Marked elevation of both indirect- and direct-reacting bilirubin levels has been reported in these infants.

DIAGNOSIS. The definitive diagnosis of erythroblastosis fetalis requires demonstration of blood group incompatibility and of corresponding antibody bound to the infant's red blood cells.

Antenatal Diagnosis. In Rh negative women a history of previous transfusions, abortion, or pregnancy should suggest the possibility of sensitization. Expectant parents' blood types should be tested for potential incompatibility, and the maternal titer of IgG antibodies to D should be assayed at 12–16, 28–32, and 36 wk. The presence of measurable antibody titer at the beginning of pregnancy, a rapid rise in titer, or a titer of 1:64 or greater suggests significant hemolytic disease, although the exact titer correlates poorly with the severity of disease. If a mother is found to have antibody against D at a titer of 1:16 or greater at any time during a subsequent pregnancy, the severity of fetal disease should be monitored by amniocentesis, percutaneous umbilical blood sampling (PUBS), and ultrasonography. If there is a history of a previously affected infant or a stillbirth, an Rh positive infant is usually equally or more severely affected than the previous infant, and the severity of disease in the fetus should be followed.

Assessment of the fetus may require information obtained from ultrasound, amniocentesis, and PUBS. Real-time ultrasound is used to detect the progression of hemolysis from mild to severe, with hydrops defined as skin or scalp edema, pleural or pericardial effusions, and ascites. Early ultrasonographic signs of hydrops include organomegaly (liver, spleen, heart), double bowel wall sign (bowel edema), and placental thickening. There may then be progression to polyhydramnios, ascites, pleural or pericardial effusions, and skin or scalp edema. If pleural effusions precede ascites and hydrops by a significant period of time, causes other than fetal anemia should be suspected (see Table 9–27). Extramedullary hematopoiesis and, less so, hepatic congestion compress the intrahepatic vessels, producing venous stasis with portal hypertension, hepatocellular dysfunction, and decreased albumin synthesis.

Hydrops is invariable when fetal hemoglobin is less than 5 g/dL, frequent when under 7 g/dL, and variable between 7 and 9 g/dL. Real-time ultrasound predicts fetal well-being by the biophysical profile (see Table 9–10), whereas Doppler ultrasound assesses fetal distress by demonstrating increased vascular resistance (see Tables 9–10 and 9–6). If there is ultrasonographic evidence of hemolysis (hepatosplenomegaly), early or late hydrops, or fetal distress, an amniocentesis or PUBS should be performed.

Amniocentesis is used to assess fetal hemolysis. Hemolysis of fetal erythrocytes produces hyperbilirubinemia before the onset of severe anemia. Bilirubin is cleared by the placenta, but a significant proportion enters the amniotic fluid and can be measured by spectrophotometry. Amniocentesis is performed if there is evidence of maternal sensitization (titer ≥ 1:16), if the father is Rh positive, or if there are ultrasonographic signs of hemolysis, hydrops, or distress. Ultrasonographic-guided transabdominal aspiration of amniotic fluid may be performed as early as 18–20 wk of gestation. Spectrophotometric scanning of amniotic fluid wavelengths demonstrates a positive optical density (OD) deviation of absorption for bilirubin from normal at 450 nm. The OD 450 is a reflection of fetal bilirubin levels, and thus hemolysis, and indicates the severity of anemia and the risk of intrauterine death. With maturity, the level of amniotic fluid bilirubin normally declines; thus the fetal risk is assessed during gestation in terms of three relative but declining zones of OD 450, with zone III representing the highest risk. However, some fetuses in zone III do not have life-threatening fetal anemia and thus do not require intrauterine transfusion. If the OD 450 is in zone III or if hydrops or other signs suggesting fetal anemia are present, PUBS should be performed to determine fetal hemoglobin levels, and packed red blood cells should be transfused if serious anemia exists (Sec. 9.13).

Postnatal Diagnosis. Immediately after the birth of any infant to an Rh negative woman, blood from the umbilical cord or from the infant should be examined for ABO blood group, Rh type, hematocrit and hemoglobin, and reaction of the direct Coombs test. If the Coombs test is positive, baseline serum bilirubin should be measured, and a commercially available red blood cell panel should be used to identify red blood cell antibodies that are present in the mother's serum, both of which tests are done not only to establish the diagnosis but also to ensure the selection of the most compatible blood for exchange transfusion should it be necessary. The direct Coombs test is usually strongly positive in clinically affected infants and may remain so for a few days up to several months.

TREATMENT. The main goals of therapy are (1) to prevent intrauterine or extrauterine death from severe anemia and hypoxia and (2) to avoid neurotoxicity from hyperbilirubinemia.

Treatment of the Unborn Infant. The survival of the severely affected fetus has been improved by the use of ultrasonographic and amniotic fluid analysis to identify the need for in utero transfusion. Intrauterine transfusion into the fetal peritoneal cavity is being replaced by direct intravascular transfusion of packed red blood cells. Hydrops or fetal anemia (hemoglobin < 8 g/dL; hematocrit < 25%) are indications for umbilical vein transfusion in infants with pulmonary immaturity (see Fig. 9–25). Intravascular transfusion is facilitated by maternal and hence fetal sedation with diazepam and by fetal paralysis with pancuronium. Packed red blood cells are given by slow-push infusion after cross-matching to the mother's serum. The cells should be obtained from a CMV-negative donor and irradiated to kill lymphocytes in order to avoid graft versus host disease. Transfusions should achieve a post-transfusion hematocrit of 40% and can be repeated every 2 wk. Indications for delivery include pulmonary maturity, fetal distress, complications of PUBS, or 35–37 wk of gestation.

Treatment of the Liveborn Infant. The birth should be attended by the physician who will care for the affected infant afterward. Fresh, low titer, group O, Rh negative blood, cross-matched against the maternal serum, should be immediately available. If clinical signs of severe hemolytic anemia (pallor, hepatosplenomegaly, edema, petechiae, or ascites) are evident at birth, immediate supportive therapy, temperature stabilization, and monitoring before proceeding with exchange transfusion may save some severely affected infants. Such therapy should include correction of acidosis with 1–2 mEq/kg of sodium bicarbonate; a small transfusion of compatible packed red blood cells to correct anemia; volume expansion for hypotension, especially in those with hydrops; and provision of assisted ventilation for respiratory failure.

Exchange Transfusion. When the infant's clinical condition at birth does not require an immediate full or partial exchange transfusion, the decision to perform one should be based on a judgment that there is a high risk of rapid development of a dangerous degree of anemia or of hyperbilirubinemia. Cord hemoglobin of 10 g/dL or less and bilirubin of 5 mg/dL or more (85 μmol/L) suggest severe hemolysis but inconsistently predict the need for immediate exchange transfusion. Some physicians consider previous kernicterus or severe erythroblastosis in a sibling, reticulocyte counts greater than 15%, and prematurity to be further factors supporting a decision for early exchange transfusion.

The hemoglobin, hematocrit, and serum bilirubin levels should be measured at 4- to 6-hr intervals at first, with extension to longer intervals if and as the rate of change diminishes. The decision to perform an exchange transfusion is based on the likelihood that the trend of bilirubin levels plotted against hours of age indicates that the serum bilirubin will reach the level indicated in Table 9–26, above which there is an increased risk of kernicterus. Ordinary transfusions of compatible Rh negative red blood cells may be necessary to correct anemia at any stage of the disease up to 6–8 wk of age, when the infant's own blood-forming mechanism may be expected to take over. Weekly determinations of hemoglobin or hematocrit should be done until a spontaneous rise has been demonstrated.

Careful monitoring of the serum bilirubin level is essential until a falling trend has been demonstrated in the absence of phototherapy (Sec. 9.45). Even then, an occasional infant, particularly if premature, may experience an unpredicted significant rise in serum bilirubin as late as the 7th day of life. Attempts to predict the attainment of dangerously high levels of serum bilirubin, based on observed levels exceeding 6 mg/dL in the first 6 hr or 10 mg/dL in the second 6 hr of life or on rates of rise exceeding 0.5–1.0 mg/dL/hr, can be unreliable. Indices of free bilirubin and bilirubin binding have not been shown to be routinely reliable aids in evaluating the risk associated with hyperbilirubinemia.

Blood for exchange transfusion should be as fresh as possible. Heparin or adenosine-citrate-phosphate-dextrose (CPD) may be used as anticoagulants. If the blood is obtained before delivery, it should be taken from a type O, Rh negative donor with a low titer of anti-A and anti-B and should be compatible with the mother's serum by indirect Coombs test. After delivery, blood should be obtained from an Rh negative donor whose cells are compatible with both the infant's and the mother's serum; when possible, type O donor cells are usually employed, but cells of the infant's ABO blood type may be used when the mother has the same type. A complete cross-match, including indirect Coombs test, should be performed prior to the second and subsequent transfusions. Blood should be gradually warmed to and maintained at a temperature between 35° and 37° C throughout the exchange transfusion. It should be kept well mixed by gentle squeezing or agitation of the bag to avoid sedimentation; otherwise, the use of supernatant serum with a low red blood cell count at the end of the exchange will leave the infant anemic. Whole blood or packed red blood cells reconstituted with fresh frozen plasma to a hematocrit of 40% should be used. The infant's stomach should be emptied prior to transfusion to prevent aspiration, body temperature should be maintained and vital signs monitored. A competent assistant should be present to help monitor, tally the volume of blood exchanged, and perform emergency procedures.

The umbilical vein is cannulated, using strict aseptic technique, with a polyvinyl catheter to a distance no greater than 7 cm in a full-term infant. When free flow of blood is obtained, the catheter is usually in a large hepatic vein or the inferior vena cava. Exchange should be carried out over a 45- to 60-min period, alternating aspirations of 20 mL of infant blood and infusions of 20 mL of donor blood. Smaller aliquots (5–10 mL) may be indicated for sick and premature infants. The goal should be an exchange of approximately 2 blood volumes of the infant (2 × 85 mL/kg). If heparinized blood is used, 0.45 mL (4.5 mg) of a 1% solution of protamine sulfate may be injected intravenously at the conclusion of the transfusion for each dL of blood exchanged.

Infants with acidosis and hypoxia from respiratory distress, sepsis, or shock may be further compromised by the significant acute acid load contained in citrated (CPD) blood, which usually has a pH between 7 and 7.2. The subsequent metabolism of citrate may result in a later metabolic alkalosis if CPD blood is used. Fresh heparinized blood avoids this problem. During the exchange, the blood pH and Pa_{O_2} should be serially monitored, since infants often become acidotic and hypoxic during exchange transfusions. Symptomatic hypoglycemia may occur before or during exchange transfusion in moderately to severely affected infants; it may also occur 1–3 hr after exchange. Acute complications, noted in 5–10% of infants, include transient bradycardia with or without calcium infusion, cyanosis, transient vasospasm, thrombosis, and apnea with bradycardia requiring resuscitation. Infectious risks include CMV, HIV, and hepatitis. Necrotizing enterocolitis is a rare complication of exchange transfusion.

After exchange transfusion the bilirubin level must be determined at frequent intervals (every 4–8 hr), as bilirubin may rebound 40–50% within hours. Repeated exchange transfusions should be carried out to keep the indirect fraction from exceeding the levels indicated in Table 9–26. Symptoms suggestive of kernicterus are mandatory indications for exchange transfusion at any time.

The risk of death from exchange transfusion performed by experienced physicians is 0.3/100 procedures. However, with the decreasing use of this procedure owing to the prevalent use of phototherapy and because sensitization is being prevented, the general level of physician competence is decreasing. Thus, it may be best to concentrate this mode of treatment in neonatal referral centers.

Late Complications. The infant who has hemolytic disease or who has had an exchange or an intrauterine transfusion must be observed carefully for the development of anemia and cholestasis. Late anemia may be hemolytic or hyporegenerative. Treatment with supplemental iron or blood transfusion may be indicated. A mild graft-versus-host reaction may be manifested as diarrhea, rash, hepatitis, and eosinophilia.

Inspissated bile syndrome refers to the rare occurrence of persistent icterus in association with significant elevations of direct as well as indirect bilirubin in infants with hemolytic disease. The cause is unclear, but the jaundice clears spontaneously within a few weeks or months.

Portal vein thrombosis may occur among children who have been subjected to exchange transfusion as newborn infants. It is probably associated with prolonged, traumatic, or septic umbilical vein catheterization.

Prevention of Rh Sensitization. The risk of initial sensitization of Rh negative mothers has been reduced from between 10 and 20% to less than 1% by intramuscular injection of 300 μg of human anti-D globulin (1 mL of RhoGAM) within 72 hr of delivery or abortion. This quantity is sufficient to eliminate approximately 10 mL of potentially antigenic fetal cells from the maternal circulation. Large fetal-to-maternal transfers of blood may require proportionately more RhoGAM. RhoGAM, administered at 28–32 wk and again at birth (40 wk), may be more effective than a single dose. The use of this technique, combined with improved methods of detecting maternal sensitization and quantitating the extent of the fetal-to-maternal transfusion, plus the use of fewer obstetric procedures that increase the risk of such fetal-to-maternal bleeding (versions, manual separation of the placenta, and so on), should further reduce the incidence of erythroblastosis fetalis.

Hemolytic Disease of the Newborn Due to A and B Incompatibility

Major blood group incompatibility between mother and fetus usually results in milder disease than does Rh incompatibility. Maternal antibody may be formed against B cells if the mother is type A or against A cells if the mother is type B. However, usually the mother is type O and the infant is type A or B. Although ABO incompatibility occurs in 20–25% of pregnancies, hemolytic disease develops in only 10% of such offspring, and usually the infants are of type A_1, which is more antigenic than A_2. Low antigenicity of the ABO factors in the fetus and newborn infant may account for the low incidence of severe ABO hemolytic disease relative to the incidence of incompatibility between the blood groups of mother and child. Although antibodies against A and B factors occur without prior immunization ("natural" antibodies), these are ordinarily present in the 19S (IgM) fraction of gamma globulin, which does not cross the placenta. However, univalent, incomplete (albumin active) antibodies to A antigen may be present in the 7S (IgG) fraction, which does cross the placenta, so that A–O isoimmune hemolytic disease may be seen in firstborn infants. Mothers who have become immunized against A or B factors from a previous incompatible pregnancy also exhibit antibody in the 7S gamma globulin fraction. These "immune" antibodies are the primary mediators in ABO isoimmune disease.

CLINICAL MANIFESTATIONS. Most cases are mild, with jaundice as the only clinical manifestation. The infant is not generally affected at birth; pallor is not present and hydrops fetalis is extremely rare. Liver and spleen are not greatly enlarged, if at all. Jaundice usually appears during the first 24 hr. Rarely, it may become severe, and symptoms and signs of kernicterus develop rapidly.

DIAGNOSIS. A presumptive diagnosis is based on the presence of ABO incompatibility, a weakly to moderately positive direct Coombs test, and spherocytes in the blood smear, which may at times suggest the presence of hereditary spherocytosis. Hyperbilirubinemia is often the only other laboratory abnormality. The hemoglobin level is usually normal but may be as low as 10–12 g/dL (100–120 g/L). Reticulocytes may be increased to 10–15%, with extensive polychromasia and increased numbers of nucleated red cells. In 10–20% of affected infants the unconjugated serum bilirubin level may reach 20 mg/dL or more unless phototherapy is employed.

TREATMENT. Phototherapy may be effective in lowering serum bilirubin levels (Sec. 9.45). Otherwise, treatment is directed at correcting dangerous degrees of anemia or hyperbilirubinemia by exchange transfusions with blood of the same group as that of the mother (Rh type should match the infant's). The indications for this procedure are similar to those previously described for hemolytic disease due to Rh incompatibility.

Other Forms of Hemolytic Disease

Blood group incompatibilities other than Rh or ABO (c, E, Kell [K], and so on) account for less than 5% of hemolytic disease of the newborn. The direct Coombs test is invariably positive, and exchange transfusion may be indicated for hyperbilirubinemia and anemia. Congenital infections, such as cytomegalic inclusion disease, toxoplasmosis, rubella, and syphilis, may present with hemolytic anemia, jaundice, hepatosplenomegaly, and thrombocytopenia, but the direct Coombs test is negative, and there are usually other distinguishing clinical findings. Homozygous α-thalassemia may present with severe hemolytic anemia and a clinical picture resembling hydrops fetalis; it can be distinguished by a negative direct Coombs test and characteristic clinical and laboratory findings (Sec. 16.26–16.28). Anemia and jaundice may occur in infancy from hereditary spherocytosis (Sec. 15.13) and, if untreated, can result in kernicterus. Hemolytic anemia producing jaundice in the 1st wk of life may also be secondary to congenital deficiencies in red blood cell enzymes, such as pyruvate kinase or G-6-PD.

9.48 PLETHORA IN THE NEWBORN INFANT

(Polycythemia)

See also Sec. 16.33.

Plethora, a ruddy, deep red-purple appearance associated with a high hematocrit, is often due to polycythemia, defined as a central hematocrit of 65% or higher. Peripheral (heelstick) hematocrits are higher than central values, whereas Coulter counter results are lower than hemotocrits determined by microcentrifugation. The incidence of neonatal polycythemia is increased at high altitude (Denver 5% vs Texas 1.6%), in postmature (3%) vs term (1–2%) infants, in SGA (8%) vs LGA (3%) vs AGA (1–2%) infants, during the 1st day of life (peak 2–3 hr), in the recipient infant of a twin-twin transfusion, after delayed clamping of the umbilical cord, in infants of diabetic mothers, in 13-, 18-, or 21-trisomy, in adrenogenital syndrome, in neonatal Graves disease, in hypothyroidism, and in Beckwith-Wiedermann syndrome. Infants of diabetic mothers and those with growth retardation may have been exposed to chronic fetal hypoxia, which stimulated erythropoietin production and increased red blood cell production.

Clinical manifestations include anorexia, lethargy, seizures, cyanosis (persistent fetal circulation), tachypnea, respiratory distress, feeding disturbances, necrotizing enterocolitis, hyperbilirubinemia, renal failure, hypoglycemia, and thrombocytopenia. Fifteen to 25% of affected infants are asymptomatic. Hyperviscosity is present in most infants with central hematocrits of 65% or more and accounts for the symptoms of polycythemia. Hyperviscosity determined at constant shear rates (e.g., 11.5 sec^{-1}) is present when whole blood viscosity is above 18 cycles/sec (cps). Hyperviscosity is accentuated because neonatal erythrocytes have decreased deformability and filterability, predisposing to stasis in the microcirculation.

The *treatment* of symptomatic plethora of the newborn is phlebotomy and replacement with saline or albumin. A partial exchange transfusion to reduce the hematocrit to 50% is a technically simpler and therapeutically more effective approach. The volume exchanged is calculated from the formula:

$$\text{Volume of exchange (mL)} = \text{Blood volume} \times \frac{\text{Observed} - \text{desired HCT}}{\text{Observed HCT}}$$

The long-term *prognosis* of polycythemic infants includes speech deficits, abnormal fine motor control, reduced IQ, and other neurologic abnormalities. Partial exchange transfusion reduces the risk of neurologic problems, poor school performance, and fine motor deficit but is associated with feeding disturbances and may increase the risk of necrotizing enterocolitis.

9.49 HEMORRHAGE IN THE NEWBORN INFANT

HEMORRHAGIC DISEASE OF THE NEWBORN. A moderate decrease of factors II, VII, IX, and X normally occurs in all newborn infants by 48–72 hr after birth, with a gradual return to birth levels by 7–10 days of age. This transient deficiency of vitamin K–dependent factors probably is due to lack of free vitamin K in the mother and absence of bacterial intestinal flora normally responsible for synthesis of vitamin K. Rarely, among term infants and more frequently among premature infants there is an accentuation and prolongation of this deficiency between the 2nd and 5th days of life, resulting in spontaneous and prolonged bleeding. Breast milk is a poor source of vitamin K, and hemorrhagic complications have appeared more commonly in breast-fed than in formula-fed infants. This form of hemorrhagic disease of the newborn, which is responsive to vitamin K therapy, must be distinguished from disseminated intravascular coagulopathy and from rarer congenital deficiencies of one or more of the other factors that are unresponsive to vitamin K (Sec. 16.71).

Hemorrhagic disease of the newborn resulting from severe transient deficiencies of vitamin K–dependent factors is characterized by bleeding that tends to be gastrointestinal, nasal, subgaleal, intracranial, or a result of circumcision. The prothrombin time, blood coagulation time, and partial thromboplastin time are prolonged, and the levels of prothrombin (II) and factors VII, IX, and X are significantly decreased. Vitamin K facilitates post-transcriptional carboxylation of factors II, VII, IX, and X. In the absence of carboxylation such factors form PIVKA (protein induced in vitamin K absence), which is a sensitive marker for vitamin K status. Bleeding time, fibrinogen, factors V and VIII, platelets, capillary fragility, and clot retraction are normal for maturity.

Administering 1 mg of natural oil-soluble vitamin K intramuscularly at the time of birth prevents the fall in vitamin K–dependent factors in full-term infants but is not uniformly effective in the prophylaxis of hemorrhagic disease of the newborn in premature infants. The disease may be effectively treated with an intravenous infusion of 1–5 mg of vitamin K_1, with improvement of coagulation defects and cessation of bleeding within a few hours. However, serious bleeding, particularly in premature infants or those with liver disease, may require a transfusion of fresh frozen plasma or whole blood. The mortality rate is low among treated patients.

A particularly severe form of deficiency of vitamin K–dependent coagulation factors has been reported in infants born to mothers receiving anticonvulsive medications during pregnancy (phenobarbital and phenytoin). There may be severe bleeding with onset within the first 24 hr of life, which is usually corrected by vitamin K_1, although in some the response is poor or delayed. A prothrombin time (PT) should be obtained on cord blood and the infant given 1–2 mg of vitamin K intravenously. If the PT is greatly prolonged and fails to improve, 10 mL/kg of fresh frozen plasma should be given.

Other forms of bleeding may be clinically indistinguishable from hemorrhagic disease of the newborn responsive to vitamin K but are neither prevented nor successfully treated with it. A clinical pattern identical to that of hemorrhagic disease of the newborn may also result from any of the **congenital defects in blood coagulation** (Sec. 16.63–16.71). Hematomas, melena, and postcircumcision and umbilical cord bleeding may be present; only 5–35% of factor VIII and IX deficiencies become clinically apparent in the newborn period. Treatment of the rare congenital deficiencies of coagulation factors requires fresh frozen plasma or specific factor replacement.

Disseminated intravascular coagulopathy in newborn infants results in consumption of coagulation factors and bleeding. The infants are often premature; the clinical course is frequently characterized by hypoxia, acidosis, shock, hemangiomas, or infection. Treatment is directed at correcting the primary clinical problem, such as infection, and at interrupting consumption and replacing clotting factors. The prognosis is poor regardless of therapy (Sec. 16.75).

Infants with central nervous system or other bleeding constituting an *immediate threat to life* should receive a small transfusion of fresh, compatible whole blood or plasma, as well as vitamin K, as soon as possible after blood has been drawn for coagulation studies, which should include determination of the number of platelets.

The so-called **swallowed blood syndrome**, in which blood or bloody stools are passed, usually on the 2nd or 3rd day of life, may be confused with hemorrhage from the gastrointestinal tract. The blood may be swallowed during delivery or from a fissure in the mother's nipple. Differentiation from gastrointestinal hemorrhage is based on the fact that the infant's blood contains mostly fetal hemoglobin, which is alkali-resistant, whereas swallowed blood from a maternal source contains adult hemoglobin, which is promptly changed to alkaline hematin upon the addition of alkali. Apt devised the following test for this differentiation:

(1) Rinse a bloodstained diaper or some grossly bloody stool with a suitable amount of water to obtain a distinctly pink supernatant hemoglobin solution. (2) Centrifuge the mixture. Decant the supernatant solution. (3) To 5 parts of the supernatant fluid add 1 part of 0.25 normal (1%) sodium hydroxide. Within 1–2 min a color reaction takes place: a yellow-brown color indicates that the blood is maternal in origin; a persistent pink, that it is from the infant. A control test with known adult or infant blood, or both, is advisable.

Widespread **subcutaneous ecchymoses** in premature infants at or immediately after birth are apparently a result of fragile superficial blood vessels rather than of a coagulation defect. Administering vitamin K_1 to the mother during labor has no effect on their incidence. Occasionally, an infant is born with petechiae or a generalized bluish suffusion limited to the face, head, and neck, which are probably the result of venous obstruction caused by a nuchal cord or sudden increases in intrathoracic pressure during delivery. It may take 2–3 wk for such suffusions to disappear.

NEONATAL THROMBOCYTOPENIC PURPURA. See Sec. 16.84.

Anonymous: Anaemia in premature infants. Lancet 1:1371, 1987.
Berkowitz RL, Chitkara U, Wilkins IA, et al: Intravascular monitoring and management of erythroblastosis fetalis. Am J Obstet Gynecol 158:783, 1988.
Black VD, Lubchenco LO, Koops BL, et al: Neonatal hyperviscosity: Randomized study of effect of partial plasma exchange transfusion on long-term outcome. Pediatrics 75:1048, 1985.
Blanchette V, Zipursky A: Assessment of anemia in newborn infants. Clin Perinatol 11:489, 1984.
Brown MS, Garcia JF, Phibbs RH, et al: Decreased response of plasma immunoreactive erythropoietin to "available oxygen" in anemia of prematurity. J Pediatr 105:793, 1984.
Buchanon G: Coagulation disorders in the neonate. Pediatr Clin North Am 33:203, 1986.
Bussel JB, Berkowitz RL, McFarland JG, et al: Antenatal treatment of neonatal alloimmune thrombocytopenia. N Engl J Med 319:1374, 1988.
Chaou W, Chou M, Eitzman DV: Intracranial hemorrhage and vitamin K deficiency in early infancy. J Pediatr 105:880, 1984.
Delaney-Black V, Camp BW, Lubchenco LO, et al: Neonatal hyperviscosity association with lower achievement and IQ scores at school age. Pediatrics 83:662, 1989.
DeMaio JG, Harris MC, Deuber C, et al: Effect of blood transfusion on apnea frequency in growing premature infants. J Pediatr 114:1039, 1989.
Desjardins L, Blaychman M, Chintu C, et al: The spectrum of ABO hemolytic disease of the newborn infant. J Pediatr 95:447, 1979.
Gibson B: Neonatal haemostasis. Arch Dis Child 64:503, 1989.
Grannum PAT, Copel JA, Moya FR, et al: The reversal of hydrops fetalis by intravascular intrauterine transfusion in severe isoimmune fetal anemia. Am J Obstet Gynecol 158:914, 1988.
Holzgreve W, Curry C, Golbus M, et al: Investigation of nonimmune hydrops fetalis. Am J Obstet Gynecol 150:805, 1984.
Lane PA, Hathaway WE: Vitamin K in infancy. J Pediatr 106:351, 1985.
Motohara K, Matsukura M, Matsuda I, et al: Severe vitamin K deficiency in breast-fed infants. J Pediatr 105:943, 1984.
Parer JT: Severe Rh isoimmunization—current methods of in utero diagnosis and treatment. Am J Obstet Gynecol 158:1323, 1988.
Phibbs RH, Johnson P, Kitterman JA, et al: Cardio-respiratory status of erythroblastotic newborn infants. III: Intravascular pressures during the first hours of life. Pediatrics 58:484, 1976.
Reece EA, Cole SW, Romero R, et al: Ultrasonography versus amniotic fluid

spectral analysis: Are they sensitive enough to predict neonatal complications associated with isoimmunization? Obstet Gynecol 74:357, 1989.
Stockman JA, Graeber JE, Clark DA, et al: Anemia of prematurity: Determinants of the erythropoietin response. J Pediatr 105:786, 1984.

9.50 GENITOURINARY SYSTEM

See also Chapter 18.

One or both kidneys are often easily palpable in the newborn infant. When both are palpable and similar, there is usually no particular diagnostic problem, but when only one kidney can be felt, the impression that it is larger than normal or is displaced by an intrinsic or extrinsic mass frequently arises. Fetal lobulation may contribute to this impression. Usually the problem resolves itself as the kidney becomes progressively less easily palpable during the early months of life. Since palpable enlargement or displacement of the kidney in the newborn may be due to hydronephrosis, neuroblastoma, embryoma, or a cystic malformation, ultrasound examination is indicated. During the neonatal period moderate elevation of the blood urea nitrogen does not necessarily signify renal disease, and elevations may occur in association with polycystic disease and hydronephrosis without necessarily implying a poor prognosis. The urine may also contain casts and cellular elements simply as a manifestation of dehydration.

THROMBOSIS OF THE RENAL VEIN. See Sec. 9.56.

9.51 THE CRANIUM

See Anencephaly, Microcephaly, Craniosynostosis, and Hydrocephalus in Chapter 20.

9.52 THE SKIN

Skin disorders of the newborn are covered in Chapter 23.

MASTITIS NEONATORUM. Engorgement of the breasts is physiologic in newborn infants. Infection may be initiated by undue manipulation of the breasts and is manifest by redness, local heat, swelling, and pain. Fever and other general symptoms may also be present. The prognosis is favorable unless septicemia develops; *Staphylococcus aureus* and *Escherichia coli* are usually the causative agents. Prophylaxis consists in avoiding the manipulation of or other trauma to the engorged breasts. Treatment includes systemic antibiotic therapy and hot compresses applied locally. If an abscess develops, it should be incised and drained.

Scar formation after infection may distort the nipple and impair the secretory power of the mammary gland in a female later in life.

THE EYE

See Chapter 22.

9.53 THE UMBILICUS

UMBILICAL CORD. The cord contains the two umbilical arteries, the vein, the rudimentary allantois, the remnant of the omphalomesenteric duct, and a gelatinous substance called Wharton jelly. The sheath of the umbilical cord is derived from the amnion. Its arteries have a strong contractile capacity; that of the vein is less so. The vein retains a fairly large lumen after birth. When the cord sloughs, portions of these structures remain in the base. The blood vessels are functionally closed but are patent anatomically for 10–20 days. The arteries become the lateral umbilical ligaments; the vein, the ligamentum teres; and the ductus venosus, the ligamentum venosum. During this interval the umbilical vessels are potential portals of entry for infection. The umbilical cord usually sloughs within 2 wk. *Delayed separation of the cord,* greater than 1 mo, has been associated with neutrophil chemotactic defects and overwhelming bacterial infection (Sec. 16.57).

A **single umbilical artery** is present in about 5–10/1,000 births; the frequency is about 35–70/1,000 twin births. Approximately one third of infants with a single umbilical artery have congenital abnormalities, usually more than one, and many such infants are stillborn or die shortly after birth. 18-Trisomy is one of the more frequent abnormalities. Since many abnormalities are not apparent on gross physical examination, it is important that at every delivery the cut cord and the maternal and fetal surfaces of the placenta be inspected. The number of arteries present should be recorded as an aid to the early suspicion and identification of abnormalities in such infants.

Patency of the omphalomesenteric duct may be responsible for an intestinal fistula, prolapse of the bowel, polyp, or a Meckel diverticulum (Sec. 13.33).

A *persistent urachus* (urachal cyst) is due to failure of closure of the allantoic duct and is associated with bladder outlet obstruction. Patency should be suspected if there is a clear, light yellow, urine-like discharge from the umbilicus.

CONGENITAL OMPHALOCELE. An omphalocele is a herniation or protrusion of abdominal contents into the base of the umbilical cord. In contrast to the more common unbilical hernia, the sac is covered with peritoneum without overlying skin. The size of the sac that lies outside the abdominal cavity depends on its contents. There is herniation of intestines into the cord in about 1 of 5,000 births, and of liver and intestines in 1 of 10,000 births. The abdominal cavity is proportionately small because the impetus to grow and develop is deficient. Immediate surgical repair, before infection has taken place and before the tissues have been damaged by drying or by rupture of the sac, is essential for survival. Silastic, Mersilene, or similar synthetic material may be used to cover the viscera if the sac has ruptured or if excessive mobilization of the skin would be necessary to cover the mass and its intact sac. Omphalocele, macrosomia, and hypoglycemia suggest Beckwith syndrome (Sec. 9.57).

TUMORS. Tumors of the umbilicus are rare; they include angioma, enteroteratoma, dermoid cyst, myxosarcoma, and cysts of urachal or omphalomesenteric duct remnants.

HEMORRHAGE. Hemorrhage from the umbilical cord may be due to trauma, to inadequate ligation of the cord, or to failure of normal thrombus formation. It may also indicate hemorrhagic disease of the newborn, septicemia, or local infection. The infant should be observed frequently during the first few days of life so that, if hemorrhage does occur, it will be detected promptly.

GRANULOMA. The umbilical cord usually dries and separates within 6–8 days after birth. The raw surface becomes covered by a thin layer of skin, scar tissue forms, and the wound is usually healed within 12–15 days. The presence of saprophytic organisms delays separation of the cord and increases the possibility of invasion by pathogenic organisms. Mild infection may result in a moist granulating area at the base of the cord with a slight mucoid or mucopurulent discharge. Good results are usually obtained by cleansing with alcohol several times daily.

The persistence of exuberant granulation tissue at the base of the umbilicus is common. The tissue is soft, vascular and granular, and dull red or pink, and it may have a seropurulent secretion. The *treatment* is cauterization with silver nitrate; it should be repeated at intervals of several days until the base is dry.

Umbilical granuloma must be differentiated from **umbilical polyp**, a rare anomaly resulting from persistence of all or part of the omphalomesenteric duct or of the urachus. The tissue of the polyp is firm and resistant, bright red, and has a mucoid secretion. If there is a communication with the ileum or bladder, small amounts of fecal material or urine may be discharged intermittently. Histologically the polyp consists of intestinal or urinary tract mucosa. Treatment is surgical excision of the *entire* omphalomesenteric or urachal remnant.

INFECTIONS. Inflammation in the umbilical region, which may be caused by any of the pyogenic bacteria, is especially serious because of the danger of hematogenous spread or extension to the liver or peritoneum. Venous phlebitis may develop, resulting in later onset of portal hypertension and cirrhosis. The general manifestations may be minimal (periumbilical erythema) even when septicemia or hepatitis has resulted. Daily baths or daily application of triple dye to the umbilical stump and surrounding skin may reduce the incidence of umbilical infection. *Treatment* includes prompt antibacterial therapy and, if there is abscess formation, surgical incision and drainage.

UMBILICAL HERNIA. Often associated with diastasis recti, umbilical hernia is due to an imperfect closure or weakness of the umbilical ring. Common especially in low birthweight and black infants, it appears as a soft swelling covered by skin that protrudes during crying, coughing, or straining and can be reduced easily through the fibrous ring at the umbilicus. The hernia consists of omentum or portions of the small intestine. The size of the defect varies from less than 1 cm in diameter to as much as 5 cm but large ones are rare.

Treatment. Most umbilical hernias that appear before the age of 6 mo will disappear spontaneously by 1 yr of age. Even large hernias (5–6 cm in all dimensions) have been known to disappear spontaneously by 5–6 yr of age. Strangulation is extremely rare. There is considerable agreement that "strapping" is ineffective. Surgery is not advised unless the hernia persists to the age of 3–5 yr, causes symptoms, becomes strangulated, or becomes progressively larger after the age of 1–2 yr.

9.54 METABOLIC DISTURBANCES

HYPERTHERMIA IN THE NEWBORN

(Transitory Fever of the Newborn; Dehydration Fever)

Elevations of temperature (38–39° C or 100–103° F) are occasionally noted on the 2nd–3rd day of life in infants whose clinical course has been otherwise satisfactory. This disturbance is especially likely to occur in breast-fed infants whose intake of fluid has been particularly low or in infants exposed to high environmental temperatures, either in an incubator or in a bassinet near a radiator or in the sun.

The infant may be restless, and there may be a precipitous drop in weight. However, there may not be a consistent relation between the fever and the extent of weight loss or inadequacy of fluid intake. The urinary output and frequency of voiding diminish. The skin may lose some of its elasticity, and the fontanel may be depressed. The infant appears unhappy and takes fluids avidly. The apparent vigor of the infant contrasts with the usual appearance of "being sick" in the presence of infection. Rarely there may be marked tachypnea and tachycardia as the infant attempts to increase heat loss by way of the respiratory tract to compensate for a sudden increase in environmental temperature. The rise in temperature may be associated with an increase in serum protein, sodium, and hematocrit. The possibility of local or systemic infection should be evaluated. Administering oral or parenteral fluids or lowering the environmental temperature leads to prompt reduction of the fever and alleviation of symptoms.

A *more severe form of neonatal hyperthermia* occurs among both newborn and older infants when they are warmly dressed for outdoor low temperatures that do not exist in their immediate indoor environment. The diminished sweating capacity of the newborn infant is a contributing factor. Warmly dressed infants left near stoves or radiators, traveling in well-heated automobiles, or left with bright sunlight shining directly on them through the windows of a closed room or automobile are likely victims. Overclothing in hot weather, especially when the infant is left in the sun, is a less common cause. Body temperature is often as high as 41–44° C (106–111° F). The skin is hot and dry, and initially the infant usually appears flushed and apathetic. This stage may be followed by stupor, grayish pallor, coma, and convulsions. Hypernatremia may contribute to the convulsions. The mortality and morbidity rates (brain damage) are high. Hyperthermia has been associated with sudden infant death and the hemorrhagic shock and encephalopathy syndrome (Sec. 25.6). The condition is prevented by dressing the infant in clothing suitable for the temperature of the *immediate* environment. In the newborn infant exposure of the body to usual room temperature or immersion in tepid water usually suffices to bring the temperature back to normal levels. Older infants may require cooling for a longer time by repeated immersions or by use of a water-cooled mattress or other apparatus for induction of hypothermia. Attention to possible fluid and electrolyte disturbance is essential.

NEONATAL COLD INJURY

Neonatal cold injury usually occurs among infants in inadequately heated homes during damp cold spells when the outside temperature is in the freezing range. The presenting features are apathy, refusal of food, oliguria, and coldness to touch. The body temperature is usually between 29.5 and 35° C (85–95° F), and immobility, edema, and redness of the extremities, especially of the hands, feet, and face, are observed. Bradycardia and apnea may also occur. The facial erythema frequently gives a false impression of health, delaying recognition that the infant is ill. Local hardening over areas of edema may lead to confusion with scleredema. Rhinitis is common, as are serious metabolic disturbances, particularly hypoglycemia and acidosis. Hemorrhagic manifestations are frequent; massive pulmonary hemorrhage is a common finding at autopsy. Treatment consists of warming and paying scrupulous attention to recognizing and correcting hypotension and metabolic imbalances, particularly hypoglycemia. Prevention consists of providing adequate environmental heat. The mortality rate is about 25%; about 10% of the survivors have evidence of brain damage.

EDEMA

Generalized edema occurs in association with hydrops fetalis and in the offspring of diabetic mothers. In the premature infant edema is often a consequence of a decreased ability to excrete water or sodium, although some have considerable edema without identifiable reason. Infants with hyaline membrane disease may become edematous without congestive heart failure. Edema of the face and scalp may result from pressure from the umbilical cord around the neck, and transient localized swellings of the hands or feet may similarly be due to intrauterine pressures. Edema may be present with heart failure due to congenital cardiac lesions; a lag in renal excretion of electrolytes and water may result in edema when there has been a sudden large increase in intake of electrolytes, particularly with feeding of concentrated cow's milk formulas. High-protein formulas also may cause edema owing to the excessive solute load, particularly in premature infants. It is difficult to show a relation between low serum protein or low hemoglobin and the occurrence of edema in older premature infants. Edema also occurs in association with anemia and vitamin E deficiency in premature infants. Rarely, *idiopathic hypoproteinemia* with edema lasting weeks or months is observed in term infants. The cause is unclear, and the disturbance is benign. Persistent edema of one or more extremities may represent congenital lymphedema (Milroy disease) or, in females, *Turner syndrome*. Generalized edema with hypoproteinemia may be seen in the neonatal period with congenital nephrosis and rarely with Hurler syndrome or after feeding hypoallergenic formulas to infants with cystic fibrosis of the pancreas. *Sclerema* is described in Sec. 23.16.

HYPOCALCEMIA (TETANY)

See Sec. 6.28.

OSTEOPENIA OF PREMATURITY. Very small premature infants with chronic illnesses often develop a rickets-like syndrome with pathologic fractures and demineralized bones. There may be associated cholestasis and vitamin D or calcium malabsorption; urine calcium loss due to diuretics; and poor calcium, phosphorus, or vitamin D intake, or aluminum toxicity. The treatment of fractures requires immobilization and administration of calcium, phosphorus, and vitamin D. Appropriate formulas for prematures should provide a more optimal intake of calcium, phosphorus, and vitamin D and promote bone mineralization. See also Sec. 4.29, 4.30, 6.28, 19.16, and 24.58.

HYPOMAGNESEMIA

Rarely, hypomagnesemia of unknown etiology may occur in the newborn infant, usually in association with hypocalcemia. It may also be associated with insufficient stores of skeletal magnesium secondary to deficient placental transfer, decreased intestinal absorption, neonatal hypoparathyroidism, hyperphosphatemia, renal loss, a defect in magnesium and calcium homeostasis, or an iatrogenic deficiency due to loss incurred during exchange transfusion or insufficient replacement during total intravenous alimentation. Infants of diabetic mothers may have serum magnesium levels that are lower than normal. The clinical manifestations of hypomagnesemia are indistinguishable from those of hypocalcemia and tetany and may, in fact, be secondary to the accompanying hypocalcemia.

Hypomagnesemia occurs when serum magnesium levels fall below 1.5 mg/dL (0.62 mmol/L), although clinical signs usually do not develop until serum magnesium levels fall below 1.2 mg/dL. During exchange transfusion with citrated blood, which is low in magnesium ion because of binding by citrate, the serum magnesium drops about 0.5 mg/dL (0.2 mmol/L); approximately 10 days are required for a return to normal. In noniatrogenic hypomagnesemia the serum magnesium may be less than 0.5 mg/dL. The serum calcium in either instance is usually at levels seen in hypocalcemic tetany, but the serum phosphorus value is normal or high. Since the hypocalcemia accompanying hypomagnesemia is inadequately corrected by administering calcium, hypomagnesemia should also be suspected in any patient with tetany not responding to calcium therapy.

Immediate *treatment* consists of the intramuscular injection of magnesium sulfate. For newborn infants 0.25 mL/kg of a 50% solution daily usually suffices. The accompanying hypocalcemia usually corrects itself as the hypomagnesemia is relieved. The same daily dose can be given for oral maintenance therapy. Four to five times higher doses may be required in malabsorptive states. In most cases the metabolic defect is transient, and treatment can be discontinued after 1–2 wk. A few patients appear to have a permanent form of the disease that requires continuous oral supplementation with magnesium to prevent recurrence of hypomagnesemia.* No residual damage to the central nervous system is evident after prompt treatment.

HYPERMAGNESEMIA

Hypermagnesemia may occur in newborn infants of mothers treated with magnesium sulfate for eclampsia. At high serum levels the central nervous system is depressed and totally paralyzed so that artificial respiration is required. Toxicity may also result from magnesium sulfate enemas. Lower levels may result in hypoventilation, hypotension, lethargy, flaccidity, and hyporeflexia. The upper limit of normal magnesium is 2.8 mg/dL (1.15 mmol/L), but serious symptoms occur at levels above 5 mg/dL (2.1 mmol/L). Hypermagnesemia may be associated with failure to pass meconium (meconium plug syndrome). Exchange transfusion has been used as a means of rapid removal of magnesium ion from the blood. Calcium salts and diuresis have also been used. Recovery appears to be complete.

OTHER METABOLIC DISEASES

A number of inborn errors of metabolism may be manifest during the neonatal period; these include phenylketonuria, galactosemia, the urea cycle defects, methylmalonic acidemia, and maple syrup urine disease (see Chapter 8). Pyridoxine deficiency and dependency are considered in Sec. 4.26.

SUBSTANCE ABUSE AND WITHDRAWALS

Physiologic addiction to narcotics or toxic effects occur in most infants born to actively addicted mothers, since opiates cross the placenta. Withdrawal may be manifest even before birth by increased activity of the fetus when the mother feels the need for the drug or develops withdrawal symptoms. Heroin and methadone are the drugs most frequently associated with withdrawal syndromes, but they also may occur with alcohol, phenobarbital, pentazocine, codeine, propoxyphene, and diazepam.

Pregnancy in an addict or alcoholic is, by definition, a high risk. Prenatal care is usually inadequate, and there is a higher incidence of sexually transmitted disease including AIDS and hepatitis, toxemia, premature rupture of the membranes, breech presentations, prolapsed cords and limbs, preterm and small for gestational age infants, and prenatal morbidity and mortality. Frequently, more than one drug is being abused in these pregnancies.

Heroin addiction results in a 50% incidence of low birthweight infants, half of whom are small for gestational age. Infections, maternal undernutrition, and a direct fetal growth inhibiting effect are associated abnormalities. The rate of stillbirths is increased, but not the incidence of congenital

---

*Four mL/kg/24 hr of the following solution: Magnesium chloride ($MgCl_2 \times 6\ H_2O$) 4g (39.6 mEq)
Magnesium citrate ($MgHC_6H_5O_7 \times 5\ H_2O$) 6g (39.6 mEq)
Water to 100 mL
Solution provides approximately 0.8 mEq of magnesium/mL.

anomalies. *Clinical manifestations* of withdrawal occur in 50–75% of infants, usually beginning within the first 48 hr, depending on the daily maternal dose (<6 mg/24 hr is associated with no or mild symptoms); duration of addiction (>1 yr has a greater than 70% incidence of withdrawal); and time of last maternal dose (there is a higher incidence if the last dose was taken within 24 hr of birth). Symptoms rarely appear as late as 4–6 wk of age. The incidence of hyaline membrane disease and hyperbilirubinemia may be decreased in low birthweight infants of heroin addicts; hyperventilation leading to respiratory alkalosis or accelerated production of surfactant may explain the former, and enzyme induction of glucuronyl transferase the latter.

Tremors and hyperirritability are the most prominent symptoms. The tremors may be fine or jittery and indistinguishable from those of hypoglycemia but are more often coarse, "flapping," and bilateral; the limbs are often rigid, hyperreflexic, and resistant to flexion and extension. Irritability and hyperactivity are generally marked and may lead to skin abrasions. Other signs include tachypnea, diarrhea, vomiting, high-pitched cry, fist sucking, poor feeding, and fever. Sneezing, yawning, myoclonic jerks, convulsions, abnormal sleep cycles, nasal stuffiness, apnea, flushing alternating rapidly with pallor, and lacrimation are less common. The *diagnosis* is generally established by the history and clinical presentation. Examining the urine for opiates may reveal only low levels during withdrawal, but quinine, which is often mixed with heroin, may be present in higher concentrations. Hypoglycemia and hypocalcemia should be excluded.

Methadone addiction has produced an increasing number of infants with withdrawal symptoms, the incidence varying from 20 to 90%. In general, mothers taking methadone have better prenatal care than those taking heroin; however, there is a high incidence of multiple drug abuse, including alcohol, barbiturates, and tranquilizers, and these mothers are often heavy smokers. There is no increased incidence of congenital anomalies. The average birthweight of infants of mothers taking methadone is higher than that of infants of heroin-addicted mothers; the *clinical manifestations* are similar except that the former group has a higher incidence of seizures (10–20%) and of late onset (2–6 wk of age) of symptoms and signs.

Alcohol withdrawal is uncommon. The infants of women who have been drinking immediately before delivery may have alcohol on their breath for several hours, since it rapidly crosses the placenta, and blood levels in the infant are similar to those in the mother. Hypoglycemia and acidosis may be present. Infants who develop withdrawal symptoms often become agitated and hyperactive with marked tremors lasting for 72 hr, followed by about 48 hr of lethargy before return to normal activity. Seizures may develop.

Phenobarbital withdrawal usually occurs in full-term, appropriate for gestational age infants of addicted mothers. Symptoms begin at a median age of 7 days (range 2–14 days). There may be a brief acute stage consisting of irritability, constant crying, sleeplessness, hiccups, and mouthing movements, followed by a subacute stage that may last 2–4 mo consisting of voracious appetite, frequent regurgitation and gagging, episodic irritability, hyperacusis, sweating, and a disturbed sleep pattern.

Cocaine addiction among pregnant women has increased significantly, but withdrawal in their infants is unusual; pregnancy may be complicated by premature labor, abruptio placentae, and fetal asphyxia. Infants may manifest intrauterine growth retardation, microcephaly, intracranial hemorrhage, cerebral cavitary and echo-dense lesions, seizures, anomalies of the gastrointestinal and renal tracts, sudden infant death syndrome (SIDS), and neurobehavioral deficits characterized by rigidity, impaired state regulation, developmental delay, and learning disabilities. Child abuse, neglect, and AIDS are common in these families.

Treatment of heroin and methadone withdrawals has been successful using various combinations of narcotics, sedatives, and hypnotics. Therapy is indicated for seizures, for diarrhea, or for such irritability that normal sleep and feeding patterns are disturbed and weight gain is poor. Methadone withdrawal may require larger amounts of medication for longer periods than heroin withdrawal to control clinical manifestations. Phenobarbital, 8–10 mg/kg/24 hr in 4 divided doses, can effectively reduce irritability and prevent seizures. It is as effective as chlorpromazine, 2.2 mg/kg/24 hr, divided into 3–4 doses. It is usually not necessary to administer either drug for more than 5 days, but on occasion it may be necessary to treat the infant for as long as 6 wk. Patients with severe autonomic symptoms may require gradually diminishing doses of methadone or paregoric for 2–10 wk. Paregoric at a beginning dose of 3–5 drops given every 3–6 hr, increased to 5–10 drops every 4 hr if necessary, depending on the size and response of the infant, will abolish most withdrawal symptoms, especially diarrhea. The dose and duration of therapy may be adjusted according to the clinical response. Parenteral administration of fluids may be necessary to prevent aspiration or dehydration until the symptoms are brought under control. Narcotic and phenobarbital withdrawal requires swaddling, frequent feedings, and protection from noxious external stimuli.

Current mortality from withdrawal is not over 5%, and with early recognition and treatment may be negligible. *Prognosis* for normal development is affected by the adverse circumstances of high-risk pregnancy and delivery and by the environment to which the infant is returned after recovery as well as by the effects of the particular drug on fetal and subsequent neonatal development.

FETAL ALCOHOL SYNDROME. High levels of alcohol ingestion during pregnancy can be damaging to embryonic and fetal development. A specific pattern of malformation identified as the *fetal alcohol syndrome* has been documented, and major and minor components of the syndrome are expressed in 1–2 infants/1,000 live births. Both moderate and high levels of alcohol intake during early pregnancy may result in alterations in growth and morphogenesis of fetus; the greater the intake, the more severe the signs. Infants born to heavy drinkers have twice the risk of abnormality compared with those born to moderate drinkers; 32% of infants born to heavy drinkers demonstrated congenital anomalies, compared with 9% in the abstinent and 14% in the moderate group.

The characteristics of the fetal alcohol syndrome include (1) prenatal onset and persistence of growth deficiency for length, weight, and head circumference; (2) facial abnormalities, including short palpebral fissures, epicanthal folds, maxillary hypoplasia, micrognathia, and thin upper lip; (3) cardiac defects, primarily septal defects; (4) minor joint and limb abnormalities, including some restriction of movement and altered palmar crease patterns; and (5) delayed development and mental deficiency varying from borderline to severe. Fetal alcohol syndrome is a common cause of mental retardation. The severity of dysmorphogenesis may range from severely affected infants with full manifestations of the fetal alcohol syndrome to those mildly affected with only a few manifestations.

The detrimental effects may be due to the alcohol itself or to one of its breakdown products. Some evidence suggests that alcohol may impair placental transfer of essential amino acids and zinc, both necessary for protein synthesis, which accounts for the intrauterine growth retardation.

The *management* of these infants may be difficult, since no specific therapy exists. The infants may remain hypotonic and tremulous despite sedation, and the prognosis is poor. Counseling with regard to recurrence is important. *Prevention* is achieved by eliminating alcohol intake after conception.

LATE METABOLIC ACIDOSIS

Between 5 and 10% of preterm low birthweight infants develop a metabolic acidosis during the 2nd or 3rd wk of life. Usually there is no history of asphyxia, respiratory distress, or other problems, and the infants are vigorous. However, they often have received cow's milk formulas of high protein and casein content shortly after birth and have had a delayed start of postnatal weight gain. Blood base excess values range from −10 to −16 mEq/L, and P_{CO_2} values are usually less than 40 mm Hg. The condition probably represents an abnormally high rate of endogenous acid formation. Treatment includes administering $NaHCO_3$ and changing to a formula of lower protein content with a whey:casein ration of 60:40.

American Academy of Pediatrics Committee on Genetics: Newborn Screening Fact Sheets. Pediatrics 83:449, 1989.

Chasnoff I, Burns W, Schnolls S, et al: Cocaine use in pregnancy. N Engl J Med 313:666, 1985.

Frank DA, Zuckerman BS, Amaro H, et al: Cocaine use during pregnancy: Prevalence and correlates. Pediatrics 82:888, 1988.

Horsman A, Ryan SW, Congdon PJ, et al: Bone mineral accretion rate and calcium intake in preterm infants. Arch Dis Child 64:910, 1989.

Horsman A, Ryan SW, Congdon PJ, et al: Osteopenia in extremely low birthweight infants. Arch Dis Child 64:485, 1989.

Kildeberg P: Late metabolic acidosis of premature infants. *In* Winters RW (ed): The Body Fluids in Pediatrics. Boston, Little, Brown, 1973.

Little BB, Snell LM, Klein VR, et al: Cocaine abuse during pregnancy: Maternal and fetal implications. Obstet Gynecol 73:157, 1989.

Lyon AJ, McIntosh N, Wheeler K, et al: Radiological rickets in extremely low birthweight infants. Pediatr Radiol 17:56, 1987.

Nervez CT, Shott RJ, Bergstrom WH, et al: Prophylaxis against hypocalcemia in low birth weight infants receiving bicarbonate infusion. J Pediatr 87:439, 1975.

Neuman L, Cohen S: The neonatal narcotic withdrawal syndrome. Clin Perinatol 2:99, 1975.

Streissguth AP, Herman CS, Smith DW: Intelligence, behavior and dysmorphogenesis in the fetal alcohol syndrome: A report of 20 patients. J Pediatr 92:363, 1978.

9.55 THE ENDOCRINE SYSTEM

The endocrinopathies are discussed in Chapter 19. The purpose of this section is to call attention to those endocrine disturbances that may be identified at birth or during the first month of life.

Pituitary dwarfism is usually not apparent at birth, although panhypopituitary male infants may present with neonatal hypoglycemia and micropenis. Conversely, constitutional dwarfs usually demonstrate length and weight consistent with prematurity when born after a normal gestational period; otherwise their physical appearance is normal.

Thyroid deficiency may be apparent at birth in genetically determined **cretinism** or in infants of mothers treated with thiouracil or its derivatives during pregnancy. Constipation, prolonged jaundice, lethargy, or poor peripheral circulation as shown by persistently mottled skin or cold extremities should suggest cretinism. The early diagnosis and treatment of congenital deficiency of thyroid hormone may be greatly facilitated by screening all newborn infants for this deficiency.

Temporary *hyperthyroidism* may occur at birth in the infants of mothers with hyperthyroidism or of those who have been receiving thyroid medication.

Transient *hypoparathyroidism* may be manifest as tetany of the newborn.

The *adrenal gland* is subject to numerous disturbances, which may become apparent and require lifesaving treatment during the neonatal period. Acute adrenal *hemorrhage* and failure may be seen after breech or other traumatic deliveries or in association with overwhelming infection. *Adrenocortical hyperplasia* is suggested by vomiting, diarrhea, dehydration, convulsions, shock, or phallic or clitoral enlargement. Since the condition is genetically determined, newborn siblings of patients with the salt-losing variety of adrenocortical hyperplasia should be observed closely for manifestations of adrenal insufficiency.

Congenitally hypoplastic adrenal glands may also give rise to adrenal insufficiency during the first few weeks of life.

Female infants with webbing of the neck, lymphangiectatic edema, hypoplasia of the nipples, cutis laxa, low hairline at the nape of the neck, low-set ears, high-arched palate, deformities of the nails, cubitus valgus, and other anomalies should be suspected of having *gonadal dysgenesis*.

Transient *diabetes mellitus* (Sec. 8.58) is rare and is seen only in the newborn. It usually presents as dehydration, loss of weight, or acidosis in small for gestational age infants.

9.56 INFANTS OF DIABETIC MOTHERS

The control of diabetes mellitus with insulin has led to the survival of increasing numbers of diabetic women who bear children. Their infants and the infants of women who later develop diabetes share certain distinctive morphologic characteristics, including large size, macrosomia, and high morbidity risks. Diabetic mothers have a high incidence of polyhydramnios, and their fetal mortality rate, which is high at all gestational ages, especially so after 32 wk, is greater than that of nondiabetic mothers. Fetal wastage throughout pregnancy is associated with poorly controlled maternal diabetes, especially ketoacidosis and congenital anomalies. Diabetic mothers produce an excess of high-birthweight infants at all gestational ages and, if complicated with vascular disease, of low birthweight infants at 37- to 40-wk gestations. The neonatal mortality rate is over 5 times that of infants of nondiabetic mothers and is higher at all gestational ages and in every birthweight for gestational age category.

PATHOPHYSIOLOGY. No single physiologic or biochemical event explains the diverse clinical manifestations. The probable pathogenic sequence is that maternal hyperglycemia causes fetal hyperglycemia, and the fetal pancreatic response leads to fetal hyperinsulinemia; fetal hyperinsulinemia and hyperglycemia then cause increased hepatic glucose uptake and glycogen synthesis, accelerated lipogenesis, and augmented protein synthesis. Related pathologic findings are the hypertrophy and hyperplasia of the pancreatic islets with a disproportionate increase in the number of β cells; increased weights of the placenta and infant organs except for the brain; myocardial hypertrophy; increased amounts of cytoplasm in liver cells; and extramedullary hematopoiesis. Hyperinsulinism produces fetal acidosis, which may result in an increased rate of stillbirth. The separation of the placenta suddenly interrupts glucose infusion into the neonate without a proportional effect on the hyperinsulinism, resulting in hypoglycemia and attenuated lipolysis during the first hours after birth.

Hyperinsulinemia has been documented in infants of gestational diabetic mothers and in those of insulin-dependent diabetic mothers without insulin antibodies. The former group also have significantly higher fasting plasma insulin levels than normal newborns despite similar glucose levels; they respond to glucose with a prompt elevation of plasma insulin and assimilate a glucose load more rapidly. Following arginine administration, they also have an enhanced insulin response and increased disappearance rates of glucose, compared with normal infants. In contrast, fasting glucose utilization rates are diminished. The lower free fatty acid levels in infants of insulin-dependent diabetic mothers probably also reflect their hyperinsulinemia. With good prenatal diabetic control, the incidence of macrosomia has decreased.

Although hyperinsulinism is probably the main cause of hypoglycemia, the diminished epinephrine and glucagon responses that occur may be contributing factors. Cortisol and human growth hormone levels are normal.

CLINICAL MANIFESTATIONS. The infants of diabetic and gestational diabetic mothers often bear a surprising resemblance to each other (Fig. 9–27). They tend to be large and plump due to increased body fat and enlarged viscera, with puffy, plethoric facies resembling those of patients who have been receiving a corticosteroid. These infants may, however, also be of normal or low birthweight, particularly if they are delivered before term or if there is associated maternal vascular disease.

The infants tend to be "jumpy," tremulous, and hyperexcitable during the first 3 days of life, although hypotonia, lethargy, and poor sucking also may occur. They may have any of the diverse manifestations of hypoglycemia. Early appearance of these signs is more likely to be related to hypoglycemia and later appearance related to hypocalcemia; these abnormalities also may occur together. Perinatal asphyxia or hyperbilirubinemia may produce similar signs. Rarely, hypomagnesemia may be associated with the hypocalcemia.

About 75% of infants of diabetic mothers and 25% of infants of mothers with gestational diabetes develop hypoglycemia (Sec. 9.57), but only a small percentage of these infants become symptomatic. The probability of an infant developing hypoglycemia increases and the glucose levels are likely to be lower at higher cord or maternal fasting blood glucose levels. Usually, the nadir in the infant's blood glucose concentration is reached between 1 and 3 hr; spontaneous recovery may begin by 4–6 hr.

Many infants of diabetic mothers develop tachypnea during the first 5 days of life, which may be a transient manifestation of hypoglycemia, hypothermia, polycythemia, cardiac failure, transient tachypnea, or cerebral edema from birth trauma or asphyxia. A greater incidence of respiratory distress syndrome appears in infants of diabetic mothers than in infants of normal mothers born at comparable gestational age; the greater incidence is possibly related to an antagonistic effect between cortisol and insulin on surfactant synthesis.

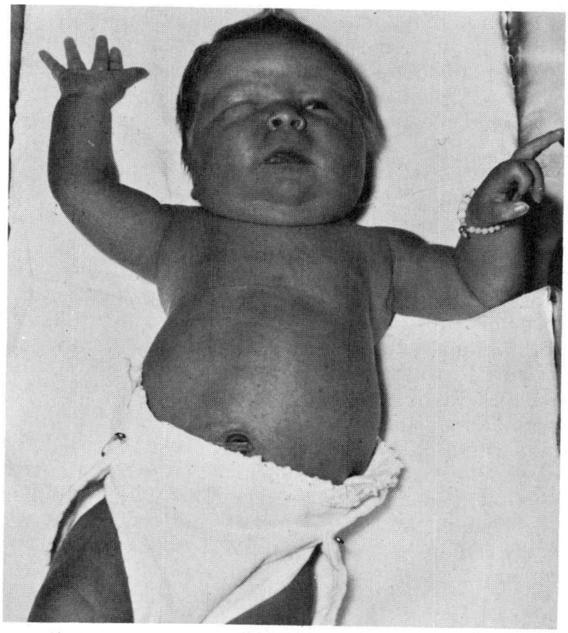

Figure 9–27. Large, plump, plethoric infant of a gestational diabetic mother. Baby was born at 38 wk of gestation but weighed 9 lb 11 oz (4,408 g). Mild respiratory distress was the only symptom other than appearance.

Cardiomegaly is common (30%), and heart failure occurs in 5–10% of infants of diabetic mothers. Asymmetric septal hypertrophy may occur, becoming manifest as idiopathic hypertrophic subaortic stenosis. Birth trauma is also common owing to fetal macrosomia.

Neurologic development and ossification centers tend to be immature and correlate with the brain size (which is not increased) and gestational age rather than with total body weight. There is also an increased incidence of hyperbilirubinemia, polycythemia, and renal vein thrombosis; the latter should be suspected in the presence of a flank mass, hematuria, and thrombocytopenia.

The incidence of congenital anomalies is increased 3-fold in infants of diabetic mothers; cardiac malformations and lumbosacral agenesis are most common. These infants may also develop abdominal distention due to a transient delay in the development of the left side of the colon, the *small left colon syndrome*.

PROGNOSIS. The subsequent incidence of diabetes mellitus in infants of diabetic mothers is increased compared with that of the general population. Physical development is normal, but oversized infants may be predisposed to obesity in childhood that may extend into adult life. Disagreement persists about whether or not a slightly increased risk of impaired intellectual development exists unrelated to hypoglycemia; symptomatic hypoglycemia probably increases the risk.

TREATMENT. Management of these infants should be initiated before birth by frequent prenatal evaluation of all pregnant women with overt or gestational diabetes, by evaluation of fetal maturity, by biophysical profile, by Doppler velocimetry, and by planning delivery of these infants in hospitals where expert obstetric and pediatric care is continuously available. Regardless of size, all infants of diabetic mothers should initially receive intensive observation and care. Asymptomatic infants should have a blood sugar determination within 1 hr of birth and then every hr for the next 6–8 hr; if clinically well and normoglycemic, oral or gavage feedings initially with 5% glucose water, followed by milk formula, should be started at 2–3 hr of age and continued at 3-hr intervals. If any question arises about an infant's ability to tolerate oral feeding, the feeding should be discontinued and glucose given by peripheral intravenous infusion at a rate of 4–8 mg/kg/min. Hypoglycemia should be treated, even in asymptomatic infants, with intravenous infusions of glucose sufficient to keep the blood levels well above this level. Bolus injections of hypertonic glucose should be avoided because they may cause further hyperinsulinemia and potentially produce rebound hypoglycemia. Managing hypoglycemia in sick or symptomatic infants is discussed in the following section. For treatment of *hypocalcemia* and *hypomagnesemia*, see Sec. 9.54; for *hyaline membrane disease* treatment, see Sec. 9.32; for treatment of *polycythemia*, see Sec. 9.48.

9.57 HYPOGLYCEMIA

See also Sec. 8.59.

Hypoglycemia is present when serum glucose levels are significantly lower than the range among postnatal age-matched normal infants. Although hypoglycemia may also be defined as the presence of neurologic (lethargy, coma, apnea, seizures) or sympathomimetic (pallor, palpitations, diaphoresis) manifestations that respond to glucose, many neonates with low serum glucose levels are asymptomatic, whereas normoglycemic infants may have nonspecific signs of hypoglycemia.

The *incidence of hypoglycemia* varies with the definition, population, method and timing of feeding, and type of glucose assay (serum levels are higher than whole blood values) (see Fig. 9–11). Early feeding decreases the incidence, whereas prematurity, hypothermia, hypoxia, maternal diabetes, maternal glucose infusion in labor, and intrauterine growth retardation increase the incidence of hypoglycemia. Serum glucose levels decline after birth until 1–3 hr of age, when levels spontaneously increase in normal infants. In healthy term term infants serum glucose values are rarely less than 35 mg/dL (1.9 mmol/L) between 1 and 3 hr of life, less than 40 mg/dL (2.2 mmol/L) from 3 to 24 hrs, and less than 45 mg/dL (2.5 mmol/L) after 24 hr. Although previous studies, performed when premature infants were fasted in the 1st day of life, suggested that premature infants have statistically lower glucose levels than term infants and that preterm infants may be unaffected by low glucose values, recent evidence does not support these conclusions. Both premature and full-term infants are at risk for serious neurodevelopmental deficits from equally low glucose levels. This risk is related to the depth and duration of the hypoglycemia.

Four pathophysiologic groups of *neonatal infants are at high risk of developing hypoglycemia*: (1) Infants of mothers with diabetes mellitus or gestational diabetes, infants with severe erythroblastosis fetalis, insulinomas, β cell nesidioblastosis, functional β cell hyperplasia, Beckwith syndrome (see below), and panhypopituitarism seem to have hyperinsulinism. (2) Infants with intrauterine growth retardation or those who are preterm may have experienced intrauterine malnutrition resulting in reduced hepatic glycogen stores and total body fat; the smaller of discordant twins (especially if discordant by 25% or more in weight with a weight of less than 2.0 kg), polycythemic infants, infants of toxemic mothers, and infants with placental abnormalities are particularly vulnerable. (Other factors in the development of hypoglycemia in this group include abnormal insulin responsiveness, impaired gluconeogenesis, diminished free fatty acid oxidation, low cortisol production rates, and possibly increased insulin levels and decreased output of epinephrine in response to hypoglycemia.) (3) Very immature or severely ill infants may develop hypoglycemia owing to increased metabolic needs disproportionate to substrate stores and calories supplied; low birth-weight infants with respiratory distress syndrome, perinatal asphyxia, polycythemia, hypothermia, and systemic infections, as well as infants in heart failure with cyanotic congenital heart disease, are at increased risk. The interruption of intravenous infusions, particularly those with high glucose concentrations, may also result in the precipitous onset of hypoglycemia. (4) Rare infants with genetic or primary metabolic defects, such as galactosemia, glycogen storage disease, fructose intolerance, propionic acidemia, methylmalonic acidemia, tyrosinemia, maple syrup urine disease, and leucine sensitivity, are also susceptible.

CLINICAL MANIFESTATIONS. In contrast to the frequency of chemical hypoglycemia, the incidence of symptomatic hypoglycemia is highest in small for gestational age infants (see Fig. 9–11). These infants usually fall into category 2 or 3 of the earlier pathophysiologic groupings, and some are referred to as having *transient symptomatic idiopathic neonatal hypoglycemia*. Because many of the symptoms also occur together with other conditions such as infections—especially sepsis and meningitis; central nervous system anomalies, hemorrhage, or edema; hypocalcemia and hypomagnesemia; asphyxia; drug withdrawal; apnea of prematurity; congenital heart disease; or polycythemia—and because some may be seen in normoglycemic well infants, the exact incidence of symptomatic hypoglycemia has been difficult to establish. It probably varies between 1 and 3 per 1,000 live births and affects about 5–15% of growth retarded infants.

The onset of symptoms varies from a few hours to a week after birth. In approximate order of frequency there are jitteriness or tremors, apathy, episodes of cyanosis, convulsions, intermittent apneic spells or tachypnea, weak or high-pitched cry, limpness or lethargy, difficulty in feeding, and eye-rolling. Episodes of sweating, sudden pallor, hypothermia, and cardiac arrest and failure also occur. There is frequently a clustering of episodic symptoms. Because these clinical manifestations may result from a variety of causes, it is critical to measure serum glucose levels and to determine whether they disappear with the administration of sufficient glucose to raise the blood sugar to normal levels; if they do not, other diagnoses must be considered.

TREATMENT. When seizures are not present, an intravenous bolus of 200 mg/kg (2mL/kg) of 10% glucose is effective in elevating the blood glucose concentration. In the presence of convulsions, 4 mL/kg of 10% glucose as a bolus injection is indicated.

Following initial therapy a glucose infusion should be given at 8 mg/kg/min. If hypoglycemia recurs, the infusion rate should be increased until 15–20% glucose is employed. If intravenous infusions of 20% glucose are inadequate to eliminate symptoms and maintain constant normal serum glucose concentrations, hydrocortisone (2.5 mg/kg/6 hr) or prednisone (1 mg/kg/24 hr) should also be administered. Serum glucose should be measured every 2 hr after initiating therapy until several determinations are above 40 mg/dL. Subsequently, levels should be obtained every 4–6 hr and the treatment gradually reduced and finally discontinued when the serum glucose has been in the normal range and the baby asymptomatic for 24–48 hr. Treatment is usually necessary for a few days to a week, rarely for several weeks. Diazoxide, epinephrine, and fructose are not of established benefit. Epinephrine and fructose may produce lactic acidosis. If neonatal hyperinsulinism is present, as in nesidioblastosis, and the infant is unresponsive to steroids and glucose given for a sufficient time, diazoxide, somatostatin, and epinephrine (Sus-Phrine) may be employed.

Surgery is the definitive treatment for *nesidioblastosis* and *islet cell adenomas*; glucagon plus somatostatin has been a helpful adjunct in some cases.

Infants who are at increased risk of developing hypoglycemia should have their serum glucose measured within 1 hr of birth and subsequently every 1–2 hr for the first 6–8 hr, then every 4–6 hr until 24 hr of life. Normoglycemic high-risk infants should receive oral or gavage feedings with formula started at 1–3 hr of age and continued at 2- to 3-hr intervals for 24–48 hr. An intravenous infusion of glucose at 4 mg/kg/min should be provided if oral feedings are poorly tolerated or if *asymptomatic transient neonatal hypoglycemia* develops.

PROGNOSIS. Prognosis for life is good. Hypoglycemia recurs in 10–15% of infants after adequate treatment. Some have been reported as late as the age of 8 mo. Recurrences are more common if intravenous fluids are extravasated or are too rapidly discontinued before oral feedings are well tolerated. Children who later develop ketotic hypoglycemia have an increased incidence of neonatal hypoglycemia. Prognosis for normal intellectual function must be guarded, since prolonged and severe hypoglycemia may be associated with neurologic sequelae. Symptomatic infants with hypoglycemia, particularly low birthweight infants and infants of diabetic mothers, have a worse prognosis for subsequent normal intellectual development than do asymptomatic infants.

Hypoglycemia with Macroglossia
(Beckwith Syndrome)

Beckwith described a syndrome of intractable neonatal hypoglycemia occurring in infants with macroglossia, large size, visceromegaly, mild microcephaly, omphalocele, facial nevus flammeus, a characteristic earlobe crease, increased risk of tumors (Wilms, hepatoblastoma, gonadoblastoma) and renal medullary dysplasia. The visceromegaly involves chiefly the liver and the kidneys in which there is a noncystic hyperplasia. Some infants are also polycythemic. Hyperinsulinemia has been demonstrated. Some infants with Beckwith syndrome have a partial duplication of chromosome 11p, a region that encodes the insulin-like growth factor II gene. Although usually sporadic, familial inheritance has been noted. Treatment is that of hypoglycemia; in this syndrome hypoglycemia may be severe and persist for several months. The prognosis is poor.

Severe hypoglycemia has also been demonstrated in extremely high birthweight infants who do not have the anomalies present in Beckwith syndrome. These *infant giants* weigh from 3.8 to 5.3 kg, and, in some, pancreatic hyperplasia has been described.

ROBERT M. KLIEGMAN
RICHARD E. BEHRMAN

Anonymous: Brain damage by neonatal hypoglycemia. Lancet 2:882, 1989.
Berk MA, Minouni F, Miodovnik M, et al: Macrosomia in infants of insulin-dependent diabetic mothers. Pediatrics 83:1029, 1989.
Binder ND, Raschko PK, Benda GI, et al: Insulin infusion with parenteral nutrition in extremely low birth weight infants with hyperglycemia. J Pediatr 114:273, 1989.
Cornblath M, Schwartz R: Carbohydrate Metabolism in the Neonate. 3rd ed. Philadelphia, WB Saunders (in press).
Heck LJ, Erenberg A: Serum glucose levels in term neonates during the first 48 hours of life. J Pediatr 110:119, 1987.
Koh THHG, Aynsley-Green A, Tarbit M, et al: Neural dysfunction during hypoglycaemia. Arch Dis Child 63:1353, 1988.
Koh THHG, Eyre JA, Aynsley-Green A: Neonatal hypoglycaemia—the controversy regarding definition. Arch Dis Child 63:1386, 1988.
Lilien L, Pildes R, Srinivasan G, et al: Treatment of neonatal hypoglycemia with minibolus and intravenous glucose infusion. J Pediatr 97:295, 1980.
Louik C, Mitchell AA, Epstein MF, et al: Risk factors for neonatal hyperglycemia associated with 10% dextrose infusion. Am J Dis Child 139:783, 1985.
Lucas A, Morley R, Cole TJ: Adverse neurodevelopmental outcome of moderate neonatal hypoglycaemia. Br Med J 297:1304, 1989.
Pildes P: Neonatal hyperglycemia. J Pediatr 109:905, 1986.
Srinivasan G, Pildes RS, Cattamanchi G, et al: Plasma glucose values in normal neonates: A new look. J Pediatr 109:114, 1986.
Swenne I: The fetus of the diabetic mother: Growth and malformations. Arch Dis Child 63:1119, 1988.

INFECTIONS OF THE NEWBORN

9.58 GENERAL CONSIDERATIONS

Infections are a frequent and important cause of morbidity and mortality in the neonatal period (Chapter 1 and Sec. 5.1). As many as 2% of fetuses are infected in utero, and up to 10% of infants are infected during delivery or the 1st mo of life. Inflammatory lesions are found in about 25% of newborn infant autopsies; these lesions are second only to hyaline membrane disease in frequency.

The uniqueness of neonatal infections is a result of a number of factors: (1) There are diverse modes of transmission of infectious agents from mother to fetus or newborn infant. Transplacental hematogenous spread may occur at different times during gestation. Manifestations of congenital infections may be present at birth or may be delayed for months or years. Vertical transmission of infection may take place in utero, just prior to delivery, or during the process of delivery. After birth, the newborn infant may be exposed to infectious diseases in the nursery or in the community. With the increasing complexity of neonatal intensive care, gestationally younger and lower birthweight newborns are surviving and remaining for a longer time in an environment with a high risk of infection. (2) The newborn infant may be less capable of responding to infection owing to one or more immunologic deficiencies involving the reticuloendothelial system, complement, polymorphonuclear leukocytes, cytokines, antibody, or cell-mediated immunity. (3) Coexisting diseases of the newborn often complicate the diagnosis and management of neonatal infections. Respiratory disorders such as hyaline membrane disease may coexist with bacterial pneumonia. Acidosis impairs functions of polymorphonuclear leukocytes. (4) The manifestations of infectious diseases in the newborn infant are extremely variable. There may be subclinical infection, congenital malformations, focal involvement, and systemic infection. The timing of exposure in utero, inoculum size, immune status, and the etiologic agent influence the expression of disease in the fetus or newborn infant. A variety of organisms, including bacteria, viruses, fungi, protozoa, and mycoplasma, are etiologic agents (Table 9–28).

The status of the mother's immunity, for example, to rubella, and her exposure to various micro-organisms, such as *Toxoplasma*, determines whether maternal infection occurs during pregnancy. Maternal infection may be clinical, often with nonspecific symptoms and signs, or subclinical, identified retrospectively by serologic methods, as part of the evaluation of suspected neonatal infection. Transplacental transmission of infection to the fetus is variable. Prenatal infections that are known to be transmitted transplacentally include syphilis, *Borrelia burgdorferi*, rubella, cytomegalovirus (CMV), parvovirus B19, human immunodeficiency virus (HIV), varicella-zoster, *Listeria monocytogenes*, and toxoplasmosis. Infection acquired in utero may result in resorption of the embryo, abortion, stillbirth, congenital malformation, intrauterine growth retardation, premature birth, acute disease in the neonatal period, or asymptomatic persistent infection with neurologic sequelae later in life.

Perinatal infections are acquired just before or during delivery with vertical transmission of the micro-organism from mother to newborn infant. The organisms may be bacteria that colonize the birth canal, such as group B streptococci, gonococci, *L. monocytogenes*, *Escherichia coli* (particularly the K1 capsular strains), *Chlamydia*, and genital mycoplasma. Other microbial species such as enteroviruses and herpes simplex may also be acquired in a similar fashion. Maternal-to-fetal transfusion at delivery is the usual mechanism of transmission of hepatitis B virus and possibly HIV also.

The *amniotic infection syndrome* refers to bacterial invasion of amniotic fluid, usually as a result of prolonged rupture of the chorioamniotic membrane. On occasion, amniotic infection occurs with apparently intact membranes. Amniotic fluid infection may be asymptomatic or may produce maternal fever and local or systemic signs of chorioamnionitis. Microscopic evidence of inflammation of membranes is uniformly present when the duration of rupture exceeds 24 hr. Difficult or traumatic delivery and premature delivery are also associated with an increased frequency of neonatal infections.

Exposure to and aspiration of bacteria in amniotic fluid lead to congenital pneumonia or systemic bacterial infection with manifestations becoming apparent prior to delivery (fetal distress, tachycardia), at delivery (perinatal asphyxia), or after a latent period of a few hours (respiratory distress, shock). Aspiration of bacteria during the birth process may lead to infection after an interval of 1–2 days. Although the term **early onset neonatal infection** has been used to refer to neonatal infections occurring as late as 1 wk of age, it should be restricted to those infections with a perinatal pathogenesis whose usual onset occurs within 72 hr.

TABLE 9–28. Viral, Parasitic, and Spirochetal Agents Associated with Fetal and Infant Morbidity and Mortality

Pathogen	Fetus	Neonatal Disease	Congenital Defects	Late Sequelae
Rubella virus	Abortion	Low birthweight, hepatosplenomegaly, petechiae, osteitis	Heart defects, microcephaly, cataracts, microphthalmia	Deafness, mental retardation, thyroid disorders, diabetes, degenerative brain tissue, autism
Cytomegalovirus	—	Anemia, thrombocytopenia, hepatosplenomegaly, jaundice, encephalitis	Microcephaly, microphthalmia, retinopathy	Deafness, psychomotor retardation, cerebral calcification
Varicella-zoster virus	—	Low birthweight, chorioretinitis, congenital chickenpox or disseminated neonatal varicella, possibly zoster	Limb hypoplasia, cortical atrophy, cicatricial skin lesions	Fatal outcome due to secondary infection
Picornaviruses				
Coxsackievirus	Abortion	Mild febrile disease, exanthems, aseptic meningitis, disseminated disease, multiple organ involvement (CNS, liver, heart), gastroenteritis	Possible congenital heart disease, myocarditis	Neurologic deficits
Echovirus	—			
Poliovirus	Abortion	Congenital poliomyelitis		Paralysis
Herpes simplex virus	Abortion	Disseminated disease, multiple organ involvement (lung, liver CNS), vesicular skin lesions, retinopathy	Possible microcephaly, retinopathy, intracranial calcifications	Neurologic deficits
Hepatitis B virus	—	Asymptomatic HB_sAg positive infection, low birthweight, rarely acute hepatitis	—	Chronic hepatitis, persistent HB_sAg positive
Human immunodeficiency virus	—	AIDS	—	AIDS
Parvovirus B19	Stillbirth Hydrops fetalis	Anemia	—	—
Borrelia burgdorferi	Stillbirth	Rash, prematurity, cortical blindness	?	?
Toxoplasma gondii	Abortion	Low birthweight, hepatosplenomegaly, jaundice, anemia	Hydrocephalus, microcephaly	Chorioretinitis, mental retardation
Treponema pallidum	Stillbirth Hydrops fetalis	Skin lesions, rhinitis, hepatosplenomegaly jaundice, osteitis, anemia	—	Interstitial keratitis, frontal bossing, saber shins, tooth changes
Malaria	Abortion	Hepatosplenomegaly, jaundice, anemia, poor feeding, vomiting	—	—
Tryponosoma cruzi (Chagas' disease)	Abortion	Low birthweight, jaundice, anemia, petechiae, heart failure, hepatosplenomegaly megoesophagus, encephalitis	Cataracts	Myocarditis, achalasia

The most important neonatal factor predisposing to infection is prematurity or low birthweight; there is a 3- to 10-fold higher incidence of sepsis in these infants than in full-term normal birthweight infants. Males have an approximately 2-fold higher incidence of sepsis than females, suggesting the possibility of a sex-linked factor in host susceptibility. Resuscitation at birth, particularly if it involves endotracheal intubation, insertion of an umbilical vessel catheter, or both, is associated with an increased risk of bacterial infection, possibly due to prematurity or the presence of infection at the time of birth.

Postnatal neonatal infections are acquired after birth during the first 28 days of life. However, similar infections are seen in infants, particularly premature infants, during the first few months of life. The term **late onset neonatal infection** is applied to these infections to differentiate them from those with a perinatal pathogenesis. The etiologic agent may be transmitted from a variety of human sources, such as the mother, family contacts, and hospital personnel or from inanimate sources such as contaminated equipment.

The majority of infants cared for in a neonatal intensive care unit are exposed to a variety of diagnostic and therapeutic procedures that may also compromise host defenses and provide a portal of entry for organisms. The extensive use of antibiotics in neonatal intensive care units may alter the low-birthweight infant's normal bacterial flora and lead to cross-infection with antibiotic-resistant organisms carried on the hands of personnel or on contaminated equipment. The

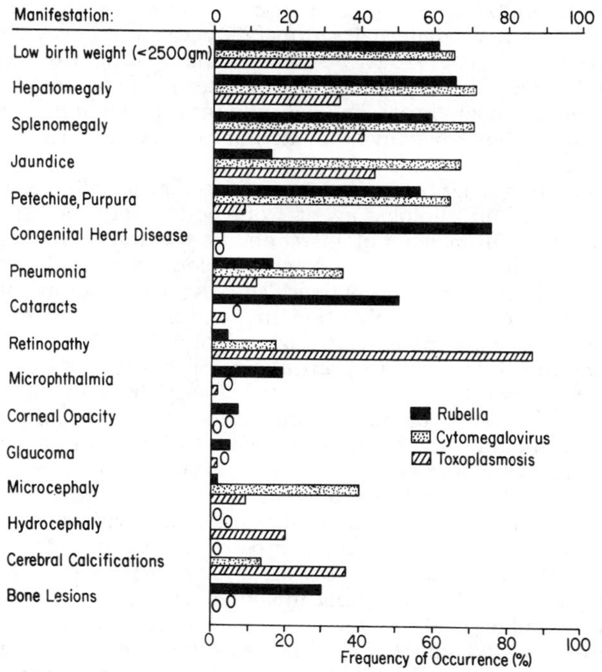

Figure 9–28. Manifestations of symptomatic congenital rubella and cytomegalovirus infections and toxoplasmosis. O indicates a manifestation not observed.

respiratory and gastrointestinal tracts and vascular catheters are common portals of entry.

CLINICAL MANIFESTATIONS. Infection in the newborn infant may be limited to a single organ or may involve multiple organs (focal or systemic); it may be mild, moderate, or severe; acute, subacute, or chronic; or it may be asymptomatic. Infections with different micro-organisms may have overlapping patterns, so that it is usually not possible to make a definitive diagnosis of a specific etiologic agent from the clinical features alone (Figs. 9–28 and 9–29). Signs consistent with infection in the newborn may also be caused by a variety of noninfectious disease processes involving different organs (Table 9–29). Hypoplastic left-sided heart syndrome, volvulus, hypoglycemia, hyperammonemia, intracranial hemorrhage, supraventricular tachycardia, and salt-losing adrenogenital syndrome are frequently confused with neonatal sepsis. The incidence of infection is higher than the incidence of many of these noninfectious disorders. An infectious etiology should always be considered in the assessment of a sick newborn infant.

DIAGNOSIS. The maternal history may provide important information about maternal infection, exposure to infection in a sexual partner, maternal immunity (natural or acquired),

TABLE 9–29. Nonspecific Clinical Manifestations of Infection in the Newborn Infant

General
- Fever, hypothermia
- "Not doing well"
- Poor feeding
- Sclerema

Gastrointestinal System
- Abdominal distention
- Anorexia, vomiting
- Diarrhea
- Hepatomegaly

Respiratory System
- Apnea, dyspnea
- Tachypnea, retraction
- Flaring, grunting
- Cyanosis

Cardiovascular System
- Pallor, mottling, cold, clammy skin
- Tachycardia
- Hypotension
- Bradycardia

Central Nervous System
- Irritability, lethargy
- Tremors, seizures
- Hyporeflexia, hypotonia
- Abnormal Moro reflex
- Irregular respirations
- Full fontanel
- High-pitched cry

Hematologic System
- Jaundice
- Splenomegaly
- Pallor
- Petechiae, purpura
- Bleeding

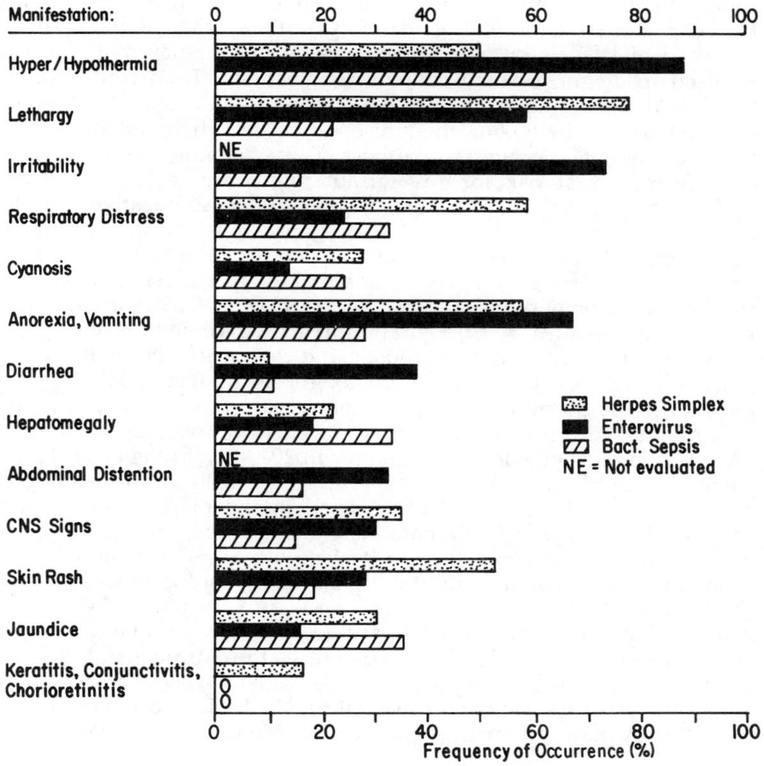

Figure 9–29. Manifestations of herpes simplex and enterovirus infections and bacterial sepsis in the neonate. O indicates a manifestation not observed.

maternal colonization, and obstetric risk factors (prematurity, prolonged ruptured membranes, and maternal chorioamnionitis). Serologic screening tests may have been performed for *Treponema pallidum*, rubella, and hepatitis B virus. Maternal cultures may have been taken for *Neisseria gonorrhoeae*, group B streptococcus, herpes simplex, or *Chlamydia*.

The acronym **TORCH** refers to toxoplasmosis, other agents, rubella, cytomegalovirus, and herpes simplex. It was modified to STORCH to include syphilis. Although the term may be helpful in remembering some of the etiologic agents of neonatal infections, the TORCH battery of serologic tests has a poor diagnostic yield, and the appropriate diagnostic studies should be selected for each etiologic agent under consideration.

Intrauterine infections due to toxoplasmosis, rubella, cytomegalovirus, herpes simplex, and syphilis present a diagnostic dilemma because (1) their clinical features overlap and may initially be indistinguishable, (2) disease may be inapparent, (3) maternal infection is often asymptomatic, (4) special laboratory studies may be needed, and (5) specific treatment for toxoplasmosis, syphilis, and herpes simplex is predicated on an accurate diagnosis and may reduce significant long-term morbidity. Common shared features that should suggest the diagnosis of an intrauterine infection include prematurity, intrauterine growth retardation, and hematologic involvement (anemia, neutropenia, thrombocytopenia, petechiae, purpura), ocular signs (chorioretinitis, cataracts, keratoconjunctivitis, glaucoma, micro-ophthalmia), central nervous system symptoms (microcephaly, hydrocephaly, intracranial calcifications), and other organ system involvement (pneumonia, myocarditis, nephritis, hepatitis with hepatosplenomegaly, and jaundice), or nonimmune hydrops.

The maternal history and physical examination of the newborn add additional diagnostic information; however, neonatal IgG titers are often difficult to interpret because IgG is acquired from the mother by transplacental passage, and neonatal IgM titers to specific pathogens are technically difficult to perform and are not universally available. IgM titers to specific pathogens have high specificity but only moderate sensitivity; they should not be employed to exclude infection. Paired maternal and fetal-neonatal IgG titers with higher newborn IgG levels or rising IgG titers during infancy may be used to diagnose some congenital infections. Total cord blood IgM, IgA (both are not actively transported across the placenta to the fetus), or the presence of IgM-rheumatoid factor in neonatal serum may be used as a screening tool to identify infants at risk for any intrauterine infection. Total IgM has a high rate of both false-positive and false-negative results.

Specific TORCH infections may be diagnosed either by culture (CMV, rubella, herpes simplex, toxoplasmosis) or serology with or without culture (Fig. 9–30). CMV titers are not helpful because 60–70% of nonpregnant women have CMV IgG; urine culture is diagnostic and demonstrates viral growth within 24–48 hr. In utero diagnosis of fetal CMV infection is made by culturing amniotic fluid or by demonstrating fetal serum CMV IgM by cordocentesis. Toxoplasma IgG may be present prior to pregnancy in 20–30% of women. Neonatal toxoplasma IgM may be absent in 10–20% of those in whom the organism is demonstrated in the placenta or cerebrospinal fluid (CSF). Prenatal diagnosis of fetal toxoplasmosis is possible by inoculation of mice with amniotic fluid or fetal blood to demonstrate the organism, by cordocentesis (20–24 wk of gestation) to identify IgM, and by fibroblast culture of amniotic fluid or fetal serum. Immunity to rubella is present in as many as 85% of women. Culture of neonatal throat, urine, or CSF samples reveals rubella virus, and cordocentesis at 19–24 wk reveals fetal rubella IgM. Chorionic villus biopsy may demonstrate early rubella infection by DNA-RNA hybridization. In utero herpes simplex infection cannot be identified by maternal serum IgG because many women have positive test results. IgM assays that distinguish herpes simplex type 1 from type 2 are helpful; neonatal culture of the conjunctivae, throat, and CSF add information if the result is positive, but if negative they do not exclude in utero herpes simplex infection.

Definitive diagnosis of a specific infection usually requires recovery of an etiologic agent from body fluids or tissues, particularly from sites of infection. In the infant with suspected bacterial infection, a complete blood count (CBC) and blood culture should be obtained. Urinalysis and culture rarely provide additional information in the first week of life. In neonatal sepsis, increases in the absolute band neutrophil count and the immature/mature neutrophil ratio and thrombocytopenia often occur within the first 24 hr after onset of symptoms. White blood cells may also contain vacuoles and toxic granulations. Thrombocytopenia also occurs in congenital cytomegalovirus, rubella, toxoplasma, and spirochetal infections. Because the prognosis and the duration of antibiotic therapy are quite different in the infant with sepsis that is without a defined source compared with the infant with sepsis that is complicated by meningits, and since neonates with late onset urinary tract infection can present a picture that resembles sepsis in the absence of bacteremia, the infant with suspected sepsis should be carefully evaluated with an assessment of the history, physical findings, and available laboratory data. Cerebrospinal fluid should be examined whenever meningitis is considered and in all patients with positive blood cultures. Gram-stained smear of spinal fluid, urine, or material from sites of infection, for example, endotracheal tubes, skin lesions, weapy umbilical stumps, or scalp monitor sites, may provide an immediate tentative diagnosis of bacterial infection and can assist in the choice of initial antibiotic therapy. Within hours, the antigens of group B streptococcus or K1 strains of *E. coli* can be identified in the spinal fluid or urine by counterimmunoelectrophoresis (CIE) or latex agglutination. Roentgenographic examination is the primary method of localizing suspected pneumonia, septic arthritis, osteomyelitis, or the osseous lesions of syphilis, rubella, or CMV.

TREATMENT. Although specific therapy should be pursued whenever possible, definitive diagnosis is often delayed. The high morbidity and mortality associated with neonatal infections and the difficulty of assessing nonspecific signs in newborn infants lead to the frequent use of empiric antimicrobial therapy. If sepsis, pneumonia, or meningitis is suspected, treatment should be initiated after appropriate cultures have been obtained and diagnostic laboratory studies performed. Antibiotics should be selected on the bases of expected antibiotic sensitivity patterns of anticipated pathogens. This judgment will depend on the age of onset of illness, the disease pattern, maternal epidemiology, and the nosocomial microbiologic agents indigenous to the nursery. Dosages of antibiotics commonly used in newborns are given in Table 9–30. The decision to continue antibiotics for a full course of therapy will depend on the results of cultures, on other laboratory tests, and on the course of the illness. Since many neonatal infections are difficult to treat despite antimicrobial agents that are effective in vitro, there is increasing interest in methods of prophylaxis (see Sec. 9.59 and 9.60). For treatment of congenital infections, see Syphilis (Sec. 12.50), Toxoplasmosis (Sec. 12.112), and Herpes simplex (Sec. 9.71).

Anonymous: TORCH syndrome and TORCH screening. Lancet 335:1559, 1990.
Baley JE: Neonatal sepsis: The potential for immunotherapy. Clin Perinatol 15:755, 1988.

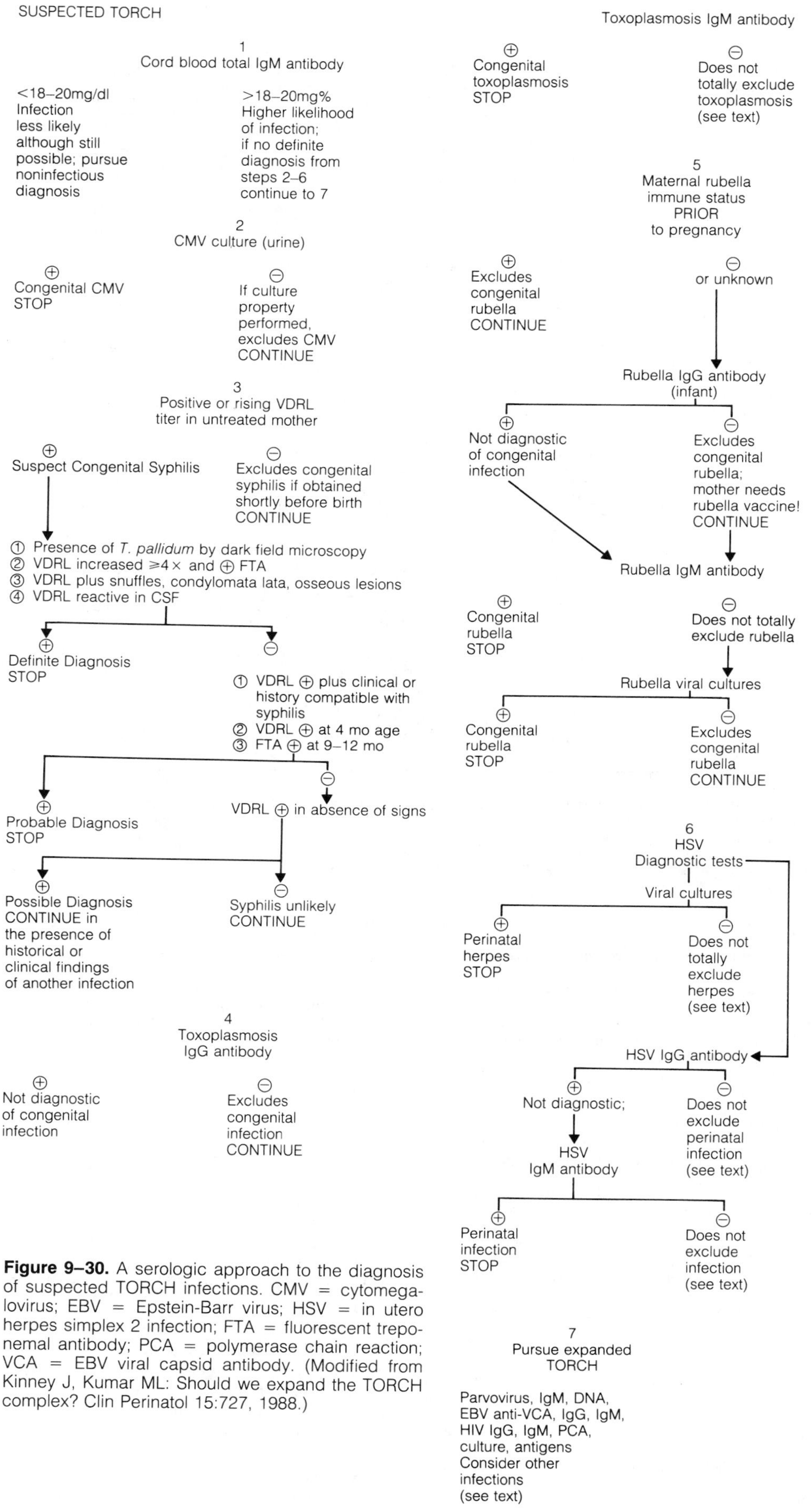

Figure 9–30. A serologic approach to the diagnosis of suspected TORCH infections. CMV = cytomegalovirus; EBV = Epstein-Barr virus; HSV = in utero herpes simplex 2 infection; FTA = fluorescent treponemal antibody; PCA = polymerase chain reaction; VCA = EBV viral capsid antibody. (Modified from Kinney J, Kumar ML: Should we expand the TORCH complex? Clin Perinatol 15:727, 1988.)

TABLE 9–30. Dosages of Antibiotics Commonly Used in Newborns*

		Dosages (mg/kg) and Intervals of Administration				
		Weight < 1200g	*Weight 1200–2000g*		*Weight > 2000g*	
Antibiotics	**Routes**	*Age 0–4 wk*	*Age 0–7 days*	*> 7 days*	*Age 0–7 days*	*> 7 days*
Amikacin†	IV, IM	7.5 q12h	7.5 q12h	7 q8h	10 q12h	10 q8h
Ampicillin,	IV, IM					
Meningitis		50 q12h	50 q12h	50 q8h	50 q8h	50 q6h
Other diseases		25 q12h	25 q12h	25 q8h	25 q8h	25 q6h
Aztreonam	IV, IM	30 q12h	30 q12h	30 q8h	30 q8h	30 q6h
Cefazolin	IV, IM	20 q12h	20 q12h	20 q12h	20 q12h	20 q8h
Cefotaxime	IV, IM	50 q12h	50 q12h	50 q8h	50 q12h	50 q8h
Ceftazidime	IV, IM	50 q12h	50 q12h	50 q8h	30 q8h	50 q8h
Ceftriaxone	IV, IM	50 q24h	50 q24h	50 q24h	50 q24h	75 q24h
Cephalothin	IV	20 q12h	20 q12h	20 q8h	20 q8h	20 q6h
Chloramphenicol‡	IV, PO	22 q24h	25 q24h	25 q24h	25 q24h	25 q12h
Clindamycin	IV, IM, PO	5 q12h	5 q12h	5 q8h	5 q8h	5 q6h
Erythromycin	PO	10 q12h	10 q12h	10 q8h	10 q12h	10 q8h
Gentamicin†	IV, IM	2.5 q18–24h	2.5 q12h	2.5 q8h	2.5 q12h	2.5 q8h
Kanamycin	IV, IM	7.5 q12h	7.5 q12h	7 q8h	10 q12h	10 q8h
Methicillin	IV, IM					
Meningitis		50 q12h	50 q12h	50 q8h	50 q8h	50 q6h
Other diseases		25 q12h	25 q12h	25 q8h	25 q8h	25 q6h
Metronidazole	IV, PO	7.5 q48h	7.5 q24h	7.5 q12h	7.5 q12h	15 q12h
Mezlocillin	IV, IM	75 q12h	75 q12h	75 q8h	75 q12h	75 q8h
Oxacillin	IV, IM	25 q12h	25 q12h	30 q8h	25 q8h	37.5 q6h
Nafcillin	IV	25 q12h	25 q12h	25 q8h	25 q8h	37.5 q6h
Netilmicin§	IV, IM	2.5 q18–24h	2.5 q12h	2.5 q8h	2.5 q12h	2.5 q8h
Penicillin G	IV					
Meningitis		50,000 U q12h	50,000 U q12h	75,000 U q8h	50,000 U q8h	50,000 U q6h
Other diseases		25,000 U q12h	25,000 U q12h	25,000 U q8h	25,000 U q8h	25,000 U q6h
Penicillin G	IM					
Benzathine			50,000 U (one dose)	50,000 U (one dose)	50,000 U (one dose)	50,000 U (one dose)
Procaine			50,000 U q24h	50,000 U q24h	50,000 U q24h	50,000 U q24h
Ticarcillin	IV, IM	75 q12h	75 q12h	75 q8h	75 q8h	75 q6h
Tobramycin†	IV, IM	2.5 q18–24h	2 q12h	2 q8h	2 q12h	2 q8h
Vancomycin‖	IV	15 q24h	10 q12h	10 q8h	15 q12h	10 q8h

Recommendations for infants weighing < 1000g based on Prober et al: Pediatr Infect Dis J 9:111, 1990.
*Adapted from Nelson JD: 1991–92 Pocketbook of Pediatric Antimicrobial Therapy, 9th ed. © 1991, The Williams & Wilkins Co., Baltimore.
†Aminoglycoside levels should be monitored if therapy continues > 3 days. Optimal peak levels 6–8 μg/mL, trough less than 2 μg/mL.
‡Serum levels are highly variable. Chloramphenicol should be given to newborns only if serum levels can be monitored.
§0.5 mg/kg/24 hr can increase to 1 mg/kg/24 hr if needed or give every other day. Treat for cumulative dose of 10–30 mg/kg.
‖Because of variable pharmacokinetics, vancomycin levels should be monitored if therapy continues > 3 days. Optimal peak levels 20–30 μg/mL, trough less than 10 μg/mL.

Davies PA, Gothefors LA: Bacterial Infections in the Fetus and Newborn Infant. Philadelphia, WB Saunders, 1984.
deLouvois J, Harvey D: Antibiotic therapy of the newborn. Clin Perinatol 15:365, 1988.
Dunkle L, Nagvi S, McCollum R, et al: Eradication of epidemic methicillin-gentamicin resistant *Staphylococcus aureus* in an intensive care nursery. Am J Med 70:455, 1981.
Feigin RD: Neonatal meningitis: Problems and prospects. Hosp Pract 18:175, 1983.
Friesen CA, Cho CT: Characteristic features of neonatal sepsis due to *Haemophilus influenzae*. Rev Infect Dis 8:777, 1986.
Gardner P, Causey WA, Beem MO: Nosocomial Infections. *In*: Feigin RD, Cherry JD (eds): Textbook of Pediatric Infectious Diseases. Philadelphia, WB Saunders, 1987.
Girardin E, Gran GE, Dayer J-M, et al: Tumor necrosis factor and interleukin-1 in the serum of children with severe infectious purpura. N Engl J Med 319:397, 1988.
Grose C, Itani O, Weiner CP: Perinatal diagnosis of fetal infections: Advances from amniocentesis to cordocentesis—congenital toxoplasmosis, rubella, cytomegalovirus, varicella virus, parvovirus, and human immunodeficiency virus. Pediatr Infect Dis J 8–459, 1989.
Hanshaw JD, Dudgeon JA, Marshall WC: Viral Diseases of the Fetus and Newborn. Philadelphia, WB Saunders, 1985.
Hill HR: Host defenses in the neonate: Prospects for enhancement. Semin Perinatol 9:2, 1985.
Kinney JS, Kumer ML: Should we expand the TORCH complex? A description of clinical and diagnostic aspects of selected old and new agents. Clin Perinatol 15:727, 1988.
Kovatch AL, Wald ER: Evaluation of the febrile neonate. Semin Perinatol 9:12, 1985.
Leland D, Morris MS, French LV, et al: The use of TORCH titers. Pediatrics 72:41, 1983.
McCracken GH Jr, Freij BJ: Perinatal bacterial diseases. *In*: Feigin RD, Cherry JD (eds): Textbook of Pediatric Infectious Diseases. Philadelphia, WB Saunders, 1987.
Noel GJ, Laufer DA, Edelson PJ: Anaerobic bacteremia in a neonatal intensive care unit: An eighteen-year experience. Pediatr Infect Dis J 7:858, 1988.
Overall JC Jr: Viral infections of the fetus and neonate. *In*: Feigin RD, Cherry JD (eds): Textbook of Pediatric Infectious Diseases. Philadelphia, WB Saunders, 1987.
Remington JS, Klein JO: Infectious Diseases of the Fetus and Newborn Infant. Philadelphia, WB Saunders, 1990.

9.59 NOSOCOMIAL NURSERY INFECTION

See also Sec. 12.9.

Neonatal infections acquired in the hospital are nosocomial. Because most early onset infections are acquired intrapartum, infections that develop later than 48–72 hr after birth are usually considered nosocomial. However, exceptions include late onset infections with organisms acquired from the mother's genital tract (e.g., some group B streptococcal infections) and nosocomial infections acquired in the delivery room (e.g., from contaminated equipment), in which signs develop soon after birth. Nosocomial infections may be sporadic or occur as epidemics, and they may occur in the hospital or after discharge.

Nosocomial infections are relatively uncommon in normal, full-term infants; the rate ranges from 0.5 to 1.7% of term infants. They usually involve the skin and are caused by *Staphylococcus aureus* or *Candida* (Sec. 12.19 and 9.75). In contrast, the rates of nosocomial infections among low-birth-weight infants in neonatal intensive care units are higher than in any other site in the hospital and range from 20 to 33%; the incidence increases with the duration of hospitalization and lower gestational ages.

Since any *pathogen* that can colonize infants, personnel, or families in the neonatal intensive care unit (NICU) and can be transmitted by direct contact or indirect contact through contaminated vehicles (intravenous fluids, medications, disinfectants, respiratory equipment, stool, breast milk, blood), the list of organisms causing nosocomial infections is long. The common causes are coagulase-negative staphylococci, gram-negative bacilli *(Klebsiella pneumoniae, Escherichia coli, Salmonella, Campylobacter, Enterobacter, Citrobacter, Pseudomonas aeruginosa, Serratia)*, enterococci, *S. aureus*, and *Candida*. Viruses contributing to nosocomial neonatal infections include enteroviruses, cytomegalovirus, hepatitis A, adenoviruses, influenza, respiratory syncytial virus, rhinovirus, parainfluenza, herpes simplex, and rotavirus. The common infections are those involving the skin, bacteremia associated with catheters, and pneumonia. Exacerbations of respiratory disease in infants with pre-existing pulmonary problems, such as bronchopulmonary dysplasia, are particularly difficult to assess, but pneumonia must be considered. Epidemics of gastroenteritis and necrotizing enterocolitis occur less commonly and may be associated with an identifiable agent or no specific pathogen.

Multiple *risk factors* influence the probability of nosocomial infection in the NICU. These include low birthweight, length of stay, invasive procedures, indwelling vascular catheters, ventricular shunts, endotracheal tubes, alterations in the skin and mucuous membrane barriers, and frequent use of broad-spectrum antibiotics. Colonization of the infant's skin, umbilicus, nasopharynx, and gastrointestinal tract by pathogenic bacteria or fungi is a common prerequisite for subsequent nosocomial infection. Antibiotics interfere with colonization resistance by the normal flora and facilitate colonization by pathogens. Crowding and inadequate infection control techniques (handwashing between patient examinations) may also contribute to the problem.

Surveillance for nosocomial infection is based on the ongoing review of nursery infections and data from the microbiology laboratory; routine surveillance to detect colonization is not indicated. Cultures should indicate the bacterial isolate and the antimicrobial sensitivity pattern. Assessment of other microbial markers (biotype, serotype, plasmid, DNA fingerprint) may be helpful in epidemics. During epidemics, investigation of possible reservoirs of infection, modes of transmission, and risk factors is necessary. Identification of colonized infants and nursery personnel may be helpful.

Prevention of neonatal nosocomial infection is complex and includes a 2-min scrub before entering the nursery, 15-sec washing between patients, scrub suits for nurses and residents, adequate nursing staff, avoidance of overcrowding, and specific isolation precautions (Sec. 12.9 and Tables 12–8 and 12–9). Control of outbreaks depends on the pathogen and epidemiology (see Sec. 12.19). Commonly used measures include investigation of the extent of colonization in infants and caretakers, a search for a common source or reservoir, cohorting of infants and caretakers, changes in handwashing solutions and protocols, and antimicrobial prophylaxis. Cord care, infant bathing practices, equipment sterilization, and hand-washing are essential, whereas gowns have not consistently been demonstrated to be effective.

Craven DE, Stager KA: Nosocomial pneumonia in the intubated patient. Infect Dis Clin North Am 3:843, 1989.

Goldmann DA: Prevention and management of neonatal infections. Infect Dis Clin North Am 3:779, 1989.

Jarvis WR: Epidemiology of nosocomial infections in pediatric patients. Pediatr Infect Dis J 6:344, 1987.

John JF: Molecular analysis of nosocomial epidemics. Infect Dis Clin North Am 3:683, 1989.

CLINICAL SYNDROMES

9.60 NEONATAL SEPSIS

The terms sepsis and septicemia are used synonymously and are not well defined. In contrast to bacteremia (bacteria in the blood), septicemia usually consists of bacteremia plus a constellation of signs and symptoms caused by micro-organisms or their toxic products in the circulation. There may be a progression of bacteremia to septicemia depending on clinical manifestations. However, septicemia, the clinical syndrome, may also occur without bacteremia, for example, culture-negative sepsis associated with pyelonephritis or pneumonia, due to endotoxemia. The best-identified clinical disorder is septic shock, which can be reproduced by intravenous administration of endotoxin from gram-negative bacteria. Since other micro-organisms such as gram-positive bacteria, viruses, fungi, rickettsiae, and protozoa have been implicated as etiologic agents in septic shock, there must be many other initiating factors in addition to endotoxin. Teichoic acids from gram-positive cocci can produce septic shock. The bacterial products result in the release of a variety of endogenous cytokines such as interleukin 1 (IL-1), tumor necrosis factor (TNF), and platelet-activating factor (PAF) from host cells. These inflammatory mediators produce physiologic effects, primarily on the cardiovascular system. Further interactions with histamine, kinins, the complement system, and other leukocyte products are being elucidated. It is now possible to demonstrate circulating bacterial products (e.g., endotoxemia) and endogenous mediators (IL-1, TNF, PAF) in some patients with septicemia (Sec. 12.14).

Neonatal sepsis (sepsis neonatorum) is a clinical syndrome resulting from the pathophysiologic effects of local or systemic infection in the 1st mo of life. Because of the lack of specificity of many of the signs associated with this syndrome and the limitations of laboratory criteria, the diagnosis will continue to be difficult to establish. For example, the asymptomatic 2-hr-old infant whose mother has chorioamnionitis may have bacteremia but not sepsis at that point in time.

EPIDEMIOLOGY. The incidence of neonatal sepsis varies from 1 to 8/1,000 live births in developed countries with considerable variability over time and geographic location. Hospital-to-hospital variability in incidence may be related to rates of prematurity, prenatal care, conduct of labor, and environmental conditions in nurseries. Attack rates of neonatal sepsis increase significantly in low-birthweight infants and in the presence of maternal (obstetric) risk factors such as prolonged rupture of membranes (>18 hr), maternal intrapartum fever (>37.5° C), maternal leukocytosis (>18,000), uterine tenderness, fetal tachycardia (>180 beats per min [BPM]), and chorioamnionitis. Inhalation of infected amniotic fluid may produce pneumonia and sepsis in utero, manifested by fetal distress or neonatal asphyxia. Exposure to adult pathogens is a risk factor after birth.

Host risk factors include male sex, developmental or congenital immune defects, galactosemia *(E. coli)*, administration of intramuscular iron *(E. coli)*, congenital anomalies (urinary tract, asplenia, myelomeningocele, sinus tracts), omphalitis, twinning (especially the second twin of an infected twin), and possibly the administration of high doses of vitamin E. Prematurity is a risk factor for early and late onset disease.

The epidemiology of neonatal sepsis is exemplified by the

extensive studies of group B streptococci (Sec. 9.67). Vertical transmission of group B streptococci and other organisms that produce early onset sepsis is well documented and is often associated with maternal risk factors. Fifty to 90% of infants whose mothers are colonized at delivery become colonized. The risk of neonatal colonization varies with the bacterial density in the maternal genital tract. However, only one in 50–75% of colonized infants develops invasive disease, again related in part to the size of the inoculum as determined by the number of sites of infant colonization.

ETIOLOGY. The agents causing neonatal sepsis vary with time and geographic area. The most common organisms associated with neonatal sepsis are shown in Table 9–31 according to the timing of infection and geographic location. All serotypes of group B streptococci and *E. coli* account for about 75% of early onset sepsis. Community-acquired late onset disease is largely due to virulent strains of group B streptococcus serotype III and *E. coli* serotype K1. Nosocomial infections in neonatal intensive care units have a different pathogenesis and are often related to the use of ventilators, vascular catheters, and other risk factors. They are most often due to coagulase-negative staphylococci, *S. aureus*, gram-negative enterics other than *E. coli*, *Pseudomonas* species, *Serratia*, and *Candida albicans*. Among the anaerobic bacteria, *Bacteroides* and *Clostridium* are established neonatal pathogens. The widespread use of antibiotics in special care nurseries has also contributed to the selection of resistant organisms such as aminoglycoside-resistant gram-negative enteric bacilli and methicillin-resistant staphylococci.

PATHOPHYSIOLOGY. An infant's immunologic status, the virulence of the micro-organism, the inoculum size, and a variety of other factors determine which infections result in the clinical syndrome of neonatal sepsis. The portals of entry for infectious agents include the skin, mucous membranes, umbilical cord, nasophyarynx, lungs, gastrointestinal tract, and urinary tract. These barriers may be breached by congenital anomalies or trauma, including instrumentation and procedures (umbilical catheterization, endotracheal intubation). In addition, the newborn infant, particularly the premature infant, has quantitative and qualitative host immune deficits that predispose to infection or adversely affect the outcome of infection. The neonate may have an antibody deficiency owing to absence of maternal antibody (IgG) that can be transferred across the placenta. Alternatively, the very low birthweight infant may have very low IgG levels (<100 mg/dL) owing to diminished passive transfer early in gestation. Levels of opsonic C3, chemotactic C5a, and factor B may further impair opsonophagocytosis and complement-mediated bacterial killing. Decreased neutrophil mobility and phagocytic activity may be due in part to decreased expression of membrane adherence protein/C3bi receptors. Neutrophil function may be further impaired by the stress response during sepsis. The frequent occurrence of granulocytopenia during neonatal sepsis, owing to neutrophil storage pool (bone marrow) depletion, predisposes the infant to a profound quantitative defect in host defenses.

Attenuated neonatal immune mechanisms may also predispose to viral infections. These compromised host defense mechanisms include deficient specific IgG, reduced production of interferon-γ by T lymphocytes, reduced interferon-γ–induced cytotoxicity, reduced nonspecific cytotoxicity, primarily due to diminished natural killer (NK) cell activity, and slightly lower antibody-dependent cell-mediated cytotoxicity.

CLINICAL MANIFESTATIONS. The initial signs of infection are often subtle or minimal. The mother or nurse may simply state that the infant "doesn't look well" or "feeds poorly." There may be temperature instability (hypothermia or hyperthermia) or signs related to one or more organ systems (see Table 9–29). Fever in full-term infants does not always signify infection. A temperature of greater than 37.8° C (axillary), as an isolated single measurement, lasting less than 1 hr, and without other manifestations of infection, is usually not due to sepsis and may be caused by increased ambient temperature, dehydration, central nervous system disorders, hyperthyroidism, familial dysautonomia, or ectodermal dysplasia. Late manifestations of sepsis may include apnea, cyanosis, hypotension, and disseminated intravascular coagulation with bleeding from multiple sites. Manifestations of sepsis may be present at birth or may appear at any time during the neonatal period. In the delivery room, sepsis with congenital consolidated pneumonia may interfere with the onset of spontaneous respirations and may be a cause of

TABLE 9–31. Patterns of Neonatal Sepsis

Feature	Early Onset	Late Onset	Nosocomial
Onset	Birth; < 7 days, usually, < 3 days	8–28 days, occasionally 60 days	1st week to discharge
Obstetric risks	Colonization, amnionitis, prematurity	Unusual	Prematurity; NICU interventions, bowel resection
Presentation	Respiratory distress, pneumonia, shock	Fever, CNS, or focal signs	Apnea, bradycardia, lethargy, temperature instability
Meningitis	30%	75%	10–20%
Other systems	Rare	Pyelonephritis, osteomyelitis, septic arthritis, cellulitis	Pneumonia, pyelonephritis, endophthalmitis, septic thrombi, phlebitis, cutaneous infections, central line sepsis, NEC
Pathogens*	Group B streptococcus types Ia, Ib, I a/c, II, III, *E. coli, Klebsiella, Listeria monocytogenes,* enterococci, nontypable *Hemophilus influenzae, S. pneumoniae*	Group B streptococcus type III, *E. coli, L. monocytogenes,* herpes simplex	*Staphylococcus epidermidis, S. aureus, Candida albicans, Pseudomonas aeruginosa, E. coli,* herpes simplex, *Klebsiella, Serratia*
Treatment	Ampicillin and gentamicin† or cefotaxime	Ampicillin and gentamicin or cefotaxime	Depends on nosocomial agents present in nursery; vancomycin or nafcillin and gentamicin
Supportive care	Mechanical ventilation, vasoactive agents, fluid resuscitation, ECMO	Mechanical ventilation, vasoactive agents, fluid resuscitation	Mechanical ventilation, vasoactive agents, fluid resuscitation
Mortality‡	15–70%	10–20%	5–10%

*Herpes simplex, enteroviruses, and cytomegalovirus can present as culture-negative late onset sepsis that is indistinguishable from severe bacterial disease.
†Dose and interval for administration vary with birthweight and postnatal age (see Table 9–30).
‡Mortality is highest when disease presents at birth and among very low birthweight (< 1,500 g) infants.

neonatal asphyxia, or it may be a separate coexisting problem. In premature infants, pneumonia may coexist with hyaline membrane disease. The presenting clinical and radiologic findings of sepsis may be difficult to differentiate from those of hyaline membrane disease. The clinical signs of infection in the newborn are often nonspecific, vary greatly in intensity and severity, and are seen in many noninfectious disorders as well (see Table 12–2).

DIAGNOSIS. Identification of a bacterial infection may be made by isolating the etiologic agent from a body fluid that is normally sterile (blood, cerebrospinal fluid, urine, joint fluid), by demonstrating endotoxin or bacterial antigen in a body fluid (cerebrospinal fluid [CSF], urine, or serum), or by demonstrating bacterial infection at autopsy. However, a positive blood culture may not always establish the diagnosis of sepsis. Cultures may be contaminated or may result from transient bacteremia secondary to focal infection. Transient group B streptococcal bacteremia also has been documented in asymptomatic infants. It is preferable to obtain two specimens by venipuncture from different sites. Interpretation of tests for bacterial antigen also may be difficult. Latex particle agglutination and counterimmunoelectrophoresis are used for identification of group B streptococcal polysaccharide and *E. coli* K1 capsular polysaccharide. The commercially available antigen detection kits are not as sensitive as blood cultures, and false-positive results may occur, particularly errors due to contamination of urine collected in bags. Since concentrated urine is an excellent fluid for use in antigen detection, this test should be confirmed with specimens collected by suprapubic aspiration or catheterization.

Although blood cultures are usually the basis for a diagnosis of sepsis, the bacteremic phase of the illness may be missed by poor timing or blood sample size (sample size may be as little as 0.2 mL, but more than 0.5–1 mL is optimal). Blood cultures performed by radiometric methods may demonstrate growth within 24–72 hr. Samples should be obtained from an umbilical catheter only at the time of initial insertion; a peripheral venous sample should be obtained when samples for cultures are drawn from central venous catheters. Focal infections producing systemic manifestations such as meningitis, arthritis, and urinary tract infections may be diagnosed by positive culture results from specific sites in the absence of positive blood cultures. Furthermore, bacterial pneumonia has been reported at autopsy in infants with negative blood cultures prior to antimicrobial therapy.

When the clinical syndrome is consistent with a diagnosis of sepsis, a full evaluation for sepsis should be performed. This includes, in addition to blood cultures, a lumbar puncture, urine examination and culture, and a chest roentgenogram (urine should be collected by catheterization or suprapubic aspiration; urine culture can be omitted in early onset sepsis because urinary tract infection is rare at this time). Demonstration of inflammation of the meninges in newborns with clinical manifestations of sepsis is generally indicative of bacterial infection, although nonbacterial infectious causes must be considered in the differential diagnosis of meningitis as well as neonatal sepsis (see Figs. 9–28 and 9–29). Demonstration of bacteria and inflammatory cells in gram-stained gastric aspirates on the 1st day of life may reflect maternal amnionitis, which is a risk factor for early onset sepsis. Examination of the buffy coat with Gram-stain or methylene blue stains may demonstrate intracellular pathogens, whereas similar stains of endotracheal secretors in infants with early onset pneumonia may demonstrate the gram-positive cocci of group B streptococci.

A number of laboratory tests, alone and in combination, have been evaluated for their utility in providing a rapid indicator of neonatal sepsis. These include the erythrocyte sedimentation rate, C-reactive protein, haptoglobin, fibrinogen, IgM, nitroblue tetrazolium dye, and leukocyte alkaline phosphatase. In general, they are not helpful. Only the total white blood cell count and differential and the ratio of immature to total neutrophils provide immediately predictive information when compared to age standards. Neutropenia is more common than neutrophilia in severe neonatal sepsis, but neutropenia also occurs in association with maternal hypertension, neonatal sensitization, necrotizing enterocolitis, periventricular hemorrhage, seizures, surgery, and possibly hemolysis. An immature neutrophil-total neutrophil ratio of 0.16 or greater suggests bacterial infection.

Diagnostic evaluations may be indicated for asymptomatic infants because of maternal risk factors. The probability of neonatal infection and subsequent neonatal sepsis correlates with the degree of prematurity and bacterial contamination of amniotic fluid. In an asymptomatic term infant whose mother has chorioamnionitis two blood cultures and a gastric aspirate should be examined to confirm the maternal diagnosis and identify presumptively the organisms by Gram stain. A lumbar puncture is not indicated because infants with meningitis are symptomatic. If the blood culture is positive or if the infant becomes symptomatic, lumbar puncture should be performed and treatment initiated immediately. Prolonged rupture of membranes for longer than 18 hr suggests the need for blood cultures in premature infants but not necessarily in asymptomatic term infants without signs of fetal distress.

TREATMENT. Once the diagnosis of neonatal sepsis has been suspected and appropriate cultures have been obtained, intravenous or intramuscular antibiotic therapy should be instituted immediately. Initial treatment of suspected neonatal sepsis is determined by the pattern of disease and the organisms that are common for the age of the infant and the flora of the nursery (see Table 9–31). Initial empiric treatment of early onset and late onset community-acquired infections should consist of ampicillin and an aminoglycoside (usually gentamicin). Nosocomial infections acquired in the NICU are more likely to be caused by staphylococci, a variety of enterobacteriaceae, *Pseudomonas*, or *Candida*. Thus, an antistaphylococcal drug, nafcillin for *S. aureus* or vancomycin for coagulase-negative staphylococci or methicillin-resistant *S. aureus*, should be substituted for ampicillin. A history of recent antimicrobial therapy or the presence of antibiotic-resistant infections in the NICU suggests the need for a different aminoglycoside agent (amikacin) and vancomycin used for methicillin-resistant staphylococcae. Doses of the commonly used antibiotics are provided in Table 9–30. When the history or the presence of necrotic skin lesions suggests *Pseudomonas* infection, initial therapy should be ticarcillin, mezlocillin, or carbenicillin and gentamicin.

Once the pathogen has been identified and the antibiotic sensitivities determined, the most appropriate drug(s) should be selected. For most of the gram-negative enteric bacteria, a 3rd-generation cephalosporin (cefotaxime or ceftazidime) should be used. Enterococcus should be treated with both a penicillin (ampicillin or piperacillin) and an aminoglycoside, since synergism has been demonstrated with this combination of antibiotics in many strains. Ampicillin alone is adequate for *Listeria monocytogenes*, and penicillin will suffice for group B streptococcus. Clindamycin or metronidazole is appropriate for anaerobic infections.

Third-generation cephalosporins such as cefotaxime are valuable additions for treating documented neonatal sepsis and meningitis because (1) the minimal inhibitory combinations need for treatment of gram-negative enteric bacilli are much lower than those for the aminoglycosides; (2) there is excellent penetration into CSF in the presence of inflamed meninges; and (3) much higher doses can be given. The end result is much higher bactericidal titers in serum and CSF than is achievable with ampicillin-aminoglycoside combinations. However, cephalosporins should not be used alone as empiric therapy or indiscriminantly because they have only modest activity against *S. aureus* and *L. monocytogenes*, and enterococci are uniformly resistant. Moreover, rapid emergence of resistant organisms is possible with frequent usage in the NICU.

Therapy should be continued for a total of 10–14 days or for at least 5–7 days after a clinical response has occurred in patients with uncomplicated bacteremia, for example, when there is no evidence of meningitis, deep tissue involvement, or abscess formation. A blood culture taken 24–48 hr after initiation of therapy should be negative. If the culture is positive, a change in therapy may be indicated, and the possibility of an infected indwelling catheter, endocarditis, an infected thrombus, an occult abscess, subtherapeutic antibiotic levels, or resistant organisms should be considered. Therapy should be continued for 14 days if sepsis is complicated by meningitis due to group B streptococcus or for a minimum of 14 days after sterilization of the CSF in gram-negative meningitis.

Supportive therapy is important in the management of neonatal sepsis. Fluids, electrolytes, and glucose should be monitored carefully with correction of hypovolemia, hyponatremia, hypocalcemia, and hypoglycemia and limitation of fluids if there is inappropriate antidiuretic hormone secretion. Shock, hypoxia, and metabolic acidosis should be identified and managed with inotropic agents, fluid resuscitation, and mechanical ventilation. Adequate oxygenation of tissues should be maintained because ventilatory support is frequently necessary for respiratory failure due to congenital pneumonia, persistent fetal circulation, or the adult respiratory distress syndrome (shock lung). Refractory hypoxia and shock may require extracorporeal membrane oxygenation, which has reduced mortality in full-term infants with septic shock and persistent fetal circulation. Hyperbilirubinemia should be monitored and treated with exchange transfusion because the risk of kernicterus increases in the presence of sepsis and meningitis. Parenteral nutrition should be considered for infants who cannot sustain enteral feedings.

Disseminated intravascular coagulation (DIC) may complicate neonatal septicemia. Platelet counts, hemoglobin, prothrombin and partial thromboplastin times, and fibrin split products should be monitored. DIC may be treated by management of the primary sepsis, but if bleeding occurs, DIC may be treated with fresh frozen plasma, platelet transfusions, or whole blood.

Because neutrophil storage pool depletion has been associated with a poor prognosis, a number of clinical trials of polymorphonuclear (PMN) replacement therapy have been conducted, with variable results. Sepsis that is unresponsive to antibiotics with persistent neutropenia may be an indication for granulocyte transfusion. The use of granulocyte-macrophage (GM) colony–stimulating factor (CSF) is under investigation. Treatment with intravenous immunoglobulins (IVIG) containing specific antibodies is currently under clinical investigation. Currently, granulocyte transfusion, G-CSF, and IVIG are experimental therapies of undetermined value.

It is important to remember that nonbacterial infectious agents can produce the syndrome of neonatal sepsis. Herpes simplex infection requires specific treatment (Sec. 9.71), as does systemic candidal infection (Sec. 9.75). Such agents should be considered in all patients who have negative cultures but whose condition continues to deteriorate despite supportive care and the use of broad-spectrum antibiotics.

PREVENTION. Aggressive management of suspected maternal chorioamnionitis with antibiotics prior to delivery and rapid delivery of the newborn infant may decrease the morbidity and mortality of neonatal sepsis. Selective intrapartum chemoprophylaxis has been shown to be effective in preventing early onset group B streptococcal infection (Sec. 9.67). IVIG is undergoing trials for prevention of late onset infections in very-low-birthweight infants, and active immunization against group B streptococcus may benefit some but not all infants.

Amon E, Lewis SV, Sibai BM, et al: Ampicillin prophylaxis in preterm premature rupture of the membranes: A prospective randomized study. Am J Obstet Gynecol 159:539, 1988.
Bennett R, Bergdahl S, Eriksson M, et al: The outcome of neonatal septicemia during fifteen years. Acta Paediatr Scand 78:40, 1989.
Decker MD, Edwards KM: Central venous catheter infections. Pediatr Clin North Am 35:579, 1988.
Dobson SRM, Baker CJ: Enterococcal sepsis in neonates: Features by age at onset and occurrence of focal infection. Pediatrics 85:165, 1990.
Evans ME, Schaffner W, Federspiel CF, et al: Sensitivity, specificity, and predictive value of body surface cultures in a neonatal intensive care unit. JAMA 259:248, 1988.
Friesen CA, Cho CT:Characteristic features of neonatal sepsis due to *Haemophilus influenzae*. Rev Infect Dis 8:777, 1986.
Gilstrap III, LC, Leveno KJ, Cox SM, et al: Intrapartum treatment of acute chorioamnionitis: Impact on neonatal sepsis. Am J Obstet Gynecol 159:579, 1988.
Kite P, Millar MR, Gorham P, et al: Comparison of five tests used in diagnosis of neonatal bacteraemia. Arch Dis Child 63:639, 1988.
Kliegman RM, Clapp DW, Berger M: Targeted immunoglobulin therapy for the prevention of neonatal infections. Rev Infect Dis 12(Suppl 4):S443, 1990.
Mason WH, Andrews R, Ross LA, et al: Omphalitis in the newborn infant. Pediatr Infect Dis J 8:521, 1989.
Morales WJ, Angel JL, O'Brien WF, et al: Use of ampicillin and corticosteroids in premature rupture of membranes: A randomized study. Obstet Gynecol 73:721, 1989.
Ohlsson A, Vearncombe M: Congenital and nosocomial sepsis in infants born in a regional perinatal unit: Cause, outcome, and white blood cell response. Am J Obstet Gynecol 156:407, 1987.
Rozycki HJ, Stahl GE, Baumgart S: Impaired sensitivity of a single early leukocyte count in screening for neonatal sepsis. Pediatr Infect Dis J 6:440, 1987.
Vesikari T, Janas M, Gronroos P, et al: Neonatal septicaemia. Arch Dis Child 60:542, 1985.
Webber S, Wilkinson AR, Lindsell D, et al: Neonatal pneumonia. Arch Dis Child 65:207, 1990.
Wilson CB: Immunologic basis for increased susceptibility of the neonate to infection. J Pediatr 108:1, 1986.

9.61 CONJUNCTIVITIS

See also Sec. 22.9.

Conjunctivitis is frequently encountered in the newborn infant, secondary to inflammation caused by silver nitrate and to infection with *Neisseria gonorrhoeae, Chlamydia trachomatis,* and *Staphylococcus aureus*. Less common causes include infection with group A or B streptococcus, *S. pneumonia, Haemophilus influenzae* (type 6 and nontypable), *Pseudomonas aeruginosa*, or Herpes simplex virus type 2. *N. gonorrhoeae, C. trachomatis*, group B streptococcus, and Herpes simplex are acquired on passage through a colonized or infected birth canal; other bacteria are usually acquired after birth. Prematurity and prolonged rupture of membranes are associated with an increased incidence of conjunctivitis due to the organisms acquired at birth. Conjunctivitis develops in 30–40% of infants born to mothers infected with *N. gonorrhoeae* or *C. trachomatis*. The incidence of gonococcal ophthalmia (4/10,000) is less than that due to chlamydia (4/1,000).

CLINICAL MANIFESTATIONS. The onset of inflammation caused by silver nitrate drops usually occurs within 6–12 hr after birth, with clearing by 24–48 hr. The usual incubation period for conjunctivitis due to *N. gonorrhoeae* is 2–5 days and for that due to *C. trachomatis*, 5–14 days. Gonococcal infection may be present at birth or delayed beyond 5 days of life owing to partial suppression by ocular prophylaxis. Gonococcal conjunctivitis may also begin in infancy following inoculation by the contaminated fingers of adults. The time of onset of disease with other bacteria is highly variable.

Gonococcal conjunctivitis begins with mild inflammation and a serosanguineous discharge. Within 24 hr the discharge becomes thick and purulent, and tense edema of the eyelids with marked chemosis occurs. If proper treatment is delayed, the infection may spread to involve the deeper layers of the conjunctivae and the cornea. Complications include corneal ulceration and perforation, iridocyclitis, anterior synechiae, and rarely panophthalmitis. Conjunctivitis caused by *C. trachomatis* (inclusion blennorrhea) may vary from mild inflammation to severe swelling of the eyelids with copious purulent discharge. The process involves mainly the tarsal conjunctivae; the corneas are rarely affected. Conjunctivitis due to *S. aureus* or other organisms is similar to that produced by *C. trachomatis*. Conjunctivitis due to *P. aeruginosa* is uncommon, is acquired in the nursery, and is a potentially serious process. It is characterized by the appearance on day 5–18 of edema, erythema of the lids, purulent discharge, pannus formation, endophthalmitis, sepsis, shock, and death.

DIAGNOSIS. Conjunctivitis appearing after 48 hr should be evaluated for a possibly infectious cause. Gram stain of the purulent discharge should be performed and the material cultured. If a viral etiology is suspected, a swab should be submitted in tissue culture media for virus isolation. In chlamydial conjunctivitis the diagnosis is made by examining Giemsa-stained epithelial cells scraped from the tarsal conjunctivae for the characteristic intracytoplasmic inclusions, by isolating the organisms from a conjunctival swab using special tissue culture techniques, by immunofluorescent staining of conjunctival scrapings for chlamydial inclusions, or by tests for chlamydial antigen. The differential diagnosis includes dacrocystitis, caused by congenital lacrimal duct obstruction with lacrimal sac distention (dacrocystocele).

TREATMENT. Treatment of the infant in whom gonococcal ophthalmia is suspected and whom Gram stain shows the characteristic intracellular gram-negative diplococci should be initiated immediately with ceftriaxone, 25–50 mg/kg/day for 7 days. Single-dose therapy also has been reported to be effective. In addition, the eye should be irrigated initially with saline every 10–30 min, gradually increasing to 2-hr intervals, until the purulent discharge has cleared. An alternate regimen includes a single dose of kanamycin (75–150 mg intramuscularly) with gentamicin eye ointment applied for 3 days. Inclusion blennorrhea is treated with oral erythromycin for 2 wk. This cures conjunctivitis and may prevent subsequent chlamydial pneumonia. *Pseudomonas* neonatal conjuctivitis is treated with systemic antibiotics, including an aminoglycoside, plus local saline irrigation and gentamicin ophthalmic ointment. Staphylococcal conjunctivitis is treated with parenteral methicillin and local saline irrigation.

PROGNOSIS AND PREVENTION. Prior to the institution of topical ophthalmic prophylaxis at birth, gonococcal ophthalmia was a common cause of blindness or permanent eye damage. If properly applied, this form of prophylaxis is highly effective unless infection is present at birth. Drops of 0.5% erythromycin or 1% silver nitrate are instilled directly into the open eyes at birth using wax or plastic single-dose containers. Saline irrigation after silver nitrate application is unnecessary. Silver nitrate is ineffective against active infection.

Identification of maternal gonococcal infection and appropriate treatment has become a standard element of routine prenatal care. An infant born to a woman who has untreated gonococcal infection should receive a single dose of ceftriaxone, 50 mg/kg (maximum 125 mg) intravenously or intramuscularly, in addition to topical prophylaxis. Dosage should be reduced for premature infants. Penicillin (50,000 units) should be used if the mother's gonococcal isolate is known to be penicillin sensitive.

Neither silver nitrate nor topical antibiotics are effective for prophylaxis for *chlamydial ophthalmia*. Furthermore, topical prophylaxis does not prevent the afebrile pneumonia that occurs in 10–20% of infants exposed to *C. trachomatis*. Although chlamydial conjunctivitis is often a self-limiting disease, chlamydial pneumonia may have serious consequences. Treatment of colonized pregnant women with erythromycin may prevent neonatal disease.

Hammerschlag MR, Cummings C, Roblin PM, et al: Efficacy of neonatal ocular prophylaxis for the prevention of chlamydial and gonococcal conjunctivitis. N Engl J Med 320:769, 1989.

Hammerschlag MR: Neonatal ocular prophylaxis. Pediatr Infect Dis J 7:81, 1988.

Schacter J: Why we need a program for the control of *Chlamydia trachomatis*. N Engl J Med 320:802, 1989.

9.62 HEPATITIS

ETIOLOGY. The agent responsible for neonatal hepatitis frequently cannot be identified (Sec. 12.79 and 13.84). Hepatitis A is transmitted across the placenta relatively rarely but has been associated with transfusions and fecal-oral contamination. Hepatitis B (HBV), on the other hand, is a common infection to which infants may be exposed during the perinatal period and presents a management problem (Sec. 12.79 and 13.83). Hepatitis C (formerly parenteral non-A–non-B hepatitis) has been recently identified; preliminary reports suggest that infants may acquire the virus from the mother and develop hepatitis 3–12 wk after birth. Hepatitis E (formerly enteral non-A–non-B hepatitis) produces severe disease in pregnant women. Other etiologic agents, enterovirus, cytomegalovirus, rubella, and herpes simplex virus (HSV) are gained through various circumstances. Hepatitis B is acquired: (1) the mother may be asymptomatic but a chronic carrier of the hepatitis surface antigen (HBsAg), (2) the mother may have active hepatitis B virus infection during pregnancy, or (3) the mother may have chronic active hepatitis. The rate of transplacental transmission varies directly with but is not consistently dependent on the presence of the e antigen (HBeAg). When maternal hepatitis occurs during the 1st and 2nd trimesters, only a small percentage of infants become infected, whereas 25–76% become infected with the virus when maternal hepatitis occurs during the 3rd trimester or near delivery. Although HBV may cross the placenta, causing infants to be born with antigenemia, most infants who acquire HBV from mothers with acute hepatitis do not have HBsAg in their cord blood but rather develop antigenemia by 6–12 wk of age, suggesting that transmission occurs at delivery or shortly thereafter. In the United States, transmission to infants is greatest following acute maternal HBV infection. In Southeast Asia, infants often acquire the virus from mothers who are asymptomatic carriers. Postpartum transmission of HBV may infrequently occur by other routes, since HBsAg has been found in saliva, breast milk, urine, and stool. Blood transfusion is another source of HBV.

CLINICAL MANIFESTATIONS. Hepatitis may be characterized by anorexia, vomiting, jaundice, and elevated hepatic enzyme levels. Mild to moderate hepatitis may be caused by any of the agents listed earlier. Severe fulminant hepatitis is characterized by very high hepatic enzyme levels, decreased production of coagulation proteins (with bleeding in approximately 25% of cases), shock, or death. Hepatic necrosis is most often associated with HSV or enteroviral infection. Infants infected with HBV usually become HBsAg positive and remain asymptomatic but develop persistent antigenemia with evidence of chronic liver involvement, or become HbsAg positive and remain asymptomatic but develop mild anicteric hepatitis and then recover with clearance of the antigenemia. Rarely, they become HBsAg-positive and develop severe fulminant hepatitis with liver necrosis and death. α_1-Antitrypsin deficiency may be present simultaneously with HBV and produces acute hepatitis. Differences in the time of exposure, the route of inoculation, the presence of HBe antigen or anti-HBe antibody, and the size of the viral inoculum may explain this wide variation in the time of antigenemia in infected neonates.

The most common sequence of events in infants who acquire HBV is to remain asymptomatic and become a chronic carrier, that is, HBsAg positive. These children have persistently elevated transaminase levels but usually show no clinical evidence of liver disease. Biopsy specimens, however, indicate persistent hepatitis and evidence of ongoing liver disease. Cirrhosis and primary adenocarcinoma of the liver may be late sequelae.

The differential diagnosis of neonatal hepatitis includes infections (bacterial sepsis, pyogenic hepatic abscess), and anatomic (biliary atresia, choledochal cyst), familial (cystic fibrosis, paucity of bile ducts, familial hepatitis), metabolic (galactosemia, tyrosinosis, α_1-antitrypsin deficiency), and toxic (drugs, hyperalimentation) disorders.

PREVENTION AND TREATMENT. Women should be tested for HBsAg during routine prenatal care, and the infants of mothers who are positive should be given hepatitis B immunoglobulin (HBIG), 0.5 ml, as soon after birth as possible, preferably within 12 hr. The first of three 0.5-mL doses (10 mg of plasma or 5 mg of genetic vaccine) of HBV vaccine should be given at the same time as HBIG in a separate syringe at a different site or within 7 days. Vaccine should be repeated at 1 and 6 mo of age; the intramuscular dose should not be given in the gluteus muscle area. To determine vaccine efficacy the infant should be tested for the presence of HBsAg (active infection) and anti-HBs (active immunization) at 12–15 mo of age. HBV vaccine should also be given to all newborn infants.

Pickering LK: Management of the infant of a mother with viral hepatitis. Pediatr Rev 9:315, 1988.

Centers for Disease Control: Prevention of perinatal transmission of hepatitis B virus: Prenatal screening of all pregnant women for hepatitis B surface antigen. MMWR 37:341, 1988.

Ip HM, Wong VC, LeLie PN, et al: Prevention of hepatitis B virus carrier state in infants according to maternal serum levels of HBV DNA. Lancet 2:406, 1989.

9.63 MENINGITIS

See also Sec 12.15.

Meningitis in the neonate is often associated with sepsis and is a cause of significant morbidity and mortality. The incidence is highest among preterm infants; overall the rate is 0.5/1,000 live births. Bacterial meningitis results from hematogenous dissemination and less often from contamination of neural tube defects, congenital sinus tracts, or following penetrating wounds from fetal scalp sampling or internal fetal electrocardiographic monitors.

ETIOLOGY. Agents that produce sepsis also commonly cause neonatal meningitis (see Sec. 9.60 and Table 9–31). *Enterobacter sakazakii*, a gram-negative bacillus, is a rare cause of severe neonatal meningitis. *Pseudomonas aeruginosa* and staphylococci may produce hematogenous meningitis but may also produce meningitis following contamination of neural tube defects. Additional pathogens include *Mycoplasma hominis, Ureaplasma urealyticum, Candida albicans* and other opportunistic fungi, *Treponema pallidum, Mycobacterium tuberculosis, Toxoplasma gondii*, and viruses (enteroviruses, Herpes simplex type 2 more often than type 1, rubella, cytomegalovirus [CMV], human immunodeficiency virus [HIV]). Bacterial meningitis may occur as part of an early onset systemic infection or as a focal late onset disease. Nonpyogenic agents produce a subacute form of meningitis. Neonatal meningitis is also characterized by a high frequency of ventriculitis, which may complicate therapy and adversely affect the outcome. Brain abscesses may precede or complicate meningitis; they are of hematogenous origin and are usually due to *Citrobacter diversus, E. sakazakii*, and *Proteus* species.

CLINICAL MANIFESTATIONS. The initial signs and symptoms may be indistinguishable from those of neonatal sepsis and those noninfectious diseases frequently confused with neonatal sepsis (see Sec. 9.60). Nonspecific manifestations include temperature instability (hypothermia in preterm, fever in term infants), apnea and bradycardia, poor feeding, emesis, high-pitched cry, cyanosis, respiratory distress, tachycardia, tachypnea, and shock. Neurologic manifestations include lethargy (50–90%), bulging or full fontanel (20–30%), focal, generalized, or subtle seizures (30–50%), nuchal rigidity (10–20%), and, rarely at initial presentation, signs of increased intracranial pressure.

DIAGNOSIS. The diagnosis is confirmed by examination of the cerebrospinal fluid (CSF) and identification of a bacteria, virus, or fungus by culture or antigen detection. Blood culture and complete blood count are part of the initial evaluation because 70–85% of neonates with meningitis will have a positive blood culture. The incidence of positive blood cultures is highest with early onset sepsis and meningitis (see Table 9–31).

Lumbar puncture is contraindicated in the presence of raised intracranial pressure (other than a bulging fontanel) or infection in the lumbar space and in a severely ill infant if the lumbar puncture would further compromise respiratory status. In these situations, blood culture and antigen detection assays should be performed and treatment initiated for presumed meningitis until a lumbar puncture can be safely performed.

Normal, uninfected neonates frequently have elevated CSF protein levels (term 90 mg/dL [range 20–170], preterm 115 mg/dL [range 65–150]), reduced glucose (term 52 mg/dL [range 34–119], preterm 50 mg/dL [range 24–63]), reduced CSF-to-blood glucose ratios (51% term, 75% preterm), and elevated CSF leukocyte counts (term 7/μL [range 0–32], preterm 8/μL [range 0–29]) with 57–61% neutrophils. In addition, preterm infants may develop elevated CSF protein levels and leukocytes and hypoglycorrhachia following intraventricular hemorrhage. Many nonpyogenic congenital infections also can produce asymptomatic alterations of CSF protein and leukocytes (toxoplasmosis, CMV, syphilis, HIV).

The Gram stain of CSF is positive in as many as 85% of patients with group B streptococcal meningitis and 78% of those with gram-negative meningitis. The leukocyte count is often elevated with a predominance of neutrophils (> 70–90%); the number is often greater than 1,000 in patients with gram-negative meningitis but may be less than 100 in those with group B streptococcal disease. Microorganisms are recovered from most patients who have not been pretreated with antibiotics. Bacteria have also been isolated from CSF that did not have an abnormal number of cells (< 25) or an abnormal protein level (< 200 mg/dL). This is more typical of group B streptococcal meningitis but emphasizes the importance of performing a culture and Gram stain on all CSF specimens. Culture-negative meningitis should suggest antibiotic pretreatment, infection with *M. hominis, U. urealyticum*, or *Bacteroidis fragilis*, a brain abscess, enterovirus infection, or Herpes simplex.

Head ultrasonography or CT scan with contrast enhancement may be helpful in diagnosing ventriculitis and brain abscess. Neonatal herpes simplex meningitis may be confirmed by isolation of the virus from the CSF or other site (skin, eye, mouth) or by herpes simplex virus antigen or DNA detection.

TREATMENT. Presumptive antimicrobial therapy of bacterial meningitis should include ampicillin and gentamicin or a cephalosporin, such as cefotaxime or ceftazidime. Most aminoglycosides administered by parenteral routes do not achieve sufficiently high antibiotic levels in the lumbar CSF or ventricles to inhibit growth of gram-negative bacilli. Although intraventricular administration of aminoglycosides has been proposed as therapy for gram-negative meningitis-ventriculitis, many authorities recommend a combination of ampicillin and a third-generation cephalosporin for the treatment of neonatal gram-negative meningitis. Cephalosporins should not be used as empiric monotherapy because *Listeria monocytogenes* is resistant to all cephalosporins. Ampicillin or penicillin is the treatment of choice for group B streptococcal meningitis, whereas ampicillin with an aminoglycoside is the treatment of choice for *L. monocytogenes*; parenteral trimethoprim-sulfamethoxazole is an alternate treatment for *L. monocytogenes* (see Table 9–30 for dosages).

Meningitis due to group B streptococci usually responds within 24–48 hr and should be treated for 14–21 days. Gram-negative bacilli may continue to grow from repeated CSF samples for 72–96 hr following therapy despite the use of appropriate antibiotics. Therapy of gram-negative meningitis should be continued for 21 days or for at least 14 days after sterilization of the CSF, whichever is longer. Persistence of positive cultures with gram-negative organisms for more than 72 hr of therapy is a poor prognostic sign and may require a change in therapy such as addition of a cephalosporin or, rarely, intraventricular instillation of gentamicin. Instillation of aminoglycosides into the lumbar intrathecal space is of no benefit; intraventricular antibiotic therapy may be associated with the development of porencephalic cysts. Current use of cefotaxime should reduce the occurrence of delayed sterilization of CSF due to gram-negative bacilli. Cure rates as high as 98–99% have been reported with cefotaxime. CSF penetration correlates best with meningeal inflammation, and cefotaxime often achieves CSF antibiotic levels that exceed the MIC for responsible organisms (except *P. aeruginosa*) by 100- to 1,000-fold. The active metabolite, deacetylcefotaxime, possesses 10–12% of the activity of cefotaxime and may be synergistic with the parent compound. Meningitis due to *P. aeruginosa* should be treated with ceftazidime. Metronidazole is the treatment of choice for infection due to *Bacteroides fragilis*. Prolonged antibiotic administration, with or without needle drainage for treatment and diagnosis, is indicated for neonatal cerebral abscesses. CT scans are indicated for patients with suspected ventriculitis, hydrocephalus, or cerebral abscess (initial and follow-up assessments) and for those with an unexpectedly complicated course (prolonged coma, seizures, focal neurologic deficits, persistent or recurrent fever).

Supportive care includes the treatment of the sepsis syndrome; anticonvulsants for seizures; management of cerebral edema, inappropriate antidiuretic hormone secretion, and hydrocephalus; and careful monitoring of bacterial sensitivities and antimicrobial drug levels.

Bell WE, McGuinness GA: Suppurative central nervous system infections in the neonate. Semin Perinatol 6:1, 1982.
Feldstein TJ, Uden DL, Larson TA: Cefotaxime for treatment of gram-negative bacterial meningitis in infants and children. Pediatr Infect Dis J 6:471, 1987.
Gandy G, Rennie J: Antibiotic treatment of suspected neonatal meningitis. Arch Dis Child 65:1, 1990.
Klein JO, Feigin RD, McCracken GH: Report of the task force on diagnosis and management of meningitis. Pediatrics 78:958, 1986.
Kline MW, Mason EO, Kaplan SL: Characterization of *Citrobacter diversus* strains causing neonatal meningitis. J Infect Dis 157:101, 1988.
Renier D, Flandin C, Hirsch E, et al: Brain abscesses in neonates. J Neurosurg 69:877, 1988.
Sarff LD, Platt LH, McCracken GH: Cerebrospinal fluid evaluation in neonates: Comparison of high risk infants with and without meningitis. J Pediatr 88:473, 1976.
Waites KB, Crouse DT, Nelson KG, et al: Chronic *Ureaplasma urealyticum* and *Mycoplasma hominis* infections of central nervous system in preterm infants. Lancet 1:17, 1988.
Willis J, Robinson JE: *Enterobacter sakazakii* meningitis in neonates. Pediatr Infect Dis J 7:196, 1988.
Wood BM, Klein JO: Therapy of bacterial sepsis and meningitis in infants and children. Pediatr Infect Dis J 8:635, 1989.

OSTEOMYELITIS AND SEPTIC ARTHRITIS

See Sec. 12.16–12.17.

9.64 OTITIS MEDIA

See also Sec. 22.22.

Acute otitis media in the newborn period presents a special diagnostic problem because the signs and symptoms of disease are subtle and nonspecific and the tympanic membrane is difficult to examine. Otitis media may be an isolated finding, but more often it is associated with bacterial infection in the sinuses and lungs. The short horizontal and wide eustachian tube in the fetus encourages the entrance of infected amniotic fluid into the middle ear; eustachian tube dysfunction or nasotracheal intubation may cause drainage of contaminated material, with subsequent development of otitis media.

In examining the eardrum it is important to determine its mobility because the tympanic membrane may appear dull and thickened in the normal infant. The diagnostic criteria for otitis media are the same as those in older infants and include inflammation, fluid in the middle ear, and signs of infection. Nonspecific signs and symptoms are similar to those that occur with other infections and include irritability or lethargy, decreased appetite or failure to thrive, mild respiratory symptoms, and low-grade fever. Infants also may be asymptomatic.

Otitis media occurs more frequently in preterm than in term infants. In contrast to older children, the etiologic agents isolated during the first 6 wk of life from about one third of infants with otitis media include *E. coli*, *K. pneumoniae*, *P. aeruginosa*, group B streptococci, and *S. aureus*, *S. pneumoniae*, and *H. influenzae*, the most common pathogens in older children, are found in approximately one third of the cases. In the remainder, nonpathogens are isolated or no organism is found. Neonatal pathogens (group B streptococci, gram-negative organisms, *S. aureus*) are most common in infants who have disease in the first 14 days of life or who are in continuous intensive care. Normal term infants > 2 wk old develop otitis media from the usual organisms (*Pneumococcus*, *H. influenzae*, *Branhamella catarrhalis*).

The initial therapy of a neonate in whom otitis media has been definitively diagnosed but in whom sepsis is also considered should be for neonatal sepsis. In an older infant ampicillin or amoxicillin may be started, but the infant should be re-evaluated carefully in 2–3 days to determine whether the middle ear disease has responded. The therapeutic regimen should be based optimally on tympanocentesis in order to identify the specific etiologic agent, and there should be careful follow-up to prevent the development of chronic middle-ear disease.

Karma PH, Pukander JS, Sipila MM, et al: Middle ear fluid bacteriology of acute otitis media in neonates and very young infants. Int J Pediatr Otorhinolaryngol 14:141, 1987.
Klein JO: Bacterial infections of the respiratory tract. *In*: Remington JS, Klein JO (eds): Infectious Diseases of the Fetus and Newborn Infant. Philadelphia, WB Saunders, 1990, p 660.
Shurin PA, Howie VM, Pelton SL, et al: Bacterial etiology of otitis media during first six weeks of life. J Pediatr 92:893, 1978.

9.65 PNEUMONIA

Pneumonia (Sec. 14.56–14.57), an important cause of morbidity and mortality in the newborn infant, is the most common inflammatory lesion found at autopsy in the neonatal period.

Although pathologic evidence of pulmonary inflammatory disease is evident in 15–20% of stillborn infants and in 20–30% of neonatal deaths, not all of the inflammatory disease is due to infection, and its role as a cause of death is often unclear.

ETIOLOGY AND EPIDEMIOLOGY. Pneumonia due to infection may be acquired transplacentally as one component of a generalized intrauterine infection caused by cytomegalovirus, rubella virus, *Toxoplasma gondii, Listeria,* or *Treponema pallidum* (Sec. 9.60, 9.73, 12.112, 12.36, and 12.50); natally by aspiration of infected amniotic fluid or birth canal secretions, with onset of illness occurring during the first few days of life (Sec. 9.58) and most commonly associated with group B streptococcus (Sec. 9.67), gram-negative enteric bacilli (Sec. 9.60), *Chlamydia* (Sec. 9.61), and herpes simplex virus (Sec. 9.71); and postnatally as a nosocomial or community-acquired infection caused by *Staphylococcus aureus* (Sec. 9.60, 12.19), *Pseudomonas aeruginosa* (Sec. 12.32), *Klebsiella, Serratia* sp. (Sec. 14.56), *B. pertussis* (Sec. 12.26), and respiratory viruses (Sec. 12.74–12.76).

Pneumonia acquired transplacentally or perinatally is often termed congenital pneumonia, is associated with bacteremia, and is frequently associated with prolonged rupture of the membranes, chorioamnionitis, prolonged labor, premature labor, or fetal distress. Pneumonia in premature infants may be superimposed on hyaline membrane disease, that in term infants may be associated with persistent fetal circulation. Pneumonia in early infancy is usually bronchopneumonia in type, occasionally interstitial or lobar. Pneumonia presenting on the 1st day of life may be indistinguishable from hyaline membrane disease.

CLINICAL MANIFESTATIONS. Infants with natal or postnatal pneumonia may initially exhibit nonspecific signs of illness such as poor feeding, lethargy, irritability, poor color, a rise or sudden fall in body temperature, abdominal distention, sudden loss or gain in weight, and the general impression that they are doing less well than before. Signs of respiratory distress, including cyanosis, tachypnea, flaring of the alae nasi, grunting, tachycardia, apnea, accentuation of periodic breathing, and retraction of the suprasternal, intercostal, and subcostal spaces, may progress rapidly or slowly.

Dullness to percussion is difficult to elicit but, when present, suggests extensive consolidation or effusion. Auscultation may reveal fine, crackling rales in any portion of the lung or decreased breath sounds, but often these may not be present, even with extensive pneumonia. It is important to auscultate the chest when the baby is crying as well as quiet, because rales frequently are heard only at the end of the deep inspirations that come with crying in the newborn. Areas of hyperresonance may indicate compensatory emphysema. Roentgenograms of the chest are often helpful and are essential to distinguish pneumonia from other causes of respiratory distress.

An acute, often fulminant, form of group B streptococcal pneumonia associated with septicemia in term or preterm infants may present during the 1st day of life or later with respiratory distress, sometimes with shock, or with the sudden deterioration of an infant receiving assisted ventilation. The roentgenogram may be typical for bronchopneumonia or may show a diffuse atelectasis resembling hyaline membrane disease.

Infants at 1–2 mo of age may present with a slowly progressive respiratory infection characterized by a persistent "staccato" cough, respiratory distress, hypoxia, rales, and apneic spells without fever. Radiologic examination of this afebrile pneumonia syndrome shows focal or diffuse interstitial pneumonitis. Peripheral blood leukocyte counts are generally not helpful; eosinophilia may be present. The etiology may be *Chlamydia trachomatis* or, less commonly, *Pneumocystis carinii*, cytomegalovirus, respiratory syncytial virus (RSV), or genital mycoplasma.

Chronically ill low-birthweight infants on ventilators often develop new infiltrates on the chest roentgenogram that are associated with deterioration in the respiratory status and sometimes are accompanied by temperature instability and elevation of the white blood cell count. Determining whether this condition is infectious pneumonia or segmental atelectasis is difficult. The infants are usually treated with antibiotics for a presumed bacterial infection, but nosocomial respiratory viral infection (adenovirus, influenza, RSV) should also be considered. If RSV infection is diagnosed ribavirin may be beneficial (Sec. 12.76).

Infants with neurologic dysfunction, congenital anomalies (tracheoesophageal fistula), or gastroesophageal reflux and those receiving mechanical ventilation may develop aspiration pneumonia. Enteric gram-negative bacteria and anaerobes may be aspirated, producing pneumonia, abscesses, empyema, or pneumatoceles.

DIAGNOSIS. Blood cultures should be obtained and tracheal secretions aspirated and examined by Gram stain and culture. Urine samples should be obtained for group B streptococcal antigen determination. In atypical cases, bronchoscopy with bronchoalveolar lavage or needle or open lung biopsy may be indicated. The differential diagnosis of congenital bacterial pneumonia includes hyaline membrane disease, meconium aspiration syndrome pneumonia, hypoplastic lungs, congenital anomalies (diaphragmatic hernia, cyanotic congenital heart disease), transient tachypnea, persistent fetal circulation, herpes simplex infection, chylothorax, and pulmonary air leaks (pneumothorax, pneumomediastinum, interstitial emphysema). Pleural fluid may be aspirated and analyzed for protein, glucose, lactic dehydrogenase (LDH), cell count, and special staining.

In the afebrile interstitial pneumonitis syndrome of young infants, tracheal aspirates or nasopharyngel swabs should be obtained for chlamydial culture or antigen identification by ELISA. Serologic tests for *Chlamydia* are helpful in diagnosing afebrile pneumonitis because infants typically have very high titers during active clinical disease.

TREATMENT. The etiologic agents of bacterial pneumonia are the same as those for neonatal sepsis, and similar antibiotic regimens are used for each depending on the pattern of presentation, the nature of the nursery's bacterial flora, and the suspected pathogen (Sec. 9.60). Because it is often difficult to distinguish *E. coli* or group B streptococcal pneumonia and sepsis from hyaline membrane disease, severely ill patients should receive broad-spectrum parenteral antibiotics for at least 72 hr pending reports of blood, CSF, and tracheal cultures.

Severe, progressive, congenital pneumonia often becomes manifest as shock and profound hypoxia that is unresponsive to conventional ventilation and antibiotics. Such patients resemble those having adult respiratory distress syndrome or persistent fetal circulation. Extracorporeal membrane oxygenation may reverse the refractory hypoxia and improve cardiac output and oxygen delivery and has increased survival rates in the severest form of pneumonia to more than 70%.

Chlamydial pneumonia is treated with oral erythromycin or trimethoprim-sulfamethoxazole.

Boyer KM, Cherry JD: Nonbacterial pneumonia. *In*: Feigin RD, Cherry JD (eds): Textbook of Pediatric Infectious Diseases. Philadelphia, WB Saunders, 1987, p 228.

Brasfield DM, Stagno S, Whitley RJ, et al: Infant pneumonitis associated with cytomegalovirus, *Chlamydia*, *Pneumocystis*, and *Ureaplasma*: Follow-up. Pediatrics 79:76, 1987.

Hubbell C, Dominguez R, Kohl S: Neonatal herpes simplex pneumonitis. Rev Infect Dis 10:2, 1988.

Klein JO: Bacterial infections of the respiratory tract. *In*: Remington JS, Klein

JO (eds): Infectious Diseases of the Fetus and Newborn Infant. Philadelphia, WB Saunders, 1990, p 664.

Overall JC Jr: Viral infections of the fetus and neonate. *In*: Feigin RD, Cherry JD (eds): Textbook of Pediatric Infectious Diseases. Philadelphia, WB Saunders, 1987, p 966.

Webber S, Wilkinson AR, Lindsell D, et al: Neonatal pneumonia. Arch Dis Child 65:207, 1990.

Wilson CW, Stevenson DK, Arvin AW: A concurrent epidemic of respiratory syncytial virus and echovirus 7 infections in an intensive care nursery. Pediatr Infect Dis J 8:24, 1989.

9.66 URINARY TRACT INFECTION

See also Sec. 18.39.

Urinary tract infection occurs in 0.1% of newborn infants. The incidence is much higher in low-birthweight infants and is about 3 times more common in males than in females. Uncircumcised males, infants having congenital anomalies of the kidney, and those with vesicoureteral reflex have a higher incidence of urinary tract infections. More than 75% of the infections are due to *E. coli*; the remainder are caused by other gram-negative enteric bacilli (*Klebsiella, Enterobacter, Pseudomonas*, and *Proteus* sp.) and gram-positive cocci (enterococci, group B streptococci, and staphylococcal species). Pyelonephritic strains of *E. coli* attach to uroepithelial cells when bacterial pili bind to specific cell receptors. Neonatal infection may be acquired by the ascending route, initially involving the bladder (cystitis), then the ureteropelvic systems and kidney (pyelonephritis), and then the bloodstream (urosepsis). It may also result from septicemia with secondary hematogenous spread to the urinary tract. The latter is unusual in early onset sepsis and most common in late onset or nosocomial disease (see Table 9–31).

CLINICAL MANIFESTATIONS. The signs are varied and nonspecific. There may be an insidious onset consisting of low-grade fever, vomiting, diarrhea, irritability, jaundice, or failure to gain weight. Some infants may be completely asymptomatic, whereas others may be feverish with or without localized signs such as balanitis, urethritis, a weak urinary stream, dysuria (cry with voiding), or a large flank mass. Premature infants and term infants in the first 1–2 wk of life may present with the sepsis syndrome (Sec. 9.60).

DIAGNOSIS. The diagnosis is confirmed by a positive urine culture. A urine culture should be included in the evaluation for sepsis of febrile or septic-appearing infants of 72 hr of age or older. A negative culture of a bagged specimen is helpful in excluding urinary tract infection. Positive bagged urine specimens have a false-positive rate of more than 30% and may yield several organisms. Since collecting a satisfactory clean-catch urine specimen is often difficult and the specimen may produce uncertain results if it is contaminated, possibly delaying therapy, an uncontaminated urine specimen obtained by catheterization or suprapubic aspiration is advised. Suprapubic aspiration is best performed in a well-hydrated infant who has not recently voided, using a 22-gauge needle on a 10-mL syringe. After Betadine cleansing of the suprapubic area, the needle is introduced above the pubic bone while constant negative pressure is applied on the syringe and the urethra is simultaneously occluded. Rare complications include transient hematuria, hematoma of the bladder, bowel perforation, and peritonitis. Contraindications include suspected bleeding disorders (thrombocytopenia, DIC, heparinization) and local undefined genital anomalies. Colony counts of greater than 10^3/mL on a catheterized specimen are strongly suggestive of infection and should be repeated. Infection is likely with greater than 10^4/mL. Any number of gram-negative bacteria in a suprapubic aspirate of urine indicate infection. A small number of gram-positive cocci may represent skin contaminants.

The urinalysis reveals more than 10 leukocytes/high power field in 50–75% and gram-negative rods in the urinary sediment of 75% of infants who have urinary tract infections. However, infection may be present without pyuria. Blood cultures are positive in 30–35% of infected infants, and meningitis is present in a small number.

TREATMENT AND PROGNOSIS. Urinary tract infection in newborns should be treated with parenteral therapy, which usually includes ampicillin and gentamicin or a cephalosporin as outlined in Sec. 9.60. The urine culture should be negative in 36–48 hr in a successfully treated patient. If cultures remain positive, an obstructive lesion, ureterocele, or abscess should be suspected. Therapy is continued for 10–14 days in the uncomplicated case. Recurrent infection may occur in 20–25% of patients, usually within the first few months after the initial episode and should be treated with a full course of antibiotics. Follow-up urine cultures should be obtained.

Every infant who is having his or her first documented urinary tract infection should undergo a renal ultrasound examination. This is a safe, noninvasive test that can be performed at the bedside, yielding information about the size and location of malformations, hydronephrosis, abscesses, or tumors. Vesicoureteral reflux can occur during the acute disease and may clear with resolution of the infection. A voiding cystourethrogram (VCUG) should be performed 2–4 wk after resolution to determine the pressure of vesicourethral reflux. Some recommend a VCUG during the acute phase, since severe reflux is rarely due to the acute infection. VCUG is indicated despite a normal renal ultrasound examination because ultrasound will not identify reflux (Sec. 18.40). Abnormalities apparent on ultrasound should prompt further evaluation of the anatomy of the urinary tract by a voiding cystourethrogram and of excretory function by means of a radionuclide scan. Infants with obstructive lesions should be referred for urologic evaluation for potential corrective surgery.

Alari U, Prey M, Davidai G, et al: Ultrasonography in the evaluation of children with urinary tract infection. Pediatrics 78:58, 1986.

Ginsburg CM, McCracken GH: Urinary tract infection in young infants. Pediatrics 69:409, 1982.

Meharzi M, Guignard J-P, Torrado A: Urinary tract infection in high risk newborn infants. Pediatrics 62:521, 1978.

Ring E, Zobel G: Urinary infection and malformations of urinary tract in infancy. Arch Dis Child 63:818, 1988.

Schoen E: The status of circumcision of newborns. N Engl J Med 322:1308, 1990.

SPECIFIC BACTERIAL INFECTIONS

CHLAMYDIA

See Sec. 12.58–12.60.

ENTERIC ORGANISMS

See Sec. 9.60 and 12.27–12.30.

9.67 GROUP B STREPTOCOCCUS (GBS)

Lancefield group B streptococcus is a major cause of severe systemic and focal infections in the newborn. Group B streptococcus has continued to be an important pathogen of neonatal sepsis and meningitis since its emergence as a dominant pathogen in the 1970s.

ETIOLOGY. *Streptococcus agalactiae*, clinically known as Lancefield group B streptococcus, is a facultative, encapsulated gram-positive diplococcus that produces a characteristic narrow zone of β-hemolysis on blood agar and a double zone of hemolysis if refrigerated an additional 18 hr. Strains of GBS are based on serotypic capsular polysaccharides or antigens and include types Ia, Ib, Ia/c, II, III, and IV. Early onset disease may be due to any serotype, whereas late onset disease is due to type III in 90% of cases (see Table 9–31). Nontypable strains are usually not associated with neonatal disease. GBS produce extracellular substances, which include hemolysin, cAMP factor, hippuricase, nucleases, protease, neuraminidase, and lipoteichoic acid. The latter two factors may be associated with increased virulence of pathogenic GBS.

EPIDEMIOLOGY. The organism is a common inhabitant of the maternal genitourinary and gastrointestinal tracts and colonizes 4–40% of pregnant women. The highest recovery rates for GBS are reported from studies that employed selective media, multiple sample sites, and sequential samples over time (see later discussion). Pregnant women are usually asymptomatic but may manifest chorioamnionitis or endometritis. Infants born of women who are heavily colonized are more likely to become colonized. Overall colonization (also called asymptomatic infection) at birth is noted in 40–70% of infants born to colonized mothers. Approximately 8% of infants born to culture-negative mothers will become colonized with GBS from other sources. Colonization rates are influenced by maternal factors including lower socioeconomic status, teenage status, and sexual activity, choice of media (selective more than nonselective, broth more than agar), and the number and location of body sites sampled in the mother (cervix, vaginal, urine, rectum), newborn infant (external auditory canal > nares, umbilicus, anorectum), or 48-hr-old neonate (throat, anorectum, umbilicus). Maternal colonization may be chronic (36%), transient (20%), intermittent (15%), or indeterminant (29%). Women colonized in the 2nd trimester may be negative at term, and women negative in the 2nd trimester may become colonized at term.

GBS is acquired by newborn infants following vertical transmission, for example, ascending infection through ruptured amniotic membranes or contamination following passage through the colonized birth canal. Infection also occurs in the absence of ruptured membranes. The rate of neonatal colonization is also influenced by prematurity, prolonged rupture of the amniotic membranes, prolonged labor, and maternal endometritis-chorioamnionitis (fever, tender uterus, leukocytosis). Neonates also may acquire GBS following horizontal transmission in the nursery or from adults other than their mothers. Infant-to-infant and adult-to-infant spread has produced colonization, late onset GBS disease, and, rarely, epidemics of GBS in nurseries.

Early onset GBS disease (mean onset, 20 hr of age) is predominatly due to serotypes present in the colonized mother, is associated with complications of pregnancy (prolonged rupture of membranes, prematurity), has an incidence of 0.7–3.7/1,000 live births, and results in bacteremia in 0.5–2% of newborn infants born to colonized mothers. Many infants with early onset GBS are infected and symptomatic at birth (50%), indicating an intrauterine infection. The highest attack rate of early onset GBS disease occurs among very low birthweight infants; the incidence is 2–2.6/1,000 in infants weighing less than 1,500 g and 0.8–1.8/1,000 in infants weighing more than 2,500 g. Nonetheless, full-term infants account for approximately 50% of cases. *Late onset* GBS disease (mean onset, 24 days of life) is due to serotypes acquired from maternal and nonmaternal sites (nursery personnel and community), is not associated with obstetric risk factors, has an incidence of 0.5–1.8/1,000 live births, and may be seen as late as the 3rd month of life.

GBS also produces maternal disease such as urinary tract infection (asymptomatic more often than symptomatic), endometritis, chorioamnionitis, bacteremia, and rarely meningitis.

PATHOGENESIS. See Sec. 9.60 and 12.14. *Early onset GBS* is associated with immature host defense mechanisms among low-birthweight infants and prolonged exposure to heavily colonized maternal genitourinary tract sites (ascending vertical transmission through ruptured amniotic membranes). GBS may cause local inflammation of intact membranes, causing subsequent weakness and rupture of amniotic fluid membranes, thus initiating premature labor. The attack rate is 0.7/1,000 with membrane rupture occurring at less than 19 hr and 18.3/1,000 with rupture occurring at 30 hr or more. Fetal infection may also develop through intact membranes. Amniotic fluid contains low levels of type-specific GBS antibodies, complement, phagocytic cells, and other nonspecific defense components and is a good culture medium for GBS. Fetal aspiration of infected amniotic fluid may initiate fetal and subsequent neonatal pneumonia, bacteremia, and septic shock.

Opsonophagocytic defects present in immature neonates are further compromised in the infant with GBS infection owing to a deficiency of maternally derived type-specific antibody. Serum levels of greater than 2 μg/mL of IgG antibody to type-specific capsular polysaccharides of GBS are associated with effective opsonophagocytosis and killing of GBS. Alveolar macrophage activity and migration of neutrophils to the lung may also be attenuated in neonates compared with adults.

Early onset GBS disease is characterized by bacteremia, pneumonia, and pulmonary hypertension. The latter may be attenuated by inhibition of thromboxane synthesis, suggesting a role for the activity of the pulmonary cyclo-oxygenase pathway in the pathogenesis of GBS-associated pulmonary hypertension. The later phase of sepsis is characterized by neutropenia, neutrophil trapping in the lung, increased vascular permeability, myocardial dysfunction, elevated central venous pressure, hypotension, and disseminated intravascular coagulation.

The pathophysiology of *late onset GBS* may be related to an initial colonization, alterations of the mucosal barrier by a prior viral respiratory tract infection, elaboration of large amounts of GBS type III capsular polysaccharide, and possibly reduced amounts of maternal antibody. The pathophysiology of late onset GBS osteomyelitis is atypical and may be due to an early onset asymptomatic bacteremia, inoculation into a traumatized bone (humerus), and subsequent late onset of a single site of osteomyelitis. These infants may have few systemic symptoms. The presence of type-specific IgG antibody to GBS type III suggests that the infant produced antibodies and restricted the infection to a metaphyseal location.

CLINICAL MANIFESTATIONS. See Sec. 9.60. The spectrum of *early onset infections* ranges from asymptomatic bacteremia to pneumonia that is indistinguishable from hyaline membrane disease, to an overwhelming infection characterized by severe perinatal asphyxia (consolidated pneumonia, coma, shock), septic shock, or persistent fetal circulation. Respiratory symptoms are prominant and include cyanosis, apnea, tachypnea, grunting, flaring, retractions, and roentgenographic findings consisting of a reticulogranular pattern (50%), patchy pneumonic infiltrates (30%), and, less commonly, pleural effusions, pulmonary edema, cardiomegaly, and increased pulmonary vascular markings.

The onset of illness may begin at birth, especially among premature infants, who may become ill within 6 hr of age, whereas term infants may occasionally have a delayed onset of more than 24 hr. Sepsis without localization is noted in 30–40%, meningitis in 30% (usually type III), and pneumonia in 30–40%. Bacteremia is present in all three presentations. Patients with meningeal involvement may have seizures, lethargy, coma, poor feeding, and a bulging fontanel. These patients cannot be identified by clinical findings; therefore, a lumbar puncture is indicated in every patient with suspected early or late onset neonatal sepsis (see Sec. 9.63). Unusual focal features of early onset GBS infection are noted in Table 9–32.

Late onset GBS infection is manifest as meningitis in 60% of patients and is predominantly due to the type III strain. Additional manifestations of late onset GBS (also type III) are noted in Table 9–32. The manifestations of late onset GBS meningitis are indistinguishable from other causes of neonatal meningitis (Sec. 9.63) and include fever, irritability, lethargy, seizures, full fontanel, and shock.

DIAGNOSIS. The *differential diagnosis* of early onset GBS infection includes hyaline membrane disease, amniotic fluid aspiration syndrome, persistent fetal circulation (PFC), sepsis from other vertically transmitted ascending infections (*E. coli*, herpes simplex), and those metabolic (hypoglycemia, hyperammonemia), anatomic (congenital heart disease, diaphragmatic hernia), or other conditions that produce cyanosis and sepsis syndrome-like manifestations (Sec. 12.80). GBS may be differentiated from some but not all cases of hyaline membrane disease by the presence of lower than expected Apgar scores, shock and apnea in the 1st day of life, prolonged rupture of membranes, cardiomegaly, pleural effusions, and a rapidly progressive deterioration in condition. PFC may be associated with GBS in term infants if hypoxia, hypotension, neutropenia, and apnea are present.

The diagnosis is established by isolation of the organism from normally sterile sites (blood, CSF, rarely urine, pleural fluid, abscess material, cellulitis aspirates, bone and joint aspirates). Isolation from skin or mucous membranes indicates colonization and not invasive infection.

Antigen detection of GBS is possible with countercurrent immunoelectrophoresis (CIE), latex particle agglutination, and staphylococcal coagglutination. Each can detect GBS antigens despite prior antibiotic therapy and can yield results in minutes (latex) or hours (CIE), and each has varying degrees of specificity and sensitivity. The latex test can detect GBS in as many as 89% of CSF samples, 60% of serum samples, and 83% of unconcentrated and 97% of concentrated urine samples. Urine samples may need to be pretreated to remove cross-reacting ABO antigens. Urine samples collected by bag may yield false-positive results in healthy but colonized neonates owing to contamination by GBS organisms, which colonize the perineum or rectum. Thus, a positive urine latex test result is highly suggestive but not diagnostic of systemic infection.

The CSF should be examined in all patients. Other findings may include an elevated serum CRP, increased band count, increased ratio of immature to total white blood cells (> 0.20),

TABLE 9–32. Unusual Focal Diseases Due to Group B Streptococcus*

Site	Predominant Time of Onset	Comment
Abdomen		
Adrenal abscess	Late > early	Prior adrenal hematoma
Gallbladder hydrops	Early > late	Nonspecific
Conjugated hyperbilirubinemia	Late > early	Nonspecific
Brain		
Abscess	Late	Associated meningitis
Subdural empyema	Late > early	Associated meningitis
Cerebritis	Late	Associated meningitis
Cardiovascular		
Endocarditis	Late > early	Recurrent bacteremia
Pericarditis	Unknown	Associated pneumonia
Myocarditis	Late	Cardiogenic shock
Ocular		
Conjunctivitis	Early > late	Rare
Ophthalmitis	Late	Local perforation or bacteremic onset
Osteoarticular		
Arthritis	Late > early	Early bacteremia with late onset
Osteomyelitis	Late	Early bacteremia with late onset
Dactylitis	Late	Uncommon
Respiratory Tract		
Ethmoiditis	Late	With or without orbital cellulitis
Otitis media	Late > early	With or without ipsilateral facial cellulitis
Mastoiditis	Late	Associated otitis media
Salivary glands	Late	Suppurative parotitis
Retropharyngeal cellulitis supraglottitis	Late	Not epiglottitis
Pleural empyema	Early > late	Associated pneumonia
"Acquired" right-sided diaphragmatic hernia	Early > late	Delayed onset respiratory distress
Skin, Soft Tissue		
Breast abscess	Late	Uncommon
Facial cellulitis, adenitis	Late > early	Facial and submandibular
Fasciitis	Late	Rare
Impetigo	Early	Rare
Purpura fulminans	Both	Septic shock, hypotension
Omphalitis	Early > late	Rare
Scalp abscess	Early > late	Fetal scalp sampling
Cystic hygroma abscess	Late	Rare
Postcircumcision bacteremia	Late	Rare
Urinary Tract Infection	Late > early	

*Modified from Baker CJ, Edwards MS: *In:* Remington JS, Klein JO: Infectious Diseases of the Fetus and Newborn Infant, 3rd ed. Philadelphia, WB Saunders, 1990.

neutropenia, leukocytosis, gram-positive cocci in the buffy coat, gastric aspirate (less specific), or tracheal secretions, and pneumonia or osteomyelitis on roentgenogram. A preterm infant who has respiratory distress after documentation of pulmonary maturity (by gastric aspirate shake test or amniotic fluid L/S ratio) or whose mother is heavily colonized by GBS should also be suspected of early onset GBS infection. However, prior to isolation of GBS from blood or CSF, none of these nonspecific clinical manifestations or laboratory tests are diagnostic for GBS and do not distinguish GBS from infection due to *E. coli*, *Listeria*, or herpes simplex. Furthermore, early onset GBS can occur in the absence of prolonged rupture of the membranes, prematurity, neutropenia, an elevated CRP or neutrophil count, and an abnormal immature-to-total white blood cell ratio.

The diagnosis of late onset GBS infection is determined by identification of GBS in blood and CSF or aspirates from infected sites (cellulitis, synovium, bone).

TREATMENT. GBS are uniformly sensitive to penicillin G, which is the treatment of choice for confirmed GBS infection. Empiric antimicrobial therapy is initiated with a penicillin (usually ampicillin) and an aminoglycoside until GBS has been differentiated from *E. coli* or *Listeria* sepsis or meningitis. In vitro, a combination of penicillin and gentamicin provides synergistic bactericidal activity against GBS despite resistance of GBS to aminoglycosides. Some authorities recommend continuation of ampicillin plus gentamicin for several days until there is a good clinical response or the CSF becomes sterile.

GBS demonstrate a minimal inhibitory concentration (MIC) (0.01–0.4 μg/mL) for penicillin G that is 4- to 10-fold greater than that of group A streptococci. An inoculum effect (higher GBS colonies/mL require more penicillin) may have clinical application because CSF may contain as many as 10^7–10^8 colony-forming units/mL. Rarely (4–6%), GBS demonstrates tolerance (minimal bactericidal concentration [MBC] > 16–32 times the MIC), which may correlate with delayed killing and recurrent infection. The significance of in vitro tolerance among GBS remains speculative.

GBS are also susceptible to vancomycin, semisynthetic pencillins, cefotaxime, ceftriaxone, and imipenem. These agents have not proved superior to penicillin or ampicillin and should not be used to treat documented GBS infection. Penicillin should be used in high doses for the treatment of GBS meningitis—300,000 units penicillin G/kg/24 hr; 300 mg ampicillin/kg/24 hr. These higher than usual doses are recommended because of a higher than usual MIC, high CSF inoculum size, reports of relapse of GBS meningitis in patients treated with 200,000 units of penicillin G/kg/24 hr, and the relative safety of penicillins in the neonate. CSF should be obtained within 48 hr of therapy of documented meningitis to determine whether persistent infection is present (> 90% are sterile within 36 hr) owing to a high inoculum effect or tolerant GBS. If GBS continues to grow from the CSF some authorities continue giving a combination of penicillin (or ampicillin) and gentamicin (for synergism) for the duration of treatment (2–3 wk). Failure to document sterile CSF within 48 hr of therapy may also signify subdural empyema, brain abscess, ventriculitis, suppurative dural sinus thrombosis, or an insufficient dose of a bactericidal antibiotic.

Recurrence or relapse is rare, but if it occurs, it is seen within 2–43 days of therapy (mean, 16 days). Prior therapy was usually too short (< 10 days for bacteremia, < 14 days for meningitis) with too low a dose of antibiotic. Antibiotic treatment may not eliminate GBS colonization from the mucosal surfaces, and prior infection may not produce protective antibody. Reinfection from maternal mastitis and neonatal brain abscess or endocarditis may occur. Repeat therapy with higher doses of pencillin, for a longer course, is effective therapy for recurrent GBS infection.

Supportive care of GBS infection has been discussed in Table 9–31 and Sec. 9.60 and 9.63. Treatment of hypoxia and shock, management of disseminated intravascular coagulation, seizures, increased intracranial pressure, and inappropriate antidiuretic hormone are discussed elsewhere. Extracorporeal membrane oxygenation may be an effective adjunctive therapy for full-term or large preterm infants with hypoxia who are unresponsive to conventional mechanical ventilation. Further information is needed about the risks and benefits of intravenous immunoglobulin therapy and granulocyte transfusion (for bacteremia and neutropenia) before these modalities can be recommended.

PREVENTION. In theory, early and possibly late onset GBS disease might be prevented by immunoprophylaxis, and early onset infection may be prevented by chemoprophylaxis. Because colonized mothers and thus infants with GBS infection often lack type-specific IgG antibody, it has been proposed that active immunization of the mother or possibly passive IgG administration to the newborn may prevent GBS disease. Sera containing type-specific antibody facilitate opsonophagocytosis against the individual GBS type in the presence of complement and neutrophils. Passive immune therapy would require development of hyperimmune type-specific GBS sera because the currently available commercial preparations of standard intravenous immunoglobulins have variable and potentially low levels of GBS IgG antibody. Type-specific active immunization is possible using purified capsular polysaccharides from type Ia, II, or III strains. Pregnant women without demonstratable antibodies to GBS at 30 wk of gestation respond to injection of type III specific polysaccharide with a significant rise in their own and, subsequently in neonatal cord sera antibody to type III GBS. Protective levels of antibody may persist for 1–2 mo in the neonate. Nonetheless, the polysaccharide antigen is not optimally immunogenic because only 54% of pregnant women demonstrate an immune response.

Chemoprophylaxis of the infant or mother has been suggested as an alternative to active or passive immune therapy. Chemoprophylaxis of the newborn, with varying regimens of intramuscular penicillin given at birth, may not be the optimal method because as many as 50% of infants may be infected in utero and are already symptomatic at birth or within 6 hr of delivery. Pencillin prophylaxis of the neonate has been demonstrated in a controlled trial to be ineffective in preventing bacteremia and death. Pencillin therapy may be indicated for the asymptomatic twin of an infected sibling.

Selective chemoprophylaxis of the high-risk, colonized pregnant woman with premature labor, fever, prolonged rupture of membranes (> 12 hr), or suspected chorioamnionitis is an effective method of preventing early onset neonatal GBS infection. Colonization is determined at 26–28 wk gestation. Intrapartum administration of intravenous ampicillin to this select group of known colonized women reduces the need to treat all mothers (only 4–5% fulfill all the criteria). Intravenous ampicillin (2 g, then 1 g every 4 hr) is given immediately to high-risk women at the onset of labor and is repeated until the infant is born. This protocol reduces both the colonization and infection of neonates. An alternate approach is to identify high-risk women at the time of labor with rapid antigen detection of vaginal GBS. Rapid tests can identify heavy maternal colonization within 5 hr and thus select the women who are at greatest risk for delivery of infected infants and in need of chemoprophylaxis with intrapartum ampicillin. Selective intrapartum ampicillin chemoprophylaxis will not benefit infants without risk factors who develop GBS disease or women with no prenatal care who deliver before the results of rapid tests are available.

PROGNOSIS. The mortality rate for early onset GBS disease ranges from 10 to 40%; mortality is highest in very low birthweight infants and in those with a low absolute neutrophil count (< 1,500), low Apgar scores, hypotension, apnea, severe cyanosis associated with persistent fetal circulation, and a delay in instituting antimicrobial therapy. The mortality from GBS-associated persistent fetal circulation has dramatically decreased owing to the use of ECMO. Factors associated with mortality following meningitis include shock, coma, CSF protein of greater than 300 mg/dL, seizures that are refractory to treatments, and neutrophil storage pool depletion. Mortality rates are lower with isolated early and late onset meningitis (10–20%). Neurologic sequelae following meningitis are severe in 20–30% of cases and include mental retardation, quadriplegia, repeated uncontrollable seizures, hypothalamic dysfunction, cortical blindness, hydrocephalus, bilateral deafness, and hemiplegia. Additional neurodevelopmental sequelae are noted in 15–25% of patients and include mild mental retardation, mild cortical atrophy, a stable seizure disorder, delay in receptive and expressive speech and language developments and other learning disabilities.

Sequelae of focal infections (arthritis-osteomyelitis) are usually localized and are not as significant as those associated with sepsis and meningitis.

Baker CJ: Immunization to prevent group B streptococcal disease: Victories and vexations. J Infect Dis 161:917, 1990.

Boyer KM, Gotoff SP: Antimicrobial prophylaxis of neonatal group B streptococcal sepsis. Clin Perinatol 15:831, 1988.

Boyer KM, Gotoff SP: Prevention of early-onset neonatal group B streptococcal disease with selective intrapartum chemoprophylaxis. N Engl J Med 314:1665, 1986.

Cabal LA, Siassi B, Cristofani C, et al: Cardiovascular changes in infants with β-hemolytic streptococcus sepsis. Crit Care Med 18:715, 1990.

Dillon HC, Khare S, Gray BM: Group B streptococcal carriage and disease: A 6-year prospective study. J Pediatr 110:31, 1987.

Gray BM, Pritchard DG, Dillon HC: Seroepidemiology of group B streptococcus type III colonization at delivery. J Infect Dis 159:1139, 1989.

Martin TR, Rubens CE, Wilson CB: Lung antibacterial defense mechanisms in infant and adult rats: Implications for the pathogenesis of group B streptococcal infections in the neonatal lung. J Infect Dis 157:91, 1988.

Noya FJ, Rench MA, Metzger TG, et al: Unusual occurrence of an epidemic of type Ib/c group B streptococcal sepsis in a neonatal intensive care unit. J Infect Dis 155:1135, 1987.

Payne NR, Burke BA, Day DL, et al: Correlation of clinical and pathologic findings in early onset neonatal group B streptococcal infection with disease severity and prediction of outcome. Pediatr Infect Dis J 7:836, 1988.

Sanchez PJ, Siegel JD, Cushion NB, et al: Significance of a positive urine group B streptococcal latex agglutination test in neonates. J Pediatr 116:601, 1990.

Tarpey MN, Graybar GB, Lyrene RK, et al: Thromboxane synthesis inhibition reverses group B streptococcus-induced pulmonary hypertension. Crit Care Med 15:644, 1987.

LISTERIA

See Sec. 12.36.

SPIROCHAETIS

See Sec. 12.50.

STAPHYLOCOCCI

See Sec. 12.19.

TUBERCULOSIS

See Sec. 12.47.

9.68 GENITAL MYCOPLASMA

Genital mycoplasma are common inhabitants of the genitourinary tracts of men and women, producing a wide variety of diseases such as nongonococcal urethritis, chorioamnionitis, endometritis and, possibly, afebrile infantile pneumonia, chronic neonatal lung disease, and meningitis.

ETIOLOGY. Mycoplasma lack a rigid cell wall, require sterols for growth, produce typical colonies on solid media (tiny 15–60 μm, *Ureaplasma urealyticum;* 200–300 μm "fried egg," *Mycoplasma hominis*), grow in cell-free media and hence are the smallest free-living micro-organisms in existence (100–300 nm in diameter), and are susceptible to antibiotics that inhibit protein synthesis. Mycoplasma are surrounded by a triple-layer membrane composed predominantly of lipids.

The important genital mycoplasma include *U. urealyticum* and *M. hominis;* of lesser importance are *M. fermentans, M. primatum,* and *M. genitalium.* There are 7 serotypes of *M. hominis;* each is susceptible to tetracycline, chloramphenicol, streptomycin (moderately susceptible to gentamicin), lincomycin, and clindamycin but resistant to erythromycin, penicillins, cephalosporins, and vancomycin. There are at least 16 serotypes of *U. urealyticum,* which have similar antimicrobial susceptibilities, except that *U. urealyticum* is sensitive to erythromycin and resistant to lincomycin or clindamycin.

EPIDEMIOLOGY. *M. hominis* and *U. urealyticum* colonize the genital and urinary tracts in 20–50% and 50–70% of sexually active women, respectively. Vertical transmission rates of 40–60% have been observed in neonates born to colonized women. Contamination by colonized amniotic fluid or during vaginal delivery is the route of neonatal acquisition. Maternal colonization usually persists throughout pregnancy. Neonatal colonization can occur in the presence of intact amniotic fluid membranes and with delivery by cesarean section; is greatest in infants weighing less than 1,500 g, in the presence of clinical chorioamnionitis, and in mothers of lower socioeconomic status; and is recovered from the newborn's throat, vagina, rectum, or, occasionally, eye for as long as 3 mo after birth.

Persistent *U. urealyticum* or *M. hominis* infection has been demonstrated in older patients with hypogammaglobulinemia and involves urinary tract infection and chronic arthritis.

PATHOGENESIS. Genital mycoplasma can produce chronic inflammation of the genitourinary tract and amniotic fluid membranes. Mycoplasma also produce phospholipases and IgA protease. Growth and, presumably, infection is inhibited by homologous antibody.

CLINICAL MANIFESTATIONS. Genital mycoplasma may be potentially responsible for neonatal disease or may be markers for premature labor with subsequent neonatal colonization rather than being specific etiologic agents of neonatal meningitis, congenital pneumonia, or chronic lung disease of premature infants. Histologic chorioamnionitis is often associated with intra-amniotic bacterial infections such as group B streptococci, *Escherichia coli,* and the genital mycoplasma. Although life-threatening fetal infection is rarely due to genital mycoplasma, the precise relationship between colonization or infection of the amniotic fluid membranes and the initiation of premature labor has not been defined.

Neonatal Central Nervous System Infection. *M. hominis* and *U. urealyticum* have been isolated from the cerebrospinal fluid (CSF) of premature and full-term infants in some but not all studies. CSF pleocytosis is not a consistent observation, and spontaneous clearance of mycoplasma has been documented without specific therapy. *U. urealyticum* meningitis has been associated with intraventricular hemorrhage and hydrocephalus; meningitis due to *M. hominis* may be benign. The day of onset of meningitis varies from 1–196 days of life; organisms may persist in the CSF without therapy for days to weeks.

Chronic Lung Disease. The role of *U. urealyticum* as a pathogen of neonatal pneumonia or as a contributing factor in the development of chronic lung disease remains unknown. *U. urealyticum* has been associated with the development of chronic lung disease in ventilator-dependent low-birthweight infants. Infants at risk weigh less than 1,000 g and are colonized at birth or have congenital *ureaplasma* pneumonia. Blood cultures may be positive in 25% of patients when *U. urealyticum* is recovered from endotracheal secretions.

DIAGNOSIS. *U. urealyticum* and *M. hominis* have been isolated from urine, blood, CSF, tracheal aspirates, pleural fluid, abscesses, and lung tissue. Most laboratories have difficulty with their identification. Organisms grow on supplemented beef heart infusion broth and agar. Identification of *U. ureaplasma* on agar requires 1–2 days of growth and visualization with the dissecting microscope, whereas *M. hominis* are apparent to the eye but may require 1 wk to grow.

TREATMENT. Therapy of neonatal genital mycoplasma infections should be limited to infections associated with a pure growth of the organism, evidence of suppuration, and evidence that the disease manifestations are compatible with an infectious process rather than colonization or the asymptomatic presence of the mycoplasma. Treatment is based on predictable antimicrobial sensitivities (see earlier section Etiology). Because the long-term consequences of asymptomatic CSF mycoplasma infection, especially in the absence of pleocytosis, are unknown and because mycoplasma may spontaneously be cleared from the CSF, therapy should involve minimal risks. If erythromycin is used in patients concurrently receiving theophylline, serum theophylline levels should be monitored carefully, since this antibiotic inhibits theophylline metabolism.

Cassell GH, Crouse DT, Canupp KP, et al: Association of *Ureaplasma urealyticum* infection of the lower respiratory tract with chronic lung disease and death in very-low-birth-weight infants. Lancet 2:240, 1988.
Cassell GH, Crouse DT, Waites KB, et al: Does *Ureaplasma urealyticum* cause respiratory disease in newborns? Pediatr Infect Dis J 7:535, 1988.
Dinsmoor MJ, Ramamurthy RS, Cassell GH, et al: Neonatal serologic response at term to the genital mycoplasmas. Pediatr Infect Dis J 8:487, 1989.
Dinsmoor MJ, Ramamaurthy RS, Gibbs RS: Transmission of genital mycoplasmas from mother to neonate in women with prolonged membrane rupture. Pediatr Infect Dis J 8:483, 1989.
Sanchez PJ, Regan JA: Vertical transmission of *Ureaplasma urealyticum* from mothers to preterm infants. Pediatr Infect Dis J 9:398, 1990.
Sanchez PJ, Regan JA: *Ureaplasma urealyticum* colonization and chronic lung disease in low birth weight infants. Pediatr Infect Dis J 7:542, 1988.
Syrogiannopoulos GA, Kapatais-Zoumbos K, Decavalas GO, et al: *Ureaplasma urealyticum* colonization of full term infants: Perinatal acquisition and persistence during early infancy. Pediatr Infect Dis J 9:236, 1990.
Waites KB, Crouse DT, Nelson KG, et al: Chronic *Ureaplasma urealyticum* and *Mycoplasma hominis* infections of central nervous system in preterm infants. Lancet 1:17, 1988.
Waites KB, Duffy LB, Crouse DT, et al: Mycoplasmal infections of cerebrospinal fluid in newborn infants from a community hospital population. Pediatr Infect Dis J 9:241, 1990.
Wang EE, Frayha H, Watts J, et al: Role of *Ureaplasma urealyticum* and other pathogens in the development of chronic lung disease of prematurity. Pediatr Infect Dis J 7:547, 1988.
Wientzen RL: Genital mycoplasmas and the pediatrician. Pediatr Infect Dis J 9:232, 1990.

SPECIFIC VIRAL INFECTIONS

9.69 CYTOMEGALOVIRUS (CMV)

See also Sec. 9.58 and 12.71.

CMV may cause serious symptomatic disease in the immunologically immature fetus or preterm newborn. Congenital CMV infection is a leading cause of mental retardation and deafness.

ETIOLOGY. CMV is a herpesvirus that produces characteristic intranuclear and intracytoplasmic inclusion bodies and an enlarged cell size (cytomegalic). It is the largest member of the herpesvirus family. The CMV genome encodes more than 25–35 structural and nonstructural proteins and can be used to identify specific strains of CMV spread by vertical or horizontal transmission through the use of restriction endonuclease fragment length DNA polymorphisms.

EPIDEMIOLOGY. Humans are the only known source of congenital, perinatal, or maternal CMV infection. The incidence of antibodies to CMV is highest in the lower socioeconomic levels, sexually active individuals, workers in day-care centers, families of children with congenitally or day-care–acquired CMV disease, multiply transfused patients, and immunocompromised patients (those with organ transplants and acquired immunodeficiency syndrome [AIDS]). One to 2% of all newborns are infected with CMV at birth; only 1–2/1,000 live births (10–15% of congenitally infected infants) have symptomatic congenital cytomegalic inclusion disease. The fetus may acquire CMV infection by vertical (transplacental) transmission following maternal viremia. Congenital infection may occur in fetuses of mothers with primary or, less likely, with a recurrent (reactivated latent) infection. Most primary and nearly all recurrent maternal CMV infections are asymptomatic. Symptomatic, clinically apparent, congenital, multiorgan system cytomegalic inclusion disease is present at birth in less than 10% of infected infants. Symptomatic disease occurs rarely among infants born to mothers with recurrent infection during pregnancy. The neonate also may acquire CMV by contamination with infected secretions or blood at the time of birth, from infected breast milk, or by blood transfused from seropositive donors. Transmission between infants or from infants to nurses in a newborn unit is quite rare.

Viral excretion, even in those with asymptomatic infection, may persist for months to years and may be present in urine, tears, blood, and oropharyngeal secretions in infants. Sexual contact in adults and close exposure to young infants in day-care centers are important sources of horizontal acquisition of CMV by mothers. Seronegative day-care workers seroconvert at a rate of 20%/yr (10 times that in the general population); close contact with infants under 3 yr of age has the greatest risk of seroconversion. Fifty per cent of seronegative family members will seroconvert within 6 mo following the introduction of CMV to the home by a newly infected infant or mother.

The risk of symptomatic congenital CMV disease may be increased with maternal infection in the first half of pregnancy. This may be due to the immaturity of fetal host defense mechanisms and inadequate placental passage of maternal CMV IgG antibody, which may be protective in recurrent maternal infections. Five to 15% of asymptomatic congenitally infected infants will develop sequelae (deafness, neurodevelopmental problems, chorioretinitis).

Perinatal acquisition from breast-feeding usually results in asymptomatic neonatal infection because transplacental passage of CMV IgG antibody may protect the infant. Nosocomial postnatal infection from seropositive blood products can produce significant disease (hepatitis, thrombocytopenia, neutropenia, sepsis syndrome) in premature seronegative infants. Exchange transfusions, multiple seropositive blood transfusions (> 50 mL) administered to seronegative very low birth-weight infants, and leukocyte transfusions are associated with the highest risk of CMV transmission.

PATHOGENESIS. Maternal viremia presumably precedes viral passage (free virus or in leukocytes) across the placenta during primary and, less often, in recurrent infection. Placental infection (villitis) is common and precedes or coincides with subsequent fetal viremia and dissemination to multiple organs, where prolonged chronic viral replication and shedding occur. CMV may produce cytopathic effects and can initiate a vasculitis in the placenta and other fetal tissues. The latter may impair placental function or produce occlusive vascular ischemia following infection of endothelial cells of the brain or other fetal organs. Infection of the central nervous system produces a focal encephalitis involving white, gray, and choroid plexus cells and a periependymitis. Healing leads to gliosis and calcification, which typically is periventricular but may appear anywhere in the brain.

Hepatitis is common and is manifest by inclusion bodies in Kupffer and biliary duct epithelial cells, cholangitis, cholestasis, extramedullary hematopoiesis, and hepatic calcification. Renal involvement is characterized by inclusion cells in the distal convoluted tubules and collecting ducts. These cells desquamate and, if identified in the urine, may aid in the early diagnosis of CMV infection.

CLINICAL MANIFESTATIONS. Symptomatic congenital CMV infection (cytomegalic inclusion disease) is a multiorgan systemic illness characterized by intrauterine growth retardation, hepatosplenomegaly, jaundice, hepatitis, petechial rash, chorioretinitis, cerebral calcifications, and microcephaly (Fig. 9–28). However, this severe form of the disease represents less than 10% of congenitally infected neonates; the majority of neonatal infections are asymptomatic. Hepatomegaly is usually associated with conjugated hyperbilirubinemia and moderate elevations of the serum transaminase and alkaline phosphatase activities. Extramedullary hematopoiesis may cause organomegaly in the absence of hepatitis. Although the duration of hepatosplenomegaly may vary from several months to several years, CMV does not cause persistent active hepatitis. Splenomegaly may occur as an isolated finding or in conjunction with hepatomegaly or petechiae. A generalized, usually pinpoint, petechial rash is found in 50–70% of severely involved infants: purpura is less common. The virus appears to affect the bone marrow directly, causing a thrombocytopenia that may clear in 48–72 hr or persist for weeks to months. Significant bleeding, however, rarely occurs. A diffuse interstitial pneumonia is rarely found in congenital disease and is more common in postnatal acquired infection in premature infants.

Infection of the central nervous system results in the most serious sequelae. Microcephaly is characteristic of severe involvement and, with cerebral calcification and chorioretinitis, is predictive of a high probability of psychomotor retardation. The cerebral calcifications are typically periventricular in distribution, in contrast to the more diffuse patterns observed in congenital *Toxoplasma* infection; these patterns, however, are not diagnostic. Microcephaly may not become apparent for several months. Meningoencephalitis, characterized by CSF pleocytosis, an elevated protein content, and the development of seizures, may also occur. The eye is less commonly involved in congenital cytomegalovirus infection than in rubella or toxoplasmosis. Chorioretinitis, sometimes indistinguishable from the same condition due to toxoplasmosis, occurs in 15–25% of severely involved infants; strabismus and optic atrophy also may occur. Microphthalmia, cataracts, and corneal opacities are rare and should suggest another pathogen. Intellectual deficits are common.

CMV can also directly infect the structure of the inner ear, resulting in hearing loss in about 60% of those infants who are symptomatic at birth and in 5–10% of asymptomatic infants. Ear involvement may be unilateral or bilateral and leads to sensorineural deafness in about 30 per cent of symptomatic infants. Dental defects are common, are seen in 25–30% of symptomatic and 4% of asymptomatic infants, and include a distinct enamel defect of the primary teeth characterized by fragile, easily chipped enamel, a yellow discoloration, and severe dental caries. A celery stalk appearance of alternately longitudinal, translucent, and radiodense bands may be noted on the distal femur or proximal tibia in CMV and other congenital infections. Congenital malformations are not associated with this infection.

Postnatal CMV infection, associated with blood transfusion, is characterized by a septic appearance, hepatitis, hepatosplenomegaly, gray pallor, afebrile pneumonitis, a deteriorating respiratory status, atypical lymphocytosis, hemolytic anemia, thrombocytopenia, and neutropenia. The disease usually occurs in sick, multiply transfused premature infants who are long-term residents of an intensive care unit; mortality is 20%. Whenever possible, only CMV-seronegative donors should be used for blood transfusions, since transfusion of seropositive blood to seronegative premature infants has been associated with this syndrome.

DIAGNOSIS. The virus can be successfully cultured from urine, saliva, or other body fluids to diagnose congenital or neonatal CMV infection. Viruria present at birth or within the 1st wk is diagnostic of congenital infection, whereas recovery of virus after this time may be suggestive of congenital or neonatally acquired infection. Viruria may persist for years, although the viral titer decreases rapidly after 3 mo of age. Refrigeration or direct inoculation of the sample is important because storage at room temperature or freezing decreases the recovery of virus. Cytopathic effects on cultured fibroblasts are noted within 24–72 hr. Rapid detection of CMV is possible by combining tissue culture and hyperimmune or monoclonal antibodies to detect CMV antigens. Direct detection of CMV antigens from urine is facilitated by the use of solid phase enzyme-linked immunosorbent assays (ELISA) or DNA hybridization.

Serum specimens for IgG antibody, one obtained in the neonatal period and one at 4–6 mo of age, may also be helpful. A falling CMV antibody titer indicates transplacental passage of antibody from mother to fetus, whereas a stable or rising titer supports a diagnosis of congenital, perinatal, or postnatal infection. Demonstration of CMV-specific IgM antibody in neonatal serum can be diagnostic, but the method has technical difficulties and may be insensitive and nonspecific. The *differential diagnosis* includes congenital rubella, toxoplasmosis, syphilis, herpes simplex, sepsis, hemolytic disease of the newborn, neonatal hepatitis, galactosemia, tyrosinemia, immune thrombocytopenia, congenital leukemia, and neuroblastoma (Sec. 9.58).

TREATMENT AND PREVENTION. There is no specific therapy for congenital CMV infection. Although ganciclovir has been used as therapy, with or without hyperimmune CMV globulin, for life- or sight-threatening CMV infections in immunocompromised hosts, there is little experience with this agent in the neonate. The use of ganciclovir in congenital CMV infection is being studied as part of a large multicenter project.

CMV is not very contagious and requires specific close contact or parenteral administration for transmission. Useful infection control measures include (1) secretion precautions in handling infants known to be infected with CMV, (2) good handwashing and personal hygiene habits in all personnel caring for infected infants, and (3) use of blood from CMV-seronegative donors, deglycerolized frozen red blood cells, or filtration removal of leukocytes from blood for neonatal transfusion. Seronegative female personnel or mothers may care for CMV-excreting infants if contact with secretions is avoided (avoid saliva, fingers in mouth, urine) and handwashing is carefully performed.

A live attenuated CMV vaccine is being developed but has not been tested in women of childbearing age.

PROGNOSIS. The outcome of symptomatic congenital CMV infection is poor; there is a 20–30% mortality and a 90–95% morbidity, characterized by psychomotor retardation, microcephaly, hearing loss, seizures, and learning disabilities. The outcome is poorest among symptomatic patients with microcephaly, intracranial calcification, and chorioretinitis. Infants with asymptomatic disease have a much lower incidence of hearing loss and learning disabilities.

Adler SP: Molecular epidemiology of cytomegalovirus: Evidence for viral transmission to parents from children infected at a day care center. Pediatr Infect Dis 5:315, 1986.

Anonymous: Screening for congenital CMV. Lancet 2:599, 1989.
Balcarek KB, Bagley R, Cloud GA, et al: Cytomegalovirus infection among employees of a children's hospital. JAMA 263:840, 1990.
Britt WJ, Vugler LG: Antiviral antibody responses in mothers and their newborn infants with clinical and subclinical congenital cytomegalovirus infections. J Infect Dis 161:214, 1990.
Conboy TJ, Pass RF, Stagno S, et al: Early clinical manifestations and intellectual outcome in children with symptomatic congenital cytomegalovirus infection. J Pediatr 111:343, 1987.
Gilbert GL, Hudson IL, Hayes K, et al: Prevention of transfusion-acquired cytomegalovirus infection in infants by blood filtration to remove leucocytes. Lancet 1:1228, 1989.
Lamberson HV, McMillan JA, Weiner LB, et al: Prevention of transfusion-associated cytomegalovirus (CMV) infection in neonates by screening blood donors for IgM to CMV. J Infect Dis 157:820, 1988.
Porath A, McNutt RA, Smiley LM, et al: Effectiveness and cost benefit of a proposed live cytomegalovirus vaccine in the prevention of congenital disease. Rev Infect Dis 12:31, 1990.
Stagno S, Pass RF, Cloud G, et al: Primary cytomegalovirus infection in pregnancy. JAMA 256:1094, 1986.
Yow MD: Congenital cytomegalovirus disease: A NOW problem. J Infect Dis 159:163, 1989.
Yow MD, Williamson DW, Leeds LJ, et al: Epidemiologic characteristics of cytomegalovirus infection in mothers and their infants. Am J Obstet Gynecol 158:1189, 1988.

9.70 ENTEROVIRUSES

See also Sec. 12.80.

The echoviruses, coxsackieviruses, polioviruses, and other numerically assigned enteroviruses are common pathogens that produce diverse and potentially serious disease in the neonate.

ETIOLOGY. Enteroviruses, one genus of Picornaviridae, are small (27–30 nm), nonenveloped, spherical, single-stranded RNA viruses. Classification was originally based on methods of isolation, and the viruses were differentiated into serotypes 1–3, polioviruses; serotypes 1–24, group A coxsackieviruses; serotypes 1–6, group B coxsackieviruses; and serotypes 1–34, echoviruses. Newer enteroviruses are numbered 68 through 71; number 72 is hepatitis A virus. Many infections are mild, nonspecific, or asymptomatic, whereas others produce characteristic illnesses such as aseptic meningitis, myocarditis, pleurodynia, or hand, foot, and mouth disease.

EPIDEMIOLOGY. Enteroviral infections produce seasonal epidemics in Northern latitudes during the summer and fall. Spread occurs by fecal-oral or oral-oral routes and also has been associated with contaminated swimming pools. Human-to-human transmission is most common; however, enteroviruses have been noted in flies, shellfish, sewage, and some domestic and wild animals. Neonatal illness is caused by the same enterovirus that is present in the community. Transplacental transmission is unusual but has been reported for poliovirus, coxsackieviruses, and echoviruses. Enteroviruses are not teratogenic. Ascending infection before labor may occur, but usually the neonate probably becomes infected during parturition or from exposure to an infected mother, relative, or caretaker after birth.

The onset of disease of perinatally acquired enterovirus infection usually occurs on the 3rd–5th day of life. The mother may be asymptomatic or may have developed a viral-like illness within 7 days of birth. The attack rate following maternal illness is 20–50%. The onset of nosocomial or community acquired disease is related to the day of exposure to symptomatic or asymptomatic contacts. Infection may be more common in patients from the lower socioeconomic classes, in males, and in formula-fed rather than human milk–fed infants.

PATHOGENESIS. The portal of entry of enteroviruses is the oropharynx or gastrointestinal tract. Within 24 hr there is direct spread to the regional lymph nodes. Viremia begins in the next 48–72 hr with dissemination to various target organs such as the brain, heart, liver, lung, skeletal muscles, skin, and mucous membranes. Multiplication of virus in these sites produces end-organ disease followed by a secondary viremia, which lasts from the 3rd–7th day of the illness and is terminated by the appearance of specific serum antibody.

The pathogenesis and severity of enterovirus illness are related to the patient's age (the very young do less well), virulence of the virus, and tissue tropism. Enteroviruses produce cytolysis with subsequent cell death and release of virus particles. This results in lymphocytic inflammation and necrosis of the muscle fibers, anterior horn cells, hepatocytes, and possibly adrenal glands.

CLINICAL MANIFESTATIONS. Poliomyelitis in neonates is similar to the disease in older children (Sec. 12.80). Echovirus and coxsackievirus infections range from subclinical to overwhelming fatal infections. Mild febrile illnesses associated with viremia or aseptic meningitis occur most commonly in full-term infants who manifest irritability, poor feeding, and fever. This pattern occurs particularly in infections due to coxsackievirus B5 and echoviruses 5, 11, and 33.

A sepsis-like illness may occur in 20% of neonates with enteroviral infections. Common agents include coxsackieviruses B2–5 and echoviruses 5, 11, and 16. The syndrome is characterized by fever, irritability, poor feeding, lethargy, jaundice, hepatitis, apnea, hypotonia, abdominal distention, vomiting, diarrhea, and rash (Fig. 9–29). Disseminated intravascular coagulation, hepatic necrosis, myocardial dysfunction, and hypotension are serious complications. Hepatic involvement is associated with echoviruses 11 and 19.

Isolated interstitial pneumonia is less common than other presentations but may occur concomitantly in patients with meningitis, myocarditis, or hepatitis. Myocarditis, manifested as cyanosis, lethargy, tachycardia, tachypnea, arrhythmias, or heart failure, may result from enteroviral infection, particularly that with coxsackieviruses B1–4.

The enteroviruses frequently produce aseptic meningitis and meningoencephalitis as focal infections or as part of the myocarditis or the systemic sepsis-like illness. Isolated meningitis is a self-limited disease that lasts for 3–5 days unless it is complicated by myocarditis. Meningitis due to enterovirus typically has a CSF profile of 50–1,000 leukocytes, which are predominantly lymphocytes, with normal glucose and protein levels. Neutrophilic pleocytosis may be seen early in the illness; elevated CSF protein levels and hypoglycorrhachia may occasionally be present. Aseptic meningitis is frequently due to coxsackieviruses B2–5 and echoviruses 3, 9, 11, and 17.

Vomiting and diarrhea may be present as part of the overall viral illness but are unusual as the only manifestations of enteroviral disease. Some authorities question the role of enteroviruses as a cause of diarrhea, suggesting that the virus is an incidental finding due to the high prevalence of virus found in asymptomatic children of the same age.

Coryza, conjunctivitis, and pharyngitis also may occur. The exanthem noted in infection with coxsackievirus B1 and B5 and echoviruses 4, 5, 7, 9, 11, 16, 17, 18, 21, and 22 is usually a minor and noncharacteristic manifestation of moderate to severe neonatal illness. The rash is noted on the 3rd–5th day of illness, disappears as the illness (fever) resolves, and is usually macular or maculopapular but rarely may be petechial.

DIAGNOSIS. Enteroviral infections may be suspected on clinical and epidemiologic considerations. The season, history of exposure, typical illness in the mother, and onset of illness beyond the period of early onset bacterial infection are helpful clues. White blood cell counts and cerebrospinal fluid results are often nonspecific and occasionally may be consistent with those characteristic of a bacterial infection and thus cannot be used to differentiate the etiology.

Viral isolation is necessary for diagnosis (see Sec. 12.7). Samples should be taken from multiple sites, for example,

nose, throat, stool, blood, urine, or cerebrospinal fluid. Acute and convalescent sera should be collected to test for neutralization titers against the isolated enterovirus. Serologic diagnosis is impractical and not useful without virus isolation because of the large number of enteroviral serotypes. Identification of viral RNA or antigen may improve identification in tissue samples such as myocardial or hepatic biopsies. The diagnosis of enteroviral meningitis has been aided by use of the polymerase chain reaction.

The *differential diagnosis* includes bacterial sepsis and meningitis, congenital heart disease, other causes of neonatal hepatitis (TORCH, hepatitis B virus), and diseases that produce the sepsis-like syndrome (see Sec. 12.3).

TREATMENT AND PREVENTION. There is no specific therapy for enteroviral infections. Intravenous immunoglobulin might be considered to neutralize viremia but has not been proved to be effective therapy for immunocompetent patients. Immunoglobulin (oral or intravenous) may also be useful in preventing disease in infants exposed to nursery outbreaks of severe infections.

Standard supportive therapy is essential for patients with meningitis, sepsis-syndrome, hepatic necrosis, and myocarditis. Such therapy includes mechanical ventilation for respiratory failure, anticonvulsant drugs for seizures, digoxin or intravenous inotropic agents for heart failure, and treatment of hepatic encephalopathy. Corticosteroids are not indicated for severe myocarditis, aseptic meningitis, or hepatic necrosis.

PROGNOSIS. Most enteroviral infections, including isolated aseptic meningitis, are self-limited, benign illnesses that have no morbidity or mortality. Long-term neurologic development is probably normal for the majority of infants with enteroviral meningoencephalitis. Mortality is high among neonates with hepatic necrosis (20–80%) and myocarditis (30–50%). Infection is usually most severe in the 1st wk of life following acquisition in utero or during birth, and in the absence of placental passage of maternal virus-specific IgG.

Amstey MS, Miller RK, Nenegus MA, et al: Enterovirus in pregnant women and the perfused placenta. Am J Obstet Gynecol 158:775, 1988.

Gilbert GL, Dickson KE, Waters MJ, et al: Outbreak of enterovirus 71 infection in Victoria, Australia, with a high incidence of neurologic involvement. Pediatr Infect Dis J 7:484, 1988.

Modlin JF: Echovirus infections of newborn infants. Pediatr Infect Dis J 7:311, 1988.

Modlin JF, Kinney JS: Perinatal enterovirus infections. Adv Pediatr Infect Dis 2:57, 1987.

Modlin JF: Perinatal echovirus infection: Insights from a literature review of 61 cases of serious infection and 16 outbreaks in nurseries. Rev Infect Dis 8:918, 1986.

Nakayama T, Urano T, Osano M, et al: Outbreak of herpangina associated with coxsackievirus B3 infection. Pediatr Infect Dis J 8:495, 1989.

Rabkin CS, Telzak EE, Ho MS, et al: Outbreak of echovirus 11 infection in hospitalized neonates. Pediatr Infect Dis J 7:186, 1988.

Rotbart HA: Diagnosis of enteroviral meningitis with the polymerase chain reaction. J Pediatr 117:85, 1990.

9.71 HERPES SIMPLEX VIRUS (HSV)

HSV type 2 and occasionally type 1 produce significant neonatal and occasionally fetal disease. Maternal infection during pregnancy or parturition is associated with intrauterine infection and, more commonly, neonatal disease acquired from the maternal genitourinary tract. It is characterized by disseminated viremia with multisystem involvement (liver, adrenal gland, brain, lung, skin) or disease localized to the brain or skin, eyes, and oropharynx.

ETIOLOGY. Herpes simplex types 1 and 2 are large, double-stranded DNA viruses, with similar electronmicrographic morphologic features. HSV 2 can be distinguished from HSV 1 on the basis of restriction endonuclease digests of viral DNA, unique surface glycoproteins, and specific serology. HSV 2 is a sexually transmitted disease infecting the cervix, vagina, labia, and perineum; HSV 1 is a common infection of the mucocutaneous margin around the mouth and the skin above the waist. Both infections occur in the oral or genital area, are neurotropic and may enter the nervous system following viremia or by retrograde neural migration, establish latency by persistence of viral DNA in the absence of obvious infection, and demonstrate reactivation of the latent state, producing local, predominantly recurrent oral or genital mucocutaneous lesions.

EPIDEMIOLOGY. The incidence of neonatal HSV infection is 1/3,000–7,500 live births. HSV 2 is the agent responsible in 75–85% of all patients and may be acquired from the mother during intrauterine and intrapartum periods or from the mother, relatives, or caretakers during the postnatal period. Approximately 80–90% of cases occur during the intrapartum period following contamination by infected genitourinary tract secretions or labial and cutaneous herpetic lesions.

The prevalence of genital herpes is about 1–2% during pregnancy and 0.1–0.4% at parturition. HSV genital lesions are present at parturition in less than 10% of cases, and a history of previous or current genital HSV infection is present in only 20–30% of mothers who deliver infected infants. Most women with HSV genital infection are asymptomatic because neither recurrent nor primary infections usually produce the typical manifestations of myalgia, headache, fever, genital pain, vaginal discharge, and visible multiple ulcerating lesions. The risk of transmission to the fetus or neonate is greater with primary infections (50%) than with recurrent disease ($< 5\%$) because the former is associated with a greater risk of viremia, higher viral titers in local lesions, longer duration of viral shedding (21 versus 5 days), a greater number of lesions (20 versus 5), and an absence of both neutralizing and antibody-dependent cellular cytotoxicity antibodies. Levels of neutralizing antibodies of greater than 1:20 are associated with a decreased risk of neonatal infection. Symptomatic primary infection has a higher risk than the more common asymptomatic primary infection, and vaginal birth or rupture of the membranes for longer than 4–6 hr before delivery, in the presence of active lesions, adds to the risk of neonatal infection.

HSV infection is associated with an increased risk of premature birth, maternal fever during parturition, the use of fetal scalp electrodes, and maternal erythema multiforme. It can be transmitted to the newborn in the absence of rupture of the amniotic membranes or after delivery by cesarean section. Additional epidemiology of neonatal HSV infection as related to the pattern of infection is noted in Table 9–33.

Postnatal HSV infection can be acquired from any adult with active herpes labialis (HSV 1). Transmission of postpartum neonatal infection has occurred by direct contact with infected material associated with breast-feeding (cutaneous lesion), endotracheal intubation and other procedures, and rarely by nosocomial spread from infant to infant. Currently, it is not recommended that employees with a cold sore be excluded from newborn units, but workers with herpetic whitlow should avoid contact with newborn infants.

PATHOGENESIS. Viral replication begins at the site of inoculation (skin, conjunctivae, or oropharynx); the disease may remain localized, enter the central nervous system by neuronal transmission, or, following viremia, may disseminate to the CNS and other tissues. Qualitative and quantitative defects in neonatal host defense mechanisms during the initial exposure (alveolar macrophages, α or γ interferon-stimulated natural killer cell cytotoxicity), and late immune response (neutralizing antibody, antibody-dependent cellular cytotoxicity effector mechanisms, γ interferon production) may predispose to dissemination. Transplacental neutralizing IgG may bind free circulating HSV, and cell-associated HSV may be attacked by the antibody-dependent cellular cytotoxicity sys-

TABLE 9–33. Patterns of Neonatal Herpes Simplex Infection*

	Disseminated	Skin-Eye-Mouth†	Central Nervous System‡
Frequency distribution (%)	25–35	30–40	30–40
Prematurity (%)	25–35	20–30	15–25
Age at diagnosis (days)	9–11	10–11	16–17
Range onset (days)	3–20	2–15	4–55
Days between onset and diagnosis	4	5	5
Vesicles (%)	70–80	85	55–65
Encephalitis (%)	70–80	0 (subclinical ?)‡	100
Pneumonia (%)	50	2–5	5
Seropositive at onset (%)	60	65	85
HSV 2 (%)	70–80	50–70	70–90
1-year treated mortality (%)	60	0	15
1-year untreated mortality (%)	80–90	0 (unless disseminated)†	50
Cause of death	Pneumonia, shock, disseminated intravascular coagulation		Brain stem involvement, cerebral edema
CNS deficits: S/P acyclovir (%)	15–20	8–10	65–75
or placebo (%)	50	25–35	65–75

*Modified from Whitley R: *In:* Remington JS, Klein JO: Infectious Diseases of the Fetus and Newborn Infant, 3rd ed. Philadelphia, WB Saunders, 1990.
†S/P = status post. As many as 70% of untreated skin, eye, mouth HSV infection may disseminate to CNS, lung, and other organs.
‡Subclinical, undetected encephalitis may be present, documented by CNS sequelae or recurrent HSV vesicles with encephalitis.

tem. Viral replication produces host cell swelling, intranuclear inclusions, cytolysis, and hemorrhagic necrosis. A lymphocytic inflammatory response is common in the CNS, meninges, and other sites of dissemination.

CLINICAL MANIFESTATIONS. Intrauterine infection due to HSV 2 is evident at birth and is characterized by cutaneous scars or vesicles, chorioretinitis, microphthalmia, keratoconjunctivitis, microcephaly, hydranencephaly, intracranial calcifications, and hepatosplenomegaly. The long-term neurodevelopmental outcome is poor for patients with intrauterine infection. A smaller number of congenitally infected infants may show only skin or eye lesions. These latter infants are usually born to mothers who have prolonged rupture of the membranes (for as long as 2 wk), and, in the absence of CNS lesions, they have a better prognosis.

Infants who acquire intrapartum or postpartum infection may have a disseminated illness, disease limited to the skin, eye, or mouth, or encephalitis (see Table 9–33 and Fig. 9–29). Disseminated disease is characterized by lesions in the skin, lungs, adrenals, CNS, trachea, esophagus, kidney, spleen, and heart. Manifestations are similar to those of severe bacterial sepsis and include respiratory distress, fever, apnea, seizures, lethargy, irritability, conjugated hyperbilirubinemia, shock, disseminated intravascular coagulation, and the characteristic localized or generalized, grouped and linear, or discrete 1–3 mm in diameter, erythematous-based vesicles. Initially appearing as erythematous macular-papular lesions, the vesicles may progress to bullous-sized lesions (> 1 cm in diameter). Unfortunately, 20–30% of patients with disseminated disease do not have vesicles at any time during their illness, thus causing a delay in diagnosis.

Skin, eye, or mouth disease may be localized if it is treated with antiviral agents but may disseminate if therapy is delayed or not provided. Cutaneous vesicles are similar to those seen in disseminated disease. They may recur during the first 6–12 mo of life, may be observed on the presenting part (vertex, buttock), or may be inoculated by a fetal scalp electrode. Ocular lesions include keratoconjunctivitis or late chorioretinitis with or without microphthalmia and cataracts. Prior to antiviral therapy, as many as 35% of infants with previously documented localized skin, eye, or mouth infection and no signs of encephalitis developed CNS defects. The latter is thought to be due to subclinical undetected CNS infection and emphasizes the importance of treating all of these patients with antiviral therapy.

Encephalitis is a third pattern of neonatal HSV 2 (occasionally HSV 1) infection, and it has different characteristics than disseminated disease or localized skin, eye, or mouth disease. Although encephalitis is present in most patients with disseminated disease, isolated CNS infection is usually of later onset and has a lower incidence of viremia and vesicles and a higher incidence of neutralizing and antibody-dependent cellular cytotoxicity antibodies. These data suggest that isolated encephalitis is due to retrograde axonal transmission of virus to the CNS rather than to viremic spread. Manifestations of encephalitis include fever, irritability, lethargy, coma, focal and generalized seizures, bulging fontanele, high-pitched cry, and focal temporal lobe lesions on CT, brain scan, or electroencephalography (EEG). HSV infection of the CNS may mimic bacterial meningitis and should be considered if the Gram stain and the culture of the CSF are negative and if the patient's condition continues to deteriorate despite appropriate antimicrobial therapy for presumed bacterial meningitis.

Occasionally isolated HSV pneumonia or disseminated disease with a predominant pneumonitic presentation may develop. Typically, a previously healthy full-term or premature infant convalescing from hyaline membrane disease becomes ill on the 4th–5th day of life with a new onset of respiratory distress or a deterioration of lung function. Fever, a paucity of cutaneous vesicles, and rapid progression to respiratory failure with an interstitial or reticulogranular appearance on roentgenogram are typical of HSV pneumonia.

DIAGNOSIS. Identification of virus is possible in 1–3 days by isolating it in tissue culture obtained from vesicles, nasopharyngeal or conjunctival swabs, urine, stool, tracheal secretions (pneumonia), duodenal aspirates (hepatitis), and CSF (encephalitis), if the usual large quantities of virus are present. Specimens must be transported in viral transport media on ice. Virus is readily isolated from active lesions (vesicles, keratoconjunctivitis, mouth ulcerations) and is present in the CSF in 25–40% of cases with encephalitis. Differentiation of HSV 2 from HSV 1 is of epidemologic and prognostic importance (see later discussion) but does not alter treatment protocols.

Cytologic examination of exfoliated cells or cells scraped from the base of the vesicle can be examined for the presence of intranuclear inclusions and multinucleated giant cells by the Tzanck test and the Wright or Papanicolaou stains. These cytologic findings may be present in 60–70% of cases of neonatal HSV infection but are not pathognomonic.

Detection of HSV antigen or DNA allows rapid diagnosis of HSV infection. Serologic diagnosis is not helpful owing to the high incidence of maternal HSV IgG antibody that crosses the placenta. Furthermore, in some mothers HSV antibody may be absent. Production of local HSV IgG antibody in CSF during meningoencephalitis is a late sign but is diagnostic.

Less specific diagnostic tests include tests for the presence of conjugated hyperbilirubinemia, elevated hepatic enzymes, coagulopathy in the presence of hepatitis, CSF pleocytosis (with erythrocytes, lymphocytes, and monocytes), elevated CSF protein, a temporal lobe focus on EEG, and a localized temporal lobe mass effect on CT or brain scan. Additional EEG findings include periodic slow and sharp waves or multiple independent foci; CT scans and magnetic resonance imaging (MRI) also demonstrate patchy areas of hemorrhage, calcification, or low attenuation in the cerebral cortex and periventricular area (see Sec. 20.1). Some authorities recommend a brain biopsy to confirm the diagnosis of HSV encephalitis, especially when cutaneous vesicles are absent and CSF cultures are negative for HSV. The presumptive diagnosis of HSV encephalitis is not confirmed by biopsy in more than 50% of suspected cases; other potentially treatable diseases may be present. Others recommend empiric therapy based on the history, physical examination, laboratory tests, and imaging information.

TREATMENT. Early diagnosis and prompt initiation of specific antiviral drugs are critical factors in improving morbidity and mortality. Two antiviral agents are recommended: vidarabine, a nonspecific inhibitor of cellular and viral replication, and acyclovir, which is selectively activated by viral thymidine kinase to a phosphorylated derivative that subsequently acts as an inhibitor of viral DNA polymerase. *Vidarabine* is relatively nontoxic, has improved survival in patients with CNS and disseminated disease, and stops the progression of local skin, eye, and mouth disease to disseminated disease if it is administered for 10–14 days in a dose of 30 mg/kg/24 hr given as a 12-hr infusion. A CNS relapse will occur in approximately 2% of patients when treated with this protocol and requires reinstitution of treatment.

Acyclovir is superior to vidarabine for the treatment of HSV encephalitis in older children and adults. It requires less fluid for administration, does not improve mortality or morbidity in neonatal HSV infection compared with vidarabine, and is equally nontoxic compared with vidarabine. Although uncommon, toxic signs of acyclovir may occur and include phlebitis, renal dysfunction and acyclovir urinary crystal formation in the presence of dehydration or prior renal insufficiency (the drug is predominantly excreted unchanged by the kidney), and lethargy, confusion, tremor, coma, or seizures. Because of the ease of administration, acyclovir is the preferred drug for the treatment of neonatal HSV infection. Acyclovir in an intravenous dose of 10 mg/kg every 8 hr is usually administered for 10–14 days. A longer course (14–21 days) may be given for encephalitis. Recurrent cutaneous vesicles have been reported in 8% of acyclovir-treated patients; these are not due to acyclovir resistance but possibly to reduced HSV antibody production during acyclovir therapy. Repeated therapy with a higher dose (15 mg/kg every 8 hr) for a longer course (21 days) is recommended after recurrent CNS disease. Because some infants with isolated skin, eye, or mouth disease who have recurrent cutaneous vesicles may also demonstrate late signs of encephalitis, some authorities suggest suppressive oral acyclovir therapy for these infants during the first few months after birth. This suggestion is currently being examined as an investigational protocol.

Ocular HSV infection should be treated with parenteral and topical therapy. Ophthalmic antiviral agents include 1% trifluorothymidine (Viroptic), idoxuridine (Stoxil), and 3% vidarabine. The last is a commonly prescribed topical therapy.

PREVENTION. Infants delivered through an infected birth canal or following rupture of membranes (> 4–6 hr) in mothers with herpetic lesions are at risk for the development of neonatal HSV disease. Conjunctival, cutaneous, and nasopharyngeal cultures should be obtained between birth and 24 hr and topical ocular therapy initiated. Some authorities recommend parenteral therapy for these infants if the mother is symptomatic with active lesions of a primary HSV infection at the time of birth. The risk of transmission to the infant in this situation may be as high as 50%. However, most infants do not require immediate prophylactic antiviral therapy because their mothers have recurrent disease; the infants can be observed carefully for vesicles or manifestations of CNS or disseminated disease, and cultures can be performed at 2- to 3-day intervals for the first 2 wk of life. Isolation of virus at birth reflects contamination and is less significant than recovery of virus after 48 hr of life, which represents viral replication and active infection. Treatment is initiated in the presence of manifestations suggestive of HSV infection (vesicles, conjunctivitis, sepsis-syndrome, encephalitis) or a positive postnatal culture for HSV. This approach has not been tested for efficacy but remains the recommended protocol for the asymptomatic HSV-exposed infant.

Protocols suggested to identify the mother with active (asymptomatic primary or recurrent) genital viral excretion have been unsuccessful. Antepartum viral cultures do not predict the presence of HSV at parturition, and such screening programs are probably not effective in preventing neonatal HSV infection. Nonetheless, if active lesions are present at the time of labor, there is a risk of neonatal infection. Cesarean section may reduce this risk, especially if it is performed within 4–6 hr of rupture of membranes.

PROGNOSIS. Despite the advent of effective antiviral therapy, disseminated neonatal HSV infections and localized encephalitis have a considerable morbidity and mortality. The outcome is improved by early identification and prompt initiation of treatment before the onset of coma, shock, or disseminated intravascular coagulation. The prognosis for neonatal encephalitis due to HSV 1 appears to be better than that for HSV 2.

Arvin AM, Hensleigh PA, Prober CG, et al: Failure of antepartum maternal cultures to predict the infant's risk of exposure to herpes simplex virus at delivery. N Engl J Med 315:796, 1986.

Barker JA, McLean SD, Jordon GD, et al: Primary neonatal herpes simplex virus pneumonia. Pediatr Infect Dis J 9:285, 1990.

Brown ZA, Ashley R, Douglas J, et al: Neonatal herpes simplex virus infection: Relapse after initial therapy and transmission from a mother with an asymptomatic genital herpes infection and erythema multiforme. Pediatr Infect Dis J 6:1057, 1987.

Brown ZA, Baker DA: Acyclovir therapy during pregnancy. Obstet Gynecol 73:526, 1989.

Brown ZA, Vontver LA, Benedetti J, et al: Effects on infants of a first episode of genital herpes during pregnancy. N Engl J Med 317:1246, 1987.

Corey L, Stone EF, Whitley RJ, et al: Difference between herpes simplex virus type 1 and type 2 neonatal encephalitis in neurological outcome. Lancet 1:1, 1988.

Dankner WM, Spector SA: Recurrent herpes simplex in a neonate. Pediatr Infect Dis 5:582, 1986.

Hutto C, Arvin A, Jacobs R, et al: Intrauterine herpes simplex virus infections. J Pediatr 110:97, 1987.

Kohl S: The neonatal human's immune response to herpes simplex virus infection: A critical review. Pediatr Infect Dis J 8:67, 1989.

Kohl S, West MS, Prober CG, et al: Neonatal antibody-dependent cellular cytotoxic antibody levels are associated with the clinical presentation of neonatal herpes simplex virus infection. J Infect Dis 160:770, 1989.

Koskiniemi M, Happonen JM, Jarvenpaa AL, et al: Neonatal herpes simplex virus infection: A report of 43 patients. Pediatr Infect Dis J 8:30, 1989.

Prober CG, Sullender WM, Yasukawa LL, et al: Low risk of herpes simplex virus infections in neonates exposed to the virus at the time of vaginal

delivery to mothers with recurrent genital herpes simplex virus infections. N Engl J Med 316:240, 1987.
Prober CG, Hensleigh PA, Boucher FD, et al: Use of routine viral cultures at delivery to identify neonates exposed to herpes simplex virus. N Engl J Med 318:887, 1988.
Rabalais GP, Nusinoff-Lehrman S, Arvin AM, et al: Antiviral susceptibilities of herpes simplex virus isolates from infants with recurrent mucocutaneous lesions after neonatal infection. Pediatr Infect Dis J 8:221, 1989.
Whitley R, Arvin A, Prober C, et al: A control trial comparing vidarabine with acyclovir in neonatal herpes simplex virus infection. N Engl J Med 324:444, 1991.
Whitley RJ, Corey L, Arvin A, et al: Changing presentation of herpes simplex virus infection in neonates. J Infect Dis 158:109, 1988.

HUMAN IMMUNODEFICIENCY VIRUS (HIV)

See Sec. 12.82.

9.72 PARVOVIRUS B19

Human parvovirus B19, a single-stranded DNA virus that replicates in erythroid progenitor cells, is the cause of erythema infectiosum, aplastic crisis in patients with hereditary hemolytic anemias, and chronic red cell aplasia in immunocompromised patients. Following symptomatic or asymptomatic maternal infection during pregnancy, fetal infection may result in asymptomatic seroconversion, no seroconversion, 2nd trimester fetal death, or stillbirth secondary to severe fetal anemia and the development of hydrops. Fetal infection occurs in 15–25% of seronegative mothers who acquire infection during pregnancy. The excess risk of fetal death in a susceptible woman due to parvovirus in the first 20 wk of pregnancy is estimated at 3–9%. The risk of fetal loss for a mother with an unknown serology is 50% of that for susceptible patients because half of women of childbearing age are seropositive for parvovirus B19. The risk of fetal loss is similar when the infection is acquired in the 1st or 2nd trimester but is less in the 3rd trimester. Teachers, day-care center workers, and pediatric health care providers are at increased risk of acquiring parvovirus infection.

CLINICAL MANIFESTATIONS. Maternal parvovirus B19 infection may be asymptomatic or associated with low-grade fever, rash, and arthralgia; thus, it may resemble rubella infection. Respiratory secretions and, rarely, blood products are the sources of human-to-human spread, but maternal viremia with transplacental passage is the mechanism for fetal infection. Parvovirus B19 infections during pregnancy have been associated with stillbirths, fatal nonimmune hydrops fetalis, subclinical infection documented by fetal IgM, or no apparaent infection (80–85%). Neonatal anemia has resulted from 3rd trimester maternal infection. Parvovirus is not a teratogen and does not produce a typical syndrome following fetal infection.

DIAGNOSIS. Parvovirus B19 virus has been detected in fetal tissues using radiolabeled cloned parvovirus DNA as a probe. IgG and IgM antibodies to B19, utilizing an antibody captive ELISA, have been used to demonstrate past and recent infection with B19.

TREATMENT. There is no specific treatment. Pregnant health care workers should not care for patients with aplastic crises because they remain infectious during this time. After the rash of erythema infectiosum appears, patients are unlikely to be contagious, and isolation is unnecessary. Exclusion of pregnant women from the workplace where erythema infectiosum is occurring is currently not recommended. Because of the widespread inapparent infection in children and adults, some risk of exposure occurs frequently, and avoidance of child care or teaching for a limited period can only reduce but not eliminate the risk of infection. Pregnant women who have been in contact with parvovirus B19 can be tested serologically and monitored with fetal ultrasound and α-fetoprotein determinations. Intrauterine management of nonimmune hydrops has been reported in a few patients; percutaneous umbilical vein blood transfusion with packed red blood cells has reversed the fetal anemia with resolution of hydrops.

Anand A, Gray ES, Brown T, et al: Human parvovirus infection in pregnancy and hydrops fetalis. N Engl J Med 316:183, 1987.
Centers for Disease Control: Risks associated with human parvovirus B19 infection. MMWR 38:81, 1989.
Committee on Infectious Disease: Parvovirus, erythema infectiosum, and pregnancy. Pediatrics 85:131, 1990.
Public Health Laboratory Service Working Party on Fifth Disease: Prospective study of human parvovirus (B19) infection in pregnancy. Br Med J 300:1166, 1990.
Soothill P: Intrauterine blood transfusion for non-immune hydrops fetalis due to parvovirus B19 infection. Lancet 336:121, 1990.
Ware R: Human parvovirus infection. J Pediatr 114:343, 1989.

9.73 RUBELLA

See also Sec 12.65.

Rubella (German measles) infection during pregnancy is associated with variable rates of fetal infection and rates of teratogenesis that are gestational age–dependent. Rubella is an RNA virus of the Togavirus family. Wild virus infection or attenuated vaccine virus immunization usually produces lifelong immunity.

EPIDEMIOLOGY. Rubella is a self-limited disease that occurs in the winter and spring and is transmitted by person-to-person contact. Mass immunization of children with attenuated vaccine has induced immunity in 80–90% of the population. Unfortunately, outbreaks continue to occur, predominantly in adolescents and young adults attending college or in workplaces with close person-to-person contact.

PATHOGENESIS. Viremia is present during symptomatic or asymptomatic primary infection in pregnant women; as many as 50% of infected women may be asymptomatic. The virus infects the placenta and is transmitted to the fetus, disseminating to multiple organs and tissues. Reinfection during pregnancy (e.g., pre-existing rubella antibodies and a significant rise in rubella IgG or the appearance of IgM) is a rare but possible cause of congenital rubella infection and teratogenesis. Inadvertent immunization of seronegative pregnant women with the current RA 27/3 vaccine rarely produces fetal infection (1–2%) and does not cause congenital anomalies or manifestations of congenital rubella syndrome. Rates of congenital infection following primary maternal rubella infection range from 75–90% in the 1st trimester, 25–39% in the 2nd, and 24–53% in the 3rd trimester. Periconceptional transmission with subsequent anomalies is uncommon. Maternal rubella may produce no fetal infection, infection alone, infection plus congenital anomalies, embryo resorption, abortion, or stillbirth.

The risk of congenital malformations depends on the gestational age at the time of maternal infection and varies from 30% between 9 and l2 wk of age to 10% from 13 to 20 wk. After 20 wk of gestation, there is little risk of congenital anomalies; however, infections may produce chronic disease and dysfunction of the eye, ear, and central nervous system. Congenital heart disease is common when infection occurs before 12 wk of gestation; deafness tends to occur with infection before 12 wk and up to 16 wk gestation.

Fetal viremia with subsequent dissemination produces a chronic infection with persistent viral excretion in utero and for months to years after birth. Rubella virus may produce fetal injury by many mechanisms, including inhibition of cell mitosis, cytolysis, placental villitis, persistent cell infection that may produce deafness (organ of Corti), myocarditis, pneumonitis, encephalitis, hepatitis, and fetal or placental vasculitis. Many of these mechanisms can limit fetal growth by reducing cell number (cytolysis, mitotic inhibition) or cell size (placentitis) or by producing anomalies (cytolysis, vasculitis). The most likely predominant factor associated with fetal injury is vascular insufficiency and tissue necrosis, since active inflammation is not observed and in vivo cytolysis is probably a rare occurrence. Chronic fetal and neonatal infection occurs despite placental transfer of maternal rubella-specific IgG and initial fetal production of IgM, followed by late fetal and neonatal production of IgG. Immune-mediated injury, due to overstimulation of the immune system, which produces immune complexes and autoantibodies in combination with persistent or reactivated viral infection, may produce the delayed sequelae of congenital rubella infection such as pneumonitis, diabetes mellitis, thyroiditis, and progressive rubella panencephalitis.

The pathology of congenital rubella infection reveals vasculitis, secondary but less extensive inflammation, and cell necrosis. The placenta demonstrates villitis with endothelial cell necrosis and edema. Cytolysis may occur, as shown by the presence of nuclear pyknosis, karyorrhexis, cytoplasmic eosinophila, and cell necrosis. Fetal tissues are hypoplastic and reveal a necrotizing angiopathy that is similar to that seen in the placenta.

CLINICAL MANIFESTATIONS. Rubella may produce transient neonatal manifestations, permanent organ malformations and tissue injury, and delayed late onset illnesses due to chronic infection or autoimmune phenomena. Late onset manifestations may occur 2 mo to 20 yr after birth (Table 9–34 and see Fig. 9–28).

Central nervous system involvement is frequent in symptomatic infants. Lethargy, irritability, disturbances of tone, and a bulging fontanel are common. Seizures may occur but often are not observed until after the neonatal period. Elevation of the protein concentration in the cerebrospinal fluid is common, but elevation of CSF cell counts is less frequent; rubella virus can often be isolated from the CSF. The extent of impairment of infants at 18 mo of age is not predictable on the basis of clinical symptomatology or virus isolation in the first few weeks of life. Severe involvement is more frequent, however, in infants with seizures and high levels of CSF protein during the neonatal period.

Cataracts, the most characteristic ocular lesion, may not be recognized until after the neonatal period. The retina also may be involved, and lesions may be widespread, mottled, or blotchy, with black pigmentary deposits that are variable in size and location—the "salt and pepper" retinitis. Retinal function is usually not adversely affected.

Bone lesions consist of small linear areas of radiolucency and increased bone density in a longitudinal axis of the metaphyseal area in the long bones of the upper and lower extremities. The abnormality usually resolves by 2–3 mo of age. The lesions may be differentiated from those observed in congenital syphilis by the absence of periosteal reaction.

Many infected infants may be asymptomatic in the newborn period. However, as many as 70% subsequently develop evidence of congenital rubella. The most significant delayed manifestations include hearing loss (87%), congenital heart disease (46%), mental retardation (39%), and cataract or glaucoma (34%). Children thought to have normal hearing when tested early in life have subsequently been found to have a hearing loss when they reached school age. The hearing loss may be profound and may be a major contributor to speech impairment and learning disabilities. Mental retardation, when present, is frequently severe. Cerebral dysfunction and psychiatric disorders, including reactive behavior disorder and infantile autism, occur.

Mortality due to congenital rubella results from prematurity, myocarditis, interstitial pneumonia, hepatitis, and progressive panencephalitis. CNS morbidity is due to chronic persistent encephalitis and sensory deficits resulting from visual and auditory impairment. Delayed onset endocrinopathies complicate the long-term management.

DIAGNOSIS. Virus can be isolated from the nasopharyngeal secretions, conjunctivae, urine, stool, CSF, circulating leukocytes, and, when available, from the lens and bone marrow. Viral excretion is most active 1–3 mo after birth; 2–20% of infants are excreting virus at 1 yr of age and 0–2% by

TABLE 9–34. Manifestations of Congenital Rubella Syndrome

Transient	Permanent	Development	Late Onset
Common			
Hepatosplenomegaly	Intrauterine growth retardation	Psychomotor retardation	Diabetes mellitis
Conjugated hyperbilirubinemia	Postnatal growth retardation	Behavioral disorders	Chronic transient rubelliform rash
Purpura	Patent ductus arteriosus	Hypotonia	
Thrombocytopenia	Peripheral pulmonic stenosis		
"Blueberry muffin" rash*	Pulmonary valve stenosis		
Adenopathy	Cataracts		
Bony radiolucencies†	Microphthalmia		
Meningoencephalitis	Retinopathy		
EEG abnormalities	Sensorineural hearing loss		
	Deafness		
	Small head circumference relative to family		
Uncommon			
Prematurity	Ventriculoseptal defect	Autism	Chronic progressive panencephalitis
Myocarditis	Atrial septal defect		Interstitial pneumonitis
Cloudy cornea	Glaucoma		Hyperthyroidism
Hepatitis	Microcephaly		Hypothyroidism
Interstitial pneumonitis	Intracranial calcifications		Thyroiditis
Hemolytic anemia	Renal artery stenosis, hypertension		Precocious puberty
Hypogammaglobulinemia	Thymic hypoplasia		Growth hormone deficiency
Large anterior fontanel	Abnormal tooth morphology		Subretinal neovascularization
Leukopenia			Keratoconus
			Lens absorption

*Dermal erythropoiesis

†Celery stalk lesions at ends of the femur and humerus (see Sec. 9.73).

2 yr of age.The Centers for Disease Control case definition for a diagnosis of congenital rubella in an infant of a mother with or without a history of a febrile rash illness includes: *confirmed cases*: typical congenital defects plus isolation of virus or detectable rubella IgM or persisting rubella hemagglutination inhibition (HI) titer; *compatible cases*: insufficient laboratory data plus two of the following: cataracts, glaucoma, heart disease, hearing loss, pigmentary retinopathy or one of the former plus one of the following: purpura, splenomegaly, jaundice, radiolucent bone lesions, meningoencephalitis, microcephaly, mental retardation; *possible cases*: some clinical findings but insufficient to meet the criteria for diagnosis; *congenital rubella infection only*: no defects visible but viral culture is positive or rubella-specific IgM antibody is present. Congenital rubella is not considered if the HI titer is absent in the mother or in a child younger than 2 yr of age and if the HI titer in the infant declines in a manner compatible with that of passively transferred maternal IgG. The usual rate of decline is 1- to 2-fold dilution/mo with an absent titer by 6–12 mo of age.

Prenatal diagnosis is possible by RNA hybridization of chorionic villus biopsy samples and culture of amniotic fluid.

TREATMENT. There is no specific chemotherapy for rubella virus infection. Careful and repeated developmental, auditory, visual, and endocrinologic assessment improves the quality of life of these children. Knowledge that this is not a static disease and that it has many late and possibly progressive life-threatening manifestations has improved the management. Corrective cardiac surgery, hearing aids, speech therapy, special education, and repeated psychologic testing are essential therapeutic and diagnostic interventions.

PREVENTION. See Sec. 5.1 and 12.65.

Best JM, Banatvala JE, Morgan-Capner P, et al: Fetal infection after maternal reinfection with rubella: Criteria for defining reinfection. Br Med J 299:773, 1989.

Centers for Disease Control: Rubella vaccination during pregnancy—United States, 1971–1986. MMWR 36:457, 1987.

De Owens CS, De Espino RT: Rubella in Panama: Still a problem. Pediatr Infect Dis J 8:110, 1989.

Enders G, Miller E, Nickerl-Pacher U, et al: Outcome of confirmed periconceptional maternal rubella. Lancet 1:1445, 1988.

Freij BJ, South MA, Sever JL: Maternal rubella and the congenital rubella syndrome. Clin Perinatol 15:247, 1988.

Munro ND, Smithells RW, Sheppard S, et al: Temporal relations between maternal rubella and congenital defects. Lancet 2:201, 1987.

Tingle AJ, Chantler JK, Pot KH, et al: Postpartum rubella immunization: Association with development of prolonged arthritis, neurological sequelae, and chronic rubella viremia. J Infect Dis 152:606, 1985.

Tokugawa K, Ueda K, Fukushige J, et al: Congenital rubella syndrome and physical growth: A 17-year, prospective, longitudinal follow-up in the Ryukyu islands. Rev Infect Dis 8:824, 1986.

9.74 VARICELLA

See also Sec. 12.69.

The incidence of varicella during pregnancy is 1-5/10,000 pregnancies. The risk of transplacental fetal infection following maternal varicella infection is approximately 25%, and congenital malformations are noted in 5% of fetuses infected in the 1st and 2nd trimesters. About 25% of newborns delivered to mothers with varicella during the last 3 wk of pregnancy will develop clinical infection, presumably acquired hematogenously following maternal and subsequent fetal viremia. If maternal varicella occurs 5–21 days prior to delivery, neonatal disease appears in the first 4 days, and the prognosis is good owing to the production and passage of maternal varicella IgG antibody. When maternal varicella presents between 5 days before to 2 days after delivery, neonatal varicella appears between 5 and 10 days of age. The illness may be mild or severe with up to a 30% mortality. The neonatal incubation period is shorter than that seen later in childhood (9–15 days compared with 14–21 days) following intrauterine infection owing to a high-grade maternal viremia that passes the placenta, causing fetal viremia without the initial nasopharyngeal viral replication that characterizes infection in postnatal varicella. Death is due to pulmonary and visceral involvement. Infants infected postnatally by the respiratory route are at no higher risk than older infants, although severe infection may be noted in some seronegative full-term infants in the 1st mo of life. Preterm infants are at increased risk because placental passage of IgG occurs late in the 3rd trimester; thus, many premature infants lack protective varicella IgG antibody. Chickenpox rather than zoster is associated with transmission to the fetus or neonate; the former is contagious owing to respiratory secretions and is accompanied by maternal viremia, but neither mechanism is relevant to zoster.

CLINICAL MANIFESTATIONS. The congenital varicella syndrome, acquired in the first half of pregnancy, is characterized by one or more of the following: cicatricial dermatomal scarring, unilateral limb hypoplasia and paresis, rudimentary digits, microcephaly, cortical and cerebellar atrophy, psychomotor retardation, seizures, chorioretinitis, cataracts, Horner's syndrome, nystagmus, and microphthalmia. Congenital varicella transmitted in the last 3 wk of pregnancy may be mild, with only a few vesicular lesions, or severe, with fever, hemorrhagic rash, pneumonia, and generalized necrotic lesions of the viscera. Neonates with congenital or postnatal varicella have a high incidence of zoster in the first 10 yr of life.

DIAGNOSIS. Diagnosis can usually be made clinically from the history and characteristic rash. Virus may be isolated with difficulty from the vesicular fluid, inclusion bodies are more often seen in Tzanck smears made from the base of lesions, and varicella-zoster antigen may be demonstrated by ELISA, counterimmunoelectrophoresis, or immunofluorescence. Serologic tests are available but are usually unnecessary. The differential diagnosis includes HSV 2 or HSV 1 infection.

TREATMENT AND PREVENTION. Acyclovir may be used for treatment of moderate to severe cases of neonatal varicella. Higher doses (15 mg/kg every 8 hr for 7 days) are used than for treatment of neonatal herpes. There are no controlled studies in neonates, but efficacy has been documented in older immunocompromised patients; very little toxicity has been observed. Acyclovir may rarely produce renal dysfunction with crystallization of the drug in the urine of patients who have had prior dehydration or renal insufficiency. Neurotoxicity is manifest as lethargy, seizures, coma, agitation, and jitteriness.

Varicella-zoster immune globulin (VZIG, in a dose of 125 units or a 1.25-ml vial given intramuscularly) is recommended for infants born to mothers who develop varicella within 5 days before to 2 days after delivery and for at-risk premature infants of less than 28 wk of gestation or weighing less than 1,000 g at birth, in order to prevent or attenuate the disease.

Varicella in newborns or mothers is highly contagious, and strict isolation is indicated, for both patients with active disease and asymptomatic patients late in the incubation period. VZIG is recommended for exposed seronegative mothers (125 units/10 kg, maximum 5 mL [625 units] given intramuscularly) but has not been demonstrated to prevent fetal-neonatal infection or teratogenesis.

Patients with active varicella should be isolated in a closed room to prevent nosocomial spread. Visitors and care providers should be seropositive, wear masks and gowns, avoid contact with respiratory secretions, and wash their hands after contact with the patient. If siblings have chickenpox at home and the mother is seronegative, both mother and newborn should avoid contact with the infected siblings; if this is not possible, they should both receive VZIG before going home. If the mother is seronegative and has no lesions but has been exposed to varicella 6–20 days prior to birth, she should be considered potentially contagious and should be discharged with her infant as soon as possible. There is a high risk of nosocomical varicella when the mother develops lesions within 5 days prior to or soon after delivery. The mother and infant should be discharged when it is clinically safe to do so, and exposed mothers and infants should also be sent home as soon as possible.

If seronegative health care workers or patients are exposed to varicella, they may become infectious within 8–21 days of exposure. Seronegative health care providers should be excluded from patient activities, and exposed seronegative patients should be isolated during this period. If maternal disease occurs 5 days before or immediately after birth and no lesions are evident in the infant, both should be isolated separately to prevent postnatal acquisition of varicella by the neonate and because approximately 50% of such neonates develop varicella from transplacental viremia within 7–15 days after the onset of maternal lesions, despite neonatal VZIG administration.

Aklalay AL, Pomerance JJ, Rimoin DL: Fetal varicella syndrome. J Pediatr 111:320, 1987.
Freij BJ, Sever JL: Herpesvirus infections in pregnancy. Clin Perinatol 15:215, 1988.
Gershon AA: Chickenpox, Measles and Mumps. *In:* Remington JS, Klein JO (eds): Infectious Diseases of the Fetus and Newborn Infant. Philadelphia, WB Saunders, 1990, p 396.
Grose C, Itani O: Pathogenesis of congenital infection with three diverse viruses: Varicella-zoster virus, human parvovirus, and human immunodeficiency virus. Semin Perinatol 13:278, 1989.
Lipton S, Brunell PA: Management of varicella exposure in a neonatal intensive care unit. JAMA 261:1782, 1989.
Miller E, Cradock-Watson JE, Ridehalgh MK: Outcome in newborn babies given antivaricella-zoster immunoglobulin after perinatal maternal infection with varicella-zoster virus. Lancet 2:371, 1989.
Wurzel CL, Rubin LG, Krilov LR: Varicella zoster immunoglobulin after postnatal exposure to varicella: Survey of experts. Pediatr Infect Dis J 6:466, 1987.

9.75 CANDIDA

Candida species are a common cause of oral mucous membrane (thrush) and perineal skin infections (diaper dermatitis) in newborn infants, but they also produce nosocomial systemic infections in premature infants in special care nurseries. Congenital intrauterine candidiasis, transmitted via the ascending route through ruptured or intact amniotic membranes, is a rare infection and is associated with cervical cerclage, intrauterine devices, and premature labor. The organisms are usually acquired during birth, and the majority of exposed infants are colonized by the end of the 1st wk of life. Clinical infection appears to be related to inoculum size. Nosocomial infection is associated with the use of broad-spectrum antimicrobial therapy, a prolonged hospital stay, indwelling vascular catheters, very low birthweight (< 1,500 g), endotracheal intubation, use of corticosteroids, and parenteral nutrition.

ETIOLOGY. *Candida* has three predominant morphologic forms. Yeast cells (blastospores) are 1.5–5 μm in diameter, bud asexually, grow on body surfaces and fluids, initiate invasive lesions, and may cause toxic or inflammatory reactions. Chlamydospores are larger (7–17 μm) and are unusual as a form of systemic illness. Hyphae (pseudomycelia) forms are the tissue, rather than the contamination, phase of *Candida* and are filamentous processes that elongate from the yeast cell.

C. albicans is the most common candidal species causing infection in the newborn (75–85%); *C. tropicalis* (10%), and *C. parapsilosis* (5%) also have been isolated. *Malassezia furfur*, a lipophilic fungus, is another cause of nosocomial fungemia in high-risk neonates who are receiving intravenous alimentation with intravenous lipids through central venous catheters. Candida are also transmitted to the fetus or newborn by ascending vaginal infection at the time of vaginal delivery or are acquired after birth from the mother or other sources.

PATHOGENESIS. Candida may rarely produce rapidly fatal aspiration fungal pneumonia immediately after birth. More often, nosocomial infection follows a period of colonization of the skin, oropharynx, and gastrointestinal tract. The high incidence of invasive candidal infection in low-birthweight infants may be due to mechanical factors (indwelling catheters disturbing the cutaneous barrier), alterations of the normal bacterial flora's inhibition of fungal growth (e.g., by broad-spectrum antibiotics), or immaturity of humoral or cellular host defense mechanisms. The precise roles of candidal IgG, neutrophil phagocytosis, and fungicidal cellular immunity as defense mechanisms for neonatal candidal infections have not been defined.

CLINICAL MANIFESTATIONS. *Thrush* consists of white curd-like plaques on the tongue, gums, or buccal mucosa. Removal of the white membrane reveals an erythematous base. The skin manifestations are erythematous (beefy red) maculopapular or vesicular scaling lesions that may coalesce and then form satellite lesions. Intertriginous areas, particularly in the perineum and diaper area, are usually involved. The infection occurs in 4–8% of term infants and peaks at 2–4 mo of age.

Congenital candidiasis presents as a generalized, intensely erythematous eruption in the first 12 hr of life. The rash may desquamate and become pustular. It contains fungi and is associated with fungal "colonies," which are visible as small yellow-white lesions on the placenta and umbilical cord. Preterm infants frequently have systemic disease characterized by pneumonia, leukocytosis, shock, and a high mortality. Parenteral theraphy is required. Full-term infants usually have disease localized to the skin and can be treated with topical antifungal agents.

The clinical manifestations of *nosocomial or delayed congenital invasive candidiasis* are similar to those of neonatal sepsis. The incidence is as high as 2–5% of very low birthweight infants in a neonatal intensive care unit. Respiratory insufficiency, apnea, bradycardia, temperature instability, glucose intolerance, feeding intolerance, and abdominal distention (necrotizing enterocolitis-like picture) are most common. Skin manifestations characteristic of congenital infection, diffuse sunburn-like erythema, and solitary or multiple subcutaneous abscesses occur in approximately 50% of cases. Clinical signs of meningeal involvement are less common than abnormal cerebrospinal fluid, which occurs in about half the infants with invasive candidal disease. Cerebrospinal fluid cultures are positive in one third of infants with systemic infection. Renal involvement is common and is manifested by positive urine cultures (in urine samples obtained by catheterization or suprapubic aspiration), renal insufficiency, or ultrasonographic abnormalities (filling defects). Endocarditis is unusual but should be considered in infants with persistent fungemia and a central venous catheter near or in the heart. Echocardiography may demonstrate valvular lesions, a thrombus, or intracardiac fungal masses. Fungal septic arthritis, osteomyelitis, and endophthalmitis may develop in association with disseminated nosocomial infection. Hepatic and possibly splenic microabscess may complicate candidal sepsis.

It is important to distinguish between catheter-associated transient candidemia and disseminated candidiasis. The former is characterized by positive blood cultures owing to contamination of in situ intravascular catheters but no evidence of focal or disseminated disease and may be treated by removing the catheter. Disseminated candidiasis is characterized by involvement of one or more organ systems, positive cultures of candida from a normally sterile fluid or tissue, or a positive culture in the absence of an intravascular catheter. Candidal sepsis is frequently indolent. Untreated patients may be fungemic for 2–3 days and occasionally appear to improve spontaneously only subsequently to develop shock, meningitis, and osteoarticular infection, leading to death. Blood cultures positive for *Candida* should be repeated and should be considered representative of infection rather than a contaminant.

DIAGNOSIS. The diagnosis of mucocutaneous infection is confirmed by scraping the membrane or skin lesion and demonstrating hyphae, pseudohyphae, or yeast forms. Diagnosis of invasive disease is made by culturing candida from normally sterile body fluids. Blood cultures should be labeled to notify the laboratory that fungemia is expected so special media can be used and incubation prolonged. Methylene blue or Gram stain of exudates or buffy coat may provide presumptive evidence of disease. Demonstration of a fungal antigen may be useful in the future, but this technique requires further study. Serologic methods are not helpful. The white blood cell counts are variable; a marked leukocytosis may be noted. Thrombocytopenia is a common early finding. Elevation of blood urea nitrogen, creatinine, bilirubin, and liver enzymes may occur in the course of systemic candidiasis. Ultrasound of catheter tip sites (to rule out infected thrombi), kidneys, heart, and the central nervous system (to rule out hydrocephalus) should be performed. Formal ophthalmologic consultation for indirect funduscopic examination is necessary to rule out chorioretinitis or endophthalmitis, which may threaten vision.

TREATMENT. Thrush should be treated with oral nystatin or gentian violet. Skin infection should respond to topical nystatin, clotrimazole, or gentian violet. Since candida are present in the gastrointestinal tract, oral nystatin may be added to decrease the inoculum and the likelihood of recurrence.

Treatment of neonates with systemic candidiasis is controversial. Most authorities use amphotericin B alone, whereas others combine intravenous amphotericin with oral flucytosine. Despite frequent resistance to flucytosine, its combination with amphotericin is synergistic against *Candida*. Amphotericin B is usually given in an initial dose of 0.25 mg/kg, with doses increased in 0.25-mg/kg increments every 24–48 hr up to a dose of 0.5–1 mg/kg/24 hr (occasionally 1.5 mg/kg/24 hr). Amphotericin is administered in a 5–10% dextrose in water infusion, without electrolytes, over 4–6 hr. Catheter-associated candidemia has been treated with a total dose of 10–15 mg/kg. Removal of the catheter is recommended, if possible, because *Candida* is difficult to eradicate from colonized central lines and the dose of amphotericin B may be reduced to 5–10 mg/kg/hr if the catheter is removed, the fungemia is rapidly cleared, and there is no evidence of metastatic disease. Disseminated candidiasis requires a total amphotericin dose of as much as 25–35 mg/kg. Toxicity to amphotericin occurs in approximately half of treated infants, with elevations of BUN and creatinine, oliguric renal failure, and hypokalemia. Potassium supplementation and adjustment in daily dosage or alternate-day antifungal therapy may be necessary. Bone marrow suppression and hepatotoxicity are less common. Toxicity is diminished in patients treated with 0.5 mg/kg/24 hr of amphotericin and 100 mg/kg/24 hr of flucytosine. Toxic effects of flucytosine include gastrointestinal dysfunction, hepatotoxicity, and bone marrow suppression.

Baley JE, Kliegman RM, Fanaroff AA: Disseminated fungal infections in very low birthweight infants: Clinical manifestations and epidemiology. Pediatrics 73:144, 1984.

Baley JE, Silverman RA: Systemic candidiasis: Cutaneous manifestations in low birthweight infants. Pediatrics 82:211, 1988.

Butler KM, Baker CJ: Candida: An increasingly important pathogen in the nursery. Pediatr Clin North Am 35:543, 1988.

Butler KM, Rench MA, Baker CJ: Amphotericin B as a single agent in the treatment of systemic candidiasis in neonates. Pediatr Infect Dis J 9:743, 1990.

Dankner WM, Spector SA, Fierer J, et al: *Malassezia* fungemia in neonates and adults: Complication of hyperalimentation. Rev Infect Dis 9:743, 1987.

Eppes SC, Troutman JL, Gutman LT: Outcome of treatment of candidemia in children whose central catheters were removed or retained. Pediatr Infect Dis J 8:99, 1989.

Weese-Mayer DE, Fondriest DW, Brouillette RT, et al: Risk factors associated with candidemia in the neonatal intensive care unit: A case-control study. Pediatr Infect Dis J 6:190, 1987.

TOXOPLASMOSIS

See Sec. 12.112.

SAMUEL P. GOTOFF

10

SPECIAL HEALTH PROBLEMS DURING ADOLESCENCE

Although adolescents (11–20 yr of age) constituted 17% of the population of the United States during 1980–1981, they were responsible for only 11% of office visits to physicians. Most visits were for acute conditions, compared with all other age groups for whom chronic illness or nonillness health care predominated (see also Sec. 3.57). The low rate of utilization of private physicians may reflect the generally good health of adolescents or an inappropriate pattern of physician utilization. Whatever the cause, the result is that physicians, and particularly pediatricians, have relatively less opportunity to evaluate and counsel teenagers than other children.

Younger adolescents had higher rates of office visits than older adolescents. Females in the 15- to 20-yr age group had higher rates than males, primarily because of gynecologic or obstetric care. For the younger adolescents, the leading diagnostic category was respiratory illness (21%), followed by routine examinations, injuries, or poisonings (16%). For older adolescents, after routine examinations, the leading diagnoses included diseases of the skin and subcutaneous tissue (14%), followed by diseases of the respiratory system (13%), injury (13%), and poisoning (13%). Thirty-five per cent of office visits of all adolescents were made to general practitioners and family physicians, whereas 29% of office visits were made to pediatricians by the 11- to 14-yr-old group, and only 8% were made by 15- to 20-yr-old patients.

Data from the National Health Examination Survey of 1966–1970 showed that 20% of presumably healthy 12–17 yr olds had previously *undiagnosed health problems*. These problems were primarily related to the rapid growth and maturation that characterizes puberty and included such problems as scoliosis (Sec. 24.15), slipped capital femoral epiphysis (Sec. 24.11), Osgood-Schlatter disease (Sec. 24.6), goiter (Sec. 19.14), and acne (Sec. 23.32). In addition, a number of health problems regarded as "adult" problems in the past are actually present during adolescence, albeit in preclinical form (e.g., hypertension, hypercholesterolemia, and carcinoma-in-situ of the cervix).

Violence, such as accidents, homicides, or suicides, accounts for 70% of all adolescent *deaths*. Neoplasms (7%), infectious diseases, or diseases of a congenital nature (7%) account for a significantly smaller proportion of adolescent deaths. Among the neoplasms, testicular tumors and tumors of bone or lymphatics are most prevalent.

The birth rate has leveled off for all other age groups but continues to rise for young adolescents; they lead the nation in cases of *sexually transmitted disease*, such as gonorrhea, chlamydia, and human papilloma viral infections. Certain nonsexually transmitted infectious diseases now have their peak incidence among adolescents, including rubella, rubeola, infectious mononucleosis, and toxic shock syndrome.

Health-destructive behavior, such as cigarette and marijuana smoking and abuse of alcohol and other drugs (often in combination with driving), continues to present serious problems for adolescents. Eating disorders, such as anorexia nervosa and bulimia, are increasing in prevalence, the former reported to affect 1% of 16- to 18-yr-old females in the United States.

10.1 ACCIDENTS

See also Sec. 6.31.

Automobile and motorcycle accidents are the leading causes of adolescent morbidity and mortality. Sixteen to 19 yr olds comprise 8% of the population and account for 17% of vehicular fatalities; 63% of automotive deaths among adolescents involve passengers in cars driven by adolescents. Sports injuries and accidental drowning are additional prominent causes of adolescent morbidity and mortality.

Alcohol is a factor underlying most vehicular fatalities, along with failure to use seat belts in cars or helmets while riding motorcycles. Most of these accidents involve male adolescents and occur between 8:00 P.M. and 4:00 A.M. Lowering the drinking age to 18 yr of age has been associated with a 5% increase in fatal automotive accidents. Driver's education classes have been associated with increased mortality rates, because they increase the number of younger drivers on the road. Pediatricians can address this problem among adolescents through anticipatory guidance and legislation aimed at raising the drinking age and enforcing the use of seat belts and helmets.

PSYCHOSOCIAL PROBLEMS

10.2 DEPRESSION

See also Sec. 3.33.

Adolescence is a time of increased emotionality, hypothetical thinking, and empathy (Sec. 3.9). As a result, it is a time for mood swings from the depth of depression to the heights of elation. It is often difficult to decide which sad-looking adolescent is at risk for true depression and even suicide. The hallmarks of the youngster who is at risk are the persistence of the depressed mood, the absence of corresponding periods of elation, the inability to function, and the expression of hopelessness and helplessness. Puig-Antich suggests that the depressed mood should be considered persistent if it lasts for at least 3 consecutive hours for three periods or more each week.

DIAGNOSIS. Assessment of the adolescent's functional status should focus on school performance and on peer and family interactions. Symptoms of depression in the adolescent may include falling school grades, an increase in school absenteeism or truancy, use of alcohol or drugs, accident-proneness, and pervasive boredom. Alternatively, persistent euphoria, if combined with acting-out behavior such as promiscuity, may mask depression (see later). Disturbances of eating and sleeping are not as pervasive in adolescents as in depressed adults but may be quite severe when present.

Initial insomnia and difficulty in falling asleep, sometimes to the extent of sleeping all day and remaining awake at night without ever feeling rested, are common signs of depression in adolescents. A family history of depressive illness increases the likelihood of depression, particularly if this history includes a suicide attempt.

Suicide (see Sec. 3.37, 5.1, and later). When severe depression is suspected, the physician should ask if the patient has ever felt so sad that death was considered to be a preferable alternative to living. If the patient answers in the affirmative, it is appropriate to inquire about the existence of a plan for self-destruction. The patient who has a suicide plan must be evaluated immediately by a psychiatrist. The adolescent who is not contemplating suicide will not be harmed by such questioning and is often relieved to have an opportunity to discuss his or her concerns with a caring physician. The physician also should not be misled by the adolescent who suddenly appears cheerful after a period of depression, because such a change may accompany the youngster's resolution of ambivalence and the decision to resolve sadness by suicide.

CLINICAL MANIFESTATIONS. Mattsson describes five forms of adolescent depression in order of increasing pathology:

1. ***Normal depressive mood swings.***
2. ***Acute depressive reactions.*** These normally occur after death or separation from a loved one and are the equivalent of a healthy grief response. Although feelings of mourning may preoccupy the adolescent for weeks or months, there is a gradual change toward resolution and restoration of normal functioning. If such an adolescent denies suicidal thoughts and if there is no increase in risk-taking behavior, he or she may be managed by close observation by the primary care physician.
3. ***Neurotic depressive disorders.*** These disorders may follow lack of resolution of a grief reaction and are characterized by feelings of hopelessness and helplessness, of self-incrimination and guilt in relationship to the lost individual, of difficulty in concentration, of withdrawal from school and social contacts, and of interference with normal sleeping, eating, and activity. A desire to join the deceased may be elicited after careful questioning. This form of depression should be managed by a psychiatrist.
4. ***Masked depression.*** In this variant of the neurotic depressive disorder, the youngster deals with his or her feelings of despair by denial and somatization. "Acting-out" behavior, such as running away from home, school truancy, multiple accidents, and substance abuse, may be the manifestations of this form of depression, as may the appearance of headaches, abdominal pain, or other physical complaints. Psychiatric management is indicated.
5. ***Psychotic depressive disorders.*** Impaired reality testing, thought distortion, and delusions of guilt may be present in addition to characteristics already described. Patients should be referred for psychiatric treatment.

10.3 SUICIDE

See Sec. 3.37 and 5.1.

Suicide is the 3rd leading cause of death among 15 to 19 yr olds in the United States and has been increasing in incidence during the last 2 decades. Females lead males in the incidence of suicide attempts, whereas male adolescents outnumber females in completed suicides. Native Americans and Asian Americans have a higher suicide rate than the general population. The chronically ill adolescent is also at increased risk for suicide as a result of feelings of impotence, diminished competence, and vulnerability to loss of a loved one; there is also often increased access to medication that may facilitate suicide.

The *method of suicide* most commonly used by teenagers is ingestion of medication. The medication may be the patient's own or often that of a parent with whom there has been conflict. The drug most often used in suicide attempts is a tricyclic antidepressant. A "bubble-pack" or similar unit-dose form of packaging should be prescribed when there is any concern that medication may be used in a suicide attempt. More violent methods, such as hanging, shooting, or wrist-slashing, are used most often by males and by those most intent on completing the act. Nevertheless, it is often difficult to assess the seriousness of the intent by the actual potency of the method. Beck and associates found medical lethality of methods to correlate poorly with seriousness of intent. There was, however, good correlation between the latter and the patient's expectation of lethality, which was often inaccurate.

Other factors to be considered in assessing the seriousness of a suicide attempt are the extent of premeditation and the likelihood of rescue. The adolescent who impulsively grabs a bottle from the medicine cabinet after announcing that he or she plans to kill himself or herself is generally less serious about commiting suicide than is the one who has carefully planned the event, particularly if rescue was unlikely. Leaving a suicide note suggests premeditation and is a sign of seriousness of intent. An attempt by a teenager with a family history of suicide is particularly significant. Any attempt or gesture should be regarded as serious, however, regardless of apparent intent, because most successful suicides occur among persons who have made earlier attempts or gestures.

Whenever an adolescent makes a suicide attempt, it is a desperate attempt at conflict resolution. Merely attending to its pharmacologic or surgical sequelae, which is usually the case in hospital emergency rooms, does little to assist in constructive resolution of the conflict. *Short-term hospitalization,* however, effectively accomplishes this latter goal by providing a secure setting for the patient, by impressing parents with the need to attend to the underlying problems, and, most important, by facilitating psychosocial assessment on which to base a recommendation for appropriate therapy or referral. Fewer than one-third of families actually follow up with recommendation for referral made after only emergency room evaluation. Consultation with a skilled psychiatrist is essential in the assessment of every teenager who makes a suicide attempt.

10.4 SUBSTANCE ABUSE

The use of mind-altering substances for medicinal, social, and religious purposes has characterized the human race throughout recorded history. The use of such agents by teenagers is also not a new phenomenon. The increased complexity of modern society, as well as the increased availability of a wide variety of drugs, has contributed to increased use by adolescents and an awareness of physical and psychosocial sequelae by health professionals. In our society, drug use may serve a variety of purposes for the adolescent. For the individual aspiring to adult status, the use of drugs may be symbolic of maturity. For those negotiating independence from parental domination, drugs may be viewed as facilitating the process. Peer group acceptance, stress reduction, escapism, and rebellion against the establishment are other functions presumably served by drug use. In addition, the developing teenager, seeking to explore the limits of his or her new cognitive abilities, may attempt to do so through hallucinogenic agents.

Intervention strategies for preventing or stopping drug use by this age group must consider alternatives that meet their developmental needs. Drug use, in the form of alcohol or marijuana, is experienced at some time by more than 90% of teenagers; accordingly, it is no longer useful to think of teenagers as either being drug users or non–drug users. Rather, the clinician should assess the role of drug use in each adolescent's life and the effects of specific drugs on physical and functional parameters in each individual. Because it is much easier to resist pressures to use drugs than to stop once begun, efforts should be focused on prevention (see also Sec. 5.1 and 5.2).

EPIDEMIOLOGY. Most data on adolescent substance abuse are based on repeated cross-sectional studies, which makes it difficult to separate effects of maturation from effects caused by changes in the availability of drugs. Johnston and associates found that the use of illicit drugs by high-school seniors in the United States declined from 1976 to 1987. Much of this decline was due to a decrease in the use of marijuana from 11% in 1978 to 3% in 1987 for daily use and from 51% to 36% for annual prevalence. Other drugs exhibiting a marked decline include amphetamines, methaqualone, and lysergic acid diethytamide (LSD). Continuation of a gradual long-term decline also occurred in the use of barbituates, tranquilizers, and phencyclidine (PCP). Heroin use dropped by one-half from 1975 to 1979 and has leveled off at less than 1%; inhalant use has been stable at 4% since 1980. In contrast, the use of *cocaine* doubled between 1975 and 1979, with significant regional differences; rates in West and Northeast sections of the United States were double those in the South and North Central regions. A one-fifth decrease in the use of cocaine was reported in 1987; the rate of use of *crack cocaine* was unchanged from that in 1986 (6%). It is probable, however, that the rate of crack cocaine use among those not in school (and therefore not surveyed) is considerably higher.

Use of *nonprescription stimulants and diet pills* has only been examined in recent years, with the finding of lifetime prevalence of 15–20% for the former and 31% for the latter. Of particular concern is a 45% lifetime prevalence for use of diet pills among adolescent females (Sec. 10.14).

Alcohol use is reported by 93% of high-school seniors, 69% within the previous month, and 5.5% daily use. The rate of binge drinking (five drinks or more in a row) during the previous 2 wk rose to 41% in 1983 and has declined since then to 37%. Data on adolescent alcohol consumption from four countries for which data are adequate and comparable with those in the United States show a recent decline in three countries and leveling off in one (Australia). In all, however, previously noted male-female differences in usage rates have narrowed.

Smoking on a daily basis by adolescents in the United States decreased from 29% in 1977 to 20% by 1981. It has been essentially unchanged through the remainder of the decade. Slightly more adolescent females smoke regularly than males (13.6% versus 13.1%, respectively), reversing earlier patterns. Future educational plans correlate significantly with smoking patterns; 8% of college-bound seniors report smoking half a packet or more daily, compared with 21% of those who do not plan to go to college. Use of "smokeless" tobacco by male adolescents is a recent and growing phenomenon.

In summary, these cross-sectional studies show that approximately two-thirds of teenagers in the United States try some illicit drug before they finish high-school; 40% have used some illicit drug other than marijuana. Daily cigarette smoking is experienced by one in every 18 high-school seniors; the same percentage drink alcohol on a daily basis.

Cohort longitudinal studies may help separate maturational from historical trends. Kandel and associates evaluated a cohort of New York State adolescents in 1971 and approximately 10 yr later. They found that the time of greatest risk for initiation of cigarette smoking or alcohol and marijuana use was before the age of 20 yr, and for illicit drugs, other than cocaine, before 21 yr of age. A decline in marijuana use began at 22.5 yr of age, whereas the use of cigarettes continued to increase through the end of the period of surveillance, at 25 yr of age. These authors believe that it is unlikely that those who have not experimented with any of these substances by 21 yr of age will do so thereafter. Jessor and Jessor evaluated 7th, 8th, and 9th grade youngsters from a city in the Rocky Mountains, first in 1969, then annually for 4 successive years, and then again in 1979 and 1981. Follow-up data extended to persons who were 25, 26, and 27 yr of age. They defined "problem drinking" as (1) having within the previous year been drunk six times or more, or (2) within the same period having on two occasions or more experienced negative consequences of drinking in three or more life areas (difficulty with teachers; difficulties with friends; trouble with parents; criticism from dates; trouble with police; or driving a car while under the influence of alcohol). By this definition, 25% of males and 16% of females in the 1972 sample of 10th, 11th, and 12th graders were problem drinkers. Among the males who were problem drinkers during adolescence, half were no longer in this category by young adulthood. For the females, only 25% of the original problem drinker group remained classified in this way during young adulthood. Among those who were nonproblem drinkers during adolescence, 40% of males and 20% of females became problem drinkers as young adults. Problem drinking during adolescence was correlated with other concurrent problem behaviors, such as smoking marijuana and sexual intercourse. On the other hand, it was not significantly correlated with negative consequences in later life. The authors concluded: "Such findings suggest that post-adolescent development and attainment are not necessarily mortgaged by adolescent problem drinking . . . (and) that premature labeling and social processing of adolescents as problem drinkers might very well set up expectations for chronicity that unnecessarily restrict the developmental options . . ."

Longitudinal studies also provide us with a better picture of the role of marijuana use as a forerunner of later use of hard drugs. Its predictive power is limited to those who begin its use at a young age. The New York study also found that alcohol use was experienced by 20% of children before 10 yr of age and by 50% by 14 yr of age, that marijuana use began to climb at approximately 13 yr of age, and that cigarette use began to rise at about 11 yr of age. The pattern for onset of use of psychedelics parallels that of marijuana, whereas that for cocaine shifts to an older age group (8% by 18 yr of age and 30% by 24 yr of age). Although males outnumber females in the magnitude of illicit drug use, psychoactive substances are prescribed more often for females, beginning in early adolescence and continuing through adulthood. These developmental observations should be used as a basis for preventive strategies.

ETIOLOGY. As indicated earlier, factors that contribute to the adolescent's initial decision to use a substance of abuse include the desire to explore the limits of emotionality; the need to try on new "adult" roles; the wish to expand one's consciousness; the availability of drugs; the desire to escape an unpleasant or stressful experience; and peer pressure. Continued use of a drug after it is first experienced usually suggests that serious problems may underlie usage or may complicate use. For example, drug use is more prevalent among depressed teenagers, as well as among those described by the Jessors as being susceptible to problem behavior. No single factor distinguishes "problem" adolescent drug users from those whose drug involvement does not portend major problems but weighing an aggregate of multiple variables may assist in this process (Table 10–1). The type of drug used (e.g., marijuana versus heroin), the circumstances of use (e.g., alone or in a group setting), the frequency and timing of use

TABLE 10–1. Assessing the Seriousness of Adolescent Drug Abuse

	0	+1	+2
Age	>15	<15	
Sex	Male	Female	
Family history of drug abuse		Yes	
Setting of drug use	In group		Alone
Affect before drug use	Happy		Sad
School performance	Good/improving	Always poor	Recently poor
Use before driving	None		Yes
History of accidents	None		Yes
Time of week	Weekend	Weekdays	
Time of day		After school	Before school
Type of drug	Marijuana, beer, wine	Hallucinogens, amphetamines	Whiskey, opiates, cocaine, barbiturates

Total score: 0–3 less worrisome; 3–8 serious; 8–18 very serious.

(e.g., daily before school versus rarely on a weekend), the premorbid personality (depressed versus happy), as well as the teenager's general functional status, should all be considered in evaluating any youngster found to be abusing a drug. In addition, apart from the existence of any high-risk factors, the use of any psychoactive substance in conjunction with operation of a motor vehicle is sufficient reason for immediate intervention to prevent harm to the teenager and to others.

PATHOPHYSIOLOGY. The process of physical growth and development that characterizes puberty may be affected adversely by the use of drugs. For example, one-third of adolescent females who use *heroin* have secondary amenorrhea, even in the absence of weight loss. The higher incidence of menstrual abnormalities in the adolescent heroin user probably results from a greater vulnerability of the hypothalamic-pituitary-ovarian axis in the maturing individual. Experiments with naloxone, the opiate antagonist, suggest that endogenous opiates block the release of gonadotropin-releasing hormone. *Amphetamines* interfere with stage 4 sleep and may impair the intimate relationship between sleep and augmentation of secretion of gonadotropins during early adolescence. To derive calories mainly from *ethanol* during the peak of the pubertal growth spurt deprives the body of the protein necessary for normal muscle growth.

The metabolism of certain prescribed drugs may be affected by coincident abuse of illicit drugs or alcohol (Table 10–2). Induction of hepatic smooth endoplasmic reticulum by barbiturates or alcohol may accelerate the metabolism and enhance the excretion of substances requiring glucuronidation. As a result of this mechanism, estrogen-containing oral contraceptives taken by an abuser of these substances may become vulnerable to pregnancy. Conversely, the use of estrogens increases the risk of intoxication from alcohol as a result of decreased ethanol metabolism. The potentiating interaction of alcohol and barbiturates must also be considered when prescribing anticonvulsant medications. Abdominal pain and vomiting occur when metronidazole is ingested by an alcohol-abusing adolescent, because of the antagonistic effect of alcohol on acetaldehyde.

PSYCHOSOCIAL SEQUELAE. Youth may engage in robbery, burglary, drug-dealing, or prostitution for the purpose of acquiring the money necessary to buy drugs or alcohol. Regular use of any drug eventually diminishes the ability to function adequately in school, to hold a job, or to operate a motor vehicle. An "amotivational" syndrome has been described in chronic marijuana users who lose interest in age-appropriate behavior.

PREVENTION. The model of prevention relevant to the problem of adolescent drug or alcohol use is one that anticipates experimentation with some agent at some point in the normal development of the adolescent and that attempts to delay that event as long as possible, to make its use as limited in amount and setting as possible, and to prevent entirely any use while operating a motor vehicle. Educational efforts based on scare techniques have not been successful, whereas those that present unemotional, factual information about medical complications of drug use have had some impact. Strategies that teach young adolescents to resist peer pressure to smoke, by the use of trained peer counselors using role-playing techniques, have significantly reduced smoking in a number of studies.

TREATMENT. Acute management is discussed in the following sections on specific agents. A variety of chronic treatment programs are available in inpatient and ambulatory settings. In general, these programs have not been adequately evaluated. Important features of successful long-term management of these adolescents are continuing medical evaluation after detoxification and the provision of developmentally appropriate psychosocial support systems.

10.5 Opiates

Opiate abuse by adolescents decreased considerably during the 1980s, but the magnitude and variety of its medical

TABLE 10–2. Interactions Between Alcohol and Prescription Drugs

Additive	Cross-Tolerant	Antagonistic
Acetaminophen	Anticoagulants (chronic intoxication)	Caffeine
Antihypertensives	Digoxin-digitoxin	Cephalosporins
Anticoagulants (acute intoxication)	Ether	Chloramphenicol
Antihistamines	Fluorinated anesthetics	Griseofulvin
Barbiturates	Impiramine	Ketoconazole
Benzodiazepines	Propranolol	Phenoformin
Chloral hydrate	Tetracyclines	
Lithium		
Nonsteroidal anti-inflammatory drugs		
Oral contraceptives		
Phenothiazines		
Propoxyphene		
Salicylates		

sequelae warrant continued attention. Moreover, a resurgence of its use in conjunction with "crack" cocaine has occurred.

PHARMACOLOGY. Heroin produces euphoria and analgesia. It is hydrolyzed to morphine, which undergoes hepatic conjugation with glucuronic acid before excretion, usually within 24 hr of administration. It can be detected in urine by thin layer chromatography up to 48 hr after administration.

The route of administration influences the timing of the onset of action. When the drug is inhaled ("snorting"), it will require almost 30 min until the desired effect is achieved. By the subcutaneous route ("skinpopping"), the effect is achieved within minutes; and when injected intravenously (IV) ("mainlining"), it has an immediate effect. A larger dose can be administered intravenously. Tolerance is developed to the euphoric effect and only rarely to the inhibitory effect on smooth muscle, which causes both constipation or miosis.

CLINICAL MANIFESTATIONS. These are determined by the pharmacologic effects of heroin or its adulterants, combined with the conditions and the route of administration.

Neuromuscular. The cerebral effects include euphoria, diminution in pain, and a sleep-like electroencephalogram (EEG) pattern. An effect on the hypothalamus is suggested by the lowering of body temperature. Transverse myelitis of the thoracic segments has been reported in patients resuming heroin use after a period of abstinence, suggesting a possible hypersensitivity reaction. Rarely, Guillain-Barré syndrome and toxic amblyopia, the latter presumably due to the quinine additive, occur in heroin addicts. Brachial and lumbosacral plexitis and polyneuropathies and mononeuropathies, the latter manifested by ankle or wrist drop, are the most common peripheral neurologic findings. Acute rhabdomyolysis with myoglobinuria may follow IV injection of heroin and is manifested by generalized muscle tenderness, edema, and marked weakness. Necrotizing fascitis is a rare complication after inadvertent subfascial injections of heroin. Other rare complications are contractures of the fingers resulting from infection and scarring medial to the proximal interphalangeal joint following injection into the small veins of the hand.

Cardiovascular. Vasodilation is a major cardiovascular manifestation related to the method of administration of the drug. Rare complications of parenteral heroin administration include arteriovenous fistula, arterial and venous thrombosis, embolism, necrotizing arteritis, and mycotic aneurysm.

Respiratory. Respiratory depression is mediated centrally and is characterized by alveolar underventilation. Particles of cotton fibers or nonsoluble adulterants inadvertently injected with the heroin are responsible for granulomatosis and pulmonary fibrosis, which may result in pulmonary hypertension and decrease in lung volume and in diffusing capacity. Pulmonary edema is common in death from the overdose syndrome, but it may also be seen as an incidental roentgenologic finding in an otherwise asymptomatic adolescent heroin abuser. Pulmonary infections have not been a prominent finding in this age group.

Dermatologic. The most common dermatologic lesions are the "tracks," the hypertrophic linear scars that follow the course of large veins. Smaller, discrete peripheral scars, resembling healed insect bites, may be easily overlooked. The adolescent who injects heroin subcutaneously may have fat necrosis, lipodystrophy, and atrophy over portions of the extremities. Attempts at concealment of these stigmata may include amateur tattoos in unusual sites. Abscesses secondary to unsterile techniques of drug administration are commonly found.

Genitourinary. There is a loss of libido; the mechanism is unknown. The female heroin user may resort to prostitution to support the habit, thus increasing the risks of sexually transmitted disease (including human immunodeficiency virus [HIV]) and of pregnancy to other hazards. Urinary retention may result from decreased tone of the detrusor muscles.

Gastrointestinal. Constipation results from decreased smooth muscle propulsive contractions and increased anal sphincter tone. The practice of concealment of heroin in a swallowed condom or balloon may cause intestinal obstruction or sudden (often fatal) overdosage if the container breaks. Hepatic enzyme activities are frequently elevated in heroin users, the majority of whom have serologic evidence suggesting viral infection with hepatitis B. Elements of chronic aggressive hepatitis on biopsy and persistence of enzyme abnormalities suggest a poor prognosis in some patients.

Infectious. The absence of sterile technique in injection may lead to cerebral microabscesses or endocarditis, usually caused by *Staphylococcus aureus*. Infection with HIV is another complication of needle use.

Immunologic. Elevations in immunoglobulin M (IgM) levels are consistently noted in parenteral heroin users, whereas IgA elevations are reported in those who inhale the drug. Abnormal serologic reactions are also common, including false-positive Venereal Disease Research Laboratory (VDRL) and latex fixation tests. Depression of lymphocyte response to stimulation by mitogens in culture has been reported but may be due to coincident acquired immunodeficiency syndrome (AIDS) (Sec. 12.82) in parenteral drug users.

Withdrawal. After a period of 8 hr or more without heroin, the addicted individual undergoes, during a period of 24–36 hr, a series of physiologic disturbances referred to collectively as "withdrawal" or the *abstinence syndrome*. The earliest sign is yawning, followed by lacrimation, mydriasis, insomnia, "gooseflesh," cramping of the voluntary musculature, hyperactive bowel sounds and diarrhea, tachycardia, and systolic hypertension. The occurrence of grand mal seizures is rare in adolescent addicts. A short course of diazepam is effective and safe treatment for heroin detoxification. An alternative for detoxification is treatment with methadone. This synthetic opiate is effective by the oral route and is pharmacologically similar to heroin, with the exception of its lack of euphoric effect. Neither the safety nor the dosage of methadone has been established for children or adolescents.

Overdose Syndrome. This is an acute reaction after the administration of an opiate. It is the leading cause of death among drug users. The rapidity of onset, the finding of eosinophilia after recovery, and the fact that it occurs only in those who have used the drug previously suggest a hypersensitivity mechanism. The clinical signs include stupor or coma, seizures, miotic pupils (unless severe anoxia has occurred), respiratory depression, cyanosis, and pulmonary edema. The differential diagnosis includes central nervous system trauma, diabetic coma, hepatic (and other) encephalopathy, Reye syndrome, as well as overdose of alcohol, barbiturates, phencyclidine piperdine (PCP), or methadone. Diagnosis of opiate toxicity is facilitated by intravenous administration of the opiate antagonist naloxone, 0.01 mg/kg (a vial of 0.4 mg usually suffices for an adolescent), which causes dilatation of pupils constricted by the opiate. Diagnosis is confirmed by the finding of morphine in the serum. *Treatment* consists of maintaining adequate oxygenation and continued administration of naloxone every 5 min, when necessary, to improve and maintain adequate ventilation. Naloxone may have to be continued for 24 hr if methadone, rather than shorter-acting heroin, has been taken.

10.6 Hallucinogens

Several naturally occurring and synthetic substances have been used by adolescents for their hallucinogenic properties. Lysergic acid diethylamide (LSD), which enjoyed popularity in the 70s, has reappeared recently. LSD flashbacks are terrifying and may be reactivated by fever. Among the other currently popular hallucinogens, PCP, certain mushrooms, and jimsonweed may cause serious toxicity and even death.

PHENCYCLIDINE

(PCP, sternyl, angel dust, "hog," "peace pill," "sheets")

Phencyclidine is an arylcyclohexalamine whose popularity is related, in part, to its ease of synthesis in home laboratories. One of the by-products of home synthesis causes cramps, diarrhea, and hematemesis. The drug is thought to potentiate adrenergic effects by inhibiting neuronal re-uptake of catecholamines. PCP is available as a tablet, liquid, or powder, which may be used alone or sprinkled on cigarettes ("joints"). The powders and tablets generally contain 2–6 mg of PCP, whereas "joints" average 1 mg for every 150 mg of tobacco leaves, or approximately 30–50 mg per "joint."

CLINICAL MANIFESTATIONS. These are dose related. Euphoria, nystagmus, ataxia, and emotional lability occur within 2–3 min after smoking 1–5 mg and last for hours. Hallucination may involve bizarre distortions of body image that often precipitate panic reactions. With doses of 5–15 mg a toxic psychosis may occur, with disorientation, hypersalivation, and abusive language lasting for more than 1 hr. After oral ingestion of 15 mg or more, the patient usually becomes comatose within 30–60 min, with alternating periods of wakefulness, with dystonic posturing, muscular rigidity, or myoclonic jerks. Hypotension, generalized seizures, and cardiac arrhythmias commonly occur with plasma concentrations from 40–200 μg/dL. Death has been reported during psychotic delirium, from hypertension, hypotension, hypothermia, seizures, and trauma. The coma of PCP may be distinguished from that of the opiates by the absence of respiratory depression; the presence of muscle rigidity, hyperreflexia, and nystagmus; and lack of response to naloxone. PCP psychosis may be difficult to distinguish from schizophrenia. In the absence of history of use, analysis of urine must be depended on for diagnosis.

TREATMENT. Management of the PCP-intoxicated patient includes placement in a darkened, quiet room on a floor pad, safe from injury. Diazepam, in a dose of 10–20 mg orally or 10 mg intramuscularly every 4 hr, may be helpful if the patient is agitated and not comatose. Ammonium chloride, 500 mg every 6 hr, may be administered orally or by nasogastric tube to maintain urinary pH at 5.5–6, which enhances urinary clearance of PCP. Supportive therapy of the comatose patient is indicated with particular attention to hydration, which may be compromised by PCP-induced diuresis.

MUSHROOMS

Mushrooms cause both cholinergic and anticholinergic effects, in addition to the sought-after euphoria and hallucinations. Most adverse effects associated with their use are usually self-limited and do not require therapy. Mushrooms containing psilocybin and related antiserotonergic indoles cause LSD-like reactions and agitation and may require treatment with diazepam. Because most hallucination-seeking adolescents are not expert mycologists, mushrooms with other toxic and even fatal effects may be ingested accidentally. Treatment is by induction of vomiting and activated charcoal (see Sec. 26.4).

JIMSONWEED

(Datura stramonium)

This is also known as "devil's weed," "locoweed," "stinkweed," and thornapple and grows wild throughout the United States. The seeds, which appear in the autumn, contain alkaloids including hyoscyamine, as well as atropine and scopolamine. One hundred seeds, the upper limit of contents of a single pod, contain the equivalent of 6 mg of atropine. Ingestion of the seeds or other plant parts produces dose-related central nervous system (CNS) and other anticholinergic effects that range from restlessness, disorientation, and the desired hallucinations, at the lower dose range, to lethargy and coma and, rarely, convulsions when larger doses are used. The presence of dry mouth, dry hot skin, fever, mydriasis, cycloplegia, urinary retention, and sinus tachycardia, in conjunction with delirium and visual or auditory hallucinations, should alert the physician to the possibility of jimsonweed intoxication.

In addition to supportive care, physostigmine salicylate, an anticholinesterase, is indicated for the treatment of hypertension, convulsions, severe hallucinations, or supraventricular tachyarrhythmias. This agent is administered slowly by the IV route for 2–5 min in an initial dose of 1–2 mg. This dose can be repeated in 20 min. If cholinergic symptoms result from physostigmine administration, atropine sulfate may be given in a dose of 0.5 mg for each milligram of physostigmine.

10.7 VOLATILE SUBSTANCES

The practice of inhalation of a variety of euphoriants has enjoyed popularity among adolescents for centuries. The first well-described documentation of this phenomenon related to an "epidemic" of ether sniffing by Irish teenagers in the 19th century. In recent history, the easy availability and low cost of substances such as airplane glue, freons, paint thinners, and gasoline has provided young adolescents with a wide range of potential hallucinogens. They have been responsible for a similarly wide range of complications, relating to chemical toxicity, to the method of administration (e.g., in plastic bags, with resultant suffocation), and to the often dangerous setting in which the inhalation occurs (e.g., inner-city roof tops).

Airplane glue enjoyed great popularity among young adolescents in the late 1960s and early 1970s and continues to be a problem in some areas of the United States. Toluene, its main ingredient, is excreted rapidly in the urine as hippuric acid, with the residual detectable in the serum by gas chromatography. The glue causes relaxation and pleasant hallucinations for up to 2 hr. Tolerance and physical dependance may occur. Its toxicity is acute, as well as chronic. Death in the acute phase may result from cerebral or pulmonary edema or myocardial involvement. Chronic use may cause pulmonary hypertension, restrictive lung defects or reduced diffusion capacity, peripheral neuropathy, acute rhabdomyosysis, hematuria, tubular acidosis, and possibly cerebral and cerebellar atrophy.

Gasoline sniffing is popular among rural adolescents and American Indian youth and may cause ataxia, nausea, and loss of consciousness. Euphoria followed by violent excitement and coma may result from prolonged or rapid inhalation. The long-term effects of chronic exposure include irreversible encephalopathy, bone marrow aplasia (from benzene), and lead encephalopathy when the gasoline contains tetraethyl lead.

Inhalation of *aerosol products,* such as hair sprays, deodorants, frypan lubricants, and cocktail glass chillants, has also become popular. The method of dispensation involves fluorocarbon propellants (freons) that have been implicated in cardiac sensitization to epinephrine, resulting in arrhythmias and death following inhalation.

A variety of *volatile nitrites,* such as amyl nitrite, butyl nitrite, and related compounds marketed as room deodorizers, are used as euphoriants, enhancers of musical appreciation, and aphrodisiacs among older adolescents and young adults. They may result in headaches, syncope, and lightheadedness; profound hypotension and cutaneous flushing followed by vasoconstriction and tachycardia; transiently inverted T waves and depressed ST segments in ECG; methemoglobinemia, increased bronchial irritation, and increased intraocular pressure.

10.8 MARIJUANA

Marijuana and alcohol, the most popular substances of abuse among adolescents, share a number of psychopharmacologic qualities. Both decrease short-term memory and fine coordination, prolong reaction time, and produce "mental clouding." About 300 mg of cannabis is equivalent to 70 g of alcohol.

PHARMACOLOGY. *Marijuana* (THC, "pot," "weed," "hash," "grass") is synthesized from the resin of the *Cannabis sativa* plant, which flourishes in temperate and hot, dry climates. The tetrahydrocannabinol (THC) fraction of the resin is responsible for its hallucinogenic properties and has been synthesized (δ-9-THC). THC is absorbed rapidly by the nasal or oral routes, producing a peak of subjective effect at 10 min and 1 hr, respectively. Marijuana is generally consumed as a "reefer" or "joint," made by rolling the crushed plant material in paper. Although there is much variation in content, each cigarette contains approximately 1 g of marijuana or 20 mg of δ-9-THC.

CLINICAL MANIFESTATIONS. In addition to the "desired" effects of elation and euphoria, marijuana may cause impairment of short-term memory, poor performance of tasks requiring divided attention (e.g., those involved in driving), loss of critical judgment, and distortion of time perception. Visual hallucinations and perceived body distortions occur rarely, but there may be "flashbacks" or recall of frightening hallucinations experienced under marijuana's influence that occur usually during stress or with fever.

Temperature may be lowered. Tachycardia is apparent within 20 min of smoking marijuana and is followed ½ hr later by transient systolic and diastolic hypertension, which disappears by 3 hr. Tachypnea is observed only in the experienced user. In placebo-controlled studies of experienced users, smoking marijuana caused hypercapnic ventilation and a decrease in forced expired volume, maximal midexpiratory flow rate, airway conductance, and diffusing capacity. Reduction in bronchospasm has also been demonstrated. Both δ-9-THC and marijuana (smoking a single "joint") cause a significant fall in intraocular pressure, lasting for up to 5 hr in normal persons, as well as in patients with glaucoma.

Kolodny demonstrated dose-related suppression of plasma testosterone levels and spermatogenesis as a result of smoking marijuana for a minimum of 4 days/wk for 6 mo, prompting concern about the potential deleterious effect of smoking marijuana before completion of pubertal growth and development. Smoking marijuana for 1 wk also decreases glucose tolerance. There is an antiemetic effect of oral THC or smoked marijuana, often followed by appetite stimulation, which is the basis of the drug's use in patients receiving cancer chemotherapy. Although the possibility of teratogenicity and carcinogenesis has been raised because of findings in animals, there is not evidence for such effects in humans at this time. There is no proof of physiologic dependency.

10.9 COCAINE

Cocaine, the most expensive of the inhalants, was not widely used by adolescents before the 1980s. However, its increased availability and decreased cost has now increased its popularity in this age group.

PHARMACOLOGY. The alkaloid extracted from the leaves of the South American *Erythroxylon coca* is supplied as the hydrochloride salt in crystalline form. It is rapidly absorbed from the nasal mucosa, detoxified by the liver, and excreted in the urine as benzoyl ecgonine. Its half-life is slightly more than 1 hr, yet social custom often dictates its repeated administration every 15 min. The perceived effect of "snorting" cocaine may be influenced by some of the many diluents now being added to or actually substituted for the drug (heroin, amphetamines, PCP, or fillers such as mannitol or quinine).

Recently, smoking the cocaine alkaloid ("free basing") in pipes or cigarettes, mixed with tobacco, marijuana, parsley, or as a paste, has become a popular method of use. The effects of smoking in this way appear to be exaggerations of those achieved by other routes. Accidental burns are potential complications of this practice.

CLINICAL MANIFESTATIONS. Cocaine causes euphoria, increased motor activity, decreased fatigability, and occasionally, paranoid ideation. Its sympathomimetic properties are responsible for tachycardia, hypertension, and hyperthermia. Binge patterns of use are common. Usage in group settings has been associated with sexual promiscuity and increased risks of sexually transmitted infections. The chronic user may develop tolerance to these physiologic effects and psychologic dependence may occur. Withdrawal symptoms upon its discontinuation have not, however, been reported suggesting that physical dependency is not a problem. Pregnant adolescents who use cocaine place their fetus at risk for premature delivery and complications of LBW, for developing urogenital tract and possibly other congenital malformations, and for developmental disorders.

TREATMENT. Intensive supportive therapy is directed at the clinical manifestations of acute intoxication. See Section 10.4 for chronic management.

10.10 CIGARETTE SMOKING

More than 13% of adolescents smoke cigarettes, and the rate among women continues to increase. The severity of atherosclerosis may be correlated with the duration of smoking, increasing its risk among those who begin smoking during adolescence. In addition, adverse health effects of smoking may occur even during adolescence itself. These adverse effects include an increased prevalence of chronic cough, phlegm production, and wheezing. Smoking during pregnancy is associated with an average decrease in fetal weight of 200 g; this, added to the already smaller size of babies born to teenagers, increases perinatal morbidity and mortality. Smoking in combination with estrogen-containing oral contraceptives is associated with increased risk of myocardial infarction. Tobacco smoke induces hepatic smooth endoplasmic reticulum and, as a result, may also influence metabolism of drugs and of endogenously produced hormones. Phenacetin, theophylline, and imipramine are examples of drugs affected in this manner. In addition, laboratory test results may be affected by smoking, for example, white blood cell count, hemoglobin, hematocrit, mean corpuscular volume (MCV), and platelet aggregation are increased and serum creatinine, albumin, globulin (in females), and uric acid (in males) are decreased.

SMOKELESS TOBACCO. Chewing tobacco may result in lesions, primarily in the mandibular mucobuccal fold. With chronic use these may become malignant.

10.11 ALCOHOL

Alcohol use among adolescents has increased during the past decade and poses a threat to the normal functioning of the teenager as well as to the lives of those potentially jeopardized by drunken drivers. The usual progression is from beer to wine to hard liquor, although regional differences may alter this pattern. Four ounces of hard liquor (86 proof) consumed on an empty stomach produces a plasma ethanol level of approximately 65 mg/dL in an adult male of average weight and 80 mg/dL in a premenstrual female of adult weight. The legal definition of intoxication in most statutes is a blood ethanol level of 100 mg/dL (0.08% or 0.10%).

PHARMACOLOGY AND PATHOPHYSIOLOGY. Alcohol (ethyl alcohol or ethanol) is rapidly absorbed from the stomach, transported to the liver, and metabolized by two pathways. The primary pathway involves removal of two hydrogen atoms to form acetaldehyde, a reaction catalyzed by alcohol dehydrogenase through reduction of a cofactor nicotinamide-adenine dinucleotide (NAD). The removed hydrogen atoms supply energy (7.1 kcal/g of alcohol) and contribute to the excess synthesis of triglycerides, a phenomenon that is responsible for producing a fatty liver, even in those who are well nourished. Engorgement of hepatocytes with fat causes necrosis, triggering an inflammatory process (alcoholic hepatitis), which is followed by fibrosis, the hallmark of cirrhosis. Early hepatic involvement may result in elevation in γ-glutamyl transpeptidase and serum glutamic-pyruvic transaminase; cirrhosis has been reported in native American adolescents. The 2nd metabolic pathway, which is utilized at high serum alcohol levels, involves the microsomal system of the liver, in which the cofactor is reduced nicotinamide-adenine dinucleotide phosphate (NADPH). The net effect of activation of this pathway is to decrease metabolism of drugs that share this system and to allow for their accumulation, enhanced effect, and possible toxicity (e.g., drinking alcohol and ingesting tranquilizers results in potentiation of each [see Table 10–2]).

CLINICAL MANIFESTATIONS. Alcohol acts primarily as a central nervous system depressant. It produces euphoria, grogginess, talkativeness, and impaired short-term memory, and it increases the pain threshold and the time needed to brake a car under simulated driving conditions. Alcohol's ability to produce vasodilation and hypothermia is also centrally mediated. At very high serum levels, respiratory depression occurs. Its inhibitory effect on pituitary antidiuretic hormone release is responsible for its diuretic effect.

The most common gastrointestinal complication of alcohol use is acute erosive gastritis, which is manifested by epigastric pain, anorexia, vomiting, and guaiac-positive stools. Less commonly, vomiting and midabdominal pain may be caused by acute alcoholic pancreatitis; diagnosis is confirmed by the finding of an elevated serum amylase and lipase activities.

Physiologic dependence upon alcohol may develop in the adolescent who uses it daily over a period of weeks. In such individuals, alcohol deprivation may precipitate a **withdrawal** or **abstinence syndrome** whose manifestations in adolescents are generally mild, occurring within 8 hr of the last dose and lasting no longer than 48 hr in the untreated patient. Anxiety, tremor, insomnia, and irritability are common symptoms. Only rarely are severe reactions found in older adolescents who have been drinking steadily for 1 yr or more; these consist of auditory or visual hallucinations, hyperthermia, delirium, and seizures occurring 48 hr or more after the last drink.

DIAGNOSIS. The *alcohol overdose syndrome* should be suspected in any teenager who appears disoriented, lethargic, or comatose. Whereas the distinctive aroma of alcohol may assist in diagnosis, confirmation by analysis of blood is recommended. There is a high correlation between results obtained by serum and breath analyses so that the latter method may be reliably used. At levels above 200 mg/dL the adolescent is at risk of death, and levels above 500 mg/dL (LD_{50}) are usually associated with a fatal outcome. When the level of depression appears excessive for the reported blood level, head trauma or ingestion of other drugs should be considered as possible confounding factors.

TREATMENT. The usual mechanism of death from the alcohol overdose syndrome is respiratory depression, and artificial ventilatory support must be provided until the liver can eliminate sufficient amounts of alcohol from the body. In a patient without alcoholism it generally takes 20 hr to reduce the blood level of alcohol from 400 mg/dL to zero. Dialysis should be considered when the blood level is higher than 400 mg/dL.

Treatment of the alcohol withdrawal or abstinence syndrome uses drugs that are cross-tolerant with alcohol but that have a longer duration of action, such as benzadiazepine derivatives, of which chlordiazepoxide (Librium) is the most popular. The usual regimen consists of an initial oral dose of 25 mg every 6 hr. If a satisfactory effect is not achieved, the dose is repeated at 2-hr intervals. Once symptomatic relief is obtained, the dose is tapered by 25 mg/day.

10.12 ANABOLIC STEROIDS

The age old quest for enhanced athletic performance has led to the phenomenon of abuse of anabolic steroids by competitive athletes of both sexes. It is estimated that 3–5% of all high-school students are users with a 10% prevalence rate among male adolescent athletes. The perception that these agents increase muscle mass and strength is not supported by objective data, but harmful side effects clearly occur. Among the adverse physical effects are abnormalities of the liver (e.g., hepatocarcinoma, peliosis hepatis, cholestasis); endocrine effects (e.g., in males: gynecomastia, lowered plasma testosterone and gonadotropin levels, testicular atrophy; in females: hirsutism, baldness, deepening of voice, breast atrophy, clitoral enlargement, acne, inhibition of ovulation, menstrual abnormalities, alopecia); effects on cardiovascular risk factors (e.g., increased levels of low-density lipoprotein and decreased levels of high-density lipoprotein cholesterol); and fluid retention. In addition to these effects that occur in individuals of all ages, the adolescent is at risk for growth retardation owing to the possibility of rapid advancement of epiphyseal closure. Serious psychologic effects also have been reported from use of high doses of these agents (often 100 times therapeutic doses), including uncontrollable rage, depression, mania, mood fluctuations, and alterations in libido.

10.13 SLEEP DISORDERS

The maturational changes in sleep patterns during adolescence indicate that between sex maturation stages (SMRs) 3 and 4 there is an increase in daytime sleepiness and a decrease in sleep latency. There is also a secretory spurt of gonadotropins and growth hormone with each completed sleep cycle during early puberty, a pattern not found at any other time of life. This normal pattern of sleep augmentation of gonadotropin secretion is disturbed in anorexia nervosa and possibly in other situations associated with significant weight loss (Sec. 10.14). The clinical association of sleep disorders with depression has long been appreciated. Shortened rapid eye movement (REM) latency appears to be common in such patients.

Narcolepsy often first becomes symptomatic during adolescence. The syndrome includes (1) attacks of REM sleep during wakefulness, with excessive daytime sleepiness; (2) hypnagogic hallucinations, frightening and recurring visual hallucinations; (3) cataplexy, the sudden inhibition of tone of a muscle group, the effects dependent on the muscle group involved; and (4) sleep paralysis, a paralysis of voluntary musculature while falling asleep. The *sleep apnea-hypersomnia syndrome* also may also first become symptomatic during adolescence and consists of increased daytime sleepiness after multiple episodes of brief night-time waking after each of the apneic spells, which results from airway obstruction.

Insomnia affects 10–20% of adolescents. The etiology may be depression or the delayed sleep phase syndrome in which the difficulty lies in falling asleep, rather than awakening once sleep has begun. According to Anders, "Adolescents may be particularly susceptible to this syndrome, because the changing social demands, which result in later bedtimes, interract with the changing neuroendocrine secretion patterns of puberty, which affect sleep state relationships."

10.14 ANOREXIA NERVOSA AND BULIMIA

EPIDEMIOLOGY. The incidence of anorexia nervosa (AN) and bulimia has increased over the last 2 decades. It is estimated that 1 in every 100 females, 16–18 yr old, has anorexia nervosa. A bimodal distribution occurs, with one peak at 14.5 and the other at 18 yr; 25% may be below the age of 13. The increased incidence has been documented in all Western countries, with sporadic reports from other nations. Affected females outnumber males by 10 to 1. Initially reported only in middle and upper socioeconomic groups, anorexia nervosa is now occurring in those from the lower socioeconomic levels. It is being diagnosed in a variety of ethnic and racial groups. Bulimia is more common than AN. An increased incidence of eating disorders among primary relatives of those with AN and bulimia suggests a familial basis.

DIAGNOSIS. The Diagnostic and Statistical Manual of Mental Disorders (DSM-IIIR) criteria for the diagnosis of AN include: (1) intense fear of becoming obese, which does not diminish as weight loss progresses; (2) disturbance in the way in which one's body weight, size, or shape is experienced (e.g., claiming to "feel fat" even when one is emanciated or believing that one area of the body is "too fat" even when obviously underweight); (3) refusal to maintain body weight over a minimal normal weight for age and height (e.g., weight loss leading to maintenance of body weight 15% below expected, failure to make expected weight gain during period of growth leading to body weight 15% below expected); and (4) in females, absence of at least three consecutive menstrual cycles when otherwise expected to occur (primary or secondary amenorrhea).

AN is characterized further by excessive physical activity in the face of apparent inanition, denial of hunger, preoccupation with food preparation, frequently accompanied by bizarre eating behaviors, and often studiousness and academic success. Most patients are described as having been "model children" before the onset of the illness. Patients who have AN are subdivided into the *restrictor* and *bulimia* subgroups, according to their method of caloric reduction. Restrictors severely limit their intake of carbohydrate and fat-containing foods, whereas bulimics tend to eat in binges and then to purge themselves of food by self-induced vomiting or the use of cathartics. The binge-purge pattern may occur in youngsters who have normal weight or are slightly obese.

DSM-IIIR separates *bulimia* from AN as a diagnostic entity, defining bulimia as (1) recurrent episodes of binge eating (rapid consumption of a large amount of food in a discrete period of time, usually less than 2 hr); (2) during the eating binges, a fear of not being able to stop eating; (3) regularly engaging in self-induced vomiting, use of laxatives, or rigorous dieting or fasting in order to counteract the effects of binge eating; and (4) a minimum average of two binge eating episodes/wk for at least 3 mo.

ETIOLOGY AND PSYCHODYNAMICS. Eating disorders commonly begin as innocent dieting behavior, not unlike that seen in many other adolescent women, but those with AN gradually progress to profound weight loss with emaciation. Premorbid psychiatric characteristics of patients with AN include excessive dependency, developmental immaturity, and isolation. Their families have been described as having difficulty with problem solving and as being intrusive and overprotective. The onset of these conditions at the time of puberty has prompted psychoanalysts to regard them as defenses against emerging sexuality, an opinion that dominated thinking until the 1950s, when Bruch conceptualized AN as a problem in identity development. Others consider that AN may represent a disorder of mood accompanied by manic or depressive symptomatology.

Recent work subdivides patients with AN on the basis of psychologic characteristics and may clarify the situation by showing that different subgroups are dynamically and prognostically different. Biogenic amine neurotransmitter abnormalities are found in some patients with AN.

CLINICAL MANIFESTATIONS. AN and bulimia are associated with disturbances in almost every organ system, although it is uncertain which may be primary and which the result of severe malnutrition. The death rate in AN is approximately 10% and is usually caused by severe electrolyte disturbance, cardiac arrhythmia, or congestive heart failure in the recovery phase. *Bradycardia and postural hypotension* are common, with pulse rates as low as 20/min. Both improve with nutritional therapy. A variety of ECG abnormalities are common, including low voltage, T wave inversion and flattening, and ST depression, as well as supraventricular and ventricular dysrhythmias, some preceded by a prolonged QT_c interval. Death from congestive heart failure is a late event and may result from unduly rapid rehydration and refeeding. On a regimen achieving a daily weight gain limited to 0.2–0.4 kg, none of our patients has experienced this complication.

Sleep disturbances occur in some anorexics and include a short REM latency time, similar to that often found in depressed patients. Problems of thermal regulation, particularly hypothermia, are very common (15% of our patients had temperatures recorded below 35 degrees). Hypothermia also occurs in some bulimics of normal weight. Disorders of the hypothalamic-pituitary-ovarian axis are manifested as amenorrhea associated with immature patterns of secretion of luteinizing hormone (LH). These findings may represent a primary hypothalamic defect rather than being secondary to weight loss (which also causes amenorrhea), in as much as amenorrhea antedates weight loss in one-third to one-half of patients with AN, and a similar proportion fail to resume menses when normal weight is restored. One-quarter of patients may be amenorrheic 8 yr later, despite weight rehabilitation. Evidence for hypothalamic-pituitary-adrenal axis dysfunction includes increased secretion of cortisol, loss of diurnal variation in its secretion, and failure of dexamethasone to suppress it. The last may also be found in starvation; however, in 44% of our patients with AN, abnormal results of dexamethasone suppression tests have persisted after weight rehabilitation. Growth hormone secretion is abnormally high in these patients, and somatomedin-C is low. TSH levels are normal, T_4 and T_3 are low, and reverse T_3 is elevated, presumably in adaptation to a lowered basal metabolic rate due to malnutrition and carbohydrate deprivation. Peripheral edema in some patients, in the absence of congestive heart failure or hypoproteinemia, has been attributed to inappropriate secretion of antidiuretic hormone (ADH).

Elevations of blood urea nitrogen (BUN) may occur reflecting dehydration and decreased glomerular filtration rate (GFR), but normal levels may be found under these same conditions because of low protein intake. Mild proteinuria, hematuria, and pyuria, with negative urine cultures, generally resolve with proper rehydration.

Bone marrow hypoplasia is common in AN, with leukopenia, anemia, and (rarely) thrombocytopenia. Low erythrocyte sedimentation rates are common, perhaps reflecting low fibrinogen production secondary to malnutrition.

Constipation is a very common complication of motility

problems in AN, as is esophagitis in those who vomit. Decreased gastrointestinal tract motility may be a cause of perforation, which has been reported to occur when a nasogastric tube has been inserted in patients who refuse to eat. Elevations in amylase levels may be associated with bilateral parotid swelling or with pancreatitis.

Electrolyte imbalance results from vomiting, "waterloading" (a practice of surreptitously drinking large amounts of water in order to achieve an agreed upon weight gain), or abuse of diuretics or laxatives. Potassium depletion, associated with a hypochloremic alkalosis, is very common. Abnormalities of calcium, magnesium, and phosphorus metabolism may result from laxative abuse, either secondary to malabsorption or to use of preparations containing phosphate.

Patients with AN appear to be remarkably resistant to infection, and the few studies of their immunologic status support this view. The fact that protein intake is relatively good in these otherwise malnourished persons may contribute to this finding. Bone density may be very abnormal. A number of possible mechanisms have been suggested to explain this finding, including low levels of estrogen and calcium and elevated cortisol levels. The skin of patients with AN is dry, and lanugo hair is often seen. Hair loss often occurs in the refeeding phase.

TREATMENT. Systematic, controlled studies of treatment in these disorders are not available. Most of the regimens in current use combine psychotherapy (individual and family), behavior modification techniques, and nutritional rehabilitation. Recently, pharmacologic therapy (primarily of antidepressant medications) has been added to treatment regimens. The success rate in short-term follow-up studies is about 70%. The frequent occurrence of medical complications and the possibility of death during the acute or rehabilitation phase require the inclusion of a medically and physiologically oriented physician in the management team.

PROBLEMS RELATED TO ADOLESCENT SEXUALITY

10.15 PREGNANCY

For women aged 15–19 the *pregnancy rate* in the United States was 96/1000 in 1981, the highest rate among developed countries. Although there has been a modest reduction in this age group's birth rate (still one-half million), this has been accomplished mainly through the increased use of abortion (39% of adolescent pregnancies), rather than through prevention of pregnancy. Additional cause for continuing concern arises from the fact that the rate of out-of-wedlock births in this age group increased by 190.1% from 1960 to 1977. Among those whose pregnancy went to term, there was an increase of 7% between 1971 and 1976 in teenaged mothers who chose to keep their babies, rather than place them for adoption. From 1973 to 1978, there was also a 5% increase in pregnancies among adolescents under 15 yr of age. This younger group is at increased risk for obstetric and perinatal complications, such as toxemia, postpartum hemorrhage, postpartum infection, infants who are small for gestational age, and stillborn infants.

Adolescent mothers are less likely to marry or to achieve a high-school education, and they are more likely to be unemployed and to have a larger number of children compared with women who postpone childbearing until after 20 yr of age. Children born to teenage mothers have an increased risk of experiencing an accident within the home and of being hospitalized before 5 yr of age.

As most pregnancies in adolescents are unintended, the challenge to pediatricians, as well as to parents and educators, is to assist in *pregnancy prevention*. Fewer than half of teenagers use any form of contraception at the time of first intercourse. The birth control methods they do use are rarely effective. The lag between becoming sexually active and seeking effective contraception usually exceeds 1 yr. As a result, almost 40% of sexually active teenagers become pregnant within 2 yr of initiating intercourse.

The pediatrician rarely has an opportunity for primary prevention of pregnancy. Discussions of abstinence are usually ignored; on the other hand, stimulating a young girl who has a boyfriend to think about whether she feels ready for intercourse may be helpful if done nonjudgmentally. For the already sexually active adolescent, information, access to, and motivation to use contraception are all necessary for successful pregnancy prevention. The last is most difficult to achieve, because many girls who have been sexually active without getting pregnant assume that they are sterile and are not in need of contraception. They are unlikely to use any contraceptive method until they are made to feel vulnerable to an unwanted pregnancy. Those who have become pregnant in the past, and thus have proved their fertility, may shun contraception after vowing that they will be abstinent or out of fear that their fertility has been impaired, as a result of an abortion, infection, or some less well-founded concern. Therefore, it is helpful to inquire about the reason why any sexually active female thinks she has not become pregnant.

Once it is established that the teenager is not pregnant, that intercourse is likely to continue, and that the patient accepts the fact that she is at risk for pregnancy, efforts should be directed toward provision of the most effective and safest contraceptive method. To enhance the likelihood of compliance once the method is prescribed, the physician must learn about the frequency and circumstances of intercourse; past experience and compliance with both contraceptive and noncontraceptive chronic medications; the partner's attitudes about various methods; and parents' knowledge and attitudes about contraception. In the United States, physicians may provide contraception to minors without parental knowledge, but it is helpful in choosing a method to know whether the parents are aware of their daughter's sexual activity.

10.16 CONTRACEPTION

The risk of any contraceptive method should be weighed against the risk of pregnancy, which for young adolescents is a significant one. If contraception is to be successful, however, every effort must be made to individualize the method to the needs of each patient. The risks, benefits, and indications for each of the available methods follow:

Barrier Methods

CONDOM. This method prevents sperm being deposited in the vagina. There are no major side effects associated with the use of a condom. Its effectiveness in preventing pregnancy is low, however, with 15 pregnancies occurring per 100 woman-years of use by adult women in the United States. No comparative figures are available for adolescents, but acceptance of this method is low in this age group. A 1979 study found that only 23% of 15- to 19-yr-old females reported that their partner ever used a condom. The recent AIDS scare appears to have increased the use of condoms only among older adolescents. Condoms used in the United States are thicker than those marketed in other countries where they enjoy widespread use. The main advantages of condoms are their low price, availability without prescription, little need for advanced planning, and most important for this age group, their effectiveness in preventing transmission of sexually transmitted diseases, including HIV (Sec. 12.82).

DIAPHRAGM. The diaphragm acts by preventing access of sperm to the cervix, while placing spermicidal jelly in a position to be effective. Other than rare cases of contact vaginitis caused by the Latex or by the powder used to preserve the diaphragm, there are no adverse side effects associated with its use. Like the condom, the diaphragm is effective in only 85% of women who use it properly. In a study of adolescents who were highly motivated to avoid pregnancy, however, use of a diaphragm was associated with only 2 pregnancies/100 woman-years. Adolescents may object to the messiness of the jelly or to the fact that the insertion of a diaphragm may interrupt the spontaneity of sex, or they may express discomfort about touching their genitalia. At Stanford University this method is currently used by 21% of sexually active women students, whereas in other studies only 3.5% of 15–19 yr olds chose this method.

A diaphragm must be fitted individually by a trained physician or nurse practitioner. Once fitted, the same diaphragm may be used for 3 yr unless extreme weight gain or loss or pregnancy occurs. After the proper diaphragm is selected, it is important that the teenager be given instructions and ample opportunity to learn to insert and remove it before leaving the office.

CERVICAL CAP. This method is currently being evaluated. The rubber cap, after proper fitting, remains affixed to the cervix by suction for 1–3 intermenstrual days. Like the diaphragm, it must be used in conjunction with spermicidal jelly.

Spermicides

A variety of agents containing the spermicide nonoxynol-9 are available as foams, jellies, creams, or effervescent vaginal suppositories. They must be placed in the vaginal cavity shortly before intercourse and reinserted before each ejaculation in order to be effective. Rare side effects consist of contact vaginitis. Effectiveness is in the range of the barrier methods (approximately 85%), but the finding that nonoxynol-9 is gonococcocidal and spirocheticidal enhances the attractiveness of these agents for adolescents because of the high incidence of sexually transmitted diseases in this group.

Combination Methods

The conjoint use of condom by the male and spermicidal foam by the female adolescent is extremely effective; the failure rate is 2%, without any of the potential side effects and complications associated with the use of other forms of contraception having comparable efficacy. This combination also prevents sexually transmitted diseases, including HIV. The contraceptive sponge, which incorporates the theoretical advantages of barrier and spermicides, has been marketed over-the-counter, but its efficacy appears to be that of either barrier or spermicide, rather than that found for the combination of foam and condom. Toxic shock syndrome has been reported in users of the sponge, a further reason that caution be used in prescribing this method for teenagers, who are at increased risk for this disease (Sec. 12.20).

Hormonal Methods

These methods currently employ either an estrogenic substance in combination with a progestin or a progestin alone. The action of the estrogen-progestin combination is to prevent the surge of LH and, as a result, to inhibit ovulation. Progestin may prevent ovulation, but this is not reliable. It does, however, affect fallopian tube transport and the composition of cervical mucus in such a way as to make fertilization or implantation less likely.

Combination oral contraceptives are commonly referred to as "the pill" and currently contain either 80, 50, or 35 μg of estrogenic substance, typically either mestranol or ethinyl estradiol, and a progestin. Thrombophlebitis, hepatic adenomas, myocardial infarction, and carbohydrate intolerance are some of the more serious potential complications of use of exogenous estrogens. These disorders are, however, exceedingly rare in adolescents.

Some long-range beneficial effects of estrogen use include decreased risks of benign breast disease, ovarian cystic disease, and anemia. However, adolescents taking estrogen-containing oral contraceptives are reported to have higher levels of high-density lipoproteins than those of controls. Inhibition of ovulation or the suppressant effect of estrogens on prostaglandin production by the endometrium make oral contraceptives effective in preventing dysmenorrhea (Sec. 10.18).

A potentially untoward effect of estrogens on epiphyseal growth does not occur, either because the amount in oral contraceptives is small or because they are taken at a time when most growth has been completed. Post-pill amenorrhea occurs with greater frequency in adolescents than in adults. It may persist for up to 18 mo after the discontinuation of use of the pill. The increased risk may not be due to age alone but may reflect oligomenorrhea or low body weight (less than 47 kg) before the initiation of use of the pill. Acne may be worsened by some and improved by other oral contraceptive preparations. Contraindications to use of estrogen-containing oral contraceptives include hepatocellular disease, migraine headaches, diabetes mellitus, and any condition in which hypercoagulability may be a problem (e.g., replaced cardiac valve, thrombophlebitis, sickle cell anemia), owing to the increased levels of factor VIII and decreased production of antithrombin III.

The pill is the most reliable contraceptive method available, with a pregnancy rate in the range of 0.8%/yr. Some side effects can, without sacrificing their efficacy, be minimized by the use of preparations of low estrogen content. With the use of the 35-μg preparation, however, there may be a higher incidence of breakthrough bleeding, which may lead to noncompliance.

All-progestin contraceptives are available for the adolescent in whom use of estrogen is potentially deleterious, for example, those with liver disease, replaced cardiac valves, or hypercoagulable states. They ("mini-pill") are less reliable in inhibiting ovulation and are associated with a 2.4%/yr pregnancy rate. Acceptance by adolescents is limited by the necessity to take the pill daily, the higher incidence of amenorrhea, and increased bleeding.

An **injectable progestin,** medroxyprogesterone (Depo-Provera), is highly effective in birth control. This substance needs to be administered only once every 3 mo and is completely reversible in its anovulatory action, furthermore the cessation of menses is coterminous with its use. This agent is particularly attractive for adolescents who have difficulty with compliance or for mentally retarded teenagers. It is not, however, now available for use as a contraceptive in the United States, because of concern about an association with increased risk of benign breast tumors in experimental animals. It is the leading birth control method in the world.

A *long-acting progestational agent,* levonorgestral (Norplant) may be contained in a small Silastic tube that is implanted subcutaneously. It can be easily removed, and the contraceptive potency remains for 5 yr. Its use in teenagers has not yet been explored.

Postcoital Contraception

Unprotected intercourse at midcycle carries a pregnancy risk of 2–30%. The risk may be reduced or eliminated by intervention within 72 hr after unprotected intercourse. The "morning-after" pill, diethylstilbestrol (DES), although effective, should be avoided because of its potential teratogenic effect (Sec. 7.34). Ethinyl estradiol, in a dose of 2.5 mg twice daily for 5 days, if begun within 72 hrs of unprotected intercourse, is equally effective, but its potential effect on a fetus is not known. Because of concern about teratogenicity, as well as the fact that this agent may produce nausea and vomiting, other approaches have been investigated. Norgestrel (Ovral), a combination oral contraceptive, may be administered in a dose of two pills initially after coitus and in two additional pills 12 hr later.

Intrauterine Devices (IUDs)

IUDs are small, flexible, plastic objects introduced into the uterine cavity through the cervix. They differ in size, shape, and the presence or absence of pharmacologically active substances (e.g., copper or progesterone). The mechanism of action of the IUD is uncertain, although they render the endometrium unsuitable for implantation by inducing a local polymorphonuclear leukocyte response, production of prostaglandins E_2 and $F_{2\alpha}$, and stimulation of uterine contractility. They are effective in preventing pregnancy in 97–99% of women. Women who become pregnant with an IUD in place, however, are at greater risk for having an ectopic pregnancy, especially if the IUD contains progesterone. Additional problems associated with the use of an IUD are increased menstrual bleeding (less so with the newer, smaller versions); increased dysmenorrhea (although those containing progesterone reportedly decrease dysmenorrhea); and of most concern, increased risk of infection, including the risks of septic abortion and death. The highest risk was associated with the use of the Dalkon Shield, which has now been removed from the market. Infection risk varies among the other types of IUDs, being highest with the progesterone-containing IUDs. The small amount of copper that leaches out of the copper-containing IUDs is bactericidal. The risk of infection also varies with characteristics of the patient; young patients and those with multiple sexual partners are at increased risk. The increased risk of infection should limit the prescription of an IUD to teenagers who require passive contraception as a last resort. IUDs were initially proscribed in nulliparous adolescents because of a high rate of expulsion. The newer, smaller types are well tolerated.

10.17 SEXUALLY TRANSMITTED DISEASES

Adolescents have the highest rate of sexually transmitted disease of any age group. This results from sexual experimentation that characterizes psychosocial development at this time, as well as from certain aspects of development. During puberty, increasing levels of estrogen cause the vaginal epithelium to thicken and cornify and cellular glycogen content to rise, the latter causing vaginal pH to fall. These changes increase the resistance of the vaginal epithelium to penetration by certain organisms (including the *gonococcus*) and increase the susceptibility to others (e.g., *Candida albicans* and *Trichomonas*). As a result of these physiologic changes, gonococcal infection becomes primarily cervical, and susceptibility to ascending infection is greatest during menses, when the pH is 6.8–7.0.

Failure to use any contraceptive method or, less frequently, the use of oral contraceptives characterizes most adolescent sexual relationships; both behaviors are conducive to the transmission of venereal organisms. Adolescents are typically reluctant to consider that a sexual partner may have a venereal disease and often lack the communication skills necessary to discuss this issue. Sexually active adolescents should be tested for sexually transmitted diseases, which are often asymptomatic. Minimizing noncompliance with treatment, finding and treating the sexual partner, and making every effort to preserve fertility are additional responsibilities. The latter often requires intensive parenteral therapy for salpingitis or tubo-ovarian abscess.

Diagnosis and therapy are often necessarily carried out within the context of a confidential relationship between the physician and the patient. Therefore, the need to report certain sexually transmitted diseases to health department authorities should be clarified at the outset. Most health departments will not violate confidentiality, if assured that treatment and case-finding have been accomplished and that the patient can be expected to follow through in a responsible, mature manner. Gonorrhea, chlamydia, and human papilloma virus are the most common sexually transmitted diseases in adolescents.

GONORRHEA (See also Sec. 12.24). Infection occurs via the urethral, cervical, anal, pharyngeal, or conjunctival route. An initial inflammatory response is followed either by resolution with a fibrous response, by extension along mucosal planes to adjacent organs (endometrium, fallopian tubes, peritoneum, liver capsule in the female, or urethra, prostate, epididymis in the male), or by hematogenous dissemination to cause arthritis, dermatitis, or rarely, meningitis or endocarditis.

Ceftriaxone has replaced penicillin as the drug of choice for the treatment of gonorrhea because of the emergence of strains resistent to the latter and because of the efficacy of a single 250 mg I.M. dose of ceftriaxone against localized gonococcal infection, as well as incubating syphilis. The patient's sexual partner also should be treated. Infection involving higher pelvic structures requires intravenous administration of cefoxitin, 2 g IV four times a day, and doxycycline, 100 mg twice a day for 10 days, to ensure compliance and to safeguard future fertility. Disseminated disease (e.g., arthritis, dermatitis) is treated with ceftriaxone 50 mg/kg/24 hr (max 0.2 g) intravenously for 7 days.

SYPHILIS (Sec. 12.50). The incidence of syphilis is rising in adolescents; accordingly, it is advisable to screen high-risk adolescents (e.g., those who are pregnant, sexually promiscuous, homosexual, delinquent, or have evidence of another sexually transmitted disease). The VDRL is the most sensitive and least specific of the serologic tests for syphilis. False-positive results may occur in intravenous abusers of drugs, as well as in those who have liver disease of any etiology, collagen-vascular disease, or infectious mononucleosis. A positive result on a test must be confirmed by the use of a more specific test, such as the treponemal immobilization test (TPI).

In the infected adolescent, the most common manifestations of syphilis are those of the secondary stage, including condyloma latum or lesions on the palms and soles. Treatment for primary and secondary syphilis is with penicillin benzathine, 2.4 million units intramuscularly (IM). Following a rape, prevention of syphilis can be accomplished with the same regimen as for the prevention of gonorrhea (250 mg of ceftriaxone IM).

CHLAMYDIA (Sec. 12.58). Cases of sexually transmitted infection with *Chlamydia* have increased dramatically in adolescents during the past decade. Most cases of urethritis, previously called "nongonococcal," are now known to be chlamydial in origin, as are approximately one-half of the cases of salpingitis. Moreover, all of the complications of gonococcal infection (e.g., perihepatitis, conjunctivitis, sterility) are potential sequelae of chlamydial infection. Therefore, a laparoscopy, with tubal puncture and culture, is the optimal approach to etiologic diagnosis in salpingitis. If this is not feasible, therapy should address the possibility of either gonococcal or chlamydial etiology (cefoxitin, 2 g IV four times a day, and doxycycline, 100 mg IV twice a day for 10 days). *Lymphogranuloma venereum (LGV)* is caused by an agent related to *Chlamydia trachomatis* (Sec. 12.62) and should be considered in the differential diagnosis of herpetiform lesions of the genitalia or of inguinal lymphadenopathy, as well as of rectal bleeding, purulent proctitis, or rectal stricture. The sexual history is, therefore, a mandatory part of the evaluation of adolescents thought to have inflammatory bowel disease, as well as a search for more obviously sexually related symptoms.

CHANCROID. The initial lesion is a vesicopustule that rapidly breaks down to form a painful, purulent, sharply delineated ulcer without induration. This latter feature, in addition to its painful nature, helps to distinguish it from the syphilitic chancre with which it shares a similar distribution in the genital region. Autoinoculation may result in multiple lesions, and unilateral painful lymphadenopathy is not uncommon. Biopsy is required for definitive diagnosis. Chancroid is treated with one dose of ceftriaxone, 250 mg IM.

HERPES PROGENITALIS (See also Sec. 12.68). The characteristic herpetic lesion may be preceded by the less-well-recognized symptom of exquisite sensitivity and sharp pain radiating from the perineum, along the course of affected nerve roots. Palliation and shortening of the symptomatic and shedding phases in primary infections may be achieved by oral administration of acyclovir, 400 mg three times a day, for 7–10 days. In recurrent cases, acyclovir is less satisfactory; patients with recurrent episodes (> 6/yr) may be given chronic treatment with 200 mg 2–5 times daily. Yearly, Papanicolaou (Pap) smears following infection with this premalignant agent are indicated. Cervical cultures may be positive in asymptomatic sexually active adolescents; Pap smears also should be obtained routinely from these adolescents.

HUMAN PAPILLOMA VIRUS (HPV). This agent is responsible for significant morbidity among adolescents, including genital warts (condyloma acuminata), subclinical infection, and the potential for oncogenic progression. Types 6, 11, and 42 are commonly expressed as warts of the anogenital area, and 16, 18, 31, 33, 35, and 39 as subclinical infections with high risk for dysplasia and cancer of the cervix. Application of a solution of 3–5% acetic acid may reveal mucosal or penile lesions as white plaques; their visualization further enhanced by use of the colposcope. All patients with genital warts and their sexual partners should have such an examination, in addition to Pap smears for females. The latter may reveal a spectrum of cytologic changes from koilocytes (cells with swollen nuclei surrounded by a halo) to cells with nuclear aneuploidy and abnormal mitotic figures (consistent with carcinoma-in-situ).

Local treatment of *condyloma acuminata* is associated with high failure rates. Application of trichloroacetic acid (85%) three times each week is the best of the chemical treatment methods; liquid nitrogen and podophyllin (20%) is preferred by some. Topical 5-fluorouracil, bleomycin, interferon, and the carbon dioxide laser are now being used for patients with extensive lesions or those who do not respond to other modes of therapy.

TRICHOMONAS. This infection is usually sexually transmitted; it may rarely occur in those who do not engage in sexual intercourse. The symptomatic female patient will have a frothy vaginal discharge. Although males may harbor the organism, they have few clinical manifestations. Diagnosis is based on identification of trichomonads on microscopic examination of a mixture of the discharge with saline. The treatment of both sexual partners with metronidazole (a single dose of 2.0 g orally) is advised, unless pregnancy is suspected. The adolescent should be cautioned about the adverse effect (abdominal pain and vomiting) of alcohol ingestion within 24 hr of metronidazole administration.

HEMOPHILUS (GARDNERELLA) VAGINALIS. This is associated with the production of an often foul-smelling vaginal discharge, which gives off a fishy odor when 10% potassium hydroxide (KOH) is added to a wet preparation, and with the appearance of "clue cells" (epithelial cells ringed with the rod-shaped organisms). The organism is frequently found in vaginal smears from asymptomatic women, but when other etiologic explanations are not found, treatment with metronidazole, 500 mg orally twice a day for 7 days may bring relief.

HUMAN IMMUNODEFICIENCY VIRUS (HIV) (Sec. 12.82). The risk factors for contraction of infection with this virus include unprotected intercourse and IV drug use, both of which occur frequently among adolescents. Therefore, it is anticipated that the numbers of AIDS cases within this age group will increase dramatically. The long incubation period of HIV infection suggests that at least half of the 20–24 yr olds diagnosed as having AIDS in 1988 contracted the infection as adolescents. Pediatricians should take responsibility for educating young people about the transmission of this infection and for screening high-risk adolescents to identify those infected so that early treatment can be initiated.

10.18 MENSTRUAL PROBLEMS OF ADOLESCENTS

AMENORRHEA

Amenorrhea, or absence of menses, may be primary or secondary. *Primary amenorrhea* indicates that menarche has never occurred, whereas *secondary amenorrhea* refers to the cessation of menses for more than 3 mo after regular menstrual cycling has been established. The diagnosis of primary amenorrhea assumes that the patient has passed the age at which menarche normally occurs, from 10 to 16 yr. Accordingly, the determination of primary amenorrhea should first be based on an assessment of the patient's stage of pubertal development; 10% of girls have menarche at SMR 2, 20% at SMR3, 60% at SMR4, and 10% at SMR5. If the patient has not entered puberty by the expected time or if pubertal development is completed without the onset of menses, she should be thoroughly evaluated, even if her chronologic age is within the normal range. Similarly, the close concordance between the age of menarche between daughters and mothers and between siblings should suggest this diagnosis when the patient is more than 1 yr older than was the mother or the sister when their menarche occurred.

The onset and continuation of normal menstrual cycling depends on the functional and anatomic integrity of (1) the hypothalamus together with higher centers, including possibly the pineal; (2) the anterior pituitary; (3) the ovary; and (4) the uterus. Evaluation of the adolescent with amenorrhea should include consideration of possible abnormalities at each of these levels.

ETIOLOGY. In *primary amenorrhea,* chromosomal or congenital abnormalities, such as gonadal dysgenesis, the triple-x syndrome, isochromosomal abnormalities, testicular feminization syndrome, and, rarely, true hermaphroditism, should be considered in addition to the conditions that cause secondary amenorrhea. Elevated levels of follicle-stimulating hormone (FSH) and LH suggest primary gonadal failure, and chromosome analysis will elucidate its cause (Sec. 19.28). Once such a diagnosis is made, management includes the use of estrogen and progesterone to produce the development of secondary sex characteristics and cyclic bleeding if a uterus is present, in order to help the patient to feel like her peers as well as to prevent later osteoporosis.

Primary or *secondary* amenorrhea also may be caused by

chronic illness, particularly that associated with malnutrition or tissue hypoxia, such as diabetes mellitus, inflammatory bowel disease, cystic fibrosis or cyanotic congenital heart disease. In most cases, the illness would have been diagnosed previously, but, occasionally, the amenorrhea is its first manifestation.

A CNS tumor, most commonly a craniopharyngioma, may present with amenorrhea (Sec. 20.74). In addition to a careful neurologic examination, the finding of a low urine specific gravity, erosion of the clinoids, calcifications in the suprasellar area, or an elevated serum prolactin level (in the case of an adenoma) support the diagnosis of pituitary neoplasm.

Abnormalities of the thyroid gland, typically hyperthyroidism, may first be suspected by delayed sexual maturation or amenorrhea, even in the absence of other signs and symptoms. Hypothyroidism more typically causes precocious puberty and menometrorrhagia. Determination of TSH, T_4, and T_3 assist in establishing this diagnosis. Anorexia nervosa, which may present with either primary or secondary amenorrhea (Sec. 10.14), is occasionally confused with hyperthyroidism because of weight loss, hyperactivity, and personality changes seen in both entities.

When primary amenorrhea occurs with advanced pubertal development, a structural anomaly of the müllerian duct system should be suspected. **Imperforate hymen** is most common and is associated with recurrent (monthly) abdominal pain and, after some time has passed, a midline lower abdominal mass, the blood-filled vagina, **hematocolpos.** Diagnosis is made by inspection of the introitus, revealing a bulging hymen with bluish discoloration. If the obstruction is at the level of the cervix, the blood-filled uterus **(hematometrium)** will be apparent on bimanual examination or ultrasonograph. Agenesis of the cervix or uterus is rare but occurs in association with sacral agenesis. Serum levels of gonadotropins are normal in such patients, and diagnosis is made by ultrasonography.

When amenorrhea occurs with signs of virilization, such as clitoromegaly, hirsutism, or excessive acne, adrenal or ovarian pathology or abuse of anabolic steroids should be suspected. The adrenal causes are discussed in Sec. 19.20 and consist of cortical tumors and, very rarely, late onset congenital adrenal hyperplasia. Determination of the 24-hr urinary 17-ketosteroid and serum testosterone levels will assist in diagnosis. Ovarian causes of virilization include the polycystic ovary syndrome (PCO) and a Sertoli-Leydig cell or lipoid cell tumor, which are both rare. In the young adolescent, PCO may present with amenorrhea or oligomenorrhea and no signs of masculinization; because 17-ketosteroids may be normal or elevated. PCO is diagnosed by the finding of normal serum levels of FSH and marked elevation of the LH level (usually 2–3 times higher). In adolescence, laparoscopic biopsy may reveal normal ovarian tissue or the histologic findings typical in the adult, consisting of cysts and thickened tunica alburginia. The adolescent may be spared the long-term masculinizing effects of this condition, as well as the risk of endometrial carcinoma from continued exposure to estrogens unopposed by progesterone, by the administration of combination oral contraceptives.

The first diagnosis to be considered in the adolescent with *secondary amenorrhea* is pregnancy. This possibility also exists, albeit rarely, as a cause of primary amenorrhea, if fertilization of the first released ovum occurred before menses. A history of sexual intercourse, nausea, and breast tenderness and physical findings of increased pigmentation of nipples and linea alba, cyanosis and softening of the cervix, and an enlarged uterus form the classic picture. A serum B-subunit HCG analysis is the most sensitive and specific pregnancy test.

Ingestion of drugs, both legal and illegal, may cause amenorrhea and in the case of phenothiazines, even a false-positive urine pregnancy test. Some drugs, including phenothiazines and certain antihypertensive agents, may cause galactorrhea, further mimicking pregnancy. A thorough drug history is, therefore, necessary.

Psychogenic factors have been implicated in amenorrhea. It is often difficult to separate psychologic factors from nutritional factors, because weight loss is a common confounding variable in many of these situations, such as depression, anorexia nervosa, or stress.

DIAGNOSIS. Evaluation of the adolescent with amenorrhea should include a thorough history and physical examination, a complete blood count, erythrocyte sedimentation rate, pregnancy test, and, if these are negative, serum levels of gonadotropins (LH, FSH), prolactin, TSH, T_4, and T_3; computed tomography (CT) or magnetic resonance imaging (MRI) of the head, if a CNS tumor is suspected; chromosome studies; and determination of urinary 17-ketosteroids. Ultrasonography often can be useful in confirming the presence and size of the uterus and ovaries and identifying tumors and cysts. Ovarian biopsy at the time of exploratory laparoscopy may assist in making a diagnosis.

TREATMENT. Determination of the etiology of amenorrhea may permit the initiation of corrective intervention. When the disorder is not amenable to remediation, consideration should be given to establishing regular pseudo-menses to allow the adolescent to feel like her peers. If the result of a vaginal smear is positive for estrogen effect, regular cycling can be accomplished using medroxyprogesterone in a dose of 10 mg orally for 5 days, every 6–12 wk. In a patient with gonadal dysgenesis, conjugated estrogens must first be given (premarin in an oral dose of 0.625 mg for the first 3 wk of each cycle) followed by medroxyprogesterone, 10 mg orally on days 17–21 of the cycle.

MENOMETRORRHAGIA

Excessive menstrual bleeding is one of the few gynecologic emergencies of adolescence. Bleeding may be so severe as to cause death, hypovolemia, and anemia in a frightened young patient. Diagnosis and therapy must be accomplished expeditiously, while providing reassurance.

DYSFUNCTIONAL UTERINE BLEEDING. Excessive menstrual bleeding is most often secondary to the anovulatory cycles that normally occur in the 1st year post menarche. Without ovulation, estrogen's effect on the endometrium is unopposed by that of progesterone, resulting in continued endometrial proliferation with eventual massive shedding. The constant estrogen effect also serves to inhibit the LH surge responsible for ovulation, thus perpetuating the problem. Imbalance between FSH and LH, such that the former is higher than the latter, often occurs. Basal body temperature determinations may indicate anovulation.

Treatment is indicated only when there is significant bleeding (i.e., when there is evidence of hypovolemia or anemia). Its goal is to correct the imbalance between estrogen and progesterone, while providing hemostasis. One approach is the immediate oral administration of 25 mg norethynodrel (Enovid). Although this may cause nausea in some patients, the effect is rapid, usually, within 2 hr. Thereafter, the dose is tapered by 5 mg/day until a dose of 5 mg/day is reached. This dose is maintained for the duration of a 21-day cycle, calculated from the day that treatment began. If bleeding recurs at any point in the tapering process, the previous day's dose is resumed, and tapering stopped until there is no further bleeding. A normal menstrual period should begin approximately 2 days after the last pill is taken. On the 5th day of bleeding, a 2-mo course of conventional dose (1/50) oral contraceptive therapy is begun. This may be continued if there is need for contraception, being cognizant of the increased risk of post-pill amenorrhea in adolescents with anovulatory cycles before ingestion of these compounds. An alternative to the use of high-dose norethynodrel consists of oral administration of norethindrone (Ortho-Novum) (2 mg) or norethynodrel (2.5 mg) every 4 hr until the bleeding slows or stops, after which it is administered twice daily until the calendar pack is finished.

In the rare case of a patient whose bleeding cannot be controlled by one of these methods, an endometrial curettage may be indicated. Although this procedure is frequently undertaken in adult women with menometrorrhagia, the rarity of endometrial carcinoma and the usual efficacy of hormonal therapy in adolescence makes this procedure unnecessarily invasive in this age group.

CONGENITAL COAGULOPATHIES. Von Willebrand disease should be considered in the adolescent whose first menstrual period is excessive. The finding of a prolonged bleeding time suggests this diagnosis, which is characterized by a defect of platelet adhesiveness and lower levels of factor VIII (Sec. 16.63). The fact that estrogen raises factor VIII levels recommends its use with this condition but underscores the necessity of performing diagnostic studies on blood obtained before the institution of this therapy. Management is the same as for dysfunctional uterine bleeding, with the exception that oral contraceptives will likely be required for the entire menstrual life of the patient.

ASPIRIN. Acquired bleeding diatheses as a result of ingestion of therapeutic doses of aspirin is relatively common and results from disruption of platelet adhesiveness secondary to the effect of the acetyl moiety on the release of adenosine diphosphate. A history of aspirin use within 14 days of menses suggests this possibility and warrants a trial of aspirin avoidance.

THROMBOCYTOPENIA. This may be secondary to toxins, marrow infiltration, hypersplenism, or idiopathic thrombocytopenic purpura (ITP) and may present with, or be complicated by, menometrorrhagia. Management is the same as that described for dysfunctional uterine bleeding, although platelet transfusions may also be necessary.

EXOGENOUS HORMONES. Improper use of oral contraceptives may cause excessive vaginal bleeding. Careful and sensitive history-taking is an important part of evaluation of a patient with this symptom.

THYROID DISORDERS. Hypothyroidism and, rarely, hyperthyroidism may cause excessive vaginal bleeding, occasionally as a presenting symptom. The characteristically low level of T_4 may be altered by the estrogen therapy used to stop the bleeding, but free T_4 should not be affected and TSH remains elevated.

OTHER CAUSES. Rarely, adrenal dysfunction, diabetes mellitus, or estrogen-secreting ovarian tumors may cause increased vaginal bleeding. The bleeding caused by adenocarcinoma of the vagina is typically scant.

In contrast with the conditions described earlier, menometrorrhagia resulting from *trauma, infection,* or *pregnancy* is typically accompanied by pain. Lacerations of the genital tract may result from first or forceful intercourse or athletics, such as waterskiing. The circumstances of the injury may be embarrassing or frightening for the patient, requiring supportive and sensitive history-taking. Surgical intervention by a gynecologist is usually needed once the cause of bleeding is identified.

As approximately 15% of pregnancies in the adolescent age group terminate in *spontaneous abortion,* this possibility should be considered in every case of painful excessive vaginal bleeding. In addition to history and physical examination, performance of a B-subunit HCG pregnancy test should be obtained because this remains positive up to 15 days after an abortion. (Other pregnancy tests revert to negative within 5–8 days.) Involvement of a gynecologist is necessary once the diagnosis is confirmed. Rarely, ectopic pregnancy may present with abnormal vaginal bleeding.

DYSMENORRHEA

Painful menstrual cramps are experienced by nearly two-thirds of post-menarcheal teenagers in the United States, according to the National Health Examination Survey. More than 10% of this group suffer sufficiently to miss school, making dysmenorrhea the leading cause of short-term school absenteeism in female adolescents. Dysmenorrhea may be primary or secondary, the former being the more common. *Secondary dysmenorrhea* results from an underlying **structural abnormality** of the cervix or uterus, a **foreign body** such as an IUD, endometriosis, or **endometritis. Endometriosis,** a condition in which implants of endometrial tissue are found at ectopic locations within the peritoneal cavity, is being diagnosed with increasing frequency among adolescents due to the use of ultrasonography and laparoscopy. Characteristically, there is severe pain at the time of menses; its specific location depends on the site of the implants. Some patients respond favorably to treatment with oral contraceptives, whereas the more severe cases are treated with danazol, an antigonadotropin.

A pelvic examination must be performed to exclude the causes of secondary dysmenorrhea, and if none is found, a diagnosis of *primary dysmenorrhea* should be considered. Prostaglandins $F_{2\alpha}$ and E_2, produced by the endometrium, stimulate the myometrium to contract, producing pain. Those suffering from dysmenorrhea have high levels of these substances and experience symptomatic relief when prostaglandin-synthetase inhibitors are administered. If given before a menstrual period (or shortly after it begins), administration of a rapidly absorbed prostaglandin-synthetase inhibitor, such as naproxen-sodium, is effective in destroying the prostaglandins before they produce pain (e.g., two tablets of 275 mg each taken with the onset of menses and one tablet taken every 6–8 hr after that for the 1st 24 hr). Medication is rarely needed beyond the 1st day. For the teenager with dysmenorrhea who requires contraception, oral contraceptive therapy may be indicated. It is not certain whether the beneficial effect of their use derives from their ability to inhibit ovulation and thus eliminate progesterone production from the corpus luteum or from their ability to limit endometrial proliferation, and therefore the production of prostaglandins.

PREMENSTRUAL SYNDROME

Premenstrual syndrome (PMS), or the late luteal phase, is a complex of physical signs and behavioral symptoms occurring during the second half of the menstrual cycle, which may resolve with the onset of menses. Clinical manifestations may include breast fullness and tenderness; bloating; fatigue; headache; increased appetite, especially for sweets and salty foods; irritability and mood swings; and depression, inability to concentrate, tearfulness, and violent tendencies. About one-third of women in the reproductive age group may have PMS, but the absence of objective findings makes this difficult to corroborate. It is not common among adolescents, and it does not relate to the presence of dysmenorrhea, which is much more common in this age group. The popular use of vitamin B_6 and progesterone supplementation is not based on evidence of their effectiveness, nor is there a theoretical basis for their use. Use of a gonadotropin-releasing hormone agonist on a short-term basis is supported by carefully controlled studies, but long-term effects and potential complications have not yet been evaluated, making its use in adolescents premature.

TOXIC SHOCK SYNDROME

See Sec. 12.20.

10.19 THE BREAST

As one of the most obvious signs of puberty (Sec. 3.9) breast development is often the focus of attention and a cause of anxiety, particularly when growth is asymmetric or if it occurs in males (gynecomastia). Rarely, the asymmetry is so marked as to create self-consciousness and interfere with self-image. Under those circumstances, consideration may be given to corrective surgery. Although both augmentation and reduction mammoplasty are possible, each has advantages and disadvantages. The former necessitates implantation of a foreign substance, whereas the latter may cause considerable loss of blood and the possibility of later cutaneous hyposensitivity. Surgery is contraindicated prior to completion of breast growth, which coincides with SMR5.

The most common of adolescent breast disorders is the presence of *a mass,* the majority of which are benign cysts or fibroadenomas. Cysts vary in size over the course of a menstrual cycle so that a patient should be re-examined 2 wk after the initial examination. Persistence of the mass or its enlargement over three menstrual cycles is an indication for surgical consultation. Aspiration is usually attempted under local anesthesia, often resulting in curative drainage if it proves to be a cyst. If no fluid is obtained, an excisional biopsy is indicated. This should be done through a circumareolar incision to prevent a disfiguring scar. In one biopsy series, 71% were found to be fibroadenomas, 11% were abscesses, and 2% were cystosarcoma phylloides, a low-grade malignancy. Carcinoma of the breast in the adolescent is rare and the possible long-term sequelae of mammography are unknown, thus this procedure is not advised for this age group.

The development of multiple small lumps in the breast is suggestive of **fibrocystic disease,** with the risk of other forms of breast disease in later years. Accordingly, these patients should be taught to examine their breasts regularly and frequently (Sec. 18.52). The use of combination oral contraceptives of low progesterone potency may be beneficial.

Gynecomastia (Sec. 19.32) occurs in approximately one third of normal males during early puberty and often causes concern that may not be openly voiced. The response should be factual information and reassurance of its usual transient nature. Rarely is it of such magnitude or persistence as to warrant surgery.

Nipple discharge in this age group is usually due to local stimulation, use of medications, including oral contraceptives, and pregnancy; rarely, it results from a pituitary or breast neoplasm or infection. Examination of the discharge assists in diagnosis; benign conditions are associated with a milky or grumous (sticky and thick) discharge, infection with a purulent one, and intraductal papilloma and cancer with a serous, serosanguineous or bloody discharge. Elevation of the serum prolactin level may occur in the amenorrhea-galactorrhea syndromes, associated with use of certain antihypertensive medications, oral contraceptives, tranquilizers, or secondary to a pituitary adenoma. The latter is evaluated with a CT scan or MRI of the head. The possibility of a breast neoplasm is an indication for cytologic examination of the discharge and surgical consultation. Infection in the non–breast-feeding adolescent is rare and may be secondary to a human bite or the initial symptom in diabetes mellitus. Culture of the discharge, followed by appropriate antibiotic therapy (usually directed against the *Staphylococcus*) is indicated, and surgical drainage is rarely necessary.

10.20 SKIN PROBLEMS

The skin responds as a secondary sex characteristic during puberty, reflecting increased levels of androgens by increased size and secretions of sebaceous follicles and of apocrine glands, the most common manifestation of which is acne. The pathogenesis, clinical picture, and management of acne are discussed in Sec. 23.32.

As adolescents become preoccupied with their appearance, acne assumes great importance. For that reason, offering treatment even to the youngster whose acne is mild may enhance self-image and is appropriate. Special considerations in the treatment of acne in adolescents include the need to be sure that the patient is not pregnant before instituting therapy with either tetracycline or *cis*-retinoic acid, is alerted to the possibility that chronic tetracycline therapy may cause vaginal infection with *Candida,* and appreciates that acne may be worsened or improved by oral contraceptives, depending on the type of estrogen or progestin.

The skin of the adolescent is influenced not only by the hormones of puberty but also by psychosocial factors occurring at this time. For example, sexual experimentation may result in a sexually transmitted disease with dermatologic manifestations (Sec. 10.17); stress may be manifested by trichotillomania; contact sports, most notably wrestling, may be associated with *herpes simplex* infection; and drug abuse may cause skin lesions (Sec. 10.4).

10.21 ORTHOPEDIC PROBLEMS

Puberty is associated with rapid growth of long bones, open epiphyses, and increased traction at sites of insertion of muscles, all of which contribute to the increased rate and unique types of orthopedic problems in this age group. Participation in sports is an additional risk factor, particularly when teams are configured on the basis of chronologic, rather than developmental, age criteria. As a result, such conditions as slipped capital femoral epiphysis, Osgood-Schlatter disease, idiopathic scoliosis, (Sec. 24.11, 24.6, and 24.15), and costochondritis of the sternoclavicular junction (Tsetse syndrome) are common in adolescents. Certain osseous neoplasms, such as osteogenic sarcoma, are also increased in incidence during adolescence. Infections of bones and joints, although generally less common in adolescents than younger children, may occur as a complication of disseminated gonococcemia or sickle cell anemia. Viral infections, such as rubella and infectious mononucleosis, are more likely to cause arthralgia in adolescents than in younger children.

10.22 DELIVERY OF HEALTH CARE TO ADOLESCENTS

In providing health care to adolescents, the physician must combine familiar elements of the "well-child" visit (Sec. 5.1) with others drawn from the practice of adult medicine that acknowledge the patient's maturation. Accordingly, prevention of physical and psychological dysfunction is addressed through examination, education, and anticipatory guidance, as well as immunization. Reimmunization against measles, mumps, and rubella (MMR) of early adolescents is recommended because of the resurgence of measles and rubella among adolescents (Sec. 12.64 and 12.65). For nonimmunocompromised older adolescents who are not pregnant, this may also be indicated. It is prudent to withhold immunization until one is satisfied that the patient is not pregnant (Sec. 10.15).

Functional status is assessed by an age-appropriate history, physical examination, and laboratory testing using instruments, techniques, and standards devised for adolescents. Dysfunction is addressed through age-appropriate interventions. Throughout, a balance is struck between the adolescents' need for autonomy, privacy, and confidentiality and parental concern and wish to be informed. Judgment is also necessary in weighing the adolescent's need to have a specific acute problem addressed and the wish to utilize a rare medical contact with the teenager for the purposes of education, prevention, and screening, often time-consuming processes.

LEGAL ISSUES

In the United States, the right of a minor to *consent* to treatment without parental knowledge is governed by state laws. Usually, the right to self-consent for treatment is granted when there is suspicion of a sexually transmitted disease. Because such diseases are often asymptomatic, this provision is generally interpreted as enabling the physician to perform a pelvic examination on any sexually active adolescent solely upon her own consent. In many states, adolescents may consent to receive care for drug abuse or mental health problems.

The minor's right to *contraceptives* has not been reviewed by the Supreme Court, although their right to privacy has been upheld (except in a decision allowing for searches in schools without due process) and accordingly, most states permit the provision of contraceptives to teenagers upon their own consent. Although attempts at restricting Title X funded programs to provision of contraception only after informing parents has not been legislated, the publicity received by the proposal has left many teenagers with the mistaken notion that their parents will be informed if they seek birth control from any physician. The right of an adolescent to obtain an *abortion* without parental consent or over parental objection is unsettled.

With the exception of Delaware, which has an age requirement of 17 yr, all other states require that an individual be 18 yr of age in order to consent to *blood donation. Organ donation* by a consenting minor generally requires parental consent as well as a court order to ensure that there is no alternative adult donor, that the transplant is absolutely necessary in order to save the life of the recipient, and that the adolescent donor will not suffer physically or psychologically as a result of the procedure.

Minors are also exempt from the requirement of parental consent for medical treatment under the following circumstances: (1) *emancipated minors.* These are children who live away from home, are no longer subject to parental control, are economically self-supporting, are married, or are members of the military. (2) *Emergencies.* In a medical emergency, a minor may be treated without consent of parents if, in the physician's judgment, the delay resulting from attempts to contact parents would jeopardize the life or health of the minor. (3) *Mature Minor Rule.* An emerging trend in the law is the recognition that many minors are sufficiently mature to understand the nature of their illness and the potential risks and benefits of proposed therapy and, therefore, should receive such treatment upon their own consent. In these cases, the physician should document that the adolescent has acted in a responsible manner. The growing number of cases involving charges of sexual misconduct against male physicians suggests that a chaparone should be present whenever an adolescent female patient is examined. The necessity for chaparoning in the situation of a female physician and a male adolescent patient has not yet become an issue.

SCREENING

Screening tests should be performed only if they are cost effective. This determination for the adolescent involves knowledge of prevalence of the condition in this age group, as well as cost (including possible psychologic and physical sequelae). Screening to detect trivial conditions or those for which there is no immediate intervention should be avoided lest their discovery further the early adolescent's natural tendency to feel flawed or imperfect. During late adolescence, however, it may be appropriate to perform screening tests for genetic disease carrier states in preparation for marriage. Reference standards for adolescents should be available before a screening test is performed to avoid an erroneous diagnosis. Gender and stage of puberty should determine the timing and choice of screening maneuvers (Tables 10–3, 10–4, and 10–5).

LABORATORY TESTS. During early adolescence, a screening *urinalysis and culture* are indicated for the female. Polymorphonuclear leukocytes in the urinary sediment suggest the possibility of either cervicitis, vaginitis, urethritis, or an asymptomatic infection of the urinary tract, the last a common finding in adolescent females. The increased incidence of iron-deficiency anemia following menarche also mandates the performance of a *hematocrit* in this group on an annual basis. The reference standard for this test changes with progression of puberty, as estrogen suppresses erythropoietin. Androgens have the opposite effect, causing the hematocrit to rise during male puberty; SMR 1 males have an average hematocrit of 39% whereas those who have completed puberty (SMR 5) have an average value of 43%. *Tuberculosis testing* on an annual basis is important in adolescents, because puberty has been shown to activate this disease in those not previously treated. Sexually active adolescents should undergo screening for *sexually transmitted diseases,* regardless of symptomatology (Sec. 10.17). *HIV testing* should be included for those at increased risk: bi- and homosexual males, female partners of bisexuals or IV drug abusers, and IV drug users. *Pap smears* are also indicated in sexually active females, regardless of age, because 5–35/1000 have early neoplastic changes. Technique is important; the practice of obtaining two successive cervical scrapes increases the yield by 26% over that obtained by a single cervical specimen. When screening tests for *genetic defect carrier states* are performed, age-appropriate counseling should be immediately available to ensure an opportunity to have questions answered and to have unspoken fears allayed. The use of *spirometry* screening for adolescents who smoke may, over time, serve as a deterrant if deterioration of respiratory status can be demonstrated.

AUDIOMETRY. Highly amplified music of the kind enjoyed by many adolescents may elevate the audiometric threshold, resulting in hearing loss. Therefore, an audiogram should be performed yearly during adolescence, even if earlier tests have been normal.

VISION TESTING. The pubertal growth spurt may involve the optic globe, resulting in its elongation and myopia in genetically predisposed individuals. Vision testing should, therefore, be performed in order to detect this problem before it affects school performance.

BLOOD PRESSURE DETERMINATION. Criteria for a diagnosis of hypertension are based on age-specific norms that increase with pubertal maturation. An individual whose

TABLE 10–3. Package of Care: The Well Adolescent Visit I and Early Adolescence (Tanner 2)

	Females	Males
Screening		
Physical	Hematocrit	—
	Urine culture screen	—
	Tuberculin	—
Psychosocial	Self-image	Self-image
	Depression	Depression
	Peer interaction (including sexuality)	Peer interaction (including sexuality)
	School performance	School performance
	Substance abuse	Substance abuse
Health promotion	Self-examination of breasts	Self-examination of scrotum
	Nutrition counseling	Nutrition counseling
Prevention	Smoking	Smoking
	Cycle safety	Cycle safety
	Automotive passenger safety	Automotive passenger safety
	Immunization update	Immunization update
Anticipatory guidance	Developing independence	Developing independence
	Dealing with peer pressure	Dealing with peer pressure
	Confidentiality	Confidentiality
	Variations in growth and development	Variations in growth and development
	Dating	Dating
	Preparation for menarche	—
Physical examination		
Special attention to:	Blood pressure	Blood pressure
	Height, weight	Height, weight
	Skinfold thickness	Skinfold thickness
	—	Grip strength
	Stage of sexual development	Stage of sexual development
	Scoliosis	—
	Goiter	—
	Acne	Acne
	—	Gynecomastia
	Tibial tubercle	Tibial tubercle
	Gait	Gait
Symptomatic treatment (anything revealed by the above +)	Acne	Acne
	Dysmenorrhea	—

blood pressure exceeds two standard deviations for his or her age is suspect for having hypertension, regardless of the absolute reading. The technique is important; false-positive results may be obtained if the cuff covers less than two-thirds of the upper arm. The patient should be seated, and an average should be taken of the 2nd and 3rd consecutive readings, using the change rather than the disappearance as the diastolic pressure. Most adolescents with elevations of blood pressure have labile hypertension (Sec. 15.81). Half of those with adolescent onset labile hypertension progress to sustained hypertension in adulthood and require close follow-up. Antihypertensive medication is not indicated and the effect of reduced salt intake in the adolescent on eventual adult hypertension is unknown. If blood pressure is below two standard deviations for age, AN and Addison disease should be considered.

SCOLIOSIS. Approximately 5% of male and 10–14% of female adolescents have a mild curvature of the spine. This is 2–4 times the rate in younger children. Scoliosis is typically manifested during the peak of the height velocity curve (Sec. 24.18), at approximately 12 yr in females and 14 yr in males. Curves measuring greater than 10 degrees should be followed by an orthopedist until growth is completed.

BREAST EXAMINATION. Examination of the female ad-

TABLE 10–4. Package of Care: The Well Adolescent Visit II and Midadolescence (Tanner 3–4)

	Females	Males
Screening		
Physical	Vision testing	Vision testing
	Hearing testing	Hearing testing
If sexually active	Papanicolaou smear	—
	VDRL* test	VDRL test
	Gonorrhea culture	Gonorrhea culture
Prevention	Automotive safety	Automotive safety
	STD† prevention	STD prevention
	Prevention of pregnancy	Prevention of pregnancy
	Vocational/educational planning	Vocational/educational planning
	Obesity/inactivity	Obesity/inactivity
Physical examination	Breast masses	Gynecomastia
	—	Testicular tumor
	Vaginal discharge	Urethral discharge
	Pregnancy	—

*VDRL = Venereal Disease Research Laboratory.
†STD = sexually transmitted diseases.

TABLE 10–5. Package of Care: The Well Adolescent Visit III and Late Adolescence (Tanner 5)

	Females	Males
Screening		
Physical		
If sexually active	Genetically transmitted diseases	Genetically transmitted diseases
	Papanicolaou smear	—
	VDRL* test	VDRL* test
If homosexual	Gonorrhea culture	Gonorrhea culture
If bisexual	HIV† test	HIV† test
Prevention	Automotive safety	Automotive safety
	STD‡ prevention	STD prevention
	Prevention of pregnancy	Prevention of pregnancy
	Obesity/inactive	Obesity/inactive
Anticipatory guidance	Planning for marriage	Planning for marriage
	Vocational/educational planning	Vocational/educational planning
	Cults	Cults
	Becoming a health care consumer	Becoming a health care consumer
	Leaving home	Leaving home
	Moving into work force/college	Moving into work force/college
	Entering military	Entering military
	Health insurance	Health insurance
Physical examination	Breast masses	—
	—	Testicular tumor
	Vaginal discharge	Urethral discharge
	Pregnancy	—
Treatment	Corrective surgery (after growth complete)	Corrective surgery (after growth complete)

*VDRL = Venereal Disease Research Laboratory.
†HIV = human immunodeficiency virus.
‡STD = sexually transmitted diseases.

olescent's breasts is performed to detect masses (Sec. 10.19), evaluate progression of sexual maturation, provide reassurance about development, and teach the technique of self-examination with the hope that this practice will continue into the higher risk later years.

SCROTUM EXAMINATION. The peak incidence of germ cell tumors of the testes is in late adolescence and early adulthood. For that reason, palpation of the testes may have an immediate yield and should serve as a model for instruction of self-examination. Because varicoceles often appear during puberty, the examination also provides an opportunity to explain and reassure the patient about this entity (Sec. 18.46).

PSYCHOSOCIAL. A few questions should be asked directed at detecting the adolescent who is having difficulty with peer relationships (e.g., "Do you have a best friend with whom you can share even the most personal secret?"); with self-image (e.g., "Is there anything you would like to change about yourself?" or "What do you consider to be your best features?"); with depression (e.g., "What do you see yourself doing 5 years from now?" or "Are you ever so sad that you think of dying?"); with school (e.g., "How are your grades this year compared with last year?" and "How many days have you been absent from school this year compared with last year?"); with personal decisions (e.g., "Are you feeling pressured to engage in any behavior for which you do not feel you are ready?" or "Is there anything you would like to change in your relationship with your boyfriend, your father, etc.?"); and with an eating disorder (e.g., "Do you ever feel that food controls you rather than visa versa?") If the responses to any of these questions suggest a problem, standardized tests are available for more thorough probing or for in-depth interviewing.

Interviewing the Adolescent

It is often difficult to establish open communication with the adolescent patient, unless a prior relationship existed with the physician. Even under that circumstance, the previously comfortable relationship may change with the advent of adolescence, as it often does with parents. The teenager may now wish more privacy than that usually available in the pediatrician's office, and the pediatrician may appear judgmental to a teenager who has some conflict with his or her own parents. Adolescents often imagine that the physician, through the process of physical examination, can detect evidence of behaviors such as smoking, drinking, or masturbation. The physician who takes time to listen, avoids judgmental statements and use of street jargon, and shows respect for the adolescent's emerging maturity will have an easier time communicating with him or her. The use of open-ended questions, rather than closed-ended questions, will further facilitate history-taking (e.g., Question = "Do you get along with your father?" Answer = "Yes." Compare with the question: "What would you like to change in your relationship with your father?" Answer = "I would like to stop him from always putting me down, especially in front of my friends."). The adolescent should be given the opportunity to express concerns and the reasons for seeking medical attention. After the teenager's agenda has been addressed, the physician may wish to define the boundaries of the physician-patient relationship. In such a relationship, the former agrees to provide confidentiality, except if the well-being of the patient or another person may be jeopardized, and the adolescent, in turn, agrees to act maturely and responsibly in terms of medical care.

HEALTH ENHANCEMENT

The health status of adolescents may be enhanced by application of principles of prevention and anticipatory guidance. Prevention of infectious disease should include immunization and counseling. Boosters of dT should be given at approximately 15 yr of age, and MMR at 11–12 yr of age. Prevention of sexually transmitted diseases (Sec. 10.17) and of pregnancy (Sec. 10.15) is an important issue to be addressed in sexually active adolescents of both sexes. Prevention of automotive accidents, the leading killer of adolescents, and of smoking, the leading killer of adults, should also be discussed.

IRIS F. LITT

PSYCHOSOCIAL PROBLEMS

Depression/Suicide

Beck AT, Beck R, Kovacs M: Classification of suicidal behaviors. 1: Quantifying intent and medical lethality. Am J Psychol 132:285, 1975.

Mattsson A: Adolescent depressions and suicide. *In:* Friedman SB, Hoekelman RA (eds): Behavioral Pediatrics. New York, McGraw-Hill, 1980.

McAnarney ER: Suicidal behavior of children and youth. Pediatr Clin North Am 22:595, 1975.

Puig-Antich J, Rabinovich H: Major child and adolescent psychiatric disorders. *In:* Levine MD, Carey WB, Crocker AC, Gross RT (eds): Developmental-Behavioral Pediatrics. Philadelphia, WB Saunders, 1983, pp 865–890.

Substance Abuse

Hallagan JB, Hallagan LF, Smyder MB: Anabolic-androgen steroid use by athletes. N Engl J Med 32:1042, 1989.

Jessor R, Chase JA, Donovan JE: Psychosocial correlates of marijuana use and problem drinking in a national sample of adolescents. Am J Public Health 70:604, 1980.

Jessor R, Jessor SL: Adolescence to young adulthood: A twelve-year prospective study of problem behavior and psychosocial development. *In:* Mednick S, Horway M (eds): Longitudinal Research in the United States. New York, Praeger, 1984.

Johnston LD, O'Malley PM, Bachman JG: Illicit drug use, smoking, and drinking by America's high school students, college students, and young adults, 1975–1987. USDHHS, PHS, Alcohol, Drug Abuse and Mental Health Administration, 1988.

Kandel DB, Logan JA: Patterns of drug use from adolescence to young adulthood. 1: Periods of risk for initiation, continued use, and discontinuation. Am J Public Health 74:660, 1984.

Kolodny RC, Masters WH, Kolodner RM, et al: Depression of plasma testosterone after chronic intensive marijuana use. N Engl J Med 290:872, 1974.

Lieber CS: The metabolism of alcohol. Sci Am 234:25, 1976.

Litt IF, Cohen MI: The drug-using adolescent as a pediatric patient. J Pediatr 77:195, 1970.

Rogol AD: Anabolic steroid hormones for athletes: efficacy or fantasy? Growth, Genetics, and Hormones 4:4, 1988.

Disorders of Sleep

Anders TF, Keener MA: Sleep-wake state development and disorders of sleep in infants, children, and adolescents. *In:* Levine MD, Carey WB, Crocker AC, et al (eds): Developmental-Behavioral Pediatrics. Philadelphia, WB Saunders, 1983.

Anorexia Nervosa

Bruch H: The Golden Cage: The Enigma of Anorexia Nervosa. Cambridge, Harvard University Press, 1978.

Palla B, Litt IF: Medical complications of eating disorders. Pediatrics 81:613, 1988.

Pregnancy and Contraception

Alan Guttmacher Institute: Teenage Pregnancy: The Problem That Hasn't Gone Away. New York, Alan Guttmacher Institute, 1981.

Hatcher RA, Guest F, Stewart F, et al: Contraceptive Technology, 1988–1989, 14th ed. New York, Irvington Publishers, 1988.

Sorensen RC: Adolescent Sexuality in Contemporary America. New York, World, 1973.

Sexually Transmitted Diseases

Davis AJ, Emans SJ: Human papilloma virus infection in the pediatric and adolescent patient. J Pediatr 115:1, 1989.

The Medical Letter: Treatment of sexually transmitted diseases. Vol. 30 (issue 757), January 15, 1988.

Menstrual Problems

Emans SJH, Goldstein DP: Pediatric and Adolescent Gynecology. Boston, Little, Brown, 1977.

Litt IF: Menstrual problems during adolescence. Pediatr Rev 4:203, 1983.

Delivery of Health Care to Adolescents

Holder AR: Legal Issues in Pediatrics and Adolescent Medicine. New York, John Wiley, 1977.

Litt IF: Adolescent health care. *In:* Green M, Haggerty RJ (eds): Ambulatory Pediatrics IV. Philadelphia, WB Saunders, 1990.

11

IMMUNITY, ALLERGY, AND DISEASES OF INFLAMMATION

11.1 THE IMMUNOLOGIC SYSTEM

The immunologic system is the segment of host defenses that includes macrophages, leukocytes, lymphocytes, and the complement system. Together with physical barriers, such as an intact integument and motile cilia, its primary function is to protect against invasion by infectious agents. The potential costs of this protection are allergy, autoimmunity, and rejection of organ transplants.

PHYSIOLOGY

SOURCE OF CELLS. The hematopoietic and lymphoid systems develop from multipotential precursors. In early intrauterine life the fetal liver serves as the repository for lymphoid precursor cells. The bone marrow is populated later, and in extrauterine life serves as the major source of the precursor cells.

DIFFERENTIATION. Lymphoid stem cells differentiate into two major lines: T cells and B cells, which have different functions in their protective roles (Table 11–1). T cells are so named because they differentiate in the thymus gland, whereas B cells mature in the bone marrow in man and the bursa of Fabricius in chickens.

TABLE 11–1. Functions of T and B Cells*

Role of T Cells
- T helper function
- T suppressor function
- T killer function
  - Containment of acidfast bacteria
  - Containment of certain viral infections after establishment (rubeola, varicella, herpes, cytomegalovirus, Epstein-Barr virus, "slow" viruses)
  - Containment of fungal infections (especially *Candida*)
  - Containment of protozoan infections
  - Rejection of allografts (and possibly tumors)
  - Graft versus host disease (GVHD)
  - Contact dermatitis

Role of B Cells
- Synthesize and secrete major classes of immunoglobulin, which:
  - Protect against staphylococcus, streptococcus, hemophilus, pneumococcus reinfection (or infection in immunized persons)
  - Neutralize viruses to prevent initial infection
  - Act as barriers along gastrointestinal and respiratory passages
  - Initiate killing of microorganisms by macrophages and other cells bearing Fc receptors
  - Cause the secretion of vasoactive amines from mast cells and basophils
  - Actively lyse cells of autologous origin or engage in antigen-antibody complex disease
  - Interfere with T killer cell activity by directly or indirectly blocking the reaction

*Adapted from Horowitz SD, Hong R: The Pathogenesis and Treatment of Immunodeficiency. Basel, S. Karger, 1977.

Differentiation of T cells in the thymus includes three major functions. Effective T cell responses to soluble antigen require that the antigen presented by the antigen-presenting cell be associated with transplantation antigens. Transplantation antigens seen in the developmental mileau of the thymus are essential components of any antigen to which the organism will develop T cell immunity. Thus, one of the important functions of early thymus differentiation is the definition of these transplantation antigens. This phenomenon is known as genetic restriction because T cell immunity is restricted to antigens presented in association with genetically determined products (i.e., the transplantation antigens); this can be thought of as our immunologic "self."

Transplantation antigens in man comprise class I and class II (Sec. 6.39). Antigens that combine with class I transplantation antigens react with T cells bearing a molecule known as CD8 on their surface, whereas antigen and class II complexes combine with CD4. During the thymic differentiation process, mature T cells bearing either CD4 or CD8 are generated from cells that transiently bear both CD4 and CD8. This process gives rise to the two major T cell subsets seen outside the thymus, the CD4+ and CD8+ cells. A former designation, T4 helper for CD4+ cells and T8 cytotoxic/suppressor cells for CD8+ cells, incorrectly associates the surface markers only with their functional capability.

For the lymphocyte to react specifically, an antigen receptor must also be created. The receptors are composed of two polypeptide chains, an α-β pair or a γ-δ pair. The γ-δ receptor develops first; mature T cells using the γ-δ receptor are found only rarely outside the thymus, and their specific role in immunity is not well understood. The majority of T cells display the α-β receptor. Receptors are formed by a process of gene rearrangement in which large, noncontiguous blocks of deoxyribonucleic acid (DNA) are spliced together. These segments, known as V (variable), D (diversity), and J (joining), each have a number of variants. VDJ segments are joined to a constant region of the α gene, and VJ segments are joined to the β gene to complete the receptor polypeptide genes. Random combinations of the segments account for much of the marked heterogeneity of the resultant receptor. Since humans must recognize 1 to 2 million different antigens throughout their lifetimes, it is necessary to generate many different specificities.

The thymus is responsible for a third important function. Many of the maturing cells have the capacity to attack the host. If these were allowed to mature and were exported from the thymus, they could result in serious autoimmune disease and even death. The thymus screens developing T cell clones and selects those needed for health. Potentially dangerous clones are destroyed in situ or at least prevented from proliferating and undergoing further differentiation and export from the gland. Only 1% of the entering precursor cells leave the thymus as mature functional effector T cells. These varied functions are accomplished by epithelial cells, dendritic cells, and macrophages of the thymus. Some of the epithelial cells elaborate hormones that play a role in differentiation, and some of these molecules have been isolated and used in treatments.

B cell differentiation takes place first in the fetal liver and later in the bone marrow. Gene rearrangement occurs that defines the B cell receptor in a way similar to the method used for the T cell receptor. The B cell receptor eventually becomes part of a secreted immunoglobulin molecule; VDJ segments are combined with constant regions of the immunoglobulin heavy chain genes, and VJ segments with constant regions of the light chain genes. Ultimately, four major immunoglobulin isotypes, IgM, IgG, IgA, and IgE, are produced, each by a B cell subset. Each cell line is ultimately derived from a pre-B cell. The direct descendant of this cell synthesizes IgM only. Subsequently, B cell switching occurs, generating a cell that produces the other isotypes. Normally, a cell line produces only one isotype.

The various stages of differentiation are marked by the acquisition of various surface markers, some of which have been described earlier. These marker systems have become useful in characterizing the lymphocyte populations, permitting enumeration of the different stages that are present. In addition, the markers are used in describing leukemias, which represent malignant expansion of normal lymphocytes at various stages of differentiation. Characterizing leukemias as of T or B cell origin and relating them to early or late stages of differentiation has important implications for therapy and prognosis.

TRAFFIC. Since the events of the immune process, from differentiation to the receipt of antigen and elaboration of immune products, take place in different areas of the body, the lymphocytes must be motile. They circulate freely through the major lymphoid channels, the thoracic duct, and the vascular tree, but their movement into and from the lymphoid organs is highly controlled. For example, cells that leave the thymic parenchyma apparently do not re-enter this site of primary differentiation. The traffic pattern appears to be controlled by chemical groupings on the surface of the lymphocytes and blood vessels. Removal of surface carbohydrate or protein moieties alters the traffic pattern.

ONTOGENY. The newborn is immunologically quite competent. Various types of T cells function beginning as early as 7.5 wk of intrauterine life. By 8–9 wk lymphoid infiltration into the thymus begins; at 12 wk the thymus resembles the mature organ. Even premature infants can reject skin grafts.

Circulating B cells are detected as early as 13 wk after conception; secretory capability is probably present for all major classes of immunoglobulins by the 20th wk. Extensive synthesis and secretion of antibody do not occur owing to the relatively sheltered antigenic environment of the fetus. IgM antibodies are first to develop; increased levels of IgM can, therefore, be taken as evidence of intrauterine infection. Serum IgM usually rises to adult levels by 1 yr of age, IgG by about 4 yr, and IgA in adolescence (Table 11–2).

CELLULAR EVENTS. The production of immune cell lines following exposure to antigen requires cellular interaction involving both T and B cells and macrophages. Physical contact between at least two of these cell types is probably necessary. Receptor molecules on the surfaces of the T and B cells combine specifically with antigens. Macrophages can adsorb antibody molecules onto their surfaces, although their usual role in antigen processing involves ingestion, partial digestion, and re-expression of the antigen on the surface in association with a transplantation antigen. Antigen can be thought of as a ligand that binds two or more cells together. Following interaction initiated by antigen exposure, the cells are rendered immune. After the immunizing event, a certain portion of the sensitized cells capable of proliferation remain in a memory pool so that cells committed to a particular antigen are available for the recall production of large numbers of cells (clones). In this way, subsequent exposures to the antigen are met with a rapid and vigorous response. Activation of the memory population allows the immune system to provide a vast array of protective capabilities yet not be burdened with maintaining such capabilities at full force by multiplying the numbers of needed responding elements quickly.

The initial external event that begins this process is the combination of antigen with the surface receptor of the B or T cell. Occupation of the receptor site initiates a cascade of events through mechanisms of cell activation now known to be utilized for many cell types in their responses to environmental stimuli. Ion fluxes, calcium mobilization, activation of kinases through the adenylate cyclase and phosphoinositol

TABLE 11–2. Levels of Immunoglobulins*

	IgG (mg/dL)	IgM (mg/dL)	IgA (mg/dL)	IgE (IU/mL)
Serum				
Newborn	1031 ± 200†	11 ± 5	2 ± 3	0–7.5
6 mo	427 ± 186	43 ± 17	28 ± 18	—
12 mo	661 ± 219	54 ± 23	37 ± 18	—
24 mo	762 ± 209	58 ± 23	50 ± 24	137 ± 147
8 yr	923 ± 256	65 ± 25	124 ± 45	251 ± 167
16 yr	946 ± 124	59 ± 20	148 ± 63	330 ± 212
Adult	1158 ± 305	99 ± 27	200 ± 61	200‡
Secretions				
Colostrum	10	61	1234	—
Stimulated parotid saliva	0.036	0.043	3.9	—
Unstimulated whole saliva	4.86	0.55	30.4	—
Jejunal fluid	34	70	—	—
Seminal fluid	510	90	116	—
Cerebrospinal fluid				
Normal	3 ± 1	0	0.4 ± 0.5	—
Purulent infection	9	4	4	—
Viral infection	4	0.5	1	—

*Adapted from Hong R: Evaluation of the immunoglobulins. Clin Immunobiol 3:1, 1976.
†Mean ± 1 standard deviation.
‡Values up to 800 IU/mL are normal.

cascades, and activation of tyrosine kinase are the important events. Special surface receptors in addition to the antigen recognition sites are important in these processes. CD45 plays an important modulating role in T cells, and CD20 has an analogous function in B cells. The T cell receptor is combined with a complex denoted CD3. Perturbation of these surface receptors in one way leads to stimulation of the immune reaction; perturbation in another way can lead to paralysis of the clone, or tolerance.

One of the events associated with activation of a clone of sensitized cells is the secretion of products that enhance proliferation, finish the differentiation events, and otherwise modulate the immune reaction. These products are known as cytokines and include interleukins, interferons, and various growth factors. Many of these substances have been produced by recombinant DNA technology and are being used in therapeutic trials (Table 11–3).

AMPLIFICATION. This term describes the augmentation, by various collaborative processes, of the protective effect of antigen-binding by B and T lymphocytes. Amplification is necessary for complete elimination of infectious agents. Common modes of amplification include processes that lyse infectious agents or produce a granulomatous response. Amplification of the protective function of B cells is accomplished chiefly by activation of the complement system, that of the T cells chiefly by lymphokines, though both B and T cells secrete lymphokines. It is doubtful that complement amplifies the protective function of T cells to any significant degree.

Lymphokines may have direct toxic effects (see Table 11–3) or act indirectly as in the case of migration inhibitory factor (MIF). MIF attracts macrophages to an area where T cells have combined with an antigen; the macrophages then destroy the infectious agent through the release of lysosomal enzymes. They also release products that may lead to the formation of granulomas and may store or carry antibody. Primary quantitative or qualitative deficiencies in macrophages, though poorly defined at present, may conceivably impair host defenses.

The biologic effects of one of the lymphokines, interleukin 1 (IL-1), have been extensively studied. IL-1 is also known as endogenous pyrogen, leukocytic endogenous mediator, lymphocyte activating factor, and mononuclear cell factor. It is unclear whether it is a single factor or a series of related factors. It is produced primarily from phagocytic cells and is responsible for many laboratory and clinical features of acute phase reactions, such as the fever and myalgias associated with many aggressive immunologic disorders.

The effect of IL-1 on the immune response is largely due to its stimulation of T cells to secrete interleukin 2 (IL-2), which supports growth of effector T cell populations. In this way, massive mobilization of T cells is brought about. IL-2 also activates T cells for nonspecific killing of tumor cells (lymphokine-activated killer cells, LAK cells). Generation of LAK cells has been used in the therapy of advanced metastatic cancer occasionally with dramatic results.

TABLE 11–3. Cytokines

Undefined (some may be included in activities of interleukins)	
	Chemotactic factor (for eosinophils, monocytes, neutrophils)
	Lymph node permeability factor
	Migration inhibition factors
	Suppressor factors
	Transfer factor
Interleukins	
	IL-1 (Endogenous pyrogen); many biologic effects, promotes IL-2 synthesis
	IL-2 (T cell growth factor); T and B cell proliferation, activation of killer cells
	IL-3 (B cell stimulatory factor-1); proliferation of activated B cells; promotes IgE production
	IL-5 (B cell growth factor); promotes IgA/IgM production, supports eosinophil growth
	IL-6 (B cell stimulatory factor-2)
	IL-7 Stimulates B cell precursor growth
	γ-Interferon; enhances IgM and IgG production, suppresses IL-4 effects

T CELL SUBPOPULATIONS. The versatility of the immune system depends on the actions of subpopulations of the T and B cells. The major T cell subgroups currently defined are helper, suppressor, and killer cells. *Helper cells* are necessary in the initial responses to antigen, especially to generate IgG and IgA; some IgM antibodies are formed in the absence of T helper cells. The immune response, because of its potential for harm as well as good, must be modulated to prevent hyperimmune reactions. It is thought that T *suppressor cells* serve a homeostatic role in keeping the immune response within a tolerable level. T *killer cells* are the effector cells of the thymus-dependent system. They combine with antigen to initiate the cytotoxic mechanisms that kill invading organisms.

T cells and their products are primarily concerned with acid-fast bacteria, certain viral infections (e.g., rubeola, varicella, herpes, cytomegalovirus), and fungi. T cells are also the major immune factor involved in rejection of organ transplants (Sec. 6.39) and are responsible for the graft-versus-host reaction (Sec. 6.39 and 11.21). The major immunopathologic mechanism in contact dermatitis is thought to be mediated by the T cell.

B CELL SUBPOPULATIONS. Subspecialization of B cells has not been as well defined as that for T cells, but surface marker analysis suggests that subpopulations also exist for B cells. The B cell products (immunoglobulins) are divided into five major classes (isotypes), each of which is produced by a different cell line. Immunoglobulins are active against staphylococci, streptococci, *Haemophilus influenzae*, and pneumococci and are important in the initial prevention of such viral infections as rubeola, varicella, and hepatitis. They can do little, however, to control an established viral disease.

Typical immediate hypersensitivity reactions such as hay fever and asthma are mediated by B cells, as are antigen-antibody complex disease and such disorders as autoimmune hemolytic anemia.

The five major classes of immunoglobulins (Igs) are IgM, IgG, IgA, IgD, and IgE. Their chemical characteristics and biologic functions are summarized in Table 11–4.

IgM can be considered the first line of defense. It is the Ig first formed in response to antigen, is found most commonly in the vascular space, and has high efficiency in the functions that enhance immunity, such as complement fixation, agglutination, and opsonic activity. IgG has a long half-life and can cross the placenta, features supporting passive immunization and recall immunity. IgA protects mainly secretory surfaces (gastrointestinal tract and eyes) where exposures to antigens are nonvascular and conditions such as acid secretion, presence of proteolytic enzyme, and intestinal motility may impair antibody activity. IgE effects the release of pharmacologically active agents from mast cells that cause asthma, hay fever, and anaphylaxis. The role of IgD is not fully known. It is primarily a lymphocyte receptor. The unique structural characteristics of IgD may promote cross-linking of receptors on cell surfaces, with potent modulation of cellular responses.

Secretory IgA and IgE play a major role in the immune status of inhabitants of underdeveloped countries, where antibiotic therapy, nutrition, and general hygiene are less than optimal. Since breast-feeding is a major means of providing long-lasting protection in these countries, weaning is followed by increased death rates from infection. In addition to secretory IgA, breast milk delivers macrophages and per-

TABLE 11–4. Properties of Immunoglobulins*

		IgA				
	IgG	*Serum*	*Secretory*	IgM	IgD	IgE
Molecular weight	140,000	160,000	370,000	900,000	160,000	197,000
Complement fixation	+	−	?	+	−	−
Placental passage	+	−	—	−	−	−
Secreted by mucous surfaces	±†	±†	+	±‡	?	±
Fixes to homologous skin and mast cells	−	−	−	−	−	+
"Blocking antibody"	+	?	+	?	?	?
Polymer formation	−	+	+	+	−	−

*From Hong R: The immunoglobulins. Immunobiology 1:29, 1972.
†In inflammatory conditions. + = positive; ± = weak or intermittent; − = negative.
‡Frequently in selective IgA deficiency.

haps T cells to the infant. IgE is a major factor in the elimination of parasites. Macrophages armed with IgE antiparasite immune complexes are especially effective in eliminating parasitic infestation. These two defenses have become less critical in developed countries, where persons with no detectable secretory IgA or IgE can sometimes enjoy normal health.

The immunoglobulins are structurally modified for these subspecialized activities. All show the same chemical structure of two heavy and two light polypeptide chains. The combining site on the antibody, where antigen combines with the antibody molecule, is formed by both chains and found in a portion of the molecule known as the *Fab fragment*. Two identical Fab fragments are found in each monomeric molecule of immunoglobulin. A third fragment (Fc) consists of two portions of heavy chain and contains the structures that determine the biologic characteristics of the immunoglobulin (complement fixation, placental passage, and so on) and the unique determinants that differentiate one Ig from another. For example, the Fab fragments of IgG and IgA are virtually identical, but the Fc portions are quite dissimilar.

IgM and secretory IgA are polymers. The polymerization is probably initiated intracellularly by a short polypeptide chain known as the *J chain*. The IgA found in secretions (gastrointestinal, genitourinary, biliary, tears, saliva) has, in addition, a fragment known as *secretory component* (SC). IgA exists in a monomeric form in serum and in dimeric form in secretions.

Each isotype includes subclasses. Four are known for IgG (IgG1, IgG2, IgG3, IgG4) and two for IgA (IgA1, IgA2). Other isotypic subclasses are less well defined. Different subclasses respond preferentially to various antigens (e.g., IgG2 to polysaccharides, IgG1 and IgG3 to Rh antigens). IgG4 cannot fix complement. Most secretory IgA is of the IgA2 subclass. The subclasses provide fine tuning of the immune response. In some patients, absence of one or more subclasses leads to clinical states somewhat different from classic panhypogammaglobulinemia (Sec. 11.11).

MACROPHAGES. Macrophages, once regarded as scavenger cells without much specificity of function, have been found to play an important role in the acquisition of immunity and tolerance and serve a key role in the effector mechanisms of T cells. Disorders of macrophages and phagocytes are considered in Sec. 11.29 to 11.33.

ASSESSMENT OF T AND B CELLS

11.2 T CELLS

A preliminary assessment of T cell function can be made from the peripheral blood lymphocyte count, lateral roentgenogram of the chest, and skin tests for delayed hypersensitivity. More definitive studies require laboratories where T cell surface markers are identified, lymphocytes are stimulated in vitro, and morphologic studies of the thymus and other lymphoid tissues can be performed. It is noteworthy that ordinary viral infections can markedly influence tests of T cell function. Repeated tests are necessary to confirm significant deficiencies of the T cell system.

Normally blood contains more than 1,500 lymphocytes/mm^3; each is less than 10 μm in diameter. In some T cell deficiencies, the number of lymphocytes may be normal or even elevated, and the lymphocytes are large (>10 μm in diameter) and have a loose chromatin network in the nucleus and a much greater amount of pale blue-staining cytoplasm. Monocytosis, eosinophilia, and neutropenia are commonly associated with T cell deficiency. In a patient who has not been stressed, the roentgenographic absence of a thymus suggests thymic deficiency, but this is often difficult to assess.

Positive delayed skin reactions (e.g., to tuberculin or *Candida*) help to establish the presence of normal T cell function if they are not the result of nonspecific irritation at the test site. Negative results on skin tests are inconclusive evidence of deficient T cell function, particularly in younger children with limited antigenic experience.

More specialized tests attempt to measure the capabilities of T cell subpopulations and can differentiate between deficiencies at various levels of T cell development or between different phases of the immune response, for example, at the stage of recognition of antigen (affector defect) or at the stage of killer cell function (effector function). Patients may lack only some of the T cell capabilities. Performance and interpretation of T cell tests requires skill, patience, and experience. No single measurement serves as an appropriate general screening test of the integrity of T cells.

The number of T cells in blood can be counted through the use of monoclonal antibodies. Sera specific for the major subsets of human mononuclear cells have been developed (see Table 11–2), and quantitative measurement of the various types is possible. These measurements generally provide the clinician with the same sort of information that is derived from quantitative measurements of immunoglobulin. Total absence of any particular subset indicates a marked deficiency; in most cases, however, there is simply a lower than normal number, the full significance of which requires further analysis. Formerly, T4 (CD4+) cells were equated with helper function and T8 (CD8+) cells were thought to be synonymous with cytotoxic/suppressor cells. The true function of the CD4 and CD8 antigens is now known and has been described earlier.

A measurement of overrated significance is the ratio of helper to suppressor cells (T4/T8 ratio). In the acquired immunodeficiency syndrome (AIDS), a major feature of advancing disease is a loss of nearly all T4 cells. Inversion of this ratio (normally >1.0) is characteristic of patients with AIDS as they move into the terminal phases of disease. A reversed T4/T8 ratio is not, however, a priori diagnostic of AIDS, nor is it an absolute sign of serious T cell deficiency. A reversal of ratio may be due to increases of T8 cells, to problems in handling of the specimen, or to mild intercurrent infections. In infants with AIDS, the T4/T8 ratio is not always depressed (Sec. 12.83).

Further assessment of T cell function is accomplished by observation of in vitro responses. The three major types of responses displayed by T cells are proliferation, cytotoxicity, and immunoregulation. The latter two can be correlated with in vivo events, but the first bears little, if any, relation to the functions of the T cell in vivo. Substances used for study of proliferation include mitogens (usually plant substances that stimulate T cells to divide), allogeneic cells (cells from unrelated persons), and antigens. Proliferative responses to mitogens merely prove that a responsive population is present, but since the biologic function of that population is not well delineated, this information provides little more than the monoclonal surface marker. Patients with profound immunodeficiency who will die of overwhelming infection may show good proliferative responses to phytohemagglutinin or to allogeneic cells. Of the proliferative responses, those to specific antigens are the best predictors of the ability to resist infection. Cytotoxic assays show the ability of the lymphocytes to kill a defined target, usually after a period of stimulation by the target in vitro (i.e., a sensitization phase). Since this process simulates fairly closely what occurs in vivo, these assays are useful in defining T cell capability. Finally, T cells can be added to mixtures of other cells engaging in an in vitro immune response. The ability of added cells to support the test is taken as an indicator of helper activity, and their ability to decrease the response as a measure of suppressor activity.

The stimulation of lymphocytes by certain substances such as concanavalin A generates a large number of T cells capable of inhibiting other T cell responses. For example, supernatants of such stimulated cultures (or the stimulated cells themselves) will inhibit a mixed leukocyte culture reaction or the synthesis of immunoglobulin by B cells. Concanavalin A-stimulated cells serve as a suppressor T cell assay.

Isolated T cells can be added to purified B cell preparations, after which T-dependent proliferative processes or the synthesis of immunoglobulin is used as a T helper cell assay.

The ability of T lymphocytes to secrete lymphokines can also be assessed. Interpretation of the results of T cell tests and assessment of T cell function are primarily functions of research laboratories.

MORPHOLOGY. The normal *thymus* consists of lobules with a rich zone of thymocytes at the outer border and a less intensely staining zone containing many epithelial elements in the center. These two areas are easily separated from each other at a corticomedullary cleavage plane. Within the medulla are whorl-like bodies known as *Hassall corpuscles*. Absence of one or more of these features is found in various abnormalities of the T cell system. In *profound defects*, there are virtually no normal areas; the gland consists only of reticular cells in a loose structure with broad fibrous bands. Hassall corpuscles and lymphoid elements (thymocytes) are conspicuously absent. The gland is very small, about 2–3% of normal size; often it does not descend into the mediastinum but remains high in the neck. In *less severe deficiency*, the thymus may appear to be involuted with a few remnants of normal structure. Some thymic abnormalities involve only mass (hypoplasia or aplasia), sometimes with a small gland of perfectly normal architecture.

In *lymph nodes*, the zone of lymphocytes situated just below the layer of follicles and germinal centers at the periphery is populated by T cells. This area is poorly developed and cell-depleted in isolated deficiency of the T cell system. In addition, although B cell follicles may sometimes be seen, formation of germinal centers does not occur. In the *spleen*, a collar of T lymphocytes surrounds the arterioles; absence of lymphocytes in this area is consistent with thymic deficiency.

11.3 B CELLS

B cells as well as T cells can be enumerated in blood. The most commonly employed markers are the IgM molecules present on the surface of B lymphocytes. Approximately 10% of mononuclear cells in the blood carry these markers and also IgD. Other immunoglobulin classes are represented rarely, if at all.

The most commonly employed test of B cell function is quantitative measurement of serum immunoglobulin levels (see Table 11–2). A common error in using the single radial diffusion method is overinterpretation of slightly low values. Normal values for immunoglobulins vary greatly (several fold) and increase over a period of several years from low values in infancy until adult levels are attained. Normal values also vary from laboratory to laboratory; it has been suggested that immunoglobulin levels be expressed in international units after comparing one's local values to an international reference standard.* The laboratory diagnosis of immunodeficiency states requires stringent standards for the diagnosis of deficiency and correlation with the clinical picture.

Most states of true B cell immunodeficiency in children show IgG values under 200 mg/dL, and IgA and IgM are undetectable. An unusual form of B cell deficiency is associated with higher than normal levels of IgM (dysgammaglobulinemia). These high values are in part artifactual due to the more rapid diffusion of some of the IgM that is present as a low molecular weight monomer (rather than as the normal heavier polymer); rapid diffusion causes a large precipitin ring to develop, suggesting a higher than actual level of IgM.

Extremely high or at least normal values of one or more of the immunoglobulins are seen also in unusual forms of combined T and B cell deficiency. In these cases, the immunoglobulins classically show restricted electrophoretic mobility resembling that of myeloma proteins. Affected patients are usually immunologically inert; no specific antibodies can be detected either before or after antigenic stimulation. In cases of IgG subclass deficiency, the total IgG levels are within normal limits, but individual subclasses are absent.

The pattern of various immunoglobulin levels in serum is diagnostically uninformative, but some hints of the underlying or associated process can occasionally be found. Markedly elevated levels of IgA are often seen with thymic deficiency. Low levels of IgG and IgA in association with near-normal IgM values, as opposed to the immunoglobulin levels typical of hypogammaglobulinemia (e.g., IgG = 150 mg/dL, IgA = 0 mg/dL, IgM = 5 mg/dL), should suggest intestinal loss of protein. In such cases the levels of albumin and transferrin will also show marked diminution. Similar changes are also seen in the hypoproteinemic states of nephrosis and in cases of lymphangiectasia.

In selective deficiency of IgA, tests utilizing radial immunodiffusion present a special problem. Because of increased permeability of the gastrointestinal tract secondary to the deficiency of IgA, more dietary antigens are absorbed. As a result, higher levels of antibodies are formed to foodstuffs, especially to milk proteins. Precipitating antibodies to bovine proteins cross-react with many antisera (e.g., goat) used as anti-immunoglobulin reagents. As a result, in the diffusion analysis a band interpreted as goat antihuman IgA precipitating with serum IgA is actually human antibovine IgG precipitating goat IgG in cross-reaction. The interpretation would be that the patient has detectable levels of IgA when in fact he or she has none. The error can be avoided by the use of rabbit antisera to human IgA for quantitation or by testing

*The standard is available from NCI Immunoglobulin Reference Center, 6715 Electronic Dr., Springfield, VA 22151. The conversion units are as follows (μg/IU): IgG, 80.4; IgA, 14.2; IgM, 8.47.

the patient's serum in immunoelectrophoretic analysis in which no arc will be seen in the IgA region.

Ambiguous values of immunoglobulins require evaluation of immunoglobulin function for full interpretation. This is accomplished by measuring antibody response to specific antigens. One can use antigens to which the patient was exposed naturally (blood group substances, common bacteria) or as a result of immunization procedures (tetanus, diphtheria), or antigens purposefully injected to measure the response. Of the latter, bacteriophage $\phi\chi$ 174* is probably most informative; in cases of suspected B cell deficiency, the diagnosis can be made even at birth because normally even newborns will eliminate the phage by immune clearance. The transferred IgG levels of the mother offer no problem in interpretation, as they might if only quantitative levels were measured. Furthermore, there are different patterns of response that serve to define more precisely the nature of the B cell defect. *It is to be emphasized that live viruses other than $\phi\chi$ 174 should never be given to a patient suspected of immunodeficiency until the immune system is known to be normal because severe disease or death may ensue.* Recently, cases of inability to respond to pneumococcal polysaccharide in the presence of normal Ig levels of all classes and subclasses have been described.

B lymphocytes stimulated with pokeweed mitogen and cultured in the presence of normal T cells will synthesize and secrete immunoglobulin. B cells that bear immunoglobulin on the surface (SIg cell) are in the early presecretory stage; the surface molecules are lost after the cell responds to the antigen and undergoes terminal differentiation, enabling it to secrete the specific antibody. A study of the lymphocyte surface markers and the response to pokeweed mitogen can define the level at which the defect occurs in many cases. For example, SIg cells are usually absent in X-linked agammaglobulinemia but present in normal numbers in late-onset common variable immunodeficiency. In the latter, pokeweed mitogen will not induce further differentiation. X-linked agammaglobulinemia can be thought of as an early defect due to lack of B cells; common variable immunodeficiency can be thought of as a failure of B cells to undergo terminal differentiation.

In some patients with common variable immunodeficiency, excessive T suppressor cell activity is found. Their T cells, incubated with normals, will completely prevent induction by pokeweed mitogen of synthesis and secretion of IgG, IgA, and IgM. In other patients deficiency of T helper cells is found. Thus, complete evaluation of B cells requires assessment of modulating influences as well as of the capability of the patient's lymphocytes to synthesize immunoglobulins.

MORPHOLOGY. The thymus can be assumed to be normal in classic "pure" B cell deficiency disorders, of which congenital hypogammaglobulinemias of the X-linked or autosomal recessive types are prime examples. The thymus is abnormal in cases associated with paraprotein-like immunoglobulins. The lymph nodes show deficient or absent follicle formation, and germinal centers are absent in cases of deficient production of immunoglobulins. In selective deficiency of IgA there may be a compensatory increase of IgM-producing cells in the lamina propria of the intestine.

INHERITANCE. The inheritance pattern of immunodeficiency diseases (X-linked or autosomal) can be determined by restriction fragment length polymorphism (RFLP) analysis of the X chromosome. Genetic counseling will be aided greatly when this analysis becomes more generally available.

PRENATAL DIAGNOSIS. With the availability of techniques for sampling fetal blood, direct evaluation of the lymphocytes can be performed on the fetus. Samples of 200 μL are adequate for a limited analysis. However, the pregnancy may be endangered by such sampling.

*Assessment is available by arrangement with R. J. Wedgwood, M.D., Department of Pediatrics, University of Washington School of Medicine, Seattle, WA 98195.

DISEASES DUE TO IMMUNOLOGIC DEFICIENCY

11.4 PRIMARY IMMUNODEFICIENCY

It is convenient to think of diseases as primarily involving the T cell or B cell systems, or both. In each case the clinical presentation and treatment are different. Generally, disorders of the T cell system are associated with a much graver prognosis than are those of the B cell system. Combined immunodeficiency involving both T and B cells carries the worst prognosis; if of the severe variety, death in the first 2 yr of life is the rule. Some patients with pure B cell disorders remain clinically well without any therapy.

Clinical differentiation between primary T or B cell deficiency cannot be made with certainty, but certain clinical features suggestive of involvement of particular systems are listed in Table 11–5.

An unusual response to usually benign infectious agents or infection with unusual organisms is a feature of immunodeficiency; this may occur in isolated T or B cell diseases or in combined disorders. The major organisms involved in immunodeficient patients are *Pneumocystis carinii*, cytomegalovirus, rubeola, and varicella; each often results in fatal pneumonia. Pneumonitis caused by any of these agents should suggest immunodeficiency. See Sec. 12.13.

There is an increased incidence of malignancy among patients with immunodeficiency. Explanations for this include increased susceptibility to infection by an oncogenic virus, the cancer as another expression of the basic genetic fault, and a failure of immune surveillance. The last explanation is based on the theory that T cells eliminate newly formed populations of malignant cells as they arise, considering them foreign transplants. An alternative hypothesis attributes the high incidence of lymphoid malignancy to failure of feedback control of antigen-induced lymphoproliferation. Since immunodeficient patients do not make antibody or other normal immune products following receipt of antigen, the stimulated aberrant lymphoid elements continue to respond by proliferation, with repeated cell divisions increasing the likelihood of random malignant mutation.

Epstein-Barr virus (EBV) is particularly associated with oncogenesis in immunodeficient states. EBV can transform human B lymphocytes into cell lines capable of long-term survival in tissue culture; premalignant clones may be perpetuated in vivo as well. In the immunodeficient host, these clones are not eliminated because of T killer cell deficiency. Genetic and other environmental factors may also play a role. In patients at risk, the appearance of markedly enlarged nodes and persistent daily fever spikes is an ominous sign. Abnormal lymphocytes can be found in the bone marrow or peripheral smear. Central nervous system symptoms of a mass lesion are common. Infiltrates of transformed B lymphocytes are often found in enlarged lymph nodes or spleen or in intestinal lymphoid nodules. These may consist of immunoblasts or small cleaved follicular center cells and may resemble malignant cells histologically. They can usually be shown to be polyclonal and may resolve spontaneously or following immunotherapy. The proliferation may be so massive that death can result from mass effects, or evolution into a monoclonal malignant tumor may occur.

11.5 PRIMARY B CELL DISEASES

Clinically, the hypogammaglobulinemic syndromes can be divided into panhypogammaglobulinemia, selective deficiencies of immunoglobulins, and deficiencies of immunoglobulin subclasses.

11.6 PANHYPOGAMMAGLOBULINEMIA
(Congenital Agammaglobulinemia; Bruton Disease)

Panhypogammaglobulinemia involving all three major classes of immunoglobulins is usually congenital in origin. X-linked (Bruton disease), autosomal recessive, sporadic, and "late-onset" forms are seen, but such differentiation is of little help in defining etiology, management, or prognosis. Since some patients with congenital deficiency remain amazingly asymptomatic until later in life, the term late-onset does not imply an acquired or secondary disorder. Most late-onset diseases are in the category termed common variable immunodeficiency (Sec. 11.7).

CLINICAL MANIFESTATIONS. Panhypogammaglobulinemia presents a history of repeated infections caused by pneumococcus, staphylococcus, and *H. influenzae.* The X-linked disorder usually presents at 6–12 mo of age with recurrent bacterial infections as the concentration of placentally transferred maternal antibody falls. Pneumonia, and persistent otitis and sinusitis are common. Gastroenteritis, pyoderma, arthritis, and meningitis also occur with increased frequency. There may also be growth failure. Conjunctivitis secondary to *H. influenzae* is especially annoying. In older patients, chronic sinusitis is common, sometimes as the only complaint. There is usually no lymphadenopathy or splenomegaly despite recurrent infections. Many children have severe dental decay. Chronic pulmonary disease, with eventual bronchiectasis, pulmonary fibrosis, and cor pulmonale, characterizes adult disease. Fatal encephalitis and chronic viremia following echovirus, type 30, and other viral infections have been reported.

Autoimmune disorders are common. An increased frequency of malignancy also occurs (Sec. 11.4).

Skin disorders are unusually frequent in patients with immunodeficiency; intractable eczema and dermatomyositis have been reported. Eczema, recurrent skin abscesses, a history of allergy, and coarse facies occur with extremely elevated serum IgE values and leukocyte dysfunction.

DIAGNOSIS. In panhypogammaglobulinemia levels of IgG seldom exceed 200 mg/dL in childhood; IgA and IgM are barely, if at all, detectable. During the first 3 mo of life, the high levels of maternally derived IgG can make the diagnosis difficult, but normal levels of IgA and IgM virtually rule out significant hypogammaglobulinemia. Inguinal lymph nodes are easily detected in normal infants, even at birth; the palpation of normal lymph nodes, along with visible tonsillar tissue, speaks strongly against the diagnosis of hypogammaglobulinemia. A rare syndrome of enlarged lymph nodes and histiocytosis-like skin lesions (Omenn disease) is discussed in Section 11.17. Criteria defining significant infections should be stringent. Upper respiratory infections are a common feature of the first few years of life, and as many as 9–10/yr may occur normally. Unless there is also a verified history of repeated bacterial pneumonias or other severe infections, frequent upper respiratory infections are not an indication for exhaustive investigation for immunodeficiency.

TREATMENT. Traditionally this consisted of the intramuscular injection of immune serum globulin (ISG) prepared by alcohol precipitation (Cohn fraction II). A dose calculated to produce a serum level of 300 mg/dL was given (a loading dose of 1.4 mL/kg, followed by 0.7 mL/kg every 4 wk).

Preparations consisting primarily of IgG are now available for intravenous administration. With these it is now possible

TABLE 11–5. Clinical Manifestations of Immunodeficiency*

Suggestive of T cell defect
Systemic illness following vaccination with any live virus or BCG†; unusual life-threatening complication following infection with ordinarily benign viruses (e.g., giant cell pneumonia with rubeola; varicella pneumonia)
Chronic oral candidiasis after 6 mo of age
Chronic mucocutaneous candidiasis
Features (fine, thin hair; short-limbed dwarfism with characteristic roentgenographic features of cartilage-hair hypoplasia [CHH])
Intrauterine graft-versus-host disease—most characteristic feature is scaling erythroderma and total alopecia (absence of eyebrows quite striking)
Graft-versus-host disease after blood transfusion
Hypocalcemia in newborn (DiGeorge anomaly, especially with characteristic facies, ears, and cardiac lesion)
Small (less than 10 μm diameter) lymphocytes: counts persistently less than 1,500/mm^3; must rule out gastrointestinal loss or loss from lymphatics
Suggestive of B cell defect
Recurrent proved bacterial pneumonia, sepsis, or meningitis
Nodular lymphoid hyperplasia
Suggestive of B and T cell defect (combined immunodeficiency disease [CID])
Features of all above except chronic mucocutaneous candidiasis and nodular lymphoid hyperplasia
Features of Wiskott-Aldrich syndrome (draining ears, thrombocytopenia, and eczema)
Features of ataxia-telangiectasia
Suggestive of immunodeficiency without clearly implicating T or B cell defect
Pneumocystis carinii pneumonia
Intractable eczema
Ulcerative colitis in infants less than 1 yr of age
Intractable diarrhea
Unexplained hematologic deficiency (RBC†, WBC†, platelet)
Severe generalized seborrheic dermatitis (Leiner disease) suggests C5 deficiency; seborrhea common in combined immunodeficiency disease
Recurrent pyogenic infections seen in C3 deficiency
Suggestive of biochemical defect
Features of combined immunodeficiency with characteristic bony lesions (adenosine deaminase deficiency)
Features of Diamond-Blackfan aplastic anemia (nucleoside phosphorylase deficiency)
Suggestive of abnormality of polymorphonuclear leukocytes
Primarily skin infections (if associated with asthma, eczema, and coarse facies, think of Buckley syndrome‡)
Chronic osteomyelitis with *Klebsiella* or *Serratia* species, draining lymph nodes (chronic granulomatous disease)
Suggestive of secondary deficiency
Concomitant or preceding viral infection
Lymphoid malignancy (chronic lymphatic leukemia, Hodgkin disease, myeloma)

*Modified from Hong R. Immunodeficiency. *In*: Rose NR, Friedman H (eds): Manual of Clinical Immunology. Washington, DC, American Society for Microbiology, 1976.

†BCG = bacille Calmette-Guérin; RBC = red blood cell; WBC = white blood cell.

‡Data from Buckley RH, et al: Extreme hyperimmunoglobulinemia E and undue susceptibility to infection. Pediatrics 49:59, 1972.

to attain near normal levels of IgG and to maintain therapeutic levels in a simple, well tolerated manner (Sec. 12.13).

Chronic infection of the central nervous system is occasionally seen in B cell deficiencies. In an affected patient daily intravenous administration of IgG resulted in dramatic control of symptoms; relapse followed cessation of therapy. Intrathecal administration of IgG may be needed. Chronic thrombocytopenia and hemolytic anemia sometimes occur as complications of hypogammaglobulinemia. Intravenous administration of gamma globulin has controlled these conditions in both immunodeficient and immunocompetent states.

Anaphylaxis may complicate either intramuscular or intravenous gamma globulin therapy, especially the latter. Close monitoring of the patient during infusion is necessary. A cause of these reactions is the existence of small aggregates of immunoglobulin that resist the chemical modification procedures. A rare cause is the paradoxical production of anti-IgA antibodies in some hypogammaglobulinemic patients. Some preparations of gamma globulin have lower amounts of IgA.

Chronic pulmonary disease is an ever-present danger in panhypogammaglobulinemia. Pulmonary function should be tested at least annually in all patients over 10 yr old unless symptoms or roentgenograms suggest that earlier assessment should be performed. Unremitting pulmonary disease is probably a sign of failure of intramuscular therapy with gamma globulin and an indication for intravenous or plasma therapy. This approach is entirely empiric. Daily prophylaxis with 10 mg/kg of trimethoprim and 50 mg/kg of sulfamethoxazole in two divided doses may also be helpful in selected cases.

11.7 COMMON VARIABLE IMMUNODEFICIENCY

This catch-all term encompasses most immunodeficiency states with a prominent B cell component and a minimal or no T cell defect. It excludes X-linked agammaglobulinemia (Bruton disease). Usually, the onset of symptoms is later than that of Bruton disease, and both sexes are involved. Otherwise, the clinical picture may be indistinguishable from that of congenital agammaglobulinemia. The later onset was originally thought to indicate an acquired cause, but examples of familial incidence and the finding of autoimmune diseases in a high percentage of 1st-degree relatives implicate a genetic mechanism. Sinopulmonary infections are a common presenting picture, and subsequent development of physical signs of chronic lung disease and bronchiectasis occur in many of these patients. Malabsorption syndromes may also occur as well as an increased frequency of autoimmune disorders.

The major difference in laboratory studies between these patients and those with Bruton disease is the finding of circulating B cells. This group of diseases does not, therefore, represent a failure of differentiation from stem cells. Inadequate T helper function, excess suppressor T cell function, and autoantibodies to T or B cells have been found. Attempts to correct some of these faults, in particular the excess T cell suppression, have not been very successful. As the patients grow older, increasingly significant T cell abnormalities develop.

About 25% of patients with common variable immunodeficiency have significant malabsorption, most commonly involving vitamin B_{12}. *Giardia lamblia* infestation is especially common. Lactose intolerance, disaccharidase deficiency, villous abnormalities, and nodular lymphoid hyperplasia may be seen. Infiltration of spleen, lung, and skin with noncaseating granulomas is common. Their cause is unknown, but corticosteroid therapy will usually cause marked reduction in their size and number.

SELECTIVE DEFICIENCIES

11.8 Selective Deficiency of IgA

IgA is the major immunoglobulin protecting the respiratory, gastrointestinal, and other secretory areas. As a result of its deficiency, recurrent respiratory infections and chronic diarrheal syndromes may occur. Many patients are asymptomatic. A striking association with autoimmune disorders, especially systemic lupus erythematosus and rheumatoid arthritis, is seen. The autoimmunity is believed to result from uncontrolled access of antigenic substances to the lymphoid system via the gastrointestinal tract, with undue stimulation causing generation of antigen-antibody complexes. Another reason for the association may be the profound dependency of the IgA system on intact thymic function, a deficiency in production of IgA implying a thymic abnormality. One such defect, the lack or deficiency of T suppressor cells, could predispose to autoimmunity.

Some patients with selective deficiency of IgA recover spontaneously. Patients with deficiency of serum IgA have gradually acquired normal levels after 3–5 yr without any specific therapy. Since all IgA-deficient patients studied to date possess normal numbers of nonsecreting lymphocytes bearing IgA molecules and since, in one study, these cells could be stimulated in vitro to become secreting cells, the potential for spontaneous recovery may exist in all patients. Selective deficiency of IgA may also be produced by external factors, for example, by administration of phenytoin.

Patients with selective *total* deficiency of IgA have normal capacity for synthesizing IgG antibody, and their B cells can respond vigorously to most antigens. If such patients receive IgA from any source, formation of anti-IgA antibody is quite likely because their immune systems treat IgA as a foreign protein. Immune serum globulin (ISG) is a common source, resulting from the frequent and, in our opinion, injudicious practice of empirically administering ISG prophylactically to children with frequent respiratory infections, which are usual in patients with total absence of IgA. ISG contains amounts of IgA that are adequate to sensitize the child with total deficiency of IgA but not to protect against agents that cause respiratory infections. If blood or blood products containing significant amounts of IgA are then administered to such IgA-sensitized patients, fatal anaphylaxis may result; ISG should not, therefore, be administered without justification to children with frequent upper respiratory infections. Furthermore, patients known to have total IgA deficiency should not receive blood or blood products without first determining that they have no anti-IgA antibodies in their sera. When possible, blood products from IgA-deficient donors should be used.

Selective IgA deficiency may be inherited in either an autosomal recessive or autosomal dominant manner. Often siblings of patients with panhypogammaglobulinemia show selective IgA deficiency. Selective IgA deficiency has an unexplained association with a chromosome 18 abnormality. The structural genes for immunoglobulins are not present on chromosome 18.

Although serum IgA and secretory IgA appear to be under separate control, virtually all patients with serum IgA deficiency also have secretory IgA deficiency. Occasionally, a patient with a deficiency of serum IgA will show IgA-staining plasma cells in the intestine. In these cases, full evaluation of the capability to produce secretory IgA in the gastrointestinal or respiratory tracts has not been carried out. It is not known, therefore, whether the number of IgA-producing cells was normal throughout the secretory system or whether their rate of synthesis of secretory IgA was adequate for protection. IgA function in the secretions is most critical, but as a practical matter in most situations measurement of serum IgA predicts the status of secretory IgA. Patients with a deficiency of secretory IgA in the presence of normal levels of serum IgA have been found to have a deficiency of secretory component (Sec. 11.9). If symptoms warrant, determination of secretory IgA status must be made regardless of the level of IgA in the serum.

It has been reported that the severity or likelihood of respiratory disease in IgA deficiency is best correlated with an associated IgG subclass defect. IgG2 or IgG4 deficiency may also increase the risk of lymphoproliferative disease. In one large series, nearly one half of patients with IgA deficiency had concomitant IgE deficiency.

IgA deficiency is probably not often an isolated defect but may be associated with a number of other defects of the T and B cell systems. Assessment of affected patients must include sufficient general evaluation of IgG subclasses and of the T cell system to determine the extent of involvement.

11.9 Selective Deficiency of Secretory Component (SC)

Secretory component is a protein produced by epithelial cells in many parts of the body. It is found on all molecules of IgA secreted into the lumen of the intestine; it may play an important role in the transport of IgA, and perhaps of IgM, from the site of synthesis in the plasma cells of the lamina propria. Absence or deficiency of secretory component has been reported in 5 of 8 children with sudden infant death syndrome (SIDS). Two children with deficiency of secretory component have had chronic diarrhea; these patients also had a deficiency of secretory IgA but normal levels of serum IgA.

11.10 Selective Deficiency of IgM

This primary deficiency state has a frequency of approximately 1 in 1000 in the general population. Affected patients tend to succumb to rapid hematogenous spread of bacterial infections; atopy and splenomegaly have also been noted. Whipple disease, regional enteritis, and lymphoid nodular hyperplasia have also been observed with increased frequency.

Patients should be treated aggressively with antibiotics at the first sign of infection. It has been recommended that their blood relatives also be treated at the first sign of infection if their serum IgM status is unknown.

11.11 IgG Subclass Deficiency

In IgG subclass deficiency the total levels of IgG are usually normal, but the heterogeneity of its electrophoretic mobility may appear restricted. When tests of specific antibody formation are done, antibody formation to some antigens but not to others appears. Clinically, the patients show the same increased susceptibility to infection that is characteristic of panhypogammaglobulinemia, and some, but not all, will respond to gamma globulin therapy.

At the present time, IgG subclass deficiency is not a clearly defined deficiency state. The clinical significance is based on the fact that many carbohydrate antibodies are of the IgG2 subclass. The inference is that those with IgG2 deficiency cannot make carbohydrate antibodies and are therefore very susceptible to bacterial infections. However, although IgG1 anticarbohydrate antibodies are made early in life and IgG2 responses represent a maturational change, there is no evidence that IgG1 antibodies are less protective. Furthermore, individuals with complete loss of the genes synthesizing IgG2, IgG4, IgA, and IgE have been discovered among normal populations. It is possible that subclass and IgA deficiencies are only markers for a potentially more serious immune deficiency state, but the important defect that determines the degree of the clinical problem has yet to be described. This would explain the fact that some individuals with these defects have no clinical disease, whereas others do.

11.12 PRIMARY T CELL DISEASES

When T cell function is compromised but B cells function normally, infections are primarily fungal or viral. Chronic interstitial pneumonia, nasal discharge, and neutropenia are other features associated with T cell deficiency. The major types of T cell defects in which the immunoglobulins are measurable (and usually functional) are the DiGeorge anomaly, Nezelof syndrome, cartilage-hair hypoplasia, some cases of adenosine deaminase deficiency, and nucleoside phosphorylase deficiency.

11.13 DiGEORGE ANOMALY

The DiGeorge anomaly (DGA, previously called the DiGeorge syndrome) was formerly thought to be an embryologic fault primarily involving the 3rd and 4th pharyngeal pouches, resulting in associated defects of the parathyroid and thymus glands. The defect is now recognized to be much more widespread and is thought to result from a field defect. Developmental fields are embryologically reactive units consisting of cells that develop with their primordia. Field defects are characterized by limited clinical expression of a disorder that has multiple causes. Thus, it is now clear why the DGA has been associated with so many different etiologies, ranging from chromosomal abnormality to the fetal alcohol syndrome. It is thought that injury to the cephalic neural crest cells, which provide important contributions to the pharyngeal pouches, is the major cause. As a consequence, the type of heart anomaly is unusually skewed to conotruncal defects and is especially associated with an interrupted aortic arch type B defect, right-sided aortic arch, persistent truncus arteriosus, aberrant left subclavian artery, right infundibular stenosis, and ventricular septal defects. Occasionally a child has no congenital heart disease. Other features of DGA include an unusual facies with micrognathia, a fishmouth deformity, hypertelorism, downward slanting eyes, and low-set posteriorly angulated auricles, bifid uvula, and high arched palate. Urinary tract abnormalities are also common. The immune deficit, due to a thymic abnormality resulting from 3rd pharyngeal pouch involvement, is variable in severity, as is the parathyroid deficiency. The DiGeorge anomaly should be considered a polytypic field defect in which the thymus and parathyroid are often but not always affected.

Neonatal hypocalcemia is frequently the initial clinical presentation, and DGA should always be considered in its differential diagnosis. Tetany may occur. Parathormone levels are usually diminished.

The immune deficiency is difficult to define because most patients have a minimal defect, and normal immunity ultimately develops. Originally, the DGA immune defect was thought to be an isolated T cell deficiency; however, as more patients have been studied, an absence of immunoglobulin production has been found to be a common feature. The degree of thymic involvement is extremely variable from patient to patient, and it is thought that when the deficit includes T helper cell function, immunoglobulin synthesis is absent. Lymphopenia is not characteristic.

Disastrous results have occurred when the possibility of DGA was not considered and fresh blood transfusions were given during the course of corrective cardiac surgery, resulting in fatal graft-versus-host disease (GVHD).

Treatment for the thymic abnormality is usually not necessary because the majority of patients with DGA have or will acquire normal immunity. Recent studies suggest that proliferative responses of lymphocytes to phytohemagglutinin and numbers of CD4+ T lymphocytes will reliably define those patients whose immunity will eventually become normal. For those who require therapy, thymus transplantation can be performed. However, some patients do not benefit from thymus transplantation. Thymic hormone therapy is not recommended. A recent success with bone marrow transplantation from a matched sibling donor has been reported. The results of therapy are confusing and suggest that our concepts of the actual fault(s) of the immune deficit are flawed.

The immune defect is usually not a reason to defer correction of the cardiac lesion if surgery is indicated. However, only irradiated blood should be used in the management of these infants until their immune status is clarified to avoid GVHD.

Hypocalcemia should be treated as indicated in Sec. 6.6.

11.14 NEZELOF SYNDROME

Originally, Nezelof syndrome was considered a variant of the DGA without involvement of the parathyroids or cardiac tissues. The presence or absence of specific antibodies was not determined in Nezelof's original studies. Newer concepts of the role of the thymus in expression of the B cell system make this an important distinction. We classify patients with immunoglobulins of known specificity in the presence of T cell deficiency as having Nezelof syndrome and believe them to be quite different from those whose immunoglobulins are measurable but are of nondefined specificity. The latter group of patients frequently do not produce all three major classes of immunoglobulins, and electrophoretic abnormalities are common. We believe that this group should be considered a variant of combined B and T cell deficiency.

11.15 CARTILAGE-HAIR HYPOPLASIA

Patients with cartilage-hair hypoplasia (CHH) have a unique form of bone dysplasia; short-limbed dwarfism; sparse, light-colored, fine hair lacking a central pigmented core; and neutropenia. At birth, short and pudgy hands, short fingernails, limited elbow extension, and redundant skin folds around the neck and extremities are noted. The patients were first found in an Amish population, but cases occur in other ethnic groups. Only a small percentage of short-limbed dwarfs show the immune defect; furthermore, even though testing implies a virtual absence of T cell function, susceptibility to infection is limited, and the major agents involved are vaccinia or varicella virus. Chronic candidosis, for example, is not a feature of this T cell deficiency.

Little information is available on the response of cartilage-hair hypoplasia to therapy. Bone marrow transplantation has been performed in one case, with complete success.

COMBINED T AND B CELL DISEASE

In these disorders, both T and B cell functions are profoundly depressed. Originally, it was thought that combined T and B cell disease was best explained by a lesion of stem cells at the point in their development immediately preceding differentiation into T and B cells. B cell differentiation is highly thymus dependent, however, and at least some combined B and T cell disorders are probably caused by a primary thymic deficiency.

11.16 COMBINED IMMUNODEFICIENCY DISEASE (CID)

The term severe combined immunodeficiency originally described a syndrome that began in infancy and usually resulted in death by 2 yr of age. Milder forms have now been observed, and early death is not inevitable. When the disorder involves both T and B cell systems, the disease is more severe than with either separate defect; the infectious processes that occur are of the varieties that characterize either deficiency state. In some of these cases there may be a specific defect in the production of interleukin-2.

If combined immunodeficiency disease (CID) is defined as a disorder in which both T and B cell functions are diminished, *absence* of products of either system is not an absolute requirement for diagnosis. For example, patients with T cells bearing mature markers but no other normal T cell functions and those with some or all classes of immunoglobulins but no detectable antibody activity ("cellular immunodeficiency with immunoglobulin") may also be included in the category of combined immunodeficiency disease. The susceptibility to infection and disease is as great in these children as in those with no detectable lymphocytes or immunoglobulins.

In addition to the *clinical manifestations* already discussed for isolated deficiencies, a number of features are characteristic of CID. Wasting, whether or not associated with chronic diarrhea, is common. If diarrhea is present, it is resistant to therapy, and total parenteral alimentation may be required. Hepatitis and gastroenteritis are common. Unusual skin eruptions, total alopecia, excessive seborrhea, cutaneous laxity manifested by redundant skin folds, large umbilical hernias, and hyperelastic joints are also seen. Chronic oral candidiasis that is refractory to treatment frequently occurs and may result in esophagitis or, rarely, systemic candidiasis. Pneumonia is common and may be severe owing to *P. carinii* or cytomegalovirus. Chronic encephalopathy also occurs. One form of CID is associated with short-limbed dwarfism, caused by metaphyseal or spondyloepiphyseal dysplasia.

Hematologic abnormalities include thrombocytosis, neutropenia, anemia, monocytosis, and eosinophilia. Monocytosis and eosinophilia may occur in response to overwhelming infections such as *Pneumocystis* pneumonia.

CID can be successfully treated with transplantation of bone marrow, resulting in apparently complete and long-lasting reconstitution of both B and T cell systems (Sec. 6.42). The successful transplants have come from siblings who are matched at the major histocompatibility locus most important in determining the severity of graft-versus-host reactions, the HLA-D locus. Only about 25% of siblings can be expected to match. Recently, two methods have been developed for transplanting marrow from haploidentical donors (usually parent to child). The mature T cells in the marrow inoculum can be removed by treatment of the marrow either with soybean lectin (usually with a sheep red blood cell-rosetting step) or with monoclonal antibody(ies) directed against mature T cells. Marrow so treated usually produces a controllable graft-versus-host disease. Failure of engraftment is more common with these techniques, suggesting that the histocompatibility differences are sufficient to incite a primitive rejection reaction by a host with virtually absent immunity. In such cases, immunosuppression of the host is necessary, even though testing of his or her T cell function indicates profound impairment. The need for T cell ablation prior to transplantation greatly complicates haploidentical bone marrow transplantation, but several successes have followed this procedure. Long-term follow-up shows equivalent results in CID treated with bone marrow from identical and haploidentical donors.

No significant benefit has resulted from treatment with

transfer factor or thymic hormone. Transplants of fetal liver, fetal liver combined with fetal thymus, fetal thymus alone, or cultured thymic epithelium (CTE) have shown promise in some cases. A child with CID has responded to injections of interleukin 2 given 3 times/wk. As diagnostic capabilities improve and cytokines become more readily available, pharmacologic therapy of many immune deficiencies may be possible.

Pneumocystis infection is responsive to either pentamidine isethionate or trimethoprim-sulfamethoxazole; prophylaxis with the latter is advisable in a patient with CID until curative transplantation of bone marrow is established. Treatment of cytomegalovirus, rubeola, and varicella infections is unsatisfactory. Zoster immunoglobulin is indicated to prevent infection upon exposure of a susceptible immunodeficient patient to varicella. In varicella pneumonia or overwhelming varicella, therapy with acyclovir is effective.

11.17 COMBINED IMMUNODEFICIENCY DISEASE AND LETTERER-SIWE SYNDROME
(Omenn Disease)

A chronic skin eruption, hepatosplenomegaly, eosinophilia, and histiocytic infiltration of the lymph nodes occur in one variety of CID. The skin eruption may take many forms but is usually papular, seborrheic, erythematous, or scaly. The marked histiocytosis has led to reports of immunodeficiency and Letterer-Siwe syndrome occurring together. However, the skin eruptions of Letterer-Siwe syndrome, with its extreme seborrhea and characteristic histiocytic infiltration, are actually quite different from any form of CID. Furthermore, in Letterer-Siwe syndrome there is no immunodeficiency unless cytotoxic drugs have been given. CID of the Omenn type is one of the few forms of severe immunodeficiency in which there is marked deficiency of both T and B cell systems but easily palpable lymph nodes. Usually, many of the tests of lymphocyte function are normal; thus, the diagnosis may require thymic biopsy for confirmation. A deficiency of the ectoenzyme 5′-nucleotidase may be characteristic of Omenn disease. *Pneumocystis* pneumonia is a common presenting symptom. The rash is often actually a manifestation of a chronic graft-versus-host disease.

11.18 WISKOTT-ALDRICH SYNDROME

This is an X-linked recessive disorder characterized by thrombocytopenia, draining ears, and eczema. The initial *clinical manifestations* may be petechiae or bleeding and/or an eczematoid rash during the first 6 mo of life. Otitis and pneumonia are common, but many other recurrent and chronic infections occur, including chronic herpes conjunctivitis. Usually these children have splenomegaly, hepatomegaly, and cervical lymphadenopathy. Serum IgA and IgE levels are markedly elevated, IgM is diminished, lymphopenia is common, and malignant reticuloendotheliosis is a common terminal event. A characteristic laboratory finding is small (approximately half-size) platelets. A defect in glycosylation of surface proteins may play a significant role in pathogenesis.

The reason for susceptibility to infection in Wiskott-Aldrich syndrome is unknown. Although the most striking immunologic abnormality consistently found is an inability to form antibodies to carbohydrate antigens, poor responses to other antigens are found as the disease progresses. Detailed study may show mild dysfunction of T cells but less than in the usual forms of T cell deficiency. The defects increase with time so that originally normal findings give way to abnormal responses; immunoglobulin levels change to a characteristic hyper-IgA, hypo-IgM pattern; and abnormalities of lymphoid tissues occur.

Bone marrow transplants have been successful in patients with Wiskott-Aldrich syndrome (Sec. 6.42). Early attempts at transplantation with minimal or modest immunosuppression were unsuccessful. Ablation equivalent to that employed for bone marrow transplantation in malignancy is required. Recent results indicate that haploidentical transplantation can be performed successfully in patients with Wiskott-Aldrich syndrome, with results similar to those seen in CID.

Splenectomy may control the thrombocytopenia in situations in which bone marrow transplantation cannot be done; for maximal benefit it must be done early in the course of the disease.

11.19 ATAXIA-TELANGIECTASIA

Ataxia-telangiectasia (AT) is characterized by ataxia, ocular and cutaneous telangiectasia, chronic sinopulmonary disease, endocrine abnormalities, and variable B and T cell deficiency. Deficiency of IgA and IgE, singly or together, constitutes the most common B cell abnormality. The disease may be due to a common embryologic fault resulting in failure of mesodermoentodermal interactions, leading to telangiectasia, neurologic disease, and lymphoid abnormalities. The finding of elevated α-fetoprotein and carcinoembryonic antigen in virtually all patients with ataxia-telangiectasia is consistent with an abnormal process of embryogenesis. Since only fetal-type cells synthesize these proteins, continued postnatal production suggests an arrest at a fetal stage. In some as yet undefined way, similar arrests involving the many and varied organ systems in ataxia-telangiectasia could lead to the manifestations observed. Some workers have found evidence for autoimmune reactivity against various organ systems, including brain and thymocytes, implying autoaggression as a factor in the pathogenesis.

Patients with AT have a defect in DNA repair mechanisms, which probably accounts for the high incidence of chromosomal breaks observed in AT karyotypes. The defect in repair is confined to x-ray–induced damage; ultraviolet radiation damage is repaired appropriately. This defect, therefore, precludes x-ray or radiomimetic therapy in the treatment of malignancy in patients with AT. It is possible that error-prone repair may be related to the clinical symptoms. It has been suggested that the defective DNA repair is indicative of the basic defect in differentiation.

The disease is inherited as an autosomal trait, probably recessive. Cerebellar ataxia is usually the first neurologic sign and progresses slowly but relentlessly to severe disability; intellectual development is normal at first but seems to stop at about the 10-yr level in many of these children. A mask-like facies with excessive drooling produces a remarkable similarity of appearance in affected patients. Variable choreoathetoid or tic-like movements and irregular eye movements occur. Muscle weakness and poor reflexes are also seen. The telangiectases are most obvious in the sclerae, although involvement of the ear, lateral aspect of the nose, and antecubital and popliteal fossae is common. This finding may occur as early as 1 yr or as late as 6 yr of age and usually becomes more prominent and appears in more areas over time. Other skin lesions include hypo- and hyperpigmentation, atopic dermatitis, cutaneous atrophy simulating scleroderma, and nummular eczema. Recurrent sinopulmonary infections lead to bronchiectasis in many patients. There is growth failure, and patients who survive to puberty often do not develop secondary sex characteristics.

Deficiency of both IgA and IgE may be seen in 50–70% of cases; isolated IgE deficiency may occur in another 20–40%. Selective IgA deficiency is also found in high frequency. Variable degrees of T cell deficiency progressively worsen with time, and death from malignant lymphoma is a common terminal event.

11.20 CHRONIC MUCOCUTANEOUS CANDIDOSIS

This chronic, indolent candidosis involves mucous membranes and spreads peripherally onto the skin. Satellite patches may occur on the trunk and extremities; onychomycosis may be present. Patients may have *Candida* granuloma and extensive skin and scalp involvement as well as oral infection. Only rarely does the candidal infection become systemic. Some patients have associated endocrine deficiencies, with hypoadrenalism, hypoparathyroidism, and hypothyroidism among the most common. Initially, these patients show increased susceptibility to infection with *Candida* only, with normal ability to resist other infectious agents. Gradually, however, their general immunity wanes, and infection occurs from other opportunistic organisms.

The early-onset presentation of this disorder is most severe, is usually associated with endocrinopathy, and may manifest *Candida* granuloma. The later-onset type of disease is usually milder and may be limited to paronychia or buccal mucosal involvement. There is also an autosomal recessive form in which endocrinopathy is uncommon. In contrast, endocrine disorders (usually hypoparathyroidism) predominate in the *Candida-endocrinopathy* syndrome, an autosomal recessive juvenile familial polyendocrinopathy with candidiasis. There is also a biotin-dependent multiple carboxylase deficiency disorder that is associated with chronic candidiasis, severe acidosis, neurologic abnormalities, and systemic bacterial and viral infections.

Endocrinopathy may be preceded by viral infection. Hypoparathyroidism and Addison disease are more common than hypothyroidism, diabetes, and pernicious anemia. Acute or chronic hepatitis may also occur.

The immunologic background for chronic mucocutaneous candidosis is varied. The usual tests may show defects of T cell immunity, deficiency of migration inhibitory factor (MIF), selective IgA deficiency, or biotin deficiency. In some patients no abnormalities have been found.

Intravenous administration of amphotericin is effective, but symptoms frequently recur upon cessation of therapy. In recalcitrant cases, clotrimazole, transfer factor, leukocyte infusions, and thymosin have all been used with variable degrees of success. An especially effective anticandidal agent is ketoconazole. It is important to remember that endocrinopathy (e.g., acute adrenal insufficiency) may occur at any time.

11.21 GRAFT-VERSUS-HOST DISEASE (GVHD)

See also Sec. 6.39.

This complication of T cell deficiency states occurs when a patient receives immunocompetent (T killer) cells with ordinary blood transfusions or transplantation of bone marrow and solid organs (Sec. 6.39). More rarely, it may occur in utero following transfusion for erythroblastosis fetalis or as a result of passage of maternal cells across the placenta into the fetal circulation. In the intrauterine situation, whether the affected fetus must be T cell deficient or not is unknown. The rarity of GVHD in the normal population and its frequent occurrence among immunodeficient patients suggest that intrauterine graft-versus-host disease probably does not occur in normal fetuses.

GVHD may be acute or chronic. The *acute* variety is usually seen in recipients of blood or bone marrow from donors who differ at the HLA-D locus; the event most often occurs when a blood transfusion is unwittingly given to a T cell deficient patient. It may rarely occur after transplants of fetal tissue. Occasionally, GVHD is associated with blood product infusions in leukemic patients. It remains a rare event, however, and probably occurs only when a number of chance events happen simultaneously. *Chronic* GVHD is seen with intrauterine transfusions, after transplantation from HLA-D matched bone marrow donors (especially in leukemia), and after transplants of fetal liver or fetal thymus.

11.22 SECONDARY IMMUNODEFICIENCY DISEASES

In these disorders the primary cause is outside the lymphoid system. The immune elements are involved either as part of a generalized process or as a result of some aspect of the primary disease which directly attacks or consumes the lymphoid products.

ADENOSINE DEAMINASE (ADA) AND NUCLEOSIDE PHOSPHORYLASE (NP) DEFICIENCY. These are the first biochemical defects in which immunodeficiency is an associated feature. Adenosine deaminase–deficient patients usually have combined immunodeficiency disease, but isolated defects of the thymus system are known. Nucleoside phosphorylase deficiency usually presents first as an isolated T cell defect, but NP deficiency eventually results in B cell deficiency as well. These biochemical defects cause immunodeficiency because products accumulated as a result of an inability to catabolize purines have a toxic effect on lymphocytes. ADA catalyzes the conversion of adenosine to inosine; in its absence, levels of lymphocyte ATP, cyclic AMP, and their deoxyanalogues increase. NP catalyzes the reversible conversion of inosine to hypoxanthine, guanosine to guanine, and xanthosine to xanthine. A breakdown in normal catabolic processes results in the accumulation of inosine and guanosine. Whether these or other metabolites are the actual toxic factors is unknown, but the notion of slow toxic attrition of the lymphoid system appears to be valid. Characteristically, a period of normal lymphoid function is followed by a gradual waning of immunity.

Most patients with these disorders have the clinical manifestations of combined immunodeficiency. ADA usually presents during the neonatal period with severe diarrhea, pneumonia, otitis media, and failure to thrive. Candidiasis is common. There may be hepatosplenomegaly. Infections with fungus, viral, bacterial, and protozoan organisms occur. The onset of ADA may be delayed, and although all patients who are homozygous for NP have been symptomatic, clinical manifestations may not appear for several years.

The diagnosis is established by measurement of enzyme levels in erythrocytes. It can also be suspected when the clinical history suggests an "acquired" defect of late onset and, in NP deficiency, from finding low serum uric acid levels. Characteristic splaying of the ends of the ribs and "squaring off" of the scapulae are seen in children with ADA deficiency. In those with NP deficiency, the metabolic defect may result in megaloblastic anemia, pure red cell aplasia, or spastic tetraparesis.

Repeated blood transfusions have shown limited benefit in some cases of ADA deficiency but not in NP deficiency. Injections of purified bovine ADA have been given as a substitute therapy; the results have been variable. Bone marrow transplantation is curative. If haploidentical transplants are performed, ablation is necessary. Gene therapy for ADA has been attempted in one patient.

LOSS OF IMMUNOLOGIC MATERIALS. Loss of protein, and hence of immunoglobulins, may occur from the genitourinary and gastrointestinal tracts and from the lymphatic system. In *nephrotic syndromes* the glomerular sieve allows the escape of IgG and IgA but retains the larger molecules of IgM, which remain at near-normal levels. Manufacture of antibody is unimpaired, and susceptibility to infection is not increased (the susceptibility of nephrotic children to pneumococcal peritonitis appears to be related, in part, to ascites and to lack of previous experience with the specific type of pneumococcus responsible for the infection in addition to factors discussed in Sec. 18.27). The situation with *protein-losing enteropathy* is analogous (Sec. 13.61). Both are characterized by hypogammaglobulinemia associated with edema or hypoalbuminemia. Loss of immunologic materials from the *lymphatic system*, whether due to congenital malformations of the lymphatic vessels or to surgical accidents, includes loss of lymphocytes as well as of circulating immunoglobulins. The lymphocyte count may drop to one third of normal, and all three major classes of immunoglobulins may fall to one half of normal levels. Tests of T cell function show abnormal lymphocyte responses in vitro and retention of allogeneic skin grafts for up to 2 yr. Resistance to infections is surprisingly unimpaired except in patients with chylothorax; lymphangiectasia involving the thoracic cavity is associated with more infectious problems than that of other areas of the body. Infants should be carefully monitored for infection and vigorously treated with appropriate antibiotics when illness is diagnosed.

NUTRITIONAL DEFICIENCY. In *protein-calorie malnutrition* (Sec. 4.17), disseminated herpes infections and gram-negative sepsis are common. Death from measles may occur. Lymphopenia is marked, in vitro lymphocyte responses are defective, and tonsils and thymus are small. Usually B cell function is only slightly diminished; IgE may be markedly elevated.

Immune cellular functions are dependent upon divalent cations. For example, internal movement of calcium ions causes proliferation of lymphocytes, and immunodeficiency has been described in association with copper, zinc, iron, and calcium abnormalities. Acrodermatitis enteropathica is due to zinc malabsorption; chronic candidosis may be associated with biotin deficiency.

CHEMICAL OR PHYSICAL IMMUNOSUPPRESSION. See Sec. 12.13.

VIRAL INFECTIONS. Intrauterine infections may cause altered development of lymphoid cells and organs, such as the thymus, in which primary differentiation takes place (Sec. 11.1). B cell deficiency may occur following infection with Epstein-Barr virus (Sec. 12.72). The disease (Duncan disease) appears to be X-linked, and the initial bout of Epstein-Barr virus infection is unusually severe and fulminant. The association of viral infection with AIDS is discussed in Sec. 12.83.

RICHARD HONG

Ammann AJ, Hong R: Disorders of the T-cell system. *In*: Stiehm ER (ed): Immunologic Disorders in Infants and Children, 3rd ed. Philadelphia, WB Saunders, 1989, p 257.

Buckley RH: Advances in the diagnosis and treatment of primary immunodeficiency diseases. Arch Intern Med 146:377, 1986.

Carbonari M, Cherchi M, Paganelli R, et al: Relative increase of T cells expressing the gamma/Delta rather than the alpha/beta receptor in ataxia-telangiectasia. N Engl J Med 322:73, 1990.

Conley ME, Lavoie A, Briggs C, et al: Nonrandom X chromosome inactivation in B cells from carriers of X chromosome-linked severe combined immunodeficiency. Proc Natl Acad Sci USA 85:3090, 1988.

Cooper MD: B lymphocytes: Normal development and function. N Engl J Med 317:1452, 1987.

Ferrara JLM, Deeg HJ: Mechanisms of disease. N Engl J Med 324:667, 1991.

Kapoor N, Kirkpatrick D, Blaese RM, et al: Reconstitution of normal megakaryocytopoiesis and immunologic functions in Wiskott-Aldrich syndrome by marrow transplantation following myeloablation and immunosuppression with busulfan and cyclophosphamide. Blood 57:692, 1981.

Marrack P, Lo D, Brinster R, et al: The effect of thymus environment on T cell development and tolerance. Cell 53:627, 1988.

Moen RC, Horowitz SD, Sondel PM, et al: Immunologic reconstitution after haploidentical bone marrow transplantation for immune deficiency disorders: Treatment of bone marrow cells with monoclonal antibody CT-2 and complement. Blood 70:664, 1987.

O'Reilly RJ, Brochstein J, Collins N, et al: Evaluation of HLA-haplotype disparate parental marrow grafts depleted of T lymphocytes by differential agglutination with a soybean lectin and E-rosette depletion for the treatment of severe combined immunodeficiency. Vox Sang 51:81, 1986.

Ochs HD, Wedgwood RD: Disorders of the B-cell system. *In*: Stiehm ER (ed): Immunologic Disorders in Infants and Children, 3rd ed. Philadelphia, WB Saunders, 1989, p 226.

Roitt I: Acquired immune response. IV. Development. *In*: Essential Immunology, 6th ed. Oxford, Blackwell Scientific Publications, 1988, p 134.

Roitt I: Recognition of antigen. I: Primary interaction. *In*: Essential Immunology, 6th ed. Oxford, Blackwell Scientific Publications, 1988, p 55.

Rosen FS, Cooper MD, Wedgwood RJP: The primary immunodeficiencies. Pt 1. N Engl J Med 311:235, 1984.

Rosen FS, Cooper MD, Wedgwood RJP: The primary immunodeficiencies. Pt 2. N Engl J Med 311:300, 1984.

Shackelford PG, Granoff DM, Polmar SH, et al: Subnormal serum concentrations of IgG2 in children with frequent infections associated with varied patterns of immunologic dysfunction. J Pediatr 116:529, 1990.

Strober W, James SP: The interleukins. Pediatr Res 24:549, 1988.

Weinberg K, Parkman R: Severe combined immunodeficiency due to a specific defect in the production of interleukin-2. N Engl J Med 322:1718, 1990.

COMPLEMENT AND ASSOCIATED DISEASES

11.23 COMPLEMENT

Complement was originally defined through the study of bacteriolysis, which requires both specific antibody and a nonspecific, heat-labile principle, now termed *complement*. By the 1960s nine complement components were known, one of which had three subcomponents. By the early 1970s a second major pathway of activation of complement, the *alternative pathway*, had been described. The latter system contains three unique factors. In addition, at least four regulators that control (decrease) activity of either or both pathways exist in serum, and at least five such regulatory proteins exist on the surface of cells. The original system of 11 components is now referred to as the classical pathway of complement. The term *complement system* generally refers to both pathways, which interact and depend on each other for their full activity. All of the 18 serum components and regulators are proteins. Together they make up about 10% of the globulin fraction of serum.

NOMENCLATURE. The terminology applied to complement is cryptic but logical and consists of only a few rules: The components have been assigned numbers in the order of their discovery and are preceded by the letter C. Unfortunately, the first four components do not interact in the sequence in which they were discovered but rather in the order C1423. The remaining components react in the appropriate numerical order, C56789. C1 has three subcomponents, C1q, C1r, and C1s. Fragments of components resulting from cleavage by other components acting as enzymes are assigned small letters (a, b, c, d, or e); with the exception of C2 fragments, the smaller piece that is released into surrounding fluids is assigned the lower case letter a, and the major part of the molecule, bound to other components or to some part of the immune complex, is assigned b, for example, C3a and C3b. When a component is activated (becomes an active enzyme), a bar is placed above the number, for example, $C\bar{1}$.

Components of the alternative pathway have been assigned upper case letters: B, D, and P (properdin). Factor B has an active form denoted $\overline{Bb}$. C3 (in particular, its major fragment, C3b) is a component of both the classical and alternative pathways.

GENERAL CONCEPTS. Complement is a *system* of interacting proteins. The biologic functions of the system depend upon the interaction of individual components, which occurs in sequential fashion. This has been referred to as a cascade, in analogy to the clotting system of blood; activation of each component (except the 1st) depends upon activation of the prior component or components in the sequence.

Interaction occurs along two pathways: the classical pathway, in the order antigen-antibody-C142356789; and the alternative pathway, in the order activator-(antibody)-properdin system-C356789. Antibody accelerates the rate of activation of the alternative pathway, but some activation can occur on appropriate surfaces in the absence of antibody. The classical and the alternative pathways interact with each other through the ability of both to activate C3.

The interaction of the early-acting components of complement (C1423) results in the generation of a series of active enzymes, $C\overline{1}$, $C\overline{42}$, and $C\overline{423}$. Thus, "activation" refers to transformation of the component into part of an active enzyme. In contrast, the interaction among C5b, C6, C7, C8, and C9 is nonenzymatic. In the case of C1, activation is a result of its interaction with antibody. Activation of C4, C2, C3, and C5, as well as factor B of the alternative pathway, is secondary to cleavage by a preceding activated component. Thus, activation of early components generates enzymes that fix to the antigen-antibody complex and catalyze a reaction on the next component, whereas later acting components (C6–C9) adsorb to the complex or the underlying cell by an interaction that depends on a change in their configuration.

These basic principles can be illustrated by a more detailed analysis of the activation sequence.

SEQUENCE OF ACTIVATION. The sequence in which the components of the classical pathway interact, the interdigitation between classical and alternative pathways, the chemical and some functional by-products of these reactions, and the regulators of the system are summarized in Figure 11–1.

The sequence begins with fixation of C1, by way of C1q, to the Fc (Sec. 11.1), nonantigen-binding part of the antibody molecule after antigen-antibody interaction. The C1 tricomplex changes configuration, and the C1s subcomponent becomes an active enzyme, $C\overline{1}$ esterase.

C-reactive protein (CRP), which reacts with C carbohydrate from micro-organisms and is elevated in certain inflammatory states, can substitute for antibody in the fixation of C1q and initiate reaction of the entire sequence. Thus, C-reactive protein functions like antibody, although it can combine with only a few specific "antigens" and its size and structure are quite different. This reaction has the potential for initiating inflammation in the absence of antibody. Other agents that can activate C1 directly, without a requirement for antibody, include certain bacteria, mycoplasma, and RNA viruses, uric acid crystals, the lipid A component of bacterial endotoxin, and the membranes of certain intracellular organelles.

In the next two steps of the classical pathway, polypeptide fragments are split from C4 and C2 during their activation and fixation by the enzymatic action of $C\overline{1}$. One of these appears to be a kinin-like peptide that can induce vascular permeability and edema through direct action on postcapillary venules. The peptide C4a has *anaphylatoxin* activity; it reacts with mast cells to release the chemical mediators of immediate hypersensitivity, including histamine. Fixation of C4b to the complex permits it to adhere to a variety of mammalian cells, including neutrophils, monocytes, and erythrocytes, a phenomenon termed *immune adherence*.

Cleavage of C3 and generation of C3b is the next step in the sequence and the most crucial in terms of biologic activity. Cleavage of C3 can be achieved through $C\overline{142}$, the C3 convertase of the classical pathway, or through the C3 convertase of the alternative pathway, $\overline{C3bBb}$ (see later). Once fixed to the complex, C3b permits adherence of the antigen-antibody complex to cells with receptors for C3b (complement receptor 1, CR1), including B lymphocytes, erythrocytes, and phagocytic cells (neutrophils, monocytes, and macrophages), leading, in the last case, to phagocytosis. Without C3 bound to them, phagocytosis of most micro-organisms in vitro, especially by neutrophils, is very inefficient. The severe pyogenic infections that occur commonly in C3-deficient patients indicate that without C3, phagocytosis is also inefficient in vivo. The biologic activity of C3b is controlled by cleavage by factor I (C3b inactivator) to iC3b, which is further degraded by factor I and serum or tissue enzymes to C3c, which is released, and to C3dg and C3d, which stay bound. iC3b promotes phagocytosis on binding to the iC3b receptor (CR3) on phagocytes. Receptors for C3dg and C3d exist on B lymphocytes (CR2) and phagocytes (CR4). Further cleavage of C3c creates C3e, which induces release of granulocytes from bone marrow.

The peptide C3a, generated when C3 is acted upon by either pathway, has anaphylatoxin activity. The action of $C\overline{423}$ or of the alternative pathway C5 convertase on C5

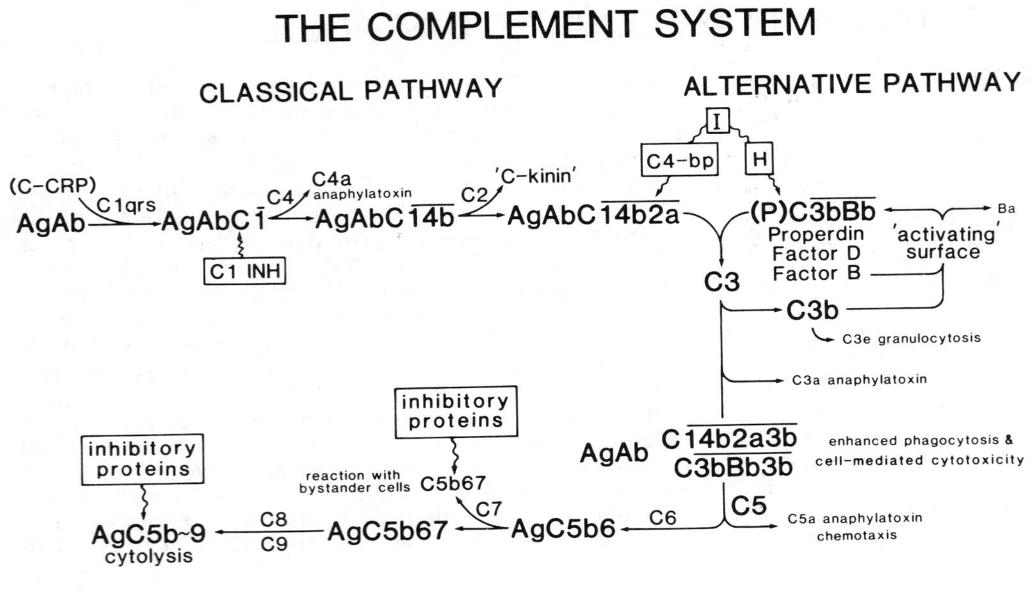

Figure 11–1. Sequence of activation of the components of the classical pathway of complement and interaction with the alternative pathway. (Ag = antigen [bacterium, virus, tumor cell, or erythrocyte]; Ab = antibody [IgG or IgM class only]; C-CRP = C carbohydrate–C-reactive protein; C1 INH = C1 inhibitor; I = factor I, C3b inactivator; C4-bp = C4-binding protein; H = factor H, β1H.) Inhibitory regulator proteins are each enclosed in a box.

releases C5a, a powerful anaphylatoxin that can react with neutrophils, macrophages, mast cells, smooth muscle cells, and certain T cells to induce release of a variety of mediators of inflammation. This same peptide serves as a potent chemical attractant for phagocytic cells.

The "membrane-attack" sequence leading to cytolysis begins with the attachment of C5b to $C\overline{423}$, the C5-activating enzyme (or to the alternative pathway enzyme). C6 is bound to C5b without being cleaved, stabilizing the activated C5b fragment. The C5b6 complex then dissociates from $C\overline{423}$ and reacts with C7. C5b67 complexes must attach to the cell membrane promptly or lose their activity and remain in the fluid phase. Next, C8 binds, and the C5b678 complex then promotes the addition of multiple C9 molecules. The C9 polymer of 12–18 molecules forms a transmembrane channel, and lysis ensues.

Control mechanisms act at several points to prevent the system's consuming itself in activity that is unnecessary or deleterious to the host. An α_2-globulin, C1 inhibitor (C1 INH), inhibits $C\overline{1s}$ enzymatic activity and, thus, the cleavage of C4 and C2. Activated C2 has a half-life of about 8 min at 37° C, and this relative instability limits the effective life of $C\overline{42}$ and $C\overline{423}$. The alternative pathway enzyme that activates C3, $\overline{C3bBb}$, also has a short half-life, though it can be prolonged by the binding of properdin (P) to the enzyme complex. Serum contains the protein "anaphylatoxin inactivator," an enzyme that cleaves the carboxyterminal arginine from both C3a and C5a, thereby markedly reducing their anaphylatoxic activity and the chemotactic activity of C5a. Factor I inactivates C4b and C3b, thus serving as an important means of controlling both pathways. Factor H(β1H) accelerates inactivation of C3b by I. An analogous factor, C4 binding protein (C4-bp), accelerates cleavage of C4b by factor I. Three protein constituents of cell membranes, CR1, membrane cofactor protein, and decay-accelerating factor (DAF), promote the disruption of C3 and C5 convertases assembled on those membranes. Other cell membrane-associated proteins can bind C8 or both C8 and C9, thereby interfering with insertion of the membrane-attack complex (C5b6789). Certain serum proteins can inhibit attachment of the C5b67 complex to cell membranes, bind C8 or C9 in a full membrane-attack complex, or otherwise interfere with the formation or insertion of this complex.

ALTERNATIVE PATHWAY. The alternative pathway can be activated by C3b generated through classical pathway activity, through leukocyte proteases released by degranulation, or perhaps through activation of thrombin or plasmin during blood coagulation. It can also be activated by a form of C3 created by low grade, spontaneous reaction of native C3 with a molecule of water, which occurs constantly in plasma. Once formed, C3b or this hydrolyzed C3 can bind to any nearby cell or to factor B. Factor B attached to C3b in the plasma or on the surface of a particle can be cleaved to Bb by D, which exists as an active proteolytic enzyme. The complex $\overline{C3bBb}$ becomes an efficient C3 convertase, which generates more C3b through an "amplification loop" (see Fig. 11–1). P can bind to $\overline{C3bBb}$, increasing stability of the enzyme and protecting it from inactivation by factors I and H, which serve to modulate the loop. Cleavage of B releases Ba, which has weak chemotactic activity.

Certain materials promote alternative pathway activation if C3b is fixed to their surface, for example, teichoic acid from bacterial cell wall, endotoxic lipopolysaccharide, or immunoglobulin aggregates, especially of the IgA class. This activation depends on the ability of the $\overline{C3bBb}$ enzyme complex to escape the efficient control otherwise exercised by factors I and H. The surface of rabbit red blood cells also protects $\overline{C3bBb}$ from inactivation. This phenomenon serves as the basis for an assay of serum alternative pathway activity. Endotoxin may alter normally "nonactivating" cell surfaces in vivo so that $\overline{C3bBb}$ is relatively protected from inactivation, which may partially explain the activation of the alternative pathway in patients with gram-negative bacteremia. Sialic acid on the surface of micro-organisms or cells prevents formation of an effective alternative pathway C3 convertase by promoting activity of I and H.

Although $\overline{C3bBb}$ can activate C3 efficiently on only a limited variety of surfaces, significant activation of C3 can occur through this pathway, and the resultant biologic activities are qualitatively the same as those achieved through activation by $C\overline{142}$, as illustrated in Figure 11–1.

PARTICIPATION IN HOST DEFENSE. Neutralization of virus by antibody can be enhanced with C1 and C4. When antibody concentrations are low, the additional fixation of C3b to the viral antigen-antibody complex through the classical or alternative pathway improves neutralization; C5 and C6 add little to the effect. Complement may, therefore, be particularly important in the early phases of a viral infection when antibody is limited. Antibody and complement can also eliminate infectivity of at least some viruses, with the production of typical complement "holes" in the virus, as seen by electron microscopy. Animal RNA tumor viruses interact directly with human C1q in the absence of antibody with resulting activation of the classical pathway and lysis of the virus. This may be a natural resistance mechanism that limits the infectivity of these viruses in humans.

C4a, C3a, and C5a can bind to mast cells and thereby trigger release of histamine and other mediators, leading to vasodilatation and to the swelling and redness of inflammation. C5a can induce monocytes to release the cytokines, tumor necrosis factor, and interleukin 1, which amplify the inflammatory response. C5a is a major chemical stimulus for the influx into inflammatory sites of neutrophils, monocytes, and eosinophils, which can efficiently phagocytize micro-organisms coated (opsonized) with C3b. Inactivation of cell-bound C3b by cleavage to C3d removes its opsonizing activity. Fixation of C3b to a target cell can enhance its lysis by a "killer" cell in an antibody-dependent, cell-mediated cytotoxicity system.

Insoluble immune complexes can be solubilized if they bind C3b, apparently because C3b disrupts the orderly antigen-antibody lattice. Binding of C3b to a complex also allows it to adhere to C3 receptors (CR1) on red cells, which then transport the complexes to fixed macrophages for removal. These findings probably are related to the immune complex disease found in patients who lack C1, C4, C2, or C3.

The complement system may be involved in certain aspects of B and T lymphocyte-mediated specific immunity. C3b– and C3d-coated particles can bind to B lymphocytes. C3a appears to suppress antibody formation, whereas C5a appears to enhance this response. C3e, a cleavage product generated during the inactivation of C3, induces an increase in circulating granulocytes.

Neutralization of endotoxin in vitro and protection from its lethal effects in experimental animals require later-acting components of complement, at least through C6. Finally, activation of the entire complement sequence can result in lysis of virus-infected cells, tumor cells, and most types of micro-organisms. Bactericidal activity of complement has not appeared to be important to host defense except for the occurrence of infections with *Neisseria* in patients lacking later-acting components of complement (Sec. 12.23).

Berger M, Frank MM: The serum complement system. *In*: Stiehm ER (ed): Immunologic Disorders in Infants and Children, 3rd ed. Philadelphia, WB Saunders, 1989, p 97.

Campbell RD, Law SK, Ried KB, et al: Structure, organization, and regulation of the complement genes. Annu Rev Immunol 6:161, 1988.

Frank MM: Complement in the pathophysiology of human disease. N Engl J Med 316:1525, 1987.

Muller-Eberhard HJ: Molecular organization and function of the complement system. Annu Rev Biochem 57:321, 1988.

DISEASES OF THE COMPLEMENT SYSTEM

11.24 PRIMARY DEFICIENCIES OF COMPLEMENT COMPONENTS

Congenital deficiencies of all 11 component proteins of the classical pathway and of factor D of the alternative pathway have been described (Table 11–6).

Complete **deficiency of C1q** has been detected in children with a syndrome of septicemia or meningitis, skin infections, and a florid maculopapular rash. Biopsies of the rash have shown deposition of immune complexes in the basal epidermis or walls of small blood vessels. **C1q dysfunction** has been found in persons with complete deficiency of C1q activity but only partially decreased amounts of an antigenically altered C1q molecule in their sera. Some family members have had a systemic lupus erythematosus-like syndrome; others were healthy. **C1r deficiency** can occur as an isolated defect or in association with C1s deficiency.

Patients with **C1q, C1r, C1r/C1s, C4, C2,** and **C3 deficiencies** have had a high incidence of vasculitis syndromes (see Table 11–6), especially systemic lupus erythematosus or a lupus-like syndrome in which antinuclear antibody may be undetectable. A few patients with **C5, C6, C7,** or **C8 deficiency** have had such a disorder, but recurrent infections are much more likely to be the major problem in this group. The reason for the concurrence of deficiencies of components of complement and these "autoimmune" diseases is not known; but if these diseases originate as infections, the association may be a result of absence of one or more of the host defense properties described in Sec. 11.23. Complement facilitates elimination of immune complexes; inefficiency of this process is another explanation.

TABLE 11–6. Genetic Deficiencies of Complement Components

Deficient Component	Associated Clinical Findings: Collagen-Vascular Disease*	Associated Clinical Findings: Infections
C1q	SLE, dermal vasculitis, MPGN, DLE	Recurrent bacterial, fungal–dermatitis, meningitis
C1q dysfunction	SLE	
C1r	CGN, SLE, dermal vasculitis	Pneumonia†, meningitis†
C1r/C1s	SLE	
C4	SLE, H-S purpura†, Sjögren syndrome†	Bacteremia†, meningitis†
C2	SLE, DLE, CGN, MPGN, H-S purpura, dermal vasculitis, dermatomyositis†, ITP†	Recurrent septicemia, especially pneumococcal; meningitis; pneumonia
C3	MPGN, SLE, dermal vasculitis	Severe, generalized bacterial
C5	SLE†	Disseminated gonococcal or meningococcal; pyoderma†; meningitis†
C6	SLE†, DLE†, MPGN†, Sjögren syndrome†	Disseminated gonococcal or meningococcal
C7	SLE†, scleroderma†, ankylosing spondylitis†, RA†	Disseminated gonococcal or meningococcal
C8	SLE†	Disseminated gonococcal or meningococcal
C9		Meningococcal meningitis†
Factor D		Recurrent sinusitis, bronchitis; bronchiectasis

*CGN = chronic glomerulonephritis; DLE = discoid lupus erythematosus; H-S = Henoch-Schönlein; ITP = idiopathic thrombocytopenic purpura; MPGN = membranoproliferative glomerulonephritis; RA = rheumatoid arthritis; SLE = systemic lupus erythematosus.

†Finding reported uncommonly in patients with this deficiency.

Several patients with **C2 deficiency** have had repeated life-threatening septicemic illnesses, most commonly due to pneumococci. Most have not had problems with increased susceptibility to infection, presumably because of the protective function of the alternative pathway. The genes for C2, factor B, and C4 are situated close to each other on chromosome 6, and a depression of factor B levels to about 50% of normal can occur in conjunction with C2 deficiency. Persons with a deficiency of both proteins might be at particular risk.

Since C3 can be activated by C142 or by the alternative pathway, a defect in the function of either pathway can be compensated, at least to some extent. Without C3, however, the chemotactic fragment from C5 is not generated, and opsonization of bacteria is inefficient. Some organisms must be well opsonized in order to be cleared, and **congenital absence of C3** has been associated with recurrent, severe pyogenic infections due to pneumococci and meningococci. Some C3-deficient patients have had sluggish neutrophilic responses to infection, in agreement with reports that a cleavage factor of C3 elicits an increase in blood neutrophils.

The first patient found to have homozygous **C5 deficiency** was a girl who developed classic systemic lupus erythematosus in late childhood and had a lifelong history of recurrent pyogenic infections, especially of the skin, perhaps because of the absence of the critical chemotactic factor split from C5. Generation of chemotaxis by her serum in vitro was markedly depressed. Other patients have had recurrent disseminated gonococcal infection or multiple episodes of meningococcal meningitis.

About half of the individuals reported to have congenital **C6, C7, C8,** or **C9 deficiencies** have had meningococcal meningitis or extragenital gonococcal infection. About 10% have had a collagen-vasular disease. In two studies of patients with systemic meningococcal disease, 10–20% had a genetic complement deficiency. It is not clear why patients with a deficiency of one of the late-acting components suffer a particular predisposition to neisserial infections; it may be that serum bacteriolysis is uniquely important in defense against this organism, but some persons with such a deficiency have had no significant illness.

Identical twin sisters had **isolated deficiency of factor D** of the alternative pathway. Both had recurrent sinusitis and bronchitis; one also had bronchiectasis. Hemolytic complement activity in their serum was normal, but alternative pathway activity was markedly deficient.

C1q dysfunction and deficiencies of C1r, C4, C2, C3, C5, C6, C7, C8, C9, factor I, and factor H are transmitted as autosomal recessive traits, of the "autosomal codominant" variety; that is, each parent transmits a gene that codes for synthesis of half the serum level of the component. The mode of transmission of C1q and C1s deficiency is probably also autosomal recessive. Properdin deficiency appears to be transmitted as an X-linked trait (Sec. 11.25). A rare form of C4 deficiency may be inherited as an autosomal dominant trait.

11.25 PRIMARY DEFICIENCIES OF COMPLEMENT CONTROL PROTEINS

Factor I deficiency was originally reported as a deficiency of C3 owing to its hypercatabolism. The first patient described had suffered a series of severe pyogenic infections similar to those seen with agammaglobulinemia or congenital deficiency of C3. Further studies indicated that the primary deficiency was that of factor I, an essential regulator of the alternative pathway. This deficiency permits prolonged existence of C3b in the C3 convertase of the alternative pathway, C3bBb, resulting in constant activation of the alternative pathway and cleavage of more C3 to C3b, in circular fashion. Intravenous infusion of plasma or purified factor I induced a prompt rise in serum C3 concentration in the patient and a return to normal of in vitro C3-dependent functions such as opsonization.

One of the first reported patients with **factor H deficiency** had hemolytic-uremic syndrome; the other was healthy. Persons with **properdin deficiency** have had a predisposition to meningococcal meningitis. All reported patients have been male, and their families have had a striking history of male deaths due to meningitis. The predisposition to infection in these patients indicates a requirement for the alternative pathway in host defense against bacterial infection. This predisposition does not exist in the presence of antibody because the classical pathway is normal in their serum. Neither the patients nor members of their families have had collagen-vascular disease.

The receptor for C3b (complement receptor 1, CR1) on cell surface membranes assists in the disruption of C4b- or C3b-bearing immune complexes that the cell encounters in the plasma or on the surface of adjacent cells. Patients with systemic lupus erythematosus (SLE) and their asymptomatic family members have a partial **deficiency of CR1,** which appears to be inherited as an autosomal recessive trait. This deficiency could increase the risk of developing immune complex disease, thereby contributing to the pathogenesis of SLE.

Hereditary angioedema occurs in persons born without the ability to synthesize normally functioning C1 inhibitor. In 85% of affected families the affected members have markedly reduced concentrations of inhibitor (5–30% of normal); in the other 15% normal or elevated concentrations of an immunologically cross-reacting but nonfunctional protein occur. Both forms of the disease are transmitted as autosomal dominant traits.

In the absence of this α_2-globulin, activation of C1 leads to uncontrolled C1s activity, with breakdown of C4 and C2 and release of a vasoactive peptide (kinin) from C2. Episodic, localized, nonpitting edema results from the vasodilatory effects of the kinin on the postcapillary venule. The mechanism by which C1 is activated in these patients is not known.

Swelling of the affected part accumulates rapidly, without urticaria, itching, discoloration, or redness, and often without severe pain. Swelling of the intestinal wall, however, can lead to intense abdominal cramping, sometimes with vomiting or diarrhea; concurrent subcutaneous edema is often absent, and patients have undergone abdominal surgery or psychiatric examination before the true diagnosis was made. Laryngeal edema can be fatal. Attacks last 2–3 days, then gradually abate. They may occur at sites of trauma, after vigorous exercise, with menses, or with emotional stress. Attacks can begin in the first 2 yr of life but are usually not severe until late childhood or adolescence. The condition can be acquired in association with lymphoid cancer or autoantibody to C1 INH. Systemic lupus erythematosus has been reported in patients with the congenital disease (Sec. 11.26 and 11.27).

11.26 SECONDARY DEFICIENCIES OF COMPLEMENT

Partial deficiency of C1q has occurred in patients with *severe combined immunodeficiency disease* or *hypogammaglobulinemia*, apparently secondary to the deficiency of IgG, which normally binds reversibly to C1q and prevents its rapid catabolism.

Serum from patients with *chronic membranoproliferative glomerulonephritis* contains a protein termed *nephritic factor* (NeF) that promotes activation of the alternative pathway. Nephritic factor is an IgG antibody to the C3-cleaving enzyme of the alternative pathway, C3bBb, that protects the enzyme from inactivation. The result is increased consumption of C3. Serum C3 concentrations vary widely from patient to patient, however. Pyogenic infections, including meningitis, may occur if the serum C3 level drops below about 10% of normal. This disorder has been found in children and adults with *partial lipodystrophy*. It is not known whether the lipodystrophy is a cause or a result of the NeF-C3 abnormality. An IgG nephritic factor that binds to and protects C42, the classical pathway C3 convertase, has been described in *acute postinfectious nephritis* and in *systemic lupus erythematosus*. The consumption of C3 that characterizes poststreptococcal nephritis and lupus could be due to this factor, to activation of complement by immune complexes, or both.

Newborn infants are known to have mild to moderate deficiencies of most components of the classical pathway of complement and of factor B and properdin. Opsonization and generation of chemotactic activity in serum from full-term newborns can be markedly deficient through either the classical or the alternative pathway. Complement activity is even lower in preterm infants than in full-term babies. Patients with *malnutrition* or *anorexia nervosa* may also have significant depletion of components and functional activity of complement. Although synthesis of components is depressed in these conditions, serum from some patients with malnutrition also appears to contain immune complexes that could accelerate depletion. Severe chronic *cirrhosis of the liver* may also result in decreased synthesis of C3.

Patients with *sickle cell disease* have normal activity of the classical pathway, but some have defective function of the alternative pathway in opsonization of pneumococci, in bacteriolysis and opsonization of salmonellae, and in lysis of rabbit erythrocytes. Similar defects have been described in about 10% of individuals who have undergone *splenectomy* and in some patients with *β-thalassemia major*. The underlying mechanism for the defects in alternative pathway function in these disorders has not been fully defined; in sickle cell disease, deficiency may be due, at least in part, to activation and consumption of the complement system. Children with *nephrotic syndrome* may have subnormal serum opsonizing activity in association with decreased serum levels of factor B.

Immune complexes, including those initiated by microorganisms or their by-products, may induce consumption of components of complement. Activation occurs primarily through fixation of C1 to antibody thereby initiating the classical pathway. In *systemic lupus erythematosus*, immune complexes activate the classical pathway, and C3 is deposited at sites of tissue damage, including kidneys and skin; depressed synthesis of C3 is also seen. Formation of immune complexes and consumption of complement have been demonstrated in *lepromatous leprosy, subacute bacterial endocarditis, infected ventriculojugular shunts, malaria, infectious mononucleosis, dengue hemorrhagic fever,* and *acute hepatitis B*. Nephritis or arthritis may develop as a result of deposition of immune complexes and activation of complement in these infections. The syndrome of *recurrent urticaria, angioedema, eosinophilia, and hypocomplementemia* secondary to activation of the classical pathway may be due to circulating immune complexes. Circulating immune complexes and decreased C3 have been reported in some patients with *dermatitis herpetiformis, celiac disease, primary biliary cirrhosis,* and *Reye syndrome.*

In patients with *bacteremic shock,* bacterial products appear to initiate direct activation of the alternative pathway. *Intravenous injection of iodinated roentgenographic contrast medium* can induce a rapid and significant activation of the alternative pathway, which may explain at least some of the occasional reactions that occur in patients undergoing this procedure.

Burns can induce massive activation of the complement system, especially the alternative pathway, within a few hours after injury. Generation of C3a and C5a occurs, which stimulates neutrophils and induces their sequestration in the lung. These events may play an important part in the development of shock lung after burn injury. Cardiopulmonary bypass, plasma exchange, or hemodialysis using cellophane membranes may be associated with a similar syndrome due to activation of plasma complement, with release of C3a and C5a. In patients with *erythropoietic protoporphyria* or *porphyria cutanea tarda* exposure of the skin to light of certain wavelengths activates complement, generating chemotactic activity. Phototoxicity is associated histologically with lysis of capillary endothelial cells, mast cell degranulation, and the appearance of neutrophils in the dermis.

Paroxysmal nocturnal hemoglobinuria results from an acquired deficiency of decay-accelerating factor in a subpopulation of erythrocytes and leukocytes. In the absence of this membrane protein, C3b that is deposited on the cells from serum in continuous low-grade fashion is not efficiently broken down by factor I. This permits the alternative pathway C3 convertase, $\overline{C3bBb}$, to develop effectively on the cell surface; the membrane-attack complex (C5~9) forms and lysis ensues.

11.27 DIAGNOSIS OF DISORDERS OF THE COMPLEMENT SYSTEM

Testing for total hemolytic complement activity (CH_{50}) is a useful screening procedure for most of the diseases of the complement system. A normal result in this assay depends on the ability of all 11 classical pathway component proteins to interact and lyse antibody-coated erythrocytes. The dilution of serum that lyses 50% of the cells determines the end-point. In congenital deficiencies of C1 through C8, the CH_{50} value will be about 0; in C9 deficiency, the value will be approximately half normal. Values in the acquired deficiencies will, of course, vary with the severity of the underlying disorder. This assay will not detect deficiencies of the alternative pathway components B, D, or P (properdin). Deficiency of factors I or H (Sec. 11.24) will permit consumption of C3, with partial reduction in the CH_{50} value.

In *hereditary angioedema,* depression of C4 and C2 during an attack significantly reduces the CH_{50}. Serum concentrations of C4 and C3 can be determined by radial immunodiffusion. In hereditary angioedema, C4 is characteristically low and C3 normal. Concentrations of C1 inhibitor can be determined with antibody, but a normal result can be anticipated in about 15% of cases (Sec. 11.25). Since C1 acts as an esterase, the specific diagnosis can be made by showing increased capacity of patients' sera to hydrolyze synthetic esters.

Decreased serum concentrations of both C4 and C3 suggest activation of the classical pathway by immune complexes. In contrast, decreased C3 and normal C4 levels suggest activation of the alternative pathway. This difference is particularly useful in distinguishing nephritis secondary to complex deposition from that due to NeF (nephritic factor). In the latter condition and in deficiency of factor I, factor B is consumed, and its serum concentration is low as measured by radial immunodiffusion. Alternative pathway activity can be measured with a relatively simple and reproducible hemolytic assay that depends on the capacity of rabbit erythrocytes to serve as both an "activating" (permissive) surface and a target of alternative pathway activity.

A defect of complement function should be suspected in any patient with collagen-vascular disease or chronic nephritis, or with recurrent pyogenic infections, neisserial infections, or septicemia. Complement disorders are frequently detected by means of the relatively simple hemolytic complement assay; this procedure should always be available as a screening test.

11.28 MANAGEMENT OF DISORDERS OF THE COMPLEMENT SYSTEM

There is no specific therapy presently available for genetic deficiencies of the complement system, but much can be done to protect patients with these disorders from serious complications. Adults with hereditary angioedema respond to danazol, a synthetic androgen with weak virilizing and mild anabolic potential. The drug, given orally, increases the level of C1 inhibitor 3- to 4-fold and prevents attacks. It can be used for short-term prophylaxis, for example, for oral surgery, by administering it for 1 wk prior to surgery. It has not been recommended for use in children.

Only supportive management is available for other primary diseases of the complement system. Purified components are not available, and if they were, the risk of inducing antibody to them would probably preclude their long-term use. It should be emphasized, however, that identification of a specific defect in the complement system may have an important impact on a patient's health. Concern for the associated complications (collagen-vascular disease and infection) should encourage vigorous diagnostic efforts and earlier institution of therapy. With the onset of unexplained fever, cultures should be obtained and antibiotic therapy instituted more quickly and with less stringent indications than in a normal child. Immunization of the patient and family members with bacterial capsular polysaccharides should also be considered. As defects are carefully characterized, the likelihood of specific therapy may improve.

RICHARD B. JOHNSTON, JR.

CONGENITAL DEFICIENCIES

Cicardi M, Bergamaschini L, Marasini B, et al: Hereditary angioedema: An appraisal of 104 cases. Am J Med Sci 284:2, 1982.

Davis AE III: C1 inhibitor and hereditary angioneurotic edema. Annu Rev Immunol 6:595, 1988.

Ellison RT III, Kohler PF, Curd JG, et al: Prevalence of congenital or acquired complement deficiency in patients with sporadic meningococcal disease. N Engl J Med 308:913, 1983.

Hauptmann G: Frequency of complement deficiencies in man, disease association and chromosome assignment of complement genes and linkage groups: A summary of the data from the literature. Complement 6:74, 1989.

Johnston RB Jr: Disorders of the complement system. *In*: Stiehm ER (ed): Immunologic Disorders in Infants and Children, 3rd ed. Philadelphia, WB Saunders, 1989, p 384.

Leggiadro RJ, Winkelstein JA: Prevalence of complement deficiencies in children with systemic meningococcal infections. Pediatr Infect Dis J 6:75, 1987.

Ross SC, Densen P: Complement deficiency states and infection: Epidemiology, pathogenesis and consequences of neisserial and other infections in an immune deficiency. Medicine 63:243, 1984.

Wilson JG, Wong WW, Schur PH, et al: Mode of inheritance of decreased C3b receptors on erythrocytes of patients with systemic lupus erythematosus. N Engl J Med 307:981, 1982.

Winkelstein JA, Colten HR: Genetically determined disorders of the complement system. *In*: Scriver CR, Beaudet AL, Sly WS, et al (eds): The Metabolic Basis of Inherited Disease, 6th ed. New York, McGraw-Hill, 1989, p 2711.

SECONDARY DEFICIENCIES

Edwards KM, Alford R, Gewurz H, et al: Recurrent bacterial infections associated with C3 nephritic factor and hypocomplementemia. N Engl J Med 308:1138, 1983.
Edwards MS: Complement in neonatal infections: An overview. Pediatr Infect Dis 5(Suppl 3):S168, 1986.
Eichenfield LF, Johnston RB Jr: Secondary disorders of the complement system. Am J Dis Child 143:595, 1989.
Halperin JA, Nicholson-Weller A: Paroxysmal nocturnal hemoglobinuria: A complement-mediated disease. Complement 6:65, 1989.
Johnston RB Jr, Altenburger KM, Atkinson AW Jr, et al: Complement in the newborn infant. Pediatrics 64:781, 1979.
Lim HW, Poh-Fitzpatrick MB, Gigli I: Activation of the complement system in patients with porphyrias after irradiation in vivo. J Clin Invest 74:1961, 1984.
Notarangelo LD, Chirico G, Chiara A, et al: Activity of classical and alternative pathways of complement in preterm and small for gestational age infants. Pediatr Res 18:281, 1984.

THE PHAGOCYTIC SYSTEMS AND ASSOCIATED DISEASES

11.29 NORMAL PHYSIOLOGY OF THE PHAGOCYTIC INFLAMMATORY RESPONSE

Understanding the disorders of phagocytic function requires a knowledge of the normal physiology of the inflammatory response of the phagocytic system. The principal phagocytes are neutrophils and monocytes; the former are more heavily involved in acute inflammation and microbial killing and the latter in chronic inflammation. Eosinophils, although capable of phagocytic microbial killing, participate in allergic and certain parasitic responses. Fixed tissue macrophages of liver, spleen, lung, and bone marrow are primed by T lymphocyte cytokines to remove immune complexes, antibody and complement-sensitized blood cells and microbes, and other particulate debris from the circulation. Neutrophils, eosinophils, and monocytes are derived from a common stem cell progenitor in the bone marrow, which is further differentiated into specific lineages defined by in vitro culture and influenced by several lymphocyte and monocyte cytokines (see also Sec. 11.1). For example, cytokine IL-3 stimulates stem cell colonies, mixed monocyte neutrophil colonies, red cell progenitor colonies called BFU-F, and megakaryocyte colonies. GM-CSF stimulates mixed monocyte neutrophil colonies as well as discrete colonies of neutrophils, monocytes, and eosinophils. G-CSF stimulates neutrophil colonies exclusively, and M-CSF stimulates monocyte colonies exclusively. Compared with monocytes, there is a large store of mature neutrophils in bone marrow that moves into the circulation in response to soluble mediators of inflammation such as endotoxin, tumor necrosis factor, interleukin 1, and activated complement by-product C3e. Following intravenous administration of 4 ng/kg endotoxin to humans, after an initial drop in peripheral blood neutrophils by 1 hr, neutrophil counts increase 3-fold by 6–8 hr with an increase in band forms. Band forms do not increase after a single oral or intravenous dose of glucocorticoids, nor are monoclonal antibody 31D4-positive bone marrow neutrophils seen in the circulation, which calls into question the notion that steroids raise the neutrophil count by causing egress of marrow neutrophils. Steroid neutrophilia may be due to delayed egress into tissues, release of a marginated pool, and increased production. Under normal conditions, neutrophils randomly exit from the circulation at a half-life rate of 4–6 hr, and the marginating pool approximates the circulating pool size. Activation of adenylate cyclase by adrenaline and other adrenergic agonists results in demargination of neutrophils and a doubling of circulating neutrophils associated with a transient elevation in cyclic AMP.

Although the ability of phagocytes to migrate to sites of infection and/or inflammation was recognized more than a century ago, the biologic nature of chemoattractants and their influences on phagocytic cell activities after binding to specific surface receptors have only recently begun to be understood. A variety of chemotactic factors are derived from cells or plasma. The activation of complement generates C5a, clotting generates thrombin, cell membrane phospholipids generate platelet-activating factor, stimulated T lymphocytes provide lymphocyte-derived chemotactic factor, and activated PMN generate leukotriene B_4. The ability of the various chemoattractant molecules to activate leukocyte responses is mediated by specific receptors, which, when occupied by a specific chemotactic factor, activate phospholipase C to produce inositol triphosphate (IP3) and diacylglycerol. IP3 in turn increases intracellular calcium-dependent responses associated with phagocyte activation, such as protein kinase C for phosphorylation of several important intracellular proteins required for cell activation and the assembly of actin and associated contractile proteins. The increased expression of a group of adherence proteins, for example, iC3b, and the assembly of actin and associated contractible proteins enable the phagocyte to attach to endothelial surfaces and move in a crawling amoeboid way to the site of infection or inflammation. The pathway is paved by an increasing gradient of chemoattractants that culminate in either a full expression of phagocytic activation or engagement of opsonized microbes. Microbes are opsonized (prepared for eating) by heat-stable and heat-labile factors in human serum that include immunoglobulin G and C3. Human leukocytes have three distinguishable receptors for each of the four immunoglobulin G subclasses (IgG1–4) and four receptors for C3 (CR1–4). CR1 and CR3 are distinct opsonin receptors on neutrophils, monocytes, and macrophages that bind C3b and iC3b, respectively, and facilitate phagocytosis of microbes and other particles or cells opsonized by them. In contrast to the IgG receptors, FcR, and the CR1 receptors, which do not require divalent cation for their ligand binding, CR3 requires 0.5 mM concentrations of calcium and magnesium ions for iC3b binding. The in vivo importance of the CR3 receptor for host defense will be discussed later. The trigger for ingestion by phagocytes of CR1- and CR3-bound microbes or cells appears to involve phosphorylation of the receptor by activated protein kinases. Adhesive proteins found in plasma and tissue matrices, such as fibronectin, laminin, or the protein kinase C stimulant phorbal myristate acetate have been shown to trigger phagocytic cell ingestion. Ingestion is an active process accompanied by further assembly and disassembly of contractile elements as the pseudopode envelopes its prey as it forms a phagosome. Granules fuse with the phagosomal membrane and discharge their contents into it. In neutrophils, specific granules interact with the phagosome earlier than do azurophilic granules. This process of degranulation occurs in all phagocytic cells and promotes the killing or digestion of microbes. On the other hand, treatment of cells with cytochalasin B disrupts assembled microfilaments, blocks ingestion, and renders the phagocytes secretory. Under such conditions, full activation induces release of the granule contents to the outside of the cell. Soluble chemotactic stimuli at sites of inflammation can induce extensive granule secretion, escalating the inflammatory process. In addition, the microbicidal and cytotoxic system of phagocytes includes the secretory products of the respiratory burst, superoxide anion, hydrogen peroxide, hydroxyl radical, and longer acting hypochlorous acid and chloramines. The azurophilic granule constituent myeloperoxidase participates in the amplification of this system by halides such as iodide and chloride. This system may also inhibit chemotactic factors and lysosomal granule components that may attenuate the inflammatory process. The respiratory burst is discussed in more detail in light of the etiology and pathogenesis of chronic granulomatous disease.

11.30 LEUKOCYTE ADHESION DEFICIENCY (LAD): A GENETIC DISORDER OF ADHESION-DEPENDENT LEUKOCYTE FUNCTION

This inherited syndrome comprises recurrent or progressive skin, mucous membrane, and subcutaneous infections characterized by diminished pus formation, poor wound healing including delayed separation of the umbilical cord, and persistent granulocytosis. The phenotypic expression of the syndrome is due to a genetic defect of a group of leukocyte membrane glycoproteins that confer adhesiveness on lymphocyte, monocyte, and granulocyte surfaces. Adhesion-dependent leukocyte functions that are vital to the protection of epithelial surfaces against microbial invasion and are involved in the normal inflammatory responses of wound healing are impaired. To date, this syndrome has been documented in 54 patients.

ETIOLOGY. This disease is defined by the defective expression of three α-β heterodimeric glycoprotein molecules unique to leukocytes called MAC-1, LFA-1, and p150,95. They share a common β subunit (95 kd, also designated CD18) but have distinctive α subunits of varying molecular weights and amino acid sequences, conferring different physicochemical properties and cell distribution. MO-1, or MAC-1 (CD11a), is a physiologically important complement receptor (CR3) that binds the iC3b component of activated complement to granulocytes and monocytes. Another site on MAC-1 is responsible for ensuring the adherence of cells to surfaces and also promotes motility, chemotaxis, and phagocytosis of complement-opsonized microbes. In contrast, LFA-1 (CD11b) is located on all lymphocytes but not on phagocytic cells, and the intercellular adhesion molecule ICAM-1 serves as one of its ligands in promoting cytotoxic T cell activity and other lymphocytic interactions with cells. The third molecule, p150,95 (CD11c), identified by monoclonal antibody LeuM5, is present on phagocytic cells and on cytotoxic and large granular lymphocytes, but its physiologic significance is unclear. The primary genetic lesion affects the common β subunit required for normal α-subunit assemblage of functionally active α-β molecules. The amino acid sequences of leukocyte adhesion receptor subunits share close homology with other receptors for extracellular matrix proteins called integrins. These include fibronectin, vitronectin, and collagen, suggesting an evolution by gene duplication from single ancestral α and β subunit genes.

EPIDEMIOLOGY. The disease has been observed in North America, Europe, North Africa, Iran, and Japan and is inherited in an autosomal recessive pattern. Family pedigrees from Hispanic, Tunisian, and English families have been described. There often is consanguinity within affected families, and asymptomatic carriers express approximately half the normal amounts of the common β subunit.

PATHOGENESIS. All signs and symptoms observed in affected patients can be related to the absence or diminished expression of adhesive glycoprotein receptors on leukocyte surfaces. The contrasting clinical picture of high blood granulocyte counts in the presence of necrotic acellular skin and soft tissue ulcers suggests defective migration of inflammatory cells from blood vessels to extravascular sites. In vivo leukocyte migration as monitored by the serial application of glass coverslips to freshly abraded skin (Rebuck skin window test) shows marked impairment of granulocyte and monocyte invasion of tissue sites. However, after granulocyte transfusion of normal cells, the skin window inflammatory response is corrected. In in vitro studies patients' phagocytic cells fail to adhere to endothelial cell monolayers or to protein-coated glass or plastic, and chemotactic stimuli do not promote increases in cellular attachment to surfaces facilitating chemotaxis. Microbes and other particles opsonized with iC3b are not phagocytized. However, LAD phagocytes are capable of both triggering a normal oxidative response that leads to microbial killing and releasing their granule constituents in response to mediators which by-pass or do not require MO-1 or CR3.

A variety of in vitro lymphocyte abnormalities dependent on normal LFA-1 expression have been observed in patients with LAD. Cytotoxic T cells, natural killer cells, and antibody-dependent cytotoxic cells are defective. Although total levels of immunoglobulin are normal, the antibody response to protein antigens such as influenza virus is blunted, but the response to polysaccharide antigens is normal. The β subunit gene has been mapped to the distal long arm of chromosome 21 (21q22.3), and studies have suggested a defect in this gene, resulting in abnormal post-translational processing of the molecule.

CLINICAL MANIFESTATIONS. Clinical expression of the disease ranging from severe to moderate correlates with the extent of deficient expression of the leukocyte adherence glycoproteins. The earliest signs occur in the neonatal period with delayed separation or infection of the umbilical cord. Surgical resection of an infected umbilicus has been needed in a few cases. Wound healing is markedly impaired. Skin and subcutaneous infections occur during early childhood. Small (<1 cm) indolent or necrotic abscesses or cellulitis may occur on any area of the body. Perirectal abscesses and lesions on the extremities leading to large ulcers with plaque formation or gangrenous bullous areas measuring between 1 and 10 cm become very difficult management problems. Puncture wounds or skin surface trauma often precipitates cellulitis and abscess formation. Surgical debridement and skin grafting may be required.

Infections of the ears, nose, and mouth are particularly prominent. Recurrent otitis media, pharyngitis, and ulcerative stomatitis are observed in almost all patients. Severe gingivitis often associated with eruption of deciduous teeth in the preschool-aged child usually progresses to generalized alveolar bone loss and severe periodontitis.

Systemic infection with life-threatening sepsis may follow episodes of perirectal abscess or other necrotizing infections of the mouth, pharynx, or intestinal tract. Recurrent bronchopneumonia as well as aseptic meningitis may occur. More than 75% of severely affected patients die before the age of 5 yr, whereas patients with a moderate phenotype are less prone to severe life-threatening infections, although more than half have died between the ages of 12 and 32 yr. Otitis, esophagitis, sinusitis, and pneumonia as well as local soft tissue infections recur in these patients. Biopsy of affected sites reveals a paucity of inflammatory cells and necrosis of tissue. This condition results from a failure of blood leukocytes, especially granulocytes and monocytes, to adhere to the vascular endothelium adjacent to the inflammatory site, inhibiting vascularization of infected tissues. As in agranulocytic patients, severe chronic gingivitis and periodontitis develop during the teenage years, leading to progressive loss of permanent dentition.

LABORATORY FINDINGS AND DIAGNOSIS. The laboratory hallmark of the disease is a persistent neutrophilia with white blood cells ranging between 15,000 and 160,000/μL, with 50–90% polymorphonuclear cells. Mild to moderate anemia parallels the extent and chronicity of the infection and inflammation. Inflammatory skin windows fail to show the expected progressive accumulation of inflammatory granulocytes and monocytes over a 24-hr period of study. In vitro studies of leukocyte functions show abnormal chemotaxis, decreased adherence to endothelial monolayers, and abnormal granulocyte aggregation but normal platelet aggregation and adherence, since platelet glycoproteins IIb/IIIa are expressed normally. Complement-coated particles (e.g., serum-treated zymosan or red cells) are not ingested, but oxidative responses (e.g., superoxide release/nitroblue tetrazolium [NBT] reduction) to the formyl-tripeptides, f-met-leu-phe, or phorbal myristate acetate (PMA) are normal. Monoclonal antibodies MO-1 or MAC-1 and LFA-1 to the leukocyte adherence glycoprotein can be employed in a flow cytometer to confirm the diagnosis by demonstrating the absence or reduction of binding of fluorescent-labeled monoclonal antibody to the leukocyte surface. LFA-1–deficient T lymphocytes have reasonably normal responses to normal concentrations of lectins (phytohemagglutinin) or antigens but impaired cytotoxicity as demonstrated by ^{51}Cr release from labeled target cells. Although no humoral deficiency has been described in most patients and serum immunoglobulin concentrations are normal to elevated, a deficiency in synthesis of specific antibody to polypeptide antigens (tetanus, influenza) but not to polysaccharide antigens (pneumococcus, *H. influenzae*) has been noted. Cultures of infected wounds and tissues yield a variety of gram-positive *(Staphylococcus aureus)* and gram-negative *(Escherichia coli, Pseudomonas* species, *Klebsiella)* bacteria or fungi (*Candida* species, *Aspergillus* species).

DIFFERENTIAL DIAGNOSIS. Patients with significant chronic and recurrent pyogenic and fungal infections usually have a disorder of phagocyte-antibody immunity. Severe forms of agranulocytosis (congenital neutropenia), deficiency of phagocyte NADPH oxidase (chronic granulomatous disease), neutrophil granule defects (specific, azurophilic, and Chédiak-Higashi syndrome [CHS]), agammaglobulinemia or other forms of hypo- and dysgammaglobulinemias, and Jobs syndrome must be considered. In general, patients with neutrophil disorders associated with chemotactic defects or in vivo inability to mount normal inflammatory responses have skin, soft tissue, mouth, and mucous membrane infections, whereas those with neutrophil bactericidal and fungicidal deficiencies experience abscess formation in subcutaneous sites, lymph nodes, lung, liver, and other abdominal viscera and bone (Table 11–7). Any patient with recurrent documented severe forms of mouth or gum infection, skin abscesses, perianal and perirectal abscesses, poor wound healing, sinopulmonary infections, or deep visceral abscesses must be considered to have a defect of phagocytic function.

The neutrophilia of LAD may be confused with (1) the reactive leukemoid reaction seen at times in collagen-vascular disorders, lung, or deep visceral abscesses, and (2) the chronic myeloproliferative disorders such as the adult form of chronic myelogenous leukemia. Patients with the latter condition usually have moderate to massive splenomegaly, an absence of leukocyte alkaline phosphatase demonstrable by special stain of a blood smear, and the presence of the Philadelphia t(9;22) chromosome. In contrast, leukemoid reactions have elevated leukocyte alkaline phosphatase scores and no leukocyte chromosomal abnormality. A source of infection or inflammation is usually demonstrable by radiologic and bacteriologic studies.

TREATMENT. Aggressive use of antibiotics for treatment of documented infections is indicated. Responses to therapy are much slower than normal. *Candida* and aspergillosis must be considered in any persistent infection not eradicated with antibiotics. Because wound healing is slow, careful attention must be paid to puncture or surgical wounds with proper local treatment and debridement. Selective use of normal granulocyte transfusions may help to eradicate acute infections but are not of value in the long-term management of these patients. Preventive dental hygiene, skin care, and attention to the perianal area often help to alleviate early signs of infection. Bone marrow transplantation has been successful in patients with severe phenotypic LAD. Eight

TABLE 11–7. Clinical and Laboratory Features of Phagocyte Disorders

Disorder	Type of Infection	WBC (μL)	Chemotaxis	O_2^- Release	Bacterial Killing
LAD*	Necrotic ulcers, no pus Skin and mucous membranes Mouth affected, gingivitis severe	50,000–100,000 60–90% PMNs‖	Decreased	Decreased—complement opsonized particles Normal—soluble (PMA, fMLP)‡	Normal
Agranulocytosis	Same	<1000 0–10% PMNs	Normal	Normal	Normal
CGD† Rare severe G-6-PD deficiency	Pustules and abscesses of soft tissue and deep viscera	10,000–20,000 60–80% PMNs	Normal	Decreased	Decreased
Neutrophil granule defects		2,000–15,000			
Myeloperoxidase deficiency	None to mild fungal infections	50–70% PMNs	Normal	Increased	Mildly decreased
Specific granule deficiency	Skin and lung abscesses		Decreased	Normal to increased	Decreased
Chédiak-Higashi syndrome	Skin and mucous membranes		Decreased	Increased	Moderately decreased
Agammaglobulinemia and related disorders	Septicemia, pneumonias	5,000–15,000 50–70% PMNs	Normal	Normal	Normal
Hyperimmunoglobulin E (Job syndrome)	Sinopulmonary Skin and subcutaneous "cold" abscesses Eczema Asthma and allergic rhinitis	5,000–15,000 20–30% eosinophils	Decreased (in some cases)	Normal	Normal

*LAD = leukocyte adhesion deficiency.
†CGD = chronic granulomatous disease.
‡PMA = phorbal myristate acetate; fMLP = f-met-leu-phe.
‖PMNs = polymorphonuclear leukocytes.

patients have received transplants, five with HLA-identical marrow. LFA-1–deficient patients seem to be able to accept HLA-partially incompatible bone marrow in a manner similar to that seen in patients with severe combined immunodeficiency (SCID) who lack T cells. Transplant candidates should be infection free and in good nutritional condition, and the procedure should be done as soon as possible after diagnosis because the early mortality in severely affected children is high.

GENETIC COUNSELING. Prenatal diagnosis of LAD is possible by obtaining fetal blood samples around 20 wk of gestation. Fetal leukocytes express leukocyte adhesion molecules, although in diminished amounts. The total absence of these adherence glycoproteins indicates the severe phenotype.

11.31 NEUTROPHIL GRANULE DEFECTS

Patients with abnormalities of the neutrophil granules either inherit or acquire them and may remain asymptomatic or experience increased susceptibility to infection. Neutrophils contain two distinct sets of granules. Peroxidase-positive azurophils and peroxidase-negative specific granules form during myeloid cell development in the bone marrow. Azurophilic granules form only during myeloblast and promyelocyte differentiation, whereas specific granules are produced during the later phases of myelocyte proliferation and maturation to the metamyelocyte and band stage. The constituents of the two sets of granules include unique bactericidal proteins, receptors, and enzymes (Table 11–8).

ETIOLOGY. Neutrophil granule defects can be separated into three phenotypic genetic disorders: (1) myeloperoxidase (MPO) deficiency of azurophilic granules, (2) specific granule deficiency (SGD), and (3) Chédiak-Higashi syndrome (CHS). Immunohistologic studies reveal the presence of a dysfunctional peroxidase protein in neutrophil and monocyte (but not eosinophil) azurophilic granules from patients with MPO deficiency. The gene, located on chromosome 17q22–23, has been cloned and sequenced. The molecular basis for the defect appears to be a pretranslational defect characterized by diminished amounts of mRNA but no gross alterations of the MPO gene. Specific granules failed to form in developing bone marrow myeloid precursors in the five unrelated patients identified with SGD. On the other hand, azurophilic granules formed normally. The molecular basis for the defect is unknown. Patients with CHS have blood neutrophils, monocytes, and lymphocytes with giant granules formed by fusion of cytoplasmic granules in bone marrow. Abnormal fusion of granules occurs in skin melanocytes, hair and retinal cells, and other cells of the central nervous system as well as in macrophages and fibroblasts of all visceral organs. The disorder is transmitted in an autosomal recessive manner and has been observed in a variety of animals.

TABLE 11–8. Contents of Neutrophil Granules

Azurophil	Specific
Bactericidal	
Peroxidase	Lysozyme
Defensins	Lactoferrin
Lysozyme	Cytochrome b
Receptors	
None identified	CR3 (iC3b)
	f-met-leu-phe
	Laminin—adherence
Acid hydrolases and neutral proteinases	
Cathepsins	Collagenase
Elastase	Plasminogen activator
	Vitamin B_{12}–binding protein

Acquired defects of granules occur in patients with refractory anemia, preleukemia, acute leukemia, and the blastic phase of chronic myelogenous leukemia. MPO and lactoferrin, constituents of azurophilic and specific granules, respectively, are diminished in some patients with acute myeloblastic leukemia and other myelodysplastic syndromes and in newborn neutrophils. Alkaline phosphatase, which is deficient in the neutrophils of patients with SGD, is either absent or diminished in the neutrophils of patients with chronic myelogenous leukemia.

PATHOGENESIS. MPO is essential for the chlorination and iodination of microbes ingested by the neutrophil. Despite a lack of peroxidation in MPO-deficient neutrophils, affected persons are generally asymptomatic, although a few patients with diabetes have experienced recurrent candidal infections. Bactericidal activity is partially compromised during the early phases of in vitro killing, but over a period of several hours effective bacterial killing is accomplished, probably by nonoxidative mechanisms. Patients with neutrophil-specific granule deficiency experience chronic recurrent skin ulcers and abscesses and lung infections, supporting the notion that the specific granule pool is probably more important for normal host defense than the azurophilic granule pool. Defensins, potent bactericidal proteins normally found in azurophilic granules, are almost completely deficient in the neutrophils of patients with SGD. Other azurophilic granule constituents, for example, cathepsin G and elastase, are normal. Conversely, neutrophils of CHS patients lack the latter two cytotoxic proteins but have a normal amount of defensins. The partial albinism, light silver-tinged hair, and extreme photophobia observed in patients with CHS are due to an abnormal dispersion of melanosomes in skin melanocytes, fibroblasts, hair roots, and retinal cells. These patients also experience recurrent infections due to functional defects of their morphologically abnormal phagocytic blood cells as well as to deficiencies of cytotoxic granule proteins.

CLINICAL MANIFESTATIONS. Hereditary MPO Deficiency. The overwhelming majority of affected persons have no obvious clinical sequelae from the deficiency. An incidence of 1 in 2,000 was found among asymptomatic persons in the United States, and a similar incidence was recorded in Western Europe. Most patients who experience severe candidiasis also have had diabetes mellitus or other compromises in host defense. Chronic mucocutaneous candidiasis is associated with neutrophils that have a normal MPO content and normal candidacidal activity.

Congenital Specific Granule Deficiency. This rare disorder is described in only five unrelated patients. A history of consanguinity was found in one patient. Clinically, all patients have recurrent infections of the skin and lung, frequently complicated by large indolent skin ulcers and repeated episodes of bronchopneumonia or lung abscesses. Also, lymphadenitis, otitis, and mastoiditis occur. The onset of infections usually occurs within the first few years of life. Both males and females have been affected, suggesting an autosomal recessive mode of inheritance. *Staphylococcus aureus* is the most frequently cultured bacterial species, but a variety of gram-negative microbes as well as *Candida albicans* have been isolated from the lesions. With careful management, these patients may survive into young adulthood.

Chédiak-Higashi Syndrome. Patients with this syndrome experience an onset of symptoms in early childhood. Presenting manifestations include photophobia, rotary nystagmus, increased red reflex, partial albinism compared with other family members, recurrent gingivitis, and periodontitis. Hair color varies from blond to dark brown but has a silvery tint that is especially noticeable in bright light. Infections involve the skin, mucous membranes, and respiratory tract and are recurrent. Gram-positive and gram-negative bacteria may be cultured from sites of infection, *S. aureus* and β-hemolytic streptococci being the most frequent causes of infection. Affected patients also have prolonged bleeding times with normal platelet counts due to a platelet aggregation defect that is related to storage pool deficiency of ADP and serotonin. If patients survive into adulthood, they develop motor and sensory neurologic defects including cranial and peripheral neuropathy. Ataxia, muscular weakness, decreased motor neuron conduction, diffuse abnormalities in electroencephalograms, and seizures may also occur. Affected patients may die at any age owing to the so-called accelerated phase of the illness, which occurs in 85% of patients. The precipitating event initiating this lethal stage may be related to infection with EBV or other lymphotrophic viruses resulting in a lymphoma-like picture with fever, widespread enlargement of lymph nodes, hepatosplenomegaly, and pancytopenia. Sepsis is frequent at this stage of the illness.

LABORATORY FINDINGS AND DIAGNOSIS. Routine complete blood count may fail to suggest a neutrophil granule defect unless particular attention is paid to the Wright stained differential. SGD is characterized by bilobed nuclei in more than 80% of the neutrophils, resembling the Pelger-Huet anomaly. The latter defect is not associated with clinical symptoms or significant functional phagocytic defects. Moreover, in SGD there is a striking decrease in cytoplasmic granularity owing to a lack of specific granules. Leukocyte alkaline phosphatase and peroxidase cytochemical stains confirm the absence of alkaline phosphatase and the presence of azurophilic granule peroxidase. Lactoferrin, another constituent of specific granules, is also absent when appropriate immunocytochemistry is employed. On the other hand, patients with hereditary or acquired myeloperoxidase deficiency have either a total or partial deficiency of peroxidase activity, but alkaline phosphatase stains are normal. Occasionally, patients with CHS are discovered because giant granules are noted on routine Wright stained differential counts. The granules are larger and less symmetric than the prominently stained toxic granules or Döhle bodies noted frequently in neutrophils of patients with infection. They result from the progressive coalescence of azurophilic and specific granules formed during myelopoiesis. Moderate neutropenia due to intramedullary destruction of myeloid cells is often noted early in the course of the disease and may contribute to the increased susceptibility to infection.

Phagocytic function is abnormal in all three granule disorders (see Table 11–7). MPO-deficient PMNs show only minor defects in the killing of *S. aureus*, whereas killing of *C. albicans* is much more impaired. The abnormal neutrophil chemotactic response of SGD is associated with impaired up-regulation of receptors for the chemoattractant f-met-leu-phe and the adherence receptor iC3b. The absence of the specific granule component cytochrome b may explain the impaired superoxide (O_2^-) release and contribute, along with lack of defensins and lactoferrin, to the impairment in bactericidal killing. CHS patients have abnormal chemotaxis, and killing is reduced because of delayed fusion of the abnormal granules with phagosomes containing ingested microbes. iC3b receptor expression is markedly reduced, a fact that probably plays an additional role in reduced motility, chemotaxis, and bactericidal activity. The cells have an increased release of superoxide (O_2^-) similar to that seen in MPO-deficient neutrophils. In addition, CHS patients have platelet aggregation defects owing to a lack of a storage pool of ADP and a prolonged bleeding time. Lymphocytes contain giant granules and function poorly in tests of antibody-dependent tumor cell lysis and natural killer cell activity.

The accelerated phase of CHS is associated with seroconversion and an abnormal antibody response to *Epstein-Barr virus*. Antibodies to viral capsid antigen and the early antigen reach high levels and persist, supporting the notion of a sustained viral infection.

DIFFERENTIAL DIAGNOSIS. The same disorders mentioned in Sec. 11.30 for any patient with significant chronic and recurrent pyogenic and fungal infections must be considered.

TREATMENT. No therapy is generally required for patients with MPO deficiency. Treatment of patients with SGD is similar to that given to other patients with a functional phagocytic defect (see Sec. 11.30). With proper use of intravenous antibiotics and drainage of abscesses, these patients may live into adulthood. Therapy for the stable phase of CHS involves the proper management of infections. Ascorbic acid has improved the clinical status and phagocytic function of some patients. Although antibiotics are valuable during acute infections, their prophylactic use has not been proved effective in patients with CHS. Corticosteroids, vincristine, and cyclophosphamide have been employed for control of the accelerated phase and have partially arrested the infiltrative process but have not been effective in arresting the progression of disease. However, acyclovir 500 mg/m^2 three times daily combined with prednisone 2 mg/kg/24 hr has provided temporary improvement in fever, pancytopenia, and coagulopathy in patients with this fatal disorder. Bone marrow transplantation has been successful in four of five patients who received HLA-compatible marrow early in their illness before the full-blown accelerated phase occurred. Mismatched transplants have not been successful.

GENETIC COUNSELING. Neutrophil granule defects include conditions of clinical diversity ranging from the asymptomatic MPO deficiency to the fatal accelerated phase of CHS. Counseling requires a knowledge of the varied clinical courses of these diseases, all inherited as autosomal recessive traits. Prenatal diagnosis of CHS is possible by examining neutrophil granules in fetal blood.

11.32 CHRONIC GRANULOMATOUS DISEASE

CGD is the most common of the inherited disorders of phagocyte function.

ETIOLOGY. The pivotal role of the respiratory burst (which follows within seconds after phagocytes are activated) in the subsequent effective killing of catalase-positive microbes became evident from studies of patients with CGD. The NADPH oxidase that catalyzes the respiratory burst is found exclusively in phagocytes and remains dormant unless activated by a variety of particulate and soluble stimuli, such as opsonized microbes and chemotactic peptides. These stimuli excite a transmembrane electron transport system in which NADPH on the cytoplasmic side of the membrane reduces oxygen through a series of reactions involving flavin adenine dinucleotide (FAD), several soluble cofactors, and membrane-associated cytochrome b. Oxygen is reduced through a univalent reduction to superoxide anion and is rapidly mutated to hydrogen perioxide and hydroxyl radicals. The latter two products are thought to be the principal means by which microbial killing or tissue damage takes place. The components of the phagocyte NADPH oxidase complex are presented in Figure 11–2. The membrane components, a hemoprotein heterodimer with subunits of 91 kd and 22 kd, require at least two cytosolic protein components of 47 kd and 67 kd to achieve maximal oxidase activity. The X-linked and autosomally inherited forms of the disease are associated with missing components or subunits (Table 11–9). The CGD gene is located on the X chromosome proximal to the muscular

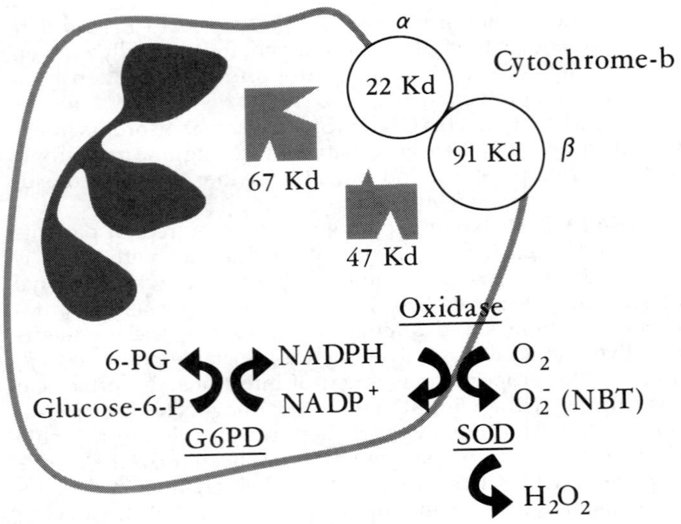

Figure 11–2. The human neutrophil NADPH oxidase complex consists of two cytochrome b membrane subunits, an α (22 kd) subunit and β (91 kd) subunit, and two cytosolic cofactors, (67 kd) and (47 kd), required for the respiratory burst. NADPH serves as substrate for reduction of oxygen to superoxide O_2, which, in turn, is rapidly dismutated either spontaneously or by superoxide dismutase (SOD) to hydrogen peroxide (H_2O_2). Superoxide is measured by the reduction of nitroblue tetrazolium (NBT). NADPH is generated from glucose-6-phosphate through the hexose monophosphate shunt by glucose-6-phosphate dehydrogenase (G-6-PD).

dystrophy gene and distal to the ornithine transcarbamylase gene on the Xp21 band. The protein encoded by the X-CGD gene is synonymous with the 91-kd subunit of the cytochrome b complex. A reservoir of cytochrome b (~ 80–90%) is found in neutrophil-specific granules and is translocated to the membrane on activation of the cell. The 22-kd membrane subunit also has been cloned.

PATHOLOGY. Characteristic granulomas, along with phagocytes, giant cells, and occasional pigmented lipid-laden histiocytes, may develop in any organ system. The lung, skin, lymph nodes, liver, spleen, and bone may be affected with abscesses or granulomas. It is likely that the fundamental defect of oxidase activation of phagocytes results in a chronic and persistent inflammatory reaction within tissues owing to seeding with viable microbes.

CLINICAL MANIFESTATIONS. Most patients develop signs and symptoms of chronic and recurrent pyogenic infections during the first 2 yr of life. Milder forms of the disease have been described with onset occurring in the teenage years or even in adulthood. Lymphadenopathy occurs in almost all cases. A common presentation is recurrent enlargement of the lymph nodes of the neck, which require incision and drainage. Hepatomegaly and splenomegaly occur later and often signify hepatic or perihepatic abscesses or granuloma formation. Chronic or recurrent pneumonia with unusual microbes, for example, *Serratia marcescens*, occurs frequently. Subcutaneous abscesses, recurrent skin furunculosis, eczematoid dermatitis, and impetigo around orifices may be presenting manifestations involving the integumentary system. Granuloma formation may lead to obstruction of the esophageal outlet, pyloris, or urethra. A history of persistent diarrhea may indicate granulomatous colitis. Perianal abscesses or rectal fistulous tracts may occur. Osteomyelitis at multiple sites or in the small bones of the hands and feet are also frequently encountered. Mucous membrane infections are less common than in patients with chemotactic disorders, but conjunctivitis, rhinitis, and stomatitis have occurred in these patients.

LABORATORY FINDINGS AND DIAGNOSIS. The neutrophils of patients with CGD demonstrate normal chemotaxis, phagocytosis, and degranulation, but they do not generate superoxide anion, nor do they kill catalase-positive microbes. Cultures from infected sites will isolate *S. aureus, Klebsiella, Aerobacter, E. coli, Shigella, Salmonella, Pseudomona, Serratia marcescens, C. albicans,* and *Aspergillus* and other fungi. Common catalase-negative peroxide-producing organisms such as *Streptococcus,* and *Haemophilus influenzae* are not isolated because the fundamental bactericidal defect in CGD is an absence of hydrogen peroxide and related reduced oxygen byproducts in the phagocytic vesicle. Bactericidal assays in vitro confirm the selective but significant defect in bacterial killing. The reduction of nitroblue tetrazolium (NBT) remains a convenient method of screening for adequate superoxide anion (O_2^-) during phagocytic activation and of detecting CGD. Quantitation of rates of superoxide generation is best carried out by using the ferricytochrome reduction method. Although most patients with CGD fail to generate superoxide, mutations of both X-linked and autosomal forms result in milder forms of the disease in which some superoxide or NBT is formed under appropriate conditions of activation of the cells.

In carriers of the X-linked form of the disease approximately half of the neutrophils are affected, whereas the other half can reduce NBT normally. This is consistent with the Lyon hypothesis (Sec. 7.24). Most female carriers are healthy and do not suffer recurrent infections. A few have had lupus-like skin lesions with photosensitivity, pleuritis, and stomatitis. The parents of children with autosomal recessive forms of CGD have normal results on NBT tests.

CBC shows appropriate neutrophilic leukocytosis during infections. Anemia of chronic infection correlates with the extent of inflammation. Sedimentation rates are usually elevated. Immunoglobulins are normal to increased. Abnormal chest roentgenograms occur in 90% of patients. Liver-spleen scans and bone scans are helpful in documenting the presence of liver abscesses and osteomyelitis, respectively. Ultrasound, endoscopy, and contrast studies usually verify suspected gastric antral obstructions. Cystourethrograms reveal granulomatous involvement of the bladder in some cases.

DIFFERENTIAL DIAGNOSIS. Because of the potential for widespread sites of infection in CGD, this entity must be considered in any child with unexplained recurrent cervical lymphadenitis, bacterial hepatic abscesses, or osteomyelitis as the basis for the primary infection. Lung abscesses or granulomas may at times be confused with tuberculosis or other fungal diseases such as histoplasmosis and coccidioidomycosis. All of the disorders discussed under Differential Diagnosis in Sec. 11.30 should also be considered. Investigations of the phagocytic functions of chemotaxis, superoxide anion release (NBT test), bacterial killing, quantitative serum immunoglob-

TABLE 11–9. Classification and Incidence of CGD Based on Molecular Defects of Neutrophil

Genetics	Incidence %	Cytochrome b	Defect
X-linked	50–55	Absent	Expression of cytochrome b 91kd subunit
	5	Present	Function of cytochrome b
Autosomal	30–35	Present	47kd cytosolic factor absent
	5	Present	67kd cytosolic factor absent
	5	Absent	? Expression of cytochrome b 22kd subunit

ulins, and complement levels should permit differentiation of this group of disorders.

TREATMENT. Although its results are still not proved, long-term trimethoprim-sulfamethoxasole (TMP-SMZ) prophylaxis appears to increase the duration of infection-free periods. One small series showed significant benefits in reducing clinical manifestations and decreasing the number of isolates causing infection when TMP-SMZ was instituted during early childhood before chronic foci of infection had developed fully. Acute episodes of infection should be managed aggressively by isolating the causative microbe, instituting appropriate intravenous antibiotics, and using short-term (average 1 wk) granulocyte transfusions selectively to achieve control of persistent infections, especially those with gram-negative bacteria. Gastric outlet obstruction and granulomatous cystitis have been successfully managed with prolonged antimicrobial therapy and prednisone.

Based on in vitro studies, which showed the ability of γ-interferon to increase the generation of superoxide anion modestly (between 1 and 10%) in the neutrophils of patients with milder CGD, in vivo treatment of these same patients with γ-interferon was associated with similar improvement in superoxide anion release by neutrophils isolated during treatment. Improved in vivo responses also were observed in a few patients with negative in vitro responses. A large multicenter study showed that γ-interferon administered subcutaneously in a dose of 0.05 mg/m^2 3 times per wk reduced the number of new infections and improved the response to existing infections.

Serious transfusion reactions have occurred in patients with CGD who lack Kell-associated red blood cell antigens, the so-called McLeod phenotype. Prior to transfusion, patients with CGD should be tested for the presence of the Kell antigen.

Bone marrow transplantation has been carried out in several patients with limited success. Graft rejection and partial engraftment have occurred. Attempts to provide somatic gene therapy employing gene transfer of the X-CGD cDNA are in progress.

GENETIC COUNSELING. Cord blood and placental blood obtained by fetoscopy have established the diagnosis of CGD using the NBT slide test. Several molecular DNA probes (Pert 84 and p754), which are capable of detecting a relatively high proportion of polymorphisms in genomic DNA and are closely linked to the X-CGD gene, may be useful in identifying an at-risk male fetus using chorionic villus biopsy. Linkage analysis requires DNA samples from three generations and restriction fragment length polymorphism of maternal DNA and maternal parent DNA. In addition, the carrier status must be identified either by NBT testing or by obtaining a history of affected offspring. Probes recognizing DNA polymorphisms in the X-CGD gene offer the most promise for improving the results of prenatal diagnosis, but these have not yet been identified.

11.33 DISORDERS OF NEUTROPHIL OXIDATIVE METABOLISM OTHER THAN CGD

SEVERE GLUCOSE-6-PHOSPHATE DEHYDROGENASE DEFICIENCY (G-6-PD). Several patients with Caucasian forms of red blood cell G-6-PD deficiency have had neutrophils with less than 5% G-6-PD activity. When activity is approximately 1%, NADPH, the substrate for the oxidase reaction, becomes rate limiting, leading to a clinical phenotype resembling CGD (see Fig. 11–2). Superoxide anion is not generated during neutrophil activation, resulting in a failure of these phagocytes to reduce NBT. G-6-PD activity of 5% results in abnormal results of in vitro tests of NBT and bacterial killing but does not usually cause clinical disease. American blacks with red blood cell G-6-PD deficiency have normal levels of the enzyme in their neutrophils.

GLUTATHIONE REDUCTASE DEFICIENCY. This flavin enzyme catalyzes the reaction of NADPH and oxidized glutathione (GSSG), and deficiencies result in hemolytic anemia. Although these children do not have infections, the respiratory burst in their neutrophils may be abbreviated when activated.

GLUTATHIONE SYNTHETASE DEFICIENCY. The synthesis of glutathione, a potent antioxidant found in high concentrations in most body cells including leukocytes, occurs in two steps: (1) glutamine and cysteine, by the action of γ-glutamyl cysteine synthetase, form glutamyl-cysteine, and (2) glycine is added by the action of glutathione synthetase to form glutathione. Absence of the latter enzyme resulted in hemolytic anemia, recurrent otitis, and an in vitro abnormality in bacterial killing in a child with this very rare defect.

HYPERIMMUNOGLOBULIN E (JOB SYNDROME). This rare disorder is characterized by extremely high serum IgE levels and recurrent serious infections of the skin and sinopulmonary tract and chronic eczema with onset in the first 8 wk of life. The infections result in deep-seated abscesses in subcutaneous tissue. Pneumonia, osteomyelitis, arthritis, and visceral abscesses may occur. Associated clinical features include allergic rhinitis, coarse facies, keratoconjunctivitis, asthma, and stunted growth. The most common organisms recovered from the abscesses are *Staphylococcus aureus* and *C. albicans*, but *H. influenzae, Streptococcus pneumoniae*, enteric gram-negative bacteria, and herpesvirus also cause infection. Laboratory studies reveal marked eosinophilia, extreme elevation of serum IgE with specificity against *S. aureus* and *C. albicans* and immune complexes containing IgE, variable chemotactic defects of neutrophils and monocytes, and absent delayed hypersensitivity on skin tests to recall antigens in vivo coupled with absent in vitro lymphocyte proliferation in response to the same antigens.

It is surmised that elevated IgE levels result from a deficiency of suppressor T cells, thereby permitting overactive T helper cells to boost IgE production. The chemotactic defect may be due to secretion of chemotactic inhibitor substances from mononuclear cells. Recurrent infection may be due to excessive amounts of nonprotective IgE directed against *S. aureus* and other infectious organisms with a concurrent inadequate synthesis of protective IgG antibody against the same organisms.

Treatment should be aggressive. Intravenous gamma globulin prophylaxis may be helpful. Abscesses should be drained surgically, and intravenous antibiotics or antifungal or antiviral agents employed based on results of cultures.

NEWBORN DYSFUNCTION OF NEUTROPHILS. Several clinical observations can be correlated with selective areas of dysfunction of newborn neutrophils: (1) the high incidence of sepsis and meningitis, particularly the poor outcome associated with severe neutropenia and depletion of marrow reserves of neutrophils, (2) the paucity of neutrophils in the alveoli of newborns dying of pneumonia, and (3) the common occurrence of skin infections with *S. aureus* and *C. albicans* in neonatal intensive care units. One of the most consistent abnormalities observed is decreased leukocyte migration, as measured by the Rebuck skin window and response to chemotactic stimuli. Motile responses of phagocytic cells depend in part on the deformability of the cell membrane and the ability of the cell to increase its adherence to endothelial cells and other surfaces in response to chemotactic signals. These are defective in newborns. The impaired movement of lectin receptors or adhesion sites on newborn neutrophil surface membranes and the impaired translocation of C3 receptors from specific granules to surface membranes probably contribute to the newborn neutrophil chemotactic defect. Bactericidal activity in neutrophils from stressed newborns is also diminished even though the respiratory burst and the ability of those cells to generate superoxide and hydrogen peroxide is preserved. The diminished content of azurophilic myeloperoxidase and specific granule contents such as lactoferrin may contribute to the dysfunction.

The administration of adult donor neutrophil transfusions for treatment of neonatal sepsis is still controversial (see Sec. 9.60). The recent observations that recombinant human GM-CSF and G-CSF stimulate neutrophil/monocyte and neutrophil marrow production, respectively; facilitate release of neutrophils from the marrow; prime the chemotactic (C3) receptor expression of the respiratory burst; and stimulate phagocytic responses in adult cells suggest that these compounds may be promising future therapies for the newborn.

ROBERT L. BAEHNER

Anderson DC: Neonatal neutrophil dysfunction. Am J Pediatr Hematol Oncol 11:224, 1989.

Anderson DC, Schmalsteig FC, Finegold MJ, et al: The severe and moderate phenotypes of heritable MAC-1, LFA-1 deficiency: Their quantitative definition and relation to leukocyte dysfunction and clinical features. J Infect Dis 152:668, 1985.

Barak Y, Nir E: Chédiak-Higashi syndrome. Am J Pediatr Hematol Oncol 9:42, 1987.

Boxer LA, Smolen JE: Neutrophil granule constituents and their release in health and disease. Hematol Oncol Clin North Am 2:101, 1988.

Cairo MS: Neutrophil transfusions in the treatment of neonatal sepsis. Review of G-CSF and GM-CSF effects on neonatal neutrophil kinetics. Am J Pediatr Hematol Oncol 11:227, 1989.

Christensen RD: Neutrophil kinetics in the fetus and neonate. Am J Pediatr Hematol Oncol 11:215, 1989.

Dana N, Clayton LK, Tennen DG: Leukocytes from four patients with complete or partial leu-CAM deficiency contain the common beta-subunit precursor and beta-subunit messenger RNA. J Clin Invest 79:1010, 1987.

Fischer A, Lisowska-Grospierre B, Anderson DC, et al: Leukocyte adhesion deficiency: Molecular basis and functional consequences. Immunodefic Rev 1:39, 1988.

Gallin JI: Neutrophil specific granule deficiency. Annu Rev Med 36:263, 1985.

Gallin JI, Goldstein IM, Snyderman R: Inflammation, Basic Principles and Clinical Correlates. New York, Raven Press, 1988.

Ganz T, Metcalf JA, Gallin JI, et al: Microbicidal cytotoxic proteins of neutrophils are deficient in two disorders: Chediak-Higashi syndrome and "specific" granule deficiency. J Clin Invest 82:552, 1988.

Hill HR: Biochemical, structural, and functional abnormalities of polymorphonuclear leukocyte in the neonate. Pediatr Res 22:375, 1987.

Nauseef WM: Myeloperoxidase deficiency. Hematol Oncol Clin North Am 2:135, 1988.

Parry MF, Root RK, Metcalf JA, et al: Myeloperoxidase deficiency: Prevalence and clinical significance. Ann Intern Med 95:293, 1981.

The International Chronic Granulomatous Disease Cooperative Study Group: A controlled trial of interferon gamma granulomatous disease. N Engl J Med 324:509, 1991.

ALLERGIC DISORDERS

Allergy is a specific, acquired change in host reactivity mediated by an immunologic mechanism and causing an untoward physiologic response. This definition precludes the use of the term allergy for disorders in which immunologic mechanisms have not been demonstrated. For example, adverse reactions following food or drug ingestion in some people may resemble typical allergic reactions, without any evidence of an immunologic basis. Sometimes there is a biochemical basis for the reaction, as in diarrhea following milk ingestion in people with disaccharidase deficiency. When there is no reason to suspect that allergy is responsible for signs or symptoms, the use of immunologic methods in diagnosis or treatment is irrational.

The terms antigen and allergen are often used interchangeably, but not all antigens are good allergens and vice versa. For example, tetanus and diphtheria toxoids are highly antigenic but are only rarely responsible for adverse reactions. On the other hand, ragweed pollen protein, one of the most potent allergens, is not a particularly potent antigen by immunologic criteria. Most naturally occurring allergens share several common characteristics. They are protein in part, are acidic with isoelectric points of 2–5.5, and have molecular weights of 10,000–70,000 daltons. Molecules smaller than 10,000 daltons would be unable to bridge the gap between adjacent IgE antibody molecules on the surface of mast cells, a requirement for release of the mediators of the allergic reaction. Molecules larger than 70,000 daltons would not easily pass through mucosal surfaces to reach IgE-forming plasma cells.

The use of the term *atopy* or *atopic* in designating an allergic reaction implies a hereditary factor expressed as susceptibility to hay fever, asthma, and eczematoid dermatitis in the families of affected individuals. The atopic patient has a predisposition to selective synthesis of IgE antibodies to common environmental antigens. IgE production is under genetic control, and there appears to be an association between HLA histocompatibility types and IgE-mediated hypersensitivity responses. In experimental models, the IgE antibody response is regulated by antigen-specific helper and suppressor T cells that secrete IgE-binding factors that potentiate or suppress the reaction. Atopic individuals may differ from nonatopic individuals in their ability to regulate IgE antibody production or to dispose of allergens coming in contact with mucosal surfaces. They may also have defective control of mediator release or generation, or have impaired mediator inactivation processes.

The formation of IgE antibodies is revealed in atopic persons by "wheal and flare" reactions on skin testing with allergenic extracts. However, the capacity to form IgE antibody is not limited to atopic individuals because IgE is found in the serum and on mast cells of virtually all normal people. Under intense allergen exposure, as in certain occupations, or in response to particular allergens, such as Ascaris, nonatopic individuals may form large quantities of allergen-specific IgE antibodies. Atopic people, however, form IgE antibodies on exposure to such common environmental substances as pollens and components of house dust, and this distinguishes them from the nonatopic. Among patients with asthma, hay fever, or eczema we can identify "highly atopic" subjects and others with lesser atopic tendencies.

11.34 IMMUNOLOGIC BASIS OF ATOPIC DISEASE

It is useful to characterize immunologic reactions in terms of the reactants involved in order to understand the mechanism by which injury occurs (Gell and Coombs classification). Immunologically mediated tissue injury may occur as a result of the interaction of humoral antibody with antigen or of the interaction of antigen with lymphocytes (cell-mediated or delayed-type hypersensitivity). There are three forms of humoral antibody-antigen reactions, two of which occur on the surface of cells and the third in the extracellular fluids.

Of the two reactions occurring on the surface of the cells, *type I hypersensitivity, mediated by IgE* (immediate type or anaphylactic hypersensitivity), is of greatest interest to the allergist. In this circumstance, circulating basophils and tissue mast cells, the latter strategically located around blood vessels, become "sensitized" through the binding of IgE antibodies to their surface receptors. This is the initial event in the production of immune tissue injury following allergen interaction with cell-bound IgE antibody molecules; the ultimate outcome of the reaction depends on a broad spectrum of secondary events involving various types of lymphoid cells, inflammatory cells, mediator-producing cells, and the soluble products derived not only from all of these cells but from other tissues (platelets, endothelial cells) at the site of the reaction. For example, in particularly intense allergen-induced reactions in the skin, the initial wheal and flare does not entirely disappear but is replaced by an inflammatory lesion that reaches its maximal size at 6–12 hr and disappears in 24–72 hr. This late cutaneous response depends upon recruitment of inflammatory cells (polymorphonuclear leukocytes, eosinophils, and mononuclear cells) by chemotactic factors released in the early response. Late-phase reactions also occur in the lung.

The terms *reaginic IgE, IgE reagins,* and *homocytotropic antibodies* refer to molecules with activities against specific allergens, such as ragweed pollen, whereas "nonspecific" IgE molecules are found in the serum and tissues of all normal individuals. The "normal" role of IgE antibody appears to be to defend the host against tissue-invasive parasites. In man the ability to induce antigen-specific release of mediators from mast cells and basophils is principally confined to antibodies of the IgE class.

IgE antibodies, like IgA antibodies, are synthesized by plasma cells located predominantly under mucosal surfaces and particularly in the respiratory and gastrointestinal tracts. IgE-forming plasma cells arise following antigen-stimulated differentiation of B cells or their precursors.

Chemical modifications of antigens used in immunotherapy of allergic diseases suppress IgE responses (Sec. 11.39). While the control of IgE antibody production is better known for animals than for man, there is good reason to believe that similar mechanisms occur in the human. The association of IgE responses with HLA-linked immune response (Ir) genes has been shown for several allergens (ragweed antigen Ra3 and HLA-A2, ragween antigen Ra5 and HLA-B7, rye grass antigen I and HLA-B8). IgE synthesis in general, and specifically hypersensitivity, is genetically determined by immune cells, probably the specific helper T cells. Bone marrow transplantation from an atopic donor to a nonatopic recipient transfers the allergic diathesis to the recipient. Helper T cells produce interleukin 4 (IL-4), which, in the presence of B cell activators (e.g., T cell cognate interaction), induces the synthesis of IgE, possibly by isotype switching of precursor B cells into IgE-synthesizing cells. Increased access of the E switch to a common recombinase may be the mechanism for the isotype switch. For optimal IgE synthesis, IL-5 (a nonisotype B cell growth factor) and IL-6 (a nonisotype B cell differentiation factor) are also needed. IL-5 also induces eosinophil differentiation. Gamma interferon, produced by another subset of T lymphocytes, can inhibit IL-4–dependent IgE synthesis and IL-4–induced expression of low-affinity IgE receptors (CD_{23}) on B cells.

Once formed, IgE antibody becomes reversibly bound or "fixed" to surface receptors of mast cells and basophils. The binding of IgE to its receptor (Fc_ER) involves the C4 and C3 domains of the Fc portion of the immunoglobulin molecule. In nonatopic individuals, only 20–50% of the receptors are occupied by IgE molecules. In atopic individuals with high serum IgE concentrations a larger percentage, up to almost 100%, of their basophil and mast cell receptors is occupied by IgE. Once binding of IgE occurs, the basophils and mast cells are "sensitized." Upon subsequent contact with this specific allergen, and if cell-bound IgE molecules are sufficiently numerous, allergen may bridge adjacent IgE molecules, causing an interaction between the IgE receptors. This causes a series of biochemical reactions (activation of methyltransferases, phospholipid methylation, Ca^{2+} influx, and activation of the phospholipid diacylglycerol cycle). This results in fusion of the mast cell granules with the mast cell plasma membrane, resulting in release of pharmacologically active substances (such as histamine), known as chemical mediators. The released mediators act on tissue receptors to cause symptoms in the patient. The reaction is largely reversible; the mast cells and basophils participating in the reaction are not lysed, and the effects of mediators are only temporary. Though aggregated IgE can fix late components of the complement system through an alternative pathway, participation of the complement system in IgE-mediated hypersensitivity disorders has not been shown. Newly synthesized chemical mediators are released by the mast cell 6–8 hr after antigenic stimulation. Thus, the late-phase reaction may last 12–48 hr.

The usual tests for inhalant or food sensitivity make use of the reaction that occurs on the surface of mast cells between antigen and IgE antibody. Small amounts of extracts of pollens, molds, danders, and foods are introduced into the patient's skin by scratch, puncture, or intradermal techniques. If IgE antibody specific for the test antigen is bound to the subject's mast cells, the interaction of injected antigen with cell-bound IgE releases histamine, a potent vasoactive agent that causes increased capillary permeability and dilatation and axon reflex stimulation, leading to the familiar wheal and flare reaction. The prototypic *anaphylactic* or *IgE-mediated* disease is ragweed hay fever. Others include anaphylactic reactions to insect venom, food-induced urticaria, and allergic conjunctivitis or rhinitis.

In *type II hypersensitivity (cytotoxic) interactions* between antigen and antibody at cell surfaces, IgG or IgM immunoglobulins react with antigenic determinants* that either are integral parts of the cell membrane or have become adsorbed to or incorporated into the membrane. In contrast to the IgE or anaphylactic type of reaction, this second kind of reaction activates the complement system in most instances, and the involved cell is destroyed. An example of this type of immunologic injury occurs after transfusion of incompatible red blood cells. The recipient's isohemagglutinins (antibodies directed against determinants on the surface of the red cells) react with the incompatible cells, the complement system is activated, and sequential action of complement proteins leads to lysis of the cell. Analogous immune injury may involve platelets or leukocytes. In the case of drug-induced immune hemolytic anemias, various other mechanisms are also involved ("innocent bystander," drug adsorption).

The *type III immunopathologic mechanism* (Arthus or immune-complex) of tissue injury involving humoral antibody and antigen occurs in the extracellular spaces. At certain ratios of antigen to antibody, antigen-antibody complexes are formed that are "toxic" to tissues in which they are deposited. For example, complexes may lodge in the filtering organs of the body (such as the kidney or lung) or infiltrate the walls of small blood vessels, activating the complement cascade. There is release of biologically active substances, including factors that are chemotactic for polymorphonuclear (PMN) leukocytes, which are attracted to the site. With phagocytosis of the complexes, the polymorphonuclear leukocytes are lysed, and basic proteins and proteolytic enzymes are released that

*An antigenic determinant or epitope is a restricted portion of an antigen molecule that determines the specificity of an antigen-antibody reaction. Antigenic determinants may consist of only four or five amino acid residues. In complex antigens found in nature, such as pollens, there may be several hundred determinants on the surface of an antigen molecule, each capable of initiating immune responses and reacting with specific antibody.

damage tissue. Immune complex disease is responsible for up to 90% of immunologic glomerulonephritis in humans.

Toxic complex injury involves cooperation between different antibodies in the production of tissue injury. The deposition of immune complexes containing IgG1, IgG2, IgG3, and IgM in small blood vessels in the kidney in experimental serum sickness in animals depends on an increase in the permeability of these vessels. This is brought about by histamine liberated in the course of a simultaneous interaction of IgE antibody and antigen, which leads to "leakiness" of the capillaries and prepares them to receive the toxic complexes. Such deposition can be largely prevented by pretreatment with antihistamine drugs in the animal model. Examples of type III reactions include serum sickness and immune complex pericarditis or arthritis following meningococcal or *Haemophilus influenzae* infection.

In *type IV, cell-mediated* or *delayed-type hypersensitivity* pathologic changes follow interaction of antigen with specifically sensitized, thymus-derived T lymphocytes. The basis for the tissue injury in classic cell-mediated immune reactions is not completely understood, but it is clear that macrophages and cytotoxic cells play major roles. Contact allergy (poison ivy, chemical-induced contact dermatitis) is the prototype of allergic disease mediated by delayed-type hypersensitivity. Drug reactions with involvement of liver, lung, and kidney may be further examples of T cell-mediated disease. Cell-mediated immunity is involved in certain infiltrative hypersensitivity lung diseases in which granuloma formation is a pathologic feature. Tuberculin reactivity, graft-versus-host disease, and tissue transplant reaction are additional type IV hypersensitivity reactions.

11.35 CHEMICAL MEDIATORS OF ALLERGIC REACTIONS AND MECHANISMS OF RELEASE

Mast cells play the central role in immediate hypersensitivity responses. Considerable heterogeneity probably exists among populations of mast cells and basophils in the human; differences among these metachromatically staining cells can be measured by morphologic, immunologic, biochemical, and functional criteria. Mast cells and basophils are involved not only in IgE-mediated reactions but also in other chronic inflammatory disorders, for example, inflammatory bowel disease, rheumatoid arthritis, and parasitic infections.

The critical triggering event in mast cell degranulation and release of chemical mediators of allergic injury is the cross-linking of receptor-bound IgE antibodies (which may be viewed as an extension of the receptor) by multivalent specific antigen. Although antigen is usually the principal factor in causing the approximation of IgE receptors, this can be accomplished in the absence of antigen or even of IgE antibody, for example, by the action of purified antibody to the IgE receptor itself. Other stimuli can also cause mast cell activation without involving antigen and cell-bound IgE. These stimuli include products of activation of the complement system (C3a, C5a), kinins, neutrophil-derived lysosomal basic proteins, and lymphokines.

Whatever the nature of the mast cell surface signal that acts as the degranulation stimulus, a series of biochemical reactions takes place that results in granule discharge. Activation of a serine esterase, utilization of intracellular energy stores, calcium influx or remobilization of intracellular calcium, and changes in the mast cell cytoskeleton such as polymerization of microtubules occur during mediator release. Changes in membrane phospholipid metabolism also occur, including methylation and activation of phospholipases and generation of phospholipid by-products, which participate in the fusion of the mast cell granules with the cell membrane, leading to extrusion of the granules. Once discharged from the mast cell, the granules, which are relatively water insoluble, may remain intact for hours. The preformed mediators, such as histamine, eosinophil chemotactic factor (ECF-A), and other chemotactic factors, are rapidly eluted from the granule matrix and act immediately on local tissues—smooth muscles and endothelial cells in blood vessels. Another set of mediators, which are preformed but granule associated (e.g., heparin, arylsulfatase B, enzymes such as trypsin and chymotrypsin, and inflammatory factors) may be involved in the immediate and late-phase reactions; these mediators express their activity either while they are still part of the intact granule or only after the granule begins to dissolve.

Bridging of adjacent, cell-bound IgE molecules also causes liberation of arachidonic acid from membrane phospholipids, either directly by action of phospholipase A_2 or indirectly by sequential actions of phospholipase C and diglyceride lipase. Metabolism of arachidonic acid by the lipoxygenase pathway leads to the new formation of 5-hydroxyeicosatetraenoic acid (5-HETE) and the leukotriene B_4, C_4, D_4, and E_4. Metabolism of arachidonic acid by the cyclooxygenase pathway results in new formation of the various prostaglandins and thromboxanes. Prostaglandin D_2 (PGD_2) is the chief prostaglandin product of mast cells. Other cells also generate prostaglandins and leukotrienes, which have various actions (Table 11–10).

Increases in intracellular concentrations of cyclic adenosine monophosphate (cAMP) are associated with inhibition of release of mediators from mast cells. Prostaglandins of the E series and β-adrenergic agonists can cause increases in cAMP.

Factors Not Mast Cell-Derived That Participate in Immediate-Type Hypersensitivity Diseases

Eosinophil-derived molecules of potent biologic activity may contribute to tissue injury in IgE-mediated and other diseases. *Eosinophil major basic protein* (MBP) causes dose-dependent epithelial damage in guinea pig trachea and in human bronchial epithelium. Immunofluorescent staining discloses extracellular deposition of MBP in areas of airway epithelial destruction in patients who have died of status asthmaticus. If MBP causes destruction of airway epithelium, it may play a role in the bronchial hyperresponsiveness characteristic of asthma. Deposition of MBP is also demonstrable in lesions of atopic dermatitis and often in those of chronic urticaria. MBP also stimulates histamine release from human basophils and causes a wheal and flare reaction when injected into human skin. In a variety of in vitro systems (bacteria, parasites, tumor cells), *eosinophil peroxidase* (EPO) causes injury. Both eosinophil-derived neurotoxin (EDN) and eosinophil cationic protein (ECP) damage myelinated cells in animals.

Kinins are another system of proteins activated in inflammatory processes that have amplifier and effector properties. Their activities include chemotaxis, increased vascular permeability, and smooth muscle contraction. Bradykinin, a nonapeptide, is the most important product of the kinin system. The kinin, complement, and clotting systems are interrelated. Activation of Hageman factor (factor XII) is the initial step in kinin generation and amplification, with positive feedback loops resembling those in the complement pathway. Hageman factor is activated by tissue injury from a number of agents, including IgG aggregates and immune complexes. Hageman factor and complexes of high molecular weight kininogen and prekallikrein and high molecular weight kininogen and factor XI are bound together. Hageman factor appears to autoactivate to form activated Hageman factor (HF_a), which converts prekallikrein to kallikrein. Kallikrein

TABLE 11–10. Chemical Mediators of Allergic Reactions

Mediator	Structural Characteristics	Actions
Histamine (preformed)	5–β–Imidazolylethylamine MW 111	H_1 receptors: Increase in venular permeability Contraction of smooth muscle Increase in cyclic GMP levels Generation of prostaglandins Increase in nasal mucus production Positive chemokinetic effect on neutrophils and eosinophils† Positive chemotactic effect on neutrophils and eosinophils Bronchial irritant receptor stimulation Pruritus H_2 receptors: Increase in vascular permeability Increase in gastric acid secretion Positive chemokinetic effect on neutrophils and eosinophils Negative chemotactic effect on neutrophils and eosinophils Inhibition of T cell responses Inhibition of basophil (not mast cell) mediator response Augmentation of gastric acid secretion Stimulation of airway mucus secretion Increase in cyclic AMP Increase in chronotropic and inotropic effects on heart
Eosinophil chemotactic factor of anaphylaxis (ECF-A tetrapeptides) (preformed)	Val/Ala-Gly-Ser-Glu MW 400–500	Chemotactic attraction and deactivation of eosinophils Increase in eosinophil complement receptors
ECF-oligopeptides (preformed)	Peptides MW 1500–3000	Chemotactic attraction and deactivation of eosinophils and mononuclear leukocytes
High molecular weight–neutrophil chemotactic factor (HMW–NCF) (preformed)	Neutral protein MW 600,000	Chemotactic attraction and deactivation of neutrophils
Platelet-activating factor (PAF) (newly formed)	AGEPC (acetyl-glyceryl-ether-phosphorylcholine) MW 551 (hexadecyl) MW 523 (octadecyl)	Aggregation of platelets and secretion of amines Neutrophil aggregation and enzyme release Production of prostaglandins and thromboxanes by platelets Increase in vascular permeability Mimics physiologic and intravascular sequelae of IgE-mediated human systemic anaphylaxis Potent chemotactic attraction and activation of eosinophils Prolonged increase in bronchial hyperresponsiveness
Heparin (preformed)	Acidic proteoglycan MW 60,000 (human)	Anticoagulation (antithrombin III binding activity) Anticomplementary activity (at several sites) Augments inactivation of histamine
Arachidonic acid (newly formed)	20-carbon fatty acid	
Cyclooxygenase products:		
PGD_2 (newly formed) (Prostaglandin D_2)		Contraction of smooth muscle Bronchoconstriction Vasodilatation (skin) Chemokinesis of granulocytes Chronotropic effect on heart Increase in vascular permeability Sneezing Rhinorrhea
PGE_2 (newly formed)		Relaxation of smooth muscle Bronchodilatation Vasodilatation
$PGF_{2\alpha}$ (newly formed)		Bronchoconstriction Constriction of microvasculature and pulmonary vasculature
PGI_2 (newly formed)		Relaxation of smooth muscle Pulmonary vasodilation
T_xA_2 (newly formed) (Thromboxane A_2)		Bronchoconstriction Constriction of microvasculature Platelet aggregation
Lipoxygenase products: LTC_4, LTD_4, LTE_4 (newly formed) (Leukotrienes)	MW 400–600	Smooth muscle contraction and bronchoconstriction, especially of peripheral airway Airway mucus secretion Dilatation and increased permeability of microvasculature Constriction of coronary and cerebral arteries Depression of myocardial contractility

Table continued on following page

TABLE 11–10. Chemical Mediators of Allergic Reactions *Continued*

Mediator	Structural Characteristics	Actions
LTB_4 (newly formed)	MW 400	Chemotactic and chemokinetic for neutrophils and eosinophils Increased leukocyte adherence to endothelium Leukocyte activation Suppression of T lymphocyte function
Hydroxyeicosatetraenoic acids (HETEs) (newly formed)		Chemotaxis and chemokinesis of eosinophils and neutrophils

*Adapted from Behrman R, et al (eds): Nelson Textbook of Pediatrics, 13th ed. Philadelphia, WB Saunders, 1986.
†Chemotactic migration requires a concentration gradient from the stimulus side. Movement in the absence of a gradient of the stimulus is termed "positive chemokinesis."

digests high molecular weight kininogen to liberate the vasoactive peptide bradykinin. Bradykinin has potent contractile effects on smooth muscle, causes increased vascular permeability, and dilates peripheral arterioles. It also stimulates pain receptors. At least two other plasma kinins have biologic activities similar to those of bradykinin. The role of bradykinin in allergic disease is uncertain. Several patients with cold urticaria have had increased concentrations of bradykinin in plasma.

Platelet-activating factor (PAF), a phospholipid, is synthesized by a variety of cells, including vascular endothelial cells, monocytes, macrophages, neutrophils, and especially eosinophils, as well as platelets. It is a potent inducer of increased vascular permeability. Its inhalation causes acute transient bronchoconstriction in both normal and asthmatic subjects. Bronchial hyperresponsiveness follows and may persist for weeks in normal subjects but may not occur in patients with asthma, possibly because of hyperresponsiveness already induced by endogenous PAF. Mediators released or formed in response to bridging of cell-bound IgE molecules, such as eosinophil chemotactic factors and LTB_4, may attract eosinophils and other cells that synthesize PAF, which in turn may cause a late-phase reaction several hours after the initial antigen-antibody reaction occurred.

Type I hypersensitivity reactions involve early (10–30 min) and late (4–8 hr) phase reactions. Early reactions after antigenic stimulation include vasodilation, edema formation from increased vascular permeability, smooth muscle constriction (bronchoconstriction), and mucus production. This response is due to the release of preformed and newly synthesized mast cell mediators. This response may be treated with antihistamines and mast cell membrane stabilizers such as cromolyn sodium. The late-phase reaction perpetuates the early changes of vascular permeability but includes the recruitment of inflammatory cell types in addition to mast cells. These recruited cells (eosinophils, neutrophils, lymphocytes) are located in the perivascular space. Erythema, edema, and induration are present, as well as airway hyperirritability to rechallenge with allergens. This late, chronic inflammatory reaction probably contributes to the hyperresponsiveness found in allergic children with asthma, rhinitis, and atopic dermatitis. Late-phase reactions respond poorly to antihistamines or bronchodilator therapy but may respond to corticosteroids.

Serotonin (5-hydroxytryptamine) is a vasoactive amine that, in experimental animals, induces contraction of smooth muscle and increases vascular permeability. Ninety percent of the body's stores of serotonin are found in the gastrointestinal tract, with the remainder divided between the central nervous system and platelets. Human mast cells lack serotonin. Serotonin has been reported to induce bronchoconstriction in asthmatics but not in normal people, but it has no significant role in immediate hypersensitivity reactions in humans. It is associated distinctively with diarrhea in the carcinoid syndrome.

While not mediators in the same sense as products released from mast cells or basophils, certain components of the *complement system* have activities that may contribute to allergic reactions. (1) Aggregated IgE can initiate complement system activity in vitro through the alternative pathway; this probably does not occur in vivo because of the large quantities of IgE required. (2) Certain "split" or "cleavage" products of the complement cascade, C3a and C5a, can induce mediator (histamine) release from basophils and from mast cells in the skin, producing wheal and flare reactions. C3a and C5a have been termed *anaphylatoxins* because they release histamine and resemble components of serum capable of causing guinea pig anaphylaxis. C5a and, to a much lesser extent, C3a are chemotactic for various leukocytes. Neutrophils attracted to the site of complement activation by C5a may degranulate, releasing basic lysosomal proteins that trigger mediator liberation from mast cells. The result in the skin is urticaria mimicking an antigen-IgE reaction. Small *N*-formylated peptides, derived from bacterial products, also possess potent granulocyte chemotactic activity and may operate in a manner similar to that of C5a to cause urticaria. (3) A kinin-like peptide derived from C2 as a result of reduced functional activity of the inhibitor of C1-esterase (C1s) is thought to mediate the angioedema observed in hereditary angioedema (HAE).

From the foregoing considerations it is evident that the signs and symptoms of typical, immediate-type allergic reactions such as anaphylaxis, though most often involving the IgE mechanism, may result from non-IgE immunologic mechanisms or from nonimmunologic mechanisms.

Chung KF, Barnes PJ: Effects of platelet activating factor on airway calibre, airway responsiveness, and circulating cells in asthmatic subjects. Thorax 44:108, 1989.
Gleich GJ, Flavahan NA, Fujisawa T, et al: The eosinophil as a mediator of damage to respiratory epithelium: A model for bronchial hyperreactivity. J Allergy Clin Immunol 81:776, 1988.
Goetzl EJ, Paxan DG, Goldman DW: Immunopathogenic roles of leukotrienes in human diseases. J Clin Immunol 4:79, 1984.
Ishizaka K: Regulation of IgE synthesis. Annu Rev Immunol 2:159, 1984.
Ishizaka T, Ishizaka K: Activation of mast cells for mediator release through IgE receptors. Prog Allergy 34:188, 1984.
Katz HR, Stevens RL, Austen KF: Heterogeneity of mammalian mast cells differentiated in vivo and in vitro. J Allergy Clin Immunol 76:250, 1985.
Leung D, Kamada M: Developments in allergy. Curr Opin Pediatr 1:27, 1989.

11.36 GENERAL AND SPECIFIC METHODS OF DIAGNOSIS

ALLERGY HISTORY. The allergy history differs from the general medical history with respect to the nature of inquiries into possible causes of the symptoms. These inquiries include a detailed history of "exposure" to potential allergens. The frequency, duration, intensity, location, and progression of symptoms are relevant to a determination of their possible causes and to decisions about the types of therapy that may be effective. Seasonal symptoms may correlate with exposure to seasonal allergens such as pollens. Exposure to the highest concentrations of house dust mites, the chief source of allergens in house dust, often occurs at the end of the summer because high humidity favors mite proliferation. Allergy to house dust mites, however, usually causes perennial symptoms. Allergy to pet dogs or cats that have access to the house also usually causes perennial symptoms. Patients may deny an association between exposure to the animal and their symptoms because they fail to recognize that contamination of the house and its furnishings with animal dander results in continual exposure to allergen despite only intermittent exposure to the animal itself. Onset or worsening of symptoms shortly after acquisition of an animal or relief when the child is away from the house should arouse suspicion.

A relationship between symptoms and the location where they occur may suggest a cause. Exposure to pollens is often more intense outdoors than indoors, especially when windows are closed and air conditioners are operating. Onset of symptoms shortly after moving to a different dwelling should suggest an environmental cause. Changes in symptoms during trips away from home may provide helpful clues to the etiology. Worsening of symptoms in a damp, musty basement should suggest allergy to fungi. An increase in symptoms at night may suggest increased exposure to allergen in the bedroom, but asthma commonly worsens at night even without exposure to allergens. Weekend remissions suggest a source of allergen at school or the workplace.

An association between symptoms and certain activities may be diagnostically helpful. Respiratory symptoms that follow exposure to freshly cut grass suggest allergy to pollen or fungi. Symptoms provoked by dusting or carpet cleaning are often due to allergy to house dust mites. Coughing or wheezing following strenuous exercise may occur in children who have asthma. Provocation of coughing by laughter, crying, or exposure to smoke or specific odors also suggests the bronchial hyperresponsiveness characteristic of asthma.

The nature of the symptoms is important. An intermittent, recurrent dry cough or a cough productive of clear mucus is consistent with asthma, but a chronic persistent cough productive of purulent sputum suggests bronchiectasis or cystic fibrosis. Aspiration of a foreign body often causes a sudden onset of coughing with choking followed by wheezing. Coughing associated with aphonia or dysphonia may be due to a hypopharyngeal or laryngeal foreign body or laryngeal papilloma. Glottic or subglottic obstruction can cause a harsh, barking cough. Paroxysmal coughing suggests pertussis or a bronchial foreign body.

Allergic rhinitis is the most common cause of a chronic or recurrent, clear nasal discharge, especially when this is associated with sneezing or conjunctival itching and injection with excessive tearing. A purulent nasal discharge suggests infection. A postnasal drip due to allergic rhinitis or sinusitis may cause frequent clearing of the throat, hoarseness, and nocturnal coughing. Intense conjunctival itching associated with photophobia and a viscid, white conjunctival discharge suggests vernal conjunctivitis.

A history of any beneficial or adverse effects of previous treatment may be helpful in establishing the diagnosis as well as guiding further therapy. Improvement of rhinitis in response to an antihistamine suggests allergy rather than infection. Antihistamines often relieve coughing due to postnasal drainage associated with allergic rhinitis, but relief of coughing by a bronchodilator suggests asthma.

The immediate family history is relevant. Atopic allergy manifested by allergic rhinitis, asthma, atopic dermatitis, or urticaria and the specific manifestations of these disorders tend to be familial. Asthma may be familial whether or not it is due to allergy. Nonetheless, any of these conditions can also occur without a positive family history.

PHYSICAL EXAMINATION. Results of the physical examination depend upon the duration and severity of the allergic disorder. *Height and weight* should be compared with normal values for age. Both severe asthma and treatment with adrenal corticosteroids can suppress growth. Poor weight gain may suggest cystic fibrosis, a consideration in the differential diagnosis of asthma.

Pulsus paradoxus, the difference in systemic arterial blood pressure during inspiration and expiration, normally does not exceed 10 mm Hg. During acute asthma it is often increased, and the extent to which it exceeds 10 mm Hg is an index of the severity of the airway obstruction. An increase to more than 20 mm Hg indicates moderate or severe airway obstruction. Other possible causes of increased pulsus paradoxus include cystic fibrosis, heart failure, and cardiac tamponade.

Cyanosis due to airway obstruction may be evident if arterial oxygen saturation is less than 85%. Need for a marked reduction in intrapleural (high negative) pressure to initiate inspiration through obstructed airways may cause *supraclavicular and intercostal retractions.* Air trapping during expiration may cause bulging of the intercostal spaces during acute asthma. *Flaring of the alae nasi* may be evident. Bobbing of the head with each inspiration indicates *dyspnea* in infants lying supine.

Mouth breathing and a dark discoloration beneath the lower eyelids *(allergic shiners)* indicate nasal obstruction, possibly due to allergic rhinitis. Frequent wrinkling of the nose and the *allergic salute* (habitual wiping of the running nose), also suggest allergic rhinitis. Frequently repeated salutes for months or years elevates the tip of the nose, causing a transverse nasal crease at the junction of the cartilaginous and bony bridge of the nose. A familial transverse nasal groove, inherited as a mendelian dominant trait, is unrelated to rhinitis. *Dennie lines* (Dennie-Morgan folds), wrinkles beneath the lower eyelids, are associated with allergic rhinitis, asthma, and atopic dermatitis.

Digital clubbing is extremely rare in patients with uncomplicated asthma. Its presence suggests a complication such as bronchiectasis or another disease (Table 11–11). Comparison of the depth of the index finger at the base of the nail with its depth at the distal interphalangeal joint is the best method of recognizing digital clubbing. The depth at the base of the nail is normally smaller. A depth at the base of the nail equal to that at the distal interphalangeal joint is 2.5 standard deviations above normal, indicating mild clubbing.

Inspection of the skin may disclose evidence of *atopic dermatitis*: an erythematous, maculopapular eruption, fine scaling, or weeping and oozing with excoriations due to frequent scratching (see also Sec. 11.42 and 23.14). Crusting may be evident if there is superimposed infection. The dermatitis may be generalized, but in infancy there is usually a predilection for the cheeks and extensor surfaces of the

TABLE 11–11. Diseases Associated with Acquired Digital Clubbing

Cardiac	Gastrointestinal
Cyanotic congenital heart disease	Celiac disease
Subacute bacterial endocarditis	Chronic dysentery
Pulmonary	Chronic ulcerative colitis
Abscess	Multiple polyposis
Bronchiectasis	Regional enteritis
Chronic pneumonia	Hepatic
Cystic fibrosis	Biliary cirrhosis
Empyema	Chronic active hepatitis
Malignant neoplasms	Other
Tuberculosis	Hodgkin disease
Pleural	Thyrotoxicosis
Mesothelioma	

extremities. In older children involvement of the antecubital spaces, popliteal spaces, and neck is most frequent. In older children lichenification and either hyperpigmentation or hypopigmentation may be evident.

Urticarial lesions may vary in appearance from multiple, 1 to 3-mm wheals with flares typical of cholinergic urticaria to giant wheals that may be associated with angioedema. Wheals are often evanescent, resolving in minutes or hours, only to appear elsewhere. There is often associated *dermographism. Contact dermatitis* is manifested by an erythematous or papulovesicular eruption in the area exposed to the contactant.

Examination of the eyes may disclose the conjunctival injection, excessive tearing, and periorbital edema of *allergic conjunctivitis*. A tenacious, ropy, mucoid conjunctival discharge associated with giant papillae on the upper palpebral conjunctiva, pseudoptosis, and photophobia should suggest *vernal conjunctivitis*.

The *nasal mucosa* may be pale, blue, or pink in children with allergic rhinitis. A profuse, clear nasal discharge is typical. Nasal turbinates are usually edematous. Hypertrophy of tonsils and adenoids is a common complication of allergic rhinitis.

Examination of the chest may disclose an increase in the *anteroposterior diameter* associated with asthma. Comparison of the depth with the width of the chest, measured with chest or obstetric calipers, permits objective evaluation of the chest configuration. The chest of the normal newborn infant is almost circular in cross-section. With growth, the width increases more than the depth (anteroposterior diameter). By the time the child's height reaches 95 cm at approximately 3 yr of age, the depth-width ratio has decreased to 0.75 and remains between 0.70 and 0.75 thereafter. Abnormal increases in the depth-width ratio occur during acute asthma attacks but return toward normal after response to a bronchodilator. A persistent increase in this ratio may occur in children with frequently recurrent or continual asthma episodes but is more characteristic of chronic conditions associated with persistent airway obstruction, such as cystic fibrosis.

In patients with asthma, ausculation of the lungs may disclose *wheezing*, more pronounced on expiration, and prolongation of the expiratory phase of respiration. Wheezing is usually generalized, but there may be minor differences in intensity from segment to segment due to segmental atelectasis.

IN VITRO TESTS. A white blood cell count and a differential count are useful in establishing whether *eosinophilia* is present. The total eosinophil count is more accurate. Eosinophils are subject to a diurnal rhythm, their numbers being highest in the early morning. Because eosinophilia may be intermittent, two or three normal results should be obtained before concluding that there is no eosinophilia. Eosinophil counts in children usually approximate 250 cells/mm^3, but as many as 700/mm^3 may be normal. Eosinophilia of respiratory tract secretions in a patient with rhinorrhea or cough is important. A smear of nasal secretions or bronchial mucus should be stained on a microscopic slide with an eosin-methylene blue stain (Hansel stain). A finding of more than 5–10% eosinophils in nasal secretions supports the diagnosis of allergic rhinitis. Eosinophils in bronchial mucus strongly suggest asthma. Blood eosinophilia in allergic conditions does not generally exceed 15–20% but may rarely be as high as 35% in allergic children in the absence of other disorders known to cause eosinophilia. Eosinophilia is also noted in drug hypersensitivity, rheumatologic disorders (periarteritis-nodosa, rheumatoid arthritis), pemphigus, dermatitis herpetiformis, inherited eosinophilia, allergic bronchopulmonary aspergillosis, various malignancies (leukemias, lymphomas, Hodgkin disease), eosinophilic fasciitis, toxic oil syndrome, and eosinophilic-myalgia syndrome (associated with L-tryptophan). Very high eosinophil counts are also noted in parasitic infections with tissue-invading helminths (*Toxocara*, trichinosis, *Echinococcus, Ascaris*) or malaria, and in hypereosinophilic syndrome (Löffler syndrome, pulmonary infiltrates, cardiomyopathy). Corticosteroids cause eosinopenia for up to 6 hr following a dose; the timing of collection of a blood specimen should be appropriately adjusted.

A number of in vitro immunologic tests are of value in allergy diagnosis, such as measurement of the *total and specific IgE content of serum* and determination of the sensitivity of the patient's leukocytes for antigen-induced histamine release. Table 11–12 shows the serum concentrations of IgE in normal Swedish subjects of different ages. Normal values vary in different populations. Mean concentrations of IgE in atopic people are often higher than normal, though a significant number of allergic individuals have normal or low IgE concentrations. Indeed, very low levels of serum IgE may be more useful in excluding atopic disease than elevated levels are in confirming this diagnosis, although patients with low IgE levels can have atopy. In patients with active atopic dermatitis, however, serum IgE levels are usually greatly elevated. Increased total IgE levels during infancy suggest the likelihood of subsequent development of atopic diseases. Table 11–13 shows some nonatopic disorders associated with increased concentrations of serum IgE.

The *radioallergosorbent test* (RAST) determines antigen-specific IgE concentrations in serum (Fig. 11–3). The correlation between RAST results and medical histories, provocation tests, or leukocyte histamine release tests is good. Correlation with allergy skin testing is also good, but RAST is somewhat less sensitive than skin testing. There has been considerable interlaboratory and intralaboratory variability in RAST results on the same specimen. Selection of a reliable laboratory is essential. More recent modifications of in vitro methods for determining specific IgE incorporate different types of solid supports for binding allergen and different types of label for anti-human IgE antibody, resulting in colored, luminescent, or fluorescent detectable products. Few direct comparisons of the results of these newer methods with RAST results have been published, but available data suggest that the newer methods are somewhat less reliable than RAST.

In vitro methods of determining specific IgE to several allergens simultaneously have been marketed as screening tests for allergy. The few published data evaluating such

Table 11–12. Levels of Serum IgE Immunoglobulin of Normal Subjects at Different Ages*

Age	Range (*IU/mL*)	Geometric Mean (± 2 SD) (*IU/mL*)
0 days	<0.1–1.5	0.22 (0.04–1.28)
6 wk	<0.1–2.8	0.69 (0.08–6.12)
3 mo	0.3–3.1	0.82 (0.18–3.76)
6 mo	0.9–28.0	2.68 (0.44–16.26)
9 mo	0.7–8.1	2.36 (0.76–7.31)
1 yr	1.1–10.2	3.49 (0.80–15.22)
2 yr	1.1–49.0	3.03 (0.31–29.48)
3 yr	0.5–7.7	1.80 (0.19–16.86)
4 yr	2.4–34.8	8.58 (1.07–68.86)
7 yr	1.6–60.0	12.89 (1.03–161.32)
10 yr	0.3–215	23.66 (0.98–570.61
14 yr	1.9–159	20.07 (2.06–195.18)
18–83 yr	1–178	21.20 (Modal values 10–20 IU/mL)†

*Ages 0–14 years adapted from Kjellman N-IM, Johansson SGO, Roth A: Clin Allergy 6:51, 1976; data on ages 18–83 years adapted from Nye L, Merrett TG, Landon J, et al: Clin Allergy 1:13, 1975. The method used was a double antibody assay.

†Modal values — the most common values observed.

‡To convert IU/mL to μg/L multiply by 2.4.

TABLE 11–13. Nonallergic Diseases Associated with Increased Serum IgE Concentrations

Parasitic Infestations		
Ascariasis	Filariasis	Schistosomiasis
Capillariasis	Hookworm	Strongyloidiasis
Echinococcosis	Onchocerciasis	Trichinosis
Fascioliasis	Paragonimiasis	Visceral larva migrans
Infections		
Allergic bronchopulmonary aspergillosis	Cytomegalovirus mononucleosis	
Candidiasis, systemic	Infectious mononucleosis (Epstein-Barr virus)	
Coccidioidomycosis	Leprosy	
Immunodeficiency		
Hyperimmunoglobulinemia E syndrome		
IgA deficiency, selective		
Nezelof syndrome		
Thymic hypoplasia (DiGeorge anomaly)		
Wiskott-Aldrich syndrome		
Neoplastic Diseases		
Hodgkin disease		
IgE myeloma		
Other Diseases and Disorders		
Burns	Kawasaki disease	
Cystic fibrosis	Liver disease	
Dermatitis, chronic acral	Pemphigoid, bullous	
Erythema nodosum, streptococcal	Polyarteritis nodosa, infantile	
Guillain-Barré syndrome	Rheumatoid arthritis	
Hemosiderosis, primary pulmonary		
Interstitial nephritis, drug-induced		

methods indicate that they are relatively insensitive and may fail to identify more than 30% of children with allergy.

Whatever the method for determining specific IgE, results must be correlated with the patient's medical history to establish clinical relevance. In vitro determination of specific IgE has both advantages and disadvantages compared with allergy skin testing (Table 11–14). For experienced clinicians, allergy skin testing remains the method of choice for most patients.

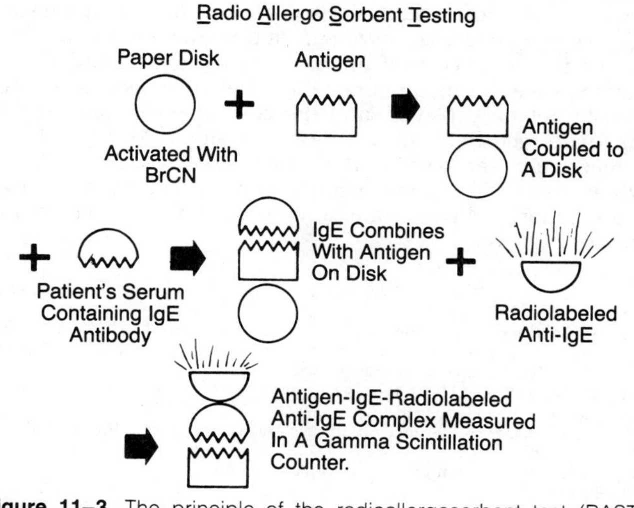

Figure 11–3. The principle of the radioallergosorbent test (RAST). After activation of some form of cellulose (e.g., a paper disk) by cyanogen bromide, antigen is coupled covalently to the disk to render the antigen insoluble. Incubation with the patient's serum permits any specific antibodies to bind to the antigen. These antibodies remain bound to antigen after washing. Addition of radiolabeled antihuman IgE results in labeling of the antigen-IgE complex. The complex is then counted in a gamma scintillation counter. The number of disintegrations per minute is proportional to the amount of specific IgE in the serum sample.

The *leukocyte histamine release test* detects specific IgE antibody attached to the surfaces of peripheral blood basophils by measuring the amount of histamine released in response to challenge with antigen. Incubation of serum with basophils from nonsensitive donors also permits detection of antibody in serum. The amount of histamine release is expressed as a percentage of the total histamine in the cells and varies with the dose of allergen. Small doses of allergen release histamine when cell sensitivity is high. Results generally correlate with allergy skin testing, but skin testing is more sensitive. Approximately 15% of subjects have basophils that do not release histamine in vitro. The complexity of this procedure limits it largely to investigational use.

IN VIVO TESTS. Determination of allergic reactivity

TABLE 11—14. Determination of Specific IgE by RAST* and Skin Testing

	Skin Test	RAST
Risk of allergic reaction	Yes	No
Sensitive†	Very	Less
Affected by antihistamines	Yes	No
Affected by corticosteroids	Usually not	No
Affected by extensive dermatitis or dermographism	Yes	No
Convenience, less patient anxiety	No	Yes
Broad selection of antigens	Yes	No
Immediate results	Yes	No
Expensive	No	Yes
Semiquantitative	No	Yes
Lability of allergens	Yes	No

*Radioallergosorbent test (RAST) as example of other in vitro tests.

†Because skin tests are more sensitive, they are more reliable than RAST in confirming life-threatening anaphylactic conditions if maximum sensitivity is required (e.g., penicillin, *Hymenoptera* hypersensitivity).

through direct *skin testing* of the patient is an important tool in the diagnosis of IgE-mediated sensitivity. A small quantity of allergenic extract is introduced into the skin by prick/puncture (epidermal or epicutaneous method) or by intradermal technique. If the patient's mast cells have IgE antibodies specific for the allergen on their surfaces, an allergen-IgE interaction triggers biochemical events that culminate in release of histamine and other mediators from the mast cell. The histamine acts upon histamine receptors in small vessels, causing increased permeability and dilatation and axon reflex stimulation, which cause a wheal and flare reaction. A positive intradermal reaction is a wheal of at least 5 mm of induration, plus surrounding erythema, occurring 15 min after injection of antigen. The immediate wheal and flare reaction usually peaks within 15–30 min and then resolves. In some patients, however, when the wheal has exceeded 10 mm in diameter, a late-phase reaction may follow. The wheal becomes less distinct, but edema and erythema persist, peak at 6–8 hr, and often resolve by 24 hr. Late-phase reactions are associated with burning, pruritus, and warmth and may become more than double the size of the antecedent immediate reaction. Histologic examination of this late-phase reaction discloses a mixed cellular infiltrate including mononuclear cells, eosinophils, and neutrophils.

The immediate wheal and flare reaction in skin indicates that specific IgE antibody is present also on the mast cells in the tissue of the clinically affected organ. *It does not indicate that the patient will necessarily have clinical symptoms on exposure to the allergen.* Some atopic people have no symptoms following natural exposure to allergens that elicit positive wheal and flare reactions on skin testing. As a general rule, the larger the size of the wheal and flare reaction, the more likely is the test antigen to be clinically relevant. But one must be cautious not to overinterpret skin test results.

Positive skin tests obtained by the puncture technique correlate better than the more sensitive intradermal tests with measurements of specific IgE antibody and with appearance of clinical symptoms upon exposure to the allergen. With the intradermal technique, only those positive tests obtained with high dilutions (weak concentrations) of extract have as high correlations. If only concentrated solutions of allergenic extract (e.g., 1–100 or 1–10 weight/volume) elicit positive intracutaneous tests, the results will more often than not be of little clinical significance. A histamine control should also be used for comparison. Overinterpretation of such reactions has led to overuse of allergenic extracts in immunotherapy.

Various drugs, extracts that contain irritant materials or substances that are too concentrated, and improper technique can induce nonimmunologic histamine release from tissue mast cells. The resulting wheal and flare reaction cannot be differentiated from that following IgE-allergen interaction, and IgE sensitivity may be mistakenly inferred. Other drugs may inhibit full expression of clinically relevant positive skin tests. Among these are certain adrenergic drugs such as epinephrine and ephedrine and the antihistamines. These drugs should be withheld prior to skin testing (ephedrine for at least 12 hr and most antihistamines for at least 72 hr, hydroxyzine for 5 days, and astemizole for 2 wk). To make sure that the skin is capable of reacting to endogenously released histamine, a positive histamine control (histamine phosphate, 1%) should always be used. Corticosteroids have no appreciable inhibitory effects on IgE-mediated wheal and flare reactions and need not be withheld before skin testing.

Because the appearance of symptoms on natural exposure may not correlate well with results of skin testing, *provocation testing* by direct exposure of the mucous membrane of the affected organ to the suspected allergen (usually in the form of an extract or aerosol of the material) has received considerable attention. Mucous membrane provocation testing has been used mostly in patients with asthma. As commonly performed, the test requires that increasing concentrations of extracts of various allergens be inhaled by the patient after nebulization with a suitable device. A positive response is manifested by an increase in airway obstruction as monitored with pulmonary function testing. The patient's degree of sensitivity should be determined by skin tests before provocation testing to permit appropriate initial concentrations of allergenic extract to be used. With reasonable precautions the method is safe, and the results of provocation testing correlate well with clinical data. It is time consuming, however, and is not suitable for general use in the office or clinic. Bronchial challenge testing may be most useful in patients who have many positive skin test results, in whom it can guide selection of those allergens that may be most clinically significant for inclusion in an immunotherapy extract mixture. Selection in this way permits a greater concentration of the more clinically significant allergens in the mixture than would be possible if all the allergens possibly implicated by skin testing were to be included. Studies have shown excellent correlations between the results of provocative bronchial challenge testing, RAST, and quantitative intradermal skin tests (end-point dilution method); accordingly, bronchial challenge testing is principally reserved for research purposes. On the other hand, bronchial provocative testing with methacholine or histamine is valuable when the degree of airway reactivity in asthma must be determined and when the diagnosis of asthma is uncertain. Methacholine bronchial challenge testing produces marked bronchoconstriction in patients with asthma compared with normal controls. Atopic children without asthma also have increased hyperresponsiveness to methacholine provocation, suggesting a predisposition to nonspecific bronchial hyperactivity.

Oral provocation should be performed in a facility capable of performing cardiopulmonary resuscitation and is contraindicated if anaphylactic reactions have occurred. Provocation testing with foods has been used to diagnose IgE-mediated food allergy and food-induced atopic dermatitis. Following an elimination diet, food antigens are introduced in a double-blind provocation trial. Skin testing may help to identify the offending food, especially in the presence of an association between ingestion and IgE-mediated events (anaphylaxis, urticaria, angioedema, eczema, abdominal cramps). Oral provocation is indicated if the history is equivocal and symptoms improve during an elimination diet. The specific food is given in gelatin capsules, and the child is evaluated for the immediate recurrence of symptoms or signs. Manifestations of allergy appear within 10–90 min and include pruritus, erythematous macular morbilliform rash, wheezing, sneezing, cough, abdominal pain, nausea, emesis, and increased serum histamine levels.

Aberg N, Engstrom I: Natural history of allergic diseases in children. Acta Pediatr Scand 79:206, 1990.
American College of Physicians: Allergy testing. Ann Intern Med 110:317, 1989.
Bierman CW, Pearlman DS (eds): Allergic Diseases from Infancy to Adulthood, 2nd ed. Philadelphia, WB Saunders, 1988.
Broadbent JB, Sampson H: Food hypersensitivity and atopic dermatitis. Pediatr Clin North Am 35:1115, 1988.
Lockey RF, Bukantz SC: Primer on allergic and immunologic diseases. JAMA 258:2829, 1987.
Ownby DR: Allergy testing: In vivo versus in vitro. Pediatr Clin North Am 35:995, 1988.
Sly RM: Textbook of Pediatric Allergy. New Hyde Park, NY, Medical Examination Publishing Co, 1985.
Van Arsdel PP, Larson E: Diagnostic tests for patients with suspected allergic disease: Utility and limitations. Ann Intern Med 110:304, 1989.

11.37 PRINCIPLES OF TREATMENT OF ALLERGIC DISORDERS

Successful management of allergic disorders is based upon four principles: avoidance of allergens or irritants, pharmacologic therapy, immunotherapy (hyposensitization or desensitization), and prophylaxis.

When clinically relevant allergens are identified by history and judicious use of allergy skin tests, their elimination or *avoidance* is all that is needed in many cases of IgE-mediated disease. If the history and skin testing indicate reactivity to house dust mites or molds, or if dog or cat allergen is contributing to the patient's symptoms, these allergens should be eliminated from the home to the greatest extent possible. The recommendation that a family pet be removed from a home is frequently difficult to implement. When the allergic disorder is a serious one, such as asthma, and when the child has a positive skin test result to the dog or cat allergen, parents can generally be persuaded to remove the animal. When skin tests to danders are negative, the problem may be more difficult; most allergists believe that elimination of potentially sensitizing pets from the household of the allergic child is desirable for prophylaxis.

Allergy to **house dust mites** requires precautions to minimize exposure to mite allergens. Avoidance in the bedroom is often sufficient because children spend more time there than in other rooms of the house. Mattresses, box springs, and pillows should be encased in airtight, allergen-proof covers.* Vacuuming the covered mattress at least weekly is necessary to remove mites. Bedding should be washed at least weekly in hot water (>70° C); cool water does not kill the mites. There should be no carpet or rug in the bedroom since either may be a rich sources of mites. A small cotton throw rug may be acceptable if it is washed at least weekly in hot water. There should be no upholstered furniture and no stuffed toys in the bedroom. When removal of carpet from a bedroom is impossible, treatment of the carpet with a solution of tannic acid inactivates mite allergens.* Repeated treatments of the carpet at intervals of 2–3 mo are necessary because the solution does not kill the mites.

Household humidity should be kept below 50% to inhibit survival of mites. It is prudent to avoid use of vaporizers. Dehumidifiers may be necessary in damp basements. Air conditioning helps to control humidity and also reduces exposure to atmospheric pollens and molds.

Avoidance of irritants is important in the control and prevention of **asthma**. Potential sources of irritants include kerosene heaters and wood-burning stoves. Smoking should not be permitted indoors, and patients with asthma should avoid public facilities where exposure to cigarette smoke is likely.

Pharmacologic therapy is a major element in management of allergic diseases (Sec. 11.38). The drugs used have specific roles in the interruption of pathways leading to tissue damage as a consequence of antigen-antibody interaction. Certain drugs, for example, modulate the antigen-induced release of mediators (histamine, leukotrienes); others affect the tension of smooth muscle; and others prevent the migration to the site of an allergic reaction of inflammatory cells having the potential for producing tissue injury. For patients whose symptoms are not mediated by an immunologic mechanism, avoidance of allergens or attempts to increase the tolerance to allergens by immunotherapy are fruitless. Drug therapy, on the other hand, may be effective whether or not an allergic mechanism is involved. Patients with nonimmunologic or nonallergic asthma may respond as well to drug treatment as those in whom allergy plays a major role.

Immunotherapy is appropriate for the treatment of allergic rhinitis or asthma mediated by IgE antibody-antigen interactions due to unavoidable inhalant allergens (Sec. 11.39).

*Allergy Control Products, 89 Danbury Road, PO Box 793, Ridgefield, CT 06877.

A predisposition to form IgE antibodies to substances of "high" allergenic potential is an important characteristic of the atopic state. Therefore, prevention of exposure of infants and children at risk has a rational basis. It is appropriate to recommend breast-feeding for infants born into families with strong histories of hay fever, asthma, or atopic dermatitis and to delay for at least 6 mo the introduction of solid foods into the diet of such infants, especially foods of highly allergenic potential, such as eggs, cow milk, wheat, fish, citrus fruit, and peanut butter. The nursing mother should avoid highly allergenic foods in her diet because there is evidence that the breast-fed infant can become sensitized to food antigens that are transmitted in breast milk. It is not definitively established whether postponing cow milk feedings in an atopic infant can prevent the development of cow milk allergy, of allergic diseases in general, or of atopic dermatitis in particular, though there is some evidence of such effects. There are no prospective studies that convincingly indicate that avoidance of environmental exposure of atopic infants and children to inhalant allergens such as dog and cat allergen lessens the likelihood of their sensitization, though such a result seems reasonable. Cord blood IgE levels greater than 1.3 IU/mL, elevated serum IgE levels, eosinophilia during infancy, and a family history of atopic dermatitis, asthma, or allergic rhinitis may predict a child at risk for future atopic disorders who might benefit from allergic avoidance.

11.38 PHARMACOLOGIC THERAPY

ADRENERGICS. These agents combine with α- and β-receptors on the surfaces of cells. With several exceptions, drugs that affect α-receptors cause physiologic responses that are excitatory (vasoconstriction), whereas drugs that influence β-receptors produce inhibitory responses (bronchodilation). In a given tissue the response to a drug depends both on the relative numbers of α- and β-receptors and upon whether the drug stimulates predominantly α-receptors, β-receptors, or both.

Variations in sensitivity of β-receptors of different organs to β-agonists (stimulants) and differences in response to β-blocking drugs of diverse chemical structure have led to separation of β-receptors into two subclasses, β_1 and β_2; β_1-receptors have approximately equal affinity for epinephrine and norepinephrine, whereas β_2-receptors have an approximately 10-fold higher affinity for epinephrine than for norepinephrine. Agents with greater β_2-selective activity (isoetharine, metaproterenol, terbutaline, albuterol, fenoterol, bitolterol) can provide effective bronchodilation in asthma without the significant increase in heart rate that may occur with isoproterenol or epinephrine, since the latter drugs stimulate both bronchial β_2-receptors and cardiac β_1-receptors, causing tachycardia. Selectivity for β_2-receptors is relative, however, and some patients develop tachycardia after administration of putative β_2-selective agents. Selective β_2 drugs have essentially no α-adrenergic activity and thus no pressor effect. These agents stimulate skeletal muscle and may induce tremors. They also stimulate glycogenolysis and may produce hypokalemia. Accordingly, such drugs do not cause the pallor that may follow epinephrine administration.

α-Adrenergic receptors have been subclassified into α_1 and α_2 subtypes; these have wide distribution and mediate different effects. Stimulation of α_1-receptors contracts vascular and airway smooth muscle.

Although experiments in vitro with human tissues have shown that adrenergic drugs can inhibit allergen-induced mediator release from mast cells and basophils, their use in allergic disorders depends principally upon their effects on smooth muscle in blood vessels and in the bronchial airways.

For example, stimulation of α-adrenergic receptors reduces edema of nasal mucous membranes through vasoconstriction and decreases the permeability of venules and capillaries, whereas β-adrenergic stimulation causes smooth muscle relaxation, which relieves at least one component of obstruction of the airway in asthma.

Adrenergic drugs include catecholamines (epinephrine, isoetharine, isoproterenol, and bitolterol) and noncatecholamines (ephedrine, albuterol, metaproterenol, terbutaline, pirbuterol, procaterol, and fenoterol). Those of the former group are rapidly inactivated by enzymes found in the gastrointestinal tract and liver; accordingly, the use of epinephrine and isoproterenol is limited largely to injection, inhalation, and topical application to mucous membranes. Ephedrine, the oldest of the noncatecholamine sympathomimetics, has relatively weak β-stimulant activity and frequently causes adverse side effects, including increased activity, insomnia, irritability, and headache. Newer noncatecholamine adrenergic agents (metaproterenol, terbutaline, and albuterol), which may also be given orally, have a somewhat longer duration of action (up to 6 hr) than ephedrine (4 hr), and have relatively selective activity on the β_2 receptors in the airways, with less of the cardiovascular effects of isoproterenol and epinephrine, especially when delivered by inhalation. Since several-fold lower doses of adrenergic drugs are effective when the agents are given by the inhalational rather than the oral route, aerosol administration is preferred wherever possible, in order to minimize adverse side effects.

Autoantibodies against β_2 adrenergic receptors have been identified in small proportions of patients with asthma, a few patients with cystic fibrosis, and a few normal controls. The presence of these autoantibodies has been associated with β-adrenergic hyporesponsiveness. Such autoantibodies may account for some of the abnormalities in autonomic function in some patients with asthma. Tolerance or desensitization to adrenergic agents may occur, but if such agents are used as prescribed, the small decrease in the duration or intensity of drug effect usually has no serious therapeutic implications.

Adverse side effects of adrenergic drugs may include skeletal muscle tremor, cardiac stimulation, worsening of hypoxemia, increased airway obstruction, headache, insomnia, irritability, nausea, vomiting, epigastric pain, flushing, and tolerance (subsensitivity, refractoriness). Metabisulfite, used as a stabilizing agent, may exacerbate bronchoconstriction due to hypersensitivity to this agent. Overreliance on metered-dose adrenergic agents or home aerosolized sympathomimetic drugs may be responsible for delay in seeking medical attention, increasing the risk of morbidity and even mortality.

THEOPHYLLINE. This is a major therapeutic agent for treatment of both acute and chronic asthma. Its mode of action is uncertain. It is no longer held that it inhibits cyclic AMP phosphodiesterase, since the concentrations necessary to demonstrate this effect are toxic in vivo. Moreover, other potent phosphodiesterase inhibitors (e.g., papaverine) are ineffective in asthma. Other possible modes of action include adenosine antagonism, an effect on calcium flux across cell membranes, prostaglandin antagonism, release of or synergistic interactions with β adrenergic agonists, and enhancement of binding of cAMP to a cAMP-binding protein. Theophylline causes bronchodilation by relaxing bronchial smooth muscle, increases concentrations of endogenous catecholamines in the circulation, and enhances the contractility of the fatigued diaphragm. It can inhibit both immediate and late-phase asthmatic responses to allergenic challenge and sometimes reduces bronchial hyperresponsiveness.

Both the therapeutic and toxic effects of theophylline are related to the serum concentration. The incidence of toxic effects increases as the serum levels progressively rise above 20 μg/mL. *Measurement of serum theophylline concentration* is an important element in effective and safe use of the drug. Methods for theophylline analysis are specific, sensitive, rapid, and require only a small serum sample; they should be available in all hospitals. A 15-min method that requires no instrument for determination of theophylline level in finger prick blood (AccuLevel) gives excellent results.

Pharmacokinetics. Both the rapidly absorbed and most (but not all) slow-release (S-R) formulations of theophylline are, for all practical purposes, completely bioavailable. Rapidly absorbed preparations may be given with food without significant effect on rate or extent of absorption, but absorption characteristics of S-R products may be altered when they are administered with a meal and either accelerated or delayed, depending upon the product. Administration of TheoDur tablets, Slo-bid Gyrocaps, or Somophyllin CRT capsules with a meal can delay attainment of peak serum concentrations by 1–2 hr usually with little or no effect on bioavailability. On the other hand, administration of TheoDur Sprinkle with a meal can reduce bioavailability by as much as 50%. Administration of Uniphyl with a meal can almost double the amount of drug absorbed. Administration of Theo-24 with meals may be followed by sudden absorption of nearly half the dose within a 4-hr period at variable times after dosing in some patients. Accordingly, unless the physician wishes to take advantage of the fact that food delays absorption of a specific S-R product (e.g., Theolair-SR), S-R products other than TheoDur tablets, Slo-bid Gyrocaps, and Somophyllin CRT are best given 60 min before meals. The ultraslow release formulations may be incompletely bioavailable when given to patients with rapid gastrointestinal transit times (especially children). The absorption from an S-R product can vary from time to time, even in the same patient, leading to confused interpretation of serum concentration data. Occasionally, a "trough" theophylline level will be higher than that in a specimen drawn at a time thought to represent a "peak" level. Peak serum concentrations usually occur 4–8 hr after administration of most S-R products (6–10 hr after TheoDur, Sustaire, or Uniphyl).

The marketed S-R products differ in theophylline-release characteristics, and care must be exercised in switching from one product to another. Substitution of a generic for a proprietary preparation without the physician's or patient's knowledge is a potential source of problems. Such unauthorized substitution by the pharmacist is legal in most states unless it is specifically forbidden on the prescription.

Despite these limitations, S-R formulations of theophylline represent an advance in dealing with the fluctuations in serum concentrations seen with rapidly absorbed products, particularly in young patients who metabolize the drug rapidly. Even with the S-R products, patients who metabolize theophylline rapidly may have unacceptable fluctuations in serum theophylline level if the drug is given at 12-hr intervals rather than 8-hr intervals. Theophylline absorption is slower during night-time hours; accordingly, administration every 12 hr may produce higher early morning levels than those later in the day. Theophylline salts such as aminophylline (theophylline ethylenediamine) do not improve efficacy and may cause adverse effects due to the development of ethylenediamine hypersensitivity.

Following its absorption, about 60% of theophylline is bound to protein (somewhat less in prematures). Free theophylline is distributed rapidly into body fluids, equilibration between serum and tissues being complete within 1 hr following intravenous injection. Salivary concentrations are about 60% of those in serum. Estimates of serum theophylline concentration derived from analysis of *appropriately collected* saliva samples are accurate enough for most clinical purposes. Theophylline distributes freely into umbilical cord blood, breast milk (not clinically significant for the infant), and cerebrospinal fluid.

TABLE 11–15. Factors that Affect Theophylline Clearance

Factor	Decreased Clearance: Increased Levels	Increased Clearance: Decreased Levels
Disease	Liver disease (cirrhosis, acute hepatitis) Congestive heart failure Acute pulmonary edema Febrile viral respiratory illness Renal failure	Hyperthyroidism Cystic fibrosis
Drugs	Troleandomycin Erythromycin Fluoroquinolones Cimetidine Ranitidine (less than cimetidine) Oral contraceptives Ketoconazole Allopurinol Thiabendazole Propranolol Influenza vaccine	Carbamazepine Phenytoin Rifampin Phenobarbital Terbutaline Isoproterenol (intravenous)
Habits		Smoking (tobacco or marijuana)
Diet	High carbohydrate, low protein Dietary xanthines	High protein, low carbohydrate Charcoal broiled meats

Theophylline is metabolized by biotransformation in the liver via a cytochrome P_{450}-dependent microsomal mixed-function oxidase. Metabolism occurs via both 1st-order (linear) and nonlinear capacity-dependent processes. Some patients show disproportionate dose-dependent changes in theophylline serum concentration, particularly at the higher doses, owing to the nonlinear elimination. About 10–15% of theophylline is excreted unchanged in urine (50% in prematures). There is substantial intersubject variation in the rate of theophylline body clearance. Intrasubject variations in clearance also occur. As with other drugs eliminated by hepatic metabolism, many environmental and disease factors alter the rate of elimination (Table 11–15). Most of the factors listed tend to decrease clearance, with increased theophylline concentration and risk of adverse effect. The clinical relevance of the factors varies: cigarette smoking, hepatic or heart disease, some drugs (macrolide antibiotics, cimetidine, allopurinol, carbamazepine, phenytoin, rifampin) have substantial effects, whereas others are probably of less clinical relevance (phenobarbital, ranitidine, protein/carbohydrate dietary content, ingestion of charcoal-broiled meats). Average theophylline clearance also varies with age, and dosage is based upon this fact (Table 11–16).

Pharmacodynamics. The logarithmic relationship between the theophylline bronchodilator effect and serum concentration in the 5–20 μg/mL range is well documented. The serum concentration that provides optimal bronchodilator effect probably varies from patient to patient. The physician should use the patient's response rather than the theophylline blood level as a guide to increases in dosage, but dosage should not exceed the average doses for the age group without determination of peak serum theophylline concentrations to ensure safety. Some patients receive good bronchodilator effect with serum concentrations less than 10 μg/mL; in such cases, there is no need to increase the theophylline dose.

TABLE 11–16. Average Theophylline Dosage Requirements after the Neonatal Period

Age (yr)	Dose (mg/kg/24 hr)
<1	8 + 0.3 × age in weeks
1–9	24
9–12	20
12–16	16–18
>16	12–13

Initial dosage should be one half to two thirds the average dose for age. Later changes in dosage should be determined by clinical response and guided by serum theophylline determinations.

Toxicity. Theophylline toxicity is a major clinical problem. Signs and symptoms of acute theophylline intoxication vary from mild nausea, insomnia, irritability, tremors, and headache to severe seizures and death. Gastrointestinal symptoms (nausea, vomiting, hematemesis, cramping) are usually the earliest to appear and generally precede the more serious central nervous system (seizures, coma) manifestations of toxicity. Uncommonly, seizures may appear as the first sign of theophylline intoxication. Disturbances in cardiac rate, most often tachycardia, rhythm disturbances (atrial and ventricular premature contractions or tachycardia), and hypotension are commonly observed with serious toxicity. Additional problems include hypokalemia, hyperglycemia, ataxia, and hallucinations. Signs and symptoms of theophylline intoxication are, by and large, serum concentration-dependent, but concentrations associated with symptoms of serious toxicity vary widely. In adults with seizures the mean serum concentration has been reported to be approximately 50 μg/mL with a range of 20–70 μg/mL. Several infants with theophylline-induced seizures have been reported to have very high serum theophylline concentrations (180 μg/mL in one case) with no apparent permanent sequelae. Healthy adolescents who ingest theophylline in suicide attempts may tolerate very high theophylline serum concentrations (over 100 μg/mL) with no permanent sequelae if treated appropriately. On the other hand, children who survive serious theophylline intoxication also may be left with severe brain damage that resembles the sequelae of anoxic encephalopathy.

Treatment of theophylline intoxication should begin with measures designed to induce emesis (e.g., administration of ipecac, if the patient is not already vomiting) or gavage, followed by a slurry of 30 g of activated charcoal to adsorb the theophylline remaining in the gastrointestinal tract. Activated charcoal can also remove serum theophylline that has already been absorbed from the gastrointestinal tract. It may be best to delay administration of charcoal until emesis has occurred when using ipecac to induce emesis, because the charcoal also adsorbs ipecac. After ingestion of S-R theophylline, repeated administration of charcoal at 2–3 hr intervals is advisable. The addition of a nonabsorbed saline cathartic is effective for decreasing intestinal transit time when S-R products have been ingested. Peritoneal dialysis can remove theophylline from intoxicated patients, but hemoperfusion using a specially prepared charcoal column is the method of choice. The indications for charcoal hemoperfusion are not completely defined; they depend both upon the serum concentration and upon clinical considerations. Diazepam is effective therapy for seizures, propranolol is helpful for treating hypotension or supraventricular or ventricular arryhthmias (lidocaine is also effective for ventricular tachycardia), and ranitidine may be helpful in controlling gastric acid-induced emesis.

Chronic theophylline use may produce or exacerbate subtle behavioral changes, such as hyperactivity and sleep disturbances.

ANTIHISTAMINES. These are drugs of diverse chemical structure that compete with histamine for receptors in various tissues. There are two histamine receptors, H_1 and H_2. Initially, only H_1-receptor blockers were used in treatment of allergic disorders. A combination of H_1 and H_2 antagonists, however, may be beneficial in some patients with chronic urticaria and in treatment of anaphylactoid reactions such as those due to intravenous injections of contrast media for urography. Cimetidine and probably ranitidine, H_2 antagonists, inhibit delayed-type hypersensitivity skin responses, suggesting that H_2-receptor blocking agents may modulate cell-mediated immune injury. The H_1-type antihistamines, as a group, are nitrogenous bases with aliphatic side chains that resemble histamine. The side chains are attached to cyclic or heterocyclic rings of various configurations. The antihistamines may be classified as follows:

Type I—ethylenediamines (tripelennamine [Pyribenzamine], methapyrilene [Histadyl]).
Type II—ethanolamines (diphenhydramine [Benadryl], carbinoxamine [Clistin, Rondec]).
Type III—alkylamines (chlorpheniramine [Chlor-Trimeton, Teldrin, Novahistine, Demazin], brompheniramine [Dimetane, Bromfed], triprolidine [Actidil, Actifed]).
Type IV—piperazines (cyclizine [Manezine], meclizine [Bonine]).
Type V—piperidines (cyproheptadine [Periactin], azatadine [Trinalin]).
Type VI—phenothiazines (promethazine [Phenergan]).

Hydroxyzine (Atarax, Vistaril), which has potent antihistaminic activity, does not belong to any of the six types listed. Two antihistaminic agents (terfenadine and astemizole) are effective in suppressing the signs and symptoms of allergic rhinitis, do not cross the blood-brain barrier (because they are lipophobic), and have less sedative effects than other antihistamines. *The antihistamines may be found alone or in combination* with decongestants in the above commercial preparations. The chemical classification of antihistamines does not usually have functional significance and, except for cyproheptadine, which also has antiserotonin activity, drugs from each class have equal activity as antihistamines.

In general, the H_1 antagonists are rapidly absorbed after oral administration, with onset of action within 30 min, peak plasma concentration within 1 hr, and complete absorption within 4 hr. Antihistamines are eliminated by biotransformation in the liver; little nonmetabolized drug is found in urine. Some antihistamines (diphenhydramine and chlorcyclizine) stimulate liver microsomal drug-metabolizing enzymes in animals and may accelerate their own metabolism and that of other drugs. There have been relatively few pharmacokinetic studies of the antihistamines; most of the prescribing patterns are empirically based upon clinical experience. Diphenhydramine (Benadryl) has a relatively short serum half-life of 3–4 hr. Yet the drug is effective in suppressing the wheal and flare response to allergy skin testing for over 24 hr. Thus, with this antihistamine there appears to be little correlation between serum concentration and therapeutic effect in the tissue. A study of chlorpheniramine in children showed a mean serum half-life of 13.7 hr (range 6–34 hr). Significant suppression of clinical symptoms of allergic rhinitis was observed for as long as 30 hr after injection of a single dose, at which time chlorpheniramine was not detectable in the serum. Data indicate that chlorpheniramine, brompheniramine, and hydroxyzine may not need to be given 3 or 4 times a day, but that twice or even once a day may suffice. In addition to histamine antagonism, the antihistamines have pharmacologic effects on exocrine secretions, the central nervous system, and the cardiovascular system. Some have anticholinergic-like side effects (Benadryl), whereas others are sedatives (hydroxyzine); both groups have the potential to produce drowsiness.

Because antihistamines act as competitive antagonists, they are more effective in preventing than in reversing the action of histamine. To be most effective, they must be administered at doses and intervals that keep tissue histamine receptor sites saturated. Histamine is released explosively at the site of an IgE-mediated reaction; accordingly, antihistamines are less potent in antagonizing the effects of endogenous than of exogenous histamine. Their relative inefficacy in patients with asthma is related both to this and to the fact that mediators of bronchoconstriction other than histamine are involved in allergic reactions in the lung. Many antihistamines possess anticholinergic activity, which is valuable in allergic rhinitis for controlling rhinorrhea. Anticholinergic activity may account for the occasional response of asthma to antihistamines. In children antihistamines usually have neither favorable nor deleterious effects on the course of asthma.

There is little reason to choose one antihistamine over another. Ethanolamines and phenothiazines usually have greater sedative effects than alkylamines; accordingly, if excessive sedation is noted, substitution of a drug from another group or of one of the newer nonsedating agents may be helpful. The physician should learn to use one or two of these drugs effectively rather than occasionally use each of a large number of different drugs.

In general, antihistamines are extraordinarily safe, and most are sold without prescription. They can have adverse effects, however, especially in high dosages. The most common side effect is sedation, to which some tolerance develops. Combinations of antihistamines with other central nervous depressants (e.g., alcohol) should be avoided. In high doses or in certain sensitive patients, the anticholinergic properties of antihistamines cause undesirable adverse reactions. These include excitation, nervousness, tachycardia, palpitations, dryness of the mouth, urinary retention, and constipation. Seizures are common in antihistamine poisoning. Skin eruptions, blood dyscrasias, fever, and neuropathy are rarely observed.

CROMOLYN SODIUM (SODIUM CROMOGLYCATE). Cromolyn sodium is the disodium salt of 1,3,-*bis* (2-carboxychromon-5-yloxy)-2-hydroxypropane. It is a chemical analog of the drug khellin, which has smooth muscle-relaxing properties. It is soluble in water but insoluble in lipids; only 1% is absorbed from the gastrointestinal tract. The drug is administered as a powder (Intal) with a special turboinhaler, the Spinhaler, or as a 1% (20 mg/2 mL) solution for nebulization, or by metered dose inhaler (800 μg/actuation). It is used principally in asthma but has some value in allergic rhinitis and conjunctivitis and in vernal conjunctivitis. It has been used with varying results in patients with aphthous ulcers, food allergy, systemic mastocytosis, ulcerative colitis, and chronic proctitis. The drug has no bronchodilator properties; it is not, therefore, effective for treatment of acute asthma but is given prophylactically, in a 20-mg dose 2–4 times/day by Spinhaler or nebulization or 1.6 mg 2–4 times each day by metered dose inhaler. Cromolyn has no antimediator or anti-inflammatory properties. It prevents both antibody-mediated and non-antibody-mediated mast cell degranulation and mediator release (from mast cells recoverable by bronchoalveolar lavage). This effect may be due to the ability of cromolyn to block antigen-stimulated calcium transport across the mast cell membrane. Cromolyn inhibition of histamine release may also occur by regulation of phosphorylation of a mast cell protein. The drug also has weak phosphodiesterase inhibitor activity. Cromolyn appears to reduce airway hyperreactivity by a mechanism that is not yet understood, and it can prevent late-phase asthmatic responses when administered before allergen challenge. It inhibits bronchoconstriction produced by nonimmunologic stimuli such as frigid air, exercise, and sulfur dioxide. Some of these stimuli do not cause release of mast cell-derived mediators; accordingly, cromolyn may directly affect neural control of the airway by inhibiting reflex bronchoconstriction through inhibition of the transmission of neural impulses by myeliniated afferent nerve fibers.

Cromolyn is of greatest value in allergic or extrinsic asthma, but patients with nonallergic or intrinsic asthma who use it may also improve. Patients with mild degrees of asthma respond more favorably than those with severe disease. About 70% of asthmatic patients receive some benefit from inhalation of the drug. The incidence of toxic reactions to cromolyn is extremely low; dry throat and transient bronchoconstriction have been the most frequently reported side effects. The latter is most likely due to inhalation of the dry powder into irritable airways and is not an intrinsic effect of the drug itself. Rare reports have associated urticaria, angioedema, and pulmonary eosinophilia with the use of cromolyn. There are no known contraindications to its use except that in some patients, during an acute attack of asthma, the powder may rarely act as an airway irritant.

Nedrocromil sodium is a pyranoquinoline dicarboxylic acid, chemically remote from cromolyn, which has antiallergic and anti-inflammatory activity. It has promise as a new agent that may effectively inhibit early- and late-phase responses after antigen challenge. Nedrocromil sodium (aerosol) inhibits antigen-, cold-, fog-, or chemically induced bronchoconstriction and reduces bronchial hyperactivity.

CORTICOSTEROIDS. Corticosteroids are the most potent drugs available for treatment of allergic disorders. Following administration of a well-absorbed tablet of prednisone, peak plasma concentration is attained at 1–2 hr. The systemic availability of the drug is more than 80% of the oral dose. Regardless of the route of administration, there is interconversion of prednisone and prednisolone (the active form), with prednisolone concentrations 4–10 times those of prednisone. There is little effect of liver disease or renal insufficiency on the conversion of prednisone to prednisolone or on prednisolone disposition. The volume of distribution, metabolic clearance, and renal clearance of prednisone increase with increasing dose owing to the partially saturable binding of prednisolone to transcortin in plasma, which provides more unbound drug at higher plasma concentrations of this steroid.

Some effects of prednisolone are evident within 2 hr after oral or intravenous administration (fall in peripheral eosinophils and lymphocytes); others may be delayed 6–8 hr or longer (e.g., hyperglycemia and improvement in pulmonary function in asthmatics). The delayed responses reflect the indirect mechanism of action of glucocorticoids. Steps leading to activity include (1) simple diffusion through the cell membrane, (2) binding to cytosol glucocorticoid receptors (found in most mammalian cells), (3) translocation of the steroid-receptor complex to the nucleus, (4) binding of the complex to chromatin, which affects nuclear gene expression, and (5) subsequent synthesis of messenger RNA and proteins with enzyme activity. It is the newly synthesized enzymes that mediate some of the effects of glucocorticoids. The biologic half-life of the steroid is determined by the turnover time of the newly synthesized enzymes, not by steroid plasma concentrations. Plasma half-lives of commonly used steroids vary from 1.5–5 hr, while biologic half-lives vary from 8–54 hr.

Pharmacokinetic studies of prednisolone have shown no differences in distribution, protein binding, plasma clearance, or disposition of unbound drug between males and females or between adults and children. Steroid-dependent asthmatics do not differ from normal individuals in prednisolone binding, distribution, or clearance. Clinically significant drug interactions occur with phenobarbital and phenytoin, both of which increase steroid clearance.

The anti-inflammatory actions of glucocorticoids result from: (1) alteration in leukocyte number and activity (redistribution, suppression of migration to sites of inflammation, decreased response to mitogens, decreased cytotoxicity, and suppression of delayed hypersensitivity responses in the skin); (2) suppression of mediator release (decreased histamine synthesis and release, decreased synthesis of prostaglandins and other products of arachidonic acid metabolism); (3) enhanced response to agents that increase cAMP (PGE_2 and histamine via the H_2 receptor); and (4) enhanced response to catecholamines (increased synthesis of β-adrenergic receptors, increased availability of epinephrine due to decreased extraneuronal uptake of catecholamines). Humoral antibody synthesis is little affected by glucocorticoids in the dosage usually given for treatment of allergic disorders. Chronic corticosteroid administration may lower total immunoglobulin concentrations.

Topical steroids have direct local effects that include decreased inflammation, edema, mucus production, vascular permeability, and mucosal IgE levels. There is also less local accumulation of neutrophils, eosinophils, basophils, and mast cells and an attenuation of mucosal hyperactivity. Topical steroids may reduce early- and late-phase reactions, whereas systemic steroids predominantly inhibit late-phase response to antigen. They reduce but do not eliminate the risk of suppression of the pituitary-adrenal axis. Topical steroids also reduce the other risks of systemic steroids.

The short-term use of *systemic corticosteroids* in self-limited allergic conditions such as contact dermatitis due to poison ivy or occasional episodes of severe asthma is not associated with significant adverse effects. Long-term use, on the other hand, especially if daily administration is required, may have substantial undesirable side effects. In children the most common adverse effect is suppression of linear growth. Posterior subcapsular cataracts develop occasionally in children receiving long-term steroid therapy. Other untoward effects of steroids include osteoporosis (vertebral collapse), hypertension, diabetes mellitus, cushingoid habitus, infections, pancreatitis, gastritis, and myopathy (see also Sec. 6.40).

Before any decision is made to initiate long-term, systemic corticosteroid therapy, all other modalities of management should be tried. Nevertheless, a small proportion of asthmatic children have severe and continuing symptoms that interfere with normal school attendance, play activities, and sports participation. The judicious use of glucocorticoids can produce substantial improvement in such children with little adverse effect, especially if they are administered as prednisone, prednisolone, or methylprednisolone, in single doses on alternate mornings.

A few considerations in the systemic use of corticosteroids bear emphasis. (1) When given in equivalent anti-inflammatory doses, available drugs do not differ qualitatively in anti-inflammatory effects. Adverse effects are related to dose, dosing interval, and duration of treatment. Prednisone or prednisolone is the preferred drug for oral administration, and methylprednisolone or hydrocortisone for intravenous use. Other steroids with longer durations of biologic activity have greater propensities for certain adverse effects, are not suitable for alternate-day therapy, and are more expensive. (2) When corticosteroid therapy is initiated, a sufficient amount should be given in 3–4 divided doses to bring the disease under control. Then an attempt should be made to adjust the dose and the dosing interval to suppress activity of the disease without adverse effects. Whenever possible, alternate-day regimens using prednisone or prednisolone should be tried. In the alternate-day regimen, the drug is given as a single dose every 48 hr between 6:00 and 8:00 A.M.. If daily steroid medication is required, a single dose is given, again between 6:00 and 8:00 A.M.; this regimen mimics endogenous cortisol secretion and causes less suppression of the hypothalamic-pituitary-adrenal axis and fewer other adverse side effects than the same daily dose of drug given in divided doses. When exacerbations of asthma occur during low-dose maintenance therapy, high-dose suppressive therapy in divided dosage is indicated for a few days, with prompt return to low-dose alternate-day treatment as soon as the acute process is under control. (3) Short-term steroid therapy (<7 days) for exacerbations of asthma or poison ivy suppresses the pituitary-adrenal axis only briefly and can be stopped abruptly without tapering the dose. Patients receiving steroids for longer periods require gradual reduction of the dose to avoid precipitating an acute adrenal crisis.

A new generation of *surface-active corticosteroids* is available for aerosol administration to corticosteroid-dependent asthmatics and patients with allergic rhinitis. Their high topical activity often permits adequate control of symptoms at very small doses that have little or no systemic effect. The administration of these compounds to a patient receiving systemic steroids frequently facilitates weaning from chronic systemic steroids. Complications of aerosol topical steroids are few and include candidiasis, dysphonia, and, rarely, subclinical suppression of the pituitary-adrenal axis.

ADDITIONAL PHARMACOLOGIC AGENTS. *Anticholinergic agents* having antimuscarinic activity may be used as adjuvant aerosol therapy for patients with severe asthma. Atropine sulfate or ipratropium bromide can be added to ongoing therapy with sympathomimetic agents and steroids for patients in status asthmaticus. Atropine methylnitrate may have less systemic effect because it is poorly absorbed. The bronchodilation effect of anticholinergic agents is not as great as that of sympathomimetic drugs. Metered dose inhalation therapy has also proved effective in adults with bronchitis.

Ketotifen, a benzocyclohepatathiophine, is an antihistamine with mast cell–stabilizing properties and a leukotriene antagonist. This drug is an antianaphylaxis agent, inhibits IgE-dependent mediator release, and attenuates platelet activating factor–induced bronchoconstriction. Ketotifen is a potentially useful drug, but limited experience with it has been recorded in allergic pediatric patients.

Investigational agents that inhibit 5-lipoxygenase enzyme activity or selectively block leukotriene D_4 receptors improve airflow, suggesting that antagonism of these mediators is a potentially new method of treating asthma.

Calcium channel blocking agents, such as nifedipine, may block bronchoconstriction owing to allergies, exercise, prostaglandin F_2, leukotrienes C_4 and D_4, cold air, histamine, and methacholine. These agents can be given by sublingual, oral, or aerosol routes. There is insufficient experience with calcium channel blockers as a therapy for allergic disorders, and such use remains experimental.

Methotrexate, an immunosuppressant antagonist of folic acid, has anti-inflammatory effects when given in low doses and has been demonstrated to reduce the dose of steroids among adult patients with severe chronic asthma. Methotrexate has also been effective in reducing the dose of steroids in patients with severe psoriasis and rheumatoid arthritis. The long-term risks of methotrexate use in children with severe allergic diseases have not been determined. Methotrexate remains an experimental therapy for older patients with severe steroid-dependent asthma.

Baker MD: Theophylline toxicity in children. J Pediatr 109:538, 1986.
Berman BA: Cromolyn: past, present and future. Pediatr Clin North Am 30:915, 1983.
Cott G, Cherniack R: Steroids and "steroid sparing" agents in asthma. N Engl J Med 318:634, 1988.
Chung K, Barnes P: New drugs. Respiratory and allergic disease I. Br Med J 296:29, 1988.
Editorial: Histamine H_1 and H_2 antihistamines, and immediate hypersensitivity reactions. J Allergy Clin Immunol 63:371, 1979.
Harper TB, Strunk RC: Techniques of administration of metered-dose aerosolized drugs in children. Am J Dis Childr 135:218, 1981.
Fraser CM, Potter PC, Venter JC, et al: Adrenergic agents. *In:* Middleton E Jr, Reed CE, Ellis EF, et al (eds): Allergy: Principles and Practice, 3rd ed. St. Louis, CV Mosby, 1988, pp 636–672.
Morris HG: Mechanisms of action and therapeutic role of corticosteroids in asthma. J Allergy Clin Immunol 75:1, 1985.
Rebuck AS, Gent M, Chapman KR: Anticholinergic and sympathomimetic combination therapy of asthma. J Allergy Clin Immunol 71:317, 1983.
Rossing TH: Methylxanthines in 1989. Ann Intern Med 110:502, 1989.
Sly RM: Textbook of Pediatric Allergy. New Hyde Park, NY, Medical Examination Publishing Co, 1985, pp 97–145, 179–184.

11.39 IMMUNOTHERAPY

IMMUNOLOGIC CHANGES. In the early weeks following the institution of regular injections of ragweed pollen extract, IgE antibody against ragweed pollen antigen increases; as treatment is continued, however, the titer of anti-ragweed IgE antibody decreases. In untreated patients with ragweed hay fever, a rise and a fall of anti-ragweed IgE occur during the year; the rise occurs with the seasonal exposure to ragweed. Injection therapy blunts this anamnestic rise. With continuing treatment, ragweed antibodies of the IgG class ("blocking" or "antigen-binding") appear in the serum; the ultimate titer achieved is related to the quantity of ragweed extract injected but does not necessarily correlate with clinical changes, if any occur.

Immunotherapy also can inhibit histamine release from leukocytes (basophils) on challenge in vitro with ragweed antigen E. Leukocytes from treated individuals require exposure to increased amounts of antigen E in order to release the same amount of histamine as they did prior to therapy. Leukocyte preparations from some treated patients behave as if they have been completely desensitized and do not release histamine upon challenge with ragweed antigen E at any concentration. The basis for this change in cell sensitivity is unknown; it does not appear to be related to titers of either anti-ragweed IgE or IgG. There may be some intrinsic change in receptors for IgE or in the biochemical pathways that cause histamine release. Changes in ratios of helper to suppressor T cells in control of B cells have been reported in experimental animals undergoing immunotherapy, and to a lesser extent in humans. Immunotherapy inhibits the late-phase asthmatic response to allergenic challenge. In animals it is possible both specifically to suppress IgE antibody production and to induce tolerance to certain chemically modified or conjugated antigens.

STUDIES OF EFFICACY. Critical review of placebo-controlled, double-blind studies of treatment of ragweed hay fever by ragweed extract injections indicates that most patients improve with immunotherapy. Data supporting the efficacy of grass and tree pollen and house dust mite immunotherapy in rhinitis induced by these allergens are less substantial, but the results appear similar to those with ragweed. Controlled, randomized, double-blind studies of treatment of asthmatic patients with extracts of ragweed, mountain cedar, house dust mites, and cat allergen have also shown beneficial effects in most patients. In other studies of asthma, most patients have improved after treatment with extracts of grass pollen and certain molds. Partly because of the multiple factors that can trigger asthma (cold, exercise, smoke, cholinergic agents), immunotherapy does not usually cause complete remission of symptoms. Immunotherapy with Hymenoptera venom in patients having anaphylactic sensitivity to such stinging insect venom protects against anaphylaxis upon subsequent sting.

The cost of immunotherapy, its inconvenience, the possibility of making the disease worse, the risk of inducing anaphylaxis, and other factors must be considered. There is no acceptable evidence for efficacy of injection therapy with allergens other than those noted above. Specifically, the injection of danders (dog, horse), most molds, bacterial vaccines, occupational allergens, synthetic antigens, whole insect extracts, or food extracts has not been shown to influence favorably the course of rhinitis, anaphylaxis, or asthma.

INDICATIONS, MATERIALS, AND PROCEDURE. Immunotherapy is indicated in patients suffering from allergic rhinitis, IgE-mediated asthma, or allergy to stinging insects. Atopic dermatitis and food allergy are not improved by immunotherapy. A patient is a candidate for a trial of immunotherapy when good correlation exists between symptoms and exposure to an inhalant allergen that cannot be adequately avoided, when the patient has evidence of IgE-mediated allergy by either in vivo (skin testing) or in vitro testing, and when disabling symptoms are not easily controlled with medication. There should also be a reasonable likelihood of good compliance with the regimen because treatment requires injections of allergenic extracts at regular intervals for several years.

Aqueous extracts are used most commonly. Extracts usually contain many different antigens in addition to the specific allergen. In ragweed pollen the allergen, antigen E, represents 8.5% of the protein extract. Salivary proteins constitute the predominant allergens for patients sensitive to a cat or dog, whereas a single protein in house dust mite feces is responsible for dust hypersensitivity. The cat salivary protein, Fel d1, is spread to the hair during grooming. Alum-precipitated pollen extracts and alum-precipitated pyridine-extracted extracts (Allpyral) do not appear to offer any substantial advantages over aqueous extract therapy. Furthermore, the immunogenicity of one Allpyral extract (ragweed) has been questioned. Allergenic extracts are considered drugs by the FDA, but standards of potency exist for only a few. Some extracts sold in the United States for diagnosis and therapy have been totally lacking in allergenic activity when tested by the RAST inhibition. Some of the antigens in allergenic extracts (e.g., ragweed antigen E) are quite labile. Methods of extraction, antigen, concentration, and storage temperature are all critical factors in determining the activity and shelf life of an allergenic extract. Pollen extracts are being modified in attempts to reduce their allergenicity without reducing their immunogenicity. Allergens polymerized with gluteraldehyde retain their immunogenicity but are less allergenic. Thus, the initial dose of extract may be substantially increased, the maintenance dose can be reached within 2 mo compared with 5–6 mo with conventional therapy, and there is a greatly reduced incidence of local and systemic reactions. Such modified extracts have not yet been approved in the United States.

In practice, immunotherapy with aqueous extracts involves the repeated injection of increasing amounts of extract until the patient reaches an "optimal" maintenance dose. The dose considered optimal is often arbitrary; clinical trials involving ragweed have reported better results with "high-dose" than with "low-dose" treatment. High-dose therapy is possible only when limited numbers of allergens are included in the extract. No more than 10 and preferably fewer than 6 allergens should be included in a single injection. Children tolerate the same doses as adults.

The injections are given 1–3 times/wk until the patient reaches the maintenance dose, usually after 5–6 mo. In the "rush" method of immunotherapy used in Scandinavia, the initial injection period is compressed into a few days with apparently satisfactory results. The interval between injections is then extended to 2, 3, and then 4 wk. If more than 1 wk has elapsed since the last dose, the dose is not increased. If more than 6 wk have elapsed between injections, the subsequent dose is reduced to avoid the possibility of a systemic reaction. There is little reason to continue weekly injections for prolonged periods of time after reaching maintenance dosage. During the course of the initial injections, the patient is observed carefully for evidence of excessive local reactions. Large local reactions may sometimes predict systemic reactions, but this is uncertain. If an extensive local reaction or a systemic reaction occurs, the subsequent dose is reduced and then cautiously increased according to the patient's tolerance. Failure to see a local reaction at any time indicates either that the patient is not allergic to the constituents of the extract or that the extract is inactive. Beneficial results often do not become evident until after 6 mo of therapy. Improvement may continue for several years.

Perennial treatment, in which injections are given throughout the year, is preferred to preseasonal treatment, in which the treatment regimen is renewed each year, beginning several months before the pollen season. During the pollen season the maintenance dose of extract is unchanged except for the patient who develops systemic reactions, presumably due to combined exposure to seasonal and injected allergen. For such patients, the dose may need to be reduced.

The optimal duration of treatment is not known and probably differs from patient to patient. Many allergists believe that if the patient is significantly improved after 3 yr of therapy, it is reasonable to discontinue the injections and observe for recurrence of symptoms. Some children have received "allergy shots" for many years with no evidence that they have been beneficial. Immunotherapy should not be continued if there is no substantial improvement in the condition for which the patient is being treated. Since skin test reactivity changes little during the early years of immunotherapy it is unnecessary to retest the child yearly.

PRECAUTIONS AND ADVERSE REACTIONS. Allergenic extracts should *always* be administered in a physician's office where treatment of a systemic reaction or of anaphylactic shock is readily available. The patient should always remain under observation for at least 30 min after each injection because life-threatening reactions are most likely to occur within this time. Occasionally children will have delayed symptoms; for example, an exacerbation of asthma may occur in the evening of the day on which an injection of extract was given. Rarely, because of distance from a physician's office, it may be necessary to administer allergenic extracts in another setting. Under such circumstances, however, the nonphysician who administers an injection must be prepared to treat a systemic reaction. Except for the possibility of constitutional reactions, no short- or long-term adverse effects of administration of allergenic extracts to children are known.

A re-evaluation of immunotherapy for asthma (Editorial). Am Rev Resp Dis 129:657, 1984.

Current status of allergen immunotherapy. Lancet 1:259, 1989.

Eggleston P: Immunotherapy for allergic respiratory disease. Pediatr Clin North Am 35:1103, 1988.

Hendrix SG: A multi-institutional trial of polymerized whole ragweed for immunotherapy of ragweed allergy. J Allergy Clin Immunol 66:486, 1980.

Sly RM: Textbook of Pediatric Allergy. New Hyde Park, NY, Medical Examination Publishing Co, 1985, p 331.

RESPIRATORY ALLERGY

The respiratory tract is the organ system most frequently affected by allergic disorders during childhood.

11.40 ALLERGIC RHINITIS

Seasonal allergic rhinitis, seasonal pollinosis, and hay fever all describe a symptom complex seen in children who have become sensitized to wind-borne pollens of trees, grasses, and weeds. Estimates indicate that 5–9% of children in unselected samples meet diagnostic criteria. Prevalence increases with age; ragweed hay fever is rarely observed before 4–5 yr of age.

In *perennial allergic rhinitis* the patient has symptoms year round. The causative agents, when they can be identified, are generally allergens to which the patient is exposed more or less continually, though exposure may vary during the year. Indoor inhalant allergens are implicated most often. These include components of house dust, feathers, allergens or danders of household pets and mold spores. In an occasional patient foods cause symptoms of allergic rhinitis. Some patients may be able to ingest certain foods with impunity except during a pollen season, when ingestion causes an aggravation of nasal symptoms.

PATHOPHYSIOLOGY. Inhaled pollens, mold spores, and animal or mite antigens are deposited on the nasal mucosa. Water-soluble antigens diffuse into the epithelium and, in genetically predisposed atopic individuals, initiate the production of local IgE. IgE-stimulated release of mast cell mediators, synthesis of new mast cell mediators, and subsequent recruitment of neutrophils, eosinophils, basophils, and lymphocytes are responsible for the early and late-phase reactions to inhalant allergens. These reactions result in mucus, edema, inflammation, pruritus, and vasodilation. Delayed inflammation may contribute to nasal hyperresponsiveness to nonspecific stimuli, a priming effect.

DIAGNOSIS. The symptoms of allergic rhinitis include sneezing, which is frequently paroxysmal; rhinorrhea, which is often watery and profuse; nasal obstruction; and itching of the nose, palate, pharynx, and ears. Itching, redness, and tearing of the eyes may also occur, causing severe discomfort.

The typical patient with allergic rhinitis presents with bilateral nasal obstruction resulting from boggy edema of the mucous membranes. Frequently, redundant mucosa is piled up on the floor of the nose. The mucous membranes are bluish in hue and rather pale, and there is a clear mucoid nasal discharge. The child often has mannerisms due to itching of the nose or attempts to improve the airway. The child wrinkles the nose (rabbit nose) and may rub it in characteristic ways (allergic salute). Rubbing in an upward direction may lead to a horizontal crease at the junction of the bulbous tip of the nose with the more rigid bridge. Dark circles under the eyes have been attributed to venous stasis resulting from interference with blood flow through edematous nasal mucous membranes. Mouth breathing is common. Fever is unusual except when bacterial sinusitis or otitis media complicates allergic rhinitis.

The diagnosis of allergic rhinitis is substantiated by the finding of a predominance of eosinophils in a smear made of the nasal secretions. A nasal smear is best prepared by having the child blow the nose into wax paper; the mucous sample is then transferred to a glass slide and stained selectively for eosinophils. There is often a personal or family history of eczema or asthma.

DIFFERENTIAL DIAGNOSIS. *Eosinophilic non-allergic rhinitis* occurs mostly in adults. Symptoms are perennial; the mucous membranes are pale, and there may be associated nasal polyps or sinus disease. Eosinophils are found in the nasal smear, but serum IgE levels are normal and allergy skin tests are generally negative. *Primary nasal mastocytosis,* with onset most often in adulthood, presents with perennial nasal blockage and rhinorrhea. Mast cells are found in the nasal smear, and allergy skin tests are negative. *Neutrophilic (infectious) rhinitis* occurs during the early years of childhood when allergic rhinitis is uncommon; there are complaints of chronic rhinorrhea and nasal blockage, mostly during cold weather. Nasal secretions are commonly mucopurulent, and the nasal smear shows neutrophils, bacteria, and debris. A posterior pharyngeal discharge is often present. X-ray studies of the maxillary sinuses frequently show evidence of sinusitis. The condition appears to result from recurrent viral respiratory illnesses complicated by bacterial infections, but the possibility of underlying disease such as humoral antibody deficiency, ciliary dyskinesia, or cystic fibrosis should be considered. *Vasomotor rhinitis* designates a poorly understood disorder, presumably due to an imbalance of autonomic nervous system control of mucosal vasculature and mucous glands, in which symptoms suggest allergic rhinitis but an allergic etiology cannot be identified. Nasal obstruction is the predominant symptom, with minimal itching, sneezing, and rhinorrhea. The obstruction is aggravated by environmental changes in temperature or humidity and by exposure to irritants such as tobacco smoke. The patients do not have eosinophils in their nasal secretions.

Other causes of nasal obstruction include *unilateral choanal atresia* in infants who have a unilateral nasal discharge, *deviated septum, hypertrophy of the adenoids, encephalocele,* and *nasal polyposis.* Nasal polyposis occurs in as many as 20% of children with cystic fibrosis. Fewer than 0.5% of patients in a typical allergy practice have nasal polyps due to allergic rhinitis. Nasal polyposis occurs in *ciliary dyskinesia* (immotile cilia syndrome, Sec. 14.53) and in *immunologic deficiencies.* The syndrome of nasal polyps, asthma, and aspirin intolerance is known as *triad asthma.* A foul-smelling, unilateral purulent, or blood-tinged purulent nasal discharge in a child suggests a *foreign body.* A persistent bloody discharge always suggests *malignancy;* nasal obstruction with epistaxis in a male in late childhood or early adolescence suggests *benign nasopharyngeal fibroma,* also known as *angiofibroma.* Nasal obstruction occurs in *hypothyroidism.* Adolescents may suffer from *rhinitis of pregnancy.* A profuse, clear nasal discharge should suggest *cerebrospinal fluid rhinorrhea,* which can be confirmed by measuring the level of glucose in the fluid. Excessive use of vasoconstrictor nose drops or sprays can lead to *rhinitis medicamentosa,* in which nasal obstruction can be severe. Reserpine can produce marked nasal congestion. Chronic cocaine abuse may produce rhinitis with or without secondary infection or nasal septum perforation. Additional rarer causes of rhinitis-like symptoms include syphilis, diphtheria, Wegener granulomatosis, sarcoidosis, and various malignancies.

Swelling of the mucous membranes of the sinuses frequently occurs with allergic rhinitis in childhood and may be seen in roentgenograms of the involved sinuses, occasionally with fluid levels. The sinuses appear abnormal so often on roentgenography, not only in children with allergic rhinitis but also in those with viral upper respiratory infections and in entirely asymptomatic children, that such examination must be carefully interpreted. Sinus infection may complicate allergic rhinitis; the symptoms generally are nocturnal coughing, fetid breath, and persistent mucopurulent nasal and pharyngeal discharge. Headache and facial pain and swelling are prominent symptoms of sinusitis in older children.

TREATMENT. Treatment of either seasonal or perennial allergic rhinitis includes avoidance of exposure to suspected allergens and irritants, immunotherapy for those who cannot avoid inhalant allergens, and drug therapy.

Avoidance. It is difficult or impractical to avoid exposure to seasonal pollens, but much can be done to eliminate exposure to such indoor inhalant factors as house dust, danders, and molds. Control of house dust, with special attention to the child's bedroom, often ameliorates symptoms in the dust-allergic child. Elimination of exposure to danders and feathers is mandatory for a child with perennial allergic rhinitis when these factors contribute to the symptoms. For the child sensitive to indoor molds, avoidance of damp basements and measures to discourage mold growth in the house frequently are beneficial. These measures include dehumidifiers, air conditioners with efficient filters, and air cleaning devices, either the electronic precipitator type or one containing an HEPA filter. A 1:750 solution of Zephiran chloride is effective in controlling mold growth. In areas that can be closed off, such as damp cellars, volatilization of paraformaldehyde (25–50 g, depending upon the size of the area to be treated) from several open jars is also frequently effective in inhibiting growth of mold. For infants with persistent rhinorrhea and nasal obstruction, dietary elimination of milk, egg, or wheat is rarely helpful unless allergy skin testing or in vitro testing has confirmed food allergy.

Immunotherapy is discussed in Sec. 11.39.

Drug Therapy. Appropriate drugs usually relieve symptoms of allergic rhinitis. *Antihistamines* are useful, especially in the treatment of seasonal allergic rhinitis (Sec. 11.38). It may be necessary to increase the dosage beyond that routinely recommended until relief of symptoms or side effects occurs. Nasal itching, sneezing, and rhinorrhea are usually well controlled by antihistamine therapy, whereas nasal obstruction is relieved to a lesser degree. The major adverse side effect of antihistamine therapy is somnolence, which usually lessens with continued use. Sometimes it requires a change to another class of antihistamine. Nonsedating antihistamines (astemizole, terfenadine) may be substituted in patients who experience undue sedation from conventional agents.

If nasal obstruction is particularly troublesome, a decongestant such as pseudoephedrine or phenylpropanolamine may be administered alone or in combination with an antihistamine. Nose drops or sprays containing sympathomimetic drugs should be avoided except for short-term use; continued use may lead to progressively severe nasal obstruction due to rebound vasodilatation. Treatment of this latter complication requires complete cessation of use of medicated nose drops and the substitution of nose drops of physiologic saline solution.

Cromolyn nasal solution (4%) is useful both in seasonal and in perennial allergic rhinitis. In children with hay fever, use of the nasal spray is best begun before the pollen season. The dose varies from 1–2 sprays in each nostril, 3–6 times/day. As with the powder, cromolyn nasal solution is used prophylactically (Sec. 11.38).

By far the most effective treatment of allergic rhinitis is topical use of *corticosteroids.* Beclomethasone (Vancenase or Beconase) or flunisolide (Nasalide) should be used in children whose nasal symptoms are resistant to antihistamine-decongestant therapy. The initial dosage is usually 1–2 inhalations in each nostril 2–3 times/day. After 3–4 days, as symptoms improve, the dose and frequency of use are reduced until a minimal effective dosage, 1–2 inhalations once or twice each day, is reached and continued as maintenance therapy. Occasionally, temporary use of corticosteroid eye drops is necessary in a child with hay fever and particularly severe eye symptoms. Treatment with 4% cromolyn eye drops (Opticrom) 4–6 times/day is safer and is often effective in preventing symptoms of allergic conjunctivitis. Complications of topical steroids include local burning, irritation, and epistaxis. There is no systemic absorption, and nasal or pharyngeal candidiasis and mucosal atrophy are not problems.

For children who suffer from persistent neutrophilic (infectious) rhinitis with or without sinusitis, a 2-wk course of a broad-spectrum antibiotic (such as amoxicillin) frequently is effective. Nasal irrigation with a warm saline solution using a bulb syringe or with an adaptation of the Water Pik device (1 tsp of salt to a full reservoir of warm water) is helpful symptomatically in patients with nonallergic chronic rhinitis.

Kaliner M, Eggleston P, Mathews K: Rhinitis and asthma. JAMA 258:2851, 1987.

Meltzer EO, Zeiger RS, Schatz M, et al: Chronic rhinitis in infants and children: Etiologic, diagnostic and therapeutic considerations. Pediatr Clin North Am 30:847, 1983.

Mullarkey MF, Hill JS, Webb DR: Allergic and non-allergic rhinitis: Their characterization with attention to the meaning of nasal eosinophilia. J Allergy Clin Immunol 65:122, 1980.

Simons FE: Allergic rhinitis: Recent advances. Pediatr Clin North Am 35:1053, 1988.

Sly RM: Textbook of Pediatric Allergy. New Hyde Park, NY, Medical Examination Publishing Co, 1985, p 168.

11.41 ASTHMA

Asthma is a leading cause of chronic illness in childhood, responsible for a significant proportion of school days lost because of chronic illness. Asthma is the most frequent admitting diagnosis in children's hospitals and results nationally in 5–7 lost school days/yr/child. As many as 10–15% of boys and 7–10% of girls may have asthma at some time during childhood. Before puberty approximately twice as many boys as girls are affected; thereafter, the sex incidence is equal. Asthma can lead to severe psychosocial disturbances in the family. With proper treatment, however, satisfactory control of symptoms is almost always possible. There is no universally accepted definition of asthma; it may be regarded as a diffuse, obstructive lung disease with (1) hyperreactivity of the airways to a variety of stimuli and (2) a high degree of reversibility of the obstructive process, which may occur either spontaneously or as a result of treatment. Also known as *reactive airway disease,* the asthma complex probably includes wheezy bronchitis, viral-associated wheezing, and atopic related asthma. In addition to bronchoconstriction, inflammation is an important pathophysiologic factor; it involves eosinophils, monocytes and immune mediators and has resulted in the alternative designation of *chronic desquamating eosinophilic bronchitis.*

Both large (>2 mm) and small (<2 mm) airways may be involved to varying degrees. Irritability or hyperreactivity of the airways, while not limited to asthmatics, appears to be an intrinsic part of the disease and is present to some degree in all subjects. This hyperresponsiveness manifests itself as bronchoconstriction following exercise; on natural exposures to strong odors or irritant fumes such as sulfur dioxide (SO_2), tobacco smoke, or cold air; and upon intentional exposures in the laboratory to inhalations of histamine or parasympathomimetic agents such as methacholine (Mecholyl). This heightened airway irritability is a sensitive objective indicator of asthma and is present to some degree when patients are asymptomatic, free of abnormal physical findings, and capable of normal findings on spirometry. Airway hyperreactivity relates to the overall severity of the disease. It varies from patient to patient but generally is relatively stable over time in the same patient except for temporary fluctuations; increased reactivity occurs during viral respiratory infections, following exposure to air pollutants and to allergens or to occupational chemicals in sensitized individuals, and following administration of β-receptor antagonists. An acute decrease in airway irritability follows administration of β-receptor agonists, theophylline, and anticholinergics, and decreased irritability follows chronic administration of cromolyn or systemic or inhaled corticosteroids.

Data on the inheritance of asthma are most compatible with polygenic or multifactorial determinants. A child with one affected parent has about a 25% risk of having asthma; the risk increases to about 50% if both parents are asthmatic. However, asthma is not universally present among monozygotic twins. Lability of bronchoconstriction with exercise is concordant in identical twins but not in dizygotic twins. Bronchial lability in response to exercise testing also has been demonstrated in healthy relatives of asthmatic children. A genetic predisposition combined with environmental factors may explain most cases of childhood asthma.

EPIDEMIOLOGY. Asthma may have its onset at any age; 30% of patients are symptomatic by 1 yr of age, whereas 80–90% of asthmatic children have their first symptoms before 4–5 yr of age. The course and severity of asthma are difficult to predict. The majority of affected children have only occasional attacks of slight to moderate severity, managed with relative ease. A minority develop severe, intractable asthma, usually perennial rather than seasonal; it is incapacitating and interferes with school attendance, play activity, and day-to-day functioning. The relationship of age of onset to prognosis is uncertain; most severely affected children have onset of wheezing during the 1st yr of life and family histories of asthma and other allergic diseases (particularly atopic dermatitis). These children may have growth retardation unrelated to corticosteroid administration, chest deformity secondary to chronic hyperinflation, and persistent abnormalities on pulmonary function testing.

The prognosis for young asthmatic children is generally good. Ultimate remission depends partly upon growth in the cross-sectional diameter of the airways. Longitudinal studies indicate that about 50% of all asthmatic children are virtually free of symptoms within 10–20 yr, but recurrences are common in adulthood. In children who have mild asthma with onset between 2 yr and puberty, the remission rate is about 50%, and only 5% develop severe disease. In contrast, children with severe asthma characterized by chronic steroid-dependent disease with frequent hospitalizations rarely improve, and about 95% become adult asthmatics. Whether the hyperirritability of their airways ever disappears is unknown; abnormal responsiveness to methacholine inhalation in former asthmatics has been found as long as 20 yr after symptoms have abated.

Both the incidence and the mortality from asthma have increased during the last 2 decades. The causes of the increased incidence are unknown, but some of the factors associated with the increased mortality have been identified. Patients who develop sudden acute severe asthma episodes and those who have chronic steroid-dependent asthma are at high risk. Additional high-risk factors are an underestimation of the severity of the illness by the patient, family, or physician, leading to a delay in treatment; underuse of steroids; noncompliance with prescribed treatment; family dysfunction and stress; severe atopic disease; and African-American race.

PATHOPHYSIOLOGY. Manifestations of the airway obstruction in asthma are due to bronchoconstriction, hypersecretion of mucus, mucosal edema, cellular infiltration, and desquamation of epithelial and inflammatory cells. Various allergic and nonspecific stimuli, in the presence of hyperreactive airways, initiate the bronchoconstriction and inflammatory response. These stimuli include inhaled allergens (dust mites, pollens, soybean or castor bean proteins), other vegetable proteins, viral infection, cigarette smoke, air pollutants, odors, drugs (nonsteroid anti-inflammatory agents, β-receptor antagonists, metabisulfite, tartrazine), cold air, and exercise.

The pathology of severe asthma includes bronchoconstriction, bronchial smooth muscle hypertrophy, mucus gland hypertrophy, mucosal edema, infiltration of inflammatory cells (eosinophils, neutrophils, basophils, macrophages), and desquamation. Pathognomonic findings include Charcot-Leyden crystals (eosinophil membranes), Curschmann spirals (bronchial mucous casts), and Creola bodies (desquamated epithelial cells).

Newly synthesized and stored mediators are released from local mucosal mast cells following nonspecific stimulation or the binding of allergens to specific mast cell–associated IgE. Mediators such as histamine, leukotrienes C_4, D_4, and E_4, and PAF initiate bronchoconstriction, mucosal edema, and the immune responses (see Sec. 11.35). The early immune response results in bronchoconstriction, is treatable with β_2-receptor agonists, and may be prevented by mast cell stabilizing agents (cromolyn). The late immune response occurs 6–8 hr later, produces a continued state of airway hyperresponsiveness with eosinophilic and neutrophilic infiltration, can be treated and prevented by steroids, and can be prevented by cromolyn.

Obstruction is most severe during expiration because the intrathoracic airways normally become smaller during expiration. Although the airway obstruction is diffuse, it is not entirely uniform throughout the lungs. Segmental or subsegmental atelectasis may occur, aggravating mismatching of ventilation and perfusion (Fig. 11–4). Hyperinflation causes decreased compliance, with consequently increased work of breathing. Increased transpulmonary pressures, necessary for expiration through obstructed airways, may cause further narrowing or complete premature closure of some airways during expiration, thus increasing the risk of pneumothorax. Increased intrathoracic pressure may interfere with venous return and reduce cardiac output, which may be manifested as a pulsus paradoxus.

Mismatching of ventilation with perfusion, alveolar hypoventilation, and increased work of breathing cause changes in blood gases (Fig. 11–4). Hyperventilation of some regions of the lung compensates initially for the higher carbon dioxide tension in blood that perfuses poorly ventilated regions. However, it cannot compensate for hypoxemia while breathing room air because of the patient's inability to increase the partial pressure of oxygen and oxyhemoglobulin saturation. Further progression of airway obstruction causes more alveolar hypoventilation, and hypercapnia may occur suddenly. Hypoxia interferes with conversion of lactic acid to carbon dioxide and water, causing metabolic acidosis. Hypercapnia increases carbonic acid, which dissociates into hydrogen ions and bicarbonate ions, causing respiratory acidosis.

Hypoxia and acidosis can cause pulmonary vasoconstriction, but cor pulmonale due to sustained pulmonary hypertension is not a common complication of asthma. Hypoxia and vasoconstriction may damage type II alveolar cells, diminishing production of surfactant, which normally stabilizes alveoli. Thus, this process may aggravate the tendency toward atelectasis.

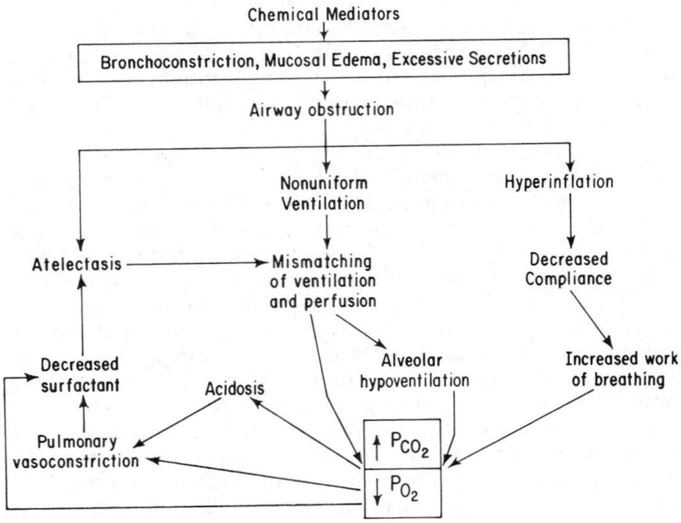

Figure 11–4. The pathophysiology of asthma. (Modified from Siegel SC: Bronchial Asthma. *In*: Kelley VC [ed]: Practice of Pediatrics. Chapter 74, Vol 2. Hagerstown, MD, Harper & Row, 1987.)

ETIOLOGY. Asthma is a complex disorder involving autonomic, immunologic, infectious, endocrine, and psychologic factors in varying degrees in different individuals. The control of the diameter of the airways may be considered a balance of neural and humoral forces. Neural bronchoconstrictor activity is mediated through the cholinergic portion of the autonomic nervous system. Vagal sensory endings in airway epithelium, termed cough or irritant receptors, depending upon their location, initiate the afferent limb of a reflex arc, which at the efferent end stimulates bronchial smooth muscle contraction. Vasoactive intestinal peptide (VIP) neurotransmission initiates bronchial smooth muscle relaxation. VIP may be a dominant neuropeptide involved in maintaining airway patency. Humoral factors favoring bronchodilation include the endogenous catecholamines that act on β-adrenergic receptors to produce relaxation in bronchial smooth muscle. When local humoral substances such as histamine and leukotrienes are released through immunologically mediated reactions, they produce bronchoconstriction, either by direct action on smooth muscle or by stimulation of the vagal sensory receptors. Locally produced adenosine, which binds to a specific receptor, may contribute to bronchoconstriction. Methyxanthines are competitive antagonists of adenosine.

Asthma may be due to abnormal β-adrenergic receptor-adenylate cyclase function, with decreased adrenergic responsiveness. Reports of decreased numbers of β-adrenergic receptors on leukocytes of asthmatics may provide a structural basis for hyporesponsiveness to β-agonists. Alternatively, increased cholinergic activity in the airway has been proposed as a defect in asthma, perhaps due to some intrinsic or acquired abnormality in irritant receptors, which seem in asthmatics to have lower than normal thresholds for response to stimulation. Neither theory reconciles all the data. In individual patients a number of factors generally contribute in varying degrees to the activity of the asthmatic process.

Immunologic Factors. In some patients with so-called *extrinsic or allergic asthma,* attacks follow exposure to environmental factors such as dust, pollens, and danders. Often but not always, such patients have increased concentrations both of total IgE and of specific IgE against the allergen implicated. In other patients with clinically similar asthma, there is no evidence of IgE involvement; skin tests are negative and IgE concentrations low. This form of asthma, which is seen most often in the first 2 yr of life and in older adults (late-onset asthma), has been called *intrinsic.* The distinction between intrinsic and extrinsic asthma may be artificial because the basic immune mediator–induced mucosal injury is similar in both groups. Extrinsic asthma may be associated with more easily identified stimuli of mediator release than intrinsic asthma. Patients of all ages with asthma usually have elevated serum IgE levels, suggesting an allergic-extrinsic component in most patients. Although increased IgE levels may be due to atopy, chronic nonspecific stimulation of the mast cell allergen–induced late-phase immune reactions create a prolonged nonspecific airway hyperreactivity, which can produce bronchospasm in the absence of identifiable extrinsic factors.

Viral agents are the most important infectious triggers of asthma. Early in life respiratory syncytial virus (RSV) and parainfluenza virus are most often involved; in older children rhinoviruses have also been implicated. Influenza virus infection assumes importance with increasing age. Viral agents may act to initiate asthma through stimulation of afferent vagal receptors of the cholinergic system in the airways. An IgE response to RSV can occur in infants and children with RSV-associated wheezing but not in those whose RSV respiratory disease is without associated wheezing. Wheezing with RSV infection may unmask a predisposition to asthma.

Endocrine Factors. Asthma may worsen in relation to pregnancy and menses, especially premenstrually, or may have its onset in women at the menopause. It improves in some children at puberty. Little else is known about the role of endocrine factors in the etiology or pathogenesis of asthma. Thyrotoxicosis increases the severity of asthma; the mechanism is unknown.

Psychologic Factors. Emotional factors can trigger symptoms in many asthmatic children and adults, but "deviant" emotional or behavioral characteristics are not more common among asthmatic children than among children with other chronic disabling illnesses. On the other hand, the effects of severe chronic illness such as asthma on children's views of themselves, their parents' views of them, or their lives in general can be devastating. Emotional or behavioral disturbances are related more closely to poor control of asthma than to the severity of the attack itself; accordingly, skillful medical intervention can have an important impact.

CLINICAL MANIFESTATIONS. The onset of an asthma attack may be acute or insidious. Acute episodes are most often caused by exposure to irritants such as cold air and noxious fumes (tobacco smoke, wet paint) or exposure to allergens or simple chemicals, for example, aspirin or sulfites. When airway obstruction develops rapidly in a few minutes, it is most likely due to smooth muscle spasm in large airways. Attacks precipitated by viral respiratory infections are slower in onset, with gradual increases in frequency and severity of cough and wheezing over a few days. Because airway patency decreases at night, many children have asthma attacks at this time. The signs and symptoms of asthma include cough, which sounds tight and is nonproductive early in the course of an attack; wheezing, tachypnea, and dyspnea with prolonged expiration and use of accessory muscles of respiration; cyanosis; hyperinflation of the chest; tachycardia and pulsus paradoxus, which may be present to varying degrees depending upon the stage and severity of the attack. Cough may be present without wheezing, or wheezing may be present without cough; tachypnea also may be present without wheezing.

When the patient is in extreme respiratory distress, the cardinal sign of asthma, wheezing, may be strikingly absent; in such patients, only after bronchodilator treatment gives partial relief of the airway obstruction can enough movement of air occur to evoke wheezing. Shortness of breath may be so severe that the child has difficulty walking or even talking. The patient with severe obstruction may assume a hunched-over, tripod-like sitting position that makes it easier to breathe. Expiration is typically more difficult because of premature expiratory closure of the airway, but many children complain of inspiratory difficulty as well. Abdominal pain is common, particularly in younger children, and is due presumably to the strenuous use of abdominal muscles and the diaphragm. The liver and spleen may be palpable because of hyperinflation of the lungs. Vomiting is common and may be followed by temporary relief of symptoms.

During a severe attack respiratory effort may be great, and the child may sweat profusely; a low-grade fever may develop simply from the enormous work of breathing; fatigue may become severe. Between attacks the child may be entirely free of symptoms and have no evidence of pulmonary disease on physical examination. A barrel chest deformity is a sign of the chronic, unremitting airway obstruction of severe asthma. Harrison sulci, an anterolateral depression of the thorax at the insertion of the diaphragm, may be present in children with recurrent severe retractions. Clubbing of the fingers is rarely observed in uncomplicated asthma, even in severe cases. Clubbing suggests other causes of chronic obstructive lung disease such as cystic fibrosis.

DIAGNOSIS. Recurrent episodes of coughing and wheezing, especially if aggravated or triggered by exercise, viral infection, or inhaled allergens, are highly suggestive of asthma. However, asthma can also cause persistent coughing in children with no history of wheezing because flow rates are insufficient to generate wheezing, airway obstruction is relatively mild, or caretakers are unable to recognize wheezing. Symptoms may have been ascribed erroneously to "allergic cough," "allergic bronchitis," "wheezy bronchitis," or "chronic bronchitis." Pulmonary function testing before and after administration of methacholine or a bronchodilator or before and after exercise may help to establish the diagnosis of asthma. Examination during an episode of severe symptoms may also be helpful if improvement occurs following bronchodilator therapy. Furthermore, when treated by measures that are specific for asthma, affected children show remarkable improvement, strongly suggesting that the cough is a sign of asthma.

Laboratory Evaluation. *Eosinophilia* of the blood and sputum occurs with asthma. Blood eosinophilia of more than 250–400 cells/mm^3 is usual. Asthmatic sputum is grossly tenacious, rubbery, and whitish. An eosin-methylene blue stain usually discloses numerous eosinophils and the granules from disrupted cells. Few diseases in children other than asthma are likely to cause eosinophilia in sputum. Sputum cultures are generally not helpful in asthmatic children because bacterial superinfection is rare and cultures are frequently contaminated with oropharyngeal organisms. Serum protein and immunoglobulin concentrations are generally normal in asthma except that IgE levels may be increased.

Allergy skin testing and RAST are useful in identifying potentially important environmental allergens (Sec. 11.36).

Inhalation bronchial challenge testing is only rarely done to explore the clinical significance of allergens implicated by skin testing, because the allergenic challenge can provoke a late-phase asthmatic response, the procedure is time consuming, and only a single allergen can be tested at a time. When the diagnosis of asthma is uncertain, testing for hyperresponsiveness to the bronchoconstrictive effect of methacholine or histamine may be helpful in children old enough to cooperate in pulmonary function testing. Methacholine provocative testing should not be performed when baseline pulmonary function is abnormal; the response to bronchodilator therapy is more appropriate.

The response of the asthmatic to *exercise testing* is quite characteristic (Sec. 14.15). Running for 1–2 min often causes bronchodilation in patients with asthma, but prolonged strenuous exercise causes bronchoconstriction in virtually all asthmatic subjects when breathing dry, relatively cold air. Demonstration of this abnormal response to exercise is diagnostically helpful and helps to convince patients and parents of the importance of preventive treatment. Treadmill running at 3–4 miles/hr up a 15% grade while breathing through the mouth for at least 6 min elicits airway obstruction in most patients with asthma, especially if the exercise has caused an increase in pulse rate to at least 180 beats/min. Measurement of pulmonary function immediately before exercise, immediately after exercise, and 5 and 10 min later usually discloses decreases in peak expiratory flow rate (PFR) or forced expiratory volume in 1 sec (FEV_1) of at least 15% without premedication. If exercise causes no airway obstruction, repeat testing on other days when relative humidity is low usually elicits a positive response in patients with asthma. Exercise testing should be deferred whenever significant airway obstruction is already present. If possible, bronchodilators and cromolyn should be withheld for at least 8 hr before testing; slow-release theophylline should not be administered 12–24 hr prior to testing.

Every child suspected of having asthma does not require *roentgenograms of the chest*, but these are often appropriate to exclude other possible diagnoses or complications, such as atelectasis or pneumonia. Lung markings are commonly increased in asthma. Hyperinflation occurs during acute attacks and may become chronic when airway obstruction is persistent. Atelectasis may occur in as many as 6% of children during acute exacerbations and is especially likely to involve the right middle lobe, where it may persist for months. Repeated chest roentgenograms during exacerbations are not indicated in the absence of fever, unless there is suspicion of a pneumothorax, or tachypnea greater than 60 beats/min, tachycardia of more than 160 beats/min, localized rales or wheezing, or decreased breath sounds.

Pulmonary function testing (Sec. 14.15) is valuable in the evaluation of children in whom asthma is suspected. In those known to have asthma, such tests are useful in assessing the degree of airway obstruction and the disturbance in gas exchange, in measuring response of the airways to inhaled allergens and chemicals or exercise (bronchial provocation testing), in assessing the response to therapeutic agents, and in evaluating the long-term course of the disease. Assessments of pulmonary function in asthma are most valuable when made before and after administration of an aerosol bronchodilator, a procedure that indicates the degree of reversibility of the airway obstruction at the time of the testing (Sec. 14.6 and 14.15). An increase of at least 10% in PFR or FEV_1 after aerosol therapy is strongly suggestive of asthma. Failure to respond does not exclude asthma and may be due to status asthmaticus or to near maximal pulmonary function.

In mild cases of asthma in remission, no abnormalities may be detected. In others a variety of abnormalities may be found. Total lung capacity (TLC), functional residual capacity (FRC), and residual volume (RV) are increased. Vital capacity (VC) is usually decreased. Dynamic tests of air flow, forced vital capacity (FVC), FEV_1, PFR, and maximum expiratory flow between 25 and 75% of the vital capacity (FEF_{25-75}) may also show reduced values, which return toward normal after administration of aerosolized bronchodilators. With the availability of small, relatively inexpensive instruments that measure peak expiratory flow rate (Mini-Wright Peak Flow Meter, Healthscan Assess Plus peak flow meter), it is feasible to monitor expiratory flow rate at home 2–3 times each day. This provides objective measurements of the degree of airway obstruction between office visits. A fall in peak expiratory flow predicts the onset of an exacerbation and encourages early intervention with additional drug therapy.

Determination of arterial blood gases and pH is important in evaluation of the patient with asthma during an exacerbation requiring hospitalization. During remission, Po_2, Pco_2, and pH may be normal. In symptomatic periods, low Po_2 is regularly found and may persist days to weeks after an acute episode is over. Pco_2 is generally low during the early stages of an asthmatic attack. As the obstruction worsens, Pco_2 rises; this is an ominous sign. Blood pH remains normal (or sometimes slightly alkalotic owing to hyperventilation) until the buffering capacity of the blood is exhausted, and then acidosis develops. As airway obstruction and hypoxia become more severe, a mixed respiratory and metabolic acidosis develops owing to hypercarbia and lactic acidosis, respectively.

DIFFERENTIAL DIAGNOSIS. Most children who have recurrent episodes of coughing and wheezing have asthma. Other causes of airway obstruction include congenital malformations (of the respiratory, cardiovascular, or gastrointestinal systems), foreign bodies in the airway or esophagus, infectious bronchiolitis, cystic fibrosis, immunologic deficiency disease, hypersensitivity pneumonitis, allergic bronchopulmonary aspergillosis, and a variety of rarer conditions that compromise the airway, including endobronchial tuberculosis, fungal diseases, and bronchial adenoma (Table 11–17). Very rarely in the United States, tropical eosinophilia and other parasitic infections may involve the lung and mimic asthma.

TABLE 11–17. Differential Diagnosis of Childhood Asthma

Disease	Comment
Infections	
Bronchiolitis (RSV)	Atopic individuals may have predisposition to wheeze with RSV
Pneumonia	Acute febrile illness
Croup	Barking cough, stridor, more than wheezing
Tuberculosis, histoplasmosis	Lymphadenopathy compresses bronchi with wheezing
Bronchiectasis	Congenital, acquired, 1st- or 2nd-degree infections
Bronchiolitis obliterans	Postinfections process (influenza, adenovirus, measles)
Bronchitis	Probably asthma
Anatomic, Congenital	
Cystic fibrosis	Persistent symptoms, clubbing, *Streptococcus aureus, Pseudomonas aeruginosa, P. cepacia*
Vascular rings	Associated esophageal abnormalities
Dysmotile cilia syndrome	Chronic, recurrent infections, situs inversus
B lymphocyte immune defect	Recurrent sinopulmonary infection
Congestive heart failure	Murmur, large left to right shunt
Laryngotracheomalacia	Stridor, noisy respirations from birth
Tumor, lymphoma	Bronchial obstruction
Repaired tracheoesophageal fistula	Patients have increased risk of reflux and wheezing, possibly asthma
H-type tracheoesophageal fistula	Rare, difficult to diagnose, recurrent aspiration pneumonia from birth
Gastroesophageal reflux	May also exacerbate true asthma
Vasculitis, Hypersensitivity	
Allergic bronchopulmonary aspergillosis	Marked eosinophilia, high serum IgE levels. Sputum positive for aspergillosis
Allergic alveolitis, hypersensitivity pneumonia	Reaction to foreign antigen (fungi, bird protein, plants); occupational
Churg-Strauss	Allergic angiitis and granulomatosis, eosinophilia
Periarteritis nodosa	Multisystem (kidney, lung, nerves), eosinophilia
Other	
Foreign body aspiration	Sudden cough, gagging, *localized* wheezing and diminished breath sounds
Pulmonary thromboembolism	Acute chest pain, hypoxia
Psychogenic cough	Absent during sleep
Sarcoidosis	Lymphadenopathy induced bronchial obstruction
Bronchopulmonary dysplasia	History of prematurity, may predispose to asthma

ASTHMA IN EARLY LIFE. Wheezing in the infant merits special mention because it is common and presents substantial diagnostic and therapeutic problems. A significant number of children subsequently shown to have asthma have had symptoms of obstructive airway disease early in life (30% under 1 yr of age and 50–55% under 2 yr of age).

A number of anatomic and physiologic peculiarities of early life predispose to obstructive airway disease: (1) a decreased amount of smooth muscle in the peripheral airways compared to adults may result in less support; (2) mucous gland hyperplasia in the major bronchi compared to adults favors increased intraluminal mucus production; (3) disproportionately narrow peripheral airways up to 5 yr of age result in decreased conductance relative to adults and render the infant and young child vulnerable to disease affecting the small airways; (4) decreased static elastic recoil of the young lung prediposes to early airway closure during tidal breathing and results in mismatching of ventilation and perfusion and hypoxemia; (5) highly compliant rib cage and mechanically disadvantageous angle of insertion of diaphragm to rib cage (horizontal vs oblique in the adult) increase diaphragmatic work of breathing; (6) decreased number of fatigue-resistant skeletal muscle fibers in the diaphragm leave the diaphragm poorly equipped to maintain high work output; and (7) deficient collateral ventilation with the pores of Kohn and the Lambert canals deficient in number and size. The infant and young child are therefore predisposed to the development of atelectasis distal to obstructed airways. The combination of the above factors with the normal susceptibility of infants and children to viral respiratory infections renders this age group particularly vulnerable to lower respiratory tract obstructive disease.

The clinical, roentgenographic, and blood gas findings in asthma and bronchiolitis are quite similar. It is helpful to remember that the incidence of bronchiolitis due to respiratory syncytial virus peaks during the first 6 mo of life, principally during the cold weather months, and that second and third attacks are uncommon. Some clinicians have proposed using the response to epinephrine to help decide whether an episode is asthma or bronchiolitis, with a favorable response favoring asthma. The validity of this test has not been established; the degree of response may be related more to the severity of the obstructive process than to its underlying nature. Trials of epinephrine or other bronchodilators are worthwhile, however, as will be discussed below.

The onset of symptoms is rather typical. Previously well infants or young children develop what may seem to be a cold with rhinorrhea, rapidly followed by irritability, cough, tachypnea, and wheezing. The symptoms may progress rapidly and often require hospitalization.

During infancy, respiratory tract infections with viruses or *Chlamydia* may cause symptoms of airway obstruction that can be confused with asthma. Bacterial infections of the lower airway are rare, and the concept that allergic reactions to bacteria cause asthma is unproved. A child with recurrent episodes of coughing and wheezing associated with bacterial infections should be investigated for cystic fibrosis or immunologic deficiency. Chronic aspiration due to swallowing dysfunction (usually in developmentally delayed children) or to gastroesophageal reflux also may cause recurrent cough and wheezing in early life. Symptoms of respiratory distress often occur with or shortly after feeding, and a chest roentgenogram is commonly abnormal. Rarer causes of obstructive airway disease in early life include obliterative bronchiolitis (usually a sequela of a severe viral insult, most often adenovirus) and bronchopulmonary dysplasia (see Table 11–17).

The role of food allergy as a major cause of obstructive airway symptoms during early life is controversial. Positive skin tests for IgE-mediated sensitivity to foods are very unusual in asthmatic infants, but when present, they indicate the need for temporary elimination of the suspected food, usually milk, wheat, or egg from the diet of the asthmatic patient. After elimination from the diet for 3 wk, challenge with the implicated food may be appropriate to confirm the clinical relevance of the positive skin test. Challenge may be necessary 2 or 3 times after temporary dietary elimination to ensure clinical relevance. Challenge is contraindicated in patients with a history of anaphylaxis after ingestion of the food. Comfirmed food allergy indicates a need for dietary elimination for at least 6 mo (Sec. 11.36).

For an infant who has had several episodes of obstructive airway disease, a history of asthma, hay fever, or atopic dermatitis in mother, father, or siblings is an important predictor of subsequent obstructive airway problems. Eczema is also frequently associated with the subsequent appearance of asthma. Eosinophilia greater than 400 cells/mm^3 (and especially greater than 700 cells/mm^3) and high serum IgE concentrations predict continuing respiratory tract problems.

TREATMENT. Asthma therapy includes basic concepts of avoiding allergens, improving bronchodilation, and reducing mediator-induced inflammation. Systemic or topical inhaled medications are used, depending upon the severity of the episode. The principles of avoidance of allergens outlined under treatment of allergic rhinitis also serve the child with asthma. The hyperreactivity of the asthmatic airway as an additional factor is dealt with by minimizing exposure to nonspecific irritants such as tobacco smoke, smoke from wood-burning stoves, and fumes from kerosene heaters and to strong odors such as wet paint and disinfectants, and by avoiding ice cold drinks and rapid changes in temperature and humidity. Maintenance of humidified air is important in dry, cold climates in the winter, but relative humidity should not exceed 50% because house dust mites thrive at higher humidity. If the clinical history suggests IgE-mediated sensitivity to inhalant factors that cannot be avoided or can be only partially avoided, immunotherapy should be considered; its indications and evidence for its efficacy in asthma are discussed in Sec. 11.39.

Pharmacologic therapy is the mainstay of treatment of asthma. Oxygen administered by mask or nasal prongs at 2–3 L/min is indicated in most children during an acute attack of asthma. Not only is the Po_2 reduced during an acute episode, but drugs used in therapy (β-adrenergic agonists or intravenous aminophylline) may cause a transient fall in Po_2 secondary to worsening of ventilation-perfusion mismatching, which occurs because these agents cause pulmonary vasodilatation and increased cardiac output. Injection of epinephrine had been the treatment of choice for acute asthma for many years, but bronchodilator aerosols are now preferable.

When epinephrine is used, a dose of 0.01 mL/kg of the 1:1,000 (1.0 mg/mL) concentration of the aqueous preparation may be given. It may be necessary to repeat the same dose once or twice at intervals of 20 min to obtain optimal relief. In infants and small children a dose of 0.05 mL is often effective. The unpleasant side effects of epinephrine (pallor, tremor, anxiety, palpitations, and headache) can frequently be minimized if doses of no more than 0.3 mL are given at any age. Terbutaline, a more selective β_2 agonist (Sec. 11.38), is available in an injectable form and is an alternative to epinephrine. The usual dose of 0.01 mL/kg of the 1:1,000 (1 mg/mL) concentration does not cause peripheral vasoconstriction and has a longer duration of activity, up to 4 hr. The maximum dose of terbutaline by subcutaneous injection is 0.25 mL; this dose may be repeated once if necessary after 20 min.

Inhalation of bronchodilator aerosols is rapidly effective in relieving the signs and symptoms of asthma. Aerosols have the advantage that substantially less drug is given than would be required by the subcutaneous route; the unpleasant side effects of injected drugs such as epinephrine are avoided. Furthermore, despite airway obstruction, which may limit aerosol deliverance to peripheral airways, aerosol therapy is probably more effective than epinephrine in reversing bronchoconstriction. Albuterol (Proventil, Ventolin) solution is safe and effective at a dose of 0.15 mg/kg (maximum 5 mg) followed by 0.05–0.15 mg/kg at intervals of 20–30 min until response is adequate. Albuterol is available as a 0.5% solution (5 mg/mL) to be diluted with 2–3 mL normal saline and as a prediluted 2.5-mg unit dose, 0.083% (0.83 mg/mL). Nebulization with oxygen at 6 L/min prevents hypoxemia that might be related to the treatment.

If the response to epinephrine or bronchodilator aerosol is not satisfactory, aminophylline may be given intravenously in a dose of 5 mg/kg for 5–15 min at a rate no greater than 25 mg/min. This dose (which will increase the serum theophylline concentration by no more than 10 μg/mL at the peak) is safe in the patient who has had no theophylline in the past few hours. If there is reason to believe that the patient may already have a significant serum theophylline concentration, the intravenous dose should be held until the theophylline level is known. Thereafter, a theophylline dose of 1 mg/kg should increase the serum level by about 2 μg/mL. There is little additional benefit to be gained from adding theophylline to optimal β_2 aerosol therapy, but this combination is associated with an increased incidence of toxicity.

Most acute exacerbations of asthma respond to this treatment regimen. Unless the patient either is corticosteroid dependent or has had corticosteroids in the recent past, administration of steroids as part of the emergency room treatment program is unnecessary. In borderline cases, however, when the decision is made to send the child home rather than to hospitalize him or her, a prescription of prednisone in decreasing doses over 5–7 days may hasten resolution of the exacerbation and causes no harm. The patient should be discharged from the emergency room with sufficient oral medication to continue therapy at home, and appropriate arrangements should be made for follow-up. Good ambulatory management will almost always reduce the need for emergency room visits for acute attacks. Overall, 70% of children treated in the emergency room remain well at home; however, 10–20% experience relapse within 10 days, and 15–20% are hospitalized. Steroid therapy reduces the relapse and hospitalization rates.

Status Asthmaticus

If a patient continues to have significant respiratory distress despite administration of sympathomimetic drugs and theophylline, the diagnosis of status asthmaticus should be considered. Status asthmaticus is a clinical diagnosis defined by increasingly severe asthma that is not responsive to drugs that are usually effective. High-risk factors for severe status asthmaticus and for death due to asthma are listed in Table 11–18. A patient in whom the diagnosis is made should be admitted to a hospital, preferably to an intensive care unit, where the condition can be carefully monitored. A respiratory score should be determined initially (Table 11–19) and monitored at regular intervals. An indwelling arterial line may be indicated. Baseline complete blood count and serum electrolytes should be measured. Since hypoxemia and acid-base disturbances predispose to cardiac arrhythmias and potentially cardiotoxic drugs (theophylline, adrenergics) will be used, cardiac monitoring is almost always indicated. Analysis of arterial blood for Po_2, Pco_2, and pH is also indicated. For these determinations well-arterialized capillary blood is adequate but less desirable than arterial blood, particularly if the patient has received epinephrine, which constricts the peripheral vascular bed.

TABLE 11–18. Factors Associated with Risk of Severe Status Asthmaticus

History
Chronic steroid-dependent asthma
Prior intensive care admission
Prior mechanical ventilation for asthma
Recurrent visits to emergency unit in past 48 hr
Sudden onset of severe respiratory distress
Poor compliance with therapy
Poor recognition by patient, family, or physician, of severity of attack
Family dysfunction, crisis
Respiratory arrest
Hypoxic seizures, encephalopathy

Physical Examination
Pulsus paradoxus >20 mm Hg
Hypotension, tachycardia, tachypnea
Cyanosis
1–2 word dyspnea
Lethargy
Agitation
Sternocleidomastoid, intercostal, suprasternal retractions
Poor air exchange (e.g., quiet chest with severe distress)

Laboratory Tests
Hypercarbia
Hypoxia with supplemental oxygen
FEV_1 <30% expected; no improvement 1 hr after aerosol therapy
Chest x-ray (pneumothorax, pneumomediastinum)

Therapy
Over-reliance on aerosol, inhaler therapy
Delayed use of systemic corticosteroids
Sedation
Delayed admission to hospital or intensive care unit

Patients in status asthmaticus are hypoxemic. Oxygen in carefully controlled concentrations is therefore always indicated to maintain tissue oxygenation. In the presence of hypercapnia, particular care should be taken to administer oxygen continuously and not intermittently. It may be administered very effectively by nasal prongs or mask at a flow rate of 2–3 L/min. A concentration of oxygen sufficient to maintain a PaO_2 of 70–90 mm Hg is optimal. A mist tent should not be used; the water does not reach the lower airway to any significant extent, and mists have an irritant effect on the airways of many asthmatics, leading to coughing and worsening of the wheezing. Furthermore, it is not possible to observe a patient who is enveloped in a dense fog.

Dehydration may be present, owing to inadequate fluid intake, greatly increased insensible water loss due to tachypnea, and the diuretic effect of theophylline. Care should be taken not to overhydrate the patient because increased secretion of antidiuretic hormone occurs during status asthmaticus, promoting fluid retention, and because the large negative peak-inspiratory pleural pressures that occur in children favor accumulation of fluid in the interstitial spaces around the small airways. No more than 1–1.5 times maintenance levels of fluid should be given usually. Sodium bicarbonate, 1.5–2 mEq/kg, should be administered every 4–6 hr or more often if the arterial pH is less than 7.3 and serum sodium is less than 145 mEq/L. Because β_2 adrenergic agents may produce hypokalemia, potassium should be added to the intravenous solution after the patient voids.

Bronchodilator sympathomimatic aerosol therapy initiated in the emergency room should be continued. Aminophylline, 4–5 mg/kg, should be given intravenously over 20 min every 6 hr. Alternatively, a 5 mg/kg loading dose followed by constant infusion in a dose of 0.75–1.25 mg/kg/hr may be administered. If the patient has received aminophylline intravenously in the emergency room, the loading dose should be omitted. It is essential to adjust the aminophylline dose by monitoring serum theophylline concentrations, since there are many physiologic derangements that occur during the course of status asthmaticus that may affect the disposition of theophylline. If the every 6-hr regimen is used, serum samples should be obtained 1 hr after the intravenous injection and just before the next dose. During constant infusion, theophylline concentration should be monitored at least at 1, 12, and 24 hr as a basis for dose adjustments. A steady-state serum concentration of approximately 12–15 μg/mL should be sought. Because age affects theophylline kinetics, the starting dose for a continuous infusion varies as follows: 0.5 mg/kg/hr at 2–6 mo, 0.9 mg/kg/hr at 6–11 mo, 1–1.5 mg/kg/hr at 1–9 yr, and 0.8 mg/kg/hr over 10 yr of age. Adrenergic drugs are best administered by aerosol as previously described. Administration of β agonists by inhalation at intervals of 20 min or continually is safer than administration by intravenous infusion and is probably equally effective.

Treatment with an antimuscarinic such as atropine sulfate given in combination with a nebulized β agonist can be more effective than treatment with either alone, although the peak bronchodilation from atropine is reached more slowly than that of the β agonist. Nebulization of atropine sulfate at doses of 0.05–0.1 mg/kg is safe for most children, but maximal doses of 0.025 mg/kg may be more appropriate for adolescents and adults because of the possible side effects, including tachycardia and mental confusion. Inhalation of nebulized atropine is usually safe at intervals of 4 hr.

Ipratropium bromide causes fewer side effects than atropine. Nebulization at doses of 0.25 mg every 6 hr is safe for children at least 6 yr old, and 0.5 mg every 6 hr is safe for children older than 12 yr.

Corticosteroids, such as methylprednisolone (Solu-Medrol), 1 mg/kg every 4–6 hr, should be administered. Because it has less effect on mineral metabolism when given in high doses and a lower cost for an equivalent anti-inflammatory dose, methylprednisolone is preferable to hydrocortisone. Corticosteroids can sometimes reverse tolerance to β agonists within 1 hr, but maximal effects of steroids are usually delayed for 6 hr. Steroids improve oxygenation, decrease airway obstruction, and shorten the time needed for recovery.

Treatment is guided by serial measurement of blood gases

TABLE 11–19. Clinical Scoring System for Children with Status Asthmaticus*

	0	1	2
PaO_2 (mm Hg) or	70–100 in room air	≤70 in room air	≤70 in 40% O_2
Cyanosis	None	In room air	In 40% O_2
Inspiratory breath sounds	Normal	Unequal	Decreased or absent
Use of accessory muscles of respiration	None	Moderate	Maximal
Expiratory wheezing	None	Moderate	Extreme or none because of poor air exchange
Cerebral function	Normal	Depressed or agitated	Comatose

*Modified from Wood DW, et al: A clinical scoring system for the diagnosis of respiratory failure. Am J Dis Child 123:227, 1972. Copyright 1972, American Medical Association.

Total score of 5 suggests impending respiratory failure. Score of 7 with arterial PCO_2 ≥65 mm Hg indicates respiratory failure.

and pH every few hours, or more often if indicated. If gas and pH analysis both indicate that respiratory failure is impending, an anesthesiologist should be alerted, and facilities and equipment should be available for tracheal intubation and respiratory support.

Mechanical ventilation should be anticipated; elective tracheal intubation with valium, vecuronium, and atropine premedication is safer than emergency intubation. Respiratory care should include patient paralysis on a volume-cycled ventilator with short inspiratory and long expiratory times, a 10- to 15-mL/kg tidal volume, 8–15 breaths/min, and peak pressures of less than 60 cm H_2O. The goals are to improve oxygenation, maintain P_{CO_2} between 40 and 60 mm Hg, and avoid barotrauma. Positive end-expiratory pressure (PEEP) is added in the recovery phase to prevent atelectasis. Sedation during mechanical ventilation may be accomplished with valium, versed, or ketamine (which at doses of 1–2.5 mg/kg/hr is a sedative-analgesic-anesthetic with bronchodilator activity). Halothane anesthesia produces prompt bronchodilation but is difficult to administer in an intensive care unit. It should be reserved for the most severe cases of status asthmaticus.

Sedation of nonventilated patients with status asthmaticus is hazardous. Tranquilizers, morphine, and other opiates are also contraindicated because of their depressant effects on the respiratory center. The best sedative for the patient is the presence of a competent, compassionate physician and nurse at the bedside and decreased airway obstruction with relief of hypoxia and hypercarbia. Chest roentgenograms should be obtained in all severe cases and repeated as indicated to detect complications such as mediastinal emphysema or pneumothorax. Routine administration of antibiotics has not been shown to alter the course of status asthmaticus in children or to reduce the incidence of infectious complications.

Daily Management of the Asthmatic Child

On the basis of the history, physical examination, laboratory data, pulmonary function testing, and need for medication, patients may be classified as having mild, moderate, or severe asthma. The daily management of these different degrees of illness varies (Sec. 11.38).

MILD ASTHMA. Children with mild asthma have attacks of varying frequency, up to once each week, that are not severe and respond to bronchodilator treatment within 24–48 hr. Generally, medication is not required between attacks when the child is essentially free of symptoms of airway obstruction. Children with mild asthma have good school attendance, good exercise tolerance, and little or no interruption of sleep by asthma. They have no hyperinflation of the chest; their chest roentgenograms are essentially normal. Pulmonary function testing may show mild, reversible airway obstruction, with little or no increase in lung volume.

MODERATE ASTHMA. Children with moderate asthma have symptoms more frequently than those with mild disease and often have cough and mild wheezing between more severe exacerbations. School attendance may be impaired, exercise tolerance will be diminished because of coughing and wheezing, and the child may lose sleep at night, particularly during exacerbations. Such children will generally require continuous rather than intermittent bronchodilator therapy to achieve satisfactory control of symptoms and may require continuous treatment with cromolyn or an inhaled corticosteroid to reverse bronchial hyperresponsiveness. Hyperinflation may be evident clinically and roentgenographically. Signs of airway obstruction on physiologic testing are more marked than in the mild group; lung volumes may be increased.

SEVERE ASTHMA. Children with severe asthma have virtually daily wheezing and more frequent and more severe exacerbations; they require recurrent hospitalization, which is rarely required for mild or moderate asthma. Severely affected children may miss significant amounts of school, have their sleep interrupted often by asthma, and have poor exercise tolerance. They have chest deformities due to chronic hyperinflation which is evident on roentgenograms. Bronchodilator medication will be required continuously, and regimens may include the regular systemic or aerosol administration of corticosteroids. Physiologic testing will show more severe airway obstruction than in mild or moderate asthma, less reversibility in response to aerosol bronchodilators, and more severe disturbances of lung volumes.

Children with mild asthma should receive bronchodilator medication only when symptomatic, and most exacerbations may be satisfactorily treated with adrenergic agents, preferably by aerosol (albuterol, metaproterenol, terbutaline, pirbuterol, or bitolterol), or, rarely, by injection (aqueous epinephrine, terbutaline). Use of a chamber such as an AeroChamber or InspirEase enhances delivery of drug to the lower airways when a metered dose inhaler is used by younger children who are unable to coordinate actuation of the inhaler with inhalation. Such chambers permit effective administration of β-agonists from metered dose inhalers to children as young as 3 yr of age. Slow inhalation also increases delivery to the lungs because a rapid inhalation causes impaction of drug particles in the pharynx. Breath holding for up to 10 sec after inhalation of the drug also favors deposition in the lungs. When moderate or severe airway obstruction is present, nebulization with an air compressor such as the DeVilbiss No. 561 Pulmo-Aide is often more effective than use of a metered dose inhaler with a chamber. Nebulization with such a compressor permits effective delivery of aerosols even to infants. β-Agonist liquids for oral administration are also available for treatment of infants and young children. Theophylline may be added to an oral regimen when indicated. Drug therapy usually can be discontinued after a few days. Exercise-induced asthma is most effectively prevented by inhalation of an adrenergic drug immediately before exercise. Inhalation of cromolyn shortly before exercise is also effective in preventing exercise-induced asthma.

For children with moderate asthma who require round-the-clock therapy, two inhalations of an adrenergic aerosol every 4–6 hr often suffices. Theophylline may be added. Dose and dosing regimen should be individualized. Some experienced allergists reserve monitoring for those patients who fail to show a favorable bronchodilator response or who have symptoms of toxicity (gastrointestinal or central nervous system) with average dosages. When slow-release (S-R) formulations of theophylline are used, the peak plasma concentration (assuming that a constant fraction of drug is absorbed, which may not be the case) occurs 4–8 hr after the dose, at which time a blood sample for monitoring should be obtained. Peak concentration may not occur until 12 hr after a bedtime dose of an S-R preparation because of delayed nocturnal absorption. Blood sampling should be delayed until after a day or so of therapy with S-R drugs to assure that a steady state has been achieved. Some children can be treated successfully on an every-12-hr schedule, but others metabolize theophylline particularly rapidly and experience marked fluctuations in serum concentration. These peaks and troughs of concentration are minimized by dividing the 24-hr dose into equal 8-hr doses.

Younger children (aged 1–9 yr) generally eliminate theophylline more rapidly than older children and adolescents and hence require a higher daily dose on a mg/kg basis. Nonetheless, it is safest to begin with a dose of 14–16 mg/kg/24 hr in most children. If this dose is well tolerated, one may increase by 25% increments at 3- to 4-day intervals to average doses for age as necessary to control symptoms (see Table 11–20). If adequate control of symptoms is not achieved at the maximum doses or if adverse effects become evident, adjustment in the dosing regimen must be guided by determination of the serum theophylline concentration.

Rapidly absorbed liquids and uncoated tablets, while suitable for children with mild asthma who require a few days of therapy for an exacerbation, have no place in the therapeutic regimen of children who require round-the-clock theophylline therapy because wide fluctuations in serum theophylline concentrations are observed when rapidly absorbed products are used. Which of the S-R products to use depends upon the dosage form (tablet vs capsule) and the amount of drug needed (Table 11–20). Capsule formulations that can be opened are virtually tasteless, should not be chewed, may be mixed with *moist* food, and are particularly suitable for young children. Crushing a slow-release tablet destroys its constant release properties. Exacerbations of asthma in patients receiving round-the-clock theophylline medication should be treated with adrenergic drugs, as described earlier for children with mild asthma.

Cromolyn powder inhaled 4 times/day from a Spinhaler or cromolyn aerosol delivered by a metered dose inhaler is useful in children with mild to moderate asthma. A solution of cromolyn is available for home nebulization regimens for young children subject to recurrent attacks of asthma. Cromolyn and albuterol or metaproterenol solutions may be mixed together in the nebulizer for ease of administration.

In certain children with moderate asthma, significant flareups occur from time to time that may require the use of corticosteroids for a few days. Early use of steroids in the child who is known to become severely ill may reduce the need for hospitalization. Early intervention with bronchodilator drugs (with or without steroids, depending upon the clinical setting) is important in the management of all asthmatic children, regardless of the severity of their conditions. Steroids should be given in adequate doses (1–2 mg/kg/24 hr of prednisone or prednisolone in 2–3 doses) and should be discontinued as quickly as possible, for example, within 5–7 days; a long "weaning" period following an acute attack of asthma is unnecessary. In patients who only rarely require steroid administration, return of normal hypothalamic-pituitary-adrenal function is hastened by the *prompt* discontinuation of the drug when the acute episode is over. Inhaled topical steroid preparations are also effective for children with moderately severe asthma.

In a minority of children who have severe asthma despite the management guidelines outlined above, unacceptable degrees of coughing and wheezing persist, severely limiting the child's play activities and school attendance. In such children the judicious administration of corticosteroids on an alternate-day basis and as an inhaled aerosol frequently results in significant amelioration of symptoms and allows the child to lead a normal life without suffering the adverse effects of corticosteroids. If alternate-day therapy is indicated because of either chronic disability or the severity or frequency of attacks of status asthmaticus, the patient is given 5–7 days of intensive daily therapy and then switched to an alternate-day regimen with a short-acting steroid (prednisone, prednisolone, or methylprednisolone). A 12-yr-old child might be given 60 mg, 40 mg, 30 mg, 20 mg, and 10 mg of prednisone/24 hr over a 5-day period for an exacerbation of asthma, to be followed by alternate-day therapy at a dose of 20 mg/24 hr given as a single dose at 7.00–8.00 A.M. every 48 hr. If the patient responds well to this regimen, the prednisone may be reduced by 5 mg per dose at 10- to 14-day intervals until the lowest dose compatible with acceptable control of symptoms is reached, usually 5–10 mg on alternate days. Concurrent therapy with aerosol adrenergic drugs, theophylline, or cromolyn should be continued because this reduces the dose of steroid required. Low-dose alternate-day therapy is associated with minimal adverse effects and thus may be justified in a disease that can be life-threatening and capable of causing chronic invalidism. Use of steroid therapy should *not*, however, substitute for or delay comprehensive management of the disease.

TABLE 11–20. Selected Slow-Release Theophylline Preparations

Preparation	Dosage Form	Anhydrous Theophylline Content (mg)
Slo-bid Gyrocaps	Capsule	50, 75, 100, 125, 200, 300
Slo-Phyllin Gyrocaps	Capsule	60, 125, 250
Somophyllin-CRT	Capsule	100, 200, 250, 300
Theo-Dur	Tablet	100, 200, 300, 450
Theolair-SR	Tablet	200, 250, 300, 500

Tablets are scored to permit adjustment of dosage.
Capsules may be opened and the contents mixed with moist food for children unable to swallow capsules or tablets.

Inhalational corticosteroids, such as beclomethasone dipropionate (Vanceril, Beclovent), flunisolide (AeroBid), and triamcinolone (Azmacort), may provide an alternative to the use of every-other-day oral corticosteroid medication. Inhalational corticosteroids may be more effective than oral steroids in reversing bronchial hyperresponsiveness and may therefore be indicated even in patients who also require continual treatment with oral steroids. Beclomethasone, which is effective in microgram (μg) doses is rapidly inactivated in the liver into metabolites devoid of glucocorticoid activity. Accordingly, systemic effects in children given less than 14 μg/kg/24 hr (usual dose is 2 inhalations or 84 μg 4 times/day) are minimal. Oropharyngeal candidiasis rarely occurs. Its frequency is diminished by rinsing the mouth after inhaling the aerosol or inhaling the aerosol through a chamber or spacer. Effective use of inhaled steroid requires a degree of compliance by the patient not often found in children under 6–7 yr of age. Studies of adults who have received beclomethasone for up to 7 yr have shown no evidence of epithelial atrophy or thinning of underlying connective tissue, and long-term adverse effects of the drug on the pharynx and airways are unknown.

Continual treatment with an inhaled corticosteroid or with cromolyn is indicated for any child with symptoms of asthma occurring as frequently as weekly.

Home monitoring of peak expiratory flow rate 2–3 times/day facilitates early detection of airway obstruction in patients with severe asthma and in patients with infrequent symptoms that may progress to severe airway obstruction. Graphing the results of monitoring will establish the child's diurnal variation and permit the physician to suggest treatment guidelines that anticipate decreases in peak expiratory flow rate. Daily changes in flow rate may also indicate a need for changes in continual treatment regimens.

Emotional tensions surrounding asthma are best handled by unhurried discussion with the parents of the child's difficulty, by avoidance of overdramatization of the child's illness, and by careful examinations with the parents of those areas in which parent and child seem to be in conflict. The use of tranquilizers or sedatives as a substitute for more direct attempts to solve emotional problems should be avoided. As the asthma is brought under control, the emotional climate is often improved.

Various factors may exacerbate asthma or make the disease difficult to treat: gastroesophageal reflux, allergic bronchopulmonary aspergillosis, nonsteroid antiinflammatory agents, pregnancy, and sinusitis. Chronic sinusitis may be due to noninfectious immune-mediated inflammation or to bacterial infection. Treatment of sinusitis with antibiotics, intranasal steroids, and oral or topical (3–5 days) decongestants for 3 wk may improve bronchoconstriction as well as sinusitis.

Asthma education programs, for example, ACT (*A*sthma *C*are *T*raining) and Superstuff, are being used in comprehensive asthma management. Their goal is to increase knowledge of asthma and its treatment on the part of both the child and parent, to improve communication within the family and with the physician and nurse, to improve compliance with the treatment plan, and to decrease the need for use of emergency room or hospital.

Prevention of Deaths from Asthma

Death from childhood asthma is rare, but asthma mortality rates have been increasing. In the United States asthma mortality rates increased from 1.2/100,000 general population in 1979 to 1.6 in 1985 and 1986. Among children 10–14 yr old the asthma mortality rate increased from 0.1 in 1979 to 0.4/100,000 in 1986, the greatest proportional increase for any age group. Rates have been 3–9 times as high in black children as in whites. Increases have also occurred in Canada and many other countries.

Reasons for these increases in mortality are unknown. Possible causes include increased prevalence of asthma; increased indoor air pollution due to tighter construction of homes with emphasis on energy conservation; delays in implementation of appropriate treatment for acute asthma; lack of access or utilization of medical care, including preventive care; over-reliance on bronchodilator inhalers leading to delayed treatment with steroids or other therapy until patients were in extremis; unavailability of epinephrine for patients unable to use inhalers effectively; inappropriate use of the metered dose inhaler and failure to provide continuity of care or education about what to do for an unusually severe episode of asthma.

Most but not all deaths from asthma are preventable with appropriate care. It is possible to identify many of those at greatest risk for death from their histories, for example, respiratory failure with hypercapnia, loss of consciousness due to asthma, or psychosocial dysfunction in the patient or family that may interfere with judgment and compliance with recommendations for management. These patients require especially close monitoring and psychotherapy when indicated. They should carry a written emergency protocol indicating current medications and recommended emergency treatment as guidance for emergency personnel who may be unfamiliar with the patient. They should also have a written crisis plan indicating what they should do in an emergency. This should include which medications to use, which doses to use at what intervals, how to reach their physicians, and where to get further assistance. A Medic-Alert emblem can be helpful if such a patient is found unconscious or unable to indicate the nature of the illness. Such patients should be provided with injectable epinephrine in a convenient preparation (e.g., EpiPen or EpiPen Jr) for use in an emergency when inhalation therapy is ineffective or inappropriate, but use of the EpiPen should not delay transport to an emergency facility.

Adinoff A, Cummings N: Sinusitis and its relationship to asthma. Pediatr Ann 18:785, 1989.
Anto J, Suryer J, Rodriquez-Roisin R, et al: Community outbreaks of asthma associated with inhalation of soybean dust. N Engl J Med 320:1097, 1989.
Attaway N, Strunk R: Death due to asthma in children: What the pediatrician can do. Pediatr Ann 18:819, 1989.
Burrows B, Martinez F, Halonen M, et al: Association of asthma with serum IgE levels and skin test reactivity to allergens. N Engl J Med 320:271, 1989.
Cheong B, Reynolds S, Rajan G, et al: Intravenous beta agonist in severe acute asthma. Br Med J 297:448, 1988.
Dworkin G, Kattan M: Mechanical ventilation for status asthmaticus in children. J Pediatr 114:545, 1989.
Ellis EF: Asthma in childhood. J Allergy Clin Immunol 72:526, 1983.
Fletcher HJ, Ibrahim SA, Speight N: Survey of asthma deaths in the Northern region, 1970–85. Arch Dis Child 65:163, 1990.
Furukawa CT, Shapiro GG, Bierman CW, et al: A double-blind study comparing the effectiveness of cromolyn sodium and sustained-release theophylline in childhood asthma. Pediatrics 74:453, 1984.
Gershel J, Goldman H, Stein R, et al: The usefulness of chest radiographs in first asthma attacks. N Engl J Med 309:336, 1983.
Isles AF, Newth CJL: Pharmacokinetics of a sustained-release theophylline preparation in infants and pre-school children with asthma. J Allergy Clin Immunol 75:377, 1985.
Lanier R (ed): Priority on pediatric asthma. J Pediatr 115:837, 1989.
Lewis CE, Rachelefsky G, Lewis MA, et al: A randomized trial of A. C. T. (Asthma Care Training) for kids. Pediatrics 74:478, 1984.
Littenberg B: Aminophylline treatment in severe acute asthma: A meta-analysis. JAMA 259:1678, 1988.
Marion RJ, Creer TL, Reynolds RVC: Direct and indirect costs associated with the management of childhood asthma. Ann Allergy 54:31, 1985.
McWilliams B, Kelley H, Murphy S: Management of acute severe asthma. Pediatr Ann 18:774, 1989.
Neddenriep D, Schumacher M, Lemen R: Asthma in childhood. Curr Probl Pediatr 19:329, 1989.
Newhouse M, Dolovich M: Control of asthma by aerosols. N Engl J Med 315:870, 1986.
Ollerenshaw S, Jarvis D, Woolcock A: Absence of immunoreactive vasoactive intestinal polypeptide in tissue from lungs of patients with asthma. N Engl J Med 320:1244, 1989.
Ratto D, Alfaro C, Sipsey J, et al: Are intravenous corticosteroids required in status asthmaticus? JAMA 260:527, 1988.
Rea HH, Scragg R, Jackson R, et al: A case-control study of deaths from asthma. Thorax 41:833, 1986.
Rock M, De LaRocha S, L'Hommedieu S, et al: Use of ketamine in asthmatic children to treat respiratory failure refractory to conventional therapy. Crit Care Med 14:514, 1986.
Schuh S, Parkin P, Rajan A, et al: High- versus low-dose, frequently administered, nebulized albuterol in children with severe, acute asthma. Pediatrics 83:513, 1989.
Shapiro GG, Furukawa CT, Pierson WE, et al: Double-blind evaluation of nebulized cromolyn, terbutaline, and the combination for childhood asthma. J Allergy Clin Immunol 81:449, 1988.
Sly RM: Mortality from asthma in children 1979–1984. Ann Allergy 60:433, 1988.
Stein R, Canny G, Bohn D: Severe acute asthma in a pediatric intensive care unit: Six years' experience. Pediatrics 83:1023, 1989.
Strachan DP: Do chesty children become chesty adults? Arch Dis Child 65:661, 1990.
Warner J, Gotz M, Landau L, et al: Management of asthma: A consensus statement. Arch Dis Child 64:1065, 1989.

11.42 ATOPIC DERMATITIS
(Infantile or Atopic Eczema)

See also Sec. 23.14.

Atopic dermatitis is an inflammatory skin disorder characterized by erythema, edema, intense pruritus, exudation, crusting, and scaling. In the acute stages intraepidermal vesiculation (spongiosis) is present. There appears to be a genetically determined predilection. Infants with atopic dermatitis tend subsequently to develop allergic rhinitis and asthma.

About 80% of patients with atopic dermatitis have serum IgE concentrations increased 5- to 10-fold above normal. There is conflicting evidence as to whether the level of IgE is related to either the severity or the extent of the dermatitis. The concentration of IgE does, however, fluctuate with the stage of the disease. The level returns to normal when the disease has been quiescent for several years. The high levels of IgE have not been satisfactorily explained. It is not established that atopic dermatitis is primarily an IgE-mediated allergic disorder; it is difficult to demonstrate consistently a role for allergens, whether foods or inhalants, in the pathogenesis of eczema. Moreover, the relationship of atopic dermatitis to allergy or immunology is made more uncertain by reports that IgE is not always increased in affected patients who have neither family history nor clinical evidence of rhinitis or asthma. Children with atopic dermatitis and food hypersensitivity have high rates of spontaneous basophil histamine release. This phenomenon returns to normal following a food elimination diet and is mediated by a monocyte cytokine (histamine-releasing factor), which interacts with a specific subtype of IgE bound to basophils.

The typical dermal manifestation of the interaction of IgE antibody with antigen is the hive (wheal and flare) rather than the erythematous papule of atopic dermatitis; and, while patients with atopic dermatitis frequently possess IgE antibody specific for inhalants or food allergens, it is not generally possible to induce skin lesions of atopic dermatitis by intradermal injection of the suspected allergen. Typical lesions of atopic dermatitis may occur in individuals with X-linked agammaglobulinemia, who have virtually no IgE.

Increased concentrations of IgE in atopic dermatitis may be related to a deficiency of IgE isotype-specific "suppressor" T cell function. Impairment of cell-mediated immunity in some patients with atopic dermatitis is indicated by (1) absence of the reactions of delayed hypersensitivity upon intradermal skin testing with certain antigens; (2) inability to be sensitized with potent contact sensitizers (e.g., poison ivy, dinitrochlorobenzene [DNCB]); (3) diminished proliferative response of lymphocytes to mitogens such as phytohemagglutinin (PHA); and (4) variable phagocytic and chemotactic defects of monocytes and neutrophils.

The hyperreactive skin of atopic dermatitis differs from normal skin in its response to a variety of physical and pharmacologic stimuli. For example, a light mechanical stroke results within 1 min in a white line with a surrounding blanched area. This phenomenon ("white dermographism") is not seen in normal skin, which becomes red. Involved skin has abnormal rates of cooling and warming in response to temperature changes, particularly in flexural areas. Paradoxical responses occur to injections of various pharmacologic agents, such as histamine, acetylcholine (blanching rather than erythema), and nicotinic acid ester. Adrenergic responses are decreased in lymphocytes and granulocytes in atopic dermatitis, suggesting that autonomic imbalance may be a basis for the abnormalities in the skin. The abnormal reactivity of the skin has a counterpart in the airway hyperreactivity of asthma; in both disorders such hyperreactivity seems to be intrinsic to the disease which may, in part, be due to the late-phase immune response (Sec. 11.35).

CLINICAL MANIFESTATIONS. Atopic dermatitis affects 2–8% of children and typically occurs in three stages with fairly distinctive features. The disease most often *begins in infancy*, usually during the first 2–3 mo of life. The onset is sometimes delayed until the 2nd or 3rd yr; 60% of patients are affected by 1 yr of age and 90% by 5 yr of age. The earliest lesions are erythematous weepy patches on the cheeks, with subsequent extension to the remainder of the face, neck, wrists, hands, abdomen, and extensor aspects of the extremities. Involvement of flexural areas characteristically appears later but may occur as popliteal and antecubital dermatitis in early life (Fig. 11–5).

Pruritus is marked; the affected infant makes incessant efforts to scratch by rubbing the face on bedclothes and against the sides of the crib. This trauma to the skin rapidly leads to weeping and crusting; secondary infection is common and may be extensive.

The onset of dermatitis frequently coincides with the introduction of certain foods into the infant's diet, especially cow milk, wheat, soy, peanut, fish, or eggs. Cutaneous symptoms develop after food challenges in 50–90% of infants and children who have dermatitis and high IgE serum concentrations. Overall, about 20–30% of patients with eczema have food hypersensitivity to one or more of the six common allergens. There is unequivocal evidence of reaginic sensitivity in certain infants who have urticaria, colic, and a diffuse erythematous flush following ingestion of the offending food. The erythematous flush appears to be accompanied by intense itching, which results in scratching and then in the appearance of the skin lesions characteristic of eczema. The major role of scratching in the production of skin lesions has been demonstrated when one extremity has been encased in surgical dressings and the other left uncovered; the lesions of atopic dermatitis occur only in the uncovered extremity.

Atopic dermatitis shows a tendency to *remission at 3–5 yr of age*. In most cases the disease becomes quiescent by the age of 5 yr; in some, a mild to moderate eczema may persist in the antecubital and popliteal fossae, on the wrists, behind the ears, and on the face and neck. During childhood, antecubital and popliteal involvement becomes common; extensor surfaces of the extremities may still be actively affected. With increasing age there is a tendency toward *drying and thickening of the skin* in the involved areas, especially in the antecubital and popliteal fossae, and on the neck, forehead, eyelids, wrists, and the dorsa of the hands and feet. The face takes on a whitish hue as increased capillary permeability and

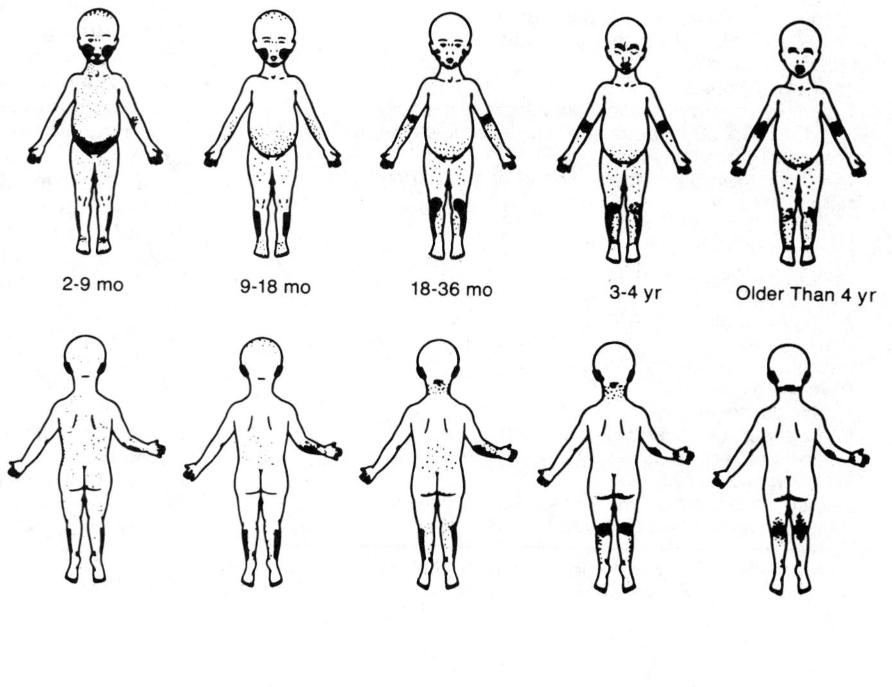

Figure 11–5. Characteristic distribution of lesions of atopic dermatitis at various ages.

dilatation result in edema and blanching of surrounding tissues, sometimes called the "mask of atopic dermatitis." Hyperpigmentation of the skin, scaling, and lichenification (a particular kind of papular thickening of the skin, with accentuation of the normal surface lines) become prominent. There is a marked tendency toward lasting remission in the 4th and 5th decades of life.

DIAGNOSIS. When pruritus is intense and the lesions characteristic, the diagnosis of atopic dermatitis may be easy. A family history of asthma, hay fever, or atopic dermatitis, the finding of elevated serum IgE concentrations and of reaginic antibodies to a variety of foods and inhalants, the presence of eosinophilia, and the demonstration of white dermographism support the diagnosis. Some patients have accentuated lines or grooves below the margin of the lower eyelids (atopic pleat, Dennie line, or Morgan fold) and an increased number of creases of the skin of the palm. The skin has an abnormal tendency to lichenify in response to chronic irritation or rubbing. Generalized dryness of the skin, even in uninvolved areas, and sparsity of the hair of the lateral portion of the eyebrows, thought to be secondary to chronic rubbing, are also characteristic. Specific diagnostic criteria are provided in Table 11–21.

DIFFERENTIAL DIAGNOSIS. The eczematoid skin reaction characterized by erythema, edema, exudation, crusting, and scaling is not specific for atopic dermatitis. In infants and children the differential diagnosis includes seborrheic dermatitis, scabies, primary irritant dermatitis, allergic contact dermatitis, infectious eczematoid dermatitis, ichthyosis, phenylketonuria, acrodermatitis enteropathica, histiocytosis X, and two primary immunologic deficiency disorders: the Wiskott-Aldrich syndrome and X-linked agammaglobulinemia. Eczematous lesions may also be noted in ataxia-telangiectasia, Job syndrome, hyper-IgE syndrome, and biotinidase deficiency.

TABLE 11–21. Diagnostic Features of Atopic Dermatitis*

Must have three or more major features:
Pruritus
Typical morphology and distribution
flexural lichenification or linearity in adults
facial and extensor involvement in infants and children
Chronic or chronically relapsing course
Personal or family history of atopy (asthma, allergic rhinitis, or atopic dermatitis)
Must also have three or more minor features:
Xerosis
Ichthyosis/palmar hyperlinearity/keratosis pilaris
Immediate (type I) skin test reactivity
Elevated serum IgE
Early age of onset
Tendency toward cutaneous infections (especially *Staphylococcus aureus* and herpes simplex)/impaired cell-mediated immunity
Tendency toward nonspecific hand or foot dermatitis
Nipple eczema
Cheilitis
Recurrent conjunctivitis
Dennie-Morgan infraorbital fold
Keratoconus
Anterior subcapsular cataracts
Orbital darkening
Facial pallor/facial erythema
Pityriasis alba
Itch when sweating
Intolerance to wool and lipid solvents
Perifollicular accentuation
Food hypersensitivity
Course influenced by environmental/emotional factors
White dermographism/delayed blanch

*From Broadbent JB, Sampson HH: Food hypersensitivity and atopic dermatitis. Pediatr Clin North Am 35(5):1115, 1988.

Seborrheic dermatitis typically begins on the scalp, often as "cradle cap," and involves the ear and contiguous skin, the sides of the nose, and eyebrows and eyelids with greasy, brownish scales. These are usually distinguished easily from the erythematous, weeping, crusted lesions of infantile atopic dermatitis, but sometimes during the first few months of life it is difficult to distinguish clearly between seborrhea and atopic dermatitis, particularly when the face is primarily involved. Seborrhea in infancy has a shorter course than that of atopic eczema and responds much more rapidly to treatment. The difficulty in differentiating the two conditions is indicated by the use of the term seborrheic eczema by some dermatologists. In infancy, *scabies* may be confused with atopic dermatitis. The location of the lesions helps to differentiate the two. Atopic dermatitis most often begins on the cheeks and does not involve the palms and soles, whereas scabies commonly starts with large papules on the upper back and with vesicles on the palms and soles. The mite of scabies or its ova can be seen in scrapings from the vesicles.

Primary irritant dermatitis is a nonallergic reaction due to various irritants and most common in infancy in the perioral (fruit juices) and diaper areas. The location and rapid response of lesions to therapy indicate the correct diagnosis.

The lesions of *allergic contact dermatitis* (poison ivy is the prototype) are usually limited to sites of exposure to the offending allergen and do not typically involve the flexural areas. Occasionally, contact dermatitis is superimposed on atopic dermatitis after sensitization to chemicals in topical agents such as neomycin, the parabens (used as preservatives in many ointments), or iodochlorohydroxyquin (Vioform).

Infectious eczematoid dermatitis may follow discharge of purulent material from a draining ear or other site of infection. The typical location of the lesions and rapid response to therapy support the diagnosis.

In *ichthyosis vulgaris,* dryness of the skin may lead to confusion with atopic dermatitis, but the scales of ichthyosis are usually larger than those of atopic dermatitis, and the pruritus of ichthyosis, if any, is generally mild. The two disorders may be associated. Infants and children with *untreated phenylketonuria* develop an eczematous dermatitis often confused with atopic eczema. The rash of phenylketonuria is responsive to a diet low in phenylalanine.

Histiocytosis X (Letterer-Siwe disease) and *acrodermatitis enteropathica* are serious systemic diseases occurring early in life. Failure to thrive is prominent. Hemorrhagic manifestations are common in the eczematous eruption of histiocytosis X. In acrodermatitis the skin around the oral, nasal, genitourinary, and rectal orifices is typically involved.

Patients with Wiskott-Aldrich syndrome and X-linked agammaglobulinemia may have an eczema that is indistinguishable from atopic dermatitis.

COMPLICATIONS. During early infancy and childhood, secondary infection of the lesions of atopic dermatitis with bacterial or viral agents is common. Staphylococci and β-hemolytic streptococci are the bacterial agents most often recovered from infected lesions. Herpes simplex (Kaposi varicelliform eruption) is also of particular concern. Infants and children with eczema should not be exposed to adults with herpes simplex infection ("cold sores"). Infections with common wart and molluscum contagiosum viruses may also occur. Keratoconus is occasionally seen in children with atopic dermatitis, perhaps owing to chronic rubbing of the eyelids. Cataracts occur in 5–10% of adults with severe atopic dermatitis but are rarely seen during childhood.

TREATMENT. Effective treatment of atopic dermatitis requires control of the environmental precipitants of the itch-scratch-itch cycle that perpetuates the disease, beginning with avoidance of ingestant, injectant, contactant, and atmospheric factors that can trigger itching or scratching. Extremes of temperature and humidity should be avoided. A warm climate of moderate humidity is optimal for most patients. Sweating leads to itching and to aggravation of the disease. Exposure to sunlight and salt water is of benefit to many patients.

Garments should be made of a smooth-textured cotton; wool should be avoided. Infants should not be allowed to crawl on wool carpeting.

For the dry skin of atopic dermatitis, use of soaps and detergents that defat the skin should be avoided as much as possible. Bathing should be kept to a minimum. The purpose of bath oil or other creams applied to the skin is to seal water into the skin; bath oil is added to the tub after the patient has soaked for 20 min, thus sealing the moisture in the hydrated skin instead of excluding it as would occur if the oil were added before the patient enters the bath. The same principle applies to application of creams and lotions; they should be applied to the damp skin following a bath. Should bathing appear to make the patient worse, a nondrying cleansing agent such as Cetaphil, a commercially available nonlipid lotion, can be used.

If a food aggravates itching, it should be excluded from the diet. Skin testing by the prick method is useful in *excluding* IgE-mediated food hypersensitivity. *Positive* skin tests must be assessed by properly controlled food challenges (Sec. 11.49). Arbitrary exclusion of numerous foods from the diets of infants with atopic dermatitis without clear evidence that they are involved in the disease is irrational and can lead to malnutrition. Double-blind food elimination and provocative testing may identify the offending food (Sec. 11.49). Subsequent elimination of the identified food from the diet will decrease symptoms (nuts, soy, egg, milk). Some children "outgrow" these food-induced symptoms. Thus, reintroducing the offending foods may be possible within 2–4 yr. Food allergen sensitization can be reduced by breast milk feeding and by delaying the introduction of solid foods until after 6 mo of age. Breast-feeding mothers should avoid ingesting high-risk foods because some food allergens appear in human milk and can potentially sensitize an atopic infant.

Local therapy is the mainstay of management of atopic dermatitis. During acute flare-ups of the disease, wet dressings (e.g., Burow solution, 1:20) have an antipruritic and anti-inflammatory effect. Topical corticosteroid lotions or creams may be applied between changes of wet dressings. The continuous application of wet dressings also has the advantage of immobilizing and protecting the affected parts and preventing scratching. Unless scratching can be controlled, it is almost impossible to manage the disease successfully, especially during infancy and early childhood. Fingernails must be kept cut as short as possible; restraints for the elbows to keep the hands from the face are sometimes necessary to control scratching at night. Itching is difficult to control with drugs. Drugs with both sedative and antihistamine activity, such as diphenhydramine (Benadryl), hydroxyzine (Atarax, Vistaril), or promethazine (Phenergan), are of greatest value. In some patients aspirin has a marked antipruritic effect.

When infection is present, antibiotics should be given systemically. Antibiotics in topical medications not only are of little therapeutic value but can lead to sensitization to the agents applied, particularly in the case of neomycin. The possibility of superimposed contact sensitization must be considered when there is sudden exacerbation of atopic dermatitis to which a topical medicament has been applied. Parabens, mercurial compounds, and lanolin can all cause contact sensitization.

After the acute phase has subsided, topical application of corticosteroid creams and ointments is of great value in managing the disease. Their cost may be a serious problem. Cost can be reduced by purchasing relatively concentrated preparations in bulk, which the pharmacist can dilute to half strength with Aquaphor or Eucerin, rather than purchasing equivalent material in 15- or 30-g amounts. Small amounts of steroid rubbed in well at frequent intervals give better results than large amounts applied only infrequently. Percutaneous absorption of corticosteroid occurs but is not generally clinically significant. Long-term topical use of steroids leads to an increase in growth of hair in some patients and to atrophy of the skin. The more potent topical steroids should not be applied to the face, nor to large areas during prolonged periods. Application of 0.5% or 1% hydrocortisone to the face is safe.

Systemic administration of corticosteroids for treatment of atopic dermatitis should be avoided except briefly in the most severely affected patients while awaiting response to other therapies.

Topical treatment with corticosteroids has largely superseded the use of coal tar preparations. Tars stain clothes and skin, and compliance of the patient in their use is often poor. However, newer preparations, Estargel (Westwood) and Psorigel (Owen), are effective and more acceptable cosmetically. Tars are considerably less expensive for long-term topical use than corticosteroids. Coal tar is photosensitizing, and occasionally its use results in a sterile, pustular folliculitis.

PROGNOSIS. With adequate control of factors known to trigger itching, appropriate local treatment, and understanding support for the parents of a child for whom no immediate cure is to be expected, reasonable control of atopic dermatitis is usually possible. Resolution occurs within 5 yr usually.

Bernhisal-Broadbent J, Sampson H: Food hypersensitivity and atopic dermatitis. Pediatr Clin North Am 35:1115, 1988.

Ferguson AC, Salinas FA: Elevated IgE immune complexes in children with atopic eczema. J Allergy Clin Immunol 74:678, 1984.

Kaplan A, Buckley R, Mathews K: Allergic skin disorders. JAMA 258:2900, 1987.

Rasmussen JE: Recent developments in the management of patients with atopic dermatitis. J Allergy Clin Immunol 74:771, 1984.

Sampson HA, Albergo R: Comparison of results in skin tests, RAST and double-blind placebo-controlled food challenge in atopic dermatitis. J Allergy Clin Immunol 74:26, 1984.

Sampson HA, Broadbent K, Bernhisal-Broadbent J: Spontaneous release of histamine from basophils and histamine-releasing factor in patients with atopic dermatitis and food hypersensitivity. N Engl J Med 321:228, 1989.

Sampson HA, Jolie PL: Increased plasma histamine concentration after food challenges in children with atopic dermatitis. N Engl J Med 311:372, 1984.

11.43 URTICARIA-ANGIOEDEMA
(Hives)

CLINICAL MANIFESTATIONS. Urticaria, or hives, is a common skin disorder characterized by usually well-circumscribed but sometimes coalescent, localized, or generalized erythematous raised skin lesions (wheals or welts) of various sizes. The lesions may be intensely pruritic or itch little, if at all. The individual hive usually resolves within 48 hr, but new ones may continue to appear singly or in crops. When urticaria persists for longer than 6 wk, the condition is arbitrarily deemed chronic. Urticaria has been attributed to edema of the upper corium due to dilatation and increased permeability of the capillaries.

In angioedema (angioneurotic edema) the deeper layers of skin or submucosa and subcutaneous or other tissues are involved; the upper respiratory tract and the gastrointestinal tract are common target organs. The distinction between urticaria and angioedema is frequently not clear; the lesions appear to differ only in the depth of tissue involvement.

INCIDENCE. As many as 20% of people experience hives at some time during life. Urticaria is somewhat more frequent in females than in males.

PATHOGENESIS. The principal noncytotoxic mechanism for urticaria and angioedema is interaction of antigen with mast cell- or basophil-bound IgE antibodies. The release of histamine from these cells causes vasodilatation and increased vascular permeability and stimulates an axon reflex, which produces a typical wheal and flare reaction. Leukotrienes may contribute to the edema of the IgE-mediated reaction. A second mediator pathway for urticaria involves the complement system. Two complement component split products, C3a and C5a, act as anaphylatoxins (Sec. 11.23) and trigger histamine release from mast cells and basophils by direct action on the cell surfaces, independent of antibodies. C3a and C5a can be generated through both the classical and the alternative complement pathways. A third mediator pathway involves the plasma kinin-forming system of the coagulation scheme. Bradykinin is at least as potent as histamine in increasing vascular permeability. Both non-IgE immunologic reactions and nonimmunologic events can cause urticaria and angioedema when they activate the complement and kinin-forming systems.

ETIOLOGY. A clinical classification of urticaria is given in Table 11–22.

DIFFERENTIAL DIAGNOSIS. With a few exceptions no laboratory tests establish or exclude the diagnosis of urticaria and angioedema. Allergy skin testing is generally not helpful except when specific drug (penicillin) or food allergies are identified. In the absence of any clue suggesting an ingestant etiology, elimination diets are not generally useful. The diagnosis is clinical and requires that the physician be aware of the various forms of urticaria. A careful history usually identifies the type. Except when there are obvious associations with IgE-mediated reactions, naming the "cause" of urticaria may be difficult. Drugs and foods are the most common causes of urticaria. The etiology of chronic urticaria is identified in only 10% of cases.

Some forms of urticaria need special mention. *Papular urticaria* usually occurs in small children, generally on the extremities and other exposed parts at the sites of insect bites. *Cholinergic urticaria* appears as wheals 1–2 mm in diameter surrounded by large areas of erythema (flares) and frequently involves the skin of the neck. It is caused by exercise, hot showers, and occasionally by anxiety. Affected people have increased sensitivity to cholinergic mediators, which can be demonstrated when an intradermal injection of 0.01 mg of methacholine (Mecholyl) in 0.1 mL of saline causes a localized hive surrounded by smaller, satellite lesions. Urticaria is probably due more often to *viral infection* than is commonly recognized. It is particularly associated with hepatitis, especially during the prodromal stages, and with infectious mononucleosis. Viral infections can also produce *erythema multiforme*, often confused with urticaria, in which typical iris or target lesions occur and mucosal involvement is common. In some patients typical hives change spontaneously into lesions of erythema multiforme, which can be a sign of drug allergy (Sec. 6.55).

Urticaria pigmentosa typically occurs during the first few years of childhood and has a distinctive presentation. *Systemic mastocytosis* is a serious form of urticaria pigmentosa in which mast cells infiltrate skeleton, liver, spleen, and lymph nodes. In adults, and rarely in children, urticaria may be associated with *malignancy* or *collagen-vascular disorders*.

Cold urticaria is the most common form due to physical factors. Urticarial lesions, which may be pruritic or painful or burning, appear upon exposure to cold and are confined to the exposed parts of the body. The lesions develop not only on exposure to cold weather but also with local application of cold. The cooling of skin associated with evaporation upon emerging from water can produce urticaria. Swimming in cold water is hazardous; death may occur in patients so exposed. There are two forms: a primary acquired form and a familial form. Cold urticaria can occur in adults with such systemic diseases as cryofibrinogenemia, cryoglobulinemia, cold-agglutinin disease, and secondary syphilis. In some cases of primary acquired urticaria, the phenomenon has been passively transferred using purified IgE and IgM fractions of serum from affected patients. After appropriate cold challenge there are also increased concentrations of histamine, eosinophil and neutrophil chemotactic factors, and platelet-activating factor in venous blood draining the challenge site. Primary acquired cold urticaria appears and disappears spontaneously; in some cases, its onset occurs with a viral illness.

Hereditary angioedema (HAE), a potentially life-threatening form of angioedema (Sec. 11.25 and 11.28), is the most important familial form of angioedema.

A syndrome of *episodic angioedema*, urticaria and fever with associated eosinophilia, has been described in both adults and children. In contrast to other hypereosinophilic syndromes, this entity has a benign course.

Exercise-induced anaphylaxis presents with varying combinations of pruritus, urticaria, angioedema, wheezing, laryngeal obstruction, or hypotension, following exercise. Cholinergic urticaria is differentiated by positive heat challenge tests and

TABLE 11–22. Types of Urticaria

Due to ingestants (IgE mechanism in some cases)
Foods, particularly fish, shellfish, nuts, eggs, and peanuts; food additives (tartrazine, azo dyes, benzoates)
Drugs (penicillin, aspirin, sulfonamides, codeine)
Due to contactants (IgE mechanism in some cases)
Plant substances (e.g., stinging nettle)
Animal–insect (tarantula hairs, Portuguese man of war, cat-scratch, mothscales)
Drugs applied to the skin
Animal saliva
Due to injectants (IgE mechanism in some cases)
Drugs (particularly penicillin), transfused blood, therapeutic antisera, insect stings and bites (papular urticaria), allergenic extracts
Due to inhalants (IgE mechanism)
Pollens, danders, and ? molds
Due to infectious agents (mechanism unknown)
Parasites
Viruses (e.g., hepatitis, infectious mononucleosis)
Bacteria (*Streptococcus*, mycoplasma)
? Fungi
Due to physical factors (mechanism mostly unknown)
Cold urticaria
Pressure urticaria
Solar urticaria
Aquagenic urticaria
Local heat urticaria
Dermographism
Exercise-induced
Vibratory angioedema
Episodic angioedema with eosinophilia (? a distinct entity)
Cholinergic urticaria (a distinct entity)
Associated with systemic diseases (mechanism mostly unknown)
Collagen-vascular (systemic lupus erythematosus, cryoglobulinuria, Sjögren syndrome)
Cutaneous vasculitis
Serum sickness-like disease
Malignancy (leukemia-lymphoma)
Hyperthyroidism
Urticaria pigmentosa (systemic mastocytosis)
Associated with genetic disorders (various mechanisms)
Familial cold urticaria
Hereditary angioedema
Amyloidosis with deafness and urticaria
C3b inactivator deficiency
Chronic urticaria and angioedema (mechanism unknown)
Psychogenic urticaria (existence as an entity uncertain)

the rare occurrence of anaphylactic shock. The combination of ingestion of various food allergens (shrimp, celery, wheat) and postprandial exercise results in cutaneous mast cell degranulation; food or exercise alone will not produce this reaction.

TREATMENT. In most instances urticaria is a self-limited illness requiring little treatment other than antihistamines. Hydroxyzine (Atarax), 0.5 mg/kg, is one of the most effective antihistamines for control of urticaria, but diphenhydramine (Benadryl), 1.25 mg/kg, and other antihistamines are also effective. These doses may be repeated at intervals of 4–6 hr if necessary.

Epinephrine 1:1,000, 0.01 mL/kg, max 0.3 mL, usually affords rapid relief of acute, severe urticaria. Hydroxyzine (0.5 mg/kg every 4–6 hr) is the drug of choice for cholinergic and chronic urticaria. The combined use of H_1- and H_2-type antihistamines is sometimes helpful to control chronic urticaria. H_2 antihistamines alone may exacerbate urticaria. Cyproheptadine (Periactin) (2–4 mg every 8–12 hr) is especially useful as a prophylactic agent for cold urticaria. Cyproheptadine can cause appetite stimulation and weight gain in some patients. Sun screens are the only effective treatment for solar urticaria. Corticosteroids have varying effects on chronic urticaria; the doses required to control the urticaria are often so large that they cause serious side effects. Chronic urticaria does not often respond favorably to dietary manipulation. Unfortunately, chronic urticaria may persist for years. For treatment of hereditary angioedema, see Sec. 11.25 and 11.28.

Casale T, Keahey T, Kaliner M: Exercise-induced anaphylactic syndromes. JAMA 255:2049, 1986.
Jorizzo JL, Smith ED: The physical urticarias: An update and review. Arch Dermatol 118:194, 1982.
Juhlin L: Recurrent urticaria: Clinical investigation of 330 patients. Br J Dermatol 104:369, 1981.
Kaplan A, Buckley R, Mathews K: Allergic skin disorders. JAMA 258:2900, 1987.
Twarog FJ: Urticaria in childhood: Pathogenesis and management. Pediatr Clin North Am 30:887, 1983.

11.44 ANAPHYLAXIS

DEFINITION. The term anaphylaxis describes sudden life-threatening reactions that are immunologic. Many anaphylactic reactions are the result of IgE-mediated sensitivity to foreign substances. Anaphylaxis is uncommon in children.

ETIOLOGY. Virtually any foreign substance is capable of producing anaphylaxis under appropriate circumstances (Table 11–23). Following IgE production in response to antigen stimulus, re-exposure to the offending antigen results in a systemic reaction.

PATHOGENESIS. In the person who has developed IgE-mediated anaphylactic sensitivity to an antigen, subsequent administration of even minute amounts of the antigen may result in an explosive antigen-antibody reaction with massive release of chemical mediators such as histamine. The action of the mediators on various tissue receptors throughout the body produces the symptoms. Histamine plays a central role in the pathogenesis of human anaphylaxis, but other vasoactive substances (arachidonic acid metabolites, kinins, platelet-activating factor) may also have roles. Decreased levels of factor V and factor VIII have been reported, suggesting consumption of coagulation factors due to intravascular coagulation. Several patients studied during severe episodes of systemic anaphylaxis have had low levels of high molecular weight kininogen, C3, and C4. When an immunologic mechanism cannot be identified (anaphylactoid reactions, see Table 11–23), it is presumed that mediator release occurs as a direct effect of the causative agent on basophils and mast cells or perhaps by activation of the alternative complement pathway, with generation of anaphylatoxins (see above).

TABLE 11–23. Etiology of Anaphylaxis

Drugs (penicillin, cephalosporins, chemotherapy, muscle relaxants)
Foods (seafood, nuts, legumes, egg, celery, milk)
Insect Stings (Hymenoptera: kissing bug, deerfly, fire ants)
Biologic Agents (L-asparaginase, allergen extracts, blood products, insulin, immunoglobulins)
Food Additives (metabisulfite, monosodium glutamate, aspartame)
Exercise-Induced
Pseudoallergic* (iodinated radiocontrast media, opiates, D-tubocurarine, thiamine, aspirin, captopril)

*Pseudoallergic or anaphylactoid is not necessarily IgE mediated. Substances can produce direct mast cell degranulation.

CLINICAL MANIFESTATIONS. Anaphylactic reactions are characteristically explosive, particularly when the antigen is injected. Surviving patients describe a "feeling of impending doom." The more rapidly symptoms appear after administration of the foreign material, the more serious is the reaction. Often the first symptom noted is a tingling sensation around the mouth or face, followed by a feeling of warmth, difficulty in swallowing, and tightness in the throat or chest. The patient becomes flushed; urticaria and angioedema then appear, along with varying degrees of hoarseness, inspiratory stridor, dysphagia, nasal congestion, itching of the eyes, sneezing, and wheezing. Abdominal cramps, diarrhea, and contractions of the uterus and other organs of smooth muscle may also occur. The patient may lose consciousness and, on examination, be hypotensive, with feeble heart sounds, bradycardia, and sometimes an arrhythmia. Cardiorespiratory arrest and death may ensue. In fatal cases death has most often resulted from acute upper airway obstruction, though profound circulatory collapse may occur without upper airway obstruction.

TREATMENT. Successful treatment of anaphylaxis depends on anticipation that the event may occur and being prepared for it. In particular, physicians who administer allergenic extracts must be ready to treat this life-threatening complication of immunotherapy. If, for example, a generalized reaction follows an injection of pollen extract into an upper extremity, aqueous epinephrine 1:1,000, 0.01 mL/kg (maximum 0.3 mL for a child or 0.5 mL for an adult) should immediately be administered subcutaneously into the other arm and a tourniquet placed above the site of injection of extract. The tourniquet can be loosened after improvement occurs or, briefly, at intervals of 3 min. An additional injection of epinephrine, half the previous dose (diluted in 2 mL normal saline), may be administered subcutaneously at the site of injection to retard absorption. An intravenous infusion should be started immediately to administer aminophylline should bronchoconstriction occur and to facilitate administration of drugs (epinephrine 1:10,000) and volume expanders for hypotension. Epinephrine may produce severe hypertension in patients receiving β-receptor blocking agents. Measurement of central venous pressure is a valuable guide to plasma volume expansion therapy. Oxygen should be administered by mask, and if there is upper airway obstruction (stridor, hoarseness), the patient may need prompt intubation or a tracheostomy. Diphenhydramine (25–50 mg) should be given intravenously, and an H_2 antihistamine, cimetidine (4 mg/kg by intravenous injection), may be helpful. Corticosteroids are not useful as emergency drugs but may be useful in preventing the recurrences of symptoms during the 12–24 hr following the acute reaction.

Serious anaphylactoid reactions to intravenous radiocontrast media are less common in children than in adults but occur occasionally. A prophylactic regimen for patients known to be at risk by virtue of previous reactions consists of prednisone, 50 mg orally every 6 hr for 3 doses, ending 1 hr before the procedure and diphenhydramine, 50 mg, given by intramuscular injection 1 hr before the procedure. This regimen prevents adverse reactions of any degree in over 90% of high-risk adult patients.

The incidence of drug-induced anaphylaxis would drop substantially if drugs were given only when indicated and only by the oral route unless some compelling reason for injection exists. Not only is anaphylactic sensitivity more easily induced by injection of drugs than by oral administration, but in the sensitized patient anaphylaxis occurs more commonly following parenteral than oral administration. The incidence of anaphylaxis following Hymenoptera stings can be reduced significantly by the appropriate use of venom immunotherapy (Sec. 11.39 and 11.47).

Sheffer AL, Tong AKF, Murphy GF, et al: Exercise-induced anaphylaxis: A serious form of physical allergy. J Allergy Clin Immunol 75:479, 1985.
Smith PL, Kagey-Sobotka A, Bleechner ER, et al: Physiologic manifestations of human anaphylaxis. J Clin Invest 66:1072, 1980.
Valentine M, Lichtenstein L: Anaphylaxis and stinging insect hypersensitivity. JAMA 258:2881, 1987.
Yunginger J, Sweeney K, Sturner W: Fatal food-induced anaphylaxis. JAMA 260:1450, 1988.

11.45 SERUM SICKNESS

The serum sickness syndrome is a characteristic systemic immunologic disorder that follows the administration of foreign antigenic material.

ETIOLOGY. The disorder was first described in 1905 by von Pirquet and Schick as a consequence of antitoxin therapy for such diseases as diphtheria and tetanus. The illness was shown to be due to an adverse reaction to the serum proteins of the animal in which the antitoxin was prepared. Therapeutic antisera of animal origin, especially equine, are still occasionally used, but today the major cause of the serum sickness syndrome is drug allergy, particularly that due to penicillin. Cases have also followed use of other therapeutic agents, including human gamma globulin and even Hymenoptera stings. Preparations of immune globulin of human origin are available for treatment of diphtheria and tetanus (and prophylaxis of rabies) in humans, but antitoxins for treatment of crotalid envenomation and clostridial intoxication (botulism, gas gangrene) are still prepared in the horse.

PATHOGENESIS. Serum sickness is the classic example of a type III hypersensitivity, "immune complex" disease in the experimental animal. After a single large dose of isotopically labeled antigen is injected into the rabbit, the symptoms of serum sickness occur coincidentally with the appearance of antibody formed against the injected antigen, at a time when the latter is still present in the circulation. Antigen-antibody complexes formed under conditions of moderate antigen excess lodge in small vessels and in filtering organs throughout the body (deposition being aided in the rabbit by the actions of IgE antibody, basophils, and platelet-activating factor and by the release of vasoactive amines that increase the permeability of blood vessels); these complexes activate the complement sequence. Complement components bound at the site of immune complex deposition promote accumulation of neutrophils through at least two general processes: adherence of neutrophils to the site of bound complement and chemotactic activity of the C567 complex and C3a and C5a fragments. Tissue injury results from the liberation of toxic molecules from the neutrophils. In this animal model, healing of the lesions occurs following elimination of the complexes from the circulation.

Serum sickness demonstrates how the differing biologic activities of the several species of antibodies formed against a complex antigen may be responsible for diverse parts of the clinical picture; the urticaria of serum sickness is thought to be due to IgE antibody molecules reacting with horse serum proteins, whereas the joint symptoms are thought to occur as a result of deposition of antigen-antibody complexes of the IgG and IgM classes. In both rabbits and humans it is suspected that histamine release from basophils and mast cells, mediated by IgE antibodies, facilitates the deposition of immune complexes through increases in vascular permeability.

CLINICAL MANIFESTATIONS. Typically the symptoms of serum sickness begin 7–12 days following injection of the foreign material but may appear as late as 3 wk afterward. If there has been earlier exposure or previous allergic reaction to the same foreign antigen, symptoms may appear in accelerated fashion, within 1–3 days following injection, or as anaphylaxis. Fever and malaise are almost always present, as are cutaneous eruptions. Urticaria, usually generalized, is a common finding. Faint erythema with a serpiginous border at the margins of palmar or plantar skin of the hands, fingers, feet, and toes may precede the generalized cutaneous eruption. This characteristic cutaneous lesion may become purpuric with time. Edema, particularly around the face and neck, facial flushing, myalgia, lymphadenopathy, arthralgia, or arthritis involving multiple joints (ankle, knee, wrist, fingers, toes), and gastrointestinal complaints (cramping, diarrhea, nausea) also occur. Intense pruritus accompanying the urticaria is the most distressing symptom in many patients. The site of injection of the foreign material generally becomes red and swollen, commonly 1–3 days before systemic symptoms appear. The disease generally runs a self-limited course, and the patient recovers in 7–10 days. Carditis and glomerulonephritis rarely occur; the most serious complications of serum sickness are Guillain-Barré syndrome and peripheral neuritis, especially involving the brachial plexus (C5–C6).

LABORATORY MANIFESTATIONS. The blood leukocyte and eosinophil counts are variable; marked thrombocytopenia is often found. Mild proteinuria, hemoglobinuria, and microscopic hematuria may be seen. Plasma cells have been found in blood. The erythrocyte sedimentation rate is often increased. A sheep cell agglutinin titer of the Forssman type is usually elevated. Serum complement levels (C3 and C4) are variably depressed and may fall to low concentrations around the 10th day. C3a anaphylatoxin may be increased. In serum sickness due to horse serum proteins, antibodies of the IgG, IgA, IgM, and IgE classes may be found directed against various horse serum proteins. Direct immunofluorescence studies of skin lesions often reveal immune deposits of IgM, IgA, IgE, or C3.

TREATMENT. Patients generally respond well to aspirin and antihistamines. When the symptoms are especially severe, corticosteroids have been used with great efficacy. High doses are given and rapidly reduced as the patient improves.

PREVENTION. The use of horse serum or other animal serum in therapy should be limited to cases for which no alternative is available. When only equine antitoxin is available, skin tests should be employed prior to administration of serum, beginning with a puncture test using a 1:10 dilution. If the reaction is negative, one may then begin intradermal testing with 0.02 mL of a 1:10,000 dilution. If there is no reaction, a subsequent skin test should be performed with a 1:1,000 dilution. If a negative result again is obtained, a final intradermal test with a 1:100 dilution of horse serum is done. A negative reaction to the strongest solution indicates that anaphylactic sensitivity to horse serum is very unlikely; skin tests do not predict the likelihood of development of serum sickness.

Occasionally patients who have evidence of anaphylactic sensitivity to horse serum by virtue of either a previous reaction or a positive immediate wheal and flare skin test require treatment with horse serum. In such a case the antitoxin can be successfully administered by a process of rapid desensitization. Some allergists medicate the patient with epinephrine and antihistamines before beginning the desensitization procedure. Others prefer not to mask possible evidence of a reaction at an early stage when it still might be of a minor degree and serve as a warning to proceed more slowly with the desensitization. The desensitization process is begun with 0.1-mL amounts of antitoxin, diluted to 1:100,000–1:10,000, depending on an estimate of the degree of the patient's sensitivity, and injected intravenously at 20-min intervals. If the patient tolerates the previous injection without adverse reactions, the amount administered may be doubled every 20 min. Generally, the entire amount of antitoxin can be administered safely over a 4- to 6-hr period. The desensitization, unfortunately, is transient, and the patient often regains the previous anaphylactic sensitivity within a few months. Administration of methylprednisolone in doses of 1–1.5 mg/kg/day has not prevented the development of serum sickness.

Bielory L, Gascon P, Lawley T, et al: Human serum sickness: A prospective analysis of 35 patients treated with equine antithymocyte globulin for bone marrow failure. Medicine 67:40, 1988.

Gilliland BG: Serum sickness and immune complexes. N Engl J Med 311:1435, 1984.

Kunnamo I, Kallio P, Pelkonen P, et al: Serum sickness-like disease is a common cause of acute arthritis in children. Acta Pediatr Scand 75:964, 1986.

Lawley TJ, Bielory L, Gascon P, et al: A prospective clinical and immunologic analysis of patients with serum sickness. N Engl J Med 311:1407, 1984.

11.46 ADVERSE REACTIONS TO DRUGS

See also Sec. 6.55.

DEFINITION. An adverse reaction to a drug may be defined as any unwanted consequence of administration of the agent during or following a course of therapy. Adverse reactions fall into two broad categories: those dependent upon pharmacologic mechanisms and those dependent upon immunologic mechanisms (Table 11–24). The majority of adverse drug reactions are pharmacologic; the Boston collaborative drug surveillance program found only 6% to have an allergic basis. In a study of hospitalized children who had adverse drug reactions, no more than 15% were thought to be of an allergic nature.

Certain generalities apply to adverse drug reactions: (1) Virtually any organ system may be involved. (2) After the neonatal period, children are less often affected than adults. (3) The incidence of reactions increases almost exponentially with the number of drugs given simultaneously. (4) Certain diseases predispose to adverse drug reactions, especially those in which multiple drug therapy is common (cardiovascular, infectious, and psychiatric illnesses). Diseases that affect organs responsible for absorption (gastrointestinal tract), metabolism (liver), or excretion of drugs (kidney) also increase the likelihood of adverse reactions. (5) The pharmacokinetic properties of a drug (for example, the extent of protein-binding) also affect the incidence of adverse reactions.

CLASSIFICATION. Adverse drug reactions can be classified in terms of their underlying mechanisms. *Toxicity* may result from a high concentration of drug in the body due to excessive intake—accidental or intentional—or to abnormalities in absorption, metabolism, or excretion of the drug. Various diseases, genetic factors, or drug interactions may permit accumulation of a drug. Some patients for unknown reasons have excessive pharmacologic responses *(intolerance)* to average drug doses. The signs and symptoms are generally intensifications of the expected pharmacologic effects of the agent.

Side effects are undesirable but essentially unavoidable effects of drugs and largely reflect the fact that a given drug rarely affects only one tissue. When theophylline is given as a bronchodilator agent in asthma, for example, central nervous system stimulation is considered a side effect, though this latter effect of theophylline warrants its use in neonatal apnea. *Secondary effects* of drugs are those not related to their primary pharmacologic actions. An example is disturbance of the bacterial flora of the intestine as a consequence of antibiotic therapy. In drug *idiosyncrasy* the signs and symptoms of the reaction are unrelated to the known pharmacologic properties of the agent, sometimes because of metabolic abnormalities. An example is the hemolytic anemia that follows ingestion of primaquine in patients with G-6-PD deficiency (Sec. 16.17).

Drug interactions are discussed in Sec. 6.55 (see Table 6–24).

Allergic drug reactions occur on the basis of recognized models of immune injury. These include (1) IgE-mediated reactions; (2) cytotoxic reactions resulting from hapten binding to cell membranes and subsequent reaction with anti-hapten antibodies; (3) immune complex reactions in which drug-antibody immune complexes with affinity for cell membranes activate the complement system, resulting in cell membrane damage; (4) reactions due to autoantibody formation; and (5) reactions due to cell-mediated mechanisms. Most drugs are simple chemicals with molecular weights of less than 1,000 and are rarely immunogenic. Substances with low molecular weights may act as haptens and become immunogenic after covalent chemical binding with tissue proteins to form drug-protein conjugates. Hapten-protein complex formation is necessary for the macrophage–T cell–B cell interaction that leads to formation of hapten-specific humoral antibodies and cellular immunity. In general, only drugs (or their degradative or metabolic products) with sufficient chemical reactivity to bind irreversibly with proteins are capable of inducing hypersensitivity reactions. The major impediment to both study and diagnosis of drug allergy is that the chemically reactive substance is often not the native drug itself but a metabolic or degradative product. Because little is known about the metabolic fate of many drugs in common use, it is often impossible to identify the chemically reactive intermediates necessary for investigative or diagnostic use.

The complexities of understanding allergic reactions to drugs are illustrated by considering the penicillin model. Benzyl penicillin (penicillin G) has produced a wide variety of allergic reactions, including systemic responses such as anaphylaxis, serum sickness, and vasculitis; hematologic disorders, including hemolytic anemia, thrombocytopenia, and granulocytopenia; a broad spectrum of cutaneous eruptions; pulmonary disease; and renal disease (Table 11–24). Under physiologic conditions, both in vivo and in vitro, a number of highly protein-reactive compounds are formed from penicillin. These metabolic products become immunogenic following conjugation with tissue proteins as described earlier. The penicilloyl group, formed by the combination of benzyl penicillenic acid with amino groups of proteins, is the antigenic determinant formed in largest amounts. Ninety-five per cent of all benzyl penicillin that conjugates with tissue proteins in vivo forms benzylpenicilloyl haptenic groups (BPO), and thus benzyl penicillin has been designated the "major" haptenic determinant of penicillin hypersensitivity. A large percentage of people who have been treated with penicillin possess antibodies to the benzylpenicilloyl determinant, but most do not develop symptoms of penicillin allergy. BPO-specific IgE antibodies can be detected through a benzylpenicilloyl-polylysine skin test reagent in which BPO haptenic groups are attached to a "backbone" of lysine. Benzylpenicilloyl polylysine is available as a skin test reagent and for coupling to cyanogen bromide-activated disks in the RAST.

TABLE 11–24. Adverse Drug Reactions

Reaction	Example	Comment
Drug Allergy		
Type I IgE-mediated hypersensitivity	Penicillin, insulin, cephalosporins	Urticaria, wheezing anaphylaxis
Type II cytotoxic antibodies	1. Penicillin—hemolytic anemia 2. Quinidine—thrombocytopenia	Drug-hapten interaction
Type III immune complex	Penicillin, sulfonamides, cephalosporins	Serum sickness
Type IV cell-mediated	Neosporin contact dermatitis, topical antihistamines	T lymphocyte dependent
Possibly Allergic–Immune		
Drug-induced systemic lupus erythematosus	Hydralazine, phenytoin, penicillamine, INH	Immune complex. Low incidence of cerebral, renal disease. Positive anti-histone antibodies
Anticonvulsant hypersensitivity	Phenytoin, phenobarbital, carbamazepine-induced rash, hepatitis, lymphadenopathy, pneumonitis, fever	Hereditary abnormal drug metabolism produces toxic metabolites that damage target cells such as lymphocytes
Sulfonamide hypersensitivity	Rash, fever, lymphadenopathy	Same as above
Drug fever	Antibiotic, phenytoin	± Eosinophilia, recurrence with rechallenge
Mucocutaneous reactions	1. Stevens-Johnson (sulfonamides) 2. Toxic epidermal necrolysis (penicillin, sulfonamides, phenytoin) 3. Fixed drug eruption (penicillin) 4. Erythema nodosum (oral contraceptive agents) 5. Photoallergic reactions (sulfonamides) 6. Trimethoprim-sulfamethoxazole induced rash, neutropenia in AIDS	Presumed allergy but mechanisms undetermined
Pulmonary hypersensitivity	1. Asthma (aspirin) 2. Pulmonary infiltrates with eosinophilia (sulfonamides)	1. Alters prostaglandin production 2. Unknown, possible lymphocyte sensitization
Hepatic hypersensitivity	1. Cholestasis (phenothiazine, sulfonamides) 2. Hepatocellular (INH, hydralazine)	Unknown
Renal hypersensitivity	Interstitial nephritis (penicillins)	High IgE, eosinophiluria
Pseudoallergic		
Anaphylactoid	Radiocontrast, D-tubocurarine, opiates	Direct mast cell degranulation
Ampicillin rash	With or without Epstein-Barr virus infection	Unknown cause; onset 7th day without EBV infection
β-Blocking agents	Asthma	Bronchoconstriction
Nonallergic		
Drug overdose	Acetaminophen	Toxic metabolite
Drug–drug interaction	Erythromycin-theophylline Toxic theophylline levels as erythromycin inhibits cytochrome P_{450} metabolism	
Drug side effect	1. Sedation-antihistamines 2. Impaired excretion	1. Predictable 2. Renal-hepatic insufficiency
Secondary effects	Antibiotics-perianal candidiasis	Predictable
Drug idiosyncrasy	1. Phenytoin 2. Glucose-6-phosphate dehydrogenase deficiency and hemolysis (sulfonamides) 3. Malignant hyperthermia (halothane)	1. May be genetically determined (see above) 2. Genetically determined enzyme deficiency 3. Genetic abnormality in muscle contraction
Drug teratogenicity	Thalidone	Maturational-differential effects in fetus
Coincidental	Development of viral rash while on therapy with antibiotics	Common in children
Psychogenic	Nausea, abdominal pain despite placebo, or drug unlikely to produce symptoms Placebo effect	

Unfortunately, the most feared consequence of **penicillin allergy**, anaphylaxis, is not due to IgE sensitization to the major BPO haptenic group but to less well defined, so-called minor haptenic determinants. These include penicilloate, penilloate, and penicillenate and its oxidation products. Though only 5% or less of the benzyl penicillin that reacts with proteins forms minor haptenic determinants, these have major clinical significance; unfortunately, antigens with minor determinant specificity are not readily available for testing either in vivo or in vitro.

Allergy to benzyl penicillin is further complicated by the development of related semisynthetic penicillins and cephalosporins that share a degree of immunologic cross-reactivity. Among the penicillins, the specificity of the antibody formed by the patient (e.g., whether directed toward the 6-aminopenicillin acid core common to all penicillins or directed toward a unique determinant on a distinctive side chain) determines the degree of cross-allergenicity. Thus, some patients allergic to benzyl penicillin can tolerate the semisynthetic penicillins and vice versa. While substantially different structurally, penicillin and cephalosporins share the highly protein-reactive β-lactam ring structure. Cases of anaphylaxis following administration of cephalosporins to patients with penicillin allergy are uncommon but have occurred.

Adverse reactions to ampicillin occur in 10% of patients who receive the drug and merit special consideration. The typical ampicillin rash is not urticarial and appears in 90% of patients with infectious mononucleosis and also in patients with hyperuricemia. That the rash causes no other ill effects and typically disappears with continuing therapy casts doubt upon its immunologic nature; the pathogenesis of ampicillin rash remains an enigma. However, allergy to ampicillin manifested by an urticarial eruption may occur in 1% of children treated with the drug.

CLINICAL MANIFESTATIONS. Cutaneous eruptions are the most common manifestation of adverse drug reactions in children. Urticarial, exanthematous, and eczematoid eruptions predominate, but almost any morphology can occur: exfoliative dermatitis (penicillin, sulfonamides, phenothiazines, anticonvulsants), bullous dermatoses (including epidermal necrolysis), erythema multiforme, Stevens-Johnson syndrome (sulfonamides, penicillin, barbiturates, anticonvulsants, phenytoin in particular), petechial eruptions, Lyell syndrome (penicillin, barbiturates, anticonvulsants, isoniazid), acneiform eruptions (iodides in postpubertal patients), lichenoid eruptions, photodermatitis (demethylchlortetracycline and phenothiazines), and fixed drug eruptions.

Renal or pulmonary disease following drug therapy rarely occurs during childhood. There have been occasional reports of interstitial nephritis associated with phenytoin with in vitro evidence of a cellular immune reaction. In a child being treated with nitrofurantoin, fever, cough, and pulmonary infiltration strongly suggest an adverse drug reaction.

When a child who has received prolonged antimicrobial therapy has persistent fever without other cause, drug fever should be considered. Drug fever is often suspected but rarely proved and does not generally occur as the sole manifestation of an adverse drug reaction. There is often a concomitant rash. The diagnosis is easily made when the drug is discontinued and defervescence occurs within 24–48 hr.

Immunologically mediated drug-induced reactions involving the liver are extremely rare in children, unlike adults. The same is true for drug-induced disorders of granulocytes and platelets; the overwhelming majority of these are toxic.

DIAGNOSIS. Diagnosis of an allergic drug reaction depends on a careful history. Urticaria or angioedema following use of a drug is more relevant than nondescript rashes, because urticaria is often due to IgE-mediated reactions. Even under the best of circumstances, however, a definitive diagnosis of an allergic drug reaction is frequently difficult to establish.

Penicillin is the only drug for which allergy skin testing is of well-established reliability in identifying anaphylactic hypersensitivity. Skin testing with benzylpenicilloyl-polylysine (BPL; PrePen) and penicillin G identifies the overwhelming majority of children who are at risk of anaphylactic reactions following penicillin administration. The BPL is tested in a concentration of 6.0×10^{-5} M (as supplied by the manufacturer), first by prick or puncture test and, if negative, then by intradermal test according to the manufacturer's instructions. Benzyl penicillin (penicillin G) supplied as potassium penicillin G for injection, USP 1,000,000 U/vial is freshly diluted with saline to a concentration of 6,000 U/mL. It is prudent to begin testing with a further 100-fold dilution of penicillin G if there is a history of a life-threatening, systemic reaction to penicillin within the previous year. Penicillin G is first tested by prick or puncture and then by intradermal technique up to a final concentration of 6,000 U/mL. If the skin tests (interpreted in the same way as skin tests with pollen or other allergenic extracts) are negative, anaphylaxis is highly unlikely, and, if there is a compelling reason to do so, treatment may be initiated with a small test dose, usually one tenth of the usual dose, given either intravenously or orally. It is, however, impossible to exclude anaphylactic sensitivity due to other haptenic determinants formed in vivo from penicillin for which no skin test reagents are available. Furthermore, penicillin skin tests are predictive only of anaphylaxis and not of serum sickness or other reactions associated with use of the drug.

Patch testing to determine delayed hypersensitivity to a drug is helpful; it should be carried out by someone familiar with the technique to avoid both false-positive and false-negative reactions due to improper procedure.

In vitro testing for drug allergy is principally carried out by RAST for detection of BPO-specific IgE antibodies. RAST for the other haptenic determinants of penicillin allergy is not available. As is the case with other allergens, the properly performed skin test is preferred to RAST because of speed, sensitivity, and cost. Search for serum antibodies to formed elements of the blood in patients with what appear to be drug-induced blood disorders is rarely productive. Assays of cellular immunity have been used in the investigation of drug allergy. Their validity in this context has not been established.

TREATMENT OF DRUG REACTIONS. Therapy depends upon the mechanism of drug reaction and the clinical manifestations. Discontinuation of the drug is indicated usually. Under certain conditions, especially in infants and small children who develop rashes while receiving antibiotics, the circumstances may support a decision to continue administration of the drug until the etiology of the rash becomes clear. If, for example, an infant or small child with a febrile illness develops an exanthematous and nonurticarial rash on first exposure to penicillin, ampicillin, or another antibiotic, the rash is more likely that of a viral illness than a cutaneous manifestation of allergy to the drug. Rather than labeling the child allergic to the drug on tenuous grounds and compromising its future use, it may be reasonable to continue therapy for a further period while the course of the rash is observed. If the history suggests that an adverse reaction has a pharmacologic basis, the drug may be introduced again at a later date, at a lower dosage or a longer interval between doses, while the serum concentration of the drug is measured, if possible. Ampicillin presents a special problem. There is little to suggest an allergic basis to the rash. If there are special circumstances that dictate the need for the drug, therapy may be continued with the expectation that the rash will disappear and no other problems develop. On the other hand, *if an allergic etiology is likely, the drug should not be reintroduced into the patient,* and an alternative drug should be sought. When treatment with penicillin is mandatory despite documented allergy to the drug, desensitization may be possible. Fatal anaphylaxis has occurred during parenteral desensitization with penicillin. Oral desensitization is probably safer (Table 11–25). No fatal or life-threatening reactions have been reported in association with oral desensitization to penicillin, but pruritus and cutaneous eruptions have occurred commonly, and serum sickness has occurred rarely. Treatment of systemic anaphylaxis is discussed in Sec. 11.44.

Cutaneous eruptions are the most common manifestation of drug allergy in children. The eruptions are generally self-limited and disappear when the drugs are discontinued. Treatment is therefore symptomatic. Antihistamines are most useful for urticarial rashes. Diphenhydramine (Benadryl) and hydroxyzine (Atarax, Vistaril) have both antihistaminic and sedative properties, which may be useful. It may be necessary to give as much as twice the usually recommended dose to achieve satisfactory control of symptoms. Epinephrine 1:1,000 in doses of 0.1–0.3 mL provides short-term relief. For a more

TABLE 11–25. Oral Desensitization to Penicillin and Other β-Lactam Antibiotics in Patients with Specific Anaphylactic Hypersensitivity to the Drug

Step	Drug Concentration (mg/mL)	Volume (mL)	Dose Administered (mg)
1	0.5	0.1	0.05
2	0.5	0.2	0.10
3	0.5	0.4	0.20
4	0.5	0.8	0.40
5	0.5	1.6	0.80
6	0.5	3.2	1.60
7	0.5	6.4	3.20
8	5.0	1.2	6.00
9	5.0	2.4	12.00
10	5.0	4.8	24.00
11	50.0	1.0	50.00
12	50.0	2.0	100.00
13	50.0	4.0	200.00
14	50.0	8.0	400.00

Dilute successive doses in 30 mL of water and administer by mouth at intervals of 15 min. Observe the patient for 30 min after completion of desensitization, and then administer 1 g of the same drug by intravenous infusion.

sustained effect, a suspension of epinephrine (Sus-Phrine) in doses of 0.1–0.2 mL may be given subcutaneously every 6 hr. Corticosteroids are reserved for severe cases not relieved by the foregoing measures. The dose and dosage interval are determined by the severity of the reaction.

PREVENTION. To minimize adverse drug reactions, physicians should use drugs only when indicated, be wary of new drugs, and know the relationships between drugs. Concurrent use of two or more drugs should be avoided unless definitely indicated. Oral administration is less sensitizing than parenteral and preferred whenever possible. Topical application should be avoided when possible because of increased risk of sensitization by this route. Drug interactions should be anticipated, and patients should be warned against self-medication.

Anderson J, Adkinson F: Allergic reactions to drugs and biologic agents. JAMA 258:2891, 1987.
Blaise M, deShazor R: Drug allergy. Pediatr Clin North Am 35:1131, 1988.
Kaplan AP: Drug-induced skin disease. J Allergy Clin Immunol 74:573, 1984.
Matthews KP: Clinical spectrum of allergic and pseudoallergic drug reactions. J Allergy Clin Immunol 74:558, 1984.
Penicillin allergy in childhood. Lancet 1:420, 1989.
Position Statement: Adverse effects and complications of treatment with beta-adrenergic agents. J Allergy Clin Immunol 75:443, 1985.
Reider M, Uetrecht J, Shear N, et al: Diagnosis of sulfonamide hypersensitivity reactions by in vitro "rechallenge" with hydroxylamine metabolites. Ann Intern Med 110:286, 1989.
Sogn DD: Penicillin allergy. J Allergy Clin Immunol 74:589, 1984.
Stark BJ, Earl HS, Gross GN, et al: Acute and chronic desensitization of penicillin-allergic patients using oral penicillin. J Allergy Clin Immunol 79:523, 1987.

11.47 INSECT ALLERGY

See also Sec. 11.39.

Allergic reactions to insects can cause (1) symptoms of respiratory allergy due to inhalation of particulate matter of insect origin, (2) local cutaneous reactions to insect bites, and (3) anaphylactic reactions to stinging insects.

ETIOLOGY. Sensitization to antigenic material found in the debris and disintegrated bodies of dead insects can cause conjunctivitis, rhinitis, or asthma. Inhalation of scales from the wings of insects such as the mayfly, caddis fly, and moths is a particularly common cause of respiratory symptoms in the Great Lakes area, where large numbers of these insects appear each summer. Local cutaneous reactions commonly follow bites by mosquitoes, flies, and various insects. Anaphylactic reactions of both immediate (IgE-mediated) and delayed (T lymphocyte) hypersensitivity due to insect allergy are almost entirely caused by Hymenoptera, including the apids (honeybee, bumblebee), the vespids (wasp, hornet, yellow jacket), and, rarely, the ant family. About 0.4–0.8% of people give histories of systemic reactions to stinging insects, which cause approximately 40 deaths each year in the United States.

PATHOGENESIS. Inhalant allergy to insects is in many cases due to IgE-mediated sensitivity to antigenic materials found in the insects' bodies. The antigenic components responsible for respiratory symptoms have not been thoroughly studied, but the allergenic material appears to reside usually in the cuticle or integument of the insect's body.

In the case of biting insects, the local reaction is frequently a wheal and flare lesion; it appears to be due to vasoactive or irritant materials deposited in the skin while the insect is feeding. There is no evidence for IgE involvement in the local reaction. The mechanism of late or persisting cutaneous reactions is unknown.

Stinging insect venoms contain at least nine components that may contribute to adverse reactions. These include vasoactive materials such as histamine, acetylcholine, and kinins, a number of enzymes (phospholipase A and B, hyaluronidase), apamine, melittin, and formic acid. Phospholipase A is the major allergen of honeybee venom. Some antigens in Hymenoptera venom and whole-body extracts are common to the Hymenoptera order; others are family-specific. There is substantial cross-reactivity among vespid venoms. The majority of patients who experience systemic reactions following Hymenoptera stings have IgE-mediated sensitivity to antigenic material in the venom. There are, however, patients with convincing histories of sting anaphylaxis in whom both skin tests and RAST to venoms are negative. Children may have a systemic reaction with the first sting.

CLINICAL MANIFESTATIONS. The clinical findings in inhalant allergy due to insects are quite similar to those seen with the usual inhalant allergens such as pollens. Rhinitis, conjunctivitis, and asthma have all been described.

The cutaneous reactions to biting insects are most often urticarial but may be papular, vesicular, and erythematous, particularly as the lesion progresses. Lesions that resemble typical delayed hypersensitivity reactions also occur.

Clinical reactions to stinging venomous insects range in severity from minimal pain and local erythema to life-threatening anaphylactic episodes. The usual reaction is swelling of less than 4–5 cm, lasting less than 24 hr. Large local reactions have more swelling and are of longer duration than the usual reaction. Systemic non–life-threatening reactions include multiple cutaneous lesions distal to the site of envenomation (e.g., generalized urticaria, angioedema, pruritus). Life-threatening, immediate systemic reactions are similar to anaphylaxis (laryngeal edema, bronchospasm, hypotension, urticaria). Children with large local or mild systemic reactions rarely develop subsequent severe anaphylaxis. A toxic nonallergic reaction of fever, malaise, emesis, and nausea often follows multiple stings and is rarely fatal. Serum sickness, nephrotic syndrome, vasculitis, neuritis, or encephalopathy may be seen as late sequelae of the reaction to stinging insects.

DIAGNOSIS. The diagnosis is usually easily made from the history and, in the case of biting insects, by examination of skin lesions. Papular urticaria, which is common in children, is almost always the result of insect bites, especially of mosquitoes, fleas, and bedbugs.

Venoms of five Hymenoptera (honeybee, yellow jacket, yellow hornet, white-faced hornet, and wasp) are available for skin testing and treatment. The skin tests should be done in accordance with the manufacturer's recommendations. There is a consensus that appropriately performed skin testing with potent materials is useful in identifying children at risk of systemic anaphylaxis, but venom skin test–negative subjects have been reported to develop anaphylaxis when stung. Moreover, as many as 40% of skin test–positive, nonimmunized subjects may *not* experience anaphylaxis upon sting challenge. In vitro testing with RAST has not substantially improved the ability to predict anaphylaxis compared with skin testing. With venom RAST there is a 20% incidence of both false-positive and false-negative results. Skin testing is indicated for children with systemic reactions.

TREATMENT. Immunotherapy is occasionally undertaken when it can be established that inhalant allergy is due to a specific insect such as the mayfly or caddis fly. Beneficial results from such treatment have not been thoroughly documented, and avoidance of the insect is the preferred management.

For cutaneous reactions due to biting insects, treatment with topical medicaments to relieve itching and local discomfort and occasionally the systemic use of an antihistamine are appropriate. Mosquito extract immunotherapy is not of established effectiveness.

In case of an anaphylactic reaction following a Hymenoptera sting, the acute treatment is essentially the same as that for anaphylaxis. Epinephrine 1:1,000 in a dose of 0.01 mL/kg, maximum 0.3 mL, by subcutaneous injection is effective for relief of laryngeal edema, bronchoconstriction, and peripheral vascular collapse. Blood volume expanders must be given for persistent hypotension. An antihistamine (e.g., diphenhydramine, 25–50 mg) may be given, although its efficacy has not been established. Corticosteroids are of little use in treatment of the acute systemic reaction but may be useful for treatment of sequelae.

Children who have had previous severe or anaphylactic reactions to Hymenoptera stings (or their parents) should be equipped with an EpiPen or EpiPen Jr, which facilitates rapid delivery of an injection of epinephrine, or with a kit that includes epinephrine for injection and an antihistamine tablet for emergency use. Patients at risk of anaphylaxis from an insect sting should also wear an identification bracelet (Medic-Alert) indicating their allergy.

Children and youth at risk from insect stings should avoid using perfumes or cosmetics and wearing bright or pastel-colored clothing when outdoors. They should always wear gloves when gardening and long pants or slacks and shoes when walking in the grass or through fields. Typical insect repellants are of little use against Hymenoptera.

Venom immunotherapy has an uncertain status because the natural history of venom reactivity is not adequately understood. IgE-mediated reactivity as measured by skin test or RAST may decline spontaneously in untreated patients. During the first months of venom therapy, venom-specific IgE antibodies increase by as much as three times but usually fall to pretreatment levels over 1–2 yr of therapy. Whether the patient's clinical sensitivity is increased during the early course of immunotherapy is unknown. Venom-specific IgG antibody, which correlates with protection against anaphylaxis in most patients, peaks at 2–4 mo following initiation of immunotherapy and declines according to the half-life of the immunoglobulin; therefore monthly injections of aqueous extracts are indicated. IgE antibodies may remain detectable for many years in the serum of treated patients. Those who experience severe systemic reactions (airway involvement or hypotension) and have a positive skin test should receive immunotherapy. Immunotherapy is not indicated for children in whom stings have caused only urticarial or local reactions. However, therapy is indicated in adolescents and adults if skin tests are positive to venom and there is a history of a non–life-threatening or life-threatening systemic reaction. Immunotherapy is not indicated in patients with a history of sting anaphylaxis and negative skin test and RAST; one would not know which venom to use. The incidence of side effects during the course of treatment is significant (50% of treated adults experience large local reactions and about 7%, systemic reactions). The incidence of both local and systemic reactions is much lower in children. A major problem is the high cost (related to the difficulty in obtaining vespid and polistes venom) of venom immunotherapy. It is uncertain how long immunotherapy with Hymenoptera venom should continue, but many adults who have received 5 yr of therapy tolerate challenge stings without systemic reactions for several years after completion of treatment.

In children with hypersensitivity to fire ant venom, systemic anaphylaxis may follow the sting of fire ants, *Solenopsis richteri* or *S. invicta*, which are members of the order Hymenoptera. Fire ants are found throughout the southeastern United States. Fire ant venom is more sensitive than whole body extract for identification of allergic patients but only whole body extract is commercially available for diagnosis by allergy skin testing and for treatment by immunotherapy. Immunotherapy has been successful, but there is considerable variation in the venom content of the commercially available whole body extracts.

Bahna SL, Strimas JH, Reed MA, et al: Imported fire ant allergy in young children: Skin reactivity and serum IgE antibodies to venom and whole body extract. J Allergy Clin Immunol 82:419, 1988.

Graft DF, Schuberth KC: Hymenoptera allergy in children. Pediatr Clin North Am 30:873, 1983.

Schuberth KC, Kwiterovich KA, Kagey-Sobotka A, et al: Starting and stopping venom immunotherapy in children with insect allergy. J Allergy Clin Immunol 81:200, 1988.

Valentine M, Lichtenstein L: Anaphylaxis and stinging insect hypersensitivity. JAMA 258:2881, 1987.

11.48 OCULAR ALLERGIES

Allergic reactions involving the eye occur much less commonly in children than in adults. The eye may be involved as part of a generalized allergic reaction in atopic dermatitis, urticaria, angioedema, for example, or the eye alone may be affected. Allergic reactions in the eye are known to occur on the basis of IgE-mediated allergy, as conjunctivitis in a child with ragweed hay fever, for example, or on the basis of a cell-mediated (delayed hypersensitivity) immune reaction, as in contact dermatitis of the eyelids.

EYELIDS. Eyelids are particularly prone to swelling because of their loose areolar connective tissue. Swelling may result from contact dermatitis to a variety of environmental substances. The lids are particularly involved because of the frequency with which offending contact sensitizers are carried to the eyelids with the hands. Occasionally, contact dermatitis appears as a result of sensitization to medication applied to the eyes. Cosmetics and topical ophthalmic medications are common sensitizing agents. Sulfonamides, neomycin, scopolamine, atropine, pilocarpine, contact lens solution, and topical anesthetics cause contact sensitization. The lids become inflamed and indurated, and a scaly eczematoid reaction is evident. The conjunctiva becomes red, and a follicular conjunctivitis may develop.

Blepharitis. This is an inflammatory eczematous reaction of the eyelid margins, which may be caused by infection, allergy, or both. A chronic staphylococcal infection has been implicated as the major cause of chronic eczema of the eyelid margins. The lid margins, particularly of the lower lids, are affected with an itchy, scaly, erythematous eruption with exudate at the base of the lashes. This gives the appearance of "granulated eyelids." The eyelids may be crusted together in the morning. The diagnosis is confirmed by slit lamp examination.

ALLERGIC CONJUNCTIVITIS. This frequently accompanies allergic rhinitis in patients with hay fever, especially when due to pollens. In affected children, both eyes itch, the conjunctivae are reddened and edematous, and there may be profuse tearing. Rubbing of the eyes aggravates the condition. There is no photophobia or other signs of corneal involvement. Occasionally edema of the conjunctiva is so severe that the conjunctiva prolapses over the lower lid in a gelatinous-appearing mass that causes great concern to parents. The secretions are frequently watery but, if persistent, may appear purulent. Even discharges that appear purulent, however, contain predominantly eosinophils; these permit differentiation from infectious conjunctivitis, in which the discharge contains mostly polymorphonuclear leukocytes and bacteria.

Atopic Keratoconjunctivitis. This condition occurs in patients with atopic dermatitis, who have extreme ocular itching, red eyes, swollen and thickened eyelids, and, when the cornea is involved, photophobia. Keratoconus, a central corneal ectasia, is thought to be due to repeated eye rubbing and cataracts are complications.

Vernal Conjunctivitis. This inflammation is more common in children, with a 3:1 male-female predominance, than in adults (80% of patients are under 14 yr old at onset). It appears most often in warm climates and during the spring and summer. The disease affects both eyes and occurs in palpebral and limbal forms. In the *palpebral* form, which is most common, the tarsal plate of the upper lid presents a characteristic "cobblestone" appearance as a result of hyperplasia and thickening of the conjunctiva. The hyperplasia may cause pseudoptosis. A thick, ropy, whitish discharge may be present over the hypertrophied, giant papillae giving the "cobblestone" appearance. In the *limbal* form, the junction of the cornea and sclera is involved, with thickening and opacity of the tissue in the area. Whitish **Trantas dots**, present on the corneoscleral limbus, which represent accumulations of eosinophils, are pathognomonic of the disease. Progression of the limbal form may scar the cornea and lead to blindness in the most severe cases. Symptoms of vernal conjunctivitis include lacrimation, extreme itching, burning, and a particularly distressing photophobia. The seasonal occurrence, the finding of eosinophils, and the frequent coexistence with other atopic diseases such as asthma, hay fever, and eczema suggest that IgE-mediated sensitivity is responsible for the condition; but detailed study of patients with the condition usually fails to identify any cause, and immunotherapy is of little if any value. The symptoms and signs of vernal conjunctivitis are mimicked in a syndrome induced by the wearing of hard or soft contact lenses, giant papillary conjunctivitis.

TREATMENT. Contact dermatitis of the lids is best managed by identification of suspected sensitizers and their elimination. A short course of topical corticosteroids is of value in managing the acute reaction.

Blepharitis is best treated by good lid hygiene, using cotton-tipped applicators and half-strength baby shampoo mixed with water to remove scales and exudate, followed by the use of antistaphylococcal ointments. If an excessive reaction to the treatment results, steroids are applied topically for a few days. Since the disease tends to recur, regular lid care is indicated, often for a lifetime.

Allergic conjunctivitis in the patient with hay fever generally responds well to topical application of sympathomimetics (naphazoline or phenylephrine) in the form of eye drops, cromolyn sodium 4% solution, or, in more severe cases, to eye drops or ointments containing corticosteroids. As noted below, steroids should be used in the eyes only with caution. Immunotherapy for allergic conjunctivitis in the absence of allergic rhinitis gives poor results.

Atopic keratoconjunctivitis requires the use of topical steroids, particularly if the cornea is involved. Referral to an ophthalmologist is indicated.

Vernal conjunctivitis may be treated with sparing use of corticosteroid eye drops or ointments. Medrysone (HMS), a topically active, poorly absorbed corticosteroid, in a dose of 1–2 drops 4 times/day, is particularly indicated in allergic conjunctivitis when there is involvement of only the superficial layers of the eye. The drug is less likely to cause increased intraocular pressure than the more readily absorbed preparations such as dexamethasone or methylprednisolone. Whenever topical steroids are used in the eye for more than a few days, intraocular pressure should be monitored. In addition, prolonged topical steroid administration may predispose the patient to cataracts and opportunistic infections. Cromolyn sodium in 4% solution, 1–2 drops 4 times/day, may provide modest relief of the symptoms of vernal conjunctivitis.

Friedlaender MH: Immunologic aspects of diseases of the eye. JAMA 258:2917, 1987.

Friedlaender MH: Clues in the diagnosis of ocular allergy. Immunol Allerg Pract 7:35, 1985.

Friedlaender MH, Akumoto M, Kelley J: Diagnosis of ocular allergy. Arch Ophthalmol 102:1198, 1984.

11.49 ADVERSE REACTIONS TO FOODS

The incidence of adverse reactions to foods is not known and unquestionably varies in different parts of the world. The average United States diet contains many food antigens, chemical food additives, antibiotics, and other substances; accordingly, a significant frequency of adverse reactions to foods should not be surprising. Food reactions caused by allergic mechanisms are estimated to occur in from 0.3–0.7% of people, but the prevalence of food allergy is a subject of substantial disagreement. Most adverse reactions to food do not have an immunologic basis. In these cases the use of immunologic methods of diagnosis (skin testing or provocative testing [injection or oral administration of food antigen]) is inappropriate. Treatment based on immunologic principles is similarly unwarranted.

ETIOLOGY. Possible mechanisms for adverse reactions to foods include not only allergy but also enzyme deficiencies and nonimmunologic reactions to tyramine, nitrites, and monosodium glutamate (Table 11–26). There is little doubt that intact macromolecules may pass through the epithelium of the gastrointestinal tract and gain access to the systemic circulation, particularly during the first few months of life. Secretory IgA limits the intestinal absorption of intact macromolecules. Children with IgA deficiency have higher levels of antibodies to cow milk proteins and of immune complexes containing milk than do normal controls. IgE-mediated reactions are characteristically rapid in onset and may present as angioedema of the lips, mouth, uvula, or glottis; as generalized urticaria; as asthma; or occasionally as shock. In such cases the patient usually recognizes that the symptoms have followed ingestion of a certain food. Persons with such IgE-mediated food allergy are at constant risk of exposure to the offending food hidden in a food mixture. For example, a nut-sensitive individual may have a serious reaction to ingestion of a cookie made with almond extract.

Individuals with IgE-mediated food reactions consistently show positive skin tests to the suspected food. In fact, skin testing itself, particularly if done by the intracutaneous technique, can precipitate the clinical reaction in individuals with anaphylactic allergy to a food. Foods that have the highest

TABLE 11–26. Differential Diagnosis of Adverse Reactions to Foods

Condition	Example
Food allergy	Anaphylaxis, urticaria-angioedema, eosinophilic colitis, eczema. nuts, eggs, seafood, milk, celery, soy
Immune-mediated	Celiac disease
Food additives	Dyes (tartrazine), flavoring (MSG*), preservatives (metabisulfite)
Food poisoning (toxins)	Botulism, *Bacillus cereus, Clostridium perfringens, Staphylococcus aureus, Scombroid, Ciguatera,* paralytic shellfish
Infections	*Salmonella, Shigella, Escherichia coli, Yersinia, Campylobacter, Giardia,* rotavirus, Norwalk agents, AIDS
Contaminants	Heavy metals, antibiotics (penicillin)
Pharmacologic agents	Caffeine, tyramine, alcohol, histamine
Gastrointestinal disorders	Gastroesophageal reflux, pyloric stenosis, tracheoesophageal fistula, malrotation, peptic ulceration, inflammatory bowel disease
Enzyme deficiencies	Galactosemia, urea cycle defects, phenylketonuria
Malabsorption syndromes	Lactose deficiency, cystic fibrosis, cholestasis
Psychologic	School phobia
Functional	Irritable bowel syndrome, chronic nonspecific diarrhea of infancy

*MSG = monosodium glutamate.

potential to cause IgE-mediated sensitivity are fish, shellfish, peanut (a legume), various nuts and seeds, eggs, cow milk, soy, wheat, and corn.

More difficult to diagnose are reactions that begin a few to 24 hr after ingestion of the offending food. Such reactions have been attributed without much convincing evidence to allergy to a digestive product of the food such as a protease or polypeptide. The roles of antigen-antibody complexes and cell-mediated immunity (delayed hypersensitivity) in the pathogenesis of these late-occurring reactions are unknown.

A variety of reactions have been reported to follow ingestion of *cow milk* by infants and children. In some cases an IgE mechanism has been established. In others, however, even with antibodies to milk proteins (particularly α-lactalbumin, β-lactoglobulin, and casein) present in sufficient quantities to be demonstrable by gel diffusion methods, no immunologic mechanism has been established. During the 1st yr of life, vomiting and watery, blood-streaked, mucoid diarrhea may follow cow milk ingestion. An enteropathy with loss of both protein and blood has been found in other young infants fed large volumes of whole pasteurized milk (but not heat-processed formula). In older infants ingestion of cow milk has been associated with occult fecal blood loss, recurrent roentgenographic pulmonary infiltrates, and multiple precipitating antibodies to cow milk proteins (Sec. 14.71). Some cases of pulmonary hemosiderosis are said to be responsive to withdrawal of milk from the diet.

Adverse reactions to milk due to *disaccharidase* deficiencies are discussed in Sec. 13.49.

A number of *enteropathies* with varying combinations of malabsorption, steatorrhea, hypoalbuminemia, and fecal blood loss have been reported due to cow milk or wheat intolerance. Despite close associations between symptoms or signs and the feeding of these foods, a precise mechanism of immunologic injury has not been identified. It is not known whether wheat-sensitive individuals who have adverse symptoms from the gluten fraction of wheat are reacting to α-gliadin as a toxin or as an antigen in an immune-complex type of injury.

During the first 3 yr of life, rashes and diarrhea following ingestion of fruits and juices are common. There is no evidence of an immunologic mechanism. Other nonimmunologic adverse reactions to foods principally in adults include headaches after ingestion of wine and cheese (tyramine), cured meat or "hot dog" headache (sodium nitrite), or the Chinese restaurant syndrome (monosodium glutamate). Affected people apparently have idiosyncratic, but not allergic, reactions to these simple chemicals. In other cases nonimmunologic adverse reactions may be due to food additives, including the dyes used in foods and drugs. A report of the National Advisory Committee on Hyperkinesis and Food Additives concluded that there was no direct causal connection between artificial food colors and flavors and hyperactivity in children.

DIAGNOSIS. An etiologic diagnosis in a child suspected of an adverse food reaction requires careful objective study. Elimination from the diet for a period of 7–10 days of a food causing difficulty should generally result in improvement in the patient's symptoms. Reintroduction of the food, initially in small quantities and then in increasing amounts, should result in the return of symptoms in a reasonable period of time, within 7 days at most. If symptoms are produced, the food is eliminated from the diet for several months. Reintroduction of the food *(except in cases of anaphylactic sensitivity)* should be attempted at regular intervals.

The critical testing of foods by the elimination and provocation method is difficult if either patient or parent anticipates an unfavorable reaction because of the emotional bias incident to the ingestion of the suspected food. Food challenges are best done in a blind manner, the food being given in a disguised form for example, in opaque capsules or mixed with another food. When symptoms have been continual, dietary elimination of the offending food should cause prompt improvement. On the other hand, when symptoms such as headache have been intermittent, results of elimination and provocation testing are frequently equivocal.

Skin testing with properly prepared food antigens reveals the presence of any IgE antibody to the test antigen. A negative prick skin test with properly prepared potent food extracts virtually excludes the possibility of IgE-mediated allergy to the test food. On the other hand, a positive skin test does not necessarily indicate that the particular food causes symptoms. Positive tests, especially if they do not correlate with the history, should be confirmed by food challenge. In anaphylactic food allergy, skin tests almost invariably show a positive reaction to the offending food, but in this instance the history alone usually establishes the diagnosis and skin testing is superfluous and may be dangerous. Occasionally, a positive result on a skin test to a food not previously suspected of causing symptoms is clinically corroborated when the history is re-examined in light of the positive test. All too often, undue attention paid to clinically irrelevant skin reactions to food extracts has led to very restricted diets with no attempt made to confirm the clinical importance of suspected foods through elimination and provocative testing. Overdiagnosis of food allergy has sometimes caused malnutrition in infants and children as well as anxiety and depression in mothers who have found it impossible to adhere to severely restrictive diets.

RAST assay has been used to detect IgE antibodies to foods. The correlation between clinical history, puncture skin test, and RAST is excellent for codfish, egg white, nuts, peanuts, and peas. Positive RAST and skin tests to cereals correlate poorly with the results of cereal challenge. RAST for soybeans and white beans is unreliable, apparently because of nonspecific binding of IgE to the RAST disk. RAST does not appear to offer any substantial advantage over skin testing with potent food extracts.

In the provocative/neutralizing method of diagnosis of food

allergy, dilutions of food extracts are injected intracutaneously in an attempt to reproduce the patient's symptoms, which are then said to be relieved by successive intracutaneous injections of other dilutions of the same extract. The techniques vary among users of the method. For example, some users both "provoke" and "neutralize" by *sublingual* administration of the antigen solutions. The validity of all of these methods has not been established, and their use in diagnosis and therapy is unwarranted and experimental at best.

TREATMENT. The treatment of an adverse food reaction is directed at the clinical manifestations, which may be anaphylaxis, urticaria, diarrhea, vomiting, rhinitis, asthma, or atopic dermatitis. Offending foods should be removed from the diet. If elimination diets are prescribed, care must be taken to ensure that they are nutritionally adequate. For reasons that are unclear, some children who are highly reactive to foods become "tolerant" as they grow older; this is especially likely to occur among infants and young children. Foods most likely to become tolerated with the passage of time are cow milk, eggs, and soy. Hypersensitivity to peanuts, nuts, and fish persists for long periods. Cautious periodic attempts to reintroduce offending foods are appropriate. Immunotherapy by injection or sublingual or oral administration of extracts of offending foods is not efficacious.

R. MICHAEL SLY

Atkins FM, Metcalfe DD: The diagnosis and treatment of food allergy. Ann Rev Nutr 4:233, 1984.

Atkins FM, Steinberg SS, Metcalfe DD: Evaluation of immediate adverse reactions to foods in adult patients. I: Correlation of demographic, laboratory and prick skin test data with responses to controlled oral food challenge. J Allergy Clin Immunol 75:348, 1985.

Atkins FM, Steinberg SS, Metcalfe DD: Evaluation of immediate adverse reactions to foods in adult patients. II: A detailed analysis of reaction patterns during oral food challenges. J Allergy Clin Immunol 75:356, 1985.

Bock SA: The natural history of food sensitivity. J Allergy Clin Immunol 69:173, 1982.

Hill DJ, Ford RPK, Skelton MJ, Hosking CS: A study of 100 infants and young children with cow's milk allergy. Clin Rev Allergy 2:125, 1984.

Savilahti E, Verkasalo M: Intestinal cow's milk allergy: Pathogenesis and clinical presentation. Clin Rev Allergy 2:7, 1984.

Simon RA: Adverse reactions to drug additives. J Allergy Clin Immunol 74:623, 1984.

RHEUMATIC DISEASES OF CHILDHOOD
(Inflammatory Diseases of Connective Tissue, Collagen Diseases)

The disorders described in these sections are grouped together because of similarities in symptomatology and pathology; in general, they are associated with inflammatory changes in various connective tissues throughout the body.

The causes of rheumatic diseases of childhood are unknown, and precise diagnostic criteria are lacking. They usually appear as distinct entities, each generally presenting characteristic clinical manifestations. For example, rheumatoid arthritis is associated with chronic arthritis, dermatomyositis with inflammation of muscle and skin, scleroderma with induration of skin, and so on. Each of these diseases, however, can affect many organs, and overlapping symptoms and signs may at times make precise diagnosis difficult.

11.50 LABORATORY STUDIES IN THE RHEUMATIC DISEASES
(Table 11–27)

Although laboratory studies are often helpful, few, if any, are diagnostic or specific for rheumatic diseases. These studies include tests for acute phase phenomena, rheumatoid factors, antinuclear and other autoantibodies, total serum complement and individual complement components, immune complexes, serum proteins and immunoglobulins, and histocompatibility antigens. Other useful tests include blood counts, urinalyses, joint fluid analyses, studies of renal and liver function, and various imaging techniques. Biopsies (skin, kidney) are frequently performed in patients with rheumatic diseases; although tissue histology may provide confirmatory evidence of tissue involvement or aid in classification of disease, it is rarely diagnostic of any specific disease.

ACUTE-PHASE REACTANTS. These are plasma constituents that appear or increase during the inflammatory state. They include the erythrocyte sedimentation rate (ESR), C-reactive protein (CRP), serum mucoproteins, various α-globulins, gamma globulins, some complement components, and certain proteins such as transferrin. Because patients with rheumatic diseases have an active inflammatory process, acute-phase phenomena or reactants are usually present during periods of active disease. Such tests are not invariably positive during inflammation, however, and their absence does not exclude the possibility of an active disease process. These tests are of little diagnostic usefulness because they may be positive in a wide variety of conditions associated with inflammation (e.g., malignancy, infection, tissue trauma, and tissue necrosis). Acute-phase phenomena are sometimes helpful in following the course of disease in individual patients. The ESR is the most readily available test.

RHEUMATOID FACTORS. These are a group of antibodies that react with the Fc portion of immunoglobulin G. These antibodies are not specific for host immunoglobulins but may react with immunoglobulin from other individuals or from other species. Rheumatoid factors detected by standard agglutination techniques such as the latex agglutination test or the sheep cell agglutination test are IgM; anti-immunoglobulin antibodies of the IgG, IgA, and IgE classes can also be identified by methods other than agglutination tests. The occurrence of rheumatoid factors in disease states such as chronic infections (*Toxocara canis,* bacterial endocarditis) or in experimental situations such as hyperimmunization of animals suggests that protracted immune stimulation, chronic infection, or inflammation may underlie their production.

Rheumatoid factors, particularly IgM detected by classic agglutination techniques, are strongly associated with classic adult rheumatoid arthritis; in such patients rheumatoid factors are present in high titer and on serial tests throughout the course of disease. A small subgroup of patients with juvenile rheumatoid arthritis resembling classic adult rheumatoid arthritis also have rheumatoid factors. However, rheumatoid factors are neither specific for nor diagnostic of rheumatoid arthritis. They also occur in other rheumatic diseases (lupus

TABLE 11–27. Laboratory Tests in the Rheumatic Diseases

Rheumatoid factors:
  Classification of JRA

Antinuclear antibodies:
  Diagnosis of SLE (DNP, DNA, Sm, etc.)
  Diagnosis of MCTD (RNP)
  Diagnosis of neonatal lupus syndrome (Ro, La)
  Course of SLE (DNA)
  Classification of JRA

HLA typing:
  Chiefly for research interest
  B27: Spondyloarthropathies

Complement studies:
  Course of SLE
  Evidence of immune complex disease

Acute phase reactants, serum proteins:
  Minor role in following disease course

Blood counts, bone marrow:
  Suspicion of malignancy

Cultures and serologic studies:
  Detect infectious disease

Radiographs, bone scans, other imaging studies:
  Detect underlying bony abnormalities (infection, trauma, malignancy, congenital, or genetic conditions), or other anatomic abnormalities

Biopsies:
  Confirm tissue involvement and sometimes permit classification; diagnosis of malignancy or infectious disease

Organ specific studies:
  Detect specific organ involvement in multisystem disease:
    Neurologic (spinal fluid, EEG, imaging)
    Cardiac (ECG, echo/Doppler)
    Pulmonary (radiograph, pulmonary function)
    Hepatic ("liver function," imaging)
    Gastrointestinal (barium studies, endoscopy)
    Renal (urinalysis, renal function)

DNA = deoxyribonucleic acid; DNP = deoxyribonucleo protein; ECG = electrocardiogram; Echo = echocardiogram; EEG = electroencephalogram; JRA = juvenile rheumatoid arthritis; MCTD = mixed connective tissue disease; RNP = ribonucleoprotein; SLE = systemic lupus erythematosus.

erythematosus, scleroderma), chronic active hepatitis, chronic infections, leukemia and lymphoid malignancies, and certain viral infections; in addition, they can be found in patients following immunizations, open heart surgery, or organ transplantation, and in normal aging human beings. Many children with transiently positive low titers on rheumatoid factor tests have probably had antecedent viral illnesses. Rheumatoid factors do not in themselves cause disease nor are they necessary for the occurrence of chronic synovitis; they may play a role in perpetuation of synovial inflammation in people with rheumatoid arthritis by forming immune complexes with immunoglobulins.

ANTINUCLEAR ANTIBODIES. The antinuclear antibodies (ANA) are a group of antibodies that react with various nuclear constituents, including deoxyribonucleoprotein (DNP), DNA, ribonucleoprotein (RNP), ribonucleic acid (RNA), Sm antigen (a soluble nuclear protein antigen), and many others. Stimuli for production of these antibodies remain unknown. ANA are not specific for organs, individuals, or species of cell origin. They are generally detected in the serum of patients by immunofluorescent staining techniques using standard in vitro frozen animal tissue sections or cell culture preparations.

ANA are neither entirely diagnostic of nor specific for any disease. They are found in almost all patients with systemic lupus erythematosus (SLE) but are also found in patients with juvenile rheumatoid arthritis (JRA), chronic active hepatitis, and scleroderma. The syndrome called *mixed connective tissue disease* is defined by the presence of antibody to RNP. Nonrheumatic conditions associated with ANA include ingestion of a wide variety of drugs (including anticonvulsants, procainamide, birth control pills); certain infections, notably Epstein-Barr infection; certain malignancies, and the normal aging process. High titers of ANA are most common in SLE and mixed connective tissue disease. Several ANA patterns may be detected on immunofluorescent preparations including speckled, homogeneous, peripheral, and nucleolar; these distinctions are of limited clinical usefulness. Antibodies to antigens such as DNA, RNP, Sm, Ro, and La are detected by individual tests utilizing specific antigens or substrates. Antibodies reactive with double-stranded DNA are reasonably specific for SLE and are indicative of active disease. Antibodies to antigens called Ro(SSA) and La(SSB) are associated with the neonatal lupus syndrome.

The lupus erythematosus (LE) cell is the result of an ANA that is reactive with DNP. When serum containing this antibody is mixed in vitro with peripheral white blood cells, their nuclei are rendered susceptible to phagocytosis; the LE cell is a granulocyte that has ingested such a nucleus. This test has been largely superseded by the more sensitive tests for ANA.

COMPLEMENT. Complement consists of a group of serum proteins that mediate certain aspects of inflammation and cell injury (Sec. 11.23). Serum complement levels can be useful in indicating the activity of SLE and other diseases with an immune complex mechanism; low serum complement levels reflect complement consumption by immune complexes and thus indicate active disease. Measurement of total serum hemolytic complement activity is the most useful test. Measurement of individual complement component C3 or C4 determines only the amount of protein without regard to its biologic activity. Complement studies are not diagnostic of any disease except the rare hereditary deficiencies of complement components.

IMMUNE COMPLEX DETERMINATIONS. Immune complexes of antigen and antibody are responsible for tissue damage in some rheumatic diseases (notably SLE) and in a wide variety of other conditions (including certain infectious diseases). Several assays can measure immune complexes in serum and other fluids; however, these tests are of uncertain clinical value.

SERUM PROTEINS AND IMMUNOGLOBULINS. Increased levels of gamma globulins and α_2-globulins are frequently found in patients with active inflammation; these tests are not specific. Elevated levels of one or more specific immunoglobulins may be found in a number of rheumatic diseases, notably SLE; however, there are no diagnostic patterns. Serum albumin levels may be low in patients with chronic inflammation of various causes. Rarely, patients with immunodeficiency states such as IgA deficiency, hypogammaglobulinemia, or various T cell or combined immunodeficiency syndromes manifest rheumatic complaints.

THE HISTOCOMPATIBILITY (HLA) SYSTEM. Associations of histocompatibility antigens (HLA antigens) with certain diseases provide valuable insights into genetically determined susceptibility to disease. Histocompatibility antigens are located on the surfaces of most human cells. Loci determining HLA antigens are located on the 6th chromosome; A, B, C, D, and DR loci are recognized. The HLA system is complex, with multiple alleles for each locus. The prevalences of various HLA alleles vary in different racial groups. HLA typing requires antisera of known specificity to type A, B, C, and DR loci and cells of known specificity to type the D locus.

Biologic roles of HLA antigens, other than those determining tissue compatibility, are not fully known. The HLA system is closely linked to several genes important to the immune system, including loci determining synthesis of various components of complement and loci determing immune responsiveness. Since the HLA antigens are genetically determined traits that can be accurately identified, they can provide information about both disease associations (the occurrence of particular diseases in association with particular HLA antigens) and disease linkages (the passage of a trait along with HLA antigens from generation to generation within the same family, implying that the genes responsible for the trait are close to those of the HLA system on the 6th chromosome).

The strongest association of human disease with the HLA system is that of HLA-B27 with ankylosing spondylitis; 95% of patients with ankylosing spondylitis have HLA-B27 compared with only 6% of the unaffected white North American population. An individual carrying HLA-B27 has a 90 times greater relative risk of developing ankylosing spondylitis than one without B27. Only an estimated 8–20% of individuals with HLA-B27 ever actually develop ankylosing spondylitis or a related disease. Reiter syndrome, the spondylitis of inflammatory bowel disease and psoriasis, acute iridocyclitis, pauciarticular arthritis of older children and adult patients, and the "reactive" arthritis following infections with *Salmonella, Shigella, Yersinia enterocolitica,* or *Campylobacter* are also associated with HLA-B27. The mechanism underlying the association between HLA-B27 and susceptibility to these diseases remains unknown. The association of these spondyloarthropathies with HLA-B27 is seen in various racial populations. No corresponding HLA-D or -DR associations have been made.

Three JRA subgroups have distinct HLA associations, suggesting that there are genetic or immunologic factors that influence the occurrence of particular types of disease. Pauciarthritis with onset in older children (pauciarticular JRA type II) is strongly associated with HLA-B27, providing laboratory evidence consistent with clinical observations that many of these children have early spondyloarthropathies. Pauciarthritis of early childhood associated with ANA and chronic iridocyclitis (pauciarticular JRA type I) has an interesting and still incompletely understood set of associations with HLA-DR8, -DR6, and -DR5. Rheumatoid factor–positive polyarticular disease has a striking association with HLA-DR4, consistent with its clinical resemblance to classic adult-onset rheumatoid arthritis, which is also associated with HLA-DR4. Closer study of DR4-positive children with seropositive arthritis reveals even stronger associations with certain HLA alleles that are detected by the broad test for DR4.

A different group of autoimmune diseases is associated with HLA-B8 and HLA-DW3/DR3 in North American and European populations. These include chronic active hepatitis, celiac sprue, dermatitis herpetiformis with malabsorption, insulin-dependent diabetes mellitus, thyroiditis, Graves disease, Addison disease, myasthenia gravis, Sjögren syndrome, childhood dermatomyositis, and perhaps SLE. All of these diseases are characterized by chronic inflammation, often associated with formation of antibodies reactive with human tissues ("autoantibodies"). Risks for any of these diseases are relatively low for individuals carrying HLA-B8 or HLA-DW3/DR3, and the D associations are stronger than the B associations. Histocompatibility studies have revealed heterogeneous subgroups in several of these diseases: for example, diabetes mellitus (only insulin-dependent diabetes is associated with B8–DW3/DR3, and there are additional associations with DR4) and dermatitis herpetiformis (only dermatitis herpetiformis with malabsorption is associated with B8–DW3/DR3). The specific HLA antigens associated with these diseases may vary among racial groups. Other human diseases, notably multiple sclerosis and psoriasis, have still other HLA-B and -D associations. Few diseases have been associated primarily with antigens in the A locus (one such disease is hemachromatosis).

Human conditions *linked* to the HLA system or transmitted along with HLA antigens from generation to generation include deficiencies of the 2nd and 4th components of complement and congenital adrenal hyperplasia.

HLA typing is not diagnostic of any disease. These studies are obviously useful in matching tissue donors to recipients. There is also a potential use in prenatal diagnosis of linked diseases such as deficiency of the 4th component of complement. Histocompatibility studies remain of great academic interest in classifying diseases, in seeking to identify genetic factors that predispose to disease, and in unraveling immunologic mechanisms in the causation of human disease.

11.51 JUVENILE RHEUMATOID ARTHRITIS

Juvenile rheumatoid arthritis (JRA) is a disease or group of diseases characterized by chronic synovitis and associated with a number of extra-articular inflammatory manifestations. A confusing number of names have been applied, including juvenile arthritis, Still disease, juvenile chronic polyarthritis, and chronic childhood arthritis. JRA encompasses several broad clinical subgroups (Table 11–28). Rheumatoid factor–positive polyarticular disease most closely resembles adult-onset rheumatoid arthritis; rheumatoid factor–negative polyarthritis also occurs in adults. Pauciarticular disease type II is related to the diseases described in adults as "spondyloarthropathies." Systemic-onset disease occurs occasionally in adults. Pauciarticular disease type I with chronic iridocyclitis has not been described in adults. Recognition of these subgroups is useful in the diagnosis, follow-up, and appropriate care of children with chronic arthritis.

ETIOLOGY AND EPIDEMIOLOGY. The etiology of rheumatoid arthritis and the mechanisms for perpetuation of chronic synovial inflammation are unknown. Two current hypotheses are that the disease results from infection with as yet unidentified micro-organisms or that it represents hypersensitivity or an "autoimmune" reaction to unknown stimuli. Attempts to link infectious agents such as rubella virus to JRA remain inconclusive. Infection with *Borrelia burgdorferi,* the spirochete of Lyme disease (Sec. 12.57), causes recurrent or chronic pauciarthritis in some children but apparently accounts for few instances of pauciarticular JRA. Organisms such as mycoplasma have also been associated with synovitis in both experimental animals and humans. The association of rheumatoid factors (antibodies reactive with IgG) with adult-onset rheumatoid arthritis suggests an immune mechanism. However these antibodies clearly do not cause the disease, although immune complexes of rheumatoid factor and immunoglobulin may perpetuate synovial inflammation and are responsible for the rheumatoid vasculitis seen in patients with seropositive rheumatoid arthritis. The low levels of complement found in the synovial fluid of some rheumatoid patients and the low serum complement levels observed in patients with rheumatoid vasculitis are consistent with an immune complex mechanism. This mechanism fails, however, to explain all instances of rheumatoid inflammation because chronic synovitis can occur in the absence of rheumatoid factors. Most children do not have classic rheumatoid factors; attempts to link "hidden rheumatoid factors" (antibodies reactive with gamma globulin detected by different methods) to the pathogenesis of JRA have been inconclusive. The occurrence of chronic arthritis in patients with IgA deficiency and hypogammaglobulinemia suggests that immunodeficiency may somehow predispose to chronic arthritis; however, no identifiable immunodeficiency has been noted in children with JRA. Clinical onset of JRA may follow an acute systemic

TABLE 11–28. Subgroups of Juvenile Rheumatoid Arthritis

	Polyarticular Rheumatoid Factor–Negative	Polyarticular Rheumatoid Factor–Positive	Pauciarticular Type I	Pauciarticular Type II	Systemic-Onset
Percentage of JRA patients	20–25	5–10	35–40	10–15	20
Sex	90% girls	80% girls	80% girls	90% boys	60% boys
Age at onset	Throughout childhood	Late childhood	Early childhood	Late childhood	Through childhood
Joints	Any multiple	Any multiple	Few large joints: knee, ankle, elbow	Few large joints: hip girdle	Any multiple
Sacroiliitis	No	Rare	No	Common	No
Iridocyclitis	Rare	No	30% chronic iridocyclitis	10–20% acute iridocyclitis	No
Rheumatoid factor	Negative	100%	Negative	Negative	Negative
Antinuclear antibodies	25%	75%	90%	Negative	Negative
HLA studies	?	HLA DR4	HLA DR5, DRW6, DRW8	HLA B27	?
Ultimate morbidity	Severe arthritis, 10–15%	Severe arthritis, >50%	Ocular damage, 10% Polyarthritis, 20%	Subsequent spondyloarthropathy, ?%	Severe arthritis, 25%

infection or physical trauma to a joint, but no direct relation to such events has been shown. Exacerbations may follow intercurrent illness or psychic stress.

Pauciarticular disease type II is frequently associated with a positive family history for ankylosing spondylitis, Reiter syndrome, acute iridocyclitis, or pauciarticular arthritis. Both pauciarticular JRA type I and rheumatoid factor–positive polyarthritis occasionally occur in one or more 1st-degree relatives of affected children. Each of these subgroups has distinct HLA associations, indicating some genetic predisposition to disease: pauciarticular disease type II with HLA-B27, pauciarticular disease type I with HLA-DR8, -DR5, and -DR6, and rheumatoid factor–positive disease with HLA-DR4. Neither systemic-onset disease nor seronegative polyarthritis has either known HLA associations or familial occurrence.

JRA is not rare; there are about a quarter million affected children in the United States. About 5% of all cases of rheumatoid arthritis begin in childhood.

PATHOLOGY. Rheumatoid arthritis is characterized by chronic nonsuppurative inflammation of the synovium. Affected synovial tissues are edematous, hyperemic, and infiltrated with lymphocytes and plasma cells. Secretion of increased amounts of joint fluid results in effusions. Projections of thickened synovial membrane form villi, which protrude into joint spaces; hyperplastic rheumatoid synovia may spread over and become adherent to articular cartilage (pannus formation). With continuing chronic synovitis and proliferation of synovia, articular cartilage and other joint structures may become eroded and progressively destroyed. The duration of synovitis before joint damage becomes permanent varies; in general, lasting articular cartilage damage occurs later in the course of JRA than in adult-onset disease, and many children with JRA never incur permanent joint damage despite prolonged synovitis. Joint destruction occurs more often in children with rheumatoid factor–positive disease or systemic-onset disease. Once joint destruction has commenced, erosions of subchondral bone, narrowing of the "joint space" (loss of articular cartilage), destruction or fusion of bones, and deformity, subluxation, or ankylosis of the joints may result. Tenosynovitis and myositis may be present. Osteoporosis, periostitis, accelerated epiphyseal growth, and premature epiphyseal closure can occur adjacent to affected joints.

Rheumatoid nodules occur less frequently in children than in adults, primarily in rheumatoid factor–positive children, and show fibrinoid material surrounded by chronic inflammatory cells. Pleura, pericardium, and peritoneum may show nonspecific fibrinous serositis; chronic constrictive pericarditis occurs rarely, if ever. The rheumatoid rash appears histologically as a mild vasculitis, with a few inflammatory cells surrounding small vessels in subepithelial tissues.

CLINICAL MANIFESTATIONS. Polyarticular-Onset Disease. This entity is characterized by involvement of multiple joints typically including the small joints of the hands (Figs. 11–6 and 11–7). Polyarticular disease unassociated with prominent systemic manifestations occurs in 35% of children with JRA. Two subgroups are included: *rheumatoid factor–negative polyarthritis* (20–25% of all patients with JRA) and *rheumatoid factor–positive polyarthritis* (5–10% of all patients with JRA). Rheumatoid factor–positive disease is characterized by onset in late childhood, more severe arthritis, frequent appearance of rheumatoid nodules, and occasional rheumatoid vasculitis. Rheumatoid factor–negative disease may begin at any time during childhood, is frequently mild, and is rarely associated with rheumatoid nodules. More girls than boys are affected in both types of disease. Both the polyarticular pattern and the nature of the rheumatoid factor tests are generally established early in the course of disease.

Onset of arthritis may be insidious, with gradual development of joint stiffness, swelling, and loss of motion, or

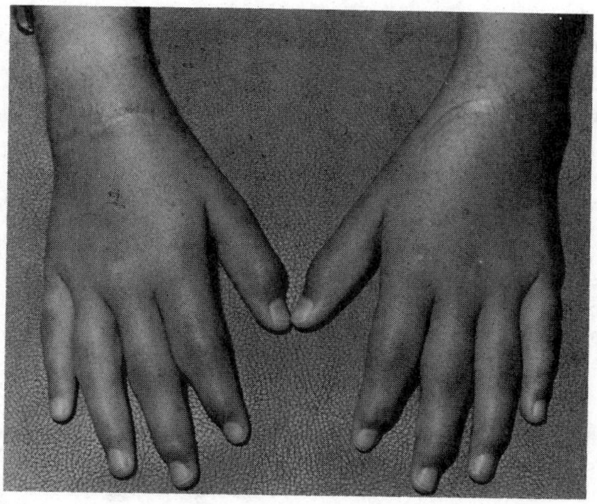

Figure 11–6. Hands and wrists of a girl with rheumatoid factor–negative polyarticular juvenile rheumatoid arthritis. Note the symmetric involvement of the metacarpophalangeal joints, proximal interphalangeal joints, and distal interphalangeal joints. Both wrists are also affected.

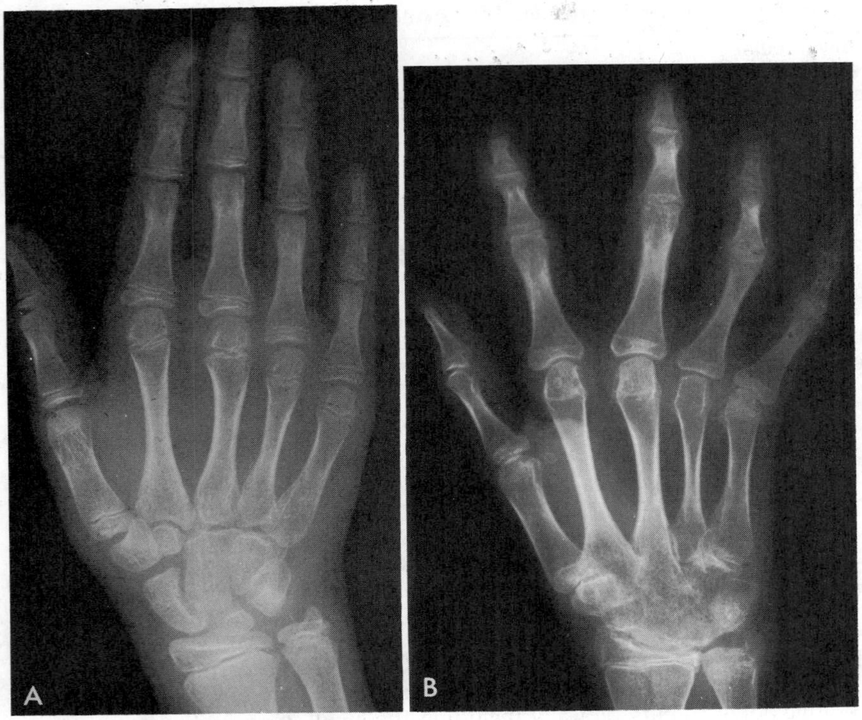

Figure 11–7. Progression of joint destruction in a girl with rheumatoid factor–positive juvenile rheumatoid arthritis despite doses of corticosteroids sufficient to suppress symptoms in the interval between *A* and *B*. *A*, Roentgenogram of the hand at onset. *B*, Roentgenogram 4 yr later, showing a loss of articular cartilage and destructive changes in the distal and proximal interphalangeal and metacarpophalangeal joints and destruction and fusion of wrist bones.

fulminant, with sudden appearance of symptomatic arthritis. Affected joints are swollen and warm but rarely red. Swelling results from periarticular edema, joint effusion, and synovial thickening. Some children have "painless" joint stiffness and discomfort before objective changes appear. Affected joints may be tender to touch and painful on motion; however, severe tenderness and pain are unusual, and many children do not complain of any pain in obviously inflamed joints. Limited joint motion is related early to muscle spasm, joint effusion, and synovial proliferation, and later to joint destruction and ankylosis or to soft tissue contracture. Pronounced synovial proliferation may produce cystic swellings about the affected joints; occasionally herniations of synovium and extravasation of synovial fluid affect the neighboring structures, particularly in the popliteal area (popliteal cyst). Morning stiffness and "gelling" following inactivity are characteristic of rheumatoid arthritis in children as in adults. Young children, particularly those with polyarthritis, are often irritable and assume a typical posture of anxious guarding of their joints against movement (Fig. 11–8).

Arthritis, which may affect any synovial joint, often begins in the large joints such as the knees, ankles, wrists, and elbows; initial involvement is often symmetric. Inflammation of proximal interphalangeal joints produces spindling or fusiform changes of the fingers; metacarpophalangeal joint involvement is equally common, and distal interphalangeal joints may also be affected (see Figs. 11–6 and 11–7). Arthritis of the cervical spine, characterized by neck stiffness and pain, occurs in about half of patients. Temporomandibular involvement with limited ability to open the mouth is common; the pain may be referred to as earache. Hip involvement occurs in at least half the children with polyarthritis, usually beginning later in the disease process. Destruction of the femoral heads may ensue; severe hip disease is a major cause of disability in late JRA (Fig. 11–9). Roentgenographic narrowing of the sacroiliac joints occurs in some patients, usually in association with hip disease. Rarely, cricoarytenoid arthritis causes hoarseness and laryngeal stridor. Involvement of the sternoclavicular joints and costochondral junctions may cause chest pain.

Growth disturbances adjacent to the inflamed joints may result in either overgrowth or undergrowth of the affected part. Increased leg length may follow chronic arthritis of the knee, and micrognathia after temporomandibular arthritis may be a late hallmark of JRA. Small, deformed feet may result from foot involvement in early childhood and shortened fingers from early hand involvement.

Extra-articular manifestations of polyarticular JRA are not as dramatic as those seen in systemic rheumatoid arthritis. Most patients with active polyarticular disease have malaise, anorexia, irritability, and mild anemia. Low-grade fever, slight

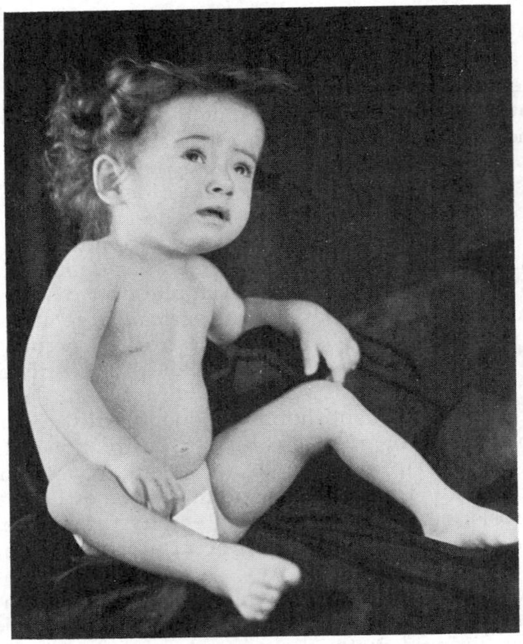

Figure 11–8. Characteristic posture of a child with juvenile rheumatoid arthritis, showing the anxious appearance and guarding of joints.

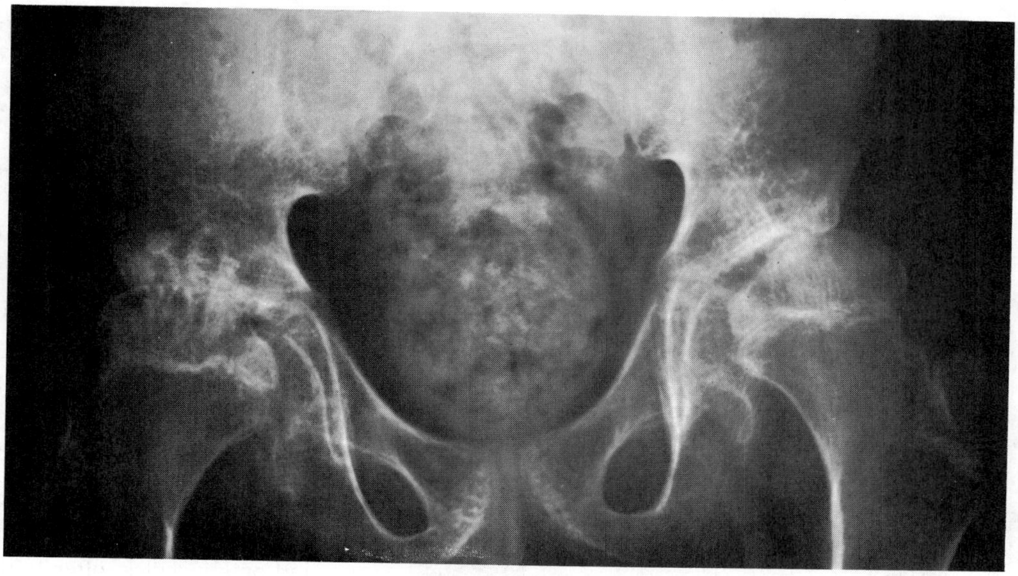

Figure 11–9. Severe hip disease in a 13-yr-old boy with long-active, systemic-onset juvenile rheumatoid arthritis, showing destruction of the femoral heads and acetabula, joint space narrowing, and subluxation of the left hip. The patient had received corticosteroids systemically for 9 yr.

hepatosplenomegaly, and lymphadenopathy may be present. Pericarditis is infrequent and iridocyclitis rare. Rheumatoid nodules may occur over pressure points, usually in patients with positive agglutination test results for rheumatoid factor. Rheumatoid vasculitis occurs at times in rheumatoid factor–positive patients, as does Sjögren syndrome. Growth may be retarded during periods of active disease; growth spurts often occur with remission.

Pauciarticular-Onset Disease. This is characterized by arthritis that remains limited to four or fewer joints for the first 6 mo after disease onset (Fig. 11–10). Large joints are primarily affected, and the distribution of arthritis is often asymmetric. There are two distinct subgroups: Type I includes primarily girls who are young at onset and are at risk for chronic iridocyclitis; type II includes primarily boys who are older at onset and who are at risk for subsequent spondyloarthropathy.

Pauciarticular disease type I is the most common form of JRA, accounting for 35–40% of all patients. The disease generally begins before the 4th birthday. As many as 90% of patients have positive tests for ANA. Neither rheumatoid factor nor HLA-B27 is associated. The most commonly affected joints are the knees, ankles, and elbows; occasionally, there is isolated involvement of other joints such as the temporomandibular joints, single toes or fingers, wrists, or neck. The hips and hip girdle are generally spared, and sacroiliitis is not associated. The clinical appearance and the synovial histology of affected joints are indistinguishable from those of polyarticular JRA. Eighty per cent of children with type I pauciarticular-onset disease continue to have limited joint involvement; and although the arthritis may be chronic or recurrent, serious disability or joint destruction is uncommon. The other 20% of children have later additional joint involvement that may result in severe polyarthritis. There is currently no way of identifying either group early in the course of the disease.

Patients with pauciarticular disease type I are at high risk for eye complications; chronic iridocyclitis occurs in about 30% at some time during the first 10 yr of the disease. *Chronic iridocyclitis* of JRA is characteristically unassociated with early symptoms or signs, activity of arthritis, or elevated ESR. Occasionally, children note early redness, pain, photophobia, or decreased visual acuity. One or both eyes may be affected; if initial involvement is unilateral, the other eye usually remains uninvolved. Iridocyclitis is sometimes the presenting manifestation of JRA, but generally it follows the onset of joint complaints by months to years. Patients with iridocyclitis frequently have positive test results for ANA. The earliest signs of inflammation of the iris and ciliary body are increased numbers of cells and amounts of protein in the anterior chamber of the eye, changes detectable only by slit-lamp examination. The ocular inflammation often remains active for years. Sequelae (Fig. 11–11) include posterior synechiae, complicated cataracts, secondary glaucoma, and phthisis bulbi (degeneration of the globe). Loss of vision may result; in severe cases permanent blindness occurs. Early detection and therapy before scarring occurs are important for preservation of vision. For this reason all children with pauciarticular disease should have slit-lamp examinations 3–4 times yearly for at least the first 5 yr of disease regardless of the activity of the joint disease.

Other extra-articular manifestations are usually mild in pauciarticular JRA; low-grade fever, malaise, modest hepatosplenomegaly and lymphadenopathy, and mild anemia may be associated with active joint disease.

Pauciarticular disease type II affects 10–15% of patients with JRA, predominantly boys older than 8 yr. Family histories often reveal relatives with pauciarticular arthritis, ankylosing spondylitis, Reiter disease, or acute iridocyclitis. Tests for both rheumatoid factors and ANA are negative; 75% of patients have HLA-B27. Large joints are affected, particularly those of the lower extremities. Toe joints, temporomandibular joints, and upper extremity joints are involved at times. Heel pain, plantar fasciitis, or Achilles tendinitis is common, and there may be inflammation at the sites of tendon insertion into bone *(enthesopathy).* Hip girdle involvement is frequent early in the disease course, and sacroiliitis can often be demonstrated by roentgenography. The peripheral arthritis is generally benign and often transient. Hip and foot pain may be incapacitating at times, although such changes are often reversible with therapy.

With time, some patients with pauciarticular disease type II develop typical ankylosing spondylitis with involvement of the lumbodorsal spine, manifestations of Reiter syndrome (hematuria, urethritis, acute iridocyclitis, or mucocutaneous manifestations), or signs of inflammatory bowel disease. The ultimate morbidity for these children lies in the possible occurrence of any of these chronic spondyloarthropathies; the risks for such occurrences are not known. Physical examination during the follow-up of children with pauciarticular disease type II should include measurements of back flexion

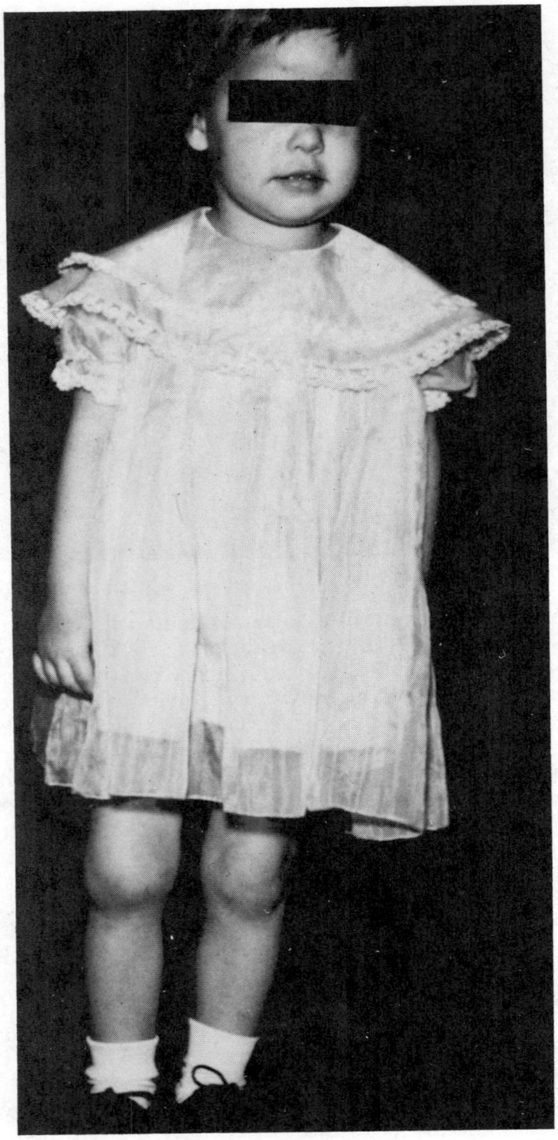

Figure 11–10. Characteristic appearance of a child with pauciarticular arthritis with onset in early childhood; note the swelling of the right knee.

and chest expansion. Ten to twenty per cent will have self-limited attacks of acute iridocyclitis, which is associated with prominent early symptoms and signs of eye inflammation but few scarring residua.

Systemic-Onset JRA. This form of disease is characterized by prominent extra-articular manifestations (Table 11–29), particularly high fevers, and rheumatoid rash. This type of disease occurs in 20% of patients with JRA. Approximately as many boys as girls are affected.

The disease generally begins with systemic symptoms. Fever is high and intermittent, with daily or twice-daily elevations to 102° F (39° C) or higher and rapid return to normal or subnormal levels (Fig. 11–12). Temperature elevations usually occur in the evening and sometimes in the morning as well. Shaking chills are frequently associated. Patients may seem alarmingly ill during the period of fever and surprisingly well during its remission. Rheumatoid rash (Figs. 11–13 and 11–14 [color plate section]) is characterized by its appearance and by its evanescent, recurrent nature. Individual lesions consist of small (several millimeters), pale,

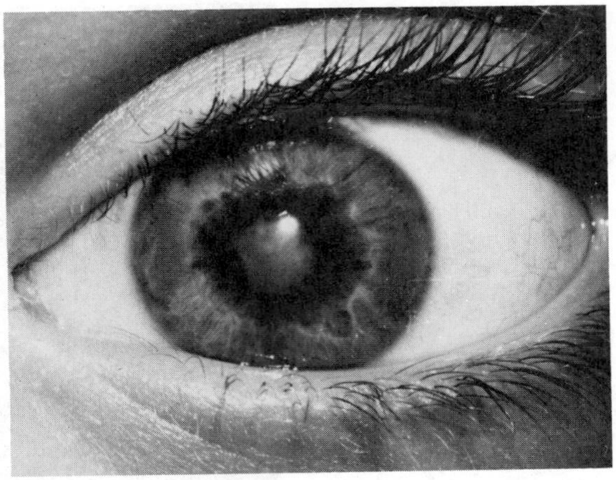

Figure 11–11. Chronic iridocyclitis of juvenile rheumatoid arthritis; extensive posterior synechiae have resulted in a small irregular pupil. There is a well-developed cataract, and early band keratopathy can be seen at the 3 and 9 o'clock positions in the cornea.

red-pink macules, often with central pallor; extensive lesions may coalesce. The rash is most frequently found on the trunk and proximal extremities but may occur anywhere on the body, including the palms and soles. It usually appears during febrile periods but may also be induced by skin trauma (isomorphic response), heat, and embarrassment. Hepatosplenomegaly and generalized lymphadenopathy occur in most children with active systemic disease. The degree of organomegaly may be marked. Mild hepatic dysfunction may be present, and lymph node histology may simulate lymphoma. About one third of affected children have pleuritis or pericarditis, often subclinical. Chest roentgenograms may show pleural thickening or small pleural effusions; pericardial effusion may be large and there may be electrocardiographic changes. The pericarditis of JRA is generally benign. Rarely, severe chest pain, dyspnea, or cardiac failure, with or without evidence of myocarditis, demands vigorous therapy. Occasionally, interstitial lung infiltrates occur with active systemic disease. A few children have episodes of severe abdominal pain during active disease, probably related to serositis or mesenteric adenopathy.

Leukocytosis and even leukemoid reactions are common. Anemia of chronic disease is also common during active disease and is occasionally profound. Disseminated intravascular coagulation and acute liver failure have been reported; relationships to drug therapies (aspirin, gold) are uncertain.

Most children with systemic JRA have joint manifestations at or within a few months of onset, but the arthritis may initially be overlooked in the presence of the overwhelming systemic symptoms. Some patients initially have only severe myalgia, athralgia, or transient arthritis. A few patients do

TABLE 11–29. Manifestations of Systemic Juvenile Rheumatoid Arthritis

	%
High intermittent fever	100
Rheumatoid rash	95
Hepatosplenomegaly or lymphadenopathy	85
Pleuritis or pericarditis	60
Abdominal pain	20
Marked leukocytosis	85
Severe anemia	40
Rheumatoid factors	0
Antinuclear antibodies	0
Arthritis/arthralgia/myalgia during febrile periods	100
Delayed-onset chronic arthritis	90
Iridocyclitis	0

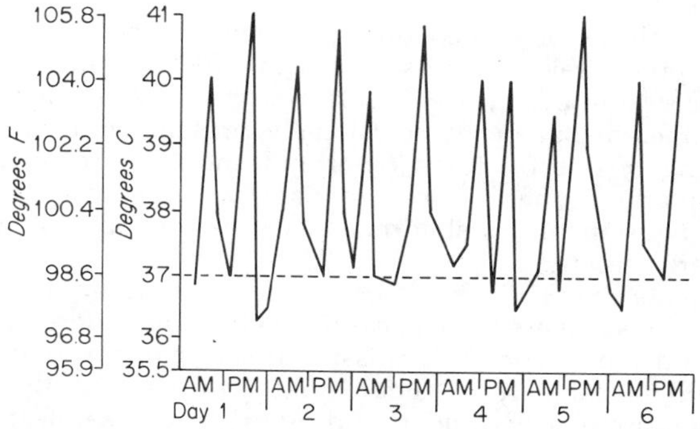

Figure 11–12. Characteristic fever of systemic juvenile rheumatoid arthritis. There are 1 or 2 daily temperature elevations to 39° C or greater, with a rapid return of temperature to normal or subnormal levels.

not develop arthritis until months or years later. The pattern of joint involvement usually resembles that described for polyarticular disease. Joints of the midcarpus and midtarsus are characteristically affected with corresponding dorsal swellings in the wrists or ankles. The systemic manifestations generally run a self-limited course for several months but may recur. The real morbidity of systemic JRA is arthritis that becomes chronic in some patients and persists after systemic symptoms have remitted. Systemic manifestations rarely recur after patients reach adulthood, even though chronic arthritis may persist.

COURSE AND PROGNOSIS. The major cause of morbidity in polyarticular and systemic JRA is chronic joint disease; in pauciarticular disease, the major morbidity is chronic iridocyclitis in type I patients and subsequent spondyloarthropathy in type II patients. The outcome is unpredictable in any individual patient. Even with severe systemic involvement, the disease is rarely life-threatening. There may be exacerbations and remissions, or symptoms may continue for years with mild arthritis causing little disability or, less commonly, with severe arthritis that progresses to joint destruction and permanent deformity. The disease does not always remit at puberty; some patients continue to have active arthritis into adulthood, and some have exacerbations after many years of apparently complete remission. Exacerbations may be associated with intercurrent illness; hepatitis and other forms of liver disease may be followed by transient remission of arthritis.

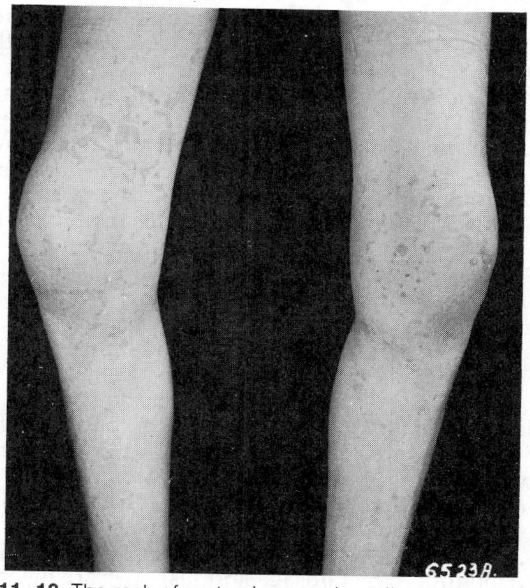

Figure 11–13. The rash of systemic-onset juvenile rheumatoid arthritis.

Patients with rheumatoid factor–positive polyarthritis and systemic-onset disease have the poorest prognosis for joint function. The overall prognosis is good, however. At least 75% of patients with JRA eventually have long remissions without significant residual deformity or loss of function; a few are left with crippling joint deformities. Severe hip disease is particularly debilitating, as is loss of vision from iridocyclitis. Secondary amyloidosis (Sec. 25.2), generally heralded by proteinuria and diagnosed by demonstration of amyloid in tissues, may cause late morbidity. In Europe, amyloidosis affects about 5% of patients with JRA; in the United States this complication is very rare.

LABORATORY FINDINGS. There are no specific diagnostic tests. The ESR and CRP are usually but not invariably elevated during active disease. Anemia is common, usually with low reticulocyte counts and a negative Coombs test. Iron deficiency, either dietary or resulting from drug-related gastrointestinal blood loss, may also be present. The white blood cell count is often elevated; leukemoid reactions sometimes occur particularly in systemic JRA, in which counts of 10,000–30,000/mm^3 are the rule, and counts may sometimes be as high as 75,000/mm^3. Thrombocytosis may occur, particularly in systemic-onset disease. Urinalyses are normal; during salicylate therapy a few erythrocytes and renal tubular cells may be seen. There may be an increase in the serum α_2 and gamma globulin fractions and a decrease in albumin. Any or all serum immunoglobulin levels may be elevated.

Antinuclear antibodies are found in some children with rheumatoid factor–negative (25%), rheumatoid factor–positive (75%), or pauciarticular type I (90%) disease but are rarely if ever present in those with systemic or pauciarticular type II disease. The finding of ANA correlates with the presence of chronic iridocyclitis but not with the severity of arthritis. *Rheumatoid factors* are found in about 5% of children with JRA and correlate with older age at onset. Test results rarely convert from negative to positive despite long-active JRA. Positive test results are most commonly associated with polyarticular disease, late childhood onset, severe destructive arthritis, and rheumatoid nodules; rheumatoid vasculitis and Sjögren syndrome are also occasionally associated.

Synovial fluid in JRA is cloudy, may clot spontaneously, and usually contains increased amounts of protein. The cell count varies from 5,000–80,000 cells/mm^3; the cells are predominantly neutrophils. Levels of glucose may be low in the joint fluid; levels of complement may be normal or decreased (see Table 12–20).

Early *roentgenographic changes* consist of soft tissue swelling, osteoporosis, and periostitis about the affected joints (Fig. 11–15). Regional epiphyseal closure may be accelerated and local bone growth increased or decreased. In long-active joint disease subchondral erosions and narrowing of cartilage spaces may occur, as may varying degrees of bony destruction and fusion. Late roentgenographic changes, for example, in the wrist and hand (see Fig. 11–7), are characteristic. Characteristic changes may occur in the neck, with narrowing and eventual fusion of the neural arch joints (most frequently seen at C2 and C3, Fig. 11–16), erosions of the odontoid process, atlantoaxial subluxation, and underdevelopment of vertebral bodies. Roentgenographic sacroiliitis resembling ankylosing spondylitis is often seen in children with pauciarticular disease type II. Specialized studies utilizing ultrasound, computed tomographic scanning, and magnetic resonance imaging may cast further light on soft tissue and bony abnormalities.

DIAGNOSIS AND DIFFERENTIAL DIAGNOSIS. See Tables 11–30 and 11–31. The diagnosis is clinical and depends

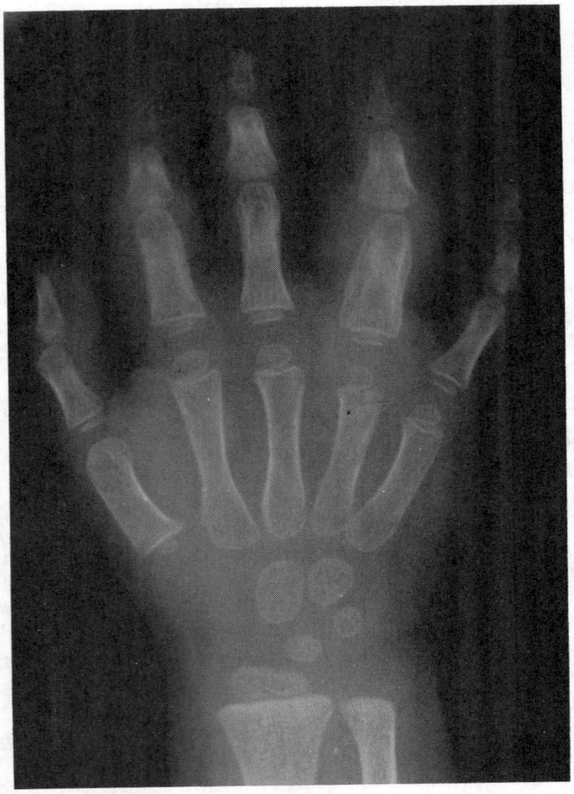

Figure 11–15. Early (6 mo duration) radiographic changes of JRA, soft tissue swelling and periosteal new bone formation appear adjacent to the 2nd and 4th proximal interphalangeal joints.

on the persistence of arthritis or typical systemic manifestations for 3 consecutive mo or more and on the exclusion of other diseases. Early in the disease pyogenic or tuberculous joint infection, osteomyelitis, sepsis, or arthritis associated with other acute infectious illnesses may be considered. Culture of joint fluid, tuberculin testing, and roentgenograms of affected joints are helpful. Lyme disease should always be considered, particularly in children with pauciarticular disease. Arthritis of limited duration may occur in association with some viral infections and with rubella immunization. Gonococcal infection may result in arthritis. Acute leukemia and other malignancies occasionally present with pain and swelling of one or more joints and should be considered, particularly if there is severe pain, or if severe anemia, thrombocytopenia, or abnormalities of peripheral white blood cells are present.

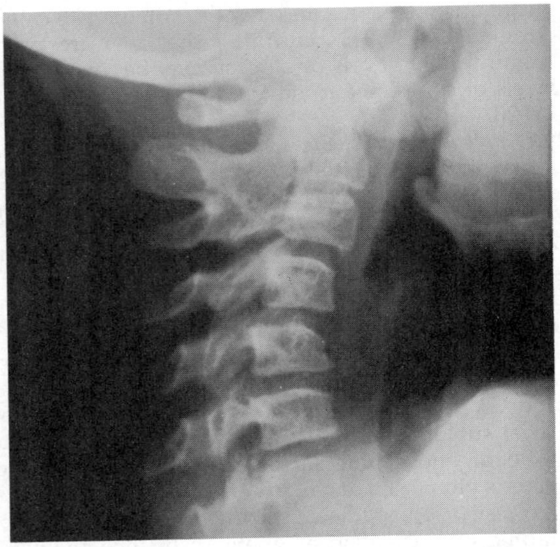

Figure 11–16. Cervical spine in long-active juvenile rheumatoid arthritis, showing fusion of neural arch between joints C2–C3, narrowing and erosions of the remaining neural arch joints, and resultant abnormal curvature.

In acute rheumatic fever the transient, migratory nature of the arthritis and evidence of carditis help in the differentiation. SLE and mixed connective tissue disease can cause arthritis indistinguishable from rheumatoid arthritis, but the joint changes are usually milder, and other clinical manifestations of SLE are usually present; however, ANA and occasionally LE cells occur in JRA as well as in SLE. Ankylosing spondylitis may present with arthritis of a few peripheral joints that is indistinguishable from JRA (pauciarticular type II) before the characteristic involvement of the spine becomes manifest; the presence of early roentgenographic sacroiliac joint changes associated with pain in the low back and hip girdle is suggestive. Reiter syndrome (arthritis, urethritis, conjunctivitis) is uncommon in children but should be considered in those with pauciarticular disease type II. The vasculitis syndromes, dermatomyositis, ulcerative colitis, regional enteritis, psoriasis, and sarcoidosis may be associated with arthritis similar to that of JRA but are generally distinguishable on clinical grounds. Immunodeficiency diseases may rarely be associated with chronic arthritis resembling JRA.

Various conditions such as joint trauma, Legg-Perthes disease, diskitis, Osgood-Schlatter disease, reflex sympathetic dystrophy, and slipped capital femoral epiphysis may initially mimic JRA. Acute toxic synovitis of the hip is a self-limited condition of uncertain origin; JRA rarely begins in or affects solely the hip. Pigmented villonodular synovitis, an uncommon synovial overgrowth, usually affects only one joint.

Synovial biopsy may be useful, especially to exclude infection in patients with monarticular disease; however, synovial histology does not distinguish among the various subgroups of JRA, various other rheumatic disorders, or even so-called postinfectious states.

TREATMENT. The aims of immediate and long-term treatment are 2-fold: (1) to preserve joint function and provide adequate care for extra-articular manifestations without causing iatrogenic harm; and (2) to support the family and child in achieving an optimal psychosocial adjustment. This requires the devoted attention of a primary physician and may require consultation with a variety of specialists. Although JRA may be of long duration and has no specific cure, the ultimate prognosis is good for most patients, and life is rarely threatened. Management of affected children and their families tests the physician's sympathy, patience, empathy, and clinical skills. Unpredictable exacerbations are discouraging and make evaluation of therapy difficult. There is an understandable tendency for parents to shop for medical help and to grasp for fad or quack cures. The chronic nature of the disease may cause the discouraged family to give up supportive efforts, which may allow unnecessary crippling disability to occur.

A number of drugs can suppress the inflammatory process. *Acetylsalicylic acid (aspirin)* in doses sufficient to maintain blood levels of 20–30 mg/dL usually alleviates both arthritic and systemic manifestations. Such blood levels can be reached by using doses of about 100 mg/kg/24 hr of aspirin for children weighing 25 kg or less and total daily doses of 2.4–3.6 g for older, heavier children. There is considerable individual variation in the dose required, and patients must be watched carefully for toxicity. Full therapeutic response may require weeks to months. When dosage and response are determined and stabilized, the medication can be continued for years.

TABLE 11–30. Diagnosis: Nonrheumatic Conditions

	Septic Arthritis	Lyme Disease	Osteomyelitis	Viral Arthritis	Childhood Malignancy	Structural, Genetic	Growing Pains, Psychogenic
SEX	Any	Any	Any	Girls > boys	Any	Any depending on condition	Growing pains; boys > girls Psychogenic; girls > boys
AGE AT ONSET	<4 yr: *H. influenzae* Teenage: Gonococcus Any age: *Staphylococcus*	Over age 2	Any	More common in older children and adults	Any	Any	Growing pains 2–8 yr Psychogenic 6 yr or older
JOINT MANIFESTATIONS	85% Monoarticular joints swollen, hot, painful	Pauciarticular; episodic, recurrent	Sterile joint effusion adjacent to the area of bone infection	Transient arthritis—often polyarticular	Severe bone/joint pain	Local bone/joint pain or dysfunction	None or bizarre Features of reflex sympathetic dystrophy
EXTRA-ARTICULAR MANIFESTATIONS	Fever, signs of sepsis, signs of gonococcal disease	Flu-like illness, erythema migranes, CNS,* neurologic, cardiac	Fever, signs of sepsis, bone pain	Those of underlying virus	Those of underlying malignancy	Those of underlying conditions, dysmorphic features, structural abnormalities	Growing pains—none; psychogenic—bizarre
LABORATORY	Cultures: joint fluid, blood, genital	Serologic: antibody to *Borrelia burgdorferi*	Culture: blood, bone: bone scan	Viral culture Serologic: Rise in antibody titers	Hematologic abnormalities, abnormal radiograph or scan	Demonstration of abnormal structure or metabolic abnormality	Normal
PATHOGENESIS	Direct synovial infection; occasional immune complex mechanism in gonococcal and meningococcal arthritis	*B. burgdorferi*—synovial and systemic infection	Direct infection of bone, sympathetic joint effusion	Direct viral synovial infection, immune complex in some	Direct primary bone tumor or periarticular or bony infiltrate of malignant cells	Idiopathic or genetic	No organic disease
DIAGNOSIS	Demonstration of organisms in joint fluid	Serologic	Demonstration of organisms: blood, bone; bone scan (early), X-ray (late)	Clinical, serologic, or viral culture	Bone marrow tissue biopsy	Recognition of condition or syndrome	Clinical
NATURAL HISTORY	Joint destruction if untreated	Chronic, recurrent; may cause long-term CNS, skin, ocular disease	Bone/joint destruction if untreated	Arthritis transient	Joint manifestations may wax/wane	Chronic	Growing pains benign, psychogenic, may become chronic and disabling
THERAPY	Specific antibiotic	Specific antibiotic	Specific antibiotic	Symptomatic	That of underlying malignancy	That of underlying conditions	Recognition, reassurance, psychosocial attention

* CNS = central nervous system.

TABLE 11–31. Differential Diagnosis: Rheumatic Disease

	Rheumatic Fever	Juvenile Rheumatoid Arthritis	Systemic Lupus Erythematosus	Kawasaki Disease	Dermatomyositis
SEX	No predilection	Dependent on subgroup	Girls > boys	No predilection	Girls 3:2
AGE AT ONSET	3 yr or older	1 yr or older	Usually over age 8	4 yr or younger	2 yr or older
JOINT MANIFESTATIONS	Transient migratory arthritis—large joints	Pauciarticular or polyarticular Chronic (6 wk or more)	Arthralgia Transient arthritis Chronic arthritis	Pain and swelling of hands and feet Arthritis occasionally	Joint contractures; arthritis occasionally
EXTRA-ARTICULAR MANIFESTATIONS	Fever Cardiac disease Chorea Rash, nodules	Dependent on subgroup: Systemic juvenile rheumatoid arthritis: fever, rash, etc. Pauciarticular: iridocyclitis	Occasionally multisystem disease, including nephritis	Fever Eye, oral, cutaneous infections Lymphadenopathy Coronary vasculitis	Rash Muscle weakness, pain Gastrointestinal, respiratory
LABORATORY	Prior streptococcal infection ECHO or ECG evidence of carditis	May have antinuclear antibodies, rheumatoid factor	Antinuclear antibodies Autoantibodies Low complement DNA antibody	Abnormal coronary vessels on ECHO	Abnormal "muscle enzymes," electromyogram, muscle biopsy
PATHOGENESIS	Post streptococcal	Unknown	Immune complex disease	Unknown	Unknown
DIAGNOSIS	Clinical (Jones criteria)	Clinical (juvenile rheumatoid arthritis criteria)	Clinical plus laboratory (systemic lupus erythematosus criteria)	Clinical (Kawasaki criteria)	Clinical Rash plus myositis Muscle biopsy
NATURAL HISTORY	Arthritis—transient carditis may cause permanent damage	Chronic: arthritis may be destructive	Chronic or recurrent may be fatal	Self-limited Coronary vasculitis May be fatal	Chronic May be fatal
THERAPY	Anti-inflammatory *Streptococcus* prophylaxis to prevent recurrence	Anti-inflammatory Physical therapy	Anti-inflammatory Corticosteroid Cytotoxic	Intravenous globulin Aspirin	Corticosteroid Cytotoxic

Chronic therapeutic salicylate administration is relatively safe even in small children if physicians, patients, and parents are aware of the potential toxic effects. Intoxication from overdosage can be avoided if the dose is calculated with care and parents watch for the rapid or heavy breathing and drowsiness or other central nervous system changes that are often the earliest signs of salicylism in children. Tinnitus, a common complaint of adults with salicylism, is rarely noted by children. Salicylates should be given with food because of the possibility of gastric irritation. If patients complain of stomach ache, antacids can be added or buffered salicylate preparations or choline salicylate substituted for ordinary aspirin. Children with persistent gastrointestinal complaints should be investigated for peptic ulcer disease. Hemorrhagic phenomena may occur secondary to effects on platelet function. Elevated serum levels of hepatic enzymes may occur in patients with rheumatic diseases receiving large doses of salicylates; association of clinically significant liver disease is unusual, but salicylates should be withdrawn if high enzyme levels occur. Epidemiologic studies suggest that aspirin ingestion is associated with Reye syndrome in children with either chickenpox or influenza, and it is advisable to discontinue aspirin use temporarily in children exposed to these infections (Sec. 13.96).

A number of *nonsteroidal anti-inflammatory agents* are available for the therapy of arthritis in adults. These drugs are of similar potency to aspirin in relieving pain and inflammation; some may provide particular relief for patients with spondyloarthropathies. Such drugs include indomethacin, tolmetin, ibuprofen, naproxen (or Naprosyn), fenoprofen, and sulindac. Only tolmetin and Naprosyn are currently labeled for routine use in children in the United States; they may be useful alternatives to aspirin. All of the nonsteroidal anti-inflammatory agents are potential gastric irritants; other potential side effects include headache and interference with platelet function. Sulfasalazine, a drug combining a salicylate and a sulfonamide, is also used in the therapy of arthritis in adults and children; this agent has long been employed in the therapy of inflammatory bowel disease. Its efficacy, if any, in JRA remains to be defined.

There are few indications for the systemic use of *corticosteroids* in JRA. These agents dramatically suppress symptoms but do not induce permanent remission or prevent the occurrence of joint damage (see Fig. 11–7). In addition, destruction of cartilage and aseptic necrosis of bone, particularly in the femoral heads, may be related to long-term steroid therapy (see Fig. 11–9). Therapeutic doses of corticosteroids also cause adrenal suppression, may suppress growth, and may produce other potentially dangerous side effects. The dose required for suppression of symptoms is unpredictable and may actually increase with prolonged therapy.

Indications for corticosteroid use in JRA include severe systemic disease unreponsive to an adequate trial of salicylates and iridocyclitis uncontrolled by topical steroids. In the former, or in rare instances of cardiac decompensation due to pericarditis or myocarditis, prednisone in initial doses of 1–2 mg/kg/24 hr is indicated. As soon as symptoms have been suppressed, the dose should be decreased and the drug gradually discontinued under a cover of salicylates. With decreasing doses there is often transient rebound of symptoms, which should be waited out. Since the systemic manifestations of JRA generally run a self-limited course, prednisone can usually be successfully discontinued within weeks or months. In patients with iridocyclitis that does not respond to topical steroid therapy, systemic steroids are indicated in doses sufficient to suppress ocular inflammation as monitored by slit-lamp examination; single doses given daily or on alternate days may be sufficient. Therapy should be managed jointly with an ophthalmologist.

Corticosteroids should rarely be used for relief of joint manifestations alone because they neither cure arthritis nor prevent joint damage, and their chronic side effects may be even less tolerable than the joint disease. Other reasonable therapeutic possibilities should always be exhausted first. If corticosteroids are used, every effort should be made to employ the lowest effective dose, to use alternate-day or single daily doses whenever possible, and to minimize the duration of treatment.

Several *alternative forms of therapy* have been advocated for severe arthritis that does not respond to nonsteroidal agents alone. These agents include gold salts (oral or intramuscular), antimalarials, D-penicillamine, methotrexate, and intravenous gamma globulin. The efficacy of methotrexate for severe JRA has been demonstrated in a double-blind placebo controlled trial, but most still consider methotrexate an experimental agent in the therapy of JRA. No efficacy of oral gold salts, D-penicillamine, or hydroxychloroquine compared to placebo has been demonstrated in similar studies. Intramuscular gold has never been tested in a controlled trial in children. Intravenous gamma globulin is currently under study. Each of these forms of therapy continues to have its advocates, however, and there is no general agreement as to order of choice.

Oral *gold therapy* is given on a daily basis; weeks to months are required for an adequate trial. Signs of toxicity include skin rash, mucosal ulcers, leukopenia, thrombocytopenia, anemia, and proteinuria. Many observers consider oral gold therapy less effective than intramuscular therapy. Intramuscular gold therapy requires weekly injections, each preceded by a careful evaluation for any signs of toxicity (rash, mucosal ulcers, leukopenia, thrombocytopenia, anemia, and proteinuria). Initial test doses should be small (2.5–5 mg of gold sodium thiomalate or gold thioglucose) with later maintenance doses no larger than 1 mg/kg/wk or a total of 25 mg/wk for children weighing over 25 kg; 50-mg doses can be given to larger teenagers (adult size). Several months are required for a therapeutic response; if no response has occurred after 24 weekly injections, the drug should be discontinued. If a response occurs, injections can be gradually spaced out to 3- to 4-wk intervals and continued indefinitely. Continuous surveillance for side effects should be maintained throughout the duration of therapy; appearance of side effects is almost always an indication for discontinuing the drug.

Hydroxychloroquine should be used with extreme care because of possible retinal toxicity; ophthalmologic examination should be made every 3 mo. *D-Penicillamine* is a potentially toxic agent that is rarely used in children with arthritis; side effects include bone marrow suppression, proteinuria, dermatologic reactions, myasthenia gravis, and various "autoimmune" phenomena.

Methotrexate is still considered by many to be an experimental drug in the therapy of JRA. It is given on a weekly basis in relatively low doses (5–10 mg/m²/wk); the route of administration may be oral, intramuscular, or intravenous. Little is known about the long-term side effects of this drug in children; hepatic toxicity is of the most immediate concern and must be carefully monitored with appropriate liver function tests. Ultimate long-term risks of decreased fertility or possible induction of malignancy are not yet defined. Other cytotoxic drugs such as cyclophosphamide, azathioprine, chlorambucil, and cyclosporine have been variously used in noncontrolled studies of patients with JRA; all are potentially dangerous and of uncertain efficacy. The potentially fatal amyloidosis of JRA has been treated with some success with chlorambucil or azathioprine (Sec. 25.2). Chlorambucil has been noted to cause chromosomal breakage in children with JRA, however, and is now rarely used. The efficacy of *intravenous gamma globulin* in patients with systemic and polyarticular JRA is under investigation.

Physical and occupational therapy are important methods of improving motion and muscular strength about the affected joints and of restoring and maintaining the functional capabilities of the patient. Patients and parents should be instructed in appropriate exercise programs to be carried out at home on a daily basis. Activities such as tricycle riding and swimming are beneficial and should be encouraged. Night splints for knees and wrists may aid in preventing and correcting deformity. Cylindric casts or prolonged immobilization of joints should be avoided. Bed rest has little role in treatment. Children can usually set their own activity levels; in general, they should avoid only those activities that cause overtiring and joint pain. Orthopedic surgery is sometimes required to correct joint deformities. Synovectomy of selected joints is occasionally helpful but not curative. Total replacement of destroyed joints, particularly hips and knees, is now possible when full growth has been attained. Injection of corticosteroids into selected joints may be helpful at times, but repeated injections should not be used. Micrognathia may require orthodontic management and oral surgery. *Functional classification* of JRA includes 4 classes: I, performs all activities; II, performs adequately with some limitations; III, limited activity, self-care only; and IV, wheelchair-bound or bedridden.

Iridocyclitis requires prompt diagnosis and therapy to preserve vision. The eyes should be examined at each medical visit, and ophthalmologic slit-lamp examinations should be performed at least once a year in children with systemic and polyarticular disease and 4 times yearly in children with pauciarticular disease. Parents should be cautioned to report at once any eye symptoms or decreased visual acuity. Therapy of iridocyclitis should be supervised by an ophthalmologist. Initially, it consists of topical use of steroids and dilating agents. Systemic steroids or subconjunctival steroid injections should be used if prompt resolution of ocular inflammation is not achieved with topical agents. Frequent and long-term follow-up of eyes is essential. Ophthalmologic surgery may be required for chronic sequelae.

Children with JRA should be encouraged to lead as normal lives as possible. They and their parents need to know what to expect and to be treated optimistically. Affected children should not be led to believe that they are invalids but should be taught to be as self-sufficient as possible. With encouragement most can lead active lives, attend school, and participate in usual activities except strenuous sports. Long hospitalizations should be avoided. Children with residual handicaps need help in vocational planning.

11.52 ANKYLOSING SPONDYLITIS

Ankylosing spondylitis is characterized by stiffness and pain in the back, involvement of the sacroiliac joints, and variable progression to the joints and periarticular tissues of the lumbodorsal and cervical spines. About half the patients have arthritis of the peripheral joints. This is usually a disease of young and middle-aged adults, but it may begin in childhood, usually in males older than 8 yr. There is a striking association between ankylosing spondylitis and HLA-B27. Pathology of synovial tissue from affected joints is similar to that described for rheumatoid arthritis.

Ankylosing spondylitis differs from rheumatoid arthritis by its (1) characteristic involvement of the sacroiliac joints and lumbodorsal spine, (2) predilection for males, (3) lack of association with rheumatoid factor or rheumatoid nodules, (4) association with acute iridocyclitis, (5) occurrence of aortitis with resulting aortic insufficiency, and (6) significant familial incidence.

CLINICAL MANIFESTATIONS. Peripheral arthritis, often transient, may be the first manifestation. Large joints, particularly those of the lower extremities, are affected most frequently. Heel pain is common, as is the occurrence of pain with or without soft tissue swelling at various other sites to which tendons and ligaments attach to bone (**enthesopathy**). Shoulders, feet, and temporomandibular joints are also involved in a significant number of patients. Affected joints may be warm, swollen, painful, and limited in motion.

Characteristic involvement of the sacroiliac joints and lumbodorsal spine may be present at the onset of disease or may appear months to years later. Pain in the lower back, hip girdles, and thighs is characteristic. The pain is often transient and more severe at night and is relieved by movement. Stiffness in the lower back with loss of normal spinal mobility follows (Fig. 11–17). Spinal involvement characteristically begins in the sacroiliac joints and ascends, involving the lumbar, dorsal, and, finally, cervical spines. In contrast, in JRA the neck is involved, but the lumbodorsal spine is spared. Decreased chest wall expansion, related to involvement of the costovertebral joints, may occur early. Low-grade fever, anemia, anorexia, fatiguability, and growth retardation may occur. The family history is frequently positive for similar arthritis or for acute iridocyclitis.

Ankylosing spondylitis may arrest at any stage, or the entire spine may become involved over a number of years with loss of virtually all vertebral mobility. Prognosis for functional outcome is usually good if good posture is maintained. Deformity of peripheral joints is uncommon; some patients develop destructive hip disease. Acute iridocyclitis occurs in about 25% of patients at some time; aortitis is rare in children but occurs in a significant number of adults.

LABORATORY FINDINGS. There are no specific laboratory tests. Although HLA-B27 is present in 95% of patients, it is not diagnostic. ESR may be elevated. Anemia similar to that of rheumatoid arthritis occurs, but neither rheumatoid factors nor ANA are noted. Involvement of the sacroiliac joints is demonstrable roentgenographically (Fig. 11–18), usually within the first 3–4 yr; destruction is progressive, with eventual obliteration of the joints. Characteristic roentgenographic changes in the lumbodorsal spine occur some years later.

DIFFERENTIAL DIAGNOSIS. Ankylosing spondylitis should be suspected in any child with persistent pain in the hips, thighs, or lower back, with or without peripheral arthritis. Roentgenographic changes in the sacroiliac joints are necessary for diagnosis, but several years may elapse before they appear. In the differential diagnosis, spinal cord tumors and other childhood malignancies, anatomic defects, infections of the vertebrae or intervertebral disks (diskitis), Scheuermann disease, and other orthopedic conditions of the spine must be considered in any child with persistent back pain. Legg-Perthes disease and slipped capital femoral epiphysis may cause persistent hip and thigh pain. Ulcerative colitis, regional enteritis, psoriasis, and Reiter syndrome may have associated spondylitis resembling ankylosing spondylitis.

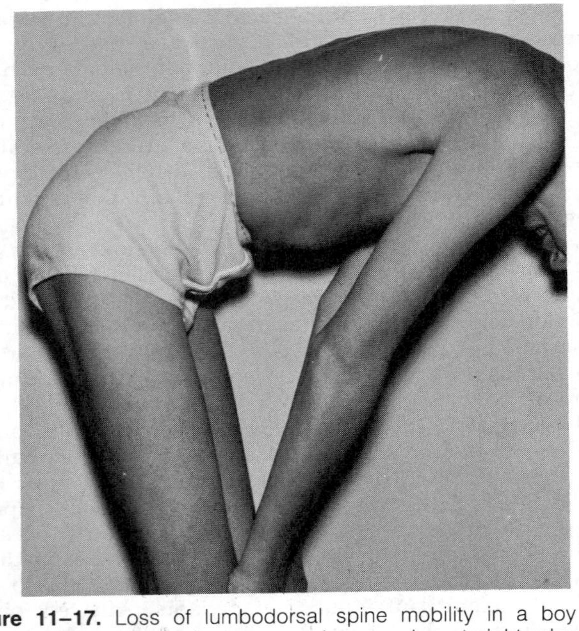

Figure 11–17. Loss of lumbodorsal spine mobility in a boy with ankylosing spondylitis: the lower spine remains straight when the patient bends forward.

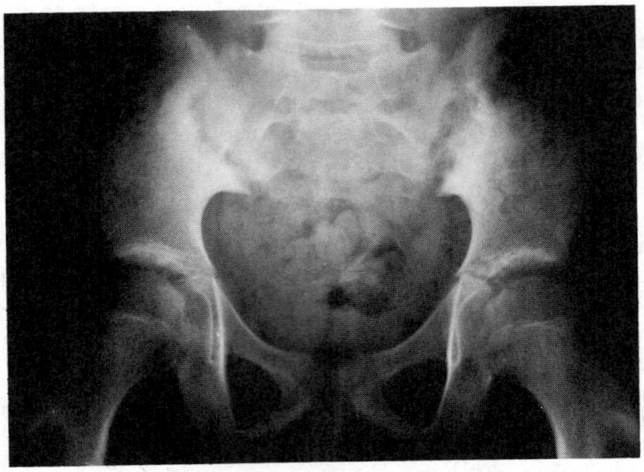

Figure 11–18. Well-developed sacroiliitis in a boy with ankylosing spondylitis; both sacroiliac joints show extensive sclerosis, erosions of joint margins, and apparent widening of the joint space.

TREATMENT. The aims of therapy are to relieve pain and to maintain good posture and function. For relief of pain, salicylates may suffice. Indomethacin or other nonsteroidal anti-inflammatory agents may be helpful. Gold salts are not considered to be effective, and corticosteroid therapy is rarely if ever indicated. Radiation therapy is contraindicated. Maintenance of good posture is essential for preservation of good function; exercises designed to promote posture and strengthen paraspinal muscles should be employed. A firm mattress or bed board should be used for sleeping and thick pillows avoided.

11.53 OTHER SPONDYLOARTHROPATHIES IN CHILDREN

The spondyloarthropathies described in adults include those seronegative types of arthritis associated with sacroiliitis and spinal arthritis: ankylosing spondylitis, Reiter disease, psoriatic arthritis, the arthritis of inflammatory bowel disease, and the "reactive arthritis" of yersiniosis and other gastrointestinal infections (Table 11–32). Although these types of arthritis are rarer in children than in adults, some of them, notably ankylosing spondylitis and Reiter disease, may sometimes be mislabeled as JRA. All of the spondyloarthropathies are associated with HLA-B27, and none are associated with rheumatoid factors or ANA. The pathology of affected synovial tissues is not distinct from that of rheumatoid arthritis. Some of the spondyloarthropathies, notably Reiter disease and reactive arthritis, may occur after identifiable environmental events such as infections with *Shigella* or *Yersinia*. Spondyloarthropathies may cluster in some families, with several family members having one or another of these types of arthritis; acute iridocyclitis also may be similarly associated. Except for psoriatic arthritis, the spondyloarthropathies affect boys and girls equally or have a male preponderance. Diagnosis rests on clinical grounds.

The pauciarticular disease type II subgroup of JRA probably represents early spondyloarthropathy in most instances. None of the three other seronegative JRA subgroups (seronegative polyarthritis, systemic-onset JRA, and pauciarticular disease

TABLE 11–32. The Spondyloarthropathies in Children

	Ankylosing Spondylitis	Reiter Syndrome	Inflammatory Bowel Disease	Reactive Arthritis	Psoriatic Arthritis
SEX	Boys > girls	Boys > girls	No predilection	Boys > girls	Girls > boys
AGE ON ONSET	8 yr or older	Occasional in young children, usually over 8 yr	Over age 4	Older children	Over age 2
JOINT MANIFESTATIONS	Pauciarticular Lower limb Sacroiliitis Axial arthritis Enthesopathy	Pauciarticular Sacroiliitis Enthesopathy	Pauciarticular Occasional spondylitis	Pauciarticular-transient	Pauciarticular or polyarticular
EXTRA-ARTICULAR MANIFESTATIONS	Eye: acute iritis Heart: aortitis	Eye Skin Genitourinary tract Fever, systemic	Those of bowel disease: erythema nodosum, growth failure, etc.	Underlying gastroenteritis: *Yersinia, Shigella, Salmonella, Campylobacter*	Psoriatic rash Nail pitting
LABORATORY	HLA B27 Radiographic sacroiliitis	HLA B27	HLA B27 in those with spondylitis	Stool culture positive HLA B27	None specific
PATHOGENESIS	Often familial	May follow infectious disease, such as *Shigella*	Arthritis related to bowel disease	Reaction to infection	Unknown
DIAGNOSIS	Clinical	Clinical	Clinical, demonstration of bowel disease	Demonstration of gastrointestinal infection	Clinical
NATURAL HISTORY	Chronic May cause spinal fusion	Episodic May recur Occasional chronic destructive arthritis	That of underlying bowel disease Peripheral arthritis, benign; spondylitis, chronic	Self-limited arthritis	Arthritis may be chronic
THERAPY	NSAIDs* Physical therapy	NSAIDs	Bowel disease NSAIDs, physical therapy	That of bowel infection	NSAIDs Remittive agents Physical therapy Skin care

*NSAID = nonsteroidal anti-inflammatory drug.

type I) is associated with sacroiliitis, HLA-B27, or subsequent spondyloarthropathy.

REITER DISEASE. In its full-blown form Reiter disease consists of sterile urethritis, arthritis, and ocular inflammation; other manifestations may include gastroenteritis and a variety of skin rashes. Males are predominantly affected. In children, Reiter disease has been reported following infections with *Shigella, Yersinia enterocolitica, Campylobacter*, and *Chlamydia*; in older children, as in adults, Reiter disease may follow sexual exposure. Reiter disease is strongly associated with HLA-B27. The arthritis is generally pauciarticular, predominantly affecting the large joints. Achilles tendinitis and other enthesopathies are common. Some cases of pauciarticular disease type II may represent "partial" Reiter disease. The long-term prognosis of childhood-onset Reiter disease is unknown. The majority of children recover within a few months. However, some individuals subsequently have ankylosing spondylitis, some have recurrent or chronic peripheral arthritis, and some have recurrent attacks of ocular or urethral inflammation. The diagnosis is clinical. Infectious urethritis and gonococcal disease must be excluded. Salicylates or one of the other nonsteroidal anti-inflammatory agents is used for treatment. Physical therapy also plays an important role in therapy. Patients should be monitored for subsequent spinal involvement.

ARTHRITIS OF INFLAMMATORY BOWEL DISEASE. Both ulcerative colitis (Sec. 13.41) and regional enteritis (Sec. 13.42) may be associated with arthritis during childhood; about 10% of children with inflammatory bowel disease will at some time have joint manifestations. Affected children are generally older than 8 yr. The arthritis generally affects a few large joints in a pauciarticular pattern. Arthritis generally begins with or after the onset of active bowel disease; in a few patients arthritis may be the first manifestation of disease. The arthritis of inflammatory bowel disease in children follows two patterns, as it does in adults. Most affected children have peripheral arthritis that waxes and wanes with activity of the bowel disease and causes neither joint destruction nor permanent joint deformity. However, a few children have disease that is inseparable from ankylosing spondylitis and that may progress to disability regardless of control of the underlying bowel disease. For this reason, it is important to follow children with inflammatory bowel disease for evidence of sacroiliitis or spinal arthritis. HLA-B27 is associated with ankylosing spondylitis but not with the peripheral arthritis of inflammatory bowel disease. Therapy for peripheral arthritis includes adequate treatment for the underlying bowel disease with the occasional additional use of salicylates or other nonsteroidal agents. If ankylosing spondylitis occurs, appropriate therapy for that condition is indicated (Sec. 11.52).

REACTIVE ARTHRITIS. Sterile arthritis may follow gastrointestinal infection with *Yersinia enterocolitica, Shigella, Salmonella*, or *Campylobacter*. Generally, only a few joints are affected. The relationship of such arthritis to Reiter disease and other spondyloarthropathies is uncertain. The arthritis is generally transient and the ultimate outcome good. However, some affected patients may subsequently develop chronic spondyloarthropathy. Any child with both gastroenteritis and arthritis should undergo appropriate stool cultures and serologic studies.

PSORIATIC ARTHRITIS. The classification of psoriatic arthritis with the spondyloarthropathies may not be appropriate; there are differences in sex ratios of affected patients and patterns of arthritis and a less strong association with HLA-B27. Although psoriasis is a relatively common skin condition of children, psoriatic arthritis is uncommon during childhood. Girls are predominantly affected in a 2.5:1 ratio. Psoriatic arthritis in childhood is similar to that seen in adults. Arthritis begins in one or several joints, often in an asymmetric fashion. More than half of patients have involvement of the distal interphalangeal joints; tendinitis is also common. In about half of the patients, psoriasis precedes arthritis by months or years; in others arthritis is the initial manifestation, with psoriasis appearing later. Nail pitting is common. The prognosis of psoriatic arthritis in children appears to be good, though there are few long-term studies. A few patients with psoriatic arthritis develop sacroiliitis and ankylosing spondylitis associated with HLA-B27. Therapy of psoriatic arthritis is similar to that seen in adults; salicylates and other nonsteroidal anti-inflammatory agents are generally used. There is little experience with agents such as methotrexate in children with psoriatic arthritis. As in JRA, physical and occupational therapy play important roles in maintaining good function.

11.54 SYSTEMIC LUPUS ERYTHEMATOSUS (SLE)

This systemic disease characteristically affects many organ systems and is associated with a variety of immune phenomena. Its natural history is unpredictable; it is often progressive, terminating in death if untreated, but may remit spontaneously or smolder for many years. SLE in children is generally more acute and severe than that in adults.

ETIOLOGY AND EPIDEMIOLOGY. The cause is unknown. Many observations support the hypothesis that SLE is a disease of altered immune regulation, perhaps genetically determined. Viruses may also play a role in pathogenesis. A variety of immune phenomena occur. Serum levels of immunoglobulins are increased. Antibodies are found that react with nuclear constituents (ANA), ribonucleic acid, gamma globulin (rheumatoid factors), red blood cells (positive Coombs test), platelets, white blood cells, antigens used in serologic tests for syphilis (biologic false-positive), coagulation factors, and phospholipids (antiphospholipid, lupus anticoagulant, anticardiolipin). There is also an association between inflammation and circulating immune complexes, particularly those consisting of DNA and antibodies reactive with DNA. Such immune complexes are deposited in tissues, fix complement, and initiate an inflammatory response that results in tissue injury such as nephritis. In SLE nephritis immunoglobulins and complement can be demonstrated in renal tissues by immunofluorescent techniques and by direct elution of DNA and anti-DNA antibodies from affected glomeruli; active SLE with nephritis is associated with decreased levels of serum complement and with circulating antibodies reactive with DNA (Sec. 18.7).

The onset of exacerbations of disease may appear to be related to intercurrent infections; there may be increased susceptibility to infections, perhaps on the basis of faulty immune mechanisms. Current evidence, including studies showing alterations in T and B lymphocyte function in patients with SLE, suggests that a state of altered immunologic reactions underlies the disease. Lupus is sometimes familial and has affected identical twins; hypergammaglobulinemia, other connective tissue diseases, antinuclear antibodies, complement component deficiency, selective IgA deficiency, and other immune abnormalities may be found in 1st-degree relatives of patients.

Lupus-like disease occurs following exposure to a number of drugs, notably hydralazine, sulfonamides, procainamide, and anticonvulsants. Drug-induced disease is generally mild and reversible when the inciting drug is withdrawn. Cutaneous manifestations of SLE and sometimes systemic manifestations may be exacerbated by sunlight.

The incidence is unknown; the disease is not rare. SLE begins in childhood in 20% of patients, usually in children over 8 yr of age. Females are predominantly affected (8:1) in all age groups; however, in prepubertal patients, the ratio is 3:1. All races may be affected, with an apparently higher prevalence in several dark-skinned racial groups including blacks, Latin Americans, Asians, and some native American tribes.

PATHOLOGY. Lesions occur at multiple sites and involve many organ systems. Characteristic masses of amorphous, purple-staining extracellular material are found with hematoxylin staining. These *hematoxylin bodies* probably represent degenerated cell nuclei similar to the inclusions of LE cells. Fibrinoid, an acellular, deeply eosinophilic material, is found in loose connective tissue or in walls of blood vessels of affected tissues. Inflammation of blood vessels (vasculitis) is common. In the spleen perivascular fibrosis results in characteristic "onion ring" lesions around affected vessels. Granulomas are sometimes found in affected tissues (see Sec. 18.7 for renal pathology).

Skin biopsy with immunofluorescent staining reveals the lupus band along the dermal-epidermal junction, and vasculitis. Linear deposits of IgG, IgM, and complement are noted in the basement membrane zone of involved skin and variably in uninvolved skin exposed to sun (30–50%) (see Sec. 23.2).

CLINICAL MANIFESTATIONS. SLE may begin insidiously or acutely. Sometimes symptoms antedate the diagnosis of SLE by years. The most frequent early symptoms in children are fever, malaise, arthritis or arthralgia, and rash (Table 11–33). Fever occurs at some time in most affected children; it may be intermittent or sustained. Malaise, anorexia, weight loss, and debility are common.

Cutaneous manifestations occur in most affected children at some time. The "butterfly" rash (Fig. 11–19 [color plate section]), consisting of bluish or scaly erythematous patches, involves the malar areas and usually extends over the bridge of the nose. The rash may be photosensitive and may spread to the face, scalp, neck, chest, and extremities; it may become bullous and secondarily infected. Isolated *diskoid lupus* (cutaneous manifestations only) is unusual in children. Other skin eruptions include erythematous macules or punctate lesions on the palms, soles, fingertips, extremities, or trunk; vasculitic rashes; livedo reticularis; and nailbed changes. Macular and often painless ulcerative lesions may occur on the palate and mucous membranes of the mouth and nose. Purpura, sometimes associated with thrombocytopenia, may appear over dependent or traumatized areas. Erythema nodosum and erythema multiforme are occasionally associated. Alopecia resulting from inflammation about the hair follicles may be patchy or generalized, and the hair may be coarse, dry, and brittle.

Raynaud phenomenon may be present. It is characterized by the triad of vasospasm-induced ischemic blanching of distal phalanges, followed by anoxic cyanosis with desaturation and then by reactive hyperemia. The phenomenon is often symmetric and painful and is precipitated by cold or emotional upset. Primary Raynaud disease (idiopathic Raynaud disease)

TABLE 11–33. Manifestations of Lupus in Children*

	% of Patients
Malaise, weight loss, growth retardation	96
Cutaneous abnormalities	96
Hematologic abnormalities	91
Fever	84
Nephritis	84
Musculoskeletal complaints	82
Pleural/pulmonary disease	67
Hepatosplenomegaly or lymphadenopathy	58
Neurologic disease	49
Cardiac abnormalities	38
Hypertension	33
Ocular abnormalities	31
Gastrointestinal symptoms	27
Raynaud phenomenon	13

*Reprinted from Arthritis and Rheumatism Journal, copyright 1978. Used by permission of the American College of Rheumatology.

is distinguished from a secondary Raynaud phenomenon (associated with SLE or, more often, systemic sclerosis) by characteristic episodes of bilateral vasospasm, normal pulsation in palpable arteries, absence of digital gangrene, absence of causal disease, and symptoms lasting 2 yr or more. Secondary Raynaud phenomenon may produce asymmetric cutaneous atrophy, necrosis, ulceration, and dystrophic nails. The interval between the onset of Raynaud phenomenon and the onset of a connective tissue disorder may be as long as 3–10 yr. It is frequently seen in women.

Arthralgia and joint stiffness are common and often occur without objective changes. Sometimes affected joints are warm and swollen; pain may be greater than expected for the clinical signs, but persistent deforming arthritis is rare. Aseptic necrosis may affect bone at a number of sites, particularly in the femoral heads. Tenosynovitis and myositis may also occur.

Polyserositis (pleurisy, pericarditis, and peritonitis) is characteristic and produces chest, precordial, or abdominal pain. Hepatosplenomegaly and generalized lymphadenopathy are common. Cardiac involvement may be manifest by variable murmurs, friction rubs, cardiomegaly, electrocardiographic changes, or congestive heart failure, with myocarditis, pericarditis, or verrucous endocarditis (Libman-Sacks endocarditis, recognized by echocardiogram or at postmortem examination). Myocardial infarctions may cause death in relatively young patients, including children. Parenchymal lung infiltrates may occur; infection must be excluded, however, before pneumonia can be ascribed to SLE. Acute pneumonia, pulmonary hemorrhage, or chronic pulmonary fibrosis may occur. Involvement of the nervous system may cause personality changes, seizures, cerebrovascular accidents, and peripheral neuritis. Gastrointestinal manifestations include abdominal pain, vomiting, diarrhea, melena, and even bowel infarction secondary to vasculitis. Ocular changes may include episcleritis, iritis, or retinal vascular changes with hemorrhages or exudates (cytoid bodies). Most children have clinical renal involvement (Sec. 18.7).

LABORATORY MANIFESTATIONS. ANA should be demonstrable in all patients with active SLE, and their demonstration provides the best screening test for the disease; however, ANA also occur in many other conditions (Sec. 11.50). ANA screening tests are generally done using a fluorescent antibody technique. Tests for specific types of ANA including Ro/SSA, La/SSB, Sm, and DNA should also be performed. Antibodies to Sm are relatively specific for SLE; antibodies to Ro/SSA and La/SSB are associated with the neonatal lupus syndrome. Antibodies to double-stranded DNA are associated with active disease, particularly nephritis; DNA antibodies thus provide a useful index of severity and activity. Serum hemolytic complement and some of its components (C3 is most frequently measured) are decreased in patients with severe active SLE, particularly in those with nephritis. Anticardiolipin (antiphospholipid) or lupus anticoagulant antibodies may be detected; these have been associated with thrombotic events (not hemorrhage) and correlate with false-positive serologic tests for syphilis. Serum gamma globulin levels are often elevated; α_2-globulin levels may be increased and albumin decreased. Levels of one or more of the individual immunoglobulins may be elevated. An increased prevalence of HLA-B8, -DW3/DR3, and -DW2/DR2 has been reported in some series.

Anemia related to chronic inflammatory disease or immune hemolysis is common. Difficulties in typing and cross-matching blood may arise from the presence of erythrocyte antibodies, detected by the Coombs test. Thrombocytopenia and leukopenia occur frequently. Platelet antibodies may be demonstrable; idiopathic thrombocytopenic purpura (ITP) may be the first manifestation of SLE. The urine may contain red blood cells, white blood cells, protein, and casts. Renal insufficiency may produce elevated levels of blood urea nitrogen or creatinine and abnormal results on renal function studies.

DIAGNOSIS AND DIFFERENTIAL DIAGNOSIS. SLE may mimic any rheumatic disease and many other diseases as well. Diagnosis is made on clinical grounds (Table 11–34) and is confirmed by laboratory tests. ANA are usually present; although they are not diagnostic, their absence makes the diagnosis unlikely. Antibodies to double-stranded DNA are virtually diagnostic but are present only in patients with severe and active disease. Hypergammaglobulinemia, positive Coombs test, false-positive test for syphilis, anemia, leukopenia or thrombocytopenia, and signs of nephritis may also be diagnostically helpful. Serum levels of hemolytic complement and some of its components are lowered in some patients with active disease; absence of measurable hemolytic complement or failure to achieve normal levels during therapy should suggest a possible complement deficiency. Renal or cutaneous biopsy may confirm the diagnosis, and renal pathologic studies will indicate the type and severity of renal involvement; however, histologic changes are not entirely specific. Thrombocytopenic purpura and hemolytic anemia may be presenting features; the differential diagnosis of these manifestations should include SLE.

Drug-induced SLE may be related to many common pharmacologic agents. This diagnosis is suggested by the absence of a history suggestive of SLE prior to drug therapy; the presence of ANA in association with drug use; the presence of antihistone antibodies (which occur in >95% of these patients but in <50% of those with idiopathic SLE); the presence of rash, arthralgia, or serositis; the absence of central nervous system (CNS) or renal disease, or lupus bands on skin biopsy; black race; and improvement in most patients after withdrawal of the drug. Many more patients develop ANA than actually show symptoms or signs of SLE. Genetic differences in drug metabolism may predispose a patient to drug-related SLE associated with use of hydralazine, procainamide, isoniazid (INH), or sulfonamides because patients who are slow hepatic acetylators have been observed to be at increased risk of being ANA positive and symptomatic. Alternatively, drug-induced photosensitivity may initiate an SLE-like syndrome.

TREATMENT. Therapy should be based on the extent and severity of disease in the individual patient. Patients must be thoroughly evaluated, particularly for renal involvement. The type and severity of the renal lesion should be determined by renal biopsy on patients with clinical evidence of nephritis. There is no specific therapy. Drugs used to treat the disease suppress inflammation and perhaps the formation of immune complexes and the activities of immunologically active effector cells (although this latter mechanism is unproved). In general, patients should be treated to maintain clinical well-being and normal serum complement levels.

In patients with mild disease without nephritis, salicylates or other nonsteroidal anti-inflammatory agents should be used to provide symptomatic relief of arthritis and other discomfort. Careful follow-up for possible development of nephritis or other major involvement is vital. The antimalarial agents chloroquine and hydroxychloroquine are used for diskoid and cutaneous manifestations of systemic lupus, but extreme care must be taken because of potential retinal toxicity. Topical use of corticosteroid preparations may suppress the facial rash.

Systemic use of steroids in doses sufficient to suppress symptoms is required in most patients. In patients with significant systemic involvement but without clinical nephritis and with normal levels of serum complement and DNA antibodies, therapy can also be symptomatic with careful follow-up. Doses of corticosteroid sufficient to suppress symp-

TABLE 11–34. 1982 Revised Criteria for Diagnosis of Systemic Lupus Erythematosus*

Criterion	Definition
Malar rash	Fixed erythema, flat or raised, over the malar eminences, tending to spare the nasolabial folds
Diskoid rash	Erythematous raised patches with adherent keratotic scaling and follicular plugging; atrophic scarring may occur in older lesions
Photosensitivity	Skin rash as a result of unusual reaction to sunlight (elicited by patient history or physician observation)
Oral ulcers	Oral or nasopharyngeal ulceration, usually painless, observed by a physician
Arthritis	Nonerosive arthritis involving two or more peripheral joints, characterized by tenderness, swelling, or effusion
Serositis	Pleuritis—convincing history of pleuritic pain or rub heard by a physician or evidence of pleural effusion
	or
	Pericarditis—documented by ECG or rub or evidence of pericardial effusion
Renal disorder	Persistent proteinuria greater than 0.5 g/day or greater than 3+ if quantitation not performed
	or
	Cellular casts—may be red blood cell, hemoglobin, granular, tubular, or mixed
Neurologic disorder	Seizures—in the absence of offending drugs or known metabolic derangements (e.g., uremia, ketoacidosis, or electrolyte imbalance)
	or
	Psychosis—in the absence of offending drugs or known metabolic derangements (e.g., uremia, ketoacidosis, or electrolyte imbalance)
Hematologic disorder	Hemolytic anemia—with reticulocytosis
	or
	Leukopenia—less than 4,000/mm^3 total on two or more occasions
	or
	Lymphopenia—less than 1,500/mm^3 on two or more occasions
	or
	Thrombocytopenia—less than 100,000/mm^3
Immunologic disorder	Positive LE cell preparation
	or
	Anti-DNA antibody to native DNA in abnormal titer
	or
	Anti-Sm—presence of antibody to Sm nuclear antigen
	or
	False-positive serologic test result for syphilis known to be positive for at least 6 mo and confirmed by *Treponema pallidum* immobilization or fluorescent treponemal antibody absorption test
Antinuclear antibody	An abnormal titer of antinuclear antibody by immunofluorescence or an equivalent assay at any point in time and in the absence of drugs known to be associated with "drug-induced lupus syndrome"

*From Tan EM, Cohen AS, Fries JF, et al: The 1982 revised criteria for the classification of systemic lupus erythematosus. Arthritis Rheum 25:1271, 1982.

The proposed classification is based on 11 criteria. For the purpose of identifying patients in clinical studies, a person shall be said to have systemic lupus erythematosus if any 4 or more of the 11 criteria are present, serially or simultaneously, during any interval of observation.

toms should be given initially (1–2 mg/kg/24 hr may be required) and then tapered to the lowest suppressive doses. Antimalarial agents may be useful adjuncts in therapy of arthritis, sparing steroids. In patients with SLE and nephritis or major systemic involvement, therapy must be geared not only to maintain the clinical well-being of the patient but also to suppress the systemic and renal disease, as reflected by return of serum complement levels to normal and reduction of circulating antibodies to DNA. Large doses of corticosteroids for prolonged periods may be required; initial doses of prednisone of 1–2 mg/kg/24 hr are usual. All the undesirable side effects of steroid therapy may be expected if large doses are required for a significant period of time. Other schedules of steroid administration may be used, including large-dose intravenous pulses or, once symptoms have been controlled, alternate-day doses. Agents such as cyclophosphamide or, less often, azathioprine may be effective adjunctive agents in suppressing severe SLE; however, such therapy must be used with extreme care. Little is known about the long-term effects of such drugs, particularly in children; side effects include increased susceptibility to severe viral and other infections, gonadal suppression, and possible induction of malignancies. Such agents should never be used in patients with mild SLE or in those whose disease can be satisfactorily controlled with corticosteroids alone. Current experience indicates that intravenous pulse therapy with cyclophosphamide (Cytoxan) offers promise in the management of severe childhood lupus; such treatment should be performed only by specialists with experience in its usage.

Seizures and other central nervous system manifestations are generally associated with severe, active disease and demand vigorous control of SLE. Central nervous system disease occurs episodically in patients with SLE and may never recur if the patient is helped over the acute episode and the disease is subsequently controlled. CNS lupus must always be distinguished from infections and steroid psychosis.

Because of the possibility of drug-induced disease, inquiry should be made about possible offending agents; drugs known to be associated with SLE should not be used in patients with the disease.

Patients with *antiphospholipid antibodies* (**lupus anticoagulants**) may manifest venous and arterial thrombosis, recurrent fetal loss, migraine, stroke, transient ischemic attacks, avascular bone necrosis, transverse myelitis, pulmonary hypertension, pulmonary embolism, livedo reticularis, and leg ulcers. Steroid or cytotoxic therapy may lower the levels of the lupus anticoagulant, and anticoagulants may be indicated in patients with thrombotic events.

Dialysis and renal transplantation are adjunct therapies for severe lupus nephritis (see Sec. 18.7).

Meticulous follow-up is of paramount importance in treating all patients with SLE and includes monitoring the patient's clinical, renal, and serologic status. Any signs of worsening disease should be promptly recognized and appropriately managed. Because there is no cure, the disease is potentially lifelong, and patients must be followed for years. Active lupus should be considered an emergency that demands prompt evaluation and vigorous therapy to bring it under control before irreparable organ system involvement ensues.

PROGNOSIS. SLE was previously considered a potentially or uniformly fatal childhood disease. Currently, children with milder disease are being recognized, and it is apparent that not all children have severe major organ involvement. Although spontaneous exacerbations and remissions occur, prolonged spontaneous remission is unusual in children. Therapy with antibiotics, corticosteroids, and cytotoxic drugs has prolonged survival and brightened the short-term prognosis for many patients with lupus. Although the 5-yr survival for children now exceeds 90%, a significant number of patients still have ongoing disease and remain at risk of future adverse sequelae. Major causes of death in SLE patients include nephritis, central nervous system complications, infections, pulmonary lupus, and myocardial infarctions. The ultimate prognosis for severe lupus with childhood onset remains to be defined.

11.55 NEONATAL LUPUS PHENOMENA

Neonatal lupus phenomena occur in infants of mothers with subclinical or active SLE or other rheumatic syndromes, notably Sjögren syndrome, and are strongly associated with the presence of maternal antibody to Ro/SSA or La/SSB. These phenomena are thought to be mediated by transplacental passage of maternal antibody; the pathogenetic mechanisms are not yet well understood. Transiently positive tests for ANA or other maternal autoantibodies in cord blood and infant serum are the most frequent abnormalities; most often there are no associated clinical manifestations, and the serologic abnormalities regress in weeks to months. Occasionally, rash, transient immune thrombocytopenia, transient hemolytic anemia, or transient leukopenia occurs in the infant as the result of maternal autoantibodies.

The most frequent clinical abnormality is a rash clinically and histologically typical of cutaneous lupus that fades over a period of several months. Lesions may occur on the trunk, extremities, or face; they often assume an erythematous circinate form that resembles that of subacute cutaneous lupus in adults, another condition associated with antibodies to Ro/SSA and La/SSB.

The heart may be permanently damaged in the form of congenital heart block. Most infants with congenital heart block, once considered a rare form of congenital heart disease, have mothers with antibodies to Ro/SSA or La/SSB with or without overt maternal lupus, Sjögren syndrome, or other rheumatic disease syndrome. The exact mechanisms of cardiac damage are unknown. Damage to the conduction system of the fetal heart with fibrosis, inflammation, and deposition of immunoglobulin has been noted in a few instances. Endocardiofibroelastosis has also been reported in these infants, and it has been claimed that fetal myocarditis is also sometimes part of the syndrome. Congenital heart block is discussed in Sec. 15.64. Sera from both infant and mother should be checked for antibodies to Ro/SSA and La/SSB in any infant with congenital heart block. The risk of congenital heart block in infants of mothers with known Ro/SSA or La/SSB antibodies is not certain, nor is there any accepted means of prevention of cardiac damage to infants of mothers known to have these antibodies. Recent observations suggest that cholestasis and hepatic fibrosis may also be concomitants of the neonatal lupus syndrome.

Few if any cases of true SLE in infants have been reported. However, several instances of later occurrence of SLE in young adults who had had "transient" manifestations of lupus in the newborn period have been reported.

11.56 VASCULITIS SYNDROMES

In these syndromes of blood vessel inflammation the various patterns of disease depend on the size and location of the affected vessels (Table 11–35). Vasculitis may be a primary disease or may be secondary to a connective tissue disorder, infection, or other process. It may be limited to the skin or exist in multiple organs. When small nonmuscular vessels are involved, the disease takes the form of Henoch-Schönlein vasculitis (anaphylactoid purpura). With involvement of the larger muscular arteries the disease is called polyarteritis nodosa; variants include Wegener granulomatosis. In Takayasu arteritis the aorta and other great vessels are sites of inflammation. Some overlap of these syndromes occurs; vessels of various sizes may sometimes be involved in the same patients. Infantile polyarteritis and Kawasaki disease are characterized by vasculitis of the large coronary arteries and to a lesser extent of other large central vessels. Inflammation of blood vessels also occurs in other rheumatic diseases in children, notably lupus erythematosus, dermatomyositis, and

TABLE 11–35. Vasculitis in Children

	Henoch-Schönlen Syndrome	Kawasaki Disease	Polyarteritis and Variants	Takayasu Disease
SEX	Boys 2:1	No predilection	Boys > girls	Girls > boys
AGE AT ONSET	Over 2 yr	Usually before age 5	Any (rare)	Older children (rare)
CLINICAL CHARACTERISTICS	Purpuric rash Angioedema Arthritis Abdominal pain Nephritis	Fever, conjunctivitis, oral changes, swelling and peeling of hands and feet, rash, cervical adenopathy, coronary vasculitis	Cutaneous or multisystem disease Granulomas of upper airway or lung (Wegeners)	Hypertension Absent pulses Various rheumatic complaints
LABORATORY CHARACTERISTICS	Elevated serum IgA in half, IgA deposits in tissues	Thrombocytosis Abnormal coronary vessels on echocardiography	None specific except histology or arteriography	None specific except histology or arteriography
PATHOGENESIS	May follow *Streptococcus* or drug exposure	Unknown	May follow infectious disease Immune complex: Hepatitis B	More common in Asians
DIAGNOSIS	Clinical	Clinical	Clinical—Demonstration of vasculitis: biopsy or arteriography	Demonstration of aortic or large central vessel involvement
NATURAL HISTORY	Self-limited Occasionally recurrent Rarely chronic: renal disease	Self-limited Fatal in 1–2% (?) Long-term coronary and large vessel damage	Chronic May be fatal	Chronic, often progressive May be fatal
THERAPY	Symptomatic Occasional corticosteroid	Intravenous gamma globulin Aspirin	Corticosteroid Cytotoxic	Corticosteroid Cytotoxic Arterectomy

scleroderma; in hypertension; and in vessels exposed to local infection, trauma, or thromboemboli.

The causes of these disorders are unknown. Both Henoch-Schönlein vasculitis and polyarteritis may follow exposure to drugs or allergens. In serum sickness (Sec. 11.45), vasculitis is caused by deposition of immune complexes. Polyarteritis nodosa has been associated with hepatitis B, vascular damage presumably being caused by immune complexes of the viral antigen and its antibody.

In contrast to most other rheumatic diseases, Henoch-Schönlein vasculitis and polyarteritis nodosa affect predominantly males. In childhood, Henoch-Schönlein vasculitis is the most commonly encountered type; polyarteritis and its variants are much rarer in children.

11.57 HENOCH-SCHÖNLEIN PURPURA (VASCULITIS)

(Anaphylactoid Purpura)

Henoch-Schönlein purpura (HSP) is characterized by non-thrombocytopenic, usually dependent, palpable purpura, arthritis, abdominal pain, and nephritis. The skin lesion is the most obvious sign; the visceral lesions are less easily recognized but are more serious. The primary manifestations are due to vasculitis of the small blood vessels.

The cause is unknown. Allergy or drug sensitivity plays a role in some patients. The disease may follow an upper respiratory tract infection, sometimes streptococcal; clustering of cases with no obvious inciting event has been noted. The syndrome may occur at any age; it is more common in children than in adults, most cases occurring in children from 2 to 8 yr of age. Boys are affected twice as often as girls.

PATHOLOGY. In the skin small vessels are surrounded by an acute leukocytoclastic inflammatory reaction of polymorphonuclear and round cells; eosinophils and varying numbers of red blood cells may be present. Dermal IgA deposits have been demonstrated. Capillaries are most frequently involved, but small arterioles and venules may be affected also. Scattered nuclear debris, edema, and swelling of collagen fibrils are found adjacent to the affected vessels. Other sites of inflammation or hemorrhage may include the synovium, the gastrointestinal tract, and the central nervous system. Edema and vasculitis of the bowel wall may lead to intussusception and, rarely, perforation and may mimic IBD. For the renal lesion, see Sec. 18.12.

CLINICAL MANIFESTATIONS. Onset may be acute, with simultaneous appearance of several manifestations, or gradual, with sequential appearance of different manifestations over a period of weeks. Various combinations of symptoms and signs may occur. Malaise and low-grade fever are present in half the patients.

Skin lesions are present in all identified patients; it is not known whether visceral manifestations occur in the absence of rash. The lesions usually appear on the lower extremities and buttocks but may involve the upper extremities, trunk, and face (Fig. 11–20 [color plate section]). Dermatologic manifestations are extremely variable. The classic lesion begins as a small wheal or erythematous maculopapule. Lesions initially blanche on pressure but later lose this feature and generally become petechial or purpuric. Purpuric areas evolve in the usual manner of ecchymoses, changing from red to purple, becoming rusty, and eventually fading. Skin lesions appear in crops, and a variety may be present at any time. In addition to these characteristic lesions, the various patterns of erythema multiforme and erythema nodosum may rarely occur and are rarely pruritic. Angioedema involving the scalp, eyelids, lips, ears, dorsa of the hands and feet, back, scrotum, and perineum is common and may be striking, especially in young children. Rarely, an entire limb segment, such as the forearm, may be transiently swollen and tender.

Arthritis occurs in two thirds of affected children. Large joints, particularly the knees and ankles, are most commonly involved. Affected joints may be swollen, tender, and painful on motion. When present, effusions reveal serous fluid; they are not hemorrhagic. Joint symptoms usually resolve after a few days without residual deformity or articular damage but may recur during periods of active disease.

Gastrointestinal symptoms appear in over half of affected children. The most common complaint is colicky abdominal pain, which may be severe and is often associated with vomiting. Stools show gross or occult blood in more than 50% of patients, and hematemesis may occur. Failure to recognize this syndrome in children with sudden onset of acute abdominal pain may lead to unnecessary laparotomy. In such cases, peritoneal exudate, enlarged mesenteric lymph nodes, segmental edema, and hemorrhage into the bowel wall may be present. Gastrointestinal roentgenograms may show decreased motility and segmental narrowing, presumably related to submucosal edema and hemorrhage. Rarely, intussusception, obstruction, or infarction with bowel perforation may occur.

Renal involvement occurs in 25–50% of children during the acute phase, the frequency depending in part on the adequacy of examination. It is usually manifest by hematuria with or without casts or proteinuria during the first few weeks of illness; sometimes renal involvement first appears later after other manifestations have become quiescent. Moderate azotemia, hypertension, oliguria, and hypertensive encephalopathy may occasionally occur. Most children with renal involvement recover, although some continue to have abnormal urinary sediment, with or without abnormal renal function; a few will experience chronic renal disease within a few years of the acute phase of HSP.

A rare but potentially serious manifestation is central nervous system involvement, with seizures, paresis, and coma. Hepatosplenomegaly and lymphadenopathy may also occur during the acute phase of the disease. Rarely, intramuscular hemorrhage, rheumatoid-like nodules, cardiac involvement, eye involvement, and testicular swelling and hemorrhage have been reported.

The *prognosis* is excellent in the absence of significant renal disease. The course varies. The disease is often mild, lasting for a few days with only transient arthritis and a few purpuric spots. In more seriously affected children the average duration is 4–6 wk, but subsequent exacerbations and remissions may occur. The illness may occasionally smolder for 1 yr or more.

LABORATORY FINDINGS. Laboratory tests are not diagnostic. The ESR may be elevated. The white blood cell count is often increased, and eosinophilia may be present. Coagulation studies are normal. With renal involvement red blood cells, white blood cells, casts, and albumin are present in the urine. There may be gross or occult blood in the stools. Neither rheumatoid factor nor ANA are present. Serum complement titers are normal or elevated. Serum levels of IgA are elevated in more than 50% of patients.

DIAGNOSIS AND DIFFERENTIAL DIAGNOSIS. The full-blown picture of HSP with rash, arthritis, and gastrointestinal and renal manifestations is characteristic. Diagnostic confusion may result when one symptom predominates or multiple system involvement is not recognized. The rash may suggest a hemorrhagic diathesis or septicemia; platelet counts, blood clotting tests, and cultures will exclude these possibilities. In addition, the patient with septicemia usually appears more acutely ill. When gastrointestinal manifestations predominate, the syndrome may suggest a number of intra-abdominal emergencies. The possibility of HSP should be considered in any child with acute abdominal pain, and inquiry should be made for associated rash, angioedema, arthritis, or nephritis. With prominent renal findings, acute glomerulonephritis may be suggested; other manifestations of Henoch-Schönlein vasculitis should allow differentiation. In children with chronic renal disease a history of acute Henoch-Schönlein vasculitis should be sought. Differentiation from other rheumatic diseases is rarely difficult. In polyarteritis nodosa peripheral neurologic changes and cardiac manifestations are more common, but clinical distinction from HSP may occasionally be difficult.

TREATMENT. There is no specific therapy. In the rare instance in which a specific allergen can be proved, the patient should avoid the antigen. When the disease follows a bacterial infection, particularly streptococcal illness, the organism should be eliminated and, if the disease recurs, prophylaxis considered. Symptomatic treatment is indicated for arthritis, rash, edema, fever, and malaise. Salicylates will often alleviate these self-limited discomforts.

Intestinal hemorrhage, obstruction, intussusception, or perforation may be life-threatening in the acute phase; these complications may be managed by the early use of corticosteroids. Therapy with prednisone, 1–2 mg/kg/24 hr, is often associated with dramatic improvement. Corticosteroid therapy is also indicated for the rare patient with central nervous system manifestations. Acute renal failure should be managed in the same way as acute glomerulonephritis (Sec. 18.12). Therapy for severe nephritis with drugs such as corticosteroids, azathioprine, and cyclophosphamide remains experimental.

PROGNOSIS. Rarely, death may occur during the acute phase from gastrointestinal complications (hemorrhage, intussusception, bowel infarction), acute renal failure, or central nervous system involvement. Chronic renal disease may cause later morbidity in a few patients. About 25% of children with initial renal involvement have persistence of abnormal urine sediment for years; the ultimate prognosis for these patients is not certain.

11.58 KAWASAKI DISEASE

(Mucocutaneous Lymph Node Syndrome, Infantile Polyarteritis)

Kawasaki disease is a febrile disease of children notable for the occurrence of vasculitis of large coronary blood vessels with potential dilatation, aneurysm formation, thrombosis, rupture, or myocardial ischemia. Kawasaki disease was first reported in Japanese children after the Second World War; however, this condition cannot be differentiated from the earlier and rare condition, which was called infantile polyarteritis. Worldwide distribution of Kawasaki disease is now recognized, affecting children of many races and apparently increasing in frequency. The condition occurs sporadically or in epidemics, generally in children 5 yr of age or younger and rarely if ever in adults. There is no evidence for person-to-person transmission. The etiology remains unknown. Early leads, which suggested a role of retroviruses or rickettsia, have not been substantiated, and no clear evidence has been found to suggest that immune aberrations have any central role in the disorder.

CLINICAL MANIFESTATIONS. Diagnosis rests on the demonstration of characteristic clinical signs (Table 11–36). Atypical cases manifesting only fever, rash, conjunctival infection, and pharyngeal signs but later demonstrating characteristic coronary artery lesions, have been reported. Atypical patients are often less than 1 yr of age, have incorrect admitting diagnoses (gastroenteritis, viral syndrome, sepsis), and have a high morbidity.

TABLE 11–36. Diagnostic Criteria for Kawasaki Disease*

A. Fever lasting for at least 5 days†
B. Presence of *four of the following five* conditions:
   1. Bilateral nonpurulent conjunctival injection
   2. Changes of the mucosa of the oropharynx, including infected pharynx, infected and/or dry fissured lips, strawberry tongue
   3. Changes of the peripheral extremities, such as edema and/or erythema of the hands or feet, desquamation, usually beginning periungually
   4. Rash, primarily truncal; polymorphous but nonvesicular
   5. Cervical lymphadenopathy
C. Illness not explained by other known disease process

*A consensus statement prepared by North American participants of the Third International Kawasaki Disease Symposium, Tokyo, Japan, December, 1988. Pediatr Infect Dis J 8:663, 1989. © by Williams & Wilkins, 1989.

†Many experts believe that, in the presence of classic features, the diagnosis of Kawasaki disease can be made (and treatment instituted) before the 5th day of fever by experienced individuals.

Onset is generally abrupt, heralded by onset of high fever (generally greater than 104° F), which is sustained, lasting for one to several weeks, and unresponsive to antibiotic therapy. Other characteristic findings include bilateral conjunctivitis without discharge, dry erythematous fissured lips, strawberry tongue (similar to that seen in streptococcal infections), and injected oral pharyngeal mucosa. Lymphadenopathy may affect one or, less often, several nodes, generally cervical, or rarely may be generalized; the nodes are nonsuppurative, can be large, and are usually nontender. Erythematous skin eruptions can affect the trunk, face, or extremities; the rash may take maculopapular, morbilliform, or erythema multiforme form. A nonspecific erythematous, desquamating perineal eruption is present in many patients during the 1st wk of the illness. After several days of disease, the hands and feet become edematous, swollen, and painful; desquamation of skin from the fingertips, toetips, palms, and soles occurs generally during the 2nd–3rd wk of illness (Table 11–37). Cutaneous desquamation may also involve other body areas. Transient arthritis may occur, particularly in older children; painful joint swelling is usually symmetric in distribution and may affect both large and small joints. Other acute manifestations include diarrhea, vomiting, abdominal pain, hydrops of the gallbladder, myositis, meatitis with sterile pyuria, tympanitis, ulcerative stomatitis, cough (sometimes associated with pulmonary infiltrates), rhinorrhea, aseptic meningitis, seizures, cranial or peripheral nerve palsies, and hepatosplenomegaly. Iridocyclitis is frequently found in children who undergo slit-lamp examination. Almost all affected children are irritable, and many may have altered mental states. Peripheral large arterial aneurysms (axillary, popliteal) and evidence of distal vascular compromise may occasionally be noted on physical examination.

Cardiac involvement is the most important manifestation of Kawasaki disease. Ten to forty per cent of children have evidence of coronary vasculitis within the first 2 wk of illness, manifested by dilatation or aneurysm formation in coronary arteries as seen by two-dimensional echocardiography. This test should be performed in all children with known or suspected Kawasaki disease at the time of presentation and again during the first 2 wk of disease. Manifestations of coronary arteritis include signs of myocardial ischemia or rarely overt myocardial infarction or rupture of an aneurysm. Pericarditis, myocarditis, endocarditis, heart failure, and arrhythmias may also occur (see Table 11–31).

LABORATORY FINDINGS. There are no diagnostic tests. Leukocytosis with a predominance of immature forms and thrombocytosis (in the 2nd–3rd wk) can be striking; anemia is also common. Sedimentation rates and C-reactive protein levels are usually greatly elevated. Tests for autoantibodies including ANA and rheumatoid factors are negative, and

TABLE 11–37. Kawasaki Syndrome: Disease Phases, Complications, and Degree of Arteritis in Untreated Patients*

	Acute	Subacute	Convalescent	Chronic
	Duration (1–11 days)	Duration (11–21 days)	Duration (21–60 days)	Duration (? yr)
Clinical findings	Fever, conjunctivitis, oral changes, extremity changes, irritability, rash, cervical lymphadenopathy, high ESR	Irritability persists Prolongation of fever may occur Normalization of most clinical findings Palpable aneurysms may develop	Most clinical findings resolve Aneurysmal dilatation of peripheral vessels may persist Conjunctivitis may persist	
Complications	Early arthritis Myocarditis Pericarditis Mitral insufficiency Congestive heart failure Iridocyclitis Meningitis Sterile pyuria	Coronary aneurysms Late-onset arthritis Mitral insufficiency Gallbladder hydrops Fingertip and toe desquamation Thrombocytosis Coronary thrombosis with infarction	Arthritis may persist Coronary and peripheral aneurysms may persist Acute phase reactant normalization	Angina pectoris, coronary stenosis, or myocardial insufficiency may develop
Arterial correlates	Perivasculitis, vasculitis of capillaries, arterioles, venules Inflammation of intima of medium and large arteries	Aneurysms, thrombi, stenosis of medium-sized arteries, panvasculitis, edema of vessel wall Myocarditis less prominent	Vascular inflammation decreases	Scar formation Intimal thickening
Cause of death	Myocarditis	Myocardial infarction Rupture of aneurysm Myocarditis	Myocardial infarction Ischemic heart disease	Myocardial infarction

*Modified from Hicks RV, Melish ME: Kawasaki syndrome. Pediatr Clin North Am 33:1151, 1986.

hemolytic complement levels are normal or high. Mild proteinuria and pyuria may be present, as may cerebrospinal fluid pleocytosis. Serum levels of hepatic transaminases and bilirubin may be slightly elevated.

Cardiac studies in the form of chest roentgenograms, electrocardiograms, and echocardiograms are vital for the initial evaluation of all patients; of these, two-dimensional echocardiography is most useful for recognizing coronary vascular disease and revealing coronary vascular dilatation or aneurysm formation. This study should be done initially and in follow-up of all patients (see Table 11–31). Arteriography of coronary vessels may also reveal lesions in patients with Kawasaki disease, but this invasive procedure is not routinely needed. Occasionally arteriography of larger central vessels may be warranted by the clinical findings.

Histologic changes at autopsy of patients with fatal lesions include intense inflammatory cell infiltrates of the media and intima of large coronary vessels and other central vessels and arterial obstruction by platelet thrombi. These changes closely resemble those of a rare condition that appears to be inseparable from Kawasaki disease and was previously called **infantile periarteritis nodosa**.

DIAGNOSIS. Diagnosis rests on the clinical features. There are no diagnostic laboratory tests, although demonstration of coronary artery involvement by echocardiography is certainly highly suggestive of this condition. Disease manifestations and diagnosis depend on the phase of Kawasaki disease (see Table 11–37). The differential diagnosis includes scarlet fever, toxic shock syndrome, leptospirosis, Epstein-Barr virus infection, juvenile rheumatoid arthritis, measles, acrodynia, Rocky Mountain spotted fever, drug reactions, Stevens-Johnson syndrome, and other vasculitic syndromes.

PROGNOSIS. Recovery is generally complete in patients who do not have detectable coronary vasculitis; second attacks occur only rarely. Most children with demonstrable cardiac involvement also appear to do well, although their long-term prognosis is not known. In the early Japanese series, 1–2% of all children with Kawasaki disease died of cardiac complications, usually within 1–2 mo of onset. A few reports now detail the later occurrence of aneurysms of large vessels other than the coronaries.

TREATMENT. Kawasaki disease may respond dramatically to therapy with intravenous gamma globulin given during the period of active febrile disease. Fever and other attendant systemic manifestations often abate within 24 hr of initial therapy. Furthermore, controlled studies show that intravenous gamma globulin therapy given early in disease prevents coronary vascular involvement as demonstrable by echocardiography. The recommended regimen consists of an intravenous infusion of 2 g/kg given as a single dose over 10–12 hr. Therapy given within 10 days of onset is effective in preventing coronary vascular damage; therapy given to symptomatic patients (febrile, high ESR) after 10 days of onset of manifestations may also be effective in providing symptomatic relief. Side effects of intravenous gamma globulin therapy are rare and include anaphylaxis, chills, fever, headache, and myalgia.

Salicylate therapy is also indicated during the febrile phase of the disease; therapeutic serum concentrations of 20–30 mg/dL are desirable but may be difficult to achieve, even with doses of salicylates as high as 100 mg/kg/24 hr. Continuance of low, single-dose (5 mg/kg/24 hr) salicylate therapy for its antithrombotic (antiplatelet) effects has been advocated for 6–8 wk after the period of active disease subsides in children without coronary lesions. Low-dose aspirin with or without dipyridamole should be continued until coronary lesions resolve. Some authorities add heparin or warfarin (Coumadin) therapy for patients with persistent large or multiple nonobstructive or obstructive aneurysms. Careful and repeated follow-up evaluations with stress testing, echocardiography, and at times angiography are warranted for those children with significant residual coronary vascular changes. The impact of such coronary vascular changes on the incidence and severity of atherosclerotic coronary artery disease in later life is not known.

Corticosteroid therapy is rarely used in Kawasaki disease, and some consider it contraindicated.

Thrombolysis with streptokinase is indicated for patients in the active phase of coronary artery thrombosis, and peripheral artery ischemia may be treated with thrombolytic drugs and prostaglandin E infusion. Aortocoronary artery bypass surgery with internal mammary artery or saphenous vein grafts has been helpful in treating symptomatic patients with severe stenotic lesions (> 75% occlusion).

RARE VASCULITIC FORMS

11.59 Polyarteritis Nodosa

Medium-sized and small arteries are the sites of inflammation in polyarteritis nodosa. This necrotizing vasculitis affects all age groups but is rare in childhood; males are affected more frequently than females. The cause is unknown, but the disease has been reported to follow drug exposure. Hepatitis B antigen has been associated with a few cases, as have streptococcal infections and serous otitis media.

Inflammation with polymorphonuclear leukocytes, eosinophils, and round cells may involve the entire vessel wall. Necrosis, thrombosis, or aneurysm formation may occur in affected vessels and result in infarction. Healed vessels become scarred or recanalized.

CLINICAL MANIFESTATIONS. These are diverse and depend on sites of vascular involvement, which typically include heart, kidney, skin, and peripheral nervous system. Signs of systemic illness such as fever, anorexia, lethargy, weakness, and weight loss are usually present. Arthralgia and arthritis are frequent; myalgia and myositis may be present. Various cutaneous manifestations are common and include erythematous rashes, nodular lesions, petechiae and purpuric spots, livedo reticularis, cutaneous ulcers, and edema. Rarely, gangrene of the extremities occurs. Peripheral neuropathy (symmetric-distal or mononeuritis multiplex), with pain, numbness, paresthesias, and muscle weakness results from involvement of the peripheral nerves adjacent to affected vessels. Abdominal pain, bleeding, ulcerations, and infarction can follow involvement of the gastrointestinal vessels. Renal involvement may result in renal failure and death. Involvement of large renal vessels results in flank pain and gross hematuria, and that of small vessels and glomeruli results in microscopic hematuria, proteinuria, and cylindruria. Associated hypertension is usual. Inflammation of pulmonary vessels may cause cough, wheezing, pulmonary infiltrates, and pleuritis. Central nervous system manifestations include seizures, encephalitic symptoms, and stroke. Cranial nerve palsies and iridocyclitis may occur. Involvement of coronary vessels may produce tachycardia, heart failure, and myocardial infarction; pericarditis may also be present. Orchitis and epididymitis are common.

LABORATORY FINDINGS. There are no specific laboratory tests. The ESR may be elevated, and acute phase reactants may be present. Anemia is common; eosinophilia and leukocytosis are sometimes found. There may be gross or microscopic hematuria, and renal function studies may be abnormal. ANA and rheumatoid factors are absent.

DIAGNOSIS. Polyarteritis nodosa is readily confused with many other diseases. Differentiation from other rheumatic diseases may be particularly difficult. The diagnosis is based primarily on clinical suspicion and on the presence of histologic changes in involved tissues on biopsy. Muscle or skin biopsies may fail to identify vasculitis. Testicular biopsies are said to be helpful but are seldom done. Mesenteric or renal arteriography may reveal arteritis and aneurysms; these are rarely seen in SLE.

PROGNOSIS. The prognosis is poor; death may result from renal failure, heart failure, or severe gastrointestinal or central nervous system disease.

TREATMENT. Corticosteroids (1–2 mg/kg/24 hr) may suppress acute manifestations and lengthen survival. Cytotoxic agents such as oral or intravenous cyclophosphamide have been reported to be effective in steroid-resistant patients.

11.60 Wegener Granulomatosis
(Lethal Midline Granuloma)

In this rare syndrome, destructive granulomatous lesions of the upper respiratory tract and lungs are associated with a systemic necrotizing vasculitis, which is most prominent in the lungs and kidneys. Upper respiratory and pulmonary granulomas may predominate in some cases, antedating recognition of systemic vasculitis by years. Males are predominantly affected (2:1). The cause is unknown; as in other vasculitis syndromes, an association with drug sensitivity and allergy has been suggested.

Respiratory symptoms are prominent *clinical manifestations*. Persistent nasal stuffiness or discharge may be an early symptom, with crusted or pustular lesions in the nares. Lesions are progressively destructive and may result in perforation of the nasal septum, obliteration of the nasal sinuses, and ulcerations of the palate, pharynx, larynx, and trachea. Cough or hemoptysis may occur; fever, weight loss, night sweats, and prostration are common. Other frequently associated manifestations include arthritis, neuropathy, rash, splenomegaly, and severe progressive glomerulitis, often terminating in renal failure. In cases with clinically inapparent systemic involvement, diffuse vasculitis may be found on post mortem examination.

There are no specific laboratory manifestations; eosinophilia may be present. Roentgenograms may reveal bone destruction in the nose and sinuses and pulmonary infiltrates suggestive of tuberculosis or neoplasm. Urinalyses usually show evidence of nephritis, and renal function studies may be abnormal.

Diagnosis is based on the clinical picture and serologic tests and is confirmed by histologic demonstration of granulomatous lesions of the respiratory tract and systemic vasculitis, particularly nephritis. The differential diagnosis includes other vasculitis syndromes, lymphoma, local or disseminated fungal infections, tuberculosis, allergic alveolitis, and Goodpasture syndrome.

Without therapy, the *prognosis* is poor. Patients with limited forms of the disease may survive for long periods, but the destructive lesions of the upper respiratory tract may be disfiguring.

Treatment with corticosteroids may suppress systemic vasculitis and prevent progression of destructive lesions in the upper respiratory tract. In adults, cyclophosphamide has been effective in the management of severe disease.

11.61 Takayasu Arteritis
(Pulseless Disease)

This uncommon condition, an inflammatory process involving the aorta and its major branches, occurs primarily in young women. Some cases have been reported in late childhood, a few in infants. Most reported patients are from Asia or Africa. The cause is unknown; associated congenital defects of the great vessels have been recorded.

The underlying pathology is a segmental panarteritis of the aorta and its major branches. Smaller vessels are generally spared. Aneurysmal dilatation and rupture may occur. Involvement of the great vessels can cause weak or absent pulses in the upper extremities, hence, the term "pulseless disease." Blood pressure in the legs may exceed that in the arms ("reverse coarctation"), in contrast to the situation seen in coarctation of the aorta. Renal arterial involvement may cause renal ischemia, resulting in hypertension. Decreased brain blood flow can result in neurologic disturbances. Visual disturbances are common.

Associated rheumatic complaints include arthritis, myalgia, pleuritis, pericarditis, fever, and rashes, sometimes antedating symptomatic aortitis by years. There are no specific laboratory data. ESR and gamma globulin levels may be elevated; LE preparations may be positive. Appropriate angiographic studies will demonstrate changes in affected vessels.

The condition should be considered in any child with obscure hypertension, particularly when fever and an elevated ESR are associated. The prognosis is variable. Some adults have survived; most children have died. Therapy with corticosteroids and cytotoxic agents has been tried. Endarterectomy may be warranted.

11.62 DERMATOMYOSITIS

This multisystem disease is characterized principally by nonsuppurative inflammation of striated muscle and distinctive cutaneous lesions.

ETIOLOGY AND EPIDEMIOLOGY. The cause of dermatomyositis is unknown. Cellular immune mechanisms may play a basic role in the pathogenesis. Lymphocytes from patients with dermatomyositis release lymphotoxins that kill muscle cells in tissue culture. Immunoglobulin and complement deposition also occur in blood vessels in affected muscle. In adults, but not in children, the disease is associated with malignancies (in 20% of patients). Preliminary studies suggest that childhood dermatomyositis may be associated with HLA-B8/DR3. Research endeavors continue to seek a link with a viral infection, notably Coxsackie virus.

Dermatomyositis is less common than rheumatoid arthritis, SLE, or HSP. It rarely begins before the 2nd birthday; the average age at onset is 8–9 yr. Girls are affected more frequently than boys (3:2), and there is no familial or racial predilection.

PATHOLOGY. Lesions in the skin, subcutaneous tissues, gastrointestinal tract, and striated muscles are irregularly distributed; care must be taken to choose an involved site if biopsies are made. The most prominent lesion in children is an occlusive vasculitis involving arterioles, venules, and capillaries in the connective tissues of the skin, nailbed, subcutaneous tissue, and muscle. In muscle, patchy degeneration, atrophy and regeneration of muscle fibers, interstitial edema, and proliferation of connective tissue occur. In affected skin, thinning of the epidermis and edema and vasculitis of the dermis are apparent. Gastrointestinal tract vasculitis may produce mucosal ulcerations and tissue infarction. Mild renal glomerular changes have also been described.

CLINICAL MANIFESTATIONS. The onset is usually insidious, with slowly developing muscle weakness, generally apparent first in the proximal muscles of the extremities and trunk. The child may develop an awkward gait and slowly lose the capacity to perform functions such as climbing stairs, rising from the floor, riding a bicycle, combing hair, and dressing. Weakness can be elicited by observing the child's inability to raise the head when lying supine (weak neck flexors) or to do a sit-up (weak abdominals) or to rise unassisted from the floor (Gower sign). Affected muscles tend to be stiff and sore and sometimes brawny, indurated, and tender. Nonpitting edema and thickening of the skin and subcutaneous tissues may be present. Although myositis is generally most pronounced in the proximal muscles, any muscles can be affected, with varying sites and degrees of atrophy or contracture formation. Severe involvement of palatorespiratory muscles may lead to respiratory difficulty, nasal regurgitation, nasal voice, aspiration, and death. Involvement of the respiratory muscles may produce hypoventilation. Cardiac involvement with conduction defects or myocarditis has been reported.

The skin lesions are characteristic and often have a distinctive violaceous (heliotrope) erythema. The upper eyelids assume a pathognomonic violaceous discoloration (heliotrope eyelids) (Fig. 11–21 [color plate section]). Periorbital and facial edema may be associated. A butterfly rash similar to that of SLE may be present. Lesions of the palatal and nasal mucous membranes may be associated with the malar rash. The skin over the extensor surfaces of the joints, particularly the knuckles (Gottron papules), knees, elbows, and medial malleoli, becomes erythematous, atrophic, and scaly (Fig. 11–22 [color plate section]). These areas later develop pigmentary changes resulting in hyperpigmentation or vitiligo. The capillaries of the nailbed, as noted by capillary microscopy, may become tortuous or occluded. A dusky erythema may cover the upper trunk and proximal extremities. Other nonspecific skin changes also may occur. The skin over the involved extremities may appear tight and glossy; in longstanding disease there may be cutaneous atrophy with binding of the skin to the underlying structures. Calcium may be deposited in affected subcutaneous tissues, muscles, and fascia; these deposits sometimes break down and are extruded in semisolid or solid form.

Gastrointestinal involvement may occur at any level, heralded by difficulty with swallowing, abdominal pain, perforation, melena, or constipation. Low-grade fever may be present. Arthritis or other evidence of systemic involvement such as lymphadenopathy and hepatosplenomegaly may occur. Pulmonary disease (interstitial, hemorrhagic, or pleuritic), ocular involvement (iritis, retinitis), and CNS manifestations (seizures) are rare concomitants of disease.

LABORATORY FINDINGS. Muscle inflammation is associated with elevated serum levels of such enzymes as transaminases (SGOT), creatine kinase (CPK), aldolase, and lactic dehydrogenase (LDH). The electromyogram of affected muscles is abnormal and should be performed after muscle enzyme studies are performed. ESR may be elevated or normal. Tests for rheumatoid factors are generally negative; ANA may be present, usually in low titers. Urinalyses are usually normal. In patients with gastrointestinal involvement there may be gross or occult blood in the stool. Roentgenograms may reveal calcium deposits in soft tissues.

DIAGNOSIS AND DIFFERENTIAL DIAGNOSIS. In its typical form dermatomyositis should present little diagnostic difficulty. The combination of proximal and axial muscle weakness, characteristic rash, elevated serum levels of enzymes, and abnormal findings on electromyography is diagnostic; muscle biopsy is helpful but is usually not necessary. In the differential diagnosis various neuromuscular disorders such as poliomyelitis, Guillain-Barré syndrome, muscular dystrophy, myasthenia gravis, and endocrine or metabolic myopathies should be considered, as should illnesses characterized by predominantly muscular lesions, such as trichinosis or toxoplasmosis. Transient rhabdomyolysis with myoglobinuria should be considered, as well as acute myositis, which has been reported in association with influenza virus and may occur with other viral infections as well. SLE, mixed connective tissue disease, JRA, and scleroderma are distinguishable clinically and by laboratory tests. When the onset is insidious, a period of observation may be needed to establish the diagnosis.

TREATMENT. During the acute phase, accurate evaluation and management of palatorespiratory function and respiratory muscle status may be lifesaving. If the swallowing mechanism is impaired, soft or liquid diets should be provided under close observation. Patients must be carefully watched for possible deterioration in respiratory function with pulmonary function tests. Constant nursing care is mandatory for any child with palatorespiratory involvement, and equipment for nasopharyngeal suction, endotracheal intubation, and tracheostomy should be available. A respirator may be required.

The possibility of serious gastrointestinal manifestations during the acute phase of disease must also be considered.

Functional recovery depends on the preservation of adequate muscle strength and the prevention of crippling contractures. Corticosteroids effectively suppress the inflammatory process in most patients. Serial serum levels of SGOT, CPK, or aldolase provide a helpful gauge of activity and therapeutic response. Prednisone in an initial dosage of 1–2 mg/kg/24 hr (or 60 mg/m^2 of body surface area/24 hr) usually reduces enzyme levels toward normal values within 1–2 wk; clinical improvement with decreased pain and swelling in muscles and increasing muscle strength usually follows. When enzyme levels have declined to normal, the steroid dosage should be slowly decreased while maintaining continuous monitoring of the clinical course and serum enzyme levels. If the steroid dosage is reduced too rapidly, rebound in enzyme levels may occur; such rebounds are followed by deterioration in the clinical condition within a few weeks unless the corticosteroid dosage is promptly increased. The lowest dose of steroids sufficient to suppress clinical symptoms and serum enzyme levels should be found and maintained for months. Steroid therapy can generally be discontinued in 1–2 yr. Steroid preparations such as triamcinolone and dexamethasone, which have been associated with "steroid myopathy," should be avoided. Salicylates may occasionally be helpful as adjunctive drugs in relieving symptoms. For patients who do not respond to steroids, pulse administration of prednisone or agents such as methotrexate, azathioprine, or cyclosporine may be beneficial.

Physical therapy is essential to avoid contractures and to rebuild muscle strength. During the acute phase when muscle weakness is pronounced, passive exercises can be used to maintain range of motion. With clinical improvement active exercises to strengthen muscles should be added. Splints to maintain good limb position may be needed. Bed rest is not necessary, and immobilization without exercise should be avoided at all times. Skin hygiene, especially around the neck, skin creases, and axillae, is important.

PROGNOSIS. The course of dermatomyositis can be favorably modified by early vigorous control of the disease, and the prognosis in adequately treated children is good. In untreated patients mortality is about 40%. Most deaths are related to palatorespiratory involvement or such gastrointestinal complications as hemorrhage or perforation and occur within 2 yr of onset. Otherwise, the disease usually becomes inactive over a period of several years, and subsequent exacerbations are unusual. Infrequently, the disease may smolder for years. Most surviving patients are able to lead active lives, although they may have residual abnormalities. A few have severe contractures and crippling deformities. Severe calcinosis can be particularly disabling; there is no satisfactory therapy. Surgical excision of calcium lesions may provide some relief. Recently, the occurrence of lipodystrophy with insulin resistance and hyperandrogenism has been recognized as a late complication of dermatomyositis.

11.63 SCLERODERMA

Scleroderma ("hard skin"), a chronic fibrotic disturbance of connective tissue, classically involves skin but may also affect the gastrointestinal tract, heart, lung, kidney, and synovium. Cutaneous involvement may occur in focal patches *(morphea)*, in a linear distribution *(linear scleroderma)*, or in a generalized, symmetric distribution. The last is usually associated with systemic involvement *(systemic sclerosis)* and is the usual adult form. Scleroderma in children usually takes the form of morphea or linear scleroderma; systemic sclerosis is uncommon (Table 11–38).

ETIOLOGY AND EPIDEMIOLOGY. The disease is rare, may begin at any time during childhood, and is subject to unpredictable slow progression or remission. Girls are affected more often than boys. There is no known familial predisposition. The etiology is not known. The histopathology of systemic sclerosis is notable for fibrosis of affected tissues, relatively little inflammatory response, and occlusive vasculitis affecting capillaries and small blood vessels.

CLINICAL MANIFESTATIONS. Morphea and Linear Scleroderma. The first signs are patchy lesions of skin and subcutaneous tissues. These often have a linear pattern similar to the distribution of peripheral nerves and may occur primarily on one side of the body. During the early phases involved areas are slightly erythematous and edematous or have an atrophic, shiny appearance. The child may complain

TABLE 11–38. Scleroderma in Children

	Focal Scleroderma	Systemic Sclerosis	Fasciitis
SEX	Girls > boys	Girls > boys	No prediction
AGE AT ONSET	2 yr or older	4 yr or older	4 yr or older
CLINICAL CHARACTERISTICS	Cutaneous fibrosis Patchy: Morphea Linear scleroderma No systemic involvement or Raynaud's phenomenon	Raynaud's phenomenon Diffuse cutaneous fibrosis: Extremities, face, trunk; arthritis; fibrosis of internal organs: heart, lungs, kidneys, gastrointestinal tract; hypertension; cardiopulmonary failure	Pain, inflammation of fascia, particularly in limbs Joint contractures—hands and others Little or no systemic disease
LABORATORY CHARACTERISTICS	May have ANA RF, increased immunoglobulins	May have ANA RF, increased immunoglobulins Capillary nailbed changes	Negative ANA, RF Eosinophilia: blood or tissue
PATHOGENESIS	Fibrosis—limited to dermal tissues	Fibrosis Cutaneous Systemic	Occasionally follows exertion Resembles syndrome following ingestion of tryptophane or toxic oil
DIAGNOSIS	Clinical, biopsy	Clinical	Clinical, fascial biopsy
NATURAL HISTORY	May progress or remit Occasionally crippling	May progress or remit May be fatal	May progress or remit
THERAPY	Uncertain: topical steroid, penicillamine	Uncertain Penicillamine Cytotoxic Control of blood pressure	Corticosteroids

ANA = antinuclear antibody; RF = rheumatoid factor.

of pain or a prickly sensation. As the disease progresses, the skin lesions become indurated with violaceous, sometimes elevated borders and pale, waxy-appearing centers. Lesions enlarge peripherally and may coalesce to involve an entire extremity or a large portion of the body. Extensive scarring and fibrosis of the involved area can occur with firm binding of cutaneous tissues to underlying structures ("hide-binding"). This may be severe enough to limit growth of the affected part and produce crippling contractures (Fig. 11–23). Chronically involved areas may be hyperpigmented or depigmented. Active disease may be arrested over a period of months to years or may smolder. Prognosis for life is good in the absence of systemic involvement.

Systemic Sclerosis. This systemic form of scleroderma is nearly always associated with Raynaud phenomenon; indeed Raynaud phenomenon is often the first manifestation of disease (Sec. 11.54). Cutaneous involvement is symmetric and includes the hands, feet, and sometimes the trunk and face as well. Induration, pigmentary changes, telangiectasia, and hide-binding of involved cutaneous tissues occur as with focal forms of the disease. Cutaneous ulcers may affect the fingertips or other areas on the limbs. Synovitis, particularly about the small hand joints, may mimic rheumatoid arthritis; tenosynovitis and nodules may occur about tendon sheaths. The disease may involve the gastrointestinal tract, heart, lungs, and kidneys. Systemic manifestations, particularly renal, cardiac, and pulmonary lesions, may be fatal. Esophageal dysfunction may result in chronic aspiration pneumonia. Severe hypertension may occur.

LABORATORY FINDINGS. There are no specific laboratory tests. The ESR is frequently normal. Rheumatoid factors and ANA may be found in both focal and systemic forms of the disease. Roentgenography may show dysfunction of esophageal and bowel motility and erosion of the distal phalanges. Pulmonary function studies, electrocardiograms, and chest roentgenograms may disclose cardiopulmonary involvement. Urinalyses and renal function studies are abnormal in the presence of renal involvement.

DIAGNOSIS AND DIFFERENTIAL DIAGNOSIS. The clinical picture is characteristic in both morphea and progressive systemic sclerosis. Eosinophilic fasciitis may be difficult to distinguish; localization of involvement to the fascial layers with relative sparing of the skin, prominent esoinophilia, and absence of Raynaud phenomenon serves to differentiate the two conditions. However, fasciitis and cutaneous scleroderma are associated in some patients and may represent overlapping conditions.

Scleroderma may bear some superficial resemblance to dermatomyositis, but the absence of severe myositis and the characteristic rash of dermatomyositis should allow differentiation. Subcutaneous fat necrosis and Weber-Christian nonsuppurative panniculitis may suggest morphea, but the course and histology are distinctive. *Scleredema adultorum*, a self-limited benign induration of subcutaneous tissues, occurs acutely, sometimes following streptococcal infection; subcutaneous tissues of the neck, upper trunk, and arms become indurated, but the skin is spared. Other sclerodermoid reactions can be distinguished by the history and specific laboratory studies (see Table 11–38).

TREATMENT. No specific therapy is known. Many therapeutic agents, including corticosteroids, salicylates, chelating agents, chloroquine, radiation, dimethyl sulfoxide, para-aminobenzoic acid, penicillamine, and immunosuppressive drugs, have been tried without clear-cut benefit. Systemic therapy with penicillamine or cytotoxic drugs may be tried for severe systemic disease. Corticosteroids may be beneficial during acute edematous phases of the disease, but are of no benefit for the other manifestations of scleroderma and may complicate the disease by exacerbating hypertension. Meticulous control of any hypertension with agents such as captopril is vital. Topical corticosteroids may be used for cutaneous lesions. Excision of local patches of morphea does not arrest the process. Vigorous physical therapy is important early in the course of cutaneous scleroderma to prevent or minimize crippling contractures. Avoidance of cold and initiation of therapy for Raynaud phenomenon with biofeedback techniques or drugs such as nifedipine are essential. Good supportive care is needed to manage the organ-specific dysfunctions.

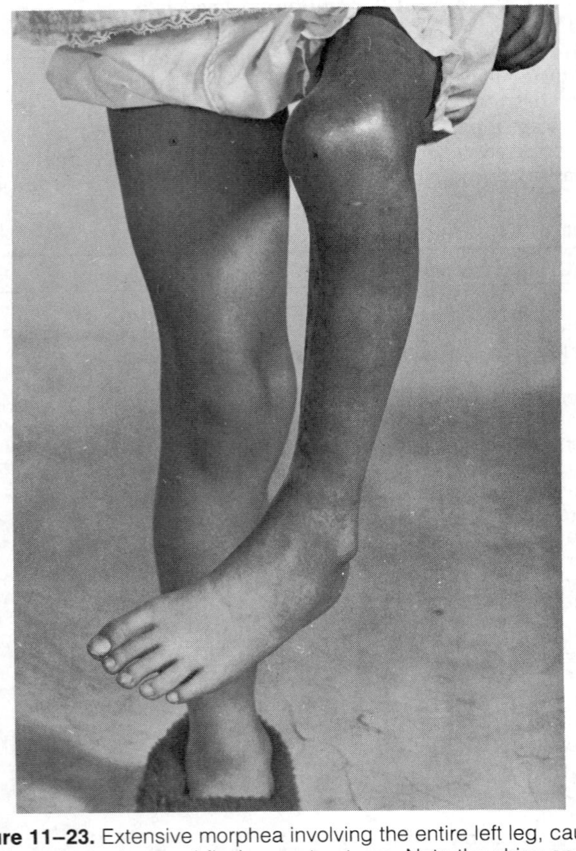

Figure 11–23. Extensive morphea involving the entire left leg, causing scarring, shortening, and flexion contractures. Note the shiny appearance and patches of hyperpigmentation and vitiligo of affected skin.

RHEUMATIC SYNDROMES OF UNCERTAIN CLASSIFICATION

11.64 MIXED CONNECTIVE TISSUE DISEASE

Mixed connective tissue disease (overlap syndrome) is a syndrome that combines the features of SLE, rheumatoid arthritis, dermatomyositis, and scleroderma. It is characterized by high serum titers of speckled ANA (to extractable nuclear antigen [ENA]) and antibody to ribonucleoprotein (RNP). The syndrome affects girls, generally over age 6. Clinical manifestations include arthritis, scleroderma-like skin changes, Raynaud phenomenon, fever, cardiac involvement (particularly pericarditis), rashes suggestive of either SLE or dermatomyositis, myositis, esophageal abnormalities, lymphadenopathy, hepatosplenomegaly, pulmonary disease, and thrombocytopenia. Renal disease occurs in some patients, and neurologic abnormalities and parotitis have also been described. The diagnosis is made over a period of time by recognizing the overlapping clinical symptoms and by demonstrating serum antibodies to RNP.

Initially this syndrome was thought to have a better prognosis than SLE and to be responsive to corticosteroid therapy. Although corticosteroid therapy does produce symptomatic improvement in many patients, and although life-threatening disease manifestations are perhaps not as common as in SLE, mixed connective tissue disease may cause severe morbidity. The ultimate prognosis is unknown. The relationships of this syndrome to other rheumatic diseases are also unclear; many observers consider it a form of SLE. Appropriate therapy consists of symptomatic treatment with corticosteroids, alertness to possible serious complications such as nephritis, physical therapy, and careful attention paid to the function of the musculoskeletal system.

11.65 FASCIITIS

(Diffuse Fasciitis, Eosinophilic Fasciitis)

This unusual disorder is characterized by diffuse inflammation of the fascial tissues. No long-term studies have yet defined the natural history of the disease. It may be a variant of scleroderma. Although most patients have been adults, the disorder does occur in children. Inflammation of fascial tissues occurs primarily in the limbs and trunk; the hands, feet, and face are generally spared. Raynaud phenomenon is not associated. Joint contractures, including contractures of the fingers, may occur. The onset may follow periods of heavy physical exertion. Affected tissues are swollen and tender; however, since the overlying skin is not affected, cutaneous tissues appear puckered. Internal organ involvement has not been described. There are no diagnostic laboratory tests; tests for rheumatoid factors and ANA are generally negative. Some patients have striking eosinophilia, and increased numbers of eosinophils may be found in affected tissues. Diagnosis is clinical and is supported by evidence on biopsy of fascial inflammation. Corticosteroid therapy may be helpful, although results of long-term follow-up studies are not available. The disease appears to be associated with morphea in children, and it overlaps somewhat with scleroderma. Rarely, eosinophilic fasciitis is associated with aplastic anemia, thrombocytopenia, leukemia, or lymphoma.

The *eosinophilia-myalgia syndrome*, which has been reported predominantly in adults, manifests striking similarities to connective tissue disorders such as eosinophilic fasciitis, scleroderma, and eosinophilic myositis. This illness is associated with the ingestion of tryptophan or a manufacturing contaminant. It is characterized by edema, pruritus, paresthesia, myalgia, eosinophilia, perivascular inflammation, and fibrotic or inflamed fascia. Treatment consists of withdrawal of tryptophan. Similar sclerodermoid illnesses have been associated with other toxic infections such as *toxic-oil syndrome*, suggesting that other agents may produce such disorders.

MISCELLANEOUS CONDITIONS ASSOCIATED WITH RHEUMATIC SYMPTOMS OR SIGNS IN CHILDREN

11.66 BENIGN RHEUMATOID NODULES

Rheumatoid nodule-like lesions unassociated with rheumatic disease occasionally occur in children. Single or multiple lesions may be present over various sites, including the pretibial areas, dorsa of the feet, scalp, hands, and elbows; they may also appear over pressure points or after trauma, as do true rheumatoid nodules. Clinically, the nodules are subcutaneous or fixed to deeper tissues and resemble rheumatoid nodules. Histologically, these lesions show central areas of fibrinoid necrosis with surrounding histiocytes and mononuclear cells; they closely resemble adult-type rheumatoid nodules or the intracutaneous lesions characteristic of granuloma annulare. Indeed, typical granuloma annulare may be associated.

The etiology is unknown. Affected children are well and have no associated rheumatic complaints. Laboratory tests are normal; tests for rheumatoid factor and ANA are negative. The nodular lesions wax, wane, and may recur, but recurrences generally cease after months or years. This is a benign condition; affected children are not at increased risk for rheumatic disease, and no therapy other than reassurance is required.

The nodules associated with rheumatic disease (rheumatoid arthritis, acute rheumatic fever, scleroderma, SLE) rarely if ever occur as sole manifestations but rather appear with other signs of active rheumatic disease. Rheumatoid nodules in rheumatoid arthritis are generally accompanied by positive test results for rheumatoid factor.

11.67 ERYTHEMA NODOSUM

Erythema nodosum is characterized by the development of painful, indurated, shiny, red, hot, elevated, ovoid nodules 1–3 cm in diameter. They are most frequently distributed symmetrically over the shins (Fig. 11–24 [color plate section]) but may also occur on the calves, thighs, buttocks, and upper extremities. Fever, malaise, and arthralgia may precede or accompany the rash, and hilar adenopathy may be present on chest roentgenograms. The skin lesions have a characteristic progression: Over a period of several days they become protuberant and violaceous; after 1–2 wk, as induration decreases, a dull purple discoloration predominates and then fades in the manner of a large bruise, leaving a brown residuum without ulceration or scar formation. The lesions come in crops, usually over a period of 3–6 wk. Erythema nodosum is uncommon in children under the age of 6 yr, becoming progressively more frequent up to the 3rd decade of life. Females are affected more frequently than males.

The lesions represent a reaction to a variety of stimuli. The eruption has been induced experimentally in patients with the disease by local injection of a single specific bacterial antigen. Epidemiologically, the disease was previously linked closely to tuberculosis, especially in Europe. In both the United States and Europe streptococcal infections are now more frequently implicated as stimuli. The eruption may also accompany sarcoidosis, leptospirosis, cat-scratch disease, Epstein-Barr virus, tularemia, psittacosis, histoplasmosis, coccidioidomycosis, and *Yersinia* infections or the administration of some drugs including sulfonamides and birth control pills. It may also occur with such systemic diseases as SLE, vasculitis, regional enteritis, ulcerative colitis, and Behçet syndrome.

Search for a precipitating infection, drug, or underlying disease should be instituted. The ESR is usually elevated, and other nonspecific evidences of inflammatory disease, such as acute phase reactants, are found. Suggestive etiologic evidence may include the demonstration of β-hemolytic streptococci in throat cultures or a rising antistreptolysin O titer; conversion of a previously negative tuberculin, histoplasmin, or coccidioidin skin reaction; roentgenographic evidence of pulmonary tuberculosis or fungus disease; or evidence of an underlying disease such as SLE, inflammatory bowel disease, or sarcoidosis.

Salicylates are usually adequate for symptomatic relief of erythema nodosum. The skin lesions and the constitutional manifestations may respond to corticosteroids, but such therapy is usually not warranted in a self-limited disease and may be contraindicated because of the presence of underlying active infection.

SARCOIDOSIS

See Sec. 25.3.

STEVENS-JOHNSON SYNDROME
(Erythema Multiforme Exudativum)

See Sec. 23.13.

GOODPASTURE SYNDROME

See Sec. 18.11.

11.68 FIBROSITIS-FIBROMYALGIA

Fibrositis-fibromyalgia is a poorly defined adult condition that has recently been described in children. There is no obvious inflammation associated with this nonarticular form of rheumatism. Little is known about its physiology or pathology; in adults a relationship to stress has been suggested. It occurs predominantly in women. There are no abnormal laboratory findings. Clinical manifestations consist of poorly defined musculoskeletal pain and discomfort that can be reproduced by soft tissue pressure on a number of so-called trigger points. Fatigue, anxiety, insomnia, and headache are frequently concomitants. This condition is neither progressive nor associated with chronic deformity. Therapy with reassurance, stress management, exercise, and perhaps nonsteroidal anti-inflammatory agents may be helpful. The ultimate prognosis is unknown.

11.69 RELAPSING NODULAR NONSUPPURATIVE PANNICULITIS
(Weber-Christian Syndrome)

This rare disorder of subcutaneous inflammation is of unknown cause and probably does not represent a single disease. Infection, drug reaction (especially to bromides and iodides), abnormal fat metabolism, and hypersensitivity have all been suggested as etiologic factors. Fat necrosis can occur in association with several rheumatic diseases, with pancreatic disease, and with corticosteroid withdrawal. Adults are affected predominantly, although the syndrome has been reported in all age groups. Females are affected more frequently than males.

Histologically, there are foci of degeneration and inflammation in subcutaneous fat. Mesenteric, perivisceral, and periarticular adipose tissues may be affected; fatty metamorphosis of the liver and reticuloendothelial hyperplasia may occur. Laboratory findings are not specific. Leukopenia and elevated ESR may be present; rheumatoid factor, ANA, and cryoglobulins have been observed.

Clinically, the disease is characterized by the appearance of crops of subcutaneous nodules on any part of the body; thighs, legs, abdomen, breasts, and arms are most frequently involved. Nodules vary in size from a few millimeters to several centimeters and may be painful, with redness and warmth of the overlying skin. Nodules regress in days to weeks, usually leaving a pigmented depression. Fever is common, and a variety of rheumatic complaints may occur, including arthritis, arthralgia, and myalgia. Hepatosplenomegaly, abdominal pain, and episcleritis have been reported. Crops of nodules and systemic symptoms generally recur over long periods of time.

Diagnosis of Weber-Christian syndrome is based on the clinical picture and the histologic changes. Differential diagnosis includes erythema induratum, sarcoidosis, postinjection subcutaneous fat necrosis, and vasculitis. Fat necrosis with subcutaneous nodules, arthritis, and visceral involvement can occur as a manifestation of pancreatic disease, presumably resulting from enzymatic action on fat cells.

No specific therapy is known. Relief may occur after therapy with corticosteroids, chloroquine, or colchicine. Patients with underlying pancreatic involvement may benefit from treatment of the pancreatic disease.

11.70 RELAPSING POLYCHONDRITIS

Relapsing polychondritis, one of the rarest of rheumatic syndromes, has been described in a few children. It is characterized by pain, swelling, destruction, and deformation of the cartilaginous elements of the ears (both external and internal structures), nose, eyes, joints, laryngotracheobronchial system, heart, and large blood vessels. Fever, malaise, and myalgia may be associated. Glomerulonephritis has been described. There are no characteristic laboratory tests. Diagnosis rests on the clinical picture and on demonstration of cartilaginous inflammation on biopsy. This condition occasionally occurs in patients who have another established rheumatic disease such as vasculitis, rheumatoid arthritis, SLE, or Sjögren syndrome. Death may result from cardiac or respiratory involvement. Therapy with corticosteroid and cytotoxic agents has been advocated, but their long-term benefits are unknown.

11.71 SYNDROME OF NEONATAL FEVER, RASH, AND ARTHROPATHY

This rare condition is characterized by high intermittent fevers, maculopapular rash, and systemic illness beginning in the first weeks of life. Other features include meningoencephalitis (with pleocytosis and elevated protein levels in CSF), progressive mental retardation, chronic iridocyclitis, hepatosplenomegaly, and lymphadenopathy. The arthropathy is manifest by swelling, pain, and warmth in one or more joints; joint roentgenograms show periostitis and destruction of the ends of the long bones. Patellar enlargement may be striking. Affected children appear to have a characteristic facies with prominent foreheads.

Nothing is known about the etiology or pathogenesis of this syndrome. Although described in one set of siblings, it has not been familial in other instances. The condition superficially resembles systemic-onset JRA; however, the neonatal onset and the association of meningoencephalopathy, mental retardation, and chronic iridocyclitis, as well as the nature of the arthropathy, are distinctive. Treatment with nonsteroidal anti-inflammatory agents and physical therapy may assist in improving musculoskeletal function but does not slow progression of the disease. Progressive mental retardation and death in the 1st or 2nd decade of life have been noted, although the true long-term prognosis is unknown.

11.72 BEHÇET SYNDROME

This disorder is characterized by recurrent oral and genital ulcers and ocular inflammation. Arthritis, thrombophlebitis, neurologic abnormalities, skin lesions, fever, and colitis are associated clinical manifestations. The condition is rare in children.

The etiology is unknown. Pathologically, there is vasculitis of small and medium-sized arteries with cellular infiltrations leading to fibrinoid necrosis and narrowing and obliteration of the vessel lumens.

The clinical course is highly variable, with recurrent exacerbations and disease-free intervals of uncertain duration. The oral ulcers develop in almost all patients, persist for days to weeks, and then heal without scarring. These painful necrotic ulcers (2–10 mm), surrounded by erythema, may occur singly or in crops over the oral-nasal cavity and upper airway. Genital ulcers occur in most patients and follow a parallel course. Ocular manifestations include anterior or posterior uveitis and retinal vasculitis, which may progress to blindness. Arthritis is common and is usually acute, recurrent, asymmetric, and polyarticular, involving the large joints. Central nervous system abnormalities such as meningoencephalitis, cranial nerve palsies, and psychosis generally occur later in the course of the disease and indicate a poor prognosis. Skin manifestations include erythema nodosum, pseudofolliculitis, papulopustular lesions, and acneiform nodules and occur in most patients. Laboratory findings are not diagnostic. Cutaneous pathergy is observed as an erythematous sterile pustule noted after 24–48 hr at a needle prick skin site.

There is no single effective treatment. Systemic prednisone, colchicine, chlorambucil, azathioprine, and cyclosporine have been effective in some patients.

11.73 SJÖGREN SYNDROME

This chronic inflammatory, autoimmune disease, rare in children, is characterized by dry eyes (keratoconjunctivitis sicca, xerophthalmia), dry mouth (xerostomia), and associated connective tissue disorders. The salivary and lacrimal glands are infiltrated by lymphocytes and plasma cells; a similar process may reduce secretions in the respiratory tract, vagina, and skin as well as in the salivary and lacrimal glands.

Clinical manifestations include photophobia, burning and itching eyes, and blurred vision; painless unilateral or bilateral enlargement of the parotid glands, decreased sense of taste, dental caries, dysphagia, fissured tongue, and angular cheilitis; decreased sense of smell and epistaxis; and hoarseness, recurrent bronchitis, pneumonia, and chronic otitis. Rheumatoid arthritis and SLE are often associated collagen-vascular diseases. Lymphoproliferative forms may also occur, with potential lymphoid malignancy. Diagnosis is based on the clinical features supported by biopsy of the lip or glands demonstrating lymphocytic infiltration; hypergammaglobulinemia, cryoglobulinemia, autoantibodies to nucleoprotein antigens (SS-B[La]), and immune complexes may be associated.

Treatment is symptomatic, with use of artificial tears, lozenges, and fluids to limit the damaging effects of decreased secretions. Corticosteroids are indicated only for severe functional disorders and life-threatening complications.

11.74 NONRHEUMATIC CONDITIONS MIMICKING RHEUMATIC DISEASES OF CHILDHOOD

A large number of "nonrheumatic" conditions that can cause musculoskeletal complaints in children, with or without accompanying signs, must be considered in the differential diagnosis of childhood rheumatic diseases (Table 11–39).

Bacterial infections of the bones and joints can cause pain and swelling about one or more joints, generally with accompanying fever and other systemic complaints (Sec. 12.16 and 12.17). Diagnosis may result from appropriate cultures, skin tests, and imaging techniques. Viral and mycoplasmal infections may be associated with transient arthritis, which should not be confused with chronic rheumatic disease. Lyme disease requires differentiation from pauciarticular JRA. Diskitis (Sec. 24.21) or inflammation of the intravertebral disks and end-plates of vertebral bodies may be confused with arthritis, although the pain in diskitis is characteristically spinal; roentgenograms or bone scans may be diagnostic.

TABLE 11–39. Conditions Other Than Rheumatic Diseases Associated with Arthritis in Children

Infectious diseases
Pyogenic arthritis
Tuberculous arthritis
Osteomyelitis with sympathetic joint effusion
Virus-related arthritis
Reactive arthritis
Lyme disease
Other (e.g., mycoplasma arthritis)
Neoplastic diseases
Leukemia
Neuroblastoma
Malignant histiocytosis
Lymphoma, Hodgkin disease, reticulum cell sarcoma
Rhabdomyosarcoma
Osteogenic sarcoma
Other primary bone tumors
"Orthopedic" conditions (noninflammatory conditions of bones and joints)
Avascular necrosis syndromes (e.g., Legg-Calvé-Perthes disease, Köhler disease, Osgood-Schlatter disease)
Toxic synovitis of the hip
Slipped capital femoral epiphysis
Trauma (child abuse fractures; joint, ligamentous, and muscle injuries, etc.)
Chondromalacia patella
Congenital anomalies and genetically determined abnormalities of musculoskeletal system (e.g., muscular dystrophies, congenital subluxation of the hips, other congenital abnormalities of bones, joints, connective tissues)
Tenosynovitis
Diskitis
Reflex sympathetic dystrophy syndrome
Limb pains of childhood (growing pains)*
Hysteria, conversion reactions, "psychogenic rheumatism"*
Miscellaneous conditions (sickle cell anemia, hemophilia, immunodeficiency-related arthritis, sarcoidosis, hypertrophic osteoarthropathy)

*These conditions may have associated symptoms suggesting arthritis; they do not produce or represent joint disease.

A number of childhood malignancies can result in musculoskeletal involvement resembling arthritis, generally through a mechanism of either infiltration of malignant cells about the joint capsules and periosteum or destruction of bone. Pain in the affected joints is often severe, and blood studies may reveal abnormal white blood cells (leukopenia or abnormal cellular forms), thrombocytopenia, anemia, or hyperuricemia. Bone roentgenograms may show metaphyseal rarefaction, periostitis, or lytic lesions. Suspicion of malignancy in a child with "arthritis" demands appropriate investigations, with oncologic consultation and biopsy of the bone marrow or other appropriate tissues.

Costochondral disease *(costochondritis)* is a relatively common disorder characterized by pain localized to the costosternal or costochondral junction. Pain may be of acute onset, sharp, darting, and of short duration, or it may evolve gradually as a dull aching pain lasting hours to days. It may be associated with a feeling of tightness due to muscle spasm and is generally not exacerbated by respiratory or other mild movements. There is often localized tenderness to palpation of one or more costal cartilages and a history of trauma or unaccustomed physical effort. The combination of pain, tenderness, swelling, and sometimes redness is referred to as the *Tietze syndrome*. Discomfort usually persists for only a few days or responds to mild analgesia and avoidance of strenuous activity.

A number of noninflammatory conditions may also mimic rheumatic diseases in children. Various orthopedic conditions such as bone fractures, soft tissue injuries, avascular necrosis syndromes, and slipped capital femoral epiphysis may mimic arthritis; roentgenograms or bone scans are generally diagnostic. In the *reflex sympathetic dystrophy syndrome* a limb or part of a limb is immobilized by severe pain; cutaneous hypersensitivity, osteoporosis, and signs of autonomic nervous dysfunction are characteristic. Successful therapy involves remobilization of the affected part. Idiopathic limb pains of childhood ("growing pains") or functional musculoskeletal pain must be differentiated from organic musculoskeletal disease.

Congenital or genetically determined conditions may superficially resemble rheumatic diseases. For example, congenital myositis ossificans (fibrodysplasia ossificans congenita) is at times confused with dermatomyositis or scleroderma, and conditions such as carpal-tarsal osteolysis or trichorhinophalangeal dysplasia may suggest JRA. A positive family history, the presence of associated dysmorphic features (e.g., digital anomalies in congenital myositis ossificans or characteristic facial anomalies in trichorhinophalangeal dysplasia), or the roentgenographic appearance of the affected bones and joints (e.g., lysis of the carpal and tarsal bones in carpal-tarsal osteolysis) will distinguish these entities (Sec. 24.27).

Many other miscellaneous conditions may mimic childhood rheumatic diseases. Noteworthy are the hand-foot syndrome of sickle cell anemia and the arthropathy of hemophilia. In general, such conditions can be differentiated on the basis of historical or physical findings that do not appear to be entirely consistent with any of the rheumatic diseases.

JANE GREEN SCHALLER

PATIENT EDUCATION

Arthritis in Children. Atlanta, Arthritis Foundation, 1987. (Obtainable from the Arthritis Foundation, 3400 Peachtree Road NE, Atlanta, GA 30326 or from the local chapter offices.)

Spencer CH, Zanga J, Passo M, et al: The child with arthritis in the school setting. Pediatr Clin North Am 33:1251, 1986.

Wetherbee LL, Neil AJ: Educational Rights for Children with Arthritis: A Manual for Parents. Atlanta, Arthritis Foundation, 1988.

White PH, McPherson M, Levinson JE: Community programs for children with rheumatic diseases. Pediatr Clin North Am 33:1239, 1986.

GENERAL

Jacobs JC: Pediatric Rheumatology for the Practitioner, 2nd ed. New York, Springer-Verlag, 1991.

Kelley WN, Harris ED, Ruddy S, et al (ed): Textbook of Rheumatology, 3rd ed. Philadelphia, WB Saunders, 1989.

McCarty DJ (ed): Arthritis and Allied Conditions: A Textbook of Rheumatology, 11th ed. Philadelphia, Lea & Febiger, 1989.

Miller ML (ed): Pediatric rheumatology. Pediatr Clin North Am 33(5):1, 1986.

Schaller JG (ed): Pediatric and heritable rheumatic disorders. Curr Opin Rheumatol 2(4):1990.

Schumacher HL, Klipple JH, Robinson DR (eds): Primer on the Rheumatic Diseases, 9th ed. Atlanta, Arthritis Foundation, 1988.

Tan EM: Interactions between autoimmunity and molecular and cell biology. Bridges between clinical and basic sciences. J Clin Invest 84:1, 1989.

JUVENILE RHEUMATOID ARTHRITIS

Bywaters EG: Heberden oration, 1966. Categorization in medicine: a survey of Still's disease. Ann Rheum Dis 26:185, 1967.

Cassidy JT, Levinson JE, Bass JC, et al: A study of classification criteria for a diagnosis of juvenile rheumatoid arthritis. Arthritis Rheum 29:274, 1986.

Harris ED: Rheumatoid arthritis. Pathophysiology and implications for therapy. N Engl J Med 322:1277, 1990.

Kanski JJ: Pediatric arthritis and uveitis. Surv Ophthalmol (in press).

Leak AM, Ansell BM, Burman SJ: Antinuclear antibody studies in juvenile chronic arthritis. Arch Dis Child 61:168, 1986.

Nepom BS, Nepom GT, Mickelson E, et al: Specific HLA-DR4-associated histocompatibility molecules characterize patients with seropositive juvenile rheumatoid arthritis. J Clin Invest 74:287, 1984.

Olson NY, Lindsley CB, Godfrey WA: Nonsteroidal antiinflammatory drug therapy in chronic childhood iridocyclitis. Am J Dis Child 142:1289, 1988.

Rosenberg AM: Advanced drug therapy for juvenile rheumatoid arthritis. J Pediatr 114:171, 1989.

Schaller JG: Juvenile rheumatoid arthritis. Pediatr Rev 2:163, 1980.

Schaller JG, Ochs HD, Thomas ED, et al: Histocompatibility antigens in childhood-onset arthritis. J Pediatr 88:926, 1976.

Schaller JG, Wedgwood RJ: Is juvenile rheumatoid arthritis a single disease? Pediatrics 50:940, 1972.

Sherry DD, Bohnsock J, Salmonson K: Painless juvenile rheumatoid arthritis. J Pediatr 116:921, 1990.

Tugwell P, Bennett K, Bell M, et al: Methotrexate in rheumatoid arthritis. Ann Intern Med 110:581, 1989.

Williams RA, Ansell BM: Radiological findings in seropositive juvenile chronic arthritis with particular reference to progression. Ann Rheum Dis 44:685, 1985.

ANKYLOSING SPONDYLITIS

Ladd JR, Cassidy JT, Martel W: Juvenile ankylosing spondylitis. Arthritis Rheum 14:579, 1971.

Schaller JG, Bitnum S, Wedgwood RJ: Ankylosing spondylitis with childhood onset. J Pediatr 74:505, 1969.

Wilkinson M, Bywaters EGL: Clinical features and course of ankylosing spondylitis: As seen in a follow-up of 222 hospital referred cases. Ann Rheum Dis 17:209, 1958.

SPONDYLOARTHROPATHIES

Calin A, Marder A, Marks S, et al: Familial aggregation of Reiter's syndrome and anykylosing spondylitis: A comparative study. J Rheumatol 11:672, 1984.

Carroll WL, Balistreri WF, Brilli R, et al: Spectrum of *Salmonella*-associated arthritis. Pediatrics 68:717, 1981.

Jacobs JC, Berdon WE, Johnston AD: HLA-B27 associated spondyloarthritis and enthesopathy in childhood: Clinical, pathologic, and radiographic observations in 58 patients. J Pediatr 100:521, 1982.

Keat A: Reiter's syndrome and reactive arthritis in perspective. N Engl J Med 309:1606, 1983.

Petty RE, Malleson P: Spondyloarthropathies of childhood. Pediatr Clin North Am 33:1079, 1986.

Rosenberg AM, Petty RE: A syndrome of seronegative enthesopathy and arthropathy in children. Arthritis Rheum 25:1041, 1982.

Russell AS: Reiter's syndrome in children following infection with *Yersinia enterocolitica* and *Shigella*. Arthritis Rheum (Suppl 2) 20:471, 1977.

Shore A, Ansell BM: Juvenile psoriatic arthritis—an analysis of 60 cases. J Pediatr 100:529, 1982.

SYSTEMIC LUPUS ERYTHEMATOSUS

Adelman DC, Saltiel E, Klinenberg JH: The neuropsychiatric manifestations of systemic lupus erythematosus: An overview. Semin Arthr Rheum 15:185, 1986.

Alarcon-Seqovia D, Deleze M, Oria C, et al: Antiphospholipid antibodies and the antiphospholipid syndrome in systemic lupus erythematosus. A prospective analysis of 500 consecutive patients. Medicine 68:353, 1989.

Austin HA 3rd, Klippel JH, Balow JE, et al: Therapy of lupus nephritis. Controlled trial of prednisone and cytotoxic drugs. N Engl J Med 314:614, 1986.

Balow JE: Lupus nephritis. Ann Intern Med 106:79, 1987.

Cardelli MB, Kleinsmith D: Raynaud's phenomenon and disease. Med Clin North Am 73:1127, 1989.

Cook CD, Wedgwood RJ: Craig JM, et al: Systemic lupus erythematosus. Description of 37 cases in children and discussion of endocrine therapy in 32 of the cases. Pediatrics 26:570, 1960.

Hess E: Drug related lupus. N Engl J Med 318:1460, 1987.

Jonsson H, Nived O, Sturfelt G: Outcome in systemic lupus erythematosus: A prospective study of patients from a defined population. Medicine 68:141, 1989.

Kaufman DB, Laxer RM, Silverman ED, et al: Systemic lupus erythematosus in childhood and adolescence—the problem, epidemiology, incidence, susceptibility, genetics, and prognosis. Curr Prob Pediatr 16:545, 1986.

Klippel JH: Systemic lupus erythematosus. Treatment related complications superimposed on chronic disease. JAMA 263:1812, 1990.

Laitman RS, Glicklich D, Sablay LB, et al: Effect of long-term normalization of serum complement levels on the course of lupus nephritis. Am J Med 87:132, 1989.

Lee HS, Mujais SK, Kasinath BS, et al: Course of renal pathology in patients with systemic lupus erythematosus. Am J Med 77:612, 1984.

Lehman TJ, McCurdy DK, Bernstein GH, et al: Systemic lupus erythematosus in the first decade of life. Pediatrics 83:235, 1989.

Lehman TJ, Sherry DD, Wagner-Weiner L, et al: Intermittent intravenous cyclophosphamide therapy for lupus nephritis. J Pediatr 114:1055, 1989.

Mandol BP: Cardiovascular involvement in systemic lupus erythematosus. Semin Arthritis Rheum 17:126, 1987.

Miller ML, Magilavy DB, Warren RW: Immunologic basis of lupus. Pediatr Clin North Am 33:1191, 1986.

Platt JL, Burke BA, Fish AJ, et al: Systemic lupus erythematosus in the first two decades of life. Am J Kidney Dis 2(Suppl 1):212, 1982.

Singsen BH, Fishman L, Hanson V: Antinuclear antibodies and lupus-like syndromes in children receiving anticonvulsants. Pediatrics 57:529, 1976.

Studenski S, Allen NB, Caldwell DS, et al: Survival in systemic lupus erythematosus: A multivariate analysis of demographic factors. Arthritis Rheum 30:1326, 1987.

Tan EM, Cohen AS, Fries JF, et al: The 1982 revised criteria for the classification of systemic lupus erythematosus. Arthritis Rheum 25:1271, 1982.

NEONATAL LUPUS PHENOMENA

Buyon J, Ben-Chetrit E, Karp S, et al: Acquired congenital heart block. Pattern of maternal antibody response to biochemically defined antigens of the SSA/Ro-SSB/La system in neonatal lupus. J Clin Invest 84:627, 1989.

Callen JP, Fowler JF, Kulick KB, et al: Neonatal lupus erythematosus occurring in one fraternal twin. Serologic and immunogenetic studies. Arthritis Rheum 28:271, 1985.

Jackson R, Gulliver M: Neonatal lupus erythematosus progressing into systemic lupus erythematosus. A 15 year follow-up. Br J Dermatol 101:81, 1979.

Laxer RM, Roberts EA, Gross KR, et al: Liver disease in neonatal lupus erythematosus. J Pediatr 116:238, 1990.

McCune AB, Weston WL, Lee LA: Maternal and fetal outcome in neonatal lupus erythematosus. Ann Intern Med 106:518, 1987.

Provost TT, Watson R, Gaither KK, et al: The neonatal lupus erythematosus syndrome. J Rheumatol 14(Suppl 13):199, 1987.

VASCULITIS

Brasile L, Kremer J, Clarke J, et al: Identification of an autoantibody to vascular endothelial cell-specific antigens in patients with systemic vasculitis. Am J Med 87:74, 1989.

Falk, RJ, Jennette SC: Anti-neutrophil cytoplasmic autoantibodies with specificity for myeloperoxidase in patients with systemic vasculitis and idiopathic necrotizing and crescentic glomerulonephritis. N Engl J Med 318:1651, 1988.

Sigal LH: The neurologic presentation of vasculitic and rheumatologic syndromes: A review. Medicine 66:157, 1987.

HENOCH-SCHÖNLEIN VASCULITIS

Allen DM, Diamond LK, Howell DA: Anaphylactoid purpura in children (Schönlein-Henoch syndrome). Review with follow up of renal complications. Am J Dis Child 99:147, 1960.

Austin HA III, Balow JE: Henoch-Schönlein nephritis: Prognostic features and the challenge of therapy. Am J Kidney Dis 2:512, 1983.

Farley TA, Gillespie S, Rasoulpour M, et al: Epidemiology of a cluster of Henoch-Schönlein purpura. Am J Dis Child 143:798, 1989.

Meadow SR, Scott DG: Berger disease: Henoch-Schönlein syndrome without the rash. J Pediatr 106:27, 1985.

Ostergaard JR, Storm K: Neurologic manifestations of Schönlein-Henoch purpura. Acta Paediatr 80:339, 1991.

Rosenblum N, Winter H: Steroid effects on the course of abdominal pain in children with Henoch-Schönlein purpura. Pediatrics 79:1018, 1987.

Saulsbury FT: The role of IgA1 rheumatoid factor in the formation of IgA-containing immune complexes in Henoch-Schönlein purpura. J Clin Lab Immunol 23:123, 1987.

POLYARTERITIS NODOSA

Fager DB, Bigler JA, Simonds JP: Periarteritis nodosa in infancy and childhood. J Pediatr 39:65, 1951.

Fink CW: Vasculitis. Pediatr Clin North Am 33:1203, 1986.

Frohnert PP, Sheps SG: Long-term follow-up study of periarteritis nodosa. Am J Med 43:8, 1967.

Gocke DJ, Hsu K, Morgan C, et al: Vasculitis in association with Australia antigen. J Exp Med 134:(Suppl:330s +), 1971.

Ronco P, Verroust P, Mignon F, et al: Immunopathological studies of polyarteritis nodosa and Wegener's granulomatosis: A report of 43 patients with 51 renal biopsies. Q J Med 52:212, 1983.

KAWASAKI DISEASE

Burns JC, Wiggins JW, Toews WH, et al: Clinical spectrum of Kawasaki disease in infants younger than 6 months of age. J Pediatr 109:759, 1986.

Dean AC, Melish ME, Hicks R, et al: An epidemic of Kawasaki syndrome in Hawaii. J Pediatr 100:552, 1982.

Engle MA, Fatica NS, Bussel JB: Clinical trial of single dose intravenous gamma globulin in acute Kawasaki disease. Am J Dis Child 143:1300, 1989.

Gidding SS, Duffy CE, Pajcic S, et al: Usefulness of echocardiographic evidence of pericardial effusion and mitral regurgitation during the acute stage in predicting development of coronary arterial aneurysms in the late stage of Kawasaki disease. Am J Cardiol 60:76, 1987.

Hicks RV, Melish ME: Kawasaki syndrome. Pediatr Clin North Am 33:1151, 1986.

Kartow H, Ichinose E, Kawasaki T: Myocardial infarction in Kawasaki disease: Clinical analysis of 195 cases. J Pediatr 108:923, 1986.

Kawasaki T, Kosaki F, Okawa S, et al: A new infantile acute febrile mucocutaneous lymph node syndrome (MLNS). Prevalence in Japan. Pediatrics 54:271, 1974.

Landing BH, Larson EJ: Are infantile periarteritis nodosa with coronary artery involvement and fatal mucocutaneous lymph node syndrome the same? Comparison of 20 patients from North America with patients from Hawaii and Japan. Pediatrics 59:651, 1977.

Leads from the MMWR: Multiple outbreaks of Kawasaki syndrome—United States. JAMA 253:959, 1985.

Leung DY, Kurt-Jones E, Newburger JW: Endothelial cell activation and high interleukin-1 secretion in the pathogenesis of acute Kawasaki disease. Lancet 2:1298, 1989.

Levy M, Korean G: Atypical Kawasaki disease: Analysis of clinical presentation and diagnostic clues. Pediatr Infect Dis J 9:122, 1990.

Newburger JW, Takahashi M, Burns JC, et al: The treatment of Kawasaki syndrome with intravenous gamma globulin. N Engl J Med 315:342, 1986.

Rowley AH, Gonzalez-Crussi F, Gidding SS, et al: Incomplete Kawasaki disease with coronary artery involvement. J Pediatr 110:409, 1987.

Salomi C, Nakamura K, Narai S, et al: Systematic visualization of coronary arteries by two-dimensional echocardiography in children and infants evaluated for Kawasaki's disease and coronary arteriovenous fistulas. Am Heart J 107:497, 1984.

Savage CO, Tizard J, Jayne D, et al: Antineutrophil cytoplasm antibodies in Kawasaki disease. Arch Dis Child 64:360, 1989.

Shulman ST, Bass JL, Bierman F, et al: Management of Kawasaki syndrome: A consensus statement prepared by North American participants of the Third International Kawasaki Disease Symposium, Tokyo, Japan, December, 1988. Pediatr Infect Dis J 8:663, 1989.

Smith L, Newburger J, Burns J: Kawasaki syndrome and the eye. Pediatr Infect Dis J 8:116, 1989.

Sundel RP, Newburger JW, McGill T, et al: Sensorineural hearing loss associated with Kawasaki disease. J Pediatr 117:371, 1990.

Suzuki A, Kamiya T, Ono Y, et al: Aortocoronary bypass surgery for coronary arterial lesions resulting from Kawasaki disease. J Pediatr 116:567, 1990.

WEGENER GRANULOMATOSIS

Fauci AS, Hayes BF, Katz P: Wegener's granulomatosis: Prospective clinical and therapeutic experience with 85 patients for 21 years. Ann Intern Med 98:76, 1983.

Hall SL, Miller LC, Duggan E: Wegener's granulomatosis in pediatric patients. J Pediatr 106:739, 1985.

Nölle B, Specks U, Lüdemann J, et al: Anticytoplasmic autoantibodies: Their immunodiagnostic value in Wegener granulomatosis. Ann Intern Med 111:28, 1989.

Orlowski JP, Clough JD, Dyment PG: Wegener's granulomatosis in the pediatric age group. Pediatrics 61:83, 1978.

TAKAYASU ARTERITIS

Danaraj TJ, Wong HO, Thomas MA: Primary arteritis of the aorta causing renal artery stenosis and hypertension. Br Heart J 25:153, 1963.

Lee KS, Sohn EY, Hong CY, et al: Primary arteritis (pulseless disease) in Korean children. Acta Paediatr Scand 56:526, 1967.

Shelhamer JH, Volkman DJ, Parrillo JE, et al: Takayasu's arteritis and its therapy. Ann Intern Med 103:121, 1985.

DERMATOMYOSITIS

Bowles N, Sewry C, Dubowitz V, et al: Dermatomyositis, polymyositis, and coxsackie-B-virus infection. Lancet 1:1004, 1987.

Bowyer SL, Blane CE, Sullivan DB, et al: Childhood dermatomyositis: Factors predicting functional outcome and development of dystrophic calcification. J Pediatr 103:882, 1983.

Ganczarczyk ML, Lee P, Amstrong SK: Nailfold capillary microscopy in polymyositis and dermatomyositis. Arthritis Rheum 31:116, 1988.

Heckmatt J, Saunders C, Peters AM, et al: Cyclosporin in juvenile dermatomyositis. Lancet 1:1063, 1989.

Pachman LM: Juvenile dermatomyositis. Pediatr Clin North Am 33:1097, 1986.

Plotz P: Current concepts in the idiopathic inflammatory myopathies: Polymyositis, dermatomyositis, and related disorders. Ann Intern Med 111:143, 1989.

Roifman CM, Schaffer FM, Wachsmuth SE, et al: Reversal of chronic polymyositis following intravenous immune serum globulin therapy. JAMA 258:513, 1987.

Sullivan DB, Cassidy JT, Petty RE, et al: Prognosis in childhood dermatomyositis. J Pediatr 80:555, 1972.

Taieb A, Guichard C, Salamon R, et al: Prognosis in juvenile dermatomyositis: A cooperative retrospective study of 70 cases. Pediatr Dermatol 2:275, 1985.

Targoff I, Arnett FC: Clinical manifestations in patients with antibody to PL-12 antigen (alanyl-t RNA synthetase). Am J Med 88:241, 1990.

SCLERODERMA: MORPHEA AND PROGRESSIVE SYSTEMIC SCLEROSIS

Bernstein RM, Pereira RS, Holden AJ, et al: Autoantibodies in childhood scleroderma. Ann Rheum Dis 44:503, 1985.
Bradford WO, Cook CD, Vawter GF, et al: Scleroderma of childhood. J Pediatr 68:391, 1966.
Claman HN: On scleroderma. Mast cells, endothelial cells, and fibroblasts. JAMA 262:1206, 1989.
Groen H, Wichers G, TerBorg E, et al: Pulmonary diffusing capacity disturbances are related to nail fold capillary changes in patients with Raynaud's phenomenon with and without an underlying connective tissue disease. Am J Med 89:34, 1990.
Singsen BH: Scleroderma in childhood. Pediatr Clin North Am 33:1119, 1986.
Steen VD, Medsgar TA Jr, Rodnan GP: D-Penicillamine therapy in progressive systemic sclerosis (scleroderma): A retrospective analysis. Ann Intern Med 97:652, 1982.
Suarez-Almazor ME, Cataggio LJ, Maldonado-Cocco JA, et al: Juvenile progressive systemic sclerosis: Clinical and serologic findings. Arthritis Rheum 28:699, 1985.

MIXED CONNECTIVE TISSUE DISEASE

Allen RC, St-Cyr C, Maddison PJ, et al: Overlap connective tissue syndromes. Arch Dis Child 61:284, 1986.
Lázaro M, Maldonado-Cocco J, Catoggio L, et al: Clinical and serologic characteristics of patients with overlap syndrome: Is mixed connective tissue disease a distinct clinical entity? Medicine 68:58, 1989.
Oetgen WJ, Boice JA, Lawless OJ: Mixed connective tissue disease in children and adolescents. Pediatrics 67:333, 1981.
Singsen BH: Mixed connective tissue disease in childhood. Pediatr Rev 7:309, 1986.

FASCIITIS

Britt WJ, Duray PH, Dahl MV, et al: Diffuse fasciitis with eosinophilia: A steroid responsive variant of scleroderma. J Pediatr 97:432, 1980.
Grisanti MW, Moore TL, Haber PL: Eosinophilic fasciitis in children. Semin Arthr Rheum 19:151, 1989.
Silver RM, Heyes MP, Maize JC, et al: Scleroderma, fasciitis, and eosinophilia associated with the ingestion of tryptophan. N Engl J Med 322:874, 1990.
Williams HJ, Ziter FA, Banta CA: Childhood eosinophilic fasciitis—progression to linear scleroderma. J Rheumatol 13:961, 1986.

BENIGN RHEUMATOID NODULES

Altman RS, Caffrey PR: Isolated subcutaneous rheumatic nodules. Pediatrics 34:869, 1964.
Burrington JD: "Pseudorheumatoid" nodules in children: Report of 10 cases. Pediatrics 45:473, 1970.
Simons FE, Schaller JG: Benign rheumatoid nodules. Pediatrics 56:29–33, 1975.

ERYTHEMA NODOSUM

Aetiology of erythema nodosum in children. Lancet 2:14, 1961.
Blomgren SE: Erythema nodosum. Semin Arthr Rheum 4:1, 1974.
Doxiadis SA: Erythema nodosum in children. Medicine 30:283, 1951.
Kirby JR, Kraft GH: Oral contraceptives and erythema nodosum. Obstet Gynecol 40:409, 1972.

FIBROSITIS-FIBROMYALGIA SYNDROMES

Yunus MB, Masi AT: Juvenile primary fibromyalgia syndrome: A clinical study of 33 patients and matched normal controls. Arthritis Rheum 28:138, 1985.
Yunus MB: Fibromyalgia syndrome: New research on an old malady. Br Med J 298:474, 1989.

RELAPSING NODULAR NONSUPPURATIVE PANNICULITIS

Case Records of the Massachusetts General Hospital: Case 17–1982. N Engl J Med 306:1035, 1982.
Sanford HN, Eubank DF, Stenn F: Chronic panniculitis with leukopenia (Weber-Christian syndrome). Am J Dis Child 83:156, 1952.
Winkelmann RK: Panniculitis in connective tissue disease. Arch Dermatol 119:336, 1983.

RELAPSING POLYCHONDRITIS

McAdam LP, O'Hanlan MA, Bluestone R, et al: Relapsing polychondritis: Prospective study of 23 patients and a review of the literature. Medicine 55:193, 1976.

SYNDROME OF NEONATAL FEVER, RASH, AND ARTHROPATHY

Prieur A, Griscelli C: Arthropathy with rash, chronic meningitis, eye lesions, and mental retardation. J Pediatr 99:79, 1981.

BEHÇET SYNDROME

Ammann AJ, Johnson A, Fyfe GA, et al: Behçet's syndrome. J Pediatr 107:41, 1985.
International Study Group for Behçet's Disease: Criteria for diagnosis of Behçet's disease. Lancet 335:1078, 1990.

OTHER CONDITIONS

Cassidy JT: Miscellaneous conditions associated with arthritis in children. Pediatr Clin North Am 33:1033, 1986.

11.75 RHEUMATIC FEVER

As recently as the 1950s and early 1960s, rheumatic fever and its major complication, valvular heart disease, were major problems worldwide. During the decades of the late 1960s and 1970s this disease almost disappeared in the United States and Western Europe, although it continues unabated in developing countries. However, the recent resurgence of acute rheumatic fever noted in the United States in the mid and late 1980s has once again emphasized the threat of this nonsuppurative sequel of group A streptococcal upper respiratory tract infections. In addition, the resurgence of rheumatic fever in the United States has also re-emphasized the need for better understanding of its pathogenesis so that appropriate public health and other preventive measures can be more effective.

ETIOLOGY. Group A β-hemolytic *Streptococcus* is the inciting agent leading to the development of acute rheumatic fever, although the exact pathogenetic mechanisms leading to rheumatic fever remain unexplained. Viral agents and cofactors have been proposed as etiologically related, but the evidence is unconvincing. Questions have been raised about whether all group A streptococci are equally capable of initiating the events leading to the clinical manifestations of acute rheumatic fever. It has been thought that all of the serotypes of group A streptococci can cause rheumatic fever. However, Kuttner and Krumweide reported that certain serotypes appeared to be more likely to cause rheumatic fever. When some strains (e.g., M type 4) were present in a very susceptible rheumatic population, no recurrences of rheumatic fever ensued. In contrast, other serotypes prevalent in the same population caused recurrence attack rates of 20–50% of those with pharyngitis. The concept of "rheumatogenicity" is further supported by studies suggesting that those serotypes of group A streptococci that were frequently associated with skin infection, usually the higher serotypes, were frequently isolated from the upper respiratory tract but seldom caused recurrences of rheumatic fever in individuals with a previous history of rheumatic fever. Further, certain serotypes of group A streptococci (e.g., M types 1, 3, 5, 6, 18, and 24) are more frequently isolated from patients with acute rheumatic fever than are other serotypes. However, since no rheumatogenic substance has been definitely identified, these epidemiologic observations remain hypothetical. Clinicians must assume that all serotypes have the capacity to cause rheumatic fever, and, especially in individuals with a previous history of rheumatic fever, all episodes of streptococcal pharyngitis should be treated accordingly.

EPIDEMIOLOGY. The epidemiology of acute rheumatic fever is essentially the epidemiology of group A streptococcal upper respiratory tract infection. Rheumatic fever is most frequently observed in the age group most susceptible to group A streptococcal infections, children from 5–15 yr of age. However, susceptibility to rheumatic fever is also evident in older age groups, as is noted by the outbreaks of acute rheumatic fever that have occurred in specific closed populations such as military recruits. Increased numbers of cases also occur in socially and economically disadvantaged groups.

This has been attributed to crowding, which is more frequent in this segment of the population. Furthermore, the increased incidence of group A streptococcal upper respiratory tract infections in fall, winter, and early spring is associated with an increased number of cases of acute rheumatic fever at these same periods of the year.

Group A streptococcal impetigo does not result in acute rheumatic fever, whereas infection of either the upper respiratory tract or the skin may lead to another nonsuppurative complication of streptococcal infection, acute poststreptococcal glomerulonephritis. The reasons for this are not fully understood. Hypotheses relating to differences in rheumatogenic potential of so-called "skin strains" and "throat strains" as well as observed differences in the immunologic response to group A streptococcal impetigo compared to streptococcal upper respiratory tract infection have been proposed to explain the contrast.

The major epidemiologic risk factor for development of acute rheumatic fever is group A streptococcal upper respiratory tract infection. The major reservoir for group A streptococci is the upper respiratory tract of man, necessitating an understanding of the epidemiology of streptococcal upper respiratory tract infection and dictating public health control of these infections in children. Suggestions that dogs and other pets might also be the reservoir for group A streptococci have never been substantiated.

The attack rate of acute rheumatic fever following group A upper respiratory tract infection is approximately 3% of individuals with untreated or inadequately treated infection. This figure has been remarkably constant, and the occasionally reported lower rates are probably due to inclusion of group A streptococcal carriers. Many children who harbor the group A *Streptococcus* are carriers of group A streptococci in the upper respiratory tract. The group A streptococcal carrier is at much reduced risk not only for development of acute rheumatic fever, but also for spread of the organism to close family or school contacts.

Of particular epidemiologic interest is the resurgence of acute rheumatic fever that occurred in the United States in the mid and late 1980s. Whereas the incidence of acute rheumatic fever in many communities in the United States was less than 1 in 100,000 population per year in the years through the 1970s and early 1980s, beginning in the mid 1980s outbreaks of acute rheumatic fever occurred in numerous areas across the United States. The initial and largest outbreak was reported from Utah, but subsequent reports from eastern states, including Ohio and Pennsylvania, indicated that this resurgence was multifocal. Since streptococcal infections and acute rheumatic fever are no longer reportable diseases in the United States, accurate data are difficult to obtain. One survey of pediatric cardiologists in large referral medical centers in the United States suggested that an increase in numbers of cases of acute rheumatic fever between 1985 and 1989 occurred in approximately 25 states. There were also at least two outbreaks of acute rheumatic fever in military recruit populations in the United States between 1985 and 1988. Current epidemiologic data from some other parts of the world are difficult to find, but reports of outbreaks have been uncommon in the Third World.

The reasons for this recurrence or resurgence of acute rheumatic fever in the United States remain unknown. Although rheumatic fever has been associated with socially and economically disadvantaged populations, the 1980s' resurgence has been associated with middle class, often suburban and rural, families. In addition, serotypes of group A streptococci that have been isolated only rarely during the previous 2 or 3 decades have emerged and spread. These serotypes began to be isolated in greater numbers when rheumatic fever cases were being reported. An increased number of isolates from either rheumatic fever patients or simultaneously from their household contacts and siblings were shown to be M types 1, 3, 5, 6, and 18. These types have historically been associated with rheumatic fever. However, very mucoid strains, especially strains of M type 18 group A streptococci, have appeared in a number of communities prior to the appearance of rheumatic fever. Mucoid strains have historically been associated with virulence.

PATHOGENESIS. Despite remarkable increases in our knowledge of the biology of the group A streptococcus and of the human host, and despite important observations about the epidemiologic association between group A streptococci and the human host, the pathogenetic mechanism responsible for the development of acute rheumatic fever remains unknown. There have been three basic groups of theories attempting to explain the development of this sequel to group A streptococcal upper respiratory tract infection. These are: (1) a direct infection of the heart and valves by group A streptococci; (2) a toxic effect produced by an extracellular toxin of group A streptococci on target organs such as myocardium, valves, synovium, and brain; and (3) an abnormal immune response by the human host. The search for the correct hypothesis has been severely hampered by the fact that there is no adequate animal model. The possibility of direct infection of the heart valves by group A streptococci has not been supported by postmortem studies or by clinical trials of large doses of penicillin given after the onset of acute rheumatic fever.

The hypotheses suggesting that rheumatic fever may be related to a direct effect of a streptococcal extracellular toxin also have not been proved. For example, although streptolysin O, an extracellular product of group A streptococci, is cardiotoxic in animals, it has not been possible to establish either a direct in vivo toxic effect by streptolysin O on the myocardium and valves or an injury of host tissue by streptolysin O resulting in "neoantigen" formation, with a subsequent immunologic response and damage to the host tissues. Of importance in this regard is the fact that group C and group G streptococci also produce streptolysin O, and these two serologic groups do not lead to acute rheumatic fever.

The most popular current hypotheses are those that postulate an abnormal immune response by the human host to some still, undefined component of the group A streptococcus. The resulting antibodies might then cause the immunologic damage leading to clinical manifestations. The latent period, usually 1–3 wk between the onset of the actual group A streptococcal infection and the onset of symptoms of acute rheumatic fever, lends support to an immunologic mechanism of tissue damage. Although the specific antigen or antigens responsible for inciting such an immune response have still to be identified, several possibilities exist. The group A streptococcus is a very complex microorganism producing a large number of both somatic and extracellular antigens that evoke brisk immune responses and therefore could initiate the onset of the immunologic response resulting in rheumatic fever. This theory is further supported by the observation that different humans appear to respond quantitatively differently to streptococcal antigens. For example, in in vitro studies with human lymphocytes, different individuals can be divided into high and low responders to streptococcal blastogen A, an extracellular product of the organism. This finding is compatible with the clinical and epidemiologic observations that not all people appear to be susceptible to developing rheumatic fever (see later).

Two streptococcal antigens are excellent examples of how an abnormal immunologic response might cause the clinical manifestations. First, the group-specific polysaccharide of the group A β-hemolytic streptococcal cell wall is antigenically similar to the glycoprotein found in human and bovine cardiac valves. There is prolonged persistence of antibody against the group A polysaccharide in individuals with chronic rheumatic valvular heart disease compared with individuals recovering from uncomplicated streptococcal infection or those with acute nephritis. Furthermore, when rheumatic mitral valves were surgically removed and replaced with prosthetic valves, serum antibody levels against the group A polysaccharide fell, as if the antigenic stimulus had been removed. However, important questions remain as to whether this antigen is responsible for the valvulitis of rheumatic heart disease. For example, it has been shown that antibodies to group-specific carbohydrate develop after group A streptococcal skin infection, and rheumatic fever does not follow group A streptococcal skin infection (pyoderma). A second so-called cross-reactive antigen was originally described in the cell wall or cell membrane. Antibodies to this (these) somatic antigen(s) are found in sera of patients with rheumatic fever (called "heart-reactive antibodies"), and it has been postulated that the myocarditis of acute rheumatic fever is related to an abnormal or autoimmune response against sarcolemma membrane. However, the significance of these observations has been questioned because these serum antibodies also develop following uncomplicated pharyngitis in individuals without evidence of rheumatic carditis.

The possibility of an abnormal immune response is also based upon cross-reactivity between group A streptococci M protein and human tissue. The M protein is the virulence factor that is responsible for the organism's ability to resist phagocytosis. In addition, following infections with group A streptococci, type-specific immunity is conferred against the specific M protein type. The group A streptococcal M protein shares certain amino acid sequences with some human tissues, and this has been proposed as a possible source of cross-reactivity between the organism and its human host, leading to the abnormal immune response. One of the two classes of M protein correlates with serotypes of group A streptococci that are frequently isolated from patients with acute rheumatic fever.

It has also been demonstrated that there are, in patients with Sydenham chorea, common antibodies to antigens found in both the group A streptococcal cell membrane and the caudate nucleus of brain. This observation further supports the concept of an abnormal autoimmune mechanism for the central nervous system manifestations of rheumatic fever and Sydenham chorea.

An understanding of the pathogenesis of rheumatic fever must encompass the fact that there are differences in human susceptibility to the development of acute rheumatic fever, including an unusual incidence of rheumatic fever and rheumatic heart disease among members of certain family groups. In regard to this genetic influence, there is a specific alloantigen present on the surface of non–T lymphocytes in 70–90% of rheumatic individuals; but fewer than 30% of "control" nonrheumatic individuals have the marker. Furthermore, the marker is more often present in family members in which there is an index case of rheumatic fever than in nonaffected members of "control" families.

Although there may be genetic differences in rheumatic susceptibility among humans, the exact mechanism remains unknown. It is unlikely that the recent outbreaks of acute rheumatic fever in the United States are due to an increasingly susceptible population based only on genetics. It is most likely that the pathogenetic mechanism for the development of rheumatic fever following upper respiratory tract infection with group A β-hemolytic streptococci involves a combination of specific characteristics of the organism and some as yet incompletely defined genetic predisposition in the human host.

CLINICAL MANIFESTATIONS AND DIAGNOSIS. There is no single specific clinical manifestation or specific laboratory test that unequivocally establishes the diagnosis of rheumatic fever. Rather, there are a number of selective clinical findings (Jones Criteria) that make the diagnosis of acute rheumatic fever highly probable and necessitate discussing the clinical manifestations and the diagnosis together. Although the Jones Criteria have been changed several times since their original publication, they have remained basically stable and are the accepted method by which the diagnosis of this disease is confirmed. The current recommendations of the American Heart Association are presented in Table 11–40 along with the three additional suggestions proposed in 1988 by the World Health Organization.

Major Criteria. The five major criteria are considered to be the most specific findings; therefore, more weight is given to major criteria.

CARDITIS (see Sec. 15.67). This important finding in acute rheumatic fever is a pancarditis that involves the pericardium, epicardium, myocardium, and endocardium. Carditis is the only residual of acute rheumatic fever that results in chronic changes. Common manifestations include evidence of valvular insufficiency, most frequently affecting the mitral valve, but both the mitral and the aortic valve may be affected. Isolated involvement of the aortic valve is rare. Tricuspid valve or pulmonary valve involvement is unusual. Valvular insufficiency is present in the acute state of the disease. Later, in the chronic stage, scarring of the valve with either typical "fishmouth" abnormality or even calcified valve tissue may lead to stenosis. Often there is a combination of both insufficiency and stenosis. Carditis is present in 40–80% of patients with rheumatic fever. In the recent outbreaks in the United States, more than 80% of patients in one of the large series had evidence of carditis.

Other manifestations of carditis include pericarditis, pericardial effusion, and arrhythmias (usually 1st-degree heart block, but 3rd-degree or complete heart block may occur). The carditis of rheumatic fever may be either mild or very severe, leading to intractable heart failure; rarely, surgical intervention, even in the acute stage of the disease, may be necessary if medical management cannot control the heart failure. These patients usually have both myocardial involvement and significant valvular insufficiency.

TABLE 11–40. The Jones Criteria Revised with Addition of World Health Organization Recommendations

Major Criteria	Minor Criteria
Carditis	Fever
Polyarthritis, migratory	Arthralgia
Erythema marginatum	Previous rheumatic fever
Chorea	Elevated acute-phase reactants (ESR, CRP)
Subcutaneous nodules	Prolonged P-R interval on an electrocardiogram
Plus	
Evidence of a preceding group A streptococcal infection (culture, rapid antigen, antibody rise/elevation, scarlet fever)	

Note: Two major criteria or one major and two minor criteria *plus* evidence of a preceding streptococcal infection indicate a high probability of rheumatic fever.

In the three special categories listed below, the diagnosis of rheumatic fever is acceptable without two major or one major and two minor criteria. However, only for a and b can the requirement for evidence of a preceding streptococcal infection be ignored. (Modified from American Heart Association and World Health Organization) See text.

a. *Chorea:* If other causes have been excluded.
b. *Insidious or late-onset carditis:* With no other explanation.
c. *Rheumatic recurrence:* In patients with documented rheumatic heart disease, the presence of one criterion, or of fever, arthralgia, or elevated acute-phase reactants suggests a presumptive diagnosis of recurrence. Evidence of previous streptococcal infection is needed here.

C = C-reactive protein; ESR = erythrocyte sedimentation rate.

Polyarthritis. This is the most confusing of the major criteria and probably leads to more diagnostic errors than any of the other manifestations. The arthritis of acute rheumatic fever is exquisitely tender. It is not uncommon for children with this form of arthritis to refuse to allow even bed sheets or clothing to cover an affected joint. The joints are red, warm, and swollen. The arthritis is migratory and affects several different joints, namely, the elbows, knees, ankles, and wrists. It rarely occurs in the fingers, toes, or spine. It need *not* be symmetric. Effusions may be present. If the joint is aspirated, a leukocytosis is usually found; polymorphonuclear leukocytes are the cells found most frequently. However, there are no specific laboratory findings in the synovial fluid.

The arthritis does *not* result in chronic joint disease. Following the initiation of anti-inflammatory therapy (see later), the arthritis may literally disappear in 12–24 hr. Untreated, it may persist for a week or more. In many patients with early arthritis of rheumatic fever, because of treatment with anti-inflammatory drugs, the classic migratory polyarthritis does not develop, thus confusing the diagnosis.

Chorea. Sydenham chorea, a unique part of the rheumatic fever syndrome, occurs much later than other manifestations. These choreoathetoid movements may begin very subtly. The latent period following streptococcal pharyngitis may be as long as several months, and the movements are often very difficult to detect at the onset. However, careful questioning of parents and teachers usually reveals evidence of increased clumsiness. One of the best signs of this in schoolchildren is a marked deterioration in their handwriting. Emotional lability is a frequent finding. Sydenham chorea may affect all four extremities or may be unilateral. Although at one time it could be seen in up to one half of patients with acute rheumatic fever, more recent evidence suggests that it is seen, at least in the United States, in 10% or less of cases. Sydenham chorea not infrequently is the only symptom of rheumatic fever. It is for this reason that the World Health Organization suggests that this symptom alone is adequate to satisfy the Jones Criteria. Sydenham chorea usually disappears within weeks to months. It may return, but in recent years this has become a rare occurrence.

Erythema Marginatum. The unique rash seen in patients with rheumatic fever is another of the major manifestations that can be very difficult to diagnose. It occurs very infrequently, and therefore few clinicians have had extensive experience in recognizing it. Although early in the disease it may become manifest as nonspecific pink macules that are usually seen over the trunk, later in its fully developed form there is blanching in the middle of the lesions, sometimes with fusing of the borders, resulting in a serpiginous-looking lesion. This rash can be made worse with application of heat, but characteristically it is evanescent. The rash does not itch. It often occurs in patients with chronic carditis. The rash of erythema marginatum can be mistaken for the rash seen with Lyme disease.

Subcutaneous Nodules. These lesions are very infrequent and are most commonly observed in patients with severe carditis. These small, pea-sized nodules are firm and nontender, and there is no inflammation. They are characteristically seen on the extensor surfaces of the joints, such as the knees and elbows, and also over the spine.

Minor Criteria. The minor manifestations are much less specific but are necessary to confirm a diagnosis of rheumatic fever. They include a previous history of documented rheumatic fever and arthralgia. Arthralgia is present if the patient feels discomfort in the joint in the absence of objective findings (pain, redness, warmth) on physical examination. (Arthralgia cannot be counted in satisfying the Jones Criteria if arthritis is present.) In addition, fever, usually no higher than 101° or 102° F, may be present. High fever of 103° or 104° F requires very careful re-evaluation and consideration of other diagnoses.

Included in the minor criteria are several laboratory tests. Acute-phase reactants, such as the ESR or CRP, may be elevated. These tests may remain elevated for prolonged periods of time (months) and are used by some clinicians as a guideline for modifying doses of anti-inflammatory drugs (see later). A prolonged P-R interval on the electrocardiogram is also included among the minor criteria. This also is a nonspecific finding and should be used only after very careful consideration.

Evidence of Group A Streptococcal Infection. This is one of the most important aspects of the Jones Criteria. There must be evidence of a preceding group A streptococcal infection documented by a positive throat culture, a history of scarlet fever, or elevated streptococcal antibodies such as antistreptolysin O (ASO), antideoxyribonuclease B (anti-DNase B), or antihyaluronidase (AH). The diagnosis of rheumatic fever should *not* be seriously considered in patients without evidence of a recent group A streptococcal infection. Approximately 80% of individuals with rheumatic fever have an elevated antistreptolysin O titer, but if the titers of two additional streptococcal antibodies are also elevated or rising, an elevation of at least one antibody will be found in more than 95% of patients with rheumatic fever.

In 1988 a World Health Organization Study Group recommended that three categories of patients be diagnosed as having acute rheumatic fever even in the absence of two major criteria or one major and two minor criteria, as required by the revised Jones Criteria, because difficulties in many developing countries have made further modifications desirable (see Table 11–40).

DIFFERENTIAL DIAGNOSIS. The differential diagnosis is extensive because so many of the clinical and laboratory findings associated with rheumatic fever are not specific and there is no single laboratory test that will confirm the diagnosis. Juvenile rheumatoid arthritis or other connective tissue diseases often need to be considered. Infective endocarditis is very frequently confused with rheumatic fever, especially in patients with recurrences of rheumatic fever. Patients with either a previous history of rheumatic fever or rheumatic valvular heart disease should be carefully evaluated for infective endocarditis before the diagnosis of recurrent rheumatic fever is made. This may be difficult because such patients may be taking an antibiotic for secondary rheumatic fever prophylaxis in a dose high enough to prevent blood cultures from becoming positive. The typical rash of Lyme disease may be confused with erythema marginatum.

COMPLICATIONS. The major complication of acute rheumatic fever is the development of rheumatic valvular heart disease. None of the other manifestations results in a chronic disease. The mitral valve is most frequently involved, but the aortic and tricuspid valves also may be affected. Usually the tricuspid valve becomes involved only in patients who have significant mitral or aortic disease resulting in pulmonary hypertension.

LABORATORY FINDINGS. No single specific laboratory test will confirm the diagnosis of acute rheumatic fever. Laboratory evidence of a previous streptococcal infection is confirmed by either a search for the organism itself (culture) or evidence of an immune response to a group A streptococcal antigen. The throat culture remains the gold standard for confirmation of the presence of group A streptococci, although rapid antigen detection tests are available. All patients suspected of having acute rheumatic fever should have at least one throat culture performed before beginning antibiotic therapy. However, because only 25–40% of individuals with acute rheumatic fever have positive throat cultures at onset and because many patients with positive throat cultures harbor only very few group A streptococci in the upper respiratory tract, two or three throat cultures should be obtained. Rapid antigen detection tests may be used as long as it is recognized that these tests have reduced sensitivity. If small numbers of group A streptococci are present, the test may be falsely "negative." On the other hand, because the specificity of most of these tests is quite good, a positive result of a rapid antigen detection test provides evidence of group A streptococci. If a rapid antigen detection test is negative, a throat culture should be obtained in patients in whom rheumatic fever is suspected.

Streptococcal antibody tests are another method of documenting the presence of a previous group A streptococcal infection. The most commonly used test is the ASO test. Other tests that may be used are the anti-DNase B test and the AH test. A commercially available agglutination test is less satisfactory because of its technical difficulties. An elevated streptococcal antibody titer is clear evidence of a previous group A streptococcal infection, but a more reliable way of demonstrating the earlier infection is by showing a rise in titer between acute and convalescent sera. The ASO test reaches its peak 3–6 wk following infection, whereas the anti-DNase B test reaches its peak slightly later (6–8 wk). If acute and convalescent sera are tested, they should be tested simultaneously. Values defining an elevated titer may vary with the age of the patient, the interval since the streptococcal infection, and the population.

Acute-phase reactants such as the ESR or CRP are always elevated at the onset of acute rheumatic fever. However, these tests are nonspecific. Determination of rheumatoid factor, tests for the presence of ANA, and determination of the complement level are rarely helpful in making a diagnosis of acute rheumatic fever. Occasionally, nonspecific elevations of serum gamma globulin may be seen.

The electrocardiogram may indicate a 1st-degree heart block (prolonged P-R interval), and on rare occasions 2nd- or 3rd-degree block may also be present. In first attacks, electrocardiograms are otherwise usually unremarkable. In patients with chronic rheumatic heart disease, however, electrocardiographic manifestations of resulting cardiac disease, such as left atrial enlargement, may be evident.

No specific findings are present on chest roentgenogram. Not infrequently, cardiomegaly is noted, especially in individuals with significant carditis.

Some individuals with subclinical evidence of valvular disease may show valvular regurgitation on two-dimensional Doppler echocardiography. This observation may explain why many patients without evidence of carditis at the time of the acute attack present in the 4th or 5th decade of life with evidence of mitral valve disease. An echocardiogram is useful in evaluating patients suspected of having rheumatic fever and/or rheumatic heart disease.

TREATMENT. Management of acute rheumatic fever can be divided into three approaches: treatment of the group A streptococcal infection that led to the disease, use of anti-inflammatory agents to control the clinical manifestations of the disease, and other supportive therapy, including management of congestive heart failure, if that has occurred.

All patients presenting with acute rheumatic fever should be treated for a group A streptococcal infection at the time the diagnosis is made, whether or not the organism is initially isolated from the patient. As mentioned earlier, it can be difficult to recover the organism from the patient at onset because of the latent period, especially in patients with chorea. Either 10 full days of an appropriate oral agent or a single intramuscular injection of 1,200,000 units of benzathine penicillin G is recommended. Treatment for group A β-hemolytic streptococcal infections is discussed in more detail in Sec. 12.19. Because some patients receiving intramuscular benzathine penicillin G may experience nonspecific rises in the ESR, some clinicians elect to treat patients initially with oral penicillin, especially if they are following the ESR as a measure of the effectiveness of anti-inflammatory therapy given for other rheumatic manifestations. Sulfadiazine is not an appropriate agent for treatment of acute streptococcal pharyngitis.

There are three systemic manifestations of acute rheumatic fever for which therapy is given acutely. These are arthritis, carditis, and Sydenham chorea. Salicylates provide prompt and dramatic relief for the patient with the arthritis of acute rheumatic fever. The exquisitely tender migratory polyarthritis can be relieved in 12–24 hr by the use of salicylates. Early administration of salicylates to a patient suspected of having rheumatic fever before the diagnosis is established with certainty may obscure the diagnosis by interrupting the development of migratory arthritis. Therefore, salicylates or other anti-inflammatory agents should be withheld until the clinical course of the disease has adequately defined itself. For those patients with very painful arthritis, comfort can be provided by the use of small doses of codeine or similar drugs because they will not interfere with the progression of the disease and its subsequent diagnosis. Corticosteroids are seldom if ever indicated for the treatment of arthritis of rheumatic fever. No studies are available documenting the efficacy of nonsteroidal anti-inflammatory agents in the treatment of rheumatic fever.

For patients with very mild carditis without evidence of congestive heart failure, salicyates alone are indicated. However, in patients with congestive heart failure or other significant manifestations of carditis, corticosteroids are required. There is no definitive evidence that the use of either salicylates or corticosteroids is beneficial in preventing the subsequent development of rheumatic heart disease. This is in contrast to the clinical impression that corticosteroids may have a beneficial effect in patients with moderate to severe carditis. It is, therefore, appropriate to restrict the use of corticosteroids to patients who have moderate or severe carditis, especially those with evidence of heart failure.

Administration of steroids should be limited both in amount and in duration to reduce their untoward side effects. For most children, a total dose of 2.5 mg/kg/24 hr divided into two doses is appropriate. A short course of steroids over 2–3 wk is usually sufficient, depending on patient response both clinically and on laboratory tests (e.g., ESR, CRP). Even with short courses of steroids in these doses, side effects may occur, including some cushingoid changes and occasionally hypertension. Alternate-day steroids may reduce the side effects, but controlled studies have not been done. The dose should be tapered rather than abruptly stopped.

Salicylates should be given in a dose that will result in blood levels of 20–25 mg/dL. Usually 90–120 mg/kg/24 hr in 4 divided doses is adequate to reach this level in children. However, serum salicylate levels should be carefully monitored to reduce the possibility of toxicity. Liver function should also be monitored. In patients who are receiving corticosteroids for therapy of carditis, it is advisable to add salicylates to the steroids, especially when the doses are being tapered in order to prevent the possibility of rheumatic rebound. The salicyates should be given during the last week of corticosteroid therapy and continued for approximately 3–4 wk after the steroids have been discontinued. The duration of salicylate therapy depends on the patient's response and clinical course.

Congestive heart failure should be treated by conventional techniques (see Sec. 15.73). Diuretics are indicated in patients with severe congestive heart failure. Cardiac glycosides such as digitalis also may be used, although usually in relatively small doses. Long periods of bed rest are not necessary for most patients. In the past, bed rest was used primarily for two groups of patients. The first were patients who had

TABLE 11–41. Primary and Secondary Prevention of Rheumatic Fever*

Route of Administration	Antibiotic	Dose	Frequency
Primary Prevention: Treatment of streptococcal pharyngitis to prevent a primary attack of rheumatic fever			
Intramuscular	Benzathine penicillin G	1,200,000 units (600,000 units if <27 kg)	Once
Oral	Penicillin V	250 mg/kg/24 hr	bid for 10 days
	Erythromycin	40 mg/kg/24 hr (not to exceed 1 g/24 hr)	tid or qid for 10 days
	Others: (e.g., clindamycin, nafcillin, ampicillin, amoxicillin, cephalexin)	Dosage varies	
Do not use tetracyclines or sulfa drugs			
Secondary Prevention: Prevention of recurrences of rheumatic fever			
Intramuscular	Benzathine penicillin G	1,200,000 units	Every 3–4 wk
Oral	Penicillin V	250 mg	bid
	Sulfadiazine	500 mg	od
	Erythromycin	250 mg	bid
Do not use tetracyclines			

*Adapted, by permission, from Rheumatic fever and heart disease: Report of a WHO Study Group. Geneva, World Health Organization, 1988.

arthritis, but this usually is not a factor after 24 hr of salicylate therapy. Strict bed rest is not needed. The second group of patients are those with carditis, especially those with congestive heart failure. Although bed rest is indicated for the therapy of patients with congestive heart failure, prolonged bed rest is usually unnecessary. It is, however, preferable to keep patients at bed rest until the ESR approaches normal and congestive heart failure has been controlled. Occasionally, steroids, bed rest, and anticongestive measures are not effective in treating the carditis of rheumatic fever. In these rare cases, cardiovascular surgery with either replacement of the valve or valvuloplasty may be required.

The treatment of Sydenham chorea has been controversial. Originally, phenobarbital or other sedatives were used; then chlorpromazine became popular. Most recently, however, diazepam, a benzodiazepine derivative, has been prescribed for patients with mild chorea. In patients with severe chorea, haloperidol has been used successfully. These children must be closely observed, however, because severe toxic reactions to this drug have been reported.

There is no specific therapy for erythema marginatum or the subcutaneous nodules of acute rheumatic fever.

PREVENTION. Prevention and treatment of group A streptococcal infection can prevent rheumatic fever. There are two forms of prevention for acute rheumatic fever, primary prophylaxis and secondary prophylaxis.

Primary prophylaxis refers to antibiotic treatment of the streptococcal upper respiratory tract infection to prevent an initial attack of rheumatic fever. Appropriate diagnosis and adequate antibiotic therapy with eradication of group A streptococci from the upper respiratory tract reduce the risk of developing rheumatic fever to near zero. It has been shown that antibiotic therapy can be delayed until approximately 1 wk after onset of the streptococcal sore throat, and rheumatic fever can still be prevented. See Sec. 12.18 for treatment of group A streptococcal infections. However, antibiotic therapy must be adequate. Ten full days of oral therapy are essential if the oral method is used. Suggested doses are shown in Table 11–41.

Secondary prophylaxis refers to the prevention of colonization and/or infection of the upper respiratory tract with group A β-hemolytic streptococci in people who have already had a previous attack of acute rheumatic fever. Patients who receive antibiotics continuously and do not have group A streptococcal infections do not have recurrences of rheumatic fever. The recommended methods of secondary prevention include either regular monthly (every 4 wk) injections of intramuscular benzathine penicillin G, daily administration of oral penicillin, daily administration of oral sulfadiazine, or daily administration of erythromycin (for individuals who cannot take any of the previously recommended antibiotics). Although sulfadiazine or other sulfa drugs should *never* be used for the treatment of group A streptococcal infections (because a high percentage of organisms are resistant to these antimicrobial agents), sulfadiazine *is* effective in preventing colonization of the upper respiratory tract and is an acceptable form of oral secondary prophylaxis. Regular injections of intramuscular benzathine penicillin G are preferable to oral secondary prophylaxis owing primarily to better compliance. Individuals at high risk for rheumatic recurrence should be given 1,200,000 units intramuscularly every 3 wk. Penicillin levels during the 4th wk following injection may be lower than the MIC for group A β-hemolytic streptococci. However, in most instances in the United States 4-wk intervals for injections are sufficient because the risk of recurrence of rheumatic fever is small.

The necessary duration of secondary prophylaxis in individuals with a documented history of rheumatic fever or with rheumatic heart disease is controversial. Recurrences of acute rheumatic fever occur less frequently 5 yr or more following the most recent attack, and for this reason, some clinicians believe that patients may not need secondary prophylaxis more than 5 yr after their most recent attack or when they reach their 18th birthday, whichever comes first. Others recommend that, in patients who have significant rheumatic heart disease or who have a significant risk of contracting group A streptococcal upper respiratory tract infection (medical professionals, school teachers, living in crowded conditions, etc.), the duration of secondary prophylaxis should be longer. Indeed, some recommend that treatment be continued for life in patients with rheumatic valvular heart disease. Recommendations for each patient must be individualized depending on the patient's condition and the environment in which he or she lives and works.

No streptococcal vaccine is presently available. Physicians and public health authorities must still depend on the accurate and timely diagnosis and therapy of group A streptococcal upper respiratory tract infections and prevention of recurrent infections in known rheumatics to prevent the crippling effects of rheumatic fever and rheumatic heart disease.

EDWARD L. KAPLAN

Bisno AL: The concept of rheumatogenic and nonrheumatogenic group A streptococci. *In*: Reed SE, Zabriskie JB (eds): Streptococcal Diseases and the Immune Response. New York, Academic Press, 1980, p 789.

Committee on Rheumatic Fever and Bacterial Endocarditis of the American Heart Association: Jones Criteria (Revised) for Guidance in the Diagnosis of Rheumatic Fever. Dallas, American Heart Association, 1982.

Committee on Rheumatic Fever, Endocarditis, and Kawasaki Disease of the American Heart Association: Prevention of rheumatic fever. Circulation 78:1082, 1988.

Committee to Revise the Jones Criteria, American Heart Association: Jones Criteria (Revised) for Guidance in the Diagnosis of Rheumatic Fever. Circulation 32:664, 1965.

Cunningham MW, Hall NK, Krisher KK, et al: A study of anti-group A streptococcal monoclonal antibodies cross-reactive with myosin. J Immunol 136:293, 1986.

Denny FW Jr, Wannamaker LW, Brink WR, et al: Prevention of rheumatic fever: Treatment of the preceding streptococcal infection. JAMA 143:151, 1950.

Dudding BA, Ayoub EM: Persistence of streptococcal group A antibody in patients with rheumatic valvular disease. J Exp Med 128:1081, 1968.

Fischetti VA: Streptococcal M protein: Molecular design and biological behavior. Clin Microbiol Rev 2:285, 1989.

Gerber MA, Wright LL, Randolph MF: Streptozyme test for antibodies to group A streptococcal antigens. Pediatr Infect Dis J 6:36, 1987.

Gray ED, Regelmann WE, Abdin Z, et al: Compartmentalization of cells bearing "rheumatic" cell surface antigens in peripheral blood and in tonsils in rheumatic heart disease. J Infect Dis 155:247, 1987.

Hosein B, McCarty M, Fischetti VA: Amino acid sequence and physicochemical similarities between streptococcal M protein and mammalian tropomyosin. Proc Natl Acad Sci USA 76:3765, 1979.

Husby G, Van de Rijn I, Zabriskie JB, et al: Antibody reacting with cytoplasm of subthalamic and caudate nuclei neurons in chorea and acute rheumatic fever. J Exp Med 144:1094, 1976.

Kaplan EL: The rapid identification of group A beta-hemolytic streptococci in the upper respiratory tract. Pediatr Clin North Am 35:535, 1988.

Kaplan EL, Berrios X, Speth J, et al: Pharmacokinetics of benzathine penicillin G: Serum levels during the 28 days after intramuscular injection of 1,200,000 units. J Pediatr 115:146, 1989.

Kaplan EL, Hill HR: Return of rheumatic fever: Consequences, implications, and needs. J Pediatr 111:244, 1987.

Kaplan EL, Johnson DR, Cleary PP: Group A streptococcal serotypes isolated from patients and sibling contacts during the resurgence of rheumatic fever in the United States in the mid 1980s. J Infect Dis 159:101, 1989.

Kavey RW, Kaplan EL: Resurgence of acute rheumatic fever. Pediatrics 84:585, 1989.

Markowitz M, Kaplan EL: Reappearance of rheumatic fever. Adv Pediatr 36:39, 1989.

Regelmann WE, Talbot R, Cairns L, et al: Distribution of cells bearing "rheumatic" antigens in peripheral blood of patients with rheumatic fever/rheumatic heart disease. J Rheumatol 16:931, 1989.

Siegel AC, Johnson EE, Stollerman GH: Controlled studies of streptococcal pharyngitis in a pediatric population: Factors related to the attack rate of rheumatic fever. N Engl J Med 265:559, 1961.

Veasy LG, Wiedmeier SE, Orsmond GS, et al: Resurgence of acute rheumatic fever in the intermountain area of the United States. N Engl J Med 316:421, 1987.

Wannamaker LW, Rammelkamp CH Jr, Denny FW Jr, et al: Prophylaxis of acute rheumatic fever by treatment of the preceding streptococcal infection with various amounts of depo penicillin. Am J Med 10:673, 1951.

Wood HF, Feinstein AR, Taranta A, et al: Rheumatic fever in children and adolescents. III. Comparative effectiveness of three prophylaxis regimens in preventing streptococcal infections and rheumatic recurrences. Ann Intern Med 60 (Suppl 5):31, 1964.

World Health Organization Study Group: Rheumatic Fever and Rheumatic Heart Disease, Technical Report Series No. 764. Geneva, World Health Organization, 1988.

12

INFECTIOUS DISEASES

GENERAL CONSIDERATIONS

12.1 FEVER

Fever occurs when various infectious and noninfectious processes interact with the host's defense mechanism. In most children fever is either due to an identifiable microbiologic agent or subsides after a short time. Fever in children may be categorized as (1) fever of short duration with localizing signs for which the diagnosis can be established by clinical history and physical examination, with or without laboratory tests; (2) fever without localizing signs, for which the history and physical examinations do not suggest a diagnosis but laboratory tests may establish an etiology; and (3) fever of unknown origin (FUO) (Sec. 12.3).

Fever is an elevation of body temperature mediated by an increase of the hypothalamic heat regulatory set-point. The hypothalamic thermoregulatory center controls body temperature by balancing signals from peripheral cold and warm neuronal receptors. Another regulatory factor is the temperature of blood circulating in the hypothalamus. The integration of these signals maintains normal core body temperature at the set-point of 37° C (98.6° F), within a narrow range of 1–1.5° C. Axillary temperature may be 1° C lower than core temperature, due in part to cutaneous vasoconstriction, and oral temperature may be falsely lowered owing to rapid respirations. Body temperature follows a circadian rhythm: Early morning temperature is low, and the highest level occurs at 4.00–6.00 P.M. Heat generation (increased cell metabolism, muscle activity, involuntary shivering) and heat conservation (vasoconstriction, heat preference behavior) are balanced against heat loss (obligate heat loss [evaporation-radiation-convection-conduction], vasodilation, sweating, and cold preference behavior).

The normal homeostatic regulation of temperature by the hypothalamus may be altered by various disease states. The causes of fever include infection, vaccines (pertussis, influenza virus, measles), biologic agents (granulocyte-macrophage colony–stimulating factor, interferon, interleukins), tissue injury (infarction, pulmonary emboli, trauma, intramuscular injections, burns), malignancy (leukemia, lymphoma, hepatoma, metastatic disease), drugs (drug fever, cocaine, amphotericin B), immunologic-rheumatologic disorders (systemic lupus erythematosus, rheumatoid arthritis), inflammatory diseases (inflammatory bowel disease), granulomatous diseases (sarcoidosis), endocrine disorders (thyrotoxicosis, pheochromocytoma), metabolic disorders (gout, uremia, Fabry disease, type 1 hyperlipidemia), and unknown or poorly understood entities (familial Mediterranean fever). Factitious (self-induced) fever may be due to intentional manipulations of the thermometer or injection of pyrogenic material.

Regardless of the etiology, the final pathway of most common causes of fever is the production of endogenous pyrogens, which then directly alter the hypothalamic temperature set-point, resulting in heat generation and heat conservation (Fig. 12–1). The sequence of cytokine generation in response to exogenous pyrogens, with subsequent hypothalamic prostaglandin E_2 (PGE_2) production, may take 60–90 min. This delayed action supports the clinical observation that blood cultures should be obtained before fever is elevated, when circulating bacteria (exogenous pyrogens) are more likely to be present. Fever is one manifestation of the inflammatory response produced by cytokine-mediated host defense mechanisms.

Except under unusual circumstances, fever by itself is not beneficial to the host response to infection. Heat production associated with fever increases oxygen consumption, carbon dioxide production, and cardiac output. Thus, it may exacerbate cardiac insufficiency in patients with heart disease or chronic anemia (e.g., sickle cell disease), pulmonary insufficiency in those with chronic lung disease, and metabolic instability in children with diabetes mellitus or inborn errors

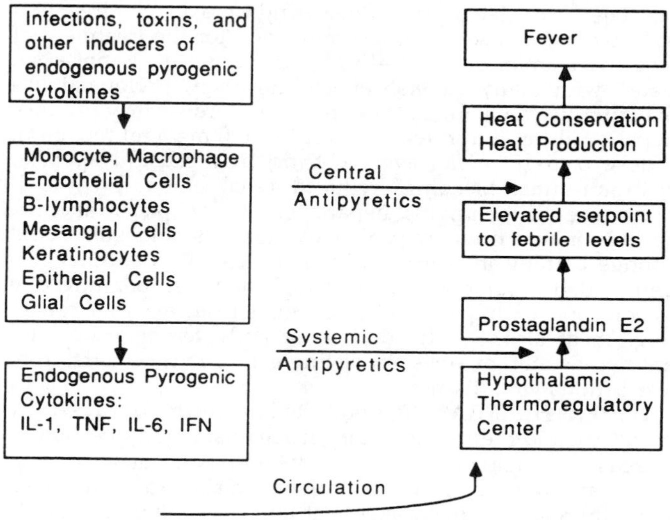

Figure 12–1. *Pathogenesis of fever.* Various infectious, immunologic, or toxin-related agents (exogenous pyrogens) induce the production of endogenous pyrogens by host inflammatory cells. These endogenous pyrogens are cytokines, such as interleukins (IL-1β, IL-1α, IL-6), tumor necrosis factors (TNF-α, TNF-β), and interferon-α (INF). Endogenous pyrogens induce fever within 10–15 min, whereas the febrile response to exogenous pyrogens (e.g., endotoxin) has a delayed onset requiring the synthesis and release of pyrogenic cytokines. Endogenous, pyrogenic cytokines directly stimulate the hypothalamus to produce prostaglandin E_2, which then resets the temperature regulatory set point; then neuronal transmission to the periphery leads to conservation and generation of heat, thus raising core body temperature. (From Dinarello C, Wolff S: Pathogenesis of fever. *In*: Mandell G, Douglas R, Bennett J: Principles and Practice of Infectious Diseases, 3rd ed. New York, Churchill Livingstone, 1990.)

of metabolism. Furthermore, children between the ages of 6 mo and 5 y are at increased risk of benign febrile seizures, whereas those with idiopathic epilepsy may have increased frequency of seizures as part of a nonspecific febrile illness (Sec. 20.20).

FEVER PATTERNS. The diurnal variation of temperature is usually preserved in patients with febrile illnesses. When this circadian rhythm is associated with tachycardia, chills (rigors), and sweating, a true rather than factitious fever should be suspected. Fever patterns may be *remittent* (daily elevated temperature returning to a baseline but above normal), *intermittent* (daily fever returning to normal), *hectic* (intermittent or remittent with temperature excursion of > 1.4° C [2.5° F]), or *sustained* or continuous (fluctuation of elevated temperature of < 0.3° C [0.5° F]). In most infectious or inflammatory processes the characteristics of the fever pattern are of little diagnostic importance. The fever associated with malaria, Hodgkin disease (Pel-Ebstein fever), and cyclic neutropenia may indicate the underlying condition.

TREATMENT. Antipyretic therapy is beneficial in high-risk patients who have chronic cardiopulmonary diseases, metabolic disorders, or neurologic diseases and in those who are at risk for febrile seizures. Other than providing symptomatic relief, antipyretic therapy does not alter the course of common infectious diseases in normal children, and thus its use remains controversial in these patients. *Hyperpyrexia* (> 41° C) places the patient at higher risk than lower temperature responses, is associated with severe infection, hypothalamic disorders, or central nervous system hemorrhage, and requires therapy (see later). High fever during pregnancy may be teratogenic.

Acetaminophen, aspirin, and nonsteroidal anti-inflammatory agents (e.g., ibuprofen) are inhibitors of hypothalamic cyclooxygenase, thus inhibiting PGE_2 synthesis. These drugs are all equally effective antipyretic agents. Because aspirin has been associated with Reye syndrome in children and adolescents, its use is not recommended for the treatment of fever. Acetaminophen, 10–15 mg/kg every 4 hr, is not associated with many adverse effects; however, prolonged use may produce renal injury, and massive overdose may produce hepatic failure. Ibuprofen (suspension 100 mg/5 mL, given in a dose of 5–10 mg/kg every 6–8 hr) may cause dyspepsia, gastrointestinal bleeding, reduced renal blood flow, and, rarely, aseptic meningitis, hepatic toxicity, or aplastic anemia. Serious injury from ibuprofen overdose is unusual. Tepid sponge bathing in warm water (not alcohol) is another recommended method of reducing high body temperature due to infection or hyperthermia resulting from external causes (e.g., heat stroke). The decline of body temperature after antipyretic therapy does not distinguish serious bacterial from less serious viral diseases.

HYPERTHERMIA. High body temperature not caused by hypothalamic thermoregulatory mechanisms may be due to increased endogenous heat production (vigorous exercise, malignant hyperthermia, neuroleptic malignant syndrome, hyperthyroidism), decreased heat loss (wrapping in multiple blanket layers, atropine intoxication), or prolonged exposure to high environmental temperatures (heat stroke) (see Sec. 6.37 and 20.52).

Malignant Hyperthermia. This autosomal dominant disorder (which has variable penetrance) may be suggested by a history of drug exposure, previously affected family members, exposure to high environmental temperature, or absence of the hypothalamic regulated circadian rhythm. It also occurs in patients with various myopathic disorders (see Sec. 21. 23).

Neuroleptic malignant syndrome occurs following exposure to phenothiazine-like agents and is indistinguishable from malignant hyperthermia. Therapy with dantrolene and supportive care are similar to the measures described for malignant hyperthermia.

DRUG FEVER. This disorder may be diagnosed when an elevated temperature coincides with drug administration and disappears when the drug is discontinued, and there is no other identified cause of the fever. Drug fever is not associated with a particular fever pattern and is not consistently associated with eosinophilia, rash, pruritus, or drug allergy. Drug fevers may develop at any time after therapy has been initiated, (median 8 days, average 21 days); the temperature elevation ranges from 38–43° C. Common agents producing drug fever include antibiotics (penicillin, cephalosporins), anticonvulsants (phenytoin, carbamazepine), antineoplastic agents (bleomycin, daunorubicin, cytarabine, L-asparaginase), and cardiovascular drugs (hydralazine, methyldopa [Aldomet], quinidine). *Treatment* includes withdrawal of the drug and, if continued therapy is needed, substitution of another agent. Fever usually resolves within 72 hr of stopping the drug. Subsequent exposure to the drug does not necessarily reproduce a drug fever.

Anonymous: Ibuprofen vs acetaminophen in children. Med Lett 31:109, 1989.
Caspe W, Nucci A, Cho S: Extreme hyperpyrexia in childhood. Presentation similar to hemorrhagic shock and encephalopathy. Clin Pediatr 28:76, 1989.
Dinarello C, Cannon J, Wolff S: New concepts on the pathogenesis of fever. Rev Infect Dis 10:168, 1988.
Guze B, Baxter L: Neuroleptic malignant syndrome. N Engl J Med 313:163, 1985.
Mackowiak P, LeMaistre C: Drug fever: A critical appraisal of conventional concepts. An analysis of 51 episodes in two Dallas hospitals and 97 episodes reported in the English literature. Ann Intern Med 106:728, 1987.
Musher D, Fainstein V, Young E, et al: Fever patterns. Their lack of clinical significance. Arch Intern Med 139:1225, 1979.
Pleet H, Graham JM, Smith DW: Central nervous system and facial defects associated with maternal hyperthermia at four to 14 weeks' gestation. Pediatrics 67:785, 1981.

12.2 FEVER AS A MANIFESTATION OF SERIOUS BACTERIAL DISEASE

Fever is a common manifestation of various infectious diseases, which have a wide range of severity. Benign febrile infections in normal hosts include bacterial diseases (otitis media, pharyngitis, impetigo) and viral disorders (rhinitis, pharyngitis, pneumonia) that respond to appropriate antibiotics and supportive therapy and are not life-threatening. Severe bacterial infections, if untreated, have a significant morbidity or mortality; such diseases include sepsis, pyogenic meningitis, bacterial pneumonia, osteoarticular infections, and pyelonephritis. Many febrile episodes are self-limited infections, which in a normal host manifesting minimal signs of toxicity require a careful history and physical examination with few if any laboratory tests. However, there are well-defined high-risk groups that, on the basis of age, associated diseases, or immunodeficiency status, require a more extensive evaluation and in certain situations prompt antibiotic therapy before a pathogen is identified (Table 12–1).

Fever Without a Focus

Fever without localizing signs or symptoms is a common diagnostic dilemma for pediatricians caring for infants less than 24 mo of age. Fever is usually of acute onset and is present for less than 1 wk. Infants less than 1 mo of age may acquire community pathogens but may also manifest late-onset bacterial diseases characteristic of neonatal sepsis (see Table 12–1). Fever and suspected sepsis among infants less than 3 mo of age are particularly difficult presenting signs to evaluate because of the high frequency of these problems in this age group, the broad range of neonatal, nosocomial, and community-acquired infections, and the many potential nonbacterial causes of a septic- or ill-appearing infant (Table 12–2).

TABLE 12–1. High-Risk Febrile Patients

Condition	Comment
Previously Normal Patients	
Neonate (< 28 days)	Group B streptococcus, *Escherichia coli*, *Listeria monocytogenes*, herpes simplex
Infants < 3 mo	Serious bacterial disease 10–15%, bacteremia 5%: seasonal viral illness—respiratory syncytial virus winter, enterovirus summer
Infants 3–24 mo	Risk of occult bacteremia increased if fever is > 40° C, WBC* < 5,000 or > 15,000, positive exposure history
Hyperpyrexia (> 41° C)	Meningitis, bacteremia, pneumonia. Heat stroke, hemorrhagic shock-encephalopathy syndrome
Fever with petechiae	Bacteremia, meningitis. Meningococcus, *Haemophilus influenzae* type b, pneumococcus
Immunocompromised Patients	
Sickle cell anemia	Pneumococcal sepsis, meningitis
Asplenia	Encapsulated bacteria
Complement/properdin deficiency	Meningococcal sepsis
Agammaglobulinemia	Bacteremia, sinopulmonary infection
AIDS†	Pneumococcus, *H. influenzae* type b, *Salmonella*
Congenital heart disease	Risk of endocarditis
Central venous line	*Staphylococcus aureus, S. epidermidis, Corynebacteria, Candida*
Malignancy	*Pseudomonas aeruginosa, S. aureus, S. epidermidis, Candida*

*WBC = white blood cell count.
†AIDS = acquired immunodeficiency syndrome.

Fever in an infant less than 3 mo of age should always suggest the possibility of serious bacterial disease. An infectious agent is identified in 70% of these infants, and the remainder are presumed to have had self-limiting nonspecific viral infections. Serious bacterial diseases are present in 10–15% of febrile infants less than 3 mo old. These infections include pyogenic meningitis, urinary tract infections, gastroenteritis, facial cellulitis, osteomyelitis, and septic arthritis. Bacteremia is present in 5% of febrile infants less than 3 mo old; organisms responsible for bacteremia include *Listeria monocytogenes* and group B streptococcus (late-onset neonatal sepsis-meningitis) and community-acquired pathogens such as *Salmonella* species (gastroenteritis), *Escherichia coli* (urinary tract infection), *Neisseria meningitidis, Haemophilus influenzae* type b (sepsis-meningitis), and *Staphylococcus aureus* (osteoarticular infection). Pyelonephritis is more common in uncircumcised male infants, neonates and infants with urinary tract anomalies, and young girls. Infants may not consistently demonstrate pyuria. Additional potential bacterial diseases in this age group include otitis media, pneumonia, omphalitis, and mastitis.

Viral pathogens are responsible for 40–60% of infections among infants less than 3 mo of age. In contrast to bacterial diseases, which have no seasonal pattern, viral diseases have a distinct pattern: respiratory syncytial virus and influenza A infections are more common during the winter, whereas enterovirus diseases (particularly aseptic meningitis) are more prevalent in the summer and fall.

The approach to the febrile patient under 3 mo of age should include a careful history and physical examination to identify specific diseases such as otitis media, gastroenteritis, cellulitis, and skeletal infection. Normal results of various laboratory tests combined with normal findings on physical examination may identify about 65% of infants who are at low risk for serious bacterial diseases. Results of these tests include a total white blood cell count of more than 5,000 or less than 15,000 cells/μL, an absolute band count of less than 1,500 cells/μL, a normal urinalysis, and a normal ESR. Nonetheless, these low-risk infants have a slightly increased risk of bacterial infection compared with nonfebrile infants even though this risk is low compared with the high-risk group.

The febrile or ill-appearing (toxic) infant less than 3 mo of age requires prompt hospitalization, cultures of blood, urine, and cerebrospinal fluid, and immediate therapy with intravenous antibiotics that are effective against age-specific pathogens. Ceftriaxone or cefotaxime and ampicillin (for *L. monocytogenes*) are effective antibiotics for the initial therapy of ill-appearing patients without focal signs. They are effective against bacterial pathogens producing meningitis, sepsis, urinary tract infection, and gastroenteritis.

Occult bacteremia (bacteremia without an obvious focus of infection) due to *Streptococcus pneumoniae, H. influenzae* type b, *N. meningitidis*, and *Salmonella* species occurs in relatively well appearing children between 3 and 24 mo of age. Although approximately 30% of febrile patients in this age group have no localizing manifestations of infection, only 4% of these children have occult bacteremia without localizing signs. Common bacterial infections among children between 3 and 24 mo who have localizing signs include otitis media, pneumonia, meningitis, osteomyelitis, gastroenteritis, and urinary tract infections. In addition, in this age group bacteremia is present in 11% of febrile children with pneumonia and in 1.5% of febrile children with otitis media or pharyngitis. *S. pneumoniae* is found on culture in 70–80% of children with occult bacteremia, whereas *H. influenzae* type b, *N. meningitidis*, and *Salmonella* species account for the remaining positive cultures.

Patients at increased risk for occult bacteremia include those with a temperature of greater than 39.4° C, a total white blood cell count of less than 5,000 or more than 15,000, and an abnormal observational score (Table 12–3). The incidence of bacteremia increases as the temperature and white blood cell counts increase: the incidence among infants between 6 and 24 mo is 10% if the temperature is higher than 40° C and the white blood cell count is more than 15,000. However, no combination of laboratory tests or clinical assessment is completely accurate in predicting the presence of occult bacteremia. Socioeconomic status, race, sex, and age (within the range of 3–24 mo) do not change the risk for occult bacteremia. The increased incidence of bacteremia among febrile 3- to 24-mo-old children may be due in part to a maturational immune deficiency in the production of opsonic IgG antibodies to the polysaccharide antigens present on these encapsulated bacteria.

Without therapy, occult bacteremia may resolve without sequelae, may persist, or may produce localized infections such as meningitis, pneumonia, cellulitis, or septic arthritis. The pattern of sequelae may be related to both host factors and the offending organism. In some children the occult bacteremic illness may represent the early signs of serious

TABLE 12–2. Differential Diagnosis of Sepsis

Infection
- Bacteremia/meningitis (pneumococcus, *Haemophilus influenzae* type b, meningococcus)
- Viral illness (influenza, enteroviruses, hemorrhagic fever group, HSV, RSV, CMV, EBV)
- Encephalitis (arbovirus, enterovirus, HSV)
- Rickettsiae (Rocky Mountain spotted fever, *Ehrlichia*, Q fever)
- Syphilis
- Vaccine reaction (pertussis, influenza virus, measles)
- Toxin-mediated reaction (toxic shock, staphylococcal scalded skin syndrome)

Cardiopulmonary
- Pneumonia (bacteria, virus, mycobacteria, fungi, allergic reaction)
- Pulmonary emboli
- Congestive heart failure
- Arrhythmia
- Pericarditis
- Myocarditis

Metabolic-Endocrine
- Adrenal insufficiency (adrenogenital syndrome, steroid withdrawal)
- Electrolyte disturbances (hypo-, hypernatremia, hypo-, hypercalcemia)
- Diabetes insipidus
- Diabetes mellitus
- Inborn errors of metabolism (organic acidosis, urea cycle, carnitine deficiency)
- Hypoglycemia
- Reye syndrome

Gastrointestinal
- Gastroenteritis with dehydration
- Volvulus
- Intussusception
- Appendicitis
- Peritonitis (spontaneous, perforation, dialysis)
- Hepatitis
- Hemorrhage

Hematologic
- Anemia (sickle cell, blood loss, nutritional)
- Methemoglobinemia
- Splenic sequestration crisis
- Leukemia-lymphoma

Neurologic
- Intoxication (drugs, carbon monoxide, intentional or accidental overdose)
- Intracranial hemorrhage
- Infant botulism
- Trauma (child abuse, nonintentional accidents)
- Guillain-Barré syndrome
- Myasthenia gravis

Other
- Anaphylaxis (food, drug, insect sting)
- Hemolytic-uremic syndrome
- Kawasaki syndrome
- Erythema multiforme
- Hemorrhagic shock-encephalopathy syndrome

HSV = herpes simplex virus; RSV = respiratory syncytial virus; CMV = cytomegalovirus; EBV = Epstein-Barr virus.

localized infection rather than a transient disease state. Bacteremia due to *H. influenzae* type b is often associated with a higher risk of localized serious infection than is bacteremia due to *S. pneumoniae. H. influenzae* bacteremia is of a higher grade, as determined by quantitative blood culture techniques than is pneumococcal bacteremia. Hospitalized children with *H. influenzae* type b bacteremia often develop focal infections such as meningitis, epiglottitis, cellulitis, or osteoarticular infection, whereas less than 5% of these bacteremias can be considered transient or occult. In contrast, among all patients with pneumococcal bacteremia (occult, symptomatic, or focal), the incidence of transient bacteremia with spontaneous resolution is 30–40%. Occult pneumococcal bacteremia, in a well-appearing child, has a higher rate of spontaneous resolution. The sequelae of occult pneumococcal bacteremia include a 1–2% incidence of meningitis, a 5% incidence of focal infections (otitis media, pneumonia), and a 15% incidence of persistent bacteremia.

The *treatment* of the toxic-appearing febrile patient between the ages of 3 and 24 mo who does not have focal signs of infection includes hospitalization, cultures of blood, urine, and cerebrospinal fluid, chest roentgenogram, and prompt institution of antibiotics in those patients considered at high risk for serious bacterial disease (septic shock, high-risk category in Table 12–1). Patients who appear well but are suspected of having occult bacteremia without an identifiable focus of infection may be sent home if careful follow-up and close observation are assured. The family should be instructed to return to the office or clinic within 24 hr if there is persistent fever or immediately if the child's condition deteriorates. Such patients can be managed as outpatients after a careful history and physical examination are performed and a blood culture is obtained. Additional helpful laboratory tests include a complete blood count, erythrocyte sedimentation rate (ESR), urinalysis, and chest roentgenogram, depending on the clinical manifestations. If indicated, a lumbar puncture should be performed. Meningitis developing after a lumbar puncture in patients with occult bacteremia does not represent inoculation of bacteria by the puncture. Rather, meningitis that occurs after the procedure is coincidental because the meningeal infection was developing prior to the lumbar puncture.

No antibiotic therapy is needed for the well-appearing child between 3 and 24 mo of age without a focus of infection who is suspected of having occult bacteremia. If pneumococcus is present in the first blood culture, the child should return to the physician as soon as the culture results have been reported. If the child appears well and is afebrile, and the physical examination is normal, a second blood culture should be obtained, and the child may return home without treatment. If the child appears ill and continues to have fever with no identifiable focus of infection, or if *H. influenzae* or *N. meningitidis* is present in the initial blood culture, the child should be evaluated for meningitis, undergo a repeat blood culture, and receive treatment in the hospital with appropriate antibiotics. If the child develops a localized infection, therapy is directed toward the specific pathogen at that particular site.

Antibiotic prophylaxis with ceftriaxone to prevent subsequent focal infection or persistent bacteremia has been proposed by some authorities. Such therapy has not been found to be consistently effective and has the added risks of producing drug allergy and antibiotic-associated diarrhea. Expectant outpatient management and close observation are indicated for well-appearing febrile patients without localizing signs who are suspected of having occult bacteremia.

Fever with Petechiae

Independent of age, fever with petechiae with or without localizing signs places the patient at high risk for life-threatening bacterial infection such as bacteremia, sepsis, and meningitis. Eight to 20% of patients with fever and petechiae have a serious bacterial infection, and 7–10% have meningococcal sepsis or meningitis. *H. influenzae* type b is less common than meningococcus but also produces serious bacterial illness. Management includes prompt hospitalization, culture of blood and cerebrospinal fluid, and administration of appropriate intravenous antibiotics that are effective against age-specific bacterial pathogens.

TABLE 12–3. Observational Scale for Prediction of Serious Illness of Bacterial and Nonbacterial Origin*

Observation Item	1 Normal	3 Moderate Impairment	5 Severe Impairment
Quality of cry	Strong with normal tone OR Content and not crying	Whimpering OR Sobbing	Weak OR Moaning OR High-pitched continual cry
Reaction to parent stimulation	Cries briefly then stops OR Content and not crying	Cries off and on	Hardly responds
State variation	If awake → stays awake OR If asleep and stimulated → wakes up quickly	Eyes close briefly → awake OR Awakes with prolonged stimulation	Falls asleep OR Will not rouse
Color	Pink	Pale extremities OR Acrocyanosis	Pale OR Cyanotic OR Mottled OR Ashen
Hydration	Skin normal, eyes normal AND Mucous membranes moist	Skin, eyes normal AND Mouth slightly dry	Skin doughy OR tented AND Dry mucous membranes AND/OR Sunken eyes
Response (talk, smile) to social overtures	Smiles OR Alerts (≤ 2 mo)	Brief smile OR Alerts briefly (≤ 2 mo)	No smile Face anxious, dull, expressionless OR No alerting (≤ 2 mo)

*From McCarthy P, Sharpe MR, Spiesel SZ, et al: Obstruction scales to identify serious illness in febrile children. Reproduced by permission of Pediatrics, Vol 70, p 802. Copyright 1982.

Fever in Patients with Sickle Cell Anemia

Infection is the most common cause of death among children with sickle cell anemia (Sec. 16.19). The incidence of infection is greatest among infants younger than 2 yr old. The increased risk of infection in these children is due in part to functional asplenia and a defect in the properdin (alternate complement) pathway. Fever without a focus is a common presenting sign of sepsis or meningitis due to pneumococcus in patients with sickle cell anemia. *H. influenzae* type b (meningitis), *Salmonella* (osteomyelitis), and *E. coli* (pyelonephritis) are additional pathogens that may present initially as fever without localizing signs.

Treatment of patients with sickle cell hemoglobinopathies requires prompt hospitalization, culture of blood and, if indicated, cerebrospinal fluid, stool, and bone, and administration of antibiotics effective against the common pathogens affecting these patients (e.g., ceftriaxone). *Prevention* of pneumococcal sepsis is possible by instituting long-term penicillin therapy continued until adolescence (oral daily or long-acting intramuscular, every 3–4 wk). Alternatively, oral daily amoxicillin has been employed to add coverage against *H. influenzae* type b. Pneumococcal and *H. influenzae* vaccines may provide additional protection, but these vaccines should not be used in place of chronic antibiotic therapy.

Hyperpyrexia

Temperatures higher than 41° C are associated with an increased risk of bacterial meningitis, pneumonia, and bacteremia. Serious bacterial diseases may be present in 10–35% of young patients; bacteremia is noted in 12% and meningitis in 10%. Although patients may have localizing signs indicative of pneumonia, sinusitus, pharyngitis, otitis media, and pyelonephritis, others may have no localizing signs, appear nontoxic, and produce normal results on laboratory tests.

The care of patients with hyperpyrexia must be individualized and is determined by age (infants < 24 mo have higher risk of bacteremia and meningitis), clinical appearance, and results of physical examination and initial laboratory tests including ESR, leukocyte count, chest roentgenogram, urinalysis, and, if indicated, cerebrospinal fluid analysis.

Fever Without a Focus in Immunosuppressed Patients

See Sec. 12.13.

ROBERT M. KLIEGMAN
RICHARD E. BEHRMAN

Anbar RD, Richardson-de Corral V, O'Malley PJ: Difficulties in universal application of criteria identifying infants at low risk for serious bacterial infection. J Pediatr 109:483, 1986.
Anonymous: Splenectomy—A long-term risk of infection. Lancet 2:928, 1985.
Baker RC, Sequin JH, Leslie N, et al: Fever and petechiae in children. Pediatrics 84:1051, 1989.
Bonadio WA, Grunske L, Smith DS: Systemic bacterial infections in children with fever greater than 41° C. Pediatr Infect Dis J 8:120, 1989.
Bonadio WA, Hegenbarth M, Zachariason M: Correlating reported fever in young infants with subsequent temperature patterns and rate of serious bacterial infections. Pediatr Infect Dis J 9:158, 1990.
Dagan R, Hall CB, Powell KR, et al: Epidemiology and laboratory diagnosis of infection with viral and bacterial pathogens in infants hospitalized for suspected sepsis. J Pediatr 115:351, 1989.
Jaffe DM, Tanz RR, Davis AT, et al: Antibiotic administration to treat possible occult bacteremia in febrile children. N Engl J Med 317:1175, 1987.
Kramer M, Naimark L, Roberts-Braver R, et al: Risks and benefits of paracetamol antipyresis in young children with fever of presumed viral origin. Lancet 337:591, 1991.
Krober MS, Bass JW, Powell JM, et al: Bacterial and viral pathogens causing fever in infants less than 3 months old. Am J Dis Child 139:889, 1985.
Marcinak JG: Evaluation of children with fever ≥ 104° F in an emergency department. Pediatr Emerg Care 4:92, 1988.
McCarthy PL, Sharpe MR, Spiesel SZ, et al: Observation scales to identify serious illness in febrile children. Pediatrics 70:802, 1982.
McLellan D, Giebink GS: Perspectives on occult bacteremia in children. J Pediatr 109:1, 1986.
Powell KR: Evaluation and management of febrile infants younger than 60 days of age. Pediatr Infect Dis J 9:153, 1990.
Zarkowsky HS, Gallagher D, Gill FM, et al: Cooperative Study of Sickle Cell Disease: Bacteremia in sickle hemoglobinopathies. J Pediatr 109:579, 1986.

12.3 FEVER OF UNKNOWN ORIGIN

Many physicians use the term fever of unknown origin (FUO) to describe the condition of any febrile child admitted to the hospital with neither an apparent site of infection nor a noninfectious diagnosis. In most of these children the development of additional clinical manifestations over a relatively short time period makes the infectious nature of the illness apparent. Therefore, the term is better reserved for children with (1) a history of fever of more than 1 wk duration (2–3 wk if an adolescent), (2) fever also documented in the hospital, and (3) no apparent diagnosis after an investigation of 1 wk in the hospital.

The principal causes of FUO in children, using more restrictive criteria, are infections and autoimmune (collagen-vascular) diseases. Neoplastic disorders should also be seriously considered, although most children with malignancies do not have fever alone. If the patient is receiving drugs, the possibility of drug fever should also be considered. The latter is not usually associated with other symptoms, and temperature remains elevated at a relatively constant level. Withdrawal of the drug is associated with resolution of the fever, generally within 72 hr (but when drugs, such as iodides, are excreted over a prolonged period of time, fever may persist for up to 1 mo after drug withdrawal).

Most fevers of unknown or unrecognized origin result from common diseases that may be atypical in their presentations. In some cases the presentation of a fever of unknown origin is typical of the disease (juvenile rheumatoid arthritis), but a definitive diagnosis can be established only after prolonged observation because there are no associated findings on physical examination and all laboratory results are negative or normal.

In the United States the systemic infectious diseases implicated most consistently in children with FUO (by the above more rigorous definition) are salmonellosis, tularemia, tuberculosis, rickettsial diseases, brucellosis, syphilis, leptospirosis, rat-bite fever, atypical prolonged presentations of common viral diseases, infectious mononucleosis, cytomegalic inclusion disease, and hepatitis. Although human immunodeficiency virus type 1 (HIV-1) infection produces fever, acquired immunodeficiency syndrome (AIDS) alone is not usually responsible for FUO. Patients who have AIDS and FUO frequently also have an opportunistic infection with a common or unusual pathogen.

Table 12–4 lists diseases that have presented as FUO in children with sufficient frequency to merit serious consideration. Specific signs and symptoms of each of these diseases and methods of diagnosis are detailed elsewhere.

Juvenile rheumatoid arthritis and systemic lupus erythematosus are the collagen diseases associated most frequently with FUO. Fever should be documented in the hospital by an individual who remains with the patient while the temperature is taken to rule out *factitious fever*. The latter may be due to inoculation (by patient or parent) of pyrogenic material or manipulation of the thermometer. Prolonged and continuous observation of the patient is imperative. FUO lasting more than 6 mo is uncommon in children and should suggest granulomatosis or autoimmune disease. Repetitive evaluation including history, physical examination, and roentgenographic studies may be required.

Diagnostic Clues in the Child with Fever of Unknown Origin

HISTORY. The age of the patient is helpful. Children under 6 yr of age often have a respiratory or genitourinary tract infection, localized infection (abscess, osteomyelitis), juvenile rheumatoid arthritis, or, rarely, leukemia. Adolescent patients are more likely to have tuberculosis, inflammatory bowel disease, autoimmune processes, and lymphoma, in addition to the causes of FUO found in younger children. A history of *exposure to wild or domestic animals* should be solicited. The incidence of zoonotic infections in the United States has been increasing, and they frequently are acquired from pets that are not overtly ill. For example, immunization of dogs against specific disorders such as leptospirosis may prevent canine disease but does not always prevent the animal from carrying and shedding leptospires, which may be transmitted to household contacts. A history of ingestion of rabbit or squirrel meat may provide a clue to the diagnosis of oropharyngeal, glandular, or typhoidal tularemia. A history of tick bite or travel to tick- or parasite-infested areas should be obtained.

A history of *pica* should be sought. Ingestion of dirt is a particularly important clue to infection with *Toxocara* (visceral larva migrans) or *Toxoplasma gondii* (toxoplasmosis).

A history of *travel* reaching back to the birth of the child should be sought. There may be re-emergence of malaria, histoplasmosis, and coccidioidomycosis years after visiting or living in an endemic area. It is important to ask about prophylactic immunizations and precautions taken by the individual against the ingestion of contaminated water or food during foreign travel (Sec. 5.6). Rocks, dirt, and artifacts from geographically distant regions that have been collected and brought into the home as souvenirs may serve as vectors of disease.

A *medication* history should be pursued rigorously. This should include over-the-counter preparations and topical agents, including eye drops (atropine-induced fever).

The *genetic background* of the patient also is important. Descendants of the Ulster Scots may have fever of unknown origin because they are afflicted with nephrogenic diabetes insipidus. Familial dysautonomia (Riley-Day syndrome, a disorder in which hyperthermia is recurrent) is more frequent among Jews than other population groups.

PHYSICAL EXAMINATION. Sweating in a febrile child should be noted. The continuing absence of sweat in the presence of an elevated or changing body temperature suggests dehydration from vomiting, diarrhea, or central or nephrogenic diabetes insipidus. It also should suggest anhidrotic ectodermal dysplasia, familial dysautonomia, or exposure to atropine.

Red, weeping eyes may be a sign of collagen-vascular disease, particularly polyarteritis nodosa. Palpebral conjunctivitis in the febrile patient may be a clue to measles, coxsackieviral infection, tuberculosis, infectious mononucleosis, lymphogranuloma venereum, or cat-scratch or Newcastle disease virus infection. In contrast, bulbar conjunctivitis in a child with fever of unknown origin suggests Kawasaki syndrome or leptospirosis. Petechial conjunctival hemorrhages suggest endocarditis. Uveitis suggests sarcoidosis, juvenile rheumatoid arthritis, systemic lupus erythematosus, Kawasaki syndrome, Behçet syndrome, and vasculitis. Chorioretinitis suggests cytomegalovirus, toxoplasmosis, and syphilis. Proptosis suggests orbital tumor, thyrotoxicosis, metastasis (neuroblastoma), orbital infection, Wegener granulomatosis, or pseudotumor. A careful ophthalmic examination is important in most patients with FUO.

Fever of unknown origin is sometimes due to hypothalamic dysfunction. A clue to this disorder is failure of pupillary constriction due to absence of the sphincter constrictor muscle of the eye. This muscle develops embryologically when hypothalamic structure and function also are undergoing differentiation.

Lack of tears or an absent corneal reflex may suggest fever resulting from familial dysautonomia. A smooth tongue may reflect absence of fungiform papillae and also suggests this diagnosis.

Tenderness to tapping over the sinuses and teeth should be sought, and the sinuses should be transilluminated.

Oral candidosis may be a clue to various disorders of the immune system.

Fever blisters are common findings in patients with pneumococcal, streptococcal, malarial, and rickettsial infection.

TABLE 12–4. Causes of Fever of Unknown Origin in Children

Infections

- ***Bacterial Diseases***
  - Specific organism causing systemic disease
    - Bartonellosis
    - Brucellosis
    - *Campylobacter*
    - Cat-scratch disease
    - Salmonellosis
    - *Streptobacillus moniliformis*
    - Tuberculosis
    - Tularemia
  - Localized infections
    - Abscesses: abdominal, dental, hepatic, pelvic, perinephric, rectal, subphrenic
    - Cholangitis
    - Endocarditis
    - Mastoiditis
    - Osteomyelitis
    - Pneumonia
    - Pyelonephritis
    - Sinusitis
- ***Spirochete***
  - *Borrelia* (borreliosis: *B. recurrentis*, *B. burgdorferi*)
  - Leptospirosis
  - Lyme disease
  - Spirillium minor
  - Syphilis
- ***Viral Diseases***
  - Cytomegalovirus
  - Hepatitis
  - Human immunodeficiency virus
  - Infectious mononucleosis (Epstein-Barr virus)
  - Unidentified presumed virus
- ***Chlamydial Diseases***
  - Lymphogranuloma venereum
  - Psittacosis
- ***Rickettsial Diseases***
  - *Ehrlichia canis*
  - Q fever
  - Rocky Mountain spotted fever
- ***Fungal Diseases***
  - Blastomycosis (nonpulmonary)
  - Coccidioidomycosis (disseminated)
  - Histoplasmosis (disseminated)
- ***Parasitic Diseases***
  - Babesiosis
  - Giardiasis
  - Malaria
  - Toxoplasmosis
  - Trypanosomiasis
  - Visceral larva migrans

Autoimmune Hypersensitivity Diseases

- Drug fever
- Hypersensitivity pneumonitis
- Juvenile rheumatoid arthritis
- Polyarteritis nodosa
- Rheumatic fever
- Serum sickness
- Systemic lupus erythematosus
- Undefined vasculitis

Neoplasms

- Atrial myxoma
- Hodgkin disease
- Leukemia
- Lymphoma
- Neuroblastoma

Granulomatous Diseases

- Granulomatous hepatitis
- Sarcoidosis
- Crohn disease

Familial-Hereditary Diseases

- Anhidrotic ectodermal dysplasia
- Fabry disease
- Familial dysautonomia
- Familial Mediterranean fever
- Hypertriglyceridemia
- Ichthyosis

Miscellaneous

- Behçet syndrome
- Chronic active hepatitis
- Diabetes insipidus (non-nephrogenic and nephrogenic)
- Factitious fever
- Hypothalamic-central fever
- Infantile cortical hyperostosis
- Inflammatory bowel disease
- Kawasaki disease
- Pancreatitis
- Periodic fever
- Pulmonary embolism
- Thyrotoxicosis

Undiagnosed Fever

- Persistent
- Recurrent
- Resolved

They also are common in children with meningococcal meningitis (which usually does not present as FUO) but rarely are seen in children with meningococcemia. Fever blisters also are rarely seen with salmonella or staphylococcal infections.

Repetitive chills and temperature spikes are common in children with septicemia (regardless of etiology), particularly when associated with renal disease, liver or biliary disease, endocarditis, malaria, brucellosis, rat-bite fever, or loculated collections of pus.

Hyperemia of the pharynx, with or without exudate, may suggest infectious mononucleosis, cytomegalic inclusion disease, toxoplasmosis, salmonellosis, tularemia, Kawasaki syndrome, or leptospirosis.

The muscles and bones should be palpated carefully. Point tenderness over a bone may suggest occult osteomyelitis or bone marrow invasion from neoplastic disease. Tenderness over the trapezius muscle may be a clue to a subdiaphragmatic abscess. Generalized muscle tenderness suggests dermatomyositis, trichinosis, polyarteritis, or mycoplasma or arboviral infection.

Rectal examination may reveal pararectal adenopathy or tenderness, which suggests a deep pelvic abscess, iliac adenitis, or pelvic osteomyelitis. A guaiac test should be obtained on any stool found on the examining finger; occult blood loss may suggest granulomatous colitis or ulcerative colitis as the cause of FUO.

The general activity of the patient and the presence or absence of rashes should be noted.

Hyperactive deep tendon reflexes may suggest thyrotoxicosis as the cause of FUO.

LABORATORY STUDIES. These should make use of the diagnostic tests most likely to provide a prompt definitive diagnosis; ordering a large number of tests in every child with fever of unknown origin according to a predetermined sequence may waste time and money. Alternatively, prolonged hospitalization for sequential tests may be more costly. The tempo of diagnostic evaluation should be adjusted to the tempo of the illness; haste may be imperative in a critically ill patient, but if the illness is more chronic, the evaluation can proceed more slowly and deliberately.

Routine *white blood cell counts* and *urinalyses* are generally of minimal diagnostic value in children who fulfill a rigorous definition of FUO. An absolute neutrophil count below 5,000 mm^3, however, is evidence against nonoverwhelming bacterial infection other than typhoid. Conversely, patients with more than 10,000 polymorphonuclear leukocytes or more than 500 nonsegmented polymorphonuclear leukocytes/mm^3 have a high chance of having a severe bacterial infection.

Direct examination of the blood smear treated with Giemsa or Wright stain may reveal malaria, trypanosomiasis, babesiosis, or relapsing fever.

An elevated *erythrocyte sedimentation rate* (>30 mm/hr, Westergren method) indicates inflammation and the need for further evaluation for infectious, autoimmune, or malignant diseases. A low ESR does not eliminate the possibility of infection or juvenile rheumatoid arthritis, but an ESR of greater than 100 suggests tuberculosis, Kawasaki syndrome, malignancy, or autoimmune disease.

Blood cultures should be obtained aerobically and anaerobically. Repeated blood cultures may be required to diagnose endocarditis, osteomyelitis, or deep-seated abscesses producing bacteremia. Polymicrobial bacteremia suggests factitious self-induced infection or gastrointestinal pathology. The isolation of leptospires, *Francisella,* or *Yersinia* may require selective media or specific conditions not routinely employed. *Urine culture* should be obtained routinely.

Tuberculin *skin testing* should be performed carefully with polysorbate 80 (Tween) stabilized purified protein derivative (PPD) that has been kept appropriately refrigerated. Other antigens (*Candida, mumps) should be placed to test for anergy.*

Roentgenographic examination of the chest, sinuses, mastoids, or gastrointestinal tract may be suggested by specific historical or physical findings. Roentgenographic evaluation of the gastrointestinal tract for inflammatory bowel disease may be helpful in evaluating selected children with FUO and no other localizing signs or symptoms.

Examination of the *bone marrow* may reveal leukemia; metastatic neoplasm; mycobacterial, fungal, or parasitic diseases; and histiocytosis or other storage diseases. If a bone marrow aspirate is performed, cultures for bacteria, *Mycobacterium,* and fungi should be obtained.

Serologic tests may aid in the diagnosis of infectious mononucleosis, cytomegaloviral disease, toxoplasmosis, salmonellosis, tularemia, brucellosis, leptospirosis, and, on some occasions, juvenile rheumatoid arthritis.

Radioactive scans may be helpful in detecting osteomyelitis and abdominal abscesses. Gallium citrate (^{67}Ga) localizes in inflammatory tissues (leukocytes) associated with tumors or abscesses. ^{99m}Tc phosphate is useful for detecting osteomyelitis before plain roentgenograms demonstrate bone lesions. Indium-III granulocytes or iodinated IgG may be useful in detecting localized pyogenic processes (see Sec. 6.56). *Echocardiograms* may suggest the presence of vegetations on the leaflets of heart valves as in subacute bacterial endocarditis. *Ultrasonography* may identify intra-abdominal abscesses of the liver, subphrenic space, pelvis, or spleen.

Total body computed tomography (CT) or MRI scanning permits the detection of neoplasms and collections of purulent material without the use of surgical exploration or radioisotopes. CT scanning is helpful in identifying lesions of the head, neck, chest, retroperitoneal spaces, liver, spleen, intra-abdominal and intrathoracic lymph nodes, kidneys, pelvis, and mediastinum. CT or ultrasound-guided aspiration or biopsy of suspicious lesions has reduced the need for exploratory laparotomy or thoracotomy.

Biopsy is occasionally helpful in establishing a diagnosis of FUO. Bronchoscopy, laparoscopy, mediastinoscopy, and gastrointestinal endoscopy may provide direct visualization and biopsy material when organ-specific manifestations are present.

TREATMENT. Fever and infection in children are not synonymous; antibiotics should not be used as antipyretics, and empiric trials of medication should generally be avoided. An exception may be the use of antituberculous treatment in critically ill children with possible disseminated tuberculosis. Empiric trials of other antibiotics may be dangerous and can obscure the diagnosis of endocarditis, meningitis, parameningeal infection, or osteomyelitis. Hospitalization may be required for laboratory or roentgenographic studies that are unavailable or impractical in an ambulatory setting, for more careful observation, or for temporary relief of parental anxiety. After a complete evaluation, antipyretics may be indicated to control fever.

PROGNOSIS. The child with FUO has a better prognosis than that reported for adults. Outcome in the child is dependent on the primary disease process, which is usually an atypical presentation of a common childhood illness. In many cases no diagnosis can be established, but fever abates spontaneously. In as many as 25% of cases in which fever persists, the cause of the fever remains unclear even after thorough evaluation.

Brusch JL, Weinstein L: Fever of unknown origin. Med Clin North Am 72:1247, 1988.
Feigin RD, Shearer WT: Fever of unknown origin in children. Curr Probl Pediatr 6:1, 1976.
Larson EB, Featherstone HJ, Petersdorf RG: Fever of undetermined origin: Diagnosis and follow-up of 105 cases, 1970–1980. Medicine 61:269, 1982.

12.4 FEVER ASSOCIATED WITH DISEASES OF THE CENTRAL NERVOUS SYSTEM

Fever may be associated with a variety of diseases that affect the central nervous system. Bacteria may produce pyogenic meningitis in the neonate (group B streptococcus, *E. coli, L. monocytogenes*) or older child (meningococcus, *H. influenzae* type b, pneumococcus). Nonpyogenic or aseptic meningitis is also associated with various infectious and noninfectious disorders (Table 12–5). In children, acute infection of the central nervous system is the most common cause of fever associated with signs and symptoms of central nervous system involvement.

Regardless of etiology, most patients with acute central nervous system infection present similar signs and symptoms, including fever, headache, nausea, vomiting, anorexia, restlessness, and irritability. Photophobia, back pain, nuchal rigidity, obtundation, stupor, coma, seizures, and focal neurologic signs also may be noted.

The neurologic expression of various parameningeal infections depends, to some extent, on the site of the lesion or lesions, which in turn is determined by the manner in which the intracranial or intraspinal infection was established. Ear infections may lead to epidural, subdural, or parenchymatous lesions of the adjacent temporal lobe or of the cerebellum. Infection of the frontal sinuses and, less often, of the maxillary sinuses may be followed by cerebral abscess, corticothrombophlebitis, or subdural empyema. Metastatic cerebral lesions may be solitary or multiple but usually occur in the distribu-

TABLE 12–5. Clinical Conditions and Infectious Agents Associated with Aseptic Meningitis*

Agents/Conditions	Example
Viruses	Enteroviruses (coxsackieviruses, echoviruses, polioviruses)
	Arboviruses (Eastern equine encephalitis, Western equine encephalitis, Venezuelan equine encephalitis, St. Louis encephalitis, California encephalitis, Colorado tick fever)
	Mumps
	Herpes simplex
	Others (HIV, varicella, Epstein-Barr virus, lymphocytic choriomeningitis, measles, rubella, rabies, influenza, parainfluenza)
Bacterial meningitis	*Mycobacterium tuberculosis*
	Pyogenic or inadequately treated
	Leptospira sp. (leptospirosis)
	Treponema pallidum (syphilis)
	Borrelia sp. (relapsing fever)
	Borrelia burgdorferi (Lyme disease)
	Nocardia sp. (nocardiosis)
	Cat-scratch disease
Bacterial parameningeal focus	Sinusitis, mastoiditis, brain abscess, subdural-epidural empyema, cranial osteomyelitis
Rickettsia	*R. rickettsii* (Rocky Mountain spotted fever), *Ehrlichia*
Mycoplasma	*M. pneumoniae, M. hominis*
Chlamydia	*C. trachomatis*
Fungi	*Coccidioides immitis* (coccidioidomycosis)
	B. dermatitidis (blastomycosis)
	Cryptococcus neoformans (cryptococcosis)
	Histoplasma capsulatum (histoplasmosis)
	Candida albicans (moniliasis)
Protozoa	*Toxoplasma gondii* (toxoplasmosis)
	Acanthamoeba; Naegleria
	Malaria
Other parasites (meningitis)	*Angiostrongylus cantonensis* (eosinophilic)
	Trichinella spiralis (trichinosis)
	Strongyloides stercoralis (hyperinfection)
	Schistosomiasis
Presumed infection	Kawasaki disease
Malignancy	Leukemia, lymphoma, CNS tumor
Postinfectious causes	Vaccines: rabies, influenza, measles; demyelinating or allergic encephalitis
Immune diseases	Sarcoidosis, Behçet syndrome, lupus erythematosus, vasculitis
Drugs	Intrathecal injections (contrast media, serum, antibiotics, antineoplastic agents)
	Nonsteroidal anti-inflammatory agents
	OKT3 monoclonal antibodies
	Carbamazepine
	Trimethoprim-sulfamethoxazole
	Azathioprine
Miscellaneous	Heavy metal poisoning
	Foreign bodies (shunt, reservoir)
	Subarachnoid hemorrhage
	Intraventricular hemorrhage (neonate)
	Familial hemophagocytic syndrome

*Modified from Cherry JD: Aseptic meningitis and viral meningitis. *In:* Feigin RD, Cherry JD (eds): Textbook of Pediatric Infectious Diseases, 2nd ed. Philadelphia, WB Saunders, 1987, p 479.

tion of the middle cerebral artery. Bacterial endocarditis leads most often to embolic occlusion of medium-sized vessels with subsequent infarction of the brain. This may result in secondary abscess formation or in the development of a mycotic aneurysm that may declare itself by a subarachnoid hemorrhage.

The diagnosis of acute bacterial meningitis and its differentiation from other central nervous system disorders associated with fever depend on careful examination of cerebrospinal fluid (CSF) obtained by lumbar puncture. If increased intracranial pressure is associated with pyogenic central nervous system infection, broad-spectrum antibiotics may be given and a CT scan of the head obtained prior to performing a lumbar puncture. Cerebrospinal fluid findings characteristic of various central nervous system disorders associated with fever are shown in Table 12–6.

A variety of chemical or immunologic tests may be performed on cerebrospinal fluid, blood, or urine to aid in differentiating bacterial from viral infections of the central nervous system in patients whose bacterial and viral cerebrospinal fluid cultures are negative. (See later sections discussing specific etiologic agents.) Cerebrospinal fluid CRP and tumor necrosis factor are usually elevated in patients with bacterial meningitis compared with levels in patients with viral meningitis.

Unfortunately, in some cases a definitive diagnosis cannot be made on the basis of either clinical or cerebrospinal fluid findings, and a thorough search for foci of infection adjacent to or remote from the meninges must be performed. The extent of dysfunction of the nervous system must be defined by repeated neurologic examinations and appropriate laboratory studies. The presence of focal neurologic findings, a lymphocytic reaction within cerebrospinal fluid in which the glucose concentration is normal, associated infection of the ears, sinuses, or lung, or the presence of bronchiectasis or cyanotic heart disease should heighten suspicion of brain abscess, epidural or subdural infection, venous thrombophlebitis, or venous sinus thrombosis.

RALPH D. FEIGIN

TABLE 12–6. Cerebrospinal Fluid Findings in Various Central Nervous System Disorders Associated with Fever

Condition	Pressure (mm H_2O)	Leukocytes mm³	Protein (mg/dL)	Glucose	Comments
Normal	50–80	<5, 75% lymphocytes	20–45	>50 mg/dL or 75% blood glucose	
Acute bacterial meningitis	Usually elevated	100–60,000+; usually a few thousand; PMNs predominate	Usually 100–500	Depressed compared with blood glucose; usually <40 mg/dL	Organism may be seen on Gram stain and recovered by culture
Partially treated bacterial meningitis	Normal or elevated	1–10,000; PMNs usual but mononuclear cells may predominate if pretreated for extended period of time	100+	Depressed or normal	Organisms may or may not be seen; in disease due to *Haemophilus influenzae,* organism may grow despite pretreatment; pretreatment may render sterile CSF of patients with pneumococcal and meningococcal disease
Tuberculous meningitis	Usually elevated; may be low due to block in advanced stages	10–500; PMNs early but lymphocytes predominate through most of course	100–500; may be higher in presence of block	<50 mg/dL usual in most cases; decreases with time if treatment is not provided	Acid-fast organisms may be seen on smear; organism can be recovered in culture
Fungal meningitis	Usually elevated	25–500; mononuclear cells predominate except PMNs early	25–500	<50 mg/dL, decreases with time if treatment is not provided	Budding yeast may be seen; organism may be recovered in culture; India ink preparation may be positive in cryptococcal disease
Syphilis (acute) and leptospirosis	Usually elevated	200–500, usually lymphocytes	50–200	Generally normal	Positive CSF serology; spirochetes not demonstrable by usual techniques of smear or culture; darkfield examination may be positive
Viral meningitis or meningo-encephalitis	Normal or slightly elevated	PMNs early; rarely more than 1,000 cells except in Eastern equine encephalomyelitis, in which counts of up to 20,000 have been recorded; mononuclear cells predominate during most of course	50–200	Generally normal; may be depressed to <40 mg/dL in various viral diseases, particularly mumps (15–20% of cases)	Enteroviruses may be recovered from CSF by appropriate viral cultures
Sarcoidosis	Normal or elevated slightly	0–100; mononuclear	40–100	Normal	No specific findings
Amebiasis	Elevated	500–20,000+; PMNs predominate	50–100	Normal or slightly depressed	Amebae may be seen rarely in CSF
Chemical (drugs, dermoids, cysts, myelography dye)	Usually elevated	100–1,000+; PMNs predominate	50–100	20–40 mg/dL	Epithelial cells may be seen within CSF in some children with dermoids by use of polarized light
Subacute bacterial endocarditis with embolism	Normal or slightly elevated	0–100; mixed PMNs and mononuclear cells	50–100	Normal	No organisms on smear or culture
Subdural empyema	Usually elevated	100–5,000; PMNs predominate	100–500	Normal	No organisms on smear or culture of CSF unless meningitis also present; organism found on tap of subdural fluid
Brain abscess	Usually elevated	10–200; fluid rarely acellular; lymphocytes predominate; if abscess ruptures into ventricle, PMNs predominate and cell count may reach >100,000	75–500	Normal unless abscess ruptures into ventricular system	No organisms on smear or culture unless abscess ruptures into ventricular system
Cerebral epidural abscess	Normal to slightly elevated	0–500; lymphocytes predominate	50–200	Normal	No organisms on smear or culture
Spinal epidural abscess	Usually low, with spinal block	10–100; lymphocytes predominate	50–400	Normal	No organisms on smear or culture
Thrombophlebitis (sometimes with subdural empyema)	Normal or elevated	0–500; PMNs and lymphocytes	50–200	Normal	No organisms on smear or culture
Acute hemorrhagic encephalitis	Usually elevated	0–1,000; PMNs predominate	100–500	Normal	No organisms on smear or culture
Collagen-vascular disease	Slightly elevated	0–500; PMNs may predominate; lymphocytes may be present	100	Normal or slightly depressed	No organisms on smear or culture; LE preparation may be positive
Tumor, leukemia	Slightly elevated to very high	0–100+; mononuclear or blast cells	50–1,000	May be depressed to 20–40 mg/dL	Cytology may be positive

PMN = polymorphonuclear leukocyte; CSF = cerebrospinal fluid; LE = lupus erythematosus cell.

Addy DP: When not to do a lumbar puncture. Arch Dis Child 62:873, 1987.
Spanos A, Harrell FE, Durack DT: Differential diagnosis of acute meningitis. An analysis of the predictive value of initial observations. JAMA 262:2700, 1989.
Talan DA, Hoffman JR, Yoshikawa TT, et al: Role of empiric parenteral antibiotics prior to lumbar puncture in suspected bacterial meningitis: State of the art. Rev Infect Dis 10:365, 1988.

12.5 RASH

Rashes with fever accompany many infectious diseases. They may be so characteristic of a particular disease that a specific diagnosis can be made without difficulty, but frequently the skin manifestations produced are common to many infections (Table 12–7). Skin lesions may be the result of direct inoculation of the skin (anthrax or tularemia); hematogenous dissemination of micro-organisms (septicemia due to meningococci, rickettsiae, or other bacteria); or contiguous spread from adjacent foci of infection (impetigo, herpetic lesions). The skin also may reflect the effect of toxins (scarlet fever), antigen-antibody reactions (rheumatic fever), or delayed hypersensitivity to the infecting agent (erythema nodosum). Responses to toxins, pathogens, or inflammation include vasodilation, vaso-occlusion, extravasation of erythrocytes, vasculitis, and necrosis.

Rashes can be classified as macular eruptions, erythematous maculopapular eruptions, papulovesicular or bullous eruptions, petechial or hemorrhagic eruptions, ulcerative eruptions, and nodular eruptions. Many infections produce skin lesions that fall into more than one of these categories. Some infectious diseases and their agents are also associated with erythema multiforme eruptions (Sec. 23.13 and Table 12–7) or with erythema nodosum.

The course of the illness and the characteristics of the rash may provide enough information to create a differential diagnosis, establish a specific etiology, or suggest tissue to be obtained for biopsy and culture. Further, the history, physical appearance, and characteristics of the rash help to differentiate acute life-threatening illnesses (meningococcemia, toxic shock syndrome) from more benign diseases (fifth disease, exanthem subitum). Important historical information includes the onset of the rash relative to the onset of the illness, the progression of the rash through various cutaneous stages (macular, papular, purpuric), its distribution and progression through various locations (trunk, face, extremities, palms and soles), the existence and nature of exposure (drugs, travel, sun, sick contacts, pets, wild animals, season, insect bites, rural vs urban environment, sexual activity), past immunizations, prior illness (congenital heart disease, immunocompromised conditions, allergies), and the severity of the current acute illness. The physical examination should focus on abnormalities of vital signs (tachycardia, hypotension, degree of fever), general appearance, signs of toxicity, characteristics of the rash (see Table 12–7); the presence of meningismus, lymphadenopathy, mucosal (oral, conjunctival, genital) lesions, hepatosplenomegaly, arthritis, signs of an underlying chronic illness (inflammatory bowel diseases, AIDS, malignancy); and signs suggestive of a noninfectious disease. A

TABLE 12–7. Differential Diagnosis of Fever and Rash

Lesion	Pathogen or Associated Factor
Maculopapular or macular rash	***Viruses:*** Measles, rubella, roseola, fifth disease (parvovirus), exanthem subitum (herpes simplex virus 6), Epstein-Barr virus, enteroviruses, hepatitis B virus (papular acrodermatitis or Gianotti-Crosti syndrome), HIV-1 ***Bacteria:*** Rheumatic fever (group A streptococcus), scarlet fever, *Arcanobacterium hemolyticum*, secondary syphilis, leptospirosis, *Pseudomonas*, meningococcus (early), *Salmonella typhi*, Lyme disease, *Listeria monocytogenes* ***Rickettsia:*** Early Rocky Mountain spotted fever, typhus (scrub, endemic) ***Other:*** Kawasaki disease
Diffuse erythroderma	***Bacteria:*** Scarlet fever (group A streptococcus), toxic shock syndrome, scalded skin syndrome *(Streptococcus aureus)* ***Fungi:*** *Candida albicans*
Urticarial rash	***Viruses:*** Epstein-Barr virus, hepatitis B ***Bacteria:*** *Mycoplasma pneumoniae*, group A streptococcus
Vesicular, bullous, pustular	***Viruses:*** Herpes simplex 1 and 2, varicella-zoster, coxsackievirus ***Bacteria:*** Staphylococcal scalded skin syndrome, staphylococcal bullous impetigo, group A streptococcal crusted impetigo, gonococcemia, *Pseudomonas aeruginosa* ***Other:*** Toxic epidermal necrolysis, erythema multiforme (Stevens-Johnson syndrome), rickettsial pox, Behçet syndrome
Petechial-purpuric	***Viruses:*** Atypical measles, congenital rubella, CMV, enterovirus, HIV-1, viral hemorrhagic fevers ***Bacteria:*** Sepsis (meningococcal, gonococcal, *Listeria*, streptococcal, staphylococcal), endocarditis ***Rickettsia:*** Rocky Mountain spotted fever, epidemic typhus ***Other:*** Vasculitis, thrombocytopenia, Henoch-Schönlein purpura
Nodules	***Bacteria:*** *Nocardia*, atypical mycobacteria ***Fungi:*** *Candida*, histoplasmosis, sporotrichosis ***Other:*** See erythema nodosum (below)
Erythema nodosum	***Viruses:*** Epstein-Barr, hepatitis B ***Bacteria:*** Group A streptococcus, tuberculosis, *Yersinia*, cat-scratch disease ***Fungi:*** Coccidioidomycosis, histoplasmosis, blastomycosis ***Other:*** Sarcoidosis, inflammatory bowel disease, systemic lupus erythematosus, cystic fibrosis, estrogen-containing oral contraceptives, pregnancy
Distinctive Rashes	
Koplik spots	Measles
Ecthyma gangrenosum	*P. aeruginosa;* rarely other bacteria or fungi
Erythema chronicum migrans	Lyme disease
Necrotic eschar	Aspergillosis, mucormycosis

rash may be a local cutaneous infection and thus may provide material for diagnostic culture and histologic stain (Gram, immunofluorescent, Tzanck). If hematogenous dissemination produces a distinct rash, as in varicella or Rocky Mountain spotted fever, histologic (Tzanck) or direct immunofluorescent staining *(Rickettsia rickettsii)* or culture, may be diagnostic aids. Skin biopsy may be helpful in differentiating infectious from noninfectious diseases (Sec. 23.2).

An appropriate list of potential diagnoses can be assembled on the basis of the appearance of the skin lesions and the use of pertinent historical data. In most cases the specific diagnosis can be made, sometimes only retrospectively, if appropriate cultures and serologic data are obtained. Antibiotic therapy for possible bacterial sepsis-meningitis should be initiated promptly but only after cultures of blood and skin lesions have been obtained. It is important to use media capable of supporting the growth of the organisms suspected of causing the infection.

ROBERT M. KLIEGMAN
RALPH D. FEIGIN
RICHARD E. BEHRMAN

Buxton PK: ABC of dermatology. Bacterial infection. Br Med J 296:189, 1988.
Buxton PK: ABC of dermatology. Viral infections. Br Med J 296:257, 1988.
Cherry JD: Cutaneous manifestations of systemic infections. *In*: Feigin RD, Cherry JD (eds): Textbook of Pediatric Infectious Diseases. Philadelphia, WB Saunders, 1987, p 786.
Kingston ME, Mackey D: Skin clues to the diagnosis of life threatening infections. Rev Infect Dis 8:1, 1986.

CLINICAL USE OF THE MICROBIOLOGY LABORATORY

12.6 LABORATORY DIAGNOSIS OF BACTERIAL INFECTIONS

GRAM STAIN. The examination of a Gram stain should be carried out on all fluids to be cultured. In addition to giving rapid results, the Gram stain may be useful in interpreting the subsequent cultural data because it allows identification of cellular exudate and the predominant organisms. The identification of cells in respiratory specimens is crucial to the interpretation of the Gram stain because the lack of cells indicates a poor quality specimen.

SPECIAL CULTURES. Most medically important bacteria can be cultivated on blood agar, chocolate agar, and eosin methylene blue or MacConkey agar. The frequency of recovery of anaerobic organisms has increased in recent years as media with low redox potentials have gained wide use. Thioglycollate broth, while an excellent general culture medium, will not foster growth of strict anaerobes. For collection of anaerobic cultures, material should be rapidly transported to the laboratory in a capped syringe, or special swabs supplied in oxygen-free tubes should be used. In some cases clinical circumstances make it advisable to consult the microbiology laboratory before sending a specimen.

BLOOD CULTURE. Culturing the blood is one of the most fruitful procedures in the diagnosis of bacterial disease. It should be done carefully *before* administration of antibiotics, using iodine-alcohol for skin disinfection. A number of different blood culture techniques are now available, most of which use 50- to 100-mL bottles containing broth nutritious for bacteria into which not more than 5–10 mL of blood are introduced. Sodium polyanethanol sulfonate is included in some modern blood culture broth media to prevent coagulation and to inactivate leukocytes; although it may be toxic to certain organisms (e.g., meningococci). Some blood culture bottles also contain an oxygen-free carbon dioxide–enriched atmosphere that allows the recovery of anaerobes. A widely used technique involves lysis of blood cells followed by inoculation of sediment obtained from centrifugation of the lysate. This method provides rapid detection, pathogen identification, and antimicrobial susceptibility data, as well as quantitative blood culture results. Another technique depends on the detection of carbon dioxide released by bacteria from substrates in the medium. Some centers use media containing resins that adsorb antibiotics that may be present in the patient's blood.

If an isolate is reported, blood cultures should be repeated to determine (1) whether treatment has been successful when the patient is already taking antibiotics, and (2) whether the isolate is a contaminant when the organism reported is usually nonpathogenic. The question of whether an organism isolated from blood is a pathogen or a contaminant should be carefully considered, since "nonpathogens" such as coagulase-negative staphylococci may cause disease in hosts with compromised immune mechanisms.

EXAMINATION OF CEREBROSPINAL FLUID (see Table 12–6). Fluid obtained by lumbar puncture or ventricular tap should be collected in sterile, capped containers and transported quickly to the laboratory, where centrifugation is done to concentrate organisms. Gram stains of CSF sediment are helpful; the presence of organisms distinguishes bacterial from viral disease, but stains should not be relied on for the identification of a specific organism. Errors are possible, even by experienced technicians; it is better to use broad-spectrum initial therapy in life-threatening disease and to wait for the culture report before ordering specific treatment. Counterimmunoelectrophoresis and agglutination of antibody-coated latex beads are additional rapid, accurate methods for diagnosis. Specific antisera can be used to detect antigens of *H. influenzae* type b, *N. meningitidis, S. pneumoniae,* group B streptococci, and *E. coli* K1.

URINE CULTURE. Urine for culture and colony count can be obtained in midstream (clean-catch), by catheterization, or by suprapubic puncture. The last method is the most reliable; urine so obtained should normally be sterile. Urine collected by catheter is likely to reflect infection if there are 10^3 organisms/mL or more. Clean-catch urine, if obtained after adequate cleansing, can be considered abnormal if 10^5 or more organisms/mL are present, and possibly abnormal if between 10^4 and 10^5 organisms/mL are counted. These limits apply only in uncomplicated urinary tract infection due to enteric gram-negative rods; different criteria may have to be used for gram-positive organisms, for yeasts, for patients in diuresis or with chronic pyelonephritis, or for patients on antibiotics. A Gram stain of unspun urine is helpful in predicting specimens with greater than 10^5 cfu/mL. Clean-catch urine specimens from girls who have inadequately washed, and specimens allowed to sit at room temperature for some time before being transported to the laboratory, may result in unreliable cultures. If delay in transporting specimens is unavoidable, dip-slides coated with bacteriologic media, dipped promptly in the urine specimen as soon as it is passed, give reliable results for urine culture.

CULTURE OF FECES. Rectal swabs or stool specimens are

cultured either to identify common bacterial pathogens such as *Salmonella* and *Shigella* or to determine the predominant flora of the intestine in a patient with weakened host defenses whose endogenous flora may become pathogenic. Since feces contain mostly anaerobic bacteria, routine cultures identify only the predominant aerobic organisms among the billions of bacteria contained in each gram of feces.

A number of organisms have recently been added to the list of bacterial pathogens found in feces, including *Helicobacter pylori, Yersinia enterocolitica, Clostridium difficile, Aeromonas* spp., *Plesiomonas* spp., *Vibrio* spp., and *E. coli* 0157:H7. DNA probes, antigen detection methods, and toxin detection have all been applied to the rapid diagnosis of enteric pathogens.

EXUDATES AND TRANSUDATES. Abscesses, pleural fluids, joint fluids, urethral exudates, and other miscellaneous exudates and transudates can be cultured directly on agar. In addition to cultures and stains, glucose and cell count determinations should be done on all transudates for the same reasons they are done on CSF.

NASOPHARYNGEAL, THROAT, AND SKIN SWABS. A dry rayon, Dacron, or calcium alginate swab is most efficient for collecting specimens from the skin and mucous membranes. Since drying rapidly destroys some pathogenic bacteria, swab specimens should be placed promptly in a transport medium. Now available are packaged swabs, which, after the specimen is taken, are inserted in a breakable ampule of transport medium.

Interpretation of results of cultures from skin and mucous membranes is difficult because microbial flora are normally recovered from these areas. Some organisms are considered pathogenic wherever found, such as *Corynebacterium diphtheriae, Bordetella pertussis,* and *Neisseria gonorrhoeae;* others, such as *Streptococcus pyogenes, N. meningitidis, H. influenzae,* or staphylococci, may be pathogenic or nonpathogenic, depending on circumstances. Still others, such as *Streptococcus viridans,* are rarely considered pathogenic. In respiratory tract disease there is little correlation between flora of the upper airway and that of the lower airway. Because sputum cultures are seldom reliable in children, bronchoalveolar lavage, tracheal aspirates, and lung punctures are sometimes necessary for accurate diagnosis. If bacteria such as *C. diphtheriae* or *Bordetella* sp. (which grow poorly in ordinary media) are suspected, the laboratory should be informed prior to receipt of the specimen.

FLUORESCENT TECHNIQUES. Fluorescent antibody (FA) techniques have increased the diagnostic scope of direct microscopy. Specific antisera are now available commercially for several common pathogens. In these sera the antibody molecules have been conjugated with a fluorescein dye. The specific dye-labeled serum is added to the smear containing the suspected organism, and the slide is microscopically examined for fluorescence under ultraviolet light. Indirect FA methods are also applicable in the absence of conjugated antibodies. FA is used principally for identifying *B. pertussis, Legionella pneumophila,* and *N. gonorrhoeae.* In the special case of *Mycobacterium tuberculosis* no antibody is used; rather, the smears are stained with auramine-rhodamine, which is taken up by the organisms and fluoresces under ultraviolet light. This acid-fast fluorescent staining procedure is more sensitive but less specific than the Ziehl-Neelsen or Kinyoun acid-fast stain.

SEROLOGIC TESTS. Bacteria are often serogrouped or serotyped through agglutination by specific antisera (sometimes attached to latex particles).

ANTIBIOTIC SENSITIVITY TESTS. Most laboratories routinely test bacterial isolates for sensitivity to various antibiotics. The most prevalent technique of antibiotic testing is the agar disk diffusion method, in which a standardized inoculum of the organism is seeded onto a plate. Filter paper disks, each impregnated with an antibiotic, are placed on the agar surface, and after 18–24 hr of incubation, the zone of inhibition of bacterial growth around each disk is measured. Standard zone diameters indicating sensitivity or resistance have been defined according to previous test results correlating zone sizes with sensitivity determined by inhibition of bacteria inoculated into dilutions of antibiotics in culture broth. However, there are some pitfalls in the disk diffusion method. Small differences in zone diameter have large implications, and control of inoculum size, rate of diffusion of antibiotics, and accurate measurement of zones are critical.

For more accurate measurement of antibiotic sensitivity, dilutions made in tubes or in wells on microtiter plates have come into wide use. Antibiotic dilutions in growth medium are prepared in steps through the range of attainable blood levels; then each tube or well is inoculated with a standardized suspension of the test organism. After 24 hr the tubes or wells are examined for turbidity; the lowest antibiotic concentration resulting in a clear tube or well indicates the bacteriostatic concentration of the particular antibiotic for the organism (minimal inhibitory concentration, or MIC). In some situations (e.g., endocarditis) it is important to measure the concentration of drug needed to kill bacteria. The tubes or wells are then subcultured to agar plates; the lowest concentration of antibiotic that yields a 99.9% decrease in organism viability is the bactericidal end-point (minimal bactericidal concentration, or MBC).

The actual concentrations of certain antibiotics in the blood can be measured by immunochemical assays. These measurements are mandatory when patients with renal disease are treated with aminoglycosides or with vancomycin. Microbiologic assays using susceptible stock strains of bacteria may be useful in special circumstances.

Office Bacteriology

Disposable materials have been developed so that rapid, inexpensive bacterial diagnosis can be made in the physician's office. Kits for detecting streptococci, gonococci, and urinary tract infection by culture are most widely used. The only additional purchase required is a small incubator. Unfortunately, quality control by testing of known positive cultures is seldom practiced. Office bacteriology may be inaccurate, unless both positive and negative results are periodically confirmed.

12.7 LABORATORY DIAGNOSIS OF VIRUSES

If viral disease is a diagnostic possibility when the patient is first seen, immediate steps should be taken to isolate the virus and obtain specimens for serologic evaluation.

MICROSCOPIC OBSERVATION. Electron microscopy and fluorescent-antibody techniques may provide rapid identification of viruses. Vesicle fluid examined by electron microscopy can distinguish a poxvirus from a herpesvirus. Smears of mucosal cells or urinary sediment stained by fluorescent antibody can identify the antigens of any virus for which there is a polyclonal or monoclonal animal antiserum, for example, influenza and respiratory syncytial viruses. The antigens of hepatitis B and the rotavirus agents, which cause infantile gastroenteritis, can be conveniently detected by *en*zyme-*l*inked *i*mmuno-*s*orbent *a*ssay (ELISA) or by radioimmunoassay (RIA) using specific antisera.

Cytologic examination aids in diagnosis when inclusion bodies or syncytia are found, for example, in the urine of patients infected with cytomegalovirus or in the noses of patients with measles. Such demonstrations should be confirmed by actual isolation of the virus.

ISOLATION. Viruses require living cells for propagation; the cells used may be in live laboratory animals, embryonated hens' eggs, or human or animal cell tissue cultures. Since some viruses are difficult to isolate and many require a variety of culture systems for their isolation, the clinician should specify the type of virus or illness suspected.

Specimens should be delivered to the laboratory promptly. Throat and stool or rectal swab specimens should be submitted routinely. The best throat specimens are taken by vigorous throat swabbing, removing some superficial cells. For certain viruses, for example, rubella, swabs should be taken from the nasal turbinates. The swab should be rinsed thoroughly in a transport medium containing antibiotics to inhibit bacterial growth, squeezed against the glass, and discarded. If the laboratory is reasonably close, specimens should be transported at 4° C.

Rectal swabs should not be heavily covered with feces because the antibiotics present in viral transport media may be insufficient to kill a large inoculum of bacteria. Rectal swabs should be collected even in patients with respiratory and central nervous system syndromes, since many viruses replicate in the intestine as well as in target organs.

Cerebrospinal fluid is often positive during the acute stages of central nervous system inflammation. An extra amount of spinal fluid for viral diagnostic studies should be obtained at the initial lumbar puncture and can be discarded if bacterial meningitis is diagnosed.

Urine culture for viruses is most useful for the isolation of cytomegalovirus, but urine is also a good source for isolation of mumps and adenoviruses. Urine should not be frozen but rather transported in ordinary ice.

Vesicular fluid can be cultured to distinguish among vaccinia, variola, varicella, herpes, and enteroviruses.

Viremia is part of cytomegalovirus, enterovirus, and other viral infections, and buffy coat cultures are often useful in the diagnosis of febrile syndromes. The diagnosis of hepatitis B is made by demonstrating that the viral antigen is present in serum.

SEROLOGIC TESTS. Serologic tests may be positive even when virus isolation fails. Correct diagnosis requires at least two blood specimens: the first should be obtained during the early acute phase of the disease ("acute serum"), and the second ("convalescent serum") 14–21 days later. If the second is taken earlier than 14 days after the first, it is advisable to take a third blood specimen 4–6 wk after the onset, since the rise of antibodies may be delayed, especially in infants. If it is not possible to send blood to the laboratory promptly, serum may be removed for preservation by freezing. Whole blood should never be frozen. To establish the etiologic diagnosis, it is necessary to demonstrate a 4-fold rise in titer of antibody to an agent in the convalescent as opposed to the acute phase serum, when all specimens are tested together.

Although the presence of a substantial titer against a suspected agent in a single late acute or convalescent specimen of serum will not differentiate between a recent and a past infection, in the following circumstances a study of a single serum specimen can support a clinical diagnosis: (1) a high antibody level in comparison with that of the population in general; (2) the presence of virus-specific antibody in the IgM fraction, particularly in neonates and in patients in the acute stage of infection; (3) antibody in the young infant not present in the mother; (4) antibody in both infant and mother that remains at the same level as the infant grows older; (5) in patients with suspected mumps, the presence of antibody to the soluble (S) fraction of the mumps virus in the acute serum (this antibody may be found as early as 2–3 days of the disease, when antibodies to the viral [V] antigen may be absent or very low); and (6) in patients with infectious mononucleosis, the presence of antibody to the early antigen found in cells infected by Epstein-Barr (EB) virus under specific conditions of preparation.

Methods of Detecting Antibody. Antibody can be detected by a variety of specific serologic methods; some are more appropriate than others for specific viruses. Complement-fixation (CF) antigens are available for a great range of viruses, and CF antibodies have the advantage of correlating with recent infection but are less useful for showing past infection. Neutralizing antibodies, on the other hand, remain for life; unless one has obtained serum early in the disease, a rise may be difficult to show. Furthermore, neutralization tests have the technical disadvantage of needing to be done in tissue cultures or in whole animals. Hemagglutination-inhibition (HI) antibodies correlate fairly well with neutralizing antibodies. Fortunately, many viruses such as the myxoviruses, rubella, and some enteroviruses can agglutinate erythrocytes. The presence of antibodies can be detected by the extent to which a particular serum specifically inhibits hemagglutination. Many of the viruses that agglutinate red blood cells also cause red blood cells to be adsorbed onto the membranes of infected cell monolayers. Inhibition of adsorption is a particularly useful test for parainfluenza virus antibodies. Fluorescent antibodies can be detected by the indirect fluorescence technique (see earlier), which requires slides bearing cells infected with the specific virus against which antibodies are being sought. Indirect hemagglutination and latex agglutination tests are now in greater use in virology; these depend on the attachment of viral antigens to glutaraldehyde- or tannic acid–treated sheep erythrocytes or to latex beads. The ELISA technique is now being used more widely, and there are now ELISA assays for antibodies to most viruses.

HIV and AIDS. The AIDS epidemic has made tests for HIV infection of great importance. Generally, ELISA tests for antibody are used to screen for infection. These are both sensitive and specific but are not 100% certain. Moreover, passive maternal antibody may confuse the diagnosis of infection in infancy. Several tests are used to confirm infection, including Western blot (a sensitive technique for demonstrating antibodies to specific viral proteins), p24 antigen detection in body fluids (this is the viral core antigen), HIV culture from blood, and detection of viral genome through polymerase chain reaction.

LABORATORY DIAGNOSIS OF OTHER ORGANISMS

These diagnoses are discussed in their respective sections in this chapter.

12.8 MOLECULAR BIOLOGY IN MICROBIOLOGIC DIAGNOSIS

ANTIGEN DETECTION. Although culture of a pathogen is the most specific method of microbiologic diagnosis, it is often a slow process, particularly in the case of viruses, and this lack of speed renders it less clinically useful. In some infections sufficient antigen is present to enable diagnosis by specific antigen detection. Examples are hepatitis B surface antigen, detected in the serum by RIA; rotavirus antigen, detected in the stool by ELISA; *Legionella* antigen, detected in the urine; and streptococcal polysaccharide antigen, detected in throat secretions by a variety of methods. Also, cell culture may be used to amplify viral agents, allowing tests for antigen to become positive within 24 hr.

ANTIBODY DETECTION USING ARTIFICIAL ANTIGENS. Sometimes cellular contaminants in the antigen preparation may confuse test results for specific antibodies. Recently, some tests have employed peptides synthesized de novo based on the derived amino acid sequence of important native epitopes. Antibodies that react with these peptides must be specific for the viral or bacterial protein.

DNA PROBES. The greatest revolution in microbiologic diagnosis to date has occurred through the use of DNA probes. Because every organism possesses a specific DNA or RNA genome, a probe constructed of complementary sequences of a portion of the genome will detect the presence of the agent.

In practice, the assays divide into those in which the hybridization is detected on some solid or semisolid support such as blotting papers or gels and those in which the DNA is detected in situ in tissue or on culture plates. Among those bacteria for which commercial probes are now available, *Mycoplasma pneumoniae, M. tuberculosis, Mycobacterium avium–intracellulare,* and enteric organisms figure prominently. Among the viruses, considerable use has been made of probes for the herpesviruses, HIV, and hepatitis B. DNA probes have not yet become as sensitive as culture. However, adaptation of the technique of polymerase chain reaction will enable amplification of the target nucleic acids and should enhance sensitivity considerably. Undoubtedly, more probe techniques will come into use in the future.

Balows A, Hausler WJ: Diagnostic Procedures for Bacterial, Mycotic and Parasitic Infections. Washington DC, American Public Health Association Inc, 1988.

Lennette EH, Balows A, Hausler WJ, et al: Manual of Clinical Microbiology. Washington, DC, American Society for Microbiology, 1985.

Lennette EH, Schmidt NJ: Diagnostic Procedures for Viral, Rickettsial and Chlamydial Infections. Washington, DC, American Public Health Association Inc, 1988.

McGowan KL: Infectious diseases: Diagnosis utilizing DNA probes. Understanding a developing clinical technology. Clin Pediatr 28:157, 1989.

Radetsky M, Solomon JA, Todd JK: Identification of streptococcal pharyngitis in the office laboratory: Reassessment of new technology. Pediatr Infect Dis J 6:556, 1987.

Todd JK: Test selection for the pediatric office laboratory. *In:* Aronoff SC, Hughes WT Jr, Kohl S, et al (eds): Advances in Pediatric Infectious Diseases, Vol 3. Chicago, Year Book Medical Publishers, 1988, pp 111–124.

12.9 INFECTION CONTROL

Approximately 5% of all children admitted to pediatric hospitals in the United States acquire an infection in the hospital (nosocomial infection). The consequences can be measured in morbidity, mortality, delayed discharge, and higher hospital costs. The aim of isolation procedures is protection of the patient, other hospitalized children, and the hospital staff. The means of prevention are surprisingly simple. For the most part, today as in the time of Semmelweis, handwashing is the most important measure that can be taken by personnel, who are the passive agents of most nosocomial infections. Indeed, efforts to contain infection will be frustrated unless there is cooperation of physicians, nurses, and other hospital personnel. Constant vigilance is required to maintain standards. Adequate separation between patients (i.e., absence of crowding) is also important in reducing nosocomial infection.

Microorganisms are transmitted in a variety of ways. Some are transmitted by direct contact with respiratory or enteric excretions; some by inhalation of small-particle aerosols; some by ingestion of contaminated food or water; some by sexual transmission; some by arthropod bites; and some by inoculation of blood. Isolation rules are tailored to fit the type of transmission that is expected and to interpose a block in that transmission (see Table 12–8).

Protective isolation is a form of isolation designed to place a barrier between exogenous microorganisms and an immunosuppressed patient, particularly one who is neutropenic (< 500 polymorphonuclear leukocytes [PMNs]/mm^3). Ideally, a patient who needs a protective environment is placed in a laminar air flow room, in which filtered air under positive pressure provides a curtain to keep contamination out. However, patients have endogenous flora that are difficult to control, even when attempts are made to sterilize them with orally administered and topical antibiotics. Moreover, hospital staff who do not practice handwashing may introduce resistant hospital flora.

Isolation is carried out by means of handwashing, private rooms, gowns, gloves, and masks. Handwashing should be practiced before and after every patient contact, whether or not the patient is known to be infected. Hospital personnel do not need to be infected themselves to infect others: Mechanical carriage is enough in the case of agents such as staphylococci and respiratory syncytial virus. Gloves are a useful additional means of reducing nosocomial infection, but they supplement rather than replace handwashing. Gowns are a means of keeping infectious materials off clothing, although in some settings they are used more as reminders that the patient is isolated.

Some patients, usually those with infections transmitted by small-particle aerosols, need to be housed in a separate room. Ideally, an isolation room has negative air pressure so that air is evacuated to the outside while new air enters around and under the door. There should be an anteroom, containing a sink and isolation supplies, which itself has a closed door. Only this type of design can contain infections like varicella and aspergillosis, which are notorious for spreading on air currents.

In contrast, many infections transmitted by large-particle aerosols can be contained by bedside isolation using gown and gloves, with masks added only for close contact with secretions or excretions (contact isolation). These methods belong in the category of *enteric and drainage secretion precautions*. Technique is important in maintaining isolation. Individual gowns must be available for each patient and must be removed before leaving the patient's area. Gloves must be put on carefully and removed and discarded without touching other surfaces.

Universal precautions (body substance isolation [BSI]) are of great significance for pediatric and other hospitals. This term means that every patient is assumed to be capable of carrying a blood-borne infection, and thus all contact with blood or other body fluids containing blood is considered potentially hazardous. Gloves are necessary for handling these fluids, and gowns, masks, and goggles are added if circumstances make splashing likely. Most pediatric centers in urban or other areas where there is a high prevalence of HIV seropositivity have adopted universal precautions routinely.

Table 12–9 summarizes the different categories of isolation. Instructions regarding specific diseases are available from several sources, notably the Report of the Committee on Infectious Diseases (Redbook) of the American Academy of Pediatrics, the Centers for Disease Control, and the American Public Health Association. In addition, each hospital should have an isolation manual, in which recommendations and procedures adapted to local circumstances are given in detail.

Some attention must be paid to *disinfection* of the physical environment. Although many microorganisms have been shown to persist on inanimate objects for long periods of time, the role of such persistence in the transmission of human infection is doubtful. Nevertheless, dust should be removed

TABLE 12–8. Recommended Isolation and Periods of Infectivity of Selected Infections

Disease	Infective	Recommended Isolation Method
AIDS (acquired immunodeficiency syndrome)	Persons seropositive for HIV* antibody must be considered potentially infective to sexual contacts and to those who have contact with their blood	Condom use during heterosexual or homosexual intercourse; avoid contact of mucous membranes or open wounds with blood or bloody body fluids of affected persons through use of "Universal Precautions"
Chickenpox (varicella)	1–2 days before rash, until 5–6 days after onset and until all lesions are crusted, longer in patients with immune deficiency; may be longer in actively or passively immunized patients	Until all lesions are crusted, usually 5–6 days; in mild cases child may return to school sooner Respiratory isolation
German measles (rubella)	Seven days before rash to 5 days after; for congenital infection time is variable, but patients are often virus positive for 10–12 mo	Contact isolation in general except that women in the 1st trimester of pregnancy should not be exposed, nor should sexually active, nonimmune women in child-bearing years who are not using contraceptive measures
Hepatitis A (infectious hepatitis)	Variable, in feces up to 3 wk before and after jaundice; disease may be most communicable 1 wk before and 1 wk after onset of jaundice	Enteric precautions; emphasize personal hygiene; infected mothers may breast feed
Hepatitis B (serum hepatitis)	Variable; probably as long as patient is HBsAg positive	Blood/body fluid precautions as part of "Universal Precautions"; emphasize personal hygiene
Measles (rubeola)	From 5th day of incubation through 4th day of rash; in immunosuppressed patients isolation lasts for length of illness	Respiratory isolation
Mumps	Up to 7 days before and 9 days after onset of parotitis or other manifestation	Until swelling subsides
Pertussis	3 wk or until cough has ceased; 5 days if treated; protect infants from exposure	Respiratory isolation
Poliomyelitis (enterovirus)	Shortly before and after onset; virus present in throat for 1 wk after onset, in feces intermittently for 3–4 wk	Enteric precautions needed for duration of illness
Respiratory syncytial (bronchiolitis)	During entire illness, particularly the 1st wk	Contact isolation for 14 days; staff may carry virus
Salmonella	Duration of illness and often afterward; variable periods	Enteric precautions needed for duration of illness
Scarlet fever (scarlatina)	Variable without therapy; 1 day after start of therapy	Drainage/secretions precautions

*HIV = human immunodeficiency virus.

and surfaces cleaned with germicidal solutions. Commercial solutions containing phenol can be used to clean isolation rooms.

Scrupulous cleanliness is needed when aqueous solutions come in contact with the patient or personnel. Water for washing may be contaminated with *Legionella*, sinks and respiratory equipment may be contaminated with gram-negative bacteria, and handwashing solutions are prone to contamination with *Pseudomonas* spp. If infections occur, water-associated sources must be examined.

Every hospital should have an infection control committee and, in addition, an infection control practitioner. The role of the latter is to survey infections on a day-to-day basis, looking for clusters or patterns that indicate epidemic or endemic nosocomial infection. An important aspect of this job is surveillance of surgical infections, which might indicate inadequate sterile technique. The infection control practitioner also attempts to improve isolation practices, institute methods of preventing infection, and educate the staff, including physicians. The role of the infection control committee is to receive reports from the practitioner and to ensure that effective actions are taken. In practice, the chairman of the committee is usually an infection disease specialist or pathologist.

STANLEY A. PLOTKIN

DISORDERS CAUSED BY A VARIETY OF INFECTIOUS AGENTS

12.10 DIARRHEA

Diarrhea, one of the most frequent problems encountered by pediatricians (Sec. 5.4, 6.20, 12.27, 12.28, and 12.30), is defined as an increase in the frequency, fluidity, and volume of feces; during the first 3 yr of life a child experiences an estimated 1–3 acute, severe episodes of diarrhea. Although most episodes of acute diarrhea subside within 72 hr with fluid administration and diet change, 1–4% of these episodes, worldwide, are fatal.

Diarrhea may follow invasion of the intestinal mucosa (e.g., with enteroinvasive *E. coli*, *Shigella*, *Y. enterocolitica*, *Entamoeba histolytica*), or it may be induced by exposure of the bowel to a microbial toxin (e.g., *Vibrio cholerae*, enterotoxigenic *E. coli*, *Shigella dysenteriae* type 1, *Clostridium perfringens*, *S. aureus*). It also may be induced by adherence of bacteria to the mucosa of the gastrointestinal tract *(E. coli)* or infestation by *Giardia*

TABLE 12–9. Recommendations for Category-Specific Isolation Precautions for Hospitalized Patients*

Category of Isolation Precautions	Handwashing for Patient Contact	Single Room	Masks	Gowns	Gloves	Other†
Strict isolation	Yes	Yes	Yes	Yes	Yes	—
Contact isolation	Yes	Yes‡	Yes for those close to patient	Yes if soiling likely	Yes for touching infective material	—
Respiratory isolation	Yes	Yes‡	Yes for those close to patient	No	No	—
Tuberculosis (AFB) isolation	Yes	Yes (with special ventilation)	Yes if patient is coughing and does not cover mouth	Only if needed to prevent gross contamination of clothing	No	—
Enteric precautions	Yes	Only if patient hygiene is poor‡	No	Yes if soiling likely	Yes for touching infective material	—
Drainage/secretion precautions	Yes	No	No	Yes if soiling likely	Yes for touching infective material	—
Blood/blood-containing body fluid precautions§	Yes (immediately) if potentially contaminated with blood or body fluids	No	No	Yes if soiling with blood or body fluids is likely	Yes for touching blood or body fluids	Avoid needle-stick injuries; clean up blood spills promptly with diluted bleach

*Modified from Report of the Committee on Infectious Diseases. Copyright © 1991 American Academy of Pediatrics. Based on recommendations of the Centers for Disease Control (Gardner JS, Simmons BP: Guidelines for isolation precautions in hospitals. Infect Control 4[Suppl]:245, 1983; Centers for Disease Control: Recommendations for prevention of HIV transmission in healthcare setting. MMWR 36[Suppl 2S]:3S, 1987; and Centers for Disease Control: Update: Universal precautions for prevention of transmission of human immunodeficiency virus, hepatitis B virus, and other bloodborne pathogens in healthcare settings. MMWR 24:377, 1988).

†In each case, articles contaminated with infective material should be discarded or bagged and labeled before being sent for decontamination and reprocessing.

‡Cohorting allowed.

§Recommended for all patients in high HIV prevalence areas (see Universal Precautions).

lamblia or cryptosporidium. The latter agent has been seen with increasing frequency as a cause of diarrhea in children in day-care centers and in those with acquired immunodeficiency syndrome (AIDS).

Viruses are the major cause of wintertime diarrhea in infants. Rotavirus is the etiologic agent in over 50% of cases of acute diarrhea in children; other viruses causing diarrhea include parvovirus-like agents (Norwalk, Hawaii, and Montgomery), coxsackie-, echo-, adeno-, and caliciviruses. More than two thirds of patients with rotavirus-associated diarrhea have a history of preceding or concurrent respiratory illness with rhinorrhea, cough, erythematous throat, or otitis media; most of these individuals are under 2 yr of age. The epidemiology of infectious diarrhea is presented in Table 12–10.

Common infections extrinsic to the gastrointestinal tract (pneumonia, otitis media) may also be accompanied by diarrhea. Diarrhea also occurs in association with a variety of anatomic defects, endocrinopathies, neoplasms, disorders accompanied by malabsorption, and inherited diseases (Table 12–11).

HISTORY AND PHYSICAL EXAMINATION. A chief complaint of diarrhea should first be verified for accuracy (increase in number, volume, or fluidity of stools). Clinical manifestations may differentiate viral from bacterial causes of diarrhea (Table 12–12). A history of recent travel to Latin America may suggest diarrhea related to shigella, enterotoxigenic *E. coli*, or amebiasis, and travel to the Rocky Mountains or the Soviet Union may suggest giardiasis. A history of blood or mucus in the stool, abdominal pain, tenesmus, fever, abdominal mass, weight loss, or consumption of dairy products or contaminated meats or water should also be sought. The degree of dehydration and state of consciousness should be described specifically (Sec. 6.16 and 6.17). The presence or absence of arthralgia, arthritis, skin rashes, and bradycardia also may suggest various etiologic diagnoses. The clinical findings coupled with a history of fluid intake, the frequency of urination, and an assessment of concurrent stool losses help to determine whether diarrhea is severe and hospitalization is required.

LABORATORY DIAGNOSIS. The total and differential white blood cell count may be normal, increased, or decreased, but more than 50% of patients with bacterial disease have 10–40% band forms in the differential counts.

The stool should be examined for volume, color, and consistency, and for the presence of mucus, blood, and leukocytes. Leukocytes may be noted by mixing a small amount of stool with 1–2 drops of methylene blue; generally, they are not seen when diarrhea is related to disease of the small bowel but are observed in patients with invasive bacteria that produce dysentery-like symptoms (see Table 12–12). The stools of various patients should be cultured: patients with fecal leukocytes, hospitalized children, patients with persistent or chronic diarrhea, and individuals who have been exposed to others having diarrhea due to a bacterial pathogen. Stool should be examined for ova and parasites when the history, physical examination, course of the illness, or negative laboratory data suggest that a parasitic disease is possible (see Table 12–10). A diagnosis of *G. lamblia* can be made by examining the stool but may require examining a duodenal aspirate or a duodenal biopsy. Stool may be sent for immunofluorescent microscopy or ELISA to confirm a diagnosis of infection by rotavirus.

Examination of stool pH, stool glucose content, and stool chloride concentration may be helpful. If the stool glucose content is low or stool pH is less than 5.5, various noninfectious causes of diarrhea should be considered. However, low stool pH may also be found in children with acquired lactase deficiency that has followed an infectious diarrheal illness. Significant stool chloride losses occur in cholera; chloride losses of greater than 90 mEq/L of stool after the fluid and

TABLE 12–10. Epidemiology of Infectious Agents Causing Diarrhea in the United States

	Percentage of Cases of Diarrhea	Epidemiology
Viruses		
Rotavirus	15–35	Person-to-person spread; winter months; infants
Enteric adenovirus	5–15	Types 40, 41. Person-to-person spread; all ages
Norwalk-like viruses (Snow Mountain, Hawaii, Ditchling)	5–15	Food- and water-borne common source, person-to-person spread; all ages
Astrovirus (Marin County agent)	1–5	Nosocomial, food-, water-borne; epidemics; all ages
Calicivirus	1–2	Year round, sporadic and epidemic cases; infants
Coronavirus	<1	Pathogenicity uncertain
Bacteria		
Campylobacter jejuni	5–15	Source: wild and domestic animals, poultry, water, raw milk; fecal-oral spread; infants and adolescents
Salmonella enteritides	3–5	May be under-reported. Source: poultry, meat, eggs, milk, pigs, turtles; fecal-oral spread; infants, young children
Shigella (sonnei, flexneri)	1–3	Person-to-person transmission, summer-fall season, dysentery; young children 1–3 yr
Escherichia coli 0157:H7	1–3	Person-to-person spread, food-borne, milk, meat; all ages
Enterotoxigenic *E. coli*	1–3	Most common cause of traveler's diarrhea
Yersinia enterocolitica	1–3	Source: animals, raw milk, tofu, bean sprouts, chitterlings; diarrhea in infants, mesenteric adenitis in adolescents
Clostridium difficile	1–2	Antibiotic associated: person-to-person nosocomial spread
Staphylococcus aureus	1	Toxin-mediated food poisoning, common source
Clostridium perfringens	1	Toxin-mediated food poisoning, common source
Aeromonas hydrophila	<1	Water-borne: shellfish, sewage, vegetables
Plesiomonas shigelloides	<1	Shellfish, foreign travel
Vibrio cholerae	<1	Gulf of Mexico, shellfish, water
Vibrio parahaemolyticus	<1	Gulf of Mexico, shellfish
Bacillus cereus	<1	Toxin-mediated food poisoning, common source
Parasites		
Giardia lamblia	High incidence in day-care centers, residential facilities	Most common parasitic cause of diarrhea, person-to-person, fecal-oral, water-borne spread; all ages
Cryptosporidium	Unknown, common in day-care centers	Water-borne, animal-human, person-to-person, AIDS spread; infants, older if AIDS is a factor
Entamoeba histolytica	<1	Person-to-person spread, Southwestern United States
Balantidium coli	<1	Pig contact, contaminated water
Strongyloides strercoralis	<1	Eosinophilia, urticaria

electrolyte balance has been corrected strongly suggest congenital chloridorrhea.

Urine cultures may help in establishing a diagnosis of shigellosis, since this disorder may be complicated by bacteremia and urinary shedding of organisms, or in excluding urinary tract infection as a cause of nonspecific diarrhea.

TABLE 12–11. Noninfectious Causes of Diarrhea

- Feeding difficulty
- Anatomic defects
  - Malrotation
  - Intestinal duplications
  - Hirschsprung disease
  - Fecal impaction
  - Short bowel syndrome
- Malabsorption
  - Disaccharidase deficiencies
  - Glucose-galactose monosaccharide malabsorption
  - Cystic fibrosis
  - Hereditary fructose intolerance
  - Abetalipoproteinemia
  - Celiac disease
- Endocrinopathies
  - Thyrotoxicosis
  - Addison disease
  - Adrenogenital syndrome
- Food poisoning
  - Heavy metals
  - Scombroid
  - Ciguaetra
  - Mushrooms
- Neoplasms
  - Neuroblastomas
  - Ganglioneuromas
  - Pheochromocytomas
  - Carcinoid
- Miscellaneous
  - Milk allergy
  - Crohn disease (regional enteritis)
  - Familial dysautonomia
  - Hemolytic-uremic syndrome
  - Immune deficiency disease
  - Protein-losing enteropathy
  - Ulcerative colitis
  - Acrodermatitis enteropathica
  - Kawasaki syndrome
  - Hartnup disease
  - Laxative abuse

Blood cultures may be helpful in selected patients with salmonellosis or shigellosis.

RALPH D. FEIGIN
MARSHALL L. STOLLER

Christensen ML: Human viral gastroenteritis. Clin Microbiol Rev 2:51, 1989.

Cohn M: The epidemiology of diarrheal diseases in the United States. Infect Dis Clin North Am 2:557, 1988.

Fontana M, Zuin G, Paccagnini S, et al: Simple clinical score and laboratory based method to predict bacterial etiology of acute diarrhea in childhood. Pediatr Infect Dis 6:1088, 1987.

Uhnoo I, Olding-Stenkuist E, Krueger A: Clinical features of acute gastroenteritis associated with rotavirus, enteric adenoviruses and bacteria. Arch Dis Child 61:732, 1986.

12.11 ACUTE ASEPTIC MENINGITIS

Acute aseptic meningitis, an inflammatory process of the meninges, is a relatively common illness caused by a large number of different factors. The cerebrospinal fluid is characterized by pleocytosis and the absence of microorganisms on Gram stain and on routine culture. In most instances the illnesses are self-limited; in some, however, the resulting diseases are severe and progressive and lead to disability and death (Sec. 12.4).

ETIOLOGY. Etiologic agents and factors in aseptic meningitis are listed in Table 12–5. Although in many instances the etiologic agent is not identified, clinical and research experience indicates that viruses are usually the responsible

TABLE 12–12. Differentiation of Bacterial and Viral Causes of Gastroenteritis

Variable	Bacterial	Viral
Temperature > 38.5° C	Yes	Unusual
Abdominal pain, tenesmus	Yes	Unusual
> 8 bowel movements/24 hr	Yes	Unusual
Emesis	Unusual	Yes
Duration > 5 days	Yes	No
Erythrocyte sedimentation rate	Elevated	Normal
Leukocytosis	Yes	No
Stool leukocytes and mucus present	Yes (*Shigella, Salmonella, Yersinia, Campylobacter,* invasive *Escherichia coli, Plesiomonas*)	
Stool leukocytes absent: secretory diarrhea	Yes (*Vibrio cholerae*, toxigenic *E. coli, Aeromonas*)	No
Hematochezia	Yes (*Shigella, Salmonella, Yersinia, Campylobacter,* enterohemorrhagic *E. coli*, pseudomembranous colitis due to *Clostridium difficile, Plesiomonas*)	No, except rotavirus in preterm infants
History of shellfish consumption	Yes (*E. coli, V. cholerae, V. parahaemolyticus,Campylobacter*)	Yes (Norwalk agent)
Traveler's diarrhea	Yes (toxigenic *E. coli, Salmonella, Shigella*)	Unusual (Norwalk agent and rotavirus)
Single-source outbreak	Yes (*Salmonella, Shigella, Streptococcus aureus, Bacillus cereus, Clostridium perfringens, Yersinia, E. coli*)	Yes (Norwalk agent)
Seasonal epidemics	Unusual (*Campylobacter*)	Yes (rotavirus)

agents. Enteroviruses account for approximately 85% of all cases of aseptic meningitis; the most common specific types are coxsackievirus B5 and echoviruses 4, 6, 9, and 11. Arboviruses account for about 5% of cases, St. Louis and California encephalitides being the most common in the United States. In regions where mumps vaccine is not routinely used, mumps is a common cause of aseptic meningitis.

The most common cause of nonviral aseptic meningitis is partially and inappropriately treated bacterial disease (see later). *M. pneumoniae* is also a frequent cause of aseptic meningitis. Of the other etiologies listed in Table 12–5, the following are those most frequently seen: tuberculosis, leptospirosis, parameningeal bacterial infection, toxoplasmosis, Kawasaki disease, and malignancy.

EPIDEMIOLOGY. Since approximately 85% of cases of aseptic meningitis are due to enteroviral infections, the basic epidemiologic pattern reflects that of these agents. Hence, in temperate climates most cases occur in the summer and fall; infection with enteroviruses is spread directly from person to person, and the incubation period is usually 4–6 days. Epidemiologic considerations in aseptic meningitis due to agents other than enteroviruses may also depend on season, geography, climatic conditions, animal exposures, and many other factors related to the specific pathogens.

CLINICAL MANIFESTATIONS. The clinical course is usually characterized at least in part by the signs and symptoms of meningitis or meningoencephalitis (Sec. 12.4 and 12.12). The onset of illness is generally acute, although it may be insidious over a week or so or may be preceded by a nonspecific acute febrile illness of a few days' duration. The presenting manifestations in older children are headache and hyperesthesia, and in infants, irritability and resentment at being handled. Headache is most often frontal or generalized; adolescents frequently note retrobulbar pain. Fever, nausea, and vomiting are frequent, but convulsions are rare. Pain in the neck, back, and legs is common, as is photophobia. Preceding or accompanying exanthems may occur, especially with the echoviruses and coxsackieviruses. Examination often reveals nuchalspinal rigidity without significant localizing neurologic changes.

The manifestations may be limited to the meningeal and/or encephalitic pattern, as often occurs with the nonpolio enteroviruses (Sec. 12.80) and in some encephalitides caused by arboviruses (Sec. 12.12); in other instances, the acute aseptic syndrome may be a phase, of varying importance, in a wide variety of clinical disorders, such as in tuberculous meningitis, congenital syphilis, leptospirosis, leukemia, and so forth (see Table 12–5). The varied clinical manifestations of enteroviral aseptic meningitis are discussed in Sec. 12.80.

LABORATORY MANIFESTATIONS. The cerebrospinal fluid contains from a few to several thousand cells/mm^3; early in the disease the cells are often polymorphonuclear; later they are chiefly mononuclear. No organisms are seen on direct smears (bacteria, mycobacteria, protozoans, nor yeasts), and there are normal to slightly elevated levels of protein. The glucose level is usually normal; decrease in glucose concentration can occur with medulloblastoma, leukemic infiltration, *M. pneumoniae* infection, inadequately treated bacterial meningitis, tuberculosis, and, rarely, certain viral infections. The spinal fluid should be cultured for viruses, bacteria, fungi, and mycobacteria, and in some instances special examinations are indicated for protozoa, mycoplasma, and other pathogens. Careful examination of the spinal fluid is most important, especially to ensure that stains used for smears do not introduce artifacts and that the tests used for glucose levels are accurate. A simultaneous blood glucose level should be taken at the time of spinal puncture. Specimens for viral culture should be obtained from the throat and feces. A serum specimen should be obtained early in the course of illness and then again 2–3 wk later for possible serologic studies. For special laboratory procedures used in the identification of viruses and other agents, refer to the sections on various diseases.

DIFFERENTIAL DIAGNOSIS. Careful analysis of the history and epidemiologic circumstances may point toward one of the specific causes listed in Table 12–5. During the summer and autumn the presence of pleurodynia, herpangina, or unexplained febrile eruptions in the community suggests the possibility of coxsackieviral or echoviral infections; the coexistence of acute paralytic disorders in other patients suggests poliomyelitis; encephalitis in horses points to the possibility of an arbovirus infection; a history of swimming in waters contaminated by urine from infected animals may suggest leptospiral infection. Knowledge of clear-cut exposure to or concurrent evidence of mumps or of one of the common exanthems may be helpful in the differential diagnosis.

The association of pneumonia or other respiratory illness preceding aseptic meningitis strongly suggests the possibility of *M. pneumoniae* as the etiologic agent.

Most difficult from the diagnostic, therapeutic, and prognostic points of view are instances of incipient or partially or inadequately treated bacterial (especially when due to *H. influenzae*) or mycobacterial meningitis. The clinical findings, the dosage of antibiotic previously used, and examination of spinal fluid by smear, latex agglutination, and other rapid antigen identification tests, culture, and glucose level may be helpful in diagnosing bacterial meningitis. When tuberculous meningitis is suspected, a careful evaluation of contacts, an examination of an appropriately stained smear from the pellicle of the cerebrospinal fluid that was allowed to settle, and a positive tuberculin reaction may confirm the diagnosis. Although combined bacterial and viral infections occur, examinations of CSF should be repeated when there is evidence of a double infection. The possibility that the observed meningeal reaction is of noninfectious origin should also be considered.

TREATMENT. Hospitalization is usually necessary because of the possibility of bacterial disease, which should be treated there, and because hydration frequently requires fluid therapy, which can be best furnished there. Treatment is symptomatic. Headache and hyperesthesia are treated with rest, nonaspirin-containing analgesics, and a reduction in room light, noise, and visitors. Acetaminophen is recommended for fever. Codeine, morphine, and the phenothiazine derivatives, often used for pain and vomiting but rarely necessary in children, should be avoided because they may induce misleading signs and symptoms.

Several weeks after apparent recovery, careful neuromuscular assessment should be conducted to ensure that muscular weakness is not a sequel. Bilateral audiometry is recommended, especially when mumps virus is involved.

Cherry JD: Aseptic meningitis and viral meningitis. *In*: Feigin RD, Cherry JD (eds): Textbook of Pediatric Infectious Diseases, 2nd ed. Philadelphia, WB Saunders, 1987.

Cherry JD: Nonpolio enteroviruses: Coxsackieviruses, echoviruses, and enteroviruses. *In*: Feigin RD, Cherry JD (eds): Textbook of Pediatric Infectious Diseases, 2nd ed. Philadelphia, WB Saunders, 1987.

12.12 ENCEPHALITIS

Encephalitis is an inflammation of the brain, and the diagnosis can be established with absolute certainty only by the microscopic examination of brain tissue. In clinical practice the diagnosis is frequently made on the basis of neurologic manifestations and epidemiologic information without the aid of histologic material. When neurologic manifestations suggest encephalitis but inflammation of the brain has not occurred (e.g., in Reye syndrome), the condition is identified by the less specific term *encephalopathy*.

When encephalitis occurs, it may be localized or other areas of the nervous system may also be involved, and diagnostic terms reflect this involvement: *acute cerebellar ataxia, meningoencephalitis, and meningoencephalomyeloradiculitis (Guillain-Barré syndrome)*.

ETIOLOGY. A classification of encephalitis by etiology and source is presented in Table 12–13. Many of the agents listed produce other illnesses and are discussed more fully elsewhere (see Index). Although only about 25% of the cases of encephalitis reported to the Centers for Disease Control have established causes, the seasonal pattern of disease in the United States indicates that the unidentified etiologic agents in the vast majority of cases are enteroviruses (Sec. 12.80) or arboviruses; viruses of the common contagious diseases, herpes viruses, and an occasional nonviral agent cause the other infections.

EPIDEMIOLOGY. Since there are many different causes of encephalitis, no unified epidemiologic pattern exists. However, the vast majority of cases occur in the summer and fall, reflecting arboviral and enteroviral infections.

Arboviruses. Arboviruses are zoonoses in which man, not being essential in the life cycle of arboviruses, is infected accidentally by an arthropod vector. Most commonly, mosquitoes or other insects acquire arboviruses by biting infected birds, which often have prolonged viremia without illness. The insect vectors, though preferring birds, bite other vertebrates, including man and horses. Encephalitis in horses and mules ("blind staggers") may be the first indication of incipient trouble in an area; veterinarians are often the first to detect an impending epidemic. Although rural exposure is most common, urban and suburban outbreaks are also frequent.

Eastern equine encephalitis has a predilection for young infants; it is devastating, with high mortality and severe sequelae.

St. Louis virus encephalitis produces inapparent infection (demonstrated only by seroconversion) as well as disease and has a lower incidence of clinical disease in young children than in adolescents and adults.

Western equine encephalitis is frequently mild or clinically inapparent, demonstrated only by seroconversion. Mortality is much lower than with Eastern equine encephalitis, but sequelae may be severe.

California virus encephalitis outbreaks occur mostly in the midwestern United States. Severe illness is common, with important sequelae.

Powassan virus encephalitis is transmitted by the bite of infected wood ticks. More cases occur in Canada than in the United States, few of them in children.

Venezuelan equine encephalitis also occurs in the United States. Thus far the incidence has been low and the illness mild, although devastating outbreaks have occurred.

Enteroviruses. Enteroviruses (Sec. 12.80) are small RNA-containing viruses; 68 specific serotypes have been identified. The severity of disease ranges from mild aseptic meningitis to severe encephalitis with death or significant sequelae. Epidemics, some devastating, have been observed among newborns in nurseries.

Herpesviruses. *Herpes simplex* types 1 and 2 are relatively frequent causes of sporadic acute encephalitis, which may occur during primary contact with the virus or after an earlier primary infection, either subclinical or long forgotten. Herpesvirus encephalitis in newborn infants (Sec. 9.71) is part of a generalized viremia; the infection may be due to either type 1 ("oral") or type 2 ("genital") herpesvirus. In older patients herpes simplex virus may produce diffuse encephalitis or simulate brain abscess or fatal bulbospinal poliomyelitis, even when the patient's serologic status indicates a nonprimary infection. Characteristically, fluid obtained by nontraumatic spinal tap may contain erythrocytes. Progressive focal neurologic signs and evidence of localization by imaging techniques or electroencephalography are frequent and are indications for prompt brain biopsy and early therapy with acyclovir (Sec. 12.68).

Varicella-zoster virus (VZV) may cause acute encephalitis in close temporal relationship with chickenpox. VZV is also capable of secluding itself in spinal and cranial nerve roots and ganglia as a latent or suppressed infection, expressing itself later as herpes zoster.

Cytomegalovirus (CMV) may produce intrauterine infection with involvement of the central nervous system (Sec. 9.69 and 12.71). Severe cases may be recognized at birth, but more often subtle evidence of brain damage is not apparent for months or several years after birth.

Epstein-Barr virus (EBV) encephalitis may occur during infectious mononucleosis (Sec. 12.72) but also occurs without hematologic changes.

TABLE 12–13. Classification of Encephalitis by Etiology and Source

I. Infections—viral
  A. Spread person to person only
    1. Mumps: frequent in an unimmunized population; often mild
    2. Measles: may have serious sequelae
    3. Enteroviruses frequent at all ages; more serious in newborns
    4. Rubella: uncommon; sequelae rare except in congenital rubella
    5. Herpesvirus group
      a. Herpes simplex (types 1 and 2): relatively common; sequelae frequent; devastating in newborns
      b. Varicella-zoster virus: uncommon; serious sequelae not rare
      c. Cytomegaloviruses—congenital or acquired: may have delayed sequelae in congenital CMV
      d. EB virus (infectious mononucleosis): not common
    6. Pox group
      a. Vaccinia and variola: uncommon, but serious CNS damage occurs
    7. Parvovirus (erythema infectiosum): not common
    8. Influenza A and B
    9. Adenoviruses
    10. Other: Reoviruses, respiratory syncytial, parainfluenza, hepatitis B
  B. Arthropod-borne agents
    Arboviruses: spread to man by mosquitoes or ticks; seasonal epidemics depend on ecology of the insect vector; the following occur in the United States:

Eastern equine	California
Western equine	Powassan
Venezuelan equine	Dengue
St. Louis	Colorado tick fever

  C. Spread by warm-blooded mammals
    1. Rabies: saliva of many domestic and wild mammalian species
    2. Herpesvirus simiae ("B" virus): monkeys' saliva
    3. Lymphocytic choriomeningitis: rodents' excreta

II. Infections—nonviral
  A. Rickettsial: in Rocky Mountain spotted fever and typhus; encephalitic component from cerebral vasculitis
  B. *Mycoplasma pneumoniae:* interval of some days between respiratory and CNS symptoms
  C. Bacterial: tuberculous and other bacterial meningitis; often has encephalitic component
  D. Spirochetal: syphilis, congenital or acquired; leptospirosis; Lyme disease
  E. Cat-scratch disease
  F. Fungal: immunologically compromised patients at special risk; cryptococcosis; histoplasmosis; aspergillosis; mucormycosis; candidosis; coccidioidomycosis
  G. Protozoal: *Plasmodium* sp.; *Trypanosoma* sp.; *Naegleria* sp.; *Acanthamoeba; Toxoplasma gondii*
  H. Metazoal: trichinosis; echinococcosis; cysticercosis; schistosomiasis

III. Parainfectious—postinfectious, allergic
  Patients in whom an infectious agent or one of its components plays a contributory role in etiology, but the intact infectious agent is not isolated in vitro from the nervous system. It is postulated that in this group the influence of cell-mediated antigen-antibody complexes plus complement is especially important in producing the observed tissue damage
  A. Associated with specific diseases (These agents may also cause direct CNS damage—see I and II above)

Measles	Rickettsial infections
Rubella	Influenza A and B
Mumps	Varicella-zoster
Mycoplasma pneumoniae	

  B. Associated with vaccines

Rabies	Measles
Vaccinia	Yellow fever

IV. Human slow-virus diseases
  Accumulating evidence that viruses frequently acquired earlier in life, not necessarily with detectable acute illness, participate in later chronic neurologic disease (similar events also known to occur in animals) (see Sec. 12.83)
  A. Subacute sclerosing panencephalitis (SSPE); measles; rubella?
  B. Creutzfeldt-Jakob disease (spongiform encephalopathy)
  C. Progressive multifocal leukoencephalopathy
  D. Kuru (Fore tribe in New Guinea only)
  E. Human immunodeficiency virus (HIV)

V. Unknown—complex group
  This group constitutes more than two thirds of the cases of encephalitis reported to the Centers for Disease Control, Atlanta, Georgia. The yearly epidemic curve of these undiagnosed cases suggests that the majority are probably due to enteroviruses and/or arboviruses.

  There is also a miscellaneous group that are based on clinical criteria: Reye syndrome is one current example. Others include the extinct von Economo encephalitis (epidemic from 1918–1928); myoclonic encephalopathy of infancy; retinomeningoencephalitis with papilledema and retinal hemorrhage; recurrent encephalomyelitis (? allergic or autoimmune); pseudotumor cerebri; and epidemic neuromyasthenia—Iceland disease.

  An encephalitic clinical pattern may follow ingestion or absorption of a number of known and unknown toxic substances. These include ingestion of lead and mercury and percutaneous absorption of hexachlorophene as a skin disinfectant and gamma benzene hexachloride as a scabicide.

PATHOGENESIS. The sequence of events varies with the agent of disease and with the host. In general, the viruses of encephalitis enter the lymphatic system, either through ingestion of an enterovirus or from a mosquito or other insect bite. There multiplication begins, and seeding of the bloodstream leads to infection of several organs. At this stage (the extraneural phase) a systemic, febrile illness is present, but if further viral multiplication takes place in the seeded organs, a secondary propagation of large amounts of virus may occur. Invasion of the central nervous system is followed by clinical evidence of neurologic disease.

It is likely that neurologic damage is caused (1) by a direct invasion and destruction of neural tissues by actively multiplying viruses, or (2) by a reaction of the patient's nervous tissue to antigens of the virus. Neuronal destruction is probably due directly to viral invasion, whereas the host's vigorous tissue response probably results in demyelinization and vascular and perivascular destruction. Vascular damage leads to impaired circulation and to signs and symptoms.

PATHOLOGY. It is difficult to determine the etiology of encephalitis at autopsy, although morphologic identification of falciparum malaria, trypanosomiasis, and fungal encephalitis is possible. In viral encephalitides, the histopathologist may recognize rabies (Negri bodies) or an agent of the herpesvirus group (intranuclear inclusion bodies), but special viral studies are usually needed. Viral isolation and identification require that tissues be collected *without fixation in preservatives*.

Tissue sections of the brain generally are characterized by meningeal congestion and mononuclear infiltration, perivascular cuffs of lymphocytes and plasma cells, some perivascular tissue necrosis with myelin breakdown, neuronal disruption in various stages including ultimately neuronophagia and endothelial proliferation or necrosis. A marked degree of demyelination with preservation of neurons and their axons is considered predominantly to represent "postinfectious" or "allergic" encephalitis. The cerebral cortex, especially the temporal lobe, is often severely affected by herpes simplex virus; the arboviruses tend to affect the entire brain; rabies has a predilection for the basal structures. Involvement of the spinal cord, nerve roots, and peripheral nerves is quite variable.

CLINICAL MANIFESTATIONS. There is a wide range of severity of clinical manifestations even with the same etiologic agent. Some children may appear to be mildly affected initially, only to lapse into coma and die suddenly. In others the illness may be ushered in by high fever, violent convulsions interspersed with bizarre movements, and hallucinations alternating with brief periods of clarity, but then leaves relatively few sequelae.

Most commonly, the initial manifestations resemble an undifferentiated acute systemic illness with fever, headache, or, in infants, screaming spells, abdominal distress, nausea, and vomiting. An associated mild nasopharyngitis is common. As the temperature rises, there may be mental dullness eventuating in stupor in combination with bizarre movements, convulsions, and nuchal rigidity, often not as pronounced as in purely meningitic illness. Focal neurologic signs may be stationary, progressive, or fluctuating. Loss of bowel and bladder control and unprovoked emotional bursts may occur.

Specific forms or complicating manifestations of encephalitis include Guillain-Barré syndrome, acute transverse myelitis, acute hemiplegia, and acute cerebellar ataxia.

Acute cerebellar ataxia is characterized by an abrupt onset of truncal ataxia resulting in varying degrees of gait disturbance. Children with this illness have tremulousness of the head and trunk when in the upright position and of the extremities when attempting to move them against gravity. The full-blown clinical pattern usually develops over 3–4 days to 1 wk, and the illness may last from a week to several months.

DIAGNOSIS AND DIFFERENTIAL DIAGNOSIS. A carefully recorded history is essential. It should take into account possible exposures during the past 2–3 wk to illnesses not only in other persons but also in animals (especially horses) and to possible contacts with mosquitos and ticks within remote areas as well as in the local community. Inquiry should also be made about recent injections of biologic substances and about the possibilities of exposure to heavy metals, pesticides, or noxious substances.

The cerebrospinal fluid should be carefully examined to exclude other disorders that may respond to specific therapy. Smears for bacteria, appropriate rapid antigen identification tests, and cultures of the cerebrospinal fluid are mandatory; the history and clinical findings may indicate the need for acid-fast stain and culture of the sediment for mycobacteria. Other circumstances may indicate the need for excluding fungal or protozoal infection; atypical cells may require cytopathologic study to exclude neural neoplasms that may have presented acutely.

In viral encephalitis the cerebrospinal fluid is generally clear; the leukocyte count may range from none to several thousand, often with a significant percentage of polymorphonuclear cells initially, moderate or no elevation of protein, and an initially normal concentration of glucose relative to the simultaneously determined blood glucose concentration.

Expert advice should be sought early for any patient suspected of having an encephalitic illness; and spinal fluid, blood, feces, and throat swabs should be collected and sent to a laboratory offering viral diagnostic services. An additional serum specimen should be collected 10–21 days later. Though these studies may not provide an immediate diagnosis, they may give early warning of an impending epidemic. If there is evidence for a specific virus, the patient can generally be assured of subsequent lasting immunity to that virus. The therapy also may be indicated by the preliminary results.

A patient with concurrent or recent mumps, measles, or similar infections (see Table 12–13, I-A) is at increased risk for developing encephalitis, and neurologic involvement may at times precede the development of other manifestations of the disease. For example, when mumps parotitis occurs without clinical evidence of involvement of the central nervous system, cerebrospinal fluid pleocytosis often indicates that such involvement is present; mumps meningoencephalitis commonly occurs without parotitis. In measles, some 40% of patients without clinical evidence of encephalitis have electroencephalograms suggestive of neurologic disturbance. The relation between acute non-neural diseases in early life and debilitating neural syndromes appearing in later life ("slow virus effects") is also important (see Table 12–13).

Occasionally patients who have traveled in Africa or Asia present with bizarre systemic and central nervous system signs and symptoms from encephalitis due to viruses, trypanosomiasis, or falciparum malaria.

Children who are immunologically compromised (e.g., by lymphoma, cytotoxic drugs, acquired immunodeficiency syndrome, immunogenetic defects) are at increased risk, especially with respect to infections in which protective cell-mediated immunity is important (e.g., chickenpox, cytomegalovirus, fungal infections). Children with leukemia who have had prophylactic radiation to the central nervous system and intrathecal drugs may develop an acute meningoencephalitis *after* cessation of such prophylaxis and despite bone marrow remission.

PREVENTION. The widespread use of effective attenuated viral vaccines for measles, mumps, and rubella has almost eliminated central nervous system complications from these diseases in the United States. The control of encephalitis due to arboviruses has been less successful because specific vaccines for the arbovirus diseases that occur in North America are not available. Control of insect vectors by suitable spraying methods and eradication of insect breeding sites is useful.

TREATMENT. With the exception of the use of acyclovir for herpes simplex encephalitis (Sec. 12.69), treatment is nonspecific and empirical, and is aimed at maintaining life and supporting each organ system. The effectiveness of various recommended regimens has not been objectively evaluated.

Until a bacterial cause and, in particular, a brain abscess is substantially excluded, parenteral antibiotic therapy should be administered.

It is crucial to anticipate and be prepared for *convulsions, cerebral edema, hyperpyrexia, inadequate respiratory exchange, disturbed fluid and electrolyte balance, aspiration and asphyxia, abrupt cardiac and respiratory arrest of central origin,* and *cardiac decompensation. Disseminated intravascular coagulation* may be a complication.

All patients with severe encephalitis should be monitored in an intensive care unit (Sec. 6.34). In patients with evidence of increased intracranial pressure, placement of a pressure transducer in the epidural space is often indicated for monitoring intracranial pressure as a guide to therapy aimed at reducing cerebral edema. The risks of cardiac and respiratory failure or arrest are high. All fluids, electrolytes, and medications are initially given parenterally. In prolonged states of coma, parenteral alimentation is indicated. *Inappropriate secretion of antidiuretic hormone* is fairly common in acute central nervous system disorders, so that constant evaluation is required for its early detection. Normal blood levels of glucose, magnesium, and calcium must be maintained in order to minimize the threat of convulsions.

Treatment of seizures and cerebral edema is discussed in Sec. 6.35, 12.15, 20.19–20.23, and 20.53–20.57. In addition, *dexamethasone*, 0.1–0.2 mg/kg IV in an initial dose followed by 0.05–0.1 mg/kg/dose IV every 4–6 hr, is given. This large dose should be reduced gradually after a few days if recovery or improvement is evident. Dexamethasone probably should not be used in patients with acute viral diseases because corticosteroids may potentiate the viral infection.

Supportive and rehabilitative efforts are very important after the patient recovers. Motor incoordination, convulsive disorders, squint, total or partial deafness, and behavioral disturbances may appear only after an interval of time. Visual disturbances due to chorioretinopathy and perceptual amblyopia may also make a delayed appearance. Special facilities and, at times, institutional placement may become necessary.

PROGNOSIS. Prognosis is guarded with respect to both immediate outcome and sequelae. Sequelae involving the central nervous system may be intellectual, motor, psychiatric, epileptic, visual, or auditory in nature. Cardiovascular, pulmonary, hepatic, intraocular, and other systems may be permanently affected. The short-term and long-term prognoses depend to some extent on etiology and age. Young infants usually have severe disease and sequelae. In general, herpes simplex viruses carry a worse prognosis for survival and residual disability than do the enteroviruses. Fetal rubella encephalitis is very ominous, as is acute generalized cytomegaloviral infection accompanied by encephalitis. The latter may be insidious, with evidence of disability deferred for some months.

JAMES D. CHERRY

Bryson YJ: Antiviral agents. *In:* Feigin RD, Cherry JD (eds): Textbook of Pediatric Infectious Diseases, 2nd ed. Philadelphia, WB Saunders, 1987.

Centers for Disease Control: Encephalitis Surveillance Annual Summary, 1978. Issued May 1981.

Cherry JD: Mycoplasma and ureaplasma. *In:* Feigin RD, Cherry JD (eds): Textbook of Pediatric Infectious Diseases, 2nd ed. Philadelphia, WB Saunders, 1987.

Cherry JD: Viral meningoencephalitis and encephalitis. *In:* Feigin RD, Cherry JD (eds): Textbook of Pediatric Infectious Diseases, 2nd ed. Philadelphia, WB Saunders, 1987.

Johnson RT: The pathogenesis of acute viral encephalitis and postinfectious encephalomyelitis. J Infect Dis 155:359, 1987.

Monath TP, Tsai T: Arbovirus diseases of North America. *In:* Feigin RD, Cherry JD (eds): Textbook of Pediatric Infectious Diseases, 2nd ed. Philadelphia, WB Saunders, 1987.

12.13 INFECTIONS IN THE COMPROMISED HOST

The compromised host has one or more defects in the normal defense mechanisms that protect him or her from infectious agents, predisposing the individual to an increased risk of severe life-threatening infection. Important nonimmunologic host defense mechanisms include local mucocutaneous mechanical barriers such as the physical integrity of the skin and mucous membranes, the biochemical nature of the mucus, mucociliary clearance, the cough reflex, and the patency of anatomic sites of mucus drainage or other body fluid excretion. The immunologic host defense mechanisms include inflammatory responses due to phagocytic cells (neutrophils, monocytes, tissue macrophages, reticuloendothelial cells) and complement or properdin activation. Specific immunologic responses include stimulation of immunoglobulin-producing B lymphocytes and the activation of cell-mediated immunity, which includes T lymphocytes, natural killer (NK) cells, and macrophages with subsequent production of immunologic-inflammatory cytokines (lymphokines) (see Sec. 11.1).

The nature of infections in the compromised host is dependent on the predominant defect present in the host defense system. Infections in immunocompetent patients are usually due to alterations of the mucocutaneous barrier following trauma, burns, surgery, or placement of an indwelling catheter (Table 12–14). Previously immunocompetent patients may also be at risk of infection if they develop a secondary immunodeficiency due to a chronic condition such as malnutrition, diabetes mellitus, or renal insuffiency (see Table 12–14). Patients with congenital or acquired defects in neutrophil number or function, cell-mediated immunity, humoral immunity, or splenic function are at particularly increased risk of severe life-threatening infections (Table 12–15). The nature of the immunodeficiency in part determines both the risk of infection with specific pathogens and the site and severity of the infection (see Table 12–15). Combinations of host defense defects, such as those produced by cancer chemotherapy (malnutrition, mucositis, granulocytopenia, and lymphopenia), together with the use of indwelling intravenous catheters (for chemotherapy infusions) predispose the patient to the highest risk of serious opportunistic infections.

Opportunistic infections involve microbial agents that are thought to have little or no pathogenic role in immunocompetent patients but readily infect debilitated patients with primary or secondary defects in one or more host defense mechanisms. Infections due to more invasive pathogens are also considered opportunistic if they affect patients with congenital or acquired defects of the immune defense system. In addition to typical patterns of infection (sepsis, pneumonia), immunocompromised patients may also demonstrate unusual manifestations of common pathogens such as cytomegalovirus-induced retinitis, enteritis in patients with AIDS, or chronic echovirus encephalitis or myositis in patients with agammaglobulinemia.

DECREASED PROTECTION BY THE SKIN OR MUCOUS MEMBRANES. The skin and mucous membranes are the first line of protection against infection. In addition to being a physical barrier that few pathogens can penetrate, the skin contains bacteriostatic and bacteriocidal fatty acids secreted by the sebaceous glands. Mucous membrane secretions contain various enzymes (lactoperoxidase, lysozyme, lactoferrin), and secretory IgA, and specific areas have unfavorable acidic environments (stomach, urine, vagina) that reduce bacterial activity. Furthermore, each mucosal surface contains a normal bacterial flora, which may prevent local colonization by pathogenic microorganisms. This *colonization resistance* is due to the local bacterial production of antimicrobial compounds (bacteriocins), alteration of the redox potential, and competition for nutrients. Additional local defense mechanisms include mucociliary clearance, the cough reflex, unobstructed flow of secretions, and the activity of tissue phagocytic cells. Interference or disruption of any of these local defense mechanisms may predispose to infection: Broad-spectrum antibiotics may alter the normal flora and reduce colonization resistance; therapy intended to increase gastric pH may increase gastric colonization with pathogenic bacteria; obstruction to the flow of urine or lung secretions may cause pyelonephritis or pneumonia, respectively; and surgical incision, burns, or trauma may alter the physical barrier. Table 12–14 lists situations in which the mucocutaneous barrier to infection may be bypassed or compromised, as well as the microorganisms frequently incriminated.

SHUNTS. Cerebrospinal fluid shunts for congenital or acquired hydrocephalus are the most common shunts em-

TABLE 12–14. Opportunistic Infections in Patients Without Primary Immunodeficiency Syndromes

Alteration of Mucocutaneous Barrier	Organism and Type of Infection
Indwelling Catheter	
Central venous catheter (Broviac, Hickman)	*Streptococcus aureus, Staphylococcus epidermidis, Corynebacterium JK, Candida:* bacteremia, fungemia
Urinary catheter	*Escherichia coli*, enterococcus, *S. saprophyticus:* pyelonephritis
Tenkhoft catheter (continuous ambulatory peritoneal dialysis)	*S. epidermidis, S. aureus, E. coli, Pseudomonas aeruginosa, Candida:* peritonitis
Cerebrospinal fluid shunts	*S. epidermidis, S. aureus*, diphtheroid: meningitis
Burns	*P. aeruginosa, S. epidermidis, Candida:* cutaneous lesions, sepsis
Inhalation Therapy	
Contaminated solutions	*P. aeruginosa, Serratia marcescens, Legionella:* pneumonia
Surgical Wounds	
Abdominal	Gram-negative bacteria, *S. aureus, S. epidermidis, Candida*
Nongastrointestinal	*S. aureus, S. epidermidis*, streptococci, gram-negative bacteria: wound abscess, sepsis
Fistula-Sinus Communications	
Neurocutaneous fistula	*S. aureus, S. epidermidis, E. coli:* meningitis
Neuroenteric fistula	Gram-negative bacteria: meningitis
Otic, facial sinus-meningeal sinus tract	Pneumococcus: meningitis
Facial sinus fracture (CSF rhinorrhea)	Pneumococcus: meningitis
Intravenous Drug Abuse	*S. aureus, P. aeruginosa*, streptococci: endocarditis, osteomyelitis, hepatitis B, C, D virus, AIDS
Prosthetic Devices	
Cardiac valves	*S. epidermidis*, streptococci, *S. aureus*, diphtheroid, *Candida:* endocarditis
Pacemaker	*S. epidermidis, S. aureus, Candida:* subcutaneous pocket endocardial infection
Chronic Disease	
Malnutrition	Measles, tuberculosis, herpes simplex; bacterial, parasitic, and viral diarrhea; gram-negative bacterial pneumonia
Cystic fibrosis	*S. aureus, Haemophilus influenzae*, mucoid *P. aeruginosa, Pseudomonas cepacia:* pneumonia
Diabetes mellitus	Urinary tract infections, *Mucor* and other fungi, sinus-orbital infection
Nephrotic syndrome	Pneumococcus, *E. coli:* peritonitis
Uremia	*S. aureus*, gram-negative bacteria, fungi: sepsis, soft tissue infection, herpes simplex, *Pneumocystis carinii*
Cirrhosis/ascites	Pneumococcus, *E. coli:* peritonitis
Chronic transfusion therapy	Hepatitis B and C viruses, Epstein-Barr virus, cytomegalovirus, parvovirus, AIDS
Prolonged broad-spectrum antibiotic therapy	*Candida*, enterococcus, multidrug-resistant gram-negative or gram-positive bacteria: sepsis
Spinal cord injury	Gram-negative or gram-positive bacteria: pneumonia, pyelonephritis, pressure sores, abscesses, osteomyelitis

ployed in children. CSF infection, with or without shunt tract infection, usually requires shunt revision and, if meningitis and ventriculitis are present, contributes to an unfavorable cognitive outcome and a possible increase in mortality. CSF-shunt infections occur in 5–15% of patients, develop within 6–8 wk of shunt placement, are more common in younger infants and following shunt revision for a previous infection, and are independent of the type of shunt (ventriculoperitoneal vs ventriculoatrial). Late infection is rare but is probably due to delayed onset of bacterial growth introduced at the time of shunt placement. External subcutaneous tract infection may occur if the catheter erodes through the skin. In addition, the distal segment may perforate the bowel, bladder, or vagina.

The predominant pathogen is *Staphylococcus epidermidis*, which produces an adherent extracellular mucoid carbohydrate slime, permitting this organism to colonize the catheter and resist phagocytosis. More than 50% of the *S. epidermidis* organisms recovered from CSF are present on the patient's skin at the time of the placement; the remaining *S. epidermidis* are environmental contaminants transmitted from the surgeon or operating room. Wound infection may be due to *S. aureus* or gram-negative bacteria, whereas true internal shunt infections are due to *S. epidermidis* and rarely to *Corynebacterium, Propionibacterium*, streptococci, gram-negative enteric bacteria, and yeasts.

The *clinical manifestations* of infections of ventriculoperitoneal shunts include indolent fever, abdominal pain, rarely peritonitis, and headache due to shunt malfunction. There may be erythema over the shunt tract and meningismus. Patients with infection of a ventriculoatrial shunt may manifest fever, shunt dysfunction, and meningismus, but they may also demonstrate hypocomplementemic glomerulonephritis due to persistent *S. epidermidis* bacteremia and antigen-antibody complex formation with deposition in the glomerulus.

The *diagnosis* of shunt infection is confirmed when a shunt CSF culture is positive or the shunt CSF white blood cell count is increased above 10 and shows a predominance of neutrophils. Bacteremia is present in more than 85% of patients with ventriculoatrial shunt infection. Signs of immune complex glomerulonephritis include hypertension, microscopic hematuria, elevated BUN and serum creatinine levels, and anemia. Infected ventriculoatrial shunts may also produce septic pulmonary emboli, pulmonary hypertension, and endocarditis. If a sample of shunt CSF cannot be obtained and there is meningismus, a lumbar puncture may reveal bacteria and a predominance of neutrophils. Occasionally, no bacterial organism is identified, and presumptive therapy must be initiated.

Treatment of shunt infection includes the use of antibiotics against the specific organism and in some situations removal of the shunt. A combination of systemic vancomycin and intraventricular gentamicin is effective initially. Resistant infections that are difficult to clear may be treated with intraventricular gentamicin plus systemic vancomycin or trimethaprim-sulfamethoxazole and rifampin. The distal end of the ventriculoperitoneal shunt should be externalized; this will usually relieve abdominal complaints within 30–60 min. If abdominal signs continue 4–6 hr after shunt externalization, other intra-abdominal pathology such as viscus perforation or appendicitis should be considered. Shunt revision may be performed according to either of two protocols: immediate revision within 24 hr of defervescence or delayed revision after three consecutive negative CSF cultures. This latter

TABLE 12–15. Risk Factors and Related Pathogens Affecting Immunocompromised Patients

Granulocytopenia (e.g., aplastic anemia, congenital myelophthisis, myelosuppressive agents, bone marrow transplant)
Bacteria
Gram-negative Organisms
Escherichia coli (sepsis, pneumonia, pyelonephritis)
Klebsiella pneumoniae (sepsis, pneumonia)
Pseudomonas aeruginosa (sepsis, pneumonia, cutaneous lesions)
Mixed anaerobic and aerobic enteric bacteria (typhlitis, perianal abscess)
Gram-positive Organisms
Staphylococcus aureus (sepsis, cellulitis, soft tissue infection)
S. epidermidis (sepsis, line infection)
Corynebacterium JK (sepsis)
α-Hemolytic streptococci (sepsis)
Fungi
Candida (sepsis, pneumonia, ophthalmitis, liver and spleen abscesses)
Aspergillus (sepsis, pneumonia, sinusitis, CNS infection, cutaneous lesions)
Mucormycosis (pneumonia, sinusitis, CNS infection)
Fusarium (sepsis, cutaneous lesions, pneumonia)
Pseudoallescheria (sepsis, cutaneous lesions, pneumonia)
Alternaria (sepsis, cutaneous lesions)
Phagocytic Dysfunction (e.g., chronic granulomatous disease, hyperimmunoglobulin E syndrome, leukocyte adhesion defects)
Bacteria
S. aureus (soft tissue, skeletal, and solid organ abscesses; pneumonia, sepsis)
Streptococci (soft tissue, skeletal, and solid organ abscesses; pneumonia, sepsis)
Serratia marcescens (soft tissue and solid organ abscesses, pneumonia, sepsis)
E. coli (soft tissue and solid organ abscesses, pneumonia, sepsis)
Pseudomonas cepacia (soft tissue abscess, pneumonia, sepsis)
Salmonella (enteritis)
Nocardia (soft tissue and solid organ abscesses, pneumonia)
Fungi
Candida (soft tissue, skeletal, and solid organ abscesses, pneumonia, sepsis)
Aspergillus (soft tissue abscess, pneumonia, sepsis)
Cellular Immune Deficiency (e.g., congenital, AIDS, immunosuppression, corticosteroid use, transplantation, Hodgkin disease)
Bacteria
Listeria monocytogenes (sepsis, meningitis)
Salmonella (sepsis)
Mycobacterium tuberculosis (pneumonia, disseminated disease)
Atypical mycobacterium *(M. avium, M. intracellulare)* (sepsis, pneumonia, disseminated disease)
Nocardia (pneumonia, CNS infection)
Legionella (pneumonia)
Fungi
Cryptococcus neoformans (sepsis, meningitis)
Histoplasma capsulatum (pneumonia, disseminated disease)
Coccidioides immitis (pneumonia, meningitis)
Viruses
Varicella-zoster (cutaneous and CNS infection, pneumonia, hepatitis)
Cytomegalovirus (bone marrow infection, hepatitis, pneumonia, retinitis, esophagitis, colitis, CNS infection)
Herpes simplex (CNS infection, pneumonia, esophagitis, hepatitis, disseminated disease)
Epstein-Barr virus (lymphoma)
Measles (pneumonia, encephalitis)
Polyomavirus BK (hemorrhagic cystitis, ureteric stenosis, renal insufficiency)
Polyomavirus JC (progressive multifocal leukoencephalopathy)
Protozoa
Pneumocystis carinii (pneumonia, rare extrapulmonary spread)
Toxoplasma gondii (CNS infection, myocarditis)
Cryptosporidium (enteritis)
Helminth
Strongyloides stercoralis (enteritis, pneumonia, sepsis, meningitis)
Humoral Defects (e.g., congenital immunoglobulin, complement, properdin deficiencies)
Bacteria
Streptococcus pneumoniae (sepsis, meningitis, sinopulmonary infection)
Haemophilus influenzae (sepsis, meningitis, arthritis, sinopulmonary infection)
Neisseria meningitidis (sepsis, meningitis, arthritis)
N. gonorrhoeae (sepsis, meningitis, arthritis)
Mycoplasma pneumoniae (arthritis)
Campylobacter (enteritis)
Virus
Enterovirus including polio vaccine (encephalitis, paralysis, myositis, arthritis)
Rotavirus (enteritis)
Protozoa
Giardia lamblia (enteritis)
Splenic Dysfunction (e.g., asplenia, sickle cell anemia, splenectomy: a combined immunoglobulin and reticuloendothelial cell deficiency)
Bacteria
S. pneumoniae (sepsis, meningitis)
H. influenzae type b (sepsis, meningitis)
N. meningitis (sepsis, meningitis)
DF-2 (sepsis, meningitis)
Protozoa
Babesiosis
Malaria

protocol is preferred for infections due to *S. aureus* and gram-negative bacteria. In either situation antibiotics should be continued for 10–14 days after shunt revision. In CSF-shunt infections due to *S. epidermidis* some centers attempt to treat the first episode with systemic and intraventricular antibiotics without performing shunt revision. This approach has been used in patients with ventriculoatrial shunts and in some patients with ventriculoperitoneal shunts (after changing the peritoneal end only).

Prevention of shunt infection includes meticulous cutaneous preparation and surgical technique. Systemic and intraventricular antibiotics and soaking the shunt tubing in antibiotics have been used to reduce the incidence of infection, with varying success (Table 12–16).

INTRAVASCULAR DEVICES. Intravenous access for the administration of nutrients, cancer chemotherapy, or blood products, for central venous pressure monitoring, and for blood sampling has become part of the routine care administered to children with various gastrointestinal disorders, malignancies, organ transplants, and cardiopulmonary distress requiring intensive care. When prolonged intravenous access is anticipated, a cuffed silicone rubber (Silastic) catheter may be inserted into the right atrium through the subclavian, cephalic, or jugular vein. The extravascular proximal segment of the catheter passes through a subcutaneous tunnel before exiting the skin, usually on the superior aspect of the chest. The Broviac or Hickman catheters are the prototype devices used for long-term venous access. The totally implanted venous access systems (Mediport, Port-a-cath, Infus-port) consist of a reservoir placed in a subcutaneous pocket with a self-sealing silicone septum that permits repeated percutaneous needle insertion and administration of drugs. The reservoir is attached to a distal catheter, which is tunneled in the subcutaneous tissue before it is inserted into the superior vena cava through the same veins as those used for the Hickman or Broviac catheter. The reservoir and catheter are totally intracorporeal and have no exit site or externalized material such as that needed for the Hickman and Broviac systems. The use of these central venous devices has improved the quality of life of high-risk patients but has also increased the risk of various infections, such as exit site and tunnel infections, as well as catheter-associated bacteremia or fungemia.

The incidence of local (exit site, tunnel, pocket) infection is 0.3–0.6 episodes/1,000 catheter days. The incidence of Broviac or Hickman catheter sepsis is 2–4/1,000 days, whereas that for implantable systems is 0.3–0.7/1,000 catheter days. The risk of catheter infection is increased among premature infants and young children, patients with neutropenia or catheter thrombosis, and those receiving total parenteral nutrition. The risk of local infection may be greatest within the 1st mo of catheter insertion, but the daily risk of catheter sepsis is constant regardless of its duration in situ. The organisms responsibile for local infection are similar to those causing catheter sepsis (see Table 12–14). Local infections due to *Pseudomonas* sp. are noted in patients permitted to swim or bathe. Right-sided endocarditis is a rare complication of an infected catheter, involves the tricuspid valve and atrial endocardium, and is associated with intracardiac thrombosis.

The pathogenesis of catheter sepsis is related to local contamination and subsequent colonization of the catheter rather than primary bacteremia seeding the intravascular device. Gram-positive bacteremia accounts for 60–70% of episodes of catheter sepsis (*S. epidermidis, S. aureus, S. pyogenes, S. faecalis*), gram-negative enteric bacteria occur in 20–30% of episodes (*Klebsiella* sp., *E. coli, Pseudomonas* sp., *Acinetobacter* sp.), and fungi account for 5–10% of catheter sepsis episodes (*Candida* sp., *Malassezia furfur*). *Mycobacterium fortuitum, Bacillus* sp., and polymicrobial sepsis are rarer causes of catheter infections.

The *clinical manifestations* of local infection include erythema, tenderness, and purulent discharge. Catheter sepsis may also present as fever without an identifiable focus or as an alternate diagnosis. All episodes of fever are not due to catheter sepsis, and all episodes of bacteremia are not related to the catheter. Catheter-related sepsis, if diagnosed early, rarely progresses to septic shock and death, whereas noncatheter-related sepsis associated with neutropenia is usually more fulminant and may progress rapidly to shock, disseminated intravascular coagulation, and death.

The *diagnosis* of catheter sepsis is confirmed by simultaneously performing blood cultures from the catheter and a peripheral vein. If quantitative blood cultures are obtained, a higher grade of bacteremia will be evident from the catheter than from the peripheral blood sample. Examination of the buffy coat from the cells in the catheter sample may help to identify the specific bacteria or fungi responsible. The *clinical manifestations* of catheter-related right-sided endocarditis include pulmonary infiltrates, fever, and persistent bacteremia. Echocardiography demonstrates tricuspid valve vegetations or mural thrombi.

The *treatment* of suspected catheter sepsis in a neutropenic patient includes initiation of broad-spectrum antibiotics such as ceftazidine with or without gentamicin or vancomycin (see later under Febrile Neutropenic Cancer Patient). Treatment of catheter sepsis in non-neutropenic patients is directed against the specific organism recovered in the blood or exit site culture. If the catheter is no longer needed, it should be removed immediately. If the catheter is required, the catheter does not need to be removed for all exit site or septic episodes; most episodes of *S. epidermidis* infection can be treated with the catheter in place. Repeated negative blood cultures through the catheter ensure that therapy has been successful. However, tunnel infections and episodes of sepsis due to fungi, *Bacillus* sp., and polymicrobial and gram-negative enteric bacteria are often difficult to treat and may require removal of the catheter.

Thrombosis complicating catheter sepsis may be treated with heparin and thrombolysis with streptokinase or urokinase. Endocarditis complicating catheter sepsis requires prolonged antibiotic therapy and ultrasound evaluation of tricuspid valve function.

Prevention of catheter-related infection includes meticulous surgical aseptic technique with gown, gloves, mask, drape, and scrub in an operating room–like environment. Use of antibacterial ointment, avoidance of occlusive or semipermeable dressings, avoidance of bathing or swimming, and detailed catheter care may reduce the incidence of catheter infection. The incidence of sepsis with totally implanted devices may be lower than that with externalized catheters owing to elimination of chronic irritation at the exit site and the intracorporeal position of implantable systems.

URETHRAL CATHETERS. Short-term use of transurethral indwelling urinary catheters is common in pediatric intensive care units and aids in the management of patients with severe cardiopulmonary compromise, coma, spinal cord injury, or urine retention. Nosocomial bacterial colonization of the bladder occurs because the catheter acts as a conduit facilitating bacterial access to the bladder. Bacteria usually travel intraluminally retrograde up the catheter or, rarely, through the extraluminal space between the urethra and the catheter. Transient uroepithelial cell dysfunction also promotes bacterial colonization, which may progress to asymptomatic bacteriuric cystitis, asymptomatic bacteremia, symptomatic pyelonephritis, and symptomatic urosepsis. Risk of bacteriuria ($\geq 10^5$ organisms/mL) may be as high as 5% daily, whereas the cumulative risk of symptomatic bacteremia is 1–2%. Risk factors for bacteriuria include the duration of catheterization, absence of systemic antibiotic use, frequent disconnection of

TABLE 12–16. Selected Prophylactic Regimens for Surgery or Following Disruption of Mucocutaneous Barriers*

Predisposing Procedure	Prophylactic Regimen	Comments
Congenital or Acquired Heart Defects		*Endocarditis Prevention*
Dental, upper respiratory	*Oral:* Amoxicillin 50 mg/kg 1 hr prior and 25 mg/kg 6 hr later, or erythromycin 20 mg/kg 2 hr prior and 10 mg/kg 6 hr later	Oral more convenient and safer than parenteral. Erythromycin or vancomycin for penicillin allergy
	Parenteral: Ampicillin 50 mg/kg IM, IV plus gentamicin 2 mg/kg IM, IV 30 min prior, *or* vancomycin 20 mg/kg IV 1 hr prior	Avoid IM injection if patient is on anticoagulants. Parenteral is most effective method and is recommended for high-risk patients with prosthetic valves, prior endocarditis, or those taking continuous penicillin for rheumatic fever prevention
Gastrointestinal, genitourinary	*Oral:* Amoxicillin 50 mg/kg 1 hr prior, 25 mg/kg 6 hr later *Parenteral:* Ampicillin 50 mg/kg IM, IV plus gentamicin 2 mg/kg IM, IV 30 min prior *or* vancomycin 20 mg/kg IV 1 hr prior plus gentamicin 2 mg/kg IM, IV 30 min prior	
Head, Neck, Oral Surgery	Cefazolin 12.5 mg/kg IV 30–60 min prior and repeated q6hr for 2 days	*Alternates:* 3rd generation cephalosporins, ampicillin, or clindamycin plus gentamicin
Cardiovascular Procedures (including pacemaker insertion)	Cefazolin 12.5 mg/kg IV q6hr or oxacillin 50 mg/kg IV q4–6hr or vancomycin 20 mg/kg IV q6hr. Begin 30–60 min prior, continue for 2 days	Vancomycin or second-generation cephalosporin may be useful if *Staphylococcus aureus* occurs despite cefazolin prophylaxis
Gastrointestinal Surgery		
Gastroduodenal-biliary	Cefazolin 12.5 mg/kg IV q6hr. Begin 30–60 min prior, continue 2 days	Can add gentamicin for biliary surgery
Colon	*Oral:* Erythromycin 15–50 mg/kg and neomycin 25 mg/kg given at 1, 2, and 11 P.M. prior to surgery	Change diet and initiate catharsis
	Parenteral: Cefoxitin 40 mg/kg IV q6hr, or metronidazole 15–50 mg/kg/24 hr, and gentamicin 2 mg/kg IV prior and q8hr for 1–2 days	Parenteral if unscheduled (emergency) surgery
Appendectomy	Cefoxitin 40 mg/kg IV q6hr for 3 doses; if perforated, cefoxitin for 3–5 days plus metronidazole 15–50 mg/kg/24 hr q6hr for 3–5 days	*Alternate:* Ampicillin, plus gentamicin plus clindamycin
Penetrating abdominal trauma	Cefoxitin ± gentamicin	*Alternate:* Ampicillin, plus gentamicin plus clindamycin
Splenectomy	Pneumococcal vaccine 1 mo prior to surgery	Daily penicillin prophylaxis if patient <10 yr old or for 1 yr postsplenectomy if older
Neurosurgical Procedures		
CSF shunt	Oxacillin 100–200 mg/kg/24 hr IV 30–60 prior and q6hr for 2 days	*Alternates:* Trimethoprim-sulfamethoxazole, vancomycin, or cefazolin ± intrathecal gentamicin
Craniotomy	Oxacillin or vancomycin 10 mg/kg IV and gentamicin 2 mg/kg IV prior to and for 2–3 days	*Alternate:* Clindamycin
Genitourinary Surgery		
Cesarean section	Cefazolin	
Premature labor with rupture of membranes, and group B streptococci carrier state	Ampicillin 1 g IV, q4hr until delivery	Prevents neonatal group B streptococcal sepsis
Chorioamnionitis	Ampicillin plus gentamicin ± clindamycin or cephalosporin IV prior to delivery	May reduce maternal and neonatal infection
Urinary tract surgery	*Oral:* Ampicillin 20 mg/kg/24 hr or nitrofurantoin 2 mg/kg/24 hr	*Alternate:* Trimethoprim-sulfamethoxazole
Other Procedures		
Dog and human bites	*Oral:* Augmentin (amoxicillin-clavulanate) may be effective but requires careful follow-up	Wound irrigation and tetanus prophylaxis indicated
Burns	*Oral:* Penicillin 50,000 U/kg/24 hr, q6hr if burn is mild *Topical:* Silver sulfadiazine (0.5%) or sulfamylon (10%) *Parenteral:* Before and after wound manipulation based on colonization and bacterial sensitivities	Removal of necrotic tissue (eschar) with early wound closure beneficial
Ocular surgery	*Topical:* Gentamicin or tobramycin *Subconjunctival:* Aminoglycoside ± cephalosporin	Parenteral antibiotics do not penetrate the aqueous or vitreous humor
Intensive care- or chemotherapy-induced neutropenia	Selective decontamination *Oral:* Polymyxin and tobramycin and amphotericin mixture by mouth or added to gastric tube. *Plus parenteral:* Cefotaxime *Alternate:* Trimethoprim-sulfamethoxazole, or ciprofloxacin	Efficacy is controversial. Risk of bacterial or fungal superinfection and antibiotic resistance. Food to be decontaminated in microwave

*Modified from Medical Letter 31:105, 1989, and 31:112, 1989; and Kaiser A: Postoperative infections and antimicrobial prophylaxis. *In:* Mandell G, Douglas R, Bennett J: Principles and Practices of Infectious Diseases, 3rd ed. New York, Churchill Livingstone, 1990, p 2254.

the catheter from the collection tube, absence of a closed collecting system, microbial colonization of the collecting bag, female patient, presence of diabetes mellitus, and periurethral colonization with potential uropathogens. Common organisms producing bacteriuria include *E. coli, Klebsiella pneumoniae, Pseudomonas mirabilis, P. aeruginosa, S. epidermidis,* and enterococci.

Clinical manifestations of symptomatic infection include fever, suprapubic pain, and pyuria.

Treatment of asymptomatic bacteriuria does not require specific antimicrobial agents but should include removal of the catheter and follow-up urine cultures to monitor the presence of persistent or recurrent bacteriuria (which may occur for as long as 1 yr). Therapy of symptomatic urinary tract infection includes use of systemic antibiotics modified to the antimicrobial sensitivities of the responsible organism. The catheter should be checked for obstruction and removed as soon as possible.

CONTINUOUS AMBULATORY PERITONEAL DIALYSIS. End-stage renal disease is frequently treated with continuous ambulatory peritoneal dialysis (CAPD) after placement of a Tenkhoft catheter in the abdominal cavity. Peritonitis is a complication of CAPD and is due to contamination of the peritoneum with organisms from the patient's endogenous cutaneous flora. Intraluminal (catheter) infection results from contamination occurring during breaks in the catheter and tubing when the system is open for changes of solutions. Periluminal infection occurs when bacteria enter the peritoneum between the catheter and the abdominal wound despite a catheter cuff, and transmural or intestinal infections occur when bacteria transgress the intestinal wall. Hematogenous infection is a rare event. Organisms responsible for peritonitis in patients on CAPD include *S. epidermidis* (30–40%), *S. aureus* (10–20%), streptococci (10–15%), *E. coli* (5–10%), *Pseudomonas* sp. (5–10%), other gram-negative bacteria (5–15%), enterococci (3–6%), fungi (2–10%) such as *Candida* sp., *Fusarium* sp., *Alternaria* sp., or *Aspergillus* sp., and rare organisms such as *Diphtheroid* sp., *Mycobacteria* sp., and anaerobic bacteria. The culture may be negative in 0–20% of episodes.

The *clinical manifestations* of peritonitis may be subtle and include low-grade fever, mild abdominal pain, and tenderness. Cloudy peritoneal dialysis fluid may be the first or predominant sign. The dialysis fluid will be cloudy when the neutrophil count exceeds 100. The cell count may be influenced by the intraperitoneal volume and the duration of time the dialysate has perfused the peritoneum. Infection is suggested by an increased number and predominance of dialysate neutrophils, a positive Gram stain and culture of peritoneal fluid, and signs of peritoneal inflammation (tenderness, guarding, rebound). Exit site and tunnel infections may occur independent of or precede CAPD peritonitis.

Treatment of peritonitis should be initiated prior to identification of the organism and then modified after culture and sensitivities are known. Intraperitoneal instillation of a 1st-generation cephalosporin or vancomycin plus an aminoglycoside is effective initial antibiotic treatment prior to identification of the pathogen. Antifungal agents usually cannot be given through the dialysis catheter because their peritoneal penetration is poor; these agents must be given by the intravenous (amphotericin B) or oral (5-fluorocytosine, ketoconazole) route. In fungal, complicated, or recurrent bacterial peritonitis the catheter may need to be removed. Treatment is continued for 7 days after the last positive culture or for 10 days for gram-positive organisms and 14 days for gram-negative organisms or for culture-negative peritonitis. Recurrent (same organism within 4 wk) peritonitis is treated for 2–4 wk.

INHALATION THERAPY EQUIPMENT. Opportunistic infection, particularly among children in neonatal and pediatric intensive care units, has been associated with the increasing use of respiratory life support systems. Reservoir nebulizers represent the greatest hazard. *P. aeruginosa, Acinetobacter* sp., *Flavobacterium* sp., and *Serratia marcescens* have been implicated most frequently. Risk of infection may be decreased by effective programs for surveillance and maintenance of respirators, nebulizers, and tubing used for inhalation therapy. Nosocomial pneumonia in mechanically ventilated patients is often due to aspiration of gram-negative bacilli that colonize the gastric and oropharyngeal mucosa. *L. pneumophila* is a common nosocomial pathogen, acquired from the water system in some hospitals. Nasotracheal intubation may cause purulent sinusitis and bacteremia if there is obstruction of the sinus orifice.

BURNS. Opportunistic infections in children with burns (Sec. 6.37) may relate to interruption of the skin and mucous membrane barriers to infection, to the presence of necrotic tissue, which serves as a culture medium, to pulmonary injury, to long-term administration of antibiotics, and to prolonged intravenous or urinary catheterization. Septicemia with *P. aeruginosa, S. aureus,* and *S. epidermidis* is frequent. Burn injury has been associated with abnormal immune response to infection, such as neutrophil dysfunction, abnormal antibody responses to specific antigens, and delayed rejection of homografts. The risk of infection is directly related to the extent of the burn, a neutrophil chemotactic defect, and an associated hypogammaglobulinemia. Prophylactic antibiotics may reduce this risk.

SURGERY. Opportunistic infection should be considered whenever fever develops postoperatively. The organisms that may produce disease postoperatively are so varied that no single specific regimen appropriate for all patients can be given, although antibiotic coverage for staphylococci should be included (Sec. 12.19). Cardiac surgery is especially associated with a significant risk of postoperative opportunistic infection, possibly related to extensive use of intravenous and intra-arterial catheters as well as of blood and blood products.

Systemic prophylaxis is indicated when the benefits of preventing a wound infection outweigh the risks of drug reactions and emergence of resistant bacteria. Procedures in which the benefits justify the risks are either those associated with a significant risk of postoperative infection or those in which the consequences of infection may be catastrophic even if the risk of infection is low. The number of micro-organisms within the wound upon completion of the procedure generally determines the probability of surgical wound infection. This has led to a classification of surgical procedures based on an estimation of bacterial contamination and risk of subsequent infection as follows:

1. Clean wounds are uninfected operative wounds in which no inflammation is noted and the respiratory, alimentary, and genitourinary tracts and the oropharynx are not entered. In addition, the procedure is elective and is performed as primarily closed or drained with closed drainage. Operative incisional wounds following nonpenetrating trauma are included in this category. *In clean wounds prophylactic antimicrobial therapy is not recommended except in circumstances in which the consequences of infection are potentially life-threatening (e.g., implantation of a prosthetic foreign body such as a prosthetic heart valve; open heart surgery for repair of structural defects; surgery in patients who are immunocompromised as a result of an inherited disease or are receiving corticosteroids or chemotherapy for malignancy; and newborn infants).* Systemic antimicrobial agents have been recommended empirically for a clean procedure in patients with infection at another site.

2. Clean but potentially contaminated wounds are operative wounds in which the respiratory, alimentary, or genitourinary tract is entered under controlled conditions and does not have unusual contamination preoperatively. These include surgery involving the biliary tract, appendix, vagina, and oropharynx in which no evidence of infection or major break in technique is encountered. In clean but potentially contaminated procedures the risk of contamination is variable. *Recommendations for pediatric patients derived from data on adults suggest that prophylaxis be provided for procedures in patients with obstructive jaundice and urinary tract surgery or instrumentation in the presence of bacteriuria or obstructive uropathy.*

3. Contaminated wounds include open, fresh, and accidental wounds; major breaks in otherwise sterile operative technique; gross spillage from the gastrointestinal tract; and incisions in which acute nonpurulent inflammation is encountered. Dirty and infected wounds include old traumatic wounds with retained devitalized tissue and those in which clinical infection is apparent or in which the viscera have been perforated. *In contaminated and dirty or infected wound procedures, antimicrobial therapy is indicated.*

Prophylactic antimicrobial therapy for surgical procedures need not be initiated until within 2 hr of the surgical procedure (except for cesarean sections). Effective prophylaxis requires adequate concentrations of antibiotics in tissues during the surgical procedure. A single dose may suffice unless the procedure is very prolonged, requiring another dose intraoperatively to maintain adequate antimicrobial concentrations. Duration of antimicrobial prophylaxis may be as brief as 12 hr and should not extend beyond 24–48 hr.

The choice of antimicrobial agents is based on knowledge of the bacteria that most commonly cause infectious complications after a specified procedure, the susceptibility of the organisms likely to be encountered to the chosen drug, and the safety and efficacy of the drug. Effective prophylaxis correlates with a decrease in the total number of organisms within a wound rather than with their complete eradication. Thus, to be effective, the chosen agent should be active against the pathogens most likely to be present, not against every potential organism. Since therapeutic concentrations are required throughout the procedure, the intravenous route of administration generally is preferred. Suggested prophylactic antimicrobial regimens for various types of surgical procedures and for other disruptions in the skin and mucous membrane are listed in Table 12–16.

DERMAL SINUS TRACTS. Children with dermal sinus tracts that communicate with the subarachnoid space or neural tissue may develop meningitis due to *S. epidermidis, S. aureus, E. coli, Pseudomonas,* or other microflora of the skin. Although such dermal sinus tracts are present in 1% of children, they usually do not communicate with the cerebrospinal fluid spaces. Local soft tissue cellulitis or an abscess may develop in a blind-ending sinus tract.

CARDIAC DEFECTS. Both congenital cardiac defects and those acquired through rheumatic fever or surgery, especially intracardiac shunts and prostheses, provide a nidus for opportunistic infection.

INHERITED OR ACQUIRED DISORDERS AFFECTING HOST DEFENSE SYSTEMS (see also Chapter 11). These disorders, the organisms recovered most frequently, and the mechanisms that may be responsible for the infections are shown in Table 12–16.

Congenital and Acquired Defects in Humoral Immunity (Sec. 11.4 and 11.5). *Antibodies* assist in host defense by opsonophagocytosis (IgG), activation of complement (IgG, IgM), interference with micro-organism adherence (IgA, IgG), neutralization of toxins or viruses (IgM, IgG, IgA), antibody-dependent cellular cytotoxicity (IgG), and basophil and mast cell degranulation (IgE). There may be qualitative and quantitative defects in all immunoglobulin types and subclasses or specific isolated defects. This variation produces different relative infectious risks, from mild (selective IgA deficiency) to severe (X-linked agammaglobulinemia, common variable hypogammaglobulinemia) and variable (selective IgG subclass deficiency). In addition, antibody deficiency may be one part of a more severe combined B and T lymphocyte immunodeficiency syndrome (severe combined immunodeficiency syndrome, acquired immunodeficiency syndrome [AIDS]), thus increasing the risk for serious opportunistic infection characteristic of both B and T cell defects (see Table 12–15). In addition to the pathogens noted in Table 12–15, patients with isolated B lymphocyte deficiencies manifest recurrent middle ear, sinopulmonary, and gastrointestinal infections, chronic conjunctivitis, bronchiectasis, malabsorption, and dental caries. Chronic mycoplasma arthritis and echovirus encephalitis or dermatomyositis also occur.

Children with isolated B cell defects are asymptomatic until 5–6 mo of age, when passively transferred maternal IgG serum levels decline to very low concentrations. Management of infections in these patients is noted in Table 12–17.

Complement and properdin are proteins involved in the inflammatory response, chemotaxis, opsonization, and direct cell lysis by the membrane-attached complex (Sec. 11.24). Deficiencies of complement components are associated with familial susceptibility to rheumatologic disorders, and increased risk for recurrent pneumococcemia, meningococcemia, and gonococcemia (Sec. 11.23). Fulminant infection due to *N. meningitidis* is also noted in patients with deficiencies of the alternate pathway (see Table 12–15). Treatment of these infections requires specific antibiotics, intensive care support for shock and disseminated intravascular coagulation, and replacement of the missing factor with fresh frozen plasma. Prevention of infection in complement- or properdin-deficient patients includes vaccination with tetravalent meningococcus, polyvalent pneumococcus, and the conjugated *H. influenzae* type b vaccines. Prophylactic antibiotics may also be useful, but the duration of such prevention is unknown.

TABLE 12–17. Management of Infections in the Host Compromised by B and T Lymphocyte Defects

Immunodeficiency Syndrome	Treatment of Infection	Prevention of Infection
Humoral defects (predominant B cell deficiency)	Intravenous immunoglobulin 0.4 g/kg Bacterial and viral culture Incision and drainage of abscess Bactericidal antibiotics based on culture and sensitivity of micro-organism Intraventricular immunoglobulin for echovirus encephalitis	Maintenance intravenous immunoglobulin 0.3–0.5 g/kg q3–4 wk Avoid live virus vaccines in patient and relatives Respiratory care, postural drainage, monitor for cor pulmonale Chronic antibiotic prophylaxis is controversial
Cellular defects (predominant T cell deficiency)	Bacterial, viral, fungal, protozoal culture, sample microscopy, and stains Incision and drainage of abscess Biopsy bronchoalveolar lavage if indicated Antibacterial, antiviral, antifungal, antiprotozoal therapy as appropriate for culture, sensitivity, sample stains, and symptoms Intravenous immunoglobulin if helper T lymphocyte–associated antibody deficiency, or if severe combined immunodeficiency syndrome	Prophylactic trimethoprim-sulfamethoxazole for *Pneumocystis carinii* No live virus vaccines or bacillus Calmette-Guérin Careful screening for tuberculosis Irradiated blood products decrease risk of GVH CMV-negative blood products Varicella-zoster immune globulin used for those with varicella exposure Immunologic reconstitution performed with: 1. Bone marrow transplant 2. Fetal thymus transplant 3. Polyethylene glycol ADA enzyme infusion 4. Potential ADA genetic reconstitution

ADA = adenosine deaminase enzyme; CMV = cytomegalovirus; GVH = graft-vs-host disease, which increases risk of infection.

Congenital and Acquired Defects in Cell-Mediated Immunity (Sec. 11.12). *T lymphocytes* aid in host defense by direct (NK cell and T cell cytotoxicity) and indirect (enhancement of neutrophil and macrophage function through stimulation of cytokine, antibody, and interferon production) mechanisms. Disorders of cell-mediated immunity may be pure T cell deficiencies (DiGeorge syndrome) or combined T and B lymphocyte defects (AIDS, severe combined immunodeficiency syndrome). Infectious complications associated with isolated T cell defects include those due to intracellular bacterial pathogens in addition to those due to the viruses, fungi, and protozoa defended by the T cell–macrophage interaction (see Table 12–15). Patients with congenital T cell or combined T and B cell immunodeficiency states develop infections after birth because T cell function is greatly reduced and is unaffected by passive transfer of maternal IgG. Early infectious complications include chronic mucocutaneous candidiasis, chronic rhinitis and otitis media, recurrent pneumonia, and diarrhea. Because of the marked heterogeneity of the immunodeficiency state in DiGeorge syndrome, some children may have minor infections, whereas others who survive after early severe infections may have less frequent or less serious infections as the immune defect spontaneously improves.

The most common acquired disorder resulting from a predominantly T lymphocyte defect is AIDS. Antibody production is also deficient in patients with AIDS due to a defect of helper T cell function. Therefore, patients with AIDS are at increased risk for infections with micro-organisms that typically infect patients with both T and B cell deficiencies (Sec. 12.83).

Treatment and prevention of infection in patients with T lymphocyte deficiencies are noted in Table 12–17. When indicated for the specific disease, immunologic reconstitution, most often accomplished by bone marrow transplantation for congenital defects, should be attempted to reduce the risk of serious opportunistic infection.

Defects of Leukocyte Function. Neutrophil functions include adhesion, chemotaxis, phagocytosis, granule production, and intracellular killing (Sec. 11.29). These functions may be compromised by intrinsic cellular defects (absent surface adhesion molecules, e.g., C3bi receptor; abnormal granule formation, e.g., Chédiak-Higashi syndrome; reduced intracellular killing, e.g., chronic granulomatous disease) or by extrinsic factors (decreased opsonization, e.g., reduced serum IgG or complement levels; reduced intracellular killing, e.g., hypophosphatemia; decreased chemotaxis, e.g., reduced complement levels or corticosteroids; acquired chemotactic inhibitors, e.g., *Capnocytophaga* gingivitis).

Patients with neutrophil defects are at increased risk of both minor bacterial infections (of skin or soft tissue) and severe pyogenic infections (sepsis, meningitis, pneumonia, skeletal disease). Infection often begins in the first 6 mo of life because intrinsic granulocyte dysfunction is inherited and is present at birth. Additional *clinical manifestations* of neutrophil dysfunction include leukocytosis, hyperimmunoglobulinemia, recurrent suppurative lymphadenitis, and hepatic abscesses in patients with chronic granulomatous disease (Sec. 11.32 and 16. 60); cold cutaneous abscesses, eczematoid skin rashes, hyperimmunoglobulin E, and defective chemotaxis in patients with Job syndrome (Sec. 16.57); and leukocytosis, omphalitis, delayed separation of the umbilical cord, fulminant sepsis, gingivitis, and ecthyma gangrenosum in patients with leukocyte adhesion defects (Sec. 11.30).

The *treatment* of patients with defects in granulocyte function includes prompt therapy of specific infections and prevention of recurrent infections (Sec. 11.32). Specific antibiotics based on the characteristic bacteria or fungi associated with the specific neutrophil defect should be instituted after appropriate cultures have been obtained. Abscesses should be drained or aspirated and the purulent material cultured and stained with Gram stain. Empiric therapy for bacterial sepsis is necessary for high-risk granulocyte disorders such as leukocyte adhesion defects. In addition to antibiotics, corticosteroids may help to resolve granulomas in patients with chronic granulomatous disease. Granulocyte transfusions should be reserved for patients with documented bacterial or fungal infections that are unresponsive to conventional therapy with intravenous bactericidal antibiotics. Although granulocyte transfusions may be beneficial, they are expensive and include the risk of transmission of cytomegalovirus, allosensitization to HLA antigens, graft-versus-host disease in immunosuppressed patients, pulmonary infiltrates and hypoxia if given in conjunction with amphotericin B, and transfusion reactions (especially in patients with X-linked chronic granulomatous disease who lack the X_k-Kell–related antigen).

Prevention of infection in patients with neutrophil functional defects may occasionally be accomplished with the use of prophylactic antibiotics such as cloxacillin. Intracellular penetration of the broad-spectrum antibiotic combination trimethoprim-sulfamethoxazole improves phagocytic killing in patients with chronic granulomatous disease. In addition, patients with chronic granulomatous disease demonstrate improved intracellular killing after therapy with interferon.

Defects of Neutrophil Number (Sec. 16.44). Neutropenia is the most common defect of phagocytic host defense. Neutrophil counts normally vary between 1,500 and 10,000 but may be as low as 1,000 in healthy black children. The risks of infection increase as the neutrophil count declines below 1,000. Neutropenia may be congenital (cyclic neutropenia, severe infantile agranulocytosis, benign familial neutropenia) or acquired (antineutrophil antibodies, e.g., autoimmune conditions, AIDS; drug reactions, e.g., phenothiazines, sulfonamides, penicillin, chloramphenicol, cancer chemotherapy). The neutropenia associated with common febrile viral illnesses is usually benign. Neutropenia may be isolated, or it may be a sign of more significant bone marrow deficiency (aplastic anemia, leukemia).

The *clinical manifestations* of infection in neutropenic patients include fever, chills, sore throat, and localizing signs and symptoms such as local erythema, tenderness, pain, swelling, and limitation of motion. Neutropenia may attenuate but may not eliminate the local manifestations of infection as noted in cellulitis, pharyngitis, catheter tract infection, and perirectal abscess. It reduces the purulent nature of local infection; pus formation is unusual at sites of cellulitis, and sputum is unusual in neutropenic patients with pneumonia. Patients with severe neutropenia (<500 neutrophils), in the absence of other host defense defects, are at high risk of fulminant bacterial sepsis, which may be asymptomatic, may be present only with fever, or may be manifest as fever, chills, disorientation, lethargy, warm-pink or cold-cyanotic extremities, and hypotension. The risk of sepsis and other serious infections in the febrile neutropenic cancer patient is excessively high (see later section on host defense defects associated with malignancy).

The *treatment* of infection in patients with congenital or acquired neutropenia depends on the micro-organisms responsible for the infection, the duration and severity of the neutropenia, the possibility of bone marrow recovery, and any associated impairment of host defense. Local infection requires a culture, Gram stain, and therapy based on the specific microorganism found. Systemic infection requires blood and other cultures with subsequent empiric administration of synergistic bactericidal antibiotics (usually a β-lactam penicillin or third-generation cephalosporin plus an aminoglycoside). Granulocyte transfusions may be indicated in neutropenic patients with a documented severe infection that does not respond to appropriate antimicrobial therapy.

Prevention of infection in neutropenic patients may be possible by increasing the neutrophil count with nonspecific (prednisone, lithium carbonate) and specific (recombinant granulocyte-macrophage colony–stimulating factor [GM-CSF]) therapy. GM-CSF and granulocyte colony–stimulating factor (G-CSF) have increased the neutrophil count in patients with congenital agranulocytosis, cyclic neutropenia, AIDS, chemotherapy-induced neutropenia, aplastic anemia, and bone marrow transplantation.

Host Defense Defects Associated with Malignancy. Malignancy is associated with multiple defects in host defense. The nature of the malignancy may directly impair immune response, as noted in patients with Hodgkin disease who have attenuated cell-mediated immunity and are at increased risk for bacterial *(L. monocytogenes, Salmonella, Nocardia)*, fungal *(Cryptococcus neoformans)*, viral (herpes simplex, varicella-zoster, cytomegalovirus, Epstein-Barr virus), and protozoan or parasitic *(Pneumocystis carinii, T. gondii, Strongyloides stercoralis)* infection. Cancer chemotherapy itself contributes additional defects in local (central venous catheter placement, surgery, mucositis, venipuncture) and systemic (neutropenia, lymphopenia, B and T lymphocyte function) host defense. Neutropenia and attenuated cell-mediated immunity are the two greatest risk factors for infection in patients with malignancy.

Neutropenia. The risk of infection in the granulocytopenic cancer patient is related to the severity of the neutropenia; it is increased if the neutrophil count is less than 500 but is highest if the count is less than 100, when the incidence of severe bacterial sepsis during febrile episodes may be as high as 10–20%. The risk is further increased when the duration of neutropenia exceeds 2 wk and the neutrophil count is decreasing owing to prior administration of chemotherapeutic agents. The risk may be higher among patients with leukemia than in patients with solid tumors. Common pathogens affecting the febrile neutropenic cancer patient are noted in Table 12–15.

The *clinical manifestations* of infection are related to the site and severity of the infection. However, the absence of physical signs does not preclude serious infections. Fever without a focus may represent gram-negative enteric bacterial sepsis following bacterial invasion and dissemination from the gastrointestinal tract damaged by chemotherapy-induced mucosal ulceration, gram-positive sepsis associated with central venous catheterization, or local or deep-seated tissue infection. Gram-negative sepsis is typically more severe than sepsis due to *S. epidermidis; E. coli* or *Pseudomonas* infection results in septic shock in 30–50% of episodes. Oropharyngeal infection manifests as ulcerating stomatitis, gingivitis, and periodontal lesions. Mucositis may be due to anaerobic bacteria, herpes simplex, or *Candida* sp., or to a mixed infection. Esophagitis may be due to these same microorganisms or to cytomegalovirus and may be associated with mucositis or may occur independently. Neutropenic enteritis may produce pneumatosis intestinalis or typhlitis. Cutaneous lesions may occur as perirectal cellulitis rather than as an abscess and may be due to polymicrobial infection. Additional sites of cutaneous infection include sites of central venous catheter exit and tracts, venipuncture, lumbar puncture, bone marrow biopsy, abrasions, sweat glands, and paronychia. Cutaneous signs of disseminated infection include ecthyma gangrenosum (*P. aeruginosa* and other microorganisms), nodules (*Candida* sp., mucormycosis), gangrenous cellulitis (*Aspergillus*, mucormycosis), and thrombotic arterial occlusion with distal ischemia due to *Aspergillus* sp.

Pulmonary infiltrates may be the primary cause of fever or may be a hematogenous complication of sepsis. Pneumonia in granulocytopenic cancer patients may be subtle and manifest as local rales, tachypnea, chest pain, or the adult respiratory distress syndrome. Pulmonary infiltrates may be absent or faint, only to appear more obvious when the neutrophil count increases above 500. Pneumonia is usually owing to gram-negative enteric bacteria but may also be due to fungi. *Aspergillus* may produce a characteristic wedge-shaped infiltrate typical of arterial invasion and subsequent thrombotic pulmonary infarction. Pulmonary cavitation is suggestive of aspergillosis, mucormycosis, and, rarely, infection with gram-negative enteric bacteria. Pulmonary infiltrates in neutropenic cancer patients may also represent noninfectious disorders such as hemorrhage, malignancy, emboli, edema, reactions to granulocyte transfusions, and radiation- or chemotherapy-induced pneumonitis.

Additional infectious complications include sinusitis with possible intracranial extension due to aspergillosis, mucormycosis, or mixed bacteria; hepatic and splenic candidiasis in the absence of candidemia; candidal endophthalmitis; and severe diarrhea due to *C. difficile*. Because of the need for recurrent transfusions of blood products, neutropenic cancer patients are also at increased risk of infection with hepatitis B and C viruses, parvovirus, cytomegalovirus, and human immunodeficiency virus.

If *diagnostic evaluation* does not distinguish infectious from noninfectious causes of fever, if the temperature is above 38° C (oral) on two consecutive readings or is above 38.5° C for one episode, and the neutrophil count is under 500, a presumptive diagnosis of bacterial sepsis should be made. Blood samples for cultures should be drawn from a peripheral vein and from each lumen of the central venous catheter. Cultures or biopsies should be made of local cutaneous lesions, and a chest roentgenogram should be examined for infiltrates, infarction, or cavitation. Nasal secretions and sputum should be cultured for the presence of *Aspergillus*. In the absence of *Aspergillus* in these secretions, sinopulmonary infection from this organism is unlikely. Sinus roentgenograms or CT may reveal asymptomatic sinusitis. Esophageal endoscopy may be indicated to identify the cause of odynophagia. If pseudohyphae are demonstrated from esophageal lesions, a presumptive diagnosis of disseminated candidiasis is suggested.

Meningitis is unusual in neutropenic febrile cancer patients, and lumbar puncture should be avoided as a routine procedure, especially in the presence of thrombocytopenia. In the presence of significant central venous system manifestations of meningitis, lumbar puncture should be obtained following platelet transfusion if needed.

In certain situtations fiberoptic bronchoscopy, bronchoalveolar lavage, transbronchial biopsy, or open lung biopsy may be required to identify the microorganism responsible for pneumonia.

Treatment of infections in febrile neutropenic cancer patients requires prompt initiation of empiric broad-spectrum, bactericidal antibiotics to decrease the risks of septic shock, the adult respiratory distress syndrome, hypotension, renal and other organ dysfunction, and death. There are several possible choices for initial empiric antibiotics for patients who do not have fulminant septic shock. Monotherapy with ceftazidime, cefoperazone, or imipenem/cilastatin, with subsequent modification by the addition of vancomycin if *S. epidermidis* is recovered, is one therapeutic approach. Monotherapy should be limited to patients who have brief episodes of mild neutropenia (500–1,000 neutrophils) when *S. epidermidis* is not considered a likely pathogen. Double β-lactam therapy with an extended gram-negative spectrum carboxy- or ureido-penicillin (carbenicillin, ticarcillin with or without clavulanic acid, mezlocillin, piperacillin) and a cephalosporin (ceftazidine, cefoperazone, cefotaxime, ceftriaxone) is another broad-spectrum bactericidal regimen that avoids potentially nephrotoxic drugs such as vancomycin and the aminoglycosides. Its disadvantages include selection of resistant bacteria, possible antibiotic antagonism, and poor antistaphylococcal coverage.

A combination of an anti-*Pseudomonas* β-lactam penicillin or cephalosporin plus an aminoglycoside avoids the risk of the emergence of resistant organisms, is synergistic, and includes anaerobic coverage. The disadvantages are the nephrotoxicity, hypokalemia, and ototoxicity resulting from aminoglycoside therapy and poor coverage of staphylococci. The traditional standard empiric antibiotic regimen includes a combination of an extended gram-negative spectrum penicillin or a cephalosporin, plus methicillin or vancomycin, plus an aminoglycoside (gentamicin, tobramycin, amikacin). This regimen is most beneficial if there is a risk of serious staphylococcal or multidrug-resistant *Pseudomonas* infection. If the patient has evidence of septic shock, a combination of a third-generation cephalosporin or an extended gram-negative spectrum penicillin plus an aminoglycoside is the treatment of choice. Pulmonary infections are initially managed with broad-spectrum antibiotics after blood and sputum cultures have been obtained. If antibacterial therapy is unsuccessful, antifungal therapy can be added. Because all antibiotic combinations may alter the enteric flora and reduce bacterial vitamin K synthesis, patients must be monitored for bleeding and given vitamin K when needed.

The duration and modification of antimicrobial therapy depend on the persistence of fever and neutropenia and on the physician's ability to identify a specific pathogen. If the patient becomes afebrile after 72 hr of antibiotic therapy and a bacterial source of infection is identified, the antimicrobial therapy should be modified based on the antibiotic sensitivity of the isolated bacteria. Nonetheless, broad-spectrum antibiotic therapy should be continued because of the high risk of breakthrough bacteremia when the antibiotic spectrum is too narrow. Antibiotic therapy should be continued for a minimum of 7 days in patients who respond to therapy, are afebrile, have negative repeat cultures, and are free of signs and symptoms of infection. Optimally, the neutrophil count should also exceed 500 when antibiotics are stopped. High-risk patients with profound neutropenia, mucositis, signs of persistent infection, central line tract infections, bleeding, impending invasive procedures, or chemotherapy may benefit from continuation of antibiotics until the neutrophil count is above 500. If bacteremia persists for 48–72 hr despite administration of appropriate antibiotics that achieve therapeutic bactericidal levels and the neutropenic patient is severely ill, granulocyte transfusions may be indicated.

If no pathogen is identified and the patient becomes afebrile within 24–72 hr and remains afebrile, antibiotics should be continued for a minimum of 7 days. If the neutrophil count recovers to above 500 or if the patient remains neutropenic but appears clinically well and has no high-risk features, antibiotics may be stopped after a minimum of 7 days of therapy. The patient should be observed closely for reappearance of the signs of infection, and treatment should be started promptly if neutropenia persists because approximately 30% of patients again become febrile after the initial empiric antibiotics are stopped. If the patient is at high risk for serious infection, antibiotics should be continued until the neutrophil count is over 500. Some clinicians recommend that antibiotics be continued until the neutrophil count is above 500 in all patients who have had fever and neutropenia regardless of defervescence or clinical well-being. In many patients neutropenia lasts 7 days unless high-dose chemotherapy immediately precedes the episode of fever.

If the patient remains febrile despite broad-spectrum antibiotic therapy and no pathogen is identified, it is important to reassess the patient's condition. The etiology of persistent fever includes a nonbacterial pathogen (*Candida, Aspergillus, Toxoplasma,* herpes simplex, cytomegalovirus, Epstein-Barr virus, enterovirus), emergence of a second resistant species of bacteria, inadequate serum or tissue antibiotic levels, drug fever, deep tissue (abscess) or catheter infection, and fever resulting from the underlying malignancy.

If no identifiable cause of the fever is evident, the fever and neutropenia remain after 5–7 days of antibiotic therapy, there is no progression or deterioration in the patient's condition, and the patient appears clinically well, the original antibiotics may be continued. If the patient appears ill or if the manifestations of infection progress, vancomycin or a third-generation cephalosporin should be added if the patient was not receiving these antibiotics as part of the initial empiric therapeutic regimen. If the patient remains neutropenic and febrile for 7 days despite modification of antibacterial therapy, intravenous amphotericin B should be started. Approximately 33% of such patients have shown evidence of invasive fungal disease that was either the primary infection or a superinfection that developed after 7 days of broad-spectrum antibiotics. Prior to the initiation of amphotericin B, an evaluation to determine the source of invasive candidiasis, aspergillosis, or mucormycosis should be performed. Biopsies of lesions should be performed, several blood and urine cultures obtained, chest and sinus roentgenograms repeated, abdominal CT performed to identify hepatic or splenic microabscesses, and an ophthalmologic examination carried out to identify candidal ophthalmitis. Amphotericin B is given daily for 2 wk if no fungal infection is identified. Antifungal therapy is then stopped and the patient's condition re-evaluated. Documented fungal infection is treated with prolonged amphotericin B and aspiration or incision and drainage of cutaneous lesions or deep abscesses. New antifungal agents such as fluconazole may be effective, especially if amphotericin is not well tolerated or if severe nephrotoxicity is present. To reduce the risk of renal impairment, concurrent administration of potentially nephrotoxic drugs should be avoided during amphotericin therapy. Third-generation cephalosporins may be substituted for aminoglycosides, and the use of chemotherapeutic agents such as cisplatin should be minimized if possible.

Catheter-related sepsis is common among neutropenic cancer patients. If a documented bacteremia occurs while a central venous catheter or implanted device is in place, antibiotics should be administered through each lumen in an attempt to sterilize the line. Most episodes of catheter-related sepsis respond to systemic antibiotics, and there is no need to remove the catheter. Difficult-to-sterilize line infections include tract infections and sepsis due to *Bacillus* sp., fungi, gram-negative enteric bacteria, and multiple organisms.

Empiric antiviral therapy for the febrile neutropenic patient is not indicated in the absence of typical mucocutaneous lesions suggestive of herpes simplex or varicella-zoster. Intravenous acyclovir is the treatment of choice for these viral infections.

Prevention of infection in neutropenic cancer patients is difficult. Methods include reverse isolation and the total protective environment (Sec. 12.9 and Table 12–16). Prophylactic oral nonabsorbable antibiotics such as colistin, nystatin, and polymyxin and oral absorbable antibiotics such as trimethoprim-sulfamethoxazole (for *P. carinii* and gram-negative enteric bacteria) and the new fluorinated quinolones (norfloxacin, ciprofloxacin) may reduce the risk of infection in severely neutropenic (< 100) patients receiving cancer chemotherapy or bone marrow transplantation. Trimethoprim-sulfamethoxazole may delay bone marrow recovery and produce drug rashes. Experimental methods for reducing the risk of infection by improving the granulocyte count without increasing the proliferation of malignant cells include treatment with GM-CSF and G-CSF.

INFECTIONS IN PATIENTS WITH MALIGNANCY AND DEFECTS OF CELL-MEDIATED IMMUNITY. Lymphocyte-monocyte interaction and function may be reduced by the underlying disease

(Hodgkin disease) or by corticosteroids, cancer chemotherapy, or radiation therapy. The common infectious agents noted in these patients, in the absence of neutropenia, are noted in Table 12–15. In addition, patients who undergo splenectomy for staging of Hodgkin disease are at increased risk of fulminant pneumococcal sepsis. *Treatment* is directed toward the specific microorganism recovered from the blood, cerebrospinal fluid, cutaneous biopsy, or pulmonary specimen (from sputum, bronchoalveolar lavage, or biopsy). Patients with Hodgkin disease who have had a splenectomy and then develop fever without a focus should receive prompt empiric therapy for possible pneumococcal sepsis. *Prevention* of infection is possible with trimethoprim-sulfamethoxazole for *P. carinii* infection, varicella vaccine for patients with leukemia who are in remission, and acyclovir for prevention of dissemination of cutaneous herpes zoster.

Infection in Patients Undergoing Transplantation (see Sec. 6.38). Transplantation has become an increasingly important therapy for patients with end-stage organ dysfunction, inborn errors of metabolism, aplastic anemia, or various pediatric malignancies. Infections in recipients of allogeneic tissue or bone marrow transplants may be due to immunosuppression with reactivation of latent infections or acquisition of microorganisms from the transplanted tissue, blood products, or the environment. In addition, neutropenia resulting from myelosuppressive drugs or CMV infection, or occurring during the pre-engraftment phase of bone marrow transplantation, also contributes to the infectious complications.

Most severe life-threatening infections occur in the first 3–4 mo after transplantation and are related to the risk of surgical wound sepsis, bacteremia occurring during neutropenia, and reactivation or acquisition of herpesviruses (cytomegalovirus, herpes simplex, Epstein-Barr virus [EBV], varicella-zoster virus), *Pneumocystis*, or *Toxoplasma*. Reactivated and primary CMV infection in transplant patients may present as fever, hepatitis, pneumonitis, neutropenia, intestinal ulceration, enteritis, esophagitis, and an infectious mononucleosis–like syndrome. The diagnosis is confirmed by culture of urine, throat, and buffy coat cells or by tissue biopsy demonstrating typical inclusion bodies. Treatment depends on the manifestations; asymptomatic viruria requires no therapy, whereas CMV pneumonitis may require ganciclovir, CMV immune globulin, and modification of the dosage of immunosuppressive agents.

Reactivated and primary EBV infection may present as mononucleosis (fever, lymphadenopathy, pharyngitis, atypical lymphocytes), but primary infection is rarely associated with the delayed (> 6 mo post-transplantation) appearance of a lymphoproliferative syndrome and lymphoma in host tissue (e.g., brain, intestine). Diagnosis of EBV infection is facilitated by observation of a rise in EBV titers, isolation of EBV from throat washings, or identification of EBV DNA or antigens in tissue. Treatment of EBV lymphoproliferative syndromes is difficult and requires a reduction in the amount of immunosuppression provided by cyclosporine.

Bacteremia may be primary or due to pneumonia, pyelonephritis, catheter infection, or a deep tissue abscess. Central nervous system infection may be due to *L. monocytogenes*, *Cryptococcus*, *Toxoplasma*, *Aspergillus*, or *Nocardia*. Additional risks for infection are related to the duration of the surgical procedure, donor organ ischemia, graft-versus-host disease, cytomegalovirus infection, and the method of immunosuppression.

Methotrexate, azathioprine, and cyclophosphamide have immunosuppressive and myelosuppressive activities and thus may produce defects of B and T lymphocytes along with neutropenia. Corticosteroids, antithymocyte globulins, and OKT3 monoclonal antibodies also impair cell-mediated immunity and increase the risk of infection. Cyclosporine is a selective immunosuppressive agent that inhibits T cell–mediated adaptive immune responses by reducing interleukin 2 and interferon synthesis. Cyclosporine does not produce neutropenia or neutrophil-macrophage dysfunction and is associated with a decreased risk of bacterial and fungal infections compared with traditional immunosuppressive agents.

The bone marrow transplant recipient is at increased risk of infection in the post-transplant period owing to the preexisting disease (malignancy, aplastic anemia, immunodeficiency syndromes), the conditioning chemotherapy needed to ablate malignant cells, the depletion of donor T cells used to reduce graft-versus-host disease, the neutropenia and lymphopenia that existed prior to engraftment, the type of immunosuppression used to prevent or treat graft-versus-host-disease, the development of acute graft-versus-host disease, and the neutrophil dysfunction and humoral immune defects noted during chronic graft-versus-host disease.

A temporal pattern of specific infections is noted following bone marrow transplantation. The immediate period of profound neutropenia lasts for 2–4 wk unless engraftment fails. During this period, the patient is at risk of enteric gram-negative and gram-positive sepsis, bacterial pneumonia, and infections due to herpes simplex and *Candida*. The period following engraftment is associated with defects in neutrophil chemotaxis, antibody production, and cell-mediated immunity and lasts approximately 100 days post transplantation. During this period, the incidence of gram-positive and gram-negative infections declines, but the incidence of cytomegalovirus and adenovirus infections, aspergillosis (if neutropenia persists), and interstitial nonbacterial pneumonia increases. Interstitial pneumonia is common in patients with leukemia, occurs about the 60th day post transplant, and may be due to cytomegalovirus, *Pneumocystis*, or respiratory syncytial virus; in 30% of patients it is idiopathic. Idiopathic interstitial pneumonia may be due to graft-versus-host disease and prior conditioning irradiation or chemotherapy, and it has a significant mortality.

The pattern of infection changes after about the 100th post-transplant day when chronic graft-versus-host–associated antibody deficiency predisposes the recipient to pneumococcal sepsis or meningitis and sinopulmonary infections. In addition, varicella-zoster infections occur with increased frequency in this late period. Additional infections include hemorrhagic cystitis due to reactivation of papovavirus BK, rotavirus enteritis, and pseudomembranous colitis due to *C. difficile*.

The *treatment* of infection after bone marrow transplantation depends on the amount of time that has elapsed since transplantation and the presence of neutropenia or of acute or chronic graft-versus-host disease. The approach to the febrile neutropenic transplant recipient is similar to that needed for the febrile neutropenic patient with malignancy and includes prompt institution of empiric bactericidal broad-spectrum antibiotics, which are usually continued until the neutrophil count is above 500.

Acyclovir is effective therapy for herpes simplex and varicella-zoster viral infections, which are usually reactivations of latent virus. Ganciclovir and CMV hyperimmune globulin have improved the survival of patients with serious primary CMV pneumonitis.

Prevention of early bacterial infection has been attempted by administering intravenous immunoglobulin and fluorinated quinolones, and by preventing acute graft-versus-host disease. Prevention of CMV infection has been attempted by instituting prophylactic administration of acylovir, avoiding administration of CMV-positive blood products and marrow in a CMV-negative recipient, and reducing the incidence of graft-versus-host disease. Trimethoprim-sulfamethoxazole is effective prophylaxis against *Pneumocystis* but is less effective against late pneumococcal infections.

Recipients of liver transplants are at increased risk of serious infection during the first 2 mo following transplantation. Operative procedures lasting more than 12 hr increase the risk of infection. Common early infections include gram-negative enteric bacterial pneumonia, soft tissue and wound infections, intra-abdominal abscesses due to enterococci and anaerobic and gram-negative enteric bacteria, peritonitis, disseminated candidiasis, and cholangitis. The latter characteristically presents with the "Charcot triad" of fever, abdominal pain, and jaundice; it should be distinguished from liver rejection by microscopic examination of a liver biopsy, Gram stain, and culture. Hepatic abscesses are often due to biliary or vascular obstruction, whereas cholangitis may be related to biliary stricture or the use of endoscopic retrograde cholangiopancreatography. Ischemic injury to the bile ducts from hepatic artery occlusion or bile duct anastomotic breakdown may produce bile leakage and gram-negative or candidal peritonitis, which will be detected by culture of the abdominal drains.

Additional infections include CMV hepatitis, which if not associated with disseminated CMV infection is often benign, mucocutaneous herpes simplex, and *P. carinii* pneumonia, which remains a risk for the first 6 mo after transplantation. Reactivation of an Epstein-Barr virus may produce a mononucleosis-like syndrome, or it may progress to a late-onset lymphoproliferative syndrome that may improve by reducing the dosage of immunosuppressive therapy.

Evaluation of the febrile liver transplant recipient for infection includes cultures of blood and abdominal drains, chest roentgenogram, abdominal ultrasound and CT imaging, and Doppler assessment of hepatic artery blood flow. Percutaneous liver biopsy is needed to diagnose cholangitis and to exclude the possibility of rejection.

Treatment is directed at the specific infectious complication present and may include broad-spectrum antibiotics and aspiration or drainage of abscesses.

Prevention of infection has been attempted by using prophylactic antibacterial agents, acyclovir, and trimethoprim-sulfamethoxazole for *P. carinii* infection, avoiding neutropenia due to azathioprine, and maintaining good surgical technique.

Renal transplantation increases the risk of infection related to the surgical procedure, the immunosuppression (see earlier), and the kidney itself. Urinary tract infections (cystitis, pyelonephritis, perinephric abscesses) are common complications of renal transplantation. Infectious agents include *E. coli, P. aeruginosa, Klebsiella, Enterococcus, Candida,* primary or reactivated CMV infection, or papovavirus BK (which produces ureteric stenosis). CMV-induced neutropenia is associated with a risk of enteric gram-negative and gram-positive sepsis or pneumonia and with renal transplant rejection.

Pulmonary infections are also common and may be acute (due to *S. pneumoniae, H. influenzae, E. coli, Pseudomonas, Klebsiella, Legionella*) or chronic (*Nocardia asteroides, Aspergillus, Cryptococcus, Candida, P. carinii*).

Treatment of infection is directed at the specific manifestation (e.g., pneumonia or urinary tract infection) and the responsible microbiologic agent. Urine, blood, and sputum should be cultured prior to antibiotic therapy. Biopsy of the transplanted kidney may be needed to differentiate infection from rejection.

Prevention of infection is similar to that used for other transplant recipients. Prophylactic trimethoprim-sulfamethoxazole may also reduce the incidence of pyelonephritis. Careful evaluation of the urinary tract for abnormalities such as urethral, ureteral, and vesicoureteral strictures, ureteral reflux, lymphocele, and neurogenic bladder may identify the cause of recurrent urinary tract infections. Primary CMV infection can be prevented by avoiding use of CMV-positive blood products as well as transplantation from a CMV-positive donor to a CMV-negative recipient.

In addition to the infectious complications inherent in immunosuppression, **heart transplant recipients** have an increased risk of pulmonary infection due to gram-positive and gram-negative enteric bacteria, *P. carinii*, and CMV and, less often, to infection due to *Aspergillus*, herpes simplex, *Legionella, Toxoplasma, Nocardia,* histoplasmosis, cryptococcosis, and tuberculosis. Mediastinitis due to *S. aureus, S. epidermidis,* and, less often, gram-negative enteric bacteria and *Mycoplasma hominis* is related to the surgical procedure. Severe bone destruction, low-grade fever, erythema, sternal tenderness, purulent drainage, and leukocytosis should suggest the diagnosis of mediastinitis. Antistaphylococcal and anti-*Pseudomonas* antibiotics, with the addition of tetracycline and clindamycin when cultures are negative (presumed *M. hominis*), together with surgical drainage and irrigation, are appropriate therapy for mediastinitis.

Additional frequent infections include toxoplasmosis (reactivated or acquired from the transplanted heart), reactivated Epstein-Barr virus producing mononucleosis, and, less often, a lymphoproliferative disease and nocardiosis.

Treatment is determined by the specific pathogen and site of infection. Prevention of infection is similar to the methods used in other transplant recipients.

Protein-Losing or Exudative Enteropathy. This may accompany gastrointestinal infection, *Menetrier syndrome* (protein loss with giant hypertrophy of gastric mucosa), gluten-induced enteropathy, intestinal lymphangiectasia, kwashiorkor, Hirschsprung disease, gastrointestinal neoplasms, allergic gastroenteritis, regional enteritis, ulcerative colitis, jejunal malformations, gastrocolic fistula, angioneurotic edema, postgastrectomy syndrome, congestive heart failure, constrictive pericarditis, and aminopterin administration. Infection with *S. pneumoniae*, enteric bacteria, and *G. lamblia* occurs with increased frequency in these patients. Increased susceptibility to infection may be related in part to the hypogammaglobulinemia that may result from intestinal protein loss. In patients with intestinal lymphangiectasia, lymphopenia and impaired homograft rejection also may occur.

ROBERT M. KLIEGMAN
RALPH D. FEIGIN
RICHARD E. BEHRMAN

Breinig MK, Zitelli B, Starzl TE, et al: Epstein-Barr virus, cytomegalovirus, and other viral infections in children after liver transplantation. J Infect Dis 156:273, 1987.

Cerebrospinal fluid shunt infections. Lancet 1:1304, 1989.

Decker MD, Edwards MK: Central venous catheter infections. Pediatr Clin North Am 35:579, 1988.

Engelhard D, Marks MI, Good RA: Infections in bone marrow transplant recipients. J Pediatr 108:335, 1986.

EORTC International Antimicrobial Therapy Cooperative Group: Empiric antifungal therapy in febrile granulocytopenic patients. Am J Med 86:668, 1989.

Glenn J, Cotton D, Wesley R, et al: Anorectal infections in patients with malignant diseses. Rev Infect Dis 10:42, 1988.

Granowetter L, Wells H, Lange BJ: Ceftazidime with or without vancomycin vs cephalothin, carbenicillin and gentamicin as the initial therapy of the febrile neutropenic pediatric cancer patient. Pediatr Infect Dis J 7:165, 1988.

Green M, Wald ER, Fricker FJ, et al: Infections in pediatric orthotopic heart transplant recipients. Pediatr Infect Dis J 8:87, 1989.

Hows JM, Brozovic B: Platelet and granulocyte transfusions. Br Med J 300:520, 1990.

Hughes WT, Armstrong D, Bodey GP, et al: Guidelines for the use of antimicrobial agents in neutropenic patients with unexplained fever. J Infect Dis 161:381, 1990.

Kahan BD: Cyclosporine. N Engl J Med 321:1775, 1989.

Kusne S, Dummer JS, Singh N, et al: Infection after liver transplantation: An analysis of 101 consecutive cases. Medicine 67:132, 1988.

Lung disease following allogeneic marrow transplantation. Lancet 2:1368, 1989.

Mouy R, Fischer A, Vilmer E, et al: Incidence, severity, and prevention of infections in chronic granulomatous disease. J Pediatr 114:555, 1989.

Patrick CC: Coagulase-negative staphylococci: Pathogens with increasing clinical significance. J Pediatr 116:497, 1990.

Ramsey PG, Rubin RH, Tolkoff-Rubin NE, et al: The renal transplant patient

with fever and pulmonary infiltrates: Etiology, clinical manifestations, and management. Medicine 59:206, 1980.
Rubin M, Hathorn JW, Marshall D, et al: Gram-positive infections and the use of vancomycin in 550 episodes of fever and neutropenia. Ann Intern Med 108:30, 1988.
Segreti J, Levin S: The role of prophylactic antibiotics in the prevention of prosthetic device infections. Infect Dis Clin North Am 3:357, 1989.
Stokes DC, Shenep JL, Parham D, et al: Role of flexible bronchoscopy in the diagnosis of pulmonary infiltrates in pediatric patients with cancer. J Pediatr 115:561, 1989.
Stuck AE, Minder CE, Frey FJ: Risk of infectious complications in patients taking glucocorticosteroids. Rev Infect Dis 11:954, 1989.
Sugarman B, Young E: Infections associated with prosthetic devices: Magnitude of the problem. Infect Dis Clin North Am 3:187, 1989.
Surveillance cultures in neutropenia. Lancet 1:1238, 1989.
Venes J: Infections of CSF shunt and intracranial pressure monitoring devices. Infect Dis Clin North Am 3:289, 1989.
Weisbart RH: Colony-stimulating factors and host defense. Ann Intern Med 110:297, 1989.
Wheeler RR, Peacock JE, Jr, Cruz JM, et al: Esophagitis in the immunocompromised host: Role of esophagoscopy in diagnosis. Rev Infect Dis 9:88, 1987.
Whimbey E, Kiehn TE, Brannon P, et al: Bacteremia and fungemia in patients with neoplastic disease. Am J Med 82:723, 1987.
Winston DJ, Ho WG, Bruckner DA, et al: Ofloxacin versus vancomycin/polymyxin for prevention of infections in granulocytopenic patients. Am J Med 88:36, 1990.

BACTERIAL INFECTIONS

12.14 BACTEREMIA AND SEPTICEMIA

The recovery of bacteria in a blood culture, *bacteremia*, may be a transient phenomenon not associated with disease or the serious extension of an invasive bacterial infection originating in the gastrointestinal *(Salmonella, Pseudomonas, E. coli, Klebsiella-Enterobacter, Enterococcus)*, genitourinary *(E. coli, Klebsiella-Enterobacter, Proteus, N. gonorrhoeae)*, or respiratory *(Pneumococcus, H. influenzae, S. aureus)* tracts or integument *(S. aureus, S. epidermidis, Streptococcus pyogenes)*. Bacteremia may precede or coincide with specific local metastatic foci of infection such as those occurring with meningitis, osteomyelitis, endocarditis, epiglottitis, and facial cellulitis. Transient or low-grade (< 100 colony-forming units/mL blood) bacteremia may follow instrumentation of the respiratory, gastrointestinal, or genitourinary tracts. Bacteremia may be asymptomatic or associated with few symptoms. Sepsis or septicemia is a severe form of bacteremia associated with active disease and may progress to septic shock. High-grade bacteremia (> 100–1,000 colony-forming units/mL) is commonly noted in patients with sepsis and in those whose condition progresses to septic shock. See Sec. 9.60 for neonatal sepsis.

EPIDEMIOLOGY. Patients at high risk for sepsis are noted in Table 12–1. Previously immunocompetent nonhospitalized patients may develop community-acquired bacteremia-sepsis from extension of local tissue infections such as pneumonia due to *S. pneumoniae* and *H. influenzae* type b, gastroenteritis due to *Salmonella*, pyelonephritis due to *E. coli*, pelvic inflammatory disease due to *N. gonorrhoeae*, and cellulitis-erysipelas with *S. pyogenes*. Alternatively, colonization and local mucosal invasion by a particularly virulent pathogen (*N. meningitidis, S. pneumoniae, H. influenzae* type b) in a previously normal host may produce primary bacteremia and sepsis. Occult pneumococcal bacteremia is discussed in Sec. 12.2.

Immunocompromised patients, as noted in Tables 12–1 and 12–15, are at increased risk for serious nosocomial sepsis. Hospitalized patients develop sepsis due to *S. aureus* or *S. epidermidis* from catheter infection or surgical wounds, whereas serious gram-negative *(E. coli, Pseudomonas, Acinetobacter, Klebsiella-Enterobacter, Serratia)* sepsis is characteristic of the immunocompromised neutropenic patient or the acutely ill patient receiving intensive care. Polymicrobial sepsis is also noted in these high-risk patients and is associated with central venous catheterization, gastrointestinal disease, neutropenia, and malignancy. Additional, less frequent causes of bacteremia or sepsis include anaerobic bacilli, *Yersinia pesti* (plague), *Salmonella typhi* (typhoid fever), *Pseudomonas pseudomallei* (melioidosis), *Vibrio vulnificus* (oyster consumption), and DF-2 (dysgonic fermentative organism from cat bites).

Pseudobacteremia may be associated with contaminated solutions such as antimicrobial disinfectants, heparinized flushes, intravenous infusates, albumin, cryoprecipitate, and contaminated equipment. Unusual water-based organisms such as *Pseudomonas cepacia* are frequently recovered, but true pathogens such as *P. aeruginosa* or *Serratia* may also be identified.

A **sepsis syndrome** may be present in the absence of documented bacteremia. It is often indistinguishable from septic shock and may be due to endotoxemia, prior antibiotic therapy, severe local infection (peritonitis), fastidious slow-growing organisms, and rickettsial or viral infection. The differential diagnosis of a septic-like appearance due to a nonbacterial etiology is noted in Table 12–2.

PATHOGENESIS OF SEPSIS AND SEPTIC SHOCK. The cardiopulmonary manifestations of gram-negative *(H. influenzae, N. meningitidis, E. coli, Pseudomonas)* sepsis can be mimicked by injection of endotoxin or tumor necrosis factor (TNF). Inhibition of TNF action by monoclonal anti-TNF antibody greatly attenuates the manifestations of septic shock in experimental models. Endotoxin and TNF can activate (1) the complement cascade and Hageman factor (factor XII), which then initiates the coagulation cascade with consumption of coagulation factors and plasmin leading to fibrinolysis, and (2) the kallikrein system, which can produce hypotension. TNF and other inflammatory mediators increase vascular permeability, producing diffuse capillary leakage, reduced vascular tone, and an imbalance between perfusion and the tissue's increased metabolic requirements. Inflammatory mediator activity or overresponsiveness may contribute to the pathogenesis of sepsis.

Peripheral vascular resistance is reduced in early septic (warm) shock but becomes greatly elevated in late (cold) shock. Tissue oxygen consumption exceeds oxygen delivery in septic shock. This imbalance is due to early peripheral vasodilation, late vasoconstriction, myocardial depression, hypotension, ventilatory insufficiency, and anemia. Although the cardiac index of children with sepsis is elevated compared with nonseptic patients, the cardiac output is insufficient for the large peripheral tissue oxygen consumption that occurs in septic shock. The resultant tissue hypoxia leads to lactic acidosis.

Pulmonary function is often severely impaired, and the development of "shock lung" or the adult respiratory distress syndrome (ARDS) is associated with a poor prognosis. ARDS is manifest as severe hypoxemia, diffuse pulmonary infiltrates, intrapulmonary right to left shunting, ventilation perfusion abnormalities, and increased pulmonary vascular resistance with a normal pulmonary wedge pressure, which implies a capillary leak from noncardiogenic pulmonary edema (see also Sec. 14.79).

CLINICAL MANIFESTATIONS. The primary signs and symptoms of septic shock include fever, shaking chills, hyperventilation, tachycardia, hypothermia, cutaneous lesions (petechiae, ecchymoses, ecthyma gangrenosum, diffuse erythema, cellulitis), and changes in mental status such as confusion, agitation, anxiety, excitation, lethargy, obtundation, or coma. Secondary manifestations include hypotension, delayed capillary refill time (> 3–5 sec), cyanosis, symmetric peripheral gangrene (purpura fulminans), oliguria or anuria, jaundice (direct-reacting hyperbilirubinemia), and signs of heart failure. Cold shock is characterized by cold, clammy, cyanotic, and pale extremities in a child unresponsive to verbal commands or painful stimuli. There may be evidence of a focus of infection such as meningitis, pneumonia, arthritis, cellulitis, and pyelonephritis or of an immunocompromised status such as malignancy, T or B lymphocyte defects, and prior splenectomy.

Laboratory manifestations of sepsis include positive blood cultures; Gram, Wright, methylene blue, or acridine orange stain of the buffy coat or petechial lesions demonstrating microorganisms; metabolic acidosis; thrombocytopenia; prolonged prothrombin and partial thromboplastin times; reduced serum fibrinogen levels; anemia; and alterations in the morphology and number of neutrophils. Vacuolization of neutrophils, toxic granulations, and Döhle bodies are also suggestive of bacterial sepsis. Elevated neutrophil and band counts (shift to the left: immature white blood cells) suggest bacterial infection, and neutropenia is an ominous sign of fulminant septic shock. Examination of the cerebrospinal fluid may reveal neutrophils and bacteria or may demonstrate only bacteria in the absence of an inflammatory response.

TREATMENT. Patients in whom sepsis or septic shock is suspected should have cultures made of blood, urine, and cerebrospinal fluid. Exudates, abscesses, and cutaneous lesions should also be cultured and stained for organisms. In addition, a complete blood count, platelet count, prothrombin and partial thromboplastin times, fibrinogen level, arterial blood gases, and chest roentgenogram should be obtained. These children should be observed in an intensive care unit where central venous pressure and continuous intra-arterial blood pressure monitoring are available (Sec. 6.33 and 6.34).

Broad-spectrum bactericidal synergistic antibiotics should be administered for presumptive sepsis. The specific antibiotic combination chosen depends on the patient's risk of having community-acquired or nosocomial sepsis. Community-acquired disease *(H. influenzae, N. meningitidis, S. pneumoniae)* can initially be treated with ceftriaxone; nosocomial sepsis should be treated with a third-generation cephalosporin or an extended gram-negative spectrum β-lactam penicillin, plus an aminoglycoside. Both intermittent and continuous intravenous administration of antibiotics have been employed, but the former is the current standard of care.

Shock should be managed by intravenous fluid resuscitation using normal saline, albumin, hetastarch, or dextran solutions. After fluid therapy, intravenous sympathomimetic agents such as dopamine and dobutamine should be employed for persistent hypotension. If hypotension remains refractory to fluids and dopamine or dobutamine administration, judicious use of a continuous intravenous infusion of epinephrine or norepinephrine, with or without sodium nitroprusside for afterload reduction, is indicated (Sec. 6.34).

Hypoxia should be treated with nasal oxygen, and, if cyanosis persists, the patient should undergo endotracheal intubation and receive mechanical ventilation. Positive end-expiratory pressures (PEEP) of between 5 and 20 cm H_2O are usually effective in improving oxygenation but may reduce venous return and thus cardiac output. "Optimal" PEEP is associated with the lowest intrapulmonary right to left shunt, improved oxygen delivery, and no impairment of cardiac output.

Disseminated intravascular coagulation (DIC) should resolve as the primary infectious disease is treated. If bleeding is noted, DIC should be treated with replacement of consumed coagulation factors by transfusion of fresh frozen plasma, cryoprecipitate, and platelets (Sec. 16.75). Heparin is indicated in the presence of thrombosis and peripheral gangrene.

Additional adjuvant therapies for severe sepsis that have had various degrees of success include intravenous immunoglobulin, monoclonal IgM to endotoxin, and granulocyte transfusion. The latter is reserved for the patient who was neutropenic prior to the septic episode, who does not respond to antibiotic therapy, and who is persistently bacteremic. Corticosteroids are not beneficial in patients with septic shock or those with ARDS. Corticosteroids may be beneficial in patients with adrenal hemorrhage that is part of the Waterhouse-Friderichsen syndrome.

PROGNOSIS. The mortality for septic shock depends on the initial site of infection, the presence of multiple organ system dysfunction, and the bacterial pathogen. It may be 40–60% for patients with gram-negative enteric sepsis. Urosepsis has a much better prognosis than primary sepsis without a focus. Poor prognostic signs in meningococcal sepsis include hypotension, coma, leukopenia (<5,000), thrombocytopenia (<100,000), low fibrinogen level (<150 mg/dL), absence of meningismus, absence of cerebrospinal fluid pleocytosis with bacteria noted on Gram stain of the CSF, rapid appearance of petechiae (in 1 hr), and hypothermia. In addition, the level of TNF, the number of bacteria/mL blood, and the level of endotoxin are related to the prognosis. Furthermore, patients who eventually survive septic shock demonstrate an increase in the cardiac index and ejection fraction during therapy compared with nonsurviving patients.

PREVENTION. Immunization against *H. influenzae* type b is recommended for all 2-mo to 4-yr-old children (Sec. 12.22). High-risk patients should receive the 23-valent pneumococcal vaccine at age 2 yr and the quadrivalent (groups A, C, Y, W-135) meningococcal vaccine (Sec. 12.21 and 12.23). Penicillin prophylaxis to prevent pneumococcal infection is recommended for patients with splenic dysfunction (sickle cell anemia) and those who have had splenectomy. Rifampin prophylaxis is recommended for close contacts of patients who may have been exposed to invasive *H. influenzae* or meningococcal disease (Sec. 12.22 and 12.33).

Prevention of sepsis in immunocompromised patients is discussed in Sec. 12.13.

ROBERT M. KLIEGMAN
RICHARD E. BEHRMAN

Brandtzaeg P, Mollness TE, Kierulf P: Complement activation and endotoxin levels in systemic meningococcal disease. J Infect Dis 160:58, 1989.

Brandtzaeg P, Kierulf P, Gaustad P, et al: Plasma endotoxin as a predictor of multiple organ failure and death in systemic meningococcal disease. J Infect Dis 159:195, 1989.

Carpenter PD, Heppner BT, Gnann JW Jr: DF-2 bacteremia following cat bites. Am J Med 82:621, 1987.

Damas P, Reuter A, Gysen P, et al: Tumor necrosis factor and interleukin-1 serum levels during severe sepsis in humans. Crit Care Med 17:975, 1989.

Davidson M, Schraer CD, Parkinson AJ: Invasive pneumococcal disease in an Alaska native population, 1980 through 1986. JAMA 261:715, 1989.

Franson TR, Hierholzer WJ Jr, LaBrecque DR: Frequency and characteristics of hyperbilirubinemia associated with bacteremia. Rev Infect Dis 7:1, 1985.

Gullberg RM, Homann SR, Phair JP: Enterococcal bacteremia: Analysis of 75 episodes. Rev Infect Dis 11:74, 1989.

Havens PL, Garland JS, Brook MM, et al: Trends in mortality in children hospitalized with meningococcal infections, 1957 to 1987. Pediatr Infect Dis J 8:8, 1989.

Hilf M, Yu VL, Sharp J, et al: Antibiotic therapy for *Pseudomonas aeruginosa* bacteremia: Outcome correlations in a prospective study of 200 patients. Am J Med 87:540, 1989.

Jacobs RF, Sowell MK, Moss MM, et al: Septic shock in children: Bacterial etiologies and temporal relationships. Pediatr Infect Dis J 9:196, 1990.

Klontz KC, Lieb S, Schreiber M, et al: Syndromes of *Vibrio vulnificus* infections: Clinical and epidemiologic features in Florida cases, 1981–1987. Ann Intern Med 109:318, 1988.

Mercier JC, Beaufils F, Hartmann JF, et al: Hemodynamic patterns of meningococcal shock in children. Crit Care Med 16:27, 1988.
Michie HR, Manogue KR, Spriggs DR, et al: Detection of circulating tumor necrosis factor after endotoxin administration. N Engl J Med 318:1481, 1988.
Parker MM, Shelhamer JH, Bacharach SL, et al: Profound but reversible myocardial depression in patients with septic shock. Ann Intern Med 100:483, 1984.
Reuben AG, Musher DM, Hamill RJ, et al: Polymicrobial bacteremia: Clinical and microbiologic patterns. Rev Infect Dis 11:161, 1989.
Sinclair JF: The management of fulminant meningococcal septicaemia in children. Intensive Care World 5:89, 1988.
Tuchschmidt J, Fried J, Swinney R, et al: Early hemodynamic correlates of survival in patients with septic shock. Crit Care Med 17:719, 1989.
Wong VK, Hitchcock W, Mason WH: Meningococcal infections in children: A review of 100 cases. Pediatr Infect Dis J 8:224, 1989.
Marshall GS, Bell LM: Correlates of high grade and low grade *Haemophilus influenzae* bacteremia. Pediatr Infect Dis J 7:86, 1988.

12.15 ACUTE BACTERIAL MENINGITIS BEYOND THE NEONATAL PERIOD

Bacterial meningitis in infants and older children is a serious clinical entity with signs and symptoms that commonly do not allow the physician to distinguish among the various etiologic agents. Initial empiric therapy and general supportive management are standard regardless of the specific pathogen, and the acute complications and chronic morbidity may be similar regardless of the etiology. The pattern of bacterial meningitis and its treatment during the neonatal period (0–28 days) are generally distinctly different from those in older infants and children, and these are therefore discussed separately (Sec. 9.63). Nonetheless, the clinical patterns of meningitis in the neonatal and postneonatal periods may overlap, especially in the 1- to 2-mo-old patient in whom group B streptococcus, *H. influenzae* type b, meningococcus, and pneumococcus may all produce meningitis.

The incidence of bacterial meningitis is sufficiently high that it should be suspected in all febrile infants who demonstrate altered mental status, irritability, and poor peripheral perfusion. The incidence of meningitis due to *H. influenzae* type b and group B streptococcus has increased during the last decade. Furthermore, *H. influenzae* has been responsible for meningitis in neonates, adolescents, and adults, and group B streptococcus has caused meningitis in infants over 1 mo of age and in postpartum mothers.

ETIOLOGY. During the first 2 mo of life the bacteria that cause meningitis in normal infants reflect the maternal flora or the environment of the infant (i.e., group B streptococci, gram-negative enteric bacilli, and *L. monocytogenes*). In addition, meningitis in this age group may occasionally be due to nontypeable *H. influenzae* or *H. influenzae* type b and the other pathogens noted in older patients.

Bacterial meningitis in children 2 mo–12 yr of age is usually due to *H. influenzae* type b, *S. pneumoniae*, or *N. meningitidis*. The incidence of disease due *H. influenzae* type b exceeds that due to *N. meningitidis*, which is slightly more common than that due to *S. pneumoniae*. In the southwestern and central regions of the United States and in some European countries the incidence of meningitis due to *N. meningitidis* exceeds that due to *H. influenzae* type b. Disease due to *H. influenzae* type b may occur at any age. Although most episodes of *H. influenzae* meningitis occur before 2 yr of age, *H. influenzae* is responsible for 40% of cases in children 6–16 yr of age and 10–20% of cases in adults. In children over 12 yr of age meningitis is usually due to *N. meningitidis* or *S. pneumoniae*. Alterations of host defense due to anatomic defects or immune deficits increase the risk of meningitis from less common pathogens such as *P. aeruginosa*, *S. aureus*, *S. epidermidis*, *Salmonella*, and *L. monocytogenes*.

EPIDEMIOLOGY. A major risk factor for meningitis is the attenuated immunologic response to specific pathogens associated with young age. The risk is greatest among infants between 1 and 12 mo of age; 95% of cases occur between 1 mo and 5 yr of age, but meningitis can occur at any age. Additional risks include recent colonization with pathogenic bacteria, close contact with individuals having invasive disease (home, day-care centers, schools, military barracks), crowding, poverty, black race, male sex, and possibly absence of breast-feeding for infants 2–5 mo of age. The mode of transmission is probably person-to-person contact through respiratory tract secretions or droplets. The risk of meningitis is increased among patients with presumed occult bacteremia; the odds ratio is greater for meningococcus (85 times) than for *H. influenzae* type b (12 times) relative to that for pneumococcus (1 time) (see Sec. 12.2). Other systemic infections are also associated with an increased risk of meningitis, as exemplified by the association of meningitis with facial cellulitis due to *H. influenzae* type b in children under 4 yr of age. Specific host defense defects due to altered immunoglobulin production in response to encapsulated pathogens may be responsible for the increased risk of bacterial meningitis seen in American Indians and Eskimos, whereas defects of the complement system (C5–C8) have been associated with recurrent meningococcal infection, and defects of the properdin system have been associated with a significant risk of lethal meningococcal disease. Splenic dysfunction (sickle cell anemia) or asplenia (due to trauma, congenital defect, staging of Hodgkin disease) is associated with an increased risk of pneumococcal, *H. influenzae* type b (to some extent), and, rarely, meningococcal meningitis and sepsis. T lymphocyte defects (congenital or acquired by chemotherapy, AIDS, or malignancy) are associated with an increased risk of *L. monocytogenes*, cryptococcal, *Toxoplasma*, and CMV infections of the central nervous system. Congenital or acquired CSF communications across the mucocutaneous barrier, such as cranial or midline facial defects (cribriform plate) and middle ear (stapedial foot plate) or inner ear fistulas (oval window, internal auditory canal, cochlear aqueduct), or CSF leakage through a rupture of the meninges due to a basal skull fracture into the cribriform plate or paranasal sinus is associated with an increased risk of pneumococcal, and, less often, *H. influenzae* type b meningitis. Lumbosacral dermal sinus and meningomyelocele are associated with staphylococcal and enteric bacterial meningitis. Penetrating cranial trauma and CSF shunt infections increase the risk of meningitis due to staphylococci and other cutaneous bacteria.

***Haemophilus influenzae* type b.** See Sec. 12.22. Nonencapsulated strains of *H. influenzae* may be found in the throat or nasopharynx of up to 80% of children and adults; 2–5% carry *H. influenzae* type b. Carriage of type b influenza occurs predominantly in children 1 mo–4 yr of age after close contact with other children who are carriers or are incubating serious *H. influenzae* disease. Invasive *H. influenzae* type b bacteremia and meningitis are most common in infants 2 mo–2 yr of age and may be associated with recent acquisition of *H. influenzae* type b colonization in patients with an age-related relative defect in production of IgG antibody to the polysaccharide capsule of the bacteria. Peak incidence occurs in infants 6–9 mo of age, and 50% of cases occur in the 1st yr of life. The annual incidence of *H. influenzae* meningitis in the United States in children under 5 yr is 30–70/100,000; the incidence is 3- to 5-fold higher among Alaskan Eskimos and Navajo Indians. The risk to children is also markedly increased among family or day-care center contacts of patients with *H. influenzae* type b disease. The highest monthly attack rates occur between November and January, although cases occur throughout the year with a smaller increase in the spring. Otitis media due to *H. influenzae* type b, human immunodeficiency virus (HIV) infection, CSF leaks, and occult bacteremia also increase the risk of *H. influenzae* meningitis.

Streptococcus pneumoniae. See Sec. 12.21. The risk of sepsis and meningitis due to *S. pneumoniae* depends in part on the serotype; types 1, 3, 6, 7, 14, 17, 18, 19, 21, and 23 commonly cause meningitis. Throat or nasopharyngeal carriage of *S. pneumoniae* is acquired from family contacts after birth, is transient (2–4 mo), is often associated with homotype antibody production, and, if recent (<1 mo), is a risk factor for serious infection. The incidence of pneumococcal meningitis is 1–3/100,000. Most episodes occur in infants under 1 yr of age. The midwinter months are the peak season. The risk of meningitis is 5- to 36-fold greater among blacks than whites. The incidence in children with sickle cell anemia is greater than that in the black population without sickle cell anemia and is more than 300-fold that in white children. Approximately 1 in 24 children with sickle cell anemia will develop pneumococcal meningitis before the age of 5 yr if they are not given prophylactic antibiotics. Additional risks for pneumococcal meningitis include an associated otitis media, sinusitis, pneumonia, CSF otorrhea or rhinorrhea, splenectomy, and chronic graft-versus-host disease following bone marrow transplantation.

Neisseria meningitidis (see Sec. 12.23). Meningococcal meningitis may be endemic and may be sporadic (groups B, C, Y organisms) or epidemic (groups A and C). Most infections are due to group B, and a small percentage are caused by group C; less than 10% are due to groups A, Y, and W135. Cases occur throughout the year but may be more common in the winter and spring. Nasopharyngeal carriage of *N. meningitidis* occurs in between 1 and 15% of the adult population. Colonization may last weeks to months; recent colonization places the nonimmune younger child at greatest risk for meningitis. The incidence of simultaneous disease occurring in association with a familial index case is 1%, a rate that is 1,000-fold the risk in the general population. The risk of secondary cases occurring in contacts at day-care centers is 1/1,000. Most infections of children are acquired from a contact in a day-care facility, a colonized adult family member, or an ill patient with meningococcal disease.

PATHOLOGY. A meningeal exudate of varying thickness may be distributed around the cerebral veins, venous sinuses, convexity of the brain, and cerebellum and in the sulci, sylvian fissures, basal cisterns, and spinal cord. Ventriculitis with bacteria and inflammatory cells in ventricular fluid may be present, as may subdural effusions and, rarely, empyema. Perivascular inflammatory infiltrates may also be present, and the ependymal membrane may be disrupted. Vascular and parenchymal cerebral changes characterized by polymorphonuclear infiltrates extending to the subintimal region of the small arteries and veins, vasospasm, vasculitis, thrombosis of small cortical veins, occlusion of major venous sinuses, necrotizing arteritis producing subarachnoid hemorrhage, and, rarely, cerebral cortical necrosis in the absence of identifiable thrombosis have been described at autopsy following pyogenic meningitis. Cerebral infarction is a frequent sequela of vascular occlusion from inflammation, vasospasm, and thrombosis.

Inflammation of spinal nerves and roots produces meningeal signs, and inflammation of the cranial nerves produces cranial neuropathies of optic, oculomotor, facial, and auditory nerves. Increased intracranial pressure also produces oculomotor nerve palsy due to the presence of temporal lobe compression of the nerve during tentorial herniation, whereas abducens palsy may be a nonlocalizing sign of raised intracranial pressure. Septic cavernous sinus thrombosis is associated with palsies of cranial nerves III–VI.

Increased intracranial pressure is due to cell death (cytotoxic cerebral edema), cytokine-induced increased capillary vascular permeability (vasogenic cerebral edema), and, possibly, increased hydrostatic pressure (interstitial cerebral edema) following obstructed reabsorption of cerebrospinal fluid in the arachnoid villus or obstruction of the flow of fluid within or exiting from the ventricles. Intracranial pressure often exceeds 300 mm H_2O; cerebral perfusion may be further compromised if the **cerebral perfusion pressure** (mean arterial pressure minus intracranial pressure) is less than 50 cm H_2O due to reduced cerebral blood flow. Inappropriate secretion of antidiuretic hormone may produce excessive water retention, increasing the risk of raised intracranial pressure. Hypotonicity of brain extracellular spaces may cause cytotoxic edema following cell swelling and lysis. Herniation syndromes occur in 5% of infants and children with meningitis and should suggest markedly raised intracranial pressure, a cerebral abscess, or subdural empyema. Tentorial, falx, or cerebellar herniation does not usually occur because the increased intracranial pressure is transmitted to the entire subarachnoid space and there is little structural displacement. Nonetheless, in the presence of severe intracranial hypertension, an epidural or cortical abscess, or subdural empyema, cerebral or cerebellar herniation may develop.

Hydrocephalus is an uncommon acute complication of meningitis occurring after the neonatal period. Most often it takes the form of a communicating hydrocephalus due to adhesive thickening of the arachnoid villi around the cisterns at the base of the brain. Less often, obstructive hydrocephalus develops following fibrosis and gliosis of the aqueduct of Sylvius or the foramina of Magendie and Luschka. Ventricular dilation follows and may be associated with cerebral necrosis due to inflammation or raised intracranial pressure and cerebral arterial or venous occlusion.

Raised CSF protein levels are due in part to increased vascular permeability of the blood-brain barrier and the loss of albumin-rich fluid from the capillaries and veins traversing the subdural space. Continued transudation may result in subdural effusions, noted in the later phase of acute bacterial meningitis. Hypoglycorrhachia (reduced CSF glucose levels) is due to decreased glucose transport by the inflamed meninges and increased glucose utilization by the cerebral tissue. The latter may produce a local lactic acidosis.

Damage to the cerebral cortex may be due to the focal or diffuse effects of vascular occlusion (infarction, necrosis), hypoxia, bacterial invasion (cerebritis), toxic encephalopathy (lactic acidosis), raised intracranial pressure, ventriculitis, and transudation (subdural effusions). The resultant manifestations of impaired consciousness, seizures, hydrocephalus, cranial nerve deficits, motor and sensory deficits, and later psychomotor retardation can be explained by one or more of the pathologic factors described earlier.

PATHOGENESIS. Bacterial meningitis most commonly results from hematogenous dissemination of microorganisms from a distant site of infection; the bacteremia usually precedes it or occurs concomitantly. Bacterial colonization of the nasopharynx with a potentially pathogenic microorganism usually precedes the bacteremia. There may be prolonged carriage of the colonizing organisms without disease or more rapid invasion of the respiratory tract and onset of illness. Prior or concurrent viral upper respiratory tract infection may enhance the pathogenicity of bacteria producing meningitis.

H. influenzae type b and meningococci attach to mucosal epithelial cell receptors by pili. Following attachment to epithelial cells, bacteria breach the mucosa and enter the circulation. *N. meningitidis* may be transported across the mucosal surface within a phagocytic vacuole following ingestion by the epithelial cell. Bacterial survival in the bloodstream is enhanced by large bacterial capsules that interfere with opsonophagocytosis and are associated with increased virulence. Host-related developmental defects in bacterial opsonophagocytosis also contribute to the bacteremia. In the young nonimmune host the defect may be due to an absence of preformed IgM or IgG anticapsular antibodies, whereas in immunodeficient patients various deficiencies of components of the complement or properdin system may attenuate opsonophagocytosis. Direct activation of the antibody-independent properdin system is one mechanism that counteracts the effects of antibody deficiency and the antiphagocytic properties of the bacterial capsule. Splenic dysfunction may also reduce opsonophagocytosis by the reticuloendothelial system.

Bacteria gain entry to the cerebrospinal fluid through the choroid plexus of the lateral ventricles and the meninges. The bacteria then circulate to the extracerebral cerebrospinal fluid and subarachnoid space and rapidly multiply because the cerebrospinal fluid concentrations of complement and antibody are inadequate to contain bacterial proliferation. Chemotactic factors then incite a local inflammatory response characterized by polymorphonuclear cell infiltration. The presence of bacterial cell wall lipopolysaccharide (endotoxin) of gram-negative bacteria (*H. influenzae* type b, *N. meningitidis*) and of pneumococcal cell wall components (teichoic acid, peptidoglycan) stimulates a marked inflammatory response with local production of tumor necrosis factor, interleukin 1, prostaglandin E_2, and other cytokine inflammatory mediators. The subsequent inflammatory response, directly related to the presence of these inflammatory mediators, is characterized by neutrophilic infiltration, increased vascular permeability, alterations of the blood-brain barrier, and vascular thrombosis. Excessive cytokine-induced inflammation continues after the cerebrospinal fluid has been sterilized and is thought to be partly responsible for the chronic inflammatory sequelae of pyogenic meningitis.

Meningitis may rarely follow bacterial invasion from a contiguous focus of infection, for example, paranasal sinusitis, otitis media, mastoiditis, orbital cellulitis, dermal sinus tracts, cranial or vertebral osteomyelitis, penetrating cranial trauma, or meningomyeloceles. Meningitis associated with otitis media is usually due not to contiguous spread but to preceding or concurrent bacteremia. Infection associated with frontal or ethmoid sinusitis (Sec. 14.30) may also produce an epidural abscess, subdural empyema, and a frontal lobe brain abscess; sphenoid sinus infection (Sec. 14.30) may produce cavernous sinus thrombosis, epidural and subdural empyemas, and infection in the area of the sella turcica; middle ear or mastoid infection (Sec. 22.22) may produce petrositis and middle fossa, temporal lobe, cerebellar, or brain stem abscesses. Meningitis may occur during endocarditis, pneumonia, or thrombophlebitis. It may also be associated with severe burns and cystic fibrosis (*S. aureus* and *P. aeruginosa*), indwelling catheters, or contaminated equipment.

CLINICAL MANIFESTATIONS. The mode of onset of acute meningitis has two predominant presentations. *Sudden onset*, with rapidly progressive manifestations of shock, purpura, disseminated intravascular coagulation, and reduced levels of consciousness, is a dramatic and often fatal presentation of meningococcal sepsis with meningitis; it may evolve to death within 24 hr. *H. influenzae* type b and pneumococcal meningitis less frequently presents as a rapidly progressive infection. More often, meningitis due to *H. influenzae* type b and pneumococcus (and some cases of meningococcal meningitis) is preceded by several days of upper respiratory tract or gastrointestinal symptoms. This *subacute presentation* may also be complicated by partial treatment with antibiotics (in 25–50% of patients) for associated otitis media or respiratory tract infections (see section on Diagnosis).

The signs and symptoms of meningitis are related to the nonspecific findings associated with a systemic infection or bacteremia and to the specific manifestations of meningeal irritation with central nervous system inflammation. The former include fever (present in 90–95%), anorexia and poor feeding, upper respiratory tract infection, myalgias, arthralgias, tachycardia, hypotension, and various cutaneous signs such as petechiae (present in 10%), purpura, or an erythematous macular rash. Meningeal irritation is manifest as nuchal rigidity, back pain, **Kernig sign** (flexion of the hip 90 degrees with subsequent pain on extension of the leg), and **Brudzinski sign** (involuntary flexion of the knees and hips following flexion of the neck while supine). In some children, particularly young infants, these signs may not occur. Increased intracranial pressure is suggested by headache, emesis, bulging fontanel or diastasis (widening) of the sutures, oculomotor or abducens nerve paralysis, a combination of hypertension and bradycardia with apnea or hyperventilation, decorticate or decerebrate posturing, stupor, coma, or signs of herniation. Papilledema is uncommon in uncomplicated meningitis and should suggest a more chronic process such as the presence of an intracranial abscess, subdural empyema, or occlusion of a dural venous sinus. Focal neurologic signs may be due to vascular occlusion or abscess formation. Cranial neuropathies of the ocular, oculomotor, abducens, facial, and auditory nerves also may be due to focal inflammation. Cortical infarction may also produce focal neurologic signs. Overall, 14% of children with bacterial meningitis have focal neurologic signs; 34% of patients with pneumococcal meningitis manifest focal deficits.

Seizures (focal or generalized) due to cerebritis, infarction, or electrolyte disturbances are noted in 20–30% of patients with meningitis. They are more frequently noted in patients with *H. influenzae* and pneumococcal meningitis than in those with meningococcal infection. Seizures that occur on presentation or within the first 4 days of onset are usually of no prognostic significance. Seizures that persist after the 4th day of illness, those that are difficult to treat, and those that appear late in the course of meningitis are associated with a poor prognosis. Seizures in a febrile infant less than 6 mo of age should suggest meningitis rather than a simple febrile seizure because the later benign seizure type is uncommon in very young infants.

Alterations of mental status and a reduced level of consciousness are common among patients with meningitis and may be due to increased intracranial pressure, cerebritis, or hypotension; manifestations include irritability, lethargy, stupor, obtundation, and coma. Comatose patients have a poor prognosis; this sign is noted more often with pneumococcal or meningococcal infection than with meningitis due to *H. influenzae*. Additional manifestations of meningitis include photophobia and tache cerebrale, which is elicited by stroking the skin with a blunt object and observing a red raised streak within 30–60 sec.

Complications. During the treatment of meningitis complications due to central nervous system or systemic effects of infection are common. Neurologic complications include seizures, increased intracranial pressure, cranial nerve palsies, stroke, cerebral or cerebellar herniation, transverse myelitis, ataxia, thrombosis of dural venous sinuses, and subdural effusions.

Collections of fluid in the subdural space develop in 10–30% of patients with meningitis and are asymptomatic in 85–90% of patients. Subdural effusions may be present in as many as 50% of cases complicated by persistent fever. They are most common in patients with *H. influenzae* type b meningitis, less common in pneumococcal infection, and rare in meningococcal meningitis. However, young age (< 12 mo) is also independently associated with a greater risk of subdural effusion. Symptomatic subdural effusions may result in a bulging fontanel, diastasis of sutures, enlarging head circumference, emesis, seizures, fever, and abnormal results of cranial transillumination. However, many of these manifestations are also present in patients with meningitis without subdural effusion. CT scanning will confirm the diagnosis of a subdural effusion. In the presence of increased intracranial pressure or a depressed level of consciousness, a symptomatic subdural effusion should be treated by aspiration through the open fontanel. Subdural empyema complicates 1% of subdural effusions. Fever alone is not an indication for subdural aspiration.

The syndrome of inappropriate secretion of antidiuretic hormone (SIADH) occurs in 30–50% of cases of meningitis. The resulting hyponatremia and reduced serum osmolality may exacerbate cerebral edema or independently produce hyponatremic seizures. Later in the course of therapy central diabetes insipidus may develop owing to hypothalamic or pituitary dysfunction.

Fever usually resolves earlier in patients with meningococcal or pneumococcal disease than in those with *H. influenzae* meningitis. By the 6th day of therapy more than 90% of patients with meningococcal or pneumococcal meningitis are afebrile compared with 70% of patients with *H. influenzae. Prolonged fever* (> 10 days) is noted in 15% of patients with *H. influenzae* meningitis, 9% of those with pneumococcal, and 6% of those with meningococcal meningitis; *persistent fever* (5–9 days) occurs in 13% of cases. Prolonged or persistent fever may be due to subdural effusions, drug reactions, nosocomial infection, phlebitis, pneumonia, pericarditis, or arthritis. The latter manifestations may represent actual pyogenic infection of the pericardium or synovial fluid if they occur within 2–4 days of onset of meningitis. Late-onset (> 5 days) pericarditis or arthritis is a sterile effusion, represents immune complex deposition, and is best managed with anti-inflammatory agents. Severe symptomatic pericarditis may require pericardiocentesis. *Secondary fever*, appearing after the patient has become afebrile, may represent subdural effusions, nosocomial infection, or breakthrough fever following the withdrawal of corticosteroids. The presence of prolonged, persistent, or secondary fever, in the absence of resistant bacteria or severe systemic infection, has no influence on the outcome of meningitis. The etiology of these fever patterns is unknown in 15–40% of patients.

Thrombocytosis, eosinophilia, and anemia may develop during therapy for meningitis. Anemia may be due to hemolysis and is most commonly noted with *H. influenzae* disease. Alternatively, anemia may be due to bone marrow suppression. Disseminated intravascular coagulation (DIC) is most often associated with the rapidly progressive pattern of presentation and is noted most commonly in patients with shock and purpura (purpura fulminans). The combination of endotoxemia and severe hypotension spontaneously initiates the coagulation cascade; the coexistence of ongoing thrombosis may produce symmetric peripheral gangrene.

Repeated episodes of meningitis are rare but have three distinct patterns. *Recrudescence* is the reappearance of infection during therapy with appropriate antibiotics. Cerebrospinal fluid culture reveals the growth of bacteria that have developed antibiotic resistance. *Relapse* occurs between 3 days and 3 wk after therapy and represents persistent bacterial infection in the central nervous system (subdural empyema, ventriculitis, cerebral abscess) or other site (mastoid, cranial osteomyelitis, orbital infection). Relapse is often associated with an inadequate choice, dose, or duration of antibiotic therapy. *Recurrence* is a new episode of meningitis due to reinfection with the same bacterial species or another pyogenic pathogen. Recurrent meningitis suggests the presence of an acquired or congenital anatomic communication between the cerebrospinal fluid and a mucocutaneous site. Defects in immune host defense also predispose to recurrent meningitis (see earlier section on Epidemiology). Patients with a deficiency of one of the late components of complement (C5, C6, C7, C8, or C9) are at increased risk for recurrent mild to moderately severe meningococcal meningitis.

DIFFERENTIAL DIAGNOSIS. Many signs and symptoms suggesting acute bacterial meningeal or intracranial infections occur with other acute or chronic infectious or noninfectious diseases; no manifestation is pathognomonic for bacterial meningitis. Pyogenic meningitis must be distinguished from the clinical conditions and infectious diseases producing aseptic meningitis (see Table 12–5). This differentiation is facilitated by careful examination of the CSF with specific stains (Kinoyoun carbol fuchin for mycobacteria, India ink for fungi), cytology, antigen detection (partial bacterial treatment, *Cryptococcus*), serology (syphilis), viral culture (herpes simplex, enterovirus, HIV), and other specific diagnostic tests such as CT or magnetic resonance imaging of the brain, blood cultures, serologic tests, and possibly brain biopsy. Acute viral meningitis is often differentiated from acute bacterial meningitis because the latter demonstrates a CSF glucose value of less than 30 mg/dL, a CSF glucose-to-blood glucose ratio of less than 0.2–0.3, a protein level of greater than 200 mg/dL, a CSF neutrophil count of more than 1,000, and a positive Gram stain (80–90% are positive); the illness also often occurs during the winter in a child less than 2 yr old (see Table 12–6).

Partial treatment, with oral or systemic antibiotics, of a patient with acute bacterial meningitis usually will not completely alter the typical bacterial CSF profile. Partially treated meningitis may reduce both the incidence of positive CSF Gram stain to less than 60% and the ability to grow microorganisms, especially the meningococcus. It does not consistently alter the CSF glucose, protein, or neutrophil profile, nor does it interfere with antigen detection methods performed on the CSF. The differential diagnosis of a CSF profile in a patient who has been partially treated, for example, no bacteria recovered but high protein and low glucose concentrations and a predominant neutrophilic pleocytosis, includes a parameningeal suppurative focus of infection such as epidural, subdural, or brain abscesses, sinusitis, mastoiditis, thrombophlebitis, cranial osteomyelitis, endocarditis, and dermal sinus tract infections.

Additional infectious and noninfectious causes of meningitis are noted in Table 12–5. Important treatable causes of bacterial meningitis other than *H. influenzae*, pneumococcus, and meningococcus include tuberculosis (Sec. 12.47), Rocky Mountain spotted fever (Sec. 12.98), *Nocardia* (Sec. 12.46), syphilis (Sec. 12.52), and Lyme disease (Sec. 12.57). Chronic meningitis lasting longer than 1 mo is unusual in children. The CSF profile in chronic meningitis varies but may resemble that in acute pyogenic meningitis. The differential diagnosis of *chronic neutrophilic meningitis* includes disease due to bacteria (*Nocardia, Actinomyces, Brucella*) fungi (*Blastomyces, Coccidioides, Candida, Aspergillus, Pseudoallescheria*), and other entities (chemical agents, carcinoma, systemic lupus erythematosus). *Chronic lymphocytic meningitis* may be due to bacteria (syphilis, *Actinomyces, Brucella*, Lyme disease, rarely tuberculosis), fungi (*C. neoformans, Candida* sp., *Coccidioides immitis, Histoplasma capsulatum, Blastomyces dermatitides, Sporothrix schenckii, Pseudoallescheria boydii*), parasites (*Toxoplasma, Cysticercus*), occasionally viruses (mumps, lymphocytic choriomeningitis, HIV, enterovirus in patients with agammaglobulinemia), and others (carcinomatosis, sarcoidosis, multiple sclerosis).

DIAGNOSIS. Early diagnosis and treatment are critical to the outcome of bacterial meningitis. The diagnosis of acute pyogenic meningitis is confirmed by analysis of the CSF, which reveals microorganisms on Gram stain and culture, a neutrophilic pleocytosis, and an elevated protein and reduced glucose content (see Table 12–6). Lumbar puncture (LP) should be performed when bacterial meningitis is suspected. *Contraindications for an immediate LP* include (1) evidence of increased intracranial pressure other than a bulging fontanel, for example, third or sixth cranial nerve palsy with a depressed level of consciousness, or hypertension and bradycardia with respiratory abnormalities; (2) severe cardiopulmonary compromise requiring prompt resuscitative measures for shock or in patients in whom positioning for the LP would further compromise cardiopulmonary function; and (3) infection of the skin overlying the site of the LP. Thrombocytopenia is a relative contraindication for immediate LP. LP is indicated in a child who shows evidence of disseminated intravascular coagulation or petechiae but may be delayed in immunosuppressed patients with chronic thrombocytopenia until platelet transfusion has been given. *If an LP is delayed by any of the above factors, immediate empiric therapy should be initiated* against the potential causative microorganisms based on the patient's age and underlying disease. CT scanning for evidence of a brain abscess or increased intracranial pressure also should not delay the onset of therapy. Lumbar puncture may be performed after increased intracranial pressure has been treated or a brain abscess has been excluded. Short-term intravenous therapy or partial treatment with oral antibiotics prior to diagnosis will not change the classic CSF profile of pyogenic bacterial meningitis but may reduce the likelihood of recovery of microorganisms by culture or Gram stain.

Countercurrent immunoelectrophoresis (CIE) may identify antigens of *H. influenzae* type b, *S. pneumoniae*, and *N. meningitidis* types A, C, Y, and W135 in the cerebrospinal fluid. *Latex particle agglutination* is more sensitive than CIE and may be used to detect antigens of group B streptococcus, *H. influenzae* type b, *S. pneumoniae*, and *N. meningitidis*. Antigen may also be detected in the serum and urine. Recent immunization with the *H. influenzae* type b polysaccharide vaccine may produce a false-positive result of the antigen test in serum and urine but not in CSF.

A *blood culture* should be performed in all patients with meningitis, especially those who will be treated empirically prior to examination of CSF. Blood cultures may reveal the responsible bacteria in 80–90% of cases of childhood meningitis.

Lumbar puncture is traditionally performed with the patient in the flexed lateral decubitus position; the styleted needle is passed into the L3–L4 or L4–L5 intervertebral space. After entry into the subarachnoid space, the patient's position is changed to a more extended one to measure the opening CSF pressure. When the pressure is high, only enough CSF is removed to permit careful examination.

The *CSF leukocyte count* in bacterial meningitis is usually elevated to more than 1,000 and reveals a neutrophilic predominance (75–95%). Turbid CSF is present when the CSF leukocyte count is greater than 200–400. Normal healthy neonates may have as many as 30 leukocytes and older children without viral or bacterial meningitis may have 5–6 leukocytes in the CSF; in both age groups there is a predominance of lymphocytes or monocytes. Although prolonged seizures may produce a CSF leukocytosis, the absolute number is usually less than 50, and neutrophilia does not occur. When seizures occur with fever and abnormal mental status, the seizures may not be the sole cause of CSF pleocytosis, and meningitis should be suspected.

A low CSF leukocyte count (< 250) may be present in as many as 20% of patients with acute bacterial meningitis; absent pleocytosis may be evident in patients with severe overwhelming sepsis and meningitis and is a poor prognostic sign. Pleocytosis with a lymphocyte predominance may be present in acute bacterial meningitis during the early stage of the illness; conversely, neutrophilic pleocytosis (total neutrophil counts usually of < 500) may be present in 20–40% of patients during the early stages of acute viral meningitis. The shift to lymphocytic-monocytic predominance in viral meningitis may be delayed 12–24 hr.

The *Gram stain* is positive in most (70–90%) patients with meningitis. This is dependent on the bacterial inoculum size; the Gram stain is positive in only 25% of patients with less than 10^3 colony-forming units (CFU) of bacteria/mL but is positive in 60% of those with 10^3–10^5 CFU/mL and in 95% of those with more than 10^5 CFU/mL. If the Gram stain is negative, an acridine orange stain, which stains bacterial DNA and is detected with a fluorescent microscope, may detect the morphology of the bacteria. Despite the identification of gram-positive or gram-negative diplococci or pleomorphic coccobacilli, treatment should not be modified on the basis of the stain but should remain empiric until a microorganism is identified by culture (see later).

Traumatic lumbar puncture complicates the diagnosis of meningitis and may be present in as many as 10% of patients. Repeat LP at another interspace may produce less hemorrhagic fluid, but the fluid usually also contains red blood cells. The Gram stain, culture, and glucose level may not be influenced by a traumatic LP. CSF obtained from a traumatic LP should not reveal xanthochromia unless the patient has a high CSF protein content, is jaundiced, or has greater than 150,000 red cells; for each 1,000 red blood cells the CSF protein content will increase 1 mg/dL. Traumatic LP interferes with the interpretation of CSF leukocytosis. The peripheral white blood cell to red blood cell ratio is usually between 1:500 and 1:750. CSF from a traumatic LP should be interpreted based on a combination of factors such as Gram stain, glucose levels, predominance of neutrophils, and any significant deviation in the standard white blood cell to red blood cell ratio.

Additional diagnostic methods used to identify the responsible pathogen or to diagnose bacterial meningitis include culture and staining of petechial lesions or the peripheral blood buffy coat and determination of CSF C-reactive protein and tumor necrosis factor levels. CT scan is not indicated for most cases of bacterial meningitis but should be considered in patients with signs of increased intracranial pressure, focal neurologic deficits, prolonged fever during therapy, increasing head circumference, and a possible suppurative parameningeal or parenchymal lesion.

TREATMENT. Initial Antibiotic Therapy. The therapeutic approach to a patient with presumed bacterial meningitis depends on the nature of the initial manifestations of the illness. A child with rapidly progressing disease of less than 24 hr duration, in the absence of increased intracranial pressure, should receive antibiotics immediately after an LP is performed. If there are signs of increased intracranial pressure or focal neurologic findings, antibiotics should be given without performing an LP and before obtaining a CT scan. Increased intracranial pressure should be treated simultaneously. In either circumstance, the patient with a rapidly progressive illness should receive antibiotics within 30–60 min of presentation. Immediate treatment of associated multiple organ system failure, such as shock and adult respiratory distress syndrome, is also indicated.

Patients who have a more protracted subacute course and become ill over a 1- to 7-day period should also be evaluated for signs of increased intracranial pressure and focal neurologic deficits. Unilateral headache, papilledema, and other signs of increased intracranial pressure suggest a focal lesion such as a brain or epidural abscess and subdural empyema. Antibiotic therapy should be initiated prior to LP and CT scanning. If no signs of increased intracranial pressure are evident, an LP should be performed. If the patient is semicomatose or comatose, antibiotic therapy is initiated before obtaining the results of the CSF analysis. If the patient is alert, treatment is based on the CSF profile. In any of these circumstances, in patients with a subacute illness, therapy should be initiated within 2 hr of presentation.

The initial (empiric) choice of therapy for meningitis in immunocompetent infants and children should be based on the antibiotic susceptibilities of *H. influenzae* type b, *S. pneumoniae*, and *N. meningitidis*. The antibiotic(s) should achieve bactericidal levels in the CSF and, if given in combination, should not be antagonistic. Antibiotics that cross the inflamed blood-brain barrier are highly lipid soluble, have a low molecular weight, and have low ionization at normal pH. The initial treatment of choice is **ceftriaxone** given either as 100 mg/kg/24 hr every day or 50 mg/kg/dose every 12 hr. This drug achieves very high bactericidal level in the CSF; the MIC is often more than 1,000 times that needed to eradicate the microorganism. Delayed bacterial killing at 24 hr is noted in 0–2% of patients treated with ceftriaxone. In contrast, 9–12% of patients receiving cefuroxime, which is no longer recommended, show evidence of delayed killing. In addition, cefuroxime is associated with an increased risk of chronic sequelae such as hearing loss. **Cefotaxime** (200 mg/kg/24 hr every 6 hr) is an alternative to ceftriaxone.

Ampicillin (300 mg/kg/24 hr every 6 hr) and **chloramphenicol** (100 mg/kg/24 hr given every 6 hr) constitute another less frequently recommended initial antibiotic regimen. Ampicillin resistance is present in 20–30% of *H. influenzae* type b organisms due to bacterial β-lactamase enzyme activity; 1–2% of isolates in the United States and about 50% in Spain are also resistant to chloramphenicol. Chloramphenicol therapy also has the potential adverse effects of aplastic anemia, shock-like gray infant syndrome, and dose-dependent bone marrow suppression. If *L. monocytogenes* infection is also suspected, as in infants 1–2 mo old or patients with a T lymphocyte deficiency, ampicillin should be given with ceftriaxone because all cephalosporins are ineffective against *L. monocytogenes*. Intravenous trimethoprim-sulfamethoxazole is an alternate treatment for *L. monocytogenes*.

If the patient is immunocompromised and gram-negative bacterial meningitis is suspected, initial therapy should include ceftazidine and an aminoglycoside.

Subsequent Antibiotic Therapy. Uncomplicated *H. influenzae* type b meningitis should be treated for 10 days with intravenous antibiotics, although 7 days of intravenous antibiotics has been effective in some studies. After determining that the organism is sensitive to ampicillin and does not produce a β-lactamase, initial antimicrobial therapy may be changed to ampicillin.

If *S. pneumoniae* is cultured from the CSF, the isolate should be tested for penicillin resistance with oxacillin. Relative resistance to penicillin (MIC 0.1–1.0 μg/mL) is present in 2–15% of *S. pneumoniae* isolates, and highly resistant organisms (MIC > 2.0 μg/mL) are found in a small number of patients. Therapy of relatively resistant *S. pneumoniae* infection includes ceftriaxone, whereas that for highly resistant pneumococci includes vancomycin. Chloramphenicol is the treatment of choice for resistant organisms if the organism is sensitive to this antibiotic. Therapy for uncomplicated penicillin-sensitive pneumococcal meningitis should be accomplished with intravenous penicillin 300,000 U/kg/24 hr, given every 4–6 hr for 10–14 days.

Intravenous penicillin 300,000 U/kg/24 hr for 7 days is the treatment of choice for uncomplicated *N. meningitidis* meningitis. Shorter therapy has been proposed (3–5 days) but is not recommended. Rare meningococcal isolates have demonstrated relative (0.25–0.5 μg/mL) and absolute (> 250 μg/mL) resistance to penicillin, and these organisms may require alternate therapy with ceftriaxone.

Patients who receive intravenous or oral antibiotics prior to LP and do not have an identifiable pathogen (on Gram stain, culture, or antigen detection) but do have evidence of an acute bacterial infection on the CSF profile should continue to receive empiric therapy with ceftriaxone for 10–14 days. If focal signs are present or the child does not respond to treatment, a parameningeal focus may be present, and a CT scan should be performed.

A repeat LP is not indicated in patients with uncomplicated meningitis due to *H. influenzae* type b, *N. meningitidis*, or *S. pneumoniae*. Repeat examination of CSF is indicated in some neonates, in patients with gram-negative bacillary meningitis, and in those who do not respond to conventional antimicrobial therapy within 48–72 hr. Improvement in the CSF profile is indicated by an increase in CSF glucose levels and the appearance of lymphocyte-monocyte cells; although the Gram stain may remain positive at this time, the CSF should be sterile.

Meningitis due to *E. coli* or *P. aeruginosa* requires therapy with ceftazidine for 3 wk or for at least 2 wk after CSF sterilization, which may occur after 2–10 days of treatment. *P. aeruginosa* may become resistant to ceftazidine during treatment due to the presence of a bacterial inducible chromosomally mediated cephalosporinase. Therefore, to prevent resistance, an aminoglycoside should be administered for at least 1 wk during treatment with ceftazidine. Ciprofloxacin is an alternate to ceftazidine for the treatment of *Pseudomonas* meningitis. Although new quinolone antibiotics are associated with bone or joint lesions in young animals, the risk of morbidity or mortality from meningitis due to a ceftazidine-resistant *P. aeruginosa* is greater than the undetermined risk of these skeletal lesions. Occasionally, daily intraventricular aminoglycoside therapy has improved the outcome for some patients with *E. coli* meningitis.

Side effects of antibiotic therapy of meningitis include phlebitis, drug fever, rash, emesis, oral candidiasis, and diarrhea. Ceftriaxone may cause reversible gallbladder pseudolithiasis, detectable by abdominal ultrasound, which is usually asymptomatic but may produce emesis and right upper quadrant pain.

Supportive Care. Repeated *medical and neurologic assessments* of the patient with bacterial meningitis are essential to enable the physician to identify early signs of cardiovascular, central nervous system, and metabolic complications. Pulse rate, blood pressure, and respiratory rate should be monitored frequently. Neurologic assessment including pupillary reflexes, level of consciousness, motor strength, cranial nerve signs, and evaluation for seizures should be determined frequently during the first 72 hr when the risk of neurologic complications is greatest. Thereafter, the neurologic assessment should be performed once a day. Important laboratory studies include an assessment of BUN, serum sodium, chloride potassium, and bicarbonate levels, urine output and specific gravity, complete blood and platelet counts, and coagulation factors (fibrinogen, prothrombin and partial thromboplastin times) in the presence of petechiae, purpura, or abnormal bleeding.

Initially, the patient should receive nothing by mouth. *Intravenous fluid administration* should be restricted to one half to one third of maintenance, or 800–1,000 mL/m²/24 hr, until it can be established that increased intracranial pressure or SIADH is not present. Fluid administration may be returned to normal (1,500–1,700 mL/m²/24 hr) when serum sodium levels are normal. Fluid restriction needs to be balanced against the need to treat systemic hypotension, since reduced blood pressure may result in a cerebral perfusion pressure of less than 50 cm H_2O with subsequent central nervous system ischemia. Therefore, shock, which occurs in the rapidly progressive pattern of meningococcal meningitis, must be treated aggressively to prevent brain and other organ dysfunction (acute tubular necrosis, adult respiratory distress syndrome). Patients with shock, a markedly raised intracranial pressure, coma, and refractory seizures require intense monitoring with central arterial and venous access and frequent vital signs, necessitating admission to a pediatric intensive care unit (Sec. 6.34). Patients with septic shock require fluid resuscitation and therapy with vasoactive agents such as dopamine, epinephrine, and sodium nitroprusside (Sec. 12.14). The goal of such therapy in patients with meningitis is avoidance of excessive increases of intracranial pressure without compromising blood flow and oxygen delivery to vital organs (brain, heart, lung, kidney).

Neurologic complications include *increased intracranial pressure* with subsequent herniation, seizures, and an enlarging head circumference due to a subdural effusion or hydrocephalus. Signs of increased intracranial pressure, other than a bulging fontanel or isolated coma, should be treated emergently with endotracheal intubation and hyperventilation (P_{CO_2} approximately 25 mm Hg). In addition, intravenous furosemide (Lasix) (1 mg/kg) and mannitol (0.5–1 g/kg) osmotherapy may reduce intracranial pressure. Furosemide may reduce brain swelling by venodilation and diuresis without increasing intracranial blood volume, whereas mannitol produces an osmolar gradient between the brain and plasma, thus shifting fluid from the central nervous system to the plasma with subsequent excretion during an osmotic diuresis. Repeated doses of mannitol may be given for signs of impending herniation; lower doses of mannitol (250 mg/kg/dose every 6 hr) are indicated for the control of chronic cerebral edema. If the serum osmolality increases to more than 320–330 mOsm/L, mannitol osmotherapy should be temporarily discontinued because the risks of hyperosmolality exceed those of increased intracranial pressure.

Seizures are common during the course of bacterial meningitis. Immediate therapy for seizures includes intravenous diazepam (0.1–0.2 mg/kg/dose) or lorazepam (0.05 mg/kg/dose), paying careful attention to the risk of respiratory suppression, which is more common with diazepam. Serum glucose, calcium, and sodium levels should be monitored to determine if hypoglycemia, hypocalcemia, or hyponatremia is causing seizures and requires specific therapy. After immediate management of seizures, the patient should receive phenytoin (15–20 mg/kg loading dose, 5 mg/kg/24 hr maintenance) for further control of seizures. Phenytoin is preferred to phenobarbital because it produces less central nervous system depression and permits assessment of the patient's level of consciousness. Because the pharmacokinetics of phenytoin are affected by age and other drugs, serum phenytoin levels should be monitored to maintain them in the therapeutic range (10–20 μg/mL).

Rapid killing of bacteria by high bactericidal antibiotic levels in the CSF effectively sterilizes the meningeal infection but releases toxic cell products following cell lysis (cell wall endotoxin), which perpetuates the cytokine-mediated inflammatory response. The resultant edema formation and neutrophilic infiltration may be in excess of that needed to contain the infection and may produce additional neurologic injury. Agents that limit the overproduction of inflammatory mediators may have a theoretical beneficial effect on the outcome of bacterial meningitis. Preliminary studies suggest that *intravenous dexamethasone* (0.15 mg/kg/dose, given every 6 hr for 4 days) may be associated with less fever, lower CSF protein and lactate levels, and a reduction in permanent auditory nerve damage as manifest by sensorineural hearing loss. Most experience with dexamethasone treatment has been gained with *H. influenzae* type b infection, and extrapolation to other bacterial pathogens should be done with caution, balancing potential benefits against risks. Dexamethasone, if used, should be given before or at the same time as antibiotics. Complications of this therapy include gastrointestinal bleeding, hypertension, hyperglycemia, leukocytosis, and rebound fever after the last dose. Patients in septic shock do not benefit from corticosteroid therapy unless the septic shock is complicated by the rare development of adrenal insufficiency due to Waterhouse-Friderichsen syndrome. Indeed, patients with sepsis and adult respiratory distress syndrome have a poorer outcome when treated with steroids.

Therapy of disseminated intravascular coagulation includes direct treatment of the inciting primary disease, correction of hypotension, replacement of coagulation factors and platelets, and, in the presence of thrombosis, the use of systemic heparinization (Sec. 16.75).

PREVENTION. Prophylaxis against meningitis is possible with antibiotic chemoprophylaxis of the index case or close contacts and vaccination of susceptible patients with specific vaccines.

***Haemophilus influenzae* type b.** *H. influenzae* type b nasopharyngeal colonization may not be eradicated despite 10 days of appropriate parenteral antibiotic therapy. Prior to discharge from the hospital, *the patient* should receive rifampin (20 mg/kg/dose every day for 4 days) to prevent introduction or reintroduction of the organism into the household or day-care center.

Rifampin prophylaxis should be given to all *household contacts*, including adults, if there are any close family members less than 4 yr old, regardless of the immunization status of the contacts. A household contact is one who lives in the residence of the index case or who has spent a minimum of 4 hr with the index case for at least 5 of 7 days preceding the patient's hospitalization. Family members should receive rifampin prophylaxis immediately after the diagnosis is confirmed in the index case because more than 50% of secondary family cases occur in the 1st wk after the index patient has been hospitalized. Rifampin prophylaxis is not needed if all family members are older than 4 yr.

The risk of secondary cases of *H. influenzae* type b infection in *day-care center contacts* is less than that for household contacts and probably greater than that for the general population. The risk is exceedingly low for day-care center children who are nonclassroom contacts and those over 2 yr old. The efficacy of chemoprophylaxis in day-care centers is uncertain, and there are difficulties in ensuring that all at-risk day-care center attendees receive the drug. Chemoprophylaxis for children and adults in day-care centers that resemble households (e.g., children $<$ 2 yr old and $>$ 25 hr/wk of close contact) should be provided. If all children are less than 2 yr old, chemoprophylaxis is not needed with one index case. Day-care center workers and parents should be educated about the signs of serious *H. influenzae* infection and the importance of seeking prompt medical attention for fever or other potential manifestations of *H. influenzae* disease. If two or more cases of *H. influenzae* type b infection occur within 60 days in a day-care center, rifampin chemoprophylaxis should be given to all adults and children. For all situations the dose of rifampin is 20 mg/kg/24 hr (maximum 600 mg) given once each day for 4 days. Rifampin discolors the urine and sweat red-orange, stains contact lenses, and reduces the efficacy of some drugs including oral contraceptives. Rifampin is contraindicated during pregnancy.

Vaccination with *H. influenzae* type b capsular polysaccharide (PRP), covalently linked to diphtheria or tetanus toxoids or the outer membrane protein of *N. meningitidis*, should be given to all children at 2, 4, 6, and 15 mo of age (Sec. 5.1–5.2). There is a theoretical risk of serious *H. influenzae* type b infection within 3 wk of vaccination. Children who have had serious *H. influenzae* type b infection before 15 mo of age should receive the vaccine at the appropriate time because they may not have produced protective antibody after the acute infection at this young age.

High-risk populations such as American Indians or Eskimos may have a lower incidence of *H. influenzae* type b infection after passive immunotherapy with bacterial polysaccharide immunoglobulin (BPIG). Currently, BPIG is only available in experimental protocols.

***Neisseria meningitidis*.** Chemoprophylaxis is recommended for all close contacts of patients with meningococcal meningitis regardless of age or immunization status. Close contacts should be treated with rifampin 10 mg/kg/dose every 12 hr for 2 days (maximum dose of 600 mg) as soon as possible after identification of a case of meningococcal meningitis or sepsis. If the organism is sensitive to sulfonamides, the contacts should receive 2 days of chemoprophylaxis with sulfasoxazole (500 mg) every 12 hr for children 1–12 yr, 500 mg/day for infants under 1 yr, and 1 g every 12 hr for contacts over 12 yr of age. Close contacts include household contacts and day-care center, nursery school, and health care workers who have direct exposure to secretions (e.g., mouth-to-mouth resuscitation, suctioning, intubation). Exposed contacts should be treated before their colonization status is known. In addition, all contacts should be educated about the early signs of meningococcal disease and the need to seek prompt medical attention if these signs develop.

Ceftriaxone and ciprofloxacin are alternative antibiotics that can be used for chemoprophylaxis in patients with rifampin-resistant meningococci. Ceftriaxone (250 mg IM for 1 dose) may be effective chemoprophylaxis in pregnant women or in adult contacts in whom *N. meningitidis* is not eliminated from the nasopharynx.

Meningococcal quadrivalent vaccine against serogroups A, C, Y, and W135 is recommended for high-risk children over 2 yr of age with asplenia, functional splenic dysfunction, or deficiencies of terminal complement proteins. The vaccine may also be used as an adjunct with chemoprophylaxis for exposed contacts and during epidemics of meningococcal disease. Unfortunately, most cases of endemic meningococcal meningitis are due to group B for which there is no current vaccine.

Streptococcus pneumoniae. No chemoprophylaxis or vaccination is required for normal hosts who may be contacts of patients with pneumococcal meningitis. High-risk patients should receive the 23-valent pneumococcal vaccine, and patients with sickle cell anemia should also receive chemoprophylaxis with daily oral penicillin or amoxicillin. Regardless of immunization or chemoprophylaxis, patients with sickle cell anemia should seek prompt medical attention for all febrile episodes.

PROGNOSIS. Appropriate recognition, prompt antibiotic therapy, and supportive care have reduced the mortality of bacterial meningitis beyond the neonatal period to 1–8%. Pneumococcal and meningococcal meningitis (not sepsis) have a higher mortality than *H. influenzae* type b meningitis. Severe neurodevelopmental sequelae may occur in 10–20% of patients, and as many as 50% have some, albeit subtle, neurobehavioral morbidity. Prognosis is poorest among infants less than 6 mo and in those with delayed sterilization of the CSF, more than 10^6 colony-forming units of bacteria/mL of CSF, a CSF glucose level of less than 20 mg/dL, seizures occurring more than 4 days into therapy, coma, focal neurologic signs on presentation, delayed or inappropriate antibiotic therapy, SIADH, infection with *E. coli* or *P. aeruginosa*, and cerebral infarction or septic shock.

Specific neurologic sequelae include mental retardation (10%), seizures (5–8%), delay in acquisition of language (15%), hearing loss (10–15%), visual impairment (2–5%), behavioral problems (10%), and additional problems such as motor deficits, ataxia, athetosis, hemiballismus, hydrocephalus, hemiparesis, transverse myelitis, and diabetes insipidus.

Sensorineural hearing loss is due to labyrinthitis following cochlear infection and occurs in as many as 30% of patients with pneumococcal meningitis, 10% with meningococcal, and 4–18% of those with *H. influenzae* type b meningitis. Hearing loss may also be due to direct inflammation of the auditory nerve. Hearing loss is associated with CSF glucose of less than 20 mg/dL, delayed sterilization of CSF, and ataxia. Ataxia may represent vestibular nerve dysfunction. Antibiotic therapy with ceftriaxone reduces the incidence of hearing loss, and adjunctive therapy with dexamethasone may reduce the incidence of severe hearing loss. Regardless of the bacterial agent, type of antibiotic therapy, or use of dexamethasone, all patients with bacterial meningitis should undergo careful audiologic assessment before or soon after discharge from the hospital. Frequent reassessment on an outpatient basis is indicated for all patients who have a hearing deficit.

Arditi M, Ables L, Yogev R: Cerebrospinal fluid endotoxin levels in children with *H. influenzae* meningitis before and after administration of intravenous ceftriaxone. J Infect Dis 160:1005, 1989.

Blazer S, Berant M, Alon U: Bacterial meningitis: Effect of antibiotic treatment on cerebrospinal fluid. J Clin Pathol 80:386, 1983.

Bonadio WA, Mannenbach M, Krippendorf R: Bacterial meningitis in older children. Am J Dis Child 144:463, 1990.

Fijen CA, Hannema AJ, Kuiper E, et al: Complement deficiencies in patients over ten years old with meningococcal disease due to uncommon serogroups. Lancet 2:585, 1989.

Hatch DL, Overturf GD: Delayed cerebrospinal fluid sterilization in infants with *Haemophilus influenzae* type b meningitis. J Infect Dis 160:711, 1989.

Havens PL, Wendelberger KJ, Hoffman GM, et al: Corticosteroids as adjunctive therapy in bacterial meningitis. Am J Dis Child 143:1051, 1989.

Infectious Diseases and Immunization Committee, Canadian Pediatric Society: Initial therapy for bacterial meningitis. Can Med Assoc J 142:305, 1990.

Kaplan SL: Recent advances in bacterial meningitis. Adv Pediatr Infect Dis 4:83, 1989.

Kim JH, van der Horst C, Mulrow CD, et al: *Staphylococcus aureus* meningitis: Review of 28 cases. Rev Infect Dis 2:698, 1989.

Klein JO, Feigin RD, McCracken GH: Report of the task force on diagnosis and management of meningitis. Pediatrics (Suppl) 78:956, 1986.

Kline MW: Review of recurrent bacterial meningitis. Pediatr Infect Dis J 8:630–634, 1989.

Mayefsky JH, Roghmann KJ: Determination of leukocytosis in traumatic spinal tap specimens. Am J Med 82:1175, 1987.

McCracken GH, Lebel MH: Dexamethasone therapy for bacterial meningitis in infants and children. Am J Dis Child 143:287, 1989.

McGravey AR: A dilated unreactive pupil in acute bacterial meningitis: Oculomotor nerve inflammation versus herniation. Pediatr Emerg Care 5:187, 1989.

Mustafa MM, Ramilo O, Saez-Llorens X, et al: Cerebrospinal fluid prostaglandins, interleukin 1β, and tumor necrosis factor in bacterial meningitis. AJDC 144:883, 1990.

Nelson JD: Management problems in bacterial meningitis. Pediatr Infect Dis 4:S41, 1985.

Peltola H, Anttila M, Renkonen OV, et al: Randomized comparison of chloramphenicol, ampicillin, cefotaxime, and ceftriaxone for childhood bacterial meningitis. Lancet 1:1281, 1989.

Radetsky M: Duration of treatment in bacterial meningitis: A historical inquiry. Pediatr Infect Dis J 9:2, 1990.

Rodriguez WJ, Khan WN, Cocchetto DM, et al: Treatment of *Pseudomonas* meningitis with ceftazidime with or without concurrent therapy. Pediatr Infect Dis J 9:83, 1990.

Saez-Llorens X, Ramilo O, Mustafa M, et al: Molecular pathophysiology of bacterial meningitis: Current concepts and therapeutic implications. J Pediatr 116:671, 1990.

Sande MA, Tauber MG, Scheld WM, et al: Report of a second workshop: Pathophysiology of bacterial meningitis. Pediatr Infect Dis J 8:901, 1989.

Schaad UB, Suter S, Gianella-Borradori A, et al: A comparison of ceftriaxone and cefuroxime for the treatment of bacterial meningitis in children. N Engl J Med 322:141, 1990.

Schaad UB, Nelson JD, McCracken GH: Recrudescence and relapse in bacterial meningitis of childhood. Pediatrics 67:188, 1981.

Spanos A, Harrell FE, Durack DT: Differential diagnosis of acute meningitis: An analysis of the predictive value of initial observations. JAMA 262:2700, 1989.

Steele RW: Cephalosporins for bacterial meningitis: Which one is best? J Pediatr 114:991, 1989.

Steele RW, McConnell JR, Jacobs RF, et al: Recurrent bacterial meningitis: Coronal thin-section cranial computed tomography to delineate anatomic defects. Pediatrics 76:950, 1985.

Syrogiannopoulos GA, Nelson JD, McCracken GH: Subdural collections of fluid in acute bacterial meningitis: A review of 136 cases. Pediatr Infect Dis 5:343, 1986.

Swartz M: Chronic meningitis—many causes to consider. N Engl J Med 317:957, 1987.

Talan DA, Guterman JJ, Overturf GD, et al: Analysis of emergency department management of suspected bacterial meningitis. Ann Emerg Med 18:856, 1989.

Talan DA, Hoffman JR, Yoshikawa TT, et al: Role of empiric parenteral antibiotics prior to lumbar puncture in suspected bacterial meningitis: State of the art. Rev Infect Dis 10:365, 1988.

Tunkel AR, Wispelwey B, Scheld WM: Bacterial meningitis: Recent advances in pathophysiology and treatment. Ann Intern Med 112:610, 1990.

Tzou-Yien L, Nelson JD, McCracken GH: Fever during treatment for bacterial meningitis. Pediatr Infect Dis 3:319, 1984.
Word BM, Klein JO: Therapy of bacterial sepsis and meningitis in infants and children: 1989 poll of directors of programs in pediatric infectious diseases. Pediatr Infect Dis J 8:635, 1989.

OSTEOMYELITIS AND SEPTIC ARTHRITIS

Bacterial infections of bones (osteomyelitis) and of joints (septic arthritis) should be suspected in infants or children who manifest fever, unexplained limp, abnormal posture or gait, or musculoskeletal pain, especially in the presence of local bone or joint tenderness, swelling, erythema, and complete (pseudoparalysis) or partial limitation of motion.

12.16 OSTEOMYELITIS

Osteomyelitis, with or without an underlying septic arthritis, may occur at any age but is diagnosed most often in children less than 1 yr and between 3 and 10 yr of age. It is 2–4 times more frequent in boys than in girls and is often preceded by a history of trauma to the involved extremity. Trauma may produce local bone injury, predisposing the site to infection. *Acute hematogenous osteomyelitis* resembles a bacteremic illness, characterized by fever, rapid development of localized bone symptoms, and a duration of less than 1 wk. *Subacute osteomyelitis* has an insidious onset over a longer period of time (1–4 wk), fewer systemic manifestations, and more pronounced local bone signs. *Chronic osteomyelitis* (lasting > 1–2 mo) may be due to infection that has spread from a contiguous focus or open fracture or to incomplete resolution of an acute or subacute osteomyelitis.

ETIOLOGY. *S. aureus* is the most common organism responsible for osteomyelitis in normal hosts (Table 12–18). The relative contribution of *S. aureus* may be modified by age (in neonates, group B streptococci or *E. coli;* in infants, *S. pneumoniae* or *H. influenzae* type b), prior medical problems, or contiguous sites of infection (see Table 12–18). *M. tuberculosis* and fungi (*Cryptococcus, Candida, Blastomyces,* sporotrichosis) are less common agents producing bone infections.

Salmonella is frequently the agent that produces osteomyelitis in patients with sickle cell anemia. This predisposition may be due to reticuloendothelial cell dysfunction and the propensity of *Salmonella* to localize in areas of necrotic tissue following a vaso-occlusive crisis. Anaerobic osteomyelitis complicates infections following human bites, decubitus ulcers, and osteomyelitis associated with cranial-facial mucosal diseases (sinusitis, mastoiditis). *Brucellosis* may produce spondylitis, and *E. coli* urinary tract infection may produce contiguous vertebral osteomyelitis and epidural abscess. *P. aeruginosa* is associated with osteomyelitis in intravenous drug users and in children wearing sneakers who suffer puncture wounds of the foot.

PATHOGENESIS AND PATHOLOGY. Hematogenous osteomyelitis usually follows a bacteremia from an unidentified site of colonization or inapparent infection (nasopharynx); less often, there may be a predisposing infection in noncontiguous soft tissue (cellulitis, abscess, furunculitis) or the respiratory tract (otitis media, pneumonia) or genitourinary tract (pyelonephritis). Hematogenous osteomyelitis begins as a metaphyseal abscess in tubular bones. The nutrient artery to the metaphysis has a high oxygen content, undergoes a 180-degree turn proximal to the growth plate, and forms a potentially stagnant sinusoidal network (Figs. 12–2 and 12–3). The afferent segment of the capillary loop lacks phagocytic lining cells, whereas the efferent loop has functionally inactive reticuloendothelial cells. The combination of stasis and reduced phagocytosis predisposes the metaphyseal area to abscess formation.

The growth plate limits spread of a metaphyseal abscess to the epiphysis and joint space in older children (see Fig. 12–3). Because of transphyseal bridging vessels in the neonate and infant, infection may more readily spread directly to the joint space. This increases the likelihood of septic arthritis and growth plate injury with arrested growth from osteomyelitis in young age groups (see Fig. 12–2). As the metaphyseal abscess enlarges, the inflammatory response produces local pressure, resulting in dissection of the infection. If the pressure reduces local arterial blood flow, distal avascular bone necrosis may occur, producing segments of dead bone (sequestrum). Lateral dissection of the metaphyseal abscess produces destruction of cortical bone with subsequent rupture through the periosteum and subperiosteal and soft tissue abscess formation. If the joint capsule inserts proximally along the metaphysis, rupture of the subperiosteal abscess into the joint space produces septic arthritis (see Fig. 12–3). Pyoarthritis due to this mechanism is common in the hip, shoulder, and elbow. Dissection of infection up the marrow cavity to the diaphysis produces reactive new bone formation and marked subperiosteal calcification *(involucrum)* along the shaft, as a response to confine the infection. Hematogenous osteomyelitis may enter a chronic phase if the abscess is confined to the metaphyseal (occasionally diaphyseal) region by an inflammatory process that walls off the infection. Production of a **Brodie abscess** in this chronic infection, usually due to *S. aureus,* is manifested by local tenderness overlying a lytic lesion with a sclerotic reaction surrounding the abscess.

Chronic osteomyelitis is often due to spread of bacteria from a contiguous infected site and from direct inoculation of organisms due to human or animal bites, puncture wounds (metal nails), or compound fractures. Chronic osteomyelitis underlying decubitus ulcers is due to direct inoculation of mixed bacteria with reduced local circulation. The organisms responsible for chronic facial or cranial osteomyelitis reflect the microbiologic flora of the adjacent infected mucosal surfaces (sinus, gingiva, mastoid).

CLINICAL MANIFESTATIONS. These vary with age and the presentation of the illness (acute, subacute, or chronic). Osteomyelitis in the neonate or infant may be an acute febrile illness resembling sepsis. Alternatively, there may be little evidence of systemic toxicity; pseudoparalysis may be the only manifestation of osteomyelitis in an infant. Multiple bones or sites within a single bone are often affected in neonates, whereas associated septic arthritis may be present in both neonates and infants (see Table 12–18).

Osteomyelitis in older children may present as an abrupt febrile illness with localizing manifestations in the long bones. Alternatively, a subacute process will have few systemic signs (30% of patients may be afebrile), and only local bone and soft tissue signs may be evident. The manifestations of acute or subacute osteomyelitis of long bones include limp, localized bone pain, and guarding of the area. When the infection is confined to the metaphyseal abscess stage there will be localized point tenderness; however, following dissection and marked periosteal abscess or involucrum formation the tenderness will be more diffuse. Passive range of motion around the contiguous joint should be minimally affected in the absence of pyoarthritis or significant abscess formation. Nonetheless, motion is voluntarily limited owing to local periosteal pain. The extremity will be warm, erythematous, and swollen in direct relation to periosteal and deep tissue abscess dissection. Osteomyelitis of the pelvis or vertebra may be indolent and may present as abdominal pain, gait disturbances, back pain, or pain referred to the thigh. Chronic osteomyelitis often presents as an indolent illness with localized pain and swelling or, if due to traumatic inoculation of bone, with a

TABLE 12–18. Epidemiology and Clinical Manifestations of Osteomyelitis

Category	Affected Sites	Symptoms and Signs	Expected Organism
Acute Hematogenous Osteomyelitis			
Neonate (0–2 mo)	Femur, humerus; multiple sites may be affected in 20–40%. Associated septic arthritis	Septic-like appearance or pseudoparalysis ± fever	Group B streptococci, *Staphylococcus aureus, Escherichia coli*
Infant (2–24 mo)	Single long bone metaphysis; femur affected most commonly, followed by tibia, humerus, fibula, radius, phalanx, in that order. May involve joint space	Fever, limp, pain, tenderness, pseudoparalysis	*S. aureus* (most common), *Streptococcus pneumoniae, Haemophilus influenzae* type b, group B streptococci
Child (2–20 yr)	Metaphysis of long bones as for infant, rarely vertebrae or pelvis	Focal pain with fever for 1–5 days, focal tenderness, swelling, rarely joint effusion	*S. aureus* (most common), streptococci, *E. coli, Salmonella,* anaerobes, rarely fungi
Intravenous drug abuse	Femur, pubis, vertebra, sternum. May be acute or chronic	Indolent, local pain, may be afebrile, swelling	*Pseudomonas aeruginosa,* methicillin-resistant *S. aureus,* streptococci, *Candida,* anaerobes
Sickle cell anemia	Diaphysis rather than metaphysis, long bones, vertebra, clavicle, calvarium, small bones of hand	Difficult to distinguish from bone vaso-occlusive crises, which are very common	*Salmonella, S. aureus,* gram-negative bacilli, *S. pneumoniae*
Chronic granulomatous disease	Metaphyseal, chronic; possibly contiguous. Possibly associated or independent septic arthritis	Indolent, local pain, limp, soft tissue swelling	*S. aureus, Aspergillus, Serratia*
Contiguous Osteomyelitis			
Fetal scalp monitoring	Scalp; acute	Open wound, drainage, swelling, may have associated meningitis	*S. aureus, S. epidermidis,* group B streptococcus, gram-negative bacilli
Neonatal heel punctures	Calcaneous; chronic	Open wound, cellulitis, drainage, tenderness, swelling	*S. aureus, S. epidermidis,* gram-negative bacilli
Decubitus ulcer	Sacrum, bony prominences; chronic	Tend to occur in patients with paraplegia (spinal cord injury, spina bifida); delayed healing of pressure sores, recurrent drainage. ESR >100, WBC >15,000	Mixed organisms, *S. aureus,* anaerobes, gram-negative bacilli, streptococci
Animal-human bites: paronychia	Hand (fist-fighting), other sites; acute	Open wound, drainage, erythema, cellulitis	*Eikenella corrodens, S. aureus,* streptococci, anaerobes, *Pasteurella multocida* (animals)
Nail puncture through sneaker	In order of frequency—calcaneous, metatarsals, cuboid, navicular, cuneiforms; acute or chronic	Open wound, cellulitis, focal tenderness, swelling, limp	*P. aeruginosa* >>> *S. aureus*
Facial-cranial injury	Bone in area contiguous to infected mucosal surface (mastoiditis, sinusitis, periodontal abscess); chronic	Pain, swelling, tenderness. Pott's puffy tumor of frontal sinus associated	*Bacteroides fragilis, B. melaninogenicus,* anaerobic cocci
Open (compound) fracture (trauma): sternotomy	Long bone (trauma); chronic	Pain, draining sinus tract, wounds fail to heal, fever in 30%	*P. aeruginosa, S. aureus, S. epidermidis* mixed organisms. Sternotomy also may be associated with atypical mycobacteria, *Mycoplasma hominis*

chronic draining sinus and local cellulitis. Acute or chronic osteomyelitis, osteochondritis, or septic arthritis of the foot develops in 5–15% of children who sustain a nail puncture wound through sneakers and is usually due to *P. aeruginosa.* These patients may have local pain, cellulitis, and a draining sinus tract (see Table 12–18).

DIAGNOSIS. The suspected diagnosis and etiologic agent of osteomyelitis should be based on the age of the patient, predisposing chronic disease state, contiguous sites of infection, and the mode of presentation (acute or chronic, see Table 12–18). Physical examination may reveal focal tenderness (metaphyseal abscess stage) or diffuse tenderness (marked periosteal reaction), soft tissue swelling, erythema, limited motion, and, if arthritis is present, a swollen joint. Laboratory studies reveal an elevated white blood cell count with a shift to the left in 70% of patients and an elevated erythrocyte sedimentation rate (ESR) and C-reactive protein in more than 90% of patients.

Blood cultures are positive in 50–60% of children with acute or subacute osteomyelitis. If long bone osteomyelitis is suspected, needle aspiration of the periosteal space is indicated to drain the periosteal abscess and obtain a sample for culture. If no exudate is aspirated, the needle is advanced into the bone to aspirate the metaphyseal abscess. Periosteal cultures reveal a pathogen in 50–60% of cases and bone aspiration is positive in 60–70%. If associated septic arthritis is present, arthrocentesis will reveal the pathogen in 70–85% of cases (Sec. 12.17). Cultures of sinus tracts, wounds, and decubitus

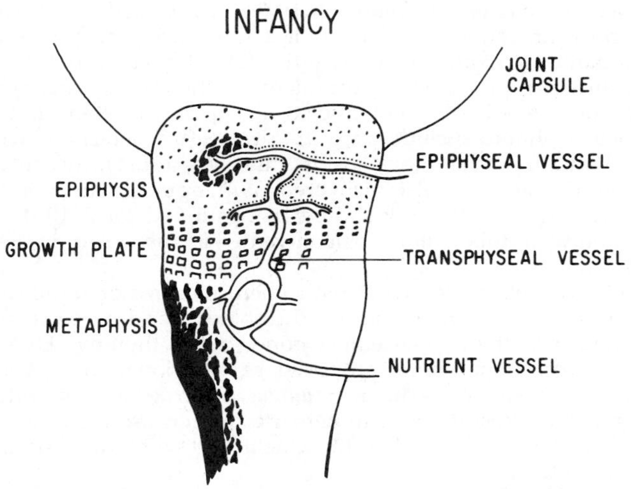

Figure 12–2. Major structures of the bone of an infant prior to maturation of the epiphyseal growth plate. Note the transphyseal vessel, which connects the vascular supply of the epiphysis and metaphysis, facilitating spread of infection between these two areas. (From Gutman LT: Acute, subacute, and chronic osteomyelitis and pyogenic arthritis in children. Curr Probl Pediatr 15[12]:1, 1985, p 6.)

ulcers do not reliably predict the responsible pathogen. Needle biopsy of the bone is therefore indicated in children with chronic draining osteomyelitis. Anaerobic cultures should be obtained in all cases of chronic draining osteomyelitis and in those associated with craniofacial infection. A tuberculosis skin test (PPD) should be placed and a chest roentgenogram obtained if tuberculosis is suspected.

Roentgenograms of the involved site are usually negative for 10–14 days in patients with acute osteomyelitis. Early roentgenographic signs include deep soft tissue swelling and loss of tissue planes, followed by periosteal elevation and later by radiolucent metaphyseal lesions of necrotic bone. *Salmonella* may also produce diaphyseal injury. Lytic lesions occur after more than 50% of the bone has been eroded by the infectious process.

Triple-phase technetium-99m diphosphate bone scans show increased uptake within 24–48 hr of infection and may remain positive despite clinical cure for many weeks owing to persistent bone remodeling and turnover. The first phase of a technetium bone scan is performed in 3- to 4-sec intervals during the 1st min and signifies blood flow. The second (blood pool) phase is performed within 5–10 min, and the third (static) phase is performed after a delay of 2–4 hr. A positive 3-phase scan suggests acute, chronic, or recurrent osteomyelitis, whereas positive blood flow and blood pool stages suggest soft tissue cellulitis. A positive static phase suggests the possibility of chronic osteomyelitis or, more likely, a noninfectious process. Technetium scanning has a lower sensitivity in neonatal osteomyelitis but is helpful in the diagnosis of discitis (see next paragraph on differential diagnosis). Computed tomography or gallium citrate (^{67}Ga) scanning may be useful in the evaluation of suspected pelvic osteomyelitis, whereas magnetic resonance imaging may reveal a secondary epidural spinal abscess associated with a vertebral osteomyelitis. Subacute or chronic hematogenous osteomyelitis (Brodie abscess) appears as a single lytic lesion with sclerotic margins on plain roentgenograms and shows positive uptake on bone scans.

DIFFERENTIAL DIAGNOSIS. Diseases that may mimic osteomyelitis include infections (cellulitis, pyomyositis, septic arthritis), trauma (sprains, fractures, child abuse), malignancy (leukemia, lymphoma, osteogenic and Ewing sarcomas, neuroblastoma), and sickle cell crisis. The latter differentiation is difficult; however, vaso-occlusive crisis is more common and is associated with diffuse generalized multifocal pain and fever (sometimes), but usually not with leukocytosis, an elevated ESR, or positive blood culture. Another noninfectious cause of bone necrosis includes Gaucher disease, which is associated with fever, bone pain, and an elevated ESR (Sec. 8.18).

Chronic multifocal osteomyelitis is a self-limited, recurrent, noninfectious illness of children characterized by remissions and exacerbations, metaphyseal involvement of multiple different bones with each episode (tibia, clavicle, fibula, spine, femur, and radius, in that order), a high ESR, normal white blood cell count, normal temperature or low-grade fever, and local pain. Associated conditions include pustulous palmoplantaris, Sweet syndrome (neutrophilic dermatosis), and vertebra plana or vertebral sclerosis. Roentgenograms reveal lytic lesions (2–18 sites) with sclerotic margins; the bone scan demonstrates multiple areas of uptake. Cultures of blood, bone, and bone marrow are negative for bacteria, fungi, or viruses; the histology reveals acute and chronic inflammation within granulation tissue. The differential diagnosis of chronic multifocal osteomyelitis includes eosinophilia granuloma, leukemia, neuroblastoma, rhabdomyosarcoma, and tuberculosis. The diagnosis is one of exclusion but requires a bone biopsy and culture. The prognosis is excellent because exacerbations respond to nonsteroidal anti-inflammatory agents. Pathologic fractures and, rarely, bone deformity may complicate chronic multifocal osteomyelitis.

Discitis should be considered in the differential diagnosis of vertebral osteomyelitis (see Sec. 24.21). Its manifestations include infectious and noninfectious inflammation of the intervertebral disk space (usually L3–L5), mild fever, irritability, back pain, limited back motion, limp, refusal to walk, abnormal back posture (excessive lordosis), high ESR, narrow disk space, and positive technetium (^{99m}Tc) or ^{67}Ga bone scans. It usually occurs in children less than 5 yr of age; discitis is unusual after this time because the disk space blood supply atrophies with age. Symptoms usually precede the diagnosis for about 10 wk. Bacteremia may be present and is often due to *S. aureus,* although gram-negative bacilli or streptococci may also be implicated; alternatively, the disk space inflam-

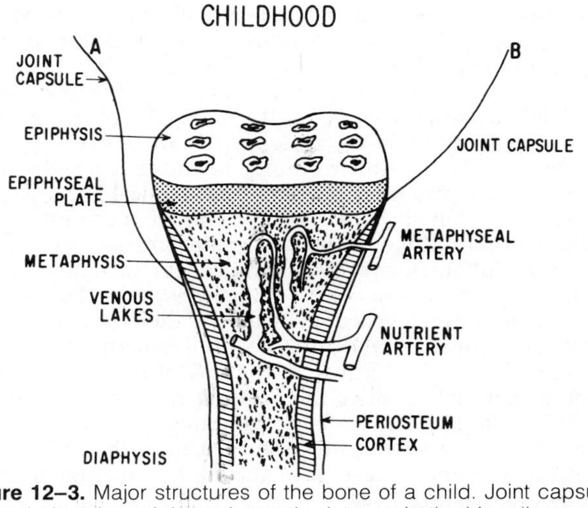

Figure 12–3. Major structures of the bone of a child. Joint capsule *A* inserts below the epiphyseal growth plate, as in the hip, elbow, ankle, and shoulder. Rupture of a metaphyseal abscess in these bones is likely to produce pyarthrosis. Joint capsule *B* inserts at the epiphyseal growth plate, as in other tubular bones. Rupture of a metaphyseal abscess in these bones is likely to lead to a subperiosteal abscess but seldom to an associated pyarthrosis. (From Gutman LT: Acute, subacute, and chronic osteomyelitis in children. Curr Probl Pediatr 15[12]:1, 1985, p 7.)

mation may be noninfectious. A PPD should be placed to test for tuberculosis. Needle biopsy is usually not needed, especially in the presence of a positive bone scan and normal neurologic examination. Discitis is usually a self-limited disease with a benign clinical course. In the presence of a positive blood culture or bone scan, discitis should be managed with bed rest and intravenous, followed by oral, antistaphylococcal antibiotics for 3–5 wk. Children who do not respond to such therapy require disk space aspiration and biopsy to identify the pathogen or noninfectious etiology of disk space necrosis. The prognosis of discitis is good, and the development of contiguous vertebral osteomyelitis or spinal fusion is unusual.

TREATMENT. Therapy varies depending on the age-specific pathogen, the acute or chronic nature of the process, the presence of dead bone, the existence of any prior chronic illness (sickle cell anemia, chronic granulomatous disease), and associated joint, sinus, or mastoid infections. Initial choice of antibiotic should be based on the most likely pathogens, and the drug should be given by the intravenous route to achieve high serum concentrations. The clinical importance of antimicrobial bone penetration and drug levels in bone has not been established. In the neonate, initial intravenous antibiotics should include an antistaphylococcal agent (nafcillin, methicillin, or oxacillin 150–200 mg/kg/24 hr, every 4–6 hr) and an aminoglycoside (gentamicin 6 mg/kg/24 hr, every 8 hr) to provide broad-spectrum bactericidal coverage. Initial therapy of the previously healthy infant needs to include coverage for *H. influenzae* type b (ceftriaxone 100 mg/kg/24 hr, given every day or every 12 hr; cefuroxime 150 mg/kg/24 hr, every 6 hr; or chloramphenicol 100 mg/kg/24 hr, every 4–6 hr; and an antistaphylococcal penicillin), especially if septic arthritis is present. Vancomycin may be substituted if methicillin-resistant *S. aureus* is suspected. Once a pathogen has been identified, antibiotic therapy should be more specific and based on the pathogen's antimicrobial sensitivities; the least toxic bactericidal antibiotic should be used. Total duration of therapy varies between 4 and 6 wk in patients with uncomplicated acute or subacute hematogenous osteomyelitis. Serum antibiotic mean bactericidal levels (MBC) against the isolated agent should be monitored during intravenous therapy, and serum trough levels of at least 1:2 in acute and at least 1:4 in chronic osteomyelitis should be achieved. Trough rather than peak levels correlate best with cure of osteomyelitis. Successful intravenous therapy, as determined by a reduction in pain, fever, swelling, ESR, and white blood cell counts should be continued for 7–14 days. Large doses of oral antibiotics (dicloxacillin 75–100 mg/kg/24 hr, given every 6 hr, or clindamycin 30–60 mg/kg/24 hr, given every 6–8 hr), sufficient to achieve MBCs similar to those reached during intravenous therapy, may be given after clinical improvement following the initial 7–14 days of intravenous antibiotics. Additional oral antibiotics include penicillin, amoxicillin, trimethoprim-sulfamethoxazole, ciprofloxacin (in adolescents), and the oral cephalosporins. Probenecid may be used to augment the serum levels of penicillins if their gastrointestinal side effects limit the oral dose. Oral antibiotic therapy should be monitored closely because of the risk of poor compliance. It should be initiated only if the patient's pathogen is available for MBC testing and there is no vomiting or diarrhea. Antimicrobial therapy should be continued until the ESR is normal, signs of active disease have abated, and roentgenograms demonstrate healing.

Surgery is indicated for osteomyelitis that does not improve with appropriate bactericidal antibiotic therapy and for that associated with septic arthritis of the hip (incision and drainage), for removal of dead necrotic bone (sequestrectomy), for curettage of a Brodie abscess, and for irrigation with debridement of chronic osteomyelitis associated with decubitus ulcers, foot punctures, and bites. Antibiotic therapy of chronic or contiguous osteomyelitis should be continued for at least 2 mo (intravenous 1–2 mo, oral 2 mo) and should include clindamycin if anaerobic bacteria are suspected, noted on Gram stain, or cultured. Antimicrobial therapy of osteomyelitis of bones in the foot due to a nail puncture through a sneaker should include an anti-*Pseudomonas* penicillin, with or without an aminoglycoside, and an antistaphylococcal agent if *S. aureus* is also recovered. With appropriate debridement, antibiotic therapy should be continued for 7–10 days. Therapy of tuberculous osteomyelitis is discussed in Sec. 12.47.

Osteomyelitis associated with open fractures or significant bone defects requires combined antibiotic and surgical (debridement, drains, cancellous bone grafts) therapy. Hyperbaric oxygen has been proposed as additional therapy for chronic osteomyelitis due to *S. aureus, P. aeruginosa,* and other organisms. Results with hyperbaric oxygen are inconsistent and may be no better than those achieved with antibiotic and surgical therapy.

PROGNOSIS. Complications of acute or subacute osteomyelitis include septic arthritis, permanent damage to the growth plate (in neonates and infants), recurrence if therapy is of less than 3 wk duration, dissection to nonosseous sites (epidural abscess), fracture through a weakened bone, and transient limb growth acceleration during healing. Young age and involvement of the hip with *S. aureus* are associated with a poor prognosis.

Chronic, poorly treated osteomyelitis is rare but may be associated with persistent or recurrent pain, limp, membranoproliferative glomerulonephritis (immune complex disease), amyloidosis, epidermoid carcinoma of the sinus tract, and antibiotic-associated side effects.

12.17 SEPTIC ARTHRITIS

Septic arthritis, a serious pyogenic infection of the joint space, is slightly more common than osteomyelitis. It occurs most often in children less than 3 yr old and in sexually active adolescent females. Septic arthritis is usually monoarticular, except in the neonate and adolescent. Infectious arthritis may be due to viral, fungal, or bacterial agents (Table 12–19), whereas septic (purulent, pyogenic, pyoarthritis) arthritis refers to infections due to bacterial pathogens, including *M. tuberculosis.* Postinfectious, reactive, and immune complex arthritides produce synovial inflammation in the absence of viable micro-organisms.

ETIOLOGY (see Table 12–19). The bacteriologic agent depends on the patient's age and the presence of alterations in host defense mechanisms such as sickle cell anemia, hypogammaglobulinemia, or chronic granulomatous disease. *S. aureus* is the most common agent found in neonatal septic arthritis and in patients more than 5 yr of age. Neonatal septic arthritis may also be due to group B streptococcus, *E. coli,* or *Candida albicans. H. influenzae* type b is the most common pathogen and *S. aureus* the second most frequent agent found in patients between 2 mo and 5 yr of age. *H. influenzae* septic arthritis is often complicated by concurrent meningitis (10–30%), osteomyelitis (5–10%), otitis media (10%), cellulitis (10–30%), and pneumonia (5%); *S. aureus* septic arthritis is often complicated by osteomyelitis (10–40%); and gonococcal arthritis is almost always associated with infection of the cervix, fallopian tubes, rectum, or pharynx. *N. gonorrhoeae* is the most frequent cause of polyarticular and monoarticular septic arthritis in sexually active adolescents.

Chronic septic arthritis in normal and immunocompromised patients may be due to *Brucella,* tuberculosis, atypical mycobacteria, *S. schenckii, C. immitis, B. dermatitides, C. albicans, P. boydii,* or *H. capsulatum.*

TABLE 12–19. Epidemiology of Infectious Arthritis

Agent	Frequency	Characteristics
Bacterial		
Staphylococcus aureus	Most common pathogen in patients <2 mo, >5 yr of age	Monoarticular; knee most commonly affected, followed by hip, ankle, elbow, in that order
Haemophilus influenzae type b	Most common pathogen in patients <5 yr and particularly <2 yr age, excluding neonates	Monoarticular; may also be reactive.
Streptococcus pneumoniae	Common in patients with sickle cell anemia and patients <2 yr of age	Monoarticular, hip affected more often than knee
Neisseria gonorrhoeae	Common in sexually active adolescent females	Monoarticular; follows a bacteremic phase with associated polyarthralgia, fever, chills, rash and tenosynovitis. Onset in 2nd–3rd trimester of pregnancy or during menstruation
Group B streptococcus	Common in neonates	Other neonatal pathogens include *S. aureus, Escherichia coli, Candida* sp.
Group A streptococcus (other streptococci)	Occurs in 10–20% of cases regardless of age	Monoarticular
Borrelia burgdorferi (Lyme arthritis)	Intermittent, migrating, polyarticular. Common in endemic areas. Chronic mono- or pauciarticular disease is uncommon	Knees: Baker cyst formation. Remote history of tick bite and erythema chronicum migrans
Brucella	Uncommon unless patient exposed to animal vector (cattle, swine, goats, sheep) including cheese, milk, carcass. 40% of children with brucellosis have arthritis	Peripheral (hip or knee) ± sacroilitis. 70% of cases are monoarticular and chronic
Pseudomonas aeruginosa	Common in intravenous drug-abusing adolescents	Other pathogens in intravenous drug-abusing population include methicillin-resistant *S. aureus, Serratia, Candida*. Joints include knee, sternoclavicular and sacroiliac joints, hip, or elbow
Mycobacterium tuberculosis	Uncommon	Chronic granulomatous monoarticular disease; knee affected most commonly followed by wrist, hip, and interphalangeal-metacarpal joints
***Reactive Bacterial* (sterile)**		
H. influenzae type b	—	Develops after 5 days of therapy; immune complexes involved
N. meningitidis	—	Develops after 5 days of therapy; immune complexes involved. May also produce septic monoarticular pyoarthritis in the absence of meningitis
Postenteric Reiter syndrome	—	Prior *Shigella, Yersinia, Campylobacter,* or *Salmonella* enteritis. Associated with HLA-B27. *Salmonella* rarely produces septic arthritis in normal patients (no more common in patients with sickle cell anemia)
Postvenereal Reiter syndrome	—	Prior nongonococcal urethritis, chlamydial disease, or sexually transmitted disease. Associated with HLA-B27
Viral		
Rubella	Common (15–30%) in postpubertal susceptible females	Polyarticular; interphalangeal-metacarpal joints affected most commonly, followed by knee, wrist, elbow
Mumps	Affects <1% of postpubertal males	Polyarticular; knees most commonly affected, asymmetric
Parvovirus B19	Common in adults (60% of patients are >20 yr old, 5% are <9 yr old). Rash may be absent	Symmetric peripheral polyarthropathy. Interphalangeal-metacarpal joints affected most commonly, then knees and wrists
Hepatitis B	Variable incidence—0–25%	Interphalangeal-metacarpal joints. Urticaria, angioedema, arthritis, circulating HBsAg immune complexes precede jaundice by days to weeks
Varicella-zoster	Uncommon	Must exclude staphylococcal cellulitis or arthritis. Monoarticular, affecting knee
Human immunodeficiency virus (AIDS)	1. AIDS-related arthritis, common 2. Reiter syndrome, common 3. Septic arthritis, uncommon	1. Etiology unknown 2. Associated with psoriatic arthritis. 3. Opportunistic agents, e.g., atypical mycobacteria, cryptococcus, histoplasmosis
Fungal		
Sporothrix schenckii	Uncommon	Chronic arthritis, knee affected most commonly, then wrist, then elbow. Occult pulmonary lesion is source, not direct inoculation
Pseudoallescheria boydii	Uncommon	Penetrating knee trauma
Blastomyces dermatitides	Uncommon	Associated with adjacent osteomyelitis
Candida albicans	Uncommon	Pathogen in neonates; affects knee, elbow, wrist
Coccidioides immitis	Uncommon	Knee involvement ± disseminated disease in other sites
Histoplasma capsulatum	Uncommon	Migratory polyarthritis, carpal tunnel syndrome, erythema nodosum
Aspergillosis	Uncommon except in chronic granulomatous disease	Other pathogens in chronic granulomatous disease include *S. aureus, Serratia*
Unknown		
Chronic aseptic arthritis in hypogammaglobulinemic patients	10–20% of cases occur in patients with Bruton agammaglobulinemia; 5–10% occur in patients with common variable immunodeficiency	Arthritis may be rheumatologic or due to *Mycoplasma pneumoniae, M. hominis, Ureaplasma urealyticum,* enterovirus. Aseptic arthritis responds to intravenous immunoglobulin therapy. Acute bacterial arthritis is due to *H. influenzae, S. aureus*

PATHOGENESIS. Septic arthritis may result from hematogenous dissemination of pathogens from an inconspicuous site of colonization or infection (nasopharynx) or during the bacteremic phase of meningitis, pneumonia, or cellulitis. Alternatively, it may be due to contiguous spread of an osteomyelitis through the epiphyseal bridging vessels present in neonates and young infants (see Fig. 12–2) or when the joint capsule insertion extends beyond the growth plate encompassing the metaphysis as occurs in the hip, shoulder, and elbow (see Fig. 12–3). Direct inoculation of pathogens by means of penetrating trauma is a rare cause of septic arthritis associated with *P. boydii* infection and the sterile but chronic pyogenic-appearing inflammation that may occur with thorn (foreign body) arthritis.

Hematogenous seeding of the highly vascular synovium initiates a marked inflammatory response. The combination of leukocyte-initiated cytokine mediators and bacterial toxins produces synovial inflammation and vascular permeability, eventually increasing fluid production and thus pressure within the joint capsule. Changes in the matrix of the superficial zone of the articular surface are noted within 24 hr of infection. More prolonged inflammation causes degeneration of chondrocytes and loosening of the articular matrix. Increased pressure in the hip joint may result in avascular necrosis of the capitular femoral epiphysis. Thrombosis of intra-articular vessels may also produce avascular necrosis.

CLINICAL MANIFESTATIONS. Septic arthritis in the neonate has a presentation similar to that of osteomyelitis. The newborn may manifest few systemic signs other than pseudoparalysis of the involved extremity. Pain when the diaper is changed is a common early manifestation of neonatal septic arthritis of the hip. Alternatively, neonatal septic arthritis may resemble a bacteremic illness with systemic manifestations (Sec. 12.16).

Septic arthritis in non-neonatal patients due to pathogens other than *N. gonorrhoeae* usually presents as a monoarticular infection (90–95%) with fever, irritability, pseudoparalysis or limited range of motion, and an antalgic gait or position of the joint. The joint is swollen, and effusion, erythema, tenderness, pain, and warmth are evident. Antalgic positioning of the hip joint reduces intracapsular pressure and hence pain; this includes abduction of the leg and flexion and external rotation of the hip. Pain from the hip may be referred to the knee, whereas pain from the pelvis or retroperitoneum is referred to the back, hip, or anterior thigh. The knee is the most commonly infected joint, followed by the hip, elbow, and ankle. Tuberculous arthritis is often chronic and involves the knee, wrist, hip, interphalangeal-metacarpal joints, spine, and ankle joints.

Viral arthritis is often polyarticular and usually involves the interphalangeal-metacarpal joints followed by the knee, wrist, ankle, and elbow (see Table 12–19). Carpal tunnel syndrome (paresthesias of the hand) results from infections due to viruses, atypical mycobacteria, *S. schenckii*, and histoplasmosis.

Gonococcal septic arthritis follows disseminated bacteremic infection and is manifested by chills, fever, migratory polyarthralgias and tenosynovitis, rash, and eventual development of a monoarticular infection of the knee, wrist, or ankle. Disseminated gonococcal infection (DGI) is more common in females (4:1) and often occurs during menstruation or the 2nd or 3rd trimester of pregnancy. Rat bite fever due to *Streptobacillus moniliformis* and Reiter syndrome may resemble DGI. Empiric therapy is often necessary to distinguish gonococcal from reactive (Reiter syndrome) arthritis. The former resolves rapidly with antibiotics, whereas continued joint symptoms and the development of new joint effusions occur in Reiter syndrome.

DIAGNOSIS. Initial laboratory studies reveal a high ESR, C-reactive protein, and peripheral total white blood cell and neutrophil counts. Roentgenograms reveal superficial and deep soft tissue swelling, swelling in the joint space, and loss of fat pads. If septic arthritis is present for longer than 10–14 days, roentgenograms may reveal osteoporosis, subluxation, and, if osteomyelitis is also present, periosteal elevation with characteristic lytic lesions. A bone scan will demonstrate increased bone uptake if osteomyelitis is present.

Arthrocentesis should be performed in every patient suspected of having septic arthritis. If possible, it is important to avoid traversing an overlying superficial cellulitis, since this may introduce organisms into a previously sterile uninvolved joint. Synovial fluid in patients with septic arthritis can be distinguished from that in other diseases that produce synovitis by the criteria shown in Table 12–20. However, patients with septic arthritis may have white blood cell counts in synovial fluid of less than 50,000. In nongonococcal infection the culture of the synovial fluid is positive in 70–80% of patients, whereas a blood culture is positive in 30–40%. Gram stain is positive in 50%; methylene blue staining may increase this yield. Because as many as 30% of patients may be partially treated owing to the use of oral antibiotics for nonspecific nonlocalizing symptoms prior to recognition of septic arthritis, serum and synovial antigen detection with counterimmunoelectrophoresis or latex agglutination methods are also useful.

It is difficult to recover *N. gonorrhoeae* from synovial fluid. Therefore, blood, cervix, rectum, and nasopharynx should be cultured to increase the chances of identifying this fastidious organism. Synovial biopsy and culture may be needed to differentiate chronic arthritis due to tuberculosis or fungi from sarcoidosis, foreign body reaction, or rheumatologic conditions.

DIFFERENTIAL DIAGNOSIS. Suppurative arthritis must be differentiated from deep cellulitis; viral, mycobacterial, fungal, and mycoplasmal arthritis; osteomyelitis; thorn or foreign body arthritis; trauma; septic bursitis (olecranon or prepatellar bursae); toxic synovitis; reactive arthritis; pyomyositis; rheumatic fever; juvenile rheumatoid arthritis; sarcoidosis; Lyme disease; inflammatory bowel disease; psoas or retroperitoneal abscess; systemic lupus erythematosus; serum sickness; leukemia; Henoch-Schönlein purpura; Kawasaki disease; and metabolic joint disease (gout, ochronosis, Farber disease). *Migratory or recurrent polyarthralgia* or arthritis may be noted in DGI, rheumatic fever, juvenile rheumatoid arthritis, Reiter syndrome, Lyme disease, and serum sickness. **Toxic synovitis** of the hip is common in children less than 5 yr of age following a viral upper respiratory tract infection. There is mild fever and few systemic manifestations other than a limp or irritability. The extremity has minimal limitation of range of motion, and the ESR and WBC counts are usually normal (see Sec. 24.10).

TREATMENT. The initial antibiotic therapy of septic arthritis is based on the Gram stain of the synovial fluid and consideration of age-specific pathogens. An antistaphylococcal penicillin (methicillin, oxacillin, or nafcillin 150–200 mg/kg/24 hr, given every 4–6 hr) should be administered intravenously (not intra-articularly) if *S. aureus* is suspected; ceftriaxone (100 mg/kg/24 hr, given every day or every 12 hr), cefuroxime (150 mg/kg/24 hr, given every 6 hr) or chloramphenicol (100 mg/kg/24 hr, given every 6 hr) plus an antistaphylococcal penicillin if *H. influenzae* type b is suspected; and ceftriaxone (1–2 g/24 hr, given every 12–24 hr) or cefoxitin (4–12 g/24 hr, every 6 hr) if *N. gonorrhoeae* is suspected. Gram-negative enteric septic arthritis is treated with an anti-*Pseudomonas* penicillin and an aminoglycoside, whereas fungal arthritis is treated with a combination of intravenous and intra-articular amphotericin B. In patients with septic arthritis due to *S. aureus*, antibiotic therapy should be continued for 4–6 wk. Septic arthritis due to *H. influenzae, S. pneumoniae,*

TABLE 12–20. Synovial Fluid Analyses in Various Joint Diseases

Condition	Appearance	Total White Blood Cell Count (/uL)	Polymorphonuclear Cells (%)	Mucin Clot	Synovial Fluid-to-Serum Glucose (mg/dL) Difference	Multiple Joints	Comments
Normal	Clear-straw colored, yellow	0–200 (200)*	<10	Good	None (<10)	—	—
Trauma	Xanthochromic, serosanguineous, sanguineous	50–4,000 (600)	<30	Good	None	No	Hemophilia or rupture of internal ligament, meniscus
Gout	Turbid	10,000–160,000 (20,000)	70	Poor	10–20	No	Synovial fluid urate, long needle-shaped crystals with negative birefringence on polarization microscope
Systemic lupus erythematosus	Clear to slightly turbid	0–9,000 (3,000)	<20	Good to fair	None	Yes	LE cell present: decreased synovial fluid complement
Rheumatoid arthritis	Turbid	250–50,000 (19,000)	50–70	Fair to poor	30	Yes	Decreased synovial fluid complement in 50%
Infectious							
Acute bacterial (septic, pyogenic, suppurative)	Very turbid, white-gray	10,000–250,000 (80,000)	90	Poor	50–90	No	Positive synovial Gram stain, culture. Positive blood culture. Prior antibiotic therapy may reduce identification of pathogen
Lyme arthritis	Turbid	500–100,000 (25,000)	>50	Poor	—	Yes	History of tick bite, erythema chronicum migrans
Tuberculosis	Turbid rice bodies†	2,500–100,000 (20,000)	60	Poor	40–70	No	Positive PPD test, plus synovial fluid culture and acid-fast stain. May require synovial biopsy
Viral	Clear, serosanguineous	5,000–10,000 (7,000)	<20	Good	None, occasionally 10–20	Yes	Small joints of hands most common sites
Postinfectious, Reactive, Sterile							
Rheumatic fever (streptococcal reactive arthritis)	Cloudy to turbid yellow	10,000–30,000 (20,000)	50	Good to fair	20–30	Yes	Positive serum group A streptococcal antibodies
Reactive arthritis (Reiter, postenteric, or postvenereal); Reiter syndrome includes, urethritis, uveitis, conjunctivitis, arthritis, rash	Cloudy to turbid; may be clear	1,000–150,000 (25,000)	65	Fair to poor	30–50	Yes	Postenteric (*Shigella, Salmonella, Campylobacter, Yersinia*), Postvenereal (*Chlamydia*). Bacterial antigen present in synovial fluid. Association with HLA-B27. Increased synovial fluid complement

*Averages in parenthesis.
†Particulate fibrinous deposits.
Synovial fluid protein content is elevated in many conditions and is nonspecific.

and group A streptococci should be treated for at least 14–21 days. Initial intravenous antimicrobial therapy may be changed to high-dose oral therapy with appropriate bactericidal antibiotics after the patient demonstrates signs of improvement (usually by day 10–14 of therapy), such as a reduction in temperature, ESR, CRP, WBC count, and size of the synovial swelling. Gonococcal arthritis should be treated for 7–10 days. If *N. gonorrhoeae* is sensitive to pencillin, oral amoxicillin (2 g/24 hr, given every 8 hr) may be initiated by day 3–5 of therapy. Doxycycline should be included to treat concurrent *Chlamydia trachomatis* genital infection. Therapy with oral antibiotics (clindamycin, dicloxacillin, amoxicillin) must be rigorously monitored as discussed in Sec. 12.16.

Despite an initial arthrocentesis, the synovial effusion may reaccumulate, necessitating repeated joint aspiration during the first 3–5 days of antibiotic therapy. Open surgical drainage is indicated for recurrent joint effusions lasting longer than 7 days, any septic arthritis of the hip at the time of presentation, and most infections involving the shoulder. Immediate open drainage of the hip joint is primarily indicated to reduce the intra-articular pressure, thus avoiding aseptic necrosis of the femoral head. Removal of necrotic bone and inflammatory mediators in this deep joint are additional benefits of open drainage of a septic hip joint. Surgery includes irrigation, drain replacement, drilling of the femoral metaphysis if osteomyelitis is suspected, and closure.

Septic arthritis treated with systemic antibiotics, rest in afunctional position, no weight bearing, and possibly immobilization usually improves within 72 hr of therapy. Thereafter, range of motion exercises may help reduce the risk of contracture.

PROGNOSIS. Poor prognostic features include young age (< 6 mo), *S. aureus*, gram-negative or fungal pathogens, hip infection, associated osteomyelitis and epiphyseal damage, and delayed therapy (delayed > 5–7 days after symptoms are apparent). Usually there is no morbidity, and few residual deficits occur if the infection is recognized early.

Barton LL, Dunkle LM, Habib FH: Septic arthritis in childhood. Am J Dis Child 141:898, 1987.

Black J, Hunt TL, Godley PJ, et al: Oral antimicrobial therapy for adults with osteomyelitis or septic arthritis. J Infect Dis 155:968, 1987.

Brook I: Anaerobic osteomyelitis in children. Pediatr Infect Dis 5:550, 1986.

Buskila D, Gladman D: Musculoskeletal manifestations of infection with human immunodeficiency virus. Rev Infect Dis 12:223, 1990.

Demopulos GA, Bleck EE, McDougall IR: Role of radionuclide imaging in the diagnosis of acute osteomyelitis. J Pediatr Orthop 8:558, 1988.

Dubey L, Krasinski K, Hernanz-Schulman M: Osteomyelitis secondary to trauma or infected contiguous soft tissue. Pediatr Infect Dis J 7:026, 1988.

Farley T, Conway J, Shulman ST: Hematogenous pelvic osteomyelitis in children. Am J Dis Child 139:946, 1985.

Fink CW, Nelson JD: Septic arthritis and osteomyelitis in children. Clin Rheumatol Dis 12:423, 1986.

Gutman LT: Acute, subacute, and chronic osteomyelitis and pyogenic arthritis in children. Curr Probl Pediatr 25:4, 1985.

Hamdan J, Asha M, Mallouh A, et al: Technetium bone scintigraphy in the diagnosis of osteomyelitis in children. Pediatr Infect Dis J 6:529, 1987.

Hansel TT, Haeney MR, Thompson RA: Primary hypogammaglobulinemia and arthritis. Br Med J 295:174, 1987.

Henley WL: Chronic recurrent multifocal osteomyelitis. J Pediatr Orthop 7:606, 1987.

Jacobs RF, McCarthy RE, Elser JM: *Pseudomonas* osteochondritis complicating puncture wounds of the foot in children: A 10-year evaluation. Infect Dis 160:657, 1989.

Kulhanjian J, Dunphy MG, Hamstra S, et al: Randomized comparative study of ampicillin/sulbactam vs. ceftriaxone for treatment of soft tissue skeletal infections in children. Pediatr Infect Dis J 8:605, 1989.

Kunnamo I, Kallio P, Pelkonen P, et al: Clinical signs and laboratory tests in the differential diagnosis of arthritis in children. Am J Dis Child 141:34, 1987.

Lewis VL, Bailey MH, Pulawski G, et al: The diagnosis of osteomyelitis in patients with pressure sores. Plast Reconstr Surg 81:229, 1988.

Rotbart HA, Glode MP: *Haemophilus influenzae* type b septic arthritis in children: Report of 23 cases. Pediatrics 75:254, 1985.

Syrogiannopoulos GA, Nelson JD: Duration of antimicrobial therapy for acute suppurative osteoarticular infections. Lancet 1:37, 1988.

Syrogiannopoulos GA, McCracken GH, Nelson JD: Osteoarticular infections in children with sickle cell disease. Pediatrics 78:1090, 1986.

Weinstein MP, Stratton CW, Hawley HB, et al: Multicenter collaborative evaluation of a standardized serum bactericidal test as a predictor of therapeutic efficacy in acute and chronic osteomyelitis. Am J Med 83:218, 1987.

Welkon CJ, Long SS, Fisher MC, et al: Pyogenic arthritis in infants and children: A review of 95 cases. Pediatr Infect Dis 5:669, 1986.

12.18 STREPTOCOCCAL INFECTIONS

Streptococci are among the most common causes of bacterial infection in infancy and childhood. Group A streptococci, the most common *bacterial* cause of acute pharyngitis, also produce a large variety of other infections and nonsuppurative sequelae such as rheumatic fever (Sec. 11.74) and glomerulonephritis (Sec. 18.5). Infection during the first 3 mo of life with group B β-hemolytic streptococci is common and may present as bacteremia, meningitis, osteomyelitis, or septic arthritis.

ETIOLOGY. Streptococci are gram-positive spherical cocci that grow in pairs or variable length chains, classified on the basis of their ability to hemolyze red blood cells: those with hemolysins producing complete hemolysis *(β-hemolytic)*, those producing partial hemolysis *(α-hemolytic)*, and those producing no hemolysis *(γ-hemolytic)*. α-Hemolysis produces a green color on sheep erythrocytes (viridans group).

Lancefield further separated the streptococci on the basis of differences in carbohydrate components (C-carbohydrate) within the cell wall; streptococcal groups A through H and K through V have been identified so far. The cell wall is composed of three distinct layers. The outer portion contains several antigenic proteins; the most important is M protein. Group A β-hemolytic streptococci can be divided into more than 80 immunologically distinct types that are based on differences in the M protein. M antigen resists phagocytosis and is the major virulence factor. Lipoteichoic acid, another cell wall constituent, is another virulence factor that promotes colonization by binding to fibronectin on the surface of epithelial cells. The hyaluronic acid capsule resists phagocytosis, further facilitating virulence. Acquired immunity is directed at the M protein. Group specificity is conferred by the cell wall carbohydrate composition; group A carbohydrate has rhamnose-*N*-acetylglycosamine, group D contains glycerol teichoic acid.

Streptococci elaborate toxins, enzymes, and hemolysins. More than 20 extracellular antigens released by group A hemolytic streptococci growing in human tissues have been identified. The extracellular products of greatest clinical significance are pyrogenic (formerly erythrogenic) toxins (A, B, and C), streptolysin O, streptolysin S, NADase, streptokinases (A and B), DNase (A, B, C, and D), hyaluronidase, proteinase, amylase, and esterase. Pyogenic toxins are responsible for the rash of scarlet fever. Generally, the elaboration of pyogenic toxin depends on bacteriophage infection (lysogeny) of the streptococcus. Streptolysin S is largely cell bound and damages the membranes of neutrophils and platelets. Streptolysin O is produced by most group A and some group G streptococci. It lyses red blood cells and is toxic to neutrophils, platelets, and mammalian heart muscle. Elaboration of streptolysins S and O produces the clear zone of hemolysis permitting classification of the organisms as β-hemolytic strains. Extracellular digestive enzymes liquify pus and, together with hyaluronidase, facilitate rapid spreading of streptococci through tissue planes. Antibodies to streptolysin O (ASO), DNase B, hyaluronidase, NADase, and streptokinase are useful in the serodiagnosis of group A streptococcal disease. M-type specific antibodies are detectable 4–8 wk after infection; antibiotic therapy oblates this response.

Separation by type of hemolysis and Lancefield typing as methods of classifying streptococci are not mutually exclusive. Table 12–21 shows classifications by both methods and outlines the relationship of streptococci to human colonization and disease.

Group A Streptococci

Sequelae of group A β-hemolytic streptococcal disease (rheumatic fever, glomerulonephritis) are discussed in Sec. 11.74 and 18.5.

EPIDEMIOLOGY. The incidence of suppurative and nonsuppurative sequelae from group A streptococci increased in the late 1980s and 1990s. The reasons for this resurgence of serious streptococcal disease are unknown. Group A streptococci are normal inhabitants of the nasopharynx; colonization rates in children vary from 15–20%. The incidence of disease depends on the age of the child, the season of the year, climate and geographic location, and the degree of contact with infected individuals.

Generally, incidence is lowest in the infant, who may be protected by transplacental acquisition of type-specific antibodies. Streptococcal infection of the skin is most common in children under 6 yr; streptococcal pharyngitis is most common between 5 and 15 yr. Streptococcal disease, including scarlet fever, is uncommon in children less than 3 yr of age, but in families with known streptococcal infection, it may present as nonspecific upper respiratory tract infection, pharyngitis, and otitis media, with or without impetigo. The incidence of

TABLE 12–21. Relationship of Streptococci Identified by Lancefield Grouping and Hemolytic Reactions to Sites of Colonization and Disease

Lancefield Antigen Group	Species	Hemolysis on Sheep Blood Agar*	Site of Colonization	Common Human Diseases
A	*Staphylococcus pyogenes* *Streptococcus anginosus* (*S. milleri*) group A†‡	β β	Pharynx, skin, rectum	Pharyngitis, tonsillitis, erysipelas, impetigo, septicemia, wound infections, necrotizing fasciitis, cellulitis, otitis media, meningitis, pneumonia, conjunctivitis, acute endocarditis, scarlet fever, toxic shock, rheumatic fever, acute glomerulonephritis
B	*S. agalactiae*	β	Pharynx, vagina	Puerperal sepsis, chorioamnionitis, endocarditis. Neonatal sepsis, meningitis, otitis media, osteomyelitis, pneumonia
C	*S. equi* *equisimilis* *dysgalactiae* *zooepidemicus* *anginosus* (*S. milleri*) group C†‡	β β α β β	Pharynx, vagina, skin, umbilicus	Wound infections, puerperal sepsis, cellulitis, food-borne pharyngitis, endocarditis, nosocomial infections, opportunistic infections
D	*S. faecalis*§ *faecium*§ *bovis*§ *equinus*	γ	Colon contents	Endocarditis, urinary tract infections, biliary tract infections, intestinal infections, peritonitis, superinfection bacteremia
E	*S. infrequens*	?	?	?
F	*S. minutus* *anginosus* (*S. milleri*) group F†‡	β	Mouth, pharynx	Sinusitis, meningitis, brain abscess, pneumonia
G	*S. cariis* *anginosus* (*S. milleri*) group G†‡	β	Pharynx, vagina, skin	Puerperal infection, skin or wound infection, endocarditis
H	*S. sanguis*‡	α	Mouth	Endocarditis, brain abscess
K	*S. salivarius*‡	α	Mouth	Endocarditis, sinusitis, meningitis, brain abscess
L	—	β or α	Mouth	Endocarditis, abscess, parotitis, neonatal sepsis
M	—	β or α	Mouth, pharynx, vagina	Endocarditis, septicemia
N	*S. lactis cremoris*	α or γ	Pharynx	?Meningitis, ?septicemia
O	—	α or β	Pharynx, conjunctiva, vagina	Pneumonia, endocarditis, septicemia
Nontypable	*S. viridans*	α	Pharynx	Endocarditis
Nontypable	*S. mutans*	α	Pharynx	Endocarditis

*α = partial hemolysis; β = complete hemolysis; γ = no hemolysis.

†*S. anginosus–milleri* group are minute β-hemolytic streptococci in contrast to true (large colony) organisms. They demonstrate α, β, or no hemolysis, are microaerophilic or anaerobic and are also called *S. intermedius* group. This group produces serious abscesses (dental, liver, brain, appendiceal, or postsurgical) and endocarditis.

‡These organisms are frequently isolated from the bloodstream as α-hemolytic streptococci. Along with many nongroupable α streptococci, they are often called *S. viridans*, a term that incorrectly implies a specific species. Nevertheless, as a group, they cause the majority of episodes of endocarditis and are usually, but not invariably, exquisitely sensitive to penicillin.

§Enterococcus.

streptococcal pharyngitis is higher in temperate climates; incidence and severity appear to increase in cold weather. Streptococcal skin disease is more prevalent in tropical climates and in warmer weather in temperate climates.

Group A β-hemolytic streptococci are spread from person to person or occasionally from animals to people. Infection may be spread by droplets; nasal and pharyngeal carriers are effective disseminators. Infection also may be spread by contact with skin lesions or transmitted by food, milk, and water.

Acquisition of streptococci generally is associated with crowding in the home, school, military installation, or other institution. Disruption of the cutaneous epithelium predisposes to streptococcal pyoderma or impetigo. Acquisition from an infected individual is most common during the acute illness (3–5 days) and decreases during the colonization stage.

Colonization (nasopharyngeal) may precede or follow (2–6 wk) overt infection. Immunity, which is type-specific, may be induced either by carriage of the organism or by overt infection. The risk of streptococcal disease diminshes during adult life as immunity develops to the more prevalent serotypes.

PATHOGENESIS. Following inhalation or ingestion, streptococci attach themselves to respiratory epithelial cells by their surface fibrils and cell wall lipoteichoic acid. Fibrils contain antiphagocytic epitopes of type-specific M proteins, which, together with capsular hyaluronic acid, resist phagocytosis. Extracellular digestive enzymes facilitate the spread of infection by interfering with local thrombosis (streptolysins) and pus formation (DNase) and enhancing connective tissue digestion (hyaluronidase). Suppurative complications follow local inflammation (peritonsillar abscess, retropharyngeal abscess), direct extension (otitis media, sinusitis), lymphangitic spread (lymphadenitis), or bacteremia (sepsis, osteomyelitis, pneumonia).

Scarlet fever–producing streptococci lead to clinical manifestations that are similar to those produced by nonpyrogenic exotoxin–containing strains except for the scarlatiniform rash. Serologically distinct pyrogenic toxins (A–C) produce the rash in nonimmune hosts. Rash production is dependent in part on a host hypersensitivity reaction and is decreased by host synthesis of specific antitoxins. These toxins also exhibit pyrogenicity, cytotoxicity, and enhancement of the effects of endotoxin. Streptococcal pyrogenic exotoxin A has partial amino acid homology with streptococcal entotoxin B; these toxins are associated with staphylococcal toxic shock and nonmenstrual staphylococcal toxic shock syndromes, respectively (see later discussion).

CLINICAL MANIFESTATIONS. The most common infections caused by group A β-hemolytic streptococci involve the respiratory tract, skin, soft tissues, and blood.

Respiratory Tract Infection (see Sec. 14.24, 14.30, and 14.56).

Scarlet Fever. This disease is the result of infection by streptococci that elaborate one of three pyrogenic (erythrogenic) toxins. The incubation period ranges from 1 to 7 days with an average of 3 days. The onset is acute and is characterized by fever, vomiting, headache, toxicity, pharyngitis, and chills. Abdominal pain may be present; when this is associated with vomiting prior to the appearance of the rash, an abdominal surgical condition may be suggested. Within 12–48 hr the typical rash appears.

Generally, temperature increases abruptly and may peak at 39.6–40° C (103–104° F) on the 2nd day and gradually returns to normal within 5–7 days in the untreated patient; it is usually normal within 12–24 hr after initiation of penicillin therapy. The tonsils are hyperemic and edematous and may be covered with a gray-white exudate. The pharynx is inflamed and covered by a membrane in severe cases. The tongue may be edematous and reddened. During the early days of illness the dorsum of the tongue has a white coat through which the red and edematous papillae project *(white strawberry tongue)*. After several days the white coat desquamates; the red tongue studded with prominent papillae persists *(red strawberry tongue)*. The palate and uvula may be edematous, reddened, and covered with petechiae.

The exanthem is red, punctate or finely papular, and blanches on pressure. In some individuals it may be palpated more readily than it is seen, having the texture of gooseflesh or coarse sandpaper. The rash appears initially in the axillae, groin, and neck but within 24 hr becomes generalized. Punctate lesions generally are not present on the face. The forehead and cheeks appear flushed, and the area around the mouth is pale *(circumoral pallor)*. The rash is most intense in the axillae and groin and at pressure sites. Petechiae may occur owing to capillary fragility. Areas of hyperpigmentation that do not blanch with pressure may appear in the deep creases, particularly in the antecubital fossae *(Pastia lines)*. In severe disease, small vesicular lesions *(miliary sudamina)* may appear over the abdomen, hands, and feet.

Desquamation begins on the face in fine flakes toward the end of the 1st wk and proceeds over the trunk and finally to the hands and feet. The duration and extent of desquamation vary with the intensity of the rash; it may continue for as long as 6 wk.

Scarlet fever may follow infection of wounds (surgical scarlet fever), burns, or streptococcal skin infection. Clinical manifestations are similar to those described above, but the tonsils and pharynx generally are not involved. A similar picture may be observed with certain strains of staphylococci that produce an erythrogenic toxin.

Scarlet fever must be distinguished from other exanthematous diseases, including measles (characterized by its prodrome of conjunctivitis, photophobia, dry cough, and Koplik spots), rubella (disease is mild, postauricular lymphadenopathy usually is present, and throat culture is negative), and other viral exanthems. With infectious mononucleosis there are generally pharyngitis, rash, lymphadenopathy, and splenomegaly as well as atypical lymphocytes. The exanthems produced by several enteroviruses can be confused with scarlet fever, but differentiation can be established by the course of the disease, the associated symptoms, and the results of culture. Roseola is characterized by the cessation of fever with the onset of rash and the transient nature of the exanthem. Kawasaki disease, drug eruption, and toxic shock syndrome must also be considered. Septic or severe scarlet fever, associated with bacteremia or toxemia, may manifest high fever and may be complicated by arthritis, jaundice, and hydrops of the gallbladder. Scarlet fever may be distinguished from Kawasaki disease by an older age of onset, absence of conjunctival involvement, and recovery of group A streptococci. Streptococcal toxic shock syndrome, associated with pyrogenic toxin A, produces toxicity, fever, shock, tissue injury (fasciitis, myositis), rash (local or diffuse erythema, maculopapular, petechial, desquamation), and multiorgan dysfunction (kidney, lung, central nervous system). The shock, local tissue injury, older age, and nonscarlatiniform rash differentiate this syndrome from scarlet fever. *Arcanobacterium haemolyticum* (formerly *Corynebacterium haemolyticum*) also produces tonsillitis, pharyngitis, and a scarlatiniform rash in adolescents and young adults. *Y. enterocolitica* and *M. pneumoniae* rarely may produce pharyngitis and rash. Severe sunburn can also be confused with scarlet fever.

Pneumonia. See Sec. 14.56.

Skin Infections. The most common form of skin infection due to group A β-hemolytic streptococci is superficial pyoderma (impetigo) (Sec. 23.26). Colonization of unbroken skin precedes pyoderma by about 10 days. Skin lesions (impetigo, ecthyma, cellulitis) develop following intradermal inoculation by insect bites, scabies, or minor trauma. Skin colonization or pyoderma may predispose the patient to later nasopharyngeal colonization with the same strain. Deeper soft tissue infections may occur secondary to impetigo. Streptococcal cellulitis is a painful, erythematous, indurated infection of the skin and subcutaneous tissues. Lymphangitis and regional lymphadenitis are common. Streptococcal soft tissue abscesses are rare but have occurred following immunization with contaminated needles. Fever and other systemic manifestations of disease may be noted. Group A streptococci also produce abscesses in underlying subcutaneous hemangiomas.

Erysipelas. Erysipelas is an acute, well-demarcated infection of the skin with lymphangitis involving the face (associated with pharyngitis) and extremities (wounds). The skin is erythematous and indurated; the advancing margins of the lesions have a raised, firm border. The skin lesion usually is associated with fever, vomiting, and irritability. In some cases streptococci break through the lymphatic barrier, and subcutaneous abscesses, bacteremia, and metastatic foci of infection are observed. Bacteremia and death have been associated with streptococcal cellulitis in the newborn infant; progression may be so rapid that there is no response to treatment with penicillin. Central clearing may be present despite continued peripheral extension. Lesions may last from days to weeks.

Bacteremia (see Sec. 12.14). Bacteremia may follow a localized cutaneous (wounds, cellulitis, varicella lesions, hemangioma, abscess) or respiratory (pharyngitis, otitis media, sinusitis, pneumonia) infection in previously healthy or immunocompromised (malnutrition, malignancy) patients. It has also occurred in children with no obvious focus of infection. Sepsis may be rapidly progressive with hypotension, fever, leukocytosis, disseminated intravascular coagulation, and peripheral gangrene. Metastatic foci may result in meningitis, brain abscess, osteomyelitis, septic arthritis, pneumonia, and peritonitis. Rarely, endocarditis may complicate group A streptococcal bacteremia. The prognosis is poorest in patients with an underlying disease such as malignancy.

Vaginitis. The β-hemolytic streptococcus is a common cause of vaginitis in prepubertal girls. There is usually a serous discharge and marked erythema and irritation of the vulvar area, accompanied by discomfort in walking and in urination. **Perianal streptococcal cellulitis** produces local itching, pain, blood-streaked stools, erythema, and proctitis. Intrafamily and nosocomial spread occurs during perianal cellulitis or colonization.

DIAGNOSIS. Although 30% of children with sore throat have a positive throat culture for group A streptococcus, only 50% of these have a positive antibody response indicative of active infection rather than colonization. Streptococcal pharyngitis is suggested by age greater than 5 yr, high fever, exudates, tender anterior cervical lymphadenopathy, scarlatiniform rash, and a history of exposure. However, only 15% of children with pharyngitis and 25% of those with exudates have streptococcal infection; 50% of those with streptococcal pharyngitis do not have tonsillar exudates. Clinical judgment does not predict which children may have streptococcal infection, which must be diagnosed by throat culture or antigen detection.

Throat culture is the most useful laboratory aid in reaching a diagnosis in patients with acute tonsillitis or pharyngitis. A positive result for a throat culture may indicate streptococcal pharyngitis, but hemolytic streptococci are common inhabitants of the nasopharynx in well children. Isolation of a group A streptococcus from the pharynx of a child with pharyngeal infection does not necessarily indicate that the disease is caused by this organism. When streptococci are isolated from children with moderate or severe exudative pharyngitis who have petechiae on the palate and cervical adenitis, the diagnosis is more secure. *Treatment is, however, recommended for all children with pharyngitis and a positive throat culture for group A streptococci, even though in some cases the streptococci represent colonization.*

The immunologic response of the host following exposure to streptococcal antigen can be assessed by measuring antistreptolysin O (ASO) titers. An increase in ASO titer to greater than 166 Todd units occurs in more than 80% of untreated children with streptococcal pharyngitis within the first 3–6 wk following infection. This response may be modified or abolished by early and effective antibiotic therapy. ASO titers may be very high in patients with rheumatic fever; in contrast, they are weakly positive or not elevated at all in patients with streptococcal pyoderma; responses in patients with glomerulonephritis are variable. Group A β-hemolytic streptococci also may be recovered from the pharynx of asymptomatic individuals who develop an antibody response to this organism, indicating that subclinical infection has occurred. Group C or G streptococcal infection also may produce a rise in ASO titer.

Individuals with impetigo may react strongly to stimulation by other streptococcal extracellular products. Anti-DNase (deoxyribonuclease) B provides the best serologic test for streptococcal pyoderma; it begins to rise 6–8 wk after infection. Most patients with streptococcal pharyngitis also develop elevated titers to this enzyme. Patients with pyoderma and pharyngitis also may develop antibody responses to hyaluronidase, but antihyaluronidase (AH) titers are elevated with less regularity than are ASO titers.

A 2-min inexpensive **Streptozyme*** slide test is designed to detect antibodies against multiple streptococcal extracellular antigens. This test detects more patients with increased antibody titers than any other single test presently available. Nonspecific (false-positive) reactions have been limited in number, and the test is capable of detecting antibody responses within 7–10 days of infection. However, the strength of the Streptozyme reagent varies from lot to lot, and it may not be specific for antibodies to extracellular products of group A streptococci. In patients with group A streptococci, the antibody response was comparable to but no greater than that achieved with the ASO or anti-DNase B tests.

A number of commercial tests that rely on detection of group A streptococcal polysaccharide antigen by specific antibody employ agglutination or enzyme immunoassays. These easily performed tests are attractive in their potential to establish a rapid diagnosis in the office setting. These tests have a high specificity (>90%), but sensitivities range from 59 to 90%. A negative test result does not indicate absence of streptococcal infection; patients who have a negative test result should then be evaluated with standard culture techniques.

The white blood cell count may or may not be elevated. Leukocytosis may be noted in many bacterial and viral diseases; hence, this finding is nonspecific. Similarly, elevations in ESR and C-reactive protein do not help to establish a specific diagnosis.

DIFFERENTIAL DIAGNOSIS. Acute pharyngitis that is indistinguishable clinically from that caused by group A β-hemolytic streptococci may be caused by many viruses, including Epstein-Barr virus (infectious mononucleosis) and cytomegalovirus. A viral etiology may be suggested by failure to isolate streptococci and can be identified specifically by viral culture and serologic studies. Infectious mononucleosis may be suggested by the clinical manifestations, the presence of atypical lymphocytes in the peripheral blood, and a rise in heterophil and Epstein-Barr viral antibody titers. Acute pharyngitis similar to that caused by β-hemolytic streptococci may be noted in patients with diphtheria, tularemia, toxoplasmosis, infection with mycoplasma or *A. haemolyticum*, and, rarely, in individuals with tonsillar tuberculosis, salmonellosis, and brucellosis or infections caused by *N. gonorrhoeae, N. meningitidis*, and *Y. enterocolitica*. These diseases can be differentiated by appropriate cultures and serologic tests. An ulcerative pharyngitis may be noted in children with agranulocytosis regardless of the etiology.

Streptococcal pyoderma must be differentiated from staphylococcal skin disease. Often these bacterial species coexist. The lesions produced are clinically indistinguishable; distinction is made only by culture.

Streptococcal septicemia, meningitis, septic arthritis, and pneumonia present signs and symptoms similar to those produced by other bacterial organisms. The offending pathogen can be established only by culture.

---

*Wampole Laboratories.

COMPLICATIONS. Complications generally reflect extension of streptococcal infection from the nasopharynx. This may result in sinusitis, otitis media, mastoiditis, cervical adenitis, retropharyngeal or parapharyngeal abscess, or bronchopneumonia. Hematogenous dissemination of streptococci may cause meningitis, osteomyelitis, or septic arthritis. Nonsuppurative late complications include rheumatic fever and glomerulonephritis.

PREVENTION. Administration of penicillin will prevent most cases of streptococcal disease if the drug is provided prior to the onset of symptoms. Indications for prophylaxis are not clear. Throat cultures should be obtained from children who are close family contacts of patients with streptococcal disease. If these cultures are positive, oral penicillin G or V (400,000 U/dose) is provided 4 times each day for 10 days. Alternatively, 600,000 U of benzathine penicillin in combination with 600,000 U of aqueous procaine penicillin may be given as a single intramuscular injection. A similar approach may be used for institutional epidemics. Children exposed to an individual case at school may be observed carefully.

Management of carriers of group A β-hemolytic streptococci is controversial. It has been suggested that treatment of the carrier precludes the development of type-specific immunity, thereby leaving the individual susceptible to reinfection later in life. It is probably unnecessary to re-treat asymptomatic convalescent patients with persistently positive throat cultures for group A streptococci, since they are generally carriers who do not have persistent or recurrent streptococcal infections.

No streptococcal vaccines are available for clinical use.

TREATMENT. The goals of therapy are to decrease symptoms and prevent septic, suppurative, and nonsuppurative complications. Penicillin is the drug of choice for the treatment of streptococcal infections. All strains of group A β-hemolytic streptococci isolated to date have been sensitive to concentrations of penicillin achievable in vivo.

Blood and tissue levels of penicillin sufficient to kill streptococci should be maintained for at least 10 days. Children with streptococcal pharyngitis should be treated with penicillin (125–250 mg/dose 3 times a day) for 10 days. Penicillin G or penicillin V may be employed; the latter is preferable because satisfactory blood levels are achieved even when the stomach is not empty. A single intramuscular injection of a long-acting benzathine penicillin G (600,000 U for children <60 lb and 1,200,000 U for children >60 lb) may be more effective for treatment or prevention of relapse and is indicated for all noncompliant patients or those having nausea, vomiting, or diarrhea.

Erythromycin (40 mg/kg/24 hr), lincomycin (40 mg/kg/24 hr), clindamycin (30 mg/kg/24 hr), or cefadroxil monohydrate (15 mg/kg/24 hr) may be used for treating streptococcal pharyngitis in patients who are allergic to penicillin. Generally, relapse rates are greater with regimens other than penicillin. Tetracyclines and sulfonamides should not be used for treatment, although sulfonamides may be used for prophylaxis of rheumatic fever.

Treatment failure, defined as persistence of streptococci after a complete course of penicillin, occurs in 5–20% of children and is more common with oral than with intramuscular therapy. It may be due to poor compliance, reinfection, the presence of β-lactamase–producing oral flora, tolerant streptococci, or presence of a carrier state. Persistent carriage of streptococci predisposes a small number of patients to symptomatic relapse. Repeating the throat culture after a course of penicillin therapy is indicated in high-risk situations, such as in patients with a history of previous rheumatic fever. If the throat culture is again positive for group A streptococcus, some clinicians recommend a second course of treatment with penicillin. Persistence after a second course of antibiotics is probably due to a carrier state, which has a low risk for the development of rheumatic fever and does not require further therapy.

Patients with severe scarlet fever, streptococcal bacteremia, pneumonia, meningitis, deep soft tissue infections, erysipelas, streptococcal toxic shock syndrome, or complications of streptococcal pharyngitis should be treated parenterally with penicillin, preferably intravenously. The dose and duration of therapy must be tailored to the nature of the disease process, with daily doses as high as 400,000 U/kg/24 hr required in the most severe infections.

PROGNOSIS. The prognosis for adequately treated streptococcal infections is excellent; most suppurative complications are prevented or readily treated. When therapy is provided promptly, nonsuppurative complications are prevented and complete recovery is the rule. In rare instances, particularly in the newborn infant or in children whose response to infection is compromised, fulminant pneumonia, septicemia, and death may occur despite usually adequate therapy.

Infections Due to Other Streptococci

In many centers the group B *Streptococcus* has become the leading cause of neonatal septicemia and meningitis (Sec. 9.67).

Human infection with streptococci of groups C to H and K to O, as well as with nontypable strains, has been reported in normal infants and children. The classification of these organisms and the infections with which they have been associated are shown in Table 12–21. Penicillin G provides effective therapy for non–group A streptococci, except for those belonging to group D (enterococci) and selected α-hemolytic strains; these organisms generally are susceptible to ampicillin. When endocarditis is caused by enterococci, therapy with ampicillin plus an aminoglycoside is recommended.

Infection with Lancefield group G streptococci has been recognized as an increasingly serious and frequent cause of human disease; endovascular infection, endocarditis, and septic arthritis are observed most frequently. Despite exquisite in vitro sensitivity to penicillin, in vivo responses have been disappointing. Therapy with ampicillin and an aminoglycoside is more efficacious than therapy with penicillin alone.

Bacterial endocarditis in children is commonly due to infection with *Streptococcus viridans.* A variant of this organism that grows slowly and requires vitamin B_6 or thiol compounds for optimal growth has also caused endocarditis in adults and children. It is important to know that supplemented media are needed for their isolation and sensitivity testing; spuriously low MICs may be reported when nonsupplemented media are used. Some of these organisms are relatively tolerant to penicillin; therapy with penicillin and an aminoglycoside is recommended until results of sensitivity studies are available. In several instances these organisms have been resistant even to this combination of drugs but have been sensitive to clindamycin and vancomycin.

Arditi M, Shulman ST, Davis AT, et al: Group C β-hemolytic streptococcal infections in children: Nine pediatric cases and review. Rev Infect Dis 11:34, 1989.

Christie CDC, Havens PL, Shapiro ED: Bacteremia with group A streptococci in childhood. Am J Dis Child 142:559, 1988.

Denny FW: Effect of treatment on streptococcal pharyngitis: Is the issue really settled? Pediatr Infect Dis 4:352, 1985.

DiNubile MJ: Treatment of endocarditis caused by relatively resistant nonenterococcal streptococci: Is penicillin enough? Rev Infect Dis 12:112, 1990.

Dobson S: Group A streptococci revisited. Arch Dis Child 64:977, 1989.

Harnden A, Lennon D: Serious suppurative group A streptococcal infections in previously well children. Pediatr Infect Dis J 7:714, 1988.

Kokx NP, Comstock JA, Facklam RR: Streptococcal perianal disease in children. Pediatrics 80:659, 1987.

Levin RM, Grossman M, Jordan C, et al: Group A streptococcal infection in children younger than three years of age. Pediatr Infect Dis J 7:581, 1988.
Miller RA, Brancato F, Holmes KK: *Corynebacterium hemolyticum* as a cause of pharyngitis and scarlatiniform rash in young adults. Ann Intern Med 105:867, 1986.
Putto A: Febrile exudative tonsillitis: Viral or streptococcal? Pediatrics 80:6, 1987.
Shulman ST: Streptococcal pharyngitis: Clinical and epidemiologic factors. Pediatr Infect Dis J 8:816, 1989.
Stevens DL, Tanner MH, Winship J, et al: Severe group A streptococcal infections associated with a toxic shock-like syndrome and scarlet fever toxin A. N Engl J Med 321:1, 1989.
Wittler RR, Yamada SM, Bass JW, et al: Penicillin tolerance and erythromycin resistance of group A β-hemolytic streptococci in Hawaii and the Philippines. Am J Dis Child 144:587, 1990.
Wong VK, Wright HT: Group A β-hemolytic streptococci as a cause of bacteremia in children. Am J Dis Child 142:831, 1988.

12.19 STAPHYLOCOCCAL INFECTIONS

Staphylococci are hardy, nonspore-forming, ubiquitous bacteria and are present in air, fomites, and dust or as normal flora of humans and animals. They are resistant to heat and drying and may be recovered from nonphysiologic environments weeks to months after inoculation. These organisms grow in clusters, aerobically or as facultative anaerobes. Strains are classified as *S. aureus* if they are coagulase positive and as *S. epidermidis* or *S. saprophyticus* (and other nonpathologic species, e.g., *S. haemolyticus*) if they are coagulase negative. Generally, *S. aureus* produces a yellow pigment and *S. epidermidis*, a white pigment. *S. aureus* generally is mannitol- deoxyribonuclease– and acid phosphatase–positive and produces β hemolysis on blood agar. *S. epidermidis* generally is mannitol and acid phosphatase negative; production of β hemolysis on blood agar is variable. *S. saprophyticus* is mannitol positive and resistant to novobiocin, which differentiates this species from *S. aureus* and *S. epidermidis*.

Infections Due to *Staphylococcus aureus*

S. aureus is the most common cause of pyogenic infection of the skin; it also may cause furuncles, carbuncles, osteomyelitis, septic arthritis, wound infection, abscesses, pneumonia, empyema, endocarditis, pericarditis, meningitis, and toxin-mediated food poisoning.

ETIOLOGY. Disease may be the result of tissue invasion or may reflect injury due to a variety of toxins and enzymes elaborated by these organisms. Strains of *S. aureus* can be identified and classified by means of bacteriophage group typing: group I (phage numbers 29, 52, 52A, 79, and 80); group II (phage numbers 3A, 3C, 55, and 71); group III (phage numbers 6, 7, 42E, 47, 53, 54, 75, 77, 83A, 84, and 85); group IV (phage number 42D); and miscellaneous (phage numbers 81 and 187).

Many strains of *S. aureus* release *exotoxins*. Four immunologically distinct hemolysins have been identified. α-Toxin acts on cell membranes and causes tissue necrosis, injures human leukocytes, and produces aggregation of platelets and spasm of smooth muscle. A β-hemolysin degrades sphingomyelin, causing hemolysis of red blood cells, and a δ-hemolysin disrupts membranes by a detergent-like action. Little is known about γ-hemolysin other than that it also appears to act on cell membranes.

Leukocidin, produced by most strains of *S. aureus*, combines with the phospholipid of the phagocytic cell membrane, producing increased permeability, leakage of protein, and eventual death of the neutrophil and macrophage.

Exfoliative toxins A and B are two serologically distinct proteins that produce localized (bullous impetigo) or generalized (scalded skin syndrome, scarlatiniform eruption) dermatologic complications (see also Sec. 12.18). Exfoliative toxin A is a chromosomal gene product and exfoliative toxin B is a plasmid gene product. Individual strains may produce one or both toxins or neither; no consistent phage type is associated with toxin production, although phage group II has been implicated in some cases. Exfoliative toxin produces scalding by splitting the desmosome and altering the intracellular matrix in the stratum granulosum.

Staphylococcal enterotoxins (types A, B, C_1, C_2, D, E, F) are elaborated by most strains of *S. aureus*. Ingestion of preformed enterotoxin A or B is associated with vomiting and diarrhea and in some cases with the development of profound hypotension (Sec. 12.20 and 26.2). Virtually all individuals by the age of 10 yr have antibodies to at least one enterotoxin. Staphylococcal enterotoxin F is now called toxic shock syndrome toxin-1 (TSST-1). It is associated with toxic shock syndrome related to menstruation. TSST-1 may occur with enterotoxin A in menstrual-related toxic shock syndrome (TSS), whereas enterotoxin B may be associated with nonmenstrual TSS. TSST-1 induces production of interleukin 1 and other inflammatory cytokines, which result in hypotension, desquamating dermatitis, fever, and multisystem involvement.

A variety of *enzymes* may be released by staphylococci. Production of coagulase differentiates *S. aureus* from *S. epidermidis* and other coagulase-negative staphylococci. Coagulase (clumping factor) causes plasma to clot by interacting with fibrinogen. Other enzymes elaborated by staphylococci include catalase (inactivates H_2O_2, promoting intracellular survival), penicillinase or β-lactamase (inactivates penicillin at the molecular level), hyaluronidase (spreading factor), lipase, and phosphodiesterase.

Most strains of *S. aureus* possess an *agglutinogen* (protein A). This material can react with the Fc fragments of IgG molecules, generates complement-derived chemotactic factors, and has antiphagocytic properties. Capsular antigens 5 and 8 account for up to 70% of strains resistant to phagocytosis by polymorphonuclear leukocytes in vitro. The cell wall peptidoglycan, a polysaccharide polymer, elicits endogenous pyrogen production from monocytes, is chemotactic, activates complement, has endotoxin-like properties, and stimulates opsonic antibody production. In addition, many staphylococci produce a loose polysaccharide capsule, or slime layer, which may interfere with opsonophagocytosis.

EPIDEMIOLOGY. Most newborn infants are colonized within the first week of life and 20–30% of normal individuals carry *S. aureus* in the anterior nares at all times.

The organisms may be transmitted from the nose to the skin, where colonization seems to be more transient. Repeated recovery of *S. aureus* from the skin suggests repeated transfer rather than persistent skin colonization. Persistent umbilical and perianal carriage has been described.

Transmission of *S. aureus* generally occurs by direct contact or by spread of heavy particles over a distance of 6 ft or less. Spread by fomites is rare. Acquisition of staphylococci is dependent on the efficiency of the disseminator and the susceptibility of the host. Heavily colonized individuals and perianal carriers are particularly effective disseminators. Newborn infants are extremely susceptible to staphylococci; the nasopharynx, skin, perineum, and umbilical stump are the most common sites of colonization. Autoinfection is common, and minor infection (styes, pustules, paronychia) may be the source of disseminations. Handwashing between contacts with patients decreases the spread of staphylococci from patient to patient. Older children and adults are more resistant than the newborn infant to colonization.

Infection may follow colonization. Antibiotic therapy with a drug to which *S. aureus* is resistant favors both colonization and the development of infection. Other factors that increase the likelihood of infection include wounds, skin disease, ventriculoatrial shunts, intravenous or intrathecal catheterization, corticosteroid treatment, starvation, acidosis, and azotemia. Viral infections of the respiratory tract also may predispose to secondary bacterial infection with staphylococci.

PATHOGENESIS. The development of staphylococcal disease is related to resistance of the host to infection and to virulence of the organism. The intact skin and mucous membranes serve as barriers to invasion by staphylococci. Defects in the mucocutaneous barriers produced by trauma, surgery, foreign surfaces (sutures, shunts, intravascular catheters), and burns increase the risk of infection. Adhesion of *S. aureus* to mucosal cells is mediated by teichoic acid in the cell wall, while exposure to the submucosa or subcutaneous sites increases adhesion to fibrinogen, fibronectin, laminin, and perhaps collagen IV. A cellular factor that appears to be a mucopeptide, which can be extracted only from virulent strains of *S. aureus*, inhibits chemotaxis and accumulation of fluid at the site of infection. The ability of virulent staphylococci to establish disease may be related directly to their capacity to inhibit chemotaxis.

Protein A, present in most strains of *S. aureus* but not in *S. epidermidis*, reacts specifically with IgG1, IgG2, and IgG4. It is located on the outermost coat of the bacterium and can absorb serum immunoglobulin, preventing antibacterial antibodies from acting as opsonins and thus inhibiting phagocytosis. Leukocidin, causing degranulation of leukocytes, and staphylococcal hemolysin that is toxic to erythrocytes and leukocytes also contribute to the virulence of *S. aureus*.

Proliferation of staphylococci in the gastrointestinal tract is also controlled by the prevalence of other bacterial species. If this balance is upset during antibiotic therapy, resistant staphylococci may proliferate and invade the bowel wall. Elaboration of enterotoxin by staphylococci within the gastrointestinal tract or ingestion of preformed enterotoxins may produce disease in the absence of tissue invasion (Sec. 26.2).

The infant may acquire type-specific humoral immunity to staphylococci transplacentally. Older children and adults develop antibodies to staphylococci as a result of intermittent minor infections of the skin and soft tissues; the antistaphylococcal titer of serum generally increases after overt staphylococcal disease. The presence of antibody, however, does not always protect the individual from staphylococcal disease. There is some indication that disseminated *S. aureus* disease in previously healthy children may occur following a viral infection that suppresses neutrophil or respiratory epithelial cell function.

Formation of antibody and delayed hypersensitivity reactions can be induced by protein components of the cell wall and by ribotol teichoic acid components of the organism. The specific protection afforded by antibodies to any of these components remains unclear.

Individuals with congenital or acquired defects in the complement system (required for chemotaxis), defective chemotaxis (Job, Chédiak-Higashi, Wiskott-Aldrich, and lazy leukocyte syndromes), defective phagocytosis, and defective humoral immunity (antibodies required for opsonization) as well as those with an impaired intracellular bactericidal capacity are at increased risk of infection with staphylococci. Patients with *chronic granulomatous disease*, in which phagocytosis proceeds normally but killing of ingested catalase-positive bacteria is severely impaired, are particularly susceptible to staphylococcal disease. Impaired mobilization of polymorphonuclear leukocytes has been documented in children with diabetic ketoacidosis and in healthy individuals following ingestion of alcohol. Patients with human immunodeficiency virus (HIV) infection have neutrophils that are defective in their ability to kill *S. aureus* in vitro.

CLINICAL MANIFESTATIONS. These vary with the location of the infection, which, though most commonly located on the skin, may involve any organ, the subcutaneous tissues, and the musculoskeletal system. Disease states of varying severity are generally the result of local suppuration, systemic dissemination with metastatic infection, or systemic effects of toxin production. Although the nasopharynx and skin of many persons may be colonized with *S. aureus*, disease due to this organism is relatively uncommon. Lesions, especially those of the skin, are considerably more prevalent among persons living in low socioeconomic circumstances and particularly among those in tropical climates.

Newborn. Nosocomial infections are discussed in Sec. 9.59, staphylococcal diseases in general sepsis and meningitis in Sec. 12.14, pneumonia in Sec. 12.15 and 14.56, otitis media in Sec. 22.22, conjunctivitis in Sec. 22.9 and 9.61, and osteomyelitis and septic arthritis in Sec. 12.16.

Skin. Pyogenic skin infections may be primary or secondary to wounds or may be a superinfection of other noninfectious skin disease (eczema), or of impetigo contagiosa.

Impetigo contagiosa, ecthyma, bullous impetigo, folliculitis, hydradenitis, furuncles, carbuncles, staphylococcal scalded skin syndrome (Ritter disease), and a syndrome resembling the rash of scarlet fever are described in Sec. 12.18. An identical clinical picture may be seen in patients with wounds, especially burns (Sec. 6.37), that are secondarily infected with staphylococci. Folliculitis (pyodermia of the hair follicle) may extend to a deep-seated furuncle or carbuncle, if more than one hair follicle is involved. *Recurrent furunculosis* is a disorder of unknown etiology and is associated with repeated episodes of pyoderma over months to years. The patient should be evaluated for immune defects associated with recurrent infection, and the family should be evaluated for nasal colonization with *S. aureus*. Nosocomial skin lesions, including pustules and cellulitis, are discussed in Sec. 9.59.

Respiratory Tract. Infections of the upper respiratory tract due to *S. aureus* are rare considering the frequency with which this area is colonized. Otitis media (Sec. 22.22) and sinusitis (Sec. 14.30) due to *S. aureus* may rarely occur. Staphylococcal sinusitis is relatively common in children with cystic fibrosis or defects in white blood cell function. Suppurative parotitis is a rare infection, but *S. aureus* is a common cause. Staphylococcal tonsillopharyngitis (Sec. 14.22) is rare except in children whose response to infection has been compromised. **Tracheitis** that clinically resembles viral croup may be caused by *S. aureus*. Patients typically have high fever, leukocytosis and evidence of severe upper airway obstruction. Direct laryngoscopy or bronchoscopy shows a normal epiglottis with subglottic narrowing and thick purulent secretions within the trachea.

Pneumonia (Sec. 14.56) due to *S. aureus* may be primary (hematogenous) or secondary following a viral infection (influenza). Hematogenous pneumonia may be secondary to septic emboli, right-sided endocarditis, or the presence of intravascular devices. Inhalation pneumonia is due to alterations of mucociliary clearance, leukocyte dysfunction, or bacterial adherence initiated by a viral infection. In children under 1 yr of age the onset may be heralded by expiratory wheeze briefly simulating bronchiolitis. More common are high fever, abdominal pain, tachypnea, dyspnea, and localized or diffuse bronchopneumonia or lobar disease. Staphylococci cause a necrotizing pneumonitis; hence empyema (Sec. 14.90), pneumatoceles, pyopneumothorax, and bronchopleural fistulas develop frequently. Occasionally, staphylococcal pneumonia produces a diffuse interstitial disease characterized by extreme dyspnea, tachypnea, and cyanosis. Cough may be nonproductive. Also see discussion of pneumonia in cystic fibrosis (Sec. 14.89).

Sepsis (see Sec. 12.14). Staphylococcal bacteremia and sepsis may be associated with any localized infection. The onset may be acute and marked by nausea, vomiting, myalgia, fever, and chills. Organisms may localize subsequently at any site but are found especially in the lung, heart, joints, bones, kidneys, and brain. If appropriate antibiotic therapy is provided, blood cultures may remain positive for 24–48 hr. The fever begins to defervesce at a median time of 22 hr (range 8–90 hr), and return of body temperature to normal occurs at a median time of 58 hr (range 12–180 hr) in patients with *S. aureus* septicemia. Differentiating sepsis from endocarditis may be difficult. Echocardiographic evidence of vegetations, intravenous drug abuse, presence of immune complexes and antistaphylococcal antibodies, and absence of a primary focus of infection suggests endocarditis.

In some instances, especially when treatment of a local infection has been inadequate, disseminated staphylococcal disease occurs, characterized by fever, bone or joint pain, and urticarial, petechial, maculopapular, or pustular rashes. Less frequently, hematuria, jaundice, seizures, nuchal rigidity, and cardiac murmurs are noted. Leukopenia or leukocytosis, proteinuria, and red and white blood cells in the urinary sediment may be noted.

Muscle. Localized staphylococcal abscesses in muscle associated with elevation of muscle enzymes but without septicemia have been called **tropical pyomyositis.** Although this disorder has been reported most frequently from tropical areas, it also has occurred in the United States in otherwise healthy children. Multiple abscesses occur in 30–40% of cases. Prodromal symptoms may include coryza, pharyngitis, diarrhea, or prior trauma at the site of the abscess. Surgical drainage and appropriate antibiotic therapy are essential.

Bones and Joints. *S. aureus* is the most common cause of osteomyelitis and septic arthritis in children (Sec. 12.16 and 12.17).

Central Nervous System. *Meningitis* (Sec. 12.15) due to *S. aureus* is associated with cranial trauma and neurosurgical procedures (craniotomy, CSF shunt placement), and less frequently with endocarditis, parameningeal foci (epidural or brain abscess), diabetes mellitus, or malignancy. The CSF profile in *S. aureus* meningitis is indistinguishable from that of other bacterial causes of meningitis.

Heart. *Acute bacterial endocarditis* (Sec. 15.66) may follow staphylococcal bacteremia. *S. aureus* is a common cause of acute virulent endocarditis on native valves. Perforation of heart valves, myocardial abscesses, heart failure, conduction disturbances, acute hemopericardium, purulent pericarditis (Sec. 15.75), and sudden death may ensue.

Kidney. *S. aureus* is a common cause of renal and perinephric abscess (Sec. 18.39). Urinary tract infection due to *S. aureus* is unusual.

Toxic Shock Syndrome. See Sec. 12.20.

Intestinal Tract. *Staphylococcal enterocolitis* follows overgrowth of normal bowel flora by staphylococci. This infection most commonly follows use of broad-spectrum oral antibiotic therapy. Diarrhea is associated with blood and mucus.

Peritonitis associated with *S. aureus* in patients receiving chronic ambulatory peritoneal dialysis usually involves the catheter tunnel. Removal of the catheter is required to achieve a bacteriologic cure.

Food poisoning (Sec. 26.2) may be caused by ingestion of enterotoxins preformed by staphylococci contaminating foods. Two to 7 hr after ingestion of the toxin, sudden, severe vomiting begins. Watery diarrhea may develop, but fever is absent or low. Symptoms rarely persist longer than 12–24 hr. Rarely, shock and death may occur.

DIAGNOSIS. The diagnosis of staphylococcal infection depends on isolation of the organisms from skin lesions, abscess cavities, blood, cerebrospinal fluid, or other sites of infection. Toxin-producing organisms may be recovered from sites of colonization (nasopharynx, vagina). The organisms can be grown readily in liquid and on solid media. Following isolation, identification is made on the basis of Gram stain and coagulase and mannitol reactivity. Patterns of sensitivity to antibiotics can be assessed and the organism phage-typed if necessary for epidemiologic reasons.

Teichoic acid, α-toxin, and peptidoglycan antibodies in patients with *S. aureus* bacteremia can be measured by functional assays (hemolysis) or by enzyme-linked immunosorbent assay. These tests may be valuable in diagnosing patients with staphylococcal endocarditis and complicated bacteremia associated with a deep tissue focus of infection.

Diagnosis of staphylococcal food poisoning generally is made on the basis of epidemiologic and clinical findings. Food suspected of contamination should be examined by Gram stain, cultured, and tested for enterotoxin. This last test can be done by the Centers for Disease Control.

DIFFERENTIAL DIAGNOSIS. Skin lesions due to *S. aureus* and those due to group A β-hemolytic streptococci may be indistinguishable. Staphylococcal pneumonia can be suspected on the basis of chest roentgenograms that may reveal pneumatoceles, pyopneumothorax, or lung abscess. These changes suggesting a necrotizing pneumonitis are not pathognomonic for staphylococcal infection and may be seen in patients with pneumonia due to other bacteria, including *Klebsiella* and many anaerobes. Fluctuant skin and soft tissue lesions also can be caused by many organisms, including *Mycobacterium, Francisella tularensis,* and various fungi and may be seen in patients with cat-scratch disease (Sec. 12.102).

PREVENTION. Staphylococcal infection is transmitted primarily by direct contact. *Strict attention to handwashing techniques* is the most effective measure for preventing the spread of staphylococci from one individual to another (Sec. 9.59). Use of a detergent containing an iodophor, chlorhexidine, or hexachlorophene is recommended. In hospitals or other institutional settings, all persons with acute staphylococcal infections should be excluded until they have been treated adequately. There should be constant surveillance for nosocomial staphylococcal infections within hospitals. Infectious disease control measures may reduce the spread of infection (Table 12–22).

Patients in an intensive care unit who received sucralfate instead of H_2 blocking agents for prophylaxis against stress ulceration were shown to have reduced gastric colonization with *S. aureus.* The reduction in colonization is secondary to the maintenance of natural gastric acidity with sucralfate. This difference in therapy was associated with a decrease in the frequency of pneumonia.

TABLE 12–22. Infectious Disease Control Measures Used to Prevent Spread of Staphylococcus Epidemics

Reinforcement of regulation for handwashing prior to examining each patient
Hand-to-elbow wash with chlorhexidine or an iodophor
Barrier precautions and/or strict isolation: gowns and/or gloves worn by staff
Isolation of cohort nurses with patients
Identification of nosocomial strain (antibiotic sensitivity, phage type, DNA profile)
Colonization surveillance of staff
Reassignment of staff with active lesions or colonization
Discharge of colonized patients as soon as possible
Notation on patient chart of colonization status if readmitted to hospital
Monitoring of fomites (e.g., instruments) for colonization
Elimination of nasal colonization with topical bacitracin or mupirocin, and oral rifampin or ciprofloxacin
Topical hexachlorophene (3%) washing during neonatal epidemics*
Triple dye to the umbilical cord

*Excessive use of topical hexachlorophene may be absorbed and may produce neurotoxicity in premature infants or patients with extensive cutaneous lesions.

Patients with recurrent staphylococcal furunculitis may be treated with hexachloraphene washes and dicloxacillin or clindamycin to prevent recurrences.

Food poisoning may be prevented by excluding individuals with staphylococcal infections of the skin from the preparation and handling of food. Prepared foods should be eaten immediately or refrigerated appropriately to prevent multiplication of staphylococci with which the food may have been contaminated.

TREATMENT. Antibiotic therapy alone is rarely effective in individuals with undrained abscesses or with infected foreign bodies. Loculated collections of purulent material should be relieved by incision and drainage. Foreign bodies should be removed, if possible. Therapy always should be initiated with a penicillinase-resistant antibiotic because more than 90% of all staphylococci isolated, regardless of source, are resistant to penicillin.

For serious infections parenteral treatment is indicated. Although clinically they are equally efficacious, methacillin and nafcillin have a more stable β-lactam ring against β-lactamase than does oxacillin. This stability is most important if there is a large bacterial burden, since the associated inoculum effect may neutralize the antibacterial activity of β-lactam antibiotics. Generally, a dose of 200 mg/kg/24 hr should be employed intravenously in 6 divided doses. Daily doses as high as 400 mg/kg/24 hr have been used without toxicity in selected patients. Serious staphylococcal infections, with or without abscesses, tend to persist and recur, necessitating prolonged therapy.

The antibiotic employed as well as the dose, route, and duration of treatment is dependent on the site of infection, the response of the patient to treatment, and the sensitivity of the organisms recovered from blood or from local sites of infection. In patients with staphylococcal pneumonia, intravenous treatment is recommended until the patient has been afebrile for 72 hr and other signs of infection have disappeared (Sec. 14.56). Oral therapy is continued for a total of 3 wk, longer in selected cases. The treatment of staphylococcal osteomyelitis (Sec. 12.16), meningitis (Sec. 12.15), and endocarditis (Sec. 15.66) are discussed in their respective sections. In all of these infections, oral treatment should be provided when parenteral therapy has been discontinued; dicloxacillin is penicillinase resistant, absorbed well orally, and quite effective. This drug is administered in a dose of 50–75 mg/kg/24 hr in 4 divided oral doses. Duration of oral therapy also depends on the response of the patient as determined by the clinical, roentgenographic, and laboratory findings and by culture results.

Skin and soft tissue infection and minor upper respiratory infection may be managed by oral therapy alone or by an initial brief course of antibiotics provided parenterally, followed by oral medication. Dicloxacillin (25–50 mg/kg/24 hr), oxacillin (100 mg/kg/24 hr), or nafcillin (100 mg/kg/24 hr), each in 4 divided oral doses, provides excellent blood and tissue concentrations of these antibiotics. Amoxicillin combined with the β-lactamase inhibitor clavulanic acid also is effective at a dose based on the amoxicillin component of 40 mg/kg/24 hr in three divided doses. In patients with very mild, localized skin infection, repeated cleansing with a mild antiseptic and use of topical antibiotics (bacitracin, mupirocin) may be effective. Penicillin should not be applied topically.

Penicillin G can be used to treat infections due to *S. aureus* if the organism proves sensitive to this antibiotic in vitro.

Individuals sensitive to penicillin and its derivatives must be treated with other antibiotics or desensitized to the penicillin derivative to be employed. About 5% of penicillin-sensitive children are also sensitive to cephalosporins. Clindamycin and lincomycin have proved effective for the treatment of skin, soft tissue, bone, and joint infections due to *S. aureus*. Clindamycin may be provided in 3–4 divided doses parenterally or orally (total daily dose 30–40 mg/kg/24 hr). Clindamycin and lincomycin should *not* be used to treat endocarditis, brain abscess, or meningitis due to *S. aureus*. Vancomycin can be used to treat penicillin-sensitive individuals with endocarditis, but serum levels of this antibiotic should be monitored when it is used. Peak serum concentrations should be 25–40 μg/mL. It can be administered in a dose of 10–15 mg/kg/dose given every 6 hr intravenously. Vancomycin or teicoplanin (a vancomycin derivative) should be used to treat bacteremic staphylococcal infections when the organism is resistant to semisynthetic penicillin derivatives. Despite in vitro susceptibility of *S. aureus* to ciprofloxacin and cephalosporins, these agents should not be used in serious staphylococcal infections because their use has not consistently been associated with high cure rates.

Staphylococcal infection of the central nervous system can be treated by intravenous methicillin or nafcillin and, in penicillin-allergic children, by vancomycin, trimethoprim-sulfamethoxazole, or imipenem. Rifampin may be added to vancomycin for synergy.

METHICILLIN-RESISTANT *STAPHYLOCOCCUS AUREUS*. Methicillin-resistant *S. aureus* (MRSA) has become a major nosocomial pathogen. Patients at risk for MRSA infection are the seriously ill (e.g., those with burns, surgical wounds, chronic venous access, lengthy hospitalizations, contact with other MRSA-infected patients, and premature infants). Most methicillin-resistant *S. aureus* strains belong to phage group II (types 77, 83A, 84, and 85); however, outbreaks with nontypable and phage group I strains have been reported.

The resistance to semisynthetic penicillins is thought to be related to a novel penicillin-binding protein that is relatively insensitive to antibiotics containing a β-lactam ring. Additionally, a low-level resistance related to enhanced production of β-lactamases may be noted. Methicillin-resistant *S. aureus* strains appear to be as virulent as their methicillin-sensitive counterparts. Vancomycin and its newer derivative, teicoplanin, are highly effective in the treatment of these infections. Vancomycin is currently the drug of choice if methicillin-resistant *S. aureus* is considered a possible cause of infection or has been isolated. MRSA is also resistant to cephalosporins and imipenem but remains sensitive to trimethoprim-sulfamethoxazole and ciprofloxacin.

When methicillin-resistant *S. aureus* is recovered, strict isolation of affected patients has been shown to be the most effective method for preventing nosocomial spread of infection. Thereafter, control measures should be directed toward identification of new isolates and strict isolation of newly colonized or infected patients. It also may be necessary to identify colonized hospital personnel and eradicate carriage in affected individuals (see Table 12–23).

PROGNOSIS. Untreated staphylococcal septicemia is associated with a mortality rate of 80% or greater. Mortality rates have been reduced to 20% by appropriate antibiotic treatment. Staphylococcal pneumonia can be fatal at any age but is more likely to be associated with high morbidity and mortality in young infants or in patients whose therapy has been delayed.

A total white blood cell count below 5,000/mm^3 or a polymorphonuclear leukocyte response of less than 50% is a grave prognostic sign. Prognosis also may be influenced by numerous host factors, including nutrition, immunologic competence, and the presence or absence of other debilitating diseases.

Infections Due to Coagulase-Negative Staphylococcus

S. epidermidis is one of 11 recognized species of coagulase-negative staphylococcus (CONS) affecting or colonizing humans. Originally thought to be avirulent commensal bacteria, CONS, particularly *S. epidermidis,* is now known to produce nosocomial infections in patients with indwelling foreign devices (intravenous catheters—sepsis; hemodialysis shunts and grafts—sepsis; cerebrospinal fluid shunts—meningitis; peritoneal dialysis catheters—peritonitis; pacemaker wires and electrodes—pocket infection; prosthetic cardiac valves—endocarditis; urinary catheters—pyelonephritis; prosthetic joints—arthritis), surgical trauma (sternal osteomyelitis, endophthalmitis), immunocompromised states (malignancy, granulocytopenia, neonates), and, rarely, community-acquired disease in patients with no underlying disease (urinary tract infection, osteomyelitis). *S. hemolyticus,* another CONS species, is also an important cause of invasive infection and may develop resistance to vancomycin and teicoplanin.

EPIDEMIOLOGY. CONS consist of normal inhabitants of the human skin, throat, mouth, vagina, and urethra. *S. epidermidis* is the most common and persistent species, representing 65–90% of staphylococci present on the skin and mucous membranes. Colonization, usually acquired from hospital staff, precedes infection; alternatively, direct inoculation during surgery may initiate infection (through CSF shunts or prosthetic valves). For epidemiologic purposes CONS can be identified on the basis of phage typing, antibiotic sensitivities, slime layer production, and molecular DNA methods (chromosomal and phage DNA hybridization—restriction enzyme analysis).

PATHOGENESIS. *S. epidermidis* produces an exopolysaccharide protective biofilm (slime) that surrounds the organism and may enhance adhesion to foreign surfaces, resist phagocytosis, and impair penetration of antibiotics. *S. epidermidis* may produce a δ-toxin, which has been recovered in some patients with neonatal necrotizing enterocolitis.

CLINICAL MANIFESTATIONS. Bacteremia. CONS, specifically *S. epidermidis,* are the most common cause of nosocomial bacteremia. In the neonate *S. epidermidis* bacteremia, with or without a central venous catheter, may be manifest as apnea, bradycardia, temperature instability, abdominal distention, hematochezia, meningitis in the absence of CSF pleocytosis, cutaneous abscesses, and persistence of positive blood cultures for as long as 2 wk despite adequate antimicrobial therapy. *S. epidermidis* bacteremia in patients with bone marrow transplantation and malignancy (leukemia, lymphoma) is associated with neutropenia, central venous access (Hickman, Broviac catheters), and gastrointestinal colonization. In most circumstances *S. epidermidis* bacteremia is indolent and is not usually associated with overwhelming septic shock.

Endocarditis. Infection of native heart valves or the right atrial wall secondary to an infected thrombosis at the end of a central line may produce endocarditis. *S. epidermidis* and other CONS may also produce native valve, subacute indolent endocarditis in previously normal patients without a central venous catheter. *S. epidermidis* is a common cause of prosthetic valve endocarditis, presumably due to inoculation at the time of surgery. Infection of the valve sewing ring, with abscess formation and dissection, produces valve dysfunction, dehiscence, arrhythmias, or valve obstruction. See Sec. 15.66 for clinical manifestations.

Central Venous Catheter Infection. Central venous catheters become infected through the exit site and subcutaneous tunnel, which provide a direct path to the bloodstream. *S. epidermidis* is the most common CONS, owing in part to its high rate of cutaneous colonization. Line sepsis is manifest as fever, leukocytosis, tenderness and erythema at the exit site or along the subcutaneous tunnel, and catheter thrombosis.

Central Nervous System CSF Shunts. *S. epidermidis,* introduced at the time of surgery, is the most common pathogen associated with CSF shunt meningitis. Most (70–80%) infections occur within 2 mo of the operation and are manifest by signs of meningeal irritation, fever, increased intracranial pressure (headache), and peritonitis due to the intra-abdominal position of the distal end of the shunt tubing.

Urinary Tract Infection. *S. epidermidis* causes asymptomatic urinary tract infection in hospitalized patients with urinary catheters and following urinary tract surgery or transplantation. *S. saprophyticus* is a common cause of symptomatic urinary tract infection in previously healthy, sexually active teenage girls following urethral colonization. Manifestations are similar to those characteristic of urinary tract infection due to *E. coli* (Sec. 18.39).

S. epidermidis is the most common pathogen producing peritonitis in patients on continuous ambulatory peritoneal dialysis. Manifestations of infection include abdominal pain, fever, more than 100 neutrophils/mm^3, and a positive culture or Gram stain.

DIAGNOSIS. Because *S. epidermidis* is a common skin inhabitant and may contaminate poorly collected blood cultures, it may be difficult to differentiate bacteremia from contamination. Similarly, it may be difficult to differentiate bacteremia due to line sepsis from sepsis not associated with central venous line colonization. Bacteremia should be suspected when blood cultures grow rapidly (within 24 hr), when two or more blood cultures are positive with the same CONS, when the peripheral venous blood culture has a higher quantitative colony count than that drawn from a central venous catheter, and when clinical and laboratory signs and symptoms compatible with CONS sepsis are present and subsequently resolve with appropriate therapy. No blood culture that is positive for *S. epidermidis* should be considered contaminated without careful assessment of the above criteria and examination of the patient.

TREATMENT. Most *S. epidermidis* are resistant to methicillin. Vancomycin is the drug of choice for methicillin-resistant *S. epidermidis.* The new quinolones and teicoplanin have some activity against CONS, and the addition of rifampin or gentamicin to vancomycin may increase antimicrobial efficacy. In many cases of CONS infection associated with foreign bodies, the catheter, valve, or shunt will need to be removed to ensure a cure. Thus, prosthetic heart valves and CSF shunts usually have to be removed to treat the infection adequately. Prior to removal of a CSF shunt, intraventricular (through the shunt) vancomycin and gentamicin should be administered; this may obviate shunt revision.

Antibiotic therapy given through an infected central venous catheter (through each lumen) may effectively cure *S. epidermidis* line sepsis. If the catheter or reservoir is no longer needed, it should be removed. Unfortunately, this is not always possible owing to the therapeutic requirements of the underlying disease (nutrition for short bowel syndrome, chemotherapy for malignancy). A trial of intravenous vancomycin is indicated to preserve the use of the central line.

Peritonitis in patients on continuous ambulatory peritoneal dialysis due to *S. epidermidis* is another infection that may be treated with intravenous or intraperitoneal antibiotics without removing the dialysis catheter. Because many *S. epidermidis* strains producing peritonitis are sensitive to methicillin, this antibiotic in routine doses may be used. If the organism is resistant to methicillin, vancomycin adjusted for renal function is appropriate therapy.

PROGNOSIS. Most episodes of CONS bacteremia respond successfully to antibiotics. Poor prognosis is associated with malignancy, neutropenia, and infected prosthetic or native heart valves. CONS increases morbidity and the duration of hospitalization as well as mortality in patients with underlying complicated illnesses.

ROBERT M. KLIEGMAN
RALPH D. FEIGIN

12.20 TOXIC SHOCK SYNDROME (TSS)

This syndrome is an acute, multisystemic disease characterized by high fever, hypotension, vomiting, abdominal pain, diarrhea, myalgias, nonfocal neurologic abnormalities, and an erythematous rash.

ETIOLOGY AND EPIDEMIOLOGY. Most cases (90%) occur in menstruating women between 15 and 25 yr of age who use hyperabsorbent tampons in the presence of vaginal colonization and/or infection with toxin-producing strains of *S. aureus*. TSS, however, also occurs in children as well as in nonmenstruating women and in men. Nonmenstrual TSS has been associated with wounds, nasal packing, sinusitis, tracheitis, pneumonia, empyema, abscesses, burns, osteomyelitis, and primary bacteremia. Without antimicrobial therapy there is a high recurrence rate (30%) in menstrual TSS, with secondary cases being milder and occurring within 3 mo of the original episode; the overall mortality rate is 3%.

A majority of *S. aureus* strains isolated from confirmed cases are phage type 29/52, are noninvasive, do not adhere to vaginal epithelium, and produce a number of extracellular toxins. Two such toxins, staphylococcal enterotoxin F (SEF) and staphylococcal pyrogenic exotoxin C (PEC), reported to be responsible for the observed clinical manifestations of TSS, have subsequently been determined to be identical and are referred to as toxic shock syndrome toxin (TSST-1). TSST-1 causes massive loss of fluid from the intravascular space directly or following production of interleukin-1 and tumor necrosis factor. However, TSS-negative strains have been isolated from patients with TSST-1, suggesting that other as yet unrecognized toxins play a role in TSS (especially nonmenstrual) and that TSST-1 production is not essential to the pathogenesis of this illness.

CLINICAL MANIFESTATIONS. The diagnosis of TSS is based on clinical manifestations (Table 12–23). The onset is abrupt with high fever, vomiting, and diarrhea and is accompanied by sore throat, headache, and myalgias. A diffuse erythematous macular rash (sunburn-like) appears within 24 hr and may be associated with hyperemia of pharyngeal, conjunctival, and vaginal mucous membranes. Petechiae may develop on day 3–4. Symptoms often include alterations in the level of consciousness, oliguria, and hypotension, which in severe cases may progress to shock and disseminated intravascular coagulation. The most frequent manifestations include diarrhea (98%), myalgia (96%), emesis (92%), fever of more than 40° C (87%), headache (72%), and sore throat (75%). Recovery occurs within 7–10 days and is associated with desquamation, particularly of palms and soles; hair and nail loss have also been observed after 1–2 mo.

TABLE 12–23. Clinical and Laboratory Criteria for Toxic Shock Syndrome*

Fever (temperature ≥ 38.9° C)
Rash (diffuse macular erythroderma) with desquamation, 1–2 wk after onset of illness, particularly of palms and soles
Hypotension (systolic blood pressure ≤ 90 mm Hg in adults or <5th percentile for age in children aged <16 years, or orthostatic syncope)
Involvement of three or more of the following organ systems:
Gastrointestinal (vomiting or diarrhea at onset of illness)
Muscular (severe myalgia or creatine kinase level ≥ twice upper limits of normal for laboratory)
Mucous membrane (vaginal, oropharyngeal, or conjunctival hyperemia)
Renal (blood urea nitrogen level or serum creatinine level ≥ twice upper limits of normal for laboratory or ≥5 leukocytes/high-power field, in the absence of urinary tract infection)
Hepatic (total bilirubin, serum aspartate aminotransaminase [AST] or serum alanine aminotransaminase [ALT] activity ≥ twice upper limits of normal for laboratory)
Hematologic (platelet count ≤ 100 × 10^9/L)
Central nervous system (disorientation or alterations in consciousness without focal neurologic signs when fever and hypotension are absent)
Negative results on the following tests:
Serologic tests for Rocky Mountain spotted fever, leptospirosis, and measles

*TSS is probable with ≥3 criteria in the presence of desquamation or when >5 criteria are met in the absence of desquamation.

There is no specific laboratory test; appropriate selective tests reveal involvement of multiple organ systems including the hepatic, renal, muscular, gastrointestinal, cardiopulmonary, and central nervous system. The most frequent laboratory signs include increased creatinine (69%), thrombocytopenia (59%), hypocalcemia (58%), azotemia (57%), hyperbilirubinemia (54%), elevated liver enzymes (50%), and leukocytosis of 15,000 or more (48%). Vaginal cultures, prior to administration of antibiotics, usually yield *S. aureus*. *S. aureus* isolates should be examined to determine their ability to produce TSST-1. Acute and convalescent sera should be tested for the presence of antibody to TSST-1.

DIFFERENTIAL DIAGNOSIS. Kawasaki disease (mucocutaneous lymph node syndrome) closely resembles TSS clinically. Both are associated with fever unresponsive to antibiotics, hyperemia of mucous membranes, and an erythematous rash with subsequent desquamation. Many of the clinical features of TSS, however, are absent or rare in Kawasaki disease, including diffuse myalgia, vomiting, abdominal pain, diarrhea, azotemia, hypotension, adult respiratory distress syndrome (Sec. 11.57), and shock. Kawasaki disease typically occurs in children under 5 yr of age; one might speculate that some cases of "adult Kawasaki disease" may be TSS. Scarlet fever, Rocky Mountain spotted fever, leptospirosis, toxic epidermal necrolysis, sepsis, and measles must also be considered in the differential diagnosis.

PREVENTION AND TREATMENT. The low risk of acquiring TSS (6.2 cases/100,000 menstruating women) can be reduced by not using high-absorbency tampons or by using them intermittently during each menstrual period.

Management of adolescents suspected of having TSS includes the careful removal of any retained tampons at the time of taking initial samples for cervical and vaginal cultures. Fluid replacement should be aggressive to prevent or treat cardiovascular collapse. Inotropic agents may be needed to treat shock; corticosteroids are reserved for severe cases.

Parenteral administration of a B-lactamase–resistant antistaphylococcal antibiotic (e.g., nafcillin, oxacillin, methicillin) is recommended after appropriate cultures have been obtained. Culture of the vagina in menstrual TSS and of infected or colonized sites in nonmenstrual TSS is indicated. Antistaphylococcal therapy with methicillin, nafcillin, or oxacillin (150–200 mg/kg/24 hr, given in 4–6 divided doses [adult: 8–10 g/24 hr]) for 10–14 days does not affect the immediate outcome but prevents recurrence in menstrual TSS. Antibiotics and drainage are indicated for specific staphylococcal infections such as sinusitis or osteomyelitis. Alternative antibiotics for patients allergic to penicillin include clindamycin, erythromycin, rifampin, and trimethoprim-sulfamethoxazole.

RALPH D. FEIGIN

STAPHYLOCOCCUS AUREUS

Brumfitt W, Hamilton-Miller J: Methicillin-resistant *Staphylococcus aureus*. N Engl J Med 320:1188, 1989.

Eng RHK, Bishburg E, Smith SM, et al: *Staphylococcus aureus* bacteremia during therapy. J Infect Dis 155:1331, 1987.

Hodes DS, Barzilai A: Invasive and toxin mediated *Staphylococcus aureus* diseases in children. Adv Pediatr Infect Dis 5:35, 1990.
Kim JH, van der Horst C, Mulrow CD, et al: *Staphylococcus aureus* meningitis: Review of 28 cases. Rev Infect Dis 2:698, 1989.
Marrack P, Kappler: The staphylococcal enterotoxins and their relatives. Science 248:705, 1990.
Ribner BS: Endemic, multiply resistant *Staphylococcus aureus* in a pediatric population. Am J Dis Child 141:1183, 1987.

COAGULASE-NEGATIVE STAPHYLOCOCCUS

Boyce MJ, Potter-Bynoe G, Opal SM, et al: A common-source outbreak of *Staphylococcus epidermidis* infections among patients undergoing cardiac surgery. J Infect Dis 161:493, 1990.
Gruskay J, Harris MC, Costarino AT, et al: Neonatal *Staphylococcus epidermidis* meningitis with unremarkable CSF examination results. Am J Dis Child 143:580, 1989.
Latham RH, Running K, Stamm WE: Urinary tract infections in young adult women caused by *Staphylococcus saprophyticus*. JAMA 250:3063, 1983.
Patrick CC: Coagulase-negative staphylococci: Pathogens with increasing clinical significance. J Pediatr 116:497, 1990.
Patrick CC, Kaplan SL, Baker CJ, et al: Persistent bacteremia due to coagulase-negative staphylococci in low birth weight neonates. Pediatrics 84:977, 1989.
Younger JJ, Christensen GD, Bartley DL, et al: Coagulase-negative staphylococci isolated from cerebrospinal fluid shunts: Importance of slime production, species identification, and shunt removal to clinical outcome. J Infect Dis 156:548, 1987.

TOXIC SHOCK SYNDROME

Buchdahl R, Levin M, Wilkins B, et al: Toxic shock syndrome. Arch Dis Child 60:563, 1985.
Chesney PJ: Clinical aspects and spectrum of illness of toxic shock syndrome: Overview.Rev Infect Dis 11:51, 1989.
Ferguson MA, Todd JK: Toxic shock syndrome associated with *Staphylococcus aureus* sinusitis in children. J Infect Dis 161:953, 1990.
Williams GR: The toxic shock syndrome: Many cases are not associated with menstruation. Br Med J 300:960, 1990.

12.21 PNEUMOCOCCAL INFECTIONS

The pneumococcus *(Streptococcus pneumoniae)*, a normal inhabitant of the upper respiratory tract, can be an invasive pathogen. *S. pneumoniae* is the most common cause of community-acquired bacterial pneumonia and otitis media and the third most common cause of meningitis. The significance of this agent is accentuated by the emergence of penicillin-resistant and multidrug-resistant strains in many communities.

ETIOLOGY. *S. pneumoniae* is a gram-positive, lancet-shaped, encapsulated diplococcus. In body fluids and culture media the organisms may be found as individual cocci or as chains. Serotypes (84) are identified by their type-specific capsular polysaccharide. Antisera to some pneumococcal capsular polysaccharides cross-react with other pneumococcal types or with other bacterial species (e.g., *E. coli*, group B streptococcus, *H. influenzae* type b). Only smooth, encapsulated strains are pathogenic for humans. Virulence is related in part to the size of the capsule, but pneumococcal types with capsules of identical size may vary widely in virulence. Fully encapsulated strains (e.g., type 3) are extraordinarily virulent. Capsular material impedes phagocytosis; the mechanism is unclear.

On solid media, the pneumococcus forms unpigmented, umbilicated colonies surrounded by a zone of incomplete (α) hemolysis. Pneumococcal capsules can be seen and the organisms typed by exposing them to homologous type-specific antisera that combine with their respective capsular polysaccharides, thus rendering the capsules refractile (quellung reaction).

C substance is a cell-wall antigen that is related to species rather than to specific pneumococcal serotypes. It is a teichoic acid–containing phosphocholine and galactosamine-6-phosphate. C substance precipitates with an acute β-globulin, the C-reactive protein, which may activate complement and stimulate phagocytosis. R antigen is a species-specific protein on or near the cell surface. A *type*-specific protein (M antigen) also has been detected, but it does not confer significant antiphagocytic properties. Antibodies to the C, R, or M antigens produce negligible immunity. Antibodies to pneumococcal surface protein A (PspA) are protective against some pneumococcal strains when tested in mice. In humans, antibodies to the capsular polysaccharide are protective. The pneumococcus produces a hemolytic toxin called pneumolysin and a toxic neuraminidase. During autolysis pneumococci release a purpura-producing factor that causes dermal and internal hemorrhages when injected into rabbits. The role of these substances, if any, in the pathogenesis of human disease is unknown.

EPIDEMIOLOGY. Many healthy individuals carry *S. pneumoniae* in their upper respiratory tracts. As many as 91% of children between 6 mo and 4.5 yr of age carry *S. pneumoniae* at some time. Serotypes 6, 19, and 23 constitute 50% of all isolates in children. These, plus types 1, 4, 9, 11, 14, 15, and 18, account for 85% of all pneumococcal isolates. Frequently, the same serotype is carried continuously for extended periods (45 days–6 mo). Carriage of a particular serotype does not consistently induce local or systemic immunity sufficient to prevent later reacquisition of the same serotype. Multiple serotypes may coexist in the same nasopharynx. Pneumococcal isolation rates peak during the first 2 yr of life and decline gradually thereafter; carriage rates are highest in institutional settings and from December to April and lowest from July to September.

S. pneumoniae is the most frequent bacterial cause of bacteremia, pneumonia, and otitis media and the third most common cause of meningitis in infants and children. The peak incidence of meningitis occurs among infants 3–5 mo of age, that of otitis media from 6 to 12 mo, and that of hospitalization for pneumonia from 13 to 18 mo of age. The decreased ability to produce antibody to polysaccharide capsule antigens in children less than 2 yr of age may explain, in part, the increased susceptibility to pneumococcal infection and the decreased vaccine effectiveness in this age group. Males are more commonly affected than females, and native Americans and blacks more than whites; the unusual susceptibility of black children is not entirely explained by the increased risk associated with sickle cell disease.

Pneumococcal disease generally occurs sporadically. *S. pneumoniae* is spread from person to person by respiratory droplet transmission. Its frequency and severity are increased in patients with sickle cell disease, asplenia, splenosis, deficiencies in humoral (B cell) immunity, AIDS, malignancy (leukemia, lymphoma), and complement deficiencies.

PATHOGENESIS AND PATHOLOGY. Pneumococci must invade to produce disease. Nonspecific host defense mechanisms, including the presence of other bacteria in the nasopharynx, generally limit the multiplication of pneumococci. Aspiration of secretions containing pneumococci is hindered by the epiglottic reflex and by the cilia of the respiratory epithelium, which continuously move infected mucus upward toward the pharynx. Whether disease develops when pneumococci reach the alveoli depends on the outcome of the interaction of the bacteria with the alveolar macrophages. Pneumococci are highly resistant to phagocytosis by alveolar macrophages.

Pneumococcal disease frequently follows a viral respiratory tract infection that may produce mucosal damage, diminish the epithelial ciliary activity, and depress the function of alveolar macrophages. Phagocytosis may be impeded by respiratory secretions and the alveolar exudate. In the tissues pneumococci multiply and spread via the lymphatics or bloodstream (bacteremia) or by direct extension from a local site of infection.

The severity of disease is related to the virulence and

number of organisms causing bacteremia and to the integrity of specific host defenses. Generally, a poor prognosis correlates with very large numbers of pneumococci or significant concentrations of capsular polysaccharide in the circulation; despite effective antibiotic therapy, patients with heavy antigenemia may have severe and protracted illness.

Deficiency of the terminal components of complement (C3–C9) has been associated classically with recurrent pyogenic infection, which includes those caused by *S. pneumoniae*. C2 deficiency also appears to be associated with *S. pneumoniae* infection. The propensity for pneumococcal disease in asplenic persons is presumed to relate to deficient opsonization of the pneumococcus as well as to absence of the filtering function of the spleen on circulating bacteria. Pneumococcal disease is more prevalent in patients with sickle cell disease (Sec. 16.19) and other hemoglobinopathies. This risk is greatest in infants less than 2 yr of age when antibody production is attenuated. Patients with sickle cell anemia have a deficit in antibody-independent properden (alternate) pathway of complement activation. Properden deficiency and deficient antibody production result in defects in antibody-independent and antibody-dependent opsonophagocytosis of pneumococcus. With advancing age, patients with sickle cell anemia produce anticapsular antibody, thus augmenting antibody-dependent opsonophagocytosis and reducing but not eliminating the risk of severe pneumococcal disease.

The efficacy of phagocytosis also is diminished in patients with B and T cell immunodeficiency syndrome because of a lack of opsonic anticapsular antibody and a failure to produce lysis and agglutination of bacteria. These observations suggest (1) that opsonization of the pneumococcus depends on both the classic and the properdin (or alternative) complement pathways and (2) that recovery from pneumococcal disease depends on the development of anticapsular antibodies that act as opsonins, thus enhancing phagocytosis and ultimately killing the pneumococcus.

In the lung and other body tissues, the spread of infection is enhanced by the antiphagocytic properties of the pneumococcal capsule. The surface fluid of the respiratory tract contains only small amounts of IgG and is deficient in complement. Both are necessary for opsonization of encapsulated microorganisms. Once inflammation has been established in the lung, there is an influx of IgG, complement, and polymorphonuclear leukocytes (PMNs). Phagocytosis of bacteria by PMNs may be noted; however, even normal human serum may not be able to opsonize pneumococci to prepare them for phagocytosis by alveolar macrophages. Macrophages eventually replace the leukocytes in the exudate, and the lesion resolves. The sequence of events evolves over a period of 7–10 days but may be modified by appropriate antibiotic therapy or by the administration of *type*-specific serum. The pathologic sequence in pneumococcal pneumonia is detailed in Sec. 14.56.

CLINICAL MANIFESTATIONS. These are related to the site of infection; see pneumonia (Sec. 14.56), otitis media (Sec. 22.22), sinusitis and pharyngitis (Sec. 14.26 and 14.30), abscesses of the upper airway (Sec. 14.27–14.29), laryngotracheobronchitis (Sec. 14.43), peritonitis (Sec. 13.103), and bacteremia (Sec. 12.2). Local spread of infection may occur, causing empyema (Sec. 14.90), pericarditis (Sec. 15.75), mastoiditis (Sec. 14.56), epidural abscess (Sec. 12.15), or, rarely, meningitis. Colonizing pneumococci may spread through the eustachean tube, producing otitis media, and aspiration of infected pharyngeal secretions may produce pneumonia. Bacteremia may be followed by meningitis (Sec. 12.15), septic arthritis (Sec. 12.16), osteomyelitis (Sec. 12.16), endocarditis (Sec. 15.66), and brain abscess (Sec. 20.72).

The incidence of pneumococcal bacteremia, meningitis, endocarditis, and endophthalmitis is increasing in infants under 1 mo of age.

Renal glomerular-capillary and cortical arteriolar thromboses have been associated with pneumococcal bacteremia. Localized gingival lesions, gangrenous areas of skin on the face or extremities, immune complex glomerulonephritis, and disseminated intravascular coagulation also occur as manifestations of pneumococcal disease.

DIAGNOSIS. This may be established by recovery of pneumococci from the site of infection or the blood. However, pneumococci found in the nose or throat of patients with otitis media, pneumonia, septicemia, or meningitis may not be related causally to their disease.

Blood cultures should be obtained in all children with pneumonia, meningitis, arthritis, osteomyelitis, peritonitis, pericarditis, or gangrenous skin lesions. It is also advisable to obtain blood cultures in children 6–24 mo of age with high fever and leukocytosis who have no localized signs of infection. Pneumococcuria, in most instances, represents seeding of the urine from a remote site of pneumococcal infection.

Pneumococci can be identified in body fluids as gram-positive, lancet-shaped diplococci. A direct quellung test utilizing pneumococcal omniserum (containing high titers of antibody to 82 pneumococcal types) may help to establish a definitive diagnosis rapidly. Early in the course of pneumococcal meningitis, many bacteria may be noted in a relatively acellular cerebrospinal fluid. Countercurrent immunoelectrophoresis (CIE) of serum, sputum, cerebrospinal fluid, and urine, utilizing pneumococcal omniserum, may be helpful in establishing the diagnosis. The latex particle agglutination test is helpful in establishing a diagnosis rapidly; it is more sensitive than CIE for the detection of pneumococcal capsular polysaccharide antigen. The latex test is highly sensitive and specific for the diagnosis of pneumococcal meningitis or bacteremia. In patients with localized disease (nonbacteremic pneumonia, otitis media), the latex particle agglutination test is usually negative. The diagnosis of pneumococcal disease also may be established by evaluation of serum using an enzyme-linked immunosorbent assay (ELISA). This test detects antibodies, IgG and IgA, to pneumococcal hemolysin and is positive in up to 82% of patients with bacteremic pneumonia and in 45% of those with nonbacteremic pneumococcal pneumonia. There is no cross-reactivity with *H. influenzae, L. pneumophilia, Chlamydia psittaci*, or influenzae A virus; however, some patients with *M. pneumoniae* infection test positive for antibodies to pneumococcal hemolysin.

Leukocytosis generally is pronounced, with total white blood cell counts of 30,000/mm^3 a common occurrence. The sedimentation rate may be elevated.

PREVENTION. Polyvalent pneumococcal vaccines have proved to be immunologic and associated with few untoward reactions. However, responsiveness to pneumococcal polysaccharide is unpredictable in children under 2 yr of age. Currently, a 23-valent pneumococcal vaccine has been licensed that contains purified polysaccharide from 23 pneumococcal serotypes responsible for more than 95% of cases of bacteremia and meningitis and for 85% of cases of otitis media seen in children. The clinical efficacy of the vaccine is controversial, with several large studies producing conflicting results. In children, the mean postimmunization antibody titers following vaccine administration are, on the average, lower than those seen in healthy adults. A minimum titer of 300 ng/mL of antibody nitrogen for each serotype is considered necessary for protection. In addition, antigen 6A, 14, 19F, and 23F are poorly immunogenic in children under 6 yr of age. Pneumococcal serotype 6A is one of the strains most likely to produce disease in children. Reimmunization has been shown to increase antibody concentrations; however, routine reimmunization is not recommended currently because of the likelihood of more frequent and severe adverse reactions.

Currently, immunization is recommended for children over 2 yr of age who have sickle cell anemia, functional or anatomic asplenia, nephrotic syndrome, splenectomy following staging laparotomy for Hodgkin disease, CSF leaks, or HIV infection. Vaccine is not recommended for prevention of recurrent otitis media or sinusitis. Reimmunization may be given to particular high-risk patients; however, the optimum time interval between initial immunization and booster immunizations is unknown. Immunization will not prevent pneumococcal disease related to serotypes not found in the vaccine and invariably will not prevent infection from a pneumococcal strain that is serotypically identical to one of the vaccine strains. There have been many reports of serious and even fatal infections in vaccinated children.

For this reason, penicillin prophylaxis is still warranted in children at risk of pneumococcal sepsis. Penicillin V potassium (125 mg twice daily) substantially decreases the incidence of pneumococcal sepsis in children with sickle cell anemia. In addition, once monthly intramuscular benzathine penicillin is efficacious in preventing overwhelming sepsis. Erythromycin may be used in children with penicillin allergy. If oral prophylaxis is used, strict compliance must be encouraged and enforced. Testing the urine of patients for penicillin at each office visit is helpful in monitoring patient compliance.

Hyperimmune bacterial polysaccharide immune globulin may reduce the incidence of invasive pneumococcal disease in high-risk infants prior to the age of vaccination.

TREATMENT. Historically, penicillin has been the treatment of choice for pneumococcal infection. The incidences of relative and complete penicillin resistance and multiple drug resistance (penicillin, tetracycline, chloramphenicol, rifampin, erythromycin, sulfonamides, clindamycin) have increased during the last decade. Relative resistance varies between 2 and 15% in North America. Multiple resistant strains have been identified in South Africa, Spain, Great Britain, Australia, and the United States. Resistance to antibiotics is seen most often in the pneumococcal serotypes 6, 14, and 19F, the serotypes that most often cause disease in children.

Problems in treatment may be encountered by organisms that are relatively resistant to penicillin (MIC 0.1–1.0 mg/L), organisms that are highly resistant to penicillin (MIC > 1.0 mg/L), and organisms that are resistant to multiple antibiotics. Because of varying patterns of resistance, all isolates should be tested for sensitivity to antibiotics. The use of an oxacillin disk is the preferred method for measuring penicillin sensitivity because it identifies moderately resistant strains more specifically. Strains identified as moderately resistant to penicillin should be tested further to establish minimum inhibitory concentrations. Vancomycin resistance has not been reported.

Treatment of pneumococcal disease should be based on knowledge of susceptibility patterns seen in specific communities. Penicillin G is the drug of choice for penicillin-susceptible strains. Oral penicillin V (50–100 mg/kg/24 hr, every 6–8 hr) for minor infections, intravenous penicillin G (200,000–250,000 U/kg/24 hr, every 4–6 hr) for bacteremia or pneumonia, and intravenous penicillin G (300,000 U/kg/24 hr, every 4–6 hr) for meningitis are recommended. For serious infections with strains that are moderately resistant to penicillin but are sensitive to chloramphenicol (100 mg/kg/24 hr, given every 6 hr), the latter would be the treatment of choice. For highly penicillin resistant and for multiply resistant strains, vancomycin (60 mg/kg/24 hr, every 6 hr) is the treatment of choice. Newer third-generation cephalosporins, such as cefotaxime and ceftriaxone, have good in vitro activity against *S. pneumoniae*. However, there is little information concerning their use in vivo. In addition, there is a substantial increase in the MICs of the cephalosporins for *S. pneumoniae* isolates that are relatively resistant to penicillin compared with isolates that are fully sensitive to penicillin.

Erythromycin, cephalosporins, and chloramphenicol provide effective, alternative therapy for individuals who are allergic to penicillin. Tetracycline should not be used because many strains of pneumococci resistant to it have been reported.

PROGNOSIS. This depends on the integrity of host defenses, the virulence of the infecting organism, the age of the host, the site of infection, and the adequacy of treatment. See sections listed under Clinical Manifestations for specific diseases.

RALPH D. FEIGIN
CARRIE BYINGTON

Alario AJ, Nelson EW, Shapiro ED: Blood cultures in the management of febrile outpatients later found to have bacteremia. J Pediatr 115:195, 1989.

Bjornson A, Lobel J: Direct evidence that decreased serum opsonization of *Streptococcus pneumoniae* via the alternative complement pathway in sickle cell disease is related to antibody deficiency. J Clin Invest 79:388, 1987.

Davidson M, Schraer CD, Parkinson AJ, et al: Invasive pneumococcal disease in an Alaska native population, 1980 through 1986. JAMA 261:715, 1989.

Hansman D: Pneumococcal carriage amongst children in Adelaide, South Australia. Epidemiol Infect 101:411, 1988.

Henderson FW, Gilligan PH, Wait K, et al: Nasopharyngeal carriage of antibiotic-resistant pneumococci by children in group day care. J Infect Dis 157:256, 1988.

Immunization Practices Advisory Committee: Pneumococcal polysaccharide vaccine. MMWR 38:64, 1989.

Jonsson S, et al: Phagocytosis and killing of common bacterial pathogens of the lung by human alveolar macrophages. J Infect Dis 152:4, 1985.

Nair P: Incidence of decreased penicillin sensitivity of *Streptococcus pneumoniae* from clinical isolates. J Clin Pathol 41:720, 1988.

O'Neill KP, Lloyd-Evans N, Campbell H, et al: Latex agglutination test for diagnosing pneumococcal pneumonia in children in developing countries. Br Med J 298:1061, 1989.

Paton JC, Toogood IR, Cockington RA, et al: Antibody response to pneumococcal vaccine in children aged 5 to 15 years. Am J Dis Child 140:135, 1986.

Westh H, Skibsted L, Korner B: *Streptococcus pneumoniae* infections of the female genital tract and in the newborn child. Rev Infect Dis 12:416, 1990.

12.22 HAEMOPHILUS INFLUENZAE

EPIDEMIOLOGY AND PATHOGENESIS. *H. influenzae* is a fastidious, gram-negative, pleomorphic coccobacillus that requires factors X (hematin, heat stable) and V (phosphopyridine nucleotide, heat labile) for growth. Encapsulated strains are classifed by the polysaccharides of the soluble capsular substance and designated as types a through f. Almost all serious invasive infections in children are due to type b. Nonencapsulated strains (nontypable) are etiologic agents principally in upper respiratory tract infections, such as otitis media and sinusitis, but may also cause systemic infection in the neonate or in the immunocompromised child. *Haemophilus* is further classified biochemically into six biotypes; biotype 1 is the most common one isolated from blood and cerebrospinal fluid. *H. influenzae* type b can be further classified, using outer membrane proteins, into six major molecular weight categories that are useful for epidemiologic investigations. For example, utilizing this classification, it has been suggested that most children having recurrent invasive *H. influenzae* type b disease are reinfected with the same organism responsible for the first infection. The lipooligosaccharide of *H. influenzae* types is also an important virulence factor for which interstrain variation can be demonstrated by electrophoretic techniques.

Pili on the outer surface of *H. influenzae* type b isolates probably enhance their ability to colonize respiratory epithelial surfaces. In an organ culture of human nasopharyngeal tissue, *H. influenzae* type b organisms attach to nonciliated columnar epithelial cells and subsequently can be seen in intercellular spaces. Once past the epithelium, the organisms probably invade small blood vessels directly, leading to bacteremia in susceptible individuals. Once a critical density of organisms has been reached in the bloodstream for a sufficient period of time, dissemination of bacteria into other tissues can occur, causing focal infections such as meningitis or arthritis.

H. influenzae is usually endemic but may be responsible for outbreaks of disease, particularly in day-care centers or chronic care facilities. Day-care attendance and household crowding are associated with an increased risk of primary *H. influenzae* type b infection. For about 30 days after onset of *H. influenzae* meningitis, the risk in household contacts is 585 times greater than the age-adjusted risk in the general population. The greatest risk of a secondary case is 6% in contacts under 1 yr of age; the risk in children under 4 yr of age is 2%. Thus, the risk of secondary cases of *H. influenzae* infection in household contacts under the age of 6 yr is very similar to the risk of secondary meningococcal disease in household contacts. The risk of secondary *H. influenzae* type b infection in day-care centers is less than that for household contacts. *H. influenzae* type b meningitis occurs more commonly in black and American Indian children than in white children; Hispanics have a rate of infection 1.6 times that of whites. The highest incidence of systemic disease occurs among Alaskan Eskimos: 491 cases/100,000 children below 5 yr of age. Children with asplenia (congenital, surgical, and functional, as in sickle cell anemia) are also at great risk of acquiring serious *H. influenzae* infections.

Antibodies directed against the capsular polysaccharide play an important role in host defense. Antipolyribophosphate (PRP) antibody is related in part to the opsonic activity of serum for *H. influenzae* type b; other antibodies directed against non-PRP antigens, such as outer membrane proteins, also play a role in opsonization. Both the classic and alternative complement pathways are important in the opsonization of *H. influenzae* type b. In addition, the macrophages of the reticuloendothelial system are critical components in the intravascular clearance of *H. influenzae* type b. Less is known about immunity to nontypable strains of *H. influenzae*, although antibody to some outer membrane proteins appear protective in animal models.

Children 18 mo of age or less demonstrate a poor or absent immunologic response to PRP antibody following either natural infection or immunization with *H. influenzae* type b capsular polysaccharide. Young children do not respond well to polysaccharide vaccines partly because purified polysaccharides are T cell–independent antigens. Anti-PRP response to both natural infection and immunization appears to be partly under genetic control. When immunized with type b polyribosephosphate vaccine, children with allotype Km(1) fail to respond with antibody production to the extent noted in children without this allotype. The converse is true for meningococcus C polysaccharide vaccine. The frequency of the erythrocyte genotype MNSs is increased in children with *H. influenzae* type b epiglottitis compared with that in children with meningitis.

INFECTIONS DUE TO HAEMOPHILUS INFLUENZAE TYPE B

H. influenzae type b accounts for approximately 95% of serious infections due to *H. influenzae.* Other typable and nontypable strains infrequently account for serious systemic diseases but are commonly isolated from children with otitis media. The rapid diagnosis of *H. influenzae* type b can be accomplished by several laboratory techniques to detect capsular polysaccharide including CIE, latex particle agglutination, staphylococcal protein A coagglutination (Co-A), and ELISA.

MENINGITIS (see Sec. 12.15). *H. influenzae* type b is the leading cause of bacterial meningitis in the United States in children between the ages of 1 mo and 4 yr. Clinically, meningitis due to *H. influenzae* cannot be distinguished from that due to *N. meningitidis* or *S. pneumoniae* and may be complicated by other infections due to this organism including pneumonia, arthritis, osteomyelitis, pericarditis, and endophthalmitis.

ACUTE EPIGLOTTITIS (see Sec. 14.43). This dramatic, potentially lethal condition usually occurs in children 2–7 yr old.

PNEUMONIA (see Sec. 14.53). The true incidence of *H. influenzae* pneumonia in children is unknown, but it appears to be more common in children 4 yr of age or less. The signs and symptoms of pneumonia due to *H. influenzae* cannot be distinguished from those due to other micro-organisms, and associated infections such as otitis media, meningitis, and epiglottitis are common.

SEPTIC ARTHRITIS (see Sec. 12.17). *H. influenzae* type b is the most common organism responsible for septic arthritis in children 2 yr of age or less. Large joints, such as knee, hip, ankle, and elbow, are affected most commonly, and associated infections such as meningitis commonly occur. The signs and symptoms of septic arthritis due to *H. influenzae* type b are indistinguishable from those due to other organisms.

CELLULITIS. *H. influenzae* type b is responsible for 5–14% of the cases of cellulitis in young children; over 85% of children with this type of cellulitis are 2 yr of age or younger. Frequently, these children have an upper respiratory infection that is followed by the acute onset of cellulitis. There is usually no prior history of trauma to the area of cellulitis. The head and neck, particularly the cheek and periorbital region, are the most common sites of infection. The lesion has generally indistinct margins and is tender and indurated. A violaceous or bluish-purple color is common but not diagnostic. In buccal cellulitis an ipsilateral otitis media may be the focus of infection. Other infections such as meningitis and septic arthritis may complicate cellulitis. Blood cultures are positive, and *H. influenzae* type b may often be recovered directly from an aspirate with or without prior injection of 0.1 mL of a nonbacteriostatic sterile solution into the cellulitis. Cellulitis should be treated with an appropriate intravenous antibiotic until the patient is afebrile and the cellulitis has resolved; antibiotics should be continued until approximately 1 wk after all signs and symptoms have resolved.

OSTEOMYELITIS (see Sec. 12.16). *H. influenzae* type b is a relatively uncommon cause of osteomyelitis in children.

PERICARDITIS (see also Sec. 15.75). *H. influenzae* type b is the etiologic agent of bacterial pericarditis in up to 15% of children with this infection. The children are most commonly 2–4 yr of age and often have had an antecedent upper respiratory infection. Fever, respiratory distress, and tachycardia are constant findings. Associated infections also are very common. The etiologic diagnosis may be established by blood culture or by culture, Gram stain, or antigen detection of pericardial fluid. Antibiotics should be provided intravenously at dosages and for a duration similar to those used for meningitis (Sec. 12.15). A pericardiectomy may be important to drain the purulent material effectively and prevent pericardial tamponade and constrictive pericarditis.

BACTEREMIA WITHOUT AN ASSOCIATED FOCUS (see Sec. 12.2 and 12.14). Bacteremia due to *H. influenzae* type b may occur without any apparent focus of infection other than signs of an upper respiratory infection or pharyngitis. Although affected children may appear only mildly ill at the initial visit, they are at substantial risk of developing a serious infection such as pneumonia or bacterial meningitis.

NEONATAL DISEASE (see Sec. 9.60 and 9.63). In the neonate nontypable *H. influenzae* is more common than type b. When illness occurs in the first 24 hr of life, especially in association with maternal amnionitis or prolonged rupture of membranes, transmission of the organism to the infant is likely through the maternal genital tract. Septicemia, pneumonia, and respiratory distress syndrome with shock, conjunctivitis, scalp abscess or cellulitis, meningitis, mastoiditis, septic arthritis, and a congenital vesicular eruption have been reported.

MISCELLANEOUS INFECTIONS. Urinary tract infection, epididymo-orchitis, cervical adenitis, acute glossitis, uvulitis, infected thyroglossal duct cysts, endocarditis, primary peritonitis, and periappendiceal abscess have been associated with *H. influenzae*.

OTITIS MEDIA (see Sec. 22.22). Otitis media and conjunctivitis occurring simultaneously are usually due to nontypable *H. influenzae*.

TREATMENT. The initial empiric antibiotic therapy of invasive infections (not otitis media or sinusitis) possibly due to *H. influenzae* type b should include an agent effective against ampicillin-resistant strains, which are almost all due to the production of a β-lactamase enzyme. Approximately 20–40% of *H. influenzae* type b strains isolated from normally sterile sites are ampicillin resistant, but the prevalence of ampicillin resistance varies throughout the United States. Isolates of *H. influenzae* type b resistant to chloramphenicol (mediated by chloramphenicol acetyltransferase) or resistant to both ampicillin and chloramphenicol are still relatively rare in the United States, although they are common in other parts of the world such as Spain.

Cefotaxime or ceftriaxone should be used as the initial antibiotic when *H. influenzae* type b is considered a likely pathogen, mainly due to their lack of serious adverse effects and ease of administration. See Sec. 12.15 for dosages.

Once the antimicrobial susceptibility of the *H. influenzae* type isolate has been determined, an appropriate parenteral agent can be selected to complete the therapy. Ampicillin remains the drug of choice for ampicillin-susceptible strains. Ceftriaxone can be administered once daily in selected circumstances, which facilitates outpatient management of patients with certain *H. influenzae* type b infections. In many instances one of several oral antibiotics (amoxicillin, amoxicillin clavulanate, cefuroxime axetil, trimethoprim-sulfamethoxazole) can be administered to complete antibiotic therapy.

PREVENTION. The *H. influenzae* type b capsular polysaccharide conjugate vaccines are more immunogenic than the polysaccharide alone in young children, presumably because of the recruitment of T cells, which help to promote antibody production by B cells. The three currently licensed conjugate vaccines are the *H. influenzae* type b capsular polysaccharide-diphtheria toxoid (PRP-D, Prohibit), *H. influenzae* type b oligosaccharide, CRM_{197}, a nontoxic mutant protein that is antigenically identical to diphtheria toxin (HbOC, HibTiter), and *H. influenzae* type b outer membrane protein capsular polysaccharide (PRP-OMP), which consists of a complex of the capsular polysaccharide of *H. influenzae* type b and outer membrane proteins of *N. meningitidis*. See Sec. 5.1 for schedules of administration.

Since the risk for secondary infection due to *H. influenzae* type b is equivalent to that of *N. meningitidis*, antibiotic prophylaxis may prevent secondary cases. Rifampin is recommended for all family contacts of individuals with *H. influenzae* type b disease if there are other children besides the index case less than 4 yr old residing in the home; children should be given rifampin orally in a 20 mg/kg dose once daily (not to exceed 600 mg/day) for 4 consecutive days. The adult dose is 600 mg once daily. Parents of children having invasive *H. influenzae* type b disease should be told that there is an increased risk of secondary infection due to this organism in other young children in the same household, should be alerted to any signs or symptoms that might be related to such an infection, and should be instructed to seek prompt medical attention when such signs do appear. Parents of children exposed to a single case of systemic *H. influenzae* type b disease in a day-care center or nursery school should be similarly warned. Rifampin should be administered to all children with invasive *H. influenzae* type b infections prior to or just after completing antibiotic therapy, since nasopharyngeal colonization is not reliably eradicated by the agents used for treatment of the infection.

SHELDON L. KAPLAN
RALPH D. FEIGIN

Bieger RC, Brewer NS, Washington JA: *Haemophilus aphrophilus:* A microbiologic and clinical review and report of 42 cases. Medicine 57:345, 1978.

Committee on Infectious Diseases: *Haemophilus influenzae* type b conjugate vaccines: Recommendations for immunization of infants and children 2 months of age and older: Update. Pediatrics 1991 (in press).

Dajani AS, Asmar BI, Thirmoorthi MC: Systemic *Haemophilus influenzae* disease: An overview. J Pediatr 94:355, 1979.

Echeverria P, Smith EWP, Ingram D, et al: *Haemophilus influenzae* b pericarditis in children. Pediatrics 56:808, 1975.

Eskola J, Peltola H, Takala AK, et al: Efficacy of *Haemophilus influenzae* type b polysaccharide-diphtheria toxoid conjugate vaccine in infancy. N Engl J Med 317:717, 1987.

Faden HS: Treatment of *Haemophilus influenzae* type b epiglottitis. Pediatrics 63:402, 1979.

Frenkel LD and the Multicenter Ceftriaxone Pediatric Study Group: Once-daily administration of ceftriaxone for the treatment of selected serious bacterial infections in children. Pediatrics 82:486, 1988.

Ginsburg CM, Howard JB, Nelson JD: Report of 65 cases of *Haemophilus influenzae* b pneumonia. Pediatrics 64:283, 1979.

Granoff DM, Boise EG, Squires JE, et al: Histocompatibility leukocyte antigen and erythrocyte MNSs specificities in patients with meningitis or epiglottitis due to *Haemophilus influenzae* type b. J Infect Dis 149:373, 1984.

Granoff DM, Daum RS: Spread of *Haemophilus influenzae* type b: Recent epidemiologic and therapeutic considerations. J Pediatr 97:854, 1980.

Kenny JF, Isburg CD, Michaels RH: Meningitis due to *Haemophilus influenzae* type b resistant to both ampicillin and chloramphenicol. Pediatrics 66:14, 1980.

Lilian LD, Yeh TF, Novack GM, et al: Early onset *Haemophilus influenzae* sepsis in newborn infants: Clinical, roentgenographic and pathologic features. Pediatrics 62:299, 1978.

Marshall R, Teele DW, Klein JD: Unsuspected bacteremia due to *Haemophilus influenzae:* Outcome in children not initially admitted to hospital. J Pediatr 95:690, 1979.

Mason EO, Kaplan SL, Lamberth LB, et al: Serotype and ampicillin susceptibility of *Haemophilus influenzae* causing systemic infections in children: 3 years of experience. J Clin Microbiol 15:543, 1982.

Ward JI, Fraser DW, Baraff LJ, et al: *Haemophilus influenzae* meningitis. A national study of secondary spread of household contacts. N Engl J Med 301:122, 1979.

12.23 MENINGOCOCCAL INFECTIONS

Neisseria meningitidis (meningococcus) is a gram-negative, biscuit-shaped diplococcus found only in man; it has not been isolated from animal or environmental sources. Most strains are fastidious, and growth is facilitated by incubation on blood, chocolate, Mueller Hinton, or trypticase soy agar in 5–10% CO_2.

ETIOLOGY. The organism is transmitted via aerosolization or contact with respiratory secretions. Disease occurs when organisms invade the bloodstream (meningococcemia) and then disseminate. The bacteria commonly are observed within polymorphonuclear leukocytes obtained from infected areas. Strains are divided into at least 13 serogroups by the surface capsular polysaccharides—A, B, C, D, 29E, H, I, K, L, W135, X, Y, and Z—and into types by the outer membrane proteins. Isolates from patients with meningococcal disease belong almost exclusively to 5 of these serogroups (A, B, C, and, less frequently, W135 and Y), whereas the other groups are isolated predominantly from carriers. The cell walls of meningococci contain lipopolysaccharide, which appears to be responsible for the endotoxin-like effect noted in some patients with meningococcemia.

EPIDEMIOLOGY. Meningococcal infections are common

in temperate and tropical climates. Epidemics of meningococcal meningitis have occurred in cyclic waves approximately every decade since the beginning of this century. Outbreaks may be due to a predominant genetic clone in the absence of herd immunity in a susceptible population. The greatest incidence occurs in winter and spring, but sporadic cases appear throughout the year in both rural and urban areas. Males are affected more often than females by a 3:2 ratio.

Carriage rates of *N. meningitidis* vary from 2–5% in healthy children to as high as 90% in groups of military personnel during epidemics. Meningococcal meningitis generally is a disease of children who acquire the organism from an adult carrier, usually in the same family. The disease has occurred following exposure to carriers or infected individuals in day-care centers and closed populations such as military camps. The estimated likelihood of meningococcal disease in family contacts, usually occurring simultaneously with the first case, is 1%. This rate is 1,000-fold greater than the risk in the community. The risk of meningitis in day-care center contacts of children with meningococcal disease is 1/1,000. Disease occurs most frequently in children less than 5 yr old, with a peak attack rate in the 6- to 12-mo age group. Children under 3 mo of age rarely develop meningococcal disease. A second peak attack rate occurs between 15 and 19 yr of age.

In the United States, serogroup A disease initially was the most prevalent. Currently, the serogroups encountered most frequently include B, C, W135, and Y. Epidemics caused by serogroups A and C occur in closed populations, whereas serogroup B disease continues to be endemic.

PATHOGENESIS. Initially, meningococci colonize the nasopharynx. Hematogenous dissemination occurs when the organism penetrates a mucosal surface and is transported by leukocytes to the bloodstream. It then localizes in other organs, including lungs, joints, meninges, heart, ears, eyes, and adrenal glands. Bactericidal antibodies directed against both capsular polysaccharide and outer membrane surface components in the form of circulating serum antibodies and specific secretory IgA seem to be important in protecting the human host from disease. Group-specific antimeningococcal antibody accumulates following prolonged carriage of meningococci. The common occurrence of antigenic shift in pilus expression and in surface antigen expression may enable meningococci to evade the host defenses and could explain the persistence of nasopharyngeal carriage despite the presence of the host immune response. Nasopharyngeal carriage of nontypable meningococci and of serogroups X, Y, and Z or lactose-fermenting meningococci also evokes the production of bactericidal antibodies against groups A, B, and C. Bactericidal antibodies that cross-react with meningococci also may be induced by contact with unrelated gram-positive and gram-negative enteric organisms. The fetus may receive antibodies transplacentally; these persist up to the 3rd mo of life, after which they are generally undetectable until approximately 8 mo of age. Subsequently, there is a gradual rise in the prevalence of antibodies; in one study 97% of children over 5 yr of age had detectable antibody levels. Group-specific, hemagglutinating antibody has been detected in nasal washings of patients following recovery from meningococcal disease. Development of group-specific, antimeningococcal secretory IgA antibody is associated with enhancement of the pharyngeal defense mechanism.

Factors that increase susceptibility to meningococcal disease include overcrowding, poor general health and living conditions, influenza, sickle cell disease, and absence of serum bactericidal activity against the meningococcus (antibody, complement, properdin). Increased virulence is associated with serogroups A, B, and C, serotypes 2 and 15/16, and resistance to sulfadiazine. Virulence factors include pili, antiphagocytic capsules, lipopolysaccharides (endotoxins), leukocyte-activating factor, a surface protein associated with decreased phagocytosis and serum-killing resistance, and possibly a major iron-related protein expressed by pathogenic *Neisseria* species. Protein and peptide hydrolases, including an IgA protease, may also be involved in the pathogenicity of the organism. These proteases may be involved in induction of disease, spread of the infecting bacteria, or maintenance of an environment suitable for proliferation of the microbial pathogen.

PATHOLOGY. Disease due to *N. meningitidis* is associated with an acute inflammatory response. Endotoxemia may be associated with release of interleukins and tumor necrosis factor, diffuse vasculitis, complement activation, and disseminated intravascular coagulation. Small blood vessels may be filled with leukocyte-rich fibrin clots. Hemorrhage and necrosis may be noted in any organ system; bleeding into the adrenals may occur in patients with septicemia and shock (Waterhouse-Friderichsen syndrome). Release of inflammatory mediators, due to endotoxemia, may produce hypotension and multisystem organ failure manifest as coma, adult respiratory distress syndrome, and acute tubular necrosis.

Meningococcal infections have been noted to occur more frequently in patients with agammaglobulinemia, inherited deficiencies of properdin components and the late terminal complement components (C5–C8, the membrane attached component), and diseases that consume complement, including systemic lupus erythematosus, multiple myeloma, and circulating C3 nephritic factor disorder. Acquired complement deficiencies, such as that noted secondary to hepatic failure, also predispose to meningococcal infections, as does absence of protective IgG or IgM antibodies or the presence of IgA antibodies that block serum bactericidal reactions. Fulminant disease also has been described in patients lacking properdin, C3, the combination of C7 and C46, and the IgG2 subclass. Statistically, the presence of the HLA B27 complex predisposes the patient to meningococcal infections.

CLINICAL MANIFESTATIONS. Patterns of meningococcal disease include bacteremia without sepsis, meningococcemic sepsis without meningitis, meningitis with or without sepsis, meningoencephalitis, and focal organ infections. The incubation period of meningococcal diseases varies from 2 to 10 days, after which varied clinical presentations occur. Upper respiratory infection with or without bacteremia is common during epidemics of meningococcal infections. It is a self-limited disorder and resolves within days and without sequelae. Some of these patients have occult or unexpected meningococcemia without sepsis. A maculopapular rubella-like exanthem may occur in some affected children. Meningococcal disease also may present with predominantly gastrointestinal symptoms including nausea, vomiting, abdominal pain, and back pain.

Acute meningococcemia may occur initially as an influenza-like illness with fever, malaise, myalgias, arthralgias, headache, and gastrointestinal complaints. Within hours petechial, purpuric, or morbilliform lesions may develop, with subsequent hypotension, disseminated intravascular coagulation, oliguria, renal failure, and coma. Fulminant meningococcemia may occur with rapidly progressive purpura and relentless shock, often with adrenal hemorrhage and extensive hematogenous dissemination that is unresponsive to treatment. Most commonly, acute meningitis is nonfulminant, varies in severity, has a low incidence of associated seizures or focal neurologic signs, and is responsive to appropriate antibiotics and supportive therapy. Meningococcemia may present as an acute immune complex vasculitis with diffuse arthralgias and myalgias that resemble drug hypersensitivity that has been treated with steroids; subsequently, some of these patients have developed fulminant disease.

Dissemination to many different sites can occur during

acute meningococcemia. If the meninges become seeded, the classic signs and symptoms of meningitis occur, including fever, malaise, headache, nuchal rigidity, nausea, vomiting, various degrees of disorientation, and mental depression leading to coma. Rare presentations include acute cerebellar ataxia, subarachnoid hemorrhage, brain abscess, and acute bilateral deafness. Rarely, brain involvement is severe and diffuse, resulting in an encephalitic picture. Endocarditis, myocarditis, myocardial failure, and pericarditis tend to be associated with acute meningococcemia. Primary meningococcal pneumonia has been described, and 15% of patients with this disorder also develop pleural effusions or empyema. Primary pericarditis may lead to tamponade. Primary arthritis, which is usually monoarticular, often involves the knee. Rarely, the eye is involved, either alone or with concomitant bacteremia; episcleritis, neonatal conjunctivitis, endophthalmitis, panophthalmitis, conjunctivitis in older children and adults, or periorbital cellulitis may occur. Also, rarely, cervicitis, vulvovaginitis, urethritis, pelvic inflammatory disease, orchitis, epididymitis, osteomyelitis, and radiculitis may be due to *N. meningitidis.*

Immunologic effects usually occur later in the course of the illness, often during recovery, when chemotherapy may have been completed. The effects probably are caused by circulating immune complexes and may be manifest by rash, polyarthropathy, fever, and pericarditis. Conus medullaris syndrome and neuropathies (of cranial nerves VI–VIII) have been noted during recovery.

Chronic meningococcemia is an unusual condition seen in both children and adults; it is characterized by low-grade fever, rash, and joint symptoms lasting longer than a week. The rash resembles that seen in disseminated gonococcal infections. Blood cultures usually are positive for *N. meningitidis.* The mean duration of illness is 6–8 wk, and it is characterized by waxing and waning symptoms including purulent arthritis, acute nonsuppurative polyarthritis, erythema nodosum, upper respiratory infections, and subacute endocarditis. Chronic meningococcal meningitis has been associated with C5 deficiency, a condition previously described only with recurrent meningococcal disease.

DIAGNOSIS. Meningococcal disease should be suspected in any patient with fever, petechiae, and abnormal mental status. The definitive diagnosis of meningococcal disease is established by a positive culture of blood, cerebrospinal fluid, skin lesion, or other site of infection. Cultures should also be taken from the nasopharynx, but isolation of meningococci from this site provides only presumptive evidence of infection. Petechial or papular lesions can be lanced and smeared to look for gram-negative diplococci. Blood cultures are positive in most patients with sepsis and in 50–60% of those with meningitis. Occasionally, bacteria can be seen on Gram stain of the buffy coat layer of a spun blood sample. Acridine orange stain is even more sensitive in detecting bacteria in any of these clinical specimens. It is particularly efficacious in detecting bacteria in body fluids obtained from partially treated patients and in normally sterile body fluids. Meningococcal organisms can be recovered from samples of peritoneal dialysis effluent that were sterile on conventional culture after lysis of the white blood cells in the fluid with 10% saponin. This technique can be applied to other body fluids in which these intracellular organisms may be present.

When meningitis is present, the morphologic and clinical characteristics of cerebrospinal fluid are those of acute bacterial meningitis (Sec. 12.15). Cerebrospinal fluid culture may be positive in the absence of clinical meningitis or CSF pleocytosis. Cerebrospinal fluid culture may be negative if the lumbar puncture has been performed early in the course of disease or if the patient has received previous antibiotic treatment. Meningococci, especially of groups A and C, show capsular swelling (quelling) upon exposure of positive CSF to specific antiserum.

Blood, CSF, and urine also can be evaluated by CIE and latex particle agglutination tests, which detect capsular antigen whether or not the organism is viable. Commercially available antisera for *N. meningitidis* types A, C, D, W135, X, Y, and Z are effective, whereas antisera for group B meningococci are unreliable. Radioimmunoassay also can be used but is not suitable as a routine test. A high-affinity IgG monoclonal antibody to meningococcal group B polysaccharide is available to evaluate serum samples from patients by different methods, including bactericidal assay, hemagglutination assay, ELISA with polysaccharide antigens, and solid-phase radioimmunosorbent assay. In patients with chronic meningococcemia, the levels of IgG and IgA antibodies against group B can be determined by ELISA using the whole bacteria as the antigen and have been found to be elevated.

Ancillary data may reveal an increased sedimentation rate and C-reactive protein, thrombocytopenia, leukocytosis, proteinuria, and hematuria. In patients with disseminated intravascular coagulation, decreased serum concentrations of prothrombin, factors V and VIII, and fibrinogen may be observed. Once the diagnosis of meningococcal disease has been established, CH_{50} screens should be obtained in all patients; if these results are abnormal, specific complement deficiencies should be determined.

DIFFERENTIAL DIAGNOSIS. This includes acute bacterial or viral meningitis, mycoplasma infection, leptospirosis, syphilis, acute hemorrhagic encephalitis, encephalopathies, serum sickness, collagen vascular diseases, Henoch-Schönlein purpura, hemolytic uremic syndrome, and ingestion of various poisons. The petechial or purpuric rash of meningococcemia is similar to that noted in any patient with a disease characterized by generalized vasculitis. These diseases include septicemia due to many gram-negative organisms; overwhelming septicemia with gram-positive organisms; bacterial endocarditis; Rocky Mountain spotted fever; epidemic typhus; *Ehrlichia canis* infection; infections with echoviruses, particularly types 6, 9, and 16; coxsackievirus infections, predominantly of types A2, A4, A9, and A16; rubella; rubeola and atypical rubeola; Henoch-Schönlein purpura; Kawasaki disease; idiopathic thrombocytopenia; and erythema multiforme or erythema nodosum due to drugs or infectious or noninfectious disease processes. The morbilliform rash occasionally observed may be confused with any macular or maculopapular viral exanthem.

COMPLICATIONS. Acute complications are due to the inflammatory response, secondary to infection, and hypoxic-ischemic organ injury, secondary to hypotension, myocardial failure, and shock. Late complications are sequelae of acute problems but may also be due to disposition of sterile immune complexes in joints or the pericardium. Meningococcal meningitis may be complicated rarely by deafness, ataxia, seizures, blindness, paresis of cranial nerves III, IV, VI, and VII, hemiparesis or quadriparesis, spinal cord infarction, obstructive hydrocephalus, transient or permanent diabetes insipidus, and brain abscess. Transient hemiballismus has been described in an infant.

Meningococcemia may be complicated by adrenal hemorrhage, encephalitis, arthritis, myocarditis, pericarditis, pneumonia, lung abscess, peritonitis, renal infarcts, disseminated intravascular coagulation, and peripheral neuropathy. The vasculitis seen with meningococcal disease can lead to skin loss, which is frequently complicated by secondary infection under the eschar and ultimately results in tissue necrosis and gangrene. Although rare, widespread bone infarctions can lead to growth disturbance and late skeletal deformities secondary to epiphyseal avascular necrosis and epiphyseal-metaphyseal defects. Vitreous collapse with secondary retinal detachment may occur.

Immune complex arthritis, vasculitis, episcleritis, and pericarditis may occur after 5 or more days of therapy and can be treated with anti-inflammatory agents and, if needed, arthrocentesis or pericardiocentesis.

PREVENTION. Exposed household, school, or day-care contacts should be observed carefully and brought to medical attention immediately if they become febrile. They should receive chemoprophylaxis as soon as possible, ideally within 24 hr of diagnosis of the primary case. Schoolroom contacts and medical personnel (except those with intimate exposure, that is, mouth-to-mouth resuscitation) do not require chemoprophylaxis. The drug of choice is rifampin (10 mg/kg [up to 600 mg] every 12 hr for 48 hr); sulfisoxazole (birth–1 yr, 500 mg/24 hr; 1–12 yr, 500 mg twice a day; 12 yr and up, 1 g twice a day; all given for 48 hr) may be used for the unusual organism that is susceptible to sulfonamides. Ceftriaxone (250 mg for adults, 125 mg for children: 1 dose) and ciprofloxacin (500 mg orally every 12 hr for 5 days in adolescents) are alternative choices for chemoprophylaxis. Meningococcal vaccine can be used with chemoprophylaxis because secondary cases may occur several weeks after the index case. Penicillin in dosage regimens practical for ambulatory patients is not effective prophylaxis for meningococcal disease.

Several meningococcal polysaccharide vaccines are licensed in the United States: monovalent A, bivalent groups A and C, and quadrivalent groups A, C, Y, and W135. An effective meningococcal serogroup B vaccine has not been prepared, but a new protein-linked vaccine is currently under investigation. Group C vaccine is effective in preventing meningococcal disease in children 2 yr of age or older and is recommended as an adjunct to chemoprophylaxis for these children if they are exposed within the household or day-care nursery to a confirmed case of serogroup C meningococcal disease. Meningococcal serogroup A vaccine is considered adjunctive therapy to chemoprophylaxis for children 3 mo of age or older who are exposed within the household or day-care facility to a confirmed case of serogroup A disease. Quadrivalent vaccine should be administered routinely to children 2 yr old and older if they are at increased risk for meningococcal disease (e.g., if they have functional or anatomic asplenia or terminal complement or properdin component deficiencies) and may be given as an adjunct to chemoprophylaxis for any exposed individual.

The quadrivalent vaccine should be used to control outbreaks of the disease caused by serogroups A, C, Y, and W135 and could benefit travelers to countries in which hyperendemic or epidemic disease has been reported. Vaccination with quadrivalent vaccine may elicit an immunologic response to type C in infants as young as 6 mo. A booster dose is needed 3 mo after the primary immunization. Quadrivalent vaccine currently is administered to all United States military recruits.

TREATMENT. *N. meningitidis* strains relatively resistant to penicillin have occasionally been recovered from blood or CSF. Therefore, cultures and sensitivities are the best method of choosing appropriate therapy. Aqueous penicillin G, 300,000 U/kg/24 hr, should be given intravenously in 6 divided doses, if the organism is sensitive to penicillin. Chloramphenicol sodium succinate, 100 mg/kg/24 hr intravenously in 4 divided doses, provides effective treatment for patients allergic to penicillin. Cefotaxime (200 mg/kg/24 hr) and ceftriaxone (100–150 mg/kg/24 hr) are effective empiric therapy for meningococcal disease and may be useful in patients who are allergic to penicillin. Therapy is continued for 7 days. Shorter courses (4–5 days) of antibiotics have been reported to be effective; however, more data are needed before short-course therapy can be recommended.

Patients with acute meningococcal infections should be monitored carefully. Supportive care and other therapy are discussed in Sec. 12.15.

PROGNOSIS. Mortality from acute meningococcemia may be as high as 15–20%. Mortality of patients with meningococcal meningitis is less than 5% in most major medical centers. Poor prognostic signs include extremes of age; development of hypotension; respiratory, cardiac, or renal failure; coma; rapidly progressive purpura; disseminated intravascular coagulation; thrombocytopenia; leukopenia; low CSF polymorphonuclear leukocyte count; high serum antigen concentrations; and a low sedimentation rate.

RALPH D. FEIGIN
REBECCA SNIDER

Brandtzaeg P, Mollnes TE, Kierulf P: Complement activation and endotoxin levels in systemic meningococcal disease. J Infect Dis 160:58, 1989.

Emparanza JI, Aldamiz-Echevarria L, Perez-Yarza EG, et al: Prognostic score in acute meningococcemia. Crit Care Med 16:168, 1988.

Havens PL, Garland JS, Brook MM, et al: Trends in mortality in children hospitalized with meningococcal infections, 1957 to 1987. Pediatr Infect Dis J 8:8, 1989.

Leggiadro RJ: Prevalence of complement deficiencies in children with systemic meningococcal infections. Pediatr Infect Dis J 6:75, 1987.

Mahdig TM, Evans-Jones G: Ophthalmitis in meningococcal disease. Arch Dis Child 63:550, 1988.

Pugsley MP, Dworzack DL, Horowitz EA, et al: Efficacy of ciprofloxacin in the treatment of nasopharyngeal carriers of *Neisseria meningitidis*. J Infect Dis 156:211, 1987.

Ross SC, Densen P: Complement deficiency states and infection: Epidemiology, pathogenesis and consequences of neisserial and other infections in an immune deficiency. Medicine 63:243, 1984.

Schwartz B, Al-Ruwais A, A'ashi J, et al: Comparative efficacy of ceftriaxone and rifampicin in eradicating pharyngeal carriage of group A *Neisseria meningitidis*. Lancet 1:1239, 1988.

Welsby PD, Golledge CL: Meningococcal meningitis: A diagnosis not to be missed. Br Med J 300:1150, 1990.

Wong VK, Hitchcock W, Mason WH: Meningococcal infections in children: A review of 100 cases. Pediatr Infect Dis J 8:224, 1989.

12.24 GONOCOCCAL INFECTIONS

Neisseria gonorrhoeae produces various forms of gonorrhea, an infection of the genitourinary tract mucous membranes and rarely of the mucosae of the rectum, oropharynx, and conjunctiva. Gonorrhea transmitted by sexual contact or perinatally is the most frequent communicable disease reported in the United States and affects children of all ages. This high prevalence and the development of antibiotic-resistant strains have produced significant morbidity in adolescents.

ETIOLOGY. *N. gonorrhoeae* is a nonmotile, aerobic, nonspore-forming, gram-negative intracellular diplococcus with flattened adjacent surfaces. Optimal growth occurs at 35–37° C and at pH 7.2–7.6 in an atmosphere of 3–5% CO_2. The specimen should be inoculated immediately into fresh, moist modified Thayer-Martin or specialized transport (Transgrow) media because gonococci do not tolerate drying. Presumptive identification may be based on colony appearance, Gram stain, and production of cytochrome oxidase. Gonococci are distinguished from other *Neisseria* species by the fermentation of glucose but not maltose, sucrose, or lactose. Gram-negative diplococci are seen in infected material, often within polymorphonuclear leukocytes.

The cell surface of the gonococcus is similar to that of other gram-negative bacteria and contains pili, outer membrane proteins, and lipopolysaccharides (endotoxin), which contribute to cell adherence, tissue invasion, and resistance to host defenses. *N. gonorrhoeae* may be subdivided on the basis of the presence of pili, serologic typing, colony appearance, and nutritional requirements. Gonococcal isolates examined by electron microscopy within 20 hr of collection are classified on the basis of pili. Piliated colonies are designated P+ or P++ (formerly T1 and T2, respectively); nonpiliated, avirulent colonies are P− (formerly T3 or T4). Piliated strains are virulent, attach to mucosal surfaces, and kill neutrophils.

EPIDEMIOLOGY. *N. gonorrhoeae* infection occurs only in humans. The organism is shed in the exudate and secretions of infected mucosal surfaces and is transmitted through intimate contact, such as sexual contact or parturition and, very rarely, by contact with fomites. Gonococcal infections in the newborn period generally are acquired during delivery. Gonococcal infections in children after the newborn period and before puberty are acquired rarely through household exposure to infected caretakers. In such cases the possibility of sexual abuse should be seriously considered.

In 1986, approximately 900,000 cases of gonorrhea were reported in the United States. About 50% of treated cases are reported; the number of undetected asymptomatic cases may be twice the number reported, placing the estimated annual United States incidence in excess of 3 million. The highest incidence of gonococcal infection is reported for men aged 20–24 yr and for women aged 15–19 yr. Risk factors include nonwhite race, homosexuality, increased number of sexual partners, prostitution, presence of other sexually transmitted diseases, unmarried status, poverty, and failure to use condoms. Peak incidence occurs in July–September, and the nadir is January–April. Techniques of auxotyping and serotyping can be utilized together to analyze the spread of individual strains of *N. gonorrhoeae* within a community.

Maintenance and subsequent spread of gonococcal infections in a community require a hyperendemic, high-risk core group such as prostitutes or inner city youth. Transmission occurs following intercourse with an asymptomatic patient or one who ignores signs of infection or has limited access to health care. Frequently, clonal transmission of one strain spreads in waves through communities. Proper education, contact identification, and local treatment clinics may limit transmission.

PATHOLOGY. Mucosal invasion by gonococci results in a local inflammatory response that produces a purulent exudate consisting of polymorphonuclear leukocytes, serum, and desquamated epithelium. The gonococcal lipopolysaccharide (endotoxin) exhibits direct cytotoxicity, causing ciliostasis and sloughing of ciliated epithelial cells. Once the gonococcus traverses the mucosal barrier, the lipopolysaccharide binds bactericidal IgM antibody and serum complement, causing an acute inflammatory response in the subepithelial space.

The purulent discharge produced by urogenital gonococcal infection may block the ducts of paraurethral (Skene) or vaginal (Bartholin) glands, causing cysts or abscesses. In the untreated patient, the inflammatory exudate is replaced by fibroblasts, and fibrous tissue may lead to stricture of the urethra. Gonococci may ascend the urogenital tract, causing acute endometritis, salpingitis, and peritonitis (collectively termed acute pelvic inflammatory disease) in postpubertal females and urethritis or epididymitis in postpubertal males. Perihepatitis **(Fitz-Hugh–Curtis syndrome)** follows dissemination through the peritoneum from the fallopian tube to the liver capsule. Gonococci that invade the lymphatics and blood vessels may lead to inguinal lymphadenopathy; to perineal, perianal, ischiorectal, and periprostatic abscesses; and to disseminated gonococcal disease.

PATHOGENESIS. A number of gonococcal virulence and host immune factors are involved in the penetration of the mucosal barrier and subsequent manifestations of local and systemic infection. A gonococcal IgA protease inactivates IgA1 by cleaving the molecule in the hinge region and may be an important factor in colonization or invasion of host mucosal surfaces. Gonococci adhere to the microvilli of nonciliated epithelial cells by hair-like protein structures (pili) that extend from the cell wall. Pili are thought to protect the gonococcus from phagocytosis and complement-mediated killing. Gonococcal attachment is accompanied by ciliostasis and sloughing of ciliated epithelial cells, which is thought to be mediated by lipopolysaccharide and degradation products of peptidoglycan.

Approximately 24 hr after attachment, the epithelial cell surface invaginates and surrounds the gonococcus in a phagocytic vacuole. This phenomenon is thought to be mediated by the gonococcal outer membrane protein I inserting into the host cell and causing alterations in membrane permeability. Subsequently, phagocytic vacuoles begin releasing gonococci into the subepithelial space by means of exocytosis. Viable organisms may then cause local disease (i.e., salpingitis) or disseminate through the bloodstream or lymphatics.

N. gonorrhoeae isolates from patients with disseminated gonococcal infection (DGI) share common features that distinguish them from other gonococci. Most gonococci that produce DGI lack the outer membrane protein II (PII−) and thus form transparent colonies (90%). They are resistant to the bactericidal activity of normal human serum. Local infections with these organisms fail to elicit an inflammatory response and are asymptomatic. The absence of protein II, which is proposed to be a binding site for bactericidal antibody, may account partially for the organism's resistance to the lethal action of normal human serum. Human IgG antibodies ("blocking antibodies") that do bind to DGI gonococci may interfere with bactericidal antibody- and complement-mediated lysis. DGI isolates have unique nutritional requirements (58% belong to the $Arg^-Hyx^-Ura^-$ auxotype), common protein I serotypes (85% belong to the WI serogroup), and greater sensitivity to penicillin.

Host factors may influence the incidence and manifestations of gonococcal infection. Prepubertal females are susceptible to vulvovaginitis and, rarely, experience salpingitis. *N. gonorrhoeae* infects noncornified epithelium, and the thin noncornified vaginal epithelium and alkaline pH of the vaginal mucin predispose this age group to infection of the lower genital tract. Estrogen-induced cornification of the vaginal epithelium in the neonate and mature female resists infection. Postpubertal females are more susceptible to salpingitis, especially during menses, when diminished bactericidal activity of the cervical mucus and the reflux of blood from the uterine cavity into the fallopian tubes facilitate passage of gonococci into the upper reproductive tract.

Populations at risk for DGI include asymptomatic carriers; neonates; menstruating, pregnant, and postpartum females; homosexuals; and immunocompromised hosts. The asymptomatic carrier state implies failure of the host immune system to recognize the gonococcus as a pathogen, the capacity of the gonococcus to avoid being killed, or both. Pharyngeal colonization has been proposed as a risk factor for DGI. The high rate of asymptomatic infection in pharyngeal gonorrhea may account for this phenomenon. Women are at greater risk for developing DGI during menstruation and pregnancy and postpartum, presumably due to the maximal endocervical shedding and decreased peroxidase bactericidal activity of the cervical mucus during these periods. A lack of neonatal bactericidal IgM antibody is thought to account for the neonate's increased susceptibility to DGI. Persons with terminal complement component deficiencies (C5–C9) are at considerable risk of developing recurrent episodes of DGI.

Advances in molecular genetics have increased our understanding of the pathogenesis of *N. gonorrhoeae*. Piliated gonococcal strains (P+) show increased uptake and incorporation of naked transforming DNA (genetic transformation) in vitro, high frequencies of biphasic switching between P+ and P− expression (phase variation), and rapid variation in expression of antigenically distinct types of pili (antigenic variation). The high degree of genotypic and phenotypic variation observed in piliated gonococci could enable these strains to escape immune surveillance and to adapt rapidly to different host environments, thus accounting for their greater virulence compared with nonpiliated strains.

An increasing number of gonococcal isolates show significant penicillin resistance, which is of two basic types: (1) plasmid-mediated β-lactamase (penicillinase) production, which confers absolute resistance (MIC 10–100 μg/mL); and (2) chromosomally mediated resistance, which does not depend on β-lactamase production and confers relative resistance (MIC 1.0–4.0 μg/mL). In 1989, penicillinase-producing *N. gonorrhoeae* (PPNG) accounted for 7.4% of all cases of gonorrhea in the United States, with local variations in the incidence of PPNG ranging from 1.5 to 32%. Gonococcal isolates showing increased levels of combined penicillin and tetracycline resistance have produced outbreaks of gonorrhea.

CLINICAL MANIFESTATIONS. Asymptomatic Gonorrhea. The incidence of this form of gonorrhea in children has not been ascertained. Gonococci have been isolated from the oropharynx of young (2–9 yr of age) children who have been abused sexually by male contacts; oropharyngeal symptoms are usually absent. In a study of 12- to 19-yr-old females in a school for delinquents, the incidence of gonorrhea was 12%, and most girls affected were asymptomatic. About 68% of infected United States military men are asymptomatic; 66% of this group remained culture positive but asymptomatic for several months. As many as 80% of sexually mature females with urogenital gonorrhea infections are asymptomatic; asymptomatic rectal carriage of *N. gonorrhoeae* has been documented in 40–60% of females with urogenital infection. At least 20% of rectal infections are asymptomatic and 78% of pharyngeal gonococcal infections are asymptomatic in homosexual men. Individuals with asymptomatic gonorrhea are an important reservoir of infection and may develop disseminated disease.

Uncomplicated Gonorrhea. Genital gonorrhea has an incubation period of 2–5 days in men and 5–10 days in women. Primary infection develops in the urethra of the male, the vulva and vagina of the prepubertal female, and the cervix of the postpubertal female. Neonatal ophthalmitis occurs in both sexes.

Urethritis is usually characterized by a purulent discharge and by burning on urination without urgency or frequency. Untreated urethritis in the male resolves spontaneously in several weeks or may be complicated by epididymitis, penile edema, lymphangitis, prostatitis, or seminal vesiculitis. Gram-negative intracellular diplococci are found in the discharge.

In the prepubertal female, vulvovaginitis usually is characterized by a purulent vaginal discharge with a swollen, erythematous, tender, and excoriated vulva. Dysuria may be noted. In the postpubertal female, symptomatic gonococcal cervicitis and urethritis are characterized by purulent discharge, suprapubic pain, dysuria, intermenstrual bleeding, and dyspareunia. The cervix may be inflamed and tender. In urogenital gonorrhea limited to the lower genital tract, pain is not enhanced by moving the cervix, and the adnexae are not tender to palpation. Purulent material may be expressed from the urethra or ducts of the Bartholin gland. Rectal gonorrhea, although often asymptomatic, may cause proctitis with symptoms of anal discharge, pruritus, and bleeding, pain, tenesmus, and constipation. Asymptomatic rectal gonorrhea may not be due to anal intercourse but may represent colonization from vaginal infection.

Gonococcal ophthalmitis may be unilateral or bilateral. It may occur in any age group following inoculation of the eye with infected secretions. Ophthalmia neonatorum due to *N. gonorrhoeae* usually appears from 1–4 days after birth (Sec. 9.61). Ocular infection in older patients results from inoculation or autoinoculation from a genital site. The infection begins with mild inflammation and a serosanguineous discharge. Within 24 hr the discharge becomes thick and purulent, and tense edema of the eyelids with marked chemosis occurs. If the disease is not treated promptly, corneal ulceration, rupture, and blindness may follow.

Disseminated Gonococcal Infection. Hematogenous dissemination occurs in 1–3% of all gonococcal infections, following asymptomatic primary infections more frequently than symptomatic infections. Women account for the majority of cases, with symptoms beginning 7–30 days after infection and within 7 days of menstruation. The most common manifestations are arthritis, tenosynovitis, dermatitis, and, rarely, carditis, meningitis, and osteomyelitis. The most common initial symptoms are acute onset of polyarthralgias with fever. Only 25% of patients complain of skin lesions. Most deny genitourinary symptoms; however, primary mucosal infection is documented by genitourinary cultures. Approximately 80–90% of cervical cultures are positive in women with DGI. In males, urethral cultures are positive in 50–60%, pharyngeal cultures are positive in 10–20%, and rectal cultures are positive in 15% of cases.

DGI has been classified into two clinical syndromes that have some overlapping features. The first and more common is the tenosynovitis-dermatitis syndrome, which is characterized by fever, chills, skin lesions, and polyarthralgias predominantly involving the wrists, hands, and fingers. Blood cultures are positive in approximately 30–40% of cases, and synovial fluid cultures are almost uniformly negative. The second syndrome is the suppurative arthritis syndrome in which systemic symptoms and signs are less prominent and a monoarticular arthritis, often involving the knee, is more common. A polyarthral phase may precede the monoarticular infection. In cases of monoarticular involvement, synovial fluid cultures are positive in approximately 45–55%, whereas blood cultures are usually negative. DGI in neonates usually occurs as a polyarticular septic arthritis.

Dermatologic lesions usually begin as painful discrete, 1- to 20-mm pink or red macules that progress to maculopapular, vesicular, bullous, pustular, or petechial lesions. The typical necrotic pustule on an erythematous base is distributed unevenly over the extremities, including the palmar and plantar surfaces, usually sparing the face and scalp. The lesions number between 5 and 40; 20–30% may contain gonococci. Although immune complexes may be present in DGI, complement levels are normal, and the role of the immune complexes in pathogenesis is uncertain.

Acute endocarditis is an uncommon (1–2%) but often fatal manifestation of DGI that usually leads to rapid destruction of the aortic valve. Acute pericarditis is a rarely described entity in patients with disseminated gonorrhea. Meningitis with *N. gonorrhoeae* has been documented. Signs and symptoms are similar to those of any acute bacterial meningitis.

COMPLICATIONS. Complications of gonorrhea result from the spread of gonococci from a local site of invasion. The time interval between primary infection and development of a complication is usually days to weeks. In postpubertal females, endometritis may occur, especially during menses. This may progress to salpingitis and peritonitis (pelvic inflammatory disease [PID]). Manifestations of PID include signs of lower genital tract infection (vaginal discharge, suprapubic pain, cervical tenderness) and upper genital tract infection (fever, leukocytosis, elevated ESR, and adnexal tenderness or mass). The differential diagnosis includes gynecologic (ovarian cyst, ovarian tumor, ectopic pregnancy) and intra-abdominal (appendicitis, urinary tract infection, inflammatory bowel disease) pathology (see Sec. 10.17).

Once inside the peritoneum, gonococci may seed the liver capsule, causing a perihepatitis. The resultant right upper quadrant pain, with or without signs of salpingitis, is known as the Fitz-Hugh–Curtis syndrome. Perihepatitis may also be due to *Chlamydia trachomatis*. Progression to PID occurs in about 20% of cases of gonococcal cervicitis. *N. gonorrhoeae* is isolated in approximately 40% of cases of PID in the United States. Untreated cases may lead to hydrosalpinx, pyosalpinx, tubo-ovarian abscess, and eventual sterility. Even with adequate treatment of PID, the risk of sterility caused by bilateral tubal occlusion approaches 20% after one episode of salpingitis and exceeds 60% with three or more episodes. In addition, the risk of ectopic pregnancy is increased approximately 7-fold after one or more episodes of salpingitis. Additional sequelae of PID include chronic pain, dyspareunia, and increased risk of recurrent PID.

Urogenital gonococcal infection acquired during the 1st trimester of pregnancy carries a high risk of septic abortion. After 16 wk, infection causes chorioamnionitis, a major cause of premature rupture of the membranes and premature delivery.

Since these patients are at high risk for other sexually transmitted disease, all patients with gonorrhea should have a serologic test for syphilis and be evaluated for recurrent *C. trachomatis* infection at the time of diagnosis. HIV testing is also indicated. The VDRL should be repeated 3 mo later.

DIAGNOSIS AND DIFFERENTIAL DIAGNOSIS. A definite diagnosis of gonococcal disease depends on isolation of *N. gonorrhoeae*. It is not possible to distinguish gonococcal from nongonococcal urethritis on the basis of symptoms and signs alone. Gonococcal urethritis and vulvovaginitis must be distinguished from other infections that produce a purulent discharge, including β-hemolytic streptococci, *C. trachomatis, Mycoplasma hominis, Trichomonas vaginalis*, and *Candida albicans*. Rarely, infection with *Herpesvirus hominis* type 2 may produce symptoms similar to those of gonorrhea.

In the male with symptomatic urethritis, a presumptive diagnosis of gonorrhea can be made by identification of gram-negative intracellular diplococci (within leukocytes) in the urethral discharge. A similar finding in females is not sufficient because *Mima polymorpha* and *Moraxella* (normal vaginal flora) have a similar appearance. The sensitivity of the Gram stain for diagnosing gonococcal cervicitis and asymptomatic infections is also low. The presence of commensal *Neisseria* species in the oropharynx prevents the use of the Gram stain for diagnosis of pharyngeal gonorrhea. Although nonpathogenic neisseria are gram-negative diplococci, they are not intracellular or associated with neutrophilia.

Bacteriologic cultures remain the gold standard for the diagnosis of *N. gonorrhoeae*. Male urethral specimens are obtained by placing a small swab 2–3 cm into the urethra. Material for cervical cultures is obtained after wiping the exocervix and placing a swab in the cervical os and rotating it gently for several seconds. For optimal culture results, specimens should be obtained with noncotton swabs, inoculated directly onto culture plates, and incubated immediately. The urethra should be cultured in heterosexual men, and the endocervix and rectum should be cultured in all females, regardless of the absence of a history of anal intercourse. Symptomatic sites plus the pharynx should be cultured in patients with orogenital exposure. Specimens from sites that normally are colonized by other organisms (i.e., cervix, rectum, pharynx) should be inoculated on a selective culture medium, such as modified Thayer-Martin medium (fortified with vancomycin, colistin, nystatin, and trimethoprim to inhibit growth of indigenous flora). Specimens from sites that are normally sterile or minimally contaminated (i.e., synovial fluid, blood, CSF) should be inoculated on a nonselective chocolate agar medium. If DGI is suspected, blood, pharynx, rectum, urethra, cervix, and synovial fluid (if involved) should be cultured. Cultured specimens should be incubated promptly at 35–37° C in 3–5% CO_2. When specimens must be transported to a central laboratory for culture plating, a reduced, nonnutrient holding medium (i.e., Amies modified Stuart medium) preserves specimens with minimal loss of viability for up to 6 hr. When transport may delay culture plating by more than 6 hr, it is preferable to inoculate the sample directly onto a culture medium and transport it at ambient temperature in a candle jar. The Transgrow and JEMBEC systems of modified Thayer-Martin medium are alternative transport systems. Colonies of *N. gonorrhoeae* are oxidase positive. Further differentiation from oxidase-positive *M. polymorpha* and *N. lactamica* (both found in normal vaginal and oral secretions) can be made by carbohydrate utilization tests; gonococci ferment glucose but not maltose, lactose, or sucrose. The organism should be tested for β-lactamase production.

When microbiology laboratory facilities are not readily available or when patients may be lost to follow-up, rapid diagnostic techniques may prove efficacious. Care must be taken in selecting and interpreting results because most rapid tests are less specific than cultures. A rapid slide coagglutination test (Phadebact) has a sensitivity of 96–98% for identification of gonococci in anogenital specimens from females and urethral specimens from males. This test cross-reacts with commensal *Neisseria* species. Enzyme immunoassay tests such as Gonozyme are comparable to Gram stain in their sensitivity and specificity for diagnosing gonococcal urethritis in males. Gonozyme is more sensitive than the Gram stain in diagnosing gonococcal cervicitis (80–92% in most studies). This test is limited by a low positive predictive value in populations with a low prevalence of gonorrhea and cannot be used for rectal or pharyngeal infections. On balance, these tests offer a more sensitive means for making a presumptive diagnosis of urogenital gonorrhea in females but have no advantage over the Gram stain for diagnosing gonococcal urethritis in males. They cannot replace bacteriologic cultures for definitive diagnosis of *N. gonorrhoeae* or for antimicrobial susceptibility testing. They may serve as useful adjuvant diagnostic tools in high-prevalence, transient populations (i.e., in adolescent sexually transmitted disease [STD] clinics), in which a rapid and accurate presumptive diagnosis is required for prompt institution of therapy.

Gonococcal arthritis must be distinguished from other forms of septic arthritis as well as from rheumatic fever, rheumatoid arthritis, Reiter syndrome, inflammatory bowel disease, and arthritis secondary to rubella or rubella immunization (Sec. 12.17). Gonococcal conjunctivitis in the newborn period must be differentiated from chemical conjunctivitis caused by silver nitrate drops as well as from conjunctivitis caused by *C. trachomatis, S. aureus*, group A or B streptococcus, *P. aeruginosa*, or *H. hominis* type 2.

PREVENTION. Efforts to develop a gonococcal pilus vaccine have been unsuccessful thus far. The high degree of inter- and intrastrain antigenic variability of pili poses a formidable deterrent to the development of a single effective pilus vaccine. In the absence of a vaccine, prevention of gonorrhea can be achieved through education, use of barrier contraceptives (especially condoms and spermicides), intensive epidemiologic and bacteriologic surveillance (screening sexual contacts), and early identification and treatment of infected contacts.

Gonococcal ophthalmia neonatorum can be prevented by instilling a 1% solution of silver nitrate into the conjunctival sac shortly after birth (see Sec. 9.61). Infants born to mothers with active gonorrhea are at high risk for developing gonococcal ophthalmitis and should be given a single 125-mg intramuscular injection of ceftriaxone for prophylaxis. For low-birthweight infants, the dosage is 25–50 mg/kg.

TREATMENT. General principles in the treatment of gonorrhea include the need to consider therapy for coexisting sexually transmitted diseases (syphilis, *Chlamydia* infection,

HIV) and infection due to PPNG and tetracycline-resistant *N. gonorrhoeae*. The incidence of *Chlamydia* coinfection is 15–25% among males and 35–50% among females. It is recommended that *Chlamydia* infection be treated simultaneously with gonorrhea (Sec. 12.58). Sexual partners exposed in the preceding 30 days should be examined, cultures should be taken, and presumptive treatment started.

Although in many communities isolates of *N. gonorrhoeae* are relatively insensitive or resistant to penicillin, in other locations penicillin is effective for initial treatment of gonorrhea. For regions in which PPNG account for 1% or more of all reported cases or when the incidence is unknown, ceftriaxone is the treatment of choice. Routine culture and antimicrobial susceptibility testing should be used as guides to therapy.

Uncomplicated urethritis or vulvovaginitis due to **penicillin-sensitive gonococci** can be treated with a single intramuscular injection of aqueous procaine penicillin G, 100,000 U/kg (4.8 million U maximum) and probenecid, 25 mg/kg orally (maximum 1.0 g). This treatment may be poorly tolerated and may be associated with psychotic reactions to procaine. Alternatively, a single oral dose of amoxicillin, 50 mg/kg (3.0 g maximum), with probenecid, 25 mg/kg (maximum 1 g), can be used. A single intramuscular injection of ceftriaxone, 125 mg for prepubertal children weighing less than 45 kg and 250 mg for adults, currently is the treatment of choice for urethral, rectal, and endocervical gonorrhea due to **insensitive or resistant gonococci.** Ceftriaxone may also be effective against incubating syphilis but is ineffective against *Chlamydia*. In sexually active individuals infected with *N. gonorrhoeae*, simultaneous infection with *C. trachomatis* is common, accounts for the majority of cases of postgonococcal urethritis, and contributes to fallopian tube scarring and infertility. Therefore, the addition of a 7-day course of tetracycline, 2 g/day in 4 divided doses, or doxycycline, 100 mg/day in 2 divided doses, is recommended. Doxycycline is tolerated better than tetracycline and the twice a day dose may improve compliance.

Several options exist for treating uncomplicated gonorrhea in penicillin-allergic individuals. A single intramuscular dose of spectinomycin may be given, 40 mg/kg for children weighing less than 45 kg and 2 g for adults. It is less effective for pharyngeal gonorrhea, is ineffective against incubating syphilis or *Chlamydia* infections, but is effective against PPNG. Spectinomycin must be followed by a course of doxycycline. Alternatively, ceftriaxone may be used because the incidence of cross-reactivity to cephalosporins is low. Additional therapy for penicillin-allergic patients, includes ciprofloxacin, 500 mg orally for 1 dose; during pregnancy erythromycin should be added to spectinomycin or ceftriaxone. Tetracyclines should not be used as single-drug therapy for gonorrhea.

Children with disseminated gonococcal disease (sensitive to penicillin) should be hospitalized and treated with intravenous aqueous penicillin G, 100,000–200,000 U/kg/24 hr in 6 divided doses for 7–10 days. For gonococcal meningitis and endocarditis, the dosages are 250,000 U/kg/24 hr for 14 days and 4 wk, respectively. Although many gonococcal isolates causing disseminated disease are sensitive to penicillin, ceftriaxone is recommended as the initial treatment of choice for DGI. A 7-day course of parenteral ceftriaxone, 50–100 mg/kg/24 hr (maximum 1 g/24 hr) intravenously or intramuscularly for children and 1 g/24 hr intravenously or intramuscularly for adults, is recommended unless the organism is sensitive to penicillin. Endocarditis or meningitis should be treated with ceftriaxone, 1–2 g intravenously every 12 hr for 4 wk and 10–14 days, respectively. Penicillin-allergic patients may be treated with ceftriaxone or spectinomycin, 2 g intramuscularly every 12 hr. Concurrent therapy with doxycycline is indicated for treatment of genital *Chlamydia* infection in sexually active patients.

Infants born to mothers with known gonococcal infection should be evaluated for sepsis with blood and CSF cultures. Ceftriaxone (50 mg/kg intramuscularly or intravenously given once, 125 mg maximum) is the drug of choice. Topical prophylaxis with this drug is not adequate. Neonates with gonococcal ophthalmitis must be hospitalized and evaluated for DGI. Cefotaxime, 25–50 mg/kg/24 hr given intravenously every 12 hr for 7 days, or ceftriaxone, 25–50 mg/kg/24 hr intravenously or intramuscularly every day for 7 days, is the treatment of choice. In the absence of systemic infection some specialists treat gonococcal ophthalmia with a single injection of ceftriaxone. Concomitant saline irrigation of the eyes is recommended.

PID requires hospitalization for evaluation and initiation of treatment. PID encompasses a spectrum of infectious diseases of the upper genital tract due to *N. gonorrhoeae, C. trachomatis*, and endogenous flora (streptococci, anaerobes, gram-negative bacilli). Therapy must cover a broad spectrum and must be given to adolescents as inpatients. A commonly recommended therapeutic regimen is cefoxitin, 2 g intravenously every 6 hr, or cefotetan, 2 g intravenously every 12 hr, plus doxycycline, 100 mg orally or intravenously every 12 hr. Therapy is continued for at least 48 hr after the patient shows improvement. Thereafter, oral doxycycline is continued for a total of 10–14 days. An alternative recommended regimen is clindamycin, 900 mg intravenously every 8 hr, plus a loading dose of gentamicin (2 mg/kg intramuscularly or intravenously), followed by maintenance gentamicin, 1.5 mg/kg every 8 hr. Therapy is then continued for 48 hr after the patient improves and is followed by oral doxycycline for 10–14 days. If an intrauterine device (IUD) is present, it must be removed and an alternative form of birth control used. Sexual partners should be examined and treated for uncomplicated gonorrhea. Follow-up culture (test of cure) of cephalosporin-doxycycline therapy of gonococcal STD is not recommended owing to the low treatment failure rate. A follow-up examination and culture is recommended in 1–2 mo to evaluate the possibility of reinfection or, rarely, treatment failure.

PROGNOSIS. Prompt diagnosis and correct therapy ensure complete recovery from uncomplicated gonococcal disease. Complications and permanent sequelae may be associated with delayed treatment, recurrent infection, metastatic sites of infection (meninges, aortic valve), and delayed or topical therapy of gonococcal ophthalmia.

RALPH D. FEIGIN
ROBERT SUGERMAN

Britigan BE, Cohen MS, Sparling PF: Gonococcal infection: A model for molecular pathogenesis. N Engl J Med 312:1683, 1985.

Cates W, Wasserheit JN: Gonorrhea, chlamydia, and pelvic inflammatory disease. Curr Opin Infect Dis 3:10, 1990.

Centers for Disease Control: Plasmid-mediated antimicrobial resistance in *Neisseria gonorrhoeae*—United States, 1988 and 1989. MMWR 39:284, 1990.

Centers for Disease Control: 1989 sexually transmitted disease treatment guidelines. MMWR 38:S-8, 1989.

Hook EW, Holmes KK: Gonococcal infections. Ann Intern Med 102:229,1985.

O'Brien JP, Goldenberg DL, Rice PA: Disseminated gonococcal infection: A prospective analysis of 49 patients and a review of pathophysiology and immune mechanisms. Medicine 62:395, 1983.

Rawstron SA, Hammerschlag MR, Gullans C, et al: Ceftriaxone treatment of penicillinase-producing *Neisseria gonorrhoeae* infections in children. Pediatr Infect Dis J 8:445, 1989.

Treatment of sexually transmitted diseases. Med Lett 32:5, 1990.

Whitington WL, et al: Incorrect identification of *Neisseria gonorrhoeae* from infants and children. Pediatr Infect Dis J 7:34, 1988.

12.25 DIPHTHERIA

Diphtheria is an acute infectious disease caused by *Corynebacterium diphtheriae*. Generalized and localized clinical manifestations follow elaboration of toxin, an extracellular protein metabolite, by toxigenic strains of *C. diphtheriae*. Records suggest that diphtheria was recognized as early as the 4th century B.C. New epidemics are being reported in Denmark, Sweden, and the United States.

ETIOLOGY. *C. diphtheriae* is an irregularly staining gram-positive, nonmotile, nonsporulating, pleomorphic bacillus. The club shape of the bacillus is not a true morphologic feature but a result of attempts to grow it under nutritionally inadequate circumstances (Loeffler medium). *C. diphtheriae* organisms demonstrate a "Chinese character," palisading morphology that differentiates it from other corynebacteria. The bacillus is recovered most readily on media containing selective inhibitors that retard the growth of other microorganisms (tellurite).

Colonies of *C. diphtheriae* appear grayish white on Loeffler medium. On tellurite media, three colony types can be distinguished: *intermedius* is the most common biotype (99% are toxigenic); *mitis* is the next most common (31% are toxigenic); *gravis* is least common (84% are toxigenic).

Infection of *C. diphtheriae* by a lysogenic β-phage carrying the gene for toxin production is required to render strains toxigenic. Multiplication of phage is not a prerequisite for toxin production because toxin occurs in the prophage stage when the phage circular DNA integrates with bacterial DNA. The synthesis of toxin depends upon both genetic and nutritional factors. Both toxigenic and nontoxigenic strains of *C. diphtheriae* can cause disease, but only strains that produce toxin are responsible for myocarditis and neuritis.

EPIDEMIOLOGY. Diphtheria occurs worldwide, but its incidence declined sharply following extensive use of diphtheria toxoid after World War II. From 1970 through 1976, an average of 248 cases of diphtheria were reported annually in the United States; since 1980, the average has been 56 cases. Mortality, however, has remained relatively constant at about 10% of cases. Humans are the only reservoir for *C. diphtheriae*.

The incidence of diphtheria peaks during the autumn and winter months. Eighty per cent of cases occur in unimmunized individuals under 15 yr of age, and the incidence is highest among the poor who reside in crowded conditions with limited access to health care. In immunized populations diphtheria occurs in susceptible adults with waning immunity, documented by antitoxin levels of less than 0.01 IU/mL.

Diphtheria is acquired by contact with either an asymptomatic carrier or a person with the disease. The bacteria may be transmitted by droplets spread by coughing, sneezing, or talking. Diphtheritic infections of the skin may predispose to respiratory colonization. Fomites and dust may also serve as vehicles of transmission.

PATHOGENESIS AND PATHOLOGY. Diphtheria is initiated predominantly by entry of *C. diphtheriae* into the nose or mouth, and the bacilli remain localized on the mucosal surfaces of the upper respiratory tract. Occasionally, the skin or the ocular or genital mucous membranes serve as the site of localization. *C. diphtheriae* is not an invasive pathogen; the main virulence factor is a potential exotoxin. Following a 2- to 4-day period of incubation, strains infected with bacteriophage may elaborate toxin. Toxin is initially adsorbed to the cell membrane and then penetrates it to interfere with mammalian but not bacterial protein synthesis. The toxin is a 62,000 dalton polypeptide consisting of a B segment (binds to susceptible cells) and an active A segment. Following proteolytic separation, segment A enters the mammalian cell and inactivates transfer RNA translocase (elongation factor), thus preventing the addition of amino acids to the growing native polypeptide chain.

Toxin-mediated tissue necrosis is severe in the vicinity of colonization. The local inflammatory response coupled with the necrotic tissue produces a patchy exudate that initially can be removed. As toxin production increases, the area of infection widens and deepens, and a fibrinous exudate develops. A tough adherent pseudomembrane is formed that varies from gray to black, depending on the amount of blood it contains. In addition to fibrin and *C. diphtheriae*, the membrane contains inflammatory, red blood, and superficial epithelial cells. Since the latter are an integral part of the membrane, attempts to remove it are followed by bleeding. The pseudomembrane sloughs spontaneously during the recovery period.

Edema of the soft tissues beneath the membrane may be extensive and may contribute to the "bull neck" appearance. Occasionally, secondary bacterial infection (usually streptococcal) develops. The membrane and edematous tissue may encroach upon the airway and may cause respiratory embarrassment or suffocation if they extend to the larynx or tracheobronchial area.

Toxin produced at the site of infection is distributed via the bloodstream throughout the body. The toxin can damage any organ or tissue, but lesions of the heart, nervous system, and kidneys are particularly susceptible. Although diphtheria antitoxin can neutralize circulating toxin or that adsorbed to cells, it is ineffective when cell penetration has occurred. There is a variable latent period before clinical manifestations appear. Myocarditis generally is observed 10–14 days after the onset of illness. Nervous system manifestations, particularly peripheral neuritis, usually do not appear for 3–7 wk.

The most prominent pathologic findings are toxic necrosis and hyaline degeneration of various organs and tissues. In the heart one may observe edema, congestion, and mononuclear cell infiltration of muscle fibers and the conducting system. A toxic neuritis with fatty degeneration of myelin sheaths may be noted. Liver necrosis may occur, possibly associated with hypoglycemia. Adrenal hemorrhage and acute tubular necrosis of the kidney are also noted in some cases.

CLINICAL MANIFESTATIONS. The signs and symptoms of diphtheria depend on the site of infection and the immunization status of the host and upon whether or not toxin escapes into the systemic circulation.

The incubation period ranges from 1–6 days. Diphtheria is classified clinically by the location of the diphtheritic membrane (nasal, tonsillar, pharyngeal, laryngeal or laryngotracheal, conjunctival, skin, and genital). More than one anatomic site may be involved.

Nasal diphtheria initially resembles a common cold and is characterized by mild rhinorrhea and a paucity of systemic symptoms. Gradually, the nasal discharge becomes serosanguineous and then mucopurulent and excoriates the nares and upper lip. A foul odor may be noticed, and careful inspection will reveal a white membrane on the nasal septum (Fig. 12–4 [color plate section]). Slow absorption of toxin, a lack of systemic symptoms, and initially mild manifestations frequently delay diagnosis. This form of the disease occurs most often in infants.

Tonsillar and/or pharyngeal diphtheria begins insidiously, and these structures are the most common site of disease. Anorexia, malaise, low-grade fever, and pharyngitis are noted initially. Within 1–2 days a membrane appears that may vary in extent according to the immune status of the host; in partially immune individuals a membrane may not develop. The membrane initially is thin and gray, resembling a spider web that gradually extends from the tonsil to the contiguous soft or hard palate; this characteristic distinguishes diphtheria from other forms of membranous tonsillitis. The adherent membrane may spread to cover the tonsils and pharyngeal wall (Fig. 12–5 [color plate section]), or it may progress into the larynx and trachea. Attempts to remove it are followed by bleeding. Cervical lymphadenitis is variable, and when associated with edema of the soft tissues of the neck it may be so severe as to give the appearance of a "bull neck." The edema may obliterate the borders of the sternocleidomastoid muscle, the mandible, and the clavicle. The edema is brawny, pitting, warm, and tender. It occurs most commonly in children over 6 yr of age.

The course of pharyngeal diphtheria depends upon the extent of the membrane and the production of toxin. In severe cases respiratory and circulatory collapse may occur. The pulse rate is increased disproportionately to the body temperature, which generally remains normal or slightly elevated (rarely > 103° F). Palatal paralysis may occur. If it is unilateral, the palate deviates away from the paralyzed side; if bilateral, paralysis may eliminate the nasal quality of the voice and cause nasal regurgitation and difficulty in swallowing. Stupor, coma, and death may follow within 7–10 days. In less severe cases, recovery may be slow or may be complicated by myocarditis or neuritis. In mild cases the membrane sloughs in 7–10 days, and recovery is uneventful.

Laryngeal diphtheria generally represents a downward extension of the membrane from the pharynx. Occasionally, only laryngeal involvement is present. The clinical findings of noisy breathing, progressive stridor, and hoarseness are indistinguishable from those seen in other types of infectious croup. Suprasternal, subcostal, and supraclavicular retractions reflect severe laryngeal obstruction, which may be fatal unless it is alleviated. Occasionally acute and fatal obstruction may occur when a partially detached piece of membrane occludes the airway. In severe cases the membrane may extend downward, covering the entire tracheobronchial tree.

Cutaneous, vulvovaginal, conjunctival, and aural diphtheria also occur and are rarely complicated by toxin-mediated organ dysfunction. *Cutaneous diphtheria* usually appears as an ulcer with a sharply defined border and a membranous base. It is more common in warmer climates and may serve as an important source of person-to-person transmission of diphtheria. *Conjunctival lesions* usually are limited to the palpebral conjunctiva, which appears red, edematous, and membranous; corneal erosion may occur. *Aural diphtheria* is characterized by otitis externa with a persistently purulent and frequently foul-smelling discharge.

DIAGNOSIS. *Diagnosis should be made as promptly as possible on the basis of clinical findings. Any delay in therapy poses a serious risk to the patient.* Clinical findings suggesting the diagnosis include membranous tonsillitis or pharyngitis extending to the uvula and soft palate, hoarseness, stridor, palatal paralysis, cervical adenopathy and edema, and serosanguineous nasal discharge. Definitive diagnosis depends upon isolation of *C. diphtheriae*. Microscopic examination of material from diphtheritic lesions is unreliable; the fluorescent antibody technique may be used but is reliable only with experienced personnel.

Material from beneath the membrane or a portion of the membrane itself should be obtained for culture. *C. diphtheriae* is relatively resistant to drying; use of non-nutritive, moisture-reducing transport medium helps to prevent the overgrowth of other microorganisms. The laboratory should be notified about the suspicion of diphtheria so that appropriate Loeffler, tellurite, and blood agar media are inoculated. Diphtheria bacilli that are recovered should be tested for toxigenicity by inoculating two guinea pigs intracutaneously with a broth suspension of the microorganism. One of the animals is given diphtheria antitoxin prior to the intracutaneous challenge. An inflammatory lesion will appear at the site of inoculation in 24 hr and will become necrotic in 72 hr in the control animal. No skin reaction should occur in the animal given antitoxin.

Other laboratory studies are of little diagnostic value. The white blood cell count may be normal or elevated. Rarely, anemia may develop as a result of rapid hemolysis. In diphtheritic neuritis there may be a slight elevation of protein and, rarely, mild pleocytosis in the cerebrospinal fluid. Hypoglycemia, glycosuria, or both may reflect hepatic toxicity. An elevation in blood urea nitrogen may develop in patients with acute tubular necrosis. Electrocardiography may reveal arrhythmias or S-T segment and T-wave changes indicative of myocarditis.

DIFFERENTIAL DIAGNOSIS. Mild forms of nasal diphtheria in the partially immunized host may resemble the common cold. When a more serosanguineous or purulent nasal discharge is present, nasal diphtheria must be distinguished from foreign body in the nose, sinusitis, adenoiditis, or the *"snuffles"* of congenital syphilis. Careful examination of the nose with a nasal speculum, sinus roentgenograms, and serologic tests for syphilis should be helpful.

Tonsillar and/or pharyngeal diphtheria must be differentiated in particular from streptococcal pharyngitis and from infectious mononucleosis. The former is generally associated with more severe pain on swallowing, higher temperature, and a relatively nonadherent membrane limited to the tonsils. Pharyngeal diphtheria and streptococcal pharyngitis may coexist. Infectious mononucleosis is usually accompanied by lymphadenopathy, splenomegaly, atypical lymphocytes, heterophilic antibodies, and a membrane that does not extend beyond the tonsils or bleed when removed.

Nonbacterial membranous tonsillitis is usually characterized by a low white blood cell count, normal throat flora, and a course unaffected by antibiotics; primary herpetic tonsillitis, by gingivitis, stomatitis, and discrete lesions of the tongue and palate; and thrush, by lesions on the buccal mucosa and tongue and by absence of constitutional symptoms. Tonsillar and pharyngeal diphtheria also must be differentiated from blood dyscrasias, such as agranulocytosis and leukemia; from post-tonsillectomy faucial membranes, in which the membranes are stationary and do not spread; and from oropharyngeal involvement by *Toxoplasma*, cytomegalovirus, *Francisella tularensis*, and salmonellae. Vincent angina may be indistinguishable.

Laryngeal diphtheria must be differentiated from croup of other causes (Sec. 14.43), aspirated foreign bodies, epiglottitis, peripharyngeal and retropharyngeal abscesses, and laryngeal papillomas, hemangiomas, or lymphangiomas. Direct laryngeal visualization in the hospital under controlled conditions should be diagnostic provided that the child's condition does not demand an emergency tracheotomy.

COMPLICATIONS. Penicillin will eradicate *C. diphtheriae* and reduce the frequency of secondary bacterial complications. Nevertheless, respiratory obstruction and death may occur suddenly in young children with laryngeal or tracheal diphtheria. Edema of the neck may also compromise the airway.

Myocarditis (Sec. 15.70) may follow both severe and mild cases of diphtheria and is most common in patients with extensive local lesions and when there has been a delay in the administration of antitoxin. Subclinical myocarditis is present in 68% of patients, and clinical manifestations develop in 10–15%. Myocarditis generally occurs in the 2nd wk of the disease but may appear as early as the 1st or as late as the 6th wk. It is potentially the gravest of the complications seen with diphtheria and demands the most careful supervision and therapy. Initial manifestations include ST-T wave changes and 1st-degree heart block. Progression to atrioventricular dissociation and left bundle branch block carries a poor prognosis, with a high risk of permanent conduction defects. Heart failure and elevated myocardial enzyme levels may also be evident. Complete bed rest is essential.

Neurologic complications generally appear after a variable latent period, are predominantly bilateral, are proportional in severity to the primary infection, and are usually motor rather than sensory. They usually resolve completely. Paralysis of the soft palate and pharyngeal muscles is common and may present as nasal regurgitation, appearing in the 1st–3rd wk. Ocular muscle and ciliary paralyses are most common during the 5th week but may appear as early as the 1st wk. They may cause blurring of vision, difficulty with accommodation, and internal strabismus. Neuritis of the phrenic nerve may cause paralysis of the diaphragm, usually between the 5th and 7th wk. Paralysis of the limbs with loss of deep tendon reflexes (at 2–7 wk) and an elevation of the cerebrospinal fluid protein level may be noted; this complication is clinically indistinguishable from signs characteristic of Guillain-Barré syndrome.

Rarely, 2–3 wk after onset of diphtheria the vasomotor centers may be affected, and hypotension and cardiac failure may ensue. Gastritis, hepatitis, and nephritis are frequent complications.

PREVENTION. Immunization. See Sec. 5.1.

Contacts. The immediate prevention of diphtheria depends upon isolation of the patient and management of his or her contacts. The patient is infectious until diphtheria bacilli can no longer be cultured from the site of infection; three consecutive negative cultures are required before the patient is released from isolation.

Cultures should be taken from close contacts, who should be observed for 7 days. If *C. diphtheria* is recovered, treatment should be instituted. Asymptomatic, immune close contacts should receive a booster of diphtheria toxoid (DT, Td), if they have not received a booster within 5 yr. If the asymptomatic close contact is not immunized or the immunization status is unknown, he or she should be closely observed and started on oral erythromycin (40 mg/kg/24 hr for 7 days, maximum 2 g/24 hr) or benzathine penicillin G (600,000–1,200,000 U given intramuscularly once); cultures should be obtained before and after antimicrobial prophylaxis and active immunization with diphtheria-pertussis-tetanus toxoid (DPT), DT, or Td (depending on age) have been given. Contacts who may be lost to follow-up should receive benzathine penicillin G and active immunization. Antitoxin is not usually recommended in this situation, but if given, the dose is 5,000–10,000 U given intramuscularly at a site other than that where the toxoid is administered and after appropriate sensitivity testing for horse serum allergy (see Sec. 11.45). The efficacy of chemoprophylaxis in preventing disease has not been established. If a contact is experiencing symptoms, treatment for diphtheria is indicated.

TREATMENT. Treatment of diphtheria is predicated upon neutralization of free toxin and eradication of *C. diphtheriae* by the use of antibiotics. The only specific treatment is antitoxin of equine origin.

Antitoxin must be administered as early as possible by the intravenous route and in a dose sufficient to neutralize all free toxin. A single dose is used to avoid the risk of sensitization from repeated doses of horse serum. *Tests for sensitivity to horse serum must be performed* prior to administration of antitoxin. For this purpose, 1 drop of a 1:10 dilution of antitoxin is placed in the conjunctival sac or 0.02 mL of a 1:100 dilution is first placed on a scratch, and, if negative, then in an intradermal site. If there is a prior history of animal allergy, the intradermal dose is reduced to 0.02 of a 1:1,000 dilution. A positive reaction (> 3 mm of erythema at the site of injection compared with a saline control within 20 min or development of conjunctivitis and tearing) necessitates desensitization. If a patient manifests sensitivity to horse serum (10% of patients have positive reactions), it should be given in slowly increasing doses at 20-min intervals. Several desensitization procedures have been recommended. They should be performed under controlled situations with preparations intended for the treatment of anaphylaxis. Some clinicians recommend pretreatment with Benadryl, prednisone, or both. The recommended regimen is:

0.1 mL of a 1:1,000 saline dilution IV followed by an increment every 15 min if there is no anaphylaxis
0.3 mL of a 1:1,000 saline dilution IV
0.6 mL of a 1:1,000 saline dilution IV
0.1 mL of a 1:100 saline dilution IV
0.3 mL of a 1:100 saline dilution IV
0.6 mL of a 1:100 saline dilution IV
0.1 mL of a 1:10 saline dilution IV
0.3 mL of a 1:10 saline dilution IV
0.6 mL of a 1:10 saline dilution IV
0.1 mL undiluted IV
0.2 mL undiluted IV
0.6 mL undiluted IV
1.0 mL undiluted IV

Another, less controlled regimen consists of initial intradermal, subcutaneous and then intramuscular injections of an increasing volume of less diluted serum. If no reaction occurs, the remaining material is given by slow intravenous infusion. Reactions should be treated with aqueous epinephrine (1:1,000) intravenously.

Antitoxin dosage is empiric and consists of 20,000–40,000 units for pharyngeal or laryngeal disease of 48 hr duration or less; 40,000–60,000 units for nasopharyngeal disease; 80,000–100,000 units for extensive disease of more than 3 days duration or presenting with brawny neck edema. Antitoxin is given for 60 min by the intravenous route. Serum sickness develops in 10% of patients (see Sec. 11.45).

Antibiotics are not a substitute for treatment with antitoxin but are needed to stop the production of diphtheria toxin, eradicate the organism, and prevent its spread. Penicillin and erythromycin are effective against most strains of *C. diphtheriae*. Penicillin may be given as aqueous procaine penicillin G, 300,000 (for patients < 10 kg)–600,000 (for patients > 10 kg) units intramuscularly once daily for 14 days. Patients sensitive to penicillin should be given erythromycin in a daily dosage of 40 mg/kg/24 hr in four divided doses for 14 days.

The end-point of therapy is three consecutive negative cultures. Each of these antibiotics is also effective in eradicating group A β-hemolytic streptococci, which may complicate up to 30% of cases of diphtheria. Amoxicillin, rifampin, and clindamycin provided in appropriate dosages also may be effective. The carrier state has been treated effectively with benzathine penicillin G or oral erythromycin.

Supportive Treatment. Because of the frequency of myocarditis, bed rest is extremely important and should be required for 2–3 wk. Serial electrocardiograms should be obtained 2–3 times each wk for 4–6 wk to detect myocarditis as early as possible.

Hydration should be maintained and a high-calorie liquid or soft diet provided. Secretions should be suctioned. The gag reflex and the quality of the voice should be checked regularly.

Laryngeal diphtheria may require relief of obstruction with a tracheostomy. This procedure should be carried out before the child has become exhausted.

Absolute bed rest must be enforced if myocarditis is detected. Sudden death has been precipitated by excessive activity. The patient with myocarditis may be digitalized if congestive heart failure develops. Digitalization for arrhythmias due to diphtheria may be contraindicated.

Palatal and pharyngeal paralysis may be complicated by aspiration. Gavage via a polyethylene tube is indicated in these patients.

Immunization is necessary following recovery of the patient. At least half of the patients who recover from diphtheria do not develop adequate immunity and remain subject to reinfection.

PROGNOSIS. Prior to the use of antitoxin and the availability of antibiotics, the mortality from diphtheria was 30–50%. Death was most common in children under 4 yr of age and often was the result of suffocation by the diphtheritic membrane. At present, the mortality is less than 5%, is most frequently associated with myocarditis, and is not associated with age.

The prognosis in all instances remains guarded until the child has recovered. The more extensive the diphtheritic membrane, the more severe the disease. Laryngeal obstruction may develop suddenly and unexpectedly. Myocarditis may be associated with congestive heart failure that responds poorly to digitalization. Occasionally, diphtheritic myocarditis is followed by permanent damage to the heart. The development of amegakaryocytic thrombocytopenia or of myocarditis with atrioventricular dissociation heralds a poorer prognosis. Phrenic nerve paralysis may occur late and produce respiratory paralysis.

The prognosis in diphtheria also depends upon the immunization status of the host, the rapidity with which medical care was sought and an accurate diagnosis suggested, the timeliness of treatment, and the adequacy of general nursing care. If specific treatment is provided on the 1st day of disease, mortality may be reduced to less than 1%; delay in treatment until the 4th day may be associated with a 20-fold increase in mortality.

Bjorkhomn B, Bottiger M, Christenson B, et al: Antitoxin antibody levels and the outcome of illness during an outbreak of diphtheria among alcoholics. Scand J Infect Dis 18:235, 1986.
Chen RT, Broome CV, Weinstein RA, et al: Diphtheria in the United States, 1971–1981. Am J Public Health 75:1393, 1985.
Karzon DT, Edwards KM: Diphtheria outbreaks in immunized populations. N Engl J Med 318:41, 1988.
Kjeldsen K, Simonsen O, Heron I: Immunity against diphtheria 25–30 years after primary vaccination in childhood. Lancet 1:900, 1985.
Rappuoli R, Perugini M, Falsen E: Molecular epidemiology of the 1984–1986 outbreak of diphtheria in Sweden. N Engl J Med 318:12, 1988.
Thisyakorn US, Wongvanich J, Kumpeng V: Failure of corticosteroid therapy to prevent diphtheritic myocarditis or neuritis. Pediatr Infect Dis J 3:126, 1984.

12.26 PERTUSSIS
(Whooping Cough)

Pertussis, meaning intensive cough, is an acute respiratory infection that can affect any susceptible host such as unimmunized children or adults with waning immunity. Called "cough of 100 days" in China, pertussis produces serious disease in young infants worldwide, but asymptomatic carriage or minor infection is also common in adults.

ETIOLOGY. Pertussis is classically caused by *Bordetella pertussis*. A similar illness has been associated with infection by *B. parapertussis* and, rarely, *B. bronchiseptica*. A sometimes indistinguishable clinical syndrome has also been associated with adenovirus infection (types 1, 2, 3, and 5). *B. pertussis* and to a lesser extent *B. parapertussis* are the etiologic agents that can be implicated in most unimmunized children with pertussis.

B. pertussis is a small, nonmotile, gram-negative coccobacillus with fastidious requirements for growth. It is recovered best on glycerin-potato-blood agar media (Bordet-Gengou) to which penicillin has been added to inhibit growth of other organisms. Freshly recovered organisms generally are an antigenic and virulent type designated phase I. Passage in culture may induce avirulent variant forms (phase II, III, or IV). This event is due to a DNA frame shift following insertion of a single nucleotide into the *vir* region of the genome. Phase I strains are required for transmission of disease and production of an effective vaccine. *B. parapertussis* and *B. bronchiseptica*, which are morphologically similar to *B. pertussis*, have similar requirements for growth but can be differentiated by specific agglutination reactions.

EPIDEMIOLOGY. Pertussis, one of the most contagious diseases, can produce attack rates of 80–100% in susceptible populations. Humans are the only known hosts. Spread occurs by direct contact or by respiratory droplets spread during coughing because the organism does not survive in the environment. Atypical symptoms or prolonged asymptomatic carriage are common among adults who serve as a major reservoir of *B. pertussis*. Intrafamily spread and epidemics among staff and patients in homes for disabled children and among housestaff exposed to infected children result in disease in adults as their immunity wanes with age. Infants less than 1 yr of age constitute 50–70% of diagnosed cases, and most deaths occur in these unimmunized infants. There is little seasonal variation. Females are affected more frequently than males.

The incidence of pertussis remains high in developing countries. In the United States the incidence has decreased dramatically since the use of pertussis vaccine began. Immunization reduces the incidence and mortality of pertussis, but immunization is neither complete nor permanent. Pertussis is endemic, but periodic 3- to 5-yr epidemics occur and are attributable to the addition of susceptible individuals into the population. Transplacental passage of maternal antibodies does not consistently protect the newborn; severe neonatal pertussis can be acquired from a mildly symptomatic mother.

PATHOLOGY. The organisms multiply only in association with ciliated epithelium and produce various active substances or virulence factors (including toxins). There is congestion and infiltration of the mucosa with lymphocytes and polymorphonuclear leukocytes, and inflammatory debris accumulates in the lumen of the bronchi. Peribronchial lymphoid hyperplasia occurs early, followed by a necrotizing process that affects the midzonal and basilar layers of the bronchial epithelium. Bronchopneumonia develops, with necrosis and desquamation of the superficial epithelium of small bronchi. Bronchiolar obstruction and atelectasis result from accumulation of mucous secretions. Bronchiectasis may develop and persist.

Pathologic changes have been described in brain and liver. Microscopic or gross cerebral hemorrhages may be noted, and cortical atrophy has been observed, possibly as the result of anoxia. Fatty infiltration of the liver may be noted with pertussis encephalopathy.

B. pertussis produces many biologically active factors that are responsible for disease; pertussis is not a single-toxin disease. *Filamentous hemagglutinin* (FHA) is a nontoxic surface component responsible for attachments to ciliated respiratory epithelium. *Fimbrial agglutinins 2 and 3/6* may also have a role in cell attachment. *Pertussis toxin* (PT), also known as lymphocytosis-promoting factor (LPF), histamine-sensitizing factor, and islet-activating factor, is a large protein that catalyzes the transfer of ADP-ribose from NAD to various regulatory guanine nucleotide-binding (G) proteins. PT functionally inactivates target G proteins, thus disrupting signal transduction in the specific cell (respiratory epithelium, neutrophil). *Adenylate cyclase toxin* is secreted by *B. pertussis*, enters mammalian cells, and, after activation by endogenous calmodulin, produces supraphysiologic levels of cyclic AMP, which results in impaired leukocyte activity and cell death. *Dermonecrotic toxin* is a heat-labile cytoplasmic toxin that causes vascular smooth muscle contractions and ischemic necrosis. *Tracheal cytotoxin* inhibits DNA synthesis, causes ciliostasis, and results in cell death. Pertussis lipopolysaccharide (endotoxin) is not important in the pathogenesis of disease.

The sequence of disease production, which includes attachment to target tissues, production of local injury, and systemic absorption of toxins, is dependent upon the disruption and evasion of host defense mechanisms (cilia and neutrophil function). *B. parapertussis* may also cause infection that is milder, due in part to the absence of PT.

CLINICAL MANIFESTATIONS. The incubation period of pertussis has a mean of 7 and a range of 6–20 days. Symptomatic illness is generally divided into three stages: catarrhal, paroxysmal, and convalescent. Illness generally lasts 6–8 wk. The clinical manifestations depend to some extent on the specific etiology of the syndrome as well as on the age and immunization status of the host. Patients less than 2 yr of age frequently have paroxysmal coughing (100%), whoops (60–70%), emesis (60–80%), dyspnea for more than 1 mo (70–80%), and seizures (20–25%); older children have a lower incidence of these manifestations and a shorter duration of illness. Seizures are uncommon in patients over 2 yr of age. In all age groups fever higher than 38.4° C is uncommon. Illness due to *B. parapertussis* or *B. bronchiseptica* is less severe and of shorter duration than that described below.

Catarrhal Stage (1–2 wk). Symptoms of an upper respiratory infection predominate. Rhinorrhea, conjunctival injection, lacrimation, mild cough, and low-grade fever are noted; a diagnosis of pertussis usually is not considered during this stage. Infants tend to have a profuse, viscid nasal discharge that may cause upper respiratory obstruction.

Paroxysmal Stage (2–4 wk or longer). Episodes of coughing increase in severity and number. Characteristically, repetitive series of 5–10 forceful coughs during a single expiration are followed by a sudden massive inspiratory effort, which produces the *whoop* as air is inhaled forcefully against a narrowed glottis. Facial redness or cyanosis, bulging eyes, protrusion of the tongue, lacrimation, salivation, and distention of neck veins are prominent during the attack. Episodes of paroxysmal coughing may recur sequentially until the mucous plug obstructing the airway is dislodged. *Post-tussive emesis* in association with the paroxysms is characteristic enough that the child should be suspected of having pertussis even in the absence of a whoop. The episodes are exhausting; it is not unusual for the patient to appear apathetic and to lose weight. Attacks may be triggered by yawning, sneezing, eating, drinking, and physical exertion or even by suggestion. Between attacks the patient may appear to be minimally ill and is usually comfortable. Some patients, especially young infants, have no whoop.

Convalescent Stage (1–2 wk). Paroxysmal episodes of coughing and vomiting gradually decrease in frequency and severity. Cough may persist for several months. Infrequently, recurrent paroxysmal cough recurs for months or years with subsequent upper respiratory infections.

Physical examination is generally uninformative. In the paroxysmal stage petechial or conjunctival hemorrhages may be noted on the head and neck. In some patients diffuse rhonchi and rales are noted.

DIAGNOSIS AND DIFFERENTIAL DIAGNOSIS. Pertussis can be recognized readily during the paroxysmal stage of disease if the diagnosis is considered. Unfortunately, very young infants, adolescents, and adults may have atypical manifestations. A history of contact with a known case is helpful, but generally the history will be negative in a highly immunized population. A cough of more than 2 wk duration with post-tussive emesis is an important diagnostic clue.

Leukocytosis (counts of 20,000–50,000 cells/mm^3 of blood) with an absolute lymphocytosis is characteristic at the end of the catarrhal and during the paroxysmal stages of the disease. The white cell count may not be helpful in infants, since they respond with lymphocytosis to many infections. Chest roentgenograms may show perihilar infiltrates, atelectasis, or emphysema.

Specific diagnosis depends on the recovery of the organism, best accomplished during the early phases of the illness by nasopharyngeal swabs that are cultured on Bordet-Gengou media at the bedside. The culture material is obtained with a Dacron or calcium alginate swab because cotton inhibits growth of *B. pertussis*. Prior antibiotic treatment may also reduce the recovery of *B. pertussis*. Direct fluorescent antibody staining of pharyngeal specimens may provide a specific diagnosis rapidly. Rapid diagnosis of pertussis also may be performed using CIE. DNA hybridization techniques are being developed to detect specific *B. pertussis* genomic DNA.

Detection of antibodies against pertussis toxin in paired serum samples may be used for serologic diagnosis of pertussis. ELISA may be used to detect serum IgM, IgG, and IgA to the filamentous hemagglutinin (FHA) and the pertussis toxin (PT). Serum levels of IgM-FHA and IgM-PT are not useful in establishing seropositivity because they represent a primary immune response and may be elicited by disease or vaccination. IgG directed toward pertussis toxin is the most sensitive and specific test for acute infection. IgA-FHA and IgA-PT are less sensitive than IgG-PT but are highly specific for natural infection and are not seen following pertussis immunization.

No single test exists today that is both highly sensitive and highly specific for detecting infection with *B. pertussis* during all phases of the illness. Cultures are most likely to be positive in the catarrhal and early paroxysmal stages and should be obtained in all suspected cases; however, rapid diagnostic techniques including fluorescent antibody staining and CIE may be helpful in making immediate clinical decisions. Serologic testing is useful in the later stages of the disease and for confirming the presence of infection in culture-negative individuals.

COMPLICATIONS. These primarily involve disorders of the respiratory and central nervous systems. Pneumonia, the most frequent complication, is responsible for more than 90% of deaths in children under 3 yr of age. It may be related to *B. pertussis* itself but is caused more commonly by secondary bacterial invaders *(H. influenzae, S. pneumoniae, S. aureus, S. pyogenes)*. Latent tuberculosis may also be activated. Atelectasis may develop secondary to viscid mucous plugs. Aspiration of mucus or vomitus may produce chemical pneumonia, which may become secondarily infected. High fever often signifies secondary bacterial infection. The forcefulness of the paroxysm can cause rupture of the alveoli, producing interstitial or subcutaneous emphysema and pneumothorax. Bronchiectasis may develop and persist.

Otitis media is common and is frequently due to *S. pneumoniae*. Other complications include ulcer of the frenulum of the tongue, epistaxis, melena, subconjunctival hemorrhages, spinal epidural hematoma, intracranial hemorrhage, rupture of the diaphragm, umbilical hernia, inguinal hernia, rectal prolapse, dehydration, and nutritional disturbances.

Convulsions and coma may occur. They are probably a reflection of cerebral hypoxia related to asphyxia, but seizures may occasionally be due to high temperature. Seizures associated with hyponatremia secondary to the syndrome of inappropriate secretion of antidiuretic hormone (SIADH) also have been reported in infants with severe pertussis. Tetanic seizures may be associated with alkalosis resulting from loss of gastric contents due to persistent vomiting.

PREVENTION. Active immunity can be induced by a total dose of 12 protective units of pertussis vaccine given in three equal doses 8 wk apart. See Sec. 5.1 for a full discussion of initial and subsequent immunization schedules and dosages. Currently available vaccines, prepared from suspensions of inactivated whole cells of *B. pertussis*, are immunogenic and protective only after the three primary immunizations are complete. Immunization is accomplished by providing pertussis, diphtheria, and tetanus toxoids in combination. Premature infants may be immunized at 2 mo postnatal age rather than waiting until 2 mo post-term (48 wk postconceptional age). If pertussis is prevalent in the community, immunization can be started at 2 wk of age and doses repeated as often as every 4 wk. Children over 7 yr are not routinely immunized. Immunity is not permanent because protection wanes during adolescence; infection in older patients is usually mild but serves as a major source of *B. pertussis* infection in nonimmune infants. Successful control of pertussis in the future may require the development of a safe booster vaccine for older patients. Adsorbed monovalent pertussis vaccine (0.25 mL, given IM) has been used to control epidemics among adults who are exposed to nonimmunized children. Children who recover from culture-documented pertussis do not require further immunization.

Adverse events following pertussis immunization include common manifestations such as erythema, induration, and tenderness at the injection site and common (fever, fretfulness, drowsiness) and uncommon (febrile or afebrile seizures, collapse or hypotonic-hyporesponsive episodes, encephalopathy and anaphylaxis) systemic complications (see Sec. 5.1). The risks associated with high fever (febrile convulsions) may potentially be attenuated by the administration of acetaminophen (15 mg/kg, given orally) at the time of immunization and every 4–6 hr for 48–72 hr. The risks of serious systemic and central nervous system complications during naturally acquired pertussis far exceed the risk following active immunization.

Reasons for deferral or omission of the first pertussis immunization include a febrile illness at the scheduled time of immunization, any progressive neurologic disorder characterized by developmental delay or changing neurologic findings (infantile spasms, progressive encephalopathy, uncontrolled epilepsy), a personal history of convulsions (until a progressive disorder is excluded), and conditions predisposing to seizures or neurologic deterioration (tuberous sclerosis, metabolic or degenerative disorders). A family history of seizures, sudden infant death syndrome (SIDS), or severe reactions to pertussis immunization is *not* a contraindication to pertussis vaccination. Contraindications to further administration of pertussis vaccine include encephalopathy within 7 days of prior vaccination, a febrile or nonfebrile convulsion within 3 days of vaccination, persistent unconsolable screaming or crying for 3 or more hr, high-pitched cry within 2 days, collapse or shock-like hypotonic-hyporesponsive state within 2 days, unexplained temperature of 40.5° C or higher within 2 days, and the uncommon occurrence of anaphylaxis.

Because of the reactogenicity of the whole-cell pertussis vaccine, new acellular preparations have been developed to improve immunogenicity without unwanted local, systemic, or central nervous system complications. "T" or Taheda acellular vaccine contains a 9:1 ratio of inactivated pertussis toxin (LPF) to FHA together with other agglutinins and proteins, whereas the "B" or Biken acellular vaccine has a 1:1 ratio of LPF to FHA. Other acellular preparations also contain LPF. Two-component vaccines are more immunogenic than single-component vaccines. Acellular vaccines may have a lower incidence of local, systemic, and CNS side effects than the whole-cell vaccine. However, more information is required about the efficacy of acellular vaccines in young infants because preliminary studies suggest that the immunologic response among young infants may be reduced.

Overinterpretation of recommended contraindications may produce a large population of nonimmune susceptible children. Therefore, the risk-benefit ratio (risk of disease far exceeds that of immunization) should be discussed with the parents, and the most recent recommendations of the American Academy of Pediatrics should be reviewed.

Contacts. Erythromycin is effective in preventing pertussis in newborn infants of mothers with pertussis. Close contacts of less than 7 yr of age who have been immunized previously against pertussis should receive a booster dose of DPT unless a booster dose has been given within the preceding 6 mo. They also should be given erythromycin, 50 mg/kg/24 hr in four divided oral doses for 14 days. Children who are more than 7 yr of age and who have been immunized also should receive prophylactic erythromycin. Early erythromycin therapy reduces the spread of infection, eliminates *B. pertussis* from the respiratory tract, and reduces symptoms of the disease. Erythromycin estolate provides the highest antibiotic levels and is the most effective agent.

Persons in contact with a patient with pertussis who have not been immunized previously should receive erythromycin for 14 days after the contact has been broken. If the contact cannot be broken, erythromycin should be given until the cough in the index patient has stopped or until the index patient has received erythromycin for 7 days. Monovalent pertussis should be given with erythromycin in institutional epidemics.

TREATMENT. Erythromycin (50 mg/kg/24 hr) for 14 days may eliminate pertussis organisms from the nasopharynx within 3–4 days, thereby shortening the period of communicability. Erythromycin may abort or eliminate pertussis when given to patients within 14 days of initial onset of the disease. Once paroxysms of coughing develop, erythromycin reduces communicability but does not usually improve symptoms, especially if it has been started late.

Supportive care includes avoidance of factors that provoke attacks of coughing and maintenance of hydration and nutrition. Oxygen should be administered for respiratory distress, acute or chronic. Gentle suction to remove profuse, viscid secretions may be required, particularly in infants with pneumonia and significant respiratory distress. Betamethasone and Salbutamol (albuterol) may reduce severe coughing paroxysms; however, their efficacy has not been tested by controlled studies. Cough suppressants are not helpful.

PROGNOSIS. Mortality rates have fallen to fewer than 10/1,000 cases in the United States; they may reach 40% in infants under 5 mo. Most deaths are due to encephalopathy and pneumonia or other pulmonary complications. The long-term respiratory sequelae following pertussis infection are uncertain. In general, infants less than 6 mo of age who have been hospitalized with severe pertussis may exhibit minor pulmonary function abnormalities and lower respiratory symptoms including wheezing during adult life.

RALPH D. FEIGIN

Ad Hoc Group for the Study of Pertussis Vaccine: Placebo-controlled trial of two acellular pertussis vaccines in Sweden—Protective efficacy and adverse events. Lancet 1:30, 1988.

Bergquist SO, Bernander S, Dahnsjo H, et al: Erythromycin in the treatment of pertussis: A study of bacteriologic and clinical effects. Pediatr Infect Dis J 6:458, 1987.

Bernbaum JC, Daft A, Anolik R, et al: Response of preterm infants to diphtheria-tetanus-pertussis immunizations. J Pediatr 107:184, 1985.

Biellik RJ, Patriarca PA, Mullen JR, et al: Risk factors for community- and household-acquired pertussis during a large-scale outbreak in central Wisconsin. J Infect Dis 157:1134, 1988.

Cherry JD: Pertussis vaccine encephalopathy: It is time to recognize it as the myth that it is. JAMA 263:1679, 1990.

Committee on Infectious Diseases, American Academy of Pediatrics: Report of the Committee on Infectious Diseases, 21st ed. 1988.

Granstrom G, Sterner G, Nord CE, et al: Use of erythromycin to prevent pertussis in newborns of mothers with pertussis. J Infect Dis 155:1210, 1987.

Griffin MR, Ray WA, Mortimer EA, et al: Risk of seizures and encephalopathy after immunization with the diphtheria-tetanus-pertussis vaccine. JAMA 263:1641, 1990.

Hoppe JE: Treatment and prevention of pertussis by antimicrobial agents (II). Infection 16:148, 1988.

Isomura S: Efficacy and safety of acellular pertussis vaccine in Aichi Prefecture, Japan. Pediatr Infect Dis J 7:258, 1988.

Long SS, Welkon CJ, Clark JL: Widespread silent transmission of pertussis in

families: Antibody correlates of infection and symptomatology. J Infect Dis 161:480, 1990.
Mortimer EA: Pertussis and its prevention: A family affair. J Infect Dis 161:473, 1990.
Sotomayor J, Weiner LB, McMillan JA: Inaccurate diagnosis in infants with pertussis. Am J Dis Child 139:724, 1985.
Steketee RW, Wassilak SGF, Adkins WN, et al: Evidence for a high attack rate and efficacy of erythromycin prophylaxis in a pertussis outbreak in a facility for the developmentally disabled. J Infect Dis 157:434, 1988.

12.27 DIARRHEAGENIC *ESCHERICHIA COLI*

ETIOLOGY AND PATHOGENESIS. Five classes of *E. coli* are currently recognized as agents associated with pediatric gastroenteritis. Because *E. coli* are normal fecal flora, demonstration of virulence characteristics is the only way by which the diarrheagenic *E. coli* can be defined. The mechanism by which *E. coli* produce diarrhea typically involves adherence of organisms to a glycoprotein or glycolipid receptor followed by production of some noxious substance that injures gut cells or disturbs their function without killing them. The genes for virulence properties and for antibiotic resistance are often carried on transferable plasmids. The current classification is summarized below.

Enterotoxigenic *E. coli* (ETEC). These *E. coli* produce a heat-labile enterotoxin (LT) and/or a heat-stable enterotoxin (ST). LT is structurally, functionally, and immunologically related to cholera toxin produced by *Vibrio cholerae*. ST is not related to LT or cholera toxin, although it is related to an enterotoxin produced by some strains of *Yersinia enterocolitica*. These toxins do not injure or kill cells; rather, they disturb cyclic nucleotide–regulated fluid and electrolyte absorption. ST stimulates guanylate cyclase, resulting in increased cyclic GMP, whereas LT (like cholera toxin) stimulates adenylate cyclase, resulting in increased cyclic AMP. The ETEC typically also possess *adherence factors (fimbria)* that allow them to adhere tightly to intestinal epithelium, thereby presumably efficiently colonizing and delivering toxin to the epithelium. A number of different colonization factor antigens (CFA) have been recognized as important in effecting the adherence of ETEC to gut mucosal cells. These CFAs are called CFA I, CFA II, E 8775, and PCF 0 159. After colonization of intestinal epithelium, the ETEC release ST and/or LT. The genes for both colonization factors and enterotoxins are typically encoded on the same plasmid. Of the more than 170 *E. coli* serogroups only a relatively small number typically are ETEC; these serogroups (06, 08, 015, 020, 025, 027, 063, 078, 080, 085, 0115, 0128ac [but not subgroups 0128ab or 0128ad], 0139, 0148, 0153, 0159, and 0167) are generally different from those found in the other diarrhea-associated *E. coli*.

Enteroinvasive *E. coli* (EIEC). These *E. coli* behave like shigellae in their capacity to invade gut epithelium and produce a dysentery-like illness. The EIEC not only adhere to gut cells, they also invade them. This *Shigella*-like behavior is due to the fact that these *E. coli* possess a large virulence plasmid that is closely related to the virulence plasmid that endows *Shigella* with its invasiveness (Sec. 12.30). A small group of polypeptides encoded on these plasmids is critical to the invasion of intestinal epithelium for both shigellae and EIEC. Invasion of epithelium causes cell death and a brisk inflammatory response (clinically recognizable as colitis). The bacterial product that kills intestinal cells is not known. EIEC encompass a small number of serogroups (028ac, 029, 0124, 0136, 0143, 0144, 0152, 0164, and 0167). These serogroups have lipopolysaccharide (LPS) antigens related to *Shigella* LPS, and, like shigellae, the organisms are nonmotile (they lack H or flagellar antigens) and are usually nonlactose fermenters.

Enteropathogenic *E. coli* (EPEC). These serogroups (O antigen or lipopolysaccharide antigen) have been associated with outbreaks of infantile gastroenteritis but do not produce conventional enterotoxins or invade epithelial cells as do the EIEC. However, organisms within these serogroups also have been isolated from well individuals. The EPEC adhere to the intestinal mucosa in a distinctive way. This pattern of adherence, seen on transmission electron microscopy, has been called "close attaching and effacing" adherence or "pedestal-forming" adherence. The lesion consists of loss of microvilli with adherence of bacteria to the epithelial cells, which form a cup or pedestal in which the bacteria can be seen. Chronic inflammation with flattened villi may also be seen on small bowel biopsy of affected children. It is not clear what toxic products the bacteria produce to cause these changes in epithelial cells. Unlike most *E. coli*, EPEC often adhere to HEp-2 cells in tissue culture; the same phenomenon that causes the changes seen on electron microscopy may be responsible for the cell adherence seen in tissue culture. The EPEC have been subdivided into two groups based on their patterns of adherence to HEp-2 cells in tissue culture and on their ability to hybridize with a 1-kilobase DNA probe (EAF probe) isolated from a 60-megadalton plasmid (pMAR2), whose presence has been associated with adherence. The serogroups that are associated with localized adherence and are EAF probe positive (055, 086, 0111, 0119, 0125, 0126, 0127, 0128ab, and 0142) have been referred to as class I EPEC, whereas those that are nonadherent or diffusely adherent to HEp-2 cells and are usually EAF probe negative (018, 044, 0112, and 0114) have been called class II EPEC.

Enterohemorrhagic *E. coli* (EHEC). These *E. coli* produce one or more toxins that kill mammalian cells. They have also been called enterocytotoxic *E. coli*, shiga-like toxin–producing *E. coli*, and verotoxin-producing *E. coli* (VTEC). Two major toxins are produced by EHEC. One is essentially identical to shigatoxin, the protein synthesis–inhibiting exotoxin of *Shigella dysenteriae* serotype 1. The second is more distantly related to shigatoxin. The first toxin is called shiga-like toxin I (or verotoxin 1) and the second, shiga-like toxin II (or verotoxin 2). Multiple variants of these toxins probably exist. They kill cells by cleaving an adenine residue from ribosomal RNA at the site where elongation factor 1–dependent attachment of aminoacyl t-RNA occurs; the result is protein synthesis inhibition and cell death. EHEC adhere to intestinal cells and produce lesions that resemble, on electron microscopy, those seen with EPEC, although they are more restricted in their distribution (being found primarily in the colon) compared with EPEC (which infest the entire intestine). The most common serotypes are *E. coli* 0157:H7 and *E. coli* 026:H11, although a number of other serotypes have also been described. *E. coli* 026:H11 was formerly considered an EPEC.

Enteroadherent *E. coli* (EAEC). These *E. coli* have the ability to adhere to HEp-2 cells in tissue culture. They are also referred to as autoagglutinating, enteroaggregative, and enteroadherent-aggregative *E. coli*. It is likely that this group will be further subdivided, and some of these organisms will be shown to be nonpathogens. Although EAEC adhere to HEp-2 cells in patterns similar to those seen with EPEC, they do not belong to classic EPEC serogroups. These organisms do not produce enterotoxins or shiga-like toxins, invade cells, or possess EAF genes. There is substantial controversy about the definition of this group in relation to slightly different assay systems; the result is that although there is agreement that some organisms adhere to HEp-2 cells in a diffuse pattern and some adhere locally, the investigators who use the designation "aggregative" *E. coli* include organisms under this term that in other assay systems are either "local" or "diffuse." It is not clear which system better recognizes the true pathogens; under the one system both locally and diffusely adherent *E. coli* are associated with diarrhea, whereas in the other system the locally adherent and aggregative *E. coli* are pathogens and the diffusely adherent organisms are not.

The nature of the bacterial products that cause fluid loss after EAEC adherence occurs is undefined. The serogroups to which these organisms belong remain to be defined.

EPIDEMIOLOGY. In the developing world the various diarrheagenic *E. coli* cause frequent infections in the first few years of life. They occur with increased frequency during the warm months in temperate climates and during rainy season months in tropical climates. Most *E. coli* (except EHEC and perhaps some EPEC) require a large inoculum of organisms to induce disease; person-to-person spread is atypical, whereas food- or water-borne illness is common. Therefore, infection is most likely when food handling or sewage disposal practices are suboptimal. Although infection occurs, in children in the United States, it is more often seen in those who live in or have recently visited the developing world. EHEC and EPEC organisms are transmitted person to person as well as by food, suggesting that ingestion of a lower number of these organisms is sufficient to cause disease. Poorly cooked meat is the most common cause of food-borne outbreaks of EHEC. If children survive the first few years of life, they develop immunity, as evidenced by the isolation of *E. coli* from the feces of well, older children.

PATHOLOGY. ETEC cause little or no structural alterations in the gut mucosa. EIEC cause colonic lesions like those of bacillary dysentery; ulcerations, hemorrhage, and infiltration of polymorphonuclear leukocytes with mucosal and submucosal edema are typical. EPEC are associated with blunting of villi, inflammatory changes and sloughing of superficial mucosal cells on light microscopy, and attaching and effacing changes on transmission electron microscopy; these lesions are found from the duodenum through the colon. EHEC lesions resemble those due to EPEC but are primarily found in the colon. Pathologic changes due to EAEC have not been studied extensively in humans.

CLINICAL MANIFESTATIONS. As might be expected from the differing mechanisms of disease production, the clinical features of *E. coli*–associated diarrhea vary from group to group. *ETEC* are a major cause of dehydrating infantile diarrhea in the developing world. The typical signs and symptoms include explosive watery diarrhea, abdominal pain, nausea, vomiting, and little or no fever. Resolution usually occurs in a matter of days. These infections have an untoward effect on infant nutritional status.

EIEC cause an illness that is indistinguishable from classic bacillary dysentery. Fever, systemic toxicity, crampy abdominal pain, tenesmus, and urgency with watery or bloody diarrhea are characteristic.

EPEC usually are isolated from infants and children in the first few years of life who have a nonbloody diarrhea with mucus; fever may occur. Unlike ETEC, EIEC, or EHEC, these organisms often cause a prolonged diarrheal disease.

EHEC may cause a nondescript diarrheal illness or an illness characterized by abdominal pain with diarrhea that is initially watery but within a few days becomes grossly bloody (hemorrhagic colitis). Although this pattern resembles that of shigellosis or EIEC disease, it differs in that fever is an uncommon manifestation. Children who have fever may be at increased risk of *hemolytic uremic syndrome*.

EAEC have not been extensively characterized in terms of the illness they cause. Significant fluid loss with dehydration is common, whereas fever, vomiting, and grossly bloody stools are relatively infrequent. These organisms, like the EPEC, are often associated with prolonged diarrhea.

COMPLICATIONS. The major complications are those related to dehydration and electrolyte loss. Some complications are related to specific pathogens. EPEC and EAEC are likely to cause persistent diarrhea. Infection with EHEC is frequently associated with the hemolytic uremic syndrome, as is infection due to *S. dysenteriae* type 1.

DIAGNOSIS. The clinical features of illness are seldom distinctive enough to allow confident diagnosis, and routine laboratory studies are of very limited value. Diagnosis currently depends heavily on laboratory studies that are not readily available to the practitioner. Routine stool cultures reveal only "normal flora." Biochemical criteria (e.g., fermentation patterns) are of minimal value. Sorbitol nonfermenting *E. coli* isolated from a child with hemorrhagic colitis suggest the possibility of the EHEC strain *E. coli* 0167:H7. Culture of duodenal fluid may be helpful in the diagnosis of EPEC because of their tendency to colonize the small intestine. This study is generally indicated only in the child with chronic diarrhea.

Other laboratory data are at best nonspecific indicators of etiology. Fecal leukocyte examination of the stool is usually positive with the EIEC but negative with all other diarrheagenic *E. coli*. Blood counts, especially with EIEC and EHEC, often show an elevated leukocyte count with a left shift. Electrolyte changes are nonspecific, reflecting only fluid loss.

The traditional methods of identification of these organisms require animal or tissue culture models that are unacceptably cumbersome and expensive for routine use by hospital laboratories. Some of these organisms, especially the EPEC, could theoretically be defined serologically. However, the frequency of cross reactions, the unavailability of suitable reagents, and the infrequency with which the serogroup alone is adequate to define a pathogen make these methods unsuitable. DNA probes for genes encoding the various virulence traits hold the greatest promise for the future; they are currently appropriate only in the research laboratory setting. Probes have been developed for ETEC, EIEC, class I EPEC, and EHEC.

Suspected organisms should be forwarded to reference or research laboratories for definitive evaluation. Such efforts are seldom necessary, but they may be critical for correct diagnosis of the child with severe or life-threatening complications or for the occasional nursery outbreak.

TREATMENT. The cornerstone of proper management is related to fluid and electrolyte therapy. In general, this therapy should include oral replacement and maintenance with rehydrating solutions such as those specified by the World Health Organization. Early refeeding with breast milk or dilute formula should be encouraged as soon as dehydration is corrected. Despite the tendency of early refeeding to aggravate diarrhea, it should be encouraged because prolonged withholding of feeding frequently leads to chronic diarrhea and malnutrition.

Specific antimicrobial therapy of diarrheagenic *E. coli* is problematic because of the difficulty of making an accurate diagnosis of these pathogens and the unpredictability of antibiotic susceptibilities. ETEC respond to antimicrobial agents such as trimethoprim-sulfamethoxazole (TMP-SMX) when the *E. coli* are susceptible. However, outside of the setting of a child recently returning from travel to the developing world, empiric treatment of severe watery diarrhea with antibiotics is seldom appropriate. Although treatment of EPEC with TMP-SMX (6.4 mg/kg/24 hr of the trimethoprim component in four divided doses intravenously or orally for 5 days) is effective in speeding resolution, the lack of a rapid diagnostic test makes treatment decisions difficult. EIEC are usually treated prior to the availability of culture results. If the organisms are susceptible, TMP-SMX is an appropriate choice. The EHEC represent a particularly difficult therapeutic dilemma. The controversial data suggest that antibiotic treatment, particularly with sulfa-containing regimens, may increase the risk of hemolytic uremic syndrome. It is too early to assess the usefulness of antibiotics in the treatment of EAEC.

Antibiotic resistance is often encoded on the same plasmids that carry virulence properties and continues to make rational decisions about antibiotic therapy difficult. Because emergence of resistance to widely used regimens is typical, new antimicrobial agents must continue to be evaluated.

Prophylactic antibiotic therapy, although effective in adult travelers, has not been studied in children and is not generally recommended. Public health measures, including sewage disposal and food-handling practices, have made pathogens that require large inocula to produce illness relatively uncommon in industrialized countries. Food-borne outbreaks of EHEC are a problem for which no adequate solution has been found. During the occasional hospital outbreak of EPEC disease, attention to enteric isolation precautions and cohorting may be critical (Sec. 12.9).

PREVENTION. In the developing world prevention of disease caused by diarrheagenic *E. coli* is probably best done by maintaining prolonged breast-feeding, paying careful attention to personal hygiene, and following proper food- and water-handling procedures. Children traveling to these places can be best protected by paying careful attention to diet (in particular, consuming only processed water and eating only foods served steaming hot).

THOMAS G. CLEARY

Cleary TG: Cytotoxin producing *E. coli* and the hemolytic uremic syndrome. Pediatr Clin North Am 35:485, 1988.

Mathewson JJ, Cravioto A: HEp-2 cell adherence as an assay for virulence among diarrheagenic *E. coli*. J Infect Dis 159:1057, 1989.

Moseley L, Echeverria P, Seriwantana J, et al: Identification of enterotoxigenic *Escherichia coli* by colony hybridization using three enterotoxin gene probes. J Infect Dis 145:863, 1982.

Rothbaum R, McAdams AJ, Giannella R, et al: A clinicopathologic study of enterocyte adherent *Escherichia coli*: A cause of protracted diarrhea in infants. Gastroenterology 83:441, 1982.

Ryder RW, Wachsmuth IK, Buxton AE, et al: Infantile diarrhea produced by heat-stable enterotoxigenic *Escherichia coli*. N Engl J Med 295:849, 1976.

Sack RB: Enterotoxigenic *Escherichia coli*: Identification and characterization. J Infect Dis 142:279, 1980.

Ulshen MH, Rollo JL: Pathogenesis of *Escherichia coli* gastroenteritis in man: Another mechanism. N Engl J Med 302:99, 1980.

12.28 INFECTIONS DUE TO SALMONELLAE

Salmonella organisms are important pathogens of humans and animals. Generally, human infections are caused by the ingestion of contaminated water or food. Currently, gastroenteritis due to *Salmonella* is one of the common infectious diseases in the United States, as it is worldwide. Although systemic infection with *Salmonella typhosa* (typhoid fever) is infrequent in the United States, it remains endemic and epidemic in many parts of the world.

ETIOLOGY. Salmonellae are motile, gram-negative, nonencapsulated, nonsporulating rods of the Enterobacteriaceae family. The principal antigens are the flagellae (H) antigens, the cell-wall (O) lipopolysaccharide antigens, and the envelope virulence (Vi) heat-labile antigens that block the O antigen-antibody agglutination. An elaborate typing scheme utilizing O and H antigens (Kaufman-White) has permitted the differentiation of over 800 *Salmonella* serotypes. A system of nomenclature has been suggested in which all salmonellae are classified into three groups (*S. enteritidis*, *S. typhi*, and *S. choleraesuis*). The first group contains all salmonellae except the latter two. Each species, then, is classified as a bioserotype such as *S. enteritidis* bio *typhimurim*. A system for "practical" naming of salmonellae treats serotypes as species. Thus, *S. typhimurium* is an acceptable notation for *S. enteritidis* bioserotype *typhimurium*.

Salmonellae are resistant to many physical agents, but they can be killed by heating to 130° F (54.4° C) for 1 hr or 140° F (60° C) for 15 min. They remain viable at ambient or reduced temperatures for days and may survive for weeks in sewage, dried foodstuffs, pharmaceutical agents, and fecal material. *Salmonella* can be differentiated from other enterobacteriaceae by its fermentation of glucose or mannose and sucrose. They can be studied, epidemiologically, by plasmid DNA fingerprinting, antibody susceptibility, and various bacteriophages.

The properties of salmonellae responsible for their pathogenicity remain incompletely defined. The O antigen (an endotoxin) enhances resistance of the organism to phagocytosis; strains deficient in it are avirulent. The effects of endotoxin in the host may be responsible for certain manifestations of the systemic disease, but no evidence supports a role in gastroenteritis. Some serotypes have distinct host preferences and produce characteristic patterns of disease. *Salmonella typhosa* infects only humans. Salmonellae of groups A and C are generally isolated from human sources, whereas *S. abortus equi* infects only horses. Despite this apparent propensity of strains to seek a particular host, 7 of the 10 types of *Salmonella* most commonly recovered from animal sources in the United States are among the 10 types most commonly isolated from humans.

NONTYPHOIDAL SALMONELLOSIS

EPIDEMIOLOGY. Opportunity to acquire an infection from contaminated food or water with one of the serotypes of *Salmonella* appears to be increasing; more than 50,000 culture-proven cases of salmonellosis are reported in the United States annually. The actual number of cases has been estimated to be 800,000–4,000,000. Of the reported cases, more than two thirds are in persons under 20 yr of age, with the highest isolation rate among infants less than 1 yr of age.

Meat, milk (raw or pasturized), poultry, and eggs are the most common sources of salmonellae infection. Modern methods of feeding, holding, and transporting farm animals lead to contamination. Animal feeds contaminated with salmonellae in bone or fishmeal are important sources of animal infection. On some farms the use of antibiotic-containing feed, especially for poultry, can lead to increased numbers of salmonellae. Large poultry processing plants must be particularly careful that a few infected birds do not contaminate conveyor belts, water baths, and other equipment, as this may cause unsuspected contamination of large numbers of chickens and turkeys.

Salmonella can infect many species of animals, but those of particular hazard to human health are meat-producing animals, poultry, and reptiles (particularly pet turtles). Most animal infections are asymptomatic. The prevalence of salmonellosis in chickens creates a high risk for contamination of eggs. Salmonellae can contaminate the shell surface, penetrate the egg, or be transmitted from an ovarian infection directly to the egg yolk. Pooling large numbers of eggs prior to freezing, drying, or use of eggs in the preparation of food materials increases the risk of human infection. All eggs utilized in processed foods should be pasteurized; up to 50% of poultry, 5% of beef, 16% of pork, and 40% of frozen egg products purchased in retail stores contain salmonellae. *Salmonella* introduced into kitchens on these contaminated foods may be transferred to other materials including utensils, table surfaces, and personnel. *Salmonella* can resist boiling within an egg for even 2–3 min. Contamination of equipment in processing plants has been responsible for outbreaks associated with baker's yeast, dried milk, dried coconut, cotton seed protein, and various dyes. Carmine red dye derived from female scale insects and larvae, sometimes used in hospitals for determination of intestinal transit time, has caused hospital outbreaks of salmonellosis. This dye is also used as an artificial coloring in drugs, foods, and cosmetics. *Salmonella* infection has also occurred following administration of platelets, use of poorly sterilized fiberoptic endoscopy equipment, inhalation of manure-contaminated marijuana, and administration of animal extracts (pituitary, liver, pancreatic, bile, thyroid, adrenal).

Humans are a less common source of *Salmonella* species than animals but can cause localized epidemics of food poisoning by contaminating food at large gatherings such as picnics. *Salmonella* species that exclusively or predominantly infect humans include *S. typhi, S. paratyphi A, S. schottmuelleri, S. hirschfield,* and *S. sendai.* Nonetheless, animal origin or human-to-human spread is often due to *S. typhimurium, S. enteritides, S. heidelberg, S. newport,* and *S. hadar.* Outbreaks in hospitals and nursing homes that are traced to a carrier are of considerable concern because of the increased morbidity and mortality observed in infants, young children, and the compromised host. Cross-contamination also can occur within institutions by means of contaminated fingers, clothes of the staff, or aerosols. Intrafamilial transmission of salmonellosis is a frequent occurrence.

During the acute stages of infection, 10^6–10^9 salmonellae/g are excreted in stool; 70–90% of infected individuals will have a positive stool culture 2 wk following infection, about 50% at 4 wk, and 10–25% at 10 wk. A large number of swallowed organisms (10^6–10^9) are thought to be needed usually to cause disease; however, as few as 20–50 organisms may be needed under optimal circumstances. The duration of *Salmonella* excretion is similar whether the infection has been asymptomatic or symptomatic, but it appears to be longer in infants than in older children. Excretion is prolonged by antibiotic therapy, and prophylactic antibiotics may increase the risk of infection. Prolonged excretion should not be confused with a chronic carrier state, defined as persistently positive stool cultures for more than 1 yr, which is rare (occurring in $< 1\%$) in persons with nontyphoidal salmonellosis.

PATHOGENESIS AND PATHOLOGY. Disease is related to the number and virulence of the organism and to various host defense mechanisms. After ingestion, salmonellae are killed by low gastric pH (< 2.0). Achlorhydria, buffering agents, fast gastric emptying (water more than food, gastroenterostomy), and a large inoculum permit passage of viable organisms into the small intestine. Local microbiologic flora may inhibit infection; prior antibiotic therapy disrupts this defense mechanism and increases the risk of *Salmonella* infection. Multiplication in the small intestine produces asymptomatic transient fecal excretion, symptomatic enterocolitis, or bacteremia. Diarrhea is the result of tissue invasion and elaboration of an enterotoxin and a cytotoxin. Colonic involvement may be more common than previously thought and is characterized by edema, inflammation, erosions, and microabscesses.

Salmonellae can penetrate the superficial layers of the mucosal lining without destroying epithelial cells. A phagosome is created around the salmonellae in the epithelial cell, but no damage to the bacteria occurs as they travel through or between cells into the lamina propria. Serotypes that usually cause diarrhea evoke a polymorphonuclear leukocyte response in the lamina propria area. The infection extends no farther, and the patient develops only diarrhea. There may be fever associated with diarrhea. The frequency of bacteremia is not known, but it is usually transient, and no metastatic phase of infection occurs in healthy individuals.

Systemic invasion by *Salmonella* is much more common in individuals at the extremes of age as well as in those with diseases that impair reticuloendothelial or cellular immune function. Children with sickle cell disease are prone to develop *Salmonella* septicemia and osteomyelitis. The numerous infarcted areas of the gastrointestinal tract, bones, and reticuloendothelial system may initially permit organisms greater access to the circulation from the intestine and then furnish an optimal environment for localization. The decreased phagocytic and opsonizing capacity of patients with SS hemoglobin disease also contributes to the enhanced infection rate. Individuals with chronic granulomatous disease of childhood or other white blood cell disorders have an increased propensity for infection. Additional risks for bacteremia include AIDS, steroid therapy, malignancy, malnutrition, bartonellosis, malaria, and infection with *S. choleraesuis.* Chronic infection is associated with cholelithiasis, *Schistosoma hematobium* urinary tract fibrosis and stone formation, and *Schistosoma mansoni* hepatosplenic involvement. Localized infections are more common in areas of necrotic tissue (effusions, tumors, hematomas) (see Table 12–24).

CLINICAL MANIFESTATIONS. Gastroenteritis due to *Salmonella* has its peak incidence in the late summer and early fall, correlating with the number of food-borne outbreaks.

TABLE 12–24. Unusual Manifestations of Salmonella Infections

Disease	Epidemiology
Meningitis	Neonatal infections, epidemics possible; ventriculitis, cerebral abscess, subdural empyema. Second most common cause of neonatal gram-negative meningitis. *S. havana, S. typhimurium, S. oranienburg, S. typhi*
Pleuropulmonary disorders	Pneumonia in immunocompromised patients. Secondary empyema of malignant pleural effusion. *S. typhimurium, S. typhi, S. choleraesuis*
Endocarditis, pericarditis	Occurs in site of pre-existing heart disease. *S. choleraesuis, S. typhimurium*
Arteritis	Atherosclerosis, arteriovenous fistulae, aneurysm; follows bacteremia
Osteomyelitis	Sickle cell anemia, pre-existing bone pathology, systemic lupus erythematosus, hematologic malignancy or normal patients. Sites affected are femur, tibia, humerus, vertebrae, in that order. *S. typhimurium, S. typhi, S. enteritides, S. choleraesuis*
Arthritis	Reactive arthritis in HLA-B27–positive patients. Rare suppurative arthritis (occurring in knee, hip, shoulder joint, in that order). *S. typhimurium, S. choleraesuis*
Splenic abscess	Pre-existing splenic cyst or post-traumatic subcapsular hematoma
Hepatic abscess	Pre-existing amebic abscess, echinococcal cysts or hematoma
Intra-abdominal abscess (pancreas, biliary)	Cholecystitis, cholangitis, subphrenic abscess. *S. typhi, S. typhimurium*
Urogenital disorders	Cystitis, pyelonephritis due to fecal contamination or bacteremic renal abscess formation. Urolithiasis, renal tumor, transplant. *S. typhi, S. typhimurium*
Soft tissue abscess	Trauma; skin or subcutaneous sites; mastitis, thyroiditis. *S. typhimurium*
Infected tumor or cyst	*S. choleraesuis* is common pathogen producing abscess in pre-existing tumor or cyst

Epidemics and sporadic cases involving small family units occur throughout the year.

The incubation period ranges from 6 to 72 hr. Onset often occurs the morning following an evening meal at which contaminated food was ingested. It is usually abrupt and is characterized by nausea, vomiting, and crampy abdominal pain followed by elimination of loose, watery stools, which occasionally contain mucus and blood. Vomiting is usually not severe and, when it does occur, is not protracted. Fever of 101–102° F is seen in as many as 70% of patients; however, chills are less frequent. Symptoms subside within 1–5 days in healthy individuals; in patients who are debilitated by the extremes of age, malignancy, or other illnesses or who are recipients of antibiotic therapy or corticosteroids, the illness may persist. Fatalities are rare (about 1%). Some patients remain afebrile and have only mild intestinal symptoms. Others develop severe disease with high fever, headache, drowsiness, confusion, meningismus, and seizures. Moderate abdominal distention and severe, even localized, pain with rebound tenderness may be manifest.

Septicemia, accompanied by chills and high fever, is more common in the first 3 mo of life than later. Symptoms of enteric fever are those described subsequently for typhoid fever but generally are shorter in duration and are associated with a lower mortality rate. Salmonellae can localize in any organ or tissue and cause a variety of disorders as noted in Table 12–24.

COMPLICATIONS. Complications of nontyphoidal salmonellosis are unusual and generally are limited to extraintestinal lesions (see Table 12–24).

DIAGNOSIS. A positive culture is necessary for diagnosis. *Salmonellae* grow readily on simple media, which are optimal for infection of usually sterile sites. Selective media are needed to inhibit the growth of normal flora in other sites. Culture of the stool is positive more frequently than are specimens collected via rectal swabs. Bacteriologic results are enhanced by the incubation of the specimen in an enriched medium (e.g., tetrathionate broth) prior to plating on selective medium. Although three consecutive negative stool cultures suggest that infection has ceased, excretion of organisms may be intermittent.

The stool of many individuals with *Salmonella* gastroenteritis contains polymorphonuclear leukocytes; these can be demonstrated by staining a freshly passed specimen with methylene blue. Mucus and red blood cells may also be present.

Serologic tests are helpful in the diagnosis of typhoid fever but are not employed for patients with simple gastroenteritis.

DIFFERENTIAL DIAGNOSIS. *Salmonella* gastroenteritis must be distinguished from other viral and bacterial causes of diarrhea, including those caused by rotavirus; enterohemorrhagic, enterotoxigenic, and enteroinvasive *E. coli; Shigella; Yersinia enterocolitica; Clostridium difficile;* and *Helicobacter pylori.* Rarely, the clinical course suggests ulcerative colitis or appendicitis.

TREATMENT. Correction of dehydration and electrolyte disturbances (Sec. 6.15–6.17) and symptomatic management of the patient are the most important aspects of therapy of *Salmonella* gastroenteritis. Antibiotics do not eliminate susceptible salmonellae from the gastrointestinal tract and rarely, if ever, alter the clinical course. Antibiotics are indicated in gastroenteritis only for individuals at high risk of dissemination of disease to other organs or tissues (infants under 3 mo of age, children with immunologic deficiency) or those suffering from a severe and protracted course.

Children with septicemia, enteric fever, or metastatic sites of infection should be treated initially with systemically administered cefotaxime (150–200 mg/kg/24 hr every 6 hr) or ceftriaxone (100 mg/kg/24 hr every 12 hr). Once the antibiotic sensitivity is known, ampicillin (200–300 mg/kg/24 hr), amoxicillin (100 mg/kg/24 hr), or chloramphenicol (50–100 mg/kg/24 hr for older children or 25 mg/kg/24 hr for newborn infants) can be given in four divided doses at 6-hr intervals. Trimethoprim-sulfamethoxazole and ciprofloxacin are alternative agents in penicillin-allergic patients. In vitro susceptibility of the organism should dictate the antibiotic to be used in each case. Resistance to chloramphenicol is unusual among salmonellae isolated in the United States but is relatively common among those recovered in other areas of the world. Twenty per cent of salmonellae isolated from humans in this country are resistant to ampicillin.

PROGNOSIS. The prognosis for patients with *Salmonella* gastroenteritis is excellent except in very young infants or debilitated children with underlying disease. The prognosis for individuals with *Salmonella* meningitis or endocarditis is poor.

Bryan JP, Rocha H, Scheld WM: Problems in salmonellosis: Rationale for clinical trials with newer β-lactam agents and quinolones. Rev Infect Dis 8:189, 1986.

Cohen JI, Bartlett JA, Corey GP: Extra-intestinal manifestations of *Salmonella* infections. Medicine 66:349, 1987.

Goldberg MB, Rubin RH: The spectrum of *Salmonella* infection. Infect Dis Clin North Am 2:571, 1988.

Hyams JS, Durbin WA, Grand RJ, et al: *Salmonella* bacteremia in the first year of life. J Pediatr 96:57, 1980.

Raucher HS, Eichenfield AH, Hodes HL: Treatment of *Salmonella* gastroenteritis in infants. Clin Pediatr 22:601, 1983.

Sharp JCM: Salmonellosis and eggs. Br Med J 297:1557, 1988.

Spika JS, Waterman SH, Soo Hoo GW, et al: Chloramphenicol-resistant *Salmonella newport* traced through hamburger to dairy farms. N Engl J Med 316:565, 1987.

St. Geme JW, Hodes HL, Marcy SM, et al: Consensus: Management of *Salmonella* infection in the first year of life. Pediatr Infect Dis J 7:615, 1988.

Torrey S, Fleisher G, Jaffe D: Incidence of *Salmonella* bacteremia in infants with *Salmonella* gastroenteritis. J Pediatr 8:718, 1986.

12.29 TYPHOID FEVER
(Enteric Fever)

EPIDEMIOLOGY. The incidence of typhoid fever has decreased from 1:100,000 in 1955 to 0.2:100,000 in 1984; 65% of cases in the United States are imported from Mexico, India, Latin and South America, and Southeast Asia. Foreign-acquired typhoid fever often occurs in students; the median age is 23 yr. Typhoid fever acquired in the United States is associated with exposure to known carriers or food-borne epidemics; the median age of patients is 20 yr. The incidence of foreign-acquired disease is highest in Hawaii and California, whereas that of domestic-acquired typhoid fever is highest in Texas and Mississippi.

The typhoid bacillus infects only humans, and infected patients excrete *Salmonella typhosa* in respiratory secretions, urine, and feces for variable periods of time. Characteristically, the implicated carrier is an asymptomatic older adult who has had contact, often as a preparer of food, with the index case. Long survival of *S. typhosa* in food facilitates transmission. Contaminated water generally involves inadequate plumbing or sanitation and is responsible for individual cases in the United States and for endemic disease in developing countries. Oysters and other shellfish cultivated in waters polluted by sewage are also a source of widespread infection. Enteric fever also may be caused by *S. paratyphi* A, *S. schottmuelleri* (formerly *paratyphi B*), and *S. hirschfield* (formerly *paratyphi* C). Disease caused by these bacteria is termed paratyphoid fever and tends to be milder than typhoid fever.

PATHOGENESIS. Infection with *S. typhosa* always results in clinical disease. Virulent *S. typhosa* contain the Vi antigen and invade the bloodstream through the Peyers patches of the distal ileum or jejunum. Multiplication occurs within monocytes in the intestinal lymph follicles. Monocytes, unable to destroy the bacilli early in the disease process, carry these organisms from the bloodstream into the mesenteric lymph nodes and other portions of the reticuloendothelial system where multiplication occurs within cells, producing inflammation in the lymph nodes, bone marrow, liver, and spleen.

The bacteria then re-enter the bloodstream from these sites. This secondary septicemia is usually prolonged, and many organs are seeded. The gallbladder is particularly susceptible and is infected from the liver via the biliary system or from the blood. Local multiplication of micro-organisms in the wall of the gallbladder produces large numbers of salmonellae, which are discharged into the large intestine.

The lipopolysaccharide portion of the cell wall of *S. typhi* may act systemically as a pyrogenic endotoxin responsible for some of the signs and symptoms of infection and may act locally to induce the histologic changes seen in the intestine, liver, skin, and other tissues. Endotoxemia is not the only factor responsible for illness because circulating levels of endotoxin are undetectable.

Cell-mediated immunity is important in protecting the human host against typhoid fever. Decreased numbers of T lymphocytes occur in patients who are critically ill with typhoid fever. Carriers show impaired cellular reactivity to *S. typhosa* antigens in the leukocyte migration inhibition test, but they do not have a generalized depression of cell-mediated immunity; the carrier state may be a consequence of a specific defect in cell-mediated immune response to *S. typhosa*. In carriers of *S. typhosa*, a large number of virulent bacilli pass into the intestine daily without entering the epithelium of the host and are excreted in the stool.

PATHOLOGY. Morphologic changes of *S. typhosa* infection are less striking in younger children than in older children and adults. The mesenteric lymph nodes, liver, and spleen are hyperemic and generally reveal areas of focal necrosis. Hyperplasia of reticuloendothelial tissue with proliferation of mononuclear cells is the predominant finding. The mucosa and lymphatic tissue of the intestinal tract are severely inflamed and necrotic. Ulceration that heals without scarring is common. Hemorrhages may occur. The inflammatory lesion may occasionally penetrate the muscularis and serosa of the intestine and produce perforation. A mononuclear response may be seen in the bone marrow associated with areas of focal necrosis. Inflammation of the gallbladder is focal, inconstant, and modest in proportion to the extent of local bacterial multiplication. Bronchitis is common. Inflammation also may be observed in the form of localized abscesses, pneumonia, septic arthritis, osteomyelitis, pyelonephritis, endophthalmitis, and meningitis.

CLINICAL MANIFESTATIONS. The clinical pattern of typhoid fever *in infants* ranges from a mild gastroenteritis to a severe septicemia. Vertical transmission may be responsible for neonatal typhoid fever that begins within 72 hr after birth. Vomiting, abdominal distention, and diarrhea are common. The temperature may be variable but can be as high as 40.5° C (106° F). Seizures may occur. Hepatomegaly, jaundice, anorexia, and weight loss can be marked.

In older children the incubation period ranges from 5 to 40 days with an average of 10–14 days. The usual inoculum size is 10^7 organisms; a larger infectious dose may decrease the incubation period. It is followed by an irregular course characterized by fever, malaise, lethargy, myalgia, headache, and abdominal pain and tenderness. Diarrhea occurs in only half of the infected children at this stage of the disease; constipation occurs less frequently. Epistaxis may occur, and cough is common. Within a week the fever rises and becomes unremitting. Fatigue, anorexia, weight loss, cough, abdominal pain, and diarrhea increase in severity. The patient may become severely obtunded. Mental depression, delirium, and stupor have been observed. The child now appears acutely ill, disoriented, and lethargic. At this stage of disease the liver and more often the spleen are enlarged, and abdominal tenderness is present. Abdominal distention may be appreciated, and rhonchi and scattered rales may be heard upon auscultation of the chest. A macular **(rose spots)** or maculopapular rash observable in 40–80% of patients occurs in the skin of the lower chest and abdomen, appearing in successive crops of lesions that are 1–6 mm in diameter and last 2–3 days. The paradoxical relationship of a high temperature and a low pulse rate is observed less commonly in children than in adults. If no complications occur, the symptoms and physical findings resolve within 2–4 wk, but malaise and lethargy may persist for an additional 1–2 mo.

COMPLICATIONS. Intestinal perforation has been observed in 0.5–3% and severe hemorrhage in 1–10% of children with typhoid fever. Most complications occur during the second stage of disease and are generally preceded by a fall in temperature and blood pressure and an increase in pulse rate. Perforation rarely occurs without preceding hemorrhage, and the site is usually in the lower ileum. Perforation is accompanied by a marked increase in abdominal pain, tenderness, vomiting, and signs of peritonitis. Toxic encephalopathy and cerebral thrombosis are other complications. Acute cerebellar ataxia, aphasia, perceptive deafness, and transverse myelitis have been observed. Permanent sequelae are rare. Peripheral and optic neuritis as well as chorea have been reported. Toxic myocarditis is manifest by arrhythmias, ST–T changes on ECG, cardiogenic shock, and fatty infiltration and necrosis of the myocardium. Acute cholecystitis has been observed, often presenting as a toxic dilatation of the gallbladder. Thrombosis and phlebitis occur rarely. Pneumonia is common during the second stage of illness but often is caused by a superinfection related to organisms other than *Salmonella*. Pyelonephritis, endocarditis, and meningitis as well as osteomyelitis and septic arthritis rarely occur in the normal host. Septic arthritis and osteomyelitis occur more frequently in individuals with hemoglobinopathies.

LABORATORY DATA. A normochromic, normocytic anemia may be associated with intestinal blood loss or toxic suppression of bone marrow. Blood leukocyte counts generally are low in relation to the fever and toxicity but seldom are less than 3,000 cells/mm^3. With pyogenic abscesses leukocytosis may reach 20,000–25,000/mm^3. Thrombocytopenia may be striking and may persist for up to a week. Melena and proteinuria are common. The chest roentgenogram is usually normal.

DIAGNOSIS. *Microscopic examination of the stool* generally reveals a large number of leukocytes, most of which are mononuclear.

Bacteriologic cultures are diagnostic, but the identification of *S. typhosa* requires 3–5 days in most laboratories. Specimens grown on selective media and examined with fluorescein-labeled antibody to the Vi antigen may provide specific and rapid identification. Blood cultures are usually positive early in the disease, whereas urine and stool cultures become positive following the secondary septicemia. Cultures are positive in as many as 40% of children during the initial stage of typhoid fever. Cultures of the bone marrow and involved lymph nodes or other reticuloendothelial tissues often remain positive after the blood has been sterilized. Aspirates of the rose spots may be culture positive. Stool and urine of chronic carriers should be cultured because bone marrow and blood cultures are not likely to be positive. Enteric carriers generally excrete 10^6–10^9 *S. typhosa* per gram of stool. In suspected cases with negative stool cultures, a culture of aspirated duodenal fluid to evaluate possible biliary infection may be helpful.

O and H antigens of *S. typhosa* are not unique to that serotype or even to salmonellae. Treatment with antibiotics may depress an antibody response; conversely, high titers of H agglutinins may result from prior typhoid immunization. An increase in O agglutinins (Widal test) in an individual immunized more than 6 mo earlier is suggestive of infection. In the nonimmunized child who has lived in a nonendemic area, O agglutinin titers of greater than 1:160 are suggestive evidence of infection during the 1st wk of symptoms. Titers of Vi agglutinins of 1:5 or greater generally identify a chronic carrier in nonendemic populations.

CIE has been used to detect serum *S. typhosa* antigen. An ELISA procedure has also been developed to detect *S. typhosa* Vi antigen in urine; its high sensitivity and specificity suggest that it may be helpful in establishing a diagnosis rapidly.

DIFFERENTIAL DIAGNOSIS. During the initial stage of typhoid fever the clinical diagnosis may be bronchitis, bronchopneumonia, gastroenteritis, or influenza. Subsequently, other infections caused by intracellular micro-organisms, including tuberculosis, systemic fungal infections, brucellosis, tularemia, and rickettsial diseases as well as shigellosis and, where applicable epidemiologically, malaria, may need to be considered. Septicemia, leukemia, lymphoma, and Hodgkin disease also may be suggested. Concern about acute surgical disease of the abdomen may lead to unnecessary operative intervention.

PROGNOSIS. The prognosis in typhoid fever depends upon the patient's age, previous state of health, and the type of complications that may occur. Individuals who are not treated with antibiotics may die (10% of infants and a smaller percentage of older children succumb). Therapy with antibiotics has reduced the mortality to less than 1% in most areas. The presence of an underlying debilitating disease, perforation of the gastrointestinal tract, or severe hemorrhage increases the chances of death. Meningitis or endocarditis may be associated with high morbidity and mortality.

Relapse occurs in 4–8% of those who are not treated with antibiotics. Clinical manifestations of relapse become apparent about 2 wk after cessation of antibiotic therapy and resemble the acute illness. The relapse, however, is generally milder and abbreviated. Multiple relapses in the same individual may occur.

Individuals who excrete *S. typhosa* 3 mo or more after infection are usually excreters at 1 yr (chronic carriers) and often for life. The risk of becoming a *chronic carrier* is low in children but increases with age. Up to 5% of acutely infected adults become chronic carriers; generally they have chronic gallbladder infections and excrete the organisms in their stool. Chronic urinary carriage also may occur but is rare except in individuals with schistosomiasis.

TREATMENT. The maintenance of appropriate fluid and electrolyte balance is essential. If shock or severe hemorrhage accompanies intestinal perforation, intravascular volume expansion and surgery may be required.

Chloramphenicol is the antibiotic preferred for the therapy of typhoid fever. It can usually be provided orally, but intravenous administration is indicated when the patient is acutely ill. Doses of 50–100 mg/kg/24 hr are given to children and 25 mg/kg/24 hr to infants under 2 wk of age, divided into four doses and given at 6-hr intervals. Most children become afebrile within 7 days, but treatment of uncomplicated cases should be continued for at least 10–14 days or for 5–7 days following defervescence. In children who have underlying significant malnutrition and a high rate of complications, results have been improved by extending therapy for a period of 21 days. Complications including intestinal hemorrhage and perforation have been observed during therapy. Treatment with chloramphenicol may increase the chance of relapse and does not prevent development of the chronic carrier state.

Ampicillin therapy results in a slower clinical response and more treatment failures than does treatment with chloramphenicol. Patients who have a favorable response to ampicillin, however, are less likely to experience relapses or become chronic carriers. The dose of ampicillin is 100–200 mg/kg/24 hr divided at 6-hr intervals. Systemic administration is preferred.

Amoxicillin (100 mg/kg/24 hr given in equal divided doses at 6-hr intervals) provides results that are superior to those for ampicillin and equivalent to those obtained with chloramphenicol.

A combination of trimethoprim and sulfamethoxazole is also effective against typhoid fever (185 mg/m^2/day TMP plus 925 mg/m^2/day SMZ orally in three equally divided doses). However, patients respond less predictably than with chloramphenicol or ampicillin.

Illness due to chloramphenicol-resistant strains has been reported from Mexico, Southeast Asia, and the Middle East. Ceftriaxone and cefoperazone produce cure rates of greater than 90% with relapse rates of 0–4% and are acceptable alternatives for treatment of multidrug-resistant *S. typhi*. *Ceftriaxone is considered the initial treatment of choice for typhoid fever by some authorities.*

Corticosteroid therapy has been suggested for individuals with severe toxemia or prolonged symptoms. It does not increase the incidence of complications if antibiotic therapy is adequate.

Platelet transfusions have been suggested for the treatment of thrombocytopenia that is sufficiently severe to cause intestinal hemorrhage in patients for whom surgery is contemplated.

Up to 80% of carriers with chronic gallbladder infection can be cured by cholecystectomy even without antibiotic therapy. High-dose ampicillin plus probenicid therapy provided for 4–6 wk has cured many carriers including some with cholecystis. Norfloxacin or ciprofloxacin may also cure the chronic carrier state.

PREVENTION. Typhoid fever stimulates host resistance by inducing a temporary nonspecific increase in phagocytic activity within the reticuloendothelial system as well as a more lasting enhancement of specific bactericidal activity in the form of type-specific antibodies. Antibodies slow extracellular bacterial multiplication and promote opsonization.

Parenteral vaccine is not indicated for routine use in children. Although available vaccines will prevent disease in most individuals exposed to small numbers of typhoid bacilli such as could occur with water-borne disease, exposure to a larger inoculum can overcome whatever immunity is induced by the vaccine. The indications for use of typhoid vaccine in the United States are as follows: (1) intimate exposure to a known household carrier; (2) an outbreak of typhoid fever in the community or an institution; and (3) travel to an endemic area, in an attempt to prevent disease acquired via contaminated water (see Sec. 5.6). For children residing in endemic areas, the vaccine may provide some protection against water-borne disease, but a booster dose is not indicated, since field tests failed to show any increased protection when more than one dose was given. Immunity lasts at least 10 yr.

Two doses of 0.5 mL administered subcutaneously 3 or more wk apart are recommended for both primary and booster immunizations of individuals 10 yr or more of age; 0.25 mL is recommended for younger children. Local reactions, including fever, are common, and prophylactic administration of antipyretics in young children may be indicated. An intradermal dose of 0.1 mL may have immunogenicity and produce fewer side reactions than the larger subcutaneous dose; it may be used as a booster injection. Unacceptable reactions occur with the intradermal administration of acetone-extracted vaccine.

An oral vaccine containing the Ty 21 attenuated mutant strains of *S. typhosa* tested in Egypt had a protection rate of 95%, suggesting the importance of local immune responses. A capsular polysaccharide Vi vaccine may also confer immunity to typhoid fever.

CONTROL OF *SALMONELLA* INFECTIONS. Attention to personal hygiene, handwashing, and sanitary practices is essential for personnel involved in the preparation of food and in patient care in order to minimize person-to-person and person-to-food transmission. Urine and feces of hospitalized patients should be handled with special precautions until three consecutive stool cultures are negative.

Every effort should be made to eradicate *S. typhosa* from carriers. When these efforts are unsuccessful, the individuals must be kept under careful surveillance by local health departments and prevented from working in food and water processing plants, in kitchens, and in occupations related to patient care. Such individuals should be made aware of their potential contagiousness and the importance of handwashing and personal hygiene.

Typhoid fever can be controlled in endemic areas only by improved sanitation and housing and by the availability of pure water. Large scale immunization programs may reduce but will not eliminate this disease.

RALPH D. FEIGIN

Acharya IL, Lowe CU, Thapa R, et al: Prevention of typhoid fever in Nepal with the Vi capsular polysaccharide of *Salmonella typhi*. N Engl J Med 317:1101, 1987.

Edelman R, Levine MM: Summary of an international workshop on typhoid fever. Rev Infect Dis 8:329, 1986.

Gotuzzo E, Guerra JG, Benavente L, et al: Use of norfloxacin to treat chronic typhoid carriers. J Infect Dis 157:1221, 1988.

Mosley JG, Chaudhuri AK: Surgery and *Salmonella*: Complications require prompt diagnosis and treatment. Br Med J 300:552, 1990.

Ryan CA, Hargrett-Bean NT, Blake PA: *Salmonella typhi* infections in the United States, 1975–1984: Increasing role of foreign travel. Rev Infect Dis 11:1, 1989.

Soe GB, Overturf GD: Treatment of typhoid fever and other systemic salmonelloses with cefotaxime, ceftriaxone, cefoperazone, and other newer cephalosporins. Rev Infect Dis 9:719, 1987.

Thisyakorn U, Mansuwan P, Taylor DN: Typhoid and paratyphoid fever in 192 hospitalized children in Thailand. Am J Dis Child 141:862, 1987.

12.30 SHIGELLOSIS

Although dysenteric syndromes have long been recognized as a scourge of man, it is only in the last 90 yr that the bacteriology of the most common form of epidemic dysentery has been appreciated. Four species of *shigella* are responsible for illness: *S. dysenteriae* (serogroup A), *S. flexneri* (serogroup B), *S. boydii* (serogroup C), and *S. sonnei* (serogroup D). There are 12 serotypes in group A, 6 serotypes and 13 subserotypes in group B, 18 serotypes in group C, and 1 serotype in group D.

PATHOPHYSIOLOGY. The basic virulence trait shared by all shigellae is the ability to invade colonic epithelial cells. This characteristic is encoded on a large (120–140 megadalton) plasmid that is responsible for synthesis of a group of polypeptides involved in cell invasion and killing. Shigellae that lose the virulence plasmid no longer act as pathogens. *E. coli* that naturally or artificially harbor this plasmid behave like shigellae. In addition to the major plasmid-encoded virulence traits, chromosomally encoded factors are also required for full virulence; some of these chromosomal traits are important for all shigellae (e.g., lipopolysaccharide synthesis), whereas others are important only in some serotypes (e.g., shigatoxin synthesis). Shigatoxin, a potent protein synthesis–inhibiting exotoxin, is produced in significant amounts only by *S. dysenteriae* serotype 1 and certain *E. coli* (enterohemorrhagic *E. coli* or shiga-like toxin–producing *E. coli*).

Shigellae require very low inocula to cause illness. Ingestion of as few as 10 *S. dysenteriae* serotype 1 organisms can cause dysentery in some susceptible individuals. This is in contrast to organisms such as *Vibrio cholerae*, which require ingestion of 10^8–10^{10} organisms to cause illness. The inoculum effect explains the ease of person-to-person transmission of shigellae in contrast to *V. cholerae*.

Immune Responses. Both secretory IgA and serum antibodies develop within days to weeks after infection with *Shigella*. Although both anti-lipopolysaccharide and antivirulence plasmid polypeptide antibodies have been described, identification of the major determinant of protection against subsequent infection remains unclear. There is evidence that protection is serotype specific, but there is also the suggestion that a degree of cross-protection against all shigellae follows infection with a given serotype. Cell-mediated immunity may also play some role in protection, although it appears to be minor.

PATHOLOGY. The pathologic changes of shigellosis take place primarily in the colon, the target organ for shigellae. The changes are most intense in the distal colon, although pancolitis may occur. Grossly, localized or diffuse mucosal edema, ulcerations, friable mucosa, bleeding, and exudate may be seen. Microscopically, ulcerations, pseudomembranes, epithelial cell death, infiltration extending from the mucosa to the muscularis mucosae by polymorphonuclear and mononuclear cells, and submucosal edema occur.

EPIDEMIOLOGY. Infection with shigellae occurs most often during the warm months in temperate climates and during the rainy season in tropical climates. The sexes are affected equally. Although infection can occur at any age, it is most common in the 2nd and 3rd yr of life. Infection in the first 6 mo is rare for reasons that are not clear. Breast milk, which in endemic areas contains antibodies to both virulence plasmid-coded antigens and lipopolysaccharides, may partially explain the age-related incidence.

In industrialized societies, *S. sonnei* is the most common cause of bacillary dysentery, with *S. flexneri* second in frequency; in preindustrial societies, *S. flexneri* is most common, with *S. sonnei* second in frequency. *S. dysenteriae serotype* 1 tends to occur in massive epidemics, although it is also endemic in Asia.

Contaminated food (often a salad or other item requiring extensive handling of the ingredients) and water are important vectors. However, person-to-person transmission is probably the major mechanism of infection in most areas of the world. Spread within families, custodial institutions, and day-care centers demonstrates the ability of low numbers of organisms to cause disease on a person-to-person basis.

CLINICAL MANIFESTATIONS. Bacillary dysentery is clinically similar regardless of whether the disease is caused by an enteroinvasive *E. coli* (Sec. 12.27) or any of the four species of *Shigella*; however, there are some clinical differences, particularly relating to the severity and risk of complications with *S. dysenteriae* serotype 1 infection.

Following ingestion of shigellae there is an incubation period of several days before symptoms ensue. Characteristically, severe abdominal pain, high fever, emesis, anorexia, generalized toxicity, urgency, and painful defecation occur. Physical examination at this point may show abdominal distention and tenderness, hyperactive bowel sounds, and a tender rectum on digital examination.

The *diarrhea* may be watery and of large volume initially, evolving into frequent small-volume, bloody mucoid stools; however, some children never progress to the stage of bloody diarrhea, whereas in others the first stools are bloody. Significant dehydration related to the fluid and electrolyte losses in both feces and emesis can occur. Untreated diarrhea may last 1–2 wk; only about 10% of patients have diarrhea persisting for more than 10 days. Chronic diarrhea is uncommon except in malnourished infants.

Neurologic findings are among the most common extraintestinal manifestations of bacillary dysentery, occurring in up to

40% of infected children. Convulsions, headache, lethargy, confusion, nuchal rigidity, or hallucinations may be present before or after the onset of diarrhea. The cause of these neurologic findings is not understood. In the past, these symptoms were attributed to the neurotoxicity of shigatoxin, but it is now clear that that explanation is wrong. Seizures sometimes occur when little fever is present, suggesting that simple febrile convulsions do not explain their appearance. Hypocalcemia or hyponatremia may be associated with seizures in a small number of patients. Although symptoms often suggest central nervous system infection, and cerebrospinal fluid pleocytosis with minimally elevated protein levels can occur, meningitis due to shigellae is rare.

The most common complication of shigellosis is dehydration with its attendant risks of renal failure and death (see Sec. 6.16). Inappropriate secretion of antidiuretic hormone with profound hyponatremia may complicate dysentery, particularly when *S. dysenteriae* is the etiologic agent.

Other major complications, particularly in very young, malnourished children, include sepsis and disseminated intravascular coagulation. Given that these organisms penetrate the intestinal mucosal barrier, these events are surprisingly uncommon. Shigellae (and a variety of other gram-negative enterics) are recovered from blood cultures in about 5% of cases in whom blood cultures are taken; since patients selected for blood cultures represent a biased sample, the risk in unselected cases of shigellosis is presumably lower. Bacteremia is more common with *S. dysenteriae* serotype 1 than with other shigellae. Mortality is high (20–50%) when sepsis occurs.

In those who have *S. dysenteriae* serotype 1 infection, hemolysis, anemia, and **hemolytic uremic syndrome** are common complications; these events may occasionally follow *S. flexneri* infection. This syndrome is thought to be related to shigatoxin, since those *E. coli* that produce toxins closely related to shigatoxin (enterohemorrhagic *E. coli*) also cause hemolytic uremic syndrome (Sec. 12.27).

Rectal prolapse, toxic megacolon or pseudomembranous colitis (usually associated with *S. dysenteriae*), cholestatic hepatitis, conjunctivitis, iritis, corneal ulcers, pneumonia, arthritis (usually 2–5 wk after enteritis), Reiter syndrome, cystitis, and vaginitis (typically with a blood-tinged discharge associated with *S. flexneri*) are uncommon events. The rare syndrome of extreme toxicity, convulsions, hyperpyrexia, and a rapidly fatal outcome without sepsis or significant dehydration **(Ekiri syndrome)** is not well understood. Death is a rare outcome in the well-nourished, older child; malnutrition and illness in patients in the first few months of life are associated with increased risk of fatal outcome.

DIAGNOSIS. Although clinical features suggest shigellosis, they are insufficiently specific to allow confident diagnosis. Infection by *Campylobacter jejuni*, *Salmonella* sp, enteroinvasive *E. coli*, enterohemorrhagic *E. coli*, *Yersinia enterocolitica*, and *Entamoeba histolytica* as well as inflammatory bowel disease may cause confusion. Unfortunately, the laboratory is often not able to confirm the clinical suspicion of shigellosis even when it is present. Presumptive data supporting a diagnosis of bacillary dysentery include the finding of fecal leukocytes (confirming the presence of colitis) and demonstration in peripheral blood of leukocytosis with a dramatic left shift (often with more bands than segmented neutrophils). The total peripheral white blood cell count is usually 5,000–15,000 cells/mm^3, although both leukopenia and leukemoid reactions occur.

Culture of both stool and rectal swab specimens optimizes the chance of diagnosing *Shigella* infection. Culture media should include MacConkey agar as well as selective media such as xylose-lysine deoxycholate (XLD) and SS agar. Transport media should be utilized if specimens cannot be cultured promptly. Appropriate media should be used to exclude *Campylobacter* and other likely agents. Culture is the gold standard for diagnosis, but it is not absolute. Stool cultures of adult volunteers with dysentery following ingestion of shigellae failed to detect the organism in nearly 20% of subjects. Studies of food-borne outbreaks suggest that a single culture allows diagnosis in about half of symptomatic patients with shigellosis. Although additional tools to improve diagnosis (e.g., gene probes) are being developed, at present the diagnostic inadequacy of cultures makes it incumbent on the clinician to use judgment in the management of clinical syndromes consistent with shigellosis. In children who appear to be toxic, blood cultures should be obtained; this is particularly important in very young or malnourished infants because of their increased risk of bacteremia.

TREATMENT. As with gastroenteritis of other causes, the first concern about a child with suspected shigellosis should be for fluid and electrolyte correction and maintenance (Sec. 6.16). Drugs that retard intestinal motility should not be used because of the risk of prolonging the illness.

The next concern is a decision about use of antibiotics. Although some authorities recommend withholding antibacterial therapy because of the self-limited nature of the infection, the cost of drugs, and the risk of emergence of resistant organisms, there is a persuasive logic in favor of empiric treatment of all children in whom shigellosis is suspected. Even if not fatal, the untreated illness may cause the child to be quite ill for 2 weeks or more; chronic or recurrent diarrhea may ensue. There is a risk of malnutrition developing or worsening during prolonged illness, particularly in children in developing countries. The risk of continued excretion and subsequent infection of family contacts also further argues against the strategy of withholding antibiotics.

There are major geographic variations in drug susceptibility. In the United States, shigellae are so frequently resistant to ampicillin that it should not be used for empiric therapy; occasional strains are also resistant to trimethoprim-sulfamethoxazole (TMP-SMX). Resistance to nalidixic acid is very rare at present. With the exception of nalidixic acid, the quinolones that have been recommended for use in adults have not been used in children (because of the putative risk of arthropathy). Treatment regimens involve a 5-day course. For strains known to be susceptible to ampicillin, this drug is given at 100 mg/kg/24 hr divided into four doses each day. The usual empiric choice prior to availability of susceptibility data is TMP-SMX, given at 5–10 mg/kg/24 hr of the TMP component in two divided doses. For strains known to be resistant to the usual drugs, nalidixic acid is administered at 55 mg/kg/24 hr in four divided doses daily. Of these agents, given a susceptible organism, TMP-SMX is preferred because of the rapidity with which it causes resolution of symptoms. In those patients too ill to take oral medications, intravenous therapy with TMP-SMX is effective if the organism is susceptible. Oral first- and second-generation cephalosporins and furazolidone are inadequate as alternative drugs. Amoxicillin is less effective than ampicillin in therapy of ampicillin-sensitive strains.

Since stool cultures are most helpful when they confirm a diagnosis of *Shigella* infection and least helpful when no pathogen is isolated, treatment of patients suspected on clinical grounds of having *Shigella* infection should be started when the patient is first examined. Stool culture is obtained primarily to assist in antibiotic selection should the child fail to respond to empiric therapy. A child who has typical dysentery and who responds to initial empiric antibiotic treatment should be continued on that drug for a full 5-day course even if the stool culture is negative. The logic of this recommendation is based not only on the difficulty of culturing *Shigella* but also on the fact that enteroinvasive *E. coli*, which cause dysentery indistinguishable from that due to shigellae, cannot be diagnosed in routine clinical microbiology laboratories. In a child who fails to respond to therapy of a dysenteric syndrome in the presence of initially negative stool cultures, cultures should be retaken and the child re-evaluated for other possible diagnoses.

PREVENTION. There are two simple measures that decrease the risk of shigellosis in children. The first is to encourage prolonged breast-feeding in settings in which shigellosis is common. Breast-feeding decreases the risk of symptomatic shigellosis and lessens its severity in infants who acquire infection despite breast-feeding. The second measure is to educate families in handwashing techniques, especially after defecation and before food preparation and consumption. Other public health measures, including water and sewage treatment, are expensive and are unlikely to be universally available in the near future in developing countries.

THOMAS G. CLEARY

Nelson JD, Kusmiesz H, Shelton S: Oral or intravenous trimethoprim-sulfamethoxazole therapy for shigellosis. Rev Infect Dis 4:546, 1982.

Salam MA, Bennish ML: Therapy for shigellosis: I. Randomized, double-blind trial of nalidixic acid in childhood shigellosis. J Pediatr 113:901, 1988.

12.31 CHOLERA

Cholera, an acute intestinal disease, is caused by an enterotoxin elaborated by *Vibrio cholerae*, serotype 01. Its clinical course ranges from asymptomatic infection to the most severe form, *cholera gravis*, in which sudden, profuse, watery diarrhea results in hypovolemic shock, metabolic acidosis, and, if untreated, death.

ETIOLOGY. *V. cholerae* is a short, slightly curved, motile, gram-negative rod with a single polar flagellum. About 70 serotypes are known, and although many of them cause acute diarrhea, only the 01 serotype causes cholera. *V. cholerae* grows readily on a variety of media. *V. cholerae* 01 (and many other *V. cholerae* serotypes) produce opaque, yellow colonies on TCBS agar and can be recognized only by reactions with specific antisera. The two biotypes of *V. cholerae* 01 are classic and El Tor; each is separable into two serotypes, Ogawa and Inaba.

EPIDEMIOLOGY. Cholera has been endemic in the Ganges delta throughout history, with annual epidemics in West Bengal and Bangladesh. From 1817 to 1926 the disease spread worldwide in six pandemics. A seventh pandemic, caused by the El Tor biotype, began in 1961 in Indonesia and by 1977 had spread to most of Southeast and South Asia, the Middle East, Africa, Southern Europe, and the Western Pacific regions. By the end of 1988, 94 countries had been involved.

In the United States only a few laboratory-acquired cases were identified from 1911 to 1973, when a single indigenous case was reported in Texas. Since 1977, 62 infections have been identified, most of which occurred in Gulf states. Most cases were traced to the consumption of seafood from the Gulf of Mexico; one outbreak was caused by rice contaminated after cooking. No other indigenous cases have been reported in other countries in the Western Hemisphere during the present pandemic, except for one acquired in Mexico in 1983.

Endemic and epidemic cholera often have a seasonal pattern. Contaminated water and food, especially shellfish, play a major role in transmission. African epidemics have often been observed following feasts and funeral gatherings at which rites were performed that facilitate transmission. Nosocomial outbreaks occur where overcrowding and poor sanitary conditions prevail. Secondary cases are rare in medical personnel who have had close contact with patients.

Persons with asymptomatic or mild infection play an important role in disseminating cholera. The ratio of asymptomatic or mild infections to severe disease is generally 5–7:1 in classic cholera and as high as 50–100:1 in El Tor cholera. A prolonged carrier state, with the gallbladder as the reservoir, has been documented in adults convalescing from El Tor cholera but has not been observed in children. Family contacts of hospitalized patients are frequently infected.

In endemic areas cholera is predominantly a disease of children; in rural Bangladesh attack rates are 5–10 times greater for children 2–9 yr than for adults. In infants, breast-feeding is protective, and cholera is rare. Increasingly high titers of vibriocidal antibody occur with advancing age, suggesting that the lower attack rate for adults is due to immunity induced by recurrent exposure to *V. cholerae* 01 and that subclinical or asymptomatic reinfection probably occurs frequently. In contrast, when cholera spreads to a previously uninfected area, attack rates are usually equal for all age groups exposed.

Both human and nonhuman reservoirs of *V. cholerae* 01 may exist in endemic areas. The organism may be transmitted as a subclinical infection during interepidemic periods by persons who are asymptomatic or have mild disease; also, the El Tor biotype may survive for a prolonged time in an aquatic environment. Animals have no role in the human disease cycle.

PATHOLOGY AND PATHOPHYSIOLOGY. The site of infection is the small intestine, primarily the jejunum. After ingestion, the vibrios multiply in the lumen and adhere to the surface of epithelial cells underneath the mucous layer; here they elaborate an enterotoxic protein. The binding subunit of this enterotoxin attaches to a receptor (GM_1 ganglioside) on the surface membrane of epithelial cells. The active subunit then enters the cells and activates adenylate cyclase to produce increased amounts of cyclic adenosine monophosphate (cAMP). This leads to a decrease in active absorption of sodium and chloride in villous cells and an increase in active secretion of chloride by crypt cells, resulting in a net loss of water and electrolyte into the bowel. At least one other "toxic" factor involved in the pathogenesis of cholera may exist; this is suggested by studies in volunteers indicating that genetically engineered strains of *V. cholerae* 01 that lack the gene for toxin production can cause diarrhea.

Biopsy of the small intestine of a patient with cholera reveals an intact epithelium with minimal cellular response; emptying of goblet cells indicates an increase in mucus secretion. Slight edema of the lamina propria and moderate dilation of the capillaries and lymphatics in the tips of villi are also seen.

The diarrheal fluid lost is isotonic with plasma and has relatively high concentrations of bicarbonate and potassium. Stools from children with cholera contain more potassium and less sodium, chloride, and bicarbonate than stools from adults. This fluid loss usually results in an isotonic deficit of sodium and water, potassium depletion, and acidosis due to deficit of base. Bicarbonate loss continues even when systemic acidosis develops. Although there is some impairment of activity of jejunal disaccharidases, including lactase, glucose absorption is usually preserved.

CLINICAL MANIFESTATIONS. Typically, after an incubation period of 6 hr–2 days, a sudden onset of painless and profuse watery diarrhea occurs. In the most severe cases stools are passed frequently and effortlessly and have a rice-water appearance (i.e., clear fluid with only flecks of mucus visible), and a slight fish-like odor. In less severe cases the stool is more yellow in appearance. Periumbilical abdominal cramps occur in about 50% of cases; tenesmus is absent. Vomiting is common in severe cases, usually occurring after the onset of diarrhea. In about 25% of children the rectal temperature is slightly elevated (38–39° C) on admission or in the first 24 hr of hospitalization.

Massive diarrhea can result in profound dehydration and circulatory collapse. In these severe cases, *cholera gravis*, the blood pressure falls and is often unobtainable, the radial pulse becomes imperceptible, respirations are rapid and deep, and urine flow ceases. The eyes and fontanel are deeply sunken; the skin is cold and clammy, with poor turgor; and the skin of the fingers becomes shriveled. Cyanosis and painful muscle cramps occur in the extremities, especially in the calves. The patient is restless and extremely thirsty. Lethargy, thick speech, and a somnolent state are common. Stool losses may continue for up to 7 days. Subsequent manifestations depend on the adequacy of replacement therapy. An early sign of recovery is usually the reappearance of bile pigment in the stool, after which the cessation of diarrhea is usually rapid.

Mild cases of cholera, considerably more common than those of cholera gravis as described above, usually present as simple diarrhea with little or no dehydration and are more common in children than in adults.

DIAGNOSIS. This depends on isolating *V. cholerae* 01 from stool. Microscopic examination of stool usually reveals fewer than 5 polymorphonuclear cells/high power field. Retrospective diagnosis is possible by determining vibriocidal, agglutinating, and toxin-neutralizing antibodies whose peak titers usually occur 7–14 days after onset of illness. Vibriocidal and agglutinating antibody titers return to baseline levels 8–12 wk after onset; antitoxin titers remain elevated for up to 12–18 mo. A 4-fold or greater rise during acute disease or a fall in titer during convalescence is usually considered diagnostic. A 4-fold rise in vibriocidal antibody also occurs after infection with other organisms, such as *Yersinia* and *Brucella*, making it imperative to interpret titers in light of clinical and epidemiologic findings. Illness with *V. cholerae* 01 is more likely to occur in persons with lower vibriocidal titers, although some with high titers have severe disease. In endemic areas asymptomatic infection may also result in 4-fold rises in vibriocidal titer.

A diagnosis of cholera should be considered in a child with severely dehydrating diarrhea, especially when the patient has been in a cholera-infected area within 5 days of onset of illness. Severe cholera may be indistinguishable clinically from severe diarrhea produced by enterotoxigenic *E. coli* or non-01 *V. cholerae*. Milder disease may be similar to that caused by other bacterial pathogens (e.g., *Salmonella, Shigella*) or certain viruses (e.g., rotavirus).

COMPLICATIONS. These are more frequent and severe in children than in adults. Inadequate fluid replacement may lead to acute renal failure from tubular necrosis. Inadequate potassium replacement can result in cardiac arrhythmias, hypokalemic nephropathy, and paralytic ileus. Rarely, pulmonary edema has occurred in children treated with excessive and rapid fluid replacement without correction of severe acidosis. Transient tetany during correction of acidosis occurs infrequently. Prolonged drowsiness, coma, or convulsions may occur before or during treatment in as many as 10% of small children; these can be caused by marked hypoglycemia, but the reason is more often unknown. Hypoglycemia is preventable by including dextrose in replacement solutions. An increase in fetal deaths during the 3rd trimester of pregnancy has been observed principally in severely dehydrated patients who delay seeking hospital care.

PREVENTION. Avoidance of contaminated food and water is the best preventive measure. Commercially available cholera vaccine containing heat- or pheno-inactivated suspensions of classic Inaba and Ogawa strains of *V. cholerae* 01 is of low efficacy and provides only limited protection of short duration. High-potency vaccines have demonstrated 50–80% protection for up to 6 mo in endemic areas; no data are available on the efficacy of vaccine in newly infected areas, but it is likely that it is less in these areas, where naturally acquired immunity is not present. Vaccine does not reduce the rate of inapparent infections and thus does not prevent transmission of cholera within families or in communities. Vaccination is not required for entry into the United States from a cholera-infected area (Sec. 5.6). Oral vaccines are being developed in an effort to enhance local immunity in the intestinal tract.

Chemoprophylaxis with tetracycline (for at least 2 days) in two daily doses of 500 mg for adults, 125 mg for children aged 4–13 yr, and 50 mg for children under 3 yr reduces infection rates in household contacts. For ease of administration doxycycline in a single dose (300 mg in adults, 6 mg/kg in children below 15 yr) is the preferred tetracycline compound. Liquid preparations of erythromycin or trimethoprim-sulfamethoxazole may also be used in the same doses recommended for the treatment of cholera (see later); however, their efficacy in chemoprophylaxis has not been evaluated. Mass chemoprophylaxis in a large community is not advisable.

TREATMENT. Successful management primarily requires prompt evaluation of dehydration (Sec. 6.16) and replacement of gastrointestinal losses of fluid and electrolytes (Sec. 6.17). Antibiotic therapy is adjunctive. Hospitalized patients do not require strict isolation but are more readily managed in a single unit. Enteric precautions should be carefully followed. When possible, patients should be weighed on admission, and subsequent stool output measured. For older children, a "cholera cot" made of canvas or burlap on a wooden frame with a plastic or rubber sheet extending through a 4- to 6-inch opening where the patient places the buttocks facilitates stool disposal and accurate measurement of stool volume.

When a cholera patient is first seen, the extent of dehydration should be quickly determined. Measurements of plasma specific gravity and serum electrolytes, especially bicarbonate, can be helpful in planning fluid replacement but are not essential to the provision of adequate care. By the time dehydration is clinically apparent, a child has lost a significant amount of body fluid and electrolytes and at least 5% of his body weight; the danger in treatment usually lies in underestimation of losses.

Patients with severe dehydration and hypovolemic shock should be given replacement fluids intravenously as promptly as possible (Sec. 6.16 and 6.17). Infants should receive about 70 mL/kg during the first 3 hr; if signs of dehydration persist, they should receive 20 mL/kg over the next 3 hr; older children and adults can usually be given the total amount of 100 mL/kg in 3–4 hr. The exact rate and amounts of fluids for replacement and maintenance should be adjusted in relation to continuous monitoring of the patient's state of hydration and stool losses. If no peripheral vein is available, the external jugular or femoral veins should be used rather than losing time by infusing fluid subcutaneously or intraperitoneally or by performing a cutdown. To avoid overhydration the neck veins should be monitored for distention, the lungs for rales of pulmonary edema, and the eyelids for edema. If Ringer lactate is used, potassium chloride should be added (10 mEq/L) or given orally. Isotonic saline can be used to correct hypovolemia if base, potassium, and glucose supplementations are given (Sec. 6.16–6.17).

Patients presenting with moderate to mild dehydration (e.g., with thirst alone or with diminished skin turgor and neck vein distention but without shock) may be given initial replacement fluid orally (Sec. 6.16 and 6.17). The solution may be made using drinking water but should be prepared daily to minimize bacterial contamination. Patients with moderate dehydration should be given 100 mL/kg of *oral rehydration salts (ORS) solution* over 4 hr; 50 mL/kg over the same time is given for mild dehydration. When a patient is tired, a nasogastric tube can be used to give fluid. Vomiting is not a contraindication to oral fluids; when it occurs, smaller amounts should be offered more frequently. In fewer than 1% of patients there is malabsorption of glucose from the oral fluid, with resultant worsening of diarrhea; in this situation the intravenous route must be used.

After replacement fluid has been given, *maintenance therapy* should be started to match insensible water loss (500–1,000 mL/m^2 of body surface/24 hr in hot climates) and continuing diarrheal losses (Sec. 6.18). During the first few hours of treatment stool output is often minimal, but once shock is corrected, the diarrheal output generally increases to as much as 200–350 mL/kg/24 hr. In older children, hourly losses may be over 800 mL. Except for patients with very high rates of stooling and those with glucose malabsorption, continuing losses can usually be replaced with the oral glucose-electrolyte solution; they should receive 10–20 mL/kg/hr until diarrhea is distinctly decreased. If signs of dehydration reappear and losses cannot be adequately replaced orally, intravenous therapy should be instituted.

For patients with mild diarrhea the oral solution can be given at home at a rate of 100/mL/kg/24 hr until diarrhea stops. Breast-fed infants should be encouraged to breast feed ad libitum during maintenance therapy; other infants can be offered water or milk formula.

Since cholera is endemic in many areas where malnutrition is common and there is evidence that most nutrients are absorbed during illness, an average diet for age should be started during maintenance therapy as soon as the patient can eat. This will help prevent further deterioration of nutritional status. Foods that are energy-rich and contain potassium should be given. For infants 4–6 mo of age or older who have not previously been given semisolid foods, this is a good time to start feeding such foods.

As soon as the patient is alert (within 2–6 hr), oral tetracycline should be given (50 mg/kg/24 hr every 6 hr for 2–3 days), although this may cause discoloration of teeth in children less than 8 yr old. Tetracycline shortens the duration and volume of diarrhea by 50–70% and the duration of carriage of *Vibrio* organisms. Tetracycline-resistant strains of *V. cholerae* 01 are uncommon. Single-dose doxycycline (6 mg/kg), furazolidone (5 mg/kg/24 hr given every 6 hr for 3 days), and erythromycin (30 mg/kg/24 hr given every 8 hr for 3 days) are as effective as tetracycline in decreasing duration and volume of diarrhea but are not as effective in shortening the period of excretion of vibrios. Both chloramphenicol (50 mg/kg/24 hr given every 6 hr for 2–3 days) and trimethoprim-sulfamethoxazole (given as 8 mg/kg/24 hr of trimethoprim and 40 mg/kg/24 hr of sulfamethoxazole in two divided doses for 3 days) are beneficial, but the latter is less so than tetracycline; most sulfonamides are ineffective. Parenteral antibiotic therapy is unnecessary. Antidiarrheal medications such as opiates, paregoric, other antimotility drugs, and steroids should not be used. Blood and plasma are not required.

PROGNOSIS. With prompt, correct treatment the outcome of cholera in infants and children should be as favorable as it is in adults, in whom the overall mortality is less than 1%. The high mortality rates (20–70%) reported in earlier studies have been dramatically reduced by improvements in fluid therapy.

MICHAEL H. MERSON

Carpenter CCJ Jr, Hirschhorn N: Pediatric cholera: Current concepts of therapy. J Pediatr 80:874, 1972.
Cholera and other vibrio associated diarrhoeas. WHO Scientific Working Group Report. Bull WHO 58:373, 1980.
Feachem R: Environmental aspects of cholera epidemiology. Parts I–III. Trop Dis Bull 78:676 and 866, 1981; 79:2, 1982.
Glass RI, Svennerholm AM, Stoll BJ, et al: Protection against cholera in breast-fed children by antibodies in breast milk. N Engl J Med 309:323, 1983.
Guidelines for Cholera Control. Document WHO CDD SER 80.4 Rev 1. Geneva, World Health Organization, 1986.
Holmgren J: Actions of cholera toxin and the prevention and treatment of cholera. Nature 292:413, 1981.
Mahalanabis D, Sack D, Moka AM: Treatment of cholera. *In* Barna D, Greenough WB (eds): Cholera. Boston, Plenum Publishers (in press).
Morris JG Jr, Black R: Cholera and other vibrioses in the United States. N Engl J Med 312:343, 1985.
World Health Organization: Treatment and Prevention of Acute Diarrhea—Practical Guidelines, 2nd ed. Geneva, World Health Organization, 1989.

12.32 INFECTIONS DUE TO *PSEUDOMONAS*

Pseudomonas lives abundantly in soil and water and is widespread throughout nature. Most infections are opportunistic and occur among low-birthweight infants and in older infants and children with impaired host defenses, such as those with cystic fibrosis, immunodeficiency disorders, malignancies, extensive burns, or malnutrition (especially in impoverished populations) and in those receiving immunosuppressive therapy (Sec. 12.13).

ETIOLOGY. There are a large number of identified *Pseudomonas* species, but only a few are pathogenic for man; of these, *P. aeruginosa* is by far the most common. Other species occasionally recognized as human pathogens include *P. cepacia, P. maltophilia, P. fluorescens, P. putrefaciens,* and *P. mallei,* the cause of glanders in horses (see later).

The pseudomonads are gram-negative rods and are strict aerobes. Since they can utilize any source of carbon, they multiply in most moist environments that contain minimal amounts of organic compounds. Strains from clinical specimens may produce β-hemolysis on blood agar; more than 90% of strains produce a bluish-green phenazine pigment (blue pus) as well as fluorescein, which is yellow-green and fluoresces. These pigments diffuse into and color the medium surrounding the colonies. Strains of *Pseudomonas* can be differentiated from one another for epidemiologic purposes by serologic, phage, and pyocin typing.

EPIDEMIOLOGY. Pseudomonads frequently enter the hospital environment on the clothes, skin, or shoes of patients or hospital personnel, in plants or vegetables brought into the hospital, and in the gastrointestinal tracts of patients. Colonization of any moist or liquid substance may ensue; for example, they may be found growing in distilled water, hospital kitchens and laundries, some antiseptic solutions, and equipment used for respiratory therapy. Colonization of patients' skin, throat, stool, and nasal mucosa is low on admission to the hospital but increases to as high as 50–70% with prolonged hospitalization and the use of broad-spectrum antibiotics, chemotherapy, mechanical ventilation, and urinary catheters.

PATHOGENESIS. The requirement of oxygen for growth may account for the lack of invasiveness of *Pseudomonas* after it has colonized or even infected the skin. It produces endotoxin that is weak compared with that of other gram-negative bacilli and exotoxin A, which produces local necrosis and systemic bacterial invasion. Exoenzyme S is another toxic virulent factor. *Pseudomonas* produces disease by three stages. Bacterial colonization and attachment are facilitated by pili or fimbriae and by opportunistic adhesion to epithelium damaged from prior injury such as ulcerating keratitis or influenzal pneumonia. A mucopolysaccharide may inhibit phagocytosis, whereas extracellular proteins, proteases, elastases, and cytotoxin (formerly leukocidin) digest cell membranes and antibodies produce capillary vascular permeabililty and inhibit leukocyte function. Dissemination and bloodstream invasion follow extension of local tissue damage and are facilitated by the antiphagocytic properties of the mucosal exopolysaccharide, protease cleavage of IgG, and other characteristics that resist serum phagocytosis. The host responds to infection by producing antibodies to *Pseudomonas* exotoxin (exotoxin A) and lipopolysaccharide. Compromised host defense mechanisms (due to trauma [cutaneous], neutropenia, mucositis, immunosuppression, impaired mucociliary transport) explain the predominant role of this organism in producing opportunistic infections.

CLINICAL MANIFESTATIONS (see Table 12–25). Although most clinical patterns relate to opportunistic infections (Sec. 12.13), *P. aeruginosa* introduced into a minor wound of a healthy child may be followed by cellulitis and a localized abscess that exudes green or blue pus. The characteristic skin lesions of *Pseudomonas*, whether due to direct inoculation or secondary to septicemia, begin as pink macules and progress to hemorrhagic nodules and eventually to areas of necrosis with eschar formation, surrounded by an intense red areola *(ecthyma gangrenosum)*.

TABLE 12–25. *Pseudomonas aeruginosa* Infections

Site	Characteristics
Endocarditis	Native right-sided (tricuspid) valve disease in intravenous drug addicts
Pneumonia	Compromised local (lung) or systemic host defense mechanisms. Nosocomial (respiratory), bacteremic (malignancy), or abnormal mucociliary clearance (cystic fibrosis) may be pathogenesis. Cystic fibrosis is associated with mucoid *P. aeruginosa* organisms producing capsular slime and *P. cepacia*
Central nervous system	Meningitis, brain abscess; contiguous spread (mastoiditis, dermal sinus tracts, sinusitis); bacteremia or direct inoculation (trauma, surgery)
External otitis	Swimmer's ear; humid warm climates, swimming pool contamination
Malignant otitis externa	Invasive, indolent, febrile toxic, destructive necrotizing lesion in young infants, immunosuppressed neutropenic patients, or diabetics. Associated 7th nerve palsy and mastoiditis
Chronic mastoiditis	Ear drainage, swelling, erythema. Perforated tympanic membrane
Keratitis	Corneal ulceration. Contact lens keratitis
Endophthalmitis	Penetrating trauma, surgery, penetrating corneal ulceration; fulminant progression
Osteomyelitis/septic arthritis	Puncture wounds of foot and osteochondritis; intravenous drug abuse; fibrocartilaginous joints, sternum, vertebrae, pelvis. Open fracture osteomyelitis. Indolent. Pyelonephritis and vertebral osteomyelitis
Urinary tract infection	Iatrogenic, nosocomial. Recurrent urinary tract infections in children, instrumented patients, and those with obstruction or stones
Gastrointestinal tract	Immunocompromised, neutropenia, typhlitis, rectal abscess, ulceration, rarely diarrhea. Peritonitis in peritoneal dialysis
Ecthyma gangrenosum	Metastatic dissemination. Hemorrhage, necrosis, erythema, eschar, discrete lesions with bacterial invasion of blood vessels. Also subcutaneous nodules, cellulitis, pustules, deep abscesses
Primary and secondary skin infections	Local infection. Burns, trauma, decubitus ulcers, toe web infection, green nail (paronychia). Whirlpool dermatitis: diffuse, pruritic, folliculitis, vesiculopustular or maculopapular, erythematous lesions

Outbreaks of dermatitis and urinary tract infections caused by *P. aeruginosa* have been reported in healthy children following use of community swimming pools, recreational whirlpools, or family-owned hot tubs. Skin lesions develop several hours to 2 days following contact with these water sources. Skin lesions may be erythematous, macular, papular, or pustular. Illness may vary from a few scattered lesions to extensive truncal involvement. In some children, malaise, fever, vomiting, sore throat, conjunctivitis, rhinitis, and swollen breasts may be associated with dermal lesions.

Pseudomonads other than *P. aeruginosa* rarely cause disease in healthy children, but pneumonia and abscesses due to *P. cepacia*, otitis media due to *P. putrefaciens* or *P. stutzeri*, abscesses due to *P. fluorescens*, and cellulitis and septicemia due to *P. maltophilia* have been reported. Septicemia and endocarditis due to *P. maltophilia* have also been associated with intravenous abuse of drugs.

Shunts, Catheters, and Equipment (see Sec. 12.13 and Table 12–25).

Burns and Wound Infection. The surfaces of wounds or burns are frequently populated by *Pseudomonas* and other gram-negative organisms; this does not necessarily imply infection but is a necessary prerequisite to invasive disease. Septicemia with *P. aeruginosa* is a major problem in the burned patient (Sec. 6.37 and 12.13). It may be related to multiplication of organisms in devitalized tissues or associated with prolonged use of intravenous or urinary catheters. Administration of antibiotics may diminish the susceptible microbiologic flora but permit selected strains of *Pseudomonas* to flourish.

Cystic Fibrosis (see Sec. 14.89).

Malignancy. Children with leukemia or other debilitating malignancies, particularly those who are receiving immunosuppressive therapy and who are neutropenic, are extremely susceptible to septicemia from invasion of the bloodstream by *Pseudomonas* with which the patient is already colonized (see Sec. 12.13). Anorexia, malaise, nausea, vomiting, diarrhea, and fever may be noted. A generalized vasculitis develops, and hemorrhagic necrotic lesions may be found in all organs, including skin, where they appear as purple nodules or ecchymotic areas that become gangrenous. Hemorrhagic or gangrenous perirectal cellulitis or abscesses may occur, associated with ileus and profound hypotension.

DIAGNOSIS AND DIFFERENTIAL DIAGNOSIS. This diagnosis depends upon recovery of the organism from the blood, cerebrospinal fluid, urine, or needle aspirate of the lung or from purulent material obtained by aspiration of subcutaneous abscesses or areas of cellulitis.

Bluish, nodular skin lesions and ulcers with ecchymotic and gangrenous centers and bright areolae (ecthyma gangrenosum) are virtually pathognomonic of *Pseudomonas* infection of the skin. Rarely, skin lesions clinically indistinguishable from those caused by *P. aeruginosa* may follow septicemia due to *Aeromonas hydrophilia*. The differential diagnosis includes local and disseminated diseases due to other gram-negative rods, fungi, or viruses.

PREVENTION. In part, this depends upon continuous surveillance of the hospital environment to identify and subsequently eradicate sources of the organism as quickly as possible. *Pseudomonas* may grow in distilled water, disinfectants, parenteral alimentation solutions, and medications. In newborn nurseries infection generally has been transmitted to the infants by the hands of personnel, from washbasin surfaces, from catheters, and from solutions used to rinse suction catheters.

Strict attention to handwashing, particularly with an iodophor-containing liquid, before and between contacts with newborn infants may prevent or interdict epidemic disease. Growth of *Pseudomonas* on suction catheters can be prevented by rinsing catheters in a 3% solution of acetic acid. Meticulous care in the preparation of solutions for total parenteral alimentation and in the insertion and care of catheters as well as daily replacement of all apparatus used for intravenous administration greatly reduces the hazard of extrinsic contamination by *Pseudomonas* and other gram-negative organisms.

Prevention of follicular dermatitis caused by *Pseudomonas* contamination of whirlpools or hot tubs is possible by maintaining pool water at a pH of 7.2–7.8 and free chlorine concentration at 70.5 mg/L.

Burn patients may be actively immunized with a polyvalent *Pseudomonas* vaccine that reduces bacteremia and mortality. The administration of specific hyperimmune globulin also prevents septicemia. Infection also may be minimized by careful protective isolation, by the topical application of sulfadiazine or 10% mafenide acetate cream, and by debridement of devitalized tissue.

Pseudomonas infection of dermal sinuses communicating with the cerebrospinal space can be prevented by early discovery and surgical repair. *Pseudomonas* infection of the urinary tract may be minimized or prevented by early identification and corrective surgery of obstructive lesions.

TREATMENT. Systemic infections with *Pseudomonas* should be treated promptly with an antibiotic to which the organism is sensitive in vitro. Response to treatment may be limited, and prolonged treatment may be necessary for systemic infection in the compromised host.

Septicemia usually should be treated with gentamicin in a dose of 5–7.5 mg/kg/24 hr in three divided doses. The higher dose may be used after the 1st wk of life. This drug may be given intramuscularly or intravenously (if it is infused slowly over a period of 1 hr). Carbenicillin (200–400 mg/kg/24 hr in six divided doses) or ticarcillin (200 mg/kg/24 hr in six divided doses intravenously) should be used concomitantly for a possible synergistic effect. Carbenicillin or ticarcillin alone is not recommended because strains of the organism rapidly become resistant to these agents. Tobramycin (3–5 mg/kg/24 hr) or amikacin (15–25 mg/kg/24 hr) in three divided doses intramuscularly or intravenously (over 1 hr) may be used to replace gentamicin in the therapeutic regimen.

Many of the newer β-lactam antibiotics possess variable degrees of activity against *P. aeruginosa*. In vitro, ceftazidime is the most active of these agents against *P. aeruginosa*, and it has also proved to be extremely effective in patients with cystic fibrosis (150–200 mg/kg/24 hr in three or four divided doses). Azlocillin and piperacillin also have proved to be effective therapy for selected strains of *P. aeruginosa* when combined with an aminoglycoside; they can be given in doses of 300 mg/kg/24 hr intravenously in three or four divided doses. Additional effective antibiotics include imipenem, aztreonam, and ciprofloxacin.

Meningitis should be treated with gentamicin and carbenicillin or ceftazidime given intravenously as above. Concomitant intraventricular or intrathecal treatment with gentamicin (1–2 mg once daily, independent of body weight, until the cerebrospinal fluid is sterile) may be required.

Abscesses should be incised and drained. Failure to do so inhibits a favorable response to systemic antibiotic treatment.

PROGNOSIS. This depends in large part on the nature of the underlying disease; for example, the leading cause of death in childhood leukemia is septicemia, and half of these cases are due to *Pseudomonas*. The outcome for patients with *P. aeruginosa* sepsis is improved by combined antimicrobial therapy, a urinary tract portal of entry, absence of neutropenia or recovery from neutropenia, and drainage of local sites of infection. *Pseudomonas* is recovered from the lungs of most children who die of cystic fibrosis and may be responsible for the slow deterioration of these patients; *P. cepacia*, which is frequently resistant to standard antimicrobial agents, has been associated with a more rapid decline in pulmonary function and lower survival. The prognosis for normal development is poor in the few infants who survive *Pseudomonas* meningitis.

Disease Due to Other Pseudomonads

GLANDERS

Glanders is a severe infectious disease of horses due to *P. mallei* that is occasionally transmitted to man. It is relatively common in Asia, Africa, and the Middle East. The clinical manifestations include acute or chronic pneumonitis and hemorrhagic necrotic lesions of the skin, nasal mucous membranes, and lymph nodes.

MELIOIDOSIS

This important disease of Southeast Asia and northern Australia is seen in the United States mainly in persons from endemic areas. The causative agent is *P. pseudomallei*, an inhabitant of soil and water in the tropics. Infection follows inhalation of dust or direct contamination of abrasions or wounds. Melioidosis may present as a single primary skin lesion (vesicle, bulla, or urticaria). Pulmonary infection may be subacute and mimic tuberculosis. Occasionally, septicemia occurs and multiple abscesses are noted in various organs of the body. Myocarditis, pericarditis, endocarditis, intestinal abscess, cholecystitis, acute gastroenteritis, urinary tract infections, septic arthritis, paraspinal abscess, osteomyelitis, and generalized lymphadenopathy have all been observed. Melioidosis may also present as an encephalitic illness with fever and seizures; generally, antibiotic therapy results in recovery. The disease may remain latent and appear when host resistance is reduced, sometimes years after the initial exposure.

Glanders is treated with tetracycline or chloramphenicol and streptomycin over a period of many months. Melioidosis is treated with ceftazidime or chloramphenicol with doxycycline and trimethoprim-sulfamethoxazole.

RALPH D. FEIGIN

Butrus SI, Klotz SA, Misra PR: The adherence of *Pseudomonas aeruginosa* to soft contact lenses. Ophthalmology 94:1310, 1987.
Chaowagul W, White NJ, Dance DAB, et al: Melioidosis: A major cause of community-acquired septicemia in northeastern Thailand. J Infect Dis 159:890, 1989.
Feder HM Jr, Grant-Kels JM, and Tilton RG: *Pseudomonas* whirlpool dermatitis. Clin Pediatr 22:638, 1983.
Fong IW, Tomkins KB: Review of *Pseudomonas aeruginosa* meningitis with special emphasis on treatment with ceftazidime. Rev Infect Dis 7:604, 1985.
Hilf M, Yu VL, Sharp JS, et al: Antibiotic therapy for *Pseudomonas aeruginosa* bacteremia: Outcome correlations in a prospective study of 200 patients. Am J Med 87:540, 1989.
Isles A, Maclusky I, Corey M, et al: *Pseudomonas cepacia* infection in cystic fibrosis: An emerging problem. J Pediatr 104:206, 1984.
Jones RJ, Roe EA, Gupta JL: Controlled trials of a polyvalent *Pseudomonas* vaccine in burns. Lancet 2:977, 1979.
Kerem E, Corey M, Gold R, et al: Pulmonary function and clinical course in patients with cystic fibrosis after pulmonary colonization with *Pseudomonas aeruginosa*. J Pediatr 116:714, 1990.
Kusne S, Eibling DE, Yu VL, et al: Gangrenous cellulitis associated with gram-negative bacilli in pancytopenic patients: Dilemma with respect to effective therapy. Am J Med 85:490, 1988.
McManus AT, Mason AD, McManus WF, et al: Twenty-five year review of

Pseudomonas aeruginosa bacteremia in a burn center. Eur J Clin Microbiol 4:219, 1985.

Olgle JW, Janda JM, Woods DE, et al: Characterization and use of a DNA probe as an epidemiologic marker for *Pseudomonas aeruginosa.* J Infect Dis 155:119, 1987.

Reed MD, Stern RC, O'Brien CA, et al: Randomized double blind evaluation of ceftazidime dose ranging in hospitalized patients with cystic fibrosis. Antimicrob Ag Chemother 31:698, 1987.

Reed RK, Larter WE, Sieber OF Jr, et al: Peripheral nodular lesions in *Pseudomonas* sepsis: The importance of incision and drainage. J Pediatr 88:977, 1976.

Salmen T, Dwyer DM, Vorse H, et al: Whirlpool associated *Pseudomonas aeruginosa* urinary tract infections. JAMA 15:2025, 1983.

Whimbey E, Kiehn TE, Brannon P, et al: Bacteremia and fungemia in patients with neoplastic disease. Am J Med 82:723, 1987.

12.33 BRUCELLOSIS

(Undulant Fever, Mediterranean Fever, Goat's Milk Fever)

Brucellosis is an acute or chronic infectious disease of animals that is transmissible to man. Human infection is usually caused by one of the four main species of *Brucella* that may be transmitted from the cow, goat, hog, or dog. *Brucella* organisms also have been recovered from wild rats, field mice, wild guinea pigs, jack rabbits, ground squirrels, rams, camels, gazelles, water buffalo, chamois, deer, elk, bison, and fowl.

ETIOLOGY. Six *Brucella* species are known to be transmissible to man: *abortus* (cows), *melitensis* (goats), *suis* (hogs), *canis* (dogs), *ovis* (sheep and hares), and *neotomae* (desert wood rats). The organisms are small, gram-negative coccobacilli or rods, nonmotile, non-spore-forming, nonencapsulated, and aerobic. Brucellae do not produce exotoxins but contain cell-wall associated endotoxin.

EPIDEMIOLOGY. In the United States, most cases of brucellosis in man result from direct contact with sick animals. Individuals working in food processing plants, dairy farmers, and others who have frequent contact with domestic animals are most commonly infected. In countries where brucellosis is endemic, ingestion of unpasteurized milk, cream, butter, cheese, or ice cream from infected animals is usually the source of infection in humans. The organism also may directly invade the eye, nasopharynx, and genital tract, but unbroken skin is resistant to invasion. Aerosol transmission is well documented. Brucellae are a common cause of laboratory-acquired infections. Brucellae may remain viable up to 3 wk in a refrigerated carcass and can survive the curing of ham. The organisms are killed by pasteurization and cooking.

As a result of compulsory pasteurization of milk, cattle vaccination, and other control measures in cattle, the number of cases in the United States has declined to less than 200 patients/yr since 1980. Texas, California, Virginia, and Florida report over 50% of these cases. Most cases associated with unpasteurized Mexican cheese have been in patients less than 20 yr of age. Human-to-human transmission of brucellosis is rare.

PATHOGENESIS AND PATHOLOGY. Brucellae are primarily intracellular parasites. The organisms are phagocytized by leukocytes and monocytes and are distributed throughout the reticuloendothelial system. Intracellular growth may take place in many cell types, including red blood cells.

Development of delayed hypersensitivity to *Brucella* antigen is characteristic and is necessary for eradication of the organism. It depends upon multiplication of living organisms; dead organisms, or fractions thereof, rarely produce sensitization, but can induce an antibody response.

The host responds to brucellosis by elaborating a variety of antibodies, including agglutinins, opsonins, bactericidins, precipitins, and complement-fixing antibodies. Multiplication of bacteria within the host appears to be essential for induction of immunity. Infection is followed by early development of specific serum IgM antibodies (increase by 1 wk, decline by 3 mo) and then shortly by the appearance of IgG antibodies (increase by 2–3 wk, persist for more than 1 yr if untreated). Cross-reacting antibodies with *Yersinia, Francisella tularensis, Vibrio cholerae,* and *Salmonella* are due to similarities of O-specific side chains of lipopolysaccharide-endotoxins.

Intracellular killing of brucellae by fixed phagocytes requires activation by specifically committed T lymphocytes. Within polymorphonuclear leukocytes, brucellae do not stimulate effective degranulation or a respiratory burst, avoiding intracellular killing. The smooth strains of *Brucella* are more virulent than the rough strains and are more resistant to the intraleukocytic killing systems. They multiply within cells, including those of immune individuals.

All species of *Brucella* may produce granulomas in the liver, spleen, lymph nodes, and bone marrow. In addition, centrilobular necrosis and cirrhosis of the liver have been described. Granulomatous inflammation of the gallbladder, interstitial orchitis with scattered areas of fibroid atrophy, endocarditis with vegetations of the valves, granulomatous lesions of the myocardium, and involvement of the brain, kidney, and skin have also been noted.

CLINICAL MANIFESTATIONS. The incubation period of brucellosis varies from a few days to several months. The manifestations are protean, and no characteristic constellation of signs is diagnostic. The onset may be sudden but most commonly is insidious. Subclinical illness in children in endemic areas is said to be relatively common. Acute manifestations and subacute complications are listed in Table 12–26.

DIAGNOSIS. The most useful method of diagnosis is the *Brucella* standard tube agglutination test; titers will be greater than 1:160 in most acute cases. The standard *Brucella* agglutination tests do not detect antibody against *B. canis;* a separate agglutination test for *B. canis* must be performed if it is suspected. Generally, the titer correlates with the activity of the infection, but *Brucella* antigen in skin tests or food may produce an anamnestic response. Inhibition by blocking antibodies may obscure serum agglutination; this can be avoided by a 1:128 dilution of the serum and repeating the agglutination. Cross-reactions occur with agglutinins against *F. tularensis, V. cholerae,* and *Y. enterocolitica;* appropriate tests should be performed to differentiate infection with these organisms. Later in the course of disease, the complement-fixation titer rises and usually is considered to be diagnostic if it is 1:16 or higher. Enzyme-linked immunosorbent assays that detect IgA, IgG, and IgM, alone or in combination, are sensitive and specific. They can distinguish acute from chronic infection and are useful in the diagnosis of neurobrucellosis. They are not yet available commercially.

Skin tests, when negative, exclude infection, but they should not be performed if serologic studies are available, because the skin test antigen may stimulate production of antibody and thereby confuse subsequent serologic results.

Isolation of *Brucella* by culture provides a definitive diagnosis. The bone marrow is the most productive source of positive cultures. Blood culture and culture of abscesses or infected tissues also may be useful. Cultures from any source are less likely to be positive in patients with chronic brucellosis. Cultures should be incubated under 10% carbon dioxide for at least 6 wk before they are discarded as negative.

DIFFERENTIAL DIAGNOSIS. Acute brucellosis can mimic many diseases, including tularemia, typhoid fever, rickettsial diseases, influenza, tuberculosis, histoplasmosis, coccidioidomycosis, and infectious mononucleosis. Chronic brucellosis may resemble malignant histiocytosis, lymphoma, or other neoplastic diseases. Appropriate historic, roentgenographic, serologic, and culture data help to differentiate these disorders. Biopsy of appropriate tissues may be required.

TABLE 12–26. Manifestations of Brucellosis

	Symptoms and Signs
Acute	
Severity greatest with *Brucella melitensis, B. suis* in nonimmune patients	Mild influenza-like illness OR Drenching sweats, chills, fever, weakness in 90%. Headache, myalgia, arthralgia, backache, weight loss in 25–50%. Temperature rises in afternoon to 39–41° C. Lymphadenopathy (20%), splenomegaly (25–35%), hepatomegaly (20–30%), elevated ESR,* CRP† (60–70%), relapses occur in 5–10%
***Complications* (1–35% of patients)**	
Skeletal (20–30%)	Arthralgia, arthritis (occurs in hip, knee, sacroiliac, ankle, elbow, in order of frequency), spondylitis, osteomyelitis, tendinitis, bursitis. Paraspinal abscess complicates spondylitis
Gastrointestinal (30%)	Hepatomegaly, granulomatous hepatitis; elevated liver enzymes (50%), cholecystitis
Spleen (35%)	Splenomegaly, abscesses, calcification
Pulmonary (15–20%)	Postinhalation or bacteremia. Cough with negative chest roentgenogram; occasional miliary x-ray pattern
Hematologic (20–30%)	Anemia, leukopenia, thrombocytopenia, pancytopenia
Cutaneous (5%)	Erythema nodosum, papules; scarlatiniform, eczematous, vasculitic rashes
Neurologic (2–5%)	Meningoencephalitis, myelitis, meningitis (lymphocytic pleocytosis), paresis, depression, psychosis
Genitourinary (2–10%)	Epididymoorchitis, interstitial nephritis, pyelonephritis
Cardiovascular (2%)	Endocarditis of aortic valve. May require valve replacement

*ESR = erythrocyte sedimentation rate.
†CRP = C-reactive protein.

COMPLICATIONS. See Table 12–26.

PREVENTION. This depends upon avoidance of exposure to brucellae. Infection of domestic animals with which man has close contact can be prevented by immunization. In addition to immunization of animals and pasteurization of milk, periodic agglutination tests of milk and blood should be used to identify infected animals. Positive reactors should be slaughtered. Ingestion of unpasteurized milk and of products derived from unpasteurized milk or cream must be avoided. There is no vaccine available for human use.

TREATMENT. Brucellosis can be treated with oral tetracycline alone for 3–4 wk, but the relapse rate can be as high as 50%. The regimen of choice is tetracycline 30–40 mg/kg/24 hr, divided into 4 oral doses for 4–6 wk (or doxycycline 5 mg/kg/24 hr twice a day), used with streptomycin 15–30 mg/kg/24 hr divided into 2 intramuscular doses for 2–3 wk (or gentamicin 5 mg/kg/24 hr twice a day for 5 days). Trimethoprim-sulfamethoxazole (10 mg/kg/24 hr trimethoprim and 50 mg/kg/24 hr sulfamethoxazole) used alone has a high relapse rate but appears to be effective in combination with streptomycin or gentamicin; this combination is the treatment of choice for children under 8 yr of age. Rifampin, 20 mg/kg/24 hr for 21 days, also has been shown to be effective, but it is preferable not to use it alone. Rifampin with doxycycline is less effective than tetracycline and streptomycin unless it is given for extended periods.

Localized abscesses should be drained. Corticosteroids may reduce the risk of a Herxheimer reaction at the onset of therapy.

PROGNOSIS. The mortality of untreated brucellosis is about 3%; recovery may require 6 mo. Prognosis following specific antibiotic therapy is excellent, and a prolonged course usually is due to a delay in diagnosis.

RALPH D. FEIGIN
MARK A. GROSHEK

Al-Eissa YA, Kambal AM, Al-Nasser MN, et al: Childhood brucellosis: A study of 102 cases. Pediatr Infect Dis J 9:74, 1990.
Lubani MM, Dudin KI, Sharda DC, et al: A multicenter therapeutic study of 1100 children with brucellosis. Pediatr Infect Dis J 8:75, 1989.
Lubani MM, Dudin KI, Araj GJ, et al: Neurobrucellosis in children. Pediatr Infect Dis J 8:79, 1989.
Mousa ARM, Muhtaseb SA, Almudallal DS, et al: Osteoarticular complications of brucellosis: A study of 169 cases. Rev Infect Dis 9:531, 1987.
Thapar MK, Young EJ: Urban outbreak of goat cheese brucellosis. Pediatr Infect Dis 5:640, 1986.

12.34 YERSINIAL INFECTIONS

Three organisms of the *Yersinia* spp. are responsible for human disease: *Y. pestis* (formerly *Pasteurella pestis*), *Y. enterocolitica*, and *Y. pseudotuberculosis*. Yersinoses are zoonotic infections of rodents, pigs, rabbits, sheep, cattle, dogs, and cats; humans are accidental hosts infected by handling contaminated animal tissues and ingesting contaminated meat, water, or milk, and by receiving flea bites *(Y. pestis)*.

Plague

Plague is a worldwide disease that is endemic in parts of China, Southeast Asia, South America, parts of Africa, and the southwestern United States (Colorado, California, New Mexico, Arizona).

ETIOLOGY. *Yersinia pestis* is a nonmotile, nonsporulating, pleomorphic, gram-negative bacillus. The characteristic "safety pin" or bipolar appearance is demonstrated best in smears of infected secretions or tissue stained by the Giemsa method.

EPIDEMIOLOGY. Plague in domestic and wild animals occurs in two forms: enzootic and epizootic. *Enzootic plague* implies a stable rodent-flea cycle of infection that is found in a relatively resistant host population. Enzootic foci are inconspicuous and serve effectively as reservoirs of infection, as in the United States. *Epizootic plague* occurs when the disease is introduced into a highly susceptible mammalian population, causing a high mortality rate among infected animals.

Plague is transmitted to man by the bite of fleas that have sucked blood from infected animals, by the skinning and evisceration of infected animals, or by inhalation of infected droplets from a patient with pneumonic plague. Infrequent portals of entry include the pharynx and the conjunctiva. Transmission from animals to man usually causes bubonic plague and is referred to as *zootic plague*. Person-to-person transmission is called *demic plague*.

In the United States reported cases of plague have been common among males, especially Native Americans. Risk factors include residence in a plague foci area, sheepherding, rabbit or prairie dog hunting, and living in dwellings (hogans) that attract rodents. Fifty to 60% of cases occur in patients younger than 20 yr of age.

PATHOLOGY AND PATHOGENESIS. Plague bacilli ingested by the flea proliferate, are regurgitated into dermal lymphatics of the human host by the flea, and are then transmitted to regional lymph nodes, which become tender and enlarged *(buboes)*. In *severe bubonic plague* the lymph nodes fail to filter out all multiplying bacilli, which gain entrance to the efferent lymphatics and disseminate to the vascular system. Once entry into the bloodstream has occurred, any organ of the body may be involved. Septicemia, meningitis, disseminated intravascular coagulation, and pneumonia (secondary) may develop. Sepsis is characterized by high-grade bacteremia with organisms present on blood smears stained by Wright stain; pneumonia is highly contagious because the sputum contains many bipolar gram-negative organisms.

Primary pulmonic plague is rare and may result from human-to-human transmission or from a laboratory accident. Droplets containing large numbers of virulent bacilli may be inhaled, causing severe pneumonia, septicemia, and, frequently, death within 24 hr.

The response of human tissues to *Y. pestis* generally is pyogenic; necrotic foci may develop within lymph nodes, spleen, and liver. Hemorrhagic lesions may also be found in many organs and tissues, particularly if disseminated intravascular coagulation develops.

CLINICAL MANIFESTATIONS. The incubation period of bubonic plague is 2–6 days, and that of pneumonic plague is 1–72 hr.

The onset of *bubonic plague* may be acute or subacute. In the subacute forms, the initial findings are a tender lymphadenitis (groin, axilla, neck) and associated lymphadenopathy. Patients are febrile but not particularly toxic in appearance. If treatment is delayed, septicemia may occur, associated with prostration, shock, and hemorrhagic pneumonitis.

Acute bubonic plague presents with high fever, tachycardia, and myalgia. The disease progresses to delirium, shock, and death within 3–5 days.

The course of *primary pneumonic plague* is even more virulent. Pulmonary signs and symptoms may be lacking until within 24 hr of death. Symptoms of plague include nausea, vomiting, abdominal pain, bloody diarrhea, and petechial and purpuric rashes.

During epidemics a *mild form* of the disease may occur in which lymphadenopathy and vesicular or pustular skin lesions develop, serious symptoms are absent, and recovery can occur without therapy.

DIAGNOSIS. The diagnosis of nonepidemic plague depends upon a high index of suspicion. Sputum, blood, purulent exudates, and aspirates of lymph nodes should be examined by smears stained with Giemsa or Wayson stain and by culture. Serologic tests may be helpful in selected patients; passive hemagglutination antibody titers to fraction I antigen of *Y. pestis* may be detectable by day 5 of illness; titers peak at 14 days.

DIFFERENTIAL DIAGNOSIS. Plague (mild form) may be confused with other disorders causing localized lymphadenitis and lymphadenopathy, including infection due to *S. aureus, S. pyogenes,* and *F. tularensis*. Septicemic plague may be indistinguishable clinically from any other form of overwhelming bacterial septicemia or from rickettsial diseases.

PREVENTION. A formalin-killed plague vaccine may produce immunity. Routine vaccination is not recommended, even for individuals living in plague enzootic areas of the United States. Immunization may be useful for those whose occupation regularly brings them into contact with infected rodents or with the organism itself in the laboratory.

If vaccinated individuals are exposed to plague, they should receive chemoprophylaxis, since the vaccine may not be completely protective even in the presence of high antibody titers.

Primary prevention consists of environmental sanitation directed toward reducing rodent populations and their fleas. In endemic areas, the public must be educated to avoid burrows, to refrain from handling sick or dead rodents, to deflea household pets, and to eliminate trash near living areas. Patients with plague should be quarantined until treated. Purulent exudates should be handled with rubber gloves. Face masks and goggles should be worn by medical personnel. *Y. pestis* may be found in feces; accordingly, stools of patients should be routinely disinfected before disposal.

TREATMENT. Streptomycin is bactericidal and can be used in a dose of 30 mg/kg/24 hr in 2–3 equally divided doses given intramuscularly for 10 days. Herxheimer reactions are not uncommon when streptomycin is given; thus this drug is usually reserved for pneumonic or septicemic forms of the disease. In children over 18 yr old tetracycline may be added after 2–3 days of streptomycin therapy in a dose of 30 mg/kg/24 hr in 4 divided oral doses and continued for 10 days.

In areas where streptomycin-resistant *Y. pestis* is found, chloramphenicol should be given to critically ill patients. Plague meningitis should be treated with chloramphenicol 100 mg/kg/24 hr in 4 divided doses intravenously for at least 10 days.

Contacts of patients with pulmonic plague should be quarantined and may be given tetracycline (20 mg/kg/24 hr) in 4 divided oral doses prophylactically for 10 days.

PROGNOSIS. The mortality of untreated bubonic plague is 60–90%. Pneumonic plague is virtually 100% fatal if untreated.

When bubonic plague is treated early, the mortality rate is less than 10%. Prognosis in primary pneumonic plague is poor if specific treatment is not provided within 18 hr of onset of symptoms.

Yersinia Enterocolitica and *Yersinia Pseudotuberculosis*

Disease from these organisms is being recognized with increasing frequency. *Yersinia* may be confused with coliform organisms. *Y. enterocolitica* organisms are oxidase-negative, urease-positive, nonlactose-fermenting, gram-negative rods that are motile at 22° C but not at 37° C. It is this last characteristic that aids in differentiating them from *Y. pestis* and Enterobacteriaceae. *Y. enterocolitica* and *Y. pseudotuberculosis* can be distinguished from each other by biochemical tests, by agglutination with specific antisera, and by the susceptibility of *Y. pseudotuberculosis* to specific bacteriophages. *Y. enterocolitica* can be separated into 50 serotypes and 5 biotypes; *Y. pseudotuberculosis* has 6 serotypes (I–VI) and four subtypes. Serotypes 3, 8, and 9 of *Y. enterocolitica* and serotype 1 of *Y. pseudotuberculosis* are the most frequent causes of disease in humans.

EPIDEMIOLOGY. *Y. enterocolitica* has been recovered from many wild and domestic animals, raw milk, oysters, and water supplies. Infection from dogs and human-to-human spread have been documented. Infants and children are most commonly infected. Chitterlings are a common source. The incubation period ranges from 1–3 wk. Disease is more common in winter and fall.

CLINICAL MANIFESTATIONS. *Y. enterocolitica* has been associated with diarrhea, acute mesenteric adenitis, pharyngitis, thyroiditis, abscesses, reactive arthritis with or without Reiter syndrome, osteomyelitis, hepatitis, carditis, meningitis, ophthalmitis, hemolytic anemia, septicemia, glomerulonephritis, and rashes, including erythema nodosum. Septicemia has been reported with diabetes, cirrhosis, malignancy, hemochromatosis, and after accidental overdose of oral iron in previously healthy children. Enhanced growth of *Y. enterocol-*

itica in the intestine after exposure of the organism to excess iron combined with damage to the intestinal mucosa by iron may play a pathogenic role in this situation. Septicemia is associated with a case-fatality rate of nearly 50%, despite antibiotic treatment.

With gastrointestinal disease, abdominal pain may be severe, simulating appendicitis. Ulceration of the small bowel has been described. Diarrhea is common and persistent, lasting 1–2 wk. The stool may be watery and mucoid, and in 15–25% of patients it contains blood. The stool of patients with diarrhea due to *Y. enterocolitica* may contain polymorphonuclear leukocytes. When disease is severe there may be hypoalbuminemia and hypokalemia, suggesting extensive disruption of the small bowel mucosa. The duration of illness generally is 2–3 wk without treatment, but occasionally diarrhea may persist for several months. The characteristic pattern of fever and diarrhea usually occurs in patients under 5 yr of age, whereas the pattern of fever, right lower quadrant pain, and leukocytosis, presenting as mesenteric adenitis or terminal ileitis, is typical of older children and adolescents and mimics inflammatory bowel disease or appendicitis.

DIAGNOSIS. This may be established by identification of the organism in the stool. Passive hemagglutination tests may also confirm the diagnosis. Antibodies are detectable 8–10 days after the onset of illness and may persist for several months. Infants are less likely to have a serologic response than are older children. Ultrasound examination of the right lower quadrant may be needed to differentiate acute appendicitis or inflammatory bowel disease.

TREATMENT. Most strains of *Y. enterocolitica* are sensitive to streptomycin, tetracycline, chloramphenicol, trimethoprim-sulfamethoxazole, third-generation cephalosporins, and quinolones. Therapy is not recommended for diarrhea or uncomplicated mesenteric adenitis but is mandatory for sepsis, which has a 50% mortality, and includes an aminoglycoside, tetracycline, or trimethoprim-sulfamethoxazole.

Y. pseudotuberculosis has been associated with mesenteric adenitis and terminal ileitis. Abdominal pain may be severe and suggest acute appendicitis. Septicemia is unusual but may occur and is associated with risk factors similar to those noted for *Y. enterocolitica*. Postdiarrheal hemolytic uremic syndrome has been reported, as have cases simulating Kawasaki disease. *Y. pseudotuberculosis* is generally sensitive to ampicillin, kanamycin, tetracycline, and chloramphenicol. Treatment is indicated for sepsis but not for uncomplicated mesenteric adenitis.

Black RE, Slome S: *Yersinia enterocolitica*. Infect Dis Clin North Am 2:625, 1988.
Boelaert JR, van Landuyt HW, Valke YJ, et al: The role of iron overload in *Yersinia enterocolitica* and *Yersinia pseudotuberculosis* bacteremia in hemodialysis patients. J Infect Dis 156:384, 1987.
Cover TL, Aber RC: *Yersinia enterocolitica*. N Engl J Med 321:16, 1989.
Mann JM, Schaudler L, Cushing A: Pediatric plague. Pediatrics 69:762, 1982.
Sato K, Ouchi K, Taki M: *Yersinia pseudotuberculosis* infection in children, resembling Izumi fever and Kawasaki syndrome. Pediatr Infect Dis 2:123, 1983.

12.35 TULAREMIA

Tularemia, a zoonotic infectious disease caused by *Francisella tularensis*, varies in its clinical patterns in relation to the virulence of the bacterium and the route of infection. Infrequently the disease may run a subclinical course. Most often, however, it assumes one of five clinical forms: ulceroglandular (80%), glandular (lymph nodes) (10%), oculoglandular (1%), oropharyngeal (relatively common in children), and typhoidal (6%).

ETIOLOGY. The organism is a short, non–spore-forming, nonmotile, unencapsulated, gram-negative pleomorphic coccobacillus. Special containment facilities are recommended in handling cultures to avoid acquisition of disease.

Strains of *F. tularensis* are antigenically homogeneous, but virulence is variable. One strain (Jellison type A), found only in North America, is highly virulent for humans. A second strain, *F. palaearctica* (Jellison type B), found in North America, Europe, and Asia, is avirulent for rabbits and causes only mild disease in man. The bacterium contains a protein antigen that reacts with endotoxin; most strains also produce β-lactamase.

EPIDEMIOLOGY. Tularemia is not an uncommon disease in the United States. No age group is immune. Most reported cases occur between May and September and are from the West–South Central States, but a large outbreak occurred in Vermont in 1968.

F. tularensis has been recovered from over 100 types of mammals and arthropods. Type A bacteria generally are acquired from cottontail rabbits or ticks. Type B strains are more commonly acquired from rats, mice, squirrels, muskrats, beavers, moles, birds, aquatic animals, and ticks. Tularemia may also be acquired from horseflies, deerflies, fleas, mosquitoes, and lice. In the United States, rabbits and ticks are important reservoirs.

Tularemia has been considered to be a disease of hunters, trappers, cooks, muskrat farmers, and others with occupational exposure to the organism. It may occur in children who have ingested food (rabbit or squirrel meat) or water contaminated with *F. tularensis* or who have been bitten by infected ticks, flies, or other vectors. In one outbreak in Baltimore, Maryland, tularemia pneumonia resulted from an aerosol established by children who beat a rabbit carcass with a stick.

PATHOLOGY AND PATHOGENESIS. The host may be infected by inoculation through broken or intact skin or mucous membranes, ingestion (including penetration of the pharyngeal mucosa by ingested organisms), inhalation, or the bite of infected arthropod vectors. Ten to 50 organisms produce disease if inhaled or injected, whereas thousands of organisms are needed if they are ingested. Within 48–72 hr after the organisms enter the skin, an erythematous maculopapular lesion may be noted, followed shortly by ulceration and regional lymphadenopathy. The organisms multiply and produce granulomas within lymph nodes. Subsequently, bacteremia may occur. Although any organ of the body may be involved, infection of the reticuloendothelial system is most prominent and common.

Pneumonia may follow inhalation of *F. tularensis*. An inflammatory reaction develops about the site of bacterial deposition, and necrosis of alveolar walls follows. The organisms that reach the lung are ingested by alveolar macrophages and enter first the hilar lymphatics and then the blood. A typhoidal form of tularemia results when the mastication of contaminated food releases *F. tularensis*, which is then inhaled.

F. tularensis is an intracellular parasite capable of surviving for extended periods of time within monocytes and other body cells. Although the immune response is usually persistent, chronic or relapsing disease may rarely occur. Cell-mediated immunity may be of greater import than are circulating antibodies in determining complete recovery.

CLINICAL MANIFESTATIONS. The incubation period varies from a few hours to a week but is usually 3–4 days. The onset is acute and characterized by myalgia, arthralgia, chills, fever of 40–41° C (104–106° F), nausea, vomiting, and diaphoresis. Headache is prominent and may be associated with photophobia. A generalized maculopapular, papular, or pustular rash occurs in 20% of patients. Hematologic data are not discriminating; even the sedimentation rate can be normal. There may be transient proteinuria.

In the *ulceroglandular* form the primary maculopapular lesion is noted within 72 hr and ulcerates within 4–5 days. The ulceration is painful, requires about a month to heal, and is located on the hands in rabbit-associated disease and on the lower extremity or perineum in tick-borne disease. Regional lymphadenopathy occurs, usually without discernible intervening lymphangitis. The lymph nodes are tender and become fluctuant in about 25% of untreated cases. Rabbit-associated disease demonstrates axillary or epitrochlear adenopathy (80–90%), whereas tick-borne disease produces inguinal or femoral adenopathy (60–70%). Generalized lymphadenopathy, splenomegaly, or both may develop.

Oropharyngeal tularemia is characterized by purulent tonsillitis and pharyngitis and occasionally by ulcerative stomatitis.

Glandular tularemia is similar to the ulceroglandular form, but no local lesion is apparent.

Oculoglandular disease is similar to the ulceroglandular form except that the primary lesion is a severe, painful conjunctivitis accompanied by preauricular or cervical lymphadenitis.

The *typhoidal* form resembles typhoid fever. Fever is protracted, and cutaneous or mucous membrane lesions may not be apparent. A dry cough, severe retrosternal chest pain, and hemoptysis are common. Clinical evidence of bronchitis, pneumonitis, and/or pleuritis may be found in 20% of cases, and roentgenographic evidence of pulmonary involvement and nodular enlargement in the mediastinum is seen in the majority of instances. Splenomegaly is common, as is hepatic enlargement.

Meningitis, encephalitis, pericarditis, endocarditis, peritonitis, thrombophlebitis, and osteomyelitis have all been observed.

DIAGNOSIS. The history and clinical manifestations may suggest the disease, particularly a history of ingestion of rabbit or squirrel meat, contact with rabbits, or bites by ticks, flies, or other vectors.

A preparation of phenolized organisms may be used for *skin testing*. Positive reactions may be observed by the 4th–7th day of infection. Skin test material may be obtained from the Rocky Mountain Laboratory of the National Institute of Allergy and Infectious Disease.

Culture of organisms is possible but requires appropriate media and is hazardous to inexperienced laboratory personnel. The organism may be isolated from blood, gastric washings, and drainage from wounds by culture or by inoculating guinea pigs intraperitoneally with these body fluids. Infected animals are even more hazardous to laboratory personnel than are cultures.

The *serum agglutination test* is reliable, although it usually is not positive until after the 1st wk of illness, and fatal cases have been reported in the absence of agglutinins. Agglutinins are first detectable between the 10th and 14th days. A titer of 1:80 or greater may be considered positive, but serially rising titers are of greater significance. Titers as high as 1:640 may be expected within another week and may be in excess of 1:1280 within the 2nd month. Low titers due to cross-reactions with *Brucella*, heterophil, OX-19, and cholera vaccine have been reported.

DIFFERENTIAL DIAGNOSIS. *Ulceroglandular tularemia* may resemble cat-scratch disease, infectious mononucleosis, sporotrichosis, plague, anthrax, melioidosis, glanders, rat-bite fever, or lymphadenitis due to *Mycobacterium tuberculosis*, atypical mycobacteria, or *Staphylococcus aureus*. *Oropharyngeal tularemia* must be differentiated from the same diseases but also from acquired cytomegaloviral disease, acquired toxoplasmosis, and infection due to adenoviruses and herpes simplex.

Tularemic pneumonitis must be differentiated from other bacterial and nonbacterial pneumonias, particularly those due to mycoplasma, *Chlamydia*, mycobacteria, fungi, and rickettsia. These distinctions can be made on the basis of isolation of the organisms.

Typhoidal tularemia must be differentiated from typhoid fever, brucellosis, and other severe septicemic illnesses.

PREVENTION. Avoidance of exposure to mammals and arthropod vectors that may be infected is most important. Rabbits that appear to be ill should be destroyed without direct handling. Rubber gloves should be worn to handle the flesh of wild animals. In areas infested with ticks, tight wristbands and boots are recommended. A careful search for ticks should be made as frequently as practical when one is within a wooded area and promptly upon departure. Ticks should be removed by an instrument or the gloved hand and should not be squeezed. The area of attachment should be cleansed with 70% ethanol.

An intradermal vaccine containing a live attenuated strain of *F. tularensis* is available. It is safe, and immunity persists for 3–5 yr. It has not been evaluated for use in children.

TREATMENT. Streptomycin, 30–40 mg/kg/24 hr in 2 divided doses intramuscularly for 7–14 days, is the treatment of choice. Tetracycline and chloramphenicol are also effective, but relapses are common with each of them, if given for less than 14 days. Retreatment with tetracycline has been effective. Gentamicin is an alternative to streptomycin.

PROGNOSIS. Untreated ulceroglandular tularemia has a fatality rate of about 5%. Untreated patients who survive experience symptoms for 2–4 wk and a subsequent period of disability of 8–12 wk. Mortality in untreated patients may reach 30% if pneumonia develops. Recovery usually provides lifelong immunity. Second attacks may occur but are mild. Prognosis following infection with Jellison type B strains may be considerably better than that reported above. If treatment is provided promptly, recovery generally is rapid and fatality exceedingly rare.

Evans ME, Gregory DW, Schattner W, et al: Tularemia: A 30 year experience with 88 cases. Medicine 64:251, 1985.

Halsted CC, Kulasinghe HP: Tularemia pneumonia in urban children. Pediatrics 61:660, 1978.

Jacobs RF, Condrey YM, Yamanchi T: Tularemia in adults and children: A changing presentation. Pediatrics 76:818, 1985.

Tyson HK: Tularemia: An unappreciated cause of exudative pharyngitis. Pediatrics 58:864, 1976.

Uhari M, Syrjala H, Salminen A: Tularemia in children caused by *Francisella tularensis* biovar *palaearctica*. Pediatr Infect Dis J 9:80, 1990.

12.36 LISTERIOSIS

Listeriosis is a septicemic or meningitic illness that most frequently affects the newborn infant, the pregnant woman, and the compromised pediatric host. Human infections with *Listeria monocytogenes*, unlike those in animals, generally are characterized by a polymorphonuclear response in blood, cerebrospinal fluid, and other body tissues.

ETIOLOGY. *L. monocytogenes* is a small, gram-positive, nonspore-forming rod displaying tumbling motility at room temperature but not at 37° C. Generally, it produces β-hemolysis on blood agar. It can occur in pairs of cocci and may be mistaken for group B streptococcus or pneumococcus; if poorly stained, it may be mistaken for *H. influenzae*. It may also be confused with contaminant diphtheroids. *Listeria* can be divided into 6 serologic types on the basis of somatic (O) and flagellar (H) antigens. Ninety per cent of human disease is due to organisms belonging to groups Ia, Ib, and IIIb.

EPIDEMIOLOGY. *Listeria* has been reported as a cause of disease in 42 domestic and feral mammalian species, 22 avian species, fish, ticks, flies, and crustaceans. Listeriosis produces abortion in domestic mammals and animal circling disease, a form of basilar meningitis. It has been isolated from soil, where survival for more than 295 days has been recorded, and from streams, sewage, silage, dust, and slaughterhouse waste. It also has been recovered from the intestinal tract, vagina, cervix, nose, ears, and, rarely, blood or urine of apparently healthy humans. *Listeria* is found in feces of 1% of normal people, 5% of slaughterhouse workers, and 25% of symptomatic patients.

Food-borne transmission of *Listeria* is well recognized. Outbreaks of listeriosis have been associated with Mexican (soft ripened) cheese, whole and 2% milk, uncooked hot dogs, undercooked chicken, raw vegetables, shellfish, and cabbage (cole slaw) contaminated with manure. *L. monocytogenes* has been cultured from pasteurizing plants and meat processing plants and has been found to survive at refrigerator temperatures. Many cases are sporadic and have no identifiable source.

In the newborn infant the organism may be acquired transplacentally or by aspiration or ingestion at the time of delivery. In some cases carriers may develop overt disease when their immune responses are altered by underlying disease (e.g., leukemia, lymphomas, Hodgkin disease) or by administration of immunosuppressive agents (transplantation, chemotherapy, steroids). Sporadic infection in immunosuppressed transplant recipients may result from invasion of the bloodstream by *Listeria* from sites of colonization in the gastrointestinal tract.

PATHOLOGY. *L. monocytogenes* produces disease in many organs, including liver, lung, adrenals, kidneys, and brain. The abscesses do not differ from those found in other pyogenic infections, but there may be granulomatous reactions and microabscess formation. Necrotizing changes may be noted in the kidneys and the lung, particularly in the bronchioles and alveolar walls.

Listeria produces a pyogenic meningitis and also may cause suppurative ependymitis, encephalitis, choroiditis, and gliosis.

PATHOGENESIS. *Listeria* is a facultative intracellular parasite, that may enter the body through the gastrointestinal tract. T lymphocytes and monocytes are important defense mechanisms, and immunoglobulins and complement-derived opsonophagocytosis play a secondary role. Any inherited or acquired disorder in which T cell function is impaired may predispose the host to infection by *Listeria*. *Listeria* hemolysin, which is antigenically related to streptolysin O, may act as a virulence factor by binding to cholesterol in cell membranes, thus interfering with monocyte function.

Listeriosis may develop at birth or be noted subsequently in the newborn infant or older child. Early-onset disease may be acquired transplacentally from a mother with subclinical or clinical infection. Infection acquired early in pregnancy may lead to abortion and, more commonly, if acquired later, to stillbirth or premature delivery.

Early-onset septicemic neonatal disease has been associated with maternal fever or other signs of maternal infection and frequently with recovery of serotypes Ia and Ib from mother and/or infant. The development of *late-onset* neonatal disease is not usually associated with maternal illness or carriage of the organism; epidemic neonatal disease has been described, presumably reflecting patient-to-patient transmission. Late-onset disease is primarily associated with recovery of serotype IVb and is predominantly a meningitis. Nonetheless, each of these serotypes may be found at either time.

At any age all organs of the body may be involved after bloodstream invasion.

CLINICAL MANIFESTATIONS. *Listeria* may cause septicemia and/or meningitis in infants and children. In the newborn infant, a spectrum of disease is apparent, and the clinical presentation depends upon the time and route of infection.

Early Onset. The liveborn infant with an infection acquired late in pregnancy may present acutely ill and expire within a few hours of birth. More often, disease becomes apparent within the 1st wk of life. Whitish granulomas may be found on the mucous membranes and disseminated erythematous papules on the skin. Posterior pharyngeal and cutaneous granulomas distinguish neonatal *Listeriosis* from other causes of early-onset neonatal sepsis. Anorexia, lethargy, vomiting, jaundice, respiratory distress, pulmonary infiltrates, cyanosis, petechial rashes, evidence of myocarditis, and hepatomegaly have been noted. These infants frequently are premature, and the mortality rate is high. Septicemia and shock are common, and there may be associated meningitis (Sec. 9.60). Severe fulminant disease, manifest at birth from in utero infection, is known as granulomatosis infantisepticum and is characterized by shock; pustular or petechial rash; hepatomegaly; disseminated lesions in the liver, kidney, lung, brain, and adrenal glands; and a high mortality.

Late Onset. The infant may appear well at birth and in the 1st wk, but septicemia or meningitis may develop later during the neonatal period, typically between 7 and 28 (mean 14) days of life. Signs and symptoms are similar to those noted in any form of pyogenic meningitis (Sec. 9.63). Meningitis often occurs alone and the course may be indolent. However, there may be associated septicemia with a more fulminant presentation.

In older children meningitis or meningoencephalitis, cerebritis, and brain, brain stem, and spinal cord abscesses may be noted. Generally, no characteristics distinguish meningitis due to *Listeria* from that due to other causes. In some cases, however, the onset is subacute and is characterized by headache, low-grade fever, and malaise of several days' duration prior to the time that symptoms and signs referable to the central nervous system are first noted.

Conjunctivitis, otitis media, hepatitis, sinusitis, pneumonia, endocarditis, and pericarditis may occur with or without meningitis in older immunocompromised or immunocompetent patients. An oculoglandular syndrome due to *Listeria*, characterized by keratoconjunctivitis, corneal ulceration, and regional lymphadenitis, has also been described. Listeriosis also may present as pneumonia, an influenza-like septicemic illness of pregnant women, endocarditis, localized abscesses, papular or pustular cutaneous lesions, conjunctivitis, and urethritis.

An infectious mononucleosis-like syndrome was the first disorder of humans with which *L. monocytogenes* was associated. The Paul-Bunnell heterophil antibody test is negative. The organism may be a secondary invader in the sense that the disease may be due to Epstein-Barr virus, but *L. monocytogenes* in some manner interferes with heterophil antibody production.

DIAGNOSIS. The possibility of animal contact should be ascertained. *Listeria* infection should be suspected in the newborn who has signs and symptoms of septicemia, pneumonia, or meningitis and in children who have malignancies and are receiving immunosuppressive therapy. Brown-stained amniotic fluid commonly is noted as a characteristic of the disease. Appropriate materials for culture vary with the clinical diagnosis. If neonatal listeriosis is sought, cultures of the blood, cerebrospinal fluid, meconium, urine, and exudate expressed from an incised skin papule should be cultured. Cultures should also be obtained from the vagina and cervix of the mother and, if possible, from the placenta and lochia. Cerebrospinal fluid findings in patients with *Listeria* meningitis show a preponderance of polymorphonuclear leukocytes, elevated protein concentration, and depressed glucose.

The microbiology laboratory should be alerted when the possibility of listeriosis is considered so that confusion with diphtheroids can be minimized. Most strains of *Listeria* can be primarily isolated on conventional media within 1–2 days. Although a rise in agglutinins may occur 2–4 wk after the onset of infection, most investigators feel that serodiagnosis is unreliable because agglutinins to *Listeria* may be found in up to 90% of animals and man.

DIFFERENTIAL DIAGNOSIS. Listeriosis must be differentiated from bacterial septicemia and meningitis of other causes. In the rare cases in which atypical lymphocytes are noted, toxoplasmosis and infection due to Epstein-Barr virus, cytomegalovirus, and hepatitis viruses must be excluded. CNS infections that may mimic listeriosis in immunocompromised non-neutropenic patients include toxoplasmosis, *Nocardia* infection, tuberculosis, and cryptococcosis. Neutropenic patients may develop meningitis from gram-negative enteric bacteria and space-occupying lesions due to aspergillosis.

TREATMENT. Therapy should be initiated with ampicillin in a dose and route appropriate for the type of infection and the age of the patient. Severe life-threatening disease should also be treated with gentamicin, which is bacteriocidal, until the sensitivity of the isolate is known. Gentamicin may be synergistic with ampicillin and may improve the outcome of patients with serious disease. Trimethoprim-sulfamethoxazole is also bacteriocidal, achieves high levels in the CSF, and may be an alternative to ampicillin in penicillin-allergic patients. The duration of therapy is at least 2 wk and may need to be prolonged (3–6 wk) in immunocompromised patients.

PROGNOSIS. If listeriosis is acquired transplacentally, the fetus is almost always aborted. The death rate of infants infected at or near term is greater than 50%. The mortality of infants with listerial pneumonia noted within 12 hr of birth approaches 100%. Mortality varies from 20 to 50% if disease develops between 5 and 30 days of birth. Early treatment of septicemia and/or meningitis in immunologically competent older infants and children may be responsible for recovery in about 95% of instances. Mental retardation, paralysis, and hydrocephalus have been noted in survivors of *Listeria* meningitis.

RALPH D. FEIGIN

Gellin BG, Broome CV: Listeriosis. JAMA 261:1313, 1989.

Kessler SL, Dajani AS: *Listeria* meningitis in infants and children. Pediatr Infect Dis J 9:61, 1990.

Linnan MJ, Mascola L, Lou XD, et al: Epidemic listeriosis associated with Mexican-style cheese. N Engl J Med 319:823, 1988.

Schwartz B, Broome CV, Brown GR, et al: Association of sporadic listeriosis with consumption of uncooked hot dogs and undercooked chicken. Lancet 2:779, 1988.

Stamm AM, Dismukes WE, Simmars BP, et al: Listeriosis in renal transplant recipients. Report of an outbreak and review of 102 cases. Rev Infect Dis 4:665, 1982.

Teberg AJ, Yonekura ML, Salminen C, et al: Clinical manifestations of epidemic neonatal listeriosis. Pediatr Infect Dis J 6:817, 1987.

12.37 TETANUS

Tetanus (lockjaw), an acute toxemic illness, is caused by a soluble exotoxin of *Clostridium tetani.*

ETIOLOGY. *C. tetani*, an obligate anaerobe, is a gram-positive, nonencapsulated, slender, motile rod that forms terminal spores resembling drumsticks. The spores are resistant to many injurious agents, including boiling, but can be destroyed by autoclaving. They survive in soil for years if not exposed to sunlight, and may be found in house dust, salt and fresh water, and feces of many animal species. Spores and vegetative organisms may be found in the intestinal contents of humans. The vegetative forms of *C. tetani* are susceptible to heat, antibodies, and disinfectants.

Tetanus bacilli are not invasive. Two toxins are produced, tetanospasmin and tetanolysin. The tetanospasmins produced by several antigenically different bacilli are immunologically identical. They are neurotoxins and are responsible for the clinical manifestations of the disease. Except for botulinum toxin, tetanospasmin is the most potent poison known; as little as 130 μg may be lethal for an adult. Tetanolysin is capable of damaging viable tissue by enlarging the volume of tissue in which the *C. tetani* organisms can multiply. It also can cause hemolysis of red blood cells.

EPIDEMIOLOGY. Tetanus occurs worldwide; in developing countries it is associated with contamination of the umbilical stump, wounds in school-age males, chronic ear infections, ear-piercing, scarification rituals, female circumcision, and pregnancy (removal of placenta, unskilled abortions). In the United States most cases occur in patients over 60 yr of age, although there are peaks between 0 and 4 yr and between 30 and 39 yr. In the United States 50–100 cases occur each year; tetanus occurs after acute lacerations, abrasions, and puncture wounds due to nails, splinters, or glass. Injury usually occurs outdoors (40–50% on farms or during gardening); however, 33% occur inside the home. Rare cases are associated with drug abuse, chronic skin ulceration or abscesses, and gangrene. No cases of neonatal tetanus have been reported in the United States.

PATHOGENESIS. *C. tetani* is usually introduced into an area of injury as spores. Disease develops only after spores are converted to vegetative organisms, which produce tetanospasmin only under conditions of reduced ambient oxygen. Contamination of the umbilical cord is the common source of infection in the newborn infant. In older children contamination usually occurs by means of a traumatic injury. The risk is greatest from a deep puncture wound or an injury associated with tissue necrosis, conditions that favor toxin elaboration. Tetanus, however, has followed minor injuries, and occasionally no portal of entry is found. Under these circumstances it is presumed that spores previously introduced persisted in normal tissue for months or years and germinated when conditions were favorable. Alternatively, the site of infection may have been the gastrointestinal tract or the tonsillar crypts. Tetanus has followed use of contaminated sera, vaccines, or suture material.

Production of the 67,000-dalton protein, *tetanospasmin*, is controlled by a plasmid and is released by cell lysis at the site of infection. Tetanospasmin binds irreversibly to neural gangliosides and enters the nervous system at the α motor neuron's neuromuscular junction. The toxin travels retrograde toward the central nervous system, migrates transsynaptically, and exerts the most profound effect by inhibiting the spinal presynaptic inhibitory synapses. The net result is a release of inhibition manifest as spasms of agonist and antagonist muscle groups. Once the toxin has been translocated into a neuron it cannot be neutralized by antitoxin. The toxin has no effect on consciousness because the mental status is not impaired; however, autonomic dysfunction can occur, characterized by tachycardia, arrhythmias, labile hypertension, diaphoresis, cutaneous vasoconstriction, and elevated urine catecholamines. Large amounts of tetanospasm may be transported via the blood and lymphatic circulations, entering neurons at a site distal from the primary lesion. This occurs in generalized disease; muscles with short neuronal distances to the central nervous system are affected first, for example, the facial, masticatory, and cervical muscles.

PATHOLOGY. *C. tetani* remain localized at the site of injury and elicit minimal tissue reaction. Local changes that may occur are secondary events.

CLINICAL MANIFESTATIONS. The incubation period is usually 3–14 days after injury but may be as short as 1 day or as long as several months. There are three clinical forms: localized, generalized, and cephalic.

Localized tetanus produces pain and continuous rigidity and spasm of muscles in proximity to the injury; these symptoms may persist for weeks and disappear without sequelae. Occasionally, this pattern precedes development of the generalized disorder. Localized as well as a mild form of generalized tetanus occurs occasionally with chronic otitis media; *C. tetani* may be recovered from the middle ear fluid. The fatality rate of localized tetanus is about 1%.

Generalized tetanus is the most common form of the disease. The onset may be insidious, but trismus is the presenting symptom in over 50% of cases. Spasm of the masseter muscle may be associated with stiffness of the neck muscles and difficulty in swallowing. Restlessness, irritability, and headache are early manifestations. Spasm of the facial muscles produces a fixed sardonic grin **(risus sardonicus)**. Shortly, tonic contractions of the somatic musculature become widespread. The lumbar and abdominal muscles may become rigid, and persistent spasm of the back muscles may result in opisthotonos. Tetanic seizures develop, characterized by sudden bursts of tonic contractions of various muscle groups, producing flexion and adduction of the arms, clenching of the fists, and extension of the lower extremities. Initially the spasms last for seconds to several minutes and are separated by periods of relaxation; with time, they become powerful and exhausting. Spasms may be precipitated by visual, auditory, or tactile stimulus. The patient is completely conscious during the clinical course and experiences intense pain. Apprehension is prominent. Spasm of the laryngeal and respiratory muscles may produce respiratory obstruction, and cyanosis and asphyxia may ensue. Dysuria or urinary retention may be secondary to spasm of the bladder sphincter. Alternatively, there may be involuntary defecation and urination. Forcefulness of the contractions may produce compression fractures of the spine and hemorrhage into muscle.

Fever is generally mild, but it may be as high as 40° C because of the energy generated by the tetanic seizures. Hyperhidrosis, tachycardia, hypertension, and cardiac arrhythmias may be manifest. Myocarditis and arrhythmias may occur owing to excess catecholamines, as noted in patients with pheochromocytomas.

Signs and symptoms increase over 3–7 days, plateau during the 2nd wk, and abate gradually. Recovery is complete in 2–6 wk.

Cephalic tetanus, a variant of localized tetanus, is unusual. The incubation period is 1–2 days following otitis media or injuries to the head and face, including foreign bodies placed in the nose by the patient. Dysfunction of cranial nerves III, IV, VII, IX, X, and XI is the most prominent feature of the disease. Cranial nerve VII is affected most frequently. The cephalic pattern may be followed by generalized tetanus. Prognosis for survival is poor; however, full neurologic recovery can be expected in those who survive.

Tetanus neonatorum usually begins within 3–10 days after birth and is generalized in type. Progressive difficulty in sucking is associated with excessive crying. Difficulty in swallowing is soon apparent; the body becomes stiff, and spasms develop. Opisthotonos may be extreme or absent. Neonatal tetanus is the result of an unhygienic birth environment and lack of maternal immunization.

DIAGNOSIS AND DIFFERENTIAL DIAGNOSIS. The diagnosis of tetanus is made on clinical grounds. Most cases occur in individuals who are not immunized or in infants of unimmunized mothers. A history of trauma within the preceding 14 days is usual. This history, in conjunction with trismus, generalized muscular stiffness or rigidity, spasms, and a clear sensorium, is strongly suggestive of tetanus.

Routine laboratory studies are of little value. The white blood cell count is not remarkable. The cerebrospinal fluid is not abnormal, except that the pressure may be elevated by the muscular contractions. The electroencephalogram is normal, and electromyography is not distinctive. Wound cultures are positive for *C. tetani* in about one third of cases. Gram stains of material from the wound may or may not show *C. tetani*. Identification of the organism by Gram stain and anaerobic cultures is presumptive evidence of tetanus, but the absence of characteristic clinical manifestations does not mean that the patient has, or will develop, tetanus.

Tetanus must be differentiated from other local and systemic diseases. Trismus may be associated with tooth, parapharyngeal, and retropharyngeal abscesses. These conditions can be differentiated by careful history, physical examination, and appropriate roentgenographic studies.

Poliomyelitis may be accompanied by stiffness and spasm early in the course of the illness; however, trismus is absent, flaccid paralysis develops, and the cerebrospinal fluid is usually abnormal (Sec. 12.80). Other forms of acute or postinfectious encephalitides rarely are associated with trismus, generally have abnormal cerebrospinal fluid findings, and display a clouded sensorium. Bacterial meningitis is also unaccompanied by trismus; examination of cerebrospinal fluid can establish or strongly suggest this diagnosis.

Both *rabies* and tetanus may follow animal bites, and trismus has been noted with the former. Rabid spasms tend to be intermittent and clonic rather than tonic, and CSF pleocytosis may be noted. *C. tetani* is not a common inhabitant of the mouth of the dog. Tetanus toxoid may be given following dogbite to prevent tetanus.

A history of ingestion of poisons containing *strychnine* is most helpful in distinguishing this intoxication. Trismus is rare and, when it occurs, develops after the onset of generalized tonic activity. Usually, there is complete relaxation between convulsions.

Tetany may be characterized by carpopedal spasm and laryngospasm, but trismus is rare. The diagnosis is confirmed by a low serum calcium concentration. The differential diagnosis also includes dystonic drug reactions, epilepsy, and narcotic withdrawal.

COMPLICATIONS. Complications of tetanus can be minimized by paying strict attention to supportive care and by instituting appropriate therapy. Respiratory muscle spasm and laryngospasm can interfere with pulmonary ventilation, which may be compromised further by accumulation of secretions, aspiration pneumonia, atelectasis, mediastinal emphysema, or pneumothorax. Lacerations of the tongue or buccal mucosa, intramuscular hematomas, and vertebral fractures may result from severe tetanic seizures. If the course is prolonged, malnutrition and dehydration may develop unless strict attention is paid to fluid balance and caloric intake. Myocarditis, arrhythmias, hypertension, hypotension, and other signs of autonomic instability have assumed great importance as factors in morbidity and mortality with improved control of spasms by paralysis, sedation, and mechanical ventilation.

PREVENTION. Routine active immunization of children is discussed in Sec. 5.1. Immunization of previously nonimmune pregnant mothers will provide the newborn infant with protection immediately following delivery; preferably, tetanus immunization should be carried out prior to pregnancy. An ELISA to detect IgG antibodies to tetanus is available and may be a useful tool for screening of pregnant women.

Children who have not been immunized by 6 yr should receive a series of 3 doses of adult-type Td intramuscularly. The second dose should be given 4–6 wk after the first, and the third 6–12 mo after the second. Thereafter, a Td booster should be given every 10 yr.

Preventive measures following injury must be dictated by the immunization status of the patient and by the characteristics of the injury. Immediate and thorough surgical treatment of wounds is mandatory. The wound should be cleansed, necrotic tissue and foreign bodies removed, and, if necessary, more extensive debridement performed. If active immunization has not been provided or if its status is unknown and the wound is not minor or clean, *human tetanus immune globulin* (TIG) should be given intramuscularly in a dose of 250–500 units. If TIG is not available, *tetanus antitoxin* (TAT) of bovine or equine origin can be given in a dose of 3,000–5,000 units intramuscularly. Careful testing for sensitivity to TAT prior to its administration is mandatory; serum sickness may follow its use. Clean or minor wounds in previously immunized patients do not require TIG. All other wounds, including those contaminated with dirt, soil, feces, or saliva, puncture wounds, avulsions, crush wounds, frostbite, and wounds from missiles, require TIG in patients who are unimmunized or whose immune status is uncertain.

Tetanus toxoid should be given to initiate active immunity. It may be given at the same time as TIG or TAT if it is administered in another site and in a separate syringe. If the child has had at least four DTP immunizations, the wound is not minor or clean, and 5 or more yr have elapsed since the fourth injection, a tetanus toxoid booster is indicated. If the wound is minor or clean, 10 yr can elapse before tetanus toxoid is needed. If the wound has been neglected for more than 24 hr, TIG or TAT should also be provided. Fluid toxoid is preferred in this case, because it produces a more rapid secondary immune response than precipitated or adsorbed tetanus toxoids. If tetanus immunization is incomplete at the time of the wound, the remainder of the series of injections should be given.

TREATMENT AND SUPPORTIVE CARE. The principal objectives of therapy are to remove the source of tetanospasmin, to neutralize circulating toxin, and to provide supportive care until tetanospasmin, which is fixed to neural tissue, can be metabolized. Supportive care must be intensive and performed meticulously.

Tetanus immune globulin of human origin, in doses varying from 500 to 3,000 units, should be given intramuscularly as soon as possible. Local instillation of antitoxin at the site of the wound may be of value if surgical excision is not possible. Intrathecal TIG (250 units) may also be effective but requires further study before it can be recommended. Administration of human TIG has not been associated with allergy or anaphylaxis; higher and more persistent titers of antitoxin are produced than with antitoxin from nonhuman sources. Protective levels are obtained rapidly and decline slowly (half-life, 24 days). Repeated doses are not required. TIG has no effect on toxin fixed to neural tissue and does not penetrate the blood–cerebrospinal fluid barrier.

If TIG is not available and skin testing shows no hypersensitivity to TAT, it can be given in a single dose of 50,000–100,000 units: half the dose is given intramuscularly and half intravenously, with careful observation of the precautions detailed in the package insert. If sensitivity to TAT is demonstrated, desensitization should be carried out as described in the package insert.

Wounds should be cleansed and debrided if necessary. Foreign bodies must be removed and the wound left open. Surgical efforts should not be delayed; however, the patient should receive both antitoxin and sedation prior to the procedure. Excision of the umbilical stump is no longer recommended.

Antibiotic therapy may eradicate vegetative *C. tetani* organisms, which grow in areas of devitalized tissue where blood supply is poor or absent. For this reason large doses of penicillin G are favored in an effort to promote diffusion into the devitalized area. Penicillin G (100,000 units/kg/24 hr) may be used intravenously in 6 divided doses for 10 days. In patients who are sensitive to penicillin, tetracycline (30–40 mg/kg/24 hr, but not more than 2 g) in 4 divided oral doses for 10 days is effective. Metronidazole also has been suggested as an effective alternative to penicillin.

Meticulous nursing care is imperative. The patient should be placed in a quiet, dark, intensive care environment and every effort made to control or eliminate auditory and visual stimuli. A respirator, oxygen, suction, and equipment for tracheotomy should be available. Although endotracheal intubation or tracheotomy need not be considered routine procedures, they should be performed prior to the development of severe involvement of respiratory muscles or laryngospasm.

Muscle relaxants should be given to all patients. Diazepam is effective in controlling hypertonicity and spasms. It may be used in an initial dose of 0.1–0.2 mg/kg every 3–6 hr intravenously; the dose is titrated to control spasms as needed. Therapy for 2–6 wk may be required; the dose may be tapered as tetanic activity decreases. Chlorpromazine, mephenesin, baclofen, dantrolene, and other benzodiazepines have been utilized with variable results. Magnesium sulfate is highly effective in controlling hypertonicity and spasms and has the additional benefit of stabilizing cardiovascular parameters; however, its use requires careful, continuous intensive care monitoring.

Neuromuscular blocking agents such as pancuronium bromide and vecuronium (0.1 mg/kg/hr continuous infusion) can be used to produce complete respiratory paralysis, which is then managed by artificial ventilation. This technique has produced the best survival rates but can be utilized only in centers where continuous intensive care and highly trained respiratory care teams are available (see Sec. 6.33 and 6.34).

Patients receiving sedation and muscle relaxants must be monitored continually and suctioned frequently. Adequate ventilation must be ensured. Respiratory depression should be avoided and treated promptly if it occurs. Sedation and nursing care must be adequate to provide minimal fluctuations in cardiovascular parameters.

Careful monitoring of daily intake and output with an adequate intake of fluid, electrolytes, and calories should be maintained. The oral route may be used in some patients; generally, however, intravenous infusion and/or nasogastric intubation are required. Meticulous care of the mouth, skin, bladder, and bowel is important. Additional complications include rhabdomyolysis with myoglubinuria and renal failure, pulmonary embolization, decubitus ulceration, gastric ulceration and hemorrhage, paralytic ileus, and autonomic instability. β-Adrenergic blocking agents (propranolol), combined β- and α-adrenergic blocking agents (labetalol), morphine, and magnesium sulfate have been used to control tachyarrhythmias and other manifestations of autonomic instability.

PROGNOSIS. Case fatality rates of tetanus approximate 5–35%; rates for neonatal tetanus are 60% or greater without intensive care but less than 10% with such care.

Prognosis is affected by a number of factors. The highest mortality is found at the extremes of life; the lowest occurs in patients 10–19 yr of age (less than 5%). Patients who have localized disease or whose disease begins after a long incubation period as well as those who remain afebrile have a better chance of recovery. Poor prognosis is associated with a short interval (< 7 days) between injury and trismus and a short progression (< 3 days) from trismus to generalized tetanospasms. Fatalities in severe cases usually occur during the 1st wk of disease. Prognosis depends mainly on the quality of supportive care.

Cerebral palsy, paralysis, mental deficit, and behavioral disturbances have been noted in a few survivors of neonatal tetanus. Apnea and anoxia resulting from prolonged episodes of spasms are possible causes of brain damage. Tetanospasm does not produce permanent damage because new synapses replace previously injured nerve terminals.

Recovery from tetanus does not confer immunity; *active immunization of the patient following recovery is imperative.*

Bleck TP: Pharmacology of tetanus. Clin Neuropharmacol 9:103, 1986.
Centers for Disease Control: Tetanus—United States, 1987 and 1988. MMWR 39:37, 1990.
Farquhar I, Hutchinson A, Curran J: Dantrolene in severe tetanus. Intensive Care Med 14:249, 1988.
Jones MFM, Manson EOM: The use of magnesium sulfate infusions in the management of very severe tetanus. Intensive Care Med 11:5, 1985.
Lau RC: Detection of tetanus toxoid antibodies in human sera in New Zealand by ELISA. Epidemiol Infect 98:199, 1987.
Powles AB, Ganta R: Use of vecuronium in the management of tetanus. Anaesthesia 40:879, 1985.
Schofield F: Selective primary health care: Strategies for control of disease in the developing world. XXII. Tetanus: A preventable problem. Rev Infect Dis 8:144, 1986.
Wright DK, Lalloo UG, Nayiager S, et al: Autonomic nervous system dysfunction in severe tetanus: Current perspectives. Crit Care Med 17:371, 1989.

12.38 OTHER CLOSTRIDIAL INFECTIONS

The genus *Clostridium* encompasses all gram-positive, anaerobic, spore-forming bacilli, which are widely distributed in nature and are responsible for a variety of infectious syndromes including bacteremia and intra-abdominal, biliary, pulmonary, genital tract, central nervous system, and soft tissue infections, including gas gangrene.

ETIOLOGY. *Clostridium* includes more than 60 species, which vary in oxygen tolerance. *C. histolyticum* and *C. tertium* are relatively aerotolerant, whereas most others are obligate anaerobes. *C. perfringens* is the most common pathologic isolate, appearing as a large boxcar-shaped organism with blunt ends, and rarely forms spores. *C. ramosum* is the next most frequent isolate, appearing as pleomorphic bacilli in chains with bulges; it rarely forms spores. *C. sporogenes, C. bifermentans, C. sordelli, C. novy, C. histolyticum, C. paraputrificum, C. butyricum, C. fallax, C. septicum,* and *C. tertium* are less frequently isolated species.

PATHOGENESIS. *C. perfringens* (formerly *C. welchii*) inhabits soil throughout the world and the intestine of most vertebrate animals and man. *C. perfringens* is divided into five types (A–E) based on the production of four lethal toxins. Only type A is found in both soil, as a replicating toxin-producing vegetative cell, and the gastrointestinal tract. α-Toxin is present in all strains, is lethal, hemolytic, necrotizing, and a lecithinase. It is probably the most important clostridial toxin and acts as a phospholipase. Following hydrolysis of lecithin to phosphorylcholine and diglyceride, there may be hemolysis, platelet consumption, and capillary injury. β-Toxin is produced by strains B and C, is lethal, and produces transmural necrosis after inoculation into the small bowel. ϵ-Toxin is produced by strains B and D, is lethal, activated by trypsin, and necrotizing, and produces increased vascular permeability and peripheral vasoconstriction. ι Toxin is produced by strain E and is a lethal binary toxin that is dependent on two proteins for binding and ADP ribosylation. Other toxins include hemolytic toxin, collagenase, gelatinase, protease, hyaluronidase, DNAase, leukocidin, neuraminidase, and an enterotoxin produced by strain A that binds to a receptor, inducing calcium-dependent intestinal cytotoxicity.

Toxin production at the site of infection, leading to local tissue damage and subsequent systemic absorption, is responsible for the pathogenesis of many infections due to *C. perfringens*. Local gas production is typical of *C. perfringens* and may result in crepitant cellulitis and emphysematous cholecystitis, gastritis, or cystitis. *E. coli*, streptococci, and mixed aerobic and anaerobic infections may also produce gas in deep soft tissue infections.

Infections

GAS GANGRENE. Myonecrosis, or gas gangrene, is a rare, serious infection of soft tissue characterized by muscle necrosis and systemic toxicity, both secondary to the elaboration of toxins. *C. perfringens* is responsible for 80% of cases; *C. novy, C. septicum, C. histolyticum, C. fallax,* and *C. bifermentans* have also been implicated. Gas gangrene follows surgical wounds (biliary or colonic resection) or traumatic injuries (automobile, farm, crush, or industrial accidents) contaminated by a *Clostridium* species. Occasionally gas gangrene may be associated with vascular gangrene, decubitus or diabetic ulcers, or septic abortions. Local tissue factors that promote replication of vegetative forms and subsequent toxin production include tissue hypoxia, foreign bodies, vascular insufficiency, necrotic tissue, and coinfection with other bacteria. Toxins produce edema, thrombosis, and necrosis, while proliferating bacteria cause local gas production, subsequent septicemia, and shock. *C. septicum*, an aerotolerant *Clostridium*, produces spontaneous gas gangrene in the absence of obvious tissue damage, most often following bloodstream dissemination from the gastrointestinal tract. Primary gastrointestinal disease (ulceration, mucositis, colitis, intussusception) or immune defects (neutropenia, leukemia, lymphoma) are predisposing factors for *C. septicum* gas gangrene.

The major *clinical manifestation* of gas gangrene is a fulminant infection with local signs of tissue infection and significant systemic toxicity. The incubation period is 1–4 days. Sudden, persistent, severe pain at the wound site is the first symptom. Local signs include tense edema, tenderness, and the presence of gas, which may also be noticed on roentgenograms or scans. The skin may be pale, bronze, or magenta; subsequently, hemorrhagic bullae appear. A characteristic sweet odor is present in the brown serosanguineous discharge, which contains many gram-positive or gram-variable rods and few or no leukocytes. Muscles at the site of infection are pale, lose contractility, and do not bleed. Systemic manifestations include the early appearance of diaphoresis, low-grade fever, tachycardia, and anxiety and the late onset of hemolytic anemia, hypotension, hemoglobinuria, renal failure, coma, and death.

The *diagnosis* of gas gangrene is based on a prior history of surgery or trauma, the physical findings of local tense edema, gas, hemorrhagic bullae, and evidence of organisms by Gram stain and culture of the exudate or blood. The *differential diagnosis* includes cellulitis, streptococcal fasciitis, mixed aerobic-anaerobic necrotizing fasciitis, and synergistic gangrene due to *S. aureus* and anaerobic streptococci.

The *treatment* of gas gangrene includes extensive surgical debridement, which may require amputation or wide excision of muscle groups. Penicillin G (250,000 units/kg/24 hr given every 6 hr) is the treatment of choice; chloramphenicol, metronidazole, and imipenem may be used if there is concern about penicillin resistance or allergy. Supportive care includes the treatment of shock, respiratory and renal failure, hemolytic anemia, and secondary infection of exposed skin. Hyperbaric oxygen has not been demonstrated to be consistently effective and may delay surgery; antitoxin is no longer available.

The *prognosis* is poor in the presence of intravascular hemolysis, renal failure, abdominal muscle involvement, and spontaneous gas gangrene. Overall mortality approaches 25%. *Prevention* is based on early, careful, and adequate debridement of wounds. There is no effective active immunization.

BACTEREMIA. *C. perfringens, C. tertium, C. septicum,* and other species rarely produce bacteremia without an obvious focus of infection. Secondary bacteremia may follow septic abortion or local infections (decubitus ulcer, gastrointestinal tract) with or without toxin production.

C. septicum bacteremia is associated with malignancies (leukemia, colon cancer) and neutropenia (chemotherapy, cyclic neutropenia). Septicemia is characterized by fever, abdominal pain, diarrhea, emesis, and shock. The intestinal pathology shows edema, hemorrhage, necrosis, and invading organisms; metastatic sites include myonecrosis, osteomyelitis, meningitis, septic arthritis, or panophthalmitis. Intravenous pencillin G is the treatment of choice.

FOCAL INFECTIONS. Other sites of infection include intra-abdominal infections (subdiaphragmatic abscess) following penetrating trauma or surgery, biliary tract infection associated with emphysematous cholecystitis, tubo-ovarian and pelvic abscesses, uterine gas gangrene following septic abortion, empyema following oropharygngeal aspiration, cerebral abscess following penetrating trauma, sinusitis or otitis, and soft tissue infections. The latter categories include suppurative myositis, common wound infections, crepitant cellulitis, and gas gangrene.

Enteric Infections

***CLOSTRIDIUM PERFRINGENS* FOOD POISONING.** Enterotoxin-producing *C. perfringens* type A causes a mild and common form of food poisoning. The enterotoxin, a structural component of the spore coat, is a protein with a molecular weight of 35,000 daltons, is resistant to trypsin digestion, binds to a brush border membrane receptor, disrupts cell integrity, and causes cell death. Food poisoning follows ingestion of contaminated cooked meats, poultry, stew, meat pies, and gravies that have undergone long periods of slow cooling and ambient temperature storage, which facilitate spore survival. Such food usually contains at least 10^8 enterotoxin-producing *Clostridium* organisms, which during intestinal passage proliferate and produce toxin.

Clinical manifestations include diarrhea (90%), abdominal cramps (80%), nausea (25%), emesis (15%), and fever (25%) with spontaneous resolution in 6–24 hr. The incubation period is brief (7–15 hr), and the history may reveal a common exposure with others who are ill. The *diagnosis* is confirmed by detection of 10^5 or more *C. perfringens* in the food source, at least 10^6 organisms/g stool within 48 hr of onset, and detection of enterotoxin with ELISA or other immunoassay. The differential diagnosis includes food poisoning from preformed toxins *(S. aureus, B. cereus, C. botulinum)*, in vivo toxin generation *(B. cereus*, toxigenic *E. coli)*, invasive enteric pathogens *(C. jejuni, Salmonella, Shigella, E. coli, Yersinia)*, heavy metals (copper, tin, zinc), scombroid (histamine), and mushrooms. *Treatment* comprises supportive care and fluid and electrolyte replacement for gastrointestinal losses caused by this self-limited enterotoxemia.

ENTERITIS NECROTICANS—PIGBEL. *C. perfringens* type C β toxin produces a severe enterotoxemia in sheep, calves, piglets, and malnourished humans. It occurs during periods of acute dietary alterations involving pig feasts and ingestion of sweet potatoes in malnourished populations of the New Guinea highlands and other areas of Asia. *C. perfringens* type C is present in the stool of asymptomatic patients and animals and in soil. The toxin, a 30,000- to 48,000-dalton protein, is sensitive to proteolytic enzymes. During pig feasts patients may be exposed to a high clostridial spore inoculum owing to inadequate heating of meat. The bacteria bind to the small bowel and produce β toxin. Proteolysis is attenuated in this population owing to malnutrition, dietary intake of trypsin inhibitors in sweet potatoes, and colonization by trypsin inhibitor–secreting *Ascaris lumbricoides*.

The illness is *clinically manifest* as a segmental disease of the small bowel with intervening patches of full-thickness hemorrhagic necrosis. Abdominal pain, distention, emesis, and bloody stools, with or without pneumatosis cystoides intestinalis (intramural gas), follow an incubation period of 1–7 days (average 2 days). Pigbel may remain a mild diarrheal illness or progress to an acute fulminant enteritis with peritonitis and death within 24 hr. The *diagnosis* is evident given the epidemiologic data and may be confirmed by identification of the organism using fluorescent antibodies to the capsular antigen. *Treatment* includes penicillin G or chloramphenicol, supportive intravenous fluid resuscitation, intestinal decompression with a nasogastric tube, and surgery for intestinal perforation, persistent severe bleeding, obstruction, or prolonged toxicity. Excluding mild enteritis, other patients have a 15–45% mortality. *Prevention* is possible with a β-toxoid vaccine.

ANTIBIOTIC-ASSOCIATED COLITIS, PSEUDOMEMBRANOUS COLITIS. Diarrhea is a common complication of antibiotic use and is usually self-limited, requires no investigation, and stops when the antibiotics are discontinued. This benign antibiotic-associated diarrhea may be due to a transient alteration of the balance of colonic microbiologic flora and does not produce obvious pseudomembranous colitis. In contrast, antibiotic-associated pseudomembranous colitis is a very serious disease due to toxigenic *Clostridium difficile*, a spore-forming, gram-positive obligate anaerobic bacillus that is part of the normal flora of 3% of adults and a much higher percentage of asymptomatic neonates (50–70%) and infants (20–50%). *C. difficile* is not invasive and produces pseudomembranous colitis following toxin production in the colon. The precise pathogenesis is not well characterized, but disease requires the presence of toxigenic strains that produce toxins A and B. Diarrhea produced by *C. difficile* toxins may be due to inflammation, protein loss, increased peristalsis, hemorrhage, increased fluid and electrolyte secretion, or cytotoxicity.

Antibiotic therapy may predispose to the growth of *C. difficile* by suppressing other micro-organisms responsible for a normal process of bacterial interference that prevents the growth of this organism. Alternatively, antibiotics may stimulate *C. difficile* to produce toxin. Other factors that predispose to pseudomembranous colitis and alter bowel function include methotrexate and other chemotherapeutic agents, antiviral drugs, dietary changes, intestinal motility disorders (Hirschsprung disease), uremia, and anesthesia.

Asymptomatic colonized or actively infected patients may be the source of new acquisition of *C. difficile*. The organism is most likely transmitted by the hands of hospital personnel; spores have been recovered from hospital and home care facilities, bed pans, toilets, sinks, floors, and endoscopes. Spores are resistant to many disinfectants but are killed by alkaline glutaraldehyde, sodium hypochlorite, and chlorine dioxide.

The *clinical manifestations* of *C. difficile* antibiotic-associated colitis include symptoms with a wide range of severity, varying from mild, nonbloody, watery-green diarrhea with abdominal cramps to a severe hemorrhagic colitis with protein-losing enteropathy, hypoalbuminemia, shock, fever, leukocytosis, abdominal tenderness and distention, toxic megacolon, colonic (cecal) perforation, peritonitis, secondary sepsis, and death. Symptoms usually begin during antibiotic therapy (days 4–8) but may be delayed as long as 21 days (average of 5 days) after antibiotics have been discontinued. Common associated antibiotics in pediatric patients include ampicillin, penicillin, cephalosporins, amoxicillin, and clindamycin; the route of administration is usually oral but may be parenteral. The duration of prior antibiotic therapy is not important because antibiotic-associated colitis has developed after a short course of antibiotics for prophylaxis or treatment of a minor infection.

The *diagnosis* of *C. difficile* pseudomembranous colitis requires detection of the organism and toxin. Stool contains leukocytes and occasionally blood but also has 10^4–10^5 organisms/g. Culture is facilitated with a selective medium containing cycloserine, cefoxitin, and fructose in agar (CCFA). The isolation of *C. difficile* alone is not proof of the pathogenesis because some adults and many neonates harbor this organism, albeit in a much lower concentration, and some *C. difficile* organisms are nontoxigenic. An ELISA or latex agglutination assay may be used to detect toxin A, but more often toxin B is detected by demonstration of cytoxicity to cultured fibroblasts. Cytopathic effects may be noted initially within 4–8 hr and become definite by 18–24 hr but may be nonspecific unless confirmed by neutralization with *C. difficile* or *C. sordellii* antitoxin. Toxin B titers in stool filtrates are usually as high as 10^{-3}–10^{-5} dilutions but do not correlate with the severity of the illness.

Colonoscopy, which is not necessary for all typical patients, demonstrates the characteristic pseudomembranous nodules or plaques in the rectum, sigmoid, and distal colon. Occasionally, lesions are present only in the cecum or transverse colon, requiring full colonoscopic examination. Lesions appear as grayish-white exudates that are poorly adherent and are surrounded by an edematous and erythematous inflammatory response.

The *differential diagnosis* includes *Staphylococcus aureus* antibiotic-associated enterocolitis, other causes of infectious diarrhea *(Salmonella, Shigella, Helicobacter, Yersinia, Entamoeba histolytica)*, hemolytic uremic syndrome (*E. coli* 0157:H7), inflammatory bowel disease, malabsorption states, and neutropenic colitis or typhlitis in immunosuppressed patients.

Treatment includes discontinuation of the associated antibiotic and fluid resuscitation if dehydration is present. Patients with mild self-limited disease often demonstrate marked improvement within 48 hr of cessation of the associated antibiotic, with complete resolution within 7–10 days. Severely ill patients and those who do not improve 48–72 hr after discontinuing the associated antibiotic require specific antimicrobial therapy against *C. difficile*. Oral vancomycin (20–40 mg/kg/24 hr every 6 hr for 7–14 days) is the treatment of choice in pediatric patients. Improvement occurs within 48 hr, as noted by a reduction in fever, abdominal cramps, diarrhea, and malaise. Oral metronidazole is an equally effective and less expensive therapy but is not recommended for routine use in children. If oral antibiotic therapy is not possible owing to toxic megacolon or adynamic ileus, a combination of intravenous vancomycin and metronidazole is recommended because neither agent alone consistently achieves sufficiently high colonic-stool levels to eradicate *C. difficile* and because this presentation of disease is very life-threatening. Oral therapy with vancomycin should be initiated as soon as possible; vancomycin may also be given through an ileostomy or colostomy or by enema. Antidiarrheal agents (opiates), cholestyramine (may bind vancomycin), and corticosteroids are not of proven benefit. Surgery is indicated for toxic megacolon, cecal perforation, or, rarely, for performance of an ileostomy through which to administer vancomycin.

The *prognosis* for severe disease is poor, with a mortality of 20–30%. Most cases can be identified early as a benign self-limiting illness. Recurrences or relapses occur in 10–20% of patients despite appropriate treatment and respond to retreatment with vancomycin or metronidazole. *Prevention* of nosocomial spread is facilitated by body substance isolation, use of appropriate disinfectants, and vinyl gloves. There is no active immunization.

Berry PR, Rodhouse JC, Hughes S, et al: Evaluation of ELISA, RPLA, and Vero cell assays for detecting *Clostridium perfringens* enterotoxin in faecal specimens. J Clin Pathol 41:458, 1988.

Brooks I: Anaerobic infections in childhood. Rev Infect Dis 6:(Suppl 1) 5187, 1984.

Camorlinga-Ponce M, Gamboa M, Barragan JJ, et al: Epidemiological aspects of *Clostridium difficile* in a pediatric hospital and its role in diarrheal disease. Eur J Clin Microbiol 6:542, 1987.

Gerding DN: Disease associated with *Clostridium difficile* infection. Ann Intern Med 110:255, 1989.

Johnson S, Gerding DN, Olson MM, et al: Prospective, controlled study of vinyl glove use to interrupt *Clostridium difficile* nosocomial transmission. Am J Med 88:137, 1990.

Kornbluth AA, Danzig JB, Bernstein LH: *Clostridium septicum* infection and associated malignancy. Medicine 68:30, 1989.

McClane BA, Synder JT: Development and preliminary evaluation of a slide latex agglutination assay for detection of *Clostridium perfringens* type A enterotoxin. J Immunol Methods 100:131, 1987.

McFarland LV, Mulligan ME, Kwok RY, et al: Nosocomial acquisition of *Clostridium difficile* infection. N Engl J Med 320:204, 1989.

Speirs G, Warren RE, Rampling A: *Clostridium tertium* septicemia in patients with neutropenia. J Infect Dis 158:1336, 1988.

Stevens DL, Musher DM, Watson DA, et al: Spontaneous, nontraumatic gangrene due to *Clostridium septicum*. Rev Infect Dis 12:286, 1990.

Styrt B, Gorbach SL: Recent developments in the understanding of the pathogenesis and treatment of anaerobic infections, Pt 1. N Engl J Med 321:240, 1989.

Styrt B, Gorbach SL: Recent developments in the understanding of the pathogenesis and treatment of anaerobic infections, Pt 2. N Engl J Med 321:298, 1989.

Teasley DG, Olson MM, Gebhard RL, et al: Prospective randomised trial of metronidazole versus vancomycin for *Clostridium difficile*-associated diarrhoea and colitis. Lancet 2:1043, 1983.

Zwiener RJ, Belknap WM, Quan R: Severe pseudomembranous enterocolitis in a child: Case report and literature review. Pediatr Infect Dis J 8:876, 1989.

12.39 BOTULISM

Three forms of botulism have been described: (1) food-borne botulism (an intoxication resulting from improperly preserved food that contains preformed botulinum toxin; see Sec. 26.2); (2) wound botulism (the result of wound infection by toxin-producing *C. botulinum* organisms); and (3) infant botulism (caused by germination of spores of *C. botulinum* in the gastrointestinal tract with toxin production in vivo). Another unclassified category among patients over 1 yr of age has no identifiable source of toxin ingestion and most probably represents in vivo toxin production in the patient's gastointestinal tract (e.g., adult-onset infant botulism).

ETIOLOGY. *C. botulinum* is a motile, anaerobic, gram-positive bacterium that produces heat-resistant spores. If the spores survive food-processing, they may germinate and elaborate toxins. Eight antigenically distinct toxins have been identified (A, B, Cα, Cβ, D, E, F, and G). Types A, B, and E have been associated with human disease. Botulinum toxins are among the most potent toxins known to man. As little as 10^{-9} mg/kg is lethal. Other clostridia (e.g., *C. baratii* and *C. butyricum*) also produce a neurotoxin and an illness indistinguishable from botulism.

EPIDEMIOLOGY. *Infant botulism* usually occurs in children under 12 mo of age, has a peak onset from 2 to 6 mo, and is most frequently caused by types A and B strains. Sources for spores include soil, house dust, vacuum cleaner dust, honey, and corn syrup. Although the distribution of cases has been widespread in the United States, the majority of patients have been reported from California, Pennsylvania, Hawaii, and Utah, clusters correlating roughly with areas where spore concentration of *C. botulinum* in the soil is high. Breast-feeding and a prior history of constipation are additional risk factors.

Food-borne botulism is a worldwide problem that also continues to result in fatalities in the United States. Improperly home-preserved foods are the most frequent cause of intoxication in the United States. Commercially prepared food and restaurant food are also responsible for outbreaks that are geographically scattered. Type A is common in the Western United States, type B is common east of the Mississippi River, and type E is associated with fish consumption and is most common in the Pacific Northwest, Alaska, Japan, Scandinavia, and Russia. Seasonal variation is noted in the United States and Canada, with most cases occurring between May and October with peaks in July. An increased incidence of botulism is seen in patients with underlying gastrointestinal disease, prolonged antibiotic use, or a history of parenteral or intranasal cocaine abuse and in individuals who reside in a household where a family member has daily contact with soil. Food contaminated by *C. botulinum* may have a normal appearance and taste; however, a small nibble can produce severe disease.

Wound botulism may follow contamination by *C. botulinum* with subsequent in vivo toxin production.

PATHOGENESIS. *Infant botulism* is caused by ingestion of spores of *C. botulinum*, which colonize and germinate in the infant's intestinal tract and elaborate toxins that are subsequently absorbed. Although spores are ubiquitous in soil and consumed regularly with foodstuffs, this sequence does not occur in older children or adults. *Food-borne botulism* usually results from intestinal absorption of preformed toxins ingested with improperly prepared foods. The toxins in *wound botulism* are produced at the sites of injury.

Toxins are probably transported by the lymphatics or blood to the motor nerve terminals and have varying affinities for binding to nervous tissue; type A is greater in binding affinity than type E, which is greater than type B. Toxins have been demonstrated in serum 3 wk after ingestion of contaminated food.

The toxin is a protein weighing about 150,000 daltons and inhibits release of acetylcholine. Toxins do not cross the blood-brain barrier or affect the adrenergic fibers.

CLINICAL MANIFESTATIONS. The course of *infant botulism* may vary from mild constipation and poor feeding to severe neurologic deterioration and sudden death. Typically, a healthy-appearing afebrile infant becomes constipated, feeds poorly owing to poor sucking and swallowing, develops weakness in crying and smiling, becomes hypotonic, and loses head control. Symmetric, descending paralysis progresses over a period of hours to days to involve sequentially the muscles innervated by cranial nerves, the trunk, and the limbs. Ileus, bladder atony, ptosis, mydriasis, the syndrome of inappropriate secretion of antidiuretic hormone, and decreased tearing and salivation occur. Infants often require ventilatory support for respiratory failure. The course in some patients may resemble that of the sudden infant death syndrome (Sec. 25.1).

Food-borne botulism usually has an incubation period of 12–36 hr, but this can range from several hours to a week. Nausea, vomiting, diplopia, dysphagia, dysarthria, and dry mouth are common manifestations. Weakness (bulbar, then descending to the trunk and limbs), postural hypotension, absent or diminished deep tendon reflexes, urinary retention, and constipation may develop. The patient remains alert at the outset but may become somnolent with time.

Physical examination generally reveals an afebrile patient with normal pulse rate. Ptosis, nystagmus, and paresis of the extraocular muscles occur. Pupils may be dilated and react sluggishly to light. Mucous membranes of the mouth, tongue, and pharynx are dry, and lacrimation may cease. Most patients have three of the characteristic pentad of manifestations: nausea and vomiting, dysphagia, diplopia, dilated fixed pupils, and dry mouth and throat. Respiratory efforts may be impaired and progress rapidly to respiratory failure. Sensory examination is normal. The severity of illness and the length of the incubation period correlate with the amount of toxin ingested.

The course of *wound botulism* may be similar to that resulting from ingestion of toxins or may be milder and more prolonged and may vary depending on the nature of the contaminated wound. The incubation period is usually 4–14 days following the injury. Sensory changes may be evident.

DIAGNOSIS AND DIFFERENTIAL DIAGNOSIS. The diagnosis of infantile botulism is established by identification of *C. botulinum* organisms and/or toxin in the feces, since they are not part of the normal bowel flora of infants. The diagnosis of food-borne botulism is confirmed by demonstrating botulinal toxin in food the patient has ingested or in the patient's serum or stool. Wound botulism is diagnosed by demonstrating the organisms in the wound and/or the toxin in the blood. Inoculation of mice with serum from the affected patient identifies the toxin by neutralization with specific known antitoxins. ELISA of feces, gastric contents, serum, or suspect foods is available to identify toxins A, B, and E. Recent development of *C. botulinum* selective media has allowed more rapid definitive diagnosis.

Infant botulism's unique clinical presentation usually differentiates it from septicemia, myasthenia gravis, poliomyelitis, spinal cord injury, and metabolic disorders in infancy that may have some similar manifestations. The electromyogram may be similar to that observed with food-borne botulism.

Food-borne botulism must be differentiated from myasthenia gravis, poliomyelitis, Guillain-Barré syndrome, tick paralysis, other forms of chemical or paralytic food poisoning, trichinosis, diphtheria, and various forms of electrolyte or mineral imbalance. A characteristic electromyographic pattern known as brief, small, abundant motor-unit action potentials (BSAP) frequently has been found. Its absence, however, does not exclude the diagnosis.

Myasthenia gravis is differentiated by the fatigability of muscle noted in this disease and by response to edrophonium chloride (Tensilon) or neostigmine. Guillain-Barré syndrome is associated with myalgia, paresthesias, ascending paralysis, sensory deficits, and an elevated concentration of cerebrospinal fluid protein. The cranial form of Guillain-Barré syndrome, Miller Fisher syndrome, may present with ophthalmoplegia and areflexia, and may be difficult to distinguish from botulism. CSF studies are normal in botulism. Cranial nerve involvement is usually absent in other forms of food poisoning, and diarrhea is more prominent. Other infectious diseases, including poliomyelitis and encephalitis, are generally accompanied by fever, and cranial nerve involvement is less prominent than that noted in patients with botulism.

PREVENTION. Boiling food for 110 min will destroy the toxin. A pressure cooker (115.5° C or 240° F for 30 min) is required to kill spores of *C. botulinum*; pressure requirements vary with the food being processed.

TREATMENT. Infant Botulism. Treatment consists of continuous monitoring of vital signs and general intensive care, including appropriate respiratory and nutritional support. Recovery usually occurs over several weeks. Antitoxin is not routinely given because of its hazards and because intensive care alone is usually sufficient. Antibiotics do not shorten the clinical course or decrease intestinal colonization; aminoglycosides may exacerbate or accelerate paralysis, including respiratory failure.

Food-Borne Botulism. All individuals known to have ingested toxin should be hospitalized. Vomiting should be induced and gastric lavage initiated. Magnesium sulfate or other cathartics may be placed in the stomach at the conclusion of lavage in the absence of ileus. A high enema should be given to facilitate elimination of unabsorbed toxin.

Cardiac and respiratory function must be monitored carefully. Endotracheal intubation and mechanical ventilation should be performed before respiratory impairment becomes severe.

Antitoxin is efficacious. Three preparations of equine origin can be obtained in the United States on a 24-hr basis from the Centers for Disease Control, Atlanta, Georgia.* The polyvalent preparation is preferred until the toxin type has been identified. Skin sensitivity testing is mandatory prior to ad-

*Call 404-639-3753 (weekdays) and 404-639-2888 (other times).

ministration because hypersensitivity reactions to equine proteins can be life-threatening. Antitoxin will neutralize only toxin not yet bound to neural receptors. If antitoxin is given within 24 hr of exposure to toxin, a shorter course of illness and a lower fatality rate can be anticipated. If it is given more than 24 hr after exposure to toxin, the length of illness is not shortened but a lower fatality rate may still be observed.

Penicillin G is recommended to kill *C. botulinum*, which may continue to produce toxin. Aqueous penicillin G should be given parenterally in a dose of 50,000 units/kg/24 hr in 4–6 divided doses. After lavage has been concluded, penicillin G also may be given orally in a dose of 1,600,000 units/24 hr in 4 divided doses and continued for 10–14 days. Fever suggests a nosocomial infection and may require specific therapy.

Hypotension should be treated with appropriate intravenous fluids; fluid and electrolyte balance must be maintained. Guanidine hydrochloride may enhance release of acetylcholine and has been beneficial in some but not all patients. It remains an experimental therapy.

Wound Botulism. Adequate debridement and drainage of the wound must be performed. Supportive intensive care and administration of antitoxin and antibiotics are similar to the treatment given for food-borne botulism, except that efforts to remove toxin from the gastrointestinal tract are not indicated.

PROGNOSIS. Infant Botulism. Most infants recover without sequelae if adequate intensive care and supportive therapy are provided. However, it has been speculated that up to 10% of sudden unexpected deaths in infancy are caused by botulism. Recovery from the clinical manifestations of infant botulism is not necessarily preceded by decreased colonization of *C. botulinum* or by a decreased quantity of toxin in the gastrointestinal tract. Recovery may require weeks to months.

Food-Borne Botulism. Severity of illness is directly proportional to the quantity of toxin ingested. A short incubation period is associated with more severe disease. The earlier the specific treatment is given, the better the prognosis. Recovery can be complete with appropriate supportive care.

Bartlett JC: Infant botulism in adults. N Engl J Med 315:254, 1986.

Critchley EM, Hayes PJ, Isaacs PE: Outbreak of botulism in northwest England and Wales, June 1989. Lancet 2:849, 1989.

Long SS: Epidemiologic study of infant botulism in Pennsylvania: Report of the Infant Botulism Study Group. Pediatrics 75:928, 1985.

MacDonald KL, Cohen ML, Blake PA: The changing epidemiology of adult botulism in the United States. Am J Epidemiol 124:794, 1986.

Sonnabend WF, Sonnabend OA, Grundler P, et al: Intestinal toxicoinfection by *Clostridium botulinum* type F in an adult. Lancet 1:357, 1987.

Spika JS, Shaffer N, Hargrett-Bean N, et al: Risk factors for infant botulism in the United States. Am J Dis Child 143:828, 1989.

Suen JC, Hatheway CL, Steigerwalt AG, et al: Genetic confirmation of identities of neurotoxigenic *Clostridium baratii* and *Clostridium butyricum* implicated as agents of infant botulism. J Clin Microbiol 26:2191, 1988.

Wainwright RB, Heyward WL, Middaugh JP, et al: Food-borne botulism in Alaska, 1947–1985: Epidemiology and clinical findings. Infect Dis Clin North Am 157:1158, 1988.

12.40 ANAEROBIC INFECTIONS OTHER THAN CLOSTRIDIAL

Advances in techniques for recovering anaerobic bacteria and an awareness of the possible role they play in clinical disease have permitted an assessment of the prevalence and significance of anaerobic microorganisms as a cause of infection.

ETIOLOGY. Anaerobic bacteria are present in soil and constitute part of the normal human flora; they are found on all mucous membranes. The ratio of anaerobic to aerobic bacteria varies at different mucocutaneous sites: 1:1 in saliva, on tooth surfaces, in stomach, small bowel, and ileum; 3–5:1 in nasal washings and the vagina; and 1,000:1 in gingival crevices and the colon. Infection is initiated by the endogenous flora rather than by acquisition of pathologic species.

Anaerobic bacteria are microorganisms to which oxygen is toxic, but strains vary considerably in their ability to tolerate oxygen. Some strains survive in the presence of oxygen but grow better when the oxygen in their environment is reduced (facultative anaerobes). Obligate anaerobes do not grow on the surface of blood agar plates incubated aerobically or even in an environment enriched with CO_2. Obligate anaerobes predominate in the normal human flora. Oxygen is directly toxic to obligate anaerobes, whereas aerotolerant strains are partially protected by the presence of the enzyme superoxide dismutase, which reduces toxic supraoxide radicals.

EPIDEMIOLOGY. Blood, intra-abdominal sources, central nervous system, respiratory tract (upper and lower), and soft tissues are the principal sites from which anaerobes are recovered during infection in infancy and childhood (Table 12–27). Except in blood cultures, several anaerobes or both anaerobes and aerobes are recovered concomitantly from sites of infection.

Symptomatic anaerobic infection occurs infrequently in a general pediatric population. Anaerobes account for 15–20% of all bacteremic episodes (8–20% in the newborn period and 5% in children over 1 yr of age). Among the newborn infants whose disease is associated with bacteremia, 10.1% of the pathogens were anaerobes unassociated with aerobic bacteria.

The major clinical settings in which anaerobic infection of children might be anticipated are (1) birth following prolonged rupture of the membranes, amnionitis, or obstetric difficulty; (2) peritonitis or septicemia associated with intestinal obstruction and perforation or with appendicitis; (3) disorders that impair the response of the host to infection; (4) subcutaneous abscesses and infections of the female genital tract; (5) orofacial infections; (6) aspiration pneumonia; and (7) chronic infection in an isolated mucous membrane location (otitis, mastoiditis, sinusitis) that predisposes to contiguous brain infection. A combination of altered physical barriers to endogenous flora, compromised tissue viability, alterations in endogenous flora, neutropenia and mucositis, mixed synergic infection, and anaerobic bacterial virulence factors contributes to infection.

PATHOGENESIS. Normally, anaerobes are of low virulence for humans. Their multiplication and invasion are favored by any means that removes oxygen from their environment or that otherwise lowers their oxidation-reduction potential. In some cases, removal of aerobes facilitates anaerobic invasion. More frequently, however, aerobes facilitate establishment of anaerobic infection by destroying previously well-oxygenated tissue.

Virulence factors include abscess-promoting capsular polysaccharides *(B. fragilis)*, production of toxic short-chain fatty acids *(B. fragilis, B melaninogenicus)*, endotoxin *(Fusobacterium)*, and digestive enzymes (hyaluronidase, collagenase, fibrinolysin). Adjuvants for infection include local tissue injury, obstruction, impaired blood flow, and a foreign body. Polymicrobial infection with interactions between aerobic *(E. coli)* and anaerobic *(B. fragilis)* organisms have been proposed to explain the early peritonitis stage *(E. coli)* and the late intra-abdominal abscess stage *(B. fragilis)* following intestinal perforation. Synergy between aerobic and anaerobic bacteria explains some disease manifestations. Synergistic gangrene involves *S. aureus*-producing hyaluronidase, which permits microaerophilic streptococci to invade the tissue space; alternatively, short-chain fatty acid production (succinic) by anaerobes may inhibit neutrophilic phagocytosis of aerobic bacteria.

Anaerobic *pleuropulmonic disease* is usually initiated by aspiration (general anesthesia, esophageal dysfunction, tonsillectomy, tooth extraction); less often by preceding extrapulmonic anaerobic infection (otitis media, pharyngitis, peritonitis), penetrating chest wounds, or open heart surgery. Polymicrobial anaerobic brain abscesses may follow chronic otitis media, mastoiditis, sinusitis, lung abscess, infections of the face or scalp, head trauma, or intracranial surgery. A brain abscess associated with congenital heart disease and a right to left shunt frequently reveals only one pathogen, usually an aerobic, microaerophilic, or anaerobic streptococci. Other anaerobic infections are noted in Table 12–27.

PATHOLOGY. Abscess formation and widespread tissue destruction are associated with anaerobic infection. The specific pathology varies with the site.

CLINICAL MANIFESTATIONS. Infections produced by anaerobic microorganisms occur in any part of the body.

Anaerobic infections of the *upper respiratory tract* are common. Periodontal infection is favored by poor dental hygiene or by malocclusion. The gingival tissues are inflamed and edematous, and a foul-smelling discharge may be elicited by pressing along the gums. **Vincent angina** (trench mouth) is an acute, fulminant, necrotizing ulcerative gingivitis characterized by pain, tissue destruction, foul odor, and pseudomembrane formation. **Noma**, a related disease of the oral mucous membranes with spread to bone and facial tissues, occurs in malnourished or chronically ill children and is fatal without appropriate therapy. Periapical abscesses or anaerobic osteomyelitis of the mandible or maxilla may develop following gingivitis.

Anaerobic microorganisms also may be involved in chronic sinusitis, otitis media, mastoiditis, peritonsillar and retropharyngeal abscesses, parotitis, and cervical lymphadenitis. Since potentially pathogenic aerobic organisms are generally recovered concomitantly, it is difficult to establish the precise role of anaerobes in these diseases.

Ludwig angina is an acute life-threatening cellulitis of the sublingual and submandibular spaces that tends to spread rapidly without lymph node involvement or abscess formation. Respiratory obstruction may require tracheotomy.

Anaerobic infection of the *lower respiratory tract* generally takes the form of necrotizing pneumonia, putrid empyema, or lung abscess. A history of aspiration can usually be elicited. Ordinarily, pneumonia develops first, and abscess formation results from liquefaction of lung tissue.

Anaerobic infection of the *central nervous system* may occur as brain abscess, subdural empyema, or septic thrombophlebitis of cortical veins and venous sinuses. The intracranial lesion may originate by direct spread from a contiguous infection or by hematogenous spread from a remote one. See Sec. 20.72 for a discussion of the signs or symptoms of brain abscess. Purulent meningitis is rarely caused by anaerobes; recovery of anaerobes from the cerebrospinal fluid suggests brain abscess or subdural empyema.

Since the concentrations of anaerobes are normally highest in the lower gastrointestinal tract, it is not surprising that peritoneal spillage of gastrointestinal contents is associated with a high incidence of anaerobic intra-abdominal infection. Generally aerobes and anaerobes are recovered from peritoneal contents concomitantly.

Anaerobic bacteremia is clinically indistinguishable from aerobic bacteremia. Fever, leukocytosis, jaundice, hemolytic anemia, and shock may occur. Anaerobic bacteremia is frequently associated with disease of the gastrointestinal (e.g., typhilitis, neutropenic mucositis) and genitourinary (e.g., calculi) systems.

Other infectious anaerobic syndromes are noted in Table 12–27.

DIAGNOSIS. The diagnosis of anaerobic infection depends upon (1) awareness of infections with which anaerobes are associated, (2) appropriate selection and collection of specimens for culture, and (3) use of media and techniques that

TABLE 12–27. Infections Associated with Anaerobic Bacteria

Site	Infection	Anaerobic Bacteria*
Central nervous system	Cerebral abscess, subdural empyema, epidural abscess, secondary to adjacent sinusitis, otitis, mastoiditis	Polymicrobial, *B. fragilis*†, *Fusobacterium, Peptostreptococcus, Veillonella*
Upper airway	Dental abscess, Ludwig angina (cellulitis of sublingual-submandibular space), Lemiere syndrome (septic jugular thrombophlebitis), necrotizing gingivitis (Vincent stomatitis), chronic otitis-mastoiditis-sinusitis, peritonsillar abscess, facial space cellulitis	*Peptostreptococcus, Fusobacterium, B. melaninogenicus*
Pleuropulmonary area	Aspiration pneumonia	Polymicrobial
	Necrotizing pneumonitis	*B. melaninogenicus*
	Lung abscess, bronchopleural fistula, empyema	*B. intermedius*
	Periodontal disease, bronchial obstruction, altered gag or consciousness predispose to infection	*Fusobacterium, Peptostreptococcus, Eubacterium, B. fragilis, Veillonella*
Intra-abdominal region	Abscess, secondary peritonitis (appendicitis, penetrating trauma: colon>>>small intestine)	Polymicrobial, *B. fragilis*, other *Bacteroides, Clostridium* sp., *Peptostreptococcus, Eubacterium, Fusobacterium*
Female genital tract	Bartholin abscess, tubo-ovarian abscess, endometritis, pelvic cellulitis or thrombophlebitis, salpingitis, septic abortion	*B. fragilis, B. bivius, Peptostreptococcus, Clostridium* sp.
	Anaerobic (nonspecific bacterial) vaginosis	*Mobiluncus* sp.
	Intrauterine device	Actinomycosis
Soft tissue	Human, animal bites, decubitus ulcers, perirectal cellulitis, abdominal wounds, pilonidal sinus	Varies with site and contamination with mouth or enteric flora
	Synergistic necrotizing cellulitis, myonecrosis	*Clostridium*, other anaerobes
Bacteremia	Secondary to intra-abdominal or genitourinary source and synergistic cellulitis	*B. fragilis, Clostridium*, anaerobic streptococci
	Immunosuppressed or neutropenic patients	*Clostridium tertium, C. septicum*
Bones and joints	Trauma, decubitus ulcers, jaw (secondary to dental pathology)	*Actinomycosis, Clostridium, Bacteroides, Fusobacterium*

*Infections may also be due to or involve aerobic bacteria as the sole or part of a mixed infection: *brain abscess* may contain aerobic streptococci; *intra-abdominal* sepsis may contain coliforms, enterococci; *salpingitis* may contain *N. gonorrhoeae, C. trachomatis.*

†*Bacteroides fragilis* is usually isolated from infections below the diaphragm except for brain abscesses.

will facilitate their recovery. Clinical specimens that should be routinely cultured for anaerobes include blood; bile; pericardial, peritoneal, pleural, or cerebrospinal fluid; abscesses; deep aspirates of wounds; transtracheal aspirates; and surgical specimens obtained from normally sterile sites.

Clinical clues to the diagnosis of anaerobic infection are noted in Table 12–28.

The following sites or specimens should not be cultured anaerobically except in rare cases: nose, mouth, throat, sputum, tracheostomy sites, gastric washings, feces, ileostomy or colostomy material, urine, vaginal swabs, or fistulas. Anaerobic microorganisms are normally found in these specimens, and it is generally impossible to implicate them in a causative relationship with any disease process. Culture specimens related to sinusitis, abscesses, empyema, and peritoneal fluid should be obtained by direct aspiration without passage through a contaminated mucosal surface if possible.

Gram stain and culture are necessary to identify pathogens (see Table 12–28). Rapid diagnosis of *Bacteroides* infection has been made utilizing an indirect immunofluorescence assay with specific antisera against the capsular polysaccharide of *B. fragilis* and pooled antisera against a number of serotypes of *Bacteroides* sp. Rapid diagnosis has also been achieved using gas-liquid chromatography of purulent material. This method identifies the characteristic fermentation profile of the specific anaerobic species.

TREATMENT. The type of infecting anaerobe can usually be predicted from a knowledge of the site of infection, and most anaerobes have predictable sensitivities to antibiotic agents. Therefore, appropriate drugs can often be selected before results of culture and sensitivity tests are available. Duration of therapy, however, varies with the nature of the disease process. A multifaceted approach to therapy should include debridement, resection, aspiration, and drainage of infected abscesses, soft tissues, or closed spaces (peritoneum, pleura, sinus).

Antibiotic therapy is most efficacious in the early inflammatory stage prior to abscess formation or deep tissue necrosis. Bacteria may survive in abscesses despite antibiotics that penetrate the lesion owing to a high bacterial inoculum, lack of bacteriocidal activity, or other local conditions. Nevertheless, some small (≤ 2 cm) abscesses can be effectively treated with antibiotics with or without needle aspiration; these include tubo-ovarian, brain, and liver abscesses. Initially, antibiotics should be given empirically, since sensitivity testing is difficult in anaerobic infections, which are often polymicrobial. Previous recommendations were to give penicillin for infections above the diaphragm, since resistant *B. fragilis* organisms are unusual in these sites (except otogenic brain abscesses), and clindamycin, metronidazole, cefoxitin, or chloramphenicol for infections below the diaphragm. Currently, this approach is modified because 15–25% of lower respiratory tract infections are due to penicillin-resistant *Bacteroides*. Antimicrobial agents that are nearly always active against anaerobes include metronidazole (except proprionibacterium, *Actinomyces*), chloramphenicol, imipenem, and β-lactamase antibiotics combined with a β-lactamase inhibitor (ticarcillin and clavulanic acid, ampicillin and sulbactam); antibiotics that are usually active against anaerobes include clindamycin (10–20% of *B. fragilis* and non-*C. perfringens* clostridia are resistant), cefoxitin (10% of *B. fragilis* and some clostridia are resistant), and anti-*Pseudomonas* penicillins (overcomes β-lactamases if high doses are administered). Variably active agents include penicillin (inactive against all *B. fragilis* and some other *Bacteroides* or clostridia) and vancomycin (active against gram-positive anaerobes). Based on epidemiology and known resistance patterns, anaerobic orofacial infections may be treated with high-dose intravenous penicillin; anaerobic pleuropulmonary infections with clindamycin; peritonitis with clindamycin, cefoxitin, and metronidazole; brain abscesses with metronidazole or chloramphenicol; salpingitis with cefoxitin; and tubo-ovarian abscesses with clindamycin, metronidazole, or cefoxitin. Serious infections can also be treated with a ticarcillin-clavulanic acid or ampicillin-sulbactam combination or with imipenem.

Antibiotic choices must also include coverage against mixed infections with aerobic bacteria such as *S. aureus* for subcutaneous soft tissue infections or *E. coli* and *P. aeruginosa* in peritonitis. Aminoglycosides, quinalones, and some broad-spectrum cephalosporins, although effective against gram-negative aerobic bacteria, are ineffective against anaerobes.

PROGNOSIS. The outcome of infection depends on the site (CNS, soft tissue), the presence and number of abscesses, delay in instituting therapy, and the underlying condition of the patient (malnutrition, neutropenia). Early treatment prior to abscess formation, drainage, aspiration, and debridement may improve the outcome. The mortality of neonatal anerobic sepsis is 15–20%. In general, mortality is related to the underlying condition.

RALPH D. FEIGIN
KATHLEEN M. FINTA

TABLE 12–28. Clues to Presumptive Diagnosis of Anaerobic Infection*

Infection that is contiguous to or in proximity with a mucosal surface colonized with anaerobic bacteria (oropharynx, intestinal-genitourinary tract)
Foul-smelling, putrid odor (present in 50% of anaerobic infections)
Severe tissue necrosis, abscesses, gangrene, or fasciitis
Gas formation in tissues
Failure to recover organisms using conventional aerobic microbiologic methods
Failure of organisms to grow after pretreatment with effective anaerobic antibiotics (clindamycin, metronidazole)
Failure of organisms to respond to antibiotics with poor efficacy against anaerobic bacteria (aminoglycosides)
Toxin-mediated syndromes (botulism, tetanus, gas gangrene, *Clostridium perfringens* food poisoning, *C. difficile* pseudomembranous colitis)
Typical infections associated with anaerobic bacteria (see Table 12–27)
Sterile pus
Septic thrombophlebitis
Septicemic syndrome with jaundice or intravascular hemolysis
Mixed polymorphic organisms on Gram stain
Typical Gram stain appearance:
Bacteroides species—small, delicate, pleomorphic, pale, gram-negative bacilli
Fusobacterium nucleatum—fusiform shape, pointed ends
F. necrophorum—pleomorphism, round ends
Peptostreptococcus—gram-positive cocci similar to aerobic cocci
C. perfringens—gram-positive bacilli, box-car-shaped

*Suspicion of anaerobic infection is critical before samples are cultured to ensure optimal microbiologic techniques and prompt, appropriate therapy.

Barlett JG: Anaerobic bacterial infections of lung. Chest 91:901, 1987.
Boom WH, Tuazon CU: Successful treatment of multiple brain abscesses with antibiotics alone. Rev Infect Dis 7:189, 1985.
Citron DM: Specimen collection and transport, anaerobic culture techniques and identification of anaerobes. Rev Infect Dis 6:551, 1984.
Cooper GS, Havlir DS, Shlaes DM, et al: Polymicrobial bacteremia in the late 1980s: Predictors of outcome and review of the literature. Medicine 69:114, 1990.
Dunn DL, Simmons RL: The role of anaerobic bacteria in intra-abdominal infections. Rev Infect Dis 6:5139, 1984.
Finegold SM: Susceptibility testing of anaerobic bacteria. J Clin Microbiol 26:1253, 1988.
Nichols RL, Smith JW, Klein DB, et al: Risk of infection after penetrating abdominal trauma. N Engl J Med 311:1065, 1984.
Spiegel CN, Eschenbach DA, Amsel R, et al: Curved anaerobic bacteria in bacterial (nonspecific) vaginosis and their response to antimicrobial therapy. J Infect Dis 148:817, 1983.

12.41 CAMPYLOBACTER ENTERITIS

Eight species of *Campylobacter* are known to cause disease in humans: (1) *C. fetus*, (2) *C. jejuni*, (3) *C. hypointestinalis*, (4) *C. coli*, (5) *C. laridis*, (6) *C. cinaedi*, (7) *C. fennelliae*, and (8) *C. upsaliensis*. *Helicobacter pylori* (formerly *C. pylori*) is a new genus, distinguished from *Campylobacter* by RNA sequence differences (Sec. 12.42).

Intestinal disease is usually associated with *C. jejuni*, whereas extraintestinal and systemic infections are associated with *C. fetus*. Less frequently, enteritis is due to *C. coli*, *C. laridis*, or *C. fetus*; systemic infections may rarely be due to *C. jejuni* or *C. coli*.

ETIOLOGY. *Campylobacter* organisms are spirally curved, thin, motile, gram-negative rods. They are either short and S-shaped or long, multispiraled, filamentous organisms. In older cultures, coccal forms may be seen. They are motile with a single unsheathed flagellum at one or both poles. They appear as small (0.5–1 mm), slightly raised, smooth colonies on solid media. Visible growth in blood culture often is not apparent until 5–14 days after initial inoculation. *Campylobacter* organisms are microaerophilic, requiring reduced oxygen tension for growth with optimal growth at 5–6% oxygen. They neither oxidize nor ferment carbohydrates. There are over 90 different serotypes of *C. jejuni* based on somatic (O) antigen pleomorphisms.

EPIDEMIOLOGY. *Campylobacter* enteritis is a worldwide zoonosis. The gastrointestinal tract of many domestic and wild animals is the main reservoir of infection. *C. jejuni* has been isolated from the feces of 30–100% of chickens, turkeys, and water fowl. Most farm animals, meat sources, and pets can harbor the organism. Transmission of *C. jejuni* occurs most commonly from animal to person via the fecal-oral route by ingestion of contaminated food, especially undercooked poultry, unpasteurized milk, and untreated water. Venereal, perinatal, and person-to-person transmission occurs but much less commonly. Homosexual men are at increased risk for *C. cinaedi* and *C. fennelleae* infections. Household transmission from young dogs and cats with diarrhea also may occur. Outbreaks of *Campylobacter* diarrhea have been reported in nurseries and day-care centers, presumably due to inadequate handwashing after handling diapers. Communicability is greatest during the acute phase of the illness and can last up to 2–3 wk, but appropriate antibiotic treatment can shorten this period to 2–3 days. *Campylobacter* enteritis is more common than that due to *Salmonella*, occurs most often in the summer and fall, and is most common in patients under 1 yr and between 15 and 29 yr of age. Asymptomatic carriage is uncommon; however, perinatal transmission may occur from an asymptomatic mother. Asymptomatic infection is also common in older children living in endemic areas of the developing world.

PATHOGENESIS AND PATHOLOGY. The pathogenesis of systemic *Campylobacter* infections is unclear. Fewer than one third of patients have documented environmental or occupational exposure. Attempts to identify pathologically significant enterotoxins or other invasive factors of *C. jejuni* have not been successful. Nonetheless, extensive hemorrhagic ulcerations of the bowel wall and edema extending from the jejunum through the rectum occur, suggesting some invasive property.

C. fetus contains a surface (S) protein capsule that disrupts C36 binding, thus inhibiting opsonophagocytosis. This resistance to serum bacteriocidal activity may explain the greater tendency toward bacteremia associated with *C. fetus* infections.

Microscopically, *Campylobacter* enteritis often mimics mucosal changes found in inflammatory bowel disease. These include the presence of mucus, pus, and blood in the lumen of the bowel and a hemorrhagic, edematous, friable mucosa.

CLINICAL MANIFESTATIONS. The vast majority (95–99%) of cases of *Campylobacter* gastroenteritis are caused by *C. jejuni; C. coli* and *C. laridis* are responsible for the other 1–5% of cases. *C. fetus* is primarily responsible for septicemic infections in humans, especially in immunocompromised individuals and neonates.

The most common clinical manifestation of *Campylobacter* infections is *gastroenteritis*. The isolation rate of *C. jejuni* from stools of children with diarrhea exceeds the rate of isolation of *Salmonella*, *Shigella*, or *Yersinia enterocolitica* and is surpassed only by rotaviruses. The incubation period of *Campylobacter* enteritis is 2–7 days. Fever, malaise, myalgias, diarrhea, and bloody stools occur in about 90% of the patients. Fever may be the only initial manifestation. Blood characteristically appears in the stools 2–4 days after the onset of symptoms. The diarrhea is generally watery, profuse, and foul-smelling. Over 90% of older children also complain of abdominal pain. The abdominal pain is periumbilical; cramping may antedate other symptoms or persist even after the stools return to normal. Abdominal pain may mimic appendicitis or intussusception. Mild infection may last only 1–2 days and may resemble viral gastroenteritis. Most patients recover in less than 1 wk, but 20% have a relapse or prolonged or severe illness. Persistent infection can also mimic acute inflammatory bowel disease. The organism may persist in stools for up to 7 wk in untreated patients but cannot be recovered after 48 hr of erythromycin therapy. The complications of *C. jejuni* enteritis include bacteremia (1%), septic and immune-mediated arthritis, meningitis, endocarditis, mesenteric adenitis, febrile convulsions, colitis, toxic megacolon, pancreatitis, cystitis, methemoglobinemia, and Guillain-Barré syndrome.

The most common manifestation of *systemic* infection is bacteremia without evidence of localized infection. The majority of bloodstream isolates are of *C. fetus*. The illness generally begins with fever, headache, and malaise. The fever, relapsing or intermittent, is associated with night sweats, chills, and weight loss when the illness is prolonged. Lethargy and confusion are common, but specific neurologic signs are unusual in the absence of cerebrovascular disease or meningitis. Abdominal pain is relatively frequent; diarrhea, jaundice, and hepatomegaly are less frequent. Cough may occur, but pulmonary parenchymal involvement is unusual. Physical examination generally is unimpressive except for the ill appearance of the child. There may be a moderate leukocytosis. Transient asymptomatic bacteremia that clears without antibiotic therapy occurs, as does rapidly fatal septicemia. Prolonged bacteremia of 8–13 wk duration also occurs, with spontaneous remissions and relapses, especially in the immunocompromised host. Vascular infections, including thrombophlebitis, have been reported in association with *C. fetus* bacteremia. A nonspecific febrile illness with prominent findings of thrombophlebitis should suggest this possibility.

Campylobacter also may produce pericarditis, spontaneous peritonitis, salpingitis, septic arthritis, lung abscess, chest wall abscess, urinary tract infection, cellulitis, vertebral osteomyelitis, and endocarditis. Endocarditis occurs primarily in adult males with pre-existing heart disease.

Both *C. fetus* and *C. jejuni* have caused meningitis in adults and neonates. Infections with *C. fetus* are often fatal, whereas *C. jejuni* infections have a better prognosis. Most patients with meningitis beyond the neonatal period survive with antibiotic therapy.

Perinatal disease is suggested by the recovery of *Campylobacter* from the placenta and fetus of a woman who has had a febrile illness during pregnancy; *Campylobacter* is associated with previous abortion and/or previous premature delivery. Maternal infection may be asymptomatic or characterized by fever, pneumonia, or bacteremia. In addition to meningitis, symptomatic gastroenteritis and asymptomatic bloody diarrhea have been reported in newborn infants.

DIAGNOSIS. The diagnosis of *Campylobacter* is confirmed by stool culture. *C. jejuni* also may be detected by specially stained stool smears and phase-contrast microscopy. Agglutination, complement fixation, and bactericidal and immunofluoroscopy assays have been used for serologic diagnosis of *C. jejuni* infection, but these have been of limited value. Several investigators have reported development of enzyme-linked immunoassays to measure antibody levels (IgG, IgM, and IgA) to *C. jejuni*. This method may help to delineate individuals with acute, chronic, or no exposure to *C. jejuni* antigens.

TREATMENT. Although uncomplicated *Campylobacter* enteritis may require only supportive therapy, oral erythromycin (50 mg/kg/24 hr) diminishes the possible spread of disease within a household, day-care center, or nursery school. If started within 3–5 days, erythromycin shortens the duration of bacterial shedding and diminishes the duration of diarrhea. *Campylobacter* enteritis also may be treated with oral tetracycline (50 mg/kg/24 hr), furazolidone (5 mg/kg/24 hr), or oral neomycin (50 mg/kg/24 hr). Treatment of diarrheal disease should be provided for at least 1 wk.

Gentamicin is the antibiotic of choice for the treatment of *Campylobacter* septicemia and nonenteric *Campylobacter* disease when the antibiotic sensitivity pattern is not known. This is especially important because several investigators have reported a number of *C. fetus* isolates resistant to erythromycin. Chloramphenicol may be considered an alternative to gentamicin and is indicated for use in patients with meningitis. Treatment of systemic infections for 4 wk is recommended. Persistent *C. jejuni* infections have been reported in patients infected with the human immunodeficiency virus; therefore, antibiotic choices should be based on sensitivities, and length of treatment may need to be modified when the host is immunocompromised. Recurrent infection in hypogammaglobulinemic patients should be managed with the addition of intravenous immunoglobulins.

PROGNOSIS. *Campylobacter* septicemia in the immunocompromised host and in the newborn is associated with a high mortality. The rarity of cases precludes a precise estimate of mortality, particularly when early effective antimicrobial therapy is provided. The prognosis for gastroenteritis caused by *Campylobacter* is good.

RALPH D. FEIGIN

Blaser MJ, Sazie E, Williams LP: The influence of immunity on raw milk-associated *Campylobacter* infection. JAMA 257:43, 1987.

Blaser MJ, Wells JG, Feldman RA, et al: *Campylobacter* enteritis in the United States. Ann Intern Med 98:360, 1983.

Centers for Disease Control: *Campylobacter* outbreak associated with raw milk provided on a dairy tour—California. MMWR 35:311, 1986.

Lee MM, Welliver RC, La Scolea LJ: *Campylobacter* meningitis in childhood. Pediatr Infect Dis 4:544, 1985.

Salazar-Lindo E, Sack RB, Chea-Woo E, et al: Early treatment with erythromycin of *Campylobacter jejuni*–associated dysentery in children. J Pediatr 109:355, 1986.

Sellu DP: *Campylobacter* enterocolitis: General and surgical aspects. Postgrad Med J 62:719, 1986.

12.42 *HELICOBACTER PYLORI (CAMPYLOBACTER PYLORIDIS)*

Spiral organisms have been described in the stomach of animals and humans since 1893. It was not until 1983 that isolation of a *Campylobacter*-like organism was recovered from gastric biopsy specimens in patients with chronic active gastritis. The organism, originally called *C. pyloridis*, has now been reclassified to a new genus, *H. pylori*.

ETIOLOGY. *H. pylori* is a gram-negative, S-shaped spiral bacterium with a smooth outer coat and multiple sheathed unipolar flagella. It grows best on moist chocolate agar under microaerophilic conditions at 37° C, producing small (1 mm), smooth, transparent colonies within 3–4 days. It loses its characteristic spiral shape in culture and assumes more coccoid forms in old colonies.

This organism has many features similar to those of *Campylobacter* strains including morphology, media requirements, antibiotic sensitivities, inability to ferment glucose, and a similar DNA base analysis. However, it also has many distinguishing features such as multiple unipolar sheathed flagella (versus a single bipolar unsheathed flagellum), high urease content (a property important for diagnostic tests), atypical protein content, distinguishing RNA sequences, and a unique structural fatty acid pattern.

EPIDEMIOLOGY. The prevalence of *H. pylori* is unknown. It is distributed widely throughout the world. There may be some genetic differences in predisposition of the human host to the organism. Higher prevalence rates are reported in China, Japan, Peru, Ethiopia, and in Polynesians in New Zealand. Its prevalence increases with age, as does the prevalence of gastritis. Children consistently show *H. pylori* less often than adults, and it has been estimated that 50% of the population above the age of 60 have serum antibody titers to *H. pylori*. The exact mode of transmission and potential reservoirs are unknown, although intrafamilial clustering of infections occurs associated with a high incidence of antibodies in parents and siblings of index cases. The host factors leading to susceptibility and chronicity of infection also have not been delineated.

PATHOGENESIS AND PATHOLOGY. *H. pylori* is found predominantly in the gastric antrum, where it has a predilection for gastric mucus-secreting cells. It is not found in areas of intestinal metaplasia in the stomach or on intestinal epithelial cells. It is highly motile in mucus, allowing it to penetrate the mucus protective layer and move toward the intercellular junctions between gastric epithelial cells where the highest concentrations of potential nutrients such as urea and hemin are present. Urease acts as a virulence factor producing ammonium from urea, thereby increasing local gastric pH, acting as a buffer, and protecting the acid-labile organism. *H. pylori* attracts and activates neutrophils. Adherence pedestals permit *H. pylori* to attach to the epithelial cell, but evidence shows that it is not an "invasive" organism. Supporting microfilaments and mucus secretory droplets within cells are disrupted, and abundant phagolysosomes are seen. *H. pylori* elaborates a protease capable of degrading gastric mucin and may also have other unknown cytotoxic effects.

In some patients acute infection is not cleared by normal immune mechanisms, thus leading to chronic infestation. The gastric mucous barrier is destroyed and inflammation results, possibly predisposing the patient to ulcer formation because the damaged cells are more susceptible to acid and peptic digestion. The inflammation may progress to involve the body of the stomach. *H. pylori* may also damage duodenal epithelium. The primary phenomenon is that antral-type epithelium (gastric metaplasia) in the duodenal cap, when colonized by *H. pylori*, results in duodenitis and subsequent ulceration.

CLINICAL MANIFESTATIONS. No diagnostic signs or symptoms are associated with active *H. pylori* infection. In children in whom endoscopy has been performed, recurrent periumbilical or epigastric pain, retrosternal chest pain, nausea, vomiting, abdominal distention, and hematemesis are associated with active gastritis and *H. pylori* infection. The symptoms are nonspecific, and resolution of infection does not necessarily correlate with symptomatic relief.

Available evidence strongly suggests an etiologic role for *H. pylori* in acute gastritis that may progress to become chronic gastritis. Numerous studies have shown that *H. pylori* is strongly associated with chronic active gastritis, characterized by neutrophil and lymphocytic infiltrates. It is seen only rarely in patients with a normal antral mucosa. A pathologic role also is supported by demonstration of significant antibody titers to the organism in patients with chronic gastritis. The chronic gastritis with which *H. pylori* is associated is commonly called type B gastritis, distinguishing it from the autoimmune gastritis associated with pernicious anemia, type A gastritis, in which the antrum is typically normal. *H. pylori* is found in most children with primary antral gastritis (no known cause) but is absent in children with a known cause of gastritis (secondary gastritis), further supporting a pathogenic role for *H. pylori* in primary or nonspecific gastritis.

Chronic antral gastritis has been shown to be present in 90–100% of adult and pediatric patients with duodenal ulcer. *H. pylori* has been isolated from the gastric antrum in up to 100% of patients with a duodenal ulcer, and the presence of an ulcer is correlated closely with the gastric lesion. There is indirect evidence favoring a pathogenic role of *H. pylori* with duodenal ulcers, but, despite the strong association, a causal role for *H. pylori* in the pathogenesis of the duodenal ulcer crater has not been proved conclusively. *H. pylori* is an important factor in recurrence and successful treatment of ulcers. When the organism is eradicated, the relapse rate is approximately 20%. If the organism is not eradicated, approximately 80% relapse.

The role of *H. pylori* in gastric ulcers is less clear. *H. pylori* has been isolated from approximately 70% of patients with gastric ulcers, but a clear etiologic role has not been defined.

DIAGNOSIS. *H. pylori* can be detected readily by many different techniques; most require flexible endoscopy for tissue biopsy. Culture of gastric or duodenal biopsy specimens will yield growth in approximately 90% of cases, but it is a fastidious, slow-growing organism. Culture of gastric brushings is less sensitive, presumably because the organism is located under the gastric mucous layer. The organism can be detected in biopsy specimens with the Gram stain, Warthin-Starry silver stain, Giemsa stain, hematoxylin-eosin stain, acridine orange stain, and phase-contrast microscopy.

A number of rapid diagnostic tests are based on the organism's ability to produce urease. One such test (CLOtest) utilizes a gel pellet containing urea, phenol red indicator, and a bacteriostatic agent into which a gastric biopsy sample is placed. If the sample contains urease, urea is split, causing a change in indicator color. A noninvasive test also has been developed using the ingestion of ^{13}C- or ^{14}C-labeled urea with release of labeled CO_2 in the breath due to bacterial urease action in the stomach.

ELISA also has been used successfully to detect antibody titers in patients. However, serum antibody titers can be detected in a large number of patients without other evidence of infection. Circulating IgA, IgG, and local IgA, but not IgM, are higher in patients with *H. pylori* infection.

TREATMENT. *H. pylori* is sensitive to a wide range of antibiotics that are ineffective in vivo: penicillin G, erythromycin, tetracycline, and gentamicin. It is sensitive to bismuth subcitrate, amoxicillin, tinidazole, and metronidazole and relatively insensitive to cimetidine, sucralfate, and antacid. Bismuth may act locally by forming a protective layer and increasing gastric mucus secretion as well as by exerting a bacteriocidal effect. Combination treatment with bismuth subcitrate for 28 days, amoxicillin for 28 days, metronidazole for days 18–28, along with continuous ranitidine, has the highest success rate in eradicating *H. pylori* and reducing the incidence of relapse. The precise timing, duration, and indications for such therapy are not agreed upon, but treatment should be considered for persistently symptomatic patients who have not responded to H_2-blocking agents.

PROGNOSIS. Combination treatment of type B gastritis with triple therapy may eradicate the organism when the histologic lesion is cleared. Long-term eradication following single-drug therapy is characterized by frequent relapses, usually caused by the same strain; relapse occurs in approximately 50% of patients with *H. pylori* infection after completion of 1 mo of treatment. Treatment of duodenal ulcers with antibiotics and/or bismuth also has been shown to eradicate the organism with resolution of the ulcer and the associated gastritis.

RALPH D. FEIGIN
AMEETA B. MARTIN

Anonymous: *Campylobacter pylori* becomes *Helicobacter pylori*. Lancet 2:1019, 1989.

Blaser MJ: *Helicobacter pylori* and the pathogenesis of gastroduodenal inflammation. J Infect Dis 161:626, 1990.

Drumm B, Perez-Perez GI, Blaser MJ, et al: Intrafamilial clustering of *Helicobacter pylori* infection. N Engl J Med 322:359, 1990.

Kilbridge PM, Dahms BB, Czinn SJ: *Campylobacter pylori*-associated gastritis and peptic ulcer disease in children. Am J Dis Child 142:1149, 1988.

Oderda G, Holton J, Altare F, et al: Amoxicillin plus tinidazole for *Campylobacter pylori* gastritis in children: Assessment by serum IgG antibody, pepsinogen I, and gastrin levels. Lancet 1:690, 1989.

Rauws EA, Tytgat GN: Cure of duodenal ulcer associated with eradication of *Helicobacter pylori*. Lancet 1:1233, 1990.

Sullivan PB, Thomas JE, Wight DG, et al: *Helicobacter pylori* in Gambian children with chronic diarrhoea and malnutrition. Arch Dis Child 65:189, 1990.

12.43 LEGIONELLOSIS
(Legionnaires' Disease and Pontiac Fever)

The term legionellosis encompasses the two recognized clinical forms of infection with *L. pneumophila*. One, first recognized in the Philadelphia outbreak, is known as **legionnaires' disease**. It is characterized by its relatively long incubation period and the severity of its virus-like pneumonic clinical pattern. The other form, known as **Pontiac fever** because of an outbreak in a Health Department in Pontiac, Michigan, has a shorter incubation period and an acute, self-limiting clinical course resembling influenza without pneumonia. No deaths from this form are known.

ETIOLOGY. Legionellaceae are small, aerobic, nonspore-forming, unencapsulated, organisms that are catalase positive and nonfermentative. The organism is gram negative but stains poorly if at all with Gram stain. It is better visualized with the Gimenez or silver (Dieterle or Warthin Starry) stains. There are 30 species of Legionellaceae; 14 are pathogenic for humans, and all are acquired from the environment. Predominant species recognized as causes of bronchopneumonia include *L. pneumophila* (14 serotypes), *L. micdadei* (see Sec.

12.44), *L. bozemanii*, *L. dumoffi*, and *L. longbeachae*. *L. pneumophila* is responsible for 90% of cases. They may be differentiated by direct fluorescence antibody staining, by biochemical reactions, and by fluorescence under ultraviolet light.

The organisms are fastidious and require L-cysteine, ferric ion, and α-ketoacids for growth. They grow poorly in standard media, requiring charcoal yeast extract buffered (pH 6.9) media with selected inhibitors of other micro-organisms to identify colonies, which take 3–5 days to appear.

EPIDEMIOLOGY. The incidence of pneumonia in adults due to *L. pneumophila* is estimated at 7–20 cases/100,000/yr in the United States. The risk of nosocomial infection is increased 2- to 3-fold in patients with cancer, organ transplantation, corticosteroid therapy, or other disorders of immunosuppression. Among patients with sporadic, community-acquired infection, diabetes mellitus, alcoholism, and chronic respiratory illness are additional predisposing factors. Legionnaires' disease may be sporadic or epidemic, whereas nosocomial disease may be endemic or hyperendemic.

The organism is found in bodies of water (rivers, lakes, streams, thermally polluted waters), cooling towers, evaporative condensors, air conditioning units, whirlpool spas, and ultrasonic humidifiers. Aerosolization occurs from showerheads or sinks and is the predominant source of infection. Direct instillation of contaminated water or aspiration of pharyngeal secretions may also produce infection. The presence of *L. pneumophila* in respiratory secretions implies that person-to-person spread may occur in some circumstances.

Numerous common-source outbreaks of legionnaires' disease have been recognized; 0.5–5.0% of those exposed have been affected. This incidence contrasts sharply with outbreaks of Pontiac fever, in which the attack rate has been 95–100%. Many of the outbreaks of legionnaires' disease have been associated with large service buildings, including hotels and hospitals.

Data on legionnaires' disease in children indicate that it is a rare cause of community-acquired pneumonia in normal hosts. In prospective studies of pneumonia in children the frequency of *Legionella* infection as determined by serologic study has ranged from 1 to 10%. Pneumonia due to *L. pneumophila* occurs more frequently in children over 4 yr of age than in younger ones. In a retrospective survey of sera from 126 children less than 10 yr of age, seroreactivity was detected as early as 1 yr of age. Approximately 25% had titers above a level considered to be presumptive evidence of previous infection. It was speculated that infection with *L. pneumophila* might also be a cause of mild respiratory disease in infants and children. *L. pneumophila* in children occurs predominantly in patients receiving corticosteroids or following organ transplantation, and in children with other immunosuppressed conditions or chronic respiratory diseases.

CLINICAL MANIFESTATIONS. Legionnaires' disease is a multi-systemic illness characterized by pneumonia, high fever, chills, cough, chest pain, myalgia, headache, confusion, and diarrhea; there is laboratory evidence of hepatic involvement and renal disease. Seizures, acute cerebellar ataxia, meningitis, and erythema nodosum have also been described. The white blood cell count is usually normal or slightly elevated with an increased proportion of segmented polymorphonuclear leukocytes. The erythrocyte sedimentation rate is elevated.

The pneumonia progresses over the 1st wk of illness with daily temperatures of 39–40° C; with treatment, subsequent resolution is gradual. Chest roentgenograms obtained early reveal patchy infiltrates that become nodular areas of consolidation and that coalesce in severe cases. Pleural effusion is usually small except in patients with impaired immunity, and in such patients pneumonic cavitation may occur. In the absence of specific therapy, mortality is about 15–20%; death usually results from progressive pneumonia. Weakness and shortness of breath may persist for months in some patients, and roentgenographic clearing of the pneumonia is slow. Extrapulmonary involvement includes shock, sinusitis, perirectal abscess, pericarditis, endocarditis (native or prosthetic valve), pyelonephritis, pancreatitis, rhabdomyolysis, and postoperative wound infections.

Pontiac fever is characterized by high fever, myalgia, headache, and extreme debilitation that may persist for 2–7 days. Cough, diarrhea, confusion, and chest pain occur but are not prominent features. All patients known to have had this form of the disease have recovered completely.

DIAGNOSIS AND DIFFERENTIAL DIAGNOSIS. *Legionella* pneumonia must be distinguished from common bacterial pneumonias and from infections caused by *Mycoplasma pneumoniae*, *Coxiella burnetii*, *Chlamydia psittaci*, TWAR agent, influenza, and other respiratory viruses. The diagnosis is established by isolating *L. pneumophila* in cultures from blood, pleural fluid, respiratory secretions, or lung tissue; by demonstrating it in respiratory secretions, lung tissue, pleural fluid, or urine by direct fluorescent antibody or enzyme-linked immunosorbent assay; or by demonstrating at least a 4-fold rise in antibody titer in paired serum specimens assayed by indirect immunofluorescence or other methods at a titer of more than 1:128. Serologic conversion commonly occurs by the 21st day but may not occur until the 6th wk. Cross reactions may occur with other gram-negative bacteria such as *Pseudomonas aeruginosa*. *Legionnella* should be suspected in the presence of pneumonia with headache, confusion, diarrhea, negative Gram stain of purulent sputum, hyponatremia, hypophosphatemia, relative bradycardia, and progression of pulmonary infiltrates while on therapy with a penicillin, cephalosporin, or aminoglycoside.

TREATMENT. The infection responds to erythromycin and to tetracycline. In epidemics mortality is reduced by therapy with erythromycin. It is administered in a dose of 40 mg/kg/24 hr in 4 divided doses intravenously for 14 days (for patients other than neonates). Oral treatment with the same dose may also be used. Relapse has been reported in several patients when treatment was stopped after 14 days; if relapse is noted, therapy should be resumed.

It is recommended that rifampin, 15 mg/kg/24 hr, be reserved for combined therapy with erythromycin when the patient is not responding to intravenous erythromycin therapy alone. Other potentially effective antibiotics include trimethoprim-sulfamethoxazole, imipenem, and ciprofloxacin. Specific therapy is apparently not required for Pontiac fever. Supportive therapy including supplemental oxygen and at times assisted ventilation may be required. Renal failure requires management of fluid and electrolyte balance and occasionally dialysis on a temporary basis. Vasoactive drugs may be of assistance in managing shock.

PREVENTION AND CONTROL. Hyperchlorisation and thermal eradication (heat flushing), in addition to culture surveillance of hospital water sources, have been used to prevent epidemics or sporadic cases of legionnaires' disease. When an epidemic is traced to a cooling tower or an evaporative condenser, the implicated source should be removed. Respiratory isolation of patients with legionnaires' disease is recommended, although person-to-person spread has not been proved.

Carlson NC, Kuskie MR, Bobyns EL, et al: Legionellosis in children: An expanding spectrum. Pediatr Infect Dis J 9:133, 1990.

Finegold S: Legionnaires' disease—still with us. N Engl J Med 318:571, 1988.

Granados A, Podzamezer D, Gudiol F, et al: Pneumonia due to *Legionella pneumophila* and pneumococcal pneumonia: Similarities and differences on presentation. Eur Respir J 2:130, 1989.

Muldoon RL, Jaecker DL, Kiefer HK: Legionnaires' disease in children. Pediatrics 67:329, 1981.

Orenstein WA, Overturf GD, Leedom JM, et al: The frequency of *Legionella* infection prospectively determined in children hospitalized with pneumonia. J Pediatr 99:903, 1981.

12.44 PITTSBURGH PNEUMONIA AGENT

The number of reported cases of pneumonia due to the Pittsburgh pneumonia agent (PPA) is increasing. Although the disease has been reported primarily in adults, it should be suspected as a cause of pneumonia in immunosuppressed children.

ETIOLOGY. In 1979 Pasculle et al reported the isolation of unique gram-negative, weakly acid-fast bacilli from the lung tissue of two renal transplant recipients who had pneumonia. This agent was designated tentatively as Pittsburgh pneumonia agent and was given the name *Legionella micdadei*. Research has shown this agent to be distinct from *L. pneumophila*. DNA hybridization studies reveal less than 20% relatedness between the two species. *L. micdadei* produces little or no β-lactamase and has differing dye uptake and pigment production compared to *L. pneumophila*. These differences have led some to suggest that *L. micdadei* be classified as a different genus and given the name, *Tatlockia micdadei*. PPA may be a contaminant of hot and cold water supplies; nosocomial infections have been traced to water storage tanks.

CLINICAL MANIFESTATIONS. Pneumonia due to *L. (Tatlockia) micdadei* has been documented in immunosuppressed patients; simultaneous infection with *L. pneumophila* and *L. micdadei* also has been reported. The patients primarily have been adults in whom pneumonia developed during hospitalization or within several days of discharge. One child has been reported with legionellosis due to *L. micdadei* complicating a relapse of acute lymphoblastic leukemia.

Initial clinical manifestations are mild. If fever is not present at onset of illness, it usually develops. There may be pleuritic pain, cough, and production of sputum. Disease has progressed in all patients despite treatment with broad-spectrum antibiotics and in several instances with antituberculous therapy as well. The hospital course of surviving patients was one of gradual, slow clinical improvement and even slower resolution of roentgenographic findings, which included patchy pneumonic infiltrates and nodular or wedge-shaped densities suggesting pulmonary embolism as well as pleural effusions.

DIAGNOSIS. This depends on an awareness of this new agent and a high index of suspicion of the possibility of this disease in patients who are immunosuppressed. Lung biopsies that reveal gram-indifferent or gram-negative bacilli that are also weakly acid-fast can be cultured in embryonated eggs or guinea pigs. *L. micdadei* can be identified by direct fluorescent antibody examination of lung tissue. Serum antibody to the PPA can be detected by an indirect fluorescent antibody (IFA) technique.

TREATMENT. Erythromycin has been suggested as the drug of choice; rifampin and trimethoprim-sulfamethoxazole appear to be efficacious in vitro. Most investigators suggest erythromycin as the drug of choice.

PROGNOSIS. The prognosis is poor, a fact that may be related to the nature of the underlying disease and the abnormal state of the host rather than to the virulence of the organism.

RALPH D. FEIGIN

Brenner DJ: Classification of *Legionella*. Semin Resp Infect 4:190, 1987.
Fang GD, Yu VL, Vickers RM: Disease due to the Legionellaceae (other than *Legionella pneumophila*): Historical, microbiological, clinical, and epidemiological review. Medicine 68:16, 1989.
Kovatch AL, Jardine DS, Dowling JN, et al: Legionellosis in children with leukemia in relapse. Pediatrics 73:811, 1984.

12.45 ACTINOMYCOSIS

Actinomycosis, a chronic granulomatous disease of man and animals characterized by abscess formation, multiple draining sinuses, and subcutaneous spread of infection, is caused by an anaerobic actinomycete of the genus *Actinomyces*.

ETIOLOGY. *Actinomyces* are slow-growing, gram-positive, filamentous bacilli that are infrequently isolated in the laboratory because of their strict anaerobic requirements. Human disease is principally due to *A. israelii*; other species, including *A. naeslundii*, *A. viscosus*, *A. odontolyticus*, and *Arachnia propionica*, have been incriminated.

EPIDEMIOLOGY. Actinomycosis is distributed worldwide but is decreasing in incidence in the United States. It is uncommon in children and more common in males than females by a ratio of 4:1. *Actinomyces* are not found free in nature but are normal inhabitants of the nasopharynx and gastrointestinal tract. Infection occurs when these bacteria enter damaged tissue following infection, trauma, or surgical instrumentation, usually producing concurrent infection with other anaerobic bacteria.

PATHOLOGY. Actinomycosis is characterized by areas of suppuration surrounded by extensive fibrosis. Sinus tract formation is common and may extend to the skin surface or into internal organs. "Sulfur granules" are scattered throughout the suppurative areas and appear in tissue secretions as rounded basophilic masses representing clumps of microorganisms cemented together and surrounded by reactive cells.

CLINICAL MANIFESTATIONS. *Cervicofacial actinomycosis*, the most common form of infection in children, is caused by microorganisms that gain access to the subcutaneous tissue of the neck from an infected tooth or after surgery or other trauma to the teeth and oral mucous membranes. An enlarging area of painless swelling is noted along the margin of the mandible from which site the fluctuance gradually extends into the neck. The overlying skin becomes tense and develops a red or purple hue, and the mass is characteristically "woody" or indurated. With time, draining cutaneous fistulas appear, and the mass may temporarily decrease in size. Involvement of lymph nodes, the thyroid gland, and underlying bone is uncommon. Pain is minimal, and the child has no evidence of systemic disease. Roentgenographic examination is typically normal; however, with longstanding disease periosteal reaction and bone destruction become apparent. "Punch" actinomycosis occurs in the hand following trauma inflicted by human teeth.

Thoracic actinomycosis is uncommon in children; it occurs following aspiration of infected oral secretions or, less commonly, after extension of esophageal disease into the mediastinum. The clinical pattern is one of chronic pulmonary infection with fever, night sweats, weight loss, chest pain, productive cough, and hemoptysis. Extension of the pulmonary disease, which most often involves the lower lobes, may lead to pleural involvement; however, massive empyema and the classic findings of a draining chest-wall sinus discharging granules are rarely seen. Involvement of the heart and other mediastinal structures is uncommon. Roentgenographic examination is not characteristic but may demonstrate an extensive pulmonary lesion (at times with cavitation) involving the chest wall that may be associated with destruction of ribs, sternum, and shoulder girdle.

Abdominal actinomycosis may follow surgical treatment of an acute appendicitis or a perforated abdominal viscus and present as abdominal pain with fever, weight loss, and a palpable mass in the ileocecal region. Intra-abdominal extension occurs, may involve the entire abdomen, and may result in draining fistulas and perirectal disease. Diagnosis is often delayed.

Colonization of the endocervix with *A. israelii* and organisms morphologically resembling actinomycetes is common in women with intrauterine contraceptive devices (IUDs) in place. However, invasive pelvic actinomycosis is rare. Removal of the foreign body from the endocervix usually results in a return to normal of the cervical cultures within a few menstrual cycles and obviates the need for antibiotic treatment. Clinical evaluation is indicated when removal of the IUD is not effective or the patient is symptomatic.

DIAGNOSIS. The diagnosis of actinomycosis is established by demonstrating sulfur granules in biopsy material and/or gram-positive filamentous bacilli with branching hyphae in an area of suppuration and by isolating the *Actinomyces* anaerobically.

TREATMENT. Actinomycosis tends to recur following short courses of therapy; thus, prolonged antibiotic treatment, surgical drainage of abscesses, and excision of infected tissue are indicated. Massive doses of penicillin (400,000 units/kg/24 hr) given intravenously for 6–8 wk followed by oral penicillin (phenoxymethyl penicillin 2–4 g/24 hr) for an additional 6–12 mo are used to treat deep-seated infections. In patients allergic to penicillin, therapeutic success has been obtained with clindamycin, erythromycin, and the tetracyclines.

Berardi RS: Abdominal actinomycosis. Surg Gynecol Obstet 149:257, 1979.
Burden P: Actinomycosis. J Infect 19:95, 1989.
Drake DD, Holt RJ: Childhood actinomycosis—report of 3 recent cases. Arch Dis Child 51:979, 1976.
Lerner PI: Susceptibility of pathogenic actinomycetes to antimicrobial compounds. Antimicrob Agents Chemother 5:302, 1974.

12.46 NOCARDIOSIS

Nocardiosis is a subacute or chronic suppurative disease of man and animals that occurs following inoculation of the skin, gastrointestinal tract, or lungs with a soil-borne actinomycete of the genus *Nocardia*. Infection in man usually presents as one of four distinct clinical syndromes: pulmonary, cutaneous, disseminated, and central nervous system disease.

ETIOLOGY. *Nocardia* species are aerobic, gram-positive, weakly acid-fast bacilli with delicate branching hyphae that appear microscopically as fragmented coccobacillary elements. These microorganisms are nonfastidious and grow over a wide temperature range (25–37° C) on a number of antibiotic-free culture media. Laboratory isolation of the microorganism poses a problem because their growth is often inhibited by more rapidly growing organisms. Accordingly, *Nocardia* sp. are more likely to be observed in media used for myobacteria and fungi, which are often observed for an extended period of time. *N. asteroides* is the dominant human pathogen in the United States and Europe and is most often responsible for systemic nocardiosis. Other human pathogens include *N. brasiliensis* and *N. caviae*, which are typically associated with localized infection of the skin and adjacent soft tissue. *N. farcinica*, an animal pathogen, may also infect man.

EPIDEMIOLOGY. Nocardiosis is being diagnosed with increasing frequency in the United States; it is estimated that 500–1,000 culture-proven cases occur annually. Nocardiosis occurs at any age but is more frequent in adults; there is no particular geographic distribution; males are affected twice as often as females; and it occurs almost exclusively as an opportunistic infection in immunosuppressed patients. The most common predisposing factor for nocardial infection is the use of high-dose corticosteroids. The respiratory tract is the initial site of involvement in 70% of cases.

PATHOLOGY. Nocardiosis produces a suppurative lesion characterized by tissue necrosis and abscess formation that microscopically resemble those of the common pyogenic bacteria. Branching filaments of *Nocardia* are often scattered throughout the area of suppuration; granule formation is uncommon. Hematogenous dissemination from a pulmonary focus occurs in approximately one third of patients. The heart, liver, and spleen are occasionally sites of secondary infection, but the central nervous system is the site most often affected; this infection presents as a poorly encapsulated multilocular brain abscess.

CLINICAL MANIFESTATIONS. In the United States nocardiosis typically presents as an acute, subacute, or chronic pulmonary infection in an immunocompromised patient with debilitating underlying disease. Pulmonary involvement begins as a confluent bronchopneumonia that progresses to consolidation, cavitation, pleural effusion, and empyema formation. The clinical findings include fever, night sweats, a productive cough, anorexia, weight loss, dyspnea, and chest pain. Without treatment, the course is chronic and may simulate tuberculosis. Clinical manifestations may also include tracheitis, bronchitis, pericarditis, and mediastinitis with obstruction of the superior vena cava. Extension through the chest wall and subcutaneous abscess formation are extremely rare. Patients whose disease is complicated by hematogenous dissemination may present with multiple subcutaneous abscesses and diffuse organ involvement. Central nervous system involvement is seen in one third of cases, and brain abscesses may dominate the clinical picture and by extension lead to purulent meningitis. The cutaneous lesion is characterized by localized swelling involving the subcutaneous tissue with multiple sinus tracts that lead to the surface as well as to the bone. The purulent drainage through the sinuses may contain granules (compact colonies of microorganisms surrounded by reactive cells); their size, shape, and color may suggest the specific nocardial strain.

DIAGNOSIS. The clinical manifestations may point to a diagnosis of nocardiosis. Branching gram-positive filamentous bacilli in sputum, bronchoscopic washings, pleural fluid, or material obtained by lung aspiration suggest the diagnosis of nocardiosis or actinomycosis. *Nocardia* are distinguished by the absence (usually) of granule formation and their acid-fast staining characteristics. Diagnosis by culture is difficult, especially in the case of heavily contaminated specimens.

TREATMENT AND PROGNOSIS. Sulfonamides (150 mg/kg/24 hr) in combination with appropriate surgical drainage of abscesses is the treatment of choice for nocardiosis. Sulfisoxazole and triple sulfonamide combinations are as effective as sulfadiazine. Antimicrobial susceptibility testing is helpful in selecting alternative therapeutic regimens when sulfonamides cannot be administered because of allergy or intolerance. Alternative drugs may be used in combination with sulfonamides in patients with serious, life-threatening infections. Imipenem and amikacin are the two most consistently active agents against *N. asteroides*. Combination therapy with amikacin and imipenem or imipenem with cefotaxime has been suggested based on in vitro observations. However, the efficacy of combination treatment for nocardiosis is not established. Therapy should be continued for a minimum of 6 wk, but sulfonamide administration is often continued for many months after apparent cure because relapse tends to occur with nocardiosis. With sulfonamide therapy, the mortality for all forms of the disease has fallen from 75 to 40%; only 35% of patients with disseminated disease survive.

Curry WA: Human nocardiosis—a clinical review with selected case reports. Arch Intern Med 140:818, 1980.

Law BJ, Marks MI: Pediatric nocardiosis. Pediatrics 70:560, 1982.
Lerner PI: Susceptibility of pathogenic actinomycetes to antimicrobial compounds. Antimicrobial Agents Chemother 4:302, 1974.
Simpson GL, Stinson EB, Egger MJ, et al: Nocardial infections in the immunocompromised host: A detailed study in a defined population. Rev Infect Dis 3:492, 1981.

12.47 TUBERCULOSIS

The incidence of tuberculosis has decreased progressively as the general standard of living and health status of children have improved in the United States, Europe, Japan, and other developed countries during the past century. In the United States tuberculosis was the 8th leading cause of death of children 1–4 yr of age in 1920; by 1960 it was not among the top 10 causes of death for any age group of children. This is in stark contrast to the persistent high incidence today in developing countries. In the United States the incidence of childhood tuberculosis has remained constant since 1976; however, there has been a recent increase in adult patients, primarily in men between 25 and 40 yr of age. This increased incidence in adults has been attributed to infection with the human immunodeficiency virus (HIV).

ETIOLOGY. Tuberculosis is caused by the tubercle bacillus, a member of the Mycobacteriaceae family, order Actinomycetales. In humans, the most common tubercle bacilli are *Mycobacterium tuberculosis*, which is responsible for most infections, and *M. bovis. M. africanum* is a rare cause of tuberculosis in West and Central Africa. Other "anonymous" or "atypical" mycobacteria exist as human pathogens and are discussed in Sec. 12.48.

All mycobacteria are aerobic, nonmotile, nonsporulating, pleomorphic rods. They are difficult to stain because of the high lipid content of their cell walls, and once stained they resist decoloration with acid-alcohol; thus they are commonly described as being acid-fast. The Ziehl-Neelsen technique stains the bacilli red with carbolfuchsin dye so that they can be identified under oil immersion (100×) against a background stained with methylene blue. The fluorochrome technique stains the mycobacteria with auramine-rhodamine dyes, which fluoresce yellow-green under ultraviolet light, allowing detection of the bacilli under low-power (25×) magnification; this increases sensitivity for identifying small numbers of bacilli in clinical specimens. The major disadvantage of the fluorochrome stain is that both viable and nonviable microorganisms are stained, preventing assessment of the specimen's infectivity.

M. tuberculosis microorganisms are slow growing; the average recovery time is 21 days, and occasional strains require 4–6 wk. Growth is best obtained using selective media, incubated aerobically at 37° C, in a carbon dioxide–enriched atmosphere. Growth can usually be detected within 2 wk by using radiolabeled nutrients in selective liquid media (Bactec radiometric system), but a major disadvantage of this system is that early speciation cannot be performed. New diagnostic techniques using RNA and DNA probes and monoclonal antibodies should allow more rapid identification of *M. tuberculosis*.

M. tuberculosis is differentiated from other mycobacterial strains by the morphology of the colony, absence of pigment, production of niacin, ability to reduce nitrates, presence of a heat-labile catalase, and sensitivity to isoniazid. (*M. tuberculosis* strains resistant to isoniazid fail to produce niacin.) "Atypical" mycobacteria grow more rapidly than *M. tuberculosis*, produce no niacin, fail to reduce nitrates, produce heat-stable catalase, and are highly resistant to isoniazid. Newer techniques for rapidly classifying mycobacteria are based upon the detection of specific antigens using either agglutination reactions or enzyme-linked immunosorbent assays.

EPIDEMIOLOGY. The principal route of infection with *M. tuberculosis* is through inhalation of contaminated droplets. (*M. bovis* can be transmitted by consumption of milk from infected cattle, but in developed countries, pasteurization of milk and elimination of diseased animals has nearly eradicated this route.) Infection with *M. tuberculosis* occurs less frequently through the oropharynx, intestine, and skin. Droplets of aerosolized pulmonary secretions, produced by coughing and sneezing, are small enough to remain suspended in air and, when inhaled, can reach the terminal bronchioles and alveoli. The infectivity of these droplets depends on the number of microorganisms present in them; the number is greatest in secretions from individuals with culture-positive sputum or cavitary pulmonary disease. Accordingly, primary infection in children (conversion to a positive tuberculin skin test) most often occurs following prolonged close contact with an untreated adult with cavitary disease. Although genitourinary secretions from infected individuals may contain microorganisms, transmission following urine aerosolization is uncommon. Similarly, transmission following contact with infectious discharges (e.g., drainage from open sinuses), contaminated objects, or household pets is uncommon.

IMMUNOLOGY. The immune response to tuberculosis involves a series of interactions between the tubercle bacilli, specific lymphocyte subpopulations, and tissue macrophages. The various classes of antibodies produced during infection play no role in inhibiting bacterial growth or creating subsequent immunity. A cellular immune response begins after viable microorganisms are inhaled; pulmonary macrophages ingest the bacilli but are ineffective in killing them, and the bacilli proliferate. Infection subsequently spreads to the regional lymph nodes; lymphatic and hematogenous dissemination and the establishment of many infected extrapulmonary foci follow.

Although the pulmonary macrophages do not kill the ingested microorganisms, macrophages are capable of processing mycobacterial antigens and presenting them to circulating T lymphocytes, which are activated by the antigens. These T lymphocytes proliferate and circulate throughout the lymphatic system, producing a number of soluble mediators, lymphokines. Lymphokines attract circulating lymphocytes and monocytes to sites of lymphocyte-antigen interaction and activate macrophages, thereby enhancing the intracellular killing of ingested microorganisms and promoting differentiation of pulmonary macrophages into epithelioid and Langerhans cells. In the presence of numerous tubercle bacilli, activated lymphocytes may also produce cytotoxic substances, which, along with hydrolytic enzymes released from living and dead pulmonary macrophages, cause incomplete or caseation necrosis. In the lungs, liquefaction of this caseous material may cause the formation of cavities and a massive increase in the number of tubercle bacilli. Normally these immunologic processes occur over a 6- to 10-wk period and contain the primary infection and eliminate metastatic foci.

A number of factors can interfere with developing natural immunity, predisposing an individual to life-threatening infection. *Genetic* factors influence morbidity and mortality. Studies of twins suggest that concordance for severe infection is present in identical twins, and recent data indicate that severe infection is more common among individuals exhibiting certain HLA histocompatibility antigens. Although certain ethnic groups (American Indians and Eskimos) are predisposed to serious infection, these populations are also affected by *demographic* and *socioeconomic* variables. *Age* also affects the severity of infection; children under 3 yr of age have a high mortality due to miliary tuberculosis and meningitis. This may be the result of an immature immunologic response, or it may reflect the relatively higher inoculum of infectious organisms received by a young child. A variety of factors that interfere with T cell function also predispose to serious illness: *malnutrition*, various *infections* including rubeola and pertussis, *pregnancy*, *reticuloendothelial disease*, and *cancer* of the lymphatic system. Initial tuberculous infection may be more severe, or dormant infection may be reactivated in patients treated with *immunosuppressive drugs*, including corticosteroids, as well as in adults and children with HIV infection.

Diagnostic Skin Tests. The tuberculin skin test, based on the detection of delayed hypersensitivity to the antigens of *M. tuberculosis*, is a reliable diagnostic technique. An infected patient responds positively within 6–10 wk of infection. The test consists of an intradermally administered antigen preparation; a positive response is indicated by the appearance of induration, which results from migration of activated lymphocytes and macrophages to the site of antigen deposition. Two antigen preparations are available, *old tuberculin* (OT) and *purified protein derivative* (PPD). OT is a crude product prepared by heat sterilization of filtrates of culture medium containing *M. tuberculosis*. It is utilized only for multiple-puncture skin tests.

The PPD is a protein precipitate derived from OT. Its dosage is expressed in terms of tuberculin units (TU) using a single lot (PPD-S) as the biologic standard against which all PPD preparations are compared. (One TU equals 0.00002 mg PPD-S.) Three dosage strengths are available: a 1st-strength PPD (1 TU/0.1 mL), an intermediate strength PPD (5 TU/0.1 mL), and a 2nd-strength PPD (250 TU/0.1 mL). Several precautions are taken to preserve the potency of PPD preparations. The protein derivative is provided as a dried powder to be diluted with buffered saline prior to use. To prevent absorption of protein to the walls of glass and plastic containers, a small amount of detergent (Tween 80) is added to the PPD diluent. In addition, after the solution has been prepared, it must be kept refrigerated (4° C) in the dark to preserve its potency. PPD, the preferred skin test antigen, is available for use in multiple-puncture skin tests and in the intracutaneous Mantoux test.

Several multiple-puncture skin tests are available and have been successfully used for mass screening of pediatric patients. Because these sensitive techniques lack specificity, patients with positive or doubtful reactions must be retested with the Mantoux test (see later). In the *tine test*, the most widely used multiple-puncture skin test, a disposable plastic unit with four stainless steel blades (tines) predipped in OT is used, usually applied to the volar surface of the forearm after the skin has been cleansed with alcohol or acetone. The test is interpreted after 48–72 hr. A positive reaction consists of vesiculation with one or more papules measuring at least 2 mm in diameter. The *Aplitest* is similar to the tine test except that the four steel prongs are coated with PPD preserved in phenol. In the *Heaf test* a special device (Heaf gun) is used that makes six simultaneous skin punctures 1 mm deep through a layer of concentrated PPD. The test is read 3–7 days afterward, and the presence of four or more papules constitutes a positive reaction. A negative multiple-puncture test does not rule out tuberculosis because false-negative results may occur. False-positive reactions are common for all of the multiple-puncture skin tests; therefore, all positive and doubtful reactions must be confirmed with a Mantoux test.

The *Mantoux test* is more difficult to administer than the multiple-puncture skin test, but because it delivers a defined amount of antigen, it is more reliable. One tenth milliliter of intermediate strength PPD (5 TU) is injected intracutaneously into the volar surface of the forearm. A single-dose plastic syringe with a short needle (26- or 27-gauge) is used, beveled side up. A wheal 6–10 mm in diameter should appear during the injection, and withdrawal of the needle is delayed briefly to minimize leakage of PPD at the puncture site. The site of antigen injection is examined for induration after 48–72 hr. A reaction of 5 mm or more after 48 hr is classified as positive in (1) individuals with HIV infection or with risk factors for HIV infection whose HIV status is unknown; (2) individuals who have had close recent contact with patients with infectious tuberculosis; and (3) individuals who have chest roentgenograms consistent with the appearance of old healed tuberculosis. A reaction of 10 mm or more is considered positive in persons who do not meet the preceding criteria but who have other risk factors for tuberculosis such as present or previous residence in high prevalence countries, use of intravenous drugs, membership in medically underserved low income populations, residence in a long-term care facility, and immunoincompetence or other disorders known to increase the risk of tuberculosis. A reaction of 15 mm or more is classified as positive in all other individuals. An induration of less than 5 mm in diameter in a well child is "negative," although anergy must be ruled out by demonstrating that the patient is able to show a positive skin test to mumps (after measles-mumps-rubella [MMR] vaccination), *Candida*, or other skin test antigens.

The most common cause of a "doubtful" response to the Mantoux test is infection with "atypical" mycobacteria (Sec. 12.48). PPD contains antigens common to nontuberculous strains of mycobacteria. This cross reactivity is seen more frequently when a dose of 250 TU is used in the test. Under certain circumstances, reactions of 5–10 mm of induration might be termed "suspicious," and might be considered an indication for therapeutic intervention. For example: In some areas of the United States, such as Alaska, atypical mycobacterial infections are uncommon, and therefore cross reactivity is an unlikely cause of the doubtful response.

False-negative responses to the Mantoux test can arise from a number of causes. A significant fraction of patients (as many as 20%) with culture-proven tuberculosis have negative skin test reactions during the early phase of the illness, even when skin testing is performed with 250 TU. The test itself can be inadequate because of loss of potency of the PPD due to improper storage or bacterial contamination, improper administration of the antigen, or inadequate concentration (1 TU) of antigen. Any factor that interferes with lymphocyte activation and the delayed hypersensitivity reaction can prevent a patient from showing a positive response, including extremes in age (infants less than 6 mo), overwhelming illness of any type (including tuberculosis), coincident viral infections (HIV, rubeola, and influenza), immunization with an attenuated virus vaccine, treatment with immunosuppressive agents (including corticosteroids), malnutrition, neoplastic disease (especially Hodgkin and non-Hodgkin lymphoma), sarcoidosis, and chronic renal failure.

False-positive responses to the Mantoux test can occur because of repeated skin testing with PPD or OT or because of prior immunization with bacillus Calmette-Guérin (BCG). Immunization with BCG may result in a tuberculin reaction that is difficult to distinguish from that due to *M. tuberculosis* infections. However, the positive response in the Mantoux test due to BCG immunization is induration, which rarely exceeds 10 mm in diameter and is strongest within the first few years after immunization. Accordingly, any reaction that exceeds 10 mm and occurs more than 3 yr following immunization should be considered an indication of tuberculous infection.

CLINICAL FORMS OF TUBERCULOSIS

Intrathoracic

PATHOGENESIS AND PATHOLOGY. Primary infection with tubercle bacilli usually occurs following inhalation of viable microorganisms. In the nonimmune child it is characterized at the cellular level by phagocytosis and intracellular multiplication of tubercle bacilli, spread from the pulmonary alveolus to the regional lymph nodes, lymphadenitis and subsequent lymphatic-hematogenous dissemination, and the establishment of metastatic infection throughout the lung, reticuloendothelial system, and other organ systems. In the absence of cell-mediated immunity, tissue damage is minimal, and signs and symptoms are absent. In most children the development of acquired immunity over 6–10 wk results in healing and calcification of pulmonary and extrapulmonary foci. The surviving bacilli remain dormant indefinitely, particularly in the apical or subapical regions of the lung. Any condition, either local or systemic, that modifies cellular immunity may permit multiplication of dormant microorganisms and reactivation of pulmonary and/or extrapulmonary foci. *Reactivation tuberculosis* is most often a localized infection occurring in the presence of cell-mediated immunity, resulting in extensive tissue damage, and producing signs and symptoms.

PRIMARY PULMONARY TUBERCULOSIS

CLINICAL MANIFESTATIONS. In *older infants* and *children* (age 3–15 yr) primary pulmonary tuberculosis is typically an asymptomatic illness identified in a child with a positive skin test and a normal chest roentgenogram. Prior to the development of tuberculin hypersensitivity, infection is asymptomatic; however, with the development of hypersensitivity, manifestations develop that often include malaise and fever and infrequently include erythema nodosum and phlyctenular keratoconjunctivitis. Cough is infrequent early in the illness but may become prominent with bronchial involvement. Hemoptysis is unusual in primary tuberculosis.

Lymph node involvement is common in primary pulmonary tuberculosis, and additional symptoms may occur secondary to massive lymph node involvement, for example, compression, obstruction, and/or erosion of mediastinal structures by enlarged lymph nodes. Nonpulmonary symptoms following subcarinal nodal enlargement and esophageal compression may include dysphagia and recurrent aspiration. Compression of major blood vessels may also occur, resulting in edema of an extremity or in the superior vena caval syndrome. Nodal compression of the recurrent laryngeal nerve or the phrenic nerve may be associated with vocal cord or diaphragmatic paralysis. Pulmonary symptoms and signs secondary to enlargement of the paratracheal-parabronchial nodes include recurrent cough, stridor, and wheezing. Prolonged compression of these latter structures may result in lobar emphysema or segmental atelectasis of one or more lobes. Complete bronchial erosion accompanied by a discharge of caseum into the adjacent or distal airways may occur, resulting in signs and symptoms of acute pneumonia. However, in most children primary pulmonary infection is a mild, asymptomatic illness that resolves over a brief period of time with or without effective chemotherapy. Late sequelae of primary infection include pleurisy with or without effusion and miliary-meningeal dissemination.

In *older children* and *adolescents*, the signs of primary pulmonary tuberculosis are similar to those observed in younger children except that there is a greater likelihood of developing progressive primary tuberculosis with or without cavitation.

DIAGNOSIS. Primary pulmonary tuberculosis is most often diagnosed in an asymptomatic infants by means of a positive tuberculin test. Routine laboratory examinations are not helpful. Roentgenographic examination of the chest is often normal; however, unilateral, often massive, hilar adenopathy with or without a small parenchymal focus in the lower or middle lung fields may be observed, and calcification may occur during the healing process. A diagnosis requires bacteriologic confirmation. Acid-fast bacilli may be found in sputum; these cultures are usually positive. However, microbial confirmation may be difficult in young infants with primary infection because infants may not cough, and sputum, when produced, is usually promptly swallowed. Pulmonary secretions may be obtained using fiberoptic bronchoscopy. Examination of gastric contents may replace sputum examination in young infants and should be carried out early in the morning in a fasting child, preferably upon awakening. Gastric contents are gently aspirated through a nasogastric tube and placed in a sterile container. Following this initial aspiration, the stomach should be lavaged with 30 mL of water and again aspirated. This material should be added to the initial specimen. This procedure should be repeated on at least two occasions on separate days. The material should be immediately transported to the laboratory for staining and culture.

PROGRESSIVE PRIMARY PULMONARY TUBERCULOSIS

Progressive primary pulmonary infection occurs when the primary focus of infection, instead of resolving, enlarges to involve the entire middle and/or lower lobes. It is uncommon except in immunosuppressed patients. Intrathoracic adenopathy is common, and cavitation, when present, may be associated with endobronchial dissemination to other portions of the lung. Clinical manifestations are prominent and include elevated temperature, malaise, anorexia, weight loss, and productive cough. Physical findings and roentgenography demonstrate hilar adenopathy, middle or lower lobe pneumonia, and cavity formation. Diagnosis depends on bacterial confirmation.

REACTIVATION TUBERCULOSIS

Reactivation tuberculosis (post-primary pulmonary tuberculosis or adult pulmonary tuberculosis) is uncommon in children, particularly when primary infection has occurred at less than 3 yr of age. Infection is often confined to the apical or posterior segments of the upper lobes or to the superior segments of the lower lobes, both of which contain conditions that favor the growth of tubercle bacilli disseminated during the lymphatic-hematogenous phase of primary infection. The initial infiltrate expands and undergoes cavitation, often in association with *endobrochial dissemination.* Intrathoracic lymphadenopathy is uncommon. The most prominent symptom is low-grade fever, which may be associated with "night sweats" when defervescence occurs during sleep. Additional manifestations include malaise, fatigue, and weight loss. With the development of caseation necrosis, liquefaction, and cavitation, a productive cough develops, often associated with mild hemoptysis. Physical findings are usually confined to the apices of the lungs and consist of fine or post-tussive rales. The earliest roentgenographic change consists of a well-circumscribed, homogeneous shadow most commonly seen in the apex of the lung. As the infiltrate enlarges, it may result in lobar consolidation. Following liquefaction necrosis, the classic thick-walled cavities that lack air-fluid levels become visible.

PLEURAL EFFUSION

Pleural effusion due to discharge of tubercle bacilli into the pleural space from a subpleural focus is an uncommon complication of primary pulmonary tuberculosis. Pleural effusions may also be secondary to miliary dissemination; these effusions are often bilateral and associated with pericarditis and peritonitis. Although the pleural effusion may resolve spontaneously, recognizing its tuberculous etiology is important; such effusions may be followed within a few years by reactivation tuberculosis, and this can be prevented by administering antituberculosis drugs. Effusions due to tuberculosis must be differentiated from effusions secondary to congestive heart failure, malignant disease, metabolic disturbances, collagen vascular disease, and the parapneumonic effusions caused by other infectious agents. Tuberculous effusions are exudates that have a specific gravity of 1.012–1.022, an elevated protein content (> 4 g/dL), high concentrations of lactic dehydrogenase (LDH) and adenosine deaminase, and a low glucose level (< 30 mg/dL). Cytologic examination reveals an absence of mesothelial cells and a predominance of lymphocytes, although neutrophils may predominate early in the course of illness. Acid-fast strains of the pleural fluid are usually negative, but positive cultures of fluid and pleural tissue may be obtained in more than half the cases. Repeated thoracentesis and centrifugation of large quantities of fluid increase the yield of positive cultures. Pleural biopsies should be obtained in all cases, preferably at the time of initial thoracentesis, since a biopsy specimen is difficult to obtain in the absence of pleural fluid. Histologic examination of the pleural tissue reveals granulomas in a majority of cases. In patients with a positive tuberculin skin test, a pleural effusion should always be considered tuberculous until proved otherwise. Similarly, an unexplained effusion in the presence of a negative tuberculin skin test mandates repetition of the test within 2–3 wk. The natural history of these effusions is gradual resorption. Repeated thoracentesis and tube drainage are contraindicated.

Extrathoracic

TUBERCULOSIS OF THE UPPER RESPIRATORY TRACT

Involvement of the upper respiratory tract (larynx, epiglottis, pharynx, and middle ear) is now rare, although prior to the availability of effective chemotherapy it was a common complication of advanced pulmonary disease. It is still observed in developing countries. Children with laryngeal tuberculosis almost always have cavitary pulmonary disease; manifestations include a croupy cough, sore throat, hoarseness, and pain on swallowing. Tuberculous otitis is associated with profound hearing loss, diffuse otorrhea, absence of pain, and pre- or postauricular adenopathy. Facial nerve involvement and mastoiditis are common. Otoscopic examination reveals a thickened tympanic membrane with one or more perforations. The treatment of upper respiratory tuberculosis depends on the extent of the concurrent pulmonary disease. Surgical intervention is indicated in tuberculous otitis in the presence of facial nerve paralysis, a subperiosteal abscess, or mastoiditis.

TUBERCULOSIS OF LYMPH NODES

The involvement of the superficial and deep lymph nodes is common in tuberculosis. In children, the hilar nodes are the principal site of lymphadenitis, and local spread may involve the paratracheal, supraclavicular, deep cervical, and abdominal nodes. Adenitis secondary to a primary focus in an extremity is less common and results in inguinal or axillary lymphadenopathy. Adenopathy may follow the hematogenous or lymphatic dissemination of tubercle bacilli during the nonimmune phase of primary infection and may affect the superficial and deep lymph nodes. *Superficial lymphadenitis,* the most common form of nonrespiratory tuberculosis, is found most often in the head and neck and usually affects multiple nodes. Bilateral involvement is common. In order of decreasing frequency, it may involve the anterior and posterior cervical (scrofula), supraclavicular, and submandibular nodes and occasionally the preauricular and submental nodes.

CLINICAL MANIFESTATIONS. The course of tuberculous lymphadenitis is insidious, but in children highly sensitive to tuberculin the illness may be acute, with elevated temperature and perinodal inflammation. The history often includes exposure to a person with active tuberculosis. The tuberculin skin test is positive in most patients (90%), and the chest roentgenogram usually demonstrates evidence of primary pulmonary tuberculous. Occasionally lymph nodes may become very large and compress adjacent structures. Thus, mediastinal hilar adenopathy may result in compression of the trachea, bronchi, major blood vessels, recurrent laryngeal nerve, or thoracic duct. Enlargement of superficial lymph nodes may lead to rupture into the surrounding tissue and formation of a cutaneous sinus tract. On physical examination, the nodes are nontender, firm, and discrete. Less often, the nodes are fluctuant and adhere to the overlying skin. Sinus tract formation is uncommon.

DIAGNOSIS. A definitive diagnosis requires histologic and bacteriologic confirmation, which is best accomplished by total excisional biopsy of the involved node(s); excision of a caseous node or nodes may also limit the need for long-term antimicrobial treatment. Partial biopsy or needle aspiration is less satisfactory and may result in sinus tract formation. Histologic examination reveals noncaseating granulomas, and acid-fast stains are usually positive. Tuberculous and atypical mycobacterial lymphadenitis cannot be differentiated histologically; therefore, all biopsy material must be cultured in appropriate media.

Tuberculous lymphadenitis can be confused with other conditions. Although *M. tuberculosis* is the predominant cause of mycobacterial cervical adenitis in adults, the atypical mycobacteria cause most cervical adenitis in children. The differential diagnosis also includes lymphadenitis due to viruses, bacteria, fungi, *Toxoplasma,* and the agent causing cat-scratch disease. Noninfectious causes of lymphadenopathy, including malignancy, sarcoidosis, and drug reaction (to phenytoin), must also be considered.

TREATMENT. Tuberculous lymphadenitis responds to therapy with isoniazid and either rifampin or ethambutol. Transient enlargement of nodes or the appearance of new nodes occurs in a minority of children during the initial phases of therapy but does not indicate failure of treatment or relapse. Residual nodes may be palpable following cure.

MILIARY TUBERCULOSIS

Miliary tuberculosis results from hematogenous spread of *M. tuberculosis* from an established focus, producing lesions that progress to necrosis and caseation in multiple organs. The granulomas are similar in size and often resemble in appearance the millet seed, hence the term "miliary." In the era before chemotherapy, this was primarily a pediatric disease resulting from massive hematogenous dissemination of tubercle bacilli at the time of primary pulmonary infection and, with meningitis, was responsible for most fatal cases of tuberculosis in infants and children. In developing countries where tuberculosis in children is common, miliary tuberculosis remains a disease of young children (more than one third of cases occur in children less than 3 yr of age) and usually presents within a year of primary infection. However, in the United States and other developed nations, miliary tuberculosis is more often secondary to reactivation of latent infection. Accordingly, disseminated infection in this country is now more common in adults (more than one third of all cases occur in individuals over 65 yr old) with chronic disease or in those receiving immunosuppressive therapy. Miliary tuberculosis also occurs in patients with the acquired immunodeficiency syndrome (AIDS).

CLINICAL MANIFESTATIONS. The onset in children is often abrupt and is characterized by temperature elevation

(102–104° F), weakness, malaise, anorexia, and weight loss. Physical findings, which include lymphadenopathy, hepatomegaly, and splenomegaly, are nonspecific. Within weeks, respiratory signs and symptoms dominate the clinical picture; tachypnea, dyspnea, and cough are common and are associated with diffuse rales over both lungs. Meningitis may be present, resulting in headache, lethargy, and nuchal rigidity. Less common physical findings include cutaneous metastasis and bilateral choroidal tubercles.

A different clinical picture is observed when small numbers of tubercle bacilli are discharged intermittently into the bloodstream over an extended period of time. This condition, occurring more commonly in adults than in children, is designated *chronic hematogenous tuberculosis* or *protracted hematogenous tuberculosis*. It is characterized by continuous or intermittent fever, weakness, and weight loss extending over a period of weeks to months. Hepatomegaly, splenomegaly, and diffuse lymphadenopathy are common. The mortality associated with disseminated miliary tuberculosis is approximately 40%. Respiratory failure due to the adult respiratory distress syndrome (ARDS) is the most serious complication of disseminated infection and when present is associated with a mortality of approximately 70%.

DIAGNOSIS. Laboratory tests help little in diagnosing miliary tuberculosis. The white blood cell count may be normal, elevated, or depressed. Anemia and an elevated erythrocyte sedimentation rate are common. Monocytosis, thrombocytopenia, and evidence of disseminated intravascular coagulation are uncommon. There may be hyponatremia and hypokalemia, and abnormalities in liver function are common. The tuberculin skin test is usually positive, but patients may be anergic owing to underlying immunosuppression or overwhelming disease. Thus, a negative skin test does not exclude the diagnosis. The chest roentgenogram is the single most important diagnostic test, typically revealing bilateral miliary infiltrates. However, it may be normal during the early stages, and roentgenographic examinations should be repeated when the index of suspicion is high.

Definitive diagnosis requires microbiologic evidence of *M. tuberculosis*. Accordingly, cultures of the urine, gastric aspirates, and cerebrospinal fluid should be obtained. A transbronchial lung biopsy with fiberoptic bronchoscopy, the diagnostic procedure of choice, will often reveal caseating and noncaseating granulomas and the presence of acid-fast bacilli. Culture of this material is usually positive.

TUBERCULOUS MENINGITIS

EPIDEMIOLOGY. The incidence of tuberculous meningitis depends on the prevalence of tuberculosis. In the United States and other developed countries, the incidence has declined, but in the developing countries it remains a significant public health problem. Tuberculous meningitis most often occurs in recently infected individuals and has traditionally been considered a disease of infants and children, with symptoms developing within 6 mo of the primary pulmonary infection. However, in developed countries, where the adult population includes a large number of tuberculin-negative individuals, it is primarily a disease of adults. Prior to the availability of effective therapy, tuberculous meningitis was invariably fatal, with most deaths occurring within weeks of initial presentation. Although antimicrobial agents have improved the survival rate, serious sequelae are common.

PATHOPHYSIOLOGY AND PATHOLOGY. Metastatic foci of mycobacteria result from the hematogenous dissemination that occurs during the nonimmune phase of primary infection and/or miliary disease. In the central nervous system (CNS) these foci (tubercles) may be solitary or may be scattered over the cerebral hemispheres and/or the meninges of the spinal cord. Tuberculous meningitis may occur during primary infection or many decades later when rupture of one or more of the subependymal tubercles or of a parameningeal focus (tuberculoma, spondylitis, otitis, or osteitis) discharges the tubercle bacilli and tuberculous antigens into the subarachnoid space. In an immune individual this results in a severe inflammatory reaction throughout the CNS. With time, a thick gelatinous exudate develops about the basal meninges, resulting in damage to cerebral arteries and veins, compression of the cranial nerves, and obliteration of the basal cisterns and ventricular foramina.

CLINICAL MANIFESTATIONS. The symptoms are insidious and involve three clinical states: stage 1, a prodromal phase with nonspecific symptomatology; stage 2, the appearance of neurologic signs and symptoms; and stage 3, an alteration in the level of consciousness proceeding from stupor to coma. In children the earlier symptoms (stage 1) include apathy, mood changes, declining school performance, loss of appetite, nausea, vomiting, and low-grade fever. Within 1–4 wk neurologic signs and symptoms appear (stage 2). Irritability is increased, and older children complain of headache. Neck stiffness accompanied by Kernig and Brudzinski signs may be present. Cranial nerve palsies are common and include ocular palsies (pupillary abnormalities, diplopia), facial palsy, decreased visual acuity, and deafness. Aphasia, slurred speech, disorientation, hemiplegia, ataxia, involuntary movements, and convulsions are not uncommon. Intracranial pressure, increased during this stage, may be associated with enlarging head circumference, a tense anterior fontanel, and, in older children, papilledema. As the disease progresses (stage 3), evidence of diffuse cerebral dysfunction increases. Thus affected, children will demonstrate stupor, coma, decerebrate or decorticate posturing, irregular respiration, and fixed and dilated pupils. It is important to recognize that the presentation in children may not be conventional, and thus cerebral tuberculosis must be considered in all children presenting with unexplained neurologic dysfunction.

DIAGNOSIS. The most important factor in rapidly diagnosing tuberculous meningitis is maintaining a high index of suspicion in children with cerebrospinal fluid pleocytosis. The history often includes exposure to an individual with active tuberculosis, and the tuberculin skin test is usually positive. A negative skin test (including a negative reaction to second-strength PPD) does not exclude the diagnosis even in a child with a positive mumps or *Candida* skin test. Many children (40–90%) have evidence of concurrent pulmonary disease (hilar adenopathy, lower lobe infiltrate). Roentgenograms of the skull are normal unless the meningitis is associated with "split sutures" due to increased pressure or a calcified tuberculoma. CT scans often reveal periventricular lucencies, edema, infarctions, and hydrocephalus. Tuberculomas have been reported before, concurrent with, or following tuberculous meningitis. Routine laboratory tests rarely help in establishing the diagnosis. Anemia and an elevated sedimentation rate are common. Hyponatremia and hypochloremia may be present when meningitis is complicated by the syndrome of inappropriate secretion of antidiuretic hormone.

Lumbar puncture reveals clear, colorless fluid under increased pressure. The cell count is elevated, although it rarely exceeds 500 cells/mm^3, and there is a predominance of lymphocytes; early in the course there may be a predominance of polymorphonuclear leukocytes. The spinal fluid glucose level is below 40 mg/dL or less than half the value of a simultaneous blood glucose determination. The protein concentration is normal or slightly elevated (100–300 mg/dL) during the initial stages but with time may exceed 1,000 mg/dL. A low spinal fluid chloride concentration reflects a low serum chloride level due to prolonged vomiting or inappropriate secretion of antidiuretic hormone. "Atypical" cerebrospinal fluid profiles are not uncommon and may include a predominance of polymorphonuclear leukocytes (in 30%) and a normal cerebrospinal fluid glucose (in 25%). Microscopic examination demonstrates acid-fast bacilli in 30% of patients. Bacilli may be best detected by allowing the cerebrospinal fluid to stand at room temperature for 24 hr and then staining the surface pellicle. Tubercle bacilli can usually be cultured from the spinal fluid. Culturing the sediment obtained following centrifugation of large volumes of cerebrospinal fluid increases the recovery of microorganisms. Measurement of cerebrospinal fluid adenosine deaminase activity, the radioactive bromide partition test, detection of bacterial metabolites by chromatographic techniques, identification of soluble antigens and/or antibody by enzyme-linked immunosorbent assay and latex particle agglutination, and DNA using polymerase chain reaction have been described but are not available in most laboratories.

TREATMENT. This consists of parenteral and/or oral administration of antituberculous drugs. Intrathecal medication (streptomycin or rifampin) is not indicated. Corticosteroids however, are recommended during the initial phase of treatment (2–4 wk) despite the absence of well-controlled studies documenting their efficacy.

PROGNOSIS. This is related to the patient's condition at the time of treatment. In stage 1 disease, a 100% cure rate and a low incidence of sequelae can be anticipated. In stage 2 illness, optimal treatment results in a cure rate of about 85%; neurologic defects can be demonstrated in approximately half the survivors. In stage 3 disease, a 50% survival has been reported, but most survivors have permanent handicaps.

TUBERCULOMA OF THE CENTRAL NERVOUS SYSTEM

Tuberculomas are single or multiple, may appear at any time during the course of tuberculosis, and often present as slowly expanding mass lesions. Symptoms include headache, visual or gait disturbances, and evidence of increased intracranial pressure. Skull reontgenograms may demonstrate calcifications in the tuberculoma (6%), and during the early stages the CT scan reveals a hypodense mass with ring enhancement and associated edema. Affected children usually have a history of exposure to active tuberculosis. A positive skin test and evidence of concurrent pulmonary disease (hilar adenopathy, lower lobe infiltrate, or pleural effusion) are present in a majority of affected children. Diagnosis is often confirmed at surgery; however, surgical removal is contraindicated, since most tuberculomas will resolve with medical management. Corticosteroids are usually administered during the first few weeks of treatment to decrease cerebral edema.

TUBERCULOSIS OF THE SKIN

See Sec. 23.26.

TUBERCULOSIS OF THE HEART AND PERICARDIUM

Tuberculous pericarditis, a rare complication of childhood tuberculosis (see also Sec. 15.75), occurs secondary to either rupture of a mediastinal lymph node into the pericardial space or hematogenous dissemination. The signs and symptoms result from decreased cardiac output. Patients often present with fever, chest pain, dyspnea, and orthopnea. Physical examination reveals tachycardia, cardiomegaly, distant heart sounds, a pericardial friction rub, and occasionally, a paradoxical pulse. Hepatomegaly and edema are common.The echocardiogram and electrocardiogram are abnormal owing to the pericardial effusion. Evidence of extracardiac tuberculosis is uncommon, but the tuberculin skin test is invariably positive. Pericardiocentesis reveals clear fluid with cytologic and chemical abnormalities similar to those described for tuberculous pleuritis. The acid-fast stain is usually negative, and the culture is positive for *M. tuberculosis* in less than half of the patients. Histologic examination and culture of pericardial tissue, which can be obtained at the time of a therapeutic pericardiocentesis, confirm the diagnosis. Treatment consists of isoniazid and either rifampin or ethambutol. Most authorities recommend a short course of corticosteroids in the hope of preventing constrictive pericarditis and the need for pericardial surgery.

ABDOMINAL TUBERCULOSIS

Gastrointestinal tuberculosis is uncommon in developed countries because of the early treatment of pulmonary tuberculosis, pasteurization of milk, and the near-eradication of bovine tuberculosis. Disease is usually secondary to swallowing infectious respiratory secretions; the extent of pulmonary involvement correlates with the incidence of gastrointestinal tuberculosis. However, it can occur in the absence of pulmonary disease, presumably owing to spread from mediastinal or peritoneal lymph nodes.

Gastrointestinal tuberculosis may produce granulomatous disease with caseation necrosis throughout the gastrointestinal tract and involvement of regional lymph nodes. Infection of the esophagus and stomach, usually secondary to spread from caseous mediastinal or peritoneal lymph nodes, may present with dysphagia, abdominal pain, or pyloric obstruction. Involvement of the small intestine is more common and may be associated with obstruction, perforation, hemorrhage, fistula formation, and malabsorption. Tuberculosis of the cecum may be associated with a painful right lower quadrant mass, hemorrhage, and obstruction or diarrhea. Tuberculosis of the colon may be diffuse or localized and may present with a clinical picture indistinguishable from that of granulomatous or ulcerative colitis, resulting in obstruction, perforation, or hemorrhage. Anal involvement is uncommon and presents with abscess formation and fistulization. Tuberculosis is the most common cause of **granulomatous hepatitis,** which may be asymptomatic. Diagnosis of gastrointestinal tuberculosis requires histologic and bacteriologic examination of biopsy material obtained by endoscopy, exploratory laparotomy, or percutaneous needle biopsy.

Tuberculous peritonitis may occur with gastrointestinal tuberculosis secondary to rupture of a caseous abdominal lymph node, or, less frequently, secondary to spread from an intestinal focus or from the female genital tract. Symptoms include fever, anorexia, and intermittent or chronic abdominal pain. Weight loss and abdominal distention are common, and evidence of extraperitoneal tuberculosis is usually absent. The skin test is usually positive. Examination of the peritoneal fluid is rarely diagnostic (an exudative response with a predominance of lymphocytes); acid-fast bacilli are usually absent, and the culture is positive in only 25% of cases. Diagnosis requires histologic and microbiologic examination of biopsy material obtained by peritoneoscopy or laparotomy.

Treatment of gastrointestinal tuberculosis requires nutritional support and administration of antituberculous antibiotics.

BONE AND JOINT TUBERCULOSIS

See Sec. 12.16 and 12.17.

UROGENITAL TUBERCULOSIS

Urogenital tuberculosis, a late manifestation of primary pulmonary disease, most commonly involves the kidneys and is rare in children. Tubercle bacilli reach the renal cortex during the nonimmune hematogenous phase of primary infection and remain dormant for many years. Reactivation may subsequently occur with multiplication of the tubercle bacilli and resultant caseation, cavitation, and extension into the renal pelvis. The discharge of viable microorganisms into the renal collecting system may cause infection of the ureters, the bladder, and the urethra. In males, secondary infection may involve the seminal vesicles, prostate, and epididymis.

CLINICAL MANIFESTATIONS. Many patients have inactive extragenital disease. Constitutional symptoms are uncommon and are usually confined to the genitourinary system. Dysuria, frequency, and urgency may be the presenting manifestations. Flank pain and renal colic are uncommon. The tuberculin skin test is invariably positive, and most patients have hematuria and pyuria; proteinuria is uncommon. Intravenous urography is often abnormal and, depending on the extent of renal involvement, demonstrates cortical calcification, calyceal blunting, reflux, and hydronephrosis. Diagnosis requires bacteriologic confirmation, which can be obtained in most patients by culturing morning urine specimens.

Tuberculosis of the *female genital system* is also uncommon in children but may involve the fallopian tubes (90%), the endometrium (50%), or the ovaries (20%). Infection of the cervix and vagina is extremely rare. Symptoms and signs include pelvic discomfort, irregular menstruation, and vaginal discharge. Diagnosis requires histologic and microbiologic examination of endometrial tissue.

TUBERCULOSIS OF THE EYE

The most common sites of ocular involvement are the choroid, retina, iris, sclera, and cornea. Ocular infection is usually secondary to hematogenous dissemination of *M. tuberculosis*, and because of its vascularity, the uvea (iris, ciliary body, and choroid) is the tissue most often involved. Choroidal tubercles are the most common form of ocular tuberculosis seen in children. They appear as solitary or multiple gray to gray-white tubercles at the posterior pole of the eye. Acute tuberculous panophthalmitis and tuberculoma of the ciliary body are very rare. Tuberculous keratoconjunctivitis presents as a severe, often bilateral conjunctival infection. Differentiation of tuberculous from viral or bacterial (nonmycobacterial) infection is facilitated by the presence of preauricular lymphadenopathy and small ulcerative lesions present on the palpebral conjunctiva. Tubercle bacilli can frequently be recovered from these palpebral ulcerations. Ocular infection resulting from exogenous inoculation or extension from contiguous sites is uncommon.

CHEMOTHERAPY OF TUBERCULOSIS

Because studies determining both the duration of therapy and the most effective agent(s) have been performed primarily in adults, optimal chemotherapeutic treatment for children is not definitely established, and this situation is unlikely to change, given the smaller number of cases in children. The application of adult treatment regimens to pediatric patients often results in overtreatment of children because of the larger number of tubercle bacilli characteristic of adult cavitary disease.

Many children with tuberculosis can be adequately managed as outpatients. Hospitalization is recommended (1) when a repeat culture or biopsy is needed to establish the diagnosis, (2) for the initial treatment of extensive or life-threatening disease, (3) for initial treatment in young infants and children, (4) when surgical intervention or corticosteroid therapy is warranted, (5) for the treatment of severe drug reaction, (6) for treatment of coexisting illness requiring hospitalization, or (7) for initial treatment when family or social circumstances prevent achievement of adequate treatment in the home. In this last situation, the child should be discharged only after arrangements have been made to administer the medication under supervised conditions.

Antituberculosis Drugs

ISONIAZID (INH). This drug of choice for tuberculosis is included in all treatment regimens unless the strain is suspected to be resistant. INH is usually administered orally as a single dose (10–20 mg/kg/24 hr) not to exceed 300 mg/24 hr. When administered twice weekly, the recommended dose is 20–40 mg/kg. The total daily dose should not exceed 900 mg. At this dosage, determining whether patients are slow or rapid inactivators of INH is not necessary. INH is well absorbed from the gastrointestinal tract, is widely distributed in body fluids and tissues, including the cerebrospinal fluid, and is metabolized in the liver and excreted via the kidneys. *Side effects* of INH therapy are uncommon. Peripheral neuritis secondary to pyridoxine deficiency has been reported in adults but is extremely rare in children, in whom simultaneous administration of pyridoxine is not indicated. Hepatotoxicity, manifested as an asymptomatic transient elevation in liver enzymes, is uncommon when INH is administered to children without pre-existing liver disease. Thus, liver function need not be monitored except in those patients who have pre-existing liver disease or who are simultaneously taking other hepatotoxic drugs (alcohol, phenytoin, rifampin). Less common side effects include gastrointestinal irritability, hypersensitivity reactions, and neurologic complications such as psychosis, confusion, and convulsions. Drug interactions with INH are uncommon; however, inhibition of the metabolism of diphenylhydantoin (phenytoin) and warfarin has been reported with high levels of INH. Rare side effects of INH include pellagra, hemolytic anemia in patients with glucose-6-phosphate dehydrogenase deficiency, systemic lupus erythematosus, and arthralgias.

RIFAMPIN (RIF). This broad-spectrum antibiotic is highly active against *M. tuberculosis*, is available in the United States in an oral preparation, and is usually administered during the fasting state as a single daily dose (10–20 mg/kg/24 hr). When administered twice weekly, the recommended dose is 10–20 mg/kg/dose, and the total daily dose should not exceed 600 mg. RIF is well absorbed from the gastrointestinal tract, penetrates into most tissues, including the cerebrospinal fluid, and is metabolized in the liver and excreted in urine and bile. *Side effects* are common and include an orange discoloration of tears (with permanent staining of soft contact lenses), urine, and saliva; gastrointestinal symptoms; and hepatotoxicity manifested as asymptomatic elevations in serum transaminase, particularly during the first few weeks of therapy. When RIF is administered with INH there is an increased risk of hepatotoxicity, which can be minimized by lowering the daily dose of INH to 10 mg/kg/24 hr. Intermittent administration of RIF has been associated with thrombocytopenia and leukopenia; an "influenza syndrome" consisting of fever, headache, and malaise; and a "respiratory syndrome" associated with dyspnea and wheezing. RIF interferes with the metabolism of a number of drugs including anticoagulants, oral contraceptives, corticosteroids, and oral hypoglycemic agents. RIF is teratogenic in laboratory animals and is contraindicated during the 1st trimester of pregnancy.

ETHAMBUTOL (ETM). This drug is active only against mycobacteria. It is administered orally as a single daily dose (15 mg/kg/24 hr) and is distributed to various body tissues but reaches low levels in the cerebrospinal fluid. In this dosage, ETM is bacteriostatic only, and its main role is to prevent the emergence of drug-resistant organisms. ETM is excreted through the kidney in an active, unchanged state, and, accordingly, high concentrations are found in the urine. Reversible ocular complications manifested as blurred vision, constriction of the visual field, and color blindness have been reported in adults and can be minimized by limiting the maximum daily dose to 20 mg/kg. Nevertheless, patients receiving this drug should be checked monthly for visual acuity, visual fields, and red-green color discrimination.

STREPTOMYCIN (STM). This antimicrobial is substantially less effective than INH or RIF but is more effective than ETM against *M. tuberculosis*. For life-threatening tuberculosis, STM is usually administered as a daily intramuscular dose (20–40 mg/kg/dose not to exceed 1 g) during the first few months of a 3-drug regimen (INH, RIF, and STM). STM diffuses rapidly into body fluids and tissues including tuberculous abscesses and caseous tissue, but it does not enter the cerebrospinal fluid unless meningitis is present. STM is filtered by the glomerulus and, unlike many other aminoglycoside antibiotics, rarely causes nephrotoxicity. The major *toxic effect* of STM is damage to the 8th cranial nerve, especially to the vestibular division, resulting in vertigo, ataxia, and, less commonly, hearing loss. STM is usually prescribed for a minimal period of time because the incidence of vestibular and cochlear damage is dose dependent.

PYRAZINAMIDE (PZA). When combined with INH, PZA is bactericidal against *M. tuberculosis*. The drug is administered orally in 2–3 divided doses (20 mg/kg/24 hr), is distributed to various body tissues, including the cerebrospinal fluid, and is excreted in the urine and bile. PZA's major limitations are its tendency to stimulate early drug resistance (which can be minimized by simultaneously administering other agents) and to cause hepatotoxicity, manifested as abnormal liver function test results and jaundice. PZA may cause arthralgias of both large and small joints, which usually responds to symptomatic treatment. This side effect may be related to inhibition of renal tubular secretion of uric acid and consequent hyperuricemia. PZA use in children has been limited because pediatric pharmacokinetic data are scarce. The total daily dose should not exceed 2 g.

PARA-AMINOSALICYLIC ACID (PAS). This principal companion drug to INH for many years has now been replaced by ETM and RIF.

ETHIONAMIDE (ETH). This is a moderately effective agent for *M. tuberculosis* and is used most often as a companion drug for the re-treatment of patients who have failed standard chemotherapy. Administered orally (15 mg/kg/24 hr) as a single daily dose, ETH is widely distributed throughout the body, including the cerebrospinal fluid. Gastrointestinal side effects are common and include nausea, vomiting, and abdominal pain due to the drug's direct effect upon the central nervous system. Use in children has been limited.

SINGLE-DRUG THERAPY

INH chemoprophylaxis is indicated for all asymptomatic tuberculin-positive infants, children, and adults under 35 yr who have a normal chest film and have never received antituberculosis therapy. Treatment for 9 mo is recommended to prevent subsequent reactivation and systemic disease. A chest roentgenogram is indicated prior to preventive treatment; if this is normal and if the child remains asymptomatic, a repeat film is not indicated. When daily INH chemoprophylaxis (10–20 mg/kg/24 hr up to 300 mg) cannot be administered owing to poor compliance, twice weekly supervised administration of INH (20–40 mg/kg/day up to 900 mg) is recommended, preferably following 1 mo of daily treatment. Hepatic dysfunction is uncommon in children receiving INH. Accordingly, in otherwise healthy children it is not necessary to obtain routine determinations of liver enzymes. However, liver function tests should be performed if one or more of the following conditions occur: (1) concurrent or recent liver disease, (2) clinical evidence of hepatic dysfunction, and (3) the higher daily dose of INH is used in combination with rifampin. Simultaneous administration of pyridoxine is recommended only for children and adolescents on meat- and milk-deficient diets and for women during pregnancy.

INH chemoprophylaxis for skin test–positive children and adolescents at risk for infection with INH-resistant microorganisms (e.g., Haitians, Asians) or for those in whom the consequences of infection are likely to be severe (e.g., young infants with household exposure to an infected adult) includes RIF (10 mg/kg/24 hr, up to 600 mg/24 hr) in addition to INH (10 mg/kg/24 hr) until susceptibility results are available. When the responsible pathogen is subsequently determined to be resistant to INH, the INH should be discontinued and RIF continued for a total of 12 mo. INH chemoprophylaxis (combined with RIF when drug resistance is suspected) is also indicated for skin test–negative, high-risk infants. In the case of children at risk (e.g., those who have household contact with an infected adult), INH and/or RIF is administered daily to the exposed infant for 3 mo, and a repeat skin test is performed. If skin test conversion occurs and the chest roentgenogram is normal, a complete 9-mo course of INH chemoprophylaxis is recommended. In those high-risk infants who continue to have a negative skin test result following 3 mo of INH and when the source of the infection is no longer contagious, INH should be discontinued. Following completion of INH chemoprophylaxis, any tuberculin-positive child who subsequently receives prolonged corticosteroid or other immunosuppressive therapy should simultaneously receive INH for the duration of this immunosuppressive therapy.

DOUBLE- OR TRIPLE-DRUG THERAPY

This treatment protocol consists of a 2-mo combination chemotherapy regimen of daily INH (10 mg/kg, up to 300 mg), RIF (10 mg/kg, up to 600 mg), and PZA (15–30 mg/kg, up to 900 mg) followed by 4 mo of twice weekly INH (20–40 mg/kg, up to 900 mg) plus RIF (10 mg/kg, up to 600 mg). This 6-mo regimen is recommended as treatment for newly diagnosed pulmonary and extrapulmonary disease in both children and adults. This treatment protocol results in rapid sterilization, is effective in the great majority of patients infected with organisms resistant to INH or STM, prevents emergence of acquired resistance during chemotherapy, and is very cost effective. Nevertheless, pediatric experience with this 6-mo regimen is limited in the United States, and, accordingly, many pediatric authorities recommend a 9-mo treatment regimen for children with newly diagnosed uncomplicated intrathoracic tuberculosis (i.e., pulmonary, pulmonary with hilar adenopathy, or positive tuberculin reaction and hilar adenopathy). This 9-mo regimen consists of daily INH (10 mg/kg, maximum 300 mg) and RIF (10–15 mg/kg, maximum 600 mg), for 3–4 wk followed by a twice weekly regimen of INH (20–40 mg/kg, maximum 900 mg) and RIF (10–20 mg/kg, maximum 600 mg) for the remainder of the 9-mo treatment period. Moreover, a third drug is recommended (e.g., PZA, STM, or ETM) when INH resistance is suspected so that the patient is treated with INH and at least two drugs to which the organism is likely to be susceptible. Therapeutic failure during chemotherapy in which resistant organisms emerge in patients with initially drug-sensitive strains is extraordinarily rare. If relapse occurs following chemotherapy, it usually occurs within 1 yr and is invariably due to drug-sensitive organisms. For treatment of extrapulmonary disease, administration of a third drug is recommended during the first 2 mo of the daily INH-RIF regimen (e.g., PZA, STM, or ETM) followed by INH-RIF for a total of 9 mo in children with isolated cervical lymphadenopathy, and 12 mo for children with miliary, meningeal, bone and joint, or renal disease.

Corticosteroid use in the treatment of pulmonary and extrapulmonary disease is limited to adults and children with pericarditis or meningitis and patients with systemic toxicity due to advanced pulmonary and/or miliary disease.

Adult patients who have *cavitary disease* and sputum that contains tubercle bacilli are noninfectious after 2 wk of chemotherapy that includes RIF. Similar criteria can be applied to infants and children. However, a longer period of isolation is suggested when close contacts include infants and children or if drug resistance is suspected; under these circumstances, the infectiousness of each child must be decided individually.

PREVENTION

The prevention of tuberculosis depends upon (1) preventing contact with those who are actively infected, (2) providing chemoprophylaxis (see earlier discussion), and (3) administering BCG to high-risk populations. General improvement in socioeconomic conditions is also an important factor in lowering the prevalence of this disease.

The indications for immunization against tuberculosis by intracutaneous inoculation with BCG remain controversial. The immunizing microorganism, an attenuated strain of *M. bovis,* was developed in the early part of the century and was subsequently demonstrated to decrease the incidence of tuberculosis, particularly in infants living in areas of high prevalence, and the mortality among tuberculosis-susceptible infants who had been immunized. However, some studies have not demonstrated this protective effect, possibly because of varying vaccine potency; improper preparation, storage, or administration of BCG; poor nutritional status of many vaccine recipients; and interference with vaccine-induced immunity by concurrent infection with nontuberculous mycobacteria.

BCG vaccination is recommended as a public health measure in developing countries with a high prevalence of tuberculosis (where skin test conversions exceed 1% annually). Pre-BCG tuberculin skin testing is usually recommended, but because this is often impractical, vaccine is usually administered without prior skin testing. (Reactions to BCG in tuberculin-positive children are rarely serious.) In countries with a low prevalence of tuberculosis, BCG vaccination is recommended for children with negative skin test results who are repeatedly exposed to untreated or inadequately treated adults and for children in subpopulations with a high infection rate and limited access to health care. BCG is *contraindicated* in children who have burns, skin infections, or cellular or combined immunodeficiencies, or who are receiving immunosuppressive agents. BCG immunization is also contraindicated in patients with AIDS. This latter contraindication is extremely important due to the increasing prevalence of HIV infection in infants and young children, particularly in Africa, where BCG vaccination is routine in infancy.

The vaccine should be stored in the dark and administered immediately following reconstitution. The recommended dose is 0.05 mL for neonates and 0.1 mL for infants and older children; it should be administered intradermally with syringe and needle. The preferred location of inoculation is the outer side of the upper arm at the insertion of the deltoid muscle. Percutaneous inoculation with a multiple-puncture apparatus and a concentrated vaccine is available. Administering BCG by jet injection is less effective and may cause several local reactions. Following successful immunization, a small papule forms at the inoculation site, gradually enlarges, crusts, and disappears in 8–12 wk. Whenever possible, a tuberculin skin test should be administered 2–3 mo following BCG and a second vaccination administered to children who have a negative skin test result. *Side effects* of BCG are uncommon and include cutaneous ulceration, localized lymphadenopathy, and, less commonly, subcutaneous abscess formation, osteomyelitis, a lupoid reaction, dissemination, and death. Severe local reactions can be controlled with antituberculous drugs; however, such treatment may inhibit the multiplication of BCG microorganisms and thus interferes with subsequent immunity; therefore, it should be discouraged.

A major theoretical disadvantage of BCG vaccination is the *production of sensitivity to tuberculin.* In developing countries with a high rate of childhood tuberculosis, most individuals become tuberculin positive during infancy, and premature production of tuberculin sensitivity due to BCG is of little consequence. In developed countries, in which there is a low risk of infection, the tuberculin skin test is an important technique for identifying cases of tuberculosis. Accordingly, the value of the skin test may outweigh the potential benefits of widespread administration of BCG, and, thus, many authorities discourage routine administration of BCG vaccine in countries such as the United States.

Skin test reactivity following BCG vaccination tends to decrease with time; by 10 yr following vaccination most individuals do not have a positive tuberculin skin test (10 mm or more of induration). Interpreting the significance of a positive tuberculin reaction in a BCG recipient is difficult and requires differentiating skin test reactivity due to BCG vaccination from reactivity due to natural infection. Most authorities recommend that a positive reaction be interpreted as indicative of acquired infection with *M. tuberculosis* and be treated accordingly. However, treatment can be withheld in asymptomatic children who have been recently (e.g., less than 5 yr) vaccinated with BCG, children with no history of exposure to tuberculosis, and children who have emigrated from a country with a low prevalence of tuberculosis.

TUBERCULOSIS DURING PREGNANCY

The potential hazards of ionizing radiation and antituberculosis chemotherapy for the pregnant woman and her unborn child have led to heavy reliance on tuberculin skin testing, limited use of roentgenographic examination, and caution in using drugs.

TUBERCULOSIS SCREENING. Since pregnancy does not inhibit cutaneous reactivity to tuberculin, all women except those with a history of a previous positive reaction should be skin tested at the first antenatal visit. A positive skin test warrants further investigation of the patient, family members, and close contacts to diagnose active disease. In asymptomatic women with a positive skin test result and normal physical findings, roentgenographic examination of the chest is deferred until after the 1st trimester. In obtaining roentgenograms during pregnancy, portable equipment, which excessively scatters radiation, should be avoided and the abdomen should be shielded to minimize the risk to the developing infant. Patients having positive skin tests and symptoms compatible with active disease or who have abnormal results on physical examination should have an immediate roentgenogram of the chest.

CHEMOPROPHYLAXIS. Pregnancy is a relative contraindication for isoniazid prophylaxis because of this drug's hepatotoxicity and because of the possible adverse effects of isoniazid on the developing fetus. Thus, asymptomatic pregnant women who have positive results on skin testing but whose chest roentgenograms show no active disease should not begin isoniazid prophylaxis until after their pregnancy. Symptomatic pregnant women or pregnant women who have roentgenographic evidence suggesting active disease should be hospitalized. Sputum and gastric aspirates should be collected, stained for acid-fast microorganisms, and cultured for *M. tuberculosis.* Women with sputum positive for acid-fast bacilli or who have clinical or radiologic findings compatible with active infection should receive treatment with INH, ETM, and pyridoxine (for 18 mo). RIF has proved to be teratogenic in animals, particularly when given in high doses, and therefore should be avoided in the treatment of women likely to become pregnant or who are less than 12 wk pregnant.

INFANTS BORN TO MOTHERS WITH ACTIVE TUBERCULOSIS. Since approximately 50% of infants born to mothers with active pulmonary tuberculosis develop disease within the 1st yr of life, prophylaxis for such infants is recommended. There is controversy, however, about whether such treatment should consist of BCG immunization or isoniazid administration. The advantages of BCG administration include probable effectiveness, lack of toxicity, and the need for only a single injection, which eliminates noncompliance and the need for follow-up examination. The disadvantages of BCG include the variability of response in immunized individuals, the limited value of subsequent tuberculin testing, and a necessary period of postimmunization separation of mother and infant prior to skin test conversion and protection. Isoniazid chemoprophylaxis has proved to be efficacious and permits continued use of tuberculin skin testing to document subsequent infection. Its major disadvantages are noncompliance in administering prophylactic medication and the lack of information on the pharmacology of isoniazid when administered during the neonatal period. Combining BCG immunization and isoniazid administration until skin test conversion occurs has been recommended. However, recent studies suggest the addition of isoniazid to the BCG regimen does not improve protection. Management of newborn infants born to mothers with a positive tuberculin skin test reaction and no evidence of active disease is less problematic. Screening of all potential household contacts is indicated. If active disease is not identified in household contacts and all others likely to be exposed to the infant, an intermediate-strength tuberculin skin test (Mantoux, 5 TU PPD) should be applied to the infant at 4–6 wk of age, at 3–4 mo of age, and again at 1 yr. The absence of skin test reactivity precludes treatment with INH.

The management approach outlined in Table 12–29 should be individualized for the newborn infant, taking into consideration the home environment and subsequent availability of the treated infant for follow-up evaluation.

WILLIAM T. SPECK

Abernathy RS, Dutt AK, Stead WW, et al: Short course chemotherapy for tuberculosis in children. Pediatrics 72:801, 1983.

Alvarez S, McCabe WR: Extrapulmonary tuberculosis revisited: A review of experience at Boston City and other hospitals. Medicine 63:25, 1984.

American Thoracic Society: Diagnostic standards and classification of tuberculosis. Am Rev Respir Dis 142:725, 1990.

American Thoracic Society and the Centers for Disease Control: Treatment of tuberculosis and tuberculosis infection in adults and children. Am Rev Respir Dis 134:355, 1986.

Comstock GW: Frost revisited: The modern epidemiology of tuberculosis. Am Rev Respir Dis 101:363, 1985.

Daniel TM: New approaches to the rapid diagnosis of tuberculous meningitis. J Infect Dis 155:599, 1987.

Fine PEM: The BCG story: Lessons from the past and implications for the future. Rev Infect Dis 2:353, 1989.

Grosset, JH: Present status of chemotherapy for tuberculosis. Rev Infect Dis 2:347, 1989.

Hsu KH: Thirty years after isoniazid. Its impact on tuberculosis in children and adolescents. JAMA 251:1283, 1984.

Kendig EL: Current status report: evolution of short-course antimicrobial treatment of tuberculosis in children, 1951–1984. Pediatrics 75:684, 1985.

Molavi A, le Frock JL: Tuberculous meningitis. Med Clin North Am 69:315, 1985.

O'Brien R, Long M, Cross F, et al: Hepatotoxicity from isoniazid and rifampin among children treated for tuberculosis. Pediatrics 72:491, 1983.

Perinatal Prophylaxis of Tuberculosis (Editorial). Lancet 336:1479, 1990.

TABLE 12–29. Management of Infants of Mothers with Positive Tuberculin Skin Test*

Mother	Management of Infant
Asymptomatic	No immediate prophylaxis necessary; tuberculin test every 3 mo for 1 yr If positive, rule out active tuberculosis If active disease, begin therapy If no active disease, begin isoniazid prophylaxis† If negative tuberculin, retest annually
Past history of treated active tuberculosis, presumably asymptomatic	Same as above
X-ray consistent with questionable or minimally active disease‡	Rule out congenital tuberculosis If present, begin therapy If not present, BCG§ vaccination or isoniazid prophylaxis
Advanced pulmonary or extrapulmonary tuberculosis, or disseminated infection	Rule out congenital tuberculosis If present, begin triple therapy If not present, isoniazid for 1 yr, or isoniazid for 3 mo followed by chest x-ray and tuberculin; if both negative, give BCG; if tuberculin reactive and chest negative, give isoniazid; if chest positive, begin total therapy for 1 yr

*After Weinstein L, Murphy T: The management of tuberculosis during pregnancy. Clin Perinatol 1:395, 1974.

†Isoniazid prophylaxis: 15–20 mg/kg/24 hr given as a single dose.

‡Mothers with active disease should be treated and separated from their infants until noncontagious.

§BCG is recommended when noncompliance and/or loss to follow-up examination is considered likely in situations in which the infant will be exposed to endemic tuberculosis in the environment.

12.48 NONTUBERCULOUS MYCOBACTERIA INFECTION

Nontuberculous, nonleprous *Mycobacterium* species (variously referred to as tuberculoid bacilli and as unclassified, anonymous, or atypical mycobacteria) are members of the family of Mycobacteriaceae, whose staining and morphologic characteristics are similar to those of *M. tuberculosis*. They differ from the tubercle bacilli in their rate of growth, nutritional requirements, ability to produce pigments, enzymatic activity, temperature sensitivity, and resistance to antituberculous agents. Although more than 100 species of atypical mycobacteria are recognized, only five *(M. kansasii, M. avium-intracellulare, M. marinum, M. scrofulaceum,* and *M. chelonei)* are commonly associated with human disease.

ETIOLOGY AND EPIDEMIOLOGY. Atypical mycobacteria are distributed worldwide and are ubiquitous in the environment, existing as saprophytes in soil and water, as pathogens in swine, birds, and cattle, and as part of the normal human pharyngeal flora. Infection, which occurs following inhalation or inoculation, is relatively common in warm, humid, rural environments; in the United States infections occur most commonly in the southern states. The AIDS epidemic has focused increasing attention on atypical mycobacteria because 20% or more of patients with AIDS die with disseminated infection caused by *M. avium-intracellulare*. Pulmonary infection in adult white males with chronic obstructive pulmonary disease is also a common clinical manifestation. Skin and soft tissue infections in infants and children occur less frequently than lymphatic infections, and disseminated disease in children is rare except when associated with compromised immune function.

CLASSIFICATION. The pathogenic and nonpathogenic atypical mycobacteria were traditionally divided into four groups: Slow-growing mycobacteria were classified as photochromogens (group I), which form pigment following exposure to light; as scotochromogens (group II), which form pigment in the dark; and as nonchromogens (group III), which fail to produce pigment. Rapid-growing atypical mycobacteria form group IV. Now, because of improved ability to identify the individual species, they are identified by species. Biochemically and immunologically closely related strains are referred to as "complexes," e.g., the *M. fortuitum-chelonei* complex or the *M. avium-intracellulare–scrofulaceum* (MAIS) complex.

PATHOLOGY AND IMMUNITY. The histologic appearances of the pathologic lesions produced by the tuberculous and nontuberculous mycobacteria are often indistinguishable. When there are differences, the histologic lesion of atypical mycobacteria may resemble "nonspecific" inflammation more than it resembles granuloma formation, and the lesion, instead of caseating, may liquefy rather quickly. Definitive diagnosis requires isolation of microorganisms from clinical specimens. The immune response to infection with atypical mycobacteria has not been extensively studied; however, it is presumed to be similar to the interactions observed between the tubercle bacilli, lymphocyte subpopulations, and tissue macrophages. Skin testing in the past has been of limited clinical value because the skin test antigens were poorly standardized and lacked sensitivity and specificity. However, the Centers For Disease Control (CDC) has recently prepared a new series of nontuberculous mycobacterium skin test antigens that are highly sensitive and specific for infection with these organisms and may hold promise as a noninvasive diagnostic test in the future.

CLINICAL MANIFESTATIONS. *Lymphadenitis* of the submandibular or anterior cervical nodes is the most frequent manifestation of atypical mycobacterial infection in children. Preauricular, posterior cervical, axillary, and inguinal nodes may also become involved. The initial pharyngeal lesion is rarely distinguished, and the cutaneous one may have disappeared or appear so insignificant that it is not recognized. Although children may appear sick and have a high temperature, affected children 1–5 yr of age usually lack constitutional symptoms and have no history of exposure to tuberculosis. Lymph node involvement is invariably unilateral, and the chest roentgenogram is normal. In the absence of treatment, the involved nodes suppurate, rupture, and form cutaneous sinus tracts; chronic drainage resembles the classic scrofula of tuberculosis. In the United States the *M. avium-intracellulare* complex and *M. scrofulaceum* are usually the responsible pathogens; however, *M. kansasii* is also recovered in a number of instances.

The differential diagnosis includes lymphadenitis due to viruses, other bacteria including *M. tuberculosis, Toxoplasma,* and the agent causing cat-scratch disease. Noninfectious causes of lymphadenopathy must also be considered; these include malignancies, sarcoidosis, and drug reactions (phenytoin). The tuberculin skin test is usually negative (less than 10 mm of induration to PPD-S), although intermediate reactions (5–10 mm) are not uncommon. Definitive diagnosis requires excision of an involved node (removal of all involved nodes is not necessary) and recovery of the responsible pathogen. Surgery without chemotherapy is curative in 95% of cases.

Cutaneous disease due to atypical mycobacteria occurs less frequently in children than superficial lymphadenitis. Infection usually follows percutaneous inoculation with fresh or salt water contaminated by *M. marinum*. Within several weeks of exposure, a solitary nodule develops at the site of minor abrasions on the elbows, knees, or feet ("swimming pool granuloma") and on the hands and fingers of fish fanciers ("fish tank granuloma"). The lesions eventually enlarge and ulcerate until they resemble the warty lesions seen in cutaneous tuberculosis. The lesions of a minority of patients resemble sporotrichosis; satellite lesions near the site of entry extend along the skin following the superficial lymphatics.

Diagnosis depends on isolating the responsible microorganisms from an excised granuloma. The cutaneous lesions usually heal spontaneously following incision and drainage, without other therapy. Heat treatment has been advocated because this pathogen is sensitive to high temperatures. Antibiotic therapy is indicated for intractable cases. All isolates are resistant to isoniazid, and drug treatment usually consists of one of three regimens: rifampin and ethambutol, trimethoprim-sulfamethoxazole, or doxycycline. Corticosteroids are contraindicated because they enhance local spread.

M. ulcerans also causes cutaneous infection in children living in tropical countries (Africa, Australia, and South America). Infection follows percutaneous inoculation and presents as a painless erythematous nodule on an extremity, which undergoes central necrosis and ulceration *(Buruli ulcers)*. The lesion, which has a characteristic undermined edge, gradually expands and may result in extensive soft tissue destruction with secondary bacterial infection. Diagnosis depends on isolation of the responsible pathogen and treatment requires extensive surgical excision.

Skin and soft tissue infections due to *M. fortuitum-chelonei* complex are rare in children and usually follow percutaneous inoculation due to puncture wounds and minor abrasions. Clinical disease usually arises after a 3- to 4-wk incubation period and presents as a localized cellulitis or a draining abscess. Superficial infections usually resolve following surgical incision and open drainage; however, deep-seated infections require initial therapy with parenteral amikacin and cefoxitin combined with oral probenecid, pending susceptibility testing.

In unusual circumstances, the atypical mycobacteria may cause *bone and joint infections* that are indistinguishable from those produced by *M. tuberculosis*. Such infections usually result from operative incision or accidental puncture wounds.

Pulmonary infection with *M. kansasii* is uncommon in children and can be mistaken for tuberculosis. The onset is usually insidious and consists of low-grade fever, cough, night sweats, and general malaise. Thin-walled cavities are characteristic, but radiographic findings may resemble those of tuberculosis. Pulmonary infection should be treated with isoniazid, rifampin, and ethambutol for 12 mo, supplemented during the first 2 mo with biweekly streptomycin.

Disseminated disease may occur in individuals who have severe immunologic defects or who are receiving immunosuppressive therapy. In children, the responsible pathogens are usually the *M. avium-intracellulare* complex. Continuous bacteremia has been described in children having acquired immunodeficiency syndrome. Empiric chemotherapy for disseminated disease due to *M. avium-intracellulare* should be initiated with at least four drugs and often six drugs. Clofazimine and rifampin in combination with isoniazid and ethambutol may be useful. Streptomycin, rifampin, and amikacin have also been used in various combinations with these drugs as empiric therapy for infection. A recent report suggests the combination of amikacin, ethambutol, rifampin, and ciprofloxacin for treatment of disseminated *M. avium-intracellulare* infections. Duration of therapy ranges from 6 to 24 mo.

WILLIAM T. SPECK
JAMES B. BESUNDER

Chiu J, Nussbaum J, Bozzehe S, et al: Treatment of disseminated *Mycobacterium avium* complex infections in AIDS with amikacin, ethambutol, rifampin, and ciprofloxacin. Ann Intern Med 113:358, 1990.

Del Beccaro MA, Mendelman PM, Nolan C: Diagnostic usefulness of mycobacterial skin test antigens in childhood lymphadenitis. Pediatr Infect Dis J 8:206, 1989.

Levin RH, Bolinger AM: Treatment of non-tuberculous mycobacterial infections in pediatric patients. Clin Pharmacy 7:545, 1988.

Ljungberg B, Christensson B, Grubb R: Failure of doxycycline treatment in aquarium-associated *Mycobacterium marinum* infections. Scand J Infect Dis 19:539, 1987.

Wallace RJ, Swenson JM, Silcox VA, et al: Spectrum of disease due to rapidly growing mycobacteria. Rev Infect Dis 5:657, 1983.

Wolinsky, E: Nontuberculous mycobacteria and associated disease. Am Rev Respir Dis 119:107, 1979.

12.49 LEPROSY (HANSEN'S DISEASE)

Leprosy is a chronic disease produced by infection with *Mycobacterium leprae* and the ensuing host response. The organs most prominently affected are the skin and the peripheral nervous system, but upper respiratory, testicular, and ocular involvement are also relatively common. Man was long believed to be the sole host of *M. leprae*, but naturally acquired infection has been documented in armadillos in the southeastern United States, and experimental infection has been established in primates, nude mice, and armadillos.

Chronic skin lesions, madarosis, sensory neuropathy resulting in the loss of digits or limbs, and paresis secondary to motor nerve dysfunction are among the sequelae of leprosy. The highly visible nature of these debilities led to the historical stigmatization of the "leper." The psychologic and sociologic sequelae of this stigma can be as debilitating as the disease itself and may result in delays in seeking medical attention. To combat this prejudice, the term "leprosy patient" has replaced the word "leper," and "Hansen's disease" has become an accepted designation.

ETIOLOGY. *M. leprae* is an acid-fast bacillus of the family Mycobacteriaceae. The exceedingly slow multiplication of *M. leprae* observed in animal models may partially explain the long incubation period seen in human disease; a period of 3–5 yr is believed to be typical. The rare occurrence of leprosy in infants as young as 3 mo of age suggests that in utero transmission may occur or that very short incubation periods may be possible in certain situations. Possible modes of transmission include contact with desquamated infected epidermis, ingestion of infected breast milk, and bites of mosquitoes or other vectors. At present, however, transmission via infected nasal secretions appears to be the basis for most infections. Extensive involvement of the nasopharynx manifested as chronic rhinitis is common in lepromatous disease.

EPIDEMIOLOGY. The World Health Organization estimated that worldwide there were 11 million cases of leprosy in 1975. This figure must be considered an underestimate because of inadequate case finding and reporting. The insidious onset of the disease and the social stigma assigned to it delay medical consultation, and the lack of an inexpensive, simple diagnostic test makes confirmation of the diagnosis difficult.

Most of the world's leprosy patients reside in Africa, India, Southeast Asia, and Central and South America. Prevalence rates vary widely between and within countries; the highest rates for entire countries are 25 or more cases per 1,000 population, but rates as high as 200 cases per 1,000 population have been found in small, hyperendemic pockets. Human-to-human transmission accounts for an overwhelming majority of cases; a high percentage of them occur in family members or in close contacts of known patients. Approximately 200 cases are reported annually in the United States, of which 90% are in immigrants. The remaining 10% develop in localized foci along the Gulf coast, in Hawaii, and in the Micronesian territories.

Leprosy occurs at all ages, but infections in infants are extremely rare; incidence rates peak during childhood and early adulthood in endemic areas.

PATHOGENESIS AND PATHOLOGY. Damage is mediated through many pathways, some of which are release of humoral mediators of inflammation by activated lymphocytes and macrophages, nerve compression by enlarging granulomata, and deposition of immune complexes. Multiple mechanisms may operate simultaneously or sequentially.

The site of entry of *M. leprae* into the human host is unknown. Primary respiratory or gastrointestinal tract involvement has not been documented prior to the appearance of lesions involving the skin and peripheral nerves. Growth and multiplication of *M. leprae* are maximal at 34–35° C. Nothing is known of the host immune responses in the initial period after infection, but skin testing (Mitsuda reaction, see later) and serologic studies suggest that up to 80–90% of those infected develop immunity without ever manifesting clinical disease. Most of the remaining patients, after a highly variable incubation period, develop typical skin lesions of *indeterminate leprosy*.

Fully developed clinical leprosy is classified into five categories that can be aligned upon a spectrum representing the range of intensity and efficacy of the cellular limb of the host immune response.

One end of the spectrum is *polar tuberculoid leprosy*, in which there is a vigorous and specific cell-mediated immune response. In tissue biopsies there are tightly organized granulomas composed of epithelioid cells and lymphocytes, but bacilli are scant or absent. Macrophages, when present, do not contain intracellular organisms. Caseation is rare. Nerve involvement is usually limited to cutaneous sensory nerve endings and to, at most, a single peripheral nerve trunk.

At the other end of the spectrum is *polar lepromatous leprosy*, in which there is total and specific anergy to *M. leprae* both by skin testing and by in vitro assays of cell-mediated immunity. Large amounts of circulating and tissue-based antibody to mycobacterial antigens are present, but they afford no protective immunity. Bacilli are found in enormous numbers in the skin, nasal mucosa, and peripheral nerves. There is continual bacillemia as well as bacillary invasion of all major organs except the central nervous system. Tissue granulomas are poorly formed and are composed chiefly of loose aggregates of foamy histiocytes. Macrophages teeming with undigested bacilli (globi) are common. There is extensive, symmetric involvement of peripheral nerves, although the cutaneous nerve endings are usually spared.

An *M. leprae*–specific suppressor T cell population is found in the circulation of patients with lepromatous leprosy, and increased numbers of suppressor T cells are found in their skin granulomas. T cells from lepromatous patients also produce less interleukin 2 and less gamma interferon following stimulation with *M. leprae* antigens than do T cells from tuberculoid patients or normal controls. These findings may relate to the underlying cellular defect that permits development of clinical leprosy in the susceptible individual.

Borderline or *dimorphous leprosy* is subdivided into three subclasses that lie between the tuberculoid and lepromatous poles on the clinical spectrum.

CLINICAL MANIFESTATIONS. Indeterminate Leprosy (I). This is the earliest clinically detectable form of leprosy. Although it is observed in only 10–20% of infected individuals, it is a stage through which most patients with advanced leprosy have passed. Usually there is a single hypopigmented macule, 2–4 cm in diameter, with a poorly defined border but having no erythema or induration. Anesthesia is minimal or absent, particularly if the lesion is on the face. Biopsies of tissue may contain granulomas, but bacilli are rarely demonstrable. The histopathology is not distinctive; the diagnosis is usually made by exclusion, in contacts (especially children) of leprosy patients. In 50–75% of patients with indeterminate leprosy, the lesions heal spontaneously; in the remainder, they progress to one of the classic forms. Thus, only 5–10 of every 100 infected individuals are likely to develop progressive leprosy.

Polar Tuberculoid (TT). There is usually a single, large (often over 10 cm in diameter) lesion with a well-demarcated, elevated erythematous rim. The interior of the lesion is flat, atrophic, hypopigmented, and anesthetic. Rarely, there may be as many as four lesions. The closest superficial nerve is often impressively thickened. The ulnar, posterior tibial, and great auricular nerves are most commonly affected. Periodic examination of all leprosy patients and their contacts should include palpation of these nerves. Without therapy, the lesion tends to enlarge slowly, but documented instances of spontaneous resolution exist. The coloration of the rim slowly fades with therapy, and the induration resolves, resulting in a flat lesion with central hypopigmentation and a ring of postinflammatory hyperpigmentation. Loss of hair follicles, sweat glands, cutaneous nerve receptors, and of sensation in the central portion of the lesion is irreversible. Marked improvement should be apparent within 1–2 mo after initiating therapy, but complete resolution may take up to 8–12 mo. There is an entity of "pure neural" tuberculoid leprosy, which presents as a mononeuropathy with prominent nerve thickening but no cutaneous lesions. Histopathology is mandatory to establish this diagnosis. Nerve trunk size varies widely, and overdiagnosis of "enlarged" nerves is common among inexperienced observers. Nodular or fusiform nerve thickening has greater diagnostic value than a palpable nerve that is smooth and symmetric.

Borderline Leprosy. The clinical and histologic criteria for the three subdivisions of borderline leprosy are less well defined than are those of the two polar categories. In contrast to the tuberculoid and lepromatous patterns, those in the borderline divisions are unstable. For example, host or bacterial factors can result in "downgrading" the clinical condition toward the lepromatous pattern or "upgrading" it toward the tuberculoid pattern. Therapy is the most common cause of upgrading reactions; downgrading can be seen in conditions that compromise host immunity, for example, pregnancy. Clinical characteristics of the three generally accepted borderline subclasses are as follows:

In *borderline tuberculoid (BT)* leprosy the lesions are greater in number but smaller in size than in tuberculoid leprosy. There may be small satellite lesions around older lesions, and the margins of the borderline tuberculoid lesions are less distinct and the center is less atrophic and anesthetic. There is usually thickening of two or more superficial nerves.

In the *borderline (BB)* pattern the lesions are more numerous and more heterogeneous in appearance. They may become confluent, and plaques may be present. The borders are poorly defined, and the erythematous rim fades into the surrounding skin. There may be anesthesia, but hypesthesia is more common. Mild to moderate nerve thickening is common, but severe muscle wasting and neuropathy are unusual.

In the *borderline lepromatous (BL)* pattern, there are a large number of asymmetrically distributed lesions that are heterogeneous in appearance. Macules, papules, plaques, and nodules may all coexist. Individual lesions are small unless confluent. Anesthesia is mild and superficial nerve trunks are spared. The initial response to therapy is often dramatic; nodules and plaques flatten within 2–3 mo. With continued therapy the lesions become macular and almost invisible.

Polar Lepromatous Leprosy (LL). The lesions are innumerable, often confluent, and symmetric. Initially there may be only vague macules or even uniform, diffuse skin infiltrations without discernible lesions. As the disease progresses, the lesions become increasingly papular and nodular, so that with the diffuse thickening and infiltration of the skin, the characteristic leonine facies accompanied by loss of the eyebrows and distortion of the earlobes becomes apparent. Anesthesia of the lesions either does not occur or is mild, but a symmetric peripheral sensory neuropathy may develop. Testicular infiltration leading to azoospermia, infertility, and gynecomastia is common in adults but not in children. Bacilli are demonstrable in most internal organs other than the central nervous system, but tissue damage or interference with function is infrequent. Glomerulonephritis, when it occurs, is felt to be secondary to immune complex deposition rather than to infection per se. The initial response to therapy may be encouraging but is often followed by a long (2–5 yr) period of very slow improvement. In true polar lepromatous leprosy, the specific anergy to the leprosy bacillus persists despite therapy, thus making the patient theoretically susceptible to relapse if even a single viable bacillus remains at the end of therapy.

Reactional States. Acute clinical exacerbations are common in leprosy and are believed to reflect abrupt changes in the host-parasite immunologic balance. Although these reactional states do occur in the absence of therapy, they are especially common during the initial years of treatment. Three major variants are recognized:

Erythema nodosum leprosum (ENL) occurs in the majority of patients with polar lepromatous leprosy and in 25–40% of borderline lepromatous cases. Tender dermal nodules, clinically resembling erythema nodosum, are the hallmark of this syndrome. High fever, migrating polyarthralgia, orchitis, and increased activity in pre-existing cutaneous lesions complete the clinical picture. Circulating and tissue-based immune complexes are frequently present and may explain the resemblance to other immune complex disorders, but the underlying mechanism appears to involve the activation of a helper T cell subset. There is a strong tendency to recurrence, and there is a risk of amyloidosis and renal failure if treatment is inadequate.

Reversal reactions are observed throughout the borderline range. Acute tenderness and inflammation at the site of existing cutaneous and neural lesions and the development of new lesions are the major manifestations. Fever and systemic toxicity are uncommon, but the acute neuritis can lead to irreversible nerve injury if it is not treated immediately. Reversal reactions constitute perhaps the only "medical emergency" related to leprosy per se. Patients should be instructed to contact their physicians immediately if signs of a reaction appear. A sudden increase in effective cell-mediated immunity with rapid killing of bacilli within nerve sheaths is the initiating event.

Lucio's phenomenon, a severe, necrotizing, cutaneous vasculitis, is uncommon; it occurs predominantly in patients of Mexican origin who have diffuse lepromatous leprosy. Conventional therapy for vasculitis has had only modest success, and fatalities are common. Experimental therapies, including plasmapheresis and cyclophosphamide, have been successful in isolated cases. The pathogenesis is unknown, although immune complexes almost certainly contribute.

DIAGNOSIS. The critical factor in the diagnosis of leprosy is its inclusion in the differential diagnosis of a skin disorder in anyone who has resided in an endemic leprosy region. Anesthetic skin lesions with or without thickened peripheral nerves are virtually pathognomonic of leprosy. A full-thickness skin biopsy from an active lesion (stained with both a standard histologic stain and an acid-fast stain such as Fite-Faraco) is the optimal procedure for confirmation of the diagnosis and accurate disease classification. Acid-fast bacilli are rarely found in patients with indeterminate or tuberculoid disease, so diagnosis in these cases is based on the clinical picture and the presence of typical dermal granulomas. Other routine clinical, microbiologic, and radiologic tests have little or no role in the diagnosis of leprosy, although they may be useful in the exclusion of other diagnoses. Various assays for serum antibodies directed against unique antigens of *M. leprae* have been developed, but current tests lack sufficient sensitivity and specificity for active disease to be useful for clinical diagnostic purposes.

Lepromin is a suspension of killed *M. leprae* obtained from infected human or armadillo tissue. Following intradermal inoculation, early (48 hr, Fernandez reaction) as well as late (3–4 wk, Mitsuda reaction) reactions may be seen. The Mitsuda reaction, a granulomatous response to the antigen, is more consistent. Patients with tuberculoid leprosy have strongly positive (5 mm) responses, whereas patients with lepromatous leprosy do not respond. The test is not useful in the diagnosis of leprosy, since the majority of the population in both endemic and nonendemic leprosy areas will be Mitsuda positive. Lepromin is not available in the United States.

Many diseases endemic in developing countries can mimic the appearance of leprosy; these include secondary syphilis, cutaneous leishmaniasis, yaws, and cutaneous fungal infections. None of these entities involves paresthesia/anesthesia localized to the skin lesions or causes thickening of peripheral nerves. The presence of nerve thickening with skin lesions also differentiates leprosy from primary neurologic disease. Indeterminate leprosy may present with minimal anesthesia, no nerve thickening, and equivocal histopathology suggesting a superficial fungal infection, particularly tinea versicolor. The diagnosis of indeterminate leprosy should be considered one of exclusion and will rarely be made in anyone other than a close contact of a known patient.

TREATMENT. Only three antimycobacterial agents have proven to be consistently effective in the treatment of leprosy.

Since the early 1940s, *dapsone* (diaminodiphenyl sulfone) has remained the cornerstone of therapy because of its low cost, minimal toxicity, and wide availability. Unfortunately, secondary resistance tends to develop when it is used as the sole agent. More worrisome is the increasing incidence of primary resistance, which has been reported in up to 30% of newly diagnosed patients in Malaysia and Ethiopia. Dermatitis, hepatitis, and methemoglobinemia are the most common side effects; granulocytopenia is rare but potentially fatal. Dose-related hemolytic anemia, which can be severe, is seen in patients with glucose-6-phosphate dehydrogenase (G-6-PD) deficiency, methemoglobin reductase deficiency, or hemoglobin M. Pregnancy studies have not shown an increased risk of fetal abnormalities.

Rifampin is the most rapidly mycobactericidal drug for *M. leprae*, achieving excellent levels inside cells, where most leprosy bacilli reside. Resistance has been reported infrequently. The widespread use of rifampin has been limited by cost more than by toxicity. Hepatitis is the most common side effect that necessitates discontinuance.

Clofazimine, a phenazine dye with both antimycobacterial and anti-inflammatory activity, is particularly useful in cases of dapsone resistance or when recurrent reactional states have developed. The pharmacokinetics are poorly understood, but the half-life is several days. The drug is avidly taken up by epithelial cells, a feature that may be important for its activity but also results in cutaneous hyperpigmentation, ichthyosis, xerosis, and enteritis. The intense reddish-brown discoloration of the skin is cosmetically a deterrent to use and often results in discontinuation or poor compliance.

The increasing incidence of drug-resistant *M. leprae* has led to an intensified search for alternative therapeutic agents. Minocycline, certain second-generation quinolones, and some new macrolide derivatives have shown promise in experimental models or preliminary human trials.

Delineation of the optimal therapeutic regimens for leprosy has been hampered by deficient patient compliance, the long durations of therapy required, and inadequacies in the long-term follow-up for late relapses. The following recommendations reflect the standard of practice among leprologists in the United States; they differ slightly from those of WHO, which largely reflect the economic realities in developing countries. The initial treatment regimen is determined by the number of bacilli in the skin (as estimated by smear or biopsy) and the histology of the skin lesions. The duration of therapy is dependent on both the initial histology and the clinical and microbiologic response.

Paucibacillary patients (bacillary index ≤2+: all indeterminate and polar tuberculoid and most borderline tuberculoid patients) should receive dapsone (2 mg/kg/24 hr up to 100 mg/24 hr) and rifampin (20 mg/kg/24 hr up to 600 mg/24 hr) for 6–12 mo (depending on the clinical response), followed by dapsone alone to complete 1 yr of therapy for patients with indeterminate leprosy and 2–3 yr for those with tuberculoid and borderline tuberculoid disease. All patients with lepromatous or borderline lepromatous disease and most patients with borderline disease have large numbers of bacilli present in the skin (multibacillary leprosy). Common practice in the United States is to initiate treatment with dapsone and rifampin (same dosages as above) for a minimum of 2 yr, followed by dapsone alone for at least 10 yr after skin smears or biopsies become negative for morphologically intact bacilli. Patients with lepromatous and borderline lepromatous disease may require therapy for life. WHO recommends the addition of clofazimine (optimal dosage has not been determined for children; adult dose ranges from 50 to 100 mg/24 hr) to the dapsone-rifampin regimen in patients with multibacillary disease, particularly in areas in which there is a high prevalence of primary dapsone resistance.

Therapy of reactional states can become very complicated and will generally require expert consultation. Erythema nodosum leprosum usually responds to corticosteroid therapy (1 mg/kg/24 hr of prednisone) but often relapses when the drug is discontinued. Clinical remission of acute and suppression of chronic erythema nodosum can be achieved with thalidomide.* *Thalidomide is absolutely contraindicated in women of child-bearing age*; otherwise it is much safer than corticosteroids for chronic use. The major side effect is fatigue. Pediatric dosages have not been established. Clofazimine is also useful in managing chronic erythema nodosum. Reversal reactions are optimally treated with corticosteroids. Alternate-day regimens may be effective in patients with frequent relapses.

Serial skin smears or repeat biopsies are useful in assessing response to therapy. Bacilli in the skin are quantitated on a logarithmic scale (bacillary index). Four to 8 yr of effective therapy are commonly required in lepromatous patients before the bacillary index becomes zero, but the appearance of the bacilli will gradually change, becoming first beaded and then fragmented. Persistence of intact bacilli in the skin or nerves during therapy suggests poor patient compliance or drug resistance and usually correlates with clinical failure or recrudescence. Drug sensitivity testing of *M. leprae* is difficult and not widely available but may be necessary to confirm suspected drug resistance.

PROGNOSIS. The prognosis for arresting progression of

---

*Thalidomide is available as an investigational agent through the Gillis W. Long Hansen's Disease Center, Carville, Louisiana. The Gillis W. Long Hansen's Disease Center and its Regional Centers are available for consultation and assistance in patient management. The use of this service is strongly encouraged.

tissue and nerve damage is good, but recovery of lost sensory and motor function is variable and generally incomplete; hyperpigmentation, hypopigmentation, and loss of skin organs persist. Intercurrent reactional states, poor compliance, and emergence of dapsone resistance can all lead to clinical exacerbations or relapses necessitating close follow-up of patients. Much of the chronic debility results from repeated trauma to anesthetic digits and limbs. Careful counseling of patients and consultation with physical and occupational therapy services is essential for an optimal outcome.

PREVENTION. Two approaches are advocated for interrupting leprosy transmission in endemic areas. The first is directed at the risk of infection among household contacts of leprosy patients, especially those with multibacillary disease. It is based on regular periodic examination of contacts and early treatment at the first evidence of leprosy. Prophylactic therapy is reserved for special circumstances so that the inappropriate treatment of the 90–95% of contacts not expected to develop leprosy can be avoided.

The second approach to leprosy control has been through vaccination. Results from clinical trials with various vaccines, including BCG, have been disappointing, but the recent cloning of the genes for the major antigens of *M. leprae* has renewed hope for the development of an effective vaccine.

One historical practice that has fortunately been abandoned is the forcing of leprosy patients into leprosariums. Mouse footpad inoculation studies have demonstrated that viability of *M. leprae* in skin biopsies falls sharply within 3 wk of initiating therapy with dapsone and rifampin. This rapid drop in infectivity combined with the high probability that family members have had prolonged exposure to the patient prior to the diagnosis makes physical isolation of leprosy patients unnecessary.

RICHARD A. MILLER

Bloom BR, Godal T: Selective primary health care. Strategies for control of disease in the developing world. V. Leprosy. Rev Infect Dis 5:765, 1983.
Brubaker ML, Meyers WM, Bourland J: Leprosy in children one year of age and under. Int J Lepr 53:517, 1985.
Chemotherapy of leprosy (Editorial). Lancet 2:487, 1988.
Neill MA, Hightower AL, Broome CV: Leprosy in the United States, 1971–1981. J Infect Dis 152:1064, 1985.
Ridley DS, Jopling WH: Classification of leprosy according to immunity: A five-group system. Int J Lepr 34:255, 1966.
Sehgal VN, Srivastava G: Leprosy in children. Int J Dermatol 26:557, 1987.
Young RA, Mehra V, Sweester D, et al: Genes for the major protein antigens of *Mycobacterium leprae*. Nature 316:450, 1985.

SPIROCHETAL DISEASES

12.50 SYPHILIS

ETIOLOGY. Syphilis is a systemic, communicable infection caused by *Treponema pallidum*, a long, slender, tightly coiled, motile spirochete with finely tapered ends belonging to the family Spirochaetaceae and the genus *Treponema*. The pathogenic members of this genus include *T. pallidum* (syphilis), *T. pertenue* (yaws), and *T. carateum* (pinta). Because these microorganisms stain poorly, detection in clinical specimens requires darkfield microscopy or immunofluorescent staining techniques. *T. pallidum* cannot be cultured in vitro, and laboratory isolation requires animal inoculation.

EPIDEMIOLOGY. Two forms of syphilis may be encountered by the pediatrician. *Congenital* (fetal) *syphilis* results from transplacental transmission of spirochetes; infant contact with a maternal chancre may rarely lead to postnatal infection. The risk of transplacental transmission varies with the stage of maternal illness. Untreated pregnant women with primary and secondary syphilis and spirochetemia are more likely to transmit infection to their unborn infants than are women with latent infection. Transmission may occur throughout pregnancy but is most likely in the 3rd trimester. The incidence of congenital syphilis has increased in the past 10 yr.

Acquired syphilis results almost exclusively from sexual contact. The incidence within the United States has increased dramatically during the 1980s, most notably among inner city minority populations in the Northeast, Southeast, and West Coast areas of the country. This spread has resulted in a concomitant increase in the rate of congenital infection. The incidence among homosexual males, another high-risk population, has decreased in the latter part of the decade owing to changes in sexual behavior related to controlling infection with HIV (Sec. 12.83).

CLINICAL MANIFESTATIONS. Congenital syphilis causes fetal or perinatal death in 40% of affected infants. Among survivors, manifestations have traditionally been divided into early and late stages. The former appear during the first 2 yr of life, whereas the latter appear gradually during the first 2 decades. *Early congenital syphilis* results from transplacental spirochetemia and is analogous to the secondary stage of acquired syphilis. There may be no manifestations during the first few weeks or months of life, or generalized symptoms such as fever, failure to gain weight, restlessness, and irritability may be present from birth or shortly thereafter. These generalized symptoms may or may not include the skin or mucous membrane lesions, and, conversely, local mucocutaneous lesions may be present in an infant who appears well. The mucocutaneous lesions of congenital syphilis are varied, and several morphologies may appear in the same patient. A vesicular or bullous eruption and an erythematous maculopapular rash are characteristic. Each is initially more common on the hands and feet and may become generalized, darken, and eventually desquamate. Wart-like moist lesions at the mucocutaneous junction of the mouth, anus, and external genitalia (analogous to the condylomata lata of acquired syphilis) may also be present. The cutaneous lesions are highly infectious, often recur over a period of weeks or months, and eventually disappear. Mucous membrane involvement may be extensive and involve the nasal mucous membranes, and in about 10% of cases it appears as a profuse, purulent, and blood-tinged nasal discharge ("snuffles") containing viable *T. pallidum*. This lesion is often associated with excoriation of the nasal structures and upper lip and heals spontaneously.

Hepatosplenomegaly is common (30%). Histologically, liver involvement includes bile stasis, fibrosis, and extramedullary hematopoiesis. Hyperbilirubinemia and elevated liver enzymes are common. Lymphadenopathy (5%) tends to be diffuse and resolve spontaneously; shotty nodes may persist.

Bone involvement occurs in 25% of infected infants. Roentgenographic abnormalities include multiple sites of osteochondritis at the wrists, elbows, ankles, and knees; periostitis of the long bones and rarely the skull; widened and serrated epiphyseal lines; and, on occasion, separation of the epiphysis. The osteochondritis is painful, may be asymmetric, and often results in irritability and refusal to move the involved extremity **(pseudoparalysis of Parrot)**. Osteochondritis of the hand (syphilitic dactylitis) resembles the hand-foot syndrome of sickle cell disease.

Histologic abnormalities involving one or all of the cellular elements of the bone marrow occur in 20% of infants with congenital syphilis. Thrombocytopenia is often associated with platelet trapping in an enlarged spleen. A Coombs-negative, hemolytic anemia is characteristic and may suggest blood group incompatibility. Leukocytosis at times may be extreme and present as a leukemoid reaction; on rare occasions, only monocytes may be involved.

Renal dysfunction, characterized by glomerulonephritis or

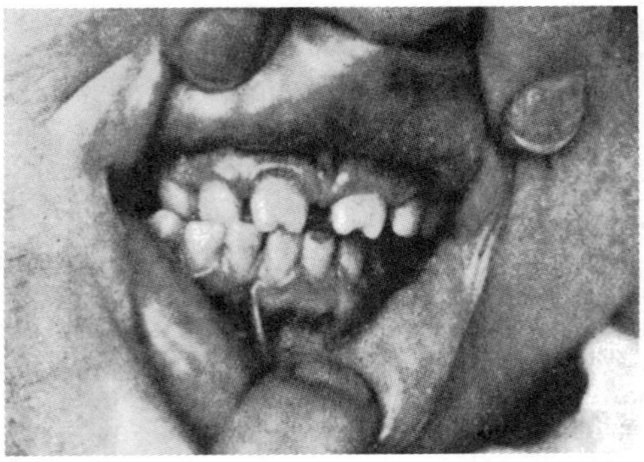

Figure 12–6. Hutchinson teeth in congenital syphilis.

the nephrotic syndrome, is noted in 5% of patients. Clinical abnormalities appear within the first few months of life and may include hypertension, hematuria, proteinuria, hypoproteinemia, hypercholesterolemia, and hypocomplementemia. They appear to be related to glomerular deposition of circulating immune complexes.

Less common clinical manifestations of early congenital syphilis include gastroenteritis, peritonitis, pancreatitis, pneumonia, eye involvement (glaucoma and chorioretinitis), nonimmune hydrops, and testicular masses.

The manifestations of *late congenital syphilis* result primarily from chronic inflammation of bone, teeth, and the central nervous system. Skeletal changes due to persistent or recurrent periostitis and associated thickening of bone include frontal bossing, a bony prominence of the forehead ("olympian brow"); unilateral or bilateral thickening of the sternoclavicular portion of the clavicle (Higoumenakis sign); an anterior bowing of the midportion of the tibia **(saber shins)**; and scaphoid scapula, a convexity along its medial border. Dental abnormalities are common and include (1) **Hutchinson teeth**, which are the peg- or barrel-shaped upper central incisors that erupt during the 6th yr of life; (2) abnormal enamel, which results in a notch along the biting surface (Fig. 12–6); and (3) mulberry molars, abnormal 1st lower (6 yr) molars, characterized by a small biting surface and an excessive number of cusps. Defects in enamel formation lead to repeated caries and eventual tooth destruction.

A **saddle nose**, a depression of the nasal root (Fig. 12–7), is a result of syphilitic rhinitis, which destroys the adjacent bone and cartilage. A perforated nasal septum is an associated abnormality. **Rhagades** are linear scars that extend in a spokelike pattern from previous mucocutaneous lesions of the mouth, anus, and genitalia (Fig. 12–8). Juvenile paresis, an uncommon latent meningovascular infection, typically presents during adolescence with behavioral changes, focal seizures, or loss of intellectual function. Juvenile tabes with spinal cord involvement and cardiovascular involvement with aortitis are extremely rare.

Other clinical manifestations of late congenital syphilis may represent a hypersensitivity phenomenon. These include unilateral or bilateral interstitial keratitis with symptoms such as intense photophobia and lacrimation, followed within weeks or months by corneal opacification and complete blindness. Less common ocular manifestations include choroiditis, retinitis, vascular occlusion, and optic atrophy. Eighth nerve deafness may be unilateral or bilateral, appears at any age, presents initially with vertigo and high tone hearing loss, and progresses to permanent deafness. The **Clutton joint** represents a unilateral or bilateral synovitis involving the lower extremities (usually the knee), which presents as painless joint swelling with sterile synovial fluid; spontaneous remission usually occurs after a period of several weeks. Soft tissue gummas (identical to those of acquired disease) and paroxysmal cold hemoglobinuria are rare hypersensitivity phenomena.

Acquired syphilis is divided into various stages: incubating, primary, secondary, latent, and late syphilis. **Primary syphilis** characteristically begins with a single painless papule at the site of inoculation 3–6 wk following contact. The papule becomes indurated and eventually erodes, leaving a shallow, clean-based, painless ulceration with a firm, raised border—the chancre. Chancres are most often located on the external genitalia and may be multiple. The lesions may also be found on the cervix, mouth, rectum, and perineum. Chancres are often associated with bilateral firm, painless, nonsuppurative local adenopathy. In untreated patients the chancre spontaneously heals within 6 wk, leaving a thin, atrophic scar.

Secondary syphilis begins 6–8 wk following the primary chancre. Clinical manifestations include a flu-like illness with low-grade fever, headache, malaise, anorexia, weight loss, sore throat, myalgias, arthralgias, and generalized lymphadenopathy. The initial cutaneous manifestation is an erythematous macular rash that begins on the trunk and upper portions of the extremities. This progresses to a generalized, nonpruritic, copper-colored, macular rash with a predilection for the palms and soles. The initial rash may also evolve into a maculopapular eruption, which may involve the hair follicles and result in localized alopecia. Pustule formation (pustular syphilis) is uncommon. In warm, moist areas of the body (e.g., axilla, perineum, breast) papules may enlarge, coalesce, and erode to produce plaque-like lesions, condylomata lata. Similar lesions may develop on mucous membranes (mucous patches), appearing as oval, slightly raised erosions covered with a grayish membrane and surrounded by a red areola. The cutaneous lesions of secondary syphilis are all highly infectious.

Noncutaneous manifestations result from multiple organ system involvement. These include meningitis (30% of all patients with secondary syphilis have cerebrospinal fluid pleocytosis and elevated spinal fluid protein, frequently without neurologic symptoms), hepatitis, glomerulonephritis

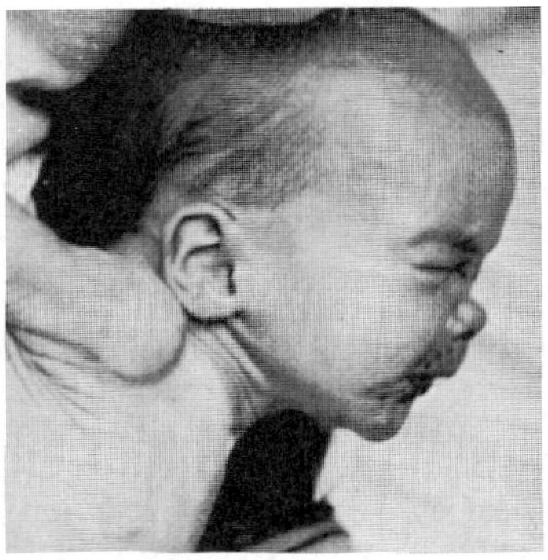

Figure 12–7. Saddle nose in early syphilis.

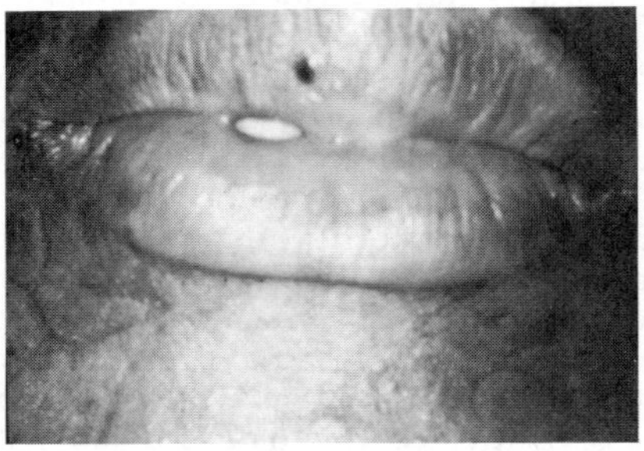

Figure 12–8. Rhagades as long-term residua of congenital syphilis.

(with or without nephrosis), bursitis, or periostitis. Laboratory abnormalities are common and reflect diffuse organ involvement.

In **latent syphilis** the patient appears to be without disease, although there is a history of prior untreated syphilis, exposure, or birth of a child with a congenital infection. In the 1st yr of the latent period, cutaneous relapses capable of infectivity occur in about 25% of patients and in as many as 85% within the first 2 yr. In the late latent phase there is no evidence of active disease, but the patient is seropositive, noninfectious, and resistant to reinfection. Approximately 60% of untreated patients with late latent syphilis remain asymptomatic; the remainder progress to late or tertiary syphilis.

Late syphilis is a slowly progressive inflammatory disease of adults that can affect any organ system. This stage of syphilis may be associated with gumma formation and the development of neurosyphilis or cardiovascular disease.

DIAGNOSIS. Serologic tests for syphilis fall into two categories: nontreponemal ("reagin") tests and specific antitreponemal tests. The former detect IgG and IgM antibody against a nonspecific lipoidal antigen of obscure origin ("cardiolipin"), and the latter measure antibody specific for *T. pallidum*. In many laboratories the traditional nontreponemal Venereal Disease Research Laboratory (VDRL) slide test and Kolmer test have been replaced by the more sensitive rapid plasma reagin card test (RPRCT) or the automated reagin test (ART). The nontreponemal tests, in addition to being rapid and inexpensive, may be quantitated and therefore used as a marker for disease activity; titers rise when disease is active (including treatment failure or reinfection) and fall when treatment is adequate (Fig. 12–9). Serum usually becomes nonreactive within 1 yr of adequate therapy for primary syphilis and within 2 yr of treatment for secondary disease. A small number of adequately treated patients, however, retain positive serology. A major disadvantage of the nontreponemal tests, particularly the VDRL, is that they are not specific for active infection and may be falsely positive, particularly in the presence of immunologic stimulation such as infection, immunization, collagen-vascular disease, pregnancy, and drug addiction. Often these "biologic false-positive tests" for syphilis have low titers, and their true nature is verified by demonstration of a negative specific antitreponemal test.

Despite their value as screening tests for primary and secondary syphilis, the nontreponemal tests may be used improperly in diagnosing congenital syphilis. Maternal antibody crosses the placenta, and accordingly a false-positive VDRL can occur in an uninfected infant delivered to a VDRL-positive mother. Passively acquired antibody is suggested when neonatal titers are significantly less (4-fold or less) than maternal titers and can be verified when antibody is no longer demonstrable by 3 mo of age. False-negative nontreponemal test results may occur in infants who acquire infections late in pregnancy; such infants become seropositive in the postnatal period.

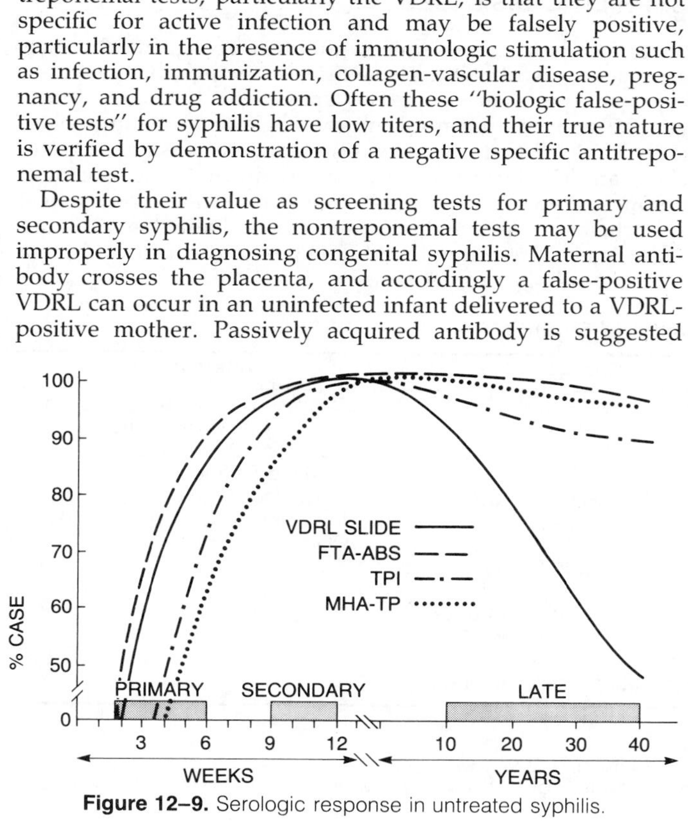

Figure 12–9. Serologic response in untreated syphilis.

Two specific antitreponemal tests capable of detecting antibody to *T. pallidum* are available. The *T. pallidum immobilization test* (TPI), against which other antitreponemal tests are compared, measures the ability of test serum (antibody) plus complement to immobilize *T. pallidum*. Few laboratories maintain the viable spirochetes necessary for this test. The principal antitreponemal antibody test in clinical use is the *fluorescent treponemal antibody absorption* (FTA-ABS) test, which is an indirect immunofluorescence test using fixed *T. pallidum* as the antigen to measure serum antitreponemal antibodies; it is both sensitive and specific. Antibodies are detected early in infection and remain detectable in latent and late infections (see Fig. 12–9). False-positive reactions are uncommon but occur in a few normal individuals during pregnancy and in patients with diseases such as lymphoproliferative disorders, cirrhosis, collagen-vascular disease, and drug addiction. The major disadvantages of this test are that its interpretation is subjective, its results cannot be quantitated, and, once positive, it remains so for life even when therapy is adequate; it should, therefore, not be used as a basis for monitoring the effectiveness of treatment. The FTA-ABS test is subject to misinterpretation during the neonatal period because seropositivity in an adequately treated mother results in a seropositive, uninfected newborn. Follow-up titers will distinguish passively acquired antibody from disease-specific antibodies, the former becoming negative after the 6th mo of life. The *T. pallidum* hemagglutination assay (TPHA-TP) may prove superior to the FTA-ABS test because it is inexpensive and easy to perform and does not require a fluorescent microscope; also, interpretation is not subjective. The test is less sensitive than the FTA-ABS test.

The significance of cerebrospinal fluid serology in both acquired and congenital syphilis remains controversial. Cerebrospinal fluid (CSF) antibodies, both reagin and antitreponemal, result from local production within the nervous system as well as passive diffusion from serum. Maternal IgG antibodies may cross the placenta into the neonatal CSF by passive diffusion, suggesting that neurosyphilis cannot be diagnosed solely on the basis of positive CSF serology during the neonatal period. Nevertheless, most authorities agree that a positive CSF-VDRL in a newborn infant warrants treatment of the infant for presumptive neurosyphilis. In patients with acquired infection, the presence of CSF abnormalities (a monocellular pleocytosis or elevated protein concentration) or positive CSF-VDRL, in the setting of neurologic symptoms, is indicative of neurosyphilis. However, as many as 25% of patients with neurosyphilis may have no elevation in either CSF cell count or protein. The FTA-ABS test has not reliably identified CNS involvement in syphilis, and its use is not widely recommended.

Darkfield microscopic examination or direct fluorescent antibody test of scrapings from primary lesions and moist, freshly scraped or swabbed congenital or secondary lesions can reveal *T. pallidum* and often permits a definitive diagnosis prior to the development of seropositivity. Antibiotics and antiseptic agents interfere with treponemal motility and accordingly interfere with th accuracy of darkfield examination. This technique is of limited value in detecting *T. pallidum* in oral lesions, since nonsyphilitic saprophytic spirochetes (*T. microdentium*) may contaminate the lesion and cannot be distinguished microscopically from *T. pallidum*. Placental examination by gross and microscopic techniques is useful in the diagnosis of congenital syphilis. The disproportionately large placentas are characterized histologically by focal proliferative villitis, endovascular and perivascular arteritis, and focal or diffuse immaturity of placental villi.

TREATMENT. Acquired Syphilis. *T. pallidum* is extremely sensitive to penicillin, and there is no evidence of increasing penicillin resistance. A serum concentration of greater than 0.03 μg/mL of penicillin is needed to ensure killing of spirochetes; microorganisms will regenerate if subinhibitory concentrations of penicillin (less than 0.0025 μg/mL) persist for more than 24 hr. Inhibitory levels of penicillin must be maintained for at least 7 days to ensure complete cure. Table 12–30 presents the currently recommended therapeutic regimens for syphilis. Although nonpenicillin regimens are available to the penicillin-allergic patient, many authorities suggest that desensitization followed by penicillin therapy is the most reliable strategy.

Single-dose benzathine penicillin at the recommended dose does not result in spirocheticidal levels of drug in the CSF. Indeed, there is growing evidence that the regimen for early syphilis may not be sufficient to preclude development of neurosyphilis in some patients, particularly those who are coinfected with HIV, in whom neurosyphilis may be difficult to cure. Although CDC guidelines continue to recommend single-dose benzathine penicillin for early acquired disease, careful follow-up and multiple-dose therapy may be required for some patients, especially HIV-infected patients.

Incubating syphilis may be effectively treated with the currently recommended penicillin regimens for gonorrhea (Sec. 12.24). Therapy with ceftriaxone and tetracycline is probably effective for incubating syphilis as well, but extensive data are lacking. In contrast, spectinomycin therapy will not cure incubating syphilis. Because of the high risk of acquiring infection, "prophylactic treatment" should be given to anyone exposed to infectious syphilis within the preceding 3 mo regardless of serology. Three additional elements of syphilis therapy are obligatory: (1) Follow-up serologic studies should be obtained in treated individuals to establish adequacy of treatment; (2) Sexual contacts should be identified and treated; and (3) Testing for other STDs, including HIV, should be performed on *all* patients.

Syphilis in Pregnancy. Routine serologic tests for syphilis should be performed during the 1st trimester and prior to delivery in high-risk populations. When clinical findings or serologic findings suggest active infection or when the diagnosis of active syphilis cannot be excluded with certainty, treatment is indicated. Women who have been adequately treated in the past do not require additional therapy unless quantitative serology suggests evidence of reinfection (4-fold increase in titer). The cephalosporins may be an effective alternative for women who are allergic to penicillin; however, experience with these agents is limited. Chloramphenicol and tetracycline should not be administered during pregnancy. Erythromycin does not effectively treat fetal infection.

Congenital Syphilis. Adequate maternal therapy eliminates the risk of congenital syphilis. Follow-up of all such infants, however, should continue until nontreponemal serologic tests are negative. The risk of giving penicillin to a newborn infant is minimal; therefore, whenever there is uncertainty concerning the adequacy of the mother's treatment, the infant should be treated, particularly if (1) there are symptoms present consistent with a diagnosis of congenital syphilis, (2) there are abnormal CSF findings or a positive CSF-VDRL, or (3) the baby has a serum VDRL titer 4-fold higher than that of the mother.

An acute systemic febrile reaction, the **Jarisch-Herxheimer reaction**, with exacerbation of lesions occurs in 15–20% of all patients with acquired or congenital syphilis who are treated with penicillin. It is not an indication for discontinuation of penicillin therapy.

Beck-Sague C, Alexander ER: Failure of benzathine penicillin G treatment in early congenital syphilis. Pediatr Infect Dis J 6:1061, 1987.

Centers For Disease Control: Sexually transmitted diseases treatment guidelines. MMWR 38:5, 1989.

Centers For Disease Control: Syphilis and congenital syphilis—United States, 1985–1988. MMWR 37:486, 1988.

Gilbert, GL: Congenital syphilis—Should we worry? Med J Aust 148:162, 1988.

Hook EW III: Treatment of syphilis: Current recommendation, alternatives, and continuing problems. Rev Infect Dis 2:1511, 1989.

Penn CW: Pathogenicity and immunobiology of *Treponema pallidum*. J Med Microbiol 24:1, 1987.

Tramont EC: Syphilis in the AIDS era. N Engl J Med 316:1600, 1987.

NONVENEREAL ENDEMIC CHILDHOOD SYPHILITIC DISEASES

Several variants of endemic syphilis are recognized by their geographic distribution. These diseases, which include yaws, bejel, and pinta, are caused by spirochetes belonging to the genus *Treponema* that are (1) morphologically and immunologically identical to *T. pallidum*, (2) extremely sensitive to penicillin, and (3) differentiated primarily on the basis of clinical findings. Yaws is the most common of the nonvenereal spirochetal diseases and occurs in Africa, Latin America, and Asia. Bejel is present in the Middle East and Africa, and pinta is found only in Latin America.

TABLE 12–30. Treatment of Syphilis*

Stage	Choice	Dosage	Alternatives
Early (primary, secondary, or latent less than 1 yr)	Penicillin G benzathine	2.4 million U IM	Tetracycline HCl (500 mg orally qid for 2 wk), or doxycycline (100 mg PO bid for 2 wk), or erythromycin (500 mg PO qid for 2 wk)
Late latent (greater than 1 yr duration)	Penicillin G benzathine	2.4 million U IM weekly for 3 doses	Tetracycline HCl (500 mg PO qid for 4 wk), or doxycycline (100 mg PO bid for 4 wk)
Neurosyphilis	Penicillin G crystalline†	12–24 million U/24 hr IV for 10–14 days	
	or		
	Penicillin G procaine‡	2.4 million U/day, IM for 10–14 days	
Congenital§	Penicillin G crystalline	50,000 U/kg/24 hr IM or IV for 14 days	
	or		
	Penicillin G procaine	50,000 U/kg/24 hr IM daily for 14 days	

*Based on MMWR 38, No. S–8, 1989.
†Followed by benzathine penicillin G, 2.4 million U/wk for 3 wk.
‡With probenecid, 500 mg PO qid for 10 days. Followed by benzathine penicillin G, 2.4 million U IM for 3 wk.
§Infants who are asymptomatic and who have a normal CSF, but who are born to an untreated mother, may receive benzathine penicillin G 50,000 U/kg IM as a one-time dose.

12.51 Yaws

Yaws is a chronic relapsing, nonvenereally transmitted disease caused by *T. pertenue*, a spirochete that cannot be differentiated microscopically or serologically from *T. pallidum*. Yaws is primarily a disease of children living in rural areas of Africa, Southeast Asia, and South America. Transmission is by direct contact with an infected lesion and is facilitated by overcrowding and poor personal hygiene. In 10% of untreated cases, there are late destructive changes involving skin, bone, and cartilage.

Infection follows penetration by the spirochete through abraded skin. After an incubation period of several weeks an initial lesion (the "mother yaw") appears at the inoculation site as either a localized maculopapular rash, a small cluster of papules, or a large exudative papilloma. This lesion ulcerates before healing spontaneously, leaving behind a small hypopigmented scar. Following a period of weeks to months, a generalized papular eruption appears, often associated with generalized lymphadenopathy, anorexia, and malaise. Individual papules may enlarge and coalesce to form large papillomas and condylomas, disappear spontaneously, or ulcerate. Ulcers, when present, are covered with a yellowish exudate containing treponemes. This polymorphic secondary eruption heals spontaneously without scarring; however, relapses are common and may extend over several years. The exacerbations are often associated with bone pain and underlying periostitis or osteomyelitis. Following the initial period of clinical activity, the patient enters a long period of latency. This is followed by the appearance of tertiary lesions at puberty, which are often solitary and destructive. These present as painful papillomas on the hands and feet, gummatous skin ulcerations, or osteitis. Bony destruction and deformity are common, as are juxta-articular nodules, depigmentation, and painful hyperkeratosis (crab yaws) of the palms and soles. Diagnosis depends on the clinical manifestations of the disease in an endemic area. Darkfield examination of cutaneous lesions and serologic tests for syphilis (VDRL, TPI, and FTA-ABS tests) are confirmatory. Treatment of patients and all contacts consists of a single intramuscular injection of benzathine penicillin (1.2 million units), which cures the lesions of active yaws, renders them noninfectious, and prevents relapse.

Eradication of yaws from endemic foci may be accomplished by treating the entire population with penicillin. Patients allergic to penicillin may be treated with erythromycin or tetracycline.

12.52 Endemic Syphilis

(Bejel, Nonvenereal Childhood Syphilis)

Bejel affects children living in the Saharan regions of Africa and the Middle East. Infection with a strain of *T. pallidum* follows penetration of the spirochete through traumatized skin or mucous membranes. In experimental infections, a primary papule forms at the inoculation site after an incubation period of 3 wk; in human infections a primary lesion is almost never visualized. The clinical manifestations of the secondary stage of bejel are confined to the skin and mucous membranes and consist of highly infectious mucous patches on the oral mucosa and condyloma-like lesions on the moist areas of the body, especially the axilla and anus. These mucocutaneous lesions resolve spontaneously over a period of several months, but recurrences are common. The secondary stage is followed by a variable latency period before the onset of late or tertiary bejel. The late complications, identical to those of yaws, include gumma formation in skin, subcutaneous tissue, and bone, resulting in painful destructive ulcerations, swelling, and deformity.

Diagnosis is suspected on epidemiologic and clinical grounds and is confirmed either by darkfield examination of the skin and mucous membrane lesions or by serologic testing (positive VDRL, TPI, and FTA-ABS tests). Differentiation from syphilis is extremely difficult in an endemic area. Bejel can be suspected by the absence of a primary chancre and lack of involvement of the central nervous and cardiovascular systems during the late stage. Treatment of early infection consists of a single intramuscular dose of benzathine penicillin (1.2 million units); late infection is treated with three injections, each of the same dose at intervals of 7 days. Patients allergic to penicillin may be treated with erythromycin or tetracycline.

12.53 Pinta

Pinta is a chronic, nonvenereally transmitted infection caused by *T. carateum*, a spirochete morphologically and serologically indistinguishable from other human treponemes. The disease is endemic in Mexico, Central America, South America, and parts of the West Indies. Infection follows direct inoculation of the treponeme through abraded skin. Following a variable incubation period of days, a primary lesion appears at the inoculation site as a small asymptomatic erythematous papule resembling localized psoriasis or eczema. The regional lymph nodes are often enlarged, and spirochetes can be visualized on darkfield examination of skin scrapings or of the involved lymph nodes. After a period of enlargement, the primary lesion disappears. Secondary lesions follow within 6–8 mo; they consist of small macules and papules on the face, scalp, and other exposed portions of the body. These pigmented lesions are scaly and nonpruritic and may coalesce to form large plaque-like elevations resembling psoriasis. In the late stage, atrophic and depigmented lesions develop on the hands, wrists, ankles, feet, face, and scalp. Hyperkeratosis of palms and soles is uncommon. Diagnosis is confirmed by darkfield examination of early lesions and a positive serologic test for syphilis. Treatment consists of a single intramuscular injection of benzathine penicillin (1.2 million units). Tetracycline and erythromycin are satisfactory alternatives for patients allergic to penicillin.

12.54 LEPTOSPIROSIS

ETIOLOGY. Leptospirosis is a generalized infection of man and animals caused by spirochetes of the genus *Leptospira*. The pathogenic leptospires belong to a single species, *L. interrogans*, which contains approximately 200 distinct serovars. A single serovar may produce a variety of distinct syndromes, and a single clinical manifestation (i.e., aseptic meningitis) may be caused by multiple serotypes.

EPIDEMIOLOGY. Leptospirosis is a zoonosis of worldwide distribution. Leptospires infect many species of wild and domestic animals and have been isolated from birds, fish, and reptiles. The rat is the principal source of human infection. Other important animal reservoirs include dogs, cats, livestock, and wild animals. Animal infection varies from inapparent to fatal. Once infected, animals excrete spirochetes in urine for an extended period of time. Leptospire survival outside the animal host is dependent upon the moisture content, temperature, and pH of the soil or water into which they are shed. The majority of human cases worldwide result from occupational exposure to rat-contaminated water or soil. Occupational groups with a high incidence of leptospirosis include agricultural workers, persons who live or work in rat-infested environments, individuals involved in animal husbandry or veterinary medicine, and laboratory workers. In the United States, the major animal reservoir is the dog, and contact with spirochetes is often associated with recreational activities that result in contact with contaminated soil or water during the summer months.

PATHOPHYSIOLOGY. Leptospires enter humans through moist and preferably abraded skin or through mucous membranes. Following penetration of the skin or mucus membranes, leptospires circulate in the bloodstream and spread to all organs of the body. The primary lesion caused by leptospires is damage to the endothelial lining of small blood vessels with resultant ischemic damage to the liver, kidneys, meninges, and muscles. After an incubation period of 7–12 days, an initial *septicemic phase* begins in which leptospires can be isolated from the blood, cerebrospinal fluid, and other tissues. Initial symptoms, which last approximately 2–7 days, may be followed by a brief period of well-being and a second symptomatic or *immune phase*. The immune phase is associated with the appearance of circulating antibody, the disappearance of organisms from the blood and cerebrospinal fluid, and the appearance of additional signs and symptoms. Despite the presence of circulating antibody, leptospires may persist in the kidney, urine, and aqueous humor. The immune or leptospiruric phase may last for several weeks.

CLINICAL MANIFESTATIONS. Most cases of human leptospirosis are subclinical, with inapparent infection particularly common in high-risk occupational groups such as farmers and their families. Symptomatic infection may present as an acute febrile illness with nonspecific signs and symptoms (70%), as meningitis (20%), or as hepatorenal dysfunction (10%). The onset is typically sudden, and the illness tends to follow a biphasic course (Fig. 12–10).

Anicteric Leptospirosis. The onset of the initial or septicemic phase is abrupt, with fever, shaking chills, severe headache, malaise, nausea, vomiting, and severe, often debiliating muscular pain. Circulatory collapse is uncommon, but some patients have bradycardia and hypotension. Typically, the child is lethargic, with mild to moderate dehydration. Additional physical findings include extreme muscle tenderness, which is most prominent in the lower extremities, the lumbosacral spine, and abdomen. Conjunctival suffusion with photophobia and orbital pain (in the absence of chemosis and purulent exudate), generalized lymphadenopathy, and hepatosplenomegaly may also be present. Cutaneous lesions are common (10%), usually consisting of a truncal erythematous maculopapular rash, but they may be urticarial, petechial, purpuric, or desquamating. Less common manifestations include pharyngitis, pneumonitis, arthritis, carditis, cholecystitis, and orchitis. The second or immune phase may follow a brief asymptomatic interlude and is characterized by recurrence of fever. Aseptic meningitis is the hallmark of this phase. Despite abnormal cerebrospinal fluid profiles in 80% of infected children, only 50% have meningeal manifestations. Spinal fluid abnormalities include a modest elevation in pressure, a mononuclear pleocytosis rarely exceeding 500 cells/mm^3 (polymorphonuclear leukocytes predominate initially), normal or slightly elevated protein, and normal glucose values. Encephalitis, cranial and peripheral neuropathies, papilledema, and paralysis are uncommon. Symptoms referable to the central nervous system resolve spontaneously within a week or so. Uveitis may occur during this phase; it can be unilateral or bilateral and is usually self-limited, rarely resulting in permanent visual impairment.

Icteric Leptospirosis (Weil Disease). This severe form of leptospirosis occurs in fewer than 10% of affected children. The initial manifestations are similar to those described for anicteric leptospirosis. The immune phase, however, is distinctive, being characterized by clinical and laboratory evidence of hepatic and renal dysfunction. In fulminating cases, hemorrhagic phenomena and cardiovascular collapse also occur. Hepatic abnormalities include right upper quadrant pain, hepatomegaly, direct and indirect hyperbilirubinemia, and modest elevation of serum liver enzymes. Renal manifestations are common, may dominate the clinical picture, and are the principal cause of death in fatal cases; all patients have abnormal findings on urinalysis (hematuria, proteinuria, and casts), and azotemia is common, often associated with oliguria or anuria. Congestive heart failure is uncommon; however, abnormal electrocardiograms are present in 90% of affected children. Hemorrhagic manifestations are rare but when present may include epistaxis, hemoptysis, and gastrointestinal and adrenal hemorrhage. Thrombocytopenia and hypoprothrombinemia also occur.

DIAGNOSIS. Leptospirosis should be considered in the differential diagnosis of any acute febrile illness when there is a history of direct contact with animals or with soil or water contaminated with animal urine, and especially when the onset is abrupt with chills, fever, severe myalgias, conjunctival suffusion, headache, nausea, and vomiting. Isolation of the infecting organism from clinical specimens or a 4-fold rise in antibody titer in the presence of clinical symptoms compatible with leptospirosis establishes the diagnosis. A presumptive diagnosis is made in symptomatic children with stable titers of 1:100 or greater in two or more specimens and in asymptomatic children with evidence of exposure and a seroconversion (i.e., a 4-fold rise in antibody titer in specimens obtained 2 or more wk apart).

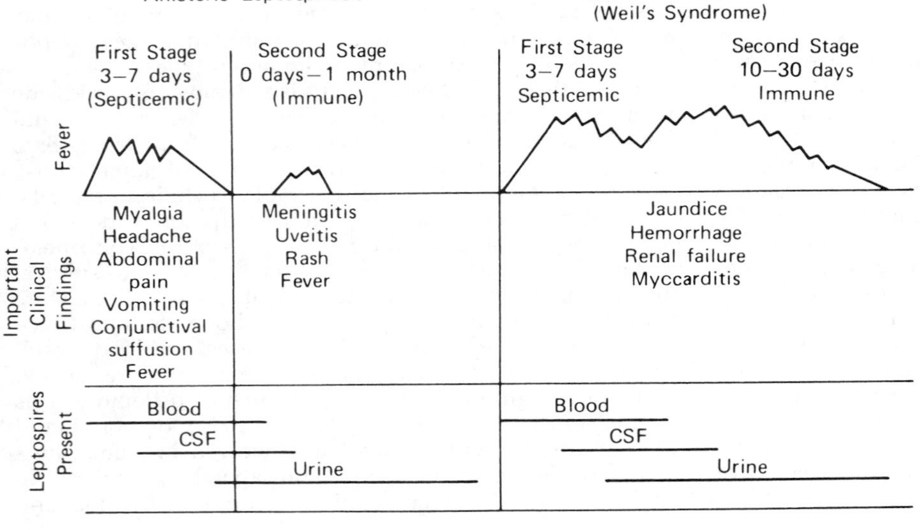

Figure 12–10. Stages of anicteric and icteric leptospirosis. Correlation between clinical findings and presence of leptospires in body fluids. (Reprinted with permission from Feigin RD, Anderson DC: CRC Crit Rev Clin Lab Sci 5:413, 1975. Copyright CRC Press, Inc., Boca Raton, FL.)

Silver impregnation and fluorescent antibody techniques permit identification of *leptospires* in infected tissue or body fluids. Spirochetes may also be demonstrated by phase-contrast or darkfield microscopy; however, the skill required and the high frequency of artifacts found with these tests limit their use. Unlike other pathogenic spirochetes, *leptospires* are easily cultured on commercially available media. They can be recovered from the blood or cerebrospinal fluid during the first 10 days of illness and from urine after the 2nd wk. Because the number of *leptospires* in clinical specimens is small and their growth rate is slow, multiple cultures should be obtained and incubated for 5–6 wk.

The diagnosis is most often established by serologic testing. A microscopic slide-agglutination test utilizing killed antigen is the most useful screening test. A microscopic slide-agglutination test with a live or formalin-treated antigen may be used to determine antibody titer and tentatively identify the infecting serotype. Agglutinins usually appear by the 12th day of illness and reach a maximum titer by the 3rd wk. Low titers may persist for years. Approximately 10% of infected persons do not have detectable agglutinins, presumably because available antisera do not identify all *Leptospira* serotypes.

TREATMENT AND PREVENTION. Despite the in vitro sensitivity of *Leptospira* to penicillin and tetracycline and the efficacy of these agents in treating experimental infection, their effectiveness in human leptospirosis remains controversial. It does appear that initiation of treatment before the 7th day will probably shorten the clinical course and decrease the severity of the infection. On this basis, treatment with penicillin or tetracycline (in children over 12 yr) should be instituted as soon as the diagnosis is suspected. Parenteral penicillin G, 6–8 million units/m^2/24 hr, in 6 divided doses for 7 days is recommended. In patients allergic to penicillin, tetracycline (10–20 mg/kg/24 hr) should be administered orally or intravenously in 4 divided doses for 7 days.

Prevention of human leptospirosis is possible by instituting rodent control measures and avoiding contaminated water and soil. Immunization of livestock and family pets has been recommended as a means of eliminating animal reservoirs, but these programs have met with limited success. A formalin-killed polyvalent human vaccine has been utilized in "at risk" occupation groups in Europe and Asia; however, there have been no clinical trials to determine its efficacy. Leptospirosis has been prevented in American servicemen stationed in the tropics by administering doxycycline, 200 mg once a week, as prophylaxis. This schedule may be similarly effective for the traveler entering a highly endemic area for a limited period of time.

Edwards GA, Domm BM: Human leptospirosis. Medicine 39:117, 1960.
Feigin RD, Anderson DC: Human leptospirosis. CRC Crit Rev Clin Lab Sci 5:413, 1975.
Heath CW Jr, Alexander AD, Galton MM: Leptospirosis in the United States. Analysis of 483 cases in man, 1949–1961. N Engl J Med 273:857, 1965.
Wong ML, Kaplan S, Dunide LM, et al: Leptospirosis: A childhood disease. J Pediatr 90:532, 1977.

12.55 RAT-BITE FEVERS

Two distinctly different diseases are categorized under the term rat-bite fever. These are spirillary and streptobacillary rat-bite fever. Both illnesses usually follow the bite or scratch of a rat; however, cases have been reported in the absence of a history of rodent exposure. Isolated case reports and several epidemics of streptobacillary rat-bite fever have been described following the ingestion of raw milk contaminated by rats *(Haverhill fever)*. The illnesses exist worldwide, with higher incidences reported in urban settings with poor sanitation and large rat populations. Infections are more common in children than adults and occur in approximately 10% of children bitten by wild rats.

Spirillary Rat-Bite Fever
(Sodoku)

The disease is caused by *Spirillum minor*, a short, tightly coiled, gram-negative spirochete that is present in the saliva of about 10% of healthy wild and laboratory rats. It cannot be grown in commercially available media; laboratory isolation requires inoculation of mice and guinea pigs. However, it can be visualized by direct darkfield examination of infected lymph obtained from the inoculation site (preferably during the ulcerative phase) or from regional lymph nodes. Occasionally, the spirochete is visualized on peripheral blood smears.

CLINICAL MANIFESTATIONS. The initial inoculation of spirochetes is followed by an asymptomatic incubation period of 14–18 days. The wound appears to heal but then becomes erythematous and indurated and eventually undergoes suppuration and eschar formation (Fig. 12–11). During this phase, localized lymphangitis and lymphadenitis are observed in about 50% of affected children. At the onset there are fever, chills, severe myalgia, and a reddish-brown or purple macular rash (80%), typically beginning at the inoculation site and spreading to involve the entire body. Arthralgia may be severe, but there is no joint effusion. In untreated children, the fever persists for 3–4 days, at which time the constitutional symptoms subside, the rash disappears, and the inoculation site heals. This asymptomatic period persists for several days and is followed by a second cycle of fever, rash, and constitutional symptoms. This relapsing pattern of illness may continue for up to a year in untreated patients; however, the disease is eventually self-limiting. Fatalities are uncommon (1%) and are usually associated with meningitis, endocarditis, and myocarditis.

DIAGNOSIS. In patients with a history of rat bite, the major differential diagnosis is etiologic—whether the infectious agent is *Streptobacillus moniliformis* or *Spirillum minor*. The long incubation period, the prompt initial healing of the primary wound followed by induration, ulceration, and eschar formation, and the absence of arthritis suggest *S. minor* infection. The laboratory diagnosis depends on the presence of negative blood and joint fluid cultures for *S. moniliformis*, the presence of spirochetes on direct darkfield examination of

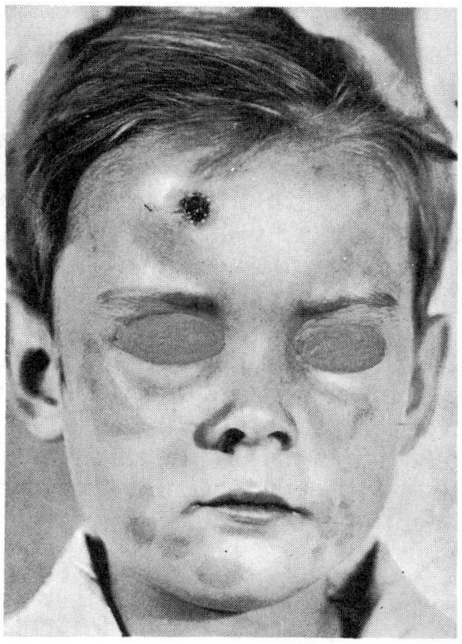

Figure 12–11. Sodoku: chancre-like indurated ulcer at a bite site on the forehead; secondary macular eruption of the face.

tissue specimens, and recovery of spirochetes following animal inoculation.

TREATMENT. *S. minor* is extremely sensitive to penicillin; however, because this illness is often confused with rat-bite fever due to *S. moniliformis*, which is more resistant to penicillin, and because dual infection has been described, large doses of procaine penicillin G (600,000 units every 12 hr for 10 days) are recommended. In patients allergic to penicillin, tetracycline, erythromycin, and cephalosporins are satisfactory alternatives.

Streptobacillary Rat-Bite Fever
(Haverhill Fever)

This form of rat-bite fever is caused by *Streptobacillus moniliformis*, an aerobic, nonmotile, pleomorphic, unencapsulated gram-negative bacillus, which can be isolated from the nasopharynx of about 50% of healthy wild and laboratory rats. The organism has also been isolated from mice, squirrels, dogs, cats, and weasels. *S. moniliformis* can be grown on commercially available artificial media. The morphologic characteristics of the pathogen, including the formation of L-forms devoid of cell walls, and the relative resistance to penicillin vary with the age of the inoculum and the components of the culture medium. Giemsa or Gram stain may reveal short rods, long chains, or long tangled filaments with fusiform swellings.

CLINICAL MANIFESTATIONS. The incubation period is short, rarely exceeding 7 days. The onset is abrupt with fever and chills. Associated symptoms include severe myalgia, weakness, headache, and upper respiratory symptoms, most notably pharyngitis. A generalized rash and joint involvement appear within several days after the onset of fever. The rash may be maculopapular, petechial, or urticarial; most often it appears as a diffuse morbilliform rash involving the hands and feet. Joint involvement occurs in approximately half the patients and consists of a polyarticular, occasionally migratory arthritis that has a predilection for knees and large joints as well as the small joints of the hands and feet. The initial inoculation site heals without suppuration, and lymphangitis and lymphadentis are uncommon. In untreated patients the symptoms spontaneously resolve after several days, whereupon the illness assumes a relapsing course of paroxysms of fever, rash, and arthritis occurring at irregular intervals for several months; the illness is eventually self-limiting, and the mortality rarely exceeds 10%. Life-threatening complications include endocarditis and pneumonitis.

DIAGNOSIS. In patients with a history of a rat bite or rodent contact, the major differential diagnosis involves the two forms of rat-bite fever. In the streptobacillary form of infection the incubation period is short, the inoculation site heals without suppuration or eschar formation, lymphangitis and lymphadenitis are uncommon, and the responsible pathogen can be readily cultured from blood and joint fluid. Other bacterial infections to be considered in the differential diagnosis include disseminated gonococcal infection, chronic meningococcemia, and leptospirosis.

TREATMENT. Since the organism is relatively resistant to penicillin, initial therapy consists of 600,000 units of procaine penicillin G every 12 hr for 7–10 days. Streptomycin or tetracycline is effective in treating infections due to penicillin-resistant strains of *S. moniliformis* and should be considered an alternative agent in children allergic to penicillin.

Brown R, McPherson J, Nunemaker JC: Rat-bite fever—A review of the American cases with re-evaluation of etiology, report of cases. Bull Johns Hopkins Hosp 70:201, 1942.

Raffin BJ, Freemark M: Streptobacillary rat-bite fever: A pediatric problem. Pediatrics 64:214, 1979.

12.56 RELAPSING FEVER
(Recurrent Fever, Louse-Borne Fever, Tick-Borne Fever)

Relapsing fever is an uncommon arthropod-borne infection characterized by recurrent episodes of fever. It is caused by spirochetes of the genus *Borrelia*, a fastidious microorganism with worldwide distribution that is transmitted to man by lice or ticks.

ETIOLOGY AND EPIDEMIOLOGY. *Epidemic relapsing fever* is caused by *B. recurrentis* and is transmitted from man to man by the human body louse *(Pediculus humanus)*. Following ingestion of an infective blood meal by the louse, the spirochetes penetrate its midgut, migrate to and multiply within the hemolymph, and remain viable throughout its life span (several weeks). Human infection occurs as a result of crushing lice during scratching, allowing infected hemolymph to enter through the abraded skin. Louse-borne disease tends to occur in epidemics, often in association with typhus. It occurs more commonly during the winter, and the major endemic focus of the disease is the highlands of Ethiopia.

Endemic relapsing fever is caused by several species of *Borrelia* and is transmitted to man by ticks (genus *Ornithodoros*). Following ingestion of an infective blood meal, spirochetes invade all tissues of their arthropod hosts including the salivary glands and reproductive tract. The latter permits transovarian passage of infected spirochetes, perpetuating arthropod infection in successive generations. Human infection occurs when saliva, coxal fluid, or excrement is released by the tick during feeding, thereby permitting spirochetes to penetrate the skin and mucous membranes. *Ornithodoros* is distributed worldwide (including the western United States), prefers warm, humid environments and high altitudes, and is found in rodent burrows, caves, and other nesting sites; rodents are the principal reservoirs. Infected ticks gain access to human dwellings on the rodent host. Human contact is often unnoticed, since these ticks are nocturnal feeders, have a painless bite, and detach immediately following a short blood meal.

PATHOPHYSIOLOGY. The cyclic nature of relapsing fever is explained by the ability of *Borrelia* organisms to continually undergo antigenic (phase) variation: Multiple variants evolve simultaneously during the first relapse, with one type becoming predominant, and spirochetes isolated during the primary febrile episode differ antigenetically from those recovered during a subsequent relapse. During febrile episodes, spirochetes enter the bloodstream, promote the development of specific IgM and IgG antibody, and undergo agglutination, immobilization, lysis, and phagocytosis. During remission, *Borrelia* spirochetes may remain in the bloodstream, but spirochetemia is insufficient to produce symptoms. The number of relapses in untreated patients depends upon the number of antigenic variants of the infecting strain.

CLINICAL MANIFESTATIONS. Louse-borne disease has a longer incubation period, longer periods of pyrexia, fewer relapses, and longer remission periods than tick-borne disease. Each illness is associated with sudden onset of high fever, headache, photophobia, nausea, vomiting, myalgia, and arthralgia. Additional symptoms may appear later and include abdominal pain, a productive cough, and mild respiratory distress. Bleeding manifestations are common and include epistaxis, hemoptysis, hematuria, and hematemesis. The child may be lethargic and often has a diffuse, erythematous, macular, or petechial rash over the trunk and shoulders. This rash is more common in louse-borne fever (25%), is of 1–2 days duration, and occurs almost exclusively during the end of the primary febrile episode. There may also be lymphadenopathy, pneumonia, and splenomegaly. Hepatic tenderness associated with hepatomegaly is a common sign.

Jaundice is not uncommon and may occur in half of affected children. Central nervous system manifestations may be the principal feature of late relapses in tick-borne disease; they include lethargy, stupor, meningismus, convulsions, peripheral neuritis, focal neurologic deficits, and cranial nerve paralysis. Myocarditis and hepatitis are not uncommon and may be responsible for death.

The initial symptomatic period characteristically ends with a crisis in 4–10 days marked by abrupt diaphoresis, hypothermia, hypotension, bradycardia, profound muscle weakness, and prostration. In untreated patients subsequent relapse occurs within 1 wk and is followed by up to five relapses with symptoms during each relapse becoming milder and shorter; the afebrile remission period lengthens. Severe manifestations include myocarditis, hepatic failure, and disseminated intravascular coagulation.

Diagnosis depends on demonstration of spirochetes in thin or thick blood smears stained with Giemsa or Wright stain. During afebrile remissions, spirochetes disappear from the blood.

TREATMENT AND PROGNOSIS. Oral or parenteral tetracycline is the drug of choice for louse-borne and tick-borne relapsing fever. In children under 12 yr of age erythromycin (50 mg/kg/24 hr) for a total of 10 days is recommended. For older children and young adults, tetracycline (500 mg every 6 hr) for 10 days has been effective. Single-dose treatment with erythromycin or tetracycline (a single 500-mg oral dose) is efficacious in adults, but experience in children is limited.

Resolution of each febrile episode either by natural crisis or as a result of antimicrobial treatment is usually accompanied within 2 hr by the Jarisch-Herxheimer reaction, which is associated with clearing of the spirochetemia. Attempts to control this reaction by prior treatment with corticosteroids or antipyretics have met with limited success.

With adequate therapy the *mortality rate* for relapsing fever is below 5%. A majority of patients recover from their illness with or without treatment after the appearance of antiborrelial antibodies, which agglutinate, kill, or opsonize the spirochete.

No vaccine is available, and disease control requires avoidance or elimination of the arthropod vectors. In epidemics of louse-borne disease, dissemination can be prevented by good personal hygiene and delousing of persons, dwellings, and clothing with commercially available insecticides.

Butler T: Relapsing fever: New lessons about antibiotic action. Ann Intern Med 102:397, 1985.

Butler T, Jones PK, Wallace CK: *Borrelia recurrentis* infection. Single dose antibiotic regimens and management of Jarisch-Herxheimer reaction. J Infect Dis 137:573, 1978.

Perine PL, Teklu B: Antibiotic treatment of louse-borne relapsing fever in Ethiopia: A report of 377 cases. Am J Trop Med Hyg 32:1096, 1983.

Stoennerita DT, Larcen C: Antigenic variation in *Borrelia hermsii*. J Exp Med 156:1297, 1982.

12.57 LYME DISEASE

(Lyme Borreliosis)

ETIOLOGY. Lyme disease, a tick-borne illness, is characterized by a distinctive skin lesion (erythema chronicum migrans), carditis, meningitis, and arthritis and is caused by a spirochete, *Borrelia burgdorferi*. These fastidious microorganisms have a worldwide distribution and are transmitted to man by ticks of the genus *Ixodes*.

EPIDEMIOLOGY. In 1975, investigators reported a number of individuals in Lyme, Connecticut with an unusual constellation of clinical signs and symptoms including carditis, arthritis, and meningitis, and referred to this illness as Lyme disease (LD). The illness is now the most common vector-borne disease in the United States. Three endemic areas of LD are recognized: the coastal areas of the Northeast, Minnesota and Wisconsin in the Midwest, and parts of California, Oregon, Texas, and Nevada in the West. These areas correspond to the distribution of the vectors (i.e., *I. damini* in the Northeast and Midwest and *I. pacificus* in the West). However, sporadic cases have been identified in 43 states, suggesting improved awareness and recognition of the disease, expansion of the vectors' range, or involvement of other hematophagous arthropods in transmission. In Europe, LD has been identified in Germany, Australia, Switzerland, and Sweden *(I. ricinus)* and has been reported in the Soviet Union and Asia *(I. persulcatus)*. The principal vector for LD in the United States is the deer tick *(I. damini)*. The life cycle of *I. damini* involves three states (larva, nymph, sexually mature adult), with each stage requiring a blood meal for survival and maturation. The white-footed mouse *(Peromyscus leucopus)* is the preferred host for the larva and nymph forms, and the white-tail deer serves as the principal host for the adult. Most cases of LD in children are acquired from ticks in the nymphal stage, and animal studies suggest that attachment for more than 48 hr is necessary for disease transmission.

CLINICAL MANIFESTATIONS. LD occurs in stages, with characteristic clinical manifestations present at each stage. In the earliest *stage 1* (localized erythema migrans), an erythematous macule or papule occurs at the site of the tick bite in a majority of children (85%). Approximately 30% of patients have a history of a tick bite at the site of the initial lesion, which within 1 wk (3–32 days) develops into an expanding erythematous annular lesion with central clearing and often reaches a diameter of about 16 cm (3–68 cm). In some patients erythema chronicum migrans (ECM) is less characteristic, with an erythematous indurated center that may become vesicular or necrotic. These asymptomatic lesions may be located anywhere; however, the thigh, groin, and axilla are common sites. Several days after the initial lesion, many patients (50%) develop multiple secondary lesions. These are generally smaller, lack indurated centers, and are not associated with previous tick bites. Secondary lesions are uncommon in European patients. Additional dermatologic findings may develop, including a malar rash, conjunctivitis, and small evanescent red macules and circles.

Except for lethargy and fatigue, which may be constant and incapacitating, initial signs and symptoms are intermittent and include headache, fever, chills, and migrating musculoskeletal pains. Lymphadenopathy, meningismus, encephalopathy, splenomegaly, hepatomegaly, and testicular swelling have also been described. During this early phase, nonspecific laboratory abnormalities include a high sedimentation rate (50%), an elevated total serum IgM (33%), an increased serum glutamic oxaloacetic transaminase (19%), microscopic hematuria, and proteinuria. Although the spirochete can often be isolated from the skin lesion(s) in stage 1 disease, positive serologic signs are present in a minority of affected children (25%). Regardless of treatment, these initial signs and symptoms resolve within 3–4 wk; however, dermatologic manifestations often recur.

Stage 2 (disseminated infection) occurs in untreated children following a latent period of several weeks to months and may involve the central nervous system (10%), the cardiovascular system (8%), or the musculoskeletal system (60%). Neurologic manifestations occur within 4 wk of the initial illness and typically resolve over 3 mo; however, symptoms may recur and less often become chronic. Thus, headache and neck stiffness are common and are often associated with meningitis and superimposed cranial or peripheral neuritis. Unilateral or bilateral facial palsy is the most common cranial neuropathy. Peripheral neuropathy, when present, is usually an asymmetric motor, sensory, or mixed radiculoneuropathy. Less common neurologic manifestations include chorea, cerebellar ataxia, Guillain-Barré syndrome, pseudotumor cerebri, demyelinating encephalopathy, hearing loss, memory impairment, and depression. In children with meningitis, the cerebrospinal fluid analysis reveals a mononuclear pleocytosis, elevated protein, and normal glucose levels. The responsible pathogen has been recovered from the cerebrospinal fluid. Neurologic manifestations have long been recognized in patients with ECM by European clinicians, and this illness has been referred to as tick-borne meningopolyneuritis, Banwarth syndrome, and lymphocytic meningoradiculitis.

Cardiac abnormalities occur within 5 wk of the initial illness and include varying degrees of atrioventricular block (1st degree, Wenckebach, or complete heart block) and electrocardiographic changes consistent with myopericarditis. Cardiac involvement is usually brief (3 days–6 wk) and rarely recurs.

Joint manifestations occur within 1 wk–2 yr following the initial illness and are more severe in children with HLA-DR-2. Early symptoms include migratory arthralgias; arthritis begins months after the onset of the illness and typically involves the large joints, especially the knee. However, both large and small joints may be affected, and a minority of patients present with symmetric polyarthritis. Musculoskeletal signs and symptoms may last for weeks to months and usually recur over several years. Synovial fluid analysis reveals white cell counts of 500–100,000 mm^3 with a predominance of polymorphonuclear leukocytes and an elevated protein level.

Stage 3 (persistent infection) occurs in a minority of patients, rarely in children, and may last for years following the initial infection. In most cases, this stage consists of progressive arthritis with subsequent erosion of cartilage and bone, often associated with permanent disability. Additional late manifestations include depression, intellectual impairment, and demyelinating disease. Acrodermatitis chronica atrophicans is a late cutaneous manifestation of LD that has been frequently observed in Europe.

Congenital infection, although rare, has been described in infants whose mothers experienced LD during the 1st trimester of pregnancy. Affected infants have had meningoencephalitis and cardiovascular abnormalities and have suffered early demise. The true incidence of congenital infection is unknown, and recent surveys reveal conflicting data.

DIAGNOSIS AND TREATMENT. Diagnosis depends on recognition of signs and symptoms in a child living in an endemic area, with or without a history of tick exposure. Clinical diagnosis may be augmented by serologic testing with indirect immunofluorescence or enzyme-linked immunosorbent assays (ELISA). However, serologic testing is not yet standardized, specificity is unreliable, and false-positive and false-negative results are relatively common. False-positive serologic tests have been reported in patients with *Treponema* and other *Borrelia* infections, Rocky Mountain spotted fever, and various autoimmune diseases. False-negative results occur during the early stages of LD (when therapy is most successful) or following effective treatment with antimicrobial agents. Thus, until more sensitive and specific laboratory diagnostic tests become available, diagnosis of LD rests on clinical features.

ECM and its associated symptoms resolve rapidly in patients treated with tetracycline, penicillin, and erythromycin. Moreover, studies suggest that early treatment with antibiotics, particularly tetracycline, prevents the late complications of LD. Thus, in older children with stage 1 or localized ECM, tetracycline (40 mg/kg/24 hr given by mouth in 4 divided doses, not to exceed 1.0 g daily) is recommended for at least 10 days and up to 20 days if symptoms persist or recur. In younger children amoxicillin (30 mg/kg/24 hr given by mouth in 4 divided doses, not to exceed 1.0 g daily) for 10 days and up to 30 days is recommended. In children with stage 2 disease involving the central nervous system (with the exception of isolated facial palsy), intravenous ceftriaxone is preferred over penicillin because it crosses the blood-brain barrier more efficiently and requires administration only once a day (2.0 g intravenously daily for 14 days.) Alternative therapy for children allergic to ceftriaxone or penicillin includes tetracycline or chloramphenicol. Treatment of stage 3 disease is problematic because clinical response, when it occurs, is slow. Nevertheless, treatment is recommended and usually consists of intravenous penicillin or ceftriaxone or oral tetracycline or amoxicillin. The optimal therapy for pregnant women with LD is not known.

PREVENTION. This includes reducing exposure to ticks, using insect repellents, wearing long-sleeved shirts and long pants, tucking pants into socks, wearing light-colored clothing, and inspecting clothing and skin frequently for ticks.

WILLIAM T. SPECK
PHILIP TOLTZIS

Steere AC: Lyme disease. N Engl J Med 321:586, 1989.

12.58 CHLAMYDIAL INFECTIONS

ETIOLOGY. Chlamydiae are obligate intracellular parasites with discrete cell walls that are similar to those of gram-negative bacteria. They contain both RNA and DNA, are inhibited by some antibiotics, and do not stain red with Gram stain. Giemsa staining reveals typical cytoplasmic inclusion bodies lying close to the nucleus.

The genus *Chlamydia* is divided into two subgroups. Group A contains *Chlamydia trachomatis* and the agent of lymphogranuloma venereum, both of which infect humans and usually produce local disease. Group B includes the agents of psittacosis/ornithosis and Reiter syndrome as well as those of feline pneumonitis, bovine encephalomyelitis, and sheep polyarthritis. Both groups have a common complement-fixing antigen, but microimmunofluorescence testing is species- and subclass-specific.

EPIDEMIOLOGY. Chlamydiae are distributed worldwide. Adult infection is spread venereally as urethritis or lymphogranuloma venereum, and from eye to hand to eye in trachoma. Infection of the newborn occurs during passage through the infected maternal birth canal. *C. pneumoniae* appears to be spread by respiratory droplets.

Trachoma is associated with crowded and unsanitary living conditions. It continues to be a problem in American Indians living on reservations. Globally it is the leading cause of acquired blindness.

Chlamydiae are the cause of about 40% of cases of nonspecific nongonococcal urethritis. *Chlamydia* also causes cervicitis, salpingitis, endometritis, and epididymitis and appears to be an important cause of tubal infertility. Infection rates of 20–30% have been observed in adolescents, many of whom were asymptomatic. A syndrome of acute salpingitis and perihepatitis (Fitz-Hugh-Curtis syndrome), also attributed to gonococcal infection, can be caused by *Chlamydia*.

Some cases of Reiter disease (Sec. 12.17) are caused by *Chlamydia*. Rarely, *Chlamydia* can cause endocarditis, otitis media, choroiditis, or erythema nodosum.

About 12% of pregnant women are infected with chlamydiae; infection is more common in young women of low socioeconomic class. Infants born through an infected cervix have a 25% incidence of conjunctivitis; 10% develop pneumonia. Fifty per cent of exposed infants are culture positive for *Chlamydia*, and 70% have seroconversion. Rectal and vaginal cultures may not become positive until the infant is 4 mo of age; untreated, these infections can persist for up to 2 yr. The incidence of *Chlamydia* infection is estimated as 28/1,000 live births. One fourth of all infants under 6 mo of age admitted to the hospital with lower respiratory tract disease and three fourths of all infants with afebrile pneumonia are infected with *Chlamydia*.

Chlamydia has been isolated from the lower respiratory tract of adults with severe bronchitis or diffuse interstitial pneumonia. Most of these patients were immunocompromised. *Chlamydia* is a rare cause of pharyngitis in school-aged children.

12.59 CHLAMYDIAL CONJUNCTIVITIS AND PNEUMONIA IN INFANTS

CLINICAL MANIFESTATIONS. *Conjunctivitis* in the newborn usually begins in the 2nd wk of life but may occur as early as 3 days or as late as 5–6 wk. Infants typically are afebrile and alert, but develop purulent discharge from one or both eyes, swollen lids, and pseudomembranes. Routine bacterial cultures are negative. If untreated, the conjunctivitis most often subsides within 2–3 wk, but chronic mild infection is common. Response to appropriate topical antibiotics is prompt, but relapse is frequent.

A distinctive syndrome of *pneumonia* has been reported in infants infected with *Chlamydia*. These patients are usually seen at 3–16 wk of age but frequently have been sick for several weeks. The infant appears well and is afebrile but develops increasing tachypnea, with prominent cough. Physical examination reveals rales and at times wheezing. Conjunctivitis is present in about 50% of these infants.

Roentgenographically, hyperinflation and diffuse interstitial or patchy infiltrates are evident. Moderate eosinophilia is common. Po_2 is decreased in arterial blood, but Pco_2 is normal. IgM and IgG are increased, sometimes to 2–4 times normal for age.

Deaths due to chlamydial pneumonia have not been reported. Organisms have been isolated from lung tissue obtained by biopsy: light microscopy shows necrotic bronchioles with alveolar and bronchiolar consolidation. Several infants with chlamydial pneumonia have also been infected with cytomegalovirus. Illness in these infants has not been clinically different from that with chlamydia alone.

Patients improve gradually without treatment, but symptoms and positive cultures for *Chlamydia* persist for weeks or months. Patients hospitalized with *Chlamydia* pneumonia or bronchiolitis show an increased incidence of chronic cough and abnormal lung function studies compared with controls.

DIAGNOSIS AND DIFFERENTIAL DIAGNOSIS. *Chlamydia* can be isolated in specially treated McCoy, hamster kidney, or HeLa cell lines. Two types of rapid antigen tests are available; one uses monoclonal antibodies for direct fluorescent staining of elementary bodies, and the second is an enzyme-linked immunosorbent assay. Both are useful for testing eye and nasopharyngeal specimens from infants and urethral and cervical specimens from adults. Because fecal flora can cross react, these tests should not be used to test rectal, vaginal, or urethral specimens from children. In cases of suspected sexual abuse of a child, culture of the organism is the only reliable method of diagnosis.

Intracytoplasmic inclusion bodies can sometimes be seen on Papanicolaou staining when *Chlamydia* cervicitis is present, but they are not pathognomonic. If conjunctivitis is present, the palpebral conjunctiva may be scraped with a blunt curette; loosened epithelial cells are fixed on glass slides and stained with Giemsa stain. Intracytoplasmic inclusions can be seen. Culture or antigen testing is more reliable. The diagnosis is usually made by a high index of suspicion in a patient with a compatible illness.

Chlamydial conjunctivitis must be differentiated from chemical conjunctivitis due to silver nitrate drops, which usually occurs while the infant is still in the nursery. Bacterial conjunctivitis caused by gonococcus or other bacteria can be identified by Gram stain and culture.

Pneumonia may be caused by a variety of bacteria or viruses. Bacterial pneumonia usually has an increased white blood cell count without eosinophilia. Blood cultures or lung taps are frequently positive for bacteria. Viral agents can be isolated with appropriate tissue culture techniques.

TREATMENT. Conjunctivitis should be treated with erythromycin (50 mg/kg/24 hr) for 14 days. Topical therapy is likely to be ineffective and does not eliminate nasopharyngeal colonization.

Chlamydial *pneumonia* responds to erythromycin in a dosage of 50 mg/kg/24 hr or to sulfisoxazole (150 mg/kg/24 hr). Improvement is seen in 5–7 days and is associated with conversions of nasopharyngeal cultures to negative. Treatment should be continued for 2 wk.

Neonatal infection that stems from maternal cervical infection can be averted by preventing or treating the maternal disease. One gram of erythromycin daily for 14 days during the 3rd trimester is effective in eradicating the mother's infection. A similar treatment of her sexual partner is also necessary. For newborn infants, topical eye prophylaxis with erythromycin is not effective in preventing conjunctivitis. When a diagnosis of chlamydial infection is made in a neonate, both parents should also receive therapy.

Genitourinary tract infections due to *Chlamydia* should be treated with tetracycline, 0.5 g 4 times a day for 7 days, or doxycycline, 100 mg twice a day for 10 days. Erythromycin for 7 days can be used in patients who are allergic to tetracycline or who are pregnant.

12.60 *CHLAMYDIA PNEUMONIAE* (TWAR)

C. pneumoniae is a distinct strain of *Chlamydia* that causes severe pharyngitis without exudate, laryngitis, fever, lymphadenopathy, and pneumonia. When pneumonia is present, usually only a single infiltrate is seen. The white blood cell count is usually normal, and the sedimentation rate is elevated. Illness is more common in late childhood and in young adults and appears to exist worldwide.

The organism can be grown in embryonated chicken eggs or HeLa cells. Complement-fixation and microimmunofluorescent tests demonstrate titer rises. Tetracycyline or erythromycin is recommended for therapy, but experience is limited. Therapy should be continued for 2–3 wk. The organism is not sensitive to sulfonamides in vitro.

12.61 PSITTACOSIS/ORNITHOSIS

This disease, caused by *Chlamydia psittaci*, is spread by psittacine and other birds. Infected particles are present in bird secretions and droppings. Infection can be present in apparently healthy birds. Those working in the poultry or pet bird industries or persons who have recently purchased a bird are especially at risk. Most cases occur in adults; mild cases are probably frequent but undiagnosed.

Onset of illness is usually abrupt, with chills, fever, severe headache, myalgia, weakness, and confusion. Pneumonia is frequent; anorexia, vomiting, photophobia, and splenomegaly are less frequent; hepatitis, pulmonary embolism, severe anemia, disseminated intravascular coagulation, erythema nodosum, and endocarditis occur rarely. The temperatures may reach 40.5° C (105° F).

Examination of the lungs may demonstrate rales; roentgenographically diffuse interstitial infiltrations are characteristic, and lobar consolidation is uncommon. The white blood cell count does not help in diagnosing the disease. Untreated, the patient may remain quite ill for 2–3 wk, gradually improving after that time. Mortality is less than 1%.

Pneumonia caused by other agents, such as *Mycoplasma*, influenza virus, or other viral agents, may present a similar clinical picture. A history of exposure to birds is suggestive. Isolation of chlamydiae from blood or sputum or a 4-fold rise in complement-fixing antibody is diagnostic. A presumptive diagnosis can be made on the basis of a single complement-fixing titer of at least 32. Relapses and reinfections occur, even in patients with high antibody titers.

Chlamydial infections are relatively infrequent in wild birds. Crowding during shipment to the United States is mainly responsible for the widespread infection of imported birds. These birds are held in quarantine on arrival in the United States, and chlortetracycline is added to their feed for prophylactic treatment. This program, however, is not well administered, and animals have been shown to be infected when released from quarantine.

Tetracycline (30–40 mg/kg/24 hr) is the treatment of choice. Erythromycin (40 mg/kg/24 hr) can be used in children less than 8 yr old, but experience with this drug is limited. Treatment should be continued for 3 wk.

Control of fever and adequate oxygenation are important. Person-to-person spread has been documented on rare occasions. Hospitalized patients should be placed in respiratory isolation.

Beem MO, Saxon E: Respiratory tract colonization and a distinctive pneumonia syndrome in infants infected with *Chlamydia trachomatis*. N Engl J Med 296:306, 1977.

Beem MO, Saxon E, Tipple MA: Treatment of chlamydial pneumonia of infancy. Pediatrics 63:198, 1979.

Bell TA, Stamm WE, Kuo CC, et al: Delayed appearance of *Chlamydia trachomatis* infections acquired at birth. Pediatr Infect Dis J 6:928, 1987.

Chacko MR, Lovchik JC: *Chlamydia trachomatis* infection in sexually active adolescents: Prevalence and risk factors. Pediatrics 73:836, 1984.

Grayston JT, Kuo C, Wang S, et al: A new *Chlamydia psittaci* strain, TWAR, isolated in acute respiratory tract infections. N Engl J Med 315:161, 1986.

Hammerschlag MR, Rettig PJ, Shields ME: False positive results with the use of chlamydial antigen detection tests in the evaluation of suspected sexual abuse in children. Pediatr Infect Dis J 7:11, 1988.

Lefebvre J, LaPerriere H, Rousseau H, et al: Comparison of three techniques for detection of *Chlamydia trachomatis* in endocervical specimens from asymptomic women. J Clin Microbiol 26:726, 1988.

Myhre EB, Mardh PA: Unusual manifestations of *Chlamydia trachomatis* infections. Scand J Infect Dis Suppl 32:122, 1982.

Potter ME, Kaufmann AK, Plikaytis BD: Psittacosis in the United States, 1979. MMWR 32:27SS, 1983.

Stamm WE: Diagnosis of *Chlamydia trachomatis* genitourinary infections. Ann Intern Med 108:710, 1988.

Wolner-Hanssen P, Westrom L, Mardh PA: Perihepatitis and chlamydial salpingitis. Lancet 1:901, 1980.

12.62 LYMPHOGRANULOMA VENEREUM
(Lymphogranuloma Inguinale)

Lymphogranuloma venereum (LGV) is usually sexually transmitted, and the majority of children and youth who have it have acquired it from an infected adult. The causative agent is related to *Chlamydia trachomatis* but differs in being more invasive.

EPIDEMIOLOGY. Lymphogranuloma venereum has been reported worldwide but most frequently occurs in Southeast Asia and Central and South America. The reported incidence is much higher in males, reaching 20:1 in some series.

PATHOLOGY. Pathologic characteristics of the primary lesion are not specific and therefore do not help in establishing the diagnosis. Primary genital ulcers have an exudate of fibrin and contain cellular debris and polymorphonuclear leukocytes. The periphery of the ulcer contains large mononuclear and plasma cells as well. The lymph nodes that drain the infected area have characteristic stellate triangular abscesses, in the centers of which are polymorphonuclear leukocytes and macrophages. In older, healing lesions scars and sinus tracts may be expected.

CLINICAL MANIFESTATIONS. If a primary genital lesion is considered the end-point, the incubation period varies from 3 to 30 days. If such a lesion is undetected, the period from sexual contact to the development of adenopathy may be much longer.

The first manifestation is a small erosion, a papule or a pustule. In men it is usually found on the coronal sulcus, frenulum, prepuce, glans, or shaft of the penis or on the scrotum. In women the most common sites are the posterior vaginal wall, cervix, and fourchette. Because the primary lesion is small and asymptomatic, it is frequently undetected. Rarely, extragenital primary lesions are noted; they too can usually be related to direct contact with infected genitals.

The secondary lesion, inguinal adenitis, develops 1–4 wk after the appearance of the primary lesion and is most often unilateral. Males often present with fever, toxicity, and inguinal adenopathy. The nodes are initially firm, tender, and movable. Later they become fixed to one another and to the overlying skin, which becomes erythematous and cyanotic, then scaly and edematous, preceding rupture of the nodes. Whether the rupture is spontaneous or surgical, a chronic sinus tract usually develops and drains for weeks or months. Rarely, the nodes resolve over a period of several months despite lack of treatment. Relapses of acute adenitis are common.

In women the anatomic site of the primary lesion determines the clinical location of the disease. Lesions of the upper third of the vagina and on the cervix drain to nodes between the external and internal iliac arteries; those of the middle third of the vagina, to nodes between the rectum and internal iliac arteries; those of the lower third of the vagina, to the pelvic and inguinal nodes.

Rectal drainage of blood, mucus, or pus secondary to rupture of perirectal nodes also occurs and may lead to fibrosis, scarring, and rectal stricture. The latter may result in periodic rectal bleeding and thin stools. Women may present initially with complications such as rectal stricture. Such symptoms are also especially common in homosexual males.

Untreated patients may develop elephantiasis of the genitalia and attendant soft tissue infections.

Like so many other sexually transmitted infections, lymphogranuloma venereum is a systemic disease and may be associated with fever, malaise, headache, anorexia, and other nonspecific symptoms. Rarely, meningoencephalitis occurs, and chlamydiae are recovered from spinal fluid.

Hypergammaglobulinemia due to elevation of IgA and IgG is common. The white blood cell count and sedimentation rate are frequently elevated. Mild anemia, decreased albumin, elevated globulin, and elevated liver enzymes can also be seen. Autoimmune serum factors such as cryoglobulins, rheumatoid factor, antinuclear factor, positive Coombs test, and anticomplementary serum factors are present in most cases. Likewise, a false-positive serologic test for syphilis is common.

DIAGNOSIS AND DIFFERENTIAL DIAGNOSIS. Lymphogranuloma venereum must be considered in patients with the typical primary lesion; with enlarged, matted, and tender inguinal lymph nodes; or with proctitis, draining inguinal or perianal fistulas, and rectal strictures. It may mimic inguinal adenopathy of any cause, such as pyogenic infections, plague, tularemia, cat-scratch disease, chancroid, granuloma inguinale, syphilis, herpes genitalis, and rectal neoplasms. Other venereal diseases can, of course, coexist. Direct examination of the tissues may reveal the somewhat characteristic pathologic lesions as well as chlamydiae in the cytoplasm of the cells, which appear as blue inclusions with Giemsa stain. Aspirates from lymph nodes should be cultured.

Serologic tests, such as the complement-fixation reaction, are carried out with heat-stable group antigens. If a test is positive in a patient with a suspicious clinical history and findings, the diagnosis is strongly supported. The indirect immunofluorescence (IF) test is more sensitive but less available.

PREVENTION. Measures for preventing sexually transmitted diseases are applicable. There is no available vaccine.

TREATMENT. Tetracycline, 500 mg every 6 hr is effective. Alternative therapies are sulfamethoxazole, 1 g twice a day, or erythromycin, 500 mg every 6 hr. Treated patients tend to have a shorter duration of the disease, less occurrence of sinus tracts, fewer relapses, and a decline in the complement-fixation titer. If there is a rise in titer after therapy, the patient should be retreated. The course of treatment should be 3–wk. Aspiration may prevent rupture. Surgical excision is contraindicated because of the possible formation of sinus tracts. Response to therapy, although variable, is better in acute cases.

CAROL F. PHILLIPS

Banou L Jr: Rectal lesions of lymphogranuloma venereum in childhood. Am J Dis Child 83:860, 1952.

McLelland BA, Anderson PC: Lymphogranuloma venereum: Outbreak in a university community. JAMA 235:56, 1976.

Thorsteinsson SB: Lymphogranuloma venereum: Review of clinical manifestations, epidemiology, diagnosis and treatment. Scand J Infect Dis Suppl 32:127, 1982.

12.63 MYCOPLASMAL INFECTIONS

RESPIRATORY MYCOPLASMAS

Among the respiratory mycoplasmas, *Mycoplasma pneumoniae* is the only known human pathogen. It is a major cause of respiratory infections in school-aged children and young adults. The incidence of illness varies greatly with the age of the patient and the epidemicity of the organism. Clinically significant disease is unusual before the age of 3–4 yr; the peak incidence occurs from 10 to 15 yr. It has been estimated that *M. pneumoniae* causes 500,000 cases of pneumonia, 11,500,000 cases of tracheobronchitis, and 3,000,000 asymptomatic infections in the United States annually.

ETIOLOGY. *M. pneumoniae*, originally thought to be a virus and called the Eaton agent, was found to be a mycoplasma in the early 1960s. Mycoplasmas have no cell wall and are intermediate in size—larger than certain viruses, smaller than others. They can be grown on lifeless media and are thus the smallest free-living microorganisms known. Methods for isolation, propagation, and specific identification are highly technical and are performed routinely in only a few laboratories.

EPIDEMIOLOGY. *M. pneumoniae* infections occur worldwide. In contrast to the acute, short-lived epidemics of some respiratory agents, *M. pneumoniae* infection is endemic in larger communities with epidemic disease occurring every 4–7 yr. Infections occur throughout the year. In smaller communities, infections are sporadic with long-lasting and smoldering outbreaks occurring at irregular intervals and having a tendency to begin in the fall.

The occurrence of mycoplasmal illness is related, in part, to the age and immune status of the patient. Overt illness is unusual before 3–4 yr of age; younger children appear to have frequent mild or subclinical infections, and reinfections appear to be common. The peak incidence of illness occurs in school-aged children; *M. pneumoniae* accounts for 33% and 70% of all pneumonias in children aged 5–9 yr and 9–15 yr, respectively. In adults, previous infections, as demonstrated by the presence of circulating antibodies, prevent or ameliorate subsequent ones.

M. pneumoniae infections are not highly communicable, as evidenced by the slow rate at which susceptible family contacts become infected; such periods may extend for weeks or months. Infection occurs through the respiratory route by large droplet spread, and the incubation period is thought to be 2–3 wk. Explosive epidemics have been reported among military recruits and summer camps for children.

PATHOLOGY, IMMUNOLOGY, AND PATHOGENESIS. Much has been learned about the attachment of *M. pneumoniae* to ciliated respiratory epithelium, the target cells of infection. Electron microscopic studies of tracheal ciliated cells show the organism to be an elongated snake-like structure with an attachment tip characterized by an electron-dense core and a trilaminar outer membrane. Attachment to the ciliary membrane is mediated by a P1 protein localized to the mycoplasma membrane of the attachment tip. Pretreatment of *M. pneumoniae* with anti-P1 antibody inhibits attachment and subsequent disease in experimental animals. The organisms attach to cell surfaces and burrow down between cells, resulting in eventual sloughing of the cells. Intracellular organisms have not been found. *M. pneumoniae* rarely invade beyond the basement membrane of the respiratory tract.

A variety of serologic responses occur following *M. pneumoniae* infection. Nonspecific cold hemagglutinins reacting to the I antigen of red blood cell glycoproteins are usually the first antibodies detected. Appearing with titers of at least 1:32 in approximately 50% of patients, cold hemagglutinins develop late in the 1st or 2nd wk of illness and increase 4-fold or more by the 3rd wk. They disappear in about 6 wk. The presence of elevated titers of cold hemagglutinins and the height of the titer correlate with the severity of the illness. Specific immunologic reactions to *M. pneumoniae* can be measured by a variety of techniques and persist for long periods of time.

Although the presence of circulating antibodies in humans can be correlated with protection against *M. pneumoniae* infections, studies in the hamster have shown that circulating antibody alone, in the absence of other forms of immunity, is incompletely protective. In hamsters, most of the peribronchial mononuclear cells are laden with antibody. However, ablation of the T cell system with antithymocyte serum completely prevents the development of pneumonia. Thus, the disease produced by *M. pneumoniae* is very complex; the immunologic response of the host may be responsible for the disease itself as well as for protection against it, depending on the qualitative and quantitative balance of humoral and cellular immunity. Patients with immunodeficiency states such as hypogammaglobulinemia and sickle cell anemia have more severe mycoplasma pneumonia than do normal hosts. *M. pneumoniae* is the most common infectious cause of acute chest syndrome in sickle cell patients but has not been prevalent in patients with AIDS.

CLINICAL MANIFESTATIONS. Respiratory and nonrespiratory sites are involved in *M. pneumoniae* infections, but the lower respiratory tract is the primary site, and tracheobronchitis and bronchopneumonia are the most commonly recognized clinical syndromes. The onset of illness is gradual and is characterized by headache, malaise, and fever; cough is prominent, and sore throat is frequent. Although the clinical course in untreated individuals is variable, coughing usually worsens during the 1st 2 wk of illness, and then all symptoms gradually resolve within 3–4 wk. The severity of symptoms is usually greater than the condition suggested by the physical signs, which appear later in the disease. Rales, which are often fine and crackling and resemble those heard in asthma and bronchiolitis, are the most prominent sign; increased sputum production occurs frequently. *M. pneumonia* can usually be isolated from the upper respiratory tract or sputum for several weeks to months after the patient recovers.

Roentgenographic findings are not specific. Pneumonia is usually described as interstitial or bronchopneumonic; involvement is most common in the lower lobes, with unilateral centrally dense infiltrates described in 75% of cases. Hilar lymphadenopathy may be described in up to 33% of patients. Significant amounts of pleural fluid are unusual, but patients with large effusions due to *M. pneumoniae* have been described. The white blood cell and differential counts are usually normal.

Additional respiratory illnesses caused infrequently by *M. pneumoniae* include undifferentiated upper respiratory tract infections, pharyngitis, croup, and bronchiolitis. In addition, otitis media and bullous myringitis have been described but are rarely seen without associated lower respiratory tract infection.

Despite the rare isolation of *M. pneumoniae* from nonrespiratory sites, patients with respiratory infections may occasionally manifest illness involving the skin, central nervous system, blood, heart, and joints. Skin lesions include a variety of exanthems, most notably maculopapular rashes, erythema multiforme, and the Stevens-Johnson syndrome. Meningoencephalitis, transverse myelitis, aseptic meningitis, cerebellar ataxia, and the Guillain-Barré syndrome have been reported. Mild degrees of hemolysis with positive Coombs test and minor reticulocytosis occurring 2–3 wk after the onset of illness is common. Severe hemolysis with high titers of cold hemagglutinins ($\geq$1:512) is rare, as are thrombocytopenia and coagulation defects. Myocarditis, pericarditis, and a rheumatic fever–like syndrome are uncommon manifestations. Transient monoarticular arthritis has been described in 1% of patients in one large series.

DIAGNOSIS. No specific clinical, epidemiologic, or laboratory observations permit a definite diagnosis of mycoplasmal infection early in the clinical course. Certain observations, however, are suggestive and can be helpful to the astute physician. For example, pneumonia in school-aged children and young adults, especially if cough is a prominent finding, is always suggestive of *M. pneumoniae* disease. Cold hemagglutinins in a titer of 1:64 or greater support the diagnosis, which can be confirmed by isolation of the organism and identification of specific antibodies. Cultures of the throat or sputum on special media may demonstrate *M. pneumoniae*, but growth is rarely detected earlier than 1 wk. Cold hemagglutinins may be determined in acute-phase serum. Complement-fixing antibody tests, in which commercially available antigen is used, are satisfactory for usual diagnostic purposes. An antibody rise (or fall) in convalescent-phase serum obtained after 10 days–3 wk is diagnostic. Rapid diagnostic testing has not proved reliable, although a DNA probe assay is available that has shown good sensitivity and specificity. When *M. pneumoniae* can be confirmed in the community in a few patients, the probability of the existence of other mycoplasmal illnesses is greatly increased.

TREATMENT. In general, *M. pneumoniae* illnesses are mild, and hospitalization is infrequent. Fatal infections are rare. Complications are unusual, as is bacterial superinfection. *M. pneumoniae* is exceptionally sensitive to erythromycin and to the tetracyclines in vitro; because of the absence of a cell wall, the organism is resistant to the penicillins. Both erythromycin and the tetracyclines are effective in shortening the course of mycoplasmal illnesses. Erythromycin is the drug of choice in small children because of the toxic effects of the tetracyclines in this age group; it should be given in full therapeutic doses for several days after defervescence, usually 7–10 days. For patients over the age of 8 yr tetracycline is an alternate choice. In spite of the efficacy of these drugs in ameliorating the clinical course, the organism is not eradicated.

GENITAL MYCOPLASMAS

Two mycoplasma species, *Mycoplasma hominis* and *Ureaplasma urealyticum*, are human urogenital pathogens. Both commonly colonize the female genital tract and are thus capable of causing perinatal infections and colonization of neonates (Sec. 9.68).

ETIOLOGY. See Sec. 9.68.

EPIDEMIOLOGY. *U. urealyticum* grows readily in the genitourinary tract of postpubertal males and females. In females, colonization is maximal in the vagina and less frequent in the endocervix, urethra, or endometrium. In the male, colonization occurs primarily in the urethra. Colonization rates are directly related to sexual activity, with colonization occurring in less than 10% of prepubertal children and sexually inactive adults. Rates are highest in those with multiple sexual partners. Colonization of pregnant females has varied from 40 to 90%. Vertical transmission of *U. urealyticum* to full-term neonates occurs in approximately 45% of infants born to colonized mothers regardless of the route of delivery. Female newborns are colonized twice as often as males because the vagina is the most frequently colonized site. Colonization rates diminish after birth and are less than 10% by 1 yr of age. Frequent maternal and neonatal colonization complicates determination of the pathogenicity of *U. urealyticum* in the perinatal period.

CLINICAL MANIFESTATIONS. The primary disease for which *U. urealyticum* is a confirmed pathogen is nongonococcal urethritis; approximately 20% of cases of this disease in males are caused by this organism either alone or together with *C. trachomatis*. Disease is most common in young adults but is also prevalent in sexually active adolescents. The average incubation period is 2–3 wk with symptoms typically consisting of scanty, mucoid-white urethral discharge, dysuria, or penile discomfort. The discharge is often evident only in the morning or after the urethra is stripped. Rare complications of nongonococcal urethritis are epididymitis, proctitis, and Reiter syndrome. There is a case report of recurring *Ureaplasma* urethritis in a prepubertal nonsexually active male. Females rarely have urethritis, and despite the high vaginal colonization rates, vaginitis or cervicitis is uncommon.

Although there is still controversy about the data, *U. urealyticum* probably contributes to premature labor, stillbirths, and congenital pneumonia (Sec. 9.68).

DIAGNOSIS. Diagnosis of an individual case of *U. urealyticum* infection is difficult because of high colonization rates. Nongonococcal urethritis is confirmed by Gram stain of urethral discharge showing at least 4 PMNs/oil-immersion field and the absence of gram-negative diplococci. Cultures of the discharge or of material obtained by a urethral swab can be done for *C. trachomatis* and *U. urealyticum*. One of the characteristic features of ureaplasmas is their close association with urethral epithelial cells in primary agar cultures of urethral exudate. Multiple *Ureaplasma* colonies are frequently observed growing into the agar media beneath infected epithelial cells. In the neonate with respiratory disease, cultures of the upper respiratory tract are probably meaningless owing to high colonization rates. Cultures of the lower respiratory tract through endotracheal aspirate or biopsy are essential. Material must be cultured immediately or frozen at $-80°$ C to avoid loss of organisms.

TREATMENT. Nongonococcal urethritis is treated with tetracycline, doxycycline, or erythromycin orally for 7 days. Since approximately 10% of *U. urealyticum* strains are tetracycline resistant, erythromycin is the drug of choice in patients in whom tetracycline treatment has failed. Sexual partners should be similarly treated to avoid recurrent disease. Data supporting the role of therapy in neonatal *Ureaplasma* infections are limited to case reports. Erythromycin is the drug of choice.

DWIGHT A. POWELL

Behan PO, Feldman RG, Segerra JM: Neurologic aspects of mycoplasmal infection. Acta Neurol Scand 74:314, 1986.

Clyde WA Jr: *Mycoplasma pneumoniae* respiratory disease symposium: Summation and significance. Yale J Biol Med 56:523, 1983.

Denny FW, Clyde WA Jr, Glezen WP: *Mycoplasma pneumoniae* disease: Clinical spectrum, pathophysiology, epidemiology, and control. J Infect Dis 123:74, 1971.

Dinsmoor MJ, Ramamurthy RS, Gibbs RS: Transmission of genital mycoplasmas from mother to neonate in women with prolonged membrane rupture. Pediatr Infect Dis J 8:483, 1989.

Dular R, Kajoika R, Kasatiya S: Comparison of Gen-Probe commercial kit and culture technique for the diagnosis of *Mycoplasma pneumoniae* infection. J Clin Microbiol 26:1068, 1988.

Fernald GW, Clyde WA Jr: Immunologic responses to *Mycoplasma pneumoniae* infection. *In*: Bienenstock JB (ed): Immunology of the Lung. New York, McGraw-Hill, 1983, p 282.

Fernald GW, Collier AM, Clyde WA Jr: Respiratory infections due to *Mycoplasma pneumoniae* in infants and children. Pediatrics 55:327, 1975.

Lucas LM, Smith DL: Nongonococcal urethritis: Diagnosis and management. J Gen Intern Med 2:199, 1987.

Murray BJ: Nonrespiratory complication of *M. pneumoniae* infection. Am Fam Physician 37:127, 1988.

Nagayama Y, Sakuri N, Yamanoto K, et al: Isolation of *Mycoplasma pneumoniae* from children with lower respiratory tract infections. J Infect Dis 157:911, 1988.

Poncz M, Kane E, Gill FM: Acute chest syndrome in sickle cell disease: Etiology and clinical correlates. J Pediatr 107:861, 1985.

Roiman CM, Rao CP, Lederman HW, et al: Increased susceptibility to mycoplasma infection in patients with hypogammaglobulinemia. Am J Med 80:590, 1986.

VIRAL INFECTIONS AND THOSE PRESUMED TO BE CAUSED BY VIRUSES

12.64 MEASLES
(Rubeola)

Measles, an acute communicable disease, is characterized by three stages: (1) an incubation stage of approximately 10–12 days with few, if any, signs or symptoms; (2) a prodromal stage with an enanthem (Koplik spots) on the buccal and pharyngeal mucosa, slight to moderate fever, mild conjunctivitis, coryza, and an increasingly severe cough; and (3) a final stage with a maculopapular rash erupting successively over the neck and face, body, arms, and legs and accompanied by high fever.

ETIOLOGY. Measles is an RNA virus of the family Paramyxoviridae, genus *Morbillivirus*. Only one antigenic type is known. During the prodromal period and for a short time after the rash appears, it is found in nasopharyngeal secretions, blood, and urine. It can remain active for at least 34 hr at room temperature.

Measles virus may be isolated in cultures of human embryonic or rhesus monkey kidney tissue. Cytopathic changes, visible in 5–10 days, consist of multinucleated giant cells with intranuclear inclusions. Circulating antibody is detectable when the rash appears.

INFECTIVITY. Maximal dissemination of virus is by droplet spray during the prodromal period (catarrhal stage). Transmission to susceptible contacts often occurs prior to diagnosis of the original case. An infected person becomes contagious by the 9th–10th day after exposure (beginning of prodromal phase), in some instances as early as the 7th day. Isolation precautions, especially in hospitals or other institutions, should be maintained from the 7th day after exposure until 5 days after the rash has appeared.

EPIDEMIOLOGY. Measles is endemic over most of the world. In the past, epidemics tended to occur irregularly, appearing in the spring in large cities at 2- to 4-yr intervals as new groups of susceptible children were exposed. Measles is very contagious; approximately 90% of susceptible family contacts acquire the disease. It is rarely subclinical. Prior to the use of measles vaccine, the age of peak incidence was 5–10 yr; most adults were immune. At present in the United States, measles occurs most often in unimmunized preschool-aged children and in teenagers and young adults who have been immunized. Epidemics have occurred in high schools and colleges where immunization levels were high. Those over age 30 are virtually all immune. Since measles is still a common disease in many countries, infective persons entering this country may infect United States citizens, and Americans traveling abroad risk exposure there.

The many similarities among the biologic features of measles and smallpox suggest the possibility that measles may be eradicable. These features are: (1) a distinctive rash, (2) no animal reservoir, (3) no vector, (4) seasonal occurrence with disease free periods, (5) no transmissible latent virus, (6) one serotype, and (7) an effective vaccine. A prevalence of more than 90% immunization of infants has been shown to produce disease-free zones. In 1980, three fourths of all counties in the United States did not report a single case of measles, but by 1988 the number of measles cases was increasing and the disease was more widespread.

Infants transplacentally acquire immunity from mothers who have had measles or measles immunization. This immunity is usually complete for the first 4–6 mo of life and disappears at a variable rate. Although maternal antibody levels are generally undetectable in the infant by the usual tests performed after 9 mo of age, some protection persists, which may interfere with immunization administered prior to 15 mo (Sec. 5.1). Most women of child-bearing age in the United States now have measles immunity by means of immunization rather than disease. Whether this antibody will have an earlier decline in the infant is not known. Infants of susceptible mothers have no such immunity and may contract the disease with the mother before or after delivery.

PATHOLOGY. The essential lesion of measles is found in the skin; in the mucous membranes of the nasopharynx, bronchi, and intestinal tract; and in the conjunctivae. Serous exudate and proliferation of mononuclear cells and a few polymorphonuclear cells occur around the capillaries. There is usually hyperplasia of lymphoid tissue, particularly in the appendix, where multinucleated giant cells of up to 100 μm in diameter (Warthin-Finkeldey reticuloendothelial giant cells) may be found. In the skin, the reaction is particularly notable about the sebaceous glands and hair follicles. Koplik spots consist of serous exudate and proliferation of endothelial cells similar to those in the skin lesions. A general inflammatory reaction of the buccal and pharyngeal mucosa extends into the lymphoid tissue and the tracheobronchial mucous membrane. Interstitial pneumonitis due to measles virus takes the form of Hecht giant cell pneumonia. Bronchopneumonia may be due to secondary bacterial infection.

In fatal cases of encephalomyelitis, perivascular demyelinization occurs in areas of the brain and spinal cord. In Dawson subacute sclerosing panencephalitis (SSPE), there may be degeneration of the cortex and white matter with intranuclear and intracytoplasmic inclusion bodies (Sec. 20.68).

CLINICAL MANIFESTATIONS. The *incubation period* is approximately 10–12 days if the first prodromal symptoms are selected as the time of onset, or approximately 14 days if the appearance of the rash is selected; rarely it may be as short as 6–10 days. A slight rise in temperature may occur 9–10 days from the date of infection and then subside for 24 hr or so.

The *prodromal phase,* which follows, usually lasts 3–5 days and is characterized by low-grade to moderate fever, a hacking cough, coryza, and conjunctivitis. These nearly always precede Koplik spots, the pathognomonic sign of measles, by 2–3 days. An enanthem or red mottling is usually present on the hard and soft palates. **Koplik spots** are grayish white dots, usually as small as grains of sand, with slight, reddish areolae; occasionally they are hemorrhagic. They tend to occur opposite the lower molars but may spread irregularly over the rest of the buccal mucosa. Rarely they are found within the midportion of the lower lip, on the palate, and on the lacrimal caruncle. They appear and disappear rapidly, usually within 12–18 hr. As they fade, red, spotty discolorations of the mucosa may remain. The conjunctival inflammation and photophobia may suggest measles before Koplik spots appear. In particular, a transverse line of conjunctival inflammation, sharply demarcated along the eyelid margin, may be of diagnostic assistance in the prodromal stage. As the entire conjunctiva becomes involved, the line disappears.

Occasionally, the prodromal phase may be severe, being ushered in by sudden high fever, at times with convulsions and even pneumonia. Usually the coryza, fever, and cough are increasingly severe up to the time the rash has covered the body.

The temperature rises abruptly *as the rash appears* and often reaches 40–40.5° C (104–105° F). In uncomplicated cases, when the rash appears on the legs and feet, within about 2 days, the symptoms subside rapidly; the subsidence includes a usually abrupt temperature drop. Patients up to this point may appear desperately ill, but within 24 hr after the temperature drop, they appear essentially well.

The rash usually starts as faint macules on the upper lateral parts of the neck, behind the ears, along the hairline, and on the posterior parts of the cheek. The individual lesions become increasingly maculopapular as the rash spreads rapidly over the entire face, neck, upper arms, and upper part of the chest within approximately the first 24 hr (Figs. 12–12 [color plate section] and 12–13). During the succeeding 24 hr it spreads over the back, abdomen, entire arms, and thighs. As it finally reaches the feet on the 2nd–3rd day, it begins to fade on the face. The fading of the rash proceeds downward in the same sequence in which it appeared. The severity of the disease is directly related to the extent and confluence of the rash. In mild measles the rash tends not to be confluent, and in very mild cases there are few, if any, lesions on the legs. In severe measles the rash is confluent, the skin being completely covered, including the palms and soles, and the face is swollen and disfigured.

The rash is often slightly hemorrhagic; in severe cases with a confluent rash, petechiae may be present in large numbers, and there may be extensive ecchymoses. Itching is generally slight. As the rash fades, branny desquamation and brownish discoloration occur and then disappear within 7–10 days.

The rash may vary markedly. Infrequently a slight urticarial, faint macular, or scarlatiniform rash may appear during the early prodromal stage and disappear in advance of the typical rash. Complete absence of rash is rare except in patients who have received human antibodies during the incubation period, some patients with AIDS, and possibly in infants under 8 mo of age who have appreciable levels of maternal antibody. In the hemorrhagic type of measles **(black measles)**, bleeding may occur from the mouth, nose, or bowel. In mild cases the rash may be less macular and more nearly pinpoint, somewhat resembling that of scarlet fever or rubella.

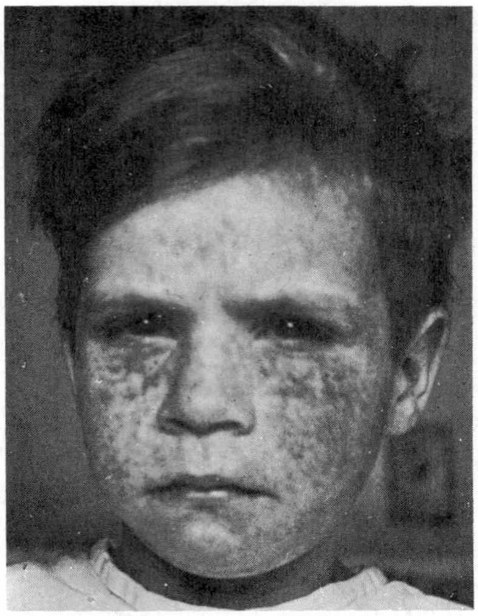

Figure 12–13. Purpuric rash of measles.

Lymph nodes at the angle of the jaw and in the posterior cervical region are usually enlarged, and slight splenomegaly may be noted. Mesenteric lymphadenopathy may cause abdominal pain. Characteristic pathologic changes of measles in the mucosa of the appendix may cause obliteration of the lumen and symptoms of appendicitis. Changes of this type tend to subside with the disappearance of Koplik spots. Otitis media, bronchopneumonia, and gastrointestinal symptoms, such as diarrhea and vomiting, are more common in infants and small children (especially malnourished ones) than in older children.

The diagnosis of measles is frequently delayed in adults because practitioners providing health care for adults are not used to encountering the disease and rarely include it in the differential diagnosis. The clinical picture is similar to that seen in children. Liver involvement, with abdominal pain, mild to moderate elevation of aspartate aminotransferase (AST) levels, and occasionally jaundice, is common in adults. In developing countries, measles frequently occurs in infants less than 1 yr old; possibly because malnutrition is concomitant there, the disease is very severe and has a high mortality.

DIAGNOSIS. This is usually made from the typical clinical picture; laboratory confirmation is rarely needed. During the prodromal stage multinucleated giant cells can be demonstrated in smears of the nasal mucosa. Virus can be isolated in tissue culture, and diagnostic rises in antibody titer can be detected between acute and convalescent sera. The white blood cell count tends to be low with a relative lymphocytosis. Lumbar puncture in patients with measles encephalitis usually shows an increase in protein and a small increase in lymphocytes. The glucose level is normal.

DIFFERENTIAL DIAGNOSIS. The rash of rubeola must be differentiated from exanthem subitum, rubella, infections due to echo-, coxsackie-, and adenoviruses, infectious mononucleosis, toxoplasmosis, meningococcemia, scarlet fever, rickettsial diseases, serum sickness, Kawasaki disease, and drug rashes.

Koplik spots are pathognomonic for rubeola, and the diagnosis of unmodified measles should not be made in the absence of cough.

Roseola infantum (exanthem subitum) is distinguished from measles in that the rash of the former appears as the fever disappears. The rashes of rubella and of enteroviral infections tend to be less striking than that of measles, as do the degree of fever and severity of illness. Although cough is present in many rickettsial infections, the rash usually spares the face, which is characteristically involved in measles. The absence of cough or the history of injection of serum or administration of a drug usually serves to identify serum sickness or drug rashes. Meningococcemia may be accompanied by a rash that is somewhat similar to that of measles, but cough and conjunctivitis are usually absent. In acute meningococcemia the rash is characteristically petechial purpuric. The diffuse, finely papular rash of scarlet fever with a "gooseflesh" texture on an erythematous base is relatively easy to differentiate.

The milder rash and clinical picture of measles modified by gamma globulin or by partial immunity induced by measles vaccine, or in infants by maternal antibody, may be difficult to differentiate.

COMPLICATIONS. The chief complications of measles are otitis media, pneumonia, and encephalitis. Noma of the cheeks may occur in rare instances. Gangrene elsewhere appears to be secondary to purpura fulminans or disseminated intravascular coagulation following measles.

Pneumonia (Sec. 14.57) may be caused by the measles virus itself; the lesion is interstitial. Measles pneumonia in patients with AIDS is often fatal and not always accompanied by rash. Bronchopneumonia is more frequent, however; it is due to secondarily invading bacteria, particularly the pneumococcus, streptococcus, staphylococcus, and *Haemophilus influenzae*. Laryngitis, tracheitis, and bronchitis are common and may be due to the virus alone.

One of the potential dangers of measles is exacerbation of an existing *tuberculous process*. There may also be a temporary loss of hypersensitivity to tuberculin.

Myocardis is an infrequent serious complication; transient electrocardiographic changes are said to be relatively common.

Neurologic complications are more common in measles than in any of the other exanthems. The incidence of *encephalomyelitis* is estimated to be 1–2/1,000 reported cases of measles. There is no correlation between the severity of the measles and that of the neurologic involvement or between the severity of the initial encephalitic process and the prognosis. Rarely, encephalitis has been reported in association with measles modified by gamma globulin or by live attenuated measles virus vaccine. Infrequently, encephalitic involvement is manifest in the pre-eruptive period, but more often the onset occurs 2–5 days after the appearance of the rash. The cause of measles encephalitis remains controversial. It is suggested that when encephalitis occurs early in the course of the disease, viral invasion plays a large role, although measles virus has rarely been isolated from brain tissue; encephalitis that occurs later is predominantly demyelinating and may reflect an immunologic reaction. In this demyelinating type the symptoms and course do not differ from those of other parainfectious encephalitides. Fatal encephalitis has occurred in children receiving immunosuppressive treatment for malignancies. Other central nervous system complications, such as Guillain-Barré syndrome, hemiplegia, cerebral thrombophlebitis, and retrobulbar neuritis, are rare.

Subacute sclerosing panencephalitis (Sec. 20.68) is due to measles virus.

PROGNOSIS. Case fatality rates in the United States have decreased in recent years to low levels for all age groups, largely because of improved socioeconomic conditions but also because of effective antibacterial therapy for the treatment of secondary infections.

When measles is introduced into a highly susceptible population, the results may be disastrous. Such an occurrence in the Faroe Islands in 1846 resulted in the deaths of about one fourth, nearly 2,000, of the total population regardless of age. At Ungava Bay, Canada, where 99% of 900 persons had measles, the mortality rate was 7%.

PROPHYLAXIS. Quarantine is of little value because of the contagiousness during its prodromal stage, when measles may not be suspected.

Active Immunization. See also Sec. 5.1.

The initial measles immunization is usually given at 15 mo but may be given earlier in areas where disease is occurring. Because the seroconversion rate following immunization is not 100% and there may be some waning of immunity with time, a second immunization against measles, usually given as MMR, is indicated. This dose can be given when the child enters school or later on entry to middle school. Adolescents entering college should also have received a second measles immunization.

The response to live measles vaccine is unpredictable if immune globulin has been administered in the 3 mo preceding immunization. Anergy to tuberculin may develop and persist for 1 mo or longer after administration of live attenuated measles vaccine. A child with active tuberculous infection should be receiving antituberculosis treatment when live measles vaccine is administered. A tuberculin test prior to or concurrent with active immunization against measles is desirable.

Use of live measles vaccine is not recommended for pregnant women or for children with untreated tuberculosis. Live vaccine is contraindicated in children with leukemia and in those receiving immunosuppresive drugs because of the risk of persistent, progressive infection such as giant cell pneumonia. After exposure of these susceptible children to measles, measles immune globulin (human) should be given intramuscularly in a dose of 0.25 mL/kg as soon as possible. A larger dose may be advisable in children with acute leukemia, even those in remission. Children with AIDS should receive measles vaccine because mortality due to measles is high in this group and they tolerate the vaccine well. Despite a history of having received measles immunization, these children should receive gamma globulin after exposure to measles in a dose of 0.5 mL/kg (maximum 15 mL). This is twice the usual recommended dose. Measles vaccine can be given following exposure to the disease. Reactions are not increased, and measles may be prevented.

The use of inactivated (killed) virus vaccine is not recommended.

Passive Immunization. Passive immunization with pooled adult serum, pooled convalescent serum, placental globulin, or gamma globulin of pooled plasma is effective for prevention and attenuation of measles. Measles can be prevented by using immune serum globulin (gamma globulin) in a dose of 0.25 mL/kg given intramuscularly within 5 days after exposure but preferably as soon as possible. Complete protection is indicated for infants, for children with chronic illness, and for contacts in hospital wards and children's institutions. Attenuation may be accomplished by the use of gamma globulin in a dosage of 0.05 mL/kg. Gamma globulin is approximately 25 times as potent in antibody titer as pooled adult serum, and it avoids the risk of hepatitis. Attenuation is variable, and the modified clinical patterns may vary from those with few or no symptoms to those with little or no modification. Encephalitis may follow measles modified by gamma globulin.

After the 7th–8th day of incubation the amounts of antibody administered must be increased greatly for any degree of protection. If the injection is delayed until the 9th, 10th, or 11th day, slight fever may already have started and only slight modification of the disease may be expected.

TREATMENT. Sedatives, antipyretics for high fever, bed rest, and an adequate fluid intake may be indicated. Humidification of the room may be necessary for laryngitis or an excessively irritating cough, and it is best to keep the room comfortably warm rather than cool. The patient should be protected from being exposed to strong light during the period of photophobia. The complications of otitis media and pneumonia require appropriate antimicrobial therapy.

With complications such as encephalitis, subacute sclerosing panencephalitis (Sec. 20.68), giant cell pneumonia, and disseminated intravascular coagulation (Sec. 16.75), each case must be assessed individually. Good supportive care is essential. Gamma globulin, hyperimmune gamma globulin, and steroids are of limited value. Currently available antiviral compounds are not effective. Treatment with oral vitamin A (400,000 IU) reduces morbidity and mortality in children with severe measles in the developing world.

Aicardi J: Acute measles encephalitis in children with immunosuppression. Pediatrics 59:232, 1977.

Brem J: Koplik spots for the record: An illustrated historical note. Clin Pediatr 11:161, 1972.

Gustafson TL, Brunell PA, Lievens AW, et al: Measles outbreak in a "fully immunized" secondary school population. N Engl J Med 316:771, 1987.

Hussey G, Klein M: A randomized trial of vitamin A in children with severe measles. N Engl J Med 323:160, 1990.

Jabbour JT, et al: Subacute sclerosing panencephalitis. JAMA 220:959, 1972.

Markowitz LE, Preblud SR, Orenstein WA, et al: Patterns of transmission in measles outbreaks in the United States, 1985–1986. N Engl J Med 320:75, 1989.

Mathias RG, Meeklson WG, Arcand TA, et al: The role of secondary vaccine failures in measles outbreaks. Am J Public Health 79:474, 1989.

McLaughlin M, Thomas P, Onorato I, et al: Live virus vaccines in human immunodeficiency virus-infected children: A retrospective study. Pediatrics 82:229, 1988.

Modlin JF: Epidemiologic studies of measles, measles vaccine, SSPE. Pediatrics 59:505, 1977.

Payne FE, Baublis JV, Itabashi HH: Isolation of measles virus from cell cultures of brain from a patient with subacute sclerosing panencephalitis. N Engl J Med 281:11, 1969.

Ruuskanen O, Salmi TT, Halonen P: Measles vaccination after exposure to natural measles. J Pediatr 98:43, 1978.

Starr S, Berkovich S: The effect of measles, gamma globulin modified measles and attenuated measles vaccine on the course of treated tuberculosis in children. Pediatrics 35:97, 1965.

12.65 RUBELLA
(German or Three-Day Measles)

Rubella is a common communicable disease of childhood characterized ordinarily by mild constitutional symptoms, a rash similar to that of mild rubeola or scarlet fever, and enlargement and tenderness of the postoccipital, retroauricular, and posterior cervical lymph nodes. In older children and adults the infection may occasionally be severe, with manifestations such as joint involvement and purpura.

Rubella in early pregnancy may cause severe congenital anomalies. The congenital rubella syndrome is an active contagious disease with multisystem involvement, a wide spectrum of clinical expression, and a long postnatal period of active infection with shedding of virus (Sec. 9.73).

ETIOLOGY. Rubella is caused by a pleomorphic, RNA-containing virus currently listed in the family Togaviridae, genus *Rubivirus*. The virus is usually isolated in tissue culture, and its presence is demonstrated by the ability of rubella-infected African green monkey kidney (AGMK) cells to resist challenge with enterovirus. During clinical illness the virus is present in nasopharyngeal secretions, blood, feces, and urine. Virus has been recovered from the nasopharynx 7 days before exanthem and 7–8 days after its disappearance. Patients with subclinical disease are also infectious.

EPIDEMIOLOGY. Humans are the only natural host of rubella virus, which is spread by oral droplet or transplacentally through congenital infection. Prior to institution of the rubella vaccine program, the peak incidence of the disease was in children 5–14 yr of age. Now most cases occur in teenagers and young adults. Large outbreaks have been reported among college students. Hospital epidemics among employees, with transmission to susceptible patients, have prompted hospitals to require that employees having contact with patients be immune to rubella. Health care personnel in physicians' offices should also be screened for rubella antibody and, if necessary, immunized. Maternal antibody is protective for the first 6 mo of life. Boys and girls are equally affected. In closed populations, such as institutions and military barracks, almost 100% of susceptible individuals may become infected. In family settings the spread of the virus is less: 50–60% of susceptible family members acquire the disease. Many infections are subclinical, with a ratio of 2:1 inapparent to overt disease. Rubella usually occurs during the spring. It can be difficult to diagnose clinically because enteroviral and other rashes may produce a similar appearance. A single attack usually confers permanent immunity. Epidemics occurred every 6–9 yr before vaccine was available. Serologic studies prior to the use of rubella vaccine showed that about 80% of adult populations in the United States and other continents had antibody to rubella. In island populations, such as those of Trinidad and Hawaii, only 20% of adults screened had detectable antibody.

The epidemiology of the congenital rubella syndrome is discussed in Sec. 9.73. Infants with rubella are a source of infection for older children who are not immune and for nonimmune adults, including pregnant women and nursery personnel.

CLINICAL MANIFESTATIONS. The incubation period is 14–21 days. The prodromal phase of mild catarrhal symptoms is shorter than that of measles and may be so mild as to go unnoticed. The most characteristic sign is retroauricular, posterior cervical, and postoccipital adenopathy. No other disease causes the tender enlargement of these nodes to the extent as does rubella. An enanthem may appear just before the onset of the skin rash. It consists of discrete rose spots on the soft palate that may coalesce into a red blush and extend over the fauces.

Lymphadenopathy is evident at least 24 hr before the *rash* appears and may remain for 1 wk or more. The exanthem is more variable than that of rubeola. It begins on the face (Fig. 12–14 [color plate section]) and spreads quickly. Its evolution is so rapid that the rash may be fading on the face by the time it appears on the trunk. Discrete maculopapules are present in large numbers; there are also large areas of flushing which spread rapidly over the entire body, usually within 24 hr. The rash may be confluent, particularly on the face. During the 2nd day the rash may assume a pinpoint appearance, especially over the trunk, resembling that of scarlet fever. Mild itching may occur. The eruption usually clears by the 3rd day. Desquamation is minimal. Rubella without a rash has been described.

The pharyngeal mucosa and the conjunctivae are slightly inflamed. In contrast to rubeola, there is no photophobia. Fever is slight or absent during the rash and persists for 1, 2, or occasionally 3 days. The temperature seldom exceeds 38.4° C (101° F). Anorexia, headache, and malaise are not common. The spleen is often slightly enlarged. The white blood cell count is normal or slightly reduced; thrombocytopenia is rare, with or without purpura. Especially in older girls and women, polyarthritis may occur with arthralgia, swelling, tenderness, and effusion but usually without any residuum. Any joint may be involved, but the small joints of the hands are affected most frequently. The duration is usually several days to 2 wk; rarely it persists for months. Paresthesia also has been reported. In one epidemic, orchidalgia was reported in about 8% of infected college-aged males.

The **congenital rubella syndrome** is discussed in Sec. 9.73.

DIFFERENTIAL DIAGNOSIS. Because similar symptoms

and rashes can occur with many other viral infections (Sec. 12.5), rubella is a difficult disease to diagnose clinically except when the patient is seen during an epidemic. A history of having had rubella or rubella vaccine is unreliable; immunity should be determined by testing for antibodies. Particularly in its more severe forms, rubella may be confused with the mild types of scarlet fever and rubeola. *Roseola infantum* (exanthem subitum) is distinguished from rubella by the severity of the fever and by the appearance of the rash at the end of the febrile episode rather than at the height of the signs and symptoms. *Drug rashes* may be extremely difficult to differentiate from rubella. The characteristic enlargement of the lymph nodes strongly supports a diagnosis of rubella. In *infectious mononucleosis* a rash may occur that resembles that of rubella, and enlargement of the lymph nodes in each disease may lead to confusion. The hematologic findings in infectious mononucleosis should be sufficient to distinguish the two diseases. Enteroviral infections accompanied by a rash can be differentiated in *some* instances by respiratory or gastrointestinal manifestations and the absence of retroauricular adenopathy.

Diagnostic tests include isolation of virus from various tissues and serologic tests. Hemagglutination-inhibition (HI) antibody has been the usual method of determining immunity to rubella. Several newer tests including latex agglutination, enzyme immunoassay, passive hemagglutination, and fluorescent immunoassay appear to be equal or superior to the HI test in sensitivity. Rubella-specific IgM can be present in the blood of affected newborn infants.

COMPLICATIONS AND PROGNOSIS. Complications are relatively uncommon in childhood. Neuritis and arthritis occur occasionally. Resistance to secondary bacterial infection is not altered significantly. Encephalitis similar to that seen with rubeola occurs in about 1/6,000 cases. The prognosis of childhood rubella is good; that of congenital rubella varies with the severity of the infection (Sec. 9.73); only about 30% of infants with encephalitis appear to escape residual neuromotor deficits, including an autistic syndrome.

PREVENTION. In a susceptible person, **passive protection** from or attenuation of the disease may or may not be afforded by intramuscular injection of immune serum globulin (ISG) given in large dosage (0.25–0.50 mL/kg or 0.12–0.20 mL/lb) within the first 7–8 days after exposure. The effectiveness of immune globulin is not predictable. It apparently depends upon the antibody content of the product used and upon unknown factors. The value of ISG has been questioned also because in some instances rash was prevented and clinical manifestations were absent or minimal though viable virus was demonstrable in the blood. This form of prevention of rubella is not indicated, except in nonimmune pregnant women.

Since 1979 live-virus vaccine RA 27/3 (human embryonic lung fibroblasts of the WI-38 line) has been used exclusively for active immunization against rubella in the United States. RA 27/3 vaccine has many advantages over other rubella vaccines used in the past because it produces nasopharyngeal antibody and a wide variety of serum antibodies, provides better protection against reinfection, and more closely resembles the protection provided by natural infection. The vaccine virus is heat and light sensitive; therefore, the vaccine should be stored in the refrigerator at 4° C and used as soon as it is reconstituted. Vaccine is administered as a single subcutaneous injection. See Sec. 5.1 for routine immunization.

Antibody develops in about 98% of those vaccinated. While virus may persist, especially in the nasopharynx, and shedding occurs from 18–25 days after vaccination, communicability does not appear to be a problem.

The duration of persistence of rubella antibody following vaccination with RA 27/3 is uncertain but is probably lifelong. Preventive measures are of the greatest importance for the protection of the fetus. It is especially important that girls have immunity to rubella before reaching child-bearing age, either by contracting the natural disease or by active immunization. The immune status can be evaluated by appropriate serologic tests.

The rubella vaccine program in the United States calls for immunization of all boys and girls between the age of 15 mo and puberty and of nonpregnant postpubertal females. Immunization is effective at 12 mo of age but is usually delayed until 15 mo and given as MMR. Rubella immunization should be offered to potentially susceptible postpubertal women at any health care visit. For women who say they might be pregnant immunization should be deferred. Pregnancy testing is not routinely necessary, but counseling about the advisability of avoiding pregnancy for 3 mo after immunization should be provided. The current immunization policy has successfully interrupted the usual epidemic cycle of rubella in the United States and decreased the reported incidence of congenital rubella syndrome. However, it has not resulted in a decrease in the percentage of women of child-bearing age who are susceptible to rubella.

Pregnant women should not be given live rubella virus vaccine, but inadvertent immunization should not ordinarily be a reason to interrupt the pregnancy. The infants of over 200 women immunized during pregnancy with RA 27/3 vaccine have been studied; no cases of clinically evident congenital rubella syndrome were found to occur. Other contraindications include immune deficiency states, severe febrile illness, hypersensitivity to vaccine components, and therapy with antimetabolites, corticosteroids, and steroid-like substances.

Clinical manifestations that may follow rubella immunization include fever, typical lymphadenopathy, rash, and arthritis and arthralgia. The last two occur more frequently in older girls and adult women and may last for weeks. Two unusual syndromes have been reported in association with rubella vaccine: one with paresthesia of the hand or arm that occurs at night lasts for up to 1 hr and may recur frequently during the night; the other is manifested by pain behind the knee and limitation of motion. Symptoms are worst in the morning, diminishing during the day. They may last for up to 5 wk. Both syndromes may recur.

Management of Pregnant Women Exposed to or Acquiring Rubella. Pregnant women, especially early in pregnancy but also during the entire gestational period, should avoid exposure to rubella regardless of history of the disease during childhood or of history of active immunization. Exposure of pregnant women to infants with congenital rubella syndrome should be especially guarded against because of prolonged shedding of virus. Risk of damage to the fetus decreases after the 14th wk of gestation.

Since approximately 80% of women in the child-bearing age are immune to rubella as a result of the natural infection or of immunization, the immune status to rubella of women who may become pregnant should be determined.

If a pregnant woman whose immune status is unknown is exposed to rubella, an antibody test should be performed *immediately as an emergency measure.* If determined to be immune, she can be reassured that the pregnancy can be continued without added risk. If she is found to be susceptible and therapeutic abortion is unacceptable or unavailable to her, passive immunization with immune serum globulin (ISG), 20–30 mL intramuscularly, should be attempted immediately. Active immunization of pregnant women is not advised.

If exposure to rubella occurs in a susceptible pregnant woman to whom abortion is available and desirable because of significant potential hazard to the fetus, it is probably advisable to withhold ISG, observe her carefully, and repeat the rubella antibody test. If rubella then develops at a stage of pregnancy at which she feels the risk is greater than she wants to assume or if serial antibody tests show that subclinical infection has occurred, abortion may be induced.

REINFECTION. The incidence of reinfection on exposure of individuals who are serologically immune to wild virus is 3–10% among those demonstrating serologic immunity without a history of immunization, and 14–18% among those immunized with RA 27/3 vaccine. Infection has been demonstrated among the fetuses of reinfected pregnant women as well as among pregnant women who had received rubella vaccine. The relevance of reinfection of serologically immune pregnant women to the production of congenital malformations remains to be determined. Until these questions are answered, *all* pregnant women should make every effort to avoid exposure to rubella.

TREATMENT. Unless bacterial complications occur, treatment is symptomatic. Adamantanamine hydrochloride (amantadine) has been reported to be effective in vitro in inhibiting early stages of rubella infection in cultured cells. An attempt to treat a child having congenital rubella with this drug was unsuccessful. *Since amantadine is not recommended for pregnant women, its usefulness is very limited.* Interferon and isoprinosine have been used with limited success.

Chang TW: Rubella reinfection and intrauterine involvement (Editorial). J Pediatr 84:617, 1974.
Clark M, et al: Effect of rubella vaccination programme on serological status of young adults in United Kingdom. Lancet 1:1224, 1979.
Immunization practices in colleges—United States. MMWR 36:209, 1987.
Miller E, Cradock-Watson JE, Pollock TM: Consequences of confirmed maternal rubella at successive stages of pregnancy. Lancet 2:781, 1982.
O'Shea S, Best JB, Banatvala JE, et al: Development and persistence of class-specific antibodies in the serum and nasopharyngeal washings of rubella vaccines. J Infect Dis 151:89, 1985.
Plotkin SA, Klaus RM, Whitely JP, et al: Hypogammaglobulinemia in an infant with congenital rubella syndrome; failure of L-adamantanamine to stop virus excretion. J Pediatr 69:1085, 1966.
Rawls WE, Desmyter J, Melnick JL: Serologic diagnosis and fetal involvement in maternal rubella. JAMA 203:627, 1968.
Rawls WE, Phillips CA, Melnick JL, et al: Persistent virus infection in congenital rubella. Arch Ophthalmol 77:430, 1967.
Rubella and congenital rubella syndrome—United States 1985–1988. MMWR 38:173, 1989.
Rubella vaccination during pregnancy—United States 1971–1986. MMWR 36:458, 1987.
Tardieu M, Grospierre B, Durandy A, et al: Circulating immune complexes containing rubella antigens in late-onset rubella syndrome. J Pediatr 97:370, 1980.
Townsend JJ: Progressive rubella panencephalitis: Late onset after congenital rubella. N Engl J Med 292:990, 1975.

12.66 EXANTHEM SUBITUM
(Roseola Infantum)

Exanthem subitum is an acute viral disease of infants and young children, usually occurring sporadically but occasionally in epidemics. It is unique in that the diagnostic rash and clinical improvement occur almost simultaneously. The disease is characterized by a period of high fever lasting 1–5 but usually 3–4 days, during which time there are insufficient clinical findings to explain the hyperpyrexia, and by an abrupt termination with a precipitous drop of the temperature to normal and the appearance of a generalized eruption, which fades quickly.

ETIOLOGY. Human herpesvirus-6 has been isolated from lymphocytes of children with roseola, and antibody titer rises against the virus have been demonstrated.

EPIDEMIOLOGY. The degree of contagiousness is not known. There is a tendency for the disease to occur in the spring and fall. It attacks both sexes equally. In the rare epidemics described, the incubation period was estimated to be 7–17 days, usually about 10 days. In one study, using a direct immunofluorescent test, the early acquisition of antibody to human herpesvirus-6 was evaluated. Most infants had maternally derived antibody for the first few months of life. By age 4 mo only 25% were antibody positive. This percentage rose to 76% by 11 mo, 90% by age 5 yr, and 98% by age 17. Most cases of clinical disease occur between 6 and 18 mo of life. Asymptomatic viral shedding in saliva of adults may be the source of infection.

CLINICAL MANIFESTATIONS. The onset is sudden with fever as high as 39.4–41.2° C (103–106° F); convulsions may occur at this time or later. Although the pharyngeal mucosa is slightly inflamed at times and there may be slight coryza, there are no typical signs. The outstanding feature is the absence of physical findings sufficient to explain the fever. Usually the child looks relatively well despite the degree of the fever. The diagnosis is suggested chiefly by excluding other infections, particularly those which at this age are the most common causes of high fever, such as otitis media, acute pyelonephritis, pneumonia, meningitis, and pneumococcal bacteremia.

During the first 24–36 hr of fever the white blood cell count may be as high as 16,000–20,000/mm^3 with an increase in neutrophils. By the 2nd day leukopenia may become evident, with counts of 3,000–5,000 on the 3rd–4th day of fever. There may be an absolute neutropenia with a relative lymphocytosis, which may be as high as 90%. Occasionally, a large number of monocytes are present. The cerebrospinal fluid is normal.

The fever falls by crisis on the 3rd–4th day. As the temperature returns to normal, a macular or maculopapular eruption appears over the body, starting on the trunk, spreading to the arms and neck, and slightly involving the face and legs. The rash soon fades, rarely remaining as long as 24 hr. Desquamation is rare, and no pigmentation remains. In the rare epidemic outbreaks, cases without a rash have been suspected. Occasionally, the lymph nodes, especially in the cervical area, are enlarged, but not to the extent that they are in rubella. Hepatitis has been reported.

DIFFERENTIAL DIAGNOSIS. Children with exanthem subitum present with the differential diagnosis of a fever of unknown origin (Sec. 12.3) until the fever drops precipitously and the rash appears. Rubella's other prodromal manifestations and the persistence of its fever after a rash appears usually distinguish it from exanthem subitum. *Rubeola* and *dengue* can be distinguished primarily by the time of appearance of their rash in relation to fever and other clinical findings. In rubeola, though there is usually a fever of variable degree for 3–4 days just before the rash, the temperature is abruptly elevated to 39.4–40° C (103–104° F) at the time the rash appears and remains elevated for the next 2 days, when the rash fades rapidly. The lack of Koplik spots, severe coryza, conjunctivitis, and cough also helps to distinguish exanthem subitum from rubeola. *Pneumococcal bacteremia* may present with high fever and a well-appearing child. The white blood count is frequently elevated, and the blood culture is positive for pneumococcus. As a rule, distinguishing exanthem subitum from entero- and adenoviral diseases and drug reactions does not present a problem.

PROGNOSIS. The prognosis is good except in the rare patient who has extreme hyperpyrexia or persistent seizures.

PROPHYLAXIS AND TREATMENT. No methods for shortening the course of the disease or for prophylaxis are known. In infants and young children who are prone to convulsions, administering a sedative at the time the sharp febrile onset of exanthem subitum appears may be effective as prophylaxis against such seizures. An antipyretic may be of help in partially reducing the fever and in allaying restlessness.

Asano Y, Yoshikawa T, Suga S, et al: Fatal fulminant hepatitis in an infant with human herpesvirus-6 infection. Lancet 335:862, 1990.
Clemens HH: Exanthem subitum (roseola infantum): A report of eighty cases. J Pediatr 26:66, 1945.
Levy J, Greenspan D, Ferro F, et al: Frequent isolation of HHV-6 from saliva and high seroprevalence of the virus in the population. Lancet 335:1047, 1990.
McEnery JT: Postoccipital lymphadenopathy as a diagnostic sign in roseola infantum (exanthem subitum). Clin Pediatr 9:512, 1970.
Yamanishi K, Skiraki K, Kondo T, et al: Identification of human herpesvirus-6 as a causal agent for exanthem subitum. Lancet 1:1065, 1988.
Yoshikawa T, Suga S, Asano Y, et al: Distribution of antibodies to a causative agent of exanthem subitum (human herpesvirus-6) in healthy individuals. Pediatrics 84:675, 1989.

12.67 ERYTHEMA INFECTIOSUM
(Fifth Disease)

Erythema infectiosum, a moderately contagious exanthematous disease affecting mainly children, is frequently called fifth disease because it was the fifth of five illnesses described exhibiting somewhat similar rashes. The other four diseases were rubella, measles, scarlet fever, and Filatov-Dukes disease, the last of which is now considered a mild atypical form of scarlet fever.

ETIOLOGY. Parvovirus B19, a single-stranded DNA–containing virus, is the etiologic agent of erythema infectiosum.

EPIDEMIOLOGY. Infants and adults are affected infrequently. There is no sex predilection. Community epidemics involving mainly school-aged children have been described. The virus is spread by the respiratory route and affects the red cell precursors in the bone marrow, producing a decrease in reticulocytes. In most people no significant anemia occurs, but children with diseases that shorten the life of the red blood cell may develop severe aplastic crises. The incubation period is about a week. Viremia and respiratory secretion of virus have cleared in normal children when the rash appears, and the patient is no longer infectious. Children with aplastic crisis are highly contagious during the period of anemia. Chronic anemia caused by parvovirus B19 may occur in immunoincompetent patients.

Distribution of the virus is worldwide; 50% of adults have antibody. Seronegative family contacts of a child with B19 infection have a 50% risk of contracting the disease; the risk for seronegative teachers in a school setting is around 20%. Fetal hydrops has been reported following B19 infections during pregnancy (Sec. 9.72).

CLINICAL MANIFESTATIONS. No prodromal symptoms usually appear. Fever is absent or low grade. The characteristic rash appears in three stages. The illness usually begins with the sudden appearance of livid erythema of the cheeks, giving the child a "slapped-cheek" appearance. An erythematous maculopapular rash then appears on the trunk and extremities; infrequently the body rash may precede the facial one. The rash fades with central clearing, giving a lacy or reticulated appearance (Fig. 12–15 [color plate section]); it is the most distinctive part of the disease. The rash lasts from 2–39 days (mean, 11 days), is frequently pruritic, and resolves without desquamation, but periodic recrudescences may occur with exercise, warm baths, rubbing of the skin, or emotional upset. Constitutional symptoms such as headache, pharyngitis, coryza, myalgia, arthralgia, arthritis, and gastrointestinal disturbance are more frequent and more severe in adults.

LABORATORY DATA. Diagnostic tests are not widely available, but specific IgM, IgG, and viral DNA determinations can be obtained from special laboratories.

DIAGNOSIS. Erythema infectiosum must be differentiated from rubella, enteroviral diseases, systemic lupus erythematosus, atypical measles, and drug rashes.

COMPLICATIONS. Complications are rare. Arthritis, hemolytic anemia, pneumonitis, and encephalopathy have been reported.

TREATMENT. No treatment is indicated. Intravenous immunoglobulin is indicated for immunoincompetent patients with chronic anemia. Isolation is not required except for patients with aplastic crises. Children with rash are not infectious.

Anderson LJ, Hurwitz ES: Human parvovirus B19 and pregnancy. Clin Perinatol 15:273, 1988.
Anderson MJ, Lewis E, Kidd IM, et al: An outbreak of erythema infectiosum associated with human parvovirus infection. J Hyg (London) 93:85, 1984.
Balfour H: Fifth disease: Full fathom five. Am J Dis Child 130:239, 1976.
Blacklock H, Mortimer P: Aplastic crisis and other effects of the human parvovirus infection. Clin Haematol 13:679, 1984.
Chorba T, Coccia R, Holman RC, et al: The role of parvovirus B19 in aplastic crisis and erythema infectiosum (fifth disease). J Infect Dis 154:383, 1986.
Hall CB, et al: Encephalopathy with erythema infectiosum. Am J Dis Child 131:65, 1977.

12.68 HERPES SIMPLEX VIRUS (HSV)

Herpesvirus hominis, a common parasite of man, has a variety of clinical manifestations involving the skin, mucous membranes, eye, central nervous system, and genital tract. It also causes generalized systemic disease. Two strains of the virus are identified: HSV-1 commonly infects skin and mucous membranes; HSV-2 primarily infects the genitalia.

Two types of infection are recognized:

1. *Primary* infection is the susceptible host's first experience with the virus, which in most instances is a subclinical infection; otherwise there are usually local superficial lesions (see below) accompanied by varying degrees of systemic reaction. In newborn infants and severely malnourished infants, a serious systemic infection, often without superficial lesions, may occur. Circulating antibodies develop in nonfatal cases.
2. *Recurrent* herpetic lesions represent reactivation of a latent infection in an immune host with circulating antibodies. Reactivation follows such nonspecific stimuli as changes in the external milieu (e.g., cold, ultraviolet light) or in the internal milieu (e.g., menstruation, fever, or emotional stress). The lesions tend to be localized and, generally, are not associated with systemic reactions.

ETIOLOGY. HSV is a DNA-containing virus. The virus readily infects a variety of animals, produces pocks on the chorioallantoic membrane of the embryonated hen's egg, and induces characteristic cytopathic changes in a variety of cells growing in monolayer tissue cultures. The two strains (HSV-1 and HSV-2) are recognized by biologic and antigenic characteristics.

EPIDEMIOLOGY. The virus develops an extremely compatible relationship with its host. In about 85% of instances the infection is subclinical; even when clinical manifestations are present, the host is only rarely seriously disabled. Under exceptional circumstances the primary infection may lead to institutional or family outbreaks of stomatitis. The incubation period is 2–12 days (average, 6 days). *The spread of infection appears to be determined by two factors: close bodily contact and trauma such as teething or a break in the skin.*

The higher incidence of HSV antibodies in lower socioeconomic groups correlates with crowded living conditions. The epidemiology differs for the two types of HSV. Detailed serologic studies have been done only in low income groups, in which most infants have transplacental antibody for about the first 6 mo of life. From 1 to 4 yr there is a sharp rise in antibodies to HSV-1 and then a much slower rate of acquisition up to 14 yr. At this time, there is a second sharp rise in antibodies, mostly to HSV-2. By adult life HSV antibodies are seen in by far the majority of persons in the lower socioeconomic groups: HSV-2 antibodies are found in up to 60% of the adults. The incidence of type 2 antibody in higher socioeconomic groups is about 10% and in nuns about 3%.

Once infected, the majority of people continue to carry the virus in a latent state and maintain an almost constant level of circulating antibodies. The initial level of antibodies reached after a primary infection may fall, and several subclinical reinfections may occur before a stable antibody level is established. Carriers may distribute the virus without having any manifest lesion. Herpes simplex virus can be isolated from the pharynx of about 5% of asymptomatic adults.

PATHOLOGY. The pathologic changes vary with the tissue infected. In general, a specific lesion is characterized by the presence of intranuclear inclusion bodies, homogeneous masses lying in the midst of a severely disorganized nucleus in which the basic chromatin has marginated to the nuclear membrane. Around the specific lesion there is always evidence of an acute inflammatory reaction. In the skin and mucous membranes the typical lesion is a unilocular vesicle. In the skin the vesicle is tense. Ballooned epithelial cells containing intranuclear inclusions can best be seen at the margins of the vesicle. The vesicular fluid contains infected epithelial cells, including multinucleated "virus" giant cells and leukocytes. In the corium there is no necrosis, but capillaries are dilated, and there is infiltration with mononuclear and polymorphonuclear cells. In the mucous membrane, because of maceration, there is early leakage of the vesicular fluid resulting in a collapsed vesicle, mainly filled with fibrin. The edematous roof cells form a gray membrane over the lesion.

In otherwise healthy persons, the lesions are confined to the skin and mucous membranes; viremia has rarely been described. Bloodstream spread of the virus with resultant widely disseminated disease is seen mainly in the newborn, in severely malnourished children, in persons with skin diseases such as eczema, and in those with defects in cell-mediated immunity. In these patients the virus spreads hematogenously from the portal of entry to susceptible organs. Virus increases within these organs, and secondary viremia occurs with evidence of extensive cell destruction. It is probable, however, that most cases of HSV-1 encephalitis other than in the newborn are caused by neurogenic transmission of the virus to the brain; HSV-2 infection is usually bloodborne. Healing begins with clearing of the viremia and a decrease in the production of virus within the cells.

CLINICAL MANIFESTATIONS. As indicated earlier, the herpesviruses characteristically produce a vesicular lesion. Only rarely is there a viremic distribution that results in widespread systemic disease or neurogenic transmission that leads to meningoencephalitis (see later and Sec. 12.12). Furthermore, although the occurrence of primary and recurrent lesions is an accepted characteristic of herpetic infection, their distinction clinically is often not possible without knowledge of the presence or absence of serum antibodies in the patient.

Lesions of the Skin and Mucous Membranes. On the skin the lesion consists of aggregates of thin-walled vesicles on an erythematous base. These rupture, scab, and heal within 7–10 days without leaving a scar except after repeated attacks or secondary bacterial infections; temporary depigmentation may occur in blacks. The local lesions may be preceded by mild irritation or burning at the local site or by severe neuralgic pain in the region. In children the vesicles often become secondarily infected, introducing *impetigo contagiosa* into the differential diagnosis. The lesions tend to recur at the same site, particularly at mucocutaneous junctions, but may occur anywhere.

Primary infection may, uncommonly, result in a generalized vesicular eruption in which the lesions are small and may continue to appear over a period of 2–3 wk. If the systemic manifestations are mild, the infection must be differentiated from varicella.

Traumatic lesions of the skin can be readily infected by the ubiquitous herpesvirus. Primary lesions can also occur on apparently unbroken skin, as, for example, on the chin of a drooling infant with herpetic stomatitis, in whom scattered isolated vesicles appear, in contrast to the grouped vesicles of recurrent attacks. When the skin of a limb is infected, vesicles appear in 2–3 days at the site of trauma. There is often centripetal spread along lymph channels causing enlargement of regional lymph nodes and scattered vesicles on the intervening undamaged skin. The final clinical picture may be mistaken for that of *herpes zoster*, especially if accompanied by neuralgic pain, unless the lesions are recognized as not being confined to a dermatome. The lesions heal slowly, often taking 3 wk; recurrences at the site of local trauma are common and may assume a bullous pattern. Wrestlers and medical personnel are prone to herpetic infections of superficial abrasions (herpes gladiatorum and herpetic whitlow). In the latter, infection of minor trauma about the nails leads to extremely painful, deep-seated spreading lesions with vesicles that resolve spontaneously in 2–3 wk. Similar lesions occur on the fingers of thumb suckers who are suffering from herpetic gingivostomatitis. Treatment is symptomatic only; the lesions should not be incised.

Acute Herpetic Gingivostomatitis (Acute Infectious Gingivostomatitis; Aphthous Stomatitis; Catarrhal Stomatitis; Ulcerative Stomatitis; Vincent Stomatitis). This primary infection, probably the most common cause of stomatitis in children 1–3 yr of age, can also occur in older children and adults. The symptoms may appear abruptly, with pain in the mouth, salivation, fetor oris, refusal to eat, and fever, often as high as 40–40.6°C (104–105°F). The onset may be insidious, fever and irritability preceding the oral lesions by 1–2 days. The initial lesion is a vesicle (Fig. 12–16), which is seldom seen because of its early rupture. The residual lesion is 2–10 mm in diameter and is covered with a yellow-gray membrane (Fig. 12–17). When this membrane sloughs, a true ulcer remains. Although the tongue and cheeks are most commonly involved, no part of the oral lining is exempt. Except in edentulous infants, acute gingivitis is characteristic of the disease and may precede the appearance of mucosal vesicles. Submaxillary lymphadenitis is common. The acute phase lasts 4–9 days and is self-limited. Pain tends to disappear 2–4 days before healing of the ulcers is complete. In some instances the tonsillar regions are involved early, and acute tonsillitis of bacterial origin or herpangina may be suspected. Failure of the lesion to respond to antibiotic therapy differentiates a bacterial infection, and the spread of the vesiculation to the buccal mucosa rules out herpangina.

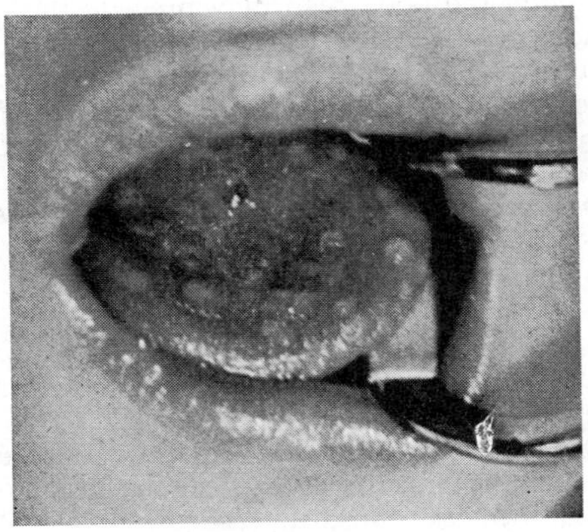

Figure 12–16. Lesions of herpetic stomatitis on the tongue.

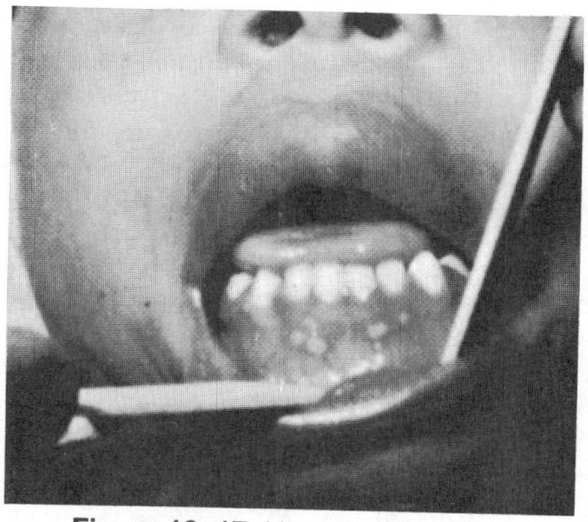

Figure 12–17. Herpetic stomatitis.

Recurrent Stomatitis. Localized lesions may occur on the palate in association with a febrile illness or on the mucosa adjacent to a lesion on the lip; recurrent aphthous ulcers, however, are not caused by herpesvirus. In some persons a generalized stomatitis recurs consistently 7–10 days after a recurrent herpetic lesion of the lip or elsewhere and is often accompanied by skin lesions of erythema multiforme.

Eczema Herpeticum (Kaposi Varicelliform Eruption; Juliusberg Pustulosis Vacciniformis Acuta). This, the most serious manifestation of "traumatic herpes," results from a widespread and usually primary infection of the eczematous skin with herpesvirus. The severity of this complication varies; the lesion may be so mild as to be overlooked, or it may be fatal. In a typical severe primary attack, vesicles develop abruptly in large numbers over the area of eczematous skin. They continue to appear in crops for as long as 7–9 days. Isolated at first, they later become grouped and may occur on adjoining areas of normal skin (Fig. 12–18). Wide denudation of the epidermis may occur. Scabs eventually form, and epithelialization occurs. The systemic reaction varies, but temperatures of 39.4–40.6° C (103–105° F) for 7–10 days are not uncommon. Recurrent attacks develop on chronic atopic skin lesions. Death may result from profound physiologic disturbances from loss of fluid, electrolytes, and protein through the skin, from dissemination of the virus to the brain and other organs, or from secondary bacterial invasion. A differentiation from *eczema vaccinatum* can usually be made by determining with reasonable certainty that the child has not been exposed to vaccinia and by the occurrence of crops of vesicles in herpes. The diagnosis can be accurately established by examination of vesicular fluid with the electron microscope. Herpes simplex virus cannot be differentiated from varicella-zoster by this method but can easily be distinguished from vaccinia and variola.

Ocular Lesions. *Conjunctivitis* and *keratoconjunctivitis* may occur as manifestations of either a primary or recurrent infection. The conjunctiva appears congested and swollen, but there is little, if any, purulent discharge. In primary infection the preauricular node is usually enlarged and tender. Cataracts, uveitis, and chorioretinitis have been described in newborn infants.

Corneal lesions may be superficial, in the form of a dendritc ulcer, or deep, as a disciform keratitis. The diagnosis is suggested by the presence of herpetic vesicles on the lids; it is established by the isolation of the virus. The highly contagious *epidemic keratoconjunctivitis* (shipyard conjunctivitis) due to any of several serotypes of adenovirus must be considered in the differential diagnosis.

Genital Herpes. Genital infections with herpesvirus occur most commonly in adolescents and young adults, are usually due to HSV-2, and are spread venereally. Five to 10% of cases are caused by HSV-1. When the patient has no antibody to either type of herpes (approximately 30% of cases), systemic symptoms such as fever, regional adenopathy, and dysuria are more likely to occur. In adult women, the vulva and vagina may be involved, but the cervix is the primary site of infection. Recurrence is common. Both primary and recurrent disease are frequently subclinical, but virus from the lesion can infect an infant during passage through the birth canal.

In males herpetic vesicles or ulcers are usually seen on the glans penis, prepuce, or shaft of the penis. The scrotum is less frequently involved.

Systemic Infection. In The Newborn Infant. See Sec. 9.71.

In Severely Malnourished Infants. The primary infection in infants who have severe protein malnutrition, as well as other *immunodeficiency disorders*, may be generalized and fatal. The clinical and pathologic findings are similar to those in the newborn infant (Sec. 9.71).

Meningoencephalitis (see also Sec. 12.12). Herpes encephalitis is seen in all age groups. HSV-2 is the usual cause in newborn infants, HSV-1 in older patients. The pathogenesis is unknown, but it can occur in patients who already possess antibody against herpes simplex. It is the most common type of nonepidemic encephalitis in the United States, has a high mortality, and in survivors frequently produces severe sequelae.

LABORATORY DATA. Microscopic examination of scrapings from lesions (Tzanck stain) reveals multinuclear giant cells and intranuclear inclusions. Immunofluorescent techniques applied to these specimens can be useful in diagnosing herpes infection and in differentiating the two types of herpes. Virus can be isolated from vesicles and from conjunctival swabs. Cerebrospinal fluid is positive for virus in about one third of infected neonates. Cerebrospinal fluid is rarely positive in older children with encephalitis; brain biopsy is required for a definitive diagnosis. Such cultures are usually positive in 1–4 days. An ELISA test for herpes simplex viral antigen has been developed and has been shown to be sensitive and specific in limited clinical studies. Polymerase chain reaction permits detection of viral DNA in CSF.

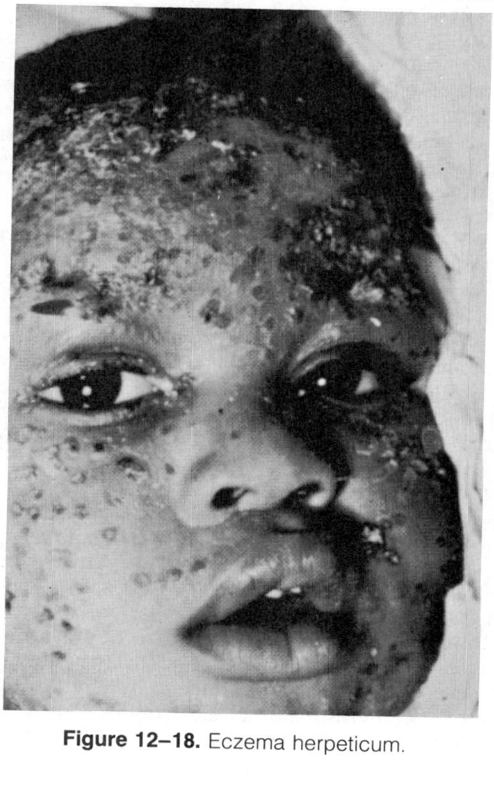

Figure 12–18. Eczema herpeticum.

Moderate polymorphonuclear leukocytosis occurs in acute herpetic gingivostomatitis, eczema herpeticum, and meningoencephalitis. In meningoencephalitis there are frequently red cells in the cerebrospinal fluid and an increase in lymphocytes, usually fewer than 100 but occasionally up to 1,000/mm^3; the protein level is elevated, and the sugar is within the normal range. EEG and CT may demonstrate a temporal lobe lesion. Thrombocytopenia often occurs with systemic infection.

DIAGNOSIS. The diagnosis is based on any two of the following: (1) a compatible clinical pattern; (2) isolation of the virus; (3) development of specific neutralizing antibodies; (4) demonstration of characteristic cells or histologic changes in scrapings or biopsy material.

COURSE AND PROGNOSIS. Primary localized infections with herpesvirus are self-limited, usually lasting 1–2 wk. Mortality rates are high in newborn infants who also have systemic infection and in older infants who are severely malnourished. In patients with meningoencephalitis the prognosis for survival or for recovery without serious permanent residuals is guarded. Otherwise the prognosis is usually good. Attacks may frequently recur, but they seldom cause more than temporary inconvenience except in the eye, where they may eventually cause scarring of the cornea and blindness. Recurrent oral herpes lesions can be a significant problem in immunocompromised patients.

TREATMENT. *Topical therapy* has been advocated for both labial and genital herpes. Topical 5-iodo-2′-deoxyuridine (IDU), adenine arabinoside (vidarabine, ara-A), ether, and 2-deoxy-D glucose are not effective. Topical acyclovir (acycloguanosine; 9-[2-hydroxyethoxymethyl] guanine) may decrease the period of viral shedding but has little effect on symptoms.

Topical acyclovir is usually effective in treating herpetic keratitis but does not reduce the recurrence rate. Topical corticosteroids may increase ocular involvement and should not be used.

Patients with primary genital infection who are treated with *oral acyclovir* (200 mg 5 times daily for 5 days) have significantly less pain, itching, and time to crusting; a shorter duration of viral shedding; and fewer new lesions compared with control patients. A dose of 800 mg twice a day appears to be just as effective and well tolerated and is easier to administer. Those with recurrent genital infections who are treated similarly with oral acyclovir have a shorter duration of viral shedding and heal faster but symptoms are not lessened; therapy of primary attacks does not prevent recurrences. However, daily prophylactic administration of oral acyclovir can diminish the number of recurrences and may be prescribed if recurrences are frequent or severe.

Acyclovir (10 mg/kg/dose given over 1 hr every 8 hr) is the treatment of choice for herpes encephalitis and local and disseminated neonatal disease. The drug is well tolerated. The best results are obtained when treatment is started early. Patients under the age of 30 yr have a better prognosis than older patients. Herpes simplex viruses are rarely resistant to acyclovir; adenine arabinoside can be used for these patients. Some infants and adults treated with acyclovir fail to develop neutralizing antibody against herpesvirus.

One study of acyclovir suspension in patients with gingivostomatitis showed that the medication did not significantly shorten the duration of disease. Patients with severe illness in Kaposi varicelliform eruption do appear to respond to intravenous acyclovir.

Symptomatic and supportive therapy is of great importance. In infants especially, eczema herpeticum and stomatitis may lead to severe dehydration, shock, and hypoproteinemia, requiring replacement of fluids, electrolytes, and proteins.

Oral lavage should be used for mouth care; Ceepryn 1:4,000 or Zephiran 1:1,000 may be useful. Local analgesics, such as viscous lidocaine or benzocaine lozenges, may allay pain and enable the older child to eat. Labial lesions may be made less painful by applying drying agents such as calamine lotion or glycerine with carbamine peroxide. Analgesics should be used systemically as required. Antibiotics are useful only in treating secondary bacterial infections.

Food and fluid intake will be facilitated by acquiescing to the child's whims. Ice-cold fluids or semisolids are often accepted when other food is refused. Recurrences are often due to emotional stress, which must be recognized and treated.

Baker DA, Gonik B, Mitch PO: Clinical evaluation of a new herpes simplex virus ELISA. Obstet Gynecol 73:322, 1989.
Brown ZA, Vontver LA, Benedetti J, et al: Effects on infants of a first episode of genital herpes during pregnancy. N Engl J Med 317:1246, 1987.
Leigh IM: Management of non-genital herpes simplex virus infections in immunocompetent patients. Am J Med 85(2A):34, 1988.
Probes CG, Kinsleigh PA, Boucher FD, et al: Use of routine viral cultures at delivery to identify neonates exposed to herpes simplex virus. N Engl J Med 318:887, 1988.
Selby PJ, Jameson B, Watson JG, et al: Parenteral acyclovir therapy for herpes virus infections in man. Lancet 2:1267, 1979.
Straus SE, Takiff HE, Seidlin M, et al: Suppression of frequently recurring genital herpes. N Engl J Med 310:1545, 1984.

12.69 VARICELLA AND HERPES ZOSTER

Herpes zoster and chickenpox are different clinical manifestations of the same virus.

ETIOLOGY. The common viral agent is *Herpesvirus varicellae*, whose structure under the electron microscope is indistinguishable from that of *Herpesvirus hominis*. The virus can be grown in a variety of primary cultures of human and simian tissues. Serum antibodies in patients recovering from varicella react equally with the viral particles derived from varicella and herpes zoster vesicles.

The reasons for different clinical manifestations of the two diseases are not understood. Varicella may be the primary response of a susceptible host, whereas herpes zoster may be the response of partial immunity when a latent infection is activated by some exogenous factor, for example, stress, trauma, malignancy, or radiation. One attack usually confers permanent immunity to generalized disease, but second episodes can occur, particularly in immunocompromised patients and in those who have received varicella vaccine. Second attacks are usually mild.

PATHOLOGY. The *skin lesions* of the two diseases are identical and cannot be distinguished histologically from those of herpes simplex. Although unusual in cases of average severity, necrosis with hemorrhage is sometimes found in the mucous membranes of the mouth, trachea, esophagus, and intestine.

In fatal cases of *varicella* intranuclear inclusions can be found in the endothelium of blood vessels. Intranuclear inclusions have been found in most organs of the body, including the salivary glands, the nervous system, and the myenteric plexus of the stomach and intestine. In the brain, perivenous demyelination is similar to that of other postinfectious encephalitides; necrosis of nerve cells and leptomeningitis have been described.

The characteristic lesions of *herpes zoster* are in the nervous system, particularly in the dorsal root ganglia. Early in the disease the cells of the dorsal ganglia of the affected dermatome contain intranuclear inclusions; later they become necrotic. As the disease progresses, evidence of inflammation and degeneration is found in the posterior roots and in the peripheral portions of the nerves. There may also be necrosis of nerve cells in the unilateral and segmental portions of the posterior horn (cf. poliomyelitis [Sec. 12.80], which involves the nerve cells of the anterior horn). Leptomeningitis occurs in the region of the involved nerves. Intranuclear inclusions have been found in the sympathetic ganglia, in the neurilemma cells of the nerve twigs in the corium, in the myenteric plexus, and in the walls of the bladder and other viscera.

VARICELLA
(Chickenpox)

Varicella is characterized by the appearance of successive crops of typical vesicles on the skin and mucous membranes, generally accompanied by a mild constitutional reaction.

EPIDEMIOLOGY. Ninety per cent of patients having this highly contagious disease are under 10 yr of age; the peak age of incidence is 5–9 yr, but the disease may occur at any age, including the neonatal period. The secondary attack rate among susceptible household contacts is about 90%. About 96% of adults in the United States are immune. The complement-fixation test is the most widely available test used to determine immunity, but it is not sensitive. Fluorescent antibody test against membrane antigen (FAMA), immunoadherence hemagglutination (IAHA), and enzyme-linked immunosorbent assay (ELISA) are more reliable but are not widely available. An intradermal skin test is being evaluated.

The disease is seen mainly between January and May. It is spread by direct contact, by droplet, or by air-borne transmission. Infectious virus is present in the vesicles but, unlike the smallpox virus, is not contained in the crusts. Patients are infectious from about 24 hr before the appearance of the rash until all lesions are crusted (usually 7–8 days). Epidemics of chickenpox have been initiated by exposure to herpes zoster.

CLINICAL MANIFESTATIONS. The incubation period varies from 11 to 21 days and most often lasts 13–17 days. Prodromal symptoms usually precede the rash by 24 hr. There may be slight fever, malaise, or anorexia, accompanied at times by a scarlatiniform or morbilliform rash. It is characteristic of the specific rash to appear rapidly. Typically, it begins as crops of small, red papules, which almost immediately develop into clear, often oval, "tear-drop" vesicles on an erythematous base; they are usually not umbilicated. The contents usually become cloudy within about 24 hr, when the vesicles are easily broken and become scabbed. Crops of widely scattered vesicles characteristically continue to appear for 3–4 days. Starting on the trunk, they spread to the face and scalp; distal parts of the extremities are involved minimally, if at all. The lesions concentrate in areas of skin pressure or irritation. Characteristically, at the height of the disease the eruption consists of papules, early and late vesicles, and crusts present at the same time (Fig. 12–19 [color plate section]). Rarely, in severe disease, the lesions appear as hard, pearly lumps (mostly at the same stage of development) and resemble those of smallpox. Pruritus is constant and annoying. Vesicles on the mucous membranes, particularly those of the mouth, rapidly become macerated and form a shallow ulcer. Less commonly, lesions are found on the genital mucous membranes and on the conjunctiva and the cornea, where they may endanger sight. Laryngeal involvement is rare. There may be generalized lymphadenopathy.

The severity of the disease varies from a few lesions and little evidence of systemic illness to many hundreds of lesions and extreme toxicity with temperatures that range from 39.4 to 40.6°C (103–105°F). Systemic manifestations occur only during the first 3–4 days, when the rash is erupting.

Infrequently, the rash becomes hemorrhagic in association with mild to severe thrombocytopenia, often with other complications, such as pneumonia, or in patients receiving immunosuppressive therapy. Purpura fulminans, which occurs about the end of the 1st wk and is associated with gangrene, probably represents a Shwartzman-like reaction.

Varicella bullosa is an uncommon variant, seen mainly in children under 2 yr of age, in which many of the lesions appear as bullae instead of vesicles. The course of the disease is not changed.

Congenital varicella may be manifest at birth or appear within a few days when the mother has an active infection (Sec. 9.74).

LABORATORY DATA. There may be a mild leukocytosis. Giant cells can be demonstrated in scrapings from the floors of fresh vesicles. The virus can be isolated in human tissue cultures.

DIAGNOSIS. Since the eradication of smallpox, the difficult distinction between mild smallpox and severe chickenpox has become moot. In contrast to smallpox, chickenpox has a short, usually mild prodrome, and the superficial nonumbilicated skin lesions begin on the trunk, spreading peripherally, and may present all stages of development at once. The viruses are easily distinguished morphologically.

COMPLICATIONS. *Secondary bacterial infection* of skin lesions is the most common complication. *Thrombocytopenia* with hemorrhage into the skin and mucous membranes may occur; rare instances of internal hemorrhage from ulcerations or into an adrenal may be fatal.

Varicella *pneumonia* is uncommon in children, but 20–30% of adults have lung involvement. Recovery is usually prompt, but roentgenographic changes may persist for 6–12 wk in the more seriously ill. Fatalities have been reported. *Purpura fulminans* (Sec. 16.75) may occur following chickenpox. Lesions on the larynx may cause edema severe enough to produce respiratory distress. Myocarditis, pericarditis, endocarditis, hepatitis, glomerulonephritis, and acute myositis of the limb muscles have been described. Keratitis and vesicular conjunctivitis are rare and usually benign. Varicella arthritis occurs, but bacterial arthritis during varicella is equally common. An increased white blood cell count and sedimentation rate are more likely to be associated with a bacterial infection. About 10% of cases of *Reye syndrome* occur following chickenpox. Infants whose mothers had varicella during the 1st trimester of pregnancy tend to be small for gestational age; have congenital malformations, skin scarring, muscular atrophy, chorioretinitis or other ocular abnormalities, seizures, and mental retardation; and tend to be unusually susceptible to infection.

Postinfectious *encephalitis* is the most common central nervous system complication (Sec. 12.12). Cerebellar signs such as ataxia, nystagmus, and tremors are common. Encephalitis that presents mainly with cerebellar signs has a much better prognosis than when it presents with cerebral symptoms of convulsions and coma. Mortality varies from 5 to 25%. About 15% of survivors have such permanent sequelae as seizures, mental retardation, or behavior disturbances. Other central nervous system complications include Guillain-Barré syndrome, transverse myelitis, facial nerve palsy, optic neuritis with transient loss of vision, and a hypothalamic syndrome with obesity and recurrent fever. In contrast to herpes zoster, chickenpox virus has not been isolated from the central nervous system of patients with chickenpox who have subsequently died.

Children receiving corticosteroids or antimetabolites are at risk for severe, often fatal, chickenpox. Children with leukemia are at great risk, but deaths have occurred in children receiving steroids for acute rheumatic fever or nephrosis.

PREVENTION. A live attenuated varicella vaccine has been developed and tested in Japan. The vaccine is well tolerated, produces measurable levels of varicella antibody, is protective if given before or immediately after exposure to a contagious patient, and does not cause severe complications in children receiving corticosteroids. In one study, about 90% of leukemic children in remission developed antibody after 1 immunization; 95% responded to 2 doses. Some children developed mild to moderate rash and were infectious to others. Vaccine efficacy was 80% in children subsequently exposed to varicella. Those who developed clinical disease had mild illness.

Passive immunity can be induced by administering zoster immune globulin (ZIG) or varicella-zoster immunoglobulin (VZIG). ZIG is a gamma globulin fraction of plasma with high titer of antibody obtained from patients recovering from herpes zoster infection; supply is very limited. VZIG is obtained from the plasma of normal donors having high levels of antibody against varicella zoster. VZIG is as effective as ZIG and is more available. VZIG is obtained through the American Red Cross. The dose is 125 units/10 kg body weight. It is effective in preventing chickenpox when given within 72 hr of exposure. The recommended dose of ZIG is at least 5 mL intramuscularly, but doses as small as 2 mL have been effective in preventing infection in normal children.

Prophylaxis is indicated only in susceptible patients who are at high risk for developing severe varicella: those with immunodeficiency diseases, leukemia, or other malignancies or those on immunosuppressive drugs. Because these children are not protected by ZIG as completely as are normal children, larger quantities of high-titer ZIG or VZIG are required. VZIG should also be given to a newborn whose mother develops varicella within 5 days of delivery. Most adults are immune to chickenpox even if they have no history of having had the disease. Management of a presumably susceptible pregnant woman exposed to varicella is controversial. If possible, antibody testing should be done immediately. If test results are positive, the woman can be reassured. If they are negative or if antibody testing cannot be done, VZIG may be offered.

TREATMENT. Symptomatic treatment should be directed toward alleviating itching by using local and systemic antipruritic agents and sedation as required. The effects of scratching will be minimized if the patient wears mittens and keeps the fingernails short. Daily changes of clothes and linen and antiseptic baths reduce the incidence of secondary bacterial infection. If secondary infection occurs, systemic antibiotic therapy is indicated. Because the use of aspirin in children with varicella increases the risk of developing Reye syndrome, other antipyretics should be used when symptomatic relief is necessary.

Acyclovir (500 mg/m^2/dose given over 1 hr every 8 hr) is effective therapy for varicella pneumonia or for immunocompromised patients who develop varicella. This dose prevents the development of pneumonia or the involvement of other viscera. The best results are obtained when therapy is begun before the 3rd day of illness.

In the hospital children with varicella should be isolated in rooms where air pressure is negative in relation to the hall. The room should have an air exhaust unit that prevents recirculation of air into the hospital, and the hall door should be kept closed.

PROGNOSIS. The prognosis is usually good; fatalities are usually the result of complications.

HERPES ZOSTER
(Shingles)

Herpes zoster, an acute infection characterized by crops of vesicles and neuralgic pain, is usually confined to a dermatome.

EPIDEMIOLOGY. Herpes zoster is relatively uncommon in children under 10 yr of age, after which its incidence increases steadily with each succeeding decade. Second attacks occur in fewer than 1% of patients. The patient usually has a history of having had varicella. In some instances a mild case of varicella may have been misdiagnosed or there may have been exposure in utero or in the neonatal period that resulted in unrecognized disease. There is an increased incidence in patients receiving immunosuppressive drugs and in children exposed to varicella in utero. The severity of herpes zoster increases with age. There is no sex, race, or seasonal predilection. The factors initiating an attack are not understood.

CLINICAL MANIFESTATIONS. Herpes zoster has a preeruptive and a posteruptive phase. The illness usually starts with pain and tenderness along the involved dermatome, often accompanied by generalized malaise and fever. Within a few days groups of red papules appear, distributed along a dermatome or two adjacent ones. The individual lesions quickly vesiculate (Fig. 12–20), become pustular, dry up, and scab in the course of 5–10 days. The lesions tend to erupt first at a point nearest the central nervous system. Successive crops appear for 1–4 days, occasionally for 7 days, extending along the course of the nerve. The eruption clears in 7–14 days in most patients under 20 yr of age, but when vesicles continue to appear for 7 days or so, healing may be delayed up to 5 wk. The lesions, except in rare instances, are unilateral. Fever, pain, and tenderness usually continue throughout the period of progression. The regional lymph nodes are invariably enlarged. Although the dermatomes of the 2nd dorsal to the 2nd lumbar nerves are the most common sites for patients under the age of 20 yr, cephalic zoster and infection of the sacral nerves, producing lesions of the leg and genitalia, do occur in children. Transient paralysis of the affected part is a rare complication.

With infection of the 5th cranial nerve, any or several of its branches may be affected. With involvement of the ophthalmic branch, lesions may occur on the forehead with local loss of hair, on the nasal tip, and on the cornea (Fig. 12–21 [color plate section]); over the cheek and the homolateral palate with infection of the maxillary branch; and over the homolateral mandible and tongue when the mandibular branch is affected. Infection of the 7th nerve or the geniculate ganglion results in the *Ramsay Hunt syndrome*, paralysis of the facial nerve and vesicles in the external ear canal. Herpes zoster occurs frequently in children with leukemia or other malignancies. Lesions may spread to involve several dermatomes or to other areas of the body and may be slow to heal.

A generalized rash may accompany herpes zoster; this tends to occur in elderly patients or in children who have had a mild attack of varicella in early infancy. Occasionally the first vesicles of varicella in children may be distributed along a dermatome.

LABORATORY DATA. A mild cerebrospinal fluid lympho-

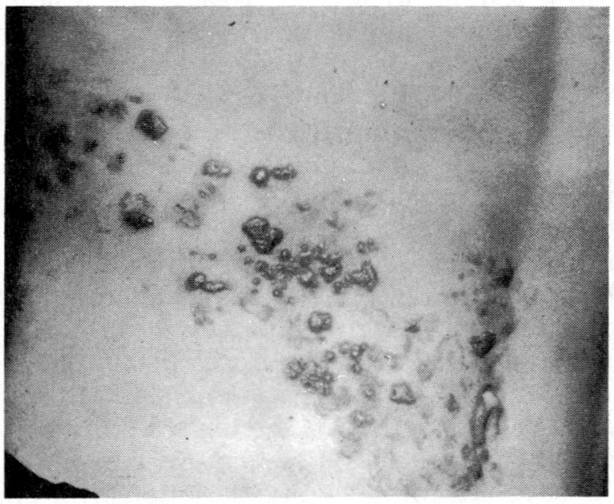

Figure 12–20. Herpes zoster. (Courtesy of Carrol S. Wright, M.D.)

cytosis often occurs. Scrapings of the floors of vesicles in their initial stage contain virus giant cells.

DIAGNOSIS. Diagnosing the disease may be difficult before the rash develops; the pain may resemble that of pleural, cardiac, or peritoneal origin, depending on the site of the lesion. When the rash appears, its distribution and characteristics together with the pain make the diagnosis relatively simple. Occasionally, herpes simplex may simulate the distribution of herpes zoster.

COMPLICATIONS. Postherpetic pain does not occur in children, and ocular complications are rare. Keratitis and uveitis may follow 5th nerve involvement in adults. Secondary bacterial infection is possible in any of the lesions.

PREVENTION. Patients with zoster are infectious to those who have not had varicella. If hospitalization is required, they should be placed in isolation.

TREATMENT. Treatment in normal children is symptomatic. Soaks and calamine or other drying lotions may be helpful. Pain is seldom a problem in children and can be controlled with analgesics; aspirin should probably be avoided because of the risk of Reye syndrome (see Sec. 12.69). Acyclovir, 500 mg/m^2/dose given over 1 hr every 8 hrs for 5 days, is effective for treatment of immunocompromised patients with severe or disseminated zoster. Antiviral therapy speeds healing of the lesions, decreases pain, shortens time of viral shedding, and prevents the development of visceral lesions. Treatment or prophylaxis with zoster immune globulin is ineffective.

COURSE AND PROGNOSIS. In children the course is usually mild, and the ultimate prognosis is good. Immunocompromised patients can have delayed healing or dissemination of the virus to other skin areas or visceral organs.

Balfour HH, Kelley JM, Suarez CS, et al: Acyclovir treatment of varicella in otherwise healthy children. J Pediatr 116:633, 1990.
Balfour HH, McMonigal KA, Bean B: Acyclovir therapy of varicella-zoster virus infections in immunocompromised patients. J Antimicrob Chemother 12(Suppl B):169, 1983.
Enders G: Varicella-zoster virus infection in pregnancy. Prog Med Virol 29:166, 1984.
Gershon AA, Steinberg SP, Gelb L, et al: Clinical reinfection with varicella-zoster virus. J Infect Dis 149:137, 1984.
Gershon AA, Steinberg SP, Gelb L, et al: Live attenuated varicella vaccine use in immunocompromised children and adults. Pediatrics 78:757, 1986.
Griffith J, et al: The nervous system diseases associated with varicella. Acta Neurol Scand 46:279, 1970.
Leclair JM, Zaia JA, Levin MJ, et al: Airborne transmission of chickenpox in a hospital. N Engl J Med 302:450, 1980.
Preblud SR, Orenstein WA, Bart KJ: Varicella: Clinical manifestations, epidemiology and health impact in children. Pediatr Infect Dis 3:505, 1984.
Triebwasser J, et al: Varicella pneumonia in adults. Medicine 46:409, 1967.

12.70 SMALLPOX*
(Variola)

Smallpox, an acute communicable viral disease that in earlier centuries was responsible for serious morbidity and high mortality worldwide and in the past century was largely eliminated in industrialized countries by means of effective vaccination measures, no longer exists throughout the world. In 1958 the World Health Organization (WHO) began a campaign to eliminate smallpox from the world; at that time there were about 250,000 cases of smallpox reported yearly. Massive organization, tireless efforts to investigate every suspected case and vaccinate susceptible contacts, and unprecedented cooperation between nations achieved this result by 1980.

The only remaining source of possible disease is laboratory accident, since seven carefully controlled laboratories in the world have stocks of variola virus. The WHO plans to stockpile large amounts of freeze-dried vaccine as insurance against any future outbreak of smallpox.

CAROL F. PHILLIPS

Kempe CH: The end of routine smallpox vaccination in the United States. Pediatrics 49:489, 1972.
Phillips CF: Smallpox; Vaccination against smallpox. *In*: Behrman RE, Vaughan VC III (eds): Nelson Textbook of Pediatrics, 12th ed. Philadelphia, WB Saunders, 1983, pp 759–763.

*In view of the current assumption that smallpox has been eliminated as a disease of man on a worldwide basis, the editors have considered it reasonable to delete the clinical description of it from this edition of the textbook. Should the assumption not prove to be correct, and we share with all mankind the hope that it is correct, then appropriate coverage of smallpox will be replaced in subsequent editions. Meanwhile, we refer the reader to the 12th edition for clinical and other pertinent information on this disease.

12.71 CYTOMEGALOVIRUS
See also Sec. 9.69.

Most cytomegalovirus (CMV) infections are inapparent, but they can cause a variety of clinical illnesses that range in seriousness from mild to fatal. CMV is the most common congenital viral infection, the most frequent debilitating viral infection in transplant recipients, and a significant complication of patients with AIDS. The most severe manifestation of congenital CMV infection is cytomegalic inclusion disease, which is characterized by low birthweight, jaundice, hepatosplenomegaly, petechiae, purpura, and microcephaly (Sec. 9.69). Frequent manifestations of CMV infection in immunosuppressed organ transplant recipients and in patients with AIDS are infectious mononucleosis syndrome, interstitial pneumonitis, retinitis, and gastrointestinal disease.

ETIOLOGY. Human cytomegalovirus is a species-specific herpesvirus, which shares two of that group's common characteristics, wide dissemination in nature and the property of remaining latent in the host. Herpesviruses contain double-stranded linear DNA, have an icosodeltahedral capsid containing 162 capsomeres that is assembled in the host cell nucleus, and have an envelope derived from the cell's nuclear membrane. Serologic tests have not defined specific serotypes of significance in epidemiologic studies; in contrast, restriction endonuclease analysis of the viral DNA has been a useful epidemiologic tool despite the fact that a homology of about 80% exists between the strains studied. A segment of the CMV genome has significant identity with the gene that encodes for the class I major histocompatibility complex molecules of primates. The virus inhibits hematopoietic colony formation, suppresses the immune response, and enhances the replication of human immunodeficiency virus type 1 (HIV-1).

EPIDEMIOLOGY. CMV infections are distributed worldwide, and most human beings have become infected by the time they reach adulthood. The incidence of congenital infections varies from less than 1% to almost 10%; it is usually higher in populations with lower standards of living. About one half (20–70%) of women of child-bearing age in the United States have serologic evidence of a previous CMV infection, 4–5% of pregnant women excrete the virus in their urine, 10% from the cervix, and 5–15% in the breast milk. The fetus may become infected during primary or secondary maternal infections. Most congenital infections occur after secondary maternal infections, but they are usually asymptomatic, and neonatal disease is extremely rare in siblings. About 10% of infants in the United States who are not congenitally infected become infected in the 1st yr of life.

The virus is present in saliva, the upper respiratory tract, semen, leukocytes, breast milk, urine, and feces, and it is probable that contact with any of these can transmit the infection. However, it is usually transmitted only after intimate contact. CMV infection is one of the sexually transmitted infectious diseases, and it is more common in sexually promiscuous individuals. Epidemics have not been described. When introduced into a household, it is likely that every susceptible member will acquire an infection eventually. Infection has been transmitted by blood transfusions and in transplanted organs (heart, kidney, and marrow). Many patients with organ transplantation who receive immunosuppressive treatment develop overt CMV infections owing either to infection acquired from the donor organ or to activation of their own latent infection. Seronegative recipients of organs harvested from seropositive donors are the most commonly infected symptomatically, although there is some evidence that more severe disease occurs in seropositive recipients who, when they receive infected organs, do develop CMV infectious disease. This may be related to the fact that individuals shed multiple strains of CMV as determined by restriction endonuclease analysis, despite the fact that no particularly pathogenic strains of CMV have been clearly identified.

Most studies have indicated that health care providers are not at increased risk for acquiring CMV infections from patients. In contrast, workers in day-care centers are at some increased risk for acquiring the infection.

PATHOLOGY. Strikingly enlarged intranuclear inclusion-bearing cells that also have cytoplasmic inclusions are pathognomonic for CMV infections and are also the reason Weller gave the virus its name. The virus induces focal mononuclear cell infiltrates, which may be present with or without cytomegalic cells. In the brain and liver the virus may induce focal necrosis; in the brain this may be extensive and accompanied by granulomatous change with calcifications. The lung, liver, kidney, and salivary glands are the most commonly infected organs, although infection has occurred in most organs at some time, and the viral genome has been found in most cell types. The extent of abnormal organ function and the quantity of virus that can be recovered from affected organs are not reflected by the number of cytomegalic inclusion–bearing cells, which may be few or absent in each organ section examined. CMV may have very subtle effects; some data indicate that it can induce atherosclerosis.

Recent evidence suggests that the pulmonary disease induced by CMV in the immunosuppressed organ transplant recipient is immunopathologically mediated. Multiplication of the virus is limited in this disease, and a host immune response is necessary for pneumonitis to appear.

CLINICAL MANIFESTATIONS. More than 90% of congenitally infected newborns appear well; those who are ill have conditions that vary greatly in severity (see Sec. 9.69).

CMV infection is usually asymptomatic when it is acquired after birth from the mother, siblings, or other contacts. However, pneumonia, bronchial or interstitial, hepatitis with mild hepatic enlargement, protracted mild diarrhea, and petechial rashes may occur when CMV infection is acquired in infancy or childhood. Rarely, the virus induces meningoencephalitis, polyneuritis, or chorioretinitis in these circumstances.

In older children and adults, apparently not immunodeficient, the virus may induce a mononucleosis-like syndrome characterized by fatigue, malaise, myalgia, headache, anorexia, abdominal pain, hepatomegaly, and splenomegaly. Abnormal results of liver function tests are common. The illness may follow transfusions of infected blood after 3–4 wk, and it may last 2 wk or longer. A morbilliform rash may appear in patients with this syndrome if ampicillin is given, as is the case in infectious mononucleosis due to Epstein-Barr virus. Abnormal serologic reactions including cold agglutinins, antinuclear antibody, rheumatoid factor, or cryoglobulins may be seen.

Interstitial pneumonitis is the most common manifestation of CMV infection in immunosuppressed individuals. This disease is present in patients with AIDS more often when *Pneumocystis carinii* and CMV are both present than when CMV alone is the infecting agent. The illness is characterized by dyspnea, fever, and nonproductive cough. If hypoxemia develops, the illness is usually fatal. Retinitis with vision loss, esophagitis, gastritis, colitis, and encephalitis also are seen frequently. *Cytomegaloviral retinitis* is the most common cause of vision loss in patients with AIDS. Gastrointestinal disease may be manifest by dysphagia, nausea, vomiting, delayed gastric emptying, abdominal pain, diarrhea, or gastrointestinal bleeding.

CMV is an apparent cause of the *vanishing bile duct syndrome* after liver transplantation. In it, the infection may precipitate rejection by inducing HLA antigen expression in patients with certain donor–recipient HLA matches.

DIAGNOSIS AND DIFFERENTIAL DIAGNOSIS. CMV can be recovered from the urine, saliva, and bronchoalveolar washings as well as from diseased tissues. Typical cytomegalic cells can be recovered from the respiratory system and the urine, but this diagnostic method is less sensitive than culture. Infants followed for several months who have sustained levels of complement-fixing, hemagglutination-inhibiting, or fluorescent antibodies, either IgM or IgG, can be presumed to have a congenital CMV infection. Antibody levels passively acquired from the mother will fall progressively and by 6 mo of age usually are 1:8 or less. The polymerase chain reaction and DNA hybridization techniques can be used to detect very small quantities of CMV in the urine, other fluids, and tissues.

When congenital CMV infection is manifest by cytomegalic inclusion disease, the differential diagnosis includes the other diseases of the TORCH group, toxoplasmosis, congenital rubella syndrome, and herpes simplex infection of the neonate (Sec. 9.58). When CMV infection is manifested by jaundice, hepatitis due to hepatitis viruses A, B, or C must be suspected. All may be characterized by atypical lymphocytosis; jaundice is more often seen in patients with the hepatitides, and in them aspartate aminotransferase (AST) levels are higher than they are in patients with CMV infection.

Patients with CMV-induced mononucleosis syndrome do not have heterophil antibody. In them serologic tests for anticytomegalovirus antibody produce more variable results than they do in the newborn period, and the CMV IgM fluorescent antibody test may be positive in both the CMV- and Epstein-Barr virus–induced sydromes, presumably because of cross-reacting antigens. Finding specific antibody to the various Epstein-Barr virus antigens is the only reliable way to distinguish between the two, but caution must be observed in assessing the reliability of these test results.

Patients with CMV pneumonia often have virus in their urine or saliva. Bronchoalveolar washings or open lung biopsy may yield cells infected with CMV that is detectable by culture, by indirect immunofluorescence techniques, or by DNA technology.

PREVENTION. Attenuated live virus vaccines are being developed. They have been shown to induce protective antibodies and have few side effects, but they have not yet been tested sufficiently to be made available. The frequency of acquisition of CMV from infected blood or organs could be significantly reduced by screening donors for antibody to CMV and selecting as donors only those who are CMV antibody negative. However, since most adults are seropositive by their 5th decade, this method of prevention has limited efficacy. Another problem is that both immunocompetent and immunodeficient individuals have frequent episodes of activation of their latent CMV infections, and in any one individual these are often associated with more than one strain of virus.

The administration of acyclovir to immunosuppressed bone marrow and renal transplant recipients is effective in reducing the frequency and severity of CMV infections in them. Similarly, anticytomegalovirus antibody containing IgG can reduce the frequency of CMV infectious disease in immunosuppressed renal allograft recipients.

Adherence to universal precaution techniques should reduce the frequency of hospital-acquired infections. Similar methods in day-care centers are probably not practical.

TREATMENT. Ganciclovir is effective in the treatment of CMV retinitis. Combined treatment of CMV pneumonitis in immunosuppressed transplant recipients with antibody and ganciclovir has been effective in reducing the frequency of death. Corticosteroids and various lymphokines are not effective in this disease.

PROGNOSIS. Congenital Disease. See Sec. 9.69.

Acquired Disease. Patients with CMV mononucleosis usually recover fully, although some may have a protracted illness lasting 2–3 yr. Many whose infections are acquired in association with immunosuppression and transplantation recover, but a significant number have severe pneumonitis, and if hypoxemia develops, the fatality rate is high. CMV infection and disease may be a terminal event in individuals with increased susceptibility to infections such as those with Hodgkin disease, lymphomas, or leukemias.

DONALD N. MEDEARIS, JR.

Alford CA Jr, Britt WJ: Cytomegalovirus. *In*: Fields BN, Knipe DM, Chanock RM, et al (eds): Virology. New York, Raven Press, 1985, pp 629–660.

Hanshaw JB: Cytomegalovirus infections. *In*: Feigin RD, Cherry JD (eds): Textbook of Pediatric Infectious Disease, Vol. 2, 2nd ed. Philadelphia, W. B. Saunders, 1987, pp 1558–1566.

Ho M: Cytomegalovirus, Biology and Infection. New York, Plenum Medical Book Co, 1982.

Plotkin SA: Cytomegalovirus vaccines. *In*: Plotkin SA, Mortimer EA Jr (eds): Vaccines. Philadelphia, W. B. Saunders, 1988, pp 513–516.

Weller TH: The cytomegaloviruses: Ubiquitous agents with protean clinical manifestations. N Engl J Med 285:203, 1971.

12.72 INFECTIOUS MONONUCLEOSIS

Infectious mononucleosis is caused by Epstein-Barr virus (EBV), a member of the herpes group. Epithelial cells of the pharynx are the initial targets of the virus, but B lymphocytes soon become infected and are disseminated throughout the lymphatic system to most of the organs, where they proliferate until checked by activated T cells.

ETIOLOGY. EBV is indistinguishable morphologically from herpes simplex virus. It was originally observed by electron microscopy in cells cultured from specimens of Burkitt lymphoma, a neoplastic disease that occurs predominantly in central Africa.

EBV is transmitted primarily to lymphocytes or lymphoblast lines. The virus also infects in vivo and in vitro several types of epithelial cells, including those of the oropharynx and uterine cervix. Although most of the atypical lymphocytes found in infectious mononucleosis are reactive T lymphocytes, EBV infects only B lymphocytes. Infection of B lymphocytes in vitro with EBV enables them to grow indefinitely in culture (immortalization). Few, if any, of the immortalized cells synthesize virus, but all harbor EBV genomes and express EBNA, the EBV-associated nuclear antigen. EBNA-positive B cell lines can be established also from the peripheral blood of seropositive donors, indicating that immortalization of B lymphocytes may also occur in vivo.

EPIDEMIOLOGY. The epidemiology of infectious mononucleosis is related to the epidemiology of EBV. Infection with EBV occurs early in life in developing countries. In central Africa almost all children are infected by 3 yr of age, and in that environment typical infectious mononucleosis is practically unknown. In western countries the age at which EBV infection occurs is related to socioeconomic group. Adolescents are 60–80% seropositive, the more affluent being less likely to have been infected. Seropositivity increases with age until in the United States nearly all adults are positive. Seroconversion is particularly high during the high school and college years in upper middle class populations; at Yale University 15% of susceptibles developed antibodies to EBV each year, and 65% of those infected had clinical infectious mononucleosis. Infectious mononucleosis occurs at all ages but appears only rarely in children under the age of 2 yr, when most EBV infections remain silent, or in adults over the age of 40 yr, when most individuals are already immune. The overall incidence is approximately 50:100,000 persons/yr, but in young adults the incidence rises to about 1:1,000/yr.

Transmission of EBV takes place by exchange of saliva from child to child, often in day-care centers, or during kissing by young adults. The source of the virus may be parotid gland ductal cells and epithelial cells of the nasopharynx. Nonintimate contact does not lead to spread of EBV. EBV is excreted in the saliva in the cell-free state, particularly before and during the clinical duration of disease, but also commonly for 6 mo after recovery and frequently longer. Healthy individuals with serologic evidence of past EBV infection excrete virus 10–20% of the time, probably intermittently. Immunosuppressed patients who are seropositive often reactivate EBV, and about 60% shed the virus.

CLINICAL MANIFESTATIONS. The incubation period of infectious mononucleosis in adolescents is 30–50 days. In children it may be shorter, but solid data are lacking. The onset is usually insidious and vague. The patient may complain of malaise, fatigue, headache, nausea, or abdominal pain. This prodromal period may last 1–2 wk. The complaints of sore throat and fever gradually increase until the patient seeks medical care. The sore throat is often accompanied by moderate to severe pharyngitis with marked tonsillar enlargement and even with exudates (Fig. 12–22 [color plate section]). The throat may resemble that characteristic of streptococcal pharyngitis, and the throat culture may be positive, but this phenomenon reflects the prevalence of inapparent streptococcal infection in normal populations. An enanthem consisting of petechiae at the junction of the hard and soft palate is frequently seen. Fever is present in about 85% of patients and is usually in the moderate range, about 39° C (102° F).

The characteristic signs, aside from sore throat, are lymphadenopathy and hepatosplenomegaly. The posterior cervical nodes are most often enlarged, but other groups are also affected. Epitrochlear lymphadenopathy is particularly consistent with infectious mononucleosis. The liver is enlarged in only about a third of patients, but elevations of enzyme activities signifying anicteric hepatitis occur in 80%; frank jaundice, much less common, is seen in only about 5%. Splenomegaly is found in about half of patients, though extension to 2–3 cm below the costal margin, rather than massive enlargement, is the rule. On the other hand, splenic enlargement may be rapid enough to cause left upper quadrant discomfort and tenderness, which may be the presenting complaint.

Other clinical findings include edema of the eyelids and rashes. Rashes are usually maculopapular and have been reported in 3–15% of patients. Eighty per cent of patients with infectious mononucleosis will develop a rash if treated with ampicillin; the reason for this phenomenon is unknown.

Symptomatic infection with EBV is more common in young

children than is generally believed. The disease may be clinically quite similar to that seen in older individuals, including development of heterophil antibodies. On the other hand, identification of current infections by viral serology (see later) has demonstrated that children may show less specific symptoms, such as tonsillitis, fever of unknown origin, or acute undifferentiated respiratory disease. Children tend to have more rashes, neutropenia, thrombocytopenia, airway obstruction, and central nervous system involvement than adults. Atypical lymphocytes are usually present, though fewer in number. In children under the age of 2 yr the great majority of primary EBV infections remain silent.

The severe symptoms usually last 2–4 wk, followed by gradual recovery. Fatigue, malaise, and some disability are common complaints for several months. Second attacks of infectious mononucleosis caused by EBV have not been documented. The prognosis for complete recovery is excellent if none of the complications described later ensue.

Chronic Mononucleosis Syndrome. In recent years a *chronic fatigue syndrome* has been frequently diagnosed in both adults and adolescents, and attempts have been made to link it to chronic EBV infection, HTLV-II, CMV, HHV-6, or unknown retroviruses. The evidence to date is that the syndrome has a variety of causes, ranging from psychoneurosis to persistent EBV infection. The latter can be distinguished by the following characteristics: an illness beginning with infectious mononucleosis and lasting 6 or more mo, with abnormal EBV antibody profiles and evidence of organ involvement such as interstitial pneumonia, lymphadenopathy, bone marrow hypoplasia, hepatitis, or splenomegaly.

The abnormal EBV profiles consist of high titers of antibodies to viral capsid antigen, VCA-IgG (>1/2,560), or to the R component of early antigen, EA (>1/320), or absence of antibody to EB nuclear antigen (EBNA) proteins, which are involved in maintenance of latency. Despite the evidence of dysregulation of EBV, this subset of patients does not benefit more from acyclovir treatment than from placebo. Supportive therapy, including psychotherapy, appears to be the soundest course until there is a clearer understanding of the cause.

ONCOGENIC ACTIVITY OF EBV. EBV is almost certainly an initiator in the induction of Burkitt lymphoma (BL) in Africa and possibly also nasopharyngeal carcinoma (NPC) in Chinese populations. BL is found in restricted areas of tropical Africa, below certain elevations, that correspond with the distribution of malarial parasites. It is a type of lymphoma, often of the jaw, that has a median onset age of 5 yr. A large prospective study in Uganda found that children who later developed BL had high titers beforehand of antibodies to EBV VCA. BL occurs sporadically in many parts of the world, including the United States, but less than 20% of these cases are associated with EBV.

NPC, mainly a disease of adults, involves the nasopharyngeal epithelial cells. It occurs at a very high rate only in Southeast Asia and among Eskimos. Occasionally, cases also occur in children 10–18 yr old. The presence of EBV genome in both BL and NPC tumor cells and the induction of lymphomas by EBV in New World monkeys strongly suggest that EBV causes these cancers, but, in addition to the requisite infection, the occurrence of BL and NPC requires the existence of environmental cofactors.

Recently, polyclonal B cell lymphomas in immunologically compromised patients were shown to be EBV associated; EBV DNA was demonstrated in the tumor and the tumor cells (expressed as EBNA). Such tumors were observed in patients with genetic and acquired immunodeficiencies (including those with AIDS) and in organ allograft recipients. Primary B cell lymphomas in the CNS, an immunologically privileged site, may be EBV associated. A decline in T cell function evidently permits EBV to escape from immune surveillance.

COMPLICATIONS. The most feared complication of infectious mononucleosis is splenic rupture, which occurs most frequently during the 2nd wk of the disease. Rupture is commonly related to trauma, which often may be mild, sometimes involving mere medical palpation.

Swelling of the tonsils and pharynx may be severe enough as to cause respiratory occlusion.

Neurologic involvement is more common than is usually appreciated and more serious. Convulsions, ataxia, and nuchal rigidity are the first signs of disease. There may be meningitis with mononuclear cells in the cerebrospinal fluid, Bell palsy, transverse myelitis, encephalitis, or Guillain-Barré syndrome. The latter can produce complete paralysis and death, at times in the absence of other signs of infectious mononucleosis. Perceptual distortions of space and size, referred to as the *Alice in Wonderland syndrome,* may be a presenting symptom.

Myocarditis and interstitial pneumonia are common complications, both resolving in 3–4 wk. Hepatitis is so common that it is considered part of the disease.

A hemolytic anemia, often with a positive Coombs test and with cold agglutinins specific for red cell antigen *i*, may occur late in the illness. Thrombocytopenic purpura and even aplastic anemia may develop, confusing the diagnosis.

Rare complications include pancreatitis, parotitis, and orchitis. Reye syndrome may occur in the wake of the disease.

Severe, persistent, and sometimes fatal EBV infection has been identified in patients with familial genetic disorders of the lymphoid system. These patients die either of disseminated lymphoproliferation involving multiple organs or of malignant lymphomas. One group of patients has been categorized as having the *X-linked lymphoproliferative syndrome* (Duncan disease), which occurs in males following EBV infection. In addition to disseminated lymphoproliferation, these patients may show unchecked fatal infectious mononucleosis, aplastic anemia, hypogammaglobulinemia, or malignant lymphoma. Other patients with a variety of cellular immune deficits, such as natural killer (NK) cell deficiency, also may suffer severe infections or EBV-induced malignancies. Rare cases of fatal disseminated infection have also been reported in previously immunocompetent hosts who developed lymphopenia during the disease.

DIAGNOSIS. Confirmation of the diagnosis of infectious mononucleosis by laboratory means has now become precise. Originally, the diagnosis could be made only on the basis of atypical lymphocytosis. Indeed, in more than 90% of cases there is leukocytosis of 10,000–20,000 cells/mm^3, of which at least two thirds are lymphocytes; atypical forms usually account for 20–40% of the total number. The atypical cells are large with an irregular shape and staining properties. They are mostly T cells, apparently responding to the presence of infected B cells. Mild thrombocytopenia (50,000–200,000/mm^3) occurs in no fewer than 50% of patients, but only rarely are values low enough to cause purpura.

The well-known serologic test for infectious mononucleosis has been the Paul-Bunnell-Davidsohn test for sheep red blood cell agglutination. This test is based on the fact that numerous abnormal antibodies, including those directed against antigens from animal tissues, are transiently found in persons with infectious mononucleosis. The antibody specific for infectious mononucleosis is in the IgM class. In order to distinguish the heterophil antibodies of infectious mononucleosis from others, serum is tested for sheep or, for greater sensitivity, horse red blood cell agglutination before and after absorption with ox red blood cells or guinea pig kidney cell suspension. In infectious mononucleosis the antibody titers to sheep or horse red blood cells remain after guinea pig kidney absorption but disappear after ox cell absorption. Titers greater than 1:28 or 1:40 (depending on the dilution system used) after absorption with guinea pig cells are considered positive. The sheep red blood cell agglutination test is likely to be positive only for several months, but the horse red blood cell agglutination test may be positive for as long as 2 yr.

Other popular tests for heterophil antibodies use formalin-treated horse or sheep red blood cells for a rapid slide agglutination with commercially produced reagents. When the clinical situation is atypical, the slide test should be confirmed by the differential heterophil tube agglutination test or by the EBV-specific serologic tests.

Most children with typical infectious mononucleosis have positive tests, but those under the age of 5 yr are more likely to be negative or to have lower titers than adults, and sensitive tests for heterophil antibodies must be used to achieve optimal results.

The specific serologic tests for EBV must be understood in the context of the structure of the virus particle. Replication of complete particles begins in the nucleus of infected cells, and virions then pass into the cytoplasm, where the viral nucleocapsid can be detected by immunofluorescence. If a patient's serum is applied to fixed-cell smears of lymphoblastoid cell lines infected with EBV, then, following exposure to fluorescein-conjugated antihuman IgG or antihuman IgM, antibodies of either class may be detected by fluorescent staining of the infected cells. IgG antibody to VCA is usually present in a titer greater than 1:160 at the time of acute disease. In addition, VCA-specific IgM antibodies are present in all cases when the patient is tested at the appropriate time, but they may occasionally be missed because the IgM response is not long-lasting. IgM antibody usually remains in evidence for 2–3 mo. Occasionally, EBV antibodies develop late; in such cases convalescent sera need to be tested.

Some lymphoblast lines do not produce viral capsid antigen or early antigens, but if these lines are superinfected with EBV, antigens are produced in the nucleus and cytoplasm by abortive infection. These have been termed early antigens because during lytic infection they precede synthesis of viral particles. Antibodies to the D, or diffuse-staining, component of the early antigens are found transiently in 80% of patients during the acute phase of infectious mononucleosis and reach high titers in patients with nasopharyngeal carcinoma. Antibodies to the R, or cytoplasmic-restricted, component emerge transiently in late convalescence from infectious mononucleosis and often attain high titers in patients with EBV-associated Burkitt lymphoma, which in the terminal stage of the disease may be exceeded by antibodies to the D component. Antibodies to D or to R may be found also in immunoincompetent patients with activated persistent EBV infections.

Another serologic test useful for diagnosis is that for EBNA antibodies. EB nuclear antigens are involved in control of latency and are detected in lymphoblasts carrying EB viral genomes by anticomplement immunofluorescence. Antibody will attach to the antigen and fix complement, which can then be detected by fluorescent antibody to complement. Antibody to EB nuclear antigen is the last to appear in infectious mononucleosis; thus, its absence when other antibodies are present implies recent infection, while its presence implies infection at least several weeks previously. Figure 12–23 summarizes the combinations of antibodies that would be expected in various situations.

DIFFERENTIAL DIAGNOSIS. The patient with atypical lymphocytosis, lymphadenopathy, hepatosplenomegaly, and a positive heterophil test presents no problems in diagnosis. If a clinical picture suggestive of infectious mononucleosis is present but the heterophil tests are negative, five conditions should be considered: EBV infection without heterophil antibody response, CMV infection, toxoplasmosis, acute HIV infection, and infectious hepatitis (hepatitis A). All five can be identified by serologic tests, including those for EBV, and virus isolation. CMV infection, a particularly common cause of an infectious mononucleosis-like illness in adults, is accompanied by negative heterophil tests.

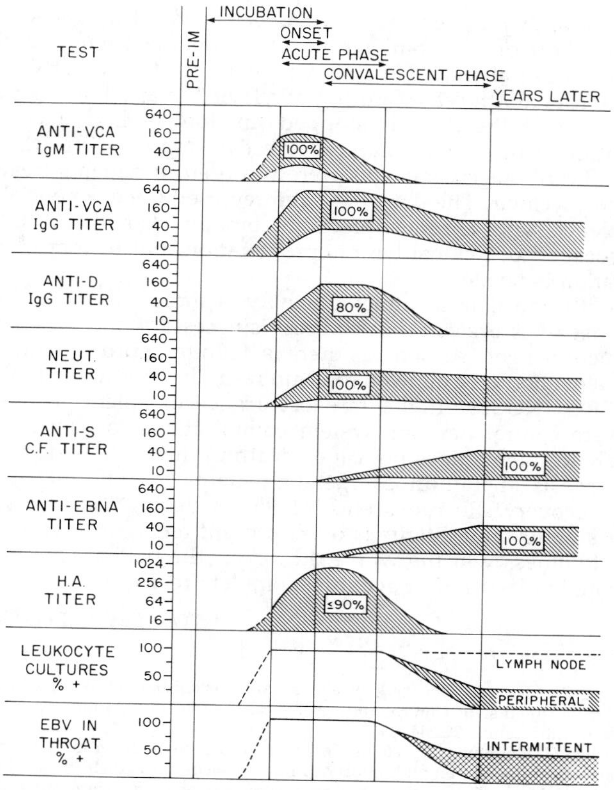

Figure 12–23. Scheme of antibody responses, leukocyte cultures, and EBV assays in throat washings during the course of infectious mononucleosis. (C.F. = complement fixing; D = diffuse-staining early antigen; EBNA = Epstein-Barr nuclear antigen; EBV = Epstein-Barr virus; H.A. = heterophile antibody; IM = infectious mononucleosis; NEUT. = neutralizing antibody; S = soluble complement-fixing antigen (probably identical with EBNA); VCA = viral capsid antigen.)

Other conditions that occasionally cause confusion are mumps, adenoviral disease, rubella, and streptococcal sore throat because of facial edema, lymphadenopathy, rash, and positive throat culture, respectively. Although throat cultures for streptococci may be positive in infectious mononucleosis, they are no more often so than in any random population. Failure of a patient with "strep throat" to improve within 48 hr should evoke suspicion of infectious mononucleosis.

The most serious problem in diagnosis arises in the occasional case with low white blood cell counts, moderate thrombocytopenia, and even hemolytic anemia. In these cases bone marrow examination and hematologic consultation are warranted to rule out leukemia. Atypical lymphocytes may be found in CMV infection, toxoplasmosis, infectious hepatitis, malaria, tuberculosis, typhoid, and mycoplasmal infection.

TREATMENT. There is no specific treatment for infectious mononucleosis. Short courses (under 14 days) of corticosteroids may be helpful if pharyngotonsillar edema threatens to obstruct the airway, in hepatitis, or in severe abdominal pain due to splenomegaly or lymphadenopathy. Longer courses may be tried in patients with hemolytic anemia, immune thrombocytopenia, or Guillain-Barré syndrome. There are no controlled data, however, showing efficacy of steroids in any of these conditions, and in view of the potential hazards of immunosuppression, steroids should not be used in the usual case of infectious mononucleosis.

The antiviral agent acyclovir is active in vitro against the replication of EBV but has no effect on the latency of the virus. Clinical trials have shown that excretion of EBV into the oropharynx ceases during acyclovir therapy but resumes as soon as the drug is stopped. In double-blind, placebo-controlled trials, more rapid subjective improvement but no significant objective effects were recorded in patients treated with acyclovir. The drug has been reported to be beneficial in patients with chronic infectious mononucleosis and EBV-associated polyclonal lymphoproliferation, but further investigation is needed.

Withdrawal from athletic activity is indicated while splenomegaly is present, but bed rest is necessary only when the patient is toxic. As soon as there is definite improvement, the patient should be allowed to begin resuming normal activities.

PROGNOSIS. If the rare occurrence of splenic rupture, severe central nervous system complications, or severe hemolytic anemia does not cause death in the acute period, the prognosis in immunocompetent patients is uniformly good for recovery. Recrudescence of illness during the first year does occur, and fatigue is often present for months after the acute illness. On the whole, however, the patient should be strongly reassured of eventual complete recovery.

STANLEY A. PLOTKIN

Biggar RJ, Henle G, Böcker J, et al: Primary Epstein-Barr virus infections in African infants. II. Clinical and serological observations during seroconversion. Int J Cancer 22:244, 1980.

Fleisher G, Lennette ET, Henle G, et al: Incidence of heterophil antibody responses in children with infectious mononucleosis. J Pediatr 94:723, 1979.

Henle W, Henle G, Horwitz CA: Epstein-Barr virus-specific diagnostic tests in infectious mononucleosis. Hum Pathol 5:551, 1974.

Miller G: Epstein-Barr herpesvirus and infectious mononucleosis. Prog Med Virol 20:84, 1975.

Naegele RF, Champion J, Murphy S, et al: Nasopharyngeal carcinoma in American children: Epstein-Barr virus–specific antibody titers and prognosis. Int J Cancer 29:209, 1982.

Niederman JC, Evans AS, Subramanyan MS, et al: Prevalence, incidence and persistence of EB virus antibody in young adults. N Engl J Med 282:361, 1970.

Straus SE: The chronic mononucleosis syndrome. J Infect Dis 157:405, 1988.

Sumaya CV, Ench Y: Epstein-Barr virus infectious mononucleosis in children. I. Clinical and general laboratory findings. Pediatrics 75:1003, 1985.

Sumaya CV, Ench Y: Epstein-Barr virus infectious mononucleosis in children. II. Heterophil antibody and viral-specific responses. Pediatrics 75:1011, 1985.

12.73 MUMPS
(Epidemic Parotitis)

Mumps is an acute, generalized viral disease in which painful enlargement of the salivary glands, chiefly the parotids, is the usual presenting sign.

ETIOLOGY. The virus is a member of the paramyxovirus group, which also includes the parainfluenza, measles, and Newcastle disease viruses. Only one serotype is known. Primary cultures of human or monkey kidney cells are used for viral isolation. Cytopathic effect is occasionally observed, but hemadsorption is the most sensitive indicator of infection. Virus has been isolated from saliva, cerebrospinal fluid, blood, urine, brain, and other infected tissues.

EPIDEMIOLOGY. Mumps is endemic in most urban populations; the virus is spread from a human reservoir by direct contact, air-borne droplets, fomites contaminated by saliva, and possibly by urine. It is distributed worldwide and affects both sexes equally; 85% of infections occurred in children under the age of 15 yr prior to widespread immunization. Now disease often occurs in young adults, producing epidemics in colleges or in the workplace. Epidemics appear to be related to lack of immunization rather than to waning of immunity. Epidemics occur at all seasons but are slightly more frequent in late winter and spring. Sources of infection may be difficult to trace because 30–40% of infections are subclinical. There has been a decrease in the incidence since the introduction of mumps vaccine.

Virus has been isolated from saliva as long as 6 days before and up to 9 days after appearance of salivary gland swelling. Transmission does not seem to occur longer than 24 hr before appearance of the swelling or later than 3 days after it has subsided. Virus has been isolated from urine from the 1st–14th day after the onset of salivary gland swelling.

Lifelong immunity usually follows clinical or subclinical infection, although second infections have been documented. Transplacental antibodies seem to be effective in protecting infants during their first 6–8 mo. Infants born to mothers who have mumps in the week prior to delivery may have clinically apparent mumps at birth or develop illness in the neonatal period. Severity ranges from mild parotitis to severe pancreatitis. The serum neutralization test is the most reliable method for determining immunity but is cumbersome and expensive. A complement-fixing antibody test is available (see Diagnosis). The presence of V antibodies alone suggests previous mumps infection.

PATHOGENESIS. After entry and initial multiplication in the cells of the respiratory tract, the virus is blood-borne to many tissues, among which the salivary and other glands are the most susceptible.

CLINICAL MANIFESTATIONS. The incubation period ranges from 14–24 days, with a peak at 17–18 days. In children, prodromal manifestations are rare but may be manifest by fever, muscular pain (especially in the neck), headache, and malaise. The onset is usually characterized by pain and swelling in one or both parotid glands. The parotid swells characteristically: it first fills the space between the posterior border of the mandible and the mastoid and then extends in a series of crescents downward and forward, being limited above by the zygoma. Edema of the skin and soft tissues usually extends further and obscures the limit of the glandular swelling, so that the swelling is more readily appreciated by sight than by palpation. Swelling may proceed extremely rapidly, reaching a maximum within a few hours, although it usually peaks in 1–3 days. The swollen tissues push the ear lobe upward and outward, and the angle of the mandible is no longer visible. Swelling slowly subsides within 3–7 days but occasionally lasts longer. One parotid gland usually swells a day or two before the other, but swelling limited to one gland is common. The swollen area is tender and painful, pain being elicited especially by tasting sour liquids such as lemon juice or vinegar. Redness and swelling about the opening of the Stensen duct are common. Edema of the homolateral pharynx and soft palate accompanies the parotid swelling and displaces the tonsil medially; acute edema of the larynx has also been described. Edema over the manubrium and upper chest wall may occur, probably due to lymphatic obstruction. The parotid swelling is usually accompanied by moderate fever; normal temperatures are common (20%), but temperatures of 40° C (104° F) or more are rare.

Although the parotid glands alone are affected in the majority of patients, swelling of the submandibular glands occurs frequently and usually accompanies or closely follows that of the parotid glands. In 10–15% of patients only the submandibular gland(s) may be swollen. Little pain is associated with the submandibular infection, but the swelling subsides more slowly than that of the parotids. Redness and swelling at the orifice of the Wharton duct frequently accompany swelling of the gland.

Least commonly the sublingual glands are infected, usually bilaterally; the swelling is evident in the submental region and in the floor of the mouth.

A maculopapular erythematous rash, most prominent on the trunk, occurs infrequently; rarely it is urticarial.

COMPLICATIONS. Viremia early in the infection probably accounts for the widespread complications.

Meningoencephalomyelitis. This is the most frequent complication in childhood. The true incidence is hard to estimate because subclinical infection of the central nervous system, as evidenced by cerebrospinal fluid pleocytosis, has been reported in over 65% of patients with parotitis. Clinical manifestations occur in over 10% of patients. The incidence of mumps meningoencephalitis is approximately 250/100,000 cases; 10% of these cases occurred in patients over 20 yr old. The mortality rate is about 2%. Males are affected 3–5 times as frequently as females. Mumps is one of the most common causes of aseptic meningitis (Sec. 12.12).

The pathogenesis of mumps meningoencephalitis has been described as (1) a primary infection of neurons and (2) a postinfectious encephalitis with demyelination. In the first type, parotitis frequently appears at the same time or following the onset of encephalitis. In the latter type, encephalitis follows parotitis by an average of 10 days. Parotitis may in some cases be absent. Aqueductal stenosis and hydrocephalus have been associated with mumps infection. Injecting mumps virus into suckling hamsters has produced similar lesions.

Mumps meningoencephalitis is clinically indistinguishable from meningoencephalitis of other origins (Sec. 12.11 and 12.12). Moderate stiffness of the neck is seen, but the remainder of the neurologic examination is usually normal. The cerebrospinal fluid (CSF) usually contains fewer than 500 cells/mm^3, although occasionally the count may exceed 2,000. The cells are almost exclusively lymphocytes, in contrast to enteroviral aseptic meningitis, in which polymorphonuclear leukocytes often predominate early in the disease. Mumps virus can be isolated from cerebrospinal fluid early in the illness.

Orchitis, Epididymitis. These lesions rarely occur in prepubescent boys but are common (14–35%) in adolescents and adults. The testis is most often infected with or without epididymitis; epididymitis may also occur alone. Rarely, there is a hydrocele. The orchitis usually follows parotitis within 8 days or so; it may also occur without evidence of salivary gland infection. In about 30% of patients both testes are affected. The onset is usually abrupt, with a rise in temperature, chills, headache, nausea, and lower abdominal pain; when the right testis is implicated, appendicitis may be suggested as a diagnostic possibility. The affected testis becomes tender and swollen, and the adjacent skin is edematous and red. The average duration is 4 days. Approximately 30–40% of affected testes atrophy. Impairment of fertility is estimated to be about 13%, but absolute infertility is probably rare.

Oophoritis. Pelvic pain and tenderness are noted in about 7% of postpubertal female patients. There is no evidence of impairment of fertility.

Pancreatitis. Severe involvement of the pancreas is rare, but mild or subclinical infection may be more common than is recognized. It may be unassociated with salivary gland manifestations and be misdiagnosed as gastroenteritis. Epigastric pain and tenderness, which are suggestive, may be accompanied by fever, chills, vomiting, and prostration. An elevated serum amylase value is characteristically present with mumps, with or without clinical manifestations of pancreatitis.

Nephritis. Viruria has been reported frequently. In one study of adults, abnormal renal function occurred at some time in every patient, and viruria was detected in 75%. The frequency of renal involvement in children is unknown. Fatal nephritis, occurring 10–14 days after parotitis, has been reported.

Thyroiditis. Although uncommon in children, a diffuse, tender swelling of the thyroid may occur about 1 wk after the onset of parotitis with subsequent development of antithyroid antibodies.

Myocarditis. Serious cardiac manifestations are extremely rare, but mild infection of the myocardium may be more common than is recognized. Electrocardiographic tracings revealed changes, mostly depression of the ST segment, in 13% of adults in one series. Such involvement may explain the precordial pain, bradycardia, and fatigue sometimes noted among adolescents and adults with mumps.

Mastitis. This is uncommon in each sex.

Deafness. Unilateral, rarely bilateral, nerve deafness may occur; although the incidence is low (1:15,000), mumps is a leading cause of unilateral nerve deafness. The hearing loss may be transient or permanent.

Ocular Complications. These include *dacryoadenitis,* painful swelling, usually bilateral, of the lacrimal glands; *optic neuritis (papillitis)* with symptoms varying from loss of vision to mild blurring with recovery in 10–20 days; *uveokeratitis,* usually unilateral, with photophobia, tearing, rapid loss of vision, and recovery within 20 days; *scleritis; tenonitis,* with resultant exophthalmos; and *central vein thrombosis.*

Arthritis. Arthralgia associated with swelling and redness of the joints is an infrequent complication; complete recovery is the rule.

Thrombocytopenic Purpura. This sign is infrequent.

Mumps Embryopathy. There is no firm evidence that maternal infection is damaging to the fetus; a possible relationship to endocardial fibroelastosis has not been established. Mumps in early pregnancy does increase the chance of abortion.

DIAGNOSIS. The diagnosis of mumps parotitis is usually apparent from the symptoms and physical examination. When the clinical manifestations are limited to those of one of the less common lesions, the diagnosis is not so clear but may be suspected, especially during an epidemic. The routine laboratory tests are nonspecific; there is usually leukopenia with relative lymphocytosis, but complications often result in polymorphonuclear leukocytosis of moderate degree. An elevation of serum amylase is common; the rise tends to parallel the parotid swelling and then to return to normal within 2 wk or so. The etiologic diagnosis depends on isolation of the virus from the saliva, urine, spinal fluid, or blood or the demonstration of a significant rise in circulating CF antibodies during convalescence. Serum antibodies to the S antigen reach their peak early in about 75% of patients and are detectable at the time of the presenting symptoms. They gradually disappear within 6–12 mo; antibodies against the V or viral antigen usually reach a peak titer in about 1 mo, remain stationary for about 6 mo, and then slowly decline during the ensuing 2 yr to a low level, at which they persist. The presence of a high anti-S titer and a low anti-V titer during the acute stage of an otherwise undiagnosed meningoencephalitis, for example, strongly suggests a mumps infection, which would be confirmed if a convalescent serum (taken 14–21 days later) revealed a 4-fold rise of anti-V antibodies accompanied by little change in the titer of anti-S antibodies.

DIFFERENTIAL DIAGNOSIS. This includes *parotitis* of other origin, as in AIDS or the rare instances of coxsackievirus A and lymphocytic choriomeningitis infections, which can be distinguished only by specific laboratory tests; *suppurative parotitis,* in which pus can often be expressed from the duct; *recurrent parotitis,* a condition of unknown origin, but possibly allergic in nature, which has frequent recurrences and a characteristic sialogram; *salivary calculus,* obstructing either a parotid or, more commonly, a submandibular duct, in which the swelling is intermittent; *preauricular* or *anterior cervical lymphadenitis* from any cause; *lymphosarcoma* or other rare *tumors* of the parotid; *orchitis due to infections other than mumps,* for example, the rare infections by coxsackievirus A or lymphocytic choriomeningitis viruses; and *parotitis due to cytomegalovirus* in immunocompromised children.

TREATMENT. Treatment of parotitis is entirely symptomatic. Bed rest should be guided by the patient's needs, but no statistical evidence indicates that it prevents complications. The diet should be adjusted to the patient's ability to chew. Orchitis should be treated with local support and bed rest. Mumps arthritis may respond to a 2-wk course of corticosteroids or a nonsteroidal anti-inflammatory agent. Salicylates do not appear to be effective.

PROPHYLAXIS. Passive. Hyperimmune mumps gamma globulin is not effective in preventing mumps or decreasing complications.

Active. The routine administration of live, attenuated mumps vaccine is discussed in Sec. 5.1. Vaccinated children usually do not develop fever or other detectable clinical reactions, do not excrete virus, and are not contagious to susceptible contacts. Rarely, parotitis can develop 7–10 days after vaccination. The vaccine induces antibody in about 96% of seronegative recipients and has a protective efficacy of about 97% against natural mumps infection. The protection appears to be long-lasting. In one outbreak of mumps, several children who had been immunized with mumps vaccine in the past developed an illness characterized by fever, malaise, nausea, and a red papular rash involving the trunk and extremities but sparing the palms and soles. The rash lasted about 24 hr. No virus was isolated from these children, but increases in the titer of mumps antibody were demonstrated.

CAROL F. PHILLIPS

Bistrian B, et al: Fatal mumps meningoencephalitis. JAMA 222:478, 1972.
Cochi SI, Preblud SR, Orenstein WA: Perspectives in the relative resurgence of mumps in the United States. Am J Dis Child 142:499, 1988.
Gordon SC, Lauter CB: Mumps arthritis: A review of the literature. Rev Infect Dis 6:338, 1984.
Quast U, Hennessen W, Widmark RM: Vaccine induced mumps-like disease. Develop Biol Standard 43:269, 1979.

12.74 INFLUENZA VIRAL INFECTIONS

Influenza viral infections create a broad spectrum of illnesses causing significant morbidity and mortality in children.

INFLUENZA VIRUSES. These are relatively large RNA *orthomyxoviruses*, which are grouped into three broad serologic types (A, B, and C), determined by the complement-fixing property of their ribonucleoprotein component (S antigen). The outer (glycoprotein) surface of influenza viruses contains spike-like projections that are responsible for antigenic characteristics that determine subtypes. On influenza A and B viruses the spike-like projections contain specific hemagglutinins and neuraminidase; neuraminidase antigen is not present on type C strains. Influenza A subtypes are identified by their hemagglutinin and neuraminidase antigens; antigens to 12 hemagglutinins (H1–H12) and 9 neuraminidases (N1–N9) are included in this system. Although antigenic variation occurs among influenza B viruses, formal subclassification utilizing neuraminidase antigens has not been done. Influenza A viruses are subject to two types of change: frequent minor antigenic changes are called antigenic "drift"; less frequent major changes are referred to as antigenic "shift." The most recent sustained shift in influenza A virus occurred in 1968 when A/Hong Kong/68 (H3N2) appeared. Subsequently, several drifts in the antigenic character of the virus have occurred; recent strains include: A/Sichuan/87 and A/Shanghai/87.

Shifts in influenza A viruses causing human disease may be cyclic; when a shift occurs, the previous viral subtype usually disappears from circulation. In the late fall of 1977 the expected shift of the influenza A subtype apparently occurred, and in early 1978 epidemics of influenza due to an H1N1 serotype (A/USSR/77) occurred in many areas of the world. However, in contrast to predictions based upon past experiences, previous H3N2 influenza serotypes did not disappear but continued to cause epidemic disease. Since 1977 both H1N1 and H3N2 viral serotypes have remained in human circulation and have caused epidemic disease. Since 1977, several drifts in the antigenic character of the H1N1 virus have also occurred (A/Brazil/78, A/England/80, A/Chile/83, and A/Taiwan/86).

Antigenic drift, the result of point mutation, allows a growth advantage in the presence of antibody. Antigenic shift may arise by recombination between human and animal influenza viruses during chance simultaneous infections.

Influenza B strains undergo antigenic drift; antigenic shift has not been demonstrated.

EPIDEMIOLOGY. Severe pandemic influenza A resulting from antigenic shift occurs every 10–40 yr. Subsequently, epidemics of generally lesser intensity occur every 2–3 yr in association with antigenic drift. Major outbreaks of influenza B are more variable but tend to occur at 4- to 7-yr intervals. Antibody studies reveal that virtually all children have experience with influenza C virus by age 10 yr, but the epidemiologic patterns of this virus have not been determined. In a large urban area there is generally some influenza viral activity each year.

Influenza viruses have no geographic restrictions. Epidemics usually occur in cooler weather in temperate climates, and during the rainy season in the tropics. Small outbreaks of infections with an influenza A virus that is antigenically distinct (significant drift) from the one responsible for a terminating epidemic frequently herald the epidemic virus for the oncoming season.

Following the appearance of a new subtype of influenza A, the highest incidence of disease occurs in children 5–14 yr old, in whom the attack rate approaches 50%. In subsequent outbreaks with variants (drifts) of the same subtype, the attack rate in children of similar age drops to about 15%. In outbreaks of influenza B, the attack rate is generally higher in children than in adults.

Respiratory secretions of infected children contain large amounts of virus, and infection is transmitted directly from person to person by the air-borne route or by fomites.

PATHOLOGY. Data about uncomplicated influenza in children are limited. The main site of cellular involvement is the mucous membrane of the respiratory tract, which shows extensive destruction of its ciliated epithelium. Influenza uncomplicated by secondary bacterial infection reveals marked desquamation of the tracheal epithelium as early as the 1st day after onset of symptoms. Cellular infiltration with lymphocytes, histiocytes, plasma cells, eosinophils, and polymorphonuclear leukocytes occurs, but to a lesser extent than might be expected on the basis of the extensive epithelial necrosis. Repair of the epithelium begins within 3–5 days. A pseudometaplastic response of undifferentiated epithelium up to 8 cell layers thick occurs, reaching its maximum within 9–15 days. After 15 days cilia reappear and mucus production resumes. With secondary bacterial involvement there is extensive inflammatory cell infiltration and destruction of the basal cell layer and the basement membrane, and consequently the regeneration of the ciliated epithelium is delayed.

In children dying of pneumonia the pulmonary findings have included peribronchiolar lymphocytic infiltration with mucus and cellular debris plugging the small bronchioles, necrosis of bronchiolar epithelium, and marked lymphocytic infiltration of the alveolar walls and interstitial lung tissue.

Although the main pathology in influenza lies in the respiratory tract, the heart, brain, or lymphoid tissues are occasionally involved in fatal cases. Toxic, focal, and diffuse forms of myocarditis have been noted. Cerebral edema is the most common central nervous system finding at autopsy. The lymph nodes of the tracheobronchial tree show extensive changes, including necrosis and disorganization of the germinal follicles.

PATHOGENESIS AND IMMUNITY. The incubation period is usually 2–3 days. The virus is commonly found in the respiratory tract, but in unusual instances viremia, viruria, and isolation of virus from extrapulmonary tissues have been noted. Immunity correlates better with secretory (IgA) nasal antibody than with circulating antibody, but high titers of serum antibody are usually protective.

Following natural infection with an influenza A virus, protection against reinfection with the particular viral subtype, even though antigenic drift may have occurred, lasts for several years. Subclinical reinfections, however, are common and tend to broaden the antibody response, allowing continued protection from disease.

When antigenic shift occurs within an influenza A virus, the previous influenza A antibody that a child may have is not protective. The duration of immunity to influenza B infections is less well known but appears quite variable. Although cell-mediated immune mechanisms can be demonstrated to be associated with influenza infections, their role in protection against and recovery from influenza viral infection is unknown. High levels of serum interferon are noted during influenza infections and may play a role in recovery.

CLINICAL MANIFESTATIONS. The predominant manifestations are respiratory, although systemic complaints are usually an integral part of the picture. In general, characteristics of influenza A and B virus illnesses are similar, but they demonstrate two distinct patterns based on age: manifestations in *older children* and those in *younger children*.

In *older children and adolescents* the manifestations are similar to those in adults (Table 12–31). The onset is abrupt with fever, flushed face, chills, headache, myalgia, and malaise. The temperature range is 39–41° C (102–106° F) and is usually inversely correlated with age; the severity of systemic symptoms generally correlates directly with age. Dry cough and coryza are also early manifestations but may be overlooked because of the severity of the systemic manifestations. Sore throat occurs in over one half of cases and is usually associated with a nonexudative pharyngitis. Ocular symptoms include tearing, photophobia, and burning and pain on eye movement. During some outbreaks, diarrhea has occurred in about one third of the children and adolescents afflicted.

Table 12–31. Relative Frequency of Symptoms and Signs during Classic Influenza in Older Children and Adolescents

	Occurrence*
Symptoms	
Chilly sensation	+ + + +
Cough	+ + +
Headache	+ + +
Sore throat	+ + +
Prostration	+ +
Nasal stuffiness	+ +
Diarrhea	+ +
Dizziness	+
Eye irritation or pain	+
Vomiting	+
Myalgia	+
Signs	
Fever	+ + + +
Pharyngitis	+ + +
Conjunctivitis (mild)	+ +
Rhinitis	+ +
Cervical adenitis	+
Pulmonary rales, wheezes or rhonchi	+

*+ + + + = 76–100%; + + + = 51–75%; + + = 26–50%; and + = 1–25%.

In uncomplicated influenza the fever usually persists for 2–3 days but may last up to 5 days. A biphasic temperature pattern may occur, however, even without secondary bacterial complications. By the 2nd–4th day, respiratory symptoms become more prominent, and the systemic complaints begin to subside. The cough is dry and hacking and usually persists for 4–10 days. Frequently, cough, in association with some degree of general malaise, persists for 1–2 wk after the illness has otherwise subsided. Illness due to influenza B virus tends to be associated with more prominent nasal and eye complaints and less prominent systemic ones than is the case with influenza A infections.

The leukocyte count and differential are usually normal, but leukopenia (<4,500 cells/mm^3) occurs in about 25% of cases. Approximately 10% of older children and adolescents have clinical and roentgenographic evidence of pulmonary involvement.

In *younger children* the manifestations of influenza viral infections are frequently similar to manifestations resulting from other respiratory viruses (parainfluenza, respiratory syncytial, rhinovirus, and adenovirus). Laryngotracheitis, bronchitis, bronchiolitis, pneumonia, and the common cold all occur. Clinical descriptions of these illnesses are presented in Sec. 14.43 and 14.44. Laryngotracheitis resulting from influenza A infection is frequently severe and associated with a thick, tenacious tracheal exudate; a greater percentage of children with croup due to influenza A virus require tracheostomy than children with similar illness resulting from other viral infections.

The onset of illness in the younger child often becomes apparent by a high fever, an appearance of moderate toxicity, and a clear nasal discharge. Febrile convulsions and vomiting are common. Mild diarrhea occurs in about 15% of cases, and otitis media occurs in almost one fourth. Fleeting erythematous, macular, or maculopapular discrete rashes occur frequently.

In the *neonate* with influenza viral infection, the sudden occurrence of fever, lethargy, poor feeding, apnea, and irritability suggests bacterial sepsis. Nasal discharge and other respiratory symptoms, however, appear early, so that the viral etiology can be suspected.

Acute myositis, particularly involving the gastrocnemius and soleus muscles, has been associated with influenza B viral infections in children. It occurs about 1 wk after onset of respiratory symptoms, usually after a brief period of clinical improvement. Acute parotitis has also occurred with influenza A infections.

Illness due to influenza C appears to be quite uncommon in children. It is characterized by fever, prolonged nasal discharge, sneezing, and cough and is generally less severe than are the influenza A and B infections.

DIAGNOSIS AND DIFFERENTIAL DIAGNOSIS. The etiologic diagnosis of a sporadic influenza viral respiratory infection is frequently difficult, although it may not be difficult during an epidemic. All age groups are clinically involved with febrile illnesses during influenza outbreaks, whereas with other agents, such as respiratory syncytial and parainfluenza viruses, illness in adults is only sporadic and is not generally associated with fever.

The virologic confirmation of influenza viral infection is easy and is accomplished relatively rapidly (72 hr) by standard virus isolation methods. Fluorescent antibody procedures and other rapid antigen identification techniques may provide a diagnosis within 24 hr. Retrospective diagnosis can be made by studying paired serum samples by complement fixation, hemagglutination inhibition, and other antibody techniques.

COMPLICATIONS. Complications frequently occur in influenza viral infections; many are variations of primary viral infection, for example, myositis, parotitis, and severe croup. Secondary or superimposed bacterial infections are most important; otitis media, purulent sinusitis, tracheitis, and pneumonia are common. One must be constantly alert for their appearance and institute appropriate antibiotic therapy should any of them occur.

Complications relating directly to the primary viral infection include hemorrhagic pneumonia, encephalitis and other neurologic syndromes, myocarditis, sudden infant death syndrome, and myoglobinuria. Reye syndrome (acute encephalopathy and fatty degeneration of the liver) is most commonly associated with epidemic influenza B viral infection, but many cases have also occurred after influenza A (H1N1) infections. Administering salicylates to children and teenagers having influenza increases the risk of their developing Reye syndrome (Sec. 13.96).

PREVENTION. Immunization with potent, antigenically up-to-date *inactivated influenza viral vaccines* is safe and effective. However, routine immunization of normal children or adults is not generally recommended. Vaccine should be given to those known to be at particularly high risk for complications, for example, the elderly and children with (1) cardiovascular disorders such as rheumatic, congenital, or hypertensive heart disease; (2) chronic bronchopulmonary disease such as tuberculosis, cystic fibrosis, asthma, bronchopulmonary dysplasia, and bronchiectasis; (3) chronic metabolic diseases such as diabetes mellitus; (4) chronic glomerulonephritis and nephrosis; (5) chronic neurologic disorders, especially those associated with weak or paralyzed respiratory muscles; and (6) sickle cell and other anemias.

Live vaccines have been successfully used in adults, and trials in children have shown some promise. Long-term studies assessing risks and benefits of more comprehensive immunization programs involving all segments of the population are needed.

Amantadine hydrochloride and *rimantadine* are effective prophylactically when administered prior to exposure to influenza A viruses. Minimal data are available supporting their pediatric efficacy and safety. The dose of amantadine hydrochloride for children 1–9 yr of age is 4.4–8.8 mg/kg/24 hr with a maximum daily dose of 150 mg. For pediatric patients over 9 yr of age, the dose is 200 mg/24 hr.

TREATMENT. Amantadine hydrochloride and rimantadine are specifically active against influenza A viruses and have benefited adults and a small number of children when given early in the course of illness. The dose of amantadine hydrochloride is the same as that for prophylaxis mentioned earlier.

Ribavirin is active against both influenza A and B viruses. When administered by aerosol it effectively shortens the course of influenza in college students. It is being evaluated for the treatment of severe influenza.

Since morbidity is frequently the result of cardiorespiratory problems, it is prudent to encourage bed rest in all but the mildest cases. Since pulmonary abnormalities may persist for a greater period of time than fever and other symptoms, it is also wise to insist upon restricted physical activity during convalescence.

Adequate fluid intake should be ensured; nonsalicylate-containing antipyretics may be used for excessive fever. Parents should be advised not to administer aspirin to children suspected of having influenza (Sec. 13.69). During convalescence the judicious use of codeine at bedtime will relieve cough. Although bacterial superinfections are common, prophylactic administration of antibiotics should be discouraged, but vigorous antibiotic therapy following appropriate culture is indicated at the first sign of bacterial infection.

PROGNOSIS. The outcome is generally good, but the prognosis must be guarded in children with underlying problems that place them in the high-risk category. Anoxia associated with severe laryngotracheitis or pneumonia can result in brain damage. Neurologic complications are frequently but not invariably associated with a poor prognosis.

Anderson EL, Belshe RB, Burk B, et al: Evaluation of cold-recombinant influenza A/Korea (CR-59) virus vaccine in infants. J Clin Microbiol 27:909, 1989.

Centers for Disease Control: Reye syndrome—United States, 1984. MMWR 34:13, 1985.

Centers for Disease Control: ACIP—Prevention and control of influenza: Part 1, Vaccines. MMWR 38:297, 1987.

Crawford SA, Clover RD, Abell TD, et al: Rimantadine prophylaxis in children: A follow-up study. Pediatr Infect Dis J 7:379, 1988.

Dagan R, Hall CB: Influenza A virus infection imitating bacterial sepsis in early infancy. Pediatr Infect Dis 3:218, 1984.

Dykes AC, Cherry JD, Nolan CE: A clinical, epidemiologic, serologic and virologic study of influenza C virus infection. Arch Intern Med 140:1295, 1980.

Farrell MK, Partin JC, Bove KE: Epidemic influenza myopathy in Cincinnati in 1977. J Pediatr 96:545, 1980.

Glezen WP, Decker M, Joseph SW, et al: Acute respiratory disease associated with influenza epidemics in Houston, 1981–1983. J Infect Dis 155:1119, 1987.

Hall CB, Dolin R, Gala CL, et al: Children with influenza A infection: Treatment with rimantadine. Pediatrics 80:275, 1987.

Hall CB, Douglas RG, Gieman JM, et al: Viral shedding patterns of children with influenza B infection. J Infect Dis 140:610, 1979.

Lennon DR, Cherry JD, Morgenstein A, et al: Longitudinal study of influenza B symptomatology and interferon production in children and college students. Pediatr Infect Dis 2:212, 1983.

Lui KJ, Kendal AP: Impact of influenza epidemics on mortality in the United States from October 1972 to May 1985. Am J Public Health 77:712, 1987.

Wilson SZ, Gilbert BE, Quarles JM, et al: Treatment of influenza A (H1N1) virus infection with ribavirin aerosol. Antimicrob Agents Chemother 26:200, 1984.

12.75 PARAINFLUENZA VIRAL INFECTIONS

Parainfluenza viruses are common causes of respiratory illnesses in children and adults and are particularly associated with croup. They are relatively large RNA paramyxoviruses. Four serologic types cause disease in humans.

EPIDEMIOLOGY. By 3 yr of age almost all children have been infected with parainfluenza type 3 virus, and the majority with types 1 and 2. Most infections with types 1, 2, and 3 are symptomatic, but the severity of illness varies markedly. Infection with type 4 virus is common, but most infections are asymptomatic. Symptomatic reinfections with types 1, 2, and 3 are common.

Infections with parainfluenza type 1 virus are frequently cyclic, with epidemics in the fall occurring every 2nd year. Type 2 infections also tend to occur in fall epidemics. However, the pattern is more sporadic than with type 1, and type 2 virus may be absent from a community for several years. Type 3 infection characteristically has been endemic, with illness noted throughout the year. However, in recent years seasonal outbreaks have occurred.

There are no geographic limitations associated with parainfluenzal infections, which are most common in young children but also frequent in adults. Serious illness is more common in boys than in girls.

Infection is transmitted from person to person, by direct respiratory contact or by exposure to infected secretions.

PATHOLOGY. The hallmark of parainfluenza viral infection is replication of virus in the respiratory epithelium, usually without deeper invasion or systemic involvement. Limited pathologic data are available, since they are drawn only from cases representing the severe end of the spectrum of illness. In laryngotracheitis a marked inflammatory response of the glottic and tracheal surfaces occurs.

PATHOGENESIS AND IMMUNITY. After experimental intranasal viral administration, the incubation period is 2–4 days. Although viremia may occur, symptomatology is mainly related to the direct involvement of the ciliated cells of the respiratory epithelium. Type 3 infections frequently occur in early life when transplacentally acquired specific serum antibody is present, and reinfection in older children and adults regularly occurs despite measurable serum antibody. Immunity correlates best with the presence of specific IgA nasal antibody, but high levels of serum antibody also reduce the risk of reinfection. The role of cell-mediated factors is unknown. However, the observation of a fatal giant cell pneumonia in children exhibiting cell-mediated defects suggests that T cell function may be important in clinical recovery. Although reinfection is common, illness is virtually always mild and affects the upper respiratory tract.

CLINICAL MANIFESTATIONS. The predominant manifestations are respiratory, although systemic manifestations are common. Eighty per cent of these infections affect the upper respiratory tract. In children hospitalized for severe respiratory illness, parainfluenza viruses account for about 50% of cases of laryngotracheitis and about 15% each of cases of bronchitis, bronchiolitis, and pneumonia. Among the parainfluenza viruses, type 1 is the most frequent cause of laryngotracheitis, whereas type 3 accounts for most cases of bronchitis, bronchiolitis, and pneumonia.

Clinical descriptions of laryngotracheitis, bronchitis, bronchiolitis, and pneumonia are presented in Sec. 14.43–14.44. The clinical manifestations of parainfluenza upper respiratory infections are listed in Figure 12–24. Sore throat is a more common complaint in the older child. Fever is observed in only 20% of cases, and its height is inversely related to age. Rashes are discrete, erythematous, maculopapular lesions of short duration. Associated otitis media is probably most often the result of secondary bacterial infection.

The duration of viral illness is quite variable, with an average of about 5 days. The persistence of fever for more than 5 days suggests the onset of a superinfection, usually bacterial, such as otitis media or pneumonia.

Types 1 and 3 parainfluenza viruses have been noted in association with acute parotitis and an illness indistinguishable from that due to mumps virus. A type 3 strain was isolated from the cerebrospinal fluid of an adolescent with Guillain-Barré syndrome. Reye syndrome has occurred in association with parainfluenza viral infections, and parainfluenza viruses have been recovered from victims of the sudden infant death syndrome.

Type 4 is associated only with mild upper respiratory illness, which is usually afebrile.

DIAGNOSIS AND DIFFERENTIAL DIAGNOSIS. In an individual case, the clinical diagnosis of the etiology of respiratory illness is difficult. The differential diagnostic considerations in young children include influenza A virus in severe laryngotracheitis, respiratory syncytial virus in bronchiolitis, influenza A virus in bronchitis, and respiratory syncytial, influenza, and adenoviruses in pneumonia. In mild upper respiratory illnesses all the common respiratory viruses need to be considered (rhinoviruses, coronaviruses, adenoviruses, respiratory syncytial virus, influenza viruses, and selected enteroviruses); in the older patient *Mycoplasma pneumoniae* infection is a further possibility.

The most important clinical differential diagnostic consideration is that between laryngotracheitis and other acute upper airway obstructive diseases such as acute epiglottitis, retropharyngeal abscess, bacterial tracheitis, angioneurotic edema, and foreign body.

The virologic confirmation of parainfluenza viral infections is relatively easy, provided proper attention is paid to the collection and transportation of the specimens for culture. Swabs containing respiratory secretions are best maintained in a small amount of transport media; they should be refrigerated and transported to the laboratory within 4 hr of collection without being exposed to sunlight. Parainfluenza viruses are isolated in monkey kidney tissue cultures; in the majority of instances results are available within 1 wk. The use of fluorescent antibody procedures on respiratory secretions may provide a diagnosis within 24 hr. Retrospective diagnosis can also be made by studying paired serum samples by complement fixation, hemagglutination inhibition, or neutralizing antibody techniques. However, serologic results may be difficult to interpret because of cross-reactions among paramyxoviruses.

COMPLICATIONS. Complications are relatively infrequent. Secondary bacterial infections are of most concern; otitis media and pneumonia are easily recognized and treated. Bacterial secondary infections in laryngotracheitis are usually manifest as tracheitis (Sec. 14.44), bronchitis (Sec. 14.51), and pneumonia (Sec. 14.56). Progressive viral pneumonia has occurred in the immunocompromised host.

PREVENTION. No satisfactory vaccine is available.

TREATMENT. Careful attention to symptomatic care is important in managing patients with severe laryngotracheitis, bronchiolitis, and pneumonia (Sec. 14.44, 14.51, and 14.56). Since the exclusion of a bacterial etiology in parainfluenza viral pneumonia and severe bronchitis and bronchiolitis is often impossible, it may be reasonable to administer antibiotics. Therapy with ceftriaxone is adequate because bacterial pneumonias would most likely be caused by *Haemophilus influenzae*, *Streptococcus pneumoniae*, and *Streptococcus pyogenes*. Secondary infection in laryngotracheitis may be caused by *Staphylococcus aureus* in addition to the above bacteria; this is also adequately treated initially with ceftriaxone. If this organism is isolated, treatment can be changed to oxacillin or another appropriate antimicrobial agent.

Ribavirin is active against parainfluenza viruses and is being investigated in children. It is administered by small-particle aerosol.

In parainfluenza viral upper respiratory illnesses, the prophylactic use of antihistamines, decongestants, and antibiotics should be discouraged because they are expensive and of unproven effectiveness.

PROGNOSIS. Parainfluenza viral infections are common, and the outcome with rare exceptions is good. Anoxia associated with severe laryngotracheitis or pneumonia can result in brain damage. Rarely, death may result from cardiorespiratory arrest.

JAMES D. CHERRY

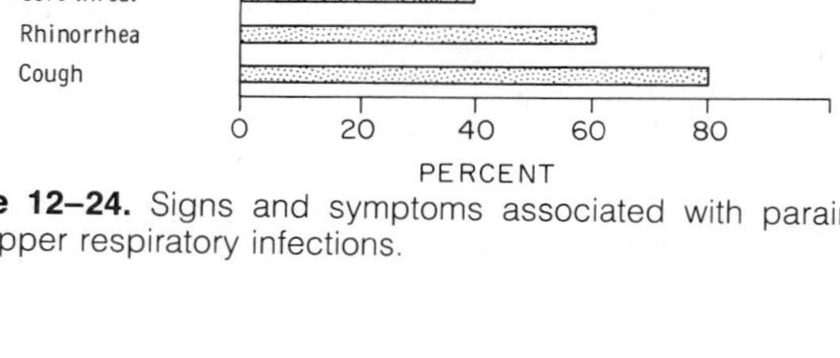

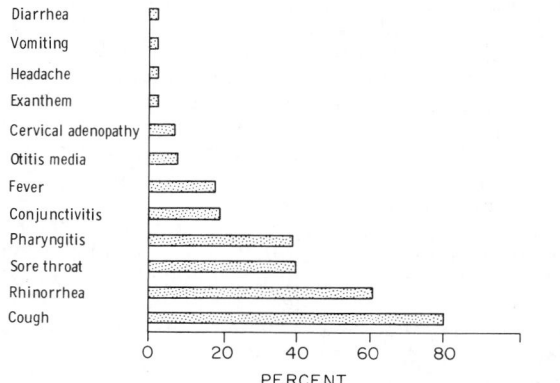

Figure 12–24. Signs and symptoms associated with parainfluenza viral upper respiratory infections.

Denny FW, Clyde WA Jr: Acute lower respiratory tract infections in nonhospitalized children. J Pediatr 108:635, 1986.

Denny FW, Murphy TF, Clyde WA Jr, et al: Croup: An 11-year study in a pediatric practice. Pediatrics 71:871, 1983.

Glezen WP, Frank AL, Taber LH, et al: Parainfluenza virus type 3: Seasonality and risk of infection and reinfection in young children. J Infect Dis 150:851, 1984.

Hall CB, Geiman JM, Breese BB, et al: Parainfluenza viral infections in children: Correlation of shedding with clinical manifestations. J Pediatr 91:194, 1977.

Korppi M, Halonen P, Kleemola M, et al: The role of parainfluenza viruses in inspiratory difficulties in children. Acta Paediatr Scand 77:105, 1988.

Putto A, Ruuskanen O, Meurman O: Fever in respiratory virus infections. Am J Dis Child 140:1159, 1986.

Ray CG, Minnich LL: Efficiency of immunofluorescence for rapid detection of common respiratory viruses. J Clin Microbiol 25:355, 1987.

12.76 INFECTIONS DUE TO RESPIRATORY SYNCYTIAL VIRUS

Respiratory syncytial virus (RSV) is the major cause of bronchiolitis (Sec. 14.54) and pneumonia in infants under 1 yr of age. It is the most important respiratory tract pathogen of early childhood.

ETIOLOGY. RSV is a medium-sized membrane-bound RNA virus that develops in the cytoplasm of infected cells and matures by budding from the plasma membrane. It belongs to the family *Paramyxoviridae*, along with parainfluenza and mumps viruses, but is classified in a separate genus, the pneumoviruses. It contains no detectable hemagglutinin or neuraminidase, and it does not grow in embryonated eggs.

Although different strains of RSV show some antigenic heterogeneity, this variation is primarily seen in only one of the two surface glycoproteins, and the virus behaves in the human host like a single serotype.

RSV grows in a number of types of tissue culture, in which it produces characteristic syncytial cytopathology. Specimens for culture should be delivered rapidly and, if possible, on wet ice to the laboratory because the virus is heat labile and very susceptible to destruction by freezing and thawing.

EPIDEMIOLOGY. The occurrence of annual outbreaks and the high incidence of infection during the first months of life are unique among human viruses. RSV is distributed worldwide and appears in yearly epidemics. In temperate climates these epidemics occur each winter and last 4–5 mo. During the remainder of the year infections are sporadic and uncommon. Epidemics usually peak in January, February, or March, but peaks have been recognized as early as December and as late as June. At these times hospital admissions for bronchiolitis and pneumonia of infants under 1 yr of age increase and decrease in proportion to the number of RSV infections in the community. In the tropics, the epidemic pattern is less clear.

Placentally transmitted antibody may have some protective effect, particularly when present in high concentration. This may account for the fact that severe infections are uncommon in the first 4–6 wk of life. Nevertheless, serum antibody is apparently not fully protective, and the age at which an infant undergoes first infection depends significantly on the opportunities for exposure. It is estimated that in an urban setting about half the susceptible infants undergo primary infection in each epidemic. Thus, infection is almost universal by the 2nd birthday. Reinfection occurs at a rate of 10–20% per epidemic throughout childhood; the frequency is lower in adults. In situations of high exposure such as day-care centers, attack rates are higher: nearly 100% for young infants and 60–80% for older infants.

Estimates of the severity of primary infections have emerged from studies of outbreaks in nurseries and institutions. Under these circumstances asymptomatic infection is rare. Most infants develop coryza and pharyngitis, usually with fever and occasionally with otitis. In 10–40% of patients the lower respiratory tract is involved to a varying degree. Bronchitis, bronchopneumonia, and bronchiolitis all occur. Calculations based on hospital admissions in the United States and Britain yield a ratio of 1–3 infants hospitalized with bronchiolitis or pneumonia for every 100 primary infections with the virus.

Reinfection may occur as early as a few weeks after recovery but usually takes place during subsequent annual outbreaks. The severity of illness during reinfection is probably as much influenced by age as by prior experience with this virus, older children being generally less ill. Nevertheless, several instances of severe RSV bronchiolitis occurring twice in succession have been recorded.

Bronchiolitis is the most common clinical diagnosis in infants hospitalized with RSV infections, although the syndrome is often indistinguishable from RSV pneumonia in infants, and, indeed, the two frequently coexist. All RSV diseases of the lower respiratory tract (excluding croup) have their highest incidence in the 2nd mo of life and decrease in frequency thereafter. The syndrome of bronchiolitis becomes uncommon after the 1st birthday; acute infective wheezing attacks after that age are often termed "wheezy bronchitis," "asthmatoid bronchitis," or, simply, asthma attacks. Viral pneumonia, on the other hand, is a persistent problem throughout childhood, although RSV becomes less prominent as the etiologic agent after the 1st year. RSV is responsible for 45–75% of cases of bronchiolitis, 15–25% of childhood pneumonias, and 6–8% of cases of croup.

Bronchiolitis and pneumonia due to RSV are more common in boys than in girls by a ratio of about 1.5:1. Racial factors make little difference. Lower respiratory tract disease, however, occurs more often and earlier in life in low socioeconomic groups and in crowded living conditions.

The incubation period from exposure to first symptoms is about 4 days. The virus is excreted for variable periods, probably depending on severity of illness and immunologic status. Most infants with lower respiratory tract illness shed virus for 5–12 days after hospital admission. Excretion for 3 wk and longer has been documented. Spread of infection occurs when large infected droplets, either air-borne or conveyed on hands, are inoculated in the nose or conjunctiva of a susceptible subject. RSV is probably introduced into most families by school children undergoing reinfection. Typically, in the space of a few days older siblings and one or both parents develop colds, while the infant becomes more severely ill with fever, otitis, or lower respiratory tract disease.

Hospital cross-infection during RSV epidemics is important. Not only do children infect one another, but also symptomatic infected adults have been implicated in the spread of the infection.

PATHOLOGY AND PATHOGENESIS. Bronchiolitis is characterized by virus-induced necrosis of the bronchiolar epithelium, hypersecretion of mucus, and round cell infiltration and edema of the surrounding submucosa. These changes result in formation of mucous plugs obstructing bronchioles with consequent hyperinflation or collapse of the distal lung tissue. In interstitial pneumonia, infiltration is more generalized, and epithelial necrosis may extend to both the bronchi and the alveoli. In both diseases, but most commonly in bronchiolitis, infants are particularly apt to develop signs and symptoms of small airway obstruction because of the small size of the normal bronchioles.

Several facts suggest immunologic injury as a factor in the pathogenesis of bronchiolitis due to RSV: (1) infants dying of bronchiolitis have shown both immunoglobulin and virus in the injured bronchiolar tissues; (2) children who received a highly antigenic, inactivated, parenterally administered RSV vaccine developed, on subsequent exposure to wild RSV, more severe and more frequent bronchiolitis than did their age-matched controls; (3) bronchiolitis merges into asthma in older infants, and RSV is a frequently recognized cause of acute asthma attacks in children 1–5 yr old; and (4) IgE antibody directed toward RSV has been found in the secretions of convalescent infants with bronchiolitis.

It is not clear what role, in addition to the destructive effect of the virus and the attendant host response, is played by superimposed bacterial infection. In most infants with bronchiolitis, with or without interstitial pneumonia, clinical experience suggests that bacteria play an insignificant role. In infants with consolidative pneumonia, the possibility of pathogenic bacterial superinfection is somewhat greater.

CLINICAL MANIFESTATIONS. The first signs of infection of the infant with respiratory syncytial virus are rhinorrhea and pharyngitis. Cough may appear simultaneously but more often appears after an interval of 1–3 days, at which time there may also be sneezing and a low-grade fever. Soon after the cough has developed, the child begins to wheeze audibly. If the disease is mild, the symptoms may not progress beyond this stage. Auscultation often reveals diffuse rhonchi, fine rales, and wheezes. Rhinorrhea usually persists throughout the illness, with intermittent fever. Roentgenograms of the chest are frequently normal.

If the illness progresses, cough and wheezing increase, and air hunger and evidence of hyperexpansion of the chest and of intercostal and subcostal retraction occur. The respiratory rate increases, and cyanosis occurs. Signs of severe, life-threatening illness are central cyanosis, tachypnea of more than 70 breaths/min, listlessness, and apneic spells. At this stage the chest may be greatly hyperexpanded and almost silent to auscultation because of poor air exchange.

Chest roentgenograms of infants hospitalized with RSV bronchiolitis are normal in about 10% of cases; air trapping or hyperexpansion of the chest occurs in about 50%. Peribronchial thickening or interstitial pneumonia is seen in 50–80%. Segmental consolidation occurs in 10–25%. Pleural effusion is rarely, if ever, seen.

In some infants the course of the illness may be more like that of pneumonia. In these instances, the prodromal rhinorrhea and cough are followed by dyspnea, poor feeding, and listlessness, with a minimum of wheezing and hyperexpansion. Although the clinical diagnosis is pneumonia, wheezing is often present intermittently and the chest roentgenogram may show air trapping. In some infants the cough may be so severe and paroxysmal that the illness may mimic the pertussis syndrome.

Fever is an inconstant sign in RSV infection. Rash and conjunctivitis each occur in a few cases. In young infants, particularly those who were born prematurely, periodic breathing and apneic spells have been distressingly frequent signs, even with relatively mild bronchiolitis. Finally, it is likely that a small portion of deaths included in the category of sudden infant death syndrome (Sec. 25.1) are due to RSV infection.

Routine laboratory tests offer little helpful information in most cases of bronchiolitis or pneumonia due to respiratory syncytial virus. The white cell count is normal or elevated, and the differential count may be normal or shifted either to the right or left. Bacterial cultures usually grow normal flora. Hypoxemia is frequent and tends to be more marked than anticipated on the basis of the clinical findings. When it is severe, it is frequently accompanied by hypercapnia and acidosis.

DIAGNOSIS. Bronchiolitis is a clinical diagnosis. The involvement of respiratory syncytial virus in any particular child's disease can be suspected with varying degrees of certainty from the season of the year and the presence of a typical outbreak at the time. Other features that may be helpful are the age of the child (aside from RSV, the only virus that attacks infants frequently during the first few months of life is parainfluenza virus type 3) and the family epidemiology (colds in siblings and parents).

The diagnostic dilemma of greatest import is the question of possible bacterial or chlamydial involvement. When bronchiolitis is mild or when infiltrates are absent by roentgenogram, there is little likelihood of a bacterial component. In infants 1–4 mo of age, interstitial pneumonitis may be caused by *Chlamydia trachomatis* (Sec. 12.59). In this instance there may be a history of conjunctivitis, and the illness tends to be of subacute onset. Coughing is prominent; wheezing is not. There may also be eosinophilia. Fever is usually absent.

Consolidation without other signs or with pleural effusion is considered of bacterial origin until proved otherwise. Other signs pointing to bacterial pneumonia are depression of the white cell count in the presence of severe disease, ileus or other abdominal signs, high fever, and circulatory collapse. In such instances there is rarely any doubt about the need for antibiotics.

Definitive diagnosis of RSV infection is based on the detection of virus or viral antigens in respiratory secretions. The specimen should be put on ice, taken directly to the laboratory, and inoculated onto susceptible cell monolayers. Nasopharyngeal or throat swabs are probably of equal value. An aspirate of mucus from the child's posterior nasal cavity is preferable. A tracheal aspirate is unnecessary.

PROGNOSIS. The mortality of hospitalized infants with RSV infection of the lower respiratory tract is about 2%. The prognosis is clearly worse in young, premature infants or those with underlying disease of the neuromuscular, pulmonary, cardiovascular, or immunologic systems.

Many children with asthma have a history of bronchiolitis in infancy. There is recurrent wheezing in 33–50% of children with typical RSV bronchiolitis in infancy. The likelihood of recurrence is increased in the presence of an allergic diathesis (eczema, hay fever, or a family history of asthma). In bronchiolitis in patients over the age of 1 yr there is an increasing probability that, though it may be virus-induced, this is the first of multiple wheezing attacks that will later be called asthma.

TREATMENT. In uncomplicated cases of bronchiolitis, treatment is symptomatic. Humidified oxygen is usually indicated for hospitalized infants, since most are hypoxic. Many infants are slightly to moderately dehydrated; therefore fluids should be carefully administered in somewhat greater than maintenance amounts. Often intravenous or tube feeding is helpful when sucking is difficult. Most infants seem to breathe better when propped up at an angle of 10–30 degrees.

Bronchodilators should not be routinely used. However, a trial of albuterol aerosols should be made in wheezing children and bronchodilators administered if aerosols are beneficial. Corticosteroids are not indicated except as a last resort in critical cases. Sedatives are rarely necessary.

In most instances antibiotics are not useful, and their indiscriminate use in presumed viral bronchiolitis and pneumonia should be discouraged. Interstitial pneumonia in infants 1–4 mo old may be chlamydial, and erythromycin (40 mg/kg/24 hr) may therefore be beneficial. When infants with interstitial pneumonia are older, or when consolidation is found, parenteral antibiotics may be indicated. In the critically ill child antibiotics may also be indicated.

The antiviral drug ribavirin, delivered by small-particle aerosol and breathed, along with the required concentration of oxygen, for 20 of 24 hr per day for 3–5 days, has a beneficial effect on the course of RSV pneumonia. It is probably indicated only in very sick infants or in high-risk infants, such as those with underlying cyanotic congenital heart disease or significant bronchopulmonary dysplasia, and should be administered early in the course of the infection (see Sec. 12.93).

PREVENTION. Within the hospital the most important preventive measures are aimed at blocking nosocomial spread. During RSV season high-risk infants should be separated from infants with respiratory symptoms. Separate gowns and gloves, and careful handwashing should be used for the care of all infants with suspected or established RSV infection.

Attempts to develop useful inactivated or attenuated vaccines have been unsuccessful. Indeed, the insufficiency of protection following natural RSV infection diminishes the likelihood that an attenuated vaccine will prevent subsequent disease. Breast milk, which contains antibody to RSV, may have some protective effect, but definitive proof is lacking to date.

Englund JA, Piedreu PA, Jefferson LS, et al: High dose, short-duration ribovirin aerosol therapy in children with suspected respiratory syncytial virus infection. J Pediatr 117:313, 1990.

Glezen WP, Paredes A, Allison JE, et al: Risk of respiratory syncytial virus infection for infants from low-income families in relationship to age, sex, ethnic group and maternal antibody level. J Pediatr 98:708, 1981.

Hall CB, Douglas RG Jr, Geiman JM, et al: Nosocomial respiratory syncytial virus infections. N Engl J Med 293:1343, 1975.

Hall CB, McBride JT, Walsh EE, et al: Aerosolized ribavirin treatment of infants with respiratory syncytial virus infection. N Engl J Med 308:1443, 1983.

Henderson FW, Collier AM, Clyde WA Jr, et al: Respiratory-syncytial-virus infections, reinfections and immunity: A prospective, longitudinal study in young children. N Engl J Med 300:530, 1979.

Loda FA, Clyde WA, Glezen WP, et al: Studies on the role of viruses, bacteria and *M. pneumoniae* as causes of lower respiratory tract infections in children. J Pediatr 72:161, 1968.

McConnochie UM, Hall CB, Walsh EE, et al: Variation in severity of respiratory syncytial virus infection with subtype. J Pediatr 117:52, 1990.

McIntosh K: Bronchiolitis and asthma: Possible common pathogenetic pathways. J Allergy Clin Immunol 57:595, 1976.

Simpson W, Hacking PM, Court SDM, et al: Radiological findings in respiratory syncytial virus infection in children. II. The correlation of radiological categories with clinical and virological findings. Pediatr Radiol 2:155, 1974.

12.77 ADENOVIRUSES

Adenoviruses cause 5–8% of acute respiratory disease in infants, plus a wide array of other syndromes including pharyngoconjunctival fever, follicular conjunctivitis, epidemic keratoconjunctivitis, hemorrhagic cystitis, acute diarrhea, and encephalomyelitis. Only a third of the 37-plus serotypes have been associated with disease. Although fatalities are rare, they are associated with infections by certain serotypes (particularly type 7) and with infections in severely immunocompromised hosts.

ETIOLOGY. Adenoviruses are DNA viruses of intermediate size, which are classified into subgenera A to G. Types 1–39 are in subgenera A to E, type 40 is subgenus F, and type 41 is subgenus G. The virion has an icosohedral coat made up of several proteins, the most abundant of which is the "hexon," a cross-reacting antigen common to all mammalian adenoviruses. The "penton" confers type specificity, and antibody to it is protective. It is also cytotoxic in tissue culture, and toxic properties have been ascribed to it in vivo as well. Adenoviruses can also be classified by the "fingerprints" their DNA make on gels after being digested with restriction endonucleases, and this classification generally conforms to their antigenic types.

All adenovirus types except types 40 and 41 grow in primary human embryonic kidney cells, and most grow in HEp-2 or HeLa cells, producing a typical destructive cytopathic effect. Types 40 and 41 (and other serotypes as well) grow in 293 cells, a line of human embryonic kidney cells into which certain "early" adenovirus genes have been introduced.

Many adenovirus types, but particularly the common childhood types (1, 2, and 5), are shed for prolonged periods from both the respiratory and gastrointestinal tracts. These types also establish low-level and chronic infection of the tonsils.

EPIDEMIOLOGY. Adenoviral infections are distributed worldwide. They occur year-round but are most prevalent in spring or early summer and again in midwinter in temperate climates. Certain types tend to occur in epidemics, notably types 4 and 7 in epidemics of febrile respiratory disease, types 3, 7, and 21 in severe pneumonia, type 3 in pharyngoconjunctival fever, type 11 in cystitis, and types 8, 19, and 37 in epidemic keratoconjunctivitis. For unexplained reasons, adenovirus types 3 and 7 cause frequent severe epidemics of pneumonia in the children of northern China, with mortality rates of 5–15%.

Over 60% of school-aged children have antibodies to the common respiratory types. Almost all adults have serum antibody to types 1–7. Infections with types 1 and 2 tend to occur during the 1st yr or 2 of life, and types 3 and 5 occur a little later. Spread occurs by the respiratory and fecal-oral routes, although it is not clear whether spread is by large- or small-particle aerosol.

PATHOLOGY AND PATHOGENESIS. Adenoviruses are one of the few "respiratory" viruses that grow well in the epithelium of the small intestine. Although mucosal surfaces are the primary target early in infection, it is likely that viremia is common, accompanying fever. Viremia is, however, of little consequence except in rare instances or in the immunocompromised patient.

Adenoviral pneumonia produces characteristic microscopic changes, with dense lymphocytic infiltrates, destruction of the bronchial and bronchiolar epithelium, focal necrosis of mucous glands, hyaline membrane formation, and several types of nuclear inclusion bodies.

CLINICAL MANIFESTATIONS. Adenoviruses cause a wide array of syndromes:

Acute Respiratory Disease. This is the most common manifestation of adenovirus infection in children and adults. Acute respiratory infections in infants and children are not clinically distinctive and are usually caused by types 1, 2, 3, 5, or 6. They are usually mild but may be complicated or severe. Primary infections in infants are frequently associated with fever and respiratory symptoms and in some series are complicated by otitis in more than half of the patients. Adenovirus respiratory infections are associated with a significant incidence of diarrhea.

Pharyngitis is a characteristic clinical syndrome, and adenoviruses can be identified in 15–20% of children with isolated pharyngitis, mostly in preschoolers and infants. The pharyngitis may be exudative and is often febrile. Most cases are due to type 1, 2, 3, or 5.

Pneumonia is uncommon but 7–9% of hospitalized children with acute pneumonia have adenovirus infection. Any of the "respiratory" types can cause pneumonia, but severe infections are most likely due to type 3, 7, or 21. Such infections have a mortality as high as 10%, and survivors may have residual airway damage, manifested by bronchiectasis, bronchiolitis obliterans, or, rarely, pulmonary fibrosis.

A *pertussis-like syndrome* has been described in association with adenovirus infections. In such instances adenoviruses frequently accompany *Bordetella pertussis* as coinfecting agents, but they may also be a causative on their own. In many cases this illness represents activation of latent or low-level chronic respiratory or tonsillar infection by the bacterium. With improved methods for detecting *B. pertussis*, doubt has increased that adenovirus (or any respiratory virus) can produce the classic pertussis syndrome on its own.

Pharyngoconjunctival fever is a clinically distinct syndrome that occurs particularly in association with type 3 adenoviral infection. Features include a high fever that lasts 4–5 days, pharyngitis with characteristic involvement of pharyngeal lymphoid tissue, conjunctivitis, preauricular and cervical adenopathy, and rhinitis. Nonpurulent conjunctivitis occurs in 75% of patients and is manifested by inflammation of both the bulbar and palpebral conjunctivae of one or both eyes; it often persists after the fever and other symptoms have resolved. Headache, malaise, and weakness are common, and there is considerable lethargy after the acute stage.

Conjunctivitis and Keratoconjunctivitis. Adenovirus is one of the most common causes of follicular conjunctivitis and keratoconjunctivitis. The former is a relatively mild illness. The latter, which may occur in epidemics, is associated with infection by adenovirus types 8, 19, and 37. The disease may cause corneal opacities that last several years.

Gastrointestinal Infections. The recent discovery of adenovirus types 40 and 41 has focused attention on the capacity of adenoviruses to cause acute diarrhea. There is some disagreement about details, but it appears that 7–9% of cases of acute diarrhea are associated with the appearance in the stool of large numbers of adenovirus particles and the development of a serum antibody response. Most instances of diarrhea are probably due to infections with the "enteric" types, 40 and 41, but some recent series include a considerable number of nonenteric types as well. Diarrhea caused by all types is often accompanied by minor respiratory symptoms and fever.

The pathogenesis of intussusception is thought by many to include enlarged lymph nodes as an initiating factor. Adenoviruses have been recovered from mesenteric lymph nodes at surgery and also from surface cultures in a higher percentage of children with intussusception than from controls. Adenoviruses have also been found in the appendices of children with appendicitis. Whether these findings represent acute etiologic relationships or are manifestations of a protracted, low-level intestinal infection analogous to that described in the tonsils is not clear.

Hemorrhagic Cystitis. This syndrome has a sudden onset of bacteriologically sterile hematuria, dysuria, frequency, and urgency lasting 1–2 wk. Infection with adenovirus types 11 and 21 has been found in some affected children and young adults.

Reye Syndrome and Reye-like Syndromes. Typical Reye syndrome has followed demonstrated adenovirus infection of several serotypes, particularly in very young children. In addition, several cases of a *Reye-like syndrome* have been reported, all of which are caused by infection with adenovirus type 7. The latter disease, which is frequently fatal, is characterized by severe bronchopneumonia, hepatitis, seizures, and disseminated intravascular coagulation. Circulating adenovirus penton antigen has been found in several patients and has been implicated in the pathogenesis.

Infections in Immunocompromised Hosts. Adenoviruses are important pathogens in the immunocompromised host. This includes those with either B or T cell deficiencies. In B cell–deficient children, a chronic meningoencephalitis very similar to that caused by enteroviruses has been described. In T cell–deficient patients, regardless of whether this deficiency is congenital, acquired, or iatrogenic, fulminant hepatitis and pneumonia, frequently with a fatal outcome, have been described.

DIAGNOSIS AND DIFFERENTIAL DIAGNOSIS. The laboratory diagnosis of adenovirus infection in children may be made by culture (or other method of identifying the presence of the virus), demonstration of a rise in serum antibody level, or some combination of the two. If virus is found in a "privileged" site, such as blood, urine, or cerebrospinal fluid, or in a biopsy of the lung or liver, the implication of infection with disease and organ damage is strong. Likewise, detection of certain adenovirus types in respiratory secretions (type 7 or 21) or stool (type 40 or 41) probably indicates their etiologic involvement in respiratory or gastrointestinal illness, respectively. The presence of untyped virus or the common childhood types in respiratory secretions or stool does not, however, indicate clinical adenovirus infection, since these viruses may be excreted chronically and asymptomatically. In these instances, discovery of a coincident rise in antibody by either complement-fixation or some more type-specific test is helpful in assigning a specific microorganism to disease. Adenovirus infection may also be considered etiologic if a rise in antibody is found between sera drawn in the acute stage and in convalescence from a patient with an appropriate illness. Adenovirus infection often results in a high ESR and WBC count.

Differential diagnosis is complex and depends on which syndrome is seen.

PREVENTION AND TREATMENT. Vaccines that contain either killed or live virus have been developed to prevent types 4 and 7 infection in military recruits. These vaccines have not, however, been used in children. There are at present no recognized antiviral agents that are effective in treating adenovirus infections. Ribavirin can inhibit viral growth of some strains in vitro, but evidence of its clinical efficacy is lacking.

Brandt CD, Kim HW, Jeffries BC, et al: Infections in 18,000 infants and children in a controlled study of respiratory tract disease. II. Adenovirus pathogenicity in relation to serologic type and illness syndrome. Am J Epidemiol 90:484, 1970.

Brandt CD, Kim HW, Rodriguez WJ, et al: Adenoviruses and pediatric gastroenteritis. J Infect Dis 151:437, 1985.

Edwards KM, Bennett SR, Garner WL, et al: Reye's syndrome associated with adenovirus infections in infants. Am J Dis Child 139:343, 1985.

Kelsey DS: Adenovirus meningoencephalitis. Pediatrics 61:291, 1978.

Koneru B, Jaffe R, Esquivel CO, et al: Adenoviral infections in pediatric liver transplant recipients. JAMA 258:489, 1987.

Ladisch S, Lovejoy FH, Hierholzer JC, et al: Extrapulmonary manifestations of adenovirus type 7 pneumonia simulating Reye syndrome and the possible role of an adenovirus toxin. Pediatrics 95:348, 1979.

Nelson KE, Gavitt F, Batt MD, et al: The role of adenoviruses in the pertussis syndrome. J Pediatr 86:335, 1975.

Numazaki Y, Kumasaki T, Yano N, et al: Further study on acute hemorrhagic cystitis due to adenovirus type H. N Engl J Med 289:344, 1973.

Ruuskanen O, Meurman O, Sarkkinen H: Adenoviral diseases in children: A study of 105 hospital cases. Pediatrics 76:79, 1985.

Similä S, Ylikorkala O, Wasz-Hockert O: Type 7 adenovirus pneumonia. J Pediatr 79:605, 1971.

12.78 RHINOVIRAL INFECTIONS

Rhinoviruses, collectively the most common cause of the "common cold" in adults, represent a smaller proportion of infections in young children because of the frequency of other viral respiratory infections. Also rhinoviral infections in young children often do not produce respiratory illness. However, rhinoviruses spread readily, producing illness in nursery and other school groups, and these children provide a major link in their spread within families.

ETIOLOGY. There are 111 serologically distinct rhinoviruses, all members of the picornavirus family of small RNA viruses. They are best identified by inoculating human embryonic kidney or human diploid cell cultures with nasal secretions from infected individuals and waiting to observe a cytopathic effect. Routine serologic testing for acquisition of antibody is not practical because of the multiplicity of types and infrequency of their cross-reactivity.

Several cross-sectional studies indicate that a low percentage of control children or children with diarrhea (1%) yield rhinoviruses at the time of sampling; similarly, only 2.2% of children with respiratory tract illness yield rhinoviruses. In longitudinal studies, however, 75% of pediatric rhinovirus infection is associated with illness, usually rhinitis or the pharyngitis-bronchitis syndrome. Rhinoviruses have also occasionally been associated with serious lower respiratory tract disease, particularly in infants with underlying illnesses. They may precipitate asthma in children and chronic bronchitis in adults.

EPIDEMIOLOGY. Rhinoviruses are distributed worldwide

with no predictable pattern of infection by serotype. Multiple types may be present in a community at one time.

In temperate climates the incidence of rhinoviral infection peaks in September and again in April or May, but some infections occur year-round. The peak incidence in the tropics occurs during the rainy season.

Rhinoviruses are recovered in highest concentration in nasal secretions, and experimental infection is most easily accomplished by nasal or conjunctival instillation. Infection via aerosol is less efficient. Virus persists for several hours in secretions on hands or other surfaces. Transmission probably occurs when infected secretions carried on contaminated fingers are rubbed into the nasal or conjunctival mucosa. More recent evidence also implicates spread through aerosols produced by talking, coughing, or sneezing.

PATHOGENESIS. The peak nasal inflammatory response occurs when virus growth is at its greatest, 2–4 days after experimental infection. Immune responses include specific nasal IgA and serum IgG antibody, which may contribute to modifying the illness and limiting viral shedding. Interferon and a nonspecific factor induced by infection with a heterotypic rhinovirus may be a part of the resistance mechanism. Usually the inflammatory response is limited to the nose, throat, and upper bronchial passages, but pneumonia has occurred.

CLINICAL MANIFESTATIONS. The primary clinical response to rhinoviral infection, like that to most respiratory viral infections, is the *common cold* (see Sec. 14.23). There is an incubation period of 2–4 days; then sneezing, nasal obstruction and discharge, and sore throat ensue. Cough and hoarseness occur in 30–40% of cases. Headache and other systemic symptoms are not as common as in influenza. Fever is neither as frequent nor as high as in primary infections with respiratory syncytial virus, parainfluenza virus, influenza virus, or adenovirus. Symptoms are worse in the first 2–3 days of illness and last for a week in a majority of patients; they persist for over 14 days in 35% of young children.

COMPLICATIONS. These are like those of any infection causing edema and inflammation in the nasopharyngeal area. They include otitis media, sinusitis, local spread down the respiratory tract, and bacterial superinfection. In one recent study rhinoviruses were the most common virus recovered from the middle ear fluids of infants and children with otitis media.

DIAGNOSIS AND DIFFERENTIAL DIAGNOSIS. Since other viral agents and β-hemolytic streptococci can produce the same manifestations, a clinical diagnosis is only presumptive. Laboratory diagnosis is not practical under ordinary circumstances. If any question exists, bacterial cultures should be taken to exclude streptococcal infection.

TREATMENT AND PREVENTION. There is no specific preventive or ameliorative treatment. Careful handwashing and avoidance of manual nose and eye manipulation is the best approach to reducing spread. For relief of acute symptoms, a mild analgesic and saline or decongestant nose drops may be used for a short time. Interferon administered by nasal spray may be of value in preventing rhinovirus infection.

KENNETH McINTOSH

Arola M, Ziegler T, Ruuskanen O, et al: Rhinovirus in acute otitis media. J Pediatr 113:693, 1988.

Dick EC, Jennings LC, Mink KA, et al: Aerosol transmission of rhinovirus colds. J Infect Dis 156:442, 1987.

Douglas RM, Moore BW, Miles HB, et al: Prophylactic efficacy of intranasal alpha$_2$-interferon against rhinovirus infections in the family setting. N Engl J Med 314:65, 1986.

Jackson GG, Muldoon RL: Viruses causing common respiratory infections in man. J Infect Dis 127:328, 1973.

Ketler A, Hall CE, Fox JP, et al: The Virus Watch Program: A continuing surveillance of viral infections in metropolitan New York families. VIII. Rhinovirus infections: Observations of virus excretion, intrafamilial spread and clinical response. Am J Epidemiol 90:244, 1969.

12.79 HEPATITIS

Hepatitis is a major health problem worldwide. In the United States there are about 60,000 reported cases yearly. The viruses of hepatitis A, hepatitis B, and at least three other viruses causing hepatitis that is neither A nor B have been identified. These may be referred to as non-A–non-B (NAN B) hepatitis viruses; they are now designated hepatitis viruses C, D, and E. Other as yet unidentified viruses may also cause hepatitis. In addition, cytomegalovirus (Sec. 12.71), Epstein-Barr virus (Sec. 12.72), rubella virus (Sec. 12.65 and 9.73), and enteroviruses (Sec. 12.80) may cause hepatitis. See also Sec. 13.94.

ETIOLOGY. Hepatitis A (HA). HA virus (HAV), a hepadnavirus, can be demonstrated in human stool by a variety of immunologic techniques; both total and specific IgM antibody against HA virus (anti-HAV) can also be measured by radioimmunoassay. Laboratory strains of HAV have been propagated in tissue culture.

Hepatitis B (HB, Hepadnavirus 1). This infection was first recognized by the detection of a viral antigen—the Australia antigen—in the blood of a hepatitis carrier. Electron microscopy initially revealed that the blood of carriers contained spherical and tubular particles, which were subsequently recognized to constitute the surface of the virion; hence, the structures originally designated Australia antigen are now referred to as hepatitis B surface antigen or HB_sAg; antibody directed against HB_s is designated anti-HB_s. A number of subtypes that have been useful in epidemiologic studies have been described for the HB_s antigen; they are referred to as a, y, w, d, r, and others.

Dane observed another larger virus-like particle in the serum of some patients with hepatitis B. This "Dane particle" is now known to represent the virion. The inner component or core of this virus is designated hepatitis B core antigen or HB_c. Antibody directed against HB_c is designated anti-HB_c.

The virus contains DNA, and DNA polymerase is found in the sera of some patients with hepatitis B, often in association with the HB_e antigen. HB_e antigen is an integral part of the core of HB virus and is associated with high infectivity. There appear to be three serotypes of HB_eAg. Antibody against HB_e is designated anti-HB.

Hepatitis D Virus (HDV). The delta (δ) virus ($HB_\delta Ag$) or HDV is an incomplete RNA virus that can multiply only in the presence of HBV. Infections may be concurrent, or δ virus can infect an individual persistently positive for HB_sAg. Transmission is usually by parenteral inoculation. Delta agent may result in fulminant hepatitis, and it also increases the likelihood of chronic liver disease in HB_sAg carriers. Epidemics have occurred among users of illicit parenteral drugs. Blood concentrates can also transmit the infection. Perinatal transmission is rare.

Hepatitis C Virus. This NANB hepatitis agent is an RNA virus with features of both flavi- and pestivirus. It is less than 80 nm in diameter and appears to contain an essential lipid in its envelope. Transmission occurs mainly by blood or blood products or by intravenous drug use, and by sexual transmission. Chronic liver disease is common in those infected.

Hepatitis E Virus. This NANB hepatitis virus appears to be water-borne. It occurs in developing countries in epidemics. The virus is about 27–30 nm in diameter, and the illness has many features of acute hepatitis.

Other. Giant cell hepatitis occurs sporadically and appears to be caused by a myxovirus.

Viruses That May Cause Hepatitis Incidentally. The liver is frequently involved in AIDS, in infectious mononucleosis, and in newborns infected with cytomegalovirus or herpesviruses. Cytomegalovirus in young adults may also cause a syndrome of hepatitis characterized by prolonged fever and development of atypical lymphocytes. Newborn infants with encephalomyocarditis due to coxsackievirus B usually have hepatic and pancreatic involvement. Coxsackieviruses have also been associated with a syndrome of hepatitis and myocarditis seen most commonly during adolescence. Fatal adenoviral pneumonia in infants has also been found to involve the liver. Hepatitis is common in congenital rubella and may occur in rare instances as a complication of varicella, mumps, measles, human herpes virus 6, and other common infections. Newborn infants infected with echovirus 11 may also develop fatal hepatitis.

EPIDEMIOLOGY. That different agents cause hepatitis with characteristic incubation periods and different modes of transmission was recognized long before the agents were identified.

Hepatitis A (Infectious Hepatitis). This highly contagious disease is transmitted by person-to-person contact, occasionally by ingestion of contaminated food or water, and on rare occasions by blood transfusion. In the United States, the number of reported cases occurring during each of the first 3 decades of life is approximately the same, but anicteric hepatitis is estimated to occur in over 80% of those infected who are under the age of 2 yr and in about half of those infected who are 3–4 yr old. The illness tends to be more severe in adults. Most infants are protected by maternal antibody during the early months of life.

The incubation period is approximately 4–6 wk from exposure until the appearance of jaundice. The highest titers of HAV in stool are found prior to onset of the rise in bilirubin.

Hepatitis A has no seasonal predilection. Seven-year cycles of peak incidence have been described. Infection appears to occur at an earlier age under conditions of poor hygiene; the disease is endemic in underdeveloped areas. Common-source outbreaks from contaminated water or infected food or food handlers have been reported. Transmission by transfused blood, although rare, has also been documented. Infection has also been contracted from primates. Spread occurs readily between homosexuals and in day-care centers. Personnel in day-care centers and household contacts of attendees are at increased risk for HAV infection.

Hepatitis A during pregnancy or at the time of delivery does not appear to result in clinical disease in the newborn, in teratogenic effects, or in increased risk of abortion.

Hepatitis B (Serum Hepatitis). The term *serum hepatitis* refers to the most common method by which it is transmitted, but percutaneous or mucous membrane inoculation may also result in infection. Transmission has been documented between sexual partners and under the conditions of institutional living. A higher rate of infection is found among children with Down syndrome living in institutions than among those living at home with their families. Hepatitis B surface antigen (HB_sAg) can be demonstrated in saliva, feces, and other body secretions.

The incubation period of hepatitis B from exposure to the onset of jaundice is 2–5 mo. There is no seasonal prevalence.

The major mechanism of transmission is by inoculation with blood of carriers, which may contain large amounts of virus. Even a prick with a needle contaminated with a minute amount of blood from a carrier of hepatitis B virus can transmit infection; shared needles probably account for the high frequency of infection among drug users. Transfusion of infected blood carried a considerable risk of serum hepatitis prior to screening of blood donors and conversion from paid to volunteer donors. Patients who required frequent use of blood products, for example, those with hemophilia or thalassemia, had high rates of infection, as did those undergoing renal dialysis. There is an increased incidence of hepatitis B in families of patients who are on dialysis or are receiving blood products frequently. Administering clotting factors prepared from pooled plasma may also transmit HBV and NANB viruses. Using heat-inactivated products and screening for HCV may reduce the risk of infection with NANB viruses. Elimination of plasma from HB_s-positive donors has reduced the risk of concentrates.

The transmission of hepatitis B from pregnant carriers of its surface antigen (HB_sAg) to their infants presents a special problem. The presence of HB_eAg mothers and absence of anti-HB_e increase the risk for an affected infant. The older siblings of affected infants also have a high rate of HB_s and HB_eAg positivity. There is no increased risk of abortion or malformations following hepatitis during the 1st trimester of pregnancy.

HB_sAg has been inconsistently demonstrated in the breast milk of infected mothers. Breast-feeding of unimmunized infants by infected mothers does not appear to confer a greater risk of hepatitis on their offspring than does artificial feeding, despite the possibility that cracked nipples may result in the ingestion of contaminated maternal blood by the nursing infant. Immunization of newborns decreases the risk.

During the neonatal period hepatitis B antigen is present in the blood of 2.5% of infants born to affected mothers, probably representing intrauterine infection. In most cases antigenemia appears later, suggesting that transmission occurred at the time of delivery; virus contained in amniotic fluid or in maternal feces or blood may be the source. Although most infants born to infected mothers become antigenemic from 2–5 mo of age, some infants of HB_sAg-positive mothers are not affected until later in the 1st or even the 2nd yr of life.

Hepatitis B tends to be relatively milder in infants and children and probably is frequently unrecognized. Although newborn infants are rarely symptomatic, about 90% of those infected become chronic carriers. The risk of developing chronic liver disease or hepatocellular carcinoma later in life is increased in these infants. The carrier and HB_eAg positivity rates appear to be highest in certain Asian and Pacific islands and among Alaskan Eskimo groups in whom perinatal transmission is the most common means of perpetuating HBV. Individuals from these groups may be at increased risk of infecting their infants even after a number of generations have lived in the United States. Women born in Haiti or sub-Saharan Africa also are at increased risk of being HB_sAg positive and infecting their newborn infants.

Hepatitis C. This disease is transmitted mainly by transfusion of blood or blood products. There is a strong association with intravenous drug use and in sexual contacts. Household spread from mother to child has been documented in one instance. Infected persons may become carriers.

Hepatitis D. This illness is transmitted by blood transfusion and intravenous drug use. Its epidemiology closely parallels that of hepatitis B, including the persistent carrier state.

Hepatitis E. Hepatitis E is largely water-borne in developing countries. It occurs in epidemics and tends to spare children.

PATHOLOGY. The acute response of the liver to virus injury from hepatitis A or B virus is similar. Initially, balloon degeneration and necrosis of single or groups of parenchymal cells occur, starting in the center of the lobules. These are followed by infiltration of the parenchyma and portal areas with lymphocytes, macrophages, plasma cells, eosinophils, and neutrophils; in the later stages, lymphocytes predominate. Regeneration of parenchymal cells is evidenced by cells or clusters of cells containing mitotic figures. Later there are striking changes in the periportal areas, with widening due to infiltration of inflammatory cells, proliferation of bile ducts, and biliary stasis. In fulminating hepatitis there is total destruction of parenchyma with only the reticular framework of the liver remaining. The newborn infant responds to hepatic injury by forming giant cells.

By 3 mo after onset of clinical illness, liver morphology is generally normal. Persistence of significant histologic changes in patients with hepatitis B usually indicates the development of chronic liver disease.

The changes in *chronic persistent hepatitis* and *chronic active hepatitis* are discussed in Sec. 13.97. Cirrhotic changes are sometimes found.

The changes in NANB hepatitis are seen mainly in the portal triads initially, with infiltration of lymphoid cells and destruction of hepatocytes. Later, more chronic changes are seen with piecemeal necrosis.

Other organ systems are affected in hepatitis. Small intestinal tissue may show changes in villous structure. Renal, joint, and skin involvement may result from circulating immune complexes. A hypoplastic bone marrow may result in aplastic anemia.

PATHOGENESIS. Jaundice results from obstruction of biliary flow and damage to parenchymal cells. Elevations of both direct and indirect serum bilirubin are found. Intrahepatic obstruction to bile flow may result in acholic stools. Resumption of flow may deliver normal or increased amounts of bilirubin to the duodenum. Urobilinogen, a metabolite of bilirubin produced in the intestine, is normally reabsorbed. Damaged liver parenchymal cells may be unable to re-excrete this material, which subsequently appears in the urine. Elevated serum alkaline phosphatase, 5′-nucleotidase, or γ-glutamyl transpeptidase activities suggest biliary obstruction.

The release into blood of serum transaminases from damaged liver cells suggests the extent and duration of injury. Serum alanine aminotransferase (ALT) provides a more specific indicator of liver cell injury than does serum aspartate aminotransferase (AST); injury to other cells such as erythrocytes, skeletal muscle cells, or myocardial cells may also cause rises in the AST. In severe liver injury, as in fulminating hepatitis, transaminases may fall to extremely low levels, indicating total destruction of parenchymal cells. Other enzymes, such as lactic dehydrogenase (LDH) may also be used to detect parenchymal cell injury.

Damage to liver cells may also be reflected in aberrations of their normal functions. Increased prothrombin time may result from their inability to synthesize proteins required for clotting. Obstruction to biliary flow reduces the flow of bile salts to the intestine, which normally facilitate fat absorption, including lipid-soluble vitamin K. Liver injury may also result in changes in carbohydrate, ammonia, and drug metabolism.

CLINICAL MANIFESTATIONS. In adolescents and older children hepatitis tends to resemble the more severe disease seen in adults. Hepatitis A tends to be acute in onset, hepatitis B, insidious.

Hepatitis A typically presents at its onset with systemic complaints of fever and malaise and digestive complaints of nausea, emesis, anorexia, intolerance of food and tobacco, and some abdominal discomfort. This prodrome may be mild or may go unnoticed in children. Dull right upper quadrant pain or epigastric fullness may be exaggerated by exercise or jolting of any kind. Jaundice and dark urine usually appear after the onset of systemic symptoms, but they may be the presenting signs in children. Jaundice may be so subtle that it can be detected only by laboratory tests, or it may last overtly as long as 2–3 wk. Light or clay-colored stools may result from obstruction of biliary flow. Constipation is more common in adults, whereas diarrhea is more common in children. Characteristic feelings of general discontent and depression are probably responsible for the cliché "a jaundiced view of life." Young infants may fail to gain weight. During convalescence, which may last several weeks, there is gradual return of appetite, exercise tolerance, and a feeling of well-being. Children tend to have less disability from hepatitis A than adults do, and their convalescence is usually shorter.

Hepatitis B may be heralded by arthralgia or skin eruptions, for example, urticarial, purpuric, macular, or maculopapular rashes. Papular acrodermatitis, *Gianotti-Crosti syndrome,* may also occur. The course tends to be insidious and lasts somewhat longer than that of hepatitis A, although it may be characterized by many of the same manifestations. In some patients hematuria or proteinuria may appear during convalescence. Mutant HBV detected by PCR may produce fulminant hepatitis.

On physical examination, skin and mucous membranes are icteric, especially the sclera and the mucosa under the tongue. The liver is usually enlarged and tender to palpation. When the liver is not palpable below the costal margin, tenderness can be demonstrated by striking the rib cage over the liver gently with a closed fist. Splenomegaly and lymphadenopathy are common.

Asymptomatic hepatitis A and B are common, particularly in the very young. Of the infants born to mothers with hepatitis B who develop demonstrable antigenemia and elevated transaminases, few have clinical evidence of hepatitis.

Hepatitis C generally is more insidious in onset than either hepatitis A or B. Transaminase elevations may be prolonged or even biphasic; clinical symptoms are generally mild.

Hepatitis E usually results in an acute illness characterized by dark urine, malaise, anorexia, abdominal pain, arthralgia, and fever. The disease is rare in children under 15 yr of age.

Hepatitis D often results in fulminant hepatitis, although most cases are indistinguishable clinically from hepatitis B.

DIAGNOSIS. A history of jaundice in family contacts, friends, schoolmates, or day-care center playmates or personnel, or travel to an endemic area may suggest the diagnosis. Accidental inoculation with blood of an infected person, drug abuse, and homosexual behavior should also arouse suspicion of hepatitis B. Children undergoing dialysis and those who receive frequent transfusions of blood products (e.g., fibrinogen, factor VIII, or factor IX particularly) are also at high risk of hepatitis B infection.

The diagnosis may be substantiated by *laboratory data* indicating liver injury. Hyperbilirubinemia may occur without clinical jaundice. Direct and indirect serum bilirubin levels are elevated, the conjugated portion more so during the early stage of disease. Later, excretion of conjugated bilirubin resumes, and there is a relative increase of indirect bilirubin. Urobilinogen is increased in serum and subsequently in urine.

Rises in serum transaminases reflect injury to hepatic cells. In hepatitis A the transaminases usually reach a higher peak, often exceeding 1,000 units, and decline more rapidly than they do in hepatitis B. Prolonged intermittent elevations are found in NANB hepatitis. With severe liver injury the prothrombin time is usually elevated. Biliary obstructive disease is manifested by elevated alkaline phosphatase, 5′-nucleotidase, or γ-glutamyl transpeptidase.

Mild leukopenia with a relative lymphocytosis and atypical lymphocytes may be observed during the first 2 wk of illness. IgM values may be elevated, particularly in hepatitis A. The sedimentation rate is usually elevated in hepatitis A and is often used as a method of following the course of the disease. *Prolongation of the prothrombin time is a serious sign mandating hospitalization.*

Acute and convalescent sera can be tested for the presence of anti-HAV. IgM anti-HAV is usually present at the onset of jaundice and is detectable for at least 6–8 wk. This test is also often useful in detecting subclinical cases among contacts of the patient. IgG anti-HAV appears a few weeks after onset and persists indefinitely. Hepatitis A virus can be demonstrated in stools for several days prior to and up to 1 wk following the onset of jaundice.

A variety of antigen-antibody systems are available for confirming the diagnosis of hepatitis B (Table 12–32). HB_sAg appears early in the disease and may disappear before the jaundice disappears. In carriers, however, HB_sAg persists indefinitely. Anti-HB_c is usually present soon after the onset of jaundice and then persists indefinitely. Anti-HB_c or IgM anti-HB_c may be the only marker present after HB_sAg has disappeared or before anti-HB_s appears, particularly in fulminant hepatitis. Anti-HB_c IgM has been less useful in young infants. DNA polymerase and HB_eAg appear early, prior to the onset of icterus. Anti-HB_e and then anti-HB_s may appear during convalescence. During exacerbations, rises in anti-HB_c are often observed. Serial samples tested simultaneously are often desirable for precise laboratory confirmation of hepatitis B.

HB_eAg in a patient's serum denotes an increased risk of transmission of HBV infection. Donors or pregnant women who are HB_sAg positive are more likely to transmit hepatitis B if they are also HB_eAg positive. Serologic tests are available for hepatitis C and D.

DIFFERENTIAL DIAGNOSIS. Physiologic jaundice, hemolytic disease, and infection in neonates are usually easily distinguished from hepatitis (Sec. 9.44 and 9.62). After the immediate newborn period, infection remains an important cause of hyperbilirubinemia, but other causes are galactosemia, hypothyroidism, congenital defects in metabolism of bilirubin, biliary atresia, hepatitis associated with α_1-antitrypsin deficiency, and choledochal cysts. The introduction of pigmented vegetables into the infant's diet may result in carotenemia, which may be mistaken for jaundice.

In later infancy and childhood hemolytic-uremic syndrome may be mistaken initially for hepatitis (Sec. 18.13). Reye syndrome may suggest acute fulminating hepatitis. Jaundice may also occur with severe infection in older children, particularly in those with malignant disorders. Malaria, leptospirosis, or brucellosis may also cause hepatitis. In adolescents as well as in children with chronic hemolytic processes, gallstones may obstruct biliary drainage and cause jaundice. Cirrhosis, which may be associated with Wilson disease, cystic fibrosis, Banti syndrome, and other causes, may sometimes present as hepatitis. The liver may be involved in collagen diseases, for example, lupus erythematosus.

A variety of *medications* may produce jaundice; for example, acetaminophen in excessive doses may cause liver damage, or other drugs may cause increased hemolysis, cholestasis, or hepatitis. Drugs well tolerated in normal children may cause problems in children with certain illnesses (Sec. 6.55).

COMPLICATIONS. Although most children recover uneventfully from hepatitis, a few suffer serious acute or chronic complications.

Acute Fulminating Hepatitis. See also Sec. 13.99. Some children develop a progressive course characterized by a rising serum bilirubin with peak levels exceeding 20 mg/dL, encephalopathy, bleeding, edema, and ascites. Drowsiness is followed by stupor and then by deep coma; clonus and hyperreflexia may be replaced later by loss of deep tendon, pupillary, and corneal reflexes. Transaminase levels may rise into the thousands and then return to normal or very low values. Blood ammonia is elevated, and the electroencephalogram is usually abnormal. The full-blown disease may develop relentlessly over 1–2 wk or more insidiously. Liver biopsy reveals "bridging necrosis," areas of parenchymal necrosis that cross limiting plates, extending from the central vein of one lobule to another.

Acute fulminating hepatitis is more frequently associated with hepatitis B when there is coinfection or superinfection with HDV than when there is infection with hepatitis B alone. The mortality is over 30%. Death from bacterial or fungal sepsis is not unusual. Treatment is aimed at sustaining the patient while providing the time needed for regeneration of hepatic cells.

Chronic Active Hepatitis (CAH). See Sec. 13.97.

Aplastic Anemia. See Sec. 16.35.

Other. Nephrosis has developed in children with HBV infection. Renal biopsy has revealed membranous glomerulonephritis with deposition of complement and HB_eAg in glomerular capillaries. Studies in Asia and Africa reveal an association of HB_sAg in mothers with the development of hepatocellular carcinoma in their offspring during young adulthood.

PREVENTION. Hepatitis A. Hospitalized infected patients who are incontinent of stool or who are in diapers should be treated with *enteric precautions*, including isolation. Patients are contagious for about 1 wk following onset of jaundice. There is no need to isolate older children, but their stool and fecally contaminated materials should be treated with precautions, and handwashing should be strictly enforced.

Household contacts should receive 0.02 mL/kg of *immune globulin* (IG) as soon as the diagnosis made. This is effective in preventing clinical hepatitis, although many recipients have rises in transaminase, indicating that the infection is probably modified rather than prevented.

Immune globulin is not routinely recommended for sporadic nonhousehold exposure (e.g., protection of hospital personnel or schoolmates). It is possible to test for anti-HAV to establish immune status, and testing may be desirable when repeated exposure is anticipated.

Mass immunization of school children has been used when epidemics have been school centered. When a single case of hepatitis occurs in a day-care center or in two families of children attending a day-care center, IG should be administered to all children and personnel. It is also advisable to immunize family members of the children in diapers. Handwashing after changing diapers should be stressed at all times in day-care centers.

HAV infection in pregnancy does not affect the newborn.

Prophylactic administration of immune serum globulin (0.06 mL/kg intramuscularly) is recommended for those traveling for extended periods in areas where hepatitis A is endemic. This larger dose will provide protection for a longer period,

TABLE 12–32. Tests for Infection with Hepatitis B Virus

Test	Preicteric	Icteric	Convalescent	Carriers
HB_s	+ + + +	+ +	+	+ +
Anti-HB_s		±	+ +	−
Anti-HB_cIgM		+ +	+ + +	
Anti-HB_c		±	+ + +	+
Anti-HB_e		+ + +	+ +	+ or −
Bilirubin	+ + + +	+ + +		+ or −
Transaminase	+ + +	±	+ +	+ or −
DNA polymerase				+ or −

obviating the need to find a local health care provider who can administer IG.

Hepatitis B. CONTROL. A major advance in controlling the spread of hepatitis B is the use for transfusion of only donated blood shown by testing to be free of HBV. Isolation of hospitalized infected patients is not mandatory, but careful handling of blood, needles, secretions, and instruments contaminated with blood of infected patients (universal precautions) is essential.

IMMUNIZATION. *Passive* immunization can be effectively provided by a dose of 0.06 mL/kg of hepatitis B immune globulin (HBIG). *Active* immunization can be provided by a vaccine prepared from a cloned DNA fragment coding for HB_sAg produced by yeast cells. All newborn infants should receive a full course of this vaccine. A 3-dose regimen should be administered; the 2nd and 3rd doses should be given 1 mo and 6 mo after the 1st dose. For those under 10 yr of age, half of the regular adult dose is recommended; a 40-μg dose should be used for patients on dialysis. The use of recombinant or pasteurized factor VIII rather than plasma-derived material should reduce the risk of HBV and HCV infections. Booster doses are required for patients on dialysis. A vaccine is available that has been approved for a schedule of 3 doses a month apart with a 4th at 1 yr.

If an infant under 1 yr of age has been exposed to an acute case of hepatitis B in the same household, 0.5 mL of HBIG and an initial dose of vaccine should be given. Other parenteral exposure (e.g., needles, bites, etc.) should be managed according to CDC recommendations.

Children or adolescents at high risk should receive HBV vaccine. This group includes those entering therapy programs that place them at increased risk, for example, those receiving dialysis or frequent administration of blood products; those who have household or institutional contact with HB_sAg-positive individuals; and homosexuals.

Testing of *all* pregnant women for HB_sAg is recommended. Efforts to test only high-risk pregnant women were unsuccessful; some HB_sAg-positive women were not in these groups.

Infants whose mothers are HB_sAg-positive or have had HBV infection during the 3rd trimester should receive 0.5 mL of HBIG after birth. The first of the 3 doses of hepatitis B vaccine should also be given at the same time at a site separate from that used for HBIG, using a different syringe. If medically indicated, the vaccine but not the HBIG may be delayed as long as 3 mo; if this is done, a 2nd dose of HBIG should be given at 3 mo. At 9 mo of age, vaccinees should be tested for HB_sAg and for anti-HB_s. Those who are antigenemic are vaccine failures and should be managed as carriers; those who are negative by both tests should receive another dose of the vaccine, and the tests should be repeated 1 mo later. Infants whose mothers are HB_eAg positive are at greatest risk of infection. The combination of passive and active immunization is 90–95% successful in preventing transmission. Cesarean section does not improve the outcome.

Although infants of HB_sAg-positive mothers do not need to be isolated, the maternal blood that may be on their skin at delivery may contain HBV and should be removed by a gloved attendant by wiping.

Infants undergoing surgery or a prolonged hospitalization should be tested for HB_sAg. About 5% of blood specimens of infants who will develop HBV infections during the first 6 mo of life are likely to be positive at birth. Testing of cord serum is unreliable and is not recommended.

Deinstitutionalized children having a tendency to bite others should be tested for HB_sAg. If positive, measures may be needed to prevent infection of persons who might be bitten.

Health care providers likely to come into frequent contact with blood should be immunized.

Immunization of high-risk groups has been poor. Immunization of those individuals born in epidemic areas, even though HB_sAg negative, should be considered. Similarly, in special circumstances, it may be desirable to immunize day-care attendees when the behavior of an HB_sAg-positive child might endanger others. Universal immunization with hepatitis B vaccine in infancy has been recommended. There are estimated to be more than 200,000 new cases of hepatitis B annually; 30% of these cases are seen in groups that are not considerd at high risk.

Hepatitis C. The effectiveness of IG for prophylaxis of hepatitis C is unclear. Some evidence supports its use in doses similar to those used for HBIG in prophylaxis of HBV infection. Pooled IG for prophylaxis of hepatitis C is not effective.

TREATMENT. Therapy for *uncomplicated hepatitis* is supportive (Sec. 13.94). Patients often find that a diet low in fat is more acceptable. Parents should be prepared to be tolerant of the child's anorexia. There is no evidence that rigid restriction of physical activity will speed recovery.

Occasionally, severe anorexia or emesis may necessitate intravenous therapy to prevent dehydration, but antiemetic preparations should be avoided because most are metabolized in the liver.

Corticosteroids are not indicated for uncomplicated hepatitis. See Sec. 13.97 for discussion of *chronic active hepatitis*.

The management of *acute fulminating hepatitis* is discussed in Sec. 13.99. The conventional strategy is to manage the patient's acute problems while awaiting the restoration of hepatic function. These problems include encephalopathy, bleeding, fluid retention and electrolyte disturbances, maintenance of adequate nutrition, and others.

PHILIP A. BRUNELL

Beasley RP, Stevens CE, Shiao IS, et al: Evidence against breast-feeding as a mechanism for vertical transmission of hepatitis B. Lancet 2:740, 1975.

Bernier RH, Sampliner R, Gerety R, et al: Hepatitis B infection in households of chronic carriers of hepatitis B surface antigen. J Epidemiol 116:199, 1982.

Centers for Disease Control: Recommendations for protection against viral hepatitis. MMWR Feb 9, 1990, Vol 39, supplement.

Choo Q-L, Kuo G, Weiner AJ, et al: Isolation of a cDNA clone derived from a blood-borne non-A, non-B viral hepatitis genome. Science 24:359, 1989.

Committee on Infectious Diseases, American Academy of Pediatrics: Prevention of hepatitis B virus infections. Pediatrics 75:362, 1985.

Derso A, Boxall EH, Tarlow MJ, et al: Transmission of HB_sAg from mother to infant in four ethnic groups. Br Med J 1:949, 1978.

Hadler SC, et al: Hepatitis in day-care centers: A community-wide assessment. N Engl J Med 302:1222, 1980.

Kumar ML, Dawson NV, McCullough AJ: Should all pregnant women be screened for hepatitis B? Ann Intern Med 107:273, 1987.

Kuo G, Choo Q-L, Alter HJ, et al: An assay for circulating antibodies to a major etiologic virus of human non-A, non-B hepatitis. Science 23:362, 1989.

Lemon SM: Type A viral hepatitis. New developments in an old disease. N Engl J Med 313:1059, 1985.

Levy RN, Sawitsky A, Florman AL, et al: Fatal aplastic anemia after hepatitis. N Engl J Med 273:1118, 1965.

Noble RL, Kane MA, Reeves SA, et al: Post transfusion hepatitis A in a neonatal intensive care unit. JAMA 252:2711, 1984.

Okada K, Kamiyama I, Inomata M: E antigen and anti-e in the serum of asymptomatic carrier mothers as indicators of positive and negative transmission of hepatitis B virus to their infants. N Engl J Med 294:746, 1976.

Phillips MJ, Blendis LM, Poucell S, et al: Syncytial giant-cell hepatitis: sporadic hepatitis with distinctive pathologic features, a severe clinical course, and paramyxoviral features. N Engl J Med 324:455, 1991.

Repsher LH, Freebern RK: Effects of early and vigorous exercise on recovery from infectious hepatitis. N Engl J Med 281:1393, 1969.

Schumacher HR, Gall EP: Arthritis in acute hepatitis and chronic active hepatitis: Pathology of the synovial membrane with evidence for the presence of Australia antigen in synovial membranes. Am J Med 57:655, 1974.

Shapiro ED: Lack of transmission of hepatitis B in a day care center. J Pediatr 110:90, 1987.

Stevens CE, Taylor PE, Tong MJ, et al: Yeast recombinant hepatitis B vaccine. JAMA 257:2612, 1987.

Storch GA, Perrillo RP, Miller P, et al: Prevalence of hepatitis B antibodies in personnel at a children's hospital. Pediatrics 76:29, 1985.

Takekoshi Y, Tanaka M, Miyakawa Y, et al: Free "small" and IgG-associated "large" hepatitis B e antigen in the serum and glomerular capillary walls of two patients with membranous glomerulonephritis. N Engl J Med 300:814, 1979.

12.80 ENTEROVIRUSES

Enteroviruses are responsible for significant and frequent human illnesses with protean clinical manifestations.

ETIOLOGY. Enteroviruses are RNA viruses belonging to the Picornaviridae family. The original enteroviral subgroups—coxsackieviruses, echoviruses, and polioviruses—were differentiated by their effects in tissue culture and animals (Table 12–33). Since 1970 new enteroviral types have been classified by enteroviral numbers. Enteroviruses retain activity for several days at room temperature and can be stored indefinitely at ordinary freezer temperatures (−20° C). They are rapidly inactivated by heat (>56° C), formaldehyde, chlorination, and ultraviolet light.

EPIDEMIOLOGY. Man is the only natural host of human enteroviruses. They are spread from person to person by fecal-oral and possibly oral-oral (respiratory) routes.

Children are immunologically susceptible, and their unhygienic habits facilitate spread. Transmission occurs from child to child (via feces to skin to mouth) and then within family groups. Recovery of enteroviruses is inversely related to age, and prevalence of specific antibodies is directly related to age. The incidence of infections and the prevalence of antibodies do not differ between boys and girls, but significant disease is more common in boys.

In temperate climates viral infection peaks in August, September, and October, although some activity does occur during the winter months. No seasonal pattern is evident in the tropics. Infection and acquisition of postinfection immunity occur with greater frequency and at earlier ages among crowded, economically deprived populations.

Although there are 68 identified enteroviral types, most illness in the United States is due to about a dozen nonpolio enteroviral types. Recently, the most prevalent types have been echoviruses 4, 6, 9, 11, and 30, coxsackieviruses A9, A16, and B2–B5, and enteroviruses 70 and 71. The universal use of live poliovaccine in the United States has virtually eliminated epidemic poliomyelitis. However, poliomyelitis still occurs in many regions of the developing world.

PATHOGENESIS. Figure 12–25 shows a schematic diagram of the events of pathogenesis. Following initial acquisition of virus by the oral or respiratory route, implantation occurs in the pharynx and the lower alimentary tract. Within 1 day the infection extends to the regional lymph nodes. On about the 3rd day minor viremia occurs, involving many secondary sites. Multiplication of virus in these sites coincides with the onset of clinical symptoms. Illness can vary from minor to fatal infections. Major viremia occurs during the period of multiplication of virus in the secondary sites, usually lasting from the 3rd to the 7th day of infection. In many enteroviral infections central nervous system involvement occurs at the same time as other secondary organ involvement, but the occasional delay of central nervous system symptoms suggests that seeding occurred later in association with the major viremia or by another pathway such as autonomic nerve fibers. Cessation of viremia correlates with the appearance of serum antibody. The viral concentration in secondary sites begins to diminish on about the 7th day. However, infection continues in the lower intestinal tract for prolonged periods.

TABLE 12–33. Human Enteroviruses

Polioviruses: Types 1–3
Coxsackieviruses A: Types A1–A24 (A23 reclassified as echovirus 9)
Coxsackieviruses B: Types B1–B6
Echoviruses: Types 1–33 (type 10 reclassified as reovirus type 1 and type 28 reclassified as rhinovirus type 1A)
Enteroviruses: Types 68–72 (hepatitis A has been provisionally classified as type 72)

PATHOLOGY AND PATHOPHYSIOLOGY. Polioviruses. The *neuropathy* of poliomyelitis is due directly to virus multiplication and is usually pathognomonic. Not all affected neurons are killed. The injury may be reversible, and function may be restored within 3–4 wk after onset. There is little histologic evidence of meningeal reaction. Perivascular cuffing and some interstitial glial infiltration are present. Histologic sections generally reveal more widespread lesions of neuronal destruction than would be estimated from the clinical findings.

Neuronal lesions occur in the (1) spinal cord (anterior horn cells chiefly and to a lesser degree the intermediate and dorsal horn and dorsal root ganglia); (2) medulla (vestibular nuclei, cranial nerve nuclei, and the reticular formation, which contains the vital centers); (3) cerebellum (nuclei in the roof and vermis only); (4) midbrain (chiefly the gray matter, but also the substantia nigra and occasionally the red nucleus); (5) thalamus and hypothalamus; (6) pallidum; and (7) cerebral cortex (motor cortex). The following areas are spared: (1) the entire cerebral cortex *except* the motor area; (2) the cerebellum except the vermis and deep midline nuclei; and (3) the white matter of the spinal cord.

Coxsackieviruses A. Records of severe illnesses associated with coxsackieviruses A are rare, and no distinctive pathology has been described.

Coxsackieviruses B. The most common findings have been

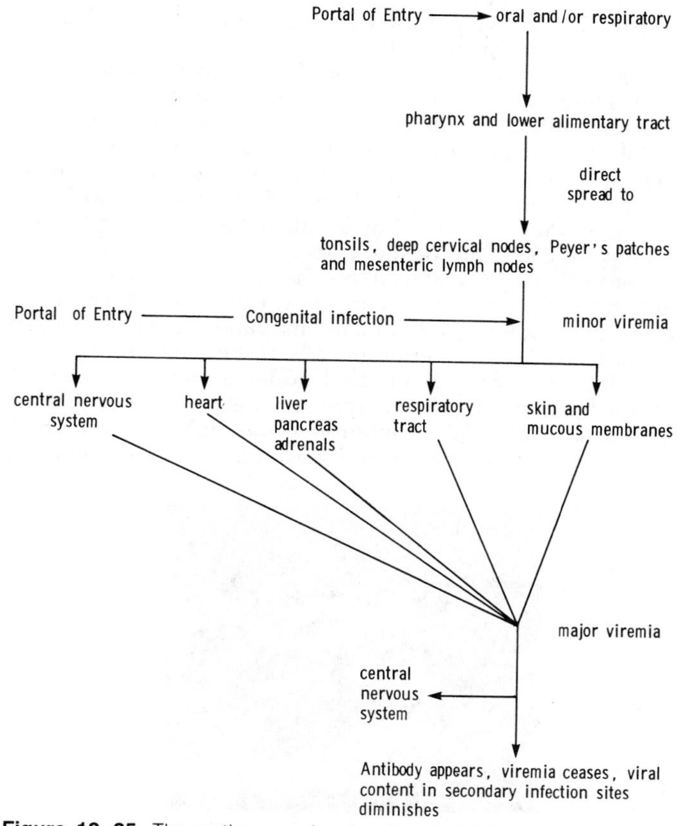

Figure 12–25. The pathogenesis of enteroviral infections. (Modified from Cherry JD. *In*: Remington JS, Klein JO [eds]: Infectious Diseases of the Fetus and Newborn Infant, 2nd ed. Philadelphia, WB Saunders, 1983.)

myocarditis and meningoencephalitis. Involvement of the adrenals, pancreas, liver, and lungs has also been noted. The *heart* is usually enlarged, with dilatation of the chambers or flabby musculature. The pericardium frequently contains some inflammatory cells; thickening, edema, and focal infiltrations of inflammatory cells may be found in the endocardium. The myocardium is congested and contains infiltrations of a wide range of inflammatory cells. The involvement of the myocardium is often patchy and focal but occasionally is diffuse. The muscle shows loss of striation as well as edema and eosinophilic degeneration. Frequently, muscle necrosis without extensive cellular infiltration is present. Lesions in *the brain and spinal cord* are focal rather than diffuse but frequently involve many different areas. The lesions consist of areas of eosinophilic degeneration of cortical cells, clusters of mononuclear and glial cells, and perivascular cuffing. The meninges are congested, edematous, and occasionally mildly infiltrated with inflammatory cells.

There are frequently areas of mild focal *pneumonitis* with peribronchiolar cellular infiltrations. The *liver* is often engorged and occasionally contains isolated foci of necrosis and mononuclear cellular infiltrations. In the *pancreas* occasional focal degeneration of the islet cells occurs. Mild to severe cortical necrosis and inflammatory cell infiltrates may be found in the *adrenals*.

Echoviruses. Hepatic necrosis has been observed in infections with echoviruses 6, 9, 11, 14, and 19. Other rare findings include adrenal and renal hemorrhage and interstitial pneumonitis.

CLINICAL MANIFESTATIONS. Poliovirus Infections. When a susceptible person has been infected with poliovirus, one of the following responses may occur, in this order of frequency: (1) inapparent infection occurs in 90–95% of those infected, (2) abortive poliomyelitis, (3) nonparalytic poliomyelitis, (4) paralytic poliomyelitis.

ABORTIVE POLIOMYELITIS. A brief febrile illness occurs with one or more of the following symptoms: malaise, anorexia, nausea, vomiting, headache, sore throat, constipation, and unlocalized abdominal pain. Coryza, cough, pharyngeal exudate, diarrhea, and localized abdominal tenderness and rigidity are uncommon. The fever seldom exceeds 39.5° C (103° F), and the pharynx shows usually little change despite the frequent complaint of sore throat.

NONPARALYTIC POLIOMYELITIS. The symptoms are those enumerated for abortive poliomyelitis, except that headache, nausea, and vomiting are more intense, and there is soreness and stiffness of the posterior muscles of the neck, trunk, and limbs. Fleeting paralysis of the bladder is not uncommon, and constipation is frequent. Approximately two thirds of the children have a short symptom-free interlude between the first phase (minor illness) and the second phase (central nervous system or major illness). This two-phase course is less common in adults, in whom the evolution of symptoms is more insidious. Nuchal and spinal rigidity should occur as a basis for the diagnosis of nonparalytic poliomyelitis during the second phase.

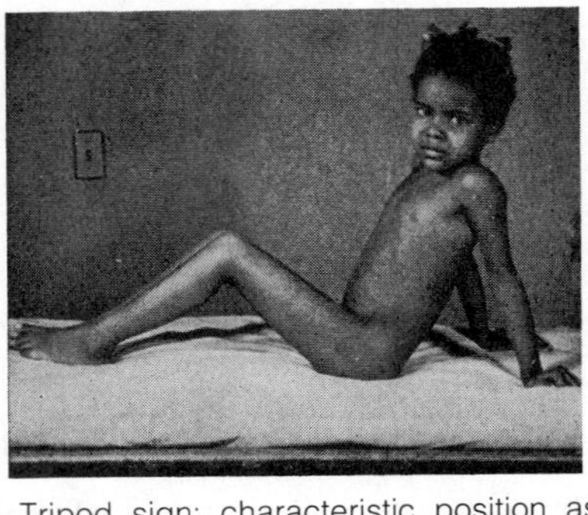

Figure 12–26. Tripod sign: characteristic position associated with stiffness of the spine. (From Steigman AJ: Diagnosis and general care of acute poliomyelitis. Pages 12–19, 1953. Pediatr Clin North Am, Vol 1, No 1A.)

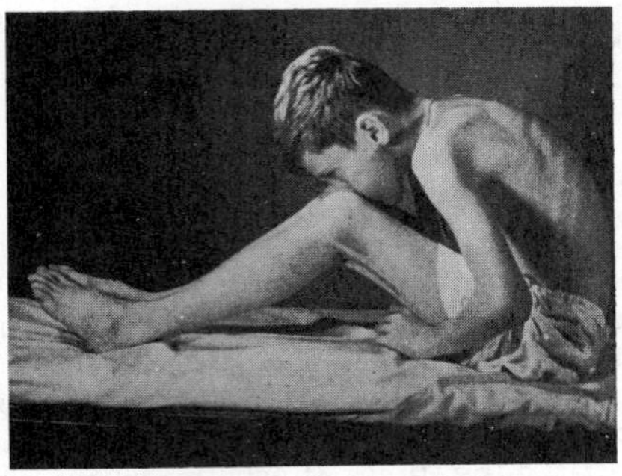

Figure 12–27. Kiss-the-knee test: ability to complete the maneuver only by flexing the knee. Note the tense appearance of the hamstrings. (From Steigman AJ: Diagnosis and general care of acute poliomyelitis. Pages 12–19, 1953. Pediatr Clin North Am, Vol 1, No 1A.)

Physical examination reveals *nuchal-spinal* signs and changes in superficial and deep reflexes. With cooperative patients the nuchal-spinal signs are first sought by active tests. The child is asked to sit up unassisted. If this causes undue effort, if the knees flex upward and the patient writhes a bit from side to side in sitting up and uses hands on the bed for the tripod supporting position, there is unmistakable spinal rigidity (Fig. 12–26). Still sitting, the patient is asked to flex chin to chest and is observed for nuchal rigidity. Alternatively, from the supine position, with knees held down gently, the patient is asked to sit up and kiss his or her knees (Fig. 12–27). If the knees draw up sharply or if the maneuver cannot be adequately completed, there is stiffness of the spine due to muscle spasm. If the diagnosis is still uncertain, attempts should be made to elicit Kernig and Brudzinski signs. Gentle forward flexion of the occiput and neck will elicit nuchal rigidity, which may precede spinal rigidity. *Head drop* may be demonstrated by placing the hands under the patient's shoulders and raising the trunk (Fig. 12–28). Normally the head follows the plane of the trunk, but in poliomyelitis it often falls backward limply. The head-drop sign is not due to true paresis of the neck flexors. In struggling infants it may be difficult to distinguish voluntary resistance from clinically important involuntary nuchal rigidity. One may place the infant's shoulders flush with the edge of the table, support the weight of the occiput in the hand, and then flex the head

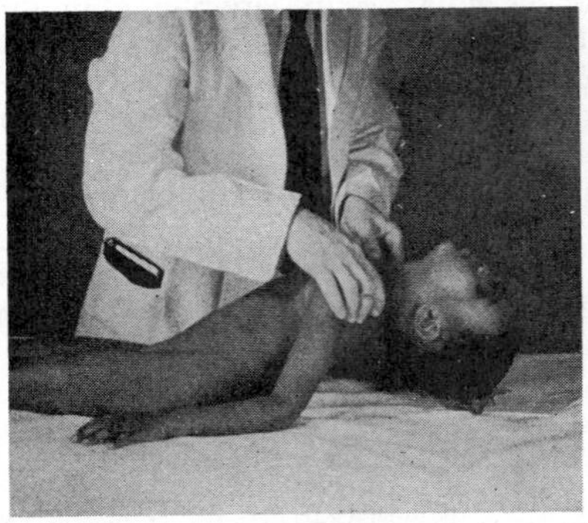

Figure 12–28. Head-drop sign: the head fails to continue in the plane of the body when the shoulders are elevated. This child had nonparalytic poliomyelitis. Tripod and head-drop signs appear in nonparalytic and paralytic poliomyelitis. (From Steigman AJ: Diagnosis and general care of acute poliomyelitis. Pages 12–19, 1953. Pediatr Clin North Am, Vol 1, No 1A.)

anteriorly (Fig. 12–29). Nuchal rigidity that persists during this maneuver may be interpreted as involuntary. When not closed, the anterior fontanel may be tense or bulging as in meningitis.

In the early stages the *reflexes* are normally active and remain so unless paralysis supervenes. Changes in reflexes, either increase or depression, may precede weakness by 12–24 hr; hence, it is important to detect them, especially in nonparalytic patients managed at home. The superficial reflexes, that is, cremasteric and abdominal reflexes and the reflexes of the spinal and gluteal muscles, are usually the first to be diminished. The spinal and gluteal reflexes may disappear before the abdominal and cremasteric ones. Changes in the deep tendon reflexes generally occur 8–24 hr after depression of superficial reflexes and indicate impending paresis of the extremities. There is absence of tendon reflexes with paralysis. Sensory defects do not occur in poliomyelitis.

Paralytic Poliomyelitis. The manifestations are those enumerated for nonparalytic poliomyelitis plus weakness of one or more muscle groups, either skeletal or cranial. These symptoms may be followed by a symptom-free interlude of several days and then a recurrence culminating in paralysis. Bladder paralysis of 1–3 days' duration occurs in approximately 20% of patients, and bowel atony is common, occasionally to the point of paralytic ileus. In some patients muscular paralysis may be the initial presentation.

Flaccid paralysis is the most obvious clinical expression of the neuronal injury. The ensuing muscular atrophy is due to denervation plus the atrophy of disuse. The pain, spasticity, nuchal and spinal rigidity, and hypertonia early in the illness are probably due to lesions of the brain stem, spinal ganglia, and posterior columns. Respiratory and cardiac arrhythmias, blood pressure and vasomotor changes, and the like are reflections of damage to vital centers in the medulla.

On physical examination the distribution of paralysis is characteristically spotty. To detect mild muscular weakness, it is often necessary to apply gentle resistance in opposition to the muscle group being tested. In the *spinal form* there is weakness of some of the muscles of the neck, abdomen, trunk, diaphragm, thorax, or extremities. In the *bulbar form* there is weakness in the motor distribution of one or more cranial nerves with or without dysfunction of the vital centers of respiration and circulation. Components of both the preceding forms occur together in *bulbospinal poliomyelitis*. In the *encephalitic form* irritability, disorientation, drowsiness, and coarse tremors not explained by inadequate ventilation are noted; peripheral or cranial nerve paralysis coexists or ensues. Hypoxia and hypercapnia due to inadequate ventilation from respiratory insufficiency may produce disorientation without true encephalitis.

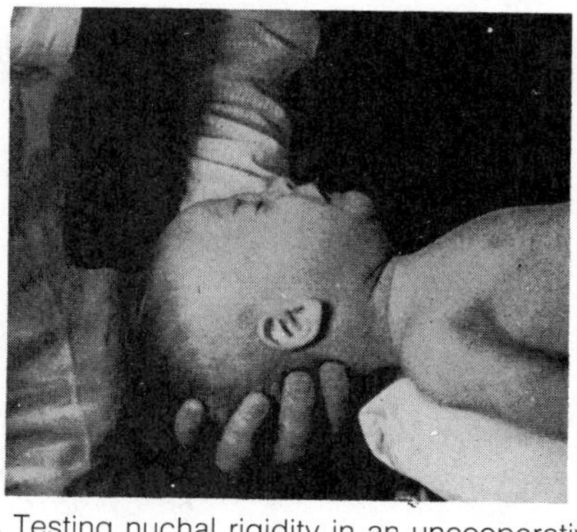

Figure 12–29. Testing nuchal rigidity in an uncooperative, struggling infant. Place the shoulders at the edge of the table, supporting the occiput manually. Flex anteriorly. Only true involuntary rigidity persists. (From Steigman AJ: Diagnosis and general care of acute poliomyelitis. Pages 12–19, 1953. Pediatr Clin North Am, Vol 1, No 1A.)

A number of components acting together may produce insufficiency of ventilation, resulting in hypoxia and hypercapnia, which may produce profound effects on many other systems. Since respiratory insufficiency may develop rapidly, continued clinical evaluation is essential. Despite weakness of the respiratory muscles, the patient may respond with so much respiratory effort (associated with anxiety and fear) that overventilation may occur at the outset, resulting in respiratory alkalosis. Such effort is fatiguing and soon leads to respiratory failure.

Certain characteristic patterns of disease occur:

1. *Pure spinal poliomyelitis with respiratory insufficiency* involves tightness, weakness, or paralysis of respiratory muscles (chiefly the diaphragm and intercostals) without discernible clinical involvement of cranial nerves or vital centers. The cervical and thoracic spinal cord segments are chiefly affected.
2. *Pure bulbar poliomyelitis* involves paralysis of motor cranial nerve nuclei with or without involvement of the vital centers that control respiration, circulation, and body temperature. Involvement of the 9th, 10th, and 12th cranial nerves results in paralysis of the pharynx, tongue, and larynx with consequent airway obstruction.
3. *Bulbospinal poliomyelitis with respiratory insufficiency* affects the respiratory muscles with coexisting bulbar paralysis.

The clinical findings resulting from *involvement of the respiratory muscles* are (1) anxious expression; (2) inability to speak without frequent pauses, resulting in short, jerky, "breathless" sentences; (3) increased respiratory rate; (4) movement of the alae nasi and of the accessory muscles of respiration; (5) inability to cough or sniff with full depth; (6) paradoxical abdominal movements due to diaphragmatic immobility from spasm or weakness of one or both leaves; (7) relative immobility of the intercostal spaces, which may be segmental, unilateral, or bilateral. When the arms are weak, and especially when deltoid paralysis occurs, there may be impending respiratory paralysis, since the phrenic nerve nuclei are in adjacent areas of the spinal cord. Observing the patient's capacity for thoracic breathing while the abdominal muscles are splinted manually will indicate minor degrees of paresis. Light manual splinting of the thoracic cage will help to assess the effectiveness of diaphragmatic movement.

The clinical findings of *bulbar poliomyelitis* with respiratory difficulty (other than paralysis of extraocular, facial, and masticatory muscles) include (1) nasal twang to the voice or cry due to palatal and pharyngeal weakness (hard-consonant words such as "cookie" or "candy" bring this out best); (2) inability to swallow smoothly, resulting in accumulation of saliva in the pharynx and indicating partial immobility (holding the larynx lightly and asking the patient to swallow will confirm immobility); (3) accumulated pharyngeal secretions, which may cause irregular respirations, since each inspiration must be "planned" to avoid aspirating; the respirations may thus appear interrupted and abnormal even to the point of falsely simulating intercostal or diaphragmatic weakness; (4) the impossibility of effective coughing, with constant fatiguing efforts to clear the throat; (5) nasal regurgitation of saliva and fluids due to palatal paralysis, with inability to separate the oropharynx from the nasopharynx during swallowing; (6) deviation of the palate, uvula, or tongue; (7) involvement of vital brain stem centers, manifested by irregularity in rate, depth, and rhythm of respiration; by cardiovascular alterations which include blood pressure changes (especially increased), alternate flushing and mottling of the skin, and cardiac arrhythmias; and by rapid changes in body temperature; (8) paralysis of one or both vocal cords causing hoarseness, aphonia, and ultimately asphyxia unless recognized by laryngoscopy and managed by immediate tracheostomy;

(9) the "rope sign," an acute angulation between the chin and larynx due to weakness of the hyoid muscles (the hyoid bone is pulled posteriorly, narrowing the hypopharyngeal inlet).

Nonpolio Enterovirus Infections (Table 12–34). Coxsackieviral and echoviral infections are exceedingly common, and their spectrum of disease is protean. Because many of the clinical-virologic associations are based upon a limited number of cases and because enteroviruses are frequently carried asymptomatically in the gastrointestinal tract for relatively long periods of time, some of the observed illnesses and coincidentally recovered viruses may not have a cause and effect relationship. However, repeated observations have confirmed many virus-illness associations, even though their occurrence has been sporadic.

Asymptomatic Infection. Coxsackieviruses and echoviruses can frequently be recovered from the stools of well children, but there are few data on the rate of asymptomatic infection with nonpolio enteroviruses. The isolation of enteroviruses from the stool cannot be equated with asymptomatic infection because illness, if it occurs, happens shortly after virus acquisition and is of short duration; a particular infection may have been associated with nonspecific illness 1–3 mo prior to collection of a stool specimen. In general, the more carefully clinical symptomatology is sought, the lower is the

TABLE 12–34. Clinical Manifestations of Nonpolio Enteroviruses

Clinical Categories	Virus Types		
	Coxsackieviruses A	*Coxsackieviruses B*	*Echoviruses and Enteroviruses*
Nonspecific febrile illness	All types	All types	All types
Respiratory			
Common cold	Mainly 21, 24; rarely other types	Mainly 1–5; rarely 6	Mainly 2, 20; rarely other types
Pharyngitis (pharyngitis, tonsillitis, tonsillopharyngitis, and nasopharyngitis)	Probably all types; mainly 9	Probably all types; mainly 1–5	Probably all types; mainly 2, 4, 6, 9, 11, 16, 19, 25, 30
Herpangina	1–10, 16, 22	1–5	6, 9, 16, 17, 25
Lymphonodular pharyngitis	10		
Stomatitis and other lesions in the anterior mouth	5, 9, 10, 16	2, 5	9, 11, 20, 71
Parotitis	Coxsackievirus A not typed	3, 4	70
Croup	9	4, 5	4, 11, 21
Bronchitis		1, 4	8, 12–14
Bronchiolitis and asthmatic bronchitis	Many types	Many types	Many types
Pneumonia	9, 16	1–5	6, 7, 9, 11, 12, 19, 20, 30
Pleurodynia	1, 2, 4, 6, 9, 16	1, 2, 3, 5, 6	1–3, 6–9, 11, 12, 14, 16, 17, 18, 19, 23, 24
Gastrointestinal			
Nausea and vomiting	9, 16	2–5	2, 4, 6, 9, 11, 16, 19, 20, 22, 30
Diarrhea	2, 4, 6, 7, 9, 10, 14, 16	1–5	3, 4, 6, 7, 9, 11–14, 16–22, 25, 30, 71
Constipation	9	3–5	4, 6, 9, 11
Abdominal pain	9, 16	2–5	4, 6, 9, 11, 19, 30
Pseudoappendicitis			1, 8, 14
Peritonitis		1	
Mesenteric adenitis		5	7, 9, 11
Appendicitis		2, 5	
Intussusception		3	7, 9
Hepatitis	4, 9, 10, 20, 24	1–5	1, 3, 4, 6, 7, 9, 11, 14, 20, 21, 30, 72
Reye syndrome	2	4	14, 22
Pancreatitis	9	3–5	
Acute hemorrhagic conjunctivitis	24		70
Pericarditis and myocarditis	1, 2, 4, 5, 7–10, 16	1–5	1, 4, 6–9, 11, 14, 17, 19, 22, 25, 30
Genitourinary			
Orchitis and epididymitis		1–5	6, 9, 11
Nephritis		4	6, 9
Hemolytic-uremic syndrome	4, 9	2–5	22
Pyuria, hematuria, or proteinuria		5	1, 6, 9
Myositis and arthritis	2, 9	4	9, 11, 18, 24
Exanthem	2, 4, 5, 7, 9, 10, 16	1–5	1–7, 9, 11, 13, 14, 16–19, 22, 25, 30, 32, 33, 71
Neurologic manifestations			
Aseptic meningitis	1–14, 16–18, 21, 22, 24	1–6	1–9, 11–27, 29–33, 71
Encephalitis	2, 4–7, 9, 10, 16	1–5	1–9, 11–25, 27, 30, 33, 71
Paralysis (lower motor neuron involvement)	2, 4–7, 9–11, 14, 21	1–6	1–4, 6–9, 11, 12, 14, 16–19, 25, 27, 30, 31, 70, 71
Guillain-Barré syndrome and transverse myelitis	2, 4–6, 9, 16	1–4	5, 6, 7, 19, 22, 70
Cerebellar ataxia	4, 7, 9	3, 4	6, 9, 16
Peripheral neuritis			9

percentage of truly asymptomatic infections. Clinical expression is also inversely related to age and varies by viral type. Overall, probably fewer than 50% of all infections are asymptomatic.

Nonspecific Febrile Illness. This is the most common manifestation of enteroviral infections. All viral types cause this clinical presentation, but the frequency varies considerably among the individual viruses. The onset of illness is usually abrupt and without prodrome. In young children the initial finding is fever and associated malaise. In older children headache and myalgia are usually also noted. The temperature ranges from 38.5 to 40° C (101–104° F) and has a mean duration of 3 days. In some instances the fever is biphasic; it occurs for 1 day, is absent for 2–3 days, and then recurs for an additional 2–4 days. In many young children the only manifestation of illness is fever, and its presence is discovered by chance by a parent. Malaise and anorexia are often related to the degree of temperature elevation, as is headache in older patients. The complaint of a sore or scratchy feeling in the throat is common, but an inflamed pharynx is not seen. Nausea and vomiting occasionally occur at the onset of illness, as does mild abdominal discomfort. A few mildly loose stools may be noted. Generalized myalgia is also noted. Findings on physical examination are generally benign. There may be minimal conjunctivitis, injection of the pharynx, and cervical lymphadenitis. The duration of illness varies from 24 hr to 6 days with an average of 3–4 days. The white blood cell count is normal.

Respiratory Manifestations (Table 12–34). Coxsackievirus A21 has produced epidemics of mild respiratory illness *(common cold)* in military populations, but epidemic disease has not been observed in children.

Pharyngitis, tonsillitis, tonsillopharyngitis, and *nasopharyngitis* are common clinical manifestations of coxsackieviral and echoviral infections; probably all enteroviruses on occasion cause mild pharyngitis. Pharyngitis is frequently associated with other clinical findings such as meningitis, pleurodynia, or exanthem. Although evidence of pharyngeal involvement may be present at the time of disease onset, the initial complaint is most often fever. Sore throat, coryza, and vomiting and/or diarrhea may also be noted. Examination of the tonsils and pharynx reveals varying degrees of erythema; in some, patches of exudate will be seen. The usual duration of uncomplicated pharyngitis is 3–6 days. The total white blood cell count may be normal or slightly elevated with a normal differential count.

Herpangina is usually characterized by the sudden onset of fever, although the initial temperature can be quite variable with a range from normal to 41° C (106° F). In general, the temperature tends to be higher in younger patients. Older children frequently complain of headache and backache. Vomiting occurs in about 25% of children under the age of 5 yr. In the majority of children the oropharyngeal lesions are present on the first examination at the time or shortly after fever is observed (Fig. 12–30 [color plate section]). The characteristic lesions are small, 1- to 2-mm vesicles and ulcers. They are usually discrete with an average of 5 per patient; some patients have only 1 or 2 lesions; in others 14 or more may be noted. When seen early, the vesicular lesions enlarge over a 2- to 3-day period to 3–4 mm in size. Each vesicular and ulcerative lesion is surrounded by an erythematous ring that varies in size up to 10 mm in diameter. The major site of the lesions is the anterior tonsillar pillars. They also occur on the soft palate, uvula, tonsils, pharyngeal wall, and occasionally the posterior buccal surfaces. Aside from these lesions, the remainder of the throat appears either normal or minimally erythematous. Although occasionally noted in association with aseptic meningitis or other more severe enteroviral illness, most cases of herpangina are mild and without complication. The usual duration of signs and symptoms is 3–6 days.

Pleurodynia (Bornholm disease) is an epidemic disease, but sporadic cases do occur. Following an incubation period of about 4 days, there is sudden onset of fever and pain. The typical pain is located in the chest or upper abdomen, is muscular in origin, and is of variable intensity. Occasionally, the pain occurs in other areas of the body. It is often excruciatingly severe and sudden and is associated with profuse sweating. The patient may appear pale and shock-like. The pain is spasmodic, with durations varying from a few minutes to several hours. Most commonly, the spasmodic periods last about 15–30 min. During spasms, the respirations are usually rapid, shallow, and grunting, suggesting pneumonia of pleural inflammation. Pleural friction rubs may be noted on auscultation, and they may appear and disappear with the coming and going of the pain episodes. Coughing, sneezing, or deep breathing makes the pain worse. In older children and adults the pain is described as stabbing or knife-like. When pain is localized to the abdomen, it is frequently crampy and suggests colic in the younger child. The child may double over and refuse to walk or move. Occasionally, the abdominal pain in association with a pale, sweaty, shock-like appearance suggests acute intestinal obstruction. Splinting and guarding of the abdomen also suggests appendicitis and peritonitis. Tenderness to some degree is present in areas of pain, but frank myositis with muscle swelling is not observed. Fever and pain usually last 1–2 days. Frequently, however, the illness is biphasic; after the initial febrile period the patient is asymptomatic for several days; then pain and fever recur. Rarely, patients have several recurrent episodes over a period of a few weeks. In these cases fever is less prominent during the recurrences.

In epidemics both children and adults are afflicted, with the majority of cases occurring in persons under 30 yr of age. Most children have other signs of enteroviral infection such as anorexia, nausea, vomiting, headache, and sore throat. Routine laboratory studies are not very helpful. The white blood cell count is variable, but an increased percentage of polymorphonuclear neutrophils and band forms is frequent. The erythrocyte sedimentation rate is also inconsistent, with normal to extremely high values observed. The chest roentgenogram is most often normal.

Complications in pleurodynia are uncommon. Aseptic meningitis has been noted, and adult males have experienced orchitis. Myocarditis and pericarditis may also complicate pleurodynia.

The major etiologic agents in epidemic pleurodynia are coxsackieviruses B3 and B5; other associated viruses include coxsackieviruses B1 and B2 and echoviruses 1 and 6. Agents associated with sporadic occurrences are listed in Table 12–34.

A variety of nonpolio enteroviruses have been associated with sporadic instances of *parotitis, croup, bronchitis, bronchiolitis, infectious asthma,* and *pneumonia* as well as outbreaks of *lymphonodular pharyngitis, stomatitis,* and other lesions in the anterior mouth (Table 12–34).

Gastrointestinal Manifestations (see Table 12–34). Gastrointestinal manifestations are common (7–30%) in enteroviral infections. *Vomiting* is a common manifestation of infections with many coxsackieviral and echoviral types, but it is rarely the major complaint of the patient or the parent. Except for the hand, foot, and mouth syndrome (coxsackievirus A16), in which vomiting is uncommon, this manifestation occurs in about 50% of all cases in epidemic enteroviral disease. Vomiting is most common in meningitis and least common in pleurodynia and uncomplicated exanthematous disease.

Diarrhea occurs commonly in coxsackieviral and echoviral infections as one of many manifestations of the systemic illness. It is rarely severe. In most instances loose stools occur for a 2- to 4-day period. The stools are rarely watery and never bloody and number at most 6–8/day.

Abdominal pain is also a common complaint in many enteroviral infections. About 10% of patients with coxsackievirus A16 (hand, foot, and mouth syndrome) complain of abdominal pain. Coxsackieviral and echoviral meningitis is associated with abdominal pain in about 25% of the cases. The severity of pain in enteroviral infections is quite variable and on occasion may suggest a surgical abdomen. The pain is most often periumbilical; it may be either constant or colicky. The associated fever is most often greater than 38.3° C (101° F).

Nonpolio enteroviruses have been associated with a variety of other gastrointestinal and abdominal complaints (see Table 12–34). In most situations the findings are just one manifestation of a more typical enteroviral illness.

Acute Hemorrhagic Conjunctivitis. Conjunctivitis may be the dominant complaint. In the majority of epidemics, enterovirus 70 has been the etiologic agent. Acute hemorrhagic conjunctivitis has a sudden onset that is accompanied by severe eye pain and associated photophobia, blurred vision, lacrimation, erythema and congestion of the eye, and edematous and chemotic lids. There are subconjunctival hemorrhages of varying size and frequently a transient punctate epithelial keratitis, conjunctival follicles, and preauricular lymphadenopathy. Eye discharge is initially serous but becomes mucopurulent with secondary bacterial infection. Systemic symptoms (including fever) are rare. Occasionally, a picture suggestive of pharyngoconjunctival fever has occurred. A small number of patients have had a polyradiculomyeloneuropathy or paralytic poliomyelitis following enterovirus 70 acute hemorrhagic conjunctivitis. Persons 20–50 yr of age have the highest attack rates, and children are less often involved. Initially most epidemics occurred in coastal areas of tropical countries toward the end of hot rainy periods. More recently, outbreaks of disease have occurred in temperate climates, including many areas of the United States. Epidemics are explosive and are spread mainly by the eye-hand-fomite-eye route.

Pericarditis and Myocarditis. These manifestations have been noted in association with 27 different nonpolio enteroviruses (see Table 12–34). The group B coxsackieviruses have been most frequently implicated, and B5 has been the most common causative agent. Of the echoviruses, type 6 has been most frequently associated with cardiac involvement. Hepatitis, pneumonia, nephritis, meningitis, and orchitis have also been occasional associated findings with coxsackievirus B. The mortality resulting from acute coxsackieviral and echoviral heart disease is significant. In nonfatal cases recovery is usually complete without residual disability; occasionally, constrictive pericarditis occurs as well as other sequelae.

Genitourinary Manifestations (see Table 12–34). Group B coxsackieviruses are second only to mumps as causative agents of *orchitis;* B5 is the most commonly associated virus, but B2 and B4 have also been implicated on many occasions. In almost all instances the orchitis is a secondary event, most commonly associated with pleurodynia. The illness is frequently biphasic; fever and pleurodynia or meningitis are followed by apparent recovery and then by orchitis about 2 wk after onset. Many patients also have *epididymitis.* In epidemics of disease due to group B coxsackieviruses, the occurrence of testicular involvement is quite variable. Generally orchitis is infrequent, but in one B2 outbreak 17% of the postpubertal males had orchitis and 7% also had epididymitis. Other genitourinary manifestations of nonpolio enteroviral infections include acute glomerulonephritis; mesangiolytic glomerulonephritis in an infant with immune deficiency; hemolytic-uremic syndrome; acute renal failure; pyuria, hematuria, or proteinuria; hemorrhagic cystitis; and vaginal ulcerative lesions.

Myositis and Arthritis (see Table 12–34). Myalgia is a common complaint accompanying many coxsackieviral and echoviral illnesses. However, there is almost no direct (demonstration of virus in muscle) or indirect (muscle enzyme elevations) evidence of muscle involvement in routine enteroviral illnesses. Coxsackievirus A2 has been associated with myositis, and coxsackievirus A9 and echovirus 18 have been associated with polymyositis. A dermatomyositis-like syndrome has been associated with immune deficiency and enteroviral infection. Arthritis has occurred rarely in enterovirus infection.

Skin Manifestations (see Table 12–34). Nonpolio enteroviruses are a common cause of a large variety of skin manifestations. In the summer and fall they are the leading cause of exanthems. There is a marked variation in the rates at which exanthems occur among the various viral types and also among different age groups of the host. In general, the frequency is inversely related to the age of the infected patient, and several different agents can produce similar skin manifestations.

Coxsackievirus A16 is the major cause of the *hand, foot, and mouth syndrome,* which has a typically enteroviral pattern, with a short incubation period (4–6 days) and a summer and fall seasonal pattern. The clinical expression rate of the enanthem-exanthem complex is high, being close to 100% in young children, 38% in school children, and 11% in adults. The intraoral lesions are ulcerative and average about 4–8 mm in size. The tongue and buccal mucosa are most frequently involved. The hands are more commonly involved than the feet. Buttock lesions are also common, but these do not usually progress to vesiculation. The lesions on the hands and feet are usually vesicular and vary in size from 3 to 7 mm; they are generally more common on the dorsal surfaces but frequently occur on the palms and soles as well. They clear by absorption of the fluid in about 1 wk. Coxsackievirus A16 is frequently associated with subacute, chronic, and recurring skin lesions. Recently, enterovirus 71 has been the etiologic agent in several outbreaks of hand, foot, and mouth syndrome. Illness with this virus is frequently more severe than with coxsackievirus A16; aseptic meningitis, encephalitis, and paralytic disease are common.

Echovirus type 9 is the most prevalent nonpolio enterovirus, and *exanthem* is a common clinical manifestation. Nonspecific febrile illness and aseptic meningitis are the usual major manifestations of echovirus 9 infection. Exanthem occurs in about one third of the cases; 57% of children under 5 yr of age have rash, whereas only 6% of those over 10 yr of age have similar cutaneous findings. The rash is most frequently rubelliform, but in addition or as the sole manifestation, petechiae frequently occur. Rash and fever usually appear at about the same time, and frequently the illness closely mimics meningococcemia. The rash usually lasts 3–5 days.

Neurologic Manifestations (see Table 12–34). *Aseptic meningitis* due to enteroviruses occurs in epidemics and as isolated cases (Sec. 12.11). Epidemics have been most common with coxsackievirus B5 and echoviruses 4, 6, 9, and 11. In general, illness is more common in children than in adults. Virtually all patients have fever, and many have mild pharyngitis; other respiratory manifestations are also common. Rash is common but varies with the specific viral agents; 30–50% of all patients with echovirus 9 meningitis have exanthem. Frequently, the rash is petechial, thus suggesting meningococcemia. Except for the occurrence of rash, herpangina, pleurodynia, or myocarditis, there is little clinical evidence that helps in identifying the etiology in a sporadic case of aseptic meningitis. Generalized muscle stiffness or spasm is usually observed, although the degree varies considerably; Kernig and Brudzinski signs are positive in fewer than half the cases. Deep tendon reflexes are usually normal.

The duration of illness is variable. In the majority of instances the temperature returns to normal within 4–6 days and disability due to neurologic involvement lasts 1–2 wk. Occasionally, a biphasic illness pattern occurs consisting of an initial period with fever, headache, nausea, vomiting, and muscle aches and pains of a few days' duration followed by general recovery; then the same symptoms return with more pronounced neurologic involvement.

About 2% of the reported cases of *encephalitis* (Sec. 12.12) in the United States are demonstrated to have an enteroviral etiology. This is probably an underestimate of the number of severe cases, which may total over 1,000/yr. Echovirus type 9 is the most common cause of enteroviral encephalitis; other commonly associated enteroviral types are echoviruses 3, 4, 6, and 11 and coxsackieviruses B2, B4, and B5. In general the prognosis in encephalitis due to enteroviral infections is good, but fatalities have occurred in association with coxsackieviruses B3 and B6, echoviruses 2, 9, 17, and 25, and enterovirus 71.

Paralysis on the basis of anterior horn cell disease occasionally results from infection with nonpolio enteroviruses. Many coxsackieviruses and echoviruses have been associated with the *Guillain-Barré syndrome. Cerebellar ataxia* has been noted in association with coxsackieviruses A4, A7, A9, B3, and B4 and with echoviruses 6, 9, and 16. *Peripheral neuritis* has been reported with echovirus 9 infection, and coxsackievirus A9 has been noted in association with a *focal encephalitis and acute hemiplegia*.

Neonatal Infections. Nonpolio enteroviral infections in neonatal infants result in a wide variety of clinical manifestations ranging from asymptomatic infection to fatal encephalitis and myocarditis (Sec. 9.70).

DIAGNOSIS. The clinical differentiation of enteroviral disease from treatable bacterial illnesses is frequently very difficult, although when all the circumstances of a particular illness are considered, enteroviral diseases often can be suspected on clinical grounds. The most important factors in clinical diagnosis are season of the year, geographic location, exposure, incubation period, and clinical symptoms. In temperate climates enteroviral prevalence is distinctly seasonal; therefore, disease is usually seen in the summer and fall and unlikely to be seen in the winter; in the tropics enteroviruses are prevalent throughout the year. A careful history of maternal illness is vitally important in neonatal disease. For example, a mother's nonspecific mild febrile illness that occurs in the summer and fall should suggest the possibility of severe neonatal illness. Certain findings (i.e., aseptic meningitis, paralysis, pleurodynia, herpangina, pericarditis, myocarditis) should alert the clinician to enteroviral illnesses. The short incubation period of enteroviral infections should be taken into consideration. Polioviral infection should be considered in any unimmunized or incompletely immunized child with nonspecific febrile illness, aseptic meningitis, or paralytic disease.

Most viral diagnostic laboratories have facilities for recovering the majority of enteroviruses that cause illness. Tissue culture systems allow the isolation of polioviruses, group B coxsackieviruses, echoviruses, and coxsackieviruses A9 and A16. Enteroviral growth in tissue culture takes only a few days in many cases and less than a week in most; identification of type frequently takes much more time. A complete diagnostic isolation spectrum can be obtained using suckling mouse inoculation. Specimens for virus isolation should be obtained from the throat and rectum (feces) and any other clinically involved site. Virus isolation from all sites except the feces can usually be considered causally related to a specific illness. Molecular biology methods may detect viral RNA. Demonstration of a rise in neutralizing antibody titer to a virus recovered from the feces indicates recent infection and tends to indicate a causal role for the isolated virus. Serum should be collected and stored frozen as soon as possible after the onset of illness and then again 2–4 wk later.

DIFFERENTIAL DIAGNOSIS. The differential diagnosis of enteroviral infections depends upon the clinical manifestations. It is most important to distinguish bacterial diseases such as those commonly associated with pharyngitis, pneumonia, pericarditis, meningitis, and septicemia, although other viral illnesses must also be considered.

Paralytic Poliomyelitis. Conditions causing muscular weakness include the following:

1. *Infectious neuronitis* (Guillain-Barré syndrome) is the most common disease and the most difficult to distinguish from poliomyelitis. Generally, the fever, headache, and meningeal signs are less notable. Paralysis is characteristically symmetric, and sensory changes and pyramidal tract signs are common but are absent in poliomyelitis. Characteristically, there are few cells but elevated globulin content in the cerebrospinal fluid.
2. *Peripheral neuritis*—postinjectional, toxic (lead, avitaminosis), paralytic cranial herpes zoster, postdiphtheritic neuropathy—is excluded by history, sensory examination, and related findings.
3. Arthropod-borne viral *encephalitis, rabies,* and *tetanus* have been confused with bulbar poliomyelitis.
4. *Botulism* may closely simulate bulbar poliomyelitis; nuchal-spinal rigidity and pleocytosis are absent.
5. *Demyelinizing types of encephalomyelitis* are associated with or follow the exanthems and other infections or occur as an untoward sequel of antirabies vaccination.
6. *Tick-bite* paralysis is uncommon; meningeal signs are absent, and removal of the tick is followed by swift recovery.
7. *Neoplasms* originating in and around the spinal cord may rarely have a fairly abrupt onset.
8. *Familial periodic paralysis, myasthenia gravis,* and *acute porphyria* are uncommon causes of weakness.
9. *Hysteria* and *malingering* are rare in children.

Conditions causing pseudoparalysis do not present with nuchal-spinal rigidity or pleocytosis and include the following:

1. *Unrecognized trauma* from contusions, sprains, fractures, and epiphyseal separation is a common cause of diagnostic confusion.
2. *Nonspecific (toxic) synovitis* produces a limp, usually unilaterally; the hip and the knee are the most common sites. There may be low-grade fever for several days.
3. *Acute osteomyelitis* has a more septic course; there is polymorphonuclear leukocytosis, with localized signs, positive blood culture, and, later, roentgenographic changes.
4. In *acute rheumatic fever* the clinical pattern is usually diagnostic.
5. *Scurvy* is revealed by a history of inadequate intake of vitamin C and by roentgenographic changes in the bones.
6. *Congenital syphilitic osteomyelitis* of the acute painful type is found only in early infancy.

Other Enteroviral Illnesses. The differential diagnoses of other enteroviral syndromes (respiratory, pericarditis/myocarditis, exanthems, meningitis/encephalitis, and so forth) are presented in the respective sections of this book relating to the clinical category.

COMPLICATIONS. Paralytic Poliomyelitis. *Melena* severe enough to require transfusion may result from single or multiple superficial intestional erosions; perforation is rare. *Acute gastric dilatation* may occur abruptly during the acute or convalescent stage, causing further embarrassment of respiration; immediate gastric aspiration and external application of ice bags are indicated. Mild *hypertension* of a few days' or weeks' duration is common in the acute stage, probably related to lesions of the vasoregulatory centers in the medulla and especially to underventilation. In the later stages, because of immobilization, hypertension may occur along with hypercalcemia, nephrocalcinosis, and vascular lesions. Dimness of vision, headache, and a light-headed feeling in association with hypertension should be regarded as premonitory of a frank *convulsion*. *Cardiac irregularities* are uncommon, but electrocardiographic abnormalities suggesting myocarditis are not rare. *Acute pulmonary edema* occurs occasionally, particularly in patients with arterial hypertension. *Pulmonary embolism* is uncommon despite the immobilization. Skeletal decalcification begins soon after immobilization and results in *hypercalciuria*, which in turn predisposes to *calculi*, especially when urinary stasis and infection are present. A high fluid intake is the only effective prophylactic measure. The patient should be mobilized as much and as early as possible.

Complications of enteroviral infections such as those associated with myocarditis or encephalitis are presented in other sections of this text.

PREVENTION. In the United States and other developed countries poliomyelitis has been virtually eliminated through the widespread use of either inactivated (IPV) or oral polio vaccines (OPV) (Sec. 5.1). However, in many areas of the world endemic and epidemic poliomyelitis is still a problem.

Attenuated viral vaccines for enteroviruses other than polioviruses are not available. However, passive protection with pooled human immune globulin (0.2 mL/kg intramuscularly) may be useful in preventing disease. This is worthwhile only in sudden and virulent nursery outbreaks. Pooled human immune globulin in most instances can be expected to contain antibodies against coxsackievirus types B1–B5, offering protection to those infants without transplacentally acquired specific antibody who have not yet become infected.

TREATMENT. Poliomyelitis. The broad principles of management are to allay fear, to minimize ensuing skeletal deformities, to anticipate and meet complications in addition to the neuromusculoskeletal ones, and to prepare the child and family for the prolonged treatment that may be required and for permanent disability when this seems likely. Patients with the nonparalytic and mildly paralytic forms of poliomyelitis may be treated at home.

For the **abortive form** simple analgesics, sedatives, an attractive diet, and bed rest until the child's temperature is normal for several days suffice. Avoidance of exertion for the ensuing 2 wk is desirable, and there should be a careful neuromusculoskeletal examination 2 mo later to detect any minor involvement.

Treatment for the **nonparalytic form** is similar to that for the abortive form, relief being indicated in particular for the discomfort of muscle tightness and spasm of the neck, trunk, and extremities. Analgesics are more effective when combined with the application of hot packs for 15–30 min every 2–4 hr. Hot tub baths are sometimes useful. A firm bed is desirable and can be improvised at home by placing table leaves or a sheet of plywood beneath the mattress. A footboard should be used to keep the feet at a right angle with the legs. Muscular discomfort and spasm may continue for some weeks, even in the nonparalytic form, necessitating hot packs and gentle physical therapy. Such patients should also be carefully examined 2 mo after apparent recovery to detect minor residuals that might cause postural problems in later years.

Most patients with the **paralytic form** require hospitalization. A calm atmosphere is desirable. Suitable body alignment is necessary to avoid excessive skeletal deformity. A neutral position with the feet at a right angle, knees slightly flexed, and hips and spine straight is achieved by use of boards, sandbags, and, occasionally, light splint shells. Active and passive motions are indicated as soon as the pain has disappeared. Opiates and sedatives are permissible only if no impairment of ventilation is present or impending. Constipation is common, and fecal impaction should be prevented. When bladder paralysis occurs, a parasympathetic stimulant such as bethanechol (Urecholine), 5–10 mg orally or 2.5–5.0 mg subcutaneously, may induce voiding in 15–30 min; some patients do not respond, and others have nausea, vomiting, and palpitation. Bladder paresis rarely lasts more than a few days. If bethanechol fails, manual compression of the bladder and the psychologic effect of running water should be tried. If catheterization must be performed, strict asepsis is essential. An interesting diet and a relatively high fluid intake should be started at once unless there is vomiting. Additional salt should be provided if the environmental temperature is high or if the application of hot packs induces sweating. Anorexia is common initially. Adequate dietary and fluid intake can be maintained by the placement of a central venous catheter. The orthopedist and the physiatrist should see these patients as early in the course of illness as possible and assume responsibility before fixed deformities develop. The management of *pure bulbar poliomyelitis* consists of maintaining the airway and avoiding all risks of inhalation of saliva, food, or vomitus. Gravity drainage of accumulated secretions is favored by using the head-low (foot of bed elevated 20–25 degrees) prone position with the face to one side. Aspirators with rigid or semirigid tips are preferred for direct oral and pharyngeal use, and soft flexible catheters may be used for nasopharyngeal aspiration. Fluid and electrolyte equilibrium is best maintained by intravenous infusion, since tube or oral feeding in the first few days may incite vomiting. In addition to close observation for respiratory insufficiency, the blood pressure should be taken at least twice daily, since hypertension is not uncommon and occasionally leads to hypertensive encephalopathy. Patients with pure bulbar poliomyelitis may require tracheostomy because of vocal cord paralysis or constriction of the hypopharynx; the majority who recover have little residual impairment, although some patients exhibit mild dysphagia and occasional vocal fatigue with slurring of speech.

Impaired ventilation must be recognized early; mounting anxiety, restlessness, and fatigue are early indications for prompt intervention (Sec. 6.34). Tracheostomy is indicated for some patients with pure bulbar poliomyelitis, spinal respiratory muscle paralysis, and bulbospinal paralysis, since these patients are generally unable to cough, sometimes for many months. Mechanical respirators are often needed.

Nonpolio Enteroviruses. There is no specific therapy for any enterovirus infection. In severe, catastrophic, and generalized neonatal infection, it is probably advisable to administer immune globulin to the infant, but there is no evidence that this therapy is beneficial. Corticosteroids should not be given during acute severe enteroviral infections, such as neonatal myocarditis or encephalitis, although some authors believe this therapy has been beneficial in patients with coxsackievirus myocarditis. These agents have had deleterious effects in experimental coxsackieviral infections of mice. Since the possibility of bacterial sepsis cannot be ruled out in many instances of enteroviral infections, antibiotics should frequently be administered for the most likely potential bacterial pathogens. Therapy of myocarditis and meningoencephalitis is discussed in Sec. 15.70 and 12.11, respectively.

PROGNOSIS. Mortality in large urban epidemics of poliomyelitis in the United States in the prevaccine era was 5–7%. Most deaths occur within the first 2 wk after onset. Mortality and the degree of disability are greater after the age of puberty. In general, the more extensive the paralysis in the first 10 days of illness, the more severe the ultimate disability. Unexpected improvement may appear soon after defervescence and again about 6 wk after onset, a time that corresponds to functional restoration of temporarily inactive neurons. The degree of functional recovery also depends upon the adequacy and promptness of therapy as related to proper body positioning, active motion, use of assistive devices, and, of great importance, the psychologic motivation of the patient to return to as full and normal a life as possible. A long-term follow-up study of adults with post-poliomyelitis neuromuscular symptoms has shown slowly progressive non–life-threatening muscle weakness, with a greater effect occurring in patients in whom poliomyelitis had caused severe disability and muscle weakness (see Sec. 21.37).

The prognosis in nonpolio enteroviral infections in the vast majority of instances is excellent. Morbidity and mortality are related almost entirely to cardiac and neurologic disease in older children and these same diseases accompanied by general disseminated infection in neonates.

JAMES D. CHERRY

GENERAL

Cherry JD: Enteroviruses. *In:* Remington JS, Klein JO (eds): Infectious Diseases of the Fetus and Newborn Infant, 3rd ed. Philadelphia, WB Saunders, 1990.

Cherry JD: Enteroviruses: Polioviruses (poliomyelitis), coxsackieviruses, echoviruses and enteroviruses. *In:* Feigin RD, Cherry JD (eds): Textbook of Pediatric Infectious Diseases, 2nd ed. Philadelphia, WB Saunders, 1987, p 1729.

Melnick JL: Enteroviruses. *In:* Evans AS (ed): Viral Infections of Humans; Epidemiology and Control, 3rd ed. New York, Plenum Medical Book Co, 1989, p 191.

SPECIFIC

Bodian D, Horstmann DM: Poliomyelitis. *In:* Horsfall FL, Tamm I (eds): Viral and Rickettsial Infections of Man, 4th ed. Philadelphia, JB Lippincott, 1965.

Dagan R, Hall CB, Powell KR, et al: Epidemiology and laboratory diagnosis of infection with viral and bacterial pathogens in infants hospitalized for suspected sepsis. J Pediatr 115:351, 1989.

Hayward JC, Gillespie SM, Kaplan KM, et al: Outbreak of poliomyelitis-like paralysis associated with enterovirus 71. Pediatr Infect Dis J 8:611, 1989.

Howard RS, Wiles CM, Spencer GT: The late sequelae of poliomyelitis. Q J Med (New Series 66) 251:219, 1988.

Kaplan MH, Klein SW, McPhee J, et al: Group B coxsackievirus infections in infants younger than three months of age: A serious childhood illness. Rev Infect Dis 5:1019, 1983.

Modlin JF: Perinatal echovirus infection: Insights from a literature review of 61 cases of serious infection and 16 outbreaks in nurseries. Rev Infect Dis 8:918, 1986.

Moore M: Enteroviral disease in the United States, 1970–1979. J Infect Dis 146:103, 1982.

Strikas RA, Anderson LJ, Parker RA: Temporal and geographic patterns of isolates of nonpolio enterovirus in the United States, 1970–1983. J Infect Dis 153:346, 1986.

Yin-Murphy M: Acute hemorrhagic conjunctivitis. Prog Med Virol 29:23, 1984.

12.81 ROTAVIRUS

Diarrhea is a significant public health problem in the developing and the developed world. Rotavirus is the most common agent responsible for infantile diarrhea throughout the world and is responsible for more than 140 million episodes per year and 1 million deaths worldwide. In the United States rotavirus causes more than 3.5 million episodes of diarrhea per year with 70,000 hospitalizations and approximately 100 deaths.

ETIOLOGY. Rotavirus is a genus in the Reoviridae family. The virus is a wheel-like, 70-nm, double-stranded RNA structure. There are seven groups (A–E), which are distinguished by different antigenic and RNA patterns. Group A is the main group affecting infants and older children and, to a lesser extent, adults, whereas group B affects mammals and has been recently identified in sick adults and children, predominantly in China. Group C has rarely been reported in humans but is found in other mammals, whereas group D (birds) and group E (pigs) have not been isolated from humans. There is no antigenic cross-reactivity or RNA cross-hybridization between the seven rotavirus groups.

Group A rotavirus has two subgroups based on antigenic differences. Group A subgroups I and II may be clinically indistinguishable except that the latter is associated with less emesis and more fever and is possibly more virulent than subgroup I.

The group A rotavirus genome is composed of 11 segments of double-stranded RNA. Strains of group A rotavirus can be identified by different migration patterns of RNA subjected to polyacrylamide electrophoresis (PAGE). The RNA genome may undergo frequent point mutations, genomic reassortments, and subsequent antigenic drifts. In a community there is often one dominant antigenic strain as determined by PAGE; however, many minor strains may also be present. During epidemics many serotypes (genotypes) appear either simultaneously or sequentially. This diversity places the patient at risk for subsequent reinfection and makes the development of a vaccine more difficult.

Vp7 and Vp4 are the major outer capsid proteins that elicit neutralizing antibodies. The serotype is determined by Vp7. Responses against Vp4 also influence immunity. Vp6 is an inner capsid protein that is a group-specific common antigen. The immune response to asymptomatic and symptomatic native and vaccine-initiated infection includes both local IgA and serum IgG antibodies. Protection against rechallenge can be induced by prior infection or vaccination, but is not definitively correlated with a specific response.

EPIDEMIOLOGY. Rotavirus infection is most common in the winter in temperate climates; epidemics spread progressively eastward from the western United States to the northeastern United States during the course of a winter.

In adults rotavirus is acquired from contact with infected infants, as an endemic illness, during water-borne epidemics, during travelers' diarrhea, or during other epidemics in closed populations. Adults infected with rotavirus may be asymptomatic. Infants less than 2 yr of age are the most commonly infected population; attack rates vary from 10 to 40/100 person years in the first 2 yr of life. Classic rotavirus enteritis is uncommon in infants less than 6 mo of age. Nonetheless, both asymptomatic primary (seroconversion) and serious (necrotizing enterocolitis, hemorrhagic colitis) infections have been reported as nosocomial infections in hospitalized preterm infants.

The incubation period is 36–48 hr, and viral shedding continues for 2–5 days (occasionally longer) after diarrhea stops. The route of transmission is predominantly fecal-oral; nosocomial infection during hospital epidemics and spread in day-care centers are common. Animal-to-human transmission is rare. As many as 10% of rotavirus-infected infants may have simultaneous infection with other gastrointestinal pathogens (*Salmonella, Shigella, E. coli*).

PATHOPHYSIOLOGY. Rotavirus replicates on the differentiated columnar epithelial cells at the apex of the small intestinal villi. Secondary disaccharidase deficiency may ensue but is not the pathogenetic mechanism of the initial diarrhea, the pathogenesis of which is unknown. A major mechanism may be decreased absorption of salt and water due to selective infection of the villous cells responsible for fluid absorption. The net result is increased intestinal fluid losses. The pathology may demonstrate cephalocaudad progression of exfoliation of mature enterocytes, villous flattening, irregularity of microvilli, and lymphocyte infiltration of the lamina propria. The acute changes are transient, and, in the absence of secondary disaccharidase deficiency or prior malnutrition, the intestinal histology returns to normal within 48–96 hr.

CLINICAL MANIFESTATIONS. Rotavirus affects infants

over 6 mo and under 2 yr of age with characteristic manifestations of fever, nonbilious emesis, and profuse watery, nonfoul-smelling diarrhea. The stool does not contain red blood cells or leukocytes. Fever (37.9–39° C) is present in as many as 50% of patients, and a smaller group may have temperatures over 39° C. In addition, infants may demonstrate rhinitis and erythema of the tympanic membranes or posterior pharynx. Additional clinical features such as irritability and lethargy are noted with similar frequency in rotavirus and nonrotavirus gastroenteritis.

Isotonic dehydration with acidosis is a common result of rotavirus infection. The duration of symptoms is 3–9 days, and, in developed countries, rotavirus infection usually is a self-limited disease, although dehydration may require hospitalization. In developing countries rotovirus infection is a major cause of death. Patients at increased risk for chronic rotavirus infection include immunocompromised hosts who have primary immunodeficiency diseases or are receiving immunosuppressive therapy (bone marrow transplantation). Rotavirus infection in malnourished infants is particularly serious and exacerbates the poor nutritional status, resulting in malabsorption, dehydration, and death.

DIAGNOSIS. Electron microscopy typically demonstrates the 72-nm wheel-like virus but is an impractical diagnostic method. Currently, various antigen-detecting immunoassays are the methods of choice for the diagnosis of group A rotavirus infection. ELISA is the most popular method because of its acceptable sensitivity and its simplicity. RNA probes and PAGE have been important epidemiologic methods in tracing epidemics, identifying different group A serotypes or subgroups, and distinguishing group A from non-group A rotaviruses (groups B–E). The differential diagnosis includes other viral, bacterial, and parasitic causes of diarrhea (see Sec. 12.10).

TREATMENT. Most cases of rotavirus infection are self-limited and can be managed by careful administration of oral fluid and electrolyte rehydration solutions. Once dehydration has been corrected, milk feeding can be reinstituted despite ongoing diarrhea. If emesis precludes enteral intake, intravenous fluids may have to be administered.

There is no specific antiviral therapy for rotavirus infection. Epidemics have been stopped by instituting good handwashing techniques and on occasion by the oral administration of intravenous human immunoglobulin. Experimental evidence suggests that protease inhibitors may be a potentially effective oral therapy for rotaviral diarrhea.

PREVENTION. Good hygiene will prevent fecal-oral spread of rotavirus, and breast-feeding may reduce the potential risk or severity of infection.

Rotavirus oral vaccines are being developed from attenuated calf (RIT 4237,WC-3) or rhesus monkey (MMU-18006) rotavirus strains. So far vaccines have given inconsistant but occasionally excellent protection.

ROBERT M. KLIEGMAN
STANLEY A. PLOTKIN

Candy DC: Viral diseases of the gastrointestinal tract. Curr Opin Infect Dis 3:263, 1990.

Hardy DB: Epidemiology of rotaviral infection in adults. Rev Infect Dis 9:461, 1987.

Kovacs A, Chan L, Hotrakitya C, et al: Rotavirus gastroenteritis: Clinical and laboratory features and use of the rotazyme test. Am J Dis Child 141:161, 1987.

LeBarron CW, Lew J, Glass RI, et al: Annual rotavirus epidemic patterns in North America: Results of a 5 year retrospective survey of 88 centers in Canada, Mexico, and the United States. JAMA 264:983, 1990.

Penaranda ME, Cubitt WD, Sinarachatanant P, et al: Group C rotavirus infections in patients with diarrhea in Thailand, Nepal, and England. J Infect Dis 160:392, 1989.

Puzzling diversity of rotaviruses (Editorial). Lancet 335:573, 1990.

Rodriguez WJ: Viral enteritis in the 1980s: Perspective, diagnosis and outlook for prevention. Pediatr Infect Dis J 1:570, 1989.

Vial PA, Kotloff KL, Losonsky GA: Molecular epidemiology of rotavirus infection in a room for convalescing newborns. J Infect Dis 157:668, 1988.

12.82 RABIES
(Hydrophobia)

Rabies is a viral infection of the central nervous system usually transmitted by contamination of a wound with saliva from a rabid animal and virtually 100% fatal once symptoms develop.

ETIOLOGY. Rabies virus belongs to the rhabdovirus group. The viral particles resemble striated bullets. Inside the cylinder is the RNA-containing nucleocapsid. Antibodies to the nucleocapsid can be detected in infected animals, but only antibodies to the surface glycoproteins are neutralizing and protective.

EPIDEMIOLOGY. Rabies is a widespread infection of warm-blooded animals. In North America rabies occurs principally in skunks, raccoons, foxes, and bats. In the United States cats are more likely than dogs to be rabid. In Central and South America dogs are the usual source of exposure. Vampire bats, which bite cattle, are an important part of the cycle of rabies in Latin America. Europe has had an epizootic of fox rabies, with many humans being bitten. In Asia and Africa the principal problem is the rabid dog. Social factors limit efforts at control of stray dogs. Human rabies is still common in the tropics as a result of canine rabies, although poor reporting precludes precise statements as to incidence. The production of numerous monoclonal antibodies (MAb) to rabies virus strains has revealed considerable antigenic variation in both the glycoprotein and nucleocapsid antigens of the virus. The result has been the identification of variant strains (called rabies-related viruses) and antigenic differences among true rabies virus that correlate with host species or geographic location. For example, strains isolated from cattle rabies in South America resemble bat strains, confirming the transmission of virus from the vampire bat to the cow.

Recently the concept of rabies-free land areas has been promulgated. This permits health authorities in certain locations to omit vaccination after most dog bites on the grounds that terrestrial rabies has been unknown there for years. Nevertheless, practically every state has rabies in rural wildlife; in 1987, 26 states reported canine rabies, and 45 states reported rabid bats. The continent of Australia and many islands, including those of the United Kingdom and Hawaii, are totally free of rabies.

PATHOGENESIS AND PATHOLOGY. The means by which rabies virus travels from the wound to the brain are only partially understood. Since the virus attaches to and penetrates cells rapidly in vitro, it is unlikely that it remains dormant in the wound for long periods of time. Moreover, although the virus has been shown to ascend axons from the periphery to the spinal cord, the speed of spread (3 mm/hr) is far too rapid to explain the long incubation period of the disease.

In animals the virus first multiplies in striated muscle. It may be hypothesized that antibody, interferon, and other host factors then act on the virus as it leaves striated muscle; if these factors are insufficiently protective, virus eventually attaches to the nerve. From then on, rabies may be inevitable. The possibility that the virus must overcome another barrier in passing from the first infected neuron to other neurons is indicated by electron microscopic studies of the brain, which demonstrate viral passage from cell to contiguous cell.

The basic lesion in the brain is neuronal destruction in the brain stem and medulla. The cerebral cortex is usually normal in the absence of prolonged anoxia before death. The hippocampus, thalamus, and basal ganglia often show neuronal destruction and glial infiltrates. The most severe pathology is evident in the pons and the floor of the 4th ventricle. The inspiratory muscle spasms that result in the striking symptom of hydrophobia may be due to destruction of brain stem neurons inhibitory to the neurons of the nucleus ambiguus, which control inspiration. Hydrophobia does not occur in other diseases, since only rabies combines brain stem encephalitis with intact cortex and maintenance of consciousness.

The Negri body, long the pathologic hallmark of rabies, is a cytoplasmic inclusion found in neurons; it consists of clumped viral nucleocapsid. The absence of Negri bodies does not exclude rabies; fluorescent antibody stains of brain sections or smears may be positive in their absence.

Transmission. In animals as in humans rabies produces encephalitis as the principal symptom. After establishment of the encephalitis, however, the virus spreads down nerves from the brain. It multiplies in many organs, but those important to transmission are the salivary glands. Not all rabid animals have virus in the saliva, and even when it is present, the quantity is variable. Skunks are particularly likely to have large amounts of virus in saliva. Although dogs may have virus in saliva for many days before symptoms occur, transmission to man from dogs who appeared normal for 10 days or more after a biting incident has not been reported. The variability of virus in saliva explains the fact that less than half of untreated bites by proven rabid animals will result in rabies.

Scratches by the claws of rabid animals are dangerous because animals lick their claws. Saliva applied to a mucosal surface such as the conjunctiva may be infectious.

Bat excreta contain enough rabies virus to pose a danger of rabies to those who enter infested caves and inhale aerosols created by bats. Aerosols of rabies virus inadvertently produced in laboratories are dangerous to laboratory workers.

In general, if a biting animal does not die within 10 days, rabies is unlikely, although rarely a rabid terrestrial animal will recover from rabies. Bats, on the contrary, are often infected for long periods without showing symptoms.

Transmission of rabies by corneal transplant from patients with undiagnosed rabies encephalitis to healthy recipients has been recorded with sufficient frequency to warrant exclusion of donors dead from unexplained neurologic disease. Human-to-human transmission is theoretically possible but is poorly documented and rare if it occurs at all.

CLINICAL MANIFESTATIONS. The incubation period of rabies is extremely variable. Exceptionally long incubation periods have been described and a 7 yr incubation period was recently confirmed by strain identification. On the other hand, an incubation period of only 9 days has followed severe exposure. Usually, the incubation period is 20–180 days with the peak at 30–60 days. It tends to be shorter in children and in vaccinated individuals who nevertheless develop rabies.

There is usually a prodromal phase of rabies, lasting 2–10 days. Common nonspecific symptoms include fever, malaise, headache, anorexia, and vomiting. The patient may be troubled by ill-defined anxiety. Characteristic symptoms at this stage are pain, pruritus, or paresthesia at the site of the wound.

The illness then enters an acute neurologic phase, of either the furious or paralytic variety, which lasts 2–10 days. In the former, *hydrophobia* is a pathognomonic sign. Attempts to swallow liquids, including saliva, result in aspiration into the trachea. Hydrophobia appears to be an exaggerated respiratory tract protective reflex, perhaps mediated by neuronal dysfunction in certain areas of the brain stem. Eventually a psychologic component exacerbates the spasms, and even the sight of water evokes terror. *Aerophobia* may be present and is considered by some also to be pathognomonic of rabies. Aerophobia is elicited by fanning a current of air across the face, which causes violent spasms of the pharyngeal and neck muscles.

The neurologic picture in the typical case may consist of bursts of hyperactivity, disorientation, and bizarre combative behavior, alternating with periods of lucidity. During the patient's lucid periods he or she may be aware of what is happening and may be able to articulate his or her fears. The facial expression of the patient is one of grim hopelessness.

Patients may also complain of pharyngeal pain, difficulty in swallowing, and hoarseness. Seizures are common, perhaps on the basis of hypoxia compounded by hyperventilation.

Some rabid patients develop meningismus or even opisthotonos. The cerebrospinal fluid may reflect meningeal irritation, with varying elevations of cells (predominantly lymphocytes) and protein, or may be normal. The peripheral white blood cell count often shows a polymorphonuclear leukocytosis.

In about 20% of patients, an ascending symmetric paralysis with flaccidity and decreased tendon reflexes dominates the entire acute phase. This course is particularly common after vampire bat bites. In the remainder of cases paralysis develops toward the end of the acute neurologic phase.

If the patient does not die of cardiorespiratory arrest during the acute stage, he or she slips into coma. With modern intensive care, life may be prolonged, but numerous complications occur during coma. Most significant is myocarditis, manifested by hypotension and arrhythmias. Rabies virus has been recovered from the heart, which shows inflammation at autopsy. Also prominent is pituitary dysfunction expressed as either diabetes insipidus or inappropriate secretion of antidiuretic hormone.

DIAGNOSIS AND DIFFERENTIAL DIAGNOSIS. When a patient has a history of having been bitten by an animal, paresthesias at the wound site, and hydrophobia, a clinical diagnosis of rabies is not difficult. Any disease in which there is encephalitis may occasionally cause confusion, such as those caused by arboviruses, enteroviruses, and *herpes simplex*. However, if one finds signs of brain stem involvement in a patient whose sensorium is basically clear and who has no signs of a space-occupying lesion, other diagnoses can usually be set aside.

Paralytic rabies may be misdiagnosed as *Guillain-Barré syndrome, poliomyelitis*, or *postrabies vaccine encephalomyelitis*. Careful neurologic examination and analysis of the cerebrospinal fluid will often help rule out these diagnoses.

The spasms of *tetanus* may cause momentary diagnostic confusion, but trismus is not seen in rabies, and hydrophobia is not seen in tetanus. *Botulism* (wound or ingestion) will cause paralysis, but the absence of sensory changes should exclude rabies.

Perhaps the most confusing differential problem is *hysteria* in an individual who thinks he or she has rabies. Normal blood gases and the absence of variation in bizarre behavior will suggest pseudorabies.

Laboratory diagnosis is now possible before death. The virus may be demonstrated by fluorescent antibody stain of smears of corneal epithelial cells or sections of skin from the neck at the hairline. These tests are positive because virus migrates down the nerves from the brain; both the cornea and hair follicles are richly innervated. Autopsy examination of the brains of patients with fatal encephalitis should include fluorescent antibody tests for rabies.

Serologic diagnosis is also possible if the patient survives beyond the acute period. Neutralizing antibodies develop eventually in both serum and cerebrospinal fluid and rapidly rise to extremely high levels, for example, more than 100 international units (IU). Vaccination, even with potent vaccine, is unlikely to raise titers above 20 IU.

TABLE 12–35. Rabies Postexposure Prophylaxis Guide–1989 (CDC Recommendations)*

Animal Species	Condition of Animal at Time of Attack	Treatment of Exposed Person†
Dog and cat	Healthy and available for 10 days observation	None, unless animal develops rabies
	Rabid or suspected rabid	Rabies-immune serum and HDCV‡ or RVA§
	Unknown (escaped)	Consult public health official. If treatment is indicated, give rabies-immune serum and HDCV or RVA
Skunk, racoon, fox, bat, and other carnivores	Regard as rabid unless proved negative by laboratory tests‖	Rabies-immune serum and HDCV or RVA
Livestock, rodents, and lagomorphs (rabbits and hares)	Consider individually. Local and state public health officials should be consulted on questions about the need for rabies prophylaxis. Bites of groundhogs, squirrels, hamsters, guinea pigs, gerbils, chipmunks, rats, mice, other rodents, rabbits, and hares almost never call for antirabies prophylaxis	

*The following recommendations are only a guide. In applying them, take into account the animal species involved, the circumstances of the exposure, the vaccination status of the animal, and the presence of rabies in the region. Local or state public health officials should be consulted if questions arise about the need for rabies prophylaxis.

†All bites and wounds should be immediately thoroughly cleansed with soap and water. If antirabies treatment is indicated, rabies-immune serum and rabies vaccine (HDCV or RVA) should be given as soon as possible, regardless of the interval from exposure. Local reactions to vaccines are common and do not contraindicate continuing treatment. Discontinue vaccine if immunofluorescene tests of the animal are negative.

During the usual holding period of 10 days, begin treatment with rabies-immune serum and HDCV or RVA at first sign of rabies in a dog or cat that has bitten someone. The symptomatic animal should be killed immediately and tested. If HRIG is not available, use equine antirabies serum. Do not use more than the recommended dosage.

‡HDCV = human diploid cell vaccine.

§RVA = rhesus monkey fibroblast cell cultures.

‖The animal should be killed and tested as soon as possible. Holding for observation is not recommended.

PROGNOSIS. Although patients can be kept alive for months with intensive care, only three patients have survived rabies, and the prognosis is bleak.

Prevention of Rabies

PRE-EXPOSURE PROPHYLAXIS. Vaccination of domestic dogs and elimination of strays have resulted in eradication of terrestrial rabies from many areas. If dog control were properly practiced, rabies could be suppressed in much of the world.

Those who are expected to be at risk, such as veterinarians, laboratory workers, and children going to rabies-enzootic areas, can be preimmunized. The cell culture vaccine (see later) will produce virtually 100% response with 3 doses given at 0, 7, and 28 days. A titer of 0.3 IU has been accepted as protective.

POSTEXPOSURE PROPHYLAXIS. First, a decision must be made about whether rabies prophylaxis is necessary. In many areas of the United States, rabies in mammals has been unknown for years. However, the unprovoked bite of a wild animal should be considered rabid if the animal belongs to a species known to be a rabies host, such as a skunk, fox, raccoon, bat, or coyote. Rodents are very rarely carriers of rabies in the United States. Knowledge of the local epidemiology of rabies is essential to the physician contemplating treatment of a human exposure. Unprovoked bites by bats or other wild animals almost always require immunization; decisions regarding bites from domestic or pet animals should be made after discussion with public health veterinarians.

If a domestic animal such as a dog or cat is the offender, consideration must be given to the question of provocation, to the clinical appearance of the animal if apprehended, and to the rabies vaccination status of the animal. Difficulty in making decisions arises when the biting animal has run away after a seemingly unprovoked attack. Whether the animal was rabid or merely ill-tempered is often impossible to decide. When the animal is under observation, rabies treatment can be withheld until the animal acts abnormally, at which point it should be sacrificed and tested for rabies. However, a wild animal should be killed immediately and its brain examined for rabies antigen by the fluorescent-antibody technique. Table 12–35 may help in making the often difficult decision about whether or not to treat.

If rabies prophylaxis is to be given after exposure, prevention depends on three complementary means of reducing the risk. Local treatment (see later) is designed to kill the virus by mechanical and virucidal action. Passive antibody (see later) then provides immediate blockage of attachment of virus to the nerve endings. However, passive antibody ultimately disappears and must be replaced by the active response provided by vaccine. The number of vaccine doses administered depends on its antigenic mass. The vaccine must not only produce a primary antibody response but also overcome the depressive effect of passive antibody on the immune response.

LOCAL TREATMENT. The chief requirement of local treatment is that it be prompt and thorough. Simple mechanical removal by soap and water should be the first step, using copious amounts of solution. Catheters should be inserted for irrigation of puncture wounds. If the mechanical trauma of the local treatment is painful, procaine-type anesthetics may be used to infiltrate the area without adding risk.

The mechanical removal of virus may be followed by application of a virucidal solution such as 1% povidone-iodine or 70% alcohol. In an emergency, any alcoholic liquor of 86 proof or higher may be used. However, most authorities eschew antisepsis and depend on soap and water irrigation.

PASSIVE ANTIBODY. Passive immunization must be given to protect the patient until vaccination produces antibodies. Passive antibody is available in the form of equine antiserum (Sclavo) or human rabies immune globulin (Cutter and Merieux). The latter avoids serum sickness reactions to equine protein, which occur in about 5% of recipients of the animal product. The dose for human rabies immune globulin is 20 IU/kg. Up to half of the dose should be infiltrated subcutaneously at the site of bite or scratch; the remainder is injected intramuscularly into the arm or buttocks. The dose for equine antirabies serum is 40 IU/kg delivered in the same manner.

Passive immunization should be performed regardless of the interval between rabies exposure and treatment. However, if vaccine was started previously there is no need for passive immunization once 8 days have elapsed. Anaphylaxis is a possibility with the equine antiserum, and tests for hypersensitivity should be carried out in the usual manner (consult package insert). Steroids should be avoided if possible in the treatment of reactions, since they cause activation of rabies virus in experimental animals.

ACTIVE IMMUNIZATION. Early rabies vaccines were prepared in the central nervous system of animals. Their antigenicity was poor and multiple injections were required. As a result postvaccination encephalitis was a frequent problem. Animal nerve tissue vaccines are still in use in many places in the world.

Human diploid cell vaccine (HDCV) was developed to increase immunogenicity and safety. HDCV has had more than 10 yr of commercial use in Europe and more recently in the United States and has withstood the challenge of severe exposures to confirmed rabid animals in Iran, West Germany, and France. HDCV is now the only vaccine licensed in this country.

HDCV is more antigenic than previous vaccines; accordingly, the number of doses can be reduced from the traditional 14 or 21. The current recommendation in the United States is 5 doses at 0, 3, 7, 14, and 28 days. For pre-exposure vaccination of high-risk groups, inoculations are given at 0, 7, and 28 days. The schedule that has been used in Europe for postexposure vaccination consists of 6 doses (1 mL intramuscularly) at 0, 3, 7, 14, 30, and 90 days.

Reaction rates have been low, and neurologic reactions have been rare, because no nerve tissue is present in the cell culture used to grow the virus. Allergic reactions have occurred in less than 0.1% after primary vaccination and systemic symptoms such as malaise and fever in only 5–15%. Nevertheless, administration of boosters results in an allergic reaction rate of 6%; accordingly, boosters are no longer routinely recommended, except following rabies exposure. A vaccine made in rhesus monkey fibroblast cell cultures (RVA) is manufactured by the Michigan State Health Department and may be useful in those who have reactions to HDCV. Several other cell culture vaccines are used outside of the United States, including one made in continuous cultures of Vero cells originating from African green monkey kidney.

TREATMENT OF CLINICAL RABIES. Large doses of interferon and antirabies serum have been advocated, but it is doubtful that these substances can affect rabies that has already spread to the brain.

STANLEY A. PLOTKIN

Anderson LJ, Sikes RK, Langkop CW, et al: Prophylactic immunization: Postexposure trial of a human diploid cell strain rabies vaccine. J Infect Dis 142:133, 1980.

Houff SA, Burton RC, Wilson RW, et al: Human-to-human transmission of rabies virus by corneal transplant. N Engl J Med 300:603, 1979.

Plotkin SA: Rabies vaccine prepared in human cell cultures: Progress and perspectives. Rev Infect Dis 2:433, 1980.

Plotkin SA, Clark HF: Committee on Immunization—prevention of rabies in man. J Infect Dis 123:227, 1971.

Plotkin SA, Clark HF: Rabies. *In*: Feigin RD, Cherry JD: Textbook of Pediatric Infectious Diseases. Philadelphia, WB Saunders, 1987, pp 1676–1684.

Public Health Service Advisory Committee on Immunization Practices: Rabies: Risk, management, prophylaxis, and immunization. MMWR, 1991.

Rupprecht CE, Dietzschold B: Perspectives on rabies virus pathogenesis (Editorial). Lab Invest 57:603, 1987.

Sureau P, Rollin P, Wiktor TJ: Epidemiologic analysis of antigenic variations of street rabies virus: Detection by monoclonal antibodies. Am J Epidemiol 117:605, 1983.

Turner GS: A review of the world epidemiology of rabies. Trans R Soc Trop Med Hyg 70:175, 1976.

Warrell DA: The clinical picture of rabies in man. Trans R Soc Trop Med Hyg 70:188, 1976.

12.83 HUMAN IMMUNODEFICIENCY VIRUS (HIV) INFECTION

(Acquired Immunodeficiency Syndrome [AIDS])

The emergence of AIDS during the past decade has generated worldwide concern. Advances in basic sciences have led to an understanding of its transmission, etiology, and pathogenesis, but prevention of spread has been variable among different high-risk groups, and therapy that is effective in prolonging life has only recently been identified. Pediatric AIDS in the 1990s may comprise a progressively larger proportion of the total cases, reflecting the increased perinatal transmission among intravenous drug abusers and other heterosexuals who are nonintravenous drug abusers. The profound effect of this disease on family structure, teenage sexuality, day-care and school attendance, pediatrician-family relationships, particularly in regard to confidentiality, legal and ethical issues, health care financing, and the development of extended ambulatory care facilities, home care, respite centers, and hospices is without recent parallel. The pediatrician's role as a coordinator of the efforts of the many different types of health care providers, the family, schools, government, religious groups, and the media and as an advocate for the patient poses unprecedented challenges.

ETIOLOGY. The human immunodeficiency virus (HIV or HIV-1), the etiologic agent of AIDS, is a retrovirus. Retroviruses are widely distributed among vertebrates, have been isolated from fish, reptiles, and birds, and have been recognized since the turn of the century as RNA tumor viruses. These viruses transfer genetic information from RNA to DNA, the reverse of the usual direction, by virtue of a unique enzyme, reverse transcriptase, which synthesizes DNA from viral RNA. Inactivation of a retrovirus is readily achieved with mild detergents, moderate pH variation, heating, or drying. Therefore, spread of these viruses requires close physical contact as in the exchange of blood or semen. Transmission is usually related to the presence of cells in fluids such as seminal or vaginal/cervical fluids. Cell-free fluids have a low frequency and low level of HIV contamination. Plasma levels are low, 10–50 infectious particles/mL compared with hepatitis B virus, which has 100 million–1 billion infectious particles/mL. This correlates with the relatively low risk of transmission of HIV compared with that of hepatitis B following needle-stick injury.

HIV has a long latency period, measured in months or years, during which the viral DNA or provirus is integrated into the host genome. Therefore, a long and unpredictable interval occurs between infection and disease manifestation. The mechanism of latency is unknown. Production of the p27 protein by the viral *nef* region, methylation of the viral genome, and variation in expression of the *tat* gene are among the possible explanations.

The virion includes an envelope, or surface glycoprotein, consisting of two proteins that coordinate HIV entrance into a cell. The larger, gp 120, is the component that specifies the target cell to be infected, particularly the CD4 receptor, or surface antigen, on T helper cells, macrophages/monocytes, Langerhans cells in the skin, glial cells, and bowel epithelium (particularly crypt cells and enterochromaffin cells). This large glycoprotein is a major target for an immune response against various infected cells. Hypervariable regions, which allow for rapid antigenic variation, are also found in the envelope. The smaller protein, gp 41 or transmembrane protein, may act as a fusion protein that interacts with a separate cellular receptor. These envelope glycoproteins are products of the *env* gene, one of the three structural genes of the virus. Another gene, the *gag* (group-specific antigen) gene, codes for several structural proteins within the oblong-shaped viral capsid. The largest of these proteins is the p24, which forms the core shell visible in electron micrographs. Others include the "matrix" protein adjacent to the membrane and a nonspecific nucleic acid–binding protein. A third gene, *pol*, synthesizes reverse transcriptase and proteases.

Other Retroviruses. A second agent, *HIV-2*, occurs in West African patients with AIDS and has been introduced into Brazil, several European countries, the United Kingdom, and the United States. The agent seems to have attenuated cytopathogenicity, and the illness may be milder than that due to HIV-1, although a fatal outcome has been described, as have dual infections with both HIV-1 and HIV-2.

HTLV-1 (human T cell lymphotropic virus type 1) is transmitted by breast-feeding, and 25% of neonates nursed by seropositive women become infected. Intrauterine and other perinatal routes are also important, as are blood transfusions and contaminated needles and syringes. Most infants remain asymptomatic for decades, but 2–4% of them develop adult T cell leukemia. Other clinical associations are *tropical spastic paraparesis* in the Caribbean, a myelopathy in Japan, and chronic relapsing polymyositis. HTLV-1 differs from HIV in morphologic and genetic structure, does not cross-react with HIV antigens, and does not cause AIDS. It may, however, serve as a cofactor in those infected with HIV and accelerate the course of the disease. Hemophiliacs who are co-infected with HIV and HTLV-1 are more likely to have AIDS if they have antibody to the *gag-env* antigen of HTLV-1. The Food and Drug Administration (FDA) recommends that whole blood and cellular components that are found to be repeatedly reactive by enzyme immunoassay (EIA) should be destroyed and the donors permanently deferred and counseled. The Western immunoblot and radioimmunoprecipitation assays provide confirmation of HTLV-1 seropositivity. The current seroprevalence rate in the United States is 0.025%. The risk of transmission by blood transfusion is 24/100,000 units.

Disease due to *HTLV-2* is of uncertain epidemiology, transmission, and clinical course. Hairy cell leukemia has been associated with this agent.

EPIDEMIOLOGY. AIDS exists worldwide, with over 215,000 cases from 153 nations reported to the World Health Organization as of January 31, 1990, including 40,500 cases from 48 African countries. In some areas of Africa 5–30% of pregnant women and 6–13% of pediatric inpatients are infected. Far fewer cases have been reported from Australia and Asia. In the United States 158,287 cases occurred in adults and adolescents and 2,786 in children less than 13 yr of age with 99,372 and 1,441 deaths, respectively (62.8% and 51.7% case fatality rates) from July 1981 to December 31, 1990. There were an estimated one million HIV infected persons in the United States and 5 million worldwide as of 1989.

In some states pediatric AIDS is virtually unknown; 63% of the total cases have occurred in New York, New Jersey, California, and Florida. Approximately 1.5% of all cases of AIDS in the United States occur in children under 13 yr of age using the classification system of the Centers for Disease Control (CDC). Perinatally acquired cases are increasing rapidly with a 38% increase in 1989 over 1988. The total number of cases is predicted to increase 3- to 20-fold from 1988 to 1991. In 75% of infected children, transmission occurred from mothers infected with HIV. Risk factors include a maternal history of AIDS, intravenous drug abuse, sexual intercourse with a high-risk male, and receipt of blood or blood products by either parent prior to April, 1985. In the remaining cases the child received infected blood or blood products, as in patients with hemophilia. An estimated 1 in 150,000 patients will contract HIV infection per unit of transfused blood components which test antibody negative. However, in high risk areas it may be as high as 1 in 42,000.

The prevalence of HIV infection in an infant born to an infected mother varies from 20 to 35%. Laboratory studies in the mother such as hemoglobin, white blood cell count, absolute lymphocytes, serum immunoglobulin levels (IgG, IgA, and IgM), and positive virus culture are not predictive of which infants will be infected. Maternal antibodies to gp120 epitopes have been correlated with reduced rates of transmission. In women with HIV infection there are often other associated perinatal risk factors such as lack of antenatal care, anemia, limited education, multigravidal status, alcohol abuse, cigarette smoking, and other sexually transmitted diseases, especially syphilis and gonorrhea. Many have antibodies to hepatitis B. Other problems such as abruptio placentae, chorioamnionitis, low birthweight, and intrauterine growth retardation and meconium staining are associated with intravenous drug abuse and are not due to HIV infection per se. If the mother has had a previously infected infant, the likelihood of recurrence of HIV infection in a subsequent pregnancy ranges from 50 to 65%, but there is no way to predict neonatal outcome in any specific case. In many instances the mother is asymptomatic and is unaware that she is HIV positive. Seroprevalence rates in pregnant women vary widely even within a given state. For example, in Massachusetts a 0.2–2.0% range was reported in rural and urban hospitals, respectively. Neonatal seroprevalence rates vary greatly, for example, 1/23 (University Hospital Newark, New Jersey), 1/61 (New York City hospitals generally), and 1/749 (New York state hospitals).

The ethnic distribution of perinatal cases is uneven, the minority community being especially devastated. Black children, who compose about 15% of the childhood population, account for 53% of all cases of pediatric AIDS. For Hispanic children the figures are 10 and 22%, respectively. Increasing heterosexual transmission, especially among female teenagers, has ominous implications for perinatal infection. Heterosexuals (nonintravenous drug abusers and intravenous drug abusers) accounted for nearly 4% of cases in the United States in 1988 compared with only 1% in 1982. Furthermore, about 80% of women with AIDS are in their peak child-bearing years, 13–39 yr. Female intravenous drug abusers also tend not to use contraceptive methods effectively and hence contribute significantly to perinatal transmission.

Adolescents account for 0.4% of the total AIDS population. HIV infection in this group is of major concern because expression of their disease may not occur for many years, and their willingness or ability to modify their high-risk sexual and drug-abusing behavior, even in response to education and counseling, is limited (also see Sec. 10.4 and 10.17). In one survey, for example, 26% practiced anal intercourse, and two thirds of those did not use condoms. About half of adolescents with HIV infection are homosexual or bisexual, and nearly a quarter have hemophilia or another coagulation disorder. Smaller proportions receive blood transfusions (6%), are intravenous drug addicts (6%), or have been infected by heterosexual contact (3%). Compared with adults, more teenage cases are acquired by heterosexual transmission, and a higher proportion are asymptomatic. Infants of infected teenage mothers pose special ethical, legal, medical, economic, and social issues. Furthermore, adolescents differ from adults in cognition, processing of information, and coping.

Rates of infection among adolescents vary widely among different groups. Military recruits have a rate of HIV seropositivity of 0.03% (range 0 to 0.6%) in 17–19 yr olds and 0.19%

(range 0 to 1.1%) age 20–24 yr. Job Corps entrants 16–21 yr old showed average seroprevalence level of 0.39% with 0.99% and 0.83% in black and Hispanic males, respectively. Among runaway and homeless youth in New York City 8% are HIV positive. The male-female ratio nationally in adolescents is 4:1 compared with 10:1 in adults. In New York City teenagers have a male-female ratio of 2.9:1, which is closer to that seen in Africa (1:1), where the disease is spread mainly via heterosexual contact. Clearly, adolescents have special needs that must be met to prevent widespread dissemination.

In the United States, childhood AIDS was the 9th leading cause of death between 1 and 4 yr of age and the 7th between the ages of 15 and 24 in 1989.

Transmission from Body Fluids Other than Blood or Semen. Postnatal transmission via breast milk has been suggested in several case reports, and HIV has been isolated from colostrum and breast milk. There are conflicting studies on whether or not breast-feeding is a major route of transmission. However, as a practical matter, breast-feeding by infected women should be avoided in industrialized nations but may be worth the potential risk in developing countries. Transmission may be enhanced if the infant has skin lesions such as impetigo or active eczema.

Saliva is unlikely to be a source of infection. Recovery of HIV is rare, and components in saliva have been shown to inactivate the agent. This issue is important in formulating guidelines for day-care attendance by children with AIDS. There is concern about such youngsters if they have biting behaviors, but the risk of transmission through biting is minimal. In instances of bites from known HIV-1–infected individuals, transmission of disease has not occurred with one possible exception. Health care workers who are occupationally exposed to saliva or who have been bitten by patients likewise rarely, if ever, have been infected by this means. The risk of infection from tears is minimal. HIV has only rarely been isolated from urine and even then in low titers.

Household or casual (nonsexual) contact has been extensively studied. No serologic or virologic evidence of transmission occurred in over 700 such contacts. However, only a limited number of children were included in these evaluations.

Incubation Period. The median incubation period in perinatally acquired infection has ranged from 8 mo to 3 yr or more. By 18 mo of age 90% were symptomatic in one survey. There may be 2 populations, one with early onset at about 4 mo and the other with onset at about 6 yr of age. Isolation of HIV from fetal tissue at 15–22 wk of gestation and from placental tissue, the occasional finding of AIDS embryopathy, and failure of cesarean section to prevent transmission suggests that some perinatal transmission occurs antepartum. The relative proportion of transmission at different times in gestation, during the intrapartum period, and postpartum is not established. Preterm birth is common but is comparable in frequency to that seen in the general high-risk population served. Monozygotic twins discordant for HIV infection have been reported. The mean incubation period for blood transfusion-acquired AIDS in children is 23–24 mo with a range of 0–82 mo. In adults the mean incubation period following transfusion has varied from 5 to 18 yr.

PATHOGENESIS AND PATHOLOGY. The initial event in HIV infection is the selective adherence of HIV to T4 lymphocytes or other cells expressing the CD4 antigen. This tropism involves the interaction of the CD4 protein of T4 lymphocytes with gp120 envelope protein. The probable location of the HIV binding site is a protruding loop on the CD4 protein. Synthetic analogs of specific CD4 residues prevent HIV-1–induced cell fusion (syncytia formation) and may be prototypes of inhibitors of HIV-receptor interaction. However, CD4-negative cells can be experimentally infected with HIV, and, reciprocally, mouse cells transfected with CD4 protein cannot be infected with HIV. Therefore, cell surface moieties other than the CD4 protein may also be important in entry of the virus into the cell.

The HIV then enters the cell by receptor-mediated endocytosis or, alternatively, by a pH-independent direct fusion of the HIV envelope to the cell membrane. HIV does not enter resting T cells; these cells must be in an activated state for infection to occur. Following entry, the virus is uncoated, and the genomic RNA is transcribed into DNA by reverse transcriptase. Some of this DNA remains unintegrated in cytoplasm. The rest is circularized and integrated into the host genome by a virus-encoded enzyme. Further stages in the cycle occur following activation of the infected cell by other pathogens (cytomegalovirus [CMV], hepatitis B virus, herpes simplex virus) or following allogeneic stimulation initiated by exposure to semen, blood, or allografts. In vitro this is achieved by mitogenic, antigenic, or allogeneic stimuli. Transcription, protein synthesis, post-translational processing, and assembly of viral proteins and genomic RNA at the cell surface then occur. With HIV replication, the host cell either is killed or survives but is permanently infected.

Another outcome of HIV infection is formation of multinucleated giant cells or syncytia that develop "ballooning" cytoplasm and die within a day. Syncytia include both infected and uninfected T4+ cells, and their formation depends on the existence of the HIV envelope with intact carbohydrate moieties and on the T4 molecule. Other mechanisms of lymphocyte killing may occur without syncytia formation. For example, coating of T4+ lymphocytes with free gp120 causes them to be recognized as "foreign"; therefore, they are cleared by the immune system. Similarly, a change in the major histocompatibility complex (MHC) class II phenotype of the HIV-infected cell would render it susceptible to immune clearance. A CD4 cell infected with HIV is susceptible to superinfection with certain other pathogens such as CMV. Since the T4 lymphocyte is the "orchestrator" of many important immune responses, its inactivation by HIV leads to many defects including those involving monocytes, macrophages, cytotoxic T cells, natural killer cells, and B cells.

It is unlikely that the regulatory genes (*tat*, *rev*, *vif*, *nef*, and *vpr*) play a role in killing cells. However, they do modify viral expression significantly. The *tat* (transactivator) gene boosts expression of viral genes 1,000-fold, leading to increased virus production. In contrast, the *nef* gene slows transcription of the viral genome, "turning off" growth and leading to dormancy. The *rev* gene has a differential effect. One of its sequences prevents transcripts from being turned into protein, but a second sequence reverses this effect. Some interactions of the regulatory genes may lead to steady-state viral growth. Other interactions cause variations in growth rate and instability and hence may determine the outcome of infection.

Biologic properties of the virus may partly determine the rate of progression of AIDS from an asymptomatic state to clinical disease. The most favorable course is associated with low-replicating, non–syncytium-inducing isolates. Such patients show the longest symptom-free interval and the most prolonged survival following diagnosis.

Monocytes and macrophages can also express the T4 antigen and hence can be infected with HIV but are relatively refractory to cell killing by syncytia formation. Thus, in these cells there is insidious viral replication, reflecting a lower surface density of CD4 receptors, and they serve as reservoirs of persisting virus. Monocytic infection also leads to a chemotactic defect and release of monokines, such as interleukin 1 or tumor necrosis factor (TNF or cachectin), which may contribute to the chronic fevers and cachexia seen in AIDS patients, since TNF is a potent catabolic agent. Elevated serum levels of TNF have been associated with progressive encephalopathy (PE), and TNF may be responsible for myelin damage found in PE due to HIV.

The infected monocyte is a vehicle for the transport of HIV to the central nervous system, but only a small proportion of monocytes are infected with HIV, 1/120–1/500 cells. HIV-infected circulating monocytes fail to stimulate resting T cells in an antigen-specific way, and this may contribute to the immunodeficient state of the patient. The opposite effect occurs in HIV-infected pulmonary macrophages, resulting in an enhanced response to nonspecific air-borne stimuli. Infected alveolar macrophages lead to the high incidence of *Pneumocystis carinii* pneumonia (PCP) and lymphoid interstitial pneumonia (LIP). B cell dysregulation may be a direct result of HIV infection or of inactivated HIV extracts. B cell activation and immunoglobulin synthesis are stimulated by neuroleukin (see later), a lymphokine homologous to gp120. The resulting polyclonal activation leads to high serum immunoglobulin levels, poor antibody response to novel antigens, and frequent, severe pyogenic infections with *Streptococcus pneumoniae* and *Haemophilus influenzae*, particularly in children. Autoimmune processes, such as immune thrombocytopenia, may also be due to the heightened production of nonspecific immunoglobulin.

CNS Involvement. See also Sec. 20.50. Several mechanisms may account for the subacute encephalitis and other neurologic manifestations characteristic of AIDS. Neuroleukin, a neurotropic factor, shows moderate sequence homology with gp120, which probably inhibits neuron growth in the presence of neuroleukin. Because gp120 is also a competitive inhibitor of neuroleukin, it may shorten the survival of certain neurons and lead to neurologic dysfunction, subacute encephalitis, vacuolar myelopathy, and peripheral neuropathy. HIV may also have a direct etiologic role. It has been isolated from the brain tissue and CSF of patients with neurologic dysfunction, often in excess of the amount recovered from blood or other tissues, and intra-blood-brain barrier HIV-specific immunoglobulins are synthesized. Such antibodies may be detected in asymptomatic, neurologically normal individuals. In contrast, HIV antigen (p24) in the CSF correlates with progressive encephalopathy and so may be of prognostic value.

Multinucleated giant cells in the brain containing HIV RNA and monocyte markers are seen in many fatal cases of AIDS. HIV is neurotropic and may find a sanctuary in the CNS, where it may survive indefinitely. The major cell type infected in the brain is the monocyte/macrophage. After the infected peripheral monocyte transports the virus across the blood-brain barrier into the CNS, HIV replicates in these infected cells, which may then release monokines or proteolytic enzymes that are toxic or chemotactic to neural cells, thereby inducing further infiltration by inflammatory cells. HIV has been isolated from the choroid plexus, brain parenchyma, and leptomeninges. The damaged glial cells and neurons are considered "innocent bystanders." However, the human brain also expresses T4 receptors, and HIV may infect glial cells. Oligodendroglia and astroglial cells have been shown to contain HIV-like particles, and HIV RNA has been detected in occasional astrocytes, microglia, and, rarely, neurons. Demyelination and neuroglial cell death may occur as a direct result of HIV infection. A patient may be neurologically asymptomatic in spite of HIV infection of the CNS.

Other Organ Pathology. Limited data are available on the histopathologic abnormalities of involved organs. In the thymus, there may be lymphocyte depletion, mononuclear or plasmacyte infiltration obscuring corticomedullary differentiation, and decreased calcified or microcystic Hassall corpuscles. Damage to the epithelial cells of Hassall corpuscles may be important in development of T cell abnormalities. Lymphoid follicles with germinal centers and multinucleated giant cells in the medulla are observed. In addition, decreased thymulin and differentiation of antigen content may occur, and immunoglobulin and complement may be deposited. Viral isolation and demonstration of the HIV antigen have been reported. In some cases the thymus may be normal.

Follicular hyperplasia, with or without lymphocyte depletion of the paracortical zone, and atrophy of follicles with lymphocyte depletion occur in lymph nodes. Lymphocytic infiltration may occur in a variety of organs. A lymphoproliferative disorder intermediate between benign and malignant, *PBLD* (polyclonal, polymorphic B cell lymphoproliferative disorder), may occur at extranodal systemic sites. Pulmonary involvement, lymphoid interstitial pneumonitis complex (LIP), is prominent in children. The pathogenesis of PBLD and of lymphoid hyperplasia may be related to Epstein-Barr virus (EBV) infection alone or in synergy with the HIV agent.

Pathologic changes occur mainly in the small and medium-sized arteries of various organs (heart, lungs, kidneys, spleen, intestine, and brain), for example, fragmentation of elastic fibers, and fibrosis and calcification of the media. The fibrocalcific lesions may be distinct from the inflammatory lesions.

Clinical Implications. Since the DNA transcribed from the HIV genome is integrated into the host cell chromosome, the organism cannot be eradicated without killing the infected cell. Most of the virus is latent or restricted and is not susceptible to immune clearance; important reservoirs such as monocytes/macrophages are resistant to cytolysis. The smaller proportion of infected, activated T4+ lymphocytes that resist lysis also constitutes a reservoir. There is considerable genomic diversity among HIV isolates, but all are recognized by the immune system. The prevalence of antigenemia (core protein p24) varies with the severity of the illness and may range as high as 80–90%.

CLINICAL MANIFESTATIONS. A wide and variable range of signs and symptoms occurs among infants and children with AIDS (Table 12–36). Poor growth, failure to thrive, interstitial pneumonia, and hepatomegaly occur in nearly all cases of pediatric AIDS. Systemic and pulmonary findings predominate in the United States, whereas chronic diarrhea, inanition, and wasting are most common in Africa, where the entity is known as "slim disease." Serious recurrent bacterial sepsis and relentlessly progressive neurologic deterioration are characteristic of pediatric AIDS and are unusual in adults. The parotid swelling seen in AIDS is suggestive of mumps but is distinguishable by its chronicity. Kaposi sarcoma, B cell lymphoma, and mononucleosis-like illnesses are unusual in children. These three findings occur in fewer than 10% of cases.

The *facial dysmorphism* is distinct from that seen in fetal alcohol syndrome and familial traits and has been observed in some centers but not in others. It includes ocular hypertelorism, prominent box-like appearance of the forehead, flat nasal bridge, obliquity of the eyes, long palpebral fissures with blue sclerae, short nose with flattened columella, well-formed triangular philtrum, and patulous lips.

Hemophilia. Progression to AIDS in seropositive hemophiliac children is slower than that in adults. Growth in some asymptomatic seropositive hemophiliac children is delayed by HIV infection. Neurodysregulation of growth hormone release occurs in some of these patients. Manifestations are variable but include lymphadenopathy, neuropsychological disorders, anemia, thrombocytopenia, and typical HIV related opportunistic infections.

Pulmonary. Pulmonary infections with pneumococcus or *H. influenzae* type b or with opportunistic agents such as *P. carinii*, *Aspergillus fumigatus*, or cytomegalovirus are common. Classic tuberculosis has been seen frequently in adults, who show an excessive prevalence of extrapulmonary manifestations and a reduced rate of tuberculin skin test positivity.

TABLE 12–36. Clinical Manifestations of Pediatric AIDS

Generalized
Fever
Failure to thrive
Lymphadenopathy
Recurrent infection
Developmental delay
Low birthweight (small for gestational age)
Specific
Embryopathy
Microcephaly
Facial dysmorphism
Hepatosplenomegaly
Lymphocytic interstitial pneumonia
Diarrhea
Gastrointestinal bleeding
Cardiomyopathy
Arteriopathy
Nephropathy
Encephalopathy
Parotitis
Kaposi sacroma
Skin rashes
Infections
Pneumocystis carinii
M. avium-intracellulare
Cytomegalovirus
Herpes simplex (types 1 and 2)
Epstein-Barr virus
Varicella-zoster virus
Cryptococcus
Cryptosporidium
Aspergillus fumigatus
Haemophilus influenzae type b
S. pneumoniae
Salmonella
Shigella
Moniliasis (oral and esophageal)
Toxoplasmosis
Giardiasis
Amebiasis

Tuberculosis is less common in children. Infections with *M. avium intracellulae* and *M. bovis* have occurred.

Lymphoid interstitial pneumonia (LIP) in children with AIDS may be associated with EBV infection; EBV DNA is typically found in lung biopsy specimens of these patients but not in those with *Pneumocystis carinii* pneumonia, CMV infection, or infection with *M. avium-intracellulare.* High titers of antibody to EBV capsid antigen also occur in these cases. LIP has a characteristic nodular infiltrative pattern on chest roentgenograms, which may permit its diagnosis without resorting to lung biopsy. Imaging with ^{67}Ga demonstrates increased uptake on chest films in both *P. carinii* pneumonia and LIP and hence does not permit a distinction between the two.

Pneumocystis carinii pneumonia is the predominant pulmonary infection among patients with AIDS and the major cause of death (see Sec. 14.58).

The classic clinical presentation includes fever, cough, tachypnea, and dyspnea. In some patients, however, these findings are absent, and physical examination may be normal. The chest roentgenogram may also be normal, at least early in the disease. Arterial blood gases may reveal hypoxia even before clinical and roentgenographic findings appear. Chest roentgenogram abnormalities include interstitial infiltration and discrete areas of pneumonia; effusions, nodules, or cavities are also occasionally seen. Gallium scanning is abnormal in nearly all cases, even with a normal chest roentgenogram, but is associated with a high false-positive rate. With the use of the flexible fiberoptic bronchoscope, bronchoalveolar lavage fluid may be obtained for identification of *P. carinii* and other organisms. This approach or deep tracheal aspirations often permits a diagnosis without resorting to open lung biopsy. Demonstration of *P. carinii* in an aspirate or lung tissue obtained by transbronchial biopsy provides a definite diagnosis. A new immunofluorescent assay using monoclonal antibodies offers the promise of accurate diagnosis based on a study of sputum and may be more sensitive than conventional stains. Immunoserologic tests (complement-fixation, latex agglutination) are of little help because most individuals have antibodies of these types prior to illness.

PCP is a major cause of early mortality with a median survival of only 1 mo among infants who were infected at 5 mo of age. Therefore, there is a need for prophylaxis as described later. Alveolar-arterial oxygen gradients and elevated lactate dehydrogenase levels distinguish survivors from nonsurvivors in adults but not in children.

Gastrointestinal and Hepatobiliary Dysfunctions (see Sec. 13.53). These are numerous and may be a manifestation of opportunistic infections with *M. avium-intracellulare* or CMV, nonspecific bleeding associated with diarrhea and thrombocytopenia, abdominal distention, biliary obstruction, pseudomembranous necrotizing jejunitis, leiomyoma, rhabdomyosarcoma, hypertrophic colonic polyps, hypergastrinemia, or hypochlorhydria. Nonspecific elevations of serum transaminases occur. Hepatitis B is less common in children with AIDS than in adults with the disease.

Cardiomyopathies. Congestive heart failure, cardiomegaly on chest roentgenogram, dyspnea, retractions, tachypnea, tachycardia, rales, hepatomegaly, and weak peripheral arterial pulses occur in some children, but others may show no clinical manifestations. At postmortem examination cardiomegaly with biventricular dilatation is seen. Microscopic examination reveals hypertrophy of the myocardial fibers, foci of vacuolization, interstitial edema, occasional small foci of myocardial fibrosis, and endocardial thickening. Specific viral infection with CMV has been reported, and EBV has been suspected. As AIDS children survive for longer periods, increased numbers with cardiac manifestations may become apparent. Anemia and nutritional deficiencies may contribute to the myocardiopathy.

Skin. Rashes may be due to specific infections such as recurrent varicella-zoster, HSV, or *Candida.* There may be urticaria, eczematoid eruptions, and genital condylomata. Epidermal hyperkeratosis with dry, scaling skin has been observed, as have prolonged episodes of scabies and tinea. Long eyelashes and sparse hair may be seen. Pyomyositis due to *S. aureus* has occurred.

Renal Disease. Four morphologic types of nephropathy occur: focal glomerulosclerosis, mesangial hyperplasia, segmental necrotizing glomerulonephritis, and minimal change disease. The first two are the most common. Endothelial tubuloreticular inclusions seen by electron microscopy may be a marker of HIV-associated nephropathy. The nephrotic syndrome has also occurred and may be the presenting sign in patients as old as 5–6 yr.

Encephalopathic Manifestations. These are common in children and have wide-ranging and potentially devastating results. The spectrum includes visual impairment (including blindness), motor abnormalities, seizures, microcephaly, speech and language disabilities, cognitive losses with delayed or lost milestones, apathy, ataxia, spasticity, and peripheral neuropathies. Intervals of stability or "plateauing" lasting for months or years occur, but the course is variable. In some cases it is insidious or indolent; in others there is steady deterioration. Mild to moderate cortical atrophy with some progression and enlarged ventricles is seen on CT scans. Calcification of the basal ganglia is an ominous sign. Abnormalities of white matter are found on magnetic resonance imaging, and cerebrovascular accidents due to hemorrhage or infarction occur. The lesions may be massive with catastrophic results. Cerebrospinal fluid analysis shows elevated protein concentration and mild pleocytosis. CNS infection may also be caused by opportunistic agents including toxoplasmosis, which appears as multiple abscess-like lesions, and cryptococcal meningitis, which occurs particularly in Africa but is less likely in children than adults. The neurologic manifestations of toxoplasmosis and cryptococcosis vary widely from subtle mild symptoms to severe, fulminant disease. In patients with cryptococcosis, severe disease may affect many extracerebral sites such as the liver, spleen, bones, lungs, and skin. Other agents involving the CNS include HSV, CMV, varicella-zoster virus, papovavirus, various bacteria, and fungi. Primary lymphoma also occurs.

DIAGNOSIS. A diagnostic classification of HIV infection in children is presented in Table 12–37.

LABORATORY FINDINGS. Elevation of serum IgG concentrations to over 1,800 mg/dL at 1 yr of age or 2,300 mg/dL at 2 yr of age is typical of AIDS and is not seen in other immunologic disorders. Subclasses IgG1 and IgG3 account for the hypergammaglobulinemia, with a relative or absolute lack of IgG2 and IgG4. Since the IgG2 subclass is essential for adequate opsonization of encapsulated organisms, its deficiency in AIDS may predispose to pyogenic infection with *pneumococcus, Staphylococcus,* and *Haemophilus*. IgD elevations are also typical and may be seen in those with normal IgG concentrations. IgM elevations are frequent but variable. Hypergammaglobulinemia may reflect abnormal T cell regulation of B cell function but may also be due to chronic infection, especially with EBV. The antibody formed is nonfunctional, and these patients usually do not respond or have a blunted response to primary or repeated immunizations with specific antibody. Hypogammaglobulinemia is less common, and in some patients is associated with rapid progression of disease, especially neurologic involvement in which cerebral calcification is probably due to HIV itself.

The laboratory abnormality most characteristic of AIDS is a reversal of the T helper-suppressor cell (T4/T8) ratio from a normal of approximately 1.5–2.3, depending on the child's age. Such a reversal also occurs in many viral infections, in intravenous drug addiction, and sometimes in pregnancy. Children are more likely to have normal helper-suppressor cell ratios and less often have peripheral lymphopenia than adults. Typical qualitative defects include poor response to mitogenic and antigenic stimuli and reduced production of various lymphokines such as interleukin 2 and interferon. Cutaneous delayed hypersensitivity reactions are reduced or absent. Other abnormalities include increased levels of circulating immune complexes, abnormal monocyte chemotaxis and antigen processing, cytotoxicity, and the production of autoantibodies.

Elevated erythrocyte sedimentation rates, anemia (iron deficiency and other), atypical lymphocytes including plasmacytoid lymphocytes, autoimmune phenomena, leukopenia, neutropenia, and lymphopenia occur in these children. Thrombocytopenia may be the initial finding, preceding other signs by a considerable time. Direct infection of megakaryocytes with HIV-1 has been demonstrated and may be one mechanism causing decreased platelet production. Leukopenia may reflect gram-negative sepsis.

Lactic dehydrogenase (LDH) elevation is indicative of unrestricted activation of B cells and is reduced by intravenous immune globulin (IVIG) administration. LDH values of 800–1,000 units/mL suggest PCP infection (in the absence of hepatitis or hemolysis). Levels below 500 units/mL are associated with LIP.

Direct toxic effects of maternal substance abuse on the fetal immune system may need to be distinguished from HIV infection. Nonspecific lymphocyte abnormalities that may occur in neonates born to intravenous drug users both at birth and during the 1st yr of life in the absence of HIV infection include poor mitogen response and decreased helper-suppressor cell ratios (OKT4/OKT8), which become worse during the 1st yr of life.

Perinatal Infection. As the prevalence of HIV infection reflected in ELISA-positive cord sera increases among high-risk populations in future years, the importance of distinguishing between passive transmission of antibody from the mother and active infection in the infant will also increase. Seropositivity alone, in neonates, does not establish a diagnosis of actual HIV infection. As many as 60–80% of antibody-positive cases represent passive transmission across the placenta, and the ELISA test will revert to negative at 10 mo of age in one half and by 15 mo of age in nearly all. A few infants who are seronegative at 15 mo and remain seronegative indefinitely are actually infected. They may become seropositive at a later date or, as occasionally happens in adults, may never seroconvert (see later). In infected infants a sequence of isotype and subclass antibodies develops during

TABLE 12–37. Classification of HIV Infection in Children Under 13 Yr of Age*

Class P–0. Indeterminate infection. Infants less than 15 mo of age with antibody to HIV. This indicates exposure to an infected mother, but the infant cannot be classified as definitely infected.

Class P–1. Asymptomatic infection. The patient meets one of the clinical or immunologic criteria without signs or symptoms of class P–2.
- Subclass A. Normal immune function
- Subclass B. Abnormal immune function
- Subclass C. Not tested

Class P–2. Symptomatic infection.

Subclass A. Nonspecific findings. Children ill for 2 mo or more. Findings include fever, failure to thrive, weight loss, organomegaly, parotitis, diarrhea, lymph node enlargement of at least 0.5 cm at 2 or more sites.

Subclass B. Progressive neurologic disease. Includes loss of developmental milestones and intellectual ability, impaired brain growth on CT or MRI scans, progressive symmetric motor deficits.

Subclass C. LIP. Typical chest roentgenogram findings or histopathlogic confirmation.

Subclass D.

Category D–1. Secondary infectious diseases listed in CDC surveillance definition for AIDS. Typical examples include TORCH agents after 1 mo of age, *Pneumocystis carinii* pneumonia, disseminated fungal infection such as coccidioidomycosis, candidiasis (esophageal, pulmonary); various other agents.

Category D–2. Recurrent serious bacterial infections: two or more within a 2-yr period including sepsis, meningitis, pneumonia, abscess of internal organs, and bone or joint infection.

Category D–3. Other specified secondary infectious diseases: oral candidiasis for 2 mo or more, two or more episodes of herpes stomatitis within a year, disseminated varicella-zoster virus infection.

Subclass E. Secondary cancers.

Category E–1. Specified secondary cancers listed in the CDC surveillance definition for AIDS. These include Kaposi sarcoma, B cell non-Hodgkin lymphoma, and primary lymphoma of the brain.

Category E–2. Other cancers possibly associated with HIV infection.

Subclass F. Other diseases possibly due to HIV infection. Included are cardiomyopathy, nephropathy, hematologic and dermatologic disorders, and hepatitis.

*Modified from MMWR 36:225, 1987.

the first 20 wk of life, namely, IgM isotype followed by IgG3 and IgG1 subclasses. However, such infants may remain asymptomatic during the first 6 mo of life. Some symptomatic infected infants who are ELISA-antibody negative will be positive by antigen capture. Immunologic markers help to identify the infected infants, who may show decreased total lymphocyte counts, decreased CD4 (helper) cells, reversed CD4/CD8 ratio, anemia (hemoglobin below 9.5 g/dL), and elevated serum IgG and IgA levels. The reduction in CD4 cells may occur as early as 5 mo of age and will be apparent in nearly all by 18 mo. Culture positivity occurs typically by 6 mo but may occur as early as 3 days of life.

Polymerase chain reaction (PCR) permits detection of an extremely small number of copies of DNA sequence, as few as 1 copy in 1 million cells. It is a promising technique in rapid, early, and definitive detection of HIV-1 in high-risk infants and children. Positive results have correlated closely with viral isolation from cultures of peripheral blood mononuclear cells. PCR has the advantages of extremely high sensitivity and specificity, fast "turnaround" time (2–3 days), and potential adaptation to detection of other viruses as well. However, it has the disadvantages of technical complexity, high cost, potential oversensitivity in picking up low levels of contamination, and potential failure to detect HIV strains resulting from a high rate of mutation. Other techniques include enzyme-linked immunospot assays for IgG antibody-secreting cells to HIV envelope recombinant protein (gp41), HIV antigen assays using p24 and whole HIV-Ag, a combination of isoelectric focusing and affinity immunoblotting to detect HIV-specific antibodies, flow cytometry with various chromophores, studies of fetal cells circulating in maternal serum, and studies of placental tissue with in situ hybridization with HIV DNA and RNA radiolabeled probes, monoclonal antibody staining against lymphocyte subsets in placental tissue, and staining of placental tissue with antibodies to envelope (gp120) and core (p24) antigens.

Prolonged seronegativity in patients from whom HIV has been isolated has been reported in adults. Infection for a period of nearly 3 yr may fail to stimulate the immune system, or there may be a loss of antiviral antibodies following transient production. Transmissibility of HIV in such cases is uncertain.

PREVENTION. The use of condoms is important in breaking the chain of transmission. Latex condoms are impermeable to HIV. Those containing nonoxynol-9, a spermicide, may inactivate HIV if slippage or breakage occurs. Protection, however, against HIV transmission is not absolute. Vaccine immunization is not available.

TREATMENT. The principal anti-HIV agent for the management of pediatric AIDS is azidothymidine (AZT or zidovudine). Other therapy is nonspecific and supportive and is designed to prevent or manage complications. Azidothymidine has been approved for use in children with AIDS. Continuous intravenous infusion of 0.4–1.8 mg/kg/hr is safe and is associated with fewer clinical reactions than in adults; it is effective in decreasing neurologic manifestations and improving IQ scores. Appetite, weight, and activity increase, as do the number of CD4 cells. Lymphadenopathy, hepatosplenomegaly, and immunoglobulin levels also decrease. Blood transfusions for complicating anemia may be required. Neutropenia also may occur and require limitation of the dose. AZT is indicated for treatment of children with symptomatic AIDS. Its administration early in the disease, even before symptoms are manifest, delays onset of frank illness and is associated with fewer hematologic side effects. A study of low (90 mg/m^2) and high (180 mg/m^2) dosage in children with mild to moderate symptoms is in progress.

A variety of other experimental agents are currently being evaluated: dideoxycytidine (DDC), dideoxyinosine (DDI), sulfated polysaccharides such as dextran sulfate, heparin, chondroitin sulfate, fucoidan, carrageenan, cholic acid derivatives, and recombinant CD4, AL721 (lipid mixture), ribavirin, foscarnet, GLQ223 (trichosanthin), and combinations of established agents such as zidovudine and acyclovir, zidovudine and interferon alpha, or zidovudine and intravenous immunoglobulin.

Nutritional support, including the use of parenteral feedings, is important. The use of central lines (Broviac or Hickman catheters) has proved valuable for both home and hospital management.

Monthly intravenous administration of IVIG in a dose of 400 mg/kg significantly prolonged infection-free survival and reduced the number of hospitalizations in symptomatic HIV-infected children with CD4 counts over 200/mm^3 compared with a placebo treated group. Survival was not affected, however. Hemophiliac children were not included in the study.

LIP has been successfully treated with oxygen, bronchodilators, and steroids. Steroids are reserved for patients with hypoxia (Pa_{O_2} <65 mm Hg) in doses as high as 2 mg/kg/24 hr of oral prednisone for several months.

Treatment of infections associated with HIV must be done on an individual basis. Multiple pathogens are frequent, and severe, wide-ranging manifestations and a high density of organisms are characteristic. Infections due to fungi, parasites, and viruses are usually not curable. They often require long-term treatment even for suppression. Appropriate antibiotic therapy is needed for bacterial infections such as those due to *S. pneumoniae, H. influenzae, Salmonella, Shigella,* and others.

Pneumocystis carinii pneumonia should be treated with trimethoprim (TMP)-sulfamethoxazole (SMX) (15–20 mg TMP/kg/24 hr intravenously and then orally) as the pneumonitis resolves. Prophylactic doses should be continued indefinitely. Corticosteroids also improve the outcome of severe PCP infection. All those with proven HIV infection from 1 mo to over 6 yr should begin PCP prophylaxis based on age and T4 cell count, in a dose of TMP 75 mg/m^2 plus SMZ 375 mg/m^2 orally. For those with adverse reactions who are able to cooperate with nebulization, aerosolized pentamidine (300 mg/mo) is an alternative. If aerosolization is not possible, intravenous pentamidine (4 mg/kg/dose, monthly) has been advised by some. Dapsone with or without TMP also may be considered but has not been extensively studied. Also see Sec. 14.58.

For disseminated or severe mucocutaneous candidiasis, amphotericin B therapy is indicated. For thrush and esophagitis, nystatin, clotrimazole, and oral ketoconazole may be effective.

There is no effective therapy for *M. avium-intracellulare* infection, which is resistant to conventional antituberculosis agents. Although it demonstrates in vitro sensitivity to rifabutin (ansamycin), clofazimine, and other agents, their administration does not reduce symptoms or lead to healing. For treatment of tuberculosis see Sec. 12.47. Isoniazid prophylaxis should be given to any HIV-infected patient with a positive tuberculin test.

Acyclovir is the agent of choice for both systemic and mucocutaneous herpes simplex infections (see Sec. 12.68). The dosage ranges from 15–30 mg/kg/24 hr intravenously in patients with visceral, disseminated, or severe mucocutaneous disease. Oral therapy is appropriate for mild mucocutaneous disease. Treatment is given for at least 10 days. Following recovery, suppressive therapy with oral acyclovir is helpful. The agent is approved for only 6 mo when given for suppression but has been administered (to adults) for up to 48 mo with neither adverse effects nor cumulative toxicity. If the strain of HSV is thymidine kinase negative (and hence resistant to acyclovir), vidarabine should be substituted in a dose of 15 mg/kg/24 hr intravenously for at least 10 days.

There is no proven therapy for CMV infection (see Sec. 12.71) DHPG (9-[2-hydroxy-1-(hydroxymethy)ethoxymethyl] guanine), ganciclovir, in a dosage of 7.5–15 mg/kg/24 hr may be effective in treatment of CMV retinitis, pneumonia, colitis, and hepatitis but not encephalitis. The results of treatment of pneumonitis are uncertain. Relapse is common. An alternative agent for treatment of ganciclovir-resistant CMV or acyclovir-resistant HSV is foscarnet (trisodium phosphonoformate), an inhibitor of HSV DNA polymerase.

Cryptococcal meningitis should be treated with amphotericin B (0.4–0.6 mg/kg/24 hr) for at least 6 wk. Relapse is common, and long-term suppressive therapy with ketoconazole or amphotericin improves survival (see Sec. 12.105).

The agents of choice for treatment of toxoplasmosis of the CNS are sulfadiazine (100 mg/kg/24 hr) and pyrimethamine (25–50 mg/kg/24 hr) given orally for 3–6 mo or longer. Bone marrow suppression or rash may necessitate discontinuation. Folinic acid is also given to prevent megaloblastic anemia. Relapses are common (see Sec. 12.117).

There is no effective treatment for cryptosporidiosis (see Sec. 12.113). In contrast, oral trimethoprim-sulfamethoxazole leads to a clinical and parasitologic cure in cases due to *Isospora belli,* although again relapse is common.

Immunization. The major difference between the immunization programs for children with HIV infection or seronegative children in the home of a patient with asymptomatic HIV infection and other children is that live polio vaccines should *not* be given. Inactivated poliovirus (IPV) vaccine should be substituted for oral poliovirus vaccine. BCG administration is not recommended in the United States for HIV infected children whether symptomatic or not. WHO recommends its administration to asymptomatic infants in areas with a high risk of tuberculosis. Diphtheria-pertussis-tetanus (DPT) vaccine and *Haemophilus* type b conjugate vaccine should be given according to the standard schedule. Pneumococcal vaccine is recommended for children 2 yr old or older whether they are symptomatic or not. Influenza vaccine is recommended for symptomatic HIV-infected children who are 6 mo of age or older and should be considered for asymptomatic HIV-infected children at 6 mo of age or older. Administration of measles-mumps-rubella (MMR) is recommended at 15 mo in accord with routine practice in both symptomatic and asymptomatic HIV-infected children. However, the vaccine is of low immunogenicity, and vaccine failure has occurred. Passive immunization with immune globulin should be given to HIV-infected children in a dose of 0.5 mL/kg if they are symptomatic or 0.25 mL/kg if they are asymptomatic. In spite of this prophylaxis measles may occur and has resulted in fatalities. See also Sec. 5.1.

Skilled nursing, social work, and psychologic support are needed in caring for these children. Medical centers that see large numbers of AIDS patients should be asked to participate in the management of virtually all cases, since they have well-trained multidisciplinary teams with the necessary clinical experience and research capabilities. Hospices, day-care centers, halfway homes, and well-organized ambulatory facilities all play a major role in offering comprehensive care.

PROGNOSIS. In one large series the average survival of patients with perinatal infection ranged from 2.5 mo to 10 yr (median 1.87 yr) with inapparent infection from 6 wk to 7.3 yr (median 0.75 yr). In another center median survival of 155 children with AIDS was 47 mo. The overall survival from the time of diagnosis was similar in those with perinatal and transfusion-acquired infection. However, in those infected by transfusion after 2 yr of age the incubation period was longer than that noted in those infected perinatally. Survival is worsened in perinatally acquired disease by the occurrence of opportunistic infections or encephalopathy. Bacterial infections and LIP, in contrast, are not associated with increased risk of death. Those diagnosed with HIV infection after 1 yr of age have more favorable survival rates than those diagnosed earlier. Among hemophiliac patients survival following the diagnosis of AIDS is similar to that of other risk groups.

HUGH E. EVANS

Epstein L, Goudsmit J, Paul DA, et al: Expression of human immunodeficiency virus in cerebrospinal fluid of children with progressive encephalopathy. Ann Neurol 21:397, 1987.

Evans LA, Moreau J, Odehouri K, et al: Characterization of a noncytopathic HIV-2 strain with unusual effects on CD4 expression. Science 249:1522, 1988.

Falloon J, Eddy J, Wiener L, et al: Human immuno-deficiency virus infection in children. J Pediatr 114:1, 1989.

Glatt AI, Chirgwin K, Landesman SH: Treatment of infections associated with human immunodeficiency virus. N Engl J Med 318:1439, 1988.

Hattori T, Kioto A, Tabatsubi K, et al: Frequent infection with human T-cell lymphotropic virus type I in patients with AIDS but not in carriers of human immunodeficiency virus type I. J Acquir Immune Defic Syndr 2:272, 1989.

Hein K: Commentary on adolescent acquired immunodeficiency syndrome: The next wave of the human immunodeficiency virus epidemic. J Pediatr 114:144, 1989.

Ho DD, Pomerantz RJ, Kaplan JC: Pathogenesis of infection with human immunodeficiency virus. N Engl J Med 317:278, 1987.

Jameson BA, Rao PE, Kong LI, et al: Location and chemical synthesis of a binding site for HIV-1 on the CD4 protein. Science 240:1335, 1988.

Joshi VV, Godal C, Connor E, et al: Dilated cardiomyopathy in children with acquired immunodeficiency syndrome. Hum Pathol 19:69, 1988.

Krasinski K, Borkowsky W: Measles and measles immunity in children infected with HIV. JAMA 261:2512, 1989.

Krasinski K, Borkowsky W, Holzman RS: Prognosis of HIV infection in children and adolescents. Pediatr Infect Dis J 8:216, 1989.

Levy JA: Human immunodeficiency viruses and the pathogenesis of AIDS. JAMA 261:2997, 1989.

Lifson AR: Do alternate modes for transmission of human immunodeficiency virus exist? A review. JAMA 259:1353, 1988.

McKinney RE, Pizzo PA, Scott GB, et al: Safety and tolerance of intermittent intravenous and oral zidovudine therapy in human immunodeficiency virus–infected pediatric patients. J Pediatr 116:640, 1990.

Mintz M, Rapaport R, Oleske J, et al: Elevated serum levels of tumor necrosis factor are associated with progressive encephalopathy in children with acquired immunodeficiency syndrome. Am J Dis Child 143:771, 1989.

Oxtoby MJ: Human immunodeficiency virus and other viruses in human milk: Placing the issues in broader perspective. Pediatr Infect Dis J 7:825, 1988.

Pizzo PA, Eddy J, Fallon J, et al: Effect of continuous intravenous infusion of zidovudine (AZT) in children with symptomatic HIV infection. N Engl J Med 319:889, 1988.

Scott GB, Hutto C, Makuch RW, et al: Survival in children with perinatally acquired human immunodeficiency virus type 1 infection. N Engl J Med 321:1791, 1989.

Tersinette M, de Gaede REY, Eeftnik-Schattenkerk JKM: Association between biological properties of human immunodeficiency virus variants and risk for AIDS and AIDS mortality. Lancet 1:983, 1989.

Weiblen BJ, Lee FK, Cooper ER, et al: Early diagnosis of HIV infection in infants by detection of IgA HIV antibodies. Lancet 1:988, 1990.

12.84 SLOW VIRAL INFECTIONS OF THE HUMAN NERVOUS SYSTEM*

Viruses cause several neurologic diseases that were once considered degenerative. The diseases have asymptomatic incubation periods of months to years and durations of overt clinical illness that may also be very long. Although the viruses may be latent in other organs of the body, pathologic changes are found only in the nervous system. Some slow viral infections of the human nervous system are caused by viruses with conventional physical properties—viruses that more often cause acute self-limited illnesses (Table 12–38). Other slow infections are caused by infectious agents of unknown structure, agents that, like viruses, are smaller than bacteria but have an array of physical properties so unlike those of conventional viruses that some authorities have suggested that they not be called viruses at all.

*All material in Sec. 12.84–12.88 is in the public domain.

Table 12–38. Slow Infections of the Nervous System Caused by Conventional Viruses

Disease	Virus	Viral Group
	RNA Viruses	
AIDS encephalopathy (dementia, myelopathy)	HIV-1	Retrovirus
Kozhevnikov epilepsy (and other chronic forms of tick-borne encephalitis)	Tick-borne encephalitis	Flavivirus
Progressive rubella panencephalitis (PRP)	Rubella	Rubivirus
Rabies	Rabies	Rhabdovirus
Subacute sclerosing panencephalitis (SSPE)	Measles	Paramyxovirus
Tropical spastic paraparesis (TSP)/HTLV-I–associated myelopathy (HAM)	HTLV-I	Retrovirus
	DNA Viruses	
Cytomegalovirus (CMV) encephalitis	CMV	Herpesvirus group
Progressive multifocal leukoencephalitis (PML)	JC (?SV40)	Papovavirus
? Rasmussen chronic encephalitis	?CMV, ?Epstein-Barr virus	Herpesvirus group

SLOW INFECTIONS WITH CONVENTIONAL VIRUSES

12.85 Subacute Sclerosing Panencephalitis (SSPE)

(Dawson Encephalitis)

ETIOLOGY. This chronic encephalitis is caused by a persistent measles virus infection. It was first clearly described and a viral etiology postulated by Dawson. Subsequently, measles virus was isolated from the brains of patients with SSPE.

EPIDEMIOLOGY. SSPE is a rare disease that occurs throughout the world. The disease has been diagnosed in patients aged 6 mo to more than 30 yr, but it affects primarily children and young adolescents. In more than 85% of cases onset occurs between 5 and 15 yr of age. The average age of onset before 1980 was about 10 yr; between 1980 and 1984 it was almost 14 yr. The risk of SSPE for boys is more than twice that for girls, and it is higher for rural children than for city children. SSPE was once especially common in the southeastern United States, and prevalences significantly higher than average were also found in the Ohio River valley and in some New England states. More recently, cases have been more common in the western United States, especially among Hispanic children. Acquisition of measles before the age of 18 mo seems to increase the risk of SSPE substantially. Exposure to birds and other animals has been reported with abnormal frequency in histories of patients with SSPE; the reason is not clear.

Mean annual incidence rates of SSPE in the United States have fallen markedly from 0.61 cases/million persons under age 20 yr in 1960 to 0.06 cases/million in 1980. Since 1982 only 4–5 new cases have been registered each year from the entire country. This drop roughly parallels the progressive decline in the annual number of measles cases diagnosed since the introduction of live attenuated measles vaccine in the United States in 1963. The risk of SSPE has been estimated at 8.5 SSPE cases/million cases of measles for a 6-yr period, during which the estimated risk after measles vaccination was only 0.7 cases/million doses of vaccine. The overwhelming advantage of measles vaccination in preventing SSPE is clear. In cases occurring in vaccinated children, it has not been determined whether SSPE resulted from persistent infection with the attenuated measles virus of the vaccine, from undiagnosed wild-type measles infection preceding vaccination, or from vaccine failure and subsequent undiagnosed measles. SSPE continues to occur in areas of the world where measles remains unchecked and may be anticipated to increase in the United States if compliance with vaccination diminishes.

PATHOLOGY. The histopathology of SSPE consists of inflammation, necrosis, and repair. Brain biopsy performed in the early stages of SSPE shows mild inflammation of meninges and a panencephalitis involving cortical and subcortical gray matter as well as white matter, with cuffs of plasma cells and lymphocytes around blood vessels and increased numbers of glia throughout. Neuronal loss may not be marked until later in the course of illness, when loss of myelin secondary to neuronal degeneration may be apparent. Intranuclear inclusion bodies surrounded by clear halos may be seen within the nuclei of neurons, astrocytes, and oligodendrocytes (Fig. 12–31). By electron microscopy the inclusions are seen to contain tubular structures typical of the nucleocapsids of paramyxoviruses. Measles viral antigens can be demonstrated by labeled-antibody techniques within the inclusions as well as in cells without inclusions. Lesions may be unevenly distributed throughout the brain, and biopsy is not always diagnostic, particularly if only a small sample of tissue is obtained. The same findings of inclusion-body panencephalitis are generally present in the brain at autopsy; however, late in the disease it may be difficult to find typical areas of inflammation, and the main histopathologic changes are necrosis and gliosis. The disease is believed to begin in the cortical gray matter, progressing then to the subcortical white and gray matter (myoclonus probably results from extrapyramidal involvement) and finally to the lower structures. Although persistent infection of lymphoid tissues with measles virus has been demonstrated, these show no pathologic changes.

PATHOGENESIS. It has been proposed that some mutation may render the measles virus more likely to establish persistent infection. The genomes of strains of measles virus isolated from patients with SSPE tend to be somewhat larger than those isolated from typical cases of measles, and multiple mutations have been found in isolates. However, no consistent genomic abnormalities have been identified in measles virus isolated from brains of SSPE patients, nor have clusters of SSPE cases suggestive of strains of special virulence been described. It has also been theorized that patients with SSPE have some subtle predisposing immune deficiency or that an infection with a second virus facilitates the chronic measles encephalitis, but neither of these hypotheses has been confirmed.

Complete measles virus particles are not found in the brains of patients with SSPE, and the matrix (M) protein required for the final assembly and budding of virus from the host cells is missing not only from brain tissues of patients but also from cells cultured from their brains; however, the full complement of genetic material needed to code for all proteins, including the M protein, is present and functional. Therefore, it has been proposed that some restriction in patients' brain cells prevents the translation of M protein, resulting in the accumulation of incomplete measles virus that cannot be cleared either by antibodies or by cell-mediated immunity.

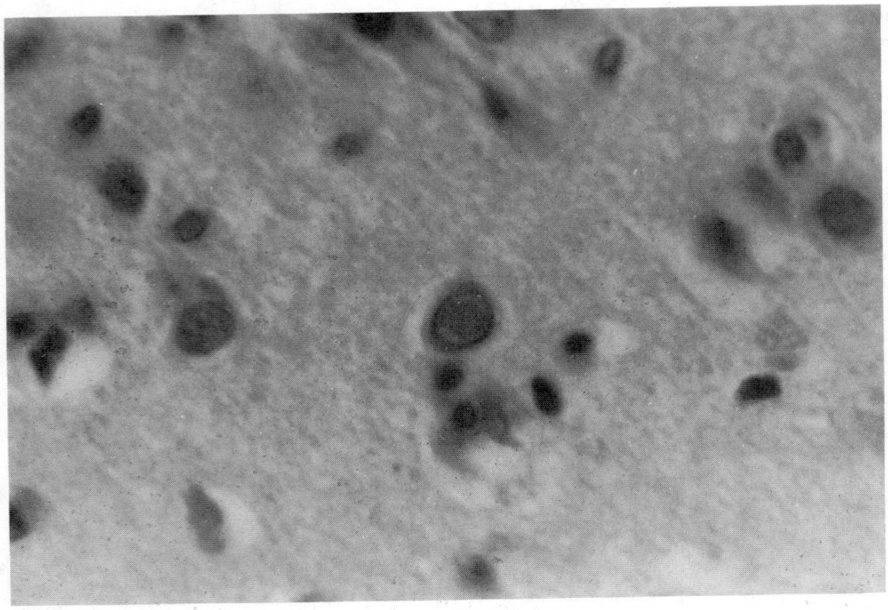

Figure 12–31. An intranuclear inclusion (cowdry type A) from the cerebral cortex of a child with subacute sclerosing panencephalitis. Same specimen as in Figure 12–30. (Courtesy of Janice Stevens, M.D., National Institute of Mental Health. The hematoxylin and eosin stained section was provided by Peggy Swoveland, M.D., University of Maryland School of Medicine.)

CLINICAL MANIFESTATIONS. Children with SSPE generally have a history of typical measles with full recovery several years before the onset of neurologic disease. Measles may have been either mild or severe. Some patients with SSPE have had measles pneumonia, but none has had a history of typical measles encephalitis. The mean interval between measles and onset of SSPE was formerly about 7 yr, but recently it has increased to 12 yr. In vaccinated patients without a history of measles, the mean interval between vaccination and onset of SSPE was 5 yr before 1980 and 7.7 yr between 1980 and 1986.

The clinical picture of SSPE tends to be quite stereotypic; almost 70% of cases have an acute, subacute, or chronic progressive course; 8% have a "stuttering" or remitting course. The onset is usually insidious, marked by subtle changes in behavior and deterioration of school work, followed by more overtly bizarre behavior and finally by frank dementia. There is no fever, photophobia, or other findings of acute encephalitis except for occasional complaints of headache. Diffuse neurologic disease becomes progressively more severe. The appearance of massive repetitive myoclonic jerks, generally symmetric, involving especially the axial musculature and occurring at 5- to 10-sec intervals, marks the onset of a second clinical stage of SSPE. The myoclonic jerks appear to be abnormal movements rather than epileptic seizures, but true convulsions can also occur at any stage of the illness. In addition to myoclonic jerks, which tend to disappear as the disease progresses, a variety of other abnormal movements and dystonias have also been observed. Cerebellar ataxia may occur. Retinopathy and optic atrophy may appear, sometimes even before behavioral changes. Dementia progresses to stupor and coma, sometimes with autonomic insufficiency. Patients may be rigid or spastic with decorticate postures, or they may be flaccid.

The speed of progression is highly variable, but in at least 60% of patients the course is inexorable and relatively rapid. The total duration of illness may be as short as a few months, but most patients survive for 1–3 yr after diagnosis, with a mean of about 18 mo. Occasional patients show some spontaneous improvement and live for more than 10 yr. In recent years the few patients diagnosed with SSPE in the United States have tended to have a relatively long survival, perhaps due to improvements in chronic care.

LABORATORY DIAGNOSIS. The blood is normal except for elevated titers of antibodies to measles virus; antibodies are of the IgG and IgM classes and are directed against all the component proteins of measles virus except the M protein. Cell content of the CSF is generally normal, although stained sediments may show plasma cells. Total protein content of the CSF is normal or only slightly elevated; however, the gamma globulin fraction is greatly elevated (usually comprising at least 20% of total protein), resulting in a paretic type of colloidal gold curve. When the CSF is examined by electrophoresis or isoelectric focusing, "oligoclonal" bands of immunoglobin are often observed. IgG and IgM antibodies to measles virus, not normally found in unconcentrated CSF, make up most of the immunoglobulin, and these can often be detected in dilutions of 1:8 or more. The complement-fixation test has been especially useful for demonstrating antibodies in CSF, but hemagglutination inhibition, immunofluorescence, and other serologic tests, including ELISA, are also satisfactory. The normal ratio of titer in serum to titer in CSF is reduced (below 200) for measles antibodies, whereas serum-CSF ratios are normal for other viral antibodies and for albumin, indicating that the increased amounts of measles antibodies in the CSF of patients with SSPE result from synthesis within the nervous system and that the blood-brain barrier is normal.

Early in the course of disease the electroencephalogram (EEG) may be normal or show only moderate nonspecific slowing. In the myoclonic stage most patients with SSPE have episodes of "suppression-burst" in which high-amplitude slow and sharp waves recur at intervals of 3–5 sec on a slow background; however, this pattern is not unique to SSPE. Later in the illness the EEG becomes increasingly disorganized and shows high-amplitude random dysrhythmic slowing; in terminal disease the amplitude may fall.

Computed tomograms or magnetic resonance images of patients with SSPE may show variable cortical atrophy and ventricular enlargement, and there may be focal or multifocal low-density lesions in white matter. However, these studies may be normal, especially early in disease.

Brain biopsy is no longer needed to diagnose SSPE. When performed, it will often show the typical histopathologic findings described earlier. Examination of frozen sections by immunofluorescence technique may demonstrate the presence of measles viral antigens. Persistence of measles virus infection in cultures may be demonstrated by labeled-antibody techniques before the complete virus appears. Many specimens fail to yield complete virus. A modification of the polymerase-chain reaction (PCR) can detect various regions of the measles virus RNA in frozen and even paraffin-embedded brain tissue specimens of patients with SSPE. Nucleic-acid hybridization techniques have also been used to demonstrate the measles viral genome.

DIFFERENTIAL DIAGNOSIS. It is most important to rule out potentially treatable illnesses such as bacterial infections and tumors. The diverse cerebral storage diseases and nonstorage poliodystrophies, leukodystrophies, and demyelinating diseases of childhood can also produce progressive dementia with seizures and paralysis resembling SSPE. Early in the course of illness, SSPE must be distinguished from atypical acute viral encephalitides. Other slow viral infections, such as Creutzfeldt-Jakob disease and progressive rubella panencephalitis, must be considered in appropriate age groups. The presence of a typical EEG pattern is suggestive of SSPE, as are unusually high levels of measles antibodies in serum. The diagnosis is practically confirmed if measles antibodies are detected in CSF.

COMPLICATIONS. Patients with SSPE have the usual secondary complications associated with incapacitating neurologic diseases, for example, pneumonias, decubitus ulcers, and others.

INFECTIVITY AND PRECAUTIONS. The persistent measles infection in SSPE does not result in complete virus particles. Patients with SSPE, therefore, pose no hazard of infection to others, and no special precautions need ordinarily be taken. If a recent report of isolation of measles virus from the blood of a patient with SSPE is confirmed, blood precautions might be justified under special circumstances.

PREVENTION. Immunization with existing attenuated measles virus vaccines prevents the large majority of cases of SSPE. Should cases of SSPE be convincingly attributed to vaccine strains of measles rather than to preceding natural measles infection or to vaccination failure, attempts to improve vaccines would be justified.

PROGNOSIS. As noted earlier, few patients live for more than 3 yr after the diagnosis of SSPE is first made, and those that do survive longer are usually disabled.

THERAPY. Administration of inosiplex may increase the number of patients with prolonged survival and may produce some clinical improvement in the degree of resulting disability (100 mg/kg/24 hr given in divided doses). Other treatments have been ineffective. The use of anticonvulsants, maintenance of nutritional status, prompt treatment of secondary bacterial infections, physical therapy, and other supportive care may also prolong survival and improve the quality of life for the patient and family. Information on current therapeutic trials should be sought through the U. S. National SSPE Registry.*

12.86 Progressive Rubella Panencephalitis (PRP)

This is an exceedingly rare chronic encephalitis, associated with persistent rubella virus infection of the brain. The 20 reported patients since the disease was first recognized in 1974 have been boys who were between the ages of 8 and 19 yr at onset; most had typical stigmata of the congenital rubella syndrome, including cataracts, deafness, and mental retardation, but two had had childhood rubella from which they made a full recovery. If the incidence of congenital and acquired rubella continues the dramatic decline that began with the advent of immunization, PRP should become even more rare.

The *clinical manifestations* at the onset of PRP resemble those of SSPE, with insidious changes in behavior and deterioration in school performance. Subsequently, frank dementia and other signs of multifocal brain disease occur, including seizures, cerebellar ataxia, and spastic weakness. Myoclonus and other abnormal movements may occur but are not as common as in SSPE. Retinopathy, similar to that seen in acute rubella, and optic atrophy may occur. The course of illness in PRP is similar to that seen in SSPE, progressing to coma, spasticity, brain stem involvement, and death in 2–5 yr.

The peripheral blood is normal in PRP except for elevated titers of antibodies to rubella virus. The CSF shows normal or slightly elevated cell content; CSF protein is slightly elevated, with a marked increase in globulin, which may make up more than 50% of the total protein. Oligoclonal electrophoretic bands of globulin are found in the CSF of PRP patients; the bands resemble those seen in SSPE but consist of antibodies to rubella virus antigens. Antibodies to rubella virus are readily detectable in CSF, often at dilutions of 1:8 or higher. The complement-fixation, hemagglutination inhibition, and ELISA techniques should be satisfactory for testing the spinal fluid. Most of the rubella antibodies in the CSF are IgG, although some IgM antibodies have also been detected early in the course of PRP. The serum-CSF ratio of antibody titers to rubella virus is reduced, whereas ratios of titers to measles and other viruses are normal.

The EEG shows a generalized slowing with occasional high-voltage activity, but the suppression-burst pattern of SSPE has not been seen in PRP. Encephalograms (computed tomograms were not available when published cases were studied) show enlargement of all ventricles, especially the 4th, with prominent atrophy of the cerebellum.

Histopathologic changes seen in the brains of patients with PRP are similar to those seen in SSPE, with cuffs of lymphocytes and plasma cells around blood vessels, glial nodules in the cortex, some loss of neurons, and an increase in astrocytes throughout the gray matter and an even greater increase in the white matter. However, in PRP there are no inclusion bodies, and deposits of material that stains with the periodic acid-Schiff reaction are found around vessels in subcortical white matter.

Rubella virus has been isolated from brain cell cultures and from separated blood lymphocytes.

Differential diagnosis of PRP is the same as that for SSPE. The stigmata of congenital rubella syndrome or a history of German measles suggests PRP. Elevated levels of rubella antibodies in serum, the presence of oligoclonal bands of gamma globulins and rubella antibodies in the spinal fluid, and a reduction in the normal serum-CSF ratio for antibodies to rubella virus establish the *diagnosis* of PRP. Isolation of rubella virus from blood lymphocytes may be attempted. Brain biopsy should not be needed to establish the diagnosis.

Patients with PRP pose no substantial risk of infection to others, although it seems reasonable to avoid exposing rubella-susceptible persons to the blood of patients with PRP. Rubella virus has not been detected in urine.

12.87 OTHER CHRONIC CONVENTIONAL VIRAL INFECTIONS OF THE NERVOUS SYSTEM

CHRONIC TICK-BORNE ENCEPHALITIS (TBE). The virus of TBE, a member of the flavivirus group of small enveloped RNA viruses, usually causes an acute meningoencephalomyelitis, also called Russian spring-summer encephalitis, that may be of variable severity. As many as 20% of patients

---

*Dr P. R. Dyken, Department of Neurology, University of South Alabama, Mobile, AL.

recover from acute encephalitis only to develop new signs of progressive neurologic disease months or even years later. Most cases of chronic progressive TBE have been reported from the Soviet Union, but two typical patients were described in Japan. Chronic progressive TBE may have the following clinical manifestations: (1) movement or seizure disorders of which epilepsia partialis continua (Kozhevnikov's epilepsy) is the most common; (2) paralytic disorders, often with brain stem involvement; (3) mixed syndromes. The seizure and movement disorders may stabilize or remit, but the progressive paralytic syndrome is usually fatal. The CSF in one patient with chronic TBE contained elevated levels of antibodies to TBE virus. Brain tissue shows panencephalitis without inclusion bodies by light microscopy and no virus-like structures by electron microscopy. Isolation of TBE virus has occasionally been reported from the brain tissue or CSF of patients with chronic post-TBE syndromes, but most attempts to isolate the virus have failed.

RASMUSSEN ENCEPHALITIS. Patients with similar types of chronic encephalitis not associated with any known viral infection have been recognized throughout the world. In North America a syndrome of seizures (especially epilepsia partialis continua), spastic paralysis, and mental retardation associated with chronic encephalitis was described by Rasmussen and colleagues in children, adolescents, and young adults. Patients had no history of preceding acute encephalitis. Computed tomography may show cerebral cortical atrophy or ventricular dilatation, and when brain tissue is resected a panencephalitis without inclusion bodies or virus-like particles is found. The Epstein-Barr virus and cytomegalovirus have occasionally been implicated in this disease. Efforts to isolate viruses from brains of patients with Rasmussen encephalitis have been unsuccessful.

PROGRESSIVE MULTIFOCAL LEUKOENCEPHALOPATHY (PML). This progressive infection of oligodendroglial cells with the JC papovavirus affects immunosuppressed subjects, in whom it is almost invariably fatal (Sec. 12.13). In children it is even more rare than in adults. Although PML is a well-recognized opportunistic infection complicating AIDS in adults, it has not yet been described in children with that disease.

PERSISTENT RETROVIRAL INFECTIONS OF THE NERVOUS SYSTEM. The lentivirus HIV-1 frequently produces both an acute encephalitis at the time of primary infection and a progressive encephalopathy that is unfortunately very common in both adults and children with AIDS (Sec. 12.83).

The human T cell leukemia-lymphoma virus (HTLV-I) has been implicated as the cause of a progressive myelopathy called both tropical spastic paraparesis (TSP) and HTLV-I-associated myelopathy (HAM). Although TSP/HAM is much more common among adults, it also occurs in children. HTLV-I may also cause meningoencephalitis and myositis, although these entities have not been observed in children. Infections with HTLV-I are usually completely asymptomatic, at least for very long periods of time. The spread of infection with HTLV-I may be reduced by excluding individuals with antibodies to the virus from donating blood.

12.88 SLOW INFECTIONS WITH UNCONVENTIONAL VIRUSES: THE SUBACUTE SPONGIFORM ENCEPHALOPATHIES

The subacute spongiform encephalopathies all have similarities in clinical manifestations and histopathology, and all are slow infections. The most striking neuropathologic change that occurs in each disease, to a greater or lesser extent is spongy degeneration of the cerebral cortical gray matter (Fig. 12–32). Kuru once affected many children and adolescents in a restricted area of Papua New Guinea; its transmission was interrupted 30 yr ago, and it is now found only in older adults. Creutzfeldt-Jakob disease (CJD), the most common human spongiform encephalopathy, was formerly thought to occur only in older adults; however, iatrogenically transmitted cases of CJD have been recognized in adolescents and young adults. Gerstmann-Sträussler syndrome (GSS), a familial spongiform encephalopathy characterized by striking amyloid plaques and more prominent cerebellar ataxia and a longer average duration than typical sporadic CJD, may be considered a variant of that disease. GSS has not been diagnosed in children or adolescents.

ETIOLOGY. The spongiform encephalopathies are all slow infections that are transmissible to susceptible animals by inoculation of tissues from affected subjects. Although the infectious agents replicate in some cell cultures, they do not achieve the high titers of infectivity found in brain tissues or cause recognizable cytopathic effects. Most studies of spongiform encephalopathy agents employ in vivo assays in which the appearance of typical scrapie or CJD in animals is taken as evidence that the agent is present and intact. Inoculation of the smallest amounts of infectivity present in very dilute preparations of all of these agents results in the accumulation in tissues of recipient animals of large amounts of an agent having the same physical and biologic properties as the original agent. Until recently the pathogens transmitting the spongiform encephalopathies were generally considered viruses, and they still are by many authorities. However, they display a spectrum of extreme resistance to inactivation by a variety of chemical and physical treatments that is unknown among other viruses. This characteristic stimulated the hypothesis that the spongiform encephalopathy agents might be unique infectious pathogens, probably subviral in size, composed of protein and devoid of nucleic acid. An alternative designation, "prions," has been suggested for these agents. However, the prion hypothesis is not universally accepted. The size and structure of the infectious agent and the presence or absence of a nucleic acid genome have not yet been established. If the spongiform encephalopathy agents ultimately prove to contain nucleic acid genomes, they might still be considered atypical viruses. Until the actual structure of the pathogens is clearly determined, it may be less contentious simply to call them agents.

"Scrapie-associated fibrils" (SAF) are found in extracts of tissues from a variety of patients and animals with spongiform encephalopathies but not in normal tissues. SAF resemble but are distinguishable from the amyloid fibrils that accumulate in the brains of patients with Alzheimer's disease. A group of antigenically related, low-molecular-weight proteins, designated the "prion protein 27–30" (PrP27–30), are components of SAF that are consistently found in the amyloid plaques seen in the brains of patients and animals with spongiform encephalopathies. It is not yet clear whether SAF/PrP27–30 constitute the complete infectious particle of spongiform encephalopathies or components of those particles, or are simply pathologic host proteins not usually separated from the actual infectious entities by currently used techniques. The demonstration that the PrP27–30 protein is encoded by a normal host gene favors the last possibility. However, other studies seem to suggest that agent-specific information can be transmitted and replicated in the absence of genetic material independent of the host.

Whatever its relationship to the actual infectious particles, SAF/PrP27–30 is extremely important in the pathogenesis of spongiform encephalopathies. It is a glycoprotein that has the physical properties of an amyloid protein. The PrP27–30 proteins of several species of animals are very similar in their amino acid sequences and antigenicity but are not identical

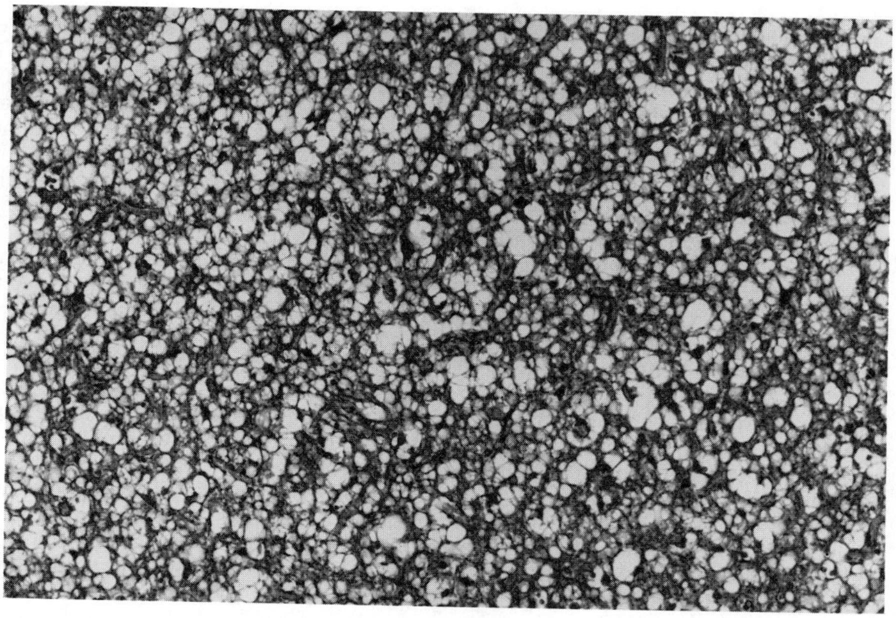

Figure 12–32. Severe vacuolation (status spongiosus) in the cerebral cortex of a patient with familial Creutzfeldt-Jakob disease.

in structure. The primary structure of PrP27–30 is encoded by the host and does not appear to be influenced by the source of the infectious agent provoking its formation. PrP27–30 is derived from a larger precursor protein, designated PrP33–35, Gp35, or scrapie amyloid precursor protein. The function of PrP33–35 in normal cells is unknown. The relationship between mutations in the gene coding for PrP and familial spongiform encephalopathies is discussed later under Genetic Counseling.

EPIDEMIOLOGY AND MECHANISMS OF TRANSMISSION. The disappearance of kuru among young people suggests that the practice of ritual cannibalism was the most important if not the only mechanism by which the infection spread in Papua New Guinea.

CJD has been recognized worldwide, at rates of 0.25–2 cases/million population/yr, with foci of considerably higher incidence among Libyan Jews in Israel, in isolated villages of Slovakia, and in other limited areas. Epidemiologic surveys have investigated several hypothetical mechanisms of spread of CJD, including contamination of meat products with scrapie agent and iatrogenic spread of infection from tissues of patients. The striking resemblance of CJD to scrapie prompted the suggestion that infected sheep tissues might be a source of spongiform encephalopathy in humans. In addition, recent recognition of bovine spongiform encephalopathy among cattle (which were apparently infected by eating scrapie-contaminated bone meal), zoo animals, and domestic cats in Great Britain raised a fear that some strain of the scrapie agent, having crossed a species barrier from sheep to cattle, may have acquired an even broader range of susceptible hosts, posing a potential danger for humans. Although no transmission of spongiform encephalopathy from animals to humans has ever been documented, it seems reasonable to avoid exposing children to meat and meat products likely to be contaminated with spongiform encephalopathy agents.

In contrast, iatrogenic transmission of CJD has been established. Accidental transmission of CJD has occurred by means of contaminated neurosurgical instruments or facilities, transplantation of contaminated cornea, contaminated cortical electrodes used during epilepsy surgery, injections of human pituitary growth hormone and human pituitary gonadotropin, and grafts of cadaver dura mater. Pharmaceuticals and grafts derived from or contaminated with human neural tissues, particularly when obtained from unselected donors and from large pools of donors, pose special risks.

Spouses and household contacts of patients are at very low risk of acquiring CJD. (A single conjugal case has been reported.) Medical personnel exposed to brains of patients with CJD may be at increased risk.

PATHOLOGY. Typical changes include vacuolation and loss of neurons (see Fig. 12–32) with hypertrophy and proliferation of glial cells, most pronounced in the cerebral cortex in patients with CJD and in the cerebellum in those with kuru. The lesions are usually most severe in or even confined to gray matter, at least early in the disease. Loss of myelin appears to be secondary to degeneration of neurons. There is usually no inflammation, but there is a marked increase in the number and size of astrocytes.

"Amyloid" plaques are found in the brains of all patients with GSS, in at least 70% of patients with kuru, and less commonly in those with CJD. They are most common in the cerebellum but occur elsewhere in the brain as well. The plaques react with antisera prepared against SAF/PrP, but even in the absence of plaques extracellular SAF/PrP has been detected by immunostaining. Tubulovesicular particles have also often been observed in the brains of patients and animals with spongiform encephalopathies.

PATHOGENESIS. The portal of entry for the kuru agent is thought to be the integument, probably through lesions rather than intact skin and mucosa. It is not known whether humans can be infected with spongiform encephalopathies through the intestinal tract. The first site of replication of the agents appears to be the tissues of the reticuloendothelial system. The CJD agent has been detected in human blood, but it is not clear whether "viremia" is responsible for the spread of infection to the nervous system. Limited evidence suggests that in mice the scrapie agent spreads to the CNS by ascending peripheral nerves. In human kuru it seems highly probable that the only portal of exit of the agent from the body, at least in quantities sufficient to infect others, was through tissues exposed during cannibalism. In iatrogenically transmitted CJD, the brain and eye of patients with CJD have been the sources of contamination. Kidney, liver, lung, lymph node, spleen, and CSF also sometimes contain the agent. At no time during the course of illness have antibodies or cell-mediated immunity to the infectious agents of the spongiform encephalopathies been convincingly demonstrated in either patients or animals.

CLINICAL MANIFESTATIONS. Kuru is a progressive degenerative disease of the cerebellum and brain stem with less obvious involvement of the cerebral cortex. The first sign of kuru is usually cerebellar ataxia followed by progressive incoordination. Coarse shivering tremors are a characteristic manifestation. Variable abnormalities in cranial nerve function appear with frequent impairment in conjugate gaze and swallowing. Patients die from inanition and pneumonia or from burns from cooking fires, usually less than a year after onset. Although changes in mentation are common, there is no frank dementia or progression to coma as in CJD. There are no signs of acute encephalitis, for example, no fever, headaches, or convulsions.

CJD occurs throughout the world. Patients initially have either sensory disturbances or confusion and inappropriate behavior, with progression over weeks or months to frank dementia and ultimately coma. Some patients have cerebellar ataxia early in disease, and most develop myoclonic jerking movements. GSS is a familial disease resembling CJD but with more prominent cerebellar ataxia and amyloid plaques; dementia may appear only late in the course. Mean survival of patients with CJD is less than 1 yr from the earliest signs of illness, although about 10% live for more than 2 yr. Patients with GSS tend to survive longer.

LABORATORY FINDINGS. Virtually all patients with CJD have abnormal EEG findings as the disease progresses; the background becomes slow and irregular with diminished amplitude. A variety of paroxysmal discharges may also appear: slow waves, sharp waves, spike and wave complexes, and these may sometimes be unilateral or focal as well as bilaterally synchronous. Paroxysmal discharges may be precipitated by loud noise. Many patients have typical periodic suppression-burst complexes of high-voltage slow activity on EEG at some time during the illness. Computed tomography may show cortical atrophy and large ventricles late in the course of CJD. There may be some elevation of CSF protein. Liver function studies sometimes suggest parenchymal disease.

DIAGNOSIS. Brain biopsy may be diagnostic of CJD, but it should be recommended only if some other potentially treatable disease remains to be excluded. The demonstration of SAF or PrP27–30 proteins in brain extracts is useful for confirming the histopathologic diagnosis. Transmission of disease to susceptible animals by inoculation of brain suspension is the ultimate diagnostic test for spongiform encephalopathy, although it is usually reserved for cases of special research interest.

PREVENTION, CONTAINMENT, AND DISINFECTION. Universal precautions should be used for handling blood and body fluids. All materials and surfaces known to be contaminated with tissues or CSF from patients suspected of having CJD must be treated with great care. Whenever possible, contaminated instruments should be discarded by careful packaging and transport to sites of incineration. Contaminated tissues and biologic products probably cannot be completely freed of infectivity without destroying their structural integrity and biologic activity; therefore, the medical and family histories of individual tissue donors should be carefully reviewed for dementia. Although no method of sterilization can be relied upon to remove all infectivity from contaminated surfaces, various heat, sodium hydroxide, and chlorine bleach disinfection methods may markedly reduce infectivity.

TREATMENT. No treatment is effective. Appropriate supportive care should be provided as for other progressive fatal neurologic diseases.

PROGNOSIS. The prognosis of spongiform encephalopathies is uniformly poor. Perhaps 10% of patients survive for a year or even longer, but their quality of life is poor.

GENETIC COUNSELING. The gene coding for PrP33–35 is closely linked if not identical to that controlling the incubation periods of scrapie in sheep and both scrapie and CJD in mice. The gene encoding the analogous protein in humans, currently designated the "PRIP" gene, is located on the short arm of chromosome 20. It has an open reading frame of some 750 nucleotides in which three different mutations linked to the occurrence of spongiform encephalopathy in families have been identified.

Spongiform encephalopathies sometimes run in families, the pattern of occurrence roughly resembling an autosomal dominant mode of inheritance. In patients with a family history of CJD the clinical and histopathologic findings are the same as those seen in sporadic cases. GSS is always familial. In several families with GSS an apparent linkage of disease to the same mutation in the PRIP gene encoding the PrP amyloid precursor protein has been found. Still other mutations in the PRIP gene linked to several cases of familial CJD have been identified.

Although the interpretation of these findings in regard to the prion hypothesis is in dispute, in affected families subjects who are heterozygous for some mutations in the PRIP gene clearly have a high probability of getting GSS and CJD. In the United States only about 10% of cases are familial; in affected families, however, about 50% of siblings and children of a CJD patient may eventually get the disease. Although in families with the autosomal dominant pattern of CJD or GSS the finding of certain mutations in the PRIP gene appears to be predictive of disease, the significance of the same or other mutations in the PRIP genes of subjects from families that have no history of spongiform encephalopathy is not known. It seems wise to avoid alarming subjects who have miscellaneous mutations in the PRIP gene or their families because the implications are not yet clear.

OTHER DEGENERATIVE DISEASES OF THE CENTRAL NERVOUS SYSTEM CAUSED BY UNCONVENTIONAL VIRUSES

It has been claimed but not confirmed that two other human diseases may be caused by infections with agents similar to those causing the spongiform encephalopathies *familial Alzheimer disease* of adults and *Alpers disease* of young children. The latter is a convulsive disorder associated with hemiatrophy and status spongiosus of the cerebral gray matter.

DAVID M. ASHER

Asher DM, Gibbs CJ Jr, Gajdusek DC: Subacute spongiform encephalopathies: Slow infections of the nervous system. Clin Microbiol Newsletter 7:129, 1985.

Asher DM, Masters CL, Gajdusek DC, et al: Familial spongiform encephalopathies. *In*: Kety SS, Rowland LP, Sidman RL, et al (eds): Genetics of Neurological and Psychiatric Disorders. New York, Raven Press, 1983, p 273.

Brown P: Human growth hormone therapy and Creutzfeldt-Jakob disease: A drama in three acts. Pediatrics 81:85, 1988.

Chen TT, Watanabe I, Zeman W, et al: Subacute sclerosing panencephalitis: Propagation of measles virus from brain biopsy in tissue culture. Science 163:1193, 1969.

Dyken PR, Cunningham SC, Ward LC: Changing character of subacute sclerosing panencephalitis in the United States. Pediatr Neurol 5:339, 1989.

Godec MS, Asher DM, Swoveland PT, et al: Detection of measles virus genomic sequences in SSPE brain tissue. J Med Virol 30:237, 1990.

Goldgaber D, Goldfarb LG, Brown P, et al: Mutations in familial Creutzfeldt-Jakob disease and Gerstmann-Sträussler-Scheinker's syndrome. Exper Neurol 106:204, 1989.

Prusiner SB: Prions and neurodegenerative diseases. N Engl J Med 317:1571, 1987.

Weil ML, Itabashi HH, Cremer NE, et al: Chronic progressive panencephalitis due to rubella virus simulating subacute sclerosing panencephalitis. N Engl J Med 292:994, 1975.

12.89 YELLOW FEVER

Yellow fever is an acute mosquito-borne infection characterized in its most severe form by fever, jaundice, proteinuria, and hemorrhage. The pediatrician practicing in North America needs to be able to provide appropriate advice regarding immunization of children travelling to endemic areas (Sec. 5.6).

ETIOLOGY. Yellow fever is a member of the flavivirus (group B arbovirus) genus of the family Flaviviridae. Virus particles are small and contain an infectious single-stranded RNA genome. Human and nonhuman primate hosts acquire the infection by the bite of infected mosquitoes. After an incubation period of 3–6 days, virus appears in the bloodstream and may serve as a source of infection for other mosquitoes. An incubation period of 1–2 wk is required in the mosquito before it is capable of transmitting the virus.

EPIDEMIOLOGY. Figure 12–33 shows the present geographic distribution of endemic yellow fever. In the 19th and early 20th centuries, the disease occurred in the Caribbean, the United States, South America, and parts of Europe; these areas, still infested with *Aedes aegypti* mosquitoes, are potentially receptive to the introduction and spread of the disease from the endemic zone. Yellow fever has never appeared in Asia. The incidence of officially reported cases in tropical South America is approximately 200/yr, but the disease is significantly underreported. In West Africa, large outbreaks have occurred periodically. In the Americas, adult males are the principal targets of yellow fever because they are exposed to infected mosquitoes while working in forested areas. In Africa, however, where epidemics occur in savannah village regions, children under 15 yr have the highest incidence; there is an increasing immune barrier with age (due to naturally acquired and vaccine immunity). Transmission is highest during the rainy season (generally December-March in tropical America and July-November in West Africa). A significant factor that promotes the occurrence of yellow fever in some areas is the migration of nonimmune laborers and other populations into endemic regions.

In tropical forests, yellow fever virus is maintained in a transmission cycle involving monkeys and tree-hole breeding mosquitoes (*Haemagogus* spp. in the Americas, *Aedes africanus* in Africa). Persons entering the forest may be exposed, resulting in sporadic cases of jungle yellow fever. In Africa, the virus activity also occurs in moist savannah and savannah-forest transition areas, where other tree-hole breeding *Aedes* vectors present in high density transmit the virus between monkeys, between monkeys and humans, and between humans. Urban yellow fever, the result of human-to-human transmission by the domestic mosquito *Aedes aegypti*, occurs in villages and towns in Africa but has not been reported in the Americas since 1942.

CLINICAL MANIFESTATIONS. Inapparent, abortive, or clinically mild infections are frequent, and some studies have suggested that children experience a milder disease than adults. Abortive infections, characterized by fever and headache, may go unrecognized except, at times, during epidemics.

In its full-blown form, yellow fever begins with sudden onset of fever, headache, myalgia, lumbosacral pain, anorexia, nausea, and vomiting. Physical findings during the early phase of illness, when virus is present in the blood, include prostration, conjunctival injection, flushing of face and neck, reddening of the tongue at the tip and edges, and a relative bradycardia. After 2–3 days, there may be a brief period of remission, followed in 6–24 hr by reappearance of fever, vomiting, epigastric pain, jaundice, dehydration, hemorrhage (particularly hematemesis), albuminuria, hypotension, signs of renal failure, delirium, convulsions, and coma. Between the 7th and 10th days death generally occurs. The fatality rate in severe cases approaches 50%. Some patients who survive the acute phase of illness may later succumb to renal failure or myocardial damage. Laboratory findings include leukopenia, prolongation of clotting, prothrombin, and partial thromboplastin times, thrombocytopenia, hyperbilirubinemia, elevation of serum transaminases, albuminuria, and azotemia. Hypoglycemia may be present in severe cases. EKG abnormalities (bradycardia, ST-T changes) have occurred.

PATHOLOGY AND PATHOPHYSIOLOGY. Histopathologic changes in the liver include: (1) coagulative necrosis of hepatocytes in the midzone of the liver lobule with sparing of cells around the portal areas and central veins; (2) eosinophilic degeneration of hepatocytes (Councilman bodies); (3) microvacuolar fatty change; and (4) minimal inflammation. The kidneys show acute tubular necrosis. Myocardial fiber degeneration and fatty infiltration are present. The brain may show edema and petechial hemorrhages. Direct viral injury to the liver, resulting in impaired biosynthesis and detoxification, is a central pathogenetic event. Hemorrhage results from decreased synthesis of vitamin K–dependent clotting factors, and, in some cases, disseminated intravascular clotting. Renal dysfunction is attributed to hemodynamic factors (prerenal failure progressing to acute tubular necrosis). The pathogenesis of shock in patients with yellow fever is not understood.

DIAGNOSIS AND TREATMENT. Yellow fever should be suspected when fever, headache, vomiting and myalgia ap-

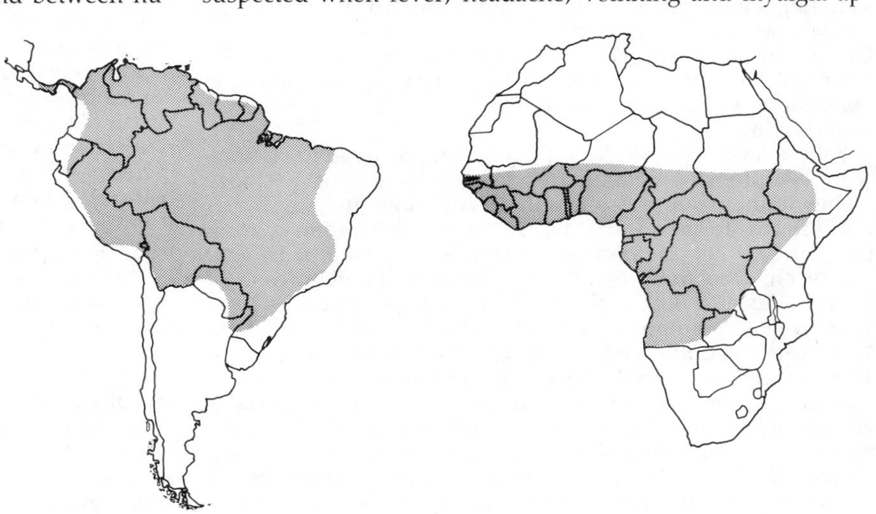

Figure 12–33. Endemic areas of yellow fever *(shaded)*. Immunization of persons traveling to these regions is recommended, whether or not national health authorities require vaccination certificates.

pear in residents of endemic areas or in unimmunized visitors who have recently traveled (within 2 wk prior to onset of symptoms) to those areas. Mild yellow fever cannot be distinguished from a wide variety of other infections. Jaundice and hemorrhage may signal the presence of any one of several other diseases that must be differentiated; such possibilities include malaria, leptospirosis, viral hepatitis, Rift Valley fever, Crimean-Congo hemorrhagic fever, typhoid, rickettsial infections, and other viral hemorrhagic fevers.

Specific diagnosis depends on tests for presence of virus or viral antigen in acute phase blood samples or on antibody determinations. The IgM enzyme immunoassay is a particularly useful serologic test. Sera obtained during the first 10 days after onset of symptoms should be kept frozen, preferably in an ultra-low-temperature freezer ($-60°$ C) and shipped on dry ice for virus testing. Convalescent-phase samples for antibody tests are managed by conventional means. In handling acutely infected blood specimens, all clinical personnel must take care to avoid contaminating unimmunized personnel as well as laboratory equipment and operations. Postmortem diagnosis is based on virus isolation from liver or blood, classic histopathologic examination, or detection of antigen or viral genome in liver tissue.

TREATMENT. Therapy is symptomatic and includes (1) careful monitoring of vital functions, (2) reduction of fever by sponging or acetaminophen (avoid aspirin because of bleeding diathesis), (3) protection of the gastric mucosa (suction, antacids, sucralfate, cimetidine), (4) adequate nutritional intake and treatment of hypoglycemia (with intravenous 10–20% glucose), (5) avoidance of CNS depressant drugs, (6) correction of acid-base disturbances, and (7) treatment of hypotension and shock. If prerenal azotemia occurs, efforts should be made to increase renal perfusion by fluid challenge or (in presence of hypotension) by dopamine or dobutamine. If oliguric acute renal failure (acute tubular necrosis) is present, peritoneal or hemodialysis may be indicated. If bacterial sepsis occurs as a complication, it should be treated with appropriate antibiotics. Bleeding diathesis, if severe, can best be managed by transfusion of fresh whole blood, fresh frozen plasma, or platelet concentrates. Heparin therapy is indicated when disseminated intravascular coagulation is diagnosed.

PREVENTION AND CONTROL. Yellow fever 17D is an extremely safe, live attenuated vaccine that should be administered as a single 0.5-mL subcutaneous injection at least 10 days before arrival in an endemic area (Fig. 12–33). All persons traveling to these areas should be considered for vaccination, but length of stay, exact locations to be visited, and likely environmental exposure may determine the specific risk and individual need for vaccination. If questions arise, information should be sought from the Centers for Disease Control, Division of Vector-Borne Diseases, Fort Collins, CO (tel. 303-221-6400). For international travel certification, vaccination is valid for 10 yr, although immunity lasts at least 40 yr and is probably lifelong.

Yellow fever vaccine should not be administered to persons with symptomatic immunodeficiency diseases or to those taking immunosuppressant drugs. Although the vaccine is not known to harm the fetus, its administration during pregnancy is contraindicated on theoretical grounds. In very young children there is an increased but ill-defined risk of encephalitis and death. Nearly all neurologic infections have been in infants immunized at 4 mo of age or less. Hence, the 17D vaccine should never be administered to infants less than 4 mo of age and should be given to infants 4–6 mo of age only if residence or travel in an ongoing epidemic area is anticipated. Travel to areas of known yellow fever activity (without an ongoing epidemic) under circumstances engendering a high risk (e.g., forested areas in the Amazon basin) warrants immunization of infants 6–9 mo of age. Routine immunization of children 9 mo and older is recommended before entry to other endemic areas is considered. In persons with a history of egg allergy, vaccination should be avoided or a skin test should be performed to determine if there is a specific allergy to the material that would preclude vaccination.

THOMAS P. MONATH

Monath TP: Yellow fever. *In:* Monath TP (ed): The Arboviruses: Epidemiology and Ecology, Vol 5. Boca Raton, FL, CRC Press, 1988, pp 139–231.

Monath TP: Yellow fever—a medically neglected disease. Rev Infect Dis 9:165, 1987.

12.90 DENGUE FEVER AND DENGUE-LIKE DISEASE

Dengue fever, a benign syndrome caused by several arthropod-borne viruses, is characterized by biphasic fever, myalgia or arthralgia, rash, leukopenia, and lymphadenopathy.

HISTORY. Epidemics were common in temperate areas of the Americas, Europe, Australia, and Asia until early in the 20th century. Dengue fever and dengue-like disease are now endemic in tropical Asia, the South Pacific Islands, Northern Australia, tropical Africa, the Caribbean, and Central and South America. Dengue fever occurs frequently among travelers.

ETIOLOGY. There are at least four distinct antigenic types of dengue virus. In addition, three other arthropod-borne (arbo) viruses cause similar or identical febrile diseases with rash (Table 12–39).

EPIDEMIOLOGY. Dengue viruses are transmitted by mosquitoes of the Stegomyia family. *Aedes aegypti*, a daytime biting mosquito, is the principal vector, and all four virus types have been recovered from it. In most tropical areas *Aedes aegypti* is highly urbanized, breeding in water stored for drinking or bathing or in rain water collected in any container. Dengue viruses have also been recovered from *Aedes albopictus*, and outbreaks in the Pacific area have been attributed to several other *Aedes* species. These species breed in water trapped in vegetation. In Malaysia, dengue may be maintained in a cycle involving canopy-feeding jungle monkeys and *Aedes niveus*, which feeds on both monkeys and man.

Dengue outbreaks in urban areas infested with *Aedes aegypti* may be explosive; up to 70–80% of the population may be involved. Most disease occurs in older children and adults. Because *Aedes aegypti* has a limited range, spread of an epidemic occurs mainly through viremic human beings and follows the main lines of transportation. Sentinel cases may infect household mosquitoes, with a large number of nearly simultaneous secondary infections giving the appearance of a contagious disease. Where dengue is endemic, children and susceptible foreigners may be the only persons to acquire overt disease, adults having become immune.

Dengue-like diseases may occur in epidemics. Epidemiologic features depend upon the vectors and their geographic distribution (see Table 12–39). Chikungunya virus is widespread in the most populous areas of the world. In Asia, *Aedes aegypti* is the principal vector; in Africa other Stegomyia may be important vectors. In Southeast Asia, dengue and chikungunya outbreaks occur concurrently. Outbreaks of o'nyong-nyong and West Nile fever usually involve villages or small towns, in contrast to the urban outbreaks of dengue and chikungunya.

PATHOLOGY. Insufficient pathologic material has been obtained from virologically confirmed cases of dengue fever to permit a comprehensive description. Fatalities are rare with chikungunya and West Nile infections; those recorded have

Table 12–39. Vectors and Geographic Distribution of Dengue-like Diseases

Genus	Virus and Disease	Vector	Geographic Distribution
Togavirus	Chikungunya	*Aedes aegypti* *Aedes africanus*	Africa, India, Southeast Asia
Togavirus	O'nyong-nyong	*Anopheles funestus*	East Africa
Flavivirus	West Nile fever	*Culex molestus* *Culex univittatus*	Africa, Middle East, India

been ascribed to viral encephalitis, hemorrhage, or febrile convulsions (Sec. 12.91).

CLINICAL MANIFESTATIONS. Manifestations vary with age and from patient to patient. In infants and young children the disease may be undifferentiated or characterized by a 1- to 5-day fever, pharyngeal inflammation, rhinitis, and mild cough. In outbreaks a majority of infected older children and adults have most of the findings described below.

After an incubation period of 1–7 days there is a sudden onset of fever, which rapidly rises to 39.4–41.1° C (103–106° F), usually accompanied by frontal or retro-orbital headache. Occasionally, back pain precedes the fever. A *transient*, macular, generalized rash that blanches under pressure may be seen during the first 24–48 hr of fever. The pulse rate may be slow relative to the degree of fever. Myalgia or arthralgia occurs soon after the onset and increases in severity. Involvement of the joints may be particularly severe in patients with chikungunya or o'nyong-nyong infection. From the 2nd–6th days of fever, nausea and vomiting are apt to occur, and generalized lymphadenopathy, cutaneous hyperesthesia or hyperalgesia, taste aberrations, and pronounced anorexia may develop.

One to 2 days after defervescence a generalized, morbilliform, maculopapular rash appears, which spares the palms and soles. It disappears in 1–5 days; desquamation may occur. Rarely there is edema of the palms and soles. About the time this second rash appears, the body temperature, which has previously fallen to normal, may become slightly elevated and establish the biphasic temperature curve.

Epistaxis, petechiae, and purpuric lesions are uncommon but may occur at any stage. Swallowed blood from epistaxis, vomited or passed by rectum, may be erroneously interpreted as gastrointestinal bleeding. Convulsions may occur during high fever, especially with chikungunya fever.

Infrequently, after the febrile stage, prolonged asthenia, mental depression, bradycardia, and ventricular extrasystoles may occur in children.

LABORATORY DATA. Pancytopenia may occur on the 3rd–4th days of illness; neutropenia may persist or reappear during the latter stage of the disease and may continue into convalescence. White blood cell counts as low as 2,000/mm^3 have been recorded. Platelets rarely fall below 100,000 cells/mm^3. Venous clotting, bleeding and prothrombin times, and plasma fibrinogen values are within normal ranges. The tourniquet test infrequently is positive. Mild acidosis, hemoconcentration, increased transaminase values, and hypoproteinemia may occur during some primary dengue virus infections. Classic dengue hemorrhagic fever/dengue shock syndrome may occur in infants born to dengue-immune mothers (Sec. 12.91). Sinus bradycardia, ectopic ventricular foci, flattened T waves, and prolongation of the P-R interval may be observed electrocardiographically.

DIAGNOSIS AND DIFFERENTIAL DIAGNOSIS. *Clinical diagnosis* derives from a high index of suspicion and a knowledge of the geographic distribution and environmental cycles of causal viruses. Exposure to dengue may occur in hotels and during daytime shopping trips in epidemic or endemic areas.

Differential diagnosis includes a number of viral respiratory and influenza-like diseases and the early stages of malaria, scrub typhus, hepatitis, and leptospirosis. Abortive forms of these latter diseases modified by therapy or vaccine may never evolve beyond a dengue-like stage.

Four arboviral diseases have dengue-like courses but without rash: Colorado tick fever, sandfly fever, Rift Valley fever, and Ross River fever. Colorado tick fever occurs sporadically among campers and hunters in the western United States; sandfly fever in the Mediterranean region, the Middle East, southern Russia, and parts of the Indian subcontinent; Rift Valley fever in North, East, Central, and South Africa; and Ross River fever is endemic in much of eastern Australia with epidemic extension to Fiji. In adults, Ross River fever often produces protracted and crippling arthralgia involving weight-bearing joints.

Because clinical findings vary and there are many possible causative agents, the term "dengue-like disease" should be used until a specific diagnosis is established. *Etiologic diagnosis* can be made by serologic study or by isolation of the virus from blood monocytes or serum. Blood for comparative antibody and viral studies should be obtained during the febrile period, preferably early, and during the convalescent phase, 14–21 days after onset. The acute phase serum or plasma may be frozen, optimally at −65° C or colder. Leukocytes should be refrigerated, not frozen. *Serologic diagnosis* depends on a 4-fold or greater increase in antibody titer in paired sera by hemagglutination-inhibition, complement-fixation, enzyme immunoassay, or neutralization test. Carefully standardized IgM and IgG-capture enzyme immunoassays permit the identification of acute phase antibodies from patients with primary or secondary dengue infections in single-serum samples. Usually such samples should be collected not earlier than 5 days nor later than 6 wk after onset. It may not be possible to distinguish the infecting virus by serologic methods alone, particularly when there has been prior infection with another member of the same arbovirus group. Virus can be recovered from tissue culture or after intrathoracic inoculation of appropriate mosquitoes.

PREVENTION AND CONTROL. Attenuated dengue types 1, 2, and 4 vaccines are under development in Thailand, and a killed vaccine for chikungunya is efficacious but not generally available. Prophylaxis consists of avoiding mosquito bite by use of insecticides, repellents, body-covering with clothing, screening of houses, and destruction of *Aedes aegypti* breeding sites. If water storage is mandatory, a tight-fitting lid or a thin layer of oil may prevent egg-laying or hatching. A larvicide, such as Abate [O,O′-(thiodi-*p*-phenylene) O,O,O,O′-tetramethyl phosphorothioate], available as a 1% sand-granule formation and effective at a concentration of 1 part/million, may be added safely to drinking water. Ultra-low-volume spray equipment effectively dispenses the adulticide malathion from truck or airplane for rapid intervention during an epidemic. Only personal antimosquito measures are effective against mosquitoes in the field, forest, or jungle.

TREATMENT. Treatment is supportive. Bed rest is advised during the febrile period. Antipyretics or cold sponging should be used to keep body temperature below 40°C (104°F).

Analgesics or mild sedation may be required to control pain. Because of its effects on hemostasis, aspirin should not be used. Fluid and electrolyte replacement is required when there are deficits due to sweating, fasting, thirsting, vomiting, or diarrhea.

PROGNOSIS. Primary infections with dengue fever and dengue-like diseases are usually self-limited and benign. Fluid and electrolyte losses, hyperpyrexia, and febrile convulsions are the most frequent complications in infants and young children. The prognosis may be adversely affected by passively acquired antibody or by prior infection with a closely related virus (Sec. 12.91).

Dengue in the Caribbean, 1977. Scientific Publication No. 375. Washington, D.C., Pan American Health Organization, 1979.

Halstead SB: Dengue: Hematologic aspects. Semin Hematol 19:116, 1982.

Halstead SB: Selective primary health care: Strategies for control of disease in the developing world. XI. Dengue. Rev Infect Dis 6:251, 1984.

12.91 DENGUE HEMORRHAGIC FEVER/DENGUE SHOCK SYNDROME

(Philippine, Thai, or Singapore Hemorrhagic Fever; Hemorrhagic Dengue; Acute Infectious Thrombocytopenic Purpura)

Dengue hemorrhagic fever, a severe, often fatal, febrile disease caused by dengue viruses, is characterized by capillary permeability, abnormalities of hemostasis, and, in severe cases, a protein-losing shock syndrome. It is currently thought to have an immunopathologic basis.

ETIOLOGY. At least four distinct types of dengue virus (types 1–4) have been isolated from patients with hemorrhagic fever.

EPIDEMIOLOGY. Dengue hemorrhagic fever occurs where multiple types of dengue virus are simultaneously or sequentially transmitted. It is endemic in tropical Asia, where warm temperatures and the practice of water storage in homes result in large, permanent populations of *Aedes aegypti*. Under these conditions infections with dengue viruses of all types are common, and second infections with heterologous types are frequent. After 1 yr of age, 99% of patients with dengue shock syndrome have a secondary rise of antibody against dengue virus, indicating a previous infection with a closely related virus. A recent outbreak in Cuba, in which children and adults were equally exposed, has shown that the acute, vascular permeability syndrome occurs almost exclusively in children 14 yr and under. In adults severe disease is more frequently associated with hemorrhagic phenomena. Dengue hemorrhagic fever can occur during primary dengue infections, most frequently in infants whose mothers are immune to dengue.

Nonimmune foreigners, adults or children, exposed to dengue virus during outbreaks of hemorrhagic fever have classic dengue fever or even milder disease. The differences in clinical manifestations of dengue infections between natives and foreigners in Southeast Asia are related more to immunologic status than to racial susceptibility. However, in the Cuban outbreak, dengue hemorrhagic fever/dengue shock syndrome attack rates were low in black children, possibly explaining the seeming absence of the syndrome in dengue-endemic areas of Africa.

PATHOLOGY. Usually no pathologic lesions are found to account for death. In rare instances, death may be due to gastrointestinal or intracranial hemorrhages. Minimal to moderate hemorrhages are seen in the upper gastrointestinal tract, and petechial hemorrhages are common in the interventricular septum of the heart, on the pericardium, and on the subserosal surfaces of major viscera. Focal hemorrhages are occasionally seen in the lungs, liver, adrenals, and subarachnoid space. The liver is usually enlarged, often with fatty changes. Yellow, watery, at times blood-tinged effusions are present in serous cavities in about three fourths of patients.

Microscopically, there is perivascular edema in the soft tissues and widespread diapedesis of red blood cells. There may be maturational arrest of megakaryocytes in bone marrow, and increased numbers of them are seen in capillaries of the lungs, in renal glomeruli, and in sinusoids of the liver and spleen.

Dengue virus is almost invariably absent in tissues at the time of death, with rare isolations reported from lymphatic tissues usually in infants under 1 yr who have experienced primary infections.

PATHOGENESIS. The pathogenesis is incompletely understood; epidemiologic studies suggest that it is usually associated with secondary dengue type 2, 3, and 4 infections. It is possible that prior exposure may promote cellular infection and enhance severity of the disease. Dengue viruses demonstrate enhanced growth in cultures of human mononuclear phagocytes prepared from dengue-immune donors or in cultures supplemented with non-neutralizing dengue antibody. Monkeys infected sequentially or receiving small quantities of enhancing antibody have enhanced viremias. Retrospective studies of sera from human mothers whose infants acquired dengue hemorrhagic fever or prospective studies on children acquiring sequential dengue infections have shown that the circulation of infection-enhancing antibodies at the time of infection is the strongest risk factor for development of severe disease. Even low levels of neutralizing antibodies, whether from earlier homotypic infection in mothers or heterotypic infections in children, protect infants or children from dengue hemorrhagic fever. Early in the acute stage of secondary dengue infections, there is rapid activation of the complement system. During shock, blood levels of C1q, C3, C4, C5–C8, and C3 proactivator are depressed, and C3 catabolic rates are elevated. The blood clotting and fibrinolytic systems are activated, and levels of factor XII (Hageman factor) are depressed. No specific mediator of vascular permeability in dengue hemorrhagic fever has been identified, although current interest centers on tumor necrosis factor or other cytokines. A mild degree of disseminated intravascular coagulation, liver damage, and thrombocytopenia may produce hemorrhage synergistically. Capillary damage allows fluid, electrolytes, protein, and, in some instances, red blood cells to leak into extravascular spaces. This internal redistribution of fluid, together with deficits due to fasting, thirsting, and vomiting, results in hemoconcentration, hypovolemia, increased cardiac work, tissue hypoxia, metabolic acidosis, and hyponatremia.

CLINICAL MANIFESTATIONS. The incubation period of dengue hemorrhagic fever is presumed to be that of dengue fever. The course is characteristic in the severely ill child. A relatively mild 1st phase with abrupt onset of fever, malaise, vomiting, headache, anorexia, and cough is followed after 2–5 days by rapid clinical deterioration and collapse. In this 2nd phase the patient usually has cold, clammy extremities, a warm trunk, flushed face, diaphoresis, restlessness, irritability, and mid-epigastric pain. Frequently, there are scattered petechiae on the forehead and extremities; spontaneous ecchymoses may appear, and easy bruisability and bleeding at sites of venipuncture are common. A macular or maculopapular rash may appear, and there may be circumoral and peripheral cyanosis. Respirations are rapid and often labored. The pulse is weak, rapid, and thready and the heart sounds faint. The liver may enlarge to 4–6 cm below the costal margin and is usually firm and somewhat tender. Fewer than 10% of patients have gross ecchymosis or gastrointestinal bleeding, usually following a period of uncorrected shock.

After a 24- to 36-hr period of crisis, convalescence is fairly rapid in the children who recover. The temperature may return to normal before or during the stage of shock. Bradycardia and ventricular extrasystoles are common during convalescence. Infrequently, there is residual brain damage due to prolonged shock or occasionally to intracranial hemorrhage. Dengue 3 virus strains circulating in mainland Southeast Asia since 1983 are associated with a particularly stormy clinical syndrome, characterized by encephalopathy, hypoglycemia, markedly elevated liver enzymes, and, occasionally, jaundice.

In contrast to the fairly characteristic pattern in the severely ill child, secondary dengue infections are relatively mild in the majority of instances, ranging from an inapparent infection through an undifferentiated upper respiratory or dengue-like disease to an illness similar to that described above but without apparent shock.

LABORATORY DATA. The most common hematologic abnormalities during clinical shock are a 20% or greater increase in hematocrit over the recovery value, thrombocytopenia, mild leukocytosis (seldom exceeding 10,000/mm^3), prolonged bleeding time, and moderately decreased prothrombin level (seldom to less than 40% of control). Fibrinogen levels may be subnormal and fibrin split-products elevated.

Other abnormalities include moderate elevations of the serum transaminase levels, mild metabolic acidosis with hyponatremia, and, at times, hypochloremia, slight elevation of serum urea nitrogen, and hypoalbuminemia. Roentgenograms of the chest reveal pleural effusions in nearly all patients.

DIAGNOSIS AND DIFFERENTIAL DIAGNOSIS. In endemic areas hemorrhagic fever should be suspected in children with a febrile illness who exhibit a positive tourniquet test, hemoconcentration, and thrombocytopenia. These may be accompanied by shock and in some instances by hemorrhagic manifestations. Appearance of pleural effusion with evidence of recent dengue infection is pathognomonic. Since many rickettsial diseases, meningococcemia, and other severe illnesses caused by a variety of agents may produce a similar clinical picture, the etiologic diagnosis should be made only when epidemiologic or serologic evidence suggests the possibility of dengue fever. Hemorrhagic manifestations have been described in other diseases of viral or presumed viral origin, including the clinically distinguishable hemorrhagic fevers described in Sec. 12.92.

In secondary dengue infections, there is a rapid and pronounced rise of both hemagglutination-inhibiting (HI) and complement-fixing (CF) antibodies to dengue antigen. There are usually high titers of HI antibody (1:640 or greater) and CF antibody (1:32 or greater) in both acute and convalescent sera. Antibodies of the IgG class dominate in paired sera.

PREVENTION. Preventive measures are described in Sec. 12.90. The possibility exists that dengue vaccination may sensitize a recipient so that ensuing dengue infection may result in hemorrhagic fever. Vaccination with yellow fever 17D strain has no effect on the severity of dengue illness, although seroconversion rates to a dengue 2 vaccine were enhanced in yellow fever–immune persons.

TREATMENT. Management requires immediate evaluation of vital signs and degrees of hemoconcentration, dehydration, and electrolyte imbalance. Close monitoring is essential for at least 48 hr because shock may occur or recur precipitously early in the disease. Patients who are cyanotic or have labored breathing should be given oxygen. Rapid intravenous replacement of fluids and electrolytes can frequently sustain patients until spontaneous recovery occurs. When elevation of the hematocrit persists after replacement of fluids, plasma or plasma colloid preparations are indicated. Care must be taken to avoid overhydration, which may contribute to cardiac failure. Transfusions of fresh blood or of platelets suspended in plasma may be required to control bleeding; they should not be given during hemoconcentration but only after evaluation of hemoglobin or hematocrit values. Salicylates are contraindicated because of their effect on blood clotting.

Paraldehyde or chloral hydrate may be required for children who are markedly agitated. Use of pressor amines, α-adrenergic blocking agents, and aldosterone has not resulted in a significant reduction of mortality compared with that observed with simple supportive therapy. See Sec. 16.75 for treatment of disseminated intravascular coagulation. Steroids do not shorten the duration of disease or improve prognosis in children receiving careful supportive therapy.

Hypervolemia during the fluid reabsorptive phase may be life-threatening and is heralded by a fall in hematocrit with wide pulse pressure. Diuretics and digitalization may be necessary.

PROGNOSIS. Death has occurred in 40–50% of patients with shock, but with adequate intensive care deaths should be less than 2%. Survival is directly related to early and intense management.

Burke DS, Nisalak A, Johnson DE, et al: A prospective study of dengue infections in Bangkok. Am J Trop Med Hyg 38:172, 1988.
Cohen SN, Halstead SB: Shock associated with dengue infection. I. The clinical and physiological manifestations of dengue hemorrhagic fever in Thailand, 1964. J Pediatr 68:448, 1966.
Halstead SB: Dengue hemorrhagic fever, a public health problem and a field for research. Bull WHO 58:1, 1980.
Halstead SB: Immune enhancement of viral infection. Prog Allergy 31:301, 1982.
Halstead SB: Pathogenesis of dengue: Challenges to molecular biology. Science 239:476, 1988.
Kliks S, Nimmannitya S, Nisalak A, et al: Evidence that maternal dengue antibodies are important in development of dengue hemorrhagic fever in infants. Am J Trop Med Hyg 38:411, 1988.
Kliks S, Nisalak A, Brandt WE, et al: Antibody-dependent enhancement of dengue virus growth in human monocytes as a risk factor for dengue hemorrhagic fever. Am J Trop Med Hyg 40:444, 1989.
Technical Guides for Diagnosis, Treatment, Surveillance, Prevention and Control of Dengue Haemorrhagic Fever. Geneva, World Health Organization, 1986.

12.92 OTHER VIRAL HEMORRHAGIC FEVERS

Viral hemorrhagic fevers are a loosely defined group of clinical syndromes in which hemorrhagic manifestations are either common or especially notable in severe illness. Both the etiologic agents and clinical features of the syndromes differ, but disseminated intravascular coaguation may be a common pathogenetic feature. A list of the more important viral hemorrhagic fevers is given in Table 12–40.

ETIOLOGY. Six of the viral hemorrhagic fevers are caused by arthropod-borne (arbo) viruses (Table 12–40). Four are toga-viruses of the flavivirus group (KFD, OHF, DHF, and YF), and three are bunyaviruses (Congo, Hantaan, and RVF). Junin (AHF), Machupo (BHF), and Lassa (LF) are arenaviruses, a morphologic and ecologic viral group. Ebola (EHF) and Marburg viruses are enveloped, filamentous RNA viruses, which are sometimes branched, unlike any other known virus, and which are now termed filoviruses.

EPIDEMIOLOGY. With rare exceptions, the viruses causing viral hemorrhagic fevers are initially transmitted through a nonhuman agency. Since a specific ecosystem is required for viral survival, these are diseases of place. Although it is commonly thought that all viral hemorrhagic fevers are arthropod-borne, eight may be contracted from environmental contamination caused by animals or animal cells or from infected humans (RVF, AHF, BHF, CHF, LF, Marburg disease, EHF, and HFRS). Laboratory and hospital infections have occurred with many of these agents. Lassa fever and Argen-

Table 12–40. Viral Hemorrhagic Fevers

Mode of Transmission	Disease	Virus
Tick-borne	Congo-Crimean HF (CHF)*	Congo
	Kyasanur Forest disease (KFD)	Kyasanur Forest disease
	Omsk HF (OHF)	Omsk
Mosquito-borne†	Dengue HF (DHF)	Dengue (4 types)
	Rift Valley fever (RVF)	Rift Valley fever
	Yellow fever (YF)	Yellow fever
Infected animals or materials to humans	Argentine HF (AHF)	Junin
	Bolivian HF (BHF)	Machupo
	Lassa fever (LF)*	Lassa
	Marburg disease*	Marburg
	Ebola HF (EHF)*	Ebola
	Hemorrhagic fever with renal syndrome (HFRS)	Hantaan

*Patients may be contagious; nosocomial infections are common.
†Chikungunya virus (Sec. 12.90) is associated at low frequency with petechiae, petechial hemorrhages, and epistaxis. More severe hemorrhagic manifestations have been reported in some studies.

tine and Bolivian hemorrhagic fevers are reportedly milder in children than in adults. Dengue hemorrhagic fever (Sec. 12.91) and yellow fever (Sec. 12.89) are well-established pediatric problems. Features of the more common viral hemorrhagic fevers are summarized below.

Tick-Borne Hemorrhagic Fevers. Congo-Crimean Hemorrhagic Fever (CHF). Sporadic human infection in Africa provided the original virus isolation. Natural foci are recognized in Bulgaria, western Crimea, and the Rostov-on-Don and Astrakhan regions; a somewhat similar disease occurs in Kazakstan and Uzbekistan. Index cases were followed by nosocomial transmission in Pakistan and Afghanistan in 1976, in the Arabian peninsula in 1983, and in South Africa in 1984. In the Soviet Union the vectors are *Hyaloma marginatum* and *H. anatolicum*, which, along with hares and birds, may serve as viral reservoirs. Disease occurs from June to September, largely among farmers and dairy workers.

Kyasanur Forest Disease (KFD). Human cases occur chiefly in adults in an area of Mysore State, India. The main vectors are two Ixodidae ticks, *Haemaphysalis turturis* and *H. spinigera*. Monkeys and forest rodents may be amplifying hosts. Laboratory infections are common.

Omsk Hemorrhagic Fever (OHF). The disease occurs throughout the south central Soviet Union and in northern Rumania. Vectors may include *Dermacentor pictus* and *D. marginatus*, but direct transmission from moles and muskrats to humans seems well established. Human disease occurs in a spring-summer-autumn pattern, paralleling the activity of vectors. Omsk hemorrhagic fever occurs most frequently in persons with outdoor occupational exposure. Laboratory infections are common.

Mosquito-Borne Hemorrhagic Fevers. Dengue Hemorrhagic Fever and Yellow Fever (DHF and YF). See Sec. 12.91 and 12.89.

Rift Valley Fever (RVF). The virus causing Rift Valley fever is responsible for epizootics involving sheep, cattle, buffalo, certain antelopes, and rodents in North, Central, East, and South Africa. The virus is transmitted to domestic animals by *Culex theileri* and several *Aedes* species. Mosquitoes may serve as reservoirs by transovarial transmission. An epizootic in Egypt in 1977–1978 was accompanied by thousands of human infections, principally among veterinarians, farmers, and farm laborers. Humans are most often infected during the slaughter or skinning of sick or dead animals. Laboratory infection is common.

Hemorrhagic Fever Transmitted Through Environmental Contamination. Arenaviral Disease. The prototype arenavirus, lymphocytic choriomeningitis virus, establishes a persistent, tolerated infection in the young of the common house mouse, *Mus musculus*, which excretes virus continuously throughout life, contaminating food and fluids and creating a risk of air-borne infection. There is evidence that Machupo and Junin viruses have similar host-parasite relationships with South American rodents as the Lassa virus has with African rodents.

Argentine Hemorrhagic Fever (AHF). Hundreds to thousands of cases occur annually from April through July in the maize-producing area northwest of Buenos Aires that reaches to the eastern margin of the Province of Cordoba. Junin virus has been isolated from the rodents *Mus musculus, Akodon arenicola*, and *Calomys laucha laucha*. It infects migrant laborers who harvest the maize and who inhabit rodent-contaminated shelters.

Bolivian Hemorrhagic Fever (BHF). The recognized endemic area consists of the sparsely populated province of Beni in Amazonian Bolivia. Sporadic cases occur in farm families who raise maize, rice, yucca, and beans. In the town of San Joaquin a disturbance in the domestic rodent ecosystem may have led to an outbreak of household infection caused by *Calomys callosus*, ordinarily a field rodent. Mortality rates are high in young children.

Lassa Fever (LF). Lassa virus has an unusual potential for human-to-human spread and has resulted in many small epidemics in Nigeria, Sierra Leone, and Liberia. Medical workers in Africa and the United States have also contracted the disease. Patients with acute Lassa fever have been transported by international aircraft, necessitating extensive surveillance among passengers and crews. The virus is probably maintained in nature in a species of African peridomestic rodent, *Mastomys natalensis*. Rodent-to-rodent transmission and infection of humans probably operate via mechanisms established for other arenaviruses.

Marburg Disease. Until recently, the world experience has been limited to 26 primary and 5 secondary cases in Germany and Yugoslavia in 1967 and to small outbreaks in Zimbabwe in 1975, in Kenya in 1980 and 1988, and in South Africa in 1983. Transmission occurs by direct contact with tissues of the African green monkey, with infected blood, or with human semen. The reservoir and mode of transmission of the virus in nature are unknown.

Ebola Hemorrhagic Fever. Ebola virus was isolated in 1976 from a devastating epidemic involving small villages in northern Zaire and southern Sudan; smaller outbreaks have occurred subsequently. Outbreaks initially have been nosocomial. Attack rates have been highest in the birth to 1-yr and 15- to 50-yr age groups. The virus resembles Marburg virus. The vertebrate reservoir and mode of transmission to man are unknown. A virus related to Ebola has been recovered from Philippine monkeys and has caused subclinical infections in workers in monkey colonies in the United States.

HEMORRHAGIC FEVER WITH RENAL SYNDROME. (epidemic hemorrhagic fever; Korean hemorrhagic fever). The endemic area includes Japan, Korea, far eastern Siberia, north and central China, European and Asian Russia, Scandinavia, Czechoslovakia, Rumania, Bulgaria, Yugoslavia, and Greece. Although the incidence and severity of hemorrhagic manifestations and the mortality are lower in Europe than in northeast Asia, the renal lesion is the same. Disease in Scandinavia, nephropathia epidemica, is caused by a different although antigenically related virus associated with *Clethrionomys glariolus*. Cases occur predominantly in the spring and summer. There appears to be no age factor in susceptibility, but because of occupational hazards, young adult men are most frequently attacked. Rodent plagues or evidences of rodent infestation have accompanied endemic and epidemic occurrences. Hantaan virus has been detected in lung tissue and excreta of *Apodemus agrarius coreae*. Antigenically related agents have been detected in laboratory rats, in urban rat populations around the world, and in the wild rodent *Microtus pennsylvanicus* in North America (Prospect Hill virus). *Rodent-to-rodent and rodent-to-man transmission presumably occurs via the respiratory route.*

Clinical, Pathologic, and Laboratory Features. OMSK HEMORRHAGIC FEVER AND KYASANUR FOREST DISEASE. After an incubation period of 3–8 days, both diseases begin with sudden onset of fever and headache. In Omsk hemorrhagic fever there is moderate epistaxis, hematemesis, and a hemorrhagic enanthem but no profuse hemorrhage; bronchopneumonia is common. Kyasanur forest disease is characterized by severe myalgia, prostration, and bronchiolar involvement; it often presents without hemorrhage, but occasionally with severe gastrointestinal bleeding. Severe leukopenia and thrombocytopenia occur in both diseases. In many patients recurrent febrile illness may follow an afebrile period of 7–15 days. This second phase takes the form of a meningoencephalitis.

In Kyasanur forest disease, acute degeneration of renal tubules may correlate with the urinary changes noted. There may be focal liver damage. In both diseases vascular dilatation, increased vascular permeability, gastrointestinal hemorrhages, and subserosal and interstitial petechial hemorrhages occur.

CRIMEAN HEMORRHAGIC FEVER. The incubation period of 3–12 days is followed by a febrile period of 5–12 days and a prolonged convalescence. Illness begins suddenly with fever, severe headache, myalgia, abdominal pain, anorexia, nausea, and vomiting. After a day or more fever may subside until the patient develops an erythematous facial or truncal flush and injected conjunctivae. A second febrile period of 2–6 days then develops with a hemorrhagic enanthem on the soft palate and a fine petechial rash on the chest and abdomen. Less frequently, there are large areas of purpura and bleeding from gums, nose, intestine, lungs, or uterus. Hematuria and proteinuria are relatively rare. During the hemorrhagic stage there is usually tachycardia with weak heart sounds, and in some cases hypotension occurs. The liver is usually enlarged, but there is no icterus. In protracted cases central nervous system signs may include delirium, somnolence, and progressive clouding of consciousness. In convalescence there may be hearing and memory loss. Mortality ranges from 2–50%. Early in the disease leukopenia with relative lymphocytosis, progressively worsening thrombocytopenia, and gradually increasing anemia occur.

RIFT VALLEY FEVER **(RVF).** Most infections have been in adults, in whom disease is dengue-like. Onset is acute, with fever, headache, prostration, myalgia, anorexia, nausea, vomiting, conjuctivitis, and lymphadenopathy. The fever lasts 3–6 days and is often biphasic. Convalescence is often prolonged. In the 1977–1978 outbreak, many patients died after showing signs that included purpura, epistaxis, hematemesis, and melena. At autopsy there was extensive eosinophilic degeneration of the parenchymal cells of the liver.

ARGENTINE AND BOLIVIAN HEMORRHAGIC FEVER AND LASSA FEVER. The incubation period is commonly 7–14 days; the acute illness lasts for 2–4 wk. Clinical illnesses range from undifferentiated fever to the characteristic severe illness. Lassa fever is most often clinically severe in whites. Onset is usually gradual, with increasing fever, headache, diffuse myalgia, and anorexia. During the 1st wk signs frequently include a sore throat, dysphagia, cough, oropharyngeal ulcers, nausea, vomiting, diarrhea, and pains in chest and abdomen. Pleuritic chest pain may persist into the 2nd–3rd wk of illness. In Argentine and Bolivian hemorrhagic fevers and less frequently in Lassa fever, a petechial enanthem appears on the soft palate 3–5 days after onset and at about the same time on the trunk. The tourniquet test may be positive.

In 35–50% of all patients these diseases may become severe, with persistent high fever, increasing toxicity, swelling of face or neck, microscopic hematuria, and frank hemorrhages from the stomach, intestines, nose, gums, and uterus. A syndrome of hypovolemic shock is accompanied by pleural effusion and renal failure. Respiratory distress due to airway obstruction, pleural effusion, or congestive heart failure may occur. Ten to 20% of patients develop late neurologic involvement characterized by intention tremor of the tongue and associated speech abnormalities. In severe cases there may be intention tremors of the extremities, seizures, and delirium. The cerebrospinal fluid is normal. In Lassa fever nerve deafness occurs in early convalescence in 25% of cases. Prolonged convalescence is accompanied by alopecia and in Argentine and Bolivian hemorrhagic fevers by signs of autonomic nervous system lability, such as postural hypotension, spontaneous flushing or blanching of the skin, and intermittent diaphoresis.

Laboratory studies reveal marked leukopenia, mild to moderate thrombocytopenia, proteinuria, and, in Argentine hemorrhagic fever, moderate abnormalities in blood clotting, decreased fibrinogen, increased fibrinogen split-products, and elevated serum transaminases. Pathologically, there is focal, often extensive eosinophilic necrosis of liver parenchyma, focal interstitial pneumonitis, focal necrosis of the distal and collecting tubules, and partial replacement of splenic follicles by amorphous eosinophilic material. Usually bleeding occurs by diapedesis with little inflammatory reaction. Mortality is 10–40%.

MARBURG DISEASE AND EBOLA HEMORRHAGIC FEVER. After an incubation period of 4–7 days, illness begins abruptly with severe frontal headache, malaise, drowsiness, lumbar myalgia, vomiting, nausea, and diarrhea. Five to 7 days later a papular eruption begins on the trunk and upper arms; becomes generalized, often hemorrhagic, and maculopapular; and exfoliates during convalescence. The exanthem is accompanied by a dark red enanthem on the hard palate, conjunctivitis, and scrotal or labial edema. Gastrointestinal hemorrhage occurs as the severity of illness increases. Late in the illness, the patient may become tearfully depressed with marked hyperalgesia to tactile stimuli. In fatal cases, patients become hypotensive, restless, and confused and lapse into coma. Convalescent patients may develop alopecia and have paresthesias of the back and trunk. There is a marked leukopenia with necrosis of granulocytes. Disseminated intravascular coagulation and thrombocytopenia are universal and correlate with severity of disease; there are moderate abnormalities in clotting proteins and elevated serum transaminases and amylase. The mortality of Marburg disease is 25%; that of Ebola hemorrhagic fever, 50–90%.

Hemorrhagic Fever with Renal Syndrome (HFRS). In most cases HFRS is characterized by fever, petechiae, mild hemorrhagic phenomena, and mild proteinuria, followed by relatively uneventful recovery. In 20% of recognized cases the disease may progress through four rather distinct phases. The *febrile phase* is ushered in with fever, malaise, and facial and truncal flushing, lasts 3–8 days, and ends with thrombocytopenia, petechiae, and proteinuria. The *hypotensive phase* of 1–3 days follows defervescence. Loss of fluid from the intravascular compartment may result in marked hemoconcentration. Proteinuria and ecchymoses increase. The *oliguric phase*, usually 3–5 days in duration, is characterized by a low output of protein-rich urine, increasing nitrogen retention, nausea, vomiting, and dehydration. Confusion, extreme restlessness, and hypertension are common. The *diuretic phase*, which may last for days or weeks, usually initiates clinical improvement. The kidneys show little concentrating ability, and rapid loss of fluid may result in severe dehydration and shock. Potassium and sodium depletion may be severe. Fatal cases manifest abundant protein-rich retroperitoneal edema and marked hemorrhagic necrosis of the renal medulla. Mortality is 5–10%.

DIAGNOSIS. Diagnosis depends upon a high index of suspicion in endemic areas. In nonendemic areas histories of recent travel, recent laboratory exposure, or exposure to an earlier case should evoke suspicion of viral hemorrhagic fever.

In all viral hemorrhagic fevers the viral agent circulates in the blood at least transiently during the early febrile stage. The diagnostic specimens required for togaviruses and bunyaviruses are the same as those described in Sec. 12.90 for dengue fever. The principles for etiologic diagnosis of Argentine and Bolivian hemorrhagic fevers are similar; acute phase blood or throat washings from patients can be inoculated intracerebrally into guinea pigs, infant hamsters, or infant mice. Lassa virus may be isolated from the same specimens by inoculation into tissue cultures. In arenavirus infections, group-reactive complement-fixing antibodies and specific neutralizing antibodies appear in convalescent serum 3–4 wk after onset of illness. For Marburg disease and EHF, acute-phase throat washings, blood, and urine may be inoculated into tissue culture, guinea pigs, or monkeys. The virus is readily visualized by electron microscopy, its filamentous structure differentiating it from all other known agents. Specific complement-fixing and immunofluorescent antibodies appear during convalescence. The virus of HFRS is recovered from acute phase serum or urine by inoculating susceptible tissue cultures and identifying virus by use of fluorescent antibody, enzyme immunoassay, or neutralization tests. A variety of antibody tests using viral subunits are becoming available. These viruses may also be detected in blood or tissues using DNA probes or first amplifying viral RNA by PCR.

Handling blood and other biologic specimens is hazardous and must be left to specially trained personnel. Blood and autopsy specimens should be placed in tightly sealed metal containers, wrapped in absorbent material inside a sealed plastic bag, and shipped on dry ice to laboratories with biocontainment level 4 facilities. Even routine hematologic and biochemical tests should be done with extreme caution.

DIFFERENTIAL DIAGNOSIS. Mild cases of hemorrhagic fever may be confused with almost any self-limited systemic bacterial or viral infection. More severe cases may suggest typhoid fever, epidemic, murine, or scrub typhus, leptospirosis, or a rickettsial spotted fever, for which effective chemotherapeutic agents are available. Many of them may be acquired in geographic or ecologic locations similar to those that may provide exposure to a viral hemorrhagic fever.

PREVENTION. A live-attenuated vaccine (Candid-I) for Argentine hemorrhagic fever is highly efficacious. A form of inactivated mouse brain vaccine is said to be effective in preventing Omsk hemorrhagic fever. Inactivated Rift Valley fever vaccines are widely used to protect domestic animals and laboratory workers. An experimental HFRS inactivated vaccine is under development in Korea, and a live-attenuated vaccine is being developed in China. A vaccinia-vector glycoprotein vaccine provides protection against Lassa fever in monkeys. Prevention of CCHF transmission by ticks includes careful examination of the skin after exposure with removal of any vectors found. Tight-fitting clothing that fully covers the extremities is helpful, as is the use of tick repellents. Disease transmitted from a rodent-infected environment can be prevented through methods of rodent control; elimination of refuse and breeding sites is particularly successful in urban or suburban areas. Congo-Crimean hemorrhagic fever, Lassa fever, Marburg disease, and Ebola hemorrhagic fever may be transmitted in hospital settings. Patients should be isolated until they are virus free or for 3 wk following illness. Patients' urine, sputum, blood, clothing, and bedding should be disinfected. Disposable syringes and needles should be used. Prompt and strict enforcement of barrier nursing may be lifesaving. The case fatality rate among medical workers contracting these diseases is 50%.

TREATMENT. The principle involved in all these diseases, especially hemorrhagic fever with renal syndrome, is the reversal of dehydration, hemoconcentration, renal failure, and protein, electrolyte, or blood losses. The contribution of disseminated intravascular coagulation to the hemorrhagic manifestations is unknown, and the management of hemorrhage should be individualized. Transfusions of fresh blood and platelets are frequently given. Good results have been reported in a few cases following the administration of clotting factor concentrates. The efficacy of steroids, ϵ-aminocaproic acid, pressor amines, or α-adrenergic blocking agents has not been established. Sedatives should be selected with regard to the possibility of kidney or liver damage. The successful management of hemorrhagic fever with renal syndrome may require renal dialysis. Dramatic improvement in some cases of Lassa fever has been reported following administration of Lassa immune serum free of infectious virus.* Ribavirin (intravenous) is being evaluated for efficacy in Lassa fever.

SCOTT B. HALSTEAD

Casals J, Henderson BE, Hoogstraal H, et al: A review of Soviet viral hemorrhagic fevers, 1969. J Infect Dis 122:437, 1970.
International symposium on arenaviral infections of public health importance, 14–16 July 1975. Bull WHO 52:381, 1975.
Johnson KM, Halstead SB, Cohen SN: Hemorrhagic fevers of Southeast Asia and South America, a comparative appraisal. Prog Med Virol 9:106, 1967.
Lee HW, Lee MC, Cho LS: Management of Korean hemorrhagic fever. Med Prog Sept:15, 1980.
Management of patients with suspected viral hemorrhagic fever. MMWR 37:Suppl 3, 1988.
Monath TP: Lassa fever and Marburg virus disease. WHO Chron 28:212, 1974.
Pattyn SR: (ed): Ebola Virus Haemorrhagic Fever. Amsterdam, Elsevier/North Holland, 1978.
Simpson DIH: Viral haemorrhagic fevers of man. Bull WHO 56:819, 1978.

12.93 ANTIVIRAL DRUGS

All currently available antiviral drugs only inhibit viral production; host defense mechanisms are extremely important in curing infection or maintaining latency of the virus. Immunodeficient patients may require repeated or prolonged

*Serum or immune serum globulin and information concerning dosage schedules may be obtained from the Centers for Disease Control, Atlanta, Georgia, or the World Health Organization, Geneva, Switzerland.

courses of therapy, which increases the possibility of developing resistance. Antiviral drugs are usually specific for a single virus or family of viruses; determination of the etiologic agent responsible for illness is important, and methods of achieving rapid viral diagnosis are being developed. Side effects are common with some of the antiviral drugs and may limit therapy. The development and clinical testing of antiviral compounds that will be useful in the treatment of infections due to HIV, CMV, and herpesvirus are progressing rapidly.

Amantadine and *rimantadine* are effective for the prophylaxsis or therapy of influenza A (Sec. 12.74). Rimantadine has been used extensively in Europe, but is not licensed in the United States. Ideally, high-risk patients and their caretakers should receive influenza immunization. Most healthy children do not require specific antiviral therapy; if treatment is to be used, it should be started within 48 hr of onset of illness. There are no data about dosage in infants under 1 yr of age. In children over a year, the suggested dose is 4.4 mg/kg/24 hr with a maximum of 150 mg/24 hr in those under 10 yr and 200 mg/24 hr in those over 10 yr of age. The drug is usually well tolerated, but seizures have been reported.

Acyclovir is the drug of choice for infections due to herpes simplex (Sec. 12.68) and varicella-zoster (Sec. 12.69). Activity depends on the presence of virus-specific thymidine kinase. Herpes simplex viruses lacking this enzyme are resistant to the drug. Although such viruses are less likely to initiate infection or develop latency, some severe infections with resistant viruses have been reported in patients with AIDS. Treatment of primary genital herpes infection with acyclovir will shorten the duration of symptoms but will not prevent latency. Prophylactic acyclovir can markedly decrease the number and severity of recurrences and is well tolerated. Such therapy should probably be reserved for severe cases because there is concern about inducing resistance. Disease recurs when prophylaxis is stopped.

Vidarabine was the first antiviral drug demonstrated to be effective in the therapy of herpes simplex encephalitis. It is poorly soluble and requires a large amount of intravenous fluids. Side effects include nausea, vomiting, anemia, leukopenia, thrombocytopenia, tremors, ataxia, and seizures. Because acyclovir has greater activity and fewer side effects, it has generally replaced vidarabine except in the rare cases when the virus is resistant.

Ribavirin has activity against a number of viruses but is currently licensed only for use in respiratory syncytial virus infections (Sec. 12.76). It is given by aerosol for 12–18 hr/24 hr and is well tolerated. The drug is teratogenic in rats but not in baboons. Human teratogenicity has not been shown, but pregnant nurses should not care for patients receiving ribavirin. The drug is recommended for use in respiratory syncytial virus-infected patients with underlying diseases such as congenital heart lesions and bronchopulmonary dysplasia, in infants less than 6 wk old, and in those with severe disease.

Zidovudine (AZT, retrovir) has been shown to be effective in adults with HIV infection. Studies in children have shown it to be useful (Sec. 12.83). Side effects in earlier studies included severe anemia, which could be controlled by transfusion, and leukopenia, which could require a reduction in dose or discontinuation of therapy. Side effects are less frequent with the lower doses currently recommended. A number of drugs can interfere with the metabolism of zidovudine and increase its toxicity; aspirin and acetaminophen should be avoided.

Ganciclovir has been used for therapy of severe cytomegalovirus infection in immunocompromised patients (Sec. 12.71). It has been shown to be effective for CMV retinitis and for gastrointestinal and liver disease; it has had variable results in the treatment of CMV pneumonia and is ineffective in patients with CMV encephalitis. Cultures become negative while the patient is on therapy but revert to positive with return of symptoms when therapy is stopped. Resistance can develop, and bone marrow toxicity occurs. Therapy with this drug should be reserved for patients with retinitis that threatens vision and potentially fatal infections.

Foscarnet is an experimental drug that inhibits herpes simplex. It has been successfully used to treat infections with herpes simplex that is resistant to acyclovir in immunocompromised patients.

CAROL F. PHILLIPS

Balfour HH, Englund JA: Antiviral drugs in pediatrics. Am J Dis Child 143:1307, 1989.

Chatis PA, Miller CH, Schrager LE, et al: Successful treatment with foscarnet of an acyclovir-resistant mucocutaneous infection with herpes simplex virus in a patient with acquired immunodeficiency syndrome. N Engl J Med 320:297, 1989.

Dolin R, Reichman RC, Madore HP, et al: A controlled trial of amantadine and rimantadine in the prophylaxis of influenza A infection. N Engl J Med 307:580, 1982.

Fischl MA, Richman DD, Grieco MH, et al: The efficacy of azidothymidine (AZT) in the treatment of patients with AIDS and AIDS-related complex. A double-blind, placebo-controlled trial. N Engl J Med 317:185, 1987.

Hall CB, McBride JT, Walsh EE, et al: Aerosolized ribavirin treatment of infants with respiratory syncytial virus infection: A randomized double-blind study. N Engl J Med 308:1443, 1983.

Merigan TC, Lane HC: Cytomegalovirus infection and treatment with ganciclovir. Rev Infect Dis 10 (Suppl 3):S457, 1988.

Nilsen AE, Aasen T, Halsos AM, et al: Efficacy of oral acyclovir in the treatment of initial and recurrent genital herpes. Lancet 2:571, 1982.

Whitley RJ, Alford CA, Hersch MS, et al: Vidarabine versus acyclovir therapy in herpes simplex encephalitis. N Engl J Med 314:144, 1986.

Zlydnekov DM, Kubas OI, Kovaleva TP, et al: Study of rimantadine in the USSR. Rev Infect Dis 3:408, 1981.

12.94 RICKETTSIAE

Rickettsiae are small, pleomorphic, coccobacillary organisms with an ultrastructure that resembles that of other gram-negative bacteria. Rickettsiae stain negative on Gram stain, red by Giemsa stain, and bright red by the Gimenéz method. Immunofluorescent techniques with specific antisera can be used to distinguish rickettsial organisms from gram-negative bacteria in tissue. Rickettsiae possess both RNA and DNA and divide by transverse binary fission inside the host cell. With the exception of *Coxiella burnetii*, the cause of Q fever, these obligate intracellular organisms cannot survive long outside the host cell, and they are readily killed by disinfectants and high temperatures (greater than 56° C).

C. burnetii is similar to rickettsiae in its obligate intracellular nature, but it differs sufficiently from other rickettsiae to be classified as a separate genus *(Coxiella)* in the family Rickettsiaceae. This organism is small, stains variably by the Gram technique, has a DNA base composition different from that of the other rickettsiae, and grows and replicates within phagolysosomes rather than in the cytoplasm of host cells. Unlike the other rickettsiae, *C. burnetii* displays host-controlled antigenic changes, referred to as phase variation, that resemble the rough-to-smooth variations of bacteria. The formation of spore-like bodies (small cell variants or endospores) may explain the ability of *C. burnetii* to survive in the environment for a long time, even when exposed to heat, cold, desiccation, sunlight, and chemicals.

Rickettsial diseases of humans are separated into groups on the basis of clinical characteristics, etiologic agent, insect vectors, and epidemiology (Table 12-41). Rickettsiae are transmitted among mammal reservoirs by arthropod vectors. Humans are not an essential link in their natural cycle but become chance hosts when they are bitten by an infected vector, scratch or rub infectious feces into the skin, or inhale

TABLE 12–41. Rickettsial Diseases of Man: Summary of Pertinent Features

Group, Disease	Causative Agent	Arthropod Vector	Hosts	Confirmatory Tests*	Geographic Distribution
Spotted fever					
Rocky Mountain spotted fever	*R. rickettsii*	Tick	Dogs, rodents	IFA, DFA	Western hemisphere
Boutonneuse fever (Mediterranean spotted fever)	*R. conorii*	Tick	Dogs, rodents	IFA, DFA	Africa, Mediterranean region, India, Middle East
Rickettsialpox	*R. akari*	Mite	Mice	IFA	North America, USSR, Korea, South Africa
Ehrlichiosis	*E. canis*	Tick	Dogs	IFA	Southeast, South Central USA
Typhus					
Epidemic typhus/Brill-Zinsser disease	*R. prowazekii*	Body louse	Humans	IFA	Highlands of Africa, Asia, Central and South America
Flying squirrel-associated typhus fever	*R. prowazekii*	Lice, fleas	Flying squirrels	IFA	Eastern United States (including Texas)
Murine (endemic) typhus	*R. typhi*	Cat or rat flea, rat louse	Rats	IFA	Worldwide
Scrub typhus					
Scrub typhus	*R. tsutsugamushi*	Mite	Rodents?	IFA, IP	Pacific Islands, Australia, and central, eastern, and southeast Asia
Others					
Q fever	*Coxiella burnetii*	Ticks?	Cattle, sheep, goats, cats	IFA, CF	Worldwide

*Although not widely available or highly sensitive, a direct fluorescent antibody (DFA) test can be used to detect rickettsiae in skin biopsies or tissue samples. Preferred confirmatory serologic tests include indirect fluorescent antibody or microimmunofluorescent assay (IFA), complement-fixation (CF), and immunoperoxidase (IP) assays. Cross-absorption of the patient's serum with specific rickettsial antigens can be done to distinguish the following infections: *R. rickettsii* versus *R. conorii* or *R. akari;* and *R. prowazekii* versus *R. typhi.*

the organism. Rocky Mountain spotted fever is the rickettsial infection most frequently encountered in the United States and accounts for nearly 90% of all rickettsial cases reported each year; small outbreaks of murine typhus, Q fever, rickettsialpox, and epidemic typhus make up the remainder. In addition, occasional cases of Boutonneuse fever or other spotted fevers are serologically confirmed in travelers who have been in southern or eastern Africa, the Mediterranean basin, India, or other rickettsia-endemic areas. Tsutsugamushi fever (scrub typhus) occurs in China, the western Pacific region, the Indian subcontinent, and Australia, where it occasionally poses a risk to travelers who venture into remote rural areas. The presence of indigenous reservoirs and vectors, plus the continuous possibility that new strains of rickettsiae may be introduced from other parts of the world, makes the threat of new outbreaks in the United States a continuing concern. Effective rickettsial vaccines are not available.

PATHOGENESIS. Rickettsemia occurs after the entry of rickettsial organisms through the skin or respiratory tract. Within minutes, the rickettsiae invade vascular and small muscle endothelial cells, probably through induced phagocytosis. In spotted fever, rickettsiae invade the media, and in typhus, the endothelium is the site where organisms are found. The rickettsiae irreparably damage endothelial and smooth muscle cells, causing widespread necrotizing vasculitis and increased capillary permeability. Any vessel may become involved, but those in skin, subcutaneous tissue, and brain are most commonly affected. The vasculitis is characterized by the presence of rickettsiae within endothelial or smooth muscle cells, endothelial swelling, and perivascular infiltrates of lymphocytic, mononuclear, and plasma cells, and macrophages. *Rickettsia*-induced alteration of the endothelial surface causes increased adherence of platelets to the cell wall, resulting in a decrease in platelet survival and formation of thrombi. The exposure of subendothelial connective tissue containing collagen can also activate Hageman factor and initiate hemostatic alterations, including activation of platelets, coagulation pathways, and the fibrinolytic system. The rickettsial vasculitis is manifested clinically by rash, an array of pathologic changes in affected organs, increased vascular permeability and edema, thrombocytopenia, hemorrhagic skin lesions, and, in severe cases, disseminated intravascular coagulation and skin necrosis.

In contrast to other rickettsial infections, humans are infected with *C. burnetii* after inhalation of infectious aerosols. The principal disease manifestation of acute Q fever is an influenza-like illness (without a rash) often accompanied by a patchy interstitial pneumonitis with a copious alveolar exudate composed primarily of histiocytes. The pathologic features of fatal Q fever pneumonia include severe intra-alveolar, focally necrotizing pneumonia with necrotizing bronchiolitis, and bronchitis.

DIAGNOSIS. If a rash is present, the rickettsial infection can be diagnosed as early as day 3–4 of illness by demonstrating a specific rickettsial antigen in vascular endothelial walls of the dermis in a biopsy specimen using a direct fluorescent antibody (DFA) technique. This method is specific but only moderately sensitive (about 50%). To avoid false-negative results, macular or petechial skin lesions should be marked with indelible ink, two or more 3- to 4-mm punch biopsies should be taken of the marked lesions, and the center of the cutaneous lesion, where the endothelial cells containing rickettsiae are usually located, should be sectioned and stained with antiserum conjugated with fluorescein isothiocyanate. The coccobacillary forms can be seen by darkfield microscopy. False-negative results are usually due to failure to perform a biopsy of the dermal lesion or to obtain a section containing the vasculitic lesion, or to obtaining the biopsy specimen too long (48 hr or more) after starting effective antibiotic treatment. Because a negative result does not rule out the diagnosis, it is important not to delay or withhold treatment in a patient suspected of having a rickettsial disease who has a negative skin test.

To confirm the diagnosis, one serum specimen should be obtained during the acute illness (acute phase) and another one 2–4 wk afterward (convalescent phase) for serologic testing, employing specific rickettsial reagents. As shown in Table 12–41, the most reliable and sensitive serologic test available is the indirect fluorescent or microimmunofluorescent antibody (IFA) assay. Other tests include the latex agglutination and complement-fixation tests, the enzyme-linked immunosorbent assay (ELISA), and the immunoperoxidase assay (IP). The IFA is used widely for most of the human rickettsioses. Like the ELISA, it is highly sensitive and specific for the diagnosis of specific rickettsial infections; both tests can be used to quantitate IgM and IgG responses, which is helpful in differentiating primary epidemic typhus infections from recrudescent typhus. The ELISA is used mainly in research or reference laboratories for seroepidemiologic studies. Latex agglutination tests are employed by some laboratories for confirmation of Rocky Mountain spotted fever. This assay is specific, but it detects mainly IgM antibody, which is short-lived. the complement-fixation test has been used for serodiagnosis of all rickettsial diseases except scrub typhus. Its main limitations are the lack of availability of reagents and its lack of sensitivity. Complement-fixation is positive in less than half of cases clearly identified as Rocky Mountain spotted fever by other serologic tests. Reasons for false-negative results include a slow rise in complement-fixation antibody titer and suppression of the antibody response by antibiotics.

All rickettsiae, with the exception of *C. burnetii* and *R. tsutsugamushi*, share antigens with other rickettsiae. When possible, washed, purified, species-specific rickettsial antigens should be employed in serologic tests to minimize the detection of cross-reacting antibodies.

Serologic confirmation by standard tests usually is not possible until 7–10 days after the onset of illness. A 4-fold rise in titer of antibody between paired acute and convalescent serum specimens generally is accepted as evidence of recent infection; occasionally, a single high titer is diagnostic if it is compatible with the clinical findings.

The Weil-Felix test, which is still used by many hospital laboratories to identify rickettsial infections, is both unreliable and nonspecific and should be replaced by more specific tests. The basis for the use of the Weil-Felix test is that it sometimes (but not always) detects antibodies in persons who are convalescing from rickettsial diseases that react with the O antigen of the *Proteus vulgaris* strains OX19, OX2, and OXK. Such patients manifest the following pattern of agglutination antibody: murine typhus or epidemic typhus, an elevated titer (≥1:320) to OX19 but low titers to OX2 or OXK; Rocky Mountain spotted fever, an elevated titer to OX19 and OX2 but little response to OXK; Tsutsugamushi disease, an elevated titer only to OXK. It is important to realize that the Weil-Felix test has major drawbacks. It is unreliable because agglutination reactions are often negative or the titers detected are not diagnostic in cases of proved disease. Moreover, the test results are always negative in cases of Q fever, trench fever, and rickettsialpox, and are frequently negative or nondiagnostic in cases of Brill-Zinsser disease (recrudescent typhus). Furthermore, Weil-Felix reactions are nonspecific; positive reactions occur in individuals with *Proteus* urinary tract infections, leptospirosis, borreliosis, and liver disease. Because strain-specific antigens and more sensitive tests are available, the Weil-Felix test should never be used as the sole diagnostic test.

Rickettsiae can be isolated by inoculation of blood or tissue specimens into guinea pigs or mice, tissue culture, or embryonated hens' eggs. However, culture of rickettsiae requires at least 4–7 days and is hazardous for laboratory personnel and therefore should be left to a special reference laboratory with proper facilities. The need to isolate rickettsiae from clinical specimens may soon be supplanted by the use of recently developed techniques, such as the polymerase chain reaction (PCR), for detection of rickettsial DNA. A recent report of the use of the PCR procedure for the detection of *R. rickettsii* and *R. conorii* in blood clots from patients with spotted fever suggests that this technique, which requires less time and is less hazardous than rickettsial isolation, can probably be adapted for use in the clinical laboratory for rapid diagnosis of rickettsial diseases.

TREATMENT. Doxycycline, tetracycline, or chloramphenicol is usually curative if begun in adequate dosage on or before the 5th day of disease. The penicillins and most other antibiotics are not effective, and the sulfonamides may make the patient worse by enhancing rickettsial replication. Final eradication of the micro-organism depends upon the immune processes of the host.

Chloramphenicol in a dose of 50–100 mg/kg/24 hr administered every 6 hr (maximum 3 g/24 hr) is the recommended treatment for children 8 yr of age and younger and for patients with poor renal function. The recommended dose of tetracycline is 25–50 mg/kg/24 hr given in 4 divided doses (maximum 2 g/24 hr) given orally or intravenously. Alternatively, doxycycline, which is potentially less destructive to tooth enamel than tetracycline, could be given to patients less than 8 yr of age if they have not taken tetracycline or doxycycline previously. Doxycycline is given in 2 loading doses (2.2 mg/kg each) given at 12-hr intervals orally or intravenously, followed by 2.2 mg/kg/24 hr in divided doses every 12 hr. The maximum dose is 300 mg. Antimicrobial therapy should continue until the patient has been afebrile for 3–5 days, usually for a total course of 7–10 days.

Early diagnosis and proper antibiotic therapy are all that are necessary in the management of most rickettsial infections. Vigorous supportive therapy, parenteral fluids, and occasionally platelet or blood transfusions and oxygen may be required for severely ill patients. Glucocorticoids are not of proven benefit.

12.95 TYPHUS FEVER

(Epidemic Typhus; Flying Squirrel-Associated Typhus Fever)

ETIOLOGY AND TRANSMISSION. Humans are the principal reservoir of *Rickettsia prowazekii*, the causative agent of epidemic typhus and its recrudescent form, Brill-Zinsser disease. The body or head louse becomes infected by feeding upon the blood of a person with rickettsemia. The ingested organisms multiply within the cells lining the alimentary tract of the insect and are eliminated in the feces. Contaminated feces may be introduced into a susceptible human host through abrasions or perforations in the skin, through the conjunctival sac, or through inhalation of dried, infected louse excreta present in the clothing, bedding, or furniture of a typhus patient. The infection usually occurs in winter and spring. In the United States there have been sporadic cases of epidemic typhus confirmed by serologic testing in which the flying squirrel *(Glaucomys volans)* is the apparent reservoir of infection. The rickettsial infection in humans might be initiated by inhalation of infected feces from squirrel lice or fleas.

CLINICAL MANIFESTATIONS. Typhus fever is usually a mild disease in children. The incubation period is less than 14 days. The clinical manifestations include fever, transient rash, and few constitutional symptoms, and are similar to those of Rocky Mountain spotted fever.

Brill-Zinsser disease is an unusual phenomenon in which a patient with a history of typhus suffers a recrudescence of the illness. Such an individual can infect lice and is a potential point of origin for a typhus epidemic.

CONTROL. The immediate destruction of vectors with an insecticide is important in the control of an epidemic. Dust containing excreta from infected lice is capable of transmitting typhus, and care must be taken to prevent its inhalation.

12.96 MURINE TYPHUS
(Endemic Typhus)

ETIOLOGY AND TRANSMISSION. Murine typhus occurs in most regions of the United States, particularly in northeastern Texas and the southeastern states. The peak incidence occurs in the summer and fall when rat populations are at their highest, except in Texas, where murine typhus occurs mainly from April to June.

Murine typhus is caused by *Rickettsia typhi* (formerly *R. mooseri*), which is transmitted from rat to rat by the rat flea. Studies of cases in Texas suggest that the cat flea may also serve as a vector. In both rat and insect vectors murine typhus is a mild disease with no apparent effect on life span. The eggs laid by infected fleas or lice do not transmit *R. typhi* to the next generation. People acquire murine typhus when rickettsiae-infected feces contaminate the bite wound or are inhaled.

CLINICAL MANIFESTATIONS. Murine typhus is similar to epidemic typhus but is a much milder illness. The incubation period is about 8 days. Prodromal symptoms such as headache, arthralgia, and myalgia are followed by a gradually increasing temperature that may reach 41.1° C (106° F) in children and last 9–14 days. The rash appears any time from the 1st–8th day of fever, most often by the 3rd–5th day. The eruption begins on the trunk and spreads toward the periphery, rarely involving the face, palms, or soles. Initially, the skin lesion is a dull red macule with ill-defined margins; it becomes slightly papular as it matures. The rash persists for 4–8 days and rarely becomes purpuric. Thirty per cent or more of children have no rash or such a transient one that it is not noticed. Pharyngitis, abdominal pain, vomiting, and diarrhea may occur, but cardiac, central nervous system, and renal complications are uncommon. The IFA serologic assay is the best confirmatory test. Because *R. typhi* shares common antigens with *R. prowazekii*, it is sometimes necessary to use antibody absorption tests to distinguish murine typhus from epidemic typhus.

CONTROL. Control of murine typhus requires elimination of the reservoir of rats and rat fleas.

12.97 SCRUB TYPHUS
(Tsutsugamushi Fever, Mite Typhus)

ETIOLOGY AND TRANSMISSION. *Rickettsia tsutsugamushi*, formerly known as *R. orientalis*, causes scrub typhus. Among its many serotypes, the Karp, Gilliam, and Kato strains cross-react with most strains that cause disease. The vectors that carry the agent are the larval forms of trombiculid mites (chiggers); both mites and rodents serve as reservoirs of *R. tsutsugamushi*. Naturally occurring scrub typhus in humans occurs in southeast Asia, China, Nepal, northeastern Australia, and Indonesia, but imported cases in the United States have also been reported.

CLINICAL MANIFESTATIONS. Scrub typhus is a mild to moderately severe illness. At the site of the mite bite, the patient usually develops a local skin ulcer, which becomes an eschar. By the end of the 1st wk of illness, a maculopapular rash develops on the chest and abdomen and gradually spreads to involve the entire body but rarely the hands and face. Diffuse, tender adenopathy, greater in the region of the primary lesion, is common. The clinical diagnosis of scrub typhus can be confirmed by using an IFA test or immunoperoxidase assay to demonstrate a 4-fold rise in antibody titer to the Karp, Gilliam, and Kato strains in acute and convalescent sera. The mortality rate when appropriate antibiotics (doxycycline or tetracycline, or chloramphenicol) are administered early is less than 5%.

CONTROL. Protective clothing is the most useful mode of prevention of scrub typhus.

12.98 ROCKY MOUNTAIN SPOTTED FEVER

EPIDEMIOLOGY. The term Rocky Mountain spotted fever is a misnomer because the disease now occurs in almost every state of the continental United States and in southwestern Canada and Mexico. States reporting the highest rates of disease in 1988 were Oklahoma, followed by North Carolina, Arkansas, Missouri, and Kansas; less than 5% of cases originated in the Rocky Mountain area. The disease occurs most commonly in wooded areas (such as rural North Carolina) and coastal grasslands or salt marshes (such as Cape Cod or Long Island), but foci of infection have also been detected in urban areas (such as the South Bronx). Cases usually occur between the months of April and September, the time of year when the tick population increases and people participate in outdoor recreational activities. The highest incidence occurs in children 5–9 yr of age.

ETIOLOGY AND TRANSMISSION. Ticks are the natural hosts, reservoirs, and vectors of *Rickettsia rickettsii*, the etiologic agent of Rocky Mountain spotted fever. Ticks become infected by feeding on infected animal hosts, such as dogs and rodents, and by transovarian infection (passage of the organism from infected ticks to their offspring). *R. rickettsii* is transmitted to dogs, other mammals, and humans by many species and genera of ticks. The principal hosts of *R. rickettsii* are *Dermacentor variabilis* (dog tick) in the eastern United States and eastern Canada; *D. andersoni* (wood tick) in the western United States and western Canada; and possibly *Amblyomma americanum*, the Lone Star tick, in the southwestern United States.

Dogs also serve as a reservoir for *R. rickettsii* and play an important role in the dissemination of infected ticks into the environment shared by humans. Results of serologic studies of patients with Rocky Mountain spotted fever in Mississippi and Ohio suggest that 39–75% of the patients contracted infection from ticks carried by a family dog. Humans usually acquire infection through the bite of an infected tick or, occasionally, by scratching or rubbing infectious tick feces into the skin. Laboratory personnel can also become infected by inoculation or inhalation of aerosolized, infectious specimens.

CLINICAL MANIFESTATIONS. The incubation period in children varies from 2 to 14 days, with a median of 7 days. The disease usually begins with such nonspecific symptoms as headache, fever, anorexia, and restlessness. Gastrointestinal symptoms such as nausea, vomiting, or diarrhea are quite common (39–63%) early in the disease. The history of tick exposure is helpful, but such information is obtained in only 50–60% of reported cases. If very carefully examined, up to 20% of patients will be found to have an indurated inflamed lesion at the site of the bite, often in the scalp or in another less visible part of the body. Discrete, pale, rose-red macules or maculopapules appear 1–5 days after the onset of illness; approximately 10% of patients have little or no rash. The rash characteristically begins peripherally on the ankles, wrists, or lower legs (Fig. 12–34) and then spreads, often rapidly, to

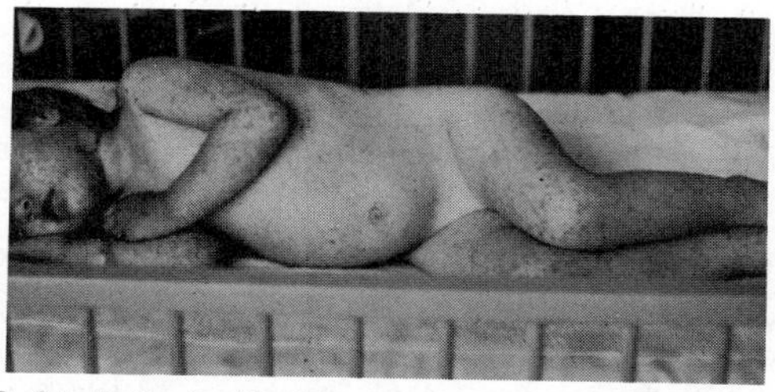

Figure 12–34. Patient with Rocky Mountain spotted fever. Note the greater concentration of skin lesions on the ankles, wrists, and lower legs. (Courtesy of William H. Wood, M.D., Cleveland.)

involve the entire body, including the palms and soles. At first the rash fades with pressure, but after 1–2 days it becomes more purple, papular, and then petechial (Fig. 12–35). Fever and severe headache persist; intense myalgia and malaise are frequent complaints. Splenomegaly and hepatomegaly are present in approximately 33% of patients. As the disease progresses, the petechiae become confluent and develop into purpura and ecchymoses that may ulcerate and become necrotic. In severe cases, thrombosis of large vessels may result in gangrene of distal parts of the body, such as the digits, ear lobes, scrotum, tip of the nose, or a limb. Other severe manifestations sometimes seen include bizarre central nervous system symptoms, edema of the face, electrocardiographic evidence of myocarditis, acute renal failure, peripheral vascular collapse, and pneumonitis.

Patients who have either inherited disorders that predispose them to develop coagulation inhibitors or a glucose-6-phosphate dehydrogenase deficiency tend to have an accelerated course of Rocky Mountain spotted fever with a profound coagulopathy, extensive thrombus formation in the vasculature, and severe damage to the kidneys, liver, lungs, and central nervous system, followed by death. Patients with multiple coagulation disturbances (disseminated intravascular coagulation) constitute the group at highest risk of death. Fatality rates before the availability of antibiotics were 10–40%; with antibiotics the case fatality rate in children is now 1–2%. Recovery in uncomplicated cases generally occurs in the 2nd wk, initiated by a fall in temperature and gradual resolution of symptoms.

LABORATORY DATA AND DIAGNOSIS. An abnormally low platelet count and low serum sodium, present in about half of the patients, may be helpful clues for early diagnosis. In general, however, the clinical laboratory findings are nonspecific and vary depending on the organ systems involved and the stage of the disease. The Centers for Disease Control has established the following criteria for serologic confirmation of Rocky Mountain spotted fever: a 4-fold rise in titer by indirect fluorescent antibody (IFA), complement-fixation (CF), microagglutination (MA), latex agglutination (LA), or indirect hemagglutination (IHA) assays; or a single elevated titer of 1:64 or higher in convalescent sera by IFA, or 1:16 or higher by CF. A case is considered probable if testing reveals a single titer of at least 1:128 by LA or MA assay, or a 4-fold rise in titer or a single titer of at least 1:320 in the Weil-Felix assay. See Sec. 12.94 for serologic tests.

DIFFERENTIAL DIAGNOSIS. The diagnosis of Rocky Mountain spotted fever should be considered in any patient presenting during the spring or summer with an acute febrile illness accompanied by headache and myalgia, particularly if he or she has been in an endemic or forested area or has had contact with a dog. A history of tick exposure and the appearance of a rash, especially on the palms or soles, together with laboratory findings of a low serum sodium concentration, normal white blood cell count with a marked left shift, and a relatively low or falling platelet count, are sometimes helpful clues in distinguishing Rocky Mountain spotted fever from some other acute infections.

The diagnosis of Rocky Mountain spotted fever can be difficult to make in patients who do not have a rash and in persons with dark skin in whom the rash may be overlooked. In atypical cases when there is no rash or when other findings predominate, the correct diagnosis can be delayed. In addition, certain manifestations of spotted fever, such as jaundice, hepatomegaly, splenomegaly, abdominal pain, vomiting, and diarrhea can be misleading.

Human disease due to *Ehrlichia canis* may resemble Rocky Mountain spotted fever. It is caused by an obligate rickettsia-like intracellular organism that infects leukocytes and usually presents as a tick-borne disease of dogs (tropical canine pancytopenia). Manifestations include fever, headache, myalgia, chills, leukopenia, thrombocytopenia, elevated transaminases, and a maculopapular or petechial rash (40–50%). Oklahoma, Arkansas, Missouri, Virginia, and surrounding states are common locales, and the onset is usually in the summer months. Diagnosis is made by fluorescent antibody, and treatment with chloramphenicol or tetracycline is effective.

Rocky Mountain spotted fever can mimic many diseases. Among the most important to consider in the differential diagnosis are meningococcemia, measles, and enteroviral exanthems. Negative blood cultures and normal spinal fluid results also aid in reaching a correct diagnosis. Other diseases sometimes included in the differential diagnosis are typhoid fever, secondary syphilis, rubella, other rickettsial diseases, Lyme disease, toxic shock syndrome, scarlet fever, rheumatic fever, Kawasaki disease, idiopathic thrombocytopenia, thrombotic thrombocytopenia purpura, Henoch-Schönlein purpura, aseptic meningitis, acute gastrointestinal illness, acute abdominal conditions (such as appendicitis), hepatitis, infectious mononucleosis, leptospirosis, and drug reactions.

CONTROL. Since no vaccines are available, prevention of Rocky Mountain spotted fever is best accomplished by elimination of tick infestations from dogs; avoidance of wooded, grassy areas where ticks reside; use of insect repellants and special protective clothing; and careful examination of children who have been playing in the woods and prompt removal of ticks. Contrary to popular beliefs, the application of petroleum jelly, 70% isopropyl alcohol, fingernail polish, or a hot match are not effective in removing ticks from persons or animals. A tick can be removed safely and effectively by grasping the tick with a pair of forceps or tweezers (or with protected fingers) and by pulling gently. After removal, the site of the bite should be disinfected. Ticks should not be squeezed, crushed, or disrupted as their fluids may be infectious. Ticks should be disposed of by soaking them in alcohol or by flushing them down the toilet after which one should wash the hands with soap and water.

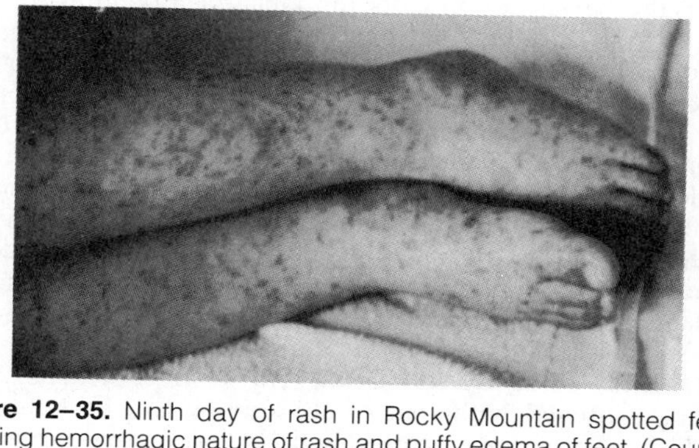

Figure 12–35. Ninth day of rash in Rocky Mountain spotted fever, showing hemorrhagic nature of rash and puffy edema of feet. (Courtesy of William H. Wood, M.D., Cleveland.)

12.99 BOUTONNEUSE FEVER

(Tick Typhus, Mediterranean Spotted Fever)

This self-limited rickettsial spotted fever is endemic in southern Europe, southern and eastern Africa, India, and the Middle East. During recent years, the incidence of human disease has increased markedly in Italy, Spain, France, and Israel. The disease that occurs in these different regions is probably caused by diverse strains of rickettsiae that are antigenically similar to *Rickettsia conorii*. The organism is transmitted to humans by the bite of the dog tick, *Rhipicephalus sanguineus*. Travelers who are exposed to ticks and dogs in endemic areas, especially those who go on safaris in high grass and bushland, are at risk. The disease is usually milder than Rocky Mountain spotted fever. Patients typically develop fever, headache, a central maculopapular or occasionally a vesicular rash (which may spread to the hands and feet and become petechial), an eschar (tach noire) at the site of the tick bite, and regional lymphadenopathy. The diagnosis can be confirmed by isolation of the organism from blood, demonstration of the organism in the eschar or macular lesion by immunofluoresence, or detection of a rise in antibody titer in paired acute and convalescent sera by IFA. Since *R. conorii* shares antigens with *R. rickettsii*, serologic tests cannot distinguish these two infections. Antibody absorption tests using different rickettsial antigens of the spotted fever group and travel history are helpful in making the correct diagnosis. Antibiotic treatment with tetracycline or chloramphenicol is usually followed by rapid clinical improvement. In vitro sensitivity of *R. conorii* to ciprofloxacin has been demonstrated, but its therapeutic efficacy has not been determined.

12.100 RICKETTSIALPOX

This febrile disease with varicelliform rash is caused by *Rickettsia akari* and is transmitted by the mouse mite, *Allodermanyssus sanguineus*. The mite vector is found in many cities of the United States. The illness is endemic in New York, and isolated cases have been reported from Boston, Philadelphia, and Cleveland.

CLINICAL MANIFESTATIONS. Rickettsialpox is a mild illness characterized by an initial skin lesion followed by fever, chills, headache, and a papulovesicular rash. The initial lesion, presumed to be the site of the mite bite, has been observed in more than 90% of cases. It may be located anywhere on the body, beginning as a nontender, nonitching, firm, red papule, 0.5–2.0 cm in diameter. A deeply entrenched vesicle develops in the center of the papule and ulcerates after several days, leaving a crusted, pigmented lesion or eschar that may persist 3 wk or longer. Adjacent lymph nodes become enlarged and tender but do not suppurate.

The initial lesion is followed in 2–7 days by fever, headache, chills, and sweating. Other symptoms may include myalgia (especially backache) and photophobia. Temperature ranges from 39 to 40° C (102–105° F), but the patient remains oriented and does not appear severely ill. Within 24–72 hr after the onset of fever, scattered erythematous maculopapules appear over the body, showing no preference for trunk, head, or extremity. The lesions enlarge, become more papular, and develop vesicles on the summit of each papule. The secondary lesions (rash) resemble the initial lesion except that they are smaller in size and heal, without leaving scars, in 4–7 days. The duration of illness seldom exceeds 7–10 days, but residual headache and lethargy may persist for 1–2 wk. Complications, sequelae, and fatalities are rare.

DIFFERENTIAL DIAGNOSIS. The rash of rickettsialpox may be confused with that of chickenpox. In the latter the vesicles are superficial, thin, dewdrop lesions that appear in successive crops beginning on the chest. These differ from the deeply seated, randomly distributed firm vesicles of the rickettsial disease. The initial lesion and the presence of chills and fever before the rash may also help in differentiation. Other diseases to be considered include infectious mononucleosis, meningococcemia, Rocky Mountain spotted fever, and typhus.

TREATMENT. Antibiotic treatment is not recommended for infants and young children with mild illness. However, a short course of tetracycline or oxytetracycline (25 mg/kg/24 hr) in 4 divided doses for 2 days is recommended for pediatric patients with severe symptoms or high fever.

CONTROL. Preventive measures should include the control of mice and their ectoparasites.

12.101 Q FEVER

Acute Q fever, a febrile disease without rash and often associated with an interstitial pneumonia, has been reported worldwide.

ETIOLOGY AND TRANSMISSION. Results from serologic surveys in the United States and elsewhere indicate that many more cases of Q fever occur each year than are recognized or reported. This is not surprising because the disease resembles an influenza-like illness, its diagnosis requires special tests, and it is not a notifiable disease. Domestic livestock (cattle, sheep, and goats), parturient cats and wild animals, and ticks serve as reservoirs for *Coxiella burnetii* infection. *C. burnetii* is highly infectious for humans and animals; even a single organism can cause infection. Disease transmission from ticks to humans or from person to person is extremely rare. Instead, the infectious agent usually is transmitted to humans in three ways: by air-borne dissemination in aerosols, dust, and straw or cloth contaminated with organisms from birth tissues, urine, or feces of infected animals; by processing of animal products (wool and hides); or by ingestion of raw milk or food. In Nova Scotia, exposure to newborn animals (chiefly kittens) has been associated with small outbreaks of Q fever in family settings. Outbreaks at medical research centers in California and Colorado have provided evidence that *C. burnetii* infections can be acquired by persons who have only casual exposure to infectious aerosols. There is also evidence suggesting that the human fetus may become infected in utero with *C. burnetii*. The organism has been isolated from placentas and breast milk of mothers who had been infected 2 mo–3 yr before delivery, and high levels of antibody to *C. burnetii* have been detected in cord blood and intracardiac blood of infants.

CLINICAL MANIFESTATIONS. Acute Q fever develops about 3 wk (range 14–39 days) after exposure to the causative agent. The severity of illness in children ranges from a subclinical (asymptomatic) infection to a febrile systemic illness with severe frontal headache, arthralgia, and myalgia, often accompanied by respiratory symptoms. In reported case series, most pediatric patients presented with fever of unknown origin and pneumonia. The pneumonitis usually resembles a viral or primary atypical pneumonia or legionnaires' disease, with a nonproductive cough. The radiologic findings with Q fever pneumonitis vary; they include multiple round segmental opacities, linear atelectasis, consolidation, and hilar adenopathy. Liver involvement with hepatomegaly, granulomatous hepatitis, and minimal liver dysfunction is common. Usually, Q fever is a self-limited disease that has a mortality rate of less than 1%. Untreated illness generally lasts for 2–3 wk, but chronic infections, particularly acute encephalitis or endocarditis, may complicate the course. Acute encephalopathy with impairment of consciousness and an abnormal pattern on EEG and CT of the brain has been reported in children with Q fever. A variety of other syndromes have been associated with Q fever, including osteomyelitis, other neurologic disorders, and Kawasaki syndrome.

Endocarditis may occur months to years after acute Q fever and may affect previously damaged aortic and mitral valves or prosthetic valves. The clinical presentation of Q fever endocarditis in children is similar to that in adults. Fever is often absent. Common features include marked clubbing of the fingers, hyperglobulinemia, hepatomegaly, and splenomegaly. A purpuric rash due to vasculitis can be seen in about 20% of patients. An elevated erythrocyte rate (>100 mm/hr), anemia, and microscopic hematuria are also common.

DIAGNOSIS AND DIFFERENTIAL DIAGNOSIS. Although it is rare in children, a diagnosis of Q fever should be considered in children with fever of unknown origin or culture-negative endocarditis, who live in rural areas or are in close contact with domestic livestock, cats, or their products. Attempts to isolate *C. burnetii* in the laboratory are hazardous and should be avoided. The diagnosis of Q fever can be confirmed serologically by significant increases in indirect fluorescent antibody levels to phase I or phase II antigens and a 4-fold rise in titer to complement-fixation antibody. Phase II antibodies appear early, whereas phase I antibodies appear later in the course of infection. It is therefore possible to differentiate acute infections from persistent or recrudescent infections by measuring phase I and phase II antibodies in serum. Elevated or rising titers of phase II antibody alone are characteristic of acute Q fever, and the appearance and persistence of elevated titers of phase I and phase II antibody are indicative of chronic Q fever. In general, the ratio of phase II to phase I antibodies is more than 1 for primary Q fever, 1 or more for granulomatous Q fever hepatitis, and 1 or less for Q fever endocarditis.

Differential diagnosis in the immunologically competent individual includes the long list of agents associated with the atypical pneumonia syndrome, such as mycoplasma, Epstein-Barr virus, psittacosis, and legionnaires' disease.

TREATMENT. To prevent complications, patients with acute Q fever should be treated promptly. The drug of choice is tetracycline. Recently, results of in vitro studies have suggested that rifampin and quinolones (ciprofloxacin) are effective, and trimethoprim, doxycycline, and chloramphenicol may also be somewhat effective. Prolonged therapy with tetracycline, usually in combination with a rickettsiacidal drug (rifampin or trimethoprim-sulfamethoxazole), is required for endocarditis. Surgery for valve replacement is indicated in patients experiencing hemodynamic difficulties or persistent or relapsing infection. The success of therapy is gauged by a fall in the erythrocyte sedimentation rate and correction of anemia and hypergammaglobulinemia. Even with proper treatment, the case fatality rate can be high.

CONTROL. Recognition of the disease in livestock should alert communities to the risk of infection. Milk from infected herds must be pasteurized at temperatures sufficient to destroy the rickettsiae. Also, 1% Lysol, 1% formaldehyde, or 5% hydrogen peroxide will destroy *C. burnetii*. Special isolation measures are not necessary because person-to-person spread of Q fever is rare.

MARY LOU CLEMENTS

Brettman LR, Lewin S, Holzman R, et al: Rickettsialpox: Report of an outbreak and a contemporary review. Medicine 60:363, 1981.

Centers for Disease Control: Rocky Mountain spotted fever—United States, 1988. MMWR 38:513, 1988.

Clements ML: Rocky Mountain spotted fever. *In*: Gorbach S, Bartlett J, Blacklow N (eds): Infectious Diseases in Medicine and Surgery. Philadelphia, WB Saunders, 1990.

Eng T, Harkess J, Fishbein D, et al: Epidemiology, clinical and laboratory findings of human ehrlichiosis in the United States, 1988. JAMA 264:2251, 1990.

McDade JE, Fishbein DB: Rickettsiaceae: The rickettsiae. *In*: Lynette EH, Haloven P, Murphy FA (eds): Laboratory Diagnosis of Infectious Diseases: Principles and Practices, Vol. 2. Viral, Rickettsial and Chlamydial Diseases. New York, Springer-Verlag, 1988, p 864.

McDonald JC, MacLean JD, McDade JE: Imported rickettsial disease. Am J Med 85:799, 1988.

Rao AK, Shapira M, Clements ML, et al: A prospective study of platelets and plasma proteolytic systems during the early stages of Rocky Mountain spotted fever. N Engl J Med 318:1021, 1988.

Richardus JH, Dumas AM, Huisman J, et al: Q fever in infancy: A review of 18 cases. Pediatr Infect Dis 4:369, 1985.

Sawyer LA, Fishbein DB, McDade JE: Q fever: Current concepts. Rev Infect Dis 9:935, 1987.

Taylor JP, Betz TG, Rawlings JA: Epidemiology of murine typhus in Texas. JAMA 255:2173, 1986.

Tzianabos T, Anderson BE, McDade JE: Detection of *Rickettsia rickettsii* DNA in clinical specimens using polymerase chain reaction technology. J Clin Microbiol 27:2866, 1989.

Walker DH (ed): Biology of Rickettsial Diseases, Vol. 1. Boca Raton, FL, CRC Press, 1981.

Walker DH: Diagnosis of rickettsial diseases. Pathol Annu 23:69, 1988.

Walker DH, Mattern WD: Rickettsial vasculitis. Am Heart J 100:896, 1980.

12.102 CAT-SCRATCH DISEASE

(Cat-Scratch Fever, Felinosis, Benign Lymphoreticulosis)

Cat-scratch disease is a self-limited, regional lymphadenitis of children and young adults that is preceded by a primary skin lesion caused by the bite or scratch of a cat.

PATHOLOGY. The microscopic appearance of the involved lymph nodes, although not diagnostic, is sufficiently characteristic to suggest cat-scratch disease. Three pathologic states have been described, progressing from reticulum cell hyperplasia to tubercle-like granuloma, which often contains Langerhans giant cells, and finally to microabscess formation; all stages may occur within a single node.

ETIOLOGY. The etiologic agent of cat-scratch disease is a small, delicate, pleomorphic gram-negative micro-organism that can be visualized with silver staining at the inoculation site and in infected tissue. This pathogen has been cultivated in artificial medium and is sensitive to a number of antimicrobial agents.

EPIDEMIOLOGY. Cat-scratch disease has been reported from most parts of the world, occurring most often in temperate climates between September and February. Eighty per cent of diagnosed cases occur in patients under 20 yr of age; 95% have a history of a cat scratch or contact. The disease also has been reported following the scratch or bite of dogs and monkeys. This illness is limited to man; cats transmitting the disease show no apparent illness and yield no infectious agent. Person-to-person transmission has not been reported.

CLINICAL MANIFESTATIONS. A primary skin lesion develops at the scratch site in 50% of patients approximately 10 days (range 7–56 days) following inoculation. This painless, nonpruritic erythematous papule may pustulate before healing without scar formation. Regional lymphadenopathy occurs within 2 wk (range 7–61 days) of the primary lesion. The involved nodes, which are superficial and may reach 8–10 cm in diameter, are painful during the early stages of the disease. The axillary and epitrochlear nodes are the most often involved, followed by lymph nodes of the head and neck and the lower extremity. Lymphangitis has not been observed. Suppuration of involved nodes occurs in 30% of cases. Within 4–6 wk the nodes become less tender, and regress within 8 wk in the majority of cases. Constitutional symptoms, including malaise, anorexia, fatigue, and low-grade fever, appear during the period of regional lymphadenopathy in half of the affected individuals. Laboratory studies are often normal, although mild elevations in the erythrocyte sedimentation rate and in the absolute eosinophil count have been reported. Atypical presentations may include unilateral swelling of the preauricular lymph node (Parinaud syndrome) or the parotid gland, erythema nodosum, osteolytic lesions, thrombocytopenia purpura, atypical pneumonia, hepatitis, splenitis, mediastinal masses, and encephalitis. Cutaneous vascular lesions and disseminated infection have been reported in patients with HIV infection.

DIAGNOSIS. The diagnosis in a child with regional lymphadenopathy has traditionally been based on fulfillment of three of the four following criteria: (1) a history of animal (usually a cat) contact, scratch, bite, and/or primary cutaneous lesion; (2) aspiration of sterile pus from an involved node; (3) characteristic histopathologic changes in an involved lymph node; and (4) a positive Hanger-Rose skin test. However, demonstration of the responsible pathogen on histologic examination and/or demonstration of an immunologic response has essentially eliminated the need for routine skin testing.

DIFFERENTIAL DIAGNOSIS. Cat-scratch disease must be differentiated from pyogenic, fungal, and tuberculous adenitis, atypical mycobacterial infection, brucellosis, plague, tularemia, lymphogranuloma venereum, rat-bite fever, sarcoidosis, and lymphoma.

TREATMENT AND PROGNOSIS. This benign illness has an excellent prognosis. Aspiration may be indicated to resolve symptoms when the involved nodes become large, fluctuant, and extremely painful. The responsible micro-organism is sensitive to a number of antimicrobial agents including aminoglycosides, cefoxitin, cefotaxime, and mezlocillin. Recent reports suggest that antibiotic treatment is associated with rapid resolution of signs and symptoms. Accordingly, treatment with gentamicin sulfate is now recommended in children with significant illness.

WILLIAM T. SPECK

Bogue CW, Wise JD, Gray GS, et al: Antibiotic therapy for Cat-scratch disease? JAMA 262:813, 1989.
Carithers HA, Margileth AM: Cat-scratch disease. AJDC 145:98, 1991.
English CK, Wear DJ, Margileth AM, et al: Cat-scratch disease: Isolation and culture of the bacterial agent. JAMA 259:1347, 1988.
Holley HP: Successful treatment of cat-scratch disease with ciprofloxacin. JAMA 265:1563, 1991.
Koehler JE, LeBoit PE, Egbert BM, et al: Cutaneous vascular lesions and disseminated cat-scratch disease in patients with the acquired immunodeficiency syndrome (AIDS) and AIDS-related complex. Ann Intern Med 109:449, 1988.
Margileth AM, Wear DJ, English CK: Systemic cat scratch disease: Report of 23 patients with prolonged or recurrent severe bacterial infection. J Infect Dis 155:390, 1987.

MYCOTIC INFECTIONS

12.103 HISTOPLASMOSIS

ETIOLOGY. Histoplasmosis is a disease of man and animals caused by *Histoplasma capsulatum*. The mycelial or saprophytic form of this dimorphic fungus is distributed worldwide in soil. It grows on Sabouraud medium at room temperature (25° C) as white or tan fluffy colonies; small, budding, oval yeast forms are found in the infected tissue.

EPIDEMIOLOGY. Histoplasmosis is the most common systemic mycosis in the United States and has emerged as an important opportunistic illness in immunocompromised patients. Human histoplasmosis follows inhalation of air-borne spores released by *H. capsulatum*. The saprophytic form grows best in soil that is heavily contaminated with avian and bat excreta. Birds, because of their high body temperature, are not infected but may carry the fungus on their feathers. However, bats may be infected and may disseminate the fungus in their excreta. Chicken, starling, or blackbird roosts and hollow trees as well as bat-infested caves, lofts, attics, and bridges may be heavily contaminated and serve as reservoirs for human infection. Histoplasmosis occurs throughout the United States, is endemic in the Mississippi, Ohio, and Missouri River valleys, and is most common in Kentucky and Tennessee, where up to 90% of the population have a positive histoplasmin skin test reaction by the age of 20 yr. Other areas of high prevalence, often very local, occur in South America, Asia, and Europe. Focal outbreaks of epidemic histoplasmosis have been reported following cave exploration, excavation, demolition, or other dust-raising activities in heavily contaminated areas. Most urban outbreaks occur at the fringes of the endemic area due to the large number of individuals at risk for primary infection. A large outbreak occurred in Indianapolis in 1979, where an estimated 100,000 persons were infected; 15 died from this disease. Histoplasmosis is not transmitted from person to person.

PATHOGENESIS AND PATHOLOGY. Human infection follows inhalation of conidia, which reach the alveoli and are transformed into small budding yeasts. During the initial period of multiplication, both local spread to adjacent lymph nodes and transient dissemination from the pulmonary focus to organs throughout the body occur. In most patients these primary lesions enlarge and undergo caseous necrosis, fibrosis, and subsequent calcification. In the lung, calcification of a primary focus and adjacent lymph nodes may resemble the Gohn complex of primary pulmonary tuberculosis. Multifocal "buckshot" areas of calcification may also occur throughout the lungs, lymphatic tissue, and spleen. Two forms of progressive histoplasmosis occur in a small proportion of infected patients. *Disseminated histoplasmosis* occurs in infants and debilitated adults with defects in cell-mediated immunity. Yeast-laden macrophages are present throughout the reticuloendothelial system with extensive involvement of bone marrow, liver, spleen, lungs, heart, adrenals, and brain. *Chronic pulmonary histoplasmosis* typically occurs in adult males and is associated with yeast invasion and multiplication in preexisting emphysematous cavities, with resultant caseous necrosis and fibrosis.

CLINICAL MANIFESTATIONS. *Acute pulmonary histoplasmosis*, the most common form of disease, is classified as primary (initial infection) or secondary (reinfection) according to previous exposure history. The primary form is most often an asymptomatic disease in infants and young children. A positive histoplasmin skin test is the only manifestation of infection. The incubation period is 10–23 days, and the severity of symptoms, when present, corresponds to the concentration of inhaled conidia. Symptomatic primary acute pulmonary histoplasmosis presents as an influenza-like illness with abrupt onset of fever, malaise, myalgia, headache, and nonproductive cough. Physical examination is often normal; however, diffuse rales and mild hepatosplenomegaly have been described. Erythema multiforme, erythema nodosum, or maculopapular rashes occur in symptomatic and asymptomatic individuals, are more common in women, and are often accompanied by arthralgias and arthritis. Roentgenographic examination of the lungs during the acute illness is usually normal (75%), but a few patients may demonstrate small, patchy infiltrates with enlargement of hilar or mediastinal lymph nodes. Abnormal chest roentgenograms may persist for several months, showing small nodular residues that eventually calcify. Less common manifestations of acute histoplasmosis include arthritis, pericarditis, and obstructive symptoms due to enlargement of mediastinal lymph nodes. The illness is self-limited in most children; abnormal signs and symptoms, when present, rarely persist for more than 3 wk. In secondary, or reinfection-type pulmonary histoplasmosis, the onset of symptoms occurs within 3 days of exposure. Symptoms are similar but less severe and of shorter duration than those seen in primary disease. The roentgenographic findings following reinfection consist of uniformly distributed miliary nodules, indistinguishable from those characteristic of miliary tuberculosis, which resolve over several months without calcification.

Epidemic histoplasmosis occurs in both endemic and nonendemic areas following massive exposure to dust heavily contaminated with spores of *H. capsulatum*. Clinical manifestations begin within 3–20 days following exposure and include an abrupt onset of high fever, chills, headache, malaise, and a nonproductive cough; pleuritic chest pain and dyspnea are common. Physical examination reveals diffuse rales often associated with minimal hepatosplenomegaly. Erythema nodosum and erythema multiforme, appearing separately or together, have been reported in young women during epidemics. Roentgenographic examination of the chest demonstrates pulmonary infiltrates, which may persist for several months. The prognosis is excellent, with spontaneous resolution of all signs and symptoms within weeks. Epidemic illness has, on rare occasions, led to disseminated disease in infants and children.

Chronic pulmonary histoplasmosis, a disease most often observed in middle-aged white male smokers with a history of chronic obstructive pulmonary disease, is uncommon in children.

Disseminated histoplasmosis is an acute illness of infants, young children, and immunosuppressed patients associated with high morbidity and mortality; untreated, the outcome is uniformly and rapidly fatal. The illness most often begins as an acute pulmonary infection with fever, cough, and dyspnea and quickly progresses to involve multiple organ systems. Affected patients appear critically ill with persistent nausea, vomiting, abdominal pain, and diarrhea. Physical findings reveal generalized rales, diffuse lymphadenopathy, and impressive hepatosplenomegaly. Roentgenographic abnormalities often include a diffuse interstitial pneumonitis. Anemia, leukopenia, and thrombocytopenia are common and predispose to bleeding or secondary bacterial infection. Death is secondary to respiratory failure, uncontrolled gastrointestinal bleeding, disseminated intravascular coagulation, or bacterial sepsis. Subacute and chronic forms of disseminated disease have been reported in adults.

Histoplasmoma and *mediastinal collagenosis* are rare in children, representing an exaggerated immune response following acute infection. Histoplasmoma presents as an enlarging, solitary pulmonary nodule with concentric layers of fibrous tissue and calcium surrounding a healed primary focus; these nodules may reach 3–4 cm in diameter and must be differentiated from neoplasms. Mediastinal collagenosis is associated with fibrocalcification originating in a mediastinal node and extending through the mediastinum, resulting in entrapment and obstruction of mediastinal structures.

DIAGNOSIS. Definitive diagnosis requires isolation of the responsible pathogen from clinical material or visualization in histopathologic specimens. The organism is rarely cultured from sputum obtained during acute pulmonary histoplasmosis but is commonly recovered from sputum in patients with chronic pulmonary infection. In disseminated disease, organisms can be cultured from blood, bone marrow, urine, and sputum. Cultures of the cerebrospinal fluid are positive in patients with meningitis. Demonstration of *Histoplasma* in tissue specimens allows rapid diagnosis in selected patients. Specifically, in disseminated infection, organisms can be identified with special stains in the buffy coat prepared from peripheral blood, in bone marrow macrophages, and in respiratory secretions or bronchial washings. The recent development of a radioimmunoassay for detection of a polysaccharide antigen of *H. capsulatum* in body fluids provides another rapid, sensitive, and specific test for histoplasmosis.

The *skin test* is rarely helpful. The test resembles the tuberculin test and is considered positive if an area of at least 5 mm of induration is observed at 48 hr. A positive reaction indicates previous sensitization to *H. capsulatum* but is not diagnostic of active disease. However, conversion from a negative to a positive reaction within a few weeks or a positive reaction in an infant suggests active infection. The limited usefulness of skin testing is due to the fact that most inhabitants in an endemic area have a positive skin test, and a large number of false-negative results have been observed in patients with disseminated disease. Moreover, skin testing may interfere with interpretation of serologic tests owing to an increase in antibody titers that occurs following skin testing in previously infected individuals.

Serologic diagnosis of histoplasmosis is possible using complement-fixation, immunodiffusion, radioimmunoassay, or enzyme-linked radioimmunoassay. Complement-fixing antibodies appear within 3–6 wk and persist for years. A 4-fold rise in paired sera or an isolated titer of 1:32 is suggestive of histoplasmosis. The immunodiffusion test measures antibodies to the M or H antigens of *H. capsulatum*. Antibodies to these antigens appear within 6 wk of exposure; however, they are not present in all infected individuals. Antibodies to the M antigen are present in approximately 50% of patients with acute histoplasmosis and are occasionally found in asymptomatic patients in endemic areas. Antibodies to the H band are more specific for acute illness but are found in only 10% of patients with acute infections. The immunodiffusion test is positive in 75% of patients with chronic pulmonary infection but in only 30% of patients with disseminated disease.

TREATMENT. Acute histoplasmosis is usually a self-limited illness and, accordingly, rarely requires treatment. Symptomatic illness in young infants may be treated with either ketoconazole or amphotericin B. In noncritically ill immunocompetent adults with nonmeningeal disease, ketoconazole is the initial treatment of choice. Experience with this oral drug in children with histoplasmosis is limited; however, ketoconazole offers an attractive alternative to parenterally administered amphotericin B. A dose of 5–10 mg/kg/24 hr of ketoconazole for 4–6 wk has been recommended for noncritically ill immunologically normal children with nonmeningeal histoplasmosis. Children who are critically ill, immunocompromised, or have disseminated disease should receive treatment with amphotericin B. The recommended total dose is 35 mg/kg for younger infants and children; a total dose of 2 g is recommended for adolescents and young adults weighing less than 60 kg. Although this regimen has proved effective in immunocompetent as well as in most immunosuppressed patients, relapse is invariable in HIV-infected patients. Accordingly, in this patient population ketoconazole or biweekly amphotericin B should be administered after an initial successful course of amphotericin B and continued indefinitely to suppress, but not cure, this infection.

Itraconazole, an oral triazole under investigation for the treatment of both superficial and deep mycotic infections, has shown promise in the treatment of histoplasmosis. This agent is less toxic, better tolerated, and more effective than ketoconazole and may become the agent of choice for all forms of histoplasmosis.

Dismukes WE, Cloud G, Bowles C, et al: Treatment of blastomycosis and histoplasmosis with ketoconazole. Ann Intern Med 103:861, 1985.
Goodwin RA, Dez Prez RM: Histoplasmosis. Am Rev Respir Dis 117:929, 1978.
Goodwin RA, Shapiro JL, et al: Disseminated histoplasmosis: Clinical pathologic correlations. Medicine 59:1, 1980.
Hughes WT: Hematogenous histoplasmosis in the immunocompromised child. J Pediatr 105:569, 1984.
Mandell W, Goldberg DM, Neu HE: Histoplasmosis in patients with acquired immune deficiency syndrome. Am J Med 81:974, 1986.
Wheat LJ: Histoplasmosis. Infect Dis Clin North Am 2:841, 1988.

12.104 BLASTOMYCOSIS

Blastomycosis is an uncommon systemic fungal infection caused by the dimorphic saprophytic fungus *Blastomyces dermatidis*.

ETIOLOGY. *Blastomyces dermatidis* in infected tissue is a round, thick-walled yeast; each daughter cell is attached to the parent by a broad-based neck.

EPIDEMIOLOGY. The epidemiology of blastomycosis is not as well defined as that of the other systemic mycoses because reporting is not required, subclinical infection is common, recovery of the fungus from soil and decayed vegetation is difficult, there is no satisfactory skin test antigen, and serodiagnosis lacks sensitivity and specificity. Blastomycosis occurs mainly in the southeastern United States and in the Mississippi, Ohio, and St. Lawrence River valleys. The endemic area includes the north central region of the United States and extends into Canada. Blastomycosis has also been reported in England, Africa, and India. Studies of epidemic infection suggest that human disease occurs following inhalation of air-borne spores from contaminated soil or decaying vegetation that reach the lower respiratory tract and, after conversion to yeast forms during a long incubation period (30–45 days), establish a primary pulmonary infection. Lymphohematogenous dissemination to multiple organ systems occurs in a minority of patients. Infection is more common in adult men with occupational or recreational exposure to contaminated soil or vegetation.

CLINICAL MANIFESTATIONS. *Primary pulmonary blastomycosis* most often presents as a mild self-limited lower respiratory infection. Thus, the child presents with low-grade fever, malaise, pleuritic chest pain, a nonproductive cough, and occasional hemoptysis. Roentgenographic examination is not diagnostic and most often reveals lobar consolidation and hilar adenopathy with or without pleural effusion. Spontaneous resolution of the acute pneumonia occurs in a majority of infected children. Less often, a progressive form of pneumonia occurs with high fever, night sweats, chills, anorexia, and dyspnea. Productive cough and hemoptysis are common. The roentgenographic examination demonstrates bilateral nodular basilar infiltrates. Cavitation and effusion are uncommon and when present may be misdiagnosed as malignancy or tuberculosis. *Disseminated blastomycosis* most often occurs in adults with chronic pulmonary infection.

The skin is the most common site of extrapulmonary involvement, and cutaneous lesions may be the presenting complaint in patients with asymptomatic or mild pulmonary disease. Solitary or multiple subcutaneous nodules of the face and trunk are characteristic of *cutaneous blastomycosis*. These lesions appear initially as papules or pustules, which, over a period of weeks or months, progress to verrucous granulomas with erythematous, indurated, raised, serpentine borders. The lesions advance centripetally with central scaring; regional lymphadenopathy does not occur. Other extrapulmonary sites include bone, joints, genitourinary tract (prostrate, epididymis, and testes) and, on rare occasions, central nervous system, adrenal glands, thyroid gland, and liver.

DIAGNOSIS. Definitive diagnosis requires identification of the fungus in tissue or in culture. Serologic tests with complement-fixation antibodies, enzyme-linked immunoassay antibodies, and immunodiffusion are useful for epidemiologic studies but lack the sensitivity and specificity necessary for clinical diagnosis. Skin testing with blastomycin has not proved sensitive or specific for blastomycosis.

TREATMENT. Acute primary pulmonary blastomycosis is a self-limited disease that rarely requires more than careful follow-up and reassurance. Treatment is indicated in children with persistent or progressive pulmonary blastomycosis or in patients with extrapulmonary infection. Amphotericin B has proved effective in the treatment of blastomycosis, and recurrences are uncommon following a total dosage of 15–30 mg/kg (2 g maximum). However, the toxicity of amphotericin B (e.g., renal dysfunction, anemia, hypokalemia, fever, and so on) is such that alternative therapeutic regimens have been sought. Ketoconazole has proved effective in nonimmunocompromised adults with blastomycosis. Accordingly, in non–life-threatening illness in children we recommend treatment with ketoconazole (5–10 mg/kg/24 hr) and reserve amphotericin B for critically ill or immunodeficient patients with systemic disease. Itraconazole has shown promise in the treatment of blastomycosis; however, experience with it is limited.

Bradsher RW: Blastomycosis. Infect Dis Clin North Am 2:877, 1988.
Laksey WK, Sarosi GA: Blastomycosis in children. Pediatrics 65:111, 1980.
Macher A: Histoplasmosis and blastomycosis. Med Clin North Am 64:447, 1980.
National Institutes of Allergy and Infectious Disease, Mycosis Study Group: Treatment of blastomycosis and histoplasmosis with ketoconazole: Results of a prospective, randomized clinical trial. Ann Intern Med 103:861, 1985.
Sarosi GA, Davis SF: Blastomycosis. Am Rev Respir Dis 120:911, 1979.

12.105 CRYPTOCOCCOSIS
(Torulosis, European Blastomycosis)

Cryptococcosis is a subacute or chronic fungal infection caused by an encapsulated budding yeast *Cryptococcus neoformans*. Clinical illness most often involves the central nervous system and usually occurs as an opportunistic infection in an immunocompromised host. The fungus is surrounded by a polysaccharide capsule that contains antigenic determinants permitting identification of four serotypes: A, B, C, and D.

EPIDEMIOLOGY. *C. neoformans* is distributed worldwide, existing in nature as a soil saprophyte. The roosting sites of birds, particularly pigeons, provide the necessary conditions for luxuriant growth, and high rates of positive skin tests occur in individuals frequently exposed to pigeons. Cryptococcosis results from inhalation of spores, which germinate in the pulmonary tissue and may disseminate through the bloodstream to brain, meninges, bone marrow, and skin. It occurs sporadically without any occupational predisposition, most often as an opportunistic infection, and is rarely associated with historical or roentgenographic evidence of respiratory involvement. Thus, there is an increased incidence of infection in patients following organ transplantation or treatment with corticosteroids and in those with lymphoreticular malignancies and insulin-dependent diabetes. Cryptococcosis is the most common life-threatening opportunistic fungal infection seen in HIV-infected individuals. This disease tends to be more common in adults, affects males more often than females (3:1), and is more common in whites.

PATHOLOGY. The characteristic lesion is a cyst-like cavity containing gelatinous material. Microscopic examination reveals clumps of cryptococci within the cyst and an inflammatory response consisting of macrophages, giant cells, and lymphocytes. In pulmonary cryptococcosis the common finding is a subpleural granuloma. In central nervous system disease multiple cystic lesions occur throughout the brain, particularly in the cortical gray matter and basal ganglia. Mass lesions are extremely rare.

CLINICAL MANIFESTATIONS. *Pulmonary cryptococcosis* is uncommon in children, occurring most often in immunosuppressed children as an influenza-like illness with low-grade fever, cough, pleuritic chest pain, and minimal sputum production. Physical examination may reveal diffuse rales. The chest roentgenogram demonstrates a varied pattern that may include a single pulmonary granuloma, apical cavities, interstitial pneumonitis, or pleural effusion. Routine laboratory studies are normal. Cultures of sputum and bronchial washings are occasionally positive, but invasive procedures may be needed to recover pathogens from tissues.

Cryptococcal meningitis is the most common form of life-threatening cryptococcal infection in children and has a subacute or chronic presentation. Symptoms are intermittent and are usually present for weeks to months; they include headache, mental changes, visual changes, nausea and vomiting, pain and stiffness of the neck and back, chills or fever, lethargy, weakness, fatigue, ataxia, and aphasia or slurred speech. Physical examination may reveal nuchal rigidity, papilledema, hearing loss, motor weakness, cerebellar signs, and coma. Cerebrospinal fluid findings are similar to those that occur in other types of chronic meningitis and include an elevated opening pressure, an elevated protein concentration, hypoglycorrhachia, and a mononuclear pleocytosis that rarely exceeds 300 cells/mm^3. The mortality rate is 50%. Treatment failure and early death are associated with underlying HIV infection, lymphoreticular malignancy, and corticosteroid therapy. Additional poor prognostic findings include a high opening CSF pressure, a low CSF glucose level, fewer than 20 leukocytes/mm^3, cryptococci seen on CSF smear, cryptococci isolated from extraneural sites, and high titers of cryptococcal antigen in CSF and serum. Forty per cent of survivors have residual neurologic deficits including visual loss, hearing defects, cranial nerve damage, motor impairment, personality change, and, on rare occasions, hydrocephalus.

Cryptococcosis may involve the skin and present as pustules or small subcutaneous masses, most often located on the face or scalp; they eventually become necrotic and ulcerate. Involvement of the musculoskeletal system is manifest as osteomyelitis and septic arthritis. Less common presentations include endocarditis, renal abscess, and adrenal insufficiency.

DIAGNOSIS. Diagnosis depends on histologic identification of cryptococci in biopsy specimens or body fluids, recovery of *C. neoformans* following appropriate cultures, or demonstration of cryptococcal antigen. Histologically, appropriately stained organisms are yeast-like with narrow-based buds. The encapsulated yeast may be visualized in 50% of patients with meningitis after mixing sediment of the cerebrospinal fluid with an adequate volume of India ink. Culture of *C. neoformans* produces creamy white mucoid colonies within 10 days of inoculation onto Sabouraud's medium. Negative cultures of cerebrospinal fluid do not necessarily exclude the diagnosis of meningitis because small numbers of organisms may necessitate repeated cultures of large volumes of centrifuged specimens. The latex agglutination technique detects cryptococcal polysaccharide capsular antigen in cerebrospinal fluid or serum in more than 90% of patients with cryptococcal meningitis.

TREATMENT. Acute pulmonary cryptococcosis in infants and children with an intact immune system is most often a self-limited disease and rarely requires treatment. However, a 1-mo course of amphotericin B plus flucytosine is recommended for symptomatic pulmonary infections in immunocompromised patients. Relapse is common in this patient population, and when it occurs, long-term suppressive therapy is recommended.

Cryptococcal meningitis is usually treated with a 6-wk course of amphotericin B (0.4–0.6 mg/kg/24 hr) plus flucytosine (100–150 mg/kg/24 hr). In immunocompromised patients, especially those with simultaneous HIV infection, CSF cultures remain positive, and symptomatic improvement is delayed. Accordingly, whenever possible immunosuppressive therapy should be eliminated or minimized in infected children and consideration given to simultaneous treatment with intraventricular amphotericin B. Nevertheless, relapse of cryptococcal meningitis is invariable in HIV-infected patients. Many authorities recommend that the initial course of amphotericin B and flucytosine be followed by long-term suppressive therapy. Most suppressive regimens require twice weekly doses of amphotericin B. The addition of flucytosine to the long-term suppressive regimen is problematic because bone marrow function may be severely compromised, especially in HIV-infected patients receiving azidothymidine.

Fluconazole has proved useful in animal models of cryptococcal meningitis and in isolated cases of meningeal and disseminated cryptococcosis. Long-term maintenance treatment with fluconazole has prevented relapse in patients with AIDS. Further experience is needed before routine use of this agent in infants and children can be recommended.

Bennett JE, Dimukes WE, et al: A comparison of amphotericin B alone and combined with flucytosine in the treatment of cryptococcal meningitis. N Engl J Med 301:126, 1979.

Diamond RD, Bennet JE: Prognostic factors in cryptococcal meningitis. Ann Intern Med 80:176, 1974.

Lewis JS, Louria DB, Chmel H: Fungal and yeast infections of the central nervous system. A clinical review. Medicine 63:108, 1984.

Sanderson PJ: Itraconazole and fluconazole: New drugs for deep fungal infections. J Antimicrob Chemother 24:275, 1989.

12.106 MUCORMYCOSIS
(Zygomycosis)

The term mucormycosis refers to a group of opportunistic mycotic infections characterized by vessel invasion, thrombosis, and necrosis that are caused by dimorphic fungi of the class Zygomycetes and the order Mucorales. The principal human pathogens, *Rhizopus, Absidia,* and *Mucor,* are distributed worldwide, commonly grow on fruit and other food (e.g., bread mold), and are easily isolated from soil. The Mucorales grow on a variety of laboratory media as fluffy white, gray, or brownish molds following incubation at 37° C. In appropriately stained clinical specimens, thick-walled, nonseptate, irregular, right-angled branching hyphae are easily visualized.

EPIDEMIOLOGY. Exposure to spores of Mucorales is universal, but disease is uncommon. The most frequent agent causing human disease is *Rhizopus oryzae.* Infection is sporadic and almost exclusively limited to children who have underlying diseases, for example, diabetes mellitus (especially with acidosis), leukemia, or lymphoma; who have undergone organ transplantation and immunosuppression; or who have burns, renal failure, or malnutrition. There is no evidence of person-to-person transmission. An unusual epidemic of cutaneous mucormycosis was associated with the use of Elastoplast bandages.

CLINICAL MANIFESTATIONS. Mucormycosis follows inhalation or ingestion of spores, subsequent germination, and invasion of the nasal, tracheal, or gastrointestinal mucosa. Infection is characterized by the tendency of these organisms to invade major blood vessels with resultant ischemia and necrosis of the surrounding tissue. *Rhinocerebral mucormycosis,* the most common form of disease, typically occurs in children with poorly controlled diabetes. Infection begins in the nasal turbinates or hard palate and presents as a black eschar. The fungus gradually extends, directly invading the paranasal sinuses. Further extension across nerves, blood vessels, cartilage, and bone leads to involvement of the face, orbit, meninges, and frontal lobes of the brain. Initial symptoms of unilateral headache, nasal stuffiness, epistaxis, and periorbital numbness may progress to include periorbital swelling, with proptosis, loss of extraocular movements, and blindness. Intracranial extension may occur, resulting in occlusion of cerebral arteries and veins. Roentgenographic examination reveals diffuse clouding of the paranasal sinuses and extensive bony destruction; computed tomography delineates orbital involvement. Diagnosis depends on histologic demonstration of hyphae in scrapings and biopsy material; cultures are positive in only 15% of cases.

Pulmonary mucormycosis is an acute, life-threatening disease that occurs in immunosuppressed children with diabetes, renal failure, leukemia, lymphoma, or severe neutropenia. Infection can occur in association with rhinocerebral mucormycosis or following inhalation of spores. Patients with isolated pulmonary disease present with pulmonary thrombosis and infarction secondary to fungal invasion and occlusion of the pulmonary vessels; symptoms are characterized by an acute onset of fever, pleuritic chest pain, and hemoptysis. Subsequent hematogenous dissemination with involvement of multiple organ systems is not uncommon. Roentgenographic examination may reveal a number of abnormalities including patchy infiltrates, lobar consolidation, cavity formation, and pleural effusion. Nodule formation, fungus balls, and mass lesions have also been reported. Examination of sputum and cultures of respiratory tract secretions are usually negative. Diagnosis requires tissue obtained by transthoracic needle aspiration, transbronchial biopsy, or open lung biopsy for culture and histologic examination.

Gastrointestinal mucormycosis is uncommon and in children is most often associated with malnutrition, kwashiorkor, or treatment with corticosteroids. Necrotic ulcers may involve the entire gastrointestinal tract, especially the stomach. Symptoms are acute, vary with the site and extent of involvement, and include abdominal pain, hematemesis, bloody diarrhea, intestinal obstruction, or perforation. Diagnosis depends on biopsy demonstration of tissue invasion or cultures of gastrointestinal tissue; secretions are invariably sterile.

Disseminated mucormycosis occurs in children with leukemia and lymphoma; is often associated with infections due to bacteria, viruses, and other pathogenic fungi; and is invariably fatal. Infection originates in the lung and disseminates to involve the brain and other organ systems. Neurologic manifestations are secondary to cerebrovascular invasion. Meningeal involvement is uncommon. Cultures of blood and cerebrospinal fluid are invariably negative, and diagnosis depends on the demonstration of fungus in the biopsy material.

Cutaneous mucormycosis occurs most often as a secondary infection following extensive burns or surgical procedures. Infection presents as an erythematous papule that ulcerates, leaving a black necrotic center. Diagnosis depends on biopsy, culture, and histologic examination of suspicious skin lesions. Dissemination is not uncommon.

Other reported infections with Mucoraceae include endocarditis, brain abscess, wound infection, and isolated renal infection.

TREATMENT. This includes control of the underlying predisposing illness, reduction or elimination of immunosuppressive therapy, surgical resection of involved tissue, and intravenous administration of amphotericin B. The optimal dosage in children has not been established; however, in adults with extensive disease, treatment consists of amphotericin 0.8–1 mg/kg/24 hr given over a 2- to 3-mo period. In superficial infection of the skin, debridement and topical therapy with amphotericin B have proved successful; however, with evidence of deep hyphal invasion, systemic therapy with amphotericin B is indicated.

Lehrer RI, Howard DH, Sypherd PS, et al: Mucormycosis. Ann Intern Med 93:93, 1989.

Meyers BR, Wormser G, Hirshman SZ, et al: Rhinocerebral mucormycosis—premortem diagnosis and therapy. Arch Intern Med 139:557, 1979.

12.107 SPOROTRICHOSIS

Sporotrichosis is an uncommon chronic fungal infection of man and animals that is caused by a dimorphic fungus, *Sporothrix schenckii*. It is distributed worldwide, and the fungus exists in its saprophytic form in living, decaying, or dead vegetation. It is commonly found in the Missouri and Mississippi River valleys. Disseminated infection is unusual, may follow inhalation or ingestion of spores, and is more common in immunocompromised patients. The cutaneous form is most common and results from intradermal inoculation of spores following contact with contaminated vegetation, for example, sphagnum moss, barberry, rosebushes, and various species of grass. Consequently, sporotrichosis is often an occupational disease of farmers, horticulturists, and others in continual contact with soil and vegetation. Epidemic sporotrichosis may occur in adults and children following contact with straw and hay heavily contaminated with spores of *S. schenckii*. Neither human-to-human nor animal-to-human transmission has been reported.

PATHOLOGY. Histologically, sporotrichosis is characterized by noncaseating granulomas and microabscess formation. Oval or cigar-shaped forms are rarely visualized in biopsy specimens because of their small number, small size, and lack of a specific staining technique.

CLINICAL MANIFESTATIONS. *Cutaneous sporotrichosis* is the most common form of disease in infants and children. *Lymphocutaneous sporotrichosis* accounts for more than 75% of reported cases and occurs after traumatic subcutaneous inoculation of spores. Following a variable and often prolonged incubation period (1–12 wk) an isolated, painless erythematous papule develops at the inoculation site, most often an extremity. The initial lesion enlarges and eventually ulcerates. Although infection may remain limited to the inoculation site (fixed cutaneous sporotrichosis), satellite lesions follow lymphangitic spread and appear as multiple, tender, subcutaneous nodules extending along the lymphatic channels draining the initial lesion. These secondary nodules represent subcutaneous granulomas that attach to the overlying skin and ulcerate. Sporotrichosis does not heal spontaneously, and ulcerative lesions may persist for years unless they are appropriately treated. Systemic signs and symptoms are uncommon. Extracutaneous sporotrichosis is rare in children; pulmonary sporotrichosis, meningitis, osteomyelitis, arthritis, and disseminated disease have been reported in adults.

DIAGNOSIS. Cutaneous sporotrichosis must be differentiated from the cutaneous forms of coccidioidomycosis, blastomycosis, histoplasmosis, tuberculosis, syphilis, *Mycobacterium marinum*, cutaneous nocardiosis, and tularemia. Histologic examination of biopsy material rarely demonstrates the organisms; a definitive diagnosis requires isolation of *S. schenckii* from infected tissue. Serologic evaluation by slide latex agglutination test and enzyme-linked immunoassays is useful in diagnosis and in monitoring response to therapy. Skin testing is available but is of little use in establishing a clinical diagnosis.

TREATMENT. Potassium iodide is the treatment of choice for cutaneous sporotrichosis. The solution is given orally (1 g/mL) beginning with 1–10 drops 3 times a day and increasing each dose by 1 drop/dose each day until a final dose of 10–40 drops 3 times a day is reached or until symptoms of iodism appear (skin eruptions, lacrimation, parotid swelling, nausea, vomiting). Treatment is continued for 1 mo after resolution of cutaneous lesions. Occasional patients have responded to oral ketoconazole. Itraconazole has more activity in vitro than ketoconazole and has cured cases of sporotrichosis. However, there are no comparative studies. Systemic administration of amphotericin B is required for extracutaneous infection.

Chandler JW, Kriel RL, Tosh FE: Childhood sporotrichosis. Am J Dis Child 115:368, 1968.
Dahl BA, Silberfarb PM, Sarosi GA, et al: Sporotrichosis in children. JAMA 215:1980, 1971.
Orr ER, Riley HD: Sporotrichosis in childhood: Report of ten cases. J Pediatr 78:951, 1971.

12.108 ASPERGILLOSIS

Aspergillosis refers to a group of diseases caused by a monomorphic fungus of the genus *Aspergillus*. Most human disease is caused by *A. fumigatus*, followed by *A. niger* and *A. flavus*. Aspergilli are distributed worldwide, and spores (conidia) are readily isolated from air, soil, water, and decaying vegetation. Although exposure to *Aspergillus* spores is frequent, disease is uncommon. Infection is most often acquired from inhalation of air-borne spores, which gain access to the paranasal sinuses or lower respiratory tract. Spores may also gain access to the body following ingestion, aspiration, surgical instrumentation, or skin and wound contamination. The three major categories of human disease are allergic aspergillosis, aspergilloma, and invasive disease.

Hypersensitivity Syndromes

Atopic asthma may be precipitated by spores from *Aspergillus* species. Inhalation triggers an IgE-mediated response and bronchospasm. The clinical manifestations are nonspecific and include acute onset of wheezing in the absence of pulmonary infiltrates or fever.

Extrinsic allergic alveolitis is a hypersensitivity pneumonitis that occurs in nonatopic individuals after repeated exposure to organic dust. *Aspergillus* is one of many organic substances that produces this syndrome ("maltworkers" or "farmers" lung). The pathogenesis is unknown; it is similar to allergic alveolitis caused by other antigens and may represent an immune complex disease of lung tissue. The clinical manifestations include fever, cough, and dyspnea, which occur within 4–6 hr following exposure to the offending antigen. Physical examination reveals rhonchi in the absence of wheezing. Sputum and blood examination do not show eosinophilia, and the chest roentgenogram reveals diffuse interstitial infiltrates. Persistent exposure gradually leads to irreversible pulmonary fibrosis.

Allergic bronchopulmonary aspergillosis often occurs in atopic children with a long history of asthma or other chronic pulmonary disease. The immune response to *Aspergillus* is mediated by IgG and IgE antibody directed against the fungus, which colonizes the airway, producing a continued supply of antigen. The diagnosis should be considered in all children with asthma and a history of unexplained pulmonary infiltrates. Symptoms include recurrent episodes of wheezing, pulmonary infiltrates, and eosinophilia. Investigations have established eight criteria that are useful in diagnosing this clinical entity: (1) paroxysmal bronchial obstruction (asthma), (2) peripheral blood eosinophilia, (3) immediate (type I) reactivity to *Aspergillus* antigens, (4) precipitating serum antibodies (precipitants) against *Aspergillus* antigen, (5) elevated serum IgE concentrations, (6) elevated serum IgE and IgG antibodies specific to *A. fumigatus*, (7) history of pulmonary infiltrates, and (8) central bronchiectasis.

Noninvasive (Saprophytic) Syndromes

Otomycosis is a benign condition characterized by pain, pruritus, and otorrhea in which *Aspergillus* species (particularly *A. niger*) grow on the cerumen and cellular debris within the external auditory canal. The tympanic membrane is usually spared. Resolution follows curettage and topical antifungal therapy.

Sinusitis (allergic *Aspergillus* sinusitis) secondary to *Aspergillus* exposure most often involves the maxillary sinuses and presents in atopic children with fever and pain over the involved sinus. Roentgenographic examination demonstrates clouding or reveals a fungus ball lying free or attached to the mucosa of a chronically infected sinus. Curettage and drainage are the treatments of choice.

Aspergillomas usually follow colonization of poorly drained bronchi or cavitary lesions within the pulmonary parenchyma by *Aspergillus* species that proliferate as a mass of hyphal elements (fungus ball). Thus, aspergillomas occur primarily in the upper lobes of the lung and have been observed in the pulmonary cavities of patients with tuberculosis, histoplasmosis, and sarcoidosis. Less often, aspergillomas are a consequence of recovery from invasive pulmonary aspergillosis. Mycelia may extend from the fungus ball into the wall of the cavity; however, extensive pulmonary invasion and hematogenous dissemination are uncommon. Affected children are often asymptomatic, although chronic cough and hemoptysis may occur. Diagnosis is established by roentgenographically demonstrating an air shadow outlining a pulmonary cavity that surrounds a solitary fungus ball. Management is controversial. Antifungal chemotherapy has little effect except in a subset of patients with resolving pulmonary aspergillosis, and most clinicians follow asymptomatic patients, reserving surgical resection for those with recurrent or life-threatening hemoptysis.

Invasive Disease

Invasive pulmonary aspergillosis is an acute life-threatening infection that occurs almost exclusively in immunosuppressed children. Predisposing factors include corticosteroid therapy, cytotoxic chemotherapy, recurrent or concurrent therapy with broad-spectrum antimicrobial agents, leukopenia ($<1,000$ cells/mm^3), acute leukemia in relapse, or rejection of an organ transplant. Infection is uncommon in children with HIV infection, reflecting the limited role of cell-mediated immunity in defense against this infection. Clinical manifestations mimic those characteristic of acute bacterial pneumonia and are secondary to alveolar proliferation of hyphae, invasion into pulmonary arterioles, and subsequent thrombosis and ischemia. Temperature elevation, nonproductive cough, and dyspnea are common. Although roentgenographic examination may reveal lobar involvement or a miliary pattern, the more common finding is a peripheral patchy bronchopneumonia. Without treatment, these densities increase in size, extend toward the periphery, and undergo cavitation or abscess formation. Histologic examination reveals areas of pulmonary infarction secondary to thrombosis resulting from vascular invasion by *Aspergillus* spp. Thus, in some cases, the clinical presentation resembles that of pulmonary embolization and infarction. Pulmonary infection is often accompanied by dissemination to the brain, heart, liver, other viscera, and skin. The clinical course is usually fulminant, with an overall mortality of 80%.

The diagnosis is suggested by the predisposing illness, the

clinical course of the illness, isolation of the fungus from pulmonary and/or nasopharyngeal secretions, negative cultures for other pathogens, and failure to respond to antibacterial therapy. Cultures of the blood, CSF, bone marrow, and urine are rarely positive in disseminated disease. Attempts to diagnose *Aspergillus* infections serologically (antibody testing) have been unrewarding, but a recent technique for detection of *Aspergillus* antigens in sera or other body fluids is encouraging.

Necrotizing pulmonary aspergillosis is a distinct clinical entity that may overlap with invasive pulmonary aspergillosis. Patients generally have underlying chronic obstructive pulmonary disease or may be mildly immunocompromised and appear chronically ill with complaints of fever, weight loss, a productive cough extending over a period of weeks to months, and signs of lower respiratory tract infection. Chest roentgenograms demonstrate infiltrative and cavitary disease typical of a chronic destructive lung process; cavity formation is often accompanied by the development of fungus balls. The diagnosis is suggested by the prolonged clinical course, the isolation of *Aspergillus* spp. from pulmonary secretions, negative cultures for other pathogens, and failure to respond to antibacterial or antimicrobial therapy. The diagnosis is confirmed by pathologic evidence of tissue invasion and response to antimycotic therapy. Surgical therapy is reserved for patients unable to tolerate chemotherapy or those who have residual lung disease.

Successful management of invasive pulmonary aspergillosis requires early diagnosis and treatment, remission of the underlying disease, and reversal, if possible, of immunosuppression. Amphotericin B is the drug of choice for invasive aspergillosis. The recommended duration of treatment is empiric, and usually at least 15–20 mg/kg are required. Data supporting the addition of other antifungal agents, tetracycline, or rifampin are based largely on in vitro studies or are anecdotal. Recent reports suggest that itraconazole may prove useful in the treatment as well as prevention of aspergillosis in immunosuppressed patients.

Sinusitis due to *Aspergillus* spp. most often involves the maxillary sinuses. Two overlapping clinical entities exist. The more common presentation is low-grade fever, purulent rhinorrhea, facial fullness, and localized or referred pain. Roentgenographic examination reveals opacification with or without a fungus ball lying free or attached to the mucosa of chronically infected sinuses. Curettage and drainage are the treatments of choice. A more invasive sinusitis, often accompanied by lower respiratory tract involvement, occurs in immunosuppressed patients. Symptoms include fever, headache, localized pain, and purulent rhinorrhea, which, when accompanied by invasion from the sinuses into the orbit or cranial vault, progress to swelling, proptosis, and paralysis of the extraocular muscles. Roentgenographic examination reveals opacification and bony destruction. Surgical drainage and parenteral administration of antimycotic therapy constitute the treatment of choice.

Ocular infection typically occurs in immunocompromised patients and produces three categories of disease: (1) mycotic keratitis, in which fungi from an external source infect the cornea following trauma or superficial disease; (2) fungal endophthalmitis in which intraocular infection is secondary to hematogenous dissemination (not an uncommon complication of intravenous drug use); and (3) extension oculomycosis, which results from the extension of fungal disease into the orbit from adjacent tissue. Treatment includes surgical drainage and systemic antifungal therapy.

Endocarditis of normal, damaged, or prosthetic heart valves may produce large, friable vegetations that obstruct the valve orifice or extend into the pulmonary or systemic arteries, resulting in metastatic foci of infection in the lungs, brain, kidney, and spleen. Treatment requires surgical removal of the infected valve and prolonged administration of amphotericin B.

WILLIAM T. SPECK
STEPHEN C. ARONOFF

Binder RE, Failing LJ, Pugath RD, et al: Chronic necrotizing pulmonary aspergillosis: A discrete clinical entity. Medicine 61:109, 1983.

Dennung DW, Tucker RM, Hanson LH, et al: Treatment of invasive aspergillosis with itraconazole. Am J Med 36:791, 1989.

Levitz SM: Aspergillosis. Infect Dis Clin North Am 3:1, 1988.

Patterson R, Greenberger PA, Radin RC, et al: Allergic bronchopulmonary aspergillosis: Staging as an aid to management. Ann Intern Med 96:286, 1982.

Rinaldi J: Invasive aspergillosis. Rev Infect Dis 5:1061, 1983.

Weiner MH, Talbot GH, Gerson SL, et al: Antigen detection in the diagnosis of invasive aspergillosis. Ann Intern Med 99:777, 1983.

12.109 COCCIDIOIDOMYCOSIS

(San Joaquin Fever, Valley Fever, Desert Rheumatism, Coccidioidal Granuloma)

ETIOLOGY. Coccidioidomycosis is an infection caused by the fungus *Coccidioides immitis* found in the soil of the New World. The minute arthroconidia of its mycelial saprophytic phase are inhaled or, rarely, enter through injured skin. In the infected host they round up into spherules, which develop endospores. Liberation of the latter leads to formation of new spherules, which spread within a host but not to a new host. Viable *C. immitis* does occur in pulmonary cavities, often in the mycelial as well as spherule form, but no cases of person-to-person infection have been discovered. Because they occur naturally, however, and on surface cultures, the arthroconidia of the saprophytic phase are highly infectious. Although isolation is unnecessary, precautions should be taken with dressings and casts over open lesions lest the mycelial arthroconidia develop in 4–5 days as they do on surface cultures. Within the arid endemic areas of California's San Joaquin Valley, in scattered regions in northern and southern California, in central and southern Arizona, and even in southwestern Texas, many long-time residents have been infected, along with cattle, sheep, dogs, and wild rodents. Recovery from infection confers permanent immunity except in those with an acquired (natural or iatrogenic) immunodeficiency. Where the population is stable, coccidioidomycosis is primarily a childhood infection.

CLINICAL MANIFESTATIONS. Human infection takes three forms: (1) a benign, self-limited, primary infection (60% of infected persons show no clinical manifestations); (2) residual pulmonary lesions; and (3) a rare, disseminating, sometimes fatal disease. The disease tends to be milder in children; however, in those requiring medical attention, dissemination to bones and meninges is fairly common and approaches the incidence of these complications in adults. Maternal-fetal or maternal-infant infection has been reported.

Primary Coccidioidomycosis. The incubation period varies from 1 to 4 wk, with an average of 10–16 days. Symptoms are influenzal in type; the onset may be insidious or abrupt with malaise, chills, and fever. Chest pain is frequent and may vary from a mere sense of constriction to excruciating pain. Night sweats and anorexia are common. On occasion, there is a persistent dry cough and there may be a painful throat. There also may be headache or backache.

A generalized, fine, macular erythema or urticarial eruption may appear within the 1st day or so. It may be evanescent and present only in the groin. Most frequently, erythema nodosum occurs with or without erythema multiforme. These lesions develop at the time sensitivity to coccidioidin is maximal, 3–21 days after onset of symptoms. Skin lesions may occur, however, in persons otherwise asymptomatic. Other allergic manifestations, arthritis, and phlyctenular conjunctivitis may occur concomitantly.

Chest examination rarely discloses positive findings, even though roentgenography reveals extensive consolidation. Infrequently dullness, a friction rub, or fine rales may be detected. Pleural effusions occur at times and may be massive enough to embarrass respiration; they may develop without preceding respiratory symptoms.

Residual Pulmonary Coccidioidomycosis. Infrequently, a cavity may develop in an area of pulmonary consolidation during the primary infection and then regress. More often, however, after a variably prolonged period a persistent cavity may form. There are often no symptoms, and the diagnosis is made roentgenographically. Occasionally there is mild to moderate hemoptysis, which may recur and be alarming. Rarely, fatal hemorrhage has occurred. Dissemination of the fungus from cavities to other areas is rare. Pulmonary residual "granulomas" sometimes persist. They are not harmful but do pose problems of differentiation from tuberculosis or neoplasms. Infrequently, a chronic progressive fibrocavitary pulmonary disease is seen.

Disseminated or Progressive Coccidioidomycosis (Coccidioidal Granuloma). Certain persons lack ability to localize coccidioidal infection. Dissemination, which is rare and occurs mainly in males, especially in Filipinos, other Asians, and blacks, usually follows the initial illness within 6 mo, often without any interlude. This is analogous to progressive primary tuberculosis. Certain immunosuppressed states enhance dissemination or bring about relapse of apparently arrested coccidioidomycosis. Dissemination is enhanced if coccidioidal infection is acquired during the later stages of pregnancy. Skin lesions and cold abscesses, both subcutaneous and osseous, occur. Meningitis is the most serious of the disseminated lesions, being clinically similar to tuberculous meningitis. In whites it is not unusual for meningitis to be the only extrapulmonary lesion. Miliary dissemination and peritonitis may be distinguishable from tuberculosis only by demonstrating the causative agent, though coccidioidal peritonitis may present as a very mild disease. The mortality rate of untreated meningitis is practically 100%, but it is variable with other forms of disseminated coccidioidomycosis.

DIAGNOSIS. Diagnosis of the disseminated infection may be established by biopsy or at autopsy. Sputum is generally so scanty in the primary infection that gastric lavage may be advisable, especially in children. If histologic examination demonstrates the characteristic double-contoured spherules with endospores and without budding, the diagnosis is certain. Demonstration of the fungus by culture and its confirmation by exoantigen test or by animal inoculation is also diagnostic. Only especially qualified laboratories should undertake such hazardous procedures.

The sedimentation rate is rapid in patients with both primary and disseminated infections and is helpful in evaluating clinical status. Eosinophilia is common and is proportionately higher with more severe infections. Serum alkaline phosphatase may be elevated in acute coccidioidomycosis even in the absence of obvious systemic dissemination.

Skin Test. Tests with coccidioidin or the newer spherulin are specific except for occasional cross-reactions with histoplasmosis and blastomycosis. A positive reaction does not distinguish between a recent and an old infection unless it has been preceded within a reasonably short time by a negative test result. However, *a negative skin test does not rule out coccidioidal infection*. Coccidioidin is administered intradermally as 0.1 mL of a 1:1,000, 1:100, or even 1:10 dilution. The reaction generally reaches its peak at 36 hr and should be read at 24 and 48 hr. An area of induration more than 5 mm in diameter is positive. Patients with suspected coccidioidal erythema nodosum are likely to be hypersensitive and should receive the 1:1,000 dilution. Patients with disseminated infections are much less sensitive; even a 1:10 dilution may not elicit a reaction. Dermal sensitivity to coccidioidin is less durable than to tuberculin. There is no danger of disseminating or activating a coccidioidal infection by a strong coccidioidin reaction, although there may be a systemic reaction as well as a local one. Coccidioidin does not evoke antibodies in the human; therefore, the skin test may precede serologic tests and will provide information useful in their interpretation. However, negative skin tests should not preclude serologic tests.

Blood and Cerebrospinal Fluid Tests. Serum precipitins (IgM) and complement-fixation (IgG) antibodies are detectable in early coccidioidomycosis and may persist with disseminated coccidioidomycosis. In general, the more severe the infection, the higher the complement-fixation titer. Antibodies are generally not demonstrable in asymptomatic acute infections. Rarely, serologic tests may be negative in active coccidioidomycosis, for example, in the patient immunosuppressed for renal transplantation or by AIDS. The cerebrospinal fluid findings are similar to those characteristic of tuberculous meningitis (Sec. 12.47). Fixation of complement by cerebrospinal fluid occurs in 95% of patients with coccidioidal meningitis and is usually diagnostic. Occasionally, epidural coccidioidal lesions may also lead to complement fixation by the cerebrospinal fluid. Complement-fixing antibody may be detected in cisternal and lumbar fluid but may be deceptively absent from the ventricular fluid. Antibodies detectable by complement fixation do not pass the blood-brain barrier (although immunodiffusion may reveal their presence) but are found in cord blood at the same titer as in the mother's blood. Passively transferred antibody disappears from the infant within 6 mo. Coccidioidal precipiten (IgM) has been detected in some neonates of mothers having coccidioidmycosis when there has been no manifestation of disease in the infants.

Roentgenography. During the primary infection roentgenograms of the chest may not reveal pulmonary changes. Hilar adenopathy is frequent, and there may be single or multiple, sharply circumscribed or soft, feathery, small pulmonary densities or larger consolidated areas. Pulmonary cavities, when present, tend to be thin-walled. Pleural effusions are of variable extent. The osseous lesions, usually multiple and with a predilection for cancellous bone, often are widespread and are generally indistinguishable from those of tuberculosis.

PREVENTION. Avoidance of exposure to the arthroconidia is the only means of preventing infection. An available vaccine is of unproved value in humans.

TREATMENT. The treatment of *primary coccidioidal infection* consists of restriction of activity and symptomatic measures until the erythrocyte sedimentation rate returns to normal, precipitins vanish, the complement-fixing titer of serum decreases, and roentgenographic improvement is noted. Pulmonary cavities frequently close spontaneously. When a cavity persists or is located peripherally or when there is recurrent bleeding or secondary infection, excision should be considered. Infrequently, bronchopleural fistulas or recurrent cavitation may occur as surgical complications; rarely, dissemination may result. When extensive thoracic surgery is required, therapy with amphotericin B may be desirable.

Antifungal chemotherapy is indicated for those at high risk of developing severe coccidioidomycosis, though there is no assurance that this will prevent dissemination. Amphotericin B, 0.5–1.0 mg/kg/24 hr given intravenously, is the mainstay of treatment of *disseminated coccidioidomycosis*. Once the full dose is achieved, it can be administered every other day or 2–3 times/wk in the face of reduced renal function owing to its toxicity. Thrombophlebitis is common. Anemia due to the drug can be effectively treated with transfusions and terminates when treatment is stopped. Agranulocytosis is rare, and hepatic insufficiency develops occasionally, mainly in those with pre-existing liver damage. The drug should not be used in primary infections except when dissemination seems imminent. Although the response is occasionally dramatic in the disseminated form of the disease, generally treatment must be continued for months and, if possible, until improvement is reflected by a significant reduction (4-fold) in complement-fixing antibodies. An increase in sensitivity to coccidioidin is evidence of a favorable immunologic response. Immunologic reconstitution with leukocyte transfer factor is of uncertain value.

Amphotericin B does not pass the blood-brain barrier in therapeutic amounts, but it may mask meningitis during intravenous treatment. Early treatment of coccidioidal meningitis is important, and intrathecal administration of the drug in doses of 0.5–1.5 mg 2–3 times/wk (gradually increased from a dose of 0.025 mg) and accompanied by a corticosteroid is usually necessary. Arachnoiditis and transverse myelitis are hazards of intraspinal administration.

Cold abscesses should be drained, infected synovial membranes removed, and, if osseous lesions are accessible, excision considered. In these cases, intravenous and local amphotericin B may be used depending on the extent of involvement.

Amphotericin B has been used to treat coccidioidomycosis during pregnancy without apparent adverse effect on the fetus.

Treatment of *coccidioidal meningitis* should begin with both intravenous and intrathecal or intraventricular administration of amphotericin B. Intrathecal administration into the cisterna magna is preferred. However, administering amphotericin in 10% glucose solution via the lumbar route with the patient's head tilted down at −30 degrees from the horizontal may reduce the incidence of serious arachnoiditis. Intravenous therapy may be discontinued when the physician feels confident that meningitis is the only extrapulmonary involvement, when the patient appears clinically well, and when laboratory findings support the clinical impression of improvement. Treatment should continue for at least 3 mo after the cerebrospinal fluid has normal cells, glucose, and protein and is negative on complement-fixation testing. Follow-up should include examination of the cerebrospinal fluid at intervals of 1–3 mo (and immediately if there is headache or any change in behavior or personality) for a period of at least 2 yr. Clinical surveillance should be continued for some years longer, as relapses have been noted as late as 3–5 yr after return of the CSF to normal.

Ketoconazole or **fluconazole** administered orally (in daily doses of approximately 3–15 mg/kg or 2–7 mg/kg, respectively) is useful in treating disseminated nonmeningeal coccidioidomycosis that is not extensive nor progressing rapidly. Ketoconazole does not prevent dissemination from the primary pulmonary disease. Cutaneous and subcutaneous lesions are most responsive to this drug, synovial lesions next, and osseous lesions least. Fluconazole (also available in intravenous preparation) has produced favorable results with these manifestations of coccidioidomycosis. Chronic pulmonary coccidioidal disease, cavitary or fibrocavitary, has not been consistently improved by azoles (or by amphotericin B). Oral ketoconazole has been used along with intrathecal amphotericin B or intraventricular miconazole for treating coccidioidal meningitis; although very high doses may penetrate the CSF, ketoconazole cannot be recommended in place of intrathecal amphotericin B or miconazole. Fluconazole readily penetrates into the CSF and has been effective in meningitis. Ketoconazole has been administered to children less than 2 yr of age, but the significance in children of the hepatic dysfunction and the inhibition of testosterone and adrenocorticoid synthesis noted in adults has not been adequately evaluated. Fluconazole, primarily excreted by the kidneys unchanged, does not significantly affect testosterone or adrenocorticoid synthesis. Relapses have occurred in some patients after favorable clinical responses following therapy for more than a year. Fluconazole and itraconazole (not released 2/91) appear to have efficacy equal to or greater than that of ketoconazole but with fewer side effects.

The sole indication for the use of parenteral miconazole is intrathecal or intraventricular administration for suppression of coccidioidal meningitis.

DEMOSTHENES PAPPAGIANIS

Ampel NM, Wieden MA, Galgiani JN: Coccidioidomycosis: a clinical update. Rev Infect Dis 11:897, 1989.

Drutz DJ: Amphotericin B in the treatment of coccidioidomycosis. Drugs 26:337, 1983.

Fluconazole is a novel advance in therapy for systemic fungal infections. Rev Inf Dis 12:Suppl 3, 1990. (several pertinent articles)

Galgiani JN: Ketoconazole in the treatment of coccidioidomycosis. Drugs 26:355, 1983.

Harrison HR, Galgiani JN, Reynolds AF Jr, et al: Amphotericin B and imidazole therapy for coccidioidal meningitis in children. Pediatr Infect Dis 2:216, 1983.

Kafka JA, Catanzaro A: Disseminated coccidioidomycosis in children. J Pediatr 98:355, 1981.

Labadie EL, Hamilton RH: Survival improvement in coccidioidal meningitis by high-dose intrathecal amphotericin B. Arch Intern Med 146:2013, 1986.

Pappagianis D: Coccidioidomycosis. *In*: Balows A, et al (eds): Laboratory Diagnosis of Infectious Diseases. New York, Springer-Verlag, 1988.

Richardson HB, Anderson JA, McKay BM: Acute pulmonary coccidioidomycosis in children. J Pediatr 70:376, 1967.

Shafai T: Neonatal coccidioidomycosis in premature twins. Am J Dis Child 132:634, 1978.

Stevens DA: Coccidioidomycosis and the indications for chemotherapy. Drugs 26:334, 1983.

Tucker RM, Williams PL, Arathoon EG, et al: Treatment of mycoses with itraconazole. Ann NY Acad Sci 544:451, 1988.

12.110 PARASITIC INFECTIONS

Infectious diseases due to protozoa and helminths are a major cause of morbidity and mortality in infants and children in many parts of the world. The major parasitic infections and their estimated prevalence, mortality, and morbidity are presented in Table 12–42. The term "parasites" has been used historically and conventionally to refer only to those infectious organisms that belong to the animal kingdom, that is, *protozoa, helminths,* and *arthropods*. Protozoa are unicellular organisms that are able to multiply within their hosts. In contrast, worms or helminths are multicellular and usually do not divide within the human host. These basic biologic differences between protozoa and helminths have important epidemiologic, clinical, and therapeutic implications.

The host-parasite relationship in protozoan and helminthic infections has several unique features. Infection and disease due to these agents must be clearly distinguished. When a parasite invades a host, it may die at once or survive without causing harm to the host (infection). Alternatively, it may survive and produce morbidity (disease) and possibly kill the host. In addition, these organisms have evolved evasive mechanisms against host immune or protective responses. In respect to the host's well-being, parasites may cause disease by their physical presence or by competition with the host for specific nutrients. Disease may also result from the host's attempts to destroy the invaders, for example, the host's immunopathologic reaction.

Warren KS, Mahmoud AAF: Tropical and Geographical Medicine. 2nd ed. New York, McGraw-Hill, 1990.

PROTOZOA

INTESTINAL PROTOZOA

Protozoan infections of the intestine cause a wide variety of clinical syndromes, ranging from asymptomatic carrier states to severe disease associated with pathologic lesions in the gastrointestinal tract or other organs (Table 12–43). Infections by the intestinal protozoa are usually acquired orally through fecal contamination of water or food, and they are more endemic in countries with unsanitary water conditions. *G. lamblia* and *Cryptosporidium,* however, have recently been recognized as a major cause of epidemics of water-borne diarrhea in North America, and particularly in day-care centers. *Cryptosporidium* infection and to a lesser extent isosporiasis have become major causes of diarrhea in patients with the acquired immunodeficiency syndrome (Sec. 12.83, 12.113, and 13.53).

TABLE 12–42. Estimated Worldwide Prevalence (In Thousands) of the Major Parasitic Infections in Relation to Associated Morbidity and Mortality

Infection	Prevalence	Morbidity	Mortality
Protozoa			
Amebiasis	500,000	40,000	70
Giardiasis	250,000	500	10
Malaria	2,600,000	150,000	1,500
Trypanosomiasis, African	1,000	10	1
Trypanosomiasis, American	24,000	1,200	60
Toxoplasmosis	800,000	10	0.1
Leishmaniasis	1,000	1,000	1
Helminths			
Ascariasis	700,000	700	10
Hookworms	800,000	1,500	50–60
Filariasis	90,000	1,000	1
Schistosomiasis	300,000	150,000	1,200

12.111 AMEBIASIS

Human infection with *Entamoeba histolytica* is prevalent worldwide; endemic foci are particularly common in areas with low socioeconomic and sanitary standards. *E. histolytica* parasitizes the lumen of the gastrointestinal tract and causes few or no disease sequelae in most infected subjects. In a small proportion of individuals the organisms invade the intestinal mucosa or may disseminate to other organs, especially the liver.

ETIOLOGY. Infection is established by ingestion of parasite cysts. These cysts measure 10–18 μm, contain 4 nuclei, and are resistant to environmental conditions such as low temperature and the concentrations of chlorine commonly used in water purification; the parasite can be killed by heating to 55° C. Upon ingestion, the cyst, which is resistant to gastric acidity and digestive enzymes, excysts in the small intestine to form 8 trophozoites. These are large, actively motile organisms that colonize the lumen of the large intestine and may invade its mucosal lining under conditions that are currently unknown. Trophozoites have an average diameter of 20 μm; their cytoplasm consists of an outer clear zone and an inner densely granular endoplasm containing a spherical nucleus, which has a small central karyosome and fine granular chromatin material. The endoplasm also contains vacuoles where, in cases of invasive amebiasis, erythrocytes may be seen. Two other species of nonpathogenic *Amoeba* may infect the human gastrointestinal tract: *E. coli* and *E. hartmanni.*

EPIDEMIOLOGY. The prevalence of amebic infections worldwide varies from 5 to 81%. It is estimated that 10% of the population worldwide is infected with *E. histolytica.* This infection is associated with 50 million cases of symptomatic disease and 70–100 thousand deaths/yr; amebiasis is the third leading parasitic cause of death on a global scale. Amebic dysentery due to invasion of the intestinal mucosa occurs in approximately 1–17% of infected subjects. Dissemination of the parasites to internal organs such as the liver occurs in an even smaller fraction of infected individuals and is less common in children than in adults.

Although highly endemic in Africa, Latin America, India,

TABLE 12–43. Important Intestinal Protozoan Infections of Children

Infection	Etiology	Transmission	Major Clinical Features	Diagnosis
Amebiasis	*Entamoeba histolytica*	Fecal-oral Water-, food-borne	Diarrhea-dysentery Liver abscess	Trophozoites or cysts in stools Serology
Giardiasis	*Giardia lamblia*	Fecal-oral Person-to-person Water-, food-borne	Diarrhea Malabsorption	Cysts in stools Cysts or trophozoites in duodenal aspirate
Cryptosporidiosis	*Cryptosporidium*	Fecal-oral Person-to-person Water-, food-borne Zoonosis	Watery diarrhea Severe diarrhea with malabsorption in AIDS patients	Oocysts in stools (acid-fast staining), small bowel biopsy
Balantidiasis	*Balantidium coli*	Fecal-oral Water-borne Zoonosis	Bloody diarrhea	Trophozoites or cysts in stools
Blastocystis	*Blastocystis hominis*	Fecal-oral Water-borne	Diarrhea Eosinophilia	Organisms in stools
Isosporiasis	*Isospora* sp.	Fecal-oral Zoonosis	Diarrhea in AIDS patients	Oocysts in stools Small bowel biopsy

and Southeast Asia, amebiasis is not exclusively limited to the tropics. In the United States, amebiasis has been estimated to occur with a prevalence of 1–4% in certain high-risk groups including chronically institutionalized persons (including mentally retarded children), promiscuous homosexual males, immigrants (especially Mexican Americans) from and travelers to endemic areas, and lower socioeconomic groups in the southern United States. The majority of children infected with *E. histolytica* fall into these risk groups.

Man is the natural host and reservoir of *E. histolytica*. The pattern of infection varies in different parts of the world. For example, infection acquired in India, Mexico, or Durban, South Africa, is apparently more virulent than that from other locations. The definition of virulence, geographic strains, and pathogenicity of different amebae, however, remains to be defined.

Infection is transmitted via contaminated food and water. Food handlers carrying amebic cysts may, therefore, play a role in spreading the infection. Direct contact with infected feces also may be responsible for person-to-person transmission.

PATHOGENESIS AND PATHOLOGY. Once *E. histolytica* trophozoites invade the intestinal mucosa, they produce tissue destruction (ulcers) with little local inflammatory response because of the cytolytic capacity of the organism. The organisms multiply and spread laterally underneath the intestinal epithelium to produce the characteristic flask-shaped ulcers. These lesions are commonly seen in the cecum, transverse, and sigmoid colon. Amebae may produce similar lytic lesions if they reach the liver (these are commonly called abscesses although they contain no granulocytes). *E. histolytica* occasionally disseminates to other extraintestinal sites such as the lungs and brain. The contrasts among the extent of tissue destruction by amebae, the absence of a local host inflammatory response, and the demonstration of systemic humoral (antibody) and cell-mediated reactions against the organisms remain a major scientific puzzle.

CLINICAL MANIFESTATIONS. Most infected individuals are asymptomatic, and cysts are found in their feces. Tissue invasion occurs in 2–8% of infected individuals and may be related to the strain of parasites or the nutritional status and intestinal flora of the host. The most common clinical manifestations of amebiasis are due to local invasion of the intestinal epithelium and dissemination to the liver.

Intestinal amebiasis may occur within 2 wk of infection or be delayed for months. The onset is usually gradual with colicky abdominal pains and frequent bowel movements (6–8 movements/24 hr). Diarrhea is frequently associated with tenesmus. Stools are blood-stained and contain a fair amount of mucus with few leukocytes. Generalized constitutional symptoms and signs are characteristically absent with fever documented in only one third of patients. Acute amebic dysentery occurs in attacks lasting a few days to several weeks; recurrence is very common in untreated individuals. Amebic colitis affects all age groups, but its incidence is strikingly high in children between the ages of 1 and 5 yr. Severe amebic colitis in infants and younger children occurs in tropical and semitropical countries. When young children become infected, they tend to have rapidly progressive illness with frequent extraintestinal involvement and high mortality rates. In contrast to this experience in endemic areas, extraintestinal amebiasis during infancy is rarely seen in the United States.

Occasionally, amebic dysentery is associated with sudden onset of fever, chills, and severe diarrhea, which may result in dehydration and electrolyte disturbances. In a few patients complications such as ameboma, toxic megacolon, extraintestinal extension, or local perforation and peritonitis may occur. The characteristic flask-shaped ulcers with healthy intervening mucosa that occur in most cases may be detected by sigmoidoscopy in 25% of patients.

Hepatic amebiasis is a very serious manifestation of disseminated infection. Although diffuse liver enlargement has been associated with intestinal amebiasis, liver abscess occurs in fewer than 1% of infected individuals and may appear in patients with no clear history of intestinal disease. In children fever is the hallmark of amebic liver abscess. It is frequently associated with abdominal pain, distention, and an enlarged, tender liver. Changes at the base of the right lung, such as elevation of the diaphragm and parenchymal compression, may also occur. Laboratory examination shows a slight leukocytosis, moderate anemia, and nonspecific elevations of liver enzymes. Stool examination for amebae is negative in more than 50% of patients with documented amebic liver abscess. In most cases, CT imaging, or isotope scans can localize and delineate the size of the abscess cavity. Most patients have a single cavity in the right hepatic lobe, although recent studies employing CT have shown an increased rate of multiple abscesses and left lobe involvement. Amebic liver abscess may be associated with rupture into the peritoneum or thorax or through the skin when diagnosis and therapy are delayed.

DIAGNOSIS. Diagnosis is based on detecting the organisms in stool samples or, rarely, in aspirates of a liver abscess. At least 3 stool samples should be examined by an experienced person. Whenever amebiasis is suspected, an additional stool sample should be preserved in polyvinyl alcohol for further identification and staining of the organisms. Material for microscopic examination may also be obtained by scraping the ulcerated areas of rectal mucosa. Endoscopy and biopsies of suspicious areas should be performed when stool samples are negative and the index of suspicion for amebic colitis remains high. The indirect hemagglutination test may be helpful in the diagnosis of invasive intestinal amebiasis and amebic liver abscess; diagnostic titers of at least 1:128 are reported in 98–100% of cases. Serologic tests may be initially negative in patients presenting with very acute disease.

TREATMENT. All individuals with *E. histolytica* trophozoites or cysts in their stools, whether symptomatic or not, should be treated. Diloxanide furoate, a luminal amebicide, is the drug of choice for asymptomatic cyst passers. The recommended dose is 10 mg/kg/24 hr orally for 10 days. Toxicity is rare, but the drug should not be used in children under 2 yr of age.

Invasive amebiasis of the intestine, liver, or other organs requires the use of metronidazole, a tissue amebicidal drug; it is administered orally in a daily dose of 50 mg/kg for 10 days. Side effects of this drug include nausea, diarrhea, metallic taste in the mouth, and leukopenia; these are uncommon and disappear on completion of therapy. Metronidazole is also a luminal amebicide but less effective than diloxanide furoate for this purpose. Patients with invasive amebiasis should therefore receive an additional course of the latter drug following metronidazole therapy. If the case is severe or if metronidazole cannot be used, dehydroemetine is the recommended alternative therapeutic agent. It is administered by the subcutaneous or intramuscular route (never intravenously) in a dose of 1 mg/kg/24 hr for 10 days. Patients should be hospitalized when this drug is given because cardiac or renal complications may occur. If tachycardia, T wave depression, arrhythmias, or proteinuria develops, the drug should be stopped. A course of diloxanide furoate is also recommended following completion of dehydroemetine therapy. Amebic liver abscesses are treated with specific therapy as outlined above; however, aspiration of large lesions or left lobe abscesses may be necessary if rupture is imminent or if the patient shows poor clinical response 4–6 days after administration of amebicidal drugs. Stool examination should be repeated 2 wk following completion of antiamebic therapy as a test of cure.

Control of amebiasis can be achieved by exercising proper sanitary measures. Regular examination of food handlers and thorough investigation of diarrhea episodes may identify the source of infection in some communities. There is no prophylactic drug for amebiasis.

12.112 GIARDIASIS

Giardia lamblia, a ubiquitous, flagellated protozoan, is a common worldwide cause of infectious diarrhea. The infection is more prevalent in children than in adults and is an important cause of morbidity in the developing world as well as in urban day-care centers and residential institutions for the mentally retarded. Giardiasis is particularly significant in people with malnutrition or immunodeficiencies.

ETIOLOGY. *Giardia lamblia* infects man through ingestion of as few as 10 cysts. The mature cyst, measuring approximately 8–10 μm, is thick walled and oval and contains 4 nuclei. They are passed in the stools of infected individuals and may remain viable in water for longer than 3 mo. Their viability is not affected by the normal concentrations of chlorine used to purify water for drinking. Upon reaching the upper small intestine, each *Giardia* cyst liberates 4 trophozoites. Trophozoites colonize the lumen of the duodenum and proximal jejunum, where they attach to the brush border of the intestinal epithelial cells and multiply by binary fusion. The body of the trophozoite is piriform, measuring 2–4 by 14 μm, and is divided longitudinally by 2 median rods and contains 2 oval nuclei anteriorly, a large sucking disk on the ventral surface, and a curved median body posteriorly. Each organism has four pairs of flagella.

EPIDEMIOLOGY. The prevalence in several parts of the world varies from 0.5–50%. Man was thought to be the only reservoir of *G. lamblia*, but it is now believed that the human parasite infects beavers and dogs as well. Person-to-person, water-borne, food-borne, and interspecies transmission may occur, possibly resulting in sporadic cases as well as in epidemics. Day-care centers probably play an important role in the transmission of urban giardiasis, with secondary attack rates in families as high as 17–30%. Giardiasis has long been recognized as an important cause of chronic diarrhea in children with agammaglobulinemia or selective IgA deficiency, suggesting the importance of immunity in controlling giardiasis. The observation that adults living in endemic areas have less symptomatic illness than infants or adult visitors provides evidence of acquired immunity to giardiasis. Human milk containing secretary IgA antibodies may provide protection to nursing infants.

CLINICAL MANIFESTATIONS. Giardiasis is more frequently symptomatic in children than in adults. Symptoms occur in 40–80% of infected children after an average incubation period of 8 days. The most common presentation is diarrhea, weight loss, crampy abdominal pain, and failure to thrive. The onset of symptoms may be abrupt or gradual; the disease may be self-limited or capable of producing severe protracted diarrhea and malabsorption. Alterations in the digestive function of the brush border are common in those with protracted symptoms. Malabsorption of sugars (such as xylose and disaccharides), fats, and fat-soluble vitamins occurs in more than half of patients who have nonspecific morphologic abnormalities of the small intestinal mucosa similar to those seen in other malabsorptive disorders.

DIAGNOSIS. *G. lamblia* trophozoites or cysts may be found in fecal samples obtained from infected children. Because cyst excretion is irregular, examination of several fecal samples may be needed but only 50% of infected individuals are identified. Evaluation by duodenal sampling or biopsy may be necessary for diagnosis. The Entero-test is an efficient, simple, and safe method for detecting *G. lamblia* in duodenal fluid of children.

TREATMENT. Furazolidone (8 mg/kg/24 hr for 10 days) is available in pediatric suspension, is well tolerated, and is considered the drug of choice for children. Tinidazole has also been evaluated for treatment of infected children; a single oral dose of 50 mg/kg resulted in an 80% cure rate. Quinicrine (6 mg/kg/24 hr for 7 days) is highly effective but is less well studied and less well tolerated by young children.

The recent increase of epidemics of giardiasis requires reexamination of sanitary practices. Water supply is the most important factor; its quality should be routinely monitored. The concentration of chlorine required for control, particularly in communities that are dependent on surface water but have no sand filtration, needs to be determined. Spread of infection in institutions may be prevented by identifying and properly treating asymptomatic carriers. No prophylactic medication prevents giardiasis.

12.113 CRYPTOSPORIDIOSIS

Cryptosporidium, a coccidian intestinal protozoan initially described as a cause of significant diarrhea in calves and other farm animals, has been recognized as an important human pathogen causing self-limited watery diarrhea in immunocompetent individuals as well as protracted and severe diarrhea in immunosuppressed patients, particularly those with AIDS (Sec. 12.83 and 13.53) or congenital immunodeficiencies. Infection is established by ingesting oocysts found in the feces of infected animals or humans. Excystation occurs in the gastrointestinal tract, and all subsequent development takes place at the surface of the intestinal epithelium. Recent stool surveys indicate that the prevalence of infection ranges from 4 to 7%. In day-care center epidemics of diarrheal illness in the United States, up to 65% of children had cryptosporidium; additionally, 10–15% of stools examined from asymptomatic children in these centers were found to have this parasite. Around the world, the prevalence of cryptosporidiosis has been 0.6–20% in developed countries and 4–32% in developing countries. Children are most susceptible to infection with *Cryptosporidium*, which is most prevalent in children less than 2 yr of age. It is quite possible that cryptosporidiosis contributes significantly to malnutrition and may slow physical and mental development in children in Third World areas.

The natural history of infection in immunocompetent patients suggests an incubation period of 2–7 days. Infection is characterized by the acute onset of watery diarrhea, nausea, and abdominal cramps. Infection is self-limited, lasting 10–14 days. In some, infection may be totally asymptomatic. In contrast, infection in immunosuppressed patients is associated with the development of profuse (1–25 L/day), watery diarrhea, resulting in weight loss (often more than 10% of total body weight) and malnutrition; diarrhea may also become chronic with unrelenting severity.

Although *Cryptosporidium* is usually found in the jejunum of infected individuals, it has also been found in the colon and biliary tract of patients with AIDS. Involvement of the biliary tree has recently been associated with cholecystitis, papillary stenosis, and pancreatitis in these patients.

Diagnosis is difficult and is based upon identification of oocysts in stool. Special stool concentration and staining methods (such as acid-fast staining) are required in the hands of experienced laboratory personnel. Parasites can also be identified on stained mucosal biopsy specimens, appearing as round eosinophilic bodies on the microvillous border.

Since the diarrheal illness due to cryptosporidiasis is self-limited in immunocompetent patients, no specific therapy is required. In some young infants supportive therapy with fluid and electrolytes may be necessary. Patients with immunodeficiencies have been treated with a wide variety of chemotherapeutic agents, but none has showed consistent antiparasitic effect. Patients with reversible immunodeficiencies can recover if immunosuppression is eliminated.

OTHER INTESTINAL PROTOZOA

Infection of children with *Balantidium coli* and other coccidia such as *Isospora* and *Sarcocystis* may be associated with vague gastrointestinal complaints such as abdominal pain, distention, and diarrhea. *B. coli* may, however, invade the intestinal mucosa, causing bloody diarrhea and ulcerations. *Isospora* has also been recognized as an increasing problem in HIV-infected individuals. Diagnosis of either infection is made by fecal examination. Therapy with metronidazole is recommended for symptomatic cases of balantidiasis.

ROBERT A. SALATA
JOHN N. AUCOTT

AMEBIASIS

Adams EB, MacLeod IN: Invasive amebiasis. I. Amebic dysentery and its complications. Medicine 56:315, 1977.

Adams EB, MacLeod IN: Invasive amebiasis. II. Amebic liver abscess and its complications. Medicine 56:325, 1977.

Dykes AC, Ruebush TK, Gorelkin L, et al: Extraintestinal amebiasis in infancy: Report of three patients and epidemiological investigations of their families. Pediatrics 4:799, 1980.

Harrison RH, Crowe PC, Fulginiti VA: Amebic liver abscess in children: Clinical and epidemiologic features. Pediatrics 64:923, 1979.

Katzenstein D, Rickerson V, Braude A: New concepts of amebic liver abscess derived from hepatic imaging, serodiagnosis, and hepatic enzymes in 67 consecutive cases from San Diego. Medicine 61:325, 1977.

Merritt RJ, Coughlin E, Thomas DW, et al: Spectrum of amebiasis in children. Am J Dis Child 136:785, 1982.

GIARDIASIS

Craft JC, Murphy T, Nelson JD: Furazolidone and quinaquine: Comparative study of therapy for giardiasis in children. Am J Dis Child 135:164, 1981.

Dupont HL, Sullivan PS: Giardiasis: The clinical spectrum, diagnosis and therapy. Pediatric Infect Dis 5:S131, 1986.

Pickening LK, Engelkirk PG: *Giardia lambia.* Pediatr Clin North Am 35:565, 1988.

Pickering LK, Woodward WE, Dupont HL, et al: Occurrence of *Giardia lambia* in children in day care centers. J Pediatr 104:522, 1984.

Rosenthal P, Liebman WM: Comparative study of stool examinations, duodenal aspiration, and pediatric Entero-test for giardiasis in children. J Pediatr 96:278, 1980.

CRYPTOSPORIDIOSIS

Alpert G, Bell LM, Kirkpatrick CE, et al: Cryptosporidiosis in day care center. N Engl J Med 311:860, 1984.

Navin TR, Juranek DD: Cryptosporidiosis: Clinical, epidemiologic, and parasitologic review. Rev Infect Dis 6:313, 1984.

Soave R, Armstron D: *Cryptosporidium* and cryptosporidiosis. Rev Infect Dis 8:1012, 1986.

SYSTEMIC PROTOZOAN INFECTIONS

12.114 MALARIA

Malaria results when erythrocytes are invaded by any of four species of protozoan parasites of the genus *Plasmodium.* It is characterized by high fever, which is often intermittent, and by anemia and splenic enlargement. Despite worldwide campaigns aimed at eradicating malaria through interruption of the life cycle of the parasite in the mosquito, the disease continues to be the principal health problem of warm climates. Frequently, malaria is imported to the temperate zone countries where, in the summer months, it may be spread by local mosquitoes.

For clinical and diagnostic purposes, malaria may be regarded as two disease entities: the more dangerous one, caused by *Plasmodium falciparum* and formerly termed "subtertian" or "malignant tertian malaria," can produce a variety of acute clinical manifestations and may, if untreated, be fatal within a few days of onset; the other, caused by *P. vivax* (benign tertian malaria), *P. ovale* (a rarity resembling *P. vivax*), or *P. malariae* (quartan malaria), is more typically paroxysmal and almost never fatal. Vivax and ovale infections may recur weeks after apparent cure of a primary attack, in contrast to the other two, which, except in the case of drug-resistant falciparum strains, rarely recrudesce after standard treatment.

ETIOLOGY. Malaria is usually acquired from the bites of previously infected female anopheline mosquitoes. In other instances, malaria has developed following transplacental passage or after the transfusion of infected blood, both of which circumvent the pre-erythrocytic phase of the parasite's development in the liver. The usual evolution of the disease is as follows:

Pre-Erythrocytic Phase. The *sporozoites* injected into the bloodstream by the biting mosquito reach the sinusoids of the liver and enter the cytoplasm of hepatic cells. Growth and nuclear division are rapid, and microscopic cysts *(schizonts)* containing *merozoites* are formed. Most of the cysts of all species rupture at the end of 6–15 days of development, liberating thousands of merozoites to penetrate red blood cells. However, a few *P. vivax* and *P. ovale* forms remain dormant in the liver for weeks or months, paving the way for relapses.

The incubation period (between the infecting mosquito bite and the presence of parasites in the blood) varies with the species; with *P. falciparum* it is 10–13 days; with *P. vivax* and *P. ovale,* 12–16 days; and with *P. malariae,* 27–37 days, depending on the size of the inoculum. Malaria transmitted by the transfusion of infected blood becomes apparent in a shorter time. Clinical manifestations of infection induced by any means may be suppressed for many months by subcurative treatment, particularly in the cases of vivax and quartan malaria.

Erythrocytic Phase. The merozoites that invade red blood cells appear first in stained smears as bluish rings or *(P. malariae)* bands of cytoplasm, with one or occasionally two red dots of nuclear chromatin. The growing parasites are named *trophozoites,* and appearing with them in the red cells are granules of yellow-brown pigment consisting of hematin derived from the hemoglobin consumed by the parasite to meet its protein requirements. The shape of the organism varies during growth until it becomes round and, with the scattered or clumped pigment, almost fills the red blood cell, which, in the case of *P. vivax,* is enlarged and stippled.

The nucleus of the parasite now divides asexually several times; its cytoplasm is arranged around the new nuclei, and the pigment aggregates into large clumps. This segmenter, or mature *schizont,* contains a varying number of merozoites, depending on the species. The erythrocytes containing these merozoites rupture, and naked merozoites, pigment, and erythrocytic debris are freed into the plasma. Those merozoites that escape inactivation by immunoglobulins or phagocytosis enter fresh red blood cells. Thus, an asexual cycle is begun each time a new crop of merozoites invades red cells. This cycle, the duration of which is of considerable clinical importance, lasts 48 hr in falciparum, vivax, and ovale malaria and 72 hr in quartan malaria. The malarial clinical paroxysm takes place only when enough cycles have occurred to produce the amount of parasitic material, pigment, and red cell debris required to induce febrile or other reactions.

Certain of the growing parasites fail to divide, the nucleus remaining intact during the period of maturation. They are differentiated into male or female forms called *gametocytes,* which are of no clinical importance but are capable of infecting mosquitoes feeding on the patient.

Mixed Infections and Broods. In mixed infections one species is usually responsible for the clinical pattern, with falciparum dominating vivax, and vivax dominating quartan; only when sufficient immunity is developed to the dominant strain does the other begin to produce clinical manifestations.

In an infection with a single species, distinct broods may develop. Since the merozoites in the liver are not released simultaneously and the erythrocytic schizonts do not all rupture at the same time, some groups of parasites begin their existence in red blood cells before or after the majority, often maturing in sufficient numbers to produce an independent clinical reaction. In vivax infections single broods will produce a febrile reaction every other day, whereas if two broods develop, there will be daily paroxysms; in falciparum malaria the classic picture of intermittent fever may likewise soon become disrupted.

EPIDEMIOLOGY. Only in regions where the people have gametocytes in their blood can anopheline mosquitoes become infected. Children may be especially important in this respect. Transmission of malaria occurs in most tropical and some temperate zones; although the United States, Canada, Europe, Australia, and Israel are at present free of indigenous malaria, focal outbreaks may occur through infection of local mosquitoes by travelers coming from endemic areas.

Congenital malaria, caused by transfer of the causative agent across the placental barrier, is rare. *Neonatal malaria,* on the other hand, is less uncommon and may result from mingling of infected maternal blood with that of the infant during the birth process.

PATHOLOGY AND PATHOPHYSIOLOGY. The extent of destruction of red blood cells depends upon the duration and severity of the infection. Hemolysis often leads to an increase in the serum bilirubin, and in falciparum malaria it may be sufficiently intense to result in hemoglobinuria (**blackwater fever**). In any malarial infection the degree of anemia is greater than that attributable solely to the destruction of cells by parasites. Autoantigenic changes produced in the red cell by the parasite probably contribute to hemolysis; these changes and increased osmotic fragility occur in all erythrocytes, whether infected or not. Hemolysis may also be induced by quinine or primaquine in persons with hereditary glucose-6-phosphate dehydrogenase deficiency.

The pigment extruded into the circulation upon red cell disintegration accumulates in the reticuloendothelial cells of the spleen, the follicles of which become hyperplastic and sometimes necrotic, in the Kupffer cells of the liver, and in the bone marrow, brain, and other organs. Deposition of sufficient pigment and of hemosiderin results in a slate-gray color of the organs.

The malignancy of falciparum malaria is peculiar to that species. The merozoites emerging from the liver are considerably more numerous than those of other species; there are as many in young children as in adults, so that children have a proportionately greater initial wave of infection. Young children are particularly prone to severe, often lethal, parasitemia.

Eight to 18 hr after the parasite has entered the red blood cells, these cells become increasingly sticky and tend to adhere to the endothelial lining of blood sinuses and vessels, especially when the circulation is slow. The sticky cell is thus fixed and unable to return to the general circulation, although the parasite within it matures in the normal manner. As more cells adhere, flow within the vessel is progressively impeded, and occlusion or even rupture may occur.

The site and extent of this interference with vascular function, coupled with a selective localization of parasitized cells in various organs or systems, are responsible for the variety of symptoms from falciparum infections. Thus, pneumonitis, encephalitis, or enteritis may be manifest when the bulk of the infection is in the lungs, brain, or intestinal tract, respectively. In the pregnant woman damage to the placenta may result in death of the fetus or in premature birth; infants born at full term to infected women have lower birth weights than those of infants born to uninfected mothers living under similar conditions.

The release of merozoites where the circulation is slowed facilitates the invasion of nearby red blood cells, so that falciparum parasitemia may be heavier than that of other species whose rupture of schizonts takes place in the active circulation. Whereas *P. falciparum* invades all erythrocytes irrespective of age, *P. vivax* attacks primarily reticulocytes, and *P. malariae* invades mature red cells, features which tend to limit parasitemia of the latter two forms to less than 20,000 red cells/mm^3. Falciparum infections in the nonimmune child may develop densities as high as 500,000 parasites/mm^3.

Successful treatment stops the proliferation of parasites. Specific antibodies are associated with increased levels of immunoglobulin G in the serum of people repeatedly infected with a particular species. Antibody facilitates the phagocytosis of naked merozoites and of parasite-laden erythrocytes, which are ingested by reticuloendothelial cells, by large lymphocytes and neutrophils, and particularly by monocytes. These antibodies do not, however, interfere with development of the parasite in the liver. Passive immunity, occurring in infants born to mothers who have the disease, limits the severity of attacks of malaria for several weeks after birth. The beneficial effect of this transplacental humoral immunity may be enhanced by persistence of fetal hemoglobin and by a diet limited to milk. Certain hemoglobinopathies are also protective and tend to be genetically selective in endemic malarious regions. *Plasmodium falciparum* may fail to mature in children with the sickle cell trait, and *P. vivax* in those with thalassemia and enzyme deficiencies; *P. falciparum* is unable to attain high densities in children deficient in glucose-6-phosphate dehydrogenase.

CLINICAL MANIFESTATIONS. Children who acquire malaria fall into two groups: those having little or no immunity because of lack of previous contact with the disease, who become seriously ill unless treated; and those having a high degree of tolerance by about 10 yr of age owing to repeated malarial infections in early childhood that they have survived, although there may be impaired growth and development. Tolerance to malaria also appears to be based on inherited factors that modify the severity of the disease; such tolerance is to be found mostly among Africans and persons of African descent. In the partially immune child heavy parasitemia may occur with few symptoms, or an intercurrent infection may initiate renewed activity of a quiescent malarial infection.

In a nonimmune child clinical signs usually appear 8–15 days after infection and may not be distinctive. Behavioral changes such as fretfulness, anorexia, unusual crying, drowsiness, or disturbances of sleep may be observed. Fever may be absent or increase gradually for 1–2 days, or the onset may be sudden with temperature up to 40.6° C (105° F) or higher, with or without prodromal chill. After varying periods of time, the temperature falls to normal or below, and sweating occurs.

The febrile paroxysm may be extremely short or may last for 2–12 hr; its characteristic pattern is usually obscured in children less than 5 yr of age. Complaints include headache, nausea, generalized aching, particularly of the back, and occasionally pain in the abdomen, when the spleen has swollen quickly and is tender. In vivax and quartan infections dominated by a single brood the fever is the characteristic manifestation, occurring at intervals of 48 hr in the former and 72 in the latter. If convulsions occur, they abate when the fever falls. Herpetic lesions of the mouth are not uncommon. The red blood cell count and hemoglobin level may decrease rapidly; leukopenia is variable, but monocytosis is common.

In falciparum infections the fever is less characteristic and may even be continuous; it may be overshadowed by severe manifestations related to the cerebral, pulmonary, intestinal, or urinary systems. Cerebral complications are evidenced by convulsions or coma, the neurologic signs of which in infants and children are those of increased intracranial pressure and symmetric upper motor neuron and brain stem disturbances such as disconjugate gaze and decerebrate and decorticate postures. Except in rare cases when bacterial or viral infections of the central nervous system are superimposed, the cerebrospinal fluid is generally normal. In cases of algid malaria, coma is preceded in the child by shock. Persistent nausea and vomiting, an enlarged and tender liver, and progressive jaundice may evolve into hepatic failure; severe diarrhea may occur; or occasionally the signs of acute appendicitis may be imitated.

The spleen is more commonly enlarged in vivax than in falciparum infections; perisplenitis, infarction, and even rupture may occur, and after repeated attacks the spleen may become very large and hard. **Tropical splenomegaly syndrome** ("hyper-reactive malarial splenomegaly") may constitute an abnormal immune response in malnourished children in developing countries. Enlargement of the spleen, without diminution following antimalarial treatment, is accompanied by lymphocytic infiltration of liver sinusoids and an elevated fluorescent antibody titer for malaria, with or without scanty parasitemia.

Disturbances of renal function are shown by oliguria, and anuria may supervene. The *nephrotic syndrome* is associated with *P. malariae* in children inhabiting endemic malarious areas; the prognosis is poor. *Blackwater fever,* now rarely seen, is associated with *P. falciparum:* hemoglobinuria results from severe and sudden intravascular hemolysis, which may lead to anuria and to death from uremia.

Hypoglycemia may be associated with falciparum malaria. In severe infections, lactic acidosis may develop, presenting with convulsions and impaired consciousness.

DIAGNOSIS. The diagnosis of malaria depends upon the identification of parasites in the blood. In falciparum malaria, only ring forms are likely to be seen initially, crescents (gametocytes) joining them after 10 days; up to 20% of the erythrocytes may be infected. All stages of the other species of parasites appear in the blood, but less than 1% of red cells will contain them.

In a blood smear the parasites within the red cells have red chromatin and bluish cytoplasm. In some leukocytes, particularly monocytes, remnants of phagocytized parasites and pigment may be seen. The parasites should first be looked for in thick blood films, since in light infections it may not be possible to find plasmodia in the thin film; the latter is best used for species differentiation. Because parasites may not be seen at the height of the fever, examinations should be repeated, preferably at intervals of 12 hr. The most suitable stain is Giemsa diluted 1:25 with distilled water preferably buffered to pH 7.0–7.2. Wright stain may be used, 0.75 g of the powder being repeatedly shaken for 2 days with 65 mL of pure methyl alcohol and 35 mL of pure glycerin.

The presence of species-specific antibodies associated with an elevated level of IgG, persisting for months or years after an acute attack, may be detected serologically, particularly by the indirect fluorescent antibody (IFA) test. A falsely positive Wassermann reaction is found in many cases.

PREVENTION. Natural infection of humans does not occur where breeding of anopheline mosquitoes is prevented, where the adult mosquitoes are kept from contact with people by screens or bed nets, or where they are killed by natural enemies or insecticides before sporozoites have had time to mature. Children visiting endemic malarious areas should be screened from mosquitoes from dusk to dawn, but as this is rarely entirely effective, they should also be given one of the chemoprophylactic drugs *regularly* throughout their stay, commencing 2 wk before the visit and terminating 8 wk after leaving the area. At least during this period, malaria should be suspected if febrile illness or chronic debility affects the child.

Chemoprophylactic drugs in common use are the following: the slightly bitter but extremely safe chlorguanide (proguanil), taken daily in amounts of 50 mg (in children up to 2 yr), 100 mg (2–6 yr), or 200 mg (older than 6); the tasteless but more toxic pyrimethamine taken weekly in amounts of 6.25 mg (to 2 yr), 12.5 mg (2–6 yr), or 25 mg; and chloroquine taken weekly in amounts of 37.5 mg of the base (to 1 yr), 75 mg (1–2 yr), 112.5 mg (2–6 yr), 150 mg (6–12 yr) or 300 mg. The bitterness of chloroquine diphosphate and sulfate may be disguised if the crushed tablet is mixed with a spoonful of jam or thick syrup. Commercially mixed syrups are available but may not remain stable for long.

Unfortunately, resistance of *P. falciparum* to pyrimethamine and chlorguanide is widely distributed; therefore chloroquine is generally preferred for prophylaxis. When resistance by *P. falciparum* to the latter compound also develops, as in most regions except western Asia and Central America, potentiating combinations of chlorguanide with dapsone (daily) or pyrimethamine with dapsone (weekly) may be indicated; however, their use for periods longer than 6 mo is discouraged because of possible side effects related to antifolate activity. Repetitive use of the combination of pyrimethamine with the long-acting sulfonamides, sulfadoxine and sulfalene, is now considered inadvisable. Children more than 8 yr old may take doxycycline orally 2 mg/kg daily for short periods, but increased photosensitivity to sunlight may occur. Chloroquine should be taken concurrently each week to protect against *P. vivax.*

TREATMENT. Therapy falls into four categories: (1) specific chemotherapy for the attack, whether fresh infection, recrudescence, or relapse; (2) supportive treatment and management of complications; (3) specific chemotherapy to prevent late relapse of vivax or ovale infections; (4) specific chemotherapy to destroy or sterilize gametocytes, and thus to protect the community if mosquitoes are present.

1. Clinical cure of all types of malaria and radical cure of falciparum and quartan malaria can be obtained by using the following drug regimens, provided that *P. falciparum* is susceptible: (1) Chloroquine phosphate or hydroxychloroquine sulfate 10 mg base/kg orally, then 5 mg base/kg 6 hr later, then 5 mg base/kg daily for 2 days; or (2) quinine sulfate orally 25 mg/kg/24 hr, in divided doses every 8 hr, for 10–14 days. Children who have inhabited malarious regions and through repeated and prolonged previous infections have acquired some immunity may be cured by using half of the quantities listed. Treatment must be repeated if vomiting occurs within 30 min of ingestion of drugs; persistent vomiting is an indication for parenteral therapy.

Although specific treatment should not usually be undertaken until the diagnosis has been established, many experienced physicians, when confronted with a critically ill or comatose child whose history is suggestive of malaria or exposure thereto, consider it advisable to administer quinine or chloroquine parenterally while awaiting the result of blood film examination.

Parenteral administration of chloroquine or quinine, although hazardous in children bordering on shock, is often essential for those who are vomiting persistently, who are in coma, or who cannot be induced to swallow the drugs even if the bitterness is concealed. Parenteral therapy with antimalarial drugs should be replaced by oral administration as soon as possible. Quinine dihydrochloride is administered intravenously in a dose of 10 mg/kg and may be repeated 12 hr later if treatment still cannot be given by mouth; it should be given well diluted in isotonic saline (1 mg/mL) and slowly (over 1 hr). When quinine is not available in an emergency situation, quinidine gluconate may be used. If neither quinine nor quinidine is available, chloroquine hydrochloride may be administered intravenously by slow drip in the quantity of 5 mg base/kg in 10 mL/kg of isotonic saline, infused over a 3- to 4-hr period; this dose may be repeated 6 hr later. The volume of saline should be adjusted to the state of hydration of the patient, dehydrated children requiring 20 mL/kg, and overhydrated children 5 mL/kg. Administration of chloroquine intramuscularly is not recommended in small children because it has occasionally precipitated convulsions and aggravated shock and resulted in death. It should not be given subcutaneously because of slow absorption by that route.

2. Supportive treatment includes that for hyperpyrexia. Particular attention should be paid to fluid and electrolyte needs (Sec. 6.15).

Metabolic requirements of the parasite rapidly deplete the reserves of glucose, vitamins, and coenzymes as well as of hemoglobin. Vitamin B_1 may be given, and when the acute phase is passed, ferrous sulfate should be prescribed for a considerable time. Transfusion of packed red cells may be beneficial to children who have had longstanding infections and consequently severe anemia (hemoglobin 5 g/dL or less).

It is essential that children with severe falciparum infections receive fluids intravenously if they are dehydrated or in shock. Rapid expansion of the circulating blood volume is more effective with whole blood than with dextran, plasma, or glucose-saline solution. Renal failure, which may require dialysis, is a rare development. When it is present, no more than one third of the conventional doses of antimalarial drugs should be given until the child is hydrated, out of shock, and urinating; quinine and primaquine are contraindicated in the presence of hemoglobinuria. The judicious use of chloroquine or amodiaquine is indicated for heavy parasitemia.

In the comatose stage of cerebral malaria, in addition to specific parenteral antimalarial treatment, dextran-75 may be useful for the prevention of intravascular sludging. Convulsions may be controlled with paraldehyde or barbiturates.

The nephrotic syndrome associated with quartan malaria is managed by the regimen described in Sec. 18.27 together with a course of chloroquine.

3. Late relapse of vivax or ovale malaria may occur up to 3 yr after the primary attack and may be prevented by treating the child with primaquine. Because primaquine given at the height of symptoms increases the tendency to vomit and may be immunosuppressive, it should not be given until the 3rd day of the concomitant clinical curative course of chloroquine, amodiaquine, or quinine. Primaquine is given for 14 days in a daily dose of 0.3 mg base/kg; for fear of possible side reactions some authorities prefer not to administer this drug to children less than 3 yr old (or to pregnant women), but to treat the acute attack with chloroquine and then place the patient on a chemoprophylactic regimen for several months.

Children receiving primaquine should be watched for toxic manifestations such as methemoglobinemia, hemolytic anemia, hemoglobinuria in children with G-6-PD deficiency, neutropenia, and renal dysfunction. Hemolytic anemia may be particularly severe in G-6-PD deficient children of eastern Mediterranean or Asian descent, for whom two approaches to anti-relapse treatment are available: primaquine may be given once each wk for 8 wk in a dose of 0.9 mg base/kg; or primaquine may be omitted entirely and chemoprophylaxis given for several months following treatment of the acute attack with chloroquine. Quinacrine (mepacrine) should not be used simultaneously with primaquine. Other synthetic antimalarial drugs are relatively nontoxic in therapeutic doses.

4. Gametocytes, however, do not give rise to symptoms and disappear from the circulation soon after destruction of their asexual precursors by chloroquine, amodiaquine, or quinine. Gametocytes can be destroyed by a single dose of primaquine, 7.5 mg base for children aged 1–3 yr, 15 mg for those aged 4–6 yr, 30 mg for those aged 6–12 yr, and 45 mg for older children; their further development in the mosquito can be inhibited by single doses of chlorguanide or pyrimethamine, provided the parasite is not resistant to these drugs.

Drug resistance is a growing concern. Many strains of *P. falciparum* are now resistant to chlorguanide and to pyrimethamine, but a greater problem is posed by the spread of resistance to chloroquine in this species to most malarious regions. Some strains are also tolerant to quinine. These strains are being introduced into areas that have been free of malaria and may cause focal summer outbreaks. Should the malarial attack not respond to chloroquine, quinine should be used immediately. If this has only a temporary effect, the course should be repeated with the addition of sulfadiazine, 35 mg/kg every 6 hr for 6 days, and pyrimethamine, given each day for 3 days, 6.25 mg (to 2 yr of age), 12.5 mg (2–6 yr), or 25 mg. An effective alternative is the full course of quinine, together with tetracycline hydrochloride, 10 mg/kg every 6 hr for 7–10 days. Tetracycline, which has a slow parasiticidal effect, should not be used unless accompanied by fast-acting quinine. In children less than 8 yr old, the potentially adverse dental effects of tetracycline should be considered.

Preparations combining sulfadoxine or sulfalene with pyrimethamine are generally effective as a single dose, the long-acting sulfonamide in the amount of 25 mg/kg and pyrimethamine in an amount of 1.25 mg/kg. Rapidity of action is enhanced if quinine is also administered. A parenteral preparation is available, each mL containing 200 mg of sulfadoxine and 10 mg of pyrimethamine; children under 5 yr may be given 1 mL, those from 5–8 yr 2 mL, and older children 3 mL. Unfortunately, *P. falciparum* in Southeast Asia and South America is developing resistance to these combinations also. A new antimalarial, mefloquine, is coming into use on a restricted basis and is effective against these parasites with multiple drug resistance.

DAVID F. CLYDE

Chongsuphajaisiddhi T: Malaria in paediatric practice. *In*: Wernsdorfer WH, McGregor I (eds): Malaria. Edinburgh, Churchill Livingstone, 1988, p 889.

Greenberg AE, Phuc Nguyen-Dinh, Davachi F, et al: Intravenous quinine therapy of hospitalized children with *Plasmodium falciparum* malaria in Kinshasa, Zaire. Am J Trop Med Hyg 40:360, 1989.

Miller RD, Greenberg AE, Campbell CC: Treatment of severe malaria in the United States with continuous infusion of quinidine gluconate and exchange transfusion. N Engl J Med 321:65, 1989.

Phillips RE, Warrell DA, White NJ, et al: Intravenous quinidine for the treatment of severe falciparum malaria: Clinical and pharmacokinetic studies. N Engl J Med 312:1273, 1985.

Snow RW, Lindsay SW, Hayes RJ, et al: Permethrin-treated bed nets (mosquito nets) prevent malaria in Gambian children. Trans R Soc Trop Med Hyg 82:838, 1988.

12.115 AMERICAN TRYPANOSOMIASIS
(Chagas' Disease)

This insect-transmitted infection is one of the major health problems of South America, largely because the primary infection, which occurs in children and young adults, frequently passes unnoticed and is essentially untreatable. In South America at least 24 million people are infected and 65 million exposed; infection occurs in every South American country and is particularly prevalent in Brazil, Argentina, Uruguay, Chile, and Venezuela. Infections also occur in Central America and in the Caribbean, and two cases have been reported in the United States, in Texans who had never left that state. No authenticated cases of natural transmission have been reported outside the Western Hemisphere. Transmission through blood transfusions has been documented in the United States.

The intermediate host infected with trypanosomes is a blood-sucking arthropod (reduviid), which is widespread in the endemic areas. In the United States, however, although infected bugs are found in all southwestern states and most southeastern states, these species are not important vectors of the disease for man because they have not become adapted to human dwellings, limiting opportunity for contact.

ETIOLOGY. American trypanosomiasis is a zoonosis caused by *Trypanosoma cruzi*, a protozoan parasite of the suborder Trypanosomatidae. It can be transmitted to man by bloodsucking insects of the genera *Triatoma*, *Rhodnius*, and *Panstrongylus*. Carlos Chagas was responsible for the initial description of the disease and the discovery of its etiology, vectors, and reservoirs.

In the invertebrate host, *T. cruzi* grows extracellularly in two distinct forms. Epimastigotes multiply in the insect gut and within 1–2 weeks differentiate in the rectum of the insect into metacyclic trypomastigotes, the infectious forms for the mammalian host. These are released with the infected insect's feces when it defecates close to the site of its bite during or after feeding on the host's blood. They enter the host via the damaged skin or through contamination of mucous membranes. Once in the vertebrate host, the metacyclic trypomastigotes readily enter cells, where they replicate as amastigotes. Amastigotes then differentiate intracellularly into trypomastigotes, which are released into the vasculatuıe, where they circulate as bloodstream-form trypomastigotes. These do not replicate until they enter another cell or are withdrawn by another insect vector.

Blood-form trypomastigotes appear in stained preparation as S-shaped flagellates 15–20 μm in length, with a flagellum emerging from the posterior end running along the parasite's body and emerging as free flagellum at the anterior end. A central nucleus and a large kinetoplast can be easily identified. Amastigotes of the vertebrate host appear as oval aflagellates of approximately 3–6 μm in diameter.

EPIDEMIOLOGY. *T. cruzi* infection originally occurred among wild mammals of the American continent and extended to humans when the reduviid insect vectors adapted to human dwellings, principally in rural and low socioeconomic areas. Reduviid bugs are variously known as wild bedbugs, conenose bugs, Mexican bedbugs, or assassin or kissing (based on the predilection to attack the face) bugs.

Adobe, mud, or cane housing with numerous cracks in the walls provides excellent shelter for reduviid bugs. Woodpiles near houses and the custom of keeping domestic animals near or within households provide easy access to human living quarters.

Animal reservoirs may play an important role in linking the wild and domestic cycles of the parasite because of their habitat and their proximity to people. Dogs and cats are important domestic reservoirs of *T. cruzi*; in Panama and Costa Rica *Rattus rattus* is the main domestic reservoir. In the United States the most important wild reservoirs are opossums and raccoons, with infection rates of 17% and 2%, respectively.

The rarity of human infection in the United States may be due to the low virulence of the organisms, the inefficiency of the insect vector, the better housing conditions of the human hosts, and the low adaptability of the North American species to human dwellings. The prevalence of infection in reduviids has been estimated at 20–25% in the Southwest, but in southern Texas only 1.8% of unselected individuals had serologic evidence of infection.

Blood transfusions and congenital transmissions may also be responsible for *T. cruzi* infection. In Brazil, for instance, 15,000 new cases/yr are attributed to transfusions, while 7,500 cases/yr are the result of transmission by the congenital route. With the increasing influx of immigrants from endemic areas into the United States, the risk of transfusion-associated Chagas' disease may become more important, particularly in immunocompromised patients. Blood banks will have to develop policies for identifying potentially infected donors and blood products as well as for screening blood donors for the likelihood of exposure to *T. cruzi*. A recent report of a child with Hodgkin disease, in remission following therapy, who developed Chagas' disease following transfusion with platelets from a *T. cruzi*–seropositive donor, highlights these risks. The donor was a 70-year-old asymptomatic woman who had emigrated from an endemic area 15 yr ago. Transfusion-acquired Chagas' disease should be considered in persistently febrile immunocompromised patients who receive blood transfusions. Accidental inoculation of laboratory workers has also occurred.

PATHOGENESIS AND PATHOLOGY. The immune mechanisms involved in resistance to *T. cruzi* and control of the parasitism during the chronic phase of infection are not completely understood. The majority of infected individuals remain asymptomatic even though serologically positive; relatively few develop late complications. Despite the establishment of strong acquired immunity, there is no parasitologic cure, and procedures known to interfere with cell-mediated immune mechanisms increase the severity of infection by *T. cruzi*.

In the nonimmune host, macrophages provide a favorable environment for the growth and replication of the organisms; there they may be protected from certain aspects of the host's immune defense system, particularly in the acute phase. In contrast, in the immune host, macrophages become activated so that they are capable of destroying the interiorized organisms. Macrophages are activated by soluble products (lymphokines) of sensitized T lymphocytes, which are stimulated by *T. cruzi* antigen.

IgG antibodies to *T. cruzi* are principally associated with protection in the chronic phase of the infection, probably primarily in mediating immunophagocytosis and killing of the organisms by activated macrophages.

Depression of humoral and cell-mediated immune mechanisms during acute *T. cruzi* infection may be mediated by a subpopulation of thymus-derived lymphocytes. Accumulation of macrophages and lymphocytes is commonly seen during the phase of parasite multiplication and active inflammatory response in the heart and in the smooth muscles of the digestive tract, when muscle fibers and peripheral ganglia of the autonomic nervous system are damaged.

The histopathologic findings in acute Chagas' myocarditis consist of an infiltrate of mononuclear cells into the interstitial space, a degenerative process in myocardial fibers, and the appearance of the so-called pseudocysts. Changes in heart morphology depend upon the intensity of the inflammatory reaction.

In chronic Chagas' cardiomyopathy there are fibrotic foci, which may vary from a few small areas to larger fibrotic plates that thin the ventricular wall; degenerating myocardial fibers, usually in fibrotic areas; and infiltrates of mononuclear cells. When fibroblastic proliferation is extensive, the size of the heart increases and there is reduction of the thickness of the ventricular wall. These alterations are frequently associated with intramural thrombi, mainly at the apex of the left ventricle. Thinning of the ventricular wall by large fibrotic plates becomes the starting point for the formation of the aneurysms often found at the apex of the left ventricle or the posterior area of the mitral valve. Autoimmune reactions have been suggested as the underlying cause of these chronic lesions; for example, antibodies against basement membrane structures could damage blood vessels and endocardium. Alternatively, the lesions could be explained by direct damage produced by the parasites and the resulting inflammation during the acute phase.

The histopathology of the hypertrophic, dilated esophagus and colon of patients with Chagas' disease shows the presence of a mononuclear cell infiltrate between smooth muscle cells and sometimes granuloma formation. A significant reduction of neurons in the myenteric plexus is also commonly seen and may produce the organomegalic syndromes. A surface antigen of the parasite that mimics mammalian nervous tissue has been identified, and this cross-reactivity might result in autoimmune damage to the host's nervous tissue.

CLINICAL MANIFESTATIONS. Initially, the infection is often asymptomatic, or the symptoms are very mild. This acute stage is followed by a long silent period, the asymptomatic chronic stage, which may last for decades. The disease may then progress to the chronic stage, presenting mainly with cardiac or intestinal manifestations. Approximately 10% of all serologically positive persons manifest chronic sequelae of the disease. There are differences in the clinical picture of disease as it occurs in different geographic localities, but the causes of these differences are unknown.

Acute American Trypanosomiasis. In most cases the clinical symptoms during the acute phase are either mild or absent, so that patients infrequently present a past history compatible with the acute disease. This rare presentation is mainly seen in children in endemic areas, particularly in those in the age range 0–2 years old, and coincides with local multiplication of the parasites at the site of entry and their subsequent hematogenous dissemination approximately 2–3 wk after infection. Initially, there may be local inflammation with heat, swelling, and redness of the area entered by the parasite. Although 25% of individuals with symptomatic acute trypanosomiasis have no local reactions, half present with unilateral swelling of the eye (Romaña sign), and one fourth develop a nodular skin lesion or a local tumor of the skin (chagoma). Enlargement of the local lymph nodes often accompanies these signs. With subsequent hematogenous dissemination of the organism, malaise, fever, muscular pain, and nontender enlargement of lymph nodes occur. A cutaneous morbilliform eruption, hepatosplenomegaly, and, less often, acute meningoencephalitis may be seen, particularly in infants. About 40% of these patients show electrocardiographic abnormalities such as tachycardia and arrhythmias. Mortality may approximate 10% and is related to heart failure or meningoencephalitis.

In transfusional transmission, the incubation period is usually 4–5 wk, but it may be as long as 4–5 mo. Fever, lymph node enlargement, and splenomegaly are frequent. Edema, tachycardia, and exanthems are often present. Symptoms usually disappear in 6–8 wk, although in some cases fever may last 4 mo or longer. Congenital transmission usually has been associated with prematurity and high mortality at birth.

The majority of acute cases of Chagas' disease evolve over 2–3 mo into a subacute stage, and from this to an asymptomatic chronic stage.

Chronic American Trypanosomiasis. The chronic phase can be divided into an asymptomatic (indeterminate) form and a symptomatic form. The latter may involve cardiac and/or digestive manifestations as well as other less frequent clinical syndromes. Over 40% of serologically positive patients are asymptomatic when assessed by routine examinations alone. However, when more sophisticated diagnostic methods are employed, or a long-term follow-up is undertaken, many of these patients are found to have clinical signs of disease. Patients within this group who have died suddenly have had foci of inflammation and fibrosis of the heart at postmortem examination. There are regional variations in the severity of the disease and in the distribution of the clinical forms. The young account for the greater number of patients in the asymptomatic group, and as age increases, the number of patients presenting with electrocardiographic abnormalities progressively increases.

Approximately 10–20% of patients with acute disease develop the chronic symptomatic form of Chagas' disease, and the prevalence of chronic cardiac and digestive manifestations is higher in patients who display the most severe acute manifestations. In endemic areas trypanosomiasis cardiomyopathy is the leading cause of cardiac disease and sudden death. In one large study, 82% of patients with chronic cardiomyopathy were 11–50 years of age. Males are more frequently affected than females.

Patients commonly present with symptoms and signs of congestive heart failure. The clinical course is one of gradually advancing myocarditis and cardiac failure with tachycardia, premature ventricular beats, enlargement of the heart, and various conduction defects. The most frequent electrocardiographic findings are partial or complete atrioventricular block and complete right bundle branch block. Signs of valvular damage and dysfunction are rare.

The incidence of organomegaly differs in the various endemic areas; it is particularly common in Brazil. Any hollow muscular viscus, but most commonly the esophagus and colon, may be involved. In 80% of 820 cases, dysphagia was the first symptom of megaesophagus. As dysphagia increases, nutritional impairment may occur. Dilation and enlargement of other hollow organs, such as the colon, ureters, or bronchi have been reported.

DIAGNOSIS. Chagas' disease should be suspected in individuals who have lived in endemic areas and show suggestive symptoms and signs. A history of insect bites and their sequelae and the probable duration of infection are suggestive. *T. cruzi* can be demonstrated in the peripheral blood of infected individuals, particularly during the acute stages of the infection. A drop of blood pressed by a cover slip and microscopically examined under high power may reveal the motile trypanosomes. Giemsa-stained blood or concentrated blood-pellet (Sec. 12.114) smears should also be examined for the characteristic C-shaped organisms. The parasites may also be isolated by blood culture or demonstrated in the blood of mice injected with the patient's blood. Xenodiagnosis, or feeding the patient's blood to laboratory-reared reduviid bugs and examining their rectal contents 30–60 days later, is also an effective diagnostic method.

Several serologic tests are available, for example, the complement-fixation test, indirect immunofluorescence, and ELISA assay. These tests are largely used in patients with chronic disease when parasitologic techniques are less likely to demonstrate the organisms. About 80% of patients with chagasic heart disease and 90% of those with megaesophagus have positive complement-fixation tests. Cross-reactivity with other infections, however, may result in false-positive reactions. The use of cloned *T. cruzi* DNA probes should allow rapid and direct detection of parasites in the blood and should provide assays of greater sensitivity and specificity in the near future.

TREATMENT. There is no established and reliable therapeutic agent against *T. cruzi*. Nifurtimox (Lampit) is a promising compound effective in eradicating parasitemia in acute and possibly chronic American trypanosomiasis, but it is associated with severe side effects and must be given for periods of up to 60 days. Symptomatic treatment is needed in patients with chronic Chagas' disease; medical or surgical intervention may be necessary.

CONTROL. This is based on educating people in endemic areas about the relation between bites from triatomine bugs and Chagas' disease. Residual insecticides such as dieldrin or lindane are highly effective in controlling the bug population when sprayed inside buildings, but these insecticides do not destroy the bug ova and therefore should be sprayed repeatedly at 2- to 4-wk intervals. Razing adobe houses that harbor the insects and replacing them with adequately screened, more modern structures is indicated when feasible. Travelers should avoid sleeping in unscreened adobe houses in endemic areas. If this is unavoidable, bed nets should be used.

NADIA NOGUEIRA

Gonzalez A, Prediger E, Huecas M, et al: Minichromosomal repetitive DNA in *Trypanosoma cruzi*: Its use in a high sensitivity parasite detection assay. Proc Nat Acad Sci USA 8:3356, 1984.

Grant IH, Gold JWM, Wittner M, et al: Transfusion associated acute Chagas' disease acquired in the USA. Ann Intern Med 111:849, 1989.

Holt R, Mott KE, Silva JR, et al: Prevalence of parasitemia and seroreactivity to *Trypanosoma cruzi* in a rural population in northeast Brazil. Am J Trop Med Hyg 28:461, 1979.

Nickerson P, Orr P, Schroeder ML, et al: Transfusion-associated *Trypanosoma cruzi* infection in a non-endemic area. Ann Intern Med 111:851, 1989.

Nogueira N, Coura JR: American trypanosomiasis (Chagas' disease). *In*: Warren K, Mahmoud A (eds): Tropical and Geographical Medicine, 2nd ed. New York, McGraw-Hill, 1989.

Sturm NR, Degrave W, Morel C, et al: Sensitive detection and schizodeme classification of *T. cruzi* cells by amplification of kinetoplast minicircle DNA sequences: Use in diagnosis of Chagas' disease. Mol Biochem Parasitol 33:205, 1989.

Van Voorhis WC, Eisen H: F-160: A surface antigen of *Trypanosoma cruzi* that mimics mammalian nervous tissue. J Exp Med 168:141, 1989.

12.116 AFRICAN TRYPANOSOMIASIS

(Sleeping Sickness)

The trypanosomiases of tropical Africa are a group of diseases of great social and economic importance. Human infections are caused by two subspecies of *Trypanosoma brucei, T. b. rhodesiense* and *T. b. gambiense*, which are morphologically indistinguishable but differ markedly in their epidemiology and the disease syndromes they cause. Infection with *T. rhodesiense* usually results in acute syndromes that run a rapid and, if untreated, fatal course, whereas *T. b. gambiense* infection usually runs a more chronic course, resulting in the typical syndrome of sleeping sickness.

Information on the distribution, prevalence, and mortality rate of African trypanosomiasis is unreliable. Human trypanosomiasis in Africa occurs primarily in the region between latitudes 15 degrees north and 15 degrees south, which corresponds roughly to the area where the annual rainfall (500 mm or more) creates optimal climatic conditions for *Glossina* flies. *T. b. rhodesiense* infection is restricted to the eastern third of the endemic area in tropical Africa, stretching from Ethiopia to the northern boundaries of South Africa; *T. b. gambiense* occurs mainly in the western half of the continent's endemic region.

ETIOLOGY. Human infection is initiated by insect bite; the organisms penetrate intact mucous membranes or skin. The infective metacyclic forms of the trypanosomes are 15 μm long and possess no free flagella. One to 3 wk after a period of local multiplication in the skin, long and slender forms (12–42 μm) can be seen in the peripheral blood; intermediate and stumpy forms also occur. These are flagellated forms with a well-developed undulating membrane. In the early stages of human infection, the organisms multiply rapidly in the blood and lymph nodes. They appear in waves in the peripheral blood, each wave being followed by a crisis. The reappearance of another population of organisms in the blood heralds the formation of a new antigenic variant. *T. brucei* are capable of producing hundreds of antigenic variants. As the infection becomes chronic, fewer organisms are seen in the peripheral blood, but they can usually be recovered from lymph nodes. Invasion of the central nervous system occurs early in *T. b. rhodesiense* infections but late in the Gambian form.

The insect intermediate vectors are species of the tsetse flies of the genus *Glossina*. Both sexes of *Glossina* feed on human blood. In nature only a small proportion of the insect population is infected. Inside the flies, the organisms localize in the posterior part of the midgut, where they multiply for about 10 days, then gradually migrate anteriorly where they attach to the walls of the salivary ducts and complete the final stages of development into the infective metacyclic forms. The life cycle within the tsetse fly takes 15–35 days; each fly infected with Rhodesian trypanosomes has been estimated to produce 40,000 infective organisms, of which only 300–450 are necessary to establish human infection.

Direct transmission to humans has also been reported. It is accomplished either mechanically through contact with the contaminated mouth parts of tsetse flies during feeding or congenitally to infants via the placenta of infected mothers.

EPIDEMIOLOGY. The insect intermediate vector plays a major role in determining the epidemiologic pattern of trypanosomiasis. Several *Glossina* species transmit the infection in different parts of tropical Africa. *Glossina* captured in endemic foci show a low rate of infection, usually under 5%. In the Rhodesian form, which usually runs an acute and often fatal course, chances of transmission to tsetse flies are greatly reduced. However, the ability of *T. b. rhodesiense* to multiply enormously in the blood stream of humans and to infect other species of mammals helps to maintain its life cycle.

T. b. gambiense infections usually run a chronic protracted course with very low levels of parasitemia. Because of low rates of infection in tsetse flies, the Gambian life cycle necessitates close and repeated contact between humans and insects to permit frequent biting. *T. b. gambiense* is found in a variety of animal reservoirs that may play an important role in the endemicity of the Gambian form of infection.

PATHOLOGY. The initial entry site of the organisms soon develops into a hard, painful, red nodule, a "trypanosomal chancre." Histologically, it contains long, thin trypanosomes multiplying beneath the dermis and is surrounded by a lymphocytic cellular infiltrate. Dissemination into the blood and lymphatic systems follows, with subsequent localization in the central nervous system. The histopathologic lesions in the brain are those of meningoencephalitis, with increased cellularity of the pia-arachnoid due to lymphocyte infiltration and perivascular cuffing of the blood vessels by the same cell type. In chronic cases the appearance of morular cells (large, strawberry-like cells, supposedly derived from plasma cells) is the most characteristic finding.

CLINICAL MANIFESTATIONS. The clinical presentations vary not only because of the two subspecies of organisms but also because of differences in host response in the indigenous population of endemic areas and in newcomers or visitors. Visitors usually suffer more from the acute symptoms and signs, but in untreated cases death is inevitable for natives and visitors alike. The clinical syndromes of African trypanosomiasis are best described as the trypanosomal chancre, hemolymphatic, and meningoencephalitic stages.

Trypanosomal Chancre. The *site of the tsetse fly bite* may be the first presenting feature. A nodule or chancre develops in 2–3 days; within 1 wk it becomes a painful, hard, red nodule surrounded by an area of erythema and swelling. These nodules are commonly seen on the lower limbs but sometimes also on the head. They subside spontaneously in about 2 wk leaving no permanent scar.

Hemolymphatic Stage. The *most common presenting features* of acute African trypanosomiasis occur at the time of invasion of the bloodstream by the parasites, approximately 2–3 wk after the infection. Irregular episodes of fever, each lasting 1–7 days, are the usual early feature. Attacks may be separated by free intervals of days or even weeks. Headache, sweating, and generalized lymphadenopathy are frequently encountered along with the fever. Enlargement of lymph nodes is one of the most constant signs, particularly in the Gambian form. It most commonly affects the posterior cervical and supraclavicular groups. The lymphadenopathy is painless; the glands are moderately enlarged and are not matted together. Another common feature of trypanosomiasis in whites is the presence of *blotchy, irregular, nonitching, erythematous macules*, which may appear any time following the first febrile episode, usually within 6–8 wk. The majority of macules have a central normal skin area, giving the rash a circinate outline. This skin rash is seen mainly on the trunk and is evanescent, fading in one place only to appear at another site. Examination of the blood during this stage may show anemia, leukopenia with relative monocytosis, and elevated levels of IgM.

Meningoencephalitic Stage. Neurologic symptoms and signs are generally nonspecific. They may precede invasion of the central nervous system by the organisms and present as irrational and inexplicable anxieties with frequent changes in mood. In untreated *T. b. rhodesiense* infections, invasion of the central nervous system occurs within 3–6 wk. It is associated with recurrent bouts of headache, fever, weakness, and signs of acute toxemia. Tachycardia from myocarditis and neurologic symptoms such as irritability, insomnia, and personality or mood changes develop. Death occurs in 6–9 mo from secondary infection or cardiac failure.

In the Gambian form cerebral symptoms can be expected to appear within 2 yr after the onset of acute symptoms, although a general increase in drowsiness during the day and insomnia at night reflect the continuous nature of the pathologic processes. Progress is characterized by increasing anemia, leukopenia, and wasting of body musculature. Patients with chronic Gambian trypanosomiasis have an increased susceptibility to secondary infections.

Involvement of the central nervous system results in a chronic diffuse meningoencephalitis with no localizing symptoms, commonly known as *sleeping sickness*. Drowsiness and an uncontrollable urge to sleep are the major features of this stage of the disease and may become almost continuous in the terminal stages. Associated signs and symptoms also point to involvement of the basal ganglia. Tremor or rigidity with stiff and ataxic gait may occur. Psychotic changes occur in almost one third of untreated patients.

DIAGNOSIS. Definitive diagnosis can be made during the early stages by examination of a fresh thick blood smear, which will allow visualization of the motile active forms. Dried, Giemsa-stained smears should be examined for the detailed morphology of the organisms. If a thick blood smear is negative, a simple concentration method may help. Ten mL of heparinized blood are added to 30 mL of 0.87% ammonium chloride and the mixture centrifuged at 1000 g for 15 minutes. The sediment can then be examined fresh or by staining dried smears. Aspiration of an enlarged lymph node can also be used to obtain material for parasitologic examination. In every positive case a sample of CSF should also be examined for the organisms. In suspected cases, when parasitologic diagnosis has failed, two rats should be inoculated intraperitoneally with 1 mL of blood; 2 wk later their blood should be examined for the parasites.

TREATMENT. The choice of chemotherapeutic agents depends on the stage of the infection and the causative organisms. The hematogenous forms of both Rhodesian and Gambian trypanosomiasis are susceptible to the action of suramin (Antrypol)*, which is available as a 10% solution for intravenous administration. A test dose of 10 mg should first be administered intravenously to detect the rare idiosyncratic reactions of shock and collapse. The dose for subsequent injections is 20 mg/kg intravenously, repeated every 5–7 days for a total of 5 injections. Suramin is nephrotoxic; therefore urine should be examined before each injection. The presence of marked proteinuria, blood, or casts is a contraindication to completion of therapy with suramin. In these rare circumstances therapy should be continued by initiation of a course of melarsoprol,* or, in early cases without central nervous system invasion, pentamidine* may be used. Pentamidine, like suramin, is effective only against the hematogenous forms of the trypanosomes; moreover, its activity may be less certain in the Rhodesian form. It is administered intramuscularly as a 10% solution on alternate days for 5 doses. The dose for each injection is 3–4 mg/kg. Side effects of pentamidine are few; hypotension, faintness, and, occasionally, collapse may occur but can be reversed by administering epinephrine.

If invasion of the central nervous system has occurred, melarsoprol should be used. Melarsoprol contains 18.8% arsenic and is formed from the original arsenical melarsen oxide by the incorporation of dimercaprol (BAL). It is effective against all stages of both Gambian and Rhodesian trypanosomiasis but because of its arsenic content is restricted to use in patients with central nervous system involvement. It is administered intravenously as a 3.6% solution beginning with 0.4 mg/kg. The drug is given in 3 courses, each consisting of an injection on each of 3 successive days with a 1-wk interval between courses. According to the tolerance of the patient, the dose should be increased gradually to reach a maximum of 3.6 mg/kg for the 3rd course. Slight reactions such as fever and pains in the chest or abdomen may occur immediately or very soon after an injection of melarsoprol, but they are generally rare. The most important and serious of its toxic effects is encephalopathy and, less commonly, exfoliative dermatitis.

CONTROL. The control of trypanosomiasis in endemic areas of Africa depends on recognition and effective therapy of human infections and on control of the vector. This is complicated by the fact that it involves cattle and humans and by the logistics of applying the available preventive measures.

Pentamidine has been used successfully as a prophylactic drug. A single injection of 3–4 mg/kg will give protection against Gambian trypanosomiasis for at least 6 mo. Its effect against the Rhodesian form, however, is not certain.

ADEL A. F. MAHMOUD

Hajduk SL, Englund PT, Smith DH: African trypanosomiasis. *In*: Warren KS, Mahmoud AAF (eds): Tropical and Geographical Medicine, 2nd ed. New York, McGraw-Hill, 1990, p 268.

Haller L, Adams H, Merouze F, et al: Clinical and pathological aspects of human African trypanosomiasis *(T.b. gambiense)* with particular reference to reactive arsenical encepholopathy. Am J Trop Med Hyg 35:94, 1986.

Greenwood BM, Whittle HC: The pathogenesis of sleeping sickness. Trans Roy Soc Trop Med Hyg 74:716, 1980.

WHO: Epidemiology and Control of African Trypanosomiasis. Technical Report Series No. 739, Geneva, WHO, 1986.

12.117 TOXOPLASMOSIS

Toxoplasma gondii, an obligate intracellular protozoan, is acquired perorally, transplacentally, or, rarely, parenterally in laboratory accidents, by transfusion, or from a transplanted organ. In the immunologically normal child, the acute acquired infection may be asymptomatic, cause lymphadenopathy, or damage almost any organ. Once acquired, the latent encysted organism persists for the lifetime of the host. In the immunocompromised infant or child, either acute acquisition or recrudescence of latent organisms most often causes signs

*Available in the United States from the Parasitic Drug Service, Centers for Disease Control, Atlanta, GA 30333.

or symptoms related to the central nervous system. Infection acquired congenitally, if untreated, almost always causes signs or symptoms in the perinatal period or later in life. The most frequent of these signs are due to chorioretinitis and central nervous system lesions. However, other manifestations such as intrauterine growth retardation, fever, lymphadenopathy, rash, hearing loss, pneumonitis, hepatitis, and thrombocytopenia also occur. Congenital toxoplasmosis in babies with HIV infection is fulminant.

ETIOLOGY. *T. gondii* is a coccidian protozoan. Its tachyzoites are oval or crescent-like, multiply only in living cells, and measure 2–4 × 4–7 μm. Tissue cysts, which are 10–100 μm in diameter, may contain thousands of parasites and remain in tissues, especially the central nervous system and skeletal and heart muscle, for the life of the host. *Toxoplasma* can multiply in all tissues of mammals and birds, and its disease spectrum is expressed with remarkable similarity in different host species, perhaps because the parasite accommodates to all cells.

Newly infected cats and other Felidae excrete *Toxoplasma* oocysts in their feces. The oocysts are infectious. *Toxoplasma* are acquired by susceptible cats by ingestion of infected meat containing encysted bradyzoites or by ingestion of oocysts excreted by other recently infected cats. The parasites then multiply through schizogonic and gametogonic cycles in the distal ileal epithelium of the cat intestine. Oocysts containing 2 sporocysts are excreted, and under proper conditions of temperature and moisture, each sporocyst matures into 4 sporozoites. For about 2 wk the cat excretes 10^5–10^7 oocysts/day, which, in a suitable environment, may retain their viability for a year or more. Oocysts sporulate 1–5 days after excretion and are then infectious. Oocysts are killed by drying, boiling, and exposure to some strong chemicals, but not to bleach. Oocysts have been isolated from soil and sand frequented by cats, and outbreaks associated with contaminated water have been reported. Oocysts and tissue cysts are the sources of animal and human infections (Fig. 12–36).

EPIDEMIOLOGY. *Toxoplasma* infection is ubiquitous in animals and is one of the most common latent infections of humans throughout the world. The incidence varies considerably among people and animals in different geographic areas. Significant antibody titers have been detected in 50–80% of residents of some localities and in fewer than 5% in others. A higher prevalence of infection usually occurs in warmer, more humid climates.

Infection is usually established by the oral route via undercooked or raw meat that contains cysts or by ingestion of oocysts. Freezing meat to −20° C or heating it to 66° C renders the cysts noninfectious. Except for transplacental infection from mother to fetus and, rarely, by organ transplant or transfusion, *Toxoplasma* are not transmitted from person to person.

Transmission to the fetus usually occurs when the infection is acquired by an immunologically normal mother during gestation. Congenital transmission from immunologically normal women infected prior to pregnancy is extremely rare. Immunocompromised women who are chronically infected have transmitted the infection to their fetuses. The incidence of congenital infection in the United States ranges from 1/1,000 to 1/8,000 live births. The incidence of newly acquired infection in a population of pregnant women depends on the risk of becoming infected in that specific geographic area and the proportion of the population that has not been previously infected.

Seronegative transplant recipients who receive an organ (e.g., heart or kidney) from a seropositive recipient have developed life-threatening illness requiring therapy. Seropositive recipients have developed increased serologic titers without associated disease when untreated.

PATHOLOGY. In the acute congenital and acquired forms of toxoplasmosis, histologic changes may occur in almost all tissues. In the congenital form, such changes are especially frequent in the central nervous system, the retina, and the choroid; retinochoroiditis occurs occasionally in acquired toxoplasmosis. During latent infection, *Toxoplasma* in tissues are seen as cysts with little or no associated tissue reaction. In acute infections, intracellular and, in areas of necrosis, extracellular tachyzoites may be noted. Gross or microscopic areas of necrosis may be present in many tissues, especially heart, lungs, skeletal muscle, liver, and spleen. Areas of calcification occur in the brain in patients with congenital toxoplasmosis. In addition, periaqueductal and periventricular vasculitis and necrosis with sloughing of brain tissue may lead to obstruction of the aqueduct of Sylvius or the foramen of Monroe and consequent hydrocephalus. Obstruction of the aqueduct of Sylvius also may occur after the perinatal period.

In acute acquired lymphadenopathic toxoplasmosis, characteristic lymph node changes include reactive follicular hyperplasia with irregular clusters of epithelioid histiocytes that encroach on and blur the margins of germinal centers. Focal distention of sinuses with monocytoid cells also occurs.

Examination of the placenta of infected newborns may reveal chronic inflammation and cysts. Tachyzoites can be seen with Wright or Giemsa stains but are best demonstrated with the immunoperoxidase technique. The tissue cyst stains well with periodic acid-Schiff (PAS) and silver stains as well as with the immunoperoxidase technique.

PATHOGENESIS. *T. gondii* is usually acquired by children and adults from eating food that contains cysts or that is contaminated with oocysts. In many areas of the world, approximately 5–35% of pork, 9–60% of lamb, and 0–9% of beef contain *T. gondii.* Oocysts are ingested in material contaminated by feces from acutely infected cats. Oocysts also may be transported to food by flies and cockroaches. When the organism is ingested, bradyzoites are released from cysts or sporozoites from oocysts, and the organisms then enter gastrointestinal cells. They multiply, rupture cells, and infect contiguous cells. They are transported via the lymphatics and disseminated hematogenously throughout the body. Tachyzoites proliferate, producing necrotic foci surrounded by a cellular reaction. With the development of a normal immune response (humoral and cell-mediated), tachyzoites disappear from tissues. In immunodeficient individuals and some apparently immunologically normal patients, the acute infection progresses and may cause potentially lethal involvement such as pneumonitis, myocarditis, or necrotizing encephalitis.

Cysts form as early as 7 days after infection and remain for the life span of the host. They produce little or no inflammatory response but cause recrudescent disease in immunocompromised patients or chorioretinitis in older children who have acquired the infection congenitally.

When a mother acquires the infection during gestation, the organism may be disseminated hematogenously to the placenta. When this occurs, infection may be transmitted to the fetus transplacentally or during vaginal delivery. If the infection is acquired by the mother in the 1st trimester and is not treated, approximately 17% of fetuses are infected and disease in the infant is usually severe. If the infection is acquired by the mother in the 3rd trimester and is not treated, approximately 65% of fetuses are infected and involvement is mild or inapparent at birth. These different rates of transmission are most likely related to placental blood flow, the virulence and amount of *T. gondii* acquired, and the immunologic ability of the mother to restrict parasitemia.

Almost all congenitally infected individuals have signs or symptoms of infection, such as chorioretinitis, by adolescence if they are not treated in the newborn period. Some more severely involved infants with congenital infection appear to

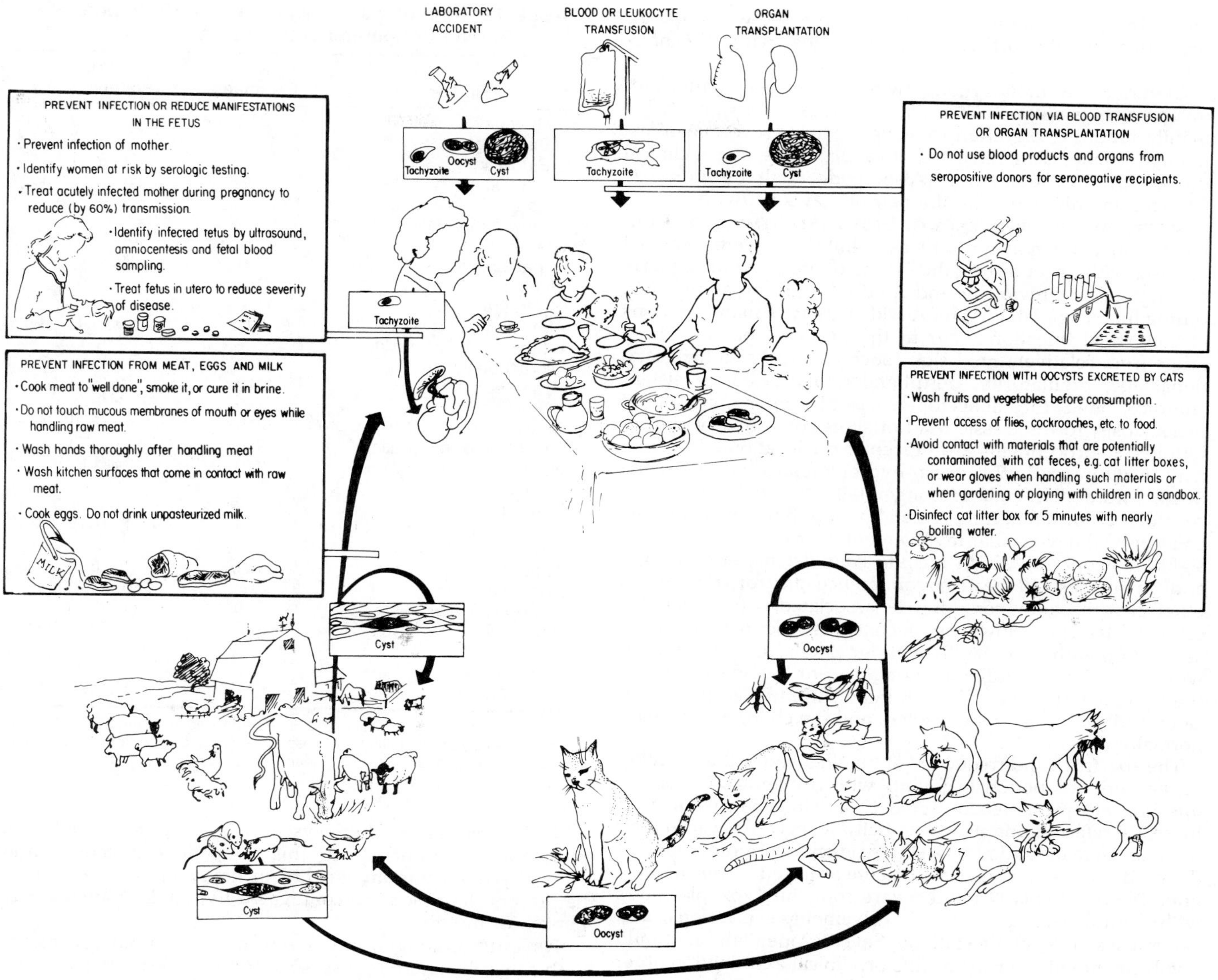

Figure 12–36. Life cycle of *Toxoplasma gondii* and prevention of toxoplasmosis by interruption of transmission to humans.

have *Toxoplasma* antigen–specific anergy of their lymphocytes, which may be important in the pathogenesis of their disease. Monoclonal gammopathy of the IgG class has been described in congenitally infected infants, and IgM levels may be elevated in newborns with congenital toxoplasmosis. Glomerulonephritis with deposits of IgM, fibrinogen, and *Toxoplasma* antigen has been reported in congenitally infected individuals. Circulating immune complexes have been detected in sera from an infant with congenital toxoplasmosis and in older individuals with systemic, febrile, and lymphadenopathic forms of toxoplasmosis, but these did not persist after signs and symptoms resolved. Diminished total serum levels of IgA may occur in congenitally infected babies, but no predilection toward associated infections has been noted. The predilection toward predominant involvement of the central nervous system and eye in this congenital infection has not been fully explained.

There are profound and prolonged alterations in T lymphocyte subpopulations during acute acquired *T. gondii* infection. These have been correlated with disease syndromes but not with disease outcome. Some patients with prolonged fever and malaise have lymphocytosis, increased suppressor T cell levels, and a decreased helper to suppressor T cell ratio. These patients may have fewer helper cells even when they are asymptomatic. In some patients with lymphadenopathy, helper cell numbers are diminished for more than 6 mo after onset of infection. Asymptomatic patients also may have abnormal ratios of T cell subpopulations. Some patients with disseminated disease have a very marked reduction in numbers of T cells and a marked depression in the ratio of helper to suppressor T lymphocytes. Depletion of inducer T lymphocytes in patients with AIDS may contribute to the severe manifestations of toxoplasmosis seen in these patients.

CLINICAL MANIFESTATIONS. Congenital Toxoplasmosis. Transmission. Approximately 50% of untreated women who acquire the infection during gestation transmit the parasite to their fetuses; the incidence of transmission is least early in gestation and greatest later in gestation, and the earlier in gestation the infection is acquired by the fetus, the more likely it is to produce severe fetal manifestations. The signs and symptoms associated with acute acquired *Toxoplasma* infection in the pregnant woman are the same as those seen in the immunologically normal child, most commonly lymphadenopathy. Congenital infection also may be transmitted by an asymptomatic immunosuppressed woman (e.g., those treated with corticosteroids, and those with HIV infection).

Genetics. In monozygotic twins the clinical pattern of involvement is most often similar, whereas in dizygotic twins manifestations often differ. In dizygotic twins severe manifestations in one twin have led to a diagnosis of subclinical disease in the other twin. Also, congenital infection has occurred in only one twin of a pair of dizygotic twins.

Spectrum and Frequency of Signs and Symptoms. Congenital infection may present as a mild or severe neonatal disease, with onset during the 1st mo of life, or with sequelae or relapse of a previously undiagnosed infection at any time during infancy or later in life. A wide variety of manifestations of congenital infection occur in the perinatal period. These range from relatively mild signs such as small size for gestational age, prematurity, peripheral retinal scars, persistent jaundice, mild thrombocytopenia, and cerebrospinal fluid pleiocytosis, to the classic triad of signs consisting of chorioretinitis, hydrocephalus, and cerebral calcifications. Infection may result in erythroblastosis, hydrops fetalis, and perinatal death. More than half of congenitally infected infants are considered normal in the perinatal period, but almost all such children will have ocular involvement later in life. Neurologic signs in neonates, which include convulsions, sunset sign, and an increase in head circumference disproportionate to other growth parameters, may be associated with substantial cerebral damage. However, such signs also may occur in association with encephalitis without extensive destruction or with relatively mild inflammation adjacent to and obstructing the aqueduct of Sylvius. If such infants are treated promptly, signs and symptoms may resolve, and the child may develop normally.

The spectrum and frequency of manifestations that develop in the perinatal period in infants with congenital *Toxoplasma* infection are presented in Table 12–44. Infection in most of these 210 referred infants was initially suspected because their mothers were identified by a serologic screening program that detected pregnant women with acute acquired *T. gondii* infection. Twenty-one (10%) had severe congenital toxoplasmosis with central nervous system involvement, eye lesions, and general systemic manifestations. Seventy-one (34%) had mild involvement with normal results on clinical examination other than retinal scars or isolated intracranial calcifications. One hundred and sixteen (55%) had no detectable manifestations. This last figure may reflect the difficulties associated with funduscopic examination of the peripheral retina in infants and young children. These figures represent an underestimation of the relative frequency of severe congenital infection for the following reasons: the most severe cases, including most of those who died, were not referred; therapeutic abortion was often performed when acute acquired infection of the mother was diagnosed early during pregnancy; in utero spiramycin therapy may have diminished the severity of infection; and only 13 infants had CT brain scans and 23% did not have a CSF examination.

The clinical spectrum and natural history of untreated congenital toxoplasmosis, which is *clinically apparent* in the 1st yr of life, is presented in Table 12–45. More than 80% of these children had IQs of less than 70, and many had convulsions and severely impaired vision.

Skin. Cutaneous manifestations in infants with congenital toxoplasmosis include petechiae, ecchymoses, or large hemorrhages secondary to thrombocytopenia, and rashes. Rashes may be fine punctate; diffuse maculopapular; lenticular, deep blue-red, sharply defined macular; and diffuse blue papules. Macular rashes involving the entire body including the palms and soles, exfoliative dermatitis, and cutaneous calcifications have been described. Jaundice due to hepatic involvement with *T. gondii* and/or hemolysis, cyanosis due to interstitial pneumonitis secondary to this congenital infection, and edema secondary to myocarditis or nephrotic syndrome may be present. Jaundice and conjugated hyperbilirubinemia may persist for months.

TABLE 12–44. Signs and Symptoms in 210 Infants with Proved Congenital Toxoplasma Infection*

Finding	No. Examined	No. Positive (%)
Prematurity	210	
Birthweight < 2,500 g		8 (3.8)
Birthweight 2,500–3,000 g		5 (7.1)
Dysmaturity (intrauterine growth retardation)		13 (6.2)
Icterus	201	20 (10)
Hepatosplenomegaly	210	9 (4.2)
Thrombocytopenic purpura	210	3 (1.4)
Abnormal blood count (anemia, eosinophilia)	102	9 (4.4)
Microcephaly	210	11 (5.2)
Hydrocephaly	210	8 (3.8)
Hypotonia	210	12 (5.7)
Convulsions	210	8 (3.8)
Psychomotor retardation	210	11 (5.2)
Intracranial calcifications on x-ray	210	24 (11.4)
Ultrasound	49	5 (10)
Computer tomography of brain	13	11 (84)
Abnormal EEG	191	16 (8.3)
Abnormal CSF	163	56 (34.2)
Microphthalmia	210	6 (2.8)
Strabismus	210	11 (5.2)
Chorioretinitis	210	
Unilateral		34 (16.1)
Bilateral		12 (5.7)

*Data are adapted from Couvreur J, et al: Ann Pediatr (Paris) 31:815, 1984. Table 1. Infants were identified by prospective study of infants born to women who acquired *Toxoplasma* infection during pregnancy.

Systemic Signs. Twenty-five to more than 50% of infants with clinically apparent disease at birth are born prematurely. Low Apgar scores also are common. Intrauterine growth retardation and instability of temperature regulation may occur. Other systemic manifestations include lymphadenopathy; hepatosplenomegaly; signs of myocarditis, pneumonitis, and nephrotic syndrome; vomiting; diarrhea; and feeding problems. Bands of metaphyseal lucency and irregularity of the line of provisional calcification at the epiphyseal plate, may occur without periosteal reaction in the ribs, femora, and vertebrae. Congenital toxoplasmosis may be confused with isosensitization causing erythroblastosis fetalis; the Coombs test is usually negative with congenital *T. gondii* infection.

Endocrine Abnormalities. Endocrine abnormalities may occur secondary to hypothalamic or pituitary involvement or end-organ involvement. The following have been reported: myxedema, persistent hypernatremia with vasopressin-sensitive diabetes insipidus without polyuria or polydipsia, sexual precocity, and partial anterior hypopituitarism.

Central Nervous System. Neurologic manifestations of congenital toxoplasmosis vary from massive acute encephalopathy to subtle neurologic syndromes. Toxoplasmosis should be considered as a cause of any undiagnosed neurologic disease in children under 1 yr of age, especially if retinal lesions are present.

Hydrocephalus may be the sole clinical neurologic manifestation of congenital toxoplasmosis and may either be compen-

TABLE 12–45. Signs and Symptoms Occurring Prior to Diagnosis or During the Course of Untreated Acute Congenital Toxoplasmosis in 152 Infants (A) and in 101 of These Same Children When They Had Been Followed 4 yrs or More (B)*

Signs and Symptoms	Frequency of Occurrence in Patients with "Neurologic" Disease†	"Generalized" Disease‡
A. Infants	*108 Patients (%)*	*44 Patients (%)*
Chorioretinitis	102 (94)§	29 (66)
Abnormal spinal fluid	59 (55)	37 (84)
Anemia	55 (51)	34 (77)
Convulsions	54 (50)	8 (18)
Intracranial calcification	54 (50)	2 (4)
Jaundice	31 (29)	35 (80)
Hydrocephalus	30 (28)	0 (0)
Fever	27 (25)	34 (77)
Splenomegaly	23 (21)	40 (90)
Lymphadenopathy	18 (17)	30 (68)
Hepatomegaly	18 (17)	34 (77)
Vomiting	17 (16)	21 (48)
Microcephalus	14 (13)	0 (0)
Diarrhea	7 (6)	11 (25)
Cataracts	5 (5)	0 (0)
Eosinophilia	6 (4)	8 (18)
Abnormal bleeding	3 (3)	8 (18)
Hypothermia	2 (2)	9 (20)
Glaucoma	2 (2)	0 (0)
Optic atrophy	2 (2)	0 (0)
Microphthalmia	2 (2)	0 (0)
Rash	1 (1)	11 (25)
Pneumonitis	0 (0)	18 (41)
B. Children, 4 yr [or more] old	*70 Patients (%)*	*31 Patients (%)*
Mental retardation	62 (89)	25 (81)
Convulsions	58 (83)	24 (77)
Spasticity and palsies	53 (76)	18 (58)
Severely impaired vision	48 (69)	13 (42)
Hydrocephalus or microcephalus	31 (44)	2 (6)
Deafness	12 (17)	3 (10)
Normal	6 (9)	5 (16)

*Adapted from Eichenwald H: A study of congenital toxoplasmosis. *In:* Siim JC (ed): Human Toxoplasmosis. Copenhagen, Munksgaard, 1960, pp 41–49. Study performed in 1947. The most severely involved institutionalized patients were not included in the later study of 101 children.

†Patients with otherwise undiagnosed central nervous system disease in the 1st yr of life.

‡Patients with otherwise undiagnosed non-neurologic diseases during the first 2 mo of life.

§Figure outside parentheses = number; figure inside parentheses = percentage.

sated or require correction with shunt placement. Hydrocephalus may present in the perinatal period, progress after the perinatal period, or, less commonly, present later in life. Patterns of seizures are protean and have included focal motor seizures, petit and grand mal seizures, muscular twitching, opisthotonus, and hypsarrhythmia (which may resolve with ACTH therapy). Spinal or bulbar involvement may be manifested by paralysis of the extremities, difficulty in swallowing, and respiratory distress. Microcephaly usually reflects severe brain damage, but some children with microcephaly due to congenital toxoplasmosis, who have been treated, appear to function normally in the early years of life. Untreated congenital toxoplasmosis that is symptomatic in the 1st yr of life can cause substantial diminution in cognitive function and developmental delays. Intellectual impairment also occurs in some children with subclinical infection despite treatment with pyrimethamine and sulfonamides for 1 mo. Seizures and focal motor defects may become apparent after the newborn period, even when infection is subclinical at birth.

Cerebrospinal fluid abnormalities occur in at least one third of infants with congenital toxoplasmosis. Local production of *T. gondii*-specific antibodies may be demonstrated in cerebrospinal fluid of congenitally infected individuals (see later under Diagnosis). CT scan of the brain with contrast enhancement is useful to detect calcifications, determine ventricular size, image active inflammatory lesions, and demonstrate porencephalic cystic structures (Fig. 12–37). Calcifications occur throughout the brain, but there appears to be a special propensity for development of such lesions in the caudate nucleus, choroid plexus, and subependyma. Ultrasonography may be useful for following ventricular size in congenitally infected babies. MRI, computed tomography with contrast enhancement, and radionucleotide brain scans may be useful for detecting active inflammatory lesions.

Eyes. Almost all untreated congenitally infected individuals will develop chorioretinal lesions by adulthood, and about 50% will have severe visual impairment. *T. gondii* causes a focal necrotizing retinitis in congenitally infected individuals (Fig. 12–38 [color plate section]). Contractures may occur with retinal detachment. Any part of the retina may be involved, either unilaterally or bilaterally, including the maculae. The optic nerve may be involved, and toxoplasmic lesions that involve projections of the visual pathways in the brain or the visual cortex also may lead to visual impairment. In association with retinal lesions and vitritis, the anterior uvea may be intensely inflamed, leading to erythema of the external eye. Other ocular findings include cells and protein in the anterior chamber, large keratic precipitates, posterior synechiae, nodules on the iris, and neovascular formation on the surface of the iris, sometimes with an associated increase in intraocular pressure and development of glaucoma. The extraocular musculature may also be involved directly, manifest as strabismus, nystagmus, visual impairment, and micro-ophthalmia. The differential diagnosis of lesions resembling ocular toxoplasmosis includes congenital colobomatous defect and other inflammatory lesions due to cytomegalovirus, *Treponema pallidum, Mycobacterium tuberculosis,* or vasculitis. Ocular toxoplasmosis is a recurrent and progressive disease that requires multiple courses of therapy. Couvreur et al have limited data that suggest that occurrence of lesions in the early years of life may be prevented by instituting antimicrobial treatment (with pyrimethamine and sulfonamides in alternate months with spiramycin) during the 1st yr of life.

Ears. Sensorineural hearing loss, both mild and severe, may occur. It is not known whether this is a static or progressive disorder.

Concomitant Infections. Congenital toxoplasmosis in infants with HIV infection usually presents as a severe and fulminant illness with substantial central nervous system involvement.

Acquired Toxoplasmosis in Immunologically Normal Individuals. Immunologically normal children who acquire the infection postnatally may have no clinically recognizable disease. The most common manifestation is enlargement of one or a few lymph nodes in the cervical region. Cases of *Toxoplasma* lymphadenopathy rarely resemble infectious mononucleosis (due to Epstein-Barr virus, cytomegalovirus, or parvovirus), Hodgkin disease, or other lymphadenopathies. In the pectoral area in older girls and women the nodes may be confused with breast neoplasms. Mediastinal, mesenteric, and retroperitoneal lymph nodes may be involved. Involvement of intra-abdominal lymph nodes may be associated with fever and mimic appendicitis. Nodes may be tender but do not suppurate. Adenopathy may appear and disappear for as long as 1 yr. When clinical manifestations are apparent, they

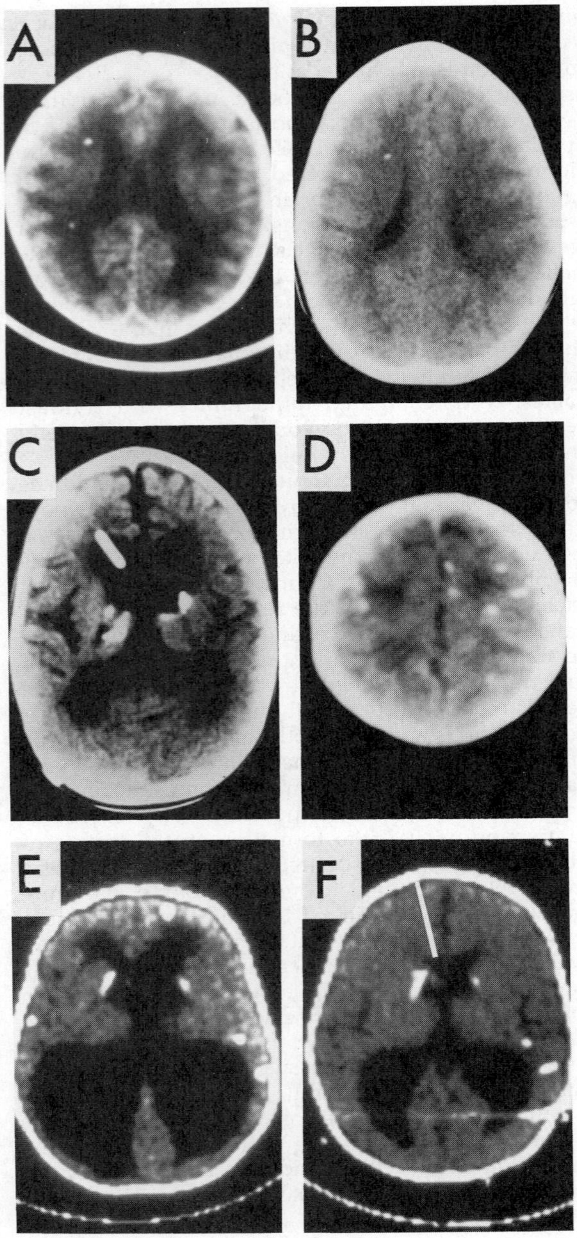

Figure 12–37. Head computed tomography (CT) scans of and historical information in babies with congenital toxoplasmosis. *A*, CT scan at birth that has areas of hypolucency, mildly dilated ventricles, and small calcifications. *B*, CT scan of the same child at 1 yr of age (after antimicrobial therapy for 1 yr). This scan is normal with the exception of two small calcifications. This child's Mental Development Index (MDI) at 1 yr of age was 140 by the Bayley Scales of Infant Development. *C*, CT scan from a 1-yr-old baby who was normal at birth. His meningoencephalitis became symptomatic in the first weeks of life but was not diagnosed correctly and remained untreated during his 1st 3 mo of life. At 3 mo of age, development of hydrocephalus and bilateral macular chorioretinitis led to the diagnosis of congenital toxoplasmosis, and antimicrobial therapy was initiated. This scan shows significant residual atrophy and calcifications. This child has substantial motor dysfunction, developmental delays, and visual impairment. *D*, CT scan obtained during the 1st mo of life of a microcephalic child. Note the numerous calcifications. This child's intelligence quotient (i.e., using the Stanford-Binet Intelligence Scale for children when she was 3 yr old and the Wechsler Preschool and Primary Scale of Intelligence when she was 5 yr old) were 100 and 102, respectively. She received antimicrobial therapy during her 1st yr of life. *E*, CT scan with hydrocephalus owing to aqueductal stenosis (before shunt). *F*, Scan from the same patient as the scan in *E*, after shunt. This child's intelligence quotient (i.e., using the Stanford-Binet Intelligence Scale for children) was approximately 100 when she was 3 and 6 yr old. (Adapted from McAuley J, Boyer K, Patel D, et al: Early outcome of congenital toxoplasmosis following therapy. [In preparation]).

may include almost any combination of fever, stiff neck, myalgia, arthralgia, maculopapular rash that spares the palms and soles, localized or generalized lymphadenopathy, hepatomegaly, hepatitis, reactive lymphocytosis, meningitis, brain abscess, encephalitis, confusion, malaise, pneumonia, polymyositis, pericarditis, pericardial effusion, and myocarditis. Chorioretinitis, usually unilateral, occurs in approximately 1% of cases. Symptoms may be present for a few days only or may persist many months.

Most patients with malaise and lymphadenopathy recover spontaneously without antimicrobial therapy. Significant organ involvement in immunologically normal individuals is uncommon, but some such individuals have suffered significant morbidity.

Ocular Involvement in the Older Child. In the United States and western Europe, *T. gondii* has been estimated to cause 35% of cases of chorioretinitis. Manifestations include blurred vision, photophobia, epiphora, and, with macular involvement, loss of central vision. Findings due to congenital ocular toxoplasmosis also include strabismus, micro-ophthalmia, microcornea, cataract, anisometropia, and nystagmus. Episodic recurrences are common. See Figure 12–38 and under Congenital Toxoplasmosis.

Toxoplasmosis in the Immunocompromised Patient. Congenital *T. gondii* infection in infants with AIDS is usually a fulminant, rapidly fatal disorder, involving brain and other organs such as the lung and heart. Disseminated *T. gondii* infections also occur in older children who are immunocompromised by AIDS, by malignancies and cytotoxic therapy or corticosteroids, or by immunosuppressive drugs given for organ transplantation. Immunocompromised individuals develop the clinical forms of *Toxoplasma* infection that occur in immunologically normal individuals. Signs and symptoms that are referable to the central nervous system are the most frequent manifestations of severe disease (occurring in 50% of patients), although other organs also may be involved.

Bone marrow transplant recipients present a special problem because active infection in these patients is difficult to diagnose. Specific antibody may not increase in serum or may be absent. In most instances, active infection occurs in a child with prior evidence of latent infection.

Individuals who have antibodies to *T. gondii* and HIV infection are at significant risk of developing toxoplasmic encephalitis, which may be the presenting manifestation of AIDS. In patients with AIDS, toxoplasmic encephalitis is fatal if not treated. Typical findings of central nervous system toxoplasmosis in patients with AIDS include fever, headache, altered mental status, psychosis, cognitive impairment, seizures, focal neurologic defects including hemiparesis, aphasia, ataxia, visual field loss, cranial nerve palsies, and dysmetric or movement disorders. Uncommon findings of central nervous system or other organ involvement include meningismus, signs referable to involvement of the heart, gastrointestinal tract, testes, panhypopituitarism, and the syndrome of inappropriate antidiuretic hormone (see Sec. 12.83). In adult patients with AIDS, toxoplasmic retinal lesions are often large with diffuse necrosis and contain many organisms but little inflammatory cellular infiltrate.

LABORATORY DIAGNOSIS. Diagnosis of acute *Toxoplasma* infection can be made by isolation of *T. gondii* from blood or body fluids and also by demonstration of tachyzoites in sections or preparations of tissues and body fluids, cysts in the placenta or tissues of a fetus or newborn, and by characteristic lymph node histology. Serologic tests also are very useful for diagnosis. The cerebrospinal fluid is often abnormal in infants with congenital toxoplasmosis.

Organisms are isolated by inoculation of body fluids, leukocytes, or tissue specimens into mice or tissue cultures. Body fluids should be processed and inoculated immediately, but *T. gondii* has been isolated from tissues and blood that have been stored at 4° C overnight. Freezing or treatment of specimens with formalin kills *T. gondii*. Six to 10 days after inoculation, or earlier if mice die, peritoneal fluids should be examined for tachyzoites. If they survive for 6 wk and there is antibody in sera of the inoculated mouse, definitive diagnosis is made by visualization of *Toxoplasma* cysts in mouse brain. If cysts are not seen, subinoculations of mouse tissue into other mice are performed.

T. gondii can also be isolated by *tissue cultures*. Under microscopic examination, the plaques in these preparations are seen to contain necrotic, heavily infected cells with numerous extracellular tachyzoites. Isolation of *T. gondii* from blood or body fluids reflects acute infection. Except in the fetus or neonate it is usually not possible to demonstrate acute infection by isolation of *T. gondii* from tissues such as skeletal muscle, lung, brain, or eye obtained by biopsy or at autopsy.

Diagnosis of acute infection can be made by *demonstration of tachyzoites* in biopsy tissue sections, bone marrow aspirate, or body fluids such as cerebrospinal fluid or amniotic fluid. Immunofluorescent antibody and immunoperoxidase staining techniques may be necessary because it is often difficult to see the tachyzoite with ordinary stains. Tissue cysts are diagnostic of infection but do not differentiate between acute and chronic infection; the presence of many cysts suggests recent acute infection. Cysts in the placenta or tissues of the newborn infant establish the diagnosis of congenital infection. Characteristic histologic features are sufficient to establish the diagnosis of toxoplasmic lymphadenitis.

The *Sabin-Feldman dye test* is sensitive and specific. It measures primarily IgG antibodies. Results should be expressed in International Units (IU/mL) based on international standard reference sera available from the World Health Organization.

The *IgG fluorescent antibody (IgG-IFA) test* measures the same antibodies as the dye test, and the titers tend to be parallel. These antibodies usually appear 1–2 wk after infection, reach high titers (≥1:1,000) after 6–8 wk and then decline over months to years. Low titers (1:4 to 1:64) usually persist for life. Antibody titer does not correlate with severity of illness. Approximately half of the commercially available IFA kits tested have been found to be improperly standardized and may yield significant numbers of false-positive and false-negative results.

An *agglutination test* (Bio-Merieux, Lyon, France) is available commercially in Europe (e.g., formalin-preserved whole parasites are used to detect IgG). This test is accurate, simple to perform, and inexpensive. The *IgM fluorescent antibody (IgM-IFA) test* is useful for the diagnosis of acute infection with *T. gondii* in the older child because IgM antibodies appear earlier (often by 5 days after infection) and disappear sooner than IgG antibodies. In most instances, IgM-IFA test antibodies rise rapidly (to levels of 1:50 to > 1:1,000) and fall to low titers (1:10 or 1:20) or disappear after weeks or months. However, for some patients they remain positive at low titers for as long as several years. The IgM-IFA test detects *Toxoplasma*-specific IgM in only approximately 25% of congenitally infected infants at birth. IgM antibodies also are often not present in sera of immunodeficient patients with acute toxoplasmosis or in most patients with active toxoplasmosis present only in the eye. Both the IgG-IFA and IgM-IFA tests may show false-positive results owing to rheumatoid factor.

The *double-sandwich enzyme-linked immunosorbent assay (DS-IgM-ELISA)* is more sensitive and specific than the IgM-IFA test for detection of *Toxoplasma* IgM antibodies. In the older child, a level of IgM antibodies against *Toxoplasma* in serum of 1.7 or greater (value of one reference laboratory; each laboratory must establish its own values) indicates that *Toxoplasma* infection has most likely been acquired recently. DS-IgM-ELISA detects approximately 75% of infants with congenital infection. DS-IgM-ELISA avoids both the false-positive results due to rheumatoid factor produced by uninfected infants in utero and false-negative results due to high levels of passively transferred maternal IgG antibody in fetal serum, as occurs in the IgM-IFA test.

The *IgM immunosorbent assay (ISAGA)* combines trapping of a patient's IgM to a solid surface and use of formalin-fixed organisms or antigen-coated latex particles. It is read like an agglutination test and is specific and sensitive. There are no false-positive results due to rheumatoid factor or antinuclear antibodies. IgM antibodies to *Toxoplasma* are detected by the IgM-IFA test for a shorter time than they are by the DS-IgM-ELISA. The IgM ISAGA is more sensitive than the IgM ELISA and may detect specific IgM antibodies before and for longer periods of time than the IgM ELISA. The *IgA ELISA* is a more sensitive test than the IgM ELISA for detection of congenital infection in the fetus and newborn as well as for detection of acute infection in some pregnant women.

Antibodies measured in *indirect hemagglutination (IHA) tests* are different from those measured in the IFA and dye tests. They may persist for years. However, the IHA test should not be used in infants with suspected congenital infection or in screening for infection acquired during pregnancy because it may be negative for too long a period early during infection.

The level of *Toxoplasma antibody in the cerebrospinal fluid or aqueous humor* demonstrates local production of antibody during active ocular or CNS toxoplasmosis as follows:

$$C = \frac{\text{antibody titer in body fluid}}{\text{antibody titer in serum}} \times \frac{\text{concentration of gamma globulin in serum}}{\text{concentration of gamma globulin in body fluid}}$$

Significant correlation coefficients [C] are 8 or more (eye), 4 or more (CNS for congenital infection), and over 1 (CNS for patients with AIDS). If the serum dye test titer is 1,000 or more, most often it is not possible to demonstrate significant local antibody production using this formula with either the dye test or the IgM-IFA test titer. IgM antibody may be present in CSF.

Toxoplasma antigen has been detected during acute *Toxoplasma* infection but not in sera of uninfected or chronically infected individuals. Antigen was present in the serum, amniotic fluid, and cerebrospinal fluid in the few infants tested with congenital infections.

Comparative *Western blot* tests of sera from a mother and baby may detect congenital infection. Infection is suspected when the mother's serum and her baby's serum contain antibodies that react with different *Toxoplasma* antigens.

Enzyme-linked immunofiltration assay (ELIFA, using micropore membranes) permits simultaneous study of antibody specificity by immunoprecipitation and characterization of antibody isotypes by immunofiltration with enzyme-labeled antibodies. This method may be capable of detecting 85% of cases of congenital infection in the first few days of life. It is still being evaluated.

Polymerase chain reaction (PCR) is used to amplify the DNA of *T. gondii*, which then can be detected using a DNA probe.

Lymphocyte blastogenesis to *Toxoplasma* antigens has been used to diagnose congenital toxoplasmosis if a question persists concerning the diagnosis and other tests are negative.

Laboratory Diagnosis of Congenital Toxoplasmosis. Fetal blood sampling, fetal ultrasound examination (performed every 2 wk during gestation), and analysis of amniotic fluid are used in *prenatal diagnosis* of congenital toxoplasmosis. Abnormalities in the following nonspecific tests suggest that fetal infection is possible: peripheral white blood cell count, number of eosinophils, platelet count, liver function tests (gamma-GTP, LDH), and total IgM. IgM specific for *T. gondii* is usually present only after 24 wk gestation, and *T. gondii* may be isolated from peripheral fetal white blood cells and cells from amniotic fluid. *T. gondii* also may be isolated from the placenta.

Serologic tests are also useful in establishing a diagnosis of congenital toxoplasmosis, for example, either persistent or rising titers in the dye test or IFA test or a positive IgM ELISA or ISAGA. The half-life of IgM is 3–5 days, so if there is a placental leak, the level of IgM antibodies in the infant's serum falls significantly within a week. Passively transferred maternal IgG antibodies may require many months to a year to disappear from the infant's serum. The length of time needed for disappearance depends on the magnitude of the original titer. IgG half-life is approximately 30 days. Synthesis of *Toxoplasma* antibody is usually demonstrable by the 3rd mo of life if the infant is untreated. If the infant is treated, synthesis may be delayed until the 9th mo of life, and, infrequently, it may not occur at all. When an infant begins to synthesize antibody, infection may be documented serologically without demonstration of IgM antibodies by computation of the specific "antibody load," that is, the ratio of specific serum antibody titer to the amount of IgG in an infected baby will increase, whereas the ratio will fall as the baby synthesizes IgG if the specific antibody has been passively transferred from the mother.

At birth, when a diagnosis of congenital toxoplasmosis is suspected, the following diagnostic studies should be performed: general, ophthalmologic, and neurologic examinations; head CT scan; attempt to isolate *T. gondii* from the placenta and the infant's white blood cells from umbilical cord blood and buffy coat; measurement of serum *Toxoplasma*-specific IgG, IgM, and IgA antibodies and the total amount of IgM and IgG in serum; lumbar puncture including analysis of CSF for cells, glucose, protein, *Toxoplasma*-specific IgG and IgM antibodies, and total amount of IgG; and evaluation of cytocentrifuge preparation of CSF for *T. gondii*. The presence of *Toxoplasma*-specific IgM in CSF that is not contaminated with blood or local antibody production of *Toxoplasma*-specific IgG antibody demonstrated in CSF establishes the diagnosis of congenital *Toxoplasma* infection.

Laboratory Diagnosis of Acute Acquired Toxoplasma Infection in the Immunocompetent Individual. Recent infection is diagnosed by seroconversion from a negative to a positive IgG antibody titer (in the absence of transfer of antibody by transfusion); a serial 2-tube rise in *Toxoplasma*-specific IgG titer when sera are obtained 3 wk apart and run in parallel; and the presence of *Toxoplasma*-specific IgM antibody.

Laboratory Diagnosis of Ocular Toxoplasmosis. IgG test titers of 1:4 to 1:64 are usual in older children with active toxoplasmic chorioretinitis. When the retinal lesions are characteristic and serologic tests are positive, the diagnosis is likely.

Laboratory Diagnosis of Toxoplasmosis in the Immunocompromised Individual. IgG antibody titers may be low, and *Toxoplasma*-specific IgM is often absent in immunocompromised individuals with toxoplasmosis. Demonstration of *Toxoplasma* antigens or DNA in serum, blood, and CSF may identify disseminated *Toxoplasma* infection in immunocompromised persons.

Resolution of central nervous system lesions during a therapeutic trial of pyrimethamine and sulfadiazine has been useful in patients with AIDS. Brain biopsy has been used to establish the diagnosis of toxoplasmic encephalitis when there is no response to this therapeutic trial or to exclude other likely diagnoses in such immunocompromised individuals.

DIFFERENTIAL DIAGNOSIS. Many manifestations of congenital toxoplasmosis occur in other perinatal diseases, especially disease caused by cytomegalovirus. Neither cerebral calcification nor chorioretinitis is pathognomonic. Fewer than 50% of children under 5 yr of age with chorioretinitis satisfy the serologic criteria for congenital toxoplasmosis; the causes of most of the other cases are unknown. The clinical picture in the newborn infant may also be compatible with sepsis, aseptic meningitis, syphilis, or hemolytic disease. In cases of acquired disease, other causes of lymphadenopathic disease must be distinguished from toxoplasmosis.

PREVENTION. Methods of prevention are outlined in Figure 12–36. Counseling women about these methods of avoiding transmission of *T. gondii* during pregnancy can substantially reduce acquisition of infection during gestation. Women who do not have specific antibody to *T. gondii* prior to pregnancy should only eat well done meat during pregnancy and avoid contact with oocysts excreted by cats. Cats that are kept indoors, maintained on prepared diets, and not fed fresh, uncooked meat should not contact encysted *T. gondii* and shed oocysts. Serologic screening, ultrasound monitoring, and treatment of pregnant women during gestation can also reduce the incidence and perhaps manifestations of congenital toxoplasmosis.

TREATMENT. Therapeutic Agents. Pyrimethamine plus sulfadiazine or trisulfapyrimidines act synergistically against *Toxoplasma*. Combined therapy is indicated to treat many of the forms of toxoplasmosis. However, use of pyrimethamine is contraindicated during the 1st trimester of pregnancy. Spiramycin should be used to prevent transmission of infection to the fetus of acutely infected pregnant women and to treat congenital toxoplasmosis. Pyrimethamine is a folic acid antagonist and therefore produces a dose-related, reversible, and usually gradual depression of the bone marrow resulting in thrombocytopenia, leukopenia, and anemia. Neutropenia is the most common side effect in treated infants. All patients treated with pyrimethamine should have platelet and peripheral blood cell counts twice weekly. Seizures may occur with overdosage of pyrimethamine. Folinic acid (calcium leukovorin) should always be administered concomitantly with pyrimethamine to prevent suppression of the bone marrow. Potential toxic effects of sulfonamides (e.g., crystalluria, hematuria, and rash) should be monitored. Hypersensitivity reactions occur, especially in patients with AIDS.

Treatment of Congenital Toxoplasmosis. All infected newborns should be treated, whether or not they have clinical manifestations of the infection. In infants with congenital infection, treatment may be effective in interrupting acute disease that damages vital organs. Infants should be treated for 1 yr. For the first 6 mo, oral pyrimethamine (1–2 mg/kg/24 hr for 2 days, then 1 mg/kg/24 hr for 2 mo, then 1 mg/kg/24 hr Monday, Wednesday and Friday), sulfadiazine or triple sulfonamides (100 mg/kg loading dose, then 100 mg/kg/24 hr in 2 divided doses), and calcium leukovorin (5–10 mg/24 hr Monday, Wednesday, Friday) should be administered. In the second 6 mo this regimen is continued or given in alternate months with spiramycin (50 mg/kg twice a day). For infants with moderate to severe involvement the first 6 mo regimen may be continued for a full year or modified to provide pyrimethamine 1 mg/kg/24 hr for the first 6 mo. Pyrimethamine, available only in tablet form, may be crushed and administered in a suspension with juice or food. The effectiveness of these regimens has not been proved, but they are considered reasonable empiric recommendations.* Prednisone (1 mg/kg/24 hr orally in divided doses) has been utilized in addition when active chorioretinitis involves the macula, CSF protein is elevated (≥1,000 mg/dL) at birth, or there is generalized infection, but its efficacy also is not established.

Treatment of Immunologically Normal Older Children with Lymphadenopathy, Severe Symptoms, or Damage to Vital Organs. Patients with lymphadenopathy do not need specific treatment unless they have severe and persistent symptoms or evidence of damage to vital organs. If such signs and symptoms occur, treatment with pyrimethamine, sulfadiazine, and leukovorin should be initiated. Although the optimal duration of therapy is unknown, patients who appear to be immunologically normal but have severe and persistent symptoms or damage to vital organs (e.g., chorioretinitis, myocarditis) need specific therapy until these specific symptoms resolve, followed by therapy for an additional 2 wk. This therapy usually lasts for at least 4–6 wk, and sometimes longer. A loading dose of pyrimethamine for older children is 2 mg/kg/24 hr (maximum 50 mg), given for the first 2 days of treatment. The maintenance dose is 1 mg/kg/24 hr (maximum 25 mg/24 hr). Folinic acid is administered orally at a dosage of 5–20 mg 3 times/wk (or even daily depending on the white blood cell count). Sulfadiazine or trisulfapyrimidine is administered to children over 1 yr of age with a loading dose of 75 mg/kg/24 hr, and thereafter 50 mg/kg/24 hr.

Treatment of Active Chorioretinitis in Older Children (also see Treatment of Congenital Toxoplasmosis). Such patients should receive pyrimethamine, sulfadiazine, and leukovorin for approximately 1 mo. Within 10 days the borders of retinal lesions should sharpen, and the vitreous haze should disappear in 60–70% of cases. Systemic corticosteroids are administered when lesions involve the macula, optic nerve head, or papillomacular bundle. Photocoagulation has been used to treat active lesions and prevent spread (i.e., most new lesions appear contiguous to old ones). Occasionally vitrectomy and removal of the lens are needed to restore visual acuity.

Treatment of Immunocompromised Patients. Serologic evidence of acute infection in an immunocompromised patient, regardless of whether signs and symptoms of infection are present or tachyzoites are present in tissue, are indications for therapy similar to that described for immunocompetent children with symptoms of organ injury. It is important to establish the diagnosis as rapidly as possible and institute treatment early. In immunocompromised patients other than those with AIDS, therapy should be continued for at least 4–6 wk beyond complete resolution of all signs and symptoms of active disease. Careful follow-up of these patients is imperative because relapse may occur, requiring prompt reinstitution of therapy. Relapse is frequent in patients with AIDS, and suppressive therapy with pyrimethamine and sulfonamides should be continued for life. Therapy usually induces a beneficial response clinically, but it does not eradicate cysts from the CNS and perhaps not from other tissues either.

Treatment of Pregnant Women with *T. gondii* Infection. The immunologically normal pregnant woman who acquired *T. gondii* before conception does not need treatment to prevent congenital infection of her fetus. Treatment of a pregnant woman who acquires infection at any time during pregnancy reduces the chance of congenital infection in her infant by approximately 60%. Spiramycin and pyrimethamine are used in combination with sulfadiazine or triple sulfonamides. Because pyrimethamine is potentially teratogenic, spiramycin is administered in the 1st trimester.* The dose of spiramycin is 1.5 g each 12 hr, given without food; lower doses are less effective.* Toxicity is infrequent. Adverse reactions include paresthesias, rash, nausea, vomiting, and diarrhea. Treatment during the remainder of pregnancy with pyrimethamine and a sulfonamide should be continued at dosages similar to those recommended for therapy of the symptomatic immunocompetent patient. Treatment of the mother of an infected fetus with pyrimethamine and a sulfonamide reduces infection in the placenta and the severity of disease in the newborn.

Chronically infected pregnant women who have been immunocompromised by cytotoxic drugs or corticosteroid therapy have transmitted *T. gondii* to their fetuses. Such women should be treated with spiramycin throughout gestation. The best approach to prevention of congenital toxoplasmosis in the fetus of a pregnant woman with HIV and inactive *T. gondii* infection is unknown. If the pregnancy is not terminated, the mother should be treated with spiramycin during the first 17 wk of gestation and then with pyrimethamine and sulfadiazine until term. In a study of adult patients with AIDS, a dose of 75 mg pyrimethamine/24 hr and high dosages of intravenously administered clindamycin (1,200 mg/6 hr intravenously) appeared equal in efficacy to sulfonamides and pyrimethamine. Other currently experimental agents include roxithromycin and azithromycin (two new macrolides). These agents have not been used in infants or children.

Azidothymidine (AZT) antagonizes in vitro the toxoplasmacidal effect of pyrimethamine and the synergy of pyrimethamine and sulfadiazine, but the clinical significance of this observation remains to be determined. Therapy with phenobarbital and pyrimethamine may reduce the half-life of pyrimethamine. Sulfadiazine interferes with the metabolism by hepatic microsomal enzymes of other agents such as phenytoin (Dilantin) and warfarin. This prolongs their half-life, and lower dosages of these drugs are therefore likely to achieve therapeutic levels.

Infants with severe systemic and neurologic manifestations of congenital toxoplasmosis, including cerebral calcifications, hydrocephalus, and chorioretinitis, do not have uniformly poor prognoses due solely to their infection, and the usual supportive measures are indicated.

PROGNOSIS. Early institution of specific treatment for

*Information concerning the U.S. National Collaborative Study evaluating these regimens can be obtained by calling 312-791-4152. Spiramycin is available in the United States only through this study or by special permission of the FDA.

*Spiramycin is available in the United States through the FDA (telephone 302-443-7580).

congenitally infected infants usually cures the manifestations of toxoplasmosis such as active chorioretinitis, meningitis, encephalitis, hepatitis, splenomegaly, and thrombocytopenia. Hydrocephalus due to aqueductal obstruction may develop or become worse during therapy. Such treatment also may reduce the incidence of some sequelae, such as chorioretinitis. Without therapy, chorioretinitis often recurs. Children with extensive involvement at birth may function normally later in life or have mild to severe impairment of vision, hearing, cognitive function, and other neurologic functions. Delays in diagnosis and therapy, perinatal hypoglycemia, hypoxia, hypotension, repeated shunt infections, and severe visual impairment are associated with a poorer prognosis. Prognosis must be guarded but is not necessarily poor for infected babies. Treatment with pyrimethamine and sulfadiazine does not eradicate the encysted parasite. No protective vaccine is available.

RIMA McLEOD
JACK S. REMINGTON

Brooks RG, McCabe RE, Remington JS: Role of serology in the diagnosis of toxoplasic lymphadenopathy. Rev Infect Dis 9:1055, 1987.
Burg JL, Grover CM, Pouletty P, et al: Direct and sensitive detection of a pathogenic protozoan. *Toxoplasma gondii*, by polymerase chain reaction. J Clin Microbiol 27:1787, 1989.
Couvreur J, Desmonts G, Tournier G, et al: Study of homogeneous genes of 210 cases of congenital toxoplasmosis in infants aged 0 to 11 months detected prospectively. Ann Pediatr 31:815, 1984.
Daffos F, Forestier F, Capella-Pavlovsky M, et al: Prenatal management of 746 pregnancies at risk for congenital toxoplasmosis. N Engl J Med 318:271, 1988.
Desmonts G, Couvreur J: Natural history of congenital toxoplasmosis. Ann Pediatr 31(10):799, 1984.
Desmonts G, Forestier F, Thulliez P, et al: Prenatal diagnosis of congenital toxoplasmosis. Lancet 1:500, 1985.
Haentjens M, Sacre L, DeMeuter F: Congenital toxoplasmosis after maternal infection before or slightly after conception. Acta Paediatr Scand 75:343, 1986.
Hohljeld P, Daffos F, Thulliez P, et al: Fetal toxoplasmosis: Outcome of pregnancy and infant follow-up after in utero treatment. J Pediatr 115:765, 1989.
Israelski DM, Remington JS: Toxoplasmic encephalitis in patients with AIDS. *In*: Sand MA, Volberding PA (eds): The Medical Management of AIDS. Philadelphia, WB Saunders, 1988, p 193–211.
Johnson D, Boyer K, McLeod R, et al: Early outcome of congenital toxoplasmosis following therapy. (In press.)
Koppe JG, Loewer-Sieger DH, De Roever-Bonnet H: Results of 20-year follow-up of congenital toxoplasmosis. Lancet 1:254, 1986.
McCabe RE, Brooks RG, Dorfman RF, et al: Clinical spectrum in 107 cases of toxoplasmic lymphadenopathy. Rev Infect Dis 9:754, 1987.
McCabe R, Remington JS: Toxoplasmosis: The time has come. N Engl J Med 318:313, 1988.
McLeod R, Hubbel J, Weller S, et al: Pyrimethamine in the treatment of congenital toxoplasmosis. (In press.)
Saxon SA, Knight W, Reynolds DW, et al: Intellectual deficits in children born with subclinical congenital toxoplasmosis: A preliminary report. J Pediatr 8:2792, 1973.
Wilson CB, Remington JS, Stagno S, et al: Development of adverse sequelae in children born with subclinical congenital *Toxoplasma* infection. Pediatr 66:767, 1980.

12.118 LEISHMANIASIS

Infection with different species of *Leishmania* can cause cutaneous lesions, ulcerations of the oronasal mucosa, or visceral dissemination resulting in fatal complications. Leishmaniasis has a vast geographic distribution involving millions of people. Effective chemotherapeutic agents are available, and drug resistance is not uncommon.

ETIOLOGY. *Leishmania* are protozoal parasites existing in two morphologically distinct forms: flagellated promastigotes, which replicate extracellularly within the sandfly vector gut and also in axenic cultures; and amastigotes, which lack flagella and are obligate intracellular parasites of mononuclear phagocytes in the mammalian host. Female vector sandflies (certain *Phlebotomus*, *Lutzomyia*, and *Psychdopygus* species) become infected by ingesting *Leishmania*-infected macrophages while taking a blood meal. In the sandfly gut, amastigotes exit from the ingested host cells, transform into promastigotes, and replicate. Transmission occurs when promastigotes are subsequently injected into a susceptible host. They enter cells (probably tissue macrophages) in the host's skin, transform into amastigotes, replicate, and infect adjacent macrophages. In cutaneous leishmaniasis only local replication of amastigotes occurs. In mucocutaneous and visceral disease, dissemination (probably hematogenous) takes place.

PATHOPHYSIOLOGY. *Leishmania* attach to mononuclear phagocyte surfaces by a complex process involving several ligands and probably requiring active participation of the parasite. Macrophage receptors for complement components, mannose, fibronectin, and (in the presence of antibody) the Fc portion of immunoglobulin G may play a role in the process. Once attached, the parasites enter by phagocytosis and become surrounded by a host plasma membrane-derived parasitophorous vacuole. Secondary lysosomes fuse with this vacuole (forming a phagolysosome) without apparent deleterious effects on the amastigotes. Different *Leishmania* species have different temperature optima for growth, which may explain why some species disseminate while others are restricted to the cooler parts of the body (skin).

Although amastigotes survive and replicate in quiescent mononuclear phagocytes, when these cells are "activated" they can inhibit parasite replication and induce death. This host defense results primarily (if not exclusively) from direct contact between effector lymphocytes and infected macrophage and from lymphocyte secretion of macrophage-activating lymphokines such as gamma interferon; the intracellular demise of the parasite occurs without damage to the host cell. In some forms of leishmaniasis (e.g., visceral and diffuse cutaneous leishmaniasis), deficiency of such host defenses permits parasite dissemination and chronicity of infection. Whether intrinsic features of the particular parasite species, the genetic composition of the host, or a complex specific interplay of parasite and host factors dictate disease outcome is unknown. Assessing this is complicated by the very large number of *Leishmania* species and by their changing taxonomy, especially at the subspecies level (complexes).

CLINICAL MANIFESTATIONS. Visceral Leishmaniasis. This disease, also called kala-azar, is caused by species of *Leishmania* (*L. donovani* complex, *L. chagasi*, *L. infantum*) that disseminate hematogenously, infecting macrophages in the liver, spleen, bone marrow, and lymph nodes. The infection is zoonotic in most areas. Dogs and other carnivores are the most common reservoirs. In India and East Africa man is thought to be the reservoir. The disease is found on all continents except Australia, and although epidemiologic features may differ widely, the important clinical features are generally similar in different geographic regions.

Typically, symptoms appear several weeks to 8 mo following the sandfly bite, although incubation periods of up to 10 yr have been reported. Lesions at the inoculation site are rarely observed when the patient first comes to medical attention. The course of the disease can be abrupt (as occurs frequently in young children) or insidious (especially in older children and adults). Oligosymptomatic and asymptomatic forms of the infection have been described in children. Fever is very common, and although it may have periodicity, the pattern is not diagnostically reliable. Vomiting, diarrhea, and a nonproductive cough accompany disease of abrupt onset. Infections with a more protracted course may be characterized by an initial 2–8 wk of fevers and nonspecific systemic complaints including weakness, anorexia, and vague abdominal problems. Thereafter, the fever may recede and the patient becomes weaker, and complains of symptoms related to an enlarged spleen, such as abdominal discomfort and early satiety. The most dramatic finding on physical examination is marked splenomegaly that may reach massive proportions. Hepatomegaly and less frequently lymphadenopathy are associated common features. With time, the hair thins and becomes brittle. The skin becomes dry and scaly and may acquire the gray, ashen appearance from which the name kala-azar ("black sickness") is derived. Petechiae, ecchymoses, and mild edema may appear; jaundice and ascites are rare.

The major complications leading to death, including hemorrhage and bacterial superinfection, result from a decrease in blood elements due to leishmanial infection of the bone marrow and hypersplenism. Anemia, leukopenia, and thrombocytopenia are common. Hypoalbuminemia, a marked polyclonal hypergammaglobulinemia (mostly IgG), circulating immune complexes and rheumatoid factor are associated laboratory findings. Immune complex glomerulonephritis with proteinuria and microscopic hematuria occurs, although renal disease is uncommon. Secondary amyloidosis and hepatic fibrosis leading to portal hypertension are unusual. Without treatment, death usually ensues within 2 yr as a result of infectious complications including pneumonia, tuberculosis, dysentery, and septicemia, or of anemia or hemorrhage.

Post kala-azar dermal leishmaniasis (PKDL) develops in 3–20% of patients after treatment of the visceral infection. The lesions range from depigmented macules on the face and trunk to firm nodules appearing mostly on the nose and around the mouth. They may persist for months or years if untreated. A history of previous kala-azar and isolation of parasites from the lesions help establish this diagnosis.

Kala-azar should be suspected in endemic areas when patients present with enlarging spleens, pancytopenia (especially anemia), and hyperglobulinemia. The infection has occurred in patients with AIDS residing in temperate regions but who travelled to areas with endemic leishmaniasis. It must be differentiated from malaria, miliary tuberculosis, salmonellosis, acute schistosomiasis, amebic liver abscess, and acute typhus. In the chronic stages it may mimic hepatosplenic schistosomiasis, brucellosis, tropical splenomegaly syndrome, chronic lymphocytic leukemia, lymphoma, malignant histiocytosis, and glycogen storage disease. PKDL may be confused with yaws, syphilis, and leprosy.

Cutaneous Leishmaniasis. This type of infection is traditionally divided into Old World (Mediterranean basin, Africa, India, China, Soviet Union, and Asia Minor) and New World (primarily Central and South America, excluding Chile and Uruguay). The former is caused by any of a number of species, including *Leishmania tropica* and *L. major*; the latter is caused by the *L. brasiliensis* and *L. mexicana* complexes. In most geographic areas, these parasites are maintained by transmission in nonhuman reservoirs, usually rodents, but human-to-human transmissions can also occur.

The characteristic skin lesion begins as an erythematous papule or macule that may ulcerate after several weeks. Unless superinfected with bacteria, the lesions are generally painless, nontender, and not pruritic. In some cases, lymphatic nodules may develop proximal to the lesion. Satellite lesions containing parasites may form adjacent to the primary one. In Old World cutaneous leishmaniasis, spontaneous healing usually occurs over a period of months.

Certain specific clinical forms are recognized in distinct geographic areas. For example, the so-called *chiclero's ulcer* is found in the northern region of Central America and the Yucatan peninsula among workers who enter the rain forests to gather chicle gum. The lesion has a propensity to form on the pinna of the ear and may be destructive. Infection acquired in the forests of northern South America can lead to hyperkeratotic or papillomatous lesions that resemble secondary yaws ("pian bois" or forest yaws). Uta, a form acquired in the Peruvian Andes and Argentinian highlands, heals spontaneously.

Diffuse cutaneous leishmaniasis (DCL) is a rare form recognized primarily in Ethiopia, Venezuela, and the Dominican Republic. Multiple lesions form on the skin in association with anergy to leishmanial antigens. Defective host defense in these patients is also revealed by a paucity of lymphocytes and a large number of heavily infected macrophages in the lesions. *Leishmania recidiva* is another rare form found in areas of endemic *L. tropica* infection and manifested by lesions (usually facial) that resemble lupus vulgaris, which may persist for years. In contrast to DCL, the parasites may be difficult to identify in these lesions.

The differential diagnosis of cutaneous leishmaniasis includes tuberculosis and atypical mycobacteriosis of the skin, fungal infections, syphilis, yaws, leprosy, basal cell carcinoma, and sarcoid.

Mucocutaneous Leishmaniasis (Espundia). This is a complication of cutaneous leishmaniasis acquired in Central and South America. The rate of this complication varies in different geographic areas, from less than 1% to as high as 30% in southern Brazil. *L. braziliensis brasiliensis* is most commonly responsible for this disease. The parasite spreads hematogenously, and the lesions in the oral and nasal mucosa may develop 1 mo–24 yr (rare cases) after the initial cutaneous lesion. Coryza, nasal stuffiness, or epistaxis can be presenting complaints. Destructive lesions can involve the lips, tongue, soft palate, nasal septum and bridge, pharynx, larynx, and trachea. Destruction of the nasal septum can lead to perforation or to collapse that gives rise to the so-called tapir nose deformity. Erosion of the nose and lips can cause grotesque facial deformities. Involvement of the larynx, pharynx, or trachea can cause dysphagia and asphyxia. Aspiration pneumonia, wound infections, and bacterial meningitis are complications. Mucocutaneous leishmaniasis may resemble syphilis, yaws, histoplasmosis, paracoccidioidomycosis, sarcoidosis, basal cell carcinoma, and midline granuloma.

DIAGNOSIS. When kala-azar is suspected, the diagnosis should be confirmed by biopsy or aspiration of an involved site. Splenic aspiration provides the highest yield (positive in > 80% of cases) but may be risky if it is attempted by an inexperienced physician. It should not be performed in patients with severe thrombocytopenia (platelets $< 40 \times 10^9/L$) or coagulopathy. Bone marrow aspiration is the second most useful procedure (54–86% positive), and liver biopsy may also be helpful (~ 70% positive). Aspiration of lymph nodes has provided the diagnosis in patients with kala-azar who have lymphadenopathy. By light microscopy, amastigotes appear in Giemsa-stained infected cells as round forms measuring about 2–5 μm in diameter with a characteristic large mitochondrion-associated mass of extrachromosomal DNA (the kinetoplast). Aspirated or homogenized biopsy material should be cultured for up to 4 wk on specialized media. Promastigotes can be observed as highly motile oblong bodies (20 μm long) in culture.

The *Montenegro skin test* (a test for cutaneous delayed type hypersensitivity response to a killed promastigote preparation called leishmanin) is negative in active kala-azar, only becoming positive after 6–8 wk of successful therapy. Leishmanin is not commercially available but can be obtained from the WHO Leishmaniasis Reference Center, Hadassah Hospital, Jerusalem, Israel. Serologic tests developed for the diagnosis of kala-azar include complement-fixation, fluorescent antibody, indirect hemagglutination, direct agglutination, and ELISA tests. The indirect immunofluorescence antibody test and direct agglutination assay are available from the Centers for Disease Control (CDC), Atlanta, GA, United States. Serologic tests should not be used to the exclusion of other diagnostic tests, since routine tests are not species-specific and may be falsely positive in patients infected with *Trypanosoma cruzi*.

Diagnosis of cutaneous leishmaniasis is best achieved by skin biopsy from the raised edge of a lesion; aspirates have also proved useful. Impression smears of biopsy material stained with Giemsa provide the most rapid diagnosis if amastigotes can be identified; identifying parasites on histologic sections may prove difficult. Some species identifiable on impression smears may fail to grow in culture. The Montenegro test generally becomes positive in 4–6 wk after infection and persists for years; in diffuse cutaneous leishmaniasis it is negative. In leishmaniasis recidiva the reaction is characteristically exuberant. Serology is unreliable in cutaneous leishmaniasis as titers are usually low. In mucocutaneous leishmaniasis organisms may be difficult to identify in tissue; the Montenegro test is generally positive. Antibody detected by immunofluorescence and direct agglutination assays are positive in 90% of such cases.

TREATMENT. The pentavalent antimonial (Sb^v) compounds sodium stibogluconate (Pentostam, 100 mg Sb/mL; available from CDC) and meglumine antimonate (Glucantime) are the preferred drugs for treating leishmaniasis. Both can be given intravenously or intramuscularly, and they appear to have similar efficacy and toxicities. Efficacy of treatment depends on the form of leishmaniasis being treated and on the geographic area where it was acquired. Resistance has been noted particularly in kala-azar acquired in East Africa, China, and the Mediterranean, and in diffuse cutaneous and mucocutaneous disease. All forms of visceral, mucocutaneous, and diffuse cutaneous leishmaniasis should be treated. Cutaneous disease acquired in the Old World usually is self-healing and requires treatment only if the lesion progresses, fails to heal in 3–5 mo, is disabling owing to its location, or is cosmetically embarrassing. The safest approach may be to treat all forms of cutaneous leishmaniasis acquired in Central and South America (except uta from Peru and Argentina), since most patients fail to heal spontaneously and some may be at risk for developing mucocutaneous disease. It is not established that treatment of the skin lesion prevents the subsequent development of mucocutaneous leishmaniasis. Therefore, patients should be followed even after successful treatment. PKDL and leishmaniasis recidiva are treated in the same way as primary infections.

Precise regimens are difficult to recommend because few careful comparisons have been reported. For most forms of leishmaniasis, 20 mg Sb^v/kg body weight (some suggest to a maximum of 850 mg/day) given once each day intramuscularly or intravenously for 20–30 days should be adequate. Shorter courses or lower doses might also be effective in some cases. For treatment failure or recurrence, repeated courses are recommended. Antimony is rapidly excreted by the kidney (80% in a few hours) with little accumulation in the tissue. Side effects of therapy occur relatively infrequently but include fever, rash, cough, and gastrointestinal irritation. Electrocardiographic changes such as T wave depression or inversion and prolonged QT_c interval may herald the onset of arrhythmias but generally are transient and well tolerated with doses of 20 mg/kg/24 hr or less for less than 20 days. Renal insufficiency may develop, and renal function should be followed; adjustment of dose or interval in patients with renal insufficiency may be advisable.

Resistant disease (such as mucocutaneous leishmaniasis) can be treated with amphotericin B or pentamidine. Amphotericin B is administered as for deep mycoses (Sec. 12.103). Patients with mucocutaneous leishmaniasis may require a total dose of 1–3 g; cutaneous disease can often be treated with less. Pentamidine administered intramuscularly, 2–4 mg/kg, 1–3 times/wk for 5–25 wk (depending on the nature of the illness) has been used as second line treatment. A variety of other agents (such as rifampin, trimethoprimsulfamethoxazole, allopurinol, and ketoconazole) have been employed successfully in isolated cases or in a small series of patients. Their routine use cannot be recommended.

Splenectomy has been reported to be effective in advanced drug-resistent kala-azar. Its indications include drug resistance in the face of massive splenomegaly and symptomatic or disabling hypersplenism, especially in small children. Appropriate management of anemia, infection, and hemorrhage as well as good nutrition are essential for optimal care during this treatment. Cryosurgery, curettage, intralesional instillation of chemotherapeutic agents, and heat treatment have all had success in treatment of isolated cases of cutaneous disease, but they cannot be recommended as replacements for antimony treatment. Restorative plastic surgery and prostheses may be of great benefit to patients with mutilating mucocutaneous disease but should be performed only after an extended period of observation following treatment so that recurrence does not cause loss of the graft.

In evaluating responses to treatment, assessing both clinical (disappearance of fever, decrease in spleen size, increase in white blood count and hemoglobin) and parasitologic parameters is important. Repeat aspirates or biopsies are useful in assessing a parasitologic "cure," but when the disease progresses despite apparent elimination of parasites, continued treatment may be necessary. On the other hand, attrition of parasites may occur even after completion of a course of therapy. Restoration of responsiveness to leishmanin and a fall in antileishmanial antibodies are useful indices of improvement in treatment of kala-azar.

PREVENTION. Prevention depends upon a detailed knowledge of the ecology of the reservoirs and vector of the various forms of leishmaniasis. Treating cases, decreasing human contact with the vector, destroying animal reservoirs, and vector control are important in reducing transmission. Insect repellents and fine mesh netting around beds can decrease exposure to sandflies. Travelers to endemic areas should be warned of the risk and instructed in methods for preventing acquisition of leishmaniasis. Spraying with residual insecticides has reduced the sandfly populations and controlled the disease in some areas; when insecticide spraying was instituted for malaria control in the Indian state of Bihar, the sandfly population was reduced to a level at which kala-azar was almost eliminated. Within a few years after such measures were ended, however, the disease returned in epidemic proportions. No chemoprophylactic agents are available. In the USSR, Iran, and Israel, a form of vaccination has been employed using live cultures of *L. tropica* or *L. major*, but complications preclude the widespread use of this measure. Since curing the infection appears to impart protection against reinfection with the homologous parasite species, developing an effective and safe vaccine should be possible. This holds the greatest promise for preventing leishmaniasis.

DAVID J. WYLER

Barado R, Jones TC, Carvalho EM, et al: New perspectives on a subclinical form of visceral leishmaniasis. J Infect Dis 154:1003, 1986.

Berman JD: Chemotherapy for leishmaniasis: Biochemical mechanisms, clinical efficacy, and future strategies. Rev Infect Dis 10:560, 1988.

Jha TK: Evaluation of diamidine compound (pentamidine isethionate) in the treatment of resistant cases of kala azar in North Bihar, India. Trans R Soc Trop Med Hyg 77:167, 1983.

Kager PA, Rees PH, Mangugu FM, et al: Clinical, hematological and parasitological response to treatment of visceral leishmaniasis in Kenya: A study of 64 patients. Trop Geogr Med 36:285, 1984.

Pearson RD, Wheeler DA, Harrison LH, et al: The immunobiology of leishmaniasis. Rev Infect Dis 5:907, 1983.

Rees PH, Kager PA, Kyambi JM, et al: Splenectomy in kala azar. Trop Geogr Med 36:285, 1984.

Sypek JP, Wyler DJ: Host defense in leishmaniasis. *In*: Leech JH, Sande MA,

Root RK (eds): Contemporary Issues in Infectious Diseases. New York, Churchill Livingstone, 1988, p 221.
Thakur CP: Epidemiological, clinical and therapeutic features of Bihar kala azar (including post kala azar dermal leishmaniasis). Trans R Soc Trop Med Hyg 78:391, 1984.
The Leishmaniases. Report of a WHO Expert Committee. WHO Tech Rep Ser 701:1, 1984.

PNEUMOCYSTIS CARINII

See Sec. 14.58.

12.119 PRIMARY AMEBIC MENINGOENCEPHALITIS

Amebic meningoencephalitis is an acute, usually fatal infection of the central nervous system occurring primarily in children and young adults. In most cases there is a history of swimming in fresh water—ponds, lakes, or even heated pools, all of which may be heavily contaminated with algae or bacteria—which has put the patient in contact with the infectious agent.

ETIOLOGY AND EPIDEMIOLOGY. Although free-living amebae occur ubiquitously in nature, the micro-organisms primarily responsible for human infection belong to the genera *Naegleria* and *Acanthamoeba*, of the families Vahlakampfiidae and Acanthamoebidae, respectively. *Naegleria* are motile, fresh water amebaeflagellates, 10–20 μm in diameter, having a large nucleus, a prominent central karyosome, and large pseudopodia, which can be cultured on a number of laboratory media and on non-nutrient agar seeded with bacteria. Various species of *Acanthamoeba*, besides those found free-living in nature, also exist as part of the normal flora of the mouth and nasopharynx. Morphologically similar to *Naegleria*, they are 6–8 μm in diameter and have an abundant cytoplasm. *Acanthamoeba* are less motile than *Naegleria* and in clinical specimens can be confused with macrophages.

Human infection with *Naegleria* has been acquired through contact with tap water in Australia, thermally polluted water in Belgium, and swimming pools in Czechoslovakia. Most cases in the United States have occurred during summer months in children and young adults after swimming, diving, or water skiing in freshwater ponds and lakes. *Acanthamoeba* infection of the central nervous system is less common but has a worldwide distribution. It is unassociated with previous aquatic activity and occurs as an opportunistic infection in a debilitated and/or immunosuppressed patient. Ocular infections with free-living amebae are produced exclusively by *Acanthamoeba* spp. Such infections often follow trauma, particularly that associated with a foreign body. Contact lenses, particularly soft lenses, may become contaminated with *Acanthamoeba* spp. prior to insertion, and this accounts for most ocular infections.

PATHOLOGY. *Naegleria* gain access to the central nervous system through the nasal mucosa covering the cribriform plate and produce diffuse and extensive damage to the brain. Hemorrhagic necrosis of the olfactory nerves, the adjacent inferior frontal lobes, and the basilar surface of the cerebrum and cerebellum is common. Amebae mixed with neutrophils and macrophages can be found in the subarachnoid space, and in the superficial substance and small perivascular spaces of the brain. The inflammatory response in the meninges, as reflected in spinal fluid, includes the presence of a large number of polymorphonuclear leukocytes and an elevated protein level but a low glucose level. *Acanthamoeba* reach the central nervous system following hematogenous dissemination. The histopathologic findings consist of a granulomatous encephalitis with foci of hemorrhagic necrosis in the occipital, parietal, temporal, and (less often) frontal lobes. The finding of characteristic cysts with silver staining establishes the diagnosis. The upper portion of the spinal cord may be involved, and visceral lesions (lung, kidney, adrenals, etc.) are not uncommon. The inflammatory response of the meninges is minimal and reflected in the cerebrospinal fluid by lymphocytic pleocytosis, an elevated protein, and a normal or borderline low glucose level.

CLINICAL MANIFESTATIONS. Ocular infection typically involves the cornea, and the infection presents as a chronic ulcerating keratitis. This infection is often confused with herpetic keratitis; however, with most acanthamoebal infections of the eye, a characteristic radial or "ring" keratoneuritis is seen. Ocular infection with *Acanthamoeba* spp. should be suspected in all patients with a chronic ulcerating keratitis that does not respond to topical antimicrobial agents and/or corticosteroids.

Naegleria meningoencephalitis is an acute and rapidly progressive illness that presents with fever, headache, neck rigidity, vomiting, and lethargy within 5 days of exposure to fresh water. Symptoms rapidly progress during the first 24 hr with increasing lethargy, convulsions, and eventual coma. The clinical course is one of rapid deterioration and death. Although *Acanthamoeba* spp. may produce an acute meningitis similar to that observed with *Naegleria*, these organisms are more often associated with a chronic granulomatous meningoencephalitis presenting with focal neurologic manifestations (e.g., hemiplegia, aphasia, visual disturbances) in an immunodeficient or immunosuppressed individual.

DIAGNOSIS. The cerebrospinal fluid in *Naegleria* infection is similar to that observed in patients with purulent bacterial meningitis with a predominance of neutrophils, elevated protein, and an extremely low glucose concentration. The Gram stain and culture fail to reveal bacteria, but the motile amebae, often mistaken for lymphocytes, can be seen in a fresh wet-mount examination of uncentrifuged and nonrefrigerated cerebrospinal fluid. *Acanthamoeba* infection shows a cerebrospinal fluid consistent with aseptic meningitis; the amebae are not present in the cerebrospinal fluid but can be demonstrated by brain biopsy. Corneal scrapings are often diagnostic for amebic keratitis because cyst can be easily visualized in stained preparations and cultured on appropriate agar.

TREATMENT. Most cases of *Naegleria* meningoencephalitis have been fatal, and numerous amebicides have been tried unsuccessfully. Therefore, prevention by avoiding contact with contaminated water is essential. Three patients have been successfully treated with intravenous and intrathecal amphotericin B (two were simultaneously treated with oral rifampin and intravenous and intrathecal miconazole). *Acanthamoeba* are more sensitive than *Naegleria* to antimicrobial agents such as sulfanilamides, clotrimazole, and 5-fluorocytosine; amphotericin B is ineffective. Although sensitive in vitro to a number of agents, the prognosis for central nervous system disease due to *Acanthamoeba* spp. is extremely poor. Ocular infections are often treated medically and surgically. Specifically, local treatment with 5-fluorocytosine and clotrimazole may prove effective; however, corneal transplantation is often necessary.

WILLIAM T. SPECK

Darby CP, Conradi SE, Holbrook TW, et al: Primary amebic meningoencephalitis. Am J Dis Child 133:1025, 1979.
Dumar RJ, Helwig WB, Martinez AJ: Meningoencephalitis and brain abscess due to free-living amoeba. Ann Intern Med 88:468, 1978.
Parlato C, Davis JC, Cohen E, et al: Acanthamoeba keratitis associated with contact lenses—United States. MMWR 35:405, 1986.
Seidel JS, Harmatz P, Visvesvara GS, et al: Successful treatment of primary amebic meningoencephalitis. N Engl J Med 306:346, 1982.

HELMINTHS

NEMATODES
(Roundworms)

INTESTINAL NEMATODES

Infection with intestinal roundworms is the most common type of helminthiasis of humans. Although these infections are more prevalent in tropical and subtropical climates, individuals residing in temperate and cold regions are not spared. Children generally are more heavily infected than adults and are therefore more likely to suffer from the pathologic consequences of these infections. Intestinal nematodes may infect humans either directly by ingestion of mature eggs or indirectly via larval penetration of skin. With the exception of *Strongyloides stercoralis,* the adult stages of these nematodes live in the lumen of the intestinal tract and do not multiply in the human host. Although intestinal nematode infections are not usually associated with peripheral blood eosinophilia, increased eosinophil counts often develop during the phase of infection when parasite larvae migrate through host tissues. The more prevalent intestinal roundworm infections of children will be discussed according to their final location in the gut: small intestine *(Ascaris lumbricoides, Ancylostoma duodenale, Necator americanus,* and *Strongyloides stercoralis),* cecum *(Enterobius vermicularis),* and large intestine (Trichuris trichiura).

12.120 Ascariasis

Infection with *Ascaris lumbricoides* is the most prevalent human helminthiasis and produces an estimated 1 billion cases worldwide. Infection is most common in children of preschool or early school age. Ascariasis is ubiquitous; the greatest number of cases occur in countries having warmer climates. Nevertheless, there are approximately 4 million infected individuals, mainly children, in North America.

ETIOLOGY. The infective stage of *A. lumbricoides* is the mature larva-containing egg. It is broadly oval, has a thick shell with an outer mamillated covering, and measures approximately 40 × 60 μm (Fig. 12–39). Eggs are passed in the feces of infected individuals and mature in 5–10 days under favorable environmental conditions to become infective. After ingestion by the human host, larvae are released from the eggs and penetrate the intestinal wall before migrating to the lungs via the venous circulation. They then break through the pulmonary tissues into the alveolar spaces, ascend the bronchial tree and trachea, and are reswallowed. Upon their arrival in the small intestine, the larvae develop into mature adult worms (males measure 15–25 cm × 3 mm and females 25–35 cm × 4 mm). Each female has a life span of 1–2 yr and is capable of producing 200,000 eggs/day.

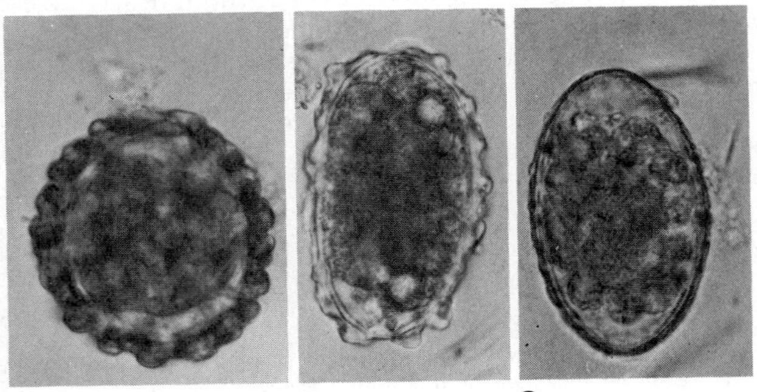

Figure 12–39. Fertilized *(A)* and unfertilized *(B, C)* eggs of *Ascaris lumbricoides* (× 400). The egg illustrated in *C* may be mistaken for that of a different nematode or of a trematode.

EPIDEMIOLOGY. Ascariasis, a soil-transmitted infection, depends on dissemination of eggs into environmental conditions that are suitable for their maturation. Promiscuous defecation and use of human manure are the two most important unhygienic practices responsible for the endemicity of ascariasis. The mode of transmission to humans is hand to mouth; the fingers are contaminated by soil contact. Alternatively, food items (particularly those commonly consumed raw) become infected by human fertilizers or by flies. Endemicity of *A. lumbricoides* is aided by the extremely high egg output of worms and their resistance to unfavorable environmental conditions. Eggs have been shown to remain infective in soil for months and may survive cooler weather (5–10° C) for 2 yr. Transmission of ascariasis may occur seasonally or throughout the year.

CLINICAL MANIFESTATIONS. Although disease sequelae occur in only a small proportion of infected individuals, they amount to a significant clinical problem because of the high incidence of ascariasis. Morbidity may be manifested during migration of the larvae through the lungs or be associated with the presence of adult worms in the small intestine. The pathogenesis of pulmonary ascariasis is not known, although a hypersensitivity phenomenon may be involved. Adult worms may cause disease by obstructing the gut or biliary tree and by affecting host nutrition. The nutritional status of children with ascariasis may be affected more by their socioeconomic and nutritional background than by the effects of the *Ascaris* infection.

Pulmonary ascariasis may occur following heavy exposure and is also common in individuals who live in areas with seasonal transmission of infection (seasonal pneumonitis). The most characteristic features are cough, blood-stained sputum, and eosinophilia. This Loeffler-like syndrome may be associated with transient pulmonary infiltrates. In children the differentiation of this syndrome from visceral larva migrans may be difficult, but abdominal symptoms or signs are very rare in pulmonary ascariasis.

The presence of adult worms in the small intestine is associated with vague complaints such as abdominal pain and distention. Intestinal obstruction, although rare, may be due to a mass of worms in heavily infected children; the peak incidence occurs in children 1–6 yr old. The onset is usually sudden with severe colicky abdominal pain and vomiting which may be bile stained; these symptoms may progress rapidly and follow a course similar to acute intestinal obstruction of any other etiology. Migration of *Ascaris* worms into the biliary tract has also been reported, particularly occurring in China and the Philippines; the likelihood of this condition increases in heavily infected children. The onset is acute with colicky abdominal pain, nausea, vomiting, and fever. Jaundice is rarely seen.

Steatorrhea and diminished vitamin A absorption have occurred in some *Ascaris*-infected children. A study of Colombian children with moderate infections (30–50 worms) showed that administration of antihelminthic drugs was followed by decreased fat and nitrogen excretion and improved xylose absorption.

DIAGNOSIS. Adult female worms deposit eggs that can be detected by direct fecal smear examination and quantified by the Kato thick smear method. Bisexual infections result in the excretion of mature fertile eggs, whereas infertile eggs are seen in individuals infected with female worms only (Fig. 12–39*B* and *C*). Diagnosis of pulmonary or obstructive ascariasis is based primarily on clinical data and a high index of suspicion.

TREATMENT. Several chemotherapeutic agents are effective against ascariasis; none, however, is useful during the pulmonary phase of the infection. Treatment, particularly of children with heavy infections, should be approached with caution. Piperazine salts (citrate, adipate, or phosphate) are administered orally in a daily dose of 50–75 mg/kg for 2 days. A single dose rather than 2-day regimens is effective in reducing worm loads in infected children. Since piperazine results in neuromuscular paralysis and a relatively rapid expulsion of the worms, it is the drug of choice for intestinal or biliary obstruction. Since sporadic hypersensitivity and neurotoxic reactions have been reported with piperazine derivatives, other drugs such as mebendazole (100 mg twice daily for 3 days) may be used for treating uncomplicated intestinal ascariasis. Rarely, surgical treatment may be needed in severe obstructive cases.

CONTROL. Although ascariasis is the most prevalent worm infection worldwide, little attention has been given to its control, partly because of controversy concerning its clinical significance and also because of its unique epidemiologic features. Attempts at reducing worm loads in humans by mass chemotherapy have shown some promise. Because of the high rate of reinfection, chemotherapy has to be repeated at 3- to 6-mo intervals. The feasibility and cost of such an undertaking will have to be evaluated before it can be widely accepted. Sanitary practices directed at treating human feces before it is used as fertilizer and providing hygienic sewage disposal facilities may be the most effective long-term preventive measures against ascariasis.

12.121 Hookworms

Three species of hookworms infect more than 900 million people: *Ancylostoma duodenale*, *Necator americanus*, and *Ancylostoma ceylanicum*. Infection is endemic in temperate, subtropical, and tropical areas of the world.

ETIOLOGY. Hookworm larvae are usually found in warm damp soil and infect the human host by penetrating the skin. Infection may also be acquired by drinking contaminated water. Larvae migrate to the venous circulation and are carried to the lungs, where they break into the alveolar spaces, migrate upward, and are then swallowed to reach their final habitat in the upper small intestine. Mature worms develop in 2–4 wk; they are grayish-white and slightly curved and measure 5–13 mm in length. The buccal cavity of *A. duodenale* has pointed, clawed teeth and that of *N. americanus* has two chitinous plates. These buccal structures help the mature worms attach to the jejunal mucosa and suck blood. In 6–9 wk worms reach sexual maturity and start to deposit eggs, which are excreted in the feces. Mature *A. duodenale* female worms produce about 30,000 eggs/day; daily egg production by *N. americanus* is 9,000. The mean life span of adult hookworms is 1–3 yr, although they may occasionally survive up to 9 yr. Hookworm eggs are ovoidal and thin-shelled and measure approximately 36 × 58 μm (Fig. 12–40). When freshly passed, these eggs contain 4 embryonic segments which mature into 1st stage larvae that hatch in 1–2 days under favorable environmental conditions. Larvae live in the soil for 1–2 wk, molt twice, and change into infective larvae capable of penetrating human skin.

EPIDEMIOLOGY. Humans are the primary host for the three species of hookworms. Endemicity of infection in any specific geographic location depends on suitability of environmental conditions for hatching of eggs and maturation of larvae, on fecal contamination of soil, and on human contact with contaminated soil. The optimal soil conditions are found in many parts of agrarian tropical countries and also in the southeastern part of the United States.

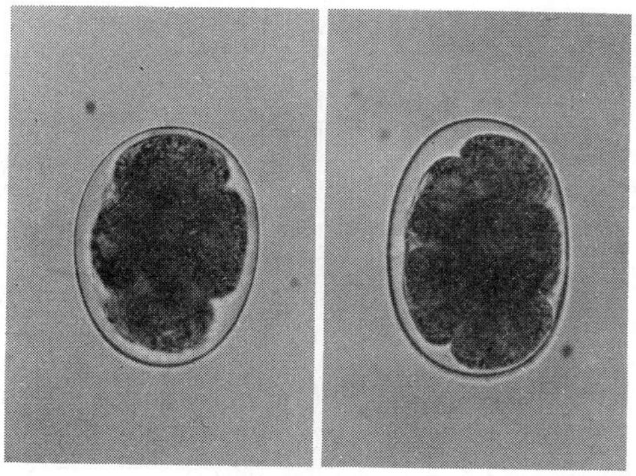

Figure 12–40. Eggs of hookworm *Necator americanus* in early cleavage as seen in freshly passed feces (× 400).

The morbidity of hookworm infections in endemic areas is sustained primarily by children. In one study half of the children were infected before age 5; 90% were infected by 9 yr of age. Intensity of infection increases up to age 6–7, then stabilizes for a few years. Newly infected children acquire a mean of 2 female worms; there is a net gain of 2.7 parasites/yr.

PATHOLOGY AND PATHOGENESIS. Several factors may contribute to the morbidity of hookworm infection; these include worm burden, diet, race, and development of immunity in chronically infected individuals. Anemia, the major pathologic manifestation of infection, is affected primarily by the worm burden and the diet of the host.

Lesions due to hookworm may occur during the migratory phase of infection or may be related to the presence of adult worms in the small intestine. Ground itch or dermatitis results from larval invasion of skin and the subsequent inflammatory response. Mild pulmonary lesions similar to those described in ascariasis may occur during lung migration of larvae; it is questionable whether a Loeffler-like syndrome occurs. The presence of adult worms in the small intestine results in anemia and hypoalbuminemia. The severity of hookworm anemia is related to the intensity of infection and the host's iron balance. Blood loss varies with hookworm species; *A. duodenale* infection causes greater losses than *N. americanus*.

CLINICAL MANIFESTATIONS. Infections are usually asymptomatic; significant clinical disease occurs in a small percentage of children in whom symptoms follow the chronologic order of worm migration in the host. Exposure of skin for the first time to infective larvae may lead to pruritus. Skin reactions vary from erythematous papules on primary exposure, which disappear within 1 wk, to vesiculation and generalized edema on subsequent infections, which may last 1–3 wk. Migration of the larvae through the lungs is associated with few, if any, specific symptoms or signs.

Symptoms of abdominal pain, loss of appetite, indigestion, postprandial fullness, and diarrhea have been attributed to the intestinal phase of hookworm infection. These clinical correlates are based primarily on observations of experimental infections in volunteers with heavy worm loads rather than on adequate studies of specific abdominal symptoms in natural hookworm infections. The significant disease sequelae of chronic hookworm infections include anemia, hypoalbuminemia, and edema. Hemoglobin concentrations under 5 g/dL have been associated with heart failure and sudden death. Hypoalbuminemia in excess of that anticipated from whole blood loss may also occur; the attendant decrease in plasma oncotic pressure may lead to edema.

DIAGNOSIS. Direct examination of fecal smears for hookworm eggs provides a qualitative assessment of infection. The Kato thick smear offers a simple technique for quantitation of infection, but since hookworm eggs disappear within 1 hr of preparation, prompt examination of these smears is mandatory. Eggs of *A. duodenale* and *N. americanus* are morphologically indistinguishable; the only way to differentiate the species is to allow the eggs to hatch and examine the released larvae.

TREATMENT. Evaluation of intensity of infection and severity of anemia should precede therapy. In children with severe anemia (hemoglobin concentration under 5 g/dL) iron therapy should be given before antihelminthic drugs. Elemental iron is administered orally at a dosage of 2 mg/kg 3 times/day until anemia is corrected. In life-threatening anemia with signs of heart failure, diuretics followed by slow transfusion of packed red cells may be indicated. Mebendazole (100 mg orally twice a day for 2 days) or tetrachlorethylene (0.1 mL/kg repeated at 4 and 8 day intervals) will eradicate or reduce the hookworm load.

CONTROL. Eradication or control of hookworm infection depends on sanitation and mass chemotherapy. To allow cost-effective application of these two principles, the rate of worm acquisition, its life span, and the rate at which infection is lost have to be determined. Seasonal variations in transmission and the hookworm species must also be taken into consideration. Eradication has been achieved in the southeast United States.

12.122 Strongyloidiasis

Infection with the nematode *Strongyloides stercoralis,* unlike that with other worms, may cause autoinfection with massive parasite invasion of the host and eventual death. This complication is more frequent in malnourished or immunosuppressed children. *S. stercoralis* infection is widely distributed throughout tropical and temperate regions, though it is less common than infection by other intestinal roundworms.

ETIOLOGY. Infected individuals pass larvae in their stools; these parasites may develop into free-living adults in the soil or change into infective filariform larvae. These latter forms penetrate human skin, pass via the bloodstream to the lungs, and follow a pathway similar to hookworm and *Ascaris* larvae until they reach their final habitat in the upper small intestine. Mature worms (2.2 mm in length) burrow into the intestinal mucosa and begin releasing eggs approximately 4 wk after infection. *S. stercoralis* eggs hatch rapidly, and small larvae (225×16 μm) are passed in feces. The larvae must undergo morphologic changes in soil to become infective, but these changes may also be accomplished as the parasites are being discharged from the body. Larvae are then capable of infecting the same individual by penetrating the intestinal wall or perianal skin. This unique feature of the *Strongyloides* life cycle allows the parasite to survive for many years inside the same host and occasionally to cause overwhelming infection.

EPIDEMIOLOGY. Humans are the primary hosts of *S. stercoralis.* Transmission of infection and its endemicity depend on suitable soil and climatic conditions and poor sanitary habits. Close contact and poor personal hygiene may be important, since the prevalence of infection is much higher in institutions for the mentally retarded. Host factors such as nutrition and immune status may play a crucial role in the development of the hyperinfection syndrome.

PATHOLOGY AND PATHOGENESIS. The initial penetration of skin by infective larvae usually produces no apparent pathologic lesions. Repeated skin invasion may, however, result in dermatitis; in cases in which autoinfection is established through the skin, a more extensive skin lesion, *larva currens,* may occur. A Loeffler-like syndrome with eosinophilia may be seen during migration of the larvae through the lungs. Eosinophilia may also occur when adult worms burrow into the intestinal mucosa. *Disseminated strongyloidiasis* is a complex pathologic entity due to larval invasion of internal organs and inducing polymicrobial gram-negative bacteremia.

CLINICAL MANIFESTATIONS. Signs and symptoms of strongyloidiasis occur in only a small percentage of infected individuals or in those with the hyperinfection syndrome. Pulmonary symptoms and skin lesions are usually mild and generally pass unnoticed. Pruritus with a papular erythematous rash may occur. *Larva currens,* a condition due to repeated skin invasion by larvae, is characterized by large erythematous urticarial lesions with rapidly moving edges. These are usually localized to an area within 30 cm of the anus and have a tendency to recur. The typical symptoms, which include abdominal pain, vomiting, and diarrhea, are caused by adult worms in the upper small intestine. These symptoms occur with uncertain frequency and may have an abrupt onset with periodic recurrences. Abdominal pain is often epigastric and may be burning, colicky, or dull in nature. Diarrhea with passage of mucus may alternate with periods of constipation. *Chronic strongyloidiasis* may result in a malabsorption-like syndrome with protein-losing enteropathy and weight loss. Blood eosinophilia is usually associated with and is often the only indication of the intestinal phase of infection.

Disseminated strongyloidiasis occurs in children with predisposing factors such as malnutrition or defects in cell-mediated immunity (lymphomas, Hodgkin disease, etc.). The onset is usually sudden, with generalized abdominal pain, distention, fever, and shock due to gram-negative septicemia. Massive invasion of internal organs by the parasite larvae causes extensive tissue destruction. Although leukocytosis may occur in these patients, eosinophilia is often absent.

DIAGNOSIS. Intestinal strongyloidiasis is diagnosed by examining feces or duodenal fluid for the characteristic larvae. Several stool samples should be examined either by direct smear or by a concentration method such as formaldehyde-ether or that of Baermann. Alternatively, duodenal fluid obtained by the pediatric Enterotest or aspiration may provide samples for definitive diagnosis. In children with hyperinfection syndrome, larvae may be found in sputum, gastric aspirates, or, rarely, in small intestinal biopsies. Strongyloidiasis should also be suspected in immunosuppressed patients who suddenly develop signs and symptoms consistent with disseminated infection. A recently described serologic test for *Strongyloides* antibodies may be more sensitive than parasitologic methods for diagnosing intestinal infection, but the utility of this assay in the hyperinfection syndrome has not been determined.

TREATMENT. The only available and effective therapeutic agent is thiabendazole. Treatment of infected children should aim at eradication of infection, and therefore subsequent stool examination is essential. Thiabendazole is administered orally in a dose of 25 mg/kg twice daily for 3 days. Courses of up to 2 wk may be needed in those with the hyperinfection syndrome.

CONTROL. Sanitary practices designed to prevent soil and person-to-person transmission are the most effective control measures. Because the infection is uncommon, case detection and treatment are also advised. Individuals who will be subjected to immunosuppressive therapy should have a screening examination for *S. stercoralis* and, if infected, be treated with thiabendazole.

12.123 Enterobiasis

(Pinworm)

Enterobius vermicularis infection occurs worldwide and affects individuals of all ages and socioeconomic levels but is especially common in children. Living in congested districts, institutions, or families with pinworm infections predisposes to enterobiasis. The infection is essentially harmless and causes more social than medical problems in affected children and their families.

ETIOLOGY. Humans are infected by ingesting embryonated eggs which are usually carried on fingernails, clothing, bedding, or house dust. Eggs hatch in the stomach and larvae migrate to the cecal region where they mature into adult worms. *E. vermicularis* are small (1 cm) white worms; the gravid females migrate by night to the perianal region to deposit masses of eggs. Pinworm ova are asymmetric, are flattened on one side, and measure 30 × 60 μm (Fig. 12–41). After a 6-hr maturation period a single-coiled larva can be seen within each ovum. These larvae may remain viable for 20 days.

EPIDEMIOLOGY. Perianal irritation during oviposition by female worms induces scratching. Eggs carried under the fingernails are transmitted directly or disseminated in the environment to infect others. Man is the only natural host of *E. vermicularis*. The prevalence and intensity of infection are low in infants and young children and reach a peak in the 5–14-yr-old age group; the prevalence decreases in adulthood because of either reduced exposure or acquisition of immunity.

CLINICAL MANIFESTATIONS. Many local and systemic signs and symptoms have been ascribed to *Enterobius* infection; however, a controlled study of infected children 2–12 yr old failed to document specific syndromes due to *E. vermicularis*. Symptomatic individuals most commonly complain of nocturnal anal pruritus and sleeplessness. The etiology and incidence of perianal and perineal irritation are unknown but may be related to the intensity of infection, to the psychiatric profile of the infected individual and his or her family, or to an allergic reaction to the parasite. Since tissue invasion does not occur in most cases of enterobiasis, eosinophilia is not observed. In a few cases, however, *E. vermicularis* has been recovered from ectopic sites such as the appendix, female genital tract, and peritoneal cavity.

DIAGNOSIS. Definitive diagnosis is established by either finding the parasite eggs or recovering worms. Eggs can be easily detected on adhesive cellophane tape pressed against the perianal region early in the morning. Repeated examinations may be necessary, and in certain situations examination of all family members may be advised. If a worm is seen in the perianal region, it should be preserved in 75% ethyl alcohol until microscopic examination can be performed.

TREATMENT. Drug therapy should be given to all infected and symptomatic individuals; mebendazole (single oral dose of 100 mg for all ages) is recommended. Piperazine salts or pyrvinium pamoate may also be used. Repeated treatments every 3–4 mo may be required in situations in which exposure is constant, for example, in children in institutions. While personal cleanliness is a useful general recommendation, there is no proof that it plays a significant role in control of enterobiasis.

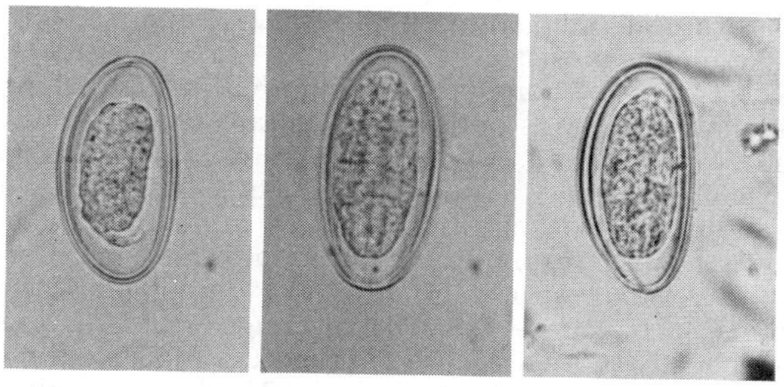

Figure 12–41. Eggs of *Enterobius vermicularis* in early developmental stages recovered from feces (× 400). One side of the shell is somewhat flat, but when viewed from above (center) it appears to be symmetric and may be mistaken for a different species. When found in human feces, which is unusual, pinworm eggs contain a tadpole-stage embryo, whereas eggs recovered on a perianal swab contain a coiled larva that is more than twice the length of the egg.

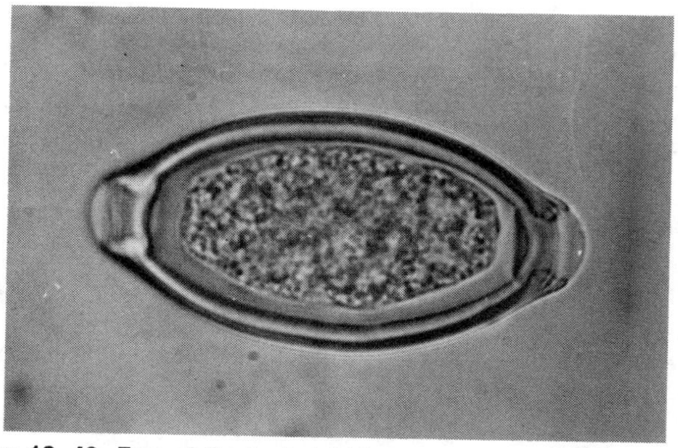

Figure 12–42. Egg of *Trichuris trichiura*, as seen in freshly passed feces (× 1,000).

12.124 Trichuriasis

Trichuris trichiura causes one of the most common worm infections of humans; approximately half a billion cases occur worldwide. Infection is more common in warm climates, but it does exist in North America.

ETIOLOGY. Infection is due to ingesting mature parasite eggs (Fig. 12–42), which are passed in the stools of infected individuals and mature in 2–4 wk if moisture and temperature conditions of the soil are optimal. Upon ingestion by man, *Trichuris* eggs hatch, and larvae penetrate the small intestinal villi where they remain for 3–10 days before slowly moving down the bowel and maturing into adult worms. The final habitats of *T. trichiura* are the cecum and ascending colon. The body is divided into an anterior whip-like portion (hence the term whipworm) and a posterior bulky part and measures approximately 40 mm in length. The worms remain in the gut by anchoring the anterior portion of their body to the intestinal mucosa. Egg deposition by maturing females begins 1–3 mo after infection.

EPIDEMIOLOGY. Trichuriasis is most common in poor rural communities lacking sanitary facilities. Man is the primary host; the highest prevalence and intensity of infection occur in children. Transmission of embryonated eggs occurs by contamination of hands, food, or drink. Eggs may also be carried by flies and other insects.

CLINICAL MANIFESTATIONS. Most infected individuals are asymptomatic; however, vague abdominal complaints, colic, and abdominal distention have been associated with infection. Adult *Trichuris* suck approximately 0.005 mL of blood/worm/day. However, only heavy childhood infections produce mild anemia, bloody diarrhea, or, rarely, rectal prolapse. These cases are referred to as massive infantile trichuriasis and are often associated with shigellosis and protozoan infections of the gastrointestinal tract.

DIAGNOSIS AND TREATMENT. Examination of stool smears reveals the characteristic eggs of *T. trichiura*. An oral course of mebendazole (100 mg twice a day for 3 days) produces a cure rate of 70–90% and reduces egg output by 90–99%.

JAMES W. KAZURA
ADEL A. F. MAHMOUD

ASCARIASIS

Louw JH: Abdominal complications of *Ascaris lumbricoides* infestation in children. Br J Surg 53:510, 1966.

Pawlowski ZS: Ascariasis. *In*: Warren KS, Mahmoud AAF (eds): Tropical and Geographical Medicine. New York, McGraw-Hill, 1990, p 369.

Spillman RK: Pulmonary ascariasis in tropical communities. Am J Trop Med Hyg 24:791, 1975.

Stephenson LS, Crompton DWT, Latham MC, et al: Relationship between *Ascaris* infection and growth of malnourished preschool children in Kenya. Am J Clin Nutr 33:1165, 1980.

HOOKWORMS

Miller TA: Hookworm infection in man. Adv Parasitol 17:315, 1979.

Nawalinski T, Schad GA, Chowdhury AB: Population biology of hookworms in children in rural West Bengal. I: General parasitological observations. Am J Trop Med Hyg 27:1152, 1978.

Nawalinski T, Schad GA, Chowdhury AB: Population biology of hookworms in children in rural West Bengal. II. Acquisition and loss of hookworms. Am J Trop Med Hyg 27:1162, 1978.

STRONGYLOIDIASIS

Burke JA: Strongyloidiasis in childhood. Am J Dis Child 132:1130, 1978.

Grove DI, Blair AJ: Diagnosis of human strongyloidiasis by immunofluorescence using *S. ratti* and *S. stercoralis* larvae. Am J Trop Med Hyg 30:344, 1981.

Scowden EB, Schaffner W, Stone WJ: Overwhelming strongyloidiasis. Medicine 57:527, 1978.

Smith JD, Goette DK, Odom RB: Larva currens: Cutaneous strongyloidiasis. Arch Dermatol 112:1161, 1976.

ENTEROBIASIS

Boyer A, Berdknikoff IK: Pinworm infestation in children; the problem and its management. Can Med Assoc J 86:60, 1962.

Weller TH, Sorensen CW: Enterobiasis: Its incidence and symptomatology in a group of 505 children. N Engl J Med 224:131, 1941.

TRICHURIASIS

Blumenthal DS: Intestinal nematodes in the United States. N Engl J Med 297:1437, 1977.

Jung RC, Beaver PC: Clinical observations on *Trichocephalus trichiurus* (whipworm) infestation in children. Pediatrics 8:548, 1951.

TISSUE NEMATODES

Tissue-dwelling nematodes infect over 800 million people worldwide. Although morbidity from these helminths primarily afflicts the populations of tropical and developing countries, inhabitants of regions with temperate climates may also be affected. These parasites have a complex life cycle which in most instances includes an intermediate invertebrate host. Childhood disease results mainly when children act either as an incidental host in whom the helminth does not undergo its normal development (*Toxocara* sp., *Dirofilaria* sp.) or as the definitive host (filariae, *Dracunculus medinensis*). Infections that are particularly common in childhood (visceral larval migrans) will be discussed first, followed by a discussion of tissue nematodes that cause disease in individuals of all ages (cutaneous larva migrans, *Trichinella spiralis, D. medinensis*) or primarily in adults (human and animal filariae).

12.125 Visceral Larva Migrans
(Toxocariasis)

Visceral larva migrans is caused by infection with larvae of *Toxocara* sp. It occurs most frequently in children under the age of 10 yr and is characterized by fever, hepatomegaly, pulmonary disease, and eosinophilia.

ETIOLOGY. *Toxocara canis, T. cati*, and *T. leonina* are common parasites of dogs and cats that infect humans when the eggs of the helminth are ingested. Adult worms of *Toxocara* sp. reside in the gastrointestinal tract of dogs and cats and release large numbers of eggs, which are passed in the feces. Ingestion of eggs by man is followed by larval penetration of the gastrointestinal tract and migration to liver, lung, and occasionally other sites (central nervous system, eye, kidney, and heart). *Toxocara* larvae do not develop beyond this stage in the human host.

EPIDEMIOLOGY. Visceral larva migrans is most common in children 1–4 yr of age, particularly those who engage in pica and have close contact with dogs and cats; ocular toxocariasis occurs most frequently in older children. Potential sources of infection are widely distributed in the canine and feline population (an estimated 20% of dogs in the United States excrete *Toxocara* eggs). These animals often defecate in areas where children play (24% of 800 soil samples taken from public parks in Great Britain were found to contain *Toxocara* eggs).

PATHOLOGY. *Toxocara* larvae usually elicit a granulomatous response characterized by large numbers of eosinophils, mononuclear cells, and tissue necrosis. These lesions are found in liver, lung, and other organs through which the helminth migrates. The inflammatory reaction is much less intense in the eye, where lesions consist mainly of mononuclear cells and a few eosinophils.

CLINICAL MANIFESTATIONS. Major symptoms include fever (80%), cough with wheezing (60–80%), and seizures (20–30%). Respiratory distress may be severe enough to warrant hospitalization. Abdominal pain has been noted in occasional patients. Physical findings include hepatomegaly (65–87%), rales and/or rhonchi (40–50%), papular or urticarial skin lesions (20%), and lymph node enlargement (8%). These manifestations subside over a period of several months. Scattered patchy infiltrates are often seen on chest roentgenograms.

Patients with ocular toxocariasis most commonly present with decreased visual acuity (in 75% of cases) and occasionally with strabismus or periorbital edema. In one study unilateral blindness was noted in 6 of 17 patients. Most children do not have concurrent signs and symptoms of visceral disease. Funduscopic examination of the eye usually reveals solitary granulomatous lesions situated in the retina near the optic disc or macula. These may be mistaken for retinoblastomas and have led to inappropriate enucleation. Peripheral retinal lesions with vitreous bands and involvement of the iris have been documented in a few cases.

DIAGNOSIS. The diagnosis is made on the basis of the clinical manifestations and serologic testing. The only reliable and specific test is an enzyme-linked immunosorbent assay (ELISA), which utilizes infective eggs of *T. canis* as antigen. This assay is positive (serum antibody titer $\geq$ 1:32) in 78% of cases of visceral larva migrans and in 45% of individuals with a clinical diagnosis of ocular toxocariasis. Eosinophilia ($>500/mm^3$ blood) occurs in nearly all subjects with the visceral syndrome but is much less common in those with ocular disease. Nonspecific findings include elevations in serum gamma globulins and isohemagglutinins. Although larvae may be found upon examination of tissue sections, biopsy of liver or other organs is generally not indicated because clinical and laboratory data provide enough evidence to make the diagnosis.

TREATMENT. Therapy is not required in the majority of cases, since the signs and symptoms are usually mild and subside over a period of weeks to months. When significant hypoxemia secondary to pulmonary disease occurs, however, the administration of anti-inflammatory drugs (prednisone, 5 mg/kg/24 hr until respiratory function improves) is beneficial. When disease is severe or when larvae lodge in critical locations, such as the eye, the use of drugs exhibiting possible larvicidal activity (diethylcarbamazine, 0.5 mg/kg/24 hr for 3 days, increased gradually to 3 mg/kg/24 hr for 21 days) has been advocated. There is disagreement about this approach, however, since dying larvae theoretically may incite an inflammatory response which produces more tissue damage than encapsulated, dormant parasites.

CONTROL. Transmission of infection may be prevented by requiring children to wash their hands after playing with pets and instructing them to avoid areas where these animals defecate, particularly children with the habit of pica. Periodic deworming of dogs, especially puppies below the age of 6 mo, also decreases the likelihood of infection.

12.126 Cutaneous Larva Migrans

(Creeping Eruption)

Cutaneous larva migrans is caused by several larval nematodes not usually parasitic for man. *Ancylostoma braziliense* (a hookworm of dogs and cats) is the most common of these helminths, but other animal hookworms *(A. caninum, Uncinaria stenocephala,* and *Bunostomum phlebotosum)* and human parasites *(Necator americanus, Ancylostoma duodenale,* and *Strongyloides stercoralis)* may produce the disease. These organisms are widely distributed throughout tropical and subtropical areas of the world. In the United States infections are most prevalent in the South. Parasite eggs are deposited in the feces of animals and hatch to form infective larvae in warm moist areas, such as near vegetation on beaches or under porches. Man is infected when the skin comes in contact with these larvae.

CLINICAL MANIFESTATIONS. After penetrating the skin, larvae localize at the epidermal-dermal junction and migrate in this plane, moving at a rate of 1–2 cm/day. The response to the parasite is characterized by raised, erythematous, serpiginous tracks which occasionally form bullae (Fig. 12–43 [color plate section]). These lesions may be single or multiple and are usually localized to an extremity, although any area of the body may be affected. As the organism migrates, new areas of involvement may appear every few days. Intense localized pruritus may be associated with the lesions.

DIAGNOSIS AND TREATMENT. Cutaneous larva migrans is diagnosed by clinical examination of the skin. Patients are often able to recall the exact time and location of exposure because the larvae produce intense itching at the site of penetration. If left untreated, the larvae die, and the syndrome resolves within a few weeks to several months. Topical application of thiabendazole oral suspension or a 0.5-g tablet triturated with 5 g petroleum jelly may be used if symptoms warrant treatment.

12.127 Trichinosis

Human infection with *Trichinella spiralis* is fairly common worldwide. Infection is transmitted by ingestion of pork or other meat carrying the parasite. Sporadic epidemics have occurred in North America following ingestion of bear meat.

ETIOLOGY. Humans are infected by eating flesh contaminated with viable *T. spiralis* larvae. This stage of the parasite excysts in the stomach and matures to form adult worms within the small intestine. Female *T. spiralis* release large numbers of newborn larvae, which penetrate the gut wall and migrate to striated muscles or occasionally to other sites such as the central nervous system and heart. Larvae that enter muscle cells eventually become encysted and may remain viable for years. The life cycle in nature is maintained by hogs or other animals that ingest garbage containing carcasses of infected rodents.

EPIDEMIOLOGY. *T. spiralis* is found in all areas of the world except Australia and some islands in the South Pacific. Although infection was common in the United States in the past (4% of diaphragms examined post mortem in 1968 contained viable larvae), recent cases have been related to outbreaks resulting from ingestion of undercooked homemade sausage, other pork products, or meat of bears, wild pigs, and walruses. Larvae are destroyed by cooking meat until there is no trace of pink fluid or flesh (this occurs at 55° C) or by storage in a freezer at −15° C for 3 wk. Smoked or salted meat may still contain viable parasites.

PATHOLOGY AND PATHOGENESIS. Adult worms localize in the upper gastrointestinal tract and induce a mucosal inflammatory reaction characterized by a reduced villous-crypt ratio and the presence of eosinophils, neutrophils, and mononuclear cells. This response peaks within the 1st wk of infection, then gradually subsides as adult worms are expelled. In muscle cells migrating larvae elicit a reaction consisting of large numbers of eosinophils and mononuclear cells. These lesions may eventually calcify.

CLINICAL MANIFESTATIONS. The signs and symptoms appear only in heavily infected individuals. Within the 1st wk adult worms in the upper gastrointestinal tract produce gastroenteritis and diarrhea associated with abdominal discomfort. Next, during larval invasion of muscle, periorbital or facial edema (80% of cases), and myalgias occur. Pain is associated with muscle activity; it is most common in the masseters, diaphragm, and intercostals. These signs and symptoms are first noted 10–14 days after infection and last for another 2–3 wk. Heart failure and arrhythmias may occur in patients with exceptionally heavy infestation.

DIAGNOSIS. Periorbital edema, myalgias, fever, and eosinophilia in an individual who gives a history of eating undercooked meat make the diagnosis of trichinosis likely. A history of similar illness in those sharing the food should be sought. Serologic studies such as the bentonite flocculation test (titer of 1:5 or greater) are confirmatory. Biopsy of muscle, usually the deltoid, may reveal larvae upon microscopic examination 3–4 wk after infection. Muscle enzymes such as creatine kinase and lactate dehydrogenase are elevated in 50% of patients.

TREATMENT. There is no clinically established therapy for the syndrome related to larval invasion of muscles. Thiabendazole (25 mg/kg/24 hr for 1 wk) is active primarily against adult worms and should therefore be given only to those individuals who are known to have acquired the infection in the preceding 1–7 days. Corticosteroids may be used in critically ill patients, such as those with myocarditis or central nervous system damage, but evidence of their beneficial effect is equivocal.

12.128 Dracunculiasis

(Guinea Worm Infection)

Dracunculiasis occurs in all areas of the tropics and is especially common in India and West Africa. The parasite, *Dracunculus medinensis,* infects man when he swallows larva-containing microscopic crustaceans (copepods) living in communal water sites. Adult worms grow to a length of 1 m or more and migrate through the subcutaneous tissues of the lower extremities (or occasionally other sites). An ulcer is produced where they penetrate the skin. The diagnosis is confirmed by identifying larvae contained in washings from the base of the lesion. Administering niridazole (12.5 mg/kg/24 hr for 10 days) or thiabendazole (50 mg/kg/24 hr for 3 days) diminishes the local inflammatory response and permits removal of the helminth. Infection may be prevented by avoiding ingestion of water that humans walk in or use for bathing. Boiling or chlorination kills the organism.

Filariases

Filariae are thread-like nematodes that may cause significant human morbidity. Disease due to infection with these organisms usually becomes evident years after exposure; it is thus uncommon for children to have clinically significant filariasis.

12.129 MALAYAN AND BANCROFTIAN FILARIASIS

Infection with *Brugia malayi, Brugia timori,* or *Wuchereria bancrofti* results in similar clinical syndromes characterized in the early stages by acute lymphangitis and lymphadenitis and later by lymphatic obstruction with hydrocele and elephantiasis. Over 200 million people in developing countries may be infected with these parasites.

ETIOLOGY. Filarial larvae are introduced into humans in secretions of biting mosquitoes. Over months to a year this stage of the helminth develops into adult worms that reside in the lymphatics. Sexually mature adult female worms release large numbers of microfilariae that circulate in the bloodstream. The life cycle of the parasite is completed when mosquitoes ingest these organisms in a blood meal.

EPIDEMIOLOGY. Although as much as 80% of the population of endemic areas may be infected, fewer than 10–20% have clinically significant morbidity. Those who work in areas where there is repeated and chronic exposure to larvae-containing mosquitoes, such as in crowded urban areas with poor sanitation, are most at risk. *W. bancrofti* infection is distributed throughout tropical and subtropical Africa, Asia, and South America, whereas infection with *B. malayi* is restricted to the South Pacific and Southeast Asia. *B. timori* infection occurs in Indonesia.

CLINICAL MANIFESTATIONS. The acute stage of infection is characterized by episodes of fever, lymphangitis of an extremity, headaches, and myalgias which last a few days to several weeks. This syndrome is most frequently observed in young people 10–20 yr old. Chronic manifestations of disease, such as hydrocele and elephantiasis, occur mostly in those over 30 yr old and are a direct result of lymphatic fibrosis and obstruction to lymph flow. The presence of larvae (microfilariae) in the blood is not thought to have any pathologic consequences, except in persons with tropical pulmonary eosinophilia.

DIAGNOSIS AND TREATMENT. Demonstrating microfilariae in the blood is the only way to diagnose lymphatic-dwelling filariasis. Two mL of blood obtained at a time of day when the number of parasites in the circulation is expected to be highest (this varies with the geographic strain of filaria) should be filtered and examined for the organisms.

The use of antifilarial drugs must be individualized. Older patients with chronic lymphatic obstruction and those who remain in endemic areas will not benefit from specific therapy. Younger individuals with acute lymphangitis should be given a course of diethylcarbamazine (50 mg on day 1, 50 mg 2 and 3 times on days 2 and 3, respectively, then 10 mg/kg on days 4–21). Recent studies indicate that a single dose of ivermectin is as effective as diethylcarbamazine in lowering microfilaremia.

12.130 ONCHOCERCIASIS, LOIASIS, AND TROPICAL PULMONARY EOSINOPHILIA

Infection with *Onchocerca volvulus* (onchocerciasis, river blindness) is a major cause of blindness in West Africa and Central America. The parasite is introduced into humans by blackflies of the genus *Simulium*, which breed in rapidly running water; people who live or work near waterways are thus most likely to be infected. Most individuals are asymptomatic; those with chronic and heavy infections (usually men over 30 yr old) may suffer from pruritic dermatitis and eye disease (punctate keratitis, corneal pannus formation, chorioretinitis) owing to the presence of microfilariae in subcutaneous and ocular tissues. Firm, nontender subcutaneous nodules containing adult parasites may also be palpable. *O. volvulus* infection is diagnosed by demonstration of parasites in skin snips removed from the buttocks or extremities or by visualization with a slit lamp of microfilariae in the cornea or anterior chamber of the eye. Children with symptomatic skin and/or eye disease should be treated with ivermectin (150 μg/kg as a single dose). The drug should not be given to persons with disorders of the central nervous system. The safety of the drug in children less than 5 yr old has not been established.

Loa loa infection occurs in the rain forests of West and Central Africa; the parasite is transmitted to humans by tabanid flies. Adult worms migrate in the subcutaneous tissues and produce painful transient areas of localized edema known as calabar swellings, which tend to appear around the joints of the legs and arms. The parasite occasionally may be directly visualized in the conjunctiva, where it produces an intense inflammatory reaction. Microfilariae are present in highest concentrations in the peripheral circulation between 10 AM and 2 PM; identification in blood samples is diagnostic. Symptomatic individuals should be given gradually increasing doses of diethylcarbamazine as described for lymphatic filariasis (Sec. 12.129). Therapy should be discontinued and corticosteroids administered if fever, headache, or joint swelling occurs.

Tropical pulmonary eosinophilia (TPE) is a syndrome of filarial etiology in which microfilariae can be found in the lung and lymph nodes. It occurs only in subjects who have lived for at least several months in endemic areas of bancroftian or Malayan filariasis and is most common in Southeast Asia and the South Pacific. Although TPE has been observed in children, 20- to 30-yr-old men are most likely to be affected. Patients present with paroxysmal nonproductive cough, occasional episodes of dyspnea, fever, weight loss, and fatigue. Rales and rhonchi are found on auscultation of the chest; roentgenographic examination may occasionally be normal but usually reveals increased bronchovascular markings, discrete opacities in the middle and basal regions of the lung, or diffuse miliary lesions. Recurrent untreated episodes may result in interstitial fibrosis and chronic respiratory insufficiency. In children hepatosplenomegaly and generalized lymphadenopathy are often seen. Eosinophilia (>2,000/mm^3 blood) with the appropriate history and symptoms suggests the diagnosis. Increased serum IgE levels (>1,000 units/mL) and high titers of antimicrofilarial antibodies in the absence of blood-borne helminths should also be documented. Although microfilariae may be found in sections of lung or lymph node, biopsy is unwarranted in most patients. The clinical response to diethylcarbamazine (5 mg/kg/24 hr for 10 days) is the final criterion for diagnosis because in the majority of patients symptoms improve with this therapy. If they recur, a second course of the drug should be administered. Subjects presenting with chronic symptoms are less likely to show improvement than those who have been ill for a short time.

12.131 INFECTION WITH ANIMAL FILARIAE

Humans may be infected with three types of animal filariae. *Dirofilaria immitis*, the heartworm, is found on all continents and is a common parasite of dogs in many parts of the United States. *D. tenuis, Brugia beaveri*, and other unclassified *Brugia* sp. have also been reported to infect man. These worms may be introduced into man by the bite of mosquitoes containing 3rd-stage larvae. The organisms, however, do not undergo normal development in the human host. *D. immitis* are trapped in the lung parenchyma after migrating for several months in the subcutaneous tissues. The pulmonary response consists of granulomas with eosinophils, neutrophils, and tissue necrosis. *D. tenuis* does not leave the subcutaneous tissues, while *B. beaveri* eventually localizes to superficial lymph nodes.

Most human infections with *D. immitis* are discovered incidentally when the chest roentgenogram reveals a solitary pulmonary nodule 1–3 cm in diameter. Definitive diagnosis and cure depend on surgical excision and identification of the nematode within the surrounding granulomatous response. *D. tenuis* and *B. beaveri* infections present as painful, rubbery 1- to 5-cm diameter nodules in the skin of the trunk, extremities, and orbit. Patients often report having been engaged in activities suggestive of exposure to infected mosquitoes, such as working in swampy areas. Diagnosis and management of these infections are similar to those of *D. immitis*.

JAMES W. KAZURA

TOXOCARIASIS

Glickman LT: Toxocariasis and related syndromes. *In*: Warren KS, Mahmoud AAf (eds): Tropical and Geographical Medicine. New York, McGraw-Hill, 1990, p 446.

Huntley CC, Costas MC, Lyerly A: Visceral larva migrans syndrome: Clinical characteristics and immunologic studies in 51 patients. Pediatrics 36:623, 1965.

Kumaraswami V, O'Hesen EA, Vijayassekeran V, et al: Ivermectin for treatment of *Wuchereria bancrofti* filariasis: Efficacy and adverse reactions. JAMA 259:3150, 1988.

Schantz PM, Glickman LT: Toxocaral visceral larva migrans. N Engl J Med 298:436, 1978.

White AT, Newland HS, Taylor HR, et al: Controlled trial and dose finding study of ivermectin for treatment of onchocerciasis. J Infect Dis 156:463, 1987.

Zinkham WH: Visceral larva migrans. A review and reassessment indicating two forms of clinical expression: Visceral and ocular. Am J Dis Child 132:627, 1978.

TREMATODES
(Flukes)

Parasitic trematodes form a group of important human infections that are endemic worldwide but are more prevalent in the less developed parts of the world. Trematodes are characterized by their complex life cycle; sexual reproduction of adult worms in the definitive host is followed by asexual multiplication by the larval stages in the intermediate host. This "alternation of generations" requires that flukes parasitize more than one host (often three) to complete their life cycle.

BLOOD FLUKES

12.132 Schistosomes

Five schistosome species infect humans; these are *Schistosoma haematobium, S. mansoni, S. japonicum, S. intercalatum,* and *S. mekongi*. Schistosomiasis infects more than 200 million people, mainly children and young adults. With the necessity of developing irrigation projects, the infection is spreading as more suitable habitats for the snail intermediate host are created. *S. haematobium* is prevalent in Africa and the Middle East; *S. mansoni* in Africa, the Middle East, Caribbean, and South America; and *S. japonicum* in China, the Philippines, and Indonesia, with some sporadic foci in parts of Southeast Asia. The other two less prevalent species are found in the Far East *(S. mekongi)* and West and Central Africa *(S. intercalatum)*.

ETIOLOGY. Humans are infected upon contact with water contaminated with cercariae, the infective forms of the parasite. These motile, forked-tail organisms emerge from infected snails and are capable of penetrating intact human skin within a few minutes. In the subcutaneous tissues cercariae change into another larval stage (schistosomula) and migrate to the lungs and finally the liver. Once they reach sexual maturation, adult worms migrate to specific anatomic sites characteristic of each schistosome species: *S. haematobium* adults are found in the vesical plexus, *S. mansoni* in the inferior mesenteric, and *S. japonicum* in the superior mesenteric veins. *S. intercalatum* and *S. mekongi* are found in the mesenteric vessels. Adult schistosome worms (1–2 cm in length) are different from most other flukes in that they exist as separate sexes; the female, however, accompanies the male in a groove formed by the lateral edges of its body. Upon fertilization, female worms begin oviposition in the small venous tributaries. The eggs of the three main schistosome species have characteristic morphologic features: *S. haematobium*, terminal spine; *S. mansoni*, lateral spine; and *S. japonicum*, smaller size with a short curved spine (Fig. 12–44). Eggs reach the lumen of urinary tract or intestines and are carried to the outside environment, where they hatch if deposited in fresh water. Motile miracidia emerge; they infect specific fresh water snail intermediate hosts and divide asexually. In 4–6 wk the infective cercariae are released in the water.

EPIDEMIOLOGY. Humans are the definitive host for the five clinically important species of schistosomes, although *S. japonicum* may infect some animals such as dogs and cattle. Transmission depends on disposal of excreta, the presence of specific intermediate snail hosts, and the patterns of water contact and social habits of the population. The distribution of infection in endemic areas shows that prevalence increases with age to a maximum in the 10- to 20-yr age group. Furthermore, measuring intensity of infection (by egg count in urine or feces) demonstrates that heavy worm loads are usually found in the younger age groups. Schistosomiasis, therefore, is most prevalent and severe in children and young adults, who are at maximal risk of suffering from its disease sequelae.

PATHOLOGY AND PATHOGENESIS. The early main manifestations are probably immunologically mediated (dermatitis). Acute schistosomiasis may be an immune complex–related disease. The major pathologic lesions are associated with retention of eggs in the host tissues during the chronic stages of infection. Eggs may be trapped at sites of deposition (urinary bladder, ureters, intestine) or be carried by the bloodstream to other organs, most commonly the liver and less often the lungs and central nervous system. The host response to these eggs involves local as well as systemic manifestations. Granulomas composed of lymphocytes, macrophages, and eosinophils surround the trapped eggs and add significantly to the size of tissue destruction. It has been shown that these granulomas are due to cell-mediated re-

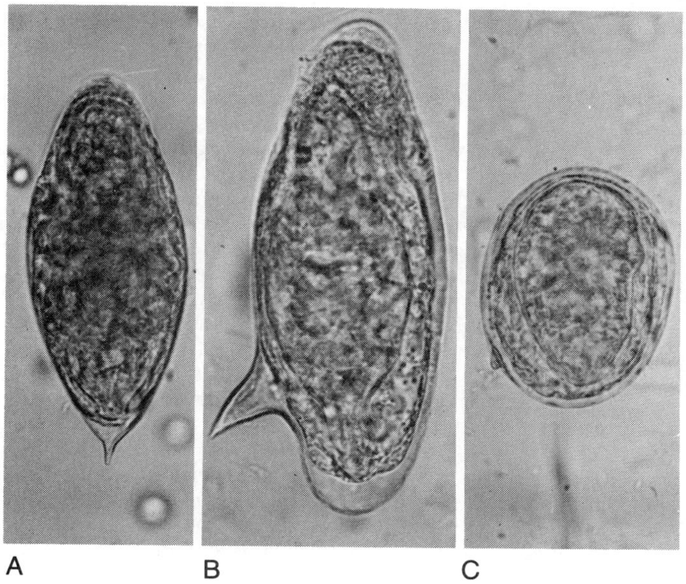

Figure 12–44. Eggs of *Schistosoma haematobium (A)*, *Schistosoma mansoni (B)*, and *Schistosoma japonicum (C)* (× 320).

sponses. Granuloma formation in the bladder wall and at the ureterovesical junction leads to the major disease manifestations of schistosomiasis hematobia: hematuria, dysuria, and obstructive uropathy. Intestinal as well as hepatic granulomas underlie the pathologic sequelae of the other schistosome infections: ulcerations and fibrosis of intestinal wall, hepatosplenomegaly, and portal hypertension due to presinusoidal obstruction of blood flow. Protective immunity against schistosomiasis has been demonstrated in some animal species and perhaps in humans.

CLINICAL MANIFESTATIONS. Most infected individuals suffer no apparent ill health; symptomatology occurs mainly in those heavily infected. Cercarial penetration of human skin may result in a papular pruritic rash (swimmer's itch). It is more pronounced in previously exposed individuals and involves edema and massive cellular infiltrates in the dermis and epidermis. *Katayama fever* (acute schistosomiasis) may occur, particularly in heavily infected individuals 4–8 wk after exposure; this is a serum sickness-like syndrome manifested by the acute onset of fever, chills, sweating, lymphadenopathy, hepatosplenomegaly, and eosinophilia. Its pathogenesis is unknown but may be due to immune complex formation.

Symptomatic children with chronic schistosomiasis haematobia usually complain of frequency, dysuria, and hematuria (often terminal). Urine examination shows erythrocytes, parasite eggs, and occasional leukocytes. In most endemic areas extensive pathologic lesions have been demonstrated in the urinary tract of more than half of infected children. The extent of disease is correlated to the intensity of infection, but significant morbidity occurs even in lightly infected children. The terminal stages of schistosomiasis haematobia are associated with chronic renal failure, secondary infections, and cancer of the bladder in some endemic areas.

Children with chronic schistosomiasis mansoni, japonica, intercalatum, or mekongi may have intestinal symptoms; colicky abdominal pain and bloody diarrhea are the most common. The intestinal phase may, however, pass unnoticed, and the syndrome of hepatosplenomegaly, portal hypertension, ascites, and hematemesis may be the initial presentation. Liver disease is due to granuloma formation and subsequent fibrosis; there is no appreciable liver cell injury, and hepatic function may be preserved for a long time. Schistosome eggs may escape into the pulmonary vasculature causing hypertension and cor pulmonale. Furthermore, *S. japonicum* worms may migrate to the brain vasculature and produce seizures. Transverse myelitis rarely has been reported in children or young adults with chronic *S. haematobium* or *S. mansoni* infection.

DIAGNOSIS. Schistosome eggs are found in the excreta of infected individuals; quantitative procedures should be used to give an indication of the intensity of infection. Urine should be collected around midday (time of maximal egg excretion) and 10 mL filtered through a nuclepore membrane for diagnosis of *S. haematobium* infection. Stool examination by the Kato thick smear procedure is the method of choice for diagnosis and quantification of other schistosome infections.

TREATMENT. Management of children with schistosomiasis should be based on an appreciation of the intensity of infection and the extent of disease. The drug of choice is praziquantel, which is effective against all schistosome species. It is administered orally as a single or divided dose of 40–60 mg/kg.

CONTROL. Transmission in endemic areas may be decreased by reducing the parasite load in the population. The availability of oral, single dose, effective chemotherapeutic agents may help achieve this goal. Other measures, particularly improved sanitation and focal application of molluscicides, may be useful. Control of schistosomiasis is closely linked to economic and social development.

12.133 LIVER FLUKES

Clonorchiasis

Infection of bile passages with the Chinese or oriental fluke *Clonorchis sinensis* is endemic in China, other parts of Southeast Asia, and Japan. Humans acquire infection by ingestion of raw or inadequately cooked freshwater fish carrying the encysted metacercariae of the parasite under its scales or skin. These metacercariae excyst in the duodenum and pass through the ampulla of Vater to the common bile duct and bile capillaries, where they mature into hermaphroditic adult worms (3 × 15 mm). *C. sinensis* worms deposit small operculated eggs (14 × 30 µm), which are discharged via the bile duct to the intestine and feces (Fig. 12–45). The eggs mature and hatch, releasing motile miracidia. If these are ingested by specific snails, numerous cercariae develop, which may escape and encyst under the skin or scales of freshwater fish.

Most *C. sinensis*-infected individuals, particularly those with light infections, are asymptomatic. Localized obstruction of a bile duct and thickening of its walls may be the result of repeated local trauma and inflammation in heavily infected individuals. In these cases cholangitis and cholangiohepatitis may lead to liver enlargement and jaundice. In Hong Kong, cholangiocarcinoma in the Chinese population is associated with *C. sinensis* infection. Clonorchiasis may be diagnosed by examining feces or duodenal aspirates for the parasite eggs. Praziquantel is the drug of choice for treating clonorchiasis (25 mg/kg tid given for 1 day).

Opisthorchiasis

Infections with species of *Opisthorchis* are clinically similar to those with clonorchiasis. *O. felineus* and *O. viverrini* are common liver flukes of cats and dogs that may occasionally infect man through ingestion of metacercariae in freshwater fish. Infection with *O. felineus* is endemic in eastern Europe and Southeast Asia, and *O. viverrini* is found mainly in Thailand. Most individuals are asymptomatic; liver enlargement, relapsing cholangitis, and jaundice may be seen in heavily infected individuals. Diagnosis is based on recovering eggs from stools or duodenal aspirates. Praziquantel, in the same dosage as for clonorchiasis, is the drug of choice.

Fascioliasis

The sheep liver fluke *Fasciola hepatica* infects cattle, other ungulates, and occasionally humans. Infection has been reported in different parts of the world, particularly South

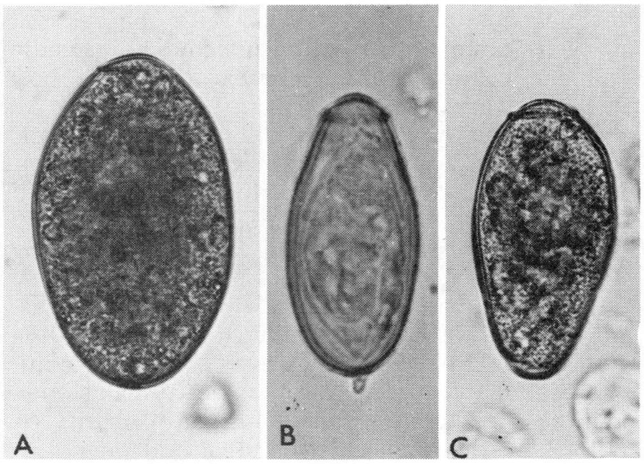

Figure 12–45. Eggs of liver flukes and a lung fluke. *A*, *Fasciola hepatica* (× 400). *B*, *Clonorchis sinensis* (× 1,000). *C*, *Paragonimus westermani* (× 400).

America, Europe, Africa, China, and Australia. Although *F. hepatica* is enzootic in North America, reported cases are extremely rare. Humans are infected by ingestion of metacercariae attached to vegetations, especially wild watercress. In the duodenum the parasites excyst; penetrate the intestinal wall, liver capsule, and parenchyma; and wander for a few weeks before entering the bile ducts, where they mature. Adult *F. hepatica* (1 × 2.5 cm) commence oviposition approximately 12 wk after infection; the eggs are large (75 × 140 μm) and operculated, pass to the intestines with bile, and leave the body in the feces (see Fig. 12–45). On reaching fresh water, the eggs mature and hatch into miracidia, which infect specific snail intermediate hosts to multiply into many cercariae. These then emerge from infected snails and encyst on aquatic grasses and plants.

Clinical manifestations usually occur either during the liver migratory phase of the parasites or after their arrival at their final habitat in bile canaliculi. The first phase is characterized by fever, right upper quadrant pain, and hepatosplenomegaly. Peripheral blood eosinophilia is usually marked. As the worms enter bile ducts, most of the acute symptoms subside. On rare occasions, patients may suffer from obstructive jaundice or biliary cirrhosis. *F. hepatica* infection is diagnosed by finding the characteristic eggs in fecal smears or duodenal aspirates. Praziquantel (25 mg/kg tid given for 1 day) is the recommended treatment.

12.134 INTESTINAL FLUKES

Several wild and domestic animal intestinal flukes, such as *Fasciolopsis buski* and *Heterophyes heterophyes*, may accidentally infect humans. The clinical significance of most of these infections is doubtful and not fully understood. *F. buski* is endemic in the Far East. Humans are infected by ingesting metacercariae encysted on aquatic plants. They hatch and produce large flukes (1 × 5 cm), which inhabit the duodenum and jejunum. Mature worms produce operculated eggs that pass with feces; the organism completes its life cycle through specific snail intermediate hosts. Individuals with *F. buski* infection are usually asymptomatic; heavily infected subjects complain of diarrhea and abdominal pain and show signs of malabsorption. Diagnosis of fasciolopsia is made by fecal examination for eggs. As in other fluke infections, praziquantel is the drug of choice.

12.135 LUNG FLUKES
(Paragonimiasis)

Human infection by the lung fluke *Paragonimus westermani* occurs throughout the Far East, in localized areas of West Africa, and in several parts of Central and South America. The highest incidence of pulmonary paragonimiasis occurs in older children and adolescents 11–15 yr of age. Although *P. westermani* is found in many carnivora, human cases are relatively rare and seem to be associated with specific dietary habits such as eating raw freshwater crayfish or crabs. These crustaceans contain the infective metacercariae in their tissues; they excyst in the duodenum, penetrate the intestinal wall, and migrate to their final habitat in the lungs. Adult worms (5 × 10 mm) encapsulate within the lung parenchyma and deposit brown operculated eggs (60 × 100 μm), which pass into the bronchioles and are coughed up (see Fig. 12–45). Ova can be detected in the sputum of infected individuals or in their feces. If eggs reach fresh water, they hatch and undergo asexual multiplication in specific snails. The cercariae encyst in the muscles and viscera of crayfish and freshwater crabs.

Most individuals infected with *P. westermani* harbor low or moderate worm loads and are asymptomatic. In symptomatic infected children hemoptysis occurs in 98% of cases; other symptoms include cough and production of rust-colored sputum. There are no characteristic physical findings, but laboratory examination usually demonstrates marked eosinophilia. Chest roentgenogram often reveals small patchy infiltrates or radiolucencies in the mid-lung fields; however, the roentgenogram may be normal in one fifth of infected individuals. In rare circumstances lung abscess, pleural effusion, or bronchiectasis may be demonstrable. Extrapulmonary localization of *P. westermani* in the brain, peritoneum, intestines, or pleura may rarely occur. Cerebral paragonimiasis is seen primarily in heavily infected individuals living in highly endemic areas of the Far East; the clinical presentation resembles jacksonian epilepsy or cerebral tumors. Definitive diagnosis of paragonimiasis is made by finding eggs in fecal or sputum smears. The treatment of choice is praziquantel (25 mg/kg) given orally three times in 1 day.

SCHISTOSOMIASIS

Jordan P, Webbe G: Schistosomiasis: Epidemiology, Treatment and Control. London, Heinemann, 1982, p 361.
King CH, Mahmoud AAF: Drugs five years later: Praziquantel. Ann Intern Med 110:290, 1989.
Mahmoud AAF: Schistosomiasis: Clinical Tropical Medicine and Communicable Diseases, Vol 2. London, Bailliere-Tindall, 1987.
Mahmoud AAF, Wahab MFA: Schistosomiasis. *In*: Warren KS, Mahmoud AAF (eds): Tropical and Geographical Medicine, 2nd ed. New York, McGraw-Hill, 1990, p 458.

OTHER FLUKES

Drugs for parasitic infections. Medical Letter 32:23, 1990.
Fischer GW, McGrew GL, Bass JW: Pulmonary paragonimiasis in childhood. JAMA 243:1360, 1980.
Harinasuta T, Bunnag D: Liver, lung, and intestinal trematodiasis. *In*: Warren KS, Mahmoud AAF (eds): Tropical and Geographical Medicine, 2nd ed. New York, McGraw-Hill, 1990, p 473.

CESTODES
(Tapeworms)

Human infection with cestodes constitutes a considerable burden of parasitism in many parts of the world. Most commonly adult worms parasitize the gastrointestinal tract, causing little or no clinical morbidity except when they interfere with host nutrition. Major clinical syndromes may occur, however, when humans are infected with the larval stages of some cestodes which disseminate and can cause disease in any internal organ.

12.136 TENIASIS AND DIPHYLLOBOTHRIASIS
(Giant Tapeworms)

There are three giant tapeworms that may cause human infection, and all three infections may be acquired by ingesting animal flesh that contains the larval stage of the parasites. *Taenia saginata* (beef tapeworm) is found in all parts of the world and is particularly common in East Africa. The exact prevalence of *T. solium* (pork tapeworm) is not known but is reportedly less than that of *T. saginata*; the infection is most endemic in India, China, South Africa, Central Europe, and some parts of South America. Teniasis solium is not endemic in North America. *Diphyllobothrium latum* (fish tapeworm) is endemic in regions with cold lakes such as Scandinavia, Northern Europe, Siberia, China, and North and South America. Parasitized fish may also be found in lakes at high altitudes in tropical areas, such as Central Africa.

ETIOLOGY. Humans are infected by ingesting raw or undercooked flesh. Infective larvae of *T. saginata* are found in

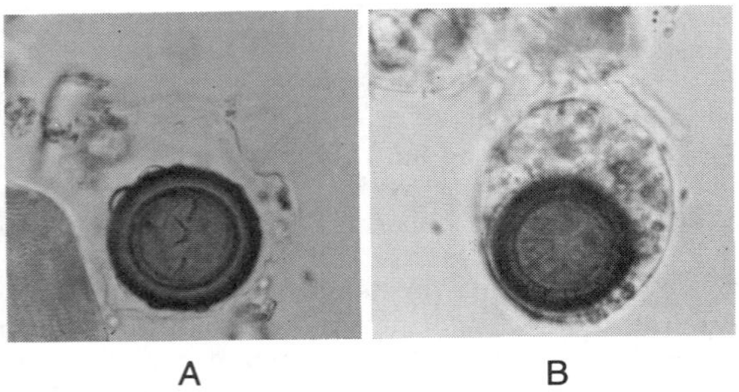

Figure 12–46. Eggs of *Taenia saginata* recovered from fresh feces (× 400). The cellular structure in which the egg develops while in the proglottid, more evident in *B* than in *A*, may be retained around the dark prismatic egg membrane that contains the larva. Usually evident in the larva are 3 pairs of hooklets *(A)*, which may occasionally be seen in motion.

beef, those of *T. solium* in pork, and those of *D. latum* in freshwater fish. These larvae start their development upon reaching the human small intestine and mature in several months. Adult tapeworms consist of ribbon-like segments, approximately 1,000 in *T. solium*, 2,000 in *T. saginata*, and 4,000 in *D. latum*. Adult worms vary in length from 4 to 10 meters. Mature segments may passively *(T. solium)* or actively *(T. saginata)* pass through the anus. Taenia eggs are rarely seen in stools. They are small (35 μm in diameter) and yellowish brown and contain hooklets in their center (Fig. 12–46). In contrast to *Taenia* sp., *D. latum* segments usually deposit their eggs within the intestinal lumen, and they are easily seen in fecal smears of infected individuals. They are operculate and measure 45 × 75 μm (Fig. 12–47). When eggs of *Taenia* sp. are ingested by cattle or pigs they are digested, and embryos disseminate throughout the tissues and develop into mature infectious cysticerci. Ingestion of *T. solium* eggs by humans may occasionally lead to cysticercosis. Further development of *D. latum* eggs takes place in fish and crustacea; the infective forms finally lodge in the tissues of freshwater fish.

EPIDEMIOLOGY. Human infection by the giant tapeworms is most common in adults. Transmission is primarily related to nutritional habits, fecal disposal practices, and the methods used to feed domestic animals. Thorough cooking or freezing destroys the infective stages of these parasites. Adult worms may live for decades; human infection is usually due to only one worm and has no adverse effects. Infection with many worms or with the larval stage of *T. solium* may, however, produce serious clinical manifestations.

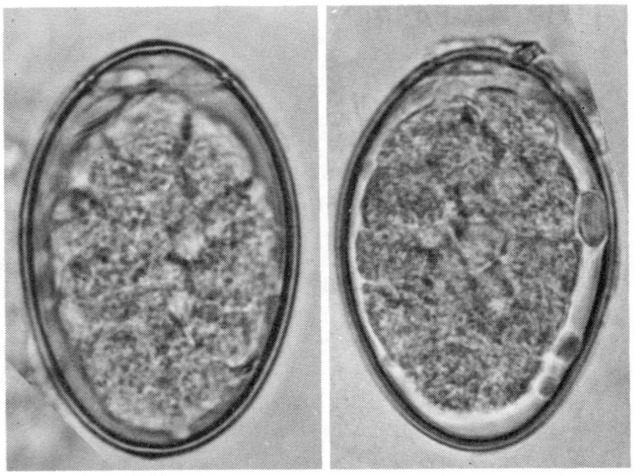

Figure 12–47. Eggs of *Diphyllobothrium latum* as seen in fresh feces (× 400). The operculum is usually evident.

CLINICAL MANIFESTATIONS. Infection with adult *T. saginata* or *T. solium* is almost always asymptomatic. These parasites do not compete to any significant degree for host nutrients. The most frequent sign in *T. saginata* infection is passage of motile segments through the anus. Although many abdominal symptoms have been associated with tapeworm infections, these correlations have not been based on properly controlled studies. Similar vague abdominal complaints have been associated with *D. latum* infection. The most important clinical sequela of this infection is vitamin B_{12} deficiency. Adult worms absorb the vitamin at a fast rate and may cause megaloblastic anemia in infected individuals.

Human infection with the cysticercus stage of *T. solium* may be asymptomatic. However, heavy infection with localization of larvae in important anatomic areas, principally the brain, may lead to generalized or focal seizures and raised intracranial pressure. Eosinophilia is variable in patients with cysticercosis.

DIAGNOSIS. Infection with *Taenia* worms is diagnosed by identification and morphologic characterization of adult segments. *D. latum* infection is usually identified by examination of feces for eggs. Cysticercosis may be diagnosed by a combination of clinical presentations, roentgenography and CT scanning to detect cysts in brain or soft tissues, and serology.

TREATMENT. All three giant tapeworm infections are treated with a single oral dose of niclosamide (2 tablets [1 g] for children weighing 11–34 kg and 3 tablets [1.5 g] for those above 34 kg). Patients with megaloblastic anemia due to *D. latum* infection should be given vitamin B_{12} and observed for neurologic complications. Symptomatic patients with cysticercosis are treated with praziquantel, 50 mg/kg/24 hr in 3 divided doses for 14 days.

12.137 HYMENOLEPIASIS
(Dwarf Tapeworms)

Infection with *Hymenolepis nana* is common in children living in warm climates; the prevalence ranges from 0.3 to 2.9% in North America. Although most children harbor light infections that are not associated with symptoms or signs, young children are more likely to develop heavy worm loads, possibly secondary to autoinfection, and may present with abdominal pain or diarrhea.

Infection is acquired by ingesting eggs passed in feces of parasitized individuals. *H. nana* eggs are spherical or ovoid, measure 40 × 50 μm, and contain embryos with characteristic hooklets (Fig. 12–48). The ova hatch in the intestinal lumen and liberate embryos that mature into adult worms (1 × 40 mm); these usually reside in the ileum and begin oviposition in a few weeks. The eggs are carried to the outside via feces

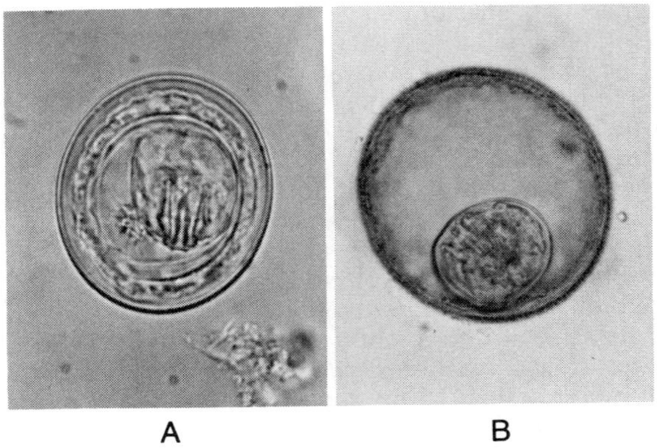

Figure 12–48. Eggs of *Hymenolepis nana (A)* (× 575) and *Hymenolepis diminuta (B)* (× 400).

but may hatch inside the same host (autoinfection), increasing the intensity of infection. *H. diminuta*, a parasite of rodents, occasionally infects man. Adult worms are larger than *H. nana*, the life cycle is similar, and eggs are identical in shape but slightly greater in size.

The characteristic eggs of *H. nana* and *H. diminuta* may be found on fecal examination by direct smear or by concentration methods. Patients may be treated with niclosamide (same dose as for tapeworms). Praziquantel is also highly effective; in one study single doses of 25 mg/kg cured 94% of infected children.

12.138 ECHINOCOCCOSIS
(Hydatid Disease)

Human infection with the larval stage of the canine tapeworm *Echinococcus granulosus* occurs worldwide but is most prevalent in countries where sheep and cattle are raised. Endemic areas include Australia, South America, South Africa, the Soviet Union, North America, and the Mediterranean region. Clinical disease occurs when hydatid cysts present as space-occupying lesions; these are most common in the liver, but other tissues, such as the lungs, brain, and bones, may also be affected.

ETIOLOGY. Domesticated dogs acquire the infection by eating parasitized viscera of sheep and cattle. Humans incidentally acquire infection with *E. granulosus* by ingesting parasite eggs that are discharged in the feces of infected dogs or wolves. Embryos escape from the eggs in the duodenum, penetrate its wall, and pass to the liver, where they are usually trapped. If the embryos escape from the liver, they may seed the lungs or travel to other organs via the systemic circulation. Wherever the parasite embryos are trapped, they may be destroyed by the host response or develop into hydatid cysts. These cysts can grow in size up to 20 cm in diameter and are lined on the inside by a germinal layer, which forms multiple larval scolices and daughter cysts.

EPIDEMIOLOGY. *E. granulosus* transmission to humans is most common in regions of the world supporting major livestock industries. Infection is usually acquired by direct contact with dogs but may also occur by ingesting contaminated soil, vegetables, and water. The prevalence is highest in children; clinical manifestations, however, occur several years later. Another cycle of transmission to man occurs in North America, particularly in some areas of Alaska and Canada. The strain of *E. granulosus* endemic in these regions is found in the wolf, and larvae are found in large deer such as moose, reindeer, or caribou.

CLINICAL MANIFESTATIONS. Most individuals with hydatid cysts are asymptomatic; clinical disease appears in a small proportion and is usually the result of the space-occupying nature of the cysts. When they occur in the liver, manifestations develop only when a cyst reaches large dimensions and presses on adjacent tissues and structures or is located in an area that obstructs blood flow, such as the porta hepatis. Since it takes several years for hydatid cysts to grow, clinical morbidity is usually detected in middle-aged or elderly patients. Symptoms occur earlier when the cysts are located in less well supported tissues like the brain and lung, where there is also an increased risk of rupture into adjacent structures. Dissemination of the daughter cysts may lead to widespread infections in the peritoneal or pleural cavities. Approximately two thirds of hydatid cysts occur in the liver and one quarter in the lungs. In contrast to liver lesions, pulmonary hydatid cysts are commonly seen in children, who may present with hemoptysis, cough, or dyspnea. The cysts may rupture into the bronchial tree and spread by discharging their contents in respiratory secretions. Hydatid disease in the brain usually presents as space-occupying lesions.

In some parts of North America, Europe, and Asia, another species of canine tapeworm, *E. multilocularis*, is found in foxes as well as domestic cats and dogs. Human infection with this parasite leads to the so-called malignant hydatid. Many small cysts occur in organs such as the liver; they multiply, spread quickly, and destroy adjacent normal tissues. The prognosis is grave, as measures to stop the spread of the infection are not available. Surgical intervention is hazardous.

DIAGNOSIS AND TREATMENT. Some cases of hydatid cyst may be discovered on routine roentgenographic examination of the chest or abdomen. Children in endemic areas with suggestive symptoms and signs should undergo roentgenographic and ultrasonic examination. The benign nature of the cyst may be confirmed by angiography. Serology is helpful, particularly when antibodies to echinococcus antigen 5 are detected.

Once a presumptive diagnosis is made, the extent of disease must be assessed. Small or calcified liver cysts should be left alone; enlarging or symptomatic cysts should be removed surgically. In patients with pulmonary or bone cysts, surgical removal is also recommended. Care should be taken during the operative procedure not to disseminate the infection. Several reports have shown the efficacy of albendazole. If these observations are confirmed, administration of this drug may provide an alternative to surgical intervention in many patients.

ADEL A. F. MAHMOUD

Kociecka W: Intestinal cestode infections. *In*: Pawlowski Z (ed): Intestinal Helminthic Infections.(Clinical Tropical Medicine and Communicable Diseases.) London, Bailliere-Tindall, 1987.

Lewall DB, McCorkell SJ: Hepatic echinococcal cysts: Sonographic appearance and classification. Radiology 155: 773, 1983.

Pawlowski ZS: Cestodiases: Taeniasis, cysticercosis, diphyllobothriasis, hymenolepiasis, and others. *In*: Warren KS, Mahmoud AAF (eds): Tropical and Geographical Medicine, 2nd ed. New York, McGraw-Hill, 1990, p 490.

Saimot AG, Meulemans A, Cremieux AC, et al: Albendazole as a potential treatment for human hydatidosis. Lancet 2:652, 1983.

Schantz PM, Okelo GBA: Echinococcosis (hydatidosis). *In*: Warren KS, Mahmoud AAF (eds): Tropical and Geographical Medicine, 2nd ed. New York, McGraw-Hill, 1990, p 505.

Stehr-Green JK, Stehr-Green PA, Schantz PM, et al: Risk factors for infection with *Echinococcus multilocularis* in Alaska. Am J Trop Med Hyg 38:380, 1988.

World Health Organization: Prevention and control of intestinal parasitic infections. Technical Report Series No. 749. Geneva, WHO, 1987.

12.139 ANTIPARASITIC DRUGS FOR CHILDREN

Pediatric parasitic infections constitute a major cause of worldwide morbidity and mortality. In the United States and other industrialized countries, parasitic infections in childhood have markedly increased in frequency. Factors involved in the resurgence of parasitic infections include increasing travel, the frequent use of immunosuppressive drugs, and the greater number of immunocompromised hosts, particularly those with HIV infection. Physicians everywhere may see infections caused by previously unfamiliar parasites.

A discussion of antiparasitic therapy is extremely complex and must take into account the numerous infecting organisms, their complicated life cycles, differences in their metabolism, and the multitude of drugs that are available. An additional problem, particularly in treating infections in pediatric age groups, relates to the paucity of controlled studies demonstrating efficacy and safety of many of the antiparasitic agents.

Taxonomically, parasites are divided into protozoa and helminths. The protozoa often have complex life cycles but are unicellular. On the other hand, the helminths have highly developed neuromuscular systems, integuments, and digestive tracts. Given those differences, it is not surprising that drugs that are effective against protozoa are not effective against helminths and vice versa. Generally, the susceptibility of parasites to therapeutic agents is associated with taxonomy and metabolism.

The dosage and duration of therapy as well as the major adverse reactions of antiparasitic drugs in treating children are provided in Tables 12–46 (antiprotozoal drugs) and 12–47 (antihelminthic drugs). In every case, the indication for treatment must be weighed against the toxicity of the drug. First-choice and alternative agents have been included. When the first choice drug is clinically ineffective but the alternative therapy is more hazardous, retreatment with the first choice may be the most prudent course.

ROBERT A. SALATA

Drugs for parasitic infections. Medical Letter 30:15, 1988.

Van Reken DE, Pearson RD: Antiparasitic agents. *In*: Mandell GL, Douglas RG, Bennett JE (eds): Principles and Practices of Infectious Diseases, 3rd ed. New York, Churchill Livingstone, 1989, pp 398–427.

12.140 ARTHROPODS AND DISEASE

Arthropods are the largest phylum in the animal kingdom, with over 900,000 species. These invertebrates share the common properties of bilateral symmetry, chitinous exoskeleton, jointed appendages, and a single body cavity filled with hemolymph. Insecta is the largest class among the arthropods and contains several orders causing disease in humans. Interactions between arthropods and humans are frequent owing to the large diversity and number of species worldwide. Only a few of these interactions result in severe morbidity or mortality. Generally, arthropods are either transient pests or persistent anthropophilic parasites recoverable from human hosts.

The categories of arthropods that cause human disease include *blood-sucking ectoparasites* such as fleas, mites, and ticks and *direct invaders of tissues*, such as those seen in myiasis and scabies. In addition, *dermatosis* results from the introduction of foreign materials (arthropod bites) and contact dermatitis (blister beetles); *envenomation* is caused by members of the classes Hymenoptera and Arachnida. Arthropods may indirectly cause other illnesses: the production of allergies and asthma, as seen with dust mites and caddis flies; bacterial infection following skin breakdown from excoriation, vesiculation, or necrosis caused by various insect bites; and foreign body reactions due to the presence of arthropod stingers or mouth parts. Last, many arthropod species serve as vectors for the transmission of *human pathogens*; these insects may serve as obligate hosts to micro-organisms (biologic transmission) or as transporters of infectious agents on body parts (mechanical transmission), although the latter role has rarely been proved.

A detailed history is critical in the evaluation of patients with suspected arthropod contact. Knowledge of the site of injury, time of day, and time course of the lesions is particularly useful. Travel history of the human host is relevant, but imported cases have occurred from bites of "stowaway" spiders or scorpions. Examination of lesions can demonstrate their location, clustering, and secondary changes. Careful inspection of skin, hair, or even clothing can sometimes produce the offending insect. However, a high degreee of suspicion for arthropod injury is necessary because often the agent cannot be recovered, the initial lesion may be minute or painless, or there may be a delay in onset of symptoms following contact.

Certain principles generally apply in arthropod injury. (1) Many species have variable effects, mostly irritating but a few severe. Some effects result from increased sensitization of the human host to foreign proteins injected into the site of bite, as in mosquito injury; some individuals have an exaggerated dermatologic response compared to other family members. (2) Envenomation may have an increased and sometimes fatal effect on the very young. (3) The incidence or severity of morbidity due to anthropophilic parasites, such as scabies or myiasis, is often increased in debilitated hosts.

BLOOD-SUCKING ECTOPARASITES

MITES (Acarinae). These are minute 6-legged insects that rarely inflict direct injury to human skin. Several species cause discomfort by inducing pruritus. Acquisition of mites follows close human-to-human or animal-to-human contact or physical exposure to fields, grains, or plants.

Scabies, the primary mite infestation of humans, represents a true infection by a human pathogen. *Sarcoptes scabiei* directly invades and reproduces in human tissues. Lesions are characteristic burrows in flexural areas such as wrists and interdigital creases. The mites require close human contact to survive. Secondary infection and hypersensitivity can occur. Scabies is discussed further in Sec. 23.31.

Trombiculidae is an order of field mites with larvae that can attach to and penetrate human skin. Known as **chiggers**, red bugs, or harvest mites, the organisms are acquired through contact with "mite islands" in fields. Microscopic larval trombuculids use a sharp spine or stylosome to pierce the dermis and digest tissue. They cause an intensely pruritic hemorrhagic bite, which can develop into pruritic wheals and papules with central vesicles resembling chickenpox. Bites tend to occur on exposed areas (e.g., legs and ankles) but may occur under close clothing (waist or genitalia). Treatments include topical application of steroids, Quotane ointment, nail polish, or an ointment of 5–10% sulfur and 1% phenol to reduce pruritis. Infestation may be prevented by tucking in clothing and reducing skin exposure. *N,N*-diethylmetatoluamide (deet) is an effective chigger repellant, as is sulfur dusted on trouser legs.

Mites are also responsible for food and animal-transmitted diseases. Contact dermatitis can result from exposure to grain itch, cheese, and produce mites. *Chleytiella* mites, transmitted from household dogs and cats, produce discrete, scattered, pruritic lesions with central pinpoint eschars. Diagnosis of infestation with these nonburrowing mites requires the presence of unexplained pruritis, other persons with similar lesions, exclusion of other types of bites (such as bedbugs, lice, fleas, mosquitoes, and spiders), absence of burrows, and a high index of suspicion.

Dust mites, *Dermatophagoides pteronyssinus* and *D. farinae*, are less than 500 μm in size and thrive on house dust. Scales, hairs, and pure extracts from these species induce bronchospasm, conjunctivitis, rhinitis, and eczema in susceptible individuals. The true extent of allergic disease caused by these

Text continued on page 914

TABLE 12–46. Drugs for Treatment of Protozoan Infections

Infection	Drug	Pediatric Dosage[a]	Adverse Effects
Amebiasis *(Entamoeba histolytica)*			
Asymptomatic			
Drug of choice:	Diloxanide furoate[b]	20 mg/kg/24 hr in 3 doses for 10 days	Frequent: flatulence Occasional: nausea, vomiting, diarrhea Rare: urticaria, pruritus
Alternatives:	Iodoquinol[c]	30–40 mg/kg/24 hr in 3 doses for 20 days	Occasional: rash, nausea, diarrhea, cramps, anal pruritus Rare: optic atrophy and loss of vision (high doses for months), iodine sensitivity
	Paromomycin	25–30 mg/kg/24 hr in 3 doses for 7 days	Frequent: GI disturbances Rare: 8th nerve dysfunction, azotemia
Intestinal disease			
Drugs of choice:	Metronidazole[d]	30–50 mg/kg/24 hr in 3 doses for 10 days	Frequent: nausea, headache, metallic taste Occasional: vomiting, diarrhea, insomnia, rash, disulfiram-like reaction with alcohol Rare: seizures, encephalopathy, ataxia, leukopenia, peripheral neuropathy
	FOLLOWED BY Diloxanide furoate[b]	20 mg/kg/24 hr in 3 doses for 10 days	See above
Alternatives:	Dehydroemetine[b, e]	1–1.5 mg/kg/24 hr (max. 90 mg/24 hr) IM in 2 doses for up to 5 days	Similar to emetine, but probably less severe
	FOLLOWED BY Diloxanide furoate[b]	20 mg/kg/24 hr in 3 doses for 10 days	See above
	OR Emetine[e]	1 mg/kg/24 hr in 2 doses (max. 60 mg/24 hr) IM for up to 5 days	Frequent: cardiac arrhythmias, precordial pain, muscle weakness, cellulitis at injection site Occasional: diarrhea, vomiting, heart failure, peripheral neuropathy
	FOLLOWED BY Diloxanide furoate[b]	20 mg/kg/24 hr in 3 doses for 10 days	See above
Hepatic abscess			
Drugs of choice:	Metronidazole	35–50 mg/kg/24 hr in 3 doses for 10 days	See above
	FOLLOWED BY Diloxanide furoate[b]	20 mg/kg/24 hr in 3 doses for 10 days	See above
Alternatives:	Dihydroemetine[b, e]	1–1.5 mg/kg/24 hr (max. 90 mg/24 hr) IM in 2 doses for up to 5 days	See above
	FOLLOWED BY Diloxanide furoate[b]	20 mg/kg/24 hr in 3 doses for 10 days	See above
	OR Emetine	1 mg/kg/24 hr in 2 doses (max. 60 mg/24 hr) IM	See above
	FOLLOWED BY Diloxanide furoate[b]	20 mg/kg/24 hr in 3 doses for 10 days	See above
Amebic Meningoencephalitis, *primary*			
Naegleria sp.			
Drug of choice	Amphotericin B[f, g]	1 mg/kg/24 hr, uncertain duration	Frequent: acute reaction (fever, rigors, occasional hypotension and tachypnea), nephrotoxicity, headache, nausea, vomiting, anemia Occasional: renal tubular acidosis, hypomagnesemia Rare: thrombocytopenia and leukopenia
Acanthamoeba spp.	See footnote[h]		

Table continued on following page

TABLE 12–46. Drugs for Treatment of Protozoan Infections *Continued*

Infection	Drug	Pediatric Dosage[a]	Adverse Effects
Babesiosis *(Babesis sp.)* Drugs of choice:	Clindamycin[g]	20–40 mg/kg/24 hr in 3 doses for 7 days	Occasional: anorexia, nausea, vomiting, mild transaminitis, rash, pseudomembranous colitis Rare: fever, eosinophilia, anaphylaxis, Stevens-Johnson syndrome
	PLUS Quinine	25 mg/kg/24 hr in 3 doses for 7 days	Frequent: cinchonism (tinnitus, headache, nausea, abdominal pain, visual disturbances) Occasional: hemolysis anemia, photosensitivity reactions, hypoglycemia, arrhythmias, hypotension, drug fever
Balantidiasis *(Balantidium coli)* Drug of choice:	Tetracycline[g]	>8 years of age: 10 mg/kg qid for 10 days (max. 2 g/24 hr)	Frequent: rash, fever, eosinophilia, GI disturbances, phototoxic reactions, in fetus and young children—staining teeth and retarding bone growth, superinfection with *Candida* Occasional: hepatotoxicity, coagulopathy, increased intracranial pressure in infancy Rare: pseudomembranous colitis
Alternatives:	Iodoquinol[c, g]	30–40 mg/kg/24 hr in 3 doses for 20 days	See above
	OR Metronidazole[d]	35–50 mg/kg/24 hr in 3 doses for 5 days	See above
Blastocystis hominis *infection* Drug of choice:	Iodoquinol[c, g]	30–40 mg/kg/24 hr in 3 doses for 20 days	See above
	OR Metronidazole[d, g]	35–50 mg/kg/24 hr in 3 doses for 10 days	See above
Cryptosporidiosis *(Cryptosporidium* sp.)	No known effective therapy		
Dientamoeba fragilis *infection* Drug of choice:	Iodoquinol[c]	40 mg/kg/24 hr in 3 doses for 20 days	See above
	OR Tetracycline[g]	10 mg/kg qid for 10 days (max. 2 g/ 24 hr)	See above
	OR Paromomycin	25–30 mg/kg/24 hr in 3 doses for 7 days	See above
Entamoeba polecki *infection* Drugs of choice:	Metronidazole[d, g]	35–50 mg/kg/24 hr in 3 doses for 10 days	See above
	FOLLOWED BY Diloxamide furoate[b]	20 mg/kg/24 hr in 3 doses for 10 days	See above
Giardiasis *(Giardia lamblia)* Drug of choice:	Furazolidone	1.25 mg/kg qid for 7–10 days	Frequent: nausea, vomiting Occasional: allergic reactions, hypotension, urticaria, fever, hypoglycemia, headache Rare: hemolytic anemia in neonates, polyneuritis, MAO-inhibitor reactions
Alternatives:	Metronidazole[d, g]	5 mg/kg tid for 5 days	See above
	OR Quinacrine HCl	2 mg/kg tid PC for 5 days (max. 300 mg/24 hr)	Frequent: dizziness, headache, vomiting Occasional: yellow staining of skin, toxic psychosis, insomnia, blood dyscrasias, psoriasis-like rash Rare: Acute hepatic necrosis, convulsions, exfoliative dermatitis, ocular effects

TABLE 12–46. Drugs for Treatment of Protozoan Infections *Continued*

Infection	Drug	Pediatric Dosage[a]	Adverse Effects
Isosporiasis *(Isospora belli)*			
Drug of choice:	Trimethoprim-sulfamethoxazole	10 mg/kg/24 hr as TMP in 4 divided oral doses for 3 wk	Frequent: GI disturbances, rash Occasional: cytopenias, hepatotoxicity, renal insufficiency, fever, skin rash, (cytopenias and hepatotoxicity occurs more frequently in patients with AIDS)
Leishmaniasis			
(*L. braziliensis, L. mexicana* and mucocutaneous leishmaniasis)			
Drug of choice:	Stibogluconate sodium[b]	20 mg/kg/24 hr IM or IV (max. 800 mg/24 hr) for 20 days	Frequent: myalgias and arthralgias, bradycardia Occasional: diarrhea, rash, pruritus Rare: hepatitis and renal failure, hemolytic anemia, shock, cardiac arrhythmias
Alternative:	Amphotericin B[b]	0.25–1.00 mg/kg/24 hr for up to 8 wk	See above
(*L. donovani*—kala azar, visceral leishmaniasis)			
Drug of choice:	Stibogluconate sodium[b, j]	20 mg/kg/24 hr IM or IV (max. 800 mg/24 hr) for 20 days	See above
Alternative:	Pentamidine sodium	2–4 mg/kg/24 hr IM or IV for up to 15 doses	Frequent: hypotension, hypoglycemia often followed by diabetes mellitus, vomiting, blood dyscrasias, GI disturbances Occasional: shock, hypocalcemia, liver failure, cardiotoxicity, rash Rare: anaphylaxis, acute pancreatitis
(*L. tropica, L. major*—oriental sore, cutaneous leishmaniasis)			
Drug of choice:	Stibogluconate sodium[b, k]	10 mg/kg/24 hr IM or IV (max. 600 mg/24 hr) for 6–10 days	See above
Alternative:	Topical therapy[l]		
Malaria			
All *Plasmodium* except chloroquine-resistant *P. falciparum*			
ORAL			
Drug of choice:	Chloroquine phosphate[m, n]	10 mg base/kg (max. 600 mg base), then 5 mg base/kg 6 hr later, then 5 mg base/kg/24 hr for 2 days	Occasional: pruritus, vomiting, headache, confusion, rash, corneal opacities, extraocular muscle paralysis, exacerbation of psoriasis, myalgia Rare: irreversible retinal injury (when total dose exceeds 100 g), discoloration of nails and mucous membranes, deafness, neuropathy and myopathy, heart block, blood dyscrasias
PARENTERAL			
Drug of choice:	Quinine dihydrochloride[b]	25 mg/kg/24 hr; give one third of daily dose over 2–4 hr, repeat every 8 hr until oral therapy can be started (max. 1,800 mg/24 hr)	See above
	OR Quinidine gluconate[g, o]	10 mg/kg IV, then 0.02 mg/kg/min IV for 72 hr	Frequent: GI disturbances, cinchonism Occasional: rash, ventricular ectopy, widening of QRS complex and prolonged QT interval, A-V block, headache, delirium, ataxia Rare: cytopenias (especially thrombocytopenia), hypotension, fever, systemic lupus erythematosus

Table continued on following page

TABLE 12–46. Drugs for Treatment of Protozoan Infections *Continued*

Infection	Drug	Pediatric Dosage[a]	Adverse Effects
Malaria *Continued* Alternative:	Chloroquine HCl[b]	Optimal dosing not determined	See above
Chloroquine-resistant *P. falciparum* ORAL Drugs of choice:	Quinine sulfate[p, q]	25 mg/kg/24 hr in 3 doses for 3 days	See above
	PLUS Pyrimethamine	<10 kg: 6.25 mg/24 hr for 3 days 10–20 kg: 12.5 mg/24 hr for 3 days 20–40 kg: 25 mg/24 hr for 3 days	Occasional: blood dyscrasias, folic acid deficiency Rare: rash, vomiting, convulsions, shock
	PLUS Sulfadiazine	100–200 mg/kg/24 hr in 4 doses for 5 days (max. 2 g/days)	See trimethoprim-sulfamethoxazole
Alternative:	Quinine sulfate[r]	25 mg/kg/24 hr in 3 doses for 3 days	See above
	PLUS Tetracycline	5 mg/kg qid for 7 days	See above
PARENTERAL Drug of choice:	Quinine dihydrochloride[b]	25 mg/kg/24 hr in 3 doses for 3 days	See above
	OR Quinidine gluconate[g, o]	10 mg/kg IV, then 0.02 mg/kg/min IV for 72 hr	See above
Prevention of Relapses *P. vivax* and *P. ovale* only Drug of choice:	Primaquine phosphate[s]	0.3 mg base/kg/24 hr for 14 days	Frequent: hemolytic anemia in G-6-PD deficiency Occasional: neutropenia, GI disturbances, methemoglobinemia in G-6-PD deficiency Rare: CNS symptoms, hypertension, arrhythymias
Prevention of Malaria[t] Chloroquine-sensitive areas Drug of choice:	Chloroquine phosphate[m, u]	5 mg/kg base (8.3 mg/kg salt) once per wk, up to maximum adult dose of 300 mg base	See above
	Mefloquine	<15 kg: not recommended 15–19 kg: ¼ tab (62.5 mg)/wk 20–30 kg: ½ tab (125 mg)/wk 31–45 kg :¾ tab (187.5 mg)/wk > 45 kg: 1 tab (250 mg)/wk	Occasional: GI disturbances, dizziness Rare: problems with fine coordination, and spacial discrimination Contraindicated in those with history of seizures, patients using beta blockers or other drugs prolonging cardiac conduction
	OR		
Chloroquine-resistant areas Drugs of choice:	Chloroquine phosphate[m]	5 mg/kg base (8.3/kg salt) once per wk, up to maximum adult dose of 300 mg base	See above
	PLUS Proguanil[v] (in Africa, south of Sahara)	<2 yr: 50 mg daily 2–6 yr: 100 mg daily 7–10 yr: 150 mg daily 10 yr: 200 mg daily	Occasional: oral ulcerations, vomiting, abdominal pain, diarrhea Rare: hematuria (with large doses)
	PLUS		

TABLE 12–46. Drugs for Treatment of Protozoan Infections *Continued*

Infection	Drug	Pediatric Dosage[a]	Adverse Effects
Malaria *Continued*			
	Pyrimethamine-sulfadoxine (Fansidar)[w]	2–11 mo: ¼ tablet 1–3 yr: ½ tablet 4–8 yr: 1 tablet 9–14 yr: 2 tablets >14 yr: 3 tablets Take single dose of above for self-treatment of febrile illness when medical care is not immediately available	See above
	OR Doxycycline[x]	>8 yr of age: 2 mg/kg/24 hr, up to adult dose of 100 mg/24 hr	See above
Pneumocystis carinii **pneumonia**			
Drug of choice:	Trimethoprim-sulfamethoxazole	TMP 20 mg/kg/24 hr, SMX 100 mg/kg/24 hr oral or IV in 4 doses for 14 days	See above
Alternatives:	Pentamadine isocyanate	4 mg/kg/24 hr IM or IV for 14 days	See above
Toxoplasmosis *(Toxoplasma gondii)*			
Drugs of choice	Pyrimethamine[y]	2 mg/kg/24 hr for 3 days, then 1 mg/kg/24 hr (max. 25 mg/24 hr) for 4 wk	See above
	PLUS Trisulfapyrimidines	100–200 mg/kg/24 hr for 3–4 wk	See above
Alternatives:	Spiramycin	50–100 mg/kg/24 hr for 3–4 wk	Occasional: GI disturbances Rare: allergic reactions
Trichomoniasis (Trichomonas vaginalis)			
Drug of choice:	Metronidazole[d, z]	15 mg/kg/24 hr orally in 3 doses for 7 days	See above
Trypanosomiasis			
(*T. cruzi,* South American trypanosomiasis, Chagas' disease)			
Drug of choice:	Nifurtimox[b]	1–10 yr: 15–20 mg/kg/24 hr in 4 divided doses for 90 days 11–16 yr: 12.5–15 mg/kg/24 hr in 4 divided doses for 90 days	Frequent: anorexia, vomiting, weight loss, loss of memory, sleep disorders, tremor, paresthesias, weakness, polyneuritis Rare: convulsions, fever, pulmonary infiltrate, pleural effusion
Alternative:	Benznidazole[aa]	5–7 mg/kg/24hr for 30–120 days	Frequent: rash, dose-dependent polyneuropathy, GI disturbances
(*T. gambiense, T. rhodesiense,* African trypanosomiasis, sleeping sickness) hemolymphatic stage			
Drug of choice[bb]:	Suramin[b]	20 mg/kg on days 1, 3, 7, 14 and 21	Frequent: vomiting, pruritus, urticaria, paresthesias, hyperesthesias, photophobia, peripheral neuropathy Occasional: renal insufficiency, blood dyscrasias, shock, optic atrophy
Alternative:	Pentamidine isocyanate	4 mg/kg/24 hr IM for 10 days	See above
Late disease with CNS involvement			
Drug of choice:	Melarsoprol[b, cc]	18–25 mg/kg total given over 1 mo; initial dose of 0.36 mg/kg IV, increasing gradually to maximum 3.6 mg/kg at intervals of 1–5 days for total of 9–10 doses	Frequent: myocardial damage, albuminuria, hypertension, Herxheimer reaction, encephalopathy, vomiting, peripheral neuropathy Rare: shock

Table continued on following page

TABLE 12–46. Drugs for Treatment of Protozoan Infections *Continued*

Infection	Drug	Pediatric Dosage[a]	Adverse Effects
Trypanosomiasis *Continued*			
Alternatives:	Tryparsamide	Unknown	Frequent: nausea, vomiting Occasional: impaired vision, optic atrophy, fever, dermatitis, tinnitus, allergic reactions
	PLUS Suramin[b]	Unknown	See above

[a]Also see appropriate sections in text.

[b]In the United States this drug is available from the CDC Drug Service, Centers for Disease Control, Atlanta, GA 30333; telephone: (404) 639–3670; evenings, weekends, and holidays: (404) 639–2888.

[c]Dosage and duration of administration should not be exceeded because of the possibility of optic neuritis; maximum dosage is 2 g/24 hr.

[d]Metronidazole is carcinogenic in rodents and mutagenic in bacteria; it should generally not be given in pregnancy (especially in the 1st trimester).

[e]Dihydroemetine is probably as effective and less toxic than emetine. Because of cardiac toxicity, patients receiving emetine should have electrocardiographic monitoring during therapy.

[f]One patient with a *Naegleria* infection was successfully treated with amphotericin B, miconazole, and rifampin (N Engl J Med 306:346, 1981).

[g]Considered an investigational drug for this condition by the U.S. Food and Drug Administration.

[h]Experimental infections with *Acanthamoeba* sp. have responded to sulfadiazine (Annu Rev Microbiol 25:231, 1971). Amebic keratitis due to *Acanthamoeba* sp. has responded to topical miconazole, propamidine isethionate, and antibiotics (Am J Ophthalmol 100:396, 1985).

[i]In sulfonamide-sensitive persons, such as many patients with AIDS, pyrimethamine 50–75 mg/day has been effective. In immunocompromised patients it may be necessary to continue therapy indefinitely.

[j]In patients with the African form of visceral leishmaniasis, therapy may have to be extended to at least 30 days and may have to be repeated.

[k]Ketoconazole 400 mg daily for 4–8 wk has been reported to be effective (Am J Trop Med Hyg 35:491, 1986).

[l]Application of heat 39–42° C directly to lesion for 20–32 hr over a period of 10–12 days has been reported to be effective in *L. tropica* minor infections (Am J Trop Med Hyg 33:800, 1984).

[m]If chloroquine phosphate is not available, hydroxychloroquine sulfate is as effective; 400 mg of hydroxychloroquine sulfate is equivalent to 500 mg of chloroquine phosphate.

[n]In *P. falciparum* malaria, if the patient has not shown a response to conventional doses of chloroquine in 48–72 hr, parasitic resistance to this drug should be considered. Intramuscular injection of chloroquine is painful and can cause abscesses.

[o]Optimal dosage for treatment of malaria is currently under investigation. For up-to-date information, telephone the Centers for Disease Control (daytime (404) 488–4046; nights, weekends, holidays (404) 639–2888). Electrocardiographic monitoring is necessary to detect arrhythmias. Some experts consider quinidine more effective than quinine.

[p]Quinine alone will usually control an attack of resistant *P. falciparum*, but in a substantial number of infections, particularly with strains from Southeast Asia, it fails to prevent recurrence; the addition of pyrimethamine and sulfadiazine lowers the rate of recurrence.

[q]For treatment of *P. falciparum* infections acquired in Thailand, quinine should be given for 7 days instead of 3, combined with 7 days of tetracycline.

[r]Quinine plus tetracycline may be the regimen of choice in areas such as Thailand, where resistance to pyrimethamine plus sulfonamides is common.

[s]Primaquine phosphate can cause hemolytic anemia, especially in patients whose red cells are deficient in G-6-PD. This deficiency is most common in blacks, Asians, and Mediterranean peoples. Patients should be screeened for G-6-PD deficiency before treatment. Primaquine should not be used during pregnancy.

[t]At present, no drug regimen guarantees protection against malaria. If fever develops within a year (particularly within the first 2 mo) after travel to malarious areas, travelers should be advised to seek medical attention. Countries with a risk of chloroquine-resistant falciparum malaria continue to increase. Travelers to any of these countries should be advised to avoid mosquito bites by using insect repellants containing diethyltoluamide (deet) and using mosquito netting when sleeping in exposed areas.

[u]For prevention of attack after departure from areas where *P. vivax* and *P. ovale* are endemic, which includes almost all areas where malaria is found (except Haiti), some experts prescribe primaquine phosphate (15 mg base (26.3 mg)/24 hr or, for children, 0.3 mg base/kg/24 hr for 14 days). Others prefer to avoid the toxicity of primaquine and rely on surveillance to detect cases when they occur, particularly when exposure was limited or doubtful. Primaquine can cause hemolytic anemia, especially in patients whose red cells are deficient in G-6-PD. This deficiency is most common in blacks, Asians, and Mediterranean peoples. Patients should be screened for G-6-PD deficiency before treatment. Primaquine should not be used during pregnancy.

[v]Proguanil (Paludrine-Ayerst, Canada; ICI) is not available in the United States.

[w]Recommended for travel to Africa south of the Sahara, the Indian subcontinent, South America (except the Amazon basin), Oceania, Hainan Island, and the southern provinces of China. Use of Fansidar, which contains 25 mg of pyrimethamine and 500 mg of sulfadoxine/tablet, is contraindicated in patients with a history of sulfonamide or pyrimethamine intolerance, in pregnancy at term, and in infants less than 2 mo old.

[x]Used in Southeast Asia and the Amazon basin. The FDA considers the use of tetracyclines as antimalarials to be investigational. Use of doxycycline is contraindicated in pregnancy and in children less than 8 yr old. Physicians who prescribe doxycycline as malaria chemoprophylaxis should advise patients to limit direct exposure to the sun to minimize the possibility of a photosensitivity reaction. Young children or other travelers who cannot take doxycycline should carry Fansidar.

[y]Pyrimethamine is teratogenic in animals. To prevent hematologic toxicity from pyrimethamine, it is advisable to give leucovorin (folinic acid) 10/mg/24 hr by injection or orally. In AIDS patients, therapy should be continued indefinitely. Most authorities would treat congenitally infected newborns for about 1 yr.

[z]Sexual partners should be treated simultaneously. Metronidazole-resistant strains have been reported.

[aa]Limited data.

[bb]In drug-resistant cases of *T. gambiense* infections, elflornithine (difluoromethylornithine, Merrell Dow) has been used successfully; field trials are now underway (Taelman H, et al: Am J Med 82:607, 1987; Doua F, et al: Am J Trop Med Hyg 37:525, 1987; Pepin J, et al: Lancet 2:1431, 1987). It is highly effective in both CNS and non-CNS infections with *T. gambiense*.

[cc]In frail patients, begin with as little as 18 mg and increase the dose progressively. Pretreatment with suramin has been advocated for debilitated patients.

mites is uncertain. Hyposensitization and reduction of mite burden (vacuuming and lowering environmental temperature and humidity) can reduce or eliminate allergic symptoms.

TICKS. These are ovoid, blood-sucking, hard- or soft-bodied acarines with 6–8 legs. They attach painlessly to the skin by means of strong teeth and secretions. Ticks in all stages in the life cycle (larval, nymph, and adult) bite humans. Ticks may cause disease directly through bites or as vectors for disease. Bites may produce local reactions or, infrequently, systemic reactions (tick fever or tick pyrexia). Chronic tick granulomas may form at sites where the mouthparts or hypostome remain imbedded in dermis. Alternatively, inflammatory dermatitis may follow continued allergic stimulation from foreign tick proteins; the resulting mononuclear and eosinophilic infiltrate can resemble lymphoma on biopsy. Finally, dermatosis occurs with an expanding circular lesion (erythema chronicum migrans) when ticks serve as vectors for Lyme disease (Sec. 12.57). Prevention of tick bites is easily accomplished with the use of 30% *N*-butyl acetanilide or other insect repellant to clothing or skin.

Tick paralysis, an unusual tick-borne disease that occurs in children, is a progressive, flaccid, ascending paralysis resembling Guillain-Barré syndrome (Sec. 21.50). This disease is believed to be caused by an ovarian neurotoxin secreted by female hard- or soft-bodied ticks. The toxin appears to affect the postsynaptic neuromuscular junction as well as conduction in the large motor nerves. In North America the most common species associated with tick paralysis are *Dermacentor*

TABLE 12–47. Drugs for Treatment of Helminthic Infections

Infection	Drug	Pediatric Dosage[a]	Adverse Effects
Angiostrongyliasis			
Angiostrongylus cantanensis			
Drug of choice:	Mebendazole[b, c, d]	100 mg bid for 5 days for children >2 yr	Occasional: diarrhea, abdominal pain Rare: leukopenia, agranulocytosis, hypospermia
Angiostrongylus costaricensis			
Drug of choice:	Thiabendazole[b, c] OR Surgical intervention	25 mg/kg tid for 3 days[e] (max. 3 g/24 hr)	Frequent: nausea, vomiting, vertigo Occasional: leukopenia, crystalluria, rash, hallucinations, olfactory disturbances, erythema multiforme, Stevens-Johnson syndrome Rare: shock, tinnitus, intrahepatic cholestasis, convulsions, angioneurotic edema
Anisakiasis (*Anisakis* sp.)			
Treatment of choice:	Surgical removal		
Ascariasis			
Ascaris lumbricoides (roundworm)			
Drug of choice:	Mebendazole OR	100 mg bid for 3 days for children >2 yr	See above
	Pyrantel pamoate	11 mg/kg once (max. 1 g)	Occasional: GI disturbances, headache, dizziness, rash, fever
Alternative:	Piperazine citrate	75 mg/kg (max. 3.5 g)/24 hr for 2 days	Occasional: dizziness, urticaria, GI disturbances Rare: exacerbation of epilepsy, ataxia, visual disturbances, hypotonia
Capillariasis			
Capillaria philippinensis			
Drug of choice:	Mebendazole[b]	200 mg bid for 20 days	See above
Alternative:	Thiabendazole[b]	25 mg/kg/24 hr for 30 days	See above
Cutaneous Larva Migrans			
Drug of choice:	Thiabendazole	25 mg/kg bid (max. 3 g/24 hr) for 2–5 days and/or topically	See above
***Dracunculus** medinensis* (Guinea worm infection)			
Drug of choice:	Metronidazole[b]	25 mg/kg/24 hr (max. 750 mg/24 hr) in 3 doses for 10 days	See Table 12–60
Alternative:	Thiabendazole[b]	25–37.5 mg/kg bid for 3 days	See above
***Enterobius** vermicularis* (Pinworm infection)			
Drug of choice:	Pyrantel pamoate	A single dose of 11 mg/kg (max. 1 g) repeated after 2 wk	See above
	OR Mebendazole	A single dose of 100 mg for children >2 yr; repeat after 2 wk	See above
Filariasis			
Wuchereria bancrofti, Brugia malayi, Mansonella, ozzardi, Loa loa			
Drug of choice:[g]	Diethylcarbamazine[h]	Day 1: 25–50 mg Day 2: 25–50 mg tid Day 3: 50–100 mg tid Day 4 thru 21: 2mg/kg tid	Frequent: severe allergic or febrile reaction, GI disturbances Rare: encephalopathy, loss of vision in onchocerciasis
Mansonella perstans			
Drug of choice:[i]	Mebendazole[b]	100 mg bid for 30 days	See above
Tropical eosinophilia			
Drug of choice:	Diethylcarbamazine[h]	2 mg/kg tid for 7–10 days	See above
Onchocerca volvulus			
Drug of choice:	Ivermectin[b, j]	150 μg/kg PO once	Occasional: fever, pruritus, tender lymph nodes Rare: hypotension
Alternatives:	Diethylcarbamazine[h]	0.5 mg/kg tid for 3 days (max. 25 mg/24 hr), then 1.0 mg/kg tid for 3–4 days (max. 50 mg/ 24 hr), then 1.5 mg/kg tid for 3–4 days (max. 100 mg/24 hr), then 2.0 mg/kg tid for 2–3 wk	See above
	FOLLOWED BY Suramin[k, l]	10–20 mg (test dose) IV, then 20 mg/kg IV at weekly intervals for 5 wk	See Table 12–60
Fluke *infection*			
Clonorchis sinensis (Chinese liver fluke)			
Drug of choice:	Praziquantel[b]	25 mg/kg tid for 2 days	Frequent: malaise, headache, dizziness Occasional: sedation, abdominal discomfort, fever, sweating, nausea, eosinophilia, fatigue

Table continued on following page

TABLE 12–47. Drugs for Treatment of Helminthic Infections *Continued*

Infection	Drug	Pediatric Dosage[a]	Adverse Effects
Fluke *infection (Continued)*			
Fasciola hepatica (sheep liver fluke) Drug of choice:	Praziquantel[m]	25 mg/kg tid for 2 days	See above
Fasciolopsis buski (intestinal fluke) Drug of choice:	Prazquantel[b]	25 mg/kg tid for 1 day	See above
	OR Niclosamide[b]	11–34 kg: a single dose of 2 tablets (1 g) >34 kg: a single dose of 3 tablets (1.5 g)	Occasional: nausea, abdominal pain
Heterophyes heterophyes (intestinal fluke) Drug of choice:	Praziquantel[b]	25 mg/kg tid for 1 day	See above
Metagonimus yokogawai (intestinal fluke) Drug of choice:	Praziquantel[b]	25 mg/kg tid for 1 day	See above
Opisthorchis viverrini (liver fluke) Drug of choice:	Praziquantel[b]	25 mg/kg tid for 1 day	See above
Paragonimus westermani (lung fluke) Drug of choice:	Praziquantel[b]	25 mg/kg tid for 2 days	See above
Alternative:	Bithionol[l]	30–50 mg/kg on alternate days for 10–15 doses	Frequent: photosensitivity, vomiting, diarrhea, abdominal pain, urticaria Rare: leukopenia, toxic hepatitis
Gnathostomiasis			
Gnathostoma spinigerum Treatment of choice:	Surgical removal OR Mebendazole[b]	Not determined	
Hookworm *infection*			
Ancylostoma duodenale, Necator americanus Drug of choice:	Mebendazole	100 mg bid for 3 days for children >2 yr	See above
	OR Pyrantel pamoate[b]	11 mg/kg (max. 1 g) for 3 days	See above
Schistosomiasis			
S. haematobium Drug of choice:	Praziquantel	20 mg/kg tid for 1 day	See above
S. japonicum Drug of choice:	Praziquantel	20 mg/kg tid for 1 day	See above
S. mansoni Drug of choice:	Praziquantel	20 mg/kg tid for 1 day	See above
Alternative:	Oxamniquine	10 mg/kg bid for 1 day[n]	Occasional: headache, fever, dizziness, somnolence, nausea, diarrhea, rash, liver enzyme changes, ECG and EEG changes, orange-red discoloration of urine Rare: convulsions, neuropsychiatric disturbances
S. mekongi Drug of choice:	Praziquantel	20/mg/kg tid for 1 day	See above
Strongyloidiasis			
Strongyloides stercoralis Drug of choice:	Thiabendazole	25 mg/kg bid (max. 3 g/24 hr) for 2 days[p]	See above
Tapeworm *infection*			
Adult or intestinal stage (*Diphyllobothrium latum* (fish), *Taenia saginata* (beef)[q] *Taenia solium* (pork), *Dipylidium caninum* (dog) Drug of choice:	Niclosamide	11–34 kg: a single dose of 2 tablets (1 g) >34 kg: a single dose of 3 tablets (1.5 g) for 1 day, then 2 tablets for 6 days	See above
Larval or tissue stage	OR	10–20 mg/kg once	See above
	Praziquantel	10–20 mg/kg once	Se above
Hymenolepsis nana (dwarf tapeworm) Drug of choice:	Praziquantel	25 mg/kg once	See above
Alternative:	Niclosamide	11–34 kg: a single dose of 2 tablets (1 g) for 1 day, then 1 tablet for 6 days >34 kg: a single dose of 3 tablets (1.5 g) for 1 day, then 2 tablets for 6 days	See above

TABLE 12–47. Drugs for Treatment of Helminthic Infections *Continued*

Infection	Drug	Pediatric Dosage[a]	Adverse Effects
Tapeworm *infection Continued*			
Echinococcus granulosus			
Treatment of choice:	Surgical resection[r]		
Echinococcus multilocularis			
Treatment of choice:	Surgical resection[s]		
Cysticercus cellulosae (cysticercosis)			
Drug of choice[t]	Praziquantel[b]	50 mg/kg/24 hr in 3 doses for 14 days	See above
Alternative:	Surgery		
Trichinosis			
Trichinella sourakus			
Drugs of choice:	Steroids for severe symptoms PLUS		
	Thiabendazole[u]	25 mg/kg for 5 days	See above
Trichostrongylus *infection*			
Drug of choice:	Thiabendazole[b]	25 mg/mg bid for 2 days	See above
Alternative:	Pyrantel pamoate[b]	11 mg/kg once (max. 1 g)	See above
Trichuriasis			
Trichuris trichiuria (whipworm)			
Drug of choice:	Mebendazole	100 mg bid for 3 days for children >2 yr	See above
Visceral Larva Migrans			
Drug of choice:	Diethylcarbamazine[b] OR	2 mg/kg tid for 7–10 days	See above
	Thiabendazole	25 mg/kg bid for 5 days (max. 3 g)	See above
Alternative:	Mebendazole[b]	100 mg bid for 5 days for children >2 yr	See above

[a]Also see specific sections.
[b]Considered an investigational drug for this condition by the U.S. Food and Drug Administration.
[c]Effectiveness documented only in animals.
[d]Analgesics, corticosteroids, and careful removal of CSF at frequent intervals can relieve symptoms. Albendazole and ivermectin have been used successfully in animals.
[e]This dose is likely to be toxic and may have to be decreased.
[f]Metronidazole is carcinogenic in rodents and mutagenic in bacteria; it should generally not be given to pregnant women, particularly in the 1st trimester.
[g]Several reports indicate that ivermectin may be effective for treatment of *W. bancrofti* (Lancet 1:1030, 1987) and *M. ozzardi* (J Infect Dis 156:662, 1987).
[h]Diethylcarbamazine should be administered with special caution in heavy infections with *Loa loa* because it can provoke ocular problems or an encephalopathy. Antihistamines or corticosteroids may be required to decrease allergic reactions owing to disintegration of microfilariae in treatment of all filarial infections, especially those caused by *Onchocerca* and *Loa loa*. Surgical excision of subcutaneous *Onchocerca* nodules is recommended by some authorities before drug therapy is started. Ivermectin may also be effective.
[i]Ivermectin may also be effective.
[j]Ivermectin in a dose of 200 μg/kg has been reported to be as effective as diethylcarbamazine in decreasing the number of microfilaria and causes fewer adverse ophthalmologic reactions (N Engl J Med 313:133, 1985; J Infect Dis 156:463, 1987). Semiannual to annual prophylaxis appears to be effective in keeping microfilarial counts at low levels.
[k]Some Medical Letter consultants use suramin only if ocular microfilariae persist after diethylcarbamazine therapy and nodulectomy.
[l]In the United States this drug is available from the CDC Drug Service, Centers for Disease Control, Atlanta, Georgia 30333; telephone (404) 639–3670; evenings, weekends, and holidays: (404) 639–2888.
[m]Unlike infections with other flukes, *Fasciola hepatica* infections may not respond to praziquantel. Limited data indicate that albendazole may be effective for this condition.
[n]In East Africa the dose should be increased to 30 mg/kg/24 hr, and in Egypt and South Africa to 30 mg/kg/24 hr for 2 days. Neuropsychiatric disturbances and seizures have been reported in some patients (Am J Trop Med Hyg 35:330, 1986).
[o]Albendazole or ivermectin has also been effective.
[p]In disseminated strongyloidiasis, thiabendazole therapy should be continued for at least 5 days. In immunocompromised patients it may be necessary to continue therapy or use other agents (see footnote *o*).
[q]Niclosamide is effective for the treatment of *T. solium*, but, since it causes distintegration of segments and release of viable eggs, its use creates a theoretical risk of causing cysticercosis. It should therefore be followed in 3 or 4 hr by a purge. Quinacrine is preferred by some clinicians because it expels *T. solium* intact.
[r]Surgical resection of cysts is the treatment of choice. When surgery is contraindicated, or when cysts rupture spontaneously during surgery, mebendazole (experimental for this purpose in the United States) can be tried (Ann Trop Parasitol 76:165, 1982; Trans R Soc Trop Med Hyg 76:510, 1982). Albendazole has also been reported to be effective (JAMA 253:2053, 1985). Flubendazole has also been used with some success. (Am J Trop Med Hyg 33:627, 1984). Praziquantel and albendazole will kill protoscolices and may be useful in case of a spill during surgery.
[s]Surgical excision is the only reliable means of treatment, although recent reports have been encouraging about the use of albendazole or mebendazole (Am J Trop Med Hyg 37:162, 1987; Bull WHO 64:383, 1986).
[t]Corticosteroids should be given for 2–3 days before and during praziquantel therapy. Praziquantel should not be used for ocular or spinal cord cysticercosis. Metrifonate 7.5 mg/kg for 5 days, repeated 6 times at 2-wk intervals, has been reported to be effective for ocular as well as cerebral and subcutaneous disease. Albendazole, 15 mg/kg for 30 days, which can be repeated, has been used successfully (Arch Intern Med 147:738, 1987).
[u]The efficacy of thiabendazole for trichinosis is not clearly established; it appears to be effective during the intestinal phase, but its effect on larvae that have migrated is questionable. In the tissue phase, mebendazole 200–400 mg tid for 3 days, then 400–500 mg tid for 10 days, may be effective. Albendazole may also be effective for this indication.

andersonii, the Rocky Mountain wood tick, and *D. variabilis*, the American dog tick. In children with suspected tick paralysis, a history of exposure to dogs or ticks or camping is important. Initially, the child may present with ataxia and areflexia mimicking the acute cerebellar ataxia of childhood. Over a period of days, ascending muscle weakness may develop; cranial nerve involvement often heralds the onset of respiratory embarrassment. Sensory deficits may be present. Diagnosis is made by a careful search of the skin, particularly in the scalp and other hair-laden regions, for the engorged tick. The tick can be covered with petrolatum and removed with forceps and gentle traction, taking care to extract the mouthparts. Use of organic solvents, such as ether or chloroform, or heat often meets with limited success. Following tick removal, there is usually a rapid recovery from neurologic deficits unless respiratory failure has occurred.

LICE (Anoplura). These arthropods cause **pediculosis**. Three types of infestation are common in humans: head lice, body lice, and pubic lice. These blood-sucking obligate parasites require human contact to complete their life cycle. Body lice are vectors for several diseases typically encountered under conditions of overcrowding and poverty. Infestations are readily treated with application of 1% lindane or pyrethrin coupled with washing of contaminated clothes and linens. A complete description of pediculosis is found in Sec. 23.31.

BED BUGS, KISSING BUGS (Hemiptera). These insects cause multiple pruritic bites that are clustered on exposed areas, often in solitary body sites. Bites are often noted upon awakening and are larger and more persistent than other insect bites. A linear pattern of hemorrhagic lesions may be seen with bed bug bites. Papular, urticarial, and occasional bullous lesions may occur; rarely, anaphylaxis may follow sensitization to foreign Hemiptera proteins. Palliative treatment of bites involves mentholated ointments and compresses; eradication of bed bugs from households can be difficult.

FLEAS (Siphonaptera). These are narrow bodied, blood-sucking, wingless insects that cause papular urticaria in children. Fleas commonly bite humans when preferred specific animal hosts are absent. Fleas may go several months without a blood meal and may reside in carpets or furniture. Consequently, flea bites may occur following a recent move into a vacant abode previously occupied by a dog or cat. Bites are papular irritant lesions with hemorrhagic punctae and are often grouped in clusters or in lines limited by tight clothing. Fleas can also induce pustular or vesicular reactions depending on the degree of host sensitization. Prevention of flea bites is best accomplished by removal of fleas and/or application of insect repellants such as deet to clothing and skin. Topical calamine lotion, mentholated ointments, or cool wet compresses can be used in combination with oral antihistamines to relieve pruritus and pain.

A burrowing flea, *Tunga penetrans* (jigger flea, chigoe), causes **tungiasis** in Central and South America and tropical Africa. The blood-sucking female flea penetrates the stratum corneum of skin between the toes, instep, and ankles and swells to the size of a pea when engorged. The initial pruritic erythematous papule becomes painful. Mature females extrude eggs through the lumen of their burrows and collapse, producing characteristic cutaneous craters. Treatment consists of removal of the intact flea with a sterile needle followed by thorough cleansing. The life cycle of the flea is interrupted by covering the feet with shoes.

MOSQUITOES, SANDFLIES, MIDGES, GNATS, BLACK FLIES, TSETSE FLIES (Diptera). These blood-sucking insects have a single pair of wings. Their bites cause pain and discomfort primarily by allergic reactions to foreign proteins injected in saliva or from local tissue damage. In addition, members of this order are vectors for several diseases characteristic of tropical and temperate climates (see later section, Transmission of Human Disease). Bites from these insects are similar to flea bites but are usually single and not clustered. More severe dermatologic reactions (bullae, induration, and lymphangitis) occasionally follow mosquito bites. Treatment is similar to therapy for flea bites and includes topical lotions and ointments, insect repellants, and removal of offending insects.

DIRECT INVASION

See also scabies and tungiasis in previous section, Blood-Sucking Ectoparasites.

MYIASIS. This refers to the invasion of host organs and tissues by the larval stage (maggot) of nonbiting flies of the order Diptera. Three types of myiasis, representing different parasitic relationships of larvae to man, occur: obligate, facultative, and accidental. Obligate Diptera, such as *Dermatobia hominis* (botfly), require the animal host for complete development. Members of this group often directly invade human tissues. Facultative Diptera are normally free-living larvae that develop in decaying vegetable or animal matter; they are semispecific for human hosts, since development is facilitated under favorable conditions. Blow flies (calliphorids), flesh flies (sarcophagids), and house flies (muscidae) are examples. Accidental myiasis results when insects are inadvertently introduced to areas of the body where larval development cannot occur. The ingestion of food contaminated with larvae or eggs from accidental Diptera produces benign and self-limited intestinal myiasis.

Pathophysiology. Maggots debride necrotic tissue, but both facultative and obligate larvae can destroy normal living tissue. Different lesions occur in myiasis depending on the species of Diptera involved and the site of oviposition. Wounds and all orifices—eyes, ears, nose, mouth, vagina, and bladder—may be infested with maggots. The skin and connective tissue are the major organ systems affected in myiasis. Furuncular lesions can result from individual obligate larvae of the tropical warble fly or human botfly *(Dermatobia hominis)*, Tumbu fly *(Cordylobia anthropophagia)*, or fox, mink, and rodent parasites. Serpiginous creeping eruptions occur when horse botflies (*Gastrophilus* sp.) move through the integument. Deep invasion, with migratory red, painful nodules, can result from the cattle botfly (*Hypoderma* spp.). The screwworms *(Cochlionyia hominivorax* and *Chrysoma bezziana)* are destructive obligate parasites that cause eroding lesions of the skin and head.

Clinical Manifestations. Myiasis frequently occurs in children after outdoor exposure and/or accidental ingestion. Wounds or other areas of injured skin (e.g., arthropod bites, sores, tracheostomy sites, or malignancies) are particularly prone to infestation by facultative larvae. Covered or neglected areas are prone to destructive lesions. *Diagnosis* is by recovery of active, white, headless larvae in tissues or fresh stools. *Treatment* requires removal of larvae by gentle squeezing or excision; debridement may be necessary to remove all invasive maggots. Application of mineral oil, turpentine, or ether will cause some larvae to back out of burrows. Wounds should be cleaned and monitored for signs of secondary infection. *Prevention* includes screening of living areas, cleaning and covering of wounds or discharges, and, in endemic areas, control of natural hosts. Fly control measures should be instituted around farms or other collections of animals.

CONTACT DERMATITIS

See also mites in earlier section, Blood-Sucking Ectoparasites.

CATERPILLARS AND MOTHS (Lepidoptera). These arthropods have irritating, hollow, nettling hairs or setae, which penetrate the dermis and release histamine and other compounds. Immediate itching and burning followed by erythema occur upon contact. Skin lesions can include papules, vesicles, eczema, and secondary infections. Commonly affected areas are the neck, forearms, and perineal region (from contaminated clothing). The puss caterpillar can also produce systemic effects. Prompt removal of hair spines with soap and water, alcohol, or adhesive tape is essential. Calomine lotion, meat tenderizer, or baking soda can be applied to affected areas, and corticosteroids and antihistamines may prove useful for hypersensitivity reactions.

BEETLES (Cleoptera). These insects can cause contact dermatitis by release of potent vesicants; severe conjunctival inflammation may follow accidental inoculation of toxin. The blister beetle (Spanish fly), *Lytta vesicatoria*, releases cantharidin when crushed on the skin, resulting in 5- to 50-mm blisters. Lesions are linear, often mirror-images where skin contacts skin, and may resemble herpetic dermatitis. Therapy is accomplished with topical steroid creams.

MILLIPEDES AND CENTIPEDES (Myriapoda). These are

multisegmented arthropods that rarely cause severe disease. Millipedes have 2 pairs of legs per body segment and are saprophagous. These insects do not bite but excrete noxious secretions from specialized glands that produce burns of the skin and mucous membranes; conjunctival irritation is particularly severe. Centipedes have a single pair of legs for each body segment and are carnivores, using powerful claws to seize prey. Centipedes possess venom glands that inject weak toxins, resulting in local warmth and pain. Occasional lymphangitis may occur. Bites from the giant desert centipede, *Scolopendra heros,* can cause serious myonecrosis and compartment syndrome of the legs. Treatment is primarily supportive, with occasional use of topical anesthetics and steroids.

ENVENOMATION

See Centipedes above.

12.141 Spiders

Spiders are members of the Arthropoda phylum and belong to the class Arachnida, along with scorpions, ticks, and mites. All spiders are members of the order Araneae, are 8-legged, and are characterized by a segmented body, paired and bisegmented cheliderae (jaws), and poison glands. In general, spiders are poisonous and bite humans; however, among the many families of spiders indigenous to the United States, few have jaws capable of penetrating human skin.

NECROTIC ARACHANIDISM. This disorder is caused by the local effects of spider venom and is characterized by the early development of a flat cutaneous lesion with central pallor and surrounding erythema at the site of a spider bite. Local cyanosis due to focal edema and arterial spasm may occur hours to days after the bite. In exceptional cases (mainly associated with *L. reclusa* bites), peripheral edema, erythema, and purpura may occur and may involve the entire limb. The central portion of the lesion becomes necrotic and develops an eschar over a period of time. In addition to the presence of the characteristic lesion, the definitive diagnosis of necrotic arachanidism requires the identification of the spider. *Treatment* is nonspecific and consists of immobilization and elevation of the affected extremity, analgesia, tetanus prophylaxis, and close observation for secondary infection. Systemic administration of corticosteroids is of unproved efficacy but may be indicated in severe cases.

TARANTULAS. These are the largest members of this class. Although the wolf spiders (Lycosidae) are the true tarantulas and are found exclusively in the areas surrounding the Mediterranean, 30–40 members of the Theraphosidae family are indigenous to the American southwest. American members of the *Dugesiella* and *Aphonopelma* genera may grow to 15–20 cm in width and produce venom consisting mainly of hyaluronidase. The danger of tarantula bites is grossly overstated, and most can be treated as necrotic arachnidism. More important, the fine, dorsal, abdominal hairs found on many tarantulas may be flung when the insect is threatened. In humans, these hairs produce pruritic, urticarial, edematous skin lesions that may take several weeks to resolve. Topical or systemic corticosteroid therapy may be required, depending on the severity of the lesions.

BROWN RECLUSE SPIDER (Loxoscelism). There are at least 6 species of the genus *Loxosceles* that cause necrotic arachanidism in humans; the best known is *L. reclusa,* the brown recluse spider. This insect is found throughout the southern and midwestern parts of the United States. The nocturnal recluse spider normally resides in caves and under rocks but is also found in dark, quiet parts of homes, warehouses, and other buildings.

The *clinical manifestations* of recluse spider bites are variable and depend on the underlying health of the victim and the amount of venom injected. Necrotic arachanidism with severe skin scarring occurs commonly with *Loxosceles* bites. Although **viscerocutaneous loxoscelism** is rare, the cases that do occur are seen predominantly in children. Following the bite and injection of venom (probably sphingomylinase D), the cutaneous lesion progresses to a diffuse rash, which may be morbilliform, urticarial, scarletiniform, or petechial in character. Within the first 72 hr, fever, generalized signs of encephalopathy, shock, disseminated intravascular coagulation, hemolysis, hemoglobinuria, and renal failure become manifest.

The *diagnosis* can be confirmed by identifying the spider and obtaining a positive result on a hemagglutination inhibition test performed on fluid expressed from the bite.

Treatment of mild bites not associated with extensive cyanosis, hyperesthesia, or bullae is similar to that given for necrotic arachanidism (see earlier). Some authorities recommend that patients sustaining extensive bites with large necrotic centers receive a short course of systemic corticosteroid therapy, particularly in the presence of early signs of loxoscelism. In one study, administration of dapsone coupled with delayed surgical excision was associated with fewer complications and better outcomes than early surgical excision of the lesion. Children with signs of evolving loxoscelism require immediate hospitalization and close monitoring. Renal function and degree of hemolysis need to be closely monitored. Prompt admission to an intensive care area is required for patients with coagulopathy and shock. Short courses of systemic steroids coupled with vigorous fluid resuscitation and replacement of blood are recommended. No antitoxin is currently available.

WIDOW SPIDERS. The red, brown, and black widow spiders are all members of the genus *Latrodectus* and are indigenous to all parts of the United States. Adult females are black, have red markings on the abdomen, and can grow to 12 mm in length; male insects are smaller. The spiders are usually found close to the ground in protected areas (e.g., under stones or in deserted rodent burrows). Although five different species are found in geographically distinct areas of the country, the neurotoxin contained in the venom of different species is similar and can be counteracted by antivenim to *L. mactans* (antivenom, Merck, Sharpe, and Dohme).

The initial bite is often painless and may go undetected. Within an hour of envenomation, dull cramping pain at the site of the bite progresses to sharp pain followed by numbness; the affected area spreads rapidly to involve the trunk, abdomen, and legs. Signs mimicking peritonitis without abdominal tenderness and distention occur within 2–3 hr and may last for several days. Other systemic symptoms include sweating, nausea, headache, hyperesthesia, muscle cramps, and lower extremity spasms suggestive of tetany. Shock, renal failure, and/or cerebral hemorrhage may occur in as many as half of young children.

For children less than 16 yr of age, hospitalization is recommended; 2.5 mL of antivenim should be administered intravenously or intramuscularly in patients without a history of sensitization to horse sera. Additional modalities include muscle relaxants and analgesics including morphine. Patients with severe pain may achieve partial relief with vigorous exercise.

12.142 Scorpions

Most scorpion stings occur in tropical and subtropical areas. In India and Israel, members of the *Buthus* genus are most commonly encountered, whereas *Androctonus* species are encountered in Africa. Scorpion envenomation in the southwestern United States is caused by *Centruroides sculpturatus*. Although the biochemical composition of venom from different genera of scorpions is variable, the target for most toxins is the neuromuscular junction. *C. sculpturatus* toxin depolarizes the presynaptic junction, causing increased Ca^{2+} permeability and release of acetylcholine. The action of scorpion toxin can be blocked in vitro by strychnine.

The site of the sting is often extremely painful. Systemic manifestations of scorpion envenomation occur most often in small children (by virtue of their size relative to the toxin load) and include tachycardia, hypertension, arrhythmias, irritability, seizures, paresthesias, hypersalivation, tachypnea, pulmonary edema, coma, and cardiac arrhythmias. Application of ice and local injections of lidocaine have been recommended to reduce pain at the site of the sting. The release of venom may be retarded by application of a tourniquet. Although the use of species- or group-specific antivenim is recommended, these preparations are of unproved efficacy.* In general, the clinical manifestations of systemic envenomation are treated supportively. Fluid support and monitoring in an intensive care setting are required. Phenobarbital (6 mg/kg) is required for seizure control; higher doses have been associated with respiratory depression in these patients.

12.143 Babesiosis
(Piroplasmosis)

This protozoan infection is caused by an intraerythrocytic parasite transmitted by hard *Ixodid* ticks. Over 70 species exist; most are confined to a single specific mammalian host. A few, transmitted by multihost ticks, are able to infect humans incidentally. These species (such as *Babesia microti*, a rodent *Babesia* species) are responsible for several emerging zoonoses. In addition, babesiosis may be acquired through blood transfusion from an asymptomatically infected host.

EPIDEMIOLOGY. The primary endemic focus of babesiosis in the United States occurs along the Northeast coastal area, centering around Nantucket Island. The small deer tick, *Ixodes dammini*, serves as the vector for *B. microti*, which is acquired from white-footed mice. Epidemiologic surveys in these areas reveal past infection in 2–7% of the population.

PATHOPHYSIOLOGY. Babesiosis parallels malaria in certain segments of its life cycle. Sporozoites are introduced by tick bites and rapidly invade host red blood cells. Budding forms develop as the protozoan matures and replicates, eventually rupturing the erythrocyte. These daughter forms or mesozoites then infect other red blood cells, and the cycle continues. Conversely, babesia lack an extraerythrocytic stage or sexual forms (gametocytes). Although a ring form may exist in erythrocytes, *Babesia* trophozoites do not contain pigment. Finally, unlike *Plasmodium* species, babesia are present in asynchronous stages in blood.

CLINICAL MANIFESTATIONS. Signs and symptoms follow a variable incubation period of 1–6 wk. A sudden or gradual onset of chills and fever is preceded by malaise, myalgias, and fatigue. Jaundice, dark urine, nausea, and vomiting occur with hemolysis. Mild splenomegaly and/or hepatomegaly occur in a quarter of infected patients. The complications of babesiosis are due to hemolysis, which can lead to renal failure from massive hemoglobinuria and capillary obstruction by parasitized erythrocytes. Laboratory studies show a mild to moderately severe hemolytic anemia, occasional thrombocytopenia, and a near normal white blood cell count; elevation of liver function test results is found in half of all cases.

Asymptomatic hosts may have low levels of parasitemia. In contrast, the most severe forms of babesiosis, including most fatalities, occur in splenectomized hosts. Thus, an intact functioning spleen is apparently necessary to prevent fulminant hemolysis and visceral invasion by babesia. Complete recovery occurs in several weeks, with or without chemotherapy.

DIAGNOSIS. Babesiosis should be suspected in a febrile individual who has travelled to an endemic area or has had a recent blood transfusion. The clinical picture may resemble that of malaria, but peripheral blood smears lack intraerythrocytic pigment, schizonts, gametocytes, or synchronous stages found with malaria. Multiple blood smears may be required to demonstrate parasitemia. An indirect immunofluorescence serologic test with good reliability is available at the Centers for Disease Control. In obscure cases, xenodiagnosis may be attempted in hamsters or gerbils.

TREATMENT. The recommended therapy for babesiosis is clindamycin (20mg/kg/24 hr) and quinine (25 mg/kg/24 hr) in combination. For life-threatening situations, exchange blood transfusions may be required. Prevention of babesiosis involves avoidance of tick-infested areas, use of protective clothing and insect repellants, and a careful search for and removal of ticks.

TRANSMISSION OF HUMAN DISEASE

Arthropods transmit pathogenic organisms either directly by mechanical means or as essential biologic hosts.

MECHANICAL TRANSMISSION. Filth flies are sarcophagous Diptera families (calliphorids, sarcophagids, muscidae) that transmit a wide range of enteric pathogens including salmonellae, shigellae, *vibrio cholera*, and *Entamoeba histolytica*. These flies are vectors of disease in epidemics and other conditions where contamination of food and water supplies by human feces occurs. Cockroaches may also transfer enteric microbes to food.

OBLIGATE TRANSMISSION. Many arthropods function as biologic vectors for human pathogens. These include the following:

Ticks: typhus, Rocky Mountain spotted fever, Q fever, Colorado tick fever, hemorrhagic fever, tularemia, viral encephalitis, Lyme disease, relapsing fever, babesiosis.
Mites: scrub typhus, murine typhus, rickettsialpox.
Body lice: epidemic typhus, trench fever, relapsing fever.
Fleas: plague, murine typhus, several other infections.
Bed bugs and *kissing bugs:* American trypanosomiasis (Chagas' disease), relapsing fever, hepatitis in vitro.
Mosquitoes: malaria, yellow fever, dengue, viral encephalitides, filariasis, tularemia.
Sandflies: leishmaniasis, bartonellosis, sandfly fever, Oroya fever, pappataci fever.
Tsetse flies: African trypanosomiasis (sleeping sickness).
Black flies: onchocerciasis (river blindness).

Interruption of the cycle of disease can be difficult. Specific vaccines reduce host susceptibility to pathogenic organisms. Insecticides reduce the likelihood of pathogen transmission by decreasing vector numbers. Simple maneuvers such as avoidance of heavily infested areas, insect repellants, or protective clothing or netting may significantly reduce the risk of disease. In epidemic conditions, destruction of the reservoir host may be necessary, such as rat vectors in plague. Control of arthropod-borne disease remains a perplexing problem worldwide.

NIRANJAN KANESA-THASAN
STEPHEN C. ARONOFF

*Contact the Information Officer at the Centers for Disease Control, Atlanta, GA.

Amitai Y, Mines Y, Aker M, et al: Scorpion sting in children. Clin Pediatr 24:136, 1984.
Diaz JD, Lockey RF, Stablein JJ, et al: Multiple stings by imported fire ants *(Solenopsis invicta)* without systemic effects. South Med J 82:775, 1989.
Ellenhorn MJ, Barceloux DG: Envenomations from bites and stings. *In:* Ellenhorn MJ, Barceloux DG (eds): Medical Toxicology: Diagnosis and Treatment of Human Poisoning. Amsterdam, Elsevier, 1988.
Guillozet N: Diagnosing myiasis. JAMA 244:698, 1980.
Haller JS, Fabara JA: Tick paralysis. Case report with emphasis on neurological toxicity. Am J Dis Child 124:915, 1972.
Harves AD, Millikan LE: Current concepts of therapy and pathophysiology in arthropod bites and stings. Parts I and II. Int J Dermatol 14:543, 621, 1975.
Honig PJ: Bites and parasites. Pediatr Clin North Am 30:563, 1983.
Insect repellants. Med Letter 31:45, 1989.
Maguire JF, Geha RS: Bee, wasp, and hornet stings. Pediatr Rev 8:5, 1986.
Platt-Mills TAE, et al: Dust mites. Immunology, allergic disease and environmental controls. J Allerg Clin Immunol 80:775, 1987.
Rachesky IJ, Banner W Jr, Dansky J, et al: Treatments for *Centruroides exilicauda* envenomation. Am J Dis Child 138:1136, 1984.
Rees RS, Altenbern P, Lynch J, et al: Brown recluse spider bites: A comparison of early surgical excision vs dapsone with delayed surgical excision. Ann Surg 202:659, 1985.
Rimsza ME, Zimmerman DR, Bergeson PS: Scorpion envenomation. Pediatrics 66:298, 1980.
Rosenthal L, Meldolesi J: Alpha-latrotoxin and related toxins. Pharmacol Ther 42:115, 1989.
Ruebush TK, Juranek DD, Spielman A, et al: Epidemiology of human babesiosis on Nantucket Island. Am J Trop Med Hyg 30:937, 1981.
Shelley ED, Shelley WB, Pula JF, et al: The diagnostic challenge of nonburrowing mite bites: *Cheyletiella yasquri*. JAMA 251:2690, 1984.
Taylor OR Jr: Health problems associated with African bees. Ann Intern Med 104:267, 1986.
Vorse H, Seccareccio P, Woodruff K, et al: Disseminated intravascular coagulopathy following fatal brown spider bite (necrotic arachnidism). J Pediatr 80:1035, 1972.
Wong RC, Hughes SE, Voorhees JJ: Spider bites. Arch Dermatol 123:98, 1987.

13

THE DIGESTIVE SYSTEM

ORAL CAVITY

The condition of the oral cavity is important to the physical and psychologic health of every child. Timely diagnosis and treatment require close cooperation between physicians and dentists. Many older children have regular dental examinations, but the oral problems of infants that require dental referral are recognized primarily through routine visits to physicians.

All parents of children should receive oral health counseling, particularly on feeding practices, from birth, but certainly before 1 yr of age. Children identified at risk for dental disease (e.g., over 1 yr of age and still sleeping with the nursing bottle) should be referred for dental care. Children should receive a visual oral inspection from a dentist by 18–24 mo of age. Once a rapport with the dentist is established, appointments should be regularly scheduled. Some children with active caries need to be followed every 3 mo. Most children should be seen every 6 mo and some once a year. Oral hygiene instruction should begin at the 1st dental visit. This provides an excellent opportunity to discuss dental disease when parental interest is high, to counsel about avoiding harmful practices, and to initiate measures to prevent dental caries (Sec. 13.6).

13.1 DEVELOPMENT OF THE TEETH

INITIATION. The primary teeth form in dental crypts that arise from a band of epithelial cells incorporated into each developing jaw. By the 12th wk of fetal life each of these epithelial bands (the dental laminae) has five areas of rapid growth on each side of the maxilla and the mandible, seen as rounded, bud-like enlargements. Organization of adjacent mesenchyme takes place in each area of epithelial growth, and the two elements together are the beginning of a tooth.

The permanent teeth form in two groups. After the formation of the primary crypts another generation of tooth buds forms lingually from each side for the permanent incisors, cuspids, and premolars, which will erupt into sites previously occupied by primary teeth. This process takes place from about the 5th gestational mo for the central incisors to about 10 mo of age for the second bicuspids. Permanent molars, on the other hand, arise from extension of the dental laminae backward, beyond the site of the second primary molars. Bud-like enlargements form for the 1st, 2nd, and 3rd permanent molars at approximately 4 mo of gestation, 1 yr of age, and 4–5 yr of age, respectively.

HISTODIFFERENTIATION-MORPHODIFFERENTIATION. As the epithelial bud proliferates, the deeper surface invaginates, and a mass of mesenchyme becomes partially enclosed. Beginning with the crown, the epithelial cells assume the shape of the tooth they represent and lay down the organic matrix for calcification of dentin. The vascular, nerve, and lymph structures (the dental pulp of the mature tooth) are confined in the mesenchyme of the hollow central portion of the tooth bud.

CALCIFICATION. The deposition of the inorganic mineral crystals of mature enamel and dentin takes place after the organic matrix has been laid down, from several sites of calcification that later coalesce. The characteristics of the inorganic portions of a tooth can be altered by (1) disturbances in formation of the matrix, (2) decreased availability of one or more of the minerals involved, or (3) the incorporation of foreign materials. Such disturbances may affect the color, texture, or thickness of the tooth surface.

ERUPTION. At the time of tooth bud formation, each tooth begins a continuous movement outward in relation to the bone. The times of eruption of the human permanent teeth and the times of eruption and shedding of the primary teeth are listed in Table 3–10. The mandibular teeth usually erupt before the maxillary teeth, and those of girls generally earlier than those of boys.

13.2 ANOMALIES ASSOCIATED WITH TOOTH DEVELOPMENT

Both failures and excesses of tooth initiation are observed. *Anodontia*, or absence of teeth, occurs when no tooth buds form. Total anodontia often occurs with ectodermal dysplasia. Partial anodontia results from disturbance of a normal site of initiation (e.g., the area of a palatal cleft), or from genetic failure (frequently familial) to code the formation of specific teeth. The third molars, maxillary lateral incisors, and mandibular second premolars are the teeth that most commonly fail to form. If the dental lamina produces more than the normal number of buds, *supernumerary teeth* occur, most often in the area of the maxillary central incisors. Because they tend to disrupt the position and eruption of the adjacent normal teeth, their identification as supernumerary teeth by roentgenographic examination is important. Supernumerary teeth occur in Gardner syndrome and orofaciodigital syndromes. *Natal teeth* must be differentiated from supernumerary teeth (see later).

Disturbances during differentiation may result in gross alterations in dental morphology, such as *macrodontia* (large teeth) or *microdontia* (small teeth). The maxillary lateral incisors may assume a slender, tapering shape ("peg-shaped laterals").

Twinning, in which two teeth are joined together, is most often observed in the mandibular incisors of the primary dentition. It may result from gemination, fusion, or concrescence. Gemination is the result of division of one tooth germ to form a bifid or cloven crown on a single root with a common pulp canal; an extra tooth is then present in the dental arch. Fusion is the joining of incompletely developed teeth that, owing to pressure or trauma or crowding, continue to develop as one tooth. Fused teeth are sometimes joined through their entire length; in other cases a single wide crown is supported on two roots. Concrescence is the attachment of the roots of closely approximated adjacent teeth by an excessive deposit of cementum. This type of twinning, unlike the others, is found most often in the maxillary molar region.

Amelogenesis imperfecta, a dominant genetic trait, results in faulty production of the organic matrix. The teeth are covered by only a thin layer of abnormally formed enamel through which the yellow underlying dentin is seen, giving a darkened appearance to the dentition. Usually both primary and permanent teeth are affected. Susceptibility to caries is low, but the enamel is subject to destruction from abrasion. Complete coverage of the crown may be indicated for dentin protection and improved appearance.

Dentinogenesis imperfecta, or hereditary opalescent dentin, is an analogous condition in which the odontoblasts fail to differentiate normally and poorly calcified dentin results. This autosomal dominant disorder may also occur in patients with osteogenesis imperfecta. The junction between the enamel and dentin is altered, the enamel has a tendency to flake away, and the exposed dentin is then susceptible to abrasion. The teeth are opaque and pearly, and the pulp chambers are obliterated by calcification. Both primary and permanent teeth are usually involved. Unless the crowns of these teeth are covered early and completely, the abrasion of chewing often reduces them to the level and contour of the supporting alveolar bone.

Localized disturbances of calcification that correlate with periods of illness or malnutrition are common and analogous to the growth disturbance lines often seen in roentgenograms of long bones. An example is the neonatal line commonly observed on the primary teeth and on the permanent central incisors and tips of cuspids at coronal levels consistent with the stage of calcification at birth. Two general disturbances of the surface of the enamel are also seen. Discoloration of the smooth surface, usually a more opaque white patch, is referred to as *hypocalcification*. A more severe disturbance, *hypoplasia*, may be manifest as pitting or as areas devoid of covering enamel. Hypoplasia is uncommon in the primary dentition because intrauterine stress is relatively infrequent compared with the frequent occurrence of illness during early infancy when the enamel of the outer third of the permanent incisors, cuspids, and first molars is forming. Enamel hypoplasia has been associated with prenatal and postnatal infection, hypothyroidism, head-neck irradiation, local trauma, and dental abscesses. Pitted enamel hypoplasia is a feature of tuberous sclerosis. Dental restoration of such areas is desirable to eliminate the sensitivity of exposed dentin, to prevent caries, and to improve the appearance.

Mottled enamel is found in persons whose early life is spent in areas where the fluoride content of the drinking water is greater than 2.0 parts per million (ppm) and is probably due to ameloblastic dysfunction. It varies from small inconspicuous white patches to severe, brownish discoloration and hypoplasia; the latter changes are usually seen with fluoride concentrations of greater than 5.0 ppm.

Disturbances due to *mineral deficiency* are rare, but irregular dentin and enlarged pulp chambers have been observed with vitamin D-resistant rickets, and hypoplasia has been observed with vitamin D-deficient rickets.

Discolored teeth may result from incorporation of foreign substances into developing enamel. Neonatal *hyperbilirubinemia* may produce blue to black discoloration of the primary teeth, beginning at the neonatal line; the tips of the permanent first molars may also be affected. Porphyria produces a red-brown discoloration. *Tetracyclines* are extensively incorporated into bones and teeth and, if administered during the period of formation of enamel, may result in brown-yellow discoloration and hypoplasia of the enamel. Such teeth fluoresce under ultraviolet light. Doxycycline has a lower risk for tooth discoloration than other tetracyclines. The period at risk extends from about the 4th mo of gestation to the 10th mo of life for primary teeth, and from about the 4th mo to the 16th yr of life for permanent teeth. Repeated or prolonged therapy with tetracycline has the highest risk. Enamel is completely formed on all but the third molars by about 8 yr of age; accordingly, tetracyclines should not be prescribed for pregnant women or for children under 8 yr of age.

As the teeth penetrate the gums, inflammation and sensitivity sometimes occur *(teething)*. The child may become irritable, and salivation may increase markedly. A blunt, firm object for the infant to bite usually provides some relief; incision of the gums is seldom indicated. There is no evidence that systemic disturbances such as low-grade fever, facial rashes, or mild diarrhea can result from teething.

Delayed eruption of all teeth may indicate systemic or nutritional disturbances such as hypopituitarism, hypothyroidism, cleidocranial dysostosis, Gardner syndrome, 21-trisomy, de Lange syndrome, progeria, and rickets. Failure of eruption of single or small groups of teeth may arise from local causes such as malpositioning of teeth, supernumerary teeth, cysts, or retained primary teeth. Premature loss of primary predecessors is the most common cause of premature eruption of teeth. If the entire dentition is advanced for age and sex, precocious puberty or hyperthyroidism should be considered.

Natal teeth are observed in approximately 1:2,000 newborn infants; usually there are two in the position of the mandibular central incisors. Natal teeth are present at birth, whereas neonatal teeth erupt in the first mo of life. Eruption cysts may precede neonatal teeth. Attachment of natal teeth is generally limited to the gingival margin, with little root formation or bony support; such teeth should not be considered supernumerary until so identified roentgenographically. A natal tooth may be a prematurely erupted primary tooth, in which case early dental eruption may be expected. Natal teeth are associated with cleft palate, Pierre Robin syndrome, Ellis-van Creveld syndrome, Hallermann-Streiff syndrome, and other anomalies. A family history of natal teeth or premature eruption is present in 15–20% of affected children.

Natal teeth may result in pain and refusal to feed, secondary to looseness and movement, and may produce maternal discomfort due to abrasion or biting of the nipple during nursing. There is danger of detachment with aspiration of the tooth. Because the tongue lies between the alveolar processes during birth, it may become lacerated, and occasionally the tip is amputated (Riga-Fede disease). Decisions regarding extraction of prematurely erupted primary teeth must be made on an individual basis; extraction requires careful dissection of the gingival attachment to prevent tearing of the tissue and excessive hemorrhage.

Exfoliation failure occurs when a primary tooth is not shed prior to the eruption of its permanent successor. The primary tooth should be extracted if the erupting permanent tooth becomes visible. This occurs most commonly in the mandibular incisor region.

13.3 DISORDERS OF THE TEETH ASSOCIATED WITH OTHER CONDITIONS

Osteogenesis imperfecta is usually accompanied by hereditary opalescent dentin, also termed "dentinogenesis imperfecta" (Sec. 13.2). Treatment usually involves covering the crowns.

In *cleidocranial dysostosis* orofacial variations include frontal bossing, mandibular prognathism, and a broadened base of the nose. Eruption of teeth is usually delayed. The primary teeth are abnormally retained, and the permanent teeth may remain unerupted. Supernumerary teeth are common, especially in the premolar area. Erupted teeth are free of hypoplasia, but variations in size and shape are common. The primary teeth and permanent teeth that do erupt should be restored if they become carious. Patients with this disorder need extensive dental therapy in order to maintain efficient chewing.

In *ectodermal dysplasia* (Sec. 23.7) the teeth are totally or partially absent. Because alveolar bone does not develop in the absence of teeth, the alveolar processes are usually either totally or partially absent, and the resultant overclosure of the mandible causes the lips to protrude. Facial development is otherwise not disturbed. Teeth, when present, are small and conical in form. Aplasia of the buccal and labial mucous glands leads to dryness and irritation of the oral mucosa. Persons with ectodermal dysplasia need either partial or full dentures. The vertical height between the jaws is thus restored, improving the position of the lips and facial contours. Masticatory function is restored, and eating habits are therefore improved.

Congenital syphilis affects differentiation of permanent teeth, resulting in screwdriver-shaped incisors, often with central notches in their incisive edges (Hutchinson incisors), and mulberry molars, with lobular occlusal surfaces and narrow, pinched crowns (Sec. 12.50). Dental problems associated with other medical conditions are noted in Table 13–1.

13.4 MALOCCLUSION

The oral cavity can be viewed as a masticatory machine. The incisal edges of the anterior teeth are brought into opposition by mandibular closure for the purpose of biting off portions of large food items. The cusps of the opposing posterior teeth interdigitate and slide across each other to reduce foodstuffs to a soft, moist bolus. The cheeks and tongue force the food onto the areas of tooth contact.

The masseter and temporal muscles are the main forces of mandibular closure. Acting in conjunction with the internal pterygoid muscles, they produce high pressures of contact on opposing teeth. If a number of teeth meet simultaneously, the force is distributed over a large area of bone-to-tooth attachment. In malocclusion, when only a few teeth touch, the same force is exerted over a much smaller area. In adulthood, occlusal deformities are a leading cause of loss of teeth. Accordingly, preventive measures in childhood should be directed at establishing proper relationships between upper and lower dental arches for physiologic as well as cosmetic reasons.

Variations in growth patterns are classified into three main types of occlusion (Fig. 13–1). The occlusal relation is determined by observing the positions of the teeth when the jaws are closed and the heads of the mandibular condyles are in the most posterior position within the glenoid fossa. In class I (normal), the cusps of the posterior mandibular teeth interdigitate ahead of and inside the corresponding cusps of the opposing maxillary teeth. This relationship provides a normal facial profile. In class II, the cusps of the posterior mandibular teeth are behind and inside the corresponding cusps of the maxillary teeth. This is the most common occlusal discrepancy; approximately 45% of the population exhibits some degree of this condition. An increased space between upper and lower anterior teeth encourages sucking and tongue-thrust habits. The appearance of a receding chin accompanies the retrognathia. In class III, the cusps of the posterior mandibular teeth interdigitate a tooth or more ahead of their opposing maxillary counterparts. The anterior teeth are directly opposed, or the mandibular incisors protrude beyond the maxillary; a protruding chin accompanies prognathia.

CROSS BITE. Normally the mandibular teeth are in a position just inside the maxillary teeth, so that the outside mandibular cusps or incisal edges meet the central portion of the opposing maxillary teeth. A reversal of this relation is referred to as a "cross bite."

OPEN AND CLOSED BITES. If the posterior mandibular and maxillary teeth make contact with each other but the anterior ones are still apart, the situation is called an "open bite." With the posterior teeth together, if the mandibular anterior teeth occlude inside the maxillary anterior teeth in an overclosed position, the situation is referred to as a "closed bite." Treatment consists of orthodontic correction; a few cases require orthognathic surgery. Optimal timing of treatment varies; earlier treatment generally allows some redirection of the growth pattern. Prognosis with early treatment is good, except in severe cases.

DENTAL CROWDING. Overlap of incisors can result when the jaws are too small for adequate alignment of the teeth. Growth of the jaws is mostly in the posterior aspects of the mandible and maxilla, and there is little growth in the anterior region; inadequate space for the permanent incisor teeth at 7 or 8 yr of age will not resolve with growth of the jaws. Moderate spacing of primary incisors is desirable for adequate alignment of successor teeth; a lack of spacing between primary incisors results in crowded permanent incisors.

THUMB SUCKING. Various and conflicting theories have explained thumb sucking in children, and there are conflicting recommendations for its correction. Prolonged thumb sucking can cause flaring of the maxillary incisor teeth. More than half of children have had a thumb-sucking habit at some time. The prevalence of thumb sucking decreases steadily from the age of 2 yr to approximately 10% by the age of 5.

TABLE 13–1. Dental Problems Associated with Selected Medical Conditions

Medical Condition	Common Associated Dental or Oral Condition
• Cleft lip and palate	Missing teeth, extra (supernumerary) teeth, shifting of arch segments, feeding difficulties
• Kidney failure	Mottled enamel (permanent teeth), facial dysmorphology
• Cystic fibrosis	Stained teeth with extensive medication, mottled enamel
• Immunosuppression	Oral candidiasis with potential for systemic candidiasis
• Low birthweight with prolonged oral intubation	Palatal groove, narrow arch
• Heart defects with SBE* susceptibility	Bacteremia from dental procedures or trauma
• Neutrophil chemotactic deficiency	Juvenile periodontitis (loss of supporting bone around teeth)
• Juvenile diabetes (uncontrolled)	Juvenile periodontitis
• Neuromotor dysfunction	Oral trauma from falling; malocclusion (open bite); gingivitis from lack of hygiene
• Prolonged illness (generalized) during tooth formation	Enamel hypoplasia of crown portions forming during illness
• Seizures	Gingival enlargement if phenytoin is used
• Vitamin D-dependent rickets	Enamel hypoplasia

*SBE = subacute bacterial endocarditis.

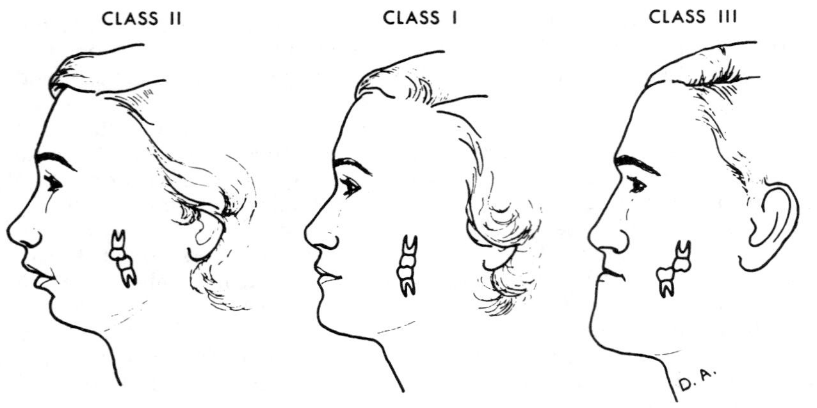

Figure 13–1. Angle classification of occlusion. The typical correspondence between the profile and molar relationship is shown.

The likelihood of long-term effect on the developing dentition and face is controversial. The prognosis is good in children with procumbent incisors and acceptable occlusion of the molar and canine teeth; discontinuation of the habit usually results in lessening of the incisor procumbency, with the possibility of an acceptable occlusion. The prognosis is mixed in children with procumbent incisors and a malrelationship of jaws or of posterior teeth; discontinuation of the habit reduces the procumbency of the incisors but will not rectify an already deviant growth pattern. The prognosis worsens with continuation of the habit beyond 6 yr of age. A variety of treatment protocols have been suggested. A common measure is the insertion of an appliance with modest extensions that serve as a reminder when the child attempts to insert the thumb. Greatest likelihood of success occurs in cases in which the child desires to stop.

13.5 DEVELOPMENTAL ABNORMALITIES WITH MULTIPLE DENTAL AND ORAL PROBLEMS

CLEFT LIP AND PALATE

Clefts of the lip and palate are distinct entities closely related embryologically, functionally, and genetically. Cleft of the lip appears to be due to hypoplasia of the mesenchymal layer, resulting in a failure of the medial nasal and maxillary processes to join. Cleft of the palate appears to represent failure of the palatal shelves to approximate or fuse.

INCIDENCE AND EPIDEMIOLOGY. The incidence of cleft lip with or without cleft palate is about 1:1,000 births; the incidence of cleft palate alone is about 1:2,500 births. The former is more common in males. Genetic factors are of more importance in cleft lip with or without cleft palate than in cleft palate alone. However, both may occur sporadically; the incidence is highest among Asians and lowest among Blacks. The incidence of associated congenital malformations and of impairment in development is increased in children with cleft defects, especially in those with cleft palate alone. These findings are partially explained by an increased incidence of conductive hearing impairment in children with cleft palate due in part to repeated middle ear infections and by the frequency of cleft defects among children with chromosomal abnormalities. The risks of recurrence of cleft defects within families are discussed in Sec. 7.10.

Animal studies suggest that nongenetic influences may be responsible for clefts in a susceptible host at a critical period of organogenesis. Associated malformations are especially frequent in structures derived from the first branchial arch.

CLINICAL MANIFESTATIONS. Cleft lip may vary from a small notch in the vermilion border to a complete separation extending into the floor of the nose. Clefts may be unilateral (more often on the left side) or bilateral and usually involve the alveolar ridge. Deformed, supernumerary, or absent teeth are associated. The nasal alar cartilage clefts of the lip are frequently associated with deficiency of the columella and elongation of the vomer, producing a protrusion of the anterior aspect of the cleft premaxillary process.

Isolated cleft palate occurs in the midline and may involve only the uvula or may extend into or through the soft and hard palates to the incisive foramen. When associated with cleft lip, the defect may involve the midline of the soft palate and extend into the hard palate on one or both sides, exposing one or both of the nasal cavities as a unilateral or bilateral cleft palate.

TREATMENT. The most immediate problem is feeding; a plastic obturator is fitted soon after birth to aid in control of fluids, provide a reference plane for suction, and provide stability for the lateral arch segments. Rapid growth of the dental arches requires the obturator to be refitted every few wk. Soft artificial nipples with large openings are beneficial to patients with cleft palate. Patients with isolated cleft lip may be breast-fed.

Surgical closure of a cleft lip is usually performed by 2 mo of age, when the infant has shown satisfactory weight gain and is free of any oral, respiratory, or systemic infection. Z-plasty is the most commonly used technique; a staggered suture line minimizes notching of the lip from retraction of scar tissue. The initial repair may be revised at 4–5 yr of age. In many instances, corrective surgery on the nose is delayed until adolescence. Nasal surgery is frequently performed at the time of the lip repair. Cosmetic results depend on the extent of the original deformity, absence of infection, and skill of the surgeon.

Because clefts of the palate vary considerably in size, shape, and degree of deformity, the timing of surgical correction should be individualized. Criteria such as width of the cleft, adequacy of the existing palatal segments, the morphology of the surrounding areas (such as width of the oropharynx), and the neuromuscular function of the soft palate and pharyngeal walls affect the decision. The goals of surgery are the union of the cleft segments, intelligible and pleasant speech, reduction of nasal regurgitation, and avoidance of injury to the growing maxilla. In an otherwise healthy child, closure of the palate is usually done prior to 1 yr of age to enhance normal speech development. When surgical correction is delayed beyond the 3rd yr, a contoured speech bulb can be attached to the posterior of a maxillary denture so that contraction of the pharyngeal and velopharyngeal muscles can bring tissues into contact with the bulb to accomplish occlusion of the nasopharynx and help the child to develop intelligible speech. Almost always the cleft crosses the alveolar ridge and interferes with the formation of teeth in the area. The missing elements of the dentition must be replaced by prosthetic devices; alterations of the positions of teeth may also be necessary.

PREOPERATIVE AND POSTOPERATIVE MANAGEMENT. Even the suspicion of infection is a contraindication to operation. If the child is in good nutritional condition and in fluid and electrolyte balance, feeding may be permitted to within 6 hr of the operation (Sec. 6.50). During the immediate postoperative period special nursing care is essential. Gentle aspiration of the nasopharynx minimizes the chances of the common complications of atelectasis or pneumonia. The primary considerations in postoperative care are maintenance of a clean suture line and avoidance of strain on the sutures. For these reasons the infant is fed with a medicine dropper, and the arms are restrained with elbow cuffs. A fluid or semifluid diet is maintained for 3 wk, and feeding is done with a dropper or spoon. The patient's hands as well as toys and other foreign bodies must be kept away from the palate.

COMPLICATIONS. Recurrent otitis media and hearing loss are frequent. Excessive dental decay is not unusual. Displacement of the maxillary arches and malpositions of the teeth usually require orthodontic correction.

Speech defects may be present or persist even after good anatomic closure of the palate. Such speech is characterized by the emission of air from the nose and by a hypernasal quality when certain sounds are made. Both before and, at times, after palatal surgery, the speech defect is due to inadequacies in function of the palatal and pharyngeal muscles. The muscles of the soft palate and the lateral and posterior walls of the nasopharynx constitute a valve that separates the nasopharynx from the oropharynx during swallowing and in the production of certain sounds. If the valve does not function adequately, it is difficult to build up enough pressure in the mouth to make such explosive sounds as p, b, d, t, h, y, or the sibilants s, sh, and ch, and such words as "cats," "boats," and "sisters" are not intelligible. After operation or the insertion of a speech appliance, speech therapy may be necessary.

A complete program of habilitation for the child with a cleft lip or palate may require years of special treatment by a team consisting of pediatrician, plastic surgeon, otolaryngologist, pediatric dentist, prosthodontist, orthodontist, speech therapist, medical social worker, psychologist, child psychiatrist, and public health nurse. Ideally, the child's physician should be responsible for coordination of the use of specialists, and for parental counseling and guidance.

PALATOPHARYNGEAL INCOMPETENCE

The speech disturbance characteristic of the child with a cleft palate can also be produced by other osseous or neuromuscular abnormalities when there is an inability to form an effective seal between oropharynx and nasopharynx during swallowing or phonation. The abnormality may be in the structures of the palate or pharynx or in the muscles attached to these structures. In a child who has previously spoken normally, adenoidectomy may precipitate the speech defect when a submucous cleft palate has not been recognized. In such cases, the adenoid mass may have facilitated a seal when the elevated soft palate made contact with it, this becoming impossible after removal of the adenoids. If there is sufficient reserve neuromuscular function, compensation in palatopharyngeal movement may take place and the speech defect may disappear, although often some symptoms of palatopharyngeal incompetence may persist. In other cases, slow involution of the adenoids may allow for gradual compensation in palatal and pharyngeal muscular function. This may explain why a speech defect does not become apparent in some children who have a submucous cleft palate or similar anomaly predisposing to palatopharyngeal incompetence.

CLINICAL MANIFESTATIONS. The symptoms of palatopharyngeal incompetence are similar to those of a cleft palate, although clinical signs vary. There may be hypernasal speech (especially noted in the articulation of pressure consonants such as p, b, d, t, h, v, f, and s); conspicuous constricting movement of the nares during speech; inability to whistle, gargle, blow out a candle, or inflate a balloon; loss of liquid through the nose when drinking with the head down; and otitis media and hearing loss. Oral inspection may reveal a cleft palate or a relatively short palate with a large oropharynx; absent, grossly asymmetric, or minimal muscular activity of the soft palate and pharynx during phonation or gagging; or a submucous cleft. The latter is suggested by a bifid uvula, by a translucent membrane in the midline of the soft palate (revealing lack of continuity of muscles), by palpable notching in the posterior border of the hard palate instead of a posterior nasal spinous process, or by forward or V-shaped displacement or grooving on the soft palate during phonation or gagging.

Palatopharyngeal incompetence may also be demonstrated roentgenographically. The head should be carefully positioned to obtain a true lateral view; one film is obtained with the patient at rest and another during continuous phonation of the vowel "u" as in "boom." The soft palate contacts the posterior pharyngeal wall in normal function, whereas in palatopharyngeal incompetence such contact is absent.

TREATMENT. In selected cases the palate may be retropositioned or pharyngoplasty performed utilizing a flap of tissue from the posterior pharyngeal wall. Dental speech appliances have also been used successfully.

SYNDROMES WITH ORAL MANIFESTATIONS

Many syndromes have distinct or accompanying facial, oral, and dental manifestations (e.g., Apert syndrome, Sec. 20.16; Crouzon disease, Sec. 20.16; Down syndrome, Sec. 7.14).

Pierre Robin sequence consists of micrognathia with glossoptosis (and pseudomacroglossia) and high arched or cleft palate. Posterior displacement of the attachment of the genioglossus muscle to the hypoplastic mandible prevents the normal anchorage of the tongue; in the supine child, under the influence of gravity, the tongue falls back, obstructing the pharynx. A postalveolar cleft of the hard and soft palates is a common but not constant feature, and in some cases the palate is high-arched.

The tongue is usually of normal size, but the floor of the mouth is foreshortened and the buccal cavity is reduced in size. Obstruction of the air passages may occur, particularly on inspiration, and usually requires treatment to prevent suffocation. The infant should be maintained in a prone or partially prone position so that the tongue falls forward to relieve respiratory obstruction. Temporary suturing of the ventral surface of the tongue to the lower lip is usually not necessary; nor is tracheostomy, because sufficient mandibular growth generally takes place within a few mo to relieve the glossoptosis. Use of splints and traction devices to pull the mandible forward has been unsuccessful. The feeding of infants with mandibular hypoplasia requires great care and patience but can usually be accomplished without resort to gavage. Often the growth of the mandible will achieve an essentially normal profile within 4–6 yr. Dental anomalies usually require individualized treatment.

In *mandibulofacial dysostosis* (Treacher Collins syndrome or Franceschetti syndrome), the facial appearance is characterized by palpebral fissures sloping downward toward the outer canthi, colobomas of the lower eyelids, sunken cheekbones, blind fistulas opening between the angles of the mouth and the ears, deformed pinnas, atypical hair growth extending toward the cheeks, receding chin, and large mouth. Facial clefts, abnormalities of the ears, and deafness are common. The disorder is autosomal dominant, often with incomplete expression. The mandible is usually hypoplastic; the undersurface is often pronouncedly concave, the ramus may be deficient, and the coronoid and condyloid processes are flat or even aplastic. The palatal vault may be either high or cleft. Infrequently, unilateral or bilateral macrostomia, or failure of embryonic fusion of the maxillary and mandibular processes, may occur. Dental malocclusions are frequent, owing to poor maxillary development and palatal deformity. The teeth may be widely separated, hypoplastic, or displaced or have an open bite. Orthodontic and routine dental treatments are indicated.

Unilateral hypoplasia of the mandible is sometimes part of a syndrome that includes partial paralysis of the facial nerve, macrostomia, blind fistulas between the angles of the mouth and the ears, and deformed ear lobes. Severe facial asymmetry and malocclusion develop because of the absence or hypoplasia of the mandibular condyle on the affected side. Congenital condylar deformity tends to increase with age. Early plastic surgery may be indicated to minimize the deformity.

Facial asymmetries resulting from excessive molding of the cranium or from displacement of the mandible during breech or face presentations are common and are usually self-correcting. Facial asymmetry owing to injury of the growing cartilage or fracture of the condylar head during birth, infancy, or early childhood may be permanent. Traumatic injuries may occur during birth from obstetric forceps placed over the area or may result from blows on the chin during infancy and childhood.

Injuries, acute infections, or arthritis of the growing condylar cartilage may result in partial (fibrous) or complete (bony) ***ankylosis of the temporomandibular joint*** and failure of that side of the mandible to grow. The normal side, meanwhile, continues to grow and pushes the midline toward the affected side. The midline deviation is exaggerated during mouth opening. Roentgenograms of the affected side reveal an increased preangular notch or displaced condylar head. Bilateral injuries to the growing cartilage result in failure of the mandible and chin to grow downward and forward, causing the entire mandible to be retruded and smaller than normal.

13.6 DENTAL CARIES

In otherwise healthy children, tooth decay is a preventable disease.

ETIOLOGY. The development of dental caries is dependent on critical inter-relationships between the tooth surface, dietary carbohydrates, and specific oral bacteria. The decay process is initiated by demineralization of the outer tooth surface, owing to formation of organic acids during bacterial fermentation of dietary carbohydrates. Incipient lesions first appear as opaque white spots; with progressive loss of tooth tissue, cavitation occurs.

An important experimental observation within the past two decades has been that dental caries have microbial specificity; that is, cariogenic potential resides in a group of oral streptococci collectively designated as *Streptococcus mutans*. Current knowledge indicates that these organisms initiate most dental caries of enamel surfaces. Once the enamel surface cavitates, other oral bacteria (in particular, the lactobacilli) invade the underlying dentin and cause further destruction of tooth structure through a mixed bacterial infection. An important approach toward prevention of dental caries would be to reduce or eliminate intraoral levels of *S. mutans*. Epidemiologic, chemotherapeutic, and immunologic approaches are currently under intense investigation.

A second important aspect of the etiology of dental caries relates to *frequency* of carbohydrate consumption. Frequency of ingestion is a more important determinant of development of dental caries than is the actual quantity of carbohydrate consumed. For example, cariogenic potential of a nursing bottle of apple juice that is sampled throughout the night or at nap times, or both, is quite different from that of the same volume of apple juice consumed at a single meal. Carbohydrates contained in food products retained orally for a long time may be more cariogenic than those in food products retained for short times (e.g., the sucrose in chewing gum is more cariogenic than the sucrose in cola beverages, as conventionally consumed).

EPIDEMIOLOGY. Recent investigations regarding the prevalence of dental caries in the developed world indicate that its severity has decreased markedly during the last 2 decades. This decrease is thought to be secondary to advances in prevention, particularly the use of fluorides.

With marked decreases in dental caries it has become apparent that the disease is not evenly distributed among children. Over half of the children in fluoridated areas are free of caries into their teens. Another group of children have dental caries or cavities limited to the grooves and fissures (defects) of the molar teeth. A smaller percentage of children persist with active smooth surface tooth decay.

CLINICAL MANIFESTATIONS. Dental caries usually begins in the pits and fissures of the occlusal (biting) surfaces of the molar teeth. Lesions of short duration cannot be diagnosed by inspection; they are usually detected by probing the affected pit or fissure. In contrast, pit and fissure caries of long duration can usually be detected by inspection and usually present extensive cavitation of the occlusal surface. The second most frequent sites of caries are contact surfaces between the teeth. These areas are difficult to examine, even for the dentist, who usually depends on intraoral radiographs. Caries lesions are least frequently detected in the necks (cervical areas) of the teeth near the gingiva. Cervical decay is uncommon in children with mild to moderate caries but is usually present in cases of *nursing bottle caries* (Fig. 13–2).

There are several significant features of *baby bottle tooth decay* (BBTD). This extensive form of tooth decay occurs from sleeping with the nursing bottle. It is relatively common, occurring in about 15% of medically underserved children in urban and rural areas and in 50% or more in some native American groups. Although an exact prevalence has not been established in suburban populations, BBTD is seen on a regular basis in private pediatric dental offices.

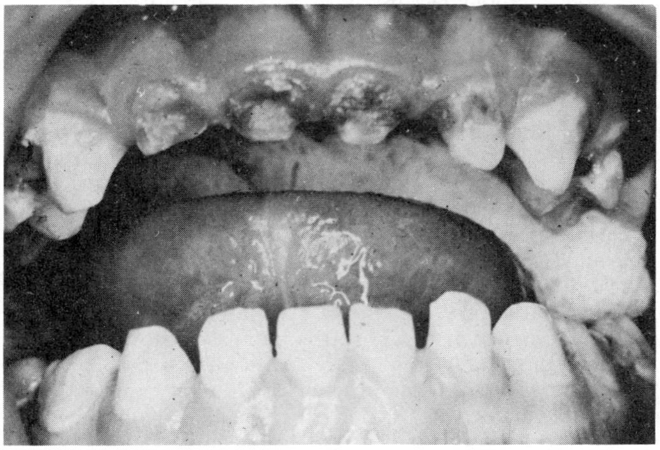

Figure 13–2. Nursing bottle caries.

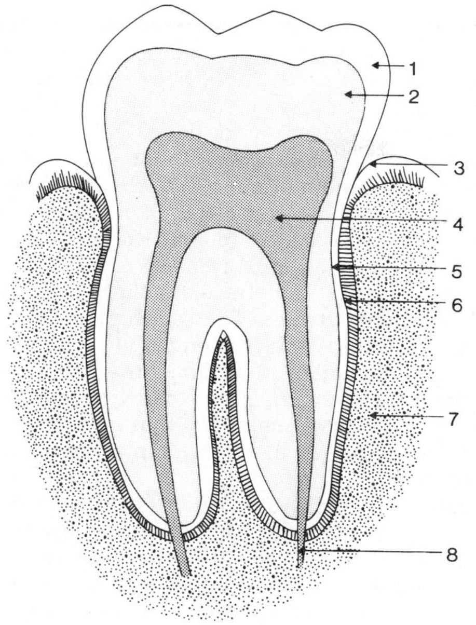

Figure 13–3. Basic dental anatomy: 1 = enamel; 2 = dentin; 3 = gingival margin; 4 = pulp; 5 = cementum; 6 = periodontal ligament; 7 = alveolar bone; 8 = neurovascular bundle.

BBTD occurs before 18 mo of age, at a time many children have not visited a dentist, but when many children have visited a pediatrician. This presents the pediatrician with the opportunity to link counseling on nutrition and dental hygiene. Breast-feeding or water bottles at night greatly reduce the occurrence of BBTD. It is the only severe dental disease common in children less than 3 yr of age. Furthermore, children with BBTD are more likely to continue to develop additional cavities on smooth surfaces of teeth. The prevention of this problem can result in the elimination of major dental problems in toddlers and less decay in later childhood. Children more than 1 yr of age who sleep with the bottle should be referred for treatment.

The age at which BBTD occurs is important in dental management. Children under 3 yr of age must often be restrained, sedated, or given general anesthesia. Beyond 3 yr of age children are more cooperative for dental care, and the caries are often less extensive.

COMPLICATIONS. If left untreated, dental caries usually destroys most of the tooth and spreads into contiguous tissues, causing pain and infection. Microbial invasion of the dental pulp (Fig. 13–3) precipitates an inflammatory response (pulpitis) that can elicit significant pain (toothache). Pulpitis can in turn progress to necrosis, with bacterial invasion of the alveolar bone (dental abscess; periapical abscess). This process may be quite painful and is associated with the complications of sepsis and facial cellulitis (Fig. 13–4). Moreover, periapical infection of a primary tooth may disrupt normal development of the successor permanent tooth.

TREATMENT. Contemporary dental therapeutics can salvage the majority of severely carious teeth. When an extraction is indicated, therapy must also address the problem that teeth surrounding the site of extraction will change their positions in the dental arch. This is particularly important in the primary and mixed dentitions in order to prevent impaction or malposition of permanent successor teeth.

Clinical management of the pain and infection associated with untreated dental caries varies with the extent of involvement and the medical status of the patient. In general, dental infection localized to the dentoalveolar unit can be managed by local measures (e.g., extraction, pulpectomy). Antibiotics are usually not indicated except in those patients with compromised host defenses, impaired wound healing, or risk for endocarditis. In contrast, antibiotics are routinely indicated for dental infections that have spread to structures outside the dentoalveolar unit. The oral route can usually be used for patients with unremarkable medical histories if the infection does not involve a vital area (e.g., buccal space). If, however, the infection involves a vital area (e.g., submandibular space, which can lead to Ludwig angina; facial triangle, which can lead to cavernous sinus thrombosis; or periorbital space, which can lead to orbital involvement), parenteral routes are indicated. Parenteral routes are also indicated for patients with compromised host defenses, with impaired wound healing, or those at risk for endocarditis. Blood cultures should be obtained prior to initiating parenteral antibiotic therapy. Areas of fluctuance should be incised and drained. Exudate should be submitted for culture and Gram stain. Penicillin is the antibiotic of choice, except in patients with a history of allergy to this agent; erythromycin, clindamycin, and vanco-

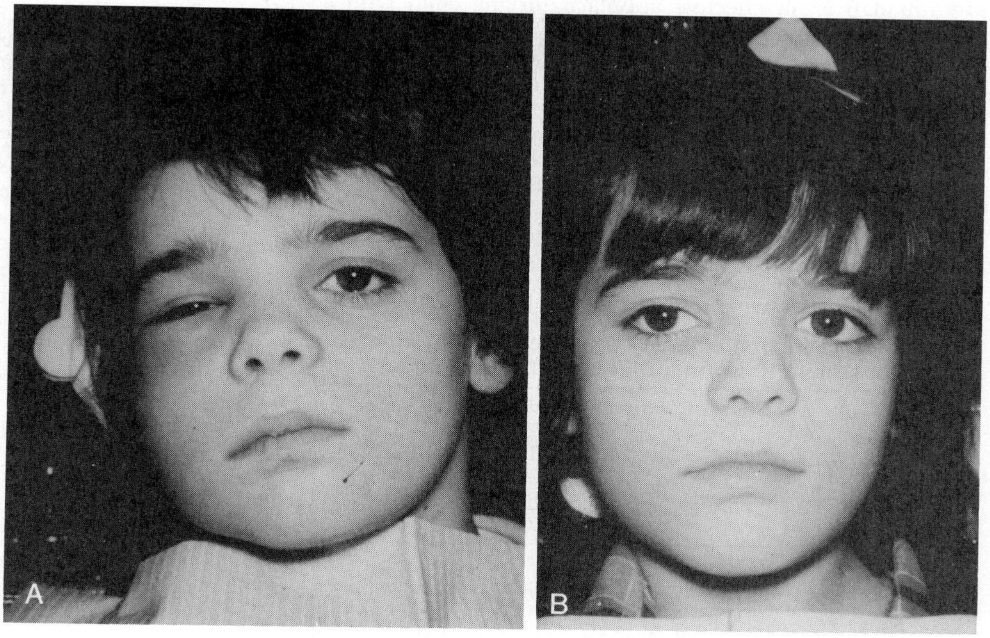

Figure 13–4. *A*, Facial cellulitis from the abscess of a maxillary primary molar. *B*, Resolution of the cellulitis in 1 wk with a course of antibiotics and extraction of the tooth.

mycin are suitable alternatives for such patients. Finally, the offending tooth must be identified and local treatment should be instituted to ensure resolution of the infection.

Measures for control of pain are adjusted to the need of the patient. Combinations of acetaminophen with codeine given orally are usually adequate.

PREVENTION

Fluoride. The most effective preventive measure against dental caries is fluoridation of communal water supplies to approximately 1.00 ppm. In fluoride-deficient areas similar caries prevention benefits are obtained from dietary fluoride supplements. The dosage schedule endorsed by the American Dental Association and the American Academy of Pediatrics is listed in Table 13–2; as indicated, dosage is based on the patient's age and the fluoride content of the water supply. The fluoride level of a water supply can usually be obtained by calling the local water board. If the patient uses a private water supply, it may be necessary for the physician or dentist to facilitate a fluoride analysis. The patient's parents should be instructed to use a plastic container for the water specimen (a glass container may impair the accuracy of the fluoride assay). No fluoride prescription should be written for more than a total of 120 mg of fluoride. This provides a daily supply of 1.0 mg of fluoride for 4 mo. Even if a child ingested this entire supply, probably only mild gastric upset would ensue, which can be alleviated by an aluminum hydroxide preparation. Finally, the topical use of fluoride agents applied either professionally or by the patient are beneficial to children at high risk for caries (e.g., with xerostomia secondary to tumoricidal doses of head and neck radiation).

Oral Hygiene. Thorough daily brushing and flossing of the teeth helps to prevent dental caries and periodontal disease. Parents should receive professional instruction regarding oral hygiene techniques for children. Studies have shown that most children under 10 yr of age do not have the eye-hand coordination required for adequate oral hygiene; accordingly, parents should assume responsibility for brushing and flossing. The degree of parental involvement should be appropriate to the child's growing ability.

Diet. Decreasing the frequency of carbohydrate ingestion prevents dental caries. Parents and children should be encouraged to avoid between-meal snacks that contain carbohydrate. The use of gum, candy, and soft drinks containing sugar substitutes (mannitol, sorbitol, and aspartame [with precautions]) is an effective approach for the child with a "sweet tooth." In addition, infants should be weaned by 1 yr of age to avoid the problems of nursing bottle caries (see Fig. 13–2). Should this not be possible, bedtime and naptime nursing bottles should contain only water.

Dental Sealants and Plastics. Excellent oral hygiene and optimal fluoride therapy have minimal effect in preventing dental caries in the pits and fissures on the occlusal surfaces of the teeth. The use of sealants has been shown to be effective in the prevention of pit and fissure caries. Sealants are plastic coatings that are professionally applied to the occlusal surfaces of the posterior teeth.

TABLE 13–2. Recommended Daily Intake of Fluoride as Supplement to Normal Diet (mg of fluoride/day)

	Concentration of F (ppm) in Water Supply		
Age (yr)	***0.0–0.3***	***0.3–0.7***	***>0.7***
Birth to 2	0.25	0*	0*
2–3	0.50	0.25	0
3 and over	1.00	0.50	0

*0.25 mg for fully breast-fed infants.

Fluoride dosage regimen accepted by the American Academy of Pediatrics and the American Dental Association (1985).

Tooth fissures are the most common sites for dental caries because they are too small to clean mechanically but may support bacterial acid production. Before the dramatic reduction in smooth surface dental caries the use of sealants was not widespread; children who developed smooth surface lesions had dental restorations placed and the sealant removed. With the combination of fluoride and dental sealants today, many children are completely caries free. Sealants are most effective when placed soon after the teeth erupt (usually within 1–2 yr) and when used in children with deep grooves and fissures in the molar teeth, teeth that are currently most susceptible to dental caries. The concept of sealant use is based on the roughening or etching of enamel surfaces with a mild acid and the subsequent attachment of plastics to the tags of enamel that remain. This etching system is also used for a variety of plastic materials that are used to restore fractured teeth, to attach orthodontic brackets, and for intratooth restorations.

Identification of High-Risk Patients. Intact salivary gland function is the major host defense against dental caries. Without it, the patient is susceptible to rampant dental caries. Appropriate preventive therapy has been shown to minimize or eliminate development of dental caries in patients with Sjögren syndrome, Mikulicz disease, chronic graft-versus-host disease, and patients receiving long-term therapy with drugs that cause xerostomia. Additional high-risk conditions for caries include gastroesophageal reflux, bulimia, rumination, mental retardation, and dystrophic epidermolysis bullosa. Hereditary fructose intolerance is associated with a reduced incidence of caries, because these patients avoid fructose-containing foods.

13.7 PERIODONTAL DISEASES

The periodontium includes the gingiva, alveolar bone, and the periodontal ligament (see Fig. 13–3). Several distinct diseases of the periodontium occur during childhood and adolescence. These include gingivitis, acute necrotizing ulcerative gingivitis, herpetic gingivostomatitis, phenytoin-induced gingival overgrowth, juvenile periodontitis, and acute pericoronitis. Whereas periodontitis has been demonstrated in adults with acquired immunodeficiency syndrome (AIDS), significant periodontal conditions have not been described in children with AIDS.

GINGIVITIS. Cessation of oral hygiene results in the accumulation of a dense bacterial mass (dental plaque) around the cervical areas of the teeth at the gingival margin (gum line). If not removed, this dental plaque will precipitate an inflammatory response of the gingiva, with reddening and swelling of the gingiva, spontaneous gingival hemorrhage, and fetor oris. These clinical signs may vary in severity. Such gingivitis may be localized or generalized; it is reversible when proper oral hygiene measures are instituted. Inability to resolve gingivitis by meticulous oral hygiene necessitates considering other problems in which gingivitis may be a presenting component (e.g., acute nonlymphocytic leukemia, diabetes mellitus, neutropenia, thrombocytopenia, scurvy, and hormonal changes associated with puberty and pregnancy).

Epidemiologic surveys indicate that over half of American school children will experience gingivitis. Gingivitis in healthy prepubertal children is much less likely to progress to periodontitis (resulting in loss of alveolar bone) than is gingivitis in adolescents and adults.

TEETHING. Teething can lead to intermittent localized discomfort in the area of an erupting tooth and subsequent irritability. Low-grade fevers may be associated with teething, but this has not been established. Many children go through teething without any apparent problem, whereas others have significant discomfort. There is no proven treatment, although an ice ring for the child to chew on may relieve some discomfort. Similar manifestations can also arise when the first permanent molars erupt at about age 6 yr. These are the largest teeth to penetrate the mucosa and, during the mucosal rearrangement, to allow eruption of the tooth; the gums can become very sore. Parents report that the child has a toothache.

ERUPTION GINGIVITIS. This is an inflammation associated with the eruption of the teeth. Gums can become sore with accompanying bleeding at the gingival margin. Gentle brushing for several days usually resolves the gingivitis. The only associated condition that has long-term consequences is the eruption of a tooth that is well out of alignment in the dental arch. In such cases, formation of normal attached gingiva may not be possible, and either alignment of the tooth orthodontically or gingival grafting can be considered.

ACUTE NECROTIZING ULCERATIVE GINGIVITIS (ANUG; Vincent Infection; Trench Mouth). ANUG is a distinct periodontal disease prone to recurrence, the etiology of which is complex and not fully understood. The dramatic clinical response in its acute phase to penicillin indicates that bacteria are involved. The associated bacteriologic flora is composed of large numbers of oral spirochetes and fusobacteria; it is not clear, however, whether bacteria initiate the disease or are secondary invaders. ANUG develops primarily in young adults and adolescents. It rarely, if ever, develops in healthy children in developed countries. It occurs with surprising frequency, however, among children in southern India and certain African countries. Affected children usually have protein malnutrition. In these children, the lesion may not confine itself to the periodontium but may extend into adjacent tissues causing necrosis of facial structures (cancrum oris, or noma).

Clinical manifestations of ANUG include (1) necrosis and ulceration of erythematous gingiva, in particular the gingiva between the teeth; (2) an adherent grayish pseudomembrane over the affected gingiva; (3) fetor oris; (4) cervical lymphadenopathy; (5) malaise; and (6) fever. The disease is usually localized, the most common site being the periodontium associated with the mandibular incisor teeth. The condition may be mistaken for acute herpetic gingivostomatitis. ANUG is confined to the periodontium, however, and vesicle formation is not a feature. Dark field microscopy will demonstrate dense spirochete populations in smears of debris obtained from ANUG lesions.

Treatment of ANUG is divided into two phases. The acute phase is managed by antibiotic therapy (penicillin or erythromycin), local debridement, oxygenating agents (direct application of 10% carbamide peroxide in anhydrous glycerol four times a day), and analgesics. Dramatic resolution usually occurs within 48 hr. A 2nd phase of treatment may be necessary if the acute phase of the disease has caused irreversible morphologic damage to the periodontium. Finally, current evidence indicates that this disease represents an endogenous rather than a communicable infection; accordingly, patients need not be managed as contagious.

HERPETIC GINGIVOSTOMATITIS. See Sec. 12.68.

PHENYTOIN-INDUCED GINGIVAL OVERGROWTH (PIGO, DILANTIN HYPERPLASIA). The use of phenytoin in anticonvulsant therapy is associated with generalized enlargement of the gingiva. The etiology is complex, and not all factors are known. Current evidence indicates that phenytoin (diphenylhydantoin [DPH]) and its metabolites are present in significant quantity in the gingiva of patients treated with DPH. DPH and its metabolites have a direct stimulatory action on gingival fibroblasts in vitro, resulting in accelerated synthesis of collagen. On the other hand, animal models and clinical studies indicate that PIGO does not complicate DPH therapy in most patients who maintain meticulous oral hygiene. This observation suggests that gingivitis plays a role in the pathogenesis of PIGO.

PIGO occurs in 10–30% of patients treated with DPH. Mild *manifestations* involve subtle gingival changes of no consequence to the patient. Severe manifestations may include (1) gross enlargement of the gingiva, sometimes to the point of covering the teeth; (2) edema and erythema of the gingiva; (3) secondary infection resulting in abscess formation; (4) migration of teeth; and (5) inhibition of exfoliation of primary teeth and subsequent impaction of permanent teeth. Severe PIGO may cause loss of optimal masticatory function and psychologic stress due to the cosmetic effects.

Treatment should be directed toward prevention. Ideally, the drug should be discontinued whenever possible. Patients treated with DPH should receive regular dental follow-up. Meticulous oral hygiene prevents or minimizes PIGO in most cases. The severe form of PIGO is usually treated by gingivectomy; the lesion will recur, however, if excellent oral hygiene cannot be maintained.

JUVENILE PERIODONTITIS (JP). This disease is characterized by rapid alveolar bone loss and is associated with a flora composed of large numbers of *Capnocytophaga, Actinobacillus, Haemophilus,* and *Bacteroides* species. Strains of *Actinobacillus* isolated from human lesions and inoculated into gnotobiotic rodents produced extensive alveolar bone loss in the experimental animals. In addition, the neutrophils of patients with JP have chemotactic and phagocytic defects; JP is associated with certain systemic diseases characterized by defects in neutrophil function (e.g., Down syndrome, diabetes mellitus, Chédiak-Higashi syndrome, Job syndrome, and cyclic neutropenia). Collectively, these data suggest that JP occurs in patients who have impaired host defenses that facilitate colonization by highly periodontopathogenic flora.

JP is exceptionally rare in preschool children who have only primary teeth. In older children it may be localized to the permanent incisors and 6-yr molars or may be generalized; the localized form may be associated with palmar and plantar hyperkeratosis (Papillon-Lefèvre syndrome). The gingiva is usually normal in appearance, but dental radiographs demonstrate alveolar bone loss. Affected teeth demonstrate mobility, which varies with the severity of alveolar bone loss.

The rate of alveolar bone loss in JP is rapid. If left untreated, affected teeth lose their attachment and exfoliate. Treatment approaches vary with the degree of involvement. Patients diagnosed at the onset of the disease are usually managed by local debridement, antibiotic therapy, and meticulous oral hygiene. Patients who have extensive alveolar bone loss at the time of initial diagnosis require extensive periodontal therapy that may include autologous osseous grafting. Prognosis depends on the degree of initial involvement and compliance with therapy.

Prevention of JP is not currently possible, but regular dental evaluations (one to two visits/yr) improve early detection and enhance the likelihood of favorable outcome. Patients with defects of neutrophil function should have such dental surveillance.

ACUTE PERICORONITIS (AP). AP is an acute inflammation of the flap of gingiva that partially covers the crown of an incompletely erupted tooth. Mandibular third molars and less often 2nd molars are common sites of AP. Accumulation of debris and bacteria between the gingival flap and tooth precipitates an inflammatory response. The flap of gingiva may become violently inflamed and edematous. Trismus and severe pain are common. Untreated cases may result in facial cellulitis and peritonsillar abscess, and fatalities have occurred in myelosuppressed patients.

Treatment of AP is in two phases. Treatment of the acute

phase includes local debridement and irrigation, hot saline rinses, antibiotic therapy, and relief of the occlusion of the inflamed flap against the opposing jaw. When the acute phase has subsided, therapy is directed at preventing recurrences. This may include extraction of the tooth or resection of the gingival flap. Early recognition of the partial impaction of mandibular 3rd molars and their subsequent extraction will prevent AP.

13.8 ORAL TRAUMA

Traumatic oral injuries may be conveniently categorized into three groups: (1) dental injuries; (2) soft tissue injuries (contusions, abrasions, lacerations, punctures, avulsions, burns); and (3) injuries to the body of the jaw bones (mandibular or maxillary fractures or both). This chapter will describe dental injuries. Basic texts of pediatric oral surgery offer complete reviews of the diagnosis and management of oral soft tissue injuries and facial fractures (see references).

DENTAL INJURIES

Approximately 10% of all young people between 18 mo and 18 yr of age will sustain significant dental trauma. There appear to be three age periods of predilection: (1) preschool (1–3 yr), usually secondary to falls or child abuse; (2) school aged (7–10 yr), usually from bicycle and playground accidents; and (3) adolescents (16–18 yr), in whom dental trauma is generally secondary to fights, athletic injuries, and automobile accidents. Dental injuries are about twice as common among children with protrusion of teeth as among children with normal occlusion. Children with craniofacial abnormalities or neuromuscular deficits or both are also at increased risk for dental injury.

Dental trauma includes injuries to the hard dental tissues and pulp and injuries to the periodontal structure.

INJURIES TO HARD DENTAL TISSUES AND PULP. Fractures of teeth are uncomplicated or complicated, in accordance with whether the fracture is confined to the hard dental tissues (uncomplicated) or extends through the pulp (complicated). Exposure of the pulp may result in its bacterial contamination, which can lead to infection and pulp necrosis. Pulp exposure complicates therapy and may lower the likelihood of a favorable outcome.

Traumatic blows to the mouth usually strike the maxillary incisor teeth, as they are the most anteriorly located. Fractures of the crowns or roots of these teeth are therefore common. Uncomplicated crown fractures are treated by covering exposed dentin and by placing an esthetic restoration. Complicated crown fractures usually require endodontic (root canal) therapy. Crown-root fractures and root fractures usually require extensive dental therapy, which in the primary dentition may interfere with normal development of the permanent dentition; accordingly, these types of injury of the primary incisor teeth are usually managed by extraction of the fractured segments.

Oral injuries resulting in fractured teeth should be referred to a dentist as soon as possible. Furthermore, even when dentition appears intact following oral trauma, the patient should be evaluated soon by a dentist. The gathering of baseline data (radiographs; mobility patterns; responses to specific stimuli [percussion, electricity, hot, and cold]) enables the dentist to assess the likelihood of future complications.

INJURIES TO PERIODONTAL STRUCTURES. These injuries usually present as mobile or displaced teeth or both. They account for approximately 20% of trauma to the permanent dentition and 70% of injuries to the primary dentition.

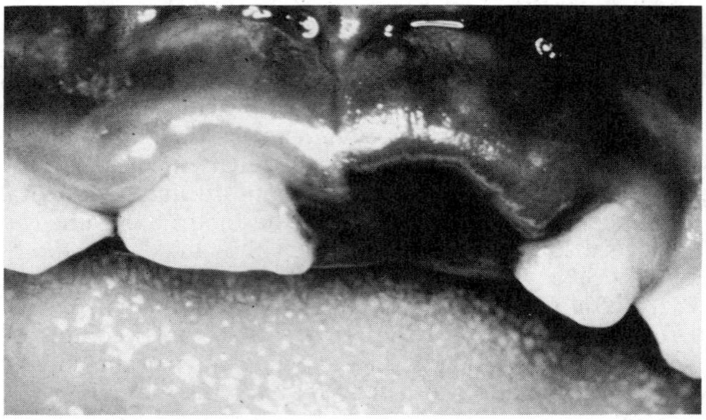

Figure 13–5. Intruded primary incisor that appears evulsed (knocked out).

Categories of trauma to the periodontium include (1) concussion, (2) subluxation, (3) intrusive luxation, (4) extrusive luxation, and (5) evulsion.

Concussion. Injuries that produce minor damage to the periodontal ligament are termed concussions. Teeth sustaining such injuries are without abnormal mobility or displacement but react markedly to percussion. This type of injury usually requires no therapy and resolves without complication. Primary incisors that sustain concussion may change color; this sign usually indicates pulpal degeneration and should be evaluated by a dentist as soon as possible.

Subluxation. This type of injury involves moderate damage to the periodontal ligament. Subluxated teeth exhibit mild to moderate horizontal mobility or vertical mobility or both. Hemorrhage is usually evident around the neck of the tooth at the gingival margin. There is no displacement of the tooth, so that a subluxated tooth retains its normal position in the dental arch. Many subluxated teeth need to be immobilized in order to ensure adequate repair of the periodontal ligament. Immobilization is facilitated by an acrylic splint. Some of these teeth will develop pulp necrosis; this type of injury should be referred to a dentist as soon as possible.

Intrusive Luxation. This type of injury is rare in the permanent dentition but is the most common injury to primary dentition. Intruded primary incisors may give the false appearance of being evulsed (Fig. 13–5). In order to rule out evulsion, an occlusal dental radiograph is indicated (Fig. 13–6). This type of injury should be referred to the dentist as soon as possible.

Extrusive Luxation. This type of injury is characterized by displacement of the tooth from its socket. The tooth is usually displaced to the lingual side, with fracture of the wall of the alveolar socket. These teeth need immediate treatment; the longer the delay, the more likely the tooth will consolidate in

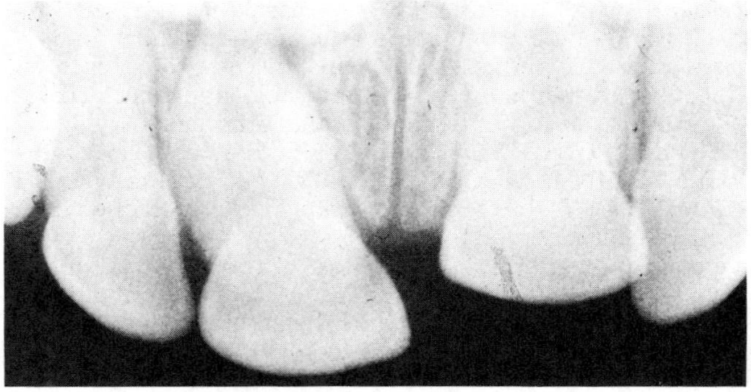

Figure 13–6. Occlusal radiograph documents intrusion of "missing tooth" presented in Figure 13–5.

its ectopic position. Therapy is directed at reduction (repositioning the tooth) and fixation (acrylic splints). In addition, many such teeth become necrotic and require endodontic therapy. Extrusive luxation in the primary dentition is usually managed by extraction, because complications of reduction and fixation may result in problems with development of permanent teeth.

Evulsion. If evulsed permanent teeth are replanted within 30 min after injury, a greater than 90% success rate may be achieved; whereas if the delay exceeds 2 hr, the failure rate approaches 95%. The likelihood that normal reattachment will follow replantation is related to the viability of the periodontal ligament, and immediate therapy is directed at applying this principle. Parents confronted with this emergency situation can be instructed to:

1. *Find the tooth.*
2. *Rinse the tooth.* (Do *not* scrub the tooth. Do *not* touch the root. After plugging the sink drain, hold the tooth by the crown and rinse it under running tap water.)
3. *Insert the tooth into the socket.* (Gently place it back into its normal position. Do not be concerned if the tooth extrudes slightly. If the parent or child is too apprehensive for replantation of the tooth, the tooth should be placed in cow's milk. Milk is the best transport medium to maintain periodontal ligament viability.)
4. *Go directly to the dentist.* (In transit, the child should hold the tooth in place with a finger. The parent should buckle a seatbelt around the child and drive safely. A quick stop may not only result in re-evulsion but may also introduce the complications of ingestion or aspiration.)

After the tooth is replanted, it must be immobilized (acrylic splint) to facilitate reattachment; endodontic therapy is usually required. The initial signs of complications associated with replantation may appear as early as 1 wk post-trauma or as late as several years later. Close dental follow-up is indicated for at least 1 yr.

PREVENTION. To minimize the likelihood of dental injuries:

1. Every child or adolescent who engages in contact sports should wear a mouth protector, which may be constructed by a dentist or purchased at any athletic goods store.
2. Helmets should be worn by children or adolescents with neuromuscular problems or seizures to protect the cranium during falls; they should also have face guards.
3. All children or adolescents with protruding incisors should be evaluated by a pediatric dentist or orthodontist.

Additional Considerations. Children with dental trauma have also sustained head trauma; accordingly, neurologic assessment is warranted. Tetanus prophylaxis should be considered with any injury that disrupts the integrity of the tissues lining the oral cavity. The possibility of child abuse should always be considered.

13.9 COMMON LESIONS OF THE ORAL SOFT TISSUES

OROPHARYNGEAL CANDIDIASIS (OPC, THRUSH, MONILIASIS) (See Sec. 9.75). Oropharyngeal infection with *Candida albicans* is not unusual in neonates who have contact with the organism in the birth canal. Transmission within the newborn nursery may reach epidemic proportions unless appropriate precautions are instituted. The lesions of OPC appear as white plaques covering all or part of the oropharyngeal mucosa. These plaques are removable from the underlying corium, which is characteristically inflamed and hemorrhagic. Discomfort associated with this infection may occasionally interfere with feeding. The diagnosis is confirmed by direct microscopic examination and culture of scrapings from lesions. OPC is usually self-limited in the healthy newborn infant, but treatment with nystatin (1,000,000 units four times a day, applied directly to the lesions) will hasten recovery and reduce the risk of spread to other infants.

OPC is also a major problem during myelosuppressive therapy. Systemic candidiasis (SC), a major cause of morbidity and mortality during myelosuppressive therapy, develops almost exclusively in patients who have had prior oropharyngeal, esophageal, or intestinal candidiasis. This observation implies that prevention of OPC should reduce the incidence of SC. The use of a multiagent regimen for OPC prophylaxis in children receiving bone marrow transplants may be effective in preventing OPC, SC, or candidal esophagitis. The multiagent regimen consists of the following:

1. Debriding all mucous membrane surfaces within the oropharyngeal cavity with one povidone-iodine swabstick four times per day.
2. Subsequently swabbing all mucous membrane surfaces within the oropharyngeal cavity with one large cotton pledget saturated with 500,000 units of nystatin four times per day.

Most of the patients are premedicated with intravenous narcotic analgesics to permit the procedure to be done thoroughly and quickly.

Finally, chronic OPC occurs in children who have certain endocrinopathies, a specific candida immunodeficiency syndrome (associated with cutaneous and nail involvement), and nutritional deficiencies or who receive broad spectrum antibiotic therapy that alters the oral flora. In these situations, successful treatment depends also on correction of the underlying problem.

APHTHOUS ULCERS (CANKER SORES). The aphthous ulcer is a distinct oral lesion, prone to recurrence. Its etiology is not known. Current data suggest that aphthous ulcers may be an autoimmune disease. They may appear as either solitary or multiple ulcers. Common sites include the floor of the mouth, the ventral surface of the tongue, and the mucobuccal fold; they are found less frequently on the palate or buccal mucosa. The aphthous ulcer is generally less than 0.5 cm in diameter, with a depressed center and erythematous periphery. The lesion is usually covered by a yellow-white fibrinous exudate. Many patients report prodromal symptoms such as burning, itching, or tenderness prior to the appearance of the ulcer. The lesions are painful and may make eating uncomfortable. Cold foods, particularly liquids, are usually better tolerated than hot. The use of oral analgesics relieves much of the discomfort associated with eating. Topical application of tetracycline to the lesion (three or four times/day) shortens healing to 2–4 days. This observation suggests that secondary infection may play a role in pathogenesis of the lesion. Lesions that persist for more than 14 days should be biopsied. The differential diagnosis is noted in Table 13–3.

BOHN NODULES. Bohn nodules are small cystic lesions located along the buccal and lingual aspects of the mandibular and maxillary ridges of the neonate. These lesions arise from remnants of mucous gland tissue. Treatment is not necessary, as the nodules disappear within a few weeks.

DENTAL LAMINA CYSTS. Dental lamina cysts are small cystic lesions located along the crest of the mandibular and maxillary ridges of the neonate. These lesions arise from epithelial remnants of the dental lamina. Treatment is not necessary; they will disappear within a few weeks.

MUCOCELE. The mucocele usually appears as a raised bluish vesicle several millimeters in diameter. It occurs most commonly in the lower lip and rarely in the upper lip, palate,

TABLE 13–3. Differential Diagnosis of Oral Ulceration

Condition	Comment
Common	
Aphthous (canker sore)	Painful
Traumatic	Accidents, chronic cheek biter
Hand, foot, mouth disease	Painful, lesions on tongue, anterior oral cavity, hands and feet
Herpangina	Painful, lesions confined to soft palate and oropharynx
Chemical burns	Alkali, acid, aspirin; painful
Uncommon	
Neutrophil defects	Agranulocytosis, leukemia, cyclic neutropenia; painful
Systemic lupus erythematosus	Recurrent, usually painless
Behçet syndrome	Resembles aphthous lesions; associated with genital ulcers, uveitis, etc.
Necrotizing ulcerative gingivostomatitis	Vincent stomatitis; painful
Syphilis	Chancre or gumma; painless
Crohn disease	Aphthous-like; painful
Histoplasmosis	Lingual

buccal mucosa, tongue, or floor of the mouth. It may persist for weeks or months prior to rupture, in which case it usually recurs. This lesion is caused by traumatic laceration of a minor salivary gland duct that permits accumulation of mucus in the soft tissues and subsequent proliferation of granulation tissue to sequester the mucus. Recurrences following surgical excision are largely the result of removing the mucocele without extirpating the minor salivary gland that produced the extravasated mucus.

FORDYCE GRANULES. Almost 80% of adults have multiple, yellow-white granules in clusters or plaque-like areas on the oral mucosa, most commonly on the buccal mucosa or lips. Histologically, normal sebaceous glands are seen in the lamina propria and submucosa. The glands are present at birth, but they hypertrophy and first appear as discrete yellowish papules during the preadolescent period in approximately 50% of children. No treatment is necessary.

HERPANGINA. See Sec. 12.80.

HERPES LABIALIS (COLD SORE, FEVER BLISTER). See Sec. 12.68.

CHEILITIS. Dryness of the lips, followed by scaling and cracking and accompanied by a characteristic burning sensation, is common in children. It is usually caused by sensitivity to contact substances (from toys and foods) plus photosensitivity to the sun's rays. It is aggravated by the alternation of wetting with the tongue and drying by the wind, especially in cold weather. Cheilitis also often occurs in association with fever. Frequent application of a bland ointment facilitates healing and is also preventive.

BLACK HAIRY TONGUE (LINGUA NIGRA). This condition is characterized by an elongation of the filiform papillae into hair-like projections. It is generally concentrated in a triangular area in front of the V-shaped line of circumvallate papillae and is associated with accumulation of debris in that region. The patch may vary from brown to black. The condition is usually chronic but will disappear with regular cleansing of the dorsal tongue.

Hairy tongue may also occur during prolonged antibiotic therapy, especially with oral troches. In addition, oral medications that contain bismuth may produce this benign condition.

GEOGRAPHIC TONGUE (MIGRATORY GLOSSITIS). This benign and asymptomatic lesion is characterized by one or more smooth, bright red patches, often showing a yellow, gray, or white membranous margin upon the dorsum of an otherwise normally roughened tongue. The patches are areas in which the filiform papillae have become completely desquamated, leaving a smooth, slick surface. The patches may be single or multiple, discrete or confluent (map-like). They travel by extension of desquamation of the papillae at one edge and regeneration of normal papillae at the other. The condition may persist for weeks or months and then regress spontaneously, only to recur later.

FISSURED TONGUE (SCROTAL TONGUE). The fissured tongue is a malformation manifested clinically by numerous small furrows or grooves on the dorsal surface. The condition is painless except when food debris collects in the grooves and produces irritation. Regular debridement of the tongue's dorsal surface with a toothbrush helps to prevent this problem.

13.10 SALIVARY GLANDS

With the exception of mumps (Sec. 12.70), disease of the salivary glands is rare in children. Bilateral enlargement of the submaxillary glands may occur in AIDS, cystic fibrosis, in malnutrition, and, transiently, during acute asthmatic attacks. Chronic vomiting and aspiration, as in achalasia or bulimia, may be accompanied by enlargement of the parotids. Benign salivary gland hypertrophy has been associated with endocrinopathies; thyroid disease, diabetes, and disorders of the pituitary-adrenal axis are the most frequently encountered.

Newborn infants discharge saliva until swallowing and lip closure are effective. Later, when the irritation of teething is accompanied by increased oral activity, drooling may occur. In some children with neurologic impairment, drooling is never overcome. Increased secretion of saliva occurs as a reflex to anticipated feeding or pain, from irritative lesions in the mouth, in conjunction with nausea, after administration of mercurial compounds, and in encephalitis and chorea.

RECURRENT PAROTITIS. Recurrent idiopathic swelling of the parotid gland may occur in otherwise healthy children. The swelling is usually unilateral, but both glands may be involved simultaneously or alternately; there may be up to 10 or more recurrences. There is little pain. The swelling is limited to the gland and usually lasts 2–3 wk. Subsidence is spontaneous and may be complete or partial. The incidence appears to be higher in the spring.

SUPPURATIVE PAROTITIS. This is usually due to *Staphylococcus aureus* and may be primary or a complication of parotitis due to another cause. It is usually unilateral and may be accompanied by fever. The gland becomes swollen, tender, and painful. Recurrent parotitis may be confused with suppurative parotitis. The latter responds to appropriate antibacterial therapy based on culture of pus obtained from the Stensen duct or by surgical drainage, which is infrequently required.

RANULA. Ranula is a cyst associated with a major salivary gland in the sublingual area. A ranula is a large, soft, mucus-containing swelling in the floor of the mouth. It occurs at any age, including infancy. The cyst should be excised, and the severed duct should be exteriorized.

XEROSTOMIA. Xerostomia (or dry mouth) may be associated with fever, dehydration, ingestion of drugs with anticholinergic activity, chronic graft-versus-host disease, Mikulicz disease, Sjögren syndrome, or tumoricidal doses of radiation when the salivary glands are within the field. Long-term xerostomia renders the patient highly susceptible to dental caries, which can be minimized or eliminated by appropriate preventive measures.

SALIVARY GLAND TUMORS. See Sec. 17.22.

13.11 DISEASES OF THE JAWS

CAFFEY DISEASE (INFANTILE CORTICAL HYPEROSTOSIS). See Sec. 24.55.

OSTEOMYELITIS (Sec. 12.16). In the newborn infant, facial osteomyelitis tends to occur in the area of the premaxillary suture, but during childhood the mandible is the more common location. The infection is marked by swelling and redness of the oral mucosa or skin and is associated with pain, fever, and lymphadenopathy. Drainage should be established and the exudate cultured so that an appropriate antibiotic may be administered. Large sequestra may require surgical removal.

RETICULOENDOTHELIOSIS (HISTIOCYTOSIS X) (Sec. 25.5). Oral lesions may occur in any of the syndromes and may be an early manifestation. Lesions of the jaws may produce pain, swelling, loosening of teeth, and fetid breath. Healing is often delayed after dental extraction.

NEOPLASMS

Benign Tumors. Ossifying fibroma is the most common benign tumor of the jaws. Growth is rapid prior to puberty, after which it may slow or cease. The lesion is painless; a unilateral soft tissue swelling is usually the first sign. Most patients do not require treatment, but if the lesion is extensive, curettage or further surgical correction may be required.

Cysts of the Jaw. These cysts occur with multiple basal cell nevoid syndrome (Sec. 23.33).

Malignant Tumors. The malignant primary tumors of the jaws in children include Burkitt lymphoma, osteogenic sarcoma, lymphosarcoma, and, more rarely, fibrosarcoma (see Chapter 17).

13.12 DIAGNOSTIC ROENTGENOGRAMS IN DENTAL ASSESSMENT

The *panoramic roentgenogram* provides a single image of the upper and lower jaws in such a way that all of the teeth and surrounding structures appear on one image. The radiograph includes the mandibular condyle, the inferior border of the mandible, and the maxillary sinuses. The x-ray beam rotates about the patient's head with corresponding movement of the radiographic film during exposure. Panoramic roentgenograms are used to show unerupted teeth, including their angulation and stage of development, cysts of the jaws, fractures, supernumerary (extra) teeth, and missing teeth.

The *cephalometric roentgenogram* positions the child's head in such a way that cranial and facial points and planes can be determined and compared with standards derived from thousands of such roentgenograms. A second major feature is that a child's facial growth can be assessed serially as cephalometric roentgenograms are taken sequentially. A similar protocol for positioning the child is used throughout the world. From the cephalometric roentgenogram the relationships of the upper and lower jaws can be determined as well as the relationships of the jaws to the cranial base, the alignment of the incisor teeth, and the relationship of the teeth to the supporting bone. This information is essential in planning orthodontic care and orthognathic surgical procedures.

Intraoral dental roentgenograms can show one section of the mouth by placing the film within the child's mouth and by directing the beam through the teeth and supporting structures. The individual intraoral roentgenograms can be used to detect dental caries and to show the extent of dental trauma. They also show the position of the supporting bone relative to the teeth as well as the stages of periodontal disease and dental anomalies immediately around the teeth.

DAVID C. JOHNSEN

Abramson JS, Givner LB: Should tetracycline be contraindicated for therapy of presumed Rocky Mountain spotted fever in children less than 9 years of age? Pediatrics 86:123, 1990.

Berkowitz RJ, Strandjord S, Jones P, et al: Stomatologic complications of bone marrow transplantation in a pediatric population. Pediatr Dent 9:105, 1987.

Enlow DH: Handbook of Facial Growth, 2nd ed. Philadelphia, WB Saunders, 1982.

Genco RJ, Van Dyke TE, Levine MJ, et al: Molecular factors influencing neutrophil defects in periodontal disease. J Dent Res 65:1379, 1986.

Greene JC, Louie R, Wycoff SJ: Preventive dentistry. I: Dental caries. JAMA 262:3459, 1989.

Greene JC, Louie R, Wycoff SJ: Preventive dentistry. II: Periodontal diseases, malocclusion, trauma and oral cancer. JAMA 263:421, 1990.

Israele V, Siegel JD: Infectious complications of craniofacial surgery in children. Rev Infect Dis 11:9, 1989.

Johnsen D, Nowjack-Raymer R: Baby bottle tooth decay: Issues, assessment, and an opportunity for the nutritionist. J Am Diet Assoc 89:1112, 1989.

King N, Lee A: Prematurely erupted teeth in newborn infants. J Pediatr 114:807, 1989.

Moss SJ: The year 2000 health objectives for the nation. Pediatr Dent 10:228, 1988.

Ross RB: Treatment variables affecting facial growth in complete unilateral cleft lip and palate. Cleft Palate J 24:5, 1987.

Tinanoff N: Dental caries: Etiology, pathogenesis, clinical manifestations, and management. *In:* Wei SHY (ed): Pediatric Dentistry: Total Patient Care. Philadelphia, Lea & Febiger, 1988, p 9.

GASTROINTESTINAL TRACT

13.13 NORMAL DIGESTIVE TRACT PHENOMENA

Normal patterns of gastrointestinal development may be interpreted as manifestations of significant disease in young children. Processes involved in *ingestion of food* are developed and coordinated at birth. The suckling infant encounters difficulties initially with solid foods, thrusting them forward with the tongue rather than back to the pharynx, but practice quickly corrects the problem. A relatively short lingual frenulum ("tongue-tie") is of no known functional significance. During suckling, infants swallow air; unlike older children they must be stimulated to burp during the course of feeding. Otherwise, gaseous gastric distention can interfere with intake. By 1 mo of age sweet and salty foods seem to be preferred.

Regurgitation of gastric content is common in infants until 9–12 mo, when they normally become upright for much of the day. This regurgitation may accompany or follow several feedings each day but it usually resolves spontaneously. If general health, growth, and development are unaffected and the complications of aspiration or esophagitis do not develop, there is no need for detailed investigation of such patients.

The *pattern of food intake and appetite* of children at different ages may seem bizarre to adults who regularly consume three meals a day. Particularly distressing to parents, but normal, is the toddler's habit of gorging himself or herself after refusing to consume the daily requirements for a few days. Appetite fluctuates enormously. In periods of rapid growth during infancy and adolescence, appetite is usually voracious, whereas during the intervening years some children appear to eat almost nothing while they grow and gain weight normally.

The *number, color, and consistency of stools* vary greatly in the same infant and between infants of similar age regardless of diet or environment. After birth the first stools consist of meconium, a dark, viscous, gum-like material. When milk feedings begin, meconium is replaced by green-brown transition stools, often containing curds, and then in 4–5 days by yellow-brown milk stools. Stool frequency may vary from one to seven per day in babies who are otherwise perfectly well. The color of the stool is of little significance unless blood is present or bilirubin is absent. Some children are 2–3 yr of age before they have formed stools. Breast-fed infants tend to have infrequent yellow stools of loose consistency. Later, husks of vegetables like corn and peas and black "worm-like" threads from the surface of the peeled banana appear in stools after these foods have been eaten (see Sec. 4.13 and 9.41).

Some *abdominal findings* in a normal young child may give rise to unnecessary concern. During the first 3–4 yr of life the abdominal musculature is relatively weak, the abdominal organs relatively large, and the lower spine lordotic so that the belly is protuberant but soft. Up to 2 yr a soft liver edge may be palpable up to 2 cm below the right costal margin. Although the spleen is not usually palpable, a soft tip may be felt in the course of an acute infection.

Blood loss from the digestive tract is never normal, but swallowed blood can be misinterpreted as enteric hemorrhage. Maternal blood may be ingested at the time of birth or later by the breast-fed baby when there is bleeding near the mother's nipple (Sec. 9.49). Also children may swallow their own blood from epistaxis or another source in the nasopharynx.

Jaundice occurs in about 20% of newborn term infants; the more prematurely born the baby, the higher will be the incidence. In most newborn infants indirect hyperbilirubinemia results not from a specific disease but from a limited capacity of the immature liver during the early weeks of life to conjugate the large quantities of hemoglobin breakdown products presented to it (Sec. 8.44). Direct hyperbilirubinemia at any age suggests a more serious condition.

13.14 MAJOR SYMPTOMS AND SIGNS OF DIGESTIVE TRACT DISORDERS

In children, symptoms strongly suggestive of a digestive tract disorder may be caused by diseases or problems involving other organs or systems (Table 13–4). An understanding of the pathogenesis of major symptoms is useful in dealing with childhood gastroenterologic disorders because in many cases the cause is unknown and specific treatment not available.

DISORDERED INGESTION. Dysfunction at different levels of the upper digestive tract can compromise dietary intake.

Transfer Dysphagia. A complex sequence of neuromuscular events is involved in the transfer of foods to the upper esophagus. Suckling requires the lips to form a tight seal about the nipple while the tongue is displaced posteriorly. As the glottis closes to guard the airway, the soft palate rises to close the nasopharynx, the cricopharyngeal muscles relax, and food passes to the back of the pharynx. Solids similarly require coordinated actions; for large chunks of solid food jaw movement and teeth become factors to consider. Salivary secretions, stimulated by the anticipation and act of ingestion, lubricate foods as they pass through the mouth. It is abnormalities of the muscles involved in the ingestion process, their innervation, strength, or coordination that usually cause transfer dysphagia in infants and children. In such cases, an oropharyngeal problem is almost always part of a more generalized neurologic or muscular problem (botulism, diphtheria, cerebral palsy). Occasionally, painful oral lesions, such as acute viral stomatitis or trauma, will interfere with ingestion. If the nasal air passage is seriously obstructed, the need for air will cause severe distress when suckling. Although severe structural, dental, and salivary abnormalities would be expected to create difficulties, ingestion proceeds relatively well in most affected children if they are hungry.

TABLE 13–4. Some Nondigestive Tract Causes of Gastrointestinal Symptoms in Children

Anorexia	
	Systemic disease (e.g., inflammatory, neoplastic)
	Iatrogenic—drug therapy, unpalatable therapeutic diets
	Depression
	Anorexia nervosa
Vomiting	
	Increased intracranial pressure
	Infection (e.g., urinary tract)
Diarrhea	
	"Parenteral" infection (e.g., respiratory, urinary)
	Uremia
Constipation	
	Hypothyroidism
	Dehydration (e.g., diabetes insipidus, renal tubular lesions)
Abdominal pain	
	Pyelonephritis, hydronephrosis, renal colic
	Pneumonia
	Pelvic inflammatory disease
	Porphyria
	Angioedema
	Familial Mediterranean fever
	Systemic lupus erythematosus
	School phobia
Abdominal mass	
	Ascites (e.g., nephrotic syndrome, neoplasm, heart failure)
	Discrete mass (e.g., Wilms tumor, hydronephrosis, neuroblastoma)
	Pregnancy
Jaundice	
	Hemolytic disease

Dysphagia, Regurgitation. Swallowing is well coordinated at birth: primary peristaltic waves, initiated by swallowing, proceed down the length of the esophagus, while secondary waves that empty the esophagus of residue are initiated by distention. Regurgitation can occur if swallowing is obstructed by an intrinsic lesion in the esophagus or by an extrinsic lesion, in which case associated compression of the trachea may lead to stridor and cough. Primary motility disorders causing impaired peristaltic function and dysphagia are rare in children.

The lower esophageal sphincter (LES) helps to prevent reflux of gastric contents into the esophagus (Sec. 13.20). In general, if LES pressure is abnormally reduced, flow of gastric content in a retrograde direction will occur. Regurgitation owing to gastroesophageal reflux is passive compared with emesis (see later). In very young symptomatic patients there is a poor correlation between sphincter pressure and occurrence of gastroesophageal reflux. Hiatal hernia (Sec. 13.21) is not an important determinant of gastroesophageal reflux.

Continued exposure of the lower esophageal mucosa to gastric juice can cause esophagitis and, as a consequence, dysphagia and chronic blood loss. The chance of aspirating gastric juice is enhanced by underlying motility problems in the esophagus, particularly by dysfunction of the upper esophageal sphincter.

Anorexia. Hunger and satiety centers are probably located in the hypothalamus; it seems likely that afferent nerves from the gastrointestinal tract to these brain centers are important determinants of the anorexia that characterizes many diseases of the stomach and intestine. For example, satiety is stimulated by distention of the stomach or upper small bowel, the signal being transmitted by sensory afferents, which are especially dense in the upper gut. Chemoreceptors in the intestine, influenced by the assimilation of nutrients, also affect afferent flow to the appetite centers. Impulses reach the hypothalamus from higher centers possibly influenced by pain or the emotional disturbance of an intestinal disease. Other regulatory factors include hormones and plasma glucose, which in turn reflect intestinal function.

VOMITING. Vomiting occurs when violent descent of the diaphragm and constriction of the abdominal muscles actively force gastric content back up the esophagus. In humans, stimulation of a center in the medulla can cause vomiting. In fact, diseases in almost any system, particularly the brain, may cause vomiting (Table 13–5).

Obstructions of the intestinal tract cause vomiting, which is probably mediated by visceral afferents reaching the vomiting center. If obstruction occurs below the second part of the duodenum, vomitus usually is bile stained. Congenital and acquired obstructing lesions are noted in Table 13–6. Nonobstructive lesions of the digestive tract can also cause vomiting; most diseases of the upper bowel, pancreas, liver, or biliary tree are capable of provoking emesis. Furthermore, metabolic derangements such as those occurring in Reye syndrome may lead to severe, persistent emesis.

DIARRHEA. Diarrhea is the excessive loss of fluid and electrolyte in stool (Sec. 6.20 and 12.10). The basis for all diarrhea is disturbed intestinal solute transport, since water movement across intestinal membranes is passive and determined by both active and passive fluxes of solutes, particularly sodium, chloride, and glucose. In most clinical situations epithelial abnormalities are known determinants of diarrhea. Hypermotility is rarely a significant factor, enteric innervation is being actively investigated, and little is known about the roles of blood and lymphatic flow to the gut in causing diarrhea. Normally, all but a small percentage of water absorption occurs in the small bowel; small bowel disease tends to cause voluminous diarrhea, whereas colonic diarrhea is less voluminous and characterized by alternating loose and formed or hard stools.

TABLE 13–5. Differential Diagnosis of Vomiting During Childhood

Infant	Child	Adolescent
Common		
Gastroenteritis	Gastroenteritis	Gastroenteritis
Gastroesophageal reflux	Systemic infection	Systemic infection
Overfeeding	Toxic ingestion	Toxic ingestion
Anatomic obstruction	Pertussis syndrome	Inflammatory bowel disease
Systemic infection	Medication	Appendicitis
		Migraine
		Pregnancy
		Medication
		Ipecac abuse/bulimia
Rare		
Adrenogenital syndrome	Reye syndrome	Reye syndrome
Inborn error of metabolism	Hepatitis	Hepatitis
Brain tumor (increased intracranial pressure)	Peptic ulcer	Peptic ulcer
Subdural hemorrhage	Pancreatitis	Pancreatitis
Food poisoning	Brain tumor	Brain tumor
Rumination	Increased intracranial pressure	Increased intracranial pressure
Renal tubular acidosis	Middle ear disease	Middle ear disease
	Chemotherapy	Chemotherapy
	Achalasia	Cyclic vomiting
	Cyclic vomiting	Biliary colic
	Esophageal stricture	Renal colic

TABLE 13–6. Causes of Gastrointestinal Obstruction*

Esophagus		
	Congenital:	Esophageal atresia
		Vascular rings
	Acquired:	Esophageal stricture
		Chagas disease
		Collagen vascular disease
		Foreign body
Stomach		
	Congenital:	Antral webs
		Pyloric stenosis
	Acquired:	Bezoars/foreign body
		Pyloric stricture (ulcer)
Small Intestine		
	Congenital:	Duodenal atresia
		Annular pancreas
		Malrotation/volvulus
		Malrotation/Ladds bands
		Ileal atresia
		Meconium ileus
		Inguinal hernia
	Acquired:	Adhesions post surgery
		Crohn disease
		Intussusception
		Meconium ileus equivalent
Colon		
	Congenital:	Meconium plug
		Hirschsprung disease
		Colonic atresia, stenosis
		Imperforate anus
		Rectal stenosis
		Pseudo-obstruction
	Acquired:	Ulcerative colitis (toxic megacolon)
		Chagas disease

*From Behrman RE, Kliegman RM: Nelson Essentials of Pediatrics. Philadelphia, WB Saunders, 1990.

Disease may cause diarrhea by damaging the bowel wall or by elaborating secretagogues, which reach the epithelium via the circulation or from the bowel lumen (Table 13–7). When the mucosa is damaged, not only may absorptive surface area be diminished but also function of the remaining cells is often compromised. For example, in rotavirus enteritis, glucose transport is defective, disaccharidase and Na^+–K^+ATPase activities are reduced, and glucose-Na^+ and alanine $-Na^+$ cotransport are impaired in the small bowel epithelium after the virus invades the intestine.

Other disorders can cause severe diarrhea without any effect on absorptive surface area or on the structure of the intestinal epithelium. Potent secretagogues produced in the gut lumen by *Vibrio cholerae* and *Escherichia coli* bind to the small intestinal brush border and stimulate adenylate cyclase activity, leading to accumulation of cyclic adenosine monophosphate (AMP) in the epithelium. The result is a massive watery diarrhea characterized by brisk chloride secretion and impaired NaCl absorption, but preservation of the glucose-stimulated Na^+ absorption and Na^+–K^+ATPase activity that are defective in viral enteritis. Other secretagogues, such as the heat-stable toxin of *E. coli*, cause cyclic GMP accumulation with a similar result. Some intraluminal fatty acids and bile salts cause the colonic mucosa to secrete; the mechanism is unknown. This phenomenon may explain the diarrhea occurring with steatorrhea and with bile salt malabsorption secondary to resection of the distal ileum. The differential diagnosis of common causes of acute and chronic diarrhea is noted in Table 13–8.

CONSTIPATION. Infrequent dry stools can arise from defects either in filling or in emptying the rectum (Table 13–9). Defective rectal filling occurs when colonic peristalsis is

TABLE 13–7. Mechanisms of Diarrhea*

Primary Mechanism	Defect	Stool Examination	Examples	Comment
Secretory	Decreased absorption Increased secretion	Watery Normal osmolality	Cholera, toxigenic *E. coli*, carcinoid, VIP†, neuroblastoma	Persists during fasting No stool leukocytes
Osmotic	Transport defects; ingestion of unabsorbable solute	Watery, acidic, and reducing substances	Lactase deficiency Glucose-galactose malabsorption Lactulose Laxative abuse	Stops with fasting Increased breath hydrogen No stool leukocytes
Increased motility	Decreased transit time	Stimulated by gastrocolic reflex	Irritable bowel syndrome Thyrotoxicosis Postvagotomy Dumping syndrome	
Combined Mechanisms				
Decreased surface area (osmotic, motility)	Decreased functional capacity	Watery	Short bowel syndrome	May require elemental diet plus parenteral alimentation
Mucosal invasion	Inflammation Decreased colonic reabsorption Increased motility	Blood and increased white blood cells in stool	*Salmonella, Shigella, Amebiasis, Yersinia, Campylobacter*	Dysentery—blood, mucus, and leukocytes

*Adapted from Behrman RE, Kliegman RM: Nelson Essentials of Pediatrics. Philadelphia, WB Saunders, 1990.
†VIP = vasoactive intestinal peptide.

ineffective (e.g., in cases of hypothyroidism or opiate use, and when there is bowel obstruction caused either by a structural anomaly or by Hirschsprung disease). The resultant colonic stasis leads to excessive drying of stool and a failure to initiate reflexes from the rectum that normally trigger evacuation. Emptying the rectum by spontaneous evacuation depends on a defecation reflex initiated by pressure receptors in the rectal muscle. Stool retention, therefore, may also result from lesions involving these rectal muscles, the sacral spinal cord afferent and efferent fibers, or the muscles of the abdomen and pelvic floor. Disorders of anal sphincter relaxation may also contribute to fecal retention.

Constipation tends to be self-perpetuating, whatever its cause. Hard, large stools in the rectum become difficult and even painful to evacuate, thus more retention occurs and a vicious circle ensues. Distention of the rectum and colon lessens the sensitivity of the defecation reflex and the effectiveness of peristalsis. Eventually, watery content from the proximal colon may percolate around hard retained stool and pass per rectum unperceived by the child. This involuntary *encopresis* may be mistaken for diarrhea. Constipation does not per se have deleterious systemic organic effects. Urinary tract stasis may accompany severe longstanding cases. Constipation may generate anxiety, having a marked emotional impact on the patient and family.

ABDOMINAL PAIN. Individuals differ greatly in tolerance for and responses to intra-abdominal events, but reported

TABLE 13–8. Common Causes of Diarrhea*

Infant	Child	Adolescent
Acute		
Gastroenteritis Systemic infection Antibiotic associated	Gastroenteritis Food poisoning Systemic infection Antibiotic associated	Gastroenteritis Food poisoning Antibiotic associated
Chronic		
Postinfectious Secondary disaccharidase deficiency Milk protein intolerance Irritable colon syndrome Cystic fibrosis Celiac disease Short bowel syndrome	Postinfectious Secondary disaccharidase deficiency Irritable colon syndrome Celiac disease Lactose intolerance Giardiasis	Inflammatory bowel disease Lactose intolerance Giardiasis Laxative abuse (anorexia nervosa)

*Adapted from Behrman RE, Kliegman RM: Nelson Essentials of Pediatrics. Philadelphia, WB Saunders, 1990.

TABLE 13–9. Important Causes of Constipation*

- Nonorganic (functional)
- Organic
  - Intestinal
    - Hirschsprung disease
    - Anal-rectal stenosis
    - Stricture
    - Volvulus
    - Pseudo-obstruction
    - Chagas disease
  - Drugs
    - Narcotic
    - Antidepressants
    - Psychoactive (thorazine)
    - Vincristine
  - Metabolic
    - Dehydration
    - Cystic fibrosis (meconium ileus equivalent)
    - Hypothyroidism
    - Hypokalemia
    - Renal tubular acidosis
    - Hypercalcemia
  - Neuromuscular
    - Absent abdominal muscle
    - Myotonic dystrophy
    - Spinal cord lesions (tumors, spina bifida, diastematomyelia)
    - Amyotonia congenita
  - Psychiatric
    - Anorexia nervosa

*Adapted from Behrman RE, Kliegman RM: Nelson Essentials of Pediatrics. Philadelphia, WB Saunders, 1990.

abdominal pain should be assumed to be real. A specific cause may be difficult to find, but the nature and location of a pain-provoking lesion can usually be determined from the clinical description. Two types of nerve fibers transmit painful stimuli in the abdomen: in skin and muscle, A fibers mediate sharp localized pain; and C fibers from viscera, peritoneum, and muscle transmit poorly localized, dull pain. These afferent fibers have cell bodies in the dorsal root ganglia, and some axons cross the mid-line and ascend to the medulla, midbrain, and thalamus. Pain is perceived in the cortex of the postcentral gyrus, which can receive impulses arising from both sides of the body.

Visceral pain tends to be experienced in the dermatome from which the affected organ receives innervation. Painful stimuli originating in liver, pancreas, biliary tree, stomach, or upper bowel are felt in the epigastrium; pain from the distal small bowel, cecum, appendix, or proximal colon is felt at the umbilicus; and pain from distal large bowel, urinary tract, or pelvic organs is usually suprapubic. When pain is referred to remote areas supplied by the same neurosegment as the diseased organ, the phenomenon usually means an increased intensity of the provoking stimuli. Parietal pain impulses travel in C fibers of nerves corresponding to dermatomes T6 to L1; such pain tends to be more localized and intense than visceral pain.

In the gut the usual stimulus provoking pain is tension or stretching. Inflammatory lesions may lower the pain threshold, but the mechanisms producing pain of inflammation are not clear. Tissue metabolites released near nerve endings probably account for the pain caused by ischemia. Perception of these painful stimuli can be modulated by input from both cerebral and peripheral sources. Psychologic factors are particularly important. Features of abdominal pain are noted in Table 13–10.

GASTROINTESTINAL HEMORRHAGE. Bleeding may occur at any site in the digestive tract, the most common being the lower esophagus, stomach, duodenum, and colon (Table 13–11). Usually, it is an erosion of the mucosa down to the vasculature that leads to hemorrhage, but vessel malformations or raised portal pressure also cause hemorrhage. Rarely, violent vomiting itself may cause mucosal tears and bleeding at the gastroesophageal junction (Mallory-Weiss syndrome). It is rare for clotting defects to cause gastrointestinal bleeding except in hemorrhagic diseases of the newborn.

When bleeding originates in the esophagus, stomach, or duodenum, it may cause *hematemesis*. When exposed to gastric or intestinal juices, blood quickly darkens to resemble coffee grounds; accordingly, the more massive and proximal the bleeding, the more likely it is to be red. Red blood in stools, *hematochezia*, signifies either a distal bleeding site or massive hemorrhage above the distal ileum. Moderate to mild bleeding from sites above the distal ileum tends to cause blackened stools of tarry consistency, *melena*, and major hemorrhages in the duodenum or above can cause melena.

Children can develop iron deficiency anemia from enteric blood loss even when occult blood is not found in stools on random testing. Gastrointestinal hemorrhage, in itself, rarely causes gastrointestinal symptoms, but brisk duodenal or gastric bleeding may lead to nausea and vomiting. The breakdown products of intraluminal blood may tip the patient into hepatic coma if liver function is already compromised.

ABDOMINAL DISTENTION AND ABDOMINAL MASSES. Enlargement of the abdomen can result from diminished tone of the wall musculature or from increased content—fluid, gas, or solid. Ascites, the accumulation of fluid in the peritoneal cavity, distends the abdomen both in the flanks and anteriorly when it is large in volume. This fluid shifts with movement of the patient and conducts a percussion wave.

Ascitic fluid is usually a transudate with a low-protein concentration resulting from reduced plasma colloid osmotic pressure of hypoalbuminemia or from raised portal venous pressure, or from both. In cases of portal hypertension the fluid leak probably occurs from lymphatics on the liver surface

TABLE 13–10. Distinguishing Features of Gastrointestinal Tract Pain in Children*

Disease	Onset	Location	Referral	Quality	Comments
Functional: Irritable bowel syndrome	Recurrent	Periumbilical	None	Dull crampy, intermittent, 2-hr duration	Family stress, school phobia, onset about 5 yr old
Esophageal reflux	Recurrent, 1 hr after meal	Substernal	Chest	Burning	Sour taste in mouth; Sandifer syndrome
Duodenal ulcer	Recurrent, between meals, at night	Epigastric	Back	Severe burning, gnawing	Relieved by food, milk, antacids
Pancreatitis	Acute	Epigastric, left upper quadrant	Back	Constant, sharp, boring	Nausea, emesis, tenderness
Intestinal obstruction	Acute or gradual	Periumbilical–lower abdomen	Back	Alternating cramping (colic) and painless periods	Distention, obstipation, emesis, increased bowel sounds
Appendicitis	Acute	Periumbilical, localized to RL quadrant	Back or pelvis if retrocecal	Sharp, steady	Nausea, emesis, local tenderness, fever
Meckel diverticulum	Recurrent	Periumbilical–lower abdomen	None	Sharp	Hematochezia
Inflammatory bowel disease	Recurrent	Lower abdomen	Back	Dull cramping, tenesmus	Fever, weight loss, hematochezia
Intussusception	Acute	Periumbilical–lower abdomen	None	Cramping, with painless periods	Hematochezia, knees in pulled up position
Lactose intolerance	Recurrent with milk products	Lower abdomen	None	Cramping	Distention, bloating, diarrhea
Urolithiasis	Acute, sudden	Back	Groin	Sharp, intermittent, cramping	Hematuria
Urinary tract infection	Acute, sudden	Back	Bladder	Dull to sharp	Fever, costochondral tenderness, dysuria, urinary frequency

*Adapted from Behrman RE, Kliegman RM: Nelson Essentials of Pediatrics. Philadelphia, WB Saunders, 1990.

TABLE 13–11. Differential Diagnosis of Gastrointestinal Bleeding in Childhood*

Infant	Child	Adolescent
Common		
Bacterial enteritis	Bacterial enteritis	Bacterial enteritis
Milk protein allergy	Anal fissure	Inflammatory bowel disease
Intussusception	Intussusception	Peptic ulcer/gastritis
Swallowed maternal blood	Peptic ulcer/gastritis	Mallory-Weiss syndrome
Anal fissure	Swallowed epistaxis	Colonic polyps
	Henoch-Schönlein purpura	
	Colonic polyps	
Rare		
Volvulus	Esophageal varices	Esophageal varices
Necrotizing enterocolitis	Esophagitis	Esophagitis
Hemorrhagic disease of newborn	Meckel diverticulum	Telangiectasia-angiodysplasia
Meckel diverticulum	Lymphonodular hyperplasia	Gay bowel disease
	Foreign body	Graft-versus-host disease
	Hemangioma, arteriovenous malformation	
	Sexual abuse	
	Hemolytic uremic syndrome	

*Adapted from Behrman RE, Kliegman RM: Nelson Essentials of Pediatrics. Philadelphia, WB Saunders, 1990.

and from visceral peritoneal capillaries, but ascites does not usually develop until the serum albumin level falls. For unknown reasons sodium excretion in the urine decreases greatly as the ascitic fluid accumulates so that additional dietary sodium goes directly to the peritoneal space, taking with it more water. When ascitic fluid contains a high protein concentration, it is usually an exudate caused by an inflammatory or neoplastic lesion.

When fluid distends the gut, either obstruction or imbalance between absorption and secretion should be suspected. Frequently, the factors causing fluid accumulation in the bowel lumen cause gas to accumulate too. The result may be audible gurgling noises. The source of gas is usually swallowed air, but endogenous flora may increase considerably in malabsorptive states and produce excessive gas when substrate reaches the lower intestine.

Gas in the peritoneal cavity, perhaps signaled by a tympanitic percussion note even over solid organs like the liver, indicates a perforated viscus.

An abdominal organ may enlarge diffusely or be affected by a discrete mass. In the digestive tract such discrete masses may occur in the lumen, in the wall, or in the mesentery. In the constipated child, mobile, nontender fecal masses are often found. The wall of the gut can be affected by anomalies, cysts, or inflammatory disease; gut wall neoplasms are extremely rare in children. The liver may enlarge diffusely in response to many disorders. Discrete liver masses may be islands of regenerating liver tissue in a cirrhotic liver or may be of inflammatory or neoplastic origin.

JAUNDICE (See Sec. 9.44 and 13.87).

J. RICHARD HAMILTON

Berman NF, Holtzapple PG: Gastrointestinal hemorrhage. Pediatr Clin North Am 22:885, 1975.

Borison HL, Wong SC: Physiology and pharmacology of vomiting. Pharmacol Rev 5:193, 1953.

Cox KC, Ament ME: Upper gastrointestinal bleeding in children and adolescents. Pediatrics 63:408, 1979.

Fitzgerald JF: Cholestatic disorders of infancy. Pediatr Clin North Am 35:357, 1988.

Grand RJ, Watkins JB, Torti FM: Development of the human gastrointestinal tract: A review. Gastroenterology 70:790, 1976.

Gupta JM: Neonatal jaundice. Med J Aust 1:745, 1977.

Hall RJC: Normal and abnormal food intake. Gut 16:744, 1975.

Hamilton JR: The pathogenesis of infectious diarrhea. Modern Concepts in Gastroenterology 1:335, 1986.

Hatch TF: Encopresis and constipation in children. Pediatr Clin North Am 35:257, 1988.

Sondheimer JM: Gastroesophageal reflux: Update on pathogenesis and diagnosis. Pediatr Clin North Am 35:103, 1988.

ESOPHAGUS

13.15 DEVELOPMENT AND FUNCTION OF THE ESOPHAGUS

The esophagus develops from primitive foregut, as two laryngotracheal grooves along its lateral wall fuse to separate the primitive esophagus from the anterior trachea. The function of the esophagus is to transport fluids and solids to the stomach and to prevent their regurgitation.

Swallowing has been observed in utero at 20 wk of gestation, and sucking and swallowing seem to be coordinated by 33–34 wk. The full-term newborn infant has short bursts of sucking followed by swallows. Within a few days (or weeks if premature) the infant is able to swallow and breathe in a coordinated, rhythmic manner during prolonged bursts of sucking.

Swallowing is initiated by a sudden elevation of the posterior portion of the tongue that propels the bolus of food or fluid toward the posterior pharynx. A simultaneous superior and anterior displacement of the larynx and positioning of the epiglottis protects the laryngeal airway, while the nasopharynx is occluded by the soft palate and uvula. The superior esophageal sphincter relaxes, and pharyngeal constrictors help to propel food into the esophagus where primary peristaltic waves propel food into the stomach. Secondary waves are usually initiated by local distention and serve to empty the esophagus of residual food or of gastric contents. Both of these waves empty the esophagus by propulsive efforts. In contrast, tertiary waves are nonpropulsive; they are abnormal if present in large numbers and can be associated with chest pains. The lower esophageal sphincter is a specialized segment of circular musculature in the distal 1–3 cm of the esophagus, where the intraluminal pressure is normally higher than that in the more proximal esophagus or in the stomach. This sphincter prevents gastroesophageal reflux but relaxes during deglutition to allow food to enter the stomach.

The *common symptoms and signs* of esophageal disease are cough or choking with swallowing, regurgitation or vomiting,

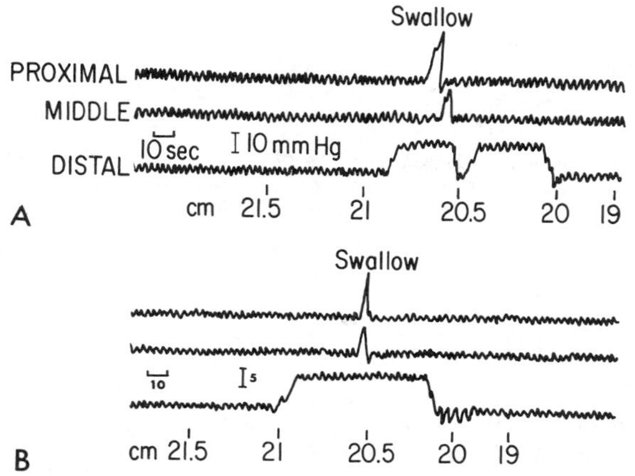

Figure 13–7. *A*, Pressures in the esophagus of a normal infant as recorded with a triple lumen catheter with recording tips 2.5 cm apart. When the distal recording tip was 21.5 cm from the gum line, it was within the lower esophageal sphincter. A swallow initiates a primary peristaltic wave. The pressure wave is detected first in the more proximal catheter and then the more distal one. A relaxation in the lower esophageal sphincter allows the food to enter the stomach. *B*, Abnormal manometric pattern in a patient demonstrating simultaneous pressure in the two proximal recording tips, characteristic of a tertiary esophageal wave. There is no relaxation of the lower esophageal sphincter. Such a pattern is seen in patients with achalasia.

dysphagia, complete inability to swallow, pain on swallowing (odynophagia), and hematemesis. Each can be attributed to one or more defects in the complex coordination of the swallowing sequence. *Diagnostic evaluations* include conventional barium swallow roentgenographic studies, which may demonstrate masses impinging on the lumen or gastroesophageal reflux. A videoesophagram can evaluate the dynamics of swallowing and reveal abnormalities that are present only transiently. Esophageal manometry permits quantitative measurements of pressures along the esophagus. The pressure in the LES is often decreased in patients with reflux, especially if esophagitis is present. In contrast, pressures are elevated, with poor relaxation, in achalasia (Fig. 13–7). Radionuclide scans can help to detect gastroesophageal reflux. In older children such scans can evaluate the efficiency of peristalsis in clearing liquid or a solid bolus from the esophagus. Measurement of intraluminal esophageal pH with a flexible 2-mm diameter pH probe in the distal esophagus is the most sensitive method to detect reflux of acid gastric contents. Esophagoscopy is especially useful in visualizing lesions on the mucosal surface and in detecting and removing foreign bodies. Flexible fiberoptic endoscopes permit direct examination and biopsy of the esophagus without general anesthesia.

13.16 DISORDERS OF THE ESOPHAGUS

13.17 ATRESIA AND TRACHEOESOPHAGEAL FISTULA

Esophageal atresia occurs in 1 in 3000–4500 live births; about one third of affected infants are born prematurely. In more than 85% of cases, a fistula between the trachea and distal esophagus accompanies the atresia (Fig. 13–8*A*). Less commonly, the esophageal atresia or tracheoesophageal fistula may occur alone (see Fig. 13–8*B*, *C*) or in unusual combinations (see Fig. 13–8*D*, *E*). These anomalies are thought to arise from defective differentiation of the primitive foregut into trachea and esophagus, defective growth of entodermal cells leading to atresia, and incomplete fusion of the lateral walls of the foregut during separation of the trachea from the foregut causing tracheoesophageal fistula.

CLINICAL MANIFESTATIONS. Atresia of the esophagus should be suspected (1) in cases of maternal polyhydramnios; (2) if a catheter used at birth for resuscitation cannot be inserted into the stomach; (3) if the infant has excessive oral secretions; or (4) if choking, cyanosis, or coughing occurs with an attempt at feeding. Suctioning of excess secretions from the mouth and pharynx frequently results in improvement, but symptoms quickly recur. Unfortunately, the diagnosis is often not made until after the baby has aspirated feedings. When a fistula connects the trachea and distal esophagus, air usually enters the abdomen, which often becomes tympanitic and may become so distended as to interfere with breathing. If a fistula connects the proximal esophagus to the trachea, the first attempt at feeding may lead to massive aspiration. Infants with atresia who have no fistula have scaphoid, airless abdomens. In the rare situation of fistula without atresia ("H type") (see Fig. 13–8*C*) the usual sign is recurrent aspiration pneumonia, and diagnosis may be delayed for days or even months. Aspiration of pharyngeal secretions is almost universal among patients with esophageal atresia, but aspiration of gastric contents via a distal fistula causes a more severe, life-threatening chemical pneumonitis.

At least 30% of infants with esophageal atresia have associated congenital anomalies, many of them potentially life-threatening. Cardiovascular anomalies are the most common. Other digestive tract defects (*duodenal stenosis*, imperforate anus, and so on) occur, along with urinary tract, skeletal, and central nervous system defects. See Sec. 7.36 for VATER anomalad.

DIAGNOSIS. Diagnosis of esophageal atresia is ideally made in the delivery room, since pulmonary aspiration is a major determinant of prognosis. Inability to pass a catheter into the stomach confirms the suspicion. The catheter usually stops abruptly 10–11 cm from the upper gum line, and roentgenograms show a coiled catheter in the upper esophageal pouch (Fig. 13–9). Occasionally, plain roentgenograms of the chest show an esophagus dilated with air. The presence of air in the abdomen indicates a fistula between the trachea and the distal esophagus. Contrast medium used for roentgenography should be water soluble; less than 1 mL given under fluoroscopic control is sufficient to outline the blind upper pouch. The contrast medium should then be withdrawn to prevent overflow into the lungs and development of chemical pneumonitis. "H type" fistulas (see Fig. 13–8*C*) may be difficult to demonstrate. A videoesophagram, while filling the esophagus with water-soluble contrast medium, is usually effective. The tracheal orifice of this type of fistula may be detectable at bronchoscopy.

TREATMENT. Esophageal atresia is a surgical emergency. Preoperatively, the patient should be kept prone to decrease any tendency of gastric contents to reach the lungs. The esophageal pouch should be kept empty by constant suction to prevent aspiration of secretions. Careful attention must be given to temperature control and respiratory function and to detection of any associated anomalies. Occasionally, the patient's condition requires that surgery be performed in stages, the first step usually being ligation of the fistula and insertion of a gastrostomy tube for feeding and the second being anastomosis of the two ends of the esophagus. Eight to 10 days after a primary anastomosis, oral feedings are usually tolerated. Esophagography at 10 days will help to determine the adequacy of the anastomosis. Stenosis at the anastomotic site is common and may require dilatations. Persistent abnormal motility is always found in the distal esophagus; it predisposes to gastroesophageal reflux, aspiration, esophagitis, and stricture formation (see Sec. 13.21). Recurrent episodes of respiratory distress may be due to aspiration pneu-

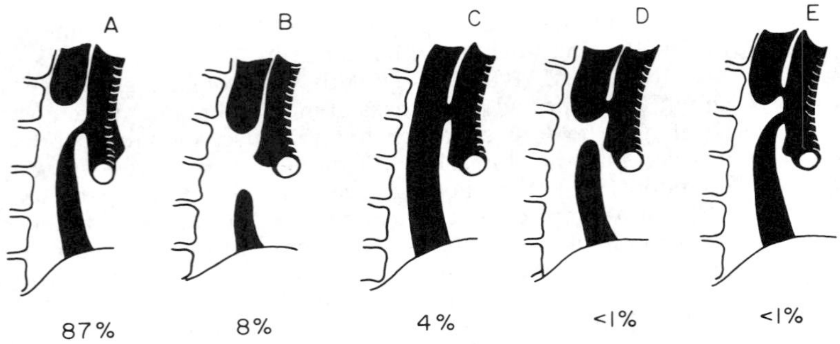

Figure 13–8. Diagrams of the five most commonly encountered forms of esophageal atresia and tracheoesophageal fistula, shown in order of frequency.

monia or reactive airway disease, a common associated problem. Failure to thrive, slow feeding, coughing, and choking are common sequelae, especially if a primary anastomosis cannot be performed in the immediate neonatal period.

13.18 OTHER DISORDERS OF THE ESOPHAGUS

LARYNGOTRACHEOESOPHAGEAL CLEFT. Rarely, the larynx and upper trachea may fail to separate completely from the esophagus for a variable distance. Symptoms of the resultant laryngotracheoesophageal cleft are similar to those of tracheoesophageal fistula; aphonia should suggest the former. Roentgenographic diagnosis using contrast material is difficult; usually endoscopy is required.

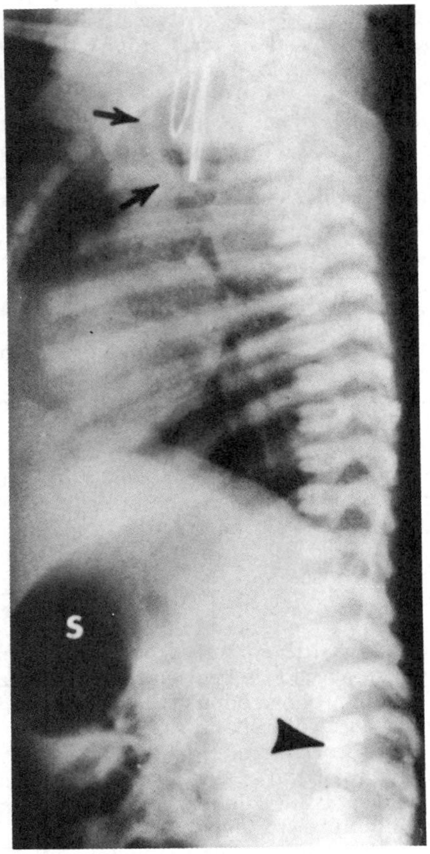

Figure 13–9. Tracheoesophageal fistula. Lateral roentgenogram demonstrating a nasogastric tube coiled *(arrows)* in the proximal segment of an atretic esophagus. The distal fistula is suggested by gaseous dilatation of the stomach (S) and small intestine. The *arrowhead* depicts vertebral fusion whereas a heart murmur and cardiomegaly suggest the presence of a ventricular septal defect. This patient demonstrated elements of the VATER anomalad. (From Balfe D, Ling D, Siegel M: The esophagus. *In:* Putman CE, Ravin CE: Textbook of Diagnostic Imaging. Philadelphia, WB Saunders, 1988.)

EXTERNAL COMPRESSION. The most common masses impinging on the esophagus are enlarged lymph nodes in the subcarinal area, which may be due to tuberculosis, histoplasmosis, other forms of pulmonary suppuration, or lymphoma. Extrinsic pressure may also be caused by vascular anomalies in the mediastinum (Sec. 15.58).

ESOPHAGEAL DUPLICATION CYSTS. These cysts may cause esophageal compression. Their epithelium may come from any portion of the intestine, and they do not communicate with the esophagus unless there is ulceration from gastric mucosa in the cyst. Two thirds are on the right side of the esophagus. Rarely, duplication cysts may extend through the diaphragm and communicate with the intestine. Diagnosis is usually made by barium esophagography. *Neurenteric cysts* are esophageal duplication cysts that contain glial elements; vertebral anomalies usually accompany these cysts.

CONGENITAL STENOSIS AND WEBS. These are rare; their embryonic development is probably similar to that of atresia. Dysphagia usually first occurs when solids are introduced into the diet. The treatment is similar to that of the more common strictures caused by peptic esophagitis, from which they must be distinguished (Sec. 13.22).

DYSPHAGIA DUE TO NEUROMUSCULAR DISEASE. Many systemic, neurologic, and muscular disorders may give rise to esophageal symptoms. These disorders are listed in Table 13–12 and discussed elsewhere (see index).

CRICOPHARYNGEAL DYSFUNCTION. Spasm of the cricopharyngeal muscle or achalasia of the superior esophageal sphincter may cause intermittent dysphagia, and the increased pressure in the pharynx and upper esophagus may lead to development of a posterior pharyngeal diverticulum. Diagnosis of this idiopathic disorder is made with a videoesophagram or manometric demonstration of a failure of the superior esophageal sphincter to relax during deglutition. Symptoms are relieved by myotomy of the cricopharyngeal muscle, analogous to the procedure used in hypertrophic pyloric stenosis (Sec. 13.27).

CRICOPHARYNGEAL INCOORDINATION OF INFANCY. This incoordination is usually evident soon after birth. Sucking is normal, but affected infants tend to choke

TABLE 13–12. Neuromuscular Disorders That May Cause Dysphagia

Cerebral palsy (more common)
Dermatomyositis
Infections—diphtheria, poliomyelitis, tetanus
Muscular dystrophy (more common)
Myasthenia gravis
Polyneuritis
Familial dysautonomia (Riley-Day) syndrome
Scleroderma
Specific cranial nerve defects (e.g., Moebius syndrome)
Werdnig-Hoffmann disease

and aspirate with deglutition; they generally have small jaws that open poorly. Videoradiography shows repetitive to-and-fro movement of the contrast medium in the posterior pharynx. Careful feedings by spoon or gavage are required until the patient is about 6 mo of age, when symptoms abate. The cause of this disorder is unknown.

BULBAR PALSY (supranuclear or lower motor neuron). This type of palsy may cause dysphagia. The child has poor sucking with liquids, and chews and swallows solid food with difficulty. With supranuclear bulbar palsy, the jaw jerk is exaggerated, and usually signs of generalized spastic cerebral palsy develop. Lower motor neuron disease with flaccid bulbar palsy and facial diplegia constitutes the Moebius syndrome.

PARALYSIS OF THE SUPERIOR LARYNGEAL NERVE. Paralysis has been reported in neonates with dysphagia, diminished esophageal motility, a preference to lie with the head turned to one side, and, in some cases, unilateral facial weakness. The syndrome is thought to be caused when an unusual intrauterine position compresses the nerve between the thyroid cartilage and the hyoid bone. Spontaneous recovery occurs during the 1st yr.

TRANSIENT PHARYNGEAL MUSCLE DYSFUNCTION. This dysfunction is often associated with palatal dysfunction and may be due to delayed normal development or associated with cerebral palsy. Choking during feeding and dribbling of formula are the main symptoms. Paralysis of pharyngeal constrictors and a flaccid soft palate are noted in videoradiographic studies. Gavage feeding can prevent aspiration (the main complication) and may be required for only a few days or for many weeks. Affected infants often have generalized hypotonia, and other nervous system dysfunctions, especially developmental delays, that often become evident later.

DIFFUSE ESOPHAGEAL SPASM. This spasm may be a cause of chest pain and dysphagia in adolescents. This primary motility disorder has characteristic esophageal contractions noted on manometry simultaneously with midchest, retrosternal pain after swallowing liquids. Tensilon testing may provoke pain. Treatment is usually not needed, except in more severe cases when nitrates or calcium channel blocking agents have been successful.

13.19 ACHALASIA
(Megaesophagus)

Achalasia, an uncommon disorder, is a lack of relaxation of the LES with swallowing. A relative obstruction at the level of the sphincter is made worse by a lack of peristaltic waves in the esophagus (see Fig. 13–7*B*). The condition affects primarily adolescents and adults; children under the age of 4 yr comprise fewer than 5% of patients. The disease has been reported in siblings. Ganglion cells are frequently decreased in number and surrounded by inflammatory cells; a heightened response of esophageal muscles to metacholine has been interpreted as evidence of denervation hypersensitivity. Only in Chagas disease has the etiology been well established.

CLINICAL MANIFESTATIONS AND DIAGNOSIS. Symptoms include difficulty in swallowing, regurgitation of food, cough from overflow of fluids into the trachea, and failure to gain weight. The diagnosis is usually made roentgenographically and is confirmed with manometry by demonstrating a persistently narrowed hypertensive gastroesophageal junction and by an absence of propulsive peristaltic waves in the esophagus. If obstruction at the gastroesophageal junction persists, esophageal dilatation may become massive and air-fluid levels are often seen on an upright roentgenogram. Pulmonary infections, even bronchiectasis, may result from persistent aspiration of esophageal contents. In patients with advanced cases, retention of fluid and food in the esophagus may cause esophagitis. In rare instances, achalasia is associated with adrenal insufficiency.

TREATMENT. Transient relief of symptoms may occur after dilating the cardioesophageal junction with a mercury bougie. Permanent relief of symptoms usually follows surgical division of muscles at the cardioesophageal junction (Heller procedure). Alternatively, the sphincter may be forcefully dilated with a pneumatic bag placed in the cardioesophageal junction under fluoroscopy. Because the esophageal dysmotility cannot be reversed, any procedure that disrupts the sphincter and relieves the obstruction may allow gastroesophageal reflux, esophagitis, and occasionally stricture formation.

13.20 HIATAL HERNIA
(Partial Thoracic Stomach)

Herniation of part of the stomach into the thorax through the esophageal hiatus may be paraesophageal or sliding type (Fig. 13–10). In the paraesophageal hernia, the gastroesophageal junction is positioned normally, but a portion of the stomach herniates into the chest through a patent esophageal hiatus. Fullness after eating and upper abdominal pain are the usual symptoms; infarction of the herniated stomach is a rare complication. In the more common sliding variety, the gastroesophageal junction and a portion of the stomach lie within the chest.

Hiatal hernia is usually congenital in children and is frequently associated with gastroesophageal reflux. An association with other congenital malformations gives evidence of genetic factors. It is unknown whether the hiatal hernias of adults represent lesions acquired in later life or ones present since infancy. Treatment is directed not at the hernia but at the gastroesophageal reflux.

13.21 GASTROESOPHAGEAL REFLUX
(Chalasia)

When the LES is not competent, excessive and passive reflux of gastric contents may cause significant symptoms. The term *chalasia* describes free reflux across a dilated sphincter. Although many infants have minor degrees of reflux, about 1:300–1:1,000 have significant reflux and associated complications.

ETIOLOGY. Many factors contribute to competency of the gastroesophageal sphincter and development of symptoms. It has been shown that reflux may occur with increased intra-abdominal pressure (crying, coughing, moving, defecating), but more important mechanisms are a chronically lax sphincter or brief but frequent, spontaneous decreases in sphincter tone. Reflux occurs frequently in normal persons after meals,

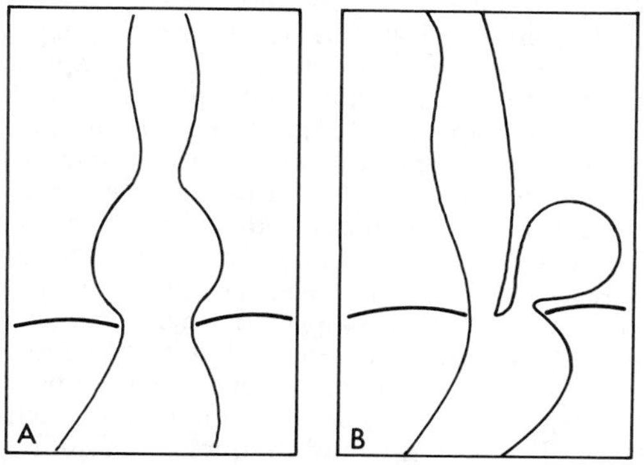

Figure 13–10. Types of esophageal hiatal hernia. *A*, Sliding hiatal hernia, the most common type; *B*, paraesophageal hiatal hernia.

and the swallowing of saliva to wash away the last traces of acid is an important mechanism for preventing esophagitis. The small reservoir capacity of the infant's esophagus predisposes to vomiting, a much less common problem in adolescents and adults. Patients with abnormal reflux may also demonstrate decreased gastric emptying and reduced acid clearance from the esophagus. Placement of a gastrostomy tube encourages reflux, probably by altering the angle by which the esophagus enters the stomach.

CLINICAL MANIFESTATIONS. The signs and symptoms relate directly to the exposure of the esophageal epithelium to refluxed gastric contents. In 85% of affected infants excessive vomiting occurs during the 1st wk of life; an additional 10% have symptoms by 6 wk. Symptoms abate without treatment in 60% by the age of 2 yr as the child assumes a more upright posture and eats solid foods, but the remainder continue to have symptoms until at least 4 yr of age. Patients with cerebral palsy, Down syndrome, and other causes of developmental delay have an increased incidence of reflux.

About two thirds of patients will have delayed gastric emptying, and vomiting occasionally may be forceful because of pylorospasm. Aspiration pneumonia occurs in about one third of patients in infancy, and in those that persist until later childhood chronic cough, wheezing, clubbing, and recurrent pneumonia are common. There may be rumination (see later). Growth and weight gain are adversely affected in about two thirds of patients.

The major manifestation of esophagitis is hemorrhage; the presence of occult blood in stool is common, hematemesis occurs in some children, but melena is rare. Iron-deficiency anemia is common in patients with severe esophagitis. (See Sec. 13.22). Complaints of substernal pain are rare, but dysphagia may cause irritability and anorexia in advanced cases. In untreated patients, esophagitis leads to stricture formation in 5% of cases, and inanition and pneumonia lead to death in another 5%.

Sandifer syndrome, opisthotonus, and other abnormal head posturing is associated with reflux. The head positioning may be a mechanism to protect the airway or reduce acid-reflux–associated pain. Methylxanthines may exacerbate reflux by lowering sphincter tone.

Reflux may rarely cause laryngospasm, apnea, and bradycardia. The relationship between reflux and acute life-threatening events (near-miss sudden infant death syndrome [SIDS]) or SIDS remains controversial and may be coincidental (Sec. 25.1).

DIAGNOSIS. In mild cases, a careful clinical assessment may be sufficient for diagnosis, which is confirmed by assessing the response to therapy. In severe or complex cases, the diagnosis can be confirmed by barium esophagography under fluoroscopic control. The finding of gastric folds above the diaphragm indicates the presence of a hiatal hernia (Fig. 13–11); in children these folds are more readily detected in a collapsed than in a full esophagus. Gastroesophageal reflux is an episodic event; accordingly, in many symptomatic patients significant reflux is not demonstrated initially by roentgenography. It is important to use enough barium to approximate the volume of a normal meal. Special maneuvering of the patient is not necessary. Normal children may have a small amount of reflux that is quickly cleared from the esophagus, but recurrent reflux is definitely abnormal. Strictures are easily demonstrated with barium esophagography. Severe esophagitis may be suspected when a ragged mucosal outline is seen on a roentgenogram, but esophagoscopy with biopsy is a superior diagnostic technique for this disorder. Gastric scintigrams can be used to demonstrate gastroesophageal reflux. The severity and frequency of reflux can be documented by continuous monitoring of esophageal pH with a probe in the distal esophagus. This technique may demonstrate that symptoms such as cough or, rarely, apnea occur at the time of reflux.

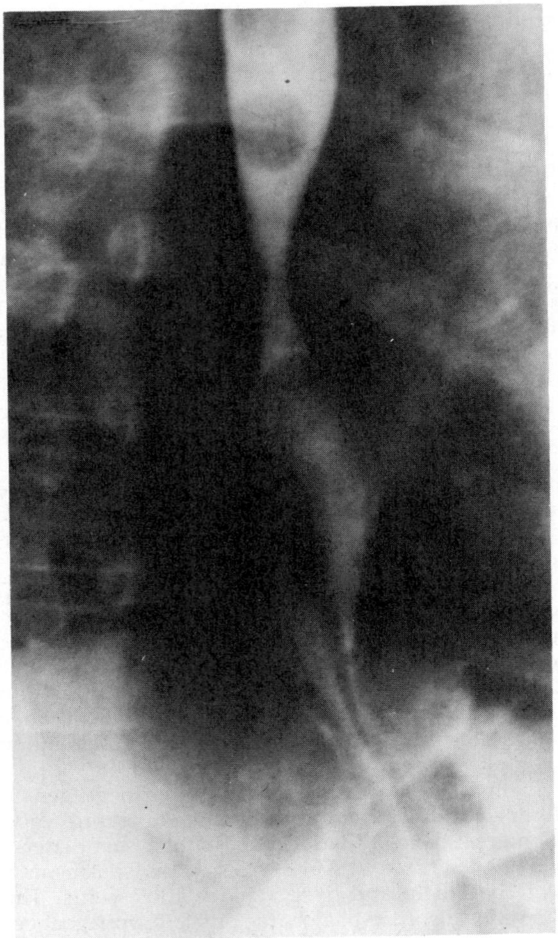

Figure 13–11. Barium esophagogram demonstrating free gastroesophageal reflux. A stricture due to peptic esophagitis is present. Longitudinal gastric folds above the diaphragm indicate the unusual presence of an associated hiatal hernia.

Biopsy of the esophagus may reveal intraepithelial eosinophils or neutrophils suggestive of esophagitis or the presence of Barrett esophagitis (columnar epithelium). The latter is associated with cellular metaplasia or, rarely, adenocarcinoma.

TREATMENT. The results of medical therapy are better in infants than in older children. In mild uncomplicated cases, keeping the child prone, thickening the feedings with cereal, and careful attention to burping are enough. In severe cases, the child should be maintained prone, with the head elevated 30 degrees. Sitting upright in an infant seat may be of no benefit for infants less than 6 mo of age. If esophagitis is present, frequent use of antacids, or cimetidine given four times a day (20–40 mg/kg/24 hr), can be helpful. Metoclopramide (0.15 mg/kg/dose) 4 times a day will accelerate gastric emptying and stimulate muscular activity in the esophagus, and thus decrease reflux. Cisapride, a non-dopamine receptor-blocking, noncholinergic agent with gastrokinetic properties enhances gastrointestinal contraction, improves antroduodenal coordination, and increases LES pressure. Preliminary evidence suggests that cisapride, 0.2 mg/kg qid, reduces the severity of reflux in infants. The response to medical therapy may not be noticeable for as long as 2 wk; increased weight gain and reduced emesis are often the first signs of improvement.

If symptoms do not respond to a 6 wk trial of intensive medical therapy, operative treatment may be indicated; the medical trial may be shortened if recurrent aspiration and apnea are major problems. When stricture has occurred with reflux esophagitis, operation is indicated without a trial of positional therapy. Bougienage of strictures can provide temporary relief of dysphagia, but unless reflux can be prevented, the stricture will recur. Repeated bougienage is usually not needed if the reflux is controlled. The Nissen fundoplication or a variation of it is most often used in children; reflux is controlled in over 90% of cases. When the esophagus is severely shortened, an intrathoracic Nissen procedure is favored. Occasionally, stricture formation is so extensive that colonic interposition is required to replace a portion of the esophagus.

RUMINATION. This uncommon but serious form of chronic regurgitation usually occurs during the latter half of the 1st yr, often with growth failure (see Sec. 3.26). The etiology is unknown. In some patients psychologic factors may be of prime importance. There are often abnormalities in the mother-child relationship, with an inability of the mother to develop a mature parental role. In some infants rumination is a repetitive self-stimulating behavior that develops when the infant has been deprived of soothing tactile, visual, or auditory stimulation. In some patients, gastroesophageal reflux or other abnormalities of esophageal function, or both, are major contributing factors; in others, abnormal esophageal function may only facilitate the development of rumination. Chewing movements and mouthing of the fingers often precede or accompany the regurgitation. Careful observation may disclose that the infant actively gags himself or herself with the tongue or fingers. A significant loss of nutrients may appear deceptively small; the infant often lies continuously in a small pool of regurgitated liquid. A barium swallow roentgenogram usually demonstrates easy reflux or a hiatal hernia and excludes other intestinal lesions such as esophageal stricture, achalasia, or duodenal ulcer.

In cases in which a warm intensive relationship with the mother is lacking, efforts should focus on providing this for the infant. The establishment of regular eye contact is often associated with decreased regurgitation. Intensive medical therapy for gastroesophageal reflux should be instituted. If the patient does not improve, surgery for gastroesophageal reflux regularly stops rumination and initiates weight gain.

13.22 ESOPHAGITIS

Peptic esophagitis due to reflux of gastric acid, with pain, blood loss, and possibly stricture formation is the most common form of esophagitis.

Retroesophageal abscess usually represents extension of a retropharyngeal abscess downward; other causes are esophageal perforations, foreign bodies, spinal osteomyelitis, pleuritis, pericarditis, ulceration from an intubation or tracheostomy tube, diphtheria of the pharynx, or suppuration of mediastinal lymph nodes. The abscess forms behind and around the esophagus and often displaces it to one side, while at the same time it compresses the more firmly seated trachea.

The symptoms are dyspnea, a brassy cough, dysphagia, and, as the trachea is pushed forward, swelling of the neck. Pain and tenderness on palpation of the neck and cervical emphysema may be present. The increased retrotracheal space can be seen on lateral roentgenograms of the neck without the use of contrast medium; if the abscess is due to esophageal perforation, barium esophagography is contraindicated.

The abscess may rupture into the pleura, trachea, or lung. Death may result from pressure of the abscess upon the trachea with consequent asphyxia, or from an erosion into the great vessels of the neck with exsanguinating hemorrhage.

Prompt surgical drainage is indicated. If the abscess is high, the retroesophageal space may be opened in the neck along the anterior border of the sternocleidomastoid muscle. Drainage here is effective to the level of the fourth dorsal vertebra; for retroesophageal abscesses below this point posterior mediastinotomy is generally indicated. Antibiotic therapy is indicated, but such therapy may mask an advancing mediastinal infection; only serial lateral roentgenograms of the neck and chest will indicate the situation in the post-tracheal area.

Esophageal candidiasis (moniliasis) usually occurs in immunosuppressed patients who have AIDS or are receiving chemotherapy for hematologic or neoplastic diseases. Oral candidiasis may be absent. Difficulty and pain on swallowing are prominent. Barium esophagography demonstrates a shaggy mucosal outline or numerous round filling defects, and esophagoscopy shows a friable mucosa with overlying whitish plaques. Treatment consists of ketoconazole 3–6 mg/kg/24 hr orally as a single daily dose, or nystatin 200,000 units orally every 2 hr. Amphotericin may be used in resistant cases. Administration of other antibiotics should be discontinued if possible. Prognosis is usually that of the underlying disease. In immunosuppressed hosts the differential diagnosis includes infection (herpes simplex virus [HSV], cytomegalovirus [CMV]), graft-versus-host disease, and chemotherapy or radiation-induced mucositis.

Diphtheria may involve the esophagus with extension of the membrane from the oropharynx (Sec. 12.25).

Tuberculosis rarely affects the esophagus; when it does, it usually extends directly from the larynx or contiguous lymph nodes.

Herpes simplex infection may cause acute esophagitis. Fever is common, and pain on swallowing is often so severe that no nutrients can be taken. Inspection usually shows typical vesicular lesions in the pharynx, and endoscopy will demonstrate the same lesions in the esophagus. The illness often lasts only a few days. Viscous 2% lidocaine, 2–3 mL every 4 hr, offers symptomatic relief. With severe cases in immunosuppressed patients, acyclovir is indicated. CMV may produce a similar picture in patients with AIDS and may occur following bone marrow transplantation.

CORROSIVE ESOPHAGITIS (See also Sec. 26.10). This injury most commonly follows ingestion of household cleaning products. Alkalis (70%), acids (20%), bleaches, detergents, microwave overheated baby bottles, and button mercuric oxide batteries are common agents. Alkalis produce a severe, deep, liquefaction necrosis that affects all layers of the esophagus. Household liquid alkali agents used as drain declogging agents contain 8–10% base, industrial strength usually contains 30–35%, whereas granular agents contain 80% base. Concentrated bases are also used to produce crack-cocaine and may be left on the table in poorly labeled containers. Alkalis have no taste; therefore, a child may ingest a significant amount.

Acidic agents include toilet bowl cleaners, drain decloggers, and rust and stain removers; they contain various acids (sulfuric, hydrochloric, oxalic, acid sulfates) with a range of concentrations (8–65%). Acids taste bitter, thus limiting the total volume of ingestion. Volatile acids (HCl) may produce respiratory symptoms. All acids produce a coagulative necrosis and a thick eschar that usually limits the depth of the esophageal injury to the mucosa and superficial muscularis layers. Both alkalis and acids (more likely) can produce severe gastritis.

The peak age of accidental corrosive ingestion is less than 5 yr of age. Corrosive solutions stored in innocuous-appearing containers (pop bottles) and in open unlocked areas are risk factors. A history of access to such substances in a child with chemical burns of the hands, mouth, or other parts of the body strongly suggests the possibility of corrosive ingestion. Mouth lesions are not universally present. Tissue injury follows a sequence of early saponification, necrosis, thrombosis (days 1–5), further necrosis (days 4–7), collagen formation (days 8–12), and healing or stricture formation (days 8–42). The time of greatest risk for esophageal perforation is days 7–26.

Clinical manifestations may or may not be present and include salivation, refusal to drink, nausea, vomiting, epigastric pain, oral burns or ulcerations, fever, and leukocytosis.

Emergency *treatment* involves the oral administration of large quantities of fluid (water or milk) to dilute the corrosive agent. Neutralization, induced emesis, and gastric lavage are contraindicated. Edema of the pharynx, larynx, or airway may require urgent endotracheal intubation or tracheostomy. The child should be hospitalized, receive nothing by mouth, and be given intravenous fluids.

Esophagogastroscopy with a flexible fiberoptic endoscope should be performed in all patients within 48 hr to assess the presence and severity of esophageal burns and gastric antral ulceration. Ampicillin may be given for suspected infection; however, perforation with acute mediastinitis requires broad-spectrum antibiotics and the placement of mediastinal drains. Although prednisone therapy was formerly thought to be effective in reducing the incidence and severity of subsequent stricture formation, a randomized controlled trial did not indicate that prednisone was effective. The risk of stricture formation is related directly to the severity of the injury as determined by circumferential ulcerations, white plaques, and sloughing of the mucosa. Intraluminal stents may reduce stricture formation in severe esophageal burns.

Early detection and dilatation of developing strictures are an important part of continuing care. Severe strictures that do not respond to dilatation and complete obliteration of the lumen can be treated by colonic interposition. Long-term sequelae, in addition to strictures, include the rare occurrence of esophageal carcinoma.

Prevention is critical because the morbidity may be great. Corrosive compounds should be kept in the original containers and out of the reach of children. Dilute formulations should be used in homes, and industrial strength solutions and solids should be kept at work or locked in a safe, hard-to-reach location.

13.24 ESOPHAGEAL PERFORATION

This is usually caused by instrumentation for pre-existing disease. Spontaneous perforation may follow sudden increases in esophageal pressure, which occur with violent retching, in automobile accidents, or even with compression in the birth canal. Ninety-five per cent of perforations occur on the left side of the distal esophagus in children but occur more commonly on the right side in neonates. Common symptoms are vomiting followed by severe substernal pain, cyanosis, and shock. Esophagography shows extraluminal water-soluble contrast material.

Violent retching can tear the esophageal mucosa and submucosa, causing hematemesis *(Mallory-Weiss syndrome)*. Esophagoscopy should differentiate this disorder from other more serious forms of upper gastrointestinal bleeding. In children, blood replacement is usually sufficient treatment for this self-limited disease.

13.24 ESOPHAGEAL VARICES

Esophageal varices may occur in children as a complication of portal hypertension. The principal signs are recurrent, profuse, bright red hematemesis, and tarry stools, with signs of intravascular volume depletion. Children with esophageal varices often have another source for acute gastrointestinal hemorrhage. Roentgenographic studies with barium may outline the varices, but esophagoscopy is more precise in diagnosis. Treatment of portal hypertension and acute gastrointestinal bleeding is discussed in Sec. 13.102.

13.25 FOREIGN BODIES IN THE ESOPHAGUS

See Sec. 13.36.

Children swallow a variety of objects that can pass through the intestinal tract without complications. Coins are commonly ingested by children less than 5 yr of age. Objects that become lodged in the esophagus usually do so at one of three areas of physiologic narrowing: below the cricopharyngeal muscle; at the level of the aortic arch; or just above the diaphragm. Lodging of material at any other site should suggest coexistent esophageal disease.

CLINICAL MANIFESTATIONS. The swallowing of a foreign body may provoke an attack of coughing, drooling, and choking. Foreign bodies in the esophagus usually cause pain, dysphagia (especially with solid foods), and occasionally dyspnea, owing to compression of the larynx. After an initial symptom-free period, edema and inflammation produce symptoms of esophageal obstruction. Pain, fever, and shock develop with perforation.

DIAGNOSIS. Radiopaque foreign bodies are easily diagnosed. Coins and other flat objects are usually seen on edge in a lateral film. Recognition of plastic and nonleaded glass objects is often difficult, but they can be detected with barium swallow roentgenography. The use of barium-soaked cotton to demonstrate the position of a foreign body is unnecessary and complicates therapy.

TREATMENT. The usual treatment is removal of the object under direct vision with esophagoscopy. Roentgenography should be repeated just prior to the procedure to make sure the foreign body has not passed into the stomach or been vomited. Asymptomatic patients with esophageal coins should be observed for 24 hr, because many will safely pass the coin to the stomach, thus obviating the need for endoscopy. An alternative procedure is usually successful for some blunt objects. A Foley catheter is inserted beyond the foreign body under fluoroscopic visualization. The balloon is inflated, and the catheter and the foreign body are removed together while taking care that the object is not aspirated. Under no circumstance should attempts be made to force the foreign object into the stomach. The patient should be observed for 24 hr after removal of the foreign body for signs of obstruction or perforation.

JOHN J. HERBST

ESOPHAGEAL ANOMALIES

Berdon WE, Baker DH: Vascular anomalies and the infant lungs: Rings, slings and other things. Semin Roentgenol 7:39, 1972.

Grossfeld JL, O'Neill JA, Clatworthy HW Jr: Enteric duplications in infancy and childhood: An 18 year review. Ann Surg 172:83, 1970.

Puntis J, Ritson D, Holden C, et al: Growth and feeding problems after repair of oesophageal atresia. Arch Dis Child 65:84, 1990.

Reyes H, Meller J, Loeff D: Management of esophageal atresia and tracheoesophageal fistula. Clin Perinatol 16:79, 1989.

HIATAL HERNIA AND GASTROESOPHAGEAL REFLUX

Byrne WJ: Reflux and related phenomena. J Pediatr Gastroenterol Nutr 8:283, 1989.

Carre IJ: The natural history of the partial thoracic stomach (hiatus hernia) in children. Arch Dis Child 34:344, 1959.

Cucchiara S, Gobio-Casali L, Balli F, et al: Cimetidine treatment of reflux

esophagitis in children: An Italian multicentric study. J Pediatr Gastroenterol Nutr 8:150, 1989.
Dodds WJ, Dent J, Hogan WJ, et al: Mechanisms of gastroesophageal reflux in patients with reflux esophagitis. N Engl J Med 307:1547, 1982.
Hoeffel JC, Nihoul-Fekete C, Schmitt M: Esophageal adenocarcinoma after gastroesophageal reflux in children. J Pediatr 115:259, 1989.
Jolley SG, Herbst JJ, Johnson DG, et al: Surgery in children with gastroesophageal reflux and respiratory symptoms. J Pediatr 96:194, 1980.
Orenstein SR: Prone positioning in infant gastroesophageal reflux: Is elevation of the head worth the trouble? J Pediatr 117:184, 1990.
Orenstein SR, Orenstein DM: Gastroesophageal reflux and respiratory disease in children. J Pediatr 112:847, 1988.
Vandenplas Y, Deneyer M, Verlinden M, et al: Gastroesophageal reflux incidence and respiratory dysfunction during sleep in infants: Treatment with cisapride. J Pediatr Gastroenterol Nutr 8:31, 1989.

RUMINATION

Richmond JB, Eddy E, Green M: Rumination: A psychosomatic syndrome of infancy. Pediatrics 22:49, 1958.
Sheagren TG, Mangurten HH, Brea F, et al: Rumination—a new complication of neonatal intensive care. Pediatrics 66:551, 1980.

ACHALASIA

Azizkhan RG, Tapper D, Eraklis A: Achalasia in childhood: A 20-year experience. J Pediatr Surg 15:452, 1980.
Nakayama DK, Shorter NA, Boyle JT, et al: Pneumatic dilatation and operative treatment of achalasia in children. J Pediatr Surg 22:619, 1987.

SWALLOWING AND DYSPHAGIA

Illingworth RS: Sucking and swallowing difficulties in infancy: Diagnostic problems of dysphagia. Arch Dis Child 44:655, 1969.
Milov D, Cynamon H, Andres J: Chest pain and dysphagia in adolescents caused by diffuse esophageal spasm. J Pediatr Gastroenterol Nutr 9:450, 1989.
Wolff PH: The serial organization of sucking in the young infant. Pediatrics 42:943, 1968.

CORROSIVE ESOPHAGITIS

Anderson KD, Rouse TM, Randolph JG: A controlled trial of corticosteroids in children with corrosive injury of the esophagus. N Engl J Med 323:637, 1990.
Hollinger PH: Management of esophageal lesions caused by chemical burns. Ann Otolaryngol 77:819, 1968.
Moore WR: Caustic ingestions: Pathophysiology, diagnosis, and treatment. Clin Pediatr 25:192, 1986.
Wijburg FA, Heymans HSA, Urbanus NAM: Caustic esophageal lesions in childhood: Prevention of stricture formation. J Pediatr Surg 24:171, 1989.

FOREIGN BODIES

Brown LP: Blind esophageal coin removal using a Foley catheter. Arch Surg 96:931, 1968.
Caravati EM, Bennett DL, McElwee NE: Pediatric coin ingestion: A prospective study on the utility of routine roentgenograms. Am J Dis Child 143:549, 1989.
Schunk JE, Corneli H, Bolte R: Pediatric coin ingestions: A prospective study of coin location and symptoms. Am J Dis Child 143:546, 1989.

STOMACH AND INTESTINES

13.26 NORMAL DEVELOPMENT, STRUCTURE, AND FUNCTION

DEVELOPMENT. The gut matures relatively early in fetal life. In the 4-wk, 3-mm embryo, the primitive foregut and hindgut form a simple tube that rotates counterclockwise around the umbilical artery as the stomach and cecum become distinct. This tube then elongates quickly and protrudes into the umbilical cord. At 8 wk the caudal end becomes continuous with the rectum, which has evolved from the cloaca, and at 10 wk the bowel rapidly re-enters the abdomen. Later, the colon achieves its mature conformation. Most structural anomalies of the stomach and intestine are attributable to a delay or aberration in this complex series of events.

The pyloric musculature of the stomach is seen by the 3rd mo of gestation, and parietal and chief cells appear by 14 wk. Intestinal-type cells found in the gastric mucosa gradually disappear during fetal life. Relatively mature villi are seen along the intestine by 12 wk, and by 20 wk the crypts are deep and the enterocytes are columnar with some microvilli. Blood vessels and the nerve supply to the gut are fully developed by 12–13 wk. Intramural ganglia appear first at the proximal end so that if their development is interrupted, the effect will be seen in the distal regions. Peristalsis has been recognized as early as 8 wk, but motility is usually not fully coordinated until near term. Lymphoid tissue has developed by 20 wk.

Some functions develop relatively early in the fetal gut; others mature in postnatal life. In the stomach acid secretion increases dramatically in the first 24 hr after birth; acid and pepsin secretion peak during the first 10 days and decrease from 10–30 days after birth. Intrinsic factor secretion rises slowly during the first 2 wk of life, but at term circulating gastrin levels are inexplicably 2- to 3-fold higher than in adults.

Small intestinal function matures throughout prenatal and postnatal life. Epithelial glucose transport is detectable in the jejunum of the human embryo by 20 wk, but adult capacity may not be achieved for years. Disaccharidase activities are measurable in the human fetus at 12 wk; sucrase and maltase achieve maximal activities by the 24th and 32nd wk, respectively; but lactase activity rises later, reaching maximal levels by 36 wk. In many children, particularly of black and oriental races, intestinal lactase activity begins to decline by 3 yr of age. Fetal intestine is involved in the daily transport of a large amount of amniotic fluid, and there is significant activity of the Na pump in 10-wk-old human fetal gut. Solute transport is probably adequate but marginal in very young infants. Accordingly, relatively severe functional disturbances in response to small intestinal diseases can be anticipated, whereas older children can be expected to have significant reserve function.

Fat absorption is less efficient in term babies than in older children and even less efficient in premature infants than in those at term. Important determinants of these age-related differences are the relatively slow rates of bile salt synthesis and transport in early life.

The human gut is capable of absorbing antigenically significant quantities of intact protein, particularly during the early weeks of life. Entry of potential protein antigens through the mucosal barrier may play a role in later food- and microbe-induced symptoms.

NORMAL STRUCTURE. The serosal layer of the bowel wall is an extension of the peritoneum that extends distally as far as the rectum. There are two muscle layers, outer longitudinal fibers and inner circular ones; in the colon the longitudinal fibers form bands, or taeniae. The submucosa is a rich matrix for lymph and vascular plexuses, containing lymphoid cells and macrophages and, in the duodenum, Brunner glands. A complex enteric nervous system is an important factor in regulating not only microvascular flow but epithelial function. The mucosa of the small bowel is well designed to absorb nutrients since its absorptive surface has a very large area owing to a multitude of constantly moving villi that extend into the lumen. In children these villi tend to be leaflike rather than finger-shaped projections; thus, the functional surface area of the small intestine probably increases with age. The colonic mucosal surface is flat, with numerous tubular crypts opening into the surface; in the rectum the surface is smooth. The lamina propria, a cellular layer just beneath the epithelium that contains cells capable of phagocytosis and immunoglobulin synthesis, provides a connective tissue core for the epithelium and its vascular supply. Lymphoid tissue is concentrated in Peyer patches, which become more numerous in the distal small bowel. There are several types of epithelial cells in the small intestine: the columnar absorptive cell dominates; goblet cells secrete mucus; endocrine cells secrete certain intestinal hormones; in the crypts there are Paneth cells, whose function is unknown; and over areas of lymphoid aggregation there are "m" cells that have a special capacity to absorb intact, potentially antigenic proteins. The columnar absorptive cell is polarized with a microvillus "brush" border at the luminal surface to which a glycocalyx or "fuzz coat" is tightly adherent. Active cell division of the enterocytes occurs in the crypts, and as cells migrate up the villi, they differentiate. The jejunal epithelium is completely renewed in 5–6 days, providing a mechanism for rapid repair after injury; but in the very young infant the process may be slow.

NORMAL FUNCTION. The stomach serves as a reservoir that delivers liquefied, blended, but minimally digested food to the intestine. It also secretes intrinsic factor, essential for the assimilation of vitamin B_{12} in the ileum. The small intestine must process not only ingested nutrients but also a large volume of water and shed epithelial cells. In adults the quantity of water entering the gut lumen is at least seven times the amount ingested.

Intraluminal digestion depends mainly on the exocrine pancreas. Synthesis and secretion of bicarbonate and digestive enzymes are stimulated by secretin and cholecystokinin, which are released by the upper intestinal mucosa in response to various intraluminal stimuli, among them components of the diet. Digestion is an efficient, fast process, usually completed in the most proximal intestinal segment. Bile salts in the lumen facilitate digestion and are essential for the efficient delivery of products of lipid hydrolysis to the absorptive surface of the epithelium. Emulsification aids digestion, and long-chain monoglycerides and fatty acids usually reach the epithelium in the form of mixed micelles with conjugated bile acids and phospholipid. Sterols such as vitamin D are particularly dependent on these micelles for their absorption; accordingly, diseases such as biliary atresia cause particular difficulties with vitamin D assimilation. Medium-chain triglycerides available in certain specially designed therapeutic diets, on the other hand, do not require micelles, emulsification, or hydrolysis for their absorption.

Carbohydrate, protein, and fat are normally absorbed by the upper half of the small intestine; the distal segments represent a vast reserve of absorptive capacity. Most of the sodium, potassium, chloride, and water is absorbed in the small bowel. Bile salts and vitamin B_{12} are selectively absorbed in the distal ileum and iron in the duodenum and proximal jejunum.

Disaccharides are hydrolyzed by disaccharidases on the outer surface of the microvillus membranes, and resultant monosaccharides are actively transported across the cell, primarily to portal venous drainage. Dipeptides and probably larger peptides can be hydrolyzed at the brush border surface, but may also enter the cell intact before they contact peptidases. The small bowel has active transport pathways for specific groups of amino acids, similar to those seen in the renal tubule. Monoglycerides and fatty acids enter the epithelium intact; triglycerides are resynthesized, incorporated with phospholipid and lipoprotein into chylomicrons, and released into lymphatics. Medium-chain triglycerides may be taken up intact and released into the portal stream.

The colon extracts additional water and ions from the luminal contents in order to render the stools partially or completely solid. Stools can then be stored in the rectum until distention triggers a defecation reflex that, when assisted by voluntary relaxation of the external sphincter, permits evacuation.

J. RICHARD HAMILTON

Grand RJ, Watkins JB, Torti FM: Development of the human gastrointestinal tract; a review. Gastroenterology 79:790, 1976.
Gryboski JD: Gastrointestinal function in the infant and young child. Clin Gastroenterol 6:253, 1976.
Watkins JB: Mechanisms of fat absorption and the development of gastrointestinal function. Pediatr Clin North Am 22:721, 1975.

CONGENITAL AND PERINATAL ANOMALIES OF THE GASTROINTESTINAL TRACT AND INTESTINAL OBSTRUCTION

Many congenital and perinatal anomalies of the gastrointestinal tract may be responsible for partial or complete obstruction. Most obstructions involve the rectum and anus or duodenum; the remainder are predominantly in the small intestine.

13.27 CONGENITAL (INFANTILE) HYPERTROPHIC PYLORIC STENOSIS

Pyloric stenosis affects approximately 1:150 male and 1:750 female infants. It occurs more frequently in first-born male infants. Familial incidence is observed in about 15% of patients, but no specific pattern of inheritance has been established. Multifactorial inheritance is likely. Male infants born to mothers who had pyloric stenosis as infants have a high incidence of pyloric stenosis. The condition sometimes occurs in miniepidemics, the reason for which is unknown.

ETIOLOGY. The cause of pyloric stenosis is not known. Favoring a congenital origin are its high concordance in monovular twins, in contrast to binovular twins, and a slight association with hiatal hernia and esophageal atresia. There is probably, however, an undetermined, acquired factor involved in pathogenesis of the lesion. High levels of serum gastrin have been found in affected infants, but it is not known whether this is a cause or a result of the condition. Pyloric stenosis has been rarely associated with eosinophilic gastroenteritis, 18-trisomy, and Turner, Smith Lemli-Opitz, and Cornelia de Lange syndromes.

PATHOLOGY AND PATHOPHYSIOLOGY. A diffuse hypertrophy and hyperplasia of the smooth muscle narrows the antrum of the stomach to a fine channel that easily becomes obstructed. The antral region is elongated, is thickened to as much as twice its normal size, and is of cartilaginous consistency. The muscular thickening is never confined to the isolated band of circular muscle fiber called the pyloric sphincter; it extends proximally well into the antrum and ends distally quite abruptly where the duodenum begins. In response to outflow obstruction and vigorous peristalsis the stomach musculature becomes uniformly hypertrophied and dilates. Gastritis with bleeding may occur after prolonged stasis. As a result of vomiting the patient may become dehydrated and develop hypochloremic alkalosis.

CLINICAL MANIFESTATIONS. Pyloric stenosis is not present at birth. Initially there is only regurgitation or occasional nonprojectile *vomiting*. The onset rarely occurs before 1 wk of age, usually in the 2nd–3rd wk; it is seldom delayed until the 2nd–3rd mo. The vomiting becomes projectile, usually within 1 wk after onset, and generally occurs during or shortly after feeding but at times up to several hours later. In some cases vomiting occurs after each feeding; in others it is intermittent. The infant is hungry and will take another feeding immediately. The vomitus consists only of gastric contents but may be blood-tinged; it is not bile-stained. The stools may become very small and infrequent, depending on the amount of food that reaches the intestinal tract.

A physical examination shows varying degrees of dehydration and lethargy depending on the metabolic state of the infant. Weight loss may occur. In advanced cases the baby may appear moribund and weight may decrease to a level below that at birth. Decreased elasticity of the skin and loss of subcutaneous tissue may occur. The eyes may be sunken and the fat pads of the cheeks lost so that the infant has a wrinkled, "old man" appearance and is obviously malnourished.

Visible peristalsis, proceeding from the left upper quadrant toward the pylorus in the right upper quadrant of the abdomen, is most prominent immediately after feeding or just before vomiting (Fig. 13–12). The infant may appear uncomfortable, but distress is not prominent. Successful palpation of the abdomen requires patience since it depends on a totally relaxed anterior abdominal wall and an empty stomach. Continuous gentle "air leak" or intermittent gastric suction with a No. 10 nasogastric tube while simultaneously feeding the baby warm sugar solution will facilitate palpation of the "tumor." Palpation is best done from the infant's left side, and if the baby has pyloric stenosis, a mass can be felt in the epigastrium to the right of or in the midline, deep to the right rectus muscle, and under the edge of the liver. The tumor is hard, mobile, and nontender and feels like an acorn or olive; it is often best felt immediately after the baby has vomited. There is no need for barium or ultrasonographic studies once the tumor has been palpated. If the diagnosis of pyloric stenosis cannot be established after several examinations and is still suspected, an ultrasonic examination may be done (Fig. 13–13). Measurements should be made of the diameter, thickness, and length of the pyloric muscle. The diagnosis is, however, essentially a clinical one, confirmed by palpating the mass.

When a barium study is necessary, the appearance of hypertrophic pyloric stenosis is characteristic. There is a vigorously peristaltic stomach with delayed or no gastric emptying, a fine elongated pyloric canal seen as a single ("string sign") or sometimes a double line of barium, and an umbrella-shaped duodenal cap stretched out over the hypertrophied pylorus. Just proximal to the canal a curious diverticulum may be seen (Fig. 13–14). The indication for barium studies is the suspicion of pyloric membranous obstruction or duodenal (supra-ampullary) blockage. If gastroesophageal reflux is suspected, medical management may be undertaken without the necessity for barium studies. Continued emesis nonetheless requires a roentgenographic examination to exclude gastric-outlet or intestinal obstruction.

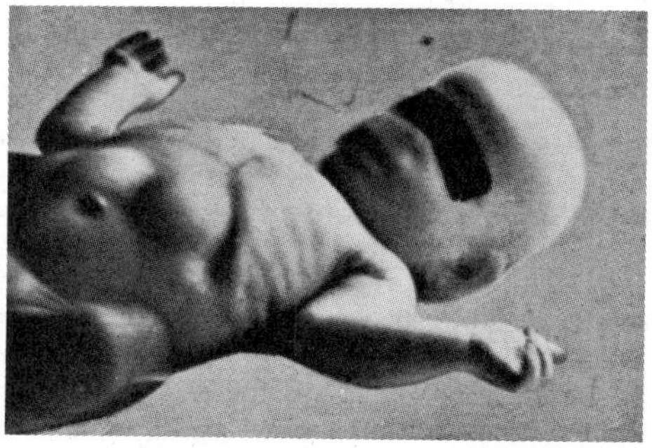

Figure 13–12. Gastric peristaltic waves of pyloric stenosis in an infant 3 wk of age. (Courtesy of Carl Wagner, M.D., Cincinnati.)

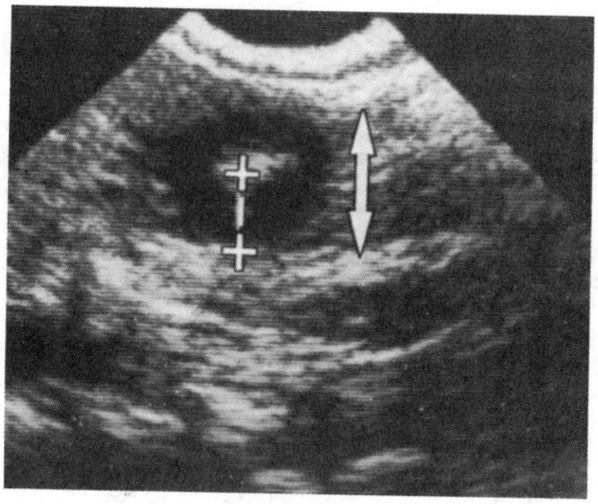

Figure 13–13. Transverse sonogram demonstrating the "target" sign of pyloric stenosis. The distance between the *crosses* demonstrates the thickness of the hypoechogenic muscle mass, whereas the *arrow* demonstrates the entire pyloric diameter. (From Rollins MD, Shields MD, Quinn RJM, et al: Pyloric stenosis: Congenital or acquired? Arch Dis Child 64:138, 1989.)

Premature infants with pyloric stenosis may demonstrate recurrent nonbilious emesis and abdominal distention without the typical olive. Pyloric stenosis, lactobezoars, and metabolic problems should be considered in these premature infants.

Two to 9% of affected infants will have jaundice; the hyperbilirubinemia is thought to result from glucuronyl transferase deficiency or an increased enterohepatic circulation of bilirubin. It usually disappears within 72 hr after operative treatment.

METABOLIC ALTERATIONS. Extensive and protracted vomiting in pyloric stenosis, as in other forms of high intestinal obstruction, may lead to critical deficits of potassium and sodium, which may be reflected by low values in the serum. Much more striking are the decrease in chloride concentration and increases in pH and in carbon dioxide content, which constitute the characteristic serum chemical changes of *hypochloremic alkalosis* (Sec. 6.21). Correction of

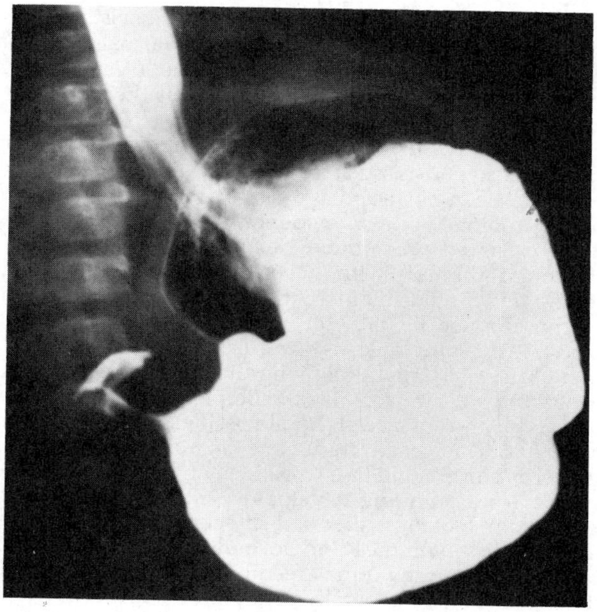

Figure 13–14. Barium in the stomach of an infant with projectile vomiting. The attenuated pyloric canal is typical of congenital hypertrophic pyloric stenosis.

these chemical changes requires replacement of sodium, chloride, and potassium. Intravenous administration of 5% glucose in isotonic sodium chloride solution, to which potassium chloride is added (to a concentration of 3–5 mEq/dL or 30–50 mEq/L), will gradually and satisfactorily replace the calculated deficits of potassium, chloride, and sodium. This also avoids the danger of hyponatremia, which may ensue if hypotonic electrolyte solutions are used for replacement of fluid and electrolytes in dehydrated infants who have had protracted vomiting. The intravenous administration of ammonium chloride solution is unnecessary. The serum chloride level, which may vary from nearly normal to as low as 70 mEq/L, may be used as a rough index of potassium deficit; if the serum chloride is normal, the potassium deficit may be minimal, and care should be taken not to overload the infant with this ion. Maintenance fluids should be given following correction of dehydration. Milder degrees of electrolyte disturbances are noted in patients with a short period of emesis (< 7 days).

DIFFERENTIAL DIAGNOSIS. The usual case can be diagnosed by the characteristic clinical pattern and the identification of a pyloric mass. Infants who are exceptionally reactive to external stimuli, those fed by inexperienced or anxious caretakers, or those for whom an adequate maternal-infant bonding relationship has not been established may vomit frequently in the early weeks of life. Such infants may come to resemble infants with pyloric stenosis; the vomiting may be persistent and even projectile. Gastric waves are occasionally visible in small, emaciated infants who do not have pyloric stenosis. Chalasia of the esophagus or hiatal hernia usually result in vomiting in the 1st wk of life and can be differentiated from pyloric stenosis by palpation and roentgenographic studies. Adrenal insufficiency may simulate pyloric stenosis, but the absence of a palpable tumor and the metabolic acidosis and elevated serum potassium and urinary sodium concentrations of adrenal insufficiency aid in differentiation. Inborn errors of metabolism may produce recurrent emesis with alkalosis (urea cycle) or acidosis (organic acidemia) and lethargy, coma, or seizures. Vomiting with diarrhea suggests gastroenteritis, but occasionally a patient with pyloric stenosis will have diarrhea. Infrequently, gastroesophageal reflux with or without a hiatal hernia may be confused with pyloric stenosis. Very rarely, a pyloric membrane or pyloric duplication may result in projectile vomiting, visible peristalsis, and, in the case of a duplication, a palpable mass. Duodenal stenosis proximal to the ampulla of Vater results in the clinical features of pyloric stenosis, but there may be no palpable mass.

TREATMENT. Surgical relief of the pyloric obstruction as soon as the diagnosis is established and the metabolic imbalances have been corrected is the treatment of choice. Well-hydrated infants without evidence of electrolyte imbalance may be operated on without delay; delays of 24–36 hr for replacement therapy without oral intake are indicated in severely dehydrated infants. At operation, after the stomach has been emptied by catheter, the seromuscular layer of the gastric antrum and pylorus is incised and the muscle split with a blunt instrument, allowing the intact mucosa to bulge between the split muscle (Fredet-Ramstedt pyloromyotomy). Four to 6 hr postoperatively, oral feedings are begun in small amounts and increased gradually. An acceptable regimen is to give 4 mL of 5% glucose in saline solution hourly for four feedings. If no vomiting develops, 8 mL is given hourly for the next four feedings; then a 4-hr schedule can be initiated with increasing volumes and formula gradually substituted for clear fluid until normal feedings are achieved, usually within 24–48 hr. We generally begin normal feedings (formula or breast milk) on the day after the operation and discharge the patient that same day. If the infant is breast-fed, it is advisable to place the infant at each breast for 1 min for the first postoperative feeding, thereafter increasing the time on each breast with each subsequent feeding. An alternative regimen is to maintain administration of intravenous fluids postoperatively, giving the infant nothing orally for 24 hr. Full feeding is then started. If vomiting occurs after feedings are begun, oral feedings are withheld for 4 hr, and feeding is then reinstituted. Persistence of vomiting beyond the 5th postoperative day suggests an incomplete pyloromyotomy or possibly concomitant hiatal hernia or chalasia; occasional episodes of vomiting are not uncommon after operation, probably as the result of persisting gastritis and this may last for 5 days. During an initial period of small feedings, intravenous administration of fluids is often required, depending on the fluid and electrolyte balance of the infant. Complete cessation of vomiting is the rule after operation, even though postoperative roentgenographic studies have shown that the pyloric canal may remain narrow for many months in the asymptomatic infant. Hospitalization is not usually required beyond 48 hr postoperatively.

NONSURGICAL TREATMENT. The slowness of improvement (2–8 mo), the higher mortality, and the current high cost and probable adverse effect on emotional development of prolonged hospitalization have led to a virtual abandonment of nonsurgical treatment for pyloric stenosis. If, for some reason, medical rather than surgical management is necessary, slow improvement may take place on a regimen of small, frequent feedings thickened with cereal, maintenance of a semi-upright position for 1 hr or so after feedings, sedation, administration of a cholinergic blocking agent, and parenteral administration of fluids as required. When there is epigastric distention before a feeding, emptying of the stomach by lavage may decrease the chance of vomiting. Balloon dilation of the pyloric canal may also be a feasible treatment.

PROGNOSIS. When the diagnosis is made early in the course of the disease and the infant is properly prepared for operation, the operative mortality is less than 1%. Medical therapy has a higher mortality. Severe and prolonged undernutrition may have an untoward effect on subsequent development.

13.28 CONGENITAL INTESTINAL OBSTRUCTION

GENERAL CONSIDERATIONS. Intestinal obstruction occurs in approximately 1:1,500 newborn infants. The cardinal signs are vomiting, abdominal distention, and failure to pass feces. Since a number of days may go by prior to full certainty that the infant has an obstructive lesion, early diagnosis depends on appreciation of the significance of vomiting and distention. *High intestinal obstruction* is characterized by vomiting, which tends to be persistent even when feedings have been stopped; gross distention is absent. *Low obstruction* is characterized principally by distention, and vomiting may be only a later manifestation. When the obstruction is in the duodenum, symptoms may become manifest within a few hours; if it is in the large intestine, symptoms may be delayed for more than 24 hr. The former is an example of a "high" obstruction; the latter is "low." The changeover level is distal to the first 15 cm of the jejunum.

From an anatomic standpoint congenital obstructive lesions of the intestines can be viewed as *intrinsic* (e.g., atresia, stenosis, meconium ileus, and aganglionic megacolon) or *extrinsic* (e.g., malrotation, constricting bands, intra-abdominal hernias, and duplications). An attempt should be made to locate the lesion preoperatively in order to guide the surgical approach.

When the obstruction is *complete*, there should be little difficulty in clinical recognition, but when it is *incomplete*, there may be considerable difficulty. Polyhydramnios is frequently an accompaniment of high intestinal obstruction, as it is of esophageal atresia. When polyhydramnios has been noted, the infant's stomach should be aspirated immediately after birth. Aspiration of 15–20 mL or more of gastric fluid, especially if it is bile-stained, is suggestive of a high intestinal obstruction.

Meconium stools may be passed initially if the obstruction is in the upper part of the small intestine or if the obstruction developed late in intrauterine life.

Obstruction in the duodenum may cause epigastric distention and, at times, gastric waves similar to those of pyloric stenosis. The distention may not be persistent, however, because it may be relieved by vomiting. The vomiting may be projectile, and the vomitus will contain bile if the obstruction is below the ampulla of Vater, as it usually is.

Obstructions in the lower ileum, colon, or rectum cause more generalized distention, often with bulging of the flanks. When percussion of liver dullness is obliterated, there is a strong possibility that intestinal perforation has occurred. Onset of vomiting with lower bowel obstruction may be delayed for 1 day. It may eventually become feculent.

When obstruction is *incomplete* (as, for example, with intestinal stenosis, constricting bands, duplications, and incomplete volvulus), signs (vomiting, abdominal distention, obstipation) may appear shortly after birth or may be delayed an indeterminate time. They may approach in severity those of a completely obstructive lesion, or they may be sufficiently mild and infrequent as to be overlooked until either an acute episode or diagnostic studies disclose the lesion. Incomplete obstruction may present as urgent a need as complete obstruction for surgical intervention.

Valuable information on the location of congenital obstructive lesions in the intestine may often be obtained from flat and upright roentgenograms of the abdomen taken without use of contrast media. With completely obstructing lesions there will be distention of the bowel above the obstruction, and there may be a series of fluid levels with superimposed gas in the distended loops in the upright or cross-table lateral position. Pneumoperitoneum may be seen, with free air in the subphrenic regions or over the liver in the left lateral decubitus position. Calcification within the peritoneal cavity usually indicates meconium peritonitis. Rarely, obstruction with intraluminal calcification may be associated with rectourinary fistula, colonic aganglionosis, or intestinal atresia. A characteristic "ground-glass" appearance in the right lower quadrant with trapped bubbles of air within the obstructing meconium may be seen in patients with meconium ileus. A study of the colon with an enema containing radiopaque material may provide additional localizing information, especially in respect to the possibility of a misplaced cecum with malrotation of the intestine. Hirschsprung disease may be noted. Air is usually demonstrable roentgenographically in the stomach of the normal infant immediately after birth; within 1 hr air may reach the proximal portion of the small intestine and segments of the colon; air may become visible in the distal parts of the colon as early as the 3rd hr or as late as 18 hr. It is difficult to accurately differentiate small from large bowel obstruction in children less than 2 yr of age.

PROGNOSIS. If a complete obstruction is not relieved promptly, the clinical course progresses rapidly. Vomiting is persistent; dehydration, loss of weight, and prostration become severe, and the infant dies within a few days. When the obstruction is not complete, the infant may survive for weeks; minor obstructions may be compatible with life even without treatment. Recovery from both complete and incomplete obstructions can be expected with early diagnosis and appropriate management.

TREATMENT. Not every obstructive lesion is amenable to surgery, but infants can withstand massive resection of the small intestine when the lesion necessitates it. Preoperative preparation (including constant gastric aspiration) and postoperative care are important, especially in respect to correction of dehydration and electrolyte deficits and to the maintenance of fluid balance and nutrition by parenteral means (Sec. 6.25 and 6.26). If a prolonged period of intravenous nutrition is anticipated, the insertion of a central venous cannula at the time of the corrective surgery is a wise precaution.

ATRESIA AND STENOSIS

Atresia (complete occlusion) and, less commonly, *stenosis* (partial occlusion) account for about one third of cases of intestinal obstruction. The obstructive lesion (excluding anorectal lesions) is more frequently in the ileum (50%) and duodenum (25%), less frequently in the jejunum, rarely in the colon, and almost never in the stomach. Infants with Down syndrome have an increased incidence of duodenal atresia and of imperforate anus. About 15% of intestinal atresias are multiple. The types of atresia are (1) a diaphragm-like occlusion of the lumen, (2) a blind end not in continuity with a distal segment, and (3) segments of bowel with cord-like connections.

13.29 CONGENITAL DUODENAL OBSTRUCTION

ETIOLOGY. Delayed vacuolization of the embryonic intestinal lumen is thought to account both for mucosal diaphragms within the duodenum and for duodenal atresia. Atresia may also be caused by vascular insufficiency.

PATHOLOGY. The atretic duodenum usually ends blindly just distal to the ampulla of Vater. Twenty to thirty per cent of affected infants have Down syndrome, an additional 20% are premature, and in 20% the common bile duct drains into the bowel beyond the site of atresia. Rarely, bile enters the bowel both proximal and distal to the site of the obstruction, especially when a duodenal diaphragm is present. After atresia, the second most common cause of congenital duodenal obstruction is incomplete rotation of the midgut, with the duodenum becoming obstructed by the misplaced peritoneal reflections of the preduodenal cecum. Volvulus neonatorum is a serious complication of malrotation and requires prompt relief. An annular pancreas, encircling the second portion of the duodenum, may compress and obstruct it partially or completely; this condition is almost always associated with an underlying duodenal stenosis. A *duodenal web*, mucosal diaphragm, or "windsock" may coexist with malrotation and should always be sought. Rarely, a preduodenal portal vein may compress and obstruct the anterior wall of the first part of the duodenum.

CLINICAL MANIFESTATIONS. Vomiting of bile-stained material may occur shortly after birth or be delayed, especially with incomplete obstruction. Early, the epigastrium may be full with peristalsis observed, although there may be no abdominal distention. Down syndrome may be present, or a history of maternal hydramnios may be obtained. With prolonged vomiting a metabolic alkalosis with dehydration and electrolyte imbalance ensues. If the duodenum is atretic proximal to the ampulla of Vater, the vomitus will not contain bile. Any incomplete duodenal obstruction may result in the onset of symptoms beyond the neonatal period. Thus, a patient with duodenal stenosis may remain well for several months, and chronic duodenal ileus associated with malrotation may become evident even later.

DIAGNOSIS. The diagnosis of duodenal obstruction may be made by in utero ultrasound and by studying the air pattern in supine and erect roentgenograms of the abdomen.

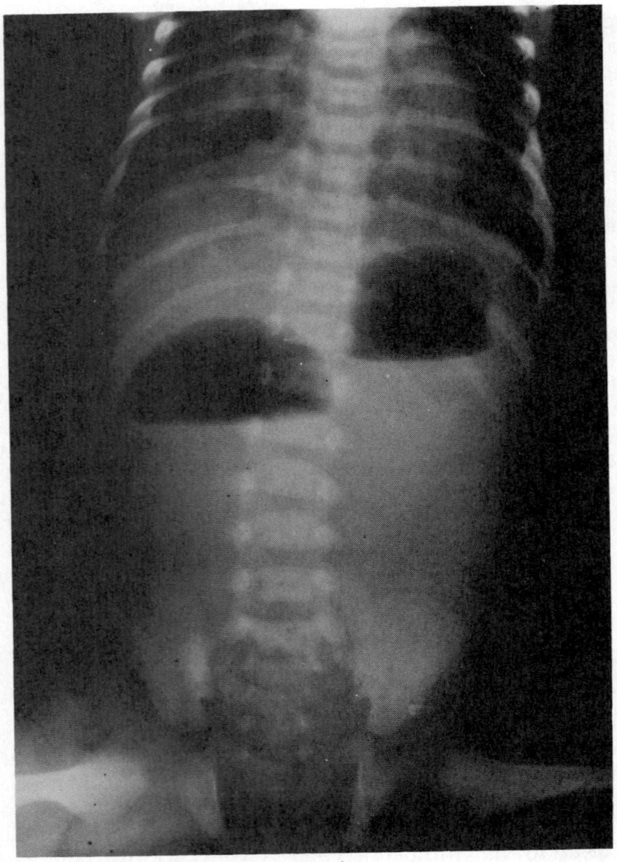

Figure 13–15. Abdominal roentgenogram of a newborn infant held upright. Note the "double bubble" gas shadow above and the absence of gas in the distal bowel in this case of congenital duodenal atresia.

Classically, a "double bubble" is seen on the upright film as the air in the stomach and the distended duodenum rises to the top of each viscus and forms level lines at the fluid-air interfaces (Fig. 13–15), with contained gastric fluid and duodenal contents. With complete atresia no gas will be seen in the rest of the abdomen. A similar appearance may occur with malrotation, annular pancreas, and severe duodenal stenosis. If there is roentgenographic evidence of duodenal obstruction, a barium enema should be done as an emergency to determine whether a malrotation is present. If the cecum is undescended, it must be assumed that the duodenal obstruction is due to Ladd bands in association with malrotation and that volvulus neonatorum of the entire midgut may coexist. Some radiologists prefer an upper intestinal contrast study to see the abnormal position of the jejunum and ligament of Treitz in the right upper quadrant.

TREATMENT. In duodenal atresia or stenosis the surgical procedures of choice are duodenoplasty, duodenoduodenostomy, or less often, duodenojejunostomy to bypass the obstruction. If obstruction is due to Ladd bands with malrotation, an operation is necessary without delay. After division of the abnormal peritoneal folds or bands, the entire large intestine is placed within the left side of the abdomen, after first removing the appendix, with the small bowel on the right—the fetal position of nonrotation. An appendectomy is done to avoid later misdiagnosis of appendicitis. Malrotation may also coexist with an intrinsic duodenal obstruction, such as a membrane or stenosis; this may be identified by passing a nasogastric balloon-tipped catheter into the jejunum below the site of obstruction, inflating the balloon, and slowly withdrawing the catheter. Annular pancreas is best treated by duodenoduodenostomy without dividing the pancreas, leaving as short a defunctioned loop as possible. Duodenal diaphragmatic obstruction is managed by duodenoplasty. The possibility exists that the common bile duct may open on the diaphragm itself.

13.30 ANOMALIES OF ROTATION
(Malrotation)

Incomplete rotation, or *malrotation of the intestine*, represents a failure of embryonic or fetal bowel to rotate to its normal position. In the normal sequence (1) the cecum rotates around the superior mesenteric artery (which acts as an axis) counterclockwise from a position in the middle of the abdomen, below the stomach; (2) the colon, which lies on the left side of the abdomen, follows the cecum into the right upper quadrant and finally into the right lower quadrant; (3) when rotation is completed, the ascending and descending mesocolons fuse with the back of the abdomen, anchoring the mesentery from the ligament of Treitz obliquely downward to the cecal area. In some cases of complete rotation, fusion of the mesentery remains incomplete so that there is abnormal mobility of the midgut and colon.

Most often in malrotation the cecum fails to move into the right lower quadrant, and the bands fixing it to the posterior abdominal wall cross over and may obstruct the duodenum (Fig. 13–16). The narrow mesenteric stalk, which suspends the small intestine in the area of the superior mesenteric vessels, is liable to volvulus, resulting in intermittent or acute obstruction that may progress to strangulation. Obstruction occurs first at the duodenum, then at the lower end of the loop. *Volvulus* accounts for more than half of operations for intestinal obstruction in patients with the cecum in the right upper portion of the abdomen. This problem usually presents symptoms of acute or recurrent intestinal obstruction at birth or in the 1st yr of life. Occasionally, a child with malrotation presents the clinical picture of malabsorption, with relief following surgical repair. Delayed recognition of volvulus may

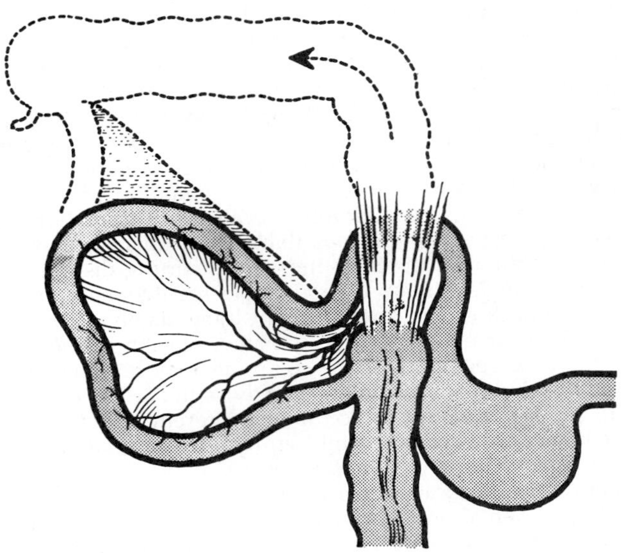

Figure 13–16. The mechanism of intestinal obstruction with incomplete rotation of the midgut (malrotation). The *dotted lines* show the course the cecum should have taken. Failure to rotate has left obstructing bands across the duodenum, and a narrow pedicle for the midgut loop, making it susceptible to volvulus. (From Nixon HH, O'Donnell B: The Essentials of Pediatric Surgery. Philadelphia, JB Lippincott, 1961.)

later present with a septic shock-like syndrome. Nonrotation is associated with midgut volvulus, gastroschisis, omphaloceles, and hernias through the foramen of Bochdalek. Malrotation may be present with annular pancreas or with congenital atresia or stenosis of the duodenum.

Roentgenograms of the abdomen may show an abnormal colonic gas pattern, and barium enema confirms the abnormal position of the cecum. An upper gastrointestinal roentgenogram may show the ligament of Treitz to be shifted to the right. In acute obstruction, diagnosis is made at laparotomy.

Management includes fluid therapy to combat shock and disturbance of body fluids and electrolytes, followed by laparotomy, at which the volvulus is unwound, transduodenal bands are divided, and the large intestine is straightened and placed in the left side of the abdomen with all the small bowel on the right. Delayed diagnosis may result in small intestinal infarction and subsequent short gut syndrome.

13.31 JEJUNAL OR ILEAL OBSTRUCTION

These obstructions may result from atresia or stenosis, meconium ileus, Hirschsprung disease, intussusception, Meckel diverticulum, intestinal duplication, or strangulated hernia.

PATHOLOGY. The bowel in *ileal* or *jejunal atresia* ends blindly proximal and distal to an interruption in its continuity; there may even be a gap in the mesentery. With stenotic or "windsock" obstructions the bowel and mesentery are in continuity. The large size of the proximal obstructed loop of bowel contrasts greatly with that of the collapsed distal bowel, which may result in an unused microcolon. Rarely, atretic segments are multiple; this form has a familial incidence. Atresias, including reabsorption of gangrenous bowel, have been experimentally produced by intrauterine ligation of mesenteric vessels of fetal bowel. The "Christmas tree" or "apple peel" deformity represents about 10% of jejunoileal atresias and is associated with an absent distal blood supply and extensive bowel necrosis. Apple peel jejunal atresia is more common in females and is associated with prematurity and, occasionally, with autosomal recessive inheritance.

Meconium ileus occurs in newborn infants with cystic fibrosis, but less than 10% of patients with the latter develop meconium ileus. The last 20–30 cm of ileum are collapsed and filled with pellets of pale-colored stool, above which a dilated loop of varying length appears obstructed by meconium with the consistency of thick syrup or glue. Peristalsis fails to propel this very viscid material forward, so that it becomes impacted in the ileum. Volvulus, atresia, or perforation of the bowel may accompany meconium ileus. Perforation in utero produces meconium peritonitis. Intraperitoneal meconium can cause dense adhesions leading postnatally to adhesive intestinal obstruction and may rapidly become calcified.

In 5% of patients with *Hirschsprung disease* the aganglionic segment involves not only the entire colon but also terminal ileum. This condition causes a dilated small intestine with ganglionated but somewhat hypertrophied walls, a funnel-shaped transitional hypoganglionic zone, and a collapsed distal aganglionic bowel.

CLINICAL MANIFESTATIONS. A history of hydramnios may be elicited with high jejunal atresias. In cystic fibrosis there may be a familial incidence. The obstructed patient may be born with abdominal distention from loops of meconium-filled bowel, or an obstruction may develop shortly after birth and progress as the result of swallowed air. Distention often results from meconium peritonitis due to intrauterine perforation and leakage of meconium into the peritoneal cavity. The site of perforation usually seals in utero so that operative intervention after birth is seldom necessary, but if the perforation is still patent, increasing abdominal distention with free intraperitoneal air develops after birth, and an operation may be required. Vomiting may occur early, with bile-stained vomitus. Infants with ileal or jejunal atresia may pass several surprisingly large meconium stools; with meconium ileus there is usually no stool. Pneumoperitoneum should be suspected if abdominal distention increases rapidly within the first 24 hr of life, if the liver is less dull to percussion, or if free fluid is evident within the abdomen.

DIAGNOSIS. In meconium ileus plain films of the abdomen show a typical hazy or "ground-glass" appearance in the right lower quadrant. Small bubbles of gas trapped in meconium are dispersed within this area. Furthermore, owing to their viscid contents, moderately dilated loops of bowel do not have the air-fluid levels usually seen roentgenographically on the erect projection. If there is meconium peritonitis, patchy calcification may be noted, usually in the flanks. Pneumoperitoneum is most readily seen as free air between the liver and the diaphragm on an upright roentgenogram of the abdomen; if there is a large amount of free air, the entire abdomen may look like a football from distention with air; the ligamentum teres is sometimes clearly visible in the midline.

It is impossible consistently to distinguish small bowel from large bowel by studying plain roentgenograms of the abdomen in newborn babies and infants. If plain roentgenograms are nonspecific, a barium or Gastrografin study of the colon may be needed to distinguish small from large intestine obstructions. A small colon, "microcolon," suggests disuse and the presence of obstruction proximal to the ileocecal valve. Gastrografin enemas should be used with caution in the diagnosis and treatment of meconium ileus, because their hyperosmolality may result in dehydration and undue injection pressure may result in perforation.

TREATMENT. Patients with small bowel obstruction should be stable and in adequate fluid and electrolyte balance before operation or roentgenographic attempts at disimpaction unless volvulus is suspected. Infections should be treated with appropriate antibiotics. Prophylactic use of antibiotics is indicated and should be given intravenously shortly before surgery.

Ileal or jejunal atresia requires resection of the dilated proximal portion of the bowel, followed by end-to-end anastomosis. If a simple mucosal diaphragm is present, jejunoplasty or ileoplasty with partial excision of the web is an acceptable alternative to resection. With meconium ileus an attempt to reduce obstruction with a Gastrografin enema containing polysorbate and a detergent (Tween 80) is usually indicated. The material should be allowed to flow around the pellets of stool in the terminal ileum and into the dilated proximal small bowel containing the obstructing meconium, where it will result in an outpouring of fluid from the bowel wall, dilution of the viscid meconium, and diarrhea. The enema may have to be repeated after 8–12 hr. Resection after reduction is not needed if there have been no ischemic complications.

About 50% of patients with meconium ileus do not adequately respond to Gastrografin enemas and will need a laparotomy. A simple small ileotomy is done within a purse-string suture just large enough to allow the insertion of a No. 10 or No. 12 French catheter. The catheter is used to irrigate and remove the viscid contents of the bowel, using acetylcysteine as a mucolytic agent in concentrations of less than 5%. Once the contents have been aspirated, the purse-string suture is tied and a small drain is placed near the ileostomy, making resections and anastomoses unnecessary.

At laparotomy for pneumoperitoneum colostomy or ileostomy may be needed at the site of perforation; if the perforation is of the stomach, duodenum, or upper jejunum, primary closure is preferred. Total parenteral nutrition will be required.

13.32 CONGENITAL MEGACOLON
(Hirschsprung Disease)

This is the most common cause of neonatal obstruction of the colon and accounts for about 33% of all neonatal obstructions. It is rare in premature infants. Occasionally there is a familial incidence. Males are affected more often than females (4:1), monozygotic twins are often concordant, and the incidence in future siblings is 3–4%. Overall the incidence is 1:5,000 live births. Hirschsprung disease is noted in 21-trisomy, Laurence-Moon-Biedl-Bardt syndrome, and Waardenburg syndrome, and with megacystis-megaureter, cryptorchidism, ventricular septal defect, and Meckel diverticulum. *Atresia* of the colon is rare.

ETIOLOGY. There may be failure of migration of cells of the embryonic neural crest into the bowel wall or failure of craniocaudal extension of the myenteric and submucous plexuses within the wall.

PATHOLOGY. This disease results from an absence of ganglion cells in the bowel wall, extending proximally from the anus for a variable distance. The aganglionic segment is limited to the rectosigmoid in 80% of patients; in 15% the colon is aganglionic from the anus to the hepatic flexure; and in 5% the entire colon lacks ganglion cells. Increased nerve endings, however, result in high concentrations of acetylcholinesterase.

Incomplete parasympathetic innervation in the aganglionic segment of bowel results in abnormal peristalsis, constipation, and a functional intestinal obstruction. Proximal to the transition zone between normally and abnormally innervated bowel, muscular hypertrophy thickens the intestinal wall, and the intestine may become enormously dilated with retained feces and gas.

CLINICAL MANIFESTATIONS. Early symptoms of megacolon range from complete acute neonatal obstruction to chronic constipation in the older child; sometimes there is diarrhea. There is often failure to thrive.

In newborn infants signs may be noted early, with failure to pass meconium, or may appear during the 1st wk and be those of partial or complete intestinal obstruction, with vomiting, abdominal distention, and failure to pass stools. Temporary relief of symptoms may occur after a rectal examination, which is characteristically followed by an explosive discharge of feces and gas. Bile-stained and even feculent vomiting may occur, and the infant may lose weight and become dehydrated. Diarrhea may be a prominent symptom in the neonatal period and be associated with symptoms of intestinal obstruction. Hypoproteinemia and edema may result from protein-losing enteropathy. Breast-fed babies with Hirschsprung disease tend not to manifest as severe clinical features as infants fed artificial formulae.

Episodes of constipation and diarrhea may alternate with periods of apparent normality. The diarrhea may develop into a fulminant *enterocolitis,* causing a profound dehydration and shock with fluid and electrolyte loss into the lumen of the obstructed bowel. This complication seems to be precipitated by gaseous and fecal colonic distention. *Clostridium difficile* has been implicated in the etiology. Unless energetically treated the condition tends to recur and may be fatal within 24 hr.

Hirschsprung disease in the older child causes chronic constipation and abdominal distention. The history often reveals increasing difficulty with the passage of stools, starting in the 1st few weeks of life. A large fecal mass is palpable in the left lower abdomen, but on rectal examination the rectum is usually empty of feces. The stools, when passed, may consist of small pellets, be ribbon-like, or have a fluid consistency; the large stools and fecal soiling of patients with functional constipation are absent. In mild cases the nutrition may not be greatly disturbed; in severe cases there is likely to be loss of subcutaneous tissue and failure to grow. The wasted extremities and large, protruding abdomen of such patients create a typical appearance, which may be confused with that of the *malabsorption syndromes* (Sec. 13.49), especially when diarrhea is present. Hypochromic anemia may be present. Intermittent attacks of intestinal obstruction from retained feces may be associated with pain and fever.

Rarely (in ultrashort-segment Hirschsprung disease) the aganglionosis is confined to the internal anal sphincter and immediately adjacent anal canal and rectum. Affected patients may have encopresis, and unless a particularly low biopsy is done, ganglion cells may be found and the patient presumed to be normal.

Hirschsprung disease must be distinguished from the more common acquired megacolon (Fig. 13–17) of colonic inertia, chronic idiopathic constipation, obstipation, and so on (Table 13–13). Small left colon syndrome in infants of diabetic mothers (Sec. 9.56), meconium plug syndrome, and ileal atresia with microcolon may mimic Hirschsprung disease in the neonatal period.

DIAGNOSIS. A rectal biopsy by the punch or suction method that finds ganglion cells absent in the submucosa and intermuscular nerve plexuses with or without increased numbers of nerve fibers is the only conclusive means of diagnosing megacolon. Because ganglion cells normally diminish in number in the more distal rectum and anal canal, biopsies should be taken no closer than 1 cm to the pectinate line. Nerve fibers in the bowel wall in Hirschsprung disease contain increased amounts of acetylcholinesterase; histochemical examination may facilitate interpretation of the biopsy.

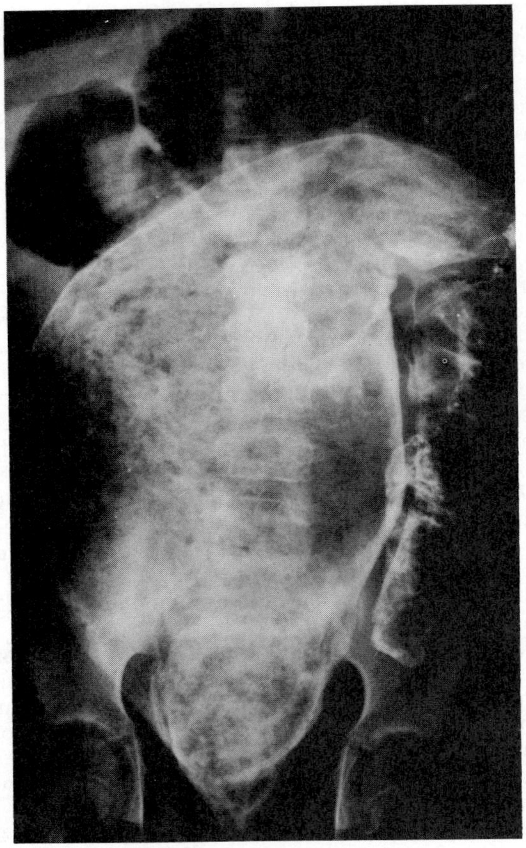

Figure 13–17. Barium enema in a 14-yr-old boy with severe constipation. The enormous dilatation of the rectum and distal colon is typical of acquired functional megacolon.

TABLE 13–13. Distinguishing Features of Hirschsprung Disease and Functional (Acquired) Constipation

	Functional (Acquired)	Hirschsprung Disease
History		
Onset constipation	After 2 yr of age	At birth
Encopresis	Common	Very rare
Forced bowel training	Usual	None
Stool size	Very large	Small, ribbon-like
Enterocolitis	None	Possible
Abdominal pain	Common	Common
Failure to thrive	Uncommon	Common
Examination		
Abdominal distention	Rare	Common
Poor growth	Rare	Common
Anal tone	Patulous	Tight
Rectal examination	Stool in ampulla	Ampulla empty
Malnutrition	Absent	Possible
Laboratory		
Barium enema	Massive amounts of stool, no transition zone	Transition zone, delayed evacuation (greater than 24 hr)
Rectal biopsy	Normal	No ganglion cells ↑ Acetylcholinesterase staining
Anorectal manometry	Distention of the rectum causes relaxation of the internal sphincter	No sphincter relaxation

Note that ultrashort-segment Hirschsprung disease may have clinical features of functional (acquired) megacolon (e.g., constipation).

Roentgenographic studies in the young infant with intestinal obstruction due to aganglionic megacolon show dilated loops of bowel throughout the abdomen on anteroposterior films taken in the erect position. In lateral erect films, rectal air, which is normally visible in the presacral area, is absent. The diagnostic findings on barium enema are (1) an abrupt change in caliber between the ganglionic and aganglionic sections of bowel (Fig. 13–18); (2) irregular "sawtooth" contractions of the aganglionic segment; (3) parallel transverse folds in the dilated proximal colon; (4) a thickened, nodular, edematous proximal colon associated with protein-losing enteropathy, if enterocolitis is present; and (5) failure to evacuate the barium. In infants a small amount of contrast material should be injected slowly through a small catheter, the tip of which is inserted barely beyond the anal sphincter while the patient, in an oblique position, is being observed under the fluoroscope; the characteristic abrupt transition in caliber may be missed if too much barium is used.

In the newborn infant with intestinal obstruction due to megacolon a barium enema will not always show the classic features as there may not have been time for the disparity in size to develop between the proximal colon and the distal aganglionic bowel. The roentgenographic appearances are even less typical when the entire colon lacks ganglion cells. There is blunting of the flexures, apparent foreshortening of the colon, and areas of spasm. Evacuation of the barium from the colon is usually delayed on a 24 hr roentgenogram in all types of Hirschsprung disease.

Anorectal manometry, measured by distention of a balloon placed within the rectal ampulla, shows a fall of pressure in the internal anal sphincter in normal individuals but a striking rise in pressure in patients with megacolon. The accuracy of this diagnostic test is more than 90% except in the neonate, in whom the test is less reliable. A normal response in the course of manometric evaluation excludes a diagnosis of congenital megacolon; an equivocal response requires a biopsy.

In the older child the diagnosis will usually be made by the history of constipation since birth and the finding of an empty rectum. Confirmation is obtained on results of the barium enema (see Fig. 13–18) and anal manometry. The roentgenographic appearance of megacolon may be misleading, however, either in terms of diagnosis or level of aganglionosis. In a suspected case, it is important not to cleanse the bowel prior to a barium enema so that the disparity in size between the ganglionic and aganglionic bowel is readily apparent.

TREATMENT. Once the diagnosis is unequivocally established in a neonate, operation is indicated. It is preferable to do a limited laparotomy with multiple biopsies, placing a colostomy in the most distal portion of normally ganglionated

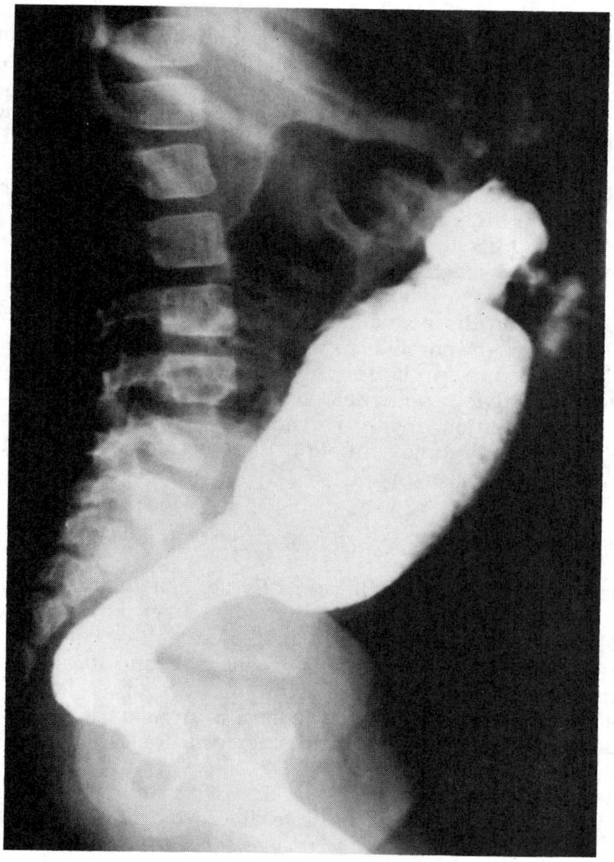

Figure 13–18. Lateral view of a barium enema in a 3-yr-old girl with Hirschsprung disease. The aganglionic distal segment is narrow with distended normal ganglionic bowel above it.

colon. Some surgeons perform a right transverse colostomy in the newborn without multiple biopsies, which is adequate for the usual case in which the aganglionic segment extends up to the rectosigmoid junction. If, however, the transition zone is at or proximal to the splenic flexure, then such a colostomy may need to be revised to bring the transverse colon down to the anus, thus avoiding excision of the intervening colon. Several excellent disposable infant stoma appliances are available to facilitate the management of the infant with a colostomy.

Attempts to postpone surgery by repeated colonic irrigations until the infant reaches a satisfactory size are not justified because of the risk of enterocolitis. With early colostomy the mortality from enterocolitis is 4%, compared with 33% if colostomy is done after the onset of enterocolitis.

When the infant is 6–12 mo of age a definitive pull-through operation is done using the Swenson (full-thickness extra-anal colorectal anastomosis), Duhamel (end-to-side colorectal anastomosis), or modified Soave (everted mucosa–full thickness colorectal anastomosis) procedure. Surgical management consists of excising the aganglionic segment, and pulling the ganglionic intestine down through the anus anastomosing it to the anal canal within 2.5 cm of the pectinate line.

In most older children a preliminary colostomy is also advisable, with its closure after the later Swenson or Duhamel types of operation.

Ultrashort-Segmental Hirschsprung Disease. If the aganglionic segment is so short as to give rise to a clinical and roentgenographic picture almost indistinguishable from acquired megacolon, major surgery is unnecessary. Excision of a strip of internal anal sphincter (internal anal myectomy) is all that is usually required if nonoperative management is unsuccessful.

Total Colon Aganglionosis. When the entire colon is aganglionic, often together with a length of terminal ileum, ileal-anal anastomosis is the treatment of choice, preserving part of the aganglionic colon to facilitate water absorption, which helps the stools to become firm. The operation of Duhamel is the best for total colon aganglionosis. The left colon is left in situ as a reservoir and it is not necessary to anastomose this left colon to the pulled through small bowel.

PROGNOSIS. Results of treatment of Hirschsprung disease are generally satisfactory, with a great majority of patients achieving fecal continence. Because most cases are diagnosed and treated in the neonatal period, immediate postoperative continence is impossible to assess. Postoperative problems include stricture, prolapse, cuff abscesses, and fecal soiling. Toilet training is usually delayed, and for several years intermittent incontinence with diarrhea may occur, but with time most children become continent. Loperamide is useful in the management of diarrhea.

13.33 DIVERTICULA AND DUPLICATIONS

These lesions consist of abnormal tissue, usually intestinal, in close relation to a part of the alimentary tract. In many there is ectopic gastric, pancreatic, duodenal, ileal, or colonic mucosa. These congenital anomalies may be due to abnormal formation of a part of an organ or duct or to failure of obliteration of one. If a diverticulum is anywhere but on the antimesenteric border, it is considered a dorsal enteric remnant.

With the exception of a Meckel diverticulum, congenital and acquired single and multiple diverticula of the intestinal tract are rare in children. *Diverticulosis* (multiple outpouchings of the intestinal tract, usually in the colon) and *diverticulitis* (inflammation of diverticula) are essentially diseases of adult life.

Meckel Diverticulum

Two to 3% of people have a Meckel diverticulum; the most common complication is bleeding. Other complications are rare.

In the embryo the intestine is linked to the yolk sac by the vitellointestinal duct. If this duct does not become completely atretic, it may persist in the form of a Meckel diverticulum. There may also be persistence of a fibrous cord from the Meckel diverticulum to the umbilicus, with cystic structures contained within the cord anywhere between the diverticulum and the peritoneal surface of the umbilicus. If the entire embryonic duct remains patent (persistent omphalomesenteric duct), there will be an enterocutaneous fistula; if the ileal end is closed, there is only mucoid secretion. A fibrous remnant of the vitelline artery may also persist as a band with the potential of causing intestinal obstruction.

PATHOLOGY. The Meckel diverticulum is usually 50–75 cm proximal to the ileocecal junction on the antimesenteric side of the intestine. The mucosal lining is the same as that of the adjacent ileum, but in at least 35% there is ectopic gastric or pancreatic tissue near the tip. This ectopic acid- or pepsin-secreting mucosa can cause an ulcer in the adjacent basal portion of the diverticulum or in the ileum to which it is attached. The erosion of the mucosa results in hemorrhage, which may be massive. Much less frequently, diverticulitis occurs, usually without demonstrable cause, though rarely a foreign body may be found. Diverticulitis may lead to perforation and peritonitis. Sometimes, the lesion is inverted and may become the apex of an ileoileal intussusception. A *Littre hernia* is seen when the Meckel diverticulum is contained within an indirect inguinal hernia. The diverticulum itself may undergo volvulus, or a band attached to it may cause a volvulus of loops of small intestine, leading to gangrene.

CLINICAL MANIFESTATIONS. Symptoms and signs from Meckel diverticulum can arise at any age but have peak incidence in the first 2 yr of life.

Painless rectal bleeding is the most common sign in children. There may be periodicity to the bleeding, as with peptic ulcer; it is usually acute, but rarely exsanguinating. Blood is often passed without stool; it is usually dark red, but if bleeding is brisk, it may be bright red. With mild recurrent bleeding iron deficiency anemia may develop that is refractory to iron therapy. Repeatedly positive results of tests for occult blood in the stools of an anemic child suggest Meckel diverticulum.

Abdominal pain, when it occurs, may be acute and due to diverticulitis, with a clinical picture resembling that of acute appendicitis, or it may be vague and recurrent. Referral of the (ileal) pain to the umbilicus may suggest the true diagnosis. Perforation of an ulcer in the diverticulum may lead to peritoneal bleeding or inflammation. A Meckel diverticulum may become the leading point of an intussusception. The signs may also be those of incarcerated hernia, volvulus, appendicitis, or intestinal obstruction. A child (other than a newborn infant) who has an intestinal obstruction without having had a previous operation, and who does not have an intussusception, most likely has a Meckel diverticulum or a fibrous remnant.

DIAGNOSIS. In infancy the Meckel diverticulum with ectopic gastric tissue often produces signs that require a rapid and accurate preoperative evaluation. The diverticulum cannot be demonstrated by barium studies, but an accurate preoperative diagnosis is possible, owing to the fact that ^{99m}technetium is excreted by gastric mucosa; a negative ^{99m}Tc scan has a high correlation with absence of a Meckel diverticulum. False-positive or false-negative results with a ^{99m}Tc scan are rare. The test is accurate and specific. A strongly positive (even bizarre) result usually denotes the presence of a tubular duplication within the alimentary tract. A patent vitellointestinal duct and its communication with a loop of bowel will be shown by injection of radiopaque material into the fistula. Patients with Meckel diverticulitis may have an incorrect preoperative diagnosis of acute appendicitis, but correct diagnosis and treatment can be carried out at surgery.

TREATMENT. Excision of the diverticulum is the treatment of choice. If there is a peptic ulcer in the adjacent ileum, it will be necessary to excise the involved bowel together with the diverticulum.

Non-Meckelian Diverticula

These may occur in the duodenum, jejunum, ileum, or colon and are usually incidental roentgenographic or necropsy findings. Rarely, they may result in a clinical problem by causing mechanical pressure, becoming inflamed or ulcerated, or perforating.

Duplications

DORSAL ENTERIC REMNANTS

Duplication may result from a failure of normal regression of embryonic diverticula, persistence of transitory intestinal diverticula, median septum formation, errors of recanalization of epithelial plugs, or traction between adhering neural tube ectoderm or notochordal mesoderm and intestinal endoderm. The latter theory would account for the frequent occurrence of a band that extends from the duplicated intestine through the diaphragm and posterior mediastinum, gaining an attachment to the thoracic or cervical spine; this is often associated with vertebral anomalies, such as hemivertebrae or anterior spina bifida.

PATHOLOGY. Duplications are saccular or tubular structures, which have a smooth muscle wall and mucous membrane similar to some parts of the gastrointestinal tract. They are found on the mesenteric side of any segment of intestine and vary widely in size and length. Tubular structures vary in length from a few centimeters to duplication of virtually the entire small bowel. Their blood supply is the same as that of the adjacent bowel, precluding selective excision of the duplication. If saccular, the duplication is not lined by gastric mucosa; nor does it communicate with the lumen of normal bowel; thus, peptic erosion of the intestine does not occur. The duplication may be so large that the intestine is stretched out over it and thereby obstructed. Less commonly, the duplication forms the apex of an intussusception or volvulus.

Tubular duplications have a gastric mucosal lining and are in communication with the adjacent bowel by one or more foramina. Acid secretion gains ready access to the unprotected normal small bowel and may cause a peptic ulcer, with bleeding or perforation.

CLINICAL MANIFESTATIONS. Symptoms and signs usually arise during infancy and early childhood and include (1) obstruction of adjoining intestine by compression; (2) intestinal bleeding from peptic ulceration; (3) pain from secretory distention of a noncommunicating duplication; (4) gangrene of the bowel from obstruction of segmental vasculature; and (5) a movable mass palpated on routine examination of the abdomen. Duplications are most frequent in the ileum, ileocecal region, and esophagus but may occur in any part of the gastrointestinal tract. Duplications of the lingual oropharynx area may resemble cystic hygromas, ectopic thyroid, or rhabdomyomas; those of the stomach may mimic pyloric stenosis; whereas those of the ileum or colon produce a mass or obstruction. Multiple duplications are noted in 10–15% of patients. Duplications in the thorax (neurenteric cysts) are usually of the esophagus or the stomach and only rarely communicate with either. They produce dysphagia and respiratory symptoms through esophageal and pulmonary compression and are demonstrable roentgenographically. Associated anomalies of vertebrae and spinal cord are common and are often at a higher level than the intrathoracic mass. Some intrathoracic duplications are lined by duodenal or jejunal mucosa.

Roentgenographic studies may show stenosis or compression of the intestinal lumen but more frequently are normal. An intrathoracic duplication is usually visible as a mediastinal mass in roentgenograms of the chest. Very rarely barium studies may fill a communicating duplication. As with Meckel diverticulum, and for the same reason, a ^{99m}Tc scan will demonstrate any ectopic gastric tissue. For intrathoracic lesions a computed tomography (CT) scan is useful. If spinal cord lesions, for example, syringomyelia, are suspected, magnetic resonance imaging should be undertaken.

CYSTIC REMNANTS OF THE TAIL GUT

These lesions are found between the anus and the sacrum or coccyx and may be derivatives of that portion of the primitive archenteron extending caudal to the cloaca. Others consider these lesions to be duplications of the rectum or even teratoma. Symptoms are produced by the presence of a mass, which, if large, may obstruct the rectum. Such lesions must be distinguished from sacrococcygeal teratoma, anterior myelomeningocele, and endodermal sinus tumor.

BILATERAL DUPLICATIONS OF COLON AND RECTUM

Several rare anomalies (''partial twinning'') consist of doubling of the alimentary tract from where a Meckel diverticulum would be found down to the anus. There may also be doubling of the vagina or penis and bladder, and even the sacrum and lumbar vertebrae may be doubled.

13.34 ACQUIRED INTESTINAL OBSTRUCTION

Paralytic ileus is a major cause of acquired intestinal obstruction. It may complicate acute infections, electrolyte imbalance, or uremia. Pneumonia and gastroenteritis are probably the most frequent causes in infants, peritonitis (especially as a complication of perforated appendicitis) most frequent in older children. Ileus is likely to present as distention, with absence of bowel sounds and minimal pain.

Incarcerated inguinal hernias, complications related to Meckel diverticulum, and intussusception are the most frequent *mechanical causes* of intestinal obstruction in infants. Intestinal obstruction may occur any time following surgery from postoperative adhesions or those following recovery from acute peritonitis, and from chronic peritonitis (e.g., tuberculous peritonitis). Other causes are duplications; foreign bodies in the intestine, including fecal concretions and inspissated meconium in the newborn infant; late obstruction by intraluminal contents in cystic fibrosis (pseudomeconium ileus); and masses of roundworms. Neonates, particularly premature infants, may rarely develop lactobezoars, also known as inspissated milk syndrome or milk bolus obstruction. A milk plug may occur in the pylorus but is more likely in the terminal ileum. An association with high medium-chain triglyceride diets and casein has been proposed.

Tumors of the bowel, including mesenteric cysts and polyps, may also be obstructive. Vomiting and abdominal distention may occur with either mechanical obstruction or ileus; severe colicky periumbilical pain and hyperactive, sometimes tinkling, bowel sounds are almost invariably found in the former.

In infants and children with intestinal obstruction, huge amounts of electrolyte-rich fluid are secreted into the lumen of the bowel. This may lead to severe fluid and electrolyte imbalances and to distention that compromises the circulation of a segment of intestine. With prolonged stasis this fluid becomes secondarily infected, often with putrefactive organisms, and the patient may have feculent vomiting (which should not be confused with true fecal vomiting, such as occurs with gastrocolic fistula or in coprophagy). A palpable distended single ("closed") loop and unexplained fever, leukocytosis, and anemia, together with abdominal tenderness, are ominous signs signifying strangulation. The development of gangrenous intestine may, however, be insidious.

13.35 INTUSSUSCEPTION

Intussusception occurs when a portion of the alimentary tract is telescoped into a segment just caudad to it. It is the most common cause of intestinal obstruction between 3 mo and 6 yr of age; it is rare under 3 mo and decreases in frequency after 36 mo. The incidence varies from 1–4/1,000 live births. The male to female ratio is 4:1. A few intussusceptions reduce spontaneously or become autoamputated; if left untreated, most would lead to death.

ETIOLOGY AND EPIDEMIOLOGY. The cause of most intussusceptions is unknown. The seasonal incidence has peaks in spring and autumn. Correlation with adenovirus infections has been noted, and the condition may complicate gastroenteritis. It is postulated that swollen Peyer patches in the ileum may stimulate intestinal peristalsis in an attempt to extrude the mass, thus causing an intussusception. At the peak age of incidence of this condition the infant's alimentary tract is also being introduced to a variety of new materials. In about 5–10% of patients recognizable causes for the intussusception are found, such as inverted Meckel diverticulum, an intestinal polyp, duplication, or lymphosarcoma. Uncommonly, the condition will complicate Henoch-Schönlein purpura, with an intramural hematoma acting as the apex of the intussusception. Rarely, intussusception is postoperative, and then always ileoileal. Unusual lesions include metastatic tumors, hemangioma, foreign bodies, parasitic infection, fecolith, and following cancer chemotherapy.

PATHOLOGY. Intussusceptions are most often ileocolic and ileoileocolic, less commonly cecocolic, and rarely exclusively ileal. Very rarely, the appendix forms the apex of an intussusception. The upper portion of bowel, the intussusceptum, invaginates into the lower, the intussuscipiens, dragging its mesentery along with it into the enveloping loop. Constriction of the mesentery obstructs venous return; engorgement of the intussusceptum follows, with edema, and bleeding from the mucosa leads to a bloody stool, sometimes containing mucus. The apex of the intussusception may extend into the transverse, descending, or sigmoid colon—even to and through the anus in neglected cases. This presentation must be distinguished from rectal prolapse. Most intussusceptions do not strangulate the bowel within the first 24 hr but may later eventuate in intestinal gangrene and shock.

CLINICAL MANIFESTATIONS. In typical cases there is sudden onset, in a previously well child, of severe paroxysmal colicky pain that recurs at frequent intervals and is accompanied by straining efforts and loud cries. Initially, the infant may be comfortable and play normally between the paroxysms of pain, but if the intussusception is not reduced, the infant becomes progressively weaker and lethargic. Eventually a shock-like state may develop, with an elevation of body temperature to as high as 41° C (106° F). The pulse becomes weak and thready, the respirations become shallow and grunting, and the pain may be manifested only by moaning sounds. Vomiting occurs in most cases and is usually more frequent early. In the later phase the vomitus becomes bile-stained. Stools of normal appearance may be evacuated during the 1st few hr of symptoms. After this time fecal excretions are small or more often do not occur, and little or no flatus is passed. Blood generally is passed in the first 12 hr, but at times not for 1–2 days and infrequently not at all; 60% of infants will pass a stool containing red blood and mucus, the *currant jelly stool.* Some patients have only irritability and alternating or progressive lethargy.

Palpation of the abdomen usually reveals a slightly tender, sausage-shaped mass, sometimes ill defined, which may increase in size and firmness during a paroxysm of pain and is most often in the right upper abdomen, with its long axis cephalocaudal. If it is felt in the epigastrium, the long axis is transverse. About 30% of patients do not have a palpable mass. It is more readily located by bimanual rectal and abdominal palpation between paroxysms of pain. The presence of bloody mucus on the finger as it is withdrawn after rectal examination supports the diagnosis of intussusception. Abdominal distention and tenderness develop as intestinal obstruction becomes more acute. On rare occasions the advancing intestine prolapses through the anus. This prolapse can be distinguished from prolapse of the rectum by the separation between the protruding intestine and the rectal wall, which does not exist in prolapse of the rectum.

Ileoileal intussusception may have a less typical clinical picture, the symptoms and signs being chiefly those of small intestinal obstruction. *Recurrent intussusception* is noted in 5–8% and is more common following hydrostatic than surgical reduction. *Chronic intussusception,* in which the symptoms exist in milder form at recurrent intervals, is more likely to occur with or following acute enteritis and may arise in older children as well as in infants.

DIAGNOSIS. The clinical history and physical findings are usually sufficiently typical for diagnosis. Plain abdominal roentgenograms may show a density in the area of the intussusception. A barium enema will show a filling defect or cupping in the head of barium where its advance is obstructed by the intussusceptum (Fig. 13–19). A central linear column

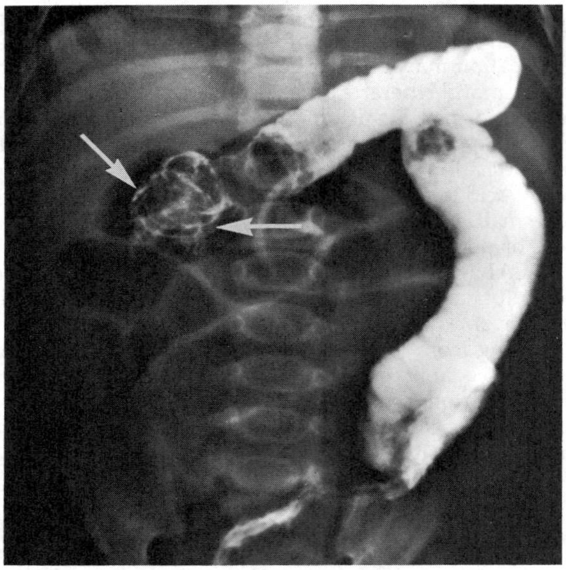

Figure 13–19. Intussusception in an infant. The obstruction is evident in the proximal transverse colon. Contrast material between the intussusceptum and the intussuscipiens is responsible for the coil-spring appearance.

of barium may be visible in the compressed lumen of the intussusceptum, and a thin rim of barium may be seen trapped around the invaginating intestine in the folds of mucosa within the intussuscipiens (coiled-spring sign), especially after evacuation. Retrogression of the intussusceptum under the pressure of the enema and gaseous distention of the small intestine from obstruction are also useful roentgenographic signs. Ileoileal intussusception is usually not demonstrable by barium enema but is suspected because of gaseous distention of the intestine above the lesion. Currently the use of an "air" enema in the diagnosis and treatment of intussusception is rapidly gaining in popularity in many centers. It is believed to be safer with less risk of perforation, at least as accurate as a barium enema, and entails less irradiation of the patient.

Real-time sonography may also provide useful diagnostic information: a target or donut configuration of bowel with hypoechoic rims and dense central echogenic core, no movement in the donut, and a rim thickness more than 0.6 cm. An exterior rim thickness more than 1.6 cm is associated with the need for surgical intervention.

DIFFERENTIAL DIAGNOSIS. It may be particularly difficult to diagnose intussusception in a child who already has *gastroenteritis;* a change in the pattern of illness, in the character of pain, or in the nature of vomiting, or the onset of rectal bleeding should alert the physician. The bloody stools and abdominal cramps that accompany *enterocolitis* can usually be differentiated from intussusception because the pain is less severe and less regular, there is diarrhea, and the infant is recognizably ill between pains. Bleeding from *Meckel diverticulum* is usually painless. The intestinal hemorrhage of *anaphylactoid purpura* is usually, but not invariably, accompanied by joint symptoms or purpura elsewhere, and the colicky pain may be similar. Since intussusception may be a complication of this disorder, a barium enema may be required.

TREATMENT. Reduction of the intussusception is an emergency procedure to be carried out immediately after diagnosis and after rapid preparation for operation with fluids and blood for shock and water and electrolytes to replace losses. In over 75% of cases of short duration, when there are no signs of prostration, shock, intestinal perforation, pneumatosis intestinalis, or peritoneal irritation, it is possible to reduce the intussusception by hydrostatic or pneumatic pressure under fluoroscopic guidance and with the consultation and close proximity of a surgeon.

A nonlubricated Foley bag catheter is placed in the rectum and inflated. The buttocks are compressed tightly and taped together with adhesive plaster. A barium solution is then allowed to flow by gravity into the colon from a height of not more than 90 cm (3 ft) above the fluoroscopic table. *The abdomen is not touched during the procedure.* The column of barium and the filling defect with it advance slowly together in a proximal direction. Full reduction of the intussusception is manifest by free filling of the small intestine, disappearance of the mass, passage of flatus or feces, and improvement in the infant's condition. If doubt remains as to the completeness of reduction, an exploratory laparotomy is done immediately.

An "air" enema requires the use of a special insufflating device. The same criteria for a successful reduction exist in terms of disappearance of the filling defect and free reflux (of air) into the ileum. Pressure of the insufflated gas (CO_2) should not exceed 80 mm Hg.

If there is clinical evidence of intestinal obstruction with abdominal distention, especially for 48 hr or longer, hydrostatic reduction of the intussusception should not be attempted because of the risk of perforating the intussuscipiens. In an ileoileal intussusception a barium enema is usually not diagnostic and reduction by the hydrostatic technique may not be possible. Such intussusceptions may develop insidiously as a complication of a laparotomy and require resection. A right-sided transverse paraumbilical or infraumbilical incision gives access to the ascending colon. If manual operative reduction is impossible or the bowel is not viable, resection of the intussusception will be necessary, with end-to-end anastomosis.

PROGNOSIS. Untreated intussusception in infants is almost always fatal; the chances of recovery are directly related to the duration of intussusception before reduction. Most infants recover if the intussusception is reduced within the first 24 hr, but the mortality rate rises rapidly after this time, especially after the 2nd day. Spontaneous reduction during preparation for operation is not uncommon.

The recurrence rate following barium enema reduction of intussusceptions is about 10%, following surgical reduction about 2–5%; none have recurred after surgical resection. It is unlikely that an intussusception caused by a lesion such as lymphosarcoma, polyp, or Meckel diverticulum will be successfully reduced by barium enema. With adequate surgical management, operative reduction carries a very low mortality rate in early cases.

Colonic Polyps

See Sec. 13.68.

HERNIAS

An *intra-abdominal* hernia occurs when loops of intestine are trapped by an anomalous fold of peritoneum created by malrotation or malfixation of the duodenum or colon to the posterior abdominal wall. Loops of intestine may also herniate through congenital defects of the mesentery, particularly near the terminal ileum. The symptoms and signs are those of intermittent or acute intestinal obstruction. Compression of the vasculature may produce gangrene of the intestine. Surgical reduction of the hernia and repair of the anomaly in order to prevent recurrence require knowledge of embryologic anatomy because of the danger of interference with intestinal blood supply. For extra-abdominal hernias, see Sec. 13.69.

13.36 FOREIGN BODIES IN THE STOMACH AND INTESTINES

If ingestion of a foreign body is suspected, plain roentgenograms of the abdomen and chest are indicated; if an object is visible above the diaphragm, esophagoscopy or bronchoscopy may be needed to retrieve it (Sec. 13.25). An object that reaches the stomach will, in most instances, pass through the gastrointestinal tract without causing injury. Certain types of foreign bodies, however, are potentially dangerous. Needles, hairpins, or bobby pins pass easily through the esophagus on their long axis, but may be unable to round the turns of the duodenum, where they become fixed and eventually perforate the intestine. Such potentially dangerous foreign bodies can usually be removed gastroscopically. If safety pins are small, they will probably pass without difficulty, whether open or closed. If they are large, either closed or open, peroral removal is safe and is indicated.

If the foreign body has passed through the pylorus into the intestine, its progress should be observed by means of infrequent roentgenograms. There is no need to have parents search the stools for the foreign body. If the object is benign (such as a coin), the second abdominal film need not be taken for a month, once it is known that there is nothing lodged in the esophagus. If serial roentgenograms show a foreign body to be moving progressively down the intestinal tract, perforation is not likely. If it remains stationary for several weeks or is long or sharp, it should be removed either endoscopically, under fluoroscopy by a magnetized nasogastric tube or at laparotomy, owing to the dangers of ulceration and perforation of the bowel. If at any time such signs of perforation as tenderness, rigidity, pain, nausea, or vomiting develop, surgery is indicated immediately. The diet should be normal, with no change from that to which the child has been accustomed. Bizarre roughage, wool, or cotton diets are valueless and may be dangerous. Laxatives are contraindicated because the accelerated activity of the intestine may increase the danger of perforation.

Bezoars

Occasionally, infants and children, particularly if emotionally disturbed or mentally retarded, acquire the habit of swallowing hair from their heads or from dolls or brushes, or they may swallow fur, wool, or cotton from wearing apparel or blankets. This material is usually passed through the intestines, but when the habit is persistent, there may be an accumulation in the stomach with formation of a *hairball* or *trichobezoar*. The symptoms are nonspecific but indigestion and gastric distress may be present. The tumor mass is often palpable and may give a soft crackling sensation on palpation. A bald spot or sparse hair may be apparent. A roentgenogram after administration of barium may disclose a mass outline by barium. A portion of the bezoar may be dislodged and subsequently become impacted in the intestine and cause obstruction. The diagnosis may be suspected from observation of the stool or of the child in the act of swallowing these materials. Surgical removal is indicated, and the child's mental and psychologic status should be evaluated.

Phytobezoars are accumulations of fibrous or mucilaginous materials as found in persimmons and various tar products. The accumulation is usually rapid compared with that of the hairball. Lactobezoars occur in the newborn (Sec. 13.34).

13.37 MOTILITY DISORDERS

Chronic Duodenal Ileus, Superior Mesenteric Artery Syndrome, Cast Syndrome

This syndrome of intermittent or chronic functional obstruction of the duodenum is thought by some to result from compression of the third part of the duodenum between the superior mesenteric artery and the aorta (although the left renal vein curiously escapes this vise). A more likely etiology is the loss of supporting fat to the 2nd and 3rd parts of the duodenum with normal or exaggerated lumbar lordosis effectively occluding the duodenum. Some cases occur as the result of incomplete rotation of the intestine.

Usually the patient is a tall, asthenic, visceroptotic adolescent female. A history of "bilious attacks" or other forms of episodic vomiting may be elicited. In many cases, the condition is encountered when the patient is in a body cast following major spinal surgery to correct scoliosis. A barium study typically shows megaduodenum and rapid, churning, to-and-fro peristaltic movements. Dilatation of the duodenum usually ends just to the right of the midline. The stomach may also be dilated. If malrotation is suspected, a barium enema should be done to locate the cecum.

If patients can be nourished and the duodenum rested, most will be relieved of their obstruction. The simplest form of treatment consists of a prone knee-elbow position after meals, which allows the duodenum to fall away from the retroperitoneal structures that may be causing obstruction. Nasojejunal intubation and jejunal feeding for a period of several seeks or total parenteral nutrition may allow periduodenal fat to accumulate, increasing the support of the duodenum and lessening the kinking at the duodenojejunal flexure. Metoclopramide and cisapride have been reported helpful in management. If there is no relief despite compliant and prolonged conservative management, operation may become necessary. A Ladd procedure is the operation of choice; duodenojejunostomy is less satisfactory.

CHRONIC IDIOPATHIC INTESTINAL PSEUDO-OBSTRUCTION

This rare condition of impaired intestinal propulsion produces persistent or recurrent episodes of nonmechanical gastrointestinal obstruction. Chronic idiopathic intestinal pseudo-obstruction (CIIP) is a heterogeneous group of disorders representing familial and nonfamilial forms of gastrointestinal neuromuscular diseases. The degenerative visceral myopathies may be familial, or more often sporadic, and demonstrate typical gastroduodenal manometric findings of absent or low-amplitude pressure phasic waves of the intestinal migrating motor complex (MMC). The familial myopathy has multiple inheritance patterns.

The visceral neuropathies have abnormal mesenteric plexus lesions (degenerative, inflammatory), are usually nonfamilial (some are autosomal dominant or recessive), and have typical intestinal manometry demonstrating MMC that are present but uncoordinated.

CIIP typically involves the small intestine and colon but may involve the stomach or esophagus (achalasia). The pathology demonstrates either (1) hyperganglionosis with hyperplasia of the Schwann cells and neurons, often associated with multiple endocrine neoplasia (MEN) syndrome with mucosal neuromas; or (2) hyperplasia of the Schwann cells without MEN. Additional cases demonstrate inflammatory and degenerative lesions.

The *clinical manifestations* include abdominal distention (>85%), emesis (60%), constipation (60%), failure to thrive (30%), diarrhea (25%), urinary tract infection (15%), and urinary tract (bladder-megacystis, ureter-megaureter, or renal pelvis) dilatation (30%), antenatal oligohydramnios (some have polyhydramnios due to gastrointestinal obstruction), and abnormal esophageal motility. The onset is often in the neonatal period; 50% of patients manifest signs before the age of 1 mo. The male-to-female ratio is equal, and overall 20% are familial. In the severe neonatal form there is fetal abdominal distention and, after birth, persistent distention, reduced or absent bowel sounds, emesis, and failure to pass meconium. Urinary stasis predisposes to urinary tract infection. Older patients demonstrate distention, emesis, and constipation.

The *differential diagnosis* includes Hirschsprung disease, other causes of mechanical obstruction, psychogenic constipation, neurogenic bladder, and superior mesenteric artery syndrome. Secondary causes of ileus or pseudo-obstruction, such as hypothyroidism, narcotics, scleroderma, Chagas disease, hypokalemia, diabetic neuropathy, amyloidosis, porphyria, angioneurotic edema, and radiation must be excluded. The diagnosis of CIIP is suggested by gastroduodenal manometry, demonstrating delayed gastric emptying by radionuclide scan, and, rarely, by exploratory laparotomy.

TREATMENT Therapy with prokinetic drugs (metoclopramide) is ineffective. A combination of home total parenteral alimentation and small enteric feedings may be effective for some patients. Others require continuous parenteral nutrition. Antibiotics are indicated for urinary tract infections and for suspected intestinal overgrowth syndrome. The *prognosis* is related to the severity of obstruction and complications of parenteral alimentation. The mortality may approach 30% during early childhood.

13.38 ANORECTAL MALFORMATIONS

Congenital anomalies of the anus and rectum are relatively common. Minor abnormalities occur in about 1:500 live births, major anomalies in 1:5,000 live births. Anomalies associated with those of the rectum include malformations of the urinary tract, esophagus, and, less commonly, the duodenum. The most useful clinical classification separates "low" and "high" lesions in accordance with whether the rectum does or does not pass through the puborectalis muscle, which is a major portion of the levator ani muscle of defecation.

EMBRYOLOGY AND PATHOGENESIS. The anus and rectum develop from the dorsal portion of the hindgut or cloacal cavity when lateral ingrowths of mesenchyme form the urorectal septum in the midline, separating the rectum and anal canal dorsally from the bladder and urethra ventrally. A small communication between the two systems, the cloacal duct, is closed by the 7th wk of gestation by a downgrowth of the urorectal septum. An ingrowth of mesoderm divides the cloacal membrane into the urogenital membrane ventrally and the anal membrane dorsally. During the 7th wk the urogenital portion of the original cloaca has acquired an external opening, but the anal membrane does not open until later. The anus develops by a fusion of the anal tubercles and an external invagination (the proctodeum), which deepens toward the rectum but is separated from it by the anal membrane. This membrane ruptures by the 8th wk of gestation.

Interference with the development of anorectal structures at varying stages gives rise to anomalies that range from anal stenosis and incomplete rupture of the anal membrane or anal agenesis (the "low" types) to complete failure of descent of the upper portion of the cloaca and failure of invagination of the proctodeum (the "high" types). Persistence of communication between the urinary and rectal portions of the cloaca results in fistulas, which are more common in the male. In the female, fistulas connect the rectum with the vagina more commonly than with the urinary system.

Since the muscle of the external anal sphincter is derived from exterior mesoderm, it is usually intact in infants with obstructive lesions of the anus and rectum.

PATHOLOGY (Fig. 13–20). Supralevator "high" anomalies occur almost exclusively in males, and there is usually a rectourethral fistula between the rectum, which ends blindly, and the prostatic urethra. The bowel ends proximal to the puborectalis muscle, with absence of the internal anal sphincter; the puborectalis muscle is relatively ineffectual in sustaining rectal continence. Associated absence of all or part of the sacrum indicates likely faulty innervation of anal and urethral musculature, with likely incontinence. When these supralevator anomalies occur in girls, there is usually a fistulous communication between the rectum and the posterior vaginal fornix. **Rectal atresia** occurs when the proctodeum (anal canal) develops normally but fails to communicate with the rectum; the rectum may be separated by a substantial gap, or there may be only a mucosal diaphragm. There is no fistula. In **rectocloacal** anomalies the urethra opens anteriorly into a common cloacal (vaginal) channel and the rectum communicates posteriorly with the same channel. There is thus a single (cloacal) orifice on the perineum with neither rectum nor urethra visible. There is often a double vagina. **Cloacal exstrophy** is a complex mixture of exstrophy of the bladder, imperforate anus, maldevelopment or absence of the colon, and grossly malformed external genitalia. There may be an associated small omphalocele.

In translevator "low" anomalies the hindgut has traversed the levator ani muscle and the internal and external anal sphincters are well developed, with normal function. In males skin or membrane covers the anus, with an anteriorly placed fistulous opening onto the skin in the midline anterior to where the anus would be. This opening may be on the perineum, scrotum, or even the under surface of the penis. In females the anus is ectopic; it may be perineal, vestibular, or even (low) vaginal in location. An intermediate translevator anomaly with rectourethral fistula may also occur.

Associated anomalies are common. Significant urinary tract and vertebral abnormalities occur in about 50% of patients with high anorectal malformation and 25% of those with low types. Sacral anomalies may be important in the prediction of later bowel or urinary functions.

DIAGNOSIS. The evaluation of the newborn infant with an anorectal malformation should be directed first toward establishing whether a low or high lesion is present, because the initial treatment, definitive treatment, and prognosis differ for these two lesions.

Low Lesions. *Stenosis of the anorectal canal* may occur at any point or extend its entire length. The constriction can be identified by digital and endoscopic examination. An *imperforate anal membrane* is readily identified as a thin translucent membrane that becomes progressively distended by the meconium just behind it.

More than 90% of the other low anomalies are associated with an external fistula of the perineum or vestibule. Fistulas may not be apparent at birth, but peristalsis gradually forces meconium through them. Repeated meticulous examinations during the first 24 hr of life will, in most cases, eventually detect a tiny speck of meconium at the opening of the fistula. Roentgenograms employing contrast media injected through a tiny catheter inserted into the fistula will confirm the diagnosis. In males, if meconium is seen at or anterior to the anus, indeed anywhere along the perineum, a low anomaly is present. Folds of skin ("bucket-handles") may accompany high or low atresias. *Perineal pearls,* cystic accumulations of inspissated green or white mucus anywhere in the midline anterior to the anus and even extending into the scrotum, always connote a covered anus. In females it is usually possible to insert a feeding tube into the ectopic anus to establish its presence and the direction of the anal canal and rectum. The presence of a dimple at the site of the anus does not indicate a low lesion.

High Lesions. A poorly developed anal dimple, a rounded perineum, or vertebral anomalies suggest a high lesion. Passage of meconium or flatus in the urine is diagnostic of a rectourinary fistula and of a rectal pouch that ends above the puborectalis muscle. In most cases a lateral roentgenogram in the upside-down position (Fig. 13–21) should be obtained when clinical distention becomes evident or after 18–24 hr of life. The infant should be held upside down for several minutes before the film is exposed, to allow the gas in the bowel to displace the meconium and proceed as far distally as possible. The level of the levator ani muscle may be represented by a line joining the symphysis pubis with the last segment of the sacrum; if the gas bubble is proximal to this line, the anomaly is a high one. Other methods of estimation involve the comparison of the level of the gas bubble with a comma-shaped ischium. A retrograde urethrocystogram usually demonstrates the rectourethral fistula.

If none of the aforementioned measures clearly identifies the level of the rectal pouch, it is safest to presume a high lesion. Blind exploration of the perineum in hopes of finding a low-lying rectal pouch should not be done.

Ultrasound should be done in all cases. A retrograde urethrogram should be done at the time of the definitive treatment or preceding the establishment of a colostomy. It will probably delineate the rectourethral fistula. A CT scan of the pelvis is useful in defining the extent of the pelvic anorectal musculature.

TREATMENT. Anal stenosis can generally be treated by

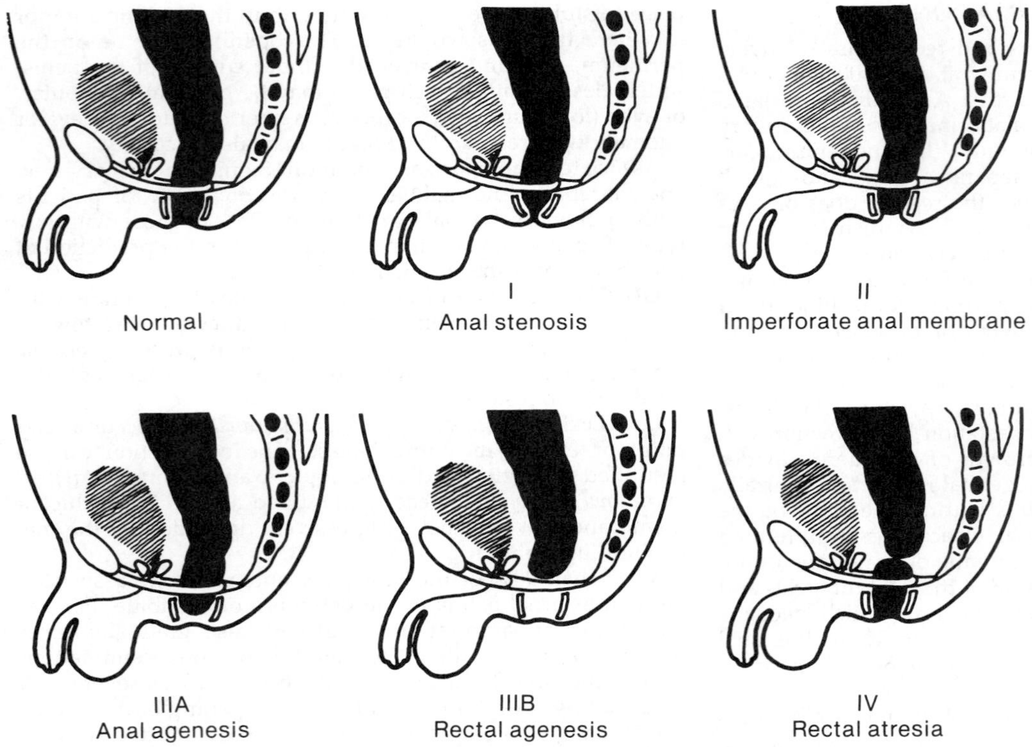

Figure 13–20. A simplified illustration of the various forms of anorectal anomalies. Types IIIA and IIIB are the most common varieties. None of the complexities of the detailed classifications are depicted, and the various fistulas are not illustrated. (From Kiesewetter WB: Anus and rectum malformation. *In:* Ravitch MM, et al: Pediatric Surgery, 3rd ed. Chicago, Year Book Medical Publishers, 1979.)

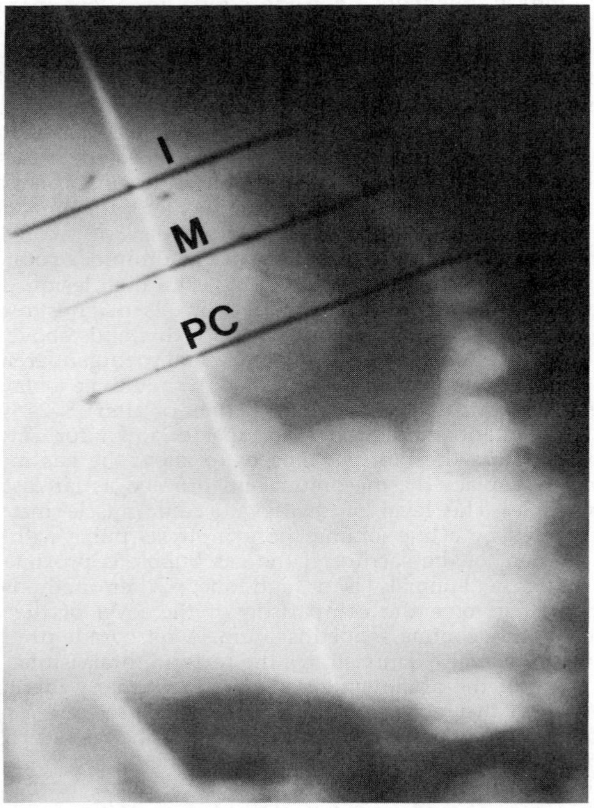

Figure 13–21. Inverted anorectogram used to determine the level of anorectal atresia. The lines represent: PC = pubococcygeus; I = most distal point of the ischium with a line drawn parallel to the PC line; M = the median or muscle line assumed to be at the level of the puborectalis sling. (From Filston HC: *In:* Sabiston DC: Textbook of Surgery, 14th ed. Philadelphia, WB Saunders, 1986.)

digital or instrumental dilatations. All other forms of imperforate anus require surgical correction.

In the low types in females, since the bowel has the proper levator relationship, repair can be managed from below. These patients will be continent unless ill-advised operations are performed. There is no evidence that an anus placed 1 cm or so anterior to its normal position results in either urinary or genital infections or in major problems with parturition. Rarely, the anus will have to be transplanted dorsally when there is a low rectovaginal fistula. The "covered anus" in males and infrequently the vestibular ectopic anus in females will need the coverings of the anus incised in a dorsal direction and the mucosa sutured to the margins of the newly created anus. Postoperative regular dilatations for 1–2 mo may be necessary.

The high types are best treated by a preliminary transverse colostomy, with definitive repair in 6–12 mo. Careful positioning of the anus in relation to the external sphincter and of the bowel in the muscle complex is essential. Fistulas are also eliminated.

Surgical treatment of imperforate anus has been advanced by the development of the Pena procedure (posterior sagittal anorectoplasty). Using an electrical muscle-stimulating device, the entire pelvic musculature is reconstructed around a tapered neorectum after closure of the rectourethral fistula. The complex cloacal abnormalities encountered with high malformations in females also respond to this procedure.

The higher the blind pouch the more extensive the operation. Significant sacral anomalies are usually associated with deficient neurologic control of defecation. In almost all cases of high imperforate anus there will be continuing problems due to stenosis, poor anal control, and lack of sensation. Both normal sphincter muscles and intact sensation are necessary in order to achieve fecal continence. Consequently, most children who have a high imperforate anus require ongoing management of their fecal incontinence. For this, the enema continence catheter is used to administer a large-volume saline enema (20 mL/kg) on alternate days, thus rendering the patient socially continent. In the postoperative period constipation rather than incontinence may be a problem. The lack of sensation of fecal material in the rectum leads to fecal impactions with paradoxic or overflow diarrheal stools and gives rise to the acquired type of megacolon. Early attention to ensure regular evacuations will prevent massive fecal impactions. As a rule, the child should be taught to defecate at a given time of day rather than await the urge. In some instances a daily enema may be needed.

PROGNOSIS. All patients with low types of anorectal malformation should be continent. Patients with high anomalies, on the other hand, may rarely be left with what is, in effect, a perineal colostomy. This form of incontinence, however, is more tolerable than abdominal colostomy in children and adolescents.

BARRY SHANDLING

PYLORIC STENOSIS

Anonymous: Is ultrasound really necessary for the diagnosis of hypertrophic pyloric stenosis? Lancet i:1146, 1988.
Beynon J, Brown R, James C, et al: Pyloromyotomy: can the morbidity be improved? J R Coll Surg Edinb 32:291, 1987.
Breaux CW Jr, Georgeson KE, Royal SA, et al: Changing patterns in the diagnosis of hypertrophic pyloric stenosis. Pediatrics 81:213, 1988.
Rollins MD, Shields MD, Quinn RJM, et al: Pyloric stenosis: Congenital or acquired? Arch Dis Child 64:138, 1989.
Tack ED, Perlman JM, Bower RJ, et al: Pyloric stenosis in the sick premature infant: Clinical and radiological findings. Am J Dis Child 142:68, 1988.
Touloukian RJ, Higgins E: The spectrum of serum electrolytes in hypertrophic pyloric stenosis. J Pediatr Surg 18:394, 1983.
Tunnell WP, Wilson DA: Pyloric stenosis: Diagnosis by real-time sonography, the pyloric muscle length period. J Pediatr Surg 19:795, 1984.

INTESTINAL ATRESIAS

Ahlgren L: Apple peel jejunal atresia. J Pediatr Surg 22:451, 1987.
Atwell JD, Klidian AM: Vertebral anomalies and duodenal atresia. J Pediatr Surg 17:237, 1982.
Doolin EJ: Motility abnormality in intestinal atresia. J Pediatr Surg 22:320, 1987.
Reyes H, Meller J, Loeff D: Neonatal intestinal obstruction. Clin Perinatol 16:85, 1989.
Smith GHH, Glasson M: Intestinal atresia: Factors affecting survival. Aust NZ J Surg 59:151, 1989.

MALROTATION

Dott NM: Anomalies of intestinal rotation: Their embryology and surgical aspects, with a report of 5 cases. Br J Surg 11:251, 1923.
Filston H, Kirks DR: Malrotation—the ubiquitous anomaly. J Pediatr Surg 16:614, 1981.
Ladd WE: Congenital obstruction of the duodenum in children. N Engl J Med 206:277, 1932.
Louw JH, Sender B, Shandling B: A rational approach to the surgical treatment of duodenal ileus. Afr J Lab Clin Med 3:249, 1957.
Stewart DR, Colodny AL, Daggett WC: Malrotation of the bowel in infants and children: A 15 year review. Surgery 79:716, 1976.

MECONIUM ILEUS

Harberg FJ, Senekjian EK, Pokorny WJ: Treatment of uncomplicated meconium ileus via T-tube ileostomy. J Pediatr Surg 16:61, 1981.
Holsclas DS, Eckstein HB, Nixon HH: Meconium ileus: A 20-year review of 109 cases. Am J Dis Child 190:101, 1965.
Miller A, Rode H, Cywes S: Management of uncomplicated meconium ileus with T-tube ileostomy. Arch Dis Child 63:390, 1988.
Rescoria FJ, Grosfeld JL, West KJ, et al: Changing patterns of treatment and survival in neonates with meconium ileus. Arch Surg 124:837, 1989.
Venugopal S, Shandling B: Meconium ileus: Laparotomy without resection, anastomosis or enterostomy. J Pediatr Surg 14:715, 1979.
Wagget J, Bishop HC, Koop CE: Experience with Gastrografin enema in the treatment of meconium ileus. J Pediatr Surg 5:649, 1970.

HIRSCHSPRUNG DISEASE

Chow CW, Campbell PE: Short-segment Hirschsprung's disease as a cause of discrepancy between histological, histochemical and clinical features. J Pediatr Surg 18:167, 1983.
Duhamel B: Retrorectal and transanal pull-through procedure for the treatment of Hirschsprung's disease. Dis Colon Rectum 7:455, 1964.
Ikeda K, Goto S: Diagnosis and treatment of Hirschsprung's disease in Japan. Ann Surg 199:400, 1984.
Joseph V, Sim C: Problems and pitfalls in the management of Hirschsprung's disease. J Pediatr Surg 23:398, 1988.
Loening-Baucke VA: Anorectal manometry: Experience with strain gauge pressure transducers for the diagnosis of Hirschsprung's disease. J Pediatr Surg 18:595, 1983.
Schofield D, Devine W, Yunis E: Acetylcholinesterase-stained suction rectal biopsies in the diagnosis of Hirschsprung's disease. J Pediatr Gastro Nutr 11:221, 1990.
Shandling B, Auldist AW: Punch biopsy of the rectum for the diagnosis of Hirschsprung's disease. J Pediatr Surg 3:386, 1968.
Sharman JO, Snyder ME, Weitzman JJ, et al: A 40-year multinational retrospective study of 880 Swenson procedures. J Pediatr Surg 24:833, 1989.
Soave F: Hirschsprung's disease: A new surgical technique. Arch Dis Child 39:116, 1964.

MECKEL DIVERTICULUM AND INTUSSUSCEPTION

Bruce J, Huh YS, Cooney DR, et al: Intussusception: Evolution of current management. J Pediatr Gastroenterol Nutr 6:663, 1987.
Campbell JB: Contrast media in intussusception. Pediatr Radiol 19:293, 1989.
Hocking M, Young DG: Duplications of the alimentary tract. Br J Surg 68:92, 1981.
Holcomb GW III, Gheissari A, O'Neill JA Jr, et al: Surgical management of alimentary tract duplications. Ann Surg 209:167, 1989.
Lee H-C, Yeh Y-J: Intussusception: The sonographic diagnosis and its clinical value. J Pediatr Gastroenterol Nutr 8:343, 1989.
Liu KW, MacCarthy J, Guiney EJ, et al: Intussusception—current trends in management. Arch Dis Child 61:75, 1986.
Mackey WC, Dineen P: A fifty year experience with Meckel's diverticulum. Surg Gynecol Obstet 156:56, 1983.
Reijnen JAM, Festen C, van Roosmalen RP: Intussusception: Factors related to treatment. Arch Dis Child 65:871, 1990.
Tamanaha K, Wimbish YB, Talwalker et al: Air reduction of intussusception in infants and children. J Pediatr 111:733, 1987.
Treves S, Grand RJ, Eraklis AJ: Pentagastrin stimulation of technetium-99m uptake by ectopic gastric mucosa in a Meckel's diverticulum. Radiology 128:711, 1978.
Vane DW, West KW, Grosfeld JL: Vitelline duct anomalies: Experience with 217 childhood cases. Arch Surg 122:542, 1987.

POLYPS

Burt RW, et al: The adenomatous polyp and the hereditary polyposis syndromes. Gastroenterol Clin North Am 17:657, 1988.
Euler AE, Seibert JJ: The role of sigmoidoscopy, radiographs, and colonoscopy in the diagnostic evaluation of pediatric age patients with suspected juvenile polyps. J Pediatr Surg 16:500, 1981.
Jagelman DG: Familial polyposis coli. Surg Clin North Am 63:117, 1983.
Louw JH: Polypoid lesions of the large bowel in children. S Afr Med J 46:1347, 1972.
Mallam AS, Thomson SA: Polyps of the rectum and colon in children. Can J Surg 3:17, 1959.
Shermeta DW, Morgan WW, Eggleston J, et al: Juvenile retention polyps. J Pediatr Surg 4:211, 1969.

MOTILITY DISORDERS

Fadda B, Maier WA, Meier-Ruge W, et al: Neuronal intestinal dysplasia—a critical 10-year analysis of clinic and bioptic results. Z Kinderchir 38:308, 1983.
Glassman M, Spivak W, Mininberg D, et al: Chronic idiopathic intestinal pseudoobstruction: A commonly misdiagnosed disease in infants and children. Pediatrics 83:603, 1989.
Nguyen L, Shandling B: Segmental dilation of the colon: A rare cause of chronic constipation. J Pediatr Surg 19:539, 1984.
Puri P, Lake BD, Gorman F, et al: Megacystic-microcolon-intestinal hypoperistalsis syndrome: A visceral myopathy. J Pediatr Surg 18:64, 1983.
Schuffler MD: Chronic intestinal pseudo-obstruction: Progress and problems. J Pediatr Gastroenterol Ntr 10:157, 1990.
Shawis RN, Rangecroft L, Cook RCM, et al: Functional intestinal obstruction associated with malrotation and short small bowel. J Pediatr Surg 19:172, 1984.
Vargas JH, Sachs P, Ament ME: Chronic intestinal pseudo-obstruction syndrome in pediatrics: Results of a national survey by members of the North American Society of Pediatric Gastroenterology and Nutrition. J Pediatr Gastroenterol Nutr 7:323, 1988.
Young LW, Yunis EJ, Girdany BR, et al: Megacystic-microcolon-intestinal hypoperistalsis syndrome: Additional clinical, radiologic, surgical and histopathologic aspects. Am J Roentgenol 137:749, 1981.

IMPERFORATE ANUS

de Vries PA, Pena A: Posterior sagittal anorectoplasty. J Pediatr Surg 17:638, 1982.

Hendren WH: Urological aspects of cloacal malformation. J Urol 140:1207, 1988.
Kiesewetter WB, Nixon HH: Imperforate anus: Its surgical anatomy. J Pediatr Surg 2:60, 1967.
Lobe TE: Fecal continence following an anterior sagittal ano-enteroplasty in a patient with cloacal exstrophy. J Pediatr Surg 19:843, 1984.
Pena A: Posterior sagittal anorectoplasty: Results in the management of 332 cases of anorectal malformation. Pediatr Surg Internat 3:94, 1988.
Pena A: Surgical management of anorectal malformations. Pediatr Surg Internat 3:82, 1988.
Pena A, de Vries PA: Posterior sagittal anorectoplasty: Important technical considerations and new applications. J Pediatr Surg 17:796, 1982.

NONINFECTIVE INFLAMMATORY GASTROINTESTINAL DISEASE

13.39 ULCER DISEASE

Ulcer disease is less common in children than in adults. Older estimates of incidences of 3.5–13.7/100,000 prior to the availability of endoscopy are certainly low, but the true incidence is much lower than the 3% noted after 45 yr of age. It is convenient to discuss peptic (primary) ulcer disease and stress (secondary) ulcers separately, although their treatment, methods of diagnosis, and biologic factors are similar.

Peptic Ulcers

Peptic ulcers occur mainly in the duodenum, less commonly in the stomach. In the 1st or 2nd yr of life, gastric and duodenal ulcers occur with similar frequency. After 6 yr, duodenal ulcers predominate and increase in adolescence.

PATHOLOGY AND PATHOPHYSIOLOGY. The etiology of peptic ulcer disease is uncertain, but a number of factors are important. A family history of ulcers can be found in 25–50% of patients with duodenal ulcers, and concordance for duodenal ulcer is 50% for monozygotic twins. Blood type O and high levels of pepsinogen I are associated with ulcer disease. Environmental factors, such as climatic conditions, dietary habits, and emotional strain, also appear to be important.

The presence of gastric acidity is very important in the development of ulcer disease. Both adults and children with duodenal ulcer disease have increased acid secretion, but there is a large overlap with the normal range, and studies do not correlate acid secretion with ulcer size or duration of symptoms. In gastric ulcer disease acid output is often normal or low. Tissue resistance is an important variable in preventing ulcer formation; factors that lower resistance include anoxia, poor perfusion, and drugs. Nonsteroidal anti-inflammatory drugs, such as salicylates, alcohol, and bile salts stimulate pepsinogen secretion, interfere with integrity of the mucosa, and favor ulcer formation, whereas prostaglandins protect mucosal integrity. The rate of cell turnover and the type and the amount of mucus secretion are also thought to be important. *Helicobacter pylori* is frequently present in gastric biopsies, but the exact relation of this bacteria to ulcer disease is unclear (see Sec. 12.42). *H. pylori* is noted in primary ulcer disease and not that due to secondary causes (e.g., salicylates). In general, factors related to acid are most important in duodenal ulcers, whereas tissue resistance appears to be of greater importance in gastric ulcers. Primary peptic ulcers are usually chronic and duodenal, whereas secondary ulcers are acute and gastric.

Histologically, the ulcer may be very superficial, may erode deeply into the mucosa and submucosa, may penetrate a blood vessel and cause hemorrhage, or may cause perforation. It is usually surrounded by an infiltration of acute and chronic inflammatory cells. A very shallow ulcer is considered an abrasion. If inflammation and edema are extensive, acute or chronic gastric outlet obstruction may occur. Occasionally, a red, granular duodenal mucosa is seen on endoscopy; it is often diagnosed as duodenitis and is treated as a developing ulcer. The relation of this lesion to symptoms or to eventual ulcer formation is unknown. Most duodenal ulcers occur in the posterior part of the bulb, and most gastric ulcers occur on the lesser curve or the antral area. Malignant gastric ulcers in children are exceedingly rare.

CLINICAL MANIFESTATIONS. The manifestations of peptic ulcer disease are variable and often nonspecific but include vomiting, gastrointestinal blood loss, pain, and a strong familial incidence. Of adults with symptoms of dyspepsia thought to be compatible with ulcer disease, only about 15% will have ulcers on investigation. In children, the frequency of abdominal pain and the infrequent finding of ulcer disease suggest a similar situation.

Although the symptoms of ulcer disease vary and are easily confused with symptoms caused by other abdominal diseases or functional problems, certain presentations are particularly common at certain ages. In the 1st mo of life, the two main presentations are gastrointestinal hemorrhage and perforation. Most such ulcers will be stress ulcers (see later); and other disorders such as sepsis, heart disease, or respiratory distress will usually be present. It is likely that many ulcers with less dramatic symptoms are not diagnosed. Between the neonatal period and 2 yr of age, recurrent vomiting, slow growth, and gastrointestinal hemorrhage are the three major symptoms. In the preschool period, pain that is typically periumbilical and worse after eating is often elicited. Recurrent vomiting and intestinal hemorrhage are also common.

After 6 yr of age the clinical features of ulcer disease are similar to those in adults and commonly include epigastric abdominal pain, acute or chronic gastrointestinal blood loss (hematemesis, hematochezia, or melena) leading to iron deficiency anemia, a preponderance of males, and a strong family history of ulcer disease. The pain is often described as dull or aching in character, rather than sharp or burning as in adults. It may last from minutes to hours, and there are frequent exacerbations and remissions lasting from weeks to months. Nocturnal pain is common. A history of typical ulcer pain with prompt relief following antacids is found in less than one third of affected patients. In patients with acute or chronic blood loss and penetration of the ulcer into the abdominal cavity or adjacent organs, symptoms of shock, anemia, peritonitis, or pancreatitis may occur.

DIAGNOSIS. An upper gastrointestinal roentgenographic examination is the most useful regularly available test if symptoms are not acute. In approximately 25% of children with duodenal ulcers, the lesion will not be detected on the first examination, and even with double contrast examination, fewer than 40% of gastric lesions will be demonstrated. The duodenal bulb is often difficult to examine in infants because of its high posterior position. The ulcer crater should be demonstrated in multiple spot films, preferably in a distended bulb so as not to be confused with barium caught in normal mucosal folds. True deformity of the bulb is a good sign of past ulcer disease but does not ensure that current symptoms are due to ulcer disease or that an ulcer is present. Spasm of the bulb that relaxes and allows filling of the bulb is common in normal patients, and radiographic interpretations such as "duodenitis," "irritability of the bulb," and "pylorospasm" should not be interpreted as ulcer disease.

Gastroduodenoscopy is indicated when roentgenographic findings are questionable or absent in symptomatic patients, when symptoms persist despite radiographic evidence of healing, or with prolonged presence of an ulcer crater. In patients with acute upper gastrointestinal hemorrhage, if gastric lavage can clear the stomach of obscuring blood and clots, endoscopy is the diagnostic procedure of choice. Direct visualization of the upper intestine has dramatically increased the precision of diagnosis of the ulcer, and use of various forms of cautery via endoscopy can control bleeding or decrease the chance of a repeat bleed. In patients with active, severe upper intestinal bleeding that precludes endoscopy, selective abdominal angiography may be indicated early in the diagnostic evaluation. Leakage of dye into the lumen from a bleeding ulcer can demonstrate the ulcer, and bleeding may be controlled by infusion of vasoconstricting agents (vasopressin 0.3–0.4 unit/1.73 m^2/min) into vessels just proximal to the bleeding site or by therapeutic embolization of the bleeding vessels. Routine gastric acid analysis is not generally useful, because the values found in normal and abnormal patients overlap widely. In patients who have recurrent severe ulcers or multiple ulcers, serum gastrin levels should be measured to detect those who have Zollinger-Ellison syndrome.

The differential diagnosis includes esophagitis, gastroesophageal reflux, Meckel diverticulum, pancreatitis, inflammatory bowel disease, cholelithiasis, appendicitis, and nonspecific abdominal pain. Functional nonspecific pain is common among school-aged children, is usually periumbilical, and is not associated with weight loss, emesis, blood loss, diarrhea, meals or night pain, but may be associated with stress related to the school or family.

TREATMENT. The goal of therapy is to hasten healing of the ulcer, relieve pain, and prevent complications. Approximately 25% of children under the age of 6 yr will have recurrence of a primary ulcer, whereas 70% of older children will have recurrences as they enter adult life. Drugs such as aspirin or alcohol that predispose to ulcer formation and hemorrhage should be avoided. Tobacco smoking is associated with delayed healing. The patient should eat a normal diet, avoiding only those foods that cause discomfort. Use of a bland diet or avoidance of cola drinks, coffee, or spiced foods has not been shown to decrease acid secretion or hasten healing.

Suppression of gastric acidity is the most important factor in the treatment of ulcer disease, and antacids are the mainstay of medical management. Large doses hasten healing of duodenal ulcers in adults. The buffering ability of antacids varies greatly, and liquid forms are more efficient than tablets, which must be chewed thoroughly for maximal efficiency. A quantity of antacid capable of buffering 100 mEq of stomach acidity/m^2 should be administered 1 and 3 hr after meals and at bedtime. This usually amounts to 15 mL/m^2 of the more concentrated liquid antacids. A bedtime snack should not be substituted, because food will stimulate acid secretion during the night. Intensive therapy with antacids should continue for 4–6 wk.

Most antacids are mixtures of magnesium hydroxide, magnesium trisilicate, and aluminum hydroxide. The magnesium compounds are effective but cause diarrhea. If diarrhea becomes a problem, intermittent use of antacids containing mainly aluminum hydroxide is warranted. Aluminum hydroxide binds with dietary phosphates and interferes with absorption. If large doses of aluminum hydroxide without phosphate are used over a prolonged period, it is possible to develop complications of phosphate depletion, including anorexia, osteomalacia, and osteoporosis. Calcium antacids can cause increased acid secretion after their buffering effect has stopped. Sodium bicarbonate is a very effective acid buffer but is not suitable for chronic use because of the large systemic alkaline and sodium load.

The H_2-blockers offer a convenient alternative even though they are not officially approved for use in children. Cimetidine 20–40 mg/kg/24 hr administered four times a day is most frequently used. Ranitidine, another H_2-blocker is also available in liquid form (4–6 mg/kg/24 hr) for twice daily dosage. Pediatric dose is not established, and it should be reserved for children over 12 yr of age. Sucralfate heals ulcers by a local coating action. The need to chew the tablets before swallowing is offset by the lack of absorption of the drug and offers an alternative in the older cooperative patient. Any therapy should be continued for at least 4 to 6 wk. Omeprazole, a potent new H^+-K^+ ATPase pump inhibitor, may completely reduce hydrogen production and has been effective in adults. The drug is not approved for children. These drugs have not been shown to be more effective in controlling gastric acidity than antacids but are more convenient and do hasten the healing of ulcers. Recurrences of primary peptic ulceration occurs in 20–60% of patients within 1 yr. A single dose at night of the H_2-blockers has been shown to be effective in preventing recurrence of ulcers.

Anticholinergic drugs can inhibit gastric acid secretion but are effective only when enough is given so that side effects of dry mouth or slightly blurred vision occur. It is often difficult to monitor these changes in children; these drugs are not, therefore, recommended as primary therapy. Antimicrobial and bismuth therapy to eradicate *H. pylori* is controversial (see Sec. 12.42).

Surgery is indicated in patients with perforation, intractable pain, chronic bleeding, or loss of over one third of the blood volume within 48 hr from a hemorrhage that could not be controlled through embolization of the bleeding vessel, as described earlier. Another indication for surgery is gastric outlet obstruction caused by edema and fibrosis around a chronic ulcer that is not improved after 72 hr of nasogastric drainage. Vagotomy and either pyloroplasty or antrectomy are the procedures most used in children. H_2-blocking agents have decreased the need for surgery.

Stress Ulcers

Stress erosions and ulcers are usually associated with physical trauma, burns, sepsis, hemorrhagic shock, or critical illness. These ulcers are usually acute; there is a lack of chronic inflammation and debris in the crater, and there are often multiple lesions. Stress ulcers occur with equal frequency in both sexes. They are more likely to occur in the duodenum and are often multiple.

Acute massive painless bleeding is frequently the first and only clinical manifestation of the ulcer. Partially because of the associated severe underlying disease, mortality is high, even if bleeding is controlled. Antacids or cimetidine can decrease the incidence of stress ulcers in adults who are at high risk. Accordingly, measures to control gastric acidity during periods of acute stress in children are recommended, especially in patients with massive burns or head injuries. Most of the ulcers that occur during the 1st 5 yr of life are stress ulcers.

The treatment for stress ulcers is similar to that for chronic peptic ulcer, especially with regard to antacid therapy. Often, bleeding stops with iced-saline lavage. Blood replacement, avoidance of aspirin, and correction of coagulation defects in the acutely ill patient are critical elements of treatment. As noted previously, selective intra-arterial infusion of Pitressin or embolization therapy may control bleeding or at least allow stabilization of these very sick patients before surgery. Suture ligature of the bleeding sites combined with a vagotomy and pyloroplasty is usually the recommended surgical procedure.

Zollinger-Ellison Syndrome

This rare syndrome can cause multiple recurrent duodenal and jejunal ulcers and is occasionally associated with diarrhea. Gastric secretion is markedly increased in volume and acidity, and hypertrophy of gastric folds is often noted on radiography. Islet cell tumor or hypertrophy causes massive elevation in serum gastrin-like activity that stimulates secretion of acid; occasionally, other hormones that cause diarrhea may also be secreted. Hypergastrinemia, albeit lower than Zollinger-Ellison syndrome, may be noted in pyloric stenosis, short bowel syndrome, hyperparathyroidism, pheochromocytoma, and multiple endocrine neoplasias. Chronic cimetidine therapy may control gastric acid secretion and reduce the need for complete gastrectomy. Symptoms can be controlled for long periods, even if these slow-growing tumors cannot be entirely removed.

JOHN J. HERBST

Caulfield M, Wyllie R, Sivak M, et al: Upper gastrointestinal tract endoscopy in the pediatric patient. J Pediatr 115:339, 1989.

Chiang B-L, Chang M-H, Lin M-I, et al: Chronic duodenal ulcer in children: Clinical observation and response to treatment. J Pediatr Gastroenterol Nutr 8:161, 1989.

DeGiacomo C, Fiocca R, Villani L, et al: *Helicobacter pylori* infection and chronic gastritis: Clinical, serological, and histologic correlations in children treated with amoxicillin and colloidal bismuth subcitrate. J Pediatr Gastroenterol Nutr 11:310, 1990.

Drumm B, Perez-Perez GI, Blaser MJ, et al: Intrafamilial clustering of *Helicobacter pylori* infection. N Engl J Med 322:359, 1990.

Drumm B, Rhoads JM, Stringer DA, et al: Peptic ulcer disease in children: Etiology, clinical findings, and clinical course. Pediatrics 82:410, 1988.

Kumar D, Spitz L: Peptic ulceration in children. Surg Gynecol Obstet 159:163, 1984.

Meyerovitz MF, Fellows KE: Angiography in gastrointestinal bleeding in children. Am J Roentgenol 143:837, 1984.

Tam PKH, Saing H: The use of H_2-receptor antagonist in the treatment of peptic ulcer disease in children. J Pediatr Gastroenterol Nutr 8:41, 1989.

13.40 INFLAMMATORY BOWEL DISEASE

Inflammatory bowel disease (IBD) encompasses two chronic idiopathic illnesses with predominant gastrointestinal and occasional extraintestinal manifestations. In Western Europe and North America, ulcerative colitis and Crohn disease (regional enteritis) are the major causes of chronic intestinal inflammation and are prominent causes of chronic illness among children and adolescents. Inflammatory bowel disease frequently has its onset in late childhood and adolescence, is characterized by unpredictable remissions and exacerbations, and has a variable response to therapy. In 85% of patients the diseases may be distinguished based on clinical, radiologic, endoscopic, and histologic features; the remaining 15% are designated as indeterminate colitis. Certain clinical and histopathologic features of these two diseases are compared in Table 13–14.

TABLE 13–14. Comparison of Crohn Disease and Ulcerative Colitis

Feature	Crohn Disease	Ulcerative Colitis
Rectal bleeding	Sometimes	Common
Abdominal mass	Common	Not present
Rectal disease	Occasional	Universal
Ileal involvement	Common	None (backwash ileitis)
Perianal disease	Common	Unusual
Strictures	Common	Unusual
Fistula	Common	Unusual
Discontinuous (skip) lesions	Common	Unusual
Transmural involvement	Common	Unusual
Crypt abscesses	Unusual	Common
Granulomas	Common	Unusual
Risk for colonic cancer	Slightly increased	Greatly increased

13.41 CHRONIC NONSPECIFIC ULCERATIVE COLITIS

This disease is characterized by recurrent bloody diarrhea associated with inflammation confined to the colonic mucosa. The estimated incidence ranges from 3 to 15/100,000, and the prevalence ranges from 40 to 225/100,000. Approximately 20% of all cases begin in adolescence or childhood. The disease is rare in infancy when milk protein allergy is a leading cause of chronic colitis. The peak age ranges from 15 to 25 yr. The sex ratio is equal, whereas the incidence is higher in whites, Jews, and in the northern hemisphere.

The intestinal lesion is characterized by distorted crypt architecture, polymorphonuclear, lymphocyte, and plasma cell infiltration of the lamina propria, crypt abscesses, and goblet cell depletion. It always involves the distal segment (rectum) and extends to a variable extent proximally. In young patients, the entire colon is involved more often than in adults. The lesion rarely extends beyond the mucosa into the deeper layers of the intestinal wall. In its typical form, therefore, ulcerative colitis is distinct from the lesion of Crohn disease.

ETIOLOGY. The cause is unknown. As with Crohn disease, the current view is that an immunologically mediated reaction is triggered in a genetically determined susceptible host. The antigen may be a microorganism. There is no evidence that dietary, environmental, allergic factors or personality disturbances predispose to this disease. Identical twins have greater concurrence than fraternal twins for ulcerative colitis, as do close family members, when compared with the community. The incidence is 2–4 times higher in Jews than in the general population and is increased in patients with ankylosing spondylitis and with Turner syndrome.

CLINICAL MANIFESTATIONS. The initial symptoms are diarrhea with fresh blood and copious mucus, fecal urgency, tenesmus, and lower abdominal cramps, particularly just before defecation. In most patients the onset is gradual; as diarrhea persists, anorexia develops with weight loss. At times, the onset is fulminant, with explosive bloody diarrhea, high fever and progression to peritonitis, and even perforation within days. If the symptoms are prolonged, particularly when nutrient intake has been poor, delayed growth and maturation occur, sometimes with secondary amenorrhea. The general impact of the disease is often reflected in the child's attendance and performance in school and at extracurricular activities.

Clinical signs of chronic ill health are usually evident at the time of diagnosis. The abdomen is tender, particularly along the left side, and bowel sounds are increased. There may be abdominal distention and tenderness on rectal examination. In fresh stools blood is usually present with masses of leukocytes and mucus; anal fissures occur, but perianal fistulas and abscesses are less common than with Crohn disease.

Extraintestinal manifestations are less common in children with ulcerative colitis than in adults; but signs of arthritis are seen in about 10% of patients, usually involving large joints that are tender, swollen, warm, and red. Usually, arthritic activity parallels colitic activity, but joint signs may be severe in the presence of subtle intestinal symptoms. Erythema nodosum occurs in fewer than 5% of cases, usually when the colitis is active. Pyoderma gangrenosum, a necrotic lesion of the skin is associated with ulcerative colitis. Iritis develops relatively late in the course of the disease. It is characterized by pain, conjunctival hyperemia in a perilimbal distribution, cells in the aqueous, deposits on the back of the cornea, and congestion of the iris. Coexisting hepatitis, also rare in children, usually causes a mixed hyperbilirubinemia with an enlarged firm liver. Unlike that of other extraintestinal features, the activity of hepatitis tends not to be related to the activity of the colonic disease. Finger clubbing occurs in fewer than 10% of patients and only in those with extensive disease. Peripheral edema (from excessive enteric protein loss), phlebitis, and hemolytic anemia are also associated with ulcerative colitis but are rare in childhood cases.

In the clinical assessment of these patients, particular attention should be paid to their psychologic status. Although emotional problems neither cause nor directly influence the course of the disease, they clearly exacerbate the child's symptoms. If the child and family are carefully evaluated initially, they can be better supported through a serious, chronic illness for which curative drug therapy is unavailable.

The usual clinical course is one of recurrent exacerbations. The disease is particularly aggressive in young patients in whom the lesion can be expected to extend with time; occasionally an adolescent patient remains in remission for many years. During periods of remission, most patients are fully active and well.

Ulcerative colitis has different modes of presentation and levels of severity initially and during acute exacerbations. An uncommon prodromal pattern (<5%) demonstrates extraintestinal (arthropathy, erythema nodosum) and inflammatory (high ESR, fever, growth failure) manifestations, in addition to nonspecific abdominal pain and bowel patterns. Mild disease seen in approximately 50% is characterized by mild rectal bleeding, less than four bowel movements per 24 hr, and abdominal pain without systemic manifestation (fever, tachycardia, anemia, extraintestinal signs). Moderate disease (~30%) demonstrates more than five bowel movements every 24 hr, more advanced rectal (tenesmus) and colonic (cramps, bloody diarrhea, abdominal tenderness) symptoms and signs, and systemic manifestation (weight loss, anorexia, fever, mild anemia). Severe disease (~10%) has more than six bloody stools every 24 hr, marked abdominal tenderness, with or without distention, tachycardia, fever, severe anemia, leukocytosis, hypoalbuminemia, and an increased risk for toxic megacolon, sepsis, acute hemorrhage, and intestinal perforations.

In general, more severe symptoms and more frequent exacerbations are associated with extensive disease, particularly pancolitis. The most serious form of exacerbation is the development of toxic megacolon, a dilatation of the diseased colon to a diameter of more than 6 cm measured roentgenographically. This very severe antecedent to perforation and sepsis, which develops in 4% or less of cases, is usually precipitated by distention of the colon resulting from investigative procedures, anticholinergic or other medications, or hypokalemia.

In patients who have had their disease for 10 yr, the risk of developing colonic carcinoma rises sharply. Studies report a 20% risk at 20 yr. The true figure may be somewhat less, but comprehensive data are not yet available. The cancer risk is highly significant and warrants repeated surveillance.

DIFFERENTIAL DIAGNOSIS. Infections are by far the most common causes of chronic intestinal inflammation (Tables 13–15 and 13–16). A careful search for infectious contacts and microbiologic studies should be completed before a diagnosis of idiopathic ulcerative colitis is made. Ulcerative colitis is rare in infants, but in this very young age group necrotizing enterocolitis and intolerance of dietary protein (particularly cow's milk) can cause colitis; furthermore, Hirschsprung disease may be complicated by colitis in infants. In older children, Crohn disease is characterized by its segmental distribution and involvement of all layers of the gut by a granulomatous inflammatory lesion. In anaphylactoid purpura, hemolytic-uremic syndrome, and Behçet syndrome, intestinal involvement may precede other manifestations, but evidence of a widespread vasculitis soon becomes apparent.

DIAGNOSIS. The clinical evaluation usually suggests the diagnosis of an inflammatory bowel lesion. Microbiologic studies should be guided by a knowledge of possible contacts (see Table 13–15).

In idiopathic ulcerative colitis, colonoscopic examination demonstrates the typical diffuse inflammatory lesion of the rectum and distal colon. The mucosa is inflamed, granular, and extremely friable; ulcers are rarely seen in children. In the typical case, biopsy shows an inflammatory lesion characterized by polymorphonuclear infiltration and crypt abscesses. However, biopsy findings alone are never sufficiently specific to establish a certain diagnosis. Even when a double-contrast technique is used, a barium enema may be normal initially, but usually the examination shows a diffuse distal lesion; the process may extend proximally to involve the entire colon. Colonoscopy is more sensitive than roentgenographic techniques in detecting minor mucosal lesions and the proximal limits of disease. This examination must be undertaken with great care in children with severe disease because of the risk of toxic megacolon.

TREATMENT. No curative medical therapy is available, but medications can reduce the activity of the inflammatory process and the incidence of recurrence.

Supportive measures are particularly important. In accordance with their ability to understand, the child and his or her parents must be given insight into the nature of the disease and supported in their efforts to cope with unpleasant symptoms, tests, and at times, unpleasant therapy. In general, dietary restrictions have little place in treatment. Diet should be nutritious and balanced. Supplementation with iron and folate are often beneficial. Some patients become seriously malnourished because of an inability to tolerate sufficient nutrient intake. Total parenteral nutrition is effective in restoring nutritional status but does not usually affect the inflammatory process in the bowel. Encouragement should be given to the patient's living as full a life as possible.

Sulfasalazine is used to reduce inflammatory activity in the colon and particularly to reduce the likelihood of exacerbation, even years after the onset of the disease. In a dose of 50–75 mg/kg/24 hr (maximum 4 g) it rarely has side effects, particularly if started in a gradually increasing dose. Anorexia or nausea can usually be reduced by using an enteric-coated drug. Occasionally, neutropenia or a hypersensitivity reaction necessitates discontinuing the medication. Sulfasalazine interferes with folic acid absorption; long-term users should either have their folate status monitored or they should receive supplemental folate. A high incidence of headache and reversible oligospermia and infertility has been associated with the long-term use of sulfasalazine.

The therapeutic response to newer drugs, containing the active portion of sulfasalazine 5-aminosalicylic acid (5-ASA), appears to be comparable with that of the sulfasalazine, and the side effects are much less. Limited experience with the rectal use of 5-ASA in children suggests a role of these enemas in active distal ulcerative colitis.

Corticosteroids are most effective for treating active disease. For mild cases, particularly those with disease confined to the distal colon, soluble hydrocortisone or prednisolone may be used as an enema, 100 mg of hydrocortisone or its equivalent for an adolescent, given slowly at bedtime for 6 wk, daily for the first 3 wk and then on alternate nights. If the patient deteriorates or does not improve within 10 days, oral administration should be added. Prednisone, 1–2 mg/kg/24 hr to a maximum daily dose of 60 mg/24 hr, is used for moderate-to-severe cases and for those that fail to respond to enema therapy. Occasionally, with fulminant disease, the patient may be too ill to tolerate oral medication and will require an equivalent intravenous dose of hydrocortisone. Once begun, a 3–4 mo course of systemic corticosteroid therapy should be given, in a full dose for 6 wk, then tapered by 5 mg/24 hr

TABLE 13–15. Infectious Agents Mimicking Inflammatory Bowel Disease

Agent	Manifestations	Diagnosis	Comments
Bacterial			
Campylobacter jejuni	Acute diarrhea, fever, fecal blood and leukocytes	Culture	Common in adolescents, may relapse
Yersinia enterocolitica	Acute→ chronic diarrhea, right lower quadrant pain, mesenteric adenitis—pseudoappendicitis, fecal blood and leukocytes Extraintestinal manifestations, mimics Crohn disease	Culture	Common in adolescents as FUO*, weight loss, abdominal pain
Clostridium difficile	Postantibiotic onset, watery diarrhea, pseudomembrane on sigmoidoscopy	Culture and cytotoxin	May be nosocomial Toxic megacolon possible
Escherichia coli 0157:H7	Colitis, fecal blood, abdominal pain	Culture and typing	Hemolytic uremic syndrome
Salmonella	Watery→ bloody diarrhea, food-borne, fecal leukocytes, cramps	Culture	Usually acute
Shigella	Watery→ bloody diarrhea, fecal leukocytes, fever, pain, cramps	Culture	Dysentery symptoms
Edwardsiella tarda	Bloody diarrhea, cramps	Culture	Ulceration on endoscopy
Aeromonas hydrophilia	Cramps, diarrhea, fecal blood	Culture	May be chronic Contaminated drinking water
Plesiomonas	Diarrhea, cramps	Culture	Shellfish source
Tuberculosis	Rarely bovine, now *Mycobacterium tuberculosis* Ileocecal area, fistula formulation	Culture, PPD†, biopsy	May mimic Crohn disease
Parasites			
Entamoeba histolytica	Acute bloody diarrhea and liver abscess, colic	Trophozoite in stool, colonic mucosal flask ulceration, serology	Travel to endemic area
Giardia lamblia	Foul-smelling, watery diarrhea, cramps, flatulence, weight loss. No colonic involvement	"Owl"-like trophozoite and cysts in stool; rarely duodenal intubation	May be chronic
AIDS‡ Associated Enteropathy			
Cryptosporidium	Chronic diarrhea, weight loss	Stool microscopy	Mucosal findings not like IBD§
Isospora belli	As in *Cryptosporidium*		Tropical location
Cytomegalovirus	Colonic ulceration, pain, bloody diarrhea	Culture, biopsy	

*FUO = fever of unknown origin.
† PPD = purified protein derivative.
‡AIDS = acquired immunodeficiency syndrome.
§IBD = inflammatory bowel disease.

TABLE 13–16. Chronic Inflammatory Intestinal Disorders

Infection—see Table 13–15
- Bacterial
- Parasite
- AIDS associated
- Toxin

Immune-Inflammatory
- Congenital immunodeficiency disorders
- Acquired immunodeficiency diseases
- Dietary protein enterocolitis
- Behçet syndrome
- Lymphoid nodular hyperplasia
- Eosinophilic gastroenteritis
- Graft-versus-host disease

Vascular-Ischemic
- Systemic vasculitis (SLE*, dermatomyositis)
- Henoch-Schönlein purpura
- Hemolytic uremic syndrome

Other
- Prestenotic colitis
- Diversion colitis
- Radiation colitis
- Neonatal necrotizing enterocolitis
- Typhlitis
- Hirschsprung colitis
- Intestinal lymphoma
- Laxative abuse

*SLE = systemic lupus erythematosus.

each wk. The changes in facial appearance and acne that occur in children receiving this medication vary in severity but are universally dreaded by young patients. Additional complications from long-term use are osteoporosis, cataracts, systemic hypertension, and growth retardation. Alternate-day administration of prednisone may avoid adrenal suppression, but it is often inadequate to control active disease.

New medications such as cyclosporine, azathioprine, and 6-mercaptopurine continue to be subjected to clinical trial but have no proven benefit.

The disease can be cured by surgical resection of the entire colon. Emergency colectomy may be indicated in cases of actual or impending perforation, massive hemorrhage, or the development of a carcinoma in the diseased bowel. The common indications of operative treatment of a child with ulcerative colitis are severe acute disease that does not respond to at least 2 wk of intensive treatment and prolonged or debilitating symptoms, particularly if there is growth or maturational delay in the face of an extended trial of medical therapy. A difficult decision must be faced when the young patient is found to have active colitis 10 yr after onset of the disease, especially if there is pancolitis. Because of the risk of carcinoma in the diseased colon, most experts advise colectomy for such patients, if the disease is extensive. There is an 11- to 19-fold increased risk (95% confidence limits of standardized incidence ratio of 15) of colorectal cancer for patients who have pancolitis. This finding suggests that perhaps prophylactic proctocolectomy should be recommended for this group, especially for patients less than 15 yr of age. Otherwise, semiannual colonoscopy with multiple biopsies is necessary for early tumor recognition to be achieved. The diagnostic reliability of regular biopsy surveillance in detecting precancerous lesions has not been well established.

The preferred operative technique for children is pancolectomy with ileoanal anastomosis and construction of a reservoir "pouch" from a segment of ileum; the anastomosis can be undertaken at the time of the initial colectomy or later on. With restoration of bowel continuity, a temporary "venting" ileostomy is fashioned and several months later, once healing has occurred, the ileostomy can be closed. Results from this surgical treatment have improved during the last 5 yr, but frequent stooling and nocturnal incontinence may occur, particularly during the 1st postoperative year. In some cases, these problems necessitate reverting to a permanent ileostomy. Inflammation may develop in the reservoir, but this problem can usually be managed with oral metronidazole. Repeated proctoscopy is required for surveillance of cancer. Perianal irritation from bile salts can be treated with sitz baths, good hygiene, and cholestyramine ointment.

PROGNOSIS. Most cases beginning in childhood are severe both in activity and in the extent of involvement. Occasionally, a fulminant onset progresses to perforation of the colon before a diagnosis is made. The usual course is one in which the patient has an initial improvement after taking medication, followed by recurrent exacerbations. Massive blood loss can occasionally be life-threatening, but the most serious acute complication is toxic megacolon. Ulcerative colitis predisposes the patient to colonic cancer; the risk is only 3% in the 1st decade after the onset but rises 20%/decade subsequently, unless the colon has been resected.

Ament M: Inflammatory disease of the colon: Ulcerative colitis and Crohn's colitis. J Pediatr 86:322, 1975.
Ekbom A, Helmick C, Zack M, et al: Ulcerative colitis and colorectal cancer. N Engl J Med 323:1228, 1990.
Kirschner BS: Inflammatory bowel disease in children. Pediatr Clin North Am 35:189, 1988.
Kleinman RE, Balistreri WF, Heyman MB, et al: Nutritional support for pediatric patients with inflammatory bowel disease. J Pediatr Gastroenterol Nutr 8:8, 1989.
Korelitz B: Considerations of surveillance, dysplasia and carcinoma of the colon in management of ulcerative colitis and Crohn's disease. Med Clin North Am 74:189, 1990.
Lightiger S, Present DH: Preliminary report: Cyclosporin in treatment of severe active ulcerative colitis. Lancet 336:16, 1990.
Markowitz RL, Ment LR, Cryboski JD: Cerebral thromboembolic disease in pediatric and adult inflammatory bowel disease: Case report and review of the literature. J Pediatr Gastroenterol Nutr 8:413, 1989.
Michener W, Wyllie R: Management of children and adolescents with inflammatory bowel disease: Med Clin North Am 74:103, 1990.
North CS, Clouse RE, Spitznagel EL, et al: The relation of ulcerative colitis to psychiatric factors: A review of findings and methods. Am J Psychol 147:947, 1990.
Olafsdottir EJ, Fluge G, Haug K: Chronic inflammatory bowel disease in children in Western Norway. J Pediatr Gastroenterol Nutr 8:454, 1989.
Peppercorn MA: Advances in drug therapy for inflammatory bowel disease. Ann Intern Med 112:50, 1990.
Tolia V, Massoud N, Klotz U: Oral 5-aminosalicyclic acid in children with colonic chronic inflammatory bowel disease: Clinical and pharmacokinetic experience. J Pediatr Gastroenterol Nutr 8:333, 1989.

13.42 CROHN DISEASE

(Regional Enteritis, Granulomatous Enterocolitis)

Crohn disease is a segmental transmural intestinal disease; it may involve one or more segments of gut from the mouth to the anus, but the distal ileum and colon are most commonly affected. Twenty-five to 40% of cases begin before 20 yr of age. The incidence rose sharply in Europe and America between 1950 and 1970, reaching 4 to 6/100,000 with a prevalence of 40–100/100,000. Recently the prevalance has reached a plateau.

The inflammatory process consists of noncaseating epithelioid granulomas with giant cell and regional lymphatic involvement. These histologic abnormalities are not specific for Crohn disease; they may not all be present in biopsy specimens or even in tissue resected at operation. Furthermore, several of these findings may be seen occasionally in cases of ulcerative colitis. A distinctive feature of Crohn disease is the development of enteric fistulas between loops of bowel or from bowel to neighboring structures such as the skin or urinary tract.

ETIOLOGY. The cause is unknown; current theories are similar to those for ulcerative colitis (Sec. 13.41). Genetic factors appear to influence vulnerability to an immunologically related inflammatory reaction. Although an increased family incidence of Crohn disease occurs, similar to that observed in ulcerative colitis, one of the two diseases predominates within a single family.

CLINICAL MANIFESTATIONS. Crohn disease rarely begins before the age of 10 yr. The onset is usually subtle; many months may pass between the 1st symptoms and diagnosis. Crampy abdominal pain is the most common initial complaint, followed by diarrhea. Unlike patients with ulcerative colitis, about half of these patients have at onset nonintestinal problems such as fever, anorexia, growth failure, general malaise, and joint symptoms. Any teenager with chronic malaise and persisting growth problems, particularly with fever, should be suspected of having this condition. Chronic perianal lesions (skin tags, fissures, abscesses, fistulas), even when there are no reasons to suspect primary bowel disease, are another early signal.

In time, most children with active Crohn disease develop abdominal pain and diarrhea. Pain from involvement of small intestine is often periumbilical or in the right lower quadrant rather than confined to the lower abdomen, as in ulcerative colitis. Stools are less explosive than in ulcerative colitis, and there is less tenesmus except when the distal segment is involved. Intestinal bleeding is rare but it can be massive.

Extraintestinal manifestations are similar to those of ulcerative colitis but are more common with Crohn disease. Arthritis, usually affecting large joints, was reported in 18% of one pediatric series. Erythema nodosum, iritis, hepatitis, and phlebitis are rare; they tend to exacerbate and remit with the activity of the intestinal lesion. Finger clubbing occurs in about a third of patients with Crohn disease. Often, the course is one of persistent malaise and fatigue, with or without pain. In time, a dominant manifestation of the impact of Crohn disease is delayed maturation and growth. These problems are particularly obvious, and they are traumatic for the adolescent.

DIFFERENTIAL DIAGNOSIS. The usual causes of inflammatory bowel lesions are summarized in Tables 13–15 and 13–16. The most important feature distinguishing Crohn disease from ulcerative colitis is that the distribution of the Crohn lesion is segmental, whereas that of ulcerative colitis is diffuse and confined to the colon. Infections that are particularly likely to be confused with Crohn disease are those that involve the distal small bowel, for example, *Yersinia enterocolitica*, which is common, and tuberculosis, which is rare in North America. *Yersinia* and anaphylactoid purpura may cause small intestinal abnormalities in barium studies similar to those found in Crohn disease. Intestinal manifestations of *Behçet syndrome* are identical to those of Crohn disease (see Sec. 11.71). Early in their courses, anaphylactoid purpura and hemolytic-uremic syndromes may closely mimic Crohn disease. All patients should be observed for skin and renal lesions.

DIAGNOSIS. A careful clinical evaluation usually suggests a diagnosis of an inflammatory bowel lesion. An elevated erythrocyte sedimentation rate gives evidence of an active inflammatory process in more than 75% of patients at the time of diagnosis. Hemoglobin levels are mildly depressed and serum albumin levels reduced in about a third of cases.

If an inflammatory lesion is suspected and microbiologic studies exclude a specific infection, barium contrast roentgenograms of small and large bowel are needed to define the segments involved. Crohn disease is characterized by irregular mucosa or a cobblestone-like pattern, thickened bowel, and enteric fistulas, but it is the lesion's segmental distribution that is diagnostic. Detail may be better seen in the small bowel by injecting barium directly by tube into the duodenum, and in the colon by using a double air-contrast technique.

Biopsies of rectal mucosa may show typical granulomas, even if there is no gross evidence of distal segment involvement on sigmoidoscopy. Because involvement of the colon is often proximal, a rigid sigmoidoscope seldom reaches the diseased area. When it is important to define the extent of colonic involvement, fiberoptic colonoscopy should be used in conjunction with air contrast barium enema.

TREATMENT. Curative medical therapy is not available. A 30-yr recurrence rate of more than 90% is reported after operative resection in Crohn disease.

Because medications are palliative at best, supportive measures are very important. The child and family must be helped to attain insight into the nature of this disease and its disabling symptoms. Therapy should be directed at enabling the patient to live as full a life as possible and creating an atmosphere in which the child does not consider himself or herself an invalid. For example, undue fatigue should be avoided but exercise should be encouraged. Generally, a full nutritious diet should be encouraged.

Placing the bowel "at rest" by use of total parenteral nutrition or by use of an elemental diet infused by nasogastric tube is usually effective in diminishing disease activity. These techniques are particularly effective for children with delayed growth and those with enteric fistulas. The enteral infusions are well tolerated unless there is very active disease, impending bowel obstruction, or severe psychologic disturbance. They can usually be given over 12-hr periods at night for 2–3 mo by patients at home.

Prednisone is indicated to treat acute exacerbations. For active small bowel disease 1–2 mg/kg/24 hr (maximum 60 mg) of prednisone should be given for 6 wk, after which gradual reduction of the dose should be attempted over a further 8–12 wk. If symptoms recur with decreased doses, the drug should be given at higher levels for a longer period. Alternate-day therapy is rarely effective in maintaining a remission. In difficult cases the concomitant use of azathioprine, 2 mg/kg/24 hr or 6-mercaptopurine, 1.5 mg/kg/24 hr, may permit reduction of steroid dose, but they should be used for no more than 1 yr, with careful monitoring of the white blood cell count. Sulfasalazine is not so beneficial in Crohn disease as in ulcerative colitis. Available data support its use (50–75 mg/kg/24 hr up to 4 g/24 hr) for colonic Crohn disease, but the drug does not increase long-term remission rates or enhance the effect of corticosteroid. Metronidazole (15 mg/kg/24 hr) may be beneficial in some cases, particularly those with fistulas and severe perianal problems. Methotrexate and cyclosporine have been used with some benefit in severe cases, but the experience with these agents is limited.

Because of high recurrence rates and in some cases extensive small bowel involvement, surgical resection for Crohn disease has less to offer than for ulcerative colitis. Massive hemorrhage, intestinal perforation, or persistent bowel obstruction demands operative intervention as lifesaving; these emergencies are rare in children with Crohn disease. The question of operative resection usually arises around the issue of persisting debility, particularly when growth and maturation are delayed. Although recurrence appears to be inevitable, resection frequently permits an interval of good health, growth, and a return to full activity. The decision to operate will be based on the severity and duration of debility, the patient's age and potential for growth, and the response of the patient and family to the disease. Every effort should be made to arrange any elective resection for a time when nutritional status is satisfactory and the inflammatory process is inactive. The current trend to undertake very limited (scar removal) rather than wide intestinal resection, such as in the past, appears to yield improved results.

PROGNOSIS. The inflammatory activity of Crohn disease remits and exacerbates through life without a consistent pattern. In most cases the region involved remains constant; when extension occurs, it often appears to be a postoperative event. The natural course of this inflammatory process is to scar resulting in narrowing and eventually in obstruction of the intestinal lumen. Ileal disease leads almost inevitably to obstructive problems, but usually 1 decade or more after the onset of the disease. The incidence of intestinal cancer is increased with longstanding Crohn disease, but not nearly to the degree seen in ulcerative colitis.

Ament M: Inflammatory disease of the colon: Ulcerative colitis and Crohn's colitis. J Pediatr 86:322, 1975.
Hamilton JR, Bruce GA, Abdourhaman M, et al: Inflammatory bowel disease in children and adolescents. Adv Pediatr 26:311, 1980.
Kelts DG, Grand RJ, Shien G, et al: Nutritional basis of growth failure in children and adolescents with Crohn's disease. Gastroenterology 76:720, 1979.
Kirschner BS: Inflammatory bowel disease in children. Pediatr Clin North Am 35:189, 1988.
Kleinman RE, Balistreri WF, Heyman MB, et al: Nutritional support for pediatric patients with inflammatory bowel disease. J Pediatr Gastroenterol Nutr 8:8, 1989.
Korelitz B: Considerations of surveillance, dysplasia and carcinoma of the colon in management of ulcerative colitis and Crohn's disease. Med Clin North Am 74:189, 1990.
Markowitz RL, Ment LR, Cryboski JD: Cerebral thromboembolic disease in pediatric and adult inflammatory bowel disease: Case report and review of the literature. J Pediatr Gastroenterol Nutr 8:413, 1989.
Mashako MNL, Cezard JP, Navarro J, et al: Crohn's disease lesions in the upper gastrointestinal tract: Correlation between clinical, radiological, endoscopic, and histological features in adolescents and children. J Pediatr Gastroenterol Nutr 8:442, 1989.
Michener W, Wyllie R: Management of children and adolescents with inflammatory bowel disease. Med Clin North Am 74:103, 1990.
Morin CL, Roulet M, Roy CC, et al: Continuous elemental enteral alimentation in children with Crohn's disease and growth failure. Gastroenterology 79:1205, 1980.
Olafsdottir EJ, Fluge G, Haug K: Chronic inflammatory bowel disease in children in Western Norway. J Pediatr Gastroenterol Nutr 8:454, 1989.
Peppercorn MA: Advances in drug therapy for inflammatory bowel disease. Ann Intern Med 112:50, 1990.
Wesson DE, Shandling B: Results of bowel resection for Crohn's disease in the young. Pediatr Surg 16:449, 1981.

NEONATAL NECROTIZING ENTEROCOLITIS (NEC)

See Sec. 9.43.

ANTIBIOTIC-ASSOCIATED PSEUDOMEMBRANOUS COLITIS

See Sec. 12.38.

13.43 GASTROINTESTINAL SYMPTOMS IN ANAPHYLACTOID PURPURA

See Sec. 11.56.

Two thirds of patients with anaphylactoid (Henoch-Schönlein) purpura have abdominal symptoms. Crampy abdominal pain may be very severe and precede any other manifestations of the disorder. The pain results from submucosal and subserosal hemorrhages, which may lead to small or large amounts of blood in the stools or to intussusception. In the acute stage of the disease, barium contrast roentgenograms may show large filling defects in the bowel wall, suggestive of Crohn disease or a neoplasm. Pancreatitis may develop. A diagnosis is made when the characteristic purpuric rash or renal manifestations develop. Systemic corticosteroids have been used to alleviate abdominal pain in these patients. There is no proof that such treatment alters the disease process. Intestinal stricture can be a late complication.

Branski D, Gross V, Gross-Kieselstein E, et al: Pancreatitis as a complication of Henoch-Schönlein purpura. J Pediatr Gastroenterol Nutr 1:235, 1982.
Goldman LP, Lindenberg RL: Henoch-Schönlein purpura: Gastrointestinal manifestations with endoscopic correlation. Am J Gastroenterol 75:357, 1972.
Lombaard KA, Shah PC, Thrasher TV, et al: Ileal stricture as a late complication of Henoch-Schönlein purpura. Pediatrics 77:396, 1986.
Silver DL: Henoch-Schönlein syndrome. Pediatr Clin North Am 19:1061, 1972.

13.44 GASTROINTESTINAL PROBLEMS IN HEMOLYTIC-UREMIC SYNDROME

See Sec. 18.13.

This potentially fatal disease may begin as an intestinal inflammatory disorder. Bloody diarrhea is frequently the first symptom. The syndrome may evolve from *Campylobacter* enterocolitis or *Shigella* dysentery. There is also an association of verotoxin-producing strains of *E. coli* (0157:H7, 026, 0111, 0121, 0145) with the hemolytic-uremic syndrome and hemorrhagic colitis. Barium contrast roentgenograms show spasm and transient early filling defects, but the lesions may progress to stenosis. Diagnosis depends on the recognition of acute renal failure, hemolytic anemia, and thrombocytopenia, none of which may be apparent in the early stages.

Karmali MA, Petric M, Kim C, et al: The association between idiopathic hemolytic-uremic syndrome and infection by verotoxin-producing *Escherichia coli*. J Infect Dis 151:775, 1985.
Sawaf H, Sharp MJ, Youn KJ, et al: Ischemic colitis and stricture after hemolytic-uremic syndrome. Pediatrics 61:315, 1978.
Tochen ML, Campbell JR: Colitis in children with hemolytic-uremic syndrome. J Pediatr Surg 12:213, 1977.
Whitington PF, Friedman AL, Chesney RW: Gastrointestinal disease in the hemolytic-uremic syndrome. Gastroenterology 76:728, 1979.

13.45 BEHÇET SYNDROME

Initial clinical descriptions of this multisystem vasculitis included reports of uveitis with severe oral mucosal and genital ulcers (Sec. 11.71). The intestine is frequently affected; segmental lesions in the colon or distal small bowel resemble those of Crohn disease. About 10% of cases of this rare syndrome begin in childhood, usually in adolescence. Iritis is uncommon in patients in North America. This disorder is distinguished from Crohn disease by the severe oral, nasopharyngeal, and genital ulcerations. Corticosteroids are the main type of treatment. Other immunosuppressives, chlorambucil, and colchicine have been reported in uncontrolled trials to have benefited patients whose disease does not respond to corticosteroid therapy. Intestinal resection is necessary when there is a progression to intestinal obstruction.

Ammann AJ, Johnson A, Fyfe GA, et al: Behçet syndrome. J Pediatr 107:41, 1985.
Stringer DA, Cleghorn GJ, Durie PR, et al: Behçet's syndrome involving the gastrointestinal tract: A diagnostic dilemma in childhood. Pediatr Radiol 16:131, 1986.

13.46 DIETARY PROTEIN INTOLERANCE
(Food Allergy)

Foods can provide gastrointestinal symptoms in children, but the mechanisms for these manifestations remain partially understood. Dietary components may cause adverse reactions because they are contaminated with microbes or toxins, because they have pharmacologic activity, or because they overload a comprised absorptive or digestive process. The immunologic basis (allergic) of gastrointestinal responses to food is especially problematic. Also see Sec. 11.49 and 26.3.

Food allergy is an immunologically mediated response to dietary antigen. Most attention has focused on cow's milk protein as the major cause of gastrointestinal food allergy in infants. Several immunologic mechanisms may be involved: immediate anaphylactic hypersensitivity involving IgE antibodies, antibody dependent cytotoxic hypersensitivity involving IgM or IgG, immune complex hypersensitivity, and cell-mediated hypersensitivity.

CLINICAL MANIFESTATIONS. Because diagnostic criteria are uncertain, the true incidence is difficult to determine; in Sweden estimates range from 0.5 to 1.5%. Food antigen may provoke respiratory, skin, or gastrointestinal symptoms. Gastrointestinal manifestations, with or without involvement of the other two systems, often dominate the clinical picture. Any region of the gastrointestinal tract can be affected.

Mouth. Recurrent shallow, mucosal ulceration and perioral dermatitis have been attributed to allergic responses to food, but usually another cause is found.

Stomach. Studies in adults suggest that intragastric antigen can provoke hemorrhagic and edematous inflammation in the gastric mucosa. Acute vomiting, presumably on the basis of this immediate hypersensitivity, can occur in infants and is usually associated with watery or even bloody diarrhea. In its most fulminant form, this rare syndrome is accompanied by glottic swelling; fatal anaphylactic shock may occur.

Small Intestine. Three syndromes are recognized. *Acute watery diarrhea* may occur as an immediate response to antigen ingestion, with or without vomiting and abdominal cramps. *Chronic diarrhea* and failure to thrive may occur after the ingestion of milk, soya, egg, or fish. A patchy villus lesion in the small intestine is associated with anorexia, chronic diarrhea, and retarded growth. Usually absorptive function is not significantly impaired. *Excessive enteric protein and blood loss* may lead to hypoproteinemia and iron deficiency, often without obvious intestinal symptoms. This occurs usually in an older infant at the time of weaning from breast milk, when milk formula feeding is withdrawn, or when ordinary dairy milk feeding is begun. Eosinophilia is common. Manifestations may resolve completely after cow's milk is withdrawn from the diet. A spontaneous "cure" may be evident after reestablishing cow's milk formula or processed milk (evaporated, dried) intake, years after the initial manifestations.

Colon. Pancolitis causing profuse bloody diarrhea may occur after cow's milk ingestion, usually in young infants. Diarrhea stools contain abundant eosinophils. This syndrome has been, rarely, seen in exclusively breast-fed infants whose mothers were ingesting cow's milk. The condition should not be confused with eosinophilic gastroenteritis (Sec. 13.47).

DIAGNOSIS. The diagnosis of dietary protein allergy is clinical. Acute symptoms should subside within 48 hr and chronic symptoms within 1 wk of complete withdrawal of the offending antigen, usually cow's milk. Caution and judgment must be exercised in rechallenging these patients with potential dietary antigens. In a young infant, particularly if an acute response is anticipated, the challenge should be carried out under observation, beginning with a small dose (e.g., 1–5 mL milk) and increasing progressively over a few days provided a response does not occur. For gastrointestinal responses to potential dietary antigens skin tests, circulating antibody titers, complement assays, and coproantibody titers are not of proven diagnostic value. In children with chronic symptoms, some centers use mucosal biopsy to evaluate the response to challenge. It is important to rule out other conditions that may cause similar symptoms, such as enteric infections, lactose intolerance, and other forms of nonspecific inflammatory bowel disease.

The syndromes described for cow's milk intolerance may occur also in response to soy protein. Some studies estimate that up to 50% of children intolerant to cow's milk are intolerant to soy. Since soy is not a commonly used food, most will not be exposed to soy unless they are first found intolerant to cow's milk. The approach to diagnosis is the same as for cow's milk.

TREATMENT. Prolonged breast-feeding reduces the likelihood of later cow's milk intolerance. Treatment consists of removing the offending food from the diet. Breast-feeding mothers may have to go on a cow's milk elimination diet if their infant has manifestations of milk protein allergy. For the young infant the non–milk-containing dietary formulas consist of various soy feedings and hydrolyzed milk protein feedings. Many children with the enteric protein and blood loss syndrome will benefit by changing from fresh milk to processed (i.e., evaporated, powdered) milk. For rare cases of intolerance to many foods, oral administration of sodium cromoglycate has been reported to suppress intestinal symptoms and permit continued ingestion of the food.

PROGNOSIS. In most cases, food protein intolerance is transitory. About 50% of infants with the conditions described earlier recover within 1 yr and most of the remainder recover within 2 yr.

Ament ME, Rubin CE: Soy protein—another cause of the flat intestinal lesion. Gastroenterology 62:227, 1972.

Eastham EJ, Walker WA: Effect of cow's milk on the gastrointestinal tract: A persistent dilemma for the pediatrician. Pediatrics 60:477, 1977.

Fontaine SL, Navarro J: Small intestinal biopsy in cow's milk protein allergy in infancy. Arch Dis Child 50:357, 1975.

Hill DJ, Firer MA, Shelton MJ, et al: Manifestations of milk allergy in infancy. J Pediatr 109:270, 1986.

Minford AMB, MacDonald A, Littlewood JM: Food intolerance and food allergy in children: A review of 63 cases. Arch Dis Child 57:742, 1982.

Patrick MK, Gall DG: Protein intolerance and immunocyte and enterocyte interaction. Pediatr Clin North Am 85:17, 1988.

Powell GK: Milk and soy-induced enterocolitis of infancy. J Pediatr 93:558, 1978.

Waldman TA, Wochner RD, Laster L, et al: Allergic gastroenteropathy: A cause of excessive gastrointestinal protein loss. N Engl J Med 276:761, 1967.

13.47 EOSINOPHILIC GASTROENTERITIS

A rare form of inflammatory involvement of the stomach and intestine is characterized by infiltrates of eosinophils. Usually, the gastric antrum and the upper small bowel are involved, but esophageal and distal intestinal lesions also occur.

The lesions normally cause abdominal pain, vomiting, diarrhea, and delayed growth and weight gain. There may be atopic symptoms, such as rhinitis and asthma and a peripheral eosinophilia, which suggest an allergic basis for the disorder. Excessive enteric protein loss may cause reduced serum albumin and immunoglobulin levels. An endoscopy reveals gastric and duodenal lesions, and a biopsy shows eosinophilic congestion of the lamina propria and patchy villus shortening. Rarely, eosinophils infiltrate more deeply to cause bowel wall thickening and granuloma formation. Mucosal involvement may produce hemorrhage, and muscularis involvement may produce strictures, whereas serosal involvement may produce ascites.

The disease usually runs a chronic debilitating course with sporadic severe exacerbations. A few patients are helped by elimination diets, but most require systemic administration of corticosteroids.

Katz AJ, Golman H, Grand RJ: Gastric mucosal biopsy in eosinophilic (allergic) gastroenteritis. Gastroenterology 73:705, 1977.

Klein NC, Hargrove RL, Sleisinger MN, et al: Eosinophilic gastroenteritis. Medicine 49:299, 1970.

Whitington PF, Whitington GL: Eosinophilic gastroenteropathy in childhood. J Pediatr Gastroenterol Nutr 7:379, 1988.

13.48 MUNCHAUSEN SYNDROME BY PROXY

This form of child abuse in which parents falsify the medical history of their child may be confused with primary gastrointestinal diseases (Sec. 3.51). Diarrhea, vomiting, and hemorrhage are common, although they are not the only symptoms. The parent induces real symptoms or apparent symptoms while denying any such involvement. The term Munchausen syndrome was used initially to describe situations in which patients falsified their own symptoms. It is now recognized as a problem inflicted on children, either unable or unwilling to identify the true offender, who is almost always the mother.

Typical patterns include the administration of laxatives like phenolphthalein to cause diarrhea and the addition of blood to stool or urine to mimic hemorrhage. The psychopathologic basis for this potentially very dangerous behavior is not understood; the afflicted relative apparently gains something from the resultant relationships formed with caregivers or with his or her family as a result of the problem.

CLINICAL MANIFESTATIONS. The symptom complex does not usually fit with a recognized disease. Cases have been reported up to 7 yr of age; the pattern varies greatly but is consistent and recurrent in each case. Diarrhea, bleeding, and vomiting are the usual gastrointestinal manifestations. Symptoms are always associated with the proximity of the mother to the child. The mother usually has a background in health care and is a "model" parent, forming close relationships with members of the health care team.

Investigations should be based on a high index of suspicion so that unpleasant, dangerous, or unnecessary tests are not undertaken. Specimens can be analyzed for potentially harmful agents and for "foreign" blood. All steps in the diagnosis should be carefully documented.

TREATMENT. The offending parent should be confronted by the physician acting in the capacity of someone who offers to help and who is not just an accuser. These cases should be reported promptly to legal authorities, because they can go on to persistent abuse, disability, and even death.

Meadow R: Management of Munchausen syndrome by proxy. Arch Dis Child 60:385, 1985.

Meadow R: Munchausen syndrome by proxy: The hinderland of child abuse. Lancet 2:343, 1977.

Richardson GF: Munchausen syndrome by proxy. Am Family Phys 36:119, 1987.

13.49 MALABSORPTIVE DISORDERS

The malabsorptive disorders are those that cause defective assimilation of ingested nutrients. The diseases that cause maldigestion or malabsorption of many nutrients tend to share certain clinical manifestations: abdominal distention; pale, foul, bulky stools; wasting of muscles, particularly the proximal muscle groups; and retarded growth and weight gain (Fig. 13–22). *Celiac syndrome* or *malabsorption syndrome* has been used to describe these diseases. Over the years specific digestive tract disorders have been identified as causes of this *celiac syndrome*. One of these, a specific *gluten-induced enteropathy*, is called *celiac disease*.

Major causes of generalized defects in absorption or digestion are summarized in Table 13–17, where diseases that tend to occur relatively frequently in North America and Europe are separated from less common disorders.

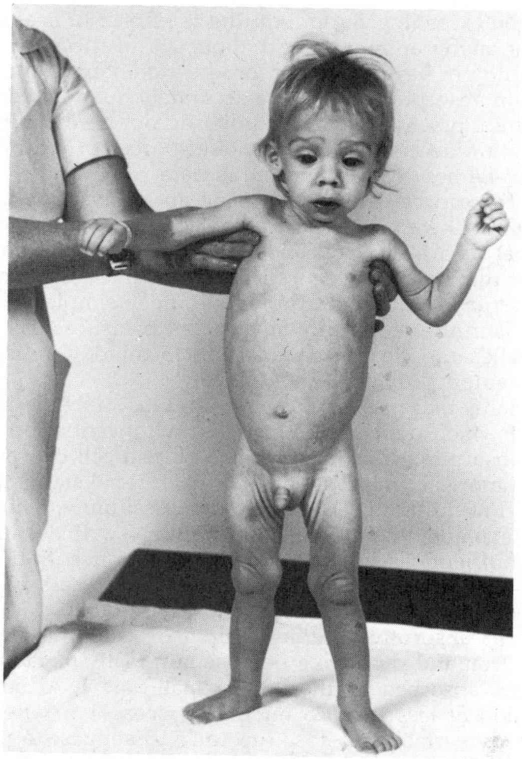

Figure 13–22. An 18-mo-old boy with active celiac disease. Note the loose skin folds, marked proximal muscle wasting, and full abdomen. The child looks ill.

Other congenital disorders have been identified that affect only a single specific intestinal transport process. The clinical features of these diseases often differ from those of the generalized malabsorptive state. Some cause intestinal symptoms, particularly diarrhea, but others may produce only nutritional deficiencies, without gastrointestinal symptoms. In Table 13–18 specific absorptive pathway defects are listed; only some of this latter group cause gastrointestinal symptoms, and all except the acquired disaccharidase deficiencies are rare.

EVALUATION OF PATIENTS SUSPECTED OF HAVING INTESTINAL MALABSORPTION

Many chronic diseases are capable of causing significant malnutrition and growth problems. Children with chronic renal disease or intracranial lesions may develop clinical manifestations very similar to those of children with malabsorptive states. Distinguishing children with true malabsorptive diseases from patients with chronic nonspecific diarrhea or nongastrointestinal diseases causing small stature depends primarily upon clinical findings. Elements in the history and physical examination that help in assessment of many of these entities are presented in this section. More detailed descriptions of specific malabsorptive diseases are presented in subsequent sections.

CLINICAL MANIFESTATIONS. Because many of the gastrointestinal diseases causing malabsorption are genetically determined, the family history may suggest the diagnosis. These inherited disorders usually cause symptoms early in infancy. The onset of symptoms may be triggered by the introduction of a new component to the diet. For example, specific intestinal transport defects affect specific nutrients, and celiac disease is caused by a general response of the mucosa to dietary glutens. Besides the time of onset of symptoms and their relationship to dietary content and intake, some aspects of the history at times offered in great detail have limited value. Descriptions of stools are highly subjective; quantity is of obvious interest, but color, odor, and consistency are of relatively little diagnostic significance. The relationship between diet and diarrhea must be logical to be meaningful; for example, if lactose is responsible for diarrhea, then one lactose-containing food should be as provocative as the next. Because diseases of many systems may produce clinical manifestations such as failure to thrive and abdominal distention suggestive of a malabsorptive state, a complete review of other systems is essential. Disorders of the central nervous system and urinary tract deserve particular attention in this regard.

The impact of symptoms on the child's general health is best assessed in terms of changes in body weight and length. Measurements should be related to earlier measurements and family patterns. Signs of malnutrition such as muscle wasting, edema, mouth sores, smooth tongue, and excessive bruising should be interpreted in the light of estimated nutrient intake. In cases of diarrhea, parents and physicians may limit the child's nutrient intake for prolonged periods, thus inducing malnutrition that may be erroneously assumed to result from malabsorption.

A rectal examination is an important step in the initial examination of children suspected of having intestinal malabsorption. In addition to assessing the anus and rectum, this procedure provides immediate access to stool for gross, microscopic, and, in some cases, chemical analysis. Children with pancreatic insufficiency who are receiving a complete diet will have excessive droplets of fat and undigested meat fibers in their stools; those with intestinal malabsorption will have crystalline aggregates of monoglyceride and fatty acid.

LABORATORY MANIFESTATIONS. Absorptive Function. Fat absorption can be quantitated by a *fecal fat balance* study comparing total losses to estimated dietary fat intake. If the patient is consuming appreciable quantities of fat (>20 g/day) and total collections are carried out for at least 4 days, excretion should not exceed 15% of intake in an infant or 10% in an older child. In the hope of supplanting the unpleasant

TABLE 13–17. Generalized Malabsorptive States in Childhood

Site	More Common	Less Common
Exocrine pancreas	Cystic fibrosis Chronic protein-calorie malnutrition	Shwachman-Diamond syndrome Chronic pancreatitis
Liver, biliary tree	Biliary atresia	Other cholestatic states
Intestine		
Anatomic defects	Massive resection Stagnant loop syndrome	Congenitally short gut
Chronic infection	Giardiasis	Immune deficiency
Others	Celiac disease	Dietary protein intolerance (milk, soy) Tropical sprue Idiopathic diffuse mucosal lesions

TABLE 13–18. Specific Defects of Digestive-Absorptive Function Occurring in Children

	Disease
Intestinal	
Fat	Abetalipoproteinemia
Protein	Enterokinase deficiency
	Amino acid transport defects (cystinuria, Hartnup disease, methionine malabsorption, blue diaper syndrome)
Carbohydrate	Disaccharidase deficiencies (congenital: sucrase-isomaltase, lactase, developmental: lactase, acquired)
	Glucose—galactose malabsorption (congenital, acquired)
Vitamin	Vitamin B_{12} malabsorption (juvenile pernicious anemia, transcobalamin II deficiency, Immerslund syndrome)
	Folic acid malabsorption
Ions, trace elements	Chloride-losing diarrhea
	Congenital sodium diarrhea
	Acrodermatitis enteropathica
	Menkes syndrome
	Vitamin D–dependent rickets
	Primary hypomagnesemia
Drug-induced	Sulfasalazine (folic acid malabsorption)
	Cholestyramine (Ca, fat malabsorption)
	Phenytoin (Dilantin) (Ca malabsorption)
Pancreatic	Specific enzyme deficiencies
	Lipase
	Trypsinogen

task of stool analysis, screening tests have been developed to assess absorption and to detect steatorrhea. The simplest is to measure fasting *serum carotene* concentration. In the presence of adequate dietary intake a result of more than 50 μg/dL suggests fat malabsorption and more than 100 μg/dL normal absorption; however, a significant number of false-positive and negative results occur with this screening test. In skilled hands, stool microscopy to assess directly the fat content of random stools compares favorably with other screening procedures for steatorrhea. ^{14}C-Triolein absorption is another test of fat digestion and pancreatic function. $^{14}CO_2$ is collected in exhaled air and reflects the metabolism of triolein following intestinal absorption.

Carbohydrate absorption cannot be quantitated by simple balance procedures because sugars are broken down in the intestinal lumen by enteric bacteria. No more than a trace of sugar is found in normal stools except for those passed by breast-fed infants. An excess of sugar in fresh stool suggests sugar intolerance, but a lack of excess does not exclude the diagnosis. Random stool samples can be tested for reducing substance quickly and easily using commercially available tablets.* A result of more than 0.5% indicates abnormal absorption if the diet contains significant amounts of a reducing sugar. Most dietary sugars, except for sucrose, are reducing sugars; if sucrose is to be tested, it must first be hydrolyzed by heating the stool sample with HCl. Usually fresh stool of a patient with sugar intolerance will have a pH of less than 6.0 because of the organic acids produced in the lumen by bacterial action on the unabsorbed sugar. A simple noninvasive indirect measure of carbohydrate malabsorption is the *breath hydrogen test. Hydrogen concentrations in expired air* may be measured after an oral dose of sugar (2 g/kg body weight to 50 g maximum). If the sugar being tested is not absorbed in the upper small bowel, it reaches the distal intestine where enteric bacteria act on it to produce hydrogen gas, which is quickly absorbed and expired quantitatively. A rise in breath hydrogen exceeding 20 ppm during the first 2 hr is abnormal. Patients taking antibiotics and about 2% of the normal population do not have hydrogen-producing enteric flora.

Protein absorption cannot be accurately quantitated in routine clinical practice. Balance studies do not necessarily reflect assimilation because of endogenous sources of fecal protein, but *fecal nitrogen* can be measured as a rough guide. *Enteric protein loss* can be quantitated using an intravenous injection of ^{51}CrCl followed by measurement of the fecal excretion of the label in a 4-day collection of stool. A result exceeding 0.8% of the injected dose indicates excessive loss. *Fecal clearance of serum α_1-antitrypsin* provides a much simpler technique for measuring enteric protein loss; as measured on a 48-hr stool collection, clearance exceeding 15 mL/day indicates excessive enteric loss.

Nutrients that may be measured in blood include iron, the level of which depends on transferrin concentration as well as on absorption; folic acid, the red blood cell concentration being a more accurate reflection of nutritional status than the serum concentration; calcium and magnesium; vitamin D and its metabolites; vitamin A; and vitamin B_{12}. If the intake of these nutrients is adequate, decreased concentrations will suggest inadequate absorption. It may take years to deplete stores of vitamin B_{12} after absorption is impaired.

Certain absorptive studies help to localize an intestinal lesion. Iron and *D-xylose*, a pentose minimally metabolized in man, are absorbed by the upper small bowel. A blood concentration of less than 25 mg/dL of xylose 1 hr after a 14.5 g/m² body surface oral dose (up to 25 g) suggests a proximal intestinal mucosal lesion, but some false-negative and false-positive results are obtained using this technique. In the distal bowel, vitamin B_{12} is absorbed and bile salts are reabsorbed. *Vitamin B_{12} absorption* can be measured directly using the *Schilling test*, in which, after body stores of the vitamin are saturated, a tracer dose of radioactive B_{12} is given by mouth, with or without intrinsic factor, and urinary excretion measured over the next 24 hr. Defective absorption in the presence of intrinsic factor, shown by urinary excretion of less than 5% of the dose, occurs when an extensive length of distal ileum is resected or diseased, or when bacterial overgrowth occurs within the bowel lumen.

Diagnostic Procedures. MICROBIOLOGIC. The only common primary infection causing chronic malabsorption is giardiasis (Sec. 12.112). Techniques to fix and stain specimens have greatly improved the diagnostic value of examining stools for *Giardia* cysts. The trophozoite may be identified in fresh duodenal contents or the duodenal mucosa. When enteric clearing of bacteria is impaired, either from stasis of luminal contents or impaired immune function, colony counts from bacterial cultures of proximal intestinal juice may be very high.

HEMATOLOGIC. A hypochromic, microcytic blood smear indicates iron deficiency; a macrocytic smear suggests deficiency and therefore malabsorption of folic acid or of vitamin B_{12}. Acanthocyte transformation of erythrocytes occurs in abetalipoproteinemia. A blood smear may also suggest a lymphocyte defect or a neutropenia associated with Shwachman-Diamond syndrome.

IMAGING PROCEDURES. Used primarily to identify local lesions in the abdomen, these procedures have limited application to the study of children with malabsorptive disorders. *Plain roentgenograms* and *barium contrast* studies may suggest a site and cause of intestinal stasis. For example, the most common anomaly causing incomplete bowel obstruction is intestinal malrotation, a condition difficult to exclude without a barium enema to locate the cecum. The small intestine should be examined with the use of large quantities of nonflocculating barium and only when a localized lesion, not diffuse disease is suspected. Although flocculation of normal

*Clinitest, Ames Co.

barium and dilated bowel with thickened mucosal folds have been attributed to diffuse malabsorptive lesions such as celiac disease, these abnormalities are nonspecific and have little diagnostic value. *Ultrasound* can detect alterations in pancreatic mass, biliary tree abnormalities, and stones, even in infants with malabsorption. *Retrograde studies of the pancreatic and biliary tree* using contrast injection via endoscopy are reserved for rare cases requiring careful delineation of the biliary tree and pancreatic ducts.

SMALL BOWEL BIOPSY. Biopsy of small intestinal mucosa is an important tool in the study of children with malabsorptive states. Now specimens may be obtained either by endoscopy or with a peroral suction instrument. The demonstration of a typical mucosal lesion is a prerequisite for the diagnosis of celiac disease; specific abnormalities are seen in the mucosa of children with abetalipoproteinemia, acrodermatitis enteropathica, eosinophilic gastroenteritis, and congenital villus atrophy. Microscopic abnormalities may also be seen in the mucosa of patients with giardiasis, lymphangiectasia, gamma globulin deficiencies, viral enteritis, tropical sprue, and cow's milk or soy intolerance.

Disaccharidase assays may be carried out on mucosa. If there is diffuse mucosal disease, there will be a generalized depression of the activities of all these enzymes but specific congenital abnormalities may also be detected.

DISEASES CAUSING GENERALIZED MALDIGESTION OR MALABSORPTION

EXOCRINE PANCREATIC INSUFFICIENCY

See Sec. 13.76.

Cystic Fibrosis

See Sec. 14.89.

Shwachman-Diamond Syndrome

(Pancreatic Hypoplasia with Neutropenia)

See Sec. 13.75 and 16.48.

13.50 DIGESTIVE TRACT IN CHRONIC MALNUTRITION

Exocrine pancreatic function is more susceptible to protein-calorie malnutrition than the intestine, and suppression of digestive enzyme secretion may occur relatively early in patients with primary malnutrition (Sec. 13.75). In developed countries where primary malnutrition is rare, chronic gastrointestinal disorders and their treatment are significant causes of malnutrition; undoubtedly, under these circumstances some degree of compromised pancreatic function develops. Children may be particularly at risk because their nutritional reserves are relatively meager. Worldwide, exocrine pancreatic insufficiency is most often attributable to malnutrition, not to a primary pancreatic disease. Because 90% of functioning exocrine tissue must be lost before significant digestive problems develop in patients who are otherwise well, malnutrition is usually severe and prolonged before pancreatic insufficiency causes clinically apparent digestive defects.

The intestine is remarkably resistant to the effects of protein-calorie malnutrition. Patients with *kwashiorkor* may have a severely flattened small intestinal villus structure, but these abnormalities probably are attributable to coexisting infections and infestations. In *marasmus* villus structure is relatively preserved, although microvillus changes and intracellular electron microscopic abnormalities have been observed. Chronic malnutrition can lead to impaired immune function; perhaps as a consequence, bacterial overgrowth of the upper intestine is seen in malnourished subjects (see Sec. 4.15–4.18).

When oral intake is withheld completely in experimental animals, intestinal mucosal mass and absorptive function diminish even when nutrient balance is maintained by the intravenous route. These changes can be reversed by small amounts of oral nutrient. Accordingly, there is a theoretical advantage in delivering nutrients via the gut rather than by vein. Also, because mucosal epithelial repair may be delayed in chronic malnutrition, convalescence from acute self-limited mucosal diseases such as viral enteritis may be prolonged in the malnourished state and shortened when nutrients are adequately provided.

Little is known about the *effect of specific nutritional deficiencies* on the pancreas or intestine; apart from potassium depletion causing ileus and severe dehydration causing constipation, available data suggest a relatively minor clinical effect of a wide range of specific deficiencies. Iron deficiency is associated with enhanced iron uptake at the mucosa and, in a few severe cases, occurrence of mucosal flattening. Deficiencies of vitamin B_{12} and folic acid may cause distortion of enterocyte morphology but no known serious functional abnormalities of the gut. Some hypocalcemic states may be accompanied by steatorrhea and even by ion and water secretion, but this poorly understood relationship is not constant. Vitamin A supplemental (8,000 IU/wk, po) has reduced the risk of death from diarrhea in children in developing countries.

13.51 LIVER AND BILIARY DISORDERS

Fat absorption is impaired whenever bile salt concentration in the duodenal lumen falls below the critical micellar concentration. In children, cholestatic disorders (biliary atresia in particular) deplete duodenal bile salts resulting in steatorrhea that can be severe. Sterols are especially dependent on bile salts for their absorption, thus vitamin D and vitamin E deficiencies are likely to be severe in advanced cholestatic states. Vitamin E malabsorption is an important determinant of the severe neuropathy associated with significant chronic cholestasis.

13.52 INTESTINAL INFECTIONS CAUSING MALABSORPTION

Malabsorption is a rare consequence of primary intestinal infection. Only parasites with a propensity to chronic infestation cause malabsorption in the host who is not immunologically compromised. *Giardia lamblia* infestation is common in children, particularly toddlers, but a very small proportion of the infected patients develop malabsorption (Sec. 12.112). *Coccidiosis* due either to *Isospora belli* or to *I. hominis* in warm climates of the Southern Hemisphere can cause malabsorption and diarrhea (Sec. 12.113). *Intestinal hookworm*, although associated with malabsorption, is not thought to cause it.

13.53 IMMUNODEFICIENCY AND THE INTESTINE

For many years, gastrointestinal symptoms and signs have been known to occur in certain congenital immunodeficiency states. Increased survival of children with malignant disease, increased use of effective immunosuppressive and myelotoxic therapies, and the global epidemic of AIDS are contributing to the rising incidence of immune deficient children and related gastrointestinal manifestations. The mechanisms for disturbed intestinal function in these children is not clear; however, the immune system contributes significantly to the intestinal barrier that protects the internal milieu from noxious enteric microbes and dietary antigens. Anorexia, diarrhea, and undernutrition are common and often serious problems in these patients, and microorganisms, both pathogenic opportunistic and nonpathogenic in the conventional sense, have an important part in causing these disabling symptoms.

Congenital Deficiencies

CONGENITAL SEX-LINKED PANHYPOGAMMAGLOBULINEMIA (BRUTON). Mild intermittent diarrhea begins early and improves after 2 yr of age. Giardiasis and chronic enteroviral infections are common. Colitic symptoms are rare, but crypt abscesses may be seen in rectal biopsies.

IgA DEFICIENCY. The most common congenital immunodeficiency, isolated IgA deficiency, is associated with gastrointestinal symptoms infrequently. Inflammatory bowel disease, nodular lymphoid hyperplasia, and celiac disease are more common in these patients than in the general population. *Giardia* infection is also relatively frequent.

COMBINED IMMUNODEFICIENCY. Severe diarrhea and malabsorption contribute to the high mortality in this group of disorders. Because these children are so sick and must be protected from ambient flora, it has been very difficult to determine the nature of their intestinal lesions. In the small intestine there is partial villus atrophy; PAS-positive macrophages are seen in the lamina propria, and diasaccharidase activities are diminished. A range of organisms can be isolated from the stools of these babies; they may harbor rotavirus for months.

NEUTROPENIA AND NEUTROPHIL DYSFUNCTION. A congenital deficiency of effective neutrophils predisposes children to at least 2 different types of gastrointestinal disorders. In patients with neutropenia, necrotizing enterocolitis may be the cause of fever and right lower quadrant pain and tenderness. This serious problem, which carries a high mortality, is also known as typhlitis; the lesion occurs most often in the lower ileum, cecum, and proximal colon where vascular compromise, mucosal ulceration, and perforation develop. A relationship of this enteropathy to *Clostridium difficile* has been postulated in some cases. In patients with chronic granulomatous disease, phagocytic function is impaired and granulomas may develop throughout the intestine, causing diarrhea and malabsorption. These granulomas, characterized by giant cells and lipid-containing histiocytes, frequently obstruct the gastric antrum.

Acquired Immunodeficiency

Whether the cause is human immunodeficiency virus (HIV), immunosuppressive therapy, or extreme disability, the immunocompromised child is susceptible to a spectrum of diseases of the alimentary tract, extending from the mouth to the anus. In general, symptoms can be traced to microorganisms, some of which are not considered to be serious pathogens in immunocompetent individuals. Clinical descriptions to date have focused on AIDS and on bone marrow transplant recipients.

In patients with AIDS, oral and esophageal lesions can be due to Candida causing typical adherent, plaque lesions; herpes simplex or cytomegalovirus causing ulceration; or Epstein-Barr virus causing hairy leukoplakia. Similar lesions are seen in other severely immunocompromised children. Potential enteric pathogens have been isolated from 55% of a series of patients with AIDS and 40% of patients with bone marrow transplants. In the former group, *C. albicans*, cytomegalovirus, *Blastocystis hominis*, *C. difficile*, *Cryptosporidium*, and *Campylobacter* were found most frequently. In the latter group, *C. difficile*, adenovirus, and rotavirus were the common pathogens found in stool. Diarrhea resulting from these infections in a patient with acquired immunodeficiency tends to persist and can be life-threatening. The offending organisms rarely clear spontaneously, and they are not amenable to direct therapy if the host remains immunosuppressed. An HIV enteropathy, with HIV DNA in the enterocyte, produces weight loss and diarrhea independent of other microbial agents.

13.54 IMMUNOPROLIFERATIVE SMALL INTESTINAL DISEASE

Initially manifesting as intermittent diarrhea in 10- to 30-yr-old males and females in developing countries, this process may progress to a high-grade small intestinal lymphoma.

EPIDEMIOLOGY. Immunoproliferative small intestinal disease is endemic in the Mediterranean basin, the Mideast, Far East, and Africa. Poverty and frequent episodes of gastroenteritis during infancy are antecedent social and medical problems. Sporadic cases occur in Europe and North or South America, predominantly in immigrants from developing countries, although occasionally in native citizens.

PATHOLOGY. Early lesions demonstrate thickened mucosal folds, duodenal or jejunal nodularity, and lymphoplasmacytic infiltrates. The process may be patchy but progresses to diffuse lymphohistiocytic nodules, mesenteric lymph node involvement, the presence of Reed-Sternberg–like cells, and eventually the development of an immunoblastic lymphoma. This process represents an IgA lymphoproliferative disorder progressing to a B cell lymphoma.

CLINICAL MANIFESTATIONS. Initially, patients have intermittent diarrhea and abdominal pain. Later stages demonstrate persistent chronic diarrhea, malabsorption, weight loss, digital clubbing, and growth failure.

DIAGNOSIS. Endoscopic biopsies of multiple duodenal and jejunal mucosal sites aid in the diagnosis. In addition, a serum marker (α heavy chain paraprotein) of IgA is present in most cases. *Giardia lamblia* may also be present but is not responsible for the lymphoproliferative disorder.

TREATMENT. The earliest lesions respond to prolonged (~6 mo) tetracycline therapy. Prelymphomatous stages may be treated with cyclophosphamide with or without prednisone and tetracycline. Lymphomas are treated with a combination of cyclophosphamide, doxorubicin, teniposide, prednisone with or without bleomycin, and vinblastine.

PROGNOSIS. Early therapy of antibiotic responsive lesions produces an excellent outcome. Treatment of the later lymphomatous lesions has resulted in a variable but usually poor outcome.

Khojasteh A, Haghighi P: Immunoproliferative small intestinal disease: Portrait of a potentially preventable cancer from the Third World. Am J Med 89:483, 1990.

13.55 STAGNANT LOOP SYNDROME

(Blind Loop Syndrome: Bacterial Overgrowth Syndrome)

These terms describe a condition associated with stasis of small intestinal contents, particularly in the upper regions. Incomplete bowel obstruction, congenital (malrotation with duodenal bands, stenosis, or a diverticulum) or acquired (postoperative intestinal adhesions, longstanding Crohn disease), impairs intestinal motility or causes loss of the normal intestinal mucosal barrier to microorganisms allowing enteric bacteria to colonize the upper small bowel. These bacteria deconjugate bile salts, which leads to inefficient intraluminal processing of dietary fat and to steatorrhea; they bind vitamin

B_{12}, interfering with its absorption; and they may damage the microvillus brush border membrane, diminishing disaccharidase activities.

In addition to symptoms of chronic incomplete bowel obstruction such as distention, pain, and vomiting, the patient may have pale, foul, bulky stools typical of steatorrhea, a megaloblastic anemia from vitamin B_{12} deficiency, or diarrhea from disaccharidase deficiency. Clinical manifestations often do not suggest chronic intestinal obstruction, but laboratory investigations find the aforementioned functional abnormalities, as well as bacterial colonization of the upper intestine and deconjugated bile salts in the upper intestinal juice after a fatty meal. Barium contrast roentgenograms may reveal neither the existence nor cause of obstruction.

Oral administration of an antimicrobial such as trimethoprim-sulfamethoxazole may be sufficient to control the problem temporarily. Definitive therapy can involve operative correction of incomplete bowel obstruction.

13.56 SHORT BOWEL SYNDROME

Short bowel syndrome is a disorder of malabsorption and malnutrition following congenital or postnatal loss of a substantial amount of small intestine, with or without loss of some large intestine.

CONGENITAL. Congenital shortness of the small bowel has been associated with intestinal malrotation, gastroschisis, and, in some cases, atresia. When the anomaly is severe, diarrhea and malabsorption begin at birth. Barium studies show a malrotated colon and a very short small bowel, in which villus structure is relatively mature. If the infant survives the early months, intestinal function improves in later years.

MASSIVE INTESTINAL RESECTION. Acute illnesses sometimes necessitate removal of large portions of the small intestine. The newborn period is particularly hazardous in this regard. Postnatal volvulus and necrotizing enterocolitis are common causes of massive intestinal resection. In young infants intestinal reserves permit loss of the colon or of short segments of small intestine, but problems in maintaining fluid and nutrient balance should be anticipated if more than 25% of the 200–300 cm of the newborn infant's small bowel is removed. Spontaneous improvement in absorptive and digestive function in the young infant can be expected over a period of at least 2 yr after intestinal resection.

In general, loss of distal small bowel is more serious than loss of the proximal segment. The jejunum is relatively incapable of compensating for ileal loss because the ileum is the sole site for absorption of bile salts and is therefore essential to the normal process of fat absorption. Preservation of the ileocecal sphincter is advantageous to infants who have had extensive bowel resections; the sphincter impedes retrograde flow of colonic flora and prolongs contact of nutrients with the mucosa of the remaining small bowel. Intestinal adaptation has been observed after 2 yr of total parenteral nutrition in infants with as little as 11–15 cm of jejunoileum with an intact ileocecal valve and with 25–30 cm without an ileocecal valve.

After massive resection, gastric acidity and retrograde bacterial contamination of the intestinal lumen may compromise absorptive function. Hyperacidity is usually transient under these circumstances. If the terminal ileum is resected, excessive bile salt losses lead to malabsorption of dietary fats and fat-soluble vitamins. Bile salts reaching the colon may also provoke increased water and electrolyte secretion. If resection includes mid and distal jejunum as well as ileum, the patient may be unable to maintain positive fluid balance. Hyperoxaluria can occur after distal small bowel resections in which the colon is preserved, but resultant nephrolithiasis is rare during early childhood. Cell-mediated immunity is normal, but circulating immunoglobulin concentrations may be reduced after massive resection.

Often oral feeding is not well tolerated for weeks after resection because of excessive stool volume but the patient can be supported by intravenous nutrition. The diet to be offered depends on the patient's age and functional deficit. Initially, liquids or liquid formulas should be isotonic and given in frequent small amounts. Constant intragastric infusion may result in greater net fluid retention than bolus feedings in the infant with an extensive resection. Excessive water intake should be avoided, particularly at times when solids are being taken. When there is severe steatorrhea, long-chain fats should be restricted and medium-chain triglycerides should be substituted. Initially, dietary glucose may be better tolerated than disaccharides, but the concentration should not exceed 5 g/dL in order to maintain relative isotonicity of the feeding. Fructose, which is passively absorbed, can be given if glucose malabsorption is present. Vitamin supplements are usually needed, and serum concentrations of calcium, magnesium, potassium, and phosphorus should be monitored and supplements given as required. If a large portion of the ileum is resected, monthly injections of 100 μg of vitamin B_{12} must be given for life, but it usually takes 2 yr or more for a deficiency to develop in the face of a severe absorptive defect. Large doses of vitamin D may be necessary to prevent rickets. Prothrombin time should also be monitored as a basis for vitamin K supplementation.

Antidiarrheal agents are rarely helpful in the management of massive bowel resection. Cholestyramine may reduce fecal water and sodium losses in infants with relatively short ileal resections by binding bile acids before they reach the colon, but if ileal resection is massive and steatorrhea is severe, cholestyramine is likely to aggravate the problem. Theoretically, antacids should benefit infants with hyperacidity, but their value in this situation is unproved. Patients with bacterial contamination and stagnant loop syndrome will derive temporary benefits from oral antibiotics, but they may require additional surgery.

Successful management of young infants after massive resection requires a coordinated team approach, often over a lengthy period. Along with the essential measures to maintain nutrient intake a concerted effort should be made to encourage mother-child bonding and to stimulate development. Studies suggest impressive preservation of intellectual function even in the most severely affected patients with early profound, prolonged malnutrition. The causes of death in patients with short bowel syndrome relate to complications of hyperalimentation and include cirrhosis, hepatic failure, and catheter-related sepsis. Small bowel transplantation is an experimental procedure that requires further experience.

13.57 CELIAC DISEASE (GLUTEN-SENSITIVE ENTEROPATHY)

This disease, a permanent intestinal intolerance to gliadin, causes severe small intestinal mucosal lesions in susceptible individuals. The incidence ranges from 1:300 (Western Ireland) to 1:5,000 (Sweden) live births. The cereals wheat, rye, and barley are toxic for patients with celiac disease. Debate persists over the toxicity of oats, which if injurious, appears to be less potent than the others. Rice and maize are nontoxic.

ETIOLOGY AND EPIDEMIOLOGY. The gliadin fraction of wheat and the prolamin fractions of the other grains are injurious to these patients. Genetic and environmental factors probably determine susceptibility. Latent gluten-sensitive enteropathy may be activated by a 2nd insult. As many as 70%

but not all monozygotic twins are concordant. Overt disease develops in 2–3% of 1st-degree relatives, whereas 10% have asymptomatic villous atrophy. The disease is associated with class I HLA antigen B8 and class II HLA antigens DR3, DR7, DQ, W2, and DR4. Eighty to 90% of patients are HLA-B8 positive. Breast-feeding appears to lower the risk for celiac disease and delay the onset of symptoms. In contrast, enteric infection with human adenovirus 12, which has a 12 amino acid sequence homology with gliadin, may trigger the disease in a susceptible host. Recent apparent decreases in prevalence may be attributable to an increase in breast-feeding and changes in wheat antigenicity.

The mechanism by which gliadin damages the small intestine is unknown, but both cellular and cell-mediated immune responses are stimulated. A glutamine, glutamate, proline-rich subfraction of molecular weight of less than 1,500 daltons is the most toxic peptide of gliadin. IgA antigliadin (AGA) and less so antireticulin or antimysium antibodies are reliable indicators of sensitization to gluten. Whether abnormalities of gliadin peptide metabolism play a role remains to be determined. Gluten-sensitive enteropathy is also evident in dermatitis herpetiformis, as determined by villus flattening and the presence of AGA.

CLINICAL MANIFESTATIONS. The clinical features of celiac disease range from generalized severe intestinal malabsorption to normal or near normal health. Major manifestations are summarized in Table 13–19. The typical patient develops irritability, anorexia, and chronic diarrhea late in the 1st yr. The stools are pale and foul, the child underweight and perhaps short, with wasted muscles, particularly in the proximal groups. In older infants with active disease, dental enamal hypoplasia is common. Additional physical signs may include mouth sores, a smooth tongue, excessive bruising, finger clubbing, and peripheral edema. However, the range of clinical findings among patients with celiac disease is extraordinarily wide. At least 30% of patients are neither irritable nor anorexic; as many have problems with vomiting as with diarrhea, and some are constipated. The most constant features are decreased rates of weight gain and linear growth, which may persist without obvious gastrointestinal symptoms. Some patients who apparently have the same disease remain well throughout infancy to develop typical symptoms as older children or adults.

LABORATORY MANIFESTATIONS. Anemia is common; usually the patient is iron deficient, but blood folate levels may also be low. Vitamin B_{12} deficiency is seen only in severe, longstanding disease. Hypoalbuminemia and reduced circulating gamma globulin levels may result from poor intake, reduced absorption, and excessive loss. Selective IgA deficiency and insulin-dependent diabetes mellitus are associated with celiac disease. In contrast with adult cases, the incidence of atopy is not increased with childhood celiac disease.

TABLE 13–19. Active Childhood Celiac Disease—42 Cases

Symptoms	No. of Patients
Failure to thrive	36
Diarrhea	30
Irritability	30
Vomiting	24
Anorexia	24
Foul stools	21
Abdominal pain	8
Excessive appetite	6
Rectal prolapse	3
Signs	**No. of Patients**
Height <25th percentile	30
Body weight <25th percentile	37
Wasted muscles	40
Abdominal distention	33
Edema	14
Finger clubbing	11

Most affected children eating significant amounts of fat have steatorrhea. A 4-day balance study usually finds fat excretion exceeding 10% of dietary intake. Stool microscopy usually reveals an excess of crystalline aggregates of fatty acid. There may also be reduced fasting serum carotene levels (<50 μg/dL), low serum 25-OH-vitamin D, calcium, and vitamin A levels, and prolonged prothrombin times. On the other hand, these latter measurements may be normal in patients with proven celiac disease.

Reflecting diffuse small bowel mucosal damage, blood xylose concentration does not exceed 25 mg/dL after an oral load in children with active celiac disease, but false-negative and false-positive results are sufficiently common to make these tests unreliable. Tests to access the permeability of the small intestinal wall based on the absorption of two nonmetabolized sugars, one a small molecule (mannitol or rhamnose) and the other larger (lactulose), have been found abnormal in celiac disease, but they lack specificity.

The measurement of serum antibodies to gliadin has had wide application. IgG antibodies are sensitive but they lack specificity; IgA antibodies are less sensitive but are more specific for untreated celiac disease, whereas antireticulin antibodies are specific, yet not sufficiently sensitive.

In barium contrast studies the small bowel is usually diffusely dilated, and the mucosal folds are coarse. Because these findings are nonspecific and inconsistent, roentgenograms are not indicated in the diagnostic evaluation of a suspected case unless a localized lesion is suspected. Bone films often show osteoporosis, but rickets is rare. Diagnosis requires intestinal mucosal biopsy.

PATHOLOGY. The diffuse lesion of the upper small intestinal mucosa that characterizes celiac disease is seen in a peroral suction biopsy specimen. Short, flat villi, deepened crypts, and irregular vacuolated surface epithelium with lymphocytes in the epithelial layer are seen by light microscopy. Similar abnormalities occur in other conditions but none is likely to be confused with celiac disease. Infections such as rotavirus enteritis, *Giardia lamblia*, or tropical sprue can cause villus flattening and elongated crypts but not the marked abnormalities of enterocytes. A flat mucosa occurs in kwashiorkor but may represent a response to infestation rather than to undernutrition. Tropical sprue, a poorly understood tropical enteropathy, can cause a lesion that is indistinguishable from that of celiac disease. Some cases of cow's milk protein or soy protein intolerance are associated with lesions similar to those of celiac disease in children. In immune deficiency and eosinophilic gastroenteritis, villi can be partially shortened. Infants with familial enteropathy have short villi, but the crypt dimensions are normal.

DIAGNOSIS. This is based on finding the characteristic duodenal or jejunal mucosal lesion in a mucosal suction biopsy; on a clinical and laboratory response to a gluten-free diet; and on the reappearance of the lesion after gluten challenge. The final test may not be appropriate in some patients because of the risk from exacerbation of the disease. No gluten challenge should be made until at least 2 yr after therapy has been started, to allow for mucosal healing. It should be noted that once the mucosa has healed, moderate quantities (1–2 slices of bread/day) can be taken for months by many children with true celiac disease without symptoms occurring. It may take 2 yr for the mucosal lesion to reappear.

Children on a Gluten-Free Diet in Whom the Diagnosis of Celiac Disease Has Not Been Proved. If a child improves after a gluten-free diet is begun without a diagnosis proved by biopsy, the question arises whether improvement was spontaneous or a response to therapy. The child can be returned to a full gluten-containing diet, and the response can be observed. If celiac disease seems a possible diagnosis, a peroral intestinal biopsy can be done when symptoms of malabsorption develop or when 2 yr have passed, at which time the diagnosis can be based on the development of a typical mucosal lesion. AGA and antireticulin antibody tests have proved useful in detecting true celiac disease in this situation. If the initial illness strongly suggests celiac disease, a gluten challenge can be deferred until the patient is at least 4 yr old when a challenge roughly equivalent to one slice of bread/day is usually tolerated without severe symptoms.

TREATMENT. All wheat, rye, and barley should be eliminated from the diet; many patients tolerate small quantities of oats. Although disaccharidase activities in the mucosa are diminished during active celiac disease, significant disaccharide intolerance is rare. A few patients who have definite lactase deficiency will benefit from a short period of disaccharide restriction. During the early months of therapy extra fat-soluble vitamins are advisable, and for those who are iron- or folate-deficient appropriate supplements should be given. Lifelong dietary treatment is a major undertaking and best carried out with the help of an experienced nutritionist and ample written instructions and recipes.

PROGNOSIS. The clinical response to a gluten-free diet of a child with celiac disease is gratifying. Improvement of mood and appetite is followed by lessening of diarrhea. In most cases changes occur within 1 wk of starting therapy, but the response may occasionally be delayed. Older patients and very ill patients tend to respond slowly, but once in remission the celiac child should be treated as a well child. During preadolescence and adolescence, children with proven celiac disease seem to tolerate considerable quantities of dietary gluten without symptoms although the typical abnormalities reappear in their mucosa. No complications from long-term gluten-free diet treatment are recognized. In adult patients the incidence of intestinal malignancy (lymphoma, adenocarcinoma) is higher than in the normal population; the scant data available do not indicate that dietary therapy prevents the development of malignancy. Additional rare complications include toxic hepatitis, neuropathies, arthritis, and uveitis.

J. RICHARD HAMILTON

13.58 POSTENTERITIS SYNDROMES

Most episodes of infectious diarrhea last for less than 1 wk. Persistent or chronic diarrhea may be caused by many factors. The definition of persistent (chronic) diarrhea is based on continued stool output (increased frequency, increased fluidity, greater than 30 g/kg/24 hr) and duration, which varies among studies from 2–4 wk. Postenteritis syndromes may have serious consequences among malnourished infants or may be confused with a benign self-limiting illness known as nonspecific diarrhea of infancy (toddler diarrhea).

13.59 CHRONIC PERSISTENT DIARRHEA

Diarrhea that persists for more than 2 wk after an apparent episode of infectious gastroenteritis occurs in 10–20% of children less than 5 yr of age in the developing world. In developed countries this may evolve into the syndrome of intractable diarrhea of infancy (see Sec. 13.60). Patients at risk in developed countries include low-birthweight infants, immigrants, those with failure to thrive, and those less than 3 mo of age with repeated episodes of diarrhea. In most infants, there is no other identifiable primary cause of diarrhea (ulcerative colitis, persistent infection, celiac disease) or malabsorption (cystic fibrosis, celiac disease). Furthermore, the initiating infectious agent may no longer be isolated from the stool, suggesting that secondary pathophysiologic mechanisms have become important in the continuation of the diarrhea.

ETIOLOGY. Acute infectious gastroenteritis usually produces a self-limited, transient, subclinical mucosal injury characterized by minimal or no protein malabsorption, mild fat malabsorption, and mild-to-moderate carbohydrate malabsorption. The latter usually affects lactose digestion, but if the gastroenteritis is severe and prolonged, there may be monosaccharide (glucose) malabsorption. If diarrhea persists for more than 2 wk and exceeds 50 g/kg/24 hr nitrogen, fat absorption usually decreases to 50%, and carbohydrate (monosaccharides and disaccharides) absorption is further impaired.

Identifiable risk factors for persistent diarrhea among children in developing countries include low birthweight, malnutrition (reduced weight for length), blood or mucus in the diarrhea, anorexia, vitamin A deficiency, other concurrent infections (lower respiratory tract), absence of breast-feeding, repeated episodes of diarrhea in children under 6 mo of age, prior antibiotic use, and various acute infectious agents such as enteropathogenic *E. coli, Salmonella, Campylobacter jejuni,* possibly *Shigella,* and rotavirus infection in infants less than 3 mo of age. The secondary immunodeficiency state associated with malnutrition may increase the potential for multiple episodes of infectious diarrhea, while the altered gut motility and local immunodeficiency predispose to bacterial overgrowth in the small intestine. The latter may exacerbate intestinal injury by direct bacterial invasion, by the effects of toxin production, or by bacterial deconjugation of bile salts. Milk protein allergy may also contribute to the initiation or prolongation of chronic intestinal injury and subsequent persistent diarrhea.

An additional risk factor associated with repeated episodes of diarrhea is the method of treatment. Protocols that call for prolonged periods of intravenous rehydration rather than early oral rehydration and subsequent slow introduction of milk may contribute to the underlying malnutrition and intestinal mucosal atrophy. Early introduction of milk may be beneficial by providing a high-calorie intake and by providing local intestinal nutrients that can reverse mucosal atrophy by stimulating intestinal villous growth.

CLINICAL MANIFESTATIONS. Chronic postinfectious diarrhea in developing countries affects males and females equally and has a peak incidence at 2 yr of age. The diarrhea persists more than 2 wk and is associated with weight loss, malabsorption, the onset or worsening of malnutrition, anorexia, and secondary infections. Prior to the episode, the child either has no diarrhea or has recovered from a previous episode of diarrhea with a normal bowel pattern intervening between episodes. If diarrhea persists for more than 1 mo and malnutrition continues, the mortality is high, especially in infants less than 1 yr of age.

DIAGNOSIS. The differential diagnosis includes *G. lamblia,* milk protein allergy, AIDS, ulcerative colitis, pseudomembranous colitis, acrodermatitis enteropathica, primary immunodeficiency syndromes, secondary or primary disaccharidase deficiencies, celiac disease, Schwachman syndrome, ganglioneuroma or other vasoactive-secreting tumors, intestinal lymphangiectasia, immunoproliferative small intestinal disease, and congenital chloride or sodium losing diarrhea. Many of these other causes of chronic diarrhea can be distinguished from chronic persistent diarrhea on the basis of history, physical, or screening laboratory examinations.

Laboratory studies include a stool culture and examination for ova and parasites. At the time of presentation there may be secondary deficits in fat and carbohydrate absorption detected by increased stool fat excretion and the presence of stool-reducing substances in an acidic diarrhea fluid, respectively. Additional tests should be based on the results of screening tests and on any suspicion of a primary disorder (sweat test: cystic fibrosis; serum zinc level: acrodermatitis enteropathica).

TREATMENT. Rehydration, correction of electrolyte and acid base disturbances, and provision of nutrition are the essential components of the therapy of chronic persistent diarrhea in developing countries. Many infants are not as dehydrated as they are malnourished, and nutritional rehabilitation should be started as soon as possible.

If oral alimentation is not possible owing to anorexia, emesis, or severe debilitation, intravenous nutrition should be provided. Oral alimentation should be started as soon as possible to provide local and systemic nutrients to reverse mucosal atrophy and malnutrition (see Sec. 4.15).

Identifiable infections should be treated when appropriate. If small intestinal bacterial overgrowth is suspected, a combination of oral gentamicin (3 days) and cholestyramine (5 days) may be effective (see Sec. 13.60).

PREVENTION. Breast-feeding should be encouraged in an attempt to reduce the incidence of chronic persistent diarrhea in developing countries.

If diarrhea develops, the child should be rehydrated rapidly with either intravenous fluids or, preferentially, oral rehydration solutions. Once rehydrated, early feeding with milk should be instituted. Breast milk or lactose-containing formula may be offered first. However, if carbohydrate intolerance exacerbates stool losses and dehydration, a non–lactose-containing formula should be substituted. Most infants have a subclinical lactose malabsorption with the 1st episode of diarrhea. This transient lactose malabsorption is usually of little clinical significance, because many infants will demonstrate adequate fluid status and weight gain on a lactose-containing formula despite a small increase in stool volume.

13.60 INTRACTABLE DIARRHEA OF INFANCY

Intractable diarrhea of infancy is defined by greater than 5 diarrhea stools/24 hr lasting more than 2 wk with the onset in infants less than 3 mo of age. The precipitating cause of diarrhea is usually unknown. Identifiable initiating events include gastrointestinal infectious agents (rotavirus, *Shigella*, *Salmonella*, enteropathogenic *E. coli*), nongastrointestinal infections (urinary tract, pneumonia), malabsorption syndromes (primary or secondary, monosaccharidase or disaccharidase deficiency, cystic fibrosis), milk protein intolerance, and adrenal insufficiency. Occasionally, a familial inflammatory autoimmune enteropathy unassociated with prior infection is the cause of chronic intractable diarrhea. *Familial enteropathy* with congenital microvillus atrophy, but no autoimmune features, presents at birth with global malabsorption, diarrhea, and severe malnutrition. This condition may be due to a defect in intestinal epithelial renewal. In contrast to celiac disease, there is little epithelial cell mitosis seen on intestinal biopsy.

Intractable diarrhea of infancy may be similar to the postenteritis chronic persistent diarrhea in the developing world. Intractable diarrhea of infancy may be seen in both developed and developing countries and is associated in both locations with small intestine mucosal injury, malabsorption, and malnutrition.

PATHOPHYSIOLOGY. A vicious circle develops in patients with intractable diarrhea of infancy that is similar to that for chronic persistent diarrhea in children in developing countries. An infant with marginal to poor nutritional status has an unidentified small intestinal mucosal injury leading to malabsorption, dehydration, secondary immunodeficiency, and, if treated with parenteral fluids, mucosal atrophy. Malnutrition, systemic or intestinal infection (small intestinal bacterial overgrowth), and absent enteral nutrients contribute to poor mucosal repair and continued villus flattening. Villus atrophy further compromises intestinal absorptive capacity leading to carbohydrate (monosaccharides and disaccharides) malabsorption and osmotic diarrhea. Milk protein allergy may initiate or contribute to the persistence of the mucosal injury. Mucosal injury may predispose to absorption of nondigested, whole foreign proteins, which may contribute to the local intestinal inflammatory (immunologic) response.

All cases have varying degrees of subtotal to total villus atrophy and nonspecific enterocolitis. Bacterial overgrowth in the small intestine is a secondary phenomenon, whereas inflammatory cells are present in patients with milk protein allergy or postinfectious diarrhea. Inflammation, autoantibodies to intestinal epithelial cells, and subtotal villus atrophy are noted in the rare disorder of familial autoimmune enteropathy. Patients with *congenital microvillus atrophy* demonstrate intracellular inclusions of microvillus structures in epithelial cells, suggesting that there is a defect in brush-border assembly and differentiation.

CLINICAL MANIFESTATIONS. Chronic intractable diarrhea for more than 2 wk produces severe loss of subcutaneous adipose tissue, weight loss, wasting of the extremities, and a marasmus-like appearance. The infant is not always severely dehydrated. The tongue may demonstrate flat filiform papillae. There may be hepatomegaly, splenomegaly, and skin manifestations of chronic malnutrition.

Laboratory studies may reveal anemia, electrolyte abnormalities, a metabolic acidosis, hypoalbuminemia, and evidence of vitamin A or K (rarely vitamin D) deficiency.

If left untreated, the infants develop varying stages of protein-energy malnutrition and secondary antibody and cellular immunodeficiencies and die of systemic bacterial infection (pneumonia, sepsis).

DIFFERENTIAL DIAGNOSIS. The differential diagnosis includes conditions that may initiate intractable diarrhea of infancy and those diseases that may mimic this disorder. Disorders associated with villus atrophy include infectious gastroenteritis, postantibiotic diarrhea, allergic milk protein enteropathy, secondary disaccharidase and monosaccharidase malabsorption, celiac disease, dermatitis herpetiformis, Hirschsprung disease, primary immunodeficiency syndromes, AIDS, and prior malnutrition. Disorders associated with persistent secretory diarrhea include vasoactive hormone secreting tumors (VIP-oma, neuroblastoma, ganglioneuroma), bacterial toxins *(E. coli, V. cholerae)*, and congenital familial chloride diarrhea. Metabolic conditions that may cause chronic diarrhea include acrodermatitis enteropathica, abetalipoproteinemia, Wolman disease, adrenogenital syndrome, hyperthyroidism, hypoparathyroidism, Hartnup disease, and niacin deficiency (pellagra). Pancreatic insufficiency (cystic fibrosis, Shwachman syndrome) and anatomic conditions (short bowel syndrome, Hirschsprung disease, malrotation, gastroschisis, lymphangiectasia) usually have other more apparent manifestations in addition to chronic diarrhea.

DIAGNOSIS. Patients with intractable diarrhea of infancy should have an initial laboratory evaluation that includes serum electrolytes, a complete blood count, stool (or blood) culture, stool-reducing substances, pH, and examination for ova and parasites, urinalysis, and abdominal roentgenograms. Subsequently, a sweat chloride, D-xylose test, and examination for immunodeficiency should be considered. A small, and possibly large, bowel biopsy performed by endoscopic examination is an important diagnostic procedure to determine the presence of primary diseases and secondary mucosal villus atrophy.

TREATMENT. Initial management includes correction of dehydration and acidosis, preferably by oral rehydration solutions. If oral therapy is not possible (e.g., because of emesis), intravenous rehydration and total parenteral nutrition should be provided until oral alimentation is feasible. Oral nutrition should be started as soon as possible to reverse the longstanding mucosal atrophy and systemic malnutrition. Resting the bowel with no oral feeding perpetuates mucosal atrophy and does not affect intestinal healing.

Early continuous nasogastric tube feeding with human milk or an elemental, isotonic formula has been successful in improving weight gain and shortening the period of diarrhea. Such elemental formulas contain glucose polymers, casein hydrolysates, and a combination of medium- and long-chain triglycerides. Underlying vitamin deficiencies require treatment, as does persistent acidosis (with oral sodium bicarbonate) and hypoalbuminemia (< 2.0 g/dL use intravenous albumin).

Treatment related problems are most commonly associated with total parenteral alimentation and include sepsis, mechanical problems of the central venous catheter, continued mucosal atrophy, and liver damage (cholestatic jaundice).

Antidiarrheal antimotility agents are not indicated. Antibiotics are not needed unless a bacterial overgrowth syndrome is suspected. Oral gentamicin (50 mg/kg/24 hr every 4 hr for 3 days) and oral cholestyramine (1 g every 6 hr for 5 days) are effective therapy of small intestinal bacterial overgrowth syndrome.

Specific initiating factors require individualized therapy. Familial autoimmune enteropathy has responded to prolonged corticosteroid or cyclosporine therapy. Nonautoimmune enteropathy requires prolonged TPN and may respond partially to long-term corticosteroid therapy. Vasoactive-secreting tumors may require resection or therapy with long-acting somatostatin analogs.

PROGNOSIS. Untreated intractable diarrhea of infancy has a 45–55% mortality. TPN and early continued elemental formula improve the chances of survival. The more chronic intractable cases that do not respond to this therapy may be rare consequences of intestinal inflammatory enteropathy, secretory diarrhea, inborn errors of metabolism, or other less common causes of chronic diarrhea.

13.61 CHRONIC NONSPECIFIC DIARRHEA: TODDLER DIARRHEA

Probably not a postenteritis syndrome, chronic nonspecific diarrhea (toddler diarrhea) is more likely an early manifestation of irritable bowel or recurrent abdominal pain syndrome.

CLINICAL MANIFESTATIONS. The patient is a healthy, usually thriving child, with 3–10 loose bowel movements (usually less than 5) per 24 hr. Males exceed females by 2:1. The onset is between 6 and 30 mo of age with spontaneous resolution by 40–50 mo of age. The diarrhea is characterized by loose, brown, watery, non–foul-smelling movements without stool blood, leukocytes, or eosinophils. When fecal blood is present, it is associated with rectal fissures or perianal excoriations, which are common. The stool contains mucus, undigested vegetable fibers, and starch granules. There is no evidence of malabsorption. The child is not adversely affected by the diarrhea, and there is no associated failure to thrive, dehydration, and electrolyte or acid-base disturbances.

PATHOPHYSIOLOGY. This syndrome may be due to enhanced intestinal autonomic reaction to stress in a vulnerable colon. The association of this syndrome and the irritable bowel or recurrent pain syndrome in families suggests a hereditary tendency. Rather than stress-induced autonomic dysfunction, the syndromes may be due to innate abnormalities in the regulation of colonic fluid resorbing capacity, pressure generation, and motility. One possible theory suggests that a rapid colonic transit time and failure to relax the rectum prevents the final desiccation of feces with resultant expulsion of watery diarrhea. The frequent gross visible appearance of undigested vegetables in the stool probably represents a rapid transit time not permitting the usual colonic bacterial digestion of plant fiber that is not digested by the human intestine. A previous history of infantile colic may be present in 40–50% of older children with irritable bowel–toddler diarrhea syndrome.

Secondary dietary factors may be important in initiating and prolonging the chronic diarrhea state. Parents frequently change formula and often increase total fluid intake, while reducing milk intake due to a belief that the diarrhea is a reflection of milk intolerance or that milk exacerbates intestinal injury. This type of diet greatly reduces fat intake, which may increase an already rapid intestinal transport time. Furthermore, the intake of very large amounts of fruit juices containing sucrose and sorbitol may produce an osmotic component to the diarrhea. Nonetheless, carbohydrate malabsorption is not the primary cause of toddler diarrhea.

DIFFERENTIAL DIAGNOSIS. The other primary and secondary causes of chronic diarrhea discussed in Sec. 13.59 and 13.60 should be considered. In chronic nonspecific (toddler) diarrhea–irritable bowel syndrome, there is no weight loss, malnutrition, malabsorption, or dehydration. Furthermore, the diarrhea starts after 6 mo of age, and there may be a family history in siblings or parents of a functional bowel syndrome.

Cystic fibrosis, celiac disease, primary carbohydrate malabsorption, bacterial (*Salmonella, Shigella, Yersinia, Campylobacter*) and parasitic (*G. lamblia*) gastrointestinal infections, and inflammatory bowel disease are usually obvious from careful history and physical examinations. A healthy child, without weight loss between 6 and 30 mo of age, with less than five watery brown stools per 24 hr, containing visibly undigested vegetable food particles most likely has chronic nonspecific diarrhea. If weight loss is present in patients with toddler diarrhea, it is probably due to parental restriction of calories in an attempt to treat the child.

Laboratory tests fail to reveal anemia, hypoproteinemia, hypocarotenemia, or acidosis, and stools usually do not contain blood, white blood cells, eosinophils, reducing substances, or a low pH. The ESR and peripheral white blood cell count, stool culture, and stool ova and parasite examination are normal.

TREATMENT. Reassuring the parents that the child has a benign self-limited, albeit disturbing condition, is essential. The child's diet should not be restricted and the parents' unrealistic dietary beliefs should be corrected to ensure a nutritionally normal diet for age, without excessive fruit juice and water intake or unnecessary restriction of milk or milk products. Because cold food may exacerbate an irritable bowel syndrome, these foods should be used cautiously.

Antispasmodic agents and antidiarrhea agents (kaolin, pectin) are not helpful. Methylcellulose, due to its hydrophilic properties, may give cohesiveness to loose stools and reduce cramping. Psyllium is also effective and is given for 2 wk at a dose of 2–3 g twice a day; a positive response may require longer therapy. Salicylate, loperamide, and cholestyramine have been used with variable results.

PROGNOSIS. Toddler diarrhea is characterized by recurrent episodes with spontaneous resolution of diarrhea by 40–50 mo of age. Many of these children develop episodes of recurrent abdominal pain or irritable bowel syndrome as adolescents. In this older age group, abdominal pain and cramps are more common than diarrhea.

ROBERT M. KLIEGMAN

13.62 OTHER MALABSORPTIVE SYNDROMES

TROPICAL SPRUE. This syndrome is confined to certain tropical regions; it occurs in some Caribbean countries but not Jamaica, in northern regions of Africa, and parts of Asia. Of unknown cause, it affects adults and children. It is characterized by generalized malabsorption associated with a diffuse lesion of the small intestinal mucosa.

Clinical Manifestations. Fever and malaise precede the onset of watery diarrhea. In a few days, acute features subside and chronic malabsorption, intermittent diarrhea, and anorexia lead eventually to severe malnutrition. Signs of malnutrition may include night blindness, glossitis, stomatitis, cheilosis, cutaneous and mucosal pigmentation, and edema. Muscle wasting is marked, and the abdomen is often distended.

Laboratory Studies. These studies usually demonstrate malabsorption of fat, sugars, and vitamin B_{12}. Biopsies of the small intestinal mucosa show varying degrees of villus shortening, increased crypt depth, round cell infiltration of the lamina propria, and irregularity and mild shortening of the surface epithelial cells. These pathologic changes are nonspecific and in their mild form are seen in healthy people in the same communities.

Treatment. Antidiarrheal agents, nutritional supplements (folic acid and vitamin B_{12}), and oral administration of broad spectrum antibiotics usually lead to rapid improvement of the intestinal lesion. This response to treatment suggests that enteric flora are involved in the pathogenesis of this syndrome.

WHIPPLE SYNDROME. This rare disease has been reported only once in a child. The disease involves many organ systems; the small intestine is always affected, and malabsorption results. Common findings are arthralgia, fever, and polyserositis. Duodenal biopsy shows focal accumulation of PAS-positive macrophages, and bacilli that may be causative are seen in the lamina propria. Antibiotics produce dramatic improvement, but long-term therapy is necessary.

INTESTINAL LYMPHANGIECTASIA. This congenital generalized defect of the lymphatic system can involve the intestine extensively, causing steatorrhea, protein-losing enteropathy, edema, and lymphocytopenia. Usually, there is slight if any disturbance of bowel habit, and edema is the major clinical manifestation. Absorptive function, except for long-chain fats and fat-soluble vitamins, is usually intact. Reduction of dietary fats may reduce enteric protein loss; medium-chain triglycerides can be substituted in the diet because they are transported by the portal stream.

Other causes of protein-losing enteropathy include celiac disease, allergic enteropathies, cystic fibrosis, graft-versus-host disease, inflammatory bowel disease, vasculitis, small intestinal lymphoma, heart failure, constrictive pericarditis, scleroderma, AIDS, intestinal tuberculosis, venous obstruction, trypsinogen and enterokinase deficiencies, and some parasites.

The *diagnosis* of protein-losing enteropathy is based on quantitation of fecal α_1-antitrypsin levels. This protein of molecular weight of about 50,000 daltons is found predominantly in serum. With increased intestinal protein loses, α_1-antitrypsin leaks into the bowel and is resistant to the proteolytic effects of human digestive enzymes and colonic bacteria. Fecal α_1-antitrypsin levels are therefore a sensitive marker for protein-losing enteropathy. Normal fecal levels in older children are approximately 1 mg/g of dry stool.

WOLMAN DISEASE. This rare lethal lipidosis leads to lipid accumulation in many organs including the small intestine. In addition to vomiting and hepatosplenomegaly there may be steatorrhea as the result of lymphatic obstruction (Sec. 8.18).

MALABSORPTION SYNDROMES

General Reviews

Ament ME: Malabsorption syndromes in infancy and childhood. J Pediatr 81:685, 1972.

Anderson CM: Malabsorption in children. Clin Gastroenterol 6:355, 1977.

Hamilton JR: Diarrhea and malabsorption in children. *In*: Sleisinger MH, Fordtran JS (eds): Gastrointestinal Disease, 2nd ed. Philadelphia, WB Saunders, 1978, p 336.

Wilson FA, Dietschy JM: Differential diagnostic approach to clinical problems of malabsorption. Gastroenterology 61:911, 1971.

Diagnostic Investigations

Ament ME, Berquist WE, Vargus J, et al: Fiberoptic upper endoscopy in infants and children. Pediatr Clin North Am 35:141, 1988.

Barr RG, Perman JA, Schoeller DA, et al: Breath tests in pediatric gastrointestinal disorders: New diagnostic opportunities. Pediatrics 62:393, 1978.

Cobden I, Pothwell J, Axon ATR: Intestinal permeability and screening tests for coeliac disease. Gut 21:512, 1980.

Ghesh SK, Littlewood JM, Goddard D, et al: Stool microscopy in screening for steatorrhea. J Clin Pathol 30:749, 1977.

Hill RE, Cutz E, Cherian G, et al: An evaluation of D-xylose absorption measurements in children suspected of having small intestinal disease. J Pediatr 99:245, 1981.

Hill RE, Hercz A, Corey MD, et al: Fecal clearance of alpha-1-antitrypsin: A reliable measure of protein loss in children. J Pediatr 99:416, 1981.

Katz AJ, Grand RJ: All that flattens is not sprue. Gastroenterology 76:375, 1979.

Murphy MS, Eastham EJ, Nelson R, et al: Non-invasive assessment of intraluminal lipolysis using a $^{13}CO_2$ breath test. Arch Dis Child 65:574, 1990.

Riddlesherger MM: Evaluation of the gastrointestinal tract in the child: CT, MRI, and isotopic studies. Pediatr Clin North Am 35:281, 1988.

Rossi T: Endoscopic examination of the colon in infancy and childhood. Pediatr Clin North Am 35:331, 1988.

Schmerling DH, Farrer JCW, Prader A: Fecal fat and nitrogen in healthy children and in children with malabsorption or maldigestion. Pediatrics 46:690, 1970.

DIGESTIVE TRACT IN CHRONIC MALNUTRITION

Brunser O: Effects of malnutrition on intestinal structure and function in children. Clin Gastroenterol 6:341, 1977.

Durie PR, Forstner GG, Gaskin KJ, et al: Elevated serum immunoreactive pancreatic cationic trypsinogen in acute malnutrition: Evidence of pancreatic damage. J Pediatr 106:233, 1985.

Romer H, Cerbach R, Gomez MA, et al: Moderate and severe protein-energy malnutrition in childhood: Effects on jejunal mucosal morphology and disaccharidase activities. J Pediatr Gastroenterol Nutr 2:459, 1983.

LIVER AND BILIARY DISORDERS

Atkinson M, Nordin BEC, Sherlock S: Malabsorption and bone disease in prolonged obstructive jaundice. QJ Med 25:299, 1956.

Hadorn B, Hess J, Troesch V, et al: Role of bile acids in the activation of trypsinogen by enterokinase: Disturbance of trypsinogen activation in patients with intrahepatic biliary atresia. Gastroenterology 66:548, 1974.

Kooh SW, Jones G, Reilly BJ, et al: Pathogenesis of rickets in chronic hepatobiliary disease in children. J Pediatr 94:870, 1979.

SHORT SMALL INTESTINE

Bohane TD, Haka-Ikse K, Biggar WD, et al: A clinical study of young infants after small intestinal resection. J Pediatr 94:552, 1979.

Caniano DA, Kanoti GA: Newborns with massive intestinal loss: Difficult choices. N Engl J Med 318:703, 1988.

Grant D, Wall W, Mimeault R, et al: Successful small-bowel/liver transplantation. Lancet 335:181, 1990.

Hamilton JR, Reilly BJ, Morecki R: Short small intestine associated with malrotation. A newly described cause of intestinal malabsorption. Gastroenterology 56:124, 1969.

Wilmore DW: Factors correlating with a successful outcome following extensive intestinal resection in newborn infants. J Pediatr 80:88, 1972.

Young WF, Swain VAJ, Pringle EM: Long term prognosis after major resection of small bowel in early infancy. Arch Dis Child 44:465, 1969.

STAGNANT LOOP SYNDROME

Bayes BJ, Hamilton JR: Blind loop syndrome in children. Acta Dis Child 44:76, 1969.

Gracey M: Intestinal microflora and bacterial overgrowth in early life. J Pediatr Gastroenterol Nutr 1:13, 1982.

Soderlund S: Anomalies of midgut rotation and fixation: Clinical aspects based on sixty-two cases in childhood. Acta Pediatr 51:135, 1966.

INFECTIONS CAUSING MALABSORPTION

Ament ME: Diagnosis and treatment of giardiasis. J Pediatr 80:663, 1972.
Liebman WM, Thaler MM, Dehorimier A, et al: Intractable diarrhea of infancy due to intestinal coccidiosis. Gastroenterology 78:579, 1980.

IMMUNODEFICIENCY STATES AND THE INTESTINE

Ament ME: Immunodeficiency syndromes and gastrointestinal disease. Pediatr Clin North Am 22:807, 1975.
Glover MT, Atherton DJ, Levinsky RJ: Syndrome of erythroderma, failure to thrive and diarrhea in infancy: A manifestation of immunodeficiency. Pediatrics 81:66, 1988.
Kotler DP, Francisco A, Clayton F, et al: Small intestinal injury and parasitic diseases in AIDS. Ann Intern Med 113:444, 1990.
Weikel CS, Gaynes BN, Roche JK: Diarrheal disease in the immunocompromised host. *In*: Guerrant R (ed): Ballière's Clinical Tropical Medicine and Communicable Diseases, Vol 3, p 401. London, Ballière Tindall, 1988.

CELIAC DISEASE

O'Mahony S, Vestey JP, Ferguson A: Similarities in intestinal humoral immunity in dermatitis herpetiformis without enteropathy and in coeliac disease. Lancet 335:1487, 1990.
Report to Working Group of European Society of Paediatric Gastroenterology and Nutrition: Revised criteria for diagnosis of coeliac disease. Arch Dis Child 65:909, 1990.
Rich EJ, Christie DL: Anti-gliadin antibody panel and xylose absorption test in screening for celiac disease. J Pediatr Gastroenterol Nutr 10:174, 1990.
Swinson CM, Slavin G, Coles EC, et al: Coeliac disease and malignancy. Lancet 1:111, 1983.
Valletta EA, Trevisiol D, Mastella G: IgA anti-gliadin antibodies in the monitoring of gluten challenge in celiac disease. J Pediatr Gastroenterol Nutr 10:169, 1990.
Yolken RH, Bishop CA, Townsend TR, et al: Infectious gastroenteritis in bone-marrow transplant recipients. N Engl J Med 306:1009, 1982.

POSTENTERITIS SYNDROMES

Ament ME: Management of chronic diarrhea with parenteral nutrition and enteral infusion techniques. Pediatrics 14:53, 1985.
Anonymous: Chronic diarrhea in children: A nutritional disease. Lancet 1:143, 1987.
Avery GB, Villavicencio O, Lilly JR, et al: Intractable diarrhea in early infancy. Pediatrics 41:712, 1968.
Bezerra JA, Duncan B, Udall J: Dietary management of acute diarrhea: Fast or feed. Intern Pediatr 5:30, 1990.
Bowie MD: Antibiotics and cholestyramine in the treatment of persistent diarrhea in infants. J Pediatr Gastroenterol Nutr 8:425, 1989.
Coulthard M, Searle J, Patrick M, et al: Cyclosporine-responsive enteropathy and protracted diarrhea. J Pediatr Gastroenterol Nutr 10:257, 1990.
Cutz E, Rhoads JM, Drumm B, et al: Microvillus inclusion disease: An inherited defect of brush border assembly and differentiation. N Engl J Med 320:646, 1989.
Hill ID, Mann MD, Med M, et al: Use of oral gentamicin, metronidazole, and cholestyramine in the treatment of severe persistent diarrhea in infants. Pediatrics 77:477, 1986.
Househam KC, Bowie DC, Mann MD, et al: Factors influencing the duration of acute diarrheal disease in infancy. J Pediatr Gastroenterol Nutr 10:37, 1990.
Larcher VF, Shepard R, Francis DEM, et al: Protracted diarrhea in infancy. Arch Dis Child 52:597, 1977.
Orenstein SR: Enteral versus parenteral therapy for intractable diarrhea of infancy: A prospective, randomized trial. J Pediatr 109:277, 1986.
Phillips AD, Jenkins P, Raafat T, et al: Congenital microvillus atrophy: Specific diagnostic features. Arch Dis Child 60:135, 1985.
Shahid NS, Sack DA, Rahman M, et al: Risk factors for persistent diarrhea. Br Med J 297:1036, 1988.

TROPICAL SPRUE

Klipstein FA, Baker SJ: Regarding the definition of tropical sprue. Gastroenterology 58:717, 1970.
Santiago-Borrero PJ, Maldonado N, Horta E: Tropical sprue in children. J Pediatr 76:470, 1970.

WHIPPLE DISEASE

Aust CH, Smith EB: Whipple's disease in a 3-month old infant. Am J Clin Pathol 37:66, 1962.

INTESTINAL LYMPHANGIECTASIA

Strober W, Wochner RD, Carbone PP, et al: Intestinal lymphangiectasia: A protein-losing enteropathy with hypogammaglobulinemia, lymphocytopenia and impaired homograft rejection. J Clin Invest 46:1643, 1967.
Vardy PA, Lebenthal E, Shwachman H: Intestinal lymphangiectasis: A reappraisal. Pediatrics 55:842, 1975.

WOLMAN DISEASE

Queloz JM, Capitanio MA, Kirkpatrick JA: Wolman's disease. Radiology 104:357, 1972.

DEFECTS OF SPECIFIC ENZYMES OR TRANSPORT PROCESSES INVOLVED IN DIGESTION OR ABSORPTION

13.63 ENZYME DEFICIENCIES

Enterokinase Deficiency

Congenital deficiency of this small-intestinal enzyme has been reported in a few children. The disease results in a complete absence of pancreatic proteolytic activity since enterokinase is an essential activator of pancreatic trypsinogens. Affected patients are ill from very early life with severe diarrhea and failure to thrive. Hypoproteinemia is common and may lead to edema. In duodenal fluid tryptic activity is missing while lipase and amylase are normal; in vitro tryptic activity of the fluid can be restored by the addition of enterokinase. Malabsorption of protein is the major defect, although mild steatorrhea has been reported. Pancreatic enzyme replacements restore normal digestive function.

Disaccharidase Deficiencies

The disaccharidases are located on the brush border membrane surface of the small bowel. Occasionally, congenital deficiencies occur, but abnormal disaccharidase activities have most often been the result of diffuse lesions of the intestinal epithelium, such as those of infection or celiac disease.

The response of the patient to significant disaccharidase deficiency (disaccharide intolerance) is similar whatever its cause or the enzymes involved. If disaccharide hydrolysis at the brush border is incomplete, the sugar accumulates in the distal intestinal lumen, where organic acids and hydrogen gas are produced by bacteria. The excess intraluminal sugar and organic acids draw water into the lumen, leading to watery osmotic diarrhea with stools that are frothy, of low pH (pH <6.0), that contain excess sugar, and tend to excoriate the buttocks. There may be bloating and borborygmi, but steatorrhea is rare. In some cases, particularly those beyond infancy, gas production causing crampy abdominal pain is the dominant problem, rather than diarrhea.

If the disaccharide involved is a reducing sugar (e.g., lactose), the standard Clinitest examination* will be 1+ or greater in most cases. Disaccharidase activities can be assayed in mucosal biopsy specimens. Breath hydrogen excretion after an oral sugar load is a useful noninvasive technique for detecting disaccharide intolerance (Sec. 13.49).

LACTASE DEFICIENCY. *Congenital* absence of lactase has been reported in very few cases. The usual mechanism for primary lactose intolerance relates to the *developmental* pattern of lactase activity. Because lactase activity rises relatively late in fetal life and begins to fall after the age of 3 yr, intolerance to lactose can be anticipated in very premature infants and in some older children and adults. Approximately 15% of adult whites, 40% of adult Orientals, and 85% of adult blacks in the United States are deficient in intestinal lactase. Since lactase activity in the mucosa is at best marginal, this enzyme is particularly likely to be depleted *secondary to diffuse mucosal diseases*.

---

*Ames Company.

Symptoms occur in response to ingestion of lactose, the sugar in milk. Explosive watery diarrhea is associated with abdominal distention, borborygmi, flatulence, and an excoriated diaper area. A syndrome of recurrent, vague, crampy abdominal pain has also been attributed to lactose intolerance. School- and preschool-aged children develop episodic mid-abdominal pain. Usually, their general health is unaffected, and there is no obvious temporal relationship of pain to milk ingestion or to diarrhea. (See also Sec. 13.49.)

Treatment consists of removal of milk from the diet. In most cases the elimination need not be total; stopping milk ingestion as a beverage is important. A lactase preparation is available for many children; when added to milk, it allows asymptomatic consumption of modest quantities of milk incubated with the added enzyme.

SUCRASE-ISOMALTASE DEFICIENCY. The only relatively common congenital deficiency of disaccharidase activities, a combined deficiency of sucrase and isomaltase, is inherited as an autosomal recessive trait and occurs in about 0.8% of North Americans. Symptoms usually begin when a sucrose-containing diet is started. There may be intolerance to starch, but because isomaltase acts only on the branch points of the starch molecule, isomaltase deficiency itself is relatively asymptomatic. The symptoms are bloating, watery diarrhea, and excoriation of buttocks. Recurrent abdominal pain has not been attributed to sucrose-isomaltose intolerance. Because sucrose is not a reducing sugar, its presence will not be detected in stool by Clinitest unless the specimen is first hydrolyzed with HCl. The morphology of the small-intestinal mucosa is normal, but enzyme assays show specific deficiencies of sucrase and isomaltase with normal levels of lactase and maltase. Breath testing usually demonstrates increased H_2 after sucrose ingestion. Affected patients improve quickly after dietary sucrose is reduced to minimal amounts.

13.64 DEFECTS OF ABSORPTION OR TRANSPORT

GLUCOSE-GALACTOSE MALABSORPTION. This rare congenital defect in brush border membrane glucose and in galactose Na^+-dependent cotransport is inherited as an autosomal recessive trait. It also affects renal tubular epithelium to a mild degree. Severe diffuse mucosal damage, particularly in a young infant, may also impair the glucose-galactose carrier sufficiently to cause intolerance to these sugars. Usually, if mucosal damage is severe enough to impair glucose transport, other absorptive processes are affected.

The symptomatic response to sugar ingestion is similar whether the defect is congenital or secondary. Watery stools follow the ingestion of glucose, breast milk, or conventional formulas because most diet sugars are polysaccharides or disaccharides with glucose or galactose moieties. The patient may be bloated, and, if diarrhea persists, dehydration and acidosis can be severe. The stools are acidic and contain sugar. Patients with the congenital defect tolerate fructose; their small bowel function and structure are normal in all other aspects.

Treatment consists of rigorous restriction of glucose and galactose and provision of a fructose-containing formula. Later in life limited amounts of glucose or sucrose may be tolerated.

ABETALIPOPROTEINEMIA (BASSEN-KORNZWEIG SYNDROME) (See also Sec. 8.34). This rare autosomal recessive disorder is characterized by steatorrhea, acanthocytosis, atypical retinitis pigmentosa, and diffuse disturbances of the central nervous system. A congenital defect in lipoprotein metabolism causes β-lipoprotein deficiency and abolishes the main route for triglyceride transport from the intestine and liver via chylomicrons.

These patients fail to thrive during the 1st year when stools are pale, foul, and bulky. The abdomen is distended, and deep tendon reflexes are absent. Intellectual development tends to be slow. After 10 yr of age, intestinal symptoms are less severe, ataxia develops, and there is a loss of position and vibration senses and the onset of intention tremors. These latter symptoms reflect involvement of the posterior columns, cerebellum, and basal ganglia. In adolescence, an atypical retinitis pigmentosa develops.

Diagnosis rests on finding acanthocytes in the peripheral blood, and very low plasma levels of cholesterol (< 50 mg/dL). Chylomicrons and VLDL are not detectable, and the LDL fraction is virtually absent from the circulation; there is marked triglyceride accumulation in villus enterocytes in the fasting duodenal mucosa. Usually, there is steatorrhea in younger patients, but other processes of assimilation are intact.

Specific therapy is not available. Large supplements of the fat-soluble vitamins A, D, E, and K should be given. Vitamin E (100 mg/kg/24 hr) and vitamin A (10,000–25,000 IU/day) may arrest the neurologic degeneration. Limiting long-chain fat intake may alleviate intestinal symptoms; medium-chain triglycerides can be used to supplement the fat intake.

HOMOZYGOUS HYPOBETALIPOPROTEINEMIA. This disorder is transmitted as an autosomal dominant trait; the homozygous form is indistinguishable from a β-lipoproteinemia. However, the parents of these patients, as heterozygotes, have reduced plasma LDL and apoprotein-β concentrations, unlike the parents of patients with β-lipoproteinemia who have normal levels.

CHYLOMICRON RETENTION DISEASE. In this rare recessive disorder, the processes leading up to the release of chylomicrons from enterocytes appear to be defective. These patients have severe intestinal symptoms with steatorrhea and failure to thrive. Acanthocytosis is rare, and neurologic manifestations are less severe than those observed in a β-lipoproteinemia. Plasma cholesterol levels are reduced, but moderately so (< 75 mg/dL), fasting triglycerides are normal, but the fat-soluble vitamins, particularly A and E, rapidly deplete. Early aggressive therapy with fat-soluble vitamins is indicated, as for a β-lipoproteinemia.

AMINO ACID TRANSPORT DEFECTS. In several of the specific congenital disorders of amino acid transport (Chapter 8) defective intestinal amino acid transport occurs. Amino acid uptake into the intestinal mucosa is defective in *cystinuria,* but these patients have no gastrointestinal symptoms. In *Hartnup disease* malabsorption of tryptophan leads to ataxia, intellectual deterioration, a pellagra-like skin rash, and at times diarrhea. *Methionine malabsorption* is associated with episodes of diarrhea in fair-complexioned, retarded children whose urine has a sweet odor and contains excess α-hydroxybutyric acid. In the *blue diaper syndrome* tryptophan absorption is defective.

VITAMIN B_{12} MALABSORPTION. Several rare congenital defects may affect assimilation of vitamin B_{12}. In *juvenile pernicious anemia* intrinsic factor production in the stomach is defective. Vitamin B_{12} malabsorption results, leading to megaloblastic anemia and growth failure. Gastric structure and function are otherwise normal.

Transcobalamin II deficiency is an inherited defect of a protein necessary for intestinal transport of vitamin B_{12}. The result is severe megaloblastic anemia, diarrhea, and vomiting.

Imerslund has described patients in whom ileal absorption of vitamin B_{12} is defective. Ileal structure and function are otherwise normal. Megaloblastic anemia develops toward the end of the 1st yr. Proteinuria is commonly associated.

Treatment of these disorders is to administer vitamin B_{12} by injection: 1,000 μg/wk for transcobalamin II deficiency, 100 μg/mo for the others.

CONGENITAL MALABSORPTION OF FOLIC ACID. A

few patients have had folic acid deficiency in infancy as the result of a specific defect in folic acid assimilation. In addition to megaloblastic anemia, they have had cerebral degeneration.

CHLORIDE-LOSING DIARRHEA. This rare specific congenital defect of ileal chloride transport is associated with maternal polyhydramnios. The dominant symptom is severe watery diarrhea beginning at birth, the result of accumulation of chloride ion in the intestinal lumen. Watery diarrhea leads to dehydration and a severe electrolyte disturbance characterized by hypokalemia, hypochloremia, and alkalosis, a most unusual pattern for a child with chronic diarrhea. Other aspects of intestinal absorption are normal. Stools contain chloride in excess of the sum of sodium and potassium. There is no adequate treatment. Potassium supplements and some restriction of chloride intake are advisable.

CONGENITAL SODIUM DIARRHEA. Two patients have been described with profuse watery diarrhea from birth. There was maternal polyhydramnios and neonatal abdominal distention; however, unlike chloride diarrhea, there was acidosis and fecal Cl^- concentration less than Na^+. Treatment with oral hydration solution was effective in maintaining normal growth. The apparent basis for this rare syndrome is a defect in Na^+/H^+ exchange in the small intestine and colon.

VITAMIN D–DEPENDENT RICKETS. In this autosomal recessive disorder a specific defect in the metabolism of vitamin D causes malabsorption of calcium (Sec. 24.62). Intestinal function is otherwise normal.

PRIMARY HYPOMAGNESEMIA. This specific intestinal transport defect in magnesium transport causes severe hypomagnesemia and, secondarily, hypocalcemic tetany in infancy. Other aspects of intestinal function are normal. The findings are reversed by large supplements of magnesium, which must be continued indefinitely.

ACRODERMATITIS ENTEROPATHICA. See also Sec. 23.13. This unusual constellation of clinical findings is due to zinc deficiency secondary to zinc malabsorption. Early in life the patient develops rashes around mucocutaneous junctions and on the extremities; alopecia, chronic diarrhea, and sometimes steatorrhea may occur. Untreated, the patient fails to thrive. Serum zinc concentration and alkaline phosphatase activity are low. Intestinal mucosal biopsies show Paneth cell inclusions that disappear after treatment. An oral supplement of zinc sulfate heptahydrate, 150 mg/24 hr, causes rapid healing of the skin lesions and improvement of diarrhea.

MENKES (KINKY HAIR) SYNDROME. This rare recessively inherited disorder is characterized by growth retardation, abnormal hair, cerebellar degeneration, and early death (Sec. 20.66). Its pathogenesis is unclear, but there is a widespread defect in cellular copper transport that affects the intestine as well as other tissues. Serum copper and ceruloplasmin levels are low, but cellular copper content is increased.

BILE ACID MALABSORPTION. Cases of primary bile acid malabsorption causing diarrhea and steatorrhea from early infancy have occurred. These patients have severe growth retardation and massive steatorrhea based on an apparent congenital defect in ileal bile salt transport.

DRUG-INDUCED ABSORPTIVE DEFECTS. Some drugs have a diffuse impact on the small intestinal epithelium. For example, methotrexate can cause arrest of enterocyte mitoses and result in a mucosal lesion; large doses of neomycin also affect mucosal structure. *Sulfasalazine* interferes with folic acid absorption. *Cholestyramine* binds bile salts and calcium in the intestinal lumen to cause hypocalcemia and steatorrhea. *Phenytoin* interferes with calcium absorption and can cause rickets.

DEFECTS OF ABSORPTION OR TRANSPORT

Isselbacher KJ, Scheig R, Plotkin GR, et al: Congenital β-lipoprotein deficiency: An heredity disorder involving a defect in the absorption and transport of lipids. Medicine 43:437, 1964.

Levy E, Chouraqui JP, Ray CC: Steatorrhea and disorders of chylomicron synthesis and secretion. Pediatr Clin North Am 35:53, 1988.

Muller DPR, Lloyd JK, Bird AC: Long-term management of abetalipoproteinemia. Arch Dis Child 52:209, 1977.

Scott BB, Miller JP, Losowsky MS: Hypobetalipoproteinemia: A variant of the Bassen-Kornzweig syndrome. Gut 20:163, 1979.

ENTEROKINASE DEFICIENCY

Hadorn B, Tarlow M, Lloyd JD, et al: Intestinal enterokinase deficiency. Lancet 1:812, 1969.

AMINO ACID TRANSPORT DEFECTS

Drummond KN, Michael AF, Ulstrom RA, et al: The blue diaper syndrome: Familial hypercalcemia with nephrocalcinosis and indicanuria. Am J Med 37:928, 1964.

Hooft G, Timmermand J, Snoeck J, et al: Methionine malabsorption syndrome. Ann Pediatr 205:73, 1965.

Milne MD: Hartnup disease. Biochemistry 111:3, 1969.

Morin CL, Thompson MW, Jackson SH, et al: Biochemical and genetic studies in cystinuria: Observations on double heterozygotes of genotype I/II. J Clin Invest 50:1961, 1971.

Whelan DT, Scriver CR: Hyperdibasicaminoaciduria: An inherited disorder of amino acid transport. Pediatr Res 2:525, 1968.

DISACCHARIDASE DEFICIENCIES

Ament ME, Perera DR, Esther L: Sucrase-isomaltase deficiency: A frequently misdiagnosed disease. J Pediatr 83:721, 1973.

Flats G: The genetics of lactose digestion in humans. Adv Hum Genet 16:1, 1987.

Harrison M, Walker-Smith JA: Reinvestigation of lactose intolerant children: Lack of correlation between continuing lactose intolerance and small intestinal morphology, disaccharidase activity and lactose tests. Gut 18:48, 1977.

Lifshitz F: Carbohydrate problems in paediatric gastroenterology. Clin Gastroenterol 6:415, 1977.

Semensa G, Auricchio S: Small intestinal disaccharidases. *In*: Scriver CS, Beaudet AL, Sly WS, et al (eds): The Metabolic Basis of Inherited Disease. New York, McGraw-Hill, 1989, p 2975.

GLUCOSE-GALACTOSE MALABSORPTION

Evans L, Grasset E, Heyman M, et al: Congenital selective malabsorption of glucose and galactose. J Pediatr Gastroenterol Nutr 4:878, 1985.

Fairclough PD, Clark ML, Dawson AM, et al: Absorption of glucose and maltose in congenital glucose-galactose malabsorption. Pediatr Res 12:1112, 1978.

Lindqvist B, Meeuwisse GW, Melin K: Glucose-galactose malabsorption. Lancet 2:666, 1962.

VITAMIN B_{12} MALABSORPTION

Chanarin I: Disorders of vitamin absorption. Clin Gastroenterol 11:73, 1982.

Hall CA: Congenital disorders of vitamin B_{12} transport and their contribution to concepts. Gastroenterology 65:684, 1973.

Hitzig WH, Dohmann V, Pluss HJ, et al: Hereditary transcobalamin II deficiency: Clinical findings in a new family. J Pediatr 85:622, 1974.

Imerslund O: Idiopathic chronic megaloblastic anaemia in children. Acta Paediatr (Suppl) 49:119, 1960.

MacKenzie IL, Donaldson RM, Trier JS, et al: Ileal mucosa in familial selective vitamin B_{12} malabsorption. N Engl J Med 286:1021, 1972.

FOLATE MALABSORPTION

Poncz M, Colman N, Herbert V, et al: Congenital folate malabsorption. J Pediatr 99:828, 1981.

Urbach J, Abrahamov A, Grossowicz N: Congenital isolated folic acid malabsorption. Arch Dis Child 62:78, 1987.

CHLORIDE-LOSING DIARRHEA

Bieberdorf FA, Gorden P, Fordtran JS: Pathogenesis of congenital alkalosis with diarrhea: Implications for the physiology of normal ileal electrolyte absorption and secretion. J Clin Invest 51:1958, 1972.

Holmberg C, Perheentupa J, Launiala K, et al: Congenital chloride diarrhea. Arch Dis Child 52:255, 1977.

CONGENITAL SODIUM DIARRHEA

Booth IW, Murer H, Strange G, et al: Defective jejunal brush border Na^+/H^+ exchange: A cause of congenital secretory diarrhea. Lancet 1:1066, 1985.

Holmberg C, Perheentupa J: Congenital Na^+ diarrhea: A new type of secretory diarrhea. J Pediatr 106:56, 1985.

VITAMIN D–DEPENDENT RICKETS

Hamilton R, Harrison J, Fraser D, et al: The small intestine in vitamin D dependent rickets. Pediatrics 45:364, 1970.

PRIMARY HYPOMAGNESEMIA

Paunier L, Radde IC, Kooh SW, et al: Primary hypomagnesemia with secondary hypocalcemia in an infant. Pediatrics 41:385, 1968.
Stromme JH, Nesbakken R, Normann T, et al: Familial hypomagnesemia. Acta Paediatr Scand 58:433, 1969.

ACRODERMATITIS ENTEROPATHICA

Bohane TD, Cutz E, Hamilton JR, et al: Acrodermatitis enteropathica, zinc and the Paneth cell. Gastroenterology 73:587, 1977.
Moynahan EJ: Acrodermatitis enteropathica: A lethal inherited human zinc-deficiency disorder. Lancet 2:399, 1974.

MENKES SYNDROME

Danks DM: Of mice and men, metals and mutations. J Med Genet 23:99, 1986.
Danks DM, Stevens BJ, Campbell PE, et al: Menkes' kinky-hair syndrome. Lancet 1:110, 1972.

PRIMARY BILE ACID MALABSORPTION

Heubi JE, Balistreri WF, Fondacaro JD, et al: Primary bile acid malabsorption: Defective in vitro ileal active bile acid transport. Gastroenterology 83:804, 1982.

DRUG-INDUCED MALABSORPTION

Franklin JL, Rosenberg HH: Impaired folic acid absorption in inflammatory bowel disease: Effects of salicylazosulfapyridine (Azulfidine). Gastroenterology 64:517, 1973.
Morijiri Y, et al: Factors causing rickets in institutionalized handicapped children on anti-convulsant therapy. Arch Dis Child 56:446, 1981.
Rogers AL, Vloedman DA, Bloom EC, et al: Neomycin-induced steatorrhea. JAMA 197:185, 1966.
Trier JS: Morphologic alterations induced by methotrexate in the mucosa of human proximal intestine. I: Serial observations by light microscopy. Gastroenterology 42:295, 1962.

13.65 RECURRENT ABDOMINAL PAIN
(Irritable Bowel Syndrome)

A common perplexing problem, particularly among teenagers and preadolescents, is abdominal pain that recurs, sometimes over an extended period. In children less than 2 yr of age, the cause is usually organic. In all cases the patient is experiencing real pain, but in older children a specific disease process is identified in fewer than 10% of patients. Ten to 15% of school-aged children are subject to recurrent attacks of abdominal pain, the origin of which is unknown. This section deals with those cases, in the majority of which no specific disease is found. Because possible mechanisms for abdominal pain are numerous and incompletely understood, the investigation and treatment of these cases are often difficult, testing not only the physicians' scientific acumen but also their skill in practicing the art of medicine. The temptation is to "overdo" the testing and the treatment when reliance on a careful clinical evaluation is the most important first step toward resolution of the problem.

ETIOLOGY. A wide range of specific lesions affecting the genitourinary or gastrointestinal tract, and disorders of the metabolic, cardiac, musculoskeletal, and central nervous systems are among the prominent known organic causes of recurrent abdominal pain (see Table 13–10). They are described in appropriate sections elsewhere in this text.

Pain in children with recurrent abdominal pain can be conceptualized as a disorder that either provokes pain pathways or an alteration in the patient's threshold to pain. A widely held plausible explanation for abdominal pain in these cases is an abnormality of the autonomic nervous system, because intestinal motility can be affected along with the occurrence of hyperalgesia and altered secretory patterns. Stress is frequently incriminated as a cause; however, it may actually be a response to the pain. There is no evidence of a consistent pattern of psychopathology among patients with idiopathic recurrent abdominal pain. Certain personality patterns have low pain thresholds, as do patients under stress. A history of depression is also at times present among close relatives. Anorexia nervosa, although not a common etiology of recurrent abdominal pain, is one specific psychiatric syndrome with which abdominal pain is often associated.

CLINICAL MANIFESTATIONS. Symptoms and signs are marked by their lack of specificity. Usually, the history and physical features distinguish or suggest patients with specific organic diseases. This crucial separation can be based on a few important findings: the specificity and consistency of the pain and its location and relationship to meals and movement; the occurrence of additional symptoms, such as vomiting or dysuria, indicating organ system involvement; the finding of specific relevant physical signs in the abdomen or elsewhere; and the general impression that the patient is ill.

The patient with nonspecific recurrent abdominal pain tends to look well, to have pain that is inconsistent in its relationship to meals and movement, to be free of major symptoms involving organ systems, and to lack significant physical signs. Erratic bowel actions with infrequent hard stools are common, as are tender, mobile fecal masses. Abdominal tenderness can be pronounced, but often it is distractible, variable in location, and associated with general tenderness of muscles. Rectal examination should be done; there may be exaggerated tenderness, but there should be no objective abnormalities. Headache and "limb tingling" are noted in one third of nonspecific cases. A preceding history of infant-feeding problems and excessive crying is noted in approximately 20%. An increased incidence of abdominal pain and other intestinal symptoms among close relatives has been suggested but not clearly defined.

Symptoms of psychologic disturbances should be elicited. Deterioration in performance and absence from school are most useful signals of worsening organic or psychologic illness. The history should suggest the severity of the pain. It is useful to determine whether the pain ever wakens the child from sleep or interrupts pleasurable activity. Both symptoms suggest organic rather than functional disease.

DIAGNOSIS. Careful examinations of urine and stool for evidence of infection, especially *G. lamblia*, are perhaps the most useful tests. Without specific clinical indicators, biochemical studies are overused and of little value. Similarly, roentgenographic imaging has not been helpful in the absence of clinical signs suggesting a specific problem. A plain abdominal roentgenogram may detect fecal retention. Abdominal ultrasound, on the other hand, is noninvasive and unexpectedly helpful at times in detecting calculi or other renal, pancreatic, or gynecologic abnormalities that are otherwise hard to identify. Measurement of breath hydrogen after administration of lactose may detect unsuspected malabsorption in a child whose symptoms suggest lactose intolerance.

Fiberoptic upper gastrointestinal endoscopic studies, as a routine investigation for nonspecific pain, have not been helpful. If the history is suggestive of peptic ulcer disease, endoscopy is indicated. Gynecologic assessment, including pelvic examination and ultrasound, should be reserved for adolescents in whom the clinical picture suggests a gynecologic problem. Pregnancy should be considered in the sexually active female and should be ruled out before any potentially hazardous roentgenographic studies are undertaken. Diagnostic procedures, particularly those that are invasive, should be guided by the clinical findings. Any potential benefit should be weighed against the additional anxiety produced by the study.

TREATMENT. Because no specific, effective treatment is available for this poorly understood functional problem, therapeutic emphasis must be on the patient's response to the pain. In most cases, unless an adolescent patient objects, these efforts should involve the parents. Initially, assurance that the problem is not life-threatening is important. Fear of cancer, often unexpressed, should be allayed. Also, one should be realistic and frank in warning the patient and family that the problem will probably persist for an extended period.

The physician should avoid prescribing medications and other therapies that can be harmful. Sedatives, antispasmodics, or analgesics have not been beneficial. These agents potentially have deleterious effects on intestinal motility and appetite and may also create dependency. Laxatives and, at times, enemas may be beneficial. With some evidence of retained stool or, in difficult cases even a suspicion of constipation, a trial of aggressive targeted treatment with mineral oil or lactulose, with or without enemas, can be effective, if combined with an appropriate approach to the whole patient.

Every effort should be made to promote full activity and a sense of normal health. A balanced, palatable nutritious diet, which is not excessive in fiber content, is recommended. For difficult patients, or those in whom a breath H_2 test suggests lactose intolerance, a 4-wk trial on a lactose-free diet is reasonable. Exercise should be promoted. Strong efforts should be made to maintain school attendance. These efforts may involve working with teachers and other school authorities. Lack of success in motivating these patients is a strong indicator of a need for additional help in exploring psychosocial factors with the aid of psychologists. Rarely, a psychiatrist is needed, if a psychiatric basis for the pain is suspected or if the pain has unmasked an underlying psychiatric problem. In some otherwise physically well patients a cycle of emotional turmoil, school or work absenteeism, and pain evolve. Breaking this cycle frequently stops the pain or makes it more tolerable. For example, the detection of unsuspected marital strife in the patient's parents and a constructive, supportive approach to that issue, involving the family with appropriate professionals, can be sufficient to arrest the pain. In general, in-hospital care should be avoided unless a separation of the patient from his or her family is important.

The prognosis for these patients is unclear. There is no significant increased risk of intra-abdominal organic disease, and in most cases symptoms improve before 20 yr of age. In adolescent females, symptoms may improve once a regular menstrual pattern is established. However, among adult patients who have nonspecific abdominal complaints (also called "spastic colon"), a previous history of abdominal pain during adolescence is often elicited. It appears that in some cases the disorder recurs during adulthood.

J. RICHARD HAMILTON

Apley J: The Child with Abdominal Pain. London, Blackwell Scientific, 1975.
Bain HW: Chronic abdominal pain in childhood. Pediatr Clin North Am 2:991, 1974.
Barbero GJ: Recurrent abdominal pain in childhood. Pediatr Rev 4:29, 1982.
Barr RG, Leone MD, Watkins JD: Recurrent abdominal pain in childhood due to lactose intolerance: A prospective study. N Engl J Med 300:1449, 1979.
Galler JR, Neustein S, Walker WA: Clinical aspects of recurrent abdominal pain in children. Adv Pediatr 27:31, 1980.
Raymer D, Weininger O, Hamilton JR: Psychological problems in children with abdominal pain. Lancet 1:439, 1984.

13.66 ACUTE APPENDICITIS

Acute appendicitis is the most common disease requiring abdominal surgery in childhood, and together with trauma to viscera, intussusception, adhesive bowel obstruction, and lesions of the ovary, it is one of the few indications for emergency surgery in children over 2 yr of age. Diagnosis in children, however, can be difficult; more often in children than in adults appendicitis progresses to perforation because a physician has failed to recognize it. The risk of perforation is greatest in 1- to 4-yr-old children (74%), is lower between 5 and 8 yr of age (66%) and is lowest in adolescents (30–40%). Preventable deaths of children from appendicitis still occur.

EPIDEMIOLOGY. The true incidence of acute appendicitis is unknown, but the annual rate of appendectomy is about 4 in every 1,000 children under the age of 14 yr. A busy physician is likely to see two to three cases each year, and an active pediatric emergency service may receive three to four each week. Males predominate in most series. Appendicitis occurs in infancy and has been reported in the neonatal period, but it is unusual under the age of 2 yr and rare under 1 yr. Peak age incidence is in the teenage and young adult years. The frequency increases in autumn and spring. Clustering of cases has occurred, and there is a familial tendency to develop appendicitis.

ETIOLOGY. Acute appendicitis is almost always caused by some obstruction of the lumen. Hard concretions (appendiceal fecalith), a crushable fecal impaction in the appendix, and appendiceal calculi (hard, noncrushable, calcified fecaliths) may be present at the site of obstruction in inflamed appendices. Formed by feces trapped in the appendiceal lumen with subsequent mineralization and inspissation, fecaliths and calculi are present in 10–12% of patients with uncomplicated appendicitis and in 20–25% of patients with complicated appendicitis. Fecaliths are not visualized on plain abdominal roentgenograms and are six times more common than the roentgenographically visible calculi. Calculi are noted more often with perforated appendicitis or periappendiceal abscess (45%) than are fecaliths (20%). The proximal portion of the appendix may be bound to the cecum by a congenital peritoneal fold (Jackson membrane), with a sharp kink and obstruction where the organ emerges from beneath the free border of this fold. The appendiceal mesentery can be so narrow that the distal portion of the appendix, with the mesentery, undergoes torsion, producing acute ischemic necrosis. Appendiceal obstruction has also been attributed to hyperplasia of the submucosal lymphoid tissue, presumably as a result of infection. Many resected appendices, both normal and diseased, contain pinworms, but parasites have not been proved to cause appendicitis. Fibrous stenosis resulting from earlier inflammation or a carcinoid tumor (argentaffinoma) may also predispose to appendicitis.

Nonobstructive appendicitis is rare; in some reported cases fecaliths have probably become dislodged. Both the clinical manifestations and the tissue changes are less severe in nonobstructive appendicitis, and resolution without perforation may occur.

Bacteriologic studies generally grow mixed intestinal organisms. Anaerobes are particularly important causes of intraperitoneal abscesses after perforation or surgery. Associated disease may delay the diagnosis of appendicitis and increase the risk of perforation, but it is doubtful that systemic infections predispose to or cause appendicitis.

PATHOLOGY. In the younger child the progression of the disease is generally so rapid that the first of three pathologic stages usually passes before medical attention is sought. First, when acute obstruction of the appendix occurs, the intraluminal pressure increases because the mucosal cells continue to elaborate mucus. Compression of mucosal vessels causes ischemia, necrosis, and ulceration. Second, bacterial invasion and infection of the appendiceal wall occur readily once the mucosa ulcerates. Inflammatory infiltrate appears within all layers, and fibrinous exudate is deposited on the serosa. Even before perforation is apparent, organisms can usually be cultured from the serosal surface of the appendix. Third, necrosis of the appendiceal wall results in perforation and fecal contamination of the peritoneum. Perforation usually occurs at the relatively ischemic tip or near the base where a fecalith has eroded through the wall.

In the older child the omentum and adjacent ileum usually adhere to the inflamed appendix prior to perforation and prevent widespread fecal spillage. The result is a localized abscess, usually in the right iliac fossa but occasionally low in the pelvis. Mesenteric venous thrombophlebitis may drain into the portal system with resultant pyogenic hepatic abscess formation. Multiple foci of intraperitoneal sepsis and pleural empyema rarely complicate general peritonitis now because diagnoses are made early when treatment is more effective. Paralytic ileus or mechanical bowel obstruction may be associated, or the abscess may rupture, usually into an adjacent, adherent loop of intestine rather than into the general peritoneal space. Spontaneous recovery follows the rupture of the abscess into the bowel lumen. In an infant or younger child, appendicitis can progress quickly to perforation and general peritonitis because at this age the omentum is small and ineffective in localizing the infection.

CLINICAL MANIFESTATIONS. Pain is invariably present. Initially, when the pathology is confined to the mucosa and muscular layers of the appendix, it is crampy and periumbilical. The colicky nature of the pain may reflect appendicular peristalsis directed at extruding the obstructing agent. When visceral and parietal peritoneal layers become involved in the inflammation, however, pain is localized to the area immediately overlying the appendix; it is commonly located in the right iliac fossa but may even be felt in the hypogastrium or within the pelvis if the appendix is pelvic, and in the loin if retrocolic. Movement such as jumping or driving over bumps in a car aggravates the pain. At this stage there is severe tenderness over the appendix, fever, tachycardia, and leukocytosis. While some older children may give the classic history described above, others locate the pain in the right iliac fossa throughout the illness. A young child will often hold a hand over the navel when asked to show where it hurts. In infancy, general irritability and a tendency to lie quietly with hips flexed may be the only indication of pain. The cramps of appendiceal obstruction are rarely severe. In fact, if an older child cries because of abdominal pain, he or she probably does not have appendicitis. The pain of peritoneal inflammation is made worse by any movement, such as a cough or a sudden turn. A patient who winces when jostled probably has peritoneal irritation.

Vomiting is almost always noted after the onset of the pain; it is not copious or frequent and is less common in older than in younger children. Anorexia is almost invariably present.

In children the duration of appendicitis before rupture is usually so short that there is insufficient time for constipation to develop. The mean time between the onset and the diagnosis for nonperforated appendicitis is 36 hr compared with 67 hr for those with perforation. If the diagnosis is delayed for more than 36 hr, the perforation rate is 65%. Risks associated with perforation include delayed diagnosis, fecaliths, young age, temperature greater than 38.6° C, leukocytosis of more than 14,000, and a positive family history of appendicitis. Diarrhea may suggest that cramps are due to gastroenteritis, but loose stools can also result from irritation of the colon by an adjacent, acutely inflamed appendix. Similarly, pelvic appendicitis can cause urinary frequency and urgency by irritating the bladder.

Sometimes a child with an acute retrocecal or retroiliac appendicitis will walk with an exaggerated lumbar lordosis and a slightly flexed hip due to spasm of the right psoas muscle.

Many children with acute appendicitis have previously had milder, self-limited attacks of a similar nature.

During history taking, it is helpful to observe the patient for pallor, flushing, physical activity, and abdominal movement. Pulse rate and rectal temperature should be obtained in advance. Jiggling the bed or gently shaking the child's thigh by a hand placed casually on the leg can suggest appendiceal inflammation if pain in the right lower abdomen results. Throughout the interview and examination it is important to proceed slowly, whenever possible distracting the child with appropriate conversation and never threatening with a sudden movement.

The physician should proceed directly to the specific abdominal examination and should leave the remainder of the examination until later. First, the abdomen should be inspected for visible swelling and movements. If the child is old enough, compliance with a request to cough or to move the abdominal wall in and out will produce pain over any site of peritoneal inflammation. Palpation in younger children may be initiated by using a stethoscope as a light palpating instrument. The pressure on the abdomen with the instrument is gradually increased, and later the hand replaces the stethoscope. There should also be an attempt to elicit increased muscle tone, pressing gently in each quadrant, observing as well as feeling the resistance. Palpation must be gentle because voluntary splinting is the response to pain and involuntary tone cannot be assessed. The site of maximum tenderness is important; in the older child it is often well localized to the McBurney point, the junction between the lateral and middle thirds of the line joining the right anterior superior iliac spine and the umbilicus. In younger children localization to the right iliac fossa is usually all that can be detected. Pain produced in the appendiceal area by pressure elsewhere in the abdomen is a valuable sign in an anxious child. Rebound tenderness is a needlessly painful sign; eliciting it serves only to destroy the carefully built-up relationship between the examiner and the child. It has also often false-positive or false-negative results. Bowel sounds may be depressed in appendicitis and silent with generalized peritonitis.

Atypical locations of the appendix cause difficulty in diagnosis. If it lies up the gutter, lateral to the cecum, the tenderness will be in the flank. A pelvic appendix may be reached only by rectal examination. Retroiliac appendicitis usually causes very poorly localized pain, thus the diagnosis is unlikely to be made before perforation occurs. A posteriorly situated appendix lying on the psoas muscle causes hip flexion, and pain may be produced by passive extension of the hip with the child lying on the left side (psoas sign). The most important physical sign is a constant, localized, significant degree of tenderness. The site of tenderness should not vary between examinations nor among examiners. An acutely inflamed but unruptured appendix should not give rise to tenderness of the entire hemiabdomen, nor should there be bilateral tenderness; an unduly extensive area of tenderness in the absence of perforation should call into question the diagnosis of appendicitis.

After the abdominal assessment the general examination is completed, leaving until last the essential rectal examination. For this, a mild hypnotic, such as one of the barbiturates, may occasionally facilitate the examination of a particularly upset child, but, if at all possible, hypnotics or sedatives should be avoided. Patience and gentle persistence are more effective aids in examination of an apprehensive child. In equivocal cases re-evaluation of the patient in 4–6 hr is helpful because the course of appendicitis is usually sufficiently rapid in children that 6 hr produces enough change to make the diagnosis. Up to 15% of operations for presumed acute appendicitis in children may lead to the removal of noninflamed appendices.

LABORATORY DATA. A high white blood cell count suggests acute suppurative disease. Usually, there is neutrophilia with a shift to the left and absence of eosinophils. The teenager with early appendicitis is unlikely to have a count higher than 15,000/mm^3, but the infant may show a leukocyte response of 20,000/mm^3 or even more before perforation. Occasionally, the white blood cell count is depressed. Pyuria usually suggests urinary tract infection, particularly if there are bacteria in a fresh specimen, but an inflamed appendix lying across the ureter or irritating the bladder can also cause pyuria. Other hematologic or biochemical tests are not diagnostically useful but may be important in assessing a patient's general state.

Roentgenograms may detect intestinal obstruction, a calcified appendicolith, or pneumonia. Scoliosis concave to the right can be caused by an inflamed appendix, and a degree of paralytic ileus may be noted.

Graded compression *ultrasound* is a rapid, safe, noninvasive, and accurate tool to diagnose nonperforated appendicitis. Acute appendicitis appears as an edematous enlarged and inflamed lesion (Fig. 13–23). Ultrasound may also demonstrate perforation and abscess formation. In addition, abdominal ultrasound is a useful method to diagnose ileocecal enteritis, thus excluding appendicitis as a cause of right lower quadrant pain. Bacterial ileocecitis appears as mural thickening of the terminal ileum and cecum with enlarged mesenteric lymph nodes due to an associated mesenteric adenitis.

A^{99m} *Tc tagged leukocyte* scan is another possible radiographic method to diagnose right lower quadrant inflammation associated with appendicitis.

Despite the improved accuracy with modern roentgenographic and ultrasonographic methods, the indication for surgery is based, in almost all cases, on abdominal physical findings suggestive of an acute abdomen due to appendicitis or other causes and not on roentgenographic signs.

DIFFERENTIAL DIAGNOSIS. The diffuse crampy pain

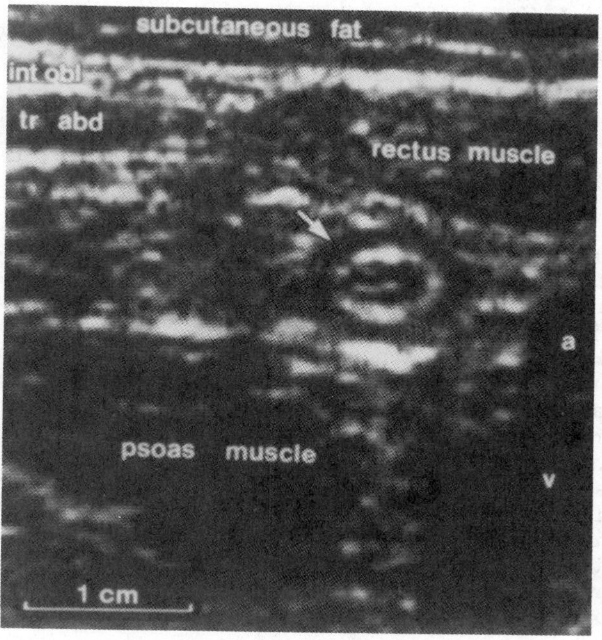

Figure 13–23. Graded compression ultrasound of acute appendicitis demonstrating edematous enlarged appendix compressed between the abdominal wall and the psoas muscle. (Int obl = internal oblique muscle; tr abd = transverse abdominus muscle; a = right iliac artery; v = right iliac vein.) (From Puylaert JB, Rutgers PH, Laisang RI, et al: A prospective study of ultrasonography in the diagnosis of appendicitis. N Engl J Med 317:666, 1987.)

and diarrhea of enteric infection usually distinguish it from appendicitis, but appendicitis may occur in a child who has had gastroenteritis for several days. The enteritis caused by *Yersinia enterocolitica* and *Campylobacter jejuni,* an acute flare-up of *Crohn disease* or regional ileitis, and, infrequently, intussusception in an older child may produce right lower abdominal symptoms highly suggestive of appendicitis. Bacterial ileocecitis manifests abdominal pain and has associated diarrhea in only 30–40% of cases. Occasionally, Crohn disease may begin by mimicking appendicitis. Inflammation rarely complicates a *Meckel diverticulum,* but when it does, the clinical findings may be identical to those of appendicitis. Many children with viral or other infections have pain and tenderness in the appendiceal area and are assumed to have *mesenteric adenitis* (see later). An infected lesion on the ipsilateral lower limb or perineum may give rise to an external iliac adenitis with tenderness low down in the right iliac fossa.

When generalized *viral infections* cause abdominal pain, it is usually midabdominal, worse upon eating, and associated with neutropenia. Early fever, headache, and chills favor a systemic infection, even if abdominal pain is noted later. *Pneumonia* involving the right lower lobe with diaphragmatic irritation may result in enough right-sided abdominal muscular rigidity and referred pain that appendicitis is suspected. Conversely, perforated appendicitis may produce subphrenic abscesses with a sympathetic ipsilateral pleural effusion. Abdominal pain occasionally accompanies acute *streptococcal tonsillitis* or *pharyngitis* and can mimic appendicitis very closely, but these disorders may also occur with true appendicitis. *Acute rheumatic fever* can cause abdominal pain in its early stages. *Urinary tract infections* occasionally cause abdominal pain and tenderness; there should always be a careful urinary tract evaluation prior to appendectomy. *Diabetic ketoacidosis* frequently causes abdominal pain and vomiting, and in the undiagnosed diabetic can be confused with appendicitis. Urinalysis should lead to the correct diagnosis and must never be omitted prior to emergency surgery. *Bleeding from the right ovary,* a graafian follicle, or a persisting corpus luteum can also simulate appendicitis. Pelvic inflammatory disease, tubo-ovarian abscess, ectopic pregnancy, ovulatory pain, and other gynecologic problems should be considered in adolescent females. *Primary peritonitis* is discussed in Sec. 13.103.

Abdominal pain is a common symptom of many hematologic disorders. It is associated with leukemia, especially in relapse. Appendicitis in patients with leukemia may be masked by immunosuppressant drugs.

Typhlitis, a necrotizing mucositis of the cecum, is encountered in neutropenic patients with leukemia who are receiving myelosuppressive anticancer therapy. Manifestations include lower abdominal pain, distention, rectal bleeding, fever, pneumatosis intestinalis, and occasionally bacteremia. Abdominal ultrasound and CT scanning demonstrate thickened bowel wall and ascites near the cecum. One should also suspect the diagnosis of appendicitis in a hemophiliac patient with abdominal pain. Sickle cell disease and anaphylactoid purpura (Henoch-Schönlein purpura) frequently cause severe abdominal pain (Sec. 16.19 and 11.56).

Patients with cystic fibrosis have a spectrum of appendiceal disease ranging from acute to chronic appendicitis to intussusception. The incidence may be as high as 1–2% and may be due to a mucous-engorged, distended appendix with or without inflammation or perforation.

TREATMENT. Emergency appendectomy is the treatment for early acute appendicitis. Only under the most extreme circumstances should operation be delayed more than a few hours. Recovery is rapid, and the child is active in 3–4 days. Most surgeons recommend that the child with a localized appendiceal abscess receive adequate external drainage after appropriate preoperative correction of any fluid and electrolyte problems; at The Hospital for Sick Children, Toronto, however, if percutaneous radiologic drainage is not possible, only supportive care is provided until spontaneous drainage of the abscess occurs into an adjacent loop of a bowel, a process that rarely takes longer than 1 wk. Then 8–12 wk later appendectomy is carried out.

The child with generalized peritonitis due to appendiceal rupture requires intravenous hydration and correction of any electrolyte disturbance before surgery, because of substantial fluid loss into the abdominal space from an inflamed peritoneum. If there are no clinical signs of dehydration, lactated Ringer solution should be administered at a volume of 5% of the body weight. Half of the calculated need should be given in the first 1–2 hr (or a bolus of 20 mL/kg should be given), followed by rest during and after the operation. If there are signs of dehydration, a volume equivalent to 7% of the body weight is administered; half of the deficit should be given preoperatively. For severe cases of dehydration 10–15% of the body weight is required as replacement. An adequate urinary output should be established before surgery.

It is essential that antibiotics be given before the operation when the appendix has ruptured to ensure adequate blood and tissue levels of the drugs used. Triple intravenous therapy using an aminoglycoside, ampicillin, and clindamycin or metronidazole or one of the newer cephalosporins is the treatment of choice. Appendectomy is necessary to limit continued fecal contamination of the peritoneum. Many surgeons use preoperative antibiotic therapy before any operation for nonperforated appendicitis, discontinuing antibiotic use postoperatively if there was no perforation. After surgery a normal fluid and electrolyte balance should be maintained, and the stomach and bowel should be kept decompressed by effective nasogastric suction until intestinal activity returns.

PROGNOSIS. The prognosis is excellent provided an appendectomy is performed before perforation has occurred and is good even after perforation. Among 550 children with generalized peritonitis from ruptured appendix managed at The Hospital for Sick Children, Toronto, three deaths (0.5%) occurred.

COMPLICATIONS. Since the institution of preoperative triple antibiotic therapy, postoperative infections have become less common. The most common postoperative complication is infection of the wound. Pelvic, subphrenic, or other intra-abdominal suppuration is especially likely to develop after operation on a gangrenous, perforated appendix. Ultrasound is a useful diagnostic aid at this stage. There is no urgent need for reoperation because of the development of intra-abdominal suppuration. Almost all pelvic abscesses will rupture into an adjacent loop of bowel and spontaneously resolve. It is virtually never necessary to drain these by the rectum. Subphrenic suppuration requires surgical drainage.

Prolonged paralytic ileus often follows generalized peritonitis; it may be aggravated by premature attempts at oral feedings.

Intestinal obstruction may occur as a postoperative complication. If this happens within 30 days of the appendectomy, nonoperative management is advisable. If an obstruction occurs more than 30 days later and there is no evidence of ischemia of the bowel, nasogastric compression may be attempted for a short period (48 hr); if this is unsuccessful, a laparotomy will be necessary. A volvulus may be present, with gangrenous bowel caused by a single adhesion in the right lower quadrant. This complication may occur many years after appendectomy. Pelvic peritonitis may result in obstruction to the fallopian tubes with consequent sterility.

APPENDIX AND CHRONIC ABDOMINAL PAIN. Obstruction of the vermiform appendix, whether by fibrous band, worms, or fecalith, used to be considered an important cause of recurrent or chronic abdominal pain, and many children were subjected to elective appendectomy for this reason. Some children may have been helped, but most continued to have pain and were belatedly diagnosed as having urinary tract pathology, gastrointestinal malfunction unrelated to the appendix, or psychophysiologic pain. Recurrent appendiceal obstruction is a rare cause of chronic or intermittent abdominal pain; an operation should be considered only after careful evaluation of these other possibilities. It is doubtful that chronic inflammation of the appendix occurs.

Rare causes of acute, recurrent abdominal pain that resembles an acute abdomen include hereditary angioedema, porphyria, and familial Mediterranean fever.

BARRY SHANDLING
JAMES C. FALLIS

Addis DG, Shaffer N, Fowler BS, et al: The epidemiology of appendicitis and appendectomy in the United States. Am J Epid 132:910, 1990.
Brender JD, Marcuse EK, Koepsell TD, et al: Childhood appendicitis: Factors associated with perforation. Pediatrics 76:301, 1985.
Browder W, Smith JW, Vivoda LM, et al: Nonperforative appendicitis: A continuing surgical dilemma. J Infect Dis 159:1088, 1989.
Cacioppo JC, Diettrich NA, Kaplan G, et al: The consequences of current constraints on surgical treatment of appendicitis. Am J Surg 157:276, 1989.
Centers for Disease Control: Investigation of a cluster of appendicitis cases—Texas. MMWR 36:340, 1987.
Coughlin JP, Gauderer MWL, Stern RC, et al: The spectrum of appendiceal disease in cystic fibrosis. J Pediatr Surg 25:835, 1990.
Henneman PL, Marcus CS, Inkelis SH, et al: Evaluation of children with possible appendicitis using technetium 99m leukocyte scan. Pediatrics 85:838, 1990.
Katz JA, Wagner ML, Gresik MV, et al: Typhlitis: An 18 year experience and post mortem review. Cancer 65:1041, 1990.
Malt RA: The perforated appendix. N Engl J Med 315:1546, 1986.
Puylaert JB, Rutgert PH, Laisang RI, et al: A prospective study of ultrasonography in the diagnosis of appendicitis. N Engl J Med 317:666, 1987.
Puylaert JB, Vermeijden RJ, van der Werf SD, et al: Incidence and sonographic diagnosis of bacterial ileocaecitis masquerading as appendicitis. Lancet 2:84, 1989.
Ravitch MM: Appendicitis. Pediatrics 70:414, 1982.
Rubin SZ, Martin DJ: Ultrasonography in the management of possible appendicitis in childhood. J Pediatr Surg 25:737, 1990.
Schwartz MZ, Tapper D, Solonberger RI: Management of perforated appendicitis in children: The controversy continues. Ann Surg 197:406, 1983.
Wilkenson RH, Bartlett RH, Eraklis AJ: Diagnosis of appendicitis in infancy. Am J Dis Child 118:687, 1969.

13.67 SURGICAL CONDITIONS OF THE ANUS, RECTUM, AND COLON

In infants and children close inspection of the anal area is as valuable as a digital rectal examination. *Fissures* can be best identified by having the mother hold the infant's hips in acute flexion so that the examiner can separate the patient's buttocks, using both thumbs, gently stretching the anus and everting the lining to expose the fissure. On the other hand, in all cases of constipation, especially when an intrinsic or extrinsic rectal obstruction is possible, a digital examination is indicated, after assessing perianal sensation. Properly done, this should cause little or no discomfort to the patient. A well-lubricated finger is passed over the anus a few times to accustom the patient to the unusual sensation. Then the pulp of the index or fifth finger is pressed against the anus with increasing flexion of the interphalangeal joints and the finger slips easily into the anal canal.

ANAL FISSURE

A small slit or crack at the mucocutaneous line is a common acquired lesion in infancy and uncommon in the school-aged child. Most anal fissures occur in the sagittal plane, usually dorsally in the midline. The cause is often not evident but may be secondary to constipation with passage of large hard stools, scratching induced by irritation from *Enterobius vermicularis* or eczema, or other perianal conditions. Chemically treated tissues used for cleansing the perianal skin may be responsible for perianal irritation in some infants.

CLINICAL MANIFESTATIONS. Pain on defecation and, frequently, refusal to defecate are the principal manifestations. Bright red blood on the surface of the stool or on toilet paper and bleeding following defecation may be observed. The diagnosis is usually made by inspection of the anal area. The skin at the peripheral end of the fissure becomes swollen and forms a "tag." A history of prolapse of some tissue suggests a rectal polyp rather than a tag. More significant, fissures also occur with Crohn disease. Sometimes, even after the fissure is healed the infant or child is afraid to defecate, anticipating anal pain; attempts are made to retain the stool, often resulting in encopresis.

TREATMENT. Most fissures heal spontaneously if the local irritation is lessened or eliminated. Anal dilatation by the mother using a well-lubricated finger twice daily for 1–2 wk will cure most anal fissures. A well-formed but not hard stool makes an excellent dilator of the anal canal and is attended by less psychic trauma than anal digital dilatation. The administration of laxatives to keep the stool fluid affords only temporary relief because eventually a more substantial stool must be passed with recurrence of the pain. If the patient is passing very hard stools, a mild stool softener may be useful, but the aim should not be to render the stools fluid. The addition of natural bran to the diet (1–3 tablespoons depending on the child's age) is of great value in softening the stool. Anesthetic ointment is traditionally prescribed, but it is often not helpful since it is most effective when applied 30 min before a bowel movement, which is impossible to predict. Washing the anal area with soap and water after every stool is important. The perianal skin is often excoriated and inflamed, and sometimes multiple superficial anal fissures occur. In such cases an ointment or cream with a triamcinolone base is useful. Care should be taken to exclude the simultaneous presence of a fungal infection.

If there is no response to medical management or if the fissure has been present for a long time, a minor operation may be indicated because excessively prolonged symptoms from a fissure may result in the development of acquired megacolon with fecal impaction and encopresis. The operation is done under general anesthesia and may consist of stretching the anus, excision of the fissure, or internal anal sphincterotomy, or of a combination of the three procedures. Minimal postoperative discomfort occurs; recurrence is unusual.

ANORECTAL ABSCESS

Perirectal abscess may occur at any age but is noted predominantly in children less than 2 yr of age. The male to female ratio is 2:1. A predisposing illness (prior rectal surgery for Hirschsprung disease or imperforate anus, drug-induced or autoimmune neutropenia, AIDS, diabetes mellitus, Crohn disease, immunosuppressive drugs) is present in more than 50% of children.

The abscess may begin as a perianal pustule or a local cellulitis. Subsequently, the infection gains entrance to the ischiorectal fossa through the anal crypts and extends to the adjacent subcutaneous tissue, usually within 1.5 cm of the anus. The bacteriology of abscess material reveals a mixed aerobic (*E. coli, Klebsiella pneumoniae, S. aureus*) and anaerobic (*Bacteroides* species, *Clostridium, Veillonella*) flora. Ten to 15% yield pure growth of either *E. coli, S. aureus*, or *B. fragilis*. Neutropenic patients may also have bacteremia that inconsistently has the same organism as the abscess. The *differential diagnosis* includes inflammatory bowel disease, foreign body, gangrenous hemorrhoids, and tuberculosis.

Clinical manifestations include fever, rectal pain, a rectal mass, pain on sitting or defecation, refusal to walk, and constipation. Neutropenic cancer patients may have fever, perirectal pain, and cellulitis without a mass. Immunocompetent patients may not have fever unless the perirectal space is infected. A tender swelling overlies the ischiorectal fossa with erythema, warmth, induration, and fluctuation.

Treatment consists of incision and drainage, and if the patient is immunocompromised, the addition of broad-spectrum antibiotics. The latter patients should receive an antibiotic combination that is effective against *S. aureus* and enteric gram-negative and fecal anaerobic bacteria. Some authorities initially treat neutropenic patients who have no obvious fluctuant abscess with antibiotics, reserving incision and drainage for patients who do not respond to this therapy.

ANAL FISTULA

Fistulas originating in the anus or rectum may be congenital or acquired and rarely may extend to and communicate with the urinary bladder, urethra, vagina, or perianal skin. Acquired fistulas are residuals of an abscess and usually open on the skin surface. There is frequently a history of one or more incisions into the abscess, of neglect, or of antibiotic treatment of the abscess.

CLINICAL MANIFESTATIONS. An acquired fistula produces a recurrent painful swelling that subsides with a purulent discharge. An opening into the skin, into which a probe may be introduced, is found beside the anal orifice, and the internal opening of the fistula is located on the pectinate line.

TREATMENT. No fistulas close spontaneously. Simple incision and unroofing of the fistulous tract are curative. Care must be taken not to injure the anal sphincter and cause incontinence.

HEMORRHOIDS

Hemorrhoids are very rare in infants and children. When they are encountered, an underlying cause may be present, such as a venacaval or mesenteric obstruction, cirrhosis, portal hypertension, or other reasons for venous obstruction. Occasionally, chronic constipation, fecal impaction, and straining at stool result in hemorrhoids. Operation is rarely indicated except for an acute external thrombus. The hemorrhoids generally subside when the primary condition is corrected.

PRURITUS ANI

Anal itching in childhood is generally secondary to enterobiasis, anal fissures, and other local inflammatory lesions, or to coarse or moist undergarments. Nocturnal itching may be the most frequent evidence of pinworm infestation. Treatment consists of eradication of the underlying cause and cleansing the anal area with a mild soap and drying it with a soft cloth or tissue. Powders or solutions such as witch hazel may be used. In small infants exposure to sunlight or dry heat is helpful when the anal area is inflamed.

PROLAPSE AND PROCIDENTIA OF THE RECTUM AND SIGMOID

Prolapse is abnormal descent of the mucous membrane of the rectum with or without protrusion through the anal orifice; *procidentia* is the abnormal descent of all the coats of the rectum or sigmoid with or without protrusion through the anus. These conditions are most common from 1–5 yr (mean, 3 yr). The anatomy of the infant's pelvis predisposes to rectal prolapse. Any sudden increase in intra-abdominal pressure, such as straining at bowel movements after prolonged sitting with the hips and knees flexed, may precipitate an abnormal descent of the bowel wall. Malnutrition with absorption of ischiorectal fat is a contributory factor. Children with chronic malabsorption, particularly cystic fibrosis, are likely to develop prolapse. Protrusion at stool initially recedes spontaneously but later requires manual replacement. Bleeding and the passage of mucus may occur. The protruding mass varies from bright to dark red; it may be as much as 6 in. long. In prolapse the striations or furrows radiate from the center of the anal aperture in contrast to the concentrically arranged rosette of procidentia. Both conditions must be differentiated from an intussusception with the apex presenting at the anus, and from juvenile rectal polyp presenting at the anus.

Rectal prolapse is also seen in patients with chronic constipation, acute diarrhea, Hirschsprung disease, ulcerative colitis, Ehlers-Danlos syndrome, meningomyelocele, pertussis, and following anorectal surgery. Ten to 20% of patients have no obvious predisposing disease. Patients with cystic fibrosis cannot be distinguished from other patients on the basis of age at onset or frequency of episodes. However, the diagnosis of cystic fibrosis is facilitated by the presence of chronic diarrhea, absence of constipation, presence of respiratory symptoms (wheezing, recurrent pneumonia), failure to thrive, family history, and an abnormal sweat chloride concentration.

Treatment should be directed to dietary correction of constipation, to proper toilet training, and to the elimination of any underlying disturbance, such as parasitic infection, diarrhea, or polyps. Oral administration of stool softeners and having the child defecate with his or her feet off the floor may be helpful. Prolonged sessions on the toilet should be discouraged.

Reduction of protrusion is aided by pressure with warm compresses. An easy method of reduction is to cover the finger with a piece of toilet paper, introduce it into the lumen of the mass, and gently push it into the rectum. The finger is then immediately withdrawn. The toilet paper adheres to the mucous membrane, permitting release of the finger; the paper, when softened, is later expelled. Submucosal injection of sclerosants into the rectal ampulla is an effective means of preventing prolapse when repetitive attempts at medical therapy have failed. For intractable cases perineal operation may, on rare occasion, be indicated. In procidentia of the rectum and sigmoid, abdominal sigmoidopexy is required.

POSTANAL DIMPLE

A *postanal dimple* is seen relatively frequently in normal babies, located behind the anus, close to the upper limit of the natal cleft. It almost never requires treatment except when it is very deep and becomes the site of minor recurrent infections. If simple hygienic measures are inadequate, excision of the dimple may be necessary.

A dermal sinus is present when there is a communication between a postanal dimple and the sacrum or coccyx. Such a tract may be attached to the dural linings of the spinal canal. This lesion requires meticulous excision to prevent the development of postoperative meningitis.

A *pilonidal sinus* is an acquired condition that is not a sequel to or a complication of a postanal dimple. It consists of one or several pits dorsal to the anus and is usually seen in hairy youths. A pilonidal sinus results from shed hairs piercing the skin in the natal cleft. This may follow undue friction of the buttocks, and during World War II it was called "jeep driver's disease." A similar condition is seen in the interdigital webs on the hands of barbers. The sinus tract may become obstructed, forming a *pilonidal cyst* or abscess. The physician is consulted when infection supervenes.

Pilonidal cysts and sinuses do not cause symptoms unless they become infected. Swelling, heat, redness, tenderness, and fluctuation over the sacrococcygeal region are characteristic of an infected sinus. Purulent material may be discharged from one or more openings. If infection occurs, drainage or total excision should be performed. Prophylaxis requires regularly washing away loose hairs.

BARRY SHANDLING

Arditi M, Yoger R: Perirectal abscess in infants and children: Report of 52 cases and review of literature. Pediatr Infect Dis J 9:411, 1990.
Parks AG: Pathogenesis and treatment of fistula-in-ano. Br Med J 1:463, 1961.
Qvist N, Rasmussen L, Klaaborg KE, et al: Rectal prolapse in infancy: Conservative versus operative treatment. J Pediatr Surg 21:887, 1986.
Stern RC, Izant RJ, Boat TF, et al: Treatment and prognosis of rectal prolapse in cystic fibrosis. Gastroenterology 82:707, 1982.
Zempsky W, Rosenstein B: The cause of rectal prolapse in children. Am J Dis Child 142:338, 1988.

13.68 TUMORS OF THE DIGESTIVE TRACT IN CHILDREN

See also Sec. 17.22.

JUVENILE COLONIC POLYP. This is the most common tumor of the bowel in childhood, present in 3–4% of the population less than 21 yr of age. It has no potential for malignancy. The lesion may appear after the first year of age. Most patients become symptomatic by 4 yr of age, and the lesion rarely persists beyond 15 yr of age. The male to female ratio is 3:2.

Approximately 80% of these hamartoms occur in the distal large bowel, within reach of an examining finger and sigmoidoscope; all except 10% are distal to the splenic flexure. Most juvenile polyps are solitary (75–85%). These oval, spherical, or flattened lesions vary in size from 0.5–4 cm; the average diameter is 1–1.5 cm. The histology demonstrates hamartomatous proliferation of glandular and stromal elements, marked vascularity, and infiltration with lymphocytes, eosinophils, and polymorphonuclear and plasma cells.

Multiple juvenile colonic polyps occur in families as a dominant trait and are associated with congenital anomalies. These lesions are identical to solitary polyps, but this rare condition may have an increased risk for colonic cancer (see later).

Typical *clinical manifestations* include bright red and painless rectal bleeding during or immediately after a bowel movement. Exsanguinating hemorrhage is rare; bleeding often stops spontaneously. Iron deficiency anemia may be present or, rarely, the initial chief complaint. Lower abdominal pain and cramps are variable and are associated with intussusception or a long pedicle. Prolapse of the polyp appears as a dark, beefy red mass in distinction to the lighter pink mucosal appearance of rectal prolapse. Spontaneous polyp infarction and self-amputation are common, whereas diarrhea and obstruction are uncommon. The *differential diagnosis* includes other forms of intestinal polyposis, Meckel diverticulum, fissure in ano, inflammatory bowel disease, intestinal infections, and coagulation disorders.

The *diagnosis* is often made by rectal examination. Confirmation or identification of more distal polyps is made by sigmoidoscopy. Polyps appear as smooth, pedunculated lesions. Fiberoptic colonoscopy of the entire colon is indicated to identify other polyps. If the polyp cannot be removed during endoscopy, the lesion should be biopsied. Air contrast barium enema may also demonstrate distal or multiple polyps.

Treatment includes the removal of the polyp during sigmoidoscopy using a cold biopsy forceps or an electrothermic snare cautery. Polyps above the peritoneal reflection can be removed at colonoscopy by snare cautery or, rarely, by transabdominal polypectomy. Recurrences are unusual and may represent overlooked smaller polyps.

FAMILIAL POLYPOSIS SYNDROMES. The rare familial syndromes associated with intestinal polyposis are important because some of them are premalignant states.

Familial Adenomatous Polyposis Coli. This mendelian dominant condition, with reduced penetrance, is premalignant and is characterized by large numbers of adenomatous lesions in the distal large bowel. The incidence is 1:8,000 persons, with usual onset late in the 1st decade of life or during adolescence. By definition there are more than 100 (often 1,000) visible adenomas present when the patient is in the 2nd or 3rd decade of life. The adenomatous polyposis coli (APC) gene is present on the long arm of chromosome 5. Some families who do not meet the criteria for adenomatous polyposis coli, but who have a high frequency of adenomatous polyps and colonic cancer, also have a mutation of the APC gene.

Initially, the polyps are asymptomatic, and many often remain so. When symptomatic, adenomatous polyps cause hematochezia, occasionally cramps, or, rarely, diarrhea. Malignancy arising from pre-existing adenomatous polyps may first appear during adolescence.

The *diagnosis* should be suspected from the family history, but no available methods predict the disorder in a young child. The diagnosis is made by direct vision through a colonoscope. The polyps are usually numerous; biopsies demonstrate the adenomatous nature without the inflammatory and cystic finding of juvenile polyps. For a child with a family history of APC, colonoscopy is recommended every 2 yr after 12 yr of age.

Management consists of a careful family survey, genetic counseling, and, for confirmed patients with APC, pancolectomy. Current anastomotic methods permit restoration of bowel continuity after resection of all colonic mucosa.

PEUTZ-JEGHERS SYNDROME. This rare dominantly inherited syndrome is characterized by mucosal pigmentation of the lips and gums, and hamartomas of the stomach and small bowel. The polyps are not premalignant. Deeply pigmented discrete freckles are seen at birth or appear during infancy on the lips and buccal mucosa, and even around the mouth. Evidence of intestinal lesions may come from bleeding or from crampy pain associated with obstruction or intussusception.

Family studies and genetic counseling are important. Relatives may be found with either partial or complete manifestations of the syndrome. Intestinal lesions should be excised if they are causing significant symptoms; involvement is usually too extensive to remove all the polyps.

GARDNER SYNDROME. This rare, dominantly inherited disorder is characterized by multiple intestinal polyps and tumors of the soft tissue and bone, particularly the mandible. Additional features include dental abnormalities, characteristic bilateral pigmented lesions in the ocular fundus, and extracolonic cancers. Patients with this syndrome have a defect in the APC gene on chromosome 5.

The soft-tissue lesions and osteomas may appear during childhood, but intestinal polyps usually do not become apparent until early adult life. These polyps may develop anywhere along the digestive tract and are premalignant. Accordingly, aggressive surgical treatment of the intestinal lesions is indicated.

HEMANGIOMA OF THE INTESTINE. These rare benign lesions can cause massive, even fatal hemorrhage. The usual clinical manifestation is painless bleeding beginning in childhood. The blood loss can be subtle and chronic, or sudden and massive. Usually, there are no additional intestinal symptoms, but if intussusception occurs, there will be obstructive symptoms. About 50% of patients have cutaneous hemangiomas, and some have a family history of similar lesions. About half of these lesions are in the colon, where they may be seen by colonoscopy. During a period of bleeding selective mesenteric arteriography may be useful in locating a lesion.

LEIOMYOMA. This rare benign tumor occurs most commonly in stomach and jejunum. It remains asymptomatic for long periods, but if it extends into the lumen, it may cause intussusception.

CARCINOMA. The fact that epithelial tumors of the digestive tract are rare in children argues against an aggressive diagnostic approach to many gastrointestinal symptoms in this age group. Several childhood conditions predispose to development of gastrointestinal adenocarcinoma in adult life; for example, familial polyposis, Gardner syndrome, idiopathic ulcerative colitis, and, to a lesser extent, Crohn disease and disorders associated with chromosomal breaks. The usual site is the colon but gastric lesions are reported. Symptoms are general ill health, abdominal pain, an abdominal mass, and, less frequently, hemorrhage. The tumors tend to be relatively undifferentiated and highly malignant.

LYMPHOSARCOMA OF THE INTESTINE. Of the malignancies of the digestive tract in children, most are lymphosarcomas and some are associated with AIDS (Sec. 17.16). The usual site is the lower small intestine. Manifestations are general ill health, abdominal pain, and anemia. Adults with longstanding celiac disease have a relatively high incidence of lymphosarcoma; a beneficial effect of dietary treatment on this relationship has not been proved.

CARCINOID TUMORS. These tumors of the enterochromaffin cells of the intestine usually occur in the appendix in children and have very low grade malignancy. They cause symptoms similar to those of appendicitis and do not recur after resection, even when the tumor has extended to the muscularis and lymphatics.

Carcinoid tumors outside the appendix commonly metastasize, and the metastatic lesions give rise to the carcinoid syndrome, which is the result of pharmacologically active secretions produced by the tumor. These produce episodic intestinal hypermotility and diarrhea, vasomotor disturbances, and bronchoconstriction. The most important active agent is serotonin, and the diagnosis is usually made by finding high urinary levels of its metabolite, 5-hydroxyindoleacetic acid. These functioning neoplasms are rare in children.

Abrahamson J, Shandling B: Intestinal hemangiomata in childhood and a syndrome for diagnosis: A collective review. J Pediatr Surg 8:487, 1973.

Bartholomew LG: Peutz-Jeghers syndrome. JAMA 183:901, 1963.

Berry CL, Keeling JW: Gastrointestinal lymphoma in childhood. J Clin Pathol 23:459, 1970.

Bodmer WF, Bailey CJ, Bodmer J, et al: Localization of the gene for familial adenomatous polyposis on chromosome 5. Nature 328:614, 1987.

Burt RW, Samowitz WS: The adenomatous polyp and the hereditary polyposis syndromes. Gastroenterol Clin North Am 17:657, 1988.

Iida M, Yao T, Itoh H, et al: Natural history of fundic gland polyposis in patients with familial adenomatosis coli/Gardner's syndrome. Gastroenterology 89:1021, 1985.

Leppert M, Burt R, Hughes JP, et al: Genetic analysis of an inherited predisposition to colon cancer in a family with a variable number of adenomatous polyps. N Engl J Med 322:904, 1990.

Postlethwait RW: Gastrointestinal carcinoid tumors—a review. Postgrad Med 40:445, 1966.

Recalde M, Holyoke ED, Elias EG: Carcinoma of the colon, rectum and anal canal in young patients. Surg Gynecol Obstet 139:909, 1974.

Traboulsi EI, Krush AJ, Gardner EJ, et al: Prevalence and importance of pigmented ocular fundus lesions in Gardner's syndrome. N Engl J Med 316:661, 1987.

DIARRHEA FROM HORMONE-SECRETING TUMORS

Certain hormone-producing tumors cause a marked increase in intestinal secretion leading to severe chronic watery diarrhea (Table 13–20). The secretory diarrhea persists when the patient is placed NPO. These tumors originate in the APUD cells (*a*mine content, *p*recursor *u*ptake, amino acid *d*ecarboxylation) of the gastroenteropancreatic endocrine system and in adrenal or extra-adrenal neurogenic sites. Neural crest cells are precursors of APUDoma and neurogenic cells.

Diarrhea is massive and results in fluid and electrolyte imbalance and weight loss. *Diagnosis* is based on the presence of secretory watery diarrhea, extraintestinal manifestations, measurement of the suspected hormone or its metabolites in serum or urine, and various imaging techniques. If possible, tumor resection is the treatment of choice. Pharmacologic therapy with hormone antagonists may be palliative (see Table 13–20).

Hamilton JR, Radde IC, Johnson G: Diarrhea associated with adrenal ganglioneuroma. New findings related to the pathogenesis of diarrhea. Am J Med 44:473, 1968.
Kaplan SJ, Holbrook CT, McDaniel HE, et al: Vasoactive intestinal peptide secreting tumors of childhood. Am J Dis Child 134:21, 1980.
Mitchell CH, Sinatra FR, Crast FW, et al: Intractable watery diarrhea, ganglioneuroblastoma and vasoactive intestinal peptide. J Pediatr 89:593, 1976.
Rambaud JC, Modigliani R, et al: Pancreatic cholera: Studies on tumor secretions and pathophysiology of diarrhea. Gastroenterology 69:110, 1975.

NODULAR LYMPHOID HYPERPLASIA. Lymphoid follicles in the lamina propria of the gut normally aggregate in Peyer patches. These areas appear as submucosal nodules which may be visible on barium contrast roentgenograms and mistaken for an abnormality. There are many more Peyer patches in the lower than the upper small bowel. In some patients lymphoid follicles become hyperplastic. The hyperplasia may occur in the colon or extend to the small bowel. Small bowel lesions are seen in cases of immunoglobulin deficiency, with and without *G. lamblia* infestation. Symptoms are mild. There may be rectal bleeding, diarrhea, and abdominal cramps beginning usually by 3 yr of age.

The major importance of this entity is the similarity of its manifestations to more serious disorders. Lymphoid hyperplasia resolves spontaneously and requires no specific treatment.

J. RICHARD HAMILTON

Hodgson JR, Hoffman HN, Huizenga KA: Roentgenologic features of lymphoid hyperplasia of the small intestine associated with dysgammaglobulinemia. Radiology 88:883, 1967.
Poley JR, Smith EL: Benign lymphatic hyperplasia of the rectum. South Med J 65:420, 1972.

13.69 HERNIAS

A hernia is a protrusion of the contents of a body compartment through the wall that normally encloses it. Hernias (or "ruptures") and hydroceles (Sec. 18.46) are the most common significant anomalies of children. The most common hernia of the groin in infancy and childhood is the indirect (congenital, infantile) inguinal hernia. Direct inguinal and femoral hernias are rare in children. Diaphragmatic and esophageal hiatal hernias are discussed in Sec. 13.103 and 13.20, omphaloceles and umbilical hernias in Sec. 9.53.

INDIRECT INGUINAL HERNIAS

PATHOLOGY AND PATHOGENESIS. Late in fetal development the processus vaginalis, an outpouching of peritoneum originating at the internal inguinal ring, extends medially down each inguinal canal. Leaving the canal at the external ring, the processus enters the scrotum in the male, where it invests the developing testicle. Its lumen is normally obliterated before birth except for the portion enveloping the testicle. This part remains as a potential sac, the tunica

TABLE 13–20. Diarrhea Due to Hormone-Secreting Tumors

Name	Site	Hormone	Manifestations	Therapy
APUDomas*				
VIPoma	Pancreas	VIP†	Watery diarrhea, achlorhydria, hypokalemia	Somatostatin Resection
Somatostatinoma	Pancreas	Somatostatin	Massive diarrhea‡	Resection
Gastrinoma	Pancreas	Gastrin	Peptic ulceration, diarrhea	Cimetidine, omeprazole Tumor resection/gastrectomy
Carcinoid	Intestinal argentaffin cells	Serotonin	Diarrhea‡, crampy abdominal pain, flushing, wheezing, cardiac valve damage	Somatostatin Resection
Mastocytoma	Cutaneous, intestine, liver, spleen	Histamine, VIP	Pruritus, flushing, apnea, If VIP is positive, diarrhea	H_1- and H_2-blocking agents, cromolyn, steroids Resection if solitary
Medullary carcinoma	Thyroid	Calcitonin, VIP, prostaglandins	Watery diarrhea	Thyroidectomy
Neurogenic				
Ganglioneuroma, ganglioneuroblastoma	Extra-adrenal sites and adrenals	Catecholamines, VIP	Massive watery diarrhea	Resection
Pheochromocytoma	Chromaffin cells; abdominal > other sites	Catecholamines, VIP	Hypertension, tachycardia, sweating, anxiety, watery diarrhea‡	Resection

*APUDoma = *a*mine *p*recursor *u*ptake and *d*ecarboxylation of amino acids. These cells are neural crest cell derivatives of the gastroenteropancreatic endocrine system.
†VIP = vasoactive intestinal polypeptide.
‡ = reported only in adults.

vaginalis. In the female the processus extends from the external ring into the labia majora. If the proximal part of the processus vaginalis fails to close, a potential hernial sac is produced, into which an abdominal viscus may herniate or fluid collect. In the male, the patent portion extends inferiorly a variable distance, sometimes into the scrotum; if it is continuous with the tunica vaginalis, a complete hernia is formed.

Inguinal hernias are particularly common in premature infants, presumably because curtailment of intrauterine development impaired the process of closure. Infants with chronic lung disease, ascites, Ehlers-Danlos syndrome, and multiple congenital anomalies of the pelvis or perineum are at increased risk for inguinal hernias. When the testicle fails to descend (is cryptorchid), there is usually a large hernial sac, probably because something has arrested both testicular descent and closure of the peritoneal process. Overall, inguinal hernias are present in 1–3% of children. Most inguinal hernias occur in males (80–90%); females should be suspected of having testicular feminization syndrome if a hernia is present.

CLINICAL MANIFESTATIONS. Usually, a swelling is noted at the external ring, but it may extend for a variable distance downward into the scrotum or labia majora. The lump may be continually present or may be apparent only with raised intra-abdominal pressure, such as when an infant cries or strains at stool. A mass will sometimes appear suddenly in an infant and will be associated with acute discomfort. In such circumstances, it may be difficult to distinguish acute hydrocele of the spermatic cord from incarcerated hernia. The former will have no gastrointestinal symptoms; in the case of the latter, an examination will reveal loops of bowel entering and leaving the internal inguinal ring. In the older child, the mass typically appears at the end of an active day or with vigorous coughing. A hernia usually disappears when a baby relaxes with a bottle or when the older child lies down.

The diagnosis of inguinal hernia in infancy and childhood may be made from the history alone, even if significant physical findings are absent when the child is seen by the physician, provided that the typical swelling is described by a competent observer. Usually, however, it is preferable that the surgeon sees and feels the lump to exclude the possibility of a retracted testis or another abnormality, and to decide whether the contents are intestinal or only fluid.

Uncomplicated inguinal hernias in children rarely cause pain; pain in the groin is more likely to represent hip disease than hernia. Occasionally, a baby will cry whenever the hernia is protruding, but usually the hernia protrudes because the child is crying. Sometimes there is fleeting inguinal discomfort or pain when the hernia or hydrocele first fills.

Intestinal obstruction may be the presenting manifestation of an inguinal hernia. All patients with intestinal obstruction should be examined for an incarcerated hernia.

The older child with a hernia may have had a hydrocele in early infancy.

The observation of an inguinal or inguinoscrotal mass that is reduced either spontaneously or with manipulation is diagnostic. If the hernia is not present on initial inspection, inducing the baby to cry while the abdomen is firmly compressed is very likely to force it out. In the older child the hernia can usually be demonstrated by having the standing patient strain as the examiner manually compresses the abdomen or by tickling the child. If these maneuvers fail to reveal a suspected hernia, the diagnosis may be supported by the finding of a thickened spermatic cord on the side in question. Introducing a finger into the external ring to detect a peritoneal impulse is of no value, because the ring may be so large and the canal may be so short that an impulse is often readily palpable in the absence of herniation. Occasionally, a full bladder may occlude the internal inguinal ring and prevent elicitation of the physical findings of the hernia; emptying the bladder will enable the hernia to be demonstrated.

TREATMENT. The treatment of choice for inguinal hernia in infancy and childhood is herniorrhaphy. Some surgeons routinely explore the opposite inguinal region in cases of clinically unilateral inguinal hernias. Risks for bilateral disease include age less than 1 yr, history of bilateral hydroceles, a thickened cord on the uninvolved side, and girls less than 5 yr of age. It is probably necessary to explore the opposite side only if a clinically detectable hernia is present; 10% of patients return with a contralateral hernia after a unilateral repair. For the older child surgical repair is carried out at the earliest convenient time. In a young infant an inguinal hernia should be repaired as soon as the patient's general condition is satisfactory, in order to remove the risk of incarceration, which is highest under the age of 12 mo. Except for premature infants under the age of 6 mo, surgical repair may be done on an outpatient basis, provided appropriate facilities are available.

Supports and trusses designed to keep the abdominal contents from protruding into a hernial sac are not indicated and are considered to potentiate strangulation.

Any inguinal hernia that cannot be reduced needs emergency surgical repair. Resection may be required if necrosis of bowel has occurred but is rarely necessary.

When associated with prematurity, a hernia should be repaired only after the infant gains strength and weight in the hospital. During this time the hernia should be carefully monitored and manually reduced as necessary. When the baby is big enough to go home, the hernia should be repaired in a facility accustomed to caring for small infants.

An incarcerated-strangulated hernia is uncommon in children; most persistent inguinal masses can be reduced by various methods. Traditional methods to reduce an apparent incarcerated inguinal hernia include sedation (morphine), ice packs, gravity in the Trendelenburg position or even in the vertical upside down position, and gentle, continuous compression of the inguinal mass toward the inguinal ring. The latter procedure may take 5–10 min. Surgery should be scheduled shortly after reduction for difficultly reduced incarcerated hernias in order to prevent recurrences. If reduction of the incarcerated hernia is not possible, urgent surgery is indicated. An infarcted intestinal incarceration will not be reduced and must be treated at surgery by local resection of necrotic bowel.

COMPLICATIONS. A hernia is incarcerated when its contents cannot be reduced and the contained bowel is obstructed. A hernia may seem irreducible on the initial examination but prove to be reducible when manipulation is carried out by an experienced physician. Incarceration of an inguinal hernia is most likely to occur at the external inguinal ring and, with time, produces obstruction of the venous return from the herniated bowel and from the testis. This results in edema and progresses to venous infarction. The risk of incarceration is greatest in the youngest children. Cramps, bilious vomiting, and distention will occur with incarceration as the picture of intestinal obstruction develops. Irritability may be the only symptom of incarcerated hernia in an infant, and the diagnosis may be missed if the infant is not examined completely undressed.

Venous infarction of the testicle is a far more common complication of strangulation than intestinal ischemia, as the spermatic cord is readily compressed between the margin of the external ring and the hernial contents. A *Richter hernia* is a rare form of incarceration in which only a part of the bowel's circumference is pinched off within the hernia and intestinal obstruction does not develop. This is rare in children. Much more common is the strangulation of some omentum within the sac, resulting in local signs but without evidence of intestinal obstruction.

INGUINAL HERNIAS IN GIRLS. About 10% of inguinal hernias in children occur in girls. In an infant girl, the ovary is the organ most likely to herniate into the inguinal canal, where it is usually easily palpable as a movable almond-sized nodule. Although uncommon, infarction of the herniated ovary may occur because of torsion or compression of the pedicle. The inflamed abscess-like lesion that then develops in the groin is easily mistaken for inguinal lymphadenitis, but there are no lymph nodes in the anterior abdominal wall immediately above the inguinal ligament. In about 1% of operations on phenotypic girls for inguinal hernial repair, a testicle is discovered in the canal, abdomen, or labia majora. Closer examination reveals normal external genitalia, with the vagina a little shorter than usual. Rectal examination fails to reveal a uterus. Laparotomy in such cases reveals an absence of female internal genital organs. The absence of chromatin bodies on buccal smear and appropriate chromosomal findings indicate the diagnosis of testicular feminization (Sec. 19.41).

PROGNOSIS. The prognosis following surgical repair of inguinal hernia in an infant or child is excellent. The complication rate is low, and recurrences should be fewer than 1% after surgery.

BARRY SHANDLING

Given JP, Rubin SZ: Occurrence of contralateral inguinal hernia following unilateral repair in a pediatric hospital. J Pediatr Surg 24:963, 1989.

Janik JS, Shandling B: The vulnerability of the vas deferens (II): The case against routine bilateral inguinal exploration. J Pediatr Surg 17:585, 1982.

Kiesewetter WB, Oh KS: Unilateral inguinal hernias in children: What about the opposite side? Arch Surg 115:1443, 1980.

McGregor DB, Halverson R, McVay CB: The unilateral pediatric inguinal hernia: Should the contralateral side be explored? J Pediatr Surg 15:313, 1980.

Rescoria FJ, Grosfeld JL: Inguinal hernia repair in the perinatal period and early infancy: Clinical considerations. J Pediatr Surg 19:832, 1984.

Shandling B, Janik JS: The vulnerability of the vas (I). J Pediatr Surg 16:461, 1981.

13.70 EXOCRINE PANCREAS

Excluding cystic fibrosis, disorders of the exocrine pancreas are uncommon in childhood. Pancreatic disease may be based on anatomic (annular pancreas, pancreas divisum), metabolic (Reye syndrome, α_1-antitrypsin deficiency), congenital (Shwachman syndrome, enzyme defects), autoimmune (diabetes mellitus), or inflammatory pathology. A comprehensive discussion of cystic fibrosis is found in Sec. 14.89.

13.71 EMBRYOLOGY AND ANATOMY

The human pancreas develops from evaginations of primitive duodenum beginning at about the 5th wk of gestation. The larger dorsal anlage, which develops into the tail, body, and part of the head of the pancreas, grows directly from the duodenum. The smaller ventral anlage develops as one or two buds from the primitive liver and eventually forms the major portion of the head of the pancreas. At about 17 wk of gestation, the dorsal and ventral anlage fuse as the buds develop and the gut rotates. The ventral duct forms the proximal portion of the major pancreatic duct of Wirsung, which opens into the ampulla of Vater. The dorsal duct forms the distal portion of the duct of Wirsung and the accessory duct of Santorini, which may empty independently in about 15% of people. Variations in fusion account for the variety of the developmental anomalies of the pancreas.

The pancreas lies transversely in the upper abdomen between the duodenum and the spleen in the retroperitoneum. The head, which rests on the vena cava and renal vein, is adherent to the C loop of the duodenum and surrounds the distal common bile duct. The tail of the pancreas reaches to the left splenic hilum and passes above the left kidney. The lesser sac separates the tail of the pancreas from the stomach.

By 13 wk of gestation both exocrine and endocrine cells can be identified. Primitive acini containing immature zymogen granules are found by 16 wk. Mature zymogen granules containing amylase, trypsinogen, chymotrypsinogen, and lipase are present at 20 wk. Centroacinar and duct cells, which are responsible for water, electrolyte, and bicarbonate secretion, are also found by 20 wk. The final three-dimensional structure of the pancreas consists of a complex series of branching ducts surrounded by grape-like clusters of epithelial cells. Cells containing glucagon are present at 8 wk. Islets of Langerhans are first observed at 12–16 wk.

13.72 Anatomic Abnormalities

An *annular pancreas* results from incomplete rotation of the left (ventral) pancreatic anlage. Patients usually present in infancy with symptoms of complete or partial bowel obstruction. There is frequently a history of maternal polyhydramnios. Some children present with chronic vomiting, pancreatitis, or biliary colic. The treatment of choice is duodenojejunostomy. Division of the pancreatic ring is not attempted, because a duodenal diaphragm or duodenal stenosis frequently accompanies annular pancreas. Annular pancreas may be associated with Down syndrome, intestinal atresia, imperforate anus, pancreatitis, and malrotation.

Ectopic pancreatic rests in the stomach or small intestine occur in approximately 3% of the population. Most cases (70%) are found in the upper intestinal tract. Recognized on barium contrast studies by their typical umbilicated appearance, they are rarely of clinical importance. On endoscopy they are typically irregular yellow nodules 2–4 mm in diameter. A pancreatic rest may occasionally be the lead point of an intussusception, produce hemorrhage, or cause bowel obstruction.

Pancreas divisum, which occurs in 5–15% of the population, is the most common pancreatic developmental anomaly. As the result of failure of the dorsal and ventral pancreatic anlagen to fuse, the tail, body, and part of the head of the pancreas drain through the small accessory duct of Santorini rather than the main duct of Wirsung. Although the clinical importance of this anomaly remains controversial, most investigators believe that this anomaly may be associated with recurrent pancreatitis, possibly due to relative obstruction of the outflow of the ventral pancreas. A variety of surgical and therapeutic endoscopic procedures have been attempted with only mixed success.

Choledochal cysts are dilatations of the biliary tract and usually cause biliary tract symptoms, such as jaundice, pain, and fever. On occasion, the presentation may be that of pancreatitis. The diagnosis is usually easily made with ultrasound, CT scanning, or biliary tract scan. Similarly, a choledochocele, an intraduodenal choledochal cyst, may present with pancreatitis. The diagnosis may be difficult and may sometimes be made only by endoscopic retrograde cholangiopancreatography (ERCP).

A number of rare conditions, such as *Ivemark syndrome*, include pancreatic dysgenesis among their many features. Many of these syndromes include renal and hepatic dysgenesis along with the pancreatic anomalies. Absence of islet cells and agenesis of the pancreas produce permanent diabetes mellitus, which begins in the neonatal period. Agenesis is also associated with malabsorption.

Newman BM, Lebenthal E: Congenital abnormalities of the exocrine pancreas. *In*: Go ELW, et al (eds): The Exocrine Pancreas: Biology, Pathology, and Diseases. New York, Raven Press, 1986, pp 773–782.
Warshaw AL: Dominant dorsal duct syndrome: Pancreas divisum redefined. J Pediatr Gastroenterol Nutr 10:281, 1990.

13.73 PHYSIOLOGY

The functional unit of the exocrine pancreas is the acinus. Acinar cells are arranged in a semicircular array around a lumen. Ducts that drain the acini are lined by centroacinar cells and ductular cells. This arrangement allows for the secretions of the various cell types to mix.

The acinar cell synthesizes, stores, and secretes more than 20 enzymes, not all of which have been characterized. These enzymes are stored in zymogen granules, some in inactive forms. The relative concentration of the various enzymes in pancreatic juice is affected, and is perhaps controlled, by the diet, probably by regulating the synthesis of specific mRNA. As a general rule, diets high in fat increase the concentration of lipase, a high-protein diet increases pancreatic content of proteases, and a high carbohydrate diet leads to increased content of amylase in the pancreatic juice.

α-Amylase splits starch into maltose, isomaltose, maltotriose, and dextrins.

Trypsin and *chymotrypsin*, both endopeptidases, and *carboxypeptidase*, an exopeptidase, are secreted by the pancreas as inactive proenzymes. Trypsinogen is activated in the gut lumen by *enterokinase*, a brush-border enzyme. Trypsin can then activate trypsinogen, chymotrypsinogen, and procarboxypeptidase into their respective active forms. Enterokinase is, thus, a key enzyme for exocrine pancreatic function.

Pancreatic *lipase* requires colipase, a coenzyme also found in pancreatic fluid, for activity. Lipase liberates fatty acids from the one and three positions of triglycerides, leaving two—monoglycerides.

The stimuli for *exocrine pancreatic secretion* are neural and hormonal. Acetylcholine mediates the cephalic phase, whereas cholecystokinin (CCK), formerly called pancreozymin, mediates the intestinal phase. CCK is released from the duodenal mucosa by luminal amino acids and fatty acids. Feedback regulation of pancreatic secretion is mediated by pancreatic proteases in the duodenum. Secretion of CCK is possibly inhibited by the digestion of a trypsin-sensitive, CCK-releasing peptide released in the lumen of the small intestine.

Centroacinar and duct cells secrete water and bicarbonate. Bicarbonate secretion is under feedback control and is regulated by duodenal intraluminal pH. The stimulus for bicarbonate production is *secretin* in concert with CCK. Secretin cells are abundant in the duodenum.

Whereas normal pancreatic function is required for digestion, maldigestion occurs only after considerable reduction in pancreatic function has occurred. For instance, lipase and colipase secretion must be decreased by 90–98% before fat maldigestion occurs.

Although amylase and lipase are present in the pancreas early in gestation, secretion of both amylase and lipase is low in the infant. Adult levels of these enzymes are not reached in the duodenum until late in the 1st yr of life. Thus, digestion of the starch found in many infant formulas depends on the low levels of salivary amylase that reach the duodenum. This explains the diarrhea that may be seen in infants who are fed formulas high in glucose polymers or starch. In contrast, neonatal secretion of trypsinogen and chymotrypsinogen is at about 70% of the level found in the 1-yr-old infant. The low levels of amylase and lipase in duodenal contents of infants may partially explain the relative starch and fat intolerance of premature babies.

Hadorn HB, Munch G: The exocrine pancreas: Development, physiology and disease. *In*: Anderson CM, Burke V, Gracey M (eds): Pediatric Gastroenterology, 2nd ed. London, Blackwell, 1987.
Lloyd-Still JD, Listernick R, Buentello G: Complex carbohydrate intolerance: Diagnostic pitfalls and approach to management. J Pediatr 112:709, 1988.
Werlin SL: The exocrine pancreas. *In*: Walker WA, Durie PR, Hamilton JE, et al (eds): Pediatric Gastrointestinal Disease. Philadelphia, BC Decker, 1990.

13.74 PANCREATIC FUNCTION TESTS

Pancreatic function can be measured by direct and indirect methods. Direct stimulation of the pancreas with a test (LUNDH) meal of corn oil, skimmed milk powder, and dextrose or with secretin plus CCK can be performed. A triple-lumen tube is used to isolate the pancreatic secretions in the duodenum. Measurement of bicarbonate concentration and enzyme activity (trypsin, chymotrypsin) is performed on the aspirated secretions. Normal values for children, excluding infants, are well established. Direct stimulation tests are uncomfortable and are not often needed.

A qualitative examination of the stool for *microscopic fat* globules is the most widely practiced screening test for malabsorption. However, analysis of random stool specimens by this method may give both false-positive and false-negative results. A 72-hr collection for *quantitative analysis of fat content* is preferable. The collection is usually performed at home, and the parent is asked to keep a careful dietary record, from which fat intake is calculated. A preweighed, sealable, plastic container is used which the parent keeps in the freezer. Freezing helps to preserve the specimen but also reduces the odor. Infants are dressed in disposable diapers with the plastic side facing the skin so that the complete sample can be transferred to the container. Normal fat absorption is greater than 93% of intake.

Pancreatic enzyme activities can be measured in stool or duodenal contents. Stool trypsin has been the most commonly measured but is not as reliable as stool chymotrypsin. Neither test is as reliable as fecal fat analysis. Similarly, a random sample of duodenal fluid can be obtained and analyzed for pancreatic enzyme content. Serum levels of trypsinogen are elevated in neonates with cystic fibrosis. With advancing pancreatic damage serum trypsinogen levels eventually fall below normal.

Bentiromide (*N*-benzoyl-L-tyrosyl-*p*-aminobenzoic acid, Chymex) is a synthetic tripeptide for noninvasive testing of pancreatic enzyme function. After oral ingestion bentiromide is cleaved by chymotrypsin, releasing para-aminobenzoic acid (PABA), which is absorbed and excreted by the kidneys. PABA may be measured in a timed 6-hr urine collection or in a serum specimen obtained at 90 min.

Pancreatic function can also be measured by *breath tests*. A labeled triglyceride, most commonly ^{14}C-triolein, is ingested and digested by pancreatic lipase in the duodenum liberating $^{14}CO_2$, which is detected in the expired air. Because of the radioactivity and long half-life of ^{14}C, this test is not appropriate for use in children. Research is now ongoing using triolein-labeled with ^{13}C, a stable, nonradioactive isotope. Although this test is safe for pediatric use, detection of $^{13}CO_2$ requires a mass spectrophotometer that is not generally available.

13.75 DISORDERS OF THE EXOCRINE PANCREAS

Disorders Associated with Pancreatic Insufficiency

Other than cystic fibrosis, conditions that cause pancreatic insufficiency are rare in children. They include Shwachman-Diamond syndrome, isolated enzyme deficiencies, enterokinase deficiency, chronic pancreatitis, and protein-calorie malnutrition (Sec. 13.50).

CYSTIC FIBROSIS

See Sec. 14.89.

Cystic fibrosis is both the most common lethal genetic disease and the most common cause of malabsorption among white American children. By the end of the 1st year of life, 90% of children with cystic fibrosis have pancreatic insufficiency, leading to malnutrition in many cases. Treatment of the associated pancreatic insufficiency follows.

SHWACHMAN-DIAMOND SYNDROME

See Sec. 16.48.

This is an autosomal recessive syndrome (1:20,000 births), consisting of pancreatic insufficiency, neutropenia which may be intermittent, neutrophil chemotaxis defects, metaphyseal dysostosis, failure to thrive, and short stature. Patients present in infancy with poor growth and greasy foul-smelling stools that are characteristic of malabsorption. These children can be readily differentiated from those with cystic fibrosis by their normal sweat chloride levels and characteristic metaphyseal lesions. Despite adequate pancreatic replacement therapy, poor growth frequently continues. Pancreatic insufficiency is often transient, and steatorrhea may spontaneously improve with age (frequently before 4 yr of age). The neutropenia may be cyclic. Recurrent pyogenic infections (otitis media, pneumonia, osteomyelitis, dermatitis, sepsis) are common and are a frequent cause of death. Thrombocytopenia is found in 70% of patients and anemia in 50% of patients. Pathologically, the pancreatic acini are replaced by fat with little fibrosis. Islet cells and ducts are normal. The fatty pancreas has a characteristic hypodense appearance on the CT scan.

ISOLATED ENZYME DEFICIENCIES

Isolated deficiencies of trypsinogen, lipase, and colipase have been reported, as has enterokinase deficiency. Although enterokinase is a brush-border enzyme, deficiency causes pancreatic insufficiency because pancreatic proteases remain inactive. Deficiencies of trypsinogen or enterokinase manifest as a protein-losing enteropathy with failure to thrive, hypoproteinemia, and edema. Isolated amylase deficiency has not been shown to exist as a primary, permanent enzyme deficiency.

Syndromes Associated with Pancreatic Insufficiency

Pancreatic agenesis, the *Johanson-Blizzard syndrome* (pancreatic insufficiency, deafness, low birthweight, microcephaly, midline ectodermal scalp defects, psychomotor retardation, hypothyroidism, dwarfism, absent permanent teeth, and aplasia of the alae nasae), the syndrome of *sideroblastic anemia* (with or without splenic atrophy) and pancreatic insufficiency, congenital pancreatic hypoplasia, and congenital rubella are rare causes of pancreatic insufficiency. Some children with both syndromic (Alagille) and nonsyndromic paucity of intrahepatic bile ducts may also have pancreatic insufficiency associated with their liver disease. Pancreatic insufficiency has also been reported in duodenal atresia and stenosis and may also be seen in the rare infant with nesidioblastosis who requires 95% pancreatectomy to control hypoglycemia.

Aggett PJ, Cavanagh NPC, Matthew DJ, et al: Shwachman's syndrome: A review of 21 cases. Arch Dis Child 55:331, 1980.

Dupont C, Sellier N, Chochillon C, et al: Pancreatic lipomatosis and duodenal stenosis or atresia in children. J Pediatr 115:603, 1989.

Gaskin KJ, Durie PR, Lee L, et al: Colipase and lipase secretion in childhood-onset pancreatic insufficiency: Delineation of patients with steatorrhea secondary to relative colipase deficiency. Gastroenterology 86:1, 1984.

Hill RE, Durie PR, Gaskin KJ, et al: Steatorrhea and pancreatic insufficiency in Shwachman syndrome. Gastroenterology 83:22, 1982.

Pearson HA, Lobel JS, Kocoshis SA, et al: A new syndrome of refractory sideroblastic anemia with vacuolization of marrow precursors and exocrine pancreatic dysfunction. J Pediatr 95:976, 1979.

Schussheim A, Choi SJ: Exocrine pancreatic insufficiency with congenital anomalies. J Pediatr 89:782, 1976.

13.76 TREATMENT OF PANCREATIC INSUFFICIENCY

Treatment of exocrine pancreatic insufficiency by oral replacement would seem rather simple. However, in practice, although creatorrhea can usually be corrected, steatorrhea is difficult to completely correct. This is due to variability of lipase activity in different commercial preparations, inadequate dosage, incorrect timing of doses, lipase inactivation by gastric acid, and the observation that chymotrypsin in the enzyme preparation digests and thus inactivates lipase. At present, Pancrease and Creon are the preparations used most widely. These products are enteric-coated preparations that resist gastric acid inactivation.

The dosage of pancreatic replacement for children depends on the amount of food eaten and, thus, can be established only by trial and error. An adequate dose is one that is followed by the return of the stools to normal fat content, size, color, and odor. Enzyme replacement should be given at the beginning of and with the meal. Tablets should be chewed; powder can be mixed with a small quantity of food. Enzyme must also be given with snacks.

When adequate fat absorption cannot be realized, gastric acid neutralization with an antacid or an H_2-receptor blocking agent will prevent gastric acid enzyme inactivation and improve delivery of lipase into the intestine. The coating of enteric-coated preparations also protects lipase from acid inactivation.

Untoward effects secondary to pancreatic enzyme replacement therapy include allergic reactions, increased uric acid levels, and kidney stones.

13.77 ACUTE PANCREATITIS

After cystic fibrosis, acute pancreatitis is probably the most common pancreatic disorder in children. Mumps, other viral illnesses, drugs, and blunt abdominal injuries account for most known etiologies; other causes are uncommon (Table 13–21). Many cases are of unknown etiology or are secondary to a systemic disease process. Child abuse is recognized with increased frequency as a cause of traumatic pancreatitis in young children. More recently defined causes of pancreatitis include the hemolytic uremic syndrome, Kawasaki syndrome, refeeding after starvation, pancreas divisum, and Reye syndrome.

PATHOGENESIS. The exact pathogenesis leading to pancreatitis is unclear, although it is assumed that after an initial insult (presumably ductal obstruction), pancreatic enzymes leak into the interstitial space. Trypsinogen is activated to trypsin, leading to autodigestion of the gland and, thus, releasing and activating more enzyme. Evidence also suggests the activation of lecithin into the toxic lysolecithin by phospholipase A. The healthy pancreas is protected from autodigestion by three factors: (1) pancreatic enzymes are synthesized as inactive proenzymes; (2) digestive enzymes are segregated into zymogen granules; and (3) the presence of protease inhibitors.

CLINICAL MANIFESTATIONS. The patient with acute pancreatitis has abdominal pain, persistent vomiting, and fever. The pain is epigastric and steady, often resulting in the

TABLE 13–21. Etiology of Acute Pancreatitis in Children

Drugs and Toxins	**Systemic Disease**
Alcohol	α_1-Antitrypsin deficiency
Acetaminophen	Cystic fibrosis
Azathioprine	Diabetes mellitus
L-Asparaginase	Henoch-Schönlein purpura
Corticosteroids	Hemochromatosis
Estrogens	Hemolytic uremic syndrome
Furosemide	Hyperlipidemia: types I, IV, and V
6-Mercaptopurine	Hyperparathyroidism
Methyldopa	Kawasaki syndrome
Pentamidine	Systemic lupus erythematosus
Scorpion bites	Malnutrition
Sulfonamides	Periarteritis nodosa
Tetracycline	Peptic ulcer
Thiazides	Postpancreatic transplantation
Valproic acid	Refeeding after malnutrition
Hereditary Pancreatitis	Uremia
Idiopathic	**Traumatic**
Infections	Blunt injury
Coxsackie B virus	Child abuse
Epstein-Barr virus	Surgical trauma
Hepatitis A	Total body cast
Influenza A	
Measles	
Mumps	
Mycoplasma	
Rubella	
Reye syndrome	
Obstructive	
Ascariasis	
Biliary tract malformation	
Cholelithiasis	
Crohn disease	
Duplication cyst	
Pancreatic pseudocyst	
Pancreas divisum	
Postoperative	
Sphincter of Oddi dysfunction	
Tumor	

child assuming an antalgic position with hips and knees flexed, sitting upright or lying on the side. The child is very uncomfortable and irritable and appears acutely ill. The abdomen may be distended and quite tender. A mass may be palpable. The pain increases in intensity for 24–48 hr, during which time vomiting may increase and the patient may require hospitalization for dehydration and need fluid and electrolyte therapy. The prognosis for the acute uncomplicated case is excellent.

Acute hemorrhage pancreatitis, the most severe form of acute pancreatitis, is rare in children. In this life-threatening condition, the patient is acutely ill with severe nausea, vomiting, and abdominal pain. Shock, high fever, jaundice, ascites, hypocalcemia, and pleural effusions may occur. A bluish discoloration may be seen around the umbilicus (Cullen sign) or in the flanks (Grey Turner sign). The pancreas is necrotic and may be transformed into an inflammatory hemorrhagic mass. The mortality rate, which is approximately 50%, is related to shock, renal failure, adult respiratory distress syndrome, disseminated intravascular coagulation, massive gastrointestinal bleeding, and systemic or intra-abdominal infection.

DIAGNOSIS. Acute pancreatitis is usually diagnosed by measurement of serum and urine amylase activities. The serum amylase level is typically elevated for up to 4 days, while urinary amylase excretion remains about three-fold elevated for 1–2 wk as a result of prolonged renal clearance. A variety of other conditions may also cause hyperamylasemia without pancreatitis (Table 13–22). The use of the ratio of renal clearances of amylase and creatinine does not improve the sensitivity and specificity of the serum amylase determination. Elevation of the salivary amylase may mislead the clinician into making the diagnosis of pancreatitis in a child with abdominal pain, but the laboratory can now separate amylase isoenzymes into pancreatic and salivary fractions. Initially, serum amylase levels are normal in 10–15% of patients. Serum lipase is more specific than amylase for acute inflammatory pancreatic disease and should be determined when pancreatitis is suspected and the amylase level is normal.

Measurement of serum immunoreactive trypsin (IRT) is a new technique that is not widely available for the diagnosis of acute pancreatitis. IRT levels increase in acute pancreatitis but decrease in pancreatic insufficiency.

Other laboratory abnormalities that may be present in acute pancreatitis include hemoconcentration, coagulopathy, leukocytosis, hyperglycemia, glucosuria, hypocalcemia, elevated gamma glutamyl transpeptidase, and hyperbilirubinemia.

Roentgenography of the chest and abdomen may demonstrate nonspecific findings. The chest roentgenogram may demonstrate plate-like atelectasis, basilar infiltrates, elevation of the hemidiaphragm, left (rarely right)-sided pleural effusions, pericardial effusion, and pulmonary edema. Abdominal roentgenograms may demonstrate a sentinel loop, dilatation of the transverse colon (cut-off sign), ileus, pancreatic calcification, blurring of the left psoas margin, a pseudocyst, diffuse abdominal haziness (ascites), and peripancreatic extraluminal gas bubbles.

Ultrasound and *CT scanning* have major roles in the diagnosis and follow-up of children with pancreatitis. Findings may include pancreatic enlargement, a hypoechoic, sonolucent edematous pancreas, pancreatic masses, fluid collections, and abscesses (Fig. 13–24). As many as 20% of children with pancreatitis initially have normal imaging studies. Endoscopic retrograde cholangiopancreatography (ERCP) may have a role in the investigation of recurrent pancreatitis, pancreas divisum, sphincter of Oddi dysfunction, and disease associated with gallbladder pathology.

TREATMENT. The aims of medical management are to relieve pain and restore metabolic homeostasis. Meperidine is the drug of choice for pain relief and should be given in adequate doses. Fluid, electrolyte, and mineral balance should

TABLE 13–22. Differential Diagnosis of Hyperamylasemia

Pancreatic Pathology
Acute or chronic pancreatitis
Complications of pancreatitis (pseudocyst, ascites, abscess)
Factitious pancreatitis
Salivary Gland Pathology
Parotitis (mumps, *Streptococcus aureus*, CMV*, HIV†, EBV‡)
Sialadenitis (calculus, radiation)
Eating disorders (anorexia nervosa, bulimia)
Intra-Abdominal Pathology
Biliary tract disease (cholelithiasis)
Peptic ulcer perforation
Peritonitis
Intestinal obstruction
Appendicitis
Systemic Diseases
Metabolic acidosis (diabetes mellitus, shock)
Renal insufficiency, transplantation
Burns
Pregnancy
Drugs (morphine)
Head injury
Cardiopulmonary bypass

*CMV = cytomegalovirus.
†HIV = human immunodeficiency virus.
‡EBV = Epstein-Barr virus.

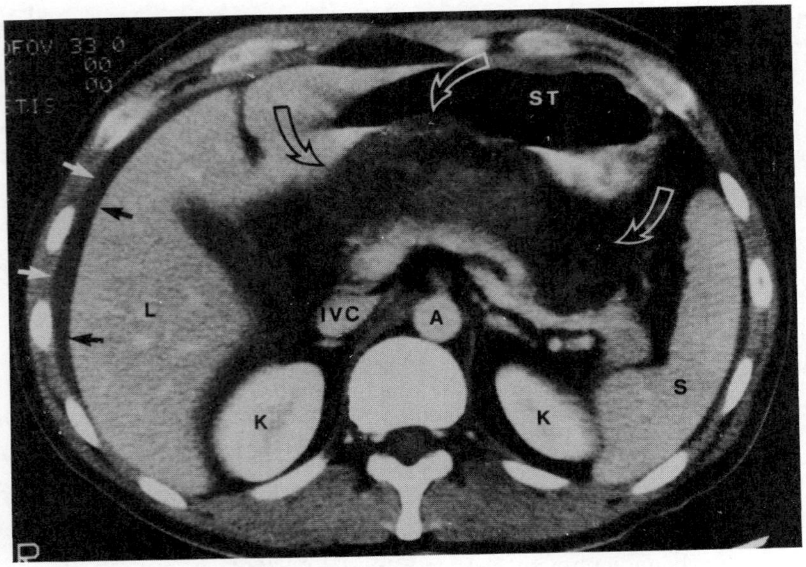

Figure 13–24. Acute pancreatitis. Computed tomography through the body of the pancreas demonstrates a halo of decreased attenuation around the pancreas that represents a peripancreatic zone of edema and fluid *(curved arrows)*. Note the pancreatic ascites most obvious lateral to the liver *(small arrows)*. If intravenous contrast was administered before the CT scan, the inflamed pancreas would appear more dense (whiter). (L = liver; A = aorta; K = kidney; PV = portal vein; S = spleen; IVC = inferior vena cava; ST = stomach). (From Freeny P, Lawson T: *In:* Putman CE, Ravin CE [eds]: Textbook of Diagnostic Imaging. Philadelphia, WB Saunders, 1988.)

be restored and maintained. Nasogastric suction is useful in patients who are vomiting. Nonetheless, the patient should be NPO. The routine use of antibiotics is of no benefit during the acute phase unless secondary infection is present. The response to treatment is usually complete over 2–4 days. Refeeding may commence when the serum amylase has normalized and clinical symptoms have resolved.

Although surgical therapy of acute pancreatitis is rarely required, the treatment of severe acute hemorrhagic pancreatitis may involve total parenteral nutrition and surgical drainage of necrotic material or abscesses. Newer modalities include peritoneal lavage to reduce the risk of secondary infection, the use of trypsin inhibitors, and, possibly, somatostatin.

PROGNOSIS. Poor prognostic factors on admission include blood glucose greater than 200 mg/dL, leukocytosis more than 16,000, serum LDH more than 700 IU, and SGOT more than 250 U. High-risk factors within the first 48 hr include a decrease in hematocrit of more than 10%, hypocalcemia less than 8 mg/dL, base deficit more than 4 mEq/L, BUN more than 50 mg/dL, hypoxia (Pa_{O_2} < 60 mm Hg), and large 3rd space losses. These poor prognostic findings are noted in lethal hemorrhagic pancreatitis.

Clavien P-A, Robert J, Meyer P, et al: Acute pancreatitis and normoamylasemia: Not an uncommon combination. Ann Surg 210:614, 1989.
Ranson JHC, Berman RS: Peritoneal lavage decreases pancreatic sepsis in pancreatitis. Ann Surg 211:708, 1990.
Weizman Z, Durie PR: Acute pancreatitis in childhood. J Pediatr 113:24, 1988.

13.78 CHRONIC PANCREATITIS

Chronic, relapsing pancreatitis in children is frequently hereditary or due to congenital anomalies of the pancreatic or biliary ductal systems. The former disease is transmitted as an autosomal dominant trait with complete penetrance but variable expressivity. Symptoms frequently begin in the 1st decade but are usually mild at the onset. Although spontaneous recovery from each attack occurs in 4–7 days, episodes may become progressively more severe. Hereditary pancreatitis is diagnosed by the presence of the disease in successive generations of a family. An evaluation during symptom-free intervals may be unrewarding until calcifications, pseudocysts, or pancreatic insufficiency develop.

Other conditions associated with chronic relapsing pancreatitis are hyperlipidemia (types I, IV, and V), hyperparathyroidism, ascariasis, and cystic fibrosis. Although it has been thought that most cases of recurrent pancreatitis in childhood are idiopathic, congenital anomalies of the ductal systems, such as pancreas divisum, are probably more common than previously recognized.

A thorough diagnostic *evaluation* of every child with more than one episode of pancreatitis is indicated. Serum lipid, calcium, and phosphorus levels are determined. Stools are evaluated for *Ascaris*, and a sweat test is performed. Plain abdominal films are evaluated for the presence of pancreatic calcifications. Abdominal ultrasound or CT scanning is performed to detect the presence of a pseudocyst. The biliary tract is evaluated for the presence of stones.

ERCP is a technique that can be used to define the anatomy of the gland and is mandatory whenever surgery is considered. This technique should be performed as part of the evaluation of any child with idiopathic, nonresolving, or recurrent pancreatitis and in patients with a pseudocyst before surgery. In these cases, ERCP may detect a previously undiagnosed anatomic defect that may be amenable to surgical therapy. ERCP is safe and can be performed successfully, even in young children, by an experienced endoscopist.

Allendorph M, Werlin SJ, Geenen JE, et al: Endoscopic retrograde cholangiopancreatography in children. J Pediatr 110:206, 1987.
Rothstein F, Wyllie R, Gauderer M: Hereditary pancreatitis and recurrent abdominal pain of childhood. J Pediatr Surg 20:535, 1985.

13.79 PANCREATIC PSEUDOCYST

Pancreatic pseudocyst formation is an uncommon sequela to acute or chronic pancreatitis. Pseudocysts are sacs delineated by a fibrous wall in the lesser peritoneal sac. They may enlarge or extend in almost any direction, thus producing a wide variety of symptoms (Fig. 13–25).

A pancreatic pseudocyst is suggested when an episode of pancreatitis fails to resolve or when a mass develops after an episode of pancreatitis. Clinical features usually include pain, nausea, and vomiting. The most common signs are a palpable mass in 50% of patients and jaundice in 10%. Other findings include ascites and pleural effusions.

The most useful diagnostic techniques are ultrasound, CT scanning, and ERCP. Because of its ease, availability, and reliability, ultrasound is the 1st choice. Sequential studies using ultrasound in adults with pancreatitis have shown that the incidence of pseudocyst formation is greater than previously thought but that most small pseudocysts resolve spontaneously. It is generally recommended that the patient with

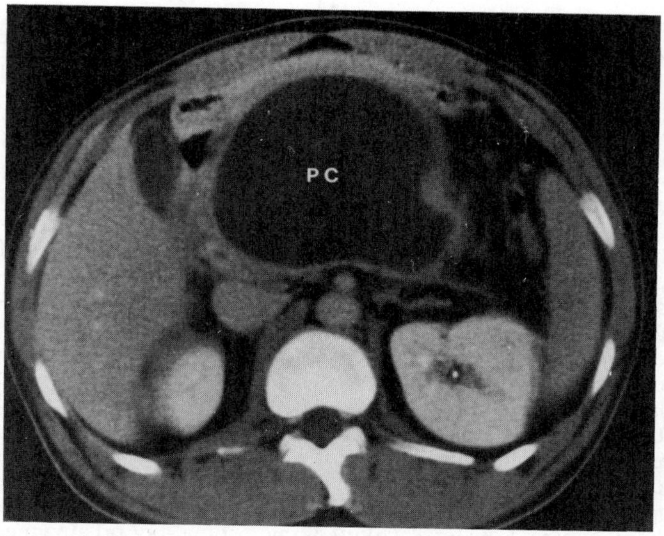

Figure 13–25. Pseudocyst. Follow-up CT scan 5 mo after the episode of acute pancreatitis demonstrates a large pseudocyst (PC). This large pseudocyst will probably not resolve spontaneously and may need drainage. (From Freeny P, Lawson T: *In:* Putman CE, Ravin CE [eds]: Textbook of Diagnostic Imaging. Philadelphia, WB Saunders, 1988.)

acute pancreatitis undergo an ultrasonographic evaluation 2 wk after resolution of the acute episode for an evaluation of possible pseudocyst formation.

Until recently, the treatment of nonresolving, large pseudocysts has been surgical. However, percutaneous drainage of pseudocysts has now been shown to be safe and effective treatment in selected patients. A pseudocyst must be allowed to mature for 4–6 wk before surgical drainage is attempted.

Millar AJW, Rode H, Studen RJ, et al: Management of pancreatic pseudocysts in children. J Pediatr Surg 23:122, 1988.

13.80 NEOPLASIA

Pancreatic tumors of childhood include both β and non-β cell tumors. Non–β cell tumors include gastrinomas and VIPomas. Secretion of gastrin by the gastrinoma produces the Zollinger-Ellison syndrome, with intractable peptic ulcer disease or diarrhea (see Table 13–20). The treatment of choice is surgical removal of the tumor. Because most tumors have metastasized by the time of diagnosis, cure is often not possible. The two options that remain are total gastrectomy and treatment with H_2 receptor (cimetidine, ranitidine) or H^+/K^+-ATPase pump (omeprazole) blocking agents that inhibit gastric acid secretion. High doses of H_2 blockers not only provide symptomatic relief but also avoid the complications of total gastrectomy.

The *watery diarrhea-hypokalemia-acidosis (WDHA) syndrome* is usually produced by the secretion of vasoactive intestinal peptide (VIP) by a non–β cell tumor (VIPoma) (see Table 13–20). VIP levels are frequently, but not always, increased in the serum. Treatment is surgical removal of the tumor. When this is not possible, symptoms may be controlled by the use of octreotide acetate (cyclic somatostatin, Sandostatin), a synthetic analog of somatostatin. Pancreatic tumors secreting a variety of hormones, including glucagon, somatostatin, and pancreatic polypeptide, have also been described.

Pancreatoblastomas, pancreatic adenocarcinomas, cystadenomas, and rhabdomyosarcomas are rarely encounted. The *Frantz tumor* is a papillary cystic tumor that is usually found in girls and young women. Presenting symptoms are usually abdominal pain, mass, or jaundice. The treatment of choice is total surgical removal.

Insulinomas and nesidioblastosis or hyperplasia of the β cells produce symptomatic hypoglycemia. Massive subtotal or total pancreatectomy is the treatment of choice when medical treatment fails (see Sec. 8.59). These children may then develop pancreatic insufficiency or diabetes as a complication of treatment.

STEVEN L. WERLIN

LIVER AND BILIARY SYSTEM

13.81 DEVELOPMENT OF HEPATIC AND BILIARY STRUCTURE AND FUNCTION

MORPHOGENESIS. The liver and biliary system originate from a cluster of cells that cap a ventral diverticulum in the primitive foregut. The hepatic anlage (pars hepatis) appears during the 4th wk of gestation as a duodenal diverticulum (Fig. 13–26). Within the ventral mesentery proliferation of cells forms anastomosing hepatic cords, with the network of primitive liver cells, sinusoids, and septal mesenchyme establishing the basic architectural pattern of liver lobule. The solid *cranial* portion of the hepatic diverticulum eventually forms hepatic glandular tissue and the intrahepatic bile ducts; the *caudal* portion (pars cystica) becomes the gallbladder, cystic duct, and common bile duct.

The hepatic lobules are identifiable at the 6th gestational wk. The liver reaches a peak relative size at the 9th wk at about 10% of the fetal weight. The bile canalicular structures that include microvilli and junctional complexes are specialized loci of the liver cell membrane; these appear very early in gestation, and by 6–7 wk large canaliculi bounded by several hepatocytes are seen. The intrahepatic bile ducts are derived through branching of the hepatic duct; formation is complete by the 3rd mo. The cystic duct and the gallbladder are fully recanalized by the 7th–8th wk.

In the hepatic excretory (biliary) system, intercellular bile canaliculi empty into the smallest bile ductules, which unite to form interlobular bile ducts that follow the terminal branches of the portal vein. At the hilum of the liver, the intrahepatic ducts leave the branches of the portal vein and merge to form the *extrahepatic* biliary system. The ducts of the right and left lobes form the common hepatic duct. The common bile duct is formed from the merger of the common hepatic duct and cystic duct; it runs along the right edge of the lesser omentum, terminating as the intramural papilla of Vater. Union of the biliary tract with the pancreatic ducts forms the ampulla of Vater, which, with the sphincter of Oddi, regulates the flow of bile into the intestine, prevents entry of bile into the pancreatic duct, and inhibits reflux of intestinal contents into the ducts.

The transport and metabolic activities of the liver are facilitated by the structural arrangement of liver cell cords (Fig. 13–26*D*), which are formed by rows of hepatocytes, separated by sinusoids that converge toward the tributaries of the hepatic vein (the central vein) located in the center of the lobule. This establishes the pathways and patterns of flow for substances to and from the liver. Plasma proteins and other plasma components are *secreted* by the liver. Absorbed and circulating nutrients arrive through the portal vein or the hepatic artery and pass through the sinusoids and past the hepatocytes to the systemic circulation at the central vein.

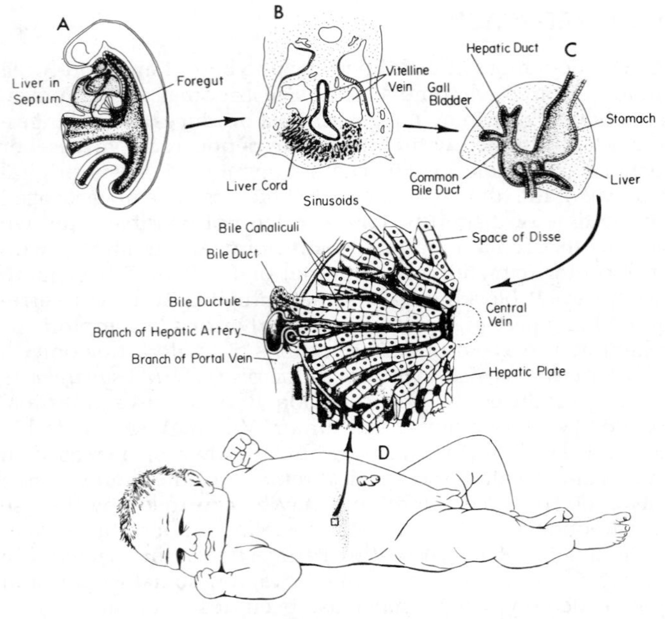

Figure 13–26. Hepatic embryogenesis. *A*, Ventral outgrowth of hepatic diverticulum from foregut endoderm in the 3.5 wk embryo. *B*, Between the two vitelline veins, the enlarging hepatic diverticulum buds off epithelial (liver) cords that become the liver parenchyma, around which the endothelium of capillaries (sinusoids) align (4-wk embryo). *C*, Hemisection of embryo at 7.5 wk demonstrating recanalization of the biliary tract. *D*, Three-dimensional representation of the hepatic lobule as present in the newborn. (From Andres JM, Mathis RK, Walker WA: Liver disease in infants. Parts I and II: Developmental hepatology and mechanisms of liver dysfunction. J Pediatr 90:686 and 964, 1977.)

Biliary components are transported via the series of enlarging channels from the bile canaliculi through the bile ductule to the common bile duct.

Bile secretion has been noted at the 12th gestational wk. The major components of bile vary with stage of development. Near term, cholesterol and phospholipid content is relatively low; and low concentrations of bile acids, the absence of bacterially derived (secondary) bile acids, and the presence of unusual bile acids reflect low rates of bile flow and immature bile acid synthesis.

Fetal hepatic blood flow is derived from the hepatic artery and from the portal and umbilical veins, which form the portal sinus. The portal venous inflow is directed mainly to the right lobe of the liver; umbilical flow is primarily to the left. The ductus venosus shunts blood from the portal and umbilical veins to the hepatic vein, bypassing the sinusoidal network. The ductus venosus becomes obliterated when oral feedings are initiated. The oxygen saturation is lower in portal than in umbilical venous blood; accordingly, the right hepatic lobe has lower oxygenation and greater hematopoietic activity than the left hepatic lobe. Sinusoidal endothelium is the site of large macrophages, which become the Kupffer (reticuloendothelial) cell network.

The liver constitutes 5% of body weight at birth but only 2% in the adult. Early in gestation (7th wk), hematopoietic cells outnumber functioning hepatocytes in the hepatic anlage. The hepatocytes are smaller (~ 20 μm) than at maturity (30–35 μm) and contain less glycogen. Near term, the hepatocytes dominate the organ, and cell size and glycogen content increase. Hematopoiesis is virtually absent by the 2nd postnatal month in full-term infants. As the density of hepatocytes increases with gestational age, the relative volume of the sinusoidal network decreases.

ULTRASTRUCTURE. Our understanding of the ultrastructural anatomy of the hepatocyte (Fig. 13–27) has been made possible through electron microscopy and cell fractionation techniques. Various regions of the hepatocyte *plasma membrane* exhibit specialized functions. For example, bidirectional transport occurs at the sinusoidal surface, where materials reaching the liver via the portal system enter and compounds secreted by the liver leave the hepatocyte. Canalicular membranes of adjacent hepatocytes form bile canaliculi, which are bounded by tight junctions preventing transfer of secreted compounds back into the sinusoid. Abundant *mitochondria* are the sites of oxidation and metabolism of heterogeneous classes of substrates, of fatty acid oxidation, of key processes in gluconeogenesis, and of storage and release of energy. The *nucleus* and *nucleolus* are surrounded by a pair of membranes, the outermost of which adjoins the *endoplasmic reticulum*. The latter is a continuous network of rough- and smooth-surfaced tubules and cisternae, which are the site of various processes, including protein and triglyceride synthesis and drug metabolism. The endoplasmic reticulum is the major part of the *microsomal* fraction obtained by ultracentrifugation of liver homogenate. Low fetal activity of microsomal-bound enzymes accounts for a relative inefficiency of xenobiotic metabolism. The *Golgi apparatus* is active in protein packaging and possibly in bile secretion. Hepatocyte microbodies *(peroxisomes)* are single-membrane–limited cytoplasmic organelles that contain enzymes such as oxidases and catalase and those that play a role in lipid and bile acid metabolism. The *cytoskeleton*, composed of actin filaments, is distributed throughout the cell and concentrated near the plasma membrane. Microfilaments and microtubules may play a role in receptor-mediated endocytosis, in bile secretion, and in maintaining the architecture and motility of the cell. *Lysosomes* contain numerous hydrolases that play a role in intracellular digestion.

In Reye syndrome, there are specific alterations in *mitochondria*; in Zellweger (cerebrohepatorenal) syndrome *peroxisomes* are absent; and in glycogenosis type II, a *lysosomal* hydrolase is absent.

FUNCTIONAL DEVELOPMENT. Functions of the liver (hepatocytes) are summarized in the following discussion. Several of these metabolic processes are immature in the healthy newborn infant, owing in part to the fetal patterns of activity of various enzymatic processes. Many hepatic functions are carried out for the fetus by the maternal liver, which provides nutrients, serves as a route of elimination of metabolic end products, and is a site of biotransformations. Fetal liver metabolism is devoted primarily to the production of proteins for growth requirements. Toward term, primary functions become production and storage of essential nutrients, excretion of bile, and establishment of processes of elimination. Extrauterine adaptation involves de novo enzyme synthesis. Modulation of these processes depends on substrate and hormonal input via the placenta, and on dietary and hormonal input in the postnatal period.

METABOLIC FUNCTIONS OF THE LIVER

CARBOHYDRATE METABOLISM. The liver stores excess carbohydrate as glycogen, a polymer of glucose readily hydrolyzed to glucose during fasting. Immediately after birth, the infant is dependent on hepatic glycogenolysis; thereafter, the infant is capable of both glycogenolysis and gluconeogenesis. Fetal glycogen synthesis begins at about the 9th wk of gestation, with glycogen stores most rapidly accumulated near term, when the liver contains two to three times the amount of glycogen of adult liver. The majority of this stored glycogen is utilized in the immediate postnatal period. Reaccumulation is initiated at about the 2nd wk of postnatal life, and glycogen stores reach adult levels at approximately the 3rd wk in

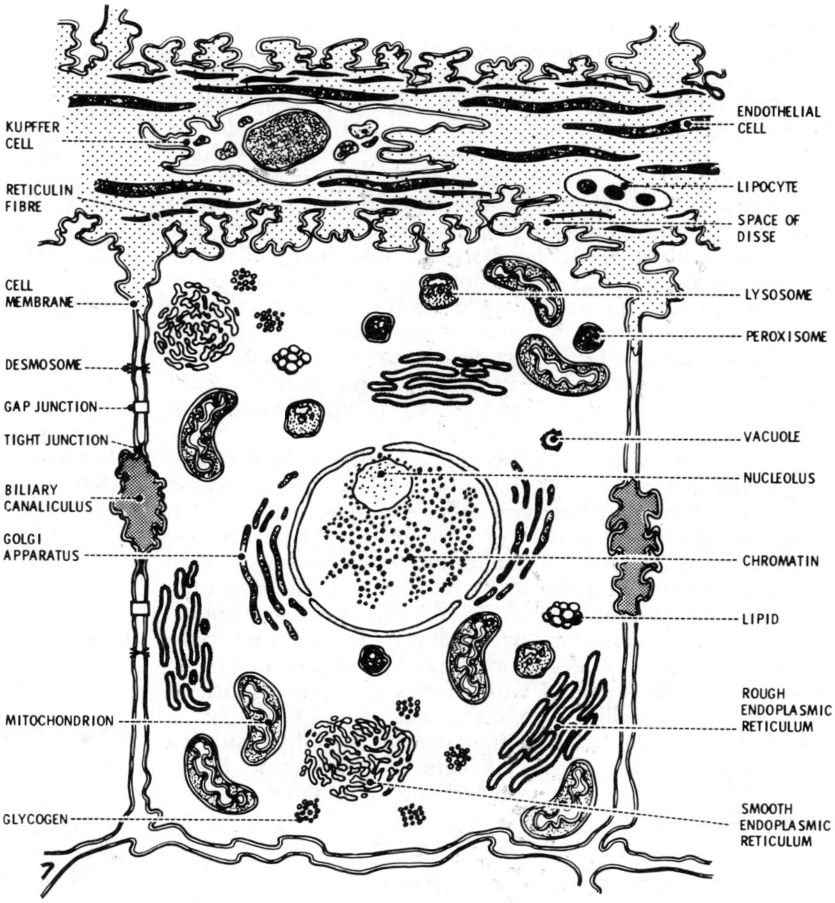

Figure 13–27. Hepatic ultrastructure, conceptualized. Electron microscopic appearance of a normal human liver cell. (From Sherlock S: *In:* Diseases of the Liver and Biliary System, Chapter 1. Oxford, Blackwell Scientific, 1981.)

healthy full-term infants. The fluctuations in serum glucose concentration in preterm infants are due in part to the fact that efficient regulation of the synthesis, storage, and degradation of glycogen develops only near the end of full-term gestation. Dietary carbohydrates such as galactose are converted to glucose, but there is a substantial dependence on gluconeogenesis for glucose in early life, especially if glycogen stores are limited. Gluconeogenic activity is not present in the fetal liver but develops rapidly after birth.

PROTEIN METABOLISM. During the rapid fetal growth phase, specific decarboxylases that are rate-limiting in the biosynthesis of physiologically important polyamines have higher activities than in the mature liver. The rate of synthesis of albumin and secretory proteins in the developing liver parallels the quantitative changes in endoplasmic reticulum. Synthesis of albumin appears at approximately the 7th–8th wk in the human fetus and increases in inverse proportion to that of α-fetoprotein, which is a dominant fetal protein. By the 3rd–4th mo of gestation, the fetal liver is able to produce fibrinogen, transferrin, and low-density lipoproteins. From this period on, fetal plasma contains each of the major protein classes, at concentrations considerably below those achieved at maturity.

The *postnatal* patterns of development of various proteins are heterogeneous. Lipoproteins of each class rise abruptly in the 1st wk after birth, to reach levels that will vary little until puberty. Albumin concentrations are low in the neonate (~ 2.5 g/dL), reaching adult levels (~ 3.5 g/dL) after several months. Levels of ceruloplasmin and complement factors increase slowly to adult values during the 1st year. In contrast, transferrin levels at birth are similar to those of the adult, decline for 3–5 mo and rise thereafter to achieve their final concentrations. Low levels of activity of specific proteins have implications for the nutrition of the infant; for example, a low level of cystathionase activity impairs the trans-sulfuration pathway by which dietary methionine is converted to cystine; accordingly, the latter must be supplied exogenously. Similar dietary requirements may exist for other sulfur-containing amino acids, such as taurine.

LIPID METABOLISM. Fatty acid oxidation provides a major source of energy in early life, complementing glycogenolysis and gluconeogenesis. The newborn infant is relatively intolerant of prolonged fasting, owing in part to a restricted capacity for hepatic ketogenesis. Rapid maturation of the ability of the liver to oxidize fatty acid occurs during the 1st few days of life. Milk provides the major source of calories in early life; this high-fat, low-carbohydrate diet mandates active gluconeogenesis to maintain blood sugar levels. When the glucose supply is limited, ketone body production from endogenous fatty acids may provide energy for hepatic gluconeogenesis and an alternative fuel for brain metabolism. Metabolic processes involving lipid and lipoprotein are predominantly hepatic; liver immaturity or disease affects lipid concentrations and lipoproteins.

BIOTRANSFORMATION. The newborn infant has a decreased capacity to metabolize and detoxify certain drugs, owing to underdevelopment of the hepatic microsomal component that is the site of the specific oxidative, reductive, hydrolytic, and conjugation reactions required for these biotransformations (Sec. 6.55). The major components of the mono-oxygenase system, such as cytochrome P-450, NADPH, and cytochrome C–reductase, are present in low concentrations in fetal microsomal preparations. In the full-term infant, hepatic uridine diphosphate (UDP) glucuronyl transferase and enzymes involved in the oxidation of polycyclic aromatic hydocarbons have very low activities. Age-related differences in pharmacokinetics vary. For example, the half-life of acetaminophen in a newborn is similar to that of an adult, whereas theophylline has a half-life of approximately 100 hr in the premature infant and 5–6 hr in the adult. These physiologic variables taken together with factors such as binding to plasma proteins and renal clearance are important in determining drug dosage and in production of toxicity. Dramatic examples of the susceptibility of the newborn infant to drug toxicity are the responses to chloramphenicol (gray syndrome) or to benzoyl alcohol and its metabolic products, which involve ineffective glucuronide and glycine conjugation, respectively. The low concentrations of vitamin E, superoxide dismutase, and glutathione peroxidase in the fetal and early newborn liver lead to increased susceptibility to deleterious effects of oxygen toxicity through lipid peroxidation.

Conjugation reactions (which convert drugs or metabolites into forms that can be eliminated in bile) also are catalyzed by hepatic microsomal enzymes. For example, the newborn infant has decreased activity of UDP-glucuronyl transferase, which converts unconjugated bilirubin to the readily excreted glucuronide conjugate and is the rate-limiting enzyme in the excretion of bilirubin (see Sec. 9.44). There is rapid postnatal development of transferase activity, even in prematurely born infants, irrespective of gestational age; this suggests that birth-related rather than age-related factors are of primary importance in the postnatal development of activity of this enzyme. Microsomal activity can be stimulated by the administration of phenobarbital or other inducers of cytochrome P-450. Alternatively, drugs such as cimetidine may inhibit microsomal P-450 activity.

HEPATIC EXCRETORY FUNCTION

Hepatic excretory function and bile flow are related closely to bile acid excretion and recirculation. Bile acids are the major product of degradation of cholesterol. Their incorporation into mixed micelles with cholesterol and phospholipid creates an efficient vehicle for the solubilization and intestinal absorption of lipophilic compounds, such as dietary fats and fat-soluble vitamins. The secretion of bile acids is the major determinant of bile flow in the mature animal. Accordingly, the maturity of bile acid metabolic processes affects overall hepatic excretory function, including biliary excretion of endogenous and exogenous compounds.

In humans, two of the bile acids (cholic and chenodeoxycholic acid—the primary bile acids) are synthesized in the liver. Before excretion, they are conjugated with glycine and taurine. In response to a meal, contraction of the gallbladder delivers bile acids to the intestine to assist in fat digestion and absorption. After mediating fat digestion, the bile acids themselves are reabsorbed from the terminal ileum through specific active transport processes. They return to the liver via portal blood, are taken up by liver cells, and are re-excreted in bile. In the adult, this enterohepatic circulation involves 90–95% of the circulating bile acid pool. Bile acids that escape ileal reabsorption reach the colon, where the bacterial flora, through dehydroxylation and deconjugation, produces the secondary bile acids, deoxycholate and lithocholate. In the adult the composition of bile reflects the excretion of not only the primary but also the secondary bile acids, which are reabsorbed from the distal intestinal tract.

In the neonate, there is inefficient ileal reabsorption and a low rate of hepatic clearance of bile acids from portal blood. The latter results in elevated serum concentrations of bile acids in healthy newborns, often to levels that would suggest liver disease in older individuals. The size of the bile acid pool in the neonate is about one half that of the adult, and the bile acid concentration in the proximal intestinal lumen is similarly decreased to levels that are frequently below the concentration required for micelle formation (2 mM); accordingly, absorption of dietary fats and fat-soluble vitamins is reduced but not sufficient to produce malabsorption. Transient phases of "physiologic cholestasis" and "physiologic steatorrhea" play a role in the nutrition of low birthweight infants but are of minor importance to healthy full-term newborns.

TABLE 13–23. Potential Sites for Disturbances in Bile Acid Metabolism

- Defective bile acid **synthesis** may result from:
  - Congenital impairment of hepatic synthesis
  - Specific defects in bile acid synthesis as seen in:
    - Cerebrotendinous xanthomatosis
    - Intrahepatic cholestasis (neonatal hepatitis)
      - Qualitative abnormalities
      - Quantitative abnormalities
  - Acquired defects in bile acid synthesis (as observed in liver diseases such as hepatitis and cirrhosis)
- Abnormalities of bile acid **delivery** to the bowel may be seen in:
  - Celiac sprue (sluggish gallbladder contraction)
  - Extrahepatic bile duct obstruction due to:
    - Biliary atresia
    - Stricture
    - Stone
    - Carcinoma
- **Interruption** of the enterohepatic circulation of bile acids may occur with:
  - An external bile fistula
  - Ileojejunal exclusion for exogenous obesity or hypercholesterolemia
  - Cystic fibrosis
  - Contaminated small bowel syndrome (with bile acid precipitation, increased jejunal absorption and "short circuiting")
  - Entrapment of bile acids in intestinal lumen by:
    - Cholestyramine
    - Trivalent cations (aluminum-containing antacids)
    - Fiber
- Bile acid malabsorption
  - Primary bile acid malabsorption (absent/inefficient ileal active transport)
    - Intractable diarrhea (infancy)
    - Irritable bowel (adults)
  - Secondary bile acid malabsorption
    - Ileal disease or resection
      - Crohn disease
      - Ileal resection
      - Ileal bypass
      - Radiation enteritis
      - Postinfectious enteritis
    - Exogenous bile acid administration (e.g., gallstone dissolution)
    - Cystic fibrosis
  - Tertiary bile acid malabsorption
    - Postcholecystectomy
    - Renal failure
    - Drugs
- Defective uptake or altered intracellular metabolism
  - Parenchymal disease (acute hepatitis, cirrhosis)
    - Regurgitation from cells
    - Portosystemic shunting
  - Cholestasis

Beyond the neonatal period, disturbances in bile acid metabolism may be responsible for diverse effects on hepatobiliary and intestinal function (Table 13–23).

13.82 MANIFESTATIONS OF LIVER DISEASE

PATHOLOGIC MANIFESTATIONS. Alterations in hepatic structure and function can be *acute* or *chronic*, with varying patterns of reaction of the liver to cell injury. The ultimate reaction is cell death, but the hepatocyte has a remarkable capacity for regeneration. Collagen is formed during the healing phase of cellular injury, with excessive growth of fibrous tissue becoming manifest as cirrhosis.

Inflammation or **necrosis** of individual hepatocytes can be due to viral infection, drugs or toxins, immunologic disorders, or hypoxia. The evolving process leads either to repair, to continuing injury with chronic changes, or in rare cases to massive hepatic damage or death.

Cholestasis is an alternative or concomitant response to injury. It is defined as the accumulation in serum of substances normally excreted in bile such as bilirubin, cholesterol, bile acids, and trace elements. A liver biopsy demonstrates accumulation of bile and bile pigment in the parenchyma. In extrahepatic obstruction, bile pigment may be visible in the intralobular bile ducts or throughout the parenchyma as bile lakes or infarcts. Cholestasis may also be seen without evidence of bile duct obstruction, when hepatocyte injury or an alteration in hepatic physiology has led to a reduction in the rate of secretion of solute and water. Likely causes may include alterations in the ultrastructure or cytoskeleton of the hepatocyte, alterations in organelles responsible for bile secretion, alterations in enzymatic activity, or alterations in permeability of the bile canalicular apparatus. The end result is clinically indistinguishable from obstructive cholestasis.

Cirrhosis (defined by the presence of bands of fibrous tissue that link central and portal areas and form parenchymal nodules) is a potential end stage of any acute or chronic liver disease. Cirrhosis may be posthepatitic or postnecrotic, or may follow chronic biliary obstruction (biliary cirrhosis). Cirrhosis may be **macronodular** with nodules of various sizes (up to 5 cm) separated by broad septae, or **micronodular**, with nodules of uniform size (< 1 cm) separated by fine septae. There may also be mixed forms. The progressive scarring of cirrhosis leads to altered hepatic blood flow, with further impairment of liver cell function. In addition, the restriction of blood flow within the liver leads to portal hypertension.

Primary tumors of the liver are discussed in Sec. 17.23.

The liver may be **secondarily** involved in neoplastic (metastatic) and non-neoplastic (storage diseases and fat infiltration) and infectious processes. The liver may also be affected by chronic passive congestion or acute hypoxia, with hepatocellular damage.

CLINICAL MANIFESTATIONS. Hepatomegaly. Enlargement of the liver can be due to several mechanisms (Table 13–24). Concepts of normal liver size have been based on age-related clinical indices, such as (1) the degree of extension of the liver edge below the costal margin, (2) the span of dullness to percussion, or (3) the length of the vertical axis of the liver, as estimated from imaging techniques. In children, the normal liver edge can be felt up to 2 cm below the right costal margin. In the newborn infant extension of the liver edge more than 3.5 cm below the costal margin in the right midclavicular line suggests hepatic enlargement. Measurement of *liver span* is carried out by percussing the upper margin of dullness and by palpating the lower edge in the right midclavicular line; it may be more reliable than an extension of the liver edge alone, and the two measurements may correlate poorly.

The liver span increases linearly with body weight and age in both sexes. If percussion is used for both the upper and lower borders, the mean liver span is related curvilinearly to age. The span ranges from about 4.5–5 cm at 1 wk of age to approximately 7–8 cm in males and 6–6.5 cm in females by 12 yr of age. The expected span of liver dullness in the midclavicular line in both sexes after 12 yr of age can be calculated as follows: in males, span (cm) = 0.032 × weight (pounds) + 0.18 × height (inches) − 7.86; in females, span (cm) = 0.027 × weight (pounds) + 0.22 × height (inches) − 10.75. These formulas are not accurate for newborns or younger children. In some persons, the lower edge of the right lobe of the liver extends downward (Riedel lobe) and may be palpable as a broad mass. Downward displacement of the liver by the diaphragm or thoracic organs can create an erroneous impression of hepatomegaly.

TABLE 13–24. Mechanisms of Hepatomegaly

- Increase in the **number** or **size** of the cells in the liver
  - Storage
    - Fat: Reye syndrome, malnutrition, obesity, metabolic liver disease, lipid infusion (total parenteral nutrition), cystic fibrosis, diabetes mellitus, medication-related
    - Specific lipid storage diseases: Gaucher, Niemann-Pick, Wolman syndromes; acyl dehydrogenase deficiencies
    - Glycogen: glycogen storage diseases (multiple enzyme defects); total parenteral nutrition; infant diabetic mother, Beckwith syndrome
    - Miscellaneous: α_1-antitrypsin deficiency, Wilson disease, hypervitaminosis A, neonatal iron storage (hemochromatosis)
- Inflammation
  - Hepatocyte enlargement (hepatitis)
    - Viral—acute and chronic
    - Bacterial (sepsis, abscess, cholangitis)
    - Toxic
  - Kupffer cell enlargement
  - Autoimmune: chronic active hepatitis, sarcoidosis, systemic lupus erythematosus
- Infiltration
  - Primary tumors
    - Hepatoblastoma
    - Hepatocellular carcinoma
    - Hemangioma
    - Focal nodular hyperplasia
  - Secondary or metastatic tumors
    - Lymphoma
    - Leukemia
    - Histiocytosis
    - Neuroblastoma
    - Wilms tumor
- Increased size of **vascular** space
  - Intrahepatic obstruction to hepatic vein outflow
    - Veno-occlusive disease
    - Hepatic vein thrombosis (Budd-Chiari syndrome)
    - Hepatic vein web
  - Suprahepatic
    - Congestive heart failure
    - Pericardial disease
    - Tamponade
    - Constrictive pericarditis
    - Hematopoietic: Sickle cell anemia, thalassemia
- Increased size of **biliary** space
  - Congenital hepatic fibrosis
  - Caroli disease
  - Extrahepatic obstruction
- Idiopathic (? "benign")

Examination of the liver should note the consistency, contour, tenderness, or the presence of any masses or bruits, as well as assessing splenic size.

Ultrasound can often help in the evaluation of unexplained hepatomegaly; size and consistency can be assessed. Hyperechogenic, bright hepatic parenchyma can be seen with metabolic disease (glycogen storage disease) or fatty liver (owing to malnutrition or hyperalimentation, or following corticosteroid therapy).

Ultrasound can also assess **gallbladder size**. Gallbladder distention may be seen in sick infants who have sepsis. Gallbladder length normally varies from 1.5–5.5 cm (average 3.0) in infants to 4–8 cm in adolescents; width ranges from 0.5–2.5 cm (mean 0.8 in neonates) at all ages.

Jaundice. Yellow discoloration of the plasma, skin, and

mucous membranes may be the earliest and only sign of hepatic dysfunction; it therefore requires urgent evaluation. Jaundice becomes clinically apparent in children and adults when the serum concentration of bilirubin reaches 2–3 mg/dL. In neonates, higher levels may be found without evident icterus. Icterus may be associated with dark urine or acholic (light-colored) stools during childhood.

Bilirubin occurs in plasma in four forms: (1) *unconjugated bilirubin* tightly bound to albumin; (2) *free or unbound bilirubin* (the form responsible for kernicterus, because it can cross cell membranes); (3) *conjugated bilirubin* (the only fraction to appear in urine); and (4) *δ fraction* (bilirubin covalently bound to albumin), which appears in serum when hepatic excretion of conjugated bilirubin is impaired in patients with hepatobiliary disease. The δ fraction permits conjugated bilirubin to persist in the circulation and delays resolution of jaundice.

Measurement of serum bilirubin is traditionally via the van den Bergh (diazo) reaction. The terms "direct-reacting" and "indirect-reacting" bilirubin correspond roughly to *conjugated* and *unconjugated* bilirubin, respectively.

Jaundice in an infant or older child may reflect accumulation of either unconjugated or conjugated bilirubin. An increase in unconjugated bilirubin may indicate increased production, hemolysis, reduced hepatic removal, or altered metabolism of bilirubin (Table 13–25). Significant accumulations of conjugated bilirubin (> 20% of total) reflect decreased excretion by damaged hepatic parenchymal cells or disease of biliary tract, which may be due to sepsis, endocrine or metabolic disease, inflammation of the liver, or obstruction. In most patients with diseases that tend to produce conjugated hyperbilirubinemia, a portion of the total bilirubin will be present in **unconjugated** form, with near-parallel rises in both fractions.

Pruritus. Intense generalized itching may occur in patients with cholestasis, presumably owing to retained components of bile such as bile acids, as pruritus responds to bile acid–binding agents such as cholestyramine or to choleretic agents such as ursodeoxycholic acid or phenobarbital. Pruritus is unrelated to the degree of hyperbilirubinemia; deeply jaundiced patients may be asymptomatic, and vice versa.

Spider Angiomas. Vascular spiders, characterized by central pulsating arterioles from which small, wiry venules radiate, may be seen in patients with chronic liver disease. These are presumably reflective of altered estrogen metabolism.

Palmar Erythema. Blotchy erythema, most noticeable over the thenar and hypothenar eminences and on the tips of the fingers, may be due to vasodilatation and increased blood flow.

Xanthomata. The elevation of serum cholesterol associated with chronic cholestasis may cause the deposition of lipid in the dermis and subcutaneous tissue. Brown nodules may develop first over the extensor surfaces of the extremities; rarely, xanthelasma of the eyelids develops.

Portal Hypertension. The portal vein drains the splanchnic area (abdominal portion of the gastrointestinal tract, pancreas, and spleen) into the hepatic sinusoids. Pressure is normally slightly higher (~ 5–10 mm Hg) in the portal vein than in other venous systems in order to overcome the resistance of the sinusoidal system. Portal hypertension is defined as an increase in portal venous pressure to greater than 20 mm Hg (see Sec. 13.102).

Ascites. Ascites may be associated with urinary tract anomalies, metabolic diseases (e.g., lysosomal storage disease), congenital or other heart disease, or hydrops fetalis. In patients with hepatic disease, sinusoidal blockade due to cirrhosis increases hydrostatic pressure and transudation of fluid; this may be worsened by hypoalbuminemia (see Sec. 13.103).

Encephalopathy. In acute or chronic liver disorders, metabolic abnormalities may produce an encephalopathy, with neuropsychiatric disturbances that may include neuromuscular dysfunction, altered mentation, altered consciousness, or coma. With chronic liver disease, hepatic encephalopathy may be recurrent and precipitated by intercurrent illness, drugs, bleeding, or electrolyte and acid-base disturbances.

Hepatic encephalopathy is characterized by profound

Table 13–25. Differential Diagnosis of Unconjugated Hyperbilirubinemia

- Increased production of unconjugated bilirubin from heme
  - Hemolytic disease (hereditary or acquired)
    - Isoimmune hemolysis (neonatal; acute or delayed transfusion reaction; autoimmune)
      - Rh-incompatibility
      - ABO-incompatibility
      - Other blood group incompatibilities
    - Congenital spherocytosis
    - Hereditary elliptocytosis
    - Erythrocyte enzyme defects:
      - Glucose-6-phosphate dehydrogenase
      - Pyruvate kinase
    - Hemoglobinopathy
      - Sickle cell anemia
      - Thalassemia
      - Others
    - Microangiopathy
      - Hemolytic uremic syndrome
      - Hemangioma
      - Mechanical trauma (heart valve)
  - Ineffective erythropoiesis
  - Drugs
    - Vitamin K
    - Maternal oxytocin
    - Phenol disinfectants
  - Infection
  - Enclosed hematoma
  - Polycythemia
    - Diabetic mother
    - Fetal tranfusion (maternal, twin)
    - Delayed cord clamping
- Decreased **delivery** of unconjugated bilirubin (in plasma) to hepatocyte
    - Right-sided congestive heart failure
    - Portacaval shunt
- Decreased bilirubin **uptake** across hepatocyte membrane
  - Presumed enzyme deficiency (e.g., Gilbert)
  - Competitive inhibition
    - Breast milk jaundice
    - Lucey-Driscoll syndrome
    - Drug inhibition (radiocontrast material)
  - Miscellaneous
    - Hypothyroidism
    - Hypoxia
    - Acidosis
- Decreased **storage** of unconjugated bilirubin in cytosol (decreased Y and Z proteins)
    - Competitive inhibition
    - Fever
- Decreased biotransformation (conjugation)
    - Neonatal jaundice (physiologic)
    - Inhibition (drugs)
    - Hereditary (Crigler-Najjar)
      - Type I (complete enzyme deficiency)
      - Type II (partial deficiency)
    - Hepatocellular dysfunction
- Enterohepatic recirculation
  - Intestinal obstruction
    - Ileal atresia
    - Hirschsprung disease
    - Cystic fibrosis
    - Pyloric stenosis
  - Antibiotic administration
- Breast milk jaundice

neural inhibition, which may be due to an interaction between γ-aminobutyric acid (GABA, the primary inhibitory neurotransmitter) and GABA receptors on postsynaptic neurons. With hepatic failure, GABA produced by bacterial flora is not cleared from the blood but crosses the blood-brain barrier and produces inhibition. There may be a simultaneous decrease in excitatory neurotransmission. Other neuroactive or vasoactive compounds, such as glycine or amines, may be synergistic. Alternative theories ascribe a pathogenetic role to ammonia, to synergistic neurotoxins, or to "false neurotransmitters" with plasma amino acid imbalance (see also Sec. 20.55).

Endocrine Abnormalities. Endocrine abnormalities are more common in adults with hepatic disease than in children. They reflect alterations in hepatic synthetic, storage, and metabolic functions, including those concerned with hormonal metabolism in the liver. For example, proteins such as those that bind hormones in plasma are synthesized in the liver, and steroid hormones are conjugated in the liver and excreted in the urine; failure of such functions may have clinical consequences. Endocrine abnormalities may also result from malnutrition or specific deficiencies.

Renal Dysfunction. There is a close relationship between liver and renal dysfunctions. Systemic disease or toxins may affect both organs simultaneously; parenchymal liver disease may produce secondary impairment of renal function, and vice versa. In hepatobiliary disorders, there may be renal alterations in sodium and water economy, impaired renal concentrating ability, and alterations in potassium metabolism. Ascites in patients with cirrhosis may be related to inappropriate retention of sodium by the kidney, with expansion of plasma volume, or to sodium retention mediated by diminished effective plasma volume.

Hepatorenal syndrome is defined as renal failure (azotemia and progressive oliguria) in a patient with cirrhosis (often with refractory ascites), in whom there is no other demonstrable cause of renal failure. This complication represent a complex sequence of compensation and decompensation in end-stage liver disease. The pathophysiology is poorly defined but seems to involve altered renal blood flow. Intense vasoconstriction of the renal cortical vessels is mediated by hemodynamic, humoral, or neurogenic mechanisms. The urinary sodium concentration is low, and the sediment is normal. In management, a trial of volume expansion is warranted in order to exclude the possibility of prerenal azotemia secondary to volume depletion.

MISCELLANEOUS MANIFESTATIONS OF LIVER DYSFUNCTION. Nonspecific signs of acute and chronic liver disease include (1) anorexia, often seen in the patient with anicteric hepatitis; (2) abdominal pain or distention; and (3) bleeding, which may be due to altered synthesis of coagulation factors (biliary obstruction with vitamin K deficiency or excessive hepatic damage) or to portal hypertension. There may be decreased synthesis of specific clotting factors, production of qualitatively abnormal proteins, or alterations in platelet number and function in the presence of hypersplenism. Altered drug metabolism may prolong the biologic half-life of commonly administered medications.

13.83 EVALUATION OF THE PATIENT WITH POSSIBLE LIVER DYSFUNCTION

Adequate evaluation of an infant, child, or adolescent with suspected liver disease involves an appropriate and accurate history, a carefully performed physical examination, and skillful interpretation of signs and symptoms. Further evaluation is aided by judicious selection of diagnostic tests, followed by a liver biopsy or the use of imaging modalities. Most "liver function tests" do not measure specific hepatic functions. A rise in serum aminotransferase activity reflects liver cell injury; an increase in immunoglobulin level reflects an immunologic response to injury; or an elevation in serum bilirubin level may reflect any of several disturbances of bilirubin metabolism. The results of any single biochemical assay provide limited information, which must be placed in the context of the entire clinical and historic picture. The most cost-efficient approach is for the clinician to become familiar with the rationale, implications, and limitations of a selected group of tests, so that specific questions can be answered.

For a patient with suspected liver disease, evaluation addresses the following issues in sequence: (1) Is liver disease present? (2) If so, what is its nature? (3) What is its severity? (4) Is specific treatment available? (5) How can we monitor the response to treatment? and (6) What is the prognosis?

BIOCHEMICAL TESTS. Laboratory tests commonly used to confirm the suspicion of liver disease include measurements of serum bilirubin level and of aminotransferase and alkaline phosphatase activities often with determinations of prothrombin time and albumin level. These tests are complementary, and provide an estimation of synthetic and excretory functions and may suggest the nature of the disturbance (e.g., inflammation or cholestasis).

Acute liver cell injury (parenchymal disease) in viral hepatitis, drug or toxin-induced liver disease, shock, hypoxemia, or metabolic disease may best be reflected in marked increases in aminotransferase activities. Cholestasis (obstructive disease) involves regurgitation of bile components into serum; accordingly, the serum levels of total and conjugated bilirubin will be elevated. Elevations in serum alkaline phosphatase and 5′ nucleotidase activities are sensitive indicators of obstructive processes or of inflammation of the biliary tract.

The **severity** of the liver disease may be reflected in (1) *clinical signs* (occurrence of encephalopathy, apparent shrinkage of liver mass owing to massive necrosis, or onset of ascites) or in (2) *biochemical alterations* (hypoglycemia, hyperammonemia, electrolyte imbalance, continued hyperbilirubinemia, marked hypoalbuminemia, or prolonged prothrombin times unresponsive to parenteral administration of vitamin K).

Measurement of the *conjugated and unconjugated fractions of serum bilirubin* help to distinguish between elevations due to hemolysis and those due to hepatic dysfunction. A predominant elevation in the conjugated fraction provides a relatively sensitive index of hepatocellular disease or hepatic excretory dysfunction. Aminotransferase activities are highly sensitive to hepatocellular damage. *Alanine aminotransferase* (ALT, SGPT) is liver specific, whereas *aspartate aminotransferase* (AST, SGOT) is derived from other organs in addition to the liver. In most cases there are parallel rises in AST and ALT, but sometimes a differential rise or fall can provide useful information. The most marked rises of aminotransferase activities occur with acute hepatocellular injury, such as viral hepatitis, hypoxia/hypoperfusion, toxic injury, or Reye syndrome. Following blunt abdominal trauma, elevations in activity of these enzymes may provide an early clue to hepatic injury. In chronic liver disease or in intrahepatic and extrahepatic biliary obstruction, rises in aminotransferase activities may be less marked. In acute hepatitis the rise in ALT may be greater than that of AST; whereas in alcohol-induced liver injury, in fulminant echovirus infection, and in various metabolic diseases, predominant rises in AST have been reported.

Hepatic synthetic function is reflected in *serum protein* levels and in *prothrombin time.* Examination of *serum globulin* concentration and of the relative amounts of the globulin fractions may be helpful. γ-Globulin levels are often high, and increased titers of smooth muscle antibody as well as antimitochondrial antibodies and antinuclear antibodies may be found in patients with chronic active hepatitis. A resurgence in *α-fetoprotein* levels may suggest hepatoma. Hypoalbuminemia due to depressed synthesis may complicate severe liver disease and serve as a prognostic factor. *Cholesterol levels* may be markedly elevated in patients with cholestasis, whether the cause be intrahepatic or extrahepatic. On the other hand, with acute liver disease, such as hepatitis, serum cholesterol levels may be depressed. Deficiencies of *factor V* and of the *vitamin K dependent factors* (II, VII, IX, and X) may occur. When the prothrombin time is prolonged as a result of nutritional input or intestinal malabsorption of vitamin K, parenteral administration of vitamin K should correct it within 12 hr; unresponsiveness to vitamin K would suggest hepatic disease. Persistently low levels of factor VII are evidence of a poor prognosis in fulminant liver disease.

Serum levels of *bile acids* are sensitive indicators of hepatobiliary disease, especially in monitoring patients at high risk for liver injury.

Interpretation of biochemical tests of hepatic structure and function must be made in the context of age-related changes. The activity of *alkaline phosphatase* varies considerably with age, reflecting predominantly the activity of the isoenzyme that originates in bone. Activity of the liver-specific isoenzyme or of *5′ nucleotidase* can be measured; the latter has a similar biliary origin and is not found in bone. An isolated increase in alkaline phosphatase may be benign if other liver function test results are normal. *γ-Glutamyl transpeptidase (GGT)* exhibits high enzyme activity in early life that declines rapidly with age. Cholesterol concentrations increase throughout life.

Interpretation of *serum ammonia* values is uncertain, owing to variability in their physiologic determinants and to inherent difficulty in laboratory measurement.

LIVER BIOPSY. The morphologic features of specific hepatic diseases are sufficiently distinctive so that liver biopsy combined with clinical data can indicate an etiologic diagnosis in most cases. Tissue obtained by percutaneous liver biopsy can be used: (1) to provide a precise histologic diagnosis (in patients with neonatal cholestasis, chronic active hepatitis, Reye syndrome, intrahepatic cholestasis (paucity of bile ducts), congenital hepatic fibrosis, or undefined portal hypertension); (2) for enzyme analysis to detect inborn errors of metabolism; and (3) for analysis of stored material (e.g., iron, copper, or specific metabolites). Serial assessments of hepatic status by liver biopsies can monitor responses to therapy or detect complications of treatment with potentially hepatotoxic agents, such as aspirin, antimetabolites, or anticonvulsants.

In infants and children, needle biopsy of the liver is easily accomplished through the percutaneous approach. The amount of tissue obtained, even in small infants, is usually sufficient for histologic interpretation, and for biochemical analyses (if the latter are deemed necessary). Percutaneous liver biopsy can be performed safely in infants as young as 1 wk of age. The patient usually requires only sedation and *local* anesthesia. Contraindications include prolonged prothrombin time, thrombocytopenia, suspicion of a vascular, cystic, or infectious lesion in the path of the needle, and severe ascites. If administration of fresh frozen plasma or of platelet transfusions fails to correct a prolonged prothrombin time or thrombocytopenia, open surgical biopsy may be considered. The risk of development of a complication such as hemorrhage, hematoma, creation of an arteriovenous fistula, pneumothorax, or bile peritonitis is very small.

HEPATIC IMAGING PROCEDURES (see also Sec. 6.56). Various techniques help define the size, shape, and architecture of the liver, including the intrahepatic and extrahepatic biliary trees. Although imaging may not provide a precise histologic and biochemical diagnosis, specific questions can be answered, such as whether hepatomegaly is related to accumulation of fat or glycogen or is due to a tumor or cyst. These studies may direct further evaluation such as percutaneous biopsy and will make possible prompt referral of patients with biliary obstruction to the surgeon. Choice of imaging procedure should be part of a carefully formulated diagnostic approach, with avoidance of redundant demonstrations by several techniques.

A *plain roentgenographic study* may suggest hepatomegaly, but a physical examination gives a more reliable assessment of liver size. The liver may appear less dense than normal in patients with fatty infiltration or more dense with deposition of heavy metals such as iron. A hepatic or biliary tract mass may displace an air-filled loop of bowel. Calcifications may be evident in the liver (parasitic and neoplastic disease), in the vasculature (with portal vein thrombosis), or in the gallbladder or biliary tree (gallstones). Collections of gas may be seen within the liver (abscess), biliary tract, or portal circulation (necrotizing enterocolitis).

Ultrasound provides information about the size, composition, and blood flow of the liver. Increased echogenicity is observed with fatty infiltration, and mass lesions as small as 1–2 cm may be shown. Ultrasound has replaced cholangiography in detecting stones in the gallbladder or biliary tree. Even in the neonate high-frequency real-time ultrasound can assess gallbladder size, detect dilatation of the biliary tract, or define a choledochal cyst. In infants with biliary atresia, the gallbladder is usually small or absent and the common duct is not visualized. In patients with portal hypertension, ultrasound can evaluate patency of the portal vein or demonstrate collateral circulation. Relatively small amounts of ascitic fluid can be detected.

Computed tomography (CT) scanning provides information similar to that obtained by ultrasound but is less suitable for use in patients under 2 yr of age because of the small size of structures, the paucity of intra-abdominal fat for contrast, and the need for heavy sedation or general anesthesia. *Magnetic resonance imaging* (MRI) has proved to be a useful alternative. The CT scan or MRI may be more accurate than ultrasound in detection of focal lesions such as tumors, cysts, and abscesses. When coupled with injection of a contrast medium, CT scanning may reveal a neoplastic mass density only slightly different from that of normal liver. When a hepatic tumor is suspected, CT scanning is the best method to define anatomic extent, solid or cystic nature, and vascularity. CT scanning can also reveal subtle differences in density of liver parenchyma, the average liver attenuation coefficient being reduced with fatty infiltration. Increases in density may occur with diffuse iron deposition or with glycogen storage. In differentiating obstructive from nonobstructive cholestasis, CT scanning or MRI identifies the precise level of obstruction more frequently than ultrasound. Either CT scanning or ultrasound may be used to guide fine needle biopsy or the aspiration of specific lesions.

Radionuclide scanning relies on selective uptake of a radiopharmaceutical agent. Commonly used agents include (1) ^{99m}Tc-labeled sulfur colloid, which undergoes phagocytosis by Kupffer cells; (2) ^{99m}Tc-iminodiacetic acid agents, which are taken up by hepatocytes and excreted into bile; and (3) ^{67}Ga, which is concentrated in inflammatory and neoplastic cells. The anatomic resolution possible with hepatic scintiscans is generally less than that obtained with CT scanning, MRI, or ultrasound.

The ^{99m}Tc-sulfur colloid scan may detect focal lesions (e.g., tumors, cysts, or abscesses) greater than 2–3 cm in diameter. This scan may help to evaluate patients with possible cirrhosis in whom hepatic uptake is patchy and in whom there is a shift of colloid uptake from liver to bone marrow.

The ^{99m}Tc-substituted iminodiacetic acid dyes may differentiate intrahepatic cholestasis from extrahepatic obstruction in the neonate. Imaging results are best when scanning is preceded by a 5- to 7-day period of treatment with phenobarbital to stimulate bile flow. Following intravenous injection, the isotope is normally detected in the bowel within 1–2 hr. In the presence of extrahepatic obstruction, excretion of the isotope is delayed; accordingly, serial scans should be made for up to 24 hr following injection. Early in the course of biliary atresia, hepatocyte function is usually good; uptake (clearance) occurs rapidly, but excretion into the intestine is absent. In contrast, uptake is poor in parenchymal liver disease, such as neonatal hepatitis, but excretion into the bile and intestine eventually ensues.

In older infants and children, scintigraphy may also help to evaluate the gallbladder, bile ducts, and bile flow in patients who have undergone liver transplantation. In patients with acute cholecystitis, the gallbladder is not visualized, but the common duct is opacified.

Cholangiography, the direct visualization of the intrahepatic and extrahepatic biliary tree following injection of opaque material, may be required in some patients to evaluate the cause, location, or extent of biliary obstruction. Percutaneous transhepatic cholangiography (PTC) with a fine needle is the technique of choice in infants and young children. The likelihood of opacifying the biliary tract is excellent in patients in whom CT scanning, MRI, or ultrasound has shown dilated ducts.

Endoscopic retrograde cholangiopancreatography (ERCP) is an alternative method of examining the bile ducts in older children. The papilla of Vater is cannulated under direct vision through a fiberoptic endoscope, and contrast material is injected into the biliary and pancreatic ducts.

Selective angiography of the celiac, superior mesenteric, or hepatic artery may be used to visualize the hepatic or portal circulation. Both arterial and venous circulatory systems of the liver can be examined. Angiography is frequently required to define the blood supply of tumors before surgery and is useful in the study of patients with known or presumed portal hypertension. The patency of the portal system, the extent of collateral circulation, and the caliber of vessels under consideration for a shunting procedure can be evaluated. MRI can provide similar information.

DISEASES OF THE LIVER

13.84 NEONATAL CHOLESTASIS

Cholestasis, the prolonged elevation of serum levels of conjugated bilirubin, is most frequently noted in the 1st months of life. Neonatal cholestasis may be due to infectious, genetic, metabolic, or undefined abnormalities giving rise either to mechanical obstruction of bile flow or to functional impairment of hepatic excretory function and bile secretion (Table 13–26). An example of the former is stricture or obstruction of the common bile duct; biliary atresia is the prototypic obstructive abnormality. Functional impairment of bile secretion may result from damage to liver cells or to the biliary secretory apparatus. Neonates with cholestasis may be divided into those with extrahepatic and those with intrahepatic disease (Fig. 13–28). The clinical features of any form of cholestasis are similar. In an affected neonate, the diagnosis of certain entities, such as galactosemia, sepsis, and hypothyroidism, is relatively simple. In most cases, however, the cause of cholestasis is more obscure. Differentiation among *extrahepatic biliary atresia,* idiopathic *neonatal hepatitis,* and *intrahepatic cholestasis* is often particularly difficult. The nosology is imprecise, and diagnostic criteria are uncertain.

Recent advances have improved our understanding of hepatic structure and function in early life, and several forms of neonatal cholestasis have been characterized within a new conceptual framework.

Mechanisms. Some of the histologic manifestations of hepatic injury in early life are not commonly seen in older individuals. For example, giant cell transformation of hepatocytes occurs frequently in infants with cholestasis and may be seen in any form of neonatal liver injury. It is more frequent and more severe, however, in intrahepatic forms of cholestasis (neonatal hepatitis or intrahepatic bile duct paucity). The clinical and histologic findings thought to exist both in neonates with neonatal hepatitis and in those with extrahepatic biliary atresia have suggested that these diseases are manifestations of a single basic process, with an undefined initiating insult causing inflammation of the liver cells or of the cells within the biliary tract. If bile duct epithelium is the predominant site of disease, cholangitis may result and lead to progressive sclerosis and narrowing of the biliary tree, the ultimate state being complete obliteration *(extrahepatic biliary atresia).* On the other hand, injury to liver cells may present the clinical and histologic picture of *neonatal hepatitis.* This concept does not account for all phenomena, but offers an explanation for well-documented cases of unexpected postnatal evolution of these disease processes; for example, infants initially regarded as having neonatal hepatitis, with a patent biliary system shown on cholangiography, have been later found to have extrahepatic biliary atresia.

Functional abnormalities in the generation of bile flow may also play a role in neonatal cholestasis. Bile flow is directly dependent on effective hepatic bile acid excretion. During the phase of relatively inefficient liver cell transport and metabolism of bile acids in early life, minor degrees of hepatic injury may further decrease bile flow and lead to production of abnormal bile acids; selective impairment of a single step in the series of events involved in hepatic excretion may produce the full expression of a cholestatic syndrome. A small number of cholestatic syndromes have a familial pattern; for example, Byler disease and benign recurrent cholestasis are presumably related to impaired metabolism or membrane transport of bile acids. Specific defects in bile acid synthesis have been found in infants with intrahepatic cholestasis, and in infants with Zellweger syndrome. A severe form of familial cholestasis has been associated with neonatal hemochromatosis and an aberration in the contractile proteins that comprise the cytoskeleton of the hepatocyte. Sepsis is known to cause cholestasis, presumably mediated by an endotoxin produced by *Escherichia coli.*

Evaluation. The clinical features of infants with neonatal cholestasis provide very few clues regarding etiology. Affected infants have icterus, dark urine, light or acholic stools, and hepatomegaly, all reflecting decreased bile flow due to either liver cell injury or bile duct obstruction. Hepatic synthetic dysfunction may lead to hypoprothrombinemia and a bleeding disorder; administration of vitamin K should be considered in the initial management of cholestatic infants, in order to prevent hemorrhage.

Most infants with neonatal cholestasis will come to medical attention in the 1st mo of life. Prompt differentiation of conjugated from unconjugated hyperbilirubinemia is imperative, because the finding of cholestasis is more ominous. The initial step in identification of cholestasis is the finding that, of the significantly elevated level of total bilirubin, more than 20% is conjugated bilirubin. The next step is the prompt recognition of any specific or treatable primary causes of cholestasis, such as *sepsis,* an *endocrinopathy* (hypothyroidism or panhypopituitarism), *nutritional hepatotoxicity* due to a specific metabolic illness (e.g., galactosemia), or other rare *metabolic diseases* (e.g., tyrosinemia). Recognition of such entities allows the institution of appropriate therapy and may possibly prevent further injury.

TABLE 13–26. Differential Diagnosis of Cholestasis in Early Life

- Infectious
  - Viral hepatitis
    - Hepatitis A, B, C
    - Cytomegalovirus
    - Rubella virus
    - Herpes simplex 1, 2, 6
    - Varicella virus
    - Coxsackievirus
    - Echovirus
    - Reovirus type 3
    - Parvovirus B19
  - Others
    - Toxoplasmosis
    - Syphilis
    - Tuberculosis
    - Listeriosis
- Toxic
  - Parenteral nutrition–related
  - Sepsis (e.g., urinary tract) with endotoxemia
  - Drug-related
- Metabolic
  - Disorders of **amino acid** metabolism
    - Tyrosinemia
    - Hypermethioninemia (?)
  - Disorders of **lipid** metabolism
    - Wolman disease
    - Niemann-Pick disease
    - Gaucher disease
  - Disorders of **carbohydrate** metabolism
    - Galactosemia
    - Fructosemia
    - Glycogenosis IV
  - Disorders of bile acid metabolism
  - Other metabolic defects
    - α_1-Antitrypsin deficiency
    - Cystic fibrosis
    - Idiopathic hypopituitarism
    - Hypothyroidism
    - Zellweger (cerebrohepatorenal) syndrome
    - Multiple acyl-CoA dehydrogenase deficiency (glutaric acid type II)
    - Neonatal iron storage disease
    - Indian childhood cirrhosis/infantile copper overload
    - Trihydroxycoprostanoic acidemia
    - Familial erythrophagocytic lymphohistiocytosis
    - Arginase deficiency
- Genetic/chromosomal
  - Trisomy E
  - Down syndrome
  - Donahue syndrome (leprechaunism)
- Intrahepatic diseases of unknown etiology
  - Intrahepatic cholestasis—persistent
    - "Idiopathic" neonatal hepatitis
    - Alagille syndrome (arteriohepatic dysplasia)
    - Intrahepatic biliary hypoplasia/paucity of intrahepatic bile ducts (nonsyndromic)
    - Byler disease
  - Intrahepatic cholestasis—recurrent
    - Familial benign recurrent cholestasis
    - Associated with lymphedema (Aagenaes)
  - Congenital hepatic fibrosis/infantile polycystic disease
  - Caroli disease (cystic dilatation of intrahepatic ducts)
- Extrahepatic diseases
  - Biliary atresia
  - Sclerosing cholangitis
  - Bile duct stenosis
  - Choledochal-pancreaticoductal junction anomaly
  - Spontaneous perforation of the bile duct
  - Choledochal cyst
  - Mass (neoplasia, stone)
  - Bile/mucous plug ("inspissated bile")
- Miscellaneous
  - Histiocytosis X
  - Shock/hypoperfusion
  - Associated with enteritis
  - Associated with intestinal obstruction
  - Neonatal lupus erythematosus
  - Myeloproliferative disease (21-trisomy)

Hepatobiliary disease may be the initial manifestation of homozygous α-antitrypsin deficiency or of cystic fibrosis. Neonatal liver disease may also be associated with infections due to agents of the TORCH complex. Hepatitis A and hepatitis B viruses rarely cause neonatal cholestasis.

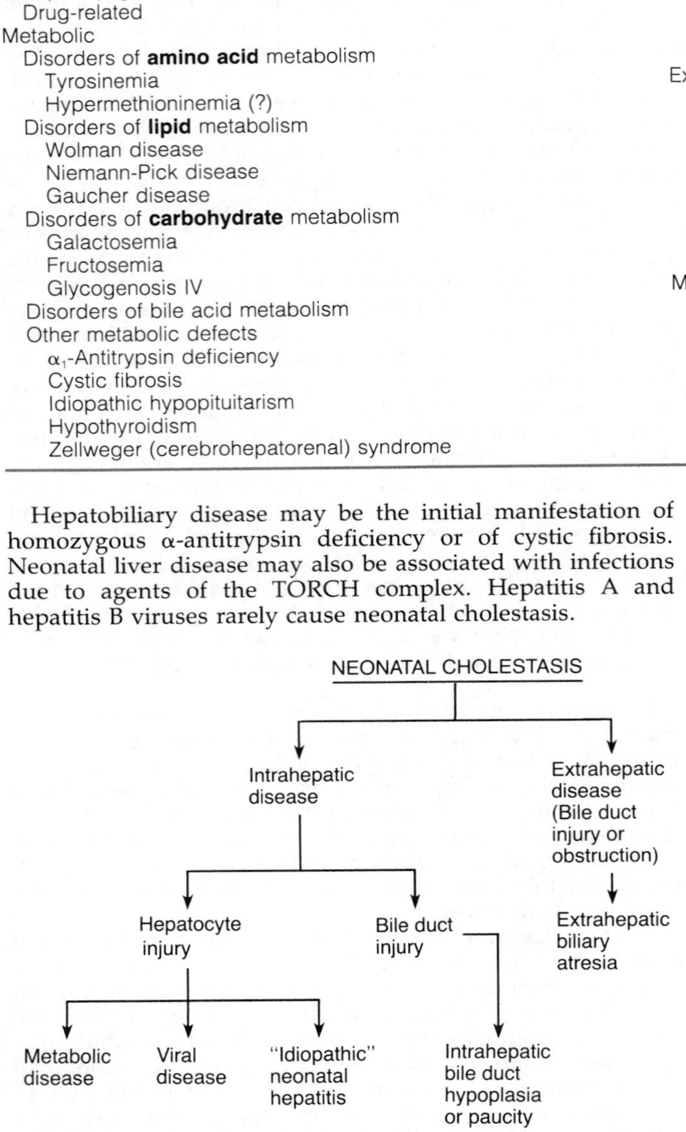

Figure 13–28. Neonatal cholestasis. Conceptual approach to the group of diseases presenting as cholestasis in the neonate. There are areas of overlap—patients with extrahepatic biliary atresia may have some degree of intrahepatic injury. Patients with "idiopathic" neonatal hepatitis may in the future be determined to have a primary metabolic or viral disease.

The final step in the evaluation of the neonate with cholestasis is to differentiate extrahepatic biliary atresia from neonatal hepatitis. Overall, in up to 80% of infants with neonatal cholestasis, extensive evaluation will establish a diagnosis of either biliary atresia or neonatal hepatitis (Table 13–27).

NEONATAL HEPATITIS SYNDROME (INTRAHEPATIC CHOLESTASIS). The term *neonatal hepatitis* implies intrahepatic cholestasis (see Fig. 13–28), of which we can designate various forms:

1. **Idiopathic neonatal hepatitis** is a disease of unknown etiology having sporadic and familial varieties. It includes most of the cases of "neonatal hepatitis." These patients presumably are afflicted with a specific, yet undefined metabolic or viral disease. In the past, patients with α_1-antitrypsin deficiency were included in this category; however following characterization of this metabolic disease, it is possible to precisely define this group of patients.
2. **Infectious hepatitis in a neonate** may be shown to be due to a specific virus, such as hepatitis B, enteroviruses, or cytomegalovirus. This accounts for a small percentage of cases of neonatal hepatitis syndrome.
3. Cases of **intrahepatic bile duct paucity** form a heterogeneous subset of cholestatic diseases that may appear as neonatal cholestasis.

INTRAHEPATIC BILE DUCT PAUCITY. Some syndromes characterized morphologically by intrahepatic cholestasis may be clinically manifest either as neonatal hepatitis (see earlier) or as cholestasis in an older child. As the patient matures, clinical and histologic features may suggest a specific syn-

TABLE 13–27. Initial Work-up for Suspected Neonatal Cholestasis

1. History and physical examination: size and consistency of liver and spleen; presence of other anomalies (cardiac, renal, skin); stool color
2. Blood and urine analysis: fractionated serum bilirubin; serum bile acids; prothrombin time; α_1-antitrypsin phenotype; metabolic screen-urine/serum amino acids, urine reducing substances; thyroxine and thyroid-stimulating hormone; sweat chloride
3. Blood, urine, spinal fluid cultures
4. Serologic studies for evidence of infection (HBsAg, TORCH, and VDRL)
5. Ultrasound
6. Hepatobiliary scintigraphy
7. Liver biopsy

drome. Many such cases are associated with bile duct "paucity" (often erroneously called intrahepatic biliary atresia), which designates an absence or marked reduction in the number of interlobular bile ducts in the portal triads, with normal-sized branches of portal vein and hepatic arteriole. This unusual histologic feature represents either (1) congenital absence or partial failure to develop or (2) progressive atrophy or disappearance due to segmental destructive processes. Biopsy in early life often reveals an inflammatory process involving the bile ducts. Subsequent biopsies then show subsidence of the inflammation with residual reduction in the number and diameter of bile ducts.

Recent observations suggest that it is possible to identify distinctive syndromes of isolated intrahepatic bile duct paucity and an intact extrahepatic biliary tree.

Alagille syndrome (arteriohepatic dysplasia) is the most common syndrome incorporating intrahepatic bile duct paucity. Serial assessment of hepatic histology often suggests progressive destruction of bile ducts. Clinical manifestations are expressed in various degrees and may be nonspecific; they include unusual *facial characteristics* (broad forehead; deep-set, widely spaced eyes; long, straight nose; and underdeveloped mandible). There may also be *ocular* abnormalities (posterior embryotoxon), *cardiovascular* abnormalities (usually peripheral pulmonic stenosis, sometimes tetralogy of Fallot), *vertebral* arch defects and failure of anterior vertebral arch fusion (butterfly vertebrae), and tubulointerstitial *nephropathy*. Other findings such as growth retardation and defective spermatogenesis may reflect nutritional deficiency. The prognosis for prolonged survival is good, but the patients are likely to have pruritus, xanthomata, and neurologic complications of vitamin E deficiency if untreated.

Zellweger (cerebrohepatorenal) syndrome is a rare autosomal recessive genetic disorder marked by progressive degeneration of the liver and kidneys. The incidence is estimated to be 1:100,000 births; the disease is usually fatal within 6–12 mo. Affected infants have severe, generalized hypotonia and markedly impaired neurologic function with psychomotor retardation. There are an abnormal shape of the head and unusual facies, hepatomegaly, renal cortical cysts, stippled calcifications of the patellae and greater trochanter, and ocular abnormalities. Hepatic cells on ultrastructural examination show an absence of peroxisomes (see Sec. 8.16).

Byler disease is a rare familial form of fetal intrahepatic cholestasis and has apparently unique structural abnormalities in the bile canalicular membrane. Affected patients present failure to thrive, steatorrhea, pruritus, and rickets. Fatal cirrhosis gradually develops. In one form of idiopathic intrahepatic cholestasis (Aagenaes), recurrent cholestasis is associated with lymphedema of the lower extremities.

Extrahepatic Biliary Atresia

The term "biliary atresia" is imprecise, because the anatomy of abnormal extrahepatic bile ducts in affected patients varies markedly. There may be distal atresia with patent extrahepatic ducts up to the portal hepatis. This is a surgically correctable lesion, but it is uncommon. The most common form of extrahepatic biliary atresia (85% of cases) is obstruction of the ducts at or above the portal hepatis, which presents much more difficult problems in management.

INCIDENCE. Biliary atresia has been detected in 1:10,000–15,000 live births, idiopathic neonatal hepatitis in 1:5,000–10,000. Intrahepatic bile duct paucity appears much less commonly, in about 1:50,000–75,000 live births.

DIFFERENTIATION OF IDIOPATHIC NEONATAL HEPATITIS FROM BILIARY ATRESIA. It may be difficult to clearly differentiate infants with extrahepatic biliary atresia (who need surgical correction) from infants with neonatal hepatitis. No single biochemical test or imaging procedure is entirely satisfactory. Diagnostic schemata incorporate clinical, historical, biochemical, and radiologic features.

Patients with idiopathic neonatal hepatitis have a familial incidence of approximately 20%, whereas extrahepatic biliary atresia is unlikely to recur within the same family. Infants with biliary atresia have an increased incidence of other abnormalities, such as the polysplenia syndrome with abdominal heterotaxia, malrotation, levocardia, and intra-abdominal vascular anomalies. Neonatal hepatitis appears to be more common in premature or small for gestational age infants. Persistently acholic stools suggest biliary obstruction, but patients with severe idiopathic neonatal hepatitis may have a transient severe retardation of bile excretion. On the other hand, consistently pigmented stools rule against biliary atresia. The finding of bile-stained fluid on duodenal intubation also excludes biliary atresia. Palpation of the liver may find an abnormal size or consistency in patients with extrahepatic biliary atresia, which is less common with neonatal hepatitis.

Imaging techniques are generally not helpful, but ultrasound should be carried out early, because it may detect a choledochal cyst or another unsuspected cause of cholestasis associated with dilatation of the biliary tract.

Hepatobiliary scintigraphy using imidodiacetic acid analogs has been used by some clinicians to differentiate biliary atresia from neonatal hepatitis. In biliary atresia, hepatocyte function is intact and uptake of the agent is unimpaired, but excretion into the intestine is absent; whereas in patients with neonatal hepatitis, uptake is sluggish, but excretion into the biliary tract and intestine eventually occurs. Oral administration of phenobarbital (5 mg/kg/day) for 5 days prior to the study enhances biliary excretion of the isotope in patients with neonatal hepatitis.

Liver biopsy provides the most reliable discriminatory evidence. In **biliary atresia**, there are bile ductular proliferation, the presence of bile plugs, and portal or perilobular edema and fibrosis, with the basic hepatic lobular architecture intact. In **neonatal hepatitis**, on the other hand, there is severe, diffuse hepatocellular disease, with distortion of lobular architecture, marked infiltration with inflammatory cells, and focal hepatocellular necrosis; the bile ductules show little alteration. Giant cell transformation is found in infants with either condition and has no diagnostic specificity.

Histologic changes similar to those in idiopathic neonatal hepatitis occur in a variety of diseases, including α_1-antitrypsin deficiency, galactosemia, and various forms of intrahepatic bile duct paucity. In the last, although paucity of intrahepatic bile ductules may be detected on liver biopsy even within the first few weeks of life, later biopsies in such patients will reveal a more characteristic pattern.

MANAGEMENT OF PATIENTS WITH SUSPECTED BILIARY ATRESIA. In infants in whom clinical features and liver biopsy suggest biliary obstruction, exploratory laparotomy and direct cholangiography should be done to determine the presence and site of obstruction. For patients in whom a

correctable lesion is present, direct drainage can be accomplished. When no correctable lesion is found, an examination of frozen sections obtained from the transected porta hepatis can detect the presence of biliary epithelium and determine the size of the residual bile ducts. In some cases, the cholangiographic finding that the biliary tract is patent but of diminished caliber suggests that the cholestasis is due to extrahepatic biliary hypoplasia or to markedly diminished flow owing to intrahepatic disease. In these cases, transection of or further dissection into the porta hepatis should be avoided.

For patients in whom **no correctable lesion** is found, the hepatoportoenterostomy procedure of Kasai can be carried out in selected cases. The rationale for this operation is that minute bile duct remnants, representing residual channels, may be present in the fibrous tissue of the porta hepatis; such channels may be in direct continuity with the intrahepatic ductule system. In such cases, transection of the porta hepatis with anastomosis of bowel mucosa to the proximal surface of the transection may allow drainage. If flow is not rapidly established within the first months of life, progressive obliteration will ensue. If microscopic channels of patency greater than 150 μm in diameter are found, postoperative establishment of bile flow is likely.

Some patients with extrahepatic biliary atresia, even of the "noncorrectable" type, derive long-term benefits from such interventions as the Kasai procedure. In most, however, a degree of hepatic dysfunction persists. Patients with extrahepatic biliary atresia usually have persistent inflammation of the intrahepatic biliary tree, which suggests that extrahepatic biliary atresia reflects a dynamic process involving the entire hepatobiliary system and which may account for the ultimate development of complications such as portal hypertension. The short-term benefit of hepatoportoenterostomy is that it may sustain the child's growth until a successful liver transplantation can be done (see Sec. 6.43).

Management of Chronic Cholestasis

With any form of neonatal cholestasis, whether the primary disease is idiopathic neonatal hepatitis, intrahepatic bile duct paucity, or extrahepatic biliary atresia, if the operation is only partially successful, patients are at increased risk for chronic complications. These reflect varying degrees of residual hepatic functional capacity and are due directly or indirectly to diminished bile flow:

1. Any substance normally excreted into bile is retained in the liver, with subsequent accumulation in tissue and in serum. Involved substances include bile acids, bilirubin, cholesterol, and trace elements.
2. Decreased delivery of bile acids to the proximal intestine leads to inadequate solubilization and malabsorption of dietary long-chain triglycerides and fat-soluble vitamins.
3. Impairment of hepatic metabolic function may alter hormonal balance and utilization of nutrients.
4. Progressive liver damage may lead to biliary cirrhosis, portal hypertension, and liver failure.

The management of such patients (Table 13–28) is empirical, and the best guide is careful monitoring. At present, no therapy is known to be effective in halting the progression of cholestasis or in preventing further hepatocellular damage and cirrhosis.

A major concern is growth failure, which is related in part to malabsorption and malnutrition due to ineffective digestion and absorption of dietary fat. Use of a medium-chain triglyceride-containing formula may improve caloric balance.

With chronic cholestasis and prolonged survival, children with hepatobiliary disease may develop deficiencies of the fat-soluble vitamins (A, D, E, and K). Inadequate absorption of fat and fat-soluble vitamins may be exacerbated by administration of the bile-acid binder, cholestyramine. Rickets is common.

A degenerative neuromuscular syndrome is found with chronic deficiency of vitamin E; affected children develop progressive areflexia, cerebellar ataxia, ophthalmoplegia, and decreased vibratory sensation. Specific morphologic lesions have been found in the central nervous system, peripheral nerves, and muscles. These lesions resemble those found in animals with vitamin E deficiency and are potentially reversible in young children (i.e., those <3–4 yr old). The deficiency may be prevented by the oral administration of large doses (up to 1,000 IU/day) of vitamin E; patients unable to absorb sufficient quantities may require administration of vitamin E (dl-α-tocopherol) intramuscularly. Serum levels may be monitored as a guide to efficacy; affected children will have low serum vitamin E concentrations, increased hydrogen peroxide hemolysis, and low ratios of serum vitamin E to total serum lipids (<0.6 mg/g for children under 12 yr of age and <0.8 mg/g for older patients).

Serum vitamin A concentrations can usually be maintained at normal levels in patients with chronic cholestasis who received oral supplementation of vitamin A esters. It is essential to monitor the vitamin A status in such patients.

Pruritus is a particularly troublesome complication of chronic cholestasis, often with the appearance of xanthomata. Both features seem to be related to the accumulation of cholesterol and bile acids in serum and in tissues. To enhance the elimination of these retained compounds is difficult when bile ducts are obstructed, but if there is any degree of bile

TABLE 13–28. Suggested Medical Management of Persistent Cholestasis

Clinical Impairment	Management
Malnutrition due to malabsorption of dietary long-chain triglyceride (LCT)	Replace with dietary formula or supplements containing medium-chain triglycerides (MCT)
Fat-soluble vitamin malabsorption	
Vitamin A deficiency (night blindness, thick skin)	Replace with *10,000–15,000 IU/day* as Aquasol A
Vitamin E deficiency (neuromuscular degeneration)	Replace with *50–400 IU/day* as oral α-tocopherol
Vitamin D deficiency (metabolic bone disease)	Replace with *5,000–8,000 IU/day of* D_2 or 3–5 μg/kg/day of 25-hydroxycholecalciferol
Vitamin K deficiency (hypoprothrombinemia)	Replace with *2.5–5.0 mg every other day* as water-soluble derivative of menadione
Micronutrient deficiency	Calcium/phosphate/zinc supplementation
Deficiency of water-soluble vitamins	Supplement with twice the recommended daily allowance
Retention of biliary constituents such as bile acids and cholesterol (itch/xanthomata)	Administer choleretics (phenobarbital *5–10 mg/kg/day)* or bile acid binders (cholestyramine *8–16 g/day*)
Progressive liver disease	
Portal hypertension (variceal bleeding, ascites, hypersplenism)	Interim management (control bleeding; salt restriction; spironolactone)
End-stage liver disease (liver failure)	Transplantation

duct patency, administration of phenobarbital and cholestyramine may increase bile flow or interrupt the enterohepatic circulation of bile acids and thus decrease the xanthomata and ameliorate the pruritus (see Table 13–28). Cholestyramine resin is unpalatable and may have side effects such as constipation, hyperchloremia, and exacerbation of fat-soluble vitamin deficiency. Ursodeoxycholic acid therapy may also decrease the degree of pruritus.

In patients with portal hypertension, variceal hemorrhage and the development of hypersplenism are common. However, episodes of gastrointestinal hemorrhage in patients who have chronic liver disease may be due not to esophageal varices but to gastritis or peptic ulcer disease. Because the managements of these various complications differ, differentiation perhaps via endoscopy is necessary before starting treatment (see Sec. 13.102).

In patients with **ascites**, initial management consists of dietary salt restriction; sodium intake is limited to 0.5 g (~ 1–2 mEq/kg/day). It is not necessary to restrict fluid intake in patients with adequate renal output. Diuresis may be maintained by the use of agents, such as thiazides, furosemide, and ethacrynic acid, alone or in combination with spironolactone (3–5 mg/kg/day in four doses). Patients with ascites, but without peripheral edema, are at risk for reduced plasma volume and decreased urine output following diuretic therapy. Tense ascites alters renal blood flow and systemic hemodynamics. Paracentesis and intravenous albumin infusions may improve hemodynamics, renal perfusion, and symptomatology. Protein intake should be limited in order to minimize the potential for hepatic encephalopathy. Follow-up includes dietary counseling and monitoring of serum and urinary electrolyte concentrations (see Sec. 13.103).

In patients with advanced chronic cholestasis, liver transplantation may have a success rate greater than 85% (Sec. 6.43). If the operation is technically feasible, it will prolong life and may correct the metabolic error in diseases such as α_1-antitrypsin deficiency, tyrosinemia, or Wilson disease. Success depends on adequate intraoperative, preoperative, and postoperative care, and on use of cyclosporine as an immunosuppressive agent. Scarcity of donors of small livers severely limits the application of liver transplantation for infants and children. However, the use of reduced size transplants has increased the ability to successfully treat small children.

Prognosis

The prognosis for infants with biliary atresia has been discussed earlier. For patients with idiopathic neonatal hepatitis, the variable prognosis may reflect the heterogeneity of the disease. In **sporadic** cases, 60–70% will recover with no evidence of hepatic structural or functional impairment. Approximately 5–10% will have persistent fibrosis or inflammation, and a smaller percentage will have more severe liver disease, such as cirrhosis. Overall mortality rate is 20–30%. Death of infants usually occurs early in the course of the illness, owing to hemorrhage or sepsis. Of infants with idiopathic neonatal hepatitis of the **familial** variety, only 20–30% will recover; 10–15% will develop chronic liver disease with cirrhosis. Mortality is 50–60%.

13.85 CHOLESTASIS IN THE OLDER CHILD

Acute viral hepatitis accounts for most cases of cholestasis after the neonatal period. Other causes include obstruction due to cholelithiasis, abdominal tumors or enlarged lymph nodes, or hepatic inflammation due to drug ingestion. Many of the conditions causing neonatal cholestasis may also cause chronic cholestasis in older patients. An adolescent with conjugated hyperbilirubinemia should be evaluated for acute and chronic hepatitis, α_1-antitrypsin deficiency, Wilson disease, liver disease associated with inflammatory bowel disease, and for the syndromes of intrahepatic bile duct paucity described above. Management will be similar to that proposed for neonatal cholestasis (see Table 13–28).

13.86 METABOLIC DISEASES OF THE LIVER

See also Chapter 8.

Because the liver plays a central role in synthetic, degradative, and regulatory pathways involving carbohydrate, protein, lipid, trace elements, and vitamin metabolism, there are many metabolic abnormalities or specific enzyme deficiencies that affect the liver primarily or secondarily (Table 13–29). Liver disease may arise when absence of an enzyme produces a block in a metabolic pathway, when unmetabolized substrate accumulates proximal to a block, when deficiency develops of an essential substance produced distal to an aberrant chemical reaction, or when synthesis of an abnormal metabolite occurs. The spectrum of pathologic changes includes: (1) *hepatocyte injury*, with subsequent failure of other metabolic functions, often eventuating in cirrhosis or liver tumors or both; (2) *storage* of lipid, glycogen, or other products; and (3) absence of structural change despite profound metabolic effects, as with urea cycle defects. The clinical manifestations of metabolic diseases of the liver mimic infections, intoxications, and hematologic and immunologic diseases (Table 13–30). Further clues are provided by family history of a similar illness or by the observation that the onset of symptoms is closely associated with a change in dietary habits (e.g., initiation of ingestion of fructose). In most cases, clinical and laboratory evidence will guide the evaluation. Liver biopsy offers morphologic study and will permit enzyme assays, as well as quantitative and qualitative assays of various other constituents. Such studies require cooperation of experienced laboratories and careful attention to collection and handling of specimens.

WILLIAM F. BALISTRERI

13.87 Inherited Deficient Conjugation of Bilirubin

(Familial Nonhemolytic Unconjugated Hyperbilirubinemia)

Hepatic glucuronyl transferase activity (Sec. 9.44) is deficient in two genetically and functionally distinct disorders producing congenital nonobstructive, nonhemolytic, unconjugated hyperbilirubinemia. Type I, which is rarer and more severe than type II, has been reported in about 100 patients.

CRIGLER-NAJJAR SYNDROME (TYPE I GLUCURONYL TRANSFERASE DEFICIENCY). This form is inherited as an autosomal recessive trait. Parents of affected children have partial defects (about 50% of normal) in conjugation by hepatic enzyme assay or by measurement of glucuronide formation, but their serum bilirubin concentrations are normal.

Clinical Manifestations. Severe unconjugated hyperbilirubinemia develops in the homozygous infant during the first 3 days of life, and without treatment serum concentrations of 25–35 mg/dL are reached during the 1st mo. Kernicterus (Sec. 9.45) usually occurs in the early neonatal period, but some treated infants have survived childhood without clinical sequelae. Stools are pale yellow. Persistence of unconjugated hyperbilirubinemia at levels above 20 mg/dL after the 1st wk of life in the absence of hemolysis should suggest the syndrome.

Diagnosis. In the bile, bilirubin concentration is less than 10 mg/dL compared with normal concentrations of 50–100 mg/dL, and there is no bilirubin glucuronide. Definitive di-

TABLE 13–29. Inborn Errors of Metabolism Manifest as Hepatobiliary Dysfunction

- Disorders of carbohydrate metabolism
  - Disorders of **galactose** metabolism
    - Galactosemia
    - Epimerase deficiency
  - Disorders of fructose metabolism
    - Hereditary fructose intolerance
    - Fructose-1,6 DP deficiency
  - **Glycogen storage** diseases:
    - Type I
      - Von Gierke (Ia)
      - Type Ib
    - Type III (Cori/Forbes)
    - Type IV (Andersen)
    - Type VI (Hers)
- Disorders of amino acid/protein metabolism
  - Disorders of **tyrosine** metabolism
    - Transient
      - Neonatal
      - Associated with severe liver disease (e.g., cirrhosis)
    - Nontransient
      - Hereditary tyrosinemia (type I)
      - Tyrosinemia, type II
        - Richner-Hanhart
        - "Medes Case"
        - Atypical forms
          - Endo
          - Giardi
        - "Hawkinsinuria"
  - Inherited **urea cycle** enzyme defects
    - CPS deficiency
    - OTC deficiency (X-linked dominant)
    - Citrullinemia
    - Argininosuccinic aciduria
    - Argininemia
    - N-AGS deficiency
- Disorders of **lipid** metabolism
  - Wolman disease
  - Cholesteryl ester storage disease
  - Gaucher disease
- Disorders of **bile acid** metabolism
  - Isomerase deficiency
  - Reductase deficiency
  - Cerebrotendinous xanthomatosis
  - "Eyssen" syndrome
  - Zellweger syndrome (cerebrohepatorenal)
- Disorders of **metal** metabolism
  - Wilson disease
  - Hepatic copper overload
  - Indian childhood cirrhosis
  - Menkes (steely-hair)
  - Neonatal iron storage disease (perinatal hemochromatosis)
- Disorders of **bilirubin** metabolism
  - Crigler-Najjar
    - Type I
    - Type II—Arias
  - Dubin-Johnson
  - Rotor
- Miscellaneous
  - α_1-Antitrypsin deficiency
  - Cystic fibrosis
  - Erythropoietic protoporphyria (EEP)

agnosis is established by measuring hepatic glucuronyl transferase activity in a liver specimen obtained by a closed biopsy; open biopsy should be avoided, because surgery and anesthesia may precipitate kernicterus. Identification of the heterozygous state in the parents is also strongly suggestive of the diagnosis. Differential diagnosis is discussed in Sec. 9.44. Type II disease may be distinguished from type I by the marked decline in serum bilirubin level that occurs in type II disease after 1 wk of treatment with phenobarbital.

Treatment. Serum bilirubin concentration should be kept below 20 mg/dL for at least the first 2–4 wk of life; in low birthweight infants the levels should be kept lower. This usually requires repeated exchange transfusions and phototherapy. Because the risk of kernicterus persists into adult life, although the serum bilirubin levels required to produce brain injury beyond the neonatal period are considerably higher (usually above 35 mg/dL), phototherapy is generally continued throughout the early years of life. In older infants and children, phototherapy is used mainly during sleep in order not to interfere with normal activities. However, despite the administration of increasing intensities of light for longer periods, the serum bilirubin decrement response to phototherapy decreases with age. Cholestyramine or agar may be used to bind photobilirubin products, thus interfering with the enterohepatic recirculation of bilirubin. Prompt treatment of intercurrent infections, febrile episodes, and other types of illness may help prevent the later development of kernicterus, which may occur at bilirubin levels of 45–55 mg/dL. All type I patients have eventually developed severe kernicterus by young adulthood, despite vigorous continuous management that maintained neurologic normality during childhood. Orthotopic hepatic transplantation will cure the disease and has been successful in a small number of patients.

GLUCURONYL TRANSFERASE DEFICIENCY TYPE II. This autosomal dominant disease with marked variability of penetrance may present in a manner similar to type I syndrome, or it may be a less severe disorder, occasionally even without neonatal manifestations.

Clinical Manifestations. When this disorder presents in the neonatal period, there is usually unconjugated hyperbilirubinemia during the first 3 days of life; serum bilirubin concentrations may be in a range compatible with physiologic jaundice or may be at pathologic levels. Characteristically, the concentrations remain elevated into and after the 3rd wk of life, persisting in a range of 1.5–22 mg/dL; concentrations in the lower part of this range may create uncertainty as to whether chronic hyperbilirubinemia is present. The onset of kernicterus is unusual. Stool color is normal, and the infants are without clinical signs or symptoms of disease. There is no evidence of hemolysis.

Diagnosis. Definitive diagnosis requires testing of the infant and the parents for the capacity to form glucuronides of bilirubin or other test substances. The former requires in vitro measurement of enzymatic activity in a percutaneous liver biopsy. The latter requires administration of substances conjugated as glucuronides, such as menthol or salicylamide, and their measurement in urine; this test is less specific and less accurate but is safer than the biopsy. The levels of conjugation are very low and not distinguishable from those found in type I syndrome. In type II syndrome, one of the parents should have a defect in conjugation; jaundice may be minimal to severe. Abnormalities in other family members may support the diagnosis. Bile bilirubin concentration is nearly normal in type II syndrome. Jaundiced infants and

TABLE 13–30. Clinical Manifestations That Suggest the Possibility of Metabolic Disease

Jaundice, hepatomegaly (± splenomegaly), fulminant hepatic failure
Hypoglycemia, organic acidemia, hyperammonemia, bleeding (coagulopathy)
Recurrent vomiting, failure to thrive, short stature, dysmorphic features
Developmental delay/psychomotor retardation, hypotonia, progressive neuromuscular deterioration, seizures
Cardiac dysfunction/failure, unusual odors, rickets, cataracts

young children having type II syndrome respond readily to 5 mg/kg/24 hr of oral phenobarbital with a decrease in serum bilirubin concentration to 2–3 mg/dL within 7–10 days. Those with type I syndrome do not respond.

Treatment. Long-term reduction in serum bilirubin levels can be achieved with chronic administration of phenobarbital at 5 mg/kg/24 hr. The cosmetic and psychosocial benefit should be weighed against the risks of an effective dose of the drug, because there is no long-term risk of kernicterus in the absence of hemolytic disease.

Inherited Conjugated Hyperbilirubinemia

In inherited conjugated hyperbilirubinemias, which are autosomal recessive disorders characterized by mild jaundice, the transfer of bilirubin and other organic anions from liver to bile is defective. Chronic mild conjugated hyperbilirubinemia is usually detected during adolescence or early adulthood but may occur as early as the 2nd year of life. The results of routine liver function tests are normal. Jaundice may be exacerbated with infection, pregnancy, oral contraceptives, alcohol, or surgery. There is usually no morbidity, and life expectancy is normal; but these disorders may initially present difficult problems in the differential diagnosis of more serious diseases.

DUBIN-JOHNSON SYNDROME. The defect is in porphyrin metabolism or excretion with more than 90% of the normal total urinary coproporphyrin excretion occurring as a coproporphyrin I isomer. Plasma bile acid and bile acid excretion are normal, but sulfabromophthalein retention is abnormal. Roentgenography of the gallbladder is also abnormal. The liver cells contain black pigment similar to melanin.

ROTOR SYNDROME. These patients have an additional deficiency in organic anion uptake. Total urinary coproporphyrin excretion is elevated with a relative increase in the amount of the coproporphyrin I isomer. The gallbladder is normal by roentgenography, and there is no black pigment in liver cells. Sulfabromophthalein excretion is often abnormal.

RICHARD E. BEHRMAN

Berk PD, Wolkoff AW, Berlin NI: Inborn errors of bilirubin metabolism. Med Clin North Am 59:803, 1975.

Shevell MI, Bernard B, Adelson JW, et al: Crigler-Najjar syndrome type I: Treatment by home phototherapy followed by orthotopic hepatic transplantation. J Pediatr 110:429, 1987.

Wolkoff AW, Cohen L, Arias IM: The inheritance of Dubin-Johnson syndrome. N Engl J Med 288:113, 1973.

Wolkoff AW, Wolpert E, Pascasio F: Rotor's syndrome: A distinct inheritable pathophysiologic entity. Am J Med 60:173, 1976.

13.88 Wilson Disease

Wilson disease (hepatolenticular degeneration) is an autosomal recessive disorder characterized by degenerative changes in the brain, cirrhosis, and Kayser-Fleischer rings in the cornea (Sec. 20.47). Incidence is 1:500,000–100,000 births. It is fatal if untreated; but specific, effective treatment is available. Rapid diagnostic investigation of the possibility of Wilson disease in a patient presenting with any form of liver disease, particularly if greater than 5 yr of age, not only will facilitate early institution of management of Wilson disease and related genetic counseling but also will allow appropriate treatment of non-Wilson liver disease once copper toxicosis is ruled out.

PATHOGENESIS. Defective copper excretion into bile leads to accumulation of copper in the liver. It may be that mutation in a controller gene perpetuates the fetal mode of copper metabolism; alternatively, defective copper excretion may be due to an abnormal metallothionein or to a specific lysosomal defect.

Fetal and neonatal liver normally contains relatively high concentrations of sulfur-rich copper-binding protein (metallothionein) and of copper; serum ceruloplasmin and copper levels are relatively low. The control mechanisms responsible for copper homeostasis in older children reach maturity by 2 yr of age; the wilsonian trait may be expressed after this time, but Wilson disease is not clinically manifest before the age of 5 yr.

Altered incorporation of copper into hepatic proteins such as ceruloplasmin is associated with diffuse accumulation of copper in the cytosol of hepatocytes. Later, as liver cells are overloaded, copper is distributed to other tissues, to which it is toxic, primarily as a potent inhibitor of enzymatic processes. Ionic copper inhibits pyruvate oxidase in brain and adenosine triphosphatase in membranes, leading to decreased ATP-phosphocreatine and potassium content of tissue. The glycolytic pathway and microsomal membrane ATPases are inhibited.

CLINICAL MANIFESTATIONS. Copper enters the circulation in a non–ceruloplasmin-bound form and accumulates in various organs. Manifestations are variable, with a tendency to familial patterns. The younger the patient, the more likely hepatic involvement will be the predominant manifestation. After the age of 20 yr, neurologic symptoms predominate. Forms of hepatic disease include asymptomatic hepatomegaly (with or without splenomegaly), subacute or chronic hepatitis, or fulminant hepatic failure. Cryptogenic cirrhosis, portal hypertension, ascites, edema, esophageal bleeding, or other effects of hepatic dysfunction (e.g., delayed puberty, amenorrhea, or coagulation defects) may be results of Wilson disease.

Neurologic and psychiatric disorders may develop insidiously or precipitously, with intention tremor, dysarthria, dystonia, deterioration in school performance, or behavioral changes. Kayser-Fleischer rings may be absent in young patients with only liver disease but are always present in patients with neurologic symptoms. Hemolysis may be an initial manifestation, possibly related to the release of large amounts of copper from damaged hepatocytes; this form of Wilson disease is usually fatal without transplantation. During hemolytic episodes urinary copper excretion and serum copper levels (non–ceruloplasmin-bound) are extraordinarily elevated. Manifestations of Fanconi syndrome and progressive renal failure with alterations in tubular transport of amino acids, glucose, and uric acid may be present. Unusual manifestations include arthritis and endocrinopathies, such as hypoparathyroidism.

PATHOLOGY. All grades of hepatic injury occur, with fatty change, ballooned hepatocytes, glycogen granules, minimal inflammation, and enlarged Kupffer cells. The lesion may be indistinguishable from that of chronic active hepatitis. Ultrastructural changes include large, dense mitochondria with altered smooth endoplasmic reticulum.

DIAGNOSIS. The clinical suspicion is confirmed by study of indices of copper metabolism. Children and teenagers with unexplained acute or chronic liver disease, neurologic symptoms of unknown cause, acute hemolysis, psychiatric illnesses, behavioral changes, Fanconi syndrome, or unexplained bone disease need to have the possibility of Wilson disease considered.

The best screening test is to measure the serum ceruloplasmin level. Most patients with Wilson disease will have decreased ceruloplasmin levels. Serum copper may be elevated in early Wilson disease, and urinary copper excretion (usually < 40 μg/day) is increased to greater than 100 μg/day, and often up to 1,000 μg or more per day. In equivocal cases the response of urinary copper output to chelation may be of diagnostic help; following a 1-g oral dose of D-penicillamine, affected patients will excrete 1,200 to 2,000 μg/day.

Liver biopsy is of value for examination of the histology and to measure the copper content (normally <10 μg/g dry weight); in Wilson disease hepatic copper content exceeds 250 μg/g dry weight. In healthy heterozygotes, levels may be intermediate.

Family members of proven cases deserve screening for presymptomatic Wilson disease. Screening includes ceruloplasmin levels, urinary copper excretion, and sometimes liver biopsy.

TREATMENT. The administration of copper-chelating agents leads to rapid excretion of excess deposited copper. A major attempt should be made to restrict copper intake to less than 1 mg/day. Foods such as liver, shellfish, nuts, and chocolate should be avoided. If the copper content of the water exceeds 0.1 mg/L, it may be necessary to demineralize the water. Chelation therapy is currently best managed with oral administration of penicillamine (β, β-dimethylcysteine) in a dose of 1 g/day in two doses before meals for adults, and 0.5–0.75 g/day for patients less than 10 yr old. In response to D-penicillamine, urinary copper excretion will markedly increase, and there may be slow clinical improvement. Urinary copper levels may become normal with continued administration of D-penicillamine, with marked improvement in hepatic and neurologic function and the disappearance of Kayser-Fleischer rings. Toxic effects of penicillamine are uncommon, and consist of hypersensitivity reactions (Goodpasture syndrome, SLE, polymyositis), interaction with collagen and elastin, deficiency of other elements such as zinc, as well as aplastic anemia and nephrosis. Because penicillamine is an antimetabolite of vitamin B_6, additional amounts of this vitamin are necessary. For those patients who are unable to tolerate penicillamine, triethylene tetramine dihydrochloride (Trien, TETA, Trientine) at a dose of 0.5–2 g/24 hr is an acceptable alternative.

PROGNOSIS. Untreated patients with Wilson disease will die from the hepatic, neurologic, renal, or hematologic complications. The prognosis in patients receiving prompt and continuous *D*-penicillamine is variable and depends on the time of initiation of and the individual responsiveness to chelation. Liver transplantation should be considered for patients with end-stage liver disease. In asymptomatic siblings of affected patients the expression of the disease can be prevented by early institution of chelation therapy.

13.89 Hepatic Copper Overload Syndrome

Recent studies have identified in American children a form of cirrhosis apparently associated with a genetic disturbance in copper metabolism. This syndrome differs from Wilson disease in its earlier onset; affected children develop progressive lethargy, abdominal distention, and jaundice and die before 6 yr of age. The hepatic histopathology resembles that of Indian childhood cirrhosis.

13.90 Indian Childhood Cirrhosis

Indian childhood cirrhosis is a fatal familial disorder that occurs predominantly in rural India in middle income Hindu families. It has been reported also in the Middle East, in West Africa, and in Central America. It affects children of both sexes, with onset usually at 1–3 yr of age. Hepatomegaly is often the 1st sign; fever, anorexia, and jaundice occur. There is in most cases rapid evolution to cirrhosis and liver failure. Serum immunoglobulin levels and hepatic copper concentrations are markedly elevated. No effective therapy is known.

It has been suggested that excessive dietary copper may play a role in etiology, owing to the use of copper and brass in cooking and for storage of water and milk. The early introduction of copper-contaminated milk into infant diets may explain the epidemiologic features. There may be a predisposing inherited susceptibility.

13.91 Neonatal Hemochromatosis

This rare, predominantly fatal disease of unknown etiology is characterized by increased iron deposition in the liver, pancreas, heart, and endocrine organs without evidence of increased iron intake (ingestion, transfusion) and without increased iron storage in the reticuloendothelial system. There may be a familial occurrence. The infants may be born premature or with intrauterine growth retardation, demonstrate a large placenta, and then manifest a rapidly fatal progressive illness characterized by hepatomegaly, hypoglycemia, hypoprothrombinemia, hypoalbuminemia, and hyperbilirubinemia. Symptoms begin in utero or in the 1st wk of life. The coagulopathy is often refractory to therapy with vitamin K or plasma.

The hepatic pathology reveals fibrosis, regenerative nodules, giant cell formation, necrosis, and hepatocellular hemosiderin deposits not unlike those in adult-type hereditary hemochromatosis. Hyperferritinemia is present.

Treatment with deferroxamine is ineffective, and liver transplantation is the only possible treatment.

13.92 Familial Hypervitaminosis A Hepatotoxicity (see Sec. 4.21)

13.93 α_1-Antitrypsin Deficiency

See also Sec. 14.77.

A small percentage of individuals homozygous for a deficiency of the major serum protease inhibitor, α_1-antitrypsin, have neonatal cholestasis and later childhood cirrhosis. α_1-Antitrypsin, a glycoprotein synthesized by the liver, accounts for 80% of the serum α_1-globulin fraction. α_1-Antitrypsin is present in more than 20 different codominant alleles, only a few of which are associated with defective protease inhibitors. The most common allele of the protease inhibitor (Pi) system is M, and the normal phenotype is PiMM. The Z allele predisposes to clinical deficiency; patients with liver disease are usually PiZZ and have serum α_1-antitrypsin levels less than 2 mg/mL (to approximately 10–20% of normal). The incidence of the PiZZ genotype is estimated at 1:2,000–4,000. Intermediate phenotypes PiMS, PiMZ, and PiSZ are not definitively associated with liver disease. The null genotype has no PAS-positive inclusions and is not associated with liver disease. Of all PiZZ persons, less than 20% will develop neonatal cholestasis. These patients are indistinguishable from other infants with "idiopathic" neonatal hepatitis, of whom they constitute approximately 5–10%.

In affected patients the course of liver disease is highly variable. Jaundice, acholic stools, and hepatomegaly are present during the 1st wk of life, but the jaundice usually clears during the 2nd–4th mo. There may follow complete resolution, persistent liver disease, or the development of cirrhosis. In older children, there may appear chronic liver disease or cirrhosis, with evidence of portal hypertension.

The fact that liver disease is not universal suggests a complex pathogenesis. The liver disease may be secondary to retention of the α_1-antitrypsin in the liver.

The diagnosis is best made by determination of α_1-antitrypsin (Pi) phenotype and confirmed by biopsy. PAS-positive diastase-resistant intracytoplasmic globules are seen in periportal hepatocytes. Immunofluorescence and immunocytochemical studies have shown this material to be antigenically related to α_1-antitrypsin. It has been suggested that abnormal biosynthesis of the protein or defective glycosylation may interfere with excretion of the product from the rough endoplasmic reticulum into the extracellular space. Electron microscopy shows amorphous deposits (glycoprotein) within dilated rough endoplasmic reticulum. The pattern of neonatal liver injury may be highly variable. There is hepatocellular damage with giant cell transformation, minimal inflammation, and bile stasis. Varying degrees of portal fibrosis with biliary duct proliferation occur.

Liver transplantation has been curative. There is no other effective therapy as yet, but replacement therapy may become possible.

13.94 INFECTIOUS DISORDERS OF THE LIVER

VIRAL HEPATITIS. This primary viral infection of the liver has been shown to be caused by any of at least five specific hepatotrophic viruses (Table 13–31). (See also Sec. 12.79.) Other infectious and noninfectious agents producing a hepatitis-like syndrome are noted in Table 13–32.

CMV infection may be transmitted by blood transfusion; the affected patient will typically have fever, lethargy, splenomegaly, and anemia with atypical mononuclear cells in the blood smear 3–6 wk following transfusion. Approximately one quarter of patients infected in this manner develop clinical evidence of hepatitis. This syndrome was identified originally in patients following heart surgery and was called "postperfusion syndrome," but exposure to smaller volumes of blood can presumably transmit CMV infection. CMV may also appear as an opportunistic infection in immunosuppressed patients, such as those undergoing renal, bone marrow, or hepatic transplantation.

Infectious Mononucleosis. This infection is accompanied by hepatic enlargement in 10–15% of uncomplicated cases; there may also be hepatic tenderness. Serum bilirubin levels may be mildly elevated in up to one third of patients with mononucleosis. Jaundice develops in about 5% of patients during the 2nd wk of the illness; it usually lasts 5–7 days. Epstein–Barr virus may rarely be the cause of transfusion-related hepatitis; outbreaks in hemodialysis units have been related to this virus.

LIVER ABSCESS. This is a common association of bacterial infections of the liver. Hepatic abscesses occur in infants in association with sepsis, umbilical vein infection, or vessel cannulation. Beyond infancy, hepatic abscesses occur most commonly in immunosuppressed patients. Of a large series of hepatic abscesses, 40% were found in patients with chronic granulomatous disease, and 20% in otherwise immunosuppressed patients (e.g., leukemia). Pyogenic hepatic abscesses may arise from (1) the portal circulation in patients with pylephlebitis or intra-abdominal sepsis (appendicitis, inflammatory bowel disease); (2) generalized sepsis; (3) cholangitis associated with biliary tract obstruction, such as by gallstones, in inflammatory bowel disease, after a Kasai procedure, and with choledochal cysts; (4) systemic spread from an intra-abdominal infection or contiguous spread (which usually produces large abscesses); and (5) cryptogenic biliary tract infections. Small abscesses (microabscesses) are most commonly secondary to bacteremia, candidemia, or cat-scratch disease. Implicated organisms include predominantly *Staphylococcus aureus*, *Escherichia coli*, *Salmonella*, and anaerobic organisms. Symptoms are nonspecific and may suggest systemic infection. There may be fever and pain in the right upper quadrant, and the liver is enlarged and may be tender to percussion. Jaundice is uncommon; serum aminotransferase and alkaline phosphatase activities may be mildly elevated. The erythrocyte sedimentation rate is high, and there is a leukocytosis. The results of blood cultures may be positive. Roentgenographic study of the chest may show elevation of the right hemidiaphragm with decreased mobility. Ultrasound or gallium scans or both may indicate the site of the abscess. In most cases, treatment requires percutaneous ultrasound or CT-guided needle aspiration and rarely surgical drainage. Antibiotics, such as nafcillin, gentamicin, or metronidazole, are administered based on the culture and Gram stain of the abscess fluid. *Entamoeba histolytica* may also cause hepatic

TABLE 13–31. Characteristics of the Agents Causing Acute Viral Hepatitis

	Hepatitis A Virus (HAV; Enterovirus 72)	Hepatitis B* Virus (HBV)	Hepatitis C† Virus (HCV; formerly post-transfusion non-A, non-B virus)	Hepatitis D Virus (HDV)	Hepatitis E Virus (HEV; formerly enteral non-A, non-B virus)
Agent	27-nm RNA virus	42-nm DNA virus	60–70 nm RNA virus Similar to flaviviruses	36-nm circular RNA hybrid particle with HBsAg coat	32–34-nm RNA virus Similar to Norwalk type viruses
Transmission	Fecal-oral Food-water	Transfusion, sexual, inoculation, vertical	Parenteral, transfusion, vertical (sexual?)	Similar to HBV	Enteral: endemic and epidemic
Incubation period	30 days	60–180 days	30–60 days	Similar to HBV	25–60 days
Serum markers	Anti-HAV	Antigens*, Anti-HBs Anti-HBc	Anti-HCV (IgG, IgM)	Anti-HDV, RNA	Anti-HEV
Fulminant liver failure	Rare	Uncommon unless with δ agent‡	Uncommon	Yes	Yes in pregnancy
Chronic liver disease	No	Yes	Yes	Yes	Uncommon
Carrier state	No	Yes§	Yes	Yes	No
Risk of hepatocellular cancer	No	Yes	Yes	No	No
Prophylaxis against	Immune serum globulin; hygiene	Hepatitis B immune globulin, vaccine Screen blood products for HBsAg	Screen blood for antibody appearing 4 mo postinfection (6 mo post-transfusion)	Screen blood for HBV markers	Screen blood for IgM, IgG antibody

*Hepatitis B whole virus particle is the Dane particle, which consists of a surface antigen HBsAg, a core antigen HBcAg, an e antigen HBeAg, and DNA with a DNA polymerase. Mutant HBV may also produce severe hepatitis.

†An unknown number of posttransfusion hepatitis cases are due to viruses other than HBV, HCV or cytomegalovirus, Epstein-Barr virus, human herpesvirus-6, or known agents and remain designated as caused by a non-A, non-B hepatitis agent.

‡δ Agent or hepatitis D virus requires hepatitis B virus coinfection or superinfection of a chronic HBV carrier for replication.

§Chronic carrier state common in Afro-Asian, Haitian, Eskimo, South Pacific immigrants, drug abusers, Down syndrome, multiply transfused patients, homosexuals, patients on hemodialysis, and dental workers.

TABLE 13–32. Causes of Acute Hepatitis In Childhood

Virus	
Hepatitis A	Lassa fever virus
Hepatitis B	Dengue
Hepatitis C	Yellow fever
Hepatitis D (with HBV)	Ebola virus
Hepatitis E	Measles
Epstein-Barr virus	Varicella-zoster virus
Cytomegalovirus	Undefined teramyxovirus (syncytial giant cells)
Enterovirus	
Human herpesvirus-6	
Bacteria	
Syphilis	Miliary tuberculosis
Leptospirosis	Gonococcus (perihepatitis)
Bacterial sepsis	*Chlamydia trachomatis* (perihepatitis)
Coxiella burnetii	
Toxic	
Isoniazid	Iron
Oral contraceptives	Erythromycin estolate
Androgens	Alcohol
Carbon tetrachloride	Mushroom poisoning *(Amanita phalloides)*
Chlorpromazine	Valproic acid
Allopurinol	Phenytoin
Acetaminophen	Carbamazepine
Salicylates	Methotrexate
Hydralazine	6-Mercaptopurine
Halothane	
Other	
α_1-Antitrypsin deficiency	Tumor
Wilson disease	Infarction
Inborn errors of metabolism (galactosemia, tyrosinemia)	Shock
Chronic active hepatitis	Heart failure
Veno-occlusive disease	Anoxia

abscesses in symptomatic or asymptomatic patients with amebic infection of the gastrointestinal tract (Sec. 12.111).

13.95 LIVER DISEASE ASSOCIATED WITH SYSTEMIC DISORDERS

Hepatobiliary disease may complicate ulcerative colitis (Sec. 13.41) *and Crohn disease* (Sec. 13.42). Both the manifestations and the severity vary. Fatty liver, pericholangitis, drug-induced injury, chronic hepatitis, portal fibrosis, cirrhosis, hepatic abscesses, infarction, portal vein thrombosis, sclerosing cholangitis, carcinoma of the biliary tract, and cholelithiasis have all been associated. These complications are more likely to occur in patients with other extraintestinal complications, but there is no correlation with the severity of the inflammatory bowel disease. The etiology of abnormalities in liver function in patients with ulcerative colitis or Crohn disease is unknown. Total colectomy has not been beneficial in management of hepatobiliary complications in patients with ulcerative colitis.

Extensive fatty change in the liver has been found, especially in patients with inflammatory bowel disease who are severely malnourished or chronically incapacitated. Most patients have no symptoms; they have only hepatomegaly as a sign. The chemical abnormalities are mild. The fatty infiltration usually subsides with therapy.

Pericholangitis may be difficult to distinguish from chronic hepatitis in patients with inflammatory bowel disease. The patients may be asymptomatic or have jaundice, pruritus, or abdominal pain. Elevation of alkaline phosphatase or 5′-nucleotidase activities is almost universal. This complication can occur any time in the course of inflammatory bowel disease. The prognosis appears to be favorable; progression to cirrhosis, however, has been reported. There has been no consistent beneficial response to various medications, such as corticosteroids.

Sclerosing cholangitis or fibrosing inflammation of various segments of the bile ducts may lead to obliteration of the duct lumen. The clinical and biochemical picture is that of cholestasis, often with intermittent attacks of acute cholangitis (fever, jaundice, right upper quadrant pain, anorexia, weight loss, and pruritus), followed by portal hypertension. This complication is associated with ulcerative colitis, and rarely with Crohn disease.

Primary sclerosing cholangitis (*not* associated with inflammatory bowel disease) is rare in children. In either case, ERCP reveals beading and irregularity of the intrahepatic and extrahepatic bile ducts. Treatment is aimed at improving biliary drainage and attempting to halt the progression of the obliterative process. Symptomatic treatment is required for such complications as pruritus, malnutrition, and infection. There is no definitive treatment; administration of corticosteroids or D-penicillamine has produced inconsistent results. The course is usually progressive to a fatal outcome if liver transplantation is not carried out.

Bacterial sepsis (Sec. 9.60 and 12.14) may be complicated by liver disease. The most frequently associated organisms are *E. coli*, *Klebsiella pneumoniae*, and *Pseudomonas aeruginosa*. It is postulated that bacterial endotoxin directly inhibits bile formation by altering the bile canalicular membrane. Clinical manifestations may be subtle and difficult to differentiate from other causes of cholestasis. There is an elevation in the serum bilirubin level, usually predominantly in the conjugated fraction. Serum alkaline phosphatase and aminotransferase activities may be elevated. Liver biopsy shows intrahepatic cholestasis with little or no hepatocyte necrosis. Kupffer cell hyperplasia and an increase in inflammatory cells are also common.

Hepatic congestion and injury may occur as a complication of severe *chronic* or *acute congestive heart failure* (Sec. 15.73) or *cyanotic heart disease* (Sec. 15.11–15.23). Hepatic dysfunction derives from hypoxemia, systemic venous congestion, and low cardiac output. Hepatic manifestations of left- and right-sided heart failure are similar. With decreased cardiac output, there is decreased hepatic blood flow and centrizonal hypoxia. Hepatic necrosis leads to lactic acidosis, elevated aminotransferase activities, jaundice, prolonged partial thromboplastin time, and possibly hypoglycemia. With right-sided heart failure, increases in right atrial and hepatic venous pressures lead to centrizonal sinusoidal distention that presents a barrier to oxygen diffusion. Hemorrhage, pressure atrophy, and necrosis follow. Jaundice and tender hepatomegaly occur. Ascites may also occur with chronic right-sided congestive heart failure. In patients with shock liver, elevated aminotransferase activities may return rapidly to normal when perfusion and cardiac function improve. A syndrome of fulminant hepatic failure may occur, particularly in patients with aortic coarctation. Hepatic necrosis may be seen in patients with hypoplastic left-sided heart syndrome.

The patient with *sickle cell anemia* (Sec. 16.19) or *sickle cell thalassemia* (Sec. 16.26) may have hepatic dysfunction owing to acute or chronic viral-associated hepatitis, iron overload, hepatic crises related to severe intrahepatic cholestasis, and ischemic necrosis. In addition, cholelithiasis and a benign form of extreme hyperbilirubinemia have been noted. Hepatic sickle cell crisis or "sickle hepatopathy" may produce intense right upper quadrant pain, fever, leukocytosis, right upper quadrant tenderness, and jaundice. Bilirubin levels may be markedly elevated; alkaline phosphatase activities may be only moderately elevated.

On occasion, children with sickle cell disease develop bilirubin levels exceeding 20 mg/dL; these levels are unaccompanied by severe pain or fever. There is no change in hematocrit or reticulocyte count nor any association with a hemolytic crisis. The clinical course is benign.

The most common metabolic complication of *total parenteral nutrition* (TPN) in premature infants is the development of liver dysfunction. Cholestasis is the most severe form and is potentially fatal. It is the major factor limiting effective use of TPN (Sec. 9.17).

In *low birthweight infants*, the incidence of TPN-associated cholestasis is inversely correlated with birthweight. It develops with TPN in almost half of infants with birthweights less than 1,000 g, in 20% of those 1,000–1,500 g, and in 5–10% of those 1,500–2,000 g. The incidence of cholestasis also correlates with the duration of TPN, with onset usually after 2 wk. Respiratory distress, acidosis, hypoxia, necrotizing enterocolitis, short bowel syndrome, and sepsis seem to enhance the likelihood and severity of cholestasis. Associated illness, the exclusion of enteral intake, and the nature of the underlying disorder that necessitates TPN may also affect the incidence.

The onset is usually insidious, with progressive jaundice and hepatic enlargement or splenomegaly. In low birthweight infants, the onset of jaundice may overlap the phase of physiologic unconjugated hyperbilirubinemia. Any icteric infant who has received TPN for more than 1 wk should have all bilirubin determinations fractionated. Cholestasis is frequently first detected through routine monitoring of infants receiving TPN. A slow progression of abnormalities is found in biochemical measurements of hepatic function. Serum bile acid concentrations may increase. Rises in serum aminotransferase activities may be a late finding. An elevation in serum alkaline phosphatase activity may be due to rickets, a common complication of TPN in low birthweight infants.

In addition to cholestasis, biliary complications of intravenous nutrition include cholelithiasis and the development of biliary sludge, associated with thick, inspissated gallbladder contents. These may be asymptomatic.

An effort must be made to differentiate TPN-associated hepatic dysfunction from benign causes of hepatomegaly, such as the deposition of glycogen or fat, which is common with TPN and with which serum bilirubin and bile acid levels will remain within the normal range. Consideration of other causes of cholestasis is also appropriate. The group in which TPN-associated cholestasis most frequently occurs (i.e., infants in the neonatal intensive care unit) often receives blood transfusions or drugs. Therefore, hepatic disease related to viral hepatitis or drug-induced liver disease is a consideration (see Table 13–32).

The most striking histologic finding in TPN-associated liver disease is canalicular cholestasis, which may begin after less than 2 wk of TPN. Bile duct proliferation may resemble that in biliary atresia. Portal fibrosis is a late finding. Progression of injury to cirrhosis is possible; late onset hepatic carcinoma has occurred in a few infants. Milder changes may be reversible with discontinuation of TPN and the initiation of oral feedings.

The pathogenesis of TPN-associated cholestasis is most likely multifactorial. The infant is of low birthweight, is receiving nothing by mouth, may have significant gastrointestinal disease, and often has other systemic complications. The administered nutrient solution has potential toxicity and may induce a specific deficiency. The omission of oral feedings and the absence of intraluminal nutrients blunt the output of the gastrointestinal hormones, which are normal stimulants to bile flow and to development of the hepatobiliary system. Potential hepatotoxins include bacterial endotoxins, specific amino acids or metabolic or degradation products, or copper or manganese; the last two are particularly hepatotoxic. The roles of specific deficiencies (of taurine, essential fatty acids, amino acid, carnitine, or vitamin E) need to be investigated.

The goal in management of the infant with TPN-associated cholestasis is to avoid progressive liver injury. It has been shown that with the administration of oral feedings gradual resolution of the liver disease occurs. The initiation of oral feedings of small volume or the infusion of nutrients by continuous nasogastric drip may enhance biliary flow and intestinal motility. This effect may occur even when the enteral intake does not provide the total caloric needs. Improved solutions that meet the specific needs of the neonate may prevent deficiencies and avoid toxicities. In the decision to continue TPN, one must weigh the risk of further hepatic injury against the risk of malnutrition.

In *older children*, TPN-associated liver dysfunction is less common and less severe than in infants, but biochemical abnormalities are not uncommon in older patients who are maintained on TPN for prolonged periods, either at home or in the hospital. Patients with chronic intestinal disease, which may be complicated by infection or bacterial overgrowth, are particularly susceptible to hepatic dysfunction. In most such patients, partial enteral alimentation reverses the abnormalities. It may be necessary at any age, when alkaline phosphatase or aminotransferase activities are elevated, to evaluate the underlying liver disease by liver biopsy. Hepatic steatosis without cholestasis is often the only abnormality.

Hepatic dysfunction is common in patients who have undergone *bone marrow transplantation*. Its genesis is multifactorial and may be related to (1) infections (viral, bacterial, or fungal), drugs, parenteral nutrition, chemotherapy, or radiation; (2) veno-occlusive disease (VOD); or (3) graft-versus-host disease (GVHD); or to any combination of these. Candidates for bone marrow transplantation have often had pre-existing liver disease, such as viral hepatitis, drug-related injury, or malignant infiltration. Percutaneous liver biopsy in such patients may show extensive bile duct injury in GVHD, viral inclusions in CMV disease, or the characteristic endothelial lesion in VOD, but the histologic distinction is often unclear. This presents a dilemma, because treatment of one suspected complication (e.g., initiation of immunosuppressive therapy for GVHD) may have a deleterious effect if the symptoms are due to another (e.g., fungal or viral infection).

VOD of the liver usually has its onset 1–3 wk after bone marrow transplantation but may appear up to 6 wk afterward. The most characteristic presentation is the onset of rapid weight gain, with ascites, hepatomegaly, right upper quadrant pain, jaundice, and oliguria. Hepatic encephalopathy and fulminant hepatic failure may follow. Less severe forms may be characterized by jaundice and ascites with a slow resolution; a mild form of VOD has histologic changes as the sole manifestation. The diagnosis rests on the exclusion of other diseases, such as congestive cardiomyopathy, constrictive pericarditis, and venous thrombosis (Budd-Chiari syndrome).

Pathologic changes in patients with VOD are best demonstrated using special (trichrome) stains to highlight the central veins. An early lesion is concentric narrowing of the lumina of small central veins, owing to edema in the subendothelial zone. There is a dense, wavy continuous band of collagen in the central veins and centrilobular hemorrhagic necrosis. The lesions may be patchy. The venular changes may progress to complete obliteration. The cause of VOD following bone marrow transplantation is not clear; it may be related to ionizing radiation or to antineoplastic drugs, or both. Risk factors for VOD include high-dose conditioning regimens, leukemia, advanced age, and pre-existing liver disease.

Budd-Chiari syndrome involves occlusion of the inferior vena cava or hepatic veins and tributaries; it may be caused by obstruction due to a web, mass, or thrombus. The disease has rarely been noted in children; however, a number of associated diseases may increase the risk. These include trauma, coagulopathies, sickle cell anemia, leukemia, polycythemia vera, hepatic abscesses, irradiation, and GVHD. The syndrome is to be regarded as distinct from VOD, which affects the centrilobular and sublobular hepatic veins, sparing the larger veins; it is not associated with thrombosis.

TABLE 13–33. Diseases That Present a Clinical/Pathologic Picture Resembling Reye Syndrome

Central nervous system infections or intoxications (meningitis, encephalitis, toxic encephalopathy)
Hemorrhagic shock with encephalopathy
Drug ingestion (salicylate, valproate)
Toxin (hypoglycin A, valproate)
Metabolic disease
- Organic acidurias/defects in hepatic fatty acid oxidation (primary or secondary)
- Urea cycle defects (carbamyl phosphate synthetase [CPS], ornithine transcarbamylase [OTC]
- Fructosemia
- Defects in fatty acid metabolism
  - Acyl-CoA dehydrogenase deficiencies
    - Long-chain (LCAD)
    - Medium-chain (MCAD)
    - Short-chain (SCAD)
  - Systemic carnitine deficiency
  - Hepatic carnitine palmitoyltransferase deficiency
  - 3-OH, 3-methylglutaryl-CoA lyase deficiency

GVHD of the liver may be acute or chronic and is generally concomitant with GVHD in other target organs (Sec. 11.21). Cholestasis and hepatic injury of various degrees occur; there may be hepatic tenderness, dark urine, acholic stools, itching, and anorexia. There are parallel rises in serum bilirubin level and alkaline phosphatase activity; AST elevation is less striking. GVHD is characterized histologically by degeneration and loss of small bile ducts and sparse inflammation, along with cholestasis.

Hepatic involvement in patients with *collagen vascular disease* is uncommon. It has been noted especially in patients with systemic lupus erythematosus. Reactive hepatitis, chronic hepatitis, steatosis, and hepatic infarction have also been described. The association of hepatic injury with drug therapy, such as salicylate use, must be differentiated.

13.96 REYE SYNDROME

See also Sec. 20.67.

The previously high incidence of this syndrome of acute encephalopathy and fatty degeneration of the liver has decreased markedly, mainly as the result of increased awareness of the highly significant association between this disorder and ingestion of aspirin-containing medications by children with influenza-like illness or varicella. However, investigations of Reye syndrome uncovered a wide variety of previously undefined metabolic diseases whose clinical picture is similar and that need to be considered in the differential diagnosis of Reye syndrome (Table 13–33).

EPIDEMIOLOGY. Case reports of Reye syndrome were sporadic until 1974, when almost 400 cases were reported in the United States, with a mortality rate of more than 40%. The incidence was increased in direct temporal and geographic relationship to viral epidemics, especially those due to influenza B and varicella. In 1988 there were 20 reported cases.

The peak incidence was at about 6 yr of age, with most cases in the 4–12 yr old range. There was no gender difference in incidence, but rural and suburban populations appeared to be more frequently affected than urban. The question that arose was whether Reye syndrome was a new disease or whether affected children had been classified as having disorders such as "postviral encephalopathy." It is very likely that mild cases were missed and recovered without event. In any case, in the late 1970s Reye syndrome was the most common potentially lethal virus-associated encephalopathy in the United States. Currently, cases mainly occur among self-medicating adolescents who use aspirin.

CLINICAL MANIFESTATIONS. The illness follows a stereotypic biphasic course. It usually occurs in a previously healthy child. A prodromal febrile illness, an upper respiratory tract infection (in 90% of the cases), or chickenpox (in 5–7%) is followed by an interval in which the child has seemingly recovered. The abrupt onset of protracted vomiting then occurs, usually within 5–7 days after the onset of the viral illness. Delirium, combative behavior, and stupor may occur simultaneously or within a few hours after the onset of vomiting. Neurologic symptoms may rapidly progress to seizures, coma, and death; focal neurologic signs are absent. There is a slight to moderate liver enlargement with abnormalities of hepatic function; the patient remains anicteric. Cerebrospinal fluid is normal except for elevated pressure.

DIAGNOSIS. The clinical features are best reflected in the system of clinical staging that has been proposed (Table 13–34); grades I through III represent mild to moderate illness, grades IV and V represent severe illness. The majority of affected children will have mild illness without progression. The cerebrospinal fluid is normal.

There is explosive release from liver and muscle of such enzymes as aminotransferases, creatine kinase (CK), and lactic dehydrogenase (LDH). The activity of the mitochondrial enzyme serum glutamate dehydrogenase (GDH) is greatly increased. Patients not in coma who have a three-fold or higher elevation in serum ammonia level are more likely to progress to coma, as are patients who have hypoprothrombinemia unresponsive to vitamin K. In younger patients, there may be hypoglycemia; however, these patients should be carefully screened for the presence of metabolic disease.

Pathology. The striking and characteristic gross pathologic feature of Reye syndrome is a yellow to white liver, reflective of a high content of triglyceride. Light microscopy shows a uniform foaminess of liver cell cytoplasm with microvesicular fatty accumulation, which may be concealed in routine preparations. Electron microscopic (EM) changes include a unique alteration of mitochondrial morphology. Biopsy should be carried out in atypical or severe cases in order to rule out metabolic or toxic liver disease, especially in patients under 1–2 yr of age. Histologic examination of brain tissue reveals a similar pattern of injury. Grossly, there is marked edema.

Pathogenesis. The major site of injury is the mitochondrion. The activities of hepatic intramitochondrial enzymes, including ornithine transcarbamylase (OTC), carbamylphosphate synthetase (CPS), and pyruvate dehydrogenase, are reduced, often to less than half of their normal values. Hyperammonemia may result from decreases in the activities of OTC and CPS.

The reasons for mitochondrial dysfunction are unknown. No toxic factor has as yet been conclusively identified, but studies have suggested an etiologic link between Reye syndrome, use of aspirin and viral infections. It is prudent to

TABLE 13–34. Clinical Staging of Reye Syndrome

Grade	*Symptoms* at Time of Admission
I	Usually quiet, **lethargic** and sleepy, vomiting, laboratory evidence of liver dysfunction
II	Deep lethargy, **confusion,** delirium, combative, hyperventilation, hyperreflexic
III	Obtunded, **light coma,** ± seizures, decorticate rigidity, intact pupillary light reaction
IV	Seizures, deepening coma, **decerebrate rigidity,** loss of oculocephalic reflexes, fixed pupils
V	Coma, loss of deep tendon reflexes, respiratory arrest, fixed dilated pupils, **flaccidity/decerebrate** (intermittent); isoelectric EEG

avoid the use of aspirin as an antipyretic in patients with influenza or varicella.

TREATMENT. Successful management of Reye syndrome requires (1) early recognition of mild cases and (2) control of increased intracranial pressure (ICP) secondary to cerebral edema, which is the major lethal factor.

Early diagnosis may be aided by a high level of clinical suspicion and by assessment of hepatic function in suspected cases. Marked elevation of aminotransferase activities, prolongation of prothrombin time, and elevation of the serum ammonia level above 125–150 μg/dL suggest the diagnosis. It is imperative that cerebral edema be identified and counteracted and that aerobic metabolism be maintained.

Management varies with the severity of the illness. Whereas observation alone may suffice in patients with grade 1 severity, more aggressive therapy will be needed in patients with more severe neurologic deterioration. All patients should initially receive glucose (10–15%) intravenously, because glycogen depletion is common. In patients with cerebral edema, the amount of fluid administered should be restricted to approximately 1500 mL/m^2 day. Hyperthermia should be avoided. Coagulopathy is managed with vitamin K, fresh frozen plasma, and platelet transfusions.

In more severely ill, comatose patients, endotracheal intubation permits adequate oxygenation; hyperventilation induces hypocarbia, which decreases cerebral blood flow by cerebral vasoconstriction. Close monitoring of ICP assists in decisions regarding management. Stimulation of the patient should be minimized, because procedures such as suctioning may generate increases in ICP.

An indwelling arterial line permits continuous assessment of cerebral perfusion pressure. Osmotherapy (mannitol 0.5–1.0 g/kg every 4–6 hr) should be used to maintain a serum osmolality of 300–320 mOsm/L and to induce cerebral dehydration; the ICP should be held to less than 20 mm Hg and the cerebral perfusion pressure to greater than 50 mm Hg. Pressure monitoring provides an effective guide to therapy with osmotic diuretics and may decrease renal complications due to hyperosmolarity. Use of pentobarbital (2.5 mg/kg) to maintain a serum barbiturate level of 20–30 μg/mL may have a protective effect on the central nervous system by decreasing cerebral metabolic demands, decreasing cerebral blood flow, and causing cerebral vasoconstriction. Excessive pentobarbital may reduce cardiac function, lowering blood pressure, and therefore cerebral perfusion pressure. Pancuronium bromide has been used with the hope of decreasing cerebral blood volume through muscular relaxation and increased peripheral blood pooling.

PROGNOSIS. The duration of disordered cerebral function during the acute stage of illness is the best predictor of eventual outcome. In patients with grade 1 disease, recovery is rapid and complete. In patients with more severe disease there may be subsequent subtle neuropsychologic defects noted (in intelligence, school achievement, visuomotor integration, and concept formation).

WILLIAM F. BALISTRERI

13.97 CHRONIC HEPATITIS

Chronic hepatitis is defined as a continuing hepatic inflammatory process manifested by elevated hepatic transaminase levels, lasting 6 mo or more. The severity is variable; the affected child may have only biochemical evidence of liver dysfunction, may have stigmata of chronic liver disease, or may present in hepatic failure.

Chronic hepatitis can be caused by persistent viral infection, drugs, and autoimmune or unknown factors. Approximately 15–20% of cases are associated with hepatitis B infection (Sec. 12.79); in this group of patients, unusually severe disease may be caused by superimposed infection with hepatitis D (a defective RNA virus that is dependent on replicating hepatitis B virus). More than 90% of infants infected during the 1st year of life develop chronic hepatitis B infection, compared with a rate of 5–10% among older children and adults. Chronic hepatitis may also follow 30–50% of hepatitis C virus infection (see Table 13–31). Patients receiving blood products or who have had massive transfusions are at increased risk. Hepatitis A virus does not cause chronic hepatitis. Drugs commonly used in children that may cause chronic liver injury include isoniazid, methyldopa, nitrofurantoin, dantrolene, and the sulfonamides (see Table 13–32).

In most cases, the cause of chronic hepatitis is unknown; in many, an autoimmune mechanism is suggested by the finding of antinuclear and antismooth muscle antibodies in serum and by multisystem involvement (including rashes, arthropathy, thyroiditis, and Coombs-positive hemolytic anemia). Histologic features have defined two major subdivisions of chronic hepatitis: *chronic persistent hepatitis* and *chronic active hepatitis*. The pathogenesis of each morphologic form is uncertain, but the criteria defining them predict a benign, self-limited course for chronic persistent hepatitis and a progressive course potentially leading to cirrhosis for chronic active hepatitis. Both forms are to be distinguished from unresolved or prolonged acute viral hepatitis in which clinical and biochemical abnormalities last 2–3 mo; liver biopsy in such cases shows predominantly single cell necrosis in the lobule, with minimal portal and lobular inflammation. In addition, disorders such as Wilson disease and α_1-antitriypsin deficiency must be considered.

Chronic Persistent Hepatitis

Chronic persistent hepatitis in childhood is a generally benign inflammatory process of the liver. It most commonly follows acute hepatitis due to hepatitis B or C viruses.

PATHOLOGY. The lobular architecture is always normal. Inflammation is limited to portal triads, and no significant fibrosis or cirrhosis is found.

CLINICAL MANIFESTATIONS. Most pediatric patients with chronic persistent hepatitis are asymptomatic or have nonspecific complaints, such as fatigue or anorexia. Some patients have minimal hepatomegaly or slight right upper quadrant tenderness. Historical features and physical stigmata of drug abuse should be sought in the adolescent.

There are mild to moderate elevations of serum aminotransferase activities and normal or only slightly increased serum bilirubin concentrations (predominantly of the direct-reacting fraction). Serum alkaline phosphatase (hepatic) activity, albumin level, and prothrombin time are normal. Serum globulin and IgG fraction concentrations are normal or only slightly increased. Tests for antismooth muscle and antinuclear antibodies have negative results. As many as one third of patients will be hepatitis B surface antigen (HBsAg) positive, whereas an unknown number are anti-HCV positive.

DIAGNOSIS. There is considerable clinical and laboratory overlap between the variants of chronic hepatitis; accordingly, liver biopsy is essential to the diagnosis of chronic persistent hepatitis. Differential diagnosis should include biliary tract disease and the pericholangitis associated with inflammatory bowel disease.

TREATMENT AND PROGNOSIS. The prognosis is good in childhood. In adults chronic persistent hepatitis B and C virus infections are more likely to progress to cirrhosis, liver failure, or hepatocellular carcinoma. Impaired immunity may be responsible for the persistent viral infection. Prednisone therapy alone is of no benefit. Interferon-α is of some benefit for chronic hepatitis B or C virus. Whether these therapies are indicated for the rare child with progression of chronic persistent hepatitis or if they will reduce the risk for hepatocellular cancer remains to be determined.

Chronic Active Hepatitis

Chronic active hepatitis is characterized by unresolving inflammation, necrosis, and fibrosis, with the possibility of progression to cirrhosis and liver failure.

ETIOLOGY. Chronic active hepatitis may be caused by chronic infection with hepatitis B or C viruses. Most patients, however, have no evidence of viral infection, drug, or metabolic liver injury as a cause for their liver disease. In many cases, clinical features strongly suggest an autoimmune mechanism.

PATHOLOGY. The histologic features common to untreated cases include (1) inflammatory infiltrates, consisting of lymphocytes and plasma cells, which expand portal areas and often penetrate the lobule; (2) moderate to severe "piecemeal" necrosis of hepatocytes extending outward from the limiting plate; and (3) variable necrosis, fibrosis, and zones of parenchymal collapse spanning neighboring portal triads or between a portal triad and central vein (bridging necrosis). Distortion of hepatic architecture may be severe; cirrhosis may be found in children at the time of diagnosis.

CLINICAL MANIFESTATIONS. The clinical features and course of chronic active hepatitis are extremely variable. Some patients develop chronic active hepatitis following a well-defined episode of hepatitis B infection or post-transfusion hepatitis C infection; and in 25–30% of patients, particularly children, the illness may mimic acute viral hepatitis. In most patients, however, the onset is insidious. About half of the patients are less than 20 yr of age; most HBsAg-negative patients are female. Patients may be asymptomatic or have fatigue, malaise, behavioral changes, anorexia, and amenorrhea, sometimes for many months before jaundice or stigmata of chronic liver disease are recognized. Extrahepatic manifestations may include arthritis, vasculitis, and nephritis in HBsAg-positive patients, presumably secondary to deposition of hepatitis B antigen-antibody immune complexes. Thyroiditis, Coombs-positive anemia, arthritis, and rash are common in patients with the autoimmune or "lupoid" variety of chronic active hepatitis. Some patients' initial clinical features may reflect cirrhosis (ascites, bleeding esophageal varices, or hepatic encephalopathy).

There is usually mild to moderate jaundice. Spider telangiectasias and palmar erythema may be present. The liver is often tender and slightly enlarged but may not be felt in patients with cirrhosis. The spleen is commonly enlarged. Edema and ascites may be present in advanced cases. Evidence of involvement of other organ systems may be found. Classic features of autoimmune hepatitis (including cushingoid appearance, acne, hirsutism, and striae) occur in a few patients.

LABORATORY MANIFESTATIONS. These reveal moderate elevation (usually less than 1,000 IU/L) of serum aminotransferase activities. Serum bilirubin concentrations (predominantly the direct reacting fraction) are commonly 2–10 mg/dL. Serum alkaline phosphatase activity is normal to slightly increased. Serum γ-globulin levels show marked polyclonal elevations in most patients but may be normal to only slightly increased in HBsAg-positive patients. Hypoalbuminemia is common. The prothrombin time is prolonged, most often as a result of vitamin K deficiency but also as a reflection of impaired hepatocellular function. A normochromic, normocytic anemia, leukopenia, and thrombocytopenia are present and usually become more severe with evolution of portal hypertension and hypersplenism. Serologic (IgG), antigenic, or genomic evidence of hepatitis B, C, or D virus infection may be evident.

All patients with autoimmune hepatitis have hypergammaglobulinemia. Serum IgG levels usually exceed 16 g/L. Characteristic patterns of serum autoantibodies have been used to define several noninfectious subgroups of chronic active hepatitis. The most common pattern is the formation of non–organ-specific antibodies, such as antiactin (smooth muscle), antinuclear, and antimitochondrial antibodies. Approximately half of these patients are 10–20 yr of age. High titers of a liver/kidney microsomal antibody are detected in another form that usually affects children 2–14 yr of age. A subgroup of primarily young women may demonstrate autoantibodies against a soluble liver antigen but not against nuclear or microsomal proteins. Some patients only demonstrate antismooth muscle or antinuclear antibodies. Additional less common autoantibodies include rheumatoid factor, antiparietal cell antibodies, and antithyroid antibodies. A Coombs-positive hemolytic anemia may be present.

DIAGNOSIS. The diagnosis of chronic active hepatitis is established by liver biopsy. The differential diagnosis should include α-antitrypsin deficiency (Sec. 13.93) and Wilson disease (Sec. 13.88). Chronic active hepatitis may occur in patients with inflammatory bowel disease, but liver dysfunction in such patients is more commonly due to pericholangitis or sclerosing cholangitis. The differential diagnosis of chronic liver disease is noted in Table 13–35.

TREATMENT. Controlled studies of the drug treatment of autoimmune forms of chronic active hepatitis have only been conducted in adults, but several retrospective studies in children and adolescents suggest that they benefit from immunosuppressive therapy. It is clear that corticosteroid therapy, with or without low doses of azathioprine, improves the clinical, biochemical, and histologic features in most patients with chronic active hepatitis and prolongs survival in most patients with severe disease. In severe chronic active hepatitis, after exclusion of HBsAg-positive and transfusion-related

TABLE 13–35. Disorders Producing Chronic Liver Disease

Genetic Disorders	**Drugs/Toxins**
Wilson disease	Aflatoxin
Galactosemia	Carbon tetrachloride
Glycogen storage disease III, IV	*Amanita* toxin
α_1-Antitrypsin deficiency	Irradiation
Tyrosinosis	Indian childhood cirrhosis
Cystinosis	**Hematologic**
Niemann-Pick disease type C	Sickle cell anemia
Gaucher disease	1° or 2° hemochromatosis
Wolman disease	Leukemia
Hepatic porphyria	Myeloproliferative disease
Zellweger syndrome	Lymphoma
Byler disease	Histiocytosis
Shwachmann syndrome	**Anatomic**
Cystic fibrosis	Biliary atresia
Familial neonatal hepatitis	Choledochal cyst
Polycystic renal disease	Intrahepatic biliary hypoplasia
Infectious Disorders	Choledocholithiasis
Hepatitis B, C, D virus	Tumors (bile duct)
CMV	Venacaval webs
Syphilis	**Immunologic**
Schistosomiasis	Chronic active hepatitis
Liver flukes	Inflammatory bowel disease
Vascular	Systemic lupus erythematosus
Veno-occlusive disease	Primary sclerosing cholangitis
Constructive pericarditis	Sarcoidosis
Epstein anomaly	Immunodeficiency diseases
Budd-Chiari syndrome	
Heart failure	

cases, the course and response to drug therapy appear to be similar whether or not autoimmune features are present.

The goal of treatment is to suppress or eliminate hepatic inflammation with minimal side effects. Prednisone is given at an initial dose of 1–2 mg/kg/day and continued until aminotransferase values return to a level twice the upper limit of normal. The dose should then be lowered in 5-mg decrements over a 4– 6-wk period, until a maintenance dose of less than 20 mg/day is achieved. In patients who respond poorly, who develop severe side effects, or who cannot be maintained on low dose steroids, azathioprine (1.5 mg/kg/day, up to 50 mg/day) may be added, with frequent monitoring for bone marrow suppression. Alternate-day corticosteroid therapy should be used with great caution. In adults, this form of treatment produced improvement or even normalization of serum aminotransferase activities, but histologic resolution did not occur.

Histologic progress should be assessed by liver biopsy 6 mo–1 yr after the initiation of treatment, because normal results of biochemical tests during therapy do not ensure histologic resolution. Disappearance of symptoms and biochemical abnormalities, and either resolution of the necroinflammatory process on biopsy or at least improvement to a pattern of chronic persistent hepatitis, justify an attempt at gradual discontinuation of medication.

Chronic hepatitis B infection usually responds poorly to corticosteroid therapy as the only treatment. Recent studies suggest an increased frequency of complications, enhanced viral replication, and a higher death rate in steroid-treated patients. Chronic hepatitis C infection, following blood transfusion, has a fluctuating clinical and biochemical course that may spontaneously improve.

Positive responses to antiviral treatment of chronic hepatitis B and C virus infections have been reported (see Chronic Persistent Hepatitis). Patients with hepatitis B who are likely to respond to treatment with interferon-α have recently acquired infection and active viral proliferation demonstrated by serum HBeAg and hepatitis B-DNA. Patients with long-standing hepatitis B infection and probable integration of viral DNA into the host genome are less likely to benefit from treatment. Unfortunately, many children with perinatal infection often fall into this category. Favorable response to interferon therapy, defined as clearance of HBeAg, hepatitis B-DNA, and DNA polymerase from serum as well as amelioration of the inflammatory liver disease, can be expected in 30–40% of patients. Remission is sustained in only 30–50% of responders, and complete eradication of the infection is unusual. Interferon-α therapy improves liver function in approximately 50% of patients with chronic hepatitis C virus infection. Half of these patients relapse after discontinuation of therapy but usually respond to retreatment.

PROGNOSIS. Treatment of autoimmune chronic active hepatitis will significantly improve survival in most HBsAg-negative patients. More than 75% of patients can be expected to respond to therapy. In patients meeting the criteria for withdrawal of treatment, 50% can be successfully weaned from medication; in the other 50%, relapse occurs after a variable period of time, but this will usually respond to retreatment. Progression to cirrhosis can occur, despite a good response to drug therapy and prolongation of life.

Orthotopic liver transplantation has been successful in patients with end-stage liver disease associated with autoimmune and post-transfusion hepatitis C forms of chronic active hepatitis. In contrast, recurrence of liver disease is likely following transplantation for chronic hepatitis B virus infection, because the virus may persist in extrahepatic sites.

13.98 DRUG- AND TOXIN-INDUCED LIVER INJURY

The liver is the main site of drug metabolism and is particularly susceptible to structural and functional injury following ingestion, parenteral administration, or inhalation of chemical agents, drugs, or environmental toxins. The possibility of drug use or toxin exposure at home or in the parental workplace should be explored for every child with liver dysfunction. The clinical spectrum of illness may vary from asymptomatic biochemical abnormalities of liver function to fulminant failure.

Hepatic metabolism of drugs and toxins is mediated by a sequence of enzymatic reactions which, in large part, transform hydrophobic, less excretable molecules into more nontoxic, hydrophilic compounds that can be readily excreted in urine or bile. *Phase 1* of the process involves the enzymatic activation of the substrate to reactive intermediates containing a carboxyl, phenol, epoxide, or hydroxyl group. Mixed function mono-oxygenase (MFO), cytochrome C-reductase, various hydrolases, and the cytochrome P450 system are involved in this process. Nonspecific induction of these enzymatic pathways, which commonly occurs with the administration of certain drugs such as anticonvulsants, may alter the metabolism of other drugs and increase the potential for hepatotoxicity. A single agent may be metabolized by more than one biochemical reaction. The reactive intermediates that are potentially damaging to the cell are enzymatically conjugated in *phase 2* reactions with glucuronic acid, sulfate, or glutathione. Some drugs may be directly metabolized by these conjugating reactions without first undergoing *phase 1* activation. Pathways for biotransformation develop early in life with the possible exception of enzymes for oxidizing polycyclic aromatic hydrocarbons and for forming glucuronide conjugates. Mechanisms for the uptake and excretion of organic ions may also be deficient early in life. Some cases of idiosyncratic hepatotoxicity may occur as a result of aberrations in *phase 1* drug metabolism producing intermediates of unusual hepatotoxic potential combined with developmental, acquired, or relative inefficiency of *phase 2* conjugating reactions. Therefore, children may be more or less susceptible than adults to hepatotoxic reactions; for example, liver injury after the use of the anesthetic halothane is rare in children, and acetaminophen toxicity is unusual in infants compared with adolescents, whereas most cases of fatal hepatotoxicity associated with sodium valproate have been reported in children. In some cases, immaturity of hepatic drug metabolic pathways may prevent degradation of a toxic agent; under other circumstances, the same immaturity might limit the formation of toxic metabolites.

Chemical hepatotoxicity may be (1) *predictable* or (2) *idiosyncratic*. *Predictable* hepatotoxicity implies a high incidence of hepatic injury in exposed individuals, with dose-dependency. The agents involved may damage the hepatocyte directly through alteration of membrane lipids (peroxidation) or through denaturation of proteins; such agents include carbon tetrachloride and trichloroethylene. Indirect injury may occur through interference with metabolic pathways essential for cell integrity or through distortion of cellular constituents by covalent binding of a reactive metabolite; examples include the liver injury produced by acetaminophen or by antimetabolites such as methotrexate or 6-mercaptopurine.

Idiosyncratic hepatotoxicity is infrequent and unpredictable. The likelihood of injury is not dose-dependent and may occur at any time during exposure to the agent. An idiosyncratic reaction may be immunologically mediated as a result of prior sensitization (hypersensitivity); extrahepatic manifestations of hypersensitivity may include fever, rash, arthralgia, and eosinophilia. Duration of exposure before reaction is generally 1–4 wk, with prompt recurrence of injury on re-exposure.

Studies indicate that arene oxides, generated through oxidative (cytochrome P450) metabolism of aromatic anticonvulsants (phenytoin, phenobarbital, carbamazepine), may initiate the pathogenesis of hypersensitivity reactions. Arene oxides, formed in vivo, may bind to cellular macromolecules, thus perturbing cell function and possibly initiating immunologic mechanisms of liver injury. Idiosyncratic drug reactions in certain patients may reflect aberrant pathways for drug metabolism, with production of toxic intermediates (isoniazid and sodium valproate may cause liver damage through this mechanism). Duration of drug usage prior to liver injury varies (weeks to 1 yr or more), and the response to re-exposure may be delayed.

The pathologic spectrum of drug-induced liver disease is extremely wide, rarely specific, and may mimic other liver diseases.

Symptoms may be mild and nonspecific, such as fever and malaise; and signs of liver dysfunction may be confused with those of the underlying disorder. The differential diagnosis should include acute and chronic viral hepatitis, biliary tract disease, septicemia, ischemic and hypoxic liver injury, malignant infiltration, and inherited metabolic liver disease.

The laboratory features of drug- or toxin-related liver disease are extremely variable. Hepatocyte damage may lead to elevations of serum aminotransferase activities and serum bilirubin levels and also to impaired synthetic function as evidenced by decreased serum coagulation factors and albumin. Hyperammonemia may occur with liver failure or with selective inhibition of the urea cycle (sodium valproate). Toxicologic screening of blood and urine specimens may aid detection of drug or toxin exposure. Percutaneous liver biopsy may be necessary to distinguish drug injury from complications of an underlying disorder or from intercurrent infection.

Slight elevation of serum aminotransferase activities (generally less than two to three times normal) may occur during therapy with drugs capable of inducing microsomal pathways for drug metabolism. Liver biopsy reveals proliferation of smooth endoplasmic reticulum but no significant liver injury. Liver test abnormalities often resolve with continued drug therapy.

Treatment of drug- or toxin-related liver injury is mainly supportive. Contact with the offending agent should be avoided. Corticosteroids may have a role in immune-mediated disease.

The *prognosis* of drug- or toxin-induced liver injury depends on its type and severity. Injury is usually completely reversible when the hepatotoxic factor is withdrawn. The mortality of submassive hepatic necrosis with fulminant liver failure may, however, exceed 50%. With continued use of certain drugs, such as methotrexate, effects of hepatoxicity may proceed insidiously to cirrhosis. Neoplasia may follow long-term androgen therapy. Rechallenge with a drug suspected of having caused previous liver injury is rarely justified and may result in fatal hepatic necrosis.

13.99 FULMINANT HEPATIC FAILURE

Fulminant hepatic failure is a clinical syndrome resulting from massive necrosis of hepatocytes or from severe functional impairment of hepatocytes in a patient who may or may not have had a pre-existing liver disease. The disorder usually evolves over a period of less than 8 wk. Synthetic, excretory, and detoxifying functions of the liver are all severely impaired, with hepatic encephalopathy an essential diagnostic criterion.

ETIOLOGY. Fulminant hepatic failure is most commonly a complication of viral hepatitis (A, B, C, or D). An unusually high risk of fulminant hepatic failure occurs in young people who have combined infections with the hepatitis B virus and hepatitis D. Epstein-Barr virus, herpes simplex virus, adenovirus, and enterovirus infections may produce fulminant hepatitis in children.

A variety of hepatotoxic drugs and chemicals may also cause fulminant hepatic failure. Predictable liver injury may occur after exposure to carbon tetrachloride, *Amanita phalloides* mushroom, or after acetaminophen overdose. Idiosyncratic damage may follow the use of drugs such as halothane or sodium valproate. Ischemia and hypoxia resulting from hepatic vascular occlusion, congestive heart failure, cyanotic congenital heart disease, or circulatory shock may produce liver failure. Metabolic disorders associated with hepatic failure include Wilson disease, acute fatty liver of pregnancy, galactosemia, hereditary tryosinemia, hereditary fructose intolerance, and neonatal iron storage disease.

PATHOLOGY. Liver biopsy usually reveals massive necrosis of hepatocytes, patchy or confluent. Multilobular or bridging necrosis may be associated with collapse of the reticulin framework of the liver. There may be little or no regeneration of hepatocytes. A zonal pattern of necrosis may be observed with certain insults (e.g., centrilobular damage is associated with acetaminophen hepatotoxicity or with circulatory shock). Evidence of severe hepatocyte dysfunction rather than cell necrosis may occasionally be the predominant histologic finding (e.g., microvesicular fatty infiltrate of hepatocytes is observed in Reye syndrome and in tetracycline toxicity).

PATHOGENESIS. The mechanisms that lead to fulminant hepatic failure are poorly understood. It is unknown why only about 1–2% of patients with viral hepatitis develop liver failure. Massive destruction of hepatocytes may represent both a direct cytotoxic effect of the virus and an immune response to the viral antigens. Formation of hepatotoxic metabolites that bind covalently to macromolecular cell constituents is involved in the liver injury produced by drugs such as acetaminophen and isoniazid; fulminant hepatic failure may follow depletion of intracellular substrates involved in detoxification, particularly glutathione. Whatever the initial cause of hepatocyte injury, a variety of factors may contribute to the pathogenesis of liver failure, including impaired hepatocyte regeneration, altered parenchymal perfusion, endotoxemia, and decreased hepatic reticuloendothelial function.

The pathogenesis of hepatic encephalopathy may relate to increased serum levels of ammonia, false neurotransmitters, amines, increased GABA receptor activity, or increased circulating levels of endogenous benzodiazepine-like compounds. Decreased hepatic clearance of these substances may produce marked central nervous system dysfunction.

CLINICAL MANIFESTATIONS. Fulminant hepatic failure may complicate previously known acute liver disease or be the presenting feature of liver disease. Progressive jaundice, fetor hepaticus, fever, anorexia, vomiting, and abdominal pain are common. A rapid decrease in liver size without clinical improvement is an ominous sign. A hemorrhagic diathesis and ascites may develop. Patients should be closely observed for hepatic encephalopathy, which is initially characterized by minor disturbances of consciousness or motor function. Irritability, poor feeding, and a change in sleep rhythm may be the only findings in infants; asterixis may be demonstrable in older children. The patient may rapidly progress to deeper stages of coma in which extensor responses and decerebrate and decorticate posturing appear. Respirations are usually increased early, but respiratory failure may occur in stage IV coma (Table 13–36).

LABORATORY FINDINGS. Serum direct and indirect bilirubin levels and serum aminotransferase activities may be markedly elevated. However, serum aminotransferase activities do not correlate well with the severity of the illness and

TABLE 13–36. Stages of Hepatic Encephalopathy

	Stages			
	I	*II*	*III*	*IV*
Symptoms	Periods of lethargy, euphoria: reversal of day-night sleeping; may be alert	Drowsiness, inappropriate behavior, agitation, wide mood swings, disorientation	Stupor but arousable, confused, incoherent speech	Coma IVa responds to noxious stimuli IVb no response
Signs	Trouble drawing figures, performing mental tasks	Asterixis, fetor hepaticus, incontinence	Asterixis, hyperreflexia, extensor reflexes, rigidity	Areflexia, no asterixis, flaccidity
EEG	Normal	Generalized slowing, θ waves	Markedly abnormal, triphasic waves	Markedly abnormal bilateral slowing, δ waves, electric-cortical silence

may actually decrease as the patient deteriorates. The blood ammonia concentration is usually increased. Prothrombin time is always prolonged and often does not improve after parenteral administration of vitamin K. Hypoglycemia can occur, particularly in infants. Hypokalemia, hyponatremia, a metabolic acidosis, or respiratory alkalosis may develop.

TREATMENT. Management of fulminant hepatic failure is supportive. No therapy is known to reverse hepatocyte injury or to promote hepatic regeneration.

The infant or child with advanced hepatic coma should be treated in an intensive care unit where continuous monitoring of vital functions is possible. Endotracheal intubation may be required to prevent aspiration, to reduce cerebral edema by hyperventilation, and facilitate pulmonary toilet. Mechanical ventilation and supplemental oxygen are often necessary in advanced coma. Electrolyte and glucose solutions should be administered intravenously to maintain urine output, to correct or prevent hypoglycemia, and to maintain normal serum potassium concentrations. Hyponatremia is common but is usually dilutional and not a result of sodium depletion. Parenteral supplementation with calcium, phosphorus, and magnesium may be required. Coagulopathy should be treated with parenteral administration of vitamin K and may require fresh frozen plasma; disseminated intravascular coagulation may also occur. Plasmapheresis may permit temporary correction of the bleeding diathesis without resulting in volume overload. Prophylactic use of antacids or H_2 receptor blockers or both should be considered because of the high risk of gastrointestinal bleeding. Hypovolemia should be avoided and treated with cautious infusions of fluids and blood products. Renal dysfunction may occur from dehydration, from acute tubular necrosis, or from functional renal failure (hepatorenal syndrome). The patient should be followed closely for infection, including sepsis, pneumonia, peritonitis, and urinary tract infections. Cerebral edema is an extremely serious complication that responds poorly to measures such as corticosteroid administration and osmotic diuresis.

Gastrointestinal hemorrhage, infection, constipation, sedatives, electrolyte imbalance, and hypovolemia may precipitate encephalopathy and should be identified and corrected. Protein intake should be restricted or eliminated. The gut should be purged with several enemas. Lactulose should be given every 2–4 hr orally or by nasogastric tube in doses (10–50 mL) sufficient to cause diarrhea. The dose is then adjusted to produce several acidic, loose bowel movements daily. Lactulose syrup diluted with 1–3 volumes of water may also be given as a retention enema every 6 hr. Lactulose, a nonabsorbable disaccharide, is metabolized to organic acids by colonic bacteria; it probably lowers blood ammonia levels through decreasing microbial ammonia production and through trapping of ammonia in acidic intestinal contents. Flumazenil, a benzodiazepine antagonist, may reverse early hepatic encephalopathy.

Controlled trials have shown a worsened outcome of fulminant hepatic failure in patients treated with corticosteroids. Orthotopic liver transplantation may be life-saving in patients who reach advanced stages of hepatic coma.

PROGNOSIS. Children with hepatic failure may do somewhat better than adults, but overall mortality exceeds 70%. The prognosis may vary considerably with the etiology of liver failure and stage of hepatic encephalopathy. With intensive medical support survival rates of 50–60% occur with hepatic failure complicating acetaminophen overdose and with fulminant hepatitis A or B virus infection. In contrast, recovery can be expected in only 10–20% of patients with liver failure caused by hepatitis C virus or an acute onset of Wilson disease. In patients who progress to stage IV coma (see Table 13–36) the prognosis is extremely poor. Major complications such as sepsis, severe hemorrhage, or renal failure increase the mortality. Studies indicate that jaundice for more than 7 days before the onset of encephalopathy, a prothrombin time more than 50 sec, and a serum bilirubin more than 17.5 mg/dL (300 μmol/L) indicate a poor prognosis irrespective of the initial stage of hepatic coma. Survival of 50–75% is being achieved in patients with the poorest prognosis following orthotopic liver transplantation. Patients who recover from fulminant hepatic failure with only supportive care do not usually develop cirrhosis or chronic liver disease.

13.100 CYSTIC DISEASES OF THE BILIARY TRACT AND LIVER

Cystic lesions of liver parenchyma or of the biliary system may be recognized initially during infancy and childhood. Their classification is not yet satisfactory. Pathologic features may be found in common among several of these disorders, but different patterns of inheritance indicate that their etiology is heterogeneous.

CHOLEDOCHAL CYSTS. These are congenital dilatations of the common bile duct that may cause progressive biliary obstruction and biliary cirrhosis. Cylindrical and spherical cysts of the extrahepatic ducts are the most common types. Segmental or diffuse dilatation can be observed. A diverticulum of the common bile duct or dilatation of the intraduodenal portion of the common duct (choledochocele) are variants. Cystic dilatation of the intrahepatic bile ducts may be associated with a choledochal cyst.

The pathogenesis of choledochal cysts remains uncertain. Some reports have suggested that junction of the common bile duct and the pancreatic duct before their entry into the sphincter of Oddi may allow reflux of pancreatic enzymes into the common bile duct, causing inflammation, localized weakness, and dilatation of the duct. Other possibilities are that choledochal cysts represent malformations of the common duct or occur as part of the disease spectrum that includes neonatal hepatitis and biliary atresia.

Approximately 75% of cases appear during childhood. The infant typically presents with cholestatic jaundice; severe liver dysfunction including ascites and coagulopathy can rapidly evolve if biliary obstruction is not relieved. An abdominal mass is rarely palpable. In the older child, the classic triad of abdominal pain, jaundice, and mass occurs in less than 33% of patients. Features of acute cholangitis (fever, right upper quadrant tenderness, jaundice, leukocytosis) may be present. The diagnosis is made by ultrasound; choledochal cysts have been identified prenatally using this technique.

The treatment of choice is primary excision of the cyst and a Roux-en-Y choledochojejunostomy. Simple drainage into the small bowel is less satisfactory owing to a risk for development of carcinoma in the residual cystic tissue. The postoperative course may be complicated by recurrent cholangitis or stricture at the anastomotic site.

CYSTIC DILATATION OF THE INTRAHEPATIC BILE DUCTS (CAROLI DISEASE). Congenital, saccular dilatation may affect multiple segments of the intrahepatic bile ducts; the dilated ducts are lined by cuboidal epithelium and are in continuity with the main duct system, which is usually normal. There is a marked predisposition to ascending cholangitis and calculus formation within the abnormal bile ducts. Choledochal cysts, features of congenital hepatic fibrosis, and renal tubular ectasia may be associated. The disorder is not thought to be familial.

Affected patients usually develop symptoms of acute cholangitis as children or young adults. Fever, abdominal pain, mild jaundice, and pruritus occur; and a slightly enlarged, tender liver is palpable. Elevated alkaline phosphatase activity, direct-reacting bilirubin levels, and leukocytosis may be observed during episodes of acute infection. Ultrasonography shows the dilated intrahepatic ducts, but definitive diagnosis and extent of disease must be determined by percutaneous transhepatic or endoscopic cholangiography.

Cholangitis and sepsis are treated with appropriate antibiotics. Calculi may require surgery. Partial hepatectomy may be curative in rare cases, when disease is confined to a single lobe. The prognosis is otherwise guarded, largely owing to difficulties in controlling cholangitis and biliary lithiasis and to a significant risk for developing cholangiocarcinoma.

CONGENITAL HEPATIC FIBROSIS. This is an autosomal-recessive disorder characterized pathologically by diffuse periportal and perilobular fibrosis in broad bands that contain distorted bile duct–like structures and that often compress or incorporate central or sublobular veins. The duct-like structures may become dilated to the point of microcyst formation but do not communicate with the biliary tract. Irregularly shaped islands of liver parenchyma contain normal-appearing hepatocytes. Caroli disease and choledochal cysts have been associated (see earlier). About 75% of patients have renal disease, such as renal tubular ectasia, nephronophthisis, or childhood polycystic disease.

The disorder usually has its clinical onset in childhood, with hepatosplenomegaly or with bleeding secondary to portal hypertension. Cholangitis may occur in patients who have associated abnormalities of bile ducts.

Hepatocellular function is well preserved. Serum aminotransferase activities and bilirubin levels are usually normal; serum alkaline phosphatase activity may be slightly elevated. The serum albumin level and prothrombin time are normal. Liver biopsy is usually required for diagnosis.

Treatment of this disorder should focus on control of bleeding from esophageal varices. Infrequent mild bleeding episodes may be managed by endoscopic sclerotherapy of the varices. Following more severe hemorrhage, portacaval anastomosis may bring relief of portal hypertension. The prognosis may be greatly improved by a shunting procedure, but survival in some patients may be limited by renal failure.

A **solitary liver cyst** (nonparasitic) rarely occurs in childhood. Abdominal distention and pain may be present, and a poorly defined right upper quadrant mass may be palpable. These benign lesions are best left undisturbed unless they compress adjacent structures or a complication occurs, such as hemorrhage into the cyst.

ADULT-TYPE POLYCYSTIC DISEASE. This disease is associated with multiple cysts of the liver, kidney, and less commonly of other organs. This disorder is autosomal dominant, with a high degree of penetrance. The cysts probably arise from defective development of intrahepatic bile ducts but do not communicate with the biliary tree. The liver may be normal-sized or markedly enlarged. Most of the affected children are asymptomatic; the prognosis is determined by the severity of the cystic renal disease. Portal hypertension and obstructive jaundice are rarely produced by large cysts.

CHILDHOOD POLYCYSTIC DISEASE OF THE KIDNEYS AND LIVER. This disease is inherited as an autosomal recessive trait. Death from renal failure is common within the first weeks or months of life in infants whose kidneys are massively enlarged with cysts. The liver lesion in these patients consists of a striking increase in the number of bile ducts, which are irregularly dilated in all portal areas; mild to moderate portal fibrosis is present.

Portal hypertension may arise in infants who survive the 1st yr. In older children, dilatation of bile ducts is less prominent, but the portal fibrosis is much more severe. The hepatic lesion at this stage may be indistinguishable from that of a congenital hepatic lesion.

Variable abnormalities of bile ducts (irregular dilatation, proliferation, cysts) and portal fibrosis may be associated with Meckel syndrome, 17–18 trisomy, tuberous sclerosis, and asphyxiating thoracic dystrophy.

13.101 DISEASES OF THE GALLBLADDER

ANOMALIES. The gallbladder is congenitally absent in about 0.1% of the population. Hypoplasia or absence of the gallbladder may be associated with extrahepatic biliary atresia or cystic fibrosis. Duplication of the gallbladder occurs rarely.

ACUTE HYDROPS. Acute noncalculous, noninflammatory distention of the gallbladder may occur in infants and children. The disorder may complicate acute infections including scarlet fever, leptospirosis, sepsis, and Kawasaki disease, but the cause is often not identified. Hydrops of the gallbladder may also develop in patients receiving long-term parenteral nutrition, presumably as a result of gallbladder stasis during the period of enteral fasting.

Affected patients usually have right upper quadrant pain with a palpable mass. Fever and jaundice may be present. Ultrasound may help in establishing the diagnosis. Acute hydrops is usually treated conservatively and rarely needs cholecystostomy and drainage. At laparotomy, a large, edematous gallbladder is found that contains white, yellow, or green bile. Obstruction of the cystic duct by mesenteric adenopathy is occasionally observed. Cholecystectomy is required if the gallbladder is gangrenous. Pathologic examination of the gallbladder wall shows edema and mild inflammation. Cultures of bile are usually sterile.

CHOLECYSTITIS AND CHOLELITHIASIS. *Acute acalculous cholecystitis* is uncommon in children and is usually caused by infection. Reported pathogens include streptococci (groups A and B) and gram-negative organisms, particularly *Salmonella*. Parasitic infestation with ascaris or *Giardia lamblia* may be found. Acalculous cholecystitis may rarely follow abdominal trauma or be associated with a systemic vasculitis, such as periarteritis nodosa. It has been reported in association with Kawasaki disease.

Clinical features include right upper quadrant or epigastric pain, nausea, vomiting, fever, and jaundice. Right upper quadrant guarding and tenderness are present. Ultrasound discloses an enlarged, thick-walled gallbladder, without calculi. Serum alkaline phosphatase activity and direct-reacting bilirubin levels are elevated. Leukocytosis is usual.

The diagnosis is confirmed at laparotomy. Cholecystectomy and treatment of the systemic infection are required.

Cholelithiasis is relatively rare in otherwise healthy children, occurring more commonly in patients with a variety of predisposing disorders. Gallstones, composed of a mixture of cholesterol, bile pigment, calcium, and inorganic matrix are the most common type. Stones of pure cholesterol or bile pigment may also occur.

The most important clinical feature is recurrent abdominal pain, which is often colicky and localized to the right upper quadrant. The older child may have intolerance for fatty foods. Acute cholecystitis may be the first manifestation, with fever, pain in the right upper quadrant, and often a palpable mass. Pain may radiate to an area just below the right scapula. A plain roentgenogram of the abdomen may reveal opaque calculi, but radiolucent (cholesterol) stones will not be visualized. Accordingly, ultrasound is the method of choice for gallstone detection. Cholecystectomy is usually curative; operative cholangiography should be done at the time of surgery to exclude common duct calculi. Dissolution of stones with oral chenodeoxycholic acid or extracorporeal lithotripsy are potential alternatives to surgery. Experience in children is limited with these nonoperative therapies.

Patients with hemolytic disease (including sickle cell anemia, the thalassemias, and red blood cell enzymopathies) and Wilson disease are at increased risk for pigmented cholelithiasis. Increasing numbers of sick premature infants are being found to have gallstones; their management is often complicated by such factors as bowel resection, necrotizing enterocolitis, prolonged parenteral nutrition without enteral feeding, cholestasis, frequent blood transfusions, and use of diuretics. Cholelithiasis in premature infants is often asymptomatic and resolves spontaneously.

Cholesterol cholelithiasis in children most frequently affects obese adolescent girls. Cholesterol gallstones are found also in children with disturbances of the enterohepatic circulation of bile acids, including patients with ileal disease and bile acid malabsorption, such as those with ileal resection, ileal Crohn disease, and cystic fibrosis. Chronic cholestasis increases the risk for cholesterol gallstones.

Cholesterol gallstone formation seems to result from an excess of cholesterol in relation to the cholesterol-carrying capacity of micelles in bile. Supersaturation of bile with cholesterol leading to crystal and stone formation could result from decreased bile acid or from an increased cholesterol concentration in bile. Other initiating factors that may be important in stone formation include gallbladder stasis, or the presence in bile of abnormal mucoproteins or bile pigments that may serve as a nidus for cholesterol crystallization.

FREDERICK J. SUCHY

DEVELOPMENT OF HEPATIC STRUCTURE AND FUNCTION

Structural Morphogenesis

Andres JM, Mathis RK, Walker WA: Liver disease in infants. Parts I and II: Developmental hepatology and mechanisms of liver dysfunction. J Pediatr 90:686 and 964, 1977.

Hutchins GM, Moore GW: Growth and asymmetry of the human liver during the embryonic period. Pediatr Pathol 8:17, 1988.

Ultrastructure of the Hepatocyte

Jones AL, Schmucker DL, Renston RH, et al: The architecture of bile secretion: A morphological perspective of physiology. Dig Dis Sci 25:609, 1980.

Functional Development

Henning SJ: Postnatal development: Coordination of feeding, digestion, and metabolism. Am J Physiol 241:G199, 1981.

Soyka LF, Redmond GP (eds): Drug Metabolism in the Immature Human. New York, Raven Press, 1981.

Hepatic Excretory Function

Balistreri WF, Heubi JE, Suchy FJ: Immaturity of the enterohepatic circulation in early life: Factors predisposing to "physiologic" maldigestion and cholestasis. J Pediatr Gastroenterol Nutr 2:346, 1983.

Oelberg DG, Lester R: Cellular mechanisms of cholestasis. Ann Rev Med 37:297, 1986.

Suchy FJ, Bucuvalas JC, Novak DA: Determinant of bile formation during development: Ontogeny of hepatic bile acid metabolism and transport. Semin Liver Dis 7:77, 1987.

Manifestations of Liver Disease

Alvarez F, Bernard O, Brunelle F, et al: Portal obstruction in children. I: Clinical investigation and hemorrhage risk: Portal obstruction in children. II: Results of surgical portosystemic shunts. J Pediatr 103:696 and 703, 1983.

Anonymous: Mechanisms and management of pediatric hepatobiliary disease. J Pediatr Gastroenterol Nutr 10:138, 1990.

Balistreri WF: The effects of liver disease on nutrition and growth. *In*: Cohen SA (ed): The Underweight Child. Norwalk CT, Appleton-Century-Crofts, 1986, pp 121–130.

Fonkalsrud EW: Shunt operations for portal hypertension in children. J Pediatr 103:741, 1983.

Ishak KF, Glunz PR: Hepatoblastoma and hepatocarcinoma in infancy and childhood: Report of 47 cases. Cancer 20:396, 1967.

Jones EA: The γ-aminobutyric acid A (GABA) receptor complex and hepatic encephalopathy. Ann Intern Med 110:532, 1989.

Oldham KT, Guice KS, Kaufman RA, et al: Blunt hepatic injury and elevated hepatic enzymes: A clinical correlation in children. J Pediatr Surg 19:457, 1984.

Reiff MI, Osborn LM: Clinical estimation of liver size in newborn infants. Pediatrics 71:46, 1983.

Stocker JH: Hepatic tumors. *In*: Balistreri WF, Stocker JT (eds): Pediatric Hepatology. Washington, Hemisphere Publishing Corp, 1989.

Evaluation of the Patient with Possible Liver Dysfunction

Laker MF: Liver function tests. Br Med J 301:250, 1990.

Riddlesberger MM Jr: Diagnostic imaging of the hepatobiliary system in infants and children. J Pediatr Gastroenterol Nutr 3:653, 1984.

Rosenthal P, Henton D, Felber S, et al: Distribution of serum bilirubin conjugates in pediatric hepatobiliary disease. J Pediatr 110:201, 1987.

Sokol RJ: Medical management of infant or child with chronic liver disease. Semin Liver Dis 7:155, 1987.

Spivak W, Sarkar S, Winter D, et al: Diagnostic utility of hepatobiliary scintigraphy with DISIDA in neonatal cholestasis. J Pediatr 110:855, 1987.

SPECIFIC DISEASES OF THE LIVER

Neonatal Cholestasis

Alagille D, et al: Syndromic paucity of interlobular bile ducts (Alagille syndrome or arteriohepatic dysplasia): Review of 80 cases. J Pediatr 110:195, 1987.

Alagille D, Odievre M, Gautier M, et al: Hepatic ductular hypoplasia associated with characteristic facies, vertebral malformation, retarded physical, mental and sexual development and cardiac murmur. J Pediatr 86:63, 1975.

Balistreri WF: Neonatal cholestasis. J Pediatr 106:171, 1985.

Danks DM, Campbell PE, Smith AL, et al: Prognosis of babies with neonatal hepatitis. Arch Dis Child 52:368, 1977.

Howard ER, Stamatakis JD, Mowat AP: Management of esophageal varices in children by injection sclerotherapy. Pediatr Surg 19:2, 1984.

Kasai M: Treatment of biliary atresia with special reference to hepatic portoenterostomy and its modifications. Progr Pediatr Surg 6:5, 1974.

Kaufman S, Murray N, Wood R, et al: Nutritional support for the infant with extrahepatic biliary atresia. J Pediatr 110:679, 1987.

Lally KP, Kanegaye J, Matsumura M, et al: Perioperative factors affecting the outcome following repair of biliary atresia. Pediatrics 83:723, 1989.

Landing BH: Consideration of the pathogenesis of neonatal hepatitis, biliary atresia, and choledochal cyst: The concept of infantile obstructive cholangiopathy. Progr Pediatr Surg 6:113, 1974.

Mieli-Vergani G, Howard ER, Portman B, et al: Late referral for biliary atresia: Missed opportunities for effective surgery. Lancet 1:421, 1989.

Mowat AP, Psacharopoulos HT, Williams R: Extrahepatic biliary atresia versus neonatal hepatitis: Review of 137 prospectively investigated infants. Arch Dis Child 51:763, 1976.

Riely CA: Familial intrahepatic cholestatic syndromes. Semin Liver Dis 7:119, 1987.

Rosenblum JL, Keating JP, Prensky AL, et al: A progressive neurologic syndrome in children with chronic liver disease. N Engl J Med 304:503, 1981.

Ryckman FC, Noseworthy J: Neonatal cholestatic conditions requiring surgical reconstruction. Semin Liver Dis 7:134, 1987.
Schweizer P: Treatment of extrahepatic bile duct atresia. Pediatr Surg Int 1:30, 1986.
Sokol RJ, Heubi JE, N Butler-Simon, et al: Treatment of vitamin E deficiency during chronic childhood cholestasis with oral D-tocopheryl polyethylene glycol-1000 succinate. Gastroenterology 93:975, 1987.
Whitington PF, Whitington GL: Partial external diversion of bile for the treatment of intractable pruritus associated with intrahepatic cholestasis. Gastroenterology 95:130, 1988.

Transplantation

Emond JC, Whitington PF, Thistlethwaite JR, et al: Reduced-size orthotopic liver transplantation: Use in the management of children with chronic liver disease. Hepatology 10:867, 1989.
Esquivel CO, Koneru B, Karrer F, et al: Liver transplantation before 1 year of age. J Pediatr 110:545, 1987.
Shaw BW Jr, Wood RP, Kaufman SS, et al: Liver transplantation therapy for children: Parts 1 and 2. Pediatr Gastroenterol Nutr 7:156 and 797, 1988.
Starzl TE, Demetris AJ, Van Thiel D: Liver transplantation. N Engl J Med 321:1014 and 1092, 1989.

Metabolic Diseases of the Liver

Colletti RB, Clemmons JJW: Familial neonatal hemochromatosis with survival. J Pediatr Gastroenterol Nutr 7:39, 1988.
Crystal RG: α_1-Antitrypsin deficiency, emphysema, and liver disease: Genetic basis and strategies for therapy. J Clin Invest 85:1343, 1990.
Czaja MJ, Weiner FR, Schwarzenberg SJ, et al: Molecular studies of ceruloplasmin deficiency in Wilson's disease. J Clin Invest 80:1200, 1987.
Dubois RS, Rodgerson DO, Hambidge KM: Treatment of Wilson's disease with triethylene tetramine hydrochloride (trientine). J Pediatr Gastroenterol Nutr 10:77, 1990.
Hubbard RC, Brantly ML, Sellers SE, et al: Anti-neutrophil-elastase defenses of the lower respiratory tract in alpha-1 antitrypsin deficiency directly augmented with an aerosol of alpha-1 antitrypsin. Ann Intern Med 111:206, 1989.
Lefkowitch JH, Honig CL, King ME, et al: Hepatic copper overload and features of Indian childhood cirrhosis in an American sibship. N Engl J Med 307:271, 1982.
Knisely AS, O'Shea PA, Stocks JF, et al: Oropharyngeal and upper respiratory tract mucosal gland siderosis in neonatal hemochromatosis: An approach to biopsy diagnosis. J Pediatr 113:871, 1988.
McCullough AJ, Fleming CR, Thistle JL, et al: Diagnosis of Wilson's disease presenting as fulminant hepatic failure. Gastroenterology 84:161, 1983.
Sarles J, Scheiner C, Sarran M, et al: Hepatic hypervitaminosis A: A familial observation. J Pediatr Gastroenterol Nutr 10:71, 1990.
Schwarzenberg SJ, Sharp HL: Pathogenesis of α_1-antitrypsin deficiency-associated liver disease, 1990. J Pediatr Gastroenterol Nutr 10:5, 1990.
Setchell DR, Street JM: Inborn errors of bile acid synthesis. Semin Liver Dis 7:85, 1987.
Setchell KDR, Suchy FJ, Welsh MB, et al: 3-Oxosteroid 5β-reductase deficiency described in identical twins with neonatal hepatitis—a new inborn error in bile acid synthesis. J Clin Invest 82:2148, 1988.
Sveger T: Liver diseases in alpha-1 antitrypsin deficiency detected by screening of 200,000 infants. N Engl J Med 294:1316, 1976.
Walshe JM: Wilson's disease presenting with features of hepatic dysfunction—A clinical analysis of 87 patients. 70:253, 1989.

Infectious Disorders of the Liver

Alter MJ: Non-A, non-B hepatitis: Sorting through a diagnosis of exclusion. Ann Intern Med 110:583, 1989.
Alter MJ, Sampliner RE: Hepatitis C: And miles to go before we sleep. N Engl J Med 321:1538, 1989.
Balistreri WF: Viral hepatitis: Pediatr Clin North Am 35:637, 1988.
Davis GL, Balart LA, Schiff ER, et al: Treatment of chronic hepatitis C with recombinant interferon-alpha: A multicenter randomized, controlled trial. N Engl J Med 321:1501, 1989.
Esteban JI, Gonzalez A, Hernandez JM, et al: Evaluation of antibodies to hepatitis C virus in a study of transfusion-associated hepatitis. N Engl J Med 323:1107, 1990.
Garson JA, Tedder RS, Briggs M, et al: Detection of hepatitis C viral sequences in blood donations by "nested" polymerase chain reaction and prediction of infectivity. Lancet 335:1419, 1990.
Gitlin N, Visveshwara, Kassel SH, et al: Fulminant neonatal hepatic necrosis associated with echovirus type II infection. West J Med 138:260, 1983.
Perrillo RP, Schiff ER, Davis GL, et al: A randomized, controlled trial of interferon alpha-2b alone and after prednisone withdrawal for the treatment of chronic hepatitis B. N Engl J Med 323:295, 1990.
Pineiro-Carrero VM, Andres JM: Morbidity and mortality in children with pyogenic liver abscess. Am J Dis Child 143:1424, 1989.
Schalm SW, Mazel JA, Degast GC, et al: Prevention of hepatitis B infection in newborns through mass screening and delayed vaccination of all infants of mothers with hepatitis-B surface antigen. Pediatrics 83:1041, 1989.
Zuckerman AJ: Hepatitis E virus: The main cause of enterically transmitted non-A, non-B hepatitis. Br Med J 300:1475, 1990.
Zuckerman AJ: The elusive hepatitis C virus: A cause of parenteral non-A, non-B hepatitis. Br Med J 299:871, 1989.

Liver Disease Associated with Systemic Disorders

Amedee-Manesme O, Bernard O, Brunelle F, et al: Sclerosing cholangitis with neonatal onset. J Pediatr 111:225, 1987.
Bernstein J, Chang C-H, Brough AJ, et al: Conjugated hyperbilirubinemia in infancy associated with parenteral alimentation. J Pediatr 90:361, 1977.
Buchanan GR, Glader BE: Benign course of extreme hyperbilirubinemia in sickle cell anemia: Analysis of six cases. J Pediatr 91:21, 1977.
Cohen JA, Kaplan MM: Left sided heart failure presenting as hepatitis. Gastroenterology 74:583, 1978.
Klion FM, Weiner JJ, Schaffner F: Cholestasis in sickle cell anemia. Am J Med 37:829, 1964.
Sisto A, Feldman P, Garel L, et al: Primary sclerosing cholangitis in children: Study of five cases and review of the literature. Pediatrics 80:918, 1987.
Weinberg AG, Bolande RP: The liver in congenital heart disease. Am J Dis Child 119:390, 1970.
Zitelli BJ, et al: Systemic disorders. *In*: Balistreri WF, Stocker JT (eds): Pediatric Hepatology. Washington, Hemisphere Publishing Corp, 1989.

Veno-Occlusive Disease/Graft-Versus-Host Disease

McDonald GB, Sharma P, Matthews DE, et al: Veno-occlusive disease of the liver after bone marrow transplantation: Diagnosis, incidence, and predisposing factors. Hepatology 4:116, 1984.
Sale GE, Shulman HM: Liver disease after marrow transplantation. *In*: Sale GE, Shulman HM (eds): The Pathology of Bone Marrow Transplantation. Chicago, Year Book Medical Publishers, 1984.
Snover DC, Weisdorf SA, Ramsay NK, et al: Hepatic graft-versus-host disease: A study of the predictive value of liver biopsy in diagnosis. Hepatology 4:123, 1984.

Reye Syndrome

Forsyth BW, Horwitz RI, Acampora D, et al: New epidemiologic evidence confirming that bias does not explain the aspirin/Reye's syndrome association. JAMA 261:2517, 1989.
Green CL, Blitzer MG, Shapira E: Inborn errors of metabolism and Reye syndrome: Differential diagnosis. J Pediatr 113:156, 1988.
Lichtenstein PK, Heubi JE, Daugherty CC, et al: Grade 1 Reye's syndrome: A frequent cause of vomiting and liver dysfunction after varicella and upper-respiratory-tract infection. N Engl J Med 309:133, 1983.
Pinsky PF, Hurwitz ES, Schonberger LB, et al: Reye's syndrome and aspirin: Evidence for a dose response effect. JAMA 260:657, 1988.
Rowe PC, Valle D, Brusilow SW: Inborn errors of metabolism in children referred with Reye's syndrome: A changing pattern. JAMA 260:3167, 1988.
Shaywitz BA, Rothstein P, Venes JL: Monitoring and management of increased intracranial pressure in Reye syndrome: Results in 29 children. Pediatrics 66:198, 1980.
Stanley CA: New genetic defects in mitochondrial fatty acid oxidation and carnitine deficiency. Adv Pediatr 34:59, 1987.

Drug-Induced Liver Disease

Kaplowitz N, Aw TY, Simon FR, et al: Drug induced hepatotoxicity. Ann Intern Med 104:826, 1986.
Shear NH, Spielberg SP: Anticonvulsant hypersensitivity syndrome: In vitro assessment of risk. J Clin Invest 82:1826, 1988.
Zimmerman HJ (ed): Drug induced liver disease. Semin Liver Dis 1:89, 1981.

Chronic Hepatitis

Brook MG, Petrovic L, McDonald JA, et al: Histologic improvement after antiviral treatment of chronic hepatitis B virus infection. J Hepatol 8:218, 1989.
Homberg J-C, Abuaf N, Bernard O, et al: Chronic active hepatitis associated with antiliver/kidney microsome antibody type 1: A second type of "autoimmune" hepatitis. Hepatology 7:1333, 1987.
Perrillo RR, Regenstein FG, Peters MG, et al: Prednisone withdrawal followed by recombinant alpha interferon in the treatment of chronic type B hepatitis: A randomized controlled trial. Ann Intern Med 109:95, 1988.
Sherlock S: Classifying chronic hepatitis. Lancet ii:1168, 1988.

Fulminant Hepatic Failure

Anonymous: Diuretics or paracentesis for ascites? Lancet ii:725, 1988.
Cade R, Wagemaker H, Vogel S, et al: Hepatorenal syndrome: Studies of the effect of vascular volume and intraperitoneal pressure on renal and hepatic function. Am J Med 82:427, 1987.
Grim G, Katzenschlager R, Schneeweiss B, et al: Improvement of hepatic encephalopathy treated with flumazenil. Lancet ii:1392, 1988.
Mullen KD, Szauter KM, Kaminsky-Russ K: "Endogenous" benzodiazepine

activity in body fluids of patients with hepatic encephalopathy. Lancet 336:81, 1990.
O'Grady JG, Alexander GJM, Hayllar KN, et al: Early indications of prognosis in fulminant hepatic failure. Gastroenterology 97:439, 1989.
Russell GJ, Fitzgerald JF, Clark JH: Fulminant hepatic failure. J Pediatr 111:313, 1987.
Stanley MM, Ochi S, Lee KK, et al: Peritoneovenous shunting as compared with medical treatment in patients with alcoholic cirrhosis and massive ascites. N Engl J Med 321:1632, 1989.

Anatomic/Cystic Malformations

Sherman P, Kolster E, Davies C, et al: Choledochal cysts: Heterogeneity of clinical presentation. J Pediatr Gastroenterol Nutr 5:867, 1986.
Summerfield JA, Nagafuchi Y, Sherlock S, et al: Hepatobiliary fibropolycystic disease: A clinical and histological review of 51 patients. J Hepatol 2:141, 1986.

13.102 PORTAL HYPERTENSION AND VARICES

ETIOLOGY. Extrahepatic portal venous obstruction causes 50–70% of portal hypertension in children, but in about two thirds of cases no specific cause can be found. In many patients it develops gradually after birth; umbilical vein catheterization and infusion are associated in about one third of such cases. Lymphatic spread of infection (omphalitis) from the umbilicus to the ductus venosus may cause portal vein thrombosis. Sludging of venous flow at the time of normal closure of the umbilical vein and ductus venosus is another suggested mechanism. In older children, abdominal trauma, pancreatitis, and tumors or inflammatory masses adjacent to the portal vein have occasionally led to portal hypertension. In Gaucher disease, arteriovenous fistulas may develop in the spleen, resulting in portal hypertension. Rarely in children, hepatic vein thrombosis (Budd-Chiari syndrome) causes raised portal venous pressure. Portal vein thrombosis may occur following splenectomy, especially for massive spleens usually associated with hematologic disorders.

Cirrhosis may also cause portal hypertension; the intrahepatic scarring and collapse distort hepatic vasculature and raise vascular resistance (Sec. 13.82). Some survivors of surgically corrected biliary atresia and all nonoperated cases develop portal hypertension. Many of the remaining known causes of childhood cirrhosis are insidious in onset and often do not progress to portal hypertension until relatively late in childhood. Examples of these conditions are α_1-antitrypsin deficiency, Wilson disease, cystic fibrosis, trypsinemia, and chronic active hepatitis (Table 13–35). Congenital hepatic fibrosis may also lead to portal hypertension. The portal pressure may also rise following right hepatic lobectomy as the entire portal flow encounters greater resistance from the reduced vascular bed.

PATHOLOGY. The liver is normal in patients with extrahepatic portal obstruction. Some portal blood does reach the liver through collateral channels in the suspensory ligaments, the diaphragmatic veins, and hepatorenal and hepatocolic veins. With intrahepatic obstruction there is no portal flow to the liver other than via the partially obstructed portal vein. A cavernomatous transformation of the portal vein is encountered in some children, with the normal vein being replaced by a number of thin-walled tortuous veins. Whether this is the result or the cause of the portal obstruction is unknown, but the portal venous pressure exceeds the pressure within the inferior vena cava by at least 150 cm of saline. Portosystemic shunts develop and lead to dilatation and varicosities in otherwise unimportant veins. Such anastomoses are found in the region of the esophagogastric junction, the retroperitoneal veins, the internal hemorrhoidal plexus in the distal rectum, and around the ligamentum teres at the umbilicus. The varicosities in the lower esophagus and cardia of the stomach are especially susceptible to erosion with consequent massive hemorrhage. Hypersplenism may complicate the picture in any patient with portal obstruction.

CLINICAL MANIFESTATIONS. Massive hematemesis is usually the initial symptom of portal hypertension in children. The blood passed per rectum varies from bright red with severe bleeding to melena. The underlying disease determines the age at which symptoms begin; younger infants tend to present with ascites first rather than hematemesis. There may be jaundice if the obstruction is hepatic. A cluster of diverging, dilated veins with centrifugal flow from the umbilicus (the caput medusae) may develop. Internal anal hemorrhoids are uncommon in children.

DIAGNOSIS. Roentgenographic demonstration of varicosities in the esophagus is relatively noninvasive and usually accurate; a barium paste is used that adheres to the esophageal mucous membrane. In children, peptic ulcer disease rarely coexists with portal hypertension. The varicosities have an unmistakable appearance when visualized directly by fiberoptic gastroesophagoscopy. Liver function should be evaluated. The portal vein is readily demonstrable by ultrasound. Splenoportography allows the measurement of splenic pulp and portal pressures and indicates the flow within the splenic and portal veins. Selective angiography allows assessment of the size of the superior mesenteric vein. If the bleeding is not from varices, this investigation may demonstrate sites of hemorrhage not associated with portal hypertension (e.g., traumatic hemobilia). It may also be useful therapeutically as a means of introducing vasopressor substances selectively into the portal system.

TREATMENT. Hematemesis from esophageal varices in children usually stops spontaneously without measures other than blood transfusion. A nasogastric tube should be inserted as a guide to the amount and rate of hemorrhage and is *not* contraindicated by a risk of precipitating or aggravating hemorrhage from varices. In many patients the bleeding is from varices at the cardia of the stomach and not from the esophagus. A central venous pressure measurement may be helpful in assessing the rate of blood volume replacement required. Vital functions must be measured frequently, including pH, arterial oxygen saturation, and electrolytes. Coagulation disorders should be corrected with vitamin K, fresh frozen plasma, or platelet transfusion. Incipient hepatic failure from cirrhosis made worse by hemorrhage is rarely seen in children. Patients who have cirrhosis will require terminal care unless hepatic transplantation is anticipated. Intravenous and local administration of vasopressin may be of use by causing splanchnic vasoconstriction with diminished blood flow to the bleeding varices. The dose is 0.3 U/kg body weight (up to 20 U) as a bolus diluted in 2 mL/kg of 5% dextrose for 10–20 min. This dose can be repeated at hourly intervals or given via continuous infusion (0.2–0.4 U/1.73 m^2 min) for 12–24 hr. Cooling the stomach is probably of no value. If bleeding persists, the passage of the triple lumen Sengstaken-Blakemore tube to produce balloon tamponade may be required. In many cases successful venous compression can be obtained without inflating the esophageal balloon, or only the distal gastric balloon needs to be inflated and with traction on the tube, bleeding is controlled; bleeding often recurs on deflation of the balloon(s). Massive pulmonary aspiration, suffocation, damage to the esophageal mucosa, and esophageal rupture are complications of this modality.

It is rarely necessary to operate upon pediatric patients with portal hypertension as an emergency to stop bleeding. Two types of procedures are currently used: those that attack the varices directly and those that divert portal blood to the systemic circulation (Sec. 13.82). Sclerotherapy is the initial treatment of choice. Inderal may reduce the risk of rebleeding once the patient has stabilized.

Repeated sclerotherapy of the bleeding varix may be successful but usually serves only as a temporizing procedure, and a more definitive operation may be required. There are many methods of diverting portal blood flow to the systemic circulation. Splenorenal shunts offer excellent means of controlling portal hypertension in children. Siguira has reported good results from a thoracoabdominal operation in which as many as 80 varicose veins or their tributaries are ligated within the thorax; the esophagus is transected and then anastomosed to interrupt intramural varicosities; within the abdomen, veins related to the upper stomach are all ligated. The Siguira procedure may be preferable to shunt operations, because it causes no increase in likelihood of subsequent encephalopathy.

Donovan TJ, Ward M, Shepard R: Evaluation of endoscopic sclerotherapy of esophageal varices in children. J Pediatr Gastroenterol Nutr 5:696, 1986.
Hassal E, Berquist WE, Ament ME, et al: Sclerotherapy for extrahepatic portal hypertension in childhood. J Pediatr 115:69, 1989.
Myburgh JA: Selective shunting procedures in portal hypertension: Current perspectives. Surg Annu 19:83, 1987.
Snady H: Acute postal vein trombosis, sclerotherapy and vasopressin: Relationships and implications. Am J Gastroenterol 82:1292, 1987.
Superina RA, Weber JL, Shandling B: A modified Siguira operation for bleeding varices in children. J Pediatr Surg 18:794, 1983.
Triger DR: Extrahepatic portal vein obstruction. GT 28:1193, 1987.

13.103 PERITONEUM AND ALLIED STRUCTURES

MALFORMATIONS OF THE PERITONEUM

Congenital peritoneal bands may be responsible for intestinal obstruction; numerous other anomalies may occur in the course of the development of the peritoneum but are rarely of clinical importance. Intra-abdominal herniations infrequently occur through ring-like formations produced by anomalous peritoneal bands. Absence of the omentum or its duplication occurs rarely. Omental cysts and torsion are unusual causes of acute abdominal crises.

ASCITES

The term "ascites" indicates an accumulation of fluid in the peritoneal cavity, but it is usually applied to accumulations of serous fluid. Renal, especially nephrotic, and cardiac conditions are most often responsible for ascites. It may be secondary to chronic adhesive pericarditis, or part of a polyserositis syndrome (SLE, familial Mediterranean fever). Other causes include obstruction of the portal circulation, due to hepatic cirrhosis (Sec. 13.82) or to enlarged lymph nodes, tumors, thrombosis, chronic tuberculous peritonitis, rheumatic peritonitis, perforation of urinary tract, or obstruction of the splenic vein.

The abdomen is distended; when distention is great, there is flattening or pouting of the umbilicus. Fluctuation can be detected on palpation; a wave-like impulse is obtained by sharp tapping on one side of the abdomen while the other hand is placed on the opposite side and an assistant's hand compresses the abdomen in the midline; shifting percussion dullness can often be shown.

Ascites must be differentiated from other conditions that cause distention of the abdomen, which may include gaseous distention of the intestine; fecal distention as occurs with megacolon; tumor masses, including cysts of the mesentery; acute or chronic peritonitis; peritoneal hemorrhage; extreme distention of the bladder; and simple obesity.

The course, prognosis, and treatment of ascites depend entirely on the cause. Patients with any type of ascites are at increased risk for spontaneous bacterial peritonitis.

CHYLOUS ASCITES

The accumulation of chyle as ascites is uncommon; this form of ascites may occur at any age of childhood and is occasionally congenital. Chylous ascites is caused by an anomaly, injury, or obstruction of the thoracic duct within its abdominal portion. In the case of anomalies the condition is present at birth or shortly thereafter. Chylothorax may be associated (Sec. 14.95). Obstructions may be produced by enlarged lymph nodes or neoplasms. The fluid has the appearance of milk because of its high-fat content. If the patient has nothing by mouth the fluid will be a serous transudate with a predominance of lymphocytes (>85%). In chronic peritonitis, peritoneal fluid may have a somewhat similar color from degeneration of inflammatory products. The fluid may even be present in scrotal hydroceles if the processus vaginalis is patent.

The accumulation of chyle can be reduced in some infants by providing a low-fat diet containing medium-chain triglycerides that are absorbed directly into the portal circulation. Because there is considerable loss of protein in this fluid, high-protein diets should be prescribed and parenteral nutrition supplementation may be indicated. Paracentesis is indicated for respiratory distress due to abdominal distention, but the efficacy of repetitive paracentesis is unknown. It may take several months for medical management to be effective. Abdominal exploration may be justified to search for the site of the leak if a trial of dietary management is unsuccessful.

Grescom NT, Colodny AH, Rosenberg HK: Diagnostic aspects of neonatal ascites: Report of 27 cases. Am J Roentgenol 128:961, 1977.
Unger SW, Chandler JG: Chylous ascites in infants and children. Surgery 93:455, 1983.

PERITONITIS

Acute infections of the peritoneum are arbitrarily designated as *primary* when their origin is outside the abdominal cavity and infection is blood- or lymph-borne. The infection is termed *secondary* when it occurs through extension from or rupture of an intra-abdominal viscus or of an abscess.

Peritonitis in the neonatal period may arise from a transplacental in utero infection; more frequently it is the result of infection acquired during or shortly after birth. It may be a manifestation of septicemia, a direct extension from an umbilical infection or from perforation of the intestine, or, rarely, the sequel of a ruptured appendix. Meconium peritonitis is described in Sec. 9.42.

ACUTE PRIMARY PERITONITIS

ETIOLOGY AND EPIDEMIOLOGY. Primary peritonitis is a bacterial infection of the peritoneal cavity without a demonstrable intra-abdominal source. This entity occurs in children with ascites secondary to nephrosis or cirrhosis and, occasionally, in otherwise healthy children. Pneumococci and group A streptococci are the predominant pathogens, with gram-negative bacteria often involved *(E. coli)*. The genders are equally affected; most cases occur before 6 yr of age.

CLINICAL MANIFESTATIONS. The onset may be insidious or rapid and is characterized by fever, abdominal pain, and vomiting. Diarrhea is common, and extreme prostration may occur. The child may appear toxic or anxious. In very ill patients, especially young infants, the temperature may be normal or subnormal. The pulse may be rapid, small, and compressible, and the respirations rapid and shallow because of the pain that abdominal respiration produces. There is usually distention of the abdomen, moderate diffuse tenderness, and a doughy resistance. Examination often reveals signs of active nephrosis or cirrhosis, including ascites. Palpation may demonstrate rebound tenderness and rigidity. Bowel sounds are hypoactive or absent.

DIAGNOSIS AND TREATMENT. Laboratory studies reveal leukocytosis with 85–95% polymorphonuclear cells. Proteinuria is present in children with active nephrosis. Roentgenographic examination of the abdomen reveals dilatation of the large and small intestines, with edema of the small intestinal wall producing an increased distance between adjacent loops of gas-filled small bowel. In most cases without a history of cirrhosis or nephrosis the clinical presentation is indistinguishable from that of appendicitis, with or without perforation; accordingly, the diagnosis of primary peritonitis can be made only at laparotomy. In a child with active nephrosis or cirrhosis, however, whose physical findings are compatible with diffuse peritonitis, an attempt should be made to establish the diagnosis of primary peritonitis by evaluation of peritoneal fluid obtained with a short-beveled needle. Cytologic and chemical analyses of the exudate are helpful. Infected ascitic fluid usually contains an elevated protein concentration and more than 300 leukocytes/mm^3, more than 25% of which are polymorphonuclear. Microscopic examination of gram-stained ascitic fluid characteristically reveals a single species of gram-positive or, less often, gram-negative bacteria; in this situation initial intravenous antibiotic therapy with ampicillin and gentamicin is indicated, with subsequent changes in antibiotics dependent upon sensitivity testing. Although resolution of all signs and symptoms characteristically occurs within 48 hr, parenteral antibiotic therapy should be continued for a minimum of 7 days. Surgical exploration is indicated if multiple organisms (gram-positive, gram-negative) are seen on Gram stain, free air is demonstrated on abdominal roentgenogram, or after 48 hr of parenteral antibiotic therapy either the child's clinical condition fails to improve or the physical findings persist and show localization.

Golden GT, Shaw A: Primary peritonitis. Surg Gynecol Obstet 133:513, 1973.
Speck WT, Dresdale SA, MacMillan RW: Primary peritonitis and the nephrotic syndrome. Am J Surg 127:267, 1974.

ACUTE SECONDARY PERITONITIS

This type of peritonitis is most often due to the entry of enteric bacteria into the peritoneal cavity through a necrotic defect in the wall of the intestines or other viscus as a result of obstruction and infarction. In children, peritonitis is most often associated with appendicitis but may occur with volvulus, incarcerated hernias, or rupture of a Meckel diverticulum. Peritonitis may also occur as a complication of intestinal mucosal disease, including peptic ulcers, ulcerative colitis, and pseudomembranous enterocolitis. Peritonitis in the neonatal period most often occurs as a complication of necrotizing enterocolitis but may be associated with meconium ileus or spontaneous rupture of the stomach or intestines. The bacteria involved are the normal aerobic and anaerobic flora of the gastrointestinal tract. Peritonitis may also complicate continuous ambulatory peritoneal dialysis (CAPD) and may be due to *S. epidermidis, S. aureus, Candida albicans,* or other skin bacteria.

CLINICAL MANIFESTATIONS. The early clinical manifestations of secondary peritonitis reflect the underlying disease process. Fever, diffuse abdominal pain, nausea, and vomiting are characteristic. Signs of peritoneal inflammation include rebound tenderness, abdominal wall rigidity, and hypoactive or absent bowel sounds. These early findings may be followed by signs and symptoms of shock due to the loss of large quantities of protein-rich fluid from the vascular compartment into the peritoneal cavity and bowel lumen, with associated intravascular volume depletion.

The manifestations of shock from a ruptured viscus or the early symptoms of acute appendicitis may merge with those of peritonitis and may be followed by an increasing toxemia, as evidenced by greater restlessness and irritability, by a higher temperature, often 39.5° C or more (103–105° F), by an increase in the pulse rate, and, at times, by chills or convulsions. In extreme situations, and especially in early infancy, the temperature may be normal or subnormal. Constipation is marked, owing to paralytic ileus.

Laboratory studies reveal white blood cell counts in excess of 12,000/mm^3 with a predominance of polymorphonuclear forms. Roentgenograms of the abdomen may reveal free air in the peritoneal cavity, evidence of ileus or obstruction, peritoneal fluid, and obliteration of the psoas shadow.

TREATMENT. The main principle of therapy is to stabilize the patient by correcting fluid and electrolyte deficiencies with parenteral fluids, by alleviating intestinal obstruction with nasal suction, and by controlling the peritoneal infection with broad-spectrum antibiotics. Numerous antibiotic regimens have been advocated depending on the presence or absence of previous illness. In the absence of previous chemotherapy, a regimen consisting of clindamycin, ampicillin, and gentamicin is indicated. Surgery should be performed to repair any damaged viscus at the earliest time after the patient is stabilized and antibiotic therapy is initiated. Cultures taken during surgery will determine whether a change in the antibiotic regimen is indicated.

ACUTE SECONDARY LOCALIZED PERITONITIS
(Peritoneal Abscess)

ETIOLOGY. A single localized pyogenic abscess, most often secondary to perforation of an inflamed appendix, is somewhat less common in children than in adults. The poor ability of young children to localize peritoneal infection of appendiceal origin has been attributed to lower general resistance and to a relatively smaller omentum. Localized peritoneal abscesses occur most often in the appendiceal region, but may occur at any site, originating from various sources; or appendiceal infections may gravitate to other areas, notably the pelvis. An abscess in the subdiaphragmatic area may originate from an appendiceal or other intra-abdominal infection or, rarely, from an empyema. A diagnostic ultrasound or CT scan may be helpful in locating an abscess.

CLINICAL MANIFESTATIONS. The general symptoms of *peritoneal abscess* are continued fever or its recurrence, poor appetite, and vomiting following ingestion of food. The white blood cell count is increased, with a predominance of polymorphonuclear cells. With *appendiceal abscess,* there is tenderness in the right lower quadrant, often with a palpable mass.

A *pelvic abscess* is suggested by abdominal distention, rectal tenesmus with or without the passage of small stools containing mucus, or bladder irritability. Rectal examination may reveal a tender mass anteriorly.

A *subphrenic abscess* is evidenced by physical signs at the base of the lung, usually on the right, due to elevation of the diaphragm and frequently to the presence of pleural fluid.

The diagnosis can be established ultrasonographically. If the infection is on the right side, the diaphragm is elevated and the liver is depressed; there is frequently a pocket of air just below the diaphragm, resulting from gas produced by bacteria. A suprahepatic or infrahepatic collection of pus may be demonstrated. CT scanning is valuable in localization of the abscess.

TREATMENT. The abscess should be drained and appropriate antibiotic therapy should be provided. Drainage may be performed under radiologic control (ultrasound or CT scan), and a drainage catheter is inserted into the abscess cavity. Initial broad-spectrum coverage with clindamycin and gentamicin should be modified, if indicated, by the results of sensitivity tests of the bacteria obtained from cultures. If the appendix cannot be removed at the initial operation, appendectomy should be done subsequently within 3 mo.

Wilson-Storey D, Scobie WG: Appendix masses—A 15-year review. Pediatr Surg Int 4:165, 1989.

TUBERCULOUS PERITONITIS

See Sec. 12.47.

INGUINAL HERNIA

See Sec. 13.69.

HYDROCELE

See Sec. 18.46.

EPIGASTRIC HERNIA

Epigastric hernias occur in the midline between the umbilicus and the lower end of the sternum. They are uncommon and, except for their location, are similar to umbilical hernias. Surgery is rarely indicated. They may become acutely painful and tender when a bit of preperitoneal fat becomes incarcerated. They should be repaired surgically only if symptomatic.

INCISIONAL HERNIA

Postoperative hernias should be repaired electively. Incisional hernias may enlarge but rarely become incarcerated.

DIAPHRAGMATIC HERNIA

Diaphragmatic hernias may be congenital or acquired. Acquired hernias are usually traumatic in origin and are not considered here. Congenital herniation of abdominal contents into the thoracic cavity may be responsible for serious respiratory distress, usually constituting a medical-surgical emergency in the immediate neonatal period. Infrequently, when little or no respiratory embarrassment occurs, the hernia may not be detected until later in infancy or childhood. The delayed presentation of a right diaphragmatic hernia should be suspected in an infant with group B streptococcal infection or signs of atelectasis, pleural effusion, or pneumonia whose condition deteriorates. The frequency of major congenital anomalies is increased in infants with diaphragmatic hernia.

In addition to herniation through a defect in the diaphragm (see later), there may be partial herniation of the stomach through the esophageal hiatus, phrenic paralysis with displacement of abdominal contents upward but not herniated, and eventration of the diaphragm. *Eventration is not a herniation* but is also an upward displacement of abdominal contents into an outpouching or sac-like structure of the diaphragm resulting from a weakness or absence of diaphragmatic musculature without an abnormal opening. The clinical manifestations of an eventration may simulate those of a diaphragmatic hernia. Complete absence of the diaphragm is rare.

ETIOLOGY. Herniation occurs most often in the posterolateral segments of the diaphragm, much more often on the left side than on the right side. The defect represents a failure of the pleuroperitoneal canal to close completely during embryonic development (foramen of Bochdalek). Much less frequently, the herniation is in the anterior portion of the diaphragm in the retrosternal area, representing failure of midline fusion of the two anlagen of the diaphragm with elements of the pericardium (foramen of Morgagni). With this defect there may be herniation of intestine into the chest, although rarely into the pericardial sac. Ectopia cordis with displacement of the heart into the peritoneal cavity is rare. Umbilical defects are commonly associated with herniation through the foramen of Morgagni.

PATHOLOGY. Protrusion of the abdominal viscera through a diaphragmatic hernia into the thoracic cavity occurs in varying degrees. In severe cases, the stomach and a large part of the intestines and the spleen, liver, and kidneys displace the lungs and heart to the opposite side. Incomplete rotation of the cecum, umbilical defects, and duodenal constricting bands may be associated. The lung on the affected side is compressed and often hyopoplastic with a decreased number of airways and blood vessels and diminished total lung volume. An increased muscularity of small pulmonary arteries may contribute to increased pulmonary vascular resistance and hypertension. Hypoplasia of the contralateral lung has also been observed. In at least one third of patients pulmonary hypertension is present. With a patent ductus arteriosus, there may be severe right-to-left shunting, thus further aggravating tissue hypoxia.

CLINICAL MANIFESTATIONS. Severe respiratory distress, including dyspnea and cyanosis, is frequently present from birth. If symptoms are not present at birth, they may appear at any time during the neonatal period or later. These include vomiting, severe colicky pain, discomfort after eating, and constipation as well as dyspnea. Symptoms and signs of acute intestinal obstruction may occur at any time. Infrequently, there are no symptoms and the condition may be discovered by chance roentgenographic examination.

Findings on physical examination depend on the degree of displacement of abdominal contents into the thoracic cavity. When there is extensive displacement in the newborn infant, the abdomen is usually small and scaphoid; the infant is cyanotic and has obvious respiratory retractions. If the respiratory embarrassment is not relieved, shock and rapidly progressive hypoxia occur. In contrast, in mildly affected patients there may be no or only minimal respiratory distress and no digestive disturbance.

The percussion note over the part of the thorax containing the stomach and intestines may be more tympanic or duller than usual, and the breath sounds may be absent. Occasionally, sounds of intestinal peristaltic movements can be heard over the chest.

The diagnosis is usually established by roentgenographic examination (Fig. 13–29). Antenatal diagnosis may be made by ultrasonography. Characteristically, in the neonatal period there are fluid- and air-filled loops of intestine in the chest that simulate cysts. The mediastinum is displaced toward the unaffected side, usually the right. Occasionally, in the case of cystic adenomatoid malformations of the lung or congenital

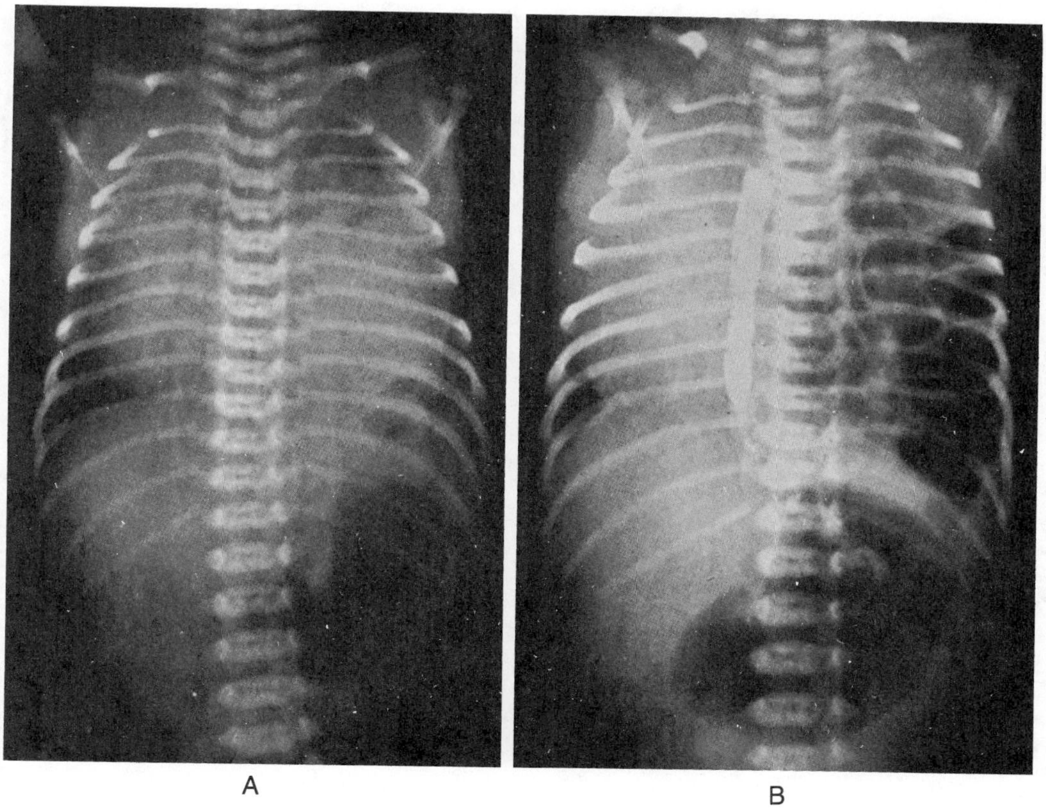

Figure 13–29. Congenital diaphragmatic hernia. *A*, Film exposed shortly after birth: distortion of shadow of the left leaf of the diaphragm with huge, mass-like density in left hemithorax displacing the heart to the right. *B*, Film exposed about 20 min after *A*. As the result of swallowed air, coils of air-filled small bowel are now demonstrated in the left hemithorax. The esophagus is outlined by swallowed contrast material. Operative correction was attempted because of extreme dyspnea. Infant died 5.5 hr after birth.

lobar emphysema, it may be necessary to use contrast material to demonstrate that the stomach and intestines are in the abdominal cavity.

TREATMENT. Resuscitation of the newborn is mandatory prior to reduction of the hernia and closure of the diaphragmatic defect. As soon as the diagnosis is suspected, the newborn infant should be positioned with head and thorax higher than the abdomen and feet to facilitate the downward displacement of the abdominal organs. Nasogastric intubation with intermittent suction will decrease entrapment of air and fluid within the herniated viscera and lessen the degree of ventilatory compromise. Positive-pressure ventilation should be administered cautiously through an endotracheal tube. Pneumothorax may result, owing to the uneven distribution of intrapulmonary pressures in the contralateral (normal) lung. This is usually a serious complication, because the ipsilateral lung is already unexpanded. Arterial blood gas measurements, including pH, should be obtained preoperatively, and metabolic and respiratory acidosis should be corrected with appropriate intravenous solutions. The patient is paralyzed and ventilated, and an immediate improvement in blood gases may be anticipated. If deterioration occurs, consideration must be given to the use of a high frequency ventilator or extracorporeal membrane oxygenation (ECMO).

Surgical correction is indicated only when the infant's condition has stabilized and maximal improvement is obtained. If the infant's condition relentlessly deteriorates, a successful operative outcome is not possible. ECMO may be of value (Sec. 9.36). A subcostal incision provides excellent exposure of the diaphragm, and the herniated contents can be reduced until the peritoneal cavities are equalized. Severely affected infants diagnosed within the 1st 24–72 hr of life have a mortality rate of approximately 50%. Most infants who do not require surgery early for respiratory distress survive. Low Apgar scores (<6) and acidosis (pH 7.2) are associated with a high mortality rate. Pulmonary hypertension with persistence of fetal circulation syndrome is a serious complication in the postoperative period, which requires careful fluid and respiratory management. It is often associated with difficulty in expanding a hypoplastic ipsilateral lung. Forceful attempts to inflate the lung may cause a pneumothorax on the opposite side.

Survivors generally can participate in normal activities through their teenage years, although they may have abnormal results on lung function studies.

BARRY SHANDLING

Anderson KD: Congenital diaphragmatic hernia. *In*: Welch KJ, et al (eds): Pediatric Surgery. Chicago, Year Book Medical Publishers, 1986, p 589.

Berman L, Stringer D, Ein SH, et al: The late-presenting pediatric Morgagni hernia: A benign condition. J Pediatr Surg 24:970, 1989.

Freyschuss U, Lannergren K, Frenckner B: Lung function after repair of congenital diaphragmatic hernia. Acta Pediatr Scand 73:589, 1985.

Geggel RL, Murphy JD, Langleben D, et al: Congenital diaphragmatic hernia: Arterial structural changes and persistent pulmonary hypertension after surgical repair. J Pediatr 107:457, 1985.

Rivilla F, de Augustin J, Lassaletta L, et al: Bilateral diaphragmatic hernia. Pediatr Surg Int 3:412, 1988.

Ruff SJ, Campbell JR, Harrison MW, et al: Pediatric diaphragmatic hernias: 11-year experience. Am J Surg 139:641, 1980.

Vacanti JP, O'Rourke PP, Lillehei CW, et al: The cardiopulmonary consequences of high-risk congenital diaphragmatic hernia. Pediatr Surg Int 3:1, 1988.

14

THE RESPIRATORY SYSTEM

14.1 DEVELOPMENT OF THE RESPIRATORY SYSTEM

Unicellular organisms exchange gases with their environment by a process of molecular diffusion. Gas diffusion across a cell layer, however, is inversely proportional to the layer's thickness. Therefore, multicellular organisms had to develop a more efficient system of gas transport. In higher organisms, this system has two components: a circulatory system, which carries oxygen and carbon dioxide to and from the milieu of individual cells, and a specialized respiratory system, which exchanges these gases with the organism's environment. Although the functions of both systems are interdependent and inseparable, the following discussion focuses on the development and function of the respiratory system.

Depending on the environment and metabolic characteristics of each organism, evolution has adopted different strategies to design the respiratory system. In air-breathing animals the gas-exchanging system derives from the endoderm; its surfaces are invaginated and form alveolar (reptiles, amphybia, and mammals) lungs or parabronchial (birds) lungs. Such an arrangement limits the loss of heat and water, while permitting a fine regulation of the temperature and humidity at the gas-exchanging surfaces. It also creates the geometric configuration needed for the function of the pulmonary surfactant. This material, which is secreted by lung cells into the gas-liquid interface, reduces surface tension and prevents the gas-exchanging surfaces from sticking to each other. Finally, the invaginated arrangement facilitates a relatively fast ventilatory response to changes in metabolic demands. Most air-breathing vertebrates aspirate air in and out of their lungs using a bellows-type pump. This mechanism can generate large and rapid variations in lung ventilation, providing the adaptability demanded by the fast metabolic pace of warm-blooded animals.

The development of the mammalian respiratory system encompasses three phases: morphogenesis or formation of the necessary respiratory structures, adaptation to atmospheric breathing, and dimensional growth. In most species, the first two phases take place primarily before birth. Growth continues after birth, generally at a pace that is dictated by the functional needs of other growing organ systems. The effects of an injury to the respiratory system depend not only on the severity of the injury but also on the time of its occurrence. Insults during the morphogenesis of the lungs, for instance, tend to produce severe and irreversible disruptions of respiratory structure and function. In contrast, injuries that interfere with lung growth are often reversible and can be compensated by the growth process.

PRENATAL DEVELOPMENT: MORPHOGENESIS

In the human, the morphogenesis of the respiratory system is divided into five periods. The first, or *embryonic period*, begins at approximately the 4th wk of gestation when the primitive airways appear as an epithelial bud arising from the foregut. This bud divides dichotomously and grows rapidly into the mesenchyma that separates the gut from the coelomic cavity. The peribronchial mesenchyma or splachnopleura plays an essential role in the shaping of the lungs during the embryonic period. First, the primitive airway buds can only divide and form a tree-like structure if they are in close contact with mesenchyma. Second, the pulmonary vasculature is a mesenchymal derivative. Both the foregut and the bronchial buds are wrapped by a vascular plexus, which originates from the aorta and drains into the major somatic veins. Although the mesenchymal plexus connects eventually with the pulmonary artery and veins to complete the pulmonary circulation, it retains some aortic connections that form the bronchial arteries. Finally, all the supporting structures of the lungs originate from the splanchnopleura. These structures include the pleura, the septal network of the lungs, and the smooth muscle, cartilage, and connective covers of the airways.

Toward the 6th wk of gestation, at the beginning of the second or *pseudoglandular period*, the lungs resemble an exocrine gland with a thick stroma crossed by narrow ducts lined by a tall epithelium. The major airways are already present and are in close association with pulmonary arteries and veins. The trachea and the foregut are now separated after the progressive fusion of epithelial ridges growing from the primitive airway. The incomplete fusion of these ridges results in a **tracheoesophageal fistula,** a relatively common malformation of the newborn. During the pseudoglandular period, the airways continue to branch until the appearance of the terminal bronchioles, while the airway high columnar epithelial cells start to differentiate into ciliated, nonciliated, globular, and basal cells. Mucous glands, cartilage, and smooth muscle can be easily distinguished in the airway walls by the 16th wk of gestation.

The diaphragm is formed during this period from two mesenchymal components. Its central tendon originates from the transverse septum, a plate of mesodermal tissue located between the pericardium and the stalk of the yolk sac. Its lateral portions are formed by the pleuroperitoneal folds, which grow from the body wall until they fuse with the esophageal mesentery and the transverse septum. The completion of this fusion closes the communication between the thorax and the abdomen and poses a limit on the caudal growth of the lungs. Its failure, usually on the left, results in the **congenital diaphragmatic hernia of Bochdalek**. This defect, which is the most frequent type of diaphragmatic hernia, allows the invasion of the primitive pleural cavity by the abdominal contents, which compress the forming lung and severely impair its growth. Initially membranous, the diaphragm is eventually invaded by striated muscle derived from cervical myotomes.

During the third or *canalicular period*, between the 16th and 28th wk of gestation, the airways complete their accessory structures (cartilage, glands, and muscle). The mesenchyma becomes thin in the vicinity of the terminal airways, which widen to form the potential airspaces. The cells that line these airspaces undergo differentiation into cuboidal type II or surfactant-producing cells and flatter alveolar type I cells. The type I cells probably originate from undifferentiated type II cells. While these transformations are occurring, the mesenchymal capillary network becomes denser and approaches the newly formed canaliculi.

Toward the 28th wk of gestation, when the lungs enter their *saccular period*, the terminal airways continue to widen and form the terminal sacs. The capillaries are now in closer proximity to the sacs and are separated from them only by a thin basement membrane. This proximity marks the creation of a potential air-blood barrier capable of supporting gas exchange, even in the absence of the typical alveolar structure of the mature lung. As the mesenchymal interstitium becomes thinner, the saccular walls appose each other, causing the septa that separate the terminal sacs to contain a double capillary network.

After the 36th wk of gestation, the beginning of the *alveolar period*, secondary crests start to appear in the terminal saccules, dividing them into typical alveoli. The capillaries in the saccular walls proliferate rapidly and fuse into a single capillary network. At birth, the human lungs contain an average of 50 million alveoli, a small number compared with the 300 million alveoli that are found in the lungs of an adult. Airway smooth muscle is present and responsive to both constricting and dilating stimuli at birth in most mammalian species, including the human.

ADAPTATION TO AIR-BREATHING

The transition from placental dependency to autonomous gas exchange through the lungs requires adaptive changes. These include the production of a surfactant system, the conditioning of the respiratory pump, the elimination of pulmonary liquid, and the establishment of parallel pulmonary and systemic circulations.

As soon as air breathing begins, a liquid-air interface forms in the airspaces. Unless reduced in some way, the surface tension forces created at this interface would threaten airspace stability, particularly at low lung volumes. The **pulmonary surfactant** accomplishes this reduction by forming a hydrophobic lipid monolayer at the surface of the peripheral airspaces. Pulmonary surfactant is a complex mixture of phospholipids and proteins and is secreted into the saccular or alveolar lining by type II cells. It is first recognized forming lamellar bodies inside these cells at about 24 wk of gestation. Surfactant lipids, however, do not appear in the amniotic fluid until 30 wk of gestation, suggesting that there is a chronologic gap between surfactant synthesis and secretion. Labor probably shortens this gap because phospholipids are uniformly found in the alveoli of infants born before 30 wk of gestation. The three apoproteins identified in pulmonary surfactant (SP-A, SP-B, and SP-C) appear to be important for the spreading and function of the material. Their synthesis and secretion follows a course similar to that of the surfactant phospholipids. Surfactant synthesis is under multiple hormonal control. Glucocorticoids and thyroid hormones increase surfactant synthesis. Only glucocorticoids, however, are known to stimulate the production of both surfactant lipids and proteins, consistent with the efficacy of these hormones in the prevention of the respiratory distress syndrome of the newborn (see Sec. 9.32).

By birth, the fetus has had the advantage of several months of breathing "exercise." Fetal breathing movements, which become more frequent as gestation advances, probably serve to condition the respiratory muscles. In addition, these movements stimulate lung development, possibly by creating a pressure gradient between the lung and the amniotic fluid.

The fetal lung is a secretory organ. Fluid and ions are actively secreted into the potential airspaces by means of a chloride ion pump. The distention of the airspaces by lung fluid appears to be important in stimulating the development of the lung acinus, because chronic drainage of this fluid in experimental animals results in lung hypoplasia. The exact mechanisms of lung fluid reabsorption are unknown. The process seems to start several days before delivery and takes place primarily through the pulmonary vasculature, even though the pulmonary lymphatic system is well developed at the end of the canalicular period. Labor accelerates lung fluid reabsorption, a phenomenom that may explain the greater incidence of transient pulmonary edema in infants born by cesarean section. β-Adrenergic hormones also increase fluid reabsorption by a mechanism that probably involves active transport of Na^+ and K^+ by the pulmonary epithelium. Glucocorticoids accelerate fluid reabsorption by inducing β-adrenergic receptors, thus increasing their sensitivity to circulating catecholamines.

At birth, the pulmonary circulation shifts from a high-resistant system to a low-resistant system, with a marked increase in pulmonary blood flow. This change results from the dilatation of the pulmonary arterial system and is, in great part, mediated by the increase in alveolar oxygen concentrations and by lung expansion. The subsequent closure of the foramen ovale and the ductus arteriosus establishes separate pulmonary and systemic circulations. As a result, arterial oxygen tension rises sharply and arterial oxygen concentration becomes homogeneous throughout the body. Remodeling of the pulmonary vasculature accounts for the gradual decrease in pulmonary vascular resistance observed during the first weeks after birth.

POSTNATAL DEVELOPMENT

Lung development during the first few months after birth is characterized by an exponential increase in the surface of the air-blood barrier. This increase is accomplished by the multiplication of pulmonary alveoli and capillaries, a process that continues at a slower pace until the ages of 5–8 yr. Thereafter, the lungs grow only by alveolar expansion. The airways increase in both diameter (particularly in the lung periphery) and length, but no new generations are added. In contrast, arteries and veins continue to increase in number. The acinary arterioles undergo a prolonged process of muscularization. At birth, muscular arteries stop at the terminal bronchioles. By 3 yr of age, the vascular smooth muscle reaches the respiratory bronchioles.

The postnatal development of the lungs is regulated by multiple factors. These factors are poorly understood, but they probably include genetic make-up, level of activity, environment, hormonal influences, and the geometric growth of the chest wall. There is a good correlation between somatic growth and lung growth; taller subjects have larger lungs. Exercise, growth hormone, and environmental hypoxia (e.g., life at high altitudes) increase the alveolar number and surface. On the other hand, most congenital or acquired deformations of the chest wall are associated with some degree of pulmonary hypoplasia, suggesting that the thoracic shape influences postnatal lung growth.

Ballard PL: Hormones and Lung Maturation. Monographs on Endocrinology. New York, Springer-Verlag, 1986.

Bucher U, Reid L: Development of the intrasegmental bronchial tree: The

pattern of branching and development of cartilage at various stages of intra-uterine life. Thorax 16:207, 1961.
Langston C, Kida K, Reed M, et al: Human lung growth in late gestation and in the neonate. Am Rev Respir Dis 129:607, 1984.
Thurlbeck WM: Postnatal growth and development of the lung. Am Rev Respir Dis 111:803, 1975.
Weibel ER: The Pathway for Oxygen: Structure and Function in the Mammalian Respiratory System. Cambridge, MA, Harvard University Press, 1984.

14.2 RESPIRATORY FUNCTION AND APPROACH TO RESPIRATORY DISEASE

The main function of the respiratory system is the provision of adequate gas exchange. Accordingly, respiratory failure is defined traditionally in terms of the concentration or partial pressure of oxygen and carbon dioxide in the arterial blood. Although this definition is useful, the clinician must remember that respiratory dysfunction frequently occurs in the absence of gas exchange aberrations. Alterations in the mechanical behavior of the respiratory system and increased work of breathing, with or without respiratory failure, are the most common manifestation of respiratory disease in children.

GAS EXCHANGE

The pressure of carbon dioxide (PCO_2) in the arterial blood is directly proportional to CO_2 production and inversely proportional to alveolar ventilation. The latter can be calculated as the difference of *minute ventilation* (the amount of gas that enters and leaves the lungs in 1 min) and *dead space ventilation* (the portion of the minute ventilation that does not contribute to alveolar gas exchange). Dead space ventilation is usually increased by respiratory disease. If the subject is unable to compensate with a sufficient increase in minute ventilation, the arterial PCO_2 rises above its normal values of 35–45 mm Hg.

The pressure of oxygen (PO_2) in the arterial blood is influenced by several variables, including the PO_2 of the inspired gas, the PO_2 of the venous blood, the hemoglobin oxygen capacity, and the respective alveolar gas and capillary blood flows in the lungs. With other factors being constant, increases in gas flow (ventilation) with respect to blood flow (perfusion) augment pulmonary capillary and arterial PO_2. Conversely, decreases in the ventilation/perfusion ratio decrease pulmonary capillary and arterial PO_2. Regional differences in *ventilation/perfusion ratios* exist in normal lungs. When exaggerated, these differences cause hypoxemia. To understand the mechanism, it is important to recognize that areas with a low ventilation/perfusion ratio cause more of a decrease in arterial oxygenation than areas with a high ventilation/perfusion ratio increase it. The reason is that, in areas with low ventilation/perfusion ratio, the hemoglobin-oxygen dissociation curve favors large decreases in the oxygen saturation and content of the capillary blood with small decrements in PO_2. In areas with a high ventilation/perfusion ratio, on the other hand, the oxygen saturation and content in the capillaries changes little even with large increases in PO_2. As a result, when the oxygen-desaturated blood from areas with low ventilation/perfusion ratio mixes with oxygenated blood from other areas in the pulmonary veins, the overall oxygen saturation and PO_2 are lower than normal.

Even though the air-blood barrier in the lungs has a lower *diffusion conductance* for oxygen than for carbon dioxide, the arterial PO_2 is close to the alveolar PO_2 because there is normally enough time for equilibration of oxygen between alveolar gas and capillary blood. However, respiratory disease frequently increases the *alveolar-arterial* PO_2 *difference*. This increase is caused by a variable combination of true intrapulmonary shunt, in areas where the ventilation/perfusion ratio is zero (e.g., with alveolar collapse), and ventilation/perfusion mismatch. Diffusion impairment may contribute to hypoxemia in interstitial lung disease in adults, but its contribution is questionable in childhood diseases. The alveolar-arterial PO_2 difference can be calculated at the bedside to quantify the amount of gas exchange impairment by measuring the arterial PO_2 and estimating the alveolar PO_2 (PAO_2) as:

$$PAO_2 = FIO_2 (P_B - 47) - PaCO_2/R$$

where FIO_2 represents the fractional concentration of inspired oxygen; P_B represents the barometric pressure; $PaCO_2$ arterial PCO_2, and R represent the respiratory exchange ratio (carbon dioxide production/oxygen consumption, which is usually close to 0.8). The alveolar-arterial PO_2 difference varies with age and is usually less than 5–6 mm Hg in room air for the adolescent and is slightly larger for the younger child and infant. This difference is caused by normal shunt pathways between the pulmonary and systemic circulations. In the term newborn, and particularly in the premature infant, the alveolar-arterial PO_2 difference is even greater. Possible explanations are the larger diffusion distance between the immature saccules and saccular capillaries, heterogeneity of ventilation/perfusion ratios, and airway closure in the supine position.

MECHANICS OF BREATHING

The respiratory system can be schematized as consisting of a gas exchanger (the alveolar-capillary interface), a pump (the lungs and chest wall), and a neural generator that controls the pump through a complicated loop of afferent and efferent connections. Similar to other systems that perform external work, the mechanical function of the pump must be analyzed in terms of work and efficiency. The work done by the pump is a relatively simple function of the volume changes and the pressure applied on the lungs. Respiratory efficiency (the ratio of work performed and energy consumed), on the other hand, is a complex function of the structural and functional state of the respiratory muscles.

The pressure that must be generated by the respiratory muscles to change lung volume during breathing has two main components. The first, or elastic component, overcomes the elastic recoil of the lungs and the chest wall. The second, or resistive component, overcomes the flow resistance of the airways and tissue. Although both components are often increased in children with respiratory illness, it is convenient to distinguish between conditions that predominantly increase the elastic pressure (restrictive respiratory disease) and those that predominantly increase the resistive pressure (obstructive respiratory disease).

RESTRICTIVE RESPIRATORY DISEASE. The pressure needed to overcome the elastic recoil of the respiratory system depends on the volume of the lungs. The volume-pressure relationship of the lungs and chest wall varies with lung volume. However, this relationship is often summarized for a given range of lung volumes by the quotient of volume and pressure changes, which defines the concept of *compliance*. When the lung compliance is decreased, the respiratory muscles must generate greater pressures and perform more work to inflate the lungs. A similar situation occurs when the chest wall compliance is decreased. In both cases, the expansion of the chest is restricted. Examples of restrictive lung parenchymal disease include conditions in which the interstitium is infiltrated with fluid (edema or infection) or when the number of available alveoli is decreased by alveolar collapse (atelectasis) or destruction. Restrictive chest wall disease occurs when the mobility of the chest wall is decreased owing to abdominal distention, congenital malformations, or neuromuscular disease.

Whether originating in the lungs or the chest wall, a decrease in compliance has two consequences. First, the work of breathing increases. Second, the increased recoil lowers the volume of the lungs. Because the alveolar structure is particularly unstable at low lung volumes, restrictive disease is commonly associated with alveolar collapse, which further decreases lung compliance and ventilation/perfusion ratios, causing hypoxemia.

OBSTRUCTIVE RESPIRATORY DISEASE. The pressure needed to overcome the resistive forces of the respiratory system depends on the rate of gas flow entering or leaving the lungs. These forces are, therefore, only present when there is gas movement. Generally, the inspiratory resistive forces are the most significant from an energetic point of view. Expiration is passive, and thus all expiratory resistive work is done by the recoil of the lungs and chest wall. The most substantial portion of the respiratory system's resistance that needs to be overcome results from the friction of the gas against the airway walls. The caliber of the airways, and thus the airway resistance, varies greatly during the respiratory cycle and depends on whether the airways are extrathoracic or intrathoracic. Understanding these variations is helpful in evaluating and diagnosing airway disease and obstruction.

The effect of the respiratory cycle phase on airway resistance is determined by the balance of pressures across the airway walls. The pressure outside the extrathoracic airways (nose, pharynx, larynx, and upper trachea) is similar to atmospheric pressure and, for practical purposes, can be considered to be zero. The pressure outside the intrathoracic airways, on the other hand, is very similar to pleural pressure, and thus it is influenced by lung volume changes. The pressure inside both extrathoracic and intrathoracic airways is negative during inspiration and is positive during expiration. The extrathoracic airways therefore narrow during inspiration, because their inside pressure (which is negative) decreases with respect to their outside pressure (zero), and widen during expiration, as the opposite becomes true. The intrathoracic airways, in contrast, widen during inspiration because the pleural pressure (outside the airways) decreases more than the pressure inside the airways and alveoli in order to overcome the elastic recoil of the lungs. During expiration, the intrathoracic airways narrow as their inside pressure increases with respect to pleural pressure.

Airway obstruction causes an exaggeration of these normal changes (Fig. 14–1). When the extrathoracic airway is obstructed (e.g., by laryngeal edema or a foreign body), the pressure inside the airways and distal to the narrowing has to become more negative during inspiration to overcome the increased resistance at the point of obstruction. Therefore, the extrathoracic airway collapses downstream from the obstruction, usually causing an audible inspiratory **stridor** as the gas rushes through. When the intrathoracic airway is obstructed, the pleural pressure must become more positive during expiration. Because the inside pressure beyond the obstruction decreases, the intrathoracic airways downstream from the obstruction point tend to collapse during expiration, producing audible expiratory **wheezes** and gas trapping. Although the subject may increase the expiratory effort, gas flow often does not increase because forced expiration increases pleural pressure and causes further collapse of the airways. This condition under which expiratory flow becomes independent of effort is known as flow limitation. Its recognition is important for diagnostic purposes because it provides a reproducible assessment of airway function.

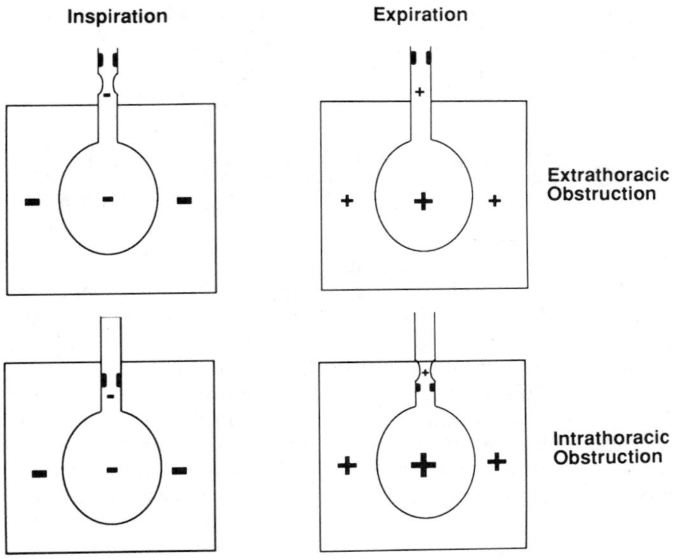

Figure 14–1. Effect of inspiration and expiration on the caliber of the airways during extrathoracic and intrathoracic obstruction. Extrathoracic airway obstruction increases during inspiration because the pressure inside the airway becomes negative with respect to the atmospheric pressure outside. Intrathoracic airway obstruction increases during expiration because, downstream from the obstruction point, the positive pleural pressure outside the airways exceeds the pressure inside. (From Pérez Fontán JJ, Lister G. *In*: Toulukian RJ [ed]: Pediatric Trauma, 2nd ed., St. Louis, CV Mosby, 1990.)

EFFICIENCY OF THE DEVELOPING RESPIRATORY SYSTEM. When the *respiratory work load* increases in the course of an illness, the respiratory system has two types of response. The first and most immediate response is to increase the force of contraction of the respiratory muscles at the cost of increased energy expenditure. The second response is to improve the efficiency of respiration and limit energy losses by introducing changes in the respiratory pattern. Because these changes depend on the mechanical derangement, their detection can help in differentiating restrictive and obstructive diseases. Children with restrictive disease breathe rapidly and shallowly, because with this pattern less work per unit of time is needed to maintain a given alveolar ventilation. In contrast, children with obstructive disorders breathe at a lower rate to minimize resistive work. In addition to respiratory pattern, other factors influence the efficiency of the respiratory system in both health and disease. These factors include the configuration of the chest wall and respiratory muscles, the chest wall compliance, and the functional state of the respiratory muscles.

The *configuration of the chest wall* and the power of the respiratory muscles are often impaired in the course of respiratory illness. The respiratory muscles can only develop their maximal force if stretched to an optimal length. The diaphragm of the adult reaches its optimal length when it adopts the shape of a dome-capped cylinder. In addition to increasing the force of the diaphragmatic contraction, this shape allows the apposition of the diaphragm to the rib cage (Fig. 14–2). The area of apposition of the diaphragm and the rib cage serves an important function during inspiration by allowing the abdominal pressures to push the lower ribs forward and laterally in the inspiratory direction. The shape of the diaphragm in the infant, and particularly in the new-

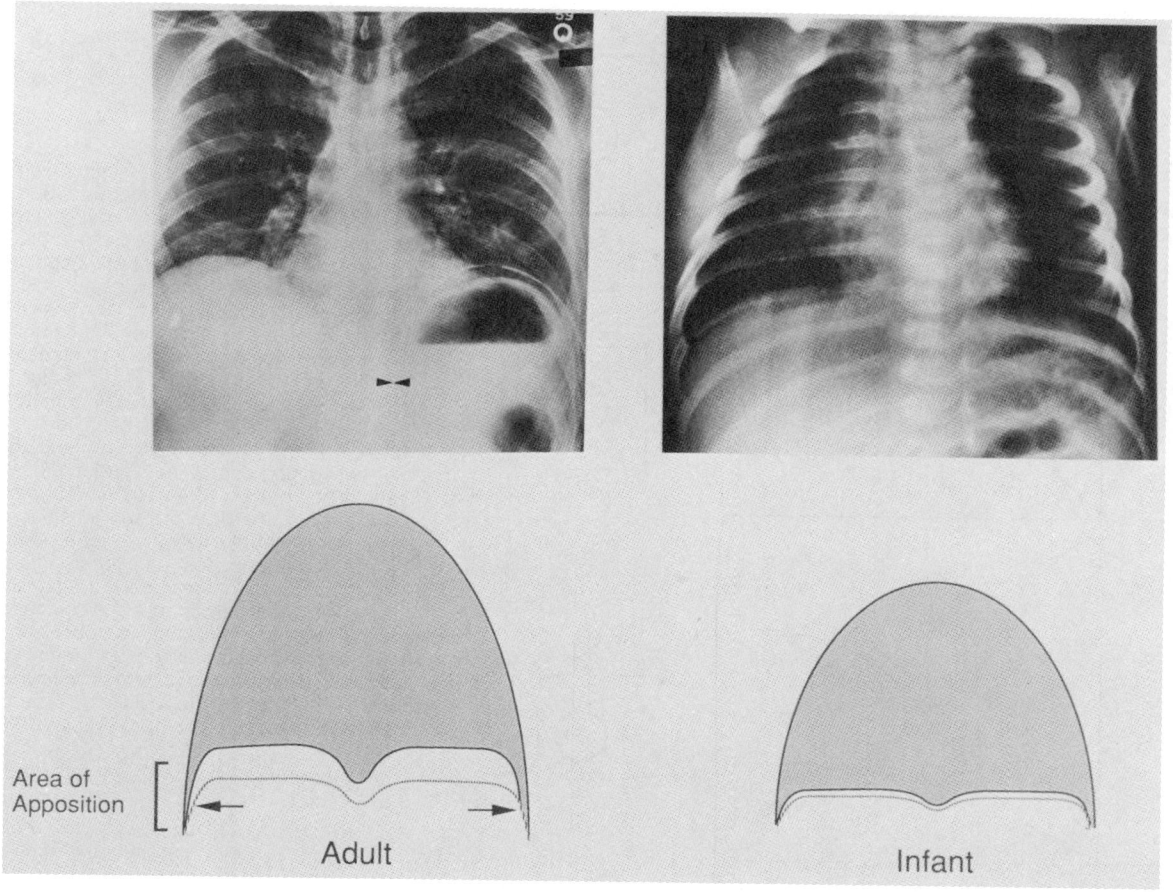

Figure 14–2. Chest radiographs and sketches illustrating the differences in the geometric shapes of the diaphragm of the adult and infant. The diaphragm of the adult *(left)* has the shape of a dome-capped cylinder whose height can be followed in the radiograph to the tip of a catheter inserted in the pleural space *(arrowheads)*. A portion of the diaphragm is apposed to the rib cage, providing a way of transforming the vertical movement of the diaphragm into the anterior and lateral movement of the rib cage in inspiration (see text). The diaphragm of the infant *(right)* is flatter and less capable of displacing large volumes in the vertical direction. In addition, it lacks a substantial area of apposition and thus has limited expanding action on the rib cage.

born, does not take advantage of these features. The lower portion of the rib cage has large anteroposterior and lateral diameters. As a result, the diaphragmatic insertions are spread out, limiting the range of lengths of the diaphragmatic fibers. In addition, the area of apposition is minimal.

The *compliance of the chest wall and lungs* varies greatly during postnatal development. The infant's chest wall is very compliant (Fig. 14–3), a feature that facilitates its deformation without injury during delivery. An increased chest wall compliance, however, has some disadvantages. First, the relaxation volume of the lungs at the end of a passive expiration is determined by the relative compliances of lungs and chest wall. The high chest wall compliance and the low pulmonary compliance cause the relaxation volume of the thorax to be low. Accordingly, to keep their functional residual capacity (the volume of gas contained in the lungs at the end of expiration during tidal breathing) within acceptable limits, newborns and small infants use various mechanisms to brake their expiratory flow. These mechanisms are easily overwhelmed when lung compliance is reduced by disease, when neurologic control is impaired, or when the chest wall compliance is very high (which occurs in premature infants). The functional residual capacity represents the largest oxygen store in the body and serves as a buffer against hypoxemia. Its reduction in infants can easily lead to hypoxemia because of the high oxygen consumption rates characteristic of early ages. The second disadvantage of a high chest wall compliance is that the chest wall undergoes regional deformation as the pleural pressures become negative. This causes chest wall retractions and limits inspiratory gas movement. The resultant loss of tidal volume is an important cause of ventilatory inefficiency.

The functional state of the respiratory muscles also influences respiratory efficiency. Sustained periods of extreme activity are likely to result in decreased muscle contractility and fatigue. Decreased availability of metabolic fuels, limitations in neuromuscular transmission, and the abundance of low-oxidative, fast-twitch fibers may render the developing diaphragm more susceptible to fatigue.

DIAGNOSTIC APPROACH TO RESPIRATORY DISEASE

PHYSICAL EXAMINATION. Respiratory dysfunction usually produces detectable alterations in the pattern of breathing. Respiratory control abnormalities may cause the child to breathe at a low rate or periodically. Mechanical abnormalities, on the other hand, produce compensatory changes that are generally directed at maintaining or increasing ventilation. These changes include variable increases in the breathing rate, chest wall retractions, and nasal flaring. In most cases, careful observation of the child's respiratory pattern provides

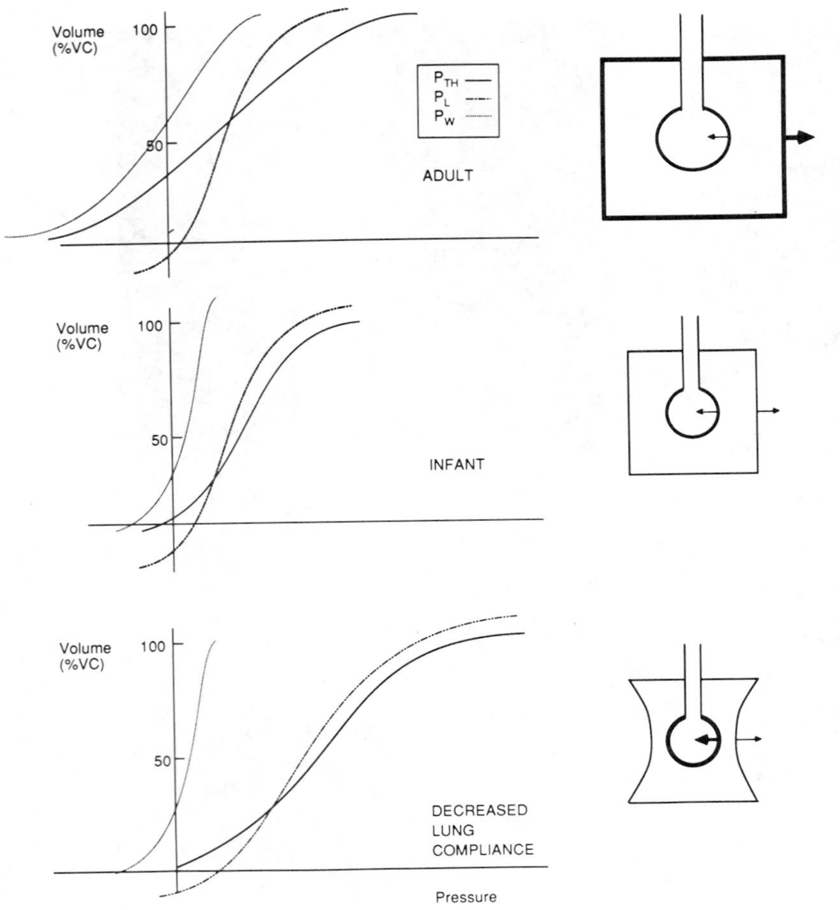

Figure 14–3. *Left,* Idealized static volume-pressure relationships of the thorax, lungs, and chest wall in the adult, infant, and infant with decreased lung compliance. Lung volume (on the ordinate axis) is expressed as a percentage of vital capacity (VC). The pressure on the abscissa indicates pressure across the thorax (P_{TH}), lungs (P_L), and chest wall (P_W), depending on the relationship. The compliance of the chest wall (calculated as the instantaneous slope of the relationship) is greater in the infant than in the adult. As a result, the chest wall contributes little to the overall volume-pressure behavior of the thorax, which is primarily determined by lung recoil (especially when lung compliance is reduced). *Right,* Representations of the chest wall and lungs corresponding to the volume-pressure relationships on the left. In the adult, the relatively large recoil *(thick arrow)* of the chest wall opposes lung recoil *(thin arrow)* and defines the functional residual capacity. In the infant, lung recoil is relatively unopposed by chest wall recoil, and therefore the functional residual capacity tends to be lower, especially when lung recoil is pathologically high (*thick arrow* in bottom drawing). (From Pérez Fontán JJ, Lister G. *In*: Toulukian RJ [ed]: Pediatric Trauma, 2nd ed., St. Louis, CV Mosby, 1990.)

information that helps in distinguishing between restrictive and obstructive forms of respiratory disease. Children with restrictive disease breathe at faster rates, and their respiratory excursions are shallow. An expiratory grunt is common, as the child attempts to raise the functional residual capacity by closing the glottis at the end of expiration. Children with obstructive disease take slower, deeper breaths. When the obstruction is extrathoracic (from the nose to the mid-trachea), inspiration is more prolonged than expiration, and an inspiratory stridor can usually be heard. When the obstruction is intrathoracic, expiration is more ostensibly prolonged and the patient often has to make use of accessory expiratory muscles. Lung percussion is usually dull in restrictive lung disease and tympanic in obstructive disease. Auscultation confirms the presence of noises and the inspiratory and expiratory prolongation and provides information about the symmetry and quality of air movement.

BLOOD GAS ANALYSIS. Cyanosis is influenced by skin perfusion and is therefore an unreliable sign of hypoxemia. Arterial hypertension, tachycardia, and diaphoresis are late and by no means exclusive signs of hypoventilation. Blood gas exchange is evaluated most accurately by the direct measurement of arterial P_{O_2}, P_{CO_2}, and pH. Although these measurements have no substitute in many conditions, they are relatively invasive and have been replaced to a great extent by noninvasive monitoring. Arterial oxygenation, for instance, can be estimated from skin surface P_{O_2} determinations, which are influenced by skin perfusion. More recently, pulse oximetry has been used to provide an assessment of arterial oxygen saturation. Arterial P_{CO_2} can be inferred from end-tidal carbon dioxide concentrations. This method, however, requires some cooperation and is inaccurate in small infants, when ventilatory rate is high, and in the presence of major airway obstruction or ventilation heterogeneity.

The age and clinical condition of the patient need to be taken into account when interpreting blood gas tensions. With the exception of very young infants, values of arterial P_{O_2} lower than 85 mm Hg are usually abnormal for a child breathing room air at sea level. Calculation of the alveolar-arterial oxygen gradient is useful in the analysis of arterial oxygenation, particularly when the patient is not breathing room air or in the presence of hypercarbia. Values of arterial P_{CO_2} exceeding 45 mm Hg usually indicate hypoventilation or severe ventilation/perfusion mismatch, unless they reflect respiratory compensation for metabolic alkalosis.

RESPIRATORY FUNCTION TESTING. The measurement of respiratory function in infants and young children is often made difficult by their lack of cooperation. Attempts have been made to overcome this limitation by creating standard tests that do not require the patient's active participation. An example is the *squeeze method* of assessing expiratory flow rates in infants, which relies on an inflatable jacket to generate a forced expiration. Although they are becoming widely used, these methods still provide only a partial insight into the mechanisms of respiratory disease at early ages.

Whether restrictive or obstructive, most forms of respiratory disease cause alterations in lung volume and its subdivisions (Fig. 14–4). Restrictive diseases typically decrease *total lung capacity* (TLC), which is the total volume of gas contained in the lungs at the end of a maximal inspiration. TLC includes *residual volume* (the volume of gas contained in the lungs at the end of a forced expiration), which is not accessible to direct determinations. It must therefore be measured indirectly by gas dilution methods or, preferably, by plethysmog-

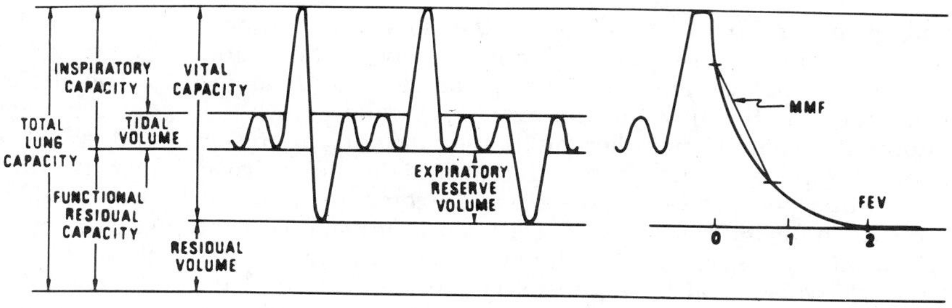

Figure 14–4. *Left*, Functional division of total lung capacity. *Right*, Flow-time relationship during a forced expiration from vital capacity. FEV represents the volume expired for a given period of time and is often measured at 1 sec. MMF represents the maximal midexpiratory flow rate and is calculated as the average flow for the middle 50% of the forced vital capacity (as shown by the cord in the drawing). (From Doershuk CF, Lough MD. *In*: Lough MD, Doershuk CF, Stern RC [ed]: Pediatric Respiratory Therapy. Chicago, Year Book Medical Publishers, 1974.)

raphy. Restrictive disease also decreases *vital capacity* (VC), which is the total amount of gas that can be inhaled after a forced expiration. VC can be measured by spirometry and is commonly used at the bedside to assess the progression of neuromuscular disorders. Obstructive diseases produce gas trapping and thus increase residual volume and *functional residual capacity* (FRC, the volume contained in the lungs at the end of a tidal expiration), particularly when these measurements are considered with respect to TLC.

Measurements of elastic recoil and respiratory compliance are poorly standardized in children, and their interpretation requires knowledge of the lung volume at which the measurements were made. Similarly, measurements of airway and total respiratory resistance are technically cumbersome and difficult to interpret because of the large and variable contribution of the upper airway (nose, pharynx, and larynx) and lung and chest wall tissues to these resistances.

Airway obstruction is more frequently evaluated from determinations of gas flow in the course of a forced expiratory maneuver. The *peak expiratory flow* is reduced in advanced obstructive disease. The wide availability of simple devices that perform this measurement at the bedside makes it useful for assessing children with airway obstruction. The clinician must remember, however, that evaluation of peak flows requires a voluntary effort and that peak flows may not be altered when the obstruction is moderate or mild. Other gas flow measurements require that the child inhale to TLC and then exhale as far and as fast as possible for several seconds. Cooperation and good muscle strength are therefore necessary for the measurements to be reproducible. The *forced expiratory volume in 1 sec* (FEV_1) correlates well with the severity of most obstructive diseases. The *maximal midexpiratory flow rate*, the average flow over the middle 50% of the forced vital capacity, is a more reliable indicator of mild airway obstruction. Its sensitivity to changes in residual volume and vital capacity, however, limits its use in children with more severe disease. The construction of flow-volume relationships during the forced vital capacity maneuvers overcomes some of these limitations by expressing the expiratory flows as a function of lung volume.

The *ventilation/perfusion ratio* can be examined in children with the help of radionuclide tracers that are inhaled simultaneously in a gas mixture and injected intravenously as albumin aggregates. This technique is useful to assess gross decreases in pulmonary perfusion (e.g., when pulmonary embolism is suspected) or in the prospective evaluation of surgical procedures such as lobectomy. *Alveolar-capillary diffusion of oxygen* is often estimated by measurement of carbon monoxide diffusion capacity. This measurement requires cooperation, and its interpretation is complicated by other factors such as lung size, pulmonary blood volume, hemoglobin concentration, and ventilation/perfusion ratios.

Exercise testing is a more direct approach to detect diffusion impairment as well as other forms of respiratory disease. Measurements of heart and respiratory rate, minute ventilation, oxygen consumption, carbon dioxide production, and arterial blood gases during incremental exercise loads often provide invaluable information about the functional nature of the disease. Often a simple assessment of the patient's exercise tolerance in conjunction with other more static forms of respiratory function testing may allow a distinction between respiratory and nonrespiratory disease in children.

The *sleep state* has an important influence on respiratory function, particularly in the newborn and young infant. Polysomonographic studies are often helpful when abnormalities of central respiratory control, muscular disorders, or respiratory complications from gastroesophageal reflux are suspected. These studies, which usually include the simultaneous assessment of ventilatory effort, airway gas flow, gas exchange, and sleep state, are also useful in the diagnosis and management of nocturnal hypoxemia and hypercarbia in children with chronic respiratory disease.

Bryan AC, Wohl MEB: Respiratory mechanics in children. *In*: Macklem PT, Mead J (eds): The Respiratory System: Mechanics of Breathing. Bethesda, American Physiological Society, 1986, pp 179–191.

Hodson AW, Alden ER, Woodrum DE: Gas exchange in the developing lung. *In*: Hodson WA (ed): Development of the Lung. New York, Marcel Dekker, 1977.

McBride JT, Wohl MEB: Pulmonary function tests. Pediatr Clin North Am 26:537, 1979.

Weibel ER: The Pathway for Oxygen: Structure and Function in the Mammalian Respiratory System. Cambridge, MA, Harvard University Press, 1984.

14.3 REGULATION OF RESPIRATION

Pediatricians need to be familiar with the general principles of the regulation of respiration for at least three reasons: (1) clinical situations involving one or more elements of the respiratory control system are very prevalent, especially in critically ill patients (e.g., apnea, upper airway obstruction, severe asthma, hypoventilation and heart failure, or hypoxemia from various causes); (2) transition from fetal to neonatal life is an extremely complex process during which there are major changes in almost every aspect of respiratory control; (3) understanding of the neural control of respiration is likely to increase significantly in the next 1–2 decades because of the explosive advances in understanding brain function in general.

THE RESPIRATORY CONTROL SYSTEM IS A NEGATIVE FEEDBACK SYSTEM WITH A CENTRAL CONTROLLER. The overall aim of the respiratory feedback system is to keep blood gas homeostasis in a normal range in the most economical way, from an energy consumption and mechanical standpoint. To accomplish this, the feedback system makes use of both an afferent limb and an efferent limb. The afferent limb is made up of tissues (e.g., the airways) that have receptor endings and can send information to the central controller about certain functional parameters, such as the magnitude of stretch of the airways. The carotid bodies that inform the central controller of the status of O_2 represent another important part of the afferent system. Both airway and carotid body sensors have a way to compare signals in order to note differences and feed this information to the central nervous system. The efferent loop is the part of the feedback system that is responsible for the execution of the decision made centrally (i.e., the respiratory muscles and their innervation). There are many muscles of respiration, and the intercostal muscles and the diaphragm are only two of them. Activity and timing of the airway muscles, as is seen later, are very crucial in determining airway resistance and, therefore, the magnitude of ventilation.

The term "negative" in this concept refers to the fact that the controller attempts to rectify the deviation from normality. If CO_2 increases, the output of the controller is increased in an attempt to increase ventilation and decrease CO_2.

The central controller has two functions that are linked: (1) integration of afferent information; and (2) generation and maintenance of respiration. These tasks are believed to be in anatomically different locations, but it is not known in precise mechanistic terms how each function takes place. For example, it is not known how the central generation of respiration takes place, where it is located, or how incoming information is integrated. The respiratory controller may be a group of neurons that either form an *emergent network* or are *endogenous* or *conditional bursters*. In the first case, respiratory neurons would not have special properties (e.g., bursting properties) that would make their membrane potential oscillate. Rather, the output of the network that they form would oscillate because of the special *interconnections* and synaptic interactions among these respiratory neurons. In the second case, similar to that of the heart, the respiratory neurons would have special properties that make them *individually* "burst" or oscillate (pacemaker), even if they are disconnected from any other neurons (endogenous burster). A conditional burster is a neuron that oscillates only when exposed to certain chemicals (e.g., neurotransmitters). The properties of the neurons also are very critical in shaping the output of the network itself, irrespective of the properties of the respiratory controller. Therefore, the study of cellular, synaptic, and network properties of neurons in the brain stem is anticipated to yield information needed to understand how the respiratory vital center paces diaphragmatic and other muscular efforts.

AFFERENT INFORMATION PLAYS AN IMPORTANT ROLE IN BREATHING. A multitude of afferent messages converge on the brain stem at any one time. Chemoreceptors and mechanoreceptors in the larynx and upper airways sense stretch, air temperature, and chemical changes over the mucosa and relay this information to the brain stem. Afferent impulses from these areas travel through the superior laryngeal nerve and the tenth cranial nerve (vagus). The superior laryngeal nerve joins and becomes part of the vagal trunk at the nodose ganglion. Changes in O_2 or CO_2 tensions are sensed at the carotid and aortic bodies, and afferent impulses travel through the carotid and aortic sinus nerves. Thermal or metabolic changes are sensed by skin or mucosal receptors or by hypothalamic neurons and are carried through spinal or central tracts to the brain stem for integrative purposes. Furthermore, afferent information to the brain stem need not be only formulated and sensed by the peripheral nervous system. As examples: (1) the major sensors of CO_2 in the body lie on the ventral surface of the medulla oblongata and therefore the main feedback about CO_2 levels comes from the brain stem itself, and (2) emotions and changes in mood that result from central nervous system processing in the limbic system influence respiration through pathways connecting higher brain centers to the brain stem.

The afferent information is probably not a prerequisite for generating and maintaining respiration. When the brain stem and spinal cord are removed from the body and maintained in vitro, rhythmic phrenic activity can be detected and measured for hours. Other experiments in vivo in which several sensory systems are blocked simultaneously (with local anesthesia to block vagal afferents, 100% O_2 to eliminate carotid discharges, sleep to eliminate wakeful stimuli, and the chronic administration of diuretics to alkalinize the blood) indicate that afferent information is not necessary to stimulate an inherent respiratory rhythm in brain stem respiratory networks. However, both in vitro and in vivo studies also demonstrate that, in the absence of afferent information, the inherent rhythm of the central generator (respiratory frequency) is slow and chemoreceptor afferents play an important part in modulating respiration and rhythmic behavior.

The neonate is more exquisitely sensitive to afferent input than the adult. Laryngeal reflexes are extremely potent in inhibiting respiration in the newborn. Aspiration and stimulation of laryngeal chemoreceptors in premature infants (who lack the ability of a strong cough), especially when these infants are anemic, hypoglycemic, or even during normal sleep, can cause life-threatening respiratory events. Similarly, when neonatal animals are deprived of carotid bodies, not only are prolonged and severe apneic episodes induced but also this can prove fatal in a large percentage of these animals.

CENTRAL INTEGRATION AND PROCESSING IN THE BRAIN STEM IS HIERARCHICAL. Respiratory muscles can be recruited to perform different tasks at different times. For example, the diaphragm and some abdominal muscles are activated not only during tidal breathing but also during expulsive maneuvers such as coughing and straining. These actions and others are recruited when an individual jumps to splint the thorax and abdomen. In other conditions, respiratory muscles can be totally inhibited. For example, when delivering a speech, CO_2 responsiveness is decreased substantially because speech muscles are recruited mostly at the expense of other respiratory muscles. Bottle or breast-feeding in the young is sometimes associated with a reduction in ventilation and a drop in arterial P_{O_2} because of partial inhibition of respiratory muscles and breathing efforts. Presented with a number of neurophysiologic signals (representing options about various needs), the central controller can enhance or reduce the response to certain stimuli. Therefore, there is a hierarchy that is used by brain stem networks for determining the response of the respiratory system at any one time.

Changes in the state of consciousness modulate the ability of the brain stem to respond to afferent stimuli. For example, trigeminal afferent impulses are less inhibited by cortical influences during quiet sleep than during rapid eye movement (REM) sleep or wakefulness. Thus, the effect of trigeminal stimulation on respiration is more pronounced in quiet sleep. Similarly, age is very important. The response of the brain stem to stimuli varies with maturation and thus with cortical input to brain stem structures.

RESPIRATORY MUSCLES AND CHEST WALL PROPERTIES (e.g., EFFERENT ORGAN) UNDERGO POSTNATAL MATURATION. Effective ventilation requires *coordinated interaction* between the respiratory muscles of the chest wall (including the diaphragm and intercostals) and those of the upper airway (including the pharynx and the larynx) under various conditions of altered respiratory drive. In infants, a specific sequential pattern of nerve and muscle activation occurs so that some upper airway muscles contract prior to and during the early part of inspiratory flow: the genioglossus muscle contracts, moving the tongue forward, which prevents pharyngeal obstruction; the vocal cords abduct, reducing inspiratory laryngeal resistance. Laryngeal muscles also modulate expiratory flow and thus may influence lung volume. Imbalance of pharyngeal and diaphragmatic activities or their responses to chemoreceptor or mechanoreceptor stimulation may contribute to obstructive apnea in infants and children.

Because the *respiratory muscles* are responsible for executing central neural responses and since muscle and chest wall properties change with age in early life, it is likely that neural responses can be influenced by pump properties. Thus, it is important to consider the maturational changes of respiratory muscles and chest wall. One of the important maturational aspects of innervation of respiratory muscles (e.g., in skeletal muscles) is its pattern of innervation. In the adult, one muscle fiber is innervated by one motoneuron. Therefore, if a motoneuron innervates certain muscle fibers (e.g., about 200 muscle fibers in the case of the diaphragm), these fibers do not receive innervation from any other motoneuron. In the newborn, however, each fiber is innervated by two or more motoneurons, and the axons of different motoneurons can synapse on the same muscle fiber, thus the term **polyneuronal innervation**. Synapse elimination takes place postnatally and in the case of the diaphragm, the adult type of innervation is reached by several weeks of age depending on the animal species. The time course of polyneuronal innervation of the diaphragm in the human newborn is not known.

The neuromuscular junctional folds, postsynaptic membranes, and acetylcholine receptors and metabolism undergo major postnatal maturational changes. The acetylcholine quantal content per end plate potential is lower in the newborn than in the adult rat diaphragm. The newborn diaphragm is also more susceptible to neuromuscular transmission failure than the adult, especially at higher frequencies of stimulation. Whether this is the result of differences in acetylcholine metabolism between the newborn and the adult or whether this is related to the neuromuscular junction itself is not known.

In addition to an increase in cross-sectional area and muscle mass, *muscle fiber types* in the diaphragm change as a function of gestational and postnatal age. However, there are conflicting reports about the composition of fiber types in young muscle, and it is not known whether human newborn muscles are more oxidative or fatigue resistant than those of the adult. The sarcoplasmic reticulum of the premature diaphragm is, however, underdeveloped compared with that of the adult. This is one major reason for the delay in the release and uptake of Ca^{2+}, which may have functional significance. The poorly developed sarcoplasmic reticulum in the newborn causes increased contraction and relaxation time in neonatal muscle fibers. This increased relaxation time may be an important factor in impeding blood flow, limiting oxidative metabolism, when the muscle is under a load.

The *chest wall* in newborn infants is highly compliant. Because of this and because young infants spend a large proportion of time in REM sleep during which the intercostal muscles are inhibited, there is little splinting of the chest wall for diaphragmatic action. Therefore, with every breath in supine infants (especially in REM sleep), the chest wall is sucked in paradoxically at a time when the abdomen expands. This creates an additional load on the respiratory system and results in a higher work of breathing per minute ventilation in the infant than in the adult. Some think that this may be an important reason for the newborn's susceptibility to muscle fatigue and respiratory failure.

THE NEWBORN AND YOUNG RESPOND DIFFERENTLY TO STIMULI COMPARED WITH THE MATURE SUBJECT. The young child and neonate respond to various stimuli in a different way compared with the adult. In response to low O_2, the newborn does not sustain an increase in ventilation, and often ventilation decreases to below baseline levels. CO_2 levels do not increase at a time when ventilation is decreasing, suggesting that ventilation is matching metabolic needs. This neonatal response to low O_2 can be considered as an intermediate response between those of the fetus and the adult; the fetus shuts off all respiratory efforts in response to O_2 deprivation, and the adult hyperventilates as long as the stimulus is present. The mechanism(s) for the lack of sustained increase in ventilation during hypoxia in the newborn is not well understood. In addition to differences in metabolic rate during hypoxemia among neonates and adults, changes in the mechanical properties of the lung and airways, maturation of carotid chemoreceptors, and alterations in the cellular and membrane properties of central neurons have all been proposed as potential individual or combined mechanisms.

CO_2 response is also reduced in the young. Whether this is a reflection of an inherent difference in their sensitivity or the result of differences in mechanical function is not known.

Although alterations in responsiveness can be secondary to a number of differences between the young and the mature organism, the central neuronal changes with maturation seem especially important. For example, the soma of lumbar and phrenic motoneurons increases with age, and their input resistance (or inverse of membrane conductance) decreases with age. The decrease in input resistance results in major part from the increase in soma size, but other mechanisms such as a change in the geometry of the dendrites and their outgrowth, a change in the number of ion channels per surface area, and an increase in the number of synapses onto motoneurons cannot be ruled out. Axonal velocity also increases with age, and action potentials of phrenic and hypoglossal motoneurons decrease in duration. There are also major maturational changes in active cellular properties in some motoneurons or premotor neurons. For example, with increasing postnatal age, neurons in the area of the nucleus tractus solitarius develop cellular properties important for repetitive firing. Changes in neuronal properties could play an important role in the integrative abilities of neuronal cells and, therefore, in their response to stimulation.

CLINICAL IMPLICATIONS

Apnea (See also Sec. 9.31). Although there are numerous studies on apnea in the newborn and adult human, there are also a number of controversies. The length of the respiratory pause that has been defined as apnea has varied (see Sec. 9.31).

Apnea can be defined statistically as a respiratory pause that exceeds 3 standard deviations of the mean breath time for an infant or a child at any particular age. This definition requires data from a population of infants at that age, lacks physiologic value, and does not differentiate between relatively shorter or longer respiratory pauses. Alternatively, the definition of apnea may be based on the fact that respiratory pauses are associated with cardiovascular or neurophysiologic changes. Such definition relies completely on the functional assessment of pauses and is, therefore, more relevant clinically. Because infants have higher O_2 consumption (per unit weight) than the adult and relatively smaller lung volume and O_2 stores, it is possible that short (e.g., seconds) respiratory pauses that may not be clinically important in the adult can present serious consequences in the very young or premature.

Independent of age group, respiratory pauses are more prevalent during sleep than during wakefulness. The frequency and duration of respiratory pauses depend on sleep state in human infants. Respiratory pauses are more frequent and shorter in REM than in quiet sleep and more frequent in the younger infants than in older infants.

Although there is a controversy regarding the pathogenesis

of respiratory pauses, there is a consensus about certain observations. Normal full-term infants, children, and adult humans exhibit respiratory pauses during sleep. Paradoxically, some believe that the presence of respiratory pauses and breathing irregularity is a "healthy" sign and that the complete absence of such pauses may be indicative of abnormalities. However, prolonged apneas can be life-threatening. The pathogenesis of these apneas may relate to the clinical condition of the patient at the time of the apneas, associated cardiovascular (systemic or pulmonary) changes, the chronicity of the clinical condition, the perinatal history, and whether the etiology is central or peripheral. Prolonged apneic spells require therapy and, optimally, treatment should be targeted to the underlying pathophysiology. A septic infant should be treated for the infection and a seizing infant with antiepileptic medication. The child with congenital hypoventilation syndrome (or Ondine curse), in the absence of pharmacologic therapy, should be placed on mechanical ventilation until properly paced with phrenic stimulators (Sec. 14.102).

Upper Airway Obstruction. Upper airway obstruction (UAO) during sleep is recognized with increasing frequency in children. In contrast to adults with UAO in whom the etiology of obstruction often remains obscure, many children have anatomic abnormalities. A common cause of UAO in children is tonsillar and adenoidal hypertrophy owing to repeated upper respiratory infections. Other associated abnormalities include craniofacial malformations, micrognathia, and muscular hypotonia. The usual site of obstruction in UAO in both infants and adults is the oropharynx, between the posterior pharyngeal wall, the soft palate, and the genioglossus. During sleep (especially REM sleep), upper airway muscles, including those of the oropharynx, lose tone, and trigger an episode of UAO.

Snoring with recurrent periods of respiratory pauses commonly occurs during sleep in children. Parents frequently describe periods of increasing chest wall movement without air flow and with cyanosis. These pauses are usually terminated by a loud snort and arousal. Disturbed sleeping habits and arousals from sleep at night are associated with UAO. In older children the syndrome may include failure to thrive, developmental delay, and poor school performance. Hypertension and daytime hypersomnolence are less common abnormalities in children than in adults. Children with longstanding signs and symptoms of UAO during sleep can present with right ventricular failure and cor pulmonale. The treatment, therefore, varies but should be targeted primarily at the underlying cause of obstruction. Some of these infants will benefit by tonsillectomy and adenoidectomy or, if obese, by a reduction in weight. In some refractory children, successful treatment has included continuous positive airway pressure applied through the nose. In infants in which other means have failed, pharmacologic interventions (respiratory stimulants) may prove worthwhile before resorting to tracheostomy.

14.4 DEFENSE MECHANISMS OF THE LUNG

The *upper airway* includes the nose, paranasal sinuses, and pharynx; the *lower airway* consists of the remainder of the system from the larynx peripherally. The nose has a relatively large surface area lined with a richly vascular, ciliated epithelium, and by the time the air column reaches the bifurcation of the trachea, up to 75% of the warming and humidification of the inspired air has occurred. During exhalation, heat and moisture are removed from the air stream. Gross filtering of particles larger than 10–15 μm is achieved by the coarse hairs at the nasal orifices, and most inhaled particles larger than 5 μm are impacted on the nasal surface.

Because the larynx is relatively narrow and ringed with cartilage, it is relatively susceptible to obstruction in young children, particularly by inflammation, because the resultant swelling of tissues rapidly encroaches on the lumen and produces inspiratory stridor.

The trachea and bronchi are lined with pseudostratified, ciliated, columnar epithelium and occasional goblet cells. Mucous glands occupy approximately one third the thickness of the airway wall and for the most part lie between the epithelial surface and the cartilage. The trachea is supported by incomplete rings of cartilage with a muscular membrane posteriorly. Irregular plates of cartilage support the bronchi, especially at bifurcations. These diminish and finally disappear in the smallest bronchi. The goblet cells and principally the submucosal glands secrete the mucous layer, which is 2–5 μm in depth and rests on the tips of the cilia. Each ciliated cell has about 275 cilia; movement results from action by microtubules within each cilium. The cilia beat within a periciliary fluid layer at about 1,000 beats/min, moving the mucous blanket toward the pharynx at a rate of approximately 10 mm/min in the trachea. In the respiratory portion of the lung the surface cells gradually become cuboidal and then flat; ciliated cells and goblet cells are usually absent.

The final 25% of the warming and humidifying of the inspired air stream occurs in the trachea and large bronchi. Failure of humidification permits dry air to reach more distal airways. Particles 1–5 μm in size precipitate out on the tracheobronchial mucous blanket so that only particles of 1 μm or less reach the respiratory bronchioles and air spaces, where some may deposit and many will be exhaled.

Respiratory tract secretions are derived primarily from mucous (glycoproteins) and serous cells of the submucosal glands that empty onto the surface epithelium; from goblet cells and Clara cells, the special secreting cells in the surface epithelium of bronchi and bronchioles, respectively; from transudation from the vascular space; and from alveolar fluid, which contributes most of the phospholipid found in tracheobronchial mucus. This mucus is about 95% water.

Beyond infancy, collateral alveolar ventilation can increasingly occur with development of the *pores of Kohn* between alveoli, which provide a means for gas to pass from one lobule to another, perhaps even between segments of lung. Bronchiolar-alveolar communications, known as the *canals of Lambert*, are also found. These anatomic connections may be helpful in preventing or delaying atelectasis.

The defenses of the respiratory system that protect the lung include the filtering of particles, the warming and humidification of inspired air, and the absorption of noxious fumes and gases by the vascular upper airway. The temporary cessation of breathing, reflexly shallow breathing, laryngospasm, or even bronchospasm limits the depth and amount of penetration of foreign matter. Spasm or decreased breathing can provide only brief protection. Aspiration of food, secretions, and foreign bodies are prevented by swallowing and closure of the epiglottis. The respiratory tract distal to the larynx is normally sterile.

CLEARANCE OF PARTICLES. Particles deposited in conducting airways are cleared within hours by the mucociliary mechanism, while clearance of those reaching the alveoli may take several days to months. The latter may be phagocytized by alveolar macrophages and removed from lungs by the mucociliary system or carried into the interstitium for clearance by the lymphocytes into regional nodes or the blood.

Some particles penetrate into the interstitium without phagocytosis. Mucociliary clearance may be aided by cough, which provides an effective means by propelling excess mucus up the airways at pressures of up to 300 mm Hg and at flows of up to 5–6 L/sec. Mucus raised by the cough mechanism is usually swallowed by young children but may be expectorated.

DEFENSE AGAINST MICROBIAL AGENTS. Phagocytosis and mucociliary clearance may not be sufficient protection from living agents, such as bacteria and viruses. Additional factors include cellular killing of organisms and immune responses to assist in the phagocytosis-killing process. Alveolar and interstitial macrophages, derived from monocytes, are an essential component of the defense system of the lung. The engulfment and killing of living particles by these macrophages may be enhanced by opsonins or by small lymphocytes. The principal antibody in respiratory secretions is secretory immunoglobulin A (IgA), which is produced by plasma cells in the submucosa of the airways (see Sec. 11.1). Two molecules of IgA combine with a polypeptide (secretory component) produced by the respiratory epithelium to yield secretory IgA, which is highly resistant to digestion by proteolytic enzymes released after lysis of bacteria and dead cells. IgA can neutralize certain viruses and toxins and help in the lysis of bacteria. IgA may also prevent antigenic substances from penetrating the epithelial surfaces. Pulmonary secretory IgA reaches adult levels in the first month of life. IgG and IgM are also found in the secretions when lung inflammation occurs.

Lysozyme, lactoferrin, and interferon may also play a defense role in respiratory secretions. In addition a small fraction of the antibodies of the respiratory surface is made up of immunoglobulin E (IgE), which plays an important role in allergic reactions (Sec. 11.34).

IMPAIRED DEFENSE MECHANISMS. The phagocytic ability of alveolar macrophages and, in most cases, the mucociliary mechanism can be impaired by ethanol ingestion, cigarette smoke, hypoxemia, starvation, chilling, corticosteroids, nitrogen dioxide, ozone, increased oxygen concentration, narcotics, and some anesthetic gases. The antibacterial killing capacity of the macrophages can be decreased by acidosis, azotemia, and recent acute viral infections, especially rubeola and influenza. Beryllium and asbestos, organic dust from cotton and sugar cane, and gases such as sulfur, nitrogen dioxide, ozone, chlorine, ammonia, and cigarette smoke are toxic to epithelial cells.

Mucociliary clearance can be reduced by hypothermia, hyperthermia, morphine, codeine, and hypothyroidism. Inhalation of dry gas by mouthbreathing during periods of nasal obstruction, after placement of a tracheostomy, or during use of poorly humidified oxygen results in drying of the mucous membrane and slowing of the ciliary beat. Cold air may irritate the tracheobronchial tree.

Damage to the respiratory epithelium may be reversible with rhinitis, sinusitis, bronchitis, bronchiolitis, acute respiratory infections associated with high levels of air pollution, and the epithelial shedding that can occur in asthma, or with some irritants, bronchospasm, edema, congestion, and perhaps mild surface ulceration. However, severe ulceration, bronchiectasis, bronchiolectasis, squamous cell metaplasia, and fibrosis represent serious injury and permanent impairment of the normal clearance mechanism. Other events that can adversely affect the lung include hyperventilation, alveolar hypoxia, pulmonary thromboembolism, pulmonary edema, hypersensitivity reactions, and certain drugs such as salicylates.

Green GM: In defense of the lung. Am Rev Respir Dis 102:691, 1970.
Newhouse MT, Bienenstock J: Respiratory tract defense mechanisms. *In:* Baum GL, Wolinsky E (eds): Textbook of Pulmonary Diseases. Boston, Little, Brown, 1989, pp 21–47.
Proctor DF: The upper airways. I: Nasal physiology and defense of the lungs. Am Rev Respir Dis 115:97, 1977.

14.5 METABOLIC FUNCTIONS OF THE LUNG

The lung contains more than 40 separate cell types. Among these heterogeneous cells, the type I and II pneumocytes, alveolar macrophage, and Clara cell are unique to the lung. The lung can synthesize lipids and proteins, including glycoproteins, secretory antibodies, interferon, proteolytic and fibrinolytic enzymes and activators, collagen, and elastin. Tissue factors such as thromboplastin are found in higher concentration in the lung than in any other organ. Megakaryocytes are concentrated in the lung.

Since the lung has the only capillary bed through which the entire blood flow must pass in the normal state, the pulmonary capillary circulation is ideally positioned to control circulating vasoactive hormones. Angiotensin II, up to 50 times more active than its precursor, is converted from angiotensin I during one passage through the pulmonary circulation. Some vasoactive materials, including serotonin; bradykinin; ATP; and prostaglandins E_1, E_2, and F_2, are almost completely removed or inactivated by one passage through the pulmonary circulation, whereas others, such as epinephrine, prostaglandin A_1 and A_2, angiotensin II, and vasopressin, may be minimally affected. Norepinephrine and histamine are taken up to a moderate degree. Failure of inactivation or periodic release of substances such as serotonin, bradykinin, histamine, slow-reacting substance of anaphylaxis (SRS-A), eosinophil chemotactic factor, platelet aggregation factor, endocrine substances, and so forth, may be important in the pathogenesis of some pulmonary disease or as a mediator of secondary effects.

GABRIEL G. HADDAD
J. PÉREZ FONTÁN

Fishman AP: Non-respiratory functions of the lung. Chest 72:84, 1977.
Fishman AP, Pietra GG: Handling of bioactive materials by the lung. N Engl J Med 291:884, 1974.
Said SI: The lung as a metabolic organ. N Engl J Med 279:1330, 1968.
Said SI: The lung in relation to vasoactive hormones. Fed Proc 32:1972, 1973.

14.6 DIAGNOSTIC PROCEDURES IN PULMONARY MEDICINE

14.7 RADIOGRAPHIC TECHNIQUES

See also Sec. 6.56.

CHEST ROENTGENOGRAMS. A posteroanterior and a lateral view, upright and at full inspiration, should be obtained in most circumstances. Films taken during expiration are often misinterpreted, but a comparison of expiratory and inspiratory films may reveal a mediastinal shift, which is helpful in evaluating bronchial obstruction (e.g., with a foreign body). Decubitus films are indicated if pleural fluid is suspected. Recumbent films may be difficult to interpret in the presence of free fluid, either within the pleural space or in a cavity. Oblique views may be helpful when evaluating the hilum and the area behind the heart, whereas the apices are best seen in a lordotic view.

COMPUTED TOMOGRAPHY. The technique of computed tomography (CT) can be useful in delineating internal structures and their relationships in greater detail than standard roentgenograms can, but it is more expensive and involves higher radiation exposure than plain films and should be used only when necessary. Because relatively long exposures are required, sedation may be needed.

UPPER AIRWAY FILMS. A lateral view of the neck can yield invaluable information about upper airway obstruction and particularly about the conditions of the retropharyngeal space, supraglottic area, and subglottic space (the latter should also be viewed in a posteroanterior projection). Knowing the phase of respiration during which the film was taken is often essential for accurate interpretation. Patients with suspected obstruction must not be sent unattended to the radiology department.

XEROGRAPHY. This gives exceptionally good soft tissue detail but requires much higher doses of radiation (especially to the thyroid) and should not be used routinely.

SINUS, NASAL FILMS. Roentgenographic examination of the sinuses is indicated when sinus disease is suspected. Because of the small size and slow development of the frontal and maxillary sinus cavities in children, transillumination is not as successful in documenting sinus disease as are roentgenograms. The need for examining the nasal passages in children is unusual and occurs most often when the neonate presents with obstruction or when tumor or occult foreign body is suspected.

FLUOROSCOPY. Fluoroscopy is especially useful for evaluating stridor and abnormal movement of the diaphragm or mediastinum. Many procedures, such as needle aspiration or biopsy of a peripheral lesion, are also best accomplished with the aid of fluoroscopy. Video tape recording, which does not increase radiation exposure, may allow detailed study, through "replay" capability, during a brief exposure to fluoroscopy.

CONTRAST STUDIES

Barium Swallow. This study is indicated in evaluating patients with recurrent pneumonia, persistent coughs of undetermined etiology, stridor, or persistent wheezing. It should be done with fluoroscopy and spot films. In the search for an "H" type of tracheoesophageal fistula, a simple barium swallow is often inadequate; the barium may have to be injected through catheters placed at several locations in the esophagus. If esophageal atresia is suspected, no more than 0.5 mL of barium should be injected into the esophagus through a soft catheter, carefully avoiding aspiration into the trachea. Many experts do not recommend contrast studies when esophageal atresia is suspected.

Bronchograms. Smaller bronchi may be delineated by instilling a contrast material directly into the airway. In small children bronchograms are usually performed through an endotracheal tube under general anesthesia. In older children and adults sedation and topical anesthesia may be sufficient. The smallest amount of contrast material necessary to coat (not fill) the airways is placed into the airways with a catheter passed transnasally, through the endotracheal tube or through a fiberoptic bronchoscope. The procedure should be performed with fluoroscopy so that the contrast material can be placed selectively in the areas and in the quantity desired. In general, bronchograms are indicated only when pulmonary surgery may be considered. Specific indications include recurrent hemoptysis, recurrent pneumonia in the same area, chronic productive cough with persistent localized physical findings, and previously demonstrated bronchiectasis unresponsive to therapy.

Pulmonary Arteriograms. These studies allow detailed evaluation of the pulmonary vasculature and are helpful in diagnosing congenital anomalies, such as lobar agenesis, unilateral hyperlucent lung, and vascular rings, and are sometimes useful in evaluating solid or cystic lesions.

Aortograms. Thoracic aortograms demonstrate the aortic arch and its major vessels, and the systemic (bronchial) pulmonary circulation. They are useful to evaluate vascular rings and suspected pulmonary sequestration. Although most hemoptysis is from the bronchial arteries, bronchial arteriography is seldom helpful in diagnosing or treating intrapulmonary bleeding in children.

Pneumoperitoneum, Pneumothorax. In selected situations, such as in the evaluation of diaphragmatic eventration, it may be advantageous to inject a small amount of air into the pleural or peritoneal cavity, outlining the limits of the diaphragm or pleural surfaces by air contrast. Rapidly absorbed, the air causes no functional impairment.

Radionuclide Lung Scans. The usual scan uses intravenous injection of material (macroaggregated human serum albumin) that will be trapped in the pulmonary capillary bed. The distribution of radioactivity, proportional to *pulmonary capillary blood flow,* is useful in evaluating pulmonary embolism and congenital cardiovascular and pulmonary defects. Acute changes in the distribution of pulmonary perfusion may reflect alterations of pulmonary ventilation.

The distribution of *pulmonary ventilation* may be determined by scanning following the inhalation of a radioactive gas such as ^{133}Xe. After the intravenous injection of ^{133}Xe dissolved in saline, both pulmonary perfusion and ventilation can be evaluated by continuous recording of the rate of appearance and disappearance of the xenon over the lung. Appearance of xenon early after injection is a measure of perfusion, whereas the rate of washout during breathing is a measure of ventilation.

14.8 ENDOSCOPY

LARYNGOSCOPY. Inspection of the glottis is often necessary when evaluating stridor and local abnormalities. In infants and small children, direct laryngoscopy is usually necessary and requires general anesthesia. While useful in older children and adults, indirect (mirror) laryngoscopy is rarely possible in infants. Direct laryngoscopy can also be done with topical anesthesia and mild sedation by passing a small flexible fiberoptic bronchoscope through the nose, allowing the glottis to be seen without the anatomic distortion that a laryngoscope blade sometimes introduces. This newer technique is also more comfortable for the patient and is especially useful for evaluating the dynamics of the larynx and upper airway.

BRONCHOSCOPY. Indications for bronchoscopy include the evaluation of recurrent pneumonia or atelectasis, the possible presence of foreign bodies, unexplained and persistent wheezes and infiltrates, hemoptysis, and suspected congenital anomalies or mass lesions. The bronchoscope is used for visual examination, for biopsy of mass lesions or for transbronchial lung biopsy, and for aspiration of secretions for culture and microscopic examination with or without bronchopulmonary lavage. Therapeutic applications include removal of foreign bodies and mucus plugs, as well as bronchial toilet and bronchopulmonary lavage. An open tube bronchoscope should be used for patients with massive pulmonary bleeding, for removal of foreign bodies, or for other operative procedures. The advantages of small flexible fiberoptic bronchoscopes include ease of insertion, greater peripheral range, a lower incidence of complications, and the elimination of the need for general anesthesia.

Complications of bronchoscopy depend on the instrument used and on the procedure performed. Transient hypoxia, cardiac arrhythmias, laryngospasm, and bronchospasm are most common, and infection, bleeding, pneumomediastinum, or pneumothorax may occur. After open tube bronchoscopy, the patient must be observed carefully for airway obstruction resulting from trauma to the subglottic space, a much less common occurrence after use of a flexible bronchoscope because of the instrument's relatively small size. Postbronchoscopy croup is treated with oxygen, mist, vasoconstrictor aerosols (racemic epinephrine), and corticosteroids as necessary.

14.9 THORACENTESIS

For diagnostic or therapeutic purposes, fluid may be removed from the pleural space by needle puncture. The site of puncture is chosen to maximize the yield of fluid and minimize the risk. The procedure is usually performed while the patient is in a sitting position. First, local anesthetic is injected using a 1.5-inch, No. 22 gauge needle passed just *above* the rib margin to avoid the neurovascular bundle. The pleura may be identified by "touch" or by withdrawing an initial volume of pleural fluid. Then a larger needle is inserted to the same depth through the inferior aspect of the intercostal space. It is often advantageous to pass a plastic catheter through the needle into the pleural space, then withdraw the needle. This allows the operator to move both catheter and patient, thus often collecting more fluid and reducing the possibility of puncture or laceration of the lung. Generally, as much fluid as possible should be withdrawn, and following the procedure, an *upright* chest roentgenogram should be obtained.

Complications of thoracentesis include infection, pneumothorax, and bleeding. Thoracentesis on the right may be complicated by puncture or laceration of the capsule of the liver, and on the left, by that of the capsule of the spleen. Specimens obtained should always be cultured, examined microscopically for evidence of bacterial infection, and evaluated for total protein and total differential cell counts. Lactic acid dehydrogenase, glucose, cholesterol, triglyceride (chylous), and amylase determinations may also be useful. If malignancy is suspected, cytologic examination is imperative.

Transudates result from mechanical factors influencing the rate of formation or reabsorption of pleural fluid and generally require no further diagnostic evaluation. *Exudates* result from inflammation or other disease of the pleural surface and underlying lung and require a more complete diagnostic evaluation. In general, transudates have a total protein of less than 3 g/dL or a ratio of pleural protein to serum protein under 0.5, a total leukocyte count of fewer than 2,000 with a predominance of mononuclear cells, and low lactate dehydrogenase levels. Exudates have high protein levels and a predominance of polymorphonuclear cells (although malignant or tuberculous effusions may have a higher percentage of mononuclear cells). Tuberculous effusions may have low glucose and high cholesterol content.

14.10 PERCUTANEOUS LUNG TAP

Using a technique very similar to that for thoracentesis, a percutaneous lung tap is the most direct method of obtaining bacteriologic specimens from the pulmonary parenchyma and is the only technique other than open lung biopsy not associated with at least some risk of contamination by oral flora. After local anesthesia, a No. 20 or 22 gauge, 1.5-inch needle attached to a 10-mL syringe containing approximately 1 mL of nonbacteriostatic sterile saline is inserted using aseptic technique through the inferior aspect of an intercostal space in the area of interest. The needle is rapidly advanced into the lung; the saline is injected and reaspirated; and the needle is withdrawn. These actions are performed as quickly as possible. This procedure usually yields a few drops of fluid from the lung, which should be cultured and examined microscopically.

Major indications for a lung tap are roentgenographic infiltrates of undetermined etiology, especially those unresponsive to therapy in immunosuppressed patients who are susceptible to unusual organisms. Complications are the same as for thoracentesis, but the incidence of pneumothorax is higher and somewhat dependent on the nature of the underlying disease process. In patients with poor pulmonary compliance, such as with pneumocystis pneumonia, the rate may approach 30%, with 5% requiring chest tubes. Bronchopulmonary lavage has replaced lung taps for the diagnosis of pneumonia in immunocompromised patients (Sec. 12.13)

14.11 LUNG BIOPSY

Lung biopsy may be the only way to establish a diagnosis, especially in protracted, noninfectious disease. In infants and small children an open surgical biopsy is the procedure of choice, and in expert hands it is associated with an extremely low morbidity. As well as ensuring that an adequate specimen can be obtained, the surgeon can inspect the lung surface and choose the site of biopsy. In older patients transbronchial biopsies can be performed using flexible forceps through an endotracheal tube or a bronchoscope, usually with fluoroscopic guidance. This technique is most appropriate when there are diffuse lung diseases such as pneumocystis pneumonia. However, because of the small specimens obtained, the diagnosis may be missed more easily than with an open biopsy.

14.12 TRANSILLUMINATION OF THE CHEST WALL

In infants up to at least 6 mo of age, a pneumothorax may often be diagnosed by transillumination of the chest wall using a fiberoptic light probe. Free air in the pleural space often results in an unusually large halo of light in the skin surrounding the probe. This test is unreliable in older patients or in those with subcutaneous emphysema.

14.13 MICROBIOLOGY

The specific diagnosis of infection in the lower respiratory tract depends on the proper handling of an adequate specimen obtained in an appropriate fashion. Nasopharyngeal or throat cultures are often used but may not correlate with cultures obtained by more direct techniques. Sputum specimens are preferred and are often obtained from patients who do not expectorate by deep throat swab immediately after coughing. Specimens may also be obtained directly from the tracheobronchial tree by nasotracheal aspiration (usually heavily contaminated), by transtracheal aspiration through the cricothyroid membrane (useful in adults and adolescents but hazardous in children), and in infants and children by a sterile catheter inserted into the trachea either during direct laryngoscopy or through an endotracheal tube. A specimen also may be obtained at bronchoscopy. A percutaneous lung tap or an open biopsy is the only way to obtain a specimen that is absolutely free of oral flora.

EXAMINATION OF SECRETIONS. A specimen obtained by direct expectoration is usually assumed to be of tracheobronchial origin, but often, especially in children, it is not from this source. The presence of alveolar macrophages—large, mononuclear cells—is the hallmark of tracheobronchial secretions. Both nasopharyngeal and tracheobronchial secretions may contain ciliated epithelial cells, which are more commonly found in sputum. Nasopharyngeal and oral secretions often contain large numbers of squamous epithelial cells. Sputum may contain both ciliated and squamous epithelial cells.

During sleep, mucociliary transport continually brings tracheobronchial secretions to the pharynx, where they are swallowed. An early morning gastric aspirate often contains material from the tracheobronchial tract that is suitable for smear and culture for acid-fast bacilli.

The absence of polymorphonuclear leukocytes in a Wright-stained smear of sputum containing adequate numbers of macrophages is significant evidence against a bacterial infectious process in the lower respiratory tract, assuming the patient has normal neutrophil counts and function. Eosinophils suggest allergic disease. Iron stains may reveal hemosiderin granules within macrophages, suggesting pulmonary hemosiderosis. Specimens should also be examined by Gram stain. Squamous epithelial cells are usually covered with bacteria, which should be ignored. Bacteria within or near macrophages and neutrophils are more significant. Viral pneumonia may be accompanied by intranuclear or cytoplasmic inclusion bodies visible on Wright-stained smears, and fungal forms may be identifiable on Gram or silver stains.

Sweat Testing

See Sec. 14.89.

14.14 BLOOD GAS ANALYSIS

An arterial blood gas analysis is probably the single most useful test of pulmonary function. If multiple samples are to be drawn over a relatively short time, an indwelling arterial line may be placed; constant perfusion with heparinized saline (1 unit/mL, 3–5 mL/hr) may prevent thrombus formation.

Arterial punctures are painful, often resulting in hyperventilation unless local anesthesia is used. The artery should be entered with a No. 21 or 23 gauge straight or scalp vein needle at an angle of approximately 45 degrees. The blood specimen is best collected anaerobically in a heparinized syringe containing only enough heparin solution to displace the air from the syringe. The syringe should be sealed, placed in ice, and carried to the laboratory for immediate analysis.

Arterialized capillary blood may be used if tissue perfusion is good and if great care is taken in collecting and handling the specimen. Under ideal conditions arterialized capillary blood correlates with arterial samples. Local vasodilation is produced in the finger, the heel, or the ear lobe by warming or by applying nitroglycerin or nicotinic acid cream. When the site has become flushed, blood is collected into a capillary tube from a free-flowing stab wound.

A pulse *oximeter* can continually measure peripheral oxygen saturation and usually correlates well with simultaneous arterial saturation. *Transcutaneous electrodes* can continuously monitor oxygen and carbon dioxide tension if tissue perfusion is adequate. *End-tidal* P_{CO_2} usually correlates well with arterial P_{CO_2} unless there is a very uneven distribution of ventilation.

Venous P_{CO_2} averages 6–8 mm Hg higher than arterial P_{CO_2}, and pH is slightly lower. Venous samples are more useful in managing chronic acid-base disturbances than in managing acute respiratory disease.

14.15 PULMONARY FUNCTION TESTING

See also Sec. 14.2.

Ventilation, perfusion, and gas exchange may all be quantified, but in clinical practice measurements of ventilation are the most commonly performed "pulmonary function test."

MEASUREMENT OF VENTILATORY FUNCTION. A *spirometer* is used to measure vital capacity (VC) and its subdivisions and expiratory (or inspiratory) flow rates (Fig. 14–4). A simple *manometer* can measure the maximal inspiratory and expiratory force a subject generates, normally at least 30 cm H_2O, which is useful in evaluating the neuromuscular component of ventilation. Expected normal values for VC, FRC, TLC, and RV are obtained from prediction equations based on body height.

Flow rates measured by spirometry usually include the volume expired in the first second (FEV_1) and the maximal midexpiratory flow rate (MMEF). More information results from a maximal expiratory flow-volume curve (MEFV), in which expiratory flow rate is plotted against expired lung volume (expressed in terms of either VC or TLC). Flow rates at lung volumes less than about 75% VC are relatively independent of effort. Expiratory flow rates at low lung volumes (less than 50% VC) are influenced much more by small airways than are flow rates at high lung volumes (FEV_1). The flow rate at 25% VC ($\dot{V}_{25}$) is a useful index of small airway function. Low flow rates at high lung volumes associated with normal flow at low lung volumes suggest upper airway obstruction (see Sec. 14.2).

Airway resistance (R_{AW}) is measured in a plethysmograph and is expressed as cm H_2O/L/sec. Alternatively, the reciprocal of R_{AW}, *airway conductance* (G_{AW}), may be used. Because airway resistance measurements vary with the lung volume at which they are taken, it is convenient to use specific airway resistance, SR_{AW} ($SR_{AW} = R_{AW} \times$ lung volume), which is nearly constant in subjects older than 6 yr (normally less than 7 sec/cm H_2O).

MEASUREMENT OF GAS EXCHANGE. The *diffusing capacity for carbon monoxide* (D_{LCO}) is measured by rebreathing from a container having a known initial concentration of CO or by using a single breath technique. Decreases in D_{LCO} reflect decreases in effective alveolar capillary surface area or decreases in diffusibility of the gas across the alveolar-capillary membrane. This test is rarely used in pediatrics because primary diffusion abnormalities are unusual in children. *Regional gas exchange* may be conveniently estimated with the perfusion/ventilation xenon scan (Sec. 14.7). Determining *arterial blood gases* will also disclose the effectiveness of alveolar gas exchange.

MEASUREMENT OF PERFUSION. Pulmonary blood flow may be measured by cardiac catheterization or by a technique employing the uptake of nitrous oxide. The distribution of blood flow may be studied in a pulmonary arteriogram or with radioisotope scans.

OTHER TESTS OF LUNG FUNCTION. Other available tests measure compliance, distribution of ventilation, dead space, elastic recoil, and closing volume. Pulmonary function tests performed before and after exercise may be useful in detecting exercise-induced bronchospasm. Sufficient exercise should be performed to elevate the pulse to 160–170/min for 5–6 min. Testing should be done 10 min after the end of the exercise period. There is poor correlation between the objective results of exercise testing and the subjective evaluation of exercise tolerance by patient or parent.

CLINICAL USE OF PULMONARY FUNCTION TESTING. Pulmonary function testing, while rarely resulting in an etiologic diagnosis, is helpful in defining the type of process (e.g., obstruction, restriction) and the degree of functional impairment in following the course and treatment of disease, and in estimating the prognosis. It is also useful in preoperative evaluation and in confirmation of functional impairment in patients having subjective complaints but a normal physical examination. In most patients with obstructive disease, a repeat test after administering a bronchodilator is warranted.

Most tests require some cooperation and understanding by the subject, and interpretation is greatly facilitated if the test conditions and the subject's behavior during the test are known. Accurate testing of children aged 3–6 yr requires great patience by the physician and training of the subject, whereas most children aged 6 yr or older can be tested reliably without excessive difficulty. Infants and young children may be studied by gas dilution and plethysmographic methods for measurement of FRC and R_{AW}, but sedation may be required.

ROBERT E. WOOD

Chernick V: Kendig's Disorders of the Respiratory Tract in Children, 5th ed. Philadelphia, WB Saunders, 1991.
Hughes WT, Buescher ES: Pediatric Procedures, 2nd ed. Philadelphia, WB Saunders, 1980.
Klein JO: Diagnostic lung puncture in the pneumonias of infants and children. Pediatrics 44:456, 1969.
Sackner MA (ed): Diagnostic Techniques in Pulmonary Disease. New York, Marcel Dekker, 1980.
Sperber M: Computerized Tomography of the Lung: Normal Anatomy and Most Common Disorders. Mount Kisco, NY, Futra Publishing Co, 1984.
Tellez DW, Galvis AG, Storgeon SA, et al: Dexamethasone in the prevention of post-extubation stridor in childhood. J Pediatr 118:289, 1991
Wood RE: Spelunking in the pediatric airways: Explorations with the flexible bronchoscope. Pediatr Clin North Am 31:785, 1984.

14.16 DISEASES OF THE RESPIRATORY SYSTEM

GENERAL CONSIDERATIONS

The patterns of respiratory tract disease in childhood are modified by age, sex, race, season, geography, and environmental and socioeconomic conditions. Intrauterine acquisition of viral infections, such as cytomegalovirus and herpes simplex virus, may result in neonatal pneumonia; cytomegalovirus, *Ureaplasma, Chlamydia trachomatis,* or group B streptococcal respiratory infection may be acquired during descent through the birth canal; immediately after birth, tuberculosis can be transmitted to the newborn, presenting after several weeks of life as a severe pneumonitis. Lung immaturity and other events related to the perinatal period predispose to hyaline membrane disease. Beyond the newborn period a lack of antibodies against common viral pathogens results in an increased incidence of respiratory tract infections that peaks at 1 yr of age. Pneumococcal lobar pneumonia is uncommon in small children, and pneumonia due to mycoplasmal infection is uncommon during the first 3–4 yr of life. The incidence of respiratory tract infection also peaks during child care or in the first 2–3 school years because of increased exposure to respiratory infections against which children have not yet developed specific immunity.

The anatomic distribution of respiratory tract disease may also change with age. Group A β-hemolytic streptococcal infections are commonly located in the nasopharynx in young children but in the tonsillar and lower pharyngeal areas of older children. A relatively short and open eustachian tube in infants and young children allows easy access of pharyngeal organisms to the middle ear cavity and is in part responsible for the higher incidence of otitis media in this group. The small size of bronchial and bronchiolar lumina in the first year of life is an important determinant in the incidence of bronchiolitis from respiratory syncytial and other virus infections. Aspiration during the first year of life most often causes lung changes in the upper lobes because during the feeding and postfeeding periods the infant is usually recumbent; thereafter most aspirations take place when children are upright, and the lung changes occur most often in the lower lobes.

The incidence or severity of respiratory tract disease based on sex varies very little: lower respiratory tract infections are slightly more common in boys than in girls under 6 yr of age; thereafter, the infection rates are equal. Noninfectious pulmonary diseases of children usually have an equal sex incidence, except for rare sex-linked recessive disorders such as chronic granulomatous disease. However, lung disease often progresses more rapidly and median survival is shorter in females with cystic fibrosis.

Seasonal variations in the incidence of respiratory tract infections and bronchial asthma are clinically important. The most common viral pathogens appear in epidemics during the winter and spring, whereas mycoplasmal infections occur more commonly in autumn and early winter. Pollen-related asthma symptoms occur most often in the spring, summer, and early fall; symptoms due to house dust and mold are more common when children are confined to the house during the cold weather; infection-related asthma also occurs more frequently during the cold weather months.

Certain fungal respiratory tract infections, such as coccidioidomycosis and histoplasmosis, have well-defined geographic distributions in the United States, but the incidence of common viral, mycoplasmal, and bacterial infections varies little with geographic location. At high altitudes, hypoxemia and cor pulmonale may play an earlier or more prominent role in the natural history of chronic lung disease, such as in cystic fibrosis. Children living in homes in which their mother or both parents smoke have more frequent respiratory tract infections. In addition, areas with high levels of air pollution predispose to frequent respiratory tract infections and episodes of asthma.

Although the frequency is not different, the severity of lower respiratory tract illness is generally less in middle class families than in lower class families, which may reflect differences in nutritional status or availability of medical care.

Finally, health disorders in other systems may influence the severity of acute respiratory tract diseases. For example, respiratory syncytial virus infections are particularly severe, not infrequently fatal, in small children with cyanotic congenital heart disease.

Chretien J, Holland W, Macklem P, et al: Acute respiratory infections in children. N Engl J Med 310:982, 1984.

Denny FW, Clyde WA: Acute lower respiratory tract infections in nonhospitalized children. J Pediatr 108:635, 1986.
Denny FW, Clyde WA, Collier AM, et al: The longitudinal approach to the pathogenesis of respiratory disease. Rev Infect Dis 1:1007, 1013, 1979.
Stagno S, Brasfield DM, Brown MB, et al: Infant pneumonitis with cytomegalovirus, chlamydia, pneumocystitis, and ureaplasma: A prospective study. Pediatrics 68:322, 1981.

14.17 ACUTE RESPIRATORY FAILURE

Acute respiratory failure may be defined as the development of hypercapnia during an acute illness. See also Sec. 14.79.

ETIOLOGY. Frequently, acute respiratory failure occurs in patients who are known to have mild to moderately severe chronic pulmonary disease with normal arterial carbon dioxide tension. During an intercurrent acute illness (e.g., influenza), such a patient may deteriorate rapidly and develop hypercapnia. Previously well children may also develop acute respiratory failure as a result of pneumonia, epiglottitis or other cause of upper airway obstruction, status asthmaticus, aspiration (including near-drowning), and certain poisonings. Patients with cystic fibrosis or severe scoliosis often develop acute respiratory failure following surgery. Acute central nervous system disease may cause respiratory failure by interfering with the central control of breathing. Severe muscle disease and thoracic abnormalities may result in respiratory failure because of inadequate alveolar ventilation. Occasionally, congenital heart lesions with large right-to-left shunts cause respiratory failure when pulmonary perfusion is too low to allow adequate excretion of carbon dioxide.

CLINICAL MANIFESTATIONS. The patient is hyperpneic and cyanotic and may use the accessory muscles of respiration; most sit up and lean forward to improve leverage for the accessory muscles and to allow easy diaphragmatic movement. Symptoms and signs of the underlying disease are also present. Hypercapnia may cause central depression accompanied by impaired consciousness and confusion. A $Pa{CO_2}$ of over 40 mm Hg suggests the possibility of developing acute respiratory failure, and a $Pa{CO_2}$ of 50 mm Hg or higher suggests it is imminent. Most patients with acute hypercapnia also have a $Pa{O_2}$ below 55 mm Hg in room air, suggesting that the oxygen content of the blood may be inadequate to meet the normal needs of the vital organs. Furthermore, at $Pa{CO_2}$ levels above 54 mm Hg, diaphragmatic function may be impaired, accelerating the patient's decline.

Acute hypoxemia and hypercapnia result in dilatation of the cerebral blood vessels and increased blood flow, often accompanied by severe headache. The sudden increased work of the accessory muscles of breathing may result in severe lower back pain. Although moderate to severe hypercapnia can cause peripheral vasodilatation, mild to moderate hypoxemia can cause peripheral vasoconstriction, and the patient may complain of cold extremities. Other symptoms of hypoxia include restlessness, dizziness, and impaired thought.

Acute respiratory failure can also result in characteristic multisystem complications. These include gastrointestinal hemorrhage (usually "stress" ulcer), cardiac arrhythmias (supraventricular arrhythmias are most common), renal failure, and malnutrition.

TREATMENT. Patients with early respiratory failure should receive maximum therapy aimed at relieving the underlying disease. Theophylline improves diaphragmatic strength and may be useful in treating respiratory failure in patients with chronic obstructive pulmonary disease. If these measures fail to reduce arterial carbon dioxide, mechanical ventilation with control of the airway is needed. If the patient is apneic or gasping, 100% oxygen is administered by bag and mask, followed immediately by endotracheal intubation (Table 14–1). When there is less urgency and there is reason to believe that several days of mechanical assistance will be required, nasotracheal intubation is preferable. Immediately after intubation, chest auscultation is important to ensure that the tube is not obstructing one of the mainstem bronchi and that there is adequate air exchange. A chest roentgenogram should be obtained to confirm proper tube placement. Patients with upper airway obstruction may not require any treatment other than intubation. For most intubated children, positive end expiration pressure (PEEP) is useful to prevent alveolar collapse.

The goal of therapy is to achieve adequate oxygen saturation and normal arterial carbon dioxide tension using the least pressure and lowest possible concentration of inspired oxygen ($Fi{O_2}$). Once artificial ventilation is undertaken, the patient must be monitored closely, by both clinical and arterial blood gas determinations, to ensure adequate ventilation. An indwelling arterial catheter is very helpful (see Sec. 14.14). Maintaining adequate tissue oxygenation is important because devastating effects of transient severe hypoxemia may persist after restoration of pulmonary function; restoration usually requires maintaining oxygen saturation above 90%. As the patient improves, the inspired oxygen concentration should be decreased as rapidly as possible to reduce the risks of oxygen toxicity. The risk of direct oxygen toxicity to the airways, although demonstrable at $Fi{O_2}$ levels above 40%, is greatly increased at $Fi{O_2}$ levels between 70 and 100%. For some patients who have very severe hypoxemia, but who can be expected to recover quickly, extracorporeal membrane oxygenation has been suggested, although it is still an experimental procedure.

Bedside measurements of tidal volume, VC, and negative inspiratory force are very helpful in predicting when the patient has a good chance of successful extubation. Ventilator assistance is then terminated, and the patient is extubated. Children with acute respiratory failure should be managed in a pediatric intensive care unit (see Sec. 6.34).

Specific treatment must also be directed at any extrapulmonary complications of acute respiratory failure, many of which (e.g., gastrointestinal hemorrhage, arrhythmia) can pose an immediate threat to life. Coping with these complications can dominate daily management decisions.

PROGNOSIS. Survival should be expected in previously normal children who develop respiratory failure with an acute illness. When acute respiratory failure is superimposed on underlying chronic illness, the prognosis is related to the nature of the chronic illness and the severity and duration of the acute process. Many of these patients regain their previous status.

Downes JJ, Fulgencio T, Raphaely RC: Acute respiratory failure in infants and children. Pediatr Clin North Am 19:423, 1972.
Juan G, Calverleg P, Talamo C, et al: Effect of carbon dioxide on diaphragmatic function in human beings. N Engl J Med 310:879, 1984.
Kumar A, Falke KJ, Geffin B, et al: Continuous positive pressure ventilation in acute respiratory failure. Effects on hemodynamics and lung function. N Engl J Med 283:1430, 1970.
Murciano D, Aubier M, Lecocquic Y, et al: Effects of theophylline on diaphragmatic strength and fatigue in patients with chronic obstructive pulmonary disease. N Engl J Med 311:349, 1984.
Pingleton SK: Complications of acute respiratory failure. Am Rev Respir Dis 137:1463, 1988.
Rogers RM, Juers JA: Physiologic considerations in the treatment of acute respiratory failure. Basics of RD 3 (No 4):1, 1975.

14.18 IATROGENIC AND DRUG-INDUCED PULMONARY DISEASE

Any patient who has had mechanical manipulation of the airway, mechanical ventilation, or prolonged drug therapy and then develops chronic respiratory symptoms or recurrent respiratory infection may have an iatrogenic disease. High oxygen concentrations and pressure ventilators can cause

TABLE 14–1. Data for Determining Inside Diameter and Length of Pediatric Endotracheal Tubes

Age	French Size	Internal Diameter (mm)	Oral Length (cm)	Nasal Length (cm)	15 mm Adapter (mm Internal Diameter)
Premature	14–16	2.5–3.0	8	11	3
Newborn–14 days	16	3.0–3.5	8.5	13	4
2–24 wk	16–18	3.5–4.0	10	15	4
6–12 mo	18–20	4.0–4.5	12	16	4–5
12–18 mo	20–22	4.5–5.0	13	16	5
18–24 mo	22–24	5.0–5.5	14	17	5–6
2–4 yr	24–26	5.5–6.0	15	18	6
4–7 yr	26–28	6.0–6.5	16	19	6–7
7–10 yr	28–30	6.5–7.0	17	21	7
10–12 yr	30–32	7.0–7.5	20	23–25	7–8

bronchopulmonary dysplasia (Sec. 9.32). Excessive infusion of blood or other plasma expanders may cause pulmonary edema. Anesthetic gases may have direct pulmonary toxicity, and atelectasis may occur as a result of both anesthetic agents and decreased deep breathing and coughing secondary to postoperative pain. Prolonged intubation has resulted in tracheal granulomas and other sequelae. Anticoagulant therapy has resulted in hemoptysis; chronic aspiration of mineral oil causes lipoid pneumonia (Sec. 14.61).

Although the pathophysiology of drug-induced pulmonary injury is better understood for some of the cancer chemotherapeutic agents, the same theoretical mechanisms apply to other drugs as well. The major metabolic processes whose disruption could lead to parenchymal injury include (1) augmented production of tissue oxidants (e.g., superoxide, hydrogen peroxide) or interference with their neutralization (e.g., superoxide dismutase, catalase); (2) acceleration, intensification, or prolongation of immunologically mediated tissue destruction (increased chemotaxis of polymorphonuclear leukocytes by the drug or by drug-induced tissue injury); (3) disruption of repair mechanisms, including the regulation of collagen deposition; (4) depression of the antiprotease system; and (5) a central nervous system (CNS) effect that causes pulmonary injury (e.g., neurogenic pulmonary edema). The knowledge needed to categorize the toxicity of individual drugs to one or more of these general mechanisms is often inadequate.

Cancer Therapy

Treatment programs based on multiple drug protocols combined with radiation therapy are used frequently in the common childhood malignancies. The increased survival time, together with the increasing total dose of many chemotherapeutic agents and radiation, has been associated with a variety of pulmonary complications (Chapter 17).

Because most protocols for cancer therapy involve multiple agents, it has been difficult to establish the exact pulmonary toxicity of individual agents or whether combined therapy is necessary for some drugs to produce pulmonary toxicity. Furthermore, other drugs administered to cancer patients may have a synergistic (or permissive) effect with regard to pulmonary injury (e.g., oxygen administration has been associated with increased toxicity of bleomycin and cyclophosphamide).

Radiation injury probably is mediated primarily by two pathophysiologic mechanisms: First, the radiation may stimulate inflammation, which ultimately leads to progressive fibrosis. Second, in children radiation has a profound long-term retarding effect on the growth of pulmonary parenchyma. Scoliosis occurs occasionally as a result of radiation, and this may further compromise pulmonary status. Radiation-induced reduction in chest wall growth may also secondarily limit growth of the lung. Because children rarely receive extensive thoracic radiation without chemotherapy, the effects of each may be difficult to distinguish. Doxorubicin and dactinomycin may potentiate or reactivate radiation toxicity.

Oncologic chemotherapeutic drugs may cause progressive pulmonary disease and limit lung size even when used without radiation. Pulmonary complications have occurred following administration of bleomycin, cyclophosphamide, busulfan, methotrexate, semustine, carmustine (BCNU), neocarzinostatin, melphalan, lomostin, chlerozotocin, cytosine arabinoside, azathioprine, mitomycin, chlorambucil, and procarbazine. Bleomycin, whose toxicity is increased by oxygen administration, causes pulmonary disease in 40% of patients. But pulmonary toxicity rarely results from 6-mercaptopurine and vincristine.

Three types of clinical syndromes are seen commonly: chronic pneumonitis/fibrosis, hypersensitivity syndromes, and noncardiogenic pulmonary edema. *Pneumonitis/fibrosis* is most common and is characterized by slowly progressive dyspnea on exertion and malaise. Physical findings include cyanosis, tachypnea, and rales. Pulmonary function testing reveals decreased diffusing capacity for carbon monoxide, evidence of restriction, and hypoxemia. Chest roentgenograms show linear interstitial densities (most common), a fine nodular pattern, or an alveolar filling process. There appears to be a total dose-risk relationship for bleomycin and busulfan but not for methotrexate. Corticosteroid treatment may be effective, especially in the form of the disease caused by mitomycin. Methotrexate-induced disease may resolve even if the drug is continued; in general, though, the suspected offending agent should be discontinued. Lung tissue shows fibrosis, interstitial infiltrates, and abnormal alveolar epithelial cells. In the case of busulfan, bizarre type II pneumocytes are a common finding.

Hypersensitivity syndromes occur with bleomycin, methotrexate, and procarbazine. Symptoms crescendo more rapidly and include dyspnea, cough, and fever. Eosinophilia may be present. Treatment with the offending agent should be discontinued, and often corticosteroids need to be administered. The prognosis is good.

Noncardiogenic pulmonary edema is a rare complication of therapy with cytosine arabinoside, methotrexate, and cyclophosphamide.

Chemotherapeutic drugs also may predispose the patient to developing a new pulmonary malignancy.

DIAGNOSIS. The principal problem is to differentiate chemotherapy-induced pulmonary disease from a pneumonia or *Pneumocystis carinii* infection and, more rarely, from diffuse tumor infiltration. Bronchoscopy and lung biopsy may be needed for definitive diagnosis.

TREATMENT AND COURSE. The natural history of the pulmonary lesion is unknown. In critically ill patients treatment with antibiotics and trimethoprim-sulfamethoxazole may be justified on an empiric basis even when lung injury from chemotherapy is strongly suspected. Patients occasionally recover even if the suspected drug is continued, but some patients have died from respiratory failure even though chemotherapy was promptly discontinued when pulmonary symptoms appeared. Adrenal corticosteroids have been used with varying success. Supportive treatment with oxygen and mechanical ventilation may be necessary.

Other Drug-Induced Pulmonary Disease

In addition to the five pathophysiologic mechanisms noted earlier, noncancer drugs have also caused bronchiolitis obliterans (penicillamine and sulfasalazine) and pulmonary renal syndrome (penicillamine), as the symptoms are similar to those of Goodpasture syndrome.

Nitrofurantoin can cause an acute or chronic pulmonary complication. This is quite rare, estimated at 237 cases in 44 million courses of therapy. Most cases have occurred in women, but they receive the drug more commonly than men. The most likely mechanism of injury is via oxygen radicals, but there is some evidence for an autoimmune abnormality as well. The most common acute reaction is characterized by fever, dyspnea, cough, and, occasionally, chest pain and cyanosis. Eosinophilia may occur transiently. Histologic findings include eosinophilia, proteinaceous edema in the air spaces, and perivasculitis. Chronic pulmonary fibrosis also occurs with prolonged treatment. Dyspnea on exertion and nonproductive cough are the most prominent symptoms. Pulmonary function testing reveals restriction and decreased carbon monoxide diffusing capacity, and the chest roentgenogram shows a diffuse interstitial pattern. Patients usually improve following discontinuation of nitrofurantoin treatment. Corticosteroids have been advocated, but there is little evidence for their effectiveness.

Anticonvulsants, including diphenylhydantoin and carbamazepine, have been reported to cause hypersensitivity pulmonary disease. The occurrence of this rare complication necessitates permanent discontinuation of the offending agent.

Opiates, including those used by drug abusers, occasionally cause noncardiogenic pulmonary edema. This may occur after the 1st dose. The mechanism(s) are unknown, but the possibilities include allergy, hypoventilation-induced hypoxemia, direct alveolar capillary toxicity, and immunologic activation of mast cells. Treatment generally includes ventilatory support; narcotic antagonists, although useful for their other effects, probably do not directly prevent or treat pulmonary edema.

Gold therapy *(chrysotherapy)* of rheumatoid arthritis results in interstitial fibrosis with dyspnea and rales. The pulmonary symptoms may be ascribed to rheumatoid lung disease. Discontinuation of gold treatments is indicated, after which some amelioration of symptoms can be expected. The pathogenesis may involve a drug-induced defect in cell-mediated immunity.

Although chronic *alcohol abuse* may have its onset during adolescence, its pulmonary sequelae (airway obstruction, decreased diffusion capacity, and alteration of ventilation-perfusion adjustment secondary to cirrhosis) will not usually be seen until adult years. The acute pulmonary toxicity of alcohol includes depression of ciliary motion (at high ethanol levels) and of pulmonary macrophage function and interference with production of surfactant. Although these changes usually do not result in clinical pulmonary problems in otherwise healthy individuals, children with chronic pulmonary disease may be at increased risk from infection.

Aspirin intolerance may be associated with nasal polyps and asthma. Pulmonary fibrosis has been reported to result from chronic use of *penicillamine* and *methysergide*. When given to patients receiving leukocyte transfusion, amphotericin B may cause severe, occasionally fatal, pulmonary toxicity.

A rare but potentially fatal toxicity, particularly for patients with pre-existing severe pulmonary disease, is produced by the *aminoglycosides* and *polymyxin* groups of antibiotics (including colistin), which can cause neuromuscular blockade and paralysis of the diaphragm and of other muscles of respiration.

ROBERT C. STERN

Cooper JAD Jr, White DA, Matthay RA: Drug-induced pulmonary disease. Part 1: Cytotoxic drugs; Part 2: Noncytotoxic drugs. Am Rev Respir Dis 133:321; 488, 1986.

Epler GR, Snider GL, Gaensler EA, et al: Bronchiolitis and bronchitis in connective tissue disease: A possible relationship to the use of penicillamine. JAMA 242:528, 1979.

Heinemann HO: Alcohol and the lung: A brief review. Am J Med 63:81, 1977.

Jacoby I: Drug-induced pulmonary disease: Confusion with infections of the lungs. Infect Dis Pract 1:1, 1978.

McCormick J, Cole S, Lahirir B, et al: Pneumonitis caused by gold salt therapy: Evidence for the role of cell-mediated immunity in its pathogenesis. Am Rev Respir Dis 122:145, 1980.

Rachelefsky GS, Coulson A, Siegel SC, et al: Aspirin intolerance in chronic childhood asthma: Detected by oral challenge. Pediatrics 56:443, 1975.

Webster DG, Robichaud KJ, Pizzo PA, et al: Lethal pulmonary reactions associated with the combined use of amphotericin B and leukocyte transfusions. N Engl J Med 304:1185, 1981.

Winterbauer RH, Wilske KR, Wheelis RF: Diffuse pulmonary injury associated with gold treatment. N Engl J Med 294:919, 1976.

Wohl MEB, Griscom NT, Traggis DG, et al: Effects of therapeutic irradiation delivered in early childhood upon subsequent lung function. Pediatrics 55:507, 1975.

14.19 UPPER RESPIRATORY TRACT

In addition to olfaction, the nose provides initial warming and humidification of inspired air. In the anterior nares turbulent air flow and coarse hairs enhance the deposition of large particulate matter; the remaining nasal airways filter out particles as small as 6 μm in diameter. In the turbinate region the air flow becomes laminar and the air stream is narrowed; thus particle deposition, warming, and humidification are enhanced. Nasal passages contribute as much as 50% of the total resistance of normal breathing. Nasal flaring, a sign of respiratory distress, reduces the resistance to inspiratory flow of air through the nose and may improve ventilation.

The nasal mucosa is more vascular, especially in the turbinate region, than that of the lower airways; however, the surface epithelium is similar, with ciliated cells, goblet cells, submucosal glands, and a covering blanket of mucus. Mucus flows toward the nasopharynx, where the air stream widens, the epithelium becomes squamous, and secretions are wiped away by swallowing; replacement of the mucous layers occurs about every 10 min. In addition to mucous glycoproteins, which provide viscoelastic properties, the nasal secretions contain lysozyme and secretory IgA, both of which have antimicrobial activity.

The *paranasal sinuses* develop in the facial bones as air cells lined with ciliated, mucous-secreting epithelium. Their ostia drain into the middle and superior meatuses and the sphenoethmoid recess of the nose. Development of the sinuses begins at 3–5 mo of gestation but occurs mostly after birth, with the maxillary and ethmoid sinuses being the earliest to form. They are seen on plain roentgenograms by 1–2 yr of age but can be identified on fine cut CT scans in the neonate.

The frontal sinuses usually begin their ascent into the frontal bone by the 2nd yr but, along with the sphenoid sinuses, are not readily visible on plain roentgenograms until 5–6 yr of age or later. Growth of the sinuses continues through adolescence; although unusual, asymmetry is most common in the frontal sinuses. Hypoplasia or septa within the maxillary sinuses are seen occasionally. Mucosal thickening greater than 4 mm, air-fluid level, or opacification seen on sinus roentgenograms suggest sinusitis, which can occur alone or in association with other conditions, such as CF, ciliary dyskinisia, or immunodeficiency.

The adenoids on the posterior nasopharyngeal wall and the tonsils at the base of the tongue are directly in line with the mucociliary flow and the air stream, enhancing their protective capabilities. The eustachian tubes, also lined with mucus-secreting, ciliated epithelium, enter the nasopharynx on the lateral walls.

Children and adults breathe through their nose unless nasal obstruction interferes, but most newborns are predominant nasal breathers.

14.20 CONGENITAL DISORDERS OF THE NOSE

Congenital structural nasal abnormalities are uncommon compared with acquired malformations. Occasionally, nasal bones are congenitally absent so that the bridge of the nose fails to develop, resulting in nasal hypoplasia. Congenital absence of the nose, complete or partial duplication, or a single centrally placed nostril occasionally occur but usually as a part of malformation syndromes incompatible with life. Rarely, supernumerary teeth may be found in the nose, or teeth may grow into it from the maxilla.

On occasion, nasal bones are sufficiently malformed to produce severe narrowing of the nasal passages. Often such narrowing is associated with a high and narrow hard palate, which is frequently associated with Down syndrome. Children with these defects may have more severe obstruction to airflow during infections of the upper airways and are more susceptible to the development of chronic or recurrent hypoventilation. Rarely, the alae nasi may be sufficiently thin and poorly supported to result in inspiratory obstruction.

A wide variety of nasal and midface abnormalities exist that may be part of more extensive craniofacial anomalies. These children are best treated by a team consisting of experienced pediatric, surgical, dental, and rehabilitation specialists.

Choanal atresia, the most common congenital anomaly of the nose, consists of a unilateral or bilateral bony or membranous septum between the nose and the pharynx. Nearly 50% of affected infants have other congenital anomalies (CHARGE syndrome). Since newborn infants have a variable ability to breath through their mouths, the obstruction does not produce the same symptoms in every infant. When only one side is affected, the infant usually does not have severe symptoms at birth and may be asymptomatic for a prolonged period, often until the first respiratory infection, when the diagnosis may be suggested by unilateral nasal discharge or disproportionately severe nasal obstruction.

Infants with bilateral choanal atresia who have difficulty with mouth breathing will make vigorous attempts to inspire, often suck in their lips, and will develop cyanosis. Distressed children then cry (which relieves the cyanosis) and become more calm, only to repeat the cycle after closing their mouths. Those who are able to mouth-breathe at once will experience difficulty when sucking and swallowing, becoming cyanotic when they attempt to nurse. Persistent mouth breathing and cyanosis when the mouth is closed (which is relieved when the infant cries) are additional manifestations.

Diagnosis is established by the inability to pass a firm catheter through each nostril 3–4 cm into the nasopharynx. The atresia plate may be seen directly with fiberoptic rhinoscopy. The anatomy is best visualized by using CT scanning.

Treatment consists of promptly providing an oral airway or maintaining the mouth in an open position. Passage of an orogastric tube is often sufficient to prevent the complete opposition of tongue and soft palate and ensure an open airway. Other techniques use a feeding nipple with large holes at the tip. Once an oral airway is established, the infant can be fed by gavage until breathing and eating without the assisted airway is learned, usually in 2–3 wk. Tracheostomy is rarely indicated. Subsequently, elective operative correction can be done weeks or months later in patients who adapt well to the obstruction. Immediate surgical correction for bilateral choanal atresia is seldom needed. Operative correction of unilateral obstruction may be deferred for several years. Stenosis necessitating reoperation is common.

Congenital defects of the nasal septum, such as *perforation* or *deviation*, are rare. Perforation can be developmental or secondary to infection, such as syphilis or tuberculosis, and to trauma. Septal deviation can be congenital or secondary to birth trauma and may be corrected with immediate realignment using blunt probes, cotton applicators, and topical anesthesia. Formal surgical correction may be required but is usually postponed to avoid disturbance of midface growth. Abnormal formation of the nasal bones is infrequent unless other malformations are also present, such as cleft lip or palate.

Congenital midline nasal masses include *dermoids, gliomas*, and *encephaloceles*. They present intranasally or extranasally and may have intracranial connections. Nasal dermoids often have a dimple on the nasal dorsum, sometimes with hair being present, and predispose to intracranial infections. Gliomas or heterotopic brain tissue are firm, whereas encephaloceles are soft and enlarge with crying or the Valsalva maneuver. Surgical excision is required, and an evaluation to determine intracranial connection is best done with magnetic resonance imaging (MRI).

Poor development of the paranasal sinuses is associated with recurrent or chronic upper airway infection in Down syndrome.

Hughes GB, Sharpino G, Hunt W, et al: Management of the congenital midline mass: A review. Head Neck Surg 2:222, 1980.
Maniglia AJ, Goodwin WJ, Arnold JE, et al: Intracranial abscesses secondary to nasal sinus and orbital infections in adults and children. Arch Otolaryngol Head Neck Surg 115:1424, 1989.
Richardson M, Osguthorpe JD: Surgical management of choanal atresia. Laryngoscope 98:915, 1988.

14.21 ACQUIRED DISORDERS OF THE NOSE

FOREIGN BODY

Food, crayons, small toys, erasers, paper wads, beads, beans, stones, and other foreign bodies are frequently introduced into the nose by children. Initial symptoms are local obstruction, sneezing, relatively mild discomfort, and, rarely, pain. Irritation results in mucosal swelling, and, because some foreign bodies are hygroscopic and increase in size as water is absorbed, signs of local obstruction and discomfort may increase with time. Infection usually follows and gives rise to a purulent, malodorous, or bloody discharge. Tetanus is a rare complication in nonimmunized children, as is toxic shock syndrome from surgical packings (Sec. 12.20). *Unilateral nasal discharge and obstruction should suggest the presence of a foreign body,* which can often be seen upon examination with a speculum. The patient may also present with a generalized body odor, bromhidrosis. The object is usually situated anteriorly at first, but through unskilled attempts at removal it may be forced deeper into the nose. Removal should be carried out promptly to minimize the danger of aspiration and to prevent local tissue necrosis. It can usually be performed with topical anesthesia, using either forceps or nasal suction. Infection usually clears promptly after the removal of the object, and generally no further therapy is necessary.

EPISTAXIS

Nosebleeds are rare in infancy, are common in childhood, and decrease in incidence after puberty. Epistaxis, when it does occur, is often transient and is not very severe; the bleeding often stops spontaneously or with minimal pressure. These isolated episodes of bleeding require no diagnostic evaluation or specific treatment. However, some children develop recurrent epistaxis with mild or moderate bleeding.

ETIOLOGY. Trauma, including picking the nose and foreign bodies, is the most common cause. There is frequently a family history of childhood epistaxis, and susceptibility is increased during respiratory infections and in the winter when dry air irritates the nasal mucosa, resulting in formation of fissures and crusting. Epistaxis is also associated with adenoidal hypertrophy, allergic rhinitis, sinusitis, polyps, and a variety of acute infections. Diseases with paroxysmal and forceful cough, such as cystic fibrosis, may also foster epistaxis. Severe bleeding may be encountered with congenital vascular abnormalities, such as telangiectasias or varicosities, and in children with thrombocytopenia, deficiency of clotting factors, hypertension, renal failure, or venous congestion. Adolescent girls may have epistaxis at the time of menarche.

CLINICAL MANIFESTATIONS. Epistaxis usually occurs without warning, with blood flowing slowly but freely from one nostril or occasionally from both. In children with nasal lesions, bleeding may follow physical exercise. When bleeding occurs at night, the blood may be swallowed and may become apparent only when the child vomits or passes blood in his stools. The source of the bleeding is usually the vascular plexus on the anterior septum (Kiesselbach plexus) or the mucosa of the anterior portions of the turbinates.

TREATMENT. Most nosebleeds stop spontaneously in a few minutes. The nares should be compressed and the child kept as quiet as possible, in an erect position until hemostasis, with the head tilted forward to avoid blood trickling posteriorly into the pharynx. If these measures do not stop the bleeding, local application of a solution of neosynephrine (0.25–1%) with or without topical thrombin may occasionally be useful. If bleeding persists, an anterior nasal pack should be inserted; if bleeding originates in the posterior nares, combined anterior and postchoanal packing is necessary. After bleeding has been controlled, and if a bleeding site is identified, its obliteration by cautery with silver nitrate may prevent further difficulties. As the septal cartilage derives its nutrition from the overlying mucoperichondrium, only one side of the septum should be cauterized at a time to reduce the chance of a septal perforation.

In patients with severe or repeated epistaxis, blood transfusions may be necessary. Otolaryngologic evaluation is indicated for these children and for those with bilateral bleeding or with hemorrhage that does not arise from the Kiesselbach plexus. Profuse epistaxis associated with a nasal mass in a boy near puberty may signal a **juvenile nasopharyngeal angiofibroma.** This unusual tumor has been reported in a 2 yr old and in 30–40 yr olds, but the incidence peaks in adolescent and preadolescent boys. The CT scan with contrast is the best initial evaluation. Arteriography, embolization, and extensive surgery may be needed. Replacement of deficient clotting factors may be required for patients who have an underlying hematologic disorder (see Sec. 16.62). If a patient lives in a dry environment, a room humidifier may prevent epistaxis.

14.22 INFECTIONS OF THE UPPER RESPIRATORY TRACT

GENERAL CONSIDERATIONS. Upper respiratory tract infections are those primarily affecting the structures of the respiratory tract above the larynx, but most respiratory illnesses affect both the upper and lower portions of the tract simultaneously or sequentially. Pathophysiologic features include inflammatory infiltrates and edema of the mucosa, vascular congestion, increased mucus secretion, and alterations of ciliary structure and function.

Many different microorganisms (chiefly viruses) are capable of causing primary upper respiratory tract disease. The same organism may cause inapparent infection or clinical symptoms of differing severity and extent in accordance with host factors such as age, sex, previous contact with the agent, allergy, and nutritional status. For example, among different members of the same family a single virus may simultaneously produce typical colds in the parents, bronchiolitis in the infant, croup in a somewhat older child, pharyngitis in another, and a subclinical infection in another.

ETIOLOGY. Most acute respiratory tract infections are caused by viruses and mycoplasma. An exception is acute epiglottitis. Streptococci and the diphtheria organisms are the major bacterial agents capable of causing primary pharyngeal disease; even in cases of acute tonsillopharyngitis, most illnesses are of nonbacterial origin. Although considerable overlapping exists, some microorganisms are more likely to produce a given respiratory syndrome than others, and certain agents have a greater tendency than others to produce severe disease. Some viruses (e.g., rubeola) may be associated with varying amounts of upper and lower respiratory tract symptomatology as part of a general clinical picture involving other organ systems.

The **respiratory syncytial virus** (RSV) is the principal single cause of bronchiolitis, accounting for about one third of all cases. It is a common cause of pneumonia, croup, and bronchitis, as well as of undifferentiated febrile disease of the upper respiratory tract (see Sec. 12.76).

The **parainfluenza viruses** account for most cases of the croup syndrome but may also produce bronchitis, bronchiolitis, and febrile upper respiratory tract disease (see Sec. 12.75). The **influenza viruses** do not play a large part in the various respiratory syndromes except during epidemics. In infants and children, influenza viruses account for more disease of the upper than the lower respiratory tract.

The **adenoviruses** account for fewer than 10% of respiratory illnesses, many of which are mild or asymptomatic. Pharyngitis and pharyngoconjunctival fever are the most common clinical manifestations in children. However, adenoviruses occasionally cause severe lower respiratory tract infection (see Sec. 12.77).

The **rhinoviruses** and **coronaviruses** usually produce symptoms limited to the upper tract, most commonly the nose, and account for a significant proportion of the "common cold" syndromes (see Sec. 12.78).

Coxsackieviruses A and B produce primarily disease of the nasopharynx (see Sec. 12.80). **Mycoplasma** can produce both upper and lower respiratory tract illness, including bronchiolitis, pneumonia, bronchitis, pharyngotonsillitis, myringitis, and otitis media (see Sec. 12.63).

Carlo WA, Martin RJ, Bruce EN, et al: Alae nasi activation (nasal flaring) decreases nasal resistance in preterm infants. Pediatrics 72:338, 1983.
Carson JL, Collier AM, Hu SS: Acquired ciliary defects in nasal epithelium of children with acute viral upper respiratory infections. N Engl J Med 312:463, 1985.

14.23 ACUTE NASOPHARYNGITIS
(Upper Respiratory Tract Infection; URI; the "Common Cold")

Acute nasopharyngitis is the most common infectious condition of children, but its significance depends primarily on the relative frequency with which complications occur. In children this syndrome is more extensive than in adults, often involving the paranasal sinuses and middle ear as well as the nasopharynx.

ETIOLOGY. The illness is caused by more than 200 serologically different viral agents. The principal agents are rhinoviruses (see Sec. 12.78), which account for more than a third of all colds; coronaviruses are responsible for about 10%. The period of infectivity lasts from a few hours prior to the appearance of symptoms to 1–2 days after the illness has appeared. Group A streptococci are the principal bacterial cause of acute nasopharyngitis. *Corynebacterium diphtheriae, Mycoplasma pneumoniae, Neisseria meningitidis,* and *N. gonorrhoeae* are also primary infectious agents. *Haemophilus influenzae, Streptococcus pneumoniae,* and *Staphylococcus aureus* may infect upper respiratory tract tissues secondarily and are responsible for complications in the sinuses, ears, mastoids, lymph nodes, and lungs. *M. pneumoniae* infections may localize to the nasopharynx and in these cases are difficult to distinguish from viral nasopharyngitis.

EPIDEMIOLOGY. Susceptibility to agents causing acute nasopharyngitis is universal, but for poorly understood reasons it varies in the same person from time to time. Although infections occur throughout the year, in the Northern Hemisphere there are peaks of occurrence in September about the time school opens, in late January, and toward the end of April. Children have an average of five to eight infections a year, and the highest number occurs during the first 2 yr of life. The frequency of acute nasopharyngitis varies directly with the number of exposures, and in nursery schools and day-care centers may be virtually epidemic. Susceptibility may be increased by poor nutrition and purulent complications by malnutrition.

PATHOLOGY. The first changes are edema and vasodilatation in the submucosa. A mononuclear cell infiltrate follows, which, within 1–2 days, becomes polymorphonuclear. Structural and functional changes of cilia result in compromised mucus clearance. In moderate to severe infection, the superficial epithelial cells separate and slough. There is profuse production of mucus, at first thin, later thicker and usually purulent.

CLINICAL MANIFESTATIONS. Colds are more severe in young children than in older children and adults. In general, children 3 mo–3 yr have fever early in the course of infection, occasionally a few hours before localizing signs appear. Younger infants are usually afebrile, and older children may have low grade fevers. Purulent complications occur with more frequency and severity at younger ages. Persistent sinusitis may occur at any age.

The initial manifestations in infants older than 3 mo of age are the sudden onset of fever, irritability, restlessness, and sneezing. Nasal discharge begins within a few hours, quickly leading to nasal obstruction, which may interfere with nursing; in small infants having a greater dependency on nose breathing, signs of moderate respiratory distress may occur. During the first 2–3 days the eardrums are usually congested, and fluid may be noted behind the drum, whether or not purulent otitis media subsequently occurs. A few infants may vomit, and some have diarrhea. The febrile phase lasts from a few hours to 3 days; fever may recur with purulent complications.

In older children the initial symptoms are dryness and irritation in the nose and not infrequently in the pharynx. These symptoms are followed within a few hours by sneezing, chilly sensations, muscular aches, a thin nasal discharge, and sometimes coughing. Headache, malaise, anorexia, and low-grade fever may be present. Within 1 day the secretions usually become thicker and eventually become purulent. The discharge is irritating, particularly during the purulent phase. Nasal obstruction leads to mouth breathing, and this, through drying of the mucous membranes of the throat, increases the sensation of soreness. In most cases, the acute phase lasts for 2–4 days.

DIFFERENTIAL DIAGNOSIS. The initial manifestations of measles and pertussis—and, to a lesser extent, of poliomyelitis, hepatitis, and mumps—are those of nasopharyngitis. A persistent nasal discharge, particularly if it is bloody, suggests a foreign body or diphtheria and, in the first week of life, choanal atresia or congenital syphilis.

Allergic rhinitis (see Sec. 11.40) differs from infectious rhinitis in that it is not accompanied by fever: its nasal discharge does not usually become purulent, and it is usually combined with persistent sneezing and itching of the eyes and nose. The nasal mucous membranes in allergic rhinitis are usually pale rather than inflamed, and nasal smears often contain many eosinophils rather than the polymorphonuclear leukocytes associated with infection. In allergic rhinitis, antihistamines may produce rapid and relatively complete disappearance of signs and symptoms; in infectious rhinitis, they produce little consistent benefit and may thicken the secretions making them harder to clear.

Drug abuse, especially with cocaine and marijuana, should also be considered in older children and adolescents.

COMPLICATIONS. These result from the bacterial invasion of the paranasal sinuses and other portions of the respiratory tract. The cervical lymph nodes may also become involved and occasionally suppurate. Mastoiditis, peritonsillar cellulitis, or periorbital cellulitis may occur. The most common complication is otitis media, which is seen in up to 25% of small infants. Although it may occur early in the course of a cold, it usually appears after the acute phase of nasopharyngitis. Thus, otitis media should be suspected if fever recurs. Most viral infections of the upper respiratory tract also involve the lower respiratory tract, and in many cases pulmonary function diminishes even though lower respiratory tract symptoms are inconspicuous or absent. On the other hand, typical laryngotracheobronchitis, bronchiolitis, or pneumonia may develop during the course of acute nasopharyngitis. Viral nasopharyngitis is also a frequent trigger for asthma symptoms in children with reactive airways.

PREVENTION. Effective vaccines are not available. Neither gamma globulin nor vitamin C reduces the frequency or severity of infections, and their use is not recommended.

Because of the ubiquity of the common cold, it is impossible to isolate children from this condition. However, because in the very young infant complications may be relatively serious, some attempt should be made to protect infants from contact with potentially infected persons.

TREATMENT. There is no specific therapy. Antibiotics do not affect the course of the illness or reduce the incidence of bacterial complications. Bed rest is generally recommended, but there is no evidence that it shortens the course of the illness or affects the outcome. Acetaminophen is usually helpful in reducing irritability, aching, and malaise for the first 1–2 days of infections, but excessive use should be avoided. Aspirin given to a child with influenza virus infection increases the risk of developing Reye syndrome and *is not recommended* for children with respiratory tract symptoms.

Most of the distress is owing to nasal obstruction. Attempts should be made to relieve this condition if it interferes with sleep or with fluid or food ingestion. Nasal instillation of medications may be an effective method for relieving nasal obstruction. In infants, instillation of sterile saline may assist with physical removal of excessive mucus. Phenylephrine (0.125–0.25%) is used widely in the United States. More potent, longer-acting nose drops, although useful to adults, tend to be irritating and occasionally are hyperexcitative or sedative to infants. Nose drops in oily vehicles should be avoided because they are readily aspirated. The addition of antibiotics, corticosteroids, or antihistamines to nose drops increases their expense and adds nothing to their effectiveness.

Nose drops are best administered 15–20 min before feeding and at bedtime. While the child is supine with the neck extended, 1–2 drops are instilled in each nostril. Because this often produces shrinkage of only the anterior mucous membranes, 1–2 drops can be instilled 5–10 min later. Introducing nasal decongestants by cotton-tipped applicators is not recommended. Older children can use a nasal spray but only under supervision, because such applications tend to be overused. In general, no medication instilled into the nose should be used for more than 4–5 days; after this time any drug may produce chemical irritation and induce nasal congestion, mimicking acute nasopharyngitis.

Nasal obstruction is difficult to treat in infants. Suction with a soft bulb syringe is occasionally essential to clear the nasal passage sufficiently to permit the young infant to nurse. The best drainage can usually be achieved by placing the infant in the prone position, if this does not further compromise respirations. A highly humidified environment provided by an efficient vaporizer prevents drying of secretions and often appears to provide substantial benefit.

Orally administered decongestants are also widely used for shrinkage of engorged nasal mucosa and for relief of obstruction. Pseudoephedrine reduces nasal resistance in older children and adults with upper respiratory tract infection; studies in infants and young children have not been reported. Many preparations combine antihistamines and adrenergic agonists. The former have been found effective in some and ineffective in other studies for relief of nasal congestion in children with acute nasopharyngitis. There is no evidence that these drugs prevent otitis media.

Most children with acute nasopharyngitis have decreased appetite, but compelling them to eat serves no purpose. Fluids of the child's choice should be offered at frequent intervals. Transient constipation is common but does not require treatment because it disappears rapidly when the child returns to a normal diet.

Doyle WJ, McBride TP, Skoner DP, et al: A double-blind, placebo-controlled trial of the effect of chlorpheniramine on the response of the nasal airway, middle ear, and eustachian tube to provocative rhinovirus challenge. Pediatr Infect Dis J 7:229, 1988.

Fleming DW, Cochi SL, Hightower AW, et al: Childhood upper respiratory tract infections: To what degree is incidence affected by day care attendance? Pediatrics 79:55, 1987.

Gaffey MJ, Kaiser DL, Hayden FG: Ineffectiveness of oral terfenadine in natural colds: Evidence against histamine as a mediator of common cold symptoms. Pediatr Infect Dis J 7:223, 1988.

Hutton N, Wilson MH, Mellits ED, et al: Effectiveness of an antihistamine-decongestant combination for young children with the common cold: A randomized, controlled clinical trial. J Pediatr 118:125, 1991.

Naclerio RM, Proud D, Kagey-Sobotka A, et al: Is histamine responsible for the symptoms of rhinovirus colds? A look at the inflammatory mediators following infection. Pediatr Infect Dis J 7:218, 1988.

14.24 ACUTE PHARYNGITIS

This term refers to all acute infections of the pharynx, including tonsillitis and pharyngotonsillitis. The presence or absence of tonsils does not affect the susceptibility, the frequency, or the course or complications of the illness. Pharyngeal involvement is part of most upper respiratory tract infections and is also found with various acute generalized infections (Chapter 12). However, in the strict sense "acute pharyngitis" refers to conditions in which the principal involvement is in the throat. The disease is uncommon under 1 yr of age. The incidence then increases to a peak from 4–7 yr but continues throughout later childhood and adult life. In diphtheria (see Sec. 12.25), herpangina (see Sec. 12.80), adenovirus infection (see Sec. 12.77), and infectious mononucleosis (see Sec. 12.72) pharyngeal involvement may be prominent.

ETIOLOGY. Acute pharyngitis, whether febrile or not, is generally caused by viruses. Group A β-hemolytic streptococcus (see Sec. 12.18) is the only common bacterial causative agent, and, except during epidemics, it accounts for probably fewer than 15% of cases. Other bacteria may proliferate during acute viral infections and may therefore be cultured in large numbers from the pharynx of an affected person. Pharyngeal gonococcal infection may occur secondary to fellatio.

CLINICAL MANIFESTATIONS. These differ somewhat, depending on whether streptococci or viruses are the cause. There is, however, much overlapping of signs and symptoms, and it is often impossible to clinically distinguish one form of pharyngitis from another.

Viral pharyngitis is generally considered a disease of relatively gradual onset, which usually has as early signs fever, malaise, and anorexia with moderate throat pain. Sore throat may be present initially but begins more commonly a day or so after the onset of symptoms, reaching its peak by the 2nd–3rd day. Hoarseness, cough, and rhinitis are also common. Even at its peak, pharyngeal inflammation may be relatively slight, but it is occasionally severe, and small ulcers may form on the soft palate and the posterior pharyngeal wall. Exudates may appear on lymphoid follicles of the palate and tonsils and may be indistinguishable from those encountered with streptococcal disease. The cervical lymph nodes are often moderately enlarged and firm and may or may not be tender. Laryngeal involvement is common, but the trachea, bronchi, and lungs are usually not sources of symptoms. White blood cell counts range from 6,000 to above 30,000, an elevated count (16,000–18,000) of predominantly polymorphonuclear cells being common in the early phase of illness. Leukocyte counts have little value in differentiating viral from bacterial disease. The entire illness may last less than 24 hr and does not usually persist for more than 5 days. Significant complications are rare.

Streptococcal pharyngitis in a child over 2 yr often begins with complaints of headache, abdominal pain, and vomiting. These symptoms may be associated with a fever as high as 40° C (104° F); occasionally, a temperature elevation is not noted for 12 hr or so. Hours after the initial complaints, the throat may become sore, and in approximately one third of patients tonsillar enlargement, exudation, and pharyngeal erythema are found. The degree of pharyngeal pain is inconstant and may vary from slight to severe, making swallowing difficult. Two thirds of patients may have only mild erythema, with no enlargement of the tonsils and with no exudate. Anterior cervical lymphadenopathy usually occurs early, and the nodes are often tender. Fever may continue for 1–4 days; in very severe cases the child may remain ill for as long as 2 wk. The physical findings most likely to be associated with streptococcal disease are diffuse redness of the tonsils and tonsillar pillars, with a petechial mottling of the soft palate, whether or not lymphadenitis or follicular exudations are found. These features, although common in streptococcal pharyngitis, are not diagnostic and occur with some frequency in viral pharyngitis.

Conjunctivitis, rhinitis, cough, and hoarseness rarely occur with proven streptococcal pharyngitis, and the presence of two or more of these signs or symptoms suggests the diagnosis of viral infection.

The term **streptococcosis** refers to systemic variations in the presentation of acute streptococcal infections, believed to be related to earlier infection with the β-hemolytic streptococcus. In infants they may take the form of an acute, usually mild episode lasting less than 1 wk and characterized by variable fever (under 39° C [102° F]), mucoserous nasal discharge, and pharyngeal infection. Usually children 6 mo–3 yr of age are most severely ill. Coryza with postnasal discharge, diffusely reddened pharynx, fever, vomiting, and loss of appetite occurs early. For a few days there is usually fever of 38–39.5° C (100–103° F), which continues irregularly for 4–8 wk, gradually becoming normal. Within a few days of onset, cervical nodes begin to enlarge and become tender; the course of the adenopathy typically parallels that of the fever. Focal complications are common.

DIAGNOSIS. Diagnosis can be made by rapid detection method for streptococcal antigens or by culture after pharyngeal swabbing. Rapid detection methods are very specific but may miss 10–15% of culture-proven infections. Therefore, antigen-negative throat swabs from children with compatible clinical features should also be cultured.

A syndrome of purulent nasal discharge, pharyngitis, and fever may also be associated with positive pharyngeal cultures for pneumococci or *H. influenzae*. Although this syndrome is probably a complication of viral pharyngitis, some of these patients respond to antibiotics.

When a membranous exudate is present on the tonsils, diphtheria should be considered. The membranous exudate of infectious mononucleosis may resemble that found in the streptococcal infection and the partially immunized child with a diphtheritic infection. Herpangina (see Sec. 12.80) is not usually associated with tonsillar exudates, but rather with many vesiculoulcerative lesions on the anterior pillars, fauces, and soft palate.

Agranulocytosis is often first manifested by symptoms of acute pharyngitis. The tonsils and posterior pharyngeal wall may be covered by a yellow or dirty white exudate. The mucous membranes under this exudate usually become necrotic, and ulceration extends into the mouth and involves the tongue. The lesions are very painful and dysphagia is severe. Enlargement of cervical lymph nodes commonly occurs, as do mucosal hemorrhages.

Children and adolescents who smoke tobacco or marijuana excessively may develop pharyngeal inflammation and sore throat. Allergic rhinitis with a nonpurulent postnasal discharge may also cause a sore throat. Gonococcal pharyngeal infections are usually asymptomatic.

Pharyngoconjunctival fever is discussed in Sec. 12.77.

COMPLICATIONS. With viral infections the complication rate is low, although purulent bacterial otitis media may occur. In debilitated children both viral and streptococcal infections may lead to large, chronic ulcers in the pharynx. With streptococcal disease, peritonsillar abscess occasionally occurs, as do sinusitis, otitis media, and, rarely, meningitis. Acute glomerulonephritis (see Sec. 18.5) and rheumatic fever (see Sec. 11.74) may follow streptococcal infections.

Mesenteric adenitis is occasionally associated with pharyngitis of either viral or bacterial origin. This may result in abdominal pain (with or without vomiting) that may closely simulate appendicitis.

TREATMENT. Since even exudative tonsillitis is usually of viral origin, for which there is no specific therapy, the use of antibiotics should be guided by the results of antigen detection tests or cultures, unless there are strong clinical and epidemiologic grounds to suspect a streptococcal infection. Streptococcal pharyngitis is best treated orally with penicillin (125–250 mg of penicillin V three times daily for 10 days). This usually produces prompt clinical response with defervescence within 24 hr and shortens the course of illness by an average of 1.5 days. Erythromycin is a satisfactory alternative if the patient is allergic to penicillin, but erythromycin resistance of group A streptococcal organisms has been documented in the United States.

Most children prefer to remain in bed during the acute phase of the disease. When throat pain is severe, acetaminophen is often helpful. Gargling with warm saline solution offers some symptomatic relief for throat pain in children old enough to cooperate; in younger children the inhalation of steam occasionally produces similar effects. Because of pain on swallowing, cool bland liquids such as ginger ale are usually more acceptable than solids or hot foods. No attempt should be made to force the child to eat.

The child with a streptococcal infection is noninfectious to others within a few hours after penicillin therapy has begun. Reculturing is not necessary if symptoms abate. A streptococcal carrier is not at risk for rheumatic fever, is unlikely to transmit infection, and does not require treatment unless there is a history of rheumatic fever in the patient or a sibling. The carrier state does make the differentiation of subsequent pharyngitis more difficult. A few children require antibiotic prophylaxis against streptococcal disease, such as those with past history of rheumatic fever (see Sec. 11.74).

Breese BB: A simple scorecard for the tentative diagnosis of streptococcal pharyngitis. Am J Dis Child 131:514, 1977.
Kim KS, Kaplan EL: Association of penicillin tolerance with failure to eradicate group A streptococci from patients with pharyngitis. J Pediatr 107:681, 1985.
Schwartz RH, Wientzen RL, Grundfart KM: Sore throat in adolescents. Pediatr Infect Dis 1:443, 1982.

14.25 ACUTE UVULITIS

Infections of the uvula are infrequent. They are characterized by fever, pain with swallowing, and drooling. Occasionally there are no symptoms or signs referrable to the pharynx. Most cases are due to group A streptococcus or *H. influenzae* type b, often in association with tonsillitis and acute epiglottis, respectively. However, isolated uvulitis has been reported. In general streptococcal uvulitis tends to occur in older children (>5 years), whereas that caused by *H. influenzae* occurs before 5 yr of age. In suspected cases blood cultures as well as cultures of the uvula and pharynx are indicated. Young children should be examined carefully for evidence of airway obstruction and treated, initially with an antibiotic that covers ampicillin-resistant *H. influenzae* administered intravenously. Older children can be treated as indicated for streptococcal pharyngitis.

14.26 CHRONIC RHINITIS AND NASOPHARYNGITIS

The child with persistent or recurring upper respiratory tract infection with or without associated chronic bronchial involvement cannot be placed in any one category; each must be studied to determine, if possible, the most important etiologic or pathophysiologic factors.

Children should recover completely after acute respiratory infections and should appear healthy between episodes. In the chronic cases the child seems to recover from one acute attack only to enter another, or there is more or less persistent rhinitis and cough and a general failure to do well. Such patterns may reflect familial or individual susceptibility or repeated exposure to respiratory infection either within the home or in a day-care school setting.

CHRONIC RHINITIS. Chronic nasal discharge, with or without acute exacerbations, may reflect an underlying disturbance, such as nasal polyps, chronic sinusitis, chronically infected adenoids, cystic fibrosis, dysmotile cilia syndrome, allergy, foreign bodies, deviated septum, various congenital malformations, nasal diphtheria, or syphilis. In addition, the possibility of a chronic debilitating infection or some nutritional, immunologic, or metabolic (as of the thyroid) deficiency must be considered.

Clinical Manifestations. Symptoms vary, but chronic nasal discharge is common to all cases. In the persistent cases the odor may be foul, and there may be excoriation of the anterior nares and upper lip. Bloody discharge is common in syphilitic and diphtheritic lesions and with foreign bodies but may also occur in other conditions, especially if there is persistent nose picking. Disturbances of taste and smell are frequent. During exacerbations or superimposed infections, fever is common but is otherwise usually absent.

Persistent *allergic rhinitis* is relatively common and may be seasonal (see Sec. 11.40). The mucous membrane tends to be pale; the soft tissues are swollen and resistant to pressure.

Chronic rhinitis may also result from prolonged or excessive use of topical nasal decongestants (rhinitis medicamentosa).

Atrophic rhinitis is uncommon and is usually associated with some general debilitating condition, or it may be a sequel to long-continued nasal infection. The sense of smell is impaired. There may be little or no discharge but considerable crusting and a sense of dryness in the nose and throat. In some cases there is a profuse, excessively foul nasal discharge **(ozena).**

Treatment. The frequent application to the nares and upper lip of a lanolin, silicone, or petrolatum-base ointment protects against skin excoriation.

In addition, providing humidified air in cold weather may prevent ongoing nasal mucosal damage and foster clearing of the chronic inflammatory state. Otherwise, treatment is directed toward the underlying disturbance. Foci of infection in sinuses, ears, adenoids, or tonsils should be eradicated, and either allergens should be removed from the environment or the patient should be desensitized. Attention should be given to nutritional status, rest, and prevention of exposure to new infections. Although mucosa-shrinking solutions such as phenylephrine and related compounds may provide symptomatic relief, they may also cause further damage. Local antibiotics should be avoided, but systemic administration may be indicated in selected cases.

CHRONIC PHARYNGITIS. Chronic pharyngitis is rare and occurs secondarily to chronic infections of the sinuses, adenoids, or tonsils, although on occasion there is no evidence of infection other than hypertrophied lymphoid tissue on the posterior pharyngeal wall and on the base of the tongue. The latter type of involvement occurs with frequency only in children whose faucial tonsils have been removed; some of these children may also have infected tonsillar tags.

Clinical Manifestations. There are likely to be repeated acute exacerbations; in the intervals there are complaints of throat discomfort such as dryness and raspy irritation. Frequent efforts to clear the throat and the presence of an irritative cough are common. The mucous membrane is usually inflamed, although it is occasionally pale, and the blood vessels are prominent. The pharyngeal wall is frequently covered with a mucopurulent secretion, and the lymphoid tissue is often hypertrophied and has a pebbled appearance.

Treatment. This should be directed toward any disturbance in the sinuses, nose (deformities), adenoids, and tonsils. Attention should also be given to the general nutrition and hygiene of the child.

14.27 RETROPHARYNGEAL ABSCESS

During early childhood the potential space between the posterior pharyngeal wall and the prevertebral fascia contains several small lymph nodes that usually disappear during the 3rd–4th year of life. The lymphatic channels that communicate with these nodes drain portions of the nasopharynx as well as the posterior nasal passages. With purulent infections of these areas the nodes may become infected; this may, in turn, progress to breakdown of the nodes and to suppuration.

ETIOLOGY. Retropharyngeal abscess may be a complication of bacterial pharyngitis. Less commonly, it occurs after extension of infection from vertebral osteomyelitis or by wound infection following a penetrating injury of the posterior pharynx. Group A hemolytic streptococci, oral anaerobes, and *S. aureus,* in this order, are the most common pathogens.

CLINICAL MANIFESTATIONS. The patient usually has a history of an acute nasopharyngitis or pharyngitis, and the clinical features of the earlier illness may still be present. There is generally an abrupt onset of high fever with difficulty in swallowing, refusal of feeding, severe distress with throat pain, hyperextension of the head, and noisy, often gurgling respirations. Respirations become increasingly labored, and secretions accumulate in the mouth and cause drooling owing to the difficulty in swallowing.

A bulge in the posterior pharyngeal wall is usually apparent. The abscess is sometimes located in an area of the nasopharynx where it may cause nasal obstruction and a bulging forward of the soft palate. A digital examination to determine whether the abscess is fluctuant must be performed with the patient in the Trendelenburg position and with provision for adequate suction in case the abscess ruptures. Retropharyngeal abscesses may not be detectable by simple inspection. However, a lateral roentgenogram of the nasopharynx or neck will reveal the retropharyngeal mass; when an abscess is present, the retropharyngeal soft tissue is more than one half the width of the adjacent vertebral bodies when the patient's neck is extended; air may be seen in the retropharynx, and there is a loss of the normal cervical lordosis.

If left untreated, the abscess may rupture into the pharynx spontaneously, resulting in aspiration of pus. It may also extend laterally and present externally on the side of the neck or dissect along fascial planes into the mediastinum. Death may occur with aspiration, airway obstruction, erosion into major blood vessels, or with mediastinitis.

DIFFERENTIAL DIAGNOSIS. Pressure on the larynx may result in stridor, making retropharyngeal abscess one of the differential diagnostic possibilities in patients with high fever and croup. Many patients have limited neck motion, which may be mistaken for meningismus. Nonfluctuant lymphadenitis may produce a tender bulge in the retropharyngeal space. Tuberculous caries of the cervical spine may occasionally produce a lateral retropharyngeal abscess; considerable rigidity of the neck and other signs of spinal involvement are usually present. A CT scan with contrast may differentiate underlying pathology or identify an early abscess, allowing earlier incision and drainage.

TREATMENT. If the abscess is recognized in the prefluctuant stage, intensive treatment with parenteral penicillin G (100,000–250,000 units/kg/24 hr) or a semisynthetic penicillin (to cover penicillinase-producing *S. aureus*) may prevent suppuration and abscess formation. Single agent treatment with clindamycin or ampicillin-sulbactam should also be effective. Analgesic drugs may be needed for pain. Because of the risk of airway obstruction, narcotics should be used only with great care. When fluctuance is present, the abscess should be incised and antibiotics should be started; the operation is best performed under general anesthesia.

14.28 LATERAL PHARYNGEAL ABSCESS

This condition occurs in the space lateral to the pharynx that extends from the hyoid bone to the base of the skull. The carotid vessels and jugular vein may be intimately associated with the abscess.

The patient usually has high fever, trismus, appears acutely ill, and has severe pain and difficulty when swallowing. The bulge in the lateral pharyngeal wall is obvious. Cervical adenitis is usually present, and torticollis toward the side of the abscess due to muscular spasm is common.

Microbiology is identical to that of retropharyngeal abscess. Treatment usually requires lateral neck drainage.

14.29 PERITONSILLAR ABSCESS

This abscess occurs in the potential space between the superior constrictor muscle and the tonsil (usually at the superior pole). It is almost always caused by group A β-hemolytic streptococci or oral anaerobes in preadolescent or adolescent patients.

CLINICAL MANIFESTATIONS. The abscess is usually preceded by an attack of acute pharyngotonsillitis. There may be an afebrile interval of several days, or the fever of the primary infection may not subside. The patient has severe throat pain, has trismus because of spasm of the pterygoid muscles, and often refuses to swallow or speak. Occasionally, there is sufficient spasm of the homolateral muscles of the neck to produce torticollis. The fever may be septic and reach 40.5° C (105° F). The affected tonsillar area is markedly swollen and inflamed; the uvula is displaced to the opposite side. In untreated patients the abscess becomes fluctuant within a few days and usually points in the region of the anterior faucial pillar. If the abscess is not incised, spontaneous rupture occurs.

TREATMENT. Antibiotics and incision and drainage or aspiration of purulence are required. Outpatient treatment is possible; however, young children usually require general anesthesia and hospitalization. If there is no history of chronic tonsillitis, the chance of recurrence is approximately 10%, and tonsillectomy is not required. If there is a prior history of tonsillitis or a previous abscess, an immediate tonsillectomy should be considered.

14.30 SINUSITIS

See also Sec. 14.19.

Starting in infancy, the maxillary antra and the anterior and posterior ethmoid cells are usually of sufficient size to harbor infection. The frontal sinus is rarely a site of significant infection until the 6th–10th yr. When there is severe ethmoidal disease in the first few years of life, the development and pneumatization of the frontal sinuses may be curtailed or even completely prevented. The sphenoidal sinus usually does not assume clinical significance until the 3rd–5th yr of life.

The paranasal sinuses are probably involved in an exudative process in practically all acute nasal infections, but, as a rule, the sinus involvement does not persist after the nasal infection has subsided unless there has been a pre-existing sinus infection. The incidence of both acute and chronic sinus infections increases in the latter part of childhood. Unrecognized allergic factors, poor sinus drainage such as might occur with septal deviation or adenoid hypertrophy, associated hereditary conditions, immunosuppression, and environmental factors may increase the possibility of sinus infection.

14.31 Acute Purulent Sinusitis

In addition to involvement of the sinuses during acute nasal infections, there may be acute empyema of one or more sinuses. Signs or symptoms often appear 3–5 days after acute rhinitis.

CLINICAL MANIFESTATIONS. Sinusitis should be suspected if a "cold" seems more severe than usual (fever >39° C, periorbital edema, facial pain) or if the "cold" lingers for more than 10 days. A night-time cough often follows a viral upper respiratory infection, but a daytime cough is more suggestive of sinusitis. Headaches, facial pain, tenderness, and edema are uncommon. An examination after topical decongestants may show pus in the middle meatus that suggests involvement of the maxillary, frontal, or anterior ethmoid sinuses; pus in the superior meatus suggests involvement of the sphenoid or posterior ethmoid cells. Postnasal discharge may result in a sore throat or a persistent cough, especially at night.

In acute *ethmoiditis*, especially in infants and small children, periorbital cellulitis with edema of the soft tissues and redness of the skin is a common manifestation.

Complications are epidural or subdural abscess, meningitis, cavernous sinus thrombosis, optic neuritis, periorbital or orbital cellulitis and abscess, and osteomyelitis.

DIAGNOSIS. Roentgenography is often used but may be misinterpreted. The most common diagnostic findings are air-fluid levels and complete opacification. Mucosa width of 4 mm or greater in children also correlates with the presence of bacteria in sinuses. CT scans are sensitive indicators of sinus disease and may be needed before surgery is planned or if a complication of sinusitis seems likely. In some centers, abbreviated CT studies have replaced the usual sinus series. Sinus roentgenograms (even CT scans) of infants are often misleading. In children it is not necessary initially to puncture a sinus to establish a diagnosis. However, antral puncture is the only reliable method of gathering material for bacterial culture. Indications for sinus aspiration include unresponsiveness to therapy, sinus disease in immunocompromised hosts, or life-threatening complications. Organisms usually recovered in children include *S. pneumoniae, M. catarrhalis,* and nontypable *H. influenzae.* Direct smear of the secretions usually reveals mostly neutrophils but may aid in detecting associated allergy if many eosinophils are present. Nasal swab cultures do not correlate well with cultures of sinus aspirates.

TREATMENT. This consists primarily of effective antimicrobial therapy. Amoxicillin is a reasonable initial choice. In areas in which *H. influenzae* and *M. catarrhalis* producing β-lactamase are common or for treatment failures, trimethoprim-sulfamethoxazole, amoxicillin with potassium clavulanate, erythromycin plus a sulfonamide, and 2nd- and 3rd-generation cephalosporins may be prescribed. Trimethoprim-sulfamethoxazole is ineffective for group A β-hemolytic streptococcus. Treatment lasts 14–21 days. Decongestants and antihistamines are not helpful. Sinus drainage and irrigation are reserved for patients who fail usual therapy, who have intraorbital, intracranial, or other complications, or who experience intense pain.

Chronic Sinusitis

Chronic infection of the paranasal sinuses should suggest the possibility of a local or generalized disturbance that facilitates persistence of the infection. A search should be made for nasal deformities, polyps, or infected and hypertrophied adenoids that might cause obstruction, for infected teeth as a source of maxillary sinusitis, for a sinus polyp or mucocele, and for such general disturbances as allergy, cystic fibrosis, and dyskinetic cilia. Chronic or recurrent sinusitis is also common in patients with absence of secretory antibodies and in other immunodeficiency states.

CLINICAL MANIFESTATIONS. Symptoms of chronic sinusitis vary considerably but frequently are not prominent. Fever, when present, is low grade. Malaise, easy fatigability, and anorexia may occur. Nasal discharge, which may be bilateral or unilateral, varies from day to day and during the day. Frequently there is sufficient swelling of the middle turbinates to cause substantial nasal obstruction. Postnasal discharge is common and, in the absence of infected adenoids or acute upper respiratory tract infection, is virtually diagnostic. When there is an associated watery nasal discharge or sneezing, the possibility of allergic rhinitis must be considered.

Any of the complications of acute sinusitis may occur with chronic sinusitis. The term *sinobronchitis* is used occasionally to designate the relationship between sinus and lower respiratory tract symptoms; children with this condition may have reactive airways, cystic fibrosis, immunodeficiency, or dyskinetic cilia as the underlying disease. Sinusitis may aggravate asthma.

TREATMENT. In addition to the organisms recovered during acute sinusitis, α-hemolytic streptococci, *S. aureus*, and anaerobes are frequently found on culture of antral aspirates. In general, appropriate antimicrobials should be given for up to 6 wks. Antihistamines and decongestants are often used in addition, especially if there are associated allergic manifestations. Surgery is frequently required.

In cystic fibrosis, panopacification of sinuses is nearly always present but symptomatic disease is unusual. In the absence of symptoms, treatment of sinus disease is not indicated.

Locally obstructive nasal deformities should be corrected, if possible, and infected or hypertrophic adenoid tissue should be removed.

14.32 NASAL POLYPS

ETIOLOGY. Nasal polyps are benign pedunculated tumors formed from edematous, usually chronically inflamed nasal mucosa. They usually originate from the ethmoid sinus and present in the middle meatus. Occasionally, they appear within the maxillary antrum and can extend to the nasopharynx (antrochoanal polyp). Very large or multiple polyps may completely obstruct the nasal passage.

Cystic fibrosis is probably the most common childhood cause of nasal polyposis; as many as 25% of patients develop polyps. Every child with nasal polyposis should be tested for cystic fibrosis, even in the absence of typical respiratory and digestive symptoms. Nasal polyposis is also associated with chronic sinusitis of other etiologies, chronic allergic rhinitis, and asthma.

CLINICAL MANIFESTATIONS. Obstruction of nasal passages with hyponasal phonation and mouth breathing is prominent. Profuse mucoid or mucopurulent rhinorrhea may also result. An examination of the nasal passages shows glistening, gray, grape-like masses squeezed between the nasal turbinates and the septum. Polyps can be readily distinguished from the well-vascularized turbinate tissue, which is pink or red. Prolonged presence of polyps may widen the bridge of the nose and erode adjacent osseous structures.

TREATMENT. Local or systemic decongestants are not usually effective in shrinking the polyps. Similarly, corticosteroid nose sprays are not usually helpful, although a trial is warranted in recurrent cases. Polyps should be removed surgically if complete obstruction, uncontrolled rhinorrhea, or deformity of the nose appears. If the underlying pathogenic mechanism cannot be eliminated (e.g., cystic fibrosis), the polyps may soon return. More aggressive surgery may reduce the recurrence rate. Antihistamines may be helpful in delaying recurrence owing to allergic causes.

14.33 TONSILS AND ADENOIDS

The term tonsils is used in its commonly accepted sense of indicating the two faucial tonsils; the term adenoids refers to the nasopharyngeal tonsil. The tonsils and adenoids are part of the lymphoid tissues that circle the pharynx and are known collectively as *Waldeyer ring*. This consists of the lymphoid tissue on the base of the tongue (lingual tonsil), the two faucial tonsils, the adenoids, and the lymphoid tissue on the posterior pharyngeal wall. This tissue serves as a defense against infection, but it may become a site of acute or chronic infection.

The principal disturbances of the tonsils and adenoids are infection and hypertrophy. The latter is usually temporary and secondary to infection. The most important issue is if and when they are to be removed. Although both tonsils and adenoids are often removed at the same operation, separate tonsillectomy or adenoidectomy may be indicated, especially in children under 4–5 yr of age. Tonsillar disturbances are uncommon in infancy.

Neoplasms of the tonsils are rare, although 7% of non-Hodgkin lymphomas present in Waldeyer ring. The nasopharynx is a common site for rhabdomyosarcomas to occur.

Acute infections of the tonsils are considered as acute pharyngitis and are discussed in Sec. 14.24.

Chronic Tonsillitis

(Chronically Hypertrophic and Infected Tonsils)

The management of tonsillitis is of special concern because of its frequency and because tonsils are potentially important to the normal development of the immune system.

CLINICAL MANIFESTATIONS. These vary considerably; the significant features are recurrent or persistent sore throat and obstruction to swallowing or breathing, most often caused by hypertrophied adenoids. There may be a sense of dryness and irritation in the throat, and the breath may be offensive. Constitutional symptoms are not prominent. Rarely, hypertrophied tonsils and adenoids obstructing the upper airway are associated with respiratory distress, chronic hypoxemia, and the development of pulmonary hypertension.

INDICATIONS FOR TONSILLECTOMY. Parents often wrongly attribute frequent respiratory infections, allergic bronchitis, mouth breathing, recurrent purulent or serous otitis, poor appetite, failure to gain weight, or recurrent or chronic fever to chronic tonsillitis. Tonsillectomy and adenoidectomy do not decrease the incidence of these problems during childhood. For children with recurrent throat infections (seven in the past year or five in each of the past 2 years), tonsillectomy decreases the number of throat infections in the subsequent 2 years, compared with no tonsillectomy. However, many children who have not had tonsillectomy also have a decline in the number of throat infections. Until better methods are available to identify those children who will truly benefit from tonsillectomy and adenoidectomy, it seems prudent to avoid surgery in most cases. Factors such as severity of illness and the frequency of missing school need to be considered.

Decision for removal of tonsils should be based on symptoms and signs related directly to hypertrophy, obstruction, and chronic infection in the tonsils and related structures. *Most hypertrophic tonsils actually are normal in size; the misinterpretation results from failure to appreciate that normally tonsils are relatively larger during childhood than in later years.*

Tonsils may virtually meet in the midline in some children who are asymptomatic; tonsils of average size are projected toward the midline when the child is gagged and may be interpreted as being hypertrophic. Alternatively, infection does not always produce hypertrophy, and chronically infected tonsils may be small and embedded behind the faucial pillars. There is no certain way to directly demonstrate whether tonsils are harboring chronic infection. The consistency or size of the tonsils and the presence of cheesy material within the crypts are not reliable guides. Persistent hyperemia of the anterior pillars is a more reliable sign, and enlargement of the cervical lymph nodes is supporting evidence. Persistent enlargement of the node just below and slightly in front of the angle of the jaw is especially significant. Hypertrophy sufficient to obstruct swallowing or breathing is readily detectable; such tonsils practically meet in the midline when the throat is examined without gagging the patient. However, before tonsillectomy is recommended, it should be ascertained that the hypertrophy is chronic and not the result of a recent acute infection. Tonsils can increase in size greatly during an acute infection and recede after its subsidence.

The only absolute indication for a tonsillectomy is to rule out tumor and severe aerodigestive tract obstruction. Tonsillectomy is of no value in the prevention or treatment of acute or chronic sinusitis, chronic otitis media, and middle ear deafness. There is also no evidence to indicate that the removal of tonsils is justified for infections in the lower respiratory tract. No systemic disturbance in itself is an indication for tonsillectomy.

Tonsillectomy in Relation to the Age of the Child. When, on rare occasions, it seems advisable to recommend tonsillectomy for a child 2–3 yr of age, every attempt should be made to postpone the operation. Frequently when the operation is postponed for reasons of age, the apparent need disappears within the next year or so. In the first few years of life the indications for adenoidectomy, although infrequent, are present more often than those for tonsillectomy. Neither procedure should be performed as a prophylaxis against the "common cold" at any age.

Tonsillectomy in Relation to Active Infection. Tonsillectomy should be postponed until 2–3 wk after subsidence of an infection, except in rare cases of acute respiratory obstruction with pulmonary artery hypertension and cor pulmonale.

COMPLICATIONS OF TONSILLECTOMY. The mean duration of postoperative sore throat is 5 days. Referred ear pain and halitosis are common. Minor hemorrhage, postoperative throat infection, or anesthetic complications occur in more than 10% of procedures. Severe hemorrhage or life-threatening complications occur occasionally and are another reason for carefully assessing the indications for surgical intervention. Pulmonary edema also not infrequently occurs after relief of upper airway obstruction with tonsillectomy or adenoidectomy. Therefore, this therapy should be reserved for settings in which postsurgical respiratory failure can be dealt with effectively. Outpatient tonsil and adenoid surgery can be performed safely and may be mandated by insurance carriers; however, surgery for airway obstruction and other conditions requires inpatient surgery and postoperative monitoring, as determined by the pediatrician and surgeon.

Adenoidal Hypertrophy

(Hypertrophy of Pharyngeal Tonsil; "Adenoids")

Disturbances of the nasopharyngeal lymphoid tissue (adenoids) tend to parallel those of the faucial tonsils. Hypertrophy and infection may occur separately but often occur together; infection is usually primary. The soft adenoid structure, which is normally widespread in the nasopharynx, especially on the posterior wall and the roof, undergoes hypertrophy, and masses of varying size are formed. These masses may almost fill the vault of the nasopharynx, interfere with the passage of air through the nose, obstruct the eustachian tubes, and block the clearance of nasal mucus.

CLINICAL MANIFESTATIONS. Mouth breathing and persistent rhinitis are the most characteristic symptoms. Mouth breathing may be present only during sleep, especially when the child lies supine, when snoring is also likely to occur. With severe adenoid hypertrophy the mouth is kept open during the day as well, and the mucous membranes of the mouth and lips are dry. Chronic nasopharyngitis may be constantly present or recur frequently. The voice is altered with a nasal, muffled quality. The breath is offensive, and taste and smell are impaired. A harassing cough may be present, especially at night, resulting from drainage of pus into the lower pharynx or irritation of the larynx by inspired air that has not been warmed and moistened by passage through the nose. Impaired hearing is common. Chronic otitis media may be associated with infected, hypertrophied adenoids and blockage of the eustachian tube orifices. Chronic mouth breathing predisposes to a narrow, high-arched palate and an elongated mandible. Referrals from orthodontists for evaluation of nasal obstruction and adenoidectomy are frequent.

A small number of young children with marked adenoidal (also tonsillar) enlargement are unable to mouth-breathe during sleep. They snort and snore loudly and often display signs of respiratory distress, such as intercostal retractions and nasal flaring. These children are at risk for respiratory insufficiency (hypoxemia, hypercapnia, acidosis) during sleep. Obstructive sleep apnea may result, and some of these children develop pulmonary arterial hypertension and, ultimately, cor pulmonale. Lymphoid tissue enlargement of the upper airway with consequent cor pulmonale has been related to cow's milk hypersensitivity in a number of preschool-aged children. Very obese children (e.g., Prader-Willi syndrome) and children with a large or posteriorly placed tongue (e.g., Pierre Robin syndrome) may also develop upper airway obstruction in sleep, mimicking the adenoidal hypertrophy syndrome. Patients with Down syndrome commonly have macroglossia, tonsillar enlargement, and skull base anomalies, which make them susceptible to obstruction.

DIAGNOSIS. During the first few years of life, the size of adenoids can be assessed by digital palpation. Indirect visualization with a pharyngeal mirror is possible in older, cooperative children. Alternatively, the fiberoptic bronchoscope can be used for visualization of the nasopharynx. Lateral pharyngeal roentgenograms are also helpful for detecting nasopharyngeal air column obliteration. The presence of adenoid hypertrophy can be suspected from such symptoms as mouth breathing, snoring, and persistent rhinitis with or without chronic otitis media.

An adenoid tissue abscess is uncommon but may be a cause of protracted fever. Identification and drainage of the abscess have been achieved by digital expression.

TREATMENT. Adenoidectomy may be indicated for symptoms such as persistent mouth breathing, nasal speech, adenoid facies, repeated attacks of otitis media (especially when accompanied by a conductive hearing loss), and persistent or recurring nasopharyngitis when these seem to be related to infected hypertrophied adenoid tissue. Tonsillectomy should not be done routinely for such problems. Chronic serous otitis media may improve after adenoidectomy in some patients. The same precautions for the complete removal and control of bleeding points, such as in tonsillectomy, should be observed.

JAMES E. ARNOLD

Boat TF, Polmar SH, Whitman V, et al: Hyperreactivity to cow milk in young children with pulmonary hemosiderosis and cor pulmonale secondary to nasopharyngeal obstruction. J Pediatr 87:23, 1975.
Carson JL, Collier AM, Collier HSS: Acquired ciliary defects in nasal epithelium of children with acute viral upper respiratory infections. N Engl J Med 312:463, 1985.
Crockett DM, McGill TJ, Healy GB, et al: Nasal and paranasal sinus surgery in children with cystic fibrosis. Ann Otol Rhinol Laryngol 96:367, 1987.
Denny FW, Clyde WA: Acute respiratory tract infections: An overview: Pediatrics 17:1026, 1983.
Dingle JH, Badger GF, Jordan WS: Illness in the Home: A Study of 25,000 Illnesses in a Group of Cleveland Families. Cleveland, Press of Western Reserve University, 1964, p 129.
Glasier CM, Ascher DP, Williams KD: Incidental paranasal sinus abnormalities on CT of children: Clinical correlation. AJNR 7:861, 1986.
Greenwald HM, Messeloff CR: Retropharyngeal abscess in infants and children. Am J Med Sci 177:767, 1929.
Johnson F: Bleeding factors and tonsils and adenoid surgery. Arch Otolaryngol 86:584, 1967.
Li K, Kiernon S, Wald ER, et al: Isolated uvulitis due to *Haemophilus influenzae* type b. Pediatrics 74:1054, 1984.
Paradise JL, Bluestone CD, Backman RZ, et al: Efficacy of tonsillectomy for recurrent throat infection in severely affected children. N Engl J Med 310:674, 1984.
Paradise JL, Bluestone CD, Backman RZ, et al: History of recurrent sore throat as an indication for tonsillectomy. N Engl J Med 298:410, 1978.
Rachelefsky GS: Chronic sinusitis, Am J Dis Child 143:886, 1989.
Shackleford PG, Polmar SH, Mayus JL, et al: Spectrum of IgG2 subclass deficiency in children with recurrent infections: Prospective study. J Pediatr 108:647, 1986.
Spires JR: Treatment of peritonsillar abscess: A prospective study of aspiration vs incision and drainage. Arch Otolaryngol Head Neck Surg 113:984, 1987.
Stern RC, Boat TF, Wood RE, et al: Treatment and prognosis of nasal polyps in cystic fibrosis. Am J Dis Child 136:1067, 1982.
Tinkelman DG, Silk HJ: Clinical and bacteriologic features of chronic sinusitis in children. Am J Dis Child 143:938, 1989.
Wald ER: Acute sinusitis in children. Pediatr Infect Dis 2:61, 1983.

14.34 LOWER RESPIRATORY TRACT

CONGENITAL ANOMALIES

14.35 CONGENITAL LARYNGEAL ANOMALIES

Complete **atresia of the larynx** is incompatible with life; only rarely can an infant in whom the diagnosis is made at birth be saved by immediate needle tracheostomy and high-pressure transtracheal ventilation. A formal tracheostomy is then performed. Subsequent successful surgical restoration of an adequate upper airway has not been reported. Patients with laryngeal atresia often have other congenital defects that also may be incompatible with life. **Laryngeal webs** are uncommon, occasionally familial, defects resulting from incomplete separation of the fetal mesenchyme between the two sides of the larynx. Most webs occur between the vocal cords. Immediate diagnosis of a complete or nearly complete web is essential to prevent asphyxiation of the newborn. Respiratory distress with severe stridor may be present, and the cry is weak and abnormal in character. The obstruction is often not complete, and there is only mild stridor and dyspnea. Direct laryngoscopy is required for prompt diagnosis and treatment. Lysis with a carbon dioxide laser is frequently successful, but surgery is occasionally necessary. Thin supraglottic webs can also be incised, but infants with thicker subglottic or intralaryngeal webs require initial incision, excision, and subsequent dilations, which may be unsuccessful because of reformation of the web. An external approach to divide and excise the web with insertion of silicone or metal is often required. Many surgically treated patients need a tracheostomy for a prolonged period thereafter.

Laryngotracheoesophageal cleft is a rare congenital lesion in which there is a long connection between the airway and the esophagus, sometimes extending to the level of the carina. The lesion is owing to failure of dorsal fusion of the cricoid, which normally is completed by the 8th wk of gestation. Other anomalies, including unilateral pulmonary hypoplasia, may be present. Symptoms of chronic aspiration, gagging during feeding, and pneumonia suggest H-type tracheoesophageal fistula, but the clinical manifestations are usually more severe and associated with abnormalities in voice. Diagnosis is extremely difficult, but careful roentgenographic studies of swallowing will show aspiration of contrast material into the trachea indicating the need for endoscopic examination of the airway and perhaps the esophagus. Successful repair has been reported but requires multiple procedures and prolonged tracheostomy.

14.36 CONGENITAL LARYNGEAL STRIDOR
(Laryngomalacia and Tracheomalacia)

Stridor persisting or appearing after the first few days of life usually results from disturbances in or adjacent to the larynx. The most common of these, **laryngomalacia** and **tracheomalacia**, are congenital deformities or flabbiness of the epiglottis and supraglottic aperture and weakness of the airway walls, leading to collapse and some airway obstruction with inspiration. Laryngomalacia is the most common congenital laryngeal abnormality. Males are affected twice as often as females. The embryologic origin of the defect is unknown.

CLINICAL MANIFESTATIONS. Noisy, crowing respiratory sounds, usually associated with inspiration, are relatively common during the neonatal period and the first year of life. Stridor, usually present from birth, may not appear until 2 mo in some patients. Symptoms can be intermittent and are worse when the infant lies on his or her back. Some infants merely have noisy breathing, whereas others have a laryngeal "crow," hoarseness or aphonia, dyspnea, and inspiratory retractions in the supraclavicular, intercostal, and subcostal space. When retractions are severe, thoracic deformity may result. Infants with severe dyspnea may have difficulty nursing, resulting in undernutrition and poor weight gain. Substantial stridor may persist for several months to 1 year after birth, occasionally becoming slightly worse in the first few months of life and then gradually disappearing with growth and development of the airway.

DIAGNOSIS. Laryngomalacia can usually be diagnosed by direct laryngoscopy. In the first few days of life, distinguishing between a congenital laryngeal disturbance and neonatal tetany or laryngeal edema secondary to trauma or aspiration at birth may be difficult. The differential diagnosis includes malformations of the laryngeal cartilages or vocal cords, intraluminal webs, generalized severe chondromalacia of the larynx and trachea, tumors of the larynx, mucus retention cysts, branchial cleft cysts, thyroglossal duct remnants, hypoplasia of the mandible, macroglossia, hemangioma, lymphangioma, Pierre Robin syndrome, congenital goiters, and vascular anomalies.

TREATMENT. Usually no specific therapy is indicated; the condition resolves spontaneously, although there may be difficulty in feeding. In one review, only 4 of 1,415 patients required tracheostomy. Parents should be reassured about the ultimate resolution and counseled to provide slow, careful feedings. A small nipple or dropper or, infrequently, gavage may be required. Most patients seem more comfortable or less noisy lying in a prone position. Severe symptoms may require nasotracheal intubation or, rarely, tracheostomy.

PROGNOSIS. Although laryngomalacia usually resolves clinically by 18 mo of age, some degree of inspiratory obstruction may persist a little longer. Sophisticated pulmonary function testing reveals that minor abnormalities persist, in some patients, into teenage, but these do not pose any clinically important problems and do not require treatment. However, some patients may develop stridor with respiratory infection, exertion, or crying throughout childhood.

OTHER ANOMALIES. Bifid epiglottis, resulting from cleavage of two thirds or more of the epiglottis, is a rare condition that may not compromise swallowing. It usually does require treatment, however, and is associated with other laryngeal anomalies and with polydactyly. Total absence of the epiglottis is extremely rare. Laryngeal cysts and laryngoceles are occasionally seen; treatment with endoscopic "unroofing" is usually successful.

Fang SH, Ocejo R, Sin M, et al: Congenital laryngeal atresia. Am J Dis Child 143:625, 1989.
Landing BH: State of the art: Congenital malformations and genetic diseases of the respiratory tract. Am Rev Respir Dis 120:151, 1979.
Macfarlane PI, Olinsky A, Phelan PD: Proximal airway function 8–16 years after laryngomalacia: Follow-up using flow-volume loop studies. J Pediatr 107:216, 1985.
Marcur CL, Crockett DM, Ward SLD: Evaluation of epiglottoplasty as treatment for severe laryngomalacia. J Pediatr 117:706, 1990.
McGill TJI, Healy BG: Congenital and acquired lesions of the infant larynx. Clin Pediatr 17:584, 1978.
McSwiney PF, Cavanagh NPC, Languth P: Outcome in congenital stridor (laryngomalacia). Arch Dis Child 52:215, 1977.
Novak RW: Laryngotracheoesophageal cleft and unilateral pulmonary hypoplasia in twins. Pediatrics 67:732, 1981.
Smith GJ, Cooper DM: Laryngomalacia and inspiratory obstruction in later childhood. Arch Dis Child 56:345, 1981.
Smith RJH, Catlin FI: Congenital anomalies of the larynx. Am J Dis Child 138:35, 1984.

TRACHEOESOPHAGEAL FISTULA

See Sec. 13.17.

VASCULAR RING

See Sec. 15.58.

14.37 AGENESIS/HYPOPLASIA OF THE LUNG

Bilateral pulmonary agenesis or hypoplasia is rare and incompatible with life; the latter is usually associated with anencephaly, diaphragmatic hernias, urinary tract abnormalities, abnormalities of the thumb, deformities of the thoracic spine and rib cage (thoracic dystrophy), renal anomalies, right-sided heart malformations, and pleural effusions. Unilateral agenesis or hypoplasia may have few symptoms and nonspecific findings, resulting in only one third of the cases being diagnosed during life. Left-sided lesions are more common. In unilateral agenesis the entire pulmonary parenchyma and supporting structures and airways are absent below the level of the carina. In pulmonary hypoplasia there is a small unexpandable lung. Persistent fetal circulation is often present when pulmonary hypoplasia presents in the newborn period (see Sec. 9.36). Occasional reports of parental consanguinity suggest a genetic basis for at least some of these cases.

There is no specific treatment. Supportive measures including mechanical ventilation and supplemental oxygen may allow sufficient pulmonary parenchymal development to permit survival (25% of the infants in one series). Older patients should be given antibiotics for pulmonary infection and receive annual influenza vaccine. Prognosis in the patients who survive infancy is extremely variable and largely dependent on the presence of associated anomalies. The contralateral lung is often larger than normal. The resultant mediastinal shift and associated mortality are greater when the hypoplasia/agenesis involves the right lung. Death may also occur from overwhelming pulmonary infection or from complications of pulmonary hypertension associated with congenital heart disease.

Kresch MJ, Markowitz RI, Smith GJW: Respiratory distress and cyanosis in a term newborn infant. J Pediatr 113:937, 1988.
Mardini MK, Nyhan WL: Agenesis of the lung: Report of four patients with unusual anomalies. Chest 87:522, 1985.
Milligan DWA, Levison H: Lung function in children following repair of tracheoesophageal fistula. J Pediatr 95:24, 1979.
Page DV, Stocker JT: Anomalies associated with pulmonary hypoplasia. Am Rev Respir Dis 125:216, 1982.
Swischuk LE, Richardson CF, Nichols MM, et al: Primary pulmonary hypoplasia in the neonate. J Pediatr 95:573, 1979.

LOBAR EMPHYSEMA

See Sec. 14.76.

14.38 PULMONARY SEQUESTRATION

A mass of nonfunctioning embryonic and cystic pulmonary tissue that receives its entire blood supply from the systemic circulation is known as a sequestration. Although most sequestrations do not communicate with functional airways, this is not always the case. Both intralobar and extralobar sequestrations arise through the same pathoembryologic mechanism as a remnant of a diverticular outgrowth of the esophagus. Gastric or pancreatic tissue may be found within the sequestration. Cysts may also be present. Other congenital anomalies, including diaphragmatic hernia and esophageal cysts, are not uncommon. Some believe that intralobar sequestration is often a manifestation of cystadenomatoid malformation and have questioned the existence of intralobar sequestration as a separate entity.

Intralobar sequestration is generally found in a lower lobe. Patients thus affected usually present with infection. In older patients, hemoptysis is fairly common. A chest roentgenogram, during a period when there is no active infection, reveals a mass lesion; an air-fluid level may be present. During infection the margins of the lesion may be blurred. There is no difference in the incidence of this lesion in each lung. Treatment is surgical removal of the lesion, a procedure that usually requires excision of the entire involved lobe. A segmental resection will occasionally suffice.

Extralobar sequestration is more common on the left. This lesion is associated strongly with diaphragmatic hernia. Many of these patients are asymptomatic when the mass is discovered by routine chest roentgenogram taken for another reason. Other patients present with respiratory symptoms or heart failure. Surgical resection of the involved area is recommended.

Physical findings in patients with sequestration include an area of dullness to percussion and decreased breath sounds over the lesion. During infection, rales may also be present. A continuous or purely systolic murmur may be heard over the back. If routine chest roentgenograms are consistent with the diagnosis, other procedures are indicated prior to surgical intervention. Bronchography reveals a mass of intrathoracic tissue without connection to the airways. Ultrasound can help rule out a diaphragmatic hernia. Aortography should be performed in these patients, since this procedure allows definitive diagnosis by demonstrating systemic blood supply from an anomalous aortic artery. Identifying the blood supply prior to surgery avoids inadvertently severing this systemic artery, which has accounted for much of the intraoperative mortality in the past.

Case Records of the Massachusetts General Hospital: Case 18–1981. N Engl J Med 304:1090, 1981.
Gottrup F, Lund C: Intralobar pulmonary sequestration: A report of 12 cases. Scand J Respir Dis 59:21, 1978.
Pryce DM: Lower accessory pulmonary artery with intralobar sequestration of lung: Report of seven cases. J Pathol Bacteriol 58:547, 1946.
Telander RL, Lennox C, Sieber W: Sequestration of the lung in children. Mayo Clin Proc 51:578, 1976.
Tolkin JB, MacAdam C, Moody S: Extralobar pulmonary sequestration. Am J Dis Child 141:1223, 1987.

14.39 BRONCHOGENIC CYSTS

These cysts are originally lined with ciliated epithelium and usually occur close to a midline structure (e.g., trachea, esophagus, carina). Once infected, the ciliated epithelium may be lost, and accurate pathologic diagnosis is then impossible. Cysts are rarely demonstrable at birth. Later, some cysts become symptomatic either by becoming infected or by enlarging in size and compromising the function of an adjacent airway. Fever, chest pain, and productive cough are the most common presenting symptoms. A chest roentgenogram reveals the cyst, which may contain an air–fluid level. Treatment for symptomatic cysts is surgical excision following appropriate antibiotic management. An asymptomatic cyst discovered incidentally by chest roentgenogram taken for another reason may not require treatment.

14.40 BRONCHOBILIARY FISTULA

This rare anomaly usually presents life-threatening problems during early infancy but, occasionally, diagnosis has been delayed until after 2 yr of age. It consists of a fistulous connection between the right middle lobe bronchus and the left hepatic ductal system. All patients have recurrent severe bronchopulmonary infection and atelectasis starting in early infancy. Definitive diagnosis requires endoscopy and bronchography or exploratory surgery. Treatment is surgical excision of the entire intrathoracic portion of the fistula. Bronchobiliary communications also occur as acquired lesions resulting from hepatic disease complicated by infection.

Pappas SC, Sasaki A, Minuk GY: Bronchobiliary fistula presenting as cough with yellow sputum. N Engl J Med 307:1027, 1982.
Weitzman JJ, Cohen SR, Woods LO Jr, et al: Congenital bronchobiliary fistula. J Pediatr 73:329, 1958.

14.41 CONGENITAL PULMONARY LYMPHANGIECTASIS

This disease, characterized by greatly dilated lymphatic ducts throughout the lung, is usually symptomatic with dyspnea and cyanosis in the newborn. Chest roentgenograms reveal both punctate and reticular densities. Respiration is compromised because of the space-occupying nature of the lesion and, possibly, because pulmonary compliance is reduced, increasing the work of breathing. Two forms of the disease—one in which the abnormality is limited to the lung and one in which the pulmonary lymphangiectasis is secondary to pulmonary venous obstruction—are always symptomatic in the neonatal period. Familial occurrence of the first type has been reported. A third form, in which the pulmonary lymphangiectasis is part of a generalized disease involving other organ systems (e.g., intestine), is associated with milder pulmonary disease and survival to midchildhood and beyond. Definitive diagnosis requires lung biopsy. There is no specific treatment.

Case Records of the Massachusetts General Hospital: Case 31–1989. N Engl J Med 321:309, 1989.
Felman AH, Rhatigan RM, Pierson KK: Pulmonary lymphangiectasis. Am J Roent 116:548, 1972.
Noonan JA, Walters LR, Reeves JT: Congenital pulmonary lymphangiectasia. Am J Dis Child 120:314, 1970.
Scott-Emuakpor AB, Warren ST, Kapur S, et al: Familial occurrence of congenital pulmonary lymphangiectasis. Am J Dis Child 135:532, 1981.

14.42 CYSTIC ADENOMATOID MALFORMATION

This is the second most common congenital lung lesion (lobar emphysema is the most common). A single lobe of one lung is enlarged and often cystic, compressing the remainder of the ipsilateral lung and frequently causing a mediastinum shift with compression of the contralateral lung. There is a slight male preponderance. The lesion probably results from an embryologic insult, usually before the 50th day of gestation, and seems to involve maldevelopment of terminal bronchiolar structures. Histologic examination reveals little normal lung and many glandular elements. Cysts are very common; cartilage is rare. The presence of cartilage may indicate a somewhat later embryologic insult, perhaps extending into the 10th–24th wk.

Most patients become symptomatic and die in the newborn period, although a few survive after emergency surgery. Rarely, patients are asymptomatic until midchildhood, when brief episodes of recurrent or persistent pulmonary infection or relatively acute chest pain occur. Breath sounds may be diminished with mediastinal shift away from the lesion on physical examination. Chest roentgenograms reveal a cystic mass with mediastinal shift. Occasionally, an air-fluid level suggests a lung abscess. The lesion may be confused with diaphragmatic hernia in the newborn. Surgical excision of the affected lobe is indicated. After surgery, long-term survival into infancy and even later into childhood has been reported, but these patients may be at increased risk for developing primary pulmonary neoplasms.

Benning TL, Godwin JD, Roggli VL, et al: Cartilaginous variant of congenital malformation of the lung. Chest 92:514, 1987.
Hartman GE, Shochat SJ: Primary pulmonary neoplasms of childhood: A review. Ann Thorac Surg 36:108, 1983.
Stocker JT, Madewell JE, Drake RM: Congenital cystic adenomatoid malformation of the lung: Classification and morphologic spectrum. Hum Pathol 8:155, 1977.

ACQUIRED DISEASE

ACUTE INFECTIONS OF THE LARYNX AND TRACHEA

GENERAL CONSIDERATIONS. Acute infections of the larynx and trachea are of great importance in infants and small children because their airway is smaller, predisposing it to a relatively greater narrowing than is produced by the same degree of inflammation in an older child.

Croup is a generic term encompassing a heterogeneous group of relatively acute infectious conditions characterized by a peculiarly brassy ("croupy") cough, which may or may not be accompanied by inspiratory stridor, hoarseness, and signs of respiratory distress due to varying degrees of laryngeal obstruction. When there is sufficient involvement of the larynx to produce symptoms, the laryngeal part of the clinical picture is likely to overshadow other manifestations.

The infection in infants and small children is rarely limited to a single area of the respiratory tract, but usually rather affects in varying degrees the larynx, trachea, bronchi, and even the upper respiratory portion. Thus, although an exact classification of these infections is not possible, identification of several clinical varieties is justified:

Acute diphtheritic laryngitis (see Sec. 12.25).
Infectious croup (acute nondiphtheritic infections)
Epiglottitis
Laryngitis
Laryngotracheobronchitis
Spasmodic laryngitis
Bacterial tracheitis

14.43 INFECTIOUS CROUP
(Acute Nondiphtheritic Infections)

ETIOLOGY AND EPIDEMIOLOGY. Viral agents account for nearly all croup except that associated with diphtheria, bacterial tracheitis, and acute epiglottitis. The parainfluenza viruses account for approximately three quarters of all cases, with the adenoviruses, respiratory syncytial, influenza, and measles viruses causing most of the remaining cases for which a viral agent can be identified. In one study, *Mycoplasma pneumoniae* was recovered from 3.6% of patients who had croup. Although *H. influenzae* type b is almost always the cause of acute epiglottitis, the group A streptococcus, the pneumococcus, and the staphylococcus are occasionally implicated. Viral epiglottitis is rare, but a milder and superficially similar picture from inflammation of the supraglottic area is probably caused by viruses.

Most patients who have viral croup are between the ages of 3 mo and 5 yr, whereas disease due to *H. influenzae* and *C. diphtheriae* is more common from 3–7 yr of age. The incidence of croup is higher in males, and it occurs most commonly during the cold season of the year. Approximately 15% of patients have a strong family history of croup, and laryngitis tends to recur in the same child.

CLINICAL MANIFESTATIONS. Croup. With progressive compromise of the upper airway, a characteristic sequence of symptoms and signs occurs. At first, there is only a mild brassy cough with intermittent respiratory stridor; the latter is sometimes preceded by 1–2 days of mild upper respiratory symptoms. As obstruction increases, stridor becomes continuous and is associated with nasal flaring and suprasternal, infrasternal, and intercostal retractions. Agitation and crying greatly aggravate the symptoms and signs, and the child prefers to sit up in bed or be held upright.

With further compromise of the airway, air hunger and restlessness occur briefly and are then superseded by severe hypoxemia and weakness, accompanied by decreased air exchange and stridor, increasing pulse, and eventual death from hypoventilation. Most patients with croup progress only as far as stridor and slight dyspnea, before they start to recover within a few hours. In the hypoxic child who may be cyanotic, pale, or obtunded, any manipulation of the pharynx, including use of a tongue depressor, may result in sudden cardiorespiratory arrest. This examination, therefore, should be deferred and oxygen should be administered until the patient is transferred to a hospital, where optimal management of the airway and shock is possible.

Acute Epiglottitis. This dramatic, potentially lethal condition usually occurs in children 2–7 yr old and the peak incidence occurs at about 3½ yr. The male:female ratio is about 3:2. It is characterized by a fulminating course of fever, sore throat, dyspnea, rapidly progressive respiratory obstruction, and prostration. Within a matter of hours, epiglottitis may progress to complete obstruction of the airway and death unless adequate treatment is administered. With adequate treatment the illness rarely lasts for more than 2–3 days. Respiratory distress is frequently the first manifestation. Often the child, particularly the younger patient, is apparently well at bedtime but awakens later in the evening with high fever, aphonia, drooling, and moderate-to-severe respiratory distress with stridor. Usually no other family members are ill with acute upper respiratory disease. The older child often complains initially of sore throat and dysphagia. Severe respiratory distress may ensue within minutes or hours of the onset, with inspiratory stridor, hoarseness, brassy cough, irritability, and restlessness. Drooling and dysphagia are common. The neck may be hyperextended, although other signs of meningeal irritation are absent. The older child may prefer a sitting position, leaning forward, with the mouth open and the tongue somewhat protruding. Some children may progress rapidly to a shock-like state characterized by pallor, cyanosis, and impaired consciousness.

The physical examination may disclose moderate-to-severe respiratory distress with inspiratory and sometimes expiratory stridor, flaring of the alae nasi, and inspiratory retractions of the suprasternal notch, supraclavicular and intercostal spaces, and subcostal area. The pharynx may be inflamed, and there may be an abundance of mucus and saliva, which may also result in rhonchi. With progression, stridor and breath sounds may be diminished as the patient tires. A brief period of air hunger with restlessness and agitation may be followed by rapidly increasing cyanosis, coma, and death. Alternatively, the child may have only mild hoarseness and a large, shiny, cherry-red epiglottis brought into view when the posterior portion of the tongue is properly depressed.

The diagnosis requires visualization of a large, swollen cherry-red epiglottis by direct examination or laryngoscopy. Laryngoscopy reveals intense inflammation of the epiglottis and surrounding area: arytenoids and arytenoepiglottic folds, vocal cords, and subglottic regions. If the diagnosis is probable on other clinical grounds, direct viewing of the epiglottis in a seriously ill child should be deferred until complete cardiorespiratory support is available and definitive treatment can be carried out because some patients may have reflex laryngospasm and acute complete obstruction, aspiration of secretions, and cardiorespiratory arrest following examination of the pharynx. Furthermore, children with suspected epiglottitis should not be placed in the supine position because of the risk of increased agitation and gravity-induced change in the position of the epiglottis with increased airway obstruction. Arterial blood gas samples should not be obtained prior to a definitive diagnosis and the establishment of an artificial airway. If epiglottitis is thought to be a reasonable possibility, however remote, in a patient with croup, the patient should have a lateral roentgenogram of the nasopharynx and upper airway prior to physical examination of the pharynx (Fig. 14–5). If a roentgenogram shows a normal epiglottis, examination of the epiglottis may be performed when appropriate equipment and personnel are available to control the airway and provide ventilatory support. Patients with suspected epiglottitis should be accompanied by a physician and intubation equipment at all times, including the trip to and from the radiology department.

Establishing an airway by either nasotracheal intubation or tracheostomy is indicated in the face of clear evidence of epiglottitis, even though the degree of apparent respiratory distress may not seem severe when the patient is initially evaluated. Fulminant pulmonary edema may be associated with acute airway obstruction. The duration of intubation depends on the clinical course of the patient and the duration of epiglottic swelling, as determined by frequent examination using direct laryngoscopy. In general, children with acute epiglottitis are intubated for 2–3 days. Bacteremia is present in most patients; therefore, parenteral antibiotic therapy including ceftriaxone or ampicillin and chloramphenicol should be instituted promptly. Concomitant infection is unusual, but meningitis, pneumonia, cervical adenitis, and otitis media may occur.

After epiglottitis, patients develop high serum antibody

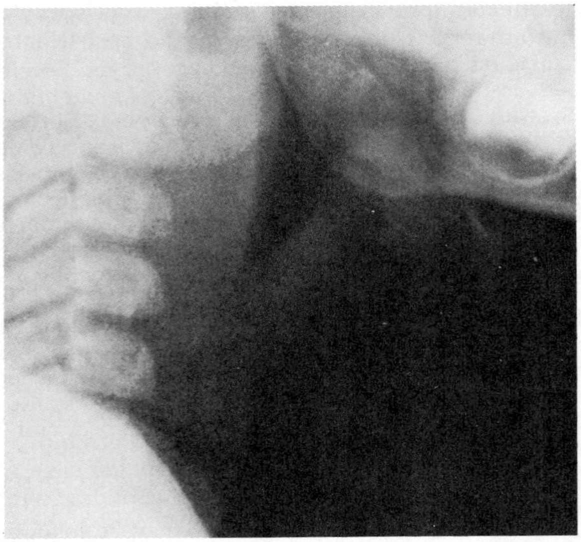

Figure 14–5. Epiglottitis. Lateral roentgenogram of the upper airway reveals the swollen-epiglottis.

titers against *H. influenzae* type b, whereas postmeningitic children do not.

Acute Infectious Laryngitis. Laryngitis is a common illness; except for diphtheria, almost all cases are caused by viruses. The onset is usually characterized by an upper respiratory tract infection during which sore throat, cough, and croup appear. The illness is generally mild; respiratory distress is unusual except in the young infant. In severe cases, however, hoarseness is marked, and the patient may present severe inspiratory stridor, retractions, dyspnea, and restlessness. As the process progresses, air hunger and fatigue become evident, and the child alternates between periods of agitation and exhaustion. The physical examination is usually not remarkable except for evidence of pharyngeal inflammation and, with respiratory distress, evidence of high respiratory obstruction. Inflammatory edema of the vocal cords and subglottic tissue may be demonstrated laryngoscopically. The principal site of obstruction is usually the subglottic area.

Acute Laryngotracheobronchitis. This most common form of croup is caused primarily by viruses. The opportunity for pathologic study is rare; the primary findings appear to be inflammatory edema, destruction of ciliated epithelium, and exudate. Secondary bacterial infection is rare. Most patients have an upper respiratory tract infection for several days before the brassy cough, inspiratory stridor, and respiratory distress become apparent. As the infection extends downward involving the bronchi and bronchioles, respiratory difficulty increases and the expiratory phase of respiration also becomes labored and prolonged. The child often appears extremely restless and frightened. The temperature may be only slightly elevated or as high as 39–40° C (102–104° F). There are usually bilaterally diminished breath sounds, rhonchi, and scattered rales. Symptoms are characteristically worse at night and often recur with decreasing intensity for several days. Children are usually not seriously ill and often have associated rhinitis, conjunctivitis, or both. Other family members may have mild respiratory illness. Occasionally, the pattern of severe laryngotracheobronchitis may be difficult to distinguish from epiglottitis despite the usually more explosive onset and rapid course of the latter; it also requires similar precautions. Roentgenographic examination of the nasopharynx and upper airway may be helpful. The duration of illness ranges from several days to several weeks, and recurrences are frequent from 3–6 yr of age, decreasing with growth of the airway.

Acute Spasmodic Laryngitis. Spasmodic croup most often occurs in children 1–3 yr of age and is clinically similar to acute laryngotracheobronchitis, except that findings of infection in the patient and family are frequent absent. The etiology is viral in most cases, but allergic and psychologic factors are important in some cases. The opportunity for pathologic study is rare; the primary findings appear to be preservation of the epithelium (unlike acute infectious laryngotracheobronchitis) and pale, watery edema. The anxious and excitable child is more susceptible to this syndrome, and in some cases there is a familial predisposition.

Occurring most frequently in the evening or night, spasmodic croup begins with a sudden onset that is usually preceded by mild-to-moderate coryza and hoarseness. The child awakens with a characteristic barking, metallic cough, noisy inspiration, and respiratory distress and appears anxious and frightened. Breathing is slow and labored, the pulse is accelerated, and the skin is cool and moist. The patient is usually afebrile. Dyspnea is aggravated by excitement, and there may be intermittent episodes of cyanosis. Usually the severity of the symptoms diminishes within several hours, and the following day the patient often appears well except for slight hoarseness and cough. Similar, but usually less severe, attacks without extreme respiratory distress may occur for another night or two, eventually concluding in complete recovery. Such episodes often recur several times.

DIFFERENTIAL DIAGNOSIS. These four syndromes must be distinguished from one another and from a variety of other entities that may present upper airway obstruction. *Bacterial tracheitis* is the most important differential diagnostic consideration (see Sec. 14.44). *Diphtheritic croup* (see Sec. 12.25) is usually preceded by an upper respiratory tract infection for several days; symptoms develop more slowly, although respiratory obstruction may occur suddenly; a serous or serosanguineous nasal discharge is occasionally present; and pharyngeal examination reveals the typical gray-white membrane. *Measles croup* almost always coincides with the full manifestations of systemic disease (see Sec. 12.64), and the course may be fulminant.

Sudden onset of respiratory obstruction may be due to *aspiration of a foreign body*. The child is generally 6 mo–2 yr of age. Choking coughing occurs suddenly, usually without signs of inflammation. A *retropharyngeal* or *peritonsillar abscess* may also present as respiratory obstruction; palpation of the posterior pharyngeal wall usually reveals a fluctuant mass. Roentgenographic examination of the upper airway and chest is essential in evaluating these possibilities as well as possible causes of *extrinsic compression* of the airway, such as a hematoma from trauma and *intraluminal obstruction* from masses (e.g., cysts or tumors).

Croup is also occasionally associated with *angioedema* of the subglottic areas as part of anaphylaxis and generalized allergic reactions, edema following *endotracheal intubation* for general anesthesia or respiratory failure, *hypocalcemic tetany*, *infectious mononucleosis*, trauma, and tumors or malformations of the larynx. A croupy cough may be an early sign of *asthma*. Psychogenic stridor can also occur. Epiglottitis, with the characteristic manifestations of drooling/dysphagia and stridor, can also result from the accidental ingestion of very hot liquid.

COMPLICATIONS. Complications occur in approximately 15% of patients with viral croup. The most common one is extension of the infectious process to involve other regions of the respiratory tract, such as the middle ear, the terminal bronchioles, or the pulmonary parenchyma. Bacterial tracheitis (see Sec. 14.44) may be a complication of viral croup rather than a distinct disease. Interstitial pneumonia may occur, but it is difficult to distinguish from patchy areas of atelectasis secondary to obstruction. Bronchopneumonia is unusual unless aspiration of stomach contents has occurred during a period of severe respiratory distress. Secondary bacterial pneumonias are rarely found; suppurative tracheobronchitis is an occasional complication of laryngotracheobronchitis (see Sec. 14.51).

Pneumonia, cervical lymphadenitis, otitis, and, rarely, meningitis and septic arthritis may occur during the course of epiglottitis. Mediastinal emphysema and pneumothorax are the most common complications of tracheotomy.

PROGNOSIS. In general, the length of hospitalization and the mortality increase as the infection extends to involve a greater portion of the respiratory tract—except in epiglottitis, in which the localized infection itself may prove fatal. Most deaths from croup are caused by a laryngeal obstruction or by the complications of tracheotomy. Untreated epiglottitis has a mortality rate of up to 25% in some series, but if the diagnosis is made and appropriate treatment is initiated before the patient is moribund, the prognosis is excellent. The outcome of acute laryngotracheobronchitis, laryngitis, and spasmodic croup is also excellent. As a group, children who need to be hospitalized for croup have somewhat increased bronchial reactivity compared with normal children when tested several years later. The differences, although statistically significant, are small and their functional importance is unclear.

TREATMENT. Therapy for infectious croup consists primarily of maintaining or providing for adequate respiratory exchange and depends in part on the primary location of the disease and its cause. In the bacterial forms, antibiotic therapy is also important.

Sleeping with a humidifier near the bedside, but out of reach, is thought by some to reduce the likelihood of development of spasmodic croup in children known to be susceptible to it.

Most afebrile children with *acute spasmodic croup* or febrile patients with mild *laryngotracheobronchitis* can usually be safely and effectively managed at home. Use of steam from a hot shower or bath in a closed bathroom, hot steam from a vaporizer, or "cold steam" from a nebulizer (which has a safety advantage) often terminates acute laryngeal spasm and respiratory distress within minutes. The same effect has been noted by many parents as they take their child out into the cold night air on the way to the physician's office. Induction of vomiting, either by coughing or by syrup of ipecac, may also break the laryngeal spasm. However, although vomiting occasionally appears to break the laryngeal spasm, there is no objective evidence for the effectiveness of ipecac, and respiratory distress may be complicated by vomiting.

Once laryngeal spasm has been broken, its return may sometimes be prevented by the use of warm or cool humidification near the child's bed until the cough has subsided, usually after 2–3 days.

Children with croup and temperatures over 39° C (102.2° F) should be hospitalized if there are any of the following: actual or suspected epiglottitis, progressive stridor, respiratory distress, hypoxia, restlessness, cyanosis, pallor, depressed sensorium, or high fever in a toxic-appearing child. In all cases the decision for hospitalization is made because of the need for reliable observation and relatively safe tracheotomy or nasotracheal intubation, if either of these becomes necessary.

At home or in the hospital, the patient with croup should be watched carefully for intensification of symptoms of respiratory obstruction. The hospitalized child is usually placed in an atmosphere of high cold humidity to lessen irritation and drying of secretions. Frequent or continuous monitoring of the respiratory rate is essential, because a rapid and rising rate may be the first sign of hypoxia and approaching total respiratory obstruction. The patient should be disturbed as little as possible; with moderate-to-severe respiratory distress, parenteral fluids should be given to lessen physical exertion and vomiting with its potential for aspiration. Sedatives are usually contraindicated because restlessness is used as one of the principal clinical indices of the severity of obstruction and the need for tracheotomy or nasotracheal intubation. Oxygen should be used to alleviate hypoxia and apprehension but, because it reduces cyanosis, which is an indication for tracheotomy or nasotracheal intubation, these patients must be observed particularly closely. Expectorants, bronchodilating agents, and antihistamines are not helpful. Opiates are contraindicated because they may depress respirations and dry secretions.

Laryngotracheobronchitis and *spasmodic croup* do not respond to antibiotics, and antibiotics are not indicated to prevent suprainfection. Nonurgent tests should be delayed owing to increased symptoms associated with agitation and anxiety. Racemic epinephrine by aerosol (2.25% solution diluted 1:8 with water in doses of 2–4 mL for 15 min) with, but usually without, positive pressure may result in transient relief of symptoms; usually close observation and repeated treatments are necessary. Rarely, there is sufficient obstruction to warrant tracheotomy or nasotracheal intubation.

The use of **corticosteroids** remains controversial; unequivocal efficacy is unproved. The theoretical basis for corticosteroid treatment in laryngotracheobronchitis is to reduce inflammatory edema and prevent destruction of ciliated epithelium; in spasmodic croup, corticosteroids could reduce edema in part by decreasing vascular permeability and by decreasing the release of edema-inducing mediators. Although many studies have been published, the relatively small number of patients, the difficulty in distinguishing spasmodic from infectious croup, and a variety of other methodologic problems have not permitted a definitive conclusion. A meta-analysis (combining data from 10 English language studies) suggests some beneficial effect; however, many of the studies on which this analysis was performed had major methodologic flaws. A more recent double-blind study of 29 hospitalized patients with acute laryngotracheitis suggested that dexamethasone is beneficial, at least for the first 24 hr after the 1st dose. There is no substantial evidence suggesting any adverse effect of corticosteroid treatment.

Epiglottitis, if diagnosed by inspection of the epiglottis or by roentgenographic examination (see Fig. 14–5) or if strongly suspected clinically in a severely ill child, should be treated immediately with an **artificial airway**; untreated patients have a substantial mortality even when observed in the hospital with appropriate intubation equipment nearby. Ceftriaxone (100 mg/kg/24 hr) or **ampicillin** (200 mg/kg/24 hr) and **chloramphenicol** (100 mg/kg/24 hr) should be given parenterally pending culture and susceptibility reports because of the increasing possibility of ampicillin-resistant strains of *H. influenzae* type b. All patients should receive **oxygen** en route to the operating room unless it is contraindicated by the increased agitation caused by the mask. Racemic epinephrine and corticosteroids are ineffective; they do not avert the need for an artificial airway and may dangerously delay definitive treatment. After insertion of the artificial airway, the patient should improve immediately, respiratory distress and cyanosis should disappear, and normal or near-normal blood gases should return. Patients usually fall asleep. The epiglottitis resolves after a few days of antibiotics, and the patient can be weaned from the tracheostomy or nasotracheal tube; antibiotics should be continued for 7–10 days.

Acute laryngeal swelling on an allergic basis responds to epinephrine (1:1,000 dilution in dosage of 0.01 mL/kg to a maximum of 0.3 mL/dose) administered subcutaneously, and isoproterenol (1:200 dilution in dosage of 0.01 mL/kg to a maximum of 0.3 mL/dose) by aerosol. After recovery, the patient and parents should be instructed in emergency administration of these drugs at home. Corticosteroids are frequently required (50–100 mg of hydrocortisone every 6 hr).

Reactive mucosal swelling, severe stridor, and respiratory distress unresponsive to mist therapy may follow *endotracheal intubation* for general anesthesia in children. Intermittent use of racemic epinephrine aerosols or, occasionally, corticosteroids may be helpful.

Tracheotomy and Endotracheal Intubation. With the introduction of routine tracheotomy for epiglottitis, mortality dropped to almost zero. Endotracheal intubation is also very effective in hospitals having special interest in and appropriate facilities for the care of intubated children. Both procedures should always be done in an operating room if time permits; prior intubation and general anesthesia greatly facilitate doing a tracheotomy without complications.

Tracheotomy or endotracheal intubation is required for patients with epiglottitis, but it is required only for those with severe laryngotracheobronchitis and for those with spasmodic croup or laryngitis who have increasing signs of respiratory failure secondary to obstruction despite appropriate treatment. Severe forms of laryngotracheobronchitis that required tracheotomy in a high proportion of patients have been reported during severe measles and influenza A virus epidemics. Assessing the need for these procedures requires experience and judgment, because they should not be delayed until cyanosis and extreme restlessness have developed; a pulse rate over 150/min and rising, and an elevated P_{CO_2}, especially in a tiring child, are indications of impending respiratory failure.

The tracheostomy or endotracheal tube must remain in place until edema and spasm have subsided and the patient is able to handle secretions satisfactorily. They should always be removed as soon as possible, usually within a few days. Adequate resolution of epiglottis inflammation that has been accurately visualized by fiberoptic laryngoscopy may permit much more rapid extubation, often within 24 hours. There is some evidence that hydrocortisone (50–100 mg/24 hr) and racemic epinephrine may be useful to facilitate extubation or to treat croup associated with extubation.

PREVENTION. See Sec. 5.1 and 12.22.

EPIGLOTTITIS

Ashcraft CK, Steele RW: Epiglottitis: A pediatric emergency. J Respir Dis 9:48, 1988.

Battaglia JD, Lockhart CH: Management of acute epiglottis by nasotracheal intubation. Am J Dis Child 120:334, 1975.

Cohen SR, Chai J: Epiglottitis: Twenty-year study with tracheostomy. Ann Otol Rhinol Laryngol 87:1, 1978.

Kulick RM, Selbst SM, Baker MD, et al: Thermal epiglottitis after swallowing hot beverages. Pediatrics 81:441, 1988.

Molteni RA: Epiglottitis: Incidence of extraepiglottic infection: Report of 72 cases and review of the literature. Pediatrics 58:526, 1976.

Nussbaum E: Fiberoptic laryngoscopy as a guide to tracheal extubation in acute epiglottitis. J Pediatrics 102:269, 1983.

Rapkin RH: The diagnosis of epiglottitis: Simplicity and reliability of radiographs of the neck in differential diagnosis of the croup syndrome. J Pediatr 80:96, 1975.

LARYNGOTRACHEOBRONCHITIS

Denny FW, Murphy TF, Clyde WA Jr, et al: Croup: An 11 year study in a pediatric practice. Pediatrics 71:871, 1984.

Gurwitz D, Corey M, Levison H: Pulmonary function and bronchial reactivity in children after croup. Am Rev Respir Dis 122:95, 1980.

Kairys SW, Olmstead EM, O'Connor GT: Steroid treatment of laryngotracheitis: A meta-analysis of the evidence from randomized trials. Pediatrics 83:683, 1989.

Singer OP, Wilson WJ: Laryngotracheobronchitis: 2 years' experience with racemic epinephrine. Can Med Assoc J 115:132, 1976.

Smith MS: Acute psychogenic stridor in an adolescent athlete treated with hypnosis. Pediatrics 72:247, 1983.

Super DM, Cartelli NA, Brooks LJ, et al: A prospective double-blind study to evaluate the effect of dexamethasone in acute laryngotracheitis. J Pediatr 115:323, 1989.

14.44 BACTERIAL TRACHEITIS

Bacterial tracheitis, an acute bacterial infection of the upper airway, does not involve the epiglottis but, like epiglottitis and croup, is capable of causing life-threatening airway obstruction. *S. aureus* is the most commonly isolated pathogen. Parainfluenza virus type 1, *Moraxilla catarrhalis* and *H. influenzae* also can be isolated. Most patients are less than 3 yr of age, although older children have occasionally been affected. There are no clear sex differences in incidence or severity. Bacterial tracheitis almost always follows an apparently viral respiratory infection (i.e., laryngotracheitis, Sec. 14.43). Thus, it may be a bacterial complication of a viral disease, rather than a primary bacterial illness. Regardless of its proper categorization, however, this life-threatening entity is probably at least as common as epiglottitis and requires prompt and appropriate intervention.

CLINICAL MANIFESTATIONS. Typically, the child develops a brassy cough, apparently as part of a viral upper respiratory infection, perhaps following typical croup. High fever and "toxicity" then occur and are associated with gradually worsening inspiratory stridor. Usual treatment for croup (i.e., mist, intravenous fluid, aerosolized racemic epinephrine) is ineffective. Intubation or tracheostomy is usually necessary. The major pathology appears to be mucosal swelling at the level of the cricoid cartilage, complicated by copious thick, purulent secretions. Suctioning these secretions, although occasionally affording temporary relief, usually does not sufficiently obviate the need for an artificial airway.

DIAGNOSIS. This is based on evidence of bacterial upper airway disease (which includes moderate leukocytosis with many band forms, high fever, and purulent airway secretions) and an absence of the classic findings of epiglottitis (which include radiologic demonstration of a swollen epiglottis, sudden catastrophic onset/rapid progression of symptoms, and typical direct laryngoscopic findings of abnormal epiglottis).

TREATMENT. Appropriate antimicrobial therapy, which usually includes antistaphylococcal agents, should be instituted in any patient with croup whose course at all suggests bacterial tracheitis. When bacterial tracheitis is diagnosed by direct laryngoscopy or strongly suspected on clinical grounds, an artificial airway is usually indicated. Oxygen should be administered if necessary.

COMPLICATIONS. Chest roentgenograms often show patchy infiltrates and may show focal densities. Subglottic narrowing can also often be demonstrated roentgenographically. When airway management is not optimal, cardiorespiratory arrest can occur. Toxic shock has occurred in association with tracheitis.

PROGNOSIS. The prognosis for well-treated patients is excellent. Most patients become afebrile within 2–3 days of instituting appropriate antimicrobial therapy. With a decrease in mucosal edema and purulent secretions, extubation can be accomplished. The mean duration of hospitalization was 12 days in one series.

Denneny JC III, Handler SD: Membranous laryngotracheobronchitis. Pediatrics 70:705, 1982.

Liston SL, Gehrz RC, Siegel LG, et al: Bacterial tracheitis. Am J Dis Child 137:764, 1983.

Nelson WE: Bacterial croup: A historical perspective. J Pediatr 105:52, 1984.

14.45 FOREIGN BODIES IN THE LARYNX, TRACHEA, AND BRONCHI

The air passages of children are frequent sites for the lodgment of foreign bodies; the carelessness of adults is occasionally a contributing factor. The symptoms and physical findings produced by foreign bodies depend on their nature, location, and the degree of obstruction of the air passage. A sharp or irritating object lodged in the larynx produces severe edema and later suppurative perichondritis, whereas an obstructive object in the bronchus produces atelectasis and later bronchiectasis, pulmonary abscess, or empyema.

Most foreign bodies aspirated into the respiratory tract are probably expelled immediately by reflex cough and never require medical attention. However, if an object too large to be eliminated by mucociliary clearance is aspirated and is not expelled by coughing, respiratory symptoms inevitably result. A large foreign body that can occlude the upper airway completely is an immediate threat to life. Smaller objects that lodge in one of the mainstem or lobar bronchi cause more chronic and usually less severe symptoms.

After the initial symptoms, which may have been forgotten, there is often a symptom-free interval that may last from hours to weeks. On occasion, dysphagia may occur from the swelling that results from a foreign body in the region of the larynx, and foreign bodies in the upper esophagus may cause symptoms referable to the air passages by compression or by the overflow of food or secretions into the larynx. Occasionally, a foreign body is not diagnosed until it is revealed by pathologic examination of a lobe that has been removed because of chronic bronchiectasis.

Laryngeal Foreign Body

CLINICAL MANIFESTATIONS. A laryngeal foreign body causes hoarseness, a cough that soon becomes croupy, and aphonia. Hemoptysis, dyspnea with wheezing, and cyanosis may occur. Obstruction resulting from the foreign body or the combination of it and the inflammatory reaction may prove fatal if the signs of high respiratory tract obstruction are not promptly recognized and appropriate treatment is not given. Hot dogs are one of the most common causes of fatal aspirations.

DIAGNOSIS. Roentgenographic and direct laryngoscopic examinations usually reveal or suggest the presence of a foreign body in the larynx (Fig. 14–6). An opaque foreign body in the neck will be clearly demonstrated on a lateral roentgenogram. When it is lodged anteriorly, it is obviously in the larynx; when it is behind the soft-tissue shadows of the larynx, it is in the hypopharynx or the cervical esophagus. The plane in which the foreign body lies is another differential point in its localization. If it lies in the sagittal plane, it is probably in the larynx. If it is in the coronal plane, it is probably in the esophagus. Even if the foreign body is not opaque, indirect evidence of its presence may be seen on the roentgenogram. Films should always be taken from both the lateral and the anteroposterior projections. In some cases, administering a small amount of opaque material may be helpful. Direct laryngoscopy confirms the diagnosis and provides access for removal of the foreign body. When there is a severe degree of dyspnea, it may be advisable to do a tracheotomy before the laryngoscopic examination.

Tracheal Foreign Body

Although a tracheal foreign body may be responsible for cough, hoarseness, dyspnea, and cyanosis, the characteristic signs are the asthmatoid wheeze and the audible slap and palpable thud produced by momentary expiratory impaction at the subglottic level. The diagnosis may occasionally be made from the symptoms, physical signs, and roentgenogram of the chest, but in most cases a definite diagnosis can be made only by bronchoscopy.

Bronchial Foreign Body

CLINICAL MANIFESTATIONS. The initial symptoms are usually similar to those of foreign bodies in the larynx or trachea. Cough, blood-streaked sputum, and metallic taste with metallic foreign bodies also may be produced by bronchial foreign bodies. The degree of obstruction and the stage in which the patient is seen are the determining factors in the symptomatology as well as in the pathologic changes. A nonobstructive, nonirritating foreign body may produce few symptoms even after a prolonged time in the lung. An obstructive foreign body quickly produces symptoms and signs and pathologic changes. When there is only a slight (bypass valve) obstruction that allows passage of air or fluid in both directions with only slight interference, a wheeze is noted. When the obstruction is of a greater degree, obstructive emphysema or obstructive atelectasis is produced; if either is allowed to persist, chronic bronchopulmonary disease may develop.

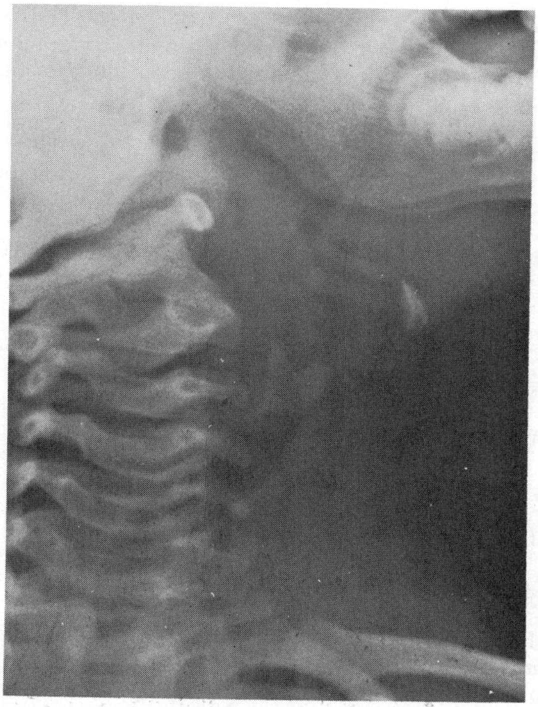

Figure 14–6. Foreign body (fragment of sea shell) in the larynx of a 2-yr-old child treated for "croup" 6 days before the object was suspected. Fortunately, tracheotomy was not required despite the presence of moderately severe laryngeal edema.

Most often, the object is aspirated into the right lung. There is usually an immediate episode of choking, gagging, and paroxysmal coughing, which may lead to medical consultation. If this acute episode does not occur or is missed, or if its importance is underestimated by the parents, a relatively long latent period may pass with only occasional cough or slight wheezing; then the patient may develop recurrent lobar pneumonia or intractable "asthma," often with bilateral wheezing and many episodes of "status asthmaticus." Occasionally, chronic wheezing starts immediately after the aspiration. Rarely, a foreign body presents with hemoptysis, occasionally months or years later. History may reveal a forgotten episode of choking while eating or while playing with small objects. Older siblings (3–6 yr old) may have supplied the aspirated object. The physical examination may reveal a tracheal shift. Breath sounds are decreased on the side of the obstruction, but this sign may not be obvious if there is diffuse wheezing.

When both main bronchi are obstructed, there may be severe dyspnea and even asphyxia. If the foreign body is vegetal (e.g., a peanut), a severe condition known as *vegetal* or *arachidic bronchitis* results. This is characterized by cough, a septic type of fever, and dyspnea. Chronic suppuration may occur when a bronchial foreign body has been present for a long time.

DIAGNOSIS. Most patients with an airway foreign body have a suggestive history. However, the possibility of a foreign body must be considered in acute or chronic pulmonary lesions whether or not there is a history of a foreign body accident. The physical signs of bronchial obstruction from foreign bodies include limited expansion, decreased vocal fremitus, impaired (atelectasis) or hyperresonant (overinflation) percussion note, and diminished breath sounds distal to the foreign body. When there is complete obstruction, with a "drowned lung" or with atelectasis, there is absence of vocal resonance and vocal fremitus, which may lead to an erroneous diagnosis of empyema. Varying degrees of tympany may be noted over areas of obstructive emphysema. Rales are more likely on the uninvaded side than on the invaded one.

If an obstructing object causes complete obstruction in the expiratory phase but allows air to pass in the inspiratory phase, air will enter the distal portion of the lung on inspiration but little or none will escape during expiration *(check valve)*. This produces obstructive overinflation (Fig. 14–7). Complete blockage of the bronchus due to the object itself or in combination with the inflammatory swelling of the bronchial mucosa results in a *stop valve* obstruction, and the air in the distal portion of the lung is soon absorbed, leaving an area of atelectasis (Fig. 14–8).

In check valve obstruction, the obstructive emphysema makes it possible to localize a bronchial foreign body by fluoroscopy. The obstructed lung remains expanded during expiration, whereas the heart and the mediastinum shift to the opposite side as the unobstructed lung empties. The diaphragm is low, flattened, and fixed on the obstructed side; its excursion is free and exaggerated on the unobstructed side. The differences between the lungs are more evident on expiration than on inspiration. With complete obstruction of the bronchus producing obstructive atelectasis, the heart and the mediastinum are drawn toward the obstructed side and remain there during both phases of respiration. The diaphragm on the obstructed side remains high, while that on the unobstructed side moves normally. Films taken at the end of inspiration and of expiration show only a slight difference resulting from the filling and emptying of the unobstructed lung. Even extensive roentgenographic procedures may not completely rule out the presence of a foreign body.

PROGNOSIS. Foreign bodies lodged in the air passages are almost invariably fatal if they are not removed. Fortunately, almost all can be removed safely by a skilled bronchoscopist. Almost all patients, who are diagnosed quickly, recover completely after removal. However, the incidence of complications, including aspiration pneumonia and airway trauma, and the need for tracheostomy because of subglottic edema, rises significantly if the diagnosis is delayed longer than 24 hr.

PREVENTION. Foreign body aspiration can be prevented by keeping small objects out of reach of children who are too young to obey restrictions; by not giving small pieces of candy, nuts, or similar food to children too young to chew them; and by not giving toys containing small or loosely attached parts to children who are still putting such objects into their mouths. Beads, button boxes, and coins should not be given to toddlers as playthings. Safety pins should always be closed and should not be left near a baby or in reach of small children. Balloons are also underestimated as potential foreign bodies.

TREATMENT. Endoscopy and removal of the foreign body under direct vision should be performed as soon as possible. Rarely a thoracotomy is necessary to "milk" the object into a position where it can be removed by bronchoscopy. Occasionally, especially with long duration vegetal foreign bodies, lobectomy may be necessary. Biplane fluoroscopy may be helpful when opaque foreign bodies are lodged in peripheral bronchi. Treatment with pulmonary physiotherapy and bronchodilators is not recommended because of the risk of impacting a dislodged foreign body at the subglottic area, which may result in acute asphyxia, and because a delay in instituting endoscopy may increase morbidity. Treating complications is important to obtaining a good outcome. Secondary infections should be treated with appropriate antibiotics. The

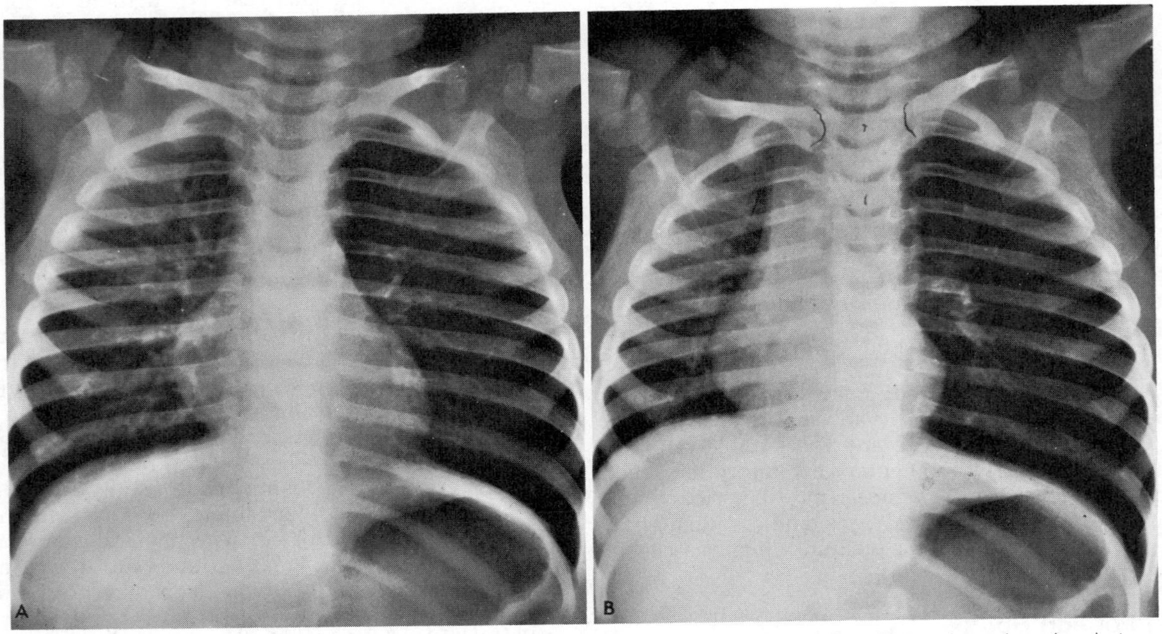

Figure 14–7. Obstructive emphysema (overinflation) due to peanut fragment in the left mainstem bronchus. Inspiratory film *(A)* appears relatively normal except for slight mediastinal shift to the right. In expiration *(B)*, the left lung remains overaerated (check the valve mechanism), and the mediastinum moves far to the right.

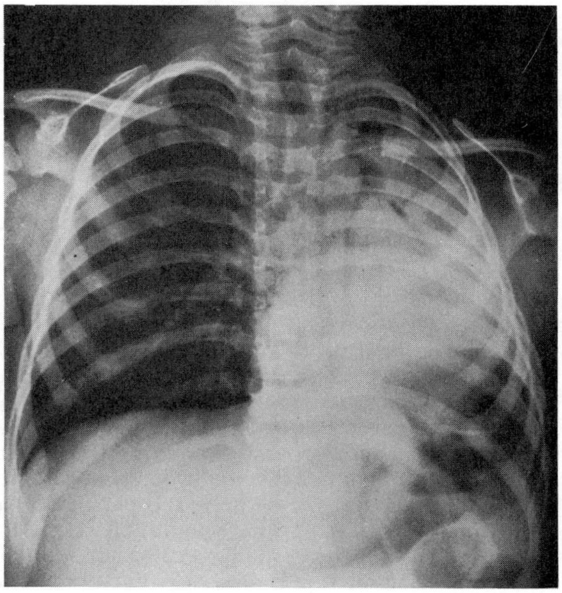

Figure 14–8. Foreign body lodged in left mainstem bronchus, producing atelectasis of the left lung. Note that the heart is drawn completely into the left side of the chest.

outcome of the aspiration of a *large foreign body* that may be immediately life-threatening depends on proper and prompt action taken at the scene of the accident.

Emergency treatment of local upper airway obstruction, as described below, is part of the "basic rescuer course" in cardiopulmonary resuscitation (CPR) of the American Heart Association (see Sec. 6.31). These procedures are used only for children who are aphonic and not breathing. The recommendations for treating infants and young children differ slightly from those for treating teenagers and adults. If the patient can breathe and is able to cough or speak, none of the maneuvers described earlier should be undertaken. For patients who are genuinely "choking," the present recommendations of the Committee on Accident and Poison Prevention of the American Academy of Pediatrics are as follows: For infants (< 1 yr), the repetitive use of four back blows and four chest thrusts is recommended. Abdominal thrusts should not be used. The back blows are delivered while holding the infant with the head lower than the trunk. Four blows are delivered with the heel of the hand between the scapulas. The purpose of this maneuver is to loosen the foreign body. After the back blows, the patient is turned and four chest thrusts are delivered using the same technique and hand positioning as is used for closed cardiac compression (i.e., over the midsternum for infants and slightly lower for older children). This maneuver increases intrathoracic pressure, which may cause expulsion of the foreign body. Blind finger sweeps should not be used in infants and young children. Instead, after the administration of the four chest thrusts, the mouth should be opened and a visualized foreign body should be grasped and removed. Following each sequence of back blows, chest thrusts, and visual attempt to remove foreign body, rescue breathing should be attempted for the unconscious patient. If unsuccessful, the sequence described above is repeated. A young child (> 1 yr) should be placed on his or her back. The rescuer kneels next to the patient and, using the heel of one hand, performs 6–10 abdominal thrusts by pushing upward and inward from the midabdomen, midway between the umbilicus and the rib cage. If unsuccessful, the victim's mouth is opened by using the tongue-jaw lift, and a visualized foreign body is removed. Blind sweeps should not be done. Rescue breathing should then be attempted before the entire sequence is repeated. Although there is controversy concerning the precise technique to be used in total upper airway obstruction by a foreign body, pediatricians should provide up-to-date information in these techniques to parents and should urge parents to expect that their babysitters (including teenagers) are familiar with the symptoms and emergency treatment of foreign body aspiration. The number of choking deaths in the 0–4 yr age group declined from 600 in 1974 to 170 in 1983.

Baker SP, Fisher RS: Childhood asphyxiation by choking or suffocation. JAMA 244:1343, 1980.

Blazer S, Naveh Y, Friedman A: Foreign body in the airway: A review of 200 cases. Am Rev Dis Child 134:68, 1980.

Blumhagen JD, Weisenberg RL, Brooks JG, et al: Endotracheal foreign bodies: Difficulties in diagnosis. Clin Pediatr 19:480, 1980.

Committee on Accident and Poison Prevention: Revised first aid for the choking child. Pediatrics 78:177, 1986.

Esclamado RM, Richardson MA: Laryngotracheal foreign bodies in children. Am J Dis Child 141:259, 1987.

Gann DS: Emergency management of the obstructed airway. JAMA 243:1141, 1980.

Greensher J, Mofenson HC: Emergency treatment of the choking child. Pediatrics 70:110, 1982.

Rothman BF, Boeckman CR: Foreign bodies in the larynx and tracheobronchial tree in children. Ann Otol Rhinol Laryngol 89:434, 1980.

14.46 TRAUMA TO THE LARYNX

BIRTH TRAUMA. Laryngeal injury during birth is not infrequent and may result in dislocation of the cricothyroid or cricoarytenoid articulations. Hoarseness and at times wheezing or fluttering respiratory sounds are heard. The diagnosis is made by direct laryngoscopic examination. Treatment by direct laryngoscopic manipulations, using a laryngeal dilator, may occasionally be effective, but tracheotomy should be done when there is evidence of hypoxia.

Unilateral or bilateral *recurrent laryngeal nerve paralysis* may also be produced by birth trauma, especially during forceps delivery. Bilateral paralysis is often associated with CNS disease. When only one cord is paralyzed, there may be only hoarseness and slight stridor without dyspnea. Unilateral paralysis is usually on the left. In bilateral paralysis there is dyspnea with stridor. In both unilateral and bilateral vocal cord paralysis, chronic aspiration can lead to recurrent pneumonia. Direct laryngoscopic examination establishes the diagnosis. Tracheotomy is usually necessary for bilateral paralysis. The older child may wear a valvular cannula, or a laryngoplasty with lateral fixation of one vocal cord may be done to improve the airway and permit decannulation if breathing through the larynx has not improved spontaneously.

POSTNATAL TRAUMA. Any trauma, such as that brought about by a fall against a hard object, may produce acute or chronic stenosis of the larynx, as may high tracheotomy and prolonged intubation. Clinically important laryngeal injury is rare in children. Penetrating injuries are usually obvious and require treatment by an otolaryngologic surgeon. Serious nonpenetrating injuries may be deceptive because substantial edema and even a compressing hematoma may give surprisingly few external clues. Laryngeal fracture should be suspected in patients who have hoarseness, hemoptysis, or subcutaneous emphysema after neck trauma. Laryngoscopy and, occasionally, surgical exploration may be indicated in patients who have relatively normal physical findings but whose history is compatible with substantial blunt neck trauma. Most patients with serious laryngeal or upper tracheal injuries require tracheostomy as part of their management; if there are signs of high obstruction, the need may be urgent. The normal voice is frequently not recovered. Similarly, severe thermal injury (e.g., following accidental inhalation of steam or smoke) is often best managed with tracheostomy. Ingestion of caustic substances has also been associated with laryngeal lesions.

Acute *overuse of the voice* (e.g., prolonged screaming at a concert or athletic event) may cause transient hoarseness. With cessation of this stress, the voice returns to normal without other treatment. The roles of resting the voice (whispering or no use of speech at all) or mist in accelerating recovery are not clear. Acute laryngitis is fairly common in older children during mild viral respiratory infections; spontaneous recovery is the rule, and the importance of steam and other therapeutic maneuvers is unknown. Occasionally, a teenager may develop chronic laryngitis from heavy cigarette smoking. The differential diagnosis of persistent hoarse voice includes vocal ("singer's" or "screamer's") nodules, papillomas, and serious tumors such as rhabdomyosarcoma. A laryngeal abscess is a rare cause of persistent hoarseness. These masses are diagnosed by laryngoscopy and may require surgical treatment, which may be followed by voice training. Otolaryngologic consultation is indicated for any child with unexplained continuous hoarseness longer than 1 wk.

Moulin D, Bertrand JM, Buts JP, et al: Upper airway lesions in children after accidental ingestion of caustic substances. J Pediatr 106:408, 1985.

14.47 ACUTE LARYNGEAL STENOSIS

Acute stenosis may result from any acute infection responsible for edema of the subglottic region or epiglottis and arytenoids; from inflammation secondary to the inspiration of a vegetal foreign body, and especially after instrumentation for the removal of such an object; from edema of an allergic reaction; or from a foreign body lodged in the larynx. Treatment consists of immediate provision of an airway by intubation or tracheotomy, followed by appropriate medical therapy.

14.48 CHRONIC LARYNGEAL STENOSIS

This is a frequent sequela of high tracheotomy in which damage of the first tracheal ring or cricoid cartilage results in perichondritis and subsequent overgrowth of cartilage or fibrous tissue. Chronic stenosis may also result from laryngeal diphtheria, syphilis, tuberculosis, radiation burns, and external trauma. The most common etiology at present, however, is neonatal intubation. Congenital laryngeal stenosis may be transmitted as an autosomal dominant trait in some patients. The clinical manifestations may include dyspnea with audible stridor and suprasternal, supraclavicular, and intercostal retractions, or may be limited to inability to decannulate a patient's tracheostomy or remove a laryngeal tube. The diagnosis is made by direct laryngoscopy, palpation of the larynx, and roentgenographic examination. Scarring and stenosis usually develop in the subglottic region, occasionally with necrosis of cartilage.

Milder cases can be treated by replacing the tracheostomy cannula with a smaller one and closure of this tube, at first partial and then complete, with a cork, thus re-educating the patient to mouthbreathe and permitting the removal of the cannula. If this method is unsuccessful, dilation through a direct laryngoscope may help but should not be done too frequently. In some patients external surgery with or without the use of an indwelling mold may be necessary. A cricoid split operation is successful in severe cases. The prognosis for eventual cure is good, but treatment may require months or years.

Fearon B: Acute airway obstruction. *In:* Ferguson CF, Kendig EL Jr (eds): Disorders of the Respiratory Tract. Vol 2: Pediatric Otolaryngology. Philadelphia, WB Saunders, 1972.
Landing BH: State of the art: Congenital malformations and genetic diseases of the respiratory tract. Am Rev Respir Dis 120:151, 1979.
McGill TJI, Healy GB: Congenital and acquired lesions of the infant larynx. Clin Pediatr 17:584, 1978.
Proctor DF: The upper airways: II. The larynx and trachea. Am Rev Respir Dis 115:315, 1977.

14.49 NEOPLASMS OF THE LARYNX

Papilloma is the most common tumor of the larynx in childhood; it rarely becomes malignant and often disappears after puberty. The pink, warty tumors may grow profusely from any portion of the larynx, although usually from the vocal cords. This disease is caused by the human papillomavirus. When maternal vaginal condyloma is present, material containing this virus may be aspirated during delivery, producing disease in a small fraction of exposed infants.

The initial symptom is hoarseness, but dyspnea is likely if the condition is allowed to persist. Asphyxia has occurred. Direct laryngoscopy accomplishes both diagnosis (confirmed histologically) and treatment, because the papilloma can be easily removed by forceps. Care should be taken not to damage normal tissue. Cure usually occurs, although at first rapid recurrence is common. Tracheostomy may be required because of recurrences and the threat of aspiration. Cryosurgery and laser surgery have been advocated as alternative or adjuvant therapy. Radical excision and radiation are contraindicated. Patients with laryngobronchial papillomatosis who fail to respond to usual treatment may improve after receiving systemic bleomycin. Human leukocyte interferon has been reported to be beneficial for patients with recurrent severe disease. However, in one controlled study, the patients in the treatment group had a better course for 6 mo, but this was not sustained for the next 6 mo. Papilloma may recur many years, even decades, after apparent cure. Malignant degeneration into squamous cell carcinoma has been reported in young children. This complication is more likely after radiation treatment.

Vocal nodules or small tumors may occur in children at the junction of the anterior and middle thirds of the cords. They are usually bilateral and produce slight hoarseness. Spontaneous regression may occur if strenuous use of the voice is avoided. They may be removed under direct laryngoscopic view or treated with laser.

Chaput M, Ninane J, Gosseye S, et al: Juvenile laryngeal papillomatosis and epidermoid carcinoma. J Pediatr 114:269, 1989.
Healy GB, Gelber RD, Trowbridge AL, et al: Treatment of recurrent respiratory papillomatosis with human leukocyte interferon. N Engl J Med 319:401, 1988.
Mehta P, Herold N: Regression of juvenile laryngobronchial papillomatosis with systemic bleomycin therapy. J Pediatr 97:479, 1980.
Steinberg BM, Topp WC, Schneider PS, et al: Laryngeal papilloma virus infection during clinical remission. N Engl J Med 308:1261, 1983.

14.50 TRACHEAL AMYLOIDOSIS

Primary amyloidosis (see Sec. 25.2) of the trachea is an extremely rare but potentially treatable lesion. Symptoms are caused by gradual reduction in the tracheal lumen secondary to progressive deposition of amyloid. Cough, dyspnea, and wheezing occur early in the course of the disease. Recurrent infection and hemoptysis are late complications. Expiratory wheezing, cough, and signs of respiratory distress may be present. The result of a chest roentgenogram may be normal. The diagnosis is made by bronchoscopy, which reveals a narrowed tracheal lumen with friable tissue lining the airways; a biopsy allows confirmation of the diagnosis. Treatment is repeated bronchoscopy for removal of amyloid until an adequate airway is restored, but improvement may be only temporary, and repeated bronchoscopic treatments are often necessary.

Gottlieb LS, Gold WM: Primary tracheobronchial amyloidosis. Am Rev Respir Dis 105:425, 1972.
Prowse CG: Amyloidosis of the lower respiratory tract. Thorax 13:308, 1958.

14.51 ACUTE BRONCHITIS

Although the diagnosis of "acute bronchitis" is frequently made, this condition may not exist in children as an isolated clinical entity. Rather, bronchitis occurs in association with a number of other conditions of the upper and lower respiratory tracts, and the trachea is nearly always involved. Bronchiolitis ("capillary bronchitis") is an entirely different illness (see Sec. 14.53).

Asthmatic bronchitis is a form of asthma that is often confused with acute bronchitis. With a variety of upper respiratory tract infections, some children have bronchial spasm and exudation similar to signs in older children with asthma.

Acute tracheobronchitis is most commonly found in association with an upper respiratory tract infection such as nasopharyngitis but is also associated with influenza, pertussis, measles, typhoid fever (and other salmonelloses), diphtheria, and scarlet fever. An acute, primary, undifferentiated tracheobronchitis also occurs, most commonly in older children and adolescents. It is likely that, except for the bacterial diseases mentioned, acute tracheobronchitis is of viral origin. Pneumococci, staphylococci, *H. influenzae*, and various hemolytic streptococci may be isolated from the sputum, but their presence does not imply a bacterial origin, and antibiotic therapy does not appreciably alter the course of the illness. Some children appear to be far more susceptible to acute tracheobronchitis than others. The reasons are unknown, but allergy, climate, air pollution, and chronic infections of the upper respiratory tract, particularly sinusitis, may be contributing factors.

The syndrome *bronchiolitis obliterans* may begin with an episode of acute bronchitis, bronchiolitis, or bronchopneumonia and then progress over several weeks to severe chronic pulmonary disease characterized by bronchiolar and bronchial obliteration and bronchiectasis (see Sec. 14.55).

CLINICAL MANIFESTATIONS. Acute bronchitis is usually preceded by a viral upper respiratory infection. Secondary bacterial infection with *S. pneumoniae* or *H. influenzae* may occur. Typically, the child presents a frequent, dry, hacking, unproductive cough of relatively gradual onset, beginning 3–4 days after the appearance of rhinitis. Low substernal discomfort or burning anterior chest pain is often present and may be aggravated by coughing. As the illness progresses, the patient may be bothered by whistling sounds during respiration (probably rhonchi), soreness of the chest, and occasionally by shortness of breath. Coughing paroxysms or gagging on secretions is associated occasionally with vomiting. Within several days the cough becomes productive, and the sputum changes from clear to purulent. Usually within 5–10 days the mucus thins and the cough gradually disappears. The considerable malaise often associated with the illness may continue for 1 wk or more after acute symptoms have subsided.

Physical findings vary with the age of the patient and the stage of the disease. Initially, the child is usually afebrile or has low-grade fever, and there are signs of nasopharyngitis, conjunctival infection, and rhinitis. Later, auscultation reveals roughening of breath sounds, coarse and fine moist rales, and rhonchi which may be high pitched, resembling the wheezing of asthma.

In otherwise healthy children complications are few, but in undernourished children or those in poor health, otitis, sinusitis, and pneumonia are common.

TREATMENT. There is no specific therapy; most patients recover uneventfully without any treatment. In small infants pulmonary drainage is facilitated by frequent shifts in position. Older children are more comfortable in high humidity, but there is no evidence that this shortens the duration of illness. Irritating and paroxysmal coughing may cause considerable distress and interfere with sleep. Although suppression of cough may increase the possibility of suppuration, judicious use of cough suppressants (including codeine) may be appropriate for symptomatic relief. Antihistamines, which dry secretions, should not be used, and expectorants are not helpful. Antibiotics do not shorten the duration of the viral illness or decrease the incidence of bacterial complications, although the fact that patients with recurrent episodes may occasionally improve with such treatment suggests that some secondary bacterial infection is present.

Children with repeated attacks of acute bronchitis should be carefully evaluated for the possibility of respiratory tract anomalies, foreign bodies, bronchiectasis, immune deficiency, tuberculosis, allergy, sinusitis, tonsillitis, adenoiditis, and cystic fibrosis.

14.52 CHRONIC BRONCHITIS

Although adult chronic bronchitis is defined as 3 mo or more of productive cough each year for 2 or more consecutive yr, there is no such accepted standard for children. Its very existence as a separate entity has been questioned, which emphasizes the importance of searching for an underlying immunologic or mucosal abnormality. A chronic or frequently recurring productive cough usually indicates an underlying pulmonary or systemic disease; affected patients should be evaluated for immune deficiencies, anatomic abnormalities, asthma, environmental disease, upper airway infection with postnasal discharge, cystic fibrosis, ciliary dyskinesis; and bronchiectasis. Cough and wheezing are common, and in one study, all 22 reported patients with chronic bronchitis had evidence of allergic disease. Rarely, bronchial irritation may be secondary to the chronic inhalation of dust or noxious fumes. Tobacco or marijuana smoking is obviously pertinent historical information. Teenagers should be similarly questioned about industrial fumes or automobile exhaust exposure at school or work.

AIR POLLUTION AND CIGARETTE SMOKING. There is a significant association between high levels of air pollution and an elevated incidence of chronic pulmonary disease including bronchitis, but a direct causal relationship has not been established. Air pollutants also aggravate pre-existent pulmonary disease and impair pulmonary function in exercising children and teenagers. Children and their parents should be advised of these relationships.

An increased incidence and exacerbations of bronchitis and other forms of acute and chronic lung disease are associated with cigarette smoking. In addition, there is increased morbidity from respiratory infections in teenagers who smoke, as reflected in school and work absences as well as in functional and pathologic evidence of small airway abnormalities. For example, cigarette smoking is a risk factor for the severity of influenza in young men. Smoking parents, and especially those whose children have chronic lung disease, should be advised that they are subjecting their children's lungs to significant amounts of "secondhand" cigarette smoke in the home; they should be urged to stop smoking.

The Committee on Genetics and Environmental Hazards of the American Academy of Pediatrics has noted that tobacco smoking is one of the most important "sources of environmental contamination and a significant threat to the health of children." It urges physicians to support legislation that would prohibit smoking in public places frequented by children, "particularly in hospitals and other health facilities."

The use of wood-burning stoves, which has increased with the rising cost of petroleum-based fuel, has been associated with a variety of pediatric pulmonary problems. Indoor wood burning results in exposure to particulate matter and polycyclic hydrocarbons. Wheezing and episodic pneumonia have been described in exposed children. In one study, 84% of children exposed to wood burning stoves (compared with 3% of controls) were reported to have at least one severe respiratory symptom. Systemic problems can also occur if the wood has been treated with toxic materials (e.g., arsenic poisoning has been reported in one family).

Clinical Manifestations. The chief symptom is cough, with or without expectoration. The child will usually also complain of chest soreness; characteristically these signs and symptoms are worse at night; wheezing may also be prominent, and physical findings are similar to those of acute bronchitis. Some patients cough up large solid, hypereosinophilic mucoid "casts" of the airways, giving rise to the term, "plastic bronchitis." These casts may be related to metaplastic bronchial epithelium, elements of which, together with inflammatory cells and noncellular material, can be found on histologic examination.

Course and Prognosis. Both the course and the prognosis depend on appropriate management or eradication of any underlying illness. Complications are those of the underlying illness.

Treatment. When an underlying cause for chronic bronchitis is found, this should receive appropriate management. Allergic management may be helpful on occasion even when no underlying cause can be discovered. Autogenous vaccines or inhalation of antibiotics is not effective.

Christensen W, Hutchins G: Hypereosinophilic mucoid impaction of bronchi in two children under two years of age. Pediatr Pulmonol 1:278, 1985.
Committee on Genetics and Environmental Hazards: The environmental consequences of tobacco smoking: Implications for public policy that affect the health of children. Pediatrics 70:314, 1982.
Kark JD, Lebiush M, Rannon L: Cigarette smoking as a risk factor for epidemic $A(H_1N_1)$ influenza in young men. N Engl J Med 307:1042, 1982.
Matsukura S, Taminato T, Kitano N, et al: Effects of environmental tobacco smoke on urinary cotinine excretion in nonsmokers: Evidence for passive smoking. N Engl J Med 311:828, 1984.
Niewoehner DE, Kleineman J, Rice DB: Pathologic changes in the peripheral airways of young cigarette smokers. N Engl J Med 291:755, 1974.
Perez-Soler A: Cast bronchitis in infants and children. Am J Dis Child 143:1024, 1989.
Samet JM, Marbury MC, Spengler JD: Health effects and sources of indoor air pollution. Parts 1 and 2. Am J Respir Dis 136:1486; 137:221, 1988.
Sheppard D: Adverse pulmonary effects of air pollution. Immunol Allergy Pract 6:25, 1984.
Smith TF, Ireland TA, Zaatari GS, et al: Characteristics of children with endoscopically proved chronic bronchitis. Am J Dis Child 139:1039, 1985.
Taussig LM, Smith SM, Blumenfield R: Chronic bronchitis in childhood: What is it? Pediatrics 67:1, 1981.
White JR, Froeb HF: Small-airways dysfunction in nonsmokers chronically exposed to tobacco smoke. N Engl J Med 203:720, 1980.

14.53 PRIMARY CILIARY DYSKINESIS

(Dyskinetic Cilia Syndrome; Ciliary Dyskinesis; Kartagener Syndrome)

In the respiratory tract the majority of the lining mucosal cells are ciliated (about 275 cilia per cell). Each cilium is anchored to the apical cytoplasm by a basal body and contains two central and nine peripheral microtubules that traverse its entire length and are loosely bound to one another by radial spokes. It is the movement of these microtubules with relation to the others that causes the typical 1,000 cycle/min beat of the cilia. The chemical basis for this movement involves an ATPase located within the cilia and visible ultrastructurally as dynein arms.

Kartagener initially described a group of patients, all of whom had situs inversus, chronic sinusitis, and chronic bronchitis with bronchiectasis. Situs inversus is also seen commonly in men with infertility secondary to sperm immotility. These observations led Afzelius to postulate that these patients have a generalized disorder of ciliary motility, some of them lacking the ATPase-containing dynein arms necessary for ciliary movement.

Cilia and their supporting structures contain at least 100 proteins. A great variety of genetic abnormalities, therefore, could lead to some form of ciliary dyskinesis and many have already been reported. The severity of the functional abnormality may vary considerably, however, among these technically different genetic diseases. Many uncommon genes are involved. Moreover, inheritance of two abnormal recessive genes, each coding for a different ciliary protein, would not be expected to result in any functional abnormality. Thus, genetic advice to prospective parents, each of whom has a family history of primary ciliary dyskinesis, is not straightforward; if the two families have different forms of the disease, the risk of an abnormal child may be zero. In any case, the overall incidence of the syndrome (i.e., the combined incidence of the different genetic variants) is about 1:20,000 persons.

CLINICAL MANIFESTATIONS. The symptoms of this disease reflect the wide distribution of cilia throughout the body. Relentless ciliary activity of embryonal tissues may be responsible for the characteristic direction of the rotation of the intestine. Impairment of ciliary movement and thus of intestinal rotation could produce situs inversus, a very common but not universal finding in the immotile cilia syndrome. Absence of ciliary clearance from the middle ears, eustachian tubes, and sinus cavities results in an increased incidence and greater severity of chronic otitis media and sinusitis in childhood. Sterility resulting from inadequate spermatozoal movement is almost always present, but motile spermatozoa have been demonstrated in a patient totally lacking dynein arms on his respiratory ciliated cells. Abnormal mucociliary clearance in children results in chronic bronchitis, usually without bronchiectasis, which is a relatively late complication. Wheezing is common, perhaps due in part to inadequate clearance of antigen from the airways. Although symptoms are often present in early childhood, they may be delayed in some patients until after age 20 yr.

DIAGNOSIS. The disease should be suspected in children who have chronic sinusitis and otitis media in addition to bronchitis. If such a patient has situs inversus, the diagnosis is a virtual certainty, but definitive testing (see later) should be done. Chronic wheezing, a family history of bronchiectasis in young adults, or male infertility are important additional clinical support for this diagnosis.

Decreased ciliary movement may be observed at bronchoscopy. Another preliminary screening test involves examining a suspension of scrapings from the nasal mucosa above the first turbinate by light microscope for evaluation of ciliary activity. The absence of ciliary activity on more than two occasions when the patient does not have an acute upper respiratory infection suggests the need for more definitive testing. However, this technique is plagued by both false-positive and false-negative results. Acute illnesses, especially viral infection, can cause transiently high percentages of nasal and airway cells with electron microscopic abnormalities and decreased ciliary activity in mucosal scrapings. This finding is one of the reasons for renaming the genetic disease as "primary ciliary dyskinesis." At present, diagnosis still depends on electron microscopic examination of cilia, obtained either by brushing or biopsy of the trachea at bronchoscopy or by nasal mucosal biopsy, preferably not obtained during or shortly after an acute illness. Spermatozoa can also be examined in older patients; however, dissociation between spermatozoal motility and respiratory ciliary function occurs.

Absence of dynein arms is probably the most common form of the disease, but other morphologic abnormalities having the same phenotypic expression (i.e., decreased or absent ciliary movement) are also possible.

The low incidence of this disease, the large number of patients who have suggestive symptoms (especially recurrent otitis, persistent bronchitis, and pansinusitis), and the lack of a good screening test make the decision about whether to proceed with the invasive, time-consuming, and expensive diagnostic biopsy a common problem in pediatric pulmonology.

TREATMENT. Treatment is symptomatic and includes close medical supervision with early and aggressive antibiotic treatment of pulmonary infection, chest physiotherapy, and bronchodilators. The efficacy of pneumococcal and *H. influenzae* vaccines is unknown. Early infection involves the *Pneumococcus* and *Haemophilus* organisms primarily. Treatment of serous otitis and sinusitis is also important.

PROGNOSIS. The average life expectancy is unknown, although normal life spans have been reported; however, there is considerable morbidity owing to bronchiectasis and other problems. The effects of early aggressive therapy are unknown. The dangers of smoking and of exposure to industrial fumes should be explained to the patient, and appropriate vocational guidance should be supplied.

Eliasson R, Mossberg B, Camner P, Afzelius BA: The immotile cilia syndrome. N Engl J Med 297:1, 1977.
Carson JL, Collier AM, Hu SS: Acquired ciliary defects in nasal epithelium of children with acute viral upper respiratory infections. N Engl J Med 312:463, 1985.
Johnson MS, McCormick JR, Gillies CG, et al: Kartagener's syndrome with motile spermatozoa. N Engl J Med 307:1131, 1982.
Rooklin AR, McGeady SJ, Mikaelian DO, et al: The immotile cilia syndrome: A cause of recurrent pulmonary disease in children. Pediatrics 66:526, 1980.
Sturgess JM, Chao J, Wong J, et al: Cilia with defective radial spokes: A cause of human respiratory disease. N Engl J Med 300:53, 1979.
Wilton LJ, Teichtahl H, Temple-Smith PD, et al: Kartagener's syndrome with motile cilia and immotile spermatozoa: Axonemal ultrastructure and function. Am Rev Respir Dis 134:1233, 1986.

14.54 ACUTE BRONCHIOLITIS

Acute bronchiolitis is a common disease of the lower respiratory tract of infants resulting from inflammatory obstruction of the small airways. It occurs during the first 2 yr of life, with a peak incidence at approximately 6 mo of age, and in many localities is the most frequent cause of hospitalization of infants. The incidence is highest during the winter and early spring. The illness occurs both sporadically and epidemically.

ETIOLOGY AND EPIDEMIOLOGY. Acute bronchiolitis is a viral illness. The respiratory syncytial virus is the causative agent in more than 50% of cases (see Sec. 12.76); the parainfluenza 3 virus, mycoplasma, some adenoviruses, and occasionally other viruses produce the remaining cases. Adenovirus may be associated with long-term complications, including bronchiolitis obliterans and unilateral hyperlucent lung syndrome (Swyer-James syndrome). There is no firm evidence that bacteria cause bronchiolitis. Occasionally, bacterial bronchopneumonia may be confused clinically with bronchiolitis.

The source of the viral infection is usually a family member with minor respiratory illness. Older children and adults tolerate bronchiolar edema better than infants and thus do not develop the clinical picture of bronchiolitis even when the smaller airways of their respiratory tract are infected by the virus.

In one report, sophisticated pulmonary function studies were performed in a large population of normal infants. The follow-up revealed that wheezy respiratory illnesses were significantly more common among infants whose initial total respiratory conductance was in the lowest third of those tested. Thus, diminished lung function may play a role in determining which infants with viral infection develop bronchiolitis.

PATHOPHYSIOLOGY. Acute bronchiolitis is characterized by bronchiolar obstruction due to edema and accumulation of mucus and cellular debris and by invasion of the smaller radicles of the bronchial tree by virus. Because resistance to airflow in a tube is inversely related to the 4th power of the radius, even minor thickening of the bronchiolar wall in infants may produce a profound effect on airflow. Airway resistance in the small air passages is increased during both the inspiratory and expiratory phases, but because the radius of an airway is smaller during expiration, the resultant ball valve respiratory obstruction leads to early air trapping and overinflation. Atelectasis may occur when an obstruction becomes complete and trapped air is absorbed.

The pathologic process impaires the normal exchange of gases in the lung. Diminished ventilation results in hypoxemia, which may occur early in the course. Carbon dioxide retention (hypercapnia) does not usually occur except in severely affected patients. Generally, the higher the respiratory rate, the lower will be the arterial oxygen tension. Hypercapnia is usually not found until respirations exceed 60/min; it then increases in proportion to the tachypnea.

CLINICAL MANIFESTATIONS. Most affected infants have a history of exposure to older children or adults with minor respiratory diseases within the week preceding onset of illness. The infant is first noted to have a mild upper respiratory tract infection with serous nasal discharge and sneezing. These symptoms usually last several days and may be accompanied by fever of 38.5–39° C (101–102° F) and diminished appetite. There is then the gradual development of respiratory distress characterized by paroxysmal wheezy cough, dyspnea, and irritability. Bottle-feeding may be particularly difficult, because the rapid respiratory rate may not permit time for sucking and swallowing. In mild cases symptoms disappear in 1–3 days. On occasion, in the more severely affected patients, symptoms may develop within several hours, and the course is protracted. Other systemic manifestations, such as vomiting and diarrhea, are usually absent. The infant is commonly afebrile, has only a low-grade fever, or may be hypothermic.

An examination reveals a tachypneic infant, often in extreme distress. Respirations range from 60–80/min; severe air hunger and cyanosis may be present. There is flaring of the alae nasi, and use of the accessory muscles of respiration results in intercostal and subcostal retractions, which are shallow because of the persistent distention of the lungs by the trapped air. The depression of the liver and spleen by the overinflated lungs may result in their being palpable below the costal margin. Widespread fine rales may be heard at the end of inspiration and in early expiration. The expiratory phase of breathing is prolonged, and wheezes are usually audible. In the most severe cases, breath sounds are barely audible when bronchiolitic obstruction is nearly complete.

Roentgenographic examination reveals hyperinflation of the lungs and an increased anteroposterior diameter on lateral view. Scattered areas of consolidation are found in about one third of patients and are due either to atelectasis secondary to obstruction or to inflammation of the alveoli. Early bacterial pneumonia cannot be excluded on radiographic grounds alone.

The white blood cell and differential counts are usually within normal limits. Lymphopenia, commonly associated with many viral illnesses, is usually not found. Nasopharyngeal cultures reveal normal bacterial flora. Virus may be demonstrated in nasopharyngeal secretions by immunofluorescence, in a rise in blood antibody titers, or in culture.

DIFFERENTIAL DIAGNOSIS. The condition most commonly confused with acute bronchiolitis is bronchial asthma. Asthma occurs uncommonly in the 1st yr of life, but frequently after this period. The presence of one or more of the following favors the diagnosis of asthma: a family history of asthma, repeated attacks in the same infant, sudden onset without preceding infection, markedly prolonged expiration, eosinophilia, and an immediate favorable response to the administration of a single small dose of epinephrine (0.01 mL/kg of 1:1,000 dilution subcutaneously). Repeated attacks represent an important differential point: fewer than 5% of recurrent attacks of clinical bronchiolitis have viral infections as a cause. Other entities that may be confused with acute bronchiolitis are congestive heart failure, foreign body in the trachea, pertussis, organic phosphorus poisoning, cystic fibrosis, and bacterial bronchopneumonias associated with generalized obstructive emphysema.

COURSE AND PROGNOSIS. The most critical phase of illness occurs during the first 48–72 hr after the onset of cough and dyspnea. During this period the infant appears desperately ill, apneic spells occur in the very small infant, and respiratory acidosis is likely to be noted. After the critical period improvement occurs rapidly and often dramatically. Recovery is complete in a few days. The case fatality rate is below 1%; death may result from prolonged apneic spells, severe uncompensated respiratory acidosis, or profound dehydration secondary to loss of water vapor from tachypnea and the inability to drink fluids. Infants with complications such as congenital heart disease or cystic fibrosis have a higher mortality. Bacterial complications, such as bronchopneumonia or otitis media, are uncommon. Cardiac failure during bronchiolitis is rare.

A significant proportion of infants with bronchiolitis have hyperreactive airways during later childhood, but the relation of these two entities, if any, is not understood. Similarly, the suggestion in some studies that even a single episode of bronchiolitis may result in very long-term small airway abnormality requires further investigation. These abnormalities may be partially explained by the finding that infants with low total respiratory conductance are more likely to develop bronchiolitis in response to viral respiratory infection.

TREATMENT. Infants with respiratory distress should be hospitalized, but only supportive treatment is indicated. The patient is commonly placed in an atmosphere of cold, humidified oxygen to relieve hypoxemia and reduce insensible water loss from tachypnea; this treatment relieves the dyspnea and cyanosis and allays anxiety and restlessness. Sedatives should be avoided whenever possible because of potential depression of respiration. The infant is usually more comfortable sitting at a 30- to 40-degree angle or with the head and chest slightly elevated so that the neck is somewhat extended. Oral intake must often be supplemented or replaced by parenteral fluids to offset the dehydrating effect of tachypnea. In the event of respiratory acidosis, electrolyte balance and pH should be adjusted by suitable intravenous solutions.

Ribavirin (Virazole), an antiviral agent, is effective in reducing the severity of bronchiolitis due to RSV infection when administered early in the course of the illness. Its use is indicated in children under 2 yr of age who have severe infection documented by fluorescent antibodies or culture or strongly suspected on epidemiologic grounds and whose hospitalization is likely to exceed 3 days. It should also be given to patients with milder bronchiolitis due to RSV infection who have underlying severe chronic illness due to cardiac disease (particularly cyanotic congenital heart disease), pulmonary disease, or immunodeficiency disease. The drug is administered by continuous inhalation as a small particle mist (Small Particle Aerosol Generator—"SPAG-II" unit) for 12–20 hr/24 hr for 3–5 days. It may be contraindicated for patients on ventilators because of the risk of mechanical interference with ventilator function, such as blockage of the expiratory port filter.

Antibiotics have no therapeutic value unless there is secondary bacterial pneumonia. The low incidence of bacterial complications is not made lower by antibiotic therapy. Corticosteroids are not beneficial and may, under certain conditions, be harmful. On the other hand, corticosteroids have not been evaluated in patients with severe adenovirus bronchiolitis in whom long-term severe sequelae (necrotizing lesions) might be more likely. Bronchodilating aerosolized drugs are frequently used empirically. Epinephrine or other α-adrenergic agents have a theoretical basis for use, but have not been adequately tested. Because the obstruction occurs at the bronchiolar level, tracheostomy is not beneficial and involves substantial risks which are not justified in these acutely ill infants. Occasional patients may progress rapidly to respiratory failure requiring ventilatory assistance.

Hall CB, McBride JT, Walsh EE, et al: Aerosolized ribavirin treatment of infants with respiratory syncytial viral infection: A randomized double blind study. N Engl J Med 308:1443, 1983.
Henderson FW, Clyde WA, Collier AM, et al: The etiologic and epidemiologic spectrum of bronchiolitis in pediatric practice. J Pediatr 95:183, 1979.
Hogg JC, Williams J, Richardson JB, et al: Age as a factor in the distribution of lower-airway conductance and in the pathologic anatomy of obstructive lung disease. N Engl J Med 282:1283, 1970.
Martinez FD, Morgan WJ, Wright AL, et al: Diminished lung function as a predisposing factor for wheezing respiratory illness in infants. N Engl J Med 319:112, 1988.
McConnochie KM, Roghmann KJ: Predicting clinically significant lower respiratory tract illness in childhood following mild bronchiolitis. Am J Dis Child 139:625, 1985.
Morgan WJ, Wright AL, et al: Diminished lung function as a predisposing factor for wheezing respiratory illness in infants. N Engl J Med 319:112, 1988.
Outwater K, Crone RK: Management of respiratory failure in infants with acute viral bronchiolitis. Am J Dis Child 138:1071, 1984.
Schuh S, Canny G, Reisman JJ, et al: Nebulized albuterol in acute bronchiolitis. J Pediatr 117:633, 1990.
Wohl MEB, Chemick V: State of the art: Bronchiolitis. A Rev Respir Dis 118:759, 1978.

14.55 BRONCHIOLITIS OBLITERANS

In this disease, the bronchioles and smaller airways are injured, and "repair" includes production of large amounts of granulation tissue that causes airway obstruction. Eventually, the airway lumens are obliterated with nodular masses of granulation and fibrosis. The precipitating injury often cannot be identified, particularly in children, but in adults, some cases are clearly related to the inhalation of the oxides of nitrogen or other chemicals. The syndrome has also been associated with connective tissue diseases, and some drugs (e.g., penicillamine) have also been reported to precipitate it. In children most cases can be temporally related to pulmonary infection; measles, influenza, adenoviral infection, mycoplasma pneumonia, and pertussis have all been reported to precede its development.

Initially, cough, respiratory distress, and, possibly, cyanosis occur and may be followed by a brief period of apparent improvement. The disease then progresses as reflected by increasing dyspnea, cough, sputum production, and wheezing. The pattern may resemble bronchitis, bronchiolitis, or pneumonia. The chest roentgenogram often suggests miliary tuberculosis. A more nonspecific diffuse infiltrate may also be seen. Bronchography shows obstruction of the bronchioles, with little or no contrast material reaching the periphery of the lung. The disease can then be confirmed by lung biopsy.

There is no specific treatment. The pathology suggests a progressive fibrotic picture that could theoretically be delayed by corticosteroid treatment. Some forms of bronchiolitis obliterans in adults, especially "bronchiolitis obliterans organizing pneumonia" respond well to corticosteroid treatment; however, no definitive data with regard to corticosteroid efficacy exist for children. Some patients deteriorate rapidly and die within weeks of the onset of the initial symptoms; others run a more chronic course; and a few may go on to develop the unilateral hyperlucent lung syndrome (see Sec. 14.76).

Azizirad H, Polgar G, Borns PF, et al: Bronchiolitis obliterans. Clin Pediatr 14:572, 1975.
Becroft DMO: Bronchiolitis obliterans, bronchiectasis and other sequelae of adenovirus type 21 infection in young children. J Clin Pathol 24:72, 1971.
Epler GR, Colby TV, McLoud TC, et al: Bronchiolitis obliterans organizing pneumonia. N Engl J Med 312:152, 1985.
Wohl MEB, Chernick V: State of the art: Bronchiolitis. Am Rev Respir Dis 118:759, 1978.

BRONCHIAL ASTHMA

See Sec. 11.41.

PNEUMONIA

The various clinical forms of pneumonia are often classified by their anatomic distribution—lobar, lobular, interstitial, bronchopneumonia—or by the agents that cause them, such as viral, bacterial, or aspiration pneumonia (see Sec. 14.59). Many of the etiologically unclassified infections which occur in infancy are probably of viral origin. Most bacterial infections are susceptible to antimicrobial therapy, whereas viral infections usually are not.

Certain lesions are commonly produced by specific causative agents. For example, the pneumococcus produces an inflammatory mucosal lesion and an alveolar exudate, usually without destruction of mucosal cells or extensive involvement of interstitial tissues. The gross lesion is a consolidation of all or part of a lobe in the lobar variety or of scattered lobules in the bronchopneumonic variety. Pneumococcal pneumonia characteristically assumes a lobar pattern in older children and young adults, but lobar consolidation is less typical in young children. In contrast, viral agents, *H. influenzae*, and certain strains of the viridans group of streptococci invade or destroy the mucous membrane and may produce principally bronchiolitis, peribronchiolitis, and interstitial lesions. Both staphylococcus and *Klebsiella* tend to destroy tissue and to produce multiple small abscesses.

The following classification is helpful in considering pneumonias in children:

I. BACTERIAL INFECTIONS
Pneumococcus (see also Sec. 12.21)
Streptococcus (see also Sec. 12.18)
Staphylococcus (see also Sec. 12.19 and 14.56)
Haemophilus influenzae (see also Sec. 12.22)
Klebsiella
Pseudomonas aeruginosa (see also Sec. 12.32)
Tubercle bacillus (see Sec. 12.47)

II. VIRAL OR PROBABLE VIRAL INFECTIONS
Interstitial pneumonitis and bronchiolitis (see e.g., respiratory syncytial virus, adenovirus, etc., in Sec. 14.57 and Chapter 12)
Cytomegalovirus (see Sec. 12.71)
Giant cell pneumonia (see also Sec. 14.57)
Influenza (see Sec. 12.74)

III. OTHER INFECTIONS
Pneumocystis carinii pneumonia (see also Sec. 14.58)
Q fever (see Sec. 12.101)
Mycoplasma pneumoniae pneumonia (see Sec. 12.63)
Treponema pallidum (see Sec. 12.50)
Nocardiosis (see Sec. 12.46)
Actinomycosis (see Sec. 12.45)
Chlamydia (see Sec. 12.59, 12.60)
Ornithosis (see Sec. 12.61)
Psittacosis (see Sec. 12.61)
Ureaplasma (see Sec. 9.68)

IV. MYCOTIC INFECTIONS
Aspergillosis (see Sec. 12.108 and 14.65)
Coccidioidomycosis (see Sec. 12.109)
Histoplasmosis (see Sec. 12.103)
Blastomycosis (see Sec. 12.104)
Mucormycosis (see Sec. 12.106)
Sporotrichosis (see Sec. 12.107)
Thrush (see also Sec. 9.75)

V. ASPIRATION OF:
Amniotic contents (see also Sec. 9.34 and 9.35)
Food and/or gastric acid (see also Sec. 14.59)
Foreign bodies (see also Sec. 14.45)
Zinc stearate
Dust
Hydrocarbons
Lipoid substances

VI. LOEFFLER SYNDROME (see also Sec. 14.66)

VII. HYPOSTATIC PNEUMONIA (see also Sec. 14.69)

VIII. DRUG/RADIATION PNEUMONIA (see Sec. 14.18 and Chapter 17)

IX. HYPERSENSITIVITY PNEUMONITIS (see also Sec. 14.64)

14.56 BACTERIAL PNEUMONIA

GENERAL CONSIDERATIONS. Primary infection of the parenchyma of the lung (pneumonia) is much less common than secondary bacterial infection complicating the acute viral bronchitis that occurs during minor upper respiratory infection. Bacterial pneumonia during childhood and recurrent pneumonia in the absence of an underlying chronic illness, such as cystic fibrosis or immunologic deficiency, is quite unusual. In infants and young children with infection of the lower respiratory tract, signs and symptoms of pulmonary involvement are often nonspecific or surprisingly few. Accordingly, roentgenographic evidence of pneumonia is frequently found in infants who clinically appear to have only upper respiratory tract infections or only tachypnea and fever without physical findings, suggesting pulmonary involvement.

The most common event disturbing the defense mechanisms of the lung (see Sec. 14.4) is a viral infection that alters the properties of normal secretions, inhibits phagocytosis, modifies the bacterial flora, and may temporarily disrupt the normal epithelial layer of the respiratory passages. A viral respiratory disease often precedes the development of bacterial pneumonia by a few days.

Children with defects in defense mechanisms or in the chain of events involved in recovery from infection experience recurrent pneumonias or fail to resolve the disease completely. These defects occur with abnormalities of antibody production (agammaglobulinemia), cystic fibrosis, cleft palate, congenital bronchiectasis, ciliary dyskinesis, tracheoesophageal fistula, abnormalities of the polymorphonuclear leukocytes, neutropenia, increased pulmonary blood flow, deficient gag reflex, and so forth. Among iatrogenic factors promoting pulmonary infection are trauma, anesthesia, and aspiration.

Pneumococcal Pneumonia

Though the incidence of pneumococcal pneumonia has declined over the last several decades, the pneumococcus *(S. pneumoniae)* is still the most common bacterial pathogen, accounting for over 90% of childhood bacterial pneumonia. See also Sec. 12.21.

PATHOLOGY AND PATHOGENESIS. Pneumococcal organisms are probably aspirated into the periphery of the lung from the upper airway or nasopharynx. Initially, a reactive edema occurs that supports proliferation of the organisms and aids in their spread into adjacent portions of the lung. The involved lobe undergoes early consolidation, a stage of *red hepatization,* with polymorphonuclear leukocytes, fibrin, red blood cells, edema fluid, and pneumococci filling the alveoli. This passes into the *gray hepatization* stage, characterized by the deposition of fibrin over the pleural surfaces and the presence of fibrin and polymorphonuclear leukocytes in the alveolar spaces where phagocytosis is rapidly taking place. With *resolution,* increasing numbers of macrophages appear in the alveolar spaces, the neutrophils degenerate, and the fibrin threads and remaining bacteria are digested and disappear. In untreated cases a clinical crisis occurs about the 7th day of illness, and resolution and re-expansion require an additional 1–3 wk. Antibiotics given in the first several days of illness interrupt the course, and the characteristic stages are not seen.

Usually one or more lobes, or parts of lobes, are involved, leaving the remaining bronchopulmonary system uninvolved. However, this pattern of lobar pneumonia is often not present in infants who may have a more patchy and diffuse disease that follows a bronchial distribution and that is characterized by many limited areas of consolidation around the smaller airways. Permanent injury is rare.

CLINICAL MANIFESTATIONS. The classic history of a shaking chill followed by a high fever, cough, and chest pain described in adults with pneumococcal pneumonia may be seen in older children, but it is rarely observed in infants and young children, in whom the clinical pattern is considerably more variable.

Infants. A mild upper respiratory tract infection characterized by stuffy nose, fretfulness, and diminished appetite usually precedes the onset of pneumococcal pneumonia in infants. This mild illness of several days' duration ends with abrupt onset of fever of 39° C or higher, restlessness, apprehension, and respiratory distress. The patient appears ill with moderate-to-severe air hunger and often cyanosis. The respiratory distress is manifest by grunting, flaring of the alae nasi, retractions of the supraclavicular, intercostal, and subcostal areas, tachypnea, and tachycardia. Cough is unusual initially but may occur later.

A physical examination of the chest is often unrevealing. Dullness is usually localized to one lobe. Auscultation may reveal diminished breath sounds and fine, crackling rales on the affected side, but these findings are less common than in older children. On the opposite side, breath sounds may be exaggerated and almost tubular in nature. On percussion, if dullness is found in young infants, the presence of pleural effusion or empyema should be suspected. Abdominal distention may be prominent, reflecting gastric distention owing to swallowed air or to ileus; it may suggest an acute surgical emergency. The liver may seem enlarged because of downward displacement of the right diaphragm or superimposed congestive heart failure. Nuchal rigidity without meningeal infection (meningismus) may also be prominent, especially with involvement of the right upper lobe. Physical findings in the lung usually change little during the course of illness, although moist rales may become audible during resolution.

Children and Teenagers. The signs and symptoms are similar to those of adults. After a brief, mild, upper respiratory infection there is often onset of a shaking chill followed by fever as high as 40.5° C. This is accompanied by drowsiness with intermittent periods of restlessness, rapid respirations, a dry, hacking, unproductive cough, anxiety, and occasionally delirium. There may be circumoral cyanosis, and many children are noted to be splinting on the affected side to minimize pleuritic pain and improve ventilation; they may lie on their side with knees drawn up to the chest. Abnormal chest findings include retractions, flaring of alae nasi, dullness, diminished tactile and vocal fremitus, diminished breath sounds, and fine and crackling rales on the affected side. On the 1st day of illness, dullness over the affected lobe is usually not evident, and the suppression of breath sounds on the affected side may lead to misinterpretation of the exaggerated breath sounds in the opposite lung as tubular breathing.

The physical findings undergo change during the course of illness. Classic signs of consolidation are noted on the 2nd–3rd day of illness and are characterized by dullness, increased fremitus, tubular breath sounds, and the disappearance of rales. As resolution occurs, moist rales are heard, and the signs of consolidation disappear. The initial dry, hacking cough loosens and becomes productive of large amounts of blood-tinged mucous material.

The development of a pleural effusion or empyema may cause a visible lag in respiration on the affected side, with exaggerated excursion on the opposite side. An examination usually reveals dullness over the area of the effusion, with diminished fremitus and breath sounds. Tubular breathing is often noted immediately above the fluid level and on the unaffected side.

LABORATORY FINDINGS. The white blood cell count is usually elevated to 15,000–40,000 cells/mm^3, with a preponderance of polymorphonuclear cells. White blood cell counts below 5000/mm^3 are often associated with a grave prognosis. The hemoglobin value is usually normal or only slightly diminished. Arterial blood samples usually show hypoxemia without hypercapnia.

In most patients pneumococci can be isolated from the nasopharyngeal secretions, but this finding cannot be considered proof of a causative relation; the isolation of pneumococci should be attempted from secretions obtained upon deep coughing, from gentle tracheal aspiration, from blood, or from pleural fluid obtained at thoracentesis. Bacteremia is found in about 30% of patients having pneumococcal pneumonia. Latex agglutination of blood, pleural fluid, or urine may be helpful in establishing the diagnosis.

ROENTGENOGRAPHIC FINDINGS. The roentgenographic changes do not always correspond with the clinical observations. Consolidation may be demonstrated by roentgenography before it can be detected by physical examination, and resolution of the infiltrate may not be complete until several weeks after the child is clinically well. Lobar consolidation is not as common in infants and young children as in the older child. Pleural reaction with the presence of fluid is not uncommon; it may be seen early in the course of illness and, even in the untreated patient, is not necessarily indicative of developing empyema. It is important that roentgenographic demonstration of complete resolution be obtained 3–4 wk after the disappearance of all symptoms. Persistence of infiltrate suggests an underlying process, such as a foreign body or immunologic deficiency. If clinical response is slow, serial roentgenograms are indicated.

DIFFERENTIAL DIAGNOSIS. Pneumococcal pneumonia cannot be differentiated from other bacterial and viral pneumonias without appropriate microbiologic studies. Conditions possibly confused with pneumonia are bronchiolitis, allergic bronchitis, congestive heart failure, acute exacerbations of bronchiectasis, aspiration of a foreign body, sequestered lobe, atelectasis, pulmonary abscess, and endotracheal tuberculosis with secondary bacterial pneumonia.

An older child with right lower lobe pneumonia may have diaphragmatic irritation with pain referred to the right lower quadrant of the abdomen. Because ileus may accompany pneumonia, right lower quadrant pain and absent bowel sounds may be misinterpreted as acute appendicitis.

When meningismus is severe and presents opisthotonos or positive Kernig and Brudzinski signs, it can be differentiated from meningitis only by examining the spinal fluid.

COMPLICATIONS. With the use of antibiotic therapy, complications of bacterial pneumonia have become unusual. Although concomitant pneumococcal infection in other locations (e.g., otitis media) may be present prior to the onset of the symptoms of pneumonia, metastatic infection after the initiation of antibiotic treatment is infrequent. Empyema and lung abscess are uncommon. Empyema results from extension of infection to the pleural surfaces and occurs most commonly in the young infant who has received medical attention late in the course of illness or who has been treated inadequately. Persistent pneumatoceles may also occur and do not usually require treatment.

PROGNOSIS. In the preantibiotic era the mortality rate in infants and small children ranged from 20–50% and in older children from 3–5%. Furthermore, the incidence of chronic empyema with altered pulmonary function was relatively high. With appropriate antibiotic therapy instituted early in the course of the illness, the mortality rate during infancy and childhood is now less than 1%, and long-term morbidity is corresponding low.

TREATMENT. See Sec. 12.21.

The majority of older children with pneumococcal pneumonia can be treated at home; the *decision to hospitalize* depends on the severity of illness, the physical adequacy of the home, and the ability of the family to supply good nursing care. Pneumonia in the young infant is best treated in the hospital, because fluids and antibiotics may have to be administered intravenously. Furthermore, the course of illness in young infants is more variable and complications are more common. Patients with pneumonia associated with pleural effusion or empyema should also be hospitalized. Liberal oral intake of *fluids* and the administration of acetaminophen for high fever are the principal adjuncts to therapy. *Oxygen* administered promptly to patients with respiratory distress greatly reduces the need for sedatives and analgesics; it should be given before the patient becomes cyanotic.

Streptococcal Pneumonia

Group A streptococci most commonly cause disease limited to the upper respiratory tract, but the organisms may spread to other areas of the body, including the lower respiratory tract. Streptococcal pneumonia and tracheobronchitis are uncommon, but certain viral infections, particularly the exanthems and epidemic influenza, predispose to these diseases, which are encountered most frequently in children 3–5 yr of age and very rarely in infants. Group B streptococcal pneumonia is discussed in Sec. 9.60 and 9.67. The group C streptococcus, an important animal pathogen, is a very rare cause of pneumonia in humans.

PATHOLOGY. Streptococcal infections of the lower respiratory tract result in tracheitis, bronchitis, or interstitial pneumonia. Lobar pneumonia is uncommon. Lesions consist of necrosis of the tracheobronchial mucosa with the formation of ragged ulcers and large amounts of exudate, edema, and localized hemorrhage. The process may extend to the interalveolar septa and involve lymphatic vessels. Infection may spread by way of the lymphatics to the mediastinal and hilar lymph nodes or may proceed in a retrograde direction in occluded vessels and reach the pleural surfaces. Pleurisy is relatively common; the effusion is often large and serous, occasionally serosanguineous, or thinly purulent, with less fibrin than the exudate of pneumococcal pneumonia.

CLINICAL MANIFESTATIONS. The signs and symptoms of streptoccal pneumonia are similar to those of pneumococcal pneumonia. The onset may be sudden, characterized by high fever, chills, signs of respiratory distress, and, at times, extreme prostration. However, it may occasionally be more insidious, which is often the case with *H. influenzae* pneumonia, and the child will appear only mildly ill with cough and low-grade fever. If an exanthem or influenza precedes the pneumonia, the onset may be seen only as an increasingly severe clinical course of the viral illness. The clinical findings may be less impressive than the disseminated interstitial infiltration noted on a roentgenogram. Pleurisy, which commonly occurs, may be evidenced by clinical findings and pleural effusion.

LABORATORY MANIFESTATIONS. Leukocytosis occurs as in pneumococcal pneumonia. A rise in serum antistreptolysin titer is supportive diagnostic evidence. The disease may be suspected if large amounts of group A β-hemolytic streptococci are isolated from throat swab, nasopharyngeal secretions, bronchial washings, or sputum, but definitive diagnosis rests on recovery of the organism from pleural fluid, blood, or lung aspirate. Bacteremia occurs in about 10% of patients.

Chest roentgenograms usually show diffuse bronchopneumonia, often with a large pleural effusion. Occasionally, there is hilar adenopathy. Final roentgenographic resolution should be demonstrated but may not be complete for up to 10 wk.

DIFFERENTIAL DIAGNOSIS. The clinical course and roentgenographic findings of streptococcal pneumonia with purulent pleurisy are often similar to those of staphylococcal pneumonia. Pneumatoceles may occur in both conditions. The roentgenographic changes of uncomplicated streptococcal pneumonia may be indistinguishable from other interstitial pneumonitides, including those caused by *M. pneumoniae.*

COMPLICATIONS. Bacterial complications and long-term morbidity are common in the untreated patient but rare after antibiotic treatment is begun. Empyema occurs in 20% of children, and occasionally septic foci develop in other areas, such as the bones or joints; otherwise extension of the disease is uncommon. Acute glomerulonephritis occurs rarely.

TREATMENT. The drug of choice is penicillin G (100,000 units/kg/24 hr). Parenteral penicillin is used initially, and a 2–3 wk course may be completed orally after clinical improvement has begun in the hospital. If empyema develops, a thoracentesis should be performed for diagnostic purposes and for removal of fluid. On occasion, repeated thoracentesis or closed drainage with indwelling chest tubes may be required if the fluid reaccumulates. Intrathoracic administration of antibiotics or enzymes to liquefy pus or dissolve fibrin is ineffective.

Staphylococcal Pneumonia

Pneumonia caused by *S. aureus* is a serious and rapidly progressive infection that, unless recognized early and treated appropriately, is associated with prolonged morbidity and high mortality. It occurs less frequently than pneumococcal or viral pneumonia and is more common in infants than in children (see Sec. 12.19).

EPIDEMIOLOGY. Most cases occur from October to May,

and, as with other bacterial pneumonias, staphylococcal pneumonia is frequently preceded by a viral upper respiratory tract infection. Although it may occur at any age, 30% of all patients are under 3 mo of age and 70% are under 1 yr. Boys are affected more commonly than girls.

PATHOGENICITY AND PATHOLOGY. Staphylococci cause confluent bronchopneumonia that is often unilateral or more prominent on one side than the other and is characterized by the presence of extensive areas of hemorrhagic necrosis and irregular areas of cavitation. The pleural surface is usually covered by a thick layer of fibrinopurulent exudate. Multiple abscesses occur, containing clusters of staphylococci, leukocytes, erythrocytes, and necrotic debris. Rupture of a small subpleural abscess may result in a pyopneumothorax, which in turn may erode into a bronchus, producing a bronchopleural fistula. Septic thrombi may form in pulmonary veins in regions of extensive destruction and inflammation.

CLINICAL MANIFESTATIONS. Most commonly, the patient is an infant under 1 yr of age, often with a history of staphylococcal skin lesions in himself or herself or in a family member and with signs and symptoms of an upper or lower respiratory tract infection for several days to 1 week. Abruptly, the infant's condition changes, with the onset of high fever, cough, and evidence of respiratory distress. Signs and symptoms include tachypnea, grunting respirations, sternal and subcostal retractions, nasal flaring, cyanosis, and anxiety. If left undisturbed, the infant is lethargic but upon arousal is irritable and appears toxic. Severe dyspnea and a shock-like state may be present. Some infants have associated gastrointestinal disturbances characterized by vomiting, anorexia, diarrhea, and abdominal distention secondary to a paralytic ileus. A rapid progression of symptoms is characteristic.

Physical findings depend on the stage of pneumonia. Early in the course of illness diminished breath sounds, scattered rales, and rhonchi are commonly heard over the affected lung. With the development of effusion, empyema, or pyopneumothorax, dullness on percussion is noted, and breath sounds and vocal fremitus are markedly diminished. A lag in respiratory excursion often occurs on the affected side. A physical examination may, however, be misleading, particularly in the young infant with meager findings disproportionate to the degree of tachypnea.

LABORATORY MANIFESTATIONS. In the older infant and child a leukocytosis of 20,000 or more cells/mm^3 usually occurs, with the increase primarily among the polymorphonuclear cells; in the young infant the white blood cell count may remain within the normal range. As in other forms of bacterial infection, a count below 5,000 cells/mm^3 is a poor prognostic sign. Mild-to-moderate anemia is common.

Material for diagnostic cultures should be obtained by tracheal aspiration or pleural tap; Gram stain frequently reveals gram-positive cocci. The finding of staphylococci in the nasopharynx is of no diagnostic value, but blood culture may be positive. Pleural fluid reveals an exudate with polymorphonuclear cell counts ranging from 300–100,000/mm^3, protein above 2.5 g/dL, and low glucose level relative to the blood level.

ROENTGENOGRAPHIC MANIFESTATIONS. Most patients with staphylococcal pneumonia have roentgenographic evidence of nonspecific bronchopneumonia early in the illness. The infiltrate may soon become patchy and limited in extent or be dense and homogeneous and involve an entire lobe or hemithorax. The right lung alone is involved in about 65% of cases; bilateral involvement occurs in fewer than 20% of patients. A pleural effusion or empyema is noted during the course in most patients; pyopneumothorax occurs in approximately 25%. Pneumatoceles of varying size are common.

Although no roentgenographic change can be considered diagnostic, progression over a few hours from bronchopneumonia to effusion or pyopneumothorax with or without pneumatoceles is highly suggestive of staphylococcal pneumonia. Chest films should be obtained at frequent intervals if the diagnosis is suspected. Clinical improvement usually precedes roentgenographic clearing by days or weeks, and pneumatoceles may persist in an asymptomatic patient for months.

DIFFERENTIAL DIAGNOSIS. Recognizing early staphylococcal pneumonia in the infant is often difficult. Abrupt onset and rapid progression of symptoms of pneumonia should be considered to be due to staphylococci until proved otherwise. A history of furunculosis, a preceding viral upper respiratory tract infection, a recent hospital admission, or maternal breast abscess should also alert the physician to the possibility of this diagnosis. Other bacterial pneumonias that cause empyema or pneumatoceles and thus may be readily confused with staphylococcal disease include streptococcal, *Klebsiella*, *H. influenzae*, and pneumococcal pneumonias and primary tuberculous pneumonia with cavitation. Occasionally, the aspiration of a nonradiopaque foreign body followed by pulmonary abscesses may lead to a similar clinical and radiologic picture. All infants with staphylococcal pneumonia should be tested for CF and screened for immunodeficiency disease.

COMPLICATIONS. Since empyema, pyopneumothorax, and pneumatoceles are so commonly seen with staphylococcal pneumonia, they are considered part of the natural course of the illness and not complications. Septic lesions outside the respiratory tract occur rarely except in the young infant, in whom staphylococcal pericarditis, meningitis, osteomyelitis, and multiple metastatic abscesses in soft tissue may occur. Metastatic infection after the initiation of appropriate antibiotic therapy is rare.

PROGNOSIS. Survival has improved substantially with present-day management, but mortality still ranges from 10–30% and varies with the length of illness prior to hospitalization, age of patient, adequacy of therapy, and the presence of other illness or complications. Children who do not have underlying disease have an excellent prognosis for complete recovery, including normal growth and development, normal pulmonary function, and no increased susceptibility to pulmonary infections. The course is usually prolonged, with hospitalizations of from 6–10 wk.

TREATMENT. Therapy consists of appropriate antibiotics and drainage of collections of pus. The infant should be given oxygen and placed in a semireclining position to relieve cyanosis and anxiety. During the acute phase, intravenous hydration and nutrition are indicated, and if the patient is severely anemic, blood transfusion may be beneficial. Assisted ventilation may occasionally be needed.

A *semisynthetic, penicillinase-resistant penicillin* should be administered intravenously immediately after culture while reports are pending (e.g., methicillin, 200 mg/kg/24 hr). Patients receiving these drugs should be closely monitored for possible nephrotoxicity. If the cultures subsequently demonstrate an organism sensitive to penicillin G, then this agent should be used in dosages of 100,000 units/kg/24 hr instead of the initial drug. In patients allergic to penicillin, a cephalosporin may be used, such as ceftriaxone (75–100 mg/kg/24 hr). From 3–4 wk of therapy is usually adequate, but the clinical response may indicate a need for longer therapy.

Although patients with staphylococcal pneumonia may occasionally recover completely without *chest tube* drainage, it is recommended even if only a small effusion or empyema is present in order to reduce the chance of bronchopleural fistula and the necessity for repeated pleural taps. Generally, pus reaccumulates so rapidly and becomes so viscous or loculated that closed drainage with a chest tube of the largest possible caliber is required. The appearance of pyopneumothorax is another indication for immediate insertion of a catheter into the pleural space. It is often necessary to use several chest tubes when loculation occurs. Once the infant begins to improve and the lung has re-expanded, the tubes may be removed, even if they are still draining small amounts of pus; in general, tubes should not remain in the chest more than 5–7 days. Decortication procedures are rarely needed (see Sec. 14.90).

Instillation of antibiotics or enzymes into the chest cavity has no beneficial effect and is associated with an increased incidence of pneumothorax and systemic toxic reactions.

Ammann AJ, Addiego J, Wara DW, et al: Polyvalent pneumococcal-polysaccharide immunization of patients with sickle-cell anemia and patients with splenectomy. N Engl J Med 297:897, 1977.

Broome CV, Facklam RR, Fraser DV: Pneumococcal disease after pneumococcal vaccine. N Engl J Med 303:549, 1980.

Ceruti E, Contreras J, Neira M: Staphylococcal pneumonia in childhood. Long-term follow-up including pulmonary function studies. Am J Dis Child 122:386, 1971.

Honig PJ, Pasquariello PS Jr, Stool SE: *H. influenzae* pneumonia in infants and children. J Pediatr 83:215, 1973.

Jay SJ, Johanson WG Jr, Pierce AK: The radiographic resolution of *Streptococcus* pneumonia. N Engl J Med 293:798, 1975.

Rebban AW, Edwards HE: Staphylococcal pneumonia: Review of 329 cases. Can Med Assoc J 82:513, 1960.

Turner RB, Lande AE, Chase P, et al: Pneumonia in pediatric outpatients: Cause and clinical manifestations. J Pediatr 111:194, 1987.

Pneumonias Caused by Gram-Negative Organisms

A small percentage of pneumonias of infants and children after the neonatal period are caused by gram-negative organisms. However, the number has been increasing in recent years, perhaps because of the widespread use of antibiotics, the contamination of hospital equipment, the increasing use of immunosuppressive agents in the treatment of malignant disorders, and the increasing survival of children with chronic pulmonary disease such as cystic fibrosis. The organisms most commonly encountered are *H. influenzae* type b (see Sec. 12.22), *Klebsiella pneumoniae*, and *Pseudomonas aeruginosa* (see Sec. 12.32). The morbidity and mortality rates of these infections are high as a result of the pathogenicity of the bacteria and the altered host resistance in many of these patients (see Sec. 12.13).

***HAEMOPHILUS INFLUENZAE* PNEUMONIA.** *H. influenzae* type b is a frequent cause of serious bacterial infection in infants and children. Nasopharyngeal infection precedes almost all clinical varieties of localized *H. influenzae* disease, such as otitis media, epiglottitis, pneumonia, and meningitis. Pneumonia is second in frequency only to meningitis in children with invasive *H. influenzae* disease; most cases occur during winter and spring.

H. influenzae pneumonias are usually lobar in distribution, but there is no characteristic chest roentgenogram. Segmental infiltrates, single or multiple lobe involvement, pleural effusion, and pneumatoceles occur. Disseminated pulmonary disease and bronchopneumonia have also been described. Males are affected slightly more often than females. Pathologically, involved areas show a polymorphonuclear or lymphocytic inflammatory reaction with extensive destruction of the epithelium of smaller airways, interstitial inflammation, and marked, often hemorrhagic, edema.

Although the *clinical manifestations* may be difficult to distinguish clinically from those of pneumococcal pneumonia, *H. influenzae* pneumonia is more often insidious in onset, and the course is usually prolonged over several weeks. Many patients are already receiving treatment for otitis media at the time of diagnosis. Although ceftriaxone or chloramphenicol and ampicillin (see later) are recommended for treatment of *H. influenzae* pneumonia, a clinical response to penicillin G is common and does not exclude this diagnosis. Cough is almost always present but may not be productive, and the patient is febrile and often tachypneic with nasal flaring and retractions. There may be localized dullness to percussion and rales and tubular breath sounds; pleural fluid is often present on roentgenogram in the young infant.

The *diagnosis* is established by isolating the organism from the blood, particularly in the young infant, from pleural fluid, or from lung aspirate. There is usually moderate leukocytosis with a relative lymphopenia. Latex agglutination tests on tracheal secretions, blood, urine, and pleural fluid may also establish an early diagnosis. If atelectasis is present, bronchoscopy may be indicated to rule out a foreign body.

Complications are frequent, particularly in the young infant, and include bacteremia, pericarditis, cellulitis, empyema, meningitis, and pyarthrosis. Meningitis occurred in 15% of the younger patients in one study; examination of cerebrospinal fluid should be strongly considered when pneumonia due to *H. influenzae* is diagnosed.

Treatment consists of the same symptomatic and supportive measures utilized in pneumococcal and staphylococcal pneumonias. When *H. influenzae* is suspected as the causative agent, ampicillin (100 mg/kg/24 hr) and chloramphenicol (100 mg/kg/24 hr) or ceftriaxone (100 mg/kg/24 hr) should be included in the initial antibiotic therapy until it is known whether the organism produces penicillinase; if the strain is sensitive, ampicillin (100 mg/kg/24 hr) alone may be administered. Appropriate in vitro susceptibility studies are essential. Effusion and pyarthrosis may require drainage. Needle thoracentesis is often adequate for effusion drainage, but the procedure may occasionally have to be repeated. Closed chest drainage may be required if purulent pleural fluid is present, but open drainage is infrequently needed. If the initial response to antibiotics is good, oral treatment can be instituted to complete a 10- to 14-day course. Roentgenographic demonstration of complete resolution should be obtained 2–4 wk later; complete resolution may require a prolonged period.

***KLEBSIELLA PNEUMONIAE* (FRIEDLÄNDER BACILLUS) PNEUMONIA.** This organism, found in the respiratory and gastrointestinal tracts of approximately 5% of normal persons, causes pneumonia in debilitated or immunosuppressed patients and frequently occurs as a secondary invader in the lungs of patients with chronic bronchiectasis, influenza, or tuberculosis. Klebsiella may be the dominant organism in cystic fibrosis, particularly during infancy, and is a common cause of pneumonia after thermal injury to the respiratory tract. Primary *K. pneumoniae* infection is unusual in infants and young children; it may occur, rarely, in nursery epidemics or as a sporadic case in neonates. During epidemics, many infants carry the organism in their nasopharynges without signs of clinical illness; only an occasional infant has severe disease. Contaminated fomites, including nursery equipment, and humidification apparatus are the primary source of nosocomial infection with the organism.

Pneumonia due to *K. pneumoniae* may be difficult to distinguish clinically from pneumonia due to other causes. In nursery epidemics, diarrhea and vomiting may be the presenting symptoms; the onset of respiratory difficulty is often abrupt. The disease may have a fulminant course characterized by copious, thick, purulent secretion and the formation of pulmonary abscesses and cavitations. A lobar infiltrate with bulging fissures on roentgenogram is suggestive of the diagnosis (Fig. 14–9). Complications are common and include bacteremia, empyema, and residual parenchymal damage. The fatality rate in sporadic cases is about 50%, but it is lower during epidemics.

Isolation of the organism from purulent tracheal secretions, blood, or lung aspirate establishes the diagnosis. Supportive

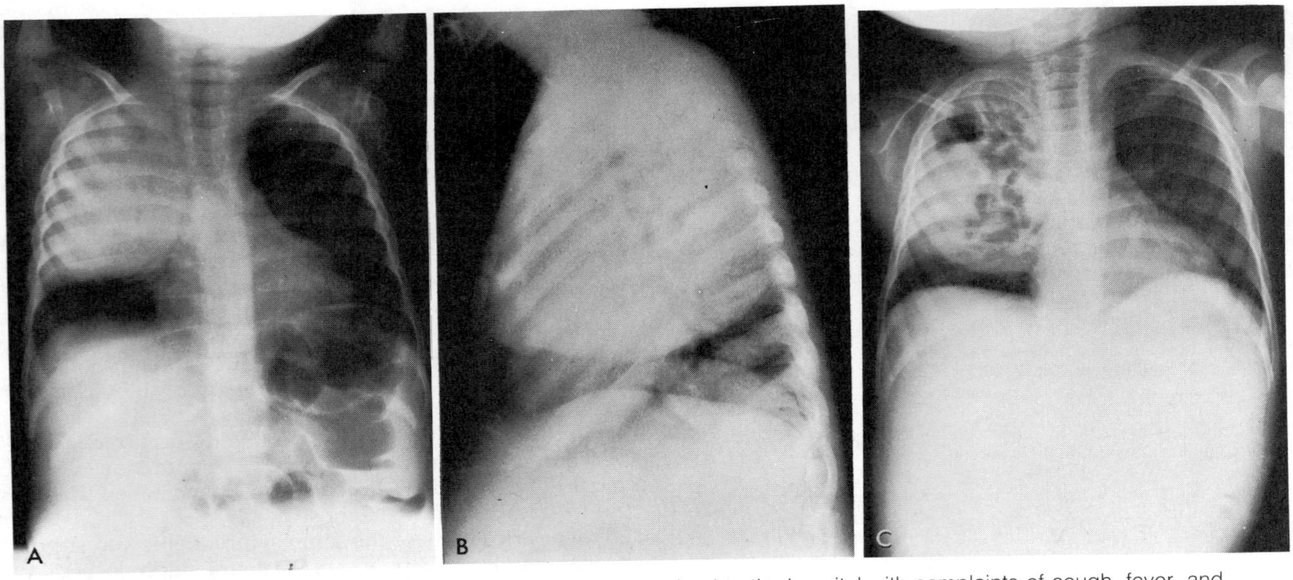

Figure 14–9. *Klebsiella* pneumonia in an 8-mo-old infant admitted to the hospital with complaints of cough, fever, and dyspnea. Roentgenograms *(A,B)* demonstrated pulmonary consolidation with characteristic bulging of fissure. Multiple pneumatoceles and abscesses appeared within 48 hr *(C)*. The patient recovered with kanamycin therapy.

treatment is similar to that of other bacterial pneumonias; drainage of empyema and abscesses may be necessary. A combination of a third generation cephalosporin and an aminoglycoside is the treatment of choice.

PSEUDOMONAS AERUGINOSA **PNEUMONIA.** (Sec. 12.32). *P. aeruginosa* produces a severe, progressive, occasionally fatal, necrotizing bronchopneumonia that is rarely a primary infection of the lung but occurs with chronic debilitating illnesses, such as CF and malignant disorders; with altered immunologic function; during prolonged antibiotic therapy; after thermal injury; and in premature infants exposed to contaminated hospital equipment. In CF a fulminant course is uncommon. Ceftazidine administered in combination with an aminoglycoside represents the most effective therapy.

Ginsburg CM, Howard JB, Nelson JD: Report of 65 cases of *Haemophilus influenzae* b pneumonia. Pediatrics 64:283, 1979.
Jacobs NM, Harris VJ: Acute *Haemophilus* pneumonia in childhood. Am J Dis Child 133:603, 1979.
Morgan HR: The enteric bacteria. *In*: Dubos R, Hirsch J (eds): Bacterial and Mycotic Infections of Man, 4th ed. Philadelphia, JB Lippincott, 1965.
Thaler MM: *Klebsiella: Aerobacter* pneumonia in infants. Pediatrics 30:206, 1962.

14.57 PNEUMONIAS OF VIRAL ORIGIN

ETIOLOGY. Many viruses cause lower respiratory tract disease in children, principally bronchiolitis and interstitial lesions. The type and severity of the illness are influenced by several factors including age, sex, season of the year, and crowding. Boys are affected slightly more often than girls. Unlike bronchiolitis where the peak attack rate is within the 1st yr, the peak attack rate for viral pneumonia is reached between the ages of 2 and 3 yr and decreases slowly thereafter. Viral pneumonia is most commonly caused by RSV (see Sec. 12.76), one of the parainfluenza viruses (see Sec. 12.75), adenovirus (see Sec. 12.77), or enterovirus (see Sec. 12.80). Less commonly, rhinovirus (see Sec. 12.78), influenza virus (see Sec. 12.74), herpes simplex virus (see Sec. 12.68), and others have also been recovered from children with pneumonia. Local epidemics may skew incidence figures for a given year or location. RSV causes a more serious disease during infancy, when it is the agent most commonly recovered.

CLINICAL MANIFESTATIONS. Most viral pneumonias are preceded by several days of respiratory symptoms, including rhinitis and cough. Often, other family members are ill. Although cough and fever are prominent, temperatures are generally lower than in bacterial pneumonia. Dyspnea with retractions and nasal flaring is more common in younger children and infants. A physical examination may be surprisingly unrevealing, although rales are present late in the illness. Wheezing, apparently related to virus-specific IgE, is frequently present with RSV pneumonia. The viral pneumonias cannot be definitely differentiated from mycoplasmal disease on purely clinical grounds and may, on occasion, be difficult to distinguish from bacterial pneumonias. Furthermore, evidence of viral infection is present in many patients who have confirmed bacterial pneumonia.

DIAGNOSIS. The chest roentgenogram is characterized by a diffuse infiltrate, especially in the perihilar areas. In some patients, transient lobar infiltrates may also be present or even dominate the picture. Hyperinflation is common. Effusion may occur. Serologic studies may allow retrospective diagnosis by demonstrating a rise in antibody titer. Respiratory viruses, including parainfluenza virus, RSV, and, less commonly, adenovirus, are occasionally found in asymptomatic children. The white blood cell count is usually under $20,000/mm^3$. Platelets may occasionally be slightly depressed.

TREATMENT. There is no specific treatment. Many patients are given antibiotic agents initially if bacterial pneumonia is suspected. Failure to respond to antibiotic treatment is additional evidence for a purely viral etiology. Usually, only minimal supportive measures are required, although some patients need hospitalization for intravenous fluids, oxygen, or even assisted ventilation. Continuously administered aerosolized ribavirin is effective in some infants with respiratory syncytial virus pneumonia (see Sec. 12.76).

PROGNOSIS. Most children with viral pneumonia recover uneventfully and have no sequelae, although the course may be prolonged, especially in infants. There is increasing evidence, however, that some patients, particularly infants, may develop bronchiolitis obliterans, unilateral hyperlucent lung, or other complications after a single episode of viral pneumonia. Adenovirus, especially types 1, 3, 4, 7, and 21, seems to be the most dangerous agent in this regard, and it has also been reported to cause a fatal acute fulminant pneumonia.

Continuing roentgenographic abnormality for 6–12 mo is not unusual. In one series bronchiectasis was present in 27% of infant survivors of adenovirus (type 7) pneumonia.

Mycoplasmal Pneumonia

(Primary Atypical Pneumonia)

See Sec. 12.63.

GIANT CELL PNEUMONIA

(Hecht Pneumonia)

See Sec. 12.64.

Denny FW, Clyde WA: Acute lower respiratory tract infections in nonhospitalized children. J Pediatr 108:635, 1986.
Henderson FW, Collier AM, Clyde WA, et al: Respiratory-syncytial-virus infections, reinfections and immunity: A prospective, longitudinal study in young children. N Engl J Med 300:530, 1979.
Hall CB, McBride JT, Walsh EF, et al: Aerosolized ribavirin treatment of infants with respiratory syncytial viral infection. N Engl J Med 308:1443, 1983.
James AG, Lang WR, Liang AY, et al: Adenovirus type 21 bronchopneumonia in infants and young children. J Pediatr 95:530, 1979.
Malatzky AJ, Cooney MK, Luce R, et al: Epidemiology of viral and mycoplasmal agents associated with childhood lower respiratory illness in a civilian population. J Pediatr 78:407, 1971.
Similä S, Linna O, Lanning P: Chronic lung damage caused by adenovirus type 7: A ten-year follow-up study. Chest 80:127, 1981.
Welliver RC, Wong DT, Sun M: The development of respiratory syncytial virus-specific IgE and the release of histamine in nasopharyngeal secretions after infection. N Engl J Med 305:841, 1981.

PNEUMONIAS OF MISCELLANEOUS CAUSES

14.58 *Pneumocystis carinii* Pneumonia

(Interstitial Plasma Cell Pneumonia)

See also Sec. 12.13 and 12.83.

EPIDEMIOLOGY. *P. carinii* organisms, ubiquitous fungi, are found only in the peripheral respiratory airways of humans and of a variety of other animals, including rodents. In the human, infection is associated with immunosuppressed or chronic debilitated states or with prematurity or severe neonatal illness (see Sec. 9.65). Most cases in the United States occur in patients with primary acquired immunodeficiency disease (AIDS) or with immunosuppression induced by malignancy or its treatment. As the treatment of malignancy has become more sophisticated and patients survive longer, the incidence of this complication has increased. In one series 4% of more than 1,200 children with malignancies had proven pulmonary pneumocystis infestation.

PATHOGENESIS AND PATHOLOGY. In newborn infants an incompletely developed immunologic responsiveness and exposure to a humidified atmosphere contaminated with the parasite may interact synergistically to produce sporadic or epidemic disease in the nursery. In some infants intensive treatment of a respiratory tract infection with antibiotics may produce activation of a latent pneumocystis infection. Infants with cytomegalic inclusion disease or children with lymphoreticular malignancies treated with cytotoxic agents, corticosteroids, or prolonged antibiotic therapy are particularly susceptible to *P. carinii* pneumonia. Infection produces a characteristic intra-alveolar exudate of lacelike appearance that contains histiocytes, lymphocytes, plasma cells, and cysts. Plasma cells are diminished or absent in agammaglobulinemia and hypogammaglobulinemia. The alveolar septa show varying degrees of edema, inflammation, and fibrosis.

CLINICAL MANIFESTATIONS. Onset in infants is usually at 3–5 wk of life, and it may be seen at any age in patients with immune deficiency syndromes or acquired, temporary, or permanent loss of host resistance. In infants the disease usually begins insidiously with cough and proceeds over a period of 1–4 wk to be characterized by low grade fever, tachypnea, and severe respiratory distress. Nasal flaring, cyanosis, and suprasternal, infrasternal, and intercostal retractions usually occur, but rales may be absent or few. In older children the onset is more abrupt with fever, tachypnea, and cough followed rapidly by retractions, nasal flaring, and cyanosis. Rales are not usually present. Fever and cough, particularly in infants, may also be absent. There is a relative paucity of pulmonary findings for the severity of distress.

The roentgenogram characteristically consists of hyperexpanded lung fields, a generalized granular pattern, and bilateral pulmonary infiltrates that originate at the hilus, extend peripherally, and eventually create a nearly solid appearance. Overaeration is most pronounced in the periphery. Arterial oxygen is reduced, but hypercapnia is uncommon.

P. carinii pneumonia usually lasts from 3–6 wk but may continue for many months.

DIAGNOSIS. Definitive diagnosis is made by demonstrating the presence of the organism in the lung by appropriate staining of tracheal or lung aspirates, bronchial washing, or lung biopsies; sputum samples or tonsillar smears may occasionally be satisfactory. Indirect immunofluorescent staining of sputum or lavage material, using monoclonal antibodies, may improve identification of the organism. If necessary, induced sputum may be used for this test. A complement fixation test may show conversion after 2–3 wk if the patient's immune system is sufficiently functional.

TREATMENT. If left untreated, the disease is often fatal; patients with cellular immune deficiency or extensive malignancy usually die within 3 wk of onset of the typical roentgenographic features. *Trimethoprim* (20 mg/kg/24 hr) and *sulfamethoxazole* (100 mg/kg/24 hr) are the treatment of choice. Treatment with *pentamidine isothionate* (4 mg/kg/24 hr intramuscularly for 2 wk) has allowed 50% of patients to recover even without restoration of immunocompetence; serious side effects of this drug include azotemia. Pentamidine may be effective despite prior unsuccessful treatment with trimethoprim-sulfamethoxazole. Prednisone may improve the outcome of PCP in patients with AIDS. In very ill patients, supplemental oxygen with or without ventilator assistance may be needed. Children over 6 yr of age may recover completely from pneumocystis pneumonia within 6 mo of treatment.

Preventive treatment with trimethoprim (5 mg/kg/24 hr) and sulfamethoxazole (20 mg/kg/24 hr) or monthly aerosolized pentamidine (in AIDS) may be useful in children who are at high risk for this disease.

Frankel LR, Smith DW, Lewiston NJ: Bronchoalveolar lavage for diagnosis of pneumonia in the immunocompromised child. Pediatrics 81:785, 1988.
Harris RE, McCallister JA, Allen SA, et al: Prevention of pneumocystis pneumonia. Am J Dis Child 134:35, 1980.
Hughes WT, Price RA, Kim HK, et al: *Pneumocystis carinii* pneumonitis in children with malignancies. J Pediatr 82:404, 1973.
Kovacs JA, Ng VL, Masure H, et al: Diagnosis of *Pneumocystis carinii* pneumonia: Improved detection in sputum with use of monoclonal antibodies. N Engl J Med 318:589, 1988.
Ognibene FP, Gill VJ, Pizzo PA, et al: Induced sputum to diagnose *Pneumocystis carinii* pneumonia in immunosuppressed pediatric patients. J Pediatr 115:430, 1989.
Sanyal SK, Mariencheck WC, Hughes WT: Course of pulmonary dysfunction in children surviving *Pneumocystis carinii* pneumonitis. Am Rev Respir Dis 124:161, 1981.
Siegel SE, Wolff LJ, Baehner RL, et al: Treatment of *Pneumocystis carinii* pneumonitis. Am J Dis Child 138:1051, 1984.

Mycotic Pulmonary Infections

See also Sec. 12.13

THRUSH PNEUMONIA

(Pulmonary Candidosis)

Pulmonary infections with *Candida albicans* are rare in children despite the relatively high incidence of oral thrush (see Sec.

9.75) in infancy. This fact has been attributed to a natural resistance of columnar epithelium to invasion by the fungus. In 17 infants under 8 wk of age, all of whom had respiratory distress, about half had oral thrush, but there was no clinical or roentgenographic characteristic to suggest it as the cause of pulmonary infection. Amphotericin B and 5-fluorocytosine are the only effective therapeutic agents.

Emanuel B, Lieberman AD, Glodin M, et al: Pulmonary candidasis in the neonatal period. J Pediatr 61:44, 1962.

14.59 Aspiration Pneumonia

ASPIRATION OF FOOD AND VOMITUS. Infants with obstructive lesions, such as tracheoesophageal fistula and duodenal obstruction, weak and debilitated infants and children with no obstructive lesions, patients with familial dysautonomia, and patients with impaired consciousness may aspirate, or regurgitate and then aspirate, an amount of food and vomitus sufficient to cause a chemical pneumonia. Aspiration may rarely be an immediate cause of death by asphyxiation. Hydrochloric acid is an important determinant of lung injury. More frequently, following aspiration of gastric contents, there is a relatively brief latent period before the onset of signs and symptoms of pneumonia. More than 90% of patients have symptoms within 1 hr, and almost all patients have symptoms within 2 hr. Fever, tachypnea, and cough are common. Apnea and shock also occur.

Physical examination reveals diffuse rales and wheezing, and many patients are cyanotic. Chest roentgenograms reveal alveolar and, occasionally, reticular infiltrates that may be localized but often are more extensive and are frequently bilateral. The irritated mucous membrane may also subsequently become the site for bacterial invasion and pneumonia. Aspiration from gastroesophageal reflux can be demonstrated sometimes by barium swallow roentgenography, but radionuclide milk scanning appears to be more sensitive.

Prophylaxis is of the greatest importance. Care should be taken to avoid amounts of feedings that will overdistend the stomach, especially in infants who are fed by gavage. After being fed, the infant should be placed on the abdomen or right side. When the infant is supine, the head should not be lower than the rest of the body. While the infant is lying face down, however, drainage from the lungs may be materially aided by lowering the head of the bed. Critically ill patients may be benefited by reduction of gastric acidity with cimetidine.

Immediate suctioning of the airway and administering oxygen are indicated for aspiration. Endotracheal intubation with suctioning and mechanical ventilation is often required in severe cases. Although prophylactic use of antibiotics and corticosteroids is advocated by some for patients who have aspirated gastric contents, evidence of their benefit is lacking. Some data suggest that corticosteroid treatment may predispose the patient to pneumonia owing to gram-negative organisms. Previously healthy unhospitalized patients may become infected with mouth flora (predominantly anaerobes); clindamycin or penicillin is effective therapy. Chronically ill hospitalized patients may be colonized with gram negative flora (*Pseudomonas, E. coli, Klebsiella*); additional coverage with an aminoglycoside may be indicated.

Prognosis depends partly on the severity of aspiration and partly on the underlying disease. Most patients demonstrate clearing of infiltrates within 2 wk; mortality before clearing of aspiration infiltrates is about 25%.

Brook I, Finegold SM: Bacteriology of aspiration pneumonia in children. Pediatrics 65:1115, 1980.
Bynium LJ, Pierce AK: Pulmonary aspiration of gastric contents. Am Rev Respir Dis 114:1129, 1976.
McVeagh P, Howman-Giles R, Kemp A: Pulmonary aspiration studied by radionuclide milk scanning and barium swallow roentgenography. Am J Dis Child 141:917, 1987.
Wolfe JE, Bone RC, Ruth WE: Effects of corticosteroids in the treatment of patients with gastric aspiration. Am J Med 83:719, 1977.

ASPIRATION OF BABY POWDER. Aspiration pneumonia resulting from inhalation of zinc stearate baby powder has become rare since the use of baby powder has decreased and since the containers still being used are now made better to control the outflow of powder. Nonetheless, these products are widely used, and catastrophic aspirations still occur. Severe respiratory distress almost immediately follows inhalation. Generalized obstructive emphysema with an expiratory type of dyspnea occurs as a result of an inflammatory reaction caused by the zinc stearate powder. Following inhalation, it is almost immediately drawn into the finer bronchioles because of its extreme lightness; for this reason bronchoscopic aspiration is useful, if at all, only to remove the secretions that may subsequently accumulate in the larger air passages. Immediate treatment is oxygen therapy in an atmosphere of high humidity.

The commonly used dusting (baby) powders today contain magnesium silicate (and other silicates), and some contain calcium undecylenate. Although not as dangerous as zinc stearate, these powders can also cause serious aspiration pneumonitis. Furthermore, talc is chemically related to asbestos, and "talcum powder" may contain microscopic asbestos particles, which may have a potential to cause malignancy. Systemic corticosteroid treatment appeared useful in one patient who had severe dyspnea after aspirating talc.

Cotton WH, Davidson PJ: Aspiration of baby powder. N Engl J Med 313:1662, 1985.
Hughes WT, Kalmer T: Massive talc aspiration. Am J Dis Child 111:653, 1966.
Mofenson HC, Caraccio TR, Okun S, et al: Hazards of baby powder. Pediatrics 78:546, 1986.

PNEUMONITIS FROM OTHER CHEMICALS. Many chemicals, particularly if inhaled in high concentrations, may cause an inflammatory reaction consisting of edema and cellular infiltrations and acute respiratory distress. Prolonged exposure to lower concentrations of these same agents or other chemicals may cause chronic interstitial pneumonitis characterized by granuloma formation. For example, shellac, polyvinylpyrrolidone (found in hair spray), gum arabic, beryllium, mercury vapors, and chlorine may cause this reaction. Corticosteroids may reduce the inflammatory reaction and prevent fibrosis.

14.60 Hydrocarbon Pneumonia

ETIOLOGY. Hydrocarbons, such as furniture polish, kerosene, charcoal lighter fluid, and gasoline, are occasionally accidentally ingested by young children, causing a secondary pneumonitis. Gasoline may be aspirated by teenagers attempting to siphon gasoline. In general, the lower the viscosity and the higher the volatility, the greater will be the pulmonary toxicity.

PATHOGENESIS. Although some controversy persists with regard to how hydrocarbons reach the lungs, they are probably aspirated during swallowing, vomiting, or gastric lavage. The low viscosity of hydrocarbons allows them to flow from the hypopharynx into the larynx. Ingestion of large quantities of these bad-tasting liquids is unusual. Therefore, gastric lavage is contraindicated unless the hydrocarbon contains poison, such as a potent insecticide. Hydrocarbons may interact with pulmonary surfactant, resulting in alveolar collapse. Alveolar macrophages may also be injured. The pulmonary changes observed in animals after hydrocarbon aspiration are edema, inflammation, and hemorrhage.

CLINICAL MANIFESTATIONS. Coughing and vomiting follow ingestion almost immediately. Within hours there may be a temperature elevation (38–40° C). However, with less extensive aspiration, the onset of pulmonary symptoms and inflammation may be delayed 12–24 hr. The pulmonary findings may include dyspnea, diminished resonance on percussion, suppressed or tubular breath sounds, and rales. Hypoxia and cyanosis, caused by inflammation and edema, may be aggravated by the displacement of alveolar gas with vaporized hydrocarbon. Pneumonic involvement is disclosed more frequently by roentgenographic examination than by physical findings. Roentgenograms may occasionally show minimal changes a few hours after ingestion only to progress rapidly after that time with extensive infiltrates. Despite what may be a stormy clinical course, which averages 2–5 days, recovery occurs in most cases. Systemic symptoms of hydrocarbon ingestion, including somnolence, convulsions, and coma, may occur and sometimes dominate the course (see Sec. 20.55 and 26.7).

COMPLICATIONS. Pneumothorax, subcutaneous emphysema of the chest wall, and pleural effusion, including empyema, have occurred. After the 1st wk, pneumatoceles may develop in areas of extensive consolidation. There may be secondary infection with bacteria or viruses.

TREATMENT. Symptoms and radiologic infiltrates may be delayed, and no patient should be sent home in less than 6 hr even if he or she is asymptomatic. Patients who are symptomatic when they are first examined or patients who become symptomatic during 6 hr of observation and all patients who ingested a particularly toxic agent (e.g., furniture polish) should be admitted to the hospital. Patients who are still asymptomatic after 6 hr and who have a normal result on a chest roentgenogram can be observed at home, but parents should be instructed to return the infant to the hospital if any respiratory symptoms occur. No pulmonary therapy is indicated prior to symptoms.

Following ingestion of small to moderate amounts of hydrocarbons, induction of vomiting or gastric lavage is contraindicated because of the risk of aspiration, especially if several hours have elapsed. If a large volume of hydrocarbon is thought to be in the stomach, nasogastric suction performed with great care to avoid aspiration may be necessary to reduce the other dangers of hydrocarbon poisoning, including CNS toxicity. The risk of aspiration during gastric lavage or suctioning can be minimized if an endotracheal tube with a balloon cuff can be inserted without inducing vomiting prior to lavage. If there is dyspnea or cyanosis or if chemical pneumonitis develops, supportive measures including oxygen, physiotherapy, and, if necessary, continuous positive airway pressure or other forms of ventilatory assistance are important components of therapy. A cathartic is usually indicated.

The routine use of antibiotics is not recommended; the occurrence of secondary infection of the affected lung can usually be readily detected by the reappearance of fever on the 3rd–5th day after ingestion and can then be suitably treated with penicillin G and tobramycin. Corticosteroids have no beneficial effect on the course of the illness and may, on occasion, be harmful. Pneumatoceles, when they occur, rarely rupture and do not require treatment. Parents must be reminded to keep cleaning fluids and kerosene in locked cabinets out of reach of children or out of the home.

PROGNOSIS. Although most children survive without complications or sequelae, some progress rapidly to respiratory failure and death. Prognosis depends on a variety of factors, including the volume of the ingestion or aspiration, the specific agent involved, and the adequacy of medical care. In one series, only 39 of 950 patients developed symptoms; 4 required assisted ventilation and 2 died. Long-term pulmonary function studies several years later are inconclusive, but if lasting damage does occur, the small airways seem to be at greatest risk.

Bergeson PS, Hales SW, Lustgarten MD, et al: Pneumatoceles following hydrocarbon ingestion. Report of three cases and review of the literature. Am J Dis Child 129:49, 1975.

Brown J III, Burke B, Dajani AS: Experimental kerosene pneumonia: Evaluation of some therapeutic regimens. J Pediatr 84:396, 1974.

Gurwitz D, Kattan M, Levison H, et al: Pulmonary function abnormalities in asymptomatic children after hydrocarbon pneumonitis. Pediatrics 62:789, 1978.

Klein BL, Simon JE: Hydrocarbon poisonings. Pediatr Clin North Am 33:411, 1986.

Nouri LA, Sordelli DO, Cerquetti C, et al: Pulmonary clearance of *Staphylococcus aureus* and plasma angiotensin-converting enzyme activity in hydrocarbon pneumonitis. Pediatr Res 17:657, 1983.

14.61 Lipoid Pneumonia

Lipoid pneumonia is a chronic, interstitial, proliferative inflammation resulting from aspiration of lipoid material; it occurs principally in debilitated infants.

PATHOGENESIS. Factors that may be responsible for aspiration of oil include (1) intranasal instillation of medicated oils; (2) any condition that interferes with swallowing, such as cleft palate, debilitation, or a horizontal position during feeding; and (3) forced feeding, and especially the administration of cod liver oil, castor oil, or mineral oil to crying children.

The severity of the pulmonary reaction depends on the kind of oil inhaled. Vegetable oils, such as olive, cottonseed, and sesame, are generally the least irritating and produce minimal if any inflammation; however, chaulmoogra, also a vegetable oil, produces extensive damage. Animal oils, owing to their high fatty acid content, are the most damaging. Milk aspirated by debilitated infants is one example; cod liver oil also belongs in this category. Liquid petrolatum is chemically inert and is not as irritative as some of the other oils but does act as a foreign body. Excessive use of lip gloss can also cause pneumonitis in teenagers.

The reaction within the lung begins as an interstitial proliferative inflammation, and there may be an exudative pneumonia. In the 2nd stage there is diffuse, chronic, proliferative fibrosis and sometimes superimposed acute infectious bronchopneumonia. In the 3rd stage there are multiple localized nodules, tumor-like paraffinomas. There are numerous macrophages in the involved areas, with giant cell formation of the foreign body type. The lipoid substance is both intracellular and extracellular. The oil-laden cells may be carried to the hilar lymph nodes.

CLINICAL MANIFESTATIONS. There are no characteristic signs or symptoms; a cough is most common, and in severe cases there may be dyspnea. Unless there is superimposed infection, there is usually no fever or physical sign, although with extensive involvement there may be some impairment to percussion and change in voice and breath sounds. Secondary bronchopneumonic infections are common.

The roentgenographic appearance is characteristic. With mild involvement there is an increase in the density and extent of the hilar shadows. With increasing involvement there is greater density of the perihilar shadows, which widen in all directions (Fig. 14–10). Pulmonary changes may be limited to the right lung, and in the infant who is recumbent most of the time, the changes may be mainly in the right upper lobe.

PROGNOSIS. The prognosis is guarded. It depends on the extent of pulmonary damage, the discontinuation of oil in-

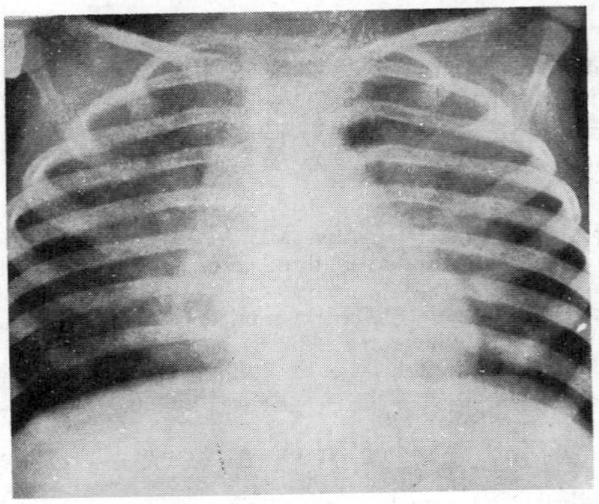

Figure 14–10. Roentgenogram showing increased density radiating from the hilus of each lung in an infant 13 mo of age after intranasal application of liquid petrolatum 3 times a day for 5 mo.

halation, the general condition of the patient, and the avoidance of intercurrent infections.

PREVENTION. Intranasal medications in an oily vehicle should not be used. Concentrated preparations of vitamins A and D in water-miscible vehicles should be substituted for cod liver oil. Administration of mineral oil and castor oil should be avoided. Infants who regurgitate or vomit frequently should be placed on their abdomens to reduce the likelihood of aspiration.

TREATMENT. There is no specific therapy other than elimination of further exposure. The infant's position should be changed frequently to reduce the chances of hydrostatic pneumonia.

Bection DL, Lowe JE, Falleta JM: Lipoid pneumonia in an adolescent girl secondary to use of lip gloss. J Pediatr 105:421, 1984.

14.62 Silo Filler Disease

This rare, acute interstitial pneumonia occurs following the inhalation of nitrogen dioxide, a gas generally encountered only in freshly filled silos. Cough and dyspnea occur immediately after exposure. An asymptomatic phase of several days follows, but then the patient suddenly experiences chills and fever associated with progressive cough, dyspnea, and cyanosis. There are rales throughout both lung fields and widespread pulmonary infiltration on roentgenogram. The interalveolar septa are widened, edematous, and filled with accumulated mononuclear cells and fibroblasts, and the epithelium is hyperplastic. The disease usually progresses rapidly to death. Corticosteroids have been used, but there is no known effective treatment.

14.63 Paraquat Lung

Paraquat, a dipyridylium compound used as a weed killer, is highly toxic, causing death from respiratory failure a few days to weeks after ingestion. The pulmonary lesion is secondary to systemic absorption through the gastrointestinal tract, skin, or lungs (smoking contaminated marijuana) and consists of proliferative bronchiolitis, alveolitis, hemorrhage causing intra-alveolar hyaline membranes and fibrosis. Gas exchange is impaired. Some of these patients probably have adult respiratory distress syndrome (ARDS) (see Sec. 14.79). It is a corrosive that also causes painful lesions of the mouth and esophagus, renal tubular damage, azotemia, and hematuria. Renal damage may result in prolongation of toxic blood levels, during which time fibroblasts proliferate, filling the terminal air spaces. There is no treatment except for general supportive measures. Oxygen may increase pulmonary toxicity. Increased incidence may be due to large-scale use of paraquat in attempts to kill marijuana plants.

Copland GM, Kolin A, Shulman HS: Fatal pulmonary intra-alveolar fibrosis after paraquat ingestion. N Engl Med 291:290, 1974.

14.64 Hypersensitivity to Inhaled Materials

Repeated inhalation of organic dusts may result in chronic pneumonitis that progressively worsens with continued exposure to the antigen. Although the syndrome is most common in adults, it has been reported frequently in children. Unlike those of asthma, the symptoms of this hypersensitivity syndrome are almost entirely unrelated to bronchospasm (see Sec. 11.41). Symptoms may result from inhalation of small particles from moldy hay (farmer's lung), maple bark (maple bark stripper's disease), sugar cane fiber (bagassosis), redwood tree bark, pigeon droppings and feathers (pigeon breeder's disease), cheese, desiccated pituitary powder, dusty output from air conditioners, and a fungus or mold associated with the specific material to which the patient is exposed.

CLINICAL MANIFESTATIONS. The signs and symptoms are similar in all of these diseases. Within several hours following exposure cough, dyspnea, chest pain, and sometimes fever occur with few physical findings, though occasional wheezes and moist rales may be audible. Roentgenograms may show minimal emphysema but are usually normal. If no further exposure occurs, the symptoms abate over a period of several days; but if contact with the responsible antigen continues, symptoms progress to severe dyspnea and cyanosis associated with diffuse, fine, interstitial or nodular densities, and peripheral alveolar infiltrates on chest roentgenogram and occasionally irreversible loss of pulmonary function. The disease should be suspected in children with relatively mild symptoms including cough, fever, and occasional dyspnea, particularly if bronchopneumonia persists despite appropriate treatment with antibiotics.

PATHOLOGY. Histologically, the infiltrate consists of subacute granulomatous inflammation with accumulation of plasma cells, lymphocytes, epithelioid cells, and giant cells of the Langhans type. With continued exposure, inflammatory lesions may be replaced by fibrosis.

DIAGNOSIS. There may be moderate to marked leukocytosis, particularly with acute attacks, elevated serum immunoglobulins (IgG, IgM, and IgA fractions), and a primary restrictive pattern on pulmonary function tests. Arterial blood gas analysis reveals moderate or marked hypoxemia, usually without hypercapnia. Skin testing with the suspected antigen may cause a vigorous delayed hypersensitivity response and is especially useful if an Arthus reaction can be demonstrated histologically by skin biopsy of the test site. Demonstration of a serum precipitin to a given antigen is frequently encountered in apparently well persons and thus is not diagnostic. Lung biopsy reveals a diffuse fibrotic or granulomatous response. If the antigen is available in purified form, an inhalation challenge may be diagnostic.

TREATMENT. Optimal therapy requires the complete elimination of exposure to the suspected (or proven) antigen, which includes thoroughly cleaning the home after the source(s) of antigen has been eliminated. The administration of adrenal corticosteroids (e.g., prednisone in initial dosage of 1–1.5 mg/kg/24 hr) usually results in prompt remission of symptoms; continued use for 1–6 mo may prevent the subsequent development of pulmonary fibrosis in cases of chronic exposure. Corticosteroid therapy may be slowly tapered down following evidence of recovery of lung function or after several weeks without exposure to a known antigen. If hypersensitivity pneumonitis is strongly suspected but the antigen remains unknown, long-term use of corticosteroid therapy, perhaps on an alternate-day regimen, may be indicated. The patient should be cautioned that re-exposure to the antigen is extremely dangerous even long after apparent complete recovery. Even if treatment is optimal and the exposure is eliminated, some fatalities occur, and a substantial percentage of patients do not completely regain their previous pulmonary status.

Allen DH, Williams GV, Woolcock AJ: Bird breeder's hypersensitivity pneumonitis. Progress studies of lung function after cessation of exposure to the provoking antigen. Am Rev Respir Dis 114:555, 1976.
Cunningham AS, Fink JN, Schlueter DP: Childhood hypersensitivity pneumonitis due to dove antigen. Pediatrics 58:436, 1976.
Katz RM, Knicker WT: Infantile hypersensitivity pneumonitis as a reaction to organic antigen. N Engl J Med 288:233, 1973.
Keith HH, Holsclaw DS, Donsky EH: Pigeon breeder's disease in children: A family study. Chest 79:107, 1981.
O'Connell EJ, Zora JA, Gillespie DN, et al: Childhood hypersensitivity pneumonitis (farmer's lung): Four cases in siblings with long-term follow-up. J Pediatr 114:995, 1989.

14.65 Pulmonary Aspergillosis

See Sec. 12.108.

A variety of species of the fungal genus *Aspergillus* are potentially pathogenic for humans. The spectrum of pulmonary manifestations is great and depends on the nature of the exposure and the condition of the host. A hypersensitivity reaction with bronchospasm is most common. The majority of these cases of *allergic bronchopulmonary aspergillosis* (ABPA) have occurred in children with chronic pulmonary diseases, particularly asthma and cystic fibrosis. In some patients the immunologic response that results in ABPA appears to be genetically determined. *Aspergillomas* (fungus balls) typically occur in an ectatic bronchus or old tuberculous cavity. Affected patients are generally asymptomatic. There have been, however, isolated case reports of parenchymal invasion by aspergillus in normal children, but *invasive aspergillosis* generally occurs in immunosuppressed patients, and any organ may be involved.

CLINICAL MANIFESTATIONS. ABPA should be suspected in an immunosuppressed or chronically ill child who presents relatively acute onset of cough, wheezing, and low-grade fever. The cough may be productive, and, occasionally, brown plugs are expectorated that on microscopic examination contain hyphae. Aspergillus can be recovered from this material on culture.

Many patients have multiple precipitin lines on diffusion of serum against aspergillus antigen. The immediate skin test reaction is often strongly positive, and a type III hypersensitivity (Arthus) reaction can usually be demonstrated after skin testing. Chest roentgenograms show transient, occasionally extensive, infiltrates. Aspergillus can be strongly suspected in a child with precipitating antibody to aspergillus antigen, a positive result on a skin test, and elevated serum IgE levels. A definite *diagnosis* should be made if there is, in addition, substantial eosinophilia or the demonstration of aspergillus-specific IgE or IgG in the patient's serum. Some believe that central bronchiectasis is always present in aspergillosis. However, aspergillus organisms are frequently recovered from cultures of respiratory tract secretions of patients with chronic pulmonary disease who do not have symptoms of ABPA. The recovery of these organisms without typical symptoms and serologic evidence of hypersensitivity is not an indication for treatment.

TREATMENT. The best approach to treatment of ABPA is not clear. Aerosolized amphotericin or direct instillation of amphotericin into the trachea has been recommended, but the correct dosage has not been established. Systemic amphotericin B (0.5–1.0 mg/kg/24hr intravenously) or 5-fluorocytosine (50–150 mg/kg/24 hr) may be effective. Although aerosolized corticosteroids have been recommended, only systemic corticosteroid (e.g., prednisone 0.5 mg/kg/24 hr for 2 wk followed by the same dose on alternate days for 3 mo) is effective and remains the treatment of choice. IgE levels should be obtained immediately after corticosteroid treatment. If, on follow-up, the IgE rises to twice this level or higher, serious consideration should be given to reinstitution of the same regimen noted earlier. In patients with underlying asthma, aerosolized bronchodilators, β-agonists, and cromolyn may be helpful.

Aspergillomas may respond to specific antifungal chemotherapy. However, surgical resection with local instillation of amphotericin is considered the treatment of choice. The prognosis, whatever the treatment, depends heavily on the underlying chronic illness. Invasive aspergillosis may be so fulminant that antifungal chemotherapy is not efficacious. Treatment generally consists of amphotericin B combined with 5-fluorocytosine. Treatment should be continued for 2–3 wk.

Bardana EJ, Sobti KL, Cianciulli FD, et al: Aspergillus antibody in patients with cystic fibrosis. Am J Dis Child 129:1164, 1975.
Berger I, Phillips WL, Shenker IR: Pulmonary aspergillosis in childhood. Clin Pediatr 11:178, 1972.
Fink J: Allergic bronchopulmonary aspergillosis. Hosp Pract 23:105, 1988.
Graves TS, Fink JN, Patterson, R, et al: A familial occurrence of allergic bronchopulmonary aspergillosis. Ann Intern Med 91:378, 1979.
Greenberger PA, Petterson R: Diagnosis and management of allergic bronchopulmonary aspergillosis. Ann Allergy 56:444, 1986.
Katz RM, Kniker WT: Infantile hypersensitivity pneumonitis as a reaction to organic antigens. N Engl J Med 288:233, 1973.
Strelling MK, Rhaney K, Simmons DAR, et al: Fatal acute pulmonary aspergillosis in two children of one family. Arch Dis Child 41:34, 1966.
Varkey B, Rose HD: Pulmonary aspergilloma: A rational approach to treatment. Am J Med 61:626, 1976.

14.66 Loeffler Syndrome
(Eosinophilic Pneumonia)

This syndrome is characterized by widespread transitory pulmonary infiltrations, which roentgenographically vary in size but may resemble those of miliary tuberculosis, and by a blood eosinophilia that may be as high as 70%. The clinical course is usually not severe and ranges from a few days to several months. There are usually paroxysmal attacks of coughing, dyspnea, pleurisy, and little or no fever. There may be associated hepatomegaly, especially in infants and young children, and biopsy sections of the liver have revealed multiple focal areas of necrosis, granuloma formation, and eosinophilic infiltration. These children have hyperglobulinemia, presumably as the result of hepatic dysfunction and in response to parasitic invasion of tissue. Autopsy studies have revealed evidences of eosinophilic infiltations in the lungs and in other organs. Localized pneumonic consolidation with an associated eosinophilia may occur.

Loeffler syndrome may be an unusual allergic manifestation of a variety of antigens and not a distinct clinical entity. In children it is most often a manifestation of helminthic infections. Perhaps the most common pathogen in this country is the larva of the dog ascarid, *Toxocara canis,* and less often of the cat ascarid, *Toxocara cati* (see Sec. 12.125). Other roundworms may also be responsible for the syndrome; these include *Ascaris lumbricoides* (usually responsible for transient pulmonary lesions), *Strongyloides stercoralis,* and hookworms (see Sec. 12.120 and 12.122). So-called tropical eosinophilia may be manifest as Loeffler syndrome and is probably caused by a number of different helminths. Paragonimiasis caused by a lung fluke (see Sec. 12.135) may produce the syndrome as well as extrapulmonary manifestations. A drug reaction may also result in this syndrome; aspirin, penicillin, sulfonamides, and imipramine are among those implicated.

A recently described variant of eosinophilic pneumonia is characterized by a more acute course of fever and a rapid progression to severe hypoxemia, in addition to the eosinophilia and diffuse pulmonary infiltrates. These young adult patients responded quickly to oral corticosteroid, and none relapsed after the dose was tapered and discontinued.

Allen JN, Pacht ER, Gadek JE, et al: Acute eosinophilic pneumonia as a reversible cause of noninfectious respiratory failure. N Engl J Med 321:569, 1989.
Beaver P: Wandering nematodes as a cause of disability and disease. Am J Trop Med Hyg 6:433, 1967.
Leitch AG: Pulmonary eosinophilia. Basics Respir Dis 7 (No 5):1, 1979.
Zuelzer WW, Apt L: Disseminated visceral lesions associated with extreme eosinophilia: Pathologic and clinical observations on a syndrome of young children. Am J Dis Child 78:153, 1948.

14.67 Pulmonary Involvement in Collagen Diseases

See Sec. 11.54, 11.58, 11.61, and 11.62.

Rheumatic pneumonia is usually a fatal, but rare, complication of acute rheumatic fever, characterized clinically by extensive pulmonary consolidation and rapidly progressive functional deterioration and pathologically by alveolar exudate, inflammatory interstitial infiltrates, and necrotizing arteritis. Physical findings are unexpectedly minimal; frequently there are no rales. Chest roentgenograms reveal transient areas of infiltrate that resemble pulmonary edema. There is no specific treatment; these patients do not respond to corticosteroids, to treatment of congestive heart failure with diuretics and digitalis, or to the antibiotic treatment of presumed infection. If the lesion is diagnosed by lung biopsy, treatment with immunosuppressive agents theoretically may be valuable but has not been reported to be effective.

Lovell D, Lindsley C, Langston C: Lymphoid interstitial pneumonia in juvenile rheumatoid arthritis. J Pediatr 105:947, 1984.
Oetgen WJ, Boice JA, Lawless OJ: Mixed connective tissue disease in children and adolescents. Pediatrics 67:333, 1981.
Park S, Nyhan WL: Fatal pulmonary involvement in dermatomyositis. Am J Dis Child 129:723, 1975.
Rajani KB, Aschbacher LV, Kinney TR: Pulmonary hemorrhage and systemic lupus erythematosus. J Pediatr 93:810, 1978.
Serlin SP, Rmisza ME, Gay JH: Rheumatic pneumonia: The need for a new approach. Pediatrics 56:1075, 1975.
Winterbauer RH, De Paso W, Lammert J: Pulmonary disease in rheumatoid arthritis patients. J Respir Dis 10(2):35, 1989.

14.68 Desquamative Interstitial Pneumonitis

This disease of unknown etiology is characterized pathologically by massive proliferation and desquamation of alveolar cells and thickening of the alveolar walls. The degree of desquamation is far greater than the degree of alveolar wall thickening. Longstanding desquamative interstitial pneumonitis may progress to chronic interstitial fibrosis. Occasionally, there are families with more than one affected child. In most children there is a history of preceding upper respiratory infection, although the relationship of the desquamative pneumonitis to these infections of probable viral origin has not been firmly established. Two infants were identified in whom desquamative interstitial pneumonitis and congenital rubella were associated. Circulating immune complexes and alveolar deposition of IgG and complement suggest an immune basis for the disease.

CLINICAL MANIFESTATIONS. Symptoms usually develop slowly. As alveolar function is compromised, tachypnea and dyspnea occur; as the disease progresses, there is a nonproductive cough, anorexia, and weight loss. Cyanosis eventually results; clubbing is not a constant feature, and fever is unusual. Physical findings include tachypnea, nasal flaring, and, occasionally, fine rales. The use of the accessory muscles of respiration is not as prominent as one would expect in obstructive diseases exhibiting an equal amount of hypoxemia.

LABORATORY MANIFESTATIONS. Chest roentgenograms reveal a diffuse, hazy, ground glass appearance, particularly at the lung bases, along with poorly defined hilar densities. Viral and bacteriologic cultures and acute and convalescent sera analyses are not helpful diagnostically. Arterial blood samples show hypoxemia; most patients seek medical care prior to the advent of hypercapnia. Definitive diagnosis requires open lung biopsy.

TREATMENT. Patients with desquamative interstitial pneumonitis often recover without specific treatment. Those suspected of having the disease can occasionally be simply observed if their respiratory symptoms are not too severe. With worsening pulmonary status or rapid deterioration shown on the chest roentgenogram, open lung biopsy is important to establish a definitive diagnosis. These patients usually respond to corticosteroid therapy with rapid resolution of symptoms and gradual improvement on roentgenogram. Occasional corticosteroid-resistant patients are reported, and a variety of other treatments, including immunosuppression, have been proposed; corticosteroid therapy may be less effective in familial cases. Chloroquine phosphate (10 mg/kg/24 hr) has been effective in some corticosteroid-resistant patients, including those with a family history of the disease. Supportive treatment including supplemental oxygen is often necessary. Corticosteroid therapy without lung biopsy diagnosis is hazardous; chronic viral pneumonitis can present with a similar clinical picture and may be worsened by corticosteroid depression of host defenses. Relapses are reported when therapy is prematurely stopped.

Bonner A, Wilmett RW, Dinwiddle R, et al: Desquamative interstitial pneumonia and antigen-antibody complexes in two infants with congenital rubella. Pediatrics 72:835, 1983.
Dreisin RB, Schwartz MI, Theofilopoulus AN, et al: Circulating immune complexes in the idiopathic interstitial pneumonias. N Engl J Med 298:353, 1978.
Farrell PM, Gilbert EF, Zimmerman JJ, et al: Familial lung disease associated with proliferation and desquamation of type II pneumocytes. Am J Dis Child 140:262, 1986.
Stillwell PC, Norris DG, O'Connell EJ, et al.: Desquamative interstitial pneumonitis in children. Chest 77:155, 1980.
Tal A, Maer E, Bar-Ziv J, et al: Fatal desquamative interstitial pneumonitis in three infant siblings. J Pediatr 104:873, 1984.

14.69 Hypostatic Pneumonia

Hypostatic pneumonia occurs after prolonged passive pulmonary congestion and may occur in any marasmic state. Lying for a long time in one position favors its development. There is dependent congestion, edema, and pneumonia. The symptoms are not characteristic. There is neither dyspnea nor fever unless these symptoms are secondary to another disorder. The physical signs are principally slight dullness on percussion, feeble respiratory sounds, and the presence of moist rales. Hypostatic congestion is usually a terminal event. There is no specific treatment. Prophylaxis is of the greatest importance; the position of any immobile patient should be changed frequently.

14.70 RESPIRATORY BURNS AND SMOKE INHALATION

Thermal and chemical injury to the lung, systemic toxicity of inhaled gases—particularly carbon monoxide—and asphyxia are important causes of morbidity and mortality in children who have been exposed to fire and should be considered in the initial treatment whether or not there are surface burns. Excessive heat may injure the respiratory mucosa, especially above the trachea. A variety of noxious gases may be generated by fires, including oxides of sulfur and nitrogen, hydrochloric acid, acetaldehyde, corrosive acids and alkalis, and carbon monoxide. Fine particles of soot carried deep within the lung may cause thermal burns or have toxic gases adsorbed on them.

Although there is usually a history of being trapped in a smoke-filled room or evidence of superficial burns around the face or singed nasal vibrissae, serious respiratory damage may occur in the absence of any of these. Exposure to steam greatly increases the chance that respiratory thermal injury has occurred. The onset of clinical manifestations of respiratory distress may be immediate or delayed several hours. Roentgenographic changes may be delayed from hours to days.

Signs of central nervous system injury from hypoxemia due to asphyxia may vary from irritability to depression. Carbon monoxide poisoning may be mild (<20% HbCO) with slight dyspnea and decreased visual acuity and higher cerebral functions; moderate (20–40% HbCO) with irritability, nausea, dimness of vision, impaired judgment, and rapid fatigue; or severe (40–60% HbCO), producing confusion, hallucination, ataxia, collapse, and coma.

Direct measurement of carboxyhemoglobin (HbCO) is important for diagnosis and prognosis, because it reflects the degree of tissue hypoxia caused by the combination of carbon monoxide and hemoglobin and the change in the shape and position of the oxygen dissociation curve. Pa_{O_2} may be normal and the oxyhemoglobin saturation values misleading because HbCO is not detected by the usual tests of saturation. Thermal injury may lead to edema, exudate, and necrosis, and to desquamation of tissue, obstruction, and atelectasis. Respiratory insufficiency may occur from asphyxia, carbon monoxide poisoning, airway obstruction due to edema and necrotic material in the airways, or bronchoconstriction.

Children who have been in fires should be hospitalized for at least 24 hr for careful observation. If carbon monoxide poisoning is suspected, humidified 100% oxygen should be administered and hyperbaric oxygen therapy considered (Sec. 6.37).

After thermal injury, respiratory complications follow a fairly predictable timetable. From *1–12 hr after exposure* acute respiratory distress secondary to bronchospasm, laryngeal edema, or lung consolidation may occur. Laryngeal obstruction, characterized by a prolonged inspiratory phase and virtually absent breath sounds, is uncommon; endotracheal intubation followed by tracheostomy is necessary in these patients. Bronchospasm, characterized by wheezing and prolonged expiration, responds best to a large intravenous bolus of corticosteroid. Bronchodilator treatment (aminophylline, albuterol aerosols) is often less effective than in asthmatics. Lung consolidation is an ominous development; in one series, 80% of affected patients died within 36 hr. Pulmonary edema occurs usually *6–72 hr after exposure*. Although fluid overload may account for some of these cases, the majority are directly due to the injury itself. Treatment includes fluid restriction and diuretics. Ventilatory assistance may be required. Cervical eschar formation and constriction of the airway may occur *60–120 hr after exposure* in patients with circumferential full-thickness burns of the neck; treatment consists of vertical division of the burn crust and immediate endotracheal intubation. Bronchopneumonia may complicate the patient's course, especially following the 4th day. At first *S. aureus* is the most common pathogen, but by the 8th day *P. aeruginosa* and *K. pneumoniae* are the dominant organisms recovered. Treatment includes encouraging cough, nasotracheal suctioning, and, on occasion, bronchoscopic suctioning. Specific antibiotic treatment based on culture results is important. Early and continuous use of intravenous corticosteroids contributes to a poor prognosis in these patients. Respiratory therapy equipment is the source of the infecting organisms in some patients.

Children who have respiratory burns and/or smoke inhalation account for most fatalities following survival of exposure to fire (see Sec. 6.37). Careful observation and specific therapy as complications develop are extremely important. Supportive care, including postural draining and encouragement of cough, are important. The demonstration that ibuprofen prevents synthetic smoke-induced pulmonary edema in rats suggests that more specific medical approaches to smoke inhalation may be possible.

The importance of strategically placed smoke detectors should be presented to families as part of well-child care.

Mellins RB, Park S: Respiratory complications of smoke inhalation in victims of fires. J Pediatr 87:1, 1975.

Pietak SP, Delahaye DJ: Airway obstruction following smoke inhalation. Can Med Assoc J 115:329, 1978.

Shinozawa Y, Hales C, Jung W, et al: Ibuprofen prevents synthetic smoke-induced pulmonary edema. Am Rev Respir Dis 134:1145, 1986.

Stone HH: Pulmonary burns in children. J Pediatr 14:48, 1979.

14.71 PULMONARY HEMOSIDEROSIS

The term "pulmonary hemosiderosis" is used to describe a number of rare conditions characterized by an abnormal accumulation of hemosiderin in the lungs. Hemosiderin deposits follow diffuse alveolar hemorrhage and may occur either as a primary disease of the lungs or as secondary to cardiac or systemic vascular disease. In children, primary hemosiderosis occurs more frequently than the secondary varieties. There are four types of primary pulmonary hemosiderosis: an idiopathic form, a form associated with cow's milk hypersensitivity (Heiner syndrome), a form occurring in association with myocarditis, and a form associated with progressive glomerulonephritis (Goodpasture syndrome). Three types of secondary pulmonary hemosiderosis are recognized: one occurs with mitral stenosis and chronic left ventricular failure of any cause; one is associated with collagen diseases; and one with hemorrhagic diseases.

IDIOPATHIC PRIMARY PULMONARY HEMOSIDEROSIS. The cause of this illness is unknown. Although the rarely reported familial incidence suggests a possible genetic basis for some cases, other explanations, such as an environmental toxin, are also possible. In one study, insecticides were suspected. Onset usually occurs in childhood, rarely later than early adult life. Most of the clinical features are related to blood in the alveoli and to the effects of chronic blood loss. Symptoms are those of recurrent or chronic pulmonary disease and include cough, hemoptysis, dyspnea, wheezing, and occasional cyanosis associated with fatigue and pallor. The cough may be productive of bloody sputum, or the infant or child may simply vomit large quantities of blood. During acute attacks, which usually last 2–4 days, the child may be febrile. Digital clubbing is often present.

The usual clinical features of fever, tachycardia, tachypnea, leukocytosis, respiratory distress, and abnormal roentgenographic findings may suggest bacterial pneumonia, and only prolonged follow-up will reveal the correct diagnosis. In some children, however, the early manifestations of illness are related to chronic iron deficiency anemia, which is often refractory to therapy, and the characteristic pulmonary symptoms do not appear until much later. Paradoxically, the child may have severe pulmonary manifestations without roentgenographic abnormalities, or the roentgenographic picture may be abnormal before pulmonary symptoms have occurred.

The anemia is typically microcytic and hypochromic; serum iron concentrations are low, and there may be elevations in bilirubin, urobilinogen, and reticulocyte count. The stool usually contains occult blood, presumably swallowed. Hemosiderin can usually be demonstrated in macrophages in smears of sputum or material obtained from tracheal or gastric aspirates. Roentgenographic changes range from minimal infiltrates resembling pneumonia to massive pulmonary involvement with secondary atelectasis, emphysema, and hilar lymphadenopathy. The findings may suggest tuberculosis or pulmonary edema, and significant changes may be seen from day to day. Open lung biopsy may be required to establish the diagnosis by histologic demonstration of intra-alveolar hemorrhage, large numbers of hemosiderin-laden macrophages, alveolar epithelial hyperplasia, interstitial fibrosis, and sclerosis of small vessels. Absence of immunoglobulin/complement deposition on the alveolar basement membrane virtually excludes Goodpasture syndrome (see later), and all biopsy specimens should be subjected to this test. Closed needle biopsy has been followed by serious complications.

Approximately half the patients die within 1–5 yr, usually from acute pulmonary hemorrhage and progressive respiratory failure. A milk-free diet is indicated, pending analysis of serum for precipitins, and also serves as a diagnostic test for cow's milk-related pulmonary hemosiderosis. Corticosteroids (prednisone, 1 mg/kg/24 hr) produce remission in some patients and are of no benefit to others. Maintenance corticosteroid therapy has been used between attacks with variable results. Immunosuppressant drugs and deferoxamine have not been adequately evaluated.

PRIMARY PULMONARY HEMOSIDEROSIS WITH HYPERSENSITIVITY TO COW'S MILK (HEINER SYNDROME). Children affected with this syndrome have the typical picture of idiopathic hemosiderosis, unusually high serum titers of precipitins to multiple constituents of cow's milk, and positive results on intradermal skin tests to various cow's milk proteins. They may also have chronic rhinitis, recurrent otitis media, gastrointestinal symptoms, and growth retardation. The symptoms improve when cow's milk is removed from the diet and return with its reintroduction. Some patients fail to improve at all on a milk-free diet, and others without multiple serum precipitins have improved. Some patients with high titers of milk precipitins and pulmonary hemosiderosis develop cor pulmonale secondary to hypertrophied nasopharyngeal lymphoid tissue. These patients should also have a tonsilloadenoidectomy. In general, patients with hemosiderosis and precipitins to cow's milk have a better prognosis than do those with other forms of the disease, and they may eventually lose their sensitivity to milk. Corticosteroids may be useful, at least during acute bleeding episodes.

PRIMARY PULMONARY HEMOSIDEROSIS WITH MYOCARDITIS. Some patients have varying degrees of inflammation of the myocardium associated with pulmonary hemosiderosis, and, if significant myocardial disease is present when pulmonary symptoms are first noted, it may be impossible to determine whether the hemosiderosis is a primary or secondary phenomenon. The clinical picture does not differ from that of the idiopathic disease except that the heart may be enlarged and there may be electrocardiographic signs compatible with myocarditis.

PRIMARY PULMONARY HEMOSIDEROSIS WITH GLOMERULONEPHRITIS (GOODPASTURE SYNDROME). This is a disease primarily of young adult males and is rarely observed in children. Initially, the presentation of the disease may be similar to idiopathic pulmonary hemosiderosis with hemoptysis and iron deficiency anemia, but careful study at the time of the initial attack usually reveals proliferative or membranous glomerulonephritis. Patients most often have progressive renal disease with hypertension and eventual renal failure and death. The pulmonary disease has improved following bilateral nephrectomy in a few patients but not in others.

SECONDARY PULMONARY HEMOSIDEROSIS. Heart disease producing a chronic increase in pulmonary capillary pressure, such as mitral stenosis, can lead to intrapulmonary hemorrhage and secondary hemosiderosis. Collagen vascular diseases may present clinical manifestations of pulmonary hemosiderosis. Occasionally, the vascular changes of polyarteritis are initially limited to the lungs. Other diseases, such as rheumatoid arthritis, may also produce pulmonary hemosiderosis as an effect of generalized diffuse vasculitis. A few patients with anaphylactoid purpura or thrombocytopenic purpura similarly have had hemosiderosis secondary to intrapulmonary hemorrhage.

Beckerman RC, Taussig LM, Pinnas JL: Familial idiopathic hemosiderosis. Am J Dis Child 133:609, 1979.
Boat TF, Polmar SH, Whitman V, et al: Hyperreactivity to cow milk in young children with pulmonary hemosiderosis and cor pulmonale secondary to nasopharyngeal obstruction. J Pediatr 87:23, 1973.
Case Records of the Massachusetts General Hospital (case 30–1988). N Engl J Med 319:227, 1988.
Cassimos CD, Chryssanthopoulos C, Panagiotidou C: Epidemiologic observations in idiopathic pulmonary hemosiderosis. J Pediatr 102:698, 1983.
Heiner DC, Sears JW, Kniker WT: Multiple precipitins to cow's milk in chronic respiratory disease. A syndrome including poor growth, gastrointestinal symptoms, evidence of allergy, iron deficiency anemia and pulmonary hemosiderosis. Am J Dis Child 103:634, 1962.
Levy J, Wilmott RW: Pulmonary hemosiderosis. Pediatr Pulmonol 2:384, 1986.

14.72 PULMONARY ALVEOLAR PROTEINOSIS

In children pulmonary alveolar proteinosis is a rare disease of unknown etiology. Occasionally there are families with two affected children, suggesting an underlying genetic basis.

CLINICAL MANIFESTATIONS. The first symptoms are usually cough and dyspnea. Fever and clubbing are each present in about a third of the patients. Hemoptysis is not uncommon. Most clinical findings result from hypoxia and include weakness, fatigue, weight loss, and cyanosis. Physical findings are relatively few unless hypoxia is severe, but roentgenographic changes generally are characteristic and consist of a fine, diffuse infiltrate radiating from the hilus to the periphery, often in a "butterfly" distribution (Fig. 14–11). Some patients demonstrate bilateral lower lobe infiltrates, while others initially show nodular densities progressing to complete lobar consolidation. Pulmonary function testing reveals a restrictive pattern, and arterial blood gases show marked hypoxemia, usually with normal CO_2 tensions. Serum IgA is frequently low, and other immunologic abnormalities are relatively common.

The diagnosis of pulmonary alveolar proteinosis must be confirmed by biopsy, although a sputum examination revealing a large amount of PAS-positive material with few or no inflammatory cells is suggestive of the disease. An amorphous lipid-protein complex progressively accumulates in the alveoli, but whether this material accumulates because of an accelerated rate of transport from the serum or because of defective clearance is unknown. Tissue sections show alveoli distended by fine, granular, eosinophilic material which stains positively with PAS stain.

Various immunologic deficiency states, including thymic alymphoplasia, have been found in some children with this disease. Not surprisingly, therefore, various fungal and bacterial superinfections also may be associated with the disease.

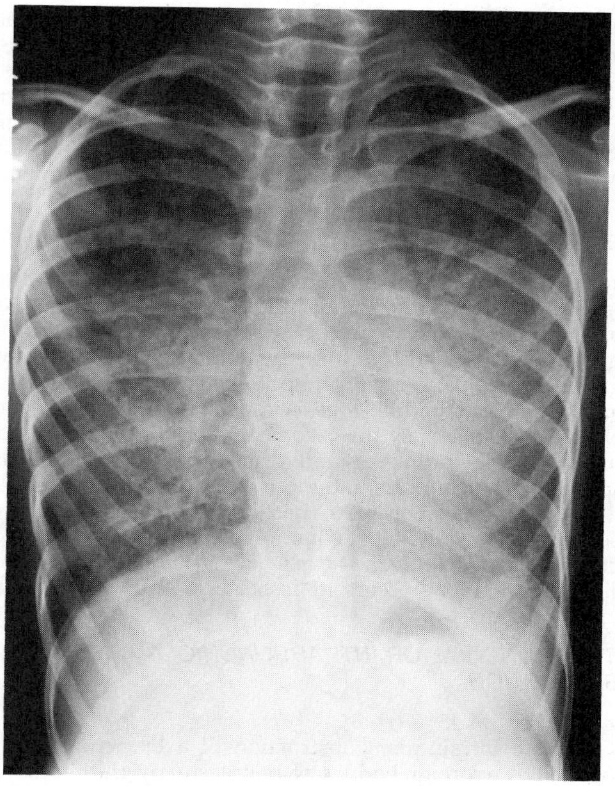

Figure 14–11. Alveolar proteinosis. PA view of the chest shows diffuse alveolar infiltrate.

No effective medical treatment exists. Corticosteroids do not alter the relentless, progressive course of the illness. Aerosols with *N*-acetylcysteine or proteolytic enzymes have been reported effective, but the mainstay of treatment is repeated pulmonary lavage to clear out the alveoli. As techniques such as the use of the fiberoptic bronchoscope are improved, lavage can be accomplished without anesthesia and may often produce transient dramatic improvement; often reaccumulation forces another series of lavages. Bacterial infection usually plays a relatively minor role in the progression of symptoms, and antibiotic therapy should be used conservatively. However, fatal fungal infections, as well as other opportunistic pathogens (including pneumocystis), have been reported. Survival has improved greatly with the introduction of modern bronchoscopic techniques. The adult form of pulmonary alveolar proteinosis has a much more favorable prognosis.

Claypool WD, Rogers RM, Matuschuk GM: Update on the clinical diagnosis, management, and pathogenesis of pulmonary alveolar proteinosis (phospholipidosis). Chest 85:550, 1984.

Case Records of the Massachusetts General Hospital (case 19–1983). N Engl J Med 308:1147, 1983.

Mazyck EM, Bonner JT, Herd HM, et al: Pulmonary lavage for childhood pulmonary alveolar proteinosis. J Pediatr 80:839, 1972.

Prakash UBS, Barham SS, Carpenter HA, et al: Pulmonary alveolar phospholipoproteinosis: Experience with 34 cases and a review. Mayo Clin Proc 62:499, 1987.

Teja K, Cooper PH, Squires JE, et al: Pulmonary alveolar proteinosis in four siblings. N Engl J Med 305:1390, 1981.

Webster JR, Battifora H, Furrey C, et al: Pulmonary alveolar proteinosis in two siblings with decreased immunoglobulin A. Am J Med 69:786, 1980.

14.73 IDIOPATHIC DIFFUSE INTERSTITIAL FIBROSIS OF THE LUNG

(Hamman-Rich Syndrome)

This is a rare, chronic, usually fatal disorder of unknown origin, ordinarily observed in adults but occasionally in infants and children. Multiple affected individuals in certain families suggest an autosomal dominant genetic basis of inheritance for some of these patients. The disease has been hypothesized to result from an uncontrolled inflammatory process following an otherwise minor insult to the lower respiratory tract. A chronic inflammatory state occurs and leads eventually to progressive fibrosis. Alveolar macrophages, perhaps stimulated by immune complexes, may play a pivotal role by releasing chemotactic factors and stimulants of fibrosis, including fibronectin and alveolar macrophage-derived growth factor. The clinical pattern is characterized by progressive pulmonary insufficiency resulting from interstitial fibrosis and alveolar-capillary block.

Onset is usually insidious, with dyspnea initially occurring only with exercise but later present even at rest. A dry cough is frequent and may be productive of blood. The patient is usually afebrile. As the disease progresses, anorexia, weight loss, and fatigability occur, and finally cyanosis, clubbing, cor pulmonale, and right-sided cardiac failure. The lungs are usually clear on auscultation, but occasionally rales are present. Most children die of respiratory failure following one of the frequent intercurrent pulmonary infections. Serial roentgenograms show progressive widespread granular or reticular mottling or small nodular densities. Hypoxemia may be present and increases with exercise. There is no increase in airway resistance, and vital capacity, compliance, and diffusion capacity are decreased. Bronchoalveolar lavage fluid contains many inflammatory cells and relatively large numbers of mast cells. ^{67}Ga scans usually have positive results, with the abnormality restricted to the lungs.

The pulmonary pathology is variable. During the early stage of the disease, fibrosis is usually not present, but there is cellular infiltration of the walls of the alveoli, alveolar ducts, and periobronchial tissue by lymphocytes, plasma cells, and occasionally eosinophils. This usually progresses to extensive and diffuse proliferation of fibrous tissue throughout all the lobes of the lung and is associated with organization of intra-alveolar exudate.

Corticosteroids may give some symptomatic relief but do not alter the progression of the disease or improve pulmonary function. Other therapy is also symptomatic. Immunosuppressant drugs have been used with benefit in some adults. A chronic inflammatory state has been demonstrated in the lungs of 50% of first-degree relatives of persons with the autosomal recessive form of the disease. If this finding is found to be predictive of subsequent clinical disease, strategies for preventive treatment might be devised.

Bitterman PB, Rennard SI, Keogh BA, et al: Familial idiopathic pulmonary fibrosis: Evidence of lung inflammation in unaffected family members. N Engl J Med 314:1343, 1986.

Bradley CA: Diffuse interstitial fibrosis of the lungs in children. J Pediatr 48:422, 1956.

Brown CH, Turner-Warwick M: The treatment of cryptogenic fibrosing alveolitis with immunosuppressant drugs. Q J Med 40:289, 1971.

Crystal RG, Bitterman PB, Rennard SI, et al: Interstitial lung disease of unknown cause: Disorders characterized by inflammation of the lower respiratory tract. N Engl J Med 310:154, 1984.

Ivemark BI, Wallgren CG: Diffuse interstitial pulmonary fibrosis (Hamman-Rich syndrome) in an infant. Report of a case with histologic and respiratory studies. Acta Paediatr 51(Suppl 135):97, 1962.

14.74 PULMONARY ALVEOLAR MICROLITHIASIS

This rare disease of unknown etiology often has its onset during childhood, but the clinical manifestations may be delayed until later years. It is characterized by widely disseminated intra–alveolar calculi, which create a characteristic pattern on the roentgenogram (Fig. 14–12). Frequently, the disease is recognized when the roentgenogram is taken for

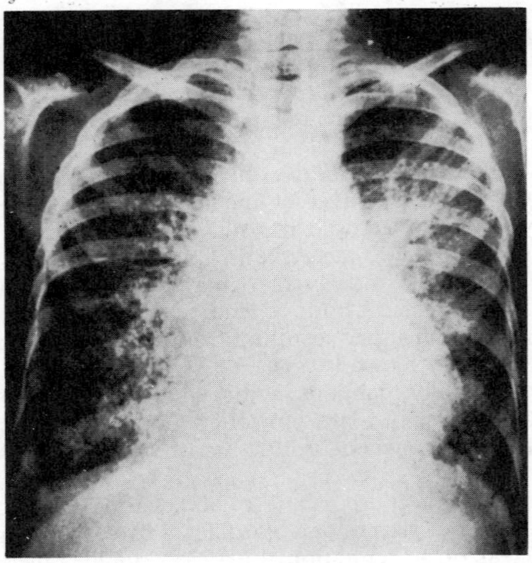

Figure 14–12. Roentgenogram of the chest of a 7-yr-old boy with pulmonary alveolar microlithiasis. (From Clark RB III, Johnson FC: Idiopathic pulmonary alveolar microlithiasis: A case report and brief review of the literature. Reproduced by permission of Pediatrics. Vol. 28, p. 650. Copyright 1961.)

an unrelated illness or when symptoms are still minimal. Definitive diagnosis requires lung biopsy.

The familial incidence strongly suggests a genetic basis, but no specific metabolic abnormalities have been identified. Serum calcium and phosphorus are normal. No treatment is available, and patients eventually die during the middle years of adulthood of slowly progressive cardiorespiratory failure, often with superimposed infection. Bronchopulmonary lavage is ineffective. Following diagnosis, other family members should be screened by chest roentgenograms, and parents should be counseled that future children are also at risk to develop the disease. These children require prompt treatment of respiratory infection and should be advised about the dangers of smoking and exposure to industrial fumes. Immunization to measles and pertussis should be completed and yearly influenza vaccine given.

Caffrey PR, Altman RS: Pulmonary alveolar microlithiasis occurring in premature twins. J Pediatr 66:758, 1965.
Kino T, Kohara Y, Tsuji S: Pulmonary alveolar microlithiasis: A report in two young sisters. Am Rev Resp Dis 105:105, 1972.
Palombini BC, da Silva Porto N, Wallace CU: Bronchopulmonary lavage in alveolar microlithiasis. Chest 80:242, 1981.
Prakash UBS, Barham SS, Rosenow EC III, et al: Pulmonary alveolar microlithiasis: A review including ultrastructural and pulmonary function studies. Mayo Clin Proc 58:290, 1983.

EOSINOPHILIC GRANULOMA OF THE LUNG

See Sec. 25.5.

14.75 ATELECTASIS

Congenital atelectasis and hyaline membrane disease are discussed in Sec. 9.32.

Acquired Atelectasis

ETIOLOGY. Atelectasis, the imperfect expansion, or collapse of air-bearing tissue is not uncommon in infants and children. Collapse results from complete obstruction of the intake of air into the alveolar sacs which persists sufficiently long to permit absorption of alveolar air into the blood. In general, the causes may be divided into three groups: (1) external pressure directly on the pulmonary parenchyma or a bronchus or bronchiole, (2) intrabronchial or intrabronchiolar obstruction, and (3) any factor responsible for a continuously decreased amplitude of respiratory excursion or for respiratory paralysis. Bronchoconstriction and increased bronchosecretion due to allergy or other stimuli including embolus and chest wall trauma may also be contributing factors. Exudate formation may be responsible for atelectasis such as in patients with cystic fibrosis.

EXTERNAL PRESSURE

External factors may be operative in one of two ways: direct interference with expansion of lungs (pleural effusion, pneumothorax, intrathoracic tumors, diaphragmatic hernia) or external compression of a bronchus completely obstructing ingress of air (enlarged lymph node, tumors, cardiac enlargement). The right middle lobe is especially likely to become atelectatic because of extrinsic compression from lymph nodes that encircle its bronchus and drain both the middle and upper lobe. Tuberculosis, although it should be considered in any patient with atelectasis, has been replaced by allergic disease/asthma as the most common cause of the right middle lobe atelectasis. In the *right middle lobe syndrome*, intermittent collapse of this lobe occurs in association with exacerbations of asthmatic disease.

INTRABRONCHIAL OR INTRABRONCHIOLAR OBSTRUCTION

See also Sec. 14.45.

Complete intraluminal obstruction of a bronchus may be produced by a foreign body; by a neoplasm; by granulomatous tissue, as in tuberculosis; or by secretions (including mucous plugs), such as with cystic fibrosis, bronchiectasis, pulmonary abscess, asthma, chronic bronchitis, or acute laryngotracheobronchitis.

Obstruction of one or more bronchioles in a given area may be produced by any of the conditions mentioned, but widespread bronchiolar obstruction is most often produced by bronchiolitis or interstitial pneumonitis and by asthma. Generalized obstructive overinflation is the initial result of such bronchiolar obstructions, but as the pathologic changes progress, some of the bronchioles may become completely obstructed, and there are then interspersed small areas of atelectasis and emphysema. Patchy atelectasis is relatively common in acute bronchiolitis or asthma and is probably always present in advanced chronic diffuse infections, such as the pulmonary infection associated with cystic fibrosis.

REDUCED AMPLITUDE OF RESPIRATORY EXCURSION OR RESPIRATORY PARALYSIS

This may result from: (1) interference with the movements of the thoracic cage (neuromuscular abnormalities as in cerebral palsy, poliomyelitis, spinal muscular atrophy, myasthenia gravis; osseous deformities caused by rickets, scoliosis, kyphosis, scleroderma, overly restrictive casts, and surgical dressings); (2) defective movement of the diaphragm (paralysis of phrenic nerve, increased abdominal pressure); or (3) restriction of respiratory effort because of postoperative pain.

PATHOLOGY. Atelectatic (airless) areas are firm in consistency and deep red.

CLINICAL MANIFESTATIONS. Symptoms vary with the cause and extent of the atelectasis. A small area is likely to be asymptomatic. When a large area of the lung becomes atelectatic, especially when it does so suddenly, dyspnea accompanied by rapid shallow respirations, tachycardia, and often cyanosis occurs. If the obstruction is removed, the symptoms disappear rapidly. Even atelectasis of an entire lobe may not result in changes in the percussion note because of compensatory expansion of adjacent lung tissue. Breath and voice sounds are decreased or absent over extensive atelectatic areas.

DIAGNOSIS. The diagnosis can usually be established by roentgenographic examination (Fig. 14–13). Small areas may be indistinguishable from pneumonic consolidations, but those that involve several lobules can usually be identified by the contraction of the area. Bronchoscopic examination will reveal a collapsed main bronchus when the obstruction is at the tracheobronchial junction and may also disclose the nature of the obstruction.

PROGNOSIS. If the obstruction disappears spontaneously or is removed, the atelectasis usually disappears unless secondary infection has occurred. The atelectatic area is more susceptible to infection because mucociliary clearance is impaired and cough is ineffective. In persistent cases bronchiectasis is a frequent complication and pulmonary abscess is occasionally a complication.

TREATMENT. *Bronchoscopic examination* is immediately indicated if atelectasis is the result of a foreign body or any other bronchial obstruction that may be relieved. It is also indicated when an isolated area of atelectasis persists for several weeks. Usually, it is advisable to suction the orifice of the involved bronchus; occasionally, a **mucous plug** can be removed, with prompt re-expansion. If no anatomic basis for atelectasis is found and no material can be obtained by suctioning, the introduction of a small amount of saline followed by suctioning allows recovery of bronchial secretions for culture and, possibly, for cytologic examination. Frequent *changes in the child's position and deep breathing* may be beneficial. *Oxygen* therapy is indicated when there is dyspnea. Morphine and atropine should be avoided if possible.

If the atelectasis is unchanged or only partially helped by bronchoscopy, *postural drainage* and, occasionally, *antibiotics* are indicated. In some situations, such as asthma, *bronchodilator* and, possibly, *corticosteroid* treatment may accelerate clearing of the atelectasis. Intermittent positive pressure breathing, incentive inspirometry, and blow bottles have been recommended, but their efficacy remains unproved.

Repeated bronchoscopies may be needed. Postural drainage should be continued at home. *Lobectomy* should not be considered unless chronic infection poses a threat to the remainder of the lung, bronchiectasis is demonstrated by bronchography, or systemic symptoms, such as anorexia or fatigue, are persistent. Occasionally, the atelectatic area becomes completely fibrosed; in this case no further treatment is needed.

Massive Pulmonary Atelectasis

Massive collapse of one or both lungs is most often a postoperative complication but occasionally results from other causes, such as trauma, asthma, pneumonia, tension pneumothorax, the aspiration of foreign material (either a solid object large enough to obstruct a mainstem bronchus or liquids such as water or blood), or paralysis, such as in diphtheria or poliomyelitis. Massive atelectasis is usually produced by a combination of factors: immobilization or decreased use of the diaphragm and the respiratory muscles, obstruction of the bronchial tree, and abolition of the cough reflex.

CLINICAL MANIFESTATIONS. The onset in postoperative cases usually occurs within 24 hr after operation but may not occur for several days, with dyspnea, cyanosis, and tachycardia. The child is extremely anxious and, if old enough, complains of chest pain. Prostration is likely. The temperature may be as high as 39.5–40° C (103–104° F).

The physical signs are characteristic. The chest appears flat on the affected side, where there is also decreased respiratory excursion, dullness to percussion, and feeble or absent breath and voice sounds. Lower lobes are more frequently involved than upper ones. The heart and the mediastinum are dis-

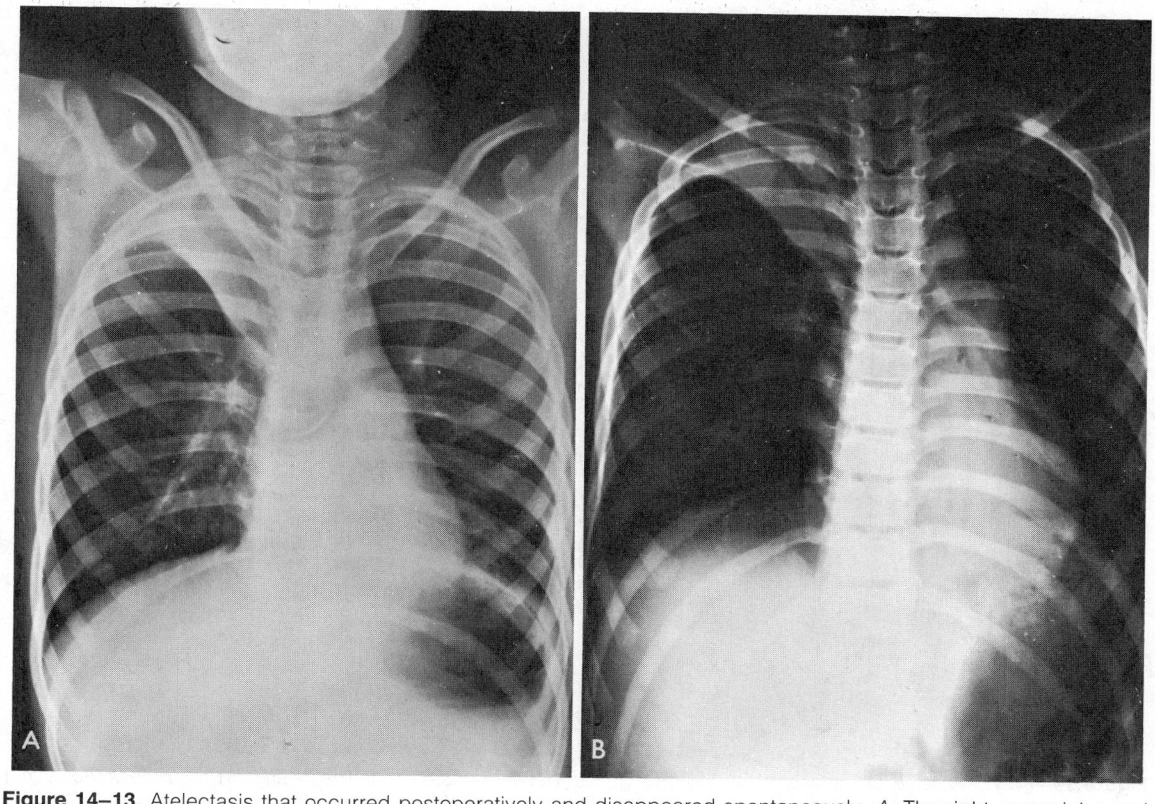

Figure 14–13. Atelectasis that occurred postoperatively and disappeared spontaneously. *A*, The right upper lobe and the left lower lobe are collapsed. The atelectasis of the left lower lobe is demonstrated on the overpenetrated film *(B)*.

placed toward the affected side. Roentgenograms show the collapsed lung, elevation of the diaphragm, narrowing of the intercostal spaces, and displacement of the mediastinal structures and heart toward the affected side (Fig. 14–14).

PROGNOSIS. Bilateral massive collapse is usually rapidly fatal, although prompt bronchoscopic aspiration and artifical respiration may be lifesaving. In the unilateral cases the prognosis is usually good.

PREVENTION. Prophylaxis is of the greatest importance. The incidence of postoperative atelectasis can be reduced by adequate ventilation during anesthesia. After operation the child's position in bed should be changed frequently, and collections of secretions in the oropharynx should be aspirated; when consciousness returns, the child should be encouraged to breathe deeply. Incentive inspirometers may be useful. Tight thoracic or abdominal binders should be avoided.

TREATMENT. When there is bilateral atelectasis, bronchoscopic aspiration should be performed immediately. When there is only unilateral atelectasis, the child should be placed on the unaffected side; forced coughing or crying while the child is lying on the unaffected side may also be helpful, as is positive pressure ventilation, but when these measures are unsuccessful, bronchoscopic aspiration should be performed.

Relapses are not infrequent, and the child should be kept under constant observation.

14.76 EMPHYSEMA AND OVERINFLATION

Pulmonary emphysema is a distention with irreversible rupture of the alveoli. It may be generalized or localized and involve part or all of a lung. Overinflation is reversible distention without alveolar rupture.

Compensatory overinflation may be either acute or chronic. It occurs in normally functioning pulmonary tissue when for any reason a sizable portion of the lung is removed or becomes partially or completely airless, which may occur with pneumonia, atelectasis, empyema, and pneumothorax.

Obstructive overinflation results from partial obstruction of a bronchus or bronchiole, when getting air out of the alveoli becomes more difficult than getting it in; there is a gradual accumulation of air distal to the obstruction, the so-called bypass or check valve type of obstruction (see Sec 14.45).

Localized Obstructive Overinflation

When a bypass type of obstruction partially occludes the mainstem bronchus, the entire lobe becomes overinflated; only individual lobules are affected when the obstruction is that of a secondary bronchus. Localized obstructions that may be responsible for overinflation include foreign bodies and the inflammatory reaction to them, intrabronchial tuberculosis or tuberculosis of the tracheobronchial lymph nodes, and intrabronchial or mediastinal tumors. When most or all of a lobe is involved, the percussion note will be hyper-resonant over the area and the breath sounds will be decreased in intensity. The distended lung may extend across the mediastinum into the opposite hemithorax. Fluoroscopically, during expiration the overinflated area does not decrease in size, and the heart and the mediastinum shift to the opposite side.

Unilateral hyperlucent lung may occur in association with a variety of cardiac and pulmonary diseases of children, but in some patients it occurs without easily demonstrable underlying active disease. Over half the cases follow one or more episodes of pneumonia; in several patients a rising titer to adenovirus has been documented. Patients may present with signs and symptoms of pneumonia, but some are discovered only when a chest roentgenogram is taken for an unrelated reason. A few patients have hemoptysis initially. Physical findings may include hyper-resonance and decreased breath sounds over the involved area. Chest roentgenogram reveals unilateral hyperlucency and an apparently small lung with the mediastinum shifted toward the more abnormal lung. Some patients show mediastinal shift away from the lesion with expiration. Bronchiectasis may be demonstrated on bronchography. There is markedly decreased perfusion on the affected side. In some patients previous chest roentgenograms have been normal or have shown only an acute

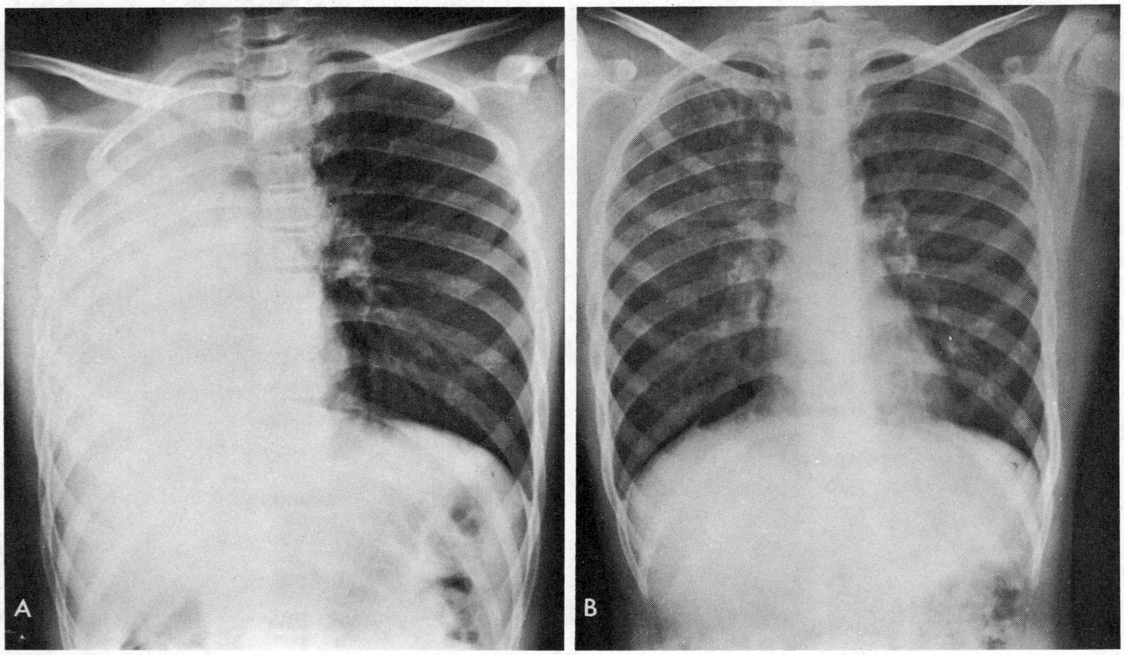

Figure 14–14. *A*, Massive atelectasis of the right lung. The patient is asthmatic. The heart and the other mediastinal structures are shifted to the right during the atelectatic phase. *B*, Comparison study after reaeration following bronchoscopic removal of a mucous plug from the right mainstem bronchus.

pneumonia, suggesting that hyperlucent lung is an acquired lesion. No specific treatment is known; it may become less symptomatic with time.

Congenital obstructive lobar emphysema may cause severe respiratory distress in early infancy. Familial occurrence has been reported. Symptoms usually become apparent in the neonatal period but may be delayed for as long as 5–6 mo in 5% of the patients. Some patients remain undiagnosed until school age or beyond. A part, but usually all, of a lobe may be involved; the left upper lobe is most often affected. In some cases the obstruction is not demonstrable, but it is assumed to be produced by a check valve type of mechanism. Such obstructions have been attributed to defective or overly compliant cartilage in the bronchi, mucosal folds that create a valve-like obstruction, bronchial stenosis, and external compression by aberrant vessels or tumors. A radiolucent lobe and a mediastinal shift are often present on roentgenographic examination. When the distention is considerable, the emphysematous lung compresses the unaffected lung below or above it and the opposite lung by extending across the mediastinum (Fig. 14–15). Immediate surgery and excision of the lobe may be lifesaving when cyanosis and severe respiratory distress are present, but some patients have responded to medical treatment.

Overinflation of all three lobes of the right lung has been produced by anomalous location of the left pulmonary artery, which partially constricts the right mainstem bronchus. A number of neonates have developed lobar overinflation while being treated for hyaline membrane disease with assisted ventilation, suggesting an acquired etiology. Medical management, sometimes with selective intubation, has occasionally been successful and lobectomy has been avoided.

Cumming GR, Macpherson RI, Chernick V: Unilateral hyperlucent lung syndrome in children. J Pediatr 78:250, 1971.

Dickman GL, Short BL, Krauss DR: Selective bronchial intubation in the management of unilateral pulmonary interstitial emphysema. Am J Dis Child 131:365, 1977.

Eigen H, Lemen RJ, Waring WW: Congenital lobar emphysema: Long-term evaluation of surgically and conservatively treated children. Am Rev Respir Dis 116:823, 1976.

McBride JT, Wohl MEB, Strieder D, et al: Lung growth and airway function after lobectomy in infancy for congenital lobar emphysema. J Clin Invest 66:962, 1980.

McKenzie SA, Allison DJ, Singh MP, et al: Unilateral hyperlucent lung: The case for investigation. Thorax 35:745, 1980.

Shannon DC, Todres ID, Moylan FMB: Infantile lobar hyperinflation: Expectant treatment. Pediatrics 59:1012, 1977.

Wall MA, Eisenberg JD, Campbell JR: Congenital lobar emphysema in a mother and daughter. Pediatrics 70:131, 1982.

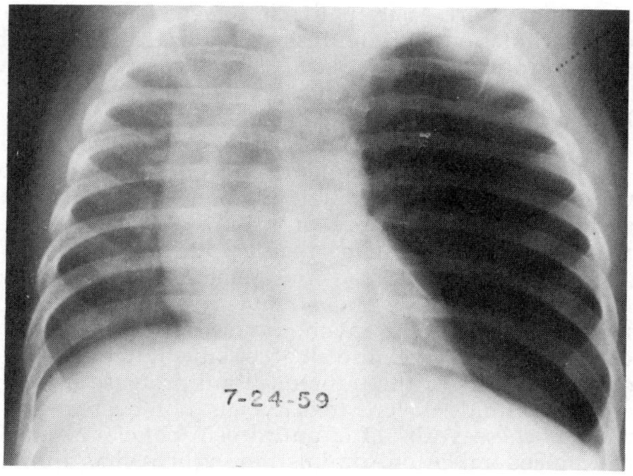

Figure 14–15. Congenital left upper lobe emphysema. Note the extension of the emphysematous lobe into the left lower lobe and its displacement of the mediastinum toward the right.

Generalized Obstructive Overinflation

Acute overinflation of the lung depends on widespread involvement of the bronchioles and is reversible. It occurs more commonly in infants than in children and may be secondary to a number of clinical conditions, including asthma, CF, acute bronchiolitis, interstitial pneumonitis, atypical forms of acute laryngotracheobronchitis, aspiration of zinc stearate powder, chronic passive congestion secondary to a congenital cardiac lesion, and miliary tuberculosis.

PATHOLOGY. In chronic overinflation many of the alveoli are ruptured and communicate with one another, producing distended saccules. Air may also enter the interstitial tissue *(interstitial emphysema)*, resulting in pneumomediastinum and pneumothorax (see Sec. 14.91).

CLINICAL MANIFESTATIONS. Generalized obstructive overinflation is characterized by an expiratory type of dyspnea. The lungs become increasingly overdistended, and the chest remains expanded during expiration. An increased respiratory rate and decreased respiratory excursions are due to the overdistention of the pulmonary alveoli and their inability to be emptied normally through the narrowed bronchioles. Air hunger is responsible for forced respiratory movements, and overaction of the accessory muscles of respiration results in retractions at the suprasternal notch, the supraclavicular spaces, the lower margin of the thorax, and the intercostal spaces. There is scarcely any reduction in size of the overdistended chest during expiration, in contrast to the flattened chest during both inspiration and expiration when there is laryngeal obstruction. There is no hoarseness or stridor as with laryngeal obstruction. Cyanosis is common in the severe cases. The percussion note is hyper-resonant, and on auscultation the inspiratory phase is usually less prominent than the expiratory phase, which is prolonged and roughened. Fine or medium rales may be present.

Roentgenographic and fluoroscopic examinations of the chest are a great help in establishing the diagnosis. Both leaves of the diaphragm are low and flattened, the ribs are farther apart than usual, and the lung fields are less dense (Fig. 14–16). The movement of the diaphragm is restricted, best demonstrated by fluoroscopic examination. The normal "doming" of the diaphragm during expiration is decreased, and the excursion of the low, flattened diaphragm in the severe cases is barely discernible. The AP diameter of the chest is increased, and the sternum may be bowed outward.

Bullous Emphysema

Bullous emphysematous blebs or cysts **(pneumatoceles)** result from overdistention and rupture of alveoli during birth or shortly thereafter, or they may be sequelae of pneumonia and of other infections. They have been observed in tuberculous lesions while the patient was being treated with specific antibacterial therapy. These emphysematous areas presumably result from rupture of distended alveoli so that a single or multiloculated cavity is formed. The cysts may become large (Fig. 14–9C) and may contain some fluid; an air-fluid level may be demonstrated on the roentgenogram. They must be differentiated from pulmonary abscesses. In most cases the cysts disappear spontaneously within a few months, although they may persist for a year or more.

There is almost never any indication for aspiration or surgery unless there is severe respiratory and cardiac embarrassment.

Subcutaneous Emphysema

This occurs whenever free air finds its way into the subcutaneous tissue. It may be a complication of fracture of the orbit

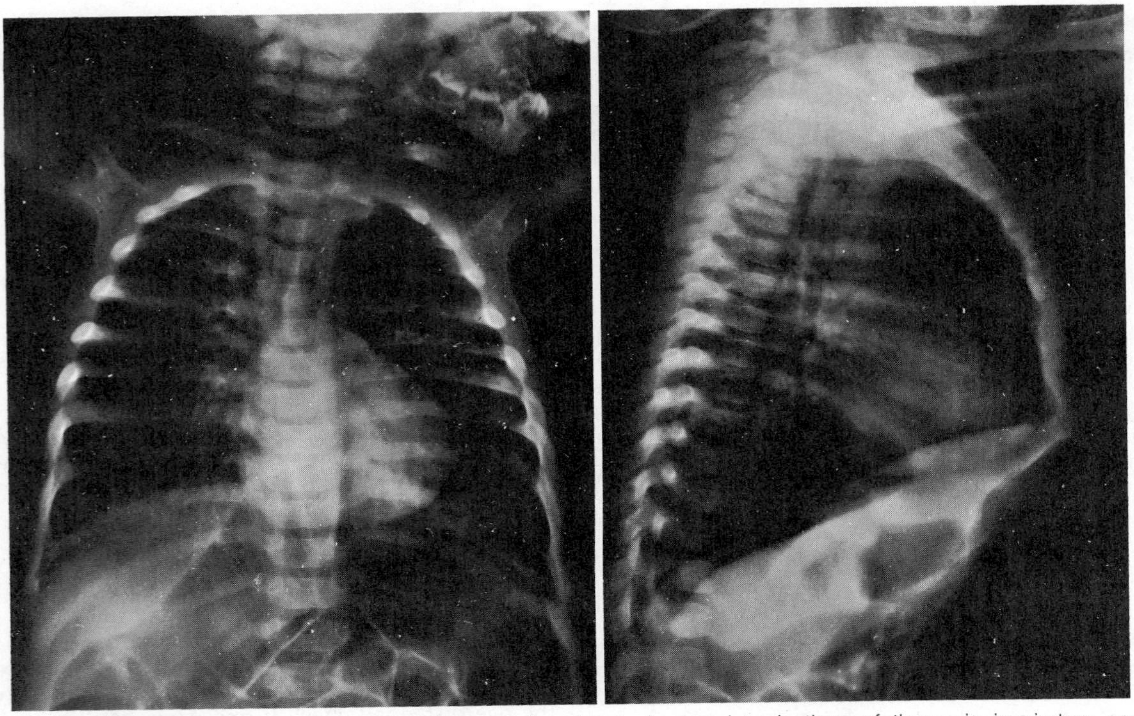

Figure 14–16. Generalized obstructive emphysema (overinflation): dorsal projections of thorax in inspiratory and expiratory phases of respiration. Notice the relative failure of the lungs to empty in the expiratory phase. The left lung is less obstructed than the right lung (empties to a greater degree in the expiratory phase). This difference between the lungs is not apparent from a study of the diaphragm, which moves very little during respiration; it is evident, however, in the upper portions of the left lung space.

permitting free air to escape from the nasal sinuses. In the neck and thorax, subcutaneous emphysema may follow tracheotomy, deep ulcerations in the pharyngeal region, esophageal wounds, or any perforating lesion of the larynx or trachea. It is an occasional complication of thoracentesis, of asthma, or of abdominal surgery. Air may also be formed in the subcutaneous tissues by gas-producing bacteria.

When the etiology is an air leak from the respiratory system, the problem is usually self-limited and requires no specific treatment. Resolution occurs by resorption of subcutaneous air following elimination of its source. Rarely, dangerous compression of the trachea by air in the surrounding soft tissue requires surgical intervention.

Kress MB, Finklestein AH: Giant bullous emphysema occurring in tuberculosis in childhood. Pediatrics 30:269, 1962.

Nelson WE, Smith LW: Generalized obstructive emphysema in infants. J Pediatr 26:36, 1945.

Victoria MS, Steiner P, Rao M: Persistent pneumatoceles in children. Chest 79:359, 1981.

14.77 α_1-Antitrypsin Deficiency and Emphysema

Homozygous deficiency of α_1-antitrypsin characterized by the early onset of severe panacinar emphysema is a rare cause of pulmonary disease in children. α_1-Antitrypsin and other serum antiproteases are thought to be important in the inactivation of proteolytic enzymes released from dead bacteria or leukocytes in the lung. Deficiency leads to accumulation of these enzymes, proteolytic destruction of pulmonary tissue, and development of emphysema. The concentration of proteases (e.g., elastase) in the patients' leukocytes may also be an important factor in determining the severity of clinical pulmonary disease with a given level of α_1-antitrypsin.

The type and concentration of α_1-antitrypsin are inherited as a series of codominant alleles; the inferred genotype is referred to as the "Pi-type." Normal persons are Pi-type MM. Types null/null and ZZ and, to a lesser extent, other abnormal Pi-types such as SZ have been associated with early onset emphysema. Some Pi-types are associated with a characteristic form of infantile cirrhosis (Sec. 13.93).

Most patients who have Pi-type ZZ have had little or no detectable pulmonary disease during childhood. A few have had very early onset of chronic pulmonary symptoms, including dyspnea, wheezing, and cough, and panacinar emphysema has been documented by lung biopsy. Physical examination may reveal growth failure, an increased anteroposterior diameter of the chest with a hyper-resonant percussion note, rales if there is active infection, and clubbing. Severe emphysema may depress the liver and spleen, making them more easily palpable. Chest roentgenograms reveal overinflation with depressed diaphragms. Serum has a low trypsin inhibitory capacity, and a immunoassay confirms the low level of α_1-antitrypsin.

Danazol, an analog of testosterone, increases hepatic α_1-antitrypsin synthesis, but masculinizing effects make it totally unacceptable for women, and overall toxicity prevents long-term administration in men. Enzyme replacement appears to be a more promising approach to treatment. α_1-Antitrypsin can be readily purified from pooled human blood and, because it is relatively heat resistant, inactivation of hepatitis and other viruses is easily accomplished. Furthermore, intravenous administration raises the blood antiprotease level into an acceptable range and results in the appearance of the transfused antiprotease in pulmonary lavage fluid. Severe toxicity has not been reported. Because of the severity of α_1-antitrypsin deficiency emphysema, the Federal Drug Administration (FDA) has approved the use of purified blood derived human enzyme for ZZ and null/null patients while a long-term study of efficacy is underway. Pure α_1-antitrypsin, produced by recombinant

DNA technology, is also available but lacks the carbohydrate side chains that protect the natural material from renal excretion. Its efficacy when aerosolized is under investigation. Replacement of the methionine of natural α_1-antitrypsin at position 358 with valine results in a substantially more stable, yet biochemically active, compound; however, considerable controversy continues over its clinical use. The possibility of more direct therapy with gene insertion has also been suggested.

Nonspecific treatment includes aggressive treatment of pulmonary infection, routine use of pneumococcal and influenza vaccines, and advice about the risks of smoking.

Treatment is also indicated for other members of the family found to be Pi-type ZZ or null/null even if they are asymptomatic. Persons with the MZ Pi-type do not have an increased risk for developing pulmonary disease. The clinical significance of the SZ Pi-type is unknown, but the nonspecific treatment seems reasonable. All persons with low levels of serum antiprotease should be warned that the eventual development of emphysema may be partially related to environmental factors, including exposure to industrial fumes and cigarette smoking.

Bruce RM, Cohen BH, Diamond EL, et al: Collaborative study to assess risk of lung disease in Pi MZ phenotype subjects. Am Rev Respir Dis 130:366, 1984.
Cox DW, Levison H: Emphysema of early onset associated with a complete deficiency of alpha-$_1$-antitrypsin (null homozygotes). Am Rev Respir Dis 137:371, 1988.
Gadek JE, Crystal RG: Experience with replacement therapy in the destructive lung disease associated with severe alpha-$_1$-antitrypsin deficiency. Am Rev Respir Dis 127(pt 2):545, 1983.
Kidokoro Y, Kravis TC, Moser KM, et al: Relationship of leukocyte elastase concentration to severity of emphysema in homozygous alpha$_1$-antitrypsin deficient persons. Am Rev Respir Dis 115:793, 1977.
Sveger T: Prospective study of children with α_1-antitrypsin deficiency: Eight-year-old follow-up. J Pediatr 104:91, 1984.

14.78 PULMONARY EDEMA

ETIOLOGY. Pulmonary edema results from the transudation of fluid from the pulmonary capillaries into the alveolar spaces and the bronchioles. It is usually associated with circulatory or neurocirculatory collapse and consequently is often a terminal event in a variety of diseases. Although pulmonary edema may vary in severity, even in its mildest stages it is an ominous finding. It is a common manifestation of left ventricular failure, the edema resulting from a rise in pulmonary venous pressure, or it may be caused by hypervolemia from too rapid or too large an intravenous infusion. It may also be a manifestation of acute or chronic nephritis or, rarely, of pneumonic and other infections with substantial degrees of toxicity. Poisoning by substances such as barbiturates, morphine, epinephrine, and alcohol may be responsible for the development of pulmonary edema, as may the inhalation of toxic gases, such as illuminating gas, ammonia, and nitrogen dioxide, or the ingestion and consequent aspiration of highly volatile hydrocarbons, such as lighter fluid. (See also Adult Respiratory Distress Syndrome, Sec. 14.60 and 14.79.)

CLINICAL MANIFESTATIONS. The onset is variable but rapid in most cases. The child often complains of difficulty in breathing or a sense of oppression or pain in the chest. Cough is usually present and often produces a frothy, pink-tinged sputum. There is tachypnea, and the pulse is rapid and feeble. The child is usually very pale and may be cyanotic. On physical examination, dullness to percussion and moist, bubbly rales are heard in the lower portions of the chest. Chest roentgenogram shows a diffuse perihilar infiltrate (butterfly distribution). Occasionally, one lung is more affected than the other. If the pulmonary edema is superimposed on another pulmonary process (e.g., pneumococcal pneumonia, left-sided heart failure in cystic fibrosis), the clinical and roentgenographic findings of the primary illness may obscure those of pulmonary edema.

TREATMENT. Treatment is directed at the primary disease causing the pulmonary edema. Administering oxygen is often useful in relieving some of the chest pain and when possible is best accomplished by intermittent positive pressure. Dyspnea can often be relieved by morphine sulfate, in a dosage of 0.1 mg/kg, and oxygen. If pulmonary edema is secondary to excessive parenteral administration of fluids or blood or to cardiac failure, administration of diuretics, such as furosemide (1 mg/kg), digitalization, or bronchodilators, the application of tourniquets or inflated blood pressure cuffs to the extremities, or the withdrawal of blood may be lifesaving.

High-Altitude Pulmonary Edema

This disease characteristically affects children and adolescents at altitudes above 2,700 meters (8,860 ft). Patients with an absent or hypoplastic right pulmonary artery appear particularly vulnerable. The pathogenesis is not fully understood; however, studies have shown large amounts of high molecular weight proteins, erythrocytes, and leukocytes in lavage fluid from mountain climbers with, but not in those without, high-altitude pulmonary edema suggesting that there is a "large-pore" leak. The extreme neutrophil invasion characteristic of other acute pulmonary injuries was not present. Microhemorrhages may also play a role. Cough, shortness of breath, vomiting, and chest pain are the most common symptoms and occur within hours of high altitude exposure. Not all persons are affected, and even affected persons may not develop symptoms after every exposure. Chest roentgenogram reveals bilateral patchy pulmonary infiltrates. Oxygen is indicated. Bed rest, diuretics, antibiotics, and corticosteroids have been used, but their efficacy has not been established. Recovery usually occurs within 48 hr, and further residence at high altitude is then tolerated without symptoms. The disease may recur, however, following return to high altitude after even a brief visit to lower levels.

Rios B, Driscoll DJ, McNamara DG: High-altitude pulmonary edema with absent right pulmonary artery. Pediatrics 75:314, 1985.
Schoene RB, Hackett PH, Henderson WR, et al: High-altitude pulmonary edema: characteristics of lung lavage fluid. JAMA 256:63, 1986.
Scoggin CH, Hyers T, Reeves JT, et al: High-altitude pulmonary edema in the children and young adults of Leadville, Colorado. N Engl J Med 297:1269, 1977.
Spring CL, Rackow EC, Fein IA, et al: The spectrum of pulmonary edema; Differentiation of cardiogenic, intermediate, and no cardiogenic forms of pulmonary edema. Am Rev Respir Dis 124:716, 1981.

14.79 Adult Respiratory Distress Syndrome (ARDS)

Noncardiogenic pulmonary edema can be precipitated by a great variety of diffuse alveolar insults, including primary pulmonary and primary extrapulmonary problems (e.g., septic or hypovolemic shock, trauma, intravascular coagulation, drug overdose, aspiration, smoke/fume/toxic gas inhalation) and, despite the name "adult respiratory distress syndrome," can occur at any age. The pulmonary edema, which is the dominant manifestation of the disease, results from increased permeability of the alveolar-capillary membrane. The exact sequence of pathophysiologic events is not completely understood and, in all likelihood, is not invariable. In most patients, however, the aggregation of leukocytes within the pulmonary circulation plays a major role by initiating a cascade of events in which potent mediators (e.g., oxygen radicals, proteolytic enzymes, arachidonic acid metabolites, fibrin degradation products, platelet activating factor) injure the vascular epithelium. Direct toxicity of inhaled gases may also be a sufficient pathophysiologic event.

CLINICAL MANIFESTATIONS. Pulmonary symptoms may be minimal immediately after the acute injury. There may be some hyperventilation. The lungs are often clear to auscultation, and there are no radiologic changes. Subsequently, however, although the patient continues to be stable clinically, a fine reticular infiltrate appears on the chest roentgenogram. At some point between 8 and 48 hr after the original insult, the patient becomes more tachypneic and dyspneic, and develops hypoxemia and a more abnormal chest roentgenogram. A large intrapulmonary shunt can be demonstrated. Gradual recovery may ensue, but many patients develop very severe disease with more severe hypoxemia and, occasionally, hypercapnia. Many do not survive these problems, but those who do often require prolonged respiratory support.

PATHOLOGY. Initially (acute stage), there is capillary congestion and evidence of interstitial pulmonary edema. The alveoli may contain nonhomogeneous fluid or blood. Leukocyte plugs may be evident. Subsequently, in patients who do not recover promptly, a chronic stage develops during which there is cuboidal cell proliferation in addition to the edema. Cellularity decreases thereafter, and evidence of fibrosis develops.

TREATMENT. These patients must be managed in an intensive care unit where appropriate monitoring (including a systemic arterial catheter, and often a pulmonary artery catheter; pulse oximetry may be useful in addition to these catheters) can be used to adjust oxygen and ventilator settings to allow adequate delivery of oxygen to the tissues. Positive end-expiratory pressure (PEEP) settings must be fine-tuned by continued surveillance of laboratory data. Very high levels of PEEP (10–20 cm H_2O) have been used. Other supportive treatment includes the maintenance of cardiac function, stabilization of the hematocrit between 35% and 40%, and attention to nutrition. Secondary infection, often with *Pseudomonas* or *Klebsiella*, but also with gram-positive organisms or viruses should be considered. Corticosteroids do not appear to be effective.

PROGNOSIS. Survival results vary, but most centers report a high mortality, usually more than 50%. For survivors, the outlook for full recovery is quite good. Most gradually return to their preillness status within 1 year, although an exercise-induced fall in Pa_{O_2} may persist. Thus, although the short-term outlook for survival is guarded and comparable with those reported for adults, the long-term outlook for return of function may be better in surviving children.

Boyall JA, Levin DL: Medical progress: Adult respiratory distress syndrome in pediatric patients. 1: Clinical aspects, pathophysiology, and mechanisms of lung injury; 2: Management. J Pediatr 112:169, 335, 1988.

Petty TL: Adult respiratory distress syndrome: Definition and historical perspective. Clin Chest Med 3:3, 1982.

Tate RM, Repine JE: Neutrophils and the adult respiratory distress syndrome. Am Rev Respir Dis 128:552, 1983.

Truog WE: ARDS in children: A critical care challenge. J Respir Dis 7:104, 1986.

14.80 PULMONARY EMBOLISM AND INFARCTION

Pulmonary embolism is uncommon in infants and children. Although it often arises from thrombi in the femoral and pelvic veins (often in the postoperative patient), emboli in children and youth can also arise from abdominal and head veins. Scoliosis surgery, in particular, may predispose to deep vein thrombosis and pulmonary embolization. Emboli are not uncommon following spinal cord injury and in severe burns. Embolization may also occur following prolonged inactivity or as a complication of intravenous infusions. Pulmonary embolism may not be uncommon in sick neonates. The most frequent underlying cause is a medical device, such as an intravenous line, arteriovenous (A-V) fistula, or other implanted device; however, emboli also occur in newborns with congenital heart disease and in infants of diabetic mothers. The original source of the embolus may be an infarcted placenta or a thrombus in the umbilical vein, perhaps dislodged by the insertion of a catheter. Asphyxia and subsequent respiratory distress may also predispose to pulmonary embolization in neonates.

In adolescence, recent abortion, drug abuse, or oral contraceptives may be the predisposing problem. As indwelling central venous catheters for home treatment of malignancies and infection become more common, the incidence of associated embolization, including both air and clotted blood, will also rise. Urokinase, a thrombolytic drug frequently used to clear these lines, may play a role in embolization if the clots are not totally lysed before the line is flushed.

Intrapulmonary thrombosis may also occur in sickle cell anemia; the subsequent infarction is often difficult to differentiate from pneumonia. Fat emboli are most likely to be derived from fractured bones; on occasion they arise from necrotic tissue in the bone marrow of patients with sickle cell disease. Multiple pulmonary infarcts resulting from small emboli may be associated with severe dehydration in diarrheal disease, cyanotic heart disease, bacterial endocarditis, ventriculoatrial shunts for the treatment of hydrocephalus, and longstanding nutritional deficiencies.

CLINICAL MANIFESTATIONS. The clinical pattern often suggests pneumonia, and the diagnosis is often made at autopsy. Emboli carrying bacteria may be responsible for multiple pulmonary abscesses. In addition to the classic physical findings of phlebothrombosis and thrombophlebitis, radiolabeled fibrinogen, impedance plethysmography, Doppler ultrasound, and contrast venography may help to define the presence and extent of deep venous thromboses.

Embolism of the pulmonary artery or its larger branches produces a variable clinical picture. Dyspnea is common, although often transient; pain and collapse are often absent. If present, pain is usually substernal, but it may be pleural and may radiate to the shoulder. Although there are often no physical signs, if the infarct is sufficiently large, there may be impaired resonance and a pleural friction rub. Breath sounds may be distant or absent, and there may be moist rales. Expectorated material, which may be profuse, often contains blood. Large emboli can cause acute right heart failure by raising pulmonary arterial pressure. However, infarction often does not occur and the classic triad of pleuritic chest pain, hemoptysis, and infiltrate is usually absent in pulmonary embolism. The case fatality rate is high, but recovery may occur even when the area of infarction is relatively large. Secondary infection may result in abscess formation.

Chest roentgenograms, although useful in ruling out other treatable causes of the patient's symptoms (e.g., pneumothorax), are often normal and rarely diagnostic. In critically ill patients in whom definitive diagnosis is urgent, pulmonary perfusion studies, ventilation scintiphotography, and pulmonary angiogram should be considered; only angiography gives unequivocal evidence of embolism, but its risk must be weighed against the risk of therapy. In children who are not gravely ill, empiric low-dose heparin therapy when scans are highly probable for pulmonary embolism may be preferable to angiography.

Exchange transfusion should precede arteriography in patients with sickle cell anemia; otherwise, massive, potentially fatal pulmonary thrombosis may occur.

Chronic showers of emboli from **ventriculoatrial shunts** may cause gradual obliteration of the pulmonary vascular bed and eventually pulmonary hypertension. Clinical findings are those of pulmonary hypertension and may include accentuation of the pulmonic component of the 2nd heart sound and the development of pulmonary or tricuspid insufficiency. In severe cases, exercise intolerance and right-sided heart failure occur, indicating that substantial compromise of lung function has already taken place. Serial electrocardiograms that show increasing right ventricular hypertrophy may give an early clue to continuing chronic embolization. Diagnosis may be confirmed by right-sided heart catheterization and determination of pulmonary arterial blood pressure. If chronic embolization is suspected, the shunt should be removed.

The diagnosis of pulmonary embolism is often missed in children, especially if the source of the emboli is not a lower extremity. Pediatricians often feel that embolism is almost exclusively an adult disease. Furthermore, children often have serious underlying diseases whose symptoms and physical findings dominate the patient's course even after embolization has occurred.

TREATMENT. Massive embolization of the larger branches of the pulmonary artery is a medical emergency. The initial treatment objective is cardiovascular support and prevention of circulatory collapse and pulmonary insufficiency by cardiotonic drugs, oxygen, and mechanical ventilation. Surgical removal of pulmonary emboli is unlikely to be successful and should be considered a desperation measure. Thrombolytic therapy may be beneficial. However, if initial treatment, including heparinization (see later) is unsuccessful, and the source of the emboli is the lower extremity, a surgical attempt to prevent their access to the inferior vena cava may be worthwhile.

After stabilization and definitive diagnosis, efforts should be made to prevent further embolization. Intravenous heparin (loading dose: 50–75 units/kg; maintenance dose: 25 units/kg/hr) should be given by continuous infusion; the dose should be adjusted to maintain the clotting time at about twice the control value (or the APTT at 1.5 times the control). After 7–10 days of intravenous heparin, 3–6 mo of oral coumarin therapy is almost always indicated, unless the source of the emboli has been definitively eliminated. In some patients, it may be prudent to reinstitute coumarin if the situation that led to the original embolus recurs (e.g., surgery, trauma, obesity).

Arnold J, O'Brodovich H, Whyte R, et al: Pulmonary thromboembolic after neonatal asphyxia. J Pediatr 106:806, 1985.
Bernstein D, Coupey S, Schonberg SK: Pulmonary embolism in adolescence. Am J Dis Child 140:667, 1986.
Bromberg PA: Pulmonary aspects of sickle cell anemia. Arch Intern Med 133:652, 1974.
Burrows PE, Leahy FA, Reed MH: Neonatal pulmonary infarction. Am J Dis Child 137:61, 1983.
Friedman S, Zita-Gozum C, Chatten J: Pulmonary vascular changes complicating ventriculovascular shunting for hydrocephalus. J Pediatr 64:305, 1964.
Uden A: Thromboembolic complications following scoliosis surgery in Scandinavia. Acta Orthrop Scand 50:175, 1979.

PULMONARY SUPPURATION

14.81 Bronchiectasis

Bronchiectasis refers to permanent dilatation of the subsegmental airways associated with inflammatory destruction of bronchial and peribronchial tissue, accumulation of exudative material in dependent bronchi, and, in some cases, distention of dependent bronchi.

ETIOLOGY. Some patients may have *congenital bronchiectasis* possibly due to an arrest in bronchial development leading to cyst formation and the destruction of the bronchial wall when the cysts become infected. Alternatively, there may be defective development of the bronchial cartilaginous supports. Tracheobronchomegaly is a rare congenital condition in which the distal trachea and main bronchi are grossly dilated; a similar condition may be associated with recurrent pneumonia.

The majority of cases of bronchiectasis are acquired after birth, usually resulting from chronic pulmonary infection, but the mechanisms involved are poorly understood. Obstruction of the bronchial tree followed by infection is one likely cause. Measles, pertussis, and pneumonia are rare causes of bronchiectasis. Cystic fibrosis is the most common underlying disease in children with generalized bronchial involvement. Other predisposing factors include aspiration of a foreign body, often a nonopaque one, enlarged bronchopulmonary nodes owing to tuberculosis, recurrent and chronic lung infections, sarcoidosis, neoplasm, lung abscess, localized cysts, emphysema with compression of the other lung parenchyma, allergy, asthma, and, rarely, extreme forms of pectus excavatum or scoliosis. Patients with immunodeficiency syndromes, especially panhypogammaglobulinemia, may have bronchiectasis, usually after repeated attacks of bacterial pneumonia and bronchitis. Recurrent aspiration pneumonitis in familial dysautonomia frequently leads to bronchiectasis. Primary ciliary dyskinesis (see Sec. 14.53) results in chronic pulmonary infection which eventually leads to bronchiectasis. Gastroesophageal reflux with chronic aspiration may be a cause of bronchiectasis. Patients with congenital heart disease may develop bronchiectasis secondary to infection related to compression of an airway by an abnormally positioned or very large blood vessel, including those used in shunting procedures.

Reversible bronchiectasis or pseudobronchiectasis occurs commonly after pertussis as well as with lobar and interstitial pneumonias. Shortly after or during these illnesses the bronchi may appear cylindrically dilated on bronchography, but if these studies are repeated months later, the changes have disappeared.

PATHOLOGY. The first destructive change is a loss of ciliated epithelium, which is regenerated as cuboidal and squamous epithelium. Concurrently the elastic tissue within the bronchial walls disappears and thickening occurs, owing to interstitial edema, fibrosis, and round cell infiltration. In adjacent parenchymal and peribronchial tissue, multiple abscesses may develop, and there is usually characteristic obstructive endarteritis of the small pulmonary vessels. Generally, bronchiectasis follows a segmental distribution, except in cystic fibrosis. The right middle lobe segments, the basal segments of the lower lobes, and the lingular segments of the left upper lobe are most frequently affected. The right lower lobe is commonly involved in aspiration of a foreign body, whereas the right middle lobe is most frequently affected by hilar lymphadenopathy.

CLINICAL MANIFESTATIONS. In symptomatic cases cough is invariably present and produces copious mucopurulent sputum during acute respiratory infections. The sputum is generally swallowed by young children. Physical activity or change in position, particularly while reclining, will often initiate a bout of coughing.

Recurrent infections of the lower respiratory tract are common; they tend to persist and are difficult to control. Anorexia, irritability, and poor weight gain are also common. Fever is much less common. Later in the course, during acute exacerbations, hemoptysis may occur, varying in severity from blood streaked sputum to exsanguinating hemorrhage. Bronchiectasis characteristically follows an intermittently improving and relapsing course.

Physical findings are absent or few. Clubbing of the fingers may be present if the patient has been symptomatic for more than 1 yr. Moist or musical rales may be heard or elicited by cough; during acute exacerbations physical signs of atelectasis or diffuse pneumonitis are often present. The usual roentgenographic examination is never pathognomonic, although mediastinal lymph nodes, radiopaque foreign bodies, and bronchovascular marking near the hilus of the lung may be suggestive. Atelectasis is relatively common.

With extensive bronchiectasis there is persistent dyspnea, and physical development is retarded. Ventilatory and diffusion studies may reveal more widespread or severe pulmonary involvement than suspected otherwise.

Every patient with suspected or proved bronchiectasis should be evaluated for sinusitis, ciliary dyskinesis, agammaglobulinemia, tuberculosis, asthma or other respiratory allergy, and cystic fibrosis. If such a diagnosis cannot be made, these patients should have bronchoscopy to exclude bronchial stenosis, strictures, tumors, and foreign bodies, and, possibly, bronchography to document the bronchiectasis and determine its extent and severity. A familial deficiency of bronchial cartilage has also been proposed as an explanation of some cases of bronchiectasis in childhood and may be suggested by marked dilatation of the 2nd–4th order bronchi during inspiration and apparent collapse during expiration. Bronchoscopic washings and sputum samples should be cultured for routine pathogens, mycobacteria, and fungi, and a tuberculin skin test should be done.

The **right middle lobe syndrome** may occur, which consists of subacute or chronic pneumonitis, bronchial obstruction, and atelectasis, and is generally caused by extrinsic compression of the middle lobe bronchus by hilar nodes, followed by peribronchitis and chronic infection. Bronchiectasis may result. On occasion this syndrome is related to asthma or congenital anomalies of the bronchi.

Young syndrome is characterized by sinusitis and bronchiectasis, often symptomatic in childhood, and by azoospermia, not detectable until later, when semen analysis can be done. Clubbing is rarely seen. Some patients develop azoospermia after a period of fertility. Urologic procedures to reestablish fertility later have been disappointing. The severity of pulmonary symptoms seems to ameliorate during adolescence or young adult life.

Yellow nail syndrome consists of pleural effusion and lymphedema, associated with discolored nails. Bronchiectasis occurred in 5 of 12 patients in one report.

TREATMENT. Therapy includes elimination of all foci of respiratory infection, effective postural drainage, and, when indicated, antibiotic therapy. Postural drainage must be carried out intensively as long as secretions are being formed and is one of the most important aspects of management.

Systemic antibiotic therapy is usually administered only during acute exacerbations in courses of 5–7 days to 2 wk. Patients with cystic fibrosis require more prolonged therapy (see Sec. 14.89). Prolonged treatment for most other patients, however, increases the risks of acquiring resistant flora and of drug reactions. The appropriate drug is selected on the basis of the antibiotic susceptibility of bacteria isolated from sputum or at bronchoscopy. If cultures contain only normal flora, antibiotics should not be used. Administering antibiotics by aerosol inhalation immediately following appropriate postural drainage may also be helpful but should not be continued for excessively long periods of time, since this encourages the establishment of a drug-resistant bacterial flora. *Pseudomonas* is particularly troublesome.

When localized severe disease progresses despite adequate medical management, segmental or lobar resection should be considered, even though the long-term results are often discouraging. Some patients with lobar bronchiectasis, especially those with the right middle lobe syndrome, do very well postlobectomy. Surgery may also be indicated when an intrinsic anatomic obstruction of the bronchus is found or when suppurative lesions exist owing to aspiration of fragmented foreign bodies, especially such vegetal objects as grass fibers or fragments of peanut which elude bronchoscopic removal.

Barker AF, Bardana EJ Jr: Bronchiectasis: Update of an orphan disease. Am Rev Respir Dis 137:969, 1988.
Becroft DMO: Bronchiolitis obliterans, bronchiectasis and other sequelae of adenovirus type 21 infection. J Clin Pathol 24:72, 1971.
Davis PB, Hubbard VS, McCoy K, et al: Familial bronchiectasis. J Pediatr 102:177, 1983.
Dees SC, Spock A: Right middle lobe syndrome in children. JAMA 197:8, 1966.
Field CE: Bronchiectasis: Third report of a follow-up study of medical and surgical cases from childhood. Arch Dis Child 44:551, 1969.
Handelsman DJ, Conway AJ, Boylan LM, et al: Young's syndrome: Obstructive azoospermia and chronic sinopulmonary infections. N Engl J Med 310:3, 1984.
Mitchell RE, Bury RG: Congenital bronchiectasis due to deficiency of bronchial cartilage (Williams-Campbell syndrome): Case report. J Pediatr 87:230, 1975.
Williams H, O'Reilly RN: Bronchiectasis in children: Its multiple clinical and pathological aspects. Arch Dis Child 34:192, 1959.

14.82 Pulmonary Abscess

A lung abscess is a suppurative process resulting in destruction of the pulmonary parenchyma and formation of a cavity containing purulent material. In children they most often result from the *aspiration of infected material* when the local defense mechanisms are overwhelmed by a large number of virulent microorganisms or are compromised by factors such as alcohol, drug abuse, recent surgery (particularly tonsillectomy or adenoidectomy), or systemic disease. Aspirated material containing bacteria that are normal inhabitants of the naso- and oropharynx reaches the most dependent portions of the lung. Thus, the posterior segments of the upper lobes and the superior segments of the lower lobes are most frequently involved, and anaerobic bacteria including bacteroides, *Fusobacterium,* and anaerobic streptococci are commonly isolated. Occasionally *pneumonia* caused by aerobic pyogenic microorganisms *(S. aureus* and *Klebsiella)* or *bronchial obstruction* due to a tumor or foreign body may be complicated by abscess formation. *Metastatic lung abscess* secondary to septic emboli from right-sided bacterial endocarditis and septic thrombophlebitis is uncommon in children. Rare causes also include amebic abscess of the lung and infections with *Nocardia,* actinomyces, and mycobacteria.

PATHOLOGY. Lung abscesses occur when pulmonary parenchyma becomes obstructed, infected, and then suppurative and necrotic. Initial inflammatory changes are followed by suppuration and thrombosis of the local blood vessels, which result in necrosis and liquefaction. Granulation tissue forms around the periphery of the abscess and may succeed in walling off the area, but more commonly the abscess ruptures into a bronchus. Contents of the abscess may then be coughed up or aspirated into other parts of the pulmonary tree with additional abscess formation. Sputum is usually fetid. Peripheral abscesses may involve the adjacent pleura, with development of an associated pleural effusion. Abscesses may rupture into the pleural cavity and produce empyema.

CLINICAL MANIFESTATIONS. The onset is generally insidious, with fever, malaise, anorexia, and weight loss. Cough, often associated with hemoptysis and producing copious amounts of foul-smelling or purulent sputum, is characteristic about 10 days after the onset in untreated patients. Lung abscess secondary to staphylococcal and *Klebsiella* pneumonia produces the acute signs and symptoms described for bacterial pneumonia. There may be respiratory distress, spiking fevers, chest pain, and marked leukocytosis. The diagnosis is generally made by roentgenographic examination when a cavity with or without a fluid level surrounded by alveolar infiltration is demonstrated. Gram stain of the sputum may reveal numerous polymorphonuclear leukocytes and findings consistent with anaerobic microorganisms, such as pleomorphic, slender, gram-negative bacilli (bacteroides, *Fusobacterium*); gram-negative rods with tapered ends (*Fusobacterium*); large gram-positive bacilli (clostridium); and tiny to small cocci (anaerobic streptococci). Sputum cultures characteristically yield a mixture of anaerobic bacteria.

TREATMENT. If a predominant aerobic organism is identified, appropriate antibiotic therapy is initiated. However, if lung abscess is secondary to aspiration and the Gram stain is compatible with anaerobic bacteria, treatment with penicillin (100,000 units/kg/24 hr) for an extended period of time (4–6 wk) is the treatment of choice pending the results of anaerobic sputum culture. This drug is effective even in patients infected with penicillin-resistant strains of *Bacteroides fragilis*. Alternative treatment in children allergic to penicillin is chloramphenicol. Experience with clindamycin and metronidazole in children is limited. Appropriate investigation for dental disease should be done in older children and adolescents.

Serial chest roentgenograms show gradual diminution in the size of the abscess cavity over a period of several weeks or months. Most patients are afebrile within 1 wk of institution of appropriate antibiotic therapy. Delayed closure is common. Bronchoscopy is indicated only to identify and remove a foreign body. The routine use of bronchoscopy to facilitate drainage or to obtain culture material is controversial. Chest tube drainage is necessary if empyema occurs. Surgical drainage of a lung abscess is almost never indicated, and resection should be considered only in children with recurrent hemoptysis, a bronchopleural fistula, repeated episodes of infection, or suspicion of malignancy.

The overall prognosis for complete recovery from primary lung abscess is excellent. In patients with secondary lung abscess, the prognosis depends heavily on the underlying disease.

Asher MI, Spier S, Beland M, et al: Primary lung abscess in childhood. Am J Dis Child 136:491, 1982.
Bartlett JG, Gorbach SL, Tally FP, et al: Bacteriology and treatment of primary lung abscess. Am Rev Respir Dis 109:510, 1974.
Brook I, Finegold JM: Bacteriology and therapy of lung abscess in children. J Pediatr 94:10, 1979.
Levine MM, Ashman R, Heald F: Anaerobic (putrid) lung abscess in adolescence. Am J Dis Child 130:77, 1976.

14.83 Pulmonary Gangrene

Gangrene of the lung is extremely rare but occasionally follows measles and is seen in persons with severe immunologic deficits. The onset is usually sudden and is associated with early pulmonary hemorrhage; there is rapid development of pneumothorax and putrid empyema, and death may occur quickly. Treatment consists of adequate pleural drainage and intensive antibiotic therapy.

14.84 HERNIA OF LUNG

Protrusion of the lung beyond its normal thoracic boundaries may be a complication of pulmonary disease in which there is frequent coughing with generation of high intrathoracic pressure, such as cystic fibrosis or asthma, or may result from a congenital weakness of the suprapleural membrane or the musculature of the neck. Over half of congenital lung hernias and almost all acquired lung hernias are cervical. Paravertebral or parasternal hernias are usually caused by rib anomalies. The presenting complaint is usually the presence of a mass in the neck while straining or coughing. Occasionally, transient pain is noted in the region of the hernia. Physical examination is normal except during a Valsalva maneuver when a soft bulge is noted in the neck. In most cases no treatment is necessary. Occasionally a surgical procedure is justified for cosmetic purposes. In patients with severe chronic pulmonary disease in whom coughing is present daily and cough suppression is contraindicated, permanent surgical correction may not be achieved.

Bronsther B, Coryllos E, Epstein B, et al: Lung hernias in children. J Pediatr Surg 3:544, 1968.
Jones JG: Cervical hernia of the lung. J Pediatr 76:122, 1970.

14.85 PULMONARY NEOPLASMS

True carcinoma of the lung is rare in children and in youth. The youngest patients were 19 yr old in one series and 20 and 25 yr old in another series. Heavy and long-duration smoking appears to be the most important risk factor even in these young patients. A great variety of primary tumors have been reported, but all are extremely rare. Fewer than 250 cases, including 150 malignancies, have been reported in English language journals. Bronchial adenoma and carcinoid are the most common primary tumors. Metastatic lesions, such as Wilms' tumor, osteogenic sarcoma, and hepatoblastoma are the most common forms of pulmonary malignancy in children (see Chapter 17). A high incidence of "inflammatory pseudotumors" clouds the statistics. Patients with symptoms, or with roentgenographic or other laboratory findings suggesting pulmonary malignancy, should be searched carefully for a tumor at another site before surgical excision is done. Pulmonary tumors may present with fever, hemoptysis, wheezing, cough, pleural effusion, chest pain, dyspnea, or recurrent or persistent pneumonia or atelectasis. Isolated primary lesions and isolated metastatic lesions discovered long after the primary tumor has been removed are best treated by excision. The prognosis varies and depends on the type of tumor involved.

Emory WB, Mitchell WT Jr, Hatch HB Jr: Mucous gland adenoma of the bronchus. Am Rev Respir Dis 108:1407, 1973.
Hartman GE, Shochat SJ: Primary pulmonary neoplasms of childhood: A review. Am Thorac Surg 36:108, 1983.
Putnam JS: Lung carcinoma in young adults. JAMA 237:35, 1977.
Roviaro GC, Varoli F, Zannini P, et al: Lung cancer in the young. Chest 87:456, 1985.
van Steensel-Moll HA, de Groot R, Neijens J, et al: Bronchial carcinoid tumor in a 12 yr old child. Pediatr Pulmonol 2:110, 1986.
Wellons HA Jr, Eggleston P, Golden GT, Allen MS: Bronchial adenoma in childhood: Two case reports and review of the literature. Am J Dis Child 130:301, 1976.

14.86 Pulmonary Hemangiomatosis

In this rare and ultimately fatal disease, uncontrolled vascular proliferation causes progressive dyspnea and eventually leads to death from massive hemoptysis or pulmonary hypertension. Its etiology is unknown, although infection may play a role. The vascular abnormality involves the smallest (capillary size) vessels in some patients and slightly larger vessels in others. The pathologic angiogenic process may also extend into other intrathoracic tissues (e.g., mediastinum, pericardium, thymus) or the spleen. The patients usually present with hemoptysis or with right-sided heart failure secondary to pulmonary hypertension. Routine chest films are often similar to those seen in interstitial lung disease. The diagnosis is made by pulmonary angiography (which also helps to exclude other forms of veno-occlusive disease) and open lung biopsy. The disease can be locally invasive but is not known to metastasize. The primary process appears to be angiogenesis. Most patients die within 1–5 yr from the onset of symptoms.

A substantial and sustained clinical improvement in a 12-yr-old boy treated with recombinant interferon α-2a (initial dose: 1 million units/m^2/24 hr and then raised rapidly to 3 million units/m^2/24 hr) has been reported. Although some hemoptysis was still present, the patient tolerated the treatment well and was still clinically stable 14 mo later. The success of this treatment is additional evidence that the primary lesion is angiogenesis.

Faber CN, Yousem SA, Dauber JH, et al: Pulmonary capillary hemangiomatosis: A report of three cases and a review of the literature. Am Rev Respir Dis 140:808, 1989.
White CW, Sondheimer HM, Crouch EC, et al: Treatment of pulmonary hemangiomatosis with recombinant interferon α-2a. N Engl J Med 320:1197, 1989.

14.87 Hiccup (Singulpus)

Hiccup (frequent or rhythmic clonic contraction of the diaphragm) is usually a transient nuisance. Prolonged hiccup, however, can be a diagnostic and therapeutic challenge and can be life-threatening. Hiccup can result from a variety of CNS diseases (e.g., posterior fossa tumors, brain injury, encephalitis), local irritation along the route of the phrenic nerve or at the diaphragm (e.g., tumor, pleurisy, pneumonia, intrathoracic adenopathy, pericarditis, esophagitis), and systemic causes (e.g., alcohol intoxication, uremia). Unusual causes for hiccup include a foreign body or insect in the ear (perhaps by stimulation of the vagus nerve). Hiccups occur frequently in young infants in whom they may be associated with apnea or hyperventilation.

A great many folklore remedies have been used for hiccup. Many of these involve maneuvers that result in aerophagia or breath-holding or that use distraction. For intractable hiccup, a variety of drugs are said to be effective (e.g., haloperidol, metoclopramide, and a variety of anesthetic agents).

ROBERT C. STERN

Brouillette RT, Thach BT, Abu-Osba YK, et al: Hiccups in infants: Characteristics and effects on ventilation. J Pediatr 96:219, 1980.
Seibert D, Al-Kawas F: Trimethoprim-sulfamethoxazole, hiccups, and esophageal ulcers. Ann Intern Med 105:976, 1986.

14.88 APPROACH TO RECURRENT OR PERSISTENT LOWER RESPIRATORY TRACT SYMPTOMS IN CHILDREN

Respiratory tract symptoms such as cough, wheeze, and stridor may occur frequently or persist for long periods of time in a substantial number of children; in others there may be persistent and recurring lung infiltrates with or without symptoms. Determining the cause of these chronic findings can be very difficult because symptoms may be due to a rapid succession of unrelated acute respiratory tract infections or to a single pathophysiologic process, and there is a paucity of easily performed, specific diagnostic tests for many acute and chronic respiratory conditions. Pressure from the affected child's family for a quick remedy because of concern over symptoms related to breathing may complicate diagnostic and therapeutic efforts.

A systematic approach to the diagnosis and treatment of these children consists of (1) assessing whether the symptoms are the manifestation of a minor problem or a life-threatening process; (2) determining the most likely underlying pathogenic mechanism; (3) selecting the simplest effective therapy for the underlying process, which may often be only symptomatic therapy; and (4) carefully evaluating the effect of therapy. Failure of this approach to identify the process responsible or to effect improvement signals the need for more extensive and perhaps invasive diagnostic efforts, including bronchoscopy.

JUDGING THE SERIOUSNESS OF CHRONIC RESPIRATORY COMPLAINTS

Clinical manifestations suggesting that a respiratory tract illness may be life-threatening or associated with the potential for chronic disability are listed in Table 14–2. If none of these are detected, the chronic respiratory process is usually benign. Active, well-nourished, and appropriately growing infants who present with intermittent noisy breathing but no other physical or laboratory abnormalities require only symptomatic treatment and parental reassurance. However, benign-appearing but persistent symptoms occasionally may be the harbinger of a serious lower respiratory tract problem, and conversely, a few children (e.g., with infection-related asthma) may have acute recurrent life-threatening episodes but few or no symptoms in the interval. Repeated examinations over an extended period, both when the child appears healthy and when the child is symptomatic, may be helpful in sorting out the severity and chronicity of lung disease.

DIFFERENTIAL DIAGNOSTIC FEATURES

RECURRENT OR PERSISTENT COUGH. Cough is a reflex response of the lower respiratory tract to stimulation of irritant or cough receptors in the airways' mucosa. The most common cause in children is reactive airways (asthma). Because cough receptors also reside in the pharynx, paranasal sinuses, stomach, and external auditory canal, the source of a persistent cough may need to be sought beyond the lungs. Specific lower respiratory stimuli include excessive secretions, aspirated foreign material, inhaled dust particles or noxious gases, and an inflammatory response to infectious agents or allergic processes. Some of the conditions responsible for chronic cough are listed in Table 14–3.

Characteristics of cough that may aid in distinguishing its origin are presented in Table 14–4. Additional useful information may include (1) a history of atopic conditions (asthma, eczema, urticaria, allergic rhinitis), a seasonal or environmental variation in frequency or intensity of cough, and a strong family history of atopic conditions, all suggesting an allergic etiology; (2) symptoms of malabsorption or family history indicative of cystic fibrosis; (3) symptoms related to feeding, suggesting aspiration; (4) a choking episode suggesting foreign body aspiration; (5) headache or facial edema associated with sinusitis; (6) a smoking history in older children and adolescents or the presence of a smoker in the house.

Considerable information pertaining to the etiology of chronic cough can be obtained during the physical examination. Posterior pharyngeal drainage combined with a night-time cough suggests chronic upper airway disease. An over-inflated chest suggests chronic airway obstruction, such as in asthma or cystic fibrosis. An expiratory wheeze, with or without diminished intensity of breath sounds, strongly suggests asthma or asthmatic bronchitis but may also be consistent with a diagnosis of cystic fibrosis, vascular ring, aspiration of foreign material, or pulmonary hemosiderosis. Careful

TABLE 14–2. Indicators of Serious Chronic Lower Respiratory Tract Disease in Children

Persistent fever
Ongoing limitation of activity
Failure to grow
Failure to gain weight appropriately
Clubbing of the digits
Persistent tachypnea and labored ventilation
Chronic purulent sputum
Persistent hyperinflation
Substantial and sustained hypoxemia
Refractory roentgenographic infiltrates
Persistent pulmonary function abnormalities

TABLE 14–3. Differential Diagnosis of Recurrent and Persistent Cough in Children

Recurrent cough
- Increased bronchial reactivity, including allergic asthma
- Drainage from upper airways
- Aspiration syndromes
- Frequently recurring respiratory tract infections
- Idiopathic pulmonary hemosiderosis

Persistent cough
- Postinfection hypersensitivity of cough receptors
- Reactive airways disease (asthma)
- Asthmatic bronchitis
- Chronic sinusitis
- Bronchitis, tracheitis owing to chronic infection, smoking (in older children)
- Bronchiectasis, including cystic fibrosis, primary ciliary dyskinesis, immunodeficiency
- Foreign body aspiration
- Recurrent aspiration owing to pharyngeal incompetence, tracheolaryngoesophageal cleft, tracheoesophageal fistula
- Gastroesophageal reflux, with or without aspiration
- Pertussis syndrome
- Extrinsic compression of the tracheobronchial tract (vascular ring, neoplasm, lymph node, lung cyst)
- Tracheomalacia, bronchomalacia
- Endobronchial or endotracheal tumors
- Endobronchial tuberculosis
- Habit cough
- Hypersensitivity pneumonitis
- Fungal infections
- Inhaled irritants, including tobacco smoke
- Irritation of external auditory canal

auscultation during forced expiration may reveal expiratory wheezes that are otherwise undetectable and that are the only indication of underlying reactive airways. Coarse crackles suggest bronchiectasis, including cystic fibrosis, but may also attend an acute or subacute exacerbation of asthma. Clubbing of the digits is seen in most patients with bronchiectasis, but in only a few with other respiratory conditions with chronic cough (see Sec. 11.41). Tracheal deviation suggests foreign body aspiration or a mediastinal mass.

It is essential to allow sufficient examination time to observe whether a spontaneous cough is present. If not spontaneous, most children by 4–5 yr of age will cough on request. Asking the child to repeatedly take a maximal breath and forcefully exhale usually induces a cough reflex. Children who cough as often as several times a minute with regularity are likely to have a habit (tic) cough. If the cough is loose, every effort should be made to obtain sputum; most older children can comply. It is sometimes possible to pick up small bits of sputum with a throat swab quickly placed into the lower pharynx while the child coughs with the tongue protruding. Clear mucoid sputum is most often associated with an allergic reaction or asthmatic bronchitis. Cloudy (purulent) sputum suggests a respiratory tract infection but may also reflect increased cellularity (eosinophilia) due to an asthmatic process. Very purulent sputum is characteristic of bronchiectasis. Malodorous expectorations suggest anerobic infection of the lungs. In cystic fibrosis the sputum, even when purulent, is rarely foul smelling.

Laboratory tests may help to evaluate a chronic cough. Only sputum specimens containing alveolar macrophages should be used for studying lower respiratory tract processes. Sputum eosinophilia suggests asthma, asthmatic bronchitis, or hypersensitivity reactions of lung, whereas a polymorphonuclear cell response suggests infection; if sputum is unavailable, the presence of eosinophilia in nasal secretions also suggests atopic disease. If most of the cells in sputum are macrophages, postinfectious hypersensitivity of cough receptors should be suspected. Sputum macrophages can be stained for hemosiderin content, diagnostic of pulmonary hemosiderosis, or for lipid content, which in large amounts suggests but is not specific for repeated aspiration. Children whose coughs persist longer than 6 wk should be tested for cystic fibrosis. Sputum culture is helpful but not specific because throat flora may contaminate the sample.

Hematologic assessment may reveal anemia that is the result of pulmonary hemosiderosis or eosinophilia that accompanies asthma and other hypersensitivity reactions of the lung. Infiltrates on chest roentgenogram may suggest cystic fibrosis, bronchiectasis, foreign body, hypersensitivity pneumonitis, or tuberculosis. When asthma equivalent cough is suspected, a trial of bronchodilator therapy may be diagnostic. After the initial evaluation, especially if the cough does not respond to initial therapeutic efforts, more specific diagnostic procedures may be indicated, including an immunologic or allergic evaluation, paranasal sinus imaging, esophagograms, tests for gastroesophageal reflux, special microbiologic studies, evaluation of ciliary morphology and function, and bronchoscopy.

RECURRENT OR PERSISTENT WHEEZE. Wheezing is a relatively frequent and particularly troublesome manifestation of obstructive lower respiratory tract disease in children. The site of obstruction may be anywhere from the intrathoracic trachea to the small bronchi or large bronchioles, but the sound is generated by turbulence in larger airways that collapse with forced expiration. Children under 2–3 yr of age are especially prone to wheezing, because bronchospasm, mucosal edema, and accumulation of excessive secretions have a relatively greater obstructive effect on their smaller airways. In addition, the very compliant airways in young children collapse more readily with active expiration. Isolated episodes of acute wheezing, such as may occur with bronchiolitis, are not uncommon, but wheezing that recurs or persists for longer than 4 wk suggests other diagnoses (Table 14–5). Most recurrent or persistent wheezing in children is the result of reactive airways disease. Nonspecific environmental factors such as cigarette smoke may be important contributors.

TABLE 14–4. Characteristics of a Chronic Cough and Their Etiologic Significance

Type of Cough	Likely Responsible Condition
Loose (discontinuous), productive	Bronchitis, asthmatic bronchitis, cystic fibrosis, other bronchiectasis
Brassy	Tracheitis, habit cough
With stridor	Laryngeal obstruction, pertussis
Paroxysmal (with or without gagging and vomiting)	Cystic fibrosis, pertussis syndrome, foreign body
Staccato	Chlamydia pneumonitis
Nocturnal	Upper and/or lower respiratory tract allergic reaction, sinusitis
Most severe on awakening in morning	Cystic fibrosis, other bronchiectasis, chronic bronchitis
With vigorous exercise	Exercise-induced asthma, cystic fibrosis, other bronchiectasis
Disappears with sleep	Habit cough, mild hypersecretory states such as in cystic fibrosis and asthma
Tight (wheezy)	Reactive airways

TABLE 14–5. Causes of Recurrent or Persistent Wheezing in Children

- Reactive airways disease
  - Atopic asthma
  - Infection associated airway reactivity
  - Exercise-induced asthma
  - Salicylate-induced asthma and nasal polyposis
  - Asthmatic bronchitis
  - Other hypersensitivity reactions:
    - Hypersensitivity pneumonitis
    - Tropical eosinophilia
    - Visceral larva migrans
    - Allergic aspergillosis
- Aspiration
  - Foreign body
  - Food, saliva, gastric contents
  - Laryngotracheoesophageal cleft
  - Tracheoesophageal fistula, H-type
  - Pharyngeal incoordination or neuromuscular weakness
- Cystic fibrosis
- Ciliary dyskinesis
- Cardiac failure
- Bronchiolitis obliterans
- Extrinsic compression of airways
  - Vascular ring
  - Enlarged lymph node
  - Mediastinal tumor
  - Lung cysts
- Tracheobronchomalacia
- Endobronchial masses
- Gastroesophageal reflux
- Pulmonary hemosiderosis
- Sequelae of bronchopulmonary dysplasia
- "Hysterical" airway closure
- Cigarette smoke, other environmental insults

Frequently recurring or persistent wheezing starting at or soon after birth suggests a variety of other diagnoses, including congenital structural abnormalities involving the lower respiratory tract or tracheobronchomalacia. Wheezing that attends cystic fibrosis is most common in the first year of life. Sudden onset of severe wheezing in a previously healthy child should suggest foreign body aspiration.

Repeated examination may be required to verify a history of wheezing in a child with episodic symptoms and should be directed toward assessing air movement, ventilatory adequacy, and evidence of chronic lung disease, such as fixed overinflation of the chest, growth failure, and digital clubbing. Clubbing suggests chronic lung infection and is rarely prominent in uncomplicated asthma. Tracheal deviation from foreign body aspiration should be sought. It is essential to rule out wheezing secondary to congestive heart failure. Allergic rhinitis, urticaria, eczema, or evidence of ichthyosis vulgaris suggests asthma or asthmatic bronchitis. The nose should be examined for polyps, which may be present in either allergic conditions or cystic fibrosis.

Sputum eosinophilia and elevated serum IgE levels suggest allergic reactions. A response to bronchodilators or related medications is confirmatory of reactive airways. Specific microbiologic studies, special imaging studies of the airways and cardiovascular structures, diagnostic studies for CF, and bronchoscopy should be considered if the response is unsatisfactory.

FREQUENTLY RECURRING OR PERSISTENT STRIDOR. Stridor, a harsh, medium-pitched, inspiratory sound associated with obstruction of the laryngeal area or the extrathoracic trachea, is often accompanied by a croupy cough and hoarse voice. Stridor is most commonly observed in children with croup; foreign bodies and trauma may also cause acute stridor. However, a small number of children develop recurrent stridor or have persistent stridor from the first days or weeks of life (Table 14–6). Most congenital anomalies of large airways that produce stridor become symptomatic soon after birth. Increase of stridor when a child is supine suggests laryngomalacia or tracheomalacia. An accompanying history of hoarseness or aphonia suggests involvement of the vocal cords.

Physical examination for recurrent or persistent stridor is usually unrewarding, although changes of its severity and intensity due to changes of body position should be assessed. Anteroposterior and lateral roentgenograms of the laryngeal and tracheal areas may demonstrate focal narrowing of the air column or extrinsic pressure on the tracheobronchial airways. Occasionally a specific lesion, such as a laryngocele, can be identified, but in most cases direct observation is necessary for diagnosis. Undistorted views of the larynx are best obtained with a fiberoptic bronchoscope positioned in the pharynx.

RECURRENT AND PERSISTENT LUNG INFILTRATES. Roentgenographic lung infiltrates due to acute pneumonia usually resolve within 1–3 wk, but a substantial number of children, particularly infants, fail to completely clear infiltrates within a 4 wk period. They may be either febrile or afebrile and may present a wide range of respiratory symptoms and signs. Persistent or recurring infiltrates present a diagnostic challenge (Table 14–7).

Symptoms associated with chronic lung infiltrates during the first several weeks of life (but not related to neonatal respiratory distress syndrome) suggest infection acquired in utero or during descent through the birth canal. Early appearance of chronic infiltrates may also be associated with cystic fibrosis or congenital anomalies, which result in aspiration or airway obstruction. A history of recurrent infiltrates, wheezing, and cough may reflect asthma, even in the first year of life.

One uncommon but characteristic syndrome appearing in

TABLE 14–6. Causes of Recurrent or Persistent Stridor in Children

Recurrent

- Allergic (spasmodic) croup
- Respiratory infections in a child with otherwise asymptomatic anatomic narrowing of the large airways
- Laryngomalacia

Persistent

- Laryngeal obstruction
  - Laryngomalacia
  - Papillomas, other tumors
  - Cysts and laryngoceles
  - Laryngeal webs
  - Bilateral abductor paralysis of the cords
  - Foreign body
- Tracheobronchial disease
  - Tracheomalacia
  - Subglottic tracheal webs
  - Endotracheal, endobronchial tumors
  - Subglottic tracheal stenosis
    - Congenital
    - Acquired
  - Extrinsic masses
    - Mediastinal masses
    - Vascular ring
    - Lobar emphysema
    - Bronchogenic cysts
    - Thyroid enlargement
    - Esophageal foreign body
  - Tracheoesophageal fistulas
- Other
  - Gastroesophageal reflux
  - Macroglossia, Pierre Robin syndrome
  - Cri du chat syndrome
  - Hysterical stridor

TABLE 14–7. Diseases Associated with Recurrent or Persistent Lung Infiltrates Beyond the Neonatal Period

Recurrent or migrating infiltrates
  Asthma*
  Repeated aspiration*
  Hypersensitivity pneumonitis
  Pulmonary hemosiderosis*
  Foreign body
  Immunodeficiency, phagocytic deficiency*
  Sickle cell disease
  Cystic fibrosis*
Persistent infiltrates
  Congenital infection*
    Cytomegalovirus
    Rubella
    Syphilis
  Acquired infection
    Cytomegalovirus*
    Tuberculosis*
    Chlamydia*
    Other viruses*
    Mycoplasma, ureaplasma*
    Pertussis*
    Fungal organisms
    *Pneumocystis carinii**
    Inadequately treated bacterial infection
  Congenital anomalies
    Lung cysts*
    Pulmonary sequestration
    Bronchial stenosis
    Vascular ring
    Congenital heart disease with large left to right shunt
  Aspiration
    Pharyngeal incompetence (e.g., cleft palate)*
    Laryngotracheoesophageal cleft*
	Tracheoesophageal fistula*
	Gastroesophageal reflux*
	Foreign body
	Lipid aspiration
	Immunodeficiency, phagocytic deficiency*
	  Humoral, cellular, combined immunodeficiency states*
	  Chronic granulomatous disease and related phagocytic defects*
	  Complement deficiency states*
	Allergy-hypersensitivity
	  Pulmonary hemosiderosis (cow's milk–related, other)*
	  Asthma
	  Hypersensitivity pneumonitis (allergic alveolitis)
	Cystic fibrosis*
	Primary ciliary dyskinesia (Kartagener)
	Other bronchiectasis
	Sarcoidosis
	Neoplasms (primary, metastatic)
	Interstitial pneumonitis and fibrosis*
	  Usual (Hamman-Rich)
	  Desquamative
	  Lymphoid (AIDS)
	Alveolar proteinosis
	Pulmonary lymphangiectasia*
	α_1-Antitrypsin deficiency
	Drug-induced, radiation-induced inflammation and fibrosis
	Collagen-vascular diseases
	Eosinophilic pneumonias
	Visceral larva migrans
	Histiocytosis
	Leukemia

*Conditions likely to cause chronic lung infiltrates in infants.

the first year of life with recurrent lung infiltrates is pulmonary hemosiderosis related to cow's milk hypersensitivity. Children with a history of bronchopulmonary dysplasia frequently have episodes of respiratory distress attended by wheezing and new lung infiltrates. Recurrent pneumonia in a child with frequent otitis media, nasopharyngitis, adenitis, or dermatologic manifestations suggests an immunodeficiency state, complement deficiency, or phagocytic defect. Particular attention must be directed to the possibility that the infiltrates represent lymphocytic interstitial pneumonitis or opportunistic infection associated with human immunodeficiency virus (HIV) infection (see Sec. 12.83). A history of paroxysmal coughing in an infant suggests pertussis syndrome or cystic fibrosis. Persistent infiltrates, especially with loss of volume, in a toddler should suggest foreign body aspiration.

Overinflation and infiltrates suggest cystic fibrosis or chronic asthma. A "silent chest" with infiltrates should arouse suspicion of alveolar proteinosis, *P. carinii* infection, desquamative interstitial pneumonitis, or tumors. Growth should be carefully assessed to determine whether the lung process has had systemic effects, indicating substantial severity and chronicity as in cystic fibrosis or alveolar proteinosis. Cataracts, retinopathy, or microcephaly suggest in utero infection. Chronic rhinorrhea may be associated with atopic disease, cow's milk intolerance, cystic fibrosis, or congenital syphilis. The absence of tonsils and cervical lymph nodes suggests a combined immunodeficiency state.

Diagnostic studies should be done selectively, based on information obtained from history and physical examination and on a thorough understanding of conditions listed in Table 14–7. Cytologic evaluation of bronchial secretions may be helpful. In patients unresponsive to antibiotics, needle aspiration of the involved area may demonstrate a pathogenic organism. Bronchography, as a rule, is most helpful in identifying surgically approachable focal bronchiectasis and should not be undertaken for routine evaluation of chronic lung infiltrates. Bronchoscopy is indicated for detecting foreign bodies, congenital or acquired anomalies of the tracheobronchial tract, and obstruction by endobronchial or extrinsic masses. In addition, bronchoscopy provides access to secretions which can be studied cytologically and microbiologically. If all appropriate studies have been completed and the condition remains undiagnosed, open lung biopsy may yield a definitive diagnosis.

Optimal medical or surgical treatment of chronic lung infiltrates frequently depends on a specific diagnosis, but chronic conditions may be self-limiting (e.g., severe and prolonged viral infections in infants); in these cases symptomatic therapy may maintain adequate lung function until spontaneous improvement occurs. Helpful measures include inhalation and physical therapy for excessive secretions, antibiotics for secondary bacterial infections, supplementary oxygen for hypoxemia, and maintenance of adequate nutrition. Because the lung of a young child has remarkable recuperative potential, normal lung function may ultimately be achieved with treatment despite the severity of pulmonary insult occurring during infancy.

Anderson VM, Haesoon L: Lymphocytic interstitial pneumonitis in pediatric AIDS. Pediatr Pathol 8:417, 1988.

Boat TF: Cystic fibrosis. *In* Behrman RE (ed): Nelson Textbook of Pediatrics, 14th ed. Philadelphia, WB Saunders, 1991.

Cloutier MM, Loughlin GM: Chronic cough in children: A manifestation of airway hyperreactivity. Pediatrics 67:6, 1981.

Eigen H: The clinical evaluation of chronic cough. Pediatr Clin North Am 29:57, 1982.

Eliasson R, Mossberg B, Camner P, et al: The immotile cilia syndrome. N Engl J Med 297:1, 1977.

Morgan WJ, Taussig LM: The child with persistent cough. Pediatr Rev 8:249, 1987.
Orenstein SR, Orenstein DM: Gastroesophageal reflux and respiratory disease in children. J Pediatr 112:847, 1988.
Skoner D, Caliquiri L: The wheezing infant. Pediatr Clin North Am 35:1011, 1988.
Stagno S, Brasfield DM, Brown MB, et al: Infant pneumonitis associated with cytomegalovirus, chlamydia, pneumocystis, and ureaplasma: A prospective study. Pediatrics 68:322, 1981.

14.89 CYSTIC FIBROSIS

CF is an inherited multisystem disorder of children and adults, characterized chiefly by chronic obstruction and infection of airways and by maldigestion and its consequences. It is the most common life-threatening genetic trait in Caucasians. A dysfunction of the exocrine glands is the predominant pathogenetic feature and is responsible for a broad, variable, and sometimes confusing array of presenting manifestations and complications.

CF is the major cause of severe chronic lung disease of children and is responsible for most exocrine pancreatic insufficiency during early life. It is also responsible for many cases of nasal polyposis, pansinusitis, rectal prolapse, and insulin-dependent hyperglycemia. In addition, CF may present as failure to thrive and occasionally as cirrhosis or other forms of hepatic dysfunction. Therefore, this disorder enters into the differential diagnosis of many pediatric conditions.

GENETICS. CF occurs in approximately 1:2,500 and 1:17,000 live births in white and black populations of the United States, respectively. The estimated incidence worldwide varies from 1:620 in a confined population with Dutch ancestry in Southwest Africa to 1:90,000 in the Oriental population of Hawaii. Generally, the CF gene is most prevalent in Northern and Central Europeans and in individuals who come from these areas.

CF is inherited as an autosomal recessive trait localized to the long arm of chromosome 7. The CF gene has a large domain coding for a protein of 1,480 amino acids, called the CF transmembrane regulator (CFTR), that is inserted into cell membranes and contains features suggestive of a regulatory function or an anion pump or channel. The most common gene mutation results in the deletion of a phenylalanine residue at amino acid 508 (ΔF508) within one of the ATP-binding sites. A sizeable number (>50) of less common mutations of the CFTR gene have been described and also cause the CF syndrome. Many of the uncommon mutations and compound heterozygous patients are associated with less frequent and/or less severe pancreatic and, possibly, lung dysfunction.

The ΔF508 mutation occurs in 70–80% of chromosomes from White and Hispanic Americans with CF, but fewer Southern Europeans (40–50%), American blacks (37%), and even fewer Ashkenazic Jews in North America (30%). Approximately 50% of individuals with CF in North America are homozygous for ΔF508, and 40% are compound heterozygotes, having one ΔF508 allele. Less frequent mutations are responsible for the other 20–30% of CF gene defects. Probes for the normal gene and some mutations are available for detection of patients and carriers from blood cell DNA.

PATHOGENESIS. The basic defect in CF has not been completely identified, but physiologic and genetic studies have narrowed the search considerably. Four observations are of fundamental importance: failure to clear mucous secretions, a paucity of water in mucous secretions, an elevated salt content of sweat and other serous secretions, and chronic infection limited to the respiratory tract. Current evidence suggests that the first three are related closely to each other and the basic genetic abnormality and that infection is a secondary event.

A physiologic basis for these observations has been constructed, starting with the observation that the potential difference across respiratory tract and other epithelia in CF is larger than that of controls. This finding was quickly followed by the determination that the apical membranes of patients with CF are relatively impermeable to chloride ions, resulting in a failure to secrete chloride, and secondarily sodium and water, onto the epithelial surface. In addition, the apical membrane of CF respiratory epithelial cells reabsorbs excessive amounts of sodium under basal conditions, leading to increased salt and water reabsorption from surface secretions. The channels that conduct sodium and chloride ions across the apical membrane are present and functional, but there is altered regulation of their activity. At present, it appears that key phosphorylation steps in cAMP-dependent and C-kinase pathways that up-regulate chloride channels and down-regulate sodium channels are defective, leading to the characteristic electrochemical, ionic, and water abnormalities at epithelial cell surfaces of the exocrine glands.

The product of the CF gene, CFTR, undoubtedly is central to the regulatory abnormality affecting salt and water translocation. A unifying pathogenetic scheme for lung dysfunction suggests that apical membrane ion transport dysfunction produces dehydrated secretions with abnormal clearance properties, which causes air flow obstruction in the lungs, duct obstruction with secondary destruction of exocrine tissue in the pancreas, and excessively sticky lumenal contents and meconium ileus in the gastrointestinal tract. Ion translocation abnormalities also cause obstructive problems in the genitourinary tract, liver, gallbladder, and perhaps other organs. The ion translocation abnormality works in reverse for the sweat gland duct. The primary fluid generated by secretory coils traverses a segment of duct that normally functions to reabsorb chloride and secondarily sodium. Because of epithelial cell membrane impermeability to chloride, this does not occur in CF and excessive amounts of salt are lost in the sweat.

Chronic infection in CF is limited to the respiratory tract. Inhaled bacteria are not promptly cleared and readily colonize the endobronchial space, which ultimately produces an inflammatory reaction. This occurs in peripheral or small airways first, probably because clearance of inspissated secretions is more difficult from these areas. Chronic bronchiolitis and bronchitis are the first lung manifestations of CF followed by bronchiolectasis and bronchiectasis. At this stage the obstruction/infection cycle feeds itself and progression of lung disease goes into an accelerated phase. The predilection of CF airways for colonization with *S. aureus* and *P. aeruginosa* is incompletely understood. Although other organisms are also found in the endobronchial space in lungs with CF, the factor(s) favoring selection of these two organisms may depend on an abnormal cell surface chemistry that promotes adherence of specific bacteria. CF cell surface and secretory glycoconjugates have been shown to be oversulfated, which is perhaps a consequence of fundamental anion translocation abnormalities of the epithelial cells. This factor or related abnormalities could play a role in abnormal surface adherence properties. Although functional deficits may occur in cellular immunity and the alternate pathway for complement as lung infection progresses to advanced stages, the immune system in CF appears to be fundamentally intact. Nutritional deficits, including fatty acid deficiency, have also been linked to a predisposition for respiratory tract infection. Indeed, the 10–15% of individuals who retain substantial exocrine pancreatic function have statistically lower sweat chloride values and delayed onset of chronic lung disease. However, nutritional factors are only in part contributory, because preservation of pancreatic function does not preclude development of typical lung disease.

PATHOLOGY. Striking changes are characteristically observed in the organs that secrete mucus. Eccrine sweat glands and parotid salivary glands, including ducts, are not involved pathologically despite abnormalities in the electrolyte content of their secretory product.

The earliest pathologic lesion in the *lung* is that of bronchiolitis (i.e., mucous plugging and an inflammatory response in the walls of the small airways). With time, mucus accumulation and inflammation extend to the larger airways (bronchitis). Goblet cell hyperplasia and submucosal gland hypertrophy become prominent pathologic expressions of a hypersecretory state, which is most likely a response to chronic airways infection. Organisms appear to be confined to the endobronchial space; invasive bacterial infection is not characteristic. With longstanding disease, evidence of airway destruction such as bronchiolar obliteration as well as bronchiolectasis and then bronchiectasis becomes prominent. Scanning electron microscopy of the airway surface remains normal, except for scattered areas of squamous cell metaplasia, but freeze fracture studies have noted alterations of tight junctions and apical membrane changes that are probably caused by chronic inflammation. Bronchiectatic cysts and emphysematous bullae or subpleural blebs are frequent with advanced lung disease, the upper lobes being most commonly involved. These enlarged air spaces may rupture and cause pneumothorax. Interstitial disease is not a prominent (common) feature, although areas of fibrosis appear eventually. True emphysema occurs but is not a general pathologic finding. Bronchial arteries are enlarged and tortuous, contributing to a propensity for hemoptysis in bronchiectatic airways. Small pulmonary arteries eventually display medial hypertrophy, which would be expected in secondary pulmonary hypertension.

The *paranasal sinuses* are uniformly filled with secretions, and the lining contains hyperplastic and hypertrophied secretory elements.

The *pancreas* is usually small, occasionally cystic, and often difficult to find at post mortem examination. The extent of involvement varies at birth. In infants, the acini and ducts are often distended and filled with eosinophilic material. In 85–90% of patients, the lesion progresses to complete or almost complete disruption of acini and replacement of exocrine pancreas with fibrous tissue and fat. Infrequently, foci of calcification may be seen on roentgenograms of the abdomen. The islets of Langerhans contain a normal number of β cells, although they may begin to show architectural disruption by fibrous tissue during the 2nd decade of life.

The *intestinal tract* shows only minimal changes. Esophageal and duodenal glands are often distended with mucous secretions. Concretions may form in the appendiceal lumen or cecum. Crypts of the appendix and rectum may be dilated and filled with secretions.

Focal biliary cirrhosis secondary to blockage of intrahepatic bile ducts is uncommon in early life, although it is responsible for occasional cases of prolonged neonatal jaundice. This lesion becomes more prevalent and extensive with age and is found in 25% or more of patients at post mortem. Infrequently, this process proceeds to symptomatic multilobular biliary cirrhosis that has a distinctive pattern of large irregular parenchymal nodules and interspersed bands of fibrous tissue. In addition, approximately 30% of patients have fatty infiltration of the liver, in some cases despite apparently adequate nutrition. At autopsy, hepatic congestion secondary to cor pulmonale is frequently observed. The gallbladder may be hypoplastic and filled with mucoid material and not infrequently contains stones. The epithelial lining often displays extensive mucous metaplasia. Atresia of the cystic duct and stenosis of the distal common bile duct have been observed.

Mucous-secreting *salivary glands* are usually enlarged and display focal plugging and dilation of ducts.

Glands of the uterine cervix are distended with mucus, and copious amounts of mucus collect in the cervical canal. Endocervicitis may be prevalent in teenagers and young women. In more than 95% of males, the body and tail of the epididymis, the vas deferens, and the seminal vesicles are obliterated or atretic.

Generalized amyloidosis has been reported rarely (Sec. 25.2).

CLINICAL MANIFESTATIONS. Mutational heterogeneity and other factors appear responsible for highly variable involvement of the lung, pancreas, and other organs. A list of presenting manifestations is lengthy (Table 14–8).

Respiratory Tract. Cough is the most constant symptom of pulmonary involvement. At first the cough may be dry and hacking, but eventually it becomes loose and productive. In older patients, the cough is most prominent on arising in the morning or after activity. Expectorated mucus is usually purulent. Some patients remain asymptomatic for long periods or seem to have only prolonged acute respiratory infections. Others develop a chronic cough within the first weeks of life or they repeatedly develop pneumonia. Extensive bronchiolitis is attended by wheezing, which is a frequent symptom during the 1st years of life. As lung disease progresses, exercise intolerance, shortness of breath, and failure to gain weight or grow are noted. Exacerbations of lung symptoms eventually require hospitalization for effective treatment. Finally, cor pulmonale, respiratory failure, and death supervene. Colonization with *P. cepacia* has been associated with particularly rapid pulmonary deterioration and death.

Early physical findings include increased anteroposterior diameter of the chest, generalized hyper-resonance, scattered or localized coarse crackles, and digital clubbing. Expiratory wheezes may be heard, especially in young children. Cyanosis is a late sign. Common pulmonary complications include atelectasis, hemoptysis, pneumothorax, and cor pulmonale and usually appear beyond the 1st decade of life.

Even though roentgenographically the paranasal sinuses are virtually always opacified, acute sinusitis is infrequent. Nasal obstruction and rhinorrhea are common, due either to inflamed, swollen mucous membranes or, in some cases, to nasal polyposis.

Intestinal Tract. In almost 10% of newborn infants with CF, the ileum is completely obstructed by meconium (meconium ileus). The frequency is greater (~30%) in siblings born subsequent to a child with meconium ileus, but there does not seem to be an association with a particular genotype. Abdominal distention, emesis, and failure to pass meconium appear within the first 24–48 hr of life (see Sec. 9.42). Abdominal roentgenograms (Fig. 14–17) show dilated loops of bowel with air/fluid levels and frequently a collection of granular, "ground-glass" material in the lower central abdomen. Rarely, meconium peritonitis results from intrauterine rupture of the bowel wall and can be detected roentgenographically by the presence of peritoneal or scrotal calcifications. Meconium plug syndrome occurs with increased frequency in infants with CF but is less specific than meconium ileus for this condition. Ileal obstruction with fecal material *(distal intestinal obstruction syndrome* or *meconium ileus equivalent)* occurs occasionally in older patients, causing cramping abdominal pain and abdominal distention.

More than 85% of children show evidence of maldigestion owing to exocrine pancreatic insufficiency. Symptoms include frequent, bulky, greasy stools and failure to gain weight even when food intake appears to be large. Characteristically, stools contain readily visible droplets of fat. A protuberant abdomen, decreased muscle mass, poor growth, and delayed maturation are typical physical signs. Excessive flatus may be a problem.

Less common gastrointestinal manifestations include intus-

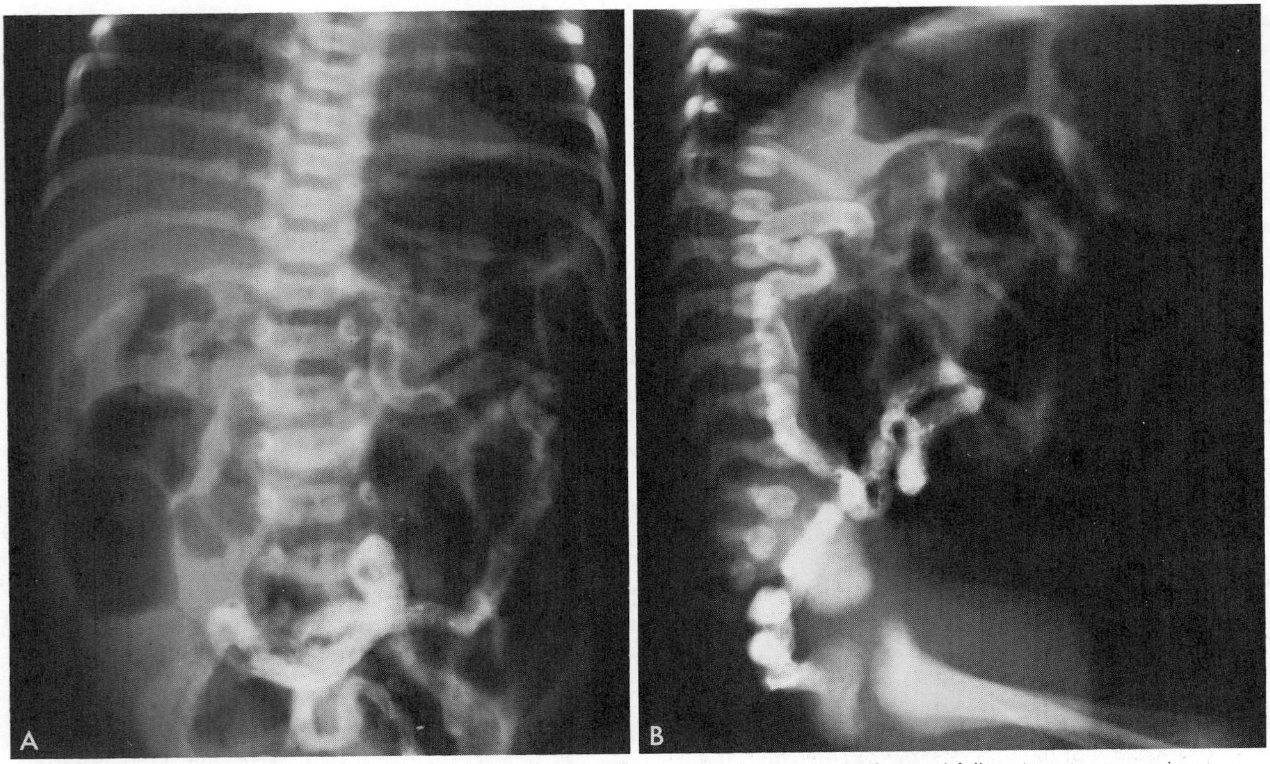

Figure 14–17. *A* and *B*, Contrast enema in a newborn infant with abdominal distention and failure to pass meconium. Note the small diameter of the sigmoid and ascending colon and dilated, air-filled loops of small intestine. Several air-fluid levels in the small bowel are seen on the upright lateral view.

susception, fecal impaction of the cecum or appendix with an asymptomatic right lower quadrant mass, and epigastric pain owing to duodenal inflammation. Subacute appendicitis and periappendiceal abscess have been encountered. Rectal prolapse is relatively frequent. Occasionally, hypoproteinemia with anasarca appears in malnourished infants, especially if children are fed soy-base preparations. Neurologic dysfunction may be accompanied by hemolytic anemia owing to vitamin E deficiency. Deficiency of fat-soluble vitamins is occasionally symptomatic. For example, hypoprothrombinemia owing to vitamin K deficiency may result in a bleeding diathesis. Clinical manifestations of other fat-soluble vitamin deficiencies, such as decreased bone density and night blindness, have been noted. Rickets is rare.

Biliary Tract. Biliary cirrhosis becomes symptomatic in only 2–3% of patients. Manifestations may include icterus, ascites, hematemesis from esophageal varices, and evidence of hypersplenism. A neonatal hepatitis-like picture and massive hepatomegaly owing to steatosis have been reported. Biliary colic secondary to cholelithiasis may occur in the 2nd decade of life.

Pancreas. In addition to exocrine pancreatic insufficiency, evidence for hyperglycemia and glycosuria including polyuria and weight loss may appear, especially after 10 yr of age when 8% of individuals develop diabetes. In most cases, ketoacidosis does not occur, but eye, kidney, and other vascular complications have been noted in patients living 10 yr or more after the onset of hyperglycemia. Recurrent acute pancreatitis occurs occasionally in individuals who have residual exocrine pancreatic function.

Genitourinary Tract. Sexual development is often delayed, but only by an average of 2 yr. More than 95% of males are azoospermic because of failure of development of wolffian duct structures, but sexual function is generally unimpaired. The incidence of inguinal hernia, hydrocele, and undescended testicle is higher than expected. Adolescent females may experience secondary amenorrhea, especially with exacerbations of pulmonary disease. Cervicitis and accumulation of tenacious mucus in the cervical canal have been noted. The female fertility rate is diminished. Pregnancy is generally tolerated well by women with good pulmonary function but may cause a progression of pulmonary disease and even death in those with moderate or advanced lung problems.

Sweat Glands. Excessive loss of salt in the sweat predisposes young children to salt depletion episodes, especially during the time of gastroenteritis and during warm weather. These children present with hypochloremic alkalosis. Frequently, parents note salt "frosting" of the skin or a salty taste when they kiss the child.

DIAGNOSIS AND ASSESSMENT. The diagnosis of CF has been based for many years on a positive quantitative sweat test in conjunction with one or more of the following: typical chronic obstructive pulmonary disease, documented exocrine pancreatic insufficiency, or a positive family history. In a few cases, the sweat test may be in the intermediate range (40–60 mEq/L), and normal range sweat concentrations have been reported in a number of patients. Therefore, for definitive diagnosis the sweat test will undoubtedly be supplemented by DNA analysis as soon as probes are available for all mutations contributing to the CF syndrome.

Sweat Testing. The sweat test, using pilocarpine iontophoresis to collect sweat and chemical analysis of its chloride content, is the only currently accepted diagnostic test. Indications are enumerated in Table 14–8. The procedure requires care and accuracy. A 3-mA electric current is used to carry pilocarpine into the skin of the forearm and locally stimulate the sweat glands. After washing the arm with distilled water, sweat is collected on filter paper or gauze or with a capillary tube that has been placed on the stimulated skin and covered to prevent evaporation. After 30–60 min, the filter paper is

TABLE 14–8. Presenting Manifestations: Indications for Sweat Testing*

Pulmonary	Gastrointestinal
Chronic or productive cough	Meconium ileus, meconium plug syndrome
Recurrent or chronic pneumonia or infiltrates	Steatorrhea, malabsorption
Recurrent bronchiolitis	Rectal prolapse
Atelectasis	Biliary cirrhosis, portal hypertension, bleeding esophageal varices
Hemoptysis	Hypoprothrombinemia beyond newborn period
Infection with *Pseudomonas* (mucoid)	Hypoproteinemia, anasarca
Staphylococcal pneumonia	Deficiency of vitamins A, D, E, or K
Other	
Family history of cystic fibrosis	
Failure to thrive	
Salty taste when kissed	
Nasal polyps	
Unexplained hypochloremic alkalosis	
Pansinusitis	
Absence of sperm in semen	

*Individuals with cystic fibrosis may present initially with any of these signs or symptoms.

removed, weighed, and eluted in distilled water. A chloridometer is recommended for the analysis of chloride in these samples. The amount of sweat collected should be measured and reported. For reliable results, at least 50 mg and preferably 100 mg of sweat should be collected. In infants, it may be necessary to use the upper back to obtain enough sweat. Reliable testing may be difficult in the first few weeks of life because of low sweat rates. Positive results on tests should be confirmed; a negative result on a test should be repeated if suspicion of the diagnosis remains.

More than 60 mEq/L of chloride in sweat is diagnostic of CF when one or more other criteria are present. Values between 40 and 60 mEq/L suggest CF and have been reported in cases with typical involvement. In healthy adults, the sweat chloride values increase slightly but 60 mEq/L chloride still adequately distinguishes CF from other conditions. Chloride concentrations in sweat are somewhat lower in individuals who retain exocrine pancreatic function but remain within the diagnostic range. False-negative results on tests may be encountered in children with hypoproteinemic edema.

Non-CF conditions associated with elevated concentrations of sweat electrolytes include untreated adrenal insufficiency, ectodermal dysplasia, hereditary nephrogenic diabetes insipidus, glucose 6-phosphatase deficiency, hypothyroidism, hypoparathyroidism, familial cholestasis, pancreatitis, mucopolysaccharidoses, fucosidosis, and malnutrition. Most of these conditions can be easily distinguished from CF by clinical criteria.

Other Diagnostic Tests. The finding of increased potential differences across nasal epithelium and the loss of this difference with topical amiloride application has been used to confirm the diagnosis in patients with equivocal or frankly normal sweat chloride values. Failure to sweat when a combination of isoproterenol and atropine is injected into the skin has also been used to characterize CF variants. Both of these tests are considered experimental; neither has been systematically assessed in large populations of CF and appropriate control subjects.

Pancreatic Function. Exocrine pancreatic dysfunction is clinically apparent in many patients. However, documentation is desirable if there are questions about the functional status of the pancreas. Measurement of fat balance with a 3-day stool collection or direct documentation of enzyme secretion after duodenal intubation and pancreozymin-secretin stimulation are reliable measures but are excessively cumbersome or invasive for children and are not used routinely. Quantitation of trypsin and chymotrypsin activity in a fresh stool sample is a useful screening test but is not definitive. Measurement of immunoreactive trypsinogen in serum reliably distinguishes patients with CF, with and without pancreatic insufficiency, after 7 yr of age but not before that time. Other indirect measures of pancreatic enzyme secretion are available but have limited clinical value. Endocrine pancreatic dysfunction may be more prevalent than previously recognized. Some have advocated yearly monitoring of glycosylated hemoglobin levels after 10 yr of age. This approach is more sensitive than spot checks of blood and urine glucose levels.

Radiology. Pulmonary radiologic findings suggest the diagnosis but are not specific. Hyperinflation of lungs occurs early and may be overlooked in the absence of infiltrates or streaky densities. Bronchial thickening and plugging and ring shadows suggesting bronchiectasis first appear in the upper lobes. Nodular densities, patchy atelectasis, and confluent infiltrates follow. Hilar lymph nodes may be prominent. With advanced disease, impressive hyperinflation with markedly depressed diaphragms, anterior bowing of the sternum, and a narrow cardiac shadow are noted. Cyst formation, extensive bronchiectasis, dilated pulmonary artery segments, and segmental or lobar atelectasis are often apparent. Bronchography is not required for the documentation of bronchiectasis, but chest CT imaging clearly delineates the distortion of conducting airways. Typical progression of lung disease is seen in Figure 14–18.

Roentgenograms of paranasal sinuses reveal panopacification and often failure of frontal sinus development.

Pulmonary Function. Pulmonary function studies are not obtained reliably until 4–6 yr of age, by which time most patients show the typical pattern of obstructive pulmonary involvement (see Sec. 14.2–14.6). Decrease in the mid-maximal flow rate is an early functional change, reflecting small airways obstruction. This lesion also affects the distribution of ventilation and increases the alveolar-arterial oxygen difference. The findings of obstructive airway disease and modest responses to a bronchodilator are consistent with the diagnosis of CF at all ages. Residual volume and functional residual capacity are increased early in the course of lung disease. Restrictive changes, characterized by declining total lung capacity and vital capacity, correlate with extensive lung injury and fibrosis and are a late finding. Testing several times a year can be used to evaluate the effect of therapy and the course of the pulmonary involvement. A few patients reach adolescent or adult life with normal routine tests and without evidence of overinflation.

Microbiology. The finding of *S. aureus* or *P. aeruginosa* on culture of the lower airways (e.g., sputum) strongly suggests a diagnosis of CF. In particular, mucoid forms of *Pseudomonas* are virtually diagnostic of CF in children.

Heterozygote Detection and Prenatal Diagnosis. Linkage analysis can usually be used to identify the presence of a CF gene mutation in siblings or a fetus but only when the entire family is available for analysis. More rapid and individual assessment can now be carried out using specific probes for CF gene mutations. The rationale for prenatal detection and termination of pregnancy is currently a matter of considerable discussion, because expected longevity is approximately 3 decades on average, with promise for even better prognosis in the future.

Newborn Screening. Most newborns with CF can be identified by determination of immunoreactive trypsinogen in blood spots. However, this test is neither sufficiently sensitive nor specific for mass screening programs. Newborn screening of the future will undoubtedly rely on genotyping procedures. However, questions continue to be raised about the advisability of this approach. Although early nutritional deficits can

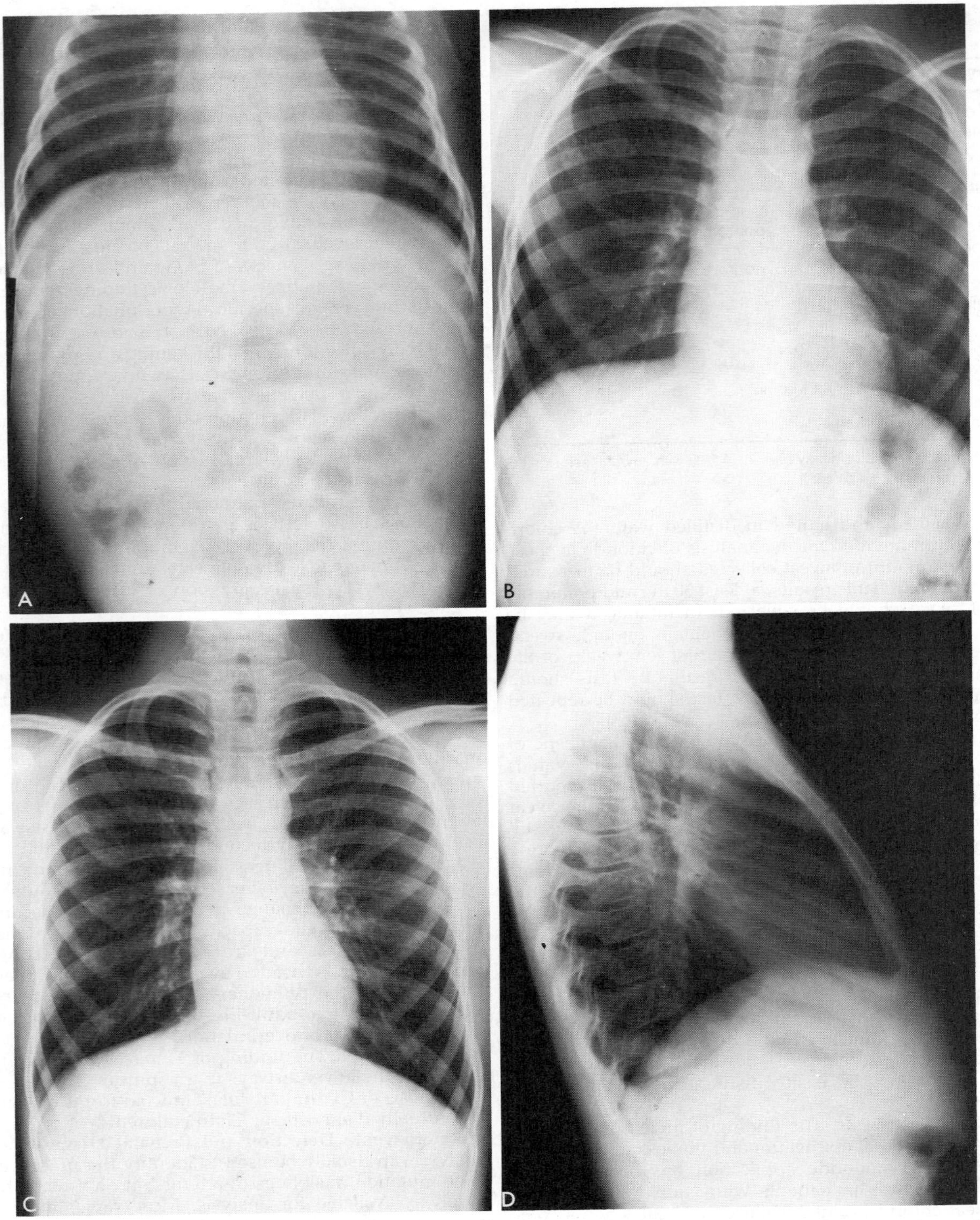

Figure 14–18. Roentgenographic progression of cystic fibrosis lung disease from the diagnosis in an infant to 17 yr of age. *A,* Admitted with cough and wheezing at 2 mo of age. Note the mild increase in bronchovascular markings especially in the upper lobe areas. *B,* At age 4 yr, cough was minimal. A mild increase in bronchovascular markings was present, and there was some improvement in the upper lobes. The wheeze never recurred. *C and D,* At age 13 yr, there was minimal cough and occasional sputum production. The bronchovascular markings were generally further increased with early bronchiectatic changes in the right upper lobe. The lateral view does not suggest overinflation.

be detected and remedied, the ability to influence longevity by early detection has not been demonstrated. This approach may have more appeal when therapeutic interventions aimed at the fundamental defect are available.

TREATMENT. The treatment plan should be comprehensive and linked to close monitoring and early, aggressive intervention.

General Approach to Care. A period of hospitalization for

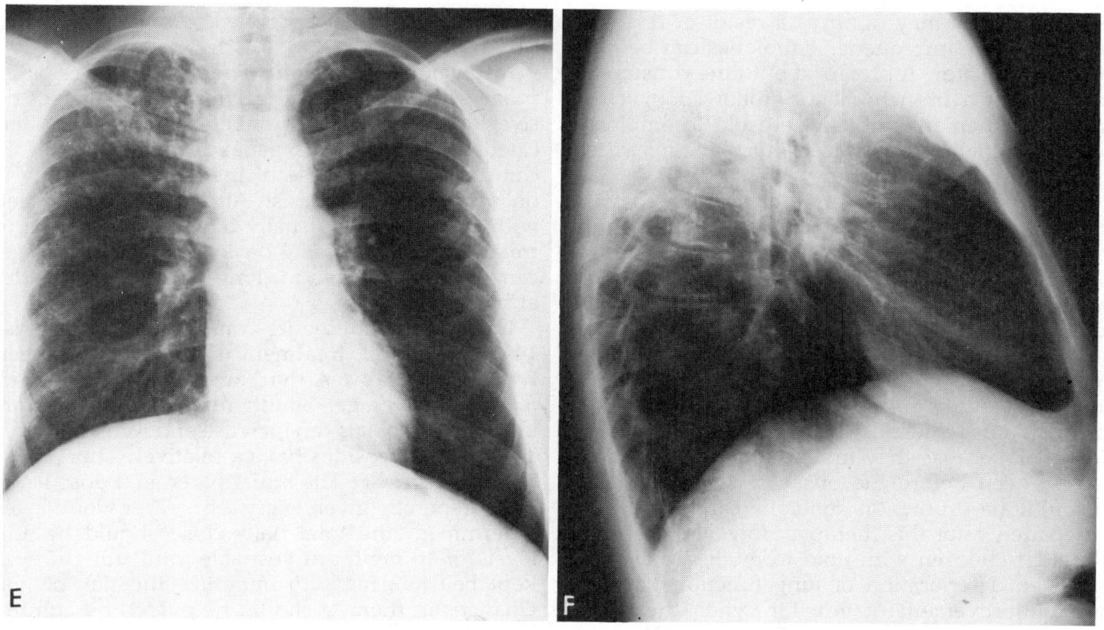

Figure 14–18 ***Continued.*** *E* and *F*, Age 18 yr. During adolescence, cough and sputum production increased even though outpatient antibiotic therapy was intensified. Small volume hemoptysis, occasional paroxysms of cough, and weight loss as well as increased nodular infiltrates (especially in the right upper lobe, and hyperinflation (as seen on the lateral view) led to the 1st hospitalization since infancy. Height and weight were maintained in the 25th–50th percentile.

accurate diagnosis, baseline assessment, initiation of treatment, clearing of the pulmonary involvement, and education of the patient and parents is recommended. The patient is hospitalized for as long as is necessary to reverse pulmonary findings and to achieve steady weight gain. Follow-up outpatient visits are scheduled at least every 2–3 mo because many aspects of the condition require careful monitoring. An interval history and physical examination should be obtained at each visit. A sputum sample or, if that is not available, a lower pharyngeal swab taken during or after a forced cough is obtained for culture and antibiotic susceptibility studies. Even asymptomatic patients may produce sputum after forced exhalations or pharyngeal stimulation with a swab. Because progressive and irreversible loss of pulmonary function from low-grade infection can occur very gradually, without acute symptoms, emphasis is placed on a thorough pulmonary history. Changes in cough frequency or productivity, the appearance of nocturnal cough, the onset of paroxysmal cough with or without vomiting, or hemoptysis all indicate exacerbation of pulmonary infection. New crackles, irritability, decreased activity, decreased appetite, and failure to gain weight may also reflect increased pulmonary infection. All suggest the need for altered or increased antibiotic and physical therapy. Immunoprophylaxis specifically against rubeola, pertussis, and influenza is essential. A nurse, respiratory therapist or physical therapist, social worker, dietitian, and psychologist should participate in the care program. Considerable education and encouragement are required if the patient and parent are to maintain an adequate level of home care.

The goal of therapy is to maintain a stable condition for prolonged periods. This can be accomplished for most patients by interval evaluation and adjustments of the home treatment program. However, some patients have episodic acute or low-grade chronic lung infection that progresses. For these patients, rehospitalization for 2 wk or more of intensive inhalation and physical therapy and intravenous antibiotics is indicated. Such admissions may be required infrequently or as often as every 2–3 mo. Significant improvement in pulmonary function and the patient's well-being is usually achieved.

The basic daily care program varies depending on the age of the patient, the degree of pulmonary involvement, other system involvement, and time available for therapy. The major components of this care are pulmonary and nutritional therapy.

Pulmonary Therapy. The object is to clear secretions from airways and to control infection. There is a divergence of opinion about specific aspects of therapy. However, the effectiveness of the overall approach, including close supervision, continuity of care, aggressive intervention, and an optimistic outlook, is more important than minor variations in the use of individual measures. When an individual patient is not doing well, every potentially useful aspect of therapy should be considered. Because of the large numbers of medications used, iatrogenic complications are frequent and deserve full consideration.

INHALATION THERAPY. Aerosol therapy is used to deliver medications and water to the lower respiratory tract. It is often given before or after segmental postural drainage. Some medications such as bronchodilators can be delivered by metered dose inhaler with or without a spacer. The mainstay is intermittent delivery using a small compressor that drives a hand-held nebulizer. Intermittent positive pressure breathing does not improve delivery of the aerosol and may aggravate the obstructive lesion. The basic aerosol solution is normal saline. In patients with reactive airways, albuterol or other β-agonists can be added. Alternatively or in addition, cromolyn sodium can be administered by this route. β-Agonists may decrease Pa_{O_2} by increasing ventilation-perfusion mismatch and decrease airway wall tone, resulting in enhanced airway collapse during expiration.

When the airway pathogens are resistant to oral antibiotics or when the infection is difficult to control at home, aerosolized antibiotics may reduce symptoms, especially those referable to tracheitis or bronchitis. Twenty to 80 mg of colistimethate, gentamicin, or tobramycin in 1–2 mL of saline has been used 2–4 times daily in home therapy and also in the hospital in conjunction with intravenous therapy. Some advocate even larger doses of aminoglycosides. Carbenicillin (1 g) and ticarcillin (0.5 g) have also been used. Sensitization or resistance to antibiotics may occur as a result of this use, but both are surprisingly infrequent. Antibiotics can be nebulized with a bronchodilator. A preferred but time-consuming regimen is delivery of a bronchodilator, followed by chest physical therapy and then an antibiotic aerosol. Recombinant DNase shows promise as an aerosolized mucolytic for assisting with clearance of purulent sputum.

Nebulization of *N*-acetylcysteine should be initiated with great caution. This mucolytic is toxic to ciliated epithelium and may do more harm than good. Prolonged administration (>2–3 days) should be avoided.

CHEST PHYSICAL THERAPY (PT). This treatment usually consists of chest percussion combined with postural drainage and derives its rationale from the idea that cough clears mucus from large airways, but that chest vibrations are required to move secretions from small airways where expiratory flow rates are low. Chest PT may be particularly useful for patients with CF because they first accumulate secretions in small airways, even before the onset of symptoms. Improvement of pulmonary function generally cannot be demonstrated immediately after this therapy. However, cessation of chest PT in older children with mild to moderate air flow limitation results in deterioration of lung function within 3 wk and prompt improvement of function when therapy is resumed. Chest PT is recommended 1–4 times a day depending on severity of lung dysfunction. Cough or forced expirations are encouraged after each lung segment is "drained." Mechanical percussors have been designed to assist with therapy and may be useful, especially for adolescents. Many care centers recommend that chest PT be preceded by inhalation therapy. Voluntary coughing, repeated forced expiratory maneuvers, and vigorous exercise have all been suggested as aids to mucus clearance but probably cannot substitute entirely for a regular regimen of chest PT.

ANTIBIOTIC THERAPY. Antibiotics are the mainstay of therapy designed to control progression of lung infection. The goal is to reduce the intensity of endobronchial infection and to delay progressive lung damage. Differentiation of colonization from infection is a recurring problem, and the usual guidelines for acute chest infections, such as fever, tachypnea, or chest pain, are often absent. Consequently, all aspects of the patient's history and examination, including anorexia, weight loss, and diminished activity, must be utilized to guide the frequency and duration of therapy. Antibiotic treatment varies from intermittent short courses of one antibiotic to continuous treatment with one or more antibiotics. Dosages are often two to three times the amount recommended for minor infections because patients with CF have proportionately more lean body mass and higher clearance rates for many antibiotics than do other individuals. In addition, it is difficult to achieve effective drug levels of many antimicrobials in respiratory tract secretions.

Oral Antibiotic Therapy. Indications include the presence of respiratory tract symptoms and identification of pathogenic organisms in respiratory tract cultures. Whenever possible, the choice of antibiotics should be guided by in vitro sensitivity testing. Common organisms include *S. aureus*, nontypeable *H. influenzae*, and *P. aeruginosa*. *P. cepacia* is encountered with increasing frequency. The first two can be eradicated from the CF respiratory tract, but *Pseudomonas* is more difficult to treat and rarely is eradicated. The usual course of therapy is 2 wk or more, and maximal doses are recommended. Low-dose, continuous antibiotic therapy is not recommended because organisms tend to develop resistance. Useful oral antibiotics are listed in Table 14–9. Some antimicrobials such as chloramphenicol are effective even when they are not indicated by microbial sensitivity testing. Use of tetracycline should be avoided in children under 9 yr of age. Ciprofloxacin, the only broadly effective oral antibiotic for *Pseudomonas* infection, is not yet approved for children less than 12 yr of age.

Intravenous Antibiotic Therapy. For the patient who has progressive or unrelenting symptoms and signs despite intensive home measures, intravenous antibiotic therapy is indicated. This therapy is usually initiated in the hospital, but completion of a course of therapy increasingly is completed on an ambulatory basis. Although many patients improve within 7 days, it is usually advisable to extend the period of treatment to at least 14 days. Permanent intravenous access can now be provided for long-term therapy in the hospital or at home.

Intravenous antibiotics commonly used are listed in Table 14–9. In general, treatment of *Pseudomonas* infection requires two drug therapy. A third agent may be required for optimal *S. aureus* coverage. Simultaneous administration of aerosolized antimicrobials can increase endobronchial concentrations. The aminoglycosides have a relatively short half-life in many patients with CF. The initial parenteral dose is noted in Table 14–9, generally given every 8 hr. After blood levels have been determined, the total daily dose should be adjusted. Peak levels of 10 mg/L are desirable, and trough levels should be kept below 2 mg/L to minimize the risk of nephrotoxicity. Changes in therapy should be guided by culture results and by lack of improvement. If patients do not improve, heart failure, reactive airways, and infection with *Aspergillus fumigatus*, *Mycobacteria*, or other unusual organisms should be considered. *P cepacia* may be a particularly resistant organism.

BRONCHODILATOR THERAPY. Reversible airway obstruction occurs in many patients with CF, sometimes in conjunction with frank asthma or acute bronchopulmonary aspergillosis. Reversible obstruction is suggested by improvement of 15% or more in flow rates after inhalation of a bronchodilator. Treatment may include use of β-adrenergic agonists by aerosol, oral sympathomimetic agents, or sustained-release oral theophylline, with the dosage adjusted after blood levels are obtained. Children with CF have a high rate of gastrointestinal symptoms on theophylline. Cromolyn sodium or ipratropium hydrochloride are alternative agents, but their efficacy has not been studied systematically.

ANTI-INFLAMMATORY AGENTS. Corticosteroids appeared to slow the progression of lung disease in children with mild or moderate lung infection in one double-blind study. The rationale for their use includes the reduction of the inflammatory response to endobronchial infection and the reduction of mucus secretion. Side effects such as hyperglycemia requiring insulin therapy have been noted and are now considered prohibitive at high doses, for example, 2 mg/kg and above on alternate days. Aerosolized corticosteroids may be useful for patients with refractory airway reactivity.

ENDOSCOPY AND LAVAGE. Treatment of obstructed airways sometimes includes tracheobronchial suctioning or lavage, especially if atelectasis or mucoid impaction is present. Bronchopulmonary lavage may be performed by the instillation of saline or by a mucolytic agent through a fiberoptic bronchoscope. Antibiotics (usually gentamicin or tobracycin) may also be directly instilled at lavage, transiently achieving a much higher endobronchial concentration than can be obtained by using intravenous therapy. There is no evidence for sustained benefit from repeated endoscopic or lavage procedures.

EXPECTORANTS. Systemic drugs, such as iodides and guaiphenesin, do not effectively assist with the removal of secretions from the respiratory tract.

Treatment of Pulmonary Complications. A number of pulmonary complications require extra attention or special measures.

ATELECTASIS. Lobar atelectasis occurs relatively infrequently; it may be asymptomatic and noted only at the time of a routine chest roentgenogram. Aggressive intravenous

TABLE 14–9. Antimicrobial Agents for CF Lung Infection

Route	Organisms	Agents	Dosage (mg/kg/24 hr)	Doses/24 hr
Oral				
	Staphylococcus aureus	Cloxacillin	50–100	3–4
		Cefaclor	40–60	3
		Clindamycin	20	3–4
		Erythromycin	50–100	3–4
		Amoxicillin/clavulanate	40	3
	Haemophilus influenzae	Amoxicillin	50–100	3
		Trimethoprim-sulfamethoxazole	20*	2–4
		Chloramphenicol	50–100	3–4
	P. aeruginosa	Ciprofloxacin	15–30	3
	Empirical	Tetracycline	50–100	3–4
Intravenous				
	S. aureus	Oxacillin	150–200	4
	P. aeruginosa	Gentamicin or Tobramycin	8–20	1–3
		Amikacin	15–30	2–3
		Netilmicin	6–12	2–3
		Carbenicillin, Ticarcillin Piperacillin, Mezlocillin, or Azlocillin	250–450	4–6
		Ticarcillin/clavulanate	250–450	4–6
		Imipenem/cilastatin	45–90	3–4
	P. aeruginosa and *cepacia*	Ceftazidime	150	3
Aerosol				
	P. aeruginosa	Gentamicin	40–80†	2–4
		Tobramycin	40–80†	
		Carbenicillin	500–1,000†	

*Quantity of trimethoprim.
†mg/dose.

therapy with antibiotics and increased chest physical therapy directed at the affected lobe may be effective. If there is no improvement in 5–7 days, bronchoscopic examination of the airways may be indicated. If the atelectasis does not resolve, continued intensive home therapy is indicated, since atelectasis may resolve during a period of weeks or months. Persistent atelectasis may be asymptomatic. However, lobectomy should be considered if expansion is not achieved and the patient has progressive difficulty from fever, anorexia, and unrelenting cough. Lobectomy should be performed only after a period of hospitalization for intensive therapy to improve the status of all remaining parts of the lung.

Hemoptysis. Endobronchial bleeding usually reflects airway wall erosion secondary to infection; dilated bronchial arteries are contributory. With increasing numbers of older patients, hemoptysis has become a relatively frequent complication. Blood streaking of sputum is particularly common. Small volume hemoptysis ($<$20 mL) should not trigger panic and is usually viewed as a need for intensified antimicrobial and chest physical therapy. When the hemoptysis is persistent or increases in severity, hospital admission is indicated. Massive hemoptysis, defined as total blood loss of 250 mL or more within a 24-hr period, requires close monitoring, including a fresh sputum culture and a blood sample for cross-match. Chest physical therapy is often discontinued until 12–24 hr after the last brisk bleeding episode and is then reinstituted gradually. Patients should receive vitamin K in the event of an abnormal prothrombin time. During brisk hemoptysis the patient requires a great deal of reassurance that the bleeding will stop. Blood transfusion is not indicated unless there is hypotension or the hematocrit is significantly reduced. Ticarcillin may interfere with platelet function and aggravate hemoptysis. Bronchoscopy has been used in an effort to localize the site of bleeding. However, usually no bleeding site is found. Lobectomy should be avoided, if possible, because functioning lung should be preserved and because it is difficult to be certain of the bleeding site. Bronchial artery embolization can be useful to control persistent, significant hemoptysis.

Pneumothorax. This is encountered, especially in older patients, and may be life-threatening. The episode may be asymptomatic but is often attended by chest and shoulder pain, shortness of breath, or hemoptysis. Even mild symptoms should be taken seriously, and a chest roentgenogram should be obtained. If the pneumothorax is smaller than 5–10%, the patient is admitted to the hospital and observed. A pneumothorax greater than 10% or under tension requires rapid, definitive treatment. Because of frequent delayed closure of the air leak and a high rate of recurrence with closed thoracotomy, an open thoracotomy through a small incision with plication of blebs, apical pleural stripping, and basal pleural abrasion is recommended after the first occurrence and within 24 hr of the diagnosis. This procedure is well tolerated even in cases of advanced lung disease. Intravenous antibiotics are begun on admission. The thoracotomy tube is removed as soon as possible, usually on the 2nd or 3rd postoperative day. The patient can then be mobilized, and full postural drainage therapy can be resumed. Recurrences, intraoperative complications, and deaths are rare as a result of this procedure. Closed thoracotomy in conjunction with a sclerosing agent continues to be used by some specialists. Rarely, bilateral simultaneous pneumothorax is encountered; in this case, control of the air leak must be achieved immediately, at least on one side.

Allergic Aspergillosis. This complication may present with wheezing, increased cough, shortness of breath, or marked hyperinflation on pulmonary function testing (see also Sec. 12.108 and 14.65). In some patients there are new, focal infiltrates on the chest roentgenogram. The presence of rust-colored sputum, the recovery of aspergillus from the sputum, the demonstration of antibodies against *Aspergillus fumigatus*, or the presence of eosinophils in fresh sputum sample support the diagnosis. The serum IgE level may be very high. Treatment is directed at controlling the inflammatory reaction with corticosteroid therapy. This condition is usually self-limited and will subside with several weeks of therapy. For refractory cases, aerosolized amphotericin B or systemic 5-fluorocytosine may be required.

Hypertrophic Osteoarthropathy. This complication causes elevation of the periosteum over the distal portions of long bones and bone pain, overlying edema, and joint effusions. Acetaminophen or ibuprofen may provide relief. Control of lung infection usually reduces symptoms. Intermittent arthropathy unrelated to other rheumatologic disorders occurs occasionally in patients, has no recognized pathogenetic basis, and usually responds to nonsteroidal anti-inflammatory agents.

Acute Respiratory Failure. Acute respiratory failure (see Sec. 14.17) in patients with mild to moderate lung disease rarely occurs and is usually the result of a severe viral illness such as influenza. Because patients with this complication usually regain their previous status, intensive therapy is indicated. In addition to the aerosol, postural drainage, and intravenous antibiotic treatment, oxygen is required to raise the arterial P_{O_2} above 50 mm Hg. A rising P_{CO_2} may require ventilatory assistance. Endotracheal or bronchoscopic suction may be necessary and can be repeated daily. Right-sided heart failure may occur and should be treated vigorously. Recovery is often slow. Intensive intravenous antibiotic therapy and postural drainage should be continued for 1–2 wk after the patient has regained baseline status.

Chronic Respiratory Failure. Patients usually develop chronic respiratory failure from prolonged slow deterioration of lung function. Although this can occur at any age, it is seen more frequently in adolescent and adult patients. Because a longstanding arterial P_{O_2} less than 50 mm Hg promotes the development of right-sided heart failure, they usually benefit from low-flow oxygen to raise arterial P_{O_2} to 55 mm Hg or above. Increasing hypercapnia may prevent the use of optimal F_{IO_2}. These patients do not benefit substantially from continuous ventilator assistance or tracheostomy. Most patients improve somewhat with intensive antibiotic and pulmonary therapy measures and can be discharged from the hospital. Low-flow oxygen therapy at home is needed, especially with sleep. These patients almost always display cor pulmonale and should be maintained on a reduced salt intake and diuretics.

Right-sided Heart Failure. Some patients develop right-sided heart failure as the result of a complication such as an acute viral infection or pneumothorax. Individuals with longstanding, advanced pulmonary disease, especially those with severe hypoxemia (Pa_{O_2} below 50 mm Hg), often develop chronic right-sided heart failure. The mechanisms include hypoxemic pulmonary arterial spasm and loss of pulmonary vasculature with destructive lung disease. Pulmonary artery wall changes contribute to increased vascular resistance with time. Some combination of cyanosis, increased shortness of breath, increased liver size with tender margin, ankle edema, jugular venous distention, an unusual weight gain, increased heart size by chest roentgenogram, or evidence for right-sided heart enlargement by electrocardiogram or echocardiography helps to confirm the diagnosis. Furosemide, 1 mg/kg administered intravenously, may result in a good diuresis and confirm the suspicion of fluid retention. Repeated doses may be required at 24- to 48-hr intervals in the initial period to reduce fluid accumulation and accompanying symptoms. Concomitant use of spironolactone may protect against potassium depletion and facilitate long-term diuresis. Hypochloremic alkalosis may complicate respiratory failure and chronic use of loop diuretics. Digitalis is not effective in pure right-sided failure, but it may be useful when there is an associated left-sided dysfunction. The arterial P_{O_2} should be maintained above 50 mm Hg if at all possible. Loss of respiratory drive may occur during the initial phases of oxygen therapy, and serial arterial blood gases or noninvasive monitoring is required to ensure the continuation of adequate ventilation. Intensive pulmonary therapy including intravenous antibiotics is most important. Initially, the salt intake should be limited to 2 g sodium/24 hr; carbenicillin may be hazardous because of its relatively high sodium content. Fluid overload should be avoided. No clear-cut long-term benefit from pulmonary vasodilators has been demonstrated. In the past, cardiac failure usually meant death within several months. However, the prognosis has been improving, and a number of patients have survived for 5 yr or more after an initial episode of cardiac failure. Combined heart-lung transplantation has been successful in a few patients with severe cor pulmonale (see Sec. 6.46).

Nutritional Therapy. Up to 90% of patients have complete loss of exocrine pancreatic function and inadequate digestion of fats and proteins. They require diet adjustment, pancreatic enzyme replacement, and supplementary vitamins.

Diet. Many infants at the time of diagnosis have nutritional deficits. Young infants who present with wheezy breathing and are fed soy protein formulas do not utilize this protein well and may develop hypoproteinemia with anasarca. Infants do well with formulas containing predigested protein and medium-chain triglycerides. A low-fat, high-protein, high-caloric diet was generally recommended in the past for older children. Some children on this diet became deficient in essential fatty acids. With the advent of improved pancreatic enzyme products, normal amounts of fat in the diet are usually tolerated well.

Most individuals have a higher than normal caloric need because of increased work of breathing and perhaps because of increased metabolic activity related to the basic defect. When anorexia of chronic infection supervenes, weight loss occurs. Further encouragement to eat high caloric foods may be useful, but weight gain generally is not realized unless lung infection is controlled. With advanced lung disease, weight stabilization or gain has been achieved by nocturnal feeding via nasogastric tube or percutaneous enterostomy or by intravenous hyperalimentation. Long-term benefits of these interventions for lung function, quality of life, and psychologic well-being are a topic of further study.

Pancreatic Enzyme Replacement. Extracts of animal pancreas given with ingested food reduce but do not fully correct stool fat and nitrogen losses. Enzyme dosage and product should be individualized for each patient. The introduction of pH-sensitive enteric-coated enzyme microspheres has been a major advance in patient care. Several strengths, based on lipase content are available. One to three capsules/meal is sufficient for most patients; infants may need only one-half capsule or may prefer pancreatin powder. The microsphere preparations usually are sufficiently effective to permit a liberal diet, which may include homogenized milk. Although patients with CF display bile salt malabsorption, enzyme preparations containing bile salts are infrequently needed. The dose of enzymes required usually increases with age, but some teenagers and young adults may later have a decrease in their requirement.

Vitamin and Mineral Supplement. Because pancreatic insufficiency results in malabsorption of fat-soluble vitamins (A, D, E, and K), vitamin supplementation is recommended. Vitamins A and D can be supplied by one of several multivitamin preparations. Vitamin E deficiency is usually corrected with daily doses of 100–200 units. Vitamin K is needed only sporadically: in the newborn period, and during periods of hemoptysis, intense antimicrobial therapy, or surgery. The usual dose is 5 mg orally given twice weekly. Infants with zinc deficiency and rash have been reported. In addition, attention should be paid to iron status; in one study almost one third of patients with CF had a low serum ferritin concentration.

Treatment of Intestinal Complications

MECONIUM ILEUS (see Sec. 9.42). When meconium ileus is suspected, a nasogastric tube is placed for suction and the infant is hydrated. In some cases Gastrografin enemas with reflux of contrast material into the ileum have resulted in the passage of a meconium plug and clearing of the obstruction. Use of this hypertonic solution requires careful replacement of water losses into the bowel. Patients who fail this procedure require operative intervention. Individuals who are successfully treated generally have a prognosis similar to that of other patients. Infants with meconium ileus should be treated as having CF until adequate sweat testing can be carried out, usually after 1–2 wk of life.

DISTAL INTESTINAL OBSTRUCTION SYNDROME (MECONIUM ILEUS EQUIVALENT) AND OTHER CAUSES OF ABDOMINAL PAIN. Despite appropriate pancreatic enzyme replacement, some patients accumulate fecal material in the terminal portion of the ileum and in the cecum, which may result in intermittent or complete obstruction. For intermittent obstruction, pancreatic enzyme replacement should be continued or even increased and laxatives or stool softeners (milk of magnesia, Colace, mineral oil) given. Increased fluid intake is also recommended. Failure to relieve symptoms signals the need for large volume bowel lavage with a balanced salt solution containing polyethyleneglycol, taken by mouth or by nasogastric tube. When there is complete obstruction, a Gastrografin enema, accompanied by large amounts of intravenous fluids, can be therapeutic. Intussusception and volvulus must also be considered in the differential diagnosis. Intussusception, usually ileocolic, occurs at any age and often follows a 1- to 2-day history of "constipation." It can often be both diagnosed and reduced by a Gastrografin enema. If a nonreducible intussusception or a voluvlus is present, laparotomy is required. Repeated episodes of intussusception may be an indication for cecectomy.

Chronic **appendicitis** with or without periappendiceal abscess may present with recurrent or persistent abdominal pain, raising the question of need for a laparotomy. A lack of acid buffering in the duodenum appears to promote **duodenitis** and **ulcer** formation in some children. **Bile reflux** into the stomach is seen in older patients. Some patients may obtain relief from antacids or H_2 antagonists.

GASTROESOPHAGEAL REFLUX. Because several factors raise intra-abdominal pressure, including cough and obstructed airways, pathologic gastroesophageal reflux is not uncommon and may exacerbate lung disease secondary to reflex wheezing and repeated aspiration. Cholinergic agonists are contraindicated because they trigger mucus secretion and progressive respiratory difficulty. Nissen fundoplication may improve lung function in selected cases.

RECTAL PROLAPSE. This occurs frequently in infants with CF and less commonly in older children. It is usually related to steatorrhea, malnutrition, and repetitive cough. The prolapsed rectum can usually be replaced manually by continuous gentle pressure with the patient in the knee-chest position. Sedation may be helpful. To prevent an immediate recurrence, the buttocks can be taped closed. Adequate pancreatin replacement, decreased fat and roughage in the diet, and control of pulmonary infection result in improvement. An occasional patient may continue to have rectal prolapse and require surgery (a rectal sling of Silastic placed around the rectum).

LIVER DISEASE. Portal hypertension with esophageal varices, hypersplenism, or ascites is the most common complication of biliary cirrhosis (see Sec. 13.85). The acute management of bleeding esophageal varices includes nasogastric suction and cold saline lavage. Sclerotherapy is recommended after an initial bleed. In the past, significant bleeding has also been treated successfully with portosystemic shunting. Splenorenal anastomosis has been the most effective. Pronounced hypersplenism may require splenectomy. The management of ascites is discussed in Sec. 13.102.

Obstructive jaundice in newborns with CF requires no specific therapy. Hepatomegaly with steatosis requires careful attention to nutrition and may respond to carnitine repletion. Rarely, biliary cirrhosis proceeds to hepatocellular failure, which should be treated as in other patients with hepatic failure (see Sec. 13.97, 13.99, and 13.102). End-stage liver disease is an indication for liver transplantation in children with CF, especially if pulmonary function is good.

PANCREATITIS. Pancreatitis may be precipitated by fatty meals, alcohol ingestion, or tetracycline therapy. Serum amylase and lipase levels may remain elevated for long periods. Treatment is discussed in Sec. 13.78.

HYPERGLYCEMIA. Onset can occur at any age and is not related to the severity of the disease; ketoacidosis is rarely encountered. If blood glucose levels are only moderately or intermittently elevated and urine glucose losses are minimal, no treatment is necessary. With more marked elevation and polyuria, insulin treatment should be instituted. Oral antidiabetic agents have not usually been effective. Exocrine pancreatic insufficiency and malabsorption make strict dietary control of hyperglycemia virtually impossible. The development of significant hyperglycemia may adversely affect prognosis.

Other Therapy

NASAL POLYPS (See also Sec. 14.21.) These occur in 15–20% of patients with CF, are most prevalent in the 2nd decade of life, and in some are a recurrent problem. Corticosteroids and nasal decongestants occasionally provide some relief. Allergy skin testing and hyposensitization may be helpful in those with allergic symptoms. When the polyps completely obstruct the nasal airway or rhinorrhea becomes constant, surgical removal is indicated; polyps may recur promptly after removal but frequently do not grow to the point of obstruction for long periods. Many adults inexplicably stop developing polyps.

SALT DEPLETION. Sweat salt losses can be high, especially in warm arid climates. Children should have free access to salt, and precautions against overdressing infants should be observed.

MATURATION. Delayed sexual maturation, often associated with short stature, occurs fairly frequently. Although many have severe pulmonary infection or poor nutrition, delayed puberty also occurs in patients with otherwise mild disease and is not well explained. Adolescents with CF should receive specific counseling through their developing years concerning sexual maturation and potential reproductive problems.

SURGERY. Minor surgical procedures, including dental work, should be performed under local anesthesia if possible. Patients with good or excellent pulmonary status can tolerate general anesthesia without any intensive pulmonary measures prior to the surgery. Those with moderate or severe pulmonary infection are usually better off with a 1- to 2-wk course of intensive antibiotic treatment before surgery. If this is impossible, prompt intravenous antibiotic therapy is indicated once it is recognized that major surgery will be required. The total time of anesthesia should be kept to a minimum. After induction, tracheal suctioning is useful and should be repeated at least at the end of the operation. Patients with severe disease require monitoring of their blood gases and may require ventilatory assistance in the immediate postoperative period.

After major surgery, cough should be encouraged and postural drainage treatments should be reinstituted as soon as possible, usually within 24 hr. Adequate analgesia is important if early effective therapy is to be achieved. For those with significant pulmonary involvement, intravenous antibiotics are continued for 7–14 postoperative days. Early ambulation and intermittent deep breathing are important; an incentive spirometer can also be helpful. Following open thoracotomy for treatment of pneumothorax or lobectomy, the chest tube is the greatest single obstacle to effective pulmonary therapy and should be removed as soon as possible so that full postural drainage therapy can resume.

PROGNOSIS. CF remains a life-limiting disorder, although survival has improved dramatically during the last 30–40 yr. Infants with severe lung disease occasionally succumb, but most children survive this difficult period and are relatively healthy into adolescence or adulthood. However, the slow progression of lung disease eventually reaches disabling proportions. National life table data now indicate a median cumulative survival approaching 30 yr. Male survival is somewhat better than female survival for reasons that are not readily apparent. Survival beyond 20 yr of treatment exceeds 90% if CF is diagnosed and treatment begun before substantial lung damage has occurred.

For the most part, children with CF have good school attendance records and do not need to be restricted in their activities. A high percentage eventually attend and graduate from college. Most find satisfactory employment, and an increasing number marry.

With increasing life span, a new set of psychosocial considerations has emerged, including dependence-independence issues, self-care, peer relationships, sexuality, sterility, substance abuse, educational and vocational planning, financial burdens, and psychologic reactions to anxiety. Many of these issues are best addressed during childhood and early adolescence, prior to the onset of psychosocial dysfunction. With appropriate medical and psychosocial support, children and adolescents with CF generally cope well. Achievement of an independent and productive adulthood is a realistic goal for many.

THOMAS F. BOAT

Boat TF, Cheng PW: Cystic fibrosis epithelial cell dysfunction: Implications for airway dysfunction. Acta Paediatr Scand Suppl 363, 1990.

Desmond KJ, Schwenk F, Thomas E, et al: Immediate and long-term effects of chest physiotherapy in patients with cystic fibrosis. J Pediatr 103:538, 1983.

Donati MA, Guenette G, Auerbach H: Prospective controlled study of home and hospital therapy of cystic fibrosis pulmonary disease. J Pediatr 111:28, 1987.

Johansen HK, Nir M, Hoiby N, et al: Severity of cystic fibrosis in patients homozygous and heterozygous for ΔF508 mutation. Lancet 337:631, 1991.

Karem E, Corey M, and Karem B, et al: The relation between genotype and phenotype in cystic fibrosis—analysis of the most common mutation (ΔF508). N Engl J Med 323:1517, 1990.

Knowles M, Gatzy J, Boucher R: Increased bioelectric potential difference across respiratory epithelia in cystic fibrosis. N Engl J Med 305:1489, 1981.

Koletzko S, Stringer DA, Cleghorn GJ, et al: Lavage treatment of distal intestinal obstruction syndrome in children with cystic fibrosis. Pediatrics, 83:727, 1989.

Lemna WK, Feldman FL, Kerem B, et al: Mutation analysis for heterozygote detection and the prenatal diagnosis of cystic fibrosis. N Engl J Med 322:291, 1990.

McColley SA, Rosenstein BJ, and Cutting GR: Differences in expression of cystic fibrosis in blacks and whites. Am J Dis Child 145:94, 1991.

Thomassen MJ, Demko AC, Klinger JD, et al: *Pseudomonas cepacia* colonization among patients with cystic fibrosis. Am Rev Respir Dis 131:791, 1985.

Tomashefski Jr, Bruce M, Goldberg HI, et al: Regional distribution of macroscopic lung disease in cystic fibrosis. Am Rev Respir Dis 133:535, 1986.

Welsh MJ, Liedtke CM: Chloride and potassium channels in cystic fibrosis airways epithelia. Nature 322:467, 1986.

DISEASES OF THE PLEURA

14.90 PLEURISY

The most common cause of pleural effusion in children is bacterial pneumonia (Sec. 14.56); heart failure and metastatic intrathoracic malignancy are the second and third. Tuberculous effusion has become much less common with improved screening procedures and chemotherapy. A variety of other diseases, including lupus erythematosus, aspiration pneumonitis, uremia, pancreatitis, subdiaphragmatic abscess, and rheumatoid arthritis, account for the remainder of the cases. Males and females are equally affected.

Inflammatory processes in the pleura are usually divided into three general types: dry or plastic, serofibrinous or serosanguineous, and purulent pleurisy or empyema.

Dry or Plastic Pleurisy

This may be associated with acute bacterial pulmonary infections or may develop during the course of an acute upper respiratory tract illness. The condition is also associated with tuberculosis and with mesenchymal diseases, such as rheumatic fever.

PATHOLOGY. The process is usually limited to the visceral pleura. There are usually small amounts of yellow serous fluid and adhesions between the pleural surfaces. In tuberculosis the adhesions develop rapidly and the pleura is often thickened. Occasionally fibrin deposition and adhesions may be sufficiently severe to produce a fibrothorax that markedly inhibits the excursions of the lung.

CLINICAL MANIFESTATIONS. Signs and symptoms are often overshadowed by the primary disease. The principal symptom is pain, which is exaggerated by deep breathing, coughing, and straining. Occasionally, pleural pain is described as a dull ache, which is less likely to vary with breathing. The pain is often localized over the chest wall and is referred to the shoulder or the back. Pain with breathing is responsible for grunting and guarding of respirations, the child often lying on the affected side in an attempt to decrease respiratory excursions. Early in the illness a leathery, rough, to-and-fro friction rub may be audible, but this usually disappears rapidly. Occasionally, increased dullness on percussion and suppressed breath sounds are heard when the layer of exudate is thick. Pleurisy may also be asymptomatic and detected only on roentgenography; a diffuse haziness at the pleural surface or a dense, sharply demarcated shadow may be noted. The latter finding may be indistinguishable from small amounts of pleural exudate. Chronic pleurisy is occasionally encountered with conditions such as atelectasis, pulmonary abscess, mesenchymal diseases, and tuberculosis.

DIFFERENTIAL DIAGNOSIS. Plastic pleurisy must be distinguished from other diseases, such as epidemic pleurodynia or trauma to the rib cage, particularly fracture of a rib, and from lesions of the dorsal root ganglia, tumors of the spinal cord, herpes zoster, gallbladder disease, and trichinosis. Even if evidence of pleural fluid is not found on physical or roentgenographic examination, a pleural tap in suspected cases often results in the recovery of a small amount of exudate, which, when cultured, usually reveals the underlying bacterial cause in cases associated with an acute pneumonia. Patients with pleurisy and pneumonia should always be screened for tuberculosis.

TREATMENT. Therapy should be aimed at the underlying disease. When pneumonia is present, neither immobilization of the chest with adhesive plaster nor therapy with drugs capable of suppressing the cough reflex is indicated. If pneumonia is not present or is under good therapeutic control, strapping of the chest to restrict expansion may afford relief from pain.

Serofibrinous Pleurisy

This is most commonly associated with infections of the lung or with inflammatory conditions of the abdomen or mediastinum. Less commonly it is found with such mesenchymal diseases as lupus erythematosus, periarteritis, or rheumatic fever. On occasion it is seen with primary or metastatic neoplasms of the lung, pleura, or mediastinum; tumors are, however, more commonly associated with a hemorrhagic pleurisy.

CLINICAL MANIFESTATIONS. Since serofibrinous pleurisy is often preceded by the plastic type, the early signs and symptoms may be those of the latter illness. As fluid accumulates, pleuritic pain may disappear and the patient becomes asymptomatic (so long as the effusion remains small), or there may be only the signs and symptoms of the underlying disease. If a large amount of fluid collects, there may be cough, dyspnea, retractions, tachypnea, orthopnea, or cyanosis. Physical findings depend to some degree on the amount of effusion. Dullness to flatness may be found on percussion. There is a decrease or absence of breath sounds, a diminution in tactile fremitus, a shift of the mediastinum away from the affected side, and, on occasion, fullness of the intercostal spaces. If the fluid is not loculated, these signs may shift with changes in position. In infants, physical signs are less definite; sometimes, instead of decreased or absent breath sounds, bronchial breathing will be heard. If extensive pneumonia is present, rales and rhonchi may also be audible. Friction rubs are usually present only during the early or late plastic stage. The process is usually unilateral.

Roentgenographic examination shows a more or less homogeneous density obliterating the normal markings of the underlying lung. Small effusions may cause only obliteration of the costophrenic or cardiophrenic angles or a widening of the interlobar septa. An examination should be performed both in the supine and in the upright positions to demonstrate a shift of the effusion with change in position; the decubitus position may also be helpful. Ultrasound examinations are very useful.

DIFFERENTIAL DIAGNOSIS. Thoracentesis should be done when pleural fluid is present or is suspected unless the effusion is very small and the patient has a classic lobar pneumococcal pneumonia. An examination of fluid is essential to identify acute bacterial infections and may disclose tubercle bacilli. Furthermore, thoracentesis can differentiate among serofibrinous pleurisy, empyema, hydrothorax, hemothorax, and chylothorax. In hydrothorax the fluid has a specific gravity below 1.015, and only a few mesothelial cells rather than leukocytes. Chylothorax and hemothorax usually have fluid distinctive in appearance; differentiating serofibrinous from purulent pleurisy is impossible without bacterial examination of the fluid. The fluid of serofibrinous pleurisy is clear or slightly cloudy and contains relatively few leukocytes and, occasionally, some erythrocytes. Protein levels greater than 3 g/dL indicate an exudate and are likely to be associated with an infectious process. Similarly, pleural fluid lactic dehydrogenase values higher than 200 IU/L suggest an exudate. Serofibrinous fluid may rapidly become purulent. A pH <7.20 suggests an exudate.

COURSE. Unless the fluid becomes purulent, it usually disappears relatively rapidly, particularly with bacterial pneumonias. It persists somewhat longer with tuberculosis and mesenchymal diseases and may remain or recur for a long time with neoplasms. As the effusion is absorbed, adhesions often develop between the two layers of the pleura, but usually little or no functional impairment results. Pleural thickening may develop and is occasionally mistaken for small quantities of fluid or for pulmonary infiltrates. Pleural thickening may persist for a long time. In general, however, the process disappears, leaving no residua.

TREATMENT. Therapy is that of the underlying diseases. When a diagnostic thoracentesis is done, as much fluid as possible should be removed for therapeutic purposes. If the underlying disease is adequately treated, further drainage is usually unnecessary, but if sufficient fluid reaccumulates to embarrass the patient's respiration, repeated thoracentesis or chest tube drainage should be performed. In older children with parapneumonic effusion, tube thoracostomy is probably necessary if the pleural fluid pH is below 7.20 or the pleural fluid glucose is below 50 mg/dL. If the fluid is clearly purulent (see later), tube drainage is usually indicated. Systemic acidosis reduces the usefulness of pleural fluid pH measurements. Patients with pleural effusions may need analgesia, particularly after thoracentesis or insertion of chest tube. Those with acute pneumonia often need supplemental oxygen in addition to antibiotic treatment.

Glasier CM, Leithiser RE, Williamson SL, et al: Extracardiac chest ultrasonography in infants and children: Radiographic and clinical implications. J Pediatr 114:540, 1989.

Light RW, Girard WM, Jenkinson SG, et al: Parapneumonic effusions. Am J Med 69:507, 1980.

Wolfe WG, Spock A, Bradford WD: Pleural fluids in infants and children. Am Rev Respir Dis 98:1027, 1968.

Purulent Pleurisy
(Empyema)

An accumulation of pus in the pleural spaces is most often associated with pneumonia due to staphylococci, less frequently with pneumococci (especially types 1 and 3) and *H. influenzae*. The relative incidence of *H. influenzae* empyema may have increased recently. In pediatric practice empyema is most frequently encountered in infants (see Sec. 14.56) and preschool children. The disease may also be produced by rupture of a lung abscess into the pleural space, by contamination introduced from trauma or thoracic surgery, or, rarely, by mediastinitis or by the extension of intra-abdominal abscesses.

PATHOLOGY. Most commonly, purulent pleurisy is an extensive process consisting of a series of loculated areas involving a large portion of one or both pleural cavities. Thickening of the parietal pleura occurs. If the pus is not drained, it may dissect through the pleura into lung parenchyma, producing bronchopleural fistulas and pyopneumothorax, or into the abdominal cavity. Pockets of loculated pus may eventually develop into thick-walled abscess cavities, or, as the exudate organizes, the lung may collapse and become surrounded by a thick, inelastic envelope.

CLINICAL MANIFESTATIONS. The initial signs and symptoms are primarily those of bacterial pneumonia. Patients treated inadequately or with inappropriate antibiotic agents may have an interval of a few days between the clinical pneumonic phase and the evidence of empyema. Most patients are febrile. In infants, there may only be a moderate exacerbation of respiratory distress. The older child is likely to appear more toxic and in greater respiratory difficulty. Physical and roentgenographic findings may be identical to those described for serofibrinous pleurisy and the two conditions differentiated only by thoracentesis, which should always be performed when empyema is suspected. (See Serofibrinous Pleurisy, earlier, and Sec. 14.9.) Roentgenographically, finding no shift of fluid with change of position indicates a loculated empyema. The maximum amount of pus obtainable should be withdrawn. The appearance of pus produced by different organisms is not distinctive; cultures must always be obtained and gram-stained smears should be examined for the presence of microorganisms. Blood cultures have a high yield (62% in one series), but latex agglutination may also be useful. Leukocytosis and an elevated sedimentation rate may occur.

COMPLICATIONS. With staphylococcal infections, bronchopleural fistulas and pyopneumothorax commonly develop. Other local complications include purulent pericarditis, pulmonary abscesses, peritonitis secondary to rupture through the diaphragm, and osteomyelitis of the ribs. Septic complications such as meningitis, arthritis, and osteomyelitis may also occur. With staphylococcal empyema, septicemia occurs infrequently; it is often encountered in *H. influenzae* and pneumococcal infections.

TREATMENT. If pus is obtained by thoracentesis, closed drainage should be instituted immediately and controlled either by an underwater seal or by continuous suction. A catheter with the largest possible internal diameter should be inserted into the site where accumulation of pus is suspected; sometimes several tubes are required to drain loculated areas. Closed drainage is usually necessary only for 1 wk or so, even though small amounts of material will continue to drain after this time, probably in response to the presence of the tube in the pleural cavity. Chest tubes that are no longer draining should be removed. When it is time to withdraw it, the entire tube should be removed all at once.

Instilling fibrinolytic agents or proteolytic enzymes into the pleural cavity commonly produces severe systemic reactions in small children and does not promote drainage. Antibiotics should not be instilled into the pleural cavity because they do not improve results obtained with systemic antibiotic therapy alone and are associated with local reactions. Controlling empyema by multiple aspirations of the pleural cavity rather than by closed continuous drainage should not be attempted.

Systemic antibiotic therapy is required; the selection of the antibiotic should be based on the in vitro sensitivities of the responsible organism. Infant staphylococcal empyema is best treated by parenteral routes with methicillin or, when applicable, with penicillin G. Pneumococcal infection usually responds to pencillin, and *H. influenzae* to ampicillin, ceftriaxone, or chloramphenicol (see Sec. 14.56). With staphylococcal infections, resolution of the process is very slow, and systemic antibiotic therapy is required for 3–4 wk. Clinical response in nonstaphylococcal empyema is also often slow, even with optimal treatment; little improvement may occur for up to 2 wk. In patients with inadequately treated empyema, extensive fibrinous changes may take place over the surface of the collapsed lungs, but decortication procedures are rarely indicated. If pneumatoceles form, no attempt should be made to treat them surgically or by aspiration, unless they reach sufficient size to embarrass respiration or become secondarily infected. The long-term clinical prognosis for adequately treated empyema is excellent, but follow-up pulmonary function studies suggest that some restrictive disease is not uncommon.

McLaughlin FJ, Goldmann DA, Rosenbaum DM, et al: Empyema in children: Clinical course and long-term follow-up. Pediatrics 73:587, 1984.
Murphy D, Lockhart CH, Todd JK: Pneumococcal empyema. Am J Dis Child 134:659, 1980.
Ravitch MM, Fein R: The changing picture of pneumonia and empyema in infants and children. A review of the experience at the Harriet Lane Home from 1934 through 1958. JAMA 175:1039, 1961.
Siegel JD, Gartner JC, Michaels RH: Pneumococcal empyema in childhood. Am J Dis Child 132:1094, 1978.

14.91 PNEUMOTHORAX

Pneumothorax in the neonatal period is discussed in Sec. 9.37. In infant staphylococcal pneumonia, the incidence of pneumothorax is relatively high, but other than the accidental introduction of air into the pleural cavity during thoracentesis, pneumothorax is uncommon during childhood. Pneumothorax may occur in pneumonia, usually in connection with empyema; it may also be secondary to pulmonary abscess, gangrene, infarct, rupture of a cyst or an emphysematous bleb (e.g., in asthma), foreign bodies in the lung, and external thoracic trauma or surgical procedures. It is found in about 5% of hospitalized asthmatic children and usually resolves without treatment. Pneumothorax is a serious complication in CF (see Sec. 14.89). In association with mediastinal emphysema it may be a complication of tracheotomy. Pneumothorax also occurs in patients with lymphoma or other malignancy. Spontaneous pneumothorax with or without exertion (valsalva) occurs occasionally in teenagers and in young adults, most frequently in males. Families have been described in which many members have had spontaneous pneumothoraces with onset ranging from birth to adulthood. Patients with collagen synthesis defects such as Ehlers-Danlos disease and Marfan syndrome are also unusually prone to develop pneumothorax. Pneumothorax may also occur after acupuncture treatment. *Catamenial pneumothorax* can result from passage of intra-abdominal air through diaphragmatic defects; therefore, when thoracotomy is performed for recurrent pneumothorax of unknown etiology, an examination of the diaphragm may be appropriate.

Pneumothorax may be associated with a serous effusion *(hydropneumothorax)* or a purulent effusion *(pyopneumothorax)*. Bilateral pneumothorax is rare beyond the neonatal period.

CLINICAL MANIFESTATIONS. The onset is usually abrupt and the severity of symptoms depend on the extent of the lung collapse and on the amount of pre-existing lung disease. Extensive pneumothorax may involve pain, dyspnea, and cyanosis. In infancy, symptoms and physical signs may be difficult to recognize. If the pneumothorax is only moderate in extent, there may be little displacement of intrathoracic organs and few or no symptoms. The severity of pain usually does not directly reflect the extent of the collapse.

Usually respiratory distress, retractions, and markedly decreased breath sounds over the involved lung are present. The percussion note over the involved area is tympanitic. Larynx, trachea, and heart may be shifted toward the unaffected side. When fluid is present, there is usually a sharply limited area of tympany above a level of flatness to percussion. It is important to determine whether the pneumothorax is under tension *(tension pneumothorax)* because this will limit expansion of the contralateral lung and may compromise cardiovascular function. The presence of amphoric breathing or, when fluid is present in the pleural cavity, of gurgling sounds synchronous with respirations suggests an open fistula connecting with air-bearing tissues. Confirmatory evidence is provided when the pneumothorax fills rapidly after it has been aspirated. The diagnosis can usually be established by roentgenographic examination (Fig. 14–19).

DIFFERENTIAL DIAGNOSIS. Pneumothorax must be differentiated from localized or generalized emphysema, from an extensive emphysematous bleb, from large pulmonary cavities or other cystic formations, from diaphragmatic hernia, from compensatory overexpansion with contralateral atelectasis, and from gaseous distention of the stomach; in most cases, a chest roentgenogram differentiates between them. Expiratory views accentuate the contrast between lung markings and the clear area of the pneumothorax. In the case of diaphragmatic hernia, however, a small amount of barium may be necessary to demonstrate that a portion of the gastrointestinal tract is in the thoracic cavity.

TREATMENT. Therapy varies with the extent of the collapse and the nature and severity of the underlying disease.

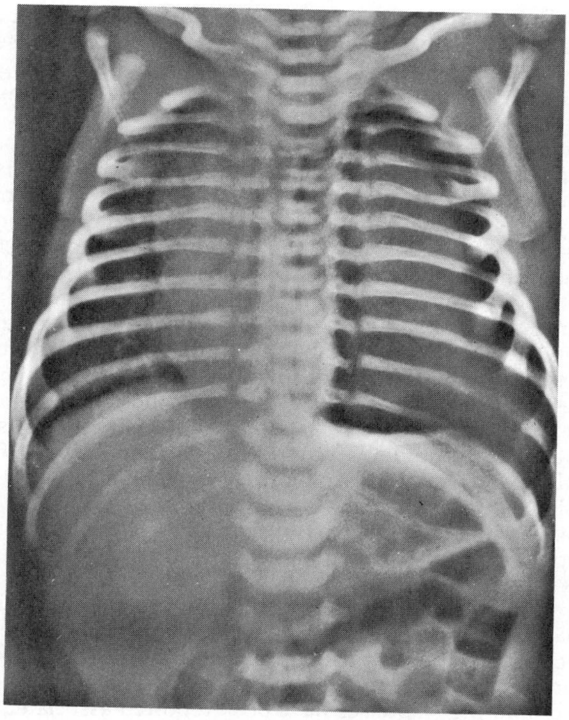

Figure 14–19. Pneumothorax in a newborn infant. The air in the left pleural cavity has partially collapsed the left lung, shifting the heart and mediastinal structures to the right.

A small or even moderately sized pneumothorax in an otherwise normal child may resolve without specific treatment usually within 1 wk or so. A small (less than 5%) pneumothorax complicating asthma may also spontaneously resolve. Administering 100% oxygen may hasten resolution by increasing the nitrogen pressure gradient between the pleural air and the blood. Patients with chronic hypoxemia should be monitored closely during the administration of supplemental oxygen. Pleural pain deserves analgesic treatment. Codeine may be justified, but its respiratory depressant effect should be considered. Occasionally, morphine or meperidine is needed. If there is more than 5% collapse or if the pneumothorax is recurrent or under tension, definitive treatment is necessary. Pneumothoraces complicating CF frequently recur, and definitive treatment may be justified with the first episode, even with less than 5% collapse. Similarly, pneumothorax complicating malignancy and its treatment, if it does not improve rapidly with observation, often necessitates treatment with chemical pleuradesis or open thoracotomy.

Closed thoracotomy (simple insertion of a chest tube) and drainage of the trapped air through a catheter, the external opening of which is kept in a dependent position under water, will be adequate to re-expand the lung in almost all patients. To prevent recurrences when there have already been many pneumothoraces, inducing the formation of strong adhesions between the lung and chest wall by a sclerosing procedure may be indicated, for example, by the introduction of tetracycline or silver nitrate into the pleural space (chemical pleurodesis). Open thoracotomy through a limited incision, with plication of blebs, closure of fistula, stripping of the pleura (usually in the apical lung where the surgeon has direct vision), and basilar pleural abrasion is also an effective treatment for recurring pneumothorax. Postoperative pain is comparable to chemical pleurodesis with silver nitrate, but the chest tube can usually be removed within 24–48 hr, compared with the usual 72 hr minimum for closed thoracotomy and pleurodesis.

Treatment of the underlying pulmonary disease should begin on admission. When open thoracotomy is planned for patients with CF, it should be done as soon as possible after the patient is admitted, because the patient's condition may gradually deteriorate because the chest tube interferes with postural drainage and physical activity.

Bernhard WF, Malcolm JA, Berry RW, et al: A study of the pathogenesis and management of spontaneous pneumothorax. Dis Chest 42:403, 1962.
Stem H, Toole AL, Merino M: Catamenial pneumothorax. Chest 78:480, 1980.
Wilson WG, Aylsworth: Familial spontaneous pneumothorax. Pediatrics 64:172, 1979.
Yellin A, Benfield JR: Pneumothorax associated with lymphoma. Am Rev Respir Dis 134:590, 1986.

14.92 PNEUMOMEDIASTINUM

Pneumomediastinum usually results from alveolar rupture during the course of an acute or chronic pulmonary disease. However, a diverse group of nonrespiratory entities can also cause pneumomediastinum, and in some of these the lung is not the source of the air. For example, pneumomediastinum has been reported following dental extractions, pneumoencephalography, normal menses, obstetric delivery, diabetes mellitus with ketoacidosis, acupuncture, and acute gastroenteritis. Pneumomediastinum can also result from esophageal perforation and penetrating chest trauma. Occasionally no underlying cause is found; in an apparently normal child the pneumomediastinum can present as chest pain associated with subcutaneous air.

Following intrapulmonary alveolar rupture, air can dissect through the perivascular sheaths and other soft-tissue planes toward the hilum and enter the mediastinum. Pneumomediastinum is rarely a major problem in older children because the mediastinum can be depressurized by escape of air into the neck or abdomen. In the newborn, however, the rate at which air can leave the mediastinum is quite limited, and pneumomediastinum can lead to dangerous cardiovascular compromise or to pneumothorax (see Sec. 9.37). Acute asthma is the most common cause of pneumomediastinum in older children and teenagers. Simultaneous pneumothorax is unusual in these patients.

The principal symptom of pneumomediastinum is transient stabbing pains in the chest that may radiate to the neck. However, isolated abdominal pain and sore throat also occur. The patient may have dyspnea, but it is difficult to know if this is really a separate symptom or if it is related to the chest pain. Pneumomediastinum is often difficult to detect by physical examination alone. Subcutaneous emphysema, if present, is virtually diagnostic. Although cardiac dullness may be decreased, many of these patients are chronically overinflated, and it is unlikely that the clinician will be sure of this finding. A mediastinal "crunch" is occasionally present but is easily confused with a friction rub. By chest roentgenogram the cardiac border, highlighted by the mediastinal air, is more distinct than normal, and on the lateral projection the posterior mediastinal structures are also clearly defined. Subcutaneous air, seen roentgenographically, confirms the pneumomediastinum.

Treatment is directed primarily at the underlying obstructive pulmonary disease. Analgesics are needed occasionally for chest pain. Rarely, subcutaneous empysema can cause sufficient tracheal compression to justify tracheotomy; the tracheotomy also decompresses the mediastinum.

Church JA, Richards W: Air leak syndromes as complications of respiratory disease in infancy and childhood. Ann Allergy 39:393, 1977.
Sandler CM, Libshitz HI, Marks G: Pneumoperitoneum, pneumomediastinum and pneumopericardium following dental extraction. Radiology 115:539, 1975.
Shahar J, Angelillo VA: Catamenial pneumomediastinum. Chest 90:776, 1986.
Sturtz GS: Spontaneous mediastinal emphysema. Pediatrics 74:431, 1984.

Tsai FY, Lee KF: Pneumopericardium and pneumomediastinum. Rare complications of pneumoencephalography. Radiology 112:95, 1974.

14.93 HYDROTHORAX

In hydrothorax the fluid is noninflammatory and has a lower specific gravity (1.015) than that of a serofibrinous exudate. It contains less protein and fewer cells and is usually associated with an accumulation of fluid in other parts of the body, such as the peritoneal cavity and the subcutaneous tissues. Hydrothorax is most often associated with cardiac or renal disease, although on occasion it may be a manifestation of severe nutritional edema, and, rarely, may result from venous obstruction by neoplasms, enlarged lymph nodes, or adhesions. Hydrothorax is usually bilateral in renal disease and in nutritional edema and may be in myocardial disease, although in this case it may be limited to the right side or greater on the right than on the left side. The physical signs are those described under Serofibrinous Pleurisy, but in hydrothorax there is more rapid shifting of the level of dullness with changes of position. The treatment is that of the primary disorder; aspiration may be necessary when pressure symptoms are notable.

Berger HW, Rammohan G, Neff MS, et al: Uremic pleural effusion. A study in 14 patients on chronic dialysis. Ann Intern Med 82:362, 1975.

14.94 HEMOTHORAX

Extensive bleeding into the pleural cavity may result from erosion of a blood vessel in association with inflammatory processes such as tuberculosis and empyema, but it is rare in children. Hemothorax may complicate a variety of congenital anomalies, including sequestration, patent ductus, and pulmonary arteriovenous malformation. It is also an occasional manifestation of intrathoracic neoplasms and blood dyscrasias and bleeding diatheses and may be the result of thoracic trauma, including surgical procedures. Rupture of an aneurysm is not likely during childhood. Hemothorax also occurs following blunt chest trauma and spontaneously, both in neonates and in older children. When a pleural hemorrhage occurs in association with a pneumothorax, it is called *hemopneumothorax*. The diagnosis of a hemothorax can be made only by thoracentesis. In every case an effort must be made to determine and treat the cause. Surgical intervention may be required to control active bleeding, and transfusion is necessary when loss of blood is excessive. Inadequate removal of blood in extensive hemothorax may lead to substantial restrictive disease secondary to deposition and organization of fibrin. A decortication procedure may then be necessary.

Berry RB, Light R: When thoracentesis yields bloody pleural fluid. J Respir Dis 7(6):18, 1986.
Block LF: Pleural disease. Basics Respir Dis 6 (May 1978):1, 1978.
Fleisher GR, Fichman KR, Honig PJ: Hemothorax in a child: An unusual cause of chest pain. Clin Pediatr 17:300, 1978.

14.95 CHYLOTHORAX

Chylothorax results from the escape of chyle from the thoracic duct into the thoracic cavity. The incidence has increased as cardiac surgery is performed on more complex congenital abnormalities; about 50% of these cases are now operative complications resulting from rupture of the thoracic duct. Most of the remainder are associated with chest injury or with primary or metastatic intrathoracic malignancy as a result of the pressure of enlarged lymph nodes or tumor. A variety of even less common causes are known and include lymphangiomatosis, restrictive pulmonary diseases, thrombosis of the duct or the subclavian vein, and congenital anomalies of the duct system. Chylothorax can occur in child abuse. In some patients, especially newborns, no specific etiology is identified. Chylothorax is rarely bilateral, usually being on the left side.

The symptoms and signs are those related to the presence of fluid in the thoracic cavity. The diagnosis is established when thoracentesis demonstrates a chylous effusion, a milky fluid containing fat, protein, lymphocytes, and other constituents of chyle. In newborn infants who have not yet been fed, the fluid may be clear. A pseudochylous milky fluid has been reported in cases of serous effusion, in which the fatty material was thought to arise from degenerative changes within the fluid and not to be due to the presence of lymph. This type of fluid may be distinguished from one containing chyle by shaking it with alkalis or ether; the fluid containing chyle tends to become clear. A more definitive test is the quantitation of fluid triglyceride (elevated in chylous fluid) and fluid cholesterol (which may be elevated in chronic serous effusions).

Spontaneous recovery has occurred in over half of the reported cases in infants under 1 yr of age. Repeated aspirations may be required to relieve the symptoms of pressure. However, chyle reaccumulates quickly, and repeated thoracenteses may cause considerable loss of calories and protein as well as large numbers of lymphocytes. Immunodeficiencies including hypogammaglobulinemia and abnormal cell-mediated immune responses have been reported associated with repeated thoracenteses for chylothorax. Attempts to prevent these problems by intravenous infusion of pleural contents are technically difficult and dangerous and of doubtful benefit. Despite large losses of T lymphocytes, clinical problems of infection are uncommon, but these patients should be protected from potentially dangerous viruses, including cytomegalovirus and live virus vaccines.

Treatment should begin in most cases with a brief period of observation on a low fat (or medium-chain triglyceride), high-protein diet. For most patients, bed rest, salt restriction, and diuresis are also indicated. The total caloric intake should be above the average requirement, and several times the daily requirements of the various vitamins, especially the fat-soluble vitamins A and D, should be added. If fluid continues to reaccumulate over 1–2 wk, a more aggressive attempt to locate and ligate the thoracic duct may be indicated. Many successful ligations have now been reported in patients with nontraumatic chylothoraces.

Dunkelman H, Sharief N, Berman L, et al: Generalized lymphangiomatosis with chylothorax. Arch Dis Child 64:1058, 1989.
Green HG: Child abuse presenting as chylothorax. Pediatrics 66:620, 1980.
Kirkland I: Chylothorax in infancy and childhood: A method of treatment. Arch Dis Child 40:186, 1965.
Macfarlane JR, Holman CW: Chylothorax. Am Rev Respir Dis 105:287, 1972.
McWilliams BC, Fan LL, Murphy SA: Transient T-cell depression in postoperative chylothorax. J Pediatr 99:595, 1981.
Van Aerde J, Campbell AN, Smyth JA, et al: Spontaneous chylothorax in newborns. Am J Dis Child 138:961, 1984.

NEUROMUSCULAR AND SKELETAL DISEASES AFFECTING PULMONARY FUNCTION

14.96 PECTUS EXCAVATUM

Midline narrowing of the thoracic cavity (pectus excavatum; "funnel chest") is usually an isolated skeletal abnormality. Rarely it is associated with rickets. It is occasionally associated with upper airway obstruction, and when this is successfully treated or resolves spontaneously, the pectus deformity may ameliorate or disappear. Substantial pectus deformity results in demonstrable restrictive pulmonary disease but usually has little or no functional effect. However, exercise testing has suggested an occasional link between pectus excavatum and exercise limitation. In some patients, cardiac function may be adversely affected. In addition, mitral valve prolapse (which may no longer be demonstrable by echocardiography following surgical correction of the pectus) and Wolff-Parkinson-White syndrome appear to be associated abnormalities. Pectus excavatum may occur in patients with segmental bronchomalacia, especially involving the left mainstem bronchus. Surgical correction of the pectus is not beneficial for most patients; however, improved exercise capability and normalization of ^{133}Xe lung perfusion scans and maximal voluntary ventilation have been reported. The functional importance of these changes is not clear. Some patients with very severe deformities may seek repair for cosmetic reasons or psychologic reasons.

Fissure of the sternum is the term used when the halves of the sternum remain separated. *Pigeon breast* is prominence of the sternum and the cartilaginous parts of the ribs, with lateral depressions of the thorax. A short sternum is a common manifestation of trisomy 18.

Beiser GD, Epstein SE, Stampfer M, et al: Impariment of cardiac function in patients with pectus excavatum, with improvement after operative correction. N Engl J Med 287:267, 1972.

Castile RG, Staats BA, Westbrook PR: Symptomatic pectus deformities of the chest. Am Rev Respir Dis 126:564, 1982.

Fan L, Murphy S: Pectus excavatum from chronic upper airway obstruction. Am J Dis Child 135:550, 1981.

Godfrey S: Association between pectus excavatum and segmental bronchomalacia. J Pediatr 96:649, 1980.

Park JM, Farmer AF: Wolff-Parkinson-White syndrome in children with pectus excavatum. J Pediatr 112:926, 1988.

Shamberger RC, Welch KJ, Sanders SP: Mitral valve prolapse associated with pectus excavatum. J Pediatr 111:404, 1987.

14.97 ASPHYXIATING THORACIC DYSTROPHY

See Sec. 24.35.

Thoracic dystrophy is one manifestation of an autosomal recessive disease that involves a generalized abnormality of skeletal growth. It usually causes life-threatening respiratory difficulties in the newborn period or early infancy. A variety of associated congenital malformations have been reported. Most patients have respiratory distress or infection before 1 yr of age. Older children are occasionally diagnosed when their parents note an abnormality in the appearance of the chest. A physical examination reveals constriction of the thorax and, usually, short extremities. There is no specific treatment. However, long-term continuous positive airway pressure was used successfully in one patient. Eventually, daytime treatment was successfully discontinued. Progressive renal failure occurs frequently among older patients. Respiratory infections should be treated promptly with antibiotics and, perhaps, physical therapy. Influenza vaccine should be administered yearly.

Herdman RC, Langer LO: Thoracic asphyxiant dystrophy and renal disease. Am J Dis Child 116:192, 1968.

Oberklaid F, Dantes DM, Mayne V, et al: Asphyxiating thoracic dysplasia: Clinical, radiological, and pathological information on 10 patients. Arch Dis Child 52:758, 1977.

Wiebicke W, Pasterkamp H: Long-term continuous positive airway pressure in a child with asphyxiating thoracic dystrophy. Pediatr Pulmonol 4:54, 1988.

14.98 RIB ANOMALIES

The absence or malformation of 1–2 ribs usually has no substantial effect on pulmonary function and does not require treatment. An absence of multiple ribs is associated with vertebral anomalies and, ultimately, scoliosis. In addition, a portion of lung can herniate through the defect in the chest wall; these hernias are most frequent at the level of the first to fifth ribs and are usually anterior. The lung may present as a soft, easily reducible, usually nontender swelling. Minor abnormalities of muscle caused by a loss of their normal attachments are also associated with this lesion. Most rib anomalies are discovered as incidental findings on chest roentgenograms obtained as part of a work-up for another illness. When the defect is large and associated with lung hernia, rib splitting and strutting techniques can provide both functional and cosmetic improvement.

Bronsther B, Coryllos E, Epstein B, et al: Lung hernias in children. J Pediatr Surg 3:544, 1968.

Rickham PP: Lung hernia secondary to congenital absence of ribs. Arch Dis Child 34:14, 1959.

14.99 NEUROMUSCULAR DISEASES WITH HYPOVENTILATION

A variety of acute (e.g., poliomyelitis, Guillain-Barré syndrome, botulism, spinal cord injury) and chronic (e.g., muscular dystrophy, progressive spinal muscular atrophy, myasthenia gravis) neuromuscular diseases can cause respiratory problems. (See Chapter 21.)

CLINICAL MANIFESTATIONS. Alveolar hypoventilation with hypoxemia and respiratory failure is easily recognized, and the need for emergency measures, including artificial ventilation, is obvious. Arterial blood gas determinations and lung volume measurements confirm its presence and are necessary for proper management. The vital capacity, which allows assessment of both the inspiratory and expiratory muscles, is particularly useful and should be carefully followed. The difference between the vital capacity obtained with the patient lying down and one obtained sitting up offers a rough guide to the strength of the diaphragm. Maximum inspiratory pressure is another easily obtained, but valuable, measure of the strength of the respiratory muscles.

Chronic, slowly progressive, neuromuscular weakness is more likely to cause the insidious onset of respiratory abnormalities that may ultimately become incapacitating and often life-limiting. With progression of weakness the patients cannot generate sufficient intrathoracic pressure for effective coughing, or they cannot hold the glottis closed well enough to allow sufficient pressure build-up in the lung. In addition, although tidal volumes may continue to be normal, the progressive decrease in vital capacity also compromises the effectiveness of the cough. Multiple minor episodes of aspiration occur as laryngeal muscles become weaker. Finally, with loss of adequate sigh and decreased ability of the diaphragm to prevent compromise of the thoracic volume by the abdominal organs, patchy microscopic atelectasis occurs accompanied by a ventilation perfusion abnormality and hypoxemia. Microscopic atelectasis also appears to be the major cause of decreased lung compliance in these patients. Recurrent or chronic infection then results and further restricts vital capacity. The increased viscosity of infected secretions also aggravates already impaired mucociliary clearance. Progressive loss of pulmonary tissue from the fibrosis associated with chronic infection and the chronic and worsening hypoxemia may lead eventually to pulmonary arterial hypertension and, ultimately, to right-sided heart failure. Finally, weakness of the pharyngeal and laryngeal muscles may result in obstruction when soft tissue, normally retracted away during inspiration, partially occludes the upper airway.

TREATMENT. All patients with chronic or progressive muscular weakness require close surveillance for, and early treatment of, respiratory complications. Prompt antibiotic treatment of upper respiratory infections is indicated. Most patients intermittently require physical therapy, including postural drainage with chest percussion, and parents should be instructed in these techniques; postural drainage is often effective when used throughout each acute respiratory illness. In some patients, an artificial cough can be accomplished by application of sudden external pressure to the thorax. The usefulness of overall respiratory muscle training in patients with Duchenne muscular dystrophy has not been demonstrated conclusively. In some patients with advanced neuromuscular disease, however, training of specific muscle groups, such as neck muscles or the pectoralis major, may help with the effectiveness of cough and may permit more sustained periods of mechanical ventilation that could be lifesaving during an electrical failure. Influenza vaccine should be administered. However, influenza vaccine should be omitted if it is suspected of playing a role in the causation of the primary disease (e.g., Guillain-Barré syndrome). Pneumococcal vaccine may be indicated.

A permanent tracheostomy to allow better access to the airway for suctioning can be very helpful. Some of these patients cannot handle secretions and may need a cuffed endotracheal tube or tracheostomy. A small tracheostomy can be plugged when suctioning is not being performed, allowing the patient to breathe and talk around the tube. A standard tracheostomy may alleviate upper airway obstruction and is useful in carefully selected patients. Patients with substantial diaphragmatic weakness may benefit from a mechanical rocking bed to reduce alveolar collapse. Intermittent positive pressure breathing has also been proposed for this purpose. Once pulmonary hypertension and overt right-sided heart failure are present, the prognosis is grave, and treatment with supplemental oxygen and other symptomatic measures allows only temporary improvement. Tolazoline is not effective. Respirator management may be appropriate for some patients whose respiratory failure is likely to be temporary (e.g., in myasthenia gravis).

Bergofsky EH: State of the art: Respiratory failure in disorders of the thoracic cage. Am Rev Respir Dis 119:643, 1979.
De Troyer A, Deisser P: The effects of intermittent positive pressure breathing on patients with respiratory muscle weakness. Am Rev Respir Dis 124:132, 1981.
De Troyer A, Estenne M, Heilporn A: The mechanism of active expiration in tetraplegic subjects. N Engl J Med 314:740, 1986.
Gilgoff IS, Barras DM, Jones MS, et al: Neck breathing: A form of voluntary respiration for the spine-injured ventilator-dependent quadriplegic child. Pediatrics 82:741, 1988.
Greenberg M, Edmonds J: Chronic respiratory problems in neuromyopathic disorders: The nature and management. Pediatr Clin North Am 21:927, 1974.
Macklem PT: Muscular weakness and respiratory function. N Engl J Med 314:775, 1986.

14.100 KYPHOSCOLIOSIS

Scoliosis, including idiopathic adolescent scoliosis, is discussed in Sec. 24.15. Mild or moderately severe scoliosis does not usually restrict the chest cage enough to seriously affect pulmonary function. Severe scoliosis, however, can dangerously impair function and may be associated with respiratory failure, cor pulmonale, or both. In addition to their restrictive lesion, these patients may also have a diffusion abnormality that aggravates hypoxemia. Minor respiratory infections may be life threatening. There is an age-related worsening of pulmonary function, but acute respiratory failure, although rare, does occur below 20 yr of age. Many of these patients can be managed without mechanical ventilation, and the intermediate term prognosis is good. Even patients with moderate scoliosis may have unexpectedly severe pulmonary problems immediately after a fusion procedure because pain and a body cast restrict breathing and interfere with coughing. In general, however, the magnitude of the postoperative impairment of pulmonary function correlates with the site and magnitude of the surgery and with the preoperative pulmonary abnormality. Patients with severe scoliosis, especially males, may have abnormalities of breathing during sleep, and the resultant periods of hypoxemia may contribute to the eventual development of pulmonary hypertension.

Patients in these categories should be treated as if they had life-threatening pulmonary disease. Influenza vaccine should be given yearly. Careful pulmonary function evaluation is essential prior to elective surgical procedures, especially before fusion. If pulmonary function is marginal (e.g., vital capacity of less than 40–50% of predicted), the patient should receive instruction in, and get experience with, positive pressure breathing prior to surgery. The possibility that the patient may awake on assisted ventilation with an endotracheal tube should be discussed prior to surgery. If possible, the patient should actually see the mechanical ventilator and understand how and why it might be used. For patients with marginal pulmonary function, careful postoperative monitoring of blood gases is essential. An occasional patient with extremely severe restrictive disease should have a tracheostomy prior to surgery. Scoliosis surgery may predispose to deep venous thrombosis and pulmonary embolus.

Kafer ER: Idiopathic scoliosis: Gas exchange and the age dependence of arterial blood gases. J Clin Invest 48:825, 1976.
Leech JA, Ernst P, Rogala EJ, et al: Cardiorespiratory status in relation to mild deformity in adolescent idiopathic scoliosis. J Pediatr 106:143, 1985.
Libby DM, Briscoe WA, Boyce B, et al: Acute respiratory failure in scoliosis or kyphosis: prolonged survival and treatment. Am J Med 73:532, 1982.
Mezon BL, West P, Israels J, et al: Sleep breathing abnormalities in kyphoscoliosis. Am Rev Respir Dis 1222:617, 1980.
Schur MS, Brown JT, Kafer ER, et al: Postoperative pulmonary function in children: Comparison of scoliosis with peripheral surgery. Am Rev Respir Dis 130:46, 1984.

14.101 OBESITY

Extreme obesity occasionally causes respiratory embarrassment with somnolence, dyspnea, cyanosis, and, possibly, right-sided heart failure. Chest and diaphragmatic excursions are limited, resulting in rapid shallow breathing; alveolar ventilation is also decreased, resulting in hypoxemia. Ventilation-perfusion abnormalities also contribute to arterial desaturation. Obstructive sleep apnea dominates the clinical picture in many patients: Hypertension and anuresis may be present. Some of these patients appear to have a diminished ventilatory response to hypoxic drive. In the *Prader-Willi syndrome*, an abnormal ventilatory response to carbon dioxide has been demonstrated in family members who are otherwise normal, suggesting that the abnormal ventilatory control adds to the respiratory problems caused by the obesity rather than results from them.

Weight loss is the primary goal of treatment (Sec. 4.20) and, if successful, it alone will reduce the pulmonary problems. Some children with hypoventilation and right-sided heart failure secondary to the extreme obesity of Prader-Willi syndrome may benefit from treatment with progesterone. Continuous positive airway pressure administered by nasal prongs may help obese patients with obstructive sleep apnea.

Lopata M, Önal E: Mass loading, sleep apnea, and the pathogenesis of obesity hyperventilation. Am Rev Respir Dis 126:640, 1982.
Orenstein DM, Boat TF, Owens RP, et al: The obesity hypoventilation syndrome in children with the Prader-Willi syndrome: A possible role for familial decreased response to carbon dioxide. J Pediatr 67:765, 1980.
Orenstein DM, Boat TF, Stern RC, et al: Progesterone treatment of the obesity hypoventilation syndrome in a child. J Pediatr 90:477, 1977.
Wilhoit SC, Brown ED, Suratt PM: Treatment of obstructive sleep apnea with continuous nasal airflow delivered through nasal prongs. Chest 85:170, 1984.

14.102 PRIMARY FAILURE OF RESPIRATORY REGULATION
(Ondine Curse)

Primary failure of CNS regulation of breathing may also occur in nonobese persons but has been infrequently reported children. Hypoventilation, which occurs more severely or exclusively during sleep, is a serious threat to life.

The ventilatory responses to oxygen and carbon dioxide are both absent during wakefulness. This suggests that, in these patients, awake breathing (and, probably, breathing during REM sleep) is mediated by "behavioral pathways," whereas regulation of breathing is seriously deranged during non-REM sleep when, in the normal person, it is dependent exclusively on "metabolic pathways." Suggested therapeutic measures include bilateral phrenic nerve pacing or tracheostomy in conjunction with assisted ventilation during sleep. Although preliminary success has been reported with both these approaches, the long-term prognosis is unknown.

Brouillette RT, Ibawi MN, Klemka-Walden L, et al: Stimulus parameters for phrenic nerve pacing in infants and children. Pediatr Pulmonol 4:33, 1988.
Hyland RH, Jones NL, Powles ACP, et al: Primary alveolar hypoventilation treated with nocturnal electrophrenic respiration. Am Rev Respir Dis 117:165, 1978.
Paton JY, Swaminathan S, Sargent CW, et al: Hypoxic and hypercapnic ventilatory responses in awake children with congenital central hypoventilation syndrome. Am Rev Respir Dis 140:368, 1989.

14.103 COUGH SYNCOPE

Cough syncope has been infrequently reported in children. During a coughing paroxysm in which high intrathoracic pressures are generated, venous obstruction, characterized by redness of the face, is followed by decreased venous return and, ultimately, by decreased cardiac output, which results in transient cerebral hypoxia and syncope. Recovery generally occurs within 10 sec to 2 min. Muscular movements and incontinence occur rarely; although these events may simulate seizures, the underlying neuronal discharges originate in the reticular formation (as opposed to the cerebral cortex in true epilepsy). Asthma is the most frequent precipitating disease. There is no specific treatment.

ROBERT C. STERN

Haslam RHA, Freigang B: Cough syncope mimicking epilepsy in asthmatic children. Can J Neurolog Sci 12:45, 1985.
Katz RM: Cough syncope in children with asthma. J Pediatr 77:48, 1970.

15

THE CARDIOVASCULAR SYSTEM

EVALUATION OF THE CARDIOVASCULAR SYSTEM

15.1 HISTORY AND PHYSICAL EXAMINATION

The importance of the history and physical examination cannot be overemphasized in the evaluation of infants and children with suspected cardiovascular disorders. After this assessment, patients may require further laboratory evaluation and eventual treatment, or the family may be reassured that no significant problem exists.

There are a number of areas of special interest in taking a *history* for a potential cardiac abnormality. Cyanosis is often overlooked by parents; it may be considered merely a "deep coloring," a normal individual variation. Blueness during exercise is more often noted as an abnormal finding by observant parents. Eliciting a history of fatigue in an older child requires specific questions about activity including stair climbing, walking various distances, bicycle riding, etc.; information should also be obtained regarding more severe manifestations such as orthopnea and nocturnal dyspnea. The history obtained from the parents of a young infant, however, should focus on the feeding process. The baby with congestive heart failure will often take less volume per feeding, become dyspneic while sucking, and perhaps perspire profusely. After falling into an exhausted sleep, the baby, inadequately fed, will awaken for the next feeding after a brief period of time. This cycle continues around the clock and must be carefully differentiated from colic or other feeding disorders.

Cardiac disease may be a manifestation of a known congenital malformation syndrome (see Table 15–7) or of a generalized disorder affecting the heart and other organ systems (Table 15–1). Extracardiac malformations may be noted in about 25% of infants with congenital heart disease; about 10% have a chromosomal abnormality. Furthermore, a family history may reveal early coronary artery disease (familial hypercholesterolemia), generalized muscle diseases (muscular dystrophy, dermatomyositis), or prior congenital heart disease.

Chest pain is usually not a manifestation of cardiac disease in the pediatric patient. Nonetheless, a careful history, subsequent physical examination, and, if indicated, laboratory or imaging tests will assist in identifying the etiology of chest pain (Table 15–2).

Physical examination begins with an assessment of growth and development. Cardiac failure results in failure to thrive manifested by poor weight gain; length remains relatively unaffected. An infant with severe congestive heart failure usually appears to be long and undernourished in contrast to an infant with cyanotic heart disease unaccompanied by cardiac decompensation, who may display normal height and weight. Failure to thrive, tachypnea, liver and less so spleen enlargement, pulmonary rales, and peripheral edema in a baby who appears to be ill are the major clinical manifestations of heart failure. Mild cyanosis may be too subtle for early detection, and clubbing of the fingers and toes is not usually manifested until late in the 1st year of life even in the presence of severe arterial oxygen desaturation. Blueness is best observed over the nail beds, lips, and mucous membranes. Differential cyanosis with blue lower extremities and pink upper torso and extremities (usually right arm) is seen with right to left shunting across a ductus arteriosus in the presence of a coarctation or interrupted aortic arch. Circumoral cyanosis or blueness about the forehead may be the result of prominent venous plexuses in these areas rather than decreased arterial oxygen saturation.

The *cardiac rate* of newborn infants is rapid and subject to wide fluctuations (Table 15–3). The average rate ranges from 120 to 140 beats/min and may increase to 170 or more during crying and activity or drop to 70–90 during sleep. As the child grows older, the average pulse rate becomes slower, as low as 40/min in athletic adolescents. Persistent tachycardia (over 200/min in neonates, 150/min in infants, or 120/min in older children), bradycardia, or irregular heart beat other than sinus arrhythmia may require investigation to exclude pathologic arrhythmias.

Careful evaluation of the *character of the pulses* is an important early step in the physical diagnosis of congenital heart disease. A wide pulse pressure with bounding pulses may suggest an aortic runoff lesion such as patent ductus arteriosus, aortic insufficiency, an arterial-venous communication, or increased cardiac output secondary to anemia, anxiety, or conditions associated with increased catecholamine secretion. Diminished pulses are associated with heart failure, pericardial tamponade, left ventricular outflow obstruction, or cardiomyopathy.

The *blood pressure* should be measured in the arms as well as in the legs, the latter on at least one occasion to be certain that coarctation of the aorta is not overlooked. Palpation of decreased femoral and/or dorsalis pedis pulses is not reliable to diagnose coarctation. In older children a mercury sphygmomanometer with a cuff that covers approximately two thirds of the upper arm or leg may be utilized for measurement. A cuff that is too small will invariably result in falsely high readings, while a cuff that is somewhat too large will record slightly decreased pressures. Three-, 5-, 7-, 12-, and 18-cm cuffs should be available to accommodate the large spectrum of pediatric patient sizes. The 1st Korotkoff sounds indicate the systolic pressure. As the cuff pressure is slowly decreased, the sounds usually become muffled before they disappear. The diastolic pressure may be recorded when the sounds are muffled (preferred) as well as when they disappear; the former is usually higher and the latter lower than the true diastolic pressure. For lower extremity blood pressure determination the stethoscope is placed over the popliteal

TABLE 15–1. Cardiac Manifestations of Systemic Diseases

Systemic Disease	Cardiac Complications
Inflammatory Disorders	
Sepsis	Hypotension, myocardial dysfunction, pericardial effusion, pulmonary hypertension
Juvenile rheumatoid arthritis	Pericarditis, rarely myocarditis
Systemic lupus erythematosus	Pericarditis, Libman-Sacks endocarditis, coronary arteritis, coronary atherosclerosis (with steroids), congenital heart block
Scleroderma	Pulmonary hypertension, myocardial fibrosis, cardiomyopathy
Dermatomyositis	Cardiomyopathy, arrhythmias, heart block
Kawasaki disease	Coronary artery aneurysm and thrombosis, myocardial infarction, myocarditis, valvular insufficiency
Sarcoidosis	Granuloma, fibrosis, amyloidosis, biventricular hypertrophy, arrhythmias
Lyme disease	Arrhythmias, myocarditis
Löffler hypereosinophilic syndrome	Endomyocardial disease
Inborn Errors of Metabolism	
Refsum	Arrhythmia, sudden death
Hunter-Hurler	Valvular insufficiency, heart failure, hypertension
Fabry	Mitral insufficiency, coronary artery disease with myocardial infarction
Glycogen storage disease IIa (Pompe disease)	Short P-R interval, cardiomegaly, heart failure, arrhythmias
Carnitine deficiency	Heart failure, cardiomyopathy
Gaucher	Pericarditis
Homocystinuria	Coronary thrombosis
Alkaptonuria	Atherosclerosis, valvular disease
Morquio-Ullrich	Aortic incompetence
Scheie	Aortic incompetence
Connective Tissue Disorders	
Arterial calcification of infancy	Calcinosis of coronary arteries, aorta
Marfan	Aortic and mitral insufficiency; dissecting aortic aneurysm, mitral valve prolapse
Congenital contractural arachnodactyly	Mitral insufficiency or prolapse
Ehlers-Danlos	Mitral valve prolapse, dilated aortic root
Osteogenesis imperfecta	Aortic incompetence
Pseudoxanthoma elasticum	Peripheral arterial disease
Neuromuscular disorders	
Friedreich ataxia	Cardiomyopathy
Duchenne dystrophy	Cardiomyopathy, heart failure
Tuberous sclerosis	Cardiac rhabdomyoma
Familial deafness	Occasionally arrhythmia, sudden death
Neurofibromatosis	Pulmonic stenosis, pheochromocytoma, coarctation of aorta
Riley-Day	Episodic hypertension, postural hypotension
von Hippel-Lindau	Hemangiomas, pheochromocytomas
Endocrine-Metabolic Disorders	
Graves	Tachycardia, arrhythmias, heart failure
Hypothyroidism	Bradycardia, pericardial effusion, cardiomyopathy, low-voltage ECG
Pheochromocytoma	Hypertension, myocardial ischemia, myocardial fibrosis, cardiomyopathy
Carcinoid	Right-sided endocardial fibrosis
Hematologic Disorders	
Sickle cell anemia	High-output heart failure, cardiomyopathy, cor pulmonale
Thalassemia major	High-output heart failure, hemochromatosis
Hemochromatosis (1° or 2°)	Cardiomyopathy
Others	
Cockayne	Atherosclerosis
Familial dwarfism and nevi	Cardiomyopathy
Jervell and Lange-Nielsen	Prolonged Q-T interval, sudden death
Leopard (lentiginosis)	Pulmonic stenosis, prolonged Q-T interval
Progeria	Accelerated atherosclerosis
Rendu-Osler-Weber	Arteriovenous fistula (lung, liver, mucous membranes)
Romano-Ward	Prolonged Q-T interval, sudden death
Weill-Marchesani	Patent ductus arteriosus
Werner	Vascular sclerosis, cardiomyopathy

TABLE 15–2. Differential Diagnosis of Pediatric Chest Pain

Musculoskeletal (common)
Trauma (accidental, abuse)
Exercise, overuse injury (strain, bursitis)
Costochondritis (Tietze syndrome)
Herpes zoster (cutaneous)
Pleurodynia
Sickle cell anemia vaso-occlusive crisis
Osteomyelitis (rare)
Primary or metastatic tumor (rare)

Pulmonary (common)
Pneumonia
Pleurisy
Asthma
Pneumothorax
Infarction (sickle cell anemia)
Foreign body
Embolism (rare)
Pulmonary hypertension (rare)
Tumor (rare)

Gastrointestinal (rare)
Esophagitis (gastroesophageal reflux)
Esophageal foreign body
Esophageal spasm
Cholecystitis
Subdiaphragmatic abscess
Perihepatitis (Fitz-Hugh–Curtis syndrome)
Peptic ulcer disease

Cardiac (rare)
Pericarditis
Postpericardiotomy syndrome
Endocarditis
Mitral valve prolapse
Aortic stenosis
Arrhythmias
Marfan syndrome (dissecting aortic aneurysm)
Anomalous coronary artery
Kawasaki disease
Cocaine, sympathomimetic ingestion
Angina (familial hypercholesterolemia)

Idiopathic (common)
Anxiety, hyperventilation

Other (rare)
Spinal cord or nerve root compression
Breast-related pathology

artery. Ordinarily, the pressure recorded in the legs with the cuff technique is about 10 mm Hg higher than in the arms.

In infants the blood pressure can be obtained by auscultation, by palpation, or by the *flush method.* The last is most feasible in a restless infant. A cuff of appropriate size is placed around the upper arm or thigh. The distal limb is squeezed and the cuff rapidly inflated so that blanching is noted. The cuff is then gradually deflated. At the point at which the limb flushes, the blood pressure reading obtained corresponds to a systolic value slightly below what would be found by the direct arterial or auscultatory method. Also available are ultrasonic (Doppler) and oscillometric (Dinamap) devices, which provide accurate measurements in infants as well as children.

The blood pressure varies with the age of the child and is closely related to height and weight. Significant increases occur during adolescence, and there are many temporary variations before the more stable levels of adult life are attained. Exercise, excitement, coughing, and straining may raise the systolic pressures of children as much as 40–50 mm above their usual levels. Variability of blood pressure among children of approximately the same age and body build should be expected, and serial measurements should always be obtained in the evaluation of a patient with hypertension (Figs. 15–1 to 15–6).

In cooperative children, inspection of the regular venous pulse wave provides information about the *venous pressure* and right atrial pressure. The veins should be inspected with the patient sitting at a 90-degree angle. Under these conditions the external jugular vein should not be visible above the clavicles unless there is elevation of venous pressure. Increased venous pressure transmitted to the internal jugular vein may appear as venous pulsations without visible distention; such pulsation does not occur in normal children reclining at an angle of 45 degrees.

The normal *jugular phlebogram* or direct tracings from the superior vena cava show three positive components corresponding to each cardiac cycle; they are termed "a," "c," and "v," respectively (Fig. 15–7). The "a" wave is synchronous with atrial systole, the "v" wave with atrial diastole, and the "c" wave with early ventricular systole. Because the great veins are in direct communication with the right atrium, changes of pressure and volume of the chamber are transmitted to the veins. For example:

1. In congestive cardiac failure the increased right atrial pressure is transmitted to the cervical veins. The main pulsation at the upper part of distribution of these veins occurs in late diastole.
2. Cardiac compression by pericardial effusion or constriction increases the jugular pressure, but the amplitude of venous pulsation is small.
3. In relatively severe pulmonary stenosis the right ventricular diastolic pressure may be elevated. Emptying of the right atrium depends upon a systolic pressure in excess of the right ventricular diastolic pressure. A conspicuous presystolic "a" wave is present under these conditions. Similar "a" waves may be detected in patients with pulmonary stenosis and right ventricular hypertrophy with a normal right ventricular end-diastolic pressure; the mechanism of the "a" wave is due to a decreased distensibility of the right ventricle during diastole.
4. A presystolic "a" wave may be present in tricuspid stenosis or atresia, and the transmission of this wave to the inferior vena cava and hepatic veins produces presystolic hepatic pulsations.
5. In tricuspid insufficiency some of the right ventricular systolic pressure is transmitted to the right atrium and results in large, conspicuous venous pulsations that correspond to ventricular systole and produce a fusion of the "c" and "v" waves.

TABLE 15–3. Pulse Rates at Rest

Age	Lower Limits of Normal		Average		Upper Limits of Normal	
Newborn	70/min		125/min		190/min	
1–11 mo	80		120		160	
2 yr	80		110		130	
4 yr	80		100		120	
6 yr	75		100		115	
8 yr	70		90		110	
10 yr	70		90		110	
	Girls	*Boys*	*Girls*	*Boys*	*Girls*	*Boys*
12 yr	70	65	90	85	110	105
14 yr	65	60	85	80	105	100
16 yr	60	55	80	75	100	95
18 yr	55	50	75	70	95	90

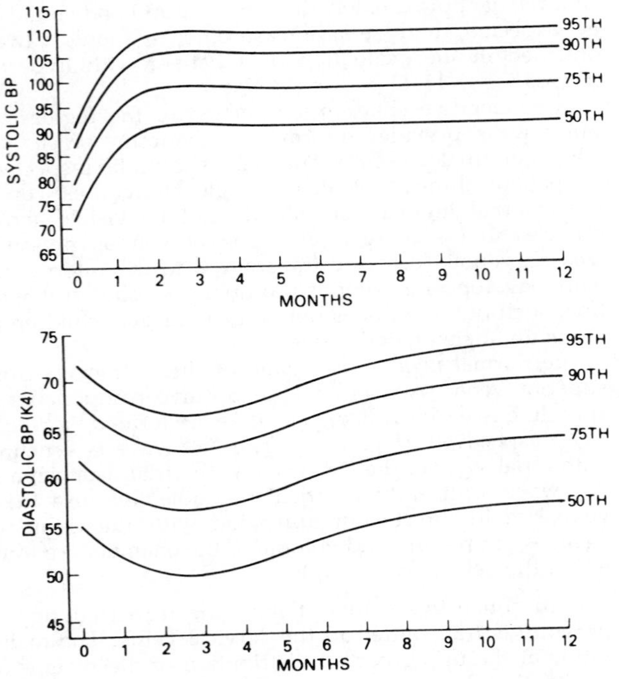

90TH PERCENTILE													
SYSTOLIC BP	87	101	106	106	106	105	105	105	105	105	105	105	105
DIASTOLIC BP	68	65	63	63	63	65	66	67	68	68	69	69	69
HEIGHT CM	51	59	63	66	68	70	72	73	74	76	77	78	80
WEIGHT KG	4	4	5	5	6	7	8	9	9	10	10	11	11

Figure 15–1. Age-specific percentiles of BP measurements in boys—birth to 12 mo of age; Korotkoff phase IV (K4) used for diastolic BP. (From National Heart, Lung, and Blood Institute, Bethesda, MD: Report of the second task force on blood pressure control in children—1987. Reproduced by permission of Pediatrics. Vol 79, p 1. Copyright © 1987.)

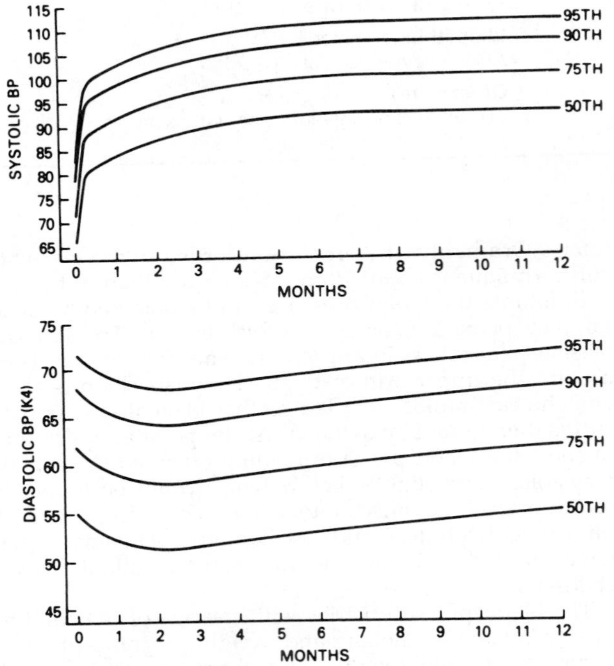

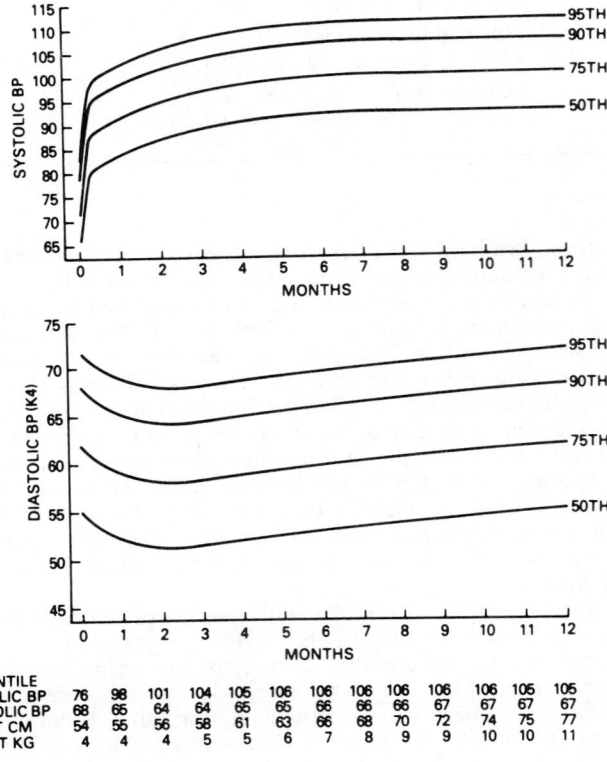

90TH PERCENTILE													
SYSTOLIC BP	76	98	101	104	105	106	106	106	106	106	106	105	105
DIASTOLIC BP	68	65	64	64	65	65	66	66	66	67	67	67	67
HEIGHT CM	54	55	56	58	61	63	66	68	70	72	74	75	77
WEIGHT KG	4	4	4	5	5	6	7	8	9	9	10	10	11

Figure 15–2. Age-specific percentiles of BP measurements in girls—birth to 12 mo of age; Korotkoff phase IV (K4) used for diastolic BP. (From National Heart, Lung, and Blood Institute, Bethesda, MD: Report of the second task force on blood pressure control in children—1987. Reproduced by permission of Pediatrics. Vol 79, p 1. Copyright © 1987.)

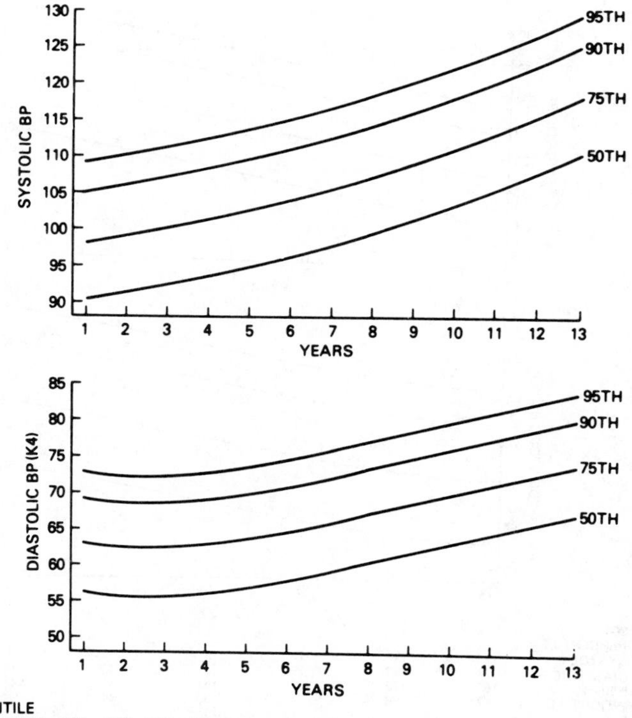

90TH PERCENTILE													
SYSTOLIC BP	105	106	107	108	109	111	112	114	115	117	119	121	124
DIASTOLIC BP	69	68	68	69	69	70	71	73	74	75	76	77	79
HEIGHT CM	80	91	100	108	115	122	129	135	141	147	153	159	165
WEIGHT KG	11	14	16	18	22	25	29	34	39	44	50	55	62

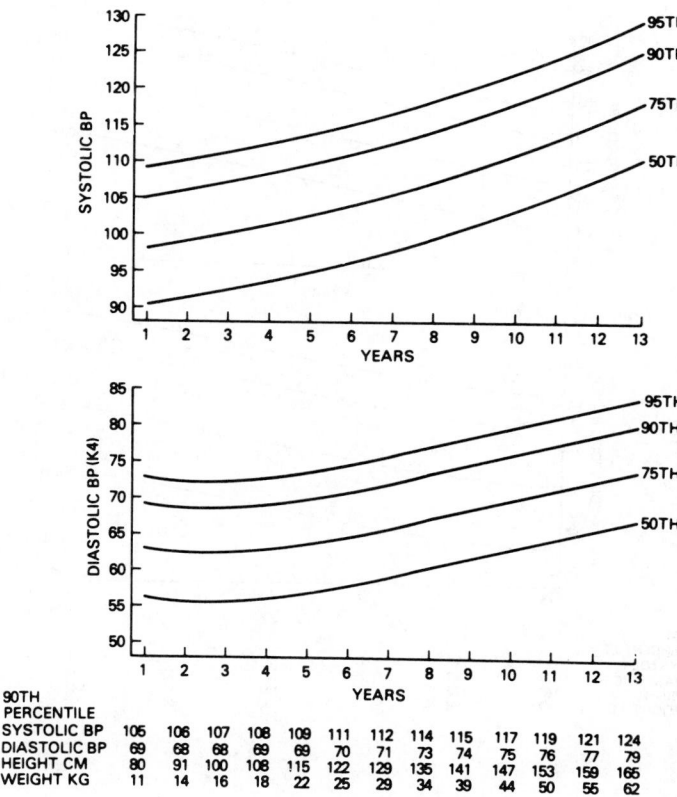

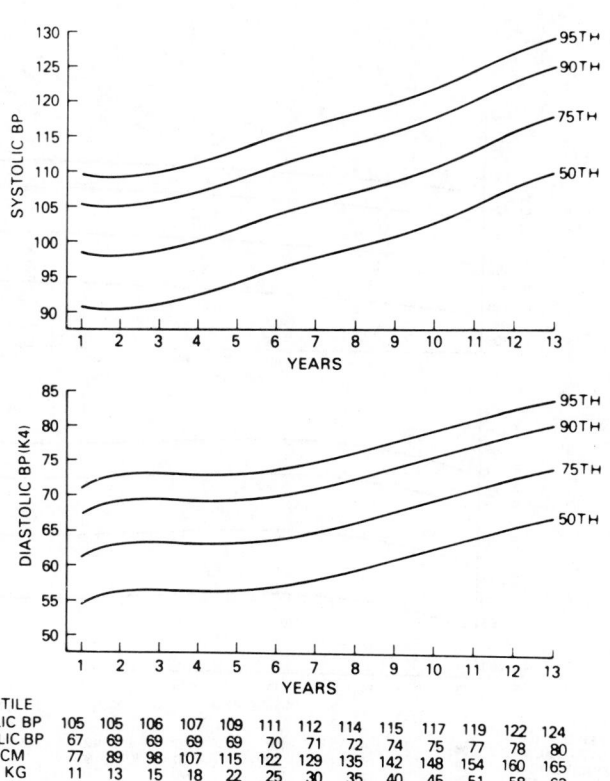

Figure 15–3. Age-specific percentiles for BP measurements in boys—1 to 13 yr of age; Korotkoff phase IV (K4) used for diastolic BP. (From National Heart, Lung, and Blood Institute, Bethesda, MD: Report of the second task force on blood pressure control in children—1987. Reproduced by permission of Pediatrics. Vol 79, p 1. Copyright © 1987.)

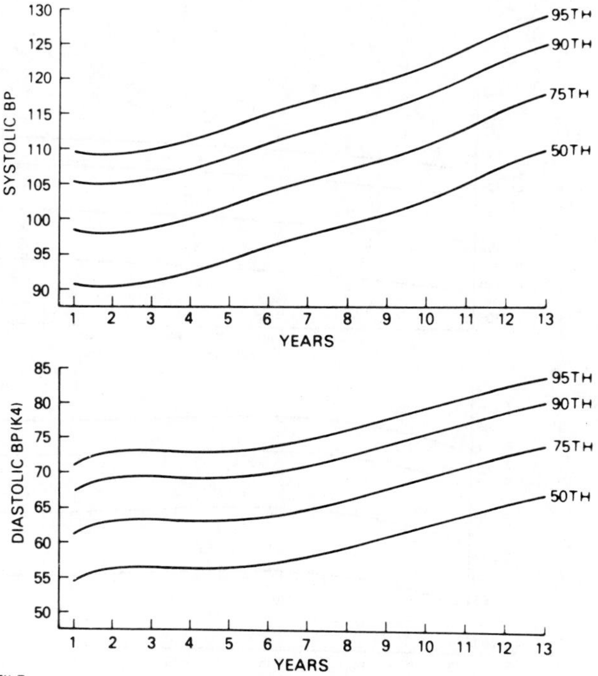

90TH PERCENTILE													
SYSTOLIC BP	105	105	106	107	109	111	112	114	115	117	119	122	124
DIASTOLIC BP	67	69	69	69	69	70	71	72	74	75	77	78	80
HEIGHT CM	77	89	98	107	115	122	129	135	142	148	154	160	165
WEIGHT KG	11	13	15	18	22	25	30	35	40	45	51	58	63

Figure 15–4. Age-specific percentiles of BP measurements in girls—1 to 13 yr of age; Korotkoff phase IV (K4) used for diastolic BP. (From National Heart, Lung, and Blood Institute, Bethesda, MD: Report of the second task force on blood pressure control in children—1987. Reproduced by permission of Pediatrics. Vol 79, p 1. Copyright © 1987.)

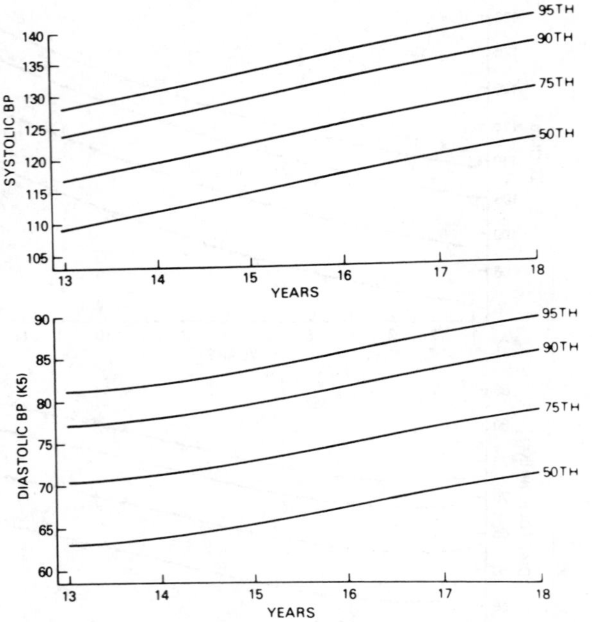

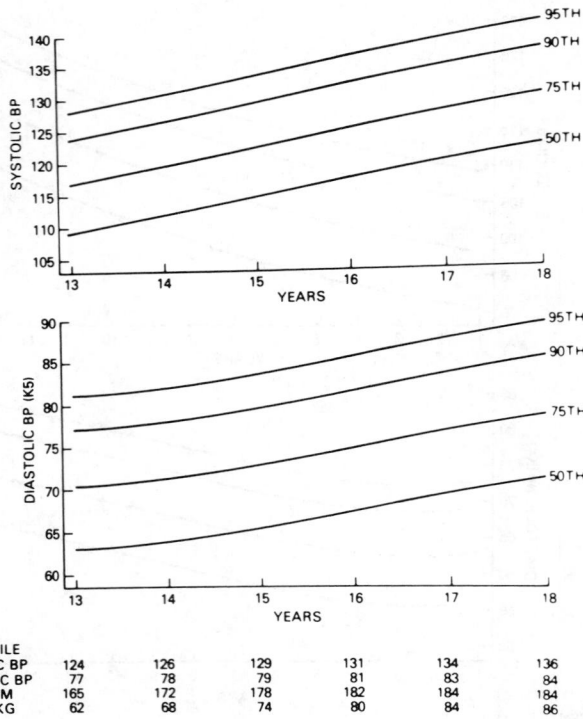

90TH PERCENTILE						
SYSTOLIC BP	124	126	129	131	134	136
DIASTOLIC BP	77	78	79	81	83	84
HEIGHT CM	165	172	178	182	184	184
WEIGHT KG	62	68	74	80	84	86

Figure 15–5. Age-specific percentiles of BP measurements in boys—13 to 18 yr of age; Korotkoff phase V (K5) used for diastolic BP. (From National Heart, Lung, and Blood Institute, Bethesda, MD: Report of the second task force on blood pressure control in children—1987. Reproduced by permission of Pediatrics. Vol 79, p 1. Copyright © 1987.)

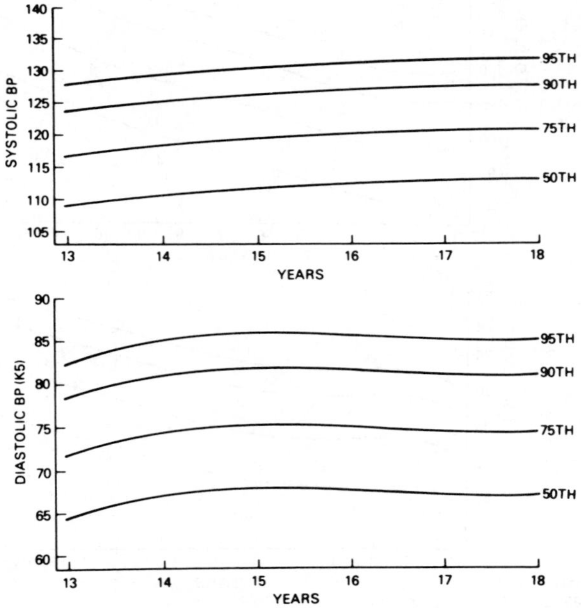

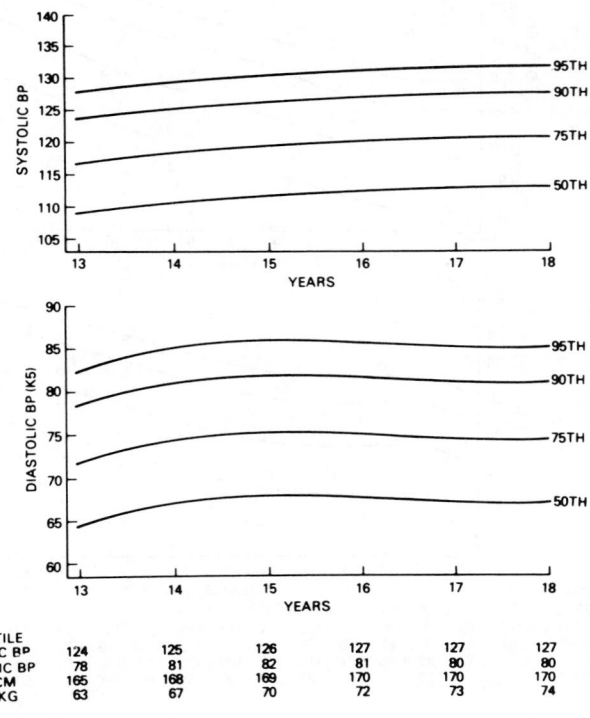

90TH PERCENTILE						
SYSTOLIC BP	124	125	126	127	127	127
DIASTOLIC BP	78	81	82	81	80	80
HEIGHT CM	165	168	169	170	170	170
WEIGHT KG	63	67	70	72	73	74

Figure 15–6. Age-specific percentiles of BP measurements in girls—13 to 18 yr of age; Korotkoff phase V (K5) used for diastolic BP. (From National Heart, Lung, and Blood Institute, Bethesda, MD: Report of the second task force on blood pressure control in children—1987. Reproduced by permission of Pediatrics. Vol 79, p 1. Copyright © 1987.)

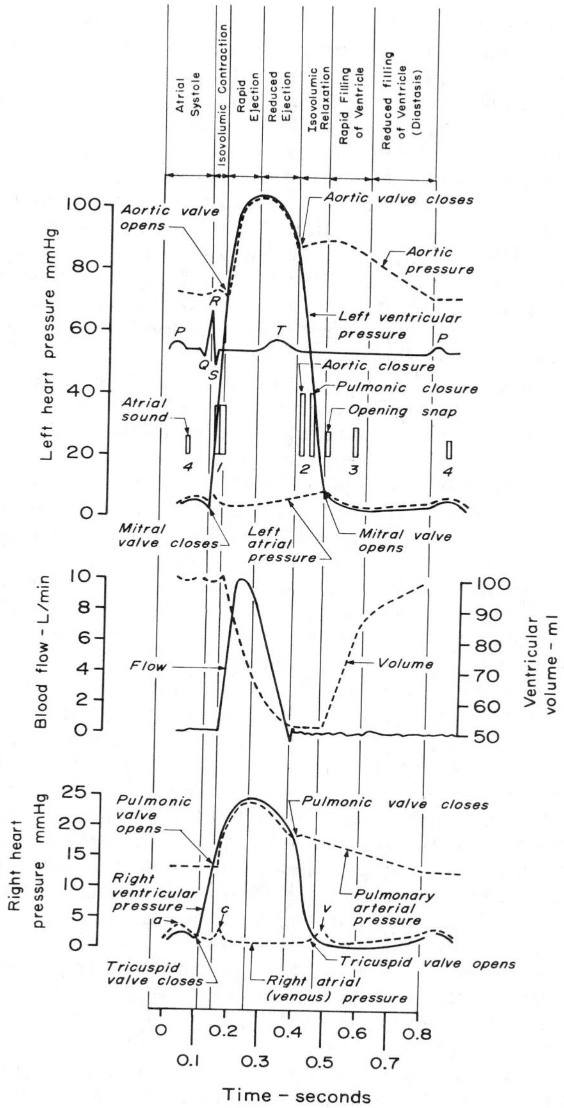

Figure 15–7. Idealized diagram of temporal events of a cardiac cycle.

6. In complete heart block the occurrence of cervical venous pulsations depends on the position of the tricuspid valve at the time of atrial systole. If the right atrium contracts when the tricuspid valve is closed, a large venous pulsation will occur.

7. In superior vena caval obstruction the jugular venous pressure is increased, but the veins do not pulsate.

CARDIAC EXAMINATION. The heart should be examined in a systematic manner concentrating on the meaning of each manifestation. Much can be learned prior to auscultation by inspection and palpation. A **precordial bulge** to the left of the sternum with increased precordial activity suggests cardiac enlargement. A **substernal thrust** indicates the presence of right ventriclular enlargement; an **apical heave** is noted with left ventricular hypertrophy. All manifestations may be present. A **hyperdynamic precordium** suggests a volume load like that found with a large left to right shunt. In contrast, a silent precordium with a barely detectable apical impulse suggests pericardial effusion or severe cardiomyopathy. The relationship of the apex beat to the midclavicular line with the child prone is also helpful in the estimation of cardiac size; the apex beat moves laterally with enlargement of the left ventricle. Right-sided apical impulses signify dextrocardia, tension pneumothorax, or left-sided thoracic space-occupying lesions (e.g., diaphragmatic hernia). **Thrills** are palpable murmurs, which should always correlate with areas of maximum intensity of the auscultatory murmurs. It is important to palpate the suprasternal notch and neck for **aortic bruits**, which may indicate the presence of aortic stenosis or, when less prominent, pulmonary stenosis. Right lower sternal border and apical systolic thrills are characteristic of ventricular septal defect and mitral insufficiency, respectively. Diastolic thrills are palpable in the presence of atrioventricular valvular stenosis. The timing and localization of thrills should be carefully noted.

Auscultation is an art that can be improved upon with practice and determination. The diaphragm of the stethoscope is placed firmly on the chest for high-pitched sounds; a lightly placed bell is optimal for low-pitched sounds. The physician should listen for one component at a time, concentrating initially on the characteristics of the individual heart sound and, later, on the murmurs. He or she must listen for the special characteristics of each heart sound and murmur. The 1st heart sound is caused by the closure of the atrioventricular valves (mitral and tricuspid); the 2nd sound is due to closure of the semilunar valves. During inspiration and increased filling of the right side of the heart, right ventricular ejection time increases and pulmonary valve closure is delayed; the variable normal splitting is thus related to respirations. The 1st heart sound is best heard at the apex, whereas the 2nd sound should be evaluated at the left upper sternal border. The patient should be supine, lying quietly, and breathing normally. The 2nd sound is split just beyond the height of inspiration and closes with expiration. The presence of splitting is more important than the intensity. The latter varies according to the age of the patient, the thickness of the chest wall, and the cardiac output. The presence of a normally split 2nd sound is strong evidence against the diagnosis of an atrial septal defect, defects associated with pulmonary artery hypertension, severe pulmonary valve stenosis, aortic and pulmonary atresia, truncus arteriosus, and transportation of the great arteries. Wide splitting is noted in pulmonary stenosis, Ebstein anomaly, total anomalous venous return, atrial septal defect, and tetralogy of Fallot. An accentuated 2nd sound with narrow splitting signifies pulmonary hypertension.

The 3rd heart sound is best heard with the bell at the apex in mid-diastole. A 4th sound, occurring in conjunction with atrial contraction, may be heard just prior to the 1st heart sound in late diastole. The 3rd sound may be normal in an adolescent with a relatively slow heart rate, but in a patient with the clinical signs of congestive heart failure and tachycardia it may be heard as a gallop rhythm and may merge with a 4th heart sound. A **gallop** rhythm is attributed to poor compliance of the ventricle with an exaggeration of the normal 3rd sound associated with ventricular filling.

Ejection clicks, which are heard in early systole, are related to dilatation of or hypertension in the aorta and pulmonary artery. They are heard so close to the 1st heart sound that they may be mistaken for a split 1st sound. Aortic systolic clicks are best heard at the left lower sternal border and are constant. They occur in conditions in which the aorta is dilated (e.g., aortic stenosis, tetralogy of Fallot, truncus arteriosus). Pulmonary ejection clicks associated with pulmonary stenosis are best heard at the left midsternal border and vary with respiration, disappearing with inspiration. A midsystolic click heard at the apex preceding a late systolic murmur suggests prolapse of the mitral valve.

Murmurs should be described as to their intensity, pitch,

timing (systolic or diastolic), area of maximal intensity, and transmission. **Systolic murmurs** are classified as ejection, pansystolic, or late systolic according to the timing of the murmur in relation to the 1st and 2nd heart sounds. The intensity of systolic murmurs is graded from I to VI: I, barely audible; II, medium intensity; III, loud but no thrill; IV, loud with a thrill; V, very loud but still requires the stethoscope to be on the chest; and VI, so loud the murmur can be heard with the stethoscope off the chest. Ejection systolic murmurs start after a well-heard 1st heart sound, increase in intensity, peak, and then decrease in intensity; they usually end before the 2nd sound. However, in patients with severe aortic or pulmonary stenosis, the murmur may extend beyond the 1st component of the 2nd sound, thus obscuring it. Pansystolic murmurs begin almost simultaneously with the 1st heart sound and continue throughout systole, on occasion becoming gradually decrescendo. In general, significant ejection murmurs imply increased flow or stenoses across a semilunar valve, whereas pansystolic murmurs are heard with ventricular septal defects or A-V valve (mitral or tricuspid) insufficiency. A "continuous murmur" is a systolic murmur that continues or "spills" into diastole and indicates continuous flow such as in the presence of a patent ductus arteriosus. This should be differentiated from a to-and-fro murmur, which indicates that the systolic component of the murmur ends at or before the 2nd sound and the diastolic murmur begins after semilunar valve closure (e.g., aortic stenosis with insufficiency). A late systolic murmur is a bruit that begins well beyond the 1st heart sound and continues until the end of systole. Such murmurs may be heard after a midsystolic click in the presence of mitral valve prolapse.

Several types of **diastolic murmurs** (graded I to IV) can be identified:

1. A high-pitched blowing diastolic murmur along the left sternal border beginning with S2 is associated with aortic insufficiency or, if pulmonary pressure is high, pulmonary valve insufficiency.
2. Early, short, lower-pitched protodiastolic murmurs along the left mid and upper sternal border are heard with pulmonary valvular insufficiency. These murmurs are typically noted after surgical repair of the pulmonary outflow tract in defects such as tetralogy of Fallot.
3. An early diastolic murmur at the left mid and lower sternal border may be due to increased blood flow across the tricuspid valve such as occurs with atrial septal defect (ASD), or less often, stenosis of this valve.
4. Rumbling mid-diastolic murmurs at the apex follow the 3rd heart sound and are due to increased left ventricular flow in conditions with large right to left shunts or with mitral insufficiency.
5. A long diastolic rumbling murmur at the apex, accentuated at the end of diastole (presystolic), indicates anatomic mitral stenosis.

The absence of a precordial murmur does not rule out significant congenital or acquired heart disease. Congenital heart defects, some of which are ductal dependent, may not demonstrate a murmur if the ductus arteriosus closes. These lesions include pulmonary or tricuspid valve atresia and transposition of the great arteries. Murmurs may seem insignificant in patients with severe aortic stenosis, ASD, anomalous pulmonary venous return, atrioventricular septal defects, coarctation of the aorta, or anomalous insertion of a coronary artery. In contrast, a murmur may be evident in patients with a large noncardiac arteriovenous malformation, myocarditis, cardiomyopathy, severe anemia, or hypertension, and can possibly delay the diagnosis of the underlying disease process.

Many murmurs are not associated with significant hemodynamic abnormalities. These are referred to as functional, "normal," insignificant, or innocent (the preferred term). During routine random auscultation, over 30% of children may have an *innocent murmur*; this percentage increases when auscultation is carried out under nonbasal circumstances (high cardiac output due to fever, infection, anxiety, etc.). The most common innocent murmur is a medium-pitched, vibratory, relatively short systolic ejection murmur, which is heard best along the left lower and midsternal border and has no significant radiation to the apex, base, or back. The short systolic ejection murmurs at the base and the continuous sound of a venous hum are other examples of common but insignificant bruits heard in childhood.

The common innocent murmur is heard most frequently from 3 to 7 yr of age. The murmur occurs during ejection and is musical, frequently sounding like the vibration of a tuning fork; it is brief in duration, may be attenuated in the sitting position, and is intensified by fever, excitement, or exercise. Innocent pulmonic murmurs are also common in children and adolescents and originate from the normal turbulence during ejection into the pulmonary artery. They are high-pitched, blowing, brief, early systolic murmurs, grades 1–2 of 6 in intensity, and best detected in the 2nd left parasternal space with the patient in the supine position. The **venous hum** is another example of a common insignificant bruit heard during childhood. This is produced by turbulence of blood in the jugular venous system; it has no pathologic significance and may be heard in the neck or anterior portion of the upper chest. It consists of a soft humming sound heard in both systole and diastole and can be exaggerated or made to disappear by varying the position of the head or can be decreased by lightly compressing the jugular venous system in the neck. These simple maneuvers are sufficient to differentiate a venous hum from the murmurs produced by organic cardiovascular disease, particularly patent ductus arteriosus.

The lack of significance of an innocent murmur should be discussed with the parents. It is important to offer complete reassurance because lingering doubts about the importance of a cardiac murmur may have profound effects on child-rearing practices, most often in the form of overprotectiveness. An underlying fear that a cardiac abnormality is present may negatively affect a child's self-image and subtly influence personality development. The physician should explain that the innocent murmur is simply a "noise" and does not indicate the presence of a significant cardiac defect. When asked, "Will it go away?" the best response is to state that since the murmur has no meaning, it does not matter whether it "goes away" or not. However, with growth, innocent murmurs are less well heard and may disappear completely.

At times, additional studies may be indicated to rule out a congenital heart defect, but "routine" electrocardiogram (ECG), x-ray, and/or ultrasound examination for well children with innocent murmurs should be avoided.

15.2 ROENTGENOGRAPHIC EXAMINATION

The chest roentgenogram may provide information about cardiac size and shape, pulmonary blood flow (vascularity), pulmonary edema, and associated lung and thorax anomalies (skeletal dysplasias, extra or deficient numbers of ribs). Variations are due to differences in body build, the phase of respiration or cardiac cycle, abnormalities of the thoracic cage, position of the diaphragm, or pulmonary disease.

The most frequently used measurement of cardiac size is the maximal width of the cardiac shadow in a midinspiration posteroanterior film: A vertical line is drawn down the middle of the sternal shadow, and perpendicular lines are drawn from the sternal line to the extreme right and left borders of the heart; the sum of the lengths of these lines is the *maximal cardiac width*. The *maximal chest width* is obtained by drawing a horizontal line between the right and left inner borders of the rib cage at the level of the top of the right diaphragm. When the maximal cardiac width is more than half the maximal chest width, the heart is usually enlarged. Cardiac size should be evaluated only when the film is taken during inspiration with the patient in an upright position. Diagnosis of "cardiac enlargement" on expiratory or prone films is a common cause of unnecessary referrals and laboratory studies.

The *cardiothoracic ratio* is a *less* useful index of cardiac enlargement in infancy than in subsequent years because the horizontal position of the heart may increase the ratio to more than half in the absence of true enlargement. Furthermore, the thymus may overlap not only the base of the heart, but virtually the entire mediastinum, thus obscuring the true cardiac silhouette.

The lateral chest roentgenogram may be helpful in infancy, as well as in older children with pectus excavatum or other conditions that result in a narrow anteroposterior chest dimension. In these situations the heart may appear quite small in the lateral view, suggesting that the apparent enlargement in the posteroanterior projection was due to either a thymic image, or flattening of the cardiac chambers as a result of a structural chest abnormality.

In the posteroanterior view, the left border of the cardiac shadow consists of three convex shadows produced from above downward by the aortic knob, the main and left pulmonary arteries, and the left ventricle, respectively (Fig. 15–8). In cases of moderate to marked left atrial enlargement the atrium may project between the pulmonary artery and the left ventricle. The outflow tract of the right ventricle or the pulmonary conus does not contribute to the shadows formed by the left border of the heart. The aortic knob is not as easily seen in infants and children as in adults. However, the side of the aortic arch (left or right) often can be inferred as being opposite to the side of the midline from which the air-filled trachea is visualized. Three structures also contribute to the right border of the cardiac silhouette; from above downward they are the superior vena cava, the ascending aorta, and the right atrium.

Interpretation of atrial or ventricular enlargement in infants by roentgenographic means is difficult, especially in the presence of a large thymic image. Abnormal roentgenographic findings should be complemented by an ECG, which is a more sensitive and accurate index of ventricular hypertrophy.

Enlargement of cardiac chambers or major arteries and veins results in prominence of areas where these structures are normally outlined on the chest roentgenogram. It is also important to assess the degree of pulmonary vascularity as represented by the intrapulmonary shadows. Angiocardiographic studies have shown that the hilar shadows are mainly vascular. Pulmonary overcirculation is usually associated with left to right shunts, and undercirculation with stenosis or atresia of the outflow tract of the right ventricle or of the pulmonary valve.

The esophagus is closely related to the great vessels, and visualization with barium helps to delineate these structures in selected situations such as coarctation of the aorta and vascular ring. However, echocardiographic examination best defines specific intracardiac chamber anatomy and enlargement. Thus, routine esophagograms and fluoroscopy are not necessary for the evaluation of most cardiac abnormalities.

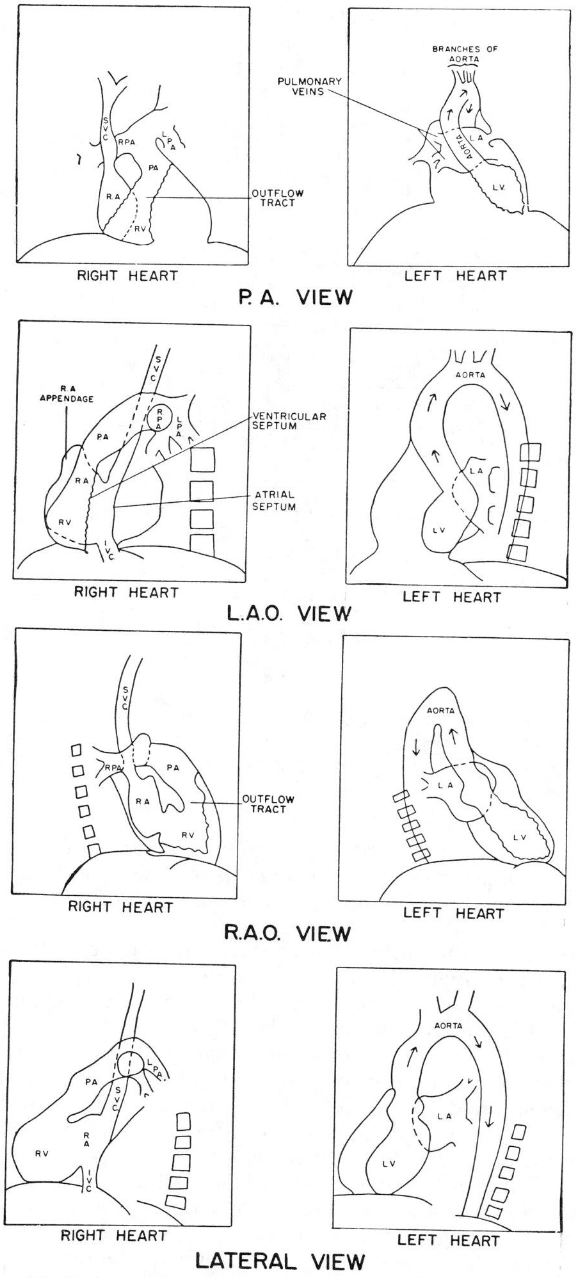

Figure 15–8. Idealized diagrams showing normal position of the cardiac chambers and great blood vessels. (P.A. = posteroanterior; L.A.O. = left anterior oblique; R.A.O. = right anterior oblique; SVC = superior vena cava; RA = right atrium; RV = right ventricle; PA = pulmonary artery; RPA = right pulmonary artery; LPA = left pulmonary artery; LA = left atrium; LV = left ventricle; IVC = inferior vena cava.) (Adapted and redrawn from Dotter and Steinberg: Radiology 53:513, 1949.)

15.3 ELECTROCARDIOGRAM

Changes in cardiac anatomy and hemodynamics soon after birth are reflected in the evolution of the ECG of the neonate. Because vascular resistances in the pulmonary and systemic circulations are nearly equal in the fetus at term, the intrauterine work of the heart results in virtually equal mass of both the right and left ventricles. After birth, systemic vascular

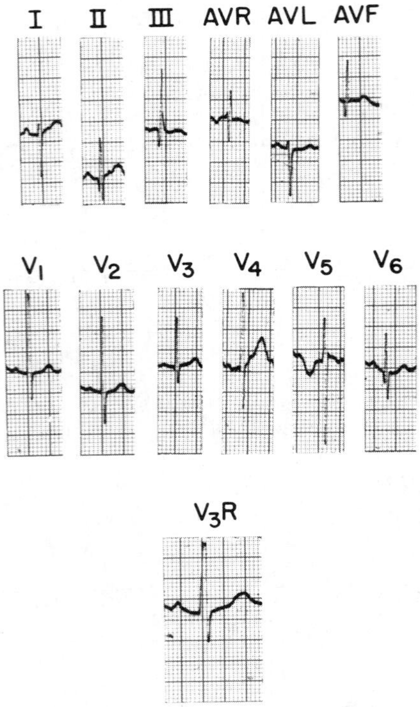

Figure 15–9. Electrocardiogram in a normal neonate less than 24 hr of age. Note the dominant R wave and upright T waves in leads V_3R and V_1. (V_3R paper speed = 50 mm/sec.)

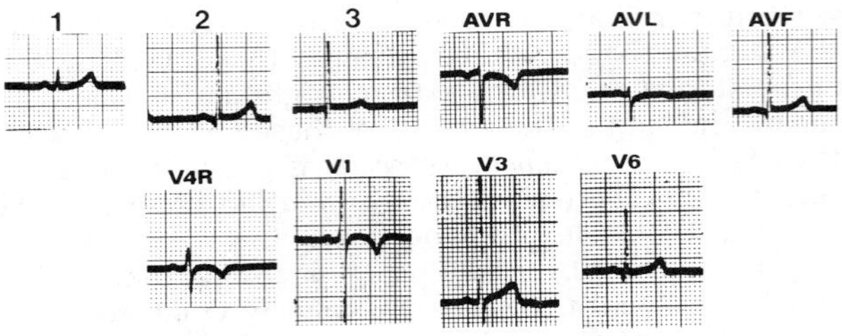

Figure 15–11. Electrocardiogram of a normal child. Note the relatively tall R waves and inversion of the T waves in V_4R and V_1.

resistance rises when the placental circulation is eliminated, and pulmonary vascular resistance falls when the lungs expand. These changes are effected over a period of hours or days.

The ECG demonstrates these anatomic and hemodynamic features principally by changes in the QRS and T wave morphology. It is *essential* that a 13-lead ECG be carried out in pediatric patients, including lead V_3R or V_4R. These right precordial leads are extremely important in the evaluation of right ventricular hypertrophy in childhood. On occasion, lead VI is positioned too far leftward to reflect right ventricular forces accurately and may display the usual R/S pattern of midprecordial lead. At the same time V_3R or V_4R may reflect a dominant R or S pattern, which is important diagnostically. During the first days of life, right axis deviation, large R waves, and upright T waves in the right precordial leads (V_3R or V_4R and V_1) are seen (Fig. 15–9). When pulmonary resistance decreases and right ventricular pressure reaches its normal level, the right precordial T waves become negative. In the great majority of instances this occurs within the first 48 hr of life, and if upright T waves persist in leads V_4R and/or V_1 beyond 1 wk, this represents an abnormal finding.

In the frontal plane leads of the standard ECG, the mean QRS axis in the newborn normally lies in the range of +110 to +180°. The right-sided chest leads reveal a larger positive (R) than negative (S) wave and may do so for months or years since the right ventricle remains relatively thick throughout infancy. Furthermore, owing to proximity, the voltage recorded by the right precordial leads is influenced to a greater extent by right ventricular depolarization. Left-sided leads (V_5 and V_6) also reflect right-sided dominance in the early neonatal period when the RS ratio may be less than 1. However, since left precordial leads are in direct proximity to the left ventricle, a dominant R wave reflecting left ventricular forces quickly becomes evident within the first few days of life (Fig. 15–10). Over the years, the QRS axis gradually shifts leftward and right ventricular forces slowly regress. As the left ventricle becomes dominant, the ECG evolves to the characteristic pattern of the older child (Fig. 15–11), and finally the typical adult electrocardiogram emerges (Fig. 15–12).

With the growth of the infant there is slow regression of right ventricular dominance and an increase in left ventricular forces. Leads V_1 and V_4R will display a prominent R wave until 6 mo–8 yr of age. The majority of children will have an RS ratio greater than 1 in lead V_4R until they are 4 yr of age. The T waves are inverted in V_4R, V_1, V_2, and V_3 during infancy and may remain so into the middle of the 2nd decade of life

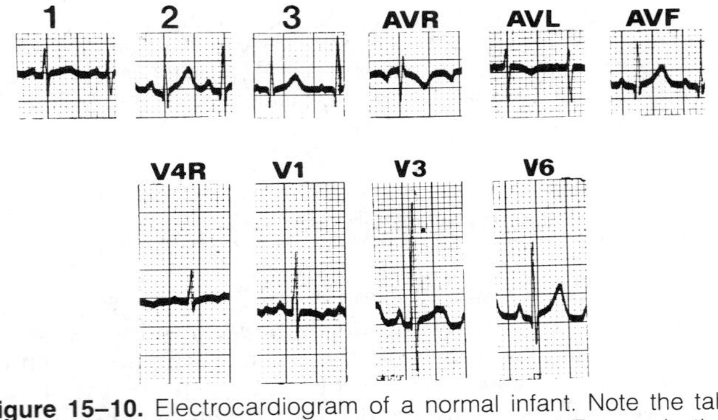

Figure 15–10. Electrocardiogram of a normal infant. Note the tall R and small S waves in V_4R and V_1 and the inverted T wave in these leads. There is also a dominant R wave in V_6.

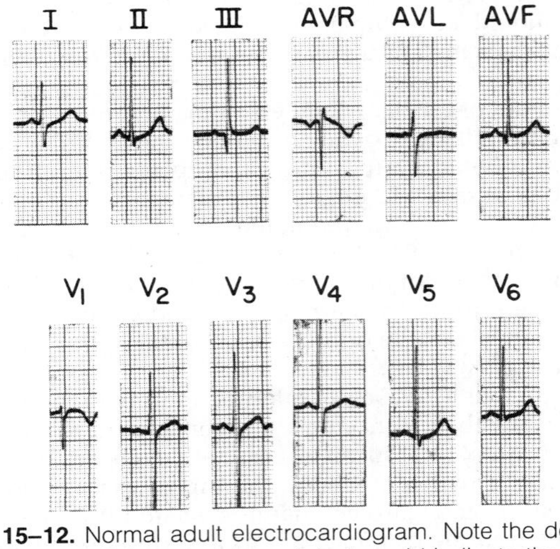

Figure 15–12. Normal adult electrocardiogram. Note the dominant S wave in lead V_1. This pattern in an infant would indicate the presence of left ventricular hypertrophy.

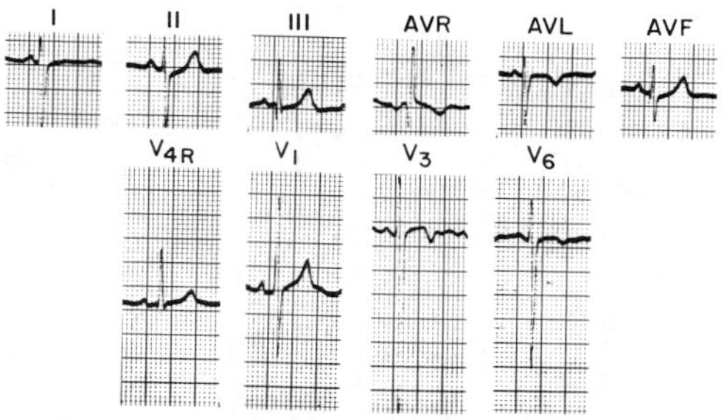

Figure 15–13. Electrocardiogram of an infant with right ventricular hypertrophy (tetralogy of Fallot). Note the tall R waves in the right precordium and deep S waves in V_6. The positive T waves in V_4R and V_1 are also characteristic of right ventricular hypertrophy.

and beyond. The processes of right ventricular thinning and left ventricular growth are best reflected in the QRS-T pattern over the right precordial leads. The diagnosis of right or left ventricular hypertrophy can be made only with an understanding of the normal states of these chambers at various ages until adulthood is reached.

Ventricular hypertrophy may result in increased voltage in the R and S waves in the chest leads. However, the height of these deflections is governed by the proximity of the exploring electrode to the surface of the heart, and by the sequence of electrical activation through the ventricles, resulting in variable degrees of cancellation of forces, as well as by hypertrophy of the myocardium. Because the chest wall in infants and children as well as in adolescents may be relatively thin, the diagnosis of ventricular hypertrophy should not be based on voltage changes alone in the entire pediatric age range.

The diagnosis of pathologic right ventricular hypertrophy is difficult in the last wk of life, as physiologic right ventricular hypertrophy is a normal finding. Serial tracings are often necessary to determine whether marked right axis deviation and potentially abnormal right precordial forces or T waves, or both, will persist (Fig. 15–13). An adult ECG pattern seen in a neonate suggests left ventricular enlargement (see Fig. 15–12). The premature infant, however, may display a more "mature" ECG than his or her full-term counterpart (Fig. 15–14) as a result of lower pulmonary resistance secondary to underdevelopment of the medial muscular layer of the pulmonary arterioles. Thus, the electrocardiogram may simulate that of the older child with left ventricular dominance manifested by a more mature R wave progression across the precordium (qR in V_6, R/S ratio in V_4R, and V_1 equal to or less than 1). Some premature infants display a pattern of generalized low voltage across the precordium.

THE P WAVE. Tall, narrow, and spiked P waves are seen in congenital pulmonary stenosis, Ebstein anomaly of the tricuspid valve, tricuspid atresia, and sometimes cor pulmonale. These abnormal waves are due to right atrial hypertrophy and/or dilatation, are usually taller than 2.5 mm, and are most obvious in standard lead II and leads V_4R, V_3R, and V_1 (Fig. 15–15*A*). Similar waves are sometimes seen in thyrotoxicosis. Widened P waves, commonly bifid, indicate left atrial enlargement (see Fig. 15–15*B*). They are seen in some patients with large ventricular septal defects, with communications between the aorta and pulmonary circulation, and with severe mitral stenosis. Flat P waves may be found in hyperkalemia.

With normal position of the atriae and sinus rhythm, the P wave should be upright in leads I and AVF. With atrial inversion (situs inversus), the P wave may be inverted in lead I. Inverted P waves in leads II and AVF are seen in nodal or junctional rhythms regardless of atrial position.

RIGHT VENTRICULAR HYPERTROPHY. Right ventricular surface leads of infants and children differ from those of adults, and tracings of the right side of the chest (V_4R or V_3R) are essential. In infants with **right ventricular hypertrophy** the following changes may occur singly or in combination (see Fig. 15–13): (1) a qR pattern in the right ventricular surface leads; (2) a positive T wave in leads V_{3-4}R through V_3 after the first 48 hr of life; (3) a monophasic R wave in V_{3-4}R and/or V_1; (4) rsR′ in right precordial leads often with a tall secondary R wave (this pattern is frequently associated with volume overload and hypertrophy of the right ventricular outflow track as typically seen in atrial septal defect); (5) age-related voltage criteria in V_{3-4}R and V_1(R), and/or V_{6-7}(S); (6) marked right axis deviation (>120 degrees); (7) a complete reversal of the normal adult precordial RS pattern; and (8) right atrial enlargement. At least two of these changes should be present to support a diagnosis of right ventricular hypertrophy. In general, if a pattern of right ventricular hypertrophy in the newborn and young infant persists or even becomes more prominent into early childhood, abnormal right ventricular hypertrophy is present. In contrast, the small infant who displays the pattern of a "normal" electrocardiogram for an older child may have left ventricular hypertrophy.

Abnormal hemodynamics can be correlated with abnormal electrocardiographic patterns. Obstruction to right ventricular and pulmonary flow (e.g., pulmonary stenosis) is associated with a systolic overload pattern characterized by tall pure R waves in the right precordial leads. In these leads the T wave is initially upright and later becomes inverted. In contrast, diastolic overload of the right ventricle (e.g., with atrial septal defect) is characterized by an rsR′ pattern and right ventricular conduction delay (Fig. 15–16). However, these patterns, al-

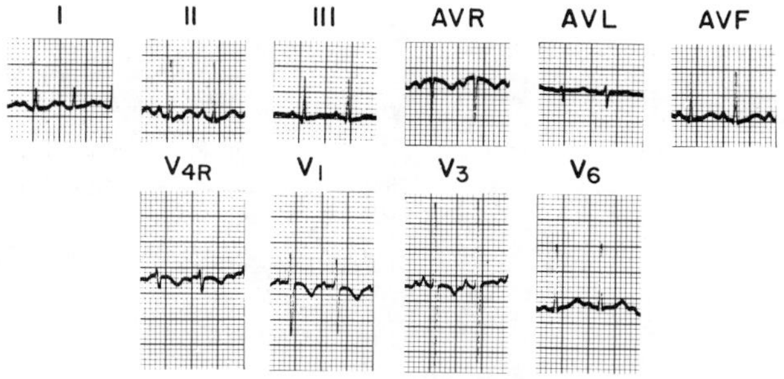

Figure 15–14. Electrocardiogram of a premature infant (weight 2 kg and age 5 wk at the time of tracing). The cardiovascular system was clinically normal. Left ventricular dominance is manifest by R wave progression across the chest simulating tracings obtained from older children. Compare with the tracing from a normal full-term infant, Figure 15–10.

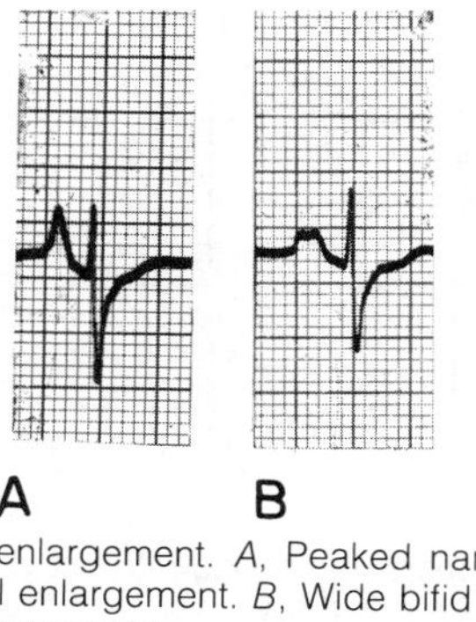

Figure 15–15. Atrial enlargement. *A*, Peaked narrow P waves characteristic of right atrial enlargement. *B*, Wide bifid M-shaped P waves typical of left atrial enlargement.

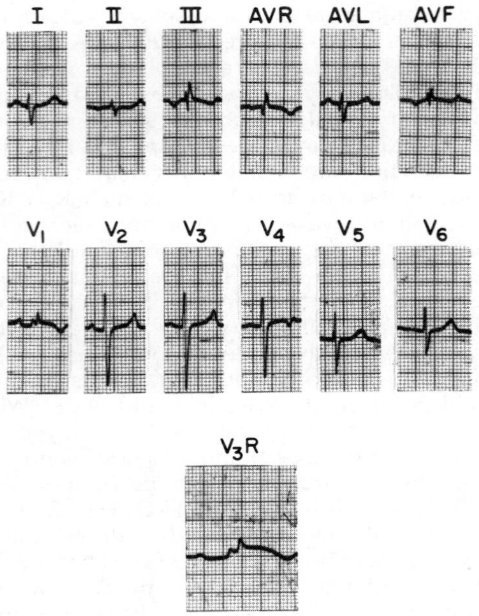

Figure 15–16. Electrocardiogram showing right ventricular conduction delay characterized by an rsR′ pattern in V_1 and a deep S wave in V_6. (V_3R paper speed = 50 mm/sec.)

though useful, may simply reflect the severity of right ventricular hypertrophy rather than serve as specific indicators of increased preload (diastolic) or afterload (systolic). For example, patients with mild to moderate pulmonary stenosis (systolic overload) often exhibit an rsR′ in the right precordial leads.

The following features indicate the presence of *left ventricular hypertrophy* (Fig. 15–17): (1) depression of the S-T segments and inversion of T waves and left precordial surface leads (V_5, V_6, and V_7), a left ventricular strain pattern; these findings suggest the presence of a severe lesion and significant myocardial abnormality; (2) increase in magnitude of initial forces to the right (i.e., deep Q in left precordial leads);

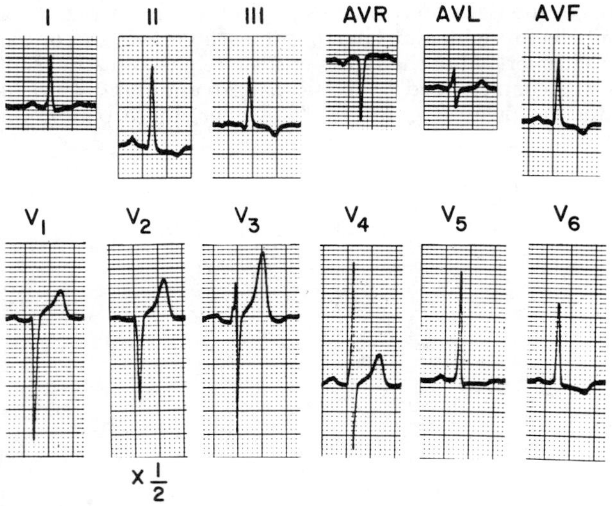

Figure 15–17. Electrocardiogram showing left ventricular hypertrophy in a 12-yr-old child with aortic stenosis. Note the deep S wave in V_1–V_3 and tall R in V_5. Also, T wave inversion is present in II, III, AVF, and V_6.

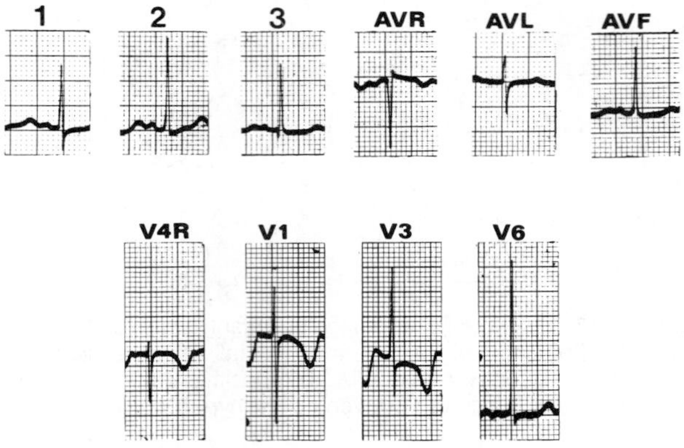

Figure 15–18. Electrocardiogram in hypocalcemia and hypokalemia (serum calcium 1.8 mEq/L; serum potassium 2.2 mEq/L at the time of tracing). Note the prolongation of electrical systole owing to long S-TU segment. This graph also shows left ventricular hypertrophy.

(3) voltage criteria in V_3R and V_1(S) and/or V_6(R). It is important to emphasize that evaluation of ventricular hypertrophy should not be based on voltage criteria alone. The concepts of systolic and diastolic overload, although not always consistent, are also useful in evaluating left ventricular enlargement. Severe systolic overload of the left ventricles is suggested by straightening of the ST segments and inverted T waves over the left precordial leads; diastolic overload may result in tall R waves, a large Q wave, and normal T waves over the left precordium.

BUNDLE BRANCH BLOCK. Complete right bundle branch block may occur as a congenital finding or be acquired after open heart surgery, especially when a right ventriculotomy has been carried out. Congenital left bundle branch block is rare; this pattern is occasionally seen with cardiomyopathy.

Q-T INTERVAL. The duration of the Q-T interval varies with the cardiac rate; a corrected Q-T interval can be calculated by dividing the measured Q-T interval by the square root of the cycle length of the R-R interval. The normal Q-TC should be less than 0.45 sec. It is often lengthened in children with hypokalemia and hypocalcemia; in the former instance a U wave may be noted at the end of the T wave (Figs. 15–18 and 15–19). Prolonged Q-T intervals (Fig. 15–20) may be seen in children who are at risk for ventricular arrhythmias and sudden death (Jervell and Lange-Nielsen syndrome with hearing loss or Romano-Ward syndrome).

ST SEGMENT AND T WAVE ABNORMALITIES. Elevation of the ST segment in normal teenagers is attributed to

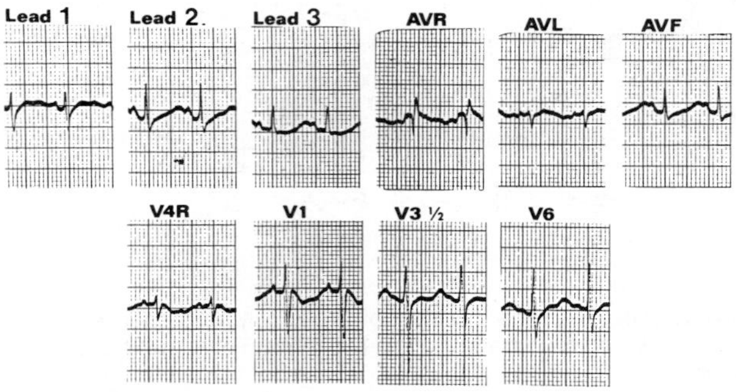

Figure 15–19. Electrocardiogram in hypokalemia (serum potassium 2.7 mEq/L; serum calcium 4.8 mEq/L at time of tracing). Note the prolongation of electrical systole as evidenced by a widened TU wave; also the depression of the ST segment in V_4R, V_1, and V_6.

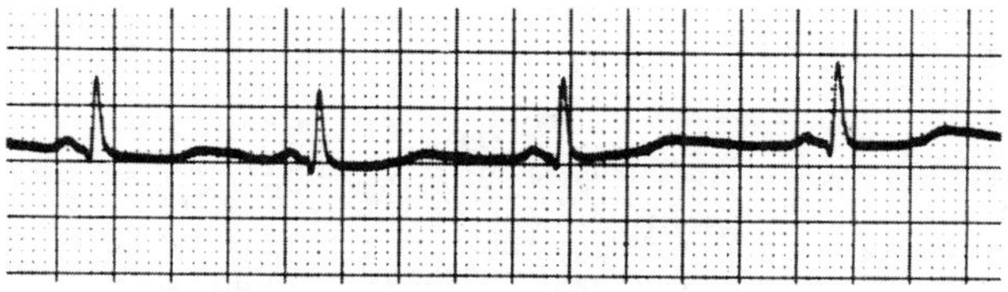

Figure 15–20. Prolonged Q-T intervals.

early repolarization of the heart. In generalized pericarditis, superficial epicardial involvement may cause elevation of the ST segment followed by abnormal T wave inversion as healing progresses. Administration of digitalis is associated with sagging of the ST segment and abnormal inversion of the T wave. Depression of the ST segment may also occur in any condition that produces myocardial damage, for example, anemia, carbon monoxide poisoning, endocardial fibroelastosis, aberrant origin of the left coronary artery from the pulmonary artery, glycogen storage disease of the heart, myocardial tumors, and mucopolysaccharidoses. Aberrant origin of the left coronary artery from the pulmonary artery may lead to changes indistinguishable from those of acute myocardial infarction in adults. Similar changes may occur in patients with other rare abnormalities of the coronary arteries and with cardiomyopathy without anatomic abnormalities of the coronary arteries.

In any form of carditis simple inversion of the T wave may occur. Hypothyroidism may produce flat or inverted T waves in association with generalized low voltage. In hyperkalemia the T waves are commonly of high voltage and are tent-shaped (Fig. 15–21).

15.4 HEMATOLOGIC DATA

Evaluation of hematologic findings as part of the assessment of the cardiovascular system should be carried out with an awareness of the normal variations in infancy (see also Sec. 16.1–16.2). Persistent polycythemia after the first month of life is frequently noted in patients with right to left shunts and cyanosis. Patients with marked polycythemia have a delicate balance between intravascular thrombosis and a bleeding diathesis; this abnormal hemostasis should be recognized and treated prior to any surgical procedure. The most frequent abnormalities are accelerated fibrinolysis, thrombocytopenia, abnormal clot retraction, hypofibrinogenemia, prolonged prothrombin time, and prolonged partial thromboplastin time. These abnormalities occur singly or in combination and may be related to the severity of the polycythemia. Abnormal coagulation may be related to the effects of hypoxia and polycythemia on platelet production and consumption combined with the effects of chronic liver dysfunction on procoagulants and fibrinolysis.

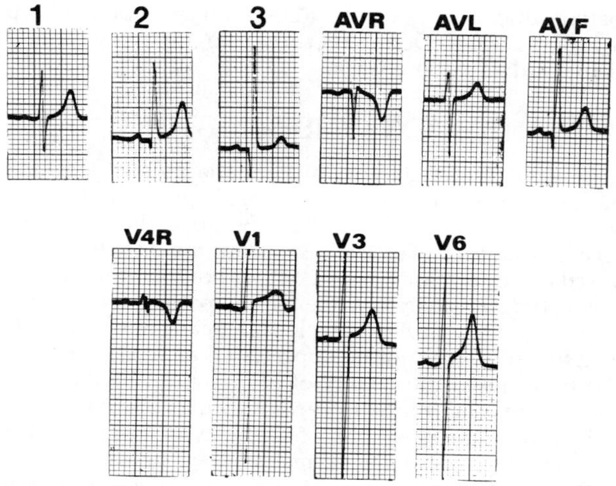

Figure 15–21. Electrocardiogram in hyperkalemia (serum potassium 6.5 mEq/L; serum calcium 5.1 mEq/L). Note the tall, tent-shaped T waves, especially in leads I, II, and V_6.

The preparation of cyanotic polycythemic patients for elective surgery such as dental extraction includes evaluation for and treatment of abnormal coagulation. Accelerated fibrinolysis has been suppressed with epsilon-aminocaproic acid. Thrombocytopenia and hypofibrinogenemia may be improved by phlebotomies.

Because of high viscosity of polycythemic blood (Hct >65%), patients having cyanotic congenital heart disease are at risk to develop vascular thrombosis, especially of cerebral veins. Polycythemic infants with iron deficiency are at even greater risk for cerebrovascular accidents, probably because thrombosis is enhanced by a decrease in velocity of blood flow as well as by altered deformability of the red cells.

Cyanotic patients should have frequent Hgb and Hct determinations. Increasing polycythemia, often associated with headache, fatigue, and/or dyspnea, is an indication for palliative or corrective surgical intervention. Among cyanotic patients with inoperable conditions, phlebotomy may be required to treat individuals whose Hct has risen to the 65–70% level or above, regardless of symptoms. This procedure is not without risk, especially in polycythemic patients with extreme elevation of pulmonary vascular resistance. Because these patients do not tolerate wide fluctuations in circulating blood volume, the phlebotomy should be performed in the same way as an exchange transfusion; blood is replaced with fresh frozen plasma or albumin. Initially, these patients require frequent phlebotomies (often weekly) until the hematocrit is stabilized at the desired level (±60%). Subsequently, phlebotomies may be necessary at intervals of only 3–5 wk.

Iron deficiency anemia is poorly tolerated by cyanotic patients with right to left shunts, especially by infants and toddlers. Such children are more susceptible to hypercyanotic spells. Iron therapy produces improvement, but surgical treatment of the cardiac anomaly is required.

15.5 ECHOCARDIOGRAPHY

Echocardiography (ultrasound) is an extremely important technique in the diagnosis of congenital and acquired cardiac disease in infants and children (see also Sec. 6.56). It can also be used to evaluate cardiac contractility (performance); gradients across stenotic valves; the direction of flow across a shunt; the patency of coronary arteries; the presence of vegetations due to endocarditis; the presence of pericardial fluid, cardiac tumors, or chamber thrombi; prosthetic valve function; septal hypertrophy; aortic root dimensions; and the effects of cardiotonic or cardiotoxic drugs. Echocardiography may also assist in performance of pericardiocentesis. Echocardiography employs M mode, two-dimensional real-time imaging, and Doppler flow studies.

M mode echocardiography identifies the motion of intracardiac structures (opening, closing of valves, movement of septa), the anatomy of valves, and the presence of endocarditis vegetations larger than 2–3 mm. M mode can define the presence or absence of individual structures and their relationships to one another (Fig. 15–22) and can evaluate cardiac function (Table 15–4). **Two-dimensional** (2-D) **echocardiography** provides a better, more coherent, realistic image of

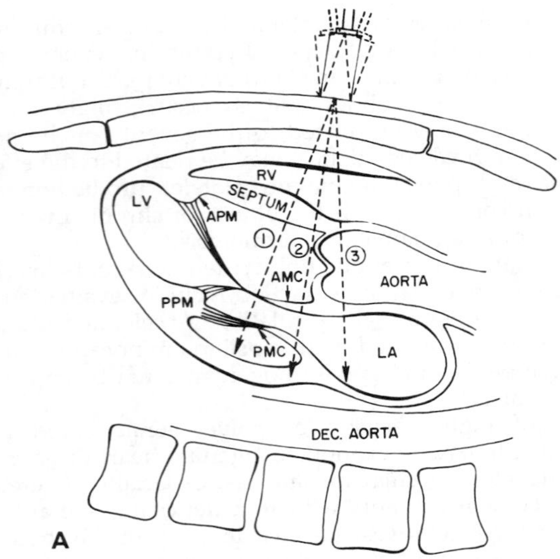

A

Figure 15–22. Normal echocardiograms. *A*, Diagram of sagittal section of heart showing structures traversed by echo beam in positions (1), (2), and (3). (AMC = anterior mitral cusp; APM = anterior papillary muscle; Dec. aorta = descending aorta; LA = left atrium; LV = left ventricle; PMC = posterior mitral cusp; PPM = posterior papillary muscle; RV = right ventricle.) *B*, Echocardiogram from transducer position (1); this is the best view to evaluate interventricular septum (S) and for measurement of the right ventricular dimension (RVED) as well as of the left ventricular dimension (LVED) in end diastole (Dd) and end systole (Ds). (CW = chest wall.) *C*, Normal septal aortic and mitral aortic relationships obtained when transducer is swept from positions (1) through (3) of A. (A = aortic valve; LA = left atrium; LV = left ventricle; MV = mitral valve; RV = right ventricle; S = interventricular septum.) Note the continuity of the anterior mitral leaflet with the posterior wall of the aorta and of the ventricular septum with the anterior wall of the aorta.

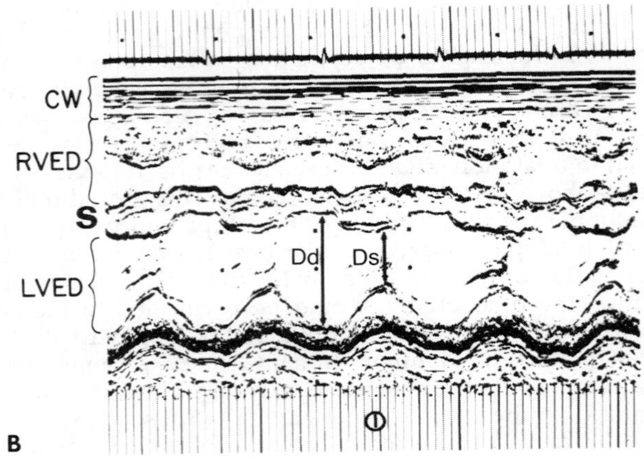

B

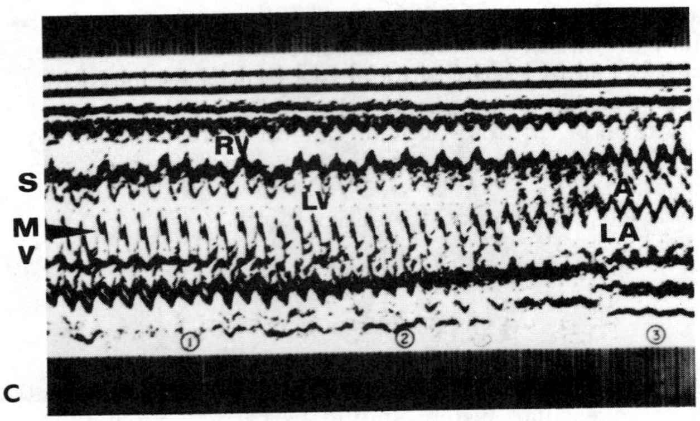

C

cardiac structures. The enhanced spatial anatomic relationships with 2-D echocardiography make this method the imaging technique of choice for diagnosing structural heart disease. With 2-D echocardiography the contracting heart is imaged by means of various views (subxiphoid, Fig. 15–23; parasagittal, Fig. 15–24; parasternal, Fig. 15–25; suprasternal, Fig. 15–26) that emphasize specific structures (e.g., chambers, valves, septa, great vessels, myocardium). Such images resemble those seen in angiography.

Doppler echocardiography is an ultrasound technique that identifies flow rather than morphology. It displays flow in cardiac chambers and vascular channels based on the change in frequency imparted to a sound wave by the movement of erythrocytes. The speed and direction of blood flow in the line of the echo beam change the transducer's reference frequency, which can be translated into volumetric (L/min) data used to estimate systemic or pulmonary blood flow and barometric (mm Hg) data used to estimate gradients across semilunar or atrioventricular valves. The directional quality of Doppler identifies abnormalities in blood flow associated with congenital heart disease (Fig. 15–27). Because small or multiple left to right or right to left shunts can be identified, color Doppler permits more accurate assessment of the presence and direction of intracardiac shunts. Valvular insufficiency is more accurately evaluated with color Doppler. Standardized colors depict flow toward (red) or away from (blue) the transducer.

Transesophageal echocardiography is a more sensitive imaging technique that produces a clearer view of smaller lesions such as vegetations in endocarditis. It is useful in visualizing the atria, aortic root dissection, mitral valve disease, and prosthetic valve dysfunction.

Used with other clinical or laboratory methods, echocardiography facilitates the selection of patients who require cardiac catheterization. Many patients with lesions such as ASD or patent ductus arteriosus (PDA) can be operated upon following 2-D and Doppler echocardiography without the need for cardiac catheterization.

15.6 EXERCISE TESTING

The normal cardiorespiratory system adapts to the extensive demands of exercise with a several-fold increase in oxygen consumption and cardiac output. Because there is a large reserve capacity for exercise, significant abnormalities of cardiovascular performance may exist without symptoms at rest or during ordinary activities. Generally, patients are evaluated in a resting state, during which significant abnormalities of cardiac function may not be appreciated or, if detected, their implications about the quality of life may not be recognized. Permission for children with cardiovascular disease to participate in various forms of physical activity is frequently based on subjective criteria. Exercise testing plays an important role in evaluating symptoms, quantitating the severity of cardiac abnormalities, and assisting in the management of these patients.

TABLE 15–4. Echographic Measurement of Cardiovascular Performance

1. Per cent shortening $= \frac{LVED - LVES}{LVED} \times 100$ (see Fig. 15–22)
   LVED = left ventricular end-diastolic dimension; LVES = left ventricular end-systolic dimension. *(Normal,* 28–38%.)
2. Mean VCF $= \frac{LVED - LVES}{LVED \times ET}$
   VCF = mean velocity of circumferential fiber shortening (expressed as circumference [circ] per second); LVED and LVES as in (1) above; ET = ejection time. (*Normal values:* neonates, 1.51 ± 0.04 [SE] circ/sec; children [5–15 yr], 1.34 ± 0.03 [SE] circ/sec.)
3. Systolic time intervals (a) $\frac{LPEP}{LVET}$ (normal range is 0.3–0.39; average, 0.35). (LPEP = left ventricular pre-ejection period; LVET = left ventricular ejection time.) (b) $\frac{RPEP}{RVET}$ (normal range is 0.16–0.30; average, 0.24). (RPEP = right ventricular pre-ejection period; RVET = right ventricular ejection time.) These ratios are indirect indices of changes in afterload, preload, contractility, and electromechanical delay.
4. Isovolemic contraction (ICT) may be derived from the following regression equation: ICT = 53 − 0.22 × heart rate (SE ± 7.3). ICT is increased in left ventricular myocardial disease and decreased in aortic runoff (e.g., patent ductus arteriosus).
5. Right and left ventricular outflow obstruction may be quantitated by Doppler estimation of the velocity of blood flow (V) across the stenotic segment. The peak systolic ejection gradient (PSEG) = $4V^2$.

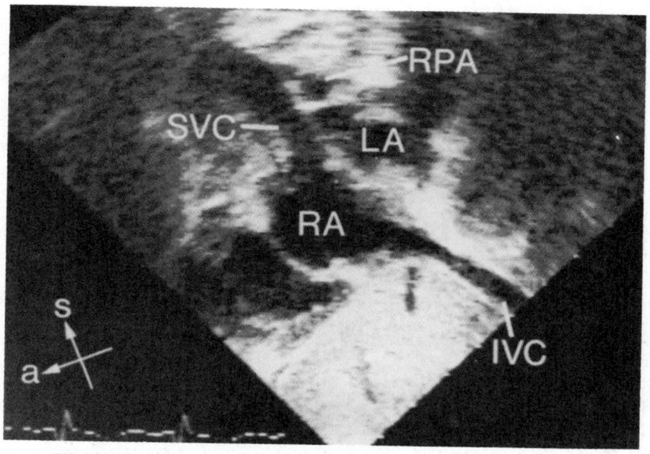

Figure 15–24. Right parasagittal normal echocardiographic plane view showing the junction of the inferior and superior venae cavae with the right atrium. (a = anterior; IVC = inferior vena cava; LA = left atrium; RA = right atrium; RPA = right pulmonary artery; s = superior; SVC = superior vena cava.) (From Sanders SP: Echocardiography. *In*: Long WA [ed]: Fetal and Neonatal Cardiology. Philadelphia, WB Saunders, 1990.)

Exercise studies are usually performed on a graded treadmill apparatus utilizing timed intervals of increasing grade and speed (Bruce protocol). Many laboratories now have the capacity to measure cardiac output and pulmonary function noninvasively during exercise.

As the child grows, the capacity for work increases with body size and skeletal muscle mass. All indices of cardiopulmonary function, however, do not increase in a uniform manner. A major response to exercise is an increase in cardiac output, principally as a result of increased heart rate, but stroke volume, systemic venous return, and pulse pressure are also increased. Systemic vascular resistance is greatly decreased as the blood vessels in working muscle dilate as a response to increasing metabolic demands. As the child becomes older and larger, the response of the heart rate to exercise remains prominent, but the cardiac output increases because of growing cardiac volume capacity and hence stroke volume. The responses to dynamic exercise are not dependent only on age. For any given body surface area, boys have a larger stroke volume than size-matched girls. This increase is mediated by posture as well as by sex. Augmentation of stroke volume with upright, dynamic exercise is facilitated by the pumping action of working muscles, which overcomes the static effect of gravity and increases systemic venous return.

Dynamic exercise testing defines not only endurance and exercise capacity, but also the effect of such exercise on myocardial blood flow and cardiac rhythm. In normal children an ECG during exercise shows a decrease in the R-R interval

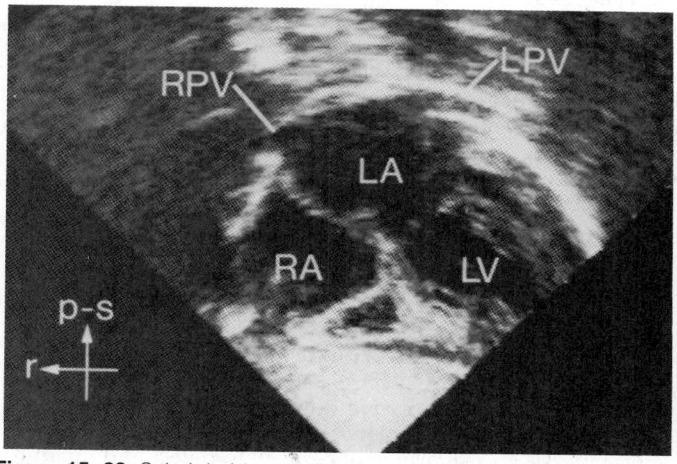

Figure 15–23. Subxiphoid normal echocardiographic view. The anterior angulation shows the mitral valve and the left ventricular inflow tract. Note the pulmonary veins connecting with the left atrium. (LA = left atrium; LPV = left pulmonary vein; RPV = right pulmonary vein; LV = left ventricle; p-s = posterior-superior; r = right; RA = right atrium.) (From Sanders SP: Echocardiography. *In*: Long WA [ed]: Fetal and Neonatal Cardiology. Philadelphia, WB Saunders, 1990.)

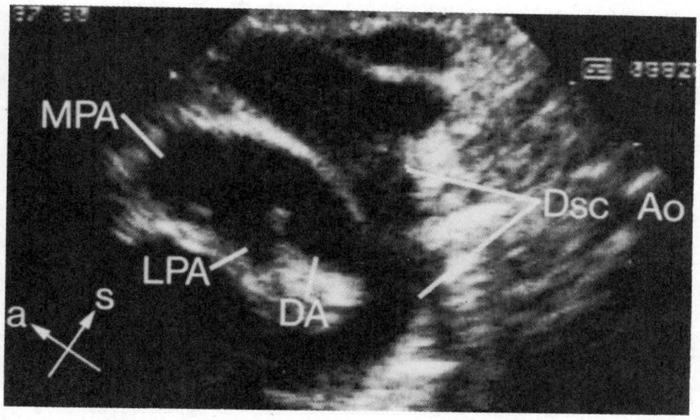

Figure 15–25. Normal high parasternal, parasagittal echocardiographic plane view for imaging the ductus arteriosus. (a = anterior; DA = ductus arteriosus; Dsc Ao = descending aorta; LPA = left pulmonary artery; MPA = main pulmonary artery; s = superior.) (From Sanders SP: Echocardiography. *In*: Long WA [ed]: Fetal and Neonatal Cardiology. Philadelphia, WB Saunders, 1990.)

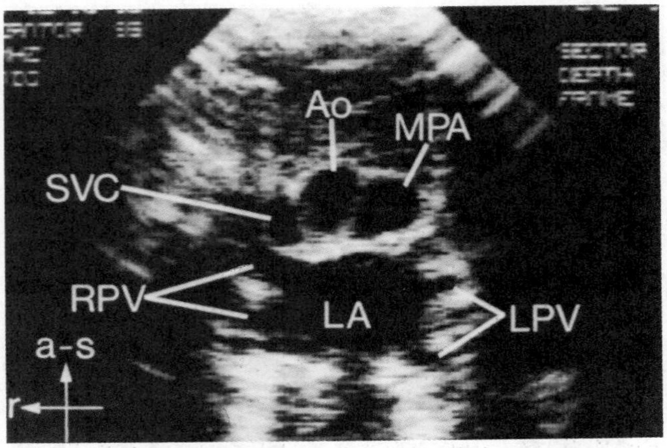

Figure 15–26. Suprasternal notch normal echocardiographic view. Pulmonary veins connecting with the left atrium. (Ao = aorta; a-s = anterior-superior; LA = left atrium; LPV = left pulmonary vein; MPA = main pulmonary artery; RPV = right pulmonary vein; r = right; SVC = superior vena cava.) (From Sanders SP: Echocardiography. *In*: Long WA [ed]: Fetal and Neonatal Cardiology. Philadelphia, WB Saunders, 1990.)

(increased heart rate) commensurate with the level of exercise. Significant ST segmental depression reflects abnormalities in myocardial perfusion. Subendocardial ischemia commonly occurs during exercise in children with hypertrophied left ventricles. The exercise electrocardiogram is considered abnormal if ST segmental depression is equal to or greater than 2 mm and extends for at least 0.06 sec after the J point (onset of ST segment) in conjunction with a horizontal, upward, or downward sloping ST segment.

Provocation of rhythm disturbances during an exercise study is an important method for evaluating selected patients with known or suspected rhythm disorders. The effect of pharmacologic management can also be tested in this manner.

Conditions in which exercise testing may be helpful include (1) left ventricular outflow obstruction, such as valvular, subvalvular, and supravalvular aortic stenosis, hypertrophic cardiomyopathy, and coarctation of the aorta; (2) chronic volume overload of the left or right ventricle, such as atrioventricular or semilunar valve incompetence and left to right shunts; (3) arrhythmias; and (4) hypertension.

A physician should be present during the exercise test to supervise its performance, and adequate emergency equipment must be immediately available (e.g., defibrillator, medications, IV fluids, etc.). Indications for termination of a study are (1) failure or inadequacy of the electocardiographic monitoring; (2) onset of serious arrhythmias, such as ventricular or supraventricular tachycardia; (3) premature beats (more than 25% of beats) precipitated or aggravated by exercise; (4) development of heart block; (5) precipitation of pain, headache, dizziness, or syncope; (6) ST segmental depression or elevation of 3 mm or more; (7) inappropriate hypertension (systolic pressure >230 mm Hg or diastolic pressure >120 mm Hg); (8) inappropriate fall of blood pressure; (9) development of cutaneous vascular insufficiency (e.g., pallor); or (10) severe fatigue.

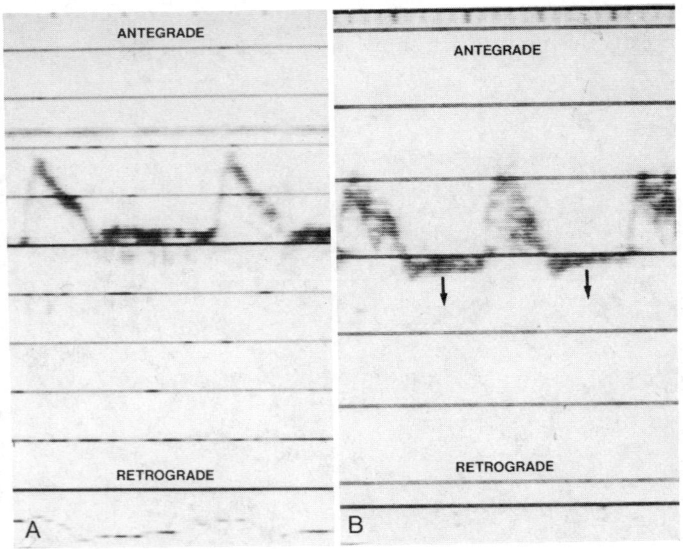

Figure 15–27. Patent ductus arteriosus. *A*, Doppler flow in the proximal descending aorta of normal infant demonstrating the normal antegrade systolic and diastolic flow. *B*, Doppler flow configuration in an infant with patent ductus arteriosus reveals antegrade systolic but retrograde diastolic flow *(arrows)*.

15.7 MAGNETIC RESONANCE IMAGING (MRI) AND RADIONUCLIDE STUDIES

Magnetic resonance imaging is helpful in the diagnosis and management of patients with congenital heart disease. It produces tomographic images of the heart in any projection (Figs. 15–28 and 15–29) by portraying the response of tissues in a homogeneous magnetic field when exposed to bursts of radiofrequency energy. The gray-scale intensity of each individual picture element in an image is related to the concentration, motion, and chemical microenvironment of hydrogen nuclei in that element. Excellent contrast resolution of fat, myocardium, and lung, as well as moving blood from blood vessel walls, is obtained.

This noninvasive method of cardiac imaging provides diagnostic imagery in malformations of the great vessels, including coarctation of the aorta, proximal branch pulmonary artery stenosis, and transposition of the great arteries, as well as simple and complex cardiac malformations, including aortic stenosis, pulmonary stenosis, ASD, ventricular septal defect (VSD), tetralogy of Fallot, single ventricle, and inversion of the ventricles.

New developments in MRI include cine MRI and in vivo magnetic resonance (MR) spectroscopy. Cine MRI allows acquisition of images in several tomographic planes. Within each plane, images are obtained at different phases of the cardiac cycle. Thus, when displayed in a dynamic "cine" format, changes in wall thickening, chamber volume, and valve function can be displayed and analyzed. Phosphorus **MR spectroscopy** provides a means of demonstrating relative concentrations of high-energy metabolites—adenosine triphosphate (ATP), adenosine diphosphate (ADP), inorganic phosphate (Pi), and phosphocreatine—within regions of myocardium.

MRI complements information provided by echocardiography and cineangiography. With further development in rapid image acquisition, and spectroscopic techniques, MRI might reduce the need for invasive angiography or tissue biopsy during cardiac catheterization.

Radionuclide angiography may be used to detect and quantify shunts and analyze the distribution of blood flow to each lung. *Gated blood pool scanning* can be used to calculate hemodynamic measurements, quantify valvular regurgitation, and detect regional wall motion abnormalities. *Thallium imaging* may be used to evaluate perfusion of cardiac muscle

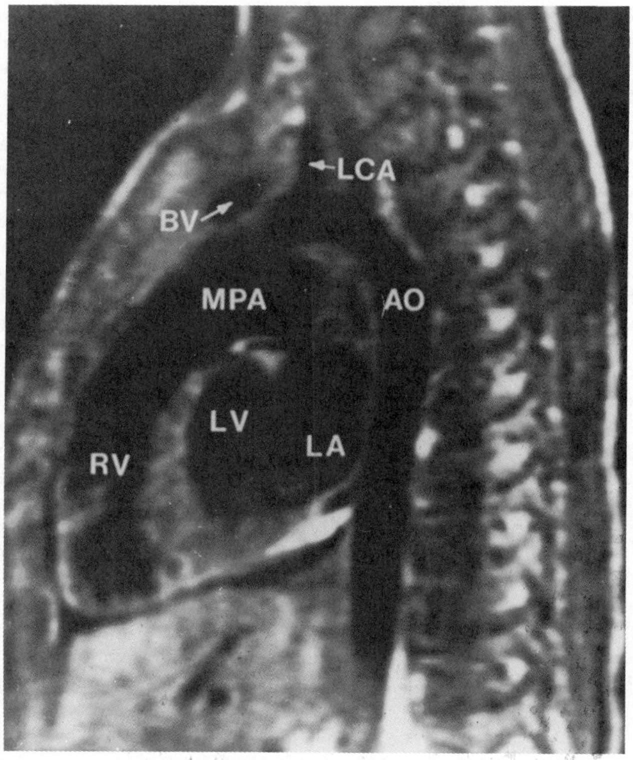

Figure 15–28. Sagittal normal MRI image. (AO = aorta; BV = brachiocephalic vein; LA = left atrium; LCA = left coronary artery; LV = left ventricle; MPA = main pulmonary artery; RV = right ventricle.) (From Bisset GS III: Cardiac and great vessel anatomy. *In*: El-Khoury GY, Bergman RA, Montgomery WJ: Sectional Anatomy by MRI/CT. New York, Churchill Livingstone, 1990, pp 219–243.)

mass. These methods can be used at the bedside of the seriously ill child and can be employed serially, with minimal discomfort and low radiation exposure.

15.8 CARDIAC CATHETERIZATION

Cardiac catheterization is an important tool in the diagnosis of congenital heart disease. With this technique the various chambers of the heart, great vessels, and veins are entered and blood samples obtained for measuring oxygen saturation. Pressures are measured, and contrast and indicator materials may be injected as required. Cardiac catheterization is usually a presurgical diagnostic test and should be utilized only when there is a reasonable expectation that an operation will be required. Although the risks are low, cardiac catheterization involves potential complications for the patient and should not be used without an opportunity for benefit. In many instances echocardiography, Doppler technique, and radionuclide studies may be used in lieu of multiple cardiac catheterizations in individual patients who require careful monitoring of their hemodynamic status.

Cardiac catheterization should be performed with the patient in a basal state; this is often not possible with children. Children are routinely sedated during these studies, but deep anesthesia is avoided if possible, as depression of cardiovascular function by various anesthetic agents may distort the calculations of hemodynamic measurements, including cardiac output, pulmonary and systemic resistance, and shunt ratios.

If cardiac catheterization is performed on a critically ill infant with congenital heart disease, a surgical team should be alerted in the event that an operation is required immediately afterward. The complication rate of cardiac catheterization and angiography is greatest among critically ill infants; they must be studied in a thermally neutral environment and treated quickly for hypothermia, acidemia, or excess blood loss. Development of soft, flow-directed balloon-tipped catheters has greatly decreased the frequency of complications from catheter manipulation, such as severe arrhythmias, cardiac perforations, and intramyocardial injection of contrast material.

In most instances catheterization involves both the left and the right sides of the heart. The catheter is passed into the heart under fluoroscopic guidance through a percutaneous entry point in the femoral vein. The left side of the heart is usually entered by passing the catheter across the foramen ovale to the left atrium and left ventricle. The left side of the heart is also catheterized by passing the catheter retrograde through the femoral artery and the aorta and across the aortic valve. The catheter is manipulated through abnormal intracardiac defects or into malpositioned great vessels. Complete hemodynamics can be calculated (Table 15–5) through data obtained at catheterization: cardiac output, intracardiac shunts, and systemic and pulmonary resistances. The normal circulatory dynamics are depicted in Figure 15–30.

INDICATOR DILUTION AND APPEARANCE TECHNIQUES. If a bolus of indicator material is injected intravenously or into the right side of the heart, it traverses the pulmonary circulation and enters the left side of the heart and then the arterial circulation. This indicator material may then be detected in the arterial blood. A continuous record of the circulation of indicator in normal subjects shows two peaks (Fig. 15–31). The time between the instant of injection and the detection of the indicator in arterial blood is known as the appearance time and is a measure of circulation time. The 1st peak of the indicator curve is due to the passage of indicator past the arterial detectors; the 2nd, to recirculation through the systemic arterial and venous systems, the pulmonary circulation, and reappearance in the arterial tree. If

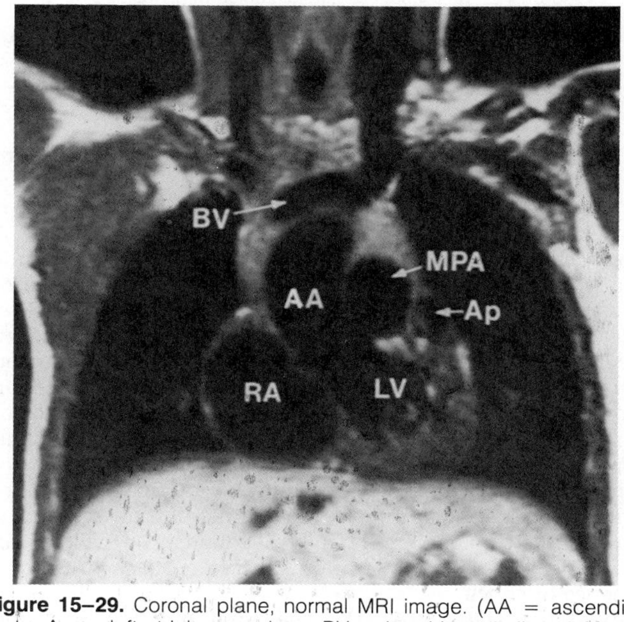

Figure 15–29. Coronal plane, normal MRI image. (AA = ascending aorta; Ap = left atrial appendage; BV = brachiocephalic vein; LV = left ventricle; MPA = main pulmonary artery; RA = right atrium.) (From Bisset GS III: Cardiac and great vessel anatomy. *In*: El-Khoury GY, Bergman RA, Montgomery WJ: Sectional Anatomy by MRI/CT. New York, Churchill Livingstone, 1990, pp 219–243.)

TABLE 15–5. Normal Values and Formulas for Determination of Hemodynamics in Cardiac Catheterization

1. Cardiac index 3.0–5.0 L/min/m^2
2. Arteriovenous oxygen difference 4.5 ± 0.7 mL/dL
3. Oxygen consumption 140–160 mL/m^2/min
4. Arterial oxygen saturation 94–100%
5. Difference in oxygen content between venae cavae and right atrium <1.9 vol %
6. Difference in oxygen content between right atrium and right ventricle <0.9 vol %
7. Difference in oxygen content between right ventricle and pulmonary artery <0.5 vol %
8. Normal mean left atrial pressure 4–8 mm Hg
9. Pulmonary arteriolar resistance 50–150 dyn sec cm^{-5} (1 unit = 80 dynes)
10. Cardiac output mL/min = $$\frac{O_2 \text{ intake (mL/min)}}{\left\{\begin{array}{l} O_2 \text{ content of arterial blood (vols \%)} \\ \text{minus } O_2 \text{ content of mixed venous blood} \end{array}\right.} \times 100$$
11. Cardiac index = cardiac output (L/min)/m^2 of body surface area
12. Pulmonary artery flow = $$\frac{O_2 \text{ intake (mL/min)}}{\left\{\begin{array}{l} O_2 \text{ content of pulmonary venous blood (vols \%)} \\ \text{minus } O_2 \text{ content of pulmonary arterial blood (vols \%)} \end{array}\right.} \times 100$$
    If a pulmonary venous sample is not available, it is assumed to be saturated to 95% of capacity
13. Systemic flow = $$\frac{O_2 \text{ intake (mL/min)}}{\left\{\begin{array}{l} \text{systemic arterial } O_2 \text{ content (vols \%)} \\ \text{minus arterial venous } O_2 \text{ content (vols \%)} \end{array}\right.} \times 100$$
14. Effective pulmonary artery flow = $$\frac{O_2 \text{ intake (mL/min)}}{\left\{\begin{array}{l} \text{pulmonary venous } O_2 \text{ content (vols \%)} \\ \text{minus mixed venous } O_2 \text{ content (vols \%)} \end{array}\right.} \times 100$$
15. Total left to right shunt = pulmonary artery flow minus effective pulmonary artery flow
16. Total right to left shunt = systemic flow minus effective pulmonary artery flow
17. Pulmonary arteriolar resistance $R = \frac{PA - PC}{PF}$

    Where R = pulmonary arteriolar resistance (resistance units)
    PA = mean pulmonary artery pressure in mm Hg
    PC = mean pulmonary "capillary" pressure in mm Hg
    PF = pulmonary flow in L/min/m^2

the concentration of circulating indicator is known, cardiac output can be computed.

The *thermodilution method* for measuring cardiac output is the most commonly used indicator dilution technique. A known change in heat content of the blood is induced at one point in the circulation (usually the right atrium or inferior vena cava), and the resultant change in temperature is detected at a point downstream (usually the pulmonary artery). The injectate is iced or room-temperature saline. This method is used to measure cardiac output in the catheterization laboratory in patients without shunts (e.g., aortic stenosis or coarctation of the aorta). When combined with the dye dilution technique, it can also be used to measure the volume of regurgitant flow across diseased mitral or aortic valves. Monitoring the cardiac output by the thermodilution method is also useful in managing critically ill infants and children in an intensive care setting after cardiac surgery or in the presence of shock.

ANGIOCARDIOGRAPHY. The great blood vessels and individual cardiac chambers may be seen by selective angiocardiography, i.e., injection of contrast material into specific cardiac chambers or great vessels. This method allows identification of specific abnormalities without interference from the superimposed shadows of normal chambers. Photofluorography with image intensification has made possible simultaneous cardiac catheterization and selective angiocardiography. The preferred method is a combination of photofluorography with closed-circuit television to monitor the fluoroscopic screen and allow visualization of the cardiac silhouette and the cardiac catheter. After the cardiac catheter is introduced into the chamber to be studied, a small amount of contrast medium is rapidly injected and moving pictures are exposed at 60 frames/sec. Biplane cineangiocardiography allows detailed evaluation of specific cardiac chambers and blood vessels in two planes with the injection of a single bolus of contrast material. Various angle views are utilized to best display anatomic features in individual lesions.

The rapid injection of contrast medium under pressure into the circulation is not without risks, and each injection should be carefully planned. Contrast agents consist of hypertonic solutions containing organic iodides, which can cause complications including nausea, a generalized burning sensation, central nervous system symptoms, and allergic rashes. Intramyocardial injection is generally avoided by careful placement of the catheter prior to injection. Hypertonicity of the contrast medium may result in transient myocardial depression and a drop in blood pressure, and soon afterward tachycardia, an increase in cardiac output, and a shift of interstitial fluid into the circulation.

"Idealized" diagrams of the normal angiocardiogram are

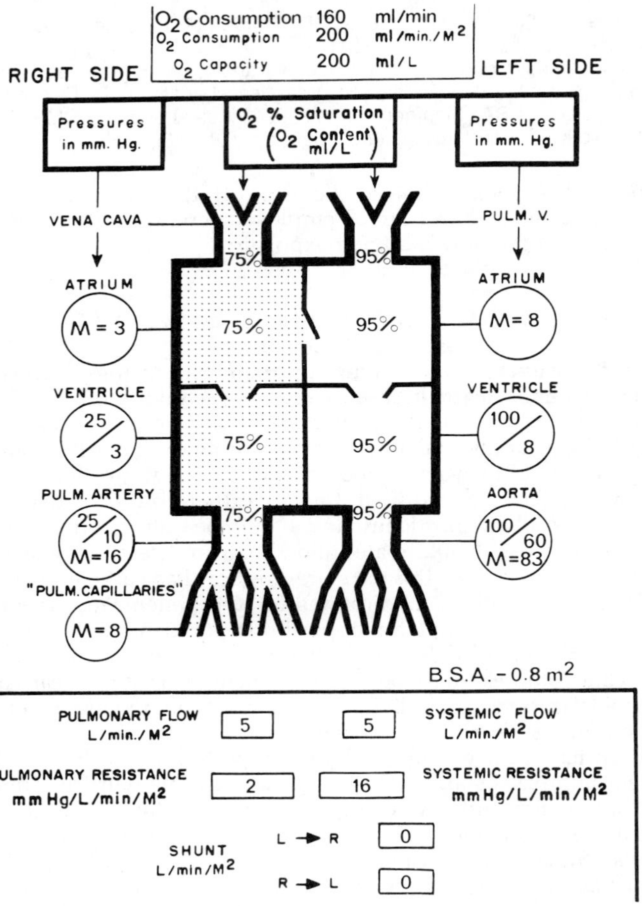

Figure 15–30. Diagram of normal circulatory dynamics with pressures, oxygen contents, and percentage of saturations. (Modified from Nadas AS, Fyler DC: Pediatric Cardiology, 3rd ed. Philadelphia, WB Saunders, 1972.)

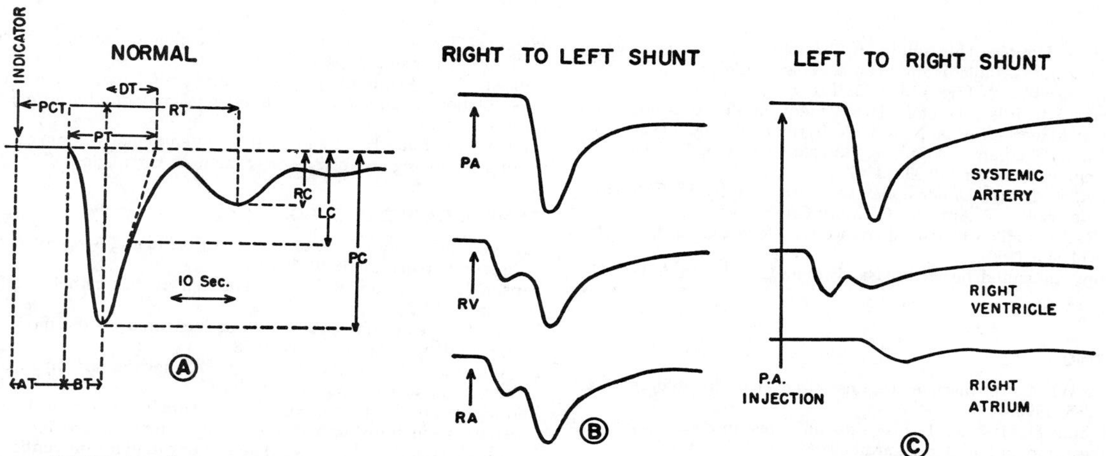

Figure 15–31. Idealized diagrams of indicator dilution curves. *A*, Normal curve showing the time and concentration components. The instant of indicator injection in the right side of the heart is shown by an *arrow* at the top left. The curve is obtained from the indicator detector in a systemic artery. (AT = appearance time; BT = build-up time; DT = disappearance time; LC = least concentration; PC = peak concentration; PCT = peak concentration time; PT = passage time; RC = maximal recirculation concentration; RT = recirculation time.) Extrapolation of declining slope of concentration is easier if the curve is plotted on a logarithmic scale. Cardiac output may be computed by the formula 601/c(PT) where 1 = amount of indicator, c = mean concentration of indicator, PT = passage time. *B*, Localization of *right to left shunt*. The instant of the injection of the indicator is shown by *arrows*. The example illustrates the shunt at ventricular levels. Site of injection: PA = pulmonary artery; RA = right atrium; RV = right ventricle. Indicator detector in systemic artery in all instances. PA injection (i.e., downstream from the shunt level) shows a normal appearance time. RV and RA injections (i.e., at and upstream from shunt level) show early appearance times. *C*, Localization of *left to right shunt*. Example illustrates shunt at ventricular level. Indicator injected into distal pulmonary artery (PA) in all instances. In the upper tracing the indicator detector is in a systemic artery, and the curve shows a prolonged disappearance time. The middle curve is from the indicator detected in the right ventricle and shows an early appearance time because of ventricular septal defect. The right atrial curve shows a normal appearance time.

shown in Figure 15–8. The indications for this study are outlined under the individual congenital lesions.

INTERVENTIONAL CATHETERIZATION. Nonsurgical treatment of certain cardiac defects that until now required intraoperative repair is possible with interventional cardiac catheterization. The procedure most often utilized is balloon valvuloplasty. A special catheter with a sausage-shaped balloon at the distal end is passed through an obstructed valve. The balloon is rapidly filled with saline solution, resulting in tearing of the stenotic valve tissue, usually at the site of inappropriately fused raphe. Valvular pulmonary stenosis can be treated by balloon angioplasty in the neonate, child, and adult. The results of this procedure appear to be similar to those obtained by open heart surgery. Although experience with balloon angioplasty for aortic stenosis is less extensive than for pulmonary stenosis, results have been excellent. Creation of significant aortic insufficiency is a more important complication than pulmonary insufficiency resulting from pulmonary valvuloplasty. There is general agreement that restenosis of a coarctation of the aorta after earlier surgery can be treated by balloon angioplasty. There is controversy as to whether the possibility of aneurysm formation is a contraindication of the procedure for a native coarctation. Other applications of the balloon technique include amelioration of mitral stenosis or subaortic stenosis, dilatation of surgical conduits (atrial baffles), relief of branch pulmonary arterial narrowing, dilatation of venous obstruction, and the long-utilized balloon atrial septostomy for transposition of the great arteries.

Interventional cardiac catheterization techniques also have been developed for obliteration of temporary arteriovenous shunts as well as of pulmonary collateral vessels, which may be detrimental after surgical repair of pulmonary atresia and VSD. There is increasing experience with catheter-introduced umbrella devices to close PDA and secundum atrial septal defects. Foam plugs may also be introduced to close a PDA. These applications remain experimental but may become available in the near future.

GENERAL

Adams FH, Emmanouilides GC, Riemerschneider T: Moss' Heart Disease in Infants, Children and Adolescents, 4th ed. Baltimore, Williams & Wilkins, 1989.
Cowgill LD: Cyanotic congenital heart disease. *In*: Cardiac Surgery, 3rd ed. New York, Wiley Medical Publishers, 1989, pp 1–277.
Dickerman JD, Lucey JF: Smith's The Critically Ill Child: Diagnosis and Medical Management. Philadelphia, WB Saunders, 1985.
Gillette PC: Congenital heart disease. Pediatr Clin North Am 37:1–239, 1990.
Pantell RH, Goodman BW Jr: Adolescent chest pain: A prospective study. Pediatrics 71:881, 1983.
Rudolph AM: Congenital Diseases of the Heart. Chicago, Year Book Medical Publishers, 1974.
Selbst SM: Chest pain in children. Pediatrics 75:1068, 1985.

CARDIAC SOUNDS AND PHONOCARDIOGRAPHY

Baragan J, Fernandez F, Thiron JM, et al (eds): Dynamic Auscultation and Phonocardiography. Bowie, MD, Charles Press Publishers, 1979.
McNamara DG: Value and limitations of auscultation in the management of congenital heart disease. Pediatr Clin North Am 37:93, 1990.
Mills P, Craige E: Echophonocardiography. Prog Cardiovasc Dis 20:337, 1989.

ELECTROCARDIOGRAM AND VECTORCARDIOGRAM

Garson A: The Electrocardiogram in Infants and Children: A Systematic Approach. Philadelphia, Lea & Febiger, 1983.
Liebman J, Plonsey R, Yoram R: Pediatric and Fundamental Electrocardiography. Boston, Martinis Nyhoff Publishers, 1987.
Lipman BF, Massey EF: Clinical Scalar Electrocardiography. Chicago, Year Book Medical Publishers, 1984.
Marriott H: Rhythm Quizlets Self Assessment. Philadelphia, Lea & Febiger, 1987.

ECHOCARDIOGRAPHY

Alverson DC, Eldridge M, Dillon T, et al: Noninvasive pulse Doppler determination of cardiac output in neonates and children. J Pediatr 101:46, 1982.
Fyfe DA, Kline CH: Fetal echocardiographic diagnosis of congenital heart disease. Pediatr Clin North Am 37:45, 1990.

Hatle L, Angelsen B: Doppler Ultrasound in Cardiology, Physical Principles and Clinical Applications. Philadelphia, Lea & Febiger, 1985.
Popp RL: Echocardiography. N Engl J Med 323:101, 1990.
Seward JB, Tajik AJ, Edwards WD, et al: Two-Dimensional Echocardiographic Atlas. I: Congenital Heart Disease. New York, Springer-Verlag, 1987.
Sherman FS, Sahn DJ: Pediatric Doppler echocardiography 1987: Major advances in technology. J Pediatr 110:333, 1987.
Silverman N, Snyder A: Two-Dimensional Echocardiography in Congenital Heart Disease. Norwalk, CT, Appleton-Century-Crofts, 1982.
Wheller JJ, Reiss R, Allen HD: Clinical experience with fetal echocardiography. Am J Dis Child 144:49, 1990.
Wiles HB: Imaging congenital heart disease. Pediatr Clin North Am 37:115, 1990.

EXERCISE TESTING

Braden DS, Strong WF: Cardiovascular responses to exercise in children. Am J Dis Child 144:1255, 1990.
Cumming GR, Everatt D, Hastman L: Bruce treadmill test in children: Normal values in a clinical population. Am J Cardiol 41:69, 1978.
James FW, Blomqvist CG, Freed MD, et al: Standards for exercise testing in the pediatric age group: American Heart Association Council on Cardiovascular Disease in the Young. Circulation 66:1377A, 1982.
James FW, Kaplan S, Glueck CJ, et al: Responses of normal children and young adults to controlled bicycle exercise. Circulation 61:902, 1980.
Rozanski JJ, Dimich I, Steinfeld L, et al: Maximal exercise stress testing in evaluation of arrhythmias in children: Results and reproducibility. Am J Cardiol 42:951, 1979.
Washington RL, et al: Normal aerobic and anaerobic exercise data for North American school-age children. J Pediatr 112:223, 1988.

MAGNETIC RESONANCE IMAGING AND NUCLEAR MEDICINE

Fletcher BD, et al: Gated magnetic resonance imaging of congenital cardiac malformations. Radiology 150:137, 1984.
Higgins CB, et al: Magnetic resonance imaging in patients with congenital heart disease. Circulation 70:851, 1984.
Hurwitz RA: Quantitation of aortic and mitral regurgitation in the pediatric population: Evaluation by radionuclide angiography. Am J Cardiol 51:252, 1983.
Slutsky R, Karliner J, Ricca D, et al: Left ventricular volume calculated by gated equilibrium angiography. A new method. Circulation 60:556, 1979.

CARDIAC CATHETERIZATION

Bargeron LM, Elliot LP, Soto B, et al: Axial cineangiography in congenital heart disease. Circulation 56:1075, 1977.
Benson LN, Freedom RM: Interventional cardiac catheterization. Curr Opin Pediatr 1:106, 1989.
Freed MD, Keane JF: Cardiac output measured by thermodilution in infants and children. J Pediatr 92:39, 1978.
Freedom RM, Culham JAG, Moes CAF: Angiocardiography of Congenital Heart Disease. New York, Macmillan, 1984.
Kan JS, White RI, Mitchell SE, et al: Treatment of restenosis of coarctation by percutaneous transluminal angioplasty. Circulation 68:1087, 1983.
Lock JE, Keane JF, Fellows KE: The use of catheter intervention procedures for congenital heart disease. J Am Coll Cardiol 7:1420, 1986.
Martin EC, Olson AP, Steeg CN, et al: Radiation exposure to the pediatric patient during cardiac catheterization and angiography. Circulation 64:153, 1981.
Mullins CE, Nihill MR, Vick GW, et al: Double balloon technique for dilatation of valvular or vessel stenosis in congenital and acquired heart disease. J Am Coll Cardiol 10:107, 1987.
Radtke W, Lick J: Balloon dilation. Pediatr Clin North Am 37:193, 1990.
Rao PS: Balloon valvuloplasty and angioplasty in infants and children. J Pediatr 114:907, 1989.
Stanger P, Heymann MA, Tarnoff H, et al: Complications of cardiac catheterization of neonates, infants, and children: A three year study. Circulation 50:595, 1974.
Suarez J, Pan M, Sancho M, et al: Percutaneous transluminal balloon dilatation for discrete subaortic stenosis. Am J Cardiol 58:619, 1986.

15.9 FETAL AND NEONATAL CIRCULATION

FETAL CIRCULATION. Much of the information concerning fetal circulation has been derived from animal studies. Although there may be some species differences, the human fetal circulation and its adjustments after birth are probably similar to those of animals. Oxygenated blood from the placenta flows to the fetus through the umbilical vein at an average rate of 175 mL/kg with a pressure close to 12 mm Hg and a P_{O_2} of about 40 mm Hg. Approximately 50% of the umbilical venous blood bypasses the liver and flows through the ductus venosus into the inferior vena cava, where it mixes with the remainder of the venous return from the caudal part of the body and enters the right atrium from the inferior vena cava. Most of this blood preferentially passes across the foramen ovale to the left atrium, flows into the left ventricle, and is ejected into the ascending aorta. The coronary and cerebral arteries and those of the upper extremities are thus perfused with blood having a higher P_{O_2} than that perfusing other parts of the body, except for the liver. The superior vena caval blood, which is considerably less oxygenated, traverses the tricuspid valve and flows primarily to the right ventricle and pulmonary arterial trunk. The major portion of this blood (which has a P_{O_2} of 19–22 mm Hg) bypasses the lungs and flows through the ductus arteriosus into the descending aorta to perfuse the caudal part of the body as well as the placenta via the umbilical arteries. The effective fetal cardiac output—that is, the sum of the left ventricular output and the ductal flow—amounts to about 220 mL/kg/min. Approximately 65% of this blood returns to the placenta; the remaining 35% perfuses the fetal organs and tissues (Fig. 15–32*A*).

Because the fetal ventricles work in parallel rather than in series, the distribution of their ejected blood depends on resistance and flow and the fact that the large ductus arteriosus equalizes aortic and pulmonary arterial pressures. Approximately 10% of the right ventricular output flows to the lungs via the pulmonary arteries, and 90% enters the descending aorta via the ductus arteriosus (see Fig. 15–32*B*). This occurs primarily because pulmonary vascular resistance in the fetus is considerably higher than systemic resistance, which is predominantly influenced by the low-resistance placental vascular bed. Left ventricular output consists of a mixture of venous return from the inferior vena cava, foramen ovale, and left atrium, as well as the minimal pulmonary venous return. Right ventricular output is approximately 50% greater than left ventricular, and thus the right ventricle is dominant during fetal life.

NEONATAL CIRCULATION. At birth the fetal circulation must immediately adapt to extrauterine life as gas exchange is transferred from the placenta to the lung (see Sec. 9.30). Some of these changes are virtually instantaneous with the first breath, and others are effected over hours or days. After an initial fall in systemic blood pressure, there is a progressive rise. The heart rate slows as a result of a baroreceptor response to an increase in systemic vascular resistance when the placental circulation is eliminated. The average central aortic pressure in the term neonate is 75/50 mm Hg. With the onset of ventilation a marked increase in pulmonary blood flow occurs because of the dilatative effect of oxygen on the pulmonary arteriolar bed. Pulmonary venous return and consequently left ventricular output are thus increased. In the normal neonate, ductal closure and fall of pulmonary vascular resistance result in a fall of pulmonary arterial and right ventricular pressures. The major decline of pressure from the high fetal levels to the low "adult" levels in the human infant at sea level usually occurs within the first 2–3 days but may be prolonged for 7 days or more.

Significant differences between the neonatal circulation and that of older infants may be summarized as follows: (1) right

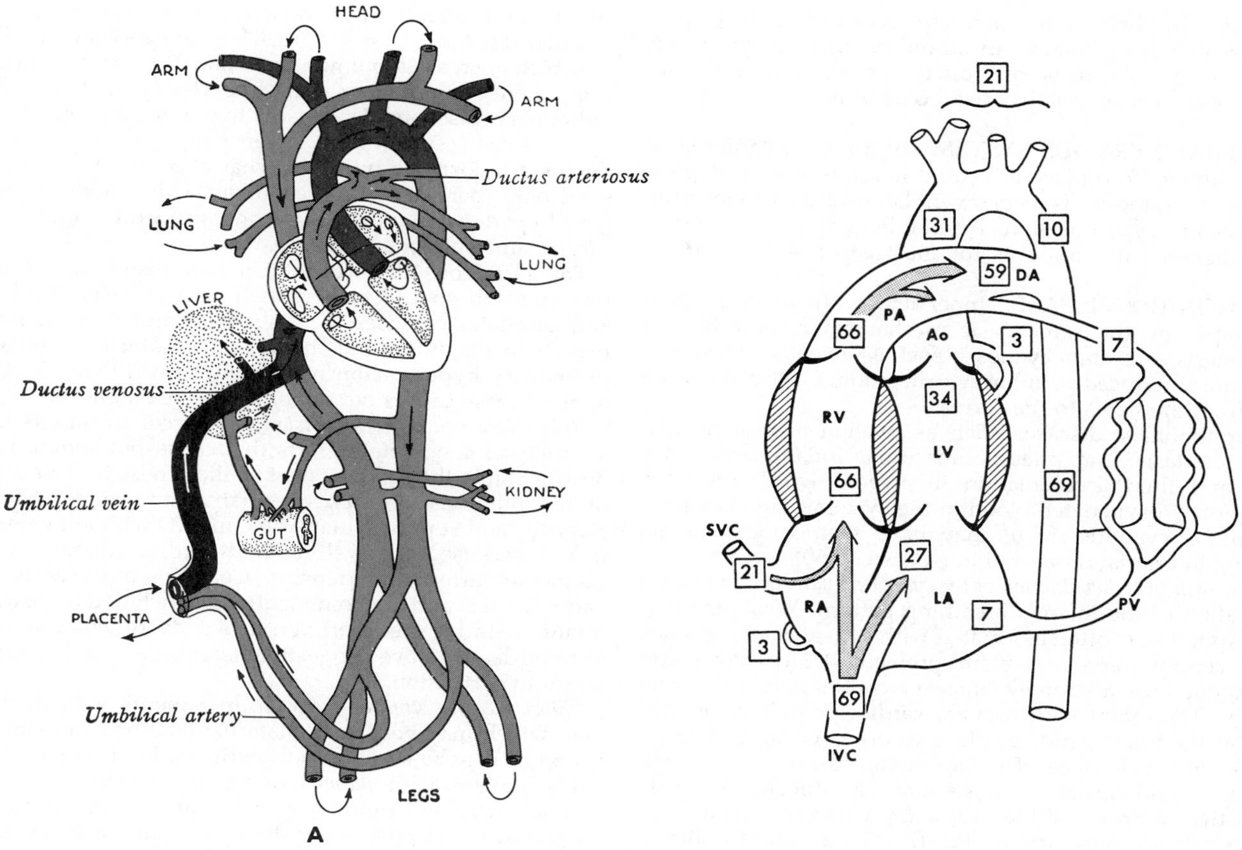

Figure 15–32. *A*, Plan of the human circulation before birth (partly after Dawes). Black shading indicates more oxygenated blood, and *arrows* indicate the direction of flow (Arey). *B*, Percentages of combined ventricular output that return to the fetal heart, that are ejected by each ventricle, and that flow through the main vascular channels. Figures are those obtained from study of late-gestation lambs. (From Rudolph AM: Congenital Diseases of the Heart. Chicago, Year Book Medical Publishers, 1974.)

to left shunting may persist across the patent foramen ovale; (2) in the presence of cardiopulmonary disease, continued patency of the ductus arteriosus may allow left to right, right to left, or bidirectional shunting; (3) the neonatal pulmonary vasculature constricts more vigorously in response to hypoxemia, hypercapnia, and acidosis; (4) the muscular mass of the left and right ventricles is almost equal; and (5) newborn infants at rest have a relatively high oxygen consumption, which is associated with their relatively high cardiac output. A high percentage of fetal hemoglobin may interfere with delivery of oxygen to the tissues since there is reduced binding of 2, 3-diphosphoglycerate in fetal hemoglobin. Under these conditions an increased cardiac output would be required for adequate delivery of oxygen to the tissues.

The foramen ovale is functionally closed by the 3rd month of life, though it is possible to pass a probe through the overlapping flaps in 25% of adults. Functional closure of the ductus arteriosus is usually complete by 10–15 hr in the normal neonate. During periods of adjustment there are rarely physical signs of patency of these structures. However, in premature newborn infants an evanescent systolic murmur with late accentuation or a continuous murmur may be audible, and in the context of the respiratory distress syndrome the patent ductus arteriosus is often important (see Sec. 9.32).

The normal ductus arteriosus differs morphologically from the adjoining aorta and pulmonary artery in that the ductus has a significant amount of circularly arranged smooth muscle in its medial layer. During fetal life, patency of the ductus arteriosus appears to be maintained by the combined relaxant effects of low oxygen tension and endogenously produced prostaglandins, specifically prostaglandin E_2 (PGE_2). It is not known whether circulating PGE_2 or that produced in ductus tissue is more important. In the neonate, oxygen is the most important factor controlling ductal closure. When the Po_2 of the blood passing through the ductus reaches about 50 mm Hg, the ductal wall constricts; the mechanisms by which oxygen activates ductal constriction are not completely understood. The effects of oxygen on the ductal smooth muscle could be direct or mediated by its effects on prostaglandin synthesis. Gestational age also appears to play a role; the ductus of the premature infant is less responsive to oxygen, even though its musculature is developed (see Sec. 9.30).

CRITICALLY ILL NEONATE WITH CYANOSIS AND RESPIRATORY DISTRESS

The severely ill neonate with cardiorespiratory distress and cyanosis presents a diagnostic challenge (see Table 9–22).

CARDIAC DISEASE. Congenital heart disease is responsible for cyanosis when obstruction to right ventricular outflow causes intracardiac right to left shunting or when complex anatomic defects, unassociated with pulmonary stenosis, cause admixture of pulmonary and systemic venous return in the heart. Cyanosis from pulmonary edema may develop in patients with heart failure. In addition, right to left shunts across the foramen ovale and ductus arteriosus due to pulmonary vascular obstruction also occur in neonates (see Sec. 9.36).

CENTRAL NERVOUS SYSTEM DISEASE. Irregular shallow breathing, secondary to central nervous system depression, results in reduced alveolar ventilation and an abnormally low alveolar oxygen tension. Arterial P_{CO_2} is elevated. Intracranial hemorrhage accounts for most cases of this type of cyanosis.

PULMONARY DISEASE. Upper airway obstructions result in cyanosis by the same basic mechanism responsible for central nervous system cyanosis, such as alveolar hypoventilation due to reduced pulmonary ventilation. Obstruction may occur from the nares to the carina.

Intrapulmonary diseases such as hyaline membrane disease, atelectasis, and pneumonitis cause inflammation, collapse, and fluid accumulation in alveoli, which result in incompletely oxygenated blood in the systemic circulation.

Rarely, a cyanotic infant may have methemoglobinemia resulting in arterial desaturation (see Sec. 8.50).

Successful *initial evaluation of the cyanotic infant* lies in careful observation of the infant's breathing pattern. Weak or irregular respiration is often associated with a weak sucking reflex and a central nervous system problem. Convulsions and general depression strongly suggest a central nervous system etiology. The infant with primary cardiac or pulmonary disease, on the other hand, displays vigorous or labored respirations with tachypnea. The differential diagnosis between pulmonary and cardiac cyanosis may be difficult, especially within the first days of life. The baby with congenital heart disease will not raise arterial P_{O_2} (Pa_{O_2}) significantly during administration of 100% oxygen (hyperoxia test), whereas patients with pulmonary disease will have an increased response as ventilation-perfusion inequalities, but not intracardiac shunts, are overcome by oxygen administration. The infant with only a central nervous system disorder will completely normalize Pa_{O_2} during artifical ventilation. If the Pa_{O_2} rises above 150 mm Hg during 100% oxygen administration, an anatomic shunt can generally be excluded.

A significant heart murmur suggests a cardiac basis for cyanosis. However, several of the more severe cardiac defects do not manifest a murmur. The chest roentgenogram may be helpful in the differentiation of pulmonary from cardiac disease and, in the latter, will indicate whether pulmonary blood flow is increased, normal, or decreased. This distinction is important in the differentiation of the various congenital heart lesions that cause cyanosis in the neonate.

Two-dimensional echocardiography has become the definitive noninvasive test to determine whether congenital heart disease is present. The information obtained by this technique is essential in avoiding an unnecessary cardiac catheterization and angiography in the absence of a cardiac defect as well as in making a specific diagnosis when congenital heart disease is present.

15.10 NEONATAL PULMONARY HYPERTENSION

(See also Sec. 9.36)

Pulmonary hypertension persists in the newborn under a variety of different circumstances and as a result of a number of different underlying mechanisms. Pulmonary arterial pressure is the product of pulmonary blood flow and pulmonary vascular resistance ($P = F \times R$). There are very few conditions in which increased pulmonary blood flow is an important component of pulmonary artery hypertension in the newborn. Pulmonary vasoconstriction and hypertension following hypoxemia can result in right to left patent foramen ovale and ductus arteriosus shunting in what appears to be a primary syndrome (persistent fetal circulation). In addition, pulmonary hypertension may be a secondary feature of a variety of cardiac and pulmonary diseases.

The numerous disease entities that result in pulmonary hypertension should be classified on the basis of anatomic and physiologic causes in order to formulate a rational approach to diagnosis and management. The term **persistent pulmonary hypertension of the newborn** (PPHN) is applied to all of these causes but is not a specific diagnosis.

Pulmonary venous hypertension may occur in infants having a variety of congenital defects that cause pulmonary venous obstruction in the first few days of life. These include stenosis of the pulmonary veins, cor triatriatum, congenital mitral stenosis, and supravalvular webs. Infants with left ventricular failure because of a well-defined cardiac lesion also have pulmonary artery hypertension. Coarction of the aorta, aortic valve disease, and cardiomyopathy are included in this group. Infants with transient left ventricular dysfunction secondary to hypoxia also have congestive heart failure and pulmonary artery hypertension.

Hyperviscosity syndrome occurs in patients with polycythemia, which may be due to maternal-fetal or fetal-fetal transfusion or may be secondary to perinatal hypoxemia.

The patient with *pulmonary vascular constriction* (with or without increased pulmonary vascular smooth muscle) and no parenchymal pulmonary disease or cardiac lesion should be diagnosed as having *persistence of the fetal circulation*. However, infants with both a pulmonary vascular constrictive component and pulmonary parenchymal disease, although also having an oxygenation defect induced in part by hypoxemia, should be classified according to the basic disease entity, for example, meconium aspiration with pulmonary vascular constriction and right to left shunting.

A *decreased pulmonary vascular bed* leads to elevated pulmonary resistance and persistent pulmonary hypertension of the newborn. This may occur with *congenital pulmonary hypoplasia* but is also seen secondary to *diaphragmatic hernia*, space-occupying *intrathoracic masses*, and other diseases. Once hypoxia occurs in these patients, the resulting pulmonary vascular constriction may add to the pulmonary resistance and exacerbate the cyanosis.

Infants with *systemic right ventricles* or *single ventricles* as a result of complex congenital heart lesions without pulmonary stenosis have pulmonary hypertension. Such infants also develop medial muscular hypertrophy of small pulmonary vessels.

Perinatal hypoxemia associated with anatomic and physiologic abnormalities results in persistent pulmonary hypertension of mixed etiologies. For example, infants with diaphragmatic hernia have ipsilateral pulmonary hypoplasia and contralateral pulmonary vasoconstriction, both of which contribute to high pulmonary resistance, hypertension, and right to left shunting. Some preterm infants with severe respiratory distress syndrome may also be cyanotic on the basis of pulmonary vasoconstriction, pulmonary hypertension, and right to left ductus arteriosus and foramen ovale shunting in the first few days of life. Later in the neonatal period ventilation-perfusion inequalities result in cyanosis, and large ductal left to right shunting may occur as pulmonary resistance falls.

CONGENITAL HEART DISEASE

INCIDENCE. Congenital heart disease occurs in approximately 8 of 1,000 live births. The incidence is higher among stillborns (2%), abortuses (10–25%), and premature infants (about 2% including VSD, excluding transient PDA). This overall incidence does not include mitral valve prolapse, the PDA of the preterm infant, and bicuspid aortic valves (present in about 0.9% of adult series). Among infants with congenital cardiac defects there is a spectrum of severity: About 2 to 3 in 1,000 infants will be symptomatic in the 1st year. The diagnosis is established by 1 wk of age in 40–50% and by 1 mo of age in 50–60% of patients with heart defects. Since palliative or corrective surgery has evolved, the number of children surviving with congenital heart disease has increased dramatically. Table 15–6 summarizes the relative frequency of specific lesions.

Most congenital defects are well tolerated during fetal life. It is only after the maternal circulation is eliminated and the cardiovascular system independently sustained that the impact of an anatomic and subsequent hemodynamic abnormality becomes apparent. The infant's circulation continues to change after birth, and later changes have a hemodynamic impact on cardiac lesions. For example, as pulmonary vascular resistance falls over the 1st weeks of life, left to right shunts become more apparent. The relative significance of various defects also changes with growth; the large ventricular septal defect may become a relatively small communication later. Aortic or pulmonary valve stenosis, which is relatively mild, may become worse if the orifice of the valve does not grow with the patient. The physician should be aware of the spectrum of severity for the various malformations, their evolution with time, and associated congenital malformations (Table 15–7).

TABLE 15–6. Relative Frequency of Congenital Heart Lesions*

Lesions	% of All Lesions
Ventricular septal defect	25–30
Atrial septal defect (secundum)	6–8
Patent ductus arteriosus	6–8
Coarctation of aorta	5–7
Tetralogy of Fallot	5–7
Pulmonary valve stenosis	5–7
Aortic valve stenosis	4–7
d-Transposition of great arteries	3–5
Hypoplastic left ventricle	1–3
Hypoplastic right ventricle	1–3
Truncus arteriosus	1–2
Total anomalous pulmonary venous return	1–2
Triscuspid atresia	1–2
Single ventricle	1–2
Double-outlet right ventricle	1–2
Others	5–10

*Excluding patent ductus arteriosus in preterm neonate, bicuspid aortic valve, peripheral pulmonic stenosis, mitral valve prolapse.

ETIOLOGY. The cause of congenital heart disease is rarely known in individual cases. Genetic factors may have a role, as certain types of VSDs (supracristal) are more common in children of Oriental than white background. Approximately 3% of patients with congenital heart disease have a single gene defect such as Marfan or Noonan syndrome. Five to eight per cent have associated chromosome anomalies: More than 90% of patients with trisomy 18, 50% with 21-trisomy, and 40% with XO (Turner syndrome) have associated congenital heart disease. Two to four per cent of cases of congenital heart disease are associated with environmental or adverse maternal conditions and teratogenic influences including maternal diabetes mellitus, phenylketonuria, systemic lupus erythematosus, congenital rubella syndrome, and drugs (lithium, ethanol, thalidomide, anticonvulsant agents) (see Table 15–1). Associated noncardiac malformations noted in identifiable syndromes may be seen in as many as 25% of patients with congenital heart disease (see Table 15–7). Most of the remaining cases are of polygenetic or multifactorial etiologies.

GENETIC COUNSELING. Parents who have a child with congenital heart disease require counseling regarding the incidence of a cardiac malformation in subsequent children (see Sec. 7.33). With the exception of syndromes due to single gene mutation, most congenital heart disease is the result of a multifactorial inheritance pattern, which results in a low risk of recurrence. There is approximately a 1% incidence of congenital heart disease in the normal population, and this incidence increases to 2–6% for a second pregnancy following the birth of a child with congenital heart disease, depending on the type of lesion in the first child. When two siblings have congenital heart disease the risk for a third affected child may reach 20–30%. In general, when a second child is found to have congenital heart disease it will tend to be similar to the lesion that was discovered in the first instance. However, the degree of severity may be disparate, and associated defects may be variable. For example, if the index patient has coarctation of the aorta, recurrences may include coarctation, aortic valvular stenosis, aortic atresia, or hypoplastic left ventricle.

The question often arises as to whether a woman with congenital heart disease, either unoperated or operated, will be able to carry a fetus to term. The major factor in determining this is the mother's cardiovascular status. In the presence of a mild congenital heart defect, or after successful repair of a more severe lesion, normal child-bearing is likely. The increased hemodynamic burden on a patient with poor cardiac function may result in significantly increased risk to the mother as well as to the fetus. The incidence of spontaneous abortion in the presence of severe congenital heart disease is high, especially when the patient is cyanotic. It is important to discuss various methods of birth control with affected young women. Prophylaxis against endocarditis is indicated at the time of delivery.

TABLE 15–7. Congenital Malformation Syndromes Associated with Congenital Heart Disease

Syndrome	Features
Chromosomal Disorders	
21-Trisomy (Down syndrome)	Endocardial cushion defect, VSD,* ASD†
22p-Trisomy (cat eye syndrome)	Miscellaneous, total anomalous pulmonary venous return
18-Trisomy	VSD, ASD, PDA,‡ coarctation of aorta, bicuspid aortic or pulmonary valve
13-Trisomy	VSD, ASD, PDA, coarctation of aorta, bicuspid aortic or pulmonary valve
9-Trisomy	Miscellaneous
XXXXY	PDA, ASD
Penta X	PDA, VSD
Triploidy	VSD, ASD, PDA
XO (Turner syndrome)	Bicuspid aortic valve, coarctation of aorta
Fragile X	Mitral valve prolapse, aortic root dilatation
Duplication 3q2	Miscellaneous
Deletion 4p	VSD, PDA, aortic stenosis
Deletion 9p	Miscellaneous
Deletion 5p (cri du chat syndrome)	VSD, PDA, ASD
Deletion 10q	VSD, TOF,§ conotruncal lesions ‖
Deletion 13q	VSD
Deletion 18q	VSD
Syndrome Complexes	
CHARGE association (coloboma, *h*eart, atresia choanae, *r*etardation, *g*enital and *e*ar anomalies)	VSD, ASD, PDA, TOF, endocardial cushion defect
DiGeorge sequence	Aortic arch anomalies, conotruncal anomalies
Alagille syndrome (arteriohepatic dysplasia)	Peripheral pulmonic stenosis
VATER association (*v*ertebral, *a*nal, *t*racheoesophageal, *r*adial, and *r*enal anomalies)	VSD, TOF, ASD, PDA
FAVS (*f*acio-*a*uriculo-*v*ertebral *s*pectrum)	TOF, VSD
CHILD (*c*ongenital *h*emidysplasia with *i*chthyosiform erythroderma, *l*imb *d*efects)	Miscellaneous
Mulibrey nanism (*mu*scle, *li*ver, *br*ain, *ey*e)	Pericardial thickening, constrictive pericarditis
Asplenia syndrome	Complex cyanotic heart lesions with decreased pulmonary blood flow, transposition of great arteries, anomalous pulmonary venous return, dextrocardia, single ventricle, single atrioventricular valve
Polysplenia syndrome	Acyanotic lesions with increased pulmonary blood flow, azygos continuation of inferior vena cava, partial anomalous pulmonary venous return, dextrocardia, single ventricle, common atrioventricular valve
Teratogenic Agents	
Congenital rubella	PDA, peripheral pulmonic stenosis
Fetal hydantoin syndrome	VSD, ASD, coarctation of aorta, PDA
Fetal alcohol syndrome	ASD, VSD
Fetal valproate effects	Coarctation of aorta, hypoplastic left side of the heart, aortic stenosis, pulmonary atresia, VSD
Maternal phenylketonuria	VSD, ASD, PDA, coarctation of aorta
Retinoic acid embryopathy	Conotruncal anomalies
Others	
Apert syndrome	VSD
Autosomal dominant polycystic kidney disease	Mitral valve prolapse
Carpenter	PDA
Conradi	VSD, PDA
Crouzon	PDA, coarctation of aorta
Cutis laxa	Pulmonary hypertension, pulmonic stenosis
de Lange	VSD
Ellis-van Creveld	Single atrium, VSD
Holt-Oram	ASD, VSD; 1st-degree heart block
Infant of diabetic mother	Hypertrophic cardiomyopathy, VSD, conotruncal anomalies
Kartagener	Dextrocardia
Meckel-Gruber	ASD, VSD
Noonan	Pulmonic stenosis, ASD, cardiomyopathy
Pallister-Hall	Endocardial cushion defect
Rubinstein-Taybi	VSD
Scimitar	Hypoplasia of the right lung, anomalous pulmonary venous return to the inferior vena cava
Smith-Lemli-Opitz	VSD, PDA
Thrombocytopenia and absent radius (TAR)	ASD, TOF
Treacher Collins	VSD, ASD, PDA
Williams syndrome	Supravalvular aortic stenosis, peripheral pulmonic stenosis

*VSD = ventricular septal defect.
†ASD = atrial septal defect.
‡PDA = patent ductus arteriosus.
§TOF = tetralogy of Fallot.
‖Conotruncal = TOF, pulmonary atresia, truncus arteriosus, transposition of the great arteries.

CONGENITAL CARDIAC DISEASE WITH CYANOSIS
(Dominant Right to Left Shunt)

15.11 TETRALOGY OF FALLOT

Tetralogy of Fallot classically consists of the combination of (1) obstruction to right ventricular outflow (pulmonary stenosis), (2) ventricular septal defect, (3) dextroposition of the aorta, and (4) right ventricular hypertrophy. Obstruction to pulmonary arterial flow is usually at the right ventricular infundibulum and pulmonary valve. The pulmonary arterial trunk may be smaller than usual, and there may be branch stenosis. Complete obstruction of right ventricular outflow with ventricular septal defect is also classified as an extreme form of tetralogy of Fallot.

PATHOLOGY. The pulmonary valve may have a small ring, is often bicuspid, and, occasionally, is the only site of stenosis. Hypertrophy of the crista supraventricularis contributes to the infundibular stenosis and results in an infundibular chamber of variable size and contour. When the right ventricular outflow tract is completely obstructed (pulmonary atresia), the anatomy of the pulmonary arteries is extremely variable; on occasion, pulmonary blood flow is supplied by collateral vessels from the aorta. The ventricular septal defect is nonrestrictive and large, just below the aortic valve, and related to the posterior and right aortic cusps. The normal continuity of the mitral and aortic valves is maintained. The aorta arches to the right in about 20% of instances; the aortic root is large and overrides the ventricular septal defect (VSD) to a varying degree.

PATHOPHYSIOLOGY. Systemic venous return to the right atrium and right ventricle is normal. When the right ventricle contracts in the presence of marked pulmonary stenosis, blood is shunted across the VSD into the aorta. Persistent arterial desaturation and cyanosis result. The pulmonary blood flow, when severely restricted by the obstruction to right ventricular outflow, may be supplemented by bronchial collateral circulation and occasionally by a patent ductus arteriosus. The peak systolic and diastolic pressures in each ventricle are similar at the systemic level, since a large pressure gradient is measured across the obstructed ventricular outflow tract, and pulmonary arterial pressure is lower than normal. The degree of right ventricular outflow obstruction determines the severity of cyanosis and the presence of right ventricular hypertrophy. When obstruction to right ventricular outflow is moderate and there is a balanced shunt across the VSD, the patient may not be visibly cyanotic (acyanotic or "pink" tetralogy of Fallot).

CLINICAL MANIFESTATIONS. *Cyanosis*, one of the most obvious manifestations of tetralogy, may not be present at birth. Right ventricular outflow obstruction may not yet be severe, and the infant may present with a large left to right shunt and even congestive heart failure. However, with time there is increasing hypertrophy of the infundibulum, and as the child grows, the obstruction is further exaggerated. Later in the 1st year cyanosis occurs, most prominently on the mucous membranes of the lips and mouth and in the fingernails and toenails. In severe cases, cyanosis is noted immediately in the neonatal period. Older children having extreme cyanosis, with a dusky blue skin surface, gray sclerae with engorged blood vessels (suggesting mild conjunctivitis), and clubbing of the fingers and toes, are rarely seen, as surgical repair of tetralogy is most often carried out in early childhood.

Dyspnea occurs on exertion. Infants and toddlers will play actively for a short time and then sit or lie down. Older children may be able to walk a block or so before stopping to rest. Characteristically, children assume a *squatting* position for the relief of dyspnea due to physical effort; the child is usually able to resume physical activity within a few minutes. These findings occur most often in patients with significant cyanosis at rest.

Paroxysmal hypercyanotic attacks (hypoxic or "blue" spells) are a particular problem during the first 2 yr of life. The infant becomes hyperpneic and restless, cyanosis increases, gasping respirations ensue, and syncope may follow. The spell occurs most frequently in the morning. Temporary disappearance or decrease in intensity of the systolic murmur is usual. The spells may last from a few minutes to a few hours but are rarely fatal. Short episodes are followed by generalized weakness and sleep. Severe spells may progress to unconsciousness and, occasionally, to convulsions or hemiparesis. The onset is usually spontaneous and unpredictable. The spells are associated with a reduction of an already compromised pulmonary blood flow, which when prolonged results in hypoxia and metabolic acidosis. The disappearance or attenuation of the systolic murmur and reduction of arterial oxygen saturation and pulmonary arterial pressure suggest that blue spells are associated with a further increase in resistance at the right ventricular outflow tract, transient decrease in systemic resistance, or both. In the presence of decreased pulmonary blood flow, the right to left shunt is increased. The resultant arterial hypoxia, metabolic acidosis, and increased P_{CO_2} further stimulate the respiratory mechanism and the hyperpnea persists. Infants who are only mildly cyanotic at rest are often more prone to develop hypoxic spells because they have not developed the homeostatic mechanisms to tolerate rapid lowering of arterial oxygen saturation.

Depending on the frequency and severity of hypercyanotic attacks, one or more of the following procedures should be instituted in sequence: (1) placement of the infant on the abdomen in the knee-chest position, making certain that there is no constricting clothing; (2) administration of oxygen; and (3) injection of morphine subcutaneously in a dose not in excess of 0.2 mg/kg. Since metabolic acidosis develops when the arterial P_{O_2} is below 40 mm Hg, rapid correction (within several minutes) is necessary if the spell is unusually severe and there is lack of response to the foregoing therapy. This may be accomplished with intravenous administration of sodium bicarbonate. Recovery from the spell is rapid once the pH has returned to normal. Repeated blood pH measurements may be necessary because rapid recurrence of acidosis may occur.

β-Adrenergic blockade by intravenous administration of propranolol (0.1 to a maximum of 0.2 mg/kg) has been used successfully in some patients with severe spells, especially spells accompanied by tachycardia. Drugs that increase systemic vascular resistance, such as intravenous methoxamine and phenylephrine, will decrease the right to left shunt and thus improve the symptoms; but their use has been limited and should not be allowed to delay needed surgery.

It is important to emphasize that calming the infant, while holding the child in a knee-chest position over the shoulder, may abort progression of an early spell. Premature attempts to obtain blood may cause further agitation and be counterproductive.

Growth and development may be delayed in severe untreated tetralogy of Fallot. Stature and nutritional status are usually below averages for age. Puberty is delayed in unoperated patients.

The *pulse* is usually normal, as are the venous and arterial pressures. The left anterior hemithorax may bulge anteriorly. The heart is usually normal in size, and there is a substernal right ventricular impulse. In 50% of cases a *systolic thrill* is felt along the left sternal border in the 3rd and 4th parasternal spaces.

The *systolic murmur* is frequently loud and harsh; it may be transmitted widely, but is most intense at the left sternal border. The murmur may be either ejection or pansystolic and may be preceded by a click. The systolic murmur is due to turbulence over the right ventricular outflow tract and tends to be less prominent with severe obstruction and large right to left shunts. The 2nd heart sound is single and is produced by closure of the aortic valve. Infrequently, the systolic murmur is followed by a diastolic murmur; this continuous murmur may be audible in any part of the chest, anteriorly or posteriorly; it is produced by enlarged bronchial collateral vessels or rarely by persistence of a patent ductus arteriosus. This finding is more frequent with pulmonary atresia.

DIAGNOSIS. *Roentgenographically*, the typical configuration as seen in the anteroposterior view consists of a narrow base, concavity of the left border in the area usually occupied by the pulmonary artery, and normal heart size. The rounded apical shadow situated rather high above the diaphragm is produced chiefly by the hypertrophied right ventricle. The cardiac silhouette has been likened to that of a wooden shoe **(coeur en sabot)** (Fig. 15–33). In the lateral projection the anterior encroachment by the hypertrophied right ventricle is usually seen. The hilar areas and lung fields are relatively clear, because of diminished pulmonary blood flow and/or small size of the pulmonary arteries.

The aorta is usually large, and its position may be important diagnostically. In about 20% of instances the aorta arches to the right instead of to the left; this may result in an indentation of the leftward positioned air-filled tracheobronchial shadow in the anteroposterior view or may be confirmed by displacement of the barium-filled esophagus to the left.

Variations from the typical roentgenographic picture include poststenotic dilatation of the pulmonary artery, which suggests valvular pulmonary stenosis. Occasionally, pulmonary vascularity is made prominent by collateral bronchial circulation that radiates from the hilus of the lungs.

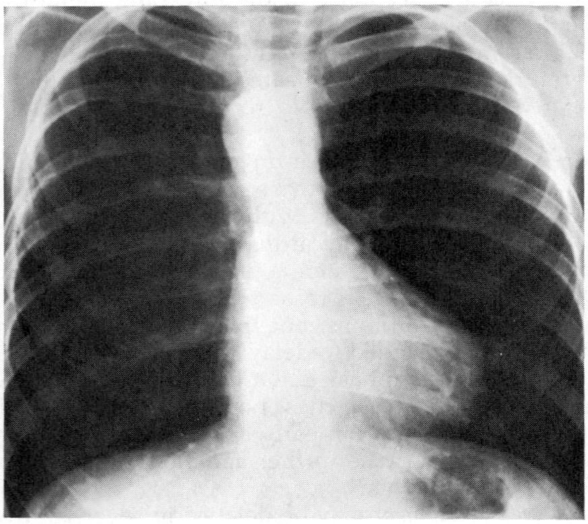

Figure 15–33. Roentgenogram of an 8-yr-old boy with tetralogy of Fallot. Note the normal heart size, some elevation of the cardiac apex, concavity in the region of the main pulmonary artery, right aortic arch, and diminished pulmonary vascularity.

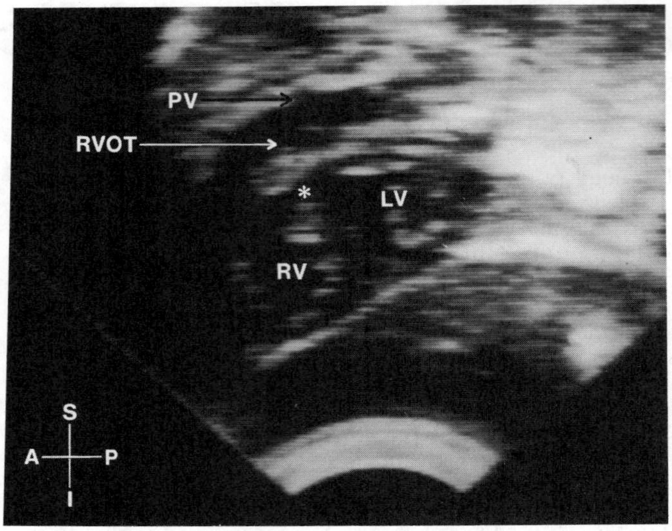

Figure 15–34. Tetralogy of Fallot. This short axis subxiphoid two-dimensional echocardiographic projection demonstrates the anterior/superior displacement of the outflow ventricular septum resulting in stenosis of the subpulmonic right ventricular outflow tract and associated anterior ventricular septal defect. (LV = left ventricle; PV = pulmonary valve; RV = right ventricle; RVOT = right ventricular outflow tract; A = anterior; P = posterior; S = superior; I = inferior; asterisk = interventricular septal defect.)

The *electrocardiogram* reveals right axis deviation and evidence of right ventricular hypertrophy. The latter, without which the diagnosis of tetralogy of Fallot is unlikely, is found in the right precordial chest leads, where the configuration of the QRS complex is Rs, R, qR, qRs, rsR′, or RS. In these leads the T wave may be positive, further evidence of right ventricular hypertrophy. The P wave is tall and peaked or sometimes bifid (see Fig. 15–13).

Two-dimensional echocardiography establishes the diagnosis (Fig. 15–34).

Cardiac catheterization reveals systolic hypertension in the right ventricle equal to systemic pressure, with a marked decrease in pressure as the catheter enters the pulmonary artery or, in some cases, the infundibular chamber beyond the obstruction.

The mean pulmonary arterial pressure is commonly 5–10 mm Hg; the right atrial pressure is usually normal. The aorta may be easily entered from the right ventricle through the ventricular septal defect. The level of arterial oxygen saturation depends on the magnitude of the right to left shunt; at rest it is usually 75–85% in a moderately cyanotic patient. Samples of blood from the venae cavae, right atrium, right ventricle, and pulmonary artery are frequently similar in oxygen content, indicating an absence of a left to right shunt.

Selective right ventriculography best demonstrates the anatomy of tetralogy of Fallot. The contrast medium outlines the heavily trabeculated right ventricle. The infundibular stenosis varies in length, width, contour, and distensibility (Fig. 15–35). An infundibular chamber may also be demonstrated. The pulmonary valve may be normal, but frequently the leaflets are thickened and domed, and the valve ring is small. Nearly simultaneous opacification of the aorta and pulmonary artery is usual. The size of the pulmonary trunk varies considerably. In severe cases it is small or hypoplastic, and localized or multiple areas of stenosis may be seen in the branches of the pulmonary artery, especially at the bifurcation. The subaortic VSD is usually large, and the aorta is well opacified.

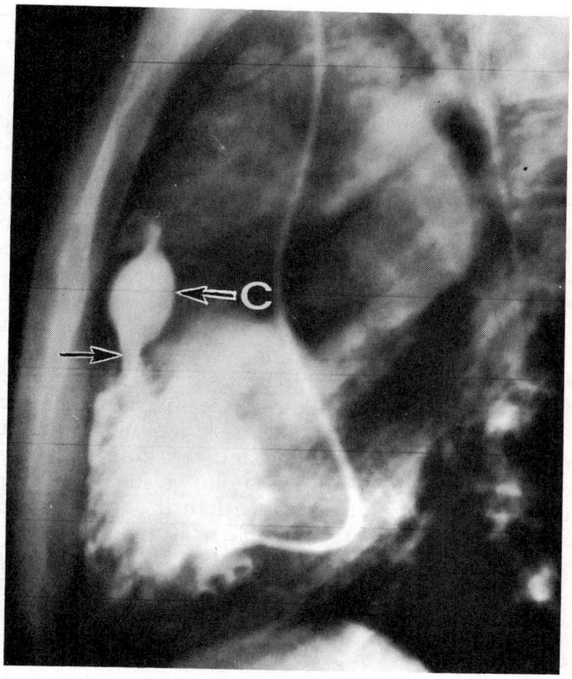

Figure 15–35. Lateral view of a selective right ventriculogram in a patient with tetralogy of Fallot. The *arrow* points to infundibular stenosis that is below the infundibular chamber (C).

Among patients with pulmonary atresia and ventricular septal defect the anatomy of the pulmonary vessels is extremely complex. There may be a central confluence of the left and right arteries with a smaller or absent main pulmonary artery. In some instances only peripheral arteries are seen, with blood entering these vessels from a patent ductus, mammary arteries, or collateral arteries arising separately or together from the descending aorta. Often, there are parallel collateral arteries, as well as the true pulmonary arteries, branching into the periphery of the lung. These vessels may have long stenotic segments as they arise from the descending aorta. The two circulations may or may not communicate. Complete and accurate information regarding the anatomy of the pulmonary arteries is very important in evaluating these children as surgical candidates.

Left ventriculography demonstrates the size of the ventricle, the position of the VSD, and the overriding aorta; it also confirms mitral-aortic continuity and rules out double-outlet right ventricle. *Aortography* or *coronary arteriography* will outline the course of the coronary arteries. In 5–10% of patients an aberrant major coronary artery crosses over the right ventricular outflow tract; this artery must be preserved during repair. Delineation of normal coronary arteries by angiography is most important when considering surgery in young infants.

COMPLICATIONS. *Cerebral thromboses,* usually occurring in the cerebral veins or dural sinuses and occasionally in the cerebral arteries, are more common in the presence of extreme polycythemia. They may also be precipitated by dehydration. *Cerebral ischemia* occurs most often in patients under the age of 2 yr. These patients may have iron deficiency anemia, frequently with hemoglobin and hematocrit levels in the normal range. Therapy consists of adequate hydration and supportive measures. Phlebotomy and volume replacement with fresh frozen plasma are indicated in the extremely polycythemic patient. Heparin is of little value, as it does not influence blood viscosity and may not prevent extension of venous thrombosis; it is contraindicated in hemorrhagic cerebral infarction. Physical therapy to the affected extremities should be instituted as early as possible.

Brain abscess is less common than cerebral vascular events. Patients are usually over the age of 2 yr. The onset of the illness is often insidious with low-grade fever. In some patients there is acute onset of symptoms, which may develop after a recent history of headache, nausea, and vomiting. Epileptiform seizures may occur; localized neurologic signs depend on the site and size of the abscess and the presence of increased intracranial pressure. The sedimentation rate and white blood cell count are usually elevated. Computed tomography, MRI, or ultrasonography confirms the diagnosis. Massive antibiotic therapy may help to keep the infection localized, but surgical drainage of the abscess is almost always necessary (see Sec. 20.74).

Bacterial endocarditis occurs in unoperated patients in the infundibulum or on the pulmonic, aortic, or, rarely, triscuspid valves. Endocarditis may complicate palliative shunts or, among patients with corrective surgery, any residual pulmonic stenosis or a VSD. Antibiotic prophylaxis is essential prior to and after dental and certain surgical procedures since the patient is at risk for developing bacteremia and subsequently endocarditis (see Sec. 15.66).

Congestive heart failure may occur in the young infant with pulmonary atresia and large collateral blood flow. This most often regresses during the first months of life, and the patient becomes cyanotic with decreased pulmonary blood flow. Heart failure is not a feature in the usual patient with tetralogy.

ASSOCIATED CARDIOVASCULAR ANOMALIES. An associated patent ductus arteriosus may be present. Associated defects in the atrial septum are occasionally seen. *Absence of the pulmonary valve* produces a distinct syndrome; cyanosis may be mild, the heart is large and hyperdynamic, and loud to-and-fro murmurs are present. Aneurysmal dilatation of the pulmonary artery often produces wheezing respiration and recurrent pneumonitis from bronchial compression. This syndrome may be lethal in the neonatal period but improves spontaneously in survivors.

Absence of a pulmonary artery should be suspected if the roentgenographic appearance of the pulmonary vasculature differs on the two sides; generally, because the left pulmonary artery is absent, the right lung appears more vascularized. Absence of a pulmonary artery will often be associated with hypoplasia of the affected lung. It may be difficult to differentiate absence of the left pulmonary artery from severe stenosis or late occlusion. It is important to recognize absence of a pulmonary artery prior to the creation of an anastomosis between the systemic circulation and the single remaining pulmonary artery, as occlusion of the latter during operation seriously compromises the already reduced pulmonary blood flow. Right aortic arch occurs in approximately 20% of cases of tetralogy of Fallot, and other anomalies of the pulmonary artery and aortic arch may also be seen. Multiple ventricular septal defects occasionally are present and must be diagnosed prior to corrective surgery. Tetralogy may occur with atrioventricular canal, often associated with Down syndrome.

TREATMENT. Although tetralogy of Fallot often presents insidiously during the 1st year with gradually increasing cyanosis, there are patients with severe tetralogy who require medical treatment and palliative surgical intervention in the neonatal period. Therapy is aimed at providing an immediate increase in pulmonary blood flow to prevent the sequelae of severe hypoxia. The infant should be transported to a medical center adequately equipped to evaluate and treat neonates under optimal conditions. It is critical that oxygenation and normal body temperature be maintained during the transfer.

Prolonged, severe hypoxia may lead to shock, respiratory failure, and intractable acidosis and will significantly reduce the chances of survival after cardiac catheterization and surgery, even when surgically amenable lesions are present. Infants with markedly reduced pulmonary blood flow deteriorate rapidly because the ductus arteriosus does not stay sufficiently patent to provide adequate pulmonary blood flow after birth. The administration of prostaglandin E_1 (0.05–0.20 μg/kg/min), a potent and specific relaxant of ductal smooth muscle, causes dilatation of the ductus arteriosus and allows adequate pulmonary blood flow to occur until a surgical procedure can be carried out in neonates with severe tetralogy of Fallot and other lesions that benefit from ductal patency. This agent is administered intravenously when the clinical diagnosis is made and continued through cardiac catheterization and surgery. Postoperatively, the infusion may be continued to augment the palliative shunt or forward flow through a surgical valvulotomy. However, it is not used for long-term therapy.

Infants with tetralogy of Fallot who are stable and awaiting surgical intervention require careful observation. The prevention or prompt treatment of dehydration is important to avoid hemoconcentration and possible thrombotic episodes. Paroxysmal dyspneic attacks in infancy may be precipitated by a relative iron deficiency; iron therapy may decrease their frequency and also improve exercise tolerance and general well-being. The hematocrit should be maintained at 55–65%. Oral propranolol (1 mg/kg every 6 hr) has been used to decrease the frequency and severity of dyspneic spells, but it is preferable to go ahead with surgical treatment if spells occur.

In general, infants presenting with symptoms and severe cyanosis in the first months of life have marked obstruction of the right ventricular outflow tract or pulmonary atresia. In such infants a systemic to pulmonary artery shunt procedure is carried out to augment pulmonary artery blood flow; it is hoped that not only will hypoxemia be allayed, but the growth of small pulmonary vessels will be augmented. Corrective open heart surgery in early infancy is being considered in critically ill patients with normal coronary artery anatomy. The benefits of corrective surgery in early versus late infancy have not been established. For infants who can be maintained until later in the 1st year of life, open correction is a reasonable primary alternative when the usual single high ventricular septal defect is present, pulmonary arteries are of sufficient size, and no other complicating great vessel abnormalities are present. In general, older patients should have open heart correction of the defect regardless of whether an earlier palliative shunt procedure was carried out.

The **Blalock-Taussig** shunt is the most useful shunt procedure and is created by anastomosis of a subclavian artery to the homolateral branch of the pulmonary artery. With the advent of microvascular surgery, the operation can be successfully performed in the newborn period. Recently, a modified procedure has been effective utilizing a polyfluorotetraethylene (Teflon) conduit side to side from the subclavian to pulmonary artery. Side-to-side anastomosis of the ascending aorta and right pulmonary artery (Waterson) and anastomosis of the upper descending aorta and left pulmonary artery (Potts) are rarely done; these procedures have a higher frequency of complicating congestive heart failure and late-onset pulmonary hypertension as well as greater technical difficulties in closing the shunt during subsequent corrective surgery.

Usually, the postoperative course of patients with a successful shunt procedure is relatively uneventful. However, postoperative complications following a thoracotomy, such as chylothorax, diaphragmatic paralysis, and Horner syndrome, may occur. *Chylothorax* may require repeated thoracocentesis and, on occasion, reoperation in order to ligate the thoracic duct. *Diaphragmatic paralysis* due to injury to the recurrent laryngeal nerve may result in a more difficult postoperative course. More prolonged respiratory support and vigorous physical therapy may be required, but diaphragmatic function will return in 1–2 mo unless the nerve was completely divided. *Horner syndrome* is usually temporary and does not require treatment. Postoperative *cardiac failure* may be due to the large size of the anastomosis; its treatment is described in Sec. 15.73. Vascular problems, other than a diminished radial pulse, are rarely seen in the upper extremity supplied by the subclavian artery used for the anastomosis.

After a successful shunt procedure, cyanosis diminishes. The development of a machinery-type murmur after the operation indicates a functioning anastomosis. However, this may not be heard for several days after surgery. The duration of symptomatic relief is variable. As the child grows, more pulmonary blood flow is needed and the shunt may eventually become inadequate. If the anatomy is such that a corrective operation can be carried out, then it should be undertaken. However, if it is not possible or if the first shunt lasts only a brief period in a small infant, a second anastomosis may be required on the opposite side. Infective endocarditis is a threat in any patient with a systemic to pulmonary artery shunt; appropriate prophylactic measures should be taken (see Sec. 15.66).

Corrective surgical therapy consists of relief of the obstruction to the right ventricular outflow tract and closure of the VSD by direct-vision intracardiac surgery with a pump oxygenator. When there is a previously established systemic to pulmonary shunt, it must be obliterated prior to cardiotomy. The surgical risk of **total correction** is currently under 5%. A right ventriculotomy is performed in most patients. In some centers a transatrial-transpulmonary approach reduces the long-term risks of ventriculotomy. Factors that have contributed to increasing success of this approach include optimal total body perfusion, adequate myocardial protection during bypass, relief of right ventricular outflow obstruction, prevention of air embolism, and meticulous postoperative care. The presence of a previous Blalock-Taussig anastomosis does not increase the operative risk. Increased bleeding in the immediate postoperative period is common in polycythemic patients but should not seriously affect the outcome. The operative risks may be higher in small infants because more complicated anatomy is likely to be encountered.

PROGNOSIS. After successful total correction patients are generally asymptomatic and able to lead unrestricted lives. Immediate postoperative problems include right ventricular failure, transient heart block, residual VSD with left to right shunting, myocardial infarction from manipulation of an aberrant coronary artery, and disproportionately increased left atrial pressure due to residual collaterals. These systemic to pulmonary shunts may need to be closed by embolization or umbrella placement during cardiac catheterization, whereas postoperative heart failure (particularly in patients with a significant outflow patch) requires inotropic agents including digoxin. The long-term effects of isolated, surgically induced pulmonary valvular incompetence are unknown, but this lesion is common when a right ventricular outflow patch is utilized and is generally well tolerated. Patients with marked pulmonary valve insufficiency have moderate to marked cardiac enlargement. A patient having severe residual gradient across the right ventricular outflow tract may require reoperation, but mild to moderate obstruction is virtually always present and does not require reintervention. Rarely, true aneurysmal dilatation of the outflow patch requires repeated surgery.

Follow-up of patients 5–20 yr after operation indicates that the marked improvement in symptomatology is generally maintained. However, even asymptomatic patients have working capacities, maximal heart rates, and cardiac outputs that are lower than those of controls. These abnormal findings may be less frequent when surgery is undertaken at an early age.

Conduction disturbances are also frequent after operation. The atrioventricular node and the bundle of His and its divisions are in close proximity to the VSD and may be injured during surgery. Permanent complete heart block following surgery is now rare. When present, it should be treated by placement of a permanently implanted pacemaker. Bifascicular block, due to injury to the anterior fascicle of the left bundle (manifested as postoperative left axis deviation) and of the right bundle (manifested as complete right bundle branch block), occurs in about 10% of patients; the long-term significance is uncertain, but in most instances there are no clinical manifestations. The additional finding of transient complete heart block in the immediate postoperative period, however, appears to be associated with an increased incidence of late-onset complete heart block and sudden death. However, unexpected cardiac arrest rarely occurs many years after surgery in patients without postoperative bifascicular block or transient complete heart block.

A number of children will display frequent premature ventricular beats following repair of tetralogy of Fallot. Usually these are benign and nonprogressive. However, 24-hr monitoring studies should be done to be certain that short episodes of ventricular tachycardia are not occurring even when the patient is asymptomatic. In addition, exercise studies may be useful in bringing out cardiac arrhythmias that are not apparent at rest. In the absence of more complex ventricular arrhythmias or severe residual hemodynamic abnormalities, prophylactic antiarrhythmia therapy often is not required. If it is decided that ventricular ectopy requires treatment, quinidine, propranolol, Dilantin, or combinations of these agents are most often used.

15.12 PULMONARY ATRESIA WITH VENTRICULAR SEPTAL DEFECT

This condition is an extreme form of tetralogy of Fallot. The pulmonary valve is atretic, rudimentary, or absent, and the pulmonary trunk is atretic or hypoplastic. The entire ventricular output is ejected into the aorta. Pulmonary blood flow is dependent on a patent ductus arteriosus or bronchial collaterals.

CLINICAL MANIFESTATIONS. These are similar to those of tetralogy but usually with earlier and more severe manifestations. Cyanosis usually appears within a few days after birth in contrast to later in the 1st yr; the systolic murmur is absent or soft; the 1st heart sound is frequently followed by an ejection click; the 2nd sound at the base is moderately loud and single; and continuous murmurs of a patent ductus arteriosus or bronchial collateral flow may be heard over the entire precordium, anteriorly and posteriorly.

The presentation of these infants in the neonatal period is variable. Some patients have congestive heart failure due to increased pulmonary blood flow via collateral vessels; others are severely cyanotic and require urgent prostaglandin E_1 infusion and palliative surgical intervention; and some infants have adequate pulmonary blood flow and can be managed like patients with uncomplicated less severe tetralogy.

The *roentgenogram* will reveal a small or enlarged heart, depending on pulmonary blood flow, a concavity at the position of the pulmonary arterial segment, and often the reticular pattern of bronchial collateral flow. The *electrocardiogram* shows right ventricular hypertrophy. The *echocardiogram* identifies the aortic override and the thick right ventricular wall and pulmonary atresia. At cardiac catheterization, *right ventriculography* reveals a large aorta, opacified immediately by passage of the contrast medium through the septal defect, and no dye entering the lungs through the right ventricular outflow tract. The pathway of pulmonary blood flow from the aorta to the lungs is also demonstrated.

TREATMENT. Systemic-pulmonary artery anastomosis may be indicated for the patient with pulmonary arteries of reasonable size. An open heart bypass from the right ventricle directly to the pulmonary artery, either by "unroofing" the outflow tract or by implanting a conduit, has been utilized in some patients. There is controversy as to whether this type of bypass may stimulate the growth of the pulmonary arteries better than a standard shunt operation. The pulmonary arteries must be of adequate size to allow the patient to become a candidate for future open heart repair, which would include closure of the VSD and an aortic homograft from the right ventricle to the pulmonary artery valve: valve-containing conduits have been used until recent years (Fig. 15–36). Previous systemic to pulmonary anastomoses are eliminated. Conduit replacement may be required later in life. Often, patients have malformations of the primary divisions of the pulmonary arteries in the form of hypoplasia, multiple branch stenoses, absence of a pulmonary artery, and large bronchial collaterals. These vessels are difficult to reconstruct surgically even after early anastomotic procedures. Some patients with extreme tetralogy of Fallot require surgical or catheter obliteration of large pulmonary collateral vessels near or at the time of a corrective surgical procedure that incorporates the true pulmonary arteries into the circulation. High-flow collaterals may cause congestive heart failure in the postoperative period.

Acquired total atresia of the right ventricular outflow tract may occur after a systemic-pulmonary anastomosis for tetralogy of Fallot. The systolic murmur due to pulmonary stenosis is attenuated or disappears. The completeness of obstruction can be confirmed by right ventriculography. Corrective surgery of the right ventricular outflow tract is similar to that utilized for tetralogy of Fallot.

15.13 PULMONARY ATRESIA WITH INTACT VENTRICULAR SEPTUM

In this anomaly the pulmonary valve leaflets are completely fused to form a membrane, and the right ventricular outflow tract is atretic. Because there is no egress of blood from the right ventricle, right atrial blood is shunted into the left atrium via the foramen ovale, mixes with pulmonary venous blood, and enters the left ventricle. The combined left and right ventricular output is pumped by the left ventricle into the aorta. Pulmonary blood flow occurs via a patent ductus arteriosus. In addition, among the great majority of patients who have small right ventricular cavities, sinusoidal channels within the right ventricle may communicate directly to the coronary arterial circulation, resulting in blood flow retrograde to the aorta. Patients with intermediate-sized or large ventricular cavities may have tricuspid insufficiency, which serves to decompress the right ventricle.

CLINICAL MANIFESTATIONS. As the ductus arteriosus closes in the first days of life, infants with pulmonary atresia and intact ventricular septum become markedly cyanotic. Untreated, most patients die within the 1st wk week of life. Physical examination reveals severe cyanosis and respiratory distress. The 2nd heart sound is single, and most often there are no murmurs.

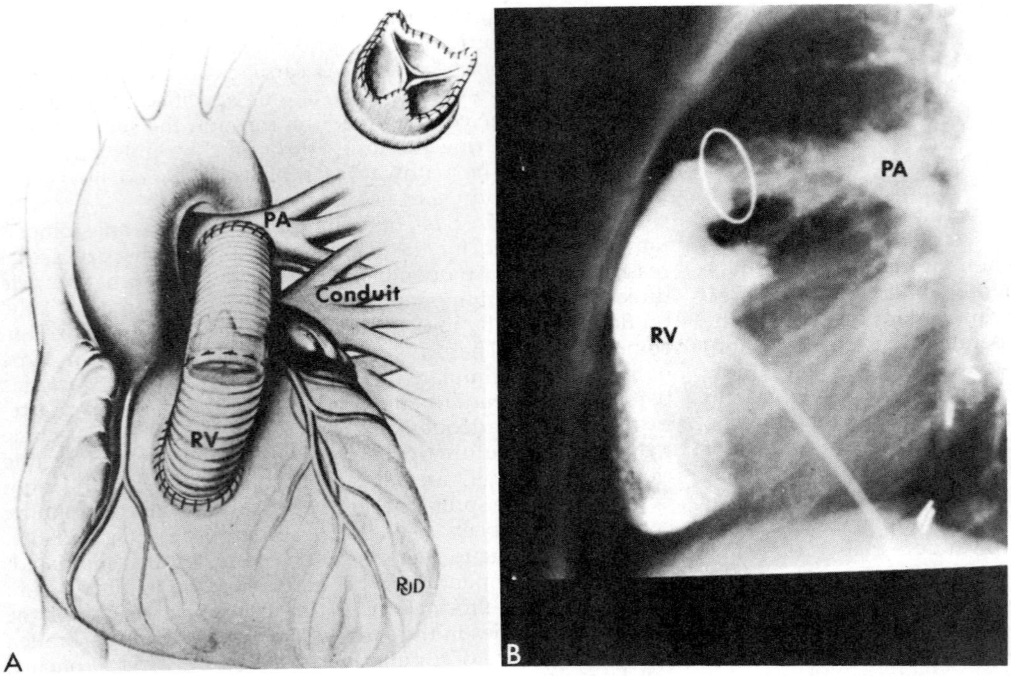

Figure 15–36. *A*, Artist's sketch of the valve-containing conduit utilized in the repair of pulmonary atresia. The porcine valve is portrayed in the inset. *B*, A right ventricular angiogram (lateral view) in a patient with pulmonary atresia and ventricular septal defect after repair with a valve-containing conduit. Recently, aortic homografts are more often utilized for this type of repair. (PA = pulmonary artery; RV = right ventricle.)

The *electrocardiogram* is helpful in that the frontal QRS axis almost always lies between 0 and +90 degrees. The tall, spiked P waves indicate right atrial enlargement. The electrocardiogram is consistent with left ventricular dominance or hypertrophy; right ventricular forces are markedly decreased in the majority of patients with small right ventricles. Occasionally, with large right ventricular cavities, right ventricular hypertrophy is seen. The chest *roentgenogram* shows the heart to be variable in size with markedly decreased pulmonary vascularity. The two-dimensional *echocardiogram* is useful in helping to estimate the right ventricular dimensions and the size of the tricuspid valve. *Cardiac catheterization* demonstrates right atrial and right ventricular hypertension. Ventriculography reveals the size of the ventricular cavity, the atretic right ventricular outflow tract, the degree of tricuspid regurgitation, and the intramyocardial sinusoids filling the coronary vessel.

TREATMENT. The prognosis for this lesion has improved with urgent medical and surgical management. Infusion of prostaglandin E_1 is usually effective in keeping the ductus open prior to intervention (see Sec. 15.11), thus reducing hypoxemia and acidemia prior to surgery. Pulmonary valvotomy is carried out to relieve outflow obstruction whenever possible, but in order to preserve adequate pulmonary blood flow, a systemic-pulmonary arterial anastomosis is done during the same procedure. Some groups have reported success by unroofing the outflow tract and patch grafting. The aim of surgery is to encourage growth in the right ventricular chamber by allowing forward flow, while utilizing the shunt to provide adequate pulmonary blood flow. Later, when possible, a more extensive valvotomy is carried out and the shunt is taken down. If the right ventricular chamber is minuscule, a Fontan procedure (see Sec. 15.14) may be utilized to allow blood to flow to the pulmonary artery directly from the right atrium. When coronary perfusion occurs via the right ventricle through myocardial sinusoids, the prognosis may be grave. Associated coronary artery abnormalities may be expected.

15.14 TRICUSPID ATRESIA

In tricuspid atresia there is no outlet from the right atrium to the right ventricle, and the entire systemic venous return enters the left heart by means of the foramen ovale. Pulmonary blood flow depends on the size of the ventricular septal defect and/or patent ductus arteriosus, the only means by which the pulmonary circulation is perfused. The inflow portion of the right ventricle is always missing in these patients, but the outflow portion is of variable size. If the ventricular septum is intact, the right ventricle is completely hypoplastic and pulmonary atresia is present. Most patients with tricuspid atresia present in the early months of life with decreased pulmonary blood flow and cyanosis. Rarely, a large ventricular septal defect in the absence of right ventricular outflow obstruction can lead to high pulmonary flow and early congestive heart failure. Variants of tricuspid atresia include associated transposition of the great arteries (TGA) and other lesions.

CLINICAL MANIFESTATIONS. Cyanosis, polycythemia, easy fatigability, exertional dyspnea, and occasional hypoxic episodes occur as a result of compromised pulmonary blood flow. Cyanosis may be evident at birth. The majority of patients have pansystolic murmurs audible along the left sternal border; the 2nd heart sound is single. The diagnosis is suspected in 85% of patients before 2 mo of age. Spontaneous VSD closure may increase cyanosis.

Roentgenographic studies show pulmonary undercirculation. Left axis deviation and left ventricular hypertrophy are almost invariably present on the *electrocardiogram* except when there is transposition of the great arteries. In the right precordial leads the normally prominent R wave is replaced by rS complex. The left precordial leads show a qR complex followed by a normal flat diphasic or inverted T wave. RV_6 is normal or tall, and SV_1 generally deep. The P waves are usually biphasic with the initial component tall and spiked in lead II. The *two-dimensional echocardiogram* reveals the absence of a tricuspid valve, the small right ventricle, and the large left ventricle and aorta.

Cardiac catheterization shows normal or slightly elevated right atrial pressure with a prominent "a" wave. If the right ventricle is entered through the ventricular septal defect, the pressure is low, reflecting the restrictive nature of the ventricular communication in most patients. With right atrial angiography there is immediate opacification of the left atrium from the right atrium followed by left ventricular filling and visualization of the aorta. Absence of direct flow to the right ventricle results in a filling defect between the right atrium and the left ventricle, but a small right ventricle usually is opacified later via a ventricular septal defect. Rarely, the pulmonary arteries are filled only through a patent ductus arteriosus. The presence or absence of associated transposition of the great vessels and pulmonary stenosis is demonstrated by selective left ventriculography.

TREATMENT. Symptomatic neonates require a surgical shunt procedure to increase pulmonary blood flow. In severe cases adequate pulmonary blood flow may be provided by maintaining ductal patency with infusion of prostaglandin. The Blalock-Taussig procedure (or its variations) is the preferred anastomosis. Some patients are benefited by a Rashkind balloon atrial septostomy (BAS). Patients with tricuspid atresia may remain stable for many years. Eventually, left ventricular dysfunction may occur, as it is this chamber that must provide blood flow to both the pulmonary and systemic circulation. In older patients the Glenn anastomosis (right superior vena cava to right pulmonary artery) has been utilized to provide more physiologic blood flow of unoxygenated systemic venous blood directly to the lungs. This type of shunt does not increase the volume work of the left ventricle. This shunt may cause superior vena cava syndrome and may close spontaneously, thereby increasing cyanosis.

The Fontan operation is the preferred approach to later surgical management. This procedure is carried out by anastomosing the right atrium to the pulmonary artery either directly or through a conduit insertion to the outflow area of the right ventricle. The atrial septal defect or foramen ovale is closed. If the right ventricle is of adequate size, a modification of this procedure has been utilized in which a valve-containing conduit is placed between the right atrium and body of the right ventricle closing the ventricular and atrial septal defects (Fig. 15–37). A four-chambered, four-valved heart is thus produced. However, at the present time, direct bicaval anastomosis to the pulmonary artery is most often done. The inferior vena cava blood flow is separated from the heart as a channel through the lateral aspect of the right atrium to the inferior portion of the superior vena cava using pericardial augmentation. Early evaluation of patients who have undergone Fontan procedures has been encouraging, and the long-term results of these types of anastomoses appear to be better than the results of systemic-pulmonary artery shunts. The Fontan procedure is contraindicated in young infants and in patients with elevated pulmonary vascular resistance (greater than 4 units/m^2) or pulmonary artery hypoplasia. For the atrial pump to function well, sinus rhythm is important as is the absence of both mitral insufficiency and elevated left ventricular end-diastolic pressure.

Postoperative problems after a Fontan procedure include marked elevated systemic venous pressure, fluid retention, and pleural or pericardial effusions. Pleural effusions may persist for more than 3 wk in 30–40% of patients. Late complications include residual obstruction, right atrial or pulmonary artery thrombi, protein-losing enteropathy, and supraventricular arrhythmias (atrial flutter, paroxysmal atrial tachycardia) occasionally associated with sudden death.

15.15. ORIGIN OF BOTH GREAT VESSELS FROM THE RIGHT VENTRICLE (DOUBLE-OUTLET RIGHT VENTRICLE), WITH PULMONARY STENOSIS

This anomaly is characterized by the aorta and pulmonary artery arising from the right ventricle; the only outlet for the left ventricle is the ventricular septal defect. The aortic and mitral valves are not in continuity, and the ventricular septal defect is inferior to the crista supraventricularis. The physiology among patients with double-outlet right ventricle and pulmonary stenosis is similar to that which occurs with tetralogy of Fallot. The history, physical examination, electrocardiogram, and roentgenograms are as described in Sec. 15.11. The two-dimensional echocardiograph demonstrates the anatomy and demonstrates the double-outlet right ventricle and mitral-aortic valve discontinuity. Selective angiocardiography shows that the aortic and pulmonary valves lie in the same horizontal body plane and that the anteriorly displaced aorta arises exclusively from the right ventricle. Surgical correction consists of creating an intraventricular channel so that the left ventricle ejects blood through the ventricular

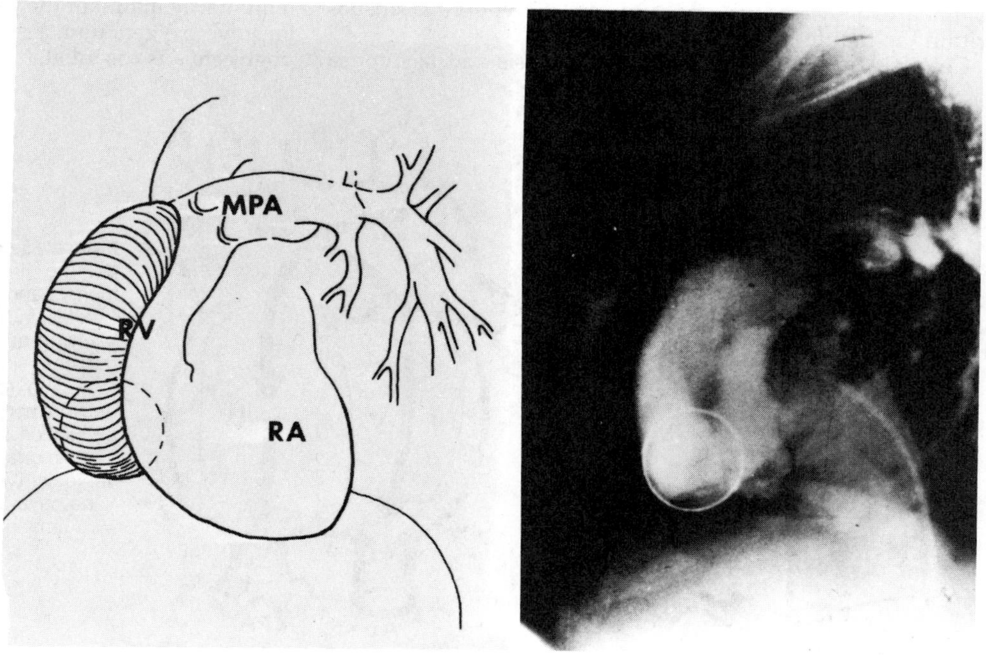

Figure 15–37. Modified Fontan operation, left lateral view. (MPA = main pulmonary artery; RV = right ventricle; RA = right atrium.)

septal defect into the aorta. The pulmonary obstruction is relieved with or without a pulmonary or aortic homograft. In small infants palliation with an aortic pulmonary shunt provides symptomatic improvement (see Sec. 15.32.)

15.16 D-TRANSPOSITION OF THE GREAT ARTERIES (TGA)

In this anomaly the aorta arises from the right ventricle and the pulmonary artery from the left ventricle. The systemic veins normally return to the right atrium, and the pulmonary veins to the left atrium. The atrial-ventricular relationships are normal (concordant). The desaturated blood from the right side of the heart inappropriately passes to the aorta, whereas the oxygenated pulmonary venous blood is returned to the lungs. Thus, the systemic and pulmonary circulation consists of two parallel circuits. The two independent circuits allow survival because the foramen ovale remains patent (with or without an associated ductus arteriosus or ventricular septal defect) to permit some mixture of blood (Fig. 15–38*A*). TGA is more common in infants of diabetic mothers and males (3:1), occurring in 1 in 5,000 live births. Prior to the modern era of corrective or palliative surgery the mortality was greater than 90% within the 1st year of life.

The aorta is usually anterior and to the right of the pulmonary trunk. The pulmonary valve is continuous with the mitral valve. Defects of the ventricular septum occur in about 50% of cases. Generally, the right coronary artery arises above the posterior sinus of Valsalva, the left, above the left sinus. (The right coronary artery normally arises above the right sinus.) The clinical presentation and hemodynamics vary in relation to the presence or absence of associated defects.

15.17 D-TRANSPOSITION OF THE GREAT ARTERIES (TGA) WITH INTACT VENTRICULAR SEPTUM

This anomaly is also referred to as simple transposition of the great arteries or isolated TGA. Prior to birth, oxygenation of the fetus is normal, but after birth the minimal mixing of the systemic and pulmonary blood at the atrial level via the patent foramen ovale is insufficient, and severe hypoxemia ensues within the first few days or weeks of life.

CLINICAL MANIFESTATIONS. Cyanosis and tachypnea are most often recognized within the first hours or days of life. Untreated, the vast majority of these infants would not survive the neonatal period. Hypoxemia is usually severe, but congestive heart failure is not a feature. This condition is a medical emergency in the neonate, and only early diagnosis and appropriate intervention can avert the sequelae of prolonged severe hypoxemia.

DIAGNOSIS. The *electrocardiogram* shows normal neonatal right-sided dominance. *Roentgenograms* of the chest may show cardiomegaly, a narrow cardiac waist, and increased pulmonary blood flow, but in most cases are virtually normal. The arterial Po_2 value is low and does not rise appreciably after the patient breathes 80–100% oxygen. *Echocardiography* confirms the diagnosis of isolated TGA. In addition, the size of the intra-atrial communication can be visualized by apical and subxiphoid two-dimensional scanning.

Cardiac catheterization shows right ventricular pressure to be systemic, as this ventricle is supporting the peripheral circulation. The catheter enters the aorta directly from the right ventricle; it also passes across the foramen ovale or an atrial septal defect into the left heart chambers and occasionally into the pulmonary artery. The blood in the left ventricle and pulmonary artery has a higher oxygen content than that in the aorta. The degree of arterial desaturation is variable, but is most often extremely low. The left ventricular and pulmonary arterial pressures are usually less than 50% of systemic pressures. *Right ventriculography* demonstrates the origin of the anteriorly placed aorta from the right ventricle, the intact ventricular septum, the closure of the ductus arteriosus, and the transposed great arteries; the aortic valve is anterior and superior to the pulmonary valve. The aortic origin of the coronary arteries is also shown. Anomalous coronary arteries are noted in 10–15%. A common coronary origin from a single right sinus of Valsalva ostium is seen in 10% and makes the arterial switch surgical repair more complicated. *Left ventriculography* shows that the pulmonary artery arises exclusively from the left ventricle and that the ventricular septum is intact.

TREATMENT. Prior to the initiation of specific therapy and during transfer to a neonatal cardiac center, particular attention must be paid to maintaining normal body temperature; hypothermia intensifies the metabolic acidosis resulting from hypoxemia. Infusions of prostaglandin E_1 (PGE_1) may temporarily maintain the patency of the ductus arteriosus and improve oxygenation. Prompt correction of acidosis and hypoglycemia is essential.

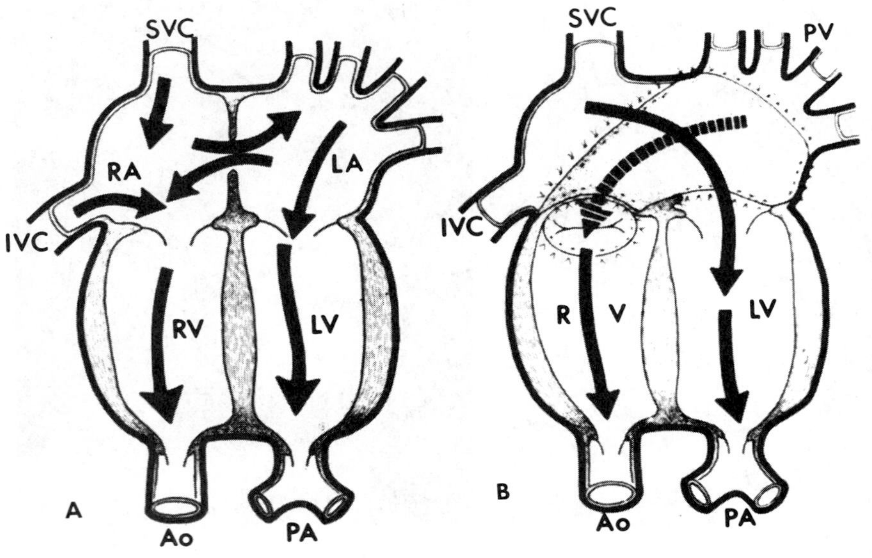

Figure 15–38. *A*, In transposition of the great arteries the circulation is in parallel. Mixing of the pulmonary and systemic circulation must occur in order to sustain life. The diagram shows bidirectional shunting at the atrial level. *B*, After intra-atrial repair (Mustard procedure), systemic venous return is routed to the left ventricle and pulmonary artery, and pulmonary venous blood reaches the systemic circulation via the right ventricle. (Ao = aorta; PA = pulmonary artery; LV = left ventricle; RV = right ventricle; IVC = inferior vena cava; SVC = superior vena cava; LA = left atrium; RA = right atrium; PV = pulmonary valve.)

After the diagnosis is established by two-dimensional echocardiography, the infant may be taken immediately to the cardiac catheterization laboratory. If echocardiography is not diagnostic, appropriate angiographic study should be carried out to confirm the diagnosis of transposition of the great arteries. In all patients in whom any delay in operation is planned, a Rashkind BAS (Fig. 15–39) is performed with as little delay as possible. At most centers the arterial (Jatene) switch operation is performed within the first 2 wk of life. If the arterial switch is planned immediately, catheterization and BAS may be avoided.

If the BAS is indicated, its success can be judged by a rise in Pa_{O_2} to 35–50 mm Hg and the elimination of the usual preseptostomy pressure gradient across the atrial septum. The rise of Pa_{O_2} indicates improved mixing of the systemic and pulmonary venous returns. Patients with transposition of the great arteries with associated anomalies should also undergo balloon septostomy. Some of the blood of these patients does not mix well at the ventricular level even in the presence of communications, and others may benefit by decompression of the left atrium to alleviate the early pulmonary symptoms of left-sided heart failure.

Some infants are so severely cyanotic and acidotic that management is required prior to the catheterization study. In this situation PGE_1 should be infused in order to maintain ductal patency or reopen a ductus arteriosus that is in the process of closing (dosage, 0.05 to 0.20 μg/kg/min). This will improve arterial oxygenation. In some instances prostaglandin administration should be prolonged, even after balloon septostomy, until Pa_{O_2} becomes stable at an acceptable level. However, infusion of PGE_1 is rarely necessary for more than a few days, and if the patient appears to be prostaglandin-dependent, surgical management should be initiated.

The arterial switch (Jatene) procedure is the surgical treatment of choice for infants preferably younger than 2 wk of age with TGA and an intact ventricular septum. The operation is occasionally done in the 3rd or 4th week. Previous experience with atrial switch (Mustard, Senning) surgery in older infants has indicated excellent immediate survival (about 85–90%) but significant long-term morbidity. Atrial switch procedures reverse blood flow patterns at the atrial level by the surgical formation of intra-atrial baffles, allowing systemic venous blood to be directed to the lungs via the left atrium, left ventricle, and pulmonary artery (see Fig. 15–38*B*). This permits oxygenated pulmonary venous blood to cross over to the right atrium, right ventricle, and aorta. Baffles are constructed with the native atrial septum, Dacron, or pericardial tissue. Elective surgery is usually performed at 4–9 mo of age. The atrial switch procedures involve significant atrial surgery and suturing and may result in atrial conduction disturbances, sick-sinus syndrome with bradytachyarrhythmias, paroxysmal atrial tachycardia, and atrial flutter. Many patients develop a junctional rhythm, which is usually well tolerated. Late sudden death may occur, especially in children with sick sinus syndrome who manifest tachyarrhythmia. Severe bradycardia requires the placement of a permanent cardiac pacemaker. An additional problem is the development of a fixed or dynamic baffle obstruction due to thrombosis, baffle or septal occlusion of venous orifices, and kinking. Such obstruction produces the superior vena cava syndrome due to obstruction of systemic venous return, or pulmonary hypertension due to obstruction of pulmonary venous return; both may reduce cardiac output. Systemic venous obstruction may also produce edema, ascites, and protein-losing enteropathy.

Atrial switch procedures require the right ventricle to assume the role of the systemic ventricle, but nevertheless can function at systemic pressures for decades. However, given the stress of infantile hypoxia, the requirement for myocardial protection at surgery, and associated cardiac defects, right ventricle performance may progressively deteriorate with time. Right ventricular dysfunction is usually manifested as exercise intolerance. Tricuspid insufficiency may also contribute to right ventricular dysfunction.

The **arterial switch procedure**, in most centers, has a survival rate of 80–90%. The arterial switch corrects the physiologic relationships of systemic and pulmonary arterial blood flow and respective ventricular performances, thus obviating the complications of the atrial switch (Fig. 15–40). The arterial switch is usually performed in the first 2 wk of life, a time prior to the regression of left ventricular muscle mass, which occurs following the normal postnatal reduction of pulmonary vascular resistance. Under optimal circumstances, systemic left ventricular pressures should be present immediately prior to surgery. This ensures adequate left ventricular function to tolerate the increased systemic arterial afterload after the switch operation.

Two-stage arterial switch procedures may be employed in patients over 2–3 wk of age who already have a reduction of left ventricular muscle mass and pressure. The 1st stage involves banding of the pulmonary artery to maintain systemic pressure in the left ventricle. However, banding may distort the pulmonary arteries and increases the operative risk with the 2nd stage, and this approach is rarely used.

Although the risk of coronary artery injury and subsequent myocardial damage is present at the time of the arterial switch procedures, complications are rare. Most often ventricular function is excellent, sinus rhythm is maintained, and most patients remain asymptomatic.

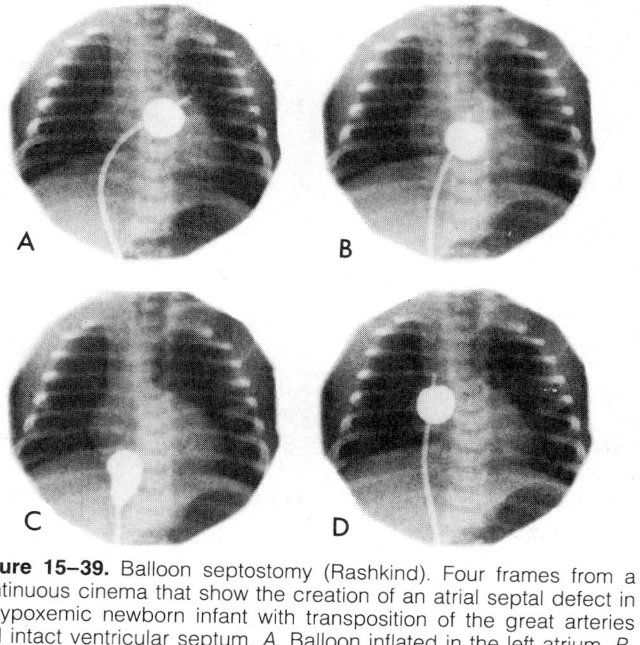

Figure 15–39. Balloon septostomy (Rashkind). Four frames from a continuous cinema that show the creation of an atrial septal defect in a hypoxemic newborn infant with transposition of the great arteries and intact ventricular septum. *A*, Balloon inflated in the left atrium. *B*, The catheter is jerked suddenly so that the balloon ruptures the foramen ovale. *C*, Balloon in the inferior vena cava. *D*, Catheter advanced to the right atrium to deflate the balloon. The time from *A* to *C* is less than 1 sec.

15.18 TRANSPOSITION OF THE GREAT ARTERIES WITH VENTRICULAR SEPTAL DEFECT

If the septal defect is small, the clinical manifestations, laboratory findings, and treatment are similar to those described above. Many of the small defects close spontaneously.

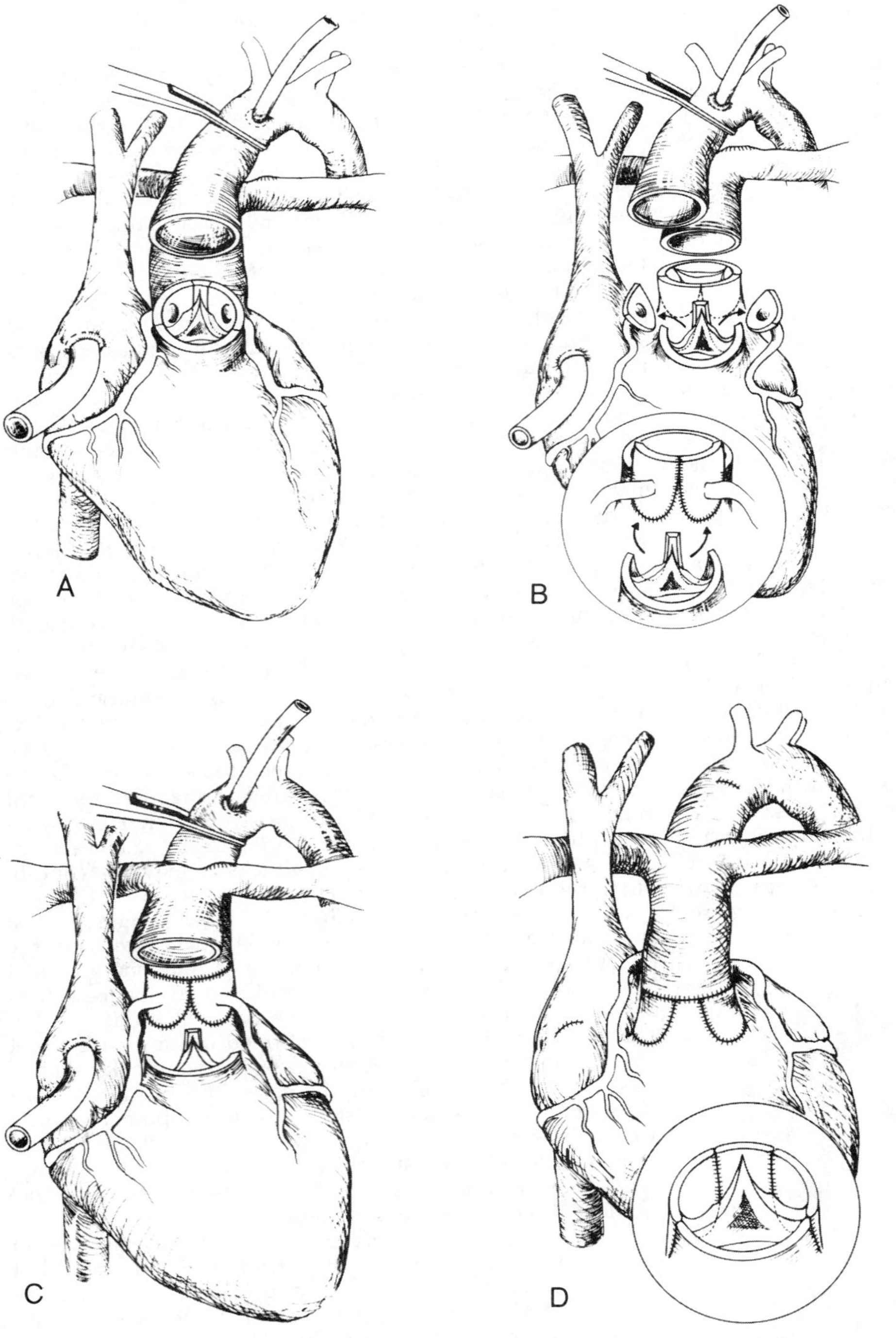

Figure 15–40. Arterial switch operation for transposition of the great arteries. *A*, Division of the ascending aorta approximately 1 cm distal to the valve commissures. The patent ductus arteriosus is divided. *B*, Excision of the left and right coronary arteries with a generous patch of the aortic wall. Division of the main pulmonary artery. Excision of segments of the pulmonary artery wall (see inset), transfer of coronary arteries, and anastomosis of both left and right coronary arteries into neoaorta. *C*, The distal pulmonary artery is brought anterior to the ascending aorta. Anastomosis of the proximal neoaorta to the distal aorta. *D*, Coronary donor site for neopulmonary artery filled with pericardial patches (see inset). End-to-end anastomosis between the proximal neopulmonary artery segment and the distal pulmonary artery. The branch pulmonary arteries were extensively mobilized at the beginning of the procedure.

When the ventricular septal defect is large and nonrestrictive to ventricular ejection, significant mixing of blood often occurs and *clinical manifestations* of congestive cardiac failure are seen. The onset of cyanosis may be subtle and frequently delayed, and its intensity is variable. With careful observation, cyanosis can usually be recognized within the 1st mo of life, but in undiagnosed infants several months elapse before it is apparent. The hypoxemia is usually associated with polycythemia but less prominently than in patients with an intact septum. The heart is significantly enlarged. The murmur is pansystolic and generally indistinguishable from that produced by a large ventricular septal defect with normally related arteries. The *electrocardiogram* shows prominent P waves, isolated right ventricular hypertrophy, or biventricular hypertrophy. Usually, the QRS axis is to the right, but sometimes it is normal or even to the left. Occasionally, dominance of the left ventricle is present. The cardiomegaly, narrow cardiac waist, and significant pulmonary vascularity are demonstrated *roentgenographically*. Pulmonary blood flow can also be assessed by *echocardiography*. (Increased flows are associated with enlargement of the left atrium and ventricle.) The diagnosis is confirmed by *cardiac catheterization* and angiocardiography. Right and left ventriculography indicates the presence of arterial transposition and demonstrates the site and size of the ventricular septal defect. The catheter may cross the ventricular septum from the right ventricle and enter the pulmonary artery. Peak systolic pressures are equal in the two ventricles, the aorta, and the pulmonary artery. The ventricular end-diastolic pressures are elevated in the presence of cardiac failure. The left atrial pressure may be much higher than right atrial pressure.

At the time of cardiac catheterization a balloon septostomy is performed to decompress the left atrium even in cases in which adequate mixing is occurring at the ventricular level. Surgical therapy is advised within the first 2–4 mo of life, as congestive heart failure and failure to thrive are difficult to manage and pulmonary vascular disease develops rapidly. Patients with this combination of defects usually require maintenance digitalis and diuretic therapy.

Without treatment, *prognosis* is poor; the majority of patients succumb in the 1st yr of life because of congestive cardiac failure, hypoxemia, and pulmonary hypertension. In the past, some survived infancy with medical therapy and without surgical intervention. The clinical picture and treatment of these patients are almost identical to those described in Eisenmenger syndrome (Sec. 15.24) with a large ventricular septal defect.

Prior to the perfection of the arterial switch procedure, patients with TGA and a VSD were initially managed with atrial septostomy or surgical septectomy and pulmonary arterial banding (to prevent development of pulmonary vascular hypertension). Correction with an atrial switch procedure and VSD closure was performed following pulmonary artery debanding at 1 yr of age (see Sec. 15.17).

Currently the patient with TGA and a VSD without pulmonic stenosis can be managed without pulmonary artery banding but with early neonatal atrial septostomy, if needed, and an arterial switch procedure. Operation in early infancy avoids the risk of developing increased pulmonary vascular resistance and eliminates the need for protective pulmonary artery banding. Because the VSD results in equal pressure in both ventricles, the left ventricle continues to face systemic pressure and there is little regression in left ventricular muscle mass, thus permitting adequate left ventricular performance against the systemic afterload following anastomosis of the aorta to the left ventricle and patch closure of the VSD.

15.19 TRANSPOSITION OF THE GREAT ARTERIES WITH VENTRICULAR SEPTAL DEFECT AND PULMONARY STENOSIS

This combination of anomalies may mimic tetralogy of Fallot. The site of obstruction is either valvular or subvalvular; the latter type may be acquired after successful atrial septostomy or pulmonary arterial banding.

The onset of *clinical manifestations* varies from soon after birth to infancy and includes cyanosis, decreased exercise tolerance, and poor physical development. The manifestations are similar to those described under tetralogy of Fallot. However, the heart may be more enlarged. The pulmonary vasculature as seen on *roentgenogram* is relatively normal. The *electrocardiogram* usually shows right axis deviation, right and left ventricular hypertrophy, and sometimes tall, spiked P waves. *Echocardiography* is useful in sequential evaluation of the degree and progression of the left ventricular outflow obstruction.

Cardiac catheterization shows that the pulmonary arterial pressure is low and as in all patients with transposition, the oxygen saturation exceeds that of the aorta. Selective right and left ventriculography demonstrates the origin of the aorta from the right ventricle, the origin of the pulmonary artery from the left ventricle, the ventricular septal defect, and the pulmonary stenosis.

The preferred *treatment* in hypoxemic infants is establishment of a systemic-pulmonary arterial shunt, when necessary, after neonatal balloon atrial septostomy. The patient can then be followed clinically until 2–6 yr of age when a Rastelli operation is the preferable corrective procedure. The Rastelli procedure achieves physiologic and anatomic correction by (1) patch closure of the VSD, directing left ventricular flow to the aorta; and (2) connection of the right ventricle to the pulmonary artery by ligating the proximal pulmonary artery and placing an extracardiac homograft between the right ventricle and the distal pulmonary artery. The conduit may eventually become stenotic or functionally restrictive with growth of the patient and require revision. Surgical correction by the Mustard operation with simultaneous closure of the ventricular septal defect and relief of left ventricular outflow obstruction may be an alternative when the position of the ventricular septal defect is not suitable for a Rastelli operation. Patients amenable to simple valvotomy can undergo correction with an arterial switch.

15.20 TOTAL ANOMALOUS PULMONARY VENOUS RETURN

Abnormal development of the pulmonary veins may result in anomalous partial (see Sec. 15.37) or complete drainage into the systemic venous circulation. The abnormal point of entry may be the right atrium, the superior or inferior vena cava or one of their major tributaries, or a persistent left superior vena cava that opens into the coronary sinus. The pulmonary veins may join a common trunk that enters the venous circulation below the diaphragm (portal vein, ductus venosus, or inferior vena cava). An associated atrial septal defect is often present; at least a patent foramen ovale is required to sustain life.

PATHOLOGY. In *total anomalous pulmonary venous return* there is no direct pulmonary venous connection into the left atrium, and all of the blood returning to the heart (the systemic and pulmonary venous blood) returns to the right atrium. Some of the blood passes into the right ventricle and pulmonary artery, and the remainder passes through an obligatory atrial septal defect or patent foramen ovale to the left atrium.

Usually, the pulmonary veins form a single trunk before entering the systemic venous circulation and join the systemic venous return through supracardiac, intracardiac, or infracardiac connections (Table 15–8). The right atrium and ventricle and the pulmonary artery may be enlarged, whereas the left atrium and ventricle are small and less compliant.

CLINICAL MANIFESTATIONS. Three types of clinical patterns are seen. Some infants present in the neonatal period with severe obstruction to pulmonary venous return. This is most prevalent in the infracardiac group (see Table 15–8). Cyanosis is prominent, and there is severe tachypnea. There may be no murmurs present on physical examination.

TABLE 15–8. Anomalous Pulmonary Venous Return

% and Site of Connection	% with Severe Obstruction
Supracardiac (50)	
Left superior vena cava (40)	40
Right superior vena cava (10)	75
Cardiac (25)	
Coronary sinus (20)	10
Right atrium (5)	5
Infracardiac (20)	95–100
Mixed (5)	

Another group of patients also presents with congestive heart failure in early life, but in these infants there is a large left to right shunt; obstruction to pulmonary venous return is only mild or moderate. Because pulmonary artery hypertension is present, the infants will be severely ill. Systolic murmurs along the left sternal border are audible, and there may be a gallop rhythm. A continuous murmur is occasionally heard along the left upper sternal border over the pulmonary area. Cyanosis is mild.

The third group of patients with total anomalous venous return are those in whom pulmonary venous obstruction is not present. In this situation, which is the least common, there is a large left to right shunt, but pulmonary hypertension is absent and the patients are unlikely to be symptomatic during infancy or early childhood. Cyanosis is absent.

DIAGNOSIS. The *electrocardiogram* demonstrates right ventricular hypertrophy (usually a qR pattern in V_4R and V_1, and the P waves are frequently tall and spiked). *Roentgenograms* are pathognomonic in older children if the pulmonary veins enter the innominate vein and persistent left superior vena cava (Fig. 15–41). There is a large supracardiac shadow with a **figure 8** or **snowman** appearance. The supracardiac shadow is produced by the dilated left superior vena cava, left innominate vein, and right superior vena cava. However, this appearance is not helpful for diagnosis in early infancy because of superimposition of the thymic image or because the pulmonary veins may drain elsewhere. In most cases of total anomalous pulmonary venous return, the heart is enlarged, the pulmonary artery and right ventricle are prominent, and the pulmonary vascularity is increased. In neonates having severe cyanosis due to marked venous obstruction (usually infradiaphragmatic), the chest roentgenograms reveal pulmonary edema with a small heart and thus commonly cause confusion with the respiratory distress syndrome. The differential diagnosis includes persistent fetal circulation, respiratory distress syndrome, pneumonia (bacterial, meconium aspiration), pulmonary lymphangiectasia, and other heart defects (hypoplastic left ventricle).

The *echocardiogram* reflects the right ventricular overload and usually identifies the pattern of pulmonary venous connections.

Cardiac catheterization shows that the oxygen saturations of blood in both atria, both ventricles, and the aorta are more or less similar and higher than the peripheral systemic venous blood proximal to the entry of the pulmonary venous trunk. In older patients the pulmonary arterial and right ventricular pressures may be only moderately elevated, but in infancy pulmonary hypertension is usual. *Selective pulmonary arteriography* shows the anatomy of the pulmonary veins and their point of entry into the systemic venous circulation (Fig. 15–42).

Without treatment, the prognosis for the great majority of patients with total anomalous pulmonary venous return is poor, and survival beyond infancy is unusual in the presence of pulmonary hypertension. Death is due to congestive heart failure. Patients who survive beyond 2 yr of age are those who do not have pulmonary arterial hypertension, and they may remain asymptomatic for many years.

Surgical correction of total anomalous pulmonary venous return during infancy is indicated. Prior to surgery, infants may be stabilized with prostaglandin (PGE_1) to dilate the ductus venosus and the ductus arteriosus; some require BAS, which is of no benefit in the presence of venous obstruction. The common pulmonary venous trunk is anastomosed to the left atrium, the atrial septal defect is closed, and the connection to the systemic venous circuit is interrupted. The surgical results have been good, even for critically ill neonates. If the postoperative hemodynamics are normal, the prognosis appears to be excellent. The postoperative period rarely may be complicated by a pulmonary vascular hypertensive crisis. Delay of surgical treatment for symptomatic infants with this lesion is not warranted.

15.21 EBSTEIN DISEASE

This anomaly consists of downward displacement of an abnormal tricuspid valve into the right ventricle. The anterior cusp of the valve retains some attachment to the valve ring, but the other leaflets are attached to the wall of the right ventricle. The latter chamber is divided into two parts by the abnormal valve; the first is continuous with the cavity of the right atrium; the second consists of thin-walled ventricular

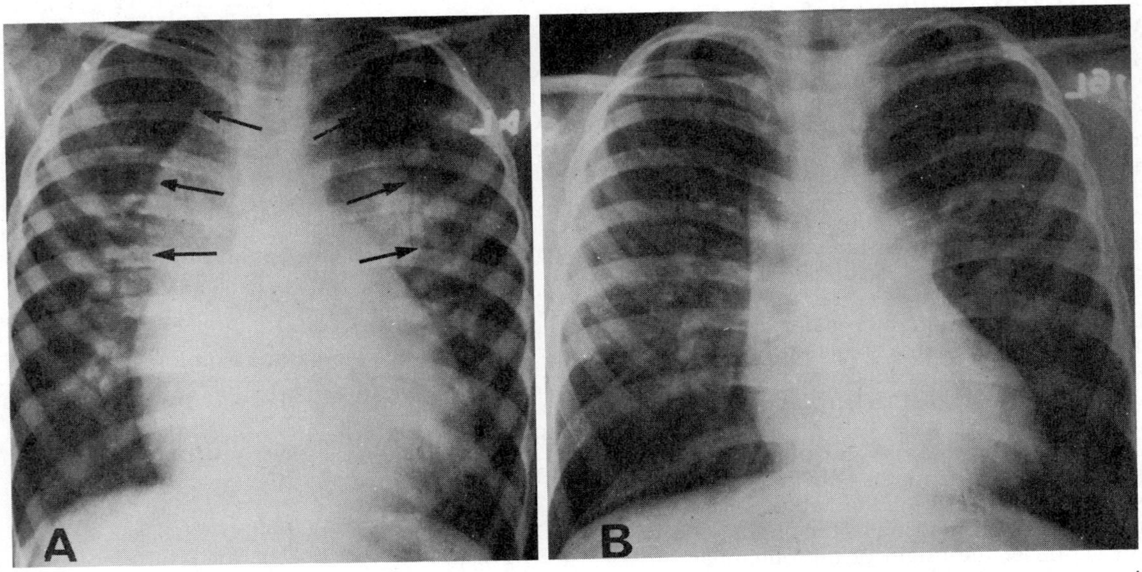

Figure 15–41. Roentgenograms in total anomalous pulmonary venous return to the left superior vena cava. *A*, Preoperative. *Arrows* point to the supracardiac shadow, which produces the snowman or figure 8 configuration. Cardiomegaly and increased pulmonary vascularity are evident. *B*, Postoperative, showing decrease in size of the heart and supracardiac shadow.

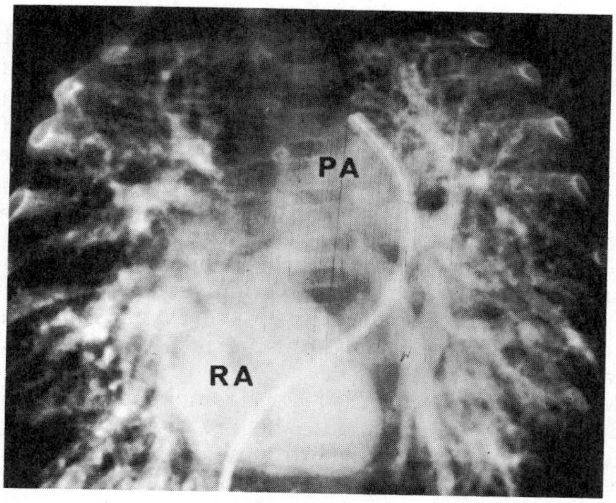

Figure 15–42. Total anomalous pulmonary venous return to the coronary sinus. Injection of contrast medium into the pulmonary artery (PA) opacifies the pulmonary arterial tree. The contrast medium returns to the coronary sinus, which drains into the densely opacified right atrium (RA).

myocardium. The right atrium is huge, and the tricuspid valve may or may not be competent. The effective output from the right side of the heart is decreased because of the poorly functioning small right ventricle and subtle obstruction produced by the large, sail-like, anterior tricuspid leaflet. Variable amounts of right to left shunting occur at the atrial level via the foramen ovale, resulting in mild to severe cyanosis.

CLINICAL MANIFESTATIONS. The severity of symptoms depends on the degree of displacement of the tricuspid valve. In many patients, symptoms are mild and the only complaint is fatigue. Cardiac dysrhythmias are frequent, the most common being numerous extrasystoles or attacks of paroxysmal tachycardia, usually supraventricular. A right to left shunt through the foramen ovale is responsible for cyanosis and polycythemia. The venous pressure is normal or increased if there is associated tricuspid insufficiency. On palpation, the precordium is quiet. A systolic murmur is audible over most of the anterior left side of the chest. Gallop rhythm is common as is a scratchy diastolic murmur at the left sternal border. This murmur is superficial and may mimic a pericardial friction rub.

Although some patients may be asymptomatic until well into adult life, newborn infants with Ebstein disease may present with cyanosis, massive cardiomegaly, and long systolic murmurs. Death may occur as a result of cardiac failure and hypoxemia. However, spontaneous improvement occurs rapidly in many symptomatic neonates as pulmonary vascular resistance falls normally and pulmonary blood flow increases.

DIAGNOSIS. The *electrocardiogram* usually shows right bundle branch block without increased right precordial voltage, normal or tall and broad P waves, and normal or prolonged P-R interval. Sometimes the pattern of the Wolff-Parkinson-White syndrome is present.

On *roentgenographic examination* the heart size varies from normal to massive cardiomegaly because of great enlargement of the right atrium and ventricle. The intrapulmonary vasculature is normal or decreased, and the aorta is small.

Echocardiography shows delayed closure and an increased amplitude of the tricuspid valve. Abnormal septal motion, retardation of the E-F slope of the tricuspid valve, and a dilated right atrium are also seen. The atrialized portion of the right ventricle and the abnormal tricuspid valve can be visualized with two-dimensional ultrasound.

Cardiac catheterization and *selective angiocardiography* confirm the presence of a large right atrium and abnormal tricuspid valve. A right to left shunt at the atrial level, if present, will be demonstrated. The right atrial pressure may be normal, but is often somewhat elevated along with the right ventricular diastolic pressure. There is a significant risk of arrhythmia during catheterization and angiographic studies.

PROGNOSIS. This is extremely variable, depending on where the patient falls within the broad spectrum of severity seen with this defect. For the neonate or infant with intractable symptoms, the prognosis is usually poor. Many patients survive into adult life.

TREATMENT. Control of hypoxemia and supraventricular dysrhythmias is of primary importance. Surgical treatment is seldom necessary in childhood. Repair or replacement of the abnormal tricuspid valve with closure of the atrial septal defect can be carried out. The results of such surgery have been inconsistent, but recently new techniques suggest a somewhat better outlook.

15.22 TRUNCUS ARTERIOSUS

In this anomaly a single arterial trunk arises from the ventricular portion of the heart and supplies the systemic, pulmonary, and coronary circulation. A ventricular septal defect is always present, and the number of semilunar valve cusps in the single truncal valve varies from two to six. The pulmonary trunk may arise from the posterior left side of the persistent truncus arteriosus (TA) and then divide into left (LPA) and right (RPA) pulmonary arteries (type I truncus arteriosus). In types II and III there is no main pulmonary trunk and the RPA and LPA arise from separate orifices in the posterior (II) or lateral (III) side of the TA. Type IV has no identifiable connection between the heart and pulmonary arteries and relies upon collateral arterial vessels from the aorta; it has been called *pseudotruncus* but is essentially a form of pulmonary atresia with a VSD.

Truncus arteriosus is seen in patients with DiGeorge syndrome and may be complicated by thymic aplasia or hypoplasia and T lymphocyte immunodeficiency, placing them at risk for infection. Parathyroid gland aplasia or hypoplasia with the subsequent appearance of hypocalcemia may also occur. Patients with DiGeorge syndrome may have TA with or without an interrupted aortic arch.

HEMODYNAMICS. Both ventricles are at systemic pressure ejecting blood into the truncus. When the pulmonary vascular resistance is relatively normal, the blood flow to the lungs is greatly increased, the arteriovenous oxygen difference is small, and cyanosis is minimal or absent. If the pulmonary resistance increases, the pulmonary blood flow decreases and cyanosis becomes more apparent. The truncal valve is occasionally incompetent.

CLINICAL MANIFESTATIONS. These vary with age, depending on pulmonary vascular resistance. In the majority of infants, pulmonary blood flow is torrential and the clinical picture is dominated by dyspnea, fatigue, heart failure, recurrent respiratory infections, poor physical development, and often death in infancy. Cyanosis is minimal or absent. The runoff of blood from the truncus to the pulmonary circulation may result in a wide pulse pressure. This may be further exaggerated by truncal valve insufficiency. The heart is usually enlarged, and the precordium is hyperdynamic. A systolic ejection murmur, sometimes accompanied by a thrill, is usually audible along the left sternal border. The murmur is frequently preceded by an ejection click. In the presence of truncal valve insufficiency, a high-pitched protodiastolic murmur is heard. The 2nd heart sound is loud and generally single. A mid-diastolic apical rumbling murmur is audible. In older children with restricted pulmonary blood flow secondary to the development of pulmonary vascular obstructive disease, progressive cyanosis, polycythemia, and clubbing develop.

DIAGNOSIS. The *electrocardiogram* is variable and shows right, left, or combined ventricular hypertrophy. There is considerable variation in the roentgenographic appearance of the chest. Cardiac enlargement is due to prominence of both ventricles. The truncus may produce a prominent shadow that follows the normal course of the ascending aorta and aortic knob; it arches to the right in almost 50% of patients. Sometimes a high bulge, left of the aortic knob, is produced by the main or left pulmonary artery. The pulmonary vascularity is increased in the presence of normal pulmonary resistance. *Echocardiography* demonstrates the large, overriding, and usually anterior truncal artery as well as VSD.

The diagnosis is confirmed by *cardiac catheterization* and by selective right ventriculography. The catheter may enter the pulmonary arteries from the truncus. A left to right shunt is demonstrated at the ventricular level, and the systolic pressures in both ventricles and the truncus are similar. Selective angiocardiography reveals the large truncus arteriosus and the origin of the pulmonary arteries. Injection of contrast medium into the truncus just above the truncal valve allows assessment of the competence of this valve.

PROGNOSIS. Without surgery, many of the patients succumb during infancy or by the 1st or 2nd yr of life. If pulmonary blood flow is restricted by development of pulmonary vascular disease, the patient may survive into adulthood.

TREATMENT. Open heart repair of truncus arteriosus has been accomplished in infants and older children. The ventricular septal defect is closed, the pulmonary arteries are separated from the truncus, and continuity is established between the right ventricle and the pulmonary arteries with a homograft. Immediate surgical results among survivors have been excellent, but after repair in infancy the conduit must be replaced as the child grows. The other option is banding of the pulmonary arteries followed by surgical correction in later years; morbidity and mortality associated with banding, however, are high, and most centers prefer early repair. In older patients with pulmonary vascular obstruction, surgical treatment is contraindicated.

15.23 SINGLE VENTRICLE

(Double-Inlet Ventricle: Univentricular Heart)

With a single ventricle, both atria empty through a common valve or two separate atrioventricular valves into a single ventricular chamber, of left, right, or indeterminate ventricular anatomic characteristics, from which the aorta and pulmonary artery arise. Associated cardiac anomalies are usual and vary considerably. Transposition of the great arteries and rudimentary outlet chamber are present in the vast majority of patients. Pulmonary stenosis or atresia is common.

CLINICAL MANIFESTATIONS. The clinical picture is variable, depending on the associated intracardiac anomalies and hemodynamics in the individual patient. If a single ventricle is associated with pulmonary stenosis, cyanosis is present in infancy and increases in intensity during childhood, when clubbing and polycythemia also appear. Dyspnea and fatigue are frequent, cardiomegaly is mild or moderate, a left parasternal lift is palpable, and a systolic thrill is common. The systolic ejection murmur is usually loud; an ejection click may be audible, and the 2nd heart sound is single and loud.

When a single ventricle is associated with an unobstructed pulmonary outflow tract, pulmonary blood flow is torrential. These patients present in early infancy with tachypnea, dyspnea, poor physical development, recurrent pulmonary infections, and congestive heart failure. Cyanosis is only mild or moderate. Cardiomegaly is generally marked, and a left parasternal lift is palpable. The systolic ejection murmur is generally not intense, and the 2nd heart sound is loud and closely split. A 3rd heart sound is common and may be followed by a short mid-diastolic murmur. The development of pulmonary vascular disease in patients who have not been operated upon may restrict pulmonary blood flow so that cyanosis increases in intensity, heart size decreases, and signs of cardiac failure appear to improve.

DIAGNOSIS. The *electrocardiogram* is nonspecific. P waves are normal, spiked, or bifid. The precordial lead pattern suggests right ventricular hypertrophy, combined ventricular hypertrophy, or sometimes left ventricular dominance. The initial QRS forces are usually to the left and anterior. *Roentgenographic examination* confirms the degree of cardiomegaly. The rudimentary systemic outflow chamber may produce a bulge on the upper left border of the cardiac silhouette in the posteroanterior projection. In the absence of pulmonary stenosis, pulmonary vasculature is increased with prominence of the major branches of the pulmonary artery. Attenuation of the size of the peripheral pulmonary arteries occurs in the presence of obstructive pulmonary vascular disease. Absence of the ventricular septum is the principal *echographic* sign. The details of the atrioventricular valve anatomy are best delineated echocardiographically.

At *cardiac catheterization* the arterial oxygen saturation is decreased in the presence of severe pulmonary stenosis or obstructive pulmonary hypertension but is near normal when pulmonary blood flow is increased. The pressure in the ventricular chamber is high; a gradient may be demonstrated across the entrance to the rudimentary outflow tract and, in the usual case, when the great arteries are transposed, this causes physiologic subvalvular aortic stenosis. Pulmonary artery stenosis is common. Severe pulmonary hypertension is present in the absence of pulmonary stenosis or pulmonary arterial banding. Selective ventriculography is diagnostic and demonstrates the single ventricle and the anatomic relationships of the pulmonary artery and aorta.

PROGNOSIS. Some patients succumb during infancy from congestive heart failure. Others may survive to adolescence and early adult life but finally succumb to the effects of chronic hypoxemia or, in the absence of pulmonary stenosis, pulmonary hypertension secondary to pulmonary vascular disease. Patients with moderate pulmonary stenosis have the best prognosis, since pulmonary blood flow, although restricted, is still adequate.

TREATMENT. If pulmonary stenosis is severe, a systemic-pulmonary arterial anastomosis is indicated. Pulmonary arterial banding is advised for patients with a large pulmonary flow to control heart failure and to prevent progressive pulmonary vascular disease. The Fontan operation is the treatment of choice for children whose pulmonary pressure and resistance are low, because of associated pulmonary stenosis or after pulmonary artery banding in infancy. Subaortic stenosis often requires surgical relief. Septation of the ventricle is an option for a rare patient.

15.24 EISENMENGER SYNDROME

The term Eisenmenger syndrome refers to patients with reversed or bidirectional shunt through a ventricular septal defect as a result of pulmonary vascular obstructive disease. This physiologic abnormality also can occur with atrial septal defect, atrioventricular canal, patent ductus arteriosus, or other communication between the aorta and pulmonary artery. Pulmonary vascular disease with isolated atrial septal defect is rare and does not occur until late in adulthood. In normal neonates, within a few weeks the structure of the pulmonary arteriole changes to that of the adult with a thin wall and a large lumen, and the pulmonary vascular resistance falls to normal adult levels. In the Eisenmenger syndrome the pulmonary vascular resistance either remains high or, after having decreased during early infancy, rises thereafter because of increased shear stress on pulmonary arterioles. This phenomenon is primarily the result of prolonged elevated pulmonary pressure, and results in severe obliterative intimal lesions in these vessels. In the Eisenmenger syndrome, pulmonary hypertension is the result of high pulmonary resistance (pulmonary vascular disease) rather than the result of markedly increased pulmonary blood flow (hyperkinetic pulmonary hypertension).

Eisenmenger physiology is due to pathologic changes in the small pulmonary arterioles and muscular arteries (<300 μm). Type 1 changes in these arteries involve medial thickening, type 2 changes consist of medial and intimal thickening, and type 3 includes both of the above plus plexiform lesions secondary to hypoplasia of the small muscular arteries' medial layer. Medial hypoplasia predisposes the arteries to aneurysmal dilatation associated with severe pulmonary arterial hypertension. Plexiform lesions indicate severe irreversible pulmonary vascular obstruction. Eisenmenger physiology is defined by an absolute elevation of pulmonary arterial pressure greater than 12 Wood units or by a ratio of pulmonary to systemic resistance greater than or equal to 1.0. Pulmonary vascular hypertension occurs sooner in patients with trisomy 21 and also significantly complicates the natural history of those patients with elevated pulmonary venous pressure, transmission of systemic pressure to the pulmonary circulation, exposure to low Po_2 (high altitude), and high pulmonary blood flow from birth.

CLINICAL MANIFESTATIONS. Symptoms usually do not occur until the 2nd or 3rd decade of life, although less often a more fulminant course is seen. Many patients survive for decades with minimal symptoms. Irreversible pulmonary vascular obstruction results in high pulmonary vascular resistance. Intra- or extracardiac communications that normally would shunt left to right allow right to left shunting as pulmonary resistance exceeds systemic resistance. Cyanosis becomes apparent, and dyspnea, fatigue, and tendency toward dysrhythmias begin to occur. In the late stages of the disease, heart failure, chest pain, syncope, and hemoptysis may be seen. Physical examination reveals a right ventricular heave and a loud, narrowly split 2nd heart sound. Only a soft ejection systolic murmur is audible along the left sternal border. Pulmonary artery pulsation may be palpable at the left upper sternal border. The degree of cyanosis depends on the stage of the disease. Functional incompetence of the pulmonary valve may result in a blowing diastolic murmur along the left sternal border (Graham Steell murmur).

DIAGNOSIS. Cyanotic patients have various degrees of polycythemia. *Roentgenographically*, the heart varies in size from normal to greatly enlarged; the latter occurs late in the course of the disease (Fig. 15–43). The main pulmonary artery is prominent. The pulmonary vessels are enlarged in the hilar areas and diminish in caliber in the peripheral branches. The right ventricle and atrium are prominent. The *electrocardiogram* shows marked right ventricular hypertrophy. The P wave may be tall and spiked. The *echocardiogram* shows a thick-walled right ventricle and demonstrates a communication between the systemic and pulmonary circulation. The right-sided systolic time interval shows a significant increase in the ratio of pre-ejection period to ejection time because of the increased pulmonary vascular resistance. Doppler studies may demonstrate the direction of the shunt and estimate the pulmonary arterial pressure.

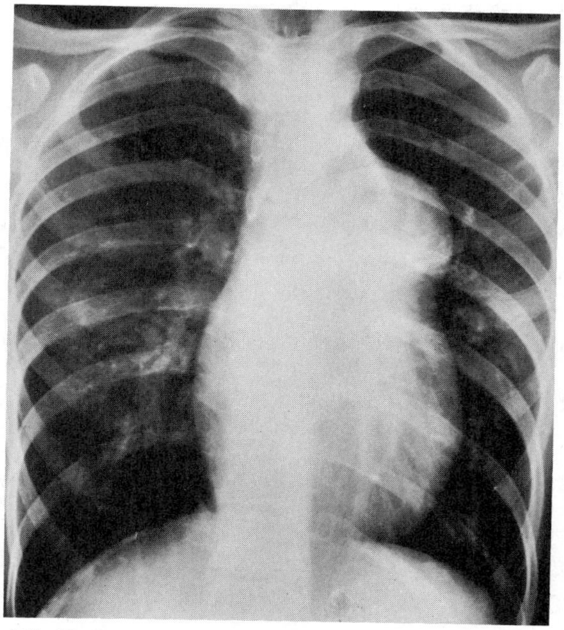

Figure 15–43. Roentgenogram in Eisenmenger syndrome due to a patent ductus arteriosus. The heart size is normal, the pulmonary artery segment is dilated, and the pulmonary vascularity is normal or slightly increased.

Cardiac catheterization usually shows a bidirectional shunt at the site of the defect. The systolic pressures are usually equal in the systemic and pulmonary circulation. The pulmonary capillary wedge pressure is normal, ruling out a left-sided heart obstructive lesion as an explanation for the pulmonary artery hypertension. The arterial oxygen saturation is decreased, reflecting the right to left shunt. Response to vasodilator therapy (oxygen, nitroprusside, prostaglandins) may identify patients with reversible pulmonary hypertension. Selective angiocardiography can locate the site of the shunt, but these studies are avoided in these patients because of increased risk with contrast media injection and the accuracy of modern echocardiography.

TREATMENT. The best management of patients who are at risk of developing late pulmonary vascular disease is *prevention* by surgical elimination of large intracardiac or great vessel communications during infancy. However, some patients will not have shown early clinical manifestations. Medical treatment of the Eisenmenger syndrome is entirely symptomatic (Table 15–9). Older children and adolescents with significant polycythemia may be improved by cautious, repeated venesections with volume replacement. Combined heart-lung or single-lung transplantation may be an option for some patients.

15.25 HYPOPLASTIC LEFT HEART SYNDROME

The term hypoplastic left heart syndrome is used to describe a closely related group of anomalies that include underdevelopment of the left side of the heart, for example, atresia of the aortic or mitral orifice, and hypoplasia of the ascending aorta. The left ventricle is small and nonfunctional; the right

TABLE 15–9. Extracardiac Complications of Cyanotic Congenital Heart Disease and Eisenmenger Physiology

Problem	Etiology	Therapy
Polycythemia	Persistent hypoxia	Phlebotomy
Relative anemia	Nutritional deficiency	Iron replacement
CNS abscess	Right to left shunting	Antibiotics, drainage
CNS thromboembolic stroke	Right to left shunting or polycythemia	Phlebotomy
Low-grade DIC, thrombocytopenia	Polycythemia	None for DIC unless bleeding, then phlebotomy
Hemoptysis	Pulmonary infarct, thrombosis or rupture of pulmonary artery plexiform lesion	Embolization
Gum disease	Polycythemia, gingivitis, bleeding	Dental hygiene
Gout	Polycythemia, diuretic agent	Allopurinol
Arthritis, clubbing	Hypoxic arthropathy	None
Pregnancy complications: abortion, fetal growth retardation, prematurity, maternal illness	Poor placental perfusion, poor ability to increase cardiac output	Bed rest
Infections	Associated asplenia, DiGeorge syndrome, endocarditis	Antibiotics
	Fatal RSV pneumonia with pulmonary hypertension	Ribavirin
Failure to thrive	Increased oxygen consumption, decreased nutrient intake	Treat heart failure; correct defect early, increased caloric intake
Psychosocial adjustment	Limited activity, cyanotic appearance, chronic disease, multiple hospitalizations	Counseling

CNS = central nervous system; DIC = disseminated intravascular coagulation; RSV = respiratory syncytial virus.

ventricle maintains both pulmonary and systemic circulations. Pulmonary venous blood passes through an atrial defect or dilated foramen ovale from the left to the right side of the heart, where it mixes with systemic venous blood. When the ventricular septum is intact, which is almost always the case, all the right ventricular blood is ejected to the pulmonary arteries; the systemic circulation is supplied retrograde via the ductus arteriosus. With a ventricular septal defect and a patent but small aortic orifice, right ventricular blood is ejected to the small left ventricle and ascending aorta as well as to the pulmonary artery. The major hemodynamic abnormalities are inadequate maintenance of the systemic circulation and pulmonary venous hypertension.

CLINICAL MANIFESTATIONS. Signs of heart failure appear within the first few weeks of life and include dyspnea, hepatomegaly, and low cardiac output. All peripheral pulses are weak or absent. Although cyanosis may not be obvious in the first 48 hr of life, a grayish blue color of the skin is soon apparent. Cardiac enlargement is usual, with a palpable right ventricular parasternal lift. A nondescript systolic murmur is usually present. Extracardiac anomalies may be present.

DIAGNOSIS. *Roentgenographically*, the heart is variable in size in the first days of life, but cardiomegaly develops rapidly and is associated with increased pulmonary vascularity. The *electrocardiogram* may show only the normal right ventricular dominance initially, but later P waves become prominent and right ventricular hypertrophy is usual.

The *echocardiogram* is diagnostic (Fig. 15–44). There is absence or gross distortion of the mitral valve, absent or small aortic root, a small left atrium and posterior ventricle, a large right atrium and anterior ventricle, and an easily identifiable tricuspid valve. The size of the atrial communication by which pulmonary venous blood leaves the left atrium is assessed. Contrast echocardiography with the transducer in the suprasternal notch identifies the small transverse aortic arch and left atrium. These findings are so characteristic that the diagnosis of aortic atresia can be made without cardiac catheterization. The hypoplastic ascending aorta can be well demonstrated by aortography, which also shows the coronary arterial system.

PROGNOSIS. Patients virtually always succumb from this anomaly during the first months of life, usually during the first week or two.

TREATMENT. There is variable success in the surgical therapy of hypoplastic left heart syndrome. Management includes palliation (Norwood procedure), heart transplantation, and, in some patients, supportive expectant care.

If a *Norwood procedure* is to be performed, preoperative medical management includes correction of acidosis and hypoglycemia, maintenance of the patency of the ductus arteriosus with prostaglandins to support systemic blood flow, and prevention of hypothermia. Balloon atrial septostomy may be indicated.

The Norwood procedure is performed in two or three stages. The first stage includes an atrial septectomy and transection and ligation of the distal main pulmonary artery; the proximal pulmonary artery is connected to the aorta and the coarcted segment of the aorta is repaired. A synthetic shunt connects the aorta to the main pulmonary artery at the bifurcation of the left and right pulmonary arteries to provide controlled pulmonary blood flow. Operative risk is high. Survival of the first stage varies greatly among centers.

The second stage may be accomplished with two operations and consists of a modified Fontan procedure connecting vena caval and right atrial flow to the pulmonary arteries. Pulmonary venous–left atrial flow is directed to the tricuspid valve and subsequently the right (systemic) ventricle. The risk is considerable and the result is a single right ventricle and a Fontan palliation. The stage 1 palliation and the later complications of the Fontan operation carry high risks.

An alternate therapy is cardiac transplantation either in the immediate neonatal period, obviating stage I of the Norwood procedure, or after a successful stage I, but in place of a stage II Fontan procedure. Cardiac function is poor following the Fontan procedure and may require cardiotonic medications; transplanted patients have the chronic risks of organ rejection and permanent immunosuppressive therapy.

15.26 ABNORMAL POSITIONS OF THE HEART: DEXTROCARDIA AND LEVOCARDIA

An approach to the classification and diagnosis of abnormal cardiac position has been suggested by Van Praagh and colleagues. *Atrial localization* is facilitated by roentgenographic

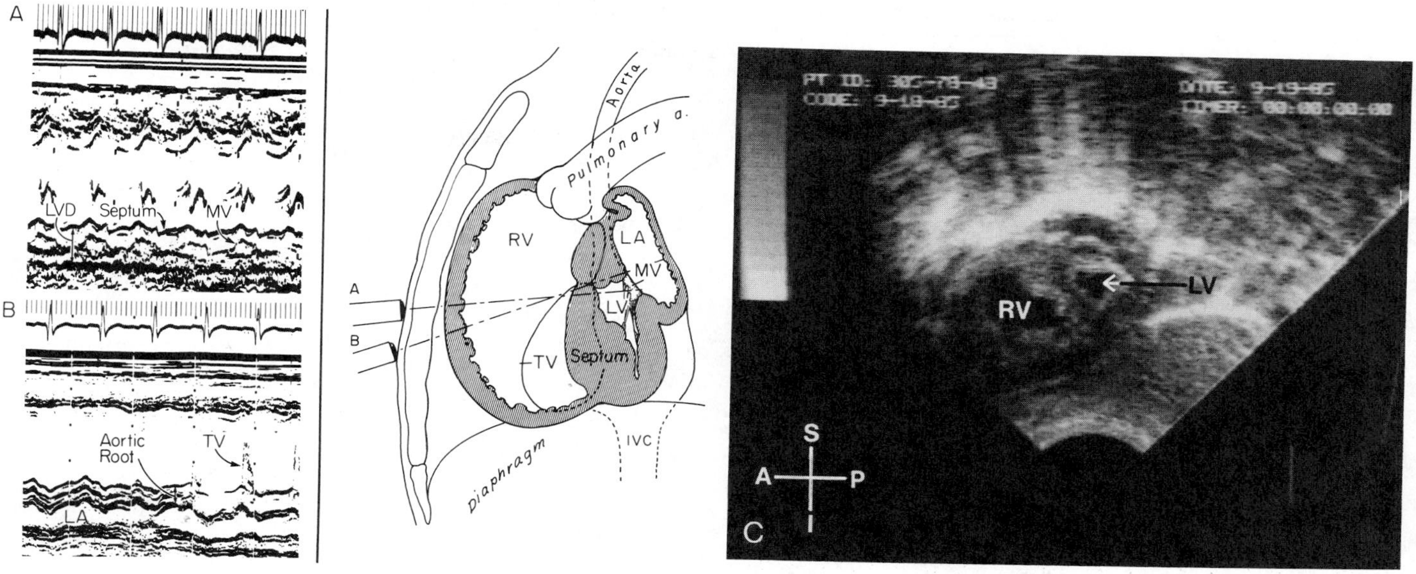

Figure 15–44. Echocardiogram from a neonate with aortic valve atresia. The idealized diagram in the center shows the small left ventricle and aorta. Echogram *A* (from transducer position *A*) shows minute left ventricular dimension (LVD) containing a small mitral valve (MV). Echogram *B* shows a small aortic root and left atrium. *C*, Subxiphoid ventricular short axis two-dimensional echocardiographic projection demonstrates thick-walled, hypoplastic left ventricle in patient with aortic atresia and severe mitral stenosis. (LV = left ventricular cavity; RV = right ventricular cavity.)

demonstration of the position of the abdominal organs and of the tracheal bifurcation for recognition of the situs of the right and left bronchi. Atrial situs is related to the visceral situs; if the viscera are in normal position, the atria have a normal position. Abdominal situs inversus is associated with the left atrium to the right and the right atrium to the left. If the abdominal situs cannot be determined, as with a centrally located liver and asplenia or rudimentary spleen, atrial localization is difficult. *Localization of the ventricles and great arteries* depends on the direction of development of the embryonic cardiac loop. Initial protrusion to the right (d-loop) carries the future right ventricle to the right, and the left ventricle remains on the left. Protrusion to the left (l-loop) carries the future right ventricle to the left, and the left ventricle is on the right. With each type of loop the relations of the great arteries may be normal or transposed. Echocardiographic and angiographic studies demonstrate the atrioventricular and ventriculoarterial relationships. The clinical manifestations of abnormal cardiac position are dominated by the associated cardiovascular anomalies.

Dextrocardia without situs inversus and **levocardia with situs inversus** are virtually always complicated by severe malformations that include various combinations of single ventricle, arterial transposition, pulmonary stenosis, ventricular and atrial septal defects, complete atrioventricular canal, anomalous pulmonary venous return, tricuspid atresia, and pulmonary arterial hypoplasia or atresia. When abdominal heterotaxia is present, the cardiac anomalies associated with polysplenia (left isomerism or bilateral left-sidedness) or asplenia (right isomerism or bilateral right-sidedness) are virtually always complex (Table 15–10). Surveys of older children and adults indicate that dextrocardia with situs inversus and with normally related great arteries (so-called mirror-image dextrocardia) is most often associated with a functionally normal heart, although congenital heart disease of a less severe nature is common.

Abnormalities of the lung, diaphragm, and thoracic cage may result in displacement of the heart to the right (dextroposition), mimicking dextrocardia. Hypoplasia of a lung may be accompanied by anomalous pulmonary venous return from that lung. The *electrocardiogram* is difficult to interpret in the presence of lesions with discordant atrial, ventricular, and great vessel anatomy. Diagnosis requires detailed echocardiographic, hemodynamic, and angiographic studies.

Prognosis and treatment of patients with one of the positional anomalies are determined by the underlying defects. Cyanotic infants with pulmonary stenosis improve after systemic to pulmonary artery shunts. Other palliative or corrective operations are utilized as indicated, depending on the anatomy and physiology. Multiple procedures are often required.

15.27 PULMONARY ARTERIOVENOUS FISTULA

Fistulous vascular communications in the lungs may be large and localized, or multiple, scattered, and small. The most common form of this unusual condition is the Rendu-Osler-Weber syndrome (hereditary hemorrhagic telangiectasia), which is also manifested by angiomas of the nasal and buccal mucous membranes, gastrointestinal tract, or liver. A direct communication between the pulmonary artery and left atrium is extremely rare.

Venous blood in the pulmonary artery is shunted through the fistula into the pulmonary vein without exposure to alveolar air, enters the left heart, and results in systemic arterial unsaturation. The shunt across the fistula is at low pressure and resistance so that pulmonary arterial pressure is normal; cardiomegaly and heart failure are not present.

The clinical picture depends on the magnitude of shunt. Dyspnea, cyanosis, clubbing, a continuous murmur, and polycythemia occur with large fistulas. Hemoptysis is rare, but may be massive. Features of the Rendu-Osler-Weber syndrome occur in about 50% of patients (or other members of their families) and include recurrent epistaxis and gastrointestinal bleeding. Transitory dizziness, diplopia, aphasia, motor weakness, or convulsions may result from cerebral thrombosis, abscess, or paradoxic emboli. Soft systolic or continuous murmurs may be audible over the site of the fistula.

TABLE 15–10. Comparison of Cardiosplenic Heterotaxia Syndromes

	Asplenia	Polysplenia
Spleen	Absent	Multiple
Sidedness (isomerism)	Bilateral right	Bilateral left
Lungs	Bilateral trilobar with eparterial bronchi	Bilateral bilobar with hyparterial bronchi
Sex	Male (65%)	Female ≥ male
Right-sided stomach	Yes	Less common
Symmetric liver	Yes	Yes
Partial intestinal rotation	Yes	Yes
Dextrocardia (%)	30–40	30–40
Pulmonary blood flow	Decreased	Increased
Severe cyanosis	Yes	No
Transposition of great arteries (%)	60–75	15
Total anomalous pulmonary venous return (%)	70–80	Rare
Common atrioventricular valve (%)	80–90	20–40
Single ventricle (%)	40–50	10–15
Absent inferior vena cava with azygos continuation	No	Characteristic
Bilateral superior vena cava	Yes	Yes
Other common defects	PA, PS	Partial anomalous pulmonary venous return, ventricular septal defect, double-outlet right ventricle
Risk of sepsis	Yes	No
Howell-Jolly and Heinz bodies, pitted erythrocytes	Yes	No
Absent gallbladder; biliary atresia	No	Yes
Mortality	High	Moderately high if symptomatic

PA = pulmonary atresia; PS = pulmonary stenosis.

The *electrocardiogram* is normal. *Roentgenographic examination* of the chest (Fig. 15–45*A*) may show opacities produced by large fistulas; multiple small fistulas may be visualized by fluoroscopy (abnormal pulsations), MRI, or tomography. Selective *pulmonary arteriography* demonstrates the site, extent, and distribution of the fistulas (Fig. 15–45*B*).

Excision of solitary or localized lesions by lobectomy or wedge resection results in complete disappearance of symptoms. However, in most instances fistulas are so widespread that surgery is not possible. If there is a direct communication between the pulmonary artery and left atrium, it can be obliterated by division and suture.

15.28 ECTOPIA CORDIS

In the most common thoracic form of ectopia cordis the sternum is split and the heart protrudes outside the chest. In others the heart protrudes through the diaphragm into the abdominal cavity or may be situated in the neck. Associated intracardiac anomalies are common. Death occurs in the first days of life in the majority of instances, usually from infection, cardiac failure, or hypoxemia. Surgical therapy for neonates without overwhelmingly severe cardiac anomalies consists of covering the heart with skin without compromising venous return or ventricular ejection. Palliation of associated defects is also often necessary. Occasional patients with the abdominal type have survived to adulthood.

15.29 DIVERTICULUM OF THE LEFT VENTRICLE

In this rare anomaly a diverticulum of the left ventricle protrudes into the epigastrium. The lesion may be isolated or associated with complex cardiovascular anomalies. A pulsat-

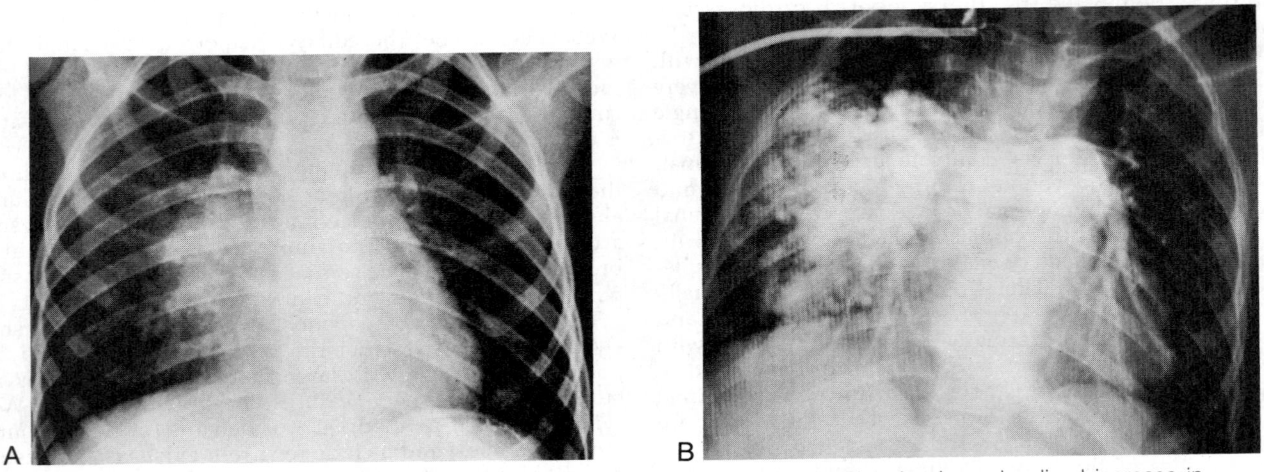

Figure 15–45. *A*, Roentgenogram of a patient with pulmonary arteriovenous fistula, showing a localized increase in pulmonary vascularity in the right lung. *B*, Angiocardiogram showing contrast medium delineating the extent of the fistula in the right lung.

ing mass is visible and palpable in the epigastrium. Systolic or systolic-diastolic murmurs produced by blood flow in and out of the diverticulum may be audible over the lower sternum and the mass. The *electrocardiogram* shows a pattern of complete or incomplete left bundle branch block. *Roentgenograms* of the chest may or may not show the mass. Associated abnormalities include defects of the sternum, abdominal wall, diaphragm, and pericardium. Surgical treatment of the diverticulum and of associated cardiac defects can be utilized in selected cases.

CONGENITAL HEART DISEASE WITH LITTLE OR NO CYANOSIS

15.30 VENTRICULAR SEPTAL DEFECT

Ventricular septal defect (VSD) is the most common cardiac malformation, accounting for 25% of congenital heart disease. The majority of defects are of the membranous type in a posteroinferior position, anterior to the septal leaflet of the tricuspid valve. Defects between the crista supraventricularis and the papillary muscle of the conus may be associated with pulmonary stenosis and the other manifestations of tetralogy of Fallot. Defects superior to the crista supraventricularis are less common; they are found just beneath the pulmonary valve and may impinge on an aortic sinus, causing aortic insufficiency. Defects in the midportion or apical region of the ventricular septum or apical area are muscular in type and may be single or multiple (Swiss-cheese type).

PATHOPHYSIOLOGY. If the defect is small (< 0.5 cm^2, pulmonary to systemic flow ratio $< 1.75:1$), the cardiac chambers and pulmonary vascular bed are normal. Large defects (> 1.0 cm^2, flow ratio $> 3:1$) produce more significant left to right shunts and result in left ventricular volume overload as well as right ventricular and pulmonary artery hypertension. The left atrium and ventricle are enlarged because of the large left to right shunt. The pulmonary arterial trunk is large. After birth, in the presence of a large VSD, pulmonary resistance may remain higher than in a normal infant and the left to right shunt may be limited. However, within a few weeks there is relatively normal involution of muscular media of the small pulmonary arteries and arterioles. A large left to right shunt ensues, and clinical symptoms become apparent. In some patients with large VSD, medial thickness remains present and, with time, intimal arteriolar pathologic changes occur; this group of patients will eventually shunt right to left and can be characterized as having the Eisenmenger syndrome (see Sec. 15.24). However, the great majority of patients with large VSD have a massive left to right shunt. Progressive increases in pulmonary resistance are rarely seen in the present era when prolonged pulmonary hypertension is prevented by early surgical intervention for large VSD.

Hemodynamics. The magnitude of the left to right shunt is determined by the size of the defect and the degree of pulmonary vascular resistance compared with systemic resistance. In most instances, pulmonary resistance is only slightly elevated, and the major contribution to pulmonary hypertension is the extremely large blood flow through the right side of the heart and pulmonary artery. When a small communication is present, the defect is restrictive and right ventricular pressure is normal.

CLINICAL MANIFESTATIONS. These vary according to the size of the defect and the pulmonary blood flow and pressure. Small defects with trivial left to right shunts and normal pulmonary arterial pressures are the most common. The patients are asymptomatic, and the cardiac lesion is usually found during routine physical examination. Characteristically, there is a loud, harsh, or blowing left parasternal pansystolic murmur, heard best over the lower left sternal border and frequently accompanied by a thrill. In a few instances the murmur ends well before the 2nd sound, presumably because of closure of the defect during late systole. The left to right shunt is limited in the neonate, and therefore systolic murmur may not be audible during the 1st days of life. In premature infants the murmur may be heard early since pulmonary vascular resistance appears to decrease more rapidly. *Roentgenograms* are usually normal, although minimal cardiomegaly and borderline increase in pulmonary vasculature may be observed. The *electrocardiogram* is usually normal but may suggest left ventricular hypertrophy.

Large defects with excessive pulmonary blood flow and pulmonary hypertension are responsible for dyspnea, feeding difficulties, poor growth, profuse perspiration, recurrent pulmonary infections, and cardiac failure in early infancy. Cyanosis is absent, but duskiness is sometimes noted during infections or crying. In the absence of heart failure, arterial and venous pulses are normal. Prominence of the left precordium and sternum is common, as are cardiomegaly, a palpable parasternal lift, an apical thrust, and a systolic thrill. The systolic murmur may be similar to that of smaller defects and is even less likely to be audible in the newborn; the sound of pulmonary valvular closure may be louder, and the 2nd sound may be virtually single. The presence of a short apical mid-diastolic rumble is caused by increased blood flow across the mitral valve, and indicates an appreciable left to right shunt. *Roentgenographically*, gross cardiomegaly is present with prominence of both ventricles, the left atrium, and pulmonary artery. The *electrocardiogram* shows biventricular hypertrophy; P waves may be notched or peaked. The *two-dimensional echocardiogram* shows volume overload of the left atrium and ventricle; the extent of their increased dimensions reflects the size of the left to right shunt. The position and size of the VSD can be visualized. Flow across the defect is demonstrated by color Doppler.

DIAGNOSIS. The effects of a VSD on the circulation may be demonstrated by cardiac catheterization. However, this diagnostic procedure usually is not required, as it is most often obvious by physical examination and echocardiography that an isolated small defect is present. When catheterization is performed, blood from the right ventricle is found to be higher in oxygen content than that from the right atrium; this increase is occasionally apparent only in pulmonary arterial blood. Small shunts may not result in a detectable increase in oxygen saturation in the right ventricle, but may be demonstrated by indicator dilution tests (see Fig. 15–31). Small defects are associated with normal right-sided heart pressure and pulmonary vascular resistance. Pulmonary blood flow in patients with large defects associated with equal pulmonary and systemic pressures may be more than three times the systemic flow. Pulmonary vascular resistance is only minimally elevated in these patients. The location and number of ventricular defects are demonstrated by left ventriculography.

Contrast medium passes across the defect(s) to opacify the right ventricle and pulmonary artery.

PROGNOSIS AND COMPLICATIONS. The natural course of VSD includes the following:

1. A significant number (30–50%) of small defects close spontaneously, most frequently during the 1st yr of life. It is less common for moderate or large defects to close spontaneously, although even defects large enough to result in heart failure may become smaller and even rarely close completely.
2. A large number of children remain asymptomatic without evidence of increase in heart size, pulmonary arterial pressure, or resistance.
3. Infective endocarditis occurs in fewer than 2%. Endocarditis is more common in adolescents and uncommon in children under 2 yr of age. The risk is independent of the VSD size.
4. A significant number of infants with large defects have repeated episodes of respiratory infection and congestive heart failure.
5. Pulmonary hypertension occurs as a result of high pulmonary blood flow. A few patients will develop elevated pulmonary vascular resistance with time if the defect is not repaired.
6. A small number acquire infundibular pulmonary stenosis, which protects the pulmonary circulation from the long-term effects of pulmonary hypertension. In these patients the clinical picture changes from VSD with large left to right shunt to VSD with pulmonary stenosis, and a diminished left to right shunt, a balanced shunt, or a right to left shunt (see Sec. 15.11). Echocardiography differentiates these cyanotic patients from those with Eisenmenger physiology.

TREATMENT. Parents should be reassured of the benign nature of the small defect, and the child should be encouraged to live a normal life. Surgical repair is not recommended. As a protection against infective endocarditis the integrity of primary and permanent teeth should be carefully maintained; antibiotic prophylaxis should be provided for dental surgery, tonsillectomy, adenoidectomy, and other oropharyngeal surgical procedures as well as for instrumentation of the genitourinary and lower intestinal tracts.

The medical management of infants with a large VSD is primarily aimed at the control of congestive cardiac failure. These patients may show signs of repeated or chronic pulmonary disease and often fail to thrive. If early treatment is successful, the shunt may diminish in size with spontaneous improvement, especially during the 1st yr of life. Because surgical closure can be carried out at low risk in most infants, medical management should not be pursued in symptomatic infants after an unsuccessful trial. Furthermore, pulmonary vascular disease is prevented when surgery is performed within the 1st yr of life. Thus, the large defects associated with pulmonary hypertension should be closed between 6–12 mo of age. Surgical complications resulting in long-term problems (e.g., heart block) are extremely rare. Surgical risks are higher for Swiss cheese–type VSDs. Pulmonary arterial banding is indicated for the symptomatic infant, with subsequent debanding and repair of multiple VSDs at an older age.

After obliteration of the left to right shunt the hyperdynamic heart becomes quiet, cardiac size decreases toward normal (Fig. 15–46), thrills and murmurs are abolished, and pulmonary artery hypertension regresses. The patient's clinical status improves markedly. The infant begins to thrive, and cardiac medications are no longer required. In some instances after successful operation, systolic ejection murmurs of low intensity persist for months. The long-term prognosis after surgery is excellent.

15.31 VENTRICULAR SEPTAL DEFECT WITH AORTIC INSUFFICIENCY

In this syndrome the VSD is complicated by prolapse of the aortic valve and aortic insufficiency. It accounts for approximately 5% of patients with VSD; a considerably larger incidence is reported among Oriental children. The septal defect, which is small or moderate in size, is usually anterior and subpulmonary (outlet septum), but in some cases the VSD is infracristal. The right or less often the noncoronary cusp prolapses into the defect. The VSD may be partially or even completely closed in this manner. Aortic insufficiency is most often not recognized until late in the first decade of life or beyond. Early congestive heart failure secondary to a large

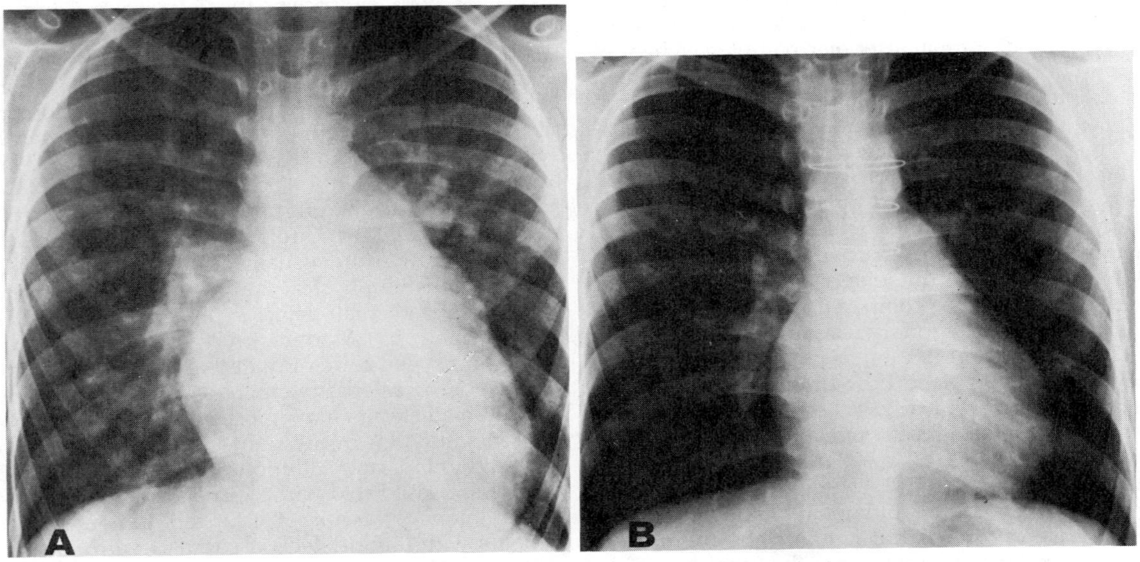

Figure 15–46. *A*, Preoperative roentgenogram in a ventricular septal defect with a large left to right shunt and pulmonary hypertension. Significant cardiomegaly, prominence of the pulmonary arterial trunk, and pulmonary overcirculation are evident. *B*, Three years after surgical closure of the defect. There is a marked decrease in the heart size, and the pulmonary vasculature is normal.

left to right shunt rarely occurs, but without operation, severe aortic insufficiency and left ventricular failure may ensue. The physical signs of aortic insufficiency (diastolic murmur and wide pulse pressure) are added to those of VSD. This entity should not be confused with patent ductus arteriosus or other defects associated with aortic runoff.

The *clinical manifestations* vary widely, from trivial aortic regurgitation and small left to right shunt in the asymptomatic child to the symptomatic adolescent with florid aortic incompetence and massive cardiomegaly. Patients having a significant aortic incompetence require surgical intervention to prevent irreversible left ventricular dysfunction. Repair of the aortic valve may be possible only with a prosthesis, but every attempt should be made to achieve a competent valve by means of valvuloplasty. The degree to which aortic insufficiency is affected by closure of the septal defect alone early in the course of the disease is questionable. The asymptomatic child with a small VSD and mild aortic valve prolapse should be observed carefully for progression of severity of the insufficiency.

15.32 DOUBLE-OUTLET RIGHT VENTRICLE WITHOUT PULMONARY STENOSIS

(Origin of Both Great Arteries from the Right Ventricle)

In this anomaly both the aorta and the pulmonary artery arise from the right ventricle (see Sec. 15.15). The only outlet from the left ventricle is a VSD. The clinical picture closely simulates that of an uncomplicated VSD with a large left to right shunt and pulmonary hypertension. The *electrocardiogram* usually shows a left superior axis and biventricular hypertrophy. *Echocardiography* is diagnostic, showing the right ventricular origin of both great vessels and their anteroposterior relationship as well as the position of the VSD. The condition may also be diagnosed by *left ventricular angiogram,* which demonstrates the commitment of the VSD to the aorta, resulting in favorable blood flow. The size of the outlet from the left ventricle confirms mitral-aortic discontinuity and shows the high position of the aortic valve, which is at the same level as the pulmonary valve. It is important to differentiate this condition from simple VSD. Surgical correction is accomplished by an intraventricular repair, which funnels the ejection of left ventricular blood via the VSD into the aorta without obstructing right ventricular outflow. Pulmonary arterial banding may be required in infancy, followed by surgical correction during the preschool years. Natural pulmonary stenosis is common (see Sec. 15.15).

In **double-outlet right ventricle with transposition of the great arteries** the VSD is supracristal and subpulmonary **(Taussig-Bing complex)** or related to both pulmonary and aortic valves (doubly committed). These patients develop cyanosis early in life and have poor physical development, pulmonary hypertension, and cardiac failure. Cardiomegaly is usual, and there is a parasternal ejection systolic murmur, sometimes preceded by an ejection click and a loud closure of the pulmonary valve. Left-sided obstructive lesions are frequently associated; these include aortic coarctation, interruption of the aortic arch, and a small VSD, which is restrictive to left ventricular ejection. The *electrocardiogram* shows right axis deviation and right, left, or biventricular hypertrophy. The *roentgenogram* documents the cardiomegaly, the large left atrium, and prominence of the pulmonary trunk and vasculature. The anatomic features of the anomaly and associated abnormalities are best demonstrated by a combination of echocardiography and selective right and left ventriculography. Palliation by pulmonary arterial banding in infancy will permit surgical correction at a later age, which may be accomplished by a Rastelli procedure (see Sec. 15.18) or by closure of the VSD incorporating the pulmonary outflow tract into the left ventricle, coupled with a Mustard or Senning procedure. Arterial switch surgery is another option (see Sec. 15.19).

15.33 L-TRANSPOSITION OF THE GREAT ARTERIES

(Corrected Transposition)

This malformation consists of discordant atrioventricular relationships (ventricular inversion) and transposition of the great arteries. Systemic blood is returned to a normal right atrium, from which it passes through a bicuspid atrioventricular valve into a right-sided ventricle that has the architecture and smooth wall appearance of the normal left ventricle. The venous blood is then ejected via the transposed pulmonary artery into the lungs. Pulmonary venous blood returns to a normal left atrium, passes through a tricuspid valve into a left-sided ventricle, which has the internal structure of a normal right ventricle, and is then ejected into the transposed aorta. The pulmonary artery lies in a medial position and the ascending aorta lies to the left and lateral, almost in the same horizontal plane. The double inversion of atrioventricular and ventriculoarterial relationships results in desaturated right atrial blood reaching the lungs, and pulmonary venous blood appropriately flowing to the aorta. Thus, the circulation is "corrected." Without other defects, the hemodynamics would be normal. However, in almost every instance, associated anomalies coexist; most common are VSD, abnormalities of the left atrioventricular valve (tricuspid), pulmonary valvular and/or subvalvular stenosis, and atrioventricular conduction disturbances (complete heart block).

Symptoms and signs are determined by the associated lesions. Posteroanterior chest *roentgenograms* may suggest the abnormal position of the great arteries; the ascending aorta occupies the upper left border of the cardiac silhouette and has a straight profile. In addition to atrioventricular conduction disturbances, *electrocardiograms* may show abnormal P waves; absent QV_6; initial Q waves in leads III, aVR, aVF, and V_1; and upright T waves across the precordium.

Surgical treatment of the associated anomalies, most often the VSD, is complicated by the position of the bundle of His, which can be injured at the time of surgery, causing heart block. Identification of the usual course of the bundle in corrected transposition (superior to the defect) has been accomplished by mapping of the conduction system at surgery. This has been an important step in eliminating this sequela in those patients who were initially in sinus rhythm, because the surgeon can avoid the bundle of His during open heart repair.

15.34 ATRIAL SEPTAL DEFECT

An isolated patent foramen ovale is of no hemodynamic significance and is not considered to be an atrial septal defect. However, if right atrial pressure is increased secondary to another defect (e.g., pulmonary stenosis or atresia, tricuspid abnormalities, right ventricular dysfunction), venous blood may be shunted across the patent foramen ovale into the left atrium with resultant cyanosis. Because of the anatomic structure of a patent foramen ovale, blood normally is not shunted from the left atrium to the right atrium. In the presence of a large volume load or a hypertensive left atrium, or both, there is enough dilatation of this communication to result in an atrial left to right shunt. An isolated patent foramen ovale does not require treatment but may be a risk for systemic emboli.

15.35 OSTIUM SECUNDUM DEFECT

This defect in the region of the fossa ovalis is associated with normal atrioventricular valves at birth. Late myxomatous changes in the mitral valve have been described, but this is only rarely an important clinical consideration. The defects may be multiple, and in symptomatic older children openings of 2 cm or more in diameter are not unusual. Large defects may extend inferiorly toward the inferior vena cava and ostium of the coronary sinus, superiorly toward the superior vena cava, or posteriorly. Females outnumber males 3:1. Partial anomalous venous return may be a common associated lesion.

HEMODYNAMICS. A considerable shunt of oxygenated blood flows from the left to the right atrium. This blood is added to the usual venous return to the right atrium and is pumped by the right ventricle to the lungs. Pulmonary blood flow is usually 2–4 times systemic flow. The principal factor that determines the direction of shunt is the diastolic compliance of the chambers of the right heart. The paucity of symptoms in infants with atrial septal defects is related to the structure of the right ventricle in early life when its muscular wall is thick and less compliant, thus limiting the left to right shunt. As the infant becomes older, the right ventricular wall becomes thinner as a result of its lower pressure-generating requirements, and the left to right shunt across the atrial defect increases. The large blood flow through the right side of the heart results in enlargement of the right atrium and ventricle and dilatation of the pulmonary artery. Despite the large pulmonary blood flow, the pulmonary arterial pressure remains normal because pulmonary vascular resistance remains extremely low. The left ventricle and aorta are normal in size. Cyanosis is extremely rare, seen only occasionally in adults with the complicating features of pulmonary vascular disease.

CLINICAL MANIFESTATIONS. A child with an ostium secundum defect is most often asymptomatic, and the lesion may be discovered inadvertently during a physical examination. Even an extremely large ASD (secundum) rarely produces heart failure in childhood; in older children varying degrees of exercise intolerance may be noted. In older infants and children the physical findings are often characteristic but require careful examination of the heart.

The pulses are normal. A right ventricular systolic lift is usually palpable from the left sternal border to the midclavicular line. The systolic murmur is of the ejection type, medium pitched, seldom accompanied by a thrill, and best heard at the left mid and upper sternal border. It is produced by the increased flow across the right ventricular outflow tract into the pulmonary artery. The murmur is preceded by a loud 1st heart sound and sometimes by a pulmonic ejection click. In most patients the 2nd heart sound at the upper left sternal edge is widely split and fixed in all phases of respiration. This auscultatory finding is characteristic and is due to constantly increased right ventricular diastolic volume and prolonged ejection time. A short early diastolic murmur produced by the high blood flow across the tricuspid valve often is audible at the lower left sternal border. This finding, which may be subtle, is an excellent diagnostic sign.

DIAGNOSIS. *Roentgenograms* show varying degrees of enlargement of the right ventricle and atrium; the left ventricle and aorta are of normal size. The pulmonary artery is large, and the pulmonary vascularity increased. These signs vary and may not be conspicuous in mild cases. Cardiac enlargement is often best appreciated on the lateral view, since the right ventricle protrudes anteriorly with increased volume.

The *electrocardiogram* shows diastolic overload of the right ventricle with right axis deviation or a normal axis, and right ventricular conduction delay (usually rsR′ in right precordial leads); the presence of an ASD is unusual in the absence of right ventricular conduction delay.

The *echocardiogram* shows findings characteristic of right ventricular volume overload, including increased right ventricular end-diastolic dimension and abnormal motion of the ventricular septum. The normal septum moves posteriorly during systole and anteriorly during diastole. With right ventricular overload and normal pulmonary vascular resistance, the septal motion is reversed, i.e., anterior movement in systole, or the motion is intermediate so that the septum remains straight. The location and size of the atrial defect are readily appreciated. Patients with classic features of ASD secundum, including echocardiographic identification of a well-defined defect, need not be catheterized prior to surgical closure.

If the diagnosis is confirmed by *cardiac catheterization*, the oxygen content of blood from the right atrium is much higher than that from the superior vena cava. This feature is not diagnostic since it may occur with anomalous pulmonary venous return to the right atrium, with ventricular septal defect and tricuspid insufficiency, with ventricular septal defects associated with left ventricular–right atrial shunts, and with aortic–right atrial communications (e.g., ruptured sinus of Valsalva). The physical signs produced by the latter three anomalies generally differ greatly from those of atrial septal defects, and their presence can usually be confirmed by selective angiocardiography. Occasionally, mixing of blood is incomplete in the right atrium, and the principal site of shunt appears to be at the ventricular level even though a VSD is not present.

The catheter often enters the left atrium from the right atrium. Indicator dilution curves may be used to demonstrate the site of the left to right shunt and the presence of anomalous pulmonary veins. Streaming of inferior vena caval blood across the defect to the left atrium may occur with uncomplicated atrial septal defects. This small right to left shunt may be demonstrated by indicator dilution curves but only rarely results in significant arterial unsaturation or cyanosis. The pressures in the right side of the heart are usually normal, but small to moderate pressure gradients may be measured across the right ventricular outflow. In the absence of associated organic pulmonary stenosis they are due to functional stenosis related to excessive blood flow. The pulmonary arteriolar resistance is almost always normal or lower than normal. The shunt is variable depending on the size of the defect, but it may be of considerable volume (as high as 20 $L/min/m^2$).

PROGNOSIS AND COMPLICATIONS. Secundum atrial septal defects are well tolerated during childhood; symptoms usually appear in the 3rd decade or later. Pulmonary hypertension, atrial dysrhythmias, tricuspid or mitral incompetence, and heart failure are late manifestations; symptoms may appear during pregnancy. Infective endocarditis is extremely rare.

Secundum atrial septal defects are usually isolated, although they may be associated with partial anomalous pulmonary venous return, pulmonary valvular stenosis, ventricular septal defect, pulmonary arterial branch stenosis, and persistent left superior vena cava, as well as mitral valve insufficiency.

TREATMENT. Closure is carried out at open heart surgery. The mortality rate from surgery is less than 1%, and surgery is advised even for asymptomatic patients prior to entry into school. It is preferred during childhood because the surgical mortality and morbidity are greater in adulthood when late signs are present. Eliminating the increased risks of pregnancy is another important reason to intervene early in females. Mild symptoms with exercise, and submaximal physical performance during sports activities are also prevented by early elective repair. Occlusional devices, implanted by cardiac catheterization, may successfully close an ASD without need for surgery.

The results after operation in children with large shunts are excellent. Symptoms disappear rapidly, and physical development frequently appears enhanced. The heart size decreases to normal, and the electrocardiogram shows decreased right ventricular forces. Late arrhythmias are less frequent and of lesser importance in patients who have had early repair.

15.36 SINUS VENOSUS DEFECT

The defect is situated in the upper part of the atrial septum in close relation to the entry of the superior vena cava. One or more pulmonary veins (usually from the right lung) drain anomalously into the superior vena cava. Sometimes the superior vena cava straddles the defect; some systemic venous blood then enters the left atrium. The abnormal hemodynamics are similar to those of secundum atrial septal defect, for example, a volume overload of the right ventricle. The clinical picture, electrocardiogram, and roentgenogram are also similar to those of secundum atrial septal defect. The diagnosis is made by two-dimensional echocardiography. If cardiac catheterization is carried out, the catheter may enter a pulmonary vein from the superior vena cava. Anatomic correction usually requires the insertion of a patch to close the defect while incorporating the entry of anomalous veins into the left atrium; surgical results are generally excellent.

15.37 PARTIAL ANOMALOUS PULMONARY VENOUS RETURN

A varying number of pulmonary veins may enter the systemic venous circulation or the right atrium and produce a left to right shunt of oxygenated blood, which may be further augmented if there is an associated atrial septal defect. Partial anomalous pulmonary venous return usually involves some or all of the veins from only one lung, more often the right. An associated atrial septal defect usually is of the sinus venosus type (see Sec. 15.36). The history, physical signs, electrocardiogram, and roentgenographic findings are indistinguishable from those of atrial septal defect (ostium secundum). Occasionally, an anomalous vein draining into the inferior vena cava is visible roentgenographically as a crescentic shadow of vascular density along the right border of the cardiac silhouette (scimitar syndrome); an atrial septal defect is usually not present. The finding of a sinus venosus atrial septal defect by echocardiography is often accompanied by the identification or suspicion of associated partial anomalous pulmonary venous return. See Sec. 15.20 for discussion of *total anomalous pulmonary venous return*.

Echocardiography confirms the diagnosis. The presence of anomalous pulmonary veins may be demonstrated by *selective pulmonary arteriography*.

The prognosis is excellent, similar to that for atrial septal defect (ostium secundum). When a large left to right shunt is present, surgical repair is carried out during cardiopulmonary bypass. The associated atrial septal defect should be closed in such a way as to direct the pulmonary venous return to the left atrium. A single anomalous pulmonary vein without an atrial communication may be difficult to redirect to the left atrium and may be left unoperated.

15.38 OSTIUM PRIMUM DEFECT AND ATRIOVENTRICULAR CANAL

(Endocardial Cushion Defects)

These abnormalities are grouped together because they represent a spectrum of a basic embryologic abnormality, a deficiency of the endocardial cushions and atrioventricular septum.

The *ostium primum defect* is situated in the lower portion of the atrial septum and overlies the mitral and tricuspid valves. In the majority of instances there is a cleft in the anterior leaflet of the mitral valve. The tricuspid valve is usually functionally normal, although some abnormality of the septal leaflet is present. The ventricular septum is intact.

Atrioventricular canal (atrioventricular septal defect) consists of a contiguous interatrial and interventricular defect with markedly abnormal atrioventricular valves. The valve, virtually single and common to both ventricles, consists of an anterior and a posterior leaflet related to the ventricular septum with a lateral leaflet in each ventricle. The lesion is common among children with Down syndrome and may occur with pulmonary stenosis (see Sec. 15.11 and 15.46).

Transitional varieties of these defects also occur. They include ostium primum defects with clefts in the anterior mitral and septal tricuspid valve leaflets, mild ventricular septal deficiencies, and, less commonly, ostium primum defects with normal atrioventricular valves. In some patients, the atrial septum is intact, but the ventricular septal defect simulates that found in the atrioventricular canal. These defects are also associated with deformities of the atrioventricular valves.

HEMODYNAMICS. The basic abnormality in patients with *ostium primum defects* is the combination of a left to right shunt across the atrial defect with mitral incompetence. The shunt is usually moderate to large. The degree of mitral incompetence is ordinarily mild to moderate. Pulmonary arterial pressures are usually normal or only mildly increased.

In *atrioventricular canal* the left to right shunt is both transatrial and transventricular. Pulmonary hypertension and increased pulmonary vascular resistance are common. Atrioventricular valvular incompetence results in regurgitation of blood from the ventricles to both atria. Some right to left shunting occurs at both atrial and ventricular levels. There may be mild but significant arterial unsaturation. Progressive pulmonary vascular disease will increase the right to left shunt so that more severe cyanosis may develop.

CLINICAL MANIFESTATIONS. Many children with *ostium primum defect* are asymptomatic, and the anomaly is discovered during a general physical examination. In patients with moderate shunts and trivial mitral incompentence, the physical signs are similar to those of atrial defect of the secundum type, but with an additional apical systolic murmur.

A history of effort intolerance, easy fatigability, and recurrent pneumonitis may be obtained, especially in infants with large left to right shunts and severe mitral incompetence. In these patients cardiac enlargement is moderate or marked and the precordium is hyperdynamic. The auscultatory signs produced by the left to right shunt include a normal or accentuated 1st sound, wide, fixed splitting of the 2nd sound, a pulmonary ejection systolic murmur sometimes preceded by a click, and a low-pitched early diastolic murmur at the lower left sternal edge and/or apex. Mitral incompetence may be manifested by an apical pansystolic murmur that radiates to the left axilla.

With *atrioventricular canal*, congestive heart failure and intercurrent pulmonary infection usually appear in infancy. During these episodes minimal cyanosis may be evident. The neck veins are prominent, the liver is enlarged, and the infant shows signs of failure to thrive. Cardiac enlargement is moderate to marked, and a systolic thrill is frequently palpable. The 1st heart sound is normal or accentuated. The 2nd heart sound is widely split if pulmonary flow is massive. A low-pitched early diastolic murmur is audible at the lower left sternal edge, and a pulmonic systolic ejection murmur is produced by the large pulmonary flow. The apical pansystolic murmur of mitral insufficiency may also be present.

DIAGNOSIS. *Roentgenograms* of children with endocardial cushion defects confirm the cardiac enlargement due to prominence of both ventricles and the right atrium. The pulmonary artery is large, and pulmonary vascularity is increased.

The *electrocardiograms* of children with endocardial cushion defects are distinctive. The principal abnormalities are (1) superior orientation of the mean frontal QRS axis with left axis deviation to the left or right upper quadrant; (2) counterclockwise inscription of the superiorly oriented QRS vector loop; (3) signs of biventricular hypertrophy or isolated right ventricular hypertrophy; (4) right ventricular conduction delay (VSR′ in leads V_3R and V_1); (5) normal or tall P waves; and (6) occasional prolongation of the P-R interval (Fig. 15–47).

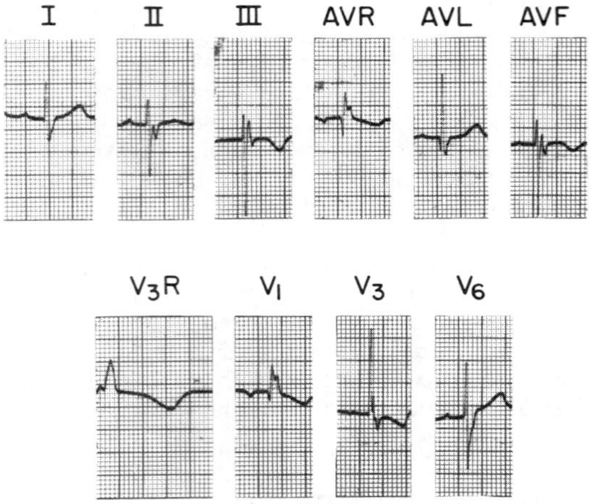

Figure 15–47. Electrocardiogram from a child with an atrioventricular canal. Note the QRS axis of −60 degrees, and the RV conduction delay; RSR′ in V_1 and V_3R. (V_3R paper speed = 50 mm/sec.)

The *echocardiogram* is characteristic and shows signs of right ventricular enlargement with encroachment of the mitral valve echo on the left ventricular outflow; this corresponds to the angiographic "goose-neck" deformity. In the atrioventricular canal, the ventricular septal echo is also deficient and the atrioventricular valve abnormalities are readily appreciated (Fig. 15–48).

Cardiac catheterization and *angiocardiography* confirm the diagnosis. These studies demonstrate the magnitude of the left to right shunt, the severity of pulmonary hypertension, the degree of elevation of pulmonary vascular resistance, and the severity of incompetence of the atrioventricular valve. The shunt is usually demonstrable at the atrial level; in some patients, increased oxygen saturations are noted only in the right ventricle, because of streaming of blood across the primum defect just proximal to the tricuspid valve. The arterial oxygen saturation is normal or mildly reduced unless severe pulmonary hypertension is present. In these patients larger right to left shunts may be demonstrable. Children with ostium primum defects usually have normal or only moderate elevation of the pulmonary arterial pressure. On the other hand, atrioventricular canal is associated with right ventricular and pulmonary hypertension as well as with an increase in pulmonary vascular resistance in older patients. The cardiac catheter readily enters the chambers of the left side of the heart from the right side, especially if there is an atrioventricular canal.

Selective left ventriculography is extremely helpful in diagnosis of endocardial cushion defects. The deformity of the mitral or common atrioventricular valve and the distortion of the outflow of the left ventricle, the goose-neck deformity, are demonstrated. The abnormal anterior leaflet of the mitral valve is serrated, and mitral incompetence is noted, usually with regurgitation of blood to both the left and right atria.

PROGNOSIS. The prognosis for endocardial cushion defects depends on the magnitude of the left to right shunt, the degree of pulmonary vascular resistance, and the severity of mitral incompetence. Death from congestive cardiac failure during infancy is frequent with atrioventricular canal not treated by operation. Patients who survive without surgery are likely to develop pulmonary vascular obstructive disease. Most patients with ostium primum defects and minimal A-V valve involvement are asymptomatic or have only minor, nonprogressive symptoms until they reach the 3rd–4th decade of life, similar to the course of patients with secundum defects.

TREATMENT. Ostium primum defects are approached surgically from an incision in the right atrium. The cleft in the mitral valve is located through the atrial defect and is repaired by direct suture. The defect in the atrial septum is usually closed by insertion of a patch prosthesis. The surgical mortality rate for primum defects is low. Surgical treatment for atrioventricular canal is more difficult, especially in infants with congestive cardiac failure and pulmonary hypertension. Pulmonary arterial banding has been successful as early palliation in severely ill infants with dominant shunts at the

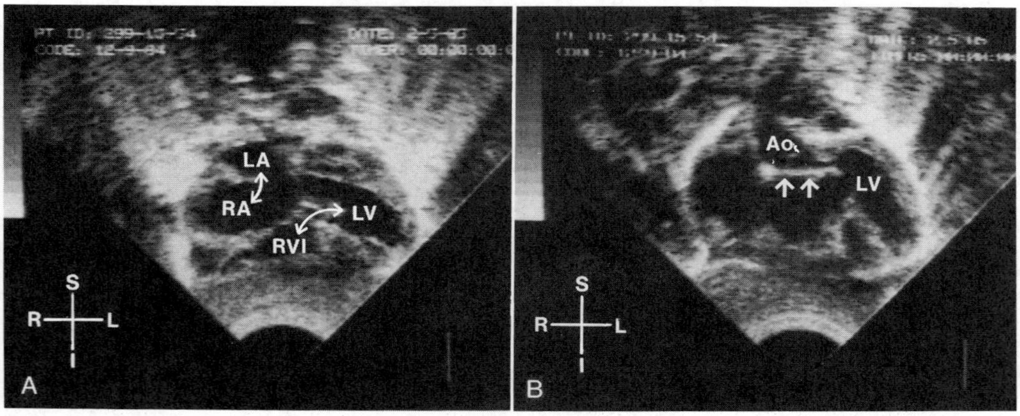

Figure 15–48. Atrioventricular defect. *A*, Four-chamber view demonstrating both an interatrial and interventricular septal defect contributing to the large central communication of this lesion *(arrows)*. *B*, Left ventricular long axis projection demonstrating the typical goose-neck deformity created by the anterior leaflet of the mitral valve *(arrows)*. (RA = right atrium; LA = left atrium; RVI = right ventricular inflow; LV = left ventricle; R = right; L = left; S = superior; I = inferior; Ao = aorta.)

ventricular level. However, successful open heart correction of these defects can be accomplished even in infancy. The atrial and ventricular defects are closed and atrioventricular valves reconstructed. Prosthetic valves are rarely required.

15.39 PATENT DUCTUS ARTERIOSUS

During fetal life most of the pulmonary arterial blood is shunted through the ductus arteriosus into the aorta (see Sec. 15.9). Functional closure of the ductus normally occurs soon after birth, but if the ductus remains patent when pulmonary vascular resistance falls, aortic blood is shunted into the pulmonary artery. The aortic end of the ductus is just distal to the origin of the left subclavian artery, and the ductus enters the pulmonary artery at its bifurcation. PDA is one of the most common congenital cardiovascular anomalies associated with maternal rubella during early pregnancy. Female patients outnumber males 2:1.

When a term infant is found to have a PDA, there is deficiency of both the mucoid endothelial layer and the muscular media of the ductus. The premature infant with a patent ductus, however, has a normal structural anatomy; patency is the result of hypoxia and immaturity. Thus a PDA in a term infant will rarely close spontaneously, whereas in the premature baby, in whom early pharmacologic or surgical intervention was not required, spontaneous closure occurs in most instances. An obligatory PDA is seen in 10% of patients with other congenital heart lesions. An isolated PDA is more common in patients born at high altitude.

HEMODYNAMICS. As a result of the higher aortic pressure, blood flow through the ductus goes from the aorta to the pulmonary artery. The extent of shunt depends on the size of the ductus and the pulmonary vascular resistance. In extreme cases 70% of the left ventricular output may be shunted through the ductus to the pulmonary circulation. The pressures within the pulmonary artery, the right ventricle, and the right atrium are normal if the PDA is small, but they may be elevated moderately or even to systemic levels with large communications. There is a wide pulse pressure due to runoff of blood into the pulmonary artery during diastole. The total blood volume is increased.

CLINICAL MANIFESTATIONS. There are usually no symptoms associated with a small patent ductus. A large defect will result in left ventricular failure similar to that in infants with large VSD and pulmonary hypertension. Retardation of physical growth may be a major manifestation in infants with large shunts.

A large PDA will result in striking physical signs attributable to the wide pulse pressure, most prominently bounding arterial pulsations. The heart is normal in size when the ductus is small but moderately or grossly enlarged in cases with a large communication. The apical impulse is prominent and, with cardiac enlargement, is heaving. A thrill, maximal in the 2nd left interspace, is often present and may radiate toward the left clavicle, down the left sternal border, or toward the apex. It is usually systolic but also may be palpated throughout the cardiac cycle. The classic murmur has been variously described as being like machinery, a humming top, a millwheel, or rolling thunder in quality. It begins soon after onset of the 1st sound, reaches maximal intensity at the end of systole, and wanes in late diastole. It may be localized to the 2nd left intercostal space or radiate down the left sternal border or to the left clavicle. When there is increased pulmonary resistance, the murmur is less prominent or absent in diastole. In patients with a large left to right shunt a low-pitched mitral diastolic murmur may be audible, owing to the large blood flow across the mitral valve.

If the left to right shunt is small, the *electrocardiogram* is normal; if the ductus is large, left ventricular or biventricular hypertrophy is present. The diagnosis of isolated, uncomplicated PDA is untenable when isolated right ventricular hypertrophy is noted.

Roentgenographic studies commonly show a prominent pulmonary artery with increased intrapulmonary vascular markings. The cardiac size depends on the degree of left to right shunt; it may be normal, or moderately to markedly enlarged. The chambers involved are the left atrium and ventricle. The aortic knob is normal or prominent and pulsates vigorously.

The *echocardiographic* view of the cardiac chambers is normal if the ductus is small. Left atrial and ventricular dimensions are increased, and isovolumic contraction time is decreased with large shunts. Scanning from the suprasternal notch allows visualization of the ductus. The aortic runoff in diastole can be identified by Doppler examination.

The clinical pattern is sufficiently distinctive to allow an accurate diagnosis in most patients. In patients with atypical findings, or when associated cardiac lesions are suspected, hemodynamic studies may be indicated.

Cardiac catheterization reveals normal or increased pressures in the right ventricle and pulmonary artery. The presence of oxygenated blood shunting into the pulmonary artery confirms a left to right shunt. Samples of blood from the venae cavae, right atrium, and right ventricle have normal oxygen contents. The catheter may pass through the ductus into the descending aorta. Injection of contrast medium into the ascending aorta shows opacification of the pulmonary artery from the aorta and identifies the ductus.

DIFFERENTIAL DIAGNOSIS. The diagnosis of uncomplicated PDA is usually not difficult. However, there are other conditions that, in the absence of cyanosis, produce systolic and diastolic murmurs in the pulmonic area and must be differentiated.

The characteristics of a *venous hum* are described in Sec. 15.1. An *aorticopulmonary septal defect* rarely may be clinically indistinguishable from a patent ductus, although in most cases the murmur is only systolic and is loudest at the right upper sternal border rather than at the left. Similarly, a *sinus of Valsalva that has ruptured into the right side of the heart or pulmonary artery, coronary arteriovenous fistulas, and an aberrant left coronary artery with massive collaterals from the right coronary* display the dynamics of an arteriovenous fistula with a continuous murmur and a wide pulse pressure. Sometimes the murmur is not maximal in the pulmonary area but is heard along the lower left sternal border. *Truncus arteriosus* with torrential pulmonary flow also has an "aortic runoff" physiology. *Pulmonary branch stenosis* is associated with systolic and diastolic murmurs, but the pulse pressure is normal. *Peripheral arteriovenous fistula* also results in a wide pulse pressure, but the distinctive murmur of a PDA is not present.

VSD with aortic insufficiency and *combined rheumatic aortic and mitral insufficiency* may be confused with PDA, but the murmurs should be differentiated by their to-and-fro rather than continous timing. The combination of a large VSD and a PDA results in findings more like those in isolated VSD.

PROGNOSIS AND COMPLICATIONS. Patients with a small PDA may live a normal span with few or no cardiac symptoms; however, late manifestations may occur. Spontaneous closure of the ductus after infancy is extremely rare.

Congestive cardiac failure most often occurs in early infancy in the presence of a large ductus, but may occur late in life with a moderate-sized communication. The chronic left ventricular volume load is less well tolerated with aging.

Infective endarteritis may be seen at any age. Pulmonary or systemic emboli may occur. Rare complications include aneurysmal dilatation of the pulmonary artery or the ductus, calcification of the ductus, noninfective thrombosis of the ductus with embolization, and paradoxic emboli. Pulmonary hypertension (Eisenmenger syndrome) can occur in patients with a large PDA who do not undergo surgical treatment.

TREATMENT. Irrespective of age, patients with PDA require surgical closure of the duct. If congestive cardiac failure develops, surgical treatment should not be postponed too long after adequate medical therapy has been instituted, even if some signs of failure persist.

Because the case fatality rate with surgical treatment is considerably less than 1% and the risk without it is greater, ligation and division of the ductus are indicated in the asymptomatic patient, preferably at 1 or 2 yr of age. Pulmonary hypertension is not a contraindication to operation at any age if it can be demonstrated that the shunt flow is from aorta to pulmonary artery and is not reversed as a result of severe pulmonary vascular obstructive disease.

Surgical closure is achieved by ligation and division. After closure, symptoms of frank or incipient cardiac failure rapidly disappear. There is usually immediate improvement in physical development of the infant who had failed to thrive. The pulse and blood pressure return to normal, and the machinery murmur disappears. A functional systolic murmur over the pulmonary area may occasionally persist; it may represent turbulence in a persistently dilated pulmonary artery. The roentgenographic signs of cardiac enlargement and pulmonary overcirculation also disappear and the electrocardiogram becomes normal. Pulmonary hypertension, if present preoperatively, also recedes.

Transcatheter closure in the cardiac catheterization laboratory using either a Teflon plug or an occlusional umbrella has been successful in selected centers and eliminates the risks of surgery.

PATENT DUCTUS ARTERIOSUS IN LOW-BIRTHWEIGHT INFANTS

See Sec. 9.32.

15.40 AORTICOPULMONARY SEPTAL DEFECT

This defect consists of a communication between the ascending aorta and main pulmonary artery. The presence of pulmonary and aortic valves and an intact ventricular septum distinguishes this anomaly from truncus arteriosus. Symptoms similar to those of a large VSD or of PDA appear during early infancy and include recurrent pulmonary infections, congestive heart failure, and, occasionally, minimal cyanosis. The defect is usually large and the cardiac murmur is systolic with a mid-diastolic rumble reflecting the increased blood flow across the mitral valve. In the rare instance when the communication is somewhat smaller and pulmonary hypertension is absent, the signs can mimic PDA; a wide pulse pressure, cardiac enlargement, and a continuous right and left upper sternal border systolic murmur may be present. The electrocardiogram shows either left or biventricular hypertrophy. Roentgenographic studies demonstrates cardiac enlargement and prominence of the pulmonary artery and intrapulmonary vascularity. The echocardiogram shows large-volume left-sided heart chambers, and the window can often be delineated.

Cardiac catheterization reveals a left to right shunt at the level of the pulmonary artery as well as hyperkinetic pulmonary hypertension because the defect is almost always large. Selective aortography with injection of contrast medium into the ascending aorta demonstrates the lesion, and manipulation of the catheter from the main pulmonary artery directly to the ascending aorta and brachiocephalic vessels is also diagnostic.

Aorticopulmonary defect is surgically corrected during infancy utilizing cardiopulmonary bypass. If surgery is not carried out in infancy, survivors carry the risk of progressive pulmonary vascular obstructive disease, similar to that of other patients who have intracardiac or great vessel communications and who have pulmonary artery hypertension.

15.41 CORONARY ARTERY FISTULA

A congenital fistula may exist between a coronary artery and an atrium, ventricle (especially the right), or pulmonary artery. Regardless of the recipient chamber, the signs are similar to those of patent ductus arteriosus, although the machinery murmur may be more diffuse. When a *coronary artery empties directly into the right side of the heart*, there is only a small left to right shunt at the atrial or ventricular level. The involved coronary artery is often dilated or aneurysmal. The anatomic abnormality is demonstrable by injection of contrast medium into the ascending aorta. Treatment consists of surgical abolition of the fistula.

15.42 RUPTURED SINUS OF VALSALVA

When one of the sinuses of Valsalva of the aorta is weakened by congenital or acquired disease, an aneurysm may form and rupture, usually into the right atrium or ventricle. This condition is extremely rare in childhood. The onset is usually sudden. The diagnosis is suspected in a patient who develops acute congestive heart failure, associated with a new loud to-and-fro murmur. Cardiac catheterization demonstrates the left to right shunt at the atrial or ventricular level. Aortography with injection of contrast medium into the ascending aorta demonstrates the site of aneurysm and rupture. Urgent surgical repair is required.

15.43 PULMONARY VALVE STENOSIS WITH INTACT VENTRICULAR SEPTUM

Various forms of right ventricular outflow obstruction with intact ventricular septum exist. The most common is valvular pulmonary stenosis. In this entity the valve cusps are deformed so that a dome-like obstruction occurs during systole. The cusps are thickened, and there is an eccentric outlet. Isolated infundibular stenosis, supravalvular pulmonary stenosis, and branch pulmonary artery stenosis are rarely encountered. In some instances when pulmonary valve stenosis is the dominant lesion, a small associated ventricular septal defect is present, but this problem is better classified as pulmonary stenosis than as tetralogy of Fallot. In addition, pulmonary stenosis and atrial septal defect are occasionally seen as associated defects. The clinical and laboratory findings reflect the dominant lesion, but it is important to make a complete diagnosis.

HEMODYNAMICS. The obstruction to outflow from the right ventricle to the pulmonary artery results in increased systolic pressure and hypertrophy of the right ventricle. The severity of these abnormalities depends on the size of the restricted valvular opening. In severe cases right ventricular pressure may be much higher than systemic systolic pressure, whereas in milder obstruction right ventricular pressure is only mildly or moderately elevated. Pulmonary arterial pressure is normal or decreased. Arterial oxygen saturation is normal except in severe cases, when a combination of decreased right ventricular compliance and intra-atrial communication leads to right to left shunting at the atrial level. This is seen most often in the neonate or small infant.

CLINICAL MANIFESTATIONS. With mild or moderate stenosis there are usually no symptoms. If the stenosis is severe, there may be exercise intolerance. In infancy, when obstruction is critical, there are signs of right ventricular failure and cyanosis. Growth and development are most often normal, and usually older infants and children with pulmonary stenosis appear to be especially well developed and healthy. Pulmonary stenosis as a result of valve dysplasia is the common cardiac abnormality of *Noonan syndrome* (see Sec. 19.29).

With mild pulmonary stenosis the venous pressure and pulse are normal. The heart is not enlarged; the apical impulse is normal, and the right ventricle is not palpable. A relatively short pulmonary systolic ejection murmur is maximally audible over the pulmonic area. The murmur is usually preceded by a pulmonic ejection click, which is heard best at the left upper sternal border during expiration. The 2nd heart sound is split with a pulmonary element of normal intensity that may be delayed. The *electrocardiogram* is normal or characteristic of mild right ventricular hypertrophy. The only abnormality demonstrable *roentgenographically* is poststenotic dilatation of the pulmonary artery. *Two-dimensional echocardiography* shows a domed valve, and Doppler studies predict a small right ventricular-pulmonary artery gradient. With more severe obstruction, the Doppler data will reflect a larger gradient.

In moderate stenosis the venous pressure may be slightly elevated with an intrinsic "a" wave noted in the jugular pulse. A right ventricular sternal lift may be palpable. The systolic ejection murmur is prolonged later into systole, and a pulmonic ejection sound may or may not be present. The 2nd heart sound is split, with a delayed and diminished pulmonary component that may not be audible. The *electrocardiogram* reveals varying degrees of right ventricular hypertrophy (systolic overload), sometimes with a prominent spiked P wave. *Roentgenographically*, the heart is normal in size or mildly enlarged because of prominence of the right ventricle; intrapulmonary vascularity may be decreased.

In severe stenosis, mild to moderate cyanosis may be noted if there is an interatrial communication. Hepatic enlargement and peripheral edema are observed in the presence of right ventricular failure. Elevation of the venous pressure is common and is due to a large presystolic jugular "a" wave. The heart is moderately or greatly enlarged, and there is a conspicuous sternal and parasternal right ventricular lift that frequently extends to the midclavicular line. A loud systolic ejection murmur, frequently accompanied by a thrill, is maximally audible in the pulmonic area and may radiate widely over the entire precordium into the neck and to the back. The murmur has late systolic accentuation, frequently encompasses the aortic component of the 2nd sound, but is not preceded by an ejection sound. The pulmonary element of the 2nd sound is usually inaudible. The *electrocardiogram* shows gross right ventricular hypertrophy, frequently accompanied by a tall spiked P wave. The *two-dimensional echocardiogram* shows a severe pulmonary valve deformity, an intact ventricular septum, and right ventricular hypertrophy. In the late stages of the disease, dysfunction of the right ventricle is seen. Doppler study predicts a large gradient across the pulmonary valve. *Roentgenographic studies* confirm the cardiac enlargement and prominence of the right ventricle and atrium. Prominence of the pulmonary artery segment is due to poststenotic dilatation (Fig. 15–49). The intrapulmonary vascularity is decreased. The classic findings of severe pulmonary stenosis in older children are now rarely seen. Critical stenosis is usually encountered in the context of cyanotic heart disease in the neonate.

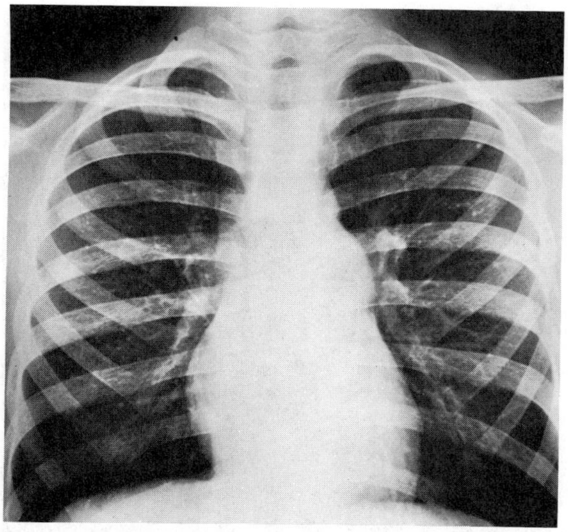

Figure 15–49. Roentgenogram in valvular pulmonary stenosis with a normal aortic root. The heart size is within normal limits, but there is poststenotic dilatation of the pulmonary artery.

Cardiac catheterization demonstrates an abrupt gradient of pressure across the pulmonary valve. The pulmonary arterial pressure is normal or low. The right ventricular systolic pressure is 30–50 mm Hg in mild cases; 50–100 mm Hg in moderate cases; and in severe cases higher than the systemic systolic pressure unless cardiac output is low or a significant right to left shunt exists across the atrial septum. In severe and in some moderate cases the right atrial pressure shows a prominent, frequently giant, "a" wave. *Selective right ventriculography* clearly demonstrates the obstruction. The flow of contrast medium through the stenotic valve in ventricular systole produces a jet of dye that fills the dilated pulmonary artery. The abnormal pulmonary valve is visible. Subvalvular hypertrophy that may intensify the obstruction may also be present (Fig. 15–50). This study also indicates whether the ventricular septum is intact.

COMPLICATIONS. Congestive cardiac failure, the most common complication, occurs only in severe cases and most often during the 1st month of life. The development of cyanosis from a right to left shunt across a foramen ovale is seen in infancy when stenosis is very severe. Infective endocarditis is not common.

COURSE AND PROGNOSIS. Children with mild or moderate stenosis can lead a normal life, but their progress should be evaluated at regular intervals. Patients who have small gradients rarely show progression and do not need intervention, but children having moderate stenosis are more likely to develop a more significant gradient as they grow. Worsening of obstruction may also be due, in part, to the development of secondary subvalvular muscular and fibrous tissue hypertrophy. Progressive electrocardiographic signs of right ventricular hypertrophy indicate increasing obstruction to right ventricular outflow. In untreated severe stenosis the course may abruptly worsen with the development of right ventricular dysfunction and cardiac failure. Infants with severe stenosis require urgent catheter balloon valvuloplasty or surgical valvotomy.

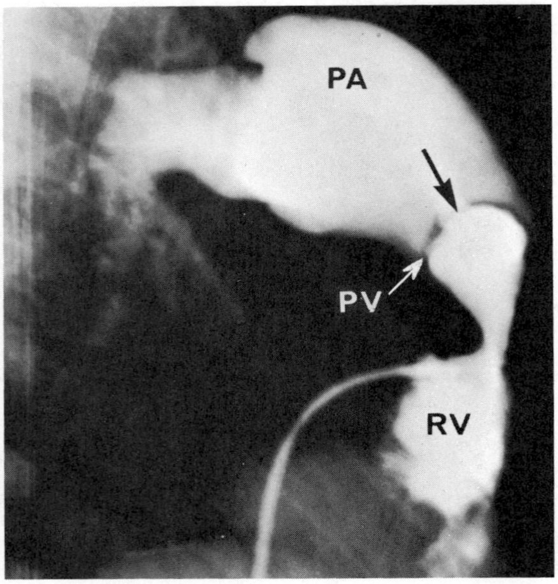

Figure 15–50. Lateral projection of a selective right ventriculogram in severe valvular pulmonary stenosis. The *black arrow* points to a jet of contrast medium through a minute opening of the pulmonary valve. Subvalvular infundibular hypertrophy is also present. (PA = poststenotic dilatation of pulmonary artery; PV = thickened pulmonary valve; RV = right ventricle.)

TREATMENT. Patients with moderate or severe isolated pulmonary stenosis require relief of obstruction. Relief of pulmonary valve stenosis is accomplished by balloon valvuloplasty, which is the treatment of choice for isolated valvular stenosis in patients in whom surgery would otherwise be indicated (Fig. 15–51). Emergency closed or open valvotomy for the neonate or infant with critical obstruction may be necessary on occasion, if catheter dilatation cannot be technically accomplished.

Excellent results are obtained in the majority of instances. The gradient across the pulmonary valve is reduced or abolished. A pulmonary diastolic murmur due to pulmonary valvular incompetence is to be expected and is not clinically significant. There appears to be no difference in the late status, regardless of method of treatment. Recurrence is unusual after successful treatment (by surgery or balloon catheter).

15.44 INFUNDIBULAR PULMONARY STENOSIS AND DOUBLE RIGHT VENTRICLE

Infundibular pulmonary stenosis is due to muscular or fibrous obstruction in the outflow tract of the right ventricle. The site of obstruction may be close to the pulmonary valve or well below it; an infundibular chamber may be present between the right ventricular cavity and the pulmonary valve. In a significant number of cases a ventricular septal defect may have been present initially and later closed spontaneously. When the pulmonary valve is also stenotic, the combined defect is primarily classified as valvular stenosis with secondary infundibular hypertrophy. The *hemodynamics* and *clinical manifestations* of patients with isolated infundibular pulmonary stenosis are similar, for the most part, to those described under simple valvular pulmonary stenosis (see Sec. 15.43).

A more common variation of right ventricular outflow obstruction below the pulmonary valve is that of *double right ventricle*. In this condition there is a muscular band in the mid right ventricular region, which divides the chamber into two parts and creates obstruction from the inlet portion to the outlet. There is often an associated ventricular septal defect that can close spontaneously. Obstruction is not seen early in life, but may progress rapidly in a similar manner to the progressive infundibular obstruction observed with tetralogy of Fallot.

The diagnosis of isolated right ventricular infundibular stenosis or double-chamber right ventricle can be made by echocardiography and/or cardiac catheterization and angiography. When contrast material is injected into the right ventricle the site of the stenosis is demonstrated. The ventricular septum must be evaluated to determine whether an associated ventricular septal defect is present. The prognosis for untreated cases of severe right ventricular outflow obstruction is similar to that for valvular pulmonary stenosis (see Sec. 15.43). When obstruction is severe, surgery is indicated. After operation the pressure gradient is abolished or markedly reduced and the outlook is excellent.

15.45 PULMONARY STENOSIS WITH LEFT TO RIGHT SHUNT

Valvular or infundibular pulmonary stenosis, or both, may be associated with a left to right shunt across an atrial septal

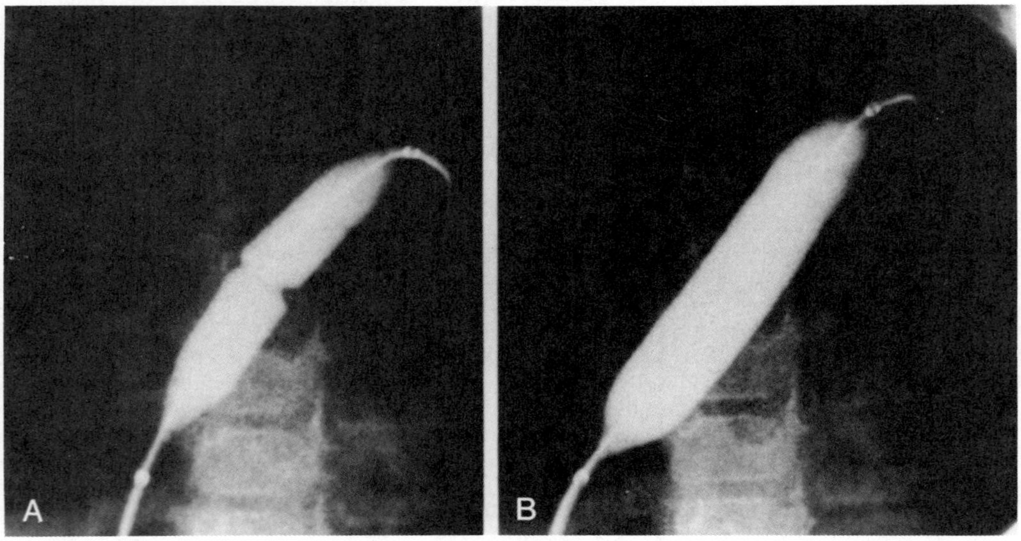

Figure 15–51. Balloon pulmonary valvuloplasty. *A*, Hourglass shape of the balloon at the start of inflation. *B*, Full balloon inflation. The left pulmonary artery is protected from the sharp tip of the catheter with a flexible-tip guidewire. (From Lababidi Z: Neonatal catheter palliations. *In*: Long WA [ed]: Fetal and Neonatal Cardiology. Philadelphia, WB Saunders, 1990, p. 707.)

defect or a VSD. The clinical features depend on the degree of stenosis and the magnitude of the left to right shunt.

The presence of a large left to right shunt at the atrial or ventricular level is evidence that the pulmonary stenosis is mild. However, worsening of obstruction will limit the shunt and perhaps even lead to right to left shunting; this more often occurs with VSD. These anomalies are repaired by cardiac surgery. Defects in the atrial or ventricular septa are closed, and the pulmonary stenosis is relieved by infundibular resection or pulmonary valvuloplasty as indicated.

15.46 PULMONARY STENOSIS WITH RIGHT TO LEFT SHUNT

See pulmonary valve stenosis with intact ventricular septum (Sec. 15.43) and tetralogy of Fallot (Sec. 15.11).

15.47 PULMONARY ARTERIAL BRANCH STENOSIS

Single or multiple constrictions may occur anywhere along the major branches of the pulmonary artery and may be mild, extensive, localized, or multiple. Frequently, this defect is associated with other types of congenital heart disease, especially pulmonary valvular stenosis, tetralogy of Fallot, patent ductus arteriosus, ventricular septal defect, atrial septal defect, and supravalvular aortic stenosis. A familial tendency has been recognized in some patients with peripheral stenosis. A high incidence has been found in infants with the congenital rubella syndrome. Supravalvular aortic stenosis with pulmonary arterial branch stenosis has also been observed with idiopathic hypercalcemia of infancy (Williams syndrome).

With a mild constriction there is little effect on the pulmonary circulation. With multiple severe constrictions there is an increase in pressure in the right ventricle and in the pulmonary artery proximal to the site of obstruction. When the anomaly is isolated, the diagnosis is suspected by the presence of murmurs in widespread locations over the chest, anteriorly or posteriorly. These murmurs are usually systolic but may be continuous. They are occasionally heard in newborn infants and will eventually disappear, suggesting that mild branch stenosis in this age group may be transient. Most often, the physical signs are dominated by the associated anomaly, such as tetralogy of Fallot. If the stenosis is severe, there is electrocardiographic evidence of right ventricular and right atrial hypertrophy.

On roentgenographic examination, cardiomegaly and prominence of the main pulmonary artery are present in severe cases. Generally, the pulmonary vasculature is normal; in some cases small intrapulmonary vascular shadows are seen, which may be shown by pulmonary arteriography to be areas of poststenotic dilatation. Pressure gradients across the areas of obstruction are demonstrable by cardiac catheterization. These gradients may not be easily identified if right ventricular outflow obstruction coexists, as the pressure in the main pulmonary artery is normal or low in such patients. Severe obstruction of the main pulmonary artery and its primary branches should be relieved during corrective surgery for tetralogy of Fallot or valvular pulmonary stenosis or may be treated by catheter balloon dilatation. Multiple peripheral intrapulmonary obstructions are not amenable to distal surgical or interventional catheterization management, but most often are mild.

15.48 PULMONARY VALVULAR INSUFFICIENCY

Pulmonary valvular insufficiency most often accompanies other cardiovascular diseases and may be secondary to severe pulmonary hypertension. Incompetence of the valve is an expected result after surgery for right ventricular outflow obstruction, for example, pulmonary valvotomy and infundibular resection. Isolated congenital insufficiency of the pulmonary valve is a rare anomaly. The patient is usually asymptomatic since the incompetence is usually mild.

The prominent physical sign is a diastolic murmur at the upper and mid left sternal border, which has a lower pitch than the murmur of aortic insufficiency. Roentgenograms of the chest show prominence of the main pulmonary artery. The electrocardiogram is normal or shows minimal right ventricular hypertrophy. Doppler studies demonstrate retrograde flow from the pulmonary artery to the right ventricle during diastole. The diagnosis can be made at cardiac catheterization if necessary. There is a low pulmonary arterial diastolic pressure. Selective pulmonary arteriography shows the incompetent valve but is difficult to evaluate in mild cases because the catheter crossing the valve results in some iatrogenic insufficiency during the injection. Isolated pulmonary valvular incompetence is usually well tolerated and does not require surgical treatment.

Absence of the pulmonary valve is usually associated with a VSD, often in the context of tetralogy of Fallot (see Sec. 15.11). In some neonates or infants, the pulmonary arteries become widely dilated and compress the bronchi, thus causing recurrent episodes of wheezing, pulmonary collapse, and pneumonitis. Florid pulmonary valvular incompetence may not be well tolerated, and death may occur from a combination of bronchial compression, hypoxemia, and heart failure. Plication of massive pulmonary arteries along with intracardiac correction has been effective in a few cases. In older patients a homograft may be inserted at the time of correction of the ventricular defect and the infundibular stenosis.

15.49 COARCTATION OF THE AORTA

Constrictions of varying length may occur at any point from the arch to the bifurcation of the aorta, but 98% occur just below the origin of the left subclavian artery at the origin of the ductus arteriosus. The anomaly occurs twice as often in males as in females. Coarctation of the aorta may be a feature of Turner (XO) syndrome (see Sec. 19.33) and is associated with bicuspid aortic valve in over 70% of patients. Mitral valve abnormalities and subaortic stenosis also are not uncommon.

PATHOLOGY. Coarctation of the aorta occurs in the form of a preductal segmental tubular hypoplasia or as a more discrete juxtaductal obstruction. Often, both components are present. It is postulated that coarctation is initiated in the presence of a cardiac abnormality that results in decreased antegrade aortic blood flow (e.g., bicuspid aortic valve) and proportionately increased flow through the pulmonary artery and ductus arteriosus. A contraductal shelf-like structure bifurcates ductal blood flow retrograde into the left subclavian and antegrade to the descending aorta (Fig. 15–52). Antegrade aortic flow supplies the innominate, left carotid, and vertebral arteries, but when very little blood reaches the aortic isthmus proximal to the left subclavian artery, isthmic tubular hypoplasia results. Occasionally, severely hypoplastic segments of the aortic isthmus may become completely atretic, resulting in an interrupted arch with the left subclavian artery arising either proximal or distal to the interruption. The nature of the coarctation lesion depends on the ultimate flow across the aortic isthmus proximal to the left carotid artery. If the segment remains patent but narrow, then the "infantile" type of coarctation occurs, usually with right to left ductal flow to the descending aorta and almost invariably with an associated ventricular septal defect. If antegrade aortic flow becomes

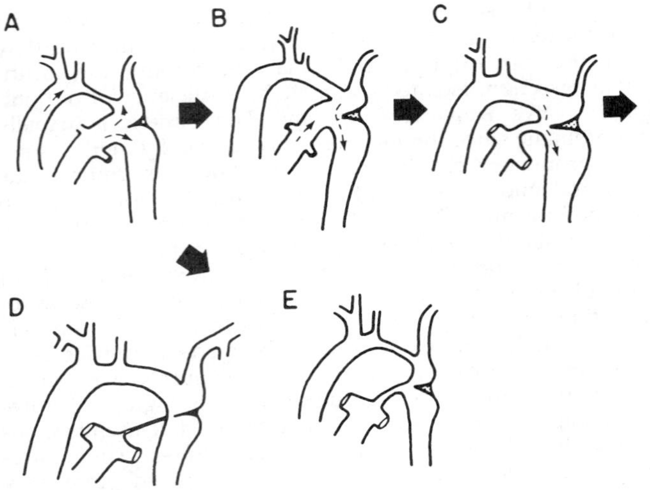

Figure 15–52. Metamorphosis of coarctation. *A*, Fetal prototype. No flow obstruction. *B*, Late gestation. The aortic ventricle increases the output and dilates the hypoplastic segment. Antegrade aortic flow bypasses the shell via a ductal orifice. *C*, Neonate. Ductal constriction initiates the obstruction by removing the bypass and by increasing antegrade arch flow. *D*, Mature juxtaductal stenosis. Bypass completely obliterated; intimal hypoplasia on the edge of the shell aggravates stenosis. Collaterals develop. *E*, Infantile-type fetal prototype persists. An intracardiac left-sided heart obstruction precludes an increase in antegrade aortic before or after birth. Both isthmal hypoplasia and contraductal shelf are present. Lower body flow often depends on patency of the ductus. (From Gersony WM: Coarctation of the aorta. *In*: Adams FH, Emmanouilides GC, Riemenschneider T: Moss Heart Disease in Infants, Children, and Adolescents, 4th ed. Copyright 1989, the Williams & Wilkins Co., Baltimore.)

normal after birth, isthmic narrowing will not be prominent, and the most common type of discrete coarctation will occur.

The blood pressure is elevated in the vessels that arise proximal to the coarctation; the blood pressure as well as pulse pressure below the constriction is lower. Hypertension is not due to the mechanical obstruction alone, but almost certainly involves renal mechanisms. Coarctation of the aorta usually results in the development of extensive collateral circulation, chiefly from the branches of the subclavian, the superior intercostal, and the internal mammary arteries. The thoracic and subscapular branches of the axillary artery may also enlarge as collateral channels. These vessels unite with the intercostal branches of the descending aorta and inferior epigastric branches of the femoral artery to create a channel for arterial blood to bypass the area of coarctation. The vessels contributing to the collateral circulation may become markedly enlarged and tortuous by early adulthood.

Coarctation of the aorta recognized after infancy rarely is associated with significant symptomatology. An occasional child will complain about weakness and/or pain in the legs after exercise, but in the great majority of instances, even patients with severe coarctation will be asymptomatic.

CLINICAL MANIFESTATIONS. The classic sign of coarctation of the aorta is disparity in pulsations and blood pressures of the arms and legs. The femoral, popliteal, posterior tibial, and dorsalis pedis pulsations are weak and delayed or absent in contrast with the bounding pulses of the arms and carotid vessels. In normal persons the systolic blood pressure in the legs obtained by the cuff method is 10–20 mm Hg higher than that in the arms. In coarctation of the aorta the blood pressure in the legs is lower than that in the arms; frequently, it is difficult to obtain. There is also a more prominent rise of systemic blood pressure in response to exercise.

This differential in blood pressures is very common in patients over 1 yr of age, about 90% of whom have systolic hypertension in the upper extremity greater than the 95th percentile for age. In one study mean upper extremity blood pressure was 145 ± 12 mm Hg; lower extremity blood pressure, when it could be obtained, was 70 ± 10 mm Hg. Although absent femoral and pedal pulses are the hallmark of the disease, in only 40% of patients were the femoral pulses completely absent. Weakly palpable femoral pulses with a pulse lag were evident in 44%; in 16% the pulses were characterized as normal. Palpable pedal pulses were noted in 23% of the patients.

It is important to determine the blood pressure in each arm; a significant difference between the right and left arms suggests involvement of the left subclavian artery in the area of coarctation.

A short systolic murmur is often heard along the left sternal border at the 3rd and 4th intercostal spaces. The murmur is well transmitted to the back and neck. An interscapular systolic murmur over the region of the coarctation is quite characteristic. Often, the typical murmur of mild aortic stenosis can be heard in the 3rd right intercostal space and an apical systolic ejection click is also common. The latter findings suggest that an aortic valve deformity is present in addition to coarctation; occasionally a significant degree of obstruction across the aortic valve is also present. Among patients with well-developed collateral blood flow, systolic or continuous murmurs may be heard over the left and right sides of the chest laterally and posteriorly.

DIAGNOSIS. The findings on *roentgenographic examination* depend on the age of the patient and on the effects of hypertension and collateral circulation. In infancy there are usually no changes except cardiac enlargement if congestive cardiac failure is present. During childhood the findings are not striking unless the left ventricle is prominent. After the 1st decade the heart tends to be mildly or moderately enlarged because of left ventricular prominence. The enlarged left subclavian artery commonly produces a prominent shadow in the left superior mediastinum. Notching of the inferior border of the ribs from pressure erosion by enlarged collateral vessels is common by late childhood except in the upper and lower 2–3 ribs. In the majority of instances there is an area of poststenotic dilatation of the descending aorta. This may be demonstrated by displacement of the barium-filled esophagus and by discontinuity of the lateral margin of the aorta below the arch.

The *electrocardiogram* is usually normal in young children but reveals evidences of left ventricular hypertrophy in older patients. Neonates and infants will display right ventricular dominance.

Most often, the diagnosis can be made simply by careful evaluation of the pulse in all major accessible peripheral arteries and by comparative blood pressure determinations in the arms and legs. The segment of coarctation can be visualized by two-dimensional *echocardiography;* associated anomalies of the aortic valve can also be demonstrated. Doppler study of the descending aorta shows a typical dampened systolic flow pattern and slightly increased diastolic flow. Coarctation of the aorta is also well demonstrated by MRI examination. *Cardiac catheterization* with selective left ventriculography and aortography is especially important in selected patients with additional anomalies, and as a means of visualizing collateral blood flow. In cases well defined by echocardiography or MRI, catheterization may not be required.

ASSOCIATED ABNORMALITIES. Abnormalities of the aortic valve are present in a majority of patients. Bicuspid aortic valves are common but usually do not produce signs unless stenosis is significant. The association of patent ductus arteriosus and coarctation of the aorta is also common. Ventricular and atrial septal defects may be suspected by signs of left to right shunt. Mitral valve abnormalities are also occasionally seen, as is subvalvular aortic stenosis.

Severe neurologic damage or even death rarely may occur from associated cerebrovascular disease. Subarachnoid or intracerebral hemorrhage may result from rupture of congenital aneurysms in the circle of Willis, of other vessels with defective elastic and medial tissue, or of normal vessels; these accidents are secondary to the hypertensive state. Abnormalities of the subclavian arteries may include involvement of the left subclavian artery in the area of coarctation, stenosis of the orifice of the left subclavian artery, and anomalous origin of the right subclavian artery.

PROGNOSIS AND COMPLICATIONS. Untreated, the great majority of patients with coarctation of the aorta would succumb between the ages of 20 and 40 yr; some live well into middle life without serious handicap. The common serious complications are related to the hypertensive state, which may result in premature coronary artery disease, congestive cardiac failure, hypertensive encephalopathy, or intracranial hemorrhage. Heart failure may be related to complicating anomalies, especially in infancy. Infective endocarditis or endarteritis is a significant complication in adults. Aneurysms of the descending aorta or of the enlarged collateral vessels are not unusual.

TREATMENT. Patients with significant coarctation of the aorta should be treated surgically. The optimal age for operation is 2–4 yr; the mortality rate at this age is less than 1%. After the 2nd decade the operation may be less successful because of decreased left ventricular function and degenerative changes. Nevertheless, if cardiac reserve is sufficient, satisfactory repair is possible well into mid adult life. Associated valvular lesions increase the hazards of late surgery.

The operation of choice is excision of the area of coarctation and primary anastomosis. A subclavian flap procedure, which incorporates the subclavian artery into the wall of the repaired coarctation, is more often utilized in the younger age group. This vertical incision may be less associated with recoarctation compared with horizontal resection and end-to-end anastomosis in this age group. Rarely, if the length of aortic constriction precludes primary anastomosis, Dacron grafts may be utilized.

After operation there is striking increase in the amplitude of pulsations in the femoral artery and dorsalis pedis and arterial tibial pulses. However, in the immediate postoperative course, "rebound" hypertension is common and may require medical management. Usually hypertension gradually subsides. Residual murmurs are common and may be due to associated cardiac anomalies, to flow across the repaired area, and/or to collateral blood flow. Additional operative problems include spinal cord injury if there are poorly developed collaterals, chylothorax, diaphragm injury, and laryngeal nerve injury. If a left subclavian flap is employed, the pulse and blood pressure in the left arm will be diminished or absent.

Repair of coarctation in the 2nd decade of life or beyond may be associated with a higher incidence of premature cardiovascular disease, even in the absence of residual cardiac abnormalities. There may be recurrence or early onset of adult hypertension, which has occurred even in patients with adequately resected coarctation. However, most follow-up studies involve young adults who were operated on several decades earlier, and the excellence of the original repair has not been documented. Most centers now advocate repair of coarctation early in the 1st decade of life in an attempt to decrease the incidence of premature cardiovascular disease during adult life. In patients with normal blood pressure following repair at 3–4 yr of age, late hypertension, early atherosclerosis, and dissecting aneurysm, all of which have been reported in the older age group, should be less likely to occur.

Although restenosis in older patients who had an adequate coarctectomy is extremely rare, a significant number of infants with end-to-end anastomoses carried out urgently in the first months of life require revision later in childhood. Balloon dilatation of restenosis has been successfully carried out, but in the opinion of some but not all centers, concerns about aneurysm formation contraindicate the use of this technique for relief of native (unoperated) coarctation. It remains to be seen whether follow-up of patients who had subclavian flap procedures in this age group will show that restenosis is much less likely. All patients should be followed carefully for an indefinite period after repair of coarctation of the aorta.

15.50 POSTCOARCTECTOMY SYNDROME

Postoperative mesenteric arteritis may be associated with hypertension and abdominal pain in the immediate postoperative period. The pain varies in severity and may be associated with anorexia, nausea, vomiting, leukocytosis, intestinal hemorrhage, bowel necrosis, and small bowel obstruction. Relief is usually obtained with antihypertensive drugs (nitroprusside, labetalol) and intestinal decompression; corticosteroids may help to alleviate the symptoms and thus avoid surgical exploration for bowel obstruction. This syndrome has been seen much less frequently in recent years.

15.51 COARCTATION IN INFANCY

Coarctation occurs in infancy associated with other cardiovascular anomalies, including patent ductus arteriosus, ventricular septal defect, severe aortic valvular disease, transposition of the great arteries, and variations of single ventricle. Severe coarctation may also be associated with endocardial sclerosis and mitral valve disease. The clinical pattern in this age group depends on the effects of the associated malformations as well as of the coarctation itself. Both anatomic and physiologic classifications have been utilized to describe all existing abnormalities and their contributions to the clinical manifestations of coarctation in infancy. These depend on the site and length of coarctation, the site of the aortic opening of the ductus, and the size of the aorta proximal to the coarctation. The direction of blood flow across the ductus depends on position, severity of obstruction at the site of the coarctation, and pulmonary vascular resistance. Virtually all coarctations are juxtaductal rather than in the preductal and postductal positions.

In infants with severe hypoplasia of the aortic isthmus or interruption of the aortic arch, right ventricular blood is ejected through the ductus to the descending aorta. Systemic flow to the lower body is dependent on right ventricular output. In this situation femoral pulses are palpable, and differential blood pressures are not helpful in the diagnosis. Such infants will have severe pulmonary hypertension and high pulmonary vascular resistance. Cyanosis, failure to thrive, and heart failure are prominent. Because the descending aorta is supplied with venous blood, differential cyanosis may be noted, but this is rarely a conspicuous sign. The heart is large, and there is a systolic murmur heard along the left sternal border with a loud 2nd heart sound. The electrocardiogram shows right ventricular hypertrophy, and the chest roentgenogram shows cardiac enlargement and prominent vascularity. In coarctation with a large right to left shunt across the ductus arteriosus the prognosis may be poor, but some cases respond well to medical management and surgical excision of the coarctation. On the other hand, the occasional infant with coarctation and a large left to right shunt through the ductus arteriosus has a much better outlook. In some of these infants, surgical repair may be delayed if response to digitalization and diuretic therapy is optimal.

Coarctation of the aorta associated with severe mitral and aortic valve disease may have to be considered within the context of hypoplastic left-sided heart syndrome. Such patients have a long segment of narrow arch with or without isolated coarctation at the site of the entrance of the ductus into the aorta. Coarctation of the aorta with transposition of the great arteries or single ventricle may be repaired alone or in combination with other palliative measures.

15.52 COARCTATION WITH VENTRICULAR SEPTAL DEFECT IN INFANCY

Isolated coarctation of the aorta is uncommonly a cause of congestive heart failure during infancy. However, coarctation in the presence of VSD results in both increased preload and afterload on the left ventricle, and patients with this combination of defects will present in the first month of life, often with intractable cardiac failure. The clinical picture is that of a seriously ill infant with tachypnea, failure to thrive, and typical findings of heart failure. Often, there is not a marked difference in blood pressures between the upper and lower extremities since cardiac output may be low. These infants present earlier in a more severely ill state than those with either VSD or coarctation alone. Although medical management may be helpful initially, early surgery is necessary. In most cases coarctation is the major anomaly causing the severe symptoms, and resection of the coarcted segment will result in marked improvement. Many centers do not band the pulmonary artery, and a number of patients will improve sufficiently so that further surgery is not required during infancy. Later repair of the VSD is carried out in some patients. However, if there is difficulty in managing the infant after surgery, open repair of the ventricular septal defect is done in infancy. When it is determined that a complicated VSD is present (multiple, muscular), pulmonary arterial banding can be done at the time of coarctation repair to avoid infant open heart surgery for complex ventricular septal abnormalities.

15.53 CONGENITAL AORTIC STENOSIS

Congenital aortic stenosis accounts for about 5% of cardiac malformations recognized in childhood, but an abnormality of the aortic valve (bicuspid) is one of the most common congenital heart lesions identified in adults. Stenosis is more common in males (3:1).

In most cases, aortic stenosis is valvular, the leaflets are thickened, and most often the commissures are fused to varying degrees. *Subvalvular (subaortic) stenosis* with a discrete fibrous shelf below the aortic valves is also an important form of left ventricular outflow obstruction. This lesion is frequently associated with other forms of congenital heart disease and is notable for rapid progression in severity. It is virtually never diagnosed during early infancy and may develop despite prior documentation of no left ventricular aortic gradient. Subvalvular aortic stenosis may become apparent after successful surgery for other congenital heart defects (e.g., coarctation of the aorta, patent ductus arteriosus, and ventricular septal defect), may develop in association with mild lesions that have not been surgically repaired, and may occur as an isolated abnormality. Although discrete subvalvular aortic stenosis may have a pre-existing substrate, the lesion can present as an "acquired" abnormality with progressive hemodynamic severity.

Supravalvular aortic stenosis, a less common type, may be sporadic, familial, or associated with a syndrome of mental retardation and an elfin facies (full face, broad forehead, flattened bridge of nose, long upper lip, and rounded cheeks). Stenoses of other arteries may also be present. This syndrome (Williams syndrome) (Fig. 15–53) is associated with idiopathic hypercalcemia of infancy (see Sec. 24.68).

CLINICAL MANIFESTATIONS. Symptomatology among patients with aortic stenosis depends on the severity of the obstruction. Aortic stenosis presents in early infancy with severe left ventricular failure. However, most children with critical aortic stenosis will remain asymptomatic and display a normal growth and development pattern. The murmur is usually discovered during routine physical examination. It is rare to see an older child with severe obstruction to left ventricular outflow with fatigue, angina, dizziness, or syncope. Sudden death has been reported with aortic stenosis but usually occurs in patients with severe left ventricular outflow obstruction manifested by electrocardiographic changes and a large gradient across the aortic valve, in whom surgical relief has been delayed.

The pulse is usually normal but may have a small volume when obstruction is critical. The heart size and apical impulse are normal when stenosis is mild or moderate. In severe cases the heart may be enlarged with a left ventricular apical thrust. A rough systolic ejection murmur, usually accompanied by a suprasternal notch thrill, is audible maximally at the right upper sternal border and radiates to the neck and down the left sternal border. In patients with subvalvular stenosis, the murmur may be maximal along the left sternal border or even at the apex. In valvular aortic stenosis the murmur is usually preceded by an aortic ejection click best heard at the apex and left sternal edge. Clicks are unusual in discrete subaortic stenosis. A diastolic murmur indicative of mild aortic insufficiency is often present when the obstruction is subvalvular, or in patients with a bicuspid aortic valve. Occasionally, an apical short mid-diastolic rumbling murmur is audible even in the presence of a normal mitral valve. The normal splitting of the 2nd heart sound is present in mild cases. In patients with severe obstruction, aortic valve closure is diminished, or, rarely in children, the 2nd sound may be split paradoxically. A 4th heart sound may be audible when the obstruction is severe.

Critical aortic stenosis in infancy is characterized by an extremely ill patient with signs of low cardiac output. Congestive heart failure, cardiomegaly, and pulmonary edema are severe, and the pulses are weak. Since cardiac output is decreased, the intensity of the murmur at the right upper sternal border may be minimal.

DIAGNOSIS. The diagnosis should be made by physical examination. Generally, a loud murmur accompanied by a right upper sternal border thrill indicates the presence of significant obstruction. If the pressure gradient across the aortic valve is small, the *electrocardiogram* is likely to be normal. The ECG may also be normal with severe obstruction, but evidence of left ventricular hypertrophy and strain is often present if severe stenosis is longstanding. *Roentgenograms* frequently show a prominent ascending aorta, but the aortic knob is normal. Heart size is usually normal. Valvular calcification has been noted in older children. *Echocardiography* identifies the anomaly and is used to evaluate both the site and the severity of obstruction. Anatomic echographic M-mode features include multiple diastolic echoes of the aortic valve, eccentric aortic valve closure, and increased thickness of the ventricular septum and the free wall of the left ventricle. Two-dimensional studies visualize the domed stenotic aortic valve or subvalvular obstruction. In the absence of left ventricular failure, the shortening fraction of the left ventricle is

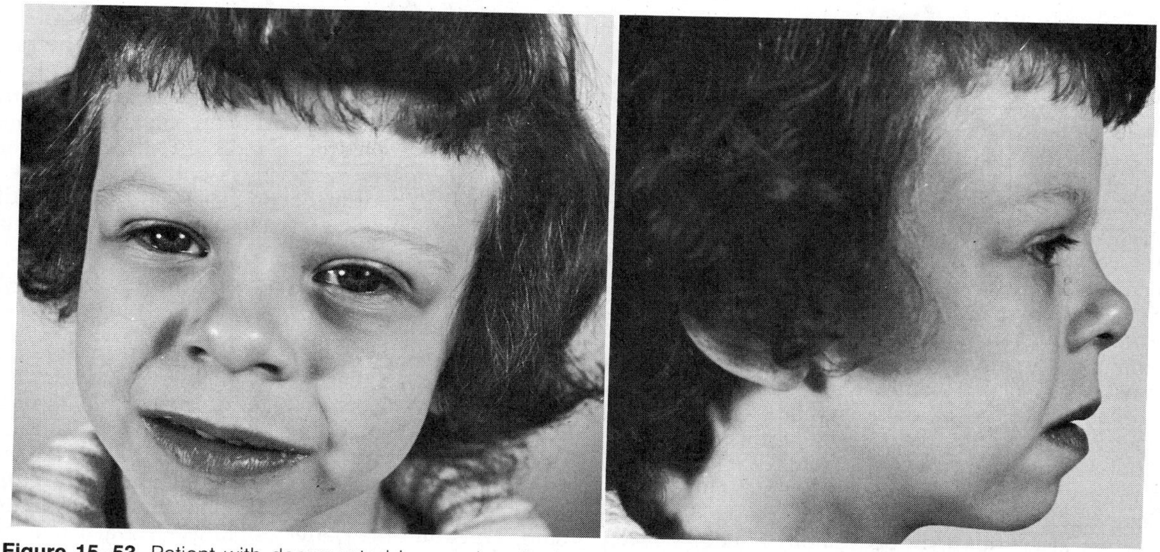

Figure 15–53. Patient with documented hypercalcemia during infancy who had supravalvular aortic stenosis relieved surgically at 8 yr of age. The upper lip is prominent, the bridge of the nose is flat, the nose is short and upturned, and hypertelorism is present.

increased since the ventricle is hypercontractile. Peak systolic left ventricular outflow gradients that exceed 45 mm Hg are usually associated with shortening fractions greater than 40%.

Graded exercise testing is useful in evaluating the severity of left ventricular outflow obstruction in older children. As the severity of the gradient increases, working capacity decreases, systolic blood pressure fails to rise adequately, diastolic blood pressure may rise, and ST segmental depression can occur. Because patients with severe aortic stenosis may deny symptoms and have normal electrocardiograms and chest roentgenograms, serial echocardiograms and graded exercise tests may be valuable in determining the timing of cardiac catheterization and surgical or balloon catheter valvuloplasty.

Left cardiac catheterization demonstrates the magnitude of pressure gradient from the left ventricle to the aorta. The site of obstruction is best identified by selective left ventriculography. The aortic pressure curve is abnormal if obstruction is severe; an early-appearing anacrotic notch, a slow, prolonged, and delayed systolic upstroke, a narrow pulse pressure, and a delayed dicrotic notch are noted. In patients with severe obstruction and decreased left ventricular compliance, the left atrial pressure is increased. Most infants with critical aortic stenosis do not require cardiac catheterization. Clinical and echocardiographic features are sufficient to make the diagnosis and plan intervention. When a critically ill infant with left ventricular outflow obstruction undergoes cardiac catheterization, left ventricular function is markedly decreased. Only a small gradient is often measured across the stenotic aortic valve because of low cardiac output.

PROGNOSIS. The prognosis is good in the majority of children with mild to moderate aortic stenosis. In a small number of patients having a severe obstruction, sudden death has occurred. In such instances there is usually evidence of gross left ventricular hypertrophy. Neonates having critical aortic stenosis who die from congestive heart failure frequently have endocardial fibroelastosis of the left ventricle. Infants who present after the first week or two of life respond well to relief of stenosis, and left ventricular function improves. Reoperations on the aortic valve are required later in childhood or in adult life.

TREATMENT. Surgical valvotomy is indicated for children having severe valvular aortic stenosis to prevent progressive left ventricular dysfunction secondary to severe afterload requirements. Balloon valvuloplasty is used successfully both in infants and older children. Whether surgical or catheter treatment has been carried out, aortic insufficiency or calcification with restenosis is likely to occur years or even decades later, resulting eventually in aortic valve replacement. Discrete subaortic stenosis can be resected without damage to the aortic valve, the anterior leaflet of the mitral valve, or the conduction system. Relief of supravalvular stenosis can be achieved if the area of obstruction is discrete and is not associated with a hypoplastic aorta.

Surgery or balloon dilatation for aortic stenosis is not indicated in the absence of definitive evidence of left ventricular hypertrophy or of a significant gradient across the aortic valve. The definition of a "significant gradient" is difficult, but it is generally agreed that surgery should be advised when the peak systolic gradient between the left ventricle and aorta exceeds 60 mm Hg at rest with a normal cardiac output. A lesser gradient is required for the more rapidly progressive subaortic obstructive lesions.

Careful follow-up is essential since severe recurrence of ventricular obstruction may not be associated with early symptoms. Electrocardiographic signs of left ventricular hypertrophy, deterioration of echocardiographic indices of left ventricular function, and recurrence of signs during graded exercise are compatible with severe restenosis.

There may be some danger in allowing patients with significant aortic stenosis to participate in active competitive sports, but otherwise they should lead normal lives. The status of each patient should be reviewed annually and intervention advised if progression of signs is definite. Prophylaxis against infective endocarditis is required.

15.54 CONGENITAL MITRAL STENOSIS

This relatively rare anomaly can be isolated or associated with other defects, the most common being patent ductus arteriosus, aortic stenosis, and coarctation of the aorta. The mitral valve is funnel shaped, with thickened leaflets and chordae tendineae that are shortened and deformed. Other mitral valve anomalies with stenosis include parachute mitral valve and double-orifice mitral valve.

Symptoms usually appear within the first 2 yr. The infants are underdeveloped and usually have obvious dyspnea secondary to congestive heart failure; cyanosis and pallor are common. Heart enlargement due to dilatation and hypertrophy of the right ventricle and left atrium is common. Most patients have rumbling diastolic murmurs followed by a loud 1st sound, but the auscultatory findings may be relatively obscure. The 2nd sound is loud and split. An opening snap of the mitral valve may be present. The *electrocardiogram* reveals right ventricular hypertrophy with normal, bifid, or spiked P waves. *Roentgenograms* usually show left atrial and right ventricular enlargement and pulmonary congestion. The *echocardiogram* is characteristic, showing thickened mitral valve leaflets, diminished E-F slope, and an enlarged left atrium with a normal or small left ventricle. Two-dimensional examinations in the short axis show a significant reduction of the mitral valve orifice in diastole; the size of the mitral valve orifice can be measured. At *cardiac catheterization* there is an increase in right ventricular, pulmonary arterial, and pulmonary capillary wedge pressures. Associated anomalies such as patent ductus arteriosus may be demonstrated. *Angiocardiography* may show delayed emptying of the left atrium and the small mitral orifice.

The prognosis for untreated patients is poor; the majority of children succumb during the first 2 yr of life. The results of surgical treatment have been variable; a mitral valve prosthesis is required.

15.55 CONGENITAL MITRAL INSUFFICIENCY

This anomaly may be isolated but is more often associated with other anomalies including patent ductus arteriosus, coarctation of the aorta, VSD, corrected transposition of the great vessels, anomalous origin of the left coronary artery from the pulmonary artery, endocardial fibroelastosis, or Marfan syndrome. Mitral incompetence is an integral part of endocardial cushion defects.

In isolated mitral insufficiency the mitral valve annulus is usually dilated; the chordae tendineae are short and may insert anomalously; and the valve leaflets are deformed. When mitral incompetence is clinically significant, the left atrium enlarges as a result of the regurgitant flow and the left ventricle becomes hypertrophied and dilated. Pulmonary venous pressure is increased and ultimately results in pulmonary hypertension and right ventricular hypertrophy and dilatation. Mild lesions produce no symptoms; the only abnormal sign is the murmur of mitral incompetence. However, severe regurgitation results in symptoms that can appear at any age. These include poor physical development, frequent respiratory infections, fatigue on exertion, and episodes of pulmonary edema or congestive heart failure. The typical apical pansystolic murmur of mitral insufficiency is present with the associated apical mid-diastolic rumbling murmur of increased diastolic flow across the mitral valve. The pulmonary component of the 2nd heart sound is accentuated in the presence of pulmonary hypertension. The *electrocardiogram* usually shows bifid P waves, signs of left ventricular hypertrophy, and sometimes signs of right ventricular hypertrophy. *Roentgenographic examination* shows enlargement of the left atrium, which at times is massive. The left ventricle is prominent, and the pulmonary vascularity is normal or prominent. *Echocardiograms* demonstrate the enlarged left atrium and ventricle. Although motion of the mitral valve is excessive with a steep E-F slope, this sign is not diagnostic.

Cardiac catheterization shows an elevated left atrial pressure measured either directly via a patent foramen ovale or by means of pulmonary capillary wedge pressure. Pulmonary artery hypertension of varying severity may be present. Selective left ventriculography reveals the presence of mitral regurgitation. *Mitral valvuloplasty* has resulted in striking improvement in symptoms and heart size, but in some patients installation of a prosthetic mechanical mitral valve may be necessary. Prior to surgery, associated anomalies must be identified. In children beyond 3–4 yr it may be difficult to exclude rheumatic fever as the cause of mitral insufficiency.

15.56 MITRAL VALVE PROLAPSE

This distinctive syndrome results from an abnormal mitral valve mechanism that causes billowing of one or both mitral leaflets, especially the posterior cusp, into the left atrium toward the end of systole. The abnormality is almost always congenital but may not be recognized until adolescence or adulthood. The syndrome is more common in girls, may be inherited as an autosomal dominant trait with variable expression, and thus may affect siblings. Mitral valve prolapse is common in patients with Marfan syndrome, straight back syndrome, pectus excavatum, and scoliosis. The dominant abnormal signs are auscultatory. The apical murmur is late systolic in timing and may be preceded by a click, but these signs vary in the same patient so that at times only the click is audible. In the standing or sitting position the click may appear earlier in systole and the murmur may be more prominent in late systole. Arrhythmias, primarily unifocal or multifocal premature ventricular contractions, may occur.

The *electrocardiogram* is usually normal, but may show diphasic T waves, especially in leads II, III, AVF, and V_6; the T wave abnormalities may vary in the same patient. The *chest roentgenogram* is normal. The *echocardiogram* shows a characteristic posterior movement of the posterior mitral leaflet during mid or late systole or pansystolic prolapse of both anterior and posterior mitral leaflets. These M-mode echographic findings must be interpreted cautiously since the appearance of minimal mitral prolapse may be a normal variant. Two-dimensional real-time echocardiography appears to be more accurate; both the free edge and the body of the mitral leaflets move posteriorly in systole toward the left atrium. The lesion is not progressive in childhood, and specific therapy is not indicated. The patient may be at risk to develop infective endocarditis. Antibiotic prophylaxis is recommended during surgery and dental procedures (see Table 15–17).

Confusion exists concerning the diagnosis of mitral valve prolapse. The frequency of mild prolapse on the echocardiogram in the absence of clinical findings suggests that true "mitral valve prolapse syndrome" is not present. The patients and their parents should be reassured to this effect, and no special recommendations should be made regarding special management or frequent laboratory studies. Otherwise, 15 to 20% of the general population would be labeled as having a significant, albeit mild, lesion. Endocarditis prophylaxis is indicated in substantiated cases.

Adults (more males than females) with mitral valve prolapse are at increased risk for cardiovascular complications (sudden death, arrhythmia, cerebrovascular accidents, progressive valve dilatation, heart failure, and endocarditis) in the presence of thickened and redundant mitral valve leaflets.

15.57 PULMONARY VENOUS HYPERTENSION

A variety of lesions may result in chronic pulmonary venous hypertension, which when extreme may result in pulmonary arterial hypertension and right-sided heart failure. These lesions include congenital mitral stenosis, mitral insufficiency, some varieties of total anomalous pulmonary venous return, left atrial myxomas, cor triatriatum (stenosis of the common pulmonary vein), individual pulmonary venous stenosis, and supravalvular mitral ring or web. In these conditions early symptoms can be confused with chronic pulmonary disease, as there may be no specific cardiac findings on physical examination. However, subtle signs of pulmonary hypertension may be present. The *electrocardiogram* shows right ventricular hypertrophy with spiked P waves. *Roentgenographic studies* reveal cardiac enlargement and prominence of pulmonary veins, the right ventricle and atrium, and the main pulmonary artery; the left atrium is normal in size or only slightly enlarged. *Echocardiograms* may demonstrate a left atrial myxoma, cor triatriatum, or a mitral valve abnormality. *Cardiac catheterization* excludes the presence of a shunt and demonstrates pulmonary hypertension with an elevated pulmonary arterial wedge pressure. The left atrial pressure is normal if the lesion is proximal. Selective pulmonary arteriography may delineate the anatomic lesion. It is important to recognize this clinical pattern since cor triatriatum, left atrial myxoma, and supravalvular mitral webs are successfully managed surgically.

The differential diagnosis includes *pulmonary veno-occlusive disease*, an idiopathic process that produces obstructive lesions in the pulmonary veins of children and young adults. Obstruction may follow local injury due to toxins or viral agents. The patient is initially thought to have left-sided heart failure on the basis of congested lungs with apparent pulmonary edema. Dyspnea, fatigue, and pleural effusions are common, whereas cyanosis, digital clubbing, syncope, and hemoptysis are variable findings. The left atrial pressure is normal, while the pulmonary arterial wedge pressure may be normal or elevated. A normal wedge pressure may be due to formation of collaterals or assessment of an uninvolved segment. Angiographically there is no evidence of anatomic abnormalities of pulmonary venous return. Lung biopsy demonstrates pulmonary venous and, occasionally, arterial involvement. Pulmonary veins and venules demonstrate fibrous narrowing or occlusion and pulmonary artery thrombi. Therapy is nonspecific and disappointing, and survival ranges from weeks to months in infants and from months to years in adults.

15.58 ANOMALIES OF THE AORTIC ARCH

RIGHT AORTIC ARCH. In this abnormality the aorta curves to the right, and, if it descends on the right side of the vertebral column, it is usually associated with other cardiac malformations. It is found in about 20% of cases of tetralogy of Fallot and is common in truncus arteriosus. A right aortic arch without another anomaly is not associated with symptoms. Right aortic arch can be visualized on roentgenograms. The trachea is deviated to the left of the midline rather than to the right as in the presence of a normal left arch. The barium-filled esophagus is indented on its right border at the level of the aortic arch.

VASCULAR RINGS. Congenital abnormalities of the aortic arch and its major branches result in the formation of vascular rings around the trachea and esophagus with varying degrees of compression. The following are the more common anomalies: (1) double aortic arch (Figs. 15–54 and 15–55), (2) right aortic arch with left ligamentum arteriosum, (3) anomalous innominate artery arising further to the left on the arch than usual, (4) anomalous left carotid artery arising further to the right than usual and passing anterior to the trachea, and (5) anomalous left pulmonary artery (vascular sling). In the latter anomaly, the abnormal vessel arises from an elongated main pulmonary artery or from the right pulmonary artery. It courses between and compresses the trachea and esophagus. Associated congenital heart disease may be present in 5–50%, depending on the vascular anomaly.

If the vascular ring produces compression of the trachea and esophagus, symptoms are frequently present during infancy. Wheezing respirations tend to be chronic and are aggravated by crying, feeding, and flexion of the neck. Extension of the neck tends to relieve the noisy respiration. Vomiting is frequent. There may be a brassy cough, and pneumonia is common. Sudden death from aspiration is a threat. Roentgenographic examination of the barium-filled esophagus and aortography identify the anomaly (see Fig. 15–55). An aberrant right subclavian artery is commonly seen but does not cause compression of the trachea. *Diagnosis* is confirmed by 2-D echocardiography, MRI, digital subtraction angiography or, more often, angiography during cardiac catheterization.

Surgery is advised for symptomatic patients who have roentgenographic evidence of tracheal compression. The anterior vessel is usually divided in patients with double aortic arch (see Fig. 15–54). Compression produced by a right aortic arch and left ligamentum arteriosum is relieved by division of the latter. Anomalous innominate or carotid arteries cannot be divided; the tracheal compression is relieved by attaching the adventitia of these vessels to the sternum. Anomalous left pulmonary artery is corrected during cardiopulmonary bypass by division at its origin and reanastomosis to the main pulmonary artery after it has been brought in front of the trachea. In this condition, severe tracheomalacia may be present and result in a poor prognosis.

15.59 ANOMALOUS ORIGIN OF CORONARY ARTERIES

ANOMALOUS ORIGIN OF THE LEFT CORONARY ARTERY FROM THE PULMONARY ARTERY. In this anomaly the blood supply to the left ventricular myocardium is compromised. Soon after birth, as the pulmonary arterial pressure falls, the perfusion pressure to the left coronary artery becomes inadequate; myocardial infarction and fibrosis may result. In some cases, interarterial collateral anastomoses develop between the right and left coronary arteries. Blood flow in the left coronary artery is then reversed, and it empties into the pulmonary artery, resulting in a "myocardial steal" syndrome. The left ventricle becomes dilated and performance is decreased as a result of myocardial injury. Mitral incompetence is a frequent complication secondary to infarction of papillary muscle. Localized aneurysms may also develop in the left ventricle. Some patients have adequate myocardial blood flow and present later in life with a continuous murmur and small left to right shunt via the dilated coronary system (aorta–right coronary–left coronary–pulmonary artery).

Evidence of congestive heart failure becomes apparent within the 1st few months of life and is often precipitated by respiratory infection. Recurrent attacks of discomfort, restlessness, irritability, sweating, dyspnea, and pallor with or without mild cyanosis could be interpreted as due to angina pectoris. Cardiac enlargement is moderate to massive. Gallop rhythm is common. If present, murmurs may be of the nonspecific, ejection type or may be regurgitant because of mitral incompetence. Older patients with abundant intercoronary anastomoses may have continuous murmurs and little or no left ventricular dysfunction. However, during adolescence they may present with angina during exercise. Rare

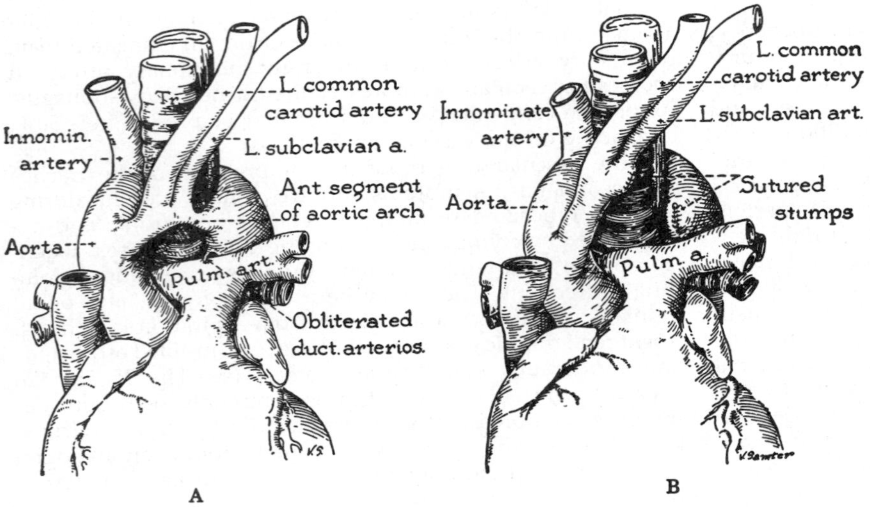

Figure 15–54. Double aortic arch. *A*, Small anterior segment of the double aortic arch (most common type). *B*, Operative procedure for the release of the vascular ring.

cases with anomalous right coronary artery may present in this manner.

Roentgenographic examination confirms the cardiomegaly, but the contour and pulsations are not specific unless there is a complicating ventricular aneurysm. The *electrocardiogram* resembles the pattern described in lateral wall myocardial infarction in adults. A QR pattern followed by inverted T waves is seen in leads I and aVL. The left ventricular surface leads (V_5 and V_6) may also show deep Q waves and exhibit elevated ST segments and inverted T waves (Fig. 15–56). In older patients, exercise study is helpful, as ST-T wave changes or symptoms, or both, occur. *Two-dimensional echocardiography* may suggest the diagnosis but is not always reliable. *Aortography* is diagnostic; there is immediate opacification of only the right coronary artery. Generally, this vessel is large and tortuous. After filling of the intercoronary anastomoses, the left coronary artery and the pulmonary artery are in turn opacified. Selective pulmonary arteriography may opacify the anomalous left coronary artery. Selective left ventriculography in the infantile type reveals a dilated left ventricle that empties poorly.

Usually death from heart failure occurs within the first 6 mo. Those who survive usually have abundant intercoronary anastomoses. Medical management includes standard therapy for heart failure (diuretics, digoxin, captopril) and for controlling ischemia (nitrates, calcium channel blockers, beta-blocking agents).

Surgical treatment consists of detaching the anomalous coronary artery from the pulmonary artery and anastomosing it to the aorta to establish normal myocardial perfusion. The seriously ill infant with a tiny left coronary artery may present a difficult technical problem. In past years ligation of the anomalous left coronary artery at its origin was carried out to prevent runoff from the coronary circuit and possibly to increase myocardial perfusion by collateral circulation. This operation occasionally may still be required in some cases.

ANOMALOUS ORIGIN OF THE RIGHT CORONARY ARTERY FROM THE PULMONARY ARTERY. This anomaly

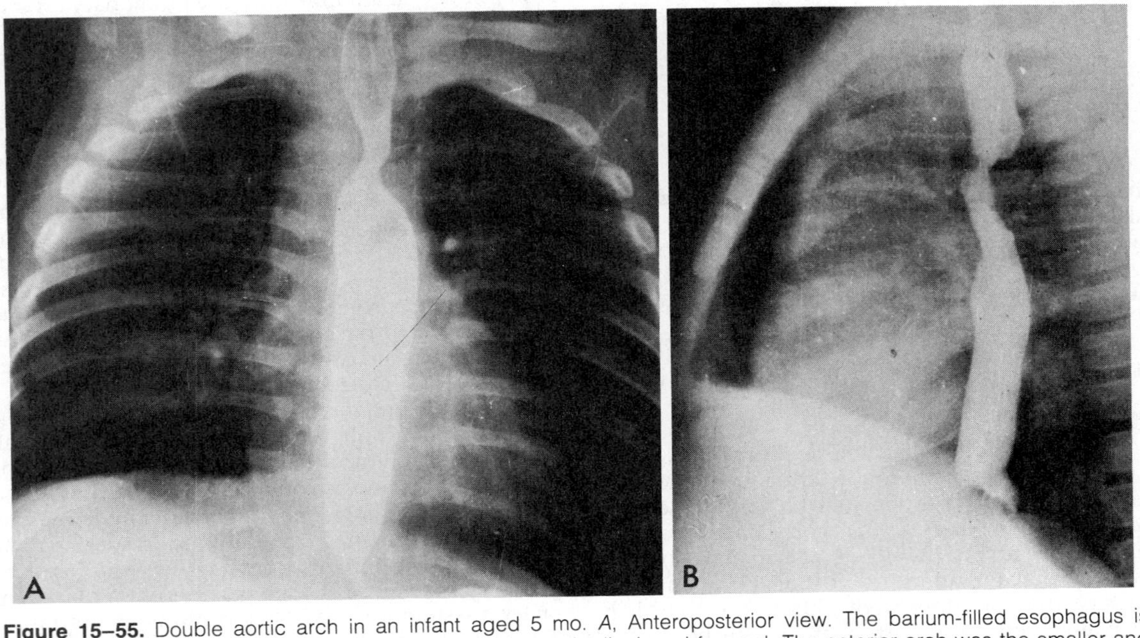

Figure 15–55. Double aortic arch in an infant aged 5 mo. *A*, Anteroposterior view. The barium-filled esophagus is constricted on both sides. *B*, Lateral view. The esophagus is displaced forward. The anterior arch was the smaller and was divided at operation.

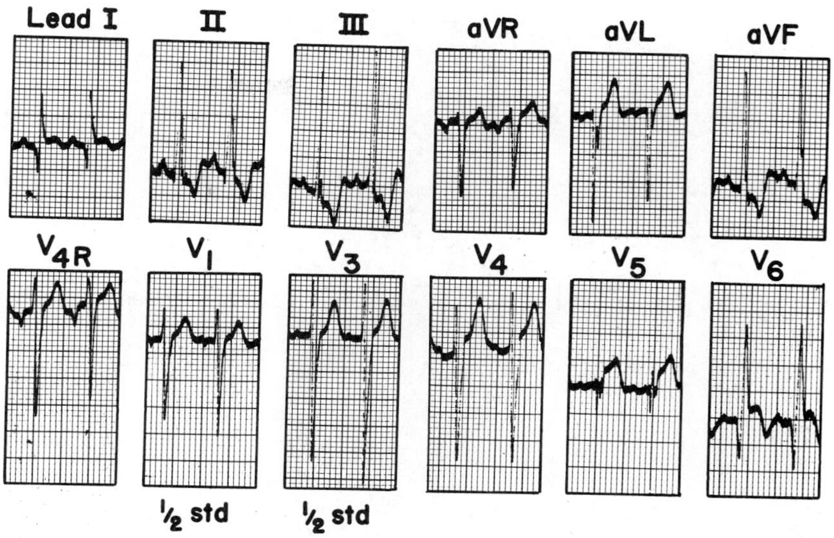

Figure 15–56. Electrocardiogram of a 3-mo-old child with anomalous origin of the left coronary artery from the pulmonary artery. Lateral myocardial infarction is present as evidenced by abnormally large and wide Q waves in leads I, V_5, and V_6, elevated ST segment in V_5 and V_6, and inversion of TV_6.

rarely manifests in infancy or early childhood. The left coronary artery is enlarged while the right is thin-walled and mildly enlarged. In early infancy perfusion of the right coronary artery is from the pulmonary artery, whereas later perfusion is from collaterals of the left coronary vessel. Angina and sudden death can occur in adolescence or adulthood. When recognized, this anomaly should be repaired by re-anastomosis of the right coronary artery to the aorta.

ECTOPIC ORIGIN OF CORONARY ARTERY FROM THE AORTA WITH ABERRANT PROXIMAL COURSE. The aberrant artery may be a left, right, or major branch coronary artery. The site of origin may be the wrong sinus of Valsalva or a proximal coronary artery. The ostium may be hypoplastic, slit-like, or of normal caliber. The aberrant vessel may pass anteriorly, posteriorly, or between the aorta and right ventricular outflow tract; it may tunnel in the conal or interventricular septal tissue. Obstruction due to hypoplasia of the ostia, tunneling between the aorta and right ventricular outflow tract or interventricular septum, and acute angulation produce focal myocardial fibrosis or myocardial infarction. Unobstructive vessels produce no symptoms. Patients with this extremely rare abnormality manifest myocardial infarction, ventricular arrhythmias, sudden death in young adult or adolescent athletes, angina pectoris, and syncope.

Diagnostic evaluation should include an electrocardiogram, stress testing, 2-D echocardiography, and cardiac catheterization with coronary angiography.

Treatment is indicated for obstructed vessels and includes aortoplasty with reanastomosis of the aberrant vessel or, more often, coronary artery bypass grafting with the internal mammary artery.

15.60 PRIMARY PULMONARY HYPERTENSION

Primary pulmonary hypertension is a disease of unknown origin characterized by hypertension of the lesser circulation and right-sided heart failure. It may occur at any age, although most pediatric patients are between 10 and 20 yr of age. A genetic component may be present, and there may be an immunologic disorder. Pulmonary hypertension is associated with precapillary obstruction of the pulmonary vascular bed due to hyperplasia of the muscular and elastic tissues and to the thickened intima of the small pulmonary arteries and arterioles. Atherosclerotic changes may be found in the larger pulmonary arteries. Other causes of pulmonary heart disease (chronic cor pulmonale) are absent, and there is no evidence of emphysema, cystic fibrosis, bronchopulmonary dysplasia, or kyphoscoliosis. Recurrent pulmonary emboli may produce the same clinical picture, but this disease is rare in childhood. Severe pulmonary hypertension may result from myriads of minute microemboli from an indwelling intravascular catheter inserted for hyperalimentation. Primary pulmonary hypertension must also be differentiated from elevated pulmonary pressure resulting from persistent obstruction of the upper airway (e.g., gross enlargement of the tonsils and adenoids), liver disease, or chronic pulmonary parenchymal disease. Female patients outnumber males 1.7:1.

HEMODYNAMICS. Pulmonary hypertension places an afterload burden on the right ventricle, which results in right ventricular hypertension. Dilatation of the pulmonary artery is present and pulmonary valve insufficiency may occur. At the late stages cardiac output is decreased.

CLINICAL MANIFESTATIONS. The predominant symptoms include effort intolerance and fatigability; occasionally, there is precordial chest pain, dizziness, or syncope. Peripheral cyanosis may be present and is associated with cold extremities; in the late stages of the disease the patient may have a gray appearance associated with low cardiac output. Arterial oxygen saturation is usually normal. If right-sided heart failure has supervened, the jugular venous pressure is elevated and hepatomegaly and edema are present. Jugular venous "a" waves are present, and when there is functional tricuspid insufficiency, a conspicuous jugular "cv" wave and systolic hepatic pulsations are manifest. The heart is moderately enlarged, and there is a right ventricular heave. The 1st heart sound is often followed by a pulmonic ejection click. The systolic murmur is soft and short and is sometimes followed by a blowing diastolic murmur due to pulmonary incompetence. The 2nd heart sound is closely split, loud, and sometimes booming; it is frequently palpable. A presystolic gallop rhythm may be audible down the left sternal border.

Roentgenograms reveal a prominent pulmonary artery and right ventricle (Fig. 15–57). The pulmonary vascularity in the hilar areas may be prominent and contrast with the peripheral lung fields, which are clear. The *electrocardiogram* shows right ventricular hypertrophy with spiked P waves.

DIAGNOSIS. At cardiac catheterization this condition must be differentiated from Eisenmenger syndrome (see Sec. 15.24), which is associated with a communication between the left and right sides of the heart or great arteries, as well as from

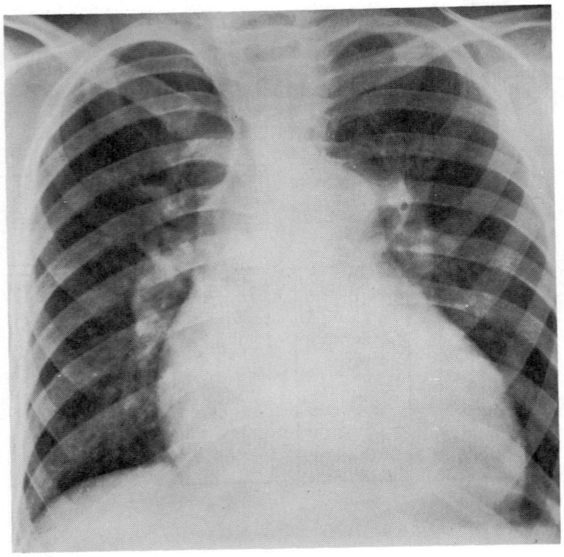

Figure 15–57. Roentgenogram in primary pulmonary hypertension. Note the moderate cardiac enlargement, dilatation of the pulmonary artery, and relative pulmonary undervascularity in the outer two thirds of the lung fields.

left-sided obstructive lesions that result in pulmonary venous hypertension (see Sec. 15.57). With left-sided heart disease, the pulmonary arterial wedge pressure is significantly elevated. The risks of cardiac catheterization may be high in severely ill patients with primary pulmonary hypertension, and syncope or death may occur after pulmonary artery angiography (which should rarely be done in the most severely ill individuals). The presence of pulmonary artery hypertension with a normal pulmonary capillary wedge pressure is diagnostic.

PROGNOSIS. Primary pulmonary hypertension is progressive, and often there is no specific treatment. Success has been reported in children with significant pulmonary vasoreactivity with the use of calcium channel blocking agents. Continuous intravenous prostacyclin may provide temporary relief. Heart/lung or lung transplantation has been carried out successfully in some adults and a few children with severe pulmonary vascular disease. The terminal event most often is sudden in a patient with low cardiac output and is related to a lethal arrhythmia.

15.61 PRINCIPLES OF TREATMENT OF CONGENITAL HEART DISEASE

Most patients who have mild congenital heart disease require no treatment. Parents and the child should be made aware that a normal life is expected and that no restriction of the child's activities is necessary. Overprotective parents may use the presence of a mild congenital lesion or even a functional heart murmur as a means to excessively control the child's activities. Although he or she may not express fears overtly, the child may become quite anxious regarding early death or debilitation, especially when an adult member of the family develops symptomatic heart disease. The family may have an unexpressed fear of sudden death, and the rarity of this manifestation should be emphasized in discussions directed at improving their understanding of the child's congenital heart defect. The difference between congenital heart disease and degenerative coronary disease in adults should be outlined. General health maintenance, including a well-balanced diet, prevention of anemia, and the usual immunization program, should be encouraged.

Even patients with moderate to severe heart disease need not be markedly restricted in physical activities. Physical education should be modified appropriately to the child's capacity to participate. Rough, competitive sports should be discouraged. Patients with severe heart disease with decreased exercise tolerance will tend to limit their own activities. Transportation to school may be helpful so that fatigue will not interfere with classroom activities. Dyspnea, headache, and fatigability in cyanotic patients may be a sign of increasing hypoxemia and may require some limitation of activities among those for whom specific medical or surgical treatment is not available.

Bacterial infections should be treated vigorously, but the presence of congenital heart disease is not an appropriate reason to utilize antibiotics indiscriminately. Prophylaxis against infective endocarditis should be carried out during extensive dental procedures, during instrumentation of the urinary tract, and prior to lower gastrointestinal manipulation. Treatment of iron deficiency anemia is especially important in cyanotic patients who will improve their exercise tolerance and general well-being with adequate hemoglobin levels. On the other hand, these patients should also be carefully observed for polycythemia. Cyanotic patients should avoid situations in which dehydration may occur. High altitudes and sudden changes in thermal environment should also be avoided. Venisection with volume replacement should be carried out at intervals in the presence of severe polycythemia (Hct $> 65\%$) in inoperable patients. Patients with severe congenital heart disease or a history of rhythm disturbance should be carefully monitored during anesthesia for even routine surgical procedures. Women should be counseled on risks associated with child-bearing and on the use of contraceptives and tubal ligation. Pregnancy may be especially dangerous for patients having chronic cyanosis and/or pulmonary artery hypertension. However, women with mild to moderate heart disease and many of those who have had corrective surgery can have normal pregnancies.

The treatment for congestive heart failure is described in

Sec. 15.73, for paroxysmal hypercyanotic attacks in Sec. 15.11, and for cardiac arrhythmias in Sec. 15.62. Appropriate surgical procedures for specific cardiac lesions are discussed in the relevant sections of this chapter.

Recently, *cardiac transplantation* has been more frequently used for children and adolescents (see Sec. 6.45). This measure may be indicated for patients in whom all medical and surgical therapy has been exhausted, and in whom the great veins and arteries are of sufficient size and in an acceptable position so that a donor heart can be implanted. In addition, pulmonary arterial vascular disease should not be present. Most pediatric candidates for cardiac transplantation have cardiomyopathy with chronic congestive heart failure and extremely poor myocardial performance. Although the long-term prognosis is unknown, some patients are living on an immunosuppressive regimen (cyclosporine) years after transplantation. The quality of life for most has been acceptable, and for selected patients with no other options, this mode of therapy may become an acceptable alternative.

POSTOPERATIVE PERIOD (Sec. 6.52). After successful open heart surgery, the postoperative course depends on numerous factors. The type of congenital defect operated upon, the age and condition of the patient prior to surgery, the events in the operating room, and the quality of the postoperative care will influence the patient's course following surgery. Many patients will have a benign postoperative period without complications, but others may be in a precarious state for hours or days after the operation.

Postoperative care should be initiated in the intensive care unit by a staff experienced with the unique problems encountered after open heart surgery (Sec. 6.52). A femoral arterial catheter is inserted prior to open heart surgery to allow direct arterial pressure measurements and arterial samplings for blood gas determinations. A second catheter positioned in the inferior vena cava via the saphenous or femoral vein is used for measuring central venous pressure. Left atrial or pulmonary artery catheters are often also utilized as are pacing wires on the atrium and ventricle.

Functional failures in one system may cause profound physiologic and biochemical changes in another (Table 15–11). Respiratory insufficiency, for example, will lead to hypoxia, acidosis, and hypercarbia, which in turn will compromise cardiac, pulmonary, vascular, and renal function. The latter problems cannot be managed successfully until adequate ventilation is re-established. Thus, it is essential that the primary source of each postoperative problem be identified and treated.

Respiratory failure is a major postoperative complication encountered after open heart surgery. Cardiopulmonary bypass carried out in the presence of pulmonary congestion results in decreased lung compliance, copious tracheal and bronchial secretions, atelectasis, and increased breathing efforts. Since fatigue and subsequently hypoventilation and acidosis may rapidly ensue, mechanical positive-pressure endotracheal ventilation is instituted immediately following open heart surgery. This is continued for a minimum of several hours in relatively stable patients and up to 2–3 days or more in severely ill patients, especially infants.

Cardiac rhythm disorders must be diagnosed quickly since a prolonged untreated arrhythmia may add a severe hemodynamic burden to the heart in the critical early postoperative period. Injury to the heart's conduction system during surgery can cause postoperative *complete heart block.* This rare complication is treated with surgically placed pacing wires that are later removed. Occasionally, heart block will become permanent, requiring insertion of implanted or venous pacemakers, but in most instances this rhythm pattern is transient, and only temporary pacing wires are needed. *Tachyarrhythmias* are more often a problem in postoperative patients.

The *electrocardiogram* should be monitored continuously during the postoperative period. A change in the heart rate may be the first indication of a serious complication, such as hemorrhage, hypothermia, hypoventilation, or congestive heart failure.

Congestive heart failure with poor cardiac output (see Table 15–11) following cardiac surgery may be secondary to respiratory failure, serious arrhythmias, myocardial injury, blood loss, hypervolemia, or significant residual hemodynamic abnormality. Specific treatment related to etiology should be instituted. Dopamine, dobutamine, digoxin, and nitroprusside are the cardioactive agents most often used in patients with myocardial dysfunction in the early postoperative period; diuretic therapy is also often required (Sec. 6.4). Epinephrine or norepinephrine is reserved for patients with severe cardiogenic shock, as are extracorporeal membrane oxygenation (ECMO) and intra-aortic balloon counterpulsation pumps.

Acidosis secondary to low cardiac output, renal failure, or hypovolemia must be prevented or promptly corrected. An arterial pH below 7.30 may result in a decrease in cardiac output with increase in lactic acid production and may be the forerunner of a series of arrhythmias or cardiac arrest.

Kidney function may be compromised by congestive heart failure and further impaired by prolonged cardiopulmonary bypass (see Table 15–11). Persistent anuria or oliguria indicates poor cardiac function, hypokalemia, and/or acute renal failure. Blood and fluid replacement and/or a cardiotonic regimen will rapidly re-establish normal urine flow in patients with hypovolemia or cardiac failure, but renal failure secondary to tubular injury may require peritoneal dialysis.

The *postcardiotomy syndrome* may occur toward the end of the first postoperative week or sometimes be delayed until weeks or months after operation. This febrile illness is characterized by pericarditis and pleurisy, which in most instances is self-limiting and associated with a benign course. When pericardial fluid accumulates, the potential danger of cardiac tamponade should be recognized. Symptomatic patients usually respond to salicylates or indomethacin and bed rest. Occasionally steroid therapy is required. A prolonged illness or late recurrences are not unusual.

Hemolysis of probable mechanical origin is rarely seen after repair of endocardial cushion defects or the insertion of an artificial prosthetic valve. It occurs secondary to unusual turbulence of blood at increased pressure. Reoperation may be necessary in rare patients with severe and progressive hemolysis who require frequent blood transfusions, but in most instances the problem slowly regresses.

INFECTION. Sepsis with infective endocarditis is an infrequent complication but can be difficult to manage, especially when prosthetic patches or valves are used (see Sec. 15.66). Other problems are noted in Table 15–11.

PROGNOSIS. Patients who have had palliative procedures for extremely complex heart disease may lead limited but productive lives. Such patients require careful follow-up and various restrictions depending on the severity of their disease. The great majority of congenital heart defects can be corrected by open heart surgery or interventional catheterization (balloon angioplasty, umbrella closure); in most patients cardiac dynamics are improved and symptoms disappear. Some patients may develop late complications or require reoperation. Children who have undergone repair of complex cardiac lesions should be followed closely with appropriate laboratory tests (e.g., Holter monitors, exercise studies, echocardiograms, radionuclide studies, and, when indicated, cardiac catheterizations). The need for special studies should be decided upon after careful clinical evaluation, electrocardiogram, and chest roentgenogram. After successful repair of simple lesions with no evidence of residual abnormalities, such as patent ductus arteriosus, atrial septal defect, or

TABLE 15–11. Systems Approach to Postoperative Care Following Surgery for Congenital Heart Disease

System and Problem	Etiology	Treatment or Prevention
Nervous System		
Coma	Global ischemia	Monitor and treat increased intracranial pressure
	Prolonged anesthetic effect	Reverse anethesia
	Hypoglycemia	Glucose
Focal lesions	Emboli (air, thrombi)	
Seizures	Metabolic (hyponatremia, hypoglycemia), ischemic, embolic disturbances	Phenytoin, correct metabolic disturbances
Diaphragm paralysis	Phrenic nerve injury	Respiratory care
Vocal cord paralysis	Traction on recurrent laryngeal nerve	Respiratory care
Horner syndrome	Dissection of subclavian artery with sympathetic chain injury	None
Paraplegia	Postcoarctation repair with spinal artery ischemia	Avoid ischemia
Pain	Surgical trauma	Fentanyl, morphine
Anxiety	Stress	Versed, Valium
Respiratory System		
ARDS* postpump syndrome	Unknown; possible release of vasoactive substances by cardiopulmonary bypass	PEEP†, mechanical ventilation, oxygen
Pulmonary edema	Heart failure, left-sided obstruction, fluid overload	Diuresis, PEEP, mechanical ventilation, inotropic agents
Pleural effusions	Hemothorax	Thoracocentesis
	Early serous effusion	Thoracocentesis
	Delayed postpericardiotomy	Anti-inflammatory agents
Chylothorax	Injury to thoracic duct	NPO‡, or medium-chain triglyceride diet Rarely surgical ligation of thoracic duct
Atelectasis	Hypoventilation, poor cough	Chest physiotherapy, PEEP
Pneumonia	Aspiration, nosocomial, bacteremia	Identify bacterial/viral (respiratory syncytial virus) etiology; specific antimicrobial therapy
Pulmonary hypertension	Repair of TAPVR, Norwood 1st stage, 21-trisomy; prior preoperative pulmonary hypertension	Hyperventilation, hyperoxia, fentanyl, nitroprusside, prostaglandins
Stridor	Vocal cord edema, paralysis	Steroids, rarely tracheotomy
Cardiovascular System		
Bradycardia, sick sinus, atrioventricular block	Injury to interatrial or interventricular conduction system	Atropine, isoproterenol, pacemaker
Right bundle branch block	Right ventriculotomy	Atrial approach to ventricular septal defect repair of tetralogy of Fallot
Tachyarrhythmias	Supraventricular, junctional tachycardia	Antiarrhythmic agents
	Ventricular tachycardia	Defibrillation, antiarrhythmic agents
Poor cardiac output	Cardiogenic—right ventriculotomy or cardiac stun (prolonged pump and cross-clamp time) or infarction	Inotropic agents, support preload, reduce afterload
	Hypocalcemia	Calcium
	Hypovolemia	Support preload
Pericardial tamponade	Pericardial effusion, acute hemorrhage	Pericardiocentesis
	Serous postpericardiotomy	Anti-inflammatory agents
Hypertension	Stress-pain	Analgesia
	Postcoarctectomy syndrome	Nitroprusside
Mesenteric arteritis	Postcoarctectomy syndrome	NPO, nitroprusside
Renal-Metabolic System		
Prerenal oliguria	Hypovolemia	Fluid administration
	Poor cardiac output	Inotropic agents
Renal failure	Hypotension, prolonged pump-cross clamp time, acute tubular necrosis	Improve blood pressure, diuretics
Edema	Fluid resuscitation, capillary leak, poor cardiac output, elevated systemic venous pressure	Diruesis, inotropic agents
Hyponatremia	Dilutional, SIADH§	Fluid restriction
	Diuretics	Fluid restriction
Hyperglycemia	Hypothermia-inhibition of insulin	None needed
Hypoglycemia	Rebound following hyperglycemia, hepatic failure	Glucose infusion
Hematologic System		
Hemorrhage	Abnormal PT,‖ PTT,** thrombocytopenia	Correct coagulopathy
	Surgical leak	Reoperation, suture
Shunt thrombosis	Poor cardiac output, hypovolemia	Fluids, heparin
Anemia (usually reflecting reduced blood volume)	Hemorrhage, hemolysis	Transfuse packed red blood cells
Graft-versus-host disease	Infusion of viable leukocytes to patients with DiGeorge syndrome	Irradiate blood products

TABLE 15–11. Systems Approach to Postoperative Care Following Surgery for Congenital Heart Disease *Continued*

System and Problem	Etiology	Treatment or Prevention
Infectious Diseases		
Wound infection (cutaneous, costochondral, sternotomy, mediastinitis, vascular lines, chest tubes)	Contamination in operating room	Antibiotics
Endocarditis	*Staphylococcus epidermidis, Corynebacterium,* contamination in operating room	Antibiotics
Cystitis, pyelonephritis	Contamination of indwelling urinary catheter	Antibiotics, remove catheter
Hepatitis	Blood borne: Cytomegalovirus, Epstein-Barr virus, hepatitis B and hepatitis C viruses	Screen blood products
Postperfusion syndrome (fever, hepatosplenomegaly, atypical lymphocytes, lymphadenopathy, transient rash)	Cytomegalovirus, Epstein-Barr virus	Screen blood products
Psychosocial Conditions		
Anxiety, separation	Age-related, fears, etc.	Preparedness (videotape, play acting); parent visitation, sedation

*ARDS = adult respiratory distress syndrome.
†PEEP = positive end-expiratory pressure.
‡NPO = nothing *per os* (by mouth).
§SIADH = syndrome of inappropriate antidiuretic hormone.
||PT = prothrombin time.
**PTT = partial thromboplastin time.

valvular pulmonary stenosis, patients require very few specific follow-up studies, and should be encouraged to lead active and full lives.

THE NEONATAL CIRCULATION

Barst RJ, Gersony WM: The pharmacological treatment of patent ductus arteriosus: A review of the evidence. Drugs 38:250, 1989.

Dawes GS: Fetal and Neonatal Physiology. Chicago, Year Book Medical Publishers, 1968.

Freed MD, Heymann MA, Lewis AB, et al: Prostaglandin E in infants with ductus arteriosus—dependent congenital heart disease. Circulation 64:899, 1981.

Friedman WF: The intrinsic physiologic properties of the developing heart. Prog Cardiovasc Dis 15:87, 1972.

Gersony WM: Neonatal pulmonary hypertension: Pathophysiology, classification, and etiology. Clin Perinatol 11:517, 1984.

Gersony WM, Peckham GJ, Ellison RC, et al: Effects of indomethacin in premature infants with patent ductus arteriosus: Results of a national collaborative study. J Pediatr 102:895, 1983.

INCIDENCE AND ETIOLOGY

Dennis NR, Warren J: Risks to offspring of patients with some common congenital heart defects. J Med Genet 18:8, 1981.

Fyler DC, Buckley LP, Hellenbrand WE, et al: Report of the New England Regional Infant Cardiac Program. Pediatrics 65(Suppl):377, 1980.

Hoffman JIE: Congenital heart disease: Incidence and inheritance. Pediatr Clin North Am 37:25, 1990.

Lin AE, Garver KL: Genetic counseling for congenital heart defects. J Pediatr 113:1105, 1988.

van Mierop LHS, Kutsche LM: Cardiovascular anomalies in DiGeorge syndrome and importance of neural crest as a possible pathogenetic factor. Am J Cardiol 58:133, 1986.

Nadas A, Ellison R, Weidman W: Report from the joint study on the natural history of congenital heart defects. Circulation 56(2):Suppl 1, Aug, 1977.

Noonan JA: Syndromes associated with cardiac defects. Cardiovasc Clin 11:97, 1980.

Nora JJ, Nora AH: Maternal transmission of congenital heart disease: New recurrence risk figures and the questions of cytoplasmic inheritance and vulnerability to teratogens. Am J Cardiol 59:459, 1987.

Somerville J: Congenital heart disease in the adolescent. Arch Dis Child 64:771, 1989.

Whittemore R, Hobbins JC, Engle MA: Pregnancy and its outcome in women with and without surgical treatment of congenital heart disease. Am J Cardiol 50:641, 1982.

TETRALOGY OF FALLOT AND PULMONARY ATRESIA

Barratt-Boyes BG, Neutze MJ: Primary repair of tetralogy of Fallot in infancy using profound hypothermia with circulatory arrest and limited cardiopulmonary bypass. Ann Surg 178:406, 1974.

Dabizzi RP, Caprioli G, Aiazzi L, et al: Distribution and anomalies of coronary arteries in tetralogy of Fallot. Circulation 61:95, 1980.

Garson A, Nihill MR, McNamara DG, et al: Status of the adult and adolescent after repair of tetralogy of Fallot. Circulation 59:1232, 1976.

Guntheroth WG, Morgan BC: Physiologic studies of paroxysmal hyperpnea in cyanotic congenital heart disease. Circulation 31:70, 1965.

Kirklin JW, Blackstone EH, Kirklin JK, et al: Surgical results and protocols in the spectrum of tetralogy of Fallot. Ann Surg 198:251, 1983.

McCaughan BC, Danielson GK, Driscoll DJ, et al: Tetralogy of Fallot with absent pulmonary valve: Early and late results of surgical treatment. J Thorac Cardiovasc Surg 89:280, 1985.

Oku H, Shirotani H, Sunakawa A, et al: Postoperative long term results in total correction of tetralogy of Fallot: Hemodynamics and cardiac function. Ann Thorac Surg 41:413, 1986.

Pinsky WW, Arciniegas E: Tetralogy of Fallot. Pediatr Clin North Am 37:179, 1990.

Rocchinl AP: Hemodynamic abnormalities in response to supine exercise in patients after operative correction of tetralogy of Fallot after early childhood. Am J Cardiol 48:325, 1981.

Zhao HX, Miller DC, Reitz BA, et al: Surgical repair of tetralogy of Fallot. J Thorac Cardiovasc Surg 89:204, 1985.

TRANSPOSITION OF THE GREAT ARTERIES

Bowyer JJ, Busst CM, Till JA, et al: Exercise ability after Mustard's operation. Arch Dis Child 65:865, 1990.

Deanfield JE: Transposition of the great arteries: To switch or not to switch? Curr Opin Pediatr 1:85, 1989.

Duncan WJ, Freedom RM, Rowe RD, et al: Echocardiographic features before and after the Jatene procedure (anatomical correction) for transposition of the great vessels. Am Heart J 102:227, 1981.

Gillette PC, Kugler JD, Gutgesell HP, et al: Mechanisms of cardiac arrhythmias after the Mustard operation for transposition of the great arteries. Am J Cardiol 45:1225, 1980.

Hagler D, Ritter D, Mair D, et al: Clinical angiographic and hemodynamic assessment of late results after Mustard operation. Circulation 57:1214, 1978.

Hayes CJ, Gersony WM: Arrhythmias after the Mustard operation for transposition of the great arteries: A long term study. J Am Coll Cardiol 7:133, 1986.

Kirklin JW, Colvin EV, McConnell ME, et al: Complete transposition of the great arteries: Treatment in the current era. Pediatr Clin North Am 37:171, 1990.

Pacifico AD, Stewart RW, Bargeron LM: Repair of transposition of great arteries with ventricular septal defect by an arterial switch operation. Circulation 68:49, 1983.

Quaegebeur JM, Rohmer J, Ottenkamp J, et al: The arterial switch operation. J Thorac Cardiovasc Surg 92:361, 1986.

Rashkind WJ, Miller WW: Creation of an atrial septal defect without thoracotomy: A palliative approach to complete transposition of the great vessels. JAMA 196:991, 1966.

Rastelli GC, McGoon DC, Wallace RB: Anatomic correction of transposition of the great arteries with ventricular septal defect and subpulmonary stenosis. J Thorac Cardiovasc Surg 58:545, 1969.

Wilcox BR, Ho SY, Macartney FJ, et al: Surgical anatomy of double-outlet right ventricle with situs solitus and atrioventricular concordance. J Thorac Cardiovasc Surg 82:405, 1981.

PULMONARY VASCULAR DISEASE

Friedman WF, Heiferman M: Clinical problems of pulmonary vascular disease. Am J Cardiol 56:31, 1982.
Heath D, Edwards JE: The pathology of hypertensive pulmonary vascular disease. Circulation 18:533, 1958.
Hoffman JIE, Rudolph AM, Heymann MA: Pulmonary vascular disease with congenital heart lesions: Pathologic features and causes. Circulation 64:873, 1981.
Wood P: Pulmonary hypertension. Mod Conc Cardiovasc Dis 28:513, 1959.

TRICUSPID ATRESIA

Fontan F, Deville C, Quaegebeur J, et al: Repair of tricuspid atresia in 100 patients. J Thorac Cardiovasc Surg 85:647, 1983.
Mair DD: The Fontan procedure: The first 20 years. Curr Opin Pediatr 1:94, 1989.
Marino B, Marcelletti C: The cavopulmonary anastomosis in congenital heart disease: A consideration of the classic and bidirectional palliations. Curr Opin Pediatr 2:973, 1990.
Sade RM, Fyfe DA: Tricuspid atresia: Current concepts in diagnosis and treatment. Pediatr Clin North Am 37:151, 1990.

EBSTEIN DISEASE

Genton E, Blount SG: The spectrum of Ebstein's anomaly. Am Heart J 73:395, 1967.
Mair DD, Seward JB, Driscoll DJ, et al: Surgical repair of Ebstein's anomaly: Selection of patients and early and later operative results. Circulation 72:70, 1985.
Zuberbuhler JR, Allwork SP, Anderson RH: The spectrum of Ebstein's anomaly of the tricuspid valve. J Thorac Cardiovasc Surg 77:202, 1979.

ATRIAL SEPTAL DEFECT AND ATRIOVENTRICULAR CANAL

Clapp SK, Perry BL, Farooki ZQ, et al: Surgical and medical results of complete atrioventricular canal: A ten-year review. Am J Cardiol 59:454, 1987.
Marino B, Vairo U, Corno A, et al: Atrioventricular canal in Down syndrome. Am J Dis Child 144:1120, 1990.
Santon E: Repair of atrioventricular septal defects in infancy. J Thorac Cardiovasc Surg 91:505, 1986.

VENTRICULAR SEPTAL DEFECT

Beerman LB, Park SC, Fischer DR, et al: Ventricular septal defect associated with aneurysm of the membranous septum. J Am Coll Cardiol 5:118, 1985.
Edwards JE: The pathology of ventricular septal defect. Semin Radiol 1:2, 1966.
Leung MP, Beerman LB, Siewers RD, et al: Long term follow up after aortic valvuloplasty and defect closure in ventricular septal defect with aortic regurgitation. Am J Cardiol 60:890, 1987.
Levin AR, Spach MS, Canent RV Jr, et al: Intracardiac pressure-flow dynamics in isolated ventricular septal defects. Circulation 35:430, 1967.
Sigman JM, Perry BL, Behrendt DM, et al: Ventricular septal defect: Results after repair in infancy. Am J Cardiol 39:66, 1977.
Weidman WH, Blount SG Jr, DuShane JW, et al: Clinical course in ventricular septal defect. Circulation 56:156, 1977.
Weidman WH, Gersony WM, Nugent EW, et al: Indirect assessment of severity in ventricular septal defect. Circulation 56(Suppl):24, 1977.

PULMONARY STENOSIS WITH NORMAL AORTIC ROOT

Benson LN, Freedom RM: Interventional cardiac catheterization. Curr Opin Pediatr 1:106, 1989.
Ellison RC, Freedom RM, Keane JF, et al: Indirect assessment of severity in pulmonary stenosis. Circulation 56(Suppl):14, 1977.
Nugent EW, Freedom RM, Nora JJ, et al: Clinical course in pulmonary stenosis. Circulation 56(Suppl):38, 1977.

TOTAL ANOMALOUS PULMONARY VENOUS RETURN

Delisle G, Masahiko A, Calder AL, et al: Total anomalous pulmonary venous connection: Report of 93 autopsied cases with emphasis on diagnostic and surgical considerations. Am Heart J 91:99, 1976.
Duff DG, Nihill MR, McNamara DG: Infradiaphragmatic total anomalous pulmonary venous return. Review of clinical and pathological findings and results of operation in 28 cases. Br Heart J 39:619, 1977.
Gersony WM: Presentation, diagnosis and natural history of total anomalous pulmonary venous drainage. *In*: Godman MJ, Marguis RM (eds): Paediatric Cardiology. Edinburgh, London and New York, Churchill Livingstone, 1979.
Turley K, Tucker WY, Ullyot DJ, et al: Total anomalous pulmonary venous connection in infancy: Influence of age and type of lesion. Am J Cardiol 45:92, 1980.
Whight CM, Barratt-Boyes BG, Calder AL, et al: Total anomalous pulmonary venous connection. Long-term results following repair in infancy. J Thorac Cardiovasc Surg 75:52, 1978.

AORTIC STENOSIS

Donner R, et al: Improved prediction of left ventricular pressure by echocardiography in children with aortic stenosis. J Am Coll Cardiol 3:349, 1984.
Doyle EF, Arumugham P, Lara E, et al: Sudden death in young patients with congenital aortic stenosis. Pediatrics 53:481, 1974.
Edmunds LH, Wagner HR, Heyman MA: Aortic valvulotomy in neonates. Circulation 61:421, 1980.
Freedom RM, Dische MR, Rowe RD: Pathologic anatomy of subaortic stenosis and atresia in the first year of life. Am J Cardiol 39:1035, 1977.
Friedman WF, Pappelbaum SJ: Indications for hemodynamic evaluation and surgery in congenital aortic stenosis. Pediatr Clin North Am 18:1207, 1971.
Leichter DA, Sullivan I, Gersony WM: "Acquired" discrete subvalvular aortic stenosis: Natural history and hemodynamics. J Am Coll Cardiol 14:1539, 1989.
McCue CM, Spicuzza TJ, Robertson LW, et al: Familial supravalvular aortic stenosis. J Pediatr 73:889, 1968.
Radtke W, Lock J: Balloon dilation. Pediatr Clin North Am 37:193, 1990.
Sandor GG, Olley PM, Trusler GA, et al: Long-term follow-up of patients after valvotomy for congenital valvular aortic stenosis in children: A clinical and actuarial follow-up. J Thorac Cardiovasc Surg 80:171, 1980.
Wagner HR, Weidman WH, Ellison RC, et al: Indirect assessment of severity in aortic stenosis. Circulation 56(Suppl):20, 1977.

MITRAL VALVE ANOMALIES

Bisset GS, Schwartz DC, Meyer RA, et al: Clinical spectrum and long-term follow-up of isolated mitral valve prolapse in 119 children. Circulation 62:423, 1980.
Devereux RB, Kramer-Fox R, Kligfield P: Mitral valve prolapse: Causes, clinical manifestations, and management. Ann Intern Med 111:305, 1989.
Glesby MJ, Pyeritz RE: Association of mitral valve prolapse and systemic abnormalities of connective tissue: A phenotypic continuum. JAMA 262:523, 1989.
John S, Krishnaswami S, Jairaj PS, et al: The profile and surgical management of mitral stenosis in young patients. J Thorac Cardiovasc Surg 69:631, 1975.
Marks AR, Choong CY, Sanfilippo AJ, et al: Identification of high-risk and low-risk subgroups of patients with mitral-valve prolapse. N Engl J Med 320:1031, 1989.
Reed GE, Pooley RW, Moggio RA: Durability of measured mitral annuloplasty: Seventeen year study. J Thorac Cardiovasc Surg 79:321, 1980.

DEXTROCARDIA AND LEVOCARDIA

Liberthson RR, Hastreiter AR, Sinha SN, et al: Levocardia with visceral heterotaxy-isolated levocardia: Pathologic anatomy and its clinical implications. Am Heart J 85:40, 1973.
Rose V, Izukawa T, Moes CAF: Syndromes of asplenia and polysplenia: A review of cardiac and non-cardiac malformations in 60 cases with special reference to diagnosis and prognosis. Br Heart J 37:840, 1975.

PRINCIPLES OF TREATMENT

Engle MA, Zabriskie JB, Seuterfit LB, et al: Viral illness and post-pericardiotomy syndrome: A prospective study in children. Circulation 62:1151, 1980.
Ferry PC: Neurologic sequelae of cardiac surgery in children. Am J Dis Child 141:309, 1987.
Gersony WM, Krongrad E: Evaluation and management of patients after surgical repair of congenital heart disease. Progr Cardiovasc Dis 18:39, 1975. Also *In*: Rosenthal EH, Sonnenblick EH, Lesch M (eds): Postoperative Congenital Heart Disease. New York, Grune & Stratton, 1975, p 145.
McCartney FT, Taylor JFN, Graham GR, et al: The fate of survivors of cardiac surgery in infancy. Circulation 62:80, 1980.
Musewe NN: The role of transesophageal echocardiography in pediatrics. Curr Opin Pediatr 2:977, 1990.
Rigby ML: The trend to primary repair of congenital heart defects in the first 3 months of life. Curr Opin Pediatr 1:82, 1989.
Schwarz SM, Gewitz MH, See CC, et al: Enteral nutrition in infants with congenital heart disease and growth failure. Pediatrics 86:368, 1990.
Thomson AH, Beardsmore CS, Firmin R, et al: Airway function in infants with vascular rings: Preoperative and postoperative assessment. Arch Dis Child 65:171, 1990.
Tynan M: Fetal and pediatric cardiac surgery. Curr Opin Pediatr 2:982, 1990.
Wiles HB: Imaging congenital heart disease. Pediatr Clin North Am 37:115, 1990.

OTHER LESIONS

Bailey LL, Gundry SR: Hypoplastic left heart syndrome. Pediatr Clin North Am 37:137, 1990.

Bertrand J-M, Chartrand C, Lamarre A, et al: Vascular ring: Clinical and physiological assessment of pulmonary function following surgical correction. Pediatr Pulmonol 2:378, 1986.
Freedom RM: The hypoplastic left heart syndrome: Evolving trends in therapy and present concerns. Curr Opin Pediatr 1:90, 1989.
Rich S, Dantzker DR, Ayres SM, et al: Primary pulmonary hypertension: A national prospective study. Ann Intern Med 107:216, 1987.
Rubin LJ, Mendoza J, Hood M, et al: Treatment of primary pulmonary hypertension with continuous intravenous prostacyclin (epoprostenol). Ann Intern Med 112:485, 1990.

15.62 DISTURBANCES OF RATE AND RHYTHM OF THE HEART

Pediatric rhythm disturbances may be transient or permanent; either congenital in a structurally normal or abnormal heart, or acquired following inflammation (rheumatic fever, myocarditis); due to ingestion of toxins (diphtheria, cocaine, theophylline, proarrhythmic antiarrhythmic drugs); or be a sequela of surgical correction of congenital heart disease.

The major risk of a cardiac rhythm disorder is that of severe tachycardia or bradycardia leading to decreased cardiac output, a more severe arrhythmia, syncope, or sudden death. When there is ectopic cardiac activity, the major issue is whether the particular rhythm disturbance noted may be prone to deteriorate into a life-threatening tachyarrhythmia or bradyarrhythmia. Some rhythm abnormalities, such as single premature atrial and ventricular beats, are common among children without heart disease and in the great majority of instances do not pose a risk.

An increasing number of pharmacologic agents are available for treating significant rhythm disturbances in adults, but all have not been used extensively in children. Problems with frequency of administration, compliance, side effects, and variable responses still remain, and selection of an appropriate agent involves a great deal of empiricism. However, most rhythm disturbances can be reliably controlled with a single agent. The most commonly used agents are listed in Table 15–12. Surgical intervention to eliminate bypass tracts associated with pre-excitation syndromes or unusually electrically active areas in the heart is available for infrequent refractory abnormalities. Implanted pacemakers have become more reliable and less prone to technical failure, while implanted defibrillators are now available for use in high-risk patients with sudden-onset ventricular tachycardia or fibrillation.

Sinus arrhythmia represents a physiologic variation in impulse discharges from within the sinus node related to respirations. There is slowing during expiration and acceleration during inspiration. Occasionally, if the sinus rate becomes slow enough there will be an escape beat from the atrioventricular junctional region (Fig. 15–58). Irregularities of sinus rhythm are commonly seen in premature infants, especially bradycardia associated with periodic apnea. Sinus arrhythmia is exaggerated during convalescence from febrile illness and by drugs that increase vagal tone, such as digitalis; it is usually abolished by exercise or by atropine. Some children have great variation in rate during sinus arrhythmia, which should not be confused with a significant rhythm disorder.

Sinus bradycardia is due to slow discharge of impulses from the sinus node. The normal resting sinus rate decreases during childhood, and the lower limit at a given rate is determined empirically. In general, a sinus rate under 90/min in neonates and under 60/min thereafter is considered to be sinus bradycardia. Sinus bradycardia is commonly seen in athletes, and in healthy individuals it is without significance. Sinus bradycardia may occur in systemic disease, for example, myxedema, and will resolve when the disorder is under control. It must be differentiated from sinoatrial and A-V blocks. Children with sinus bradycardia will significantly increase their heart rate with exercise to well over 100/min, whereas patients with A-V block are unable to do so. *Low-birthweight infants* display great variation in sinus rate. Sinus bradycardia is common and may be associated with junctional escape beats. Premature atrial contractions are frequent. These rhythm changes, especially bradycardia, appear more commonly during sleep and are not associated with symptoms. No therapy is necessary.

Wandering atrial pacemaker (Fig. 15–59) is defined as an intermittent shift in the pacemaker of the heart from the sinus node to another part of the atrium. This is common in childhood and usually represents a normal variant. Wandering atrial pacemaker may be seen in patients with central nervous system disturbances, for example, subarachnoid hemorrhage.

Extrasystoles are produced by the discharge of an ectopic focus that may be situated anywhere in atrial, junctional, or ventricular tissue. In the majority of instances extrasystoles are of no clinical or prognostic significance. Under certain circumstances premature beats may be due to organic heart disease (inflammatory, ischemic, fibrotic, etc.). Drug toxicity, especially with digitalis, may also produce extrasystoles.

Premature atrial complexes are not uncommon in childhood, even in the absence of cardiac disease. Depending on the degree of prematurity and the preceding cycle length, some premature atrial complexes result in a normal QRS configuration. In other instances they may be conducted to the ventricle while the specialized ventricular conducting system is partially refractory and may result in an abnormal QRS configuration (Fig. 15–60), which then must be distinguished from premature ventricular systoles. Careful scrutiny of the electrocardiogram for a premature P wave, preceding the QRS, that has a different contour from sinus P waves is essential for diagnosis.

Premature ventricular complexes (PVCs) may arise in any region of the ventricles. They are characterized by premature, widened, bizarre QRS complexes that are not preceded by a P wave (Fig. 15–61). When they have identical contours, they are classified as unifocal in origin. When PVCs vary in contour, they are designated as multifocal.

Extrasystoles are usually followed by a compensatory pause as they interfere with the next sinus beat. In the majority of instances extrasystoles disappear during the tachycardia of exercise. If they remain or become exaggerated during exercise, the arrhythmia may have greater significance. Extrasystoles produce a smaller stroke and pulse volume than normal and, if very premature, may not be audible with a stethoscope or palpable at the radial pulse. Extrasystoles may assume a definite rhythm, for example, alternating with normal beats (pulsus bigeminus) or occurring after 2 normal beats (pulsus trigeminus). The following criteria are indications for further investigation of PVCs, which could require suppressive therapy: (1) sequential ventricular depolarizations without intervening sinus beats, (2) multiform origin, (3) increased ventricular ectopia with exercise, (4) R on T phenomenon (premature ventricular depolarization occurs on the T wave

TABLE 15–12. Commonly Used Antiarrhythmic Drug Schedules in Pediatric Patients

		Oral Administration		Intravenous Administration*		Comments and Side Effects				
Drug	**Indications**	***Maintenance Dose***	***Maximal Maintenance Dose***	***Loading Dose***	***Maximal Dose***	***Comments***	***Side Effects***	***Drug Interactions***	***Proarrhythmias***	***Drug Level***
Digoxin	SVT,[1] atrial flutter, atrial fibrillation	0.01–0.02 mg/kg/24 hr q 12 hr	0.5 mg	0.025–0.05 mg/kg/24 hr q 4–8 hr	0.5 mg	Oral loading dose 0.04–0.07 mg/kg/24 hr q 8 hr; see text for age-related differences	APC, VPC, bradycardia, AV block, nausea, vomiting, anorexia; prolongs P-R interval	Quinidine, amiodarone, verapamil, increase digoxin levels. Diuretic, amphotericin-induced hypokalemia increases digoxin arrhythmia.	Induces APC, VPC, accelerated AV junctional tachycardia	1–2 ng/mL
Quinidine sulfate	SVT,[1] atrial fibrillation, atrial flutter, VPC.	20–60 mg/kg/24 hr q 6 hr	2.4 g	—	—	—	Nausea, vomiting, diarrhea, fever, cinchonism, QRS and Q-T prolongation, AV block, asystole, syncope, thrombocytopenia, hemolytic anemia, SLE, blurred vision, convulsions, allergic reactions, exacerbation of periodic paralysis	Enhances digoxin effects	Yes, torsades de pointes	2–7 μg/mL
Quinidine gluconate	Digoxin, verapamil or propranolol must be given first to prevent ventricular tachycardias, as quinidine slows atrial rate.	20–60 mg/kg/24 hr q 8–12 hr	2.0 g	10–15 mg/kg as 250 μg/kg/min	20 mg/min to 1.0 g	Oral test dose 2 mg/kg				
Procainamide	SVT,[1] atrial fibrillation, atrial flutter. VPC, ventricular tachycardia[2]	50–100 mg/kg/24 hr q 4–6 hr or q 6 hr†	6.0 g	10–20 mg/kg as 300 μg/kg/min	20 mg/min to 1.0 g	Intravenous maintenance 20–80 μg/kg/min	P-R, QRS, Q-T interval prolongation, anorexia, nausea, vomiting, rash, fever, agranulocytosis, thrombocytopenia, Coombs-positive hemolytic anemia, SLE, hypotension, exacerbation of periodic paralysis	Toxicity increased by amiodarone, cimetidine	Yes, torsades de pointes	4–10 μg/mL
Disopyramide	SVT,[1] atrial fibrillation, atrial flutter, VPC	8–12 mg/kg/24 hr q 6 hr or q 12 hr†	1.2 g	—	—	—	Anticholinergic effects, urinary retention, blurred vision, dry mouth, Q-T and QRS prolongation, hepatic toxicity, negative inotropic effects, agranulocytosis, psychosis, hypoglycemia	—	Yes, torsades de pointes	2–8 μg/mL
Phenytoin	Digoxin-induced arrhythmias with heart block	3–6 mg/kg 24 hr q 12 hr	600 mg	10–15 mg/kg as 250 μg/kg/min	20 mg/min to 1.0 g	—	Rash, gingival hyperplasia, ataxia, lethargy, vertigo, tremor, macrocytic anemia, bradycardia with rapid push	Amiodarone, oral anticoagulants, cimetidine, nifedipine, disopyramide increase toxicity. Phenytoin decreases effect of quinidine, mexiletine, furosemide, disopyramide.	No	5–20 μg/mL
Lidocaine	VPC, ventricular tachycardia,[2] ventricular fibrillation[3]	—	—	1 mg/kg; repeat q 5 min for 3 times	50–75 mg	Intravenous maintenance 30–50 μg/kg/min	CNS effects, confusion, convulsions, high-degree AV block, asystole, coma, paresthesias, respiratory failure	Propranolol, cimetidine, tocainide increase toxicity	No	1.5–6 μg/mL
Verapamil	SVT[1]	4–10 mg/kg/24 hr q 8 hr	480 mg	0.075–0.15 mg/kg q 20 min for 2 times	5 mg	Contraindicated in ventricular tachycardia, severe CHF, and atrial fibrillation with WPW. Use with caution in infants.	Bradycardia, asystole, high-degree AV block, P-R prolongation, hypotension, CHF	Use with beta-blocking agent or disopyramide exacerbates or precipitates CHF. Increases digoxin levels and toxicity.	No, but may increase AV block	—

TABLE 15–12. Commonly Used Antiarrhythmic Drug Schedules in Pediatric Patients *Continued*

		Oral Administration		Intravenous Administration*		Comments and Side Effects				
Drug	**Indications**	***Maintenance Dose***	***Maximal Maintenance Dose***	***Loading Dose***	***Maximal Dose***	***Comments***	***Side Effects***	***Drug Interactions***	***Proarrhythmias***	***Drug Level***
Propranolol	SVT,[1] VPC	1–4 mg/kg/24 hr q 6 hr	Not established	0.1–0.15 mg/kg	1 mg/min to 10 mg	Long-acting beta blocking agents (nadolol, atenolol) are preferred for long-term therapy (less frequent administration and fewer CNS side effects)	Bradycardia, loss of concentration or memory, bronchospasm, hypoglycemia, hypotension, heart block, CHF	Use with disopyramide or verapamil exacerbates or precipitates CHF	No	—
Adenosine	SVT[1]	—	—	50–300 μg/kg; begin with 50 μg/kg and increase by 50–100 μg/kg/dose if no effect; 6–12 mg in adolescents	Must be given as rapid IV push, repeat at higher dose if no effect	Because of short half-life adverse effects (chest pain, dyspnea, facial flushing) last <1 min. May see transient bradycardia, rarely transient asystole, VPC	May be less effective in patients receiving theophylline. Increased heart block with carbamazepine	—	—	
Bretylium	Ventricular tachycardia,[2] ventricular fibrillation[3]	—	—	5 mg/kg, then 5–10 mg/kg q 6 hr	30 mg/kg	—	Hypotension, sinus bradycardia, increased sensitivity to catecholamines with transient arrhythmias	Possible hypertension with concurrent sympathomimetic amines	No	—

[1]Vagotonic maneuvers (placing face in iced saline or ice bag over the face) may be attempted first. If the patient is severely compromised and critically ill, cardioversion is treatment of choice for SVT, atrial flutter, and atrial fibrillation.
[2]Cardioversion is treatment of choice for sustained ventricular tachycardia with significant hemodynamic compromise. Some cardiologists try chest thump and/or IV lidocaine. If heart block is present, a temporary ventricular pacemaker may be needed.
[3]Defibrillation is treatment of choice.
*intravenous administration of antiarrhythmic drugs should always be given slowly with constant monitoring of blood pressure and an electrocardiogram, particularly in patients with compromised cardiac, renal, or hepatic function. The dose must be modified in patients wih abnormal renal or hepatic function.
†Sustained-release preparations available for clinical use.
AV = atrioventricular node.
SVT = supraventricular tachycardia.
SLE = systemic lupus erythematosus–like illness, ANA positive.
VPC = ventricular premature contraction.
APC = atrial premature contraction.
IV = intravenous.
WPW = Wolff-Parkinson-White pre-excitation.
CHF = congestive heart failure.
CNS = central nervous system.

of the preceding beat), (5) presence of underlying heart disease, and (6) unusual patient awareness of beats associated with marked anxiety.

Most patients are unaware of premature contractions, although some may be aware of a "skipped beat" or a sudden "turnover" or "tickle" over the precordium. This is due to the increased cardiac output from the normal beat following a compensatory pause. Anxiety, a febrile illness, or ingestion of various drugs or stimulants causes premature ventricular beats. The basis of therapy for benign PVCs is convincing reassurance that the arrhythmia is not the result of structural heart disease; sedatives or suppressive agents may be used in selected cases.

15.63 TACHYARRHYTHMIAS

SUPRAVENTRICULAR TACHYARRHYTHMIAS (SVT)

Paroxysmal Atrial Tachycardia (PAT)

Re-entry within the A-V node is the most common mechanism of paroxysmal atrial tachycardia. The tachycardia is initiated by a premature atrial beat that is conducted through a tract within the A-V node. The ventricular response induces an atrial echo beat via a retrograde tract within the A-V node, which in turn is transmitted back to the ventricle and so on.

In older children paroxysmal atrial tachycardia is characterized by abrupt onset and cessation; the attack may be precipitated by an acute infection and usually when the patient is at rest. Attacks may last only a few seconds or may persist for hours. The cardiac rate usually exceeds 180/min and occasionally may be as rapid as 300/min. The only complaint may be awareness of the rapid cardiac rate. Many children tolerate these episodes extremely well, and it is unlikely that short paroxysms are a danger to life. If the rate is exceptionally rapid or if the attack is prolonged, precordial discomfort and congestive cardiac failure may supervene.

In young infants, the diagnosis may be more obscure because the cardiac rate at this age is normally rapid and increases greatly with crying. A baby having PAT may present with congestive heart failure, if the precipitating severe tachycardia was not recognized for a long time. The cardiac rate during paroxysms is frequently in the range of 200–300/min. If the attack lasts 6–24 hr or more with an extremely fast heart rate, the infant may become acutely ill, with an ashen color, and be restless and irritable. Tachypnea and hepatomegaly are the prominent signs of cardiac failure, and there may be fever and leukocytosis. Intrauterine tachycardia can cause severe cardiac failure and be responsible for hydrops fetalis (Fig. 15–62).

SVT in neonates presents with a narrow QRS complex (less than 0.08 sec), unless there is the rare occurrence of aberrant

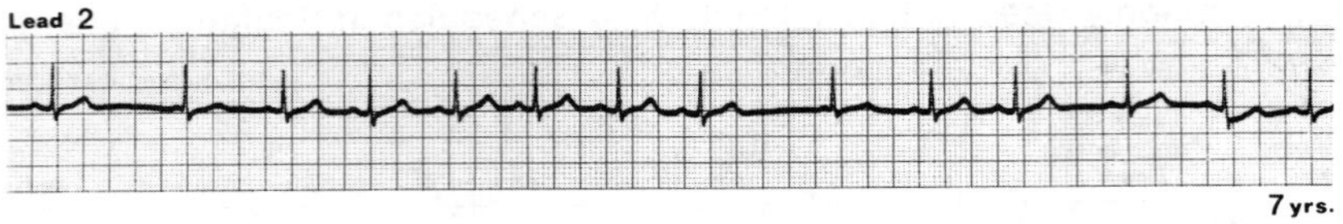

Figure 15–58. Sinus arrhythmia with junctional escape beat: note the variation in P-P interval with little change in P morphology or P-R interval. When the sinus rate is slow enough, the atrioventricular junction takes over and produces escape beats. This rhythm is normal.

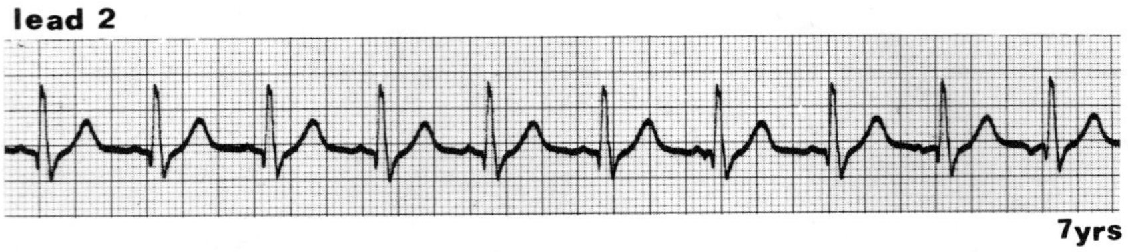

Figure 15–59. Wandering atrial pacemaker: note the change in P wave configuration in the 7th, 9th, and 10th beats. The 7th P wave may represent a fusion between the sinus P and the ectopic atrial pacemaker seen in the 10th beat.

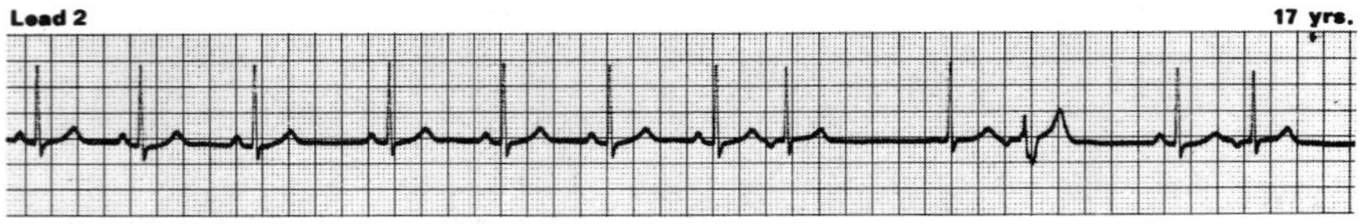

Figure 15–60. Premature atrial contraction (PAC): QRS complexes, the 8th, 10th, and final, in this strip are preceded by a P wave that is inverted, denoting an ectopic origin of atrial depolarization. Note that the 8th and final QRS complexes resemble those of sinus origin, whereas the 10th is aberrantly conducted. This is a function of the preceding cycle length that influences the refractory period of the bundle branches. Note that the pause after the PAC is longer than 2 P-P intervals, implying that the premature atrial depolarization has invaded and discharged the sinus node, and reset it, so that it fires later.

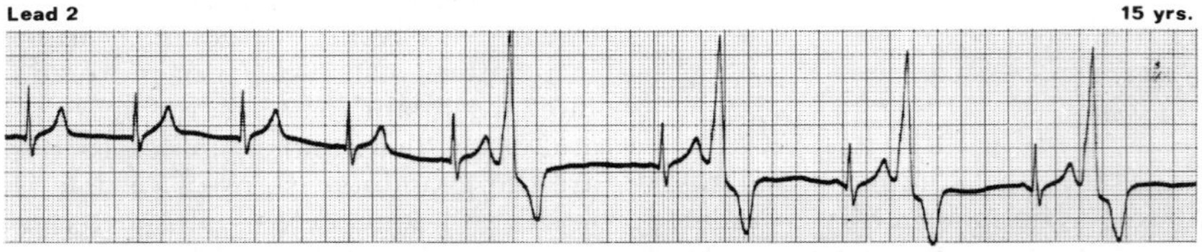

Figure 15–61. Premature ventricular contractions (PVC) induced by hyperventilation: Note that the premature beat is wide and has a completely different morphology from that of the sinus beat. The premature beat is not preceded by a P wave, and the pause following it is fully compensatory (i.e., the P-P interval containing the PVC equals 2 sinus cycles); this indicates that the sinus mechanism has not been disturbed by the premature beats.

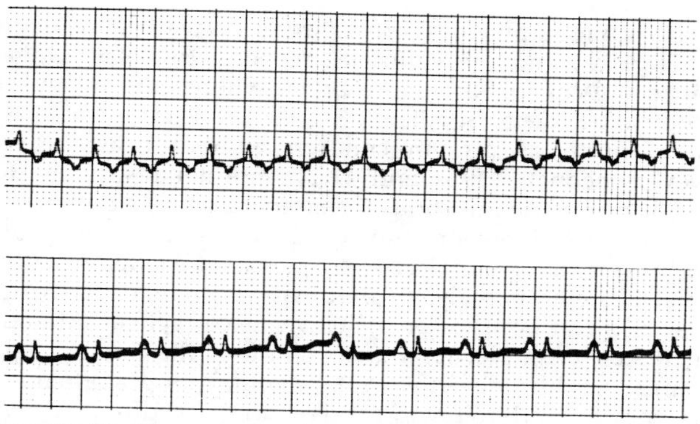

Figure 15–62. The upper tracing shows paroxysmal supraventricular or atrial tachycardia (PAT) with a ventricular rate of 230/min. The lower tracing shows sinus rhythm after D-C cardioversion. Note that during the tachycardia, the T wave is deformed by an inverted, presumably retrograde, P wave. The QRS morphology is unchanged during the tachycardia. Low voltage is due to peripheral edema in a 1-day-old infant who had intrauterine tachycardia and hydrops fetalis.

conduction. The P wave is visible on a standard electrocardiogram in 50–60% of neonates with SVT but is visible with a transesophageal lead in most patients. Differentiation from sinus tachycardia may be difficult; if the rate is greater than 230 beats/min and there is an abnormal P wave axis (normal positive P wave in leads I and AVF), SVT is more likely. Differentiation from ventricular tachycardia is critical, because digoxin precipitates ventricular fibrillation in patients with ventricular tachycardia. The absence of P waves and presence of wide QRS complexes that are dissimilar to the QRS complex during sinus rhythm are diagnostic of ventricular tachycardia. SVT may be noted in the anatomically normal heart, or may be associated with Wolff-Parkinson-White pre-excitation syndrome or exposure to sympathomimetic amines (decongestants).

TREATMENT. Vagal stimulation by a simple procedure, such as iced saline facial submersion or an ice bag over the face, may abort the attack. Older children may be taught vagotonic maneuvers to abolish the paroxysm, such as straining, the Valsalva maneuver, breathholding, drinking ice water, or the adoption of a particular posture. When these measures fail and the child is symptomatic enough to warrant treatment, several alternatives are available (see Table 15–12). In urgent situations when congestive heart failure has occurred, electrical synchronized cardioversion (1–2 watt-sec/kg) is recommended as initial management. Pharmacotherapy should be considered as the initial approach under other circumstances. Digoxin has been the mainstay of therapy for patients with supraventricular tachycardia. Conduction is slowed within the A-V node and the re-entrant circuit is interrupted. Digoxin is effective in 95% of cases but often requires several hours to take effect. In neonates, digoxin therapy may be instituted even if the paroxysm has been abolished by other means since the recurrence rate is high; therapy in infants should be maintained for 3–6 mo or longer.

Other drugs that have been used to abolish PAT (or SVT, a term that is used interchangeably) include infusions of phenylephrine (Neo-Synephrine) or edrophonium (Tensilon) and oral administration of quinidine sulfate or propranolol. Calcium channel blockers have also been used in the initial treatment of paroxysmal supraventricular tachyarrhythmias in older children. When verapamil (Isoptin, Cordan) is administered intravenously 92–96% of children can be converted to normal sinus rhythm within 5 min of an initial 0.1–0.2 mg/kg dose. No side effects are experienced by patients whose supraventricular tachycardias are due to re-entrant mechanisms (see Table 15–12). Verapamil may reduce cardiac output and produce hypotension and cardiac arrest in infants under 1 yr of age; therefore, digoxin is the initial drug of choice for the acute therapy of SVT in this age group. Verapamil is the drug of choice in older patients. Intravenous adenosine is an effective initial agent to terminate SVT in infants and older patients (see Table 15–12). Because of adenosine's short half-life and intravenous formulation, chronic therapy with another agent is required. For maintenance therapy digoxin remains the treatment of choice for most patients.

In most instances of paroxysmal atrial tachycardia there is no underlying structural cardiac disease. If cardiac failure occurs during prolonged tachycardia in an infant with a normal heart, cardiac function rapidly returns to normal after sinus rhythm is reinstituted.

Between attacks some children may exhibit the electrocardiographic changes of the *Wolff-Parkinson-White (pre-excitation) syndrome*: short P-R interval and slow upstroke of the QRS (delta wave) (Fig. 15–63). Although most often present in a normal heart, this syndrome may also be associated with Ebstein anomaly, corrected transposition (ventricular inversion), and cardiomyopathy. The syndrome causes a predilection for a re-entrant tachycardia. The anatomic substrate comprising the re-entrant circuit is the A-V node and an accessory pre-excitation pathway, a muscular bridge connecting atrium to ventricle on the right or left lateral cardiac border or within the ventricular septum (Fig. 15–64). During sinus rhythm the impulse is carried over both the A-V node and the accessory pathway; it produces some degree of fusion of the two depolarization fronts that results in an abnormal QRS. During tachycardia an impulse is usually carried anterogradely over the A-V node, resulting in a normal QRS complex, and in retrograde fashion through the accessory pathway, reaching the atrium and perpetuating the tachycardia. Only after cessation of the tachycardia are the typical features of Wolff-Parkinson-White syndrome recognized (see Fig. 15–63). When rapid antegrade conduction occurs through the pre-excitation pathway during tachycardia and the retrograde re-entry pathway to the atrium is via the A-V node, the potential for more serious arrhythmias is greater, especially should atrial fibrillation occur. Digoxin or verapamil should not be administered for chronic treatment; procainamide or quinidine may be used. Surgical excision of bypass tracts can be successfully carried out in selected patients with life-threatening arrhythmias, and early results of radiofrequency

A

B

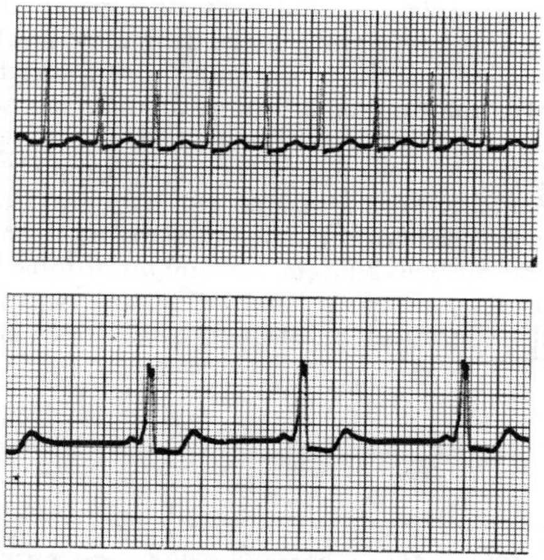

Figure 15–63. *A*, PAT in a child with Wolff-Parkinson-White (WPW) syndrome. Note the normal QRS complexes during the tachycardia. *B*, Later the typical features of WPW are apparent (short P-R interval, δ wave, and wide QRS).

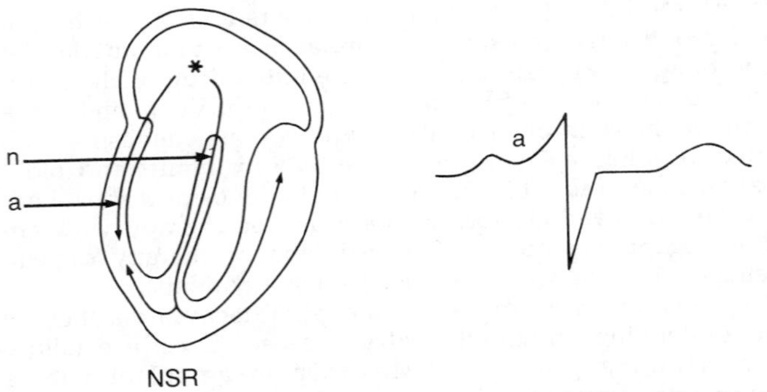

Figure 15–64. Schematic representation of the heart with a right-sided anomolous pathway. The *asterisk* indicates the initiation of the sinus beat. The *arrows* indicate the direction and spread of excitation. The electrocardiographic complex shown represents a fusion beat that combines activation over the normal (n) and accessory (a) pathways. The latter inscribes the δ wave.

ablation in the cardiac catheterization laboratory have been promising.

Ectopic atrial tachycardia is an uncommon tachycardia in childhood. It is characterized by a variable rate (seldom greater than 200), identifiable P waves with abnormal frontal plane axis, and chronicity in either a sustained or intermittent tachycardia. There is an automatic focus rather than the more usual re-entry mechanism. It is usually more difficult to control pharmacologically than the more common paroxysmal supraventricular tachycardias. Suppression of the ectopic atrial focus is difficult; therapy should, therefore, be directed to slowing atrioventricular conduction with digitalis or propranolol rather than relying on drugs that suppress atrial automaticity, such as quinidine and disopyramide. In some cases no treatment is necessary.

Chaotic or multifocal atrial tachycardia is characterized by two or more ectopic P waves with two or more different ectopic P-P cycles, frequent blocked P waves, and varying P-R intervals of conducted beats. This arrhythmia usually occurs in the absence of cardiac disease and usually terminates spontaneously after weeks or months. If the patient is asymptomatic, no treatment is necessary. Digitalis may be used to control the ventricular rate.

Accelerated junctional tachycardia is an arrhythmia in which the junctional rate exceeds that of the sinus node so that atrioventricular dissociation results. This arrhythmia is most often recognized in the early postoperative period following cardiac surgery and may be difficult to control. It often disappears spontaneously without specific treatment. Junctional tachycardia may be a sign of digitalis intoxication, and when this occurs, the drug should be discontinued.

Atrial flutter is a regular or regularly irregular tachycardia due to atrial activity at a rate of 250–400/min. These contractions may be due to a circus movement in the atria and produced by an irritable focus in the atrial muscle similar to that responsible for paroxysmal atrial tachycardia and atrial extrasystoles. Because the atrioventricular node cannot transmit such rapid impulses, there is virtually always some degree of A-V block, and the ventricles respond to every 2nd–4th atrial beat. Occasionally, the response will be variable and the rhythm will appear irregular.

Atrial flutter is rare in children without heart disease; however, neonates frequently have normal hearts. It may occur during acute infectious diseases, but is most often seen in patients with large stretched atria, such as those associated with longstanding mitral or tricuspid insufficiency, tricuspid atresia, Ebstein anomaly, or rheumatic mitral stenosis. Atrial flutter also can occur after palliative or corrective intra-atrial surgery, for example, for transposition of the great arteries, ostium secundum defect, or total anomalous pulmonary venous return, and following a Fontan procedure. As with supraventricular tachycardia, uncontrolled atrial flutter may precipitate congestive cardiac failure. Carotid sinus pressure or iced saline submersion usually produces a temporary slowing of the cardiac rate. The diagnosis is confirmed by electrocardiography, which demonstrates the rapid and regular atrial saw-toothed flutter waves. Digitalis slows the ventricular response in atrial flutter by prolonging conduction time through the A-V node. Occasionally, the rhythm will then convert to atrial fibrillation. After full digitalization, quinidine or procainamide may be added to convert to sinus rhythm. However, atrial flutter usually converts immediately to sinus rhythm by cardioversion, and this has become the treatment of choice. Neonates with normal hearts, who respond to digoxin, may be treated for 1 yr.

Atrial fibrillation is produced by a mechanism similar to that causing atrial flutter; the atrial excitation is irregularly irregular and more rapid (300–500/min) (Fig. 15–65). The arrhythmia occurs most frequently in older children with rheumatic mitral valve disease. It also is seen rarely as a complication of intra-atrial surgery (e.g., Mustard operation), with left atrial enlargement secondary to left atrioventricular valve incompetence, in conditions producing atrial flutter, and in patients with Wolff-Parkinson-White syndrome. This rhythm disorder is most often the result of chronically stretched atrial myocardium. Thyrotoxicosis, pulmonary emboli, and pericarditis should be suspected in a previously normal older child or adolescent. The best initial treatment is digitalization, which restores the ventricular rate to normal, although the atrial fibrillation persists. Digoxin is not given if Wolff-Parkinson-White syndrome is present. Normal sinus rhythm may then be restored with quinidine sulfate, procainamide or electrical cardioversion. However, reinstitution of sinus rhythm may not be possible in the patient whose atrial fibrillation is associated with florid atrioventricular valve disease and cardiomegaly. In such cases, chronic therapy with digitalis is usually required.

VENTRICULAR TACHYARRHYTHMIAS

Ventricular tachycardia is more common than had been thought in the past, but is less often seen than supraventricular tachycardia. Ventricular tachycardia is defined as at least 3 PVCs at greater than 120 beats/min. It may be paroxysmal or incessant (present most of the day). It may be associated

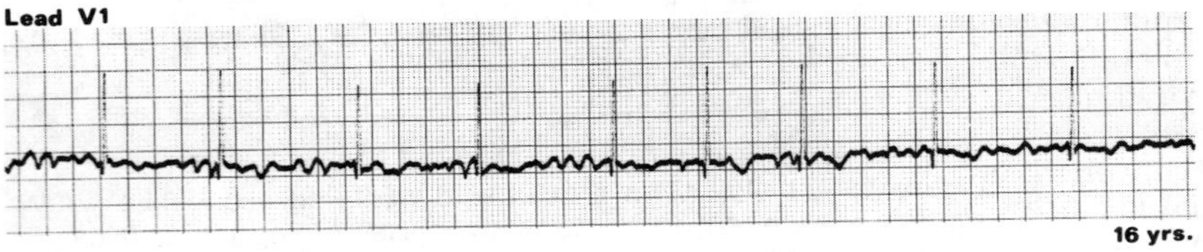

Figure 15–65. Atrial fibrillation, characterized by absence of P waves; presence of fibrillatory waves, which are grossly irregular, rapid undulations; and an irregular ventricular response. Fibrillatory waves may not be visible in all leads and should be carefully sought in every tracing with irregular R-R intervals. (The coexisting qR in V_1 is diagnostic of right ventricular hypertrophy in this patient with Eisenmenger syndrome.)

with myocarditis, anomalous origin of a coronary artery, arrhythmogenic right ventricular dysplasia, mitral valve prolapse, primary cardiac tumors, cardiomyopathy, congenital or acquired (proarrhythmic drugs) prolonged Q-T interval, Wolff-Parkinson-White syndrome, or drugs (cocaine, amphetamine); develop many years after intraventricular surgery (tetralogy of Fallot, VSD); or occur without obvious organic heart disease. It must be distinguished from supraventricular tachycardia with aberrancy or rapid conduction over an accessory pathway. The presence of capture and fusion beats confirms the diagnosis. In the absence of these features, diagnosis is more difficult. Right precordial and/or esophageal leads are helpful in identifying P waves. Although some children tolerate rapid ventricular rates for many hours, this arrhythmia should be promptly treated because hypotension and ventricular fibrillation may result. Lidocaine and cardioversion (1–2 watt-sec/kg) are methods of choice for rapid treatment. Bretylium is an alternative drug (see Table 15–12). Quinidine, procainamide, and propranolol are most useful for chronic therapy. Neonates may have a myocardial tumor; resection is usually curative.

Ventricular fibrillation results in death unless an effective ventricular beat is restored. A thump on the chest sometimes restores sinus rhythm. Usually external cardiac massage with artificial ventilation and electrical defibrillation are necessary. Implanted defibrillators are inserted in selected patients who are refractory to pharmacologic preventive therapy.

DIFFERENTIAL DIAGNOSIS OF TACHYARRHYTHMIAS. It is important from the standpoint of prognosis and treatment to accurately identify the type of tachyarrhythmia that is present (Table 15–13). Often the diagnosis is clear on a clinical and electrocardiographic basis, but in some instances differential diagnosis may be difficult.

First, it should be determined whether the patient is actually in sinus tachycardia. Time for treating an infection, acute anemia, or other illness that results in sinus tachycardia may be lost while a tachyarrhythmia is being considered, wrongly diagnosed, or even treated. Heart rates greater than 225/min are too rapid for sinus tachycardia, but rates in the 140–220 range could signify either an arrhythmia or sinus tachycardia. Ventricular tachycardia is almost invariably slower than supraventricular tachycardia.

Second, the configuration of the P waves should be evaluated. Although it is possible to have a supraventricular tachycardia with P waves of normal configuration (upright in leads I, II, and AVF), in most instances P waves will be abnormal. In many cases of supraventricular tachycardia with rapid ventricular response, the P wave will not be visible on the standard electrocardiogram, and it may be necessary to obtain Lewis-Golub leads (exploring right chest electrodes) or an esophageal lead to identify obscure P waves. The distinctive saw-toothed atrial waves produced by atrial flutter are best recognized in lead V_1. During atrial fibrillation atrial activity is represented by a chaotic baseline. During ventricular tachycardia the P wave is either absent or noted to be out of phase with the QRS deflections (**atrioventricular dissociation**).

Third, an extremely narrow QRS suggests that the rhythm comes from either the supraventricular area or the region of the A-V node. However, prolonged QRS duration (usually > 0.120 sec) may be seen with a QRS aberrancy in the face of a supraventricular tachycardia as well as with ventricular arrhythmias. In the former the QRS morphology is almost always of the right bundle branch block type. Most wide complex tachycardia in children is ventricular tachycardia unless a prior ventriculotomy is present (tetralogy of Fallot repair). The QRS complex in neonatal ventricular tachycardia may be greater than or equal to 0.08 sec.

Finally, the rhythmicity should be determined. In sinus tachycardia the rate will vary every few seconds and will gradually slow with vagotonic maneuvers, only to speed up again when they are discontinued. Atrial tachycardia is extremely regular, except at the onset or just prior to ending, whereas ventricular tachycardia displays slight beat-to-beat variations. Either atrial flutter will be regular or, with block, the ventricular response will consistently be some multiple of the interval between the flutter waves. In atrial fibrillation the ventricular response will be irregularly irregular.

15.64 BRADYARRHYTHMIAS

Sinus arrest and sinoatrial block may cause a sudden pause in the heart beat. The former is presumed to be due to failure of impulse formation within the sinus node; the latter, to a block between the sinus impulse and the surrounding atrium. These arrhythmias are rare in childhood except as manifestations of digitalis intoxication or in patients who have had extensive atrial surgery.

Atrioventricular block may be divided into *1st-degree block*, in which the P-R interval is prolonged but all of the atrial impulses are not conducted to the ventricle; *2nd-degree block*, in which some impulses are not conducted to the ventricle; and *3rd-degree block* (complete heart block), in which no impulses from the atria reach the ventricles. In a variant of 2nd-degree block, known as the *Wenckebach type* (also called Mobitz type I), the P-P interval remains constant, the P-R interval increases until a P wave is not conducted, and, in the cycle following the pause, the P-R is again shorter (Fig. 15–66). In Mobitz II, occasional atrial beats are not conducted to the ventricle; this conduction defect has more potential to cause syncope, and may be progressive.

Congenital complete atrioventricular block in children is

Table 15–13. Diagnosis of Tachyarrhythmias

	Electrocardiographic Findings			
	Heart Rate/Min	*P Wave*	*QRS Duration*	*Regularity*
Sinus tachycardia	<225	Always present Normal axis	Normal	Rate varies with respiration
Atrial tachycardia	180–320	Present—50% Superior axis common	Normal or prolonged (RBBB* pattern)	Regular
Atrial fibrillation	120–180	Fibrillatory waves	Normal or prolonged (RBBB pattern)	Irregularly irregular
Atrial flutter	Atrial: 250–400 Ventricular response variable: 100–320	Saw-toothed flutter waves	Normal or prolonged (RBBB pattern)	Regular ventricular response (e.g., 2:1, 3:1, 3:2, etc.)
Ventricular tachycardia	120–240	Absent or atrioventricular dissociation	Usually prolonged	Slightly irregular

*RBBB = right bundle branch block.

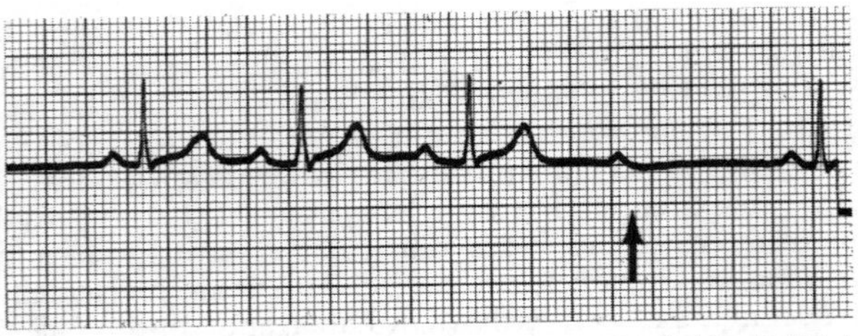

Figure 15–66. Wenckebach phenomenon (Mobitz I). The P-R interval gradually lengthens until the 4th P wave in the cycle is not conducted to the ventricle *(arrow)*. The ensuing P-R interval is once again normal.

most often due to autoimmune injury of the fetal conduction systems by maternal-derived IgG antibodies (anti-SSA/Ro, anti-SSB/La) in a mother with overt or, more often, asymptomatic systemic lupus erythematosus (SLE). Rarely rheumatoid arthritis, dermatomyositis, or Sjögren syndrome is the primary autoimmune process. Autoimmune disease accounts for 60–70% of all congenital heart block and about 80% of cases with structurally normal hearts. Complete heart block is also seen in patients with complex congenital heart disease (corrected *l*-loop transposition of the great arteries, single ventricle), abnormal embryonic development of the conduction system, myocardial tumors, myocarditis, myocardial abscess due to endocarditis, long QT syndrome, postsurgical repair of congenital heart disease involving the ventricular septum, and **Kearns-Sayer syndrome** (external ophthalmoplegia, pigmentary retinal degeneration, mitochondrial myopathy). The incidence of congenital complete heart block is 1 in 20,000–25,000 live births; a high fetal wastage rate causes an underestimation of its incidence. In some infants of mothers with SLE, complete heart block is not present at birth but develops within the first 3–6 mo of birth. The arrhythmia is occasionally suspected in the fetus and may produce hydrops. At greatest risk are infants with associated congenital heart disease who, in the first weeks of life, were in congestive cardiac failure, with atrial rates exceeding 150/min and ventricular rates lower than 55.

In older children with otherwise normal hearts the condition is commonly asymptomatic, although attacks of syncope may occur. Older infants may develop night terrors, tiredness with frequent naps, and irritability. The peripheral pulse is prominent as a result of the large ventricular stroke volume and the peripheral vasodilatation; the systolic blood pressure is elevated. Jugular venous pulsations occur irregularly and may be large when the atrium contracts against a closed tricuspid valve (cannon wave). Exercise and atropine produce an acceleration of 10–20 beats/min or more in the child. Systolic murmurs are frequent along the left sternal border, and apical mid-diastolic murmurs are not unusual. Heart block in itself results in cardiac enlargement simply on the basis of increased diastolic ventricular filling.

The diagnosis is confirmed by electrocardiogram; the P waves and QRS complexes have no constant relation (Fig. 15–67). The QRS duration may be prolonged or may be normal if the heart beat is initiated high in the His bundle.

The prognosis for congenital heart block is usually favorable; patients who have been observed to the age of 30–40 yr have lived normally active lives. However, some patients have episodes of dizziness with or without syncope (**Stokes-Adams attacks**); this complication requires the implantation of a permanent cardiac pacemaker.

Neonates with ventricular rates lower than or equal to 50–55 beats/min, evidence of hydrops, or the development of heart failure after birth require cardiac pacing. Atropine or isoproterenol may be used to try to increase the heart rate

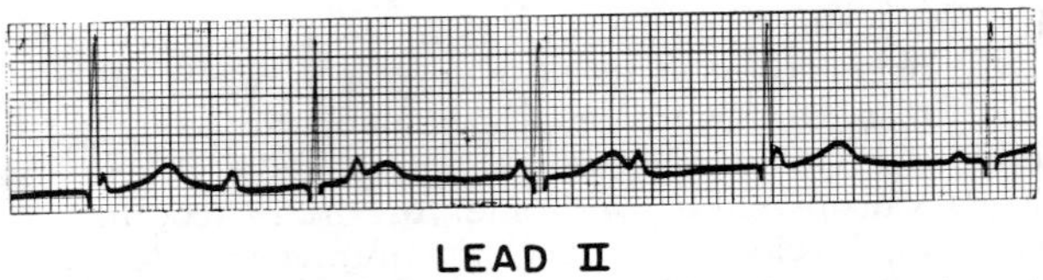

Figure 15–67. Complete atrioventricular block: The ventricular rate is regular at 53/min. The atrial rate varied from 65–95/min (probably sinus arrhythmia). The QRS morphology is normal, which is usual in congenital A-V block.

while arranging for pacemaker placement. Patients with complete heart block and a wide QRS ventricular response should be paced prior to receiving antiarrhythmia drugs, as these may suppress the escape focus. Transthoracic epicardial pacemaker implants have been traditionally employed; however, transvenous placement of pacemaker leads is gaining acceptance for infants and young children.

15.65 SICK-SINUS SYNDROME

The sick-sinus syndrome is the result of abnormalities in the sinus node and/or atrial conduction pathways as outlined in Figure 15–68. This syndrome may occur in the absence of congenital heart disease and has been reported in siblings, but is most commonly seen after surgical correction of congenital heart defects, especially the Mustard procedure for transposition of the great arteries. Clinical presentation depends on the heart rate. Most patients remain asymptomatic without treatment. Dizziness and syncope can occur during periods of marked sinus slowing with failure of junctional escape (Fig. 15–69). Supraventricular tachycardias may alternate with bradycardia (bradycardia-tachycardia syndrome) causing palpitations, exercise intolerance, or dizziness. Treatment must be individualized. In general, aside from digitalis, drug therapy to control tachyarrhythmia (e.g., propranolol, quinidine, procainamide) may suppress sinus and atrioventricular nodal function to the degree that symptomatic bradycardia may be produced. Therefore, an insertion of a demand ventricular pacemaker in conjunction with drug therapy is necessary for symptomatic patients.

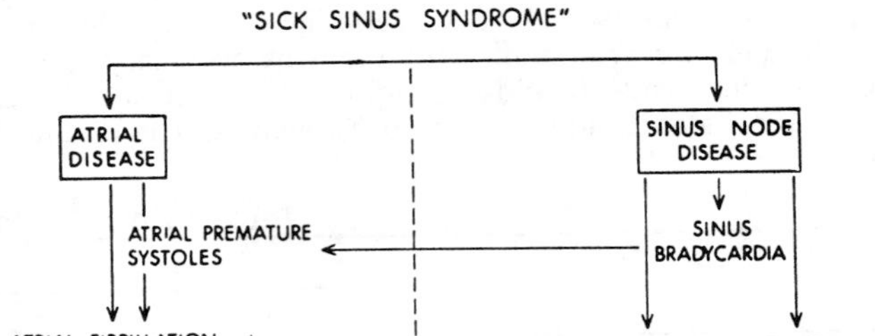

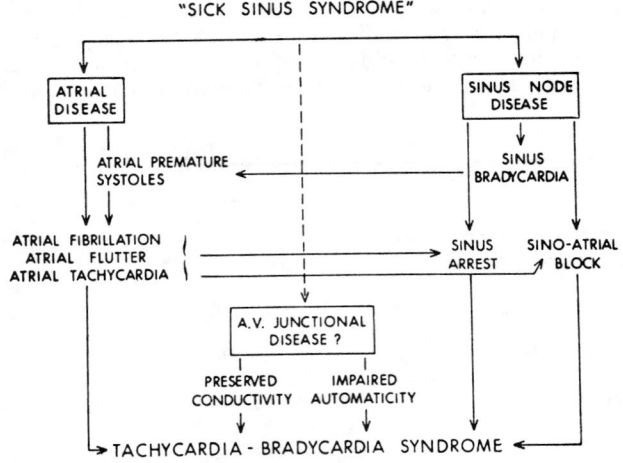

Figure 15–68. Factors resulting in the sick-sinus syndrome. (From Kaplan BM, Langendorf R, Lev M, et al: Am J Cardiol 31:497, 1973. Reproduced by permission of Technical Publishing Company.)

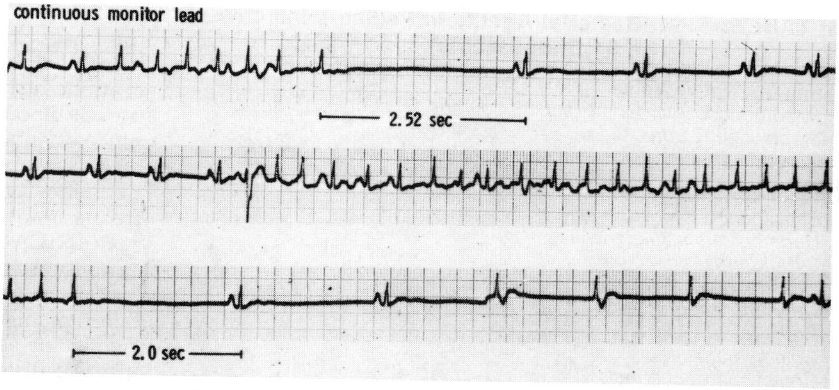

Figure 15–69. Sick-sinus syndrome with bradytachycardia: Note the bursts of supraventricular tachycardia, probably multifocal in origin, followed by long periods of sinus arrest and by sinus bradycardia.

Akhtar M, Shenasa M, Jazayeri M, et al: Wide QRS complex tachycardia: Reappraisal of a common clinical problem. Ann Intern Med 109:905, 1988.

Benson DW Jr, Smith WM, Dunnigan A, et al: Mechanisms of regular, wide QRS tachycardia in infants and children. Am J Cardiol 49:1778, 1982.

Brooks R, Burgess JH: Idiopathic ventricular tachycardia: A review. Medicine 67:271, 1988.

Case C, Crawford F, Gillette P: Surgical treatment of dysrhythmias. Pediatr Clin North Am 37:79, 1990.

Dewey RC, Capeless MA, Levy AM: Use of ambulatory electrocardiographic monitoring to identify high-risk patients with congenital complete heart block. N Engl J Med 316:835, 1987.

Dick M: Complete heart block in children. Curr Opin Pediatr 2:957, 1990.

DiMarco JP, Miles W, Akhtar M, et al: Adenosine for paroxysmal supraventricular tachycardia: Dose ranging and comparison with verapamil. Ann Intern Med 113:104, 1990.

Dungan WT, Garson A Jr, Gillette PC: Arrhythmogenic right ventricular dysplasia: A cause of ventricular tachycardia in children with apparently normal hearts. Am Heart J 102:745, 1981.

Dunnigan A, Benson DW Jr, Banditt DG: Atrial flutter in infancy: Diagnosis, clinical features, and treatment. Pediatrics 75:725, 1985.

Garson A, Gillette PC, McNamara DG: Supraventricular tachycardia in children: Clinical features, response to treatment and long-term follow-up in 217 patients. J Pediatr 98:875, 1981.

Garson A Jr, Gillette PC, Titus JL, et al: Surgical treatment of ventricular tachycardia in infants. N Engl J Med 310:1443, 1984.

Gillette PC, Garson A, Kugler JD: Wolff-Parkinson-White syndrome in children: Electrophysiologic and pharmacologic characteristics. Circulation 60:1487, 1979.

Gillette PC, Shannon C, Blair H, et al: Transvenous pacing in pediatric patients. Am Heart J 105:843, 1983.

Gow R: Ventricular arrhythmias in infants and children. Curr Opin Pediatr 2:963, 1990.

Griffith MJ, Linker NJ, Garratt CJ, et al: Relative efficacy and safety of intravenous drugs for termination of sustained ventricular tachycardia. Lancet 336:670, 1990.

Hayes CJ, Gersony WM: Arrhythmias after the Mustard operation for transposition of the great arteries: A long-term study. J Am Coll Cardiol 7:133, 1986.

Johnson WH, Dunnigan A, Fehr P, et al: Association of atrial flutter with orthodromic reciprocating fetal tachycardia. Ann J Cardiol 59:374, 1987.

Josephson ME: Antiarrhythmic agents and the danger of proarrhythmic events. Ann Intern Med 111:101, 1989.

Kirk CR, Gibbs JL, Thomas R: Cardiovascular collapse after verapamil in supraventricular tachycardia. Arch Dis Child 62:1265, 1987.

Marchlinski FE: Treatment of sustained ventricular arrhythmias: Which therapy to use? Ann Intern Med 109:522, 1988.

Perry JC, Garson A Jr: Diagnosis and treatment of arrhythmias. Adv Pediatr 36:177, 1989.

Pongiglione G: The role of the pediatric electrophysiologist in the diagnosis and treatment of supraventricular tachydysrhythmias. Curr Opin Pediatr 1:124, 1989.

Porter CJ, Gillette PC, McNamara DG: Twenty-four hour ambulatory ECG's in the detection and management of cardiac dysrhythmias in infants and children. Pediatr Cardiol 1:203, 1980.

Ross B: Congenital complete atrioventricular block. Pediatr Clin North Am 37:69, 1990.

Scheinman M: Catheter and surgical treatment of cardiac arrhythmias. JAMA 263:79, 1990.

Sreeram N, Wren C: Supraventricular tachycardia in infants: Response to initial treatment. Arch Dis Child 65:127, 1990.

Tchou PJ, Kadri N, Anderson J, et al: Automatic implantable cardioverter defibrillators and survival of patients with left ventricular dysfunction and malignant ventricular arrhythmias. Ann Intern Med 109:529, 1988.

Till J, Shinebourne EA, Rigby ML, et al: Efficacy and safety of adenosine in the treatment of supraventricular tachycardia in infants and children. Br Heart J 62:204, 1989.

Wellens HJJ, Brugada P, Penn OC: The management of preexcitation syndromes. JAMA 257:2325, 1987.

15.66 INFECTIVE ENDOCARDITIS

The term infective endocarditis includes the entities referred to as acute and subacute bacterial endocarditis (see Sec. 12.18–12.19) as well as infections of nonbacterial endocarditis such as those caused by viruses, fungi, and other agents. The disease remains a significant cause of morbidity and mortality among children and adolescents despite the advances in the management and prophylaxis of the disease with antimicrobial agents. The inability to eradicate infective endocarditis by prevention or early treatment stems from several factors: The nature of the infecting organism has changed over the years; physicians, dentists, and the public are not sufficiently aware of the threat of infective endocarditis and the preventive measures available; diagnosis may be difficult when delayed; and special risk groups have emerged, which include an increasing number of narcotics users, survivors of cardiac surgery, and patients with lowered resistance to infection who require intravascular catheters. Brain abscess, which is rarely seen among patients with cyanotic heart disease, is virtually never associated with endocarditis.

ETIOLOGY. *Streptococcus viridans* is responsible for approximately 50% of cases of infective endocarditis. Staphylococcal endocarditis has become more common over the past 2 decades and is now responsible for almost one third of the cases. Other organisms cause endocarditis less frequently, and in approximately 10% of cases blood cultures are negative (Table 15–14). No relationship exists between the infecting organism and the type of congenital defect, duration of the illness, or age of the child. However, staphylococcal endocarditis is more common in patients who do not have underlying heart disease; *S. viridans* is noted after dental procedures, group D enterococcus after lower bowel or genitourinary manipulation; and *Pseudomonas aeruginosa* or *Serratia marcescens* among intravenous drug users.

EPIDEMIOLOGY. Infective endocarditis is most often a

TABLE 15–14. Bacterial Agents in Pediatric Infective Endocarditis

Common: Native Valve
Streptococcus viridans group (*S. mutans, S. sanguis, S. mitis*)
Staphylococcus aureus
Group D streptococcus (enterococcus) (*S. bovis, S. faecalis*)
Uncommon: Native Valve
Streptococcus pneumoniae
Haemophilus influenzae
S. epidermidis
Coxiella burnetii (Q fever)*
Neisseria gonorrhoeae
*Brucella**
*Chlamydia psittaci**
*Chlamydia trachomatis**
*Chlamydia pneumoniae**
HACEK group†
*Streptobacillus moniliformis**
*Pasteurella multocida**
Campylobacter fetus
Culture negative (10% of cases)
Prosthetic Valve
Staphylococcus epidermidis
S. aureus
S. viridans
Pseudomonas aeruginosa
Serratia marcescens
Diphtheroids
Legionella species*
HACEK group†
Fungi‡

*These fastidious bacteria plus some fungi may produce culture-negative endocarditis. Detection may require special media, incubation for more than 7 days, or serology.

†HACEK grup includes *Haemophilus* species (*H. paraphrophilus, H. parainfluenzae, H. aphrophilus*), *Actinobacillus actinomycetemcomitans, Cardiobacterium hominis, Eikenella corrodens, Kingella* species.

‡*Candida* species, *Aspergillus* species, *Pseudoallescheria boydii, Histoplasma capsulatum.*

complication of congenital or rheumatic heart disease but can also occur in children who do not have a cardiac malformation. In developed countries, congenital heart disease is the overwhelming predisposing factor. The disease is extremely rare in infancy.

Patients with a lesion that is associated with a high velocity of blood injected into a chamber or vessel are most susceptible to the infection. Vegetation is usually formed at the site of the endocardial or intimal erosion that results from the turbulent flow. Thus, children with ventricular septal defect, left-sided valvular disease, and systemic-pulmonary arterial communications are at the highest risk for developing infective endocarditis, while a very low incidence is reported in secundum atrial septal defect, a lesion characterized by low velocity flow across the interatrial defect. The risk of endocarditis in surgically uncorrected VSD (2–5%) and aortic stenosis (5–10%) increases with advancing age. Tetralogy of Fallot, VSD, aortic stenosis, PDA, transposition of the great arteries, and palliative shunts are the most frequent structural lesions associated with pediatric endocarditis. In older patients congenital bicuspid aortic valves and mitral valve prolapse pose additional risks for endocarditis. Surgical correction of heart disease reduces but does not eliminate the risk of endocarditis, except for repair of a simple ASD and PDA (risk is minimal 6 mo after repair). However, children who have had valve replacement and valve conduit repairs remain at risk.

In approximately 30% of patients with infective endocarditis a predisposing factor is recognized. A surgical or dental procedure can be implicated in approximately two thirds of the cases in which the potential source of bacteremia is identified. Furthermore, poor dental hygiene in children with cyanotic heart disease results in a greater risk for contamination of blood and eventually of the endocardium. The occurrence of endocarditis directly following cardiac catheterization or heart surgery is relatively low. However, on the basis of frequency of the performance of these procedures, they are frequent antecedent events.

CLINICAL MANIFESTATIONS (Table 15–15). The early symptoms and signs are usually mild, especially when *S. viridans* is the infecting organism. Prolonged fever, without other manifestations (except occasionally weight loss), persisting for as long as several months may often be the only medical history that can be elicited. Alternatively, the onset may be acute and severe, with high, intermittent fever and prostration. Usually, however, the onset and course vary within a range between these two extremes. The symptoms are usually nonspecific and consist of low-grade fever with afternoon elevations, fatigue, myalgia, arthralgia, headache,

TABLE 15–15. Manifestations of Infective Endocarditis

History
Prior congenital or rheumatic heart disease
Preceding dental, urinary, or intestinal procedure
Intravenous drug use
Central venous catheter
Prosthetic heart valve
Symptoms
Fever
Chills
Chest pain
Arthralgia/myalgia
Dyspnea
Malaise
Night sweats
Weight loss
CNS* manifestations (stroke, seizures, headache)
Signs
Elevated temperature
Tachycardia
Embolic phenomena (Roth spots, petechiae, splinter nailbed hemorrhages, Osler nodes, CNS or ocular lesions)
Janeway lesions
New or changing murmur
Splenomegaly
Arthritis
Heart failure
Arrhythmias
Metastatic infection (arthritis, meningitis, mycotic arterial aneurysm, pericarditis, abscesses, septic pulmonary emboli)
Clubbing
Laboratory
Positive blood culture
Elevated erythrocyte sedimentation rate; may be low with heart or renal failure
Elevated C-reactive protein
Anemia
Leukocytosis
Immune complexes
Hypergammaglobulinemia
Hypocomplementemia
Cryoglobulinemia
Rheumatoid factor
Hematuria
Azotemia, high creatinine (glomerulonephritis)
Echocardiographic evidence of valve vegetations, prosthetic valve dysfunction or leak, or myocardial abscess

*CNS = central nervous system.

and at times chills, nausea, and vomiting. Depending on the virulence of the agent the clinical findings may include signs of embolization and changes in the cardiac examination. Splenomegaly is relatively common, and petechiae may occur. New or changing heart murmurs are common, especially when there is destruction of valves and when there is associated congestive heart failure.

Serious neurologic complications, such as emboli, cerebral abscesses, mycotic aneurysms, and hemorrhage, that are manifested by meningismus, increased intracranial pressure, altered sensorium, and focal neurologic signs are most often associated with staphylococcal disease.

Myocardial abscesses may also occur with staphylococcal disease and may rupture into the pericardium. Pulmonary and other systemic emboli are infrequent except with fungal disease. Many of the classic skin manifestations develop late in the course of the disease; hence, they are seldom seen in the appropriately treated patient. These are *Osler nodes* (tender pea-sized intradermal nodules in the pads of the fingers and toes), *Janeway lesions* (painless small erythematous or hemorrhagic lesions on the palms and soles), and *splinter hemorrhages* (linear lesions beneath the nails). These lesions probably represent vasculitis produced by circulating antigen-antibody complexes.

The identification of infective endocarditis will most often be based on a high index of suspicion in the evaluation of an infection in a child with an underlying contributory factor.

LABORATORY DATA (see Table 15–15). *The critical information for appropriate treatment of infective endocarditis is obtained from blood cultures.* All other laboratory data are secondary in importance. Mild to moderate leukocytosis can be expected; the erythrocyte sedimentation rate is commonly elevated, and a mild hemolytic anemia (hemoglobin value seldom <9 g/dL) is not unusual. Microscopic hematuria, when present, is usually a manifestation of immune complex glomerulonephritis. Autoantibodies may develop as the disease progresses, and rheumatoid factors (antiglobulins) and cryoglobulins may be demonstrable at times.

Blood cultures must be obtained as promptly as possible in each child in whom infective endocarditis is a diagnostic possibility. These must be drawn even if the child feels well and has no other physical findings. Three to five separate blood collections should be obtained after careful preparation of the phlebotomy site. Contamination presents a special problem, as bacteria found on the skin may themselves cause infective endocarditis. The timing of collections is not important because bacteremia can be expected to be relatively constant. In 90% of cases of endocarditis the etiologic agent is recovered from the first two blood cultures. The laboratory should be notified that endocarditis is suspected as the blood may need to be cultured on enriched media for a longer than usual time (>7 days) to detect nutritionally deficient and fastidious bacteria or fungi. Antimicrobial pretreatment of the patient reduces the yield of blood cultures to 50–60%. The microbiology laboratory should be notified if the patient received antibiotics so that more sophisticated methods can be used to recover the offending agent. Other sites that may be cultured include cutaneous lesions, urine, synovial fluid, abscesses, and, in the presence of manifestations of meningitis, the cerebrospinal fluid (CSF). Serologic diagnosis is needed in patients with unusual or fastidious microorganisms (see Table 15–14).

The combination of M-mode, two-dimensional, and transesophageal echocardiography has enhanced the diagnosis of endocarditis. M mode can detect valvular vegetations larger than 2–3 mm. Two-dimensional echocardiography can identify the size, shape, location, and mobility of the lesion; when combined with Doppler studies the presence of valve dysfunction (regurgitation, obstruction) can be determined.

Transesophageal echocardiography has a much higher resolution than transthoracic techniques and detects even smaller vegetations. Echocardiography may help predict embolic complications, as lesions greater than 1 cm and fungating masses are at greatest risk for embolization. Echocardiography is particularly helpful in diagnosing endocarditis in patients with negative blood cultures and in bacteremic (but not necessarily endocarditis) patients with congenital heart disease or prosthetic valves. Nonetheless, the absence of vegetations does not exclude endocarditis, and vegetations are often not visualized in the early phases of the disease.

The effects of mitral and aortic valvular incompetence and prosthetic valve instability on left ventricular performance can also be evaluated by ultrasound techniques.

PROGNOSIS AND COMPLICATIONS. In the preantibiotic era infective endocarditis was a fatal disease. Mortality remains at 20–25%. Complications occur in 50–60% of children with documented infective endocarditis; the most common is cardiac failure due to vegetations involving the aortic or mitral valve. Myocardial abscesses and toxic myocarditis may also lead to congestive heart failure but without characteristic changes in auscultatory findings.

Superimposed on left-sided heart or aortic lesions, systemic emboli, often with central nervous system manifestations, are a major threat in patients with infective endocarditis. Pulmonary emboli may occur in children with ventricular septal defect or tetralogy of Fallot, although massive life-threatening pulmonary embolization is rare. Mycotic aneurysms, ruptured sinus of Valsalva, obstructive valve disease secondary to large vegetations, acquired ventricular septal defect, and heart block as a result of involvement of the specialized conduction system have all been reported as a result of infective endocarditis.

TREATMENT. Antibiotic therapy should be instituted immediately on diagnosis of infective endocarditis. When virulent organisms are responsible, small delays may result in progressive endocardial damage and a greater likelihood of severe complications. The choice of antibiotics, method of administration, and length of treatment are outlined in Table 15–16. High serum bactericidal levels must be maintained long enough to eradicate organisms that are growing in relatively inaccessible avascular vegetations. From 5 to 20 times the minimum in vitro inhibiting concentration must be produced at the site of infection to destroy bacteria growing at the core of these lesions. Several weeks are required for a vegetation to organize completely; thus, therapy must be continued through this period so that recrudescence can be avoided. A total of 4–6 wk of treatment is recommended, with serumcidal levels by tube dilution of at least 1:8 after a dose of antibiotic. Depending on the clinical and laboratory responses, antibiotic therapy may require modification, and in some instances more prolonged treatment is required. With highly sensitive *S. viridans* infections, shortened regimens including oral penicillin have been recommended.

Bed rest should be instituted and should be extended if congestive heart failure occurs. Similarly, digitalis, restriction of sodium, and diuretic therapy should be utilized when indicated.

Surgical intervention during the course of infective endocarditis is an integral part of management in cases in which severe aortic or mitral valve involvement leads to intractable heart failure. Rarely, a mycotic aneurysm or a rupture of an aortic sinus requires emergency operation. Other surgical indications include failure to sterilize the blood despite adequate antibiotic levels, a myocardial abscess, recurrent emboli, and failure of medical management. Although antibiotic therapy should be administered for as long as possible prior to surgical intervention, active infection is not a contraindication

TABLE 15–16. Treatment of Infective Endocarditis

Etiologic Agent	Drug	Dose	Route	Duration of Therapy (Weeks)
Streptococcus viridans, S. bovis (Minimal inhibitory concentration [MIC] ≤0.1 μg/mL)	(1) Penicillin G	200,000–300,000 U/kg/24 hr q 4 hr not to exceed 20 million U/24 hr	IV	4–6
	or			
	(2) Penicillin G	As above No. 1	IV	2–4
	plus gentamicin	2–4 mg/kg/24 hr q 8 hr not to exceed 80 mg/24 hr	IV	2
S. viridans, S. bovis (MIC ≥0.1 μg/mL)	(3) Penicillin G	As above No. 2	IV	4–6
	plus gentamicin	As above No. 2	IV	2
S. viridans or enterococcus (*S. bovis* or *S. faecalis*) (MIC >0.5 μg/mL)	(4) Penicillin G	As above No. 2	IV	4–6
	or ampicillin	300 mg/kg/24 hr q 4–6 hr not to exceed 12 g/24 hr	IV	4–6
	plus gentamicin	As above No. 2	IV	4–6
*S. viridans, S. bovis** (penicillin allergy†)	(5) Vancomycin	40–60 mg/kg/24 hr q 8–12 hr not to exceed 2 g/24 hr*	IV	4–6
	plus (6) gentamicin if resistant*	As above No. 2	IV	4–6
Staphylococcus aureus	(7) Nafcillin *or* oxacillin	200 mg/kg/24 hr q 4–6 hr not to exceed 12 g/24 hr	IV	6–8
	plus optional gentamicin	As above No. 2	IV	1–2
S. aureus (methicillin resistant) (penicillin allergy)	(8) Vancomycin	As above No. 5	IV	6–8
	plus optional trimethoprim-sulfamethoxazole	12 mg/kg/24 hr trimethoprim q 8 hr not to exceed 1 g/24 hr	IV, PO	4–8
S. aureus (with prosthetic device, methicillin sensitive)‡	(9) Nafcillin	As above No. 7	IV	6–8
	plus gentamicin	As above No. 2	IV	2
	plus optional rifampin	15–30 mg/kg/24 hr q 12 hr not to exceed 600 mg/24 hr	PO	≥6
S. aureus (with prosthetic device, methicillin resistant)	(10) Vancomycin	As above No. 5	IV	6–8
	plus gentamicin	As above No. 9	IV	2
	plus optional rifampin	As above No. 9	PO	≥6
S. epidermidis	(11) Vancomycin	As above No. 5	IV	6–8
	plus optional rifampin	As above No. 9	PO	6–8
Haemophilus species	(12) Ampicillin	As above No. 4	IV	4–6
	plus optional gentamicin	As above No. 2	IV	2–4
Unknown Postoperative	(13) Vancomycin	As above No. 5	IV	6–8
	plus gentamicin	As above No. 2	IV	2–4
Nonoperative	(14) Nafcillin	As above No. 7	IV	6–8
	or vancomycin	As above No. 5	IV	6–8
	plus gentamicin	As above No. 2	IV	2–4
	plus optional ampicillin	As above No. 4	IV	6–8

*Add gentamicin for relatively resistant organisms. Monitor vancomycin peaks one hour after infusion (30–45 μg/mL). Adjust dose according to vancomycin levels.

†Desensitization should be considered for patients who are allergic to penicillin. Cephalosporins are not recommended.

‡May require valve (device) replacement.

TABLE 15–17. Recommendations for Prevention of Bacterial Endocarditis*

Dental Procedures and Surgery of Upper Respiratory Tract	
(1) For most patients: Oral amoxicillin	*Adults:* 3 g 1 hr before a procedure and 1.5 g 6 hr after the initial dose *Children:* 50 mg/kg 1 hr before a procedure and 25 mg/kg 6 hr after the initial dose†
(2) Penicillin allergy: Oral erythromycin	*Adults:* 1 g 2 hr before a procedure and 500 mg 6 hr after the initial dose *Children:* 20 mg/kg 2 hr before a procedure and 10 mg/kg 6 hr after the initial dose†
or Oral clindamycin	*Adults:* 300 mg 1 hr before a procedure and 150 mg 6 hr after the initial dose *Children:* 10 mg/kg 1 hr before a procedure and 5 mg/kg 6 hr after the initial dose†
(3) High-risk patients:‡ Parenteral ampicillin plus gentamicin (IV or IM)	*Adults:* Ampicillin 2 g 30 min before a procedure§ Gentamicin 1.5 mg/kg 30 min before a procedure§ *Children:* Ampicillin 50 mg/kg 30 min before a procedure†§ Gentamicin 2 mg/kg 30 min before a procedure§
(4) High-risk penicillin-allergic patients: Vancomycin (IV)	*Adults:* 1 g infused slowly in 1 hr, initiated 1 hr before a procedure; no repeat dose needed *Children:* 20 mg/kg infused as adults; no repeat dose needed†
Gastrointestinal and Genitourinary Tract Surgery and Instrumentation	
(1) For most patients: Parenteral ampicillin plus gentamicin (IV or IM)	*Adults:* Ampicillin 2 g 30 min before a procedure§ Gentamicin 1.5 mg/kg 30 min before a procedure§ *Children:* Ampicillin 50 mg/kg 30 min before a procedure†§ Gentamicin 2 mg/kg 30 min before a procedure
(2) Penicillin allergy: Parenteral vancomycin plus gentamicin	*Adults:* Vancomycin 1 g infused slowly over 1 hr before a procedure‖ Gentamicin 1.5 mg/kg 30 min before a procedure‖ *Children:* Vancomycin 20 mg/kg infused slowly over 1 hr before a procedure† Gentamicin 2 mg/kg 30 min before a procedure‖
(3) Oral regimen for low-risk patients: Amoxicillin	*Adults:* 3 g 1 hr before a procedure and 1.5 g 6 hr later *Children:* 50 mg/kg 1 hr before a procedure and 25 mg 6 hr later†

Adapted from JAMA 264:2919, 1990, Copyright 1990, American Medical Association, and from Med Lett Drug Ther 31:112, 1989.

Oral regimens are less expensive, more convenient, and safer than parenteral routes. Amoxicillin is recommended because of excellent bioavailability and good activity against streptococci and enterococci. Parenteral routes are more effective and are recommended by some authorities for high-risk patients.

*Prophylaxis is recommended for patients with previous endocarditis, valvular heart disease, prosthetic heart devices, idiopathic hypertrophic subaortic stenosis, mitral valve prolapse with regurgitation, cardiac transplantation (possibly), and congenital heart disease except for an isolated secundum atrial septal defect and for patients who have recovered at least 6 mo from surgery for a patent ductus arteriosus or simple atrial septal defect without a patch.

†Maximal doses for children should not exceed adult doses.

‡High risk includes prosthetic valves, previous endocarditis, continuous penicillin prophylaxis for rheumatic fever, surgically constructed systemic-pulmonary shunts or conduits.

§Additional parenteral (ampicillin and gentamicin), or more often oral dose (amoxicillin), should be given 6–8 hr after the initial dose in high-risk patients. The dose of gentamicin should not exceed 80 mg.

‖Additional dose may be repeated 8 hr after the initial dose.

if the patient is critically ill as a result of severe hemodynamic deterioration from infective endocarditis. Removal of vegetations and, in some instances, valve replacement may be lifesaving, and sustained antibiotic administration will most often prevent reinfection. Replacement of infected prosthetic valves carries a higher risk.

Fungal endocarditis is difficult to manage and most often has a poor prognosis regardless of treatment. It has been encountered after cardiac surgery in severely debilitated patients, or in the immunosuppressed patient. The drugs of choice are amphotericin B and flucytosine, but surgery to excise infected tissue is occasionally attempted with limited success.

PREVENTION. Antimicrobial prophylaxis prior to and after various procedures, including tooth extractions and other forms of dental manipulation, reduces the incidence of infective endocarditis in susceptible patients. However, proper general dental care and oral hygiene are most important in decreasing the risk of infective endocarditis in susceptible individuals. Vigorous treatment of sepsis and local infections and careful asepsis during cardiac surgery and catheterization will also reduce the incidence of infective endocarditis.

Recommendations for specific antibiotic regimens for prevention of infective endocarditis under various circumstances are listed in Table 15–17.

Bisno AL, Dismukes WE, Durack DT, et al: Antimicrobial treatment of infective endocarditis due to viridans streptococci, enterococci, and staphylococci. JAMA 261:1471, 1989.

Dinubile MJ: Surgery in active endocarditis. Ann Intern Med 96:650, 1982.

Elward K, Hruby N, Christy C: Pneumococcal endocarditis in infants and children: Report of a case and review of the literature. Pediatr Infect Dis J 9:652, 1990.
Geva T, Frand M: Infective endocarditis in children with congenital heart disease: The changing spectrum, 1965–1985. Eur Heart J 9:1244, 1988.
van Hare GF, Ben-Shachar G, Liebman J, et al: Infective endocarditis in infants and children during the past 10 years: A decade of change. Am Heart J 107:1235, 1984.
Heimberger TS, Duma RJ: Infections of prosthetic heart valves and cardiac pacemakers. Infect Dis Clin North Am 3:221, 1989.
O'Callaghan C, McDougall P: Infective endocarditis in neonates. Arch Dis Child 63:53, 1988.
Shulman ST, Amren DP, Bisno AL, et al: Prevention of bacterial endocarditis. Am J Dis Child 139:232, 1985.
Stanton BF, Baltimore RS, Clemens JD: Changing spectrum of infective endocarditis in children. Am J Dis Child 138:720, 1984.
Wall TC, Peyton RB, Corey GR: Gonococcal endocarditis: A new look at an old disease. Medicine 68:375, 1989.
Walterspiel JN, Kaplan SL: Incidence and clinical characteristics of "culture-negative" infective endocarditis in a pediatric population. Pediatr Infect Dis 5:328, 1986.
Weinstein MP, Stratton CW, Ackley A, et al: Multicenter collaborative evaluation of a standardized serum bactericidal test as a prognostic indicator of infective endocarditis. Am J Med 78:262, 1985.

15.67 RHEUMATIC HEART DISEASE

Rheumatic involvement of the valves and endocardium is the most important manifestation of rheumatic fever (see Sec. 11.74). The lesions begin as small verrucae composed of fibrin and blood cells along the borders of one of the heart valves; the mitral valve is affected most often. The aortic valve is next in frequency; right-sided heart manifestations are rare. As the inflammation subsides, the verrucae tend to disappear and leave scar tissue. With a repeated attack of rheumatic fever, new verrucae form near the previous ones, and the mural endocardium and chordae tendineae become involved.

CLINICAL PATTERNS OF VALVULAR DISEASE. Mitral Insufficiency. This is the result of structural changes that usually include some loss of valvular substance and shortening and thickening of the chordae tendineae. During acute rheumatic fever with severe cardiac involvement, congestive heart failure is most often due to a combination of the mechanical effects of severe mitral insufficiency coupled with inflammatory disease that may involve the pericardium, myocardium, endocardium, and epicardium. Because of the high volume load and inflammatory process, the left ventricle becomes large and inefficient. The left atrium dilates as blood regurgitates into this chamber. Increased left atrial pressure results in pulmonary congestion and symptoms of left-sided heart failure. In patients with severe chronic mitral insufficiency the pulmonary arterial pressure becomes elevated, and enlargement of the right ventricle and atrium and subsequent right-sided heart failure will occur. However, in most cases mitral insufficiency is mild or moderate. Even in those patients in whom incompetence is severe at the onset, there is spontaneous improvement with time. The resultant chronic lesion is most often mild or moderate in severity, and the patient will be asymptomatic. Over half of patients with mitral insufficiency during an acute attack will no longer have the murmur of mitral involvement 1 yr later.

The principal physical signs of mitral insufficiency include a heaving apical left ventricular precordial impulse with a pansystolic murmur at the apex radiating to the axilla and the sternal edge. A mid-diastolic rumble at the apex suggests severe insufficiency. There is rarely a midsystolic ejection click as seen in patients with nonrheumatic mitral valve prolapse. In a young child with mitral insufficiency and no history suggestive of acute rheumatic fever, the differential diagnosis between a congenitally abnormal valve and rheumatic mitral involvement on the basis of the physical examination or echocardiography may be difficult. With severe mitral insufficiency, signs of chronic congestive heart failure, including fatigue, weight gain, weakness, and dyspnea on exertion, may be noted. The heart is enlarged with an apical systolic thrill. The 1st heart sound is normal; the 2nd heart sound may be accentuated if pulmonary hypertension is present. A 3rd heart sound is prominent. In addition to the pansystolic murmur a short diastolic rumble follows the 3rd sound; it is due to increased blood flow from the volume-loaded left atrium across the mitral valve as a result of the massive insufficiency. This murmur is associated with mitral incompetence and does not mean that mechanical mitral stenosis is present. The latter lesion takes many years to develop and is characterized by a diastolic murmur of greater length with presystolic accentuation.

The *electrocardiogram* and *roentgenograms* are normal if the lesion is mild. With more severe insufficiency the electrocardiogram shows prominent bifid P waves, signs of left ventricular hypertrophy, and sometimes associated right ventricular hypertrophy. Roentgenographically, there is prominence of the left atrium and ventricle. When pulmonary hypertension or congestive heart failure is present, the pulmonary artery segment and right-sided heart chambers are prominent. Signs of pulmonary venous hypertension may also be evident. Calcification of the mitral valve is rare in children. *Echocardiography* shows enlargement of the left atrium and ventricle, and Doppler study demonstrates mitral regurgitation. The left ventricular shortening fraction may be normal even with poor ventricular function. This is because of the "unloading" effect of the retrograde flow to the low-pressure left atrium. The signs of classic mitral valve prolapse are usually absent.

Cardiac catheterization and *left ventriculography* are considered *only* if there is rapid progression of the disease and surgical treatment is contemplated, and if diagnostic questions regarding other valves are not totally resolved on the basis of noninvasive assessment. The cardiac output is normal or decreased in severe lesions. The left atrial pressure is frequently but not always increased. The pulse curve of the left atrium shows a steep rise in early systole to the peak of the "v" wave and is followed by a rapid "y" descent. A diastolic flow gradient may be measured across the mitral valve even in the absence of mitral stenosis. The left ventricular end-diastolic pressure rises during exercise or in the presence of left ventricular failure. Left ventriculography results in opacification of the left atrium. The degree of opacification is used as a qualitative assessment of the severity of incompetence.

Complications. Severe mitral incompetence may result in cardiac failure that may be precipitated by progression of the rheumatic process, the onset of atrial fibrillation with rapid ventricular response, or infective endocarditis. After many years, the effects of chronic mitral insufficiency may become manifest without a new event. Right-sided heart failure may be accompanied by tricuspid or pulmonary valve incompetence. Occasional atrial or ventricular extrasystoles are seen. Atrial fibrillation is more common when mitral incompetence is associated with a large left atrium. Patients with atrial fibrillation may need to receive low-dose warfarin therapy (target prothrombin time ratio, 1.2:1.5) for prevention of thromboemboli and stroke.

Treatment. In most patients with mitral insufficiency, prophylaxis against recurrences of rheumatic fever is all that is required since the lesions are mild and well tolerated (Sec.

11.74). The treatment of complicating heart failure, dysrhythmias, and infective endocarditis is described elsewhere in this chapter. Afterload-reducing agents (captopril) may be especially useful. Surgical treatment is indicated in patients who, despite adequate medical therapy, suffer from recurrent episodes of heart failure, dyspnea with moderate activity, and progressive cardiomegaly, often with pulmonary hypertension. Although annuloplasty gives good results in some children and adolescents, valve replacement may be required. Activity should not be restricted in children having mild mitral incompetence.

Mitral Stenosis. Congenital mitral stenosis has been described in Sec. 15.54.

Mitral stenosis of rheumatic origin results from fibrosis of the mitral ring, commissural adhesions, and contracture of the valve leaflets, chordae, and papillary muscles over a significant period of time. It usually takes 10 yr or more for the lesion to become fully established, although the process may occasionally be accelerated. Rheumatic mitral stenosis is seldom encountered prior to adolescence, and usually is not recognized until adult life.

Mitral stenosis is recognized clinically if the valvular orifice is reduced to 25% or less of the expected normal. Such reductions result in increased pressure and hypertrophy of the left atrium. The increased pressure causes pulmonary venous hypertension, increased pulmonary vascular resistance, and pulmonary hypertension. Right ventricular and atrial dilatation and hypertrophy ensue and are followed by right-sided heart failure.

Generally, there is a good correlation between symptoms and severity of obstruction. Patients with mild lesions are asymptomatic. More severe degrees of obstruction are associated with effort intolerance and dyspnea. Critical lesions can result in orthopnea, paroxysmal nocturnal dyspnea, and overt pulmonary edema. These symptoms may be precipitated by uncontrolled tachycardia, atrial fibrillation, or pulmonary infections. Congestive heart failure is usually but not invariably associated with moderate or severe pulmonary hypertension. Right ventricular dilatation may result in functional tricuspid incompetence, hepatomegaly, ascites, and edema. Hemoptysis due to ruptured bronchial or pleurohilar veins and, occasionally, pulmonary infarction may occur. Blood-streaked sputum occurs during episodes of pulmonary edema. With chronic severe mitral stenosis, cyanosis and a malar flush are noted.

The jugular venous pressure is increased in the presence of congestive heart failure, tricuspid valve disease, or severe pulmonary hypertension. The heart size is normal with minimal disease. Moderate cardiomegaly is usual with severe mitral stenosis and sinus rhythm, but cardiac enlargement can be great, especially when atrial fibrillation and heart failure supervene. The apical impulse is normal, but a parasternal right ventricular lift is palpable when pulmonary pressure is high. The principal auscultatory findings are a loud 1st heart sound, an opening snap of the mitral valve, and a long, low-pitched, rumbling mitral diastolic murmur with presystolic accentuation at the apex. The mitral diastolic murmur may be virtually absent in patients who are in congestive heart failure. A systolic murmur due to tricuspid incompetence may be audible. In the presence of pulmonary hypertension, pulmonary valvular closure is accentuated. An early diastolic murmur may be due to associated aortic incompetence or secondary pulmonary valvular incompetence (Graham Steell murmur).

Electrocardiograms and *roentgenograms* are normal if the lesion is mild; as severity increases, there are prominent and notched P waves and varying degrees of right ventricular hypertrophy. Atrial fibrillation is a common late manifestation. Moderate or severe lesions are associated with roentgenographic signs of left atrial enlargement, prominence of the pulmonary artery and right-sided heart chambers, and a normal or small aorta and left ventricle (Fig. 15–70); there may be calcifications

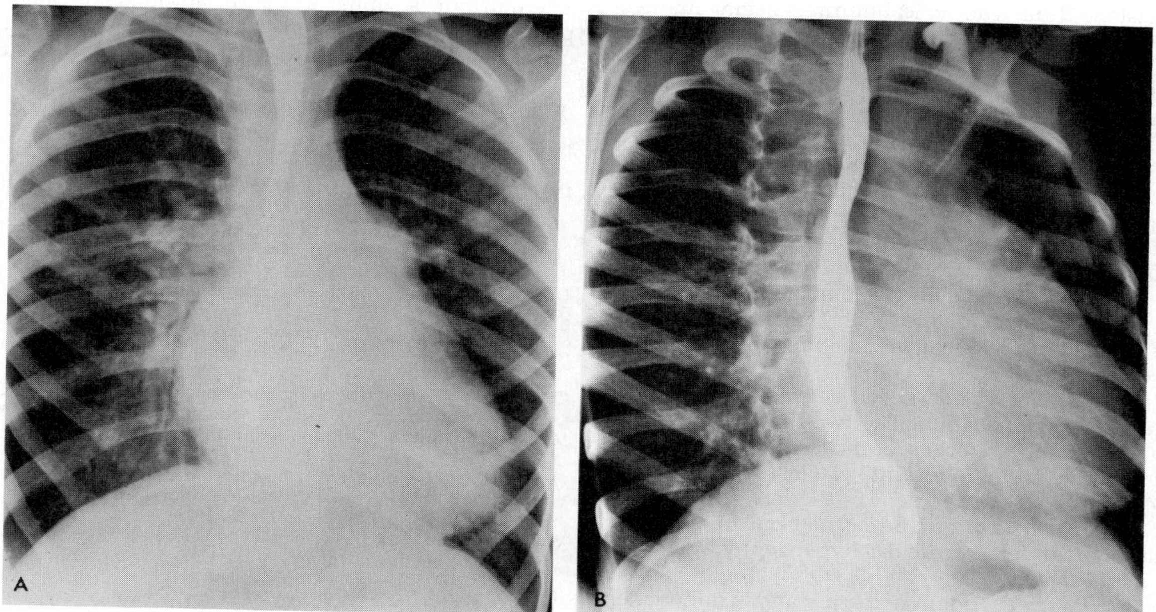

Figure 15–70. Roentgenograms in isolated rheumatic mitral stenosis. *A*, Posteroanterior view showing cardiomegaly and prominent main pulmonary artery. Vascular shadows in the lungs are due to prominent pulmonary arteries and veins. *B*, Right anterior oblique view showing indentation of the esophagus by the large left atrium. This patient required a valvotomy at 8 yr of age.

noted in the region of the mitral valve. Severe obstruction is associated with a redistribution of pulmonary blood flow so that the apices of the lung have a greater perfusion (i.e., reverse of normal). Septal lines at the costophrenic angles may also be present. *Echocardiography* shows distinct narrowing of the mitral orifice during diastole and left atrial enlargement. A Doppler diastolic gradient can be calculated. *Cardiac catheterization* quantitates the diastolic gradient across the mitral valve and the pulmonary arterial pressure.

TREATMENT. Surgical treatment is undertaken when there are clinical signs and hemodynamic evidence of severe obstruction, but prior to the severe manifestations outlined earlier. Since extreme valvular distortion and calcification are rare, surgical or balloon catheter mitral valvotomy generally yields good results in rheumatic mitral stenosis; valve replacement is avoided unless absolutely necessary. Balloon valvuloplasty is indicated in symptomatic, stenotic pliable noncalcified valves of patients without atrial arrhythmias or thrombi.

Aortic Insufficiency. In chronic rheumatic aortic insufficiency, sclerosis of the aortic valves results in distortion and retraction of the cusps. Regurgitation of blood results in a volume overload with dilatation and hypertrophy of the left ventricle. *Combined mitral and aortic insufficiency are more common than aortic involvement alone.* Left ventricular failure may eventually occur.

Symptoms are unusual except in gross aortic incompetence. The large stroke volume and forceful left ventricular contractions may result in palpitations. Excessive sweating and heat intolerance are related to vasodilatation. Dyspnea on effort can progress to orthopnea and pulmonary edema; angina may occur during heavy exertion. In adolescents with severe incompetence, nocturnal attacks with sweating, tachycardia, chest pain, and hypertension may occur. In the United States patients with the classic clinical picture of florid mitral or aortic disease are rarely encountered.

Because of the reflux of blood through the aortic valve during diastole, the pulse pressure is wide with bounding peripheral pulses. The systolic blood pressure is elevated, the diastolic lowered. In severe aortic insufficiency, the heart is enlarged and there is a left ventricular apical heave. There may be a diastolic thrill. The typical murmur begins immediately with the 2nd heart sound and continues until late in diastole. The murmur is heard over the upper and middle left sternal border with radiation to the apex and to the aortic area. Characteristically, it has a hollow, high-pitched blowing quality. Generally, the murmur is more easily audible in full expiration, with the diaphragm of the stethoscope placed firmly on the chest and the patient leaning forward. Occasionally, it may be louder in the recumbent position. A systolic ejection murmur sometimes preceded by a click is frequent and is produced by the large stroke volume. An apical presystolic murmur (Austin Flint) resembling that of mitral stenosis is sometimes heard and is the result of the large regurgitant aortic flow in diastole that prevents the mitral valve from opening fully.

The *echocardiogram* shows a large left ventricle and diastolic mitral valve flutter or oscillation. The two-dimensional echocardiogram shows the abnormal aortic valve, and Doppler studies demonstrate aortic runoff into the left ventricle.

Roentgenograms show enlargement of the left ventricle and aorta. The *electrocardiogram* may be normal but in advanced cases reveals signs of left ventricular hypertrophy and strain with prominent P waves.

Cardiac catheterization is seldom necessary and is undertaken only when surgery is contemplated because of a progressive lesion. The degree of elevation of left ventricular end-diastolic, left atrial, and pulmonary arterial pressures is established, and ascending aortography demonstrates the aortic insufficiency.

Mild and moderate lesions are well tolerated. Many adolescents with severe regurgitation are symptom-free and tolerate advanced lesions into the 3rd–4th decades. Unlike mitral incompetence, aortic insufficiency does not regress. Patients with combined lesions at the time of acute rheumatic fever may have only aortic involvement 1–2 yr later. Surgical intervention should be carried out well in advance of the onset of congestive heart failure, pulmonary edema, or angina, when there are signs of decreasing myocardial performance. When there are early symptoms, ST-T wave changes on the electrocardiogram and/or decreasing left ventricular ejection fraction, surgery is considered.

Treatment in most cases consists of prophylaxis against the recurrence of acute rheumatic fever and occurrence of infective endocarditis. The patient is encouraged to lead as active and normal a life as possible. Surgical treatment (valve replacement) is undertaken when there is progressive cardiomegaly and early signs of left ventricular dysfunction.

Tricuspid Valvular Disease. Primary tricuspid involvement is rare following rheumatic fever. *Tricuspid insufficiency* secondary to right ventricular dilatation resulting from severe left-sided lesions can occur in patients with severe cases in whom surgery is not carried out. The signs produced by tricuspid insufficiency include prominent pulsations of the jugular veins with a "c-v" wave, systolic pulsations of the liver, and blowing systolic murmur in the 4th and 5th left parasternal spaces that increases in intensity during inspiration. Concomitant signs of mitral or aortic valve disease, with or without atrial fibrillation, are frequent. Signs of tricuspid incompetence decrease or disappear when heart failure produced by the left-sided lesions is successfully treated. However, tricuspid valvuloplasty may be required in some cases.

Pulmonary Valvular Disease. Pulmonary insufficiency occurs on a functional basis secondary to pulmonary hypertension or dilatation of the pulmonary artery. This is a late finding with severe mitral stenosis (Graham Steell murmur). The murmur is similar to that of aortic insufficiency, but the peripheral arterial signs are absent. The correct diagnosis is confirmed by 2-D echocardiography and Doppler studies.

Anonymous: Acute rheumatic fever at a Navy training center—San Diego, California. MMWR 37:101, 1988.

Barnett LA, Cunningham MW: A new heart-cross-reactive antigen in *Streptococcus pyogenes* is not M protein. J Infect Dis 162:875, 1990.

Dajani AS, Bisno AL, Chung KJ, et al: Prevention of rheumatic fever: A statement for health professionals by the Committee on Rheumatic Fever, Endocarditis and Kawasaki Disease of the Council on Cardiovascular Disease in the Young, the American Heart Association. Pediatr Infect Dis J 8:263, 1989.

Durack DT, Kaplan EL, Bisno AL: Apparent failures of endocarditis prophylaxis. JAMA 205:2218, 1983.

Gersony WM, Hayes CJ: Bacterial endocarditis in patients with pulmonary stenosis, aortic stenosis, or valvular septal defect. Circulation 56(Suppl): 84, 1977.

Griffiths SP, Gersony WM: Acute rheumatic fever in New York City (1969 to 1988): A comparative study of two decades. J Pediatr 116:882, 1990.

Markowitz M, Kaplan EL: Reappearance of rheumatic fever. Adv Pediatr 36:39, 1989.

Quinn RW: Comprehensive review of morbidity and mortality trends for rheumatic fever, streptococcal disease, and scarlet fever: The decline of rheumatic fever. Rev Infect Dis 11:928, 1989.

Veasy LG, Wiedmeier SE, Orsmond GS, et al: Resurgence of acute rheumatic fever in the intermountain area of the United States. N Engl J Med 316:421, 1987.

Westlake RM, Graham TP, Edwards KM: An outbreak of acute rheumatic fever in Tennessee. Pediatr Infect Dis J 9:97, 1990.

15.68 DISEASES OF THE MYOCARDIUM

15.69 CONDITIONS CAUSING MYOCARDIAL DAMAGE

The status of the myocardium is a critical factor in the prognosis of cardiac disease. If, in spite of congenital cardiac malformations, acquired valvular disease, or arrhythmias, the myocardium is still able to provide satisfactory circulation of blood, the child will be able to maintain adequate nutrition, growth, and activity. In addition to injury resulting from chronic volume or pressure load, the myocardium may be directly affected by infections, mesenchymal diseases, endocrine disorders, metabolic and nutritional diseases, neuromuscular diseases, blood diseases, tumors, hypertension, and congenital anomalies (Table 15–18).

BACTERIAL INFECTIONS. In **diphtheria** (see Sec. 12.25) the toxin of the bacillus may produce peripheral circulatory failure or toxic myocarditis. Peripheral circulatory failure occurs within the first 2 wk of the disease and is associated with a rapid, thready pulse; cold, pale, and clammy skin; and hypotension. In addition to therapy for diphtheria, treatment for cardiogenic shock is essential. This disease is especially prone to affect the conduction system.

Toxic myocarditis is characterized by the development of atrioventricular block, bundle branch block, or extrasystoles. Congestive cardiac failure occurs later and is associated with cardiac enlargement and gallop rhythm. In addition to the arrhythmia, the electrocardiogram shows ST segment depression and T wave inversion in most leads. The immediate prognosis is grave (about 50% mortality). Treatment includes strict bed rest until all signs of myocarditis have disappeared and management of arrhythmias, including cardiac pacing. Digitalis is reserved for patients with frank congestive heart failure but must be used with care because of the possibility of increased sensitivity.

In **bacterial infections**, circulatory involvement is manifested as peripheral circulatory collapse or toxic myocarditis. Toxic myocarditis as evidenced by tachycardia, gallop rhythm, and cardiac enlargement may complicate pneumonia, infective endocarditis, and septicemia. A myocardial depressant factor may produce an acute toxic cardiomyopathy. The prognosis depends on control of the primary infection.

RICKETTSIAL DISEASES. Rocky Mountain spotted fever (see Sec. 12.89), in particular, may be complicated by hypotension and peripheral vascular collapse. This complication has been attributed to the general vasculitis characteristic of the disease, but acute myocarditis may be a contributing factor.

VIRAL INFECTIONS. A viral etiology has been implicated in many patients with acute myocarditis (see Sec. 15.70).

TABLE 15–18. Etiology of Myocardial Disease

Familial-Hereditary
- Carnitine deficiency syndromes*
- Mitochondrial myopathy syndromes*
- Hypertrophic cardiomyopathy*
- Duchenne muscular dystrophy*
- Other muscular dystrophies (Becker, limb girdle)
- Myotonic dystrophy
- Kearns-Sayre (progressive external ophthalmoplegia)
- Friedreich ataxia
- Mucopolysaccharidosis
- Hemochromatosis
- Fabry disease
- Pompe disease
- Primary endocardial fibroelastosis

Infection
- *Virus:* coxackievirus A and B,* human immunodeficiency virus (AIDS), echovirus, rubella, varicella, influenza, mumps, Epstein-Barr, measles, poliomyelitis
- *Rickettsiae:* psittacosis, coxiella, Rocky Mountain spotted fever
- *Bacteria:* diphtheria, mycoplasma, meningococcus, leptospirosis, Lyme disease, typhoid fever, tuberculosis, streptococcus, listeriosis
- *Parasites:* Chagas disease, toxoplasmosis, Loa loa, *Toxocara canis,* schistosomiasis, cysticercosis, *Echinococcus,* trichinosis
- *Fungi:* histoplasmosis, coccidioidomycosis, actinomycosis

Metabolic, Nutritional, Endocrine
- Beriberi (thiamine deficiency)
- Keshan disease (selenium deficiency)
- Kwashiorkor
- Hypothyroidism
- Hyperthyroidism
- Carcinoid
- Pheochromocytoma
- Hypercholesterolemia
- Infant of diabetic mother*

Connective Tissue–Granulomatous Disease
- Systemic lupus erythematosus
- Scleroderma
- Churg-Strauss vasculitis
- Rheumatoid arthritis
- Rheumatic fever
- Sarcoidosis
- Amyloidosis
- Dermatomyositis
- Periarteritis nodosa

Drugs-Toxins
- Adriamycin*
- Cyclophosphamide
- Chloroquine
- Ipecac (emetine)
- Iron overload (hemosiderosis)
- Sulfonamides
- Mesalezine
- Chloramphenicol
- Hypersensitivity reaction
- Alcohol
- Irradiation

Coronary arteries
- Kawasaki disease*
- Medial necrosis
- Anomalous left coronary artery

Other
- Anemia*
- Sickle cell anemia (sickling)*
- Hypereosinophilic syndrome (Löffler syndrome)
- Endomyocardial fibrosis
- Ischemia-hypoxia
- Peripartum cardiomyopathy
- Idiopathic dilated cardiomyopathy (familial, enteroviral, autoimmune)
- Arrhythmogenic right ventricular dysplasia (familial and nonfamilial)
- Uhl right ventricular anomaly
- Histiocytoid (oncocytic, lipidosis) cardiomyopathy
- Acute eosinophilic necrotizing myocarditis

*Relatively common etiology of myocarditis-cardiomyopathy.

PARASITIC AND FUNGAL INFECTIONS. Lesions in the myocardium have been described in association with *histoplasmosis, coccidioidomycosis, toxoplasmosis,* and *trichinosis.* In these conditions the cardiac lesion seldom produces clinical signs of myocarditis. *Actinomycosis* may involve the pericardium and myocardium by direct contiguity to, for example, a pulmonary abscess. *Hydatid cysts* of the pericardium may be found on routine roentgenograms of the chest and usually produce symptoms only when they rupture. *Schistosomiasis* may produce pulmonary hypertension and cor pulmonale. *Cruz trypanosomiasis* (Chagas disease) may produce acute or subacute myocarditis and sudden death.

MUCOCUTANEOUS LYMPH NODE SYNDROME (KAWASAKI DISEASE). See Sec. 11.57. Arteritis disease initially involves small arterioles, but in the 2nd and 3rd weeks of illness medium-sized arteries become inflamed and aneurysmal dilatation of the coronary arteries may occur. Myocarditis is uncommon but manifests as congestive heart failure. During the healing phase alternate areas of coronary dilatation and stenosis may result and have led to myocardial infarction and death.

MESENCHYMAL DISEASES. *Rheumatic carditis* is described in Sec. 15.67, and the cardiovascular manifestations of *rheumatoid arthritis, disseminated lupus erythematosus, periarteritis nodosa, dermatomyositis,* and *scleroderma* are described in Chapter 11.

ENDOCRINE DISORDERS. *Hyperthyroidism* (Sec. 19.12) produces tachycardia, vasodilatation, wide pulse pressure, cardiac enlargement, and, rarely, atrial fibrillation. *Cretinism* seldom produces gross cardiac involvement, but the electrocardiogram is characterized by bradycardia, low voltage of all complexes—especially of the P and T waves, left axis deviation, and prolonged electrical systole. These signs may disappear within 1 mo after initiation of adequate thyroid therapy.

METABOLIC AND NUTRITIONAL DISEASES. Among vitamin deficiency diseases, *beriberi* (Sec. 4.7) causes the most conspicuous cardiac damage. In patients with malnutrition the deficiencies are often multiple, and it is difficult to separate the cardiac lesion of one nutritional disease from that of another. (See Blood Diseases later and Sec. 16.10 and 16.11.)

NEUROMUSCULAR DISEASES. Heart disease is common in *Friedreich ataxia.* In most cases cardiac symptoms are less intense than the neurologic component (Sec. 20.58), which limits physical activities. In some patients effort intolerance, chest pain, and heart failure have been the presenting symptoms. These are due to primary myocardial disease that chiefly affects the left ventricle and results in congestive or restrictive cardiomyopathy. The electrocardiogram shows generalized T wave inversion or signs of left ventricular hypertrophy. Myocardial dysfunction is demonstrated by 2-D echocardiography. Arrhythmias may also occur and consist of atrial tachycardia or fibrillation or extrasystoles. Varying degrees of cardiomegaly, left ventricular prominence, and pulmonary congestion are demonstrable roentgenographically.

In *progressive muscular dystrophy* (Sec. 21.11) 50% of children have postmortem evidence of myocardial involvement similar to that of the striated muscle. Cardiac symptoms, however, are not common, but the electrocardiogram is frequently abnormal and may reveal tachycardia, abnormalities of the P waves, short P-R interval, and abnormal Q and T waves. Minimal evidence of right or left ventricular hypertrophy also may be noted, and some patients have congestive heart failure.

BLOOD DISEASES. In infants and children anemia is the most common blood disease associated with cardiac involvement. Although cardiac output increases when the hemoglobin is below about 7 g/dL, cardiac enlargement in infants with or without congestive heart failure occurs only with an extreme reduction in hemoglobin, to 3–4 g or less. The heart rate is rapid, the pulse pressure widened, and the venous pressure increased. A systolic murmur at the apex or along the left sternal border is usual; diastolic murmurs may occur in the same areas, and gallop rhythm is common. The electrocardiographic changes include depressed ST segments and flat T waves. Occasionally, only minimal signs and symptoms are present when extreme states of anemia have developed gradually.

Treatment is directed toward the cause of the anemia. If blood transfusions are indicated in the presence of cardiomegaly or cardiac failure, small volumes (4–5 mL/kg) of packed cells should be administered. (See Sec. 16.10 and 16.11–16.36.) Often, it is more prudent to use exchange transfusion to avoid an acute increase in blood volume.

GLYCOGEN STORAGE DISEASE. Cardiac as well as skeletal muscle is affected in the generalized form of glycogen storage disease known as type II or Pompe disease (Sec. 8.40). Cardiomegaly is massive; murmurs are insignificant. Pulmonary atelectasis with secondary infection is common and is related to compression by the large heart. The *electrocardiogram* is characteristic and shows prominent P waves, short P-R interval, massive QRS voltage, signs of isolated left or biventricular hypertrophy, and intraventricular conduction defects. *Roentgenograms* confirm the striking cardiomegaly with prominence of the left ventricle. The prognosis is poor.

HURLER SYNDROME (Sec. 8.43). The lesion in the heart and great vessels is the same as that in the connective tissue elsewhere in the body. The most pronounced lesions are found in the valves and coronary arteries, but abnormalities in the pericardium and aorta are not uncommon. The heart may be moderately enlarged, with electrocardiographic signs of left ventricular hypertrophy. Cardiac murmurs may result from incompetence and stenosis of the mitral and aortic valves. Sometimes the pulmonary and tricuspid valves are also involved. Coronary arterial disease may result in angina and perhaps explain the frequent occurrence of sudden death. The prognosis is poor.

CALCINOSIS OF THE CORONARY ARTERIES. This is a rare disease of infancy. The coronary arteries are tortuous and calcareous, and the ventricles, especially the left, are hypertrophied. Other blood vessels may be similarly involved. The onset of cardiac failure is sudden; death usually occurs in infancy.

DOXORUBICIN HYDROCHLORIDE ADRIAMYCIN CARDIOTOXICITY. Severe, dose-dependent cardiomyopathy occurs in about 30% of patients when the total cumulative dose of doxorubicin hydrochloride exceeds 550 mg/m^2. Cardiomegaly is due principally to left ventricular and left atrial enlargement. If congestive cardiac failure develops, the case fatality rate is 30–50%. T wave flattening or inversion is nonspecific evidence of cardiac involvement; early cardiac changes may be detected by serial echocardiograms that show progressive decrease in myocardial contractility, even in asymptomatic patients. The child's condition may remain clinically stable for many years.

IPECAC CARDIAC TOXICITY. This is noted in patients with chronic intentional ipecac abuse secondary to anorexia nervosa or bulimia nervosa. Manifestations are probably due to the emetine component of ipecac and include chest pain, tachycardia, dyspnea, hypotension, arrhythmias, flattening and inversion of T waves, ST segment abnormalities, prolongation of Q-T and P-R intervals, cardiac failure, and death. Differentiating the cardiac abnormalities due to ipecac from those of chronic starvation, abnormal diets, and electrolyte abnormalities may be difficult.

15.70 MYOCARDITIS

Myocarditis refers to inflammation, necrosis, or myocytolysis that may be due to many infectious, connective tissue, granulomatous, toxic, or idiopathic processes affecting the myocardium with or without associated systemic manifestations of the disease process or involvement of the endocardium or pericardium (see Table 15–18). Coronary pathology is uniformly absent. The most common manifestation is congestive heart failure, although arrhythmias and sudden death may be the first sign of myocarditis. Acute or chronic infection due to coxsackievirus B is the prototype of viral myocarditis.

EPIDEMIOLOGY. The incidence of myocarditis in children is unknown. Viral myocarditis is typically a sporadic but occasionally epidemic illness, noted as an acute potentially fulminant disease of 1- to 4-wk-old infants, as an acute but more benign myopericarditis of toddlers and young children, and as a precursor to idiopathic dilated cardiomyopathy in infants but more often adolescents and young adults.

PATHOGENESIS. Acute viral myocarditis may produce a fulminant inflammatory process characterized by cellular infiltrates, cell degeneration and necrosis, and subsequent fibrosis. Viral myocarditis may also become a chronic process with persistence of coxsackievirus RNA (but not infectious virus particles) in the myocardium. Chronic inflammation is then perpetuated by the host immune response, which includes T lymphocytes activated against viral-host antigenic alterations. Such cytotoxic lymphocytes and natural killer cells together with persistent and possibly defective viral replication may impair myocyte function without obvious cytolysis. Alternatively, the persistent viral infection may alter major histocompatibility complex antigen expression, with resultant exposure of neoantigens to the immune system. In addition, some viral proteins may share antigenic epitopes with host cells, resulting in autoimmune damage to the antigenically related myocyte. The net final result of chronic viral-associated inflammation may be dilated cardiomyopathy.

CLINICAL MANIFESTATIONS. The presentation depends on the age and acute or chronic nature of infection. The neonate with coxsackievirus myocarditis may present with fever, severe heart failure, respiratory distress, cyanosis, distant heart sounds, weak pulses, tachycardia out of proportion to the fever, mitral insufficiency due to dilatation of the valve annulus, a gallop rhythm, shock, acidosis with evidence of viral hepatitis, aseptic meningitis, rash, and death within 1–7 days of the onset of symptoms. The chest roentgenograms reveal a large heart and pulmonary edema; the electrocardiogram reveals sinus tachycardia, reduced QRS complex voltage, and ST segment and T wave abnormalities. Arrhythmias may be the first manifestation and in the presence of fever with a large heart should suggest myocarditis.

The older patient, with persistent presence of the coxsackievirus genome in the myocardium, will present with the gradual onset of congestive heart failure or the sudden onset of ventricular arrhythmias (see Sec. 15.72).

DIAGNOSIS. The sedimentation rate and heart enzymes (CPK, LDH) may be elevated in acute or chronic myocarditis. Coxsackievirus IgM is present transiently in 50–60% of acute myocarditis and may persist for 5–10 yr in some patients with dilated cardiomyopathy. Echocardiography will demonstrate poor ventricular function and possibly the presence of a pericardial effusion, mitral valve regurgitation, and the absence of coronary artery or other congenital lesions.

Myocarditis may be confirmed by percutaneous endomyocardial biopsy. This is performed during cardiac catheterization and can also detect other causes of cardiomyopathy (carnitine deficiency, storage disease, mitochondrial defects); approximately 50% of clinically suspected cases of myocarditis have another diagnosis. Specimens obtained are sent for light and electron microscopy, immunologic studies, examination for inborn errors of metabolism, and molecular biology assays to detect products of the viral genome. Initial findings suggestive of active myocarditis include an inflammatory infiltrate with damage to adjacent myocytes, with or without fibrosis. Three tissue specimens are taken, as the early process may be focal rather than generalized. The uninvolved myocardium is normal while damage consists of necrosis, vacuolization, irregular cell outlines, or cellular disruption with closely associated lymphocytes near the cell surface. Subsequent follow-up biopsy findings of persistent myocarditis include the same or worsening features as in the original biopsy, whereas resolving myocarditis reveals less inflammation and cellular pathology. Resolved myocarditis demonstrates no inflammatory cells or ongoing cell necrosis.

DIFFERENTIAL DIAGNOSIS. The predominant diseases mimicking myocarditis include carnitine deficiency, mitochondrial defects, cardiomyopathy (idiopathic dilated or hypertrophic), pericarditis, endocardial fibroelastosis, and anomalies of the coronary arteries or left side of the heart (see Table 15–18).

TREATMENT. Therapy of severe congestive heart failure is discussed in Sec. 15.73 and includes diuretics, sodium and fluid restriction, digoxin, dobutamine, amrinone, and afterload reduction (nitroprusside, captopril). Dopamine or epinephrine may be helpful if there is poor cardiac output with systemic hypotension. Pericardiocentesis should be performed if there is evidence of cardiac tamponade. Arrhythmias should be treated as noted in Table 15–12; patients with myocarditis may be more susceptible to the arrhythmogenic properties of digoxin and to sympathomimetic inotropic agents.

The role of corticosteroids for acute neonatal myocarditis due to coxsackievirus has not been established. However, prednisone (60 mg daily; later 60 mg every other day) may be beneficial in adolescent or adult patients with reactive immune-mediated dilated cardiomyopathy. Cardiac transplantation is the treatment of choice in patients with refractory heart failure (see Sec. 6.45).

PROGNOSIS. The outcome of the symptomatic neonate with acute viral myocarditis remains poor, with a mortality between 50 and 70%. These patients may be at the end of a spectrum while other neonates may manifest minimal cardiac signs and symptoms.

The outcome of the biopsy-proven chronic dilated cardiomyopathy associated with coxsackievirus is poor without therapy. Patients continue to have inflammation fibrosis and deteriorating cardiac function (ejection fraction). Spontaneous resolution may occur in 10–20%. As many as 50% of untreated older patients die within 2 yr of presentation and 80% die within 8 yr.

15.71 ENDOCARDIAL FIBROELASTOSIS

This condition has been called fetal endocarditis, endocardial fibrosis, prenatal fibroelastosis, elastic tissue hyperplasia, and endocardial sclerosis.

It is classified into two general types: primary and secondary. In *primary* endocardial fibroelastosis (EFE) there is no apparent predisposing valvular lesion or other congenital abnormality. Genetic forms have been described. In the *secondary* type severe congenital heart disease of the left-sided obstructive type (e.g., aortic stenosis or atresia, forms of hypoplastic left side of the heart, and severe coarctation of the aorta) is present. In secondary EFE the ventricular cavity is often contracted, whereas in the primary disease a dilated left ventricular chamber is seen in the infant. However, in young adults a primary contracted type of EFE has been observed.

No etiology for primary EFE has been established; possibilities include inflammation or infection before or after birth, maldevelopment, and inadequate blood supply to the endocardium. The endocardial changes could also be secondary to myocardial disease which, resulting in cardiac dilatation and in stretching of the endocardium, initiates fibroelastic proliferation. The disease has occurred in siblings.

Pathologically, there is a white, opaque fibroelastic thickening of the endocardium, virtually always in the left ventricle, which frequently obscures the trabeculation of the inner surfaces of the cardiac chamber. The lesion may spread to involve the valves. Microscopically, the lesion consists of a fibroelastic thickening of the endocardium and may result in subendocardial degeneration or necrosis of muscle with vacuolation of muscle fibers. The involved valve leaflets are characterized by a myxomatous proliferation with an increase in collagenous elements.

The *clinical manifestations* are variable. Infants, usually younger than 6 mo of age, who apparently have been in good health develop severe congestive cardiac failure, often precipitated by a respiratory infection. The prognosis is poor unless there is a significant response to therapy for cardiac failure. Other infants have similar milder symptoms with periods of remission. Affected infants may manifest some dyspnea, refusal to feed, failure to gain weight adequately, and recurrent pulmonary infections. Chronic congestive cardiac failure can be controlled for some time by digitalis and diuretics. Most patients eventually succumb. Infants in whom valvular lesions or associated congenital cardiovascular defects are predominant expire in the first months of life.

During episodes of congestive cardiac failure the infant with primary EFE is acutely ill with dyspnea, cough, and anorexia. The jugular venous pressure is elevated, the liver greatly enlarged, and edema of the extremities, sacral area, or face may be present. Pulmonary rales and rhonchi are due to intercurrent pulmonary infection and congestion. The heart is moderately or greatly enlarged and has a normal or left ventricular impulse. Murmurs of mitral incompetence are frequent.

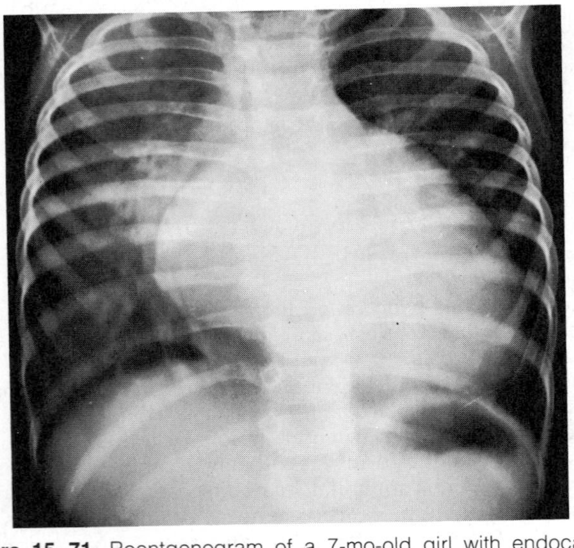

Figure 15–71. Roentgenogram of a 7-mo-old girl with endocardial fibroelastosis. Note the enlargement of the heart, without a distinctive contour and clear lung fields.

Roentgenograms confirm the cardiac enlargement (Fig. 15–71). There may be signs of intercurrent pulmonary infection or edema. The *electrocardiogram* is abnormal, with changes indicative of left atrial and ventricular hypertrophy with strain. The *echocardiogram* shows the hyperechogenic endocardial fibroelastosis and a dilated, poorly functioning left ventricle.

The short-term *prognosis* has improved because of the availability of potent diuretics and peripheral vasodilator therapy. In patients who have survived with clinical findings and a course suggestive of primary EFE, the clinical diagnosis is inferential, since it is not possible to be certain that the original cardiac involvement was that of EFE or of another myocardial disease.

Treatment is directed toward alleviation of congestive cardiac failure and prevention of intercurrent infections. EFE that appears to be end-stage, with decreased cardiac output on a maximal medical regimen, is an indication for cardiac transplantation.

15.72 CARDIOMYOPATHY

Heart muscle disease, in the absence of congenital heart disease, hypertension, acquired valve processes, or abnormal coronary arteries, may be classified as a primary disease or may be secondary to other systemic illnesses that also involve the myocardium (see Table 15–18). Primary cardiomyopathy may be classified as hypertrophic (obstructive and nonobstructive), dilated/congestive (idiopathic dilated, endocardial fibroelastosis), or restrictive (endomyocardial fibrosis, Löffler eosinophilic endomyocardial syndrome, hemochromatosis, Fabry disease, pseudoxanthoma elasticum). Other possible categories include arrhythmogenic right ventricular dysplasia and oncocytic cardiomyopathy, which predominantly manifest with ventricular arrhythmias or sudden cardiac death. The three major categories manifest with an insidious onset of congestive heart failure, chest pain, dyspnea, arrhythmias, or sudden death.

HYPERTROPHIC CARDIOMYOPATHY. This condition is also known as *idiopathic hypertrophic subaortic stenosis* and *asymmetric septal hypertrophy*. Massive ventricular hypertrophy with principal involvement of the ventricular septum characterizes the disease, but all portions of the left ventricle and sometimes of the right are affected. Varying degrees of myocardial fibrosis are also present. The mitral valve is displaced anteriorly by the hypertrophy of papillary muscle, and the left ventricular cavity is distorted by the massive generalized hypertrophy. Microscopically, patchy areas of abnormally thick and short muscle fibers are arranged in circular collections and interspersed among normal as well as hypertrophied muscle fibers. Electron microscopy shows disarray of myofibrils and myofilaments. An excessive response to calcium or to excessive calcium ion channels may be responsible for myocyte hypertrophy in some patients. Increased calcium action may augment intramyocardial wall stress, leading to myofibril disarray and hypertrophy.

Hemodynamics. The hypertrophic, fibrosed, stiff muscle has a decreased distensibility so that there is resistance to left ventricular filling, but systolic pumping function remains good until late in the course of the disease. Obstruction to left ventricular outflow may develop owing to apposition of the abnormally placed anterior mitral leaflet against the hypertrophied septum. Peak systolic pressure gradients across the left ventricular outflow may be constantly or intermittently present or may be absent. Varying degrees of mitral valve regurgitation are common.

Epidemiology. The disease has been recognized in all age groups, even in neonates, and may occur in many members of the same family, although overt manifestations are present in only about one third of affected individuals discovered through a screening process. Familial studies, using echocardiographic evidence of disproportionate ventricular septal hypertrophy and DNA probes, suggest that in some patients disease is transmitted in an autosomal dominant pattern with a high degree of penetrance, whereas in different families the disease is genetically heterogeneous.

Often hypertrophic cardiomyopathy occurring in a child is not typical of the adult disease, although clinically and dynamically the disease seems similar. In childhood, there is a greater tendency for right ventricular outflow obstruction to occur; the disease may be more diffuse through the left ventricular muscularity, as opposed to being restricted more or less to the ventricular septum; and a pure disease form with autosomal dominant inheritance is less often seen.

Clinical Manifestations. Many children are asymptomatic and are first evaluated only because of a heart murmur. In others the clinical pattern is dominated by weakness, fatigue, dyspnea on effort, palpitations, angina pectoris, dizziness, and syncope. There is risk of sudden death even in asymptomatic children. The pulse is brisk because of the early systolic ejection of blood from the ventricle. There is a prominent left ventricular lift and double apical impulse. The 1st and 2nd heart sounds are usually normal. The rarity of systolic ejection clicks helps to differentiate hypertrophic obstructive cardiomyopathy from valvular aortic stenosis. A 3rd sound is not common, but a 4th sound may be audible in older patients. The systolic murmur is ejection in type and of medium intensity; it is heard maximally at the left sternal edge and apex. The *electrocardiogram* shows left ventricular hypertrophy with or without ST segment depression and T wave inversion. The Wolff-Parkinson-White syndrome and other intraventricular conduction defects may be present. *Roentgenograms* show mild cardiomegaly with prominence of the left ventricle. The ascending aorta and aortic knob are usually normal. The *echocardiogram* shows asymmetric ventricular septal hypertrophy, systolic anterior motion of the anterior leaflet of the mitral valve, and premature closure of the aortic valve.

At *cardiac catheterization*, left ventricular outflow obstruction may or may not be present. When a systolic gradient is present, its severity may be variable even during a relatively short study. The obstruction may be intensified by digitalis glycosides, isoproterenol, amyl nitrite, and nitroglycerin. The gradient may increase shortly after exercise is discontinued, during the Valsalva maneuver, or during assumption of the erect position. Left ventriculography shows encroachment on the left ventricular cavity by the hypertrophied muscle, especially by the interventricular septum. During systole the anterior mitral leaflet is drawn into the left ventricular outflow tract. Mitral regurgitation is common. It is extremely important to rule out a discrete obstruction with secondary muscular hypertrophy in patients with left ventricular outflow gradients, as surgical management of discrete subaortic stenosis is standardized and effective (see Sec. 15.53).

The prognosis is unpredictable, especially in the asymptomatic patient, who may remain stable for years.

Treatment. There is no standardized therapy. Competitive sports and strenuous physical activity should be discouraged. Digitalis is not appropriate, and in most patients is contraindicated. Brisk diuresis or the infusion of isoproterenol should also be avoided. Beta-adrenergic blocking agents (propranolol) and calcium channel blocking agents (verapamil) have been used with apparent success in decreasing the degree of outflow obstruction, but obliteration of an LV-AO gradient does not necessarily affect prognosis. Surgical ventricular septal myotomy or resection of the left ventricular outflow tract has been successfully accomplished in some patients, especially in those with disabling angina or syncope and in some with severe obstruction at rest (a gradient exceeding 70 mm Hg). Mitral valve replacement may be needed if obstruction cannot be alleviated.

IDIOPATHIC DILATED (CONGESTIVE) CARDIOMYOPATHY (see Sec. 15.69). This condition is characterized by massive cardiomegaly as a result of the extensive dilatation of the ventricles, especially the left. Associated ventricular hypertrophy is present. The etiology is unknown and is probably multifactorial; a remote history of viral disease in some patients suggests that the disease may be a sequela of a previous myocarditis. Some patients have this condition as a result of carnitine deficiency; urine and serum levels should be obtained. Genetic mitochondrial disease and other metabolic abnormalities affecting the myocardium may result in congestive cardiomyopathy as a final common pathway. However, a specific etiology is rarely found when hearts are examined after longstanding disease. Myocardial biopsy with special investigative techniques early in the disease process may be more useful (see Sec. 15.70). Myocardial performance is poor as evidenced by reduced stroke volume, low ejection fraction, and increased systolic and diastolic volumes. All age groups are affected, even infants. Usually the onset is insidious, but sometimes symptoms of congestive cardiac failure occur suddenly. Irritability, anorexia, cough due to pulmonary congestion, and dyspnea with mild exertion are common. When the disease is fully established, the skin is cool and pale, the arterial pulse volume is decreased, the pulse pressure is reduced, and tachycardia is present. Jugular venous pressure is increased, and hepatomegaly and edema are common. The heart is enlarged, and pansystolic murmurs of mitral and tricuspid incompetence are present. A gallop rhythm is audible in the presence of severe congestive heart failure.

The *electrocardiogram* shows a combination of atrial enlargement, varying degrees of left ventricular hypertrophy, and nonspecific T wave abnormalities. The *roentgenogram* confirms the cardiomegaly; and pulmonary congestion and pleural effusions may be present. The *echocardiogram* shows the inordinate dilatation of the left ventricle and poor contractions. A relatively enlarged left atrium and displaced mitral valve are noted.

The course of the disease is usually downhill, although some patients remain stable for years. Vigorous treatment for heart failure may result in remissions, but relapses are common, and in time patients tend to become resistant to therapy. The prognosis is poor. Cardiac transplantation has been utilized successfully in this group of patients as well as in patients with other forms of cardiomyopathy (see Sec. 6.45). Complications include arrhythmias as well as pulmonary and/or systemic emboli from intracardiac thrombi.

RESTRICTIVE CARDIOMYOPATHY. Poor ventricular compliance is the major abnormality, and in this type of cardiomyopathy inadequate filling of the ventricular cavities occurs during diastole. This results in a clinical pattern that closely simulates that of constrictive pericarditis. In its full-blown form restrictive cardiomyopathy results in dyspnea, edema, ascites, hepatomegaly, increased venous pressure, and pulmonary congestion. The heart is mildly or moderately enlarged, and murmurs are nonspecific. The electrocardiogram shows prominent P waves, often normal QRS voltage, ST segment depression, and T wave inversion. Roentgenographic examination shows slight or moderate cardiomegaly. Differential diagnosis from constrictive pericarditis is critical, as the latter can be treated surgically with dramatic success. **Löffler hypereosinophilic syndrome** produces serious multisystem dysfunction (skin, lung, nervous system, liver), but the predominant cause of death is cardiomyopathy. This restrictive cardiomyopathy produces endocardial fibrosis of the mitral and tricuspid valves and the right and left ventricles. Subsequent formation of endocardial thrombi results in embolization. Löffler syndrome should be distinguished from nonrestrictive, nonfibrotic acute **eosinophilic necrotizing myocarditis**, an acute rapidly fatal illness, and from **hypersensitivity myocarditis** (characterized by fever, rash, tachycardia, eosinophilia, drug allergy, and arrhythmias). Steroids and cytotoxic agents (hydroxyurea) may be beneficial in hypereosinophilic syndromes. Anticoagulant therapy may reduce the incidence of thromboembolism.

The prognosis for restrictive cardiomyopathy is generally poor. Treatment is directed toward relief of edema with diuretics, and calcium channel blocking agents may be used to increase diastolic compliance. Cardiac transplantation is the last management option.

Anonymous: Cardiac biopsy in myocarditis. Lancet 336:283, 1990.
Anonymous: Dilated cardiomyopathy and enteroviruses. Lancet 336:971, 1990.
Bowles NE, Richardson PJ, Olsen EGJ, et al: Detection of coxsackie-B-virus-specific RNA sequences in myocardial biopsy samples from patients with myocarditis and dilated cardiomyopathy. Lancet 1:1120, 1986.
Caforio ALP, Stewart JT, McKenna WJ: Idiopathic dilated cardiomyopathy: Rational treatment awaits better understanding of pathogenesis. Br Med J 300:890, 1990.
Chen S-C, Tsai CC, Nouri S: Carditis associated with *Mycoplasma pneumoniae* infection. Am J Dis Child 140:471, 1986.
Chow LC, Dittrich HC, Shabetai R: Endomyocardial biopsy in patients with unexplained congestive heart failure. Ann Intern Med 109:535, 1988.
Dunnigan A, Staley NA, Smith SA, et al: Cardiac and skeletal muscle abnormalities in cardiomyopathy: Comparison of patients with ventricular tachycardia or congestive heart failure. J Am Coll Cardiol 10:608, 1987.
Gilbert EM, Anderson JL, Deitchman D, et al: Long-term β-blocker vasodilator therapy improves cardiac function in idiopathic dilated cardiomyopathy: A double-blind, randomized study of bucindolol versus placebo. Am J Med 88:223, 1990.
Imperato-McGinley J, Gautier T, Ehlers K, et al: Reversibility of catecholamine-induced dilated cardiomyopathy in a child with a pheochromocytoma. N Engl J Med 316:793, 1987.
Katz AM: Cardiomyopathy of overload: A major determinant of prognosis in congestive heart failure. N Engl J Med 322:100, 1990.
Maron BJ, Tajik AJ, Ruttenberg HD, et al: Hypertrophic cardiomyopathy in infants: Clinical features and natural history. Circulation 65:7, 1982.
McCaffrey FM, Braden DS, Strong WB: Sudden cardiac deaths in young athletes. Am J Dis Child 145:177, 1991.
Parrillo JE: Heart disease and the eosinophil. N Engl J Med 323:1560, 1990.
Parrillo JE, Cunnion RE, Epstein SE, et al: A prospective, randomized, controlled trial of prednisone for dilated cardiomyopathy. N Engl J Med 321:1061, 1989.
Scott GB, Hutto C, Makuch RW, et al: Survival in children with perinatally acquired human immunodeficiency virus type 1 infection. N Engl J Med 321:1791, 1989.
Solomon SD, Jarcho JA, McKenna W, et al: Familial hypertrophic cardiomyopathy is a genetically heterogeneous disease. J Clin Invest 86:993, 1990.
Spicer RL, Rocchini AP, Crowley DC, et al: Hemodynamic effects of verapamil in children and adolescents with hypertrophic cardiomyopathy. Circulation 67:413, 1983.
Thiene G, Nava A, Corrado D, et al: Right ventricular cardiomyopathy and sudden death in young people. N Engl J Med 318:129, 1988.
de Vivo DC, Tein I: Primary and secondary disorders of carnitine metabolism. Int Pediatr 5:134, 1990.
Wagner JA, Sax FL, Weisman HF, et al: Calcium-antagonist receptors in the atrial tissue of patients with hypertrophic cardiomyopathy. N Engl J Med 320:755, 1989.
Young LHY, Joag SV, Zheng L-M, et al: Perforin-mediated myocardial damage in acute myocarditis. Lancet 336:1019, 1990.

15.73 CONGESTIVE HEART FAILURE

Heart failure is that state in which the heart cannot produce the cardiac output required to sustain the metabolic needs of the body without evoking certain compensatory mechanisms (cardiac reserve). As these mechanisms become ineffective, increasingly severe clinical manifestations result.

Cardiac output can be calculated as the product of heart rate and stroke volume (HR × SV). There are several types of pathophysiologic derangements that, when sufficiently severe, compromise stroke volume and thus lead to cardiac decompensation. These include *afterload* (pressure work), *preload* (volume work), and *myocardial* abnormalities. In addition, *tachyarrhythmias* shorten the diastolic time interval for filling of the ventricles, compromising stroke volume and cardiac output.

PATHOPHYSIOLOGY. The heart can be viewed as a pump whose output is directly proportional to its filling volume. As end-diastolic volume increases, the healthy heart will increase cardiac output in a linear fashion until a maximum is reached (Frank-Starling principle) and cardiac output can no longer be augmented (Fig. 15–72). The increased stroke volume obtained in this manner is due to increased myocardial contractility associated with stretching of muscle fibers, but also requires increased wall tension and increased myocardial oxygen. Hearts functioning under various types of stress will produce different types of Frank-Starling curves (see Fig. 15–72). Cardiac muscle whose contractility is compromised will require greater dilatation to produce increased stroke volume but will not achieve the cardiac output of the normal myocardium. If a cardiac chamber is already dilated because of a lesion causing an increased preload (e.g., left to right shunt, valve insufficiency, anemia, etc.), there will be little room for further dilatation and augmentation of cardiac output. The presence of lesions that result in severe afterloads will also markedly compromise the usual Frank-Starling relationships between filling volume and cardiac output.

High-output failure is the development of signs and symptoms of congestive heart failure when there is no basic

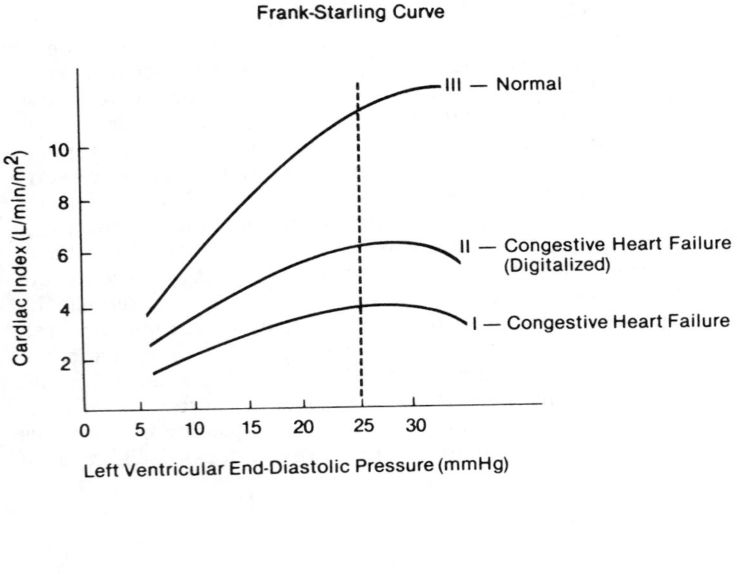

Figure 15–72. As the left ventricular end-diastolic pressure (LVED) increases, cardiac index increases, even in the presence of congestive heart failure, until a critical level of LVED is reached. Adding an inotropic agent (digoxin) shifts the curve from I to II. (From Gersony WM, Steep CN: *In*: Dickerman JD, Lucey JF [eds]: Smith's The Critically Ill Child: Diagnosis and Medical Management, 3rd ed. Philadelphia, WB Saunders, 1984.)

abnormality in myocardial function and the cardiac output is greater than normal. It is caused by conditions such as profound anemia, severe hyperthyroidism, and large systemic arteriovenous fistulas. These diseases reduce peripheral vascular resistance and cardiac afterload and increase myocardial contractility. Heart "failure" results when the demands for cardiac output exceed the ability of the heart to respond. Chronic severe high-output failure may eventually result in a decrease in myocardial performance as the metabolic requirements of the myocardium itself are not met.

CLINICAL MANIFESTATIONS. The clinical manifestations of congestive heart failure depend on the degree of cardiac reserve under various conditions. A critically ill infant or child who has exhausted his compensatory mechanisms to the point where he can no longer achieve sufficient cardiac output to meet the basal metabolic needs of the body will be symptomatic at rest. Other patients may be comfortable when quiet but are incapable of increasing cardiac output in response to even mild activity without developing significant symptoms. On the other hand, it may take rather vigorous exercise to compromise cardiac function in children who have less severe heart disease.

A thorough history is extremely important both in making the diagnosis of heart failure and in evaluating the possible causes. Parents who are observing their infant on a daily basis may not recognize subtle changes that have occurred over the course of days or weeks. Cyanosis may be considered merely "a deep coloring" and not recognized as an abnormal finding. The history obtained from the parents of a young infant should focus on the feeding process (see Sec. 15.1 and Table 15–1). The infant having congestive heart failure often takes less volume per feeding, becomes dyspneic while sucking, and perhaps perspires profusely. After falling into an exhausted sleep, the infant, inadequately fed, will soon awaken for the next feeding. This cycle continues around the clock and must be carefully differentiated from colic or other feeding disorders. Eliciting a history of fatigue in an older child requires specific questions about activity, including stair climbing, walking various distances, bicycle riding, etc. Inquiry should also be made regarding orthopnea and nocturnal dyspnea.

In children the signs and symptoms of congestive heart failure are similar to those in adults. These include fatigue, effort intolerance, anorexia, abdominal pain, and cough. Dyspnea is a reflection of pulmonary congestion. Elevation of systemic venous pressure may be gauged by clinical assessment of the jugular venous pressure, and liver enlargement. Orthopnea and basal rales may be present; edema is usually discernible in dependent portions of the body, or anasarca may be present. Cardiomegaly is invariably noted. Gallop rhythm is common; other auscultatory findings are those produced by the basic lesion.

In infants congestive heart failure may be more difficult to identify. Prominent manifestations include tachypnea, feeding difficulties, poor weight gain, excessive perspiration, irritability, weak cry, and noisy, labored respiration with costal and subcostal retractions as well as flaring of the alae nasi and sternal retractions. Pulmonary congestion may be indistinguishable from signs and symptoms of bronchiolitis. Pneumonitis with or without atelectasis of part of the lung is common. Hepatomegaly nearly always occurs, and cardiomegaly is invariably present. In spite of pronounced tachycardia, gallop rhythm can frequently be recognized. The other auscultatory signs are those produced by the cardiac lesion that resulted in heart failure. Clinical assessment of the jugular venous pressure in infants may be difficult because of the shortness of the neck and the difficulty of observing a relaxed state. Edema, especially in infants, is frequently not clinically detectable; when present, the edema may be generalized, involving the eyelids as well as the sacrum, legs, and feet. The differential diagnosis is age dependent (Table 15–19).

LABORATORY DATA. *Roentgenograms of the chest* show cardiac enlargement. The pulmonary vascularity is variable depending on the etiology of the heart failure. Infants and children having large left to right shunts will have exaggeration of the pulmonary arterial vessels to the periphery of the lung fields, whereas patients having cardiomyopathy may have a relatively normal pulmonary vascular bed early in the course of their disease. Fluffy pulmonary markings suggestive of venous congestion and acute pulmonary edema are usually not seen in childhood except in the most extreme circumstances.

The diagnosis of specific chamber enlargement by *electrocardiography* may be helpful in assessing the etiology of congestive heart failure but does not establish the diagnosis. Left or right ventricular ischemic changes may correlate well with clinical and other noninvasive parameters of ventricular function. Low voltage QRS morphology with ST-T wave abnormalities may suggest myocardial inflammatory disease and can also be seen with pericarditis. The electrocardiogram is the best tool for evaluating rhythm disorders as a cause of cardiac failure.

Echocardiographic techniques to determine the relationship between end-systolic and end-diastolic diameters (shortening fraction) are useful in assessing ventricular function. The normal shortening fraction should be 28–36%, compared with

TABLE 15–19. Etiology of Heart Failure

Fetal
Severe anemia (hemolysis, fetal-maternal transfusion, parvovirus B19–induced anemia, hypoplastic anemia)
Supraventricular tachycardia
Ventricular tachycardia
Complete heart block

Premature Neonate
Fluid overload
Patent ductus arteriosus
Ventricular septal defect
Cor pulmonale (bronchopulmonary dysplasia)
Hypertension

Full-Term Neonate
Asphyxial cardiomyopathy
Arteriovenous malformation (vein of Galen, hepatic)
Left-sided obstructive lesions (coarctation of aorta, hypoplastic left side of the heart)
Large mixing cardiac defects (single ventricle, truncus arteriosus)
Viral myocarditis

Infant-Toddler
Left to right cardiac shunts (ventricular septal defect)
Hemangioma (arteriovenous malformation)
Anomalous left coronary artery
Metabolic cardiomyopathy
Acute hypertension (hemolytic-uremic syndrome)
Supraventricular tachycardia
Kawasaki disease

Child-Adolescent
Rheumatic fever
Acute hypertension (glomerulonephritis)
Viral myocarditis
Thyrotoxicosis
Hemochromatosis-hemosiderosis
Cancer therapy (radiation, Adriamycin)
Sickle cell anemia
Endocarditis
Cor pulmonale (cystic fibrosis)
Cardiomyopathy (hypertrophic, dilated, postviral)

the normal ejection fraction of 55–65% measured by angiography. The pre-ejection/ejection period ratio (PEP/EP) should be less than 40%. A long pre-ejection time with a very short ejection time usually denotes myocardial failure. *Radionuclide studies* are also useful, since the ejection fraction can be determined by injecting a radioisotope (e.g., ^{99m}Tc) into a vein and measuring end-diastolic volume and systolic volume by counts over the ventricles.

Arterial Blood Gases and Electrolytes. Arterial oxygen levels may be decreased when ventilation/perfusion inequalities occur secondary to pulmonary edema. When heart failure is severe, mild respiratory acidemia may be present. Infants with severe heart failure and decreased cardiac output will demonstrate metabolic acidemia. In contrast, infants with marked tachypnea associated with decreased pulmonary compliance secondary to interstitial congestion without alveolar edema may have mild respiratory alkalosis.

Infants with congestive heart failure often display hyponatremia owing to water retention. Although serum sodium is low, total body sodium is increased. An abnormal steady state is reached in which relatively more water is retained.

TREATMENT. The underlying cause of cardiac failure must be removed or alleviated if possible. If the etiology is a congenital cardiovascular anomaly amenable to surgery, medical treatment is indicated for a time before the surgical procedure and should usually be continued in the immediate postoperative period. For many patients with cardiomyopathies only medical management can be provided unless cardiac transplantation is indicated.

General Measures. Strict bed rest is rarely necessary except in extreme cases, but it is important that the child rest often and sleep adequately. Most patients feel better in a semi-upright position, and an infant chair is advisable for infants with chronic congestive heart failure. When patients are responding to treatment, restrictions on activities should be within the context of the patient's ability to be relatively active.

For patients with pulmonary edema, bed rest, positive-pressure ventilation, and morphine (0.1 mg/kg) may be required along with other drug therapy. In extreme situations, beta agonists such as dopamine and dobutamine along with peripheral vasodilators (e.g., nitroprusside, captopril) may be required in an intensive care setting.

Digitalis. *Digoxin* is the digitalis glycoside used most often in the pediatric patient. The half-life of 36 hr is long enough to allow daily or twice daily administration, and short enough to limit toxic effects from overdosage. Digoxin is absorbed by the gastrointestinal tract. When taken with or after meals the rate of absorption may be somewhat retarded, but the amount of digoxin absorbed is almost always unchanged. Following oral administration, approximately 60–85% of digoxin is absorbed. Absorption is greater for the elixir than for tablets. The peak effect for oral digoxin is approximately 2–6 hr; an initial effect can be seen as early as 30 min after administration. When the drug is administered intravenously the initial effect is seen in 15–30 min and the peak effect occurs at 1–4 hr. The drug crosses the placenta, and therefore the fetus can be treated via administration to the mother. Digoxin is eliminated by the kidney and the rate of excretion is proportional to the glomerular filtration rate. After intravenous administration, 50–70% is excreted unchanged in the urine. The half-life of digoxin is 1–2 days in children who have normal renal function but is 6 days in patients with renal shutdown, who must utilize slower hepatic excretion pathways.

Rapid digitalization of infants and children in congestive heart failure may be carried out intravenously. The dose depends on the patient's age (Table 15–20), and various regimens are utilized. The recommended schedule is to give one third of the total digitalizing dose immediately and the succeeding two doses 8–16 hr later. In cases of profound congestive failure, more rapid digitalization using narrower intervals and a larger initial loading dose may be required. The electrocardiogram must be closely monitored and rhythm strips obtained prior to each of the three digitalizing doses. Digoxin should be discontinued if a new rhythm disturbance is noted. A prolongation of the PR interval is not in itself an indication to withhold digitalis, but a delay in administering the next dose or a reduction in the dosage should be considered depending on the patient's clinical status. Serum digoxin determination is helpful when digitalis toxicity is suspected. ST segments or T wave changes are commonly noted with digitalis administration and should not affect the digitalization regimen. Baseline serum electrolyte levels should be measured prior to and after digitalization.

Maintenance digitalis therapy is started approximately 12 hr after full digitalization. The daily dosage is divided in two and given at 12-hr intervals for more consistent blood levels and more flexibility in case of toxicity. The dosage is one quarter to one third of the full digitalizing dose. For patients who are initially digitalized intravenously, maintenance digoxin can be given orally once oral feedings are tolerated. Since absorption from the gastrointestinal tract is less certain, the oral maintenance dose is approximately 25% higher than when digoxin is utilized parenterally (see Table 15–20). The

TABLE 15–20. Dosage of Drugs Commonly Used for the Treatment of Congestive Heart Failure

Drug	Dosage
Digoxin	
Digitalization (PO) (3 doses q 8 hr)	Premature 0.02–0.025 mg/kg Neonate (≤ 1 mo) 0.03–0.04 mg/kg Infant or child 0.04–0.06 mg/kg Adolescent or adult 1.0–1.5 mg in divided doses
Digitalization (IV) (Timing of dosage variable, depending on clinical indications)	75% of PO dose
Maintenance	¼–⅓ of digitalizing dose, divided q 12 hr
Furosemide	
IV	1–2 mg/dose, prn
PO	1–4 mg/kg/24 hr, qd, bid, or qid
Bumetanide	
IV	0.01–0.2 mg/kg/dose
PO	0.04–0.8 mg/kg/24 hr q 6–8 hr
Chlorothiazide (PO)	20–50 mg/kg/24 hr, bid, or qid
Spironolactone (PO)	2–3 mg/kg/24 hr, bid
β Agonists (IV)	
Isoproterenol	0.01–0.5 μg/kg/min
Dopamine	2–20 μg/kg/min
Dobutamine	2–20 μg/kg/min
Amrinone (IV)	0.75 mg/kg bolus 5–10 μg/kg
Afterload-reducing agents	
Nitroprusside (IV)	0.5–8 μg/kg/min
Hydralazine	
IV	0.5 mg/kg
PO	0.5–7.5 mg/kg/24 hr, tid
Captopril (PO)	0.5–6 mg/kg/24 hr, qid

normal daily dosage of digoxin for older children (>5 yr of age) calculated by body weight should not exceed the usual adult dose of 0.2–0.5 mg/24 hr.

Patients who are not critically ill may be digitalized initially using the oral regimen (see Table 15–20), and in most instances digitalization should be completed within 24 hr. When slow digitalization is acceptable, initiation of a maintenance digoxin schedule without loading dosage will achieve full digitalization in 7–10 days. This often can be carried out on an outpatient basis.

If an infant improves significantly on digitalis over a period of a few months and the need for the drug appears to be lessening (e.g., a VSD that is becoming smaller), dosage is not increased as the child gains weight. If the clinical status warrants, the drug is eventually discontinued.

If there are questions as to the effectiveness or toxicity of digitalis, plasma digoxin levels should be measured. Blood should be drawn at least 4 hr after the last dose so that tissue/plasma equilibration has occurred. A normal blood level in an infant is approximately 2–4 ng/mL and in older children 1–2 ng/mL. Exceeding these levels will not generally add significantly to the management of congestive heart failure.

Measurement of *serum digoxin levels* is useful under four circumstances: (1) when a standard dose of digoxin is not having beneficial therapeutic effects; (2) when an unknown amount of digoxin has been administered or ingested accidentally; (3) when renal function is impaired or if drug interactions are possible; and (4) when a toxic response is suspected. In this last situation, *elevated serum digoxin levels are not in themselves diagnostic of toxicity but must be interpreted as an adjunct to other clinical and electrocardiographic findings*. A finding of toxicity is primarily based on rhythm and conduction disturbances; nausea and vomiting are not frequent in the pediatric patient. Hypokalemia, hypomagnesemia, and hypercalcemia, cardiac inflammation, and prematurity may potentiate digoxin toxicity. A cardiac arrhythmia that develops in a child with congestive heart failure who is taking digitalis also may be related to cardiac disease rather than to the drug. However, *any form of arrhythmia occurring following the institution of digitalis therapy must be considered to be drug related until proven otherwise*. Succeeding dosage should be withheld until the question is resolved.

Diet. Infants having congestive heart failure are calorically deprived because of increased metabolic requirements and decreased caloric intake. Increasing daily calories is an important aspect of their management. Often as other therapeutic measures take effect, the child will have an improved appetite. However, increasing calories per ounce of feeding may occasionally be beneficial, for example, using formulas containing 24 calories per ounce. Some infants will not tolerate increased concentration of calories because of gastrointestinal disturbances, particularly diarrhea. These formulas may also provide too large a solute load for compromised kidneys, which may then fail to maintain adequate sodium and water balance.

Severely ill infants in congestive heart failure may lack sufficient strength for effective sucking because of extreme fatigue, rapid respirations, and generalized weakness. Nasogastric feedings may be helpful. When congestive heart failure continues unabated, however, an increased caloric diet will frequently be of no avail. Indeed, continued malnutrition may be an important factor in the decision to undertake early surgical intervention in patients who have an operable congenital heart lesion.

The use of very low sodium formulas in the routine management of infants with congestive heart failure is not recommended, since these preparations are often poorly tolerated and thus, although sodium intake is decreased, caloric needs are less well met than with standard formulas. The use of more potent diuretic agents allows more palatable standard formulas to be utilized for nutrition while controlling salt and water balance by chronic diuretic administration. Some infants and children can be managed with "no added salt" diets and abstinence from foods containing large amounts of sodium. A strict extremely low sodium diet is rarely required.

Diuretics. Diuretic agents interfere with reabsorption of water and sodium by the kidneys, which results in the reduction of circulating blood volume and thereby reduces ventricular filling pressures. These agents are most often used in conjunction with digitalis therapy in patients with severe congestive heart failure.

Furosemide is the most commonly used diuretic in patients with cardiac failure. It inhibits the reabsorption of sodium and chloride, not only in the distal tubules but also in the loop of Henle. Patients requiring acute diuresis should be given intravenous or intramuscular furosemide at an initial dose of 1–2 mg/kg. This often results in rapid diuresis and prompt improvement in clinical status, particularly if symptoms of pulmonary congestion are present. Chronic furosemide therapy is then prescribed at a dose of 1–4 mg/kg/24 hr or every other day, usually as a single morning oral dose. Careful monitoring of electrolytes is necessary with long-term diuretic therapy, since there may be significant loss of potassium. Potassium chloride supplementation and/or spironolactone may be administered in conjunction with chronic diuretic therapy to preserve potassium. Spironolactone is given orally in divided doses of 2–3 mg/kg/24 hr in order to enhance potassium retention and inhibit aldosterone. When furosemide is administered every other day, dietary potassium supplementation may be adequate to maintain normal serum potassium levels. Chronic administration of furosemide rarely may cause contraction of the extracellular fluid compartment resulting in a "contraction alkalosis" (see Sec. 6.8). Under these circumstances, substitution of acetazolomide, a carbonic anhydrase inhibitor, may be useful

Chlorothiazide is used occasionally for diuresis in children with less severe chronic congestive heart failure. It is less immediate in action and less potent than furosemide, and it affects the reabsorption of electrolytes only in the renal tubules. The usual dose is 20–50 mg/kg/24 hr or every other day in divided doses. Potassium supplementation may also be utilized concurrently with this diuretic agent.

Afterload-Reducing Agents. A group of drugs are available that reduce ventricular afterload by decreasing peripheral vascular resistance, thereby improving myocardial contractility. Some of these agents also decrease systemic venous tone, significantly reducing preload. Afterload reducers are of greatest benefit to children with congestive heart failure secondary to a cardiomyopathy, but they are also effective in patients with severe mitral regurgitation or aortic insufficiency. Congestive heart failure secondary to left to right shunts or stenotic lesions is less often treated with afterload-reducing agents. This therapy has not been used often in the management of large left to right shunts because of uncertain effects on pulmonary vascular resistance. If heart failure is the result of a fixed obstructive cardiac lesion, peripheral vasodilatation beyond the site of stenosis will not significantly affect total ventricular afterload. Afterload-reducing agents are most often used in conjunction with other anticongestive drugs, such as digoxin and diuretics. In pediatrics, these drugs are rarely first-line therapeutic modalities, but are added to treatment in specific situations when decreasing peripheral vascular resistance will add significantly to optimal management. Only a few afterload-reducing agents have been used extensively in children (see Table 15–20).

Nitroprusside directly dilates arterial and venous vessels and is a potent intravenous medication that should be administered only in an intensive care setting. Peripheral arterial vasodilatation and afterload reduction are the major effects, but venodilatation causing a decrease in venous return is also beneficial to the patient on the basis of preload reduction. Blood pressure must be continuously monitored by means of an intra-arterial line, as sudden hypotension can occur with overdosage. Nitroprusside is contraindicated when hypotension pre-exists. As the drug is metabolized, small amounts of circulating cyanide are produced, which are detoxified in the liver to thiocyanate, which is excreted in the urine. However, when high doses of nitroprusside are administered for several days, toxic symptoms related to thiocyanide poisoning may occur, such as fatigue, nausea, disorientation, and muscular spasm. If nitroprusside use is prolonged, blood thiocyanate levels should be monitored; values greater than 10 μg/dL are consistent with clinical symptoms of toxicity. Nitroprusside should be utilized only in the most critically ill patients and for as short a period of time as possible.

Hydralazine is a direct arteriolar smooth muscle relaxant and has virtually no effects on preload. Therefore, it is occasionally administered together with a venodilating agent such as a nitrate derivative. The usual oral dose of hydralazine is 0.5–7.5 mg/kg/24 hr in three divided doses. In some cases it may be advantageous to evaluate the acute effects of intravenous hydralazine; if increased cardiac output, decreased peripheral vascular resistance, and decreased left ventricular filling pressure are observed, then chronic oral therapy is instituted. Many patients require increasing dosage with time in order to maintain the peripheral dilating effects (tachyphylaxis).

Adverse reactions with hydralazine include headache, palpitations, nausea, and vomiting. In addition, systemic lupus erythematosus occasionally occurs after administration of large doses of hydralazine over prolonged periods; these manifestations are reversible when the drug is discontinued.

Captopril is an orally active angiotensin-converting-enzyme inhibitor that produces marked arterial dilatation by blocking the production of angiotensin II, resulting in significant afterload reduction. Venodilatation and consequent preload reduction have also been reported. This agent also interferes with aldosterone production and thereby also helps control salt and water retention. The oral dose is 0.5–6 mg/kg/24 hr given in 2–4 divided doses. Some patients who initially do not show significant improvement on captopril have clinical benefits when the drug is administered on a long-term basis. However, the converse occurs in some patients.

The adverse reactions to captopril include hypotension and its sequelae (e.g., syncope, weakness, and dizziness). A maculopapular pruritic rash is encountered in 5–8% of patients, but the drug may be continued since the rash often disappears spontaneously with time. Neutropenia and proteinuria have also been reported.

β-Agonists. *Isoproterenol*, an intravenous preparation used for treating low cardiac output, has central and peripheral beta-adrenergic effects, and therefore both enhances myocardial contractility and reduces cardiac afterload. The drug is administered in an intensive care setting, where the dose is titrated between 0.01 and 0.5 μg/kg/min depending on the heart rate response. Continuous determinations of arterial blood pressure and heart rate are mandatory, and measuring cardiac output at the bedside also may be helpful in assessing drug efficacy. Since isoproterenol has a marked chronotropic effect, it should not be used in patients who have significant tachycardia. Children receiving isoproterenol must be carefully monitored for atrial or ventricular premature depolarizations, as they may lead to supraventricular or ventricular tachycardia. As the patient's clinical condition improves, the drug is gradually tapered, usually over 1–2 days. Often, as isoproterenol treatment is withdrawn, digoxin therapy is added for continued inotropic effect.

Dopamine is an effective β-adrenergic agent that is less chronotropic and arrhythmogenic than isoproterenol. In addition, it is a selective renal vasodilator, particularly useful in patients with the compromised kidney function that is often associated with low cardiac output. At a dose of 2–10 μg/kg/min, dopamine results in increased contractility. However, if the dose must be increased beyond 15 μg/kg/min, peripheral α-adrenergic effects may result in vasoconstriction.

Dobutamine, a derivative of dopamine, is used to treat low cardiac output. It has the advantage of causing direct inotropic effects with some (albeit less than isoproterenol) reduction in peripheral vascular resistance. Dobutamine can be used as an effective substitute for high-dose dopamine therapy in order to avoid vasoconstrictive effects, and it is unlikely to cause cardiac rhythm disturbances even at maximal dosage. The usual dose is similar to that of dopamine (2–20 μg/kg/min).

Amrinone, a new inotropic agent, is useful in treating patients with low cardiac output who are refractory to standard therapy. It is representative of a new class of cardiac inotropic agents that are different from the cardiac glycosides and catecholamines in structure and mechanism of action. Amrinone has both positive inotropic effects on the heart and significant peripheral vasodilatory effects. The agent has generally been used as an adjunct to dopamine or dobutamine therapy in an intensive care unit and is given at an initial loading dose of 0.75 mg/kg intravenously followed by an intravenous infusion of 5–10 μg/kg/min. A major side effect is hypotension secondary to peripheral vasodilatation. The hypotension can usually be managed by the administration of intravenous fluids to restore adequate vascular volume. A second side effect of amrinone administration is thrombocytopenia; the degree of severity appears to be related to both the rate of amrinone infusion and the duration of therapy. The thrombocytopenia is reversed when the drug is discontinued or the rate of infusion decreased.

15.74 CARDIOGENIC SHOCK

See also Sec. 6.35.

Cardiogenic shock may occur as a complication of (1) severe cardiac dysfunction, often following surgery; (2) septicemia; (3) severe burns; (4) immunologic disease (anaphylaxis); (5) hemorrhage or dehydration; (6) severe debilitation; and (7) acute central nervous system disorders. It is characterized by low cardiac output and hypotension resulting in inadequate tissue perfusion.

Treatment is aimed at reinstitution of adequate cardiac output and peripheral perfusion to prevent the untoward effects of prolonged ischemia to vital organs as well as management of the underlying cause. Under physiologic conditions, the cardiac output is increased as a result of sympathetic discharge, which increases heart rate. However, in the presence of cardiogenic shock with marked tachycardia, a further increase in heart rate will not increase and may reduce cardiac output by decreasing diastolic filling time. Cardiac output must be increased by increasing stroke volume. If fluid administration is increased, the Starling mechanism results in increased stroke volume by increasing central venous pressure and ventricular filling pressure (preload). When central venous pressure is low, infusion of volume will reliably increase cardiac output. Optimal filling pressure is variable and depends on a number of extracardiac factors including ventilatory support with high positive end-expiratory pressure, peak inspiratory pressure, and intra-abdominal pressure. The increased pressure necessary to fill relatively noncompliant right ventricles should also be considered, particularly after open heart surgery. If incremental fluid administration does not result in improved cardiac output, abnormal myocardial contractility and/or high afterload must be implicated as the cause of low cardiac output.

Myocardial contractility will improve when treatment of the basic cause of shock is instituted, hypoxia eliminated, and acidosis corrected. However, dopamine, epinephrine, and dobutamine are catecholamines, which will also improve cardiac contractility, increase heart rate, and ultimately increase cardiac output. The major differences among these agents lie in their effects on the peripheral vascular bed. *Dopamine* has no significant peripheral beta effects on vascular resistance at a dosage of 2–10 μg/kg/min. However, at higher doses (>15 μg/kg/min) it causes significant dose-dependent increases in systemic vascular resistance via alpha receptors similar to those seen with norepinephrine. Dopamine also has specific effects on the renal vascular system and increases renal blood flow out of proportion to other vascular beds at doses <5 μg/kg/min. At high doses dopamine may cause an increase in pulmonary vascular resistance, particularly in patients with extremely reactive pulmonary vascular circulations. *Epinephrine* also causes a dose-dependent increase in systemic vascular resistance via the alpha-adrenergic receptors. All of these agents may cause tachycardias and, particularly in the presence of hypoxia and/or acidosis, may be arrhythmogenic. Norepinephrine may produce less tachycardia with enhanced systemic blood pressure and has been used in patients with septic shock. A major advantage of the catecholamines is their very short half-lives; therefore, positive inotropic effects are virtually immediate, and untoward effects can be reversed quickly by discontinuation of the drug. *Dobutamine* has "pure" central beta effects with some peripheral vasodilatation. Along with dopamine, dobutamine has less chronotropic effect than isoproterenol and is more advantageous when a marked tachycardia is present prior to initiation of an inotropic agent. These drugs may be used in various combinations.

The use of cardiac glycosides to treat acute low cardiac output states should be avoided. Digoxin has a slower effect than the catecholamines, even with intravenous administration. In addition, adverse effects may result from larger doses, and toxicity is less predictable, depending on myocardial and serum potassium and calcium levels. Since it is quite common for patients with cardiovascular shock to have compromised renal perfusion, the administration of digoxin may result in high persistent blood levels because it is excreted in the kidneys. When digoxin is required for such patients, a lower dosage scale should be used and serum digoxin levels frequently monitored.

Patients with cardiogenic shock may have a marked increase in systemic vascular resistance resulting in high afterload and poor peripheral perfusion. If high systemic vascular resistance is persistent and the administration of positive inotropic agents alone does not improve tissue perfusion, the use of afterload-reducing agents may be appropriate, for example, nitroprusside used in combination with dopamine.

Postoperative patients with cardiogenic shock may benefit from intra-aortic balloon counterpulsation; these and other patients may benefit from extracorporeal membrane oxygenation.

Sequential evaluation and management of cardiovascular shock is mandatory (see Sec. 6.34). Table 15–21 outlines the treatment of acute cardiac circulatory failure under most circumstances. The treatment of infants and children with low cardiac output following cardiac surgery depends on the nature of the operative procedure and the patient's status after surgery (see Sec. 15.61 and Table 15–11).

Artman M, Graham T: Guidelines for vasodilator therapy of congestive heart failure in infants and children. Am Heart J 113:121, 1987.
Awan NA, Miller RR, Mason DT: Comparison of effects of nitroprusside and prazosin on left ventricular function and the peripheral circulation in chronic refractory congestive heart failure. Circulation 57:152, 1978.
Benzing G III, Helmsworth JA, Schreiber JT, et al: Nitroprusside after open-heart surgery. Circulation 54:467, 1976.
Dickerman JD, Lucey JF: Smith's The Critically Ill Child, 3rd ed. Philadelphia, WB Saunders, 1985.
Doering W: Quinidine-digoxin interaction: Pharmacokinetics, underlying mechanism and clinical implications. N Engl J Med 301:401, 1979.
Friedman WF, George BL: Medical progress: Treatment of congestive heart failure by altering loading conditions of the heart. J Pediatr 106:697, 1985.
Goodwin JF: Prospects and predictions for the cardiomyopathies. Circulation 50:210, 1974.
Greenwood RD, Nadas AS, Fyler DC: The clinical course of primary myocardial disease in infants and children. Am Heart J 92:549, 1976.
Harris LC, Nghiem QX: Cardiomyopathies in infants and children. Prog Cardiovasc Dis 25:255, 1972.
Hayes CJ, Butler VP Jr, Gersony WM: Serum digoxin studies in infants and children. Pediatrics 52:561, 1973.
Hernandez A, Burton RM, Pagtakhan RD, et al: Pharmacodynamics of ^{3}H-digoxin in infants. Pediatrics 44:418, 1969.
Lang D, von Bernuth G: Serum concentration and serum half-life of digoxin in premature and mature infants. Pediatrics 59:902, 1977.
Loggie JMH, Kleinman LI, VanMaanen EF: Renal function and diuretic therapy in infants and children. J Pediatr 86:485, 657, 825, 1975.
Perkin RM, Levin DL: Shock in the pediatric patient. Part I. J Pediatr 101:163, 1982.
Perkin RM, Levin DL: Shock in the pediatric patient. Part II. Therapy. J Pediatr 101:319, 1982.
Zaritsky A, Chernow B: Use of catecholamines in pediatrics. J Pediatr 105:341, 1984.

TABLE 15–21. Treatment of Cardiogenic Shock

Goal—to improve peripheral perfusion by increasing cardiac output

Cardiac output = Heart rate × stroke volume

	Determinants of Stroke Volume		
	Preload	***Contractility***	***Afterload***
Parameters measured	CVP, PCWP	CO, BP	CO, BP
Abnormal physiologic manifestations	Low CVP or PCWP ↓ CO ↓ BP	Elevation of CVP or PCWP ↓ CO ↓ BP	Elevation of CVP or PCWP ↓ CO →↑ BP
Treatment to improve cardiac output	Volume expansion Crystalloid, colloids Whole blood	Catecholamines Dopamine, 5–20 μg/kg/min Dobutamine, 2.5–20 μg/kg/min	Vasodilatation Nitroprusside, 0.5–8 μg/kg/min Hydralazine, 0.5 mg/kg

CVP = central venous pressure; PCWP = pulmonary capillary wedge pressure; CO = cardiac output; BP = blood pressure; ↓ = Decreased; → = Normal; ↑ = Increased.

15.75 DISEASES OF THE PERICARDIUM

Major diseases that involve the pericardium are noted in Table 15–22. In some instances the involvement of the pericardium is only one manifestation of a more generalized illness, and the prominence of the pericardial component will vary depending on the disease entity.

HEMODYNAMICS. Pericardial inflammation results in an accumulation of fluid in the pericardial space. The fluid varies according to the etiology of the pericarditis and may be serous, fibrinous, purulent, or hemorrhagic. Cardiac tamponade occurs when the amount of pericardial fluid reaches a level that compromises cardiac function. In a healthy child there is 10–15 mL of fluid in the pericardial space, whereas in an adolescent with pericarditis an excess of 1,000 mL of fluid may accumulate. For every small increment of fluid the pericardial pressure rises slowly, but once a critical level is reached, there is a rapid rise in pressure culminating in severe cardiac compression. Inhibition of ventricular filling during diastole, elevated systemic and pulmonary venous pressures, and, if untreated, eventual compromised cardiac output and shock occur.

CLINICAL MANIFESTATIONS. The first symptom of pericardial disease is often precordial pain. The major complaint is a sharp, stabbing sensation of the left shoulder; the chest, shoulder, and back pain that occurs may be exaggerated by lying and relieved by sitting, especially leaning forward. Because there is no sensory innervation of the pericardium, the pain is probably referred pain from diaphragmatic and pleural irritation. Cough, dyspnea, and fever may also occur. The presence of symptoms or signs associated with other organs and systems depends on the basic etiology of the pericarditis.

On physical examination, many of the findings relate to the degree of fluid accumulation in the pericardial sac. The presence of a friction rub is helpful but may be a late sign in acute pericarditis, becoming apparent only after the effusion is reduced. Narrow pulses, tachycardia, enlarged percussible heart, quiet precordium, distant heart sounds, neck vein distention, and a paradoxic pulse suggest significant fluid accumulation.

Greater than 20 mm Hg of *paradoxic pulse* in a child with pericarditis is a reliable indicator of the presence of cardiac tamponade; a 10–20 mm Hg change is equivocal. There is normally a slight decrease in systolic arterial pressure during inspiration. With cardiac tamponade this normal phenomenon is exaggerated, probably because of decreased filling of the left side of the heart with the inspiratory phase of respiration. In order to determine the degree of pulsus paradoxus, one first measures the exact systolic blood pressure during normal expiration. The manometer is then slowly allowed to fall. The point when the systolic pressure is heard equally well during inspiration and expiration is then recorded. The difference between the two determinations represents the degree of paradox. Significant pulsus paradoxus may also be present with severe dyspnea of any origin and is not infrequent in patients who have emphysema or asthma or who are being ventilated with a positive-pressure respirator. In these patients the paradoxic pulse is due to a marked increase in intrathoracic pressure. The etiology of paradoxic pulse in a child on a ventilator after cardiac surgery may therefore be difficult to assess.

LABORATORY DATA. The specific findings depend on the underlying disease. The effects of pericarditis on the *electrocardiogram* are multiple. Low voltage of the QRS complexes results from a damping effect of pericardial fluid. Pressure on the myocardium by fluid or exudate produces a current of injury that results in mild elevation of ST segments. Generalized T wave inversion occurs as a consequence of associated myocardial inflammation. The ST segment and T wave changes with pericarditis are more generalized than those seen with myocardial infarction, and the ST segment elevations tend to precede the T wave changes. Electrical alternans demonstrated by variable QRS complex amplitude may be present. There may be an interval when the electrocardiogram is in a transitional phase and appears to be normal. This may occur during the acute phase of the illness prior to diagnosis. In some instances clear-cut abnormalities are never identified.

A relatively large pericardial effusion must be present to cause an enlarged cardiac shadow with the usual "water-bottle" configuration on *chest roentgenogram* (Fig. 15–73). In most instances the lung fields are clear. With constrictive disease the heart is relatively small and calcification may be present.

The *echocardiogram* is a sensitive technique for evaluating the size and progression of pericardial effusions. Normally, the pericardium is closely adherent to the epicardium, and the two layers can be only narrowly separated by the ultrasound beam. In patients with pericardial effusion a clear echofree space is recorded between the epicardium and pericardium. A posterior effusion is recorded behind the left ventricular epicardium and ends at the junction of the left ventricle and left atrium. An anterior effusion will be recorded between the chest wall and the anterior right ventricular wall. The presence of both an anterior and posterior effusion generally indicates that a large collection of fluid is present.

TABLE 15–22. Etiology of Pericardial Disease

Congenital Anomalies
Absence (partial, complete)
Cysts
Mulibrey nanism (*mu*scle, *li*ver, *bre*in, *ey*e) with congenital pericardial thickening and constriction
Infectious
Viral (coxsackievirus B, Epstein-Barr virus)
Bacterial (streptococcus, pneumococcus, staphylococcus, meningococcus, mycoplasma, tularemia)
Immune complex (meningococcus, *H. influenzae*)
Tuberculosis
Fungal (histoplasmosis, actinomycosis)
Parasitic (toxoplasmosis, echinococcus)
Connective Tissue Diseases
Rheumatoid arthritis
Rheumatic fever
Systemic lupus erythematosus
Systemic sclerosis
Sarcoidosis
Metabolic-Endocrine
Uremia
Hypothyroidism
Chylopericardium
Hematology-Oncology
Bleeding diathesis
Malignancy (primary, metastatic)
Radiotherapy induced
Other
Trauma (penetrating or blunt injury)
Postpericardiotomy (cardiac surgery)
Aortic dissection
Idiopathic
Familial Mediterranean fever

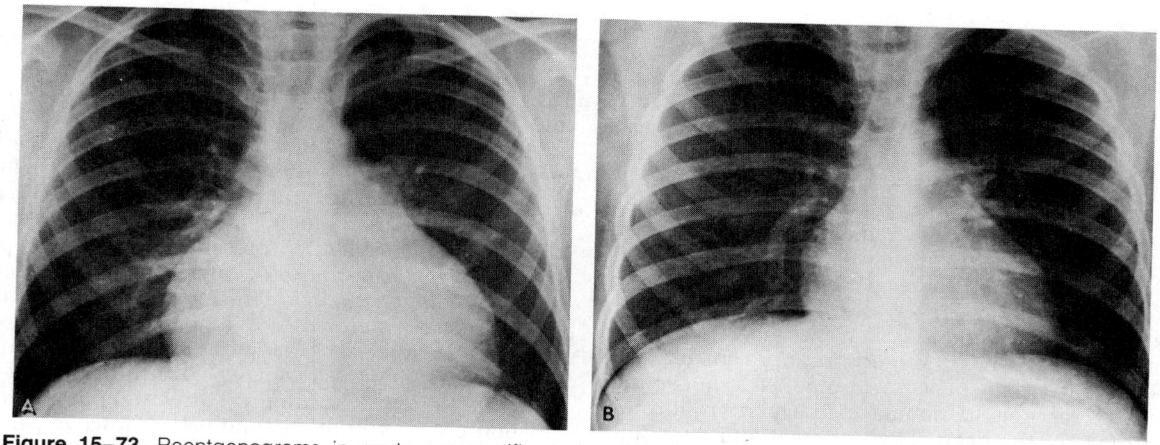

Figure 15–73. Roentgenograms in acute nonspecific pericarditis. *A,* Increase in cardiopericardial shadow due to pericardial effusion. *B,* One month later after complete recovery.

DIFFERENTIAL DIAGNOSIS. **Viral and Acute Benign Pericarditis.** These entities are considered synonymous since most episodes of acute benign pericarditis follow or coincide with viral illness. Viruses recognized to cause pericarditis include coxsackievirus B, influenza, echovirus, and adenovirus. The pathogenesis is unclear but may be related to a hypersensitivity reaction to a viral disease. However, pericardial inflammation is not necessarily the precursor of a generalized inflammatory process. Most cases are mild, and recovery occurs within several weeks.

Only symptomatic therapy is indicated. In rare instances the patient will be severely ill, and cardiac tamponade may ensue. There are also patients in whom a chronic relapsing illness occurs. The differential diagnosis between these patients and those with collagen vascular disease may be difficult. These patients respond dramatically to corticosteroids or nonsteroidal anti-inflammatory agents such as indomethacin; milder forms may be controlled with aspirin. The clinical course may vary from months to 1–2 yr, during which time the patients are dependent on drug therapy for suppression of the pericarditis. Ultimately, the patients improve and the prognosis is good.

The clinical differential diagnosis between acute pericarditis and myocarditis may be difficult. Indeed, in patients with pericarditis there is usually a myocardial inflammatory component, and the reverse is also true. However, management of these conditions is quite different; anti-inflammatory treatment and urgent response to cardiac tamponade are appropriate in the former, and therapy for congestive heart failure is required in the latter. The echocardiogram is useful in the differential diagnosis, as it will demonstrate large pericardial effusions and can also indicate the presence of myocardial dysfunction.

Purulent Pericarditis. This is most often associated with bacterial infections such as pneumonia, epiglottitis, meningitis, or osteomyelitis. There may be signs and symptoms of the primary infection. Once the purulent process is established, the course is fulminant, terminated by acute cardiac tamponade and death. Open pericardial drainage is required, along with appropriate intravenous antibiotics. Although closed pericardial aspiration provides exudate for diagnostic purposes and may be lifesaving in the face of severe cardiac compression, it should not be considered final therapy. Without open drainage, tamponade will recur almost invariably because with large effusions only a small reaccumulation of pericardial fluid may markedly increase intrapericardial pressure. Open pericardial drainage has significantly increased survival in patients with this disease. Rarely, with infections that are identified extremely early and with pericardial fluid that is more of a transudate than an exudate, multiple pericardial taps and antibiotic therapy have been successful; in the vast majority of cases, this approach should not be considered. The most common organisms implicated in purulent pericarditis are *Staphylococcus aureus, Haemophilus influenzae* type b, and *Neisseria meningitidis.* (For treatment, see Sec. 12.19, 12.22, and 12.23, respectively.) Tuberculous pericarditis rarely occurs in children outside of underdeveloped countries. Extensive treatment with antituberculous chemotherapy is required (see Sec. 12.47), and late constriction may occur. Immune complex mediated pericarditis may occur 5–7 days after the initiation of therapy for severe systemic or meningeal infection with meningococcus or *H. influenzae* type b. Therapy includes anti-inflammatory agents and pericardiocentesis, if tamponade develops. The pericardial fluid is sterile.

Acute Rheumatic Fever. Pericarditis occurs in acute rheumatic fever as a component of pancarditis (see Sec. 11.74 and 15.67). Rheumatic pericarditis is associated with acute valvulitis, and a murmur of mitral or aortic regurgitation will be audible. Pericarditis and other manifestations of acute rheumatic pancarditis respond to therapy with steroids. Cardiac tamponade is extremely rare.

Rheumatoid Arthritis. Pericarditis is not an uncommon manifestation of rheumatoid arthritis in children (see Sec. 11.51). Rarely, pericarditis may be the only manifestation of rheumatoid arthritis and precede the onset of arthritis by months or even years. Differentiation of rheumatoid pericarditis from that seen with other collagen vascular disease, particularly lupus erythematosus, may be difficult. Treatment consists of steroids or salicylates, which may be needed on a long-term basis to suppress the disease process.

Uremia. Uremic pericarditis occurs only in the presence of prolonged severe renal failure and results from chemical irritation of the pericardium secondary to the metabolic abnormalities. In most instances it is an incidental part of end-stage chronic renal disease. However, with the advent of chronic hemodialysis, uremic pericarditis has been recognized as a more chronic problem, culminating in cardiac tamponade. Pericardial effusion has also been implicated in the etiology of recurrent hypotension during hemodialysis. If adequate relief of uremic pericarditis does not occur with hemodialysis, pericardiectomy is recommended.

Neoplastic Disease. Neoplastic pericardial effusion is seen in patients with Hodgkin disease, lymphosarcoma, and leukemia and results from direct neoplastic invasion of the pericardium. Cardiac tamponade may occur late in the course of the illness. Rarely, pericardial infiltration is the initial manifestation of neoplastic disease, and the diagnosis can be made by examination of the pericardial fluid for neoplastic cells.

Patients with malignancy may also develop pericarditis as a result of radiation therapy to the mediastinum. This manifestation may be related to the radiation dose and to the technique utilized.

Postpericardiotomy Syndrome. Postpericardiotomy syndrome is characterized by fever, chest pain, pleural and pericardial effusion, and fluid retention (Sec. 15.61). It is seen 1–2 wk following open heart surgery in approximately 15% of postoperative patients. The syndrome is a nonspecific hypersensitivity reaction to trauma to the pericardium and epicardial surface of the heart. High titers of anti-heart antibody have been reported to correlate with clinical signs of the syndrome.

In most patients, postpericardiotomy syndrome is a relatively short illness, and affected children will generally respond well to anti-inflammatory therapy with aspirin. Corticosteroids are very rarely needed. Treatment is maintained for 1–3 mo, but recurrences may be seen as long as 1 yr postoperatively and require reinstitution of therapy.

CONSTRICTIVE PERICARDITIS. This disease represents a special problem in terms of both the clinical picture and the differential diagnosis. Predisposing pericardial diseases include purulent pericarditis, tuberculous pericarditis, acute benign or viral pericarditis, mediastinal irradiation for intrathoracic malignancy, neoplastic invasion of the pericardium, and trauma. In most instances constriction occurs months or years after the initial insult, but occasionally it may be an acute, rapidly progressive process. Constrictive pericarditis most often occurs without a preceding illness or generalized systemic disease.

The *clinical manifestations* occur as a result of impairment of diastolic ventricular filling, compromise of myocardial contractility, and resultant depression of cardiac function. Hepatomegaly and ascites may be out of proportion to the other signs and symptoms and thus suggest chronic liver disease. However, liver function studies are only mildly abnormal, and careful physical examination reveals other sometimes subtle findings of constriction including neck vein distention, narrow pulses, quiet precordium, distant heart sounds, faint pericardial friction rub, and paradoxic pulse. Typical findings become apparent gradually and thus may be easily overlooked. The auscultatory presence of an early pericardial knock and the appearance of calcification of the pericardium on chest roentgenogram are the more obvious manifestations. Protein-losing enteropathy with hypoproteinemia and lymphopenia may be seen in association with constriction.

Constrictive pericarditis may be difficult to distinguish from chronic restrictive cardiomyopathy. Impaired myocardial function occurs with both conditions. However, the myocardial disease of constrictive pericarditis is almost always reversible with pericardiectomy. At times, a definite diagnosis can be made only by exploratory thoracotomy and direct examination of the pericardium.

Radical pericardiectomy with decortication of the pericardium over a wide area of the heart, including the systemic and pulmonary veins, is the only therapy for constrictive pericarditis. In most patients surgical intervention elicits a rapid response characterized by increased cardiac output and prompt diuresis. The long-term prognosis is usually excellent.

Gersony WM, Hordof AH: Infective endocarditis and diseases of the pericardium. Pediatr Clin North Am 25:831, 1978.

Hara KS, Ballard DJ, Ilstrup DM, et al: Rheumatoid pericarditis: Clinical features and survival. Medicine 69:81, 1990.

Muir P, Nicholson F, Tilzey AJ, et al: Chronic relapsing pericarditis and dilated cardiomyopathy: Serological evidence of persistent enterovirus infection. Lancet 1:804, 1989.

Nishimura RA, Connolly DC, Parkin TW, et al: Constrictive pericarditis: Assessment of current diagnostic procedures. Mayo Clin Proc 60:397, 1985.

Sinzobahamvya N, Ikeogu MO: Purulent pericarditis. Arch Dis Child 62:696, 1987.

15.76 DISEASES OF THE BLOOD VESSELS

15.77 ANEURYSMS AND FISTULAS

Aneurysms are not common in children and occur most frequently in the aorta in association with coarctation of the aorta, patent ductus arteriosus, and Marfan syndrome and in intracranial vessels (see Sec. 20.71). They may also occur secondary to an infected embolus; infection contiguous to a blood vessel; trauma; congenital abnormalities of structure, especially of the medial coat; and arteritis, for example, polyarteritis nodosa (see Sec. 11.58) and Takayasu arteritis (see Sec. 11.60). Aneurysm of the coronary arteries, rarely with thrombosis and myocardial infarction, may complicate Kawasaki disease (see Sec. 11.57 and 15.68).

Arteriovenous fistulas may be limited to small cavernous hemangiomas or may be extensive (see Sec. 20.71 and 23.8). The most common sites in infants and children are intracranial, hepatic, and pulmonary sites and the extremities. They have also been described in other parts of the body, especially in vessels in or near the thoracic wall. The fistulas, though usually congenital, may follow trauma or be a manifestation of hereditary hemorrhagic telangiectasia (Rendu-Osler-Weber syndrome).

Cardiovascular manifestations occur only in association with large communications when arterial blood flows into a low-pressure venous system, increasing local venous pressure and decreasing arterial flow beyond the fistula. Systemic arterial resistance falls because of the runoff of blood through the fistula. Compensatory mechanisms include tachycardia and increased stroke volume so that cardiac output rises. Blood volume is also increased. Cardiac failure may develop with large arteriovenous fistulas.

The clinical manifestations of arteriovenous fistulas depend on the size of the shunt across the fistula. In extensive fistulas, left ventricular hypertrophy and dilatation, a widened pulse pressure, and congestive heart failure occur. Arteriograms after injection of contrast material into an artery proximal to the fistula confirm the diagnosis.

Large *intracranial arteriovenous fistulas* most often occur in the newborn infant in association with a vein of Galen malformation. The large intracranial left to right shunt results in congestive heart failure secondary to the demand for extremely high cardiac output. Patients with smaller communications may not have cardiovascular manifestations, but later develop hydrocephalus (see Sec. 20.71) or seizure disorders. The newborn infant with a large symptomatic intracranial arteriovenous fistula has a grave prognosis; some will survive with medical management but are subject to later complications due to the intracranial mass. Older patients with more diffuse intracranial arteriovenous malformations may be recognized on the basis of intracranial calcification and a high cardiac output, without frank cardiac failure.

Hepatic arteriovenous fistulas may be localized or generalized in the liver. The fistula may be located between the hepatic artery and ductus venosus or portal vein. Congenital hemorrhagic telangiectasia may also be associated. Large arteriovenous fistulas are associated with a large cardiac output and heart failure. Hepatomegaly is usual, and systolic or continuous murmurs may be audible over the liver.

Peripheral arteriovenous fistulas usually involve the extremities. These lesions are associated with disfigurement, swelling of the extremity, and visible hemangiomas. Some are located in areas that result in upper airway obstruction. Because only a small minority result in large arterial runoff, cardiac failure is not common.

TREATMENT. Surgical removal of a large arteriovenous fistula is often not possible, especially in the most severe cases with large arterial runoffs, such as intracranial and hepatic types. Medical management of congestive heart failure is initially helpful in the neonate with these conditions; with time the size of the shunt may diminish and symptoms spontaneously regress. Hemangiomas of the liver often completely disappear with time. This abnormality is occasionally treated by steroid, epsilon-aminocaproic acid, or interferon administration, local compression, embolization, or local radiation; the beneficial effects of this management are not established but this approach may be worth a trial. Individual patients display marked variations in clinical course without treatment. Surgical removal of a large fistula may be attempted in the presence of severe cardiac failure and the lack of improvement with medical treatment. However, surgical treatment may be unsuccessful when the lesion is extensive and diffuse or is located in a position where adjoining tissue may be injured during the surgery or related procedures.

15.78 COLD INJURY

See also Neonatal Cold Injury, Sec. 9.54.

FROSTBITE. Frostbite may occur especially in the face or extremities from exposure to cold. Cellular injury is due to intravascular thrombosis or ice crystal formation in the tissues. The skin initially becomes red and then pale or, rarely, cyanotic as the arterioles remain in spasm in an effort to preserve body heat. During thawing, hyperemia occurs, and blisters may form on the skin. Gangrene may occur if early relief is not obtained.

Treatment consists of rapidly rewarming the skin of the affected area that is still white. Analgesics are usually necessary. Massage of the **damaged area** or rubbing with snow or ice is contraindicated. Other therapeutic measures that have yielded equivocal results include anticoagulants (especially heparin), low molecular weight dextran, and sympathectomy. Meticulous local care to the injured area is essential. Recovery of an extremity from severe frostbite can be striking and, in the absence of infection, amputation or excision of tissue should be postponed as long as possible to make certain that it is necessary.

CHILBLAIN (PERNIO). This form of cold injury, presumably vascular in origin, consists of a (sometimes blistering) localized erythema, which itches, may be painful, and frequently results in swelling and in scabbing ulcerations of the affected areas. The mechanism is unknown, but it is probably related to prolonged constriction of peripheral arterioles, which is manifested by pallor and coldness of the subsequently affected areas during cold, particularly damp, weather.

The tops of the ears and tips of the fingers and toes are most frequently affected; the exposed legs of girls wearing skirts and no stockings may also be affected. Without further exposure the lesions usually clear in 1–2 wk but may persist longer.

Avoiding prolonged chilling or protecting susceptible areas with woolen caps, gloves, and stockings can be preventive. Therapeutic measures include dermal corticosteroid preparations for itching and antibiotics for infection.

15.79 TUMORS OF THE HEART

Primary tumors of the heart are rare in infancy and childhood and are most often benign. Clinical manifestations depend primarily upon the location of the tumor and, to a lesser extent, upon the histologic type.

The most common benign cardiac tumors in children are rhabdomyomas, fibromas, and myxomas. *Rhabdomyomas* occur as single or usually multiple nodules embedded in chamber walls. They may remain clinically unimportant or even regress but also may cause mechanical obstruction, heart failure, or arrhythmias. Rhabdomyomas may be familial and are often found in association with tuberous sclerosis. Most rhabdomyomas are seen in infants under 1 yr of age. Incessant ventricular tachycardia in an infant younger than 2 yr of age should raise suspicion of a small endocardial or epicardial rhabdomyoma or Purkinje cell tumor. *Fibromas* are usually solitary unencapsulated nodules, located in the ventricles; they can be massive. The treatment of rhabdomyomas and fibromas depends on their location and size. Small asymptomatic tumors in the myocardial wall or ventricular septum may be observed for growth. Large tumors that show signs of obstructing blood flow and those producing ventricular arrhythmias should be removed. Large and diffuse tumors may interfere with cardiac performance. Removal of large lesions is difficult because insufficient normal myocardium may remain. Cardiac transplantation is the only recourse for patients with extensive tumors.

Myxomas develop in intracavitary locations, most frequently (90%) in the left atrium. Most occur in females (75%). These tumors are solid, smooth, pedunculated masses (1–8 cm) that attach to the interatrial septum, protrude into the atrial chamber and, by their position relative to the mitral valve, cause intermittent obstruction and a clinical picture consistent with mitral stenosis (syncope, heart failure, atrial fibrillation). A myxoma should be considered in the presence of fainting spells, a positional character (supine versus erect) to the murmur, or evidence of systemic embolization. Atrial myxomas also manifest fever, malaise, arthralgias, and systemic emboli mimicking endocarditis, rheumatic fever, or systemic lupus erythematosus. Laboratory features include a high sedimentation rate, hematuria, and echocardiographic evidence of the tumor. Atrial myxomas may be associated with multiple pigmented skin lesions (lentiginosis), myxoid fibroadenomas of the breast, cutaneous myxomas, and adrenal pigmented nodules. Some are associated with various cutaneous and connective tissue lesions and testicular tumors or pituitary adenomas. Treatment consists of surgical excision, which must include all of the base of the tumor to prevent recurrence.

Other benign tumors include *papillomas*, which are attached to valve leaflets and may present in the neonate; *lipomas*, which are situated in ventricular walls; and *mesotheliomas*, which may involve the atrioventricular node and cause abnormalities of electrical conduction, including complete heart block.

Primary malignant cardiac tumors in children are almost exclusively *sarcomas*. These tumors are usually located in the right side of the heart, atrial septum, right atrial wall, or root of the pulmonary artery. They may extend either into the adjacent chamber to cause obstruction to blood flow or into the pericardial cavity to produce effusion or tamponade.

The heart may be involved in the metastatic dissemination of a noncardiac malignancy, such as leukemia or lymphoma, or by direct extension via the inferior vena cava (Wilms tumor).

Physical examination of the heart reflects the location and size of the tumor as it interferes with blood flow. Conduction system involvement can be assessed by electrocardiography. Two-dimensional echocardiography allows excellent visualization of the location and extent of the tumor. Cardiac catheterization, including pressure measurement and angiography, provides further information about the anatomy of the tumor and the hemodynamic effects.

When indicated, surgical intervention is directed toward complete removal of the tumor, relief of obstruction, and control of arrhythmia. Long-term outcome depends upon the type of tumor, completeness of surgical removal, and the postsurgical integrity of the normal cardiac structures and myocardium.

WELTON M. GERSONY

Bini RM, Westaby S, Bargeron LM, et al: Investigation and management of primary cardiac tumors in infants and children. J Am Coll Cardiol 2:351, 1983.
Birnbaum S, McGahan JP, Janos GG, et al: Fetal tachycardia and intramyocardial tumors. J Am Coll Cardiol 6:1358, 1985.
Coltart DJ, Billingham ME, Popp RL, et al: Left atrial myxoma: Diagnosis, treatment and cytological observations. JAMA 234:950, 1975.
Danoff A, Jarmark S, Lorber D, et al: Adrenocortical micronodular dysplasia, cardiac myxomas, lentigines, and spindle cell tumors: Report of a kindred. Arch Intern Med 147:443, 1987.
Felner JM, Knopf WD: Echocardiographic recognition of intracardiac and extracardiac masses. Echocardiography 2:1, 1985.
Garson A Jr, Gillette PC, Titus JL, et al: Surgical treatment of ventricular tachycardia in infants. N Engl J Med 310:1443, 1984.

15.80 SYSTEMIC HYPERTENSION

Systemic hypertension, a sign of underlying pathophysiology, is recognized more commonly in adults (the prevalence is 10–15% in the adult population) than in children and adolescents. Untreated essential or primary hypertension increases the risk of myocardial infarction, stroke, and renal failure in affected individuals. To increase early detection of hypertension, blood pressure measurement should be a part of the periodic physical examination in children, and careful inquiry of family history of hypertension should be undertaken.

Blood pressure is the product of peripheral vascular resistance and cardiac output. Accurate measurement of blood pressure requires attention to the comfort of the patient and is dependent on the quality of the equipment and the skill of the observer. Many patients of all ages have some level of anxiety associated with initial measurements of blood pressure. Depending upon age and desire, the patient may be seated or supine, but subsequent measurements taken for comparison should be obtained with the patient in the same position. Especially in young children, careful attention to cuff size is necessary. The bladder of the pressure cuff should nearly encircle the upper arm, but its ends should not overlap; the cuff should cover at least two thirds of the length of the upper arm. Although systolic pressure is indicated by the appearance of the 1st Korotkoff sound, the true diastolic pressure probably lies between the muffling and the disappearance of sound as the cuff pressure is decreased. Doppler and oscillometric techniques may be used satisfactorily in infants and young children. Because blood pressure often decreases as the patient becomes comfortable with the procedure, repeated measurements are necessary for accuracy.

Because systemic blood pressure gradually increases with age and correlates with weight and height throughout childhood and adolescence, reference standards (see Figs. 15–1, 15–2, 15–3, 15–4, 15–5, and 15–6) are necessary for interpretation of values obtained during physical examinations. Pressure that is consistently above the 95th percentile for age is abnormal and requires further evaluation. Unless there is need for urgency because of marked elevation of pressure or evidence of a systemic complication, sequential measurements of blood pressure should be obtained over a period of weeks before concluding that the patient has systemic hypertension.

ETIOLOGY AND PATHOPHYSIOLOGY. An increase in cardiac output or peripheral resistance results in an increase in blood pressure. When the cause of the increase in pressure can be explained by an associated disease, the hypertension is referred to as secondary; the term primary or essential hypertension implies that no known underlying disease is present. However, it is recognized that many factors, such as heredity, salt intake, stress, and obesity, may play a role in the development of essential hypertension.

Essential hypertension is probably not a single entity, so it is likely that several pathogenic mechanisms are involved. In experimental settings, normotensive children of hypertensive parents may show abnormal physiologic responses that are similar to those of their parents. When subjected to stress or competitive tasks, the offspring of hypertensive adults, as a group, respond with greater increases in heart rate and blood pressure than do children of normotensive parents. Similarly, some children of hypertensive parents may excrete higher levels of urinary catecholamine metabolites or may respond to sodium loading with greater weight gain and increases in blood pressure than those without a family history of hypertension. The abnormal responses in children with affected parents tend to be greater in the black population than in white subjects. As other possible markers for the development of subsequent hypertension, erythrocyte sodium transport, free calcium concentration in platelets, urine kallikrein excretion, and sympathetic nervous system receptors are under investigation.

Categorization of essential hypertension according to the level of plasma renin activity (high, normal, low) has been useful in understanding the pathophysiology and developing treatment regimens in adults; similar large studies have not been conducted in adolescents with primary hypertension. Investigations are under way to define the role of atrial natriuretic peptides in the maintenance of normal blood pressure and the development of hypertension. These peptides stimulate sodium excretion by the kidney and have vasodilating properties. With changes in sodium intake, there often are reciprocal changes in the secretion of renin and the atrial natriuretic peptides.

Tracking of blood pressure is likely to occur as children develop, so that over time individuals maintain their relative ranking of blood pressure with respect to their peers. Therefore, children and young adolescents with pressure above the 90th percentile for age often become adults with elevated pressure. Adolescents with essential hypertension may progress from a high cardiac output and normal systemic vascular resistance state to the adult pattern of normal cardiac output with elevated systemic vascular resistance. There are racial differences, however, and black adults with hypertension have greater elevations in peripheral resistance, whereas hypertensive white adults show predominantly an increase in cardiac output.

Secondary hypertension is more common than essential hypertension in infants and children. Both transient and chronic hypertension may accompany diseases, as listed in Tables 15–23 and 15–24. The etiology of hypertension varies with age. For example, elevated pressure in the newborn is most often associated with high umbilical artery catheterization and renal artery obstruction due to thrombus formation. Hypertension during childhood is also usually secondary, but primary hypertension occurs with increasing frequency in later childhood and adolescence. The level of blood pressure is also helpful in distinguishing secondary from primary hypertension; in general, adolescents with essential hypertension have diastolic pressures at or slightly above the 95th percentile for age.

Approximately 75–80% of children with secondary hypertension have a *renal abnormality*. Urinary tract infection is present in 25–50% of these patients and is often related to an obstructive lesion of the urinary tract. This hypertension may be associated with sodium retention, renin secretion, or a decrease in bradykinin production. A proportion of children with chronic pyelonephritis do not develop hypertension until they become azotemic. Other children, however, demonstrate elevated blood pressure during an episode of acute pyelonephritis; the infection may simply unmask essential hypertension.

Other renal parenchymal lesions associated with hypertension include acute and chronic glomerulonephritis, congenital lesions, tumors, and trauma. The reduced glomerular filtration rate of nephritis results in salt and water accumulation, whereas mass lesions (cysts, solid tumors, hematoma) may impair perfusion of portions of the kidney and stimulate renin production by the juxtaglomerular apparatus. There is also evidence that both Wilms tumor and juxtaglomerular cell tumor (hemangiopericytoma) secrete renin or a pressor substance without feedback control.

Renovascular lesions result in hypertension through stimulation of the *renin-angiotensin-aldosterone system*. Renin is a proteolytic enzyme secreted by juxtaglomerular cells that converts the α_2-globulin, angiotensinogen, to angiotensin I.

TABLE 15–23. Conditions Associated with Transient or Intermittent Hypertension in Children

Renal
Acute postinfectious glomerulonephritis
Anaphylactoid (Henoch-Schönlein) purpura with nephritis
Hemolytic-uremic syndrome
Acute tubular necrosis
After renal transplant (immediate and during episodes of rejection)
After blood transfusion in patients with azotemia
Hypervolemia
After surgical procedures on genitourinary tract
Pyelonephritis
Renal trauma
Leukemic infiltration of kidney
Obstructive uropathy associated with Crohn disease

Drugs and Poisons
Cocaine
Oral contraceptives
Sympathomimetic agents
Amphetamines
Phencyclidine
Corticosteroids and ACTH
Cyclosporine treatment post-transplantation
Licorice (glycyrrhizic acid)
Lead, mercury, cadmium, thallium
Antihypertensive withdrawal (clonidine, methyldopa, propranolol)
Vitamin D intoxication

Central and Autonomic Nervous System
Increased intracranial pressure
Guillain-Barré syndrome
Burns
Familial dysautonomia
Stevens-Johnson syndrome
Posterior fossa lesions
Porphyria
Poliomyelitis
Encephalitis

Miscellaneous
Pre-eclampsia
Fractures of long bones
Hypercalcemia
Postcoarctation repair
White cell transfusion
Extracorporeal membrane oxygenation (ECMO)
Chronic upper airway obstruction

TABLE 15–24. Conditions Associated with Chronic Hypertension in Children

Renal
Chronic pyelonephritis
Chronic glomerulonephritis
Hydronephrosis
Congenital dysplastic kidney
Multicystic kidney
Solitary renal cyst
Vesicoureteral reflux nephropathy
Segmental hypoplasia (Ask-Upmark kidney)
Ureteral obstruction
Renal tumors
Renal trauma
Rejection damage following transplantation
Postirradiation damage
Systemic lupus erythematosus (other connective tissue diseases)

Vascular
Coarctation of thoracic or abdominal aorta
Renal artery lesions (stenosis, fibromuscular dysplasia, thrombosis, aneurysm)
Umbilical artery catheterization with thrombus formation
Neurofibromatosis (intrinsic or extrinsic narrowing of vascular lumen)
Renal vein thrombosis
Vasculitis
Arteriovenous shunt
Williams Beuren syndrome

Endocrine
Hyperthyroidism
Hyperparathyroidism
Congenital adrenal hyperplasia (11β-hydroxylase and 17-hydroxylase defect)
Cushing syndrome
Primary aldosteronism
Dexamethasone-suppressible hyperaldosteronism
Pheochromocytoma
Other neural crest tumors (neuroblastoma, ganglioneuroblastoma, ganglioneuroma)
Diabetic nephropathy

Central Nervous System
Intracranial mass
Hemorrhage
Residual following brain injury
Quadriplegia

Essential Hypertension
Low renin
Normal renin
High renin

Renin production is affected to some extent by the sympathetic nervous system, renal blood flow, prostaglandin synthesis, and urine/plasma sodium concentration. Angiotensin I, a decapeptide, possesses little physiologic activity and is rapidly converted to angiotensin II by angiotensin-converting enzyme (ACE). This converting enzyme is also responsible for the metabolic degradation of vasodilating kinins. Angiotensin II is a potent vasoconstrictor and also stimulates aldosterone secretion; both effects lead to increased blood pressure.

Although probably not the primary cause of hypertension in patients with coarctation of the aorta, activation of the renin-angiotensin-aldosterone system may contribute to the postoperative hypertension frequently seen in those patients. Intracranial hemorrhage may occur because of elevated pressure in the cerebral vessels and associated congenital aneurysms in the circle of Willis.

Endocrinopathies linked with hypertension involve the thyroid, parathyroid, and adrenal glands. Systolic hypertension and tachycardia are common in hyperthyroidism, but diastolic pressure is usually not elevated. Hypercalcemia, whether secondary to hyperparathyroidism or other causes, often results in mild elevation in pressure because of an increase in vascular tone. Adrenocortical disorders may produce hypertension if there is an increased mineralocorticoid effect due to an increased amount of active precursors, aldosterone, or cortisol.

Catecholamine-secreting tumors give rise to hypertension because of the cardiac and vascular effects of epinephrine and norepinephrine. Children with pheochromocytoma usually have sustained hypertension (see Sec. 19.26). The tumor may be unilateral or bilateral and may arise in the adrenal medulla or in other chromaffin cells. Approximately 5% of patients with neurofibromatosis will develop pheochromocytoma. Hypertension is much less frequent with other neural crest tumors but may result from catecholamine secretion or interference with renal perfusion.

Excess catecholamines appear to play a role in intermittently elevating blood pressure in patients with Guillain-Barré syndrome, poliomyelitis, burns, and Stevens-Johnson syndrome. Autonomic instability is suggested by episodic increases in urinary excretion of catecholamine metabolites. Sympathetic outflow from the central nervous system is also affected by intracranial lesions.

A number of *drugs of abuse, therapeutic agents,* and *toxins* may increase blood pressure. Inhalation or mucosal application of cocaine may provoke rapid increase in blood pressure and result in seizures or intracranial hemorrhage. Transient hypertension often accompanies phencyclidine use and may become persistent in chronic abusers of amphetamines. Sympathomimetic agents used as nasal decongestants, appetite suppressants, and stimulants for attention deficit disorder produce peripheral vasoconstriction and varying degrees of cardiac stimulation. Individuals vary in their susceptibility to these effects. Oral contraceptives are a common cause of hypertension in adolescent females. Although as many as 15% of patients who take oral contraceptives may develop hypertension, it is not certain that the incidence can be reduced through the use of low-estrogen preparations. The pathogenesis of the elevated blood pressure may be due to stimulation of the renin-angiotensin-aldosterone system or to a direct effect of estrogen on salt and water retention. The nephrotoxicity of cyclosporine used as an immunosuppressant is the likely explanation for the hypertension observed in patients after cardiac, bone marrow, and, in some cases, renal and liver transplantation. The coadministration of steroids appears to increase the incidence of hypertension in such patients. Licorice, not licorice flavoring, contains glycyrrhizic acid, which acts on the distal tubule in a manner similar to that of aldosterone. Blood pressure may be elevated in patients with poisoning by a heavy metal; there is also interest in the effect of subtoxic levels of lead on vascular tone.

CLINICAL MANIFESTATIONS. Preadolescents and adolescents with primary hypertension rarely have clinical evidence of disease until the blood pressure elevation is detected, usually at the time of a routine examination or during physical evaluation prior to athletic participation. In addition to having a mild elevation in pressure, many affected individuals are somewhat overweight. Blood pressure is often at the highest level in such patients while they are supine.

The pressure in children with secondary hypertension may be only a few millimeters above the 95th percentile for age or may be markedly elevated. Unless the pressure has been sustained or is rising rapidly, hypertension will usually not produce symptoms. Therefore clinical manifestations of the underlying disease, such as growth failure in children with chronic renal disease, most frequently draw attention to the blood pressure. With substantial elevation, however, headache, dizziness, changes in vision, and seizures may occur. Hypertensive encephalopathy is suggested by the presence of vomiting, temperature elevation, ataxia, stupor, and seizures. Regardless of the cause of the hypertension, cardiac and renal function deteriorate in the face of marked increases in blood pressure.

Young children and infants with unexplained heart failure or seizures should have their blood pressure measured. Such patients often cannot communicate symptoms such as headache, and their behavior may not be considered abnormal until the complications of hypertension are present. Often, in retrospect, after blood pressure has been lowered, parents of hypertensive infants will comment that their child had been increasingly irritable before the hypertension was recognized.

Specific manifestations of the diseases associated with hypertension (see Tables 15–23 and 15–24) are discussed in their respective sections. Routinely measuring and recording blood pressure in infants, children, and adolescents will result in identification of affected patients before symptoms of hypertension develop.

DIAGNOSIS. Essential hypertension is suggested by the patient's age, level of blood pressure, weight, family history, and the paucity of signs and symptoms of underlying disease. It is uncommon to make this diagnosis in children younger than 10 yr of age. Before a patient is diagnosed as hypertensive, several recordings of blood pressure should be obtained. If the pressure is only mildly elevated on the first visit, measurement on two or three occasions over the ensuing weeks may reveal that the initial elevation was related to apprehension; such patients, however, need annual evaluation, as they may subsequently develop sustained hypertension. Excess body weight is associated with essential hypertension; except with disorders of the adrenal cortex, patients with secondary hypertension are rarely obese. Heredity is also a strong determinant of blood pressure; therefore, an adolescent with mild elevation of pressure and a definite family history of essential hypertension rarely needs evaluation for underlying disease. Adolescents suspected of having essential hypertension require regular measurement of blood pressure to determine the course of the evaluation over time. If the pressure continues to rise over several weeks or months of observation, additional diagnostic studies are indicated.

If age, level of blood pressure, or symptomatology suggests that secondary hypertension is likely, the initial focus should be the urinary tract. Measures of growth are important, as is a history of intermittent febrile illnesses, which might suggest recurring infection of the urinary tract. Physical examination should determine the presence of flank masses or abdominal bruits. Screening tests should include complete blood count, urinalysis, serum electrolytes, blood urea nitrogen, serum creatinine, and uric acid. Urine culture should be obtained even if the sediment is unremarkable. Chest roentgenography and electrocardiography are helpful in assessing cardiac response to the elevated pressure.

Renal imaging is discussed in Sec. 6.56. Whereas a renal ultrasound will provide a comparison of kidney size and a view of the anatomy of the collecting system, an intravenous pyelogram is not adequate for detecting differences in renal perfusion. A radionuclide scan is helpful in distinguishing variation in perfusion of the two kidneys. Renal angiography can demonstrate lesions in the main arteries or in the segmental branches; at angiography, venous blood samples should be collected from both renal veins and the inferior vena cava for assay of plasma renin activity. Doppler ultrasound may demonstrate arterial and venous blood flow.

Peripheral plasma renin activity is a useful screening test for both renovascular and renal parenchymal disease. Normal values gradually decrease with age and vary between laboratories. A suppressed value suggests excess mineralocorticoid effect, and an elevated value is associated with renal or renovascular involvement. One approach to the adolescent with hypertension is noted in Figure 15–74.

COURSE AND PROGNOSIS. The natural history of essential hypertension that is first detected during adolescence is under investigation; many such patients will probably continue to have essential hypertension as adults. Collaborative studies in adults with essential hypertension have shown the value of drug therapy in reducing the incidence of congestive heart failure, renal failure, and stroke. A similar reduction in incidence of myocardial infarction has not been proved. That lack of effect is most likely due to antecedent coronary artery disease that is well established before blood pressure is controlled. Drug-induced alteration of serum lipids may exacerbate this problem. Detection and intervention at an earlier age with drugs that do not increase serum lipids should improve outcome.

Prognosis for secondary hypertension is primarily determined by the nature of the underlying disease and its responsiveness to specific therapy. For example, survival in patients with underlying chronic renal diseases is often determined by the patients' response to dialysis and transplant programs. In patients with hyper-reninemic hypertension (e.g., renovascular disease), evaluation of renal vein renin activity may help predict prognosis. A discrepancy in renin secretion between the two kidneys of more than 1.5:1 suggests that the kidney producing the higher level is primarily responsible for the hypertension. Surgical correction of the lesion on the involved side yields a high probability of marked improvement or resolution of the hypertension. The prognosis after surgical repair of coarctation is variable. Although the majority of patients will establish normal systemic blood pressure following surgery, some will have persistently elevated pressure that may become more prominent during exercise. The long-term outcome is favorable for neonates who develop hypertension as a complication of umbilical artery catheterization. Few of these infants require therapy beyond 12 mo of age, and most show marked improvement in renal perfusion.

PREVENTION. The prevention of high blood pressure may be viewed as a part of the prevention of cardiovascular disease. Several risk factors for cardiovascular disorders have been identified and include obesity, elevated serum cholesterol, high dietary sodium intake, sedentary life style, alcohol abuse, and tobacco use. Beginning in childhood and continuing through adolescence, it is especially important to discourage cigarette smoking because of the pulmonary and cardiovascular consequences. The increase in arterial wall rigidity and increase in blood viscosity that are associated with cigarette smoking may contribute to the adverse effect of tobacco use on blood pressure.

TREATMENT. Both nonpharmacologic and pharmacologic

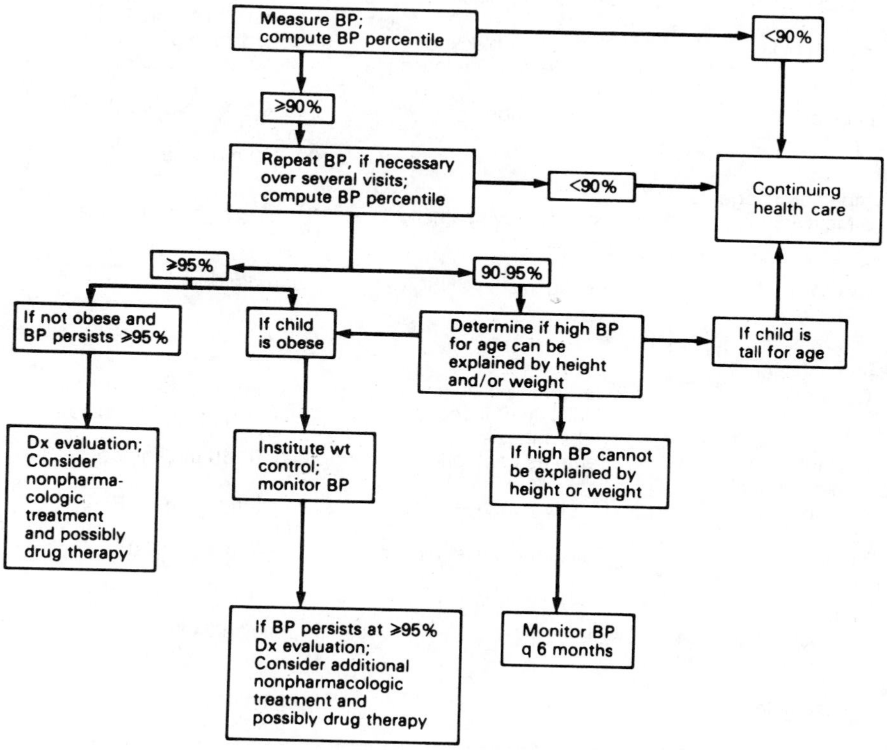

Figure 15–74. Algorithm for identifying children with high BP. Note that whenever BP measurement is stipulated, the average of at least two measurements should be used. (From National Heart, Lung, and Blood Institute, Bethesda, MD: Report of the second task force on blood pressure control in children—1987. Reproduced by permission of Pediatrics. Vol 79, p 1. Copyright © 1987.)

approaches to treatment are useful in managing a patient with elevated blood pressure. Adolescents with essential hypertension are usually best managed initially with *nonpharmacologic* therapy. Intervention will focus on the factors that were cited as important in prevention. Because many patients with mild elevation of pressure are overweight, weight reduction may result in up to 5–10 mm Hg reduction in systolic pressure and 5 mm Hg reduction in diastolic pressure. A reduction in sodium intake will often lower elevated pressure by about 5 mm Hg. A consistent program of aerobic exercise also has been noted to reduce blood pressure in groups of patients with mild essential hypertension. In view of these benefits and the undesirable effects of many antihypertensive drugs, a well-supervised program of nonpharmacologic therapy should be enthusiastically prescribed for most young patients with essential hypertension. When the patient will not cooperate with the nondrug approach or the reduction of pressure is not adequate, antihypertensive agents should be prescribed. If, however, the adolescent complies poorly with changes in diet and activity, it is likely that long-term compliance with a drug regimen will be unsatisfactory.

For children with secondary hypertension and for selected patients with essential hypertension, *pharmacologic* therapy will be required. A number of antihypertensive drugs are available for hypertensive emergencies and for chronic therapy (Table 15–25). Rapid reduction of blood pressure in patients with hypertensive crisis is best achieved with an intravenously administered agent. An agent with minimal central nervous system side effects is preferred if hypertensive encephalopathy is present. Parenteral hydralazine has had

Table 15–25. Antihypertensive Drugs*

Drug	Mechanism of Action	Dosage Range	Route	Duration	Side Effects
Vasodilators					
Hydralazine	Relax arteriolar smooth muscle	0.4–0.8 mg/kg/dose 0.5–2 mg/kg and increase to max 200 mg/24 hr	IV PO	2–4 hr 6–8 hr	Tachycardia, nausea Drug-induced lupus
Diazoxide	Relax smooth muscle	2–5 mg/kg/dose, max 100 mg	IV	6–24 hr	Tachycardia, hypotension, hyperglycemia
Nitroprusside	Dilatation of arterioles and venules	0.5–8.0 μg/kg/min	IV	With infusion	Thiocyanate production, rarely hypothyroidism
Minoxidil	Arteriolar dilatation	0.2–1.0 mg/kg/24 hr, max 50 mg/24 hr	PO	12–24 hr	Hypertrichosis, fluid retention
Adrenergic blockade					
Phentolamine	α-Receptor blockade	0.1 mg/kg/dose, max 5 mg	IV	1 hr	Reflex tachycardia
Phenoxybenzamine	α-Receptor blockade	2–5 mg/24 hr	PO	6–12 hr	Tachycardia may progress to arrhythmia
Prazosin	α-Receptor blockade	1-mg initial dose, may increase to 15 mg/24 hr	PO	8–12 hr	First-dose orthostatic hypotension
Propranolol	β-Receptor blockade Reduces renin release	0.025–0.1 mg/kg/dose 0.25–1.0 mg/kg/dose	IV PO	6–8 hr	Bronchospasm, bradycardia, vivid dreams
Labetalol	α-β Blockade	titrate 0.2–2 mg/kg/hr (based on adult dose) 100–400 mg (adult)	IV PO	With infusion 12 hr	Orthostasis, dizziness, bronchospasm
Sympatholytic agents					
α-Methyldopa	Decrease sympathetic tone	10 mg/kg/24 hr and increase	PO	6–8 hr	Sedation, hepatic dysfunction, positive Coombs reaction
Clonidine	2-α Agonist in CNS	3–5 μg/kg/dose	PO	6–8 hr	Sedation, constipation, rebound withdrawal, hypertension
Renin-angiotension					
Captopril	Converting-enzyme inhibition of angiotensin II synthesis	0.1–0.3 mg/kg/dose and increase to max 2 mg/kg/dose	PO	8 hr	Proteinuria, neutropenia, rash, dysgeusia
Enalaprilat	Same as captopril	0.005–0.010 mg/kg/dose	IV	8–12 hr	Transient hypotension
Calcium channel					
Nifedipine	Calcium channel blocker	0.2–0.5 mg/kg, max 10–20 mg	PO Sub†	Repeat q 30–60 min	Facial flushing, tachycardia
Verapamil	Calcium channel blocker	120–240 mg (adults)	PO	12–24 hr	Limited pediatric experience
Diuretic agents					
Hydrochlorothiazide	Diuresis	1–2 mg/kg/24 hr	PO	12–24 hr	Hypokalemia, hyperuricemia, hypercalcemia
Furosemide	Diuresis	1 mg/kg/dose 2 mg/kg/dose	IV PO	4–6 hr 4–6 hr	Hypokalemia, alkalosis

*Adapted from Med Lett Drugs Ther 1:25, 1989; 31:31, 1989.
†Sublingual.

widespread use in children with acute onset of moderate hypertension. Marked elevation in pressure and impending encephalopathy may be treated with intravenous diazoxide or sodium nitroprusside infusion. Alternatively, the sympathetic blocker labetalol or the calcium channel blocker nifedipine may be used for rapid onset of action. Labetalol blocks both the α_1 receptor and β receptors; after intravenous bolus administration or with continuous infusion, pressure may be rapidly controlled. Because nifedipine is available only as a liquid within a capsule, administration to children has presented some difficulty. Onset of action is somewhat more rapid if the preparation is absorbed from the sublingual space rather than from the gastrointestinal tract. Most patients with hypertensive crisis have chronic or acute renal disease; management of blood pressure also requires careful attention to fluid balance and requires diuresis. Intravenous furosemide is usually effective even though glomerular filtration may be impaired.

In selecting a drug regimen for long-term use, an understanding of the underlying pathophysiology is helpful. Drugs with different sites and mechanisms of action are available to specifically alter that pathology. For example, excessive activity of the renin-angiotensin-aldosterone system may be affected by a β-blocking drug (e.g., propranolol) for suppression of renin secretion, an ACE inhibitor (e.g., captopril), or, rarely, an aldosterone antagonist (e.g., spironolactone). ACE inhibitors are useful, not only in patients with high renin hypertension that is secondary to renovascular or renal parenchymal disease but also in patients with high renin essential hypertension. Excess angiotensin production is the likely cause of most hypertension in the neonate that follows partial occlusion of a renal vessel by thrombus. Captopril is an effective agent in most of these patients, but it must be used with careful attention to renal function. α-Blocking agents (phentolamine, phenoxybenzamine) are beneficial in patients with neural crest tumors and high circulating levels of catecholamines. In such patients, β-blocking drugs are also needed to control cardiac rate, or an agent with dual blocking action (labetalol) may be used. Sympathetic blockade with labetalol is also efficacious in patients who experience marked stimulation of the cardiovascular system from high doses of cocaine. Patients in whom the underlying pathophysiology is not understood may be successfully managed with other agents that affect the sympathetic nervous system through various mechanisms (α-methyldopa, clonidine).

Young patients with essential hypertension who require drug therapy may be treated initially with a diuretic or a β-blocking agent. Patients with volume-dependent hypertension usually respond adequately to diuretics; those with high-renin, high cardiac output physiology respond best to β-blockers. If the pressure is not lowered adequately, a calcium channel blocker may be added to the diuretic and an ACE inhibitor may replace the β-blocker. Chronic use of diuretics may result in elevation of serum lipids, but long-term investigations of that effect in children are not available. β-Blocking agents have also been associated with changes in serum lipids, and some studies suggest a reduction in exercise tolerance in patients treated with propranolol.

In patients with longstanding or poorly controlled hypertension, the underlying pathophysiology is often complex. Such patients frequently require trials of combinations of antihypertensive agents in order to gain control of markedly elevated or labile pressure. The basic principle of combination antihypertensive therapy is the coadministration of drugs with different sites or mechanisms of action. Because compliance may become a problem, the drug regimen should be as simple as possible and should take advantage of longer-acting agents when available. Drug calendars, parental supervision, and close patient-physician communication also will help to ensure that the medications are taken as prescribed.

Percutaneous transluminal dilatation of lesions that produce renal artery stenosis may cure as many as 50% of patients with fibromuscular dysplasia. Angioplasty is not successful for renal artery stenosis because of atherosclerotic plaques. If angioplasty is unsuccessful for fibromuscular dysplasia, the kidney may be removed and the renal artery repaired and then reimplanted to maintain renal function.

ALBERT W. PRUITT

Anderson EA, Mahoney LT, Laurer RM, et al: Enhanced forearm blood flow during mental stress in children of hypertensive parents. Hypertension 10:544, 1987.

Anonymous: Drugs for hypertension. Med Lett Drugs Ther 31:25, 1989.

Anonymous: Drugs for hypertensive emergencies. Med Lett Drugs Ther 31:31, 1989.

Anonymous: Screening for hypertension in childhood. Lancet 1:918, 1988.

Calhoun DA, Oparil S: Treatment of hypertensive crisis. N Engl J Med 323:1177, 1990.

Cangiano JL: Rational treatment of essential hypertension. Semin Nephrol 8:185, 1988.

Capalan MS, Cohn RA, Langman CB, et al: Favorable outcome of neonatal aortic thrombosis and renovascular hypertension. J Pediatr 115:291, 1989.

Devereux RB: Does increased blood pressure cause left ventricular hypertrophy or vice versa? Ann Intern Med 112:157, 1990.

Farine M, Arbus GS: Management of hypertensive emergencies in children. Pediatr Emerg Care 5:51, 1989.

Feld LG, Springate JE: Hypertension in children. Curr Probl Pediatr 18:317, 1988.

Ganguly A: Glucocorticoid-suppressible hyperaldosteronism: An update. Am J Med 88:321, 1990.

Mirkin BL, Newman TJ: Efficacy and safety of captopril in the treatment of severe childhood hypertension: Report of the International Collaborative Study Group. Pediatrics 75:1091, 1985.

Ogborn MR, Crocker JFS: Investigation of pediatric hypertension: Use of a tailored protocol. Am J Dis Child 141:1205, 1987.

Ramsay LE, Waller PC: Blood pressure response to percutaneous transluminal angioplasty for renovascular hypertension: An overview of published series. Br Med J 300:569, 1990.

Sinaiko AR, Gomez-Marin O, Prineas RJ: "Significant" diastolic hypertension in pre-high school black and white children. Am J Hyperten 1:178, 1988.

Tack ED, Perlman JM: Renal failure in sick hypertensive premature infants receiving captopril therapy. J Pediatr 112:805, 1988.

Task Force on Blood Pressure Control in Children: Report of the second task force on blood pressure control in children—1987. Pediatrics 79:1, 1987.

Welsh P, Repetto R: Renovascular hypertension in pediatric patients. J Cardiovasc Surg 28:505, 1987.

Wilson PD, Ferencz C, Dischinger PC, et al: Twenty-four-hour ambulatory blood pressure in normotensive adolescent children of hypertensive and normotensive parents. Am J Epidemiol 127:946, 1988.

16

DISEASES OF THE BLOOD

DEVELOPMENT OF THE HEMATOPOIETIC SYSTEM

Blood formation in the human embryo can be recognized as early as the 3rd wk after conception. Large, primitive hematopoietic elements are then widely scattered throughout mesodermal tissues, intimately associated with developing vascular channels. By 2 mo active hematopoiesis is established in the liver, which is the main site of blood formation during the middle portion of fetal life. After about 6 mo hematopoiesis shifts gradually to the medullary spaces, and by birth most blood formation normally takes place in bone marrow.

Active hematopoietic tissue (red marrow) fills the medullary spaces of the bones of infants. During childhood fatty tissue (yellow marrow) gradually replaces hematopoietic tissue in the long bones, active blood formation in the older child and adult being concentrated in the ribs, sternum, vertebrae, pelvis, skull, clavicles, and scapulas. The yellow marrow of the extremities can resume active hematopoiesis in response to certain severe hematologic stresses.

Study of the bone marrow provides valuable information for evaluating many hematologic diseases. *Marrow aspiration* is safe and technically simple. Although the marrow aspirate represents only a minute sample of the entire hematopoietic tissue, there is usually a striking uniformity of aspirates taken simultaneously from multiple sites. In the infant the preferred sites for aspiration are the proximal tibia and posterior iliac crest. In older children the posterior iliac crest provides a large marrow-bearing space that is not near major blood vessels or vital organs. *Marrow biopsy* using special instruments (e.g., the Jamshidi needle) permits more accurate assessment of marrow cellularity than is possible through simple aspiration. Biopsy is also useful for detecting focal involvement of marrow in metastatic or granulomatous processes. Table 16–1 lists the types and proportions of cells that occur in marrow of normal infants and children.

16.1 RED BLOOD CELLS

Synthesis of red blood cells requires a constant supply of amino acids, iron, certain vitamins, and other trace nutrients. Production of red cells is regulated by a specific hormone—erythropoietin. The prohormone of erythropoietin is produced in the epithelial cells of the glomerular tuft; a serum factor activates it to biologically active erythropoietin. The process is stimulated by decreases in tissue oxygenation. The principal action of erythropoietin is to induce differentiation of stem cells into an erythrocytic sequence. The early erythroid-committed progenitor cells then undergo successive cellular division. Studies of bone marrow in tissue culture have added to the understanding of red blood cell development. After culture of small mononuclear, lymphocyte-like marrow cells in semi-solid media for 5–6 days, small numbers of erythropoietin-sensitive precursors form recognizable clusters of red cells called colony-forming units, erythroid (CFUe). At 12–14 days larger burst-forming erythroid units (BFUe) appear, which are believed to be the most primitive committed erythroid precursors (no longer erythropoietin-sensitive). Cellular differentiation as the red blood cell attains maturity includes condensation and extrusion of the nucleus and production of hemoglobin. Ninety per cent of the dry weight of the mature red cell is hemoglobin.

16.2 HEMOGLOBIN

The combustion that is essential to life requires that tissues receive a constant supply of oxygen. The evolutionary development of oxygen-carrying proteins, the hemoglobins, has increased the ability of blood to give fluid transport to this gas. Furthermore, the combination of oxygen with and its dissociation from hemoglobin are accomplished without expenditure of metabolic energy.

Hemoglobin is a complex protein consisting of iron-containing heme groups and the protein moiety, globin. A dynamic interaction between heme and globin gives hemoglobin its unique properties in the reversible transport of oxygen. The hemoglobin molecule is a tetramer made up of two pairs of polypeptide chains, each chain having a heme group attached.

TABLE 16–1. Differential Counts of Bone Marrow During Infancy and Childhood

Age	Blasts (%)	Promyelocytes (%)	Myelocytes and Metamyelocytes (%)	Bands and Polymorphonuclears (%)	Eosinophils (%)	Lymphocytes (%)	Nucleated Red Blood Cells (%)	Myeloid: Erythroid (M:E) Ratio
Birth	1	2	5	40	1	10	40	1.2:1
7 days	1	2	10	40	1	20	25	2.1:1
6 mo–2 yr	0.5	0.5	8	30	1	40	20	2.0:1
6 yr	1	2	15	35	1	25	20	2.7:1
12 yr	1	2	20	40	1	15	20	3.2:1
Adult	1	2	21	44	2	10	20	3.5:1

The polypeptide chains of various hemoglobins are of chemically different types. For example, the major hemoglobin (Hb) of the normal adult (Hb A) is made up of alpha (α) and beta (β) polypeptide chains, one pair of each. Hb A can therefore be represented as $\alpha_2\beta_2$. α and β chains differ in both the number and sequence of amino acids, and their synthesis is directed by separate genes.

Within the red blood cells of the embryo, fetus, child, and adult, six different hemoglobins may normally be detected: the embryonic hemoglobins, Gower-1, Gower-2, and Portland; the fetal hemoglobin, Hb F; and the adult hemoglobins, Hb A and A_2. The electrophoretic mobilities of hemoglobins vary with their chemical structures. The time of appearance and quantitative relationships among the hemoglobins are determined by complex developmental processes (Fig. 16–1). Two sets of genes for α polypeptide chains are located on human chromosome 16. β, γ, and δ genes are closely linked on chromosome 11. Two pairs of alleles, located on chromosome 16, provide the genetic information for the structure of the α chain.

EMBRYONIC HEMOGLOBINS. The blood of early human embryos contains two slowly migrating hemoglobins, Gower-1 and Gower-2, and Hb Portland, which has Hb F–like mobility. The zeta (ζ) chains of Hb Portland and Gower-1 are structurally quite similar to α chains. Both Gower hemoglobins contain a unique type of polypeptide chain, the epsilon (ϵ) chain. Hb Gower-1 has the structure $\zeta_2\epsilon_2$ and Gower-2, $\alpha_2\epsilon_2$. Hb Portland has the structure $\zeta_2\gamma_2$. In embryos of 4–8 wk gestation the Gower hemoglobins predominate, but by the 3rd mo they have disappeared.

FETAL HEMOGLOBIN. Hb F contains γ polypeptide chains in place of the β chains of Hb A and can be represented as $\alpha_2\gamma_2$. Its resistance to denaturation by strong alkali is usually used in its quantitation. After the 8th gestational wk Hb F is the predominant hemoglobin; in the 6-mo-old fetus it constitutes 90% of the total hemoglobin. Then a gradual decline occurs, so that at birth Hb F averages 70% of the total. Synthesis of Hb F decreases rapidly postnatally, and by 6–12 mo of age only a trace is present. Less than 2.0% can be detected by alkali denaturation in older children and adults. Hb F is heterogeneous because of two types of γ chains, whose synthesis is directed by two sets of genes. The chains differ at position 136 in the presence of either a glycine (Gγ) or an alanine (Aγ) residue. In the newborn the relative proportion or ratio of Gγ to Aγ chain is 3:1.

ADULT HEMOGLOBINS. Some Hb A ($\alpha_2\beta_2$) can be detected in even the smallest embryos. Accordingly, it is possible as early as 16–20 wk gestation to make a prenatal diagnosis of major β-chain hemoglobinopathies, such as thalassemia major. Prenatal diagnosis is based on techniques that examine the rates of synthesis of β chains or the structure of newly synthesized β chains. Earlier diagnosis is possible using molecular biology techniques and sampling of chorionic villus tissue or amniotic fluid if DNA structural defects are a cause of the hemoglobinopathies. Similarly, gene deletion disorders such as the α-thalassemias are detectable by the same method.

By the 6th mo of gestation there is about 5–10% of Hb A present. A steady increase follows so that at term Hb A averages 30%. By 6–12 mo of age the normal adult hemoglobin pattern appears. The minor adult hemoglobin component Hb A_2 contains delta (δ) chains and has the structure $\alpha_2\delta_2$. It is seen only when significant amounts of Hb A are also present. At birth less than 1.0% of Hb A_2 is seen, but by 12 mo of age the normal level of 2.0–3.4% is attained. Throughout life the normal ratio of Hb A to A_2 is about 30:1.

NORMAL RELATIONSHIPS AMONG THE HEMOGLOBINS. During fetal life and early childhood the rates of synthesis of γ and β chains and the amounts of Hb A and Hb F are inversely related. This relationship has been attributed to a "switch mechanism" similar to genetic regulatory mechanisms in bacteria, but the genetic, biologic, and developmental processes that direct a switchover from predominantly γ-chain synthesis in utero to predominantly β-chain synthesis after birth are unclear. It is not certain whether the mechanisms involve selective genetic inhibition or facilitation. It has been shown that differential selection and amplified production of red blood cell precursors derived from BFUe result in considerable Hb F production. This may be the basis for the increased levels of Hb F that occur in many anemias when there is severe erythropoietic stress. Alternative explanations involve more basic genetic regulators in the DNA sequences that flank the hemoglobin gene complexes.

ALTERATIONS OF THE HEMOGLOBINS BY DISEASE. Because hemoglobins containing epsilon chains are normally present only very early in intrauterine life, they are largely of theoretic interest. Small amounts of the Gower hemoglobins have been detectable in a few newborn infants with 13/15-trisomy. Increased levels of Hb Portland have been found in cord blood of stillborn infants with homozygous α-thalassemia.

Levels of fetal hemoglobin may be influenced by various factors. Because the fetal hemoglobin level is elevated during the 1st year of life, a knowledge of its normal decline is important (Fig. 16–2). In persons heterozygous for β-thalassemia (β-thalassemia trait) the postpartum decrease of Hb F is retarded; about 50% of such persons have elevated levels of Hb F (more than 2.0%) in later life. In homozygous thalassemia (Cooley anemia) and in hereditary persistence of fetal hemoglobin, large amounts of Hb F are characteristically found. In patients with major β-chain hemoglobinopathies (e.g., Hb SS, SC), Hb F is usually increased, particularly during childhood. Finally, moderate elevations of Hb F may

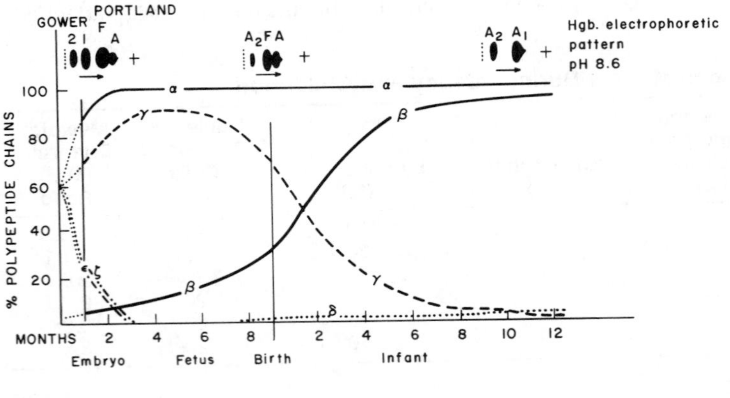

Figure 16–1. Proportions of the various human hemoglobin polypeptide chains through early life. The hemoglobin electrophoretic pattern typical for each period is also shown. (Modified from Pearson HA: Recent advances in hematology. J Pediatr 69:466, 1966.)

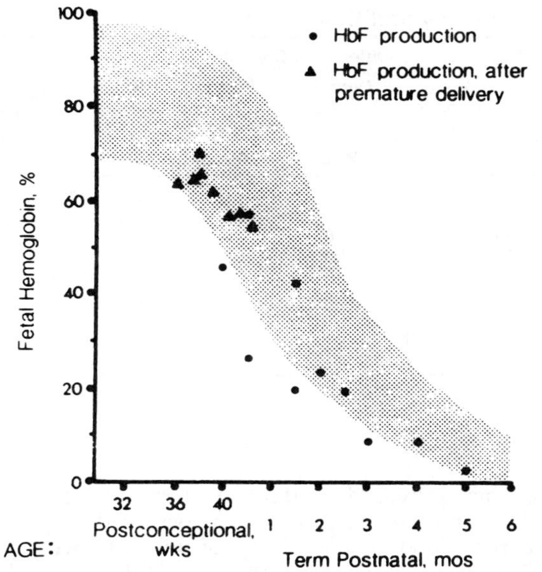

Figure 16–2. Postnatal changes in percentage of fetal hemoglobin (Hb F) *(shaded area)*. The triangles represent postnatal production by reticulocytes in premature infants, and the dots represent cord and postnatal reticulocyte production in term infants. The percentage Hb F present reflects Hb F production over the previous weeks, whereas the rate of Hb F production is a result of the current proportion of Hb F produced by reticulocytes present, and is thus lower as the Hb F to adult hemoglobin (Hb A) switch progresses. (From Brown MS: Fetal and neonatal erythropoiesis. *In*: Stockman JA, Pochedly C [eds]: Developmental and Neonatal Hematology. New York, Raven Press, 1988, p 258.)

be seen in many diseases accompanied by hematologic stress, such as hemolytic anemias, leukemia, and aplastic anemia, because of a minor population of red blood cells that contains increased amounts of Hb F, as can be demonstrated by the acid-elution staining technique of Kleihauer and Betke. Tetramers of γ chains (γ_4 or Hb Barts) or β chains (β_4, Hb H) may be seen in α-thalassemia syndromes.

The normal adult level of Hb A_2 (2.4–3.4%) is seldom altered. Levels of Hb A_2 exceeding 3.4% are found in most persons with the β-thalassemia trait and in those with megaloblastic anemias secondary to vitamin B_{12} and folic acid deficiency. Decreased Hb A_2 levels are found in those with iron deficiency anemia and α-thalassemia.

16.3 METABOLISM OF THE RED BLOOD CELL

The nucleated red blood cells in bone marrow participate in various metabolic functions, including active protein synthesis. After extrusion of the nucleus much of this metabolic ability is lost, including the ability to synthesize proteins. Loss of the nucleus makes the red blood cell a better vessel for oxygen transport, but it imposes on the red blood cell a finite life span, because the cell cannot replace or repair its vital enzymatic proteins. The mature red cell contains more than 40 enzymes. Many of these are essential for cellular viability, but genetically determined deficiencies of others, such as catalase, do not interfere with normal survival.

The mature red blood cell is not metabolically inert. It has no mitochondria, however, and ATP generation cannot occur by oxidative phosphorylation in Krebs cycle reactions. Rather, glucose is taken up and lactic acid produced mostly by anaerobic glycolysis (Embden-Meyerhof pathway); about 10% of glucose is metabolized oxidatively through the pentose phosphate pathway. At least five functions for ATP generated by glucose metabolism are essential to normal cell viability:

1. Maintenance of electrolyte gradients. The principal intracellular cation of the red blood cell is potassium, whereas that in plasma is sodium. Reversal of the constant tendency for sodium to enter the red blood cell and concomitantly for potassium to leak out, with preservation of normal ionic gradients, is accomplished by an energy (ATP)-dependent membrane mechanism, the cation pump. When the cation pump fails, sodium and water enter the red blood cell, causing it to swell and ultimately to hemolyze. Energy is also used to maintain low intracellular levels of calcium ion.
2. Initiation of energy production. ATP is required for the initial reaction of glycolysis involving phosphorylation of glucose to glucose-6-phosphate.
3. Maintenance of red blood cell membrane and shape. Energy is required to maintain the complex phospholipid structure of the red blood cell membrane. Maintenance of the biconcave shape is probably also energy-dependent.
4. Maintenance of heme iron in the reduced (ferrous) form. Oxidative potentials within the red blood cell may cause oxidation of the iron of hemoglobin. Hemoglobin containing ferric iron (methemoglobin) is ineffective in oxygen transport. Moreover, if perioxides and other oxidant substances are not inactivated, hemoglobin may be denatured and precipitated. Cells containing such denatured hemoglobin (Heinz bodies) are rapidly removed from the circulation. Protection of the red cell from the effects of oxidation ultimately depends on NADPH and NADH. These compounds are continually regenerated by activities of the glycolytic pathway and pentose shunt. In many genetically determined deficiencies of glycolytic and pentose pathway enzymes, hemolytic states occur because the energy necessary to perform these vital functions cannot be generated.
5. Maintenance of the levels of organic phosphates such as 2,3-diphosphoglycerate (2,3-DPG) and ATP within the red blood cells. These compounds interact with hemoglobin and have profound effects on oxygen affinity.

THE ANEMIAS

Anemia is defined as a reduction of the red blood cell volume or hemoglobin concentration below the range of values occurring in healthy persons. Table 16–2 lists the means and ranges for hemoglobin and hematocrit values by age groups of well-nourished children. Extensive studies of American children suggest that there may be racial differences in hemoglobin levels. Black children have levels that average about 0.5 g/dL lower than those of white and Oriental children of comparable age and socioeconomic status, possibly in part because of the relatively high incidence of α-thalassemia and nutritional anemias in blacks. Alternatively, higher levels of red blood cell 2,3-diphosphoglycerate (2,3-DPG) have been found in black children that, if not an adaptive mechanism to anemia, would permit better oxygen delivery and a lower hemoglobin.

Although a reduction in the amount of circulating hemo-

TABLE 16–2. Hematologic Values During Infancy and Childhood

Age	Hemoglobin (g/DL)		Hematocrit (%)		Reticulocytes (%)	Leukocytes (WBC/mm³)		Differential Counts: Neutrophils (%)		Lymphocytes (%)	Eosinophils (%)	Monocytes (%)	Nucleated Red Blood Cells/ 100 WBC†
	Mean	Range	Mean	Range	Mean	Mean	Range	Mean	Range	Mean*	Mean	Mean	
Cord blood	16.8	13.7–20.1	55	45–65	5.0	18,000	(9,000–30,000)	61	(40–80)	31	2	6	7.0 (3–10)
2 wk	16.5	13.0–20.0	50	42–66	1.0	12,000	(5,000–21,000)	40		48	3	9	0
3 mo	12.0	9.5–14.5	36	31–41	1.0	12,000	(6,000–18,000)	30		63	2	5	0
6 mo–6 yr	12.0	10.5–14.0	37	33–42	1.0	10,000	(6,000–15,000)	45		48	2	5	0
7–12 yr	13.0	11.0–16.0	38	34–40	1.0	8,000	(4,500–13,500)	55		38	2	5	0
Adult													
Female	14	12.0–16.0	42	37–47	1.6	7,500	(5,000–10,000)	55	(35–70)	35	3	7	0
Male	16	14.0–18.0	47	42–52									

*Relatively wide range.
†WBC = white blood cells.

globin decreases the oxygen-carrying capacity of the blood, few physiologic disturbances occur until the hemoglobin level falls below 7–8 g/dL. Below this level pallor becomes evident in the skin and mucous membranes. Physiologic adjustments to anemia include tachycardia, increased cardiac output, a shift in the dissociation curve, which makes oxygen more readily available to the tissues, and a deviation of blood flow toward vital organs and tissues. In response to anemia or hypoxia the concentration of 2,3-DPG increases within the red blood cell. The resultant "shift to the right" of the oxygen dissociation curve, by reducing the affinity of hemoglobin for oxygen, results in more complete transfer of oxygen to the tissues. The same shift may also occur at high altitude in response to a decrease in the oxygen content of inspired air. When moderately severe anemia develops slowly, surprisingly few symptoms or objective findings may be evident, but weakness, tachypnea, shortness of breath on exertion, tachycardia, cardiac dilatation, and congestive heart failure ultimately result from increasingly severe anemia, regardless of its cause.

Anemia is not a specific entity but an indication of an underlying pathologic process or disease. A useful physiologic (erythrokinetic) classification of the anemias of childhood divides them into two large groups: (1) those resulting primarily from decreased production of red blood cells or hemoglobin; and (2) those in which increased destruction or loss of red blood cells is the predominant mechanism. In Table 16–3 the important anemias of childhood are classified by these criteria. In addition, a morphologic classification is often used, the red blood cells being characterized by their mean corpuscular volume (MCV) as microcytic (MCV $<$ 75 fL), macrocytic (MCV $>$ 100 fL), or normocytic (75–100 fL). The MCV changes with age and, before an anemia can be specifically characterized with respect to red blood cell size, developmental changes should be understood. Anemias in childhood may also be classified by variations in cell size and shape, as reflected by alterations in the red blood cell distribution width (RDW). The RDW, as determined by the use of electronic cell counting technology, is the coefficient of variation of red blood cell size (standard deviation of the MCV divided by the mean MCV times 100). A knowledge of both the MCV and the RDW can be helpful in the initial classification of the anemias of childhood (Table 16–4). In every case of significant anemia it is essential to describe the morphologic characteristics of the red blood cells, to determine the relative importance of defective red blood cell production and of cell destruction in the genesis of the anemia and, when possible, to identify the basic etiologic process.

ANEMIAS RESULTING FROM INADEQUATE PRODUCTION OF RED BLOOD CELLS

These anemias result when the bone marrow cannot produce sufficient numbers of new red blood cells to replace those removed from the circulation. A slight reduction in the red blood cell life span may occur, but generally this is insufficient to cause anemia if hematopoiesis is adequate. Low reticulocyte counts are observed in most anemias of this group.

16.4 CONGENITAL PURE RED BLOOD CELL ANEMIA

(Congenital Hypoplastic Anemia; Diamond-Blackfan Syndrome)

This rare condition usually becomes symptomatic in early infancy. The most characteristic diagnostic feature is a deficiency of red blood cell precursors in an otherwise normally cellular bone marrow.

ETIOLOGY. A genetic basis is suggested by instances of familial occurrence. Males and females are affected in equal numbers. An ill-defined abnormality of tryptophan metabolism has been reported in some patients. Adenosine deaminase (ADA) activity has been reported to be increased in the red blood cells of patients with this disorder but not in those with other types of hypoplastic anemia. A consistent finding is low numbers of CFUe and BFUe in the bone marrow. High levels of erythropoietin are present in serum and urine.

CLINICAL MANIFESTATIONS. About half of affected infants appear pale even in the 1st few days of life, but hematopoiesis must be generally adequate in fetal life. Profound anemia usually becomes evident by 2–6 mo of age, occasionally somewhat later. Unless blood transfusions are given, the anemia progresses to heart failure and death. The liver and spleen are not enlarged initially. Some cases of pure red blood cell anemia have been associated with congenital anomalies, including triphalangeal thumbs; others have had the Turner syndrome phenotype with normal karyotypes.

TABLE 16–3. Classification of the Anemias*

Anemias resulting primarily from inadequate production of red blood cells or hemoglobin
Decreased numbers of red blood cell precursors in the marrow
"Pure red blood cell" anemias
Congenital pure red blood cell anemia
Acquired pure red blood cell anemias (e.g., TEC†)
Inadequate production despite normal numbers of red blood cell precursors
Anemia of infection, inflammation, and cancer
Anemia of chronic renal disease
Congenital dyserythropoietic anemias
Deficiency of specific factors
Megaloblastic anemias
Folic acid deficiency or malabsorption
Vitamin B_{12} deficiency, malabsorption, or transport
Orotic aciduria
Microcytic anemias
Iron deficiency
Pyridoxine-responsive and X-linked hypochromic anemias
Lead poisoning
Copper deficiency
Thalassemia trait
Hemolytic anemias
Intrinsic abnormalities of the red blood cell
"Structural" defects
Hereditary spherocytosis
Hemolytic elliptocytosis
Paroxysmal nocturnal hemoglobinuria
Pyropyknocytosis
Enzymatic defects (nonspherocytic hemolytic anemias)
Enzymes of glycolytic pathway—pyruvate kinase, hexokinase, and others
Enzymes of the pentose phosphate pathway and glutathione complex
Defects in synthesis of hemoglobin
Hb S, C, D, E, etc, alone and in combination
Thalassemia
Extrinsic (extracellular) abnormalities
Immunologic disorders
Passively acquired antibodies (hemolytic disease of the newborn)
Rh isoimmunization
A or B isoimmunization
Other blood group families
Active antibody formation
Idiopathic autoimmune hemolytic anemia; cold agglutinin diseases
Symptomatic—lupus, lymphoma
Drug-induced
Nonimmunologic disorders
Toxic from drugs, chemicals
Infections—malarial, clostridial

*See also anemia in pancytopenias and leukemia.
†TEC = transient erythropenia of childhood.

LABORATORY FINDINGS. The red blood cells are normochromic and macrocytic. Assay of red blood cell enzymes reveals a pattern characteristic of a "young" erythrocyte population. The level of Hb F is increased for age; in more chronic cases the fetal membrane antigen i is found on the red blood cells. These findings may help distinguish congenital red blood cell aplasia from acquired transient erythroblastopenia of childhood (Sec. 16.6). Thrombocytosis and occasionally neutropenia may also be present initially. The most important feature is the lack of erythropoietic activity in blood and bone marrow despite high levels of erythropoietin. Reticulocytes are diminished, even when the anemia is severe. Red blood cell precursors are markedly reduced in the marrow, and myeloid-erythroid ratios are 10–200:1. In some cases a few pronormoblasts may be present, but not more mature forms. A normal complement of other marrow elements is usually present. Serum iron levels are elevated, with a decrease in the iron-binding ability. Red blood cell survival is normal. Bone marrow culture shows markedly reduced numbers of CFUe and BFUe. In a few cases incubation of the marrow cells with T cell antibodies prior to culture has restored normal red blood cell maturation in vitro.

DIFFERENTIAL DIAGNOSIS. Congenital hypoplastic anemia must be differentiated from other anemias in which blood shows low reticulocyte counts. The anemia of the convalescent phase of hemolytic disease of the newborn may, on occasion, be associated with markedly reduced erythropoiesis. This terminates spontaneously at 5–8 wk of age, whereas congenital hypoplastic anemia is not usually recognized before this time. Aplastic crises characterized by reticulocytopenia and by decreased numbers of red blood cell precursors may complicate various types of hemolytic disease. These transient episodes of "aplastic crisis" may be related to parvovirus-like infections (Sec. 16.5).

The syndrome of transient erythroblastopenia may be differentiated from Diamond-Blackfan syndrome by its relatively late onset and by biochemical differences in the red blood cells (Sec. 16.6).

PROGNOSIS. Unless corticosteroid therapy produces remission of hypoplastic anemia, survival depends on blood transfusions. By late childhood affected children may have had 100 or more transfusions, and hemosiderosis is an inevitable consequence. The liver and spleen enlarge, and secondary hypersplenism with leukopenia and thrombocytopenia may occur. Growth retardation is usual, and puberty may not occur. Diabetes mellitus resulting from hemosiderosis is common.

Unless modified by the use of iron chelation therapy, death usually occurs in the 2nd decade. Chronic congestive heart failure resulting from ischemic and siderotic myocardial disease is a common terminal event.

TREATMENT. When anemia becomes severe, blood transfusions must be given. Corticosteroid therapy is frequently beneficial if begun early; the mechanism of its effect is unknown. Relatively large doses, 2–4 mg/kg/24 hr, of prednisone or its equivalent are administered initially. Red blood cell precursors appear in bone marrow 1–3 wk after therapy is begun, and then a brisk peripheral reticulocytosis occurs. The hemoglobin may reach normal levels in 4–6 wk. The dose of corticosteroid may then be reduced gradually until the lowest effective dose is found. This is often a very small amount, such as 2.5 mg/24 hr of prednisone or less, which may produce no adverse side effects or growth suppression. Intermittent administration every other day or for 3 or 4 consecutive days each week may also be effective. Therapy should be discontinued periodically to determine whether the child is still dependent on steroids, because many responsive patients ultimately outgrow the dependence on steroid therapy.

About 10–15% of patients do not respond to corticosteroid therapy, and transfusions at intervals of 4–8 wk are necessary to sustain life. Other therapies, including hematinics, cobalt, and testosterone, have had no beneficial effect. Reports of late responses to immunosuppressive therapy (cyclosporine) need further evaluation before this can be recommended, but this might be considered in refractory cases with abnormal T cell function. Splenectomy is usually of no value but may decrease the need for transfusion if hypersplenism or isoimmunization has developed. Because spontaneous remission occasionally occurs, children refractory to corticosteroid therapy should be maintained as long as possible by transfusions, preferably of freshly drawn, packed red blood cells. The use of chelating agents to induce excretion of excess iron is discussed later for thalassemia major (Sec. 16.27). The role of bone marrow transplantation is currently undefined.

TABLE 16–4. Proposed Classification of Anemic Disorders Based on Red Blood Cell Mean (MCV) and Heterogeneity (RDW)*†‡

Microcytic Homogeneous (MCV low, RDW normal)†	Microcytic Heterogeneous (MCV low, RDW high)	Normocytic Homogeneous (MCV normal, RDW normal)	Normocytic Heterogeneous (MCV normal, RDW high)	Macrocytic Homogeneous (MCV high, RDW normal)	Macrocytic Heterogeneous (MCV high, RDW high)
Heterozygous thalassemia	Iron deficiency	Normal	Mixed deficiency	Aplastic anemia	Folate deficiency
Chronic disease	Hb S–β-thalassemia; hemoglobin H; red cell fragmentation	Chronic disease, chronic liver disease; nonanemic hemoglobinopathy (e.g., AS, AC); transfusion; chemotherapy; chronic lymphocytic leukemia; chronic myelocytic leukemia; hemorrhage; hereditary spherocytosis	Early iron deficiency anemia; anemic hemoglobinopathy (e.g., SS, SC); myelofibrosis; sideroblastic	Preleukemia	Vitamin B_{12} deficiency; immune hemolytic anemia; cold agglutinin; chronic lymphocytic leukemia, high count

*Modified from Bessman JD, Gilmer P, Gardener F: Improved classification of anemias by MCV and RDW. Am J Clin Pathol 80:322, 1983.
†MCV = mean corpuscular volume.
‡RDW = red blood cell distribution width.

16.5 ACQUIRED PURE RED BLOOD CELL ANEMIAS

A number of forms of acquired anemia with reticulocytopenia and reduced red blood cell precursors in the marrow have been described. The causes of most of them are uncertain. In some cases, in adults, remission has followed removal of a tumor of the thymus. Association with thymoma has been reported in a child. In other cases an erythropoietin-inhibiting antibody, antibodies to erythroblasts, or inhibitors of heme synthesis have been found in plasma. The presence of a complement-dependent antibody cytotoxic for erythroblasts in some adults has suggested their need for immunosuppressive therapy. The acquired pure red blood cell anemias may respond to therapy with corticosteroids, and a trial is indicated in any chronic case. Immunosuppressive therapy with cyclophosphamide or azathioprine may be given a trial if corticosteroids are ineffective.

Large doses of chloramphenicol inhibit erythropoiesis. Reticulocytopenia, erythroid hypoplasia, and vacuolated pronormoblasts in the marrow are reversible effects of this drug.

Episodes of acute failure of erythropoiesis may follow various viral infections. During these episodes a marked reduction in circulating reticulocytes (<0.1%) and an elevation of the serum iron level occur. Bone marrow aspiration shows markedly reduced numbers of erythrocytic precursors. These episodes are self-limited, last only 10–14 days, and are of no consequence to a child with a normal red blood cell survival. In a patient with a shortened red blood cell survival, however, profound anemia may ensue; this is the basis of the so-called *aplastic crises* of some hemolytic anemias (Sec. 16.12).

16.6 TRANSIENT ERYTHROBLASTOPENIA OF CHILDHOOD (TEC)

This increasingly recognized syndrome of severe, reversible aregenerative anemia involves previously normal children, 6 mo–5 yr of age, who slowly develop anemia with reticulocytopenia and decreased numbers of red blood cell precursors in the bone marrow. The serum iron level and iron saturation are increased. The level of Hb F is normal, and the profile of red blood cell enzymes is consistent with an "old" red blood cell population. The MCV is normal, as is ADA activity. Marrow culture studies suggest varying pathogenetic mechanisms: in some cases, a serum inhibitor of erythroid stem cells; in others, abnormalities of erythroid stem cells, either in number or in responsiveness to erythropoietin. It is likely that this is an autoimmune disease directed at the primitive red blood cell precursors rather than at the mature red blood cell. Spontaneous remission occurs; corticosteroid therapy is not necessary or indicated. Transfusions may be necessary until recovery occurs.

16.7 ANEMIAS OF CHRONIC INFECTION, INFLAMMATION, AND RENAL DISEASE

Anemia complicates a number of chronic systemic diseases associated with infection, inflammation, or tissue breakdown. Examples of such conditions include chronic pyogenic infections such as bronchiectasis and osteomyelitis; chronic inflammatory processes such as rheumatic fever, rheumatoid arthritis, and ulcerative colitis; and advanced renal disease. Despite diverse underlying causes the erythrokinetic abnormalities are similar. Red blood cell life span is moderately decreased, reflecting increased red blood cell destruction by a hyperactive reticuloendothelial system. This increased hemolysis is less important, however, than a relative failure of bone marrow response, reflecting both hypoactivity of marrow and an erythropoietin production inadequate for the degree of anemia. Furthermore, there are abnormalities of iron metabolism, including defective iron release from the tissues into the plasma. In renal failure accumulation of toxic nondialyzable substances in the blood can directly inhibit erythropoiesis.

CLINICAL MANIFESTATIONS. Few symptoms are attributable to the usually moderate degree of anemia present; the important symptoms and signs are those of the underlying disease.

LABORATORY FINDINGS. Hemoglobin concentrations usually range from 6–9 g/dL. The anemia is usually normochromic and normocytic; occasionally, modest hypochromia and microcytosis are observed. Reticulocyte counts are normal or low, and leukocytosis is common. Free erythrocyte protoporphyrin (FEP) levels are moderately elevated (>35 μg/dL whole blood). The serum iron level is low, averaging 30 μg/dL;

there is, however, no increase in total iron-binding ability as in iron deficiency (average 200 μg/mL). This pattern of serum iron and iron-binding protein is a regular and valuable diagnostic feature. Serum ferritin is often elevated. The elevation of the serum ferritin level reflects the fact that ferritin is an acute phase reactant. The bone marrow has normal cellularity; the red blood cell precursors are adequate, and granulocytic hyperplasia may be present. An increased hemosiderin level can often be seen in marrow. A frequent clinical challenge is to identify iron deficiency in the patient with an inflammatory disease. Such patients may have normal levels of serum ferritin, which are inappropriately low in the presence of an inflammatory process. A trial of iron therapy may be needed to resolve the issue. This is a common problem, particularly in disorders such as juvenile rheumatoid arthritis, for which treatment may result in gastrointestinal blood loss and consequent iron deficiency.

TREATMENT AND PROGNOSIS. Because these anemias are secondary to other disease processes, they do not respond to iron or hematinics unless there is concomitant deficiency. Transfusions raise the hemoglobin concentration only temporarily and are rarely indicated. If the underlying systemic disease can be controlled, the anemia is spontaneously corrected. Recombinant erythropoietin can increase the hemoglobin level and improve activity and sense of well-being in patients with end-stage renal failure. Associated problems include exacerbation of hypertension, thrombosis, and increased iron requirements (see Sec. 18.37).

16.8 CONGENITAL DYSERYTHROPOIETIC ANEMIAS

These rare normocytic or macrocytic anemias display multinuclearity and abnormal chromatin patterns in red blood cell precursors. Four types have been distinguished, with considerable variation within each type and overlap among them. Type I (about 15% of cases) is defined by binuclearity of erythroblasts and megaloblastic morphology. Type II (more than 60% of cases) has erythroblastic multinuclearity and a positive acidified serum (Ham) test, but only with some normal serum added. Red blood cells in type II are strongly agglutinated by anti-i antibody. Types I and II appear to be inherited as autosomal recessive traits. Type III (about 15% of cases) has pronounced multinuclearity and huge red blood cell precursors in marrow. It appears to be inherited as an autosomal dominant trait. Type IV is rare; it resembles type II morphologically but does not have associated serologic abnormalities. In all types there are variable degrees of anemia (sometimes only in adults), ineffective erythropoiesis, and abnormal uptake of iron. Findings of chronic hemolysis, such as intermittent jaundice, gallstones, and splenomegaly, are common. There is no treatment other than blood transfusion for anemia. Splenectomy has been advocated for patients with anemia severe enough to require chronic transfusions.

16.9 PHYSIOLOGIC ANEMIA OF INFANCY

The normal newborn has higher hemoglobin and hematocrit levels than older children and adults. Within the 1st wk of life a progressive decline in hemoglobin level begins, which persists for approximately 6–8 wk. This decline is generally referred to as a physiologic anemia of infancy. The term is a misnomer, because at its nadir the hemoglobin level in the full-term infant rarely falls below 9 g/dL.

Several factors are operative. First, there is abrupt cessation of erythropoiesis with onset of respiration when the arterial oxygen saturation rises toward 95%. Concomitantly, the high fetal levels of erythropoietin drop to undetectable levels. A shortened survival of the fetal red blood cell also contributes to the development of physiologic anemia. Furthermore, the sizable expansion of blood volume that accompanies rapid weight gain during the 1st 3 mo of life creates a situation that has aptly been described as "bleeding into the circulation." When the hemoglobin level has fallen to 9–11 g/dL at 2–3 mo of age, erythropoiesis resumes. This "anemia" should be viewed as a physiologic adaptation to extrauterine life.

The premature infant also develops a physiologic anemia; the same factors are operative as in term infants, but they are exaggerated. The decline in hemoglobin level is both more extreme and more rapid. Minimal hemoglobin levels of 7–9 g/dL commonly occur by 3–6 wk of age and, in very small premature infants, levels may be even lower (see Sec. 9.46).

In preterm infants, the inability to produce compensatory amounts of erythropoietin may account for the greater decline in hemoglobin concentrations. When premature infants are transfused with adult blood containing Hb A, the shift of the oxygen dissociation curve as a result of the Hb A facilitates delivery of oxygen to the tissues. Accordingly, the definition of anemia and the need for transfusion in the premature infant must be based not only on hemoglobin level but also on oxygen requirements and the affinity of the infant's circulating hemoglobin for oxygen.

The marginal erythropoietic equilibrium responsible for physiologic anemia can aggravate processes associated with increased hemolysis such as congenital hemolytic states which may be associated with severe anemia in the early weeks of life.

Dietary factors may also aggravate physiologic anemia. Deficiencies of folic acid or vitamin E superimposed on the physiologic process may result in more severe anemia.

In premature infants vitamin E has an important role in red blood cell stability. Such infants are born with a small reserve of vitamin E and frequently become deficient, with serum vitamin E levels falling to less than 0.5 mg/L during the 1st months of life. If the diet contains a high proportion of polyunsaturated fatty acids (as in many proprietary formulas), and especially if an iron supplement is given, hemolytic anemia, thrombocytosis, and edema may occur. Red blood cells include many bizarre acanthocytes (burr cells). Vitamin E prophylaxis, 5 mg/24 hr, should be considered for the small premature infant, with therapeutic doses (50 mg) indicated for established deficiency. The composition of most proprietary formulas is such that hemolysis does not occur even when iron supplementation at a concentration of 10–12 mg/L is used. Larger doses of medicinal iron are not indicated in the newborn; they may not only provoke hemolysis but could also predispose to serious infections, particularly if parenteral iron preparations are used. In patients with malabsorption of fat, vitamin E deficiency may lead to significant hemolytic anemia, as occurs in cystic fibrosis.

Infantile pyknocytosis, a self-limited hemolytic process with large numbers of acanthocytes in blood, probably represents vitamin E deficiency.

Unless there has been significant perinatal blood loss, iron deficiency should not be considered as a cause of anemia in the 1st 3 mo of life. Assuming an infant is born with adequate iron stores, dietary iron deficiency cannot be a cause of anemia until these iron stores have been exhausted. In the absence of blood loss, this cannot occur until the birthweight has approximately doubled.

TREATMENT. As a developmental process, physiologic anemia usually requires no therapy other than ensuring that the diet of the infant contains the essential nutrients for normal hematopoiesis, especially folic acid and vitamin E. A premature infant who is feeding well and growing normally rarely needs transfusion. Occasionally, very low hemoglobin levels (<7 g/dL) or complicating medical conditions requiring frequent blood samples for testing may necessitate small transfusions of packed red blood cells. If so, only enough blood should be given to raise the hemoglobin level to about 9 g/dL. Larger transfusions may delay spontaneous recovery by suppressing normal erythropoiesis. Apnea and failure to gain weight may sometimes be an indication for transfusion. Neither iron nor any other hematinic substance has any effect on physiologic anemia. Because the anemia seen in very low birthweight preterm infants may be related to a relative deficiency of erythropoietin, clinical trials using recombinant erythropoietin are underway to evaluate its potential benefit.

16.10 MEGALOBLASTIC ANEMIAS

The megaloblastic anemias all have in common certain diagnostic abnormalities of red blood cell morphology and maturation. The red blood cells at every stage of development are larger than normal and have a peculiar open, finely dispersed arrangement of nuclear chromatin and an asynchrony between the maturation of nucleus and cytoplasm. Megaloblastic tissues have an increased amount of RNA in proportion to DNA. Megaloblastic morphology may be seen in a number of conditions; almost all cases in children result from a deficiency of folic acid, of vitamin B_{12}, or of both. Both substances are cofactors required in the synthesis of nucleoproteins. Megaloblastic anemias are uncommon in the United States.

FOLIC ACID DEFICIENCIES

Megaloblastic Anemia of Infancy

This disease is caused by a deficient intake or absorption of folic acid (see also Sec. 4.7). Dietary deficiency is usually compounded by rapid growth or infection, which may increase folic acid requirements. The normal daily requirement is small, estimated at 20–50 μg/24 hr. Human and cow milks provide adequate amounts of folic acid. Goat milk is clearly deficient; folic acid supplementation must be given when it is the main food. Unless supplemented, powdered milk may also be a poor source of folic acid. Ascorbic acid deficiency probably impairs the availability of dietary folic acid conjugates.

CLINICAL MANIFESTATIONS. Mild megaloblastic anemia has been reported in very low birthweight infants and routine folic acid supplementation advised. Megaloblastic anemia has its peak incidence at 4–7 mo of age, somewhat earlier than iron deficiency anemia. Besides having the usual features of severe anemia, affected infants are irritable, fail to gain weight adequately, and have chronic diarrhea. Thrombocytopenic hemorrhages occur in advanced cases. Concomitant signs and symptoms of scurvy may be present. Folic acid deficiency may accompany kwashiorkor or marasmus.

LABORATORY FINDINGS. The anemia is progressive. The red blood cell count is disproportionately lower than the hematocrit; accordingly, the anemia is macrocytic (MCV > 100 fL). Variations in red blood cell shape and size are common (Fig. 16–3*B*). The reticulocyte count is low, but nucleated red blood cells demonstrating megaloblastic morphology are often seen in the blood. Neutropenia and thrombocytopenia may be present. The neutrophils are large, with hypersegmented nuclei; more than 5% of neutrophils have five or more nuclear segments. Normal serum folic acid levels are 5–20 ng/mL; deficiency is accompanied by levels of less than 3 ng/mL. Levels of red blood cell folate are a better indicator of chronic deficiency. The normal red blood cell folate level is 150–600 ng/mL of packed cells. Levels of iron and vitamin B_{12} in serum are normal or elevated. Formiminoglutamic acid is excreted in the urine, especially after an oral dose of histidine. Serum activity of lactic acid dehydrogenase (LDH) is markedly elevated. The bone marrow is hypercellular because of erythroid hyperplasia. Megaloblastic changes are prominent, although some normal red blood cell precursors may also be found. Large, abnormal neutrophilic forms (giant metamyelocytes) with cytoplasmic vacuolization are seen, as well as hypersegmentation of the nuclei of megakaryocytes.

TREATMENT. Initially, folic acid may be administered parenterally in a dose of 2–5 mg/24 hr. Because a hematologic response can be expected within 72 hr, transfusions are indicated only when the anemia is severe or the child is very ill. Folic acid therapy should be continued for 3–4 wk. Satisfactory responses have been obtained with doses of folic acid as low as 50 μg/24 hr. These "physiologic" doses have no effect on primary vitamin B_{12} deficiencies; a therapeutic test using such low amounts may be used, therefore, to differentiate between primary folic acid and vitamin B_{12} deficiencies. If juvenile pernicious anemia is present or if the anemia recurs after therapy, the prolonged use of folic acid should be avoided, because in pernicious anemia folic acid may produce a partial response of anemia without benefiting the neurologic abnormalities. If signs of scurvy are present, therapeutic doses of ascorbic acid should be given. Antibiotic therapy should be used for superimposed bacterial infection.

Megaloblastic Anemia of Pregnancy

Folate requirements increase markedly during pregnancy, in part to meet fetal needs. Decreases in serum and red blood cell folate levels occur in as many as 25% of pregnant women at term and may be aggravated by infection. Folate supplementation, 1 mg/24 hr, is often advocated, particularly during the last trimester.

Folic Acid Deficiency of Malabsorption Syndromes

Folic acid is absorbed throughout the small intestine, and diffuse inflammatory or degenerative disease of the intestine may reduce intestinal polyglutamate deconjugase activity as well as markedly impair absorption. Celiac disease, chronic infectious enteritis, and enteroenteric fistulas may lead to folic acid deficiency and megaloblastic anemia. Measurement of serum folate is widely used to assess small intestinal absorptive functions in malabsorptive disorders. Oral folic acid supplements of 1 mg/24 hr may be indicated in these states (see also Chapter 13).

Congenital Defect of Folic Acid Absorption

A specific congenital defect in the intestinal absorption of folic acid and an associated inability to transfer folate from the plasma to the central nervous system have been associated with megaloblastic anemia, convulsions, mental retardation, and cerebral calcifications. Treatment with oral folic acid, 15–50 mg/24 hr, was necessary to maintain normal hematologic values.

Folic Acid Deficiency Complicating Hemolytic Anemias

Chronic hemolytic processes may increase the requirement for folic acid, probably more often in adults than in children. Frank megaloblastic erythropoiesis may lead to more severe

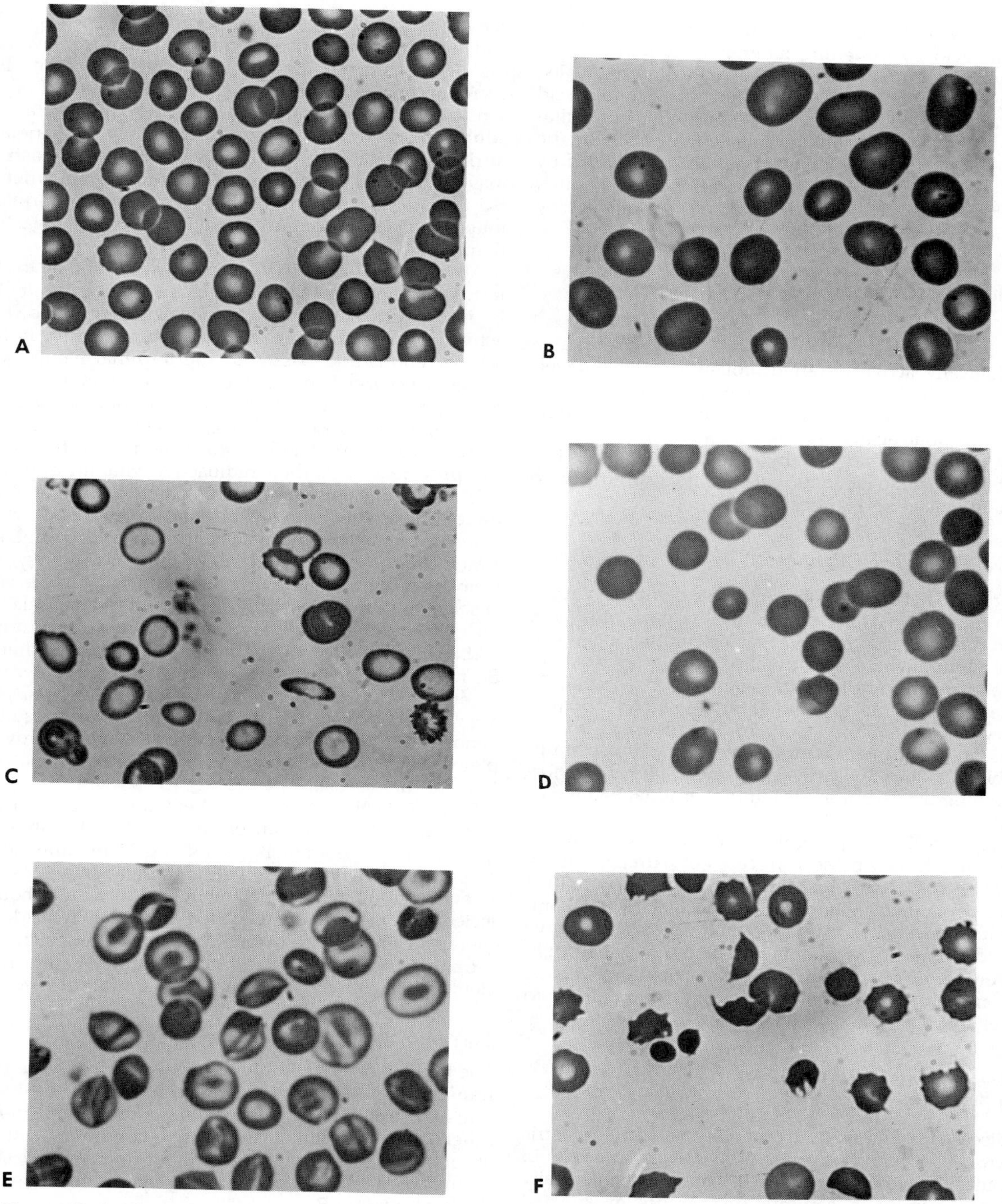

Figure 16–3. Morphologic abnormalities of the red blood cell. *A*, Normal. *B*, Macrocytes (folic acid deficiency). *C*, Hypochromic microcytes (iron deficiency). *D*, Spherocytes (hereditary spherocytosis). *E*, Target cells (Hb CC disease). *F*, Schizocytes (hemolytic-uremic syndrome).

anemia and increased need for transfusion. The bone marrow should be examined for megaloblastic changes if there is an unexplained worsening of chronic anemia or increased transfusion requirements in chronic hemolytic states. Continuous folic acid supplementation is not ordinarily necessary for such patients if their diets are normal, at least during childhood.

Folic Acid Deficiency Associated with Anticonvulsants and Other Drugs

Many patients have low serum levels of folic acid during therapy with certain anticonvulsant drugs (e.g., phenytoin, primidone, phenobarbital), but they usually have no anemia or symptoms. Frank megaloblastic anemia is rare and responds to folic acid therapy even if administration of the offending drug is continued. Malabsorption of folic acid induced by anticonvulsant drugs is the probable mechanism; displacement by the drug of folate from its serum carrier has also been suggested. Megaloblastic anemia, probably a result of folic acid malabsorption, has been seen in users of oral contraceptives.

A number of drugs have antifolic acid activity as their primary pharmacologic effect and regularly produce megaloblastic anemia. Methotrexate and aminopterin prevent the uptake of folic acid by inhibiting its enzymatic reduction to active coenzymatic forms. Pyrimethamine (Daraprim), which is used in the therapy of toxoplasmosis, may induce folic acid deficiency and megaloblastic anemia. Trimethoprim-sulfamethoxazole, which is also being increasingly used for the treatment of urinary infections and of pneumonia caused by *Pneumocystis carinii*, may also cause megaloblastic anemia. Therapy with folic acid (rescue) or folinic acid (not used by microorganisms) may be beneficial.

Congenital Dihydrofolate Reductase Deficiency

This has been reported in several patients who were unable to form biologically active tetrahydrofolate and who developed severe megaloblastic anemia in early infancy. These patients were successfully treated with large doses of folic acid or tetrahydrofolic acid.

Deficiency of methylene tetrahydrofolate reductase has been described in some patients with homocystinuria who had no hematologic abnormalities.

VITAMIN B_{12} DEFICIENCIES

To be absorbed, dietary vitamin B_{12} must combine with a glycoprotein (intrinsic factor) secreted by the parietal cells of the gastric fundus. The B_{12}-intrinsic factor complex passes to the terminal ileum, where specific absorptive sites exist. In the presence of intrinsic factor and ionic calcium, vitamin B_{12} traverses the intestinal mucosa and enters the blood. Vitamin B_{12} deficiency may therefore result from inadequate intake, lack of secretion of intrinsic factor by the stomach, consumption or inhibition of the B_{12}-intrinsic factor complex, or abnormalities involving the receptor sites in the terminal ileum (see also Sec. 4.7).

Because vitamin B_{12} is present in many foods, dietary deficiency is rare. It may be seen in cases of extreme dietary restriction ("vegans") in which no milk, eggs, or animal products are consumed. Vitamin B_{12} deficiency is not commonly seen in kwashiorkor or infantile marasmus. Cases have been reported in breast-fed infants whose mothers had deficient diets or pernicious anemia. Because vitamin B_{12} is so ubiquitous, most cases of deficiency stem from failure to absorb the vitamin.

Juvenile Pernicious Anemia

(Congenital Pernicious Anemia)

This rare disease results from an inability to secrete gastric intrinsic factor. It differs from the typical disease in adults in that the stomach secretes acid normally and is histologically normal. Consanguinity is common in parents of affected children and suggests mendelian recessive inheritance.

CLINICAL MANIFESTATIONS. The symptoms of juvenile pernicious anemia become prominent at 9 mo–10 yr of age. This interval is consistent with exhaustion of the stores of vitamin B_{12} acquired in utero. As the anemia becomes severe, irritability, anorexia, and listlessness occur. The tongue is smooth, red, and painful. Neurologic manifestations include ataxia, paresthesias, hyporeflexia, Babinski responses, clonus, and coma.

LABORATORY FINDINGS. The anemia is macrocytic, with prominent macro-ovalocytosis of the red blood cells. The neutrophils are large and hypersegmented. In advanced cases neutropenia and thrombocytopenia are seen. Serum vitamin B_{12} levels are below 100 pg/mL. Concentrations of serum iron and serum folic acid are normal or elevated. Serum LDH activity is markedly increased, primarily because of the 1st and 2nd heat-stable isoenzymes. Moderate elevations (2–3 mg/dL) of serum bilirubin levels may be seen. Excessive excretion of methylmalonic acid in the urine is a reliable and sensitive index of vitamin B_{12} deficiency. In contrast to many adult cases, serum antibodies directed against parietal cells or intrinsic factor cannot be detected in children. Gastric acidity may be reduced initially but returns to normal when vitamin B_{12} therapy is instituted. Biopsy reveals a normal gastric mucosa, but intrinsic factor activity is absent in gastric secretion.

Absorption of vitamin B_{12} is usually assessed by the Schilling test. When a normal person ingests a small amount of vitamin B_{12} into which ^{57}Co or ^{60}Co has been incorporated, the radioactive vitamin combines with the intrinsic factor in the stomach secretions and passes to the terminal ileum, where absorption occurs. Because the absorbed vitamin is bound to blood proteins and tissues, none is normally excreted in the urine. If a large dose (1,000 μg) of *nonradioactive* vitamin B_{12} is then injected parenterally ("flushing dose"), from 10–30% of the previously absorbed radioactive vitamin appears in the urine. Patients with pernicious anemia excrete 2% or less under these conditions. That malabsorption of vitamin B_{12} results from lack of intrinsic factor can be confirmed through a modification of the standard Schilling test: 30 mg of intrinsic factor is administered along with the radioactive vitamin. If absence of intrinsic factor is the basis of the B_{12} malabsorption, normal amounts of radioactive vitamin should now be absorbed and flushed out. On the other hand, when vitamin B_{12} malabsorption results from disease of ileal receptor sites or other intestinal causes, no improvement in absorption is seen with intrinsic factor. The Schilling test result remains abnormal in pernicious anemia, even when therapy has completely reversed the hematologic and neurologic manifestations of the disease.

TREATMENT. A prompt hematologic response follows parenteral administration of vitamin B_{12}. The physiologic requirement for vitamin B_{12} is 1–5 μg/24 hr, and hematologic responses have been observed with these small doses. If there is evidence of neurologic involvement, 1 mg should be injected intramuscularly daily for at least 2 wk. Maintenance therapy is necessary throughout the patient's life; monthly intramuscular administration of 1 mg of vitamin B_{12} is sufficient. Attempts at oral therapy are contraindicated.

Transcobalamin Deficiency

The two major vitamin B_{12}–binding proteins in the plasma are transcobalamins I and II. Transcobalamin II is the principal transport vehicle for vitamin B_{12}; a congenital deficiency is inherited as an autosomal recessive condition, with failure to absorb and transport vitamin B_{12}. Severe megaloblastic anemia occurs in early infancy; therapy requires massive parenteral doses of vitamin B_{12}.

Vitamin B_{12} Deficiency in Older Children

In some cases of vitamin B_{12} malabsorption in late childhood atrophy of the gastric mucosa and achlorhydria have been seen; in others the stomach is normal. Malabsorption of vitamin B_{12} may also occur in combination with a familial syndrome of cutaneous candidosis, hypoparathyroidism, and other endocrine deficiencies; the serum contains antibodies against intrinsic factor and parietal cells; an abnormal Schilling test result is corrected by addition of exogenous intrinsic factor. Parenteral vitamin B_{12} should be administered regularly to these patients to prevent the development of megaloblastic anemia. A case of megaloblastic anemia with a structurally abnormal intrinsic factor has been reported.

Vitamin B_{12} Malabsorption of Intestinal Causes

A few cases have been reported of familial occurrence of a specific intestinal defect in the absorption of vitamin B_{12}, in some instances associated with proteinuria (Imerslund syndrome); histology of the stomach is normal, and intrinsic factor and acid are present in gastric secretions.

Surgical resection of the terminal ileum or such inflammatory diseases as regional enteritis, neonatal necrotizing enterocolitis, or tuberculosis may also impair absorption of vitamin B_{12}. When the terminal ileum has been removed, lifelong parenteral administration should be considered if the Schilling test indicates that vitamin B_{12} is not absorbed. An overgrowth of intestinal bacteria within diverticula or duplications of the small intestine may cause vitamin B_{12} deficiency by consumption of or competition for the vitamin or by splitting of its complex with intrinsic factor. In these cases hematologic response may follow broad-spectrum antibiotic therapy. Similar mechanisms may operate when the fish tapeworm *Diphyllobothrium latum* infests the upper small intestine. When megaloblastic anemia occurs in these situations the serum vitamin B_{12} level is low, the gastric juice contains intrinsic factor, and the abnormal Schilling test result is not corrected by addition of exogenous intrinsic factor.

RARE MEGALOBLASTIC ANEMIAS

Orotic aciduria is a genetically determined defect in pyrimidine biosynthesis associated with a severe megaloblastic anemia, neutropenia, and crystalluria caused by excretion of orotic acid (Sec. 8.45). Physical and mental retardation may be frequently present. The anemia is refractory to vitamin B_{12} or folic acid but responds promptly to administration of the nucleic acid precursor, uridine, or yeast. The basic defect appears to be a deficiency of orotate phosphoribosyl transferase and orotidine-5-phosphate decarboxylase, which involves many tissues. Inheritance is autosomal recessive. Megaloblastic anemia can also occur in the Lesch-Nyhan syndrome, in which regeneration of purine nucleotides is blocked (Sec. 8.44).

Two cases of thiamine-responsive and thiamine-dependent megaloblastic anemia have been reported. Administration of thiamine, 100 mg/24 hr, produced a brisk reticulocyte response and a sustained increase in hemoglobin level. Sensorineural deafness and diabetes mellitus were associated. The pathogenesis of this disorder is unclear.

MICROCYTIC ANEMIAS

16.11 IRON DEFICIENCY ANEMIA

Anemia resulting from lack of sufficient iron for synthesis of hemoglobin is the most common hematologic disease of infancy and childhood. Its frequency is related to certain basic aspects of iron metabolism and nutrition. The body of the newborn infant contains about 0.5 g of iron, whereas the adult content is estimated at 5.0 g. To make up this 4.5-g discrepancy, an average of 0.8 mg of iron must be absorbed each day during the 1st 15 yr of life. In addition to this growth requirement a small amount is necessary to balance normal losses through excretion of iron. Accordingly, to maintain positive iron balance in childhood, 0.8–1.5 mg of iron must be absorbed each day. Because less than 10% of dietary iron is absorbed, a diet containing 8–15 mg of iron is necessary for optimal nutrition. Iron is absorbed more efficiently from human milk than from cow's milk; breast-fed infants may, therefore, require less from other foods. During the 1st years of life, because relatively small quantities of iron-rich foods are taken, it is often difficult to attain these amounts. For this reason the diet should include such foods as infant cereals or formulas that have been fortified with iron. At best, the infant is in a precarious situation with respect to iron. Should the diet become inadequate or external blood loss occur, anemia ensues rapidly.

ETIOLOGY. Most of the iron of the newborn is contained in the circulating hemoglobin. Total body iron at birth averages 75 mg/kg body weight. Low birthweight and significant perinatal hemorrhage are associated with decreases in neonatal hemoglobin mass and stores of iron. As the high hemoglobin concentration of the newborn falls during the 1st 2–3 mo of life, considerable iron is reclaimed and stored (Sec. 16.9). These reclaimed stores are usually sufficient for blood formation in the 1st 6–9 mo of life in term infants. Transplacental iron stores are exhausted by the time the birthweight approximately doubles. In low-birthweight infants or those with perinatal blood loss, stored iron may be depleted earlier, and dietary sources become of paramount importance. Anemia caused solely by inadequate dietary iron is unusual during the 1st 4–6 mo but becomes common from 9–24 mo of age. Thereafter, it is relatively infrequent. The usual dietary pattern observed in infants with iron deficiency anemia is the consumption of large amounts of milk and of carbohydrates unsupplemented with iron.

Blood loss must be considered a possible cause in every case of iron deficiency anemia, particularly in the older child. Chronic iron deficiency anemia from occult bleeding may be caused by a lesion of the gastrointestinal tract, such as peptic ulcer, Meckel diverticulum, polyp, or hemangioma. In some geographic areas hookworm infestation is an important cause.

As many as one third of infants with severe iron deficiency in the United States have chronic intestinal blood loss induced by exposure to a heat-labile protein in whole cow's milk. Loss of 1–7 mL of blood in the stools each day is not influenced by iron replacement or transfusion but can be prevented either by reducing the quantity of whole cow's milk to 1 pint/day or less or by using heated or evaporated milk or a milk substitute. This gastrointestinal reaction is not related to enzymatic abnormalities in the mucosa, such as lactase deficiency, or to typical "milk allergy." Characteristically, involved infants develop anemia that is more severe and occurs earlier than would be expected simply from an inadequate intake of iron.

Histologic abnormalities of the mucosa of the gastrointestinal tract are present in advanced iron deficiency anemia. The morphologic changes may be a direct manifestation of tissue deficiency of iron.

CLINICAL MANIFESTATIONS. Pallor is the most important clue to iron deficiency. In mild to moderate iron deficiency (hemoglobin levels of 6–10 g/dL) compensatory mechanisms, including increased levels of 2,3-DPG and a shift of the oxygen dissociation curve, may be so effective that few symptoms of anemia are noted. When the hemoglobin level falls below 5 g/dL, irritability and anorexia are prominent. Tachycardia and cardiac dilatation occur, and systolic murmurs are often present.

The spleen is palpably enlarged in 10–15% of patients and in longstanding cases, widening of the diploë of the skull similar to that seen in congenital hemolytic anemias may occur. These changes resolve slowly with adequate replacement therapy. The child with iron deficiency anemia may be obese or may be underweight with other evidences of undernutrition. Pica is sometimes prominent. The irritability and anorexia characteristic of advanced cases may reflect deficiency in tissue iron, because with iron therapy striking improvement in behavior frequently occurs before significant hematologic improvement.

Monoamine oxidase (MAO), an iron-dependent enzyme, plays a crucial role in neurochemical reactions in the central nervous system. MAO can also be measured in platelets. Iron deficiency produces decreases in the activities of enzymes such as catalase and cytochromes. Catalase and peroxidase contain iron, but their biologic essentiality is not well established. It is not possible to measure in vivo iron in the enzymatic compartment easily and accurately, and yet this is perhaps the most vital area of iron metabolism. In the past the intracellular enzyme iron component was held to be tenaciously maintained even in the presence of marked depletion in the other iron compartments, including in severe anemia, but this view is being questioned.

Iron deficiency may also have effects on neurologic and intellectual function. A number of reports suggest that iron deficiency anemia and even iron deficiency without significant anemia affect attention span, alertness, and learning of both infants and adolescents.

LABORATORY FINDINGS. In progressive iron deficiency a sequence of biochemical and hematologic events occurs. First, the tissue iron stores represented by liver and bone marrow hemosiderin disappear. It is possible to measure in the serum small amounts of ferritin, the iron-storage protein of the tissues. The level of serum ferritin provides a relatively accurate estimate of body iron stores. During infancy and childhood the mean level of serum ferritin is 35 ng/mL. Levels less than 10 ng/mL accompany iron deficiency. Next, there is a decrease in serum iron to less than 30 μg/dL, the iron-binding capacity of the serum increases to more than 350 μg/dL, and the per cent saturation falls below 15%. At a level of transferrin saturation of 10–15%, the availability of iron becomes rate-limiting for hemoglobin synthesis, and a moderate accumulation of the heme precursors called free erythrocyte protoporphyrins (FEP) results. Normal FEP levels are 1.9 ± 0.4 μg/g Hb (<35 μg/dL, whole blood); a characteristic level in iron deficiency is 10.9 ± 6.2 μg/g Hb (>50 μg/dL, whole blood).

As the deficiency progresses, the red blood cells become smaller than normal and their hemoglobin content decreases. The morphologic characteristics of red blood cells are best quantified by the determination of mean corpuscular volume (MCV) and mean corpuscular hemoglobin (MCH). Developmental changes in MCV require the use of age-related standards for diagnosis of microcytosis (Table 16–5). With increasing severity the red blood cells become deformed and misshapen and present characteristic microcytosis, hypochromia, and poikilocytosis (see Fig. 16–3C), without which a diagnosis of significant iron deficiency anemia is untenable.

TABLE 16–5. Mean Corpuscular Volume in Children*

Age	MCV (fL) Mean (Range)
Birth	119 (110–128)
6–24 mo	77 (70–85)
2–6 yr	81 (75–90)
6–12 yr	85 (78–95)
Adult	90 (80–100)

*Modified from Koerper MA, Mentzer WC, Brecher G, et al: J Pediatr 89:580, 1976.

The reticulocyte count is normal or minimally elevated; nucleated red blood cells may occasionally be seen in the peripheral blood. White blood cell counts are normal. Thrombocytosis, sometimes of a striking degree (600,000–1,000,000/mm^3) may occur or, in a few cases, significant thrombocytopenia. The mechanisms of these platelet abnormalities are not clear; they appear to be a direct consequence of iron deficiency, and they return to normal with iron therapy. The bone marrow is hypercellular with erythroid hyperplasia. The normoblasts have scanty, fragmented cytoplasm with poor hemoglobinization. Leukocytes and megakaryocytes are normal. Hemosiderin cannot be demonstrated in marrow specimens by the Prussian blue staining techniques. In about a third of cases occult blood can be detected in the stools. Certain iron-containing enzymes may be functionally decreased at varying degrees of iron deficiency anemia.

DIFFERENTIAL DIAGNOSIS (see Table 16–3). Iron deficiency must be differentiated from other hypochromic microcytic anemias. In lead poisoning the red cells are morphologically similar, but coarse basophilic stippling of the red blood cells is prominent. Very marked elevations of the blood lead, free erythrocyte protoporphyrin, and urinary coproporphyrin levels are seen (Sec. 26.16). Many patients with lead poisoning have concomitant iron deficiency. The blood changes of the β-thalassemia trait resemble those of iron deficiency, but characteristic elevations in the levels of Hb A_2 and Hb F are usually present, which do not occur in iron deficiency (Sec. 16.28). α-Thalassemia trait occurs in about 3% of blacks and in many Southeast Asian peoples. The diagnosis requires complicated tests after the newborn period; the diagnosis can be assumed when a case of familial hypochromic microcytic anemia with normal levels of Hb A_2 is refractory to iron therapy. In the newborn period infants with α-thalassemia trait have 3–5% Barts hemoglobin and the MCV is 94 fL (Sec. 16.2). Thalassemia major, with its pronounced erythroblastosis and hemolytic component, should present no diagnostic confusion. The red blood cell morphology of chronic inflammation and infection, though usually normochromic, may be microcytic, but in these conditions both the serum iron level and iron-binding ability are reduced, and serum ferritin levels are normal or elevated. Elevations of the FEP level are not specific to iron deficiency. Elevations are observed in those with lead poisoning, chronic hemolytic anemias, the anemia associated with chronic disorders, and some of the porphyrias.

TREATMENT. The regular response of iron deficiency anemia to adequate amounts of iron is an important diagnostic and therapeutic feature. Oral administration of simple ferrous salts (sulfate, gluconate, fumarate) provides inexpensive and satisfactory therapy. There is no evidence that addition of any trace metal, vitamin, or other hematinic substance significantly increases the response to simple ferrous salts. On the other hand, absorption of some iron chelates may be suboptimal. For routine clinical use the physician should be familiar with an inexpensive preparation of one of the simple ferrous compounds. The therapeutic dose should be calculated in terms of elemental iron; ferrous sulfate is 20% and ferrous gluconate is 10–12% elemental iron by weight. A daily total of 6 mg/kg of elemental iron in three divided doses provides an optimal amount of iron for the stimulated bone marrow to use. Doses of elemental iron in excess of 6 mg/kg/24 hr do not result in a more rapid hematologic response. Better absorption may result when medicinal iron is given between meals. Ingestion of large amounts of milk may significantly decrease absorption of iron. Intolerance to oral iron is extremely rare; malabsorption of oral iron is more frequently suspected than proved. A parenteral iron preparation (iron-dextran) is an effective form of iron, safe when given in a properly calculated dose, but the response to parenteral iron is no more rapid or complete than that obtained with proper oral administration of iron; in most cases the indication for parenteral iron therapy is a social one (to ensure compliance).

While adequate iron medication is given the family must be educated about the patient's diet and the consumption of milk limited to a reasonable quantity, preferably 500 mL (1 pt)/day or less. This reduction has a dual effect: the amount of iron-rich foods in the diet is increased, and gastrointestinal blood loss from intolerance to cow's milk proteins is prevented. When the re-education of child and parent is not successful, parenteral iron medication may be indicated. Iron deficiency can be prevented in high-risk populations by providing iron-fortified formula or cereals during infancy.

The expected clinical and hematologic responses to iron therapy are described in Table 16–6.

Within 72–96 hr after administration of iron to the anemic child, peripheral reticulocytosis is seen. The height of this response is inversely proportional to the severity of the anemia. Reticulocytosis is followed by a rise in the hemoglobin level, which may increase as much as 0.5 g/dL/24 hr. Iron medication should be continued for 4–6 wk after blood values are normal. Failures of iron therapy occur when the child does not receive the prescribed medication, when it is given in a form that is poorly absorbed, or when there is continuing unrecognized blood loss. *An incorrect original diagnosis of nutritional iron deficiency anemia may be revealed by therapeutic failure of iron medication.*

Because a rapid hematologic response can be confidently predicted in typical iron deficiency, blood transfusion is indicated only when the anemia is very severe or when superimposed infection may interfere with the response. It is not necessary to attempt rapid correction of severe anemia by transfusion and may be dangerous because of associated hypervolemia and cardiac dilatation. Packed or sedimented red cells, which are relatively fresh or are preserved in citrate-phosphate-dextrose (CPD) anticoagulant to ensure normal oxygen-hemoglobin affinity, should be administered slowly in an amount sufficient to raise the hemoglobin to a safe level at which the response to iron therapy can be awaited. In general, severely anemic children with hemoglobins under 4 g/dL should be given only 2–3 mL/kg of packed cells at any one time. If there is evidence of frank congestive heart failure, a modified exchange transfusion employing fresh packed red blood cells should be considered. Furosemide may also be administered. Digitalis is usually unnecessary.

TABLE 16–6. Responses to Iron Therapy in Iron Deficiency Anemia

Time After Iron Administration	Response
12–24 hr	Replacement of intracellular iron enzymes; subjective improvement; decreased irritability; increased appetite
36–48 hr	Initial bone marrow response; erythroid hyperplasia
48–72 hr	Reticulocytosis, peaking at 5–7 days
4–30 days	Increase in hemoglobin level
1–3 mo	Repletion of stores

OTHER MICROCYTIC ANEMIAS

SIDEROBLASTIC ANEMIAS

The sideroblastic anemias are a heterogeneous group of hypochromic microcytic anemias whose basic defects may be abnormalities of iron or heme metabolism. Serum iron levels are increased. In the bone marrow ringed sideroblasts are found; these are nucleated red blood cells with a perinuclear collar of coarse hemosiderin granules that represent iron-laden mitochondria.

A form of sideroblastic anemia transmitted as an X-linked recessive trait becomes symptomatic by late childhood. Splenomegaly is usually present. FEP levels are not elevated. In some cases an enzymatic deficiency of ALA synthetase has been postulated. A syndrome of refractory sideroblastic anemia with vacuolization of marrow precursor cells and exocrine pancreatic dysfunction has been reported. Acquired sideroblastic anemias occur in adults with various inflammatory and malignant processes or with alcoholism.

Some cases of sideroblastic anemia are partially responsive to pyridoxine (vitamin B_6) given in doses of 200–500 mg/24 hr, though abnormalities of tryptophan metabolism may not occur and other findings of vitamin B_6 deficiency are not observed.

LEAD POISONING

See Sec. 26.16.

RARE TYPES OF HYPOCHROMIC MICROCYTIC ANEMIA

Isolated cases are known of hypochromic microcytic anemia with other abnormalities of iron metabolism; some cases have had defects in iron mobilization or reutilization. Congenital absence of the iron-binding protein (atransferrinemia) is associated with severe hypochromic anemia, and requires lifelong transfusions. Iron is absorbed normally and is deposited in the visceral organs rather than in bone marrow.

Several patients have had refractory hypochromic anemia associated with lymphatic tumors or lymphoid hyperplasia. Correction of the anemia followed removal of the abnormal lymphatic tissue in these patients.

See also Thalassemia, Sec. 16.26.

16.12 HEMOLYTIC ANEMIAS

The fundamental basis of the hemolytic anemias is a shortened survival time of the red blood cells. Red blood cells normally spend 100–120 days in the circulation; about 1% of red cells (senescent ones) are removed from the blood each day and are replaced by an equal number of new cells released from the bone marrow.

In response to a shortened survival of red blood cells, the activity of bone marrow increases, and the reticulocyte count exceeds 2%. Sustained reticulocytosis in conjunction with an unchanging hemoglobin level is presumptive evidence of a hemolytic disorder. Hyperplasia of the erythropoietic marrow elements occurs, with lowering or reversal of the myeloid-erythroid ratio from the normal ranges of 2:1–4:1. In the chronic hemolytic processes of childhood, hypertrophy of the marrow may expand the medullary spaces, producing striking roentgenographic changes, particularly in the skull, metacarpals, and phalanges.

Elevations of the unconjugated (indirect) bilirubin level may accompany many hemolytic states, but overt jaundice is unusual if hepatic function is not impaired. Accelerated destruction of red blood cells increases the biliary excretion of heme pigments, which can be quantitated by measurement of fecal urobilinogen. Pigmented gallstones composed of calcium bilirubinate may be formed as early as the 4th yr of life. A chronic hemolytic process should be considered possible in any case of pigmentary cholelithiasis in childhood, but only about 15% of cases of gallstones in children are a consequence of hemolytic anemia. Plasma concentrations of hemoglobin increase in hemolytic anemias, and the free hemoglobin combines irreversibly with specific binding proteins (haptoglobins). The large haptoglobin-hemoglobin complex is cleared from the circulation by reticuloendothelial activity. Normal levels of serum haptoglobin are 20–200 mg/dL. In severe hemolytic states the loss of haptoglobin exceeds the synthesizing ability of the liver, and serum haptoglobin is decreased or absent. The level of hemopexin, another plasma protein that binds hemoglobin, is also reduced in hemolytic states. Catabolism of hemoglobin results in the formation of carbon monoxide (CO), and quantitation of CO in blood or expired air can provide a dynamic indicator of hemolysis. The assay is difficult, however, and not often used.

In addition to these indirect indicators of hemolysis, isotopic techniques can estimate red blood cell survival directly. Sodium chromate ($Na_2{}^{51}CrO_4$) and diisofluorophosphate ($DF^{32}P$) are the radioactive compounds most often used as red blood cell "tags." After injection of ^{51}Cr–tagged red blood cells, blood radioactivity normally decreases to 50% of its initial level in 25–35 days ($^{51}Cr\ t_{1/2}$ or half-life). A shortened red blood cell survival is likely when the $^{51}Cr\ t_{1/2}$ is reduced below 20 days. $DF^{32}P$ is expensive and more difficult to count but permits an actual measurement of red blood cell survival. In practice it is rarely necessary to use these techniques.

The stimulated normal bone marrow can ordinarily increase its output 6- to 8-fold; accordingly, red blood cell survival can theoretically be reduced to 15–20 days without producing anemia, but in childhood chronic hemolysis usually results in some degree of anemia. Patients with hemolytic anemias of whatever type may have transient episodes of bone marrow failure. These *aplastic crises* are characterized by reticulocytopenia and markedly decreased numbers of red blood cell precursors in the marrow. Occasionally, hugh abnormal erythroid precursors ("gigantoblasts") are seen. Profound and life-threatening anemia may develop quickly because the shortened red blood cell survival is no longer even partially compensated. These episodes of acute marrow failure are self-limited and last 10–14 days. Aplastic crises appear to be associated usually with parvovirus infection and may occur within a few days in several affected members of a family (Sec. 12.67). They constitute a potentially serious, life-threatening complication of any chronic hemolytic process.

The hemolytic anemias may be generally divided into two large classes: (1) those with premature destruction resulting from intrinsic abnormalities of the red blood cell; and (2) those caused by noxious extraerythrocytic factors. Table 16–3 lists the important hemolytic anemias of childhood. In hemolytic states associated with intrinsic defects, red blood cell survival is short in normal persons receiving transfusions of the patient's red cells, as well as in patients themselves. In contrast, red blood cells from patients with anemias resulting from extrinsic factors survive normally in healthy recipients.

HEMOLYTIC ANEMIAS CAUSED BY INTRINSIC ABNORMALITIES OF THE RED BLOOD CELL

16.13 HEREDITARY SPHEROCYTOSIS

(Congenital Hemolytic Anemia; Congenital Acholuric Jaundice)

Other than glucose-6-phosphate dehydrogenase deficiency (G-6-PD), this is the most common hereditary hemolytic state in which there is no abnormality of hemoglobin. The classic features are a congenital and familial hemolytic process associated with splenomegaly and with red blood cells that are spherical in shape. Cases have been reported in most ethnic groups, but the disease is most common among persons of northern European origin.

ETIOLOGY. Hereditary spherocytosis is usually transmitted as an autosomal dominant and occasionally as an autosomal recessive trait; about 25% of cases are sporadic and presumably represent new mutations. The basic defect is an abnormality of spectrin, the protein lattice that underlies the red blood cell lipid bilayer and provides stability to the erythrocyte membrane shape. Either the amount or function of the spectrin may be abnormal. Affected cells are unduly permeable to sodium and acquire the characteristic spherocytic shape because of loss of membrane function and increases in volume. An increased intracellular concentration of sodium is believed to lead to an increased uptake of ATP to drive the "cation pump." Premature senescence and destruction are thought to result from metabolic overwork and loss of red blood cell membrane.

The spleen is intimately involved in the hemolytic process. The splenic circulation imposes a metabolic environment that is stressful to spherocytic cells, and repeated passages through this unfavorable environment result in their sequestration and destruction. The spherocyte is relatively rigid and passes with difficulty through the minute apertures between the splenic cords and sinuses. The hemolytic process abates after splenectomy, though the biochemical and morphologic abnormalities persist.

CLINICAL MANIFESTATIONS. The disease has its onset in infancy and may present in the neonatal period with anemia and hyperbilirubinemia severe enough to require phototherapy or exchange transfusions. The anemia varies considerably in severity during infancy and childhood but tends to be similar within families. Some patients with relatively severe anemia during the 1st 6–8 mo of life show more satisfactory compensation thereafter. Slight jaundice is usually present. Moderate expansion of the marrow cavity of the skull may occur, but to a lesser extent than in thalassemia or other hemoglobinopathies. After infancy the spleen is almost always palpably enlarged. Pigmentary gallstones have been reported as early as 4–5 yr of age, but they usually do not develop until late childhood or adolescence. Approximately 50% of unsplenectomized patients ultimately form gallstones. Aplastic crises associated with parvovirus infections are the most serious complications during childhood.

LABORATORY FINDINGS. Evidence of hemolysis include reticulocytosis, anemia, and hyperbilirubinemia. The hemoglobin level usually ranges from 6–10 g/dL and the reticulocyte count from 5–20%, averaging 10%. The characteristic spherocytic red cell is smaller than the normal erythrocyte and lacks the central pallor of the biconcave disk (Fig. 16–3*D*). This morphologic change may be subtle, and only a relatively small proportion of the cells may be spherocytic. The mean corpuscular hemoglobin concentration (MCHC) may be elevated. There is erythroid hyperplasia in marrow, but the red blood cell precursors are not spherocytic. There are no abnormal hemoglobins.

The abnormality of the red blood cell membrane can be demonstrated by osmotic fragility studies. When red blood cells are placed in hypotonic saline solutions, water and sodium enter the cells, causing them to swell. The normal red blood cell of biconcave shape can increase its volume, but the spherical cell already has the maximal volume for its surface area. Imbibition of small amounts of water causes the spherocyte to rupture. In 10–20% of cases of hereditary spherocytosis the abnormality may be demonstrated only if the blood is incubated at 37° C for 24 hr before determining osmotic fragility. The autohemolysis test is also useful. When normal blood is incubated under sterile conditions for 48 hr at 37° C, fewer than 5% of the red blood cells hemolyze. Red blood cells of patients with hereditary spherocytosis have markedly increased rates of autohemolysis (15–45%). Abnormal autohemolysis can be corrected by the addition of small amounts of glucose to the blood before incubation.

DIFFERENTIAL DIAGNOSIS. Hereditary spherocytosis must be differentiated from other congenital hemolytic states. The family history, blood smear, and studies of osmotic fragility and autohemolysis are of most diagnostic value. Acquired spherocytosis of the red blood cells is seen in autoimmune hemolytic anemias; here the spherocytosis is more noticeable than in hereditary spherocytosis, and the Coombs test result is usually positive. It may be difficult to differentiate hereditary spherocytosis in the newborn infant from hemolytic disease because of A or B incompatibility when an appropriate blood group incompatibility is coincidentally present. A period of observation may be necessary to clarify the diagnosis. Acquired spherocytosis may follow thermal injury to red blood cells during extensive burns. Newborn red blood cells are osmotically resistant, so if an osmotic fragility curve is determined at this age to establish a diagnosis of hereditary spherocytosis, age-specific normative fragility curves must be used. In subjects with hereditary spherocytosis and iron deficiency the osmotic fragility curve may be normal. Iron deficiency is also associated with increased osmotic resistance.

TREATMENT. Splenectomy invariably produces a clinical cure. Splenectomy should be deferred whenever possible until the patient is 5–6 yr of age or older. If anemia is severe enough to impair growth or if aplastic crises are frequent, the operation may be considered earlier; an extended period of observation is indicated before splenectomy can be justified in infancy. Splenectomy prevents gallstones and eliminates the threat of aplastic crises. Hemochromatosis and hepatic failure have occurred in adults with hereditary spherocytosis who have not had splenectomy. After splenectomy jaundice and reticulocytosis rapidly disappear, and the hemoglobin level attains the normal range, though the spherocytosis and osmotic fragility become more pronounced. Thrombocytosis may occur in the immediate postoperative period, but anticoagulation therapy is not routinely indicated. Overwhelming sepsis after splenectomy is not a frequent threat to older patients, but after splenectomy the febrile child should be carefully evaluated and therapy initiated on the presumption of life-threatening infection. Polyvalent pneumococcal vaccine should be given prior to splenectomy. Prophylactic penicillin therapy afterward is advocated by many authorities (Sec. 16.92).

16.14 HEREDITARY ELLIPTOCYTOSIS

An oval or elliptic shape of the red blood cells occurs as a benign, dominantly inherited morphologic curiosity in about 1 in 2,000 persons (Fig. 16–4*A*). A less common variant, associated with spherocytes as well as elliptocytes, results in a moderate, usually compensated, hemolysis. Elliptocytes may be seen in other conditions, such as thalassemia and iron deficiency anemia, but in these they are far fewer in number than in hereditary elliptocytosis. Hemolysis is usually mild or absent, but about 10% of patients have a significant hemolytic anemia.

ETIOLOGY. Family studies of affected children usually reveal one parent with elliptocytosis without hemolysis, whereas the other parent is normal. A few cases may have represented homozygous inheritance. The gene for elliptocytosis is sometimes linked with the Rh locus. No biochemical abnormality of the red blood cell has been defined; a primary membrane abnormality involves spectrin dimer interactions. In hereditary pyropoikilocytosis (heat instability of red blood cells), children probably inherit an elliptocytotic gene from one parent and an unknown abnormal gene from the other. These patients have elliptocytes, spherocytes, fragmented red blood cells, and striking microcytosis, indicating significant hemolysis (Sec. 16.15).

CLINICAL MANIFESTATIONS. Hemolytic elliptocytosis may produce neonatal jaundice even though characteristic elliptocytosis may not be evident at that time; the blood of the affected newborn may show bizarre poikilocytes and pyknocytes. The usual features of a chronic hemolytic process are seen later as anemia, jaundice, splenomegaly, and osseous changes. Cholelithiasis may occur in later childhood, and aplastic crises have been reported.

LABORATORY FINDINGS. The morphology of the red blood cells is the most important diagnostic feature (see Fig. 16–4*B*). Elliptic cells are prominent, but in those with overt hemolysis many bizarre poikilocytes, microcytes, and spherocytes are also present. The reticulocyte count is increased. Erythroid hyperplasia is present in the bone marrow, but red blood cell precursors are not elliptic. There is no abnormal hemoglobin. The genes for abnormal hemoglobin, thalassemia, or G-6-PD deficiency do not interact with the gene for elliptocytosis to produce more severe disease.

TREATMENT. Splenectomy decreases the hemolytic component of this disease, although some degree of hemolysis may continue. It should be considered if there is significant chronic hemolysis. The red blood cell morphology is not corrected by the operation and may become more abnormal after splenectomy.

16.15 OTHER STRUCTURAL DEFECTS

Paroxysmal Nocturnal Hemoglobinuria

Paroxysmal nocturnal hemoglobinuria is a rare chronic anemia with prominent intravascular hemolysis. The hemolysis is characteristically worse during sleep, and nocturnal and morning hemoglobinuria is a classic finding. The disease is not congenital; it results from an ill-defined acquired dysplastic defect of the red cell membrane that renders it susceptible to hemolysis by serum complement (Sec. 11.26). In addition to chronic hemolysis there may be thrombocytopenia or leukopenia. Pyogenic infection, thrombosis, and thromboembolic phenomena are serious complications. Abdominal, back, and head pain may be prominent complaints. Some cases have been associated with hypoplastic or aplastic pancytopenia. The diagnosis of either disorder may precede the other. The diagnosis is established by a positive result in the acid serum (Ham) or thrombin tests. The sucrose lysis test is also useful. Markedly reduced levels of red blood cell acetylcholinesterase activity are found. Reduced levels of decay accelerating factor are diagnostic (Sec. 11.26). Splenectomy is not indicated. Prolonged anticoagulation therapy may be of benefit when thromboses occur. Because there is chronic loss of

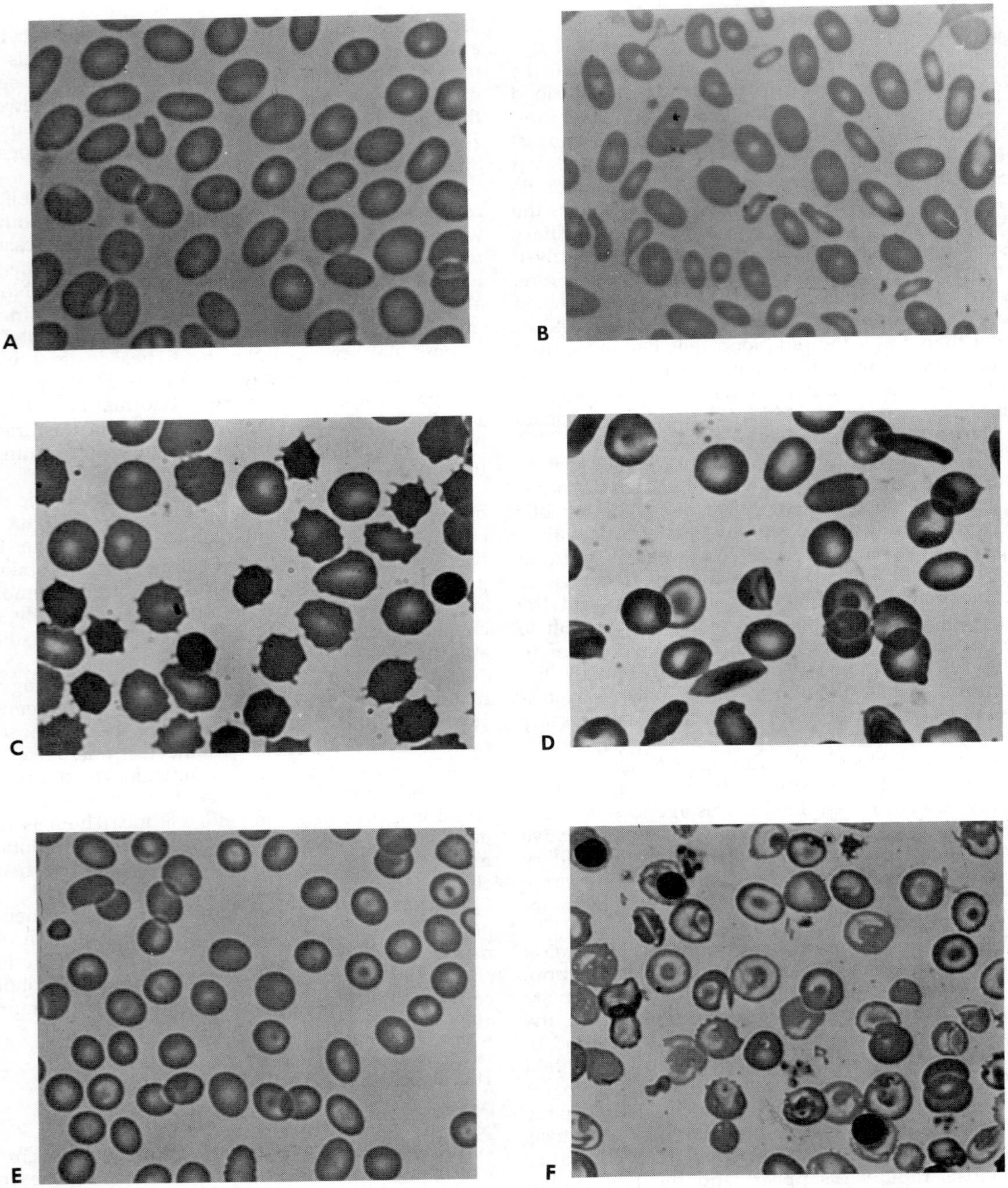

Figure 16–4. Morphologic abnormalities of the red blood cell. *A*, Elliptocytes (hereditary elliptocytosis). *B*, Bizarre elliptocytes (hemolytic elliptocytosis). *C*, Acanthocytes (abetalipoproteinemia). *D*, Sickle cells (Hb SS disease). *E*, Thalassemia trait. *F*, Thalassemia major.

iron in the urine, iron therapy may be necessary. Bone marrow transplantation has been successful in some cases.

Hereditary Stomatocytosis

Hereditary stomatocytosis is a rare condition in which the red blood cells are swollen and cup-shaped; on stained smears they present a mouth-like slit in place of the usual circular area of central pallor. There may be hemolytic anemia. Extreme permeability of the red blood cell membrane to cations has been observed. Splenectomy is not consistently effective but may be indicated in patients with severe hemolysis. Acquired stomatocytosis may be seen in several conditions, especially liver disease.

Acanthocytosis

This rare defect of lipid metabolism is characterized by malabsorption, neuromuscular abnormalities, and retinitis pigmentosa. The distorted red blood cells have sharp projections (see Fig. 16–4C), but there is usually no significant hemolytic anemia. The morphologic changes presumably result from decreased levels of cholesterol and β-lipoprotein in the serum. (See Abetalipoproteinemia, Sec. 8.34, 13.62, and 20.58.)

Pyropoikilocytosis

This rare, recessively transmitted, hemolytic anemia is characterized by bizarre fragmented and poikilocytic red blood cells and spherocytes that have reduced thermal stability. Osmotic fragility is abnormal. In some families there is an association between pyropoikilocytosis and elliptocytosis. Splenectomy may be helpful; the morphologic abnormalities are more pronounced after the operation.

HEMOLYTIC ANEMIAS CAUSED BY ENZYMATIC DEFECTS OF THE RED BLOOD CELLS

Within a group of diseases known collectively as congenital nonspherocytic hemolytic anemias because they lack spherocytosis and have normal osmotic fragility, the quantitation of various red cell enzymes has permitted the identification of a number of specific entities. Abnormal enzymes have been found in the major pathways of glucose catabolism, the anaerobic Embden-Meyerhof pathway and the oxidative pentose phosphate shunt. Disorders involving G-6-PD affect more than 100 million people throughout the world; patients with pyruvate kinase deficiency probably number in the thousands; all the other reported red blood cell enzyme deficiencies probably affect only a few hundred individuals.

16.16 PYRUVATE KINASE DEFICIENCY

A congenital hemolytic anemia occurs in persons homozygous for an autosomal recessive gene that causes either a marked reduction in red blood cell content of pyruvate kinase or production of an abnormal enzyme with decreased activity. Generation of ATP within the red cell is impaired and low levels of ATP, pyruvate, and NAD are seen. Concentrations of 2,3-DPG are increased. As a consequence of decreased ATP, potassium leaks from the red blood cell at a markedly increased rate and the cell's life span is considerably reduced.

CLINICAL MANIFESTATIONS AND LABORATORY FINDINGS. The clinical manifestations vary from a severe, congenital hemolytic process to a mild, well-compensated one noted first in adulthood. Jaundice and anemia may occur in the neonatal period, and kernicterus has been reported. The later severity of the hemolytic component varies from patient to patient, but pallor, jaundice, and splenomegaly are usually present. A severe form of the disease has a relatively high incidence among the Amish of the midwestern United States.

Macrocytosis and polychromatophilia reflect the elevated reticulocyte count. Spherocytes are uncommon, but a few spiculated pyknocytes are usually present. Nonincubated osmotic fragility is normal. Autohemolysis is moderately or markedly increased, but addition of glucose does not regularly correct the abnormality as it does in hereditary spherocytosis.

Diagnosis relies on demonstration of marked reductions of pyruvate kinase (PK) activity in the red blood cells. Other red blood cell enzyme activities are normal or elevated. There are no abnormalities of hemoglobin. The white blood cells have normal PK activity and must be excluded from hemolysates used to measure PK activity. Heterozygous carriers usually have moderately reduced levels of PK activity.

TREATMENT. Exchange transfusions may be indicated for hyperbilirubinemia in the newborn. Transfusions of packed red blood cells are necessary for severe anemia or for aplastic crises. If the anemia is consistently severe or if frequent transfusions are required, splenectomy should be performed after 5–6 yr of age. Although not curative, the operation may be followed by higher hemoglobin levels and by strikingly high (30–60%) reticulocyte counts. Deaths resulting from overwhelming pneumococcal sepsis have followed splenectomy (Sec. 16.92).

DEFICIENCIES OF OTHER GLYCOLYTIC ENZYMES

Congenital nonspherocytic anemias may stem from defects in hexokinase, glucose phosphate isomerase, phosphofructokinase, glyceraldehyde 3-phosphate dehydrogenase, triose phosphate isomerase, aldolase, and 2,3-diphosphoglycerate kinase and mutase; these defects are transmitted as autosomal recessive traits. Phosphoglycerate kinase deficiency caused by an X-linked defect has been reported in a mentally retarded boy. In homozygous triose phosphate isomerase deficiency, progressive neurologic dysfunction, mental retardation, and cardiac abnormalities occur in infants who live to more than a few months of age.

In these conditions the red blood cell morphology is not strikingly abnormal except for polychromasia and macrocytosis. Nonincubated osmotic fragility is normal. Splenectomy has been of variable benefit and is indicated when the hemolytic process is severe.

In addition to these glycolytic enzymopathies, rare cases of hemolytic anemia caused by pyrimidine-5′ nucleotidase or ATPase have been reported, as well as deficiencies of other red cell enzymes (e.g., lactic hydrogenase, methemoglobin reductase, catalase) without hemolysis.

DEFICIENCIES OF ENZYMES OF THE PENTOSE PHOSPHATE PATHWAY AND RELATED COMPOUNDS

The most important function of the pentose pathway, through which about 10% of the glucose taken up by the red blood cell passes, is to provide the NADPH, or reduced triphosphopyridine nucleotide (TPNH), necessary for conversion of oxidized to reduced glutathione. This is essential for the physiologic inactivation of oxidant compounds, such as hydrogen peroxide, that accumulate within the red blood cell. If glutathione or any compound or enzyme necessary for maintaining it in the reduced state is decreased, hemoglobin may become denatured and may precipitate into red blood cell inclusions called *Heinz bodies*. Once Heinz bodies have formed, the red blood cell is rapidly removed from the circulation; an acute hemolytic process may result from damage to the red blood cell membrane by the precipitated hemoglobin and the action of the spleen.

16.17 GLUCOSE-6-PHOSPHATE DEHYDROGENASE (G-6-PD) DEFICIENCY

G-6-PD deficiency, the most important disease in this group, is responsible for two clinical syndromes: an episodic hemolytic anemia induced by infections or certain drugs and a spontaneous chronic nonspherocytic hemolytic anemia. The deficiency is caused by inheritance of any of a large number of abnormal alleles of the gene responsible for the synthesis of the G-6-PD molecule. The normal enzyme found in most populations is designated G-6-PD B^+. A normal variant designated G-6-PD A^+ is common in American blacks. More than 100 distinct enzyme variants of G-6-PD have been found to be associated with a wide spectrum of hemolytic disease.

Drug-Induced Hemolytic Anemia
(Primaquine Sensitivity)

Synthesis of red blood cell G-6-PD is determined by genes borne on the X chromosome. Diseases involving this enzyme occur, therefore, more frequently in males than in females. About 13% of American black males and 2% of black females have a mutant enzyme (G-6-PD A⁻) that results in a deficiency of red blood cell G-6-PD activity (to 5–15% or less of normal). Italians, Greeks, and other Mediterranean, Middle Eastern, African, and Oriental ethnic groups also have a high incidence, ranging from 5–40% of a variant designated G-6-PD B⁻ (G-6-PD Mediterranean). The G-6-PD activity of the homozygous female or the heterozygous male is less than 5% of normal. The heterozygous female has an intermediate enzymatic activity and, as an example of random X chromosome inactivation (Lyon hypothesis), has two populations of red blood cells—one is normal, the other deficient in G-6-PD activity. The heterozygous female does not, however, have clinical hemolysis after exposure to oxidant drugs.

There is considerable variation in the defect among various racial groups; the defect in blacks is less severe than in affected whites. In blacks, the electrophoretically distinct enzyme variant is unstable in vivo, and its activity is decreased in the older red cells in the circulation. The activity of red blood cells containing the white variant enzyme (G-6-PD B⁻) is very low, often under 1% of normal. A third common mutant enzyme with markedly reduced activity (G-6-PD Canton) occurs in about 5% of Chinese. A number of other rare enzyme variants have been associated with drug-induced hemolysis. The basic defect appears to be production of an unstable enzyme that becomes inactive more rapidly than normal.

CLINICAL MANIFESTATIONS. In the usual pattern of G-6-PD deficiency no evidence of hemolysis is apparent until 48–96 hr after the patient has ingested a substance that has oxidant properties. Drugs that have these properties include antipyretics, sulfonamides, antimalarials, and naphthaquinolones. The fava bean, a Mediterranean dietary staple, is also particularly potent, producing an acute and severe hemolytic syndrome called *favism*. The degree of hemolysis varies with the agent, the amount ingested, and the severity of the enzyme deficiency in the patient. In severe cases hemoglobinuria and jaundice result, and the hemoglobin concentration may decrease by 60–70%. Death may occur as a consequence of severe hemolysis. Even if administration of the responsible drug is continued, recovery is the rule, with evidence of a compensated hemolytic process. Infection may result in hemolysis. This defect is an important cause of neonatal hyperbilirubinemia and kernicterus in Greek and Chinese newborn infants with the G-6-PD B⁻ and Canton variants. Significant hemolysis may occur even when no exposure to drugs can be documented. In the G-6-PD A⁻ variant the hemolytic process after drug exposure is usually self-limited and mild because the younger red blood cells in the circulation have nearly normal enzyme activity and resist hemolytic destruction. In black newborns spontaneous hemolysis may occur in premature, but not term, infants with G-6-PD deficiency. When a pregnant woman ingests drugs such as sulfonamides or naphthalene, they may be transmitted to her G-6-PD–deficient fetus, and hemolytic anemia and jaundice may ensue after birth.

LABORATORY FINDINGS. Hemoglobinemia and hemoglobinuria are manifested in severe acute cases, with falls in hemoglobin of 2–10 g/dL. Unstained or supravital preparations of red blood cells reveal Heinz bodies, which are not visible on Wright-stained blood smears. Because cells containing these inclusions are rapidly removed from the circulation, they are not seen after the 1st 3–4 days of illness. Recovery is heralded by reticulocytosis and an increase in hemoglobin concentration.

DIAGNOSIS. Diagnosis depends on direct or indirect demonstration of reduced G-6-PD activity in red blood cells. By direct measurement, enzyme activity in affected persons is 10% of normal or less, and the reduction of enzyme is more extreme in whites and Orientals than in blacks. Satisfactory screening tests are based on decoloration of methylene blue and on reduction of methemoglobin. Immediately after a hemolytic episode reticulocytes and young red blood cells predominate. These young cells have significantly higher enzyme activity than older cells; testing may, therefore, have to be deferred for a few weeks before a diagnostically low level of enzyme can be shown. The diagnosis can be suspected when the G-6-PD activity is within the low normal range in the presence of a high reticulocyte count. G-6-PD variants can also be detected by electrophoretic analysis.

TREATMENT. Prevention of hemolysis constitutes the most important therapeutic measure. When possible, males belonging to ethnic groups in which there is a significant incidence of G-6-PD deficiency (e.g., Greeks, southern Italians, Sephardic Jews, Filipinos, southern Chinese, blacks, and Thais) should be tested for the defect before known oxidant drugs are given. When hemolysis has occurred, supportive therapy may include blood transfusions. Spontaneous recovery is the rule.

OTHER HEMOLYTIC ANEMIAS ASSOCIATED WITH DEFICIENCIES OF G-6-PD OR OF RELATED SUBSTANCES

Rare instances of chronic hemolytic anemia have been associated with profound deficiencies of G-6-PD caused by enzyme variants particularly defective in quantity, activity, or stability. Occasionally and unaccountably, persons with G-6-PD B⁻ (Mediterranean) enzyme deficiency have chronic hemolysis; the condition is X-linked recessive and has affected many males of northern European origin. Chronic hemolytic anemia is maintained, and worsening of the hemolytic process may follow ingestion of oxidant drugs. Splenectomy is of little value. A mild, chronic nonspherocytic anemia has also been reported in association with a genetically determined deficiency of red blood cell glutathione. 6-Phosphogluconate dehydrogenase deficiency has been associated with drug hemolysis. Hyperbilirubinemia has been related to a deficiency of glutathione peroxidase in several newborn infants.

JAMES A. STOCKMAN III

16.18 HEMOGLOBIN DISORDERS

The clinical disorders that result from abnormalities of the globin genes comprise a diverse group of hematologic diseases. Normal hemoglobins are tetrameric molecules containing pairs of α or α-like and β or β-like globin-heme subunits. The normal postnatal hemoglobins include hemogoblin (Hb) A ($\alpha_2\beta_2$), Hb F ($\alpha_2\gamma_2$), and Hb A_2 ($\alpha_2\delta_2$). The embryonic hemoglobins, which usually disappear before birth, include Hb Gower-1 ($\zeta_2\epsilon_2$), Hb Gower-2 ($\alpha_2\epsilon_2$), and Hb Portland ($\zeta_2\gamma_2$) (see also Sec. 16.2.) The genes for the α and ζ chains are encoded on chromosome 16; those for the β group have been localized to chromosome 11. The nucleotide sequences of all these genes have been determined, and many globin-gene abnormalities have been characterized at the molecular level.

The hemoglobin disorders are subdivided into three major groups. The structural abnormalities, or hemoglobinopathies, result from changes in the amino acid sequences of the globin chains. Most have a single amino acid substitution; in others, however, amino acids may be deleted or inserted, or other, more complex, structural changes may be present. The thalassemias are expressed as quantitative defects, in which the synthesis of one or more of the globin chains is decreased or, in the most severe forms, is totally suppressed. The hereditary persistence of fetal hemoglobin (HPFH) syndromes are characterized by elevated levels of Hb F continuing throughout adult life. Almost all these abnormalities result from the same types of molecular defects: nucleotides may be substituted, deleted, or inserted into globin-gene DNA.

HEMOGLOBIN STRUCTURAL ABNORMALITIES
(Hemoglobinopathies)

Approximately 500 structural variants of hemoglobin have been identified. Most are rare but a few, including some severely pathologic forms, occur with high frequency in certain populations. Many abnormal hemoglobins are readily identified by electrophoresis, but some are electrophoretically "silent" and require other laboratory studies for identification. Many hemoglobin variants that have abnormal electrophoretic mobility, including benign and pathologic forms, exhibit very similar electrophoresis findings and cannot be specifically identified by this means alone.

16.19 SICKLE CELL HEMOGLOBINOPATHIES

Sickle hemoglobin (Hb S) differs from normal adult hemoglobin by a substitution of glutamic acid at the 6th position of its β chains by valine. In the oxygenated state Hb S functions normally. When this hemoglobin is deoxygenated, an interaction between the β6 valine and a complementary region on the β chains of an adjacent molecule results in the formation of highly ordered molecular polymers; these elongate to form filamentous structures, which aggregate into rigid, crystal-like rods. This process of molecular polymerization is responsible for the spiny, brittle character of sickle erythrocytes under conditions of decreased oxygenation. Certain other abnormal hemoglobins, notably Hb C, Hb D Los Angeles, and Hb O Arab, participate in the molecular polymerization of deoxy-Hb S. Hb A does so to a smaller degree, but fetal hemoglobin (Hb F) does not.

Erythrocytes of heterozygous (sickle cell trait) individuals have been shown to resist invasion by malarial parasites, which appears to have provided protection against the frequently lethal *Plasmodium falciparum* form of the disease. The β^s gene is found in high frequency in those living in regions in which *P. falciparum* malaria has been endemic, including many parts of Africa, the Mediterranean area, and parts of Turkey, the Middle East, and India. In individuals from several geographic areas the sickle mutation has been shown to exist in genetic linkage with discrete sets of closely associated markers. Some of these Hb S "haplotypes" appear to be predictive of the degree of severity of the sickle cell disease. Those associated with particularly mild disease have additional closely linked mutations that promote the production of higher levels of fetal hemoglobin.

Hb S is readily identified by electrophoresis. A confirmatory solubility test excludes other abnormal hemoglobins with similar electrophoretic mobility. Although affected newborns express only small quantities of Hb S, because of the predominance of Hb F at birth, the sickle cell syndromes can nevertheless be identified reliably in the newborn by electrophoretic methods. Neonatal screening programs for the detection of infants with sickle cell disease are widely established in the United States. These disorders can also be determined antenatally using amniocyte or chorionic villus DNA by methods that identify the specific β^s nucleotide substitution.

SICKLE CELL ANEMIA
(Homozygous Hb S)

This disorder is characterized by severe chronic hemolytic disease resulting from premature destruction of the brittle, poorly deformable erythrocytes. Other manifestations of sickle cell anemia are attributable to ischemic changes resulting from vascular occlusion by masses of sickled cells. The clinical course of affected children is typically associated with intermittent episodic events, often referred to as "crises."

CLINICAL MANIFESTATIONS. Affected newborns usually exhibit none of the characteristic clinical features of sickle cell disease; hemolytic anemia gradually develops over the 1st 2–4 mo, parallelling the replacement of much of the fetal hemoglobin by Hb S. Other clinical manifestations are uncommon prior to 5–6 mo of age. Acute sickle dactylitis, presenting as the hand-foot syndrome, is frequently the 1st overt evidence that sickle cell disease is present in the infant. Its associated findings include painful, usually symmetric, swelling of the hands and feet. The underlying abnormality is ischemic necrosis of the small bones, believed to be caused by a choking off of the blood supply as a result of the rapidly expanding bone marrow. Roentgenograms are not informative in the acute phase, but later show evidence of extensive bony destruction and repair (Fig. 16–5).

Acute painful vaso-occlusive episodes represent the most frequent and prominent manifestation of sickle cell disease. Most patients experience some pain on a nearly daily basis. Episodes of severe pain that require hospitalization and parenteral narcotic administration average about one per year in children with Hb SS but this interval varies considerably, with some patients never experiencing severe pain and others requiring hospital admission with such frequency as to become seriously disabled. In young children pain often involves the extremities; in older patients head, chest, abdominal, and back pain occur more commonly. In an individual patient pain tends to recur in a limited number of sites. Intercurrent illnesses accompanied by fever, hypoxia, and acidosis, all of which promote the deoxygenation of Hb S, may precipitate sickle pain episodes, but acute pain also develops frequently without an apparent antecedent event. Sickle-related abdominal pain may mimic that of an acute surgical condition.

More extensive vaso-occlusive events in these patients can produce gross ischemic damage. Acute pain episodes may progress to infarction of bone marrow or bone. Splenic infarcts are common in children between 6 and 60 mo, causing pain and contributing to the process of "autosplenectomy." Pulmonary infarction, often occurring in association with pneumonitis, may produce the severe clinical picture of *acute chest syndrome.* Strokes caused by cerebrovascular occlusion are among the most catastrophic acute events and are a frequent cause of hemiplegia. As many as 10% of children with sickle cell anemia, mainly pre-adolescent and older patients, exhibit sequelae of cerebrovascular occlusion. Ischemic damage may also affect the myocardium, liver, and kidneys. Renal function is progressively impaired by diffuse glomerular and tubular fibrosis, and hyposthenuria accompanied by polyuria are characteristic findings in patients over 5 yr of age. Renal papillary necrosis and nephrotic syndrome also develop occasionally. Priapism is a relatively frequent complication that results from the pooling of blood in the corpora cavernosa, causing obstruction of the venous outflow.

Young children with Hb SS may have splenic enlargement associated with their hemolytic disease, with progression to the syndrome of hypersplenism accompanied by worsening anemia and sometimes thrombocytopenia. *Acute splenic sequestration* is a distinct and episodic event that occurs in infants and young children with sickle cell anemia. For unknown reasons large amounts of blood become acutely pooled in the spleen, which becomes massively enlarged, and signs of circulatory collapse rapidly develop. Blood transfusions in the acute phase may be lifesaving.

Altered splenic function in young children with sickle cell disease is a significant factor leading to their increased sus-

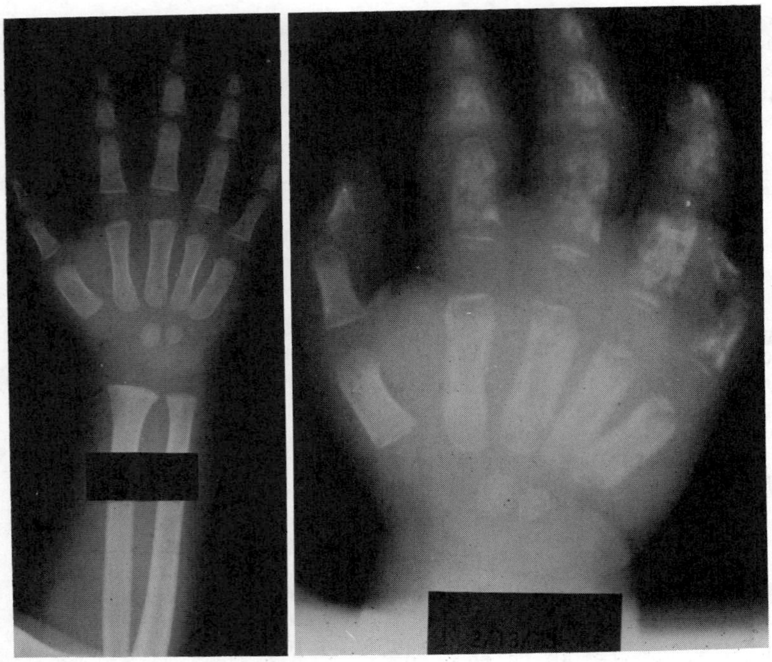

A B

Figure 16–5. Roentgenograms of an infant with sickle cell anemia and acute dactylitis. *A*, The bones appear normal at the onset of the episode. *B*, Destructive changes and periosteal reaction are evident 2 wk later.

ceptibility to meningitis, sepsis, and other serious infections, mainly caused by pneumococci and *Haemophilus influenzae*. In the absence of specific antibody to the polysaccharide capsular antigens of these organisms, splenic activity is essential for removing these bacteria when they invade the blood. In spite of frequent enlargement of the spleen in young patients with Hb SS, its phagocytic and reticuloendothelial functions have been shown to be markedly reduced. As an additional risk factor, children with sickle cell disease have also been shown to have deficient levels of serum opsonins (Properdin) against pneumococci. Children with sickle cell disease also have increased susceptibility to *Salmonella* osteomyelitis due, in part, to bone necrosis.

In common with patients having other forms of chronic hemolytic anemia, children with Hb SS are at risk of developing a rapid decrease in their hemoglobin level (aplastic episodes) in association with parvovirus infection (see Sec. 16.18).

An additional group of sickle cell sequelae is attributable primarily to the hemolytic anemia that accompanies this disorder. *Hemolytic crisis* may occur with concomitant G-6-PD deficiency (Sec. 16.17). Cardiomegaly is invariably present in older children, often caused partly by sickle-related cardiomyopathy. Increased iron absorption contributes to parenchymal damage of the liver, pancreas, and heart. Symptomatic gallstone formation is common in adolescent and adult patients, occasionally occurring in children as young as 5 yr of age.

By midchildhood most patients are underweight, and puberty is frequently delayed. Chronic leg ulcers are relatively uncommon in children, usually occurring only in late adolescence.

LABORATORY FINDINGS. Hemoglobin concentrations usually range from 5–9 g/dL. The peripheral blood smear typically contains target cells, poikilocytes, and irreversibly sickled cells (Fig. 16–6*A*). These findings allow Hb SS and most of the other forms of sickle cell disease to be readily distinguished from sickle cell trait and other clinically benign conditions. Reticulocyte counts usually range from 5 to 15%, and nucleated red cells and Howell-Jolly bodies are often present. The total white blood cell count is elevated to 12,000–20,000/mm^3, with a predominance of neutrophils. The platelet count is usually increased; the sedimentation rate is slow. Other changes include abnormal liver function test results, hyperbilirubinemia, and diffuse hypergammaglobulinemia. The bone marrow is markedly hyperplastic and shows erythroid predominance. Roentgenograms show expanded marrow spaces and osteoporosis.

DIAGNOSIS. The diagnosis is established by hemoglobin studies. Electrophoresis at an alkaline pH demonstrates a characteristic mobility, intermediate between those of Hb A and Hb A_2. To distinguish Hb S from other hemoglobins with similar electrophoretic properties, another (confirmatory) test is required, such as electrophoresis at an acidic pH, a sickle cell preparation in which sickling is observed when the cells are deoxygenated or, most commonly, a hemoglobin solubility test. In the Hb S solubility test a measured amount of hemoglobin is added to a concentrated buffer that contains a reducing agent; a turbid precipitate forms when more than about 15% Hb S is present. Beyond infancy, red cells from patients with Hb SS contain Hb with between 2 and 20% Hb F and normal quantities of Hb A_2. Hb A is notably absent. The identification of Hb S in each parent provides additional supportive evidence for the diagnosis of sickle cell anemia.

DIFFERENTIAL DIAGNOSIS. The various clinical manifestations of sickle cell disease, including limb pain, heart murmurs, hepatosplenomegaly, and anemia, may suggest a number of other diagnoses, including rheumatic fever or rheumatoid arthritis, osteomyelitis, and leukemia. In patients who have a Hb SS electrophoresis pattern and concomitant microcytosis (MCV less than 78 fL), possibilities that require consideration include iron deficiency or a combination of Hb S with α- or β°-thalassemia (Table 16–7).

TREATMENT. Measures directed toward the prevention of serious complications of sickle cell disease are among the most important elements of patient management. Maintaining full immunization status of these children is particularly important. Administration of a polyvalent pneumococcal vaccine may be beneficial, but unfortunately the forms of these vaccines currently available appear to be poorly immunogenic in children with Hb SS who are under the age of 5 yr. *H. influenzae* and hepatitis B immunizations are indicated. Pro-

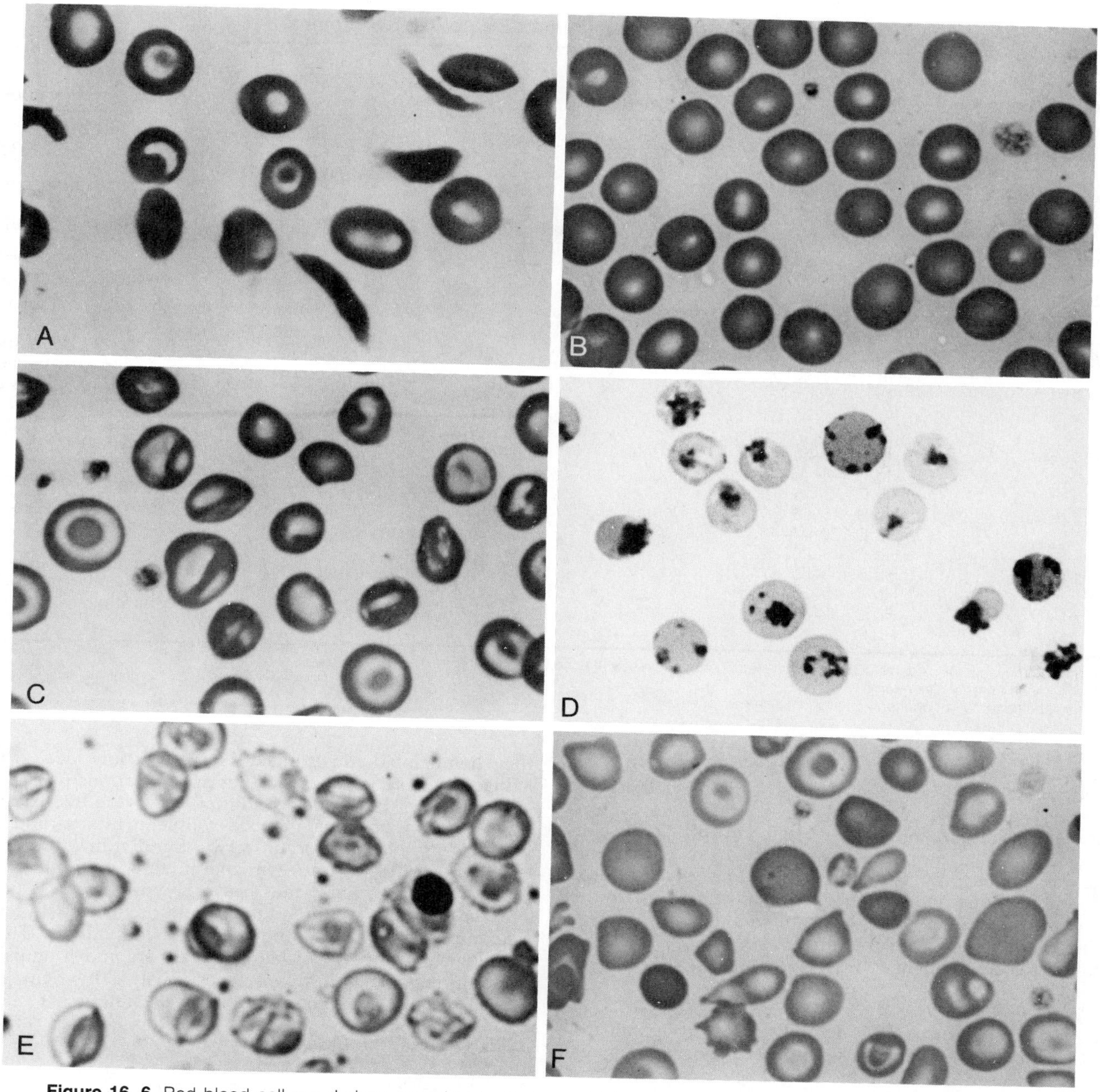

Figure 16–6. Red blood cell morphology associated with hemoglobin disorders. *A*, Sickle cell anemia (Hb SS): target cells and fixed (irreversibly sickled) cells. *B*, Sickle cell trait (Hb AS): normal red blood cell morphology. *C*, Hemoglobin CC: target cells and occasional spherocytes. *D*, Congenital Heinz body anemia (unstable hemoglobin): red blood cells stained with supravital stain (brilliant cresyl blue) reveal intracellular inclusions. *E*, Homozygous β^0-thalassemia: severe hypochromia with deformed red blood cells and normoblasts. *F*, Hemoglobin H disease (α-thalassemia): anisopoikilocytosis with target cells.

phylactic penicillin G (or amoxicillin for *H. influenzae*) is highly efficacious in preventing serious pneumococcal infections and should be administered to all young children with sickle cell disease. The penicillin is given orally, twice daily, starting in early infancy and continuing at least to the age of 6 yr. Parents of these children also need to be aware of the need to bring the child promptly to medical attention for acute illness, especially with fever above 39° C. Because of the substantial risk of life-threatening bacterial infections, prompt parenteral antibiotic therapy should be considered for patients with an acute onset of high fever. Parents and caretakers of these children should also be informed about the manifestations of acute splenic sequestration and the need for immediate medical attention for the child with rapid splenic enlargement and pallor.

Painful episodes can frequently be managed with oral acetaminophen, alone or with codeine. More severe episodes may require hospitalization and the parenteral administration of narcotics. Any dehydration and/or acidosis should be rapidly corrected by the intravenous route. Blood transfusions are seldom indicated for painful episodes, and it is doubtful whether transfusion can ameliorate the course of a pain crisis. For patients with disabling chronic pain, for those with ischemic organ damage or stroke, or in preparation for major

TABLE 16–7. Clinically Important Sickle Cell Syndromes*

Sickle Cell Disorder	Hemoglobin Composition (%)	Hb A_2 Level	Erythrocyte Volume (MCV)†	Clinical Severity	Clinical Features
Hb SS	Hb S: 80–95 Hb F: 2–20	Normal	Normal	+ + to + + + +	(See text)
Hb S–β^0-thalassemia	Hb S: 75–90 Hb F: 5–25	Increased	Decreased	+ + to + + + +	Generally indistinguishable from SS
Hb S–β^+-thalassemia	Hb S: 55–85 Hb A: 10–30 Hb F: 5–10	Increased	Decreased	+ to + + +	Generally milder than SS
Hb SS with α-thalassemia trait (− ,α/ − ,α)	Hb S: 80–90 Hb F: 10–20	Normal	Decreased	+ + to + + + +	May be milder than SS
Hb SC	Hb S: 45–50 Hb C: 45–50 Hb F: 2–5	Normal	Normal	+ to + + +	Generally milder than SS; higher frequency of bone infarcts and proliferative retinal disease
Hb SO Arab	Hb S: 50–55 Hb O: 40–45 Hb F: 2–15	Normal	Normal	+ + to + + + +	Generally indistinguishable from SS
Hb SD Los Angeles	Hb S: 45–50 Hb D: 30–40 Hb F: 5–20	Normal	Normal	+ + to + + + +	May be as severe as SS
Hb S/HPFH‡	Hb S: 65–80 Hb F: 15–30	Normal	Normal	0 to +	Usually asymptomatic
Hb AS‡	Hb S: 32–45 Hb A: 52–65	Normal	Normal	0 to +	Asymptomatic

*Adapted from Honig GR, Adams JG III: Human Hemoglobin Genetics. Vienna, Springer-Verlag, 1986.
†MCV = mean corpuscular volume.
‡These conditions do not ordinarily produce sickle cell disease.

surgery, however, transfusions of normal red blood cells can provide symptomatic relief and prevent further ischemic complications. Packed red blood cell transfusions are specifically indicated for acute splenic sequestration and aplastic episodes. Repeated episodes of splenic sequestration are also an indication for splenectomy. Infection is the leading cause of death in children. Bone marrow transplantation from a normal donor provides a cure for aplastic anemia, but the risks and morbidity associated with this procedure limit its application to highly selected patients with sickle cell disease.

OTHER SICKLE CELL SYNDROMES

Sickling disorders of varying degrees of severity result from Hb S existing in combination with other abnormal hemoglobins or thalassemias (see Table 16–7). Several of these syndromes, including Hb SD Los Angeles, Hb SO Arab, and Hb S—β^0-thalassemia, present a clinical picture virtually indistinguishable from that of sickle cell anemia. Most of the others produce less severe manifestations.

Hb SC disease results from the concurrence of genes for Hb S and Hb C. Painful episodes and other vaso-occlusive manifestations are usually less severe in this condition than those associated with Hb SS. Most affected children have persistent splenomegaly, and bone infarcts occur more frequently than in those with Hb SS. Retinal vascular changes, predominantly in adolescents and adults, may lead to hemorrhage with retinal detachment. The hemoglobin concentration averages 9–10 g/dL, with the blood smear showing target cells and characteristic spindle-shaped red cells.

16.20 SICKLE CELL TRAIT
(Heterozygous Hb S; Hb AS)

Heterozygous expression of the sickle hemoglobin gene is usually associated with a totally benign clinical course. About 8% of American Blacks have sickle cell trait, with 35–45% of their hemoglobin consisting of Hb S. This low level of Hb S is insufficient to produce sickling manifestations under usual circumstances, but under conditions of severe hypoxia vaso-occlusive complications may occur. Splenic infarcts and other ischemic sequelae may occur in Hb AS individuals after flying at high altitudes in unpressurized aircraft and from hypoxia associated with general anesthesia. Hyposthenuria is usually present in older children and adults. Occasionally, gross hematuria develops in otherwise well individuals. The hematologic findings in sickle cell trait are indistinguishable from normal. The diagnosis is established by hemoglobin electrophoresis, with confirmatory sickle testing.

16.21 OTHER HEMOGLOBINOPATHIES

HEMOGLOBIN C

Hemoglobin C ($\alpha_2\beta_2{}^6$lysine) occurs in about 2% of American Blacks. In the heterozygous state (Hb AC) no anemia or disease is present, but increased numbers of target cells are seen in the peripheral blood. In the homozygous individual (Hb CC disease) a moderately severe hemolytic anemia with hemoglobin levels from 8 to 11 g/dL, a reticulocytosis of 5–10%, and splenomegaly are regularly observed. The peripheral blood contains striking numbers of target cells and occasional spherocytes (see Fig. 16–6C).

HEMOGLOBIN E

Hemoglobin E ($\alpha_2\beta_2{}^{26}$lysine) is prevalent in populations from Southeast Asia, particularly Thailand and Cambodia. Homozygous Hb E disease is characterized by hemolytic anemia with prominent target cells, microcytosis, and moderate to severe splenomegaly. The syndrome of Hb E—β^0-thalassemia may be expressed as a severe Cooley anemia-like disorder; electrophoresis shows the presence of only Hb E and Hb F.

16.22 UNSTABLE HEMOGLOBIN DISORDERS (Congenital Heinz Body Anemia)

A substantial group of abnormal hemoglobins, most of which are uncommon or rare, are characterized by molecular instability leading to denaturation and precipitation of hemoglobin within the red cells. In the more severe forms of these disorders amorphous masses of the denatured hemoglobin, known as Heinz bodies, attach to the red blood cell membrane, damaging the cell and shortening its survival. The Heinz bodies, which are particularly prominent following splenectomy, can be visualized by supravital staining of the red blood cells with brilliant cresyl blue (see Fig. 16–6-*D*). These hemolytic anemias are inherited in an autosomal dominant mode, but many of the severe abnormalities apparently occur as new mutations.

Most of the severe forms involve the hemoglobin β chains, and hemolysis first becomes apparent at 3–6 mo after birth, when Hb F is replaced by adult hemoglobin. Anemia with increased reticulocytes, jaundice, and splenomegaly are characteristically present, becoming more pronounced with infections or following exposure to oxidant drugs or chemicals. With some of the unstable β-chain abnormalities, hemolysis is accompanied by excretion of darkly pigmented dipyrrolic compounds in the urine. In contrast to the clinical picture of chronic hemolytic disease typically associated with the highly unstable hemoglobins, some of the less severe abnormalities (e.g., Hb Zurich and Hb Hasharon) produce mild and usually inapparent anemia. With fever, infections, or exposure to oxidant conditions, however, these individuals may experience acute hemolytic episodes similar to those associated with G-6-PD deficiency.

Some unstable hemoglobins can be detected by electrophoresis, but many of them comigrate with Hb A. Heating at 50° C or treating the hemolysate with a 17% buffered solution of isopropanol produces a precipitate of the unstable hemoglobin, and screening tests based on these methods are used to detect these abnormalities. Examples include Hb Koln, Hb Hammersmith, and Hb Abraham Lincoln. Splenectomy is sometimes of benefit in these patients, particularly those with severe splenomegaly.

16.23 ABNORMAL HEMOGLOBINS WITH INCREASED OXYGEN AFFINITY

Almost 100 different rare, abnormal hemoglobins have been identified that have increased oxygen affinity, as indicated by a leftward displacement of their oxygen dissociation curves. Because of their increased oxygen affinity these hemoglobins release oxygen poorly to the tissues, resulting in hypoxia at the tissue level. The hypoxic stimulus increases erythropoietin production, with the development of secondary erythrocytosis. Hemoglobin levels in affected individuals typically range from 16 to 19 g/dL. Some of these variants can be demonstrated by electrophoresis, but many of them have normal electrophoretic properties (e.g., Hb Chesapeake, Hb Malmo, Hb Kempsey).

16.24 ABNORMAL HEMOGLOBINS CAUSING CYANOSIS

Several rare hemoglobin variants with markedly decreased oxygen affinity have been identified. The oxygen dissociation curves of blood from affected individuals are significantly displaced to the right. Examples of these abnormalities, which produce benign cyanosis, include Hb Kansas and Hb Beth Israel.

An additional group of abnormal hemoglobins that cause cyanosis is the Hb M group. These variants all have amino acid substitutions at positions in the molecule that are close to the heme groups. The structural changes in these hemoglobins have the effect of stabilizing the heme iron atoms in the ferric (Fe^{3+}) state, rendering them incapable of binding oxygen. The Hb M syndromes are characterized by a brown color of the blood, even when fully oxygenated, and by cyanosis. Two of the Hb M variants, Hb M Saskatoon and Hb M Hyde Park, are also unstable and produce chronic hemolytic anemia. The Hb M variants that result from β-chain substitutions, such as Hb M Saskatoon, have an onset of cyanosis beginning at 4–6 mo of age, whereas the α-chain variants, such as Hb M lwate, produce cyanosis that is apparent at birth. The autosomal dominant mode of inheritance of these abnormalities helps distinguish them from other causes of congenital cyanosis.

Methemoglobinemias resulting from Hb M can be differentiated from other forms of methemoglobinemia by characteristic changes in the spectral absorption patterns of hemoglobin solutions and by the presence of normal levels of methemoglobin reductase (diaphorase) (see Sec. 8.50). Electrophoresis can demonstrate some (but not all) of the Hb M variants. These are clinically benign abnormalities, except for the hemolytic disease that accompanies two of the Hb M group, and no treatment is required.

16.25 SYNDROMES OF HEREDITARY PERSISTENCE OF FETAL HEMOGLOBIN (HPFH)

These disorders are characterized by the production of elevated levels of Hb F beyond the neonatal period. At least 20 distinct forms of HPFH have been identified, affecting many different ethnic groups. Various molecular abnormalities have been determined as the cause for these conditions; for example, the common African forms result from extensive DNA deletions that encompass the entire β-globin gene. The normal changeover from γ-globin synthesis to β-chain synthesis consequently cannot take place in individuals with these affected chromosomes. In heterozygotes for the common African types, the level of Hb F is 15–30%. These types are characterized by a uniform distribution of Hb F in the red cells (pancellular HPFH) as compared with some of the other forms, in which the Hb F is unevenly distributed (heterocellular HPFH). Rare homozygotes for the African deletion HPFH forms have 100% Hb F in their red blood cells. Except for mild microcytosis they have normal hematologic findings. Individuals who have genes for both sickle hemoglobin and African pancellular HPFH have levels of Hb S in their red blood cells that are similar to those in patients with sickle cell anemia (see Table 16–7). This combination, however, is clinically benign, presumably because the elevated Hb F in all the red blood cells inhibits the sickling process.

16.26 THALASSEMIA SYNDROMES

The thalassemias are a heterogeneous group of heritable hypochromic anemias of varying degrees of severity. Underlying genetic defects include total or partial deletions of globin chain genes and nucleotide substitutions, deletions, or insertions. The consequences of these various changes are a decrease or absence of mRNA for one or more of the globin chains or the formation of functionally defective mRNA. The result is a decrease or total suppression of hemoglobin polypeptide chain synthesis. Approximately 100 distinct mutations are known that produce thalassemia phenotypes; many of these mutations are unique to localized geographic regions. In general, the globin chains synthesized in thalassemic red blood cells are structurally normal. In severe forms of α-thalassemia abnormal homotetramer hemoglobins (β_4, γ_4) are formed, but their component globin polypeptides have a normal structure. Conversely, a number of abnormal hemoglobins also produce thalassemia-like hematologic changes. In characterizing the expression of the various thalassemia genes, superscript designations are used to distinguish those that produce a demonstrable globin chain product, although at decreased levels (e.g., β^+-thalassemia), from those in which the synthesis of the affected globin chain is totally suppressed (e.g., β^0-thalassemia).

Thalassemia genes are remarkably widespread, and these abnormalities are believed to be the most prevalent of all human genetic diseases. Their main distribution includes areas bordering the Mediterranean Sea, much of Africa, the Middle East, the Indian subcontinent, and Southeast Asia. From 3 to 8% of Americans of Italian or Greek ancestry and 0.5% of black Americans carry a gene for β-thalassemia. In some regions of Southeast Asia as many as 40% of the population have one or more thalassemia genes. The geographic areas in which thalassemia is prevalent closely parallel the regions in which *Plasmodium falciparum* malaria was formerly endemic. Resistance to lethal malarial infections by carriers of thalassemia genes apparently represented a strong selective force that favored their survival in these areas of endemic disease.

16.27 HOMOZYGOUS β^0-THALASSEMIA
(Cooley Anemia; Thalassemia Major)

CLINICAL MANIFESTATIONS. Homozygous β^0-thalassemia usually becomes symptomatic as a severe, progressive hemolytic anemia during the 2nd 6 mo of life. Regular blood transfusions are necessary in these patients to prevent the profound weakness and cardiac decompensation caused by the anemia. Without transfusion life expectancy is no more than a few years. In untreated cases or in those receiving infrequent transfusions at times of severe anemia, hypertrophy of erythropoietic tissue occurs in medullary and extramedullary locations. The bones become thin and pathologic fractures may occur. Massive expansion of the marrow of the face and skull (Fig. 16–7) produces characteristic facies. Pallor, hemosiderosis, and jaundice combine to produce a greenish-brown complexion. The spleen and liver are enlarged by extramedullary hematopoiesis and hemosiderosis. In older patients the spleen may become so enlarged that it causes mechanical discomfort and secondary hypersplenism. Growth is impaired in older children; puberty is delayed or absent because of secondary endocrine abnormalities. Diabetes mellitus resulting from pancreatic siderosis may also occur. Cardiac complications, including intractable arrhythmias and chronic congestive failure caused by myocardial siderosis, are common terminal events. With modern regimens of comprehensive care for these patients, many of these complications can be prevented and others ameliorated and delayed in their onset.

LABORATORY FINDINGS. The red cell morphologic abnormalities in untransfused patients with homozygous β^0-thalassemia are extreme. In addition to severe hypochromia and microcytosis (see Fig. 16–6*E*) many bizarre, fragmented poikilocytes and target cells are present. Large numbers of nucleated red blood cells circulate, especially after splenectomy. Intraerythrocytic inclusions, which represent precipitated excess α chains, are also seen after splenectomy. The hemoglobin level falls progressively to lower than 5 g/dL unless transfusions are given. The unconjugated serum bilirubin level is elevated. The serum iron level is high, with saturation of the iron-binding capacity. LDH activities are also very high, reflecting ineffective erythropoiesis. A striking biochemical feature is the presence of very high levels of fetal hemoglobin in the red blood cells (Table 16–8). Hemoglobin A_2 is usually less than 3%. Dipyrrolic compounds render the urine dark brown, especially after splenectomy.

TREATMENT. Transfusions are given on a regular basis to maintain the hemoglobin level above 10 g/dL. This "hypertransfusion" regimen has striking clinical benefits: it permits normal activity with comfort, prevents progressive marrow expansion and cosmetic problems associated with facial bone changes, and minimizes cardiac dilatation and osteoporosis. Transfusions of 15–20 mL/kg of packed cells are usually necessary every 4–5 wk. Cross-matching should be performed to forestall alloimmunization and prevent transfusion reactions. The use of packed red blood cells that are relatively fresh (less than 1 wk in CPD anticoagulant) is desirable. Even with meticulous care, febrile reactions to transfusions are common. These can be minimized with the use of erythrocytes reconstituted from frozen blood or leukocyte-poor red blood cell preparations, and by the administration of antipyretics before transfusions.

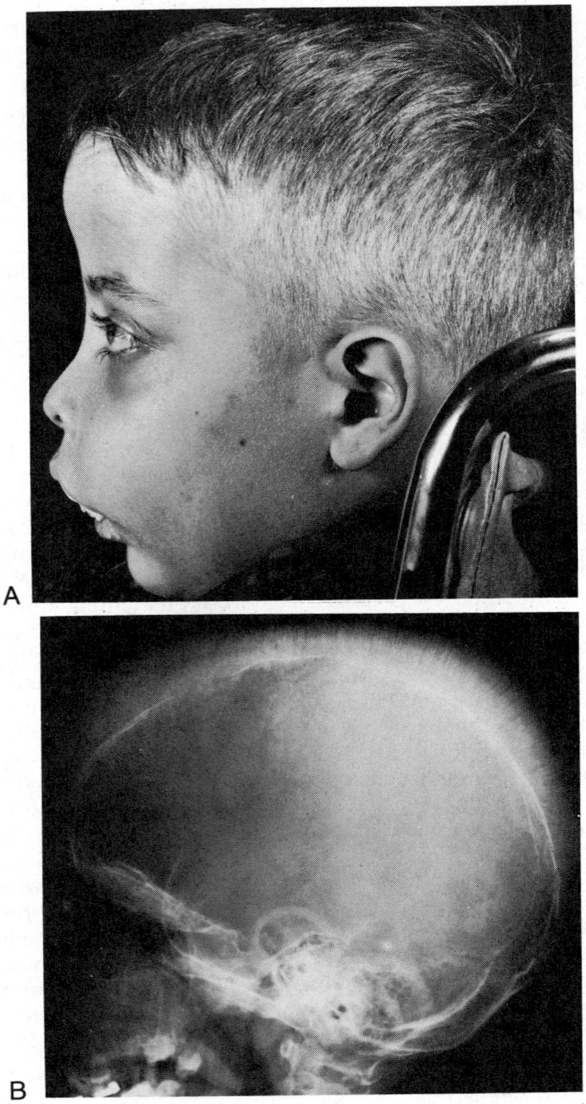

Figure 16–7. *A*, Facial deformities in an inadequately transfused patient with thalassemia major (Cooley anemia). Severe maxillary hyperplasia and malocclusion are present. *B*, Roentgenogram of the skull demonstrates the maxillary overgrowth and shows prominent widening of the diploic spaces, with the "hair-on-end" appearance caused by vertical trabeculae. These changes can be prevented by an appropriate transfusion regimen.

Hemosiderosis is an inevitable consequence of prolonged transfusion therapy because each 500 mL of blood delivers about 200 mg of iron to the tissues that cannot be excreted by

TABLE 16–8. Clinical and Hematologic Features of the Principal Forms of Thalassemia*

Type of Thalassemia	Globin-Gene Expression	Hematologic Features	Clinical Expression	Hemoglobin Findings
β-Thalassemias				
β^0 homozygous	β^0/β^0	Severe anemia; normoblastemia (see Fig. 16–6*E*)	Cooley anemia	Hb F > 90% no Hb A Hb A_2 increased
β^+ homozygous	β^+/β^+	Anisocytosis, poikilocytosis; moderately severe anemia	Thalassemia intermedia	Hb A: 20–40% Hb F: 60–80%
β^0 heterozygous	β/β^0	Microcytosis, hypochromia, mild to moderate anemia	May have splenomegaly, jaundice	Increased Hb A_2 and Hb F
β^+ heterozygous	β/β^+	Microcytosis, hypochromia, mild anemia	Normal	Increased Hb A_2 and Hb F
β silent carrier, heterozygous	β/β^+	Normal	Normal	Normal
δβ heterozygous	$\delta\beta/(\delta\beta)^0$	Microcytosis, hypochromia, mild anemia	Usually normal	Hb F: 5–20% Hb A_2: normal or low
γδβ heterozygous	$\gamma\delta\beta/(\gamma\delta\beta)^0$	Newborn: microcytosis hemolytic anemia normoblastemia Adult: similar to heterozygous δβ	Newborn: hemolytic disease with splenomegaly Adult: similar to heterozygous δβ	Normal
α-Thalassemias				
α silent carrier	$-,\alpha/\alpha,\alpha$	Mild microcytosis or normal	Normal	Normal
α trait	$-,\alpha/-,\alpha$ or $-,-/\alpha,\alpha$	Microcytosis, hypochromia, mild anemia	Usually normal	Newborn: Hb Barts (γ_4), 5–10% Child or adult: normal
Hb H disease	$-,\alpha/-,-$	Microcytosis, inclusion bodies by supravital staining; moderately severe anemia (see Fig. 16–7*F*)	Thalassemia intermedia	Newborn: Hb Barts (γ_4), 20–30% Child or adult: Hb H (β_4), 4–20%
α-Hydrops fetalis	$-,-/-,-$	Anisocytosis, poikilocytosis; severe anemia	Hydrops fetalis; usually stillborn or neonatal death	Hb Barts (γ_4), 80–90%; no Hb A or Hb F

*Adapted from Honig GR, Adams JG III: Human Hemoglobin Genetics. Vienna, Springer-Verlag, 1986.

physiologic means. Myocardial siderosis is a significant contributing factor in the early death of these patients. Hemosiderosis can be decreased or even prevented with the parenteral administration of the iron-chelating drug, deferoxamine, which forms an iron complex that can be excreted in the urine. A sustained high blood level of deferoxamine is needed for adequate iron excretion. It is administered subcutaneously over an 8 to 12-hr period using a small portable pump (during sleep), 5 or 6 nights/wk. Patients who adhere to this regimen can maintain serum ferritin levels of lower than 1,000 ng/mL, which is well below the toxic range. Lethal complications of hepatic and myocardial siderosis can thus be prevented or significantly delayed.

Hypertransfusion therapy prevents massive splenomegaly resulting from extramedullary erythropoiesis. Splenectomy eventually becomes necessary, however, because of the size of the organ or because of secondary hypersplenism. Splenectomy increases the risk of severe, overwhelming sepsis, and therefore the operation should be performed only for significant indications (see Sec. 16.92) and should be deferred as long as possible. The most important indication for splenectomy is an increased need for transfusions, indicating an element of hypersplenism. A transfusion requirement exceeding 240 mL/kg of packed red blood cells/yr is usually evidence of hypersplenism and is an indication for considering splenectomy. Immunization of these patients with hepatitis B vaccine and pneumococcal polysaccharide vaccine is desirable, and prophylactic penicillin therapy is also advocated.

Bone marrow transplantation is curative in these patients and has been performed with increasing success, even in patients who have been transfused extensively. This procedure, however, carries considerable risks of morbidity and mortality and can only be used for patients who have nonaffected histocompatible siblings.

16.28 OTHER β-THALASSEMIA SYNDROMES

The homozygous expression of milder (β^+) thalassemia genes produces a Cooley anemia-like syndrome of lesser severity ("thalassemia intermedia"; see Table 16–8). Skeletal deformities and hepatosplenomegaly develop in these patients, but their hemoglobin levels are usually maintained at 6–8 g/dL without transfusion. Nevertheless, they may develop severe hemosiderosis, attributable to their greatly increased gastrointestinal iron absorption. For such patients, who do not receive deferoxamine chelation therapy, a low-iron diet is indicated.

Several structurally abnormal hemoglobins produce β-thalassemia–like hematologic changes and, when present in combination with a gene for β-thalassemia, also result in a thalassemia intermedia syndrome. The most prevalent are the Hb Lepore variants, which are composed of α chains and hybrid δβ fusion globin chains. The Lepore hemoglobins are identified by electrophoresis, in which they exhibit Hb S–like mobility.

Most forms of heterozygous β-thalassemia are associated with mild anemia. The hemoglobin concentration typically averages 2–3 g/dL lower than age-related normal values. The red blood cells are hypochromic and microcytic, with poikilocytosis, ovalocytosis, and often coarse basophilic stippling. Target cells may be present but usually are not prominent and are not specific for thalassemia. The MCV is low, averaging 65 fL, and the mean corpuscular hemoglobin (MCH) values are also low (<26 pg). A mild decrease in red blood cell survival can be shown, but overt signs of hemolysis are usually absent. The serum iron level is normal or elevated.

The individuals with thalassemia trait are often misdiagnosed as having iron deficiency anemia and may be inappropriately treated with iron for extended periods. More than 90% of persons with β-thalassemia trait have diagnostic elevations of Hb A_2 of 3.4–7%. About 50% of these individuals also have slight elevations of Hb F, about 2–6%. In a small number of otherwise typical cases, normal levels of Hb A_2 with Hb F levels ranging from 5 to 15% are found, representing the δβ type of thalassemia (see Table 16–8). The "silent carrier" form of β-thalassemia produces no demonstrable abnormality in heterozygous individuals (see Table 16–8) but the gene for this condition, when inherited together with a gene for β^0-thalassemia, results in a thalassemia intermedia syndrome.

A rare type of deletion defect, which involves the γ-, δ-, and β-globin genes, produces a clinical picture similar to that of δβ thalassemia trait in heterozygous individuals. In the newborn period, however, this defect is accompanied by significant hemolytic disease with microcytosis, normoblastemia, and splenomegaly (see Table 16–8). The hemolytic process is self-limited, but supportive transfusions may be required.

16.29 α-THALASSEMIA

Microcytic anemias resulting from deficient synthesis of α-globin chains are prevalent in those in Africa, Mediterranean area countries, and much of Asia. Deletions of α-globin genes account for most of these abnormalities. Four α-globin genes are present in normal individuals, and four distinct forms of α-thalassemia have been identified corresponding to deletions of one, two, three, or all four of these genes (see Table 16–8).

Deletion of a single α-globin gene produces the silent carrier α-thalassemia phenotype. No hematologic abnormality is usually evident, except for mild microcytosis. Approximately 25% of African-Americans have this form of α-thalassemia.

Individuals lacking two α-globin genes exhibit the features of α-thalassemia trait, with mild microcytic anemia. In affected newborns, small quantities of Hb Barts (γ_4) can be identified by hemoglobin electrophoresis. Beyond about 1 mo of age Hb Barts is no longer detectable, and the levels of Hb A_2 and F are characteristically normal. Inclusions of precipitated hemoglobin may be visualized in red blood cell smears, however, following supravital staining.

The deletion of three of the four α-globin genes is associated with a thalassemia intermedia–like syndrome, Hb H disease. Microcytic anemia in this condition is accompanied by abnormal red blood cell morphology (see Fig. 16–6*F*), with prominent intracellular inclusions present in the red blood cells following supravital staining. Hemoglobin H (β_4) is highly unstable; it can be readily identified by electrophoresis, but, unless special measures are taken to prevent its precipitation during sample preparation, it may escape detection.

The most severe form of α-thalassemia, resulting from deletion of all the α-globin genes, is accompanied by a total absence of α-chain synthesis. Because hemoglobins F, A, and A_2 all contain α chains, none of these hemoglobins are produced. Hb Barts (γ_4) accounts for most of the hemoglobin in affected infants, and, because γ_4 has a high oxygen affinity and therefore cannot transport oxygen to the tissues, these infants are severely hypoxic. Their red blood cells also contain small quantities of the normal embryonic Hb Portland ($\zeta_2\gamma_2$), which functions as an oxygen transporter. Most of these infants are stillborn, and most who are born alive die within a few hours. These infants are severely hydropic, with congestive heart failure and massive generalized edema. Those that survive with aggressive neonatal management are also transfusion-dependent.

The types of α-thalassemia genes vary among affected populations, and these differences account for the α-thalassemia syndromes that predominate in specific population groups. In African-Americans α-thalassemia genes are prevalent, with almost all affected individuals having the deletion arrangement (–,α) that produces a single α-locus chromosome. In this population, therefore, α-thalassemia occurs mainly as the silent carrier phenotype (–,α/α,α) or as the α-thalassemia trait (–,α/–,α). Chromosomes with deletions of both of the α loci (–,–) are prevalent in both Mediterranean and Asian populations, and Hb H disease (–,α/–,–) therefore occurs with significant frequency in both groups. The two α-locus deletion defects in Asians are often accompanied by retention of the ζ-globin genes (i.e., ζ,–,–), whereas those from Mediterranean countries usually are not (–,–,–). The latter type of defect, therefore, cannot support the synthesis of Hb Portland ($\zeta_2\gamma_2$), which appears to be essential for the intrauterine survival of fetuses with the hydrops fetalis form of α-thalassemia. Accordingly, the hydrops fetalis form is seen almost exclusively in infants of Asian ancestry.

A number of abnormal hemoglobins also produce α-thalassemia–like changes. The α-chain variant Hb Constant Spring occurs commonly in far Eastern populations and is frequently observed in patients with Hb H disease, who have the genotype ($\alpha^A,\alpha^{Co\ Sp}/-,-$). The gene for Hb G Philadelphia, which is the most prevalent α-chain abnormality of African-Americans, usually occurs on a single-locus chromosome ($-,\alpha^G$). Individuals who express this abnormal hemoglobin therefore also exhibit α-thalassemia–like hematologic changes.

GEORGE R. HONIG

HEMOLYTIC ANEMIAS RESULTING FROM ABNORMALITIES OF THE RED BLOOD CELL PRODUCED BY EXTRINSIC FACTORS

A number of agents with the ability to damage red blood cells may lead to their premature destruction. Among the most clearly defined are antibodies associated with immune hemolytic anemias. These antibodies, directed against specific intrinsic antigens, so damage the red blood cell that viability is compromised and rapid destruction ensues in the reticuloendothelial tissues of the spleen and liver. The hallmark of this group of diseases is a positive result of the Coombs test, which detects a coating of immunoglobulin or components of complement on the red blood cell surface. The most important immune hemolytic disorder in pediatric practice is hemolytic disease of the newborn (erythroblastosis fetalis), caused by transplacental transfer of maternal antibody active against the red blood cells of the fetus (Sec. 9.47).

16.30 AUTOIMMUNE HEMOLYTIC ANEMIAS ASSOCIATED WITH "WARM" ANTIBODIES

In the autoimmune hemolytic anemias, abnormal antibodies directed against red blood cells are produced by the patient. The pathogenic mechanisms are uncertain. One theory postulates autonomous proliferation of a forbidden clone of immunologically competent cells that do not recognize self-antigens. Alternative explanations suggest that drugs or infectious agents in some way alter the red blood cell membrane so that it becomes "foreign" or antigenic to the host.

Autoimmune hemolytic anemias associated with an underlying disease process such as lymphoma, lupus erythematosus, or immunodeficiency are said to be secondary or symptomatic. In other instances (idiopathic) no underlying cause can be found. In as many as 20% of cases of immune hemolysis, drugs may be implicated. A number of drugs, such as penicillin and cephalosporins, attach to the red blood cell membrane, changing antigenicity and evoking production of antibodies directed against the red blood cell–drug complex. Other drugs, such as phenacetin and quinidine, form immune complexes that become attached to the red blood cell, causing its destruction. α-Methyldopa produces an autoimmune hemolytic process by unknown mechanisms.

CLINICAL MANIFESTATIONS. Autoimmune hemolytic anemias occur in two general clinical patterns. The first is an acute transient type that occurs predominantly in infants and younger children and is frequently preceded by an infection, usually respiratory. The onset is acute, with prostration, pallor, jaundice, pyrexia, and hemoglobinuria. The spleen is usually markedly enlarged. Underlying systemic disorders are unusual in this group. A consistent response to corticosteroid therapy, low mortality, and full recovery within 3 mo are characteristic of the acute form.

The other type pursues a prolonged and chronic course. Hemolysis continues for many months or years. Abnormalities involving other blood elements are common, and the response to corticosteroids is variable and inconsistent. Mortality is about 10%, often attributable to an underlying systemic disease.

LABORATORY FINDINGS. In many cases the anemia is profound, with hemoglobin levels under 6 g/dL. Considerable spherocytosis and polychromasia are present. More than 50% of the circulating red blood cells may be reticulocytes, and nucleated red blood cells are usually present. In some cases an initially low reticulocyte count may reflect a process so acute that the bone marrow has not yet had time to respond. Leukocytosis is common. The platelet count is usually normal; occasionally, there is a concomitant immune thrombocytopenic purpura (*Evans syndrome*). The prognosis of Evans syndrome is poor; many cases become chronic.

The direct Coombs test result is strongly positive, and free antibody can sometimes be demonstrated in the serum. These antibodies are active at 37° C ("warm" antibodies) and belong to the IgG class. They do not require complement for activity and may not produce agglutination in vitro. Antibodies from the serum and those eluted from the red blood cells react with red blood cells of many persons in addition to the patient. They have often been regarded as nonspecific panagglutinins, but careful studies have revealed many to have specificity for certain red blood cell antigens, usually those of the Rh system. A number of such antibodies have had anti-e(Rh) specificity. Because more than 95% of the population have the red blood cell e antigen, the antibody might be considered a panagglutinin unless careful tests are performed. In other cases antibodies specific for the ubiquitous antigen LW are found. Sometimes spontaneous agglutination of the patient's own red blood cells occurs in all testing sera so that the patient may be mistakenly blood-typed as group AB Rh-positive. In many cases only complement is found on the red blood cells, chiefly the C3 and C4 components. A "broad-spectrum" Coombs serum must be used to detect complement-coated red blood cells. In 80% of acute transient cases only complement-type positive Coombs tests are found, whereas in the chronic variety an IgG or mixed type of Coombs response occurs in over 80% of cases. Occasionally, the Coombs test is negative because of the limited sensitivity of the Coombs reaction. A minimum of 250–500 molecules of IgG is necessary on the red blood cell membrane to produce a positive reaction. Special tests are required to detect the antibody in cases of "Coombs test negative" autoimmune hemolytic anemia.

TREATMENT. Transfusions are usually only of transient benefit but may be required by the severity of the anemia. It may be extremely difficult to find compatible blood; blood in which the red blood cells give the least positive in vitro reaction by the Coombs technique should be chosen. Sometimes it is necessary to give blood that is "incompatible" as judged by the cross-matching. Failure to transfuse a profoundly anemic infant may lead to serious morbidity and even death.

Prednisone or its equivalent should be administered in a dose of 2.5 mg/kg/24 hr. In some patients with severe hemolysis doses up to 6 mg/kg/24 hr of prednisone may be required to reduce the rate of hemolysis. Treatment should be continued until the evidence of hemolysis decreases, and then the dose is gradually reduced. If relapse occurs, resumption of full dosage may be necessary. The disease tends to remit spontaneously within a few weeks or months. The Coombs test result may remain positive even after hemolysis has subsided. When hemolytic anemia remains severe despite corticosteroid therapy or if very large doses are necessary to maintain a reasonable hemoglobin level, splenectomy may be beneficial. Intravenous immunoglobulin and danazol should be tried before splenectomy. Immunosuppressive agents have been of some benefit in chronic cases refractory to conventional therapy. Various plasmaphoresis techniques may be used in refractory cases.

COURSE AND PROGNOSIS. The acute variety of idiopathic autoimmune hemolytic disease in childhood may be severe but is self-limited. The disease may be fulminating; severe cases have been refractory to corticosteroids, immunosuppressive agents, splenectomy, and thymectomy. In immune hemolytic anemia secondary to lymphoma or lupus erythematosus the status of the basic disease determines the prognosis.

16.31 AUTOIMMUNE HEMOLYTIC ANEMIAS ASSOCIATED WITH "COLD" ANTIBODIES

Red blood cell antibodies that are more active at low body temperatures have been called "cold" antibodies. They are of the IgM class and require complement for activity.

Cold Agglutinin Disease

Cold antibodies may be present in low levels in normal blood. Following viral infections or mycoplasmal pneumonia, the levels may increase considerably and occasionally enormous increases may occur, titers of 1:30,000 or greater being recorded. The antibody has specificity for the I antigen and reacts poorly with human cord blood cells possessing the i antigen. Spontaneous agglutination and rouleaux formation are seen on the blood smear. The MCV may be spuriously elevated because of cell agglutination.

When very high titers of cold antibodies are present, severe episodes of intravascular hemolysis with hemoglobinemia and hemoglobinuria may follow exposure of the patient to cold.

Occasionally, patients with infectious mononucleosis develop acute immunohemolytic anemia. The antibodies in these patients have anti-i specificity.

Paroxysmal Cold Hemoglobinuria

This form of hemolytic anemia is associated with a specific type of cold antibody, the Donath-Landsteiner hemolysin, which has anti-P specificity. About one third of cases are associated with either congenital or acquired syphilis. Transfusions are given for severe anemia. Chilling of the patient should be avoided.

16.32 HEMOLYTIC ANEMIAS OF INTOXICATIONS AND INFECTIONS

In sufficiently large doses arsenic and phenylhydrazine produce hemolysis.

Hemolytic anemias may complicate various infections. Direct red blood cell damage by microorganisms or their toxins may be the basis of hemolysis observed in septicemia. Actual parasitism of the red blood cell occurs in malaria and bartonellosis.

JAMES A. STOCKMAN III

GENERAL

Miller DR, Bachner RE, McMillan O: Blood Diseases of Infancy and Childhood, 5th ed. St. Louis, CV Mosby, 1984.
Nathan DG, Oski FA: Hematology of Infancy and Childhood, 3rd ed. Philadelphia, WB Saunders, 1987.
Oski FA, Naiman JL: Hematologic Problems of the Newborn, 3rd ed. Philadelphia, WB Saunders, 1982.
Stockman JA III, Pochedly C: Developmental and Neonatal Hematology. New York, Raven Press, 1988.

RED BLOOD CELLS

Harris JW, Kellermeyer RW: The Red Cell, 2nd ed. Cambridge, Harvard University Press, 1970.

PURE RED BLOOD CELL ANEMIAS

Alter BP: Childhood red cell aplasia. Am J Pediatr Hematol 2:121, 1980.
Glader B, Backer K, Diamond LK: Elevated erythrocyte adenosine deaminase activity in congenital hypoplastic anemia. N Engl J Med 309:1486, 1983.
Halperin DS, Freedman MH: Diamond-Blackfan anemia: Etiology, pathophysiology, and treatment. Am J Pediatr Hematol Oncol 11:380, 1989.
Nathan DG, Clarke BJ, et al: Erythroid precursors in congenital hypoplastic (Diamond-Blackfan) anemia. J Clin Invest 61:489, 1978.
Wang WC, Mentzer WC: Differentiation of transient erythroblastopenia of childhood from congenital hypoplastic anemia. J Pediatr 88:784, 1976.

ANEMIAS OF CHRONIC INFECTIONS, INFLAMMATION, AND RENAL DISEASE

Douglas SW, Adamson JW: The anemia of chronic disorders: Studies of marrow regulation and iron metabolism. Blood 45:55, 1975.
Koerper MA, Stempel DA, Dallmar PR: Anemia in patients with juvenile rheumatoid arthritis. J Pediatr 91:878, 1978.

PHYSIOLOGIC ANEMIA OF INFANCY

Stockman JA, Graeber JE, Clark DA, et al: Anemia of prematurity: Determinants of the erythropoietin response. J Pediatr 105:786, 1984.
Williams ML, Shott RJ, O'Neal PL, et al: Role of dietary iron and fat in vitamin E deficiency of infancy. N Engl J Med 292:887, 1975.

MEGALOBLASTIC ANEMIAS

Haggard ME, Lockhart LH: Megaloblastic anemia and orotic aciduria: An hereditary disorder of pyrimidine metabolism responsive to uridine. Am J Dis Child 113:733, 1967.
Hakami N, Neiman PE: Neonatal megaloblastic anemia due to inherited transcobalamin II deficiency in two siblings. N Engl J Med 285:1163, 1971.
Heisil MA, Siegel SE, Falk RE, et al: Congenital pernicious anemia: Report of seven patients with study of an extended family. J Pediatr 105:564, 1984.
Higgenbottom MC, Swertman L, Nyhan WL: A syndrome of methylmalonic aciduria, homocystinuria megaloblastic anemia and neurologic abnormalities in a vitamin B_{12}-deficient breast-fed infant of a strict vegetarian. N Engl J Med 299:317, 1978.
Hoffbrand AV: Megaloblastic anaemia. Clin Haematol 5:52, 1976.
Lampkin BC, Shore NA, Chadwick D: Megaloblastic anemia of infancy secondary to maternal pernicious anemia. N Engl J Med 274:1168, 1966.
Vrana MB, Carvalho RJ: Thiamine responsive megaloblastic anemia. Sensorineural deafness and diabetes mellitus: A new syndrome. J Pediatr 93:235, 1978.

MICROCYTIC ANEMIA

Committee on Nutrition (AAP): Iron-fortified formulas. Pediatrics 84:1114, 1989.
Humbert JR, Moore LL: Iron deficiency and infection. A dilemma. J Pediatr Gastroenterol Nutr 2:403, 1983.
Oski FA, Honig AS, Helu B: Effect of iron therapy on behavior performance in nonanemic, nondeficient infants. Pediatr 71:877, 1983.
Reeves JD, Vichinsky E, Addiego J Jr, et al: Iron deficiency in health and disease. Adv Pediatr 30:281, 1983.
Wilson JF, Lahey ME, Heiner DC: Studies on iron metabolism. V. Further observations on cow's milk-induced gastrointestinal bleeding. J Pediatr 84:355, 1974.

HEMOLYTIC ANEMIAS

Dacie JV: The Haemolytic Anemias, 3rd ed. New York, Grune & Stratton, 1985.

HEREDITARY SPHEROCYTOSIS

Eber SW, Armbrust R, Schröter W: Variable clinical severity of hereditary spherocytosis: Relation to erythrocytic spectrum concentration, osmotic fragility, and autohemolysis. J Pediatr 117:409, 1990.
Kelleher JH, Lerban NLC, Mortimer PP: Human serum "parvovirus": A specific cause of aplastic crisis in children with hereditary spherocytosis. J Pediatr 102:722, 1983.
Kruger HC, Burgert EO: Hereditary spherocytosis in 100 children. Mayo Clin Proc 41:921, 1966.
Manno CS, Cohen AR: Splenectomy in mild hereditary spherocytosis: Is it worth the risk? Am J Pediatr Hematol Oncol 11:300, 1989.
Trucco JT, Brown AK: Neonatal manifestations of hereditary spherocytosis. Am J Dis Child 113:263, 1967.

HEREDITARY ELLIPTOCYTOSIS

Austin RF, Desforges JF: Hereditary elliptocytosis: An unusual presentation of hemolysis in the newborn associated with transient morphologic abnormalities. Pediatrics 44:196, 1969.
Pearson HA: The genetic basis of hereditary elliptocytosis with hemolysis. Blood 32:972, 1968.

PAROXYSMAL NOCTURNAL HEMOGLOBINURIA

Dacie JV, Lewis SM: Paroxysmal noctural hemoglobinuria: Clinical manifestations, hematology and nature of the disease. Ser Haematol 5:3, 1972.
Miller DR, Baehner RL, Diamond LK: Paroxysmal nocturnal hemoglobinuria in childhood and adolescence. Pediatrics 39:675, 1967.

HEREDITARY STOMATOCYTOSIS

Mentzer WC, Smith WB, Goldstone J, et al: Hereditary stomatocytosis: Membrane and metabolism studies. Blood 46:659, 1975.

ENZYMATIC DEFECTS OF THE RED BLOOD CELL

Beutler E: Abnormalities of the hexose monophosphate shunt. Semin Hematol 8:311, 1971.
Gilman PA: Hemolysis in the newborn resulting from deficiencies of red blood cell enzymes: Diagnosis and management. J Pediatr 84:625, 1974.
Jaffe ER: Hereditary hemolytic disorders and enzymatic deficiencies of human erythrocytes. Blood 35:116, 1970.
Tanaka KR, Paglia DE: Deficiency of pyruvate kinase. Semin Hematol 8:367, 1971.

AUTOIMMUNE HEMOLYTIC ANEMIA

Buchanan GR, Boxer LA, Nathan DG: The acute and transient nature of idiopathic immune hemolytic anemia in childhood. J Pediatr 88:780, 1976.
Garratty G, Petz LD: Drug-induced immune hemolytic anemia. Am J Med 58:398, 1975.
Habibi B, Homberg JC, Schaison G, et al: Autoimmune hemolytic anemia in children. Am J Med 56:61, 1974.
Zuelzer WW, Mastrangelo R, Shulberg CS, et al: Autoimmune hemolytic anemia; natural history and viral-immunologic interactions in childhood. Am J Med 49:80, 1970.

HEMOGLOBIN DISORDERS

Cohen PS, Israel MA: Basic molecular biology for the pediatric hematologist/oncologist. Am J Pediatr Hematol Oncol 11:467, 1989.
Honig GR, Adams JG III: Human Hemoglobin Genetics. Vienna, Springer-Verlag, 1986.

Weatherall DJ, Clegg JB, Higgs DR, et al: The Hemoglobinopathies. *In*: Scriver CR, Beaudet AL, Sly WS, et al (eds): The Metabolic Basis of Inherited Disease, 6th ed. New York, McGraw-Hill, 1989.

SICKLE CELL DISEASE

Charache S, Lubin B, Reid CD (eds): Management and Therapy of Sickle Cell Disease. Washington, DC, United States Department of Health and Human Services, NIH Publ. No. 84-2117, 1984.
Gaston MH, Verter JI, Woods G, et al: Prophylaxis with oral penicillin in children with sickle cell anemia. N Engl J Med 314:1593, 1986.
Honig GR: Sickling syndromes in children. Adv Pediatr 23:271, 1976.
Kinney TR, Ware RE, Schultz PA-C, et al: Long term management of splenic sequestration in children with sickle cell disease. J Pediatr 117:194, 1990.
O'Brien RT, McIntosh S, Aspnes GT, et al: Prospective study of sickle cell anemia in infancy. J Pediatr 89:205, 1976.
Pearson HA, Spencer RP, Cornelius EA: Functional asplenia in sickle cell anemia. N Engl J Med 281:293, 1969.
Saiki RK, Chang C, Levenson CH, et al: Diagnosis of sickle cell anemia and β-thalassemia with enzymatically amplified DNA and nonradioactive allele-specific oligonucleotide probes. N Engl J Med 319:537, 1988.
Scott MT, Hammerschlag MR, Chirgwin SP, et al: Rule of chlamydia pneumoniae in acute chest syndrome of sickle cell disease. J Pediatr 118:30, 1991.
Serjeant GR: Sickle Cell Disease. Oxford, England, Oxford University Press, 1985.
Tsevat J, Wong JB, Pauker SG, et al: Neonatal screening for sickle cell disease: A cost-effectiveness analysis. J Pediatr 118:546, 1991.
Vermylen C, Fernandez Robles E, Ninane J, et al: Bone marrow transplantation in five children with sickle cell anemia. Lancet 1:1427, 1988.
Wethers D, Pearson H, Gaston M: Newborn screening for sickle cell disease and other hemoglobinopathies. Pediatrics 83:813, 1989.

THALASSEMIA

Ehlers RH, Giardena PJ, Lesser ML, et al: Prolonged survival in patients with beta-thalassemia major treated with deferoxamine. J Pediatr 118:540, 1991.
Lucarelli G, Galimberti M, Polchi P, et al: Marrow transplantation in patients with advanced thalassemia. N Engl J Med 316:1050, 1987.
Modell B, Berdoukas V: The Clinical Approach to Thalassaemia. London, Grune & Stratton, 1984.
Piomelli S, Hart D, Graziano J, et al: Current strategies in the management of Cooley's anemia. Ann NY Acad Sci 445:256, 1985.
Weatherall DJ, Clegg JB: The Thalassaemia Syndromes, 3rd ed. Oxford, England, Blackwell Scientific Publications, 1981.
Wolfe L, Olivieri N, Sallan D, et al: Prevention of cardiac disease by subcutaneous deferoxamine in patients with thalassemia major. N Engl J Med 312:1600, 1985.

16.33 POLYCYTHEMIA
(Erythrocytosis)

Polycythemia exists when the red blood cell count, the hemoglobin and hematocrit levels, and the total red blood cell volume significantly exceed the upper limits of normal. In the older child the levels of hemoglobin and hematocrit that can be considered to represent polycythemia are 16 g/dL and 55%, respectively, corresponding to a total red blood cell mass exceeding 35 mL/kg. A decrease in plasma volume, such as occurs in acute dehydration and burns, may result in disproportionately high levels of hemoglobin and hematocrit, but these situations are more accurately designated hemoconcentration than relative polycythemia. The volume of red blood cell mass is not increased; expansion of the plasma volume or rehydration restores the hematocrit to normal levels.

Measurement of the total red blood cell volume by radioisotopic techniques is essential in the differential diagnosis of polycythemia. True polycythemia is characterized by increases of both the total red blood cell and total blood volumes.

SECONDARY POLYCYTHEMIA

Polycythemia may be present in any clinical situation associated with chronic arterial oxygen desaturation. Hypoxia of the kidney results in increased production of erythropoietin, which stimulates increased production of red blood cells and ultimately results in an expanded red blood cell mass. Cardiovascular defects involving right to left shunts and pulmonary diseases interfering with proper oxygenation are the most common causes of secondary polycythemia. Examples of such conditions are cyanotic congenital heart disease, emphysema, and bronchiectasis (Sec. 15.24). Clinical findings usually include cyanosis, hyperemia of sclerae and mucous membranes, and clubbing of the fingers. The red blood cell count and hemoglobin and hematocrit values are all increased. The oxygen saturation of arterial blood is decreased. In children with cardiac lesions causing severe cyanosis, as the hematocrit rises above 65%, symptoms of hyperviscosity may require phlebotomy. On the other hand, such children may also have iron deficiency (as indicated by microcytosis and relatively low hemoglobin levels). The polycythemia associated with cyanotic congenital heart disease is frequently associated with an elevation in the MCV, and an MCV less than or equal to that of the 90th percentile for age is usually microcytic in this circumstance. The risk of intracranial thrombosis has been reported to be increased by such anemia, and iron therapy is indicated. Living at high altitudes also causes a secondary polycythemia; the hemoglobin level increases about 4% for each rise of 1,000 m in altitude.

More subtle forms of hypoxia may also cause polycythemia. Congenital methemoglobinemia resulting from a deficiency of NADH-reactive diaphorase may cause familial cyanosis and polycythemia. This condition is transmitted as an autosomal recessive. Dominantly transmitted cyanosis and polycythemia may be associated with the hemoglobins that have altered oxygen affinity (Sec. 16.23). Transient benign polycythemia is said to occur in otherwise healthy adolescents; this syndrome has not been studied sufficiently to determine its frequency or cause. In several families benign polycythemias seem to have been transmitted as dominant or recessive conditions, the bases of which are not known.

Polycythemia has also been associated with renal tumors and cysts and with vascular tumors of the cerebellum when these tumors have secreted erythropoietin.

When the hematocrit exceeds 65–70% there is a marked increase in blood viscosity, and periodic phlebotomies may be done, blood being replaced with plasma or saline solution.

POLYCYTHEMIA RUBRA VERA
(Erythremia)

This disorder, characterized by polycythemia, leukocytosis, thrombocytosis, and hyperplasia of the bone marrow, has been reported in only a few children. High leukocyte alkaline phosphatase activities and elevated serum vitamin B_{12} levels are characteristic. In contrast to those of normal persons, in vitro cultures of erythroid precursors of affected persons do not require added erythropoietin to stimulate growth.

PLETHORA OF THE NEWBORN

See Sec. 9.48.

THE PANCYTOPENIAS

Aplasia of bone marrow, or replacement of its hematopoietic elements by other tissue, results in profound depression of all the formed elements of the blood. The clinical manifestations that result are anemia, thrombocytopenic hemorrhage, and decreased resistance to infection because of neutropenia. The pancytopenias have traditionally been classified with the anemias, but the consequences of the thrombocytopenia and the neutropenia are much more striking and serious than the anemias. The pancytopenias may be constitutional and genetically determined; may be acquired as a result of damage to the marrow by various chemical or other agents, including viruses; or may result from invasion by abnormal tissue. In these conditions underproduction of blood cells is a result of hypocellularity or replacement of marrow. Examination of an adequate sample of marrow obtained by needle or surgical biopsy is essential to diagnosis.

16.34 CONSTITUTIONAL APLASTIC PANCYTOPENIA

(Fanconi Syndrome)

The constitutional aplastic anemias are familial disorders, believed to be inherited as autosomal recessive conditions with variable penetrance, whose expression may be modified by other genetic and environmental factors. About two thirds of affected children have evident congenital anomalies; especially common are microcephaly, microphthalmia, and absence of the radii and thumbs (Fig. 16–8); abnormalities of the heart and kidney are also relatively common. Short stature is found in more than two thirds of patients, as is generalized hyperpigmentation of the skin. Some affected children have no serious anatomic defects.

Pancytopenia is not usually present at birth or during early infancy. The clinical onset occurs from 1½–22 yr, with an average of 6–8 yr. Bruising caused by thrombocytopenia is noted first, followed by progressively severe anemia and leukopenia.

LABORATORY. Severe pancytopenia is evident in peripheral blood. The red blood cells are macrocytic, with an MCV of 95–105 fL. Macrocytosis may precede the development of aplasia by many years. The bone marrow is strikingly hypocellular, with depression of all cell types and an increase in fatty tissue. Reticulum, plasma, and mast cells are prominent.

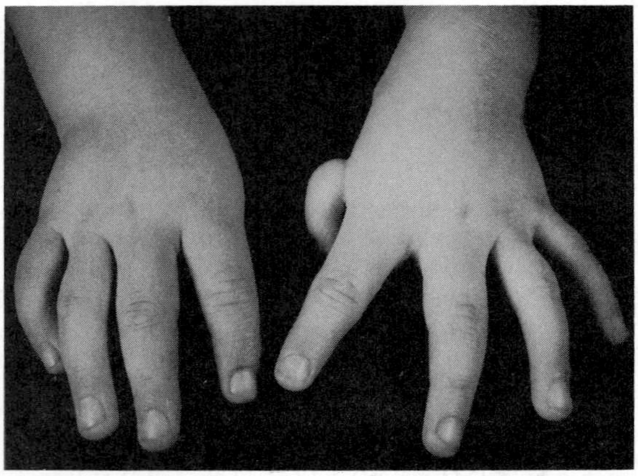

Figure 16–8. Hands of a child with constitutional aplastic pancytopenia. The thumb is absent on the right hand, and is rudimentary on the left hand.

A surgical or needle biopsy of the bone marrow is useful as an adjunct to aspiration, because it provides a large specimen in which to judge cellularity. There is an increase in the percentage of Hb F of 5–15%, which may antedate development of marrow aplasia and cytopenia. A patchy distribution of Hb F within each cell is shown by Kleihauer-Betke preparations. In vitro cultures of bone marrow show decreased numbers of precursors of both erythroid and granulocytic series. Chromosomal studies of blood lymphocytes reveal an abnormally high percentage (10–70%) of chromatid breaks, gaps, rearrangements, exchanges, and endoreduplications (changes seen in fewer than 10% of chromosomes of normal individuals); these changes, too, precede frank pancytopenia. Prenatal diagnosis is often possible once an index case has been detected.

TREATMENT. In addition to symptomatic treatment with blood transfusions and antibiotics, therapy with androgenic steroids is beneficial. Testosterone propionate is given as sublingual tablets in a dose of 1–2 mg/kg/24 hr to a maximum of 60 mg/24 hr. Alternatively, 400–600 mg may be given as an intramuscular injection every 4 wk. Synthetic androgen derivatives such as oxymetholone and stanozolol are also effective. Relatively small doses of corticosteroids, such as 5–10 mg of prednisone or its equivalent, are also given to reduce the tendency to bruising and bleeding and to retard acceleration of bone age. In most patients a hematologic response becomes evident within 2–4 mo. The marrow develops greater cellularity, and the hemoglobin rises. The response of the neutrophils is usually less complete, and platelets may show only moderate increases in numbers. When the hemoglobin has reached normal levels, it is sometimes possible to reduce the dose of androgen, but, if the drug is too rapidly or drastically decreased, relapse occurs. Most patients require continuous therapy to maintain hematologic response, and many ultimately become refractory to androgen therapy.

These effective doses of androgen regularly produce signs and symptoms of masculinization, including acne, hirsutism, deepening of the voice, and enlargement of the penis or clitoris. Synthetic androgen derivatives have fewer of these side effects, but some degree of masculinization is probably inevitable. Some of the testosterone preparations have hepatic toxicity. Prior to the advent of testosterone therapy these patients usually died during late childhood of hemorrhage, infection, or the complications of multiple transfusions. Hemorrhagic cysts of the liver (peliosis hepatis) and malignant hepatomas occur with increased frequency in patients receiving prolonged treatment with large doses of oral synthetic androgens. Bone marrow transplantation can be considered when a histocompatible sibling is available. Acute myelogenous leukemia (AML) develops in 5–10% of patients with Fanconi anemia, and their close relatives are at increased risk of AML.

Fanconi anemia must be differentiated from dyskeratosis congenita, a rare form of ectodermal dysplasia. Cutaneous hyperpigmentation, pancytopenia, and short stature occur in both conditions. Skeletal and renal anomalies do not regularly occur in dyskeratosis congenita.

16.35 ACQUIRED APLASTIC PANCYTOPENIAS

A number of physical, chemical, and infectious agents may severely damage the bone marrow and lead to severe pancytopenia. Some of these agents produce marrow aplasia in any person who is exposed to them in a sufficient dose. Such obligate marrow depressants include ionizing radiation; chemotherapeutic drugs, such as nitrogen mustard, 6-mercaptopurine, and methotrexate; and certain organic solvents, especially benzene. A 2nd group of agents produces aplastic pancytopenia only in a small (often remarkably small) number of persons exposed to them. In these persons the adverse hematologic reactions must reflect idiosyncrasies. The drug most frequently associated with aplastic pancytopenia is chloramphenicol. It has been estimated that only 1 in 24,000–60,000 patients taking chloramphenicol suffers marrow aplasia, but this drug has been involved in more than 50% of drug-related aplastic pancytopenias. Other drugs associated with appreciable incidences of marrow aplasia are sulfonamides, phenylbutazone, and certain anticonvulsants. Severe infections may also produce severe marrow damage, but it is often difficult to decide whether the infection represents cause or effect. Some cases of marrow aplasia or hypoplasia have followed instances of apparent infectious hepatitis (usually non-A–non-B hepatitis), as well as parvovirus infection, and it has been reported to follow infectious mononucleosis or appear as a complication of pregnancy. In about 50% of cases of aplastic pancytopenia no history of exposure to toxins or other agents can be elicited; these cases are usually called idiopathic, but the possibility of an environmental factor cannot be excluded.

CLINICAL AND LABORATORY FINDINGS. Hemorrhage secondary to thrombocytopenia is usually the 1st clinical manifestation. The signs and symptoms of anemia and neutropenia become apparent later. The spleen and lymph nodes are not enlarged. Profound decreases in red cells, platelets, and neutrophils are observed. The marrow aspirate is scanty; the particles are fatty; and lymphocytes, plasma cells, and reticulum cells predominate. Culture of bone marrow reveals decreased numbers of progenitor stem cells of the erythroid and granulocytic series. Chromosome configuration is normal. Levels of Hb F may be above 2%; reports that elevated levels of Hb F indicate a good prognosis are not confirmed. T-lymphocyte suppressor cells active against both erythroid and granulocytic colony growth have been found in some patients.

TREATMENT. The patient must immediately be removed from contact with any potentially toxic drugs or agents. When the onset of the disease is acute, with massive hemorrhage and serious sepsis, aggressive therapy with platelet concentrates and antibiotics is necessary; the choice of antibiotic should be based on bacterial culture and sensitivity tests. Even with the best of supportive therapy the prognosis of severe aplastic pancytopenia is grave. As many as two thirds of patients succumb within 6 mo of diagnosis, and fewer than 10–20% recover. Reports of success with androgen and corticosteroid therapy in acquired aplastic pancytopenia have not been confirmed by more recent studies. Other forms of therapy are of dubious value.

Controlled studies indicate that when an HLA-compatible sibling is available as a donor, bone marrow transplantation is effective (Sec. 6.42). Siblings of patients with severe pancytopenia who have markedly hypocellular bone marrows should be examined for both HLA and MLC compatibility. If compatibility between patient and sibling is established, bone marrow transplantation, after suitable immunosuppression, can be considered. About 50–80% of transplanted patients accept the donor marrow and have restoration of normal peripheral blood values. Graft-versus-host disease is common and may be severe. Currently, bone marrow transplantation, when possible, is the treatment of choice in refractory severe cases.

Hematologic improvement in severe aplastic pancytopenia after unsuccessful marrow transplantation and intense immunosuppressive therapy indicates that some patients may have an immunologic basis for their bone marrow depression. Criteria identifying patients who should be treated with immunosuppressive therapy alone have not been defined, but successful treatment with anti-thymocyte globulin (ATG), anti-lymphocyte globulin (ALG), high-dose dexamethasone, and cyclosporine is being increasingly reported. Alternatively, clinical trials are now underway to determine the effectiveness of granulocyte-macrophage colony-stimulating factor (GM-CSF), produced by recombinant technology, in cases of moderate to severe aplastic anemia.

COURSE. Unless marrow engraftment is possible or the patient responds to immunotherapy, approximately a third of patients die quickly as a result of hemorrhage and infection. *Pseudomonas* and staphylococcal septicemias are common causes of death (Sec. 12.13). The remaining two thirds of children have a subacute clinical course. In some of these androgen therapy may be beneficial. Half of this group ultimately recover completely; the other half have a chronic course, many succumbing to sepsis and hemorrhage months or years after onset. Leukemia and paroxysmal nocturnal hemoglobinuria have developed in some children after recovery from aplastic pancytopenia.

16.36 PANCYTOPENIA CAUSED BY MARROW REPLACEMENT

Diffuse replacement of bone marrow by nonhematopoietic tissue results in peripheral pancytopenia. Neuroblastoma is the childhood tumor that most frequently metastasizes to the bone marrow. Osteopetrosis is frequently associated with anemia and thrombocytopenia because of marrow obliteration; an element of hypersplenism may also be present. In these diseases the red blood cell morphology is frequently abnormal, showing teardrop forms and ovalocytes. Nucleated red blood cells are noted in the blood. Bone marrow transplantation has been used successfully in a small number of patients with severe osteopetrosis. Acute leukemia occasionally presents pancytopenia with a reticular appearance of the initially aspirated marrow. Adequate sampling or biopsy of the marrow from other sites will usually provide the correct diagnosis. A short trial of corticosteroid therapy that results in rapid return of the blood counts to normal favors a diagnosis of leukemia.

Myelofibrosis has occurred in a few infants and children, presenting as severe anemia with abnormal forms (teardrops, ovalocytes), nucleated red blood cells, and high white blood cell counts (leukoerythroblastic anemia), and with enlarged liver and spleen resulting from extramedullary erythropoiesis. Pancytopenia also occurs in familial and acquired (CMV, EBV) *hemophagocytic syndromes.*

TRANSFUSIONS

The most important indications for transfusions are restoration of blood volume and treatment of shock following acute blood loss, and provision of red blood cells for maintenance of the blood hemoglobin level. An individual component of blood, such as red blood cells, platelets, plasma, or specific plasma proteins, may often be used effectively in place of whole blood.

16.37 INDICATIONS FOR TRANSFUSION

ACUTE HEMORRHAGE

The signs and symptoms accompanying hemorrhage vary with the magnitude and rapidity of the blood loss. When 15–20% or more of the circulating blood volume is acutely lost, tachycardia, hypotension, and shock may develop, accompanied by weakness, restlessness, and syncope. Immediately after acute hemorrhage the hemoglobin or hematocrit level may be deceptively high, but hemodilution soon reduces this to a value that reflects the magnitude of the blood loss. Thrombocytosis and neutrophilia occur within a few hours and reticulocytosis within a few days of an acute bleeding episode. The most common causes of severe acute hemorrhage are trauma and gastrointestinal bleeding from peptic ulcers, Meckel diverticulum, and esophageal varices. In patients with defects of the hemostatic mechanism, exsanguinating hemorrhage may occur from nosebleeds or gastritis.

Severe bleeding in the perinatal period may result in the clinical picture of asphyxia pallida. Pallor, shock, tachycardia, and low venous pressures are seen. External hemorrhage may occur from the umbilicus or the gastrointestinal tract. The fetus may bleed before and during birth into the maternal circulation, and fetofetal transfusions may occur between identical twins.

LABORATORY FINDINGS. The anemia of acute blood loss is usually normochromic and normocytic. Depending on the duration of the hemorrhage and timing of the tests, compensatory reticulocytosis and normoblastemia may be seen. In the newborn infant with hemorrhage, the Coombs test result is generally negative and the level of serum bilirubin low. With loss of blood from fetus to mother, maternal blood contains a minor population of red blood cells that contain Hb F (Kleihauer-Betke technique).

TREATMENT. When possible, local measures to control the hemorrhage should be taken. Whole blood transfusions should be given to restore blood volume and treat shock; 20 mL/kg of blood should be administered initially. The need for additional blood is determined by the clinical response and by physical and laboratory findings. Plasma or plasma expanders may be used to sustain the patient in shock until blood can be made available, but, if the blood loss has been great, red cell replacement will be necessary.

CHRONIC ANEMIAS

With anemias that develop slowly and stabilize at hemoglobin levels of 6–9 g/dL, the patient may have remarkably few symptoms, and transfusions are not routinely indicated. When such anemias result from deficiency of a specific factor, such as folic acid or iron, a rapid response follows replacement therapy. Transfusion is indicated only if the anemia is profound or if infections or other complications are present. No firm rule can be made as to the hemoglobin level at which transfusion is recommended. Some children with iron deficiency anemia may have hemoglobin levels of 4–5 g/dL with few signs of clinical or cardiorespiratory distress. A reasonable estimate of the effect of transfusion of packed red blood cells is that the increase in hematocrit (%) equals the mL/kg of packed cells given. For example, if 5 mL/kg of packed cells is given, the recipient's hematocrit rises about 5%. The formula assumes a recipient blood volume of about 75 mL/kg and a hematocrit of about 75% for packed red blood cells.

In progressive refractory anemias such as thalassemia major and pure red blood cell anemias, transfusions are necessary to sustain life. Packed red blood cells, especially leukocyte-poor or glycerol-frozen preparations, are preferred for control of such chronic anemias because they reduce the frequency of febrile reactions secondary to development of leukoagglutinins. The maximal dose of packed red blood cells to be given in one transfusion is 15 mL/kg; if signs suggestive of incipient congestive heart failure are present, considerably smaller amounts should be used. In extreme anemia with secondary heart failure, multiple small transfusions of 2–4 mL/kg of packed red blood cells may be helpful, and the simultaneous use of furosemide may be considered. If frank congestive heart failure is present, exchange transfusion should be considered, replacing the patient's blood isovolumetrically with packed red cells. Digitalis is of limited value.

16.38 USE OF BLOOD FRACTIONS

PLATELET TRANSFUSIONS

Platelets may be transfused to attain temporary hemostasis in some patients with thrombocytopenic hemorrhage. The life span of transfused platelets is normally 9–10 days. Although administration of fresh whole blood produces inconsequential rises in the recipient's platelet count, clinical hemorrhage may be controlled. Use of platelet-rich plasma or platelet concentrates prepared from fresh blood drawn in plastic equipment permits attainment of more nearly normal platelet counts. It is desirable to use platelets that are ABO- and Rh-compatible, but it is frequently impossible to do so. Infusion of platelet concentrates from incompatible donors rarely produces problems, but, because these concentrates contain red cells, those from Rh-positive donors should not be given to Rh-negative recipients. Transfusion of platelets that are HLA-compatible does not readily evoke isoimmunization and results in more satisfactory platelet survival. Platelet transfusions are temporarily beneficial in thrombocytopenias because of inadequate production, such as hypoplastic pancytopenia and leukemia, but are useless or of only transient value in states characterized by peripheral hyperdestruction of platelets such as idiopathic thrombocytopenic purpura. In addition, isoantibodies to platelet antigens are frequently formed after transfusions of platelets from multiple donors. With successive platelet transfusions, decreasing therapeutic responses are noted. Transfusion of 1 unit of platelet concentrate can be expected to produce an increment in platelet count of about $100{,}000/mm^3$ in the newborn and about $10{,}000\ mm^3$ in the adult.

GRANULOCYTE TRANSFUSIONS

Because of the brief intravascular life span and low concentration of granulocytes in normal blood, transfusions of normal whole blood have no practical value in supplying white blood cells. Extraction of large numbers of polymorphonuclear leukocytes from normal donors can be accomplished with continuous flow blood separators employing differential centrifugation or nylon fiber filter systems. Double-flow plasmapheresis and continuous flow centrifugation techniques are also used to harvest large numbers of granulocytes from single donors. Administration of granulocytes lowers mortality in profoundly leukopenic patients with gram-negative sepsis and is used in the management of febrile and infected patients with severe potentially self-limited neutropenia resulting from cancer chemotherapy or bone marrow transplantation. Granulocyte transfusions have been used for treatment of septic newborns who have neutropenia and depletion of granulocyte reserves (Sec. 9.60).Granulocyte colony stimulating factor augmentation of neutrophil production may be an alternate to granulocyte transfusion.

PLASMA AND PLASMA CONCENTRATES

In acute dehydration, in which the plasma volume is decreased but the red blood cell mass is adequate, plasma can be used effectively to expand the blood volume and to restore circulation and renal blood flow. The usual dose of plasma is 10 mL/kg. Other solutions (crystalloids, colloids) are also recommended, as they are equally effective but have no risks of infection. The use of fresh plasma and of concentrates of plasma such as factor VIII and fibrinogen preparations for bleeding disorders is described elsewhere.

16.39 SPECIAL CONSIDERATIONS

CHOICE OF BLOOD FOR TRANSFUSION

Storage of blood at 4° C results in a decrease in red blood cell viability that is proportional to the length of storage time. When blood is given for acute hemorrhage, this is of no consequence, but for children who must receive transfusions repeatedly the blood selected should be as fresh as possible.

A citrate-phosphate-dextrose mixture with added adenine (CPDA) has supplanted ACD as the standard anticoagulant because it better maintains red cell viability and function.

Blood for transfusion should be of the same blood group (O, A, B, or AB) as the recipient's. The donor red blood cells should always be tested for compatibility with the recipient's plasma (major cross-matching) by the Coombs technique. Compatibility for the Rh antigens between donor and recipient is desirable. Rh-negative (d/d) persons should never receive Rh-positive blood, but the reverse is permissible. Considerable battlefield experience indicates that the use of so-called universal donor blood (group O Rh-negative blood with a low titer of anti-A and anti-B isohemagglutinins) is safe but, with adequate modern blood banking facilities, this is rarely necessary except in an emergency.

RISKS OF BLOOD TRANSFUSION

Although modern technology has made blood transfusion a generally safe procedure, a definite risk is involved. Transfusions should be given, therefore, only when the benefit to the patient exceeds the inherent danger of the procedure. It has been estimated that 1 of every 2,000 persons receiving a blood transfusion has a severe reaction as a result of the immediate procedure or its consequences. Problems may arise for various reasons.

CLERICAL ERRORS. The mislabeling or faulty identification of containers may lead to a patient's receiving the wrong blood. If a type O patient receives type A or B blood, fatal intravascular hemolysis may occur.

RED BLOOD CELL ISOIMMUNIZATION. In almost every blood transfusion the donor red blood cells have some antigen factor that the recipient does not possess. Many such factors are poor antigens, but some evoke intense antibody formation, the immunized persons being at increased risk if another transfusion is given.

HEPATITIS (see Sec. 12.79 and 13.94). A small proportion of the normal population are asymptomatic carriers of agents for serum hepatitis. In the United States the routine screening of blood for hepatitis B surface antigen (HB_sAg) prior to transfusion has significantly reduced the risk for transfusion-related hepatitis B, but only about one third of donors who can transmit serum hepatitis have demonstrable hepatitis B-associated antigen (Australia antigen, HB_sAg) in their blood. Currently, the most common cause of transfusional hepatitis is designated hepatitis C virus (see Sec. 12.79 and 13.94); it has a variable incubation period and is usually clinically mild. It seems to be fairly common and is often manifested by elevated levels of AST (SGOT) and ALT (SGPT). The incidence of post-transfusion hepatitis C may be reduced by prescreening donor units. Use of frozen red blood cells is believed to reduce the risk of hepatitis. Syphilis, malaria, toxoplasmosis, Chagas disease, cytomegalovirus, and other infections can also be transmitted by blood transfusion (see Sec. 13.94)..

ACQUIRED IMMUNODEFICIENCY SYNDROME (AIDS). AIDS was first reported in homosexual men and intravenous drug users. Later, cases were found among recipients of blood transfusions and hemophiliacs who had received factor VIII concentrate. The cause of AIDS is human immunodefiency virus (HIV) (see Sec. 12.83).

In the spring of 1985 blood banks in the United States began testing all donor blood for antibodies against HIV, using an enzyme-linked immunosorbent assay (ELISA) that is believed to identify almost all potentially infectious blood. This procedure, with the exclusion of high-risk persons from the donor population, markedly reduces the risk of contracting this disease through transfusions.

CYTOMEGALOVIRUS (CMV) INFECTION. Severe transfusion-transmitted CMV infections characterized by pneumonia, hepatitis, thrombocytopenia, and hemolytic anemia have been described in premature infants receiving blood from CMV-seropositive donors. Use of seronegative donors markedly reduces the incidence of this disease (see Sec. 9.69 and 12.71).

WHITE BLOOD CELL, PLATELET, AND PLASMA PROTEIN IMMUNIZATION. White blood cells, platelets, and some of the serum proteins have polymorphic antigens; multiple transfusions may be associated with development of antibodies against these components.

CIRCULATORY OVERLOAD. Patients with chronic anemia have expanded plasma volume and increased cardiac output, so infusion of blood or plasma may precipitate congestive heart failure; rapid administration of large volumes of blood should be avoided.

DEPLETION OF LABILE SUBSTANCES. Storage of blood is associated with loss of platelets and decreasing activities of the labile coagulation factors, such as factor VIII, 75% of which is lost after 7 days of storage. When massive or exchange transfusions of stored blood are given, a complex disturbance of hemostasis may ensue. The use of fresh blood avoids these complications. As a general rule, when multiple transfusions are given in a short period of time, every 4th unit of blood should be fresh. Reconstitution of packed red cells with fresh-frozen plasma is also effective. Acute citrate toxicity may occur.

IRON OVERLOAD. Each 500 mL of blood contains about 200 mg of iron. Patients with refractory anemias who need frequent transfusion ultimately have hemosiderosis. Iron deposited in skin, liver, spleen, and other organs may interfere with normal function (Sec. 16.27).

REACTIONS TO BLOOD TRANSFUSION

ALLERGIC REACTIONS. These are associated with 1–2% of transfusions. The most common manifestation is urticaria with itching; occasionally, wheezing and arthralgia occur. The mechanism of these reactions is not certain, but they may be caused by the presence of allergenic substances or by antibodies in the donor plasma. The development of urticaria alone does not necessitate discontinuing the transfusion; therapy with antihistamines or corticosteroids is effective in treating or preventing this type of reaction.

FEBRILE REACTIONS. The use of disposable plastic equipment has eliminated most external pyrogenic substances. Sensitization to white blood cell antigens may produce febrile reactions characterized by shaking chills and an increase in temperature of 1–2° C (2–4° F) beginning during or shortly after the transfusion and lasting only a few hours. The use of washed, leukocyte-poor packed cells excluding the buffy coat, and liberal dosage of salicylates may reduce these reactions. White blood cell filters may be used at transfusion in patients with a prior history of transfusion reactions. Use of reconstituted frozen red blood cells may greatly ameliorate severe febrile reactions. Rarely, a unit of blood may be contaminated with bacteria. Severe febrile reactions, shock, and death may occur if infected blood is transfused. Because it is difficult to differentiate febrile from hemolytic reactions, blood transfusions should be promptly discontinued if fever and chills occur during their administration.

HEMOLYTIC TRANSFUSION REACTIONS. Hemolytic reactions result in massive intravascular destruction of red blood cells, manifested clinically by fever, chills, headache, and back pain. These symptoms do not appear when the patient is anesthetized. In severe reactions, shock and acute renal failure may ensue. Hemoglobinemia and hemoglobinuria are usually observed. When a hemolytic reaction is suspected, the transfusion should be *terminated immediately*. Diagnosis is proved by re-examining the blood types of donor cells and of the recipient, repeating the cross-matching, and examining plasma and urine for free hemoglobin. A diuresis should be established by fluid therapy and administration of mannitol. The patient generally survives the initial acute episode; if a period of renal failure can be adequately managed, recovery is the rule. Less acute reactions are possible and suggested by a poor increment in post-transfusion hemoglobin.

GRAFT-VERSUS-HOST DISEASE. This may occur in patients having primary or acquired immunodeficiency states. Irradiation of donor units eliminates this risk. Because of the relative immaturity of the immune system of neonates, some centers routinely irradiate all donor units of blood or blood components containing any lymphocytes before infusion into these infants.

JAMES A. STOCKMAN III

POLYCYTHEMIA

Hathaway WE: Neonatal hyperviscosity. Pediatrics 72:567, 1983.
Michael AF Jr, Mauer AM: Maternal-fetal transfusion as a cause of plethora in the neonatal period. Pediatrics 28:458, 1961.
Natelson EA, Lynch EC: Polycythemia vera in childhood. Am J Dis Child 122:241, 1971.
Ramamurthy RS, Brans YW: Neonatal polycythemia. 1. Criteria for diagnosis and therapy. Pediatrics 68:168, 1981.
Weinberger MM, Oleinick A: Congenital marrow dysfunction in Down's syndrome. J Pediatrics 77:273, 1970.

THE PANCYTOPENIAS

Alter BP, Potter NU: Classification and aetiology of the aplastic anemias. Clin Haematol 7:431, 1978.
Baron F, Sybert VP, Andrews RG: Cutaneous neutrophilic infiltrates (Sweet syndrome) in three patients with Fanconi anemia. J Pediatr 115:726, 1989.
Bloom GE, Warner S, Gerald PS, et al: Chromosome abnormalities in constitutional aplastic anemia. N Engl J Med 274:8, 1966.
Champlain R, Ho W, Gale RP: Antithymocyte globulin treatment in patients with aplastic anemia. N Engl J Med 308:113, 1983.
Gordon-Smith EC: Treatment of aplastic anemias. Hosp Pract 20:69, 1985.
Nienhuis AW: Hematopoietic growth factors: Biologic complexity and clinical promise. N Engl J Med 318:916, 1988.
Storb R: Bone marrow transplantation for severe aplastic anemia. Semin Hematol 21:27, 1984.
Vowels MR: Recent advances in bone marrow transplantation. Aust Pediatr J 23:315, 1987.
Williams DM, Lynch RE, Cartwright GE: Drug-induced aplastic anemia. Semin Hematol 10:195, 1973.

TRANSFUSIONS

Bove JR: Practical Blood Transfusion, 3rd ed. Boston, Little, Brown, 1986.
Bucholz DM: Pediatric transfusion therapy. J Pediatr 84:1, 1974.
Christiansen RD, Rothstern G, Anstall HB: Granulocyte transfusions in neonates with bacterial infection, neutropenia, and depletion of mature marrow neutrophils. Pediatrics 70:1, 1982.
Frickhofen N, Kaltwasser JP, Schrezenmeier H, et al: Treatment of aplastic anemia with antilymphocyte globulin and methylprednisolone with or without cyclosporine. N Engl J Med 324:1297, 1991.
Herzig RH, Herzig GP, Graw RG, et al: Successful granulocyte transfusion therapy for gram-negative septicemia. N Engl J Med 296:701, 1977.
Mollison PL: Blood Transfusion in Clinical Medicine, 7th ed. London, Blackwell, 1983.
Platelet transfusion therapy (Editorial). Lancet 2:490, 1987.
Wheeler JG: Buffy coat transfusions in neonates with sepsis and neutrophil storage depletion. Pediatrics 79:422, 1987.
Yeager AS, Grumet FC, Hafleigh EB: Prevention of transfusion-acquired cytomegalovirus infections in newborn infants. J Pediatr 98:281, 1981.
Zuck TF: Transfusion-transmitted AIDS revisited. N Engl J Med 318:511, 1988.

16.40 DISORDERS OF THE LEUKOCYTES

See also Sec. 11.29–11.33.

The leukocytes are divided into major classes: the granulocytes, consisting of the neutrophils, eosinophils, and basophils, and the mononuclear nongranulated lymphocytes and monocytes. Leukocytes have cellular antigens distinct from those of the erythrocyte. The most important leukocyte functions are concerned with resistance to infection and disposal of products of cellular breakdown. Because characteristic changes occur in many diseases, the leukocyte and differential counts are important as general screening tests. The normal values are listed in Table 16–2.

16.41 TYPES OF LEUKOCYTES

See Sec. 11.29.

NEUTROPHILS. The neutrophils are the predominating type of granulocyte. The nuclei of the cells have one to five segments, the the designation polymorphonuclear leukocytes. Qualitatively, neutrophils are the most important phagocytic cells that defend the host against acute bacterial infection. They are formed in the bone marrow and are released to circulate in the bloodstream.

The mechanisms by which the neutrophil is attracted to, identifies, and destroys its target are beginning to be understood. Antigens or pathogens interact with protein in the serum to form chemotactic factors, and the diffusion of these factors creates a gradient that mechanically attracts neutrophils to the involved site. Many substances can attract neutrophils. An activated complement fragment, C5a, is the most potent chemotactic factor; other factors include platelet products (e.g., platelet-activating factor, PAF) and products released by the neutrophil itself, such as leukotriene B_4 (LTB_4). The neutrophil responds to these stimuli through specific receptors on its surface. Following activation of the receptor, the neutrophils change their shape and the number of receptors increases, which may amplify the process. After attachment of a chemotactic factor to its receptor, the surface potential of the cell changes within 10 sec. There is also an increase in intracellular calcium, which precedes the functional responses.

Receptor stimulation is probably transduced into functional responses by guanine nucleotide binding proteins that regulate the activation of phospholipase C. Activated phospholipase C cleaves 1-phosphatidyl-D-myoinositol 4,5-bisphosphate (PIP_2) into the secondary messengers inositol triphosphate and diacylglycerol, which cause the activation of protein kinase C and increase intracellular calcium. Another consequence of PIP_2 hydrolysis is the release of arachidonic acid. The generation of LTB_4 increases calcium flux, and it also functions as a chemotaxin. These events lead to shape changes, motility, degranulation, adhesiveness, and the respiratory burst.

The mechanism by which the neutrophil moves is unclear, but it involves a change in the configuration of actin, myosin, and microtubules within the cell cytoplasm. These substances are also important in degranulation, in which products of primary (azurophilic) and secondary (specific) granules are released into phagosomes and externally. Primary granules contain enzymes important for the bactericidal action of the neutrophil (e.g., elastase, myeloperoxidase, defensins). Secondary granules contain receptors that are transferred to the cell surface (e.g., C3bi) and substances crucial to the inflammatory response (e.g., collagenase, lactoferrin, complement activators). The membranes of the specific granules contain the glycoprotein receptors involved in neutrophil adhesion and ingestion of complement-coated microbes (e.g., C3bi). In addition to degranulating within seconds of stimulation, the neutrophil increases its oxygen consumption and generates toxic oxygen metabolites (respiratory burst). These toxic metabolites are important in killing bacteria and in activating antiproteases. A plasma membrane enzyme (NADPH oxidase) generates superoxide ($O_2^{\cdot-}$). $O_2^{\cdot-}$ is converted to hydrogen peroxide by superoxide dismutase. More toxic oxygen metabolites such as hypochlorous acid can also then be generated through the interaction with myeloperoxidase.

Disorders of adherence, cell motility, chemotaxis, opsonization, ingestion, degranulation, and the respiratory burst have been described. Generally, these disorders are suggested by recurrent continuous, peridontal, respiratory, or soft-tissue infections. Infections occur secondary to *Staphylococcus aureus*, gram-negative bacilli, and occasionally *Candida albicans*. Treatment involves surgical drainage and antibiotics.

Neutrophils become available to the blood and tissues as a result of an intricately regulated kinetic pattern. The enormous total body neutrophil pool is divided into two compartments: a bone marrow compartment contains the stem cells from which the myeloid series originates; the blood compartment is divided almost equally into a circulating blood-neutrophil pool and a marginated blood-neutrophil pool. In the marginated pool, cells adhere to postcapillary venules and are in constant equilibrium with the circulating pool. Therefore, the total measurable neutrophil pool of blood at any given time usually reflects only a minor portion of the cells available for host defenses. In addition, the body provides a steady supply of neutrophils from the bone marrow reserve pool. The size of the marrow reserve pool is 10 times that of the circulating pool. This is essential, because neutrophils have a rapid turnover rate and a relatively short half-life in the blood (6–7 hr). It has been estimated that it takes 6–11 days for a cell to pass through the various stages of differentiation, from a myeloblast to a mature neutrophil emerging into the peripheral blood.

Although the mechanisms involved in the normal disappearance of neutrophils in the circulation are poorly understood, more is known about the mechanisms that allow neutrophils to migrate from the blood into the tissues at the site of inflammation. Within minutes of tissue damage or pathogenic invasion, neutrophils adhere to the endothelium of vessel walls and subsequently migrate into involved tissues. The neutrophils pass through blood vessel walls by projecting pseudopods between the vascular endothelial cells and actually forcing their way out. The migration of neutrophils out of the circulation into the tissue is considered an end stage of kinetics, because there is no substantial return of these cells to the blood. Labelled neutrophils appear in the liver, spleen, lung, gastrointestinal tract, and urine, which represent sites where neutrophils are normally lost from the circulation.

Leukocytosis occurs rapidly during infection and persists as a result of several changes in the kinetics of myelopoiesis. During acute infection neutrophils arise from the bone marrow reserve pool, which can temporarily augment the supply of circulating neutrophils in response to an infection before an increased number of mature cells can be derived from dividing myeloid cells. Mitotic division also occurs in the myeloblast, promyelocytes, and myelocytes in the bone marrow. The transit time through the maturational pool (i.e., from myelocyte to segmented forms) decreases from 6 to 2 days, and there is also increased mitosis and decreased transit time in the proliferating pool of neutrophil precursors in the bone marrow. Increased stem cell division leads to more mature neutrophils, but there is a 9 to 11-day lag before peripheral blood neutrophilia occurs from this source.

Adequacy of the marrow storage compartment can be estimated by changes in the blood leukocyte count after intravenous administration of corticosteroids. Normally, a 2 to 4-fold increase in the numbers of circulating neutrophils results from such stimulated release of cells from the marrow storage compartment. In states of marrow hypoplasia no release occurs.

Neutrophil formation and regulation can be assessed by culturing cells in semisolid agar gel. Normal bone marrow contains a small number of colony-forming units—granulocyte-macrophage (CFU-GM) and colony-forming units—granulocyte (CFU-G). In tissue culture the CFU resembles a primitive blast cell and forms aggregates of granulocytes when under stimulation of a hormone-like glycoprotein that has been designated granulocyte colony-stimulating factor (G-CSF). The CFU-GM can often be distinguished from eosinophil progenitors and appear to arise independently from primitive pleuripotential stem cells. Diversity is the hallmark of the progenitor cell population because some stem cells give rise not only to individual colonies of neutrophils and eosinophils, but also to mixed colonies of neutrophils and macrophages or neutrophils and eosinophils under stimulation of the hormone-like protein granulocyte-macrophage colony-stimulating factor (GM-CSF). Both GM-CSF and G-CSF are now available as recombinant proteins and are being evaluated in the therapy of patients with neutropenia.

EOSINOPHILS. Eosinophils are characterized by large coarse granules of prominent red color (with Romanowsky stain) and by a nucleus with one or two segments. They normally account for fewer than 5% of circulating leukocytes. Eosinopenia may be produced by at least two mechanisms: (1) acute stress, with the resultant stimulation of adrenocorticoids or release of epinephrine, or both; and (2) acute inflammatory states. Eosinophil counts are increased in parasitic infections, allergic phenomena, or dermatologic conditions. Other causes of eosinophilia include gastrointestinal disorders, Hodgkin's disease, and immune deficiency diseases, and it can occur during convalescence from viral diseases. The most pronounced eosinophilia encountered in the United States accompanies invasion of the tissues by parasitic helminths, and from such diseases as visceral larva migrans and trichinosis. Hypereosinophilic syndrome refers to a broad continuum of illnesses varying from Loeffler syndrome (Sec. 14.66) to severe chronic and ultimately fatal eosinophilic leukemia.

BASOPHILS. These leukocytes are distinguished by coarse, deep blue granules that fill the cytoplasm and obscure the nucleus. The granules contain large amounts of heparin and histamine. Basophils account for 0.5% of total leukocytes. Increases occur in those with chronic myelogenous leukemia, ulcerative colitis, juvenile rheumatoid arthritis, iron deficiency, and chronic renal failure, and following radiation therapy.

LYMPHOCYTES. Lymphocytes constitute 30–60% of the blood leukocytes. Most are small cells measuring 9 μm in diameter with a round, dark, blue-black nucleus and thin blue cytoplasm. Lymphocytes are actively motile but not phagocytic. Lymphocytes can be characterized as T or B lymphocytes or natural killer cells on the basis of physical and immunologic properties (Sec. 11.2). Marked absolute lymphocytosis can be seen in certain acute infections such as pertussis, infectious mononucleosis, and acute infectious lymphocytosis. Acute infections with moderate relative lymphocytosis include the common childhood exanthems and other viral illnesses, brucellosis, and typhoid and paratyphoid fevers. Chronic infections, drug and allergic reactions, leukemia, thyrotoxicosis, and Addison disease may also be associated with lymphocytosis. Thymic alymphoplasia is associated with profound lymphopenia.

MONOCYTES. These large phagocytic cells are characterized by a large lobulated nucleus and abundant gray cytoplasm that contains fine azurophilic granules. They normally account for 1–5% of the circulating leukocytes. The blood monocyte is an important component of the body's phagocytic system and is derived from the bone marrow stem cell. There is no substantial bone marrow reserve pool of monocytes, and mature monocytes are released into the bloodstream several days earlier than the bone marrow neutrophils. Consequently, during recovery from bone marrow aplasia or hypoplasia, a relative monocytosis of the peripheral blood may herald the return of neutrophils. This is most commonly noted in patients recovering from the use of chemotherapeutic agents.

In the bloodstream the monocyte functions as a phagocytic cell, similarly to the neutrophil. The half-life of blood monocytes is 8 hr. Unlike the neutrophil, monocytes at inflammatory sites undergo a wide variety of phagocytic functions in response to bacterial products, particularly lipopolysaccharides. Despite its impressive ability to enhance its phagocytic function, the monocyte cannot replace the neutrophil as the primary phagocytic cell, because it moves more slowly than the neutrophil.

After leaving the bloodstream monocytes enter tissues, where they differentiate into tissue macrophages. These long-lived tissue macrophages remain for as long as 2 yr to carry out macrophage functions such as scavenging of debris and ingesting bacteria. In addition to their usually phagocytic functions, tissue macrophages are particularly adept at handling microorganisms and parasites such as *Legionalla pneumophila, Listeria monocytogenes,* and *Toxoplasma gondii.* Monocytes are increased in such diseases as tuberculosis, systemic mycosis, bacterial endocarditis, chronic inflammatory bowel disease, and certain protozoan infections. Elevated monocyte counts are also frequently seen in patients with isolated neutropenia.

16.42 QUANTITATIVE DISORDERS OF THE NEUTROPHILS

Absolute neutrophil counts vary widely in normal subjects. The relative proportion of neutrophils and lymphocytes in the blood varies with age (see Table 16–2). Neutrophils predominate at birth but decrease rapidly in the 1st few days of life. During infancy they constitute 20–30% of the circulating leukocytes. Similar proportions of neutrophils and lymphocytes occur by about 5 yr of age, but the approximately 70% predominance of neutrophils characteristic of the adult is not attained until puberty. In normal healthy children, therefore, from 20–70% of the total circulating white blood cells may be neutrophils. In absolute terms they number 1,500–2,500/mm^3. Levels exceeding this range are designated neutrophilia or polymorphonuclear leukocytosis.

16.43 NEUTROPHILIA

An increase in circulating neutrophils is the result of a disturbance of the equilibrium involving neutrophil bone marrow production, movement in and out of the bone marrow compartments into the circulation, and neutrophil destruction. Three mechanisms, either alone or in combination, largely account for neutrophilia.

1. Increased numbers of neutrophils may be mobilized from either the bone marrow storage compartment or peripheral marginating pools into the circulating pool.
2. There may be increased blood neutrophil survival because of impaired neutrophil egress into tissue.
3. There may be expansion of the circulating neutrophil pool as a result of increased progenitor cell proliferation and terminal differentiation through the neutrophilic series, increased mitotic activity of neutrophilic cell precursors, or shortening of the cell mitotic cycle of neutrophil precursors.

Acute neutrophilia accompanies physical exercise or an epinephrine-induced reaction, such as a panic response. Epinephrine-induced reactions reflect mobilization of the marginating pool of the neutrophils into the circulating pool. Slower onset of acute neutrophilia can occur following glucocorticosteroid administration or in response to inflammation or infection associated with the generation of endotoxins. Maximal response usually occurs within 4–24 hr and is probably secondary to the release of neutrophils into the circulation from the marrow storage compartments. Glucocorticoids may also impede the release of neutrophils from the circulation into the tissue.

Chronic neutrophilia may be associated with continuous stimulation of neutrophil production, probably through inhibition of marrow feedback mechanisms. Chronic neutrophilia may be associated with prolonged administration of glucocorticoids, chronic inflammatory reactions, or chronic anxiety.

Leukemoid reactions or reactive leukocytosis resembling the blood picture of leukemia have been associated with sepsis, systemic mycotic and protozoan infections, hepatic failure, diabetic acidosis, azotemia, and with disorders associated with malignancy involving the bone marrow. Occasionally, leukemoid reactions may resemble those of chronic myelogenous leukemia. The neutrophils in leukemoid reactions, however, have elevations in alkaline phosphatase activity, whereas this enzyme activity is low in chronic myelogenous leukemia.

Neutrophilia may also accompany various hematologic disorders such as chronic hemolytic anemia, hemorrhage, transfusion reactions, post-splenectomy reactions, and myeloproliferative disorders. Neutrophilia has also been reported in the functional disorder of neutrophils associated with deficiency of the C3bi receptor on the neutrophil (leukocytic adhesion deficiency). Lack of the C3bi glycoprotein results in compromise of neutrophil adhesion to endothelium and in inability of the neutrophil to ingest complement-coated microbes.

16.44 NEUTROPENIA

See also Sec. 12.13.

Neutropenia is defined as an absolute decrease in the number of circulating neutrophils in the blood. Normal neutrophil levels should be stratified for age and race. For whites, the lower limit for normal neutrophil counts (neutrophils and bands) is 1,500/mm^3. Blacks have somewhat lower neutrophil counts, and the lower limits of normal can be considered to range from 100 to 200/mm^3 less than the count for whites. These relatively low counts are probably secondary to a relative decrease of neutrophils in the storage compartment of the bone marrow. Because the methods of characterizing the neutropenias kinetically are still crude, the neutropenic syndromes are generally described in terms of clinical characteristics or according to etiology, when possible.

Individual patients may be characterized as having mild neutropenia with neutrophil counts of 1,000–1,500/mm^3, moderate neutropenia with counts of 500–1,000/mm^3, and severe neutropenia with counts generally below 500/mm^3. This stratification is useful for predicting the risks of pyogenic infections, because only patients with severe neutropenia have an increased susceptibility to life-threatening infections. Endogenous bacteria are the most frequent invaders, but colonization with various organisms of nosocomial origin is often observed.

Susceptibility to bacterial infections, even with severe neutropenia, varies. Some patients having chronic neutropenia with counts below 200/mm^3 do not experience serious infections, probably because they have an intact immune system. Patients receiving anticancer immunosuppressant drugs who develop neutropenia are more prone to developing serious bacterial infections than those with isolated neutropenia because of a compromised immune system. The most frequently occurring types of pyogenic infections in patients with significant neutropenia are cutaneous cellulitis, superficial or deep cutaneous abscesses, furunculosis, pneumonia, and septicemia. Stomatitis, gingivitis, perirectal inflammation, and otitis media also occur. Isolated neutropenia does not heighten patients' susceptibility to viral, fungal, or parasitic infections, or to bacterial meningitis. The most common organisms isolated from neutropenic patients are *Staphylococcus aureus* and gram-negative organisms. The usual signs and symptoms of local infections, such as exudates, fluctuation, ulcerations, fissure formation, and regional adenopathy, are generally less evident in neutropenic patients than in non-neutropenic individuals. The basic approach to evaluating patients with neutropenia includes a history and physical examination emphasizing related phenotypic abnormalities and detection of bacterial infections of the skin and mucous membranes, lymphadenopathy, hepatosplenomegaly, and other signs of underlying associated chronic illnesses (Sec. 12.13).

DISORDERS OF PROLIFERATION OF COMMITTED STEM CELLS

16.45 Chronic Idiopathic Neutropenia

This common group of disorders involves stem cells of the myeloid series. There are normal numbers of red blood cell and platelet precursors. Compensatory monocytosis and eosinophilia are usually present. Investigation of granulopoiesis suggests that a decreased or ineffective production of neutrophils may be the principal mechanism of neutropenia in more severely affected individuals. The underlying basis for the defective myelopoiesis is not well characterized, although in some instances it has been attributed to the altered expression of receptors on myeloid cells for growth factors or an abnormal marrow microenvironment. The degree of susceptibility to infection in chronic idiopathic neutropenia is roughly proportional to the neutrophil count. Blood neutrophil counts often remain stable over a course of years.

BENIGN NEUTROPENIA

Other than infection, chronic idiopathic neutropenia has few serious sequelae, and, thus, if neutropenia is mild to moderate, this disorder may be benign. Some neutropenic patients have a non–X-linked dominant familial pattern, whereas others have acquired isolated neutropenia. Genetically transmitted benign neutropenias are also found in a large number of Yemenite Jews.

The spleen size is usually normal. The bone marrow morphology may vary both among patients and among marrow aspirates obtained from the same patient at different times. The marrow morphology may reveal adequate numbers of myeloid precursors associated with an impaired arrest in development at any stage of maturation from promyelocytes through juvenile neutrophil forms. The marrow response to intravenous corticosteroids has some predictive value. Children with a normal number of myeloid elements in the bone marrow and a normal bone marrow response to steroid stimulation generally have a benign course with relatively few infections, whereas patients who fail to respond to steroids by increasing their levels of circulating neutrophils tend to have a higher frequency of bacterial infections. In some affected children, total remissions occur in late childhood. These patients' infections can be controlled by appropriate antibiotic therapy.

Neutropenia may occur in patients with myelokathexis, a form of moderate neutropenia with a bizarre morphologic disturbance of granulocyte nuclei. Most of the blood neutrophils have cytoplasmic vacuoles and an abnormal nuclei with thin filaments connecting the nuclear lobes.

Disorders of immunoglobulin production have also been associated with neutropenic syndromes. One third of males with sex-linked agammaglobulinemia have neutropenia at some time during the course of their disease. Dysgammaglobulinemia type I (absence of IgA, IgG and normal to elevated IgM levels) may be associated with persistent neutropenia. Neutropenia may also be seen with hypogammaglobulinemia. In children having neutropenia, hypogammaglobulinemia, and recurrent infections treatment with intravenous gammaglobulin and G-CSF to correct both the humoral deficiency and the neutrophil count may be successful.

16.46 SEVERE CONGENITAL NEUTROPENIA

In Scandinavia this disorder is inherited as an autosomal recessive disorder known as Kostmann disease; in the United States it occurs sporadically. Patients chronically maintain an absolute neutrophil count below 200/mm^3 in spite of an accompanied monocytosis and moderate eosinophilia. With onset of disease in early infancy these children have recurrent, severe pyogenic infections, especially of the skin, mouth, and rectum. Bone marrow morphology reveals normal development only up to the promyelocytic or myelocytic stage and marked depletion of mature neutrophils. The platelet count is normal, and often these patients have anemia associated with chronic inflammatory disease. The severe neutropenia of this disorder is often associated with fatal infections. Restoration of a normal neutrophil count may occur following the subcutaneous administration of G-CSF and can lead to a marked decrease in the number of infections. Infections should be treated with appropriate antimicrobial agents.

16.47 Cyclic Neutropenia

This ill-defined disease is characterized by periodic episodes of fever and oral ulcerations, with profound neutropenia. Cyclic neutropenia occurs with increased frequency among family members; 25–33% of patients have a family history consistent with an autosomal dominant pattern of inheritance. Onset usually occurs by 10 yr of age. Neutropenia persists for 3–6 days, after which the neutrophil count returns to normal and symptoms abate. Such episodes occur in cycles, generally of 21 days. The bone marrow exhibits a period of intense myelopoiesis, which begins with the period of neutropenia. The blood monocyte count is typically elevated at the nadir of the neutrophil count. Bacterial infections should be treated with antibiotics. The administration of G-CSF may shorten the duration of the low neutrophil count from 5 days to 1 day.

PHENOTYPIC ABNORMALITIES

16.48 Schwachman Syndrome

This familial syndrome of chronic moderate neutropenia and pancreatic insufficiency is a result of atrophy and fatty replacement. The disorder is probably transmitted as an autosomal recessive trait. It is differentiated from cystic fibrosis by normal sodium and chloride levels in the sweat and by the absence of pulmonary disease. The blood count and smear reveal decreased numbers of neutrophils and, occasionally, thrombocytopenia and anemia. The bone marrow is markedly hypocellular. Roentgenograms may reveal metaphyseal dysostosis. The most prominent symptoms are related to pancreatic insufficiency, which causes malabsorption, diarrhea, and growth failure. No therapy has been effective in improving the hemotologic abnormalities, although restoration of neutrophil counts might be induced with the administration of G-CSF. Pancreatic enzyme replacements ameliorate the malabsorption (Sec. 13.76).

16.49 Cartilage-Hair Hypoplasia

This autosomal recessive disorder is frequently found in the Amish population and is characterized by short limb dwarfism, fine hair, moderate neutropenia, and increased susceptibility to infections. Many of these patients also have impaired cellular immune functions. Appropriate treatment of infections is indicated.

16.50 Dyskeratosis Congenita

This X-linked recessive disorder is characterized by nail dystrophy, leukoplakia and reticulated hyperpigmentation of the skin. Many of these patients have associated marrow hypoplasia, including one third who have neutropenia. Most patients do not have serious infections and survive into adulthood. Infections should be treated appropriately.

DISORDERS OF NEUTROPHIL SURVIVAL

16.51 Infection

The most common cause of transient neutropenia in childhood is viral infections. Viruses that commonly cause neutropenia include those of hepatitis A and B, respiratory syncytial virus, influenza A and B, measles, rubella, and varicella. Neutropenia develops during the 1st 24–48 hr of the illness and may persist for 3–6 days. It usually corresponds to the period of acute viremia and may relate to virus-induced redistribution of neutrophils from the circulating to the marginating granulocyte pool, sequestration, or increased neutrophil uptake following tissue damage by the viruses. Sepsis is one of the more serious causes of neutropenia. The neutropenia in patients with bacteremia and endotoxemia may result from excessive destruction of neutrophils following phagocytosis of microbes and release of metabolites of arachidonic acid. Neutropenia may also result from activation of the complement system that leads to the generation of C5a, which can activate neutrophils and render them hyperadhesive to endothelial surfaces. C5a-induced neutropenia occurs transiently during hemodialysis, continuous flow leukapheresis, and following thermal injury. Underlying infections should be treated appropriately. Rarely, neutrophil infusion may be used to treat severe, persistent neutropenia.

Isoimmune Neonatal Neutropenia

Neonatal isoimmune neutropenia, analogous to Rh-hemolytic anemia, occurs in about 3% of live births. During gestation maternal sensitization to fetal neutrophil antigens inherited from the father produces an IgG antibody that crosses the placenta and destroys the infant's neutrophils. Affected infants frequently develop fever after a few days of life. Diagnosis is established by identifying an antibody in the maternal or neonatal serum that is reactive to the father's neutrophils.

Cutaneous infections predominate, usually secondary to *S. aureus* and less frequently to *E. coli* or β-hemolytic *Streptococcus*. By a median age of 7 wk, the infant's neutrophil count usually has returned to normal, as would be expected based on the half-life of the maternal IgG. Bacterial infections usually respond to antibiotic therapy, but in life-threatening infections, plasma exchange to remove the offending antibodies may be useful. This exchange should be followed by an infusion of the maternal neutrophils that are known to lack the antigen toward which the antibody is directed.

16.52 Autoimmune Neutropenia

Neutropenia may be acquired on an autoimmune basis. Immune neutropenia occurring in the absence of other diseases is uncommon in adults but occurs more frequently in infants from 5 to 24 mo of age. Children having this syndrome of autoimmune neutropenia present with severe neutropenia (counts $< 200/mm^3$) that is usually discovered coincidentally during mild infections. The neutropenia may persist for 6–24 mo and then undergo spontaneous remission. The diagnosis is based on the demonstration of neutrophil antibodies by direct and indirect immunofluorescence assays or by assays that quantitate surface-bound IgG directly. Therapy with corticosteroids may be effective in increasing the numbers of circulating neutrophils in patients with autoimmune neutropenia and recurrent pyogenic infections. Steroids should be used for no more than 4–6 wk. Administration of intravenous gammaglobulin usually only produces a transient restoration of the neutrophil count to normal. Infections should be treated with antimicrobial agents and/or drainage.

Acquired immune mediated neutropenia may also occur in systemic lupus erythematosus and rheumatoid arthritis.

16.53 Reticuloendothelial Sequestration

Splenic enlargement caused by portal hypertension or splenic hyperplasia can lead to neutropenia. Often, moderate neutropenia is accompanied by moderate thrombocytopenia and anemia. The reduced neutrophil survival corresponds with spleen size, and the extent of neutropenia is inversely proportional to the compensatory response of the bone marrow. Bed rest alone may lead to restoration of neutrophil counts because it reduces splenic pressure. In certain cases splenectomy may be necessary to restore the neutrophil count to normal, but this approach predisposes the patient to infections by encapsulated organisms.

16.54 Acquired Neutropenia

Malignancies such as leukemia or lymphoma that infiltrate the bone marrow may result in a leukoerythroblastic peripheral blood smear. Tumor-induced myelofibrosis may accentuate the neutropenia further. Myelofibrosis can also result from granulomatous infections, Gaucher disease, osteopetrosis, drugs with a benzene ring structure, fluoride, or x-irradiation.

Ineffective granulopoiesis may result from nutritional deficiencies of vitamin B_{12} or folic acid that cause megaloblastic pancytopenia and elevated serum nuramidase levels. Neutropenia also occurs as a result of starvation in conditions such as anorexia nervosa and marasmus and in patients receiving parenteral feedings. Neutropenia and marrow megaloblastosis have been observed in patients thought to have a copper deficiency. In these patients serum copper levels are low and hematologic responses occur with oral copper replacement. Treatment of the acquired neutropenias consists of management of the underlying disorders.

16.55 Drug-Induced Neutropenia

Drugs can induce severe neutropenia by an idiosyncratic or hypersensitivity reaction. This form of neutropenia should be distinguished from similar hematologic presentations seen with viral infections and from the severe neutropenia that is normally seen after the administration of large doses of cytotoxic drugs or of radiation.

The idiosyncratic reactions, by definition, are unpredictable. With some drugs, such as the phenothiazines, there appears to be an abnormal sensitivity of myeloid precursors to the agent. In this form of neutropenia there is a latency period of 20–40 days after the patient has received 10–12 g of the drug before neutropenia is detected on routine blood counts.

Hypersensitivity-mediated neutropenia is rare and occasionally may involve arene oxide metabolites of aromatic anticonvulsants (e.g., phenytoin, phenobarbital). Hypersensitivity reactions have a delayed onset after the initiation of drug therapy and may also be associated with febrile illness, skin rash, lymphadenopathy, hepatitis, nephritis, pneumonitis, or aplastic anemia. Hypersensitivity can be corroborated by individual challenge or by a history of drug sensitivity.

Immune neutropenia is thought to arise from drugs that act as a hapten antibody stimulus causing an accelerated destruction of the neutrophils (e.g., aminopyrine, penicillin, propylthiouracil, and gold). If neutropenia occurs, it usually begins abruptly 7–14 days after 1st exposure to the drug or immediately after re-exposure. Fevers, chills, or severe prostation are common in these patients.

In drug-induced neutropenia the bone marrow can vary from hypocellular to hypercellular, and myeloid precursors can be absent, normal, or increased. Mature marrow myeloid elements are usually severely reduced because of the release of stored marrow elements into the blood and the relative expansion of the proliferative cell compartments, leading to a picture of myeloid maturation arrest. Following drug withdrawal the previously hypercellular marrow becomes repopulated with early myeloid forms within a few days. The marrow mitotic compartment then expands over the next few days and the cells mature in a synchronized fashion. Bone marrow examination performed at this time may give the false impression of maturation arrest. Within 1–2 wk the marrow appears morphologically normal. Increasing numbers of lymphocytes, monocytes, and immature neutrophils herald recovery in the peripheral blood.

The duration of drug-induced neutropenia varies greatly. Acute hypersensitivity drug reactions may last for only a few days, whereas chronic idiosyncratic reactions may last for months or years. By contrast, immune-mediated neutropenia usually last for 6–8 days. Because neutropenia usually occurs suddenly its occurrence cannot be predicted by sequential blood counts.

Once neutropenia occurs, the most important therapeutic measure is withdrawal of all drugs that are not essential, particularly drugs suspected to be myeloid-toxic. Infections should be treated with therapeutic doses of antibiotics, the choice of which should be determined by cultures and sensitivity studies; when feasible, bactericidal antibiotics should be employed. Prophylactic antibiotics are not indicated. Corticosteroids are generally not beneficial.

16.56 Inherited Leukocyte Abnormalities

Of the neutrophils in the blood of normal persons, 90% have two to four segments. Only about 5% are unsegmented (bands), and fewer than 5% have five or more segments. An increase in unsegmented forms, or a shift to the left, usually indicates infection or inflammation, whereas hypersegmented forms or a shift to the right usually occurs in megaloblastic anemias secondary to folic acid or vitamin B_{12} deficiency.

HEREDITARY HYPERSEGMENTATION OF NEUTROPHILS AND HEREDITARY GIANT NEUTROPHIL LEUKOCYTE

Neutrophil hypersegmentation is inherited as an autosomal dominant trait; no other associated clinical abnormalities have been described. Homozygotes with this condition have a mean nuclear index exceeding four lobes/cell, as opposed to a normal number of slightly less than three.

Giant neutrophils may be inherited as an autosomal dominant trait with no other disorders associated. Giant neutrophils have a volume twice that of normal neutrophils. These cells are also hypersegmented, with six to ten lobes/neutrophil.

HEREDITARY HYPOSEGMENTATION (Pelger-Huët Anomaly)

This anomaly is characterized by a failure in the normal lobe development of granulocytic cells. Typically, these mature neutrophils have one or two lobes/nucleus and take on a round, dumbbell, or peanut shape. The disorder is inherited as an autosomal dominant trait, is usually not associated with any other congenital abnormality, and does not appear to affect neutrophil function. Patients with specific granule deficiency (Sec. 11.31) also demonstrate the Pelger-Huët anomaly, and this disorder is associated with impaired neutrophil function and clinical infections.

ALDER-REILLY ANOMALY

In this condition, which is probably transmitted as an autosomal recessive trait, neutrophil granulations are larger and stain more prominently than normal ones. The granules are distinctly lavender or blue, and are thus easily differentiated from eosinophils. A small proportion of patients with mucopolysaccharidosis may show similar granulations in their neutrophils, although more commonly they have metachromatic granules in their lymphocyte cytoplasm.

MAY-HEGGLIN ANOMALY

This rare, dominantly transmitted anomaly involves neutrophils and platelets. Most of the neutrophils contain irregular blue cytoplasmic inclusions similar to Döhle bodies, which consist of precipitated messenger RNA. Almost all the individuals known to have this disorder have been in good health despite mild leukopenia, thrombocytopenia, and bizarre giant platelets.

QUALITATIVE ABNORMALITIES OF THE NEUTROPHILS

Patients with certain syndromes involving intracellular defects of the neutrophils display increased susceptibility to infection despite adequate numbers of neutrophils in their circulation. Neutrophil dysfunction may arise from abnormalities in the adherent, motile, degranulation, or bactericidal responses of the cells or from a combination of these functions. See also Sec. 11.30–11.33.

16.57 DISORDERS OF CELL MOTILITY AND CHEMOTAXIS

The migration of neutrophils from the circulation to inflammatory sites leads to the accumulation of an exudate responsible for the clinical signs of inflammation and infection. The attraction of cells to chemical substances is known as chemotaxis. For normal chemotaxis to occur, a complex series of events must be carefully coordinated. Chemotactic factors must be generated in sufficient quantities to establish a long-range chemotactic gradient. The neutrophils, in turn, must have receptors for the various chemotactic agents and mechanisms for discerning the direction of the chemotactic gradient. Because of the complexity of the chemotactic response, it is not surprising that depressed neutrophil chemotaxis is observed in a large number of clinical conditions. These disorders are classified according to the presumed derangement of chemotaxis (Table 16–9). However, the chemotactic defects encountered in many of these disorders contribute little to the decreased resistance to bacterial infections.

Patients with chemotactic disorders may be infected by various microorganisms, including gram-positive and gram-negative bacteria and fungi. *Staphylococcus aureus* is the most common bacteria involved. Typically, the skin, gingiva, mucosa, and regional lymph nodes are involved. Respiratory tract infections are frequent, but sepsis is uncommon. Although the cells move slowly in chemotactic chambers, they do accumulate in sufficient numbers to produce pus at inflammatory sites. It is not uncommon to see delayed signs and symptoms of infections, because phagocyte arrival is often delayed. Infections should be appropriately treated.

16.58 DISORDERS OF NEUTROPHIL INGESTION

Patients with leukocyte adherence deficiency lack the C3bi receptor in both their neutrophils and monocytes (see Sec. 11.30). The absence of the C3bi receptor results in a substantial defect in particle ingestion and in oxidative metabolism triggered by the occupancy of the C3bi receptor.

Another disorder characterized by a profound defect in ingestion is the neutrophil actin dysfunction syndrome. Infants with this disorder, like patients with C3bi deficiency, have recurrent pyogenic infections from birth. Their neutrophils are deficient in both chemotactic and phagocytic re-

TABLE 16–9. Disorders of Neutrophil Chemotaxis

Defects in the generation of chemotactic factors
Familial deficiency of C1r, C2, C4 (classic complement components)
Familial deficiency of C3, C5, properdin
Acquired C3 deficiency (systemic lupus erythematosus, chronic hemolytic anemia, glomerulonephritis, immunoglobulin deficiency)
Enhanced generation of normal chemotactic inactivators
Hodgkin disease
Sarcoidosis
Malignancy
Lepromatous leprosy
Cirrhosis
Direct inhibitors of the neutrophil itself
Immune complex disease (rheumatoid arthritis)
Bone marrow transplantation
C5a generation in plasma (sepsis, hemodialysis, thermal injury)
Wiskott-Aldrich syndrome
Drugs (corticosteroids, tetracycline, amphotericin B, ethanol, antithymocyte globulin)
Juvenile periodontitis *(Capnocytophaga)*
Hyperimmunoglobulin IgE syndrome
IgA myeloma
Intrinsic defects of neutrophils
Neonatal neutrophils
Leukocyte adhesion defect
Neutrophil-actin dysfunction
Chédiak-Higashi syndrome
Specific granule deficiency
Hypophosphatemia
Shwachman syndrome
Glycogenosis, type 1b
Kartagener syndrome
Hyperimmunoglobulin E
Chromosome 7 abnormalities
Zinc deficiency (acrodermatitis enteropathica)
Alcoholism
Increased microtubule assembly

sponses, which is related to impaired neutrophil actin assembly. Infections should be promptly and adequately treated.

16.59 DISORDERS OF DEGRANULATION

CHÉDIAK-HIGASHI SYNDROME

This rare autosomal recessive disorder was initially recognized as one in which leukocytes contained giant cytoplasmic granules (see Sec. 11.31). It is now recognized as a generalized cellular disease affecting all granule-bearing cells.

ETIOLOGY. The basic abnormalities underlying neutrophil function in the Chédiak-Higashi syndrome are unknown, but altered membrane fusion is probably important. One unifying hypothesis for the functional aberrations of this disorder is that abnormal membrane fluidity leads to uncontrolled granule fusion and to other defects, including the inability of the neutrophils to move normally and to concentrate seritonin into platelets and hydrolytic enzymes into neutrophil lysosomes.

CLINICAL MANIFESTATIONS. Melanocytes contain giant melanosomes, leading to a failure to dispense pigment. The patients therefore display a partial albinism involving the hair and skin. Schwann cells also contain giant granules, presumably contributing to striking central and peripheral neuropathies that affect many of these patients in later years. Other features of the disease include the presence of giant azurophils and specific granules in circulating neutrophils. These giant granules form in the cytoplasm during myelopoiesis of myeloid precursors, but most of the myeloid precursors die within the bone marrow, producing moderate neutropenia. An increased susceptibility to infection can be explained in part by the neutropenia and in part by defective chemotaxis, degranulation, and bactericidal activity of the remaining neutrophils. The infections usually encountered in those with Chédiak-Higashi syndrome involve the skin, respiratory tract, and mucous membranes and are caused by gram-positive and gram-negative bacteria. Lymphocytes contain giant cytoplasmic granules and function poorly in antibody dependent–cell-mediated cytolysis of tumor cells. Natural killer cell function is also compromised, which may be related to the deranged secretion of the abnormal granules found in these cells.

Patients with Chédiak-Higashi syndrome have a prolonged bleeding time in spite of a normal platelet count because of impaired platelet aggregation and associated with a deficiency of granules containing adenosine diphosphate and serotonin. There is also a peculiar propensity for lymphohistiocytic proliferation (known as the **accelerated phase**) to occur in the reticuloendothelial system, which intensifies the already existing neutropenia and leads to pancytopenia. This proliferation is associated with recurrent bacterial and viral infections, fever, and prostation. It usually results in death. The onset of the accelerated phase may relate to the inability of these patients to contain and control Epstein-Barr virus and produces features simulating those of the viral-mediated hemophagocytic syndrome.

TREATMENT. Management of the stable phase of Chédiak-Higashi syndrome primarily involves the treatment of infectious complications. High doses of ascorbic acid may result in clinical improvement and improved in vitro function of neutrophils in some patients, but not all.

Management of the accelerated phase is more difficult. Corticosteroids, vincristine, and antithymic serum have not proven useful in preventing death during the accelerated phase. In contrast, bone marrow transplant using HLA-compatible siblings has led to restoration of normal hematopoietic and immunologic function.

See Sec. 11.31 for a discussion of specific granule deficiency.

16.60 DISORDERS OF OXIDATIVE MICROBICIDAL ACTIVITY

CHRONIC GRANULOMATOUS DISEASE

Chronic granulomatous disease (CGD) is an inherited disorder in which phagocytic cells ingest but do not kill catalase-positive microorganisms, because the cells fail to generate oxygen metabolites that normally kill these microbes (see Sec. 11.32.)

The manner in which the metabolic deficiency of the CGD neutrophil predisposes the host to infection relates to the inability of the neutrophil to accumulate hydrogen peroxide (H_2O_2) in the phagosome containing ingested microorganisms. Normally, H_2O_2 and myeloperoxidase delivered to the phagosome by degranulation kill incorporated microbes. The quantity of H_2O_2 produced by normal neutrophils is sufficient to exceed the ability of catalase, an enzyme produced by many aerobic organisms, to metabolize H_2O_2. *Staphylococcus aureus,* most gram-negative enteric bacteria, *Candida albicans,* and *Aspergillosis* spp. are prominent catalase-producing organisms. When these organisms gain entry to CGD neutrophils, however, they are not exposed to endogenous H_2O_2 because the neutrophil does not produce it and the H_2O_2 generated by the microbes themselves is destroyed by the accompanying catalase. The catalase-producing microbes can multiply intracellularly, where they are protected from most circulating antibiotics, and can be transported by the neutrophils to distant sites and released to establish new sites of infections. The granulomatous nature of the lesion of CGD is similar to that of infections by organisms that survive intracellularly in normal phagocytes, such as microbacteria. CGD neutrophils can ingest pneumococci and kill them because the organisms do not contain catalase.

The biochemical events that participate in the respiratory burst that generates the oxygen metabolites toxic to bacteria are initiated by a pyridine nucleotide oxidase (NADPH oxidase). This enzyme catalyzes the one-electron reduction of oxygen to O_2^-. The NADPH oxidase may be composed of several components, one of which traverses the membrane completely and conducts electrons from the pyridine nucleotides on the cytoplasmic site to oxygen in the external environment (see Fig. 11–2). Some sort of lipid appears to be essential for this oxidase activity. Cytochrome b is probably the terminal component of this oxidase chain and binds oxygen, the final electron acceptor. Cytochrome b is composed of two subunits, one of molecular weight 90,000 and the other 22,000. The high molecular weight subunit is probably located on the internal surface of the plasma membrane; the superoxide is released from this surface. Another subunit is a 47,000-molecular-weight phosphoprotein located in the cytosol of the neutrophil. It is phosphorylated on activation of the cell, after which it moves into the membranes, where it attaches to the binding site on the cytochrome b. It may be an electron-transporting molecule or may play a structural or regulatory role in integrating the activation of the electron transport chain. Finally, there is a 66,000-molecular-weight cytosolic protein that moves into the membrane on activation of the neutrophil. This protein may be a flavoprotein that contains flavine adenine nucleotide (FAD) as the prosthetic group and, in turn, binds to an NADPH-containing protein.

In X-linked CGD a defective gene codes for the large subunit of the cytochrome b. The most common result of an abnormality of this gene is failed transcription of its message, as

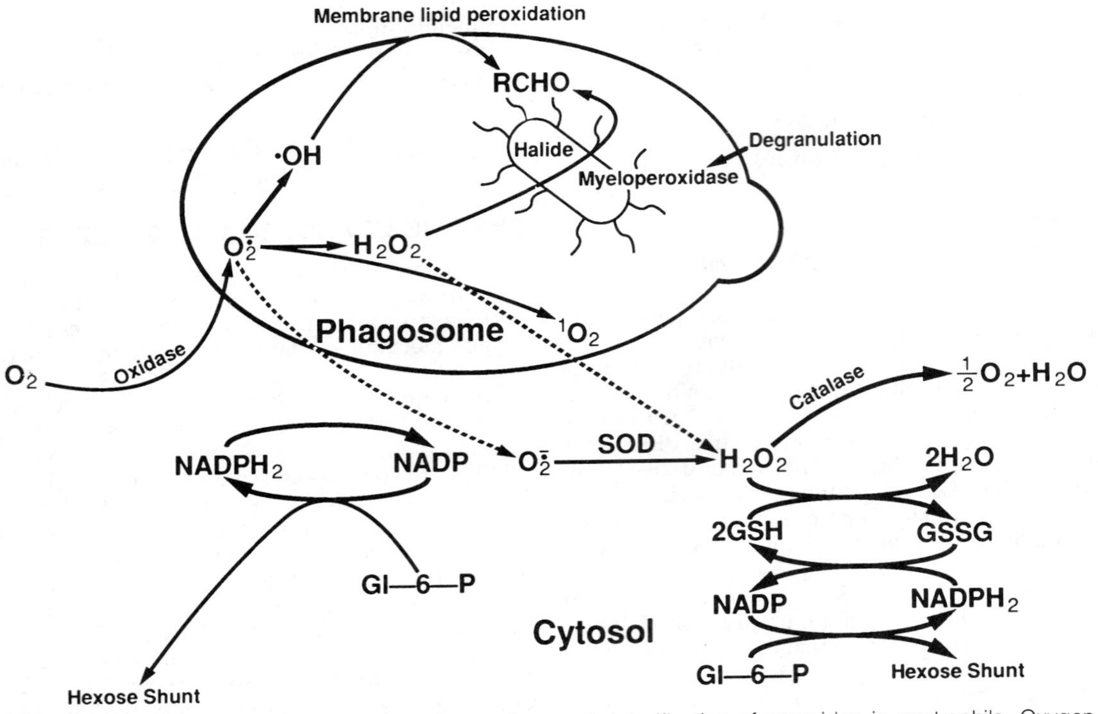

Figure 16–9. The mechanisms for the production, action, and detoxification of peroxides in neutrophils. Oxygen is reduced to superoxide ($O_2^{\bar{\cdot}}$) by an oxidase. NADPH is regenerated from NADP by the hexose monophosphate shunt. Superoxide may spontaneously decompose to hydrogen peroxide and singlet oxygen ($^1O_2$). Hydrogen peroxide can react with superoxide to form hydroxyl radicals and generate bactericidal aldehydes (RCHO) by oxidizing bacterial constituents in the presence of halide ions and myeloperoxidase that delivered to the phagosome by degranulation. Hydroxyl radicals (OH·) can peroxidize unsaturated fatty acids of the phagosomal membrane and thus yield the potentially bactericidal aldehydes. Superoxide leaking out of the phagosome may be converted rapidly to hydrogen peroxide by superoxide dismutase (SOD). Hydrogen peroxide in the cytosol is destroyed by catalase or reduced glutathione (GSH). Reduced GSH is regenerated by coupled reactions that stimulate the flow of glucose-6-phosphate (G-6-P) into the hexose monophosphate shunt.

well as that of the smaller subunit of cytochrome b, and the complete absence of both proteins from the patient's phagocytes. Most of the autosomal recessive patients have an abnormality of the 47,000-molecular-weight phosphoprotein, thereby blocking the transport of electrons to the cytochrome. Additionally, rare patients with the autosomal recessive disorder lack the 66,000-molecular-weight flavoprotein.

Chronic granulomatous disease can be diagnosed by any of several laboratory tests. The inability of CGD neutrophils to undergo the respiratory burst forms the basis for diagnostic tests that measure oxygen consumption, H_2O_2 production, chemiluminescence, and superoxide production. A more convenient assay is the nitroblue tetrazolium (NBT) test, in which neutrophils are stimulated to undergo a respiratory burst in the presence of NBT. The yellow dye forms a purple precipitate on the membrane of those cells that generate superoxide. CGD cells can reduce NBT because they cannot generate superoxide (see Sec. 11.32).

16.61 GLUCOSE-6-PHOSPHATE DEHYDROGENASE DEFICIENCY

The clinical manifestations of this rare syndrome are similar to those of classic CGD. The G-6-PD level is less than 5% of normal. The biochemical relationship between G-6-PD deficiency and the defect of respiratory burst relates to the role of NADPH as the physiologic substrate for the NADPH oxidase in the neutrophil. Failure to convert NADP to NADPH in severe G-6-PD deficiency compromises the ability of the oxidase to use substrate, even though the oxidase appears to be activated normally. Despite similarity between the erythrocyte and leukocyte G-6-PD enzymes, only rare patients with erythrocyte G-6-PD deficiency develop the leukocyte disorder.

See Sec. 11.31 for a description of myeloperoxidase deficiency.

16.62 DISORDERS OF OXIDANT REMOVAL

GLUTATHIONE REDUCTASE AND GLUTATHIONE SYNTHETASE DEFICIENCY

See also Sec. 11.33.

Normal neutrophils have enzymes to inactivate potentially damaging reduced oxygen by-products. Much of the O_2^- and H_2O_2 generated by NADPH oxidase is delivered directly into phagosomes because of the membrane location of the oxidase. Some of these reactive compounds defuse into the cytoplasm, where they may cause serious cellular damage. The neutrophils are equipped with various enzymes and antioxidants to remove potentially damaging oxygen derivatives from the cytoplasm (Fig. 16–9). Superoxide dismutase converts superoxide (O_2^-) to H_2O_2. Hydrogen peroxide is detoxified by catalase and by a glutathione peroxidase-glutathione reductase system, which uses reduced glutathione to convert H_2O_2 to water and oxygen. Insufficient reduced glutathione resulting from deficiencies of glutathione reductase or of glutathione synthetase, both inherited as autosomal recessive traits, can lead to oxidative damage of the membrane and microtubules, as well as to decreased bactericidal activity of neutrophils. Congenital deficiency in neutrophil catalase can result in surface damage from external sources of H_2O_2. The glutathione redox cycle not only decomposes H_2O_2, as does catalase, but is also involved in repairing components of oxidized cells, such as microtubules.

Patients with glutathione reductase and glutathione synthetase deficiency have relatively mild clinical susceptibility to recurrent bacterial infections. In patients with glutathione deficiency, α-tocopherol can function as an oxygen radical scavenger and has been shown to protect neutrophils from oxidant damage.

DIAGNOSTIC EVALUATION OF THE PATIENT WITH RECURRENT INFECTIONS

Susceptibility to pyogenic infections is determined by the adequacy of the host's defenses against microbes to which the host is exposed and the conditions of the exposure. It is difficult to diagnose a specific neutrophil dysfunction on clinical grounds alone. The similarity in the clinical presentation of many of the phagocyte disorders, such as recurrent pyogenic infections, may complicate attempts to establish the diagnosis, even when appropriate phagocytic function tests are used. Test results can be difficult to interpret because of intrinsic biologic or laboratory variability. A useful algorithm for diagnosing these patients is presented in Figure 16–10.

LAURENCE A. BOXER

GENERAL

Curnutte JT, Boxer LA: Disorders of granulopoiesis and granulocyte function. *In*: Nathan DG, Oski FA (eds): Hematology of Infancy and Childhood, 3rd ed. Philadelphia, WB Saunders, 1987, pp 797–847.

Lasslo J, Rundles RW: Morphology of neutrophils and neutrophil precursors. *In*: Williams WJ, Butler E, Erslev AJ, et al (eds): Hematology, 3rd ed. New York, McGraw-Hill, 1983, pp 719–725.

NEUTROPENIA

Bonilla MA, Gillio AP, Ruggeiro M, et al: Effects of recombinant human granulocyte colony-stimulating factor on neutropenia in patients with congenital agranulocytosis. N Engl J Med 320:1574, 1989.

Boxer LA, Greenberg MS, Boxer GJ, et al: Autoimmune neutropenia. N Engl J Med 293:748, 1975.

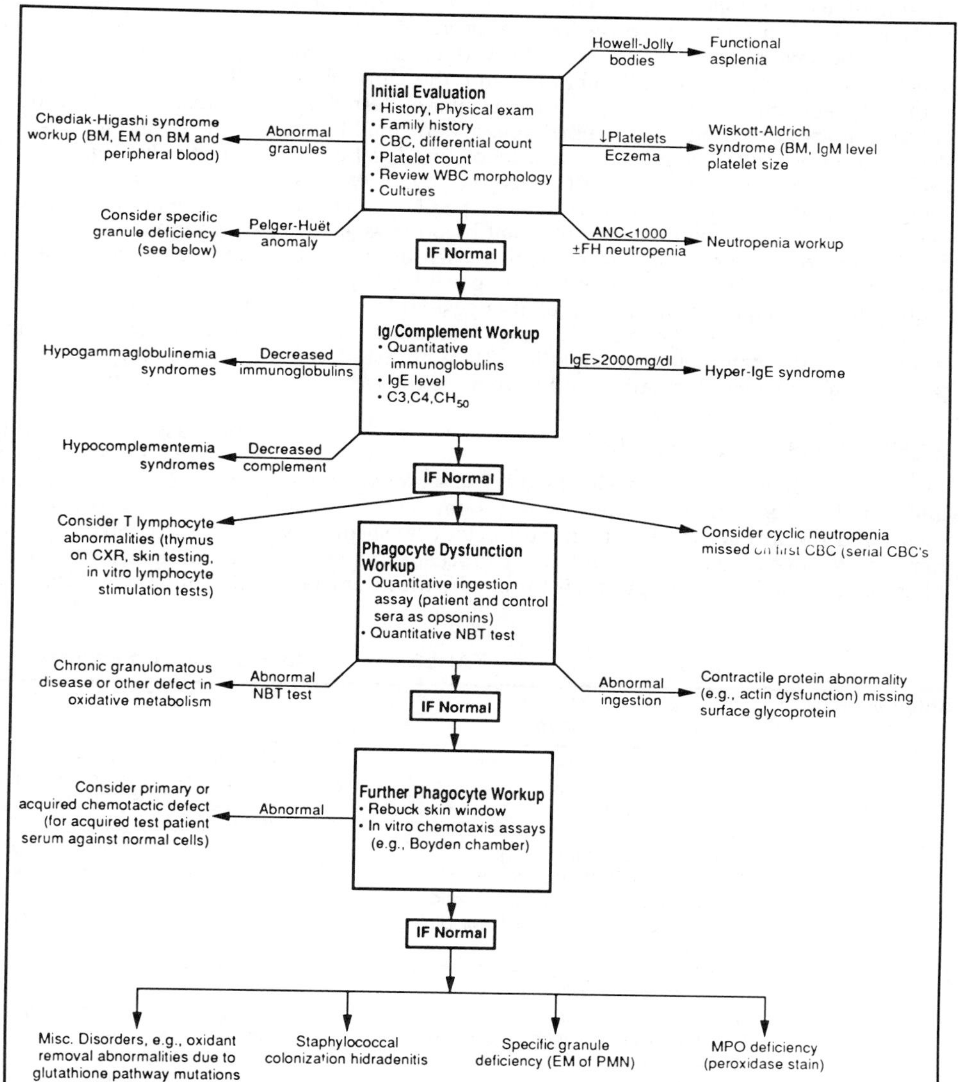

Figure 16–10. Algorithm for the work-up of a patient with recurrent infections. (ANC = absolute neutrophil counts; FH = family history; BM = bone marrow aspirate; CBC = complete blood count; CXR = chest x-ray; EM = electron microscopy; MPO = myeloperoxidase; NBT = nitroblue tetrazolium; PMN = neutrophils; WBC = white blood cell.) (Adapted from Curnutte JT, Boxer LA: Disorders of granulopoiesis and granulocyte function. *In*: Nathan DJ, Oski FA [eds]: Hematology of Infancy and Childhood, 3rd ed. Philadelphia, WB Saunders, 1987, pp 797–847.)

Bussel JB, Abboud MR: Autoimmune neutropenia of childhood. Crit Rev Oncol Hematol 7:37, 1987.
Dale DC, Hammond WP, IV: Cyclic neutropenia: A clinical review. Blood Rev 2:178, 1988.
Hutchinson R, Boxer LA: Disorders of granulocyte and monocyte production. *In*: Benz EJ, Cohen HJ, Furie B, et al (eds): Hematology: Basic Principles and Practice. New York, Churchill Livingstone, 1990, pp 193–204.
Jonsson OG, Buchanan GR: Chronic neutropenia in a single institution. AJDC 145:232, 1991.
Shear NH, Spielberg SP: Anticonvulsant hypersensitivity syndrome. In vitro assessment of risk. J Clin Invest 82:1826, 1988.

QUALITATIVE ABNORMALITIES

Anderson DC, Schmalstieg FC, Finegold MJ, et al: The severe and moderate phenotypes of heritable Mac-1, LFA-1 deficiency: Their quantitative definition and relation to leukocyte function in clinical features. J Infect Dis 152:668, 1985.
Boxer LA, Morganroth ML: Neutrophil function disorders. DM 33:683, 1987.
Brown CC, Gallin JI: Chemotactic disorders. Hematol Oncol Clin North Am 2:61, 1988.
Curnutte JT: Classification of chronic granulomatous disease. Hematol Oncol Clin North Am 2:241, 1988.
Forrest CB, Forehand JR, Axtell RA, et al: Clinical features and current management of chronic granulomatous disease. Hematol Oncol Clin North Am 2:253, 1988.
Nauseef WM: Myeloperoxidase deficiency. Hematol Oncol Clin North Am 2:135, 1988.
Orkin SH: Molecular genetics in chronic granulomatous disease. Ann Rev Immunol 7:277, 1989.
Segal AW: The electron transport chain on the microbicidal oxidase of phagocytic cells and its involvement in the molecular pathology of chronic granulomatous disease. J Clin Invest 83:785, 1989.
Shurin SB: Pathologic states associated with activation of eosinophils and with eosinophilia. Hematol Oncol Clin North Am 2:171, 1988.

16.63 HEMORRHAGIC AND THROMBOTIC DISEASES

The blood is in dynamic equilibrium between fluidity and coagulation. This balance must be precisely maintained to ensure that neither excessive bleeding nor thrombosis occurs spontaneously or following trivial trauma. The hemostatic mechanism is complex: it involves local reactions of the blood vessels, the several activities of the platelet, the interaction of specific coagulation factors, inhibitors, and the fibrinolytic proteins that circulate in the blood. The vascular endothelium is the primary barrier against hemorrhage. When small blood vessels are transected, active vasoconstriction and local tissue pressure control minute areas of bleeding, even without mobilization of the coagulation process. The platelet, however, is essential for maintenance of small blood vessels and for the control of hemorrhage from small-vessel injury. More extensive injury and involvement of larger blood vessels require the participation of the coagulation system to provide a firm, stable, fibrin clot. Within this process natural inhibitors in plasma and a competent fibrinolytic system are needed to prevent excessive clot formation and to remove the clot.

SCHEMA OF HEMOSTASIS

The classic schema of hemostasis includes vascular response and platelet plug formation (the primary hemostatic mechanism) and the formation of a stable fibrin clot (the secondary hemostatic mechanism). Coagulation proceeds in three phases: in phase I, thromboplastin is formed by the interaction of certain coagulation factors, phospholipids, and tissue juice (which contains tissue factor); in phase II prothrombin (factor II) is converted to thrombin (factor IIa); and in phase III, soluble fibrinogen is converted by thrombin to fibrin. This simple scheme has been expanded, but retention of the concept as a basic three-phase reaction has merit. Table 16–10 lists the more common coagulation factors and their synonyms. A comprehensive representation of hemostasis is depicted in Fig. 16–11.

Following vascular injury, vasoconstriction occurs and a platelet plug forms. The platelets must first stick to the injured endothelium (adhesion). They require a plasma factor (von Willebrand factor) to be adhesive. After adhesion, the platelets undergo a release reaction in which certain intraplatelet factors (e.g., adenosine diphosphate [ADP], thromboxane A_2) are released into the surrounding area. These materials cause aggregation of platelets and the eventual formation of the platelet plug. In phase I of the coagulation scheme there are two pathways to the formation of thromboplastin (factor Xa, and factor V plus phospholipid complex) called the intrinsic (or plasma) and extrinsic (or tissue) pathways. The intrinsic pathway involves the successive enzymatic conversion of the inactive forms of factors XII, XI, and IX. (Two other plasma proteins are also involved in the activation of factor XII and factor XI—prekallikrein for factor XII and high-molecular-weight kininogen for factor XI.) The activated factor IX (factor IXa) interacts with factor VIII, calcium, and phospholipid to

TABLE 16–10. The Coagulation Factors

International Numbers	Synonyms	Comment
I	Fibrinogen	Number rarely used—congenital deficiency known (afibrinogenemia)
II	Prothrombin	Number rarely used—congenital deficiency known
III	Thromboplastin	No specific factor identified
IV	Calcium	Number rarely used
V	Labile factor, proaccelerin	Congenital deficiency known (parahemophilia, Owren disease)
VI	Activated labile factor, accelerin	No longer differentiated from factor V
VII	Stable factor, SPCA, proconvertin	Congenital deficiency known
VIII	Antihemophilic factor (AHF) or globulin (AHG)	Hemophilia A (classic hemophilia)—results from congenital deficiency
IX	Christmas factor, plasma thromboplastin component (PTC)	Hemophilia B—results from congenital deficiency
X	Stuart-Prower factor	Congenital deficiency known
XI	Plasma thromboplastin antecedent, PTA	Congenital deficiency known
XII	Hageman factor	No clinical symptoms associated with congenital deficiency
XIII	Fibrin-stabilizing factor	Congenital deficiency known

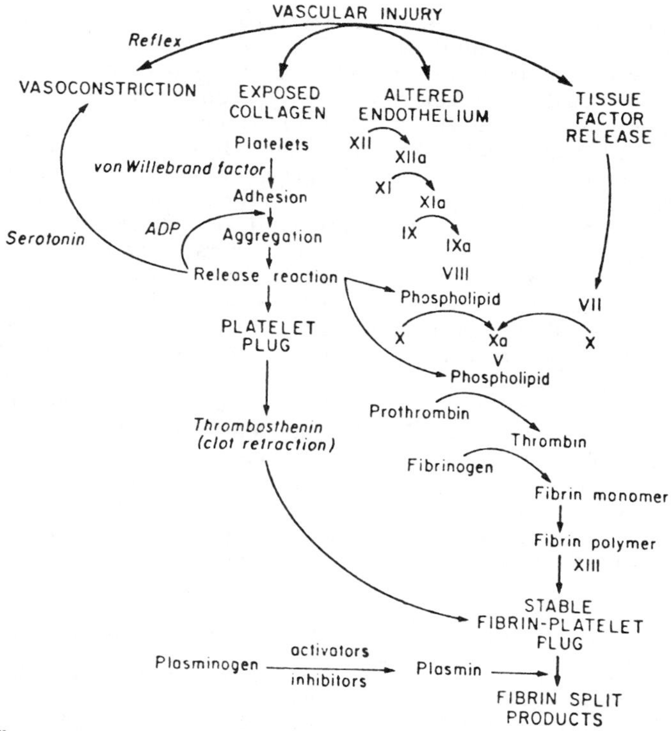

Figure 16–11. Diagrammatic representation of the hemostatic mechanism. (From Nathan DG, Oski FA: Hematology of Infancy and Childhood, 3rd ed. Philadelphia, WB Saunders, 1987, p 1294.)

activate factor X. Factor Xa interacts with factor V, calcium, and phospholipid and becomes the active complex that converts prothrombin (factor II) to thrombin. This active complex has been called prothrombinase (preferred), prothrombin activator, and thromboplastin. The extrinsic pathway involves the conversion of factor VII to factor VIIa by tissue factor (a phospholipid protein complex). In the extrinsic pathway factor VIIa activates factor X directly.

Phase II of coagulation involves the enzymatic cleavage of factor II into smaller molecules, one of which is thrombin (factor IIa). This step requires factor II as substrate for the factor Xa-factor V-phospholipid-calcium complex.

In phase III thrombin splits four small peptides (two fibrinopeptide A and two fibrinopeptide B) from fibrinogen-producing fibrin monomers. These monomers then polymerize spontaneously to form fibrin. Factor XIIIa (formed by the action of thrombin on factor XIII) causes covalent bonding of the fibrin strands, which produces a stable clot.

There are at least three clinically important, naturally occurring coagulation inhibitors: antithrombin III, protein C, and protein S. Antithrombin III inhibits activated coagulation factors that have a serine moiety in their active site, such as thrombin, factor Xa, factor IXa, factor XIa, and factor XIIa. Protein C, when activated (protein Ca), inhibits factor V and factor VIII, using protein S as its cofactor.

The fibrinolytic system is composed of plasminogen, activators, and inhibitors. Plasminogen must be converted to plasmin, which is the active proteolytic enzyme, by activators (such as tissue-type plasminogen activator and urinary-type plasminogen activator). This reaction is modulated by plasminogen activator inhibitors (PAIs) and by α_2-antiplasmin (α_2-plasmin inhibitor). Plasmin's function is to lyse fibrin, a process that produces soluble fibrin degradation (split) products.

16.64 EVALUATION OF THE PATIENT WITH A SUSPECTED HEMOSTATIC DEFECT

HISTORY AND PHYSICAL EXAMINATION. The focus of the history and physical examination is to determine whether the suspected defect is acquired or congenital (inherited) and which mechanism appears to be affected (primary or secondary hemostatic mechanism). The history should determine the site or sites of bleeding, the severity and duration of the hemorrhage, the age of onset, what was done to control the bleeding, whether the bleeding was spontaneous or induced, the family history, a drug history, the patient's experiences with prior trauma (e.g., surgical procedures, biopsies, venipunctures, dental extraction) and, in females, a detailed menstrual history. The physical examination should determine the characteristics of the bleeding (e.g., petechiae, ecchymoses, hematomas, hemarthroses, mucous membrane bleeding) and identify signs of a primary systemic disease. The characteristic bleeding manifestations in a patient with a defective primary hemostatic mechanism (platelet–blood vessel interaction) are mucous membrane bleeding (e.g., epistaxis, hematuria, menorrhagia, gastrointestinal), petechiae in the skin and mucous membranes, and multiple, small, ecchymotic lesions. The typical bleeding signs in a patient with a defective secondary hemostatic mechanism (coagulation system) are deep bleeding into joints and muscles, large spreading ecchymotic lesions, and hematomas.

LABORATORY TESTS. Patients who are hemorrhaging or who have a history suggestive of a hemostatic disorder should have a platelet count, bleeding time, prothrombin time, and activated partial thromboplastin time (APTT) performed. These screening studies should identify most hemostatic defects, although there are exceptions. More specific tests may be needed to define the defect more precisely.

Certain previously used tests are no longer employed either because they lack sensitivity and specificity or because the current techniques are less cumbersome and the results are easier to interpret. Tests that are now rarely used are the tourniquet test, whole blood clotting time, prothrombin consumption time, and thromboplastin generation test.

Bleeding Time. The bleeding time is the best test for assessing the vascular and platelet phases of hemostasis. It has been standardized by the use of a template that regulates the length and depth of the skin incision. A blood pressure cuff is applied to the arm and inflated to 40 mm Hg for children, 30 mm Hg for term newborns, and 20 mm Hg for preterm babies, and an incision is made using a template and scalpel blade. At 30-sec intervals drops of blood are blotted from the margin of the incision. Normally, blood flow stops within 4–8 min.

Platelet Count. A platelet count is essential in the evaluation, because thrombocytopenia is the most common cause of a defective primary hemostatic mechanism that produces a significant bleeding diathesis in children. There is a linear relationship between the bleeding time and the platelet count—that is, the lower the platelet count, the more prolonged the bleeding time. Using a template, bleeding time in this relationship can be determined as

$$\text{Bleeding time (min)} = 30.5 - \frac{\text{platelet count (per } \mu\text{L)}}{3{,}850}$$

If the bleeding time is disproportionate to the platelet count, a qualitative platelet defect should be suspected. Patients with a platelet count above 50×10^9/L rarely have significant bleeding.

Platelet Aggregation and Other Tests. If a platelet function defect is detected, further in vitro studies can be carried out, including platelet aggregation tests using activators (e.g.,

ADP, collagen, epinephrine, thrombin, and/or ristocetin), clot retraction, prothrombin consumption test (for platelet factor 3), ATP and serotonin release, and others.

The three phases of coagulation can be individually assessed by simple, reliable tests.

Thrombin Time. Phase III can be evaluated by the thrombin time, the time required for plasma to clot after the addition of bovine or human thrombin (factor IIa). The normal thrombin time ranges from 15 to 20 sec in most laboratories. Prolongation of the thrombin time occurs with hypofibrinogenemia, or dysfunctional fibrinogen (dysfibrinogenemia), or by substances that interfere with fibrin polymerization (e.g., heparin, certain fibrinolytic degradation products). If heparin contamination is the cause, the heparin can be inactivated by various neutralizing agents and the test repeated, or the thrombin time can be determined using a snake venom (reptilase) in place of the thrombin. Reptilase is a thrombin-like enzyme that is not affected by heparin. Fibrinogen also can be measured by chemical, immunologic, and heat precipitation methods.

Prothrombin Time. Phase II of coagulation is assessed by the prothrombin time, the time taken for plasma to clot after the addition of exogenous thromboplastin (tissue factor) and calcium. The normal prothrombin time ranges from 11.5 to 14 sec. If phase III is intact, a prolonged prothrombin time indicates a deficiency involving factors II, V, VII, and/or X. Specific assays are available for all these factors. The prothrombin time, however, does not reflect the activity of factors XII, XI, IX, VIII, or XIII.

Activated Partial Thromboplastin Time. Phase I, the most complex part of the coagulation mechanism, is evaluated by the activated partial thromboplastin time (APTT). The APTT is the time required for the clotting of plasma that has been activated by incubation with an inert activator (e.g., kaolin, celite, ground glass, ellagic acid) when calcium and platelets (or a lipid substitute for platelets) are added. The normal APTT ranges from 25 to 40 sec. This test is a simple, inexpensive, and reliable way to assess the adequacy of factors XII (and prekallikrein, high-molecular-weight kininogen), XI, IX, and VIII. The APTT does not assess factor VII or factor XIII activity. If phase III and phase II are intact, a prolonged APTT represents either a deficiency or an inhibitor in the intrinsic pathway.

Mixing Study. The next test to be performed is a mixing study. In this study, normal plasma is added to the patient's plasma and the APTT is carried out on the mixture. If the resulting APTT is normal (i.e., the patient's abnormal APTT is corrected), then a deficiency state is present. If, however, the mixture's APTT remains prolonged, an inhibitor is present. Correction of the abnormal APTT in the mixing study in a patient with a bleeding disorder indicates a deficiency of factor VIII, IX, or XI or, in a patient without a bleeding disorder, indicates a deficiency of factor XII, prekallikrein, high-molecular-weight kininogen. If the mixing study does not correct (or worsens with incubation) and the patient has a bleeding disorder, an inhibitor against factors VIII, IX, or XI should be suspected. If the patient has no hemorrhagic manifestations, the inhibitor is probably the so-called "lupus anticoagulant." Assays for each coagulation factor are available and are needed to identify the specific factor involved and the severity of the defect. Severity is graduated as follows: severe—activity less than 1% of normal (also reported as less than 1 unit/dL or less than 0.01 unit/mL); moderate—activity greater than 1% but less than 5% of normal (or 1–5 units/dL); and mild—activity greater than 5% of normal (or greater than 5 units/dL). Normal levels in most laboratories for these factors is between 50 and 150% (50–150 units/dL).

Other Tests. There are no screening tests for the natural inhibitors of the coagulation mechanism. Specific functional and immunologic assays are available for measuring the plasma levels of antithrombin III, protein C, and protein S.

Screening tests for overall fibrinolysis are insensitive. Such tests include the whole blood clot lysis time and the plasma clot lysis time. The euglobulin clot lysis time (ELT) is used by most laboratories to assess fibrinolysis. In this test a euglobulin fraction of plasma is made (usually by acetic acid precipitation) and the fraction is clotted with calcium or thrombin. The time for clot lysis is determined (usually from 2 to 4 hr). The euglobulin fraction has clotting factors, fibrinogen, plasminogen, and plasminogen activators, but no inhibitors. A short ELT can be a result of increased activators and/or reduced fibrinogen; a prolonged ELT is seen with reduced plasminogen, reduced activator, or with extremely increased fibrinogen concentration. Other tests for assessing the fibrinolytic mechanisms include assays for plasminogen, plasminogen activators and inhibitors, and immunologic assays for fibrinolytic split (degradation) products.

The levels of the components of the hemostatic mechanism are different in the normal newborn when compared to those of adults (Table 16–11). Generally, the more preterm the infant, the more marked are the differences.

Bleyer WA, Hakami N, Shepard TH: The development of hemostasis in the human fetus and newborn infant. J Pediatr 79:838, 1971.

Corrigan JJ, Jr: Hemorrhagic and Thrombotic Diseases in Childhood and Adolescence. New York, Churchill Livingstone, 1985.

Feusner JH: Normal and abnormal bleeding times in neonates and young children utilizing a fully standardized template technique. Am J Clin Pathol 74:73, 1980.

Harker LA, Slichter SJ: The bleeding time as a screening test for evaluation of platelet function. N Engl J Med 287:155, 1972.

Hilgartner MW, Pochedly C: Hemophilia in the Child and Adult, 3rd ed. New York, Raven Press, 1989.

Hathaway WE, Bonnar J: Hemostatic Disorders of the Pregnant Woman and Newborn Infant. New York. Elsevier, 1987.

Johnston M, Zipursky A: Microtechnology for the study of the blood coagulation system in newborn infants. Can J Med Technol 42:159, 1980.

Mielke CH: Measurement of the bleeding time. Thromb Haemost 52:210, 1984.

Oski FA, Naiman JL: Hematologic Problems in the Newborn, 3rd ed. Philadelphia. WB Saunders, 1982.

Stamatoyannopoulos G, Nienhuis AW, Leder P, et al: The Molecular Basis of Blood Diseases. Philadelphia, WB Saunders, 1987.

Williams CE, Short PE, George AJ, et al: Critical Factors in Haemostasis. Evaluation and Development. Chichester, England, Ellis Horwood, 1988.

TABLE 16–11. Hemostatic Mechanisms of the Newborn*

Component	Newborn Level
Coagulation factors	
Fibrinogen	Lower limit of normal
Factors II, VII, IX, X, XI, XII, high molecular weight kininogen, and prekallikrein	Very low
Factors V and XIII	Normal
Factor VIII and von Willebrand factor	Normal to increased
Inhibitors	
Antithrombin III	Low
Proteins C and S	Low
Fibrinolytic components	
Plasminogen	Low
Plasminogen activators	Low
Plasminogen activator inhibitors	Normal
Plasmin inhibitors	Normal to increased
Platelets	
Quantitative	Normal
Qualitative (function)	Impaired

*Compared with those of older children and adults.

HEMORRHAGIC DISORDERS

CONGENITAL AND INHERITED COAGULATION DISORDERS

PHASE I DISORDERS: THE HEMOPHILIAS

The hemophilias are the most common and serious of the congenital coagulation disorders. They are associated with genetically determined deficiencies of factors VIII, IX, or XI.

16.65 Factor VIII Deficiency

(Classic Hemophilia; Hemophilia A; Antihemophilic Factor [AHF] Deficiency)

About 80% of cases of hemophilia are hemophilia A, which is caused by a defective gene carried on the X chromosome. This results in a profound depression of the level of factor VIII coagulation activity in the plasma. Factor VIII is complexed with von Willebrand protein (called the factor VIII–von Willebrand complex) in plasma, with the von Willebrand protein acting as a carrier protein. Patients with hemophilia A and women who are carriers for the disorder have reduced factor VIII activity but normal plasma levels of the von Willebrand protein (in contrast to classic von Willebrand disease, in which both levels are reduced). In the normal population the plasma ratio of factor VIII activity to von Willebrand protein is 1.0. Thus, most female carriers have a ratio less than one, which can be used for carrier detection and genetic counseling. Recently, carrier and fetal detection has become more precise by measuring restriction fragment length polymorphism using DNA probes or markers.

In 80% of cases the family history is positive for the disease. Sporadic cases may represent a new mutation. The clinical severity depends on the level of factor VIII activity in the plasma: severe cases have less than 1% (1 unit/dL) of normal activity; moderate cases have 1–5% (1–5 units/dL); and mild cases have 6–30% (6–30 units/dL). The degree of severity tends to be consistent within a given family.

CLINICAL MANIFESTATIONS. Because factor VIII does not cross the placenta, a bleeding tendency may be evident in the neonatal period. Hematomas after injections and bleeding from circumcision are common, but many affected newborns exhibit no clinical abnormalities. As ambulation begins, excessive bruising occurs. Large intramuscular hematomas result from minor trauma. A relatively minor traumatic laceration, as of the tongue or lip, which bleeds persistently for hours or days, is frequently the event that leads to diagnosis. Of patients with severe disease, 90% have had clear clinical evidence of increased bleeding by 1 yr of age.

The hallmark of hemophilia is hemarthrosis. Hemorrhages into the elbows, knees, and ankles cause pain and swelling and limit movement of the joint; these may be induced by relatively minor trauma but often appear to be spontaneous. Repeated hemorrhages may produce degenerative changes, with osteoporosis, muscle atrophy and, ultimately, a fixed, unusable joint. Spontaneous hematuria is a troublesome but not usually serious complication. Intracranial hemorrhage and bleeding into the neck constitute life-threatening emergencies.

Patients with factor VIII activities greater than 6% (6 units/dL) do not have spontaneous symptoms. These patients, with "mild hemophilia," may experience only prolonged bleeding following tooth extractions or dental work, surgery, or injury.

LABORATORY FINDINGS. The only significant laboratory abnormalities occur in coagulation tests and reflect a serious deficiency of factor VIII. The partial thromboplastin time (PTT) is greatly prolonged. The platelet count, bleeding time, and prothrombin time are normal. Mixing studies using normal plasma show a correction of the PTT. A specific assay for factor VIII activity confirms the diagnosis.

TREATMENT. Prevention of trauma is an important aspect of care for the hemophilic child. During early life the crib and playpen should be padded, and the child should be carefully supervised while learning to walk. As he or she becomes older, physical activities that do not entail a risk of trauma should be encouraged. It is important that a course between overprotection and permissiveness be followed. Aspirin and other drugs that affect platelet function may provoke hemorrhage and must be avoided by hemophilic patients. Because children with severe hemophilia are exposed to blood products throughout life, they should be immunized against hepatitis B virus. The vaccine may be given in the newborn period.

Replacement Therapy. When bleeding episodes occur, replacement therapy is essential to prevent pain, disability, or life-threatening hemorrhage. The aim of therapy is to increase factor VIII activity in the plasma to a level that secures hemostasis. Currently, this can be done only by the intravenous infusion of fresh-frozen plasma or of plasma concentrates.

Therapy of the hemophilic patient has been considerably facilitated by the development of factor VIII concentrates; these permit fairly precise estimation of the dosage necessary to attain hemostatic levels. By definition, 1 mL of normal plasma contains 1 unit of factor VIII. Because the plasma volume is about 45 mL/kg, it is necessary to infuse 45 units/kg of factor VIII to increase its level in the hemophilic recipient from 0–100% (0–100 units/dL). A dose of 25–50 units/kg of factor VIII is usually given to raise the recipient's level to 50–100% (50–100 units/dL) of normal. Because the half-life of factor VIII in the plasma is about 8–12 hr, repeated infusions can be given, as necessary, to maintain the desired level of activity.

Several factor VIII concentrates are available. The most inexpensive of these is cryoprecipitate, which can be prepared in the blood bank from fresh plasma. The yield from 250 mL of fresh plasma is one bag of cryoprecipitate, which usually contains 75–125 units of factor VIII; there may, however, be marked variability in the content of bags. One bag of cryoprecipitate/5 kg of body weight raises the recipient's level to about 50% (50 units/dL) of normal. Because cryoprecipitate is produced from single units of whole blood, the risk of blood-borne diseases such as hepatitis B and AIDS (Sec. 12.79 and 12.83) is lower than with concentrates prepared from large plasma pools. New factor VIII concentrates that are heat- or detergent-treated are prepared by monoclonal antibody techniques. These products (Monoclate; Hemofil M) are more expensive than cryoprecipitate but are safer with regard to transmission of infectious organisms. These are dispensed as lyophilized powders in bottles of 250–500 units that can be reconstituted just prior to use; they are tremendously useful and convenient. Their potency and relatively low protein content permit rapid restoration of normal hemostatic levels with very small volumes. Commercial factor VIII concentrates also contain anti-A and anti-B isohemagglutinins; when massive amounts are given to persons of blood group A or B, hemolysis may occur.

When the hemophilic child has significant bleeding, replacement therapy should be promptly instituted. Local measures should include application of cold and pressure, but these should not substitute for adequate replacement therapy. For ordinary hemarthroses, it is necessary to raise the factor VIII level to about 50% (50 units/dL) and to maintain it at least above 5% (5 units/dL) for 48–72 hr. A single infusion of 20–30 units/kg of factor VIII concentrate suffices, permitting the "one-shot" therapy of ordinary bleeding episodes. Immobilization is initially indicated, but passive exercise should be started within 48 hr to prevent joint stiffness and fibrosis. The need for aspiration of blood from the joint is controversial. When the skin overlying the joint is tense because therapy has been delayed the aspiration of blood, after adequate factor VIII has been given, may provide relief of pain. Replacement therapy is the most important aspect of the management of hemarthrosis, because equally good results have been obtained by some who routinely practice joint aspiration and by others who do not. Aggressive replacement therapy with factor VIII and careful orthopedic management of hemarthroses can prevent much severe deformity and crippling, which are now less common than in the past.

When hemorrhage occurs in vital areas such as the brain or neck, or when major surgery is contemplated, intensive therapy using factor VIII concentrates is indicated to maintain the plasma level above 50% (50 units/dL) for 2 wk. ε-Aminocaproic acid, 50–100 mg/kg every 6 hr, may be indicated in conjunction with replacement therapy for oral mucous membrane hemorrhage and dental extraction. Venipuncture should be performed only from superficial veins; aspiration from femoral or internal jugular veins is hazardous and has led to some deaths. There is compelling evidence that early treatment with factor VIII concentrates reduces disability and deformity as well as the amount and duration of replacement treatment necessary for bleeding episodes. Parents, or the older patient, can be trained to give intravenous infusions or concentrates at home, with substantial decreases in hospitalization, morbidity, and risk of blood-transmitted diseases.

Home treatment with periodic assessment and counsel from the physician represents optimal or ideal management for the hemophilic child and family, and this enlightened management may permit the present generation of hemophilic children to enter adult life without major physical or psychologic crippling. On the other hand, some long-term complications may result from modern therapy. Abnormalities of hepatic enzyme activities are found in 50% of patients. Instances of chronic active hepatitis and cirrhosis have been reported. A high proportion of patients now have antibodies against hepatitis B and C viruses, and many have antibodies against the AIDS virus (human immunodeficiency virus, HIV). These findings are the basis for recommending active immunization against HBV. Hypertension and renal disease with hematuria occur in many adult patients; their causes have not been defined.

Desmopressin (DDAVP; Stimate) causes an increase in factor VIII in patients with mild hemophilia A and in some patients with moderate disease. The recommended dose is 0.3 μg/kg body weight, which raises the factor VIII level 25–50% above the baseline. It should only be given once every 1–2 days and only for minor bleeding episodes such as oral bleeding, dental extractions, and small hematomas. It is ineffective in hemarthrosis, central nervous system bleeding, and for sustaining factor VIII levels after major surgery.

Factor VIII Inhibitors. Ten to 15% of patients with hemophilia become refractory to factor VIII therapy because a circulating inhibitor or antibody develops. The development of inhibitors is not related to the number of plasma transfusions, and replacement therapy should not be withheld in hope of avoiding this. These inhibitors are IgG globulins and are specifically active against factor VIII. The inhibitors may be of low titer and transient, or of extremely higher titer and very persistent. The "Bethesda unit" of inhibition is the amount of inhibitory activity in 1 mL of plasma that reduces the factor VIII level in 1 mL of normal plasma from 1 to 0.5 unit. It is almost impossible to overpower a high-titer inhibitor but, when life-threatening hemorrhage occurs, massive doses of factor VIII concentrates or plasmapheresis with replacement with factor VIII should be given and may be of temporary benefit. Immunosuppressive therapy is of no value.

Another attempt at therapy of the hemophilic child who has developed a factor VIII inhibitor involves the use of factor IX concentrates (Konyne; Autoplex; FEIBA), which apparently contain amounts of a factor VIII bypassing principle. These activated coagulants enter the coagulation cascade distal to the level of factor VIII (see Fig. 16–11) and thus bypass the effects of the inhibitor. The activities of various preparations, however, and even of different lots of the same preparation, vary markedly. Thrombosis is a possible combination.

Porcine factor VIII (Hyate C) is effective in hemophilia A patients with inhibitors. This animal factor VIII provides adequate factor VIII activity in patients with less than 50 Bethesda units of inhibitor. The usual starting dose is 100–150 porcine units/kg. Reported side effects include mild fever, nausea, headache, flushing, and occasional vomiting.

Immune tolerance may potentially be achieved with combined therapy including intravenous immunoglobulin, cyclophosphamide, and factor VIII.

PRENATAL DIAGNOSIS. Each male fetus of a mother who carries hemophilia has a 50% risk of having the disease. Prenatal diagnosis is possible through examination of the blood of the (male) fetus, which can be obtained at fetoscopy at 20–22 wk of gestation. Fetal plasma is assayed for von Willebrand protein and for factor VIIIc; as in the older patient, a markedly higher von Willebrand protein level compared to the factor VIIIc level identifies an affected male. It is now possible to identify a fetus with hemophilia by examining DNA polymorphisms in amniotic fluid fibroblasts. Trophoblastic biopsy in fetuses at risk may permit the diagnosis of hemophilia as early as 10–12 wk of gestation.

16.66 Factor IX Deficiency

(Christmas Disease; Hemophilia B)

Factor IX is produced by the liver and is one of the vitamin K-dependent coagulation factors. About 12–15% of the hemophilias result from a genetically determined deficiency of factor IX.

CLINICAL MANIFESTATIONS. This disease is clinically indistinguishable from factor VIII deficiency (hemophilia A); joint and muscle hemorrhages are characteristic. It is transmitted as an X-linked recessive trait, and the severity is related to the level of coagulant activity of the factor in plasma. Factor IX is normally reduced in the plasma of newborns and slowly increases into the adult range after several months. Thus, unlike factor VIII, which is at normal or above-normal levels at birth, mild or moderate hemophilia B is difficult to diagnose in the newborn period, but severe hemophilia B (less than 1% factor IX activity) can be diagnosed in the newborn. Although female carriers can be identified by factor IX coagulation assays, detection is more specific by using monoclonal antibody or DNA analysis techniques.

LABORATORY FINDINGS. The partial thromboplastin time is usually abnormally prolonged. The bleeding time and prothrombin time are normal. Specific factor IX assay is necessary to distinguish the deficiency from that of hemophilia A and to define the severity of the defect.

TREATMENT. Replacement of factor IX is accomplished by infusions of fresh frozen plasma (FFP) or a factor IX concentrate. Because the half-life of factor IX is longer than factor VIII (about 24 hr), it may be administered less frequently. Also, the dose-response relationship to factor IX is different than that for factor VIII. One unit of factor IX/kg raises the plasma factor IX from 1.0–1.2% of normal (factor

TABLE 16–12. Genetic and Laboratory Findings in Von Willebrand Disease

Type	Parameter						
	BT	*VIII-C*	*vW-Ag*	*R-Cof*	*RIPA*	*Multimer Structure*	*Mode of Inheritance*
I (classic)	P†	R	R	R	R	N	AD
II							
A	P	N/R	N/R	R	R	Abn	AD
B	P	N/R	N/R	N/R	I	Abn	AD
III	P	R	R	R	R	Variable	AR

BT = bleeding time; VIII-C = factor VIII coagulant activity; vW-Ag = von Willebrand antigen (protein); R-Cof = ristocetin cofactor; RIPA = ristocetin-induced platelet aggregation (agglutination); P = prolonged; R = reduced; N = normal; I = increased; N/R = normal or reduced; Abn = abnormal; AD = autosomal dominant; AR = autosomal recessive.

VIII, 1 unit/kg, can raise the plasma factor VIII by 2%). Thus, to achieve 100% (100 units/dL) activity in a patient with severe hemophilia B, an infusion of 100 units of factor IX/kg is needed. Fresh-frozen plasma has about 1 unit of factor IX/mL, whereas the concentrates contain considerably more factor IX in less volume. Concentrates that are heat-treated continue to have the risk of transmitting hepatitis B and C viruses. Their use is preferred when levels of factor IX greater than 30% (30 units/dL) are needed. All patients with hemophilia B should receive the hepatitis B vaccine.

Episodes of thrombosis have occurred after use of the concentrates, especially in the postoperative patient with underlying liver disease, presumably because the concentrates contain coagulants.

16.67 Factor XI Deficiency
(Hemophilia C)

Factor XI deficiency is the least common type of hemophilia and is found in 2–3% of all hemophilia patients. Factor XI deficiency is transmitted as an incomplete autosomal recessive disease that affects males and females. Only homozygous patients have a bleeding diathesis. Postoperative and post-trauma hemorrhage is characteristic. Patients may also have epistaxis, hematuria, and menorrhagia. Spontaneous bleeding is rare.

Homozygous patients with factor XI deficiency have a prolonged partial thromboplastin time, and normal bleeding and prothrombin times. The factor XI level is 1–10% (1–10 units/dL), whereas heterozygous patients have factor XI levels of 30–65% (30–65 units/dL).

The half-life of factor XI in vivo is from 40 to 80 hr. Replacement therapy for bleeding episodes is carried out with fresh-frozen plasma. Plasma therapy in a dose of 10–15 mL/kg every 24 hr is effective.

16.68 Factor XII Deficiency
(Hageman Factor Deficiency)

Homozygous occurrence of an autosomal gene results in a profound deficiency of factor XII. Despite markedly abnormal test results of the 1st phase of coagulation (PTT and clotting times), affected persons have no clinical abnormalities of bleeding; in fact, some patients have a thrombotic tendency.

16.69 Von Willebrand Disease
(Vascular Hemophilia)

This disease is not as common as hemophilia A (factor VIII deficiency) but is probably more frequent than hemophilia B (factor IX deficiency). It occurs in both sexes and is inherited as an autosomal dominant trait. A few families with severe disease have been described in which the genetic transmission was autosomal recessive. The disease is caused by underproduction of von Willebrand protein or, in some families, by the synthesis of a dysfunctional protein. The von Willebrand protein contains a platelet-adhesive component (von Willebrand factor) and also the protein functions to carry factor VIII in the plasma.

There are at least three major varieties of von Willebrand disease, based on genetic and laboratory studies (Table 16–12). Types I and II are autosomal dominant and type III is autosomal recessive. Types I (classic von Willebrand disease) and III show reduced factor VIII activity, reduced von Willebrand protein and function, and usually a normal multimer structure of the von Willebrand protein on gel electrophoresis. Type II can have normal or reduced factor VIII activity, normal or reduced von Willebrand protein, reduced von Willebrand factor activity, and a loss of large and intermediate-sized multimers on electrophoresis.

CLINICAL MANIFESTATIONS. These include nosebleeds, bleeding from gums, menorrhagia, prolonged oozing from cuts, and increased bleeding after trauma or surgery. Spontaneous hemarthroses are very rare.

LABORATORY FINDINGS. The bleeding time is prolonged in all von Willebrand syndromes. The platelet count and prothrombin time are normal. The partial thromboplastin time may be normal but usually is mildly to moderately prolonged. Type I patients (classic von Willebrand disease) have reduced plasma levels of von Willebrand protein, von Willebrand factor activity, and factor VIII activity. The platelets in von Willebrand disease have decreased adhesiveness and do not aggregate when the antibiotic ristocetin is added to platelet-rich plasma (because von Willebrand factor is missing), unlike platelets from normal individuals. Rare patients may show increased reactivity to ristocetin (type II B).

TREATMENT. Therapy consists of replacement of the von Willebrand factor using fresh-frozen plasma or cryoprecipitate. Cryoprecipitate is the preferred form of therapy for serious bleeding or for preparation for surgery. The recommended dose is two–four bags of cryoprecipitate/10 kg, which can be repeated every 12–24 hr, depending on the bleeding episode to be treated or prevented. Patients with mild to moderate type I von Willebrand disease who have minor bleeding manifestations (e.g., epistaxis), or who are to undergo certain surgical procedures (e.g., dental extraction), may be given DDAVP as for those with hemophilia A.

16.70 PHASE II DISORDERS

Factors II (prothrombin), V, VII, and X are involved in the 2nd phase of coagulation and are designated the prothrombin complex. These factors are produced in the liver, and all except factor V require vitamin K for normal synthesis. The vitamin is necessary for the γ-carboxylation of glutamic acid residues, which converts the inactive precursors into their biologically active forms. These precursors are also known as PIVKA (protein induced by vitamin K absence) and preprotein. For example, factor II's precursor is called PIVKA-II, or prefactor II.

Deficiency of a factor in the prothrombin complex is rare and is inherited in an autosomal recessive manner. The production of a functionally abnormal factor II (dysprothrombinemia) is inherited as an autosomal dominant trait. Patients with a deficiency in one or more of these factors have bleeding manifestations similar to those of the hemophilias, except that there is a high prevalence of spontaneous central nervous system bleeding in those with factor VII deficiency.

LABORATORY FINDINGS. The laboratory tests reveal a prolonged prothrombin time in these patients. Patients with factors II, V, and X deficiency also have a prolonged partial thromboplastin time (PTT). In contrast, patients with factor VII deficiency have a normal PTT. Bleeding time, platelet count, and platelet function tests are normal.

TREATMENT. Therapy consists of replacement of the deficient factor or factors with fresh-frozen plasma. There is no factor concentrate available for factor V replacement. Severe cases of factor II, VII, or X deficiency may need a prothrombin complex concentrate (Proplex) for control of hemostasis. These deficiencies are refractory to vitamin K therapy.

16.71 PHASE III DISORDERS

Congenital Afibrinogenemia

This rare hemorrhagic disorder is caused by an autosomal recessive gene. Despite totally incoagulable blood, these patients usually do not have severe spontaneous hemorrhages or hemarthroses, but trauma or surgery may be followed by severe bleeding. Therapy with 100 mg/kg of fibrinogen provides a hemostatic plasma level. Because the plasma half-life of fibrinogen is 3–5 days, frequent infusions are not necessary. Cryoprecipitate contains fibrinogen and is used effectively for therapy. Each cryoprecipitate bag contains between 225 and 250 mg of fibrinogen/bag. Thus, four to five bags provide 1 g of fibrinogen.

Congenital Dysfibrinogenemias

A number of abnormal fibrinogens with defective function may be associated with thrombotic and bleeding states. Inheritance is as a dominant trait. The thrombin time is prolonged, but chemical or immunologic methods reveal normal levels of fibrinogen.

Factor XIII Deficiency
(Fibrin-Stabilizing Factor Deficiency)

Deficiency of factor XIII has its onset most often in infancy, with bleeding after separation of the umbilical cord stump. Gastrointestinal, intracranial, and intra-articular hemorrhages are the most common clinical manifestations. Routine coagulation studies are normal. Factor XIII deficiency is diagnosed by finding an abnormal solubility of the clot in 5 M urea solution and a short euglobulin lysis time. These patients can be treated with fresh frozen plasma or cryoprecipitate.

Corrigan JJ Jr: The vitamin K-dependent proteins. *In*: Barness LA (ed): Advances In Pediatrics. Chicago, Year Book Medical Publishers, 1981, p 57.
Geddes VA, MacGillivray RTA: The molecular genetics of hemophilia B. Transfusion Med Rev 1:161, 1987.
Hilgartner MW, Pochedly C (ed): Hemophilia in the Child and Adult, 3rd ed. New York, Raven Press, 1989.
Kasper CK: Treatment of factor VIII inhibitors. Prog Hemost Thromb 9:57, 1989.
Kogan SC, Doherty M, Gitschier J: An improved method for prenatal diagnosis of genetic diseases by analysis of amplified DNA sequences. Application to hemophilia A. N Engl J Med 317:985, 1987.
Mammen EF: Congenital coagulation disorders. Semin Thromb Hemost 9:1, 1983.
Mannucci PM: Desmopressin: A nontransfusional form of treatment for congenital and acquired bleeding disorders. Blood 72:1449, 1988.
Oster H, Hejtmancik F: Prenatal diagnosis and carrier detection of genetic diseases by analysis of deoxyribonucleic acid. J Pediatr 112:670, 1988.
Zimmerman TS, Ruggeri ZM, Fulcher CA: Factor VIII/von Willebrand factor. Prog Hematol 13:279, 1983.

ACQUIRED COAGULATION DISORDERS

VITAMIN K DEFICIENCY

16.72 Hemorrhagic Disease of the Newborn

See Sec. 9.49.

16.73 Postneonatal Vitamin K Deficiency

Vitamin K deficiency rarely occurs after the neonatal period, although "late" hemorrhagic disease has been reported in breast-fed children. Intestinal malabsorption of fats and prolonged administration of broad-spectrum antibiotics may result in vitamin K deficiency, and cystic fibrosis and biliary atresia may be complicated by disorders of the prothrombin complex. Prophylactic administration of water-soluble vitamin K orally is indicated in these situations (2–3 mg/24 hr for children and 5–10 mg for adolescents and adults). In those with advanced liver disease synthesis of the factors of the prothrombin complex may be compromised by hepatocellular damage, so vitamin K therapy is often ineffective in correcting these disorders if advanced liver disease is present. The anticoagulant properties of dicumarol and related anticoagulants depend on interference with vitamin K and the formation of factors II, VII, and X. Rat poison (superwarfarin) produces a similar deficiency. Vitamin K is a specific antidote.

The laboratory manifestations of vitamin K deficiency are prolonged prothrombin and partial thromboplastin times. The platelet count, bleeding time, and plasma fibrinogen level are normal. If needed, specific assays for factors II, VII, IX, and X or for detecting the noncarboxylated protein precursors of the vitamin K-dependent coagulation factors can be performed.

16.74 LIVER DISEASE

Coagulation abnormalities are common in patients with liver disease, estimated to be as high as 85%. Only 15% of patients, however, have significant clinical bleeding states. The severity of the coagulation abnormality appears to be directly proportional to the extent of hepatic cell damage. The most common mechanism causing the defect is decreased synthesis of the coagulation factors. Almost all the coagulation factors are produced only in the liver except, apparently, factor VIII, which can be produced in other organs. Severe liver disease characteristically has normal to increased (not reduced) levels of factor VIII activity in plasma. More rare causes of coagulation defects in hepatic disease are disseminated intravascular coagulation or hyperfibrinolysis.

The treatment of the coagulopathy of liver disease consists of replacement with fresh frozen plasma and cryoprecipitates. Fresh frozen plasma (10–15 mL/kg) can be expected to correct all clotting factor defects except fibrinogen. For fibrinogen correction, cryoprecipitates are recommended (four to five bags/10 kg). Because a reduction in the vitamin K dependent coagulation factors is common in those with acute and chronic liver disease, vitamin K therapy can be given a trial. The vitamin can be given orally, subcutaneously, or intravenously (not intramuscularly) in a dose of 1 mg/24 hr of vitamin K for

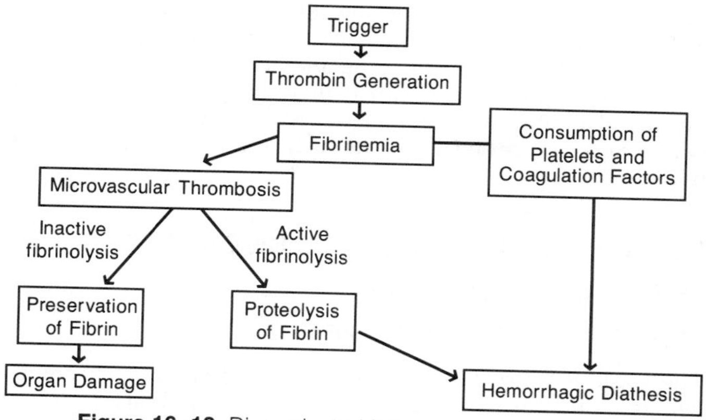

Figure 16–12. Disseminated intravascular coagulation.

infants, 2–3 mg for children, and 5–10 mg for adolescents and adults. An inability to correct the coagulopathy indicates that the coagulopathy may be caused by a reduction in one or more of the non–vitamin K dependent proteins, or because the liver is severely impaired and cannot produce the precursor vitamin K proteins.

16.75 INHIBITORS

Acquired circulating anticoagulants (inhibitors) are defined as abnormal endogenous components of blood that inhibit the coagulation of normal blood. These anticoagulants are usually specific types of gamma globulin and may represent autoantibodies. The circulating anticoagulant may affect coagulation either by neutralizing a specific coagulation factor, directly or by acting against certain reaction sites in the coagulation pathway. When the anticoagulant acts against a specific coagulation factor (e.g., factor VIII or IX), the patient has a clinical bleeding picture similar to that of the congenital deficiency state. Usually no or minimal bleeding is noted in patients in whom the anticoagulant is directed toward a reaction site.

Circulating anticoagulants are uncommon in otherwise normal children. They are found in patients with systemic lupus erythematosus (SLE) or lymphomas, or in those with penicillin or other drug reactions. Spontaneous inhibitors have been reported in children following incidental viral infections.

LABORATORY FINDINGS. Inhibitors against specific coagulation factors usually affect factor VIII, IX, or XI (a phase I defect). The PTT is prolonged and the test does not correct with the addition of normal plasma. The prothrombin time is normal. Specific factor assays determine which factor is involved.

The most common inhibitor against a reaction site is the so-called lupus anticoagulant. Although this inhibitor is found in patients with SLE, it may also occur spontaneously and in other disease states. This anticoagulant does not cause bleeding but paradoxically has been reported to be associated with a thrombotic tendency. It produces a prolonged PTT and it may also result in a prolonged prothrombin time. The addition of normal, platelet-poor plasma does not correct the abnormal tests, but the addition of platelets neutralizes the anticoagulant.

TREATMENT. Management of the patient with an inhibitor against a coagulation factor is the same as for the hemophilia patient who develops an alloantibody against factor VIII or IX. Infusions of a prothrombin complex concentrate (Konyne) or activated prothrombin complex concentrate (Autoplex; FEIBA) may be needed to control significant bleeding manifestations. Spontaneous inhibitors, usually following a viral infection, tend to disappear with a few weeks to months. Inhibitors seen with an underlying disease disappear when the primary disease is treated.

16.76 CONSUMPTION COAGULOPATHY
(Disseminated Intravascular Coagulation Syndromes)

Consumption coagulopathy refers to a large group of conditions, including disseminated intravascular coagulation (DIC). Consequences of this process include widespread intravascular deposition of fibrin, which may lead to tissue ischemia and necrosis, a generalized hemorrhagic state, and hemolytic anemia.

ETIOLOGY. A number of pathologic processes may incite episodes of DIC, including hypoxia, acidosis, tissue necrosis, shock, and endothelial damage (Fig. 16–12). Accordingly, it is not surprising that a large number of diseases have been reported to be associated with DIC, including incompatible blood transfusions, septic shock (especially gram-negative), rickettsial infections, snakebite, purpura fulminans, giant hemangioma, malignancies, and acute promyelocytic leukemia.

CLINICAL MANIFESTATIONS. Most frequently DIC accompanies a severe systemic disease process. Bleeding frequently first occurs from sites of venipuncture or surgical incision, with associated petechiae and ecchymoses. Tissue thrombosis may involve many organs and can be most spectacular as infarction of large areas of skin and subcutaneous tissue or of kidneys. Anemia caused by hemolysis may develop rapidly.

LABORATORY FINDINGS. There is no well-defined sequence of events. The consumption coagulation factors (II, V, VIII, and fibrinogen) and platelets may be consumed by the ongoing intravascular clotting process, with prolongation of the prothrombin, partial thromboplastin, and thrombin times. Platelet counts may be profoundly depressed. The blood contains fragmented burr and helmet-shaped red blood cells (schizocytes), changes referred to as microangiopathic. In addition, because the fibrinolytic mechanism is activated, fibrin split products (FSP) appear in the blood. Table 16–13 presents the laboratory findings in children with the three common acquired coagulation defects.

TREATMENT. The most important component of therapy is control or reversal of the process that initiated the DIC. Infection, shock, acidosis, and hypoxia must be treated promptly and vigorously. If the underlying problem can be controlled bleeding quickly ceases, and there is improvement of the abnormal laboratory findings. Blood components are used for replacement therapy in patients who have hemorrhage. This may consist of platelet infusions (for thrombocy-

TABLE 16–13. Laboratory Findings in Disseminated Intravascular Coagulation, Vitamin K Deficiency, and Liver Disease

	Disorder		
Test	*DIC*	*Vitamin K Deficiency*	*Liver Disease*
PTT	P	P	P
PT	P	P	P
TT	P	N	P
Platelet count	L	N	N/L
FSPs	+	−	±
Fibrinogen	L	N	L
Factor VIII	L	N	N/I

DIC = disseminated intravascular coagulation; PTT = partial thromboplastin time; PT = prothrombin time; TT = thrombin time; FSPs = fibrinolytic split products; P = prolonged; N = normal; L = low; N/L = normal or low; + = present; − = absent; ± = present or absent; I = increased.

topenia), cryoprecipitates (for hypofibrinogenemia), and/or fresh-frozen plasma (for replacement of other coagulation factors and natural inhibitors).

In some patients the treatment of the primary disease may be inadequate or incomplete, or the replacement therapy may not be effective in controlling the hemorrhage. When this occurs the DIC may be treated with anticoagulants. Heparin is the drug of choice and can be administered on an intermittent or continuous intravenous treatment schedule. Using the intermittent intravenous schedule, heparin is given in a dose of 75–100 units/kg every 4 hr. With the continuous schedule, 50–75 units of heparin/kg is given as a bolus followed by a continuous infusion of 15–25 units/kg/hr. The duration and effectiveness of heparin therapy can be judged by serial measurements of the platelet count and plasma fibrinogen concentration.

Heparin has been found to be an effective drug in children with DIC associated with purpura fulminans and promyelocytic leukemia. Lower doses (10–15 units/kg/hr without loading dose) are used for those with progranulocytic leukemia. Heparin is not indicated and has been reported to be ineffective in septic shock, snake envenomation, heat stroke, massive head injury, and incompatible blood transfusion reaction.

Corrigan JJ Jr: Coagulation inhibitors. Am J Pediatr Hematol Oncol 2:281, 1980.
Hathaway WE, Bonnar J: Hemostatic Disorders of the Pregnant Woman and Newborn Infant. New York. Elsevier, 1987.
Corrigan JJ Jr: Disseminated intravascular coagulation: Pathogenesis, diagnosis, and management. *In*: Lusher JM, Barnhart MI (eds): Acquired Bleeding Disorders in Children: Abnormalities of Hemostasis. New York. Masson, 1981, p 27.
Owen CA Jr: Coagulation disorders associated with hepatocellular disease. *In*: Lusher JM, Barnhart MI (eds): Acquired Bleeding Disorders in Children: Abnormalities of Hemostasis. New York, Masson, 1981, p 41.

16.77 PLATELET AND BLOOD VESSEL DISORDERS

Platelets are non-nucleated, cellular fragments produced by the megakaryocytes of the bone marrow. The large size of the megakaryocyte reflects its polyploidy. As the megakaryocyte reaches maturity, fragmentation of the cytoplasm occurs and large numbers of platelets are liberated. In the circulation they have a life span of 7–10 days. The platelet has a number of intrinsic antigens, which are distinct from those of the red blood cell, and some are shared by the leukocytes.

The platelets are intimately involved in both the vascular and clotting aspects of hemostasis. They are necessary for integrity of the vascular endothelium—when small blood vessels are transected, platelets accumulate at the site of injury, forming a hemostatic plug. Platelet adhesion is initiated by contact with extravascular components such as collagen. Release of thromboxane (a prostaglandin derivative) and endogenous ADP causes firm aggregation. Serotonin and histamine liberated during these processes increase local vasoconstriction. Platelets have a phospholipid with partial thromboplastin activity, which makes an important contribution to coagulation. They also transport other blood coagulation factors through absorption to the platelet surface. Finally, the platelet is necessary for normal clot retraction.

The normal platelet count is 150–400 × 10^9/L. Lower counts indicate thrombocytopenia, either caused by inadequate production or by excessive destruction or removal of platelets. Inadequate production is almost always a result of marrow dysfunction, with decreases in the number of megakaryocytes. By contrast, in the thrombocytopenias caused by increased destruction, the megakaryocytes are quantitatively normal or increased. The hypomegakaryocytic thrombocytopenias result from aplasia of the marrow or from its infiltration by abnormal or neoplastic tissue. Because of the grave prognosis of such disorders, bone marrow aspiration is indicated in those with significant, unexplained thrombocytopenia. Bone marrow aspirations can usually be performed without serious bleeding, even in patients with severe thrombocytopenia, because thromboplastins in tissue juice usually effect hemostasis.

CONGENITAL AND INHERITED DISORDERS

16.78 Thrombocytopenias

WISKOTT-ALDRICH SYNDROME

The Wiskott-Aldrich syndrome consists of eczema, thrombocytopenic hemorrhage, and increased susceptibility to infection because of an immunologic defect that is transmitted as an X-linked recessive trait (see Sec. 11.18). The bone marrow contains a normal number of megakaryocytes, but many have bizarre nuclear morphology. Homologous platelets survive normally when transfused into these patients, but autologous platelets have a shortened life span and are small in size. Wiskott-Aldrich syndrome may represent an unusual circumstance in which thrombocytopenia results from abnormal platelet formation or release, despite quantitatively adequate numbers of megakaryocytes. Splenectomy has often been followed by overwhelming sepsis and death, but significant improvement in thrombocytopenia occurs after splenectomy. Prophylactic use of penicillin is essential postsplenectomy. About 5% of patients with Wiskott-Aldrich syndrome develop lymphoreticular malignancies. A few cases have been reported to benefit from the administration of transfer factor or from bone marrow transplantation.

OTHER INHERITED THROMBOCYTOPENIAS

Other types of inherited thrombocytopenias have been described. Some are X-linked and some have autosmal transmission. Responses to therapy, including splenectomy, have usually been disappointing. The inordinately high mortality of young males splenectomized for presumed idiopathic thrombocytopenic purpura (ITP) suggests that, even without other stigmata, X-linked thrombocytopenia may represent a variant of Wiskott-Aldrich syndrome. Thus, the young thrombocytopenic male must be carefully studied before a diagnosis of ITP is made. A platelet survival study may be indicated in such patients.

THROMBOPOIETIN DEFICIENCY

A few patients have had chronic thrombocytopenia attributed to deficiency of a megakaryocyte maturation factor contained in normal plasma. Plasma infusions repeatedly produced a sustained rise in the platelet count. In somewhat similar cases, episodic thrombocytopenia and microangiopathic hemolysis were reversed by infusions of plasma.

THROMBOCYTOPENIA WITH CAVERNOUS HEMANGIOMA
(Kasabach-Merritt Syndrome)

Some infants with large, cavernous hemangiomas of the trunk, extremities, or abdominal viscera have severe thrombocytopenia and other evidence of intravascular coagulation (see also Sec. 23.8). Histologic and isotopic studies indicate that platelets are trapped and destroyed within the extensive vascular bed of the tumor. The peripheral blood reveals thrombocytopenia and red blood cell fragments, and the bone marrow contains adequate numbers of megakaryocytes. Spontaneous thrombosis within the tumor may lead to obliteration of the vascular channels and spontaneous recovery; radiation therapy in a single dose of 600–800 rad (6–8 Gy) may accelerate this process, but repeated courses may be necessary. When anatomically feasible, external compression or total excision may be attempted, but surgery can be associated with uncontrollable hemorrhage. Corticosteroids and interferon may hasten involution and warrant trial, especially in the young infant. Splenectomy is contraindicated.

CONGENITAL HYPOPLASTIC THROMBOCYTOPENIA WITH ASSOCIATED MALFORMATIONS
(Thrombocytopenia Absent Radius [TAR] Syndrome)

Severe thrombocytopenia associated with aplasia of radii and thumbs, and with cardiac and renal anomalies, occurs as a familial condition. Severe hemorrhagic manifestations are evident in the 1st days of life. Hemoglobin levels are normal; leukocytosis and even leukemoid reactions have been found in some patients. Megakaryocytes are absent from the bone marrow.

The anomalies in this disease are similar to those observed in Fanconi pancytopenia, in which the hematologic abnormalities are not usually observed until the 3rd–4th year of life. In this disorder chromosomes do not reveal the abnormalities found in Fanconi syndrome. No infants with congenital hypoplastic thrombocytopenia have been reported to develop full-blown Fanconi syndrome, nor have both conditions been observed in the same family.

16.79 Platelet Function Defects

Hemorrhagic disease resulting from congenital disorders of platelet function are not common. The inheritance pattern is not known for many of these disorders. The defects can be in adhesion, aggregation, and platelet coagulant activity.

CLINICAL MANIFESTATIONS. The clinical manifestations are similar to those encountered in patients with thrombocytopenia and consist of mucous membrane bleeding (epistaxis, oral cavity bleeding, menorrhagia, gastrointestinal and genitourinary hemorrhage), skin petechiae, and small ecchymoses.

LABORATORY FINDINGS. The laboratory test results are variable and reflect the functional defect, but all functional defects have a prolonged bleeding time, normal prothrombin time, normal PTT, and either a normal or moderately reduced platelet count. The defects can be defined by specific in vitro platelet function tests. Patients with platelet factor 3 deficiency, however, have a normal bleeding time but abnormal prothrombin consumption test.

TREATMENT. Treatment of the bleeding disorders in these patients is difficult. Platelet transfusions are usually required to control significant hemorrhage.

BERNARD-SOULIER SYNDROME

This autosomal recessive inherited platelet adhesion defect is characterized by moderate thrombocytopenia, large platelets, and decreased ristocetin-induced platelet agglutination (aggregation) that is not corrected by the addition of von Willebrand factor.

GLANZMANN THROMBASTHENIA

This autosomal recessive inherited platelet disorder is characterized by a normal platelet count, absent in vitro aggregation with all agonists, and absent clot retraction.

OTHER DEFECTS

Defects in the normal platelet release reaction have been described, caused by platelet granule deficiency, impaired platelet arachidonic acid metabolism, or an impaired secretion of intraplatelet agonists. Laboratory studies reveal a normal platelet count and abnormal in vitro aggregation. The deficient granule variety can be detected by using electron microscopic techniques.

16.80 Blood Vessel Defects

Bleeding secondary to defective blood vessels is uncommon in childhood. Disorders such as hereditary hemorrhagic telangiectasia and Ehlers-Danlos syndrome can cause significant mucous membrane and skin bleeding. All laboratory tests for hemostasis are usually normal in these patients.

ACQUIRED DISORDERS

Thrombocytopenias

16.81 IDIOPATHIC THROMBOCYTOPENIC PURPURA

Acute idiopathic thrombocytopenic purpura (ITP), the most common of the thrombocytopenic purpuras of childhood, is associated with petechiae, mucocutaneous bleeding and, occasionally, hemorrhage into tissues. There is a profound deficiency of circulating platelets, despite adequate numbers of megakaryoctyes in the marrow.

ETIOLOGY. The disease often appears to be related to sensitization by viral infections; in about 70% of cases there is an antecedent disease such as rubella, rubeola, or viral respiratory infection. The interval between infection and onset of purpura averages 2 wk. As with the adult form, it seems probable that an immune mechanism is the basis for the thrombocytopenia. Platelet antibodies can be detected in some acute cases. Increased amounts of IgG have been found bound to platelets, and may represent immune complexes absorbed on the platelet surface. No consistently reliable test currently exists for the serologic diagnosis of ITP.

CLINICAL MANIFESTATIONS. The onset is frequently acute. Bruising and a generalized petechial rash occur 1–4 wk after a viral infection or without antecedent illness. The bleeding is typically asymmetric and may be most prominent over the legs. Hemorrhages in mucous membranes may be prominent, with hemorrhagic bullae of the gums and lips. Nosebleeds may be severe and difficult to control. The most serious complication is intracranial hemorrhage, which occurs in fewer than 1% of cases. The liver, spleen, and lymph nodes are not enlarged. Except for the signs of bleeding the patient appears clinically well. The acute phase of the disease associated with spontaneous hemorrhages lasts for only 1–2 wk. Thrombocytopenia may persist, but spontaneous mucocutaneous hemorrhages subside. Sometimes the onset is more insidious, with moderate bruising and few petechiae.

LABORATORY FINDINGS. The platelet count is reduced below 20×10^9/L. The few platelets observed on blood smear are large (megathrombocytes) and reflect increased marrow production. Those tests that depend on platelet function, such as the bleeding time and clot retraction, yield abnormal results. The white count cell count is normal, and anemia is not present unless significant blood loss has occurred.

Bone marrow aspiration reveals normal granulocytic and erythrocytic series and, frequently, modest eosinophilia. Normal or increased numbers of megakaryocytes are seen. Some of these are immature, with deep basophilic cytoplasm; platelet budding may be scanty, but there is no pathognomonic or diagnostic megakaryocyte morphology. The changes seen reflect increased megakaryocytic turnover.

DIFFERENTIAL DIAGNOSIS. ITP must be differentiated from aplastic or infiltrative processes of the bone marrow. Marrow aplasia or replacement is unlikely if the physical examination and blood count are normal, except for thrombocytopenia. Significant enlargement of the spleen suggests primary liver disease with congestive splenomegaly, lipidosis, or reticuloendotheliosis. Thrombocytopenic purpura may be an initial manifestation of systemic lupus erythematosus, AIDS, or lymphoma, but this sequence is unusual in young children. In adolescents the possibility is greater, and serologic studies for systemic lupus erythematosus and AIDS are indicated. Genetically determined thrombocytopenias must be considered in infants (particularly males) found to have low platelet counts.

TREATMENT. ITP has an excellent prognosis, even when no specific therapy is given. Within 3 mo 75% of patients recover completely, most within 8 wk. Severe spontaneous hemorrhages and intracranial bleeding are usually confined to the initial phase of the disease. After the initial acute phase, spontaneous manifestations tend to subside. About 90% of affected children have regained normal platelet counts 9–12 mo after onset, and relapses are unusual.

Fresh blood or platelet concentrates have transient benefit because transfused platelets survive only briefly, but they should be administered when life-threatening hemorrhage occurs.

When the disease is mild and hemorrhages of the retina or mucous membranes are not present, no specific therapy may be indicated. The affected child should be protected from falls or trauma. Vitamins K and C have no therapeutic effect.

Gamma Globulin. Infusions of intravenous gamma globulin (Sandoglobulin; Gamimune N) are followed by sustained rises of platelet count. Large doses of intravenous gamma globulin (400 mg/kg for 5 days) induce remission of many cases of acute and, occasionally, chronic ITP.

Corticosteroid Therapy. Although corticosteroid therapy has not decreased the number of chronic cases, it is benefical because it reduces the severity and shortens the duration of the initial phase. In more severe cases, therapy with a corticosteroid, such as prednisone in a dose of 1–2 mg/kg/24 hr in divided doses or its equivalent, is indicated. The necessity for corticosteroid therapy in mild cases has been debated, although the platelet count returns to a hemostatic level more rapidly with such therapy. This therapy is continued until the platelet count is normal or for 3 wk, whichever comes first. At this point steroid therapy should be discontinued, even if the platelet count remains low. Prolonged corticosteroid therapy is not indicated and may depress the bone marrow, in addition to producing cushingoid changes and growth failure. If thrombocytopenia persists for 4–6 mo, a 2nd short course of corticosteroid therapy or intravenous immunoglobulin may be given.

Whether the initial therapy of choice in acute ITP is no therapy, intravenous gamma globulin, or corticosteroids is now being reassessed. Splenectomy should be reserved for chronic patients, defined as thrombocytopenia persistent for more than 1 yr, and for severe cases that do not respond to corticosteroids. Considerable improvement can usually be expected. If the hemorrhagic manifestations are severe, or if intracranial hemorrhage is suspected, larger doses of prednisone (5–10 mg/kg/24 hr) and intravenous gamma globulin can be used. Platelet transfusions may provide temporary control of bleeding, but sustained platelet counts are rarely achieved.

16.82 DRUG-INDUCED THROMBOCYTOPENIAS

A number of drugs can cause thrombocytopenia, either as a result of an immune-mediated process (with the drug functioning as a hapten) or of megakaryocyte injury. Drugs commonly used in pediatrics that can cause thrombocytopenia include carbamazepine (Tegretol), phenytoin (Dilantin), sulfonamides, trimethoprim-sulfamethoxazole, and chloramphenicol.

16.83 HEMOLYTIC-UREMIC SYNDROME

See also Sec. 18.13.

This acute disease of infancy and early childhood usually follows an episode of acute gastroenteritis. Shortly thereafter signs and symptoms of hemolytic anemia, thrombocytopenia, and acute renal insufficiency develop. Bilateral renal cortical necrosis may occur, and case fatality rates as high as 30% have been reported. Its occasional epidemic occurrence suggests that an infectious agent may be involved.

LABORATORY FINDINGS. The hemolytic anemia is associated with characteristically bizarre red blood cell morphology. Many of the red blood cells are contracted and distorted, with a prominence of spherocytes, burr cells, and helmet-shaped forms (see Fig. 16–3*F*). A depressed platelet count, despite normal numbers of megakaryocytes in the marrow, indicates excessive peripheral destruction. Tests of the coagulation mechanism are usually normal. Protein, red blood cells, and casts are present in the urinary sediment, and grave renal damage is reflected by anuria and azotemia.

TREATMENT. For a discussion of the management of uremia and anuria, see Sec. 18.13. Transfusions are indicated for severe anemia. Corticosteroid and heparin therapy do not affect survival or prognosis.

16.84 THROMBOTIC THROMBOCYTOPENIC PURPURA

This rare and serious disease is similar to the hemolytic–uremic syndrome. Diffuse embolism and thrombosis of the small blood vessels of the brain are evidenced by shifting neurologic signs such as aphasias, blindness, and convulsions. The prognosis is grave. Laboratory findings include thrombocytopenia and a hemolytic anemia associated with distorted and fragmented red blood cell microangiopathy. Plasmapheresis and plasma infusions are effective in 60–70% of cases. Corticosteroids and splenectomy are reserved for refractory cases.

OTHER CAUSES

Thrombocytopenia is a common complication of viral and bacterial (especially septicemia) infections, disseminated intravascular coagulation, and, rarely, heparin therapy.

16.85 NEONATAL THROMBOCYTOPENIA

Thrombocytopenia of the newborn may indicate primary disease in the infant's hematopoietic system or may be a result of the transfer of abnormal factors from the mother.

ASSOCIATION WITH INFECTION

Thrombocytopenia may occur in various fetal and neonatal infections and may be responsible for serious spontaneous bleeding. These include viral infections (especially rubella and cytomegalic inclusion disease), protozoal infections (e.g., toxoplasmosis), syphilis, and bacterial infections, especially those caused by gram-negative bacilli. Hemolysis is usually also present in infants with prominent anemia and jaundice. The liver and spleen are considerably enlarged. The bone marrow changes are variable, but reduced numbers of megakaryocytes may be seen.

IMMUNE NEONATAL THROMBOCYTOPENIA

About 30% of infants born of mothers with active idiopathic thrombocytopenic purpura have thrombocytopenia resulting from the transplacental transfer of antiplatelet antibodies. Rarely, infants with neonatal disease have been born of mothers with past histories of ITP who have normal platelet counts, and whose disease has been inactive for many years. Petechiae are not present initially but appear in a generalized distribution within a few minutes after birth. Bleeding from the bowel or kidney and intracranial hemorrhage may occur. In mild cases there may be few abnormal findings. Hepatosplenomegaly is not present. The duration of the thrombocytopenia is 2–3 mo.

Therapy is not strikingly successful, but intravenous immunoglobulin, exchange transfusions, or platelet transfusions may be of temporary value in arresting acute bleeding. Corticosteroid therapy has not been proved beneficial. Because of the self-limited nature of the disease, splenectomy is contraindicated. Corticosteroid therapy given to the mother 1 wk prior to delivery or administration of intravenous gamma globulin to the mother late in pregnancy may reduce the severity of the disease in the mother and perhaps in the infant.

When the fetus has platelet antigens that the mother does not have, alloimmunization may occur. If maternal antibodies to fetal platelet antigens reach a sufficiently high titer, enough may cross the placenta to produce thrombocytopenia in the fetus. The disease may be familial, and first-born infants are frequently affected. Clinical signs include petechiae and other hemorrhagic manifestations. Antiplatelet antibodies can be demonstrated in about 50% of cases using sensitive tests. The PLA-1 antigen is most frequently involved. Exchange transfusion is temporarily effective in stopping bleeding. Intravenous gamma globulin given to the affected newborn may be helpful. If compatible platelets can be obtained (these are most easily procured by preparing washed platelet concentrates from the mother), they offer specific, effective therapy. Infants born of successive pregnancies may be affected. Elective cesarean section has been advocated to spare the infant's head the trauma of delivery.

When the mother has drug-induced thrombocytopenia, both antibody and drug may cross the placenta and cause neonatal thrombocytopenia. Corticosteroid therapy, and especially exchange transfusions, should be considered when bleeding manifestations are severe.

16.86 Platelet Function Disorders

Acquired disorders of platelet function are caused by toxic metabolic products (e.g., in uremia), autoantibodies, immune complexes, fibrin split (degradation) products (FSPs), and drugs. These patients have a prolonged bleeding time and abnormalities in platelet aggregation tests.

The most common acquired defect is caused by drugs. Some drugs produce an irreversible reduction of prostaglandin synthesis within the platelet by inhibition of cyclo-oxygenase enzymes. This prevents the release of endogenous ADP and of the prostaglandin derivative thromboxane, which are essential for platelet aggregation. The abnormality can be most easily demonstrated with a platelet aggregometer, by which an ablation of the so-called secondary wave of platelet aggregation can be demonstrated. The most important drug that produces this effect is aspirin. The effect is not dose-related. Abnormal platelet aggregation can be demonstrated in adults within 1 hr of ingestion of as little as 300 mg of aspirin. The abnormality persists for 4–6 days, or until the platelets that have been exposed to the drug have been replaced. Usually the effects of these drugs produce no clinical problems, although prolongation of bleeding time is frequently seen. If the patient has an underlying bleeding disorder such as hemophilia or undergoes surgery, however, hemorrhage may occur. Aspirin or other drugs that inhibit platelet aggregation are contraindicated in these circumstances and should be replaced with other agents, such as acetaminophen, when indicated. Aspirin may have transplacental effects on platelet function in the newborn, producing neonatal hemorrhage; maternal aspirin consumption should be avoided during the last trimester of pregnancy.

16.87 Vascular Disorders

The most common cause of a vascular type of nonthrombocytopenic purpura is Schönlein-Henoch syndrome or anaphylactoid purpura (Sec. 11.56). This acute inflammatory process of unknown origin involves the small blood vessels of the skin, joints, gut, and kidney. The striking centrifugal distribution of the rash and involvement of the legs and buttocks are characteristic, particularly when combined with arthritis, nephritis, or gastrointestinal bleeding. The petechiae should be differentiated from those of early meningococcemia or of septicemia caused by other micro-organisms. Toxic vasculitis may produce a hemorrhagic rash as a reaction to drugs such as arsenicals and iodides. Similar findings may occur during viral or rickettsial infections.

Treatment of this self-limited condition is supportive. Corticosteroids can be effective in controlling the painful edema, gastrointestinal pain, and arthritis, but not the vasculitic skin rash.

16.88 Thrombocytosis

Platelet counts in excess of $750 \times 10^9/L$ may be designated as thrombocytosis. Markedly elevated counts may accompany hemorrhage, iron deficiency anemia, hemolytic anemias, and primary myeloproliferative disorders. Acute and chronic inflammatory states may be accompanied by elevated platelet counts. Platelet counts exceeding $600 \times 10^9/L$ are regularly observed in those with Kawasaki disease. Persons with asplenia and children with sickle cell anemia often have somewhat elevated platelet counts. After splenectomy for ITP or hemolytic anemia the platelet count often rises precipitously and may exceed $1{,}000 \times 10^9/L$ 10–14 days postoperatively. Generally, no specific therapy such as anticoagulation is necessary, because thrombosis is extremely rare. The use of aspirin (or dipyridamole), which inhibits platelet function, may be considered if factors predisposing to thrombosis are present.

A case of primary thrombocytosis associated with thrombotic episodes and myocardial infarction has been described.

Ballin A, Andrew M, Ling E, et al: High-dose intravenous gamma globulin therapy for neonatal autoimmune thrombocytopenia. J Pediatr 112:789, 1988.

Buchanan GR: Childhood acute idiopathic thrombocytopenic purpura: How many tests and how much treatment required? J Pediatr 106:928, 1985.

George JN, Nurden AT, Phillips DR: Molecular defects in interactions of platelets with the vessel wall. N Engl J Med 311:1084, 1984.

Halperin DS, Doyle JJ: Is bone marrow examination justified in idiopathic thrombocytopenic purpura? Am J Dis Child 142:508, 1988.

Heath HW, Pearson HA: Thrombocytosis in pediatric outpatients. J Pediatr 114:805, 1989.

Imbach P, Barandum S, Hirt A, et al: Intravenous immunoglobulin for idiopathic thrombocytopenic purpura (ITP) in childhood. Am J Pediatr Hematol Oncol 2:171, 1984.

Imbach P: A multicenter European trial of intravenous immune globulin in immune thrombocytopenic purpura in childhood. Vox Sang 49:25, 1985.

Weiss HJ: Congenital disorders of platelet function. Semin Hematol 17:228, 1980.

Vain NE, Bedros AA: Treatment of isoimmune thrombocytopenia of the newborn with transfusion of maternal platelets. Pediatrics 63:107, 1979.

16.89 THROMBOTIC DISORDERS

CLINICAL MANIFESTATIONS AND DIAGNOSIS. The occlusion of a blood vessel with a platelet plug or fibrin clot may occur in vessels of any size. Capillary and small-vessel occlusion are seen in vasculitic diseases and as complications of disseminated intravascular coagulation; in medium-sized vessels, in homocystinuria, cyanotic congenital heart disease, dehydration, and polyarteritis nodosa; and in larger vessels, such as in aortic thrombosis, superior vena cava thrombosis in the newborn, deep venous thrombosis, sickle cell anemia, and pulmonary embolism. The mechanism leading to the thrombosis is vessel injury in addition to one or all of the following: abnormal platelet adhesiveness-aggregation; an activated coagulation mechanism; an inactive inhibitor system; an inactive fibrinolytic mechanism; and reduced blood flow. Arterial thrombosis appears to depend on vascular injury and platelet activation, whereas venous thrombosis generally occurs in low-flow conditions associated with activation of the coagulation mechanism or with an impaired inhibitor-fibrinolytic system.

The clinical manifestations reflect organ or tissue injury resulting from the absence or a severe reduction in blood perfusion. In general, vascular occlusive events in children have an acute or sudden onset. The diagnosis is made by angiography. Ultrasound and radionuclide scanning techniques can be used for screening purposes. Other laboratory studies are rarely helpful in diagnosing a thromboembolic event except in two settings: when the event is a result of DIC (in which case the patient demonstrates thrombocytopenia, hypofibrinogenemia, reduced factors II, V, and VIII, and positive FSPs) and or, in rare patients, of congenital deficiencies of natural inhibitors.

CONGENITAL AND INHERITED DEFECTS

The formation of a fibrin clot is regulated by a complex inhibitor system that involves antithrombin III, protein C, and protein S. By regulating clot formation, these plasma inhibitors prevent spontaneous intravascular coagulation, limit the thrombotic response of the body to injury, and control the extension of existing clots. Reduced plasma levels of any one of these inhibitors leads to a propensity to excessive thrombosis. Also, a reduced ability to remove fibrin clots (congenital hypoplasminogenemia and dysplasminogenemia) and the formation of an unusual fibrin clot (congenital dysfibrinogenemia) can lead to thrombotic diseases. The thromboembolic diseases reported in deficient patients predominantly affect the venous system; arterial forms are rare. Deep vein thrombosis of the legs, pulmonary embolism, thromboses of the pelvic veins and mesenteric veins, and saggital sinus thrombosis are frequent manifestations. The 1st thromboembolic event usually occurs from 10 yr to 25 yr of age. A severe neonatal form (see later) has been reported.

Antithrombin III Deficiency

Antithrombin III (AT III) is a plasma inhibitor protein that blocks the enzymatic activity of some serine protease coagulation factors. The activity of this inhibitor is increased by heparin (formally called heparin cofactor activity). Antithrombin III is therefore necessary for heparin's anticoagulant activity. Antithrombin III is synthesized in the liver, is not vitamin K-dependent, and can be consumed during the process of extensive intravascular clotting. Patients with AT III deficiency have AT III activity levels between 20 and 60% of normal. Normal newborns have reduced AT III activity.

Congenital AT III deficiency is an autosomal dominant trait that affects both sexes and has been observed in all races. Homozygous patients have not been described. Diagnosis is by detection of reduced AT III activity in plasma. There are at least two types of hereditary AT III deficiency: type I patients (most common) lack both AT III functional activity and protein, and type II patients lack functional activity but have the protein (a dysfunctional protein).

Treatment of thrombotic events in these patients can be difficult. Mildly deficient patients may respond to intravenous heparin but patients with severe deficiency do not. An infusion of plasma (as a source of AT III) plus heparin can be tried for acute therapy. Early initiation of long-term warfarin therapy is recommended for such patients. Danazol, a synthetic weak androgen, may raise AT III levels in selected patients. The efficacy and safety of this drug have not been established in children.

Protein C Deficiency

Protein C is a plasma inhibitor protein that, once activated, inhibits clot formation and enhances fibrinolysis. It is synthesized in the liver and is vitamin K-dependent. Protein C is converted into an active enzyme by a thrombin-thrombomodulin complex on the endothelial cell surface. Activated protein C (protein Ca) inhibits a plasminogen activator inhibitor, which results in enhanced fibrinolysis and, with protein S as a cofactor, inhibits the clotting ability of factors V and VIII. Thromboembolic disease has been reported in patients with levels that are from 38 to 49% of normal, but not all patients with protein C deficiency have thromboembolic disease. Clinical thrombotic events appear in adolescence.

Congenital protein C deficiency is an autosomal dominant trait. Diagnosis is by detection of reduced protein C activity in plasma. There are two types: type I patients (most common) have both activity and protein reduced, and type II patients have functionally reduced activity but a normal amount of protein.

Treatment includes heparin anticoagulation for thrombosis and chronic oral anticoagulation with warfarin to prevent recurrence of thrombosis. Androgenic drugs (e.g., danazol) have been shown to increase the protein C protein level to normal levels within 10–20 days, but the functional activity remains significantly lower than the antigenic level. Thus, its efficacy has not been established.

Purpura Fulminans Neonatalis

Homozygous protein C-deficient infants are characterized by the abrupt, early onset of subcutaneous ecchymoses and necrosis and by the widespread thrombosis of blood vessels. The thrombosis is accompanied by evidence of disseminated intravascular coagulation. These patients have undetectable levels of protein C, and the parents have values consistent with the heterozygous state. Treatment of this rare, severe condition includes fresh-frozen plasma and long-term anticoagulation with warfarin. A similar condition has occurred in an infant with homozygous protein S deficiency.

Protein S Deficiency

Protein S, a vitamin K-dependent plasma protein, is synthesized in the liver and by endothelial cells. It functions as a cofactor for the anticoagulant effect of activated protein C. Protein S exists in the protein-bound and free forms in the plasma; the free form is biologically active. Protein S-deficient patients have been identified by immunologic and functional assays. Patients with recurrent thrombosis have protein S free levels from 15 to 37% of normal.

Congenital protein S deficiency is inherited as an autosomal dominant trait. Homozygous deficiency has been described. Thromboembolic disease may or may not occur in the heterozygotes. Treatment consists of heparin anticoagulation for thrombosis and oral anticoagulants for the prevention of further thrombosis.

Plasminogen and Fibrinogen Abnormalities

Both qualitative and quantitative plasminogen abnormalities have been observed in rare patients with thromboembolic disorders. The inheritance pattern for these abnormalities is not known. Many abnormal fibrinogens (dysfibrinogenemia) have been discovered that form abnormal clots; the dysfibrinogens appear to be inherited as an autosomal dominant trait. Treatment of thromboses in these disorders consists of the administration of heparin and long-term warfarin to prevent subsequent thrombotic events.

ACQUIRED DEFECTS

Acquired thrombotic and embolic events are usually uncommon in children, in general. But there are increasing reports of thromboembolic disease (TED) in newborns and in patients with specific diseases (Table 16–14). Arterial events usually present as stroke (at any age), a cold and pulseless lower extremity, with or without renal involvement (aortic thrombosis in the newborn), and myocardial infarction, although any arterialized organ can be affected. Venous events usually present as deep venous thrombosis with or without phlebitis, pulmonary embolism, and renal vein thrombosis.

Treatment of TED is designed to remove the thrombus or embolus (e.g., by thrombectomy or thrombolytic agents) or to inhibit the formation and propagation of a thrombus with drugs (anticoagulants).

Venous Thrombosis and Thrombophlebitis

Superficial thrombophlebitis is treated by anti-inflammatory drugs (e.g., aspirin), heat compresses, rest, and elevation of the affected part. Patients with deep venous thrombosis or thrombophlebitis are treated with anticoagulation and sometimes with thrombolytic agents. Heparin anticoagulation should be used in a full dose for 7–10 days, with warfarin added for an additional 2–3 mo in those patients with proximal venous thrombosis. Patients with calf vein thrombosis should be treated with heparin for 7 days and then with warfarin or subcutaneous heparin for an additional 6 wk. Acute iliofemoral venous thrombosis in adults is treated with thrombolytic agents followed by anticoagulation with heparin and warfarin. Experience with thrombolytic therapy is limited in children, so its usefulness is unknown.

TABLE 16–14. Acquired Thromboembolic Disease in Newborns, Children, and Adolescents

Newborn: umbilical catheter-related; renal vein thrombosis; aortic thrombosis; vena cava thrombosis
Nephrotic syndrome: venous thrombosis
Cyanotic heart disease: venous thrombosis
Acyanotic heart disease: arterial embolism from prosthetic valves, mitral valve prolapse, mural thrombi; coronary artery thrombosis in Kawasaki disease and polyarteritis nodosa
Vessel injury: arterial and venous thrombosis
DIC syndromes: microvascular thrombosis
Sickle cell anemia: arterial and venous thrombosis
Homocystinuria: arterial and venous thrombosis
Drugs: L-asparaginase
Pregnancy and oral contraceptives: venous thrombosis
Paroxysmal nocturnal hemoglobinuria
Diamond-Blackfan syndrome

Pulmonary Embolism

(See Sec. 14.80 and 15.79)

The patient with pulmonary embolism (PE) can be treated with heparin or thrombolytic drugs. Thrombolytic therapy produces a more rapid clinical improvement than heparin therapy, but the overall survival and long-term pulmonary function abnormalities appear to be the same in both treatment groups. If maximal medical management is not successful within 1 hr, embolectomy should be strongly considered.

Arterial Thrombosis

Surgical removal of the clot is the treatment of choice in acute arterial thrombosis or embolism. Surgery may not be possible, however, because of the location of the clot, size of the artery, or clinical condition of the patient. In such patients, intra-arterial or intravenous thrombolytic drugs have been used, along with successful removal or partial removal of the clot. The therapeutic plan should include prevention of new clot formation by anticoagulation. Platelet-inhibiting drugs may be beneficial in some patients with arterial diseases that predispose to thrombosis, such as aneurysms, cardiomyopathies (mural thrombi), and cardiac prosthesis.

Stroke

Arterial occlusion in the brain occurs when there is a vascular injury or anomaly or, more commonly, embolization from the heart. Venous thrombosis of cerebral vessels can be seen in those with cyanotic heart disease, inflammatory lesions of the brain, or hyperviscosity states. The therapeutic approach is directed toward the cause of the occlusion. Anticoagulation and/or platelet inhibitor drugs may be used. The presence of a hemorrhagic infarct is a contraindication for anticoagulant therapy. It is not known whether thrombolytic therapy is effective or safe in these children.

ANTICOAGULANT AND THROMBOLYTIC THERAPY

ANTICOAGULANTS

Heparin

Heparin enhances the rate by which antithrombin III neutralizes the activities of several of the activated clotting proteins, especially thrombin. The average half-life of intravenously administered heparin is about 60 min in adults and can be as short as 30 min in the newborn. Heparin does not cross the placenta. The half-life of heparin is dose-dependent—that is, the higher the dose, the longer the circulating half-life. In thrombotic disease the half-life may be shorter than normal in patients with significant TED (such as pulmonary embolism) and longer than normal in patients with cirrhosis and uremia.

Anticoagulation with heparin is contraindicated in the following circumstances: a pre-existing coagulation defect or bleeding abnormality; a recent central nervous system hemorrhage; bleeding from inaccessible sites; malignant hypertension; bacterial endocarditis; previous surgery of the eye, brain, or spinal cord; and current administration of regional or lumbar block anesthesia. In spite of these precautions, the frequency of bleeding in patients given heparin anticoagulation is about 5–10%.

Heparin can be given as an intravenous or subcutaneous injection. It is not effective when taken orally and should not be given as an intramuscular injection. Two techniques can be used to administer the drug intravenously, intermittent bolus or continuous infusion. Using intermittent schedule, the patient is given 75–100 units/kg of heparin intravenously by bolus every 4 hr. Using the continuous infusion schedule, the patient is given a bolus injection of 50–75 units/kg followed by a continuous infusion of 10–25 units/kg/hr. Both schedules provide adequate anticoagulation, but the continuous method has been reported to have the effect of less anticoagulant-related bleeding.

Various coagulation tests are available to measure the action of heparin, including the activated partial thromboplastin time (APTT), the thrombin clotting time (TCT), and the factor Xa inhibition assay. The APTT is the most frequently used test for monitoring heparin therapy. It is sensitive to small amounts of heparin, is rapid and reproducible, and can be performed in most clinical laboratories. Clinical studies suggest that the APTT should be maintained at 1.5–2 times the patient's own preheparin control APTT.

After initiation of heparin therapy, an APTT should be performed periodically to ensure that adequate anticoagulation has occurred and that the patient's requirements for the drug have not changed. In patients receiving the intermittent bolus schedule, the APTT should be determined 1 hr after the initial infusion and should be greatly prolonged at that time. The next APTT should be performed at the 4th hr—that is, just prior to the next dose of heparin; at that time it should be 5–10 sec longer than the normal control time for the laboratory. If the APTT is very prolonged, the dose of the drug should be reduced by 10%, or, if the APTT is within the normal range, the dose of the heparin should be increased 10% and the test repeated 4 hr later. Using the continuous schedule, the APTT can be performed at any time 4 hr after the continuous infusion has begun. The desired result is an APTT 1.5–2 times the patient's pretreatment value. Dose adjustments of 5–10% can be made during this period to achieve adequate anticoagulation.

Heparin can be neutralized immediately by using protamine sulfate. Because of the rapid clearance rate of heparin, however, most patients can be treated by stopping the infusion. As a general rule, 1 mg of protamine sulfate neutralizes between 90 and 110 units of heparin. Because heparin has a rapid in vivo metabolic decay, only half of the total dose of protamine should be administered. A clotting test is performed to determine whether adequate neutralization has occurred; if not, the additional protamine can be given. Protamine itself is an anticoagulant, so if too much is given the clotting time may be prolonged. Although excess protamine has an anticoagulant effect, it rarely (if ever) is a cause of clinical bleeding.

Warfarin

The coumarin derivatives are oral anticoagulant drugs that act by decreasing the rate of synthesis of the vitamin K-dependent coagulation factors II, VII, IX, and X. In addition, protein C and protein S (the vitamin K-dependent anticoagulants) are also affected. These drugs inhibit vitamin K-dependent carboxylation of the precursor coagulation proteins. Warfarin probably acts by competitively inhibiting vitamin K metabolism. Following the administration of warfarin, the levels of factors II, VII, IX, and X decrease gradually, according to their half-life. Because factor VII has the shortest half-life, its level is the first to decrease, followed by factor IX, X, and finally II. It generally takes about 4–5 days to provide a reduction in all four coagulation factors to a level consistent with anticoagulation.

The prothrombin time (PT) is the clotting test used to assess warfarin anticoagulation. The previously recommended therapeutic range of maintaining the patient(s) PT at 2.0–2.5 times the normal control should not be used when commercial rabbit brain is used as the clotting reagent. Current recommendations are for mechanical prosthetic heart valves and recurrent systemic embolism, 1.5–2.0, for treatment of deep vein thrombosis or pulmonary embolism, 1.3–1.5, and for prevention of systemic embolism in patients with atrial fibrillation, valvular heart disease, or tissue heart valves, 1.3–1.5 times the control plasma.

The most serious side effect of warfarin is hemorrhage. This is often related to changes in the dose or metabolism of the drug. The addition or removal of certain drugs to the patient's therapeutic regimen can have significant effects on oral anticoagulation. For example, warfarin's effect can be enhanced by the administration of antibiotics, salicylates, anabolic steroids, chloral hydrate, laxatives, allopurinol, vitamin E, and methylphenidate HCl; its effect can be diminished by barbiturates, vitamin K, oral contraceptives, phenytoin, and others. Warfarin-induced bleeding is treated by discontinuation of the drug and the administration of vitamin K. Generally the amount of vitamin K given is equal to the amount of the daily warfarin dose. The vitamin can be administered orally, subcutaneously, or intravenously (not intramuscularly). Correction of the coagulopathy begins within 6–8 hr and should be complete in 24–48 hr. If the patient is having a significant bleeding problem, fresh frozen plasma (15 mL/kg) should be given at the same time the vitamin K is administered.

Coumarin anticoagulants are contraindicated in essentially the same circumstances as those for heparin therapy. The oral anticoagulants cross the placenta and should not be given during pregnancy. Although breast milk contains warfarin, the quantity is insignificant and the drug can be used in the lactating mother.

THROMBOLYTIC THERAPY

Thrombolytic therapy involves the removal of blood clots by enzymatic digestion. It is accomplished by the in vivo generation of plasmin through the administration of plasminogen activators such as streptokinase, urokinase, and tissue-type plasminogen activator (TPA). Urokinase and TPA act as direct activators, whereas streptokinase acts by binding to plasminogen, and the streptokinase-plasminogen complex becomes the plasminogen activator. For this therapy to be effective, the patient must have a relatively fresh clot (<7–10 days old), the clot must be accessible to the lytic agent, there must be an adequate amount of plasminogen, and the fibrinolytic inhibitors must not interfere with the reaction. Once plasmin has been formed, it lyses fibrin. The plasmin generated by urokinase and streptokinase can produce a systemic hyperfibrinolytic state; when this occurs, the plasmin can degrade other plasma proteins, including fibrinogen, and factors V and VIII, resulting in a hemorrhagic disorder. TPA is fibrin-specific—it acts as an activator within or on a fibrin clot. Clinical trials with TPA suggest that a systemic hyperfibrinolytic state is rarely produced.

Thrombolytic therapy has been reported to be beneficial in those with pulmonary embolism, deep venous thrombosis, certain arterial occlusive events, and occluded access shunts. However, there are few published studies on its use in the pediatric age group.

JAMES J. CORRIGAN, JR.

Bithel T: Hereditary dysfibrinogenemia. Clin Chem 31:509, 1985.
Comp PC: Hereditary disorders predisposing to thrombosis. Prog Hemost Thromb 8:71, 1986.
Comp PC, Nixon RR, Cooper MR, et al: Familial protein S deficiency is associated with recurrent thrombosis. J Clin Invest 74:2082, 1984.
Corrigan JJ Jr: Thrombosis and thromboembolism. *In*: Corrigan JJ (ed): Hemorrhagic and Thrombotic Diseases in Childhood and Adolescence. New York, Churchill Livingstone. 1985, pp 147–176.
Corrigan JJ Jr: Neonatal thrombosis and the thrombolytic system: Pathophysiology and therapy. Am J Pediatr Hematol Oncol 10:83, 1988.
Esmon CT: The regulation of natural anticoagulant pathways. Science 235:1348, 1987.
Hirsh J, Levine MN: The optimal intensity of oral anticoagulant therapy. JAMA 258:2723, 1987.
Mahasandana C, Suvatte V, Chuansumrit TA, et al: Homozygous protein S deficiency in an infant with purpura fulminans. J Pediatr 117:750, 1990.
Marciniak E, Farley CH, DeSimone PA: Familial thrombosis due to antithrombin III deficiency. Blood 43:219, 1974.
McDonald MM, Hathaway WE: Anticoagulant therapy by continuous heparinization in newborn and older infants. J Pediatr 101:451, 1982.
Peters C, Casella JF, Marlar RA, et al: Homozygous protein C deficiency: Observations on the nature of the molecular abnormality and the effectiveness of warfarin therapy. Pediatrics 81:272, 1988.
Samama MM: Thrombolytic agents and treatments. Semin Thromb Hemost 13:127, 1987.

16.90 THE SPLEEN

The spleen is a large mass of lymphoid and phagocytic reticuloendothelial cells with a complex network of tortuous capillaries and fenestrated sinusoids. These impart the important properties of a biologic filter.

FUNCTIONS. A number of functions can be assigned to the spleen, some of which are germane to hematologic processes and diseases.

Reservoir Function. In lower animals the spleen is a contractile organ because considerable smooth muscle is present in the capsule and trabeculae. In humans little muscle is present, and the reservoir function is normally not very great. The spleen releases both factor VIII and platelets following infusion of epinephrine. The normal spleen contains only about 25 mL of blood but, when the spleen enlarges for any reason, its content of blood increases. The sequestration crisis of sickle cell states is an exaggeration of reservoir function.

Hematopoiesis. The spleen is a site of active blood formation during fetal life, but by about 6 mo gestation hematopoiesis disappears unless a condition such as hemolytic disease of the newborn is present. In a few exceptional diseases such as thalassemia and osteopetrosis, hematopoiesis persists or is resumed postnatally. The stimulus for this is not known.

"Culling." This term is used to describe the ability of the spleen, because of its unique circulation and structure. This function is demonstrated by the fact that red blood cells and platelets lightly coated by antibodies are selectively sequestered and destroyed by the spleen. The spleen's activity in destroying spherocytes is another example of culling.

"Pitting." The spleen has the ability to remove or "pit" intracytoplasmic inclusions such as Howell-Jolly bodies or siderotic granules from within the red blood cell without destroying the cell. The blood of a person with no spleen contains relatively large numbers of these intracellular inclusions.

Destruction of Old Red Blood Cells. The spleen is probably the principal site of destruction of senescent red blood cells. This function is easily assumed by other portions of the reticuloendothelial system, however, and red blood cell life span is not significantly increased in the absence of spleen.

Membrane Effect. The normal spleen is postulated to have an ill-defined effect on the red blood cell membrane. When the spleen is absent, red blood cells are flatter and thinner than normal, increased numbers of target cells are seen, and osmotic fragility is decreased. Examination of red blood cells by interference phase contrast microscopy shows membrane indentations resembling craters in 20% or more of the cells of asplenic persons. Fewer than 1% of the red blood cells of individuals with normal spleen have these depressions or "pocks," which may be small vesicles.

Filtering and Immunologic Functions. Because of the intimate relation of the circulating blood with lymphoid and reticuloendothelial elements within the spleen, this organ plays an important role in the primary defense against bacteria that gain access to the circulation. The spleen is especially vital in the immature and nonimmune person, for it constitutes the primary site of clearance of organisms such as pneumococci in the absence of specific antibody. The spleen has a relatively minor role in overall antibody formation as long as the antigen is administered by intramuscular or subcutaneous routes, but the spleen is essential to antibody formation in response to small doses of particulate intravenous antigens.

The spleen is an important participant in the synthesis of IgM, properdin, and "tuftsin," a phagocytosis-promoting tetrapeptide. Levels of these humoral factors are depressed in the splenectomized child.

Hormonal Function. It has been postulated that the spleen produces a hormonal substance ("splenin") that exerts an effect on bone marrow activity. There is little evidence for such a hormone, and hypersplenism is better explained on the basis of excessive filtering or culling activities. The spleen can be functionally inactive despite clinical enlargement, as in young children with sickle cell anemia (functional hyposplenism).

Clinical Examination. Careful and gentle palpation of the relaxed abdomen provides reliable information about the size of the spleen. The tip can be felt at the left costal margin in 5–10% of normal children and in a higher proportion of children with viral infections. The spleen must be increased to 2 to 3 times its average size before it can be regularly felt on physical examination. Lesser degrees of enlargement can be detected radiographically. An enlarged spleen must be differentiated from other masses in the left upper quadrant. Useful physical characteristics that aid in identifying the spleen include concealment of its upper margin by the rib cage, the presence of a palpable notch, and the absence of overlying bowel. When it is impossible to be certain of the identity of a mass, isotopic scanning studies are of value. Short-lived isotopes such as technetium-99m (^{99m}Tc) may be used to label gelatinous sulfur colloid particles. Injected intravenously, this radioactive colloid is rapidly cleared by reticuloendothelial elements in the liver, spleen and, to a lesser extent, bone marrow; scanning permits definition of the size and configuration of spleen and liver. This technique has proved of great value in demonstrating anatomic abnormalities of the spleen; it is noninvasive and involves a very low radiation exposure.

The spleen has vascular, lymphatic, and reticuloendothelial components; pathologic processes involving any of these may produce splenomegaly. Table 16–15 lists important causes of splenic enlargement.

TABLE 16–15. Some Causes of Splenomegaly in Children

Hematologic diseases
- Hemolytic anemias—caused by extramedullary hematopoiesis and reticuloendothelial hyperplasia
- Congenital and acquired hemolytic anemias
- Hemoglobinopathies and thalassemia

Infections
- Bacterial: septicemias, typhoid, endocarditis, abscess
- Viral: Epstein-Barr, cytomegalovirus, etc.
- Protozoal: malaria, toxoplasmosis

Congestive splenomegaly
- Secondary to portal or splenic vein obstruction
- Secondary to intrahepatic disease—cirrhosis
- Chronic congestive heart failure

Infiltrations
- Lipidoses—Niemann-Pick, Gaucher diseases
- Nonlipid reticuloendothelioses

Cysts
- Congenital—epidermoid cysts
- Acquired—pseudocysts

Neoplasms
- Leukemia and lymphosarcoma
- Hodgkin disease
- Hemangioma and lymphangioma

Miscellaneous
- Rheumatoid arthritis (Still disease)
- Lupus erythematosus

16.91 CONGESTIVE SPLENOMEGALY
(Banti Syndrome)

The venous outflow from the spleen may be obstructed within the liver or in the portal or splenic veins (Sec. 13.102). This vascular obstruction produces congestion and ultimately splenomegaly. Liver diseases associated with parenchymal inflammation, fibrosis, and vascular constriction include postnecrotic cirrhosis, galactosemia, Wilson disease, cystic fibrosis, biliary atresia, α_1-antitrypsin deficiency, and microcystic disease of liver and kidney. Septic omphalitis, either primary or following umbilical vein cannulation, may progress to portal vein thrombophlebitis and thrombosis. Rarely, congenital or acquired anomalies of the splenic or portal veins may cause obstruction and secondary splenomegaly. In some areas of the world schistosomiasis and malaria are important causes of splenomegaly.

CLINICAL MANIFESTATIONS. Observation or palpation of an enlarged spleen may be the initial indication of the disease process. The enlarged spleen may filter out and destroy excessive numbers of blood cells and platelets and thus cause thrombocytopenic hemorrhage and anemia. In response to portal vein obstruction, collateral circulation develops through the short gastric, esophageal, superficial abdominal, and hemorrhoidal veins. In some cases massive hemorrhage from ruptured esophageal varices is the 1st clinical manifestation of congestive splenomegaly.

LABORATORY FINDINGS. Pancytopenia of varying degree is seen. The bone marrow shows active hematopoiesis with abundant megakaryocytes. Liver function tests may indicate hepatocellular disease. It is possible to measure the portal venous pressure, and injection of radiopaque dyes into the spleen permits radiologic visualization of the splenic and portal veins. This should usually be done under direct vision, because percutaneous needling may lacerate the splenic capsule. In cases of hepatic fibrosis and cirrhosis, ^{99m}Tc scan may show a contracted liver with massive splenomegaly.

TREATMENT. The site of obstruction must be determined. If only the splenic vein is involved, splenectomy is curative. In patients in whom the portal vein is extensively involved or in which intrahepatic obstruction is present, splenectomy corrects pancytopenia but does not relieve portal hypertension. On the other hand, because generalized bleeding or infection rarely results from thrombocytopenia or neutropenia, these hematologic findings do not mandate splenectomy. Portacaval anastomosis, which in general is preferred to splenorenal shunting in the young child, is indicated when portal hypertension is clearly shown or when repeated episodes of life-threatening hemorrhage have occurred. Successful relief of portal hypertension may result in a decrease in splenic size and improvement of pancytopenia. It may also result in metabolic complications, especially hyperammonemia.

16.92 ANOMALIES AND TRAUMA

SPLENIC CYSTS

Cysts of the spleen are of two general types: epidermoid cysts are lined with stratified columnar epithelium, and pseudocysts, presumably of post-traumatic or post-infarction origin, have no epithelial lining and are filled with necrotic material and blood. Diagnosis is suggested by an asymptomatic smooth mass in the left upper quadrant, displacing the stomach medially. Isotopic scans with ^{99m}Tc–gelatin colloid indicate that the cystic mass is within the substance of the spleen. Ultrasonography and computed tomography (CT scan) effectively demonstrate splenic cysts.

ACCESSORY SPLEENS

Multiple and accessory spleens are not uncommon. Of 1,413 children subjected to splenectomy, 229 (16%) had one or more accessory spleens (145 had only 1; 10 had five or more). Accessory spleens are usually located close to the hilum or adjacent to the tail of the pancreas. A congenital syndrome of polysplenism is characterized by left-sided visceral isomerism and cardiac defects. Affected children have a high rate of intrahepatic biliary atresia (Sec. 15.26).

CONGENITAL ABSENCE OF THE SPLEEN

Absence of the spleen occurs as part of an unusual group of anomalies, including complex abnormalities of the heart and great vessels with severe cyanotic congenital heart disease (Sec. 15.26). Apparent dextrocardia and varying degrees of heterotopia of the abdominal viscera are seen (Ivemark syndrome). The condition can be suspected from examination of the blood; target cells, increased numbers of spherocytes, intraerythrocytic inclusions (such as Howell-Jolly and Heinz bodies), and hemosiderin granules are easily demonstrated. The incidence of overwhelming sepsis is increased in congenital asplenia.

HYPERSPLENISM

This is not a specific diagnosis but is a descriptive term for a clinical complex that includes the following: (1) depression of one or more of the cellular elements of the blood; (2) active formation of that element in the bone marrow; (3) an enlarged spleen, which may be the result of a large number of causes (see Table 16–15); and (4) correction of the hematologic abnormalities by splenectomy. A diagnosis of primary hypersplenism is difficult to establish; other causes of splenomegaly with secondary pancytopenia should be excluded.

FUNCTIONAL HYPOSPLENIA

Occasionally, anatomically enlarged spleens may be devoid of reticuloendothelial system (RES) activity. This has been most clearly demonstrated in infants and young children with sickle cell anemia. In the great majority of these children, after 6–18 mo of age ^{99m}Tc scan fails to demonstrate RES activity of the anatomically enlarged organ. Howell-Jolly and Heinz bodies are seen in the blood. Young children with sickle cell anemia are 600 times more likely to develop pneumococcal meningitis and sepsis than their normal peers, and this propensity to infection is, in part, caused by defective splenic function. Functional hyposplenia can be temporarily reversed by the transfusion of normal red blood cells; after years, autoinfarction ultimately reduces the spleen to a siderofibrotic nubbin.

RUPTURE OF THE SPLEEN

Traumatic injury of the spleen may result from a hard, direct blow to the left flank or left side of the abdomen, such as may occur during automobile accidents or contact sports. If the tear in the splenic capsule is small, the symptoms may be moderate and include left upper quadrant or left shoulder pain and signs of peritoneal irritation as a result of the presence of blood. In more extreme cases shock may develop rapidly. When the spleen is pathologically enlarged, rupture may occur after relatively minor trauma. This occurs in the neonate with hemolytic disease and in the older child with infectious mononucleosis. Radionuclide and CT scanning are valuable in demonstrating lacerations and hematomas of the spleen.

Laparotomy and splenectomy are indicated when rupture leads to severe intra-abdominal bleeding and hypotension, but splenectomy is not always mandatory for splenic laceration. In the child, bleeding from the lacerated splenic surface often stops spontaneously. If the child's vital signs are stable or controlled with relatively small amounts of blood transfusion (<25 mL/kg) during the 1st 48 hr after splenic injury, nonoperative management may be safely attempted. This observational period requires a surgeon in attendance who can act rapidly if deterioration occurs. Serial examinations of the spleen with ^{99m}Tc scans, ultrasonography, or computed tomography are needed to show that the splenic lesion is not expanding. The child should be watched carefully in the hospital for 10–14 days and maintained on restricted activities for several months. Late rupture or splenic pseudocysts have not been observed; scans reveal complete healing of the lesion.

Nonoperative management is not indicated if other abdominal organs are damaged or if severe shock develops. If laparotomy is necessary, it may be possible to repair the damaged spleen or to leave some splenic tissue in situ (see later).

SPLENOSIS

Heterotopic autotransplantations of splenic tissue onto the surface of the peritoneum, with its subsequent growth, occur frequently after splenic injury requiring splenectomy. Changes in the circulating red blood cells (Howell-Jolly bodies, membrane craters) are not found in affected patients. ^{99m}Tc spleen scans show extrahepatic uptake of the radionuclide by small masses of regenerated splenic tissue that may be protective to some degree against severe bacterial infections. The degree of protection can vary, however, with the amount of splenic tissue and its arterial blood supply; death from overwhelming infection has occurred in patients with splenosis.

16.93 SPLENECTOMY

INDICATIONS. Removal of the spleen is a common operation performed for various indications. Primary surgical indications include the following: (1) rupture of the spleen; (2) removal of tumors, cysts, or vascular anomalies involving the spleen; (3) need for adequate surgical exposure of the left upper portion of the abdomen; (4) certain shunting procedures; (5) relief of mechanical distress resulting from massive enlargement in thalassemia major or Gaucher disease; and (6) the need for staging procedures for Hodgkin disease and other lymphoreticular malignancies (Sec. 17.9 and 17.10).

Hematologic indications include the following: (1) congenital hemolytic states, such as hereditary spherocytosis and elliptocytosis, and some cases of nonspherocytic anemias, such as pyruvate kinase deficiency; (2) autoimmune hemolytic anemia when chronic and refractory to corticosteroid therapy; (3) chronic idiopathic thrombocytopenia purpura (ITP); and (4) hypersplenism.

OVERWHELMING SEPSIS FOLLOWING SPLENECTOMY. Removal of the spleen alters host resistance, and overwhelming and often fatal meningitis and septicemia are seen with increased frequency in asplenic persons. The risks vary with the reasons for which splenectomy was done, and especially with the age of the patient.

The risk of overwhelming sepsis is low (0.5–1%) when splenectomy is done for traumatic rupture, hereditary spherocytosis, or ITP. A higher incidence of infection is seen when the indication is thalassemia major, histiocytosis, or lipidosis. The risk is high when there is an underlying disease that in itself has a predisposition to infection, such as the Wiskott-Aldrich syndrome. The risk is higher in all categories for younger infants and children. Sepsis has occurred at all ages, regardless of the indication for splenectomy or the interval after the operation. Severe infections after splenectomy (usually meningitis and septicemia) are characterized by an acute and fulminating course, with death often occurring within 12–24 hr after onset of symptoms. In more than 60% of patients, pneumococci are the responsible agents; *H. influenzae* and meningococci are responsible for a smaller number of infections. Because of this risk splenectomy should be performed only for clear indications and, when possible, the operation should be deferred until after 5–6 yr of age or even later if the condition of the patient is well compensated. Prophylactic use of penicillin has been advocated for the young child after splenectomy, and many centers use this routinely. There are no adequately controlled studies assessing the effectiveness of such management, except for patients with sickle cell anemia.

Immunization with polyvalent capsular polysaccharide antigens of pneumococci, *H. influenzae*, and meningococci probably reduces the frequency of postsplenectomy infection but is generally ineffective before 18–24 mo.

In any case, patients whose spleens have been removed, and their families, should know that splenectomy carries a risk of development of a life-threatening infection at any time, and that any febrile illness calls for immediate medical evaluation.

Eraklis AJ, Filler RM: Splenectomy in childhood: A review of 1413 cases. J Pediatr Surg 7:382, 1972.
Likhite VV: Immunological impairment and susceptibility to infection after splenectomy. JAMA 236:1376, 1976.
Pearson HA: The born-again spleen. N Engl J Med 298:1373, 1978.
Pearson HA: Splenectomy, its risk and role. Hosp Pract 94:85, 1980.
Pearson HA, Spencer RP, Cornelius E: Functional asplenia in sickle cell anemia. N Engl J Med 281:923, 1969.
Pearson HA, Spencer RP, Touloukian R: The binary spleen: A radioisotopic scan sign of splenic pseudocyst. J Pediatr 77:216, 1970.
Pochedly C, Sills RH, Schwartz AD: Disorders of the Spleen. New York, Marcel Dekker, 1989. Prevention of serious infection after splenectomy. Med Lett 19:2, 1977.
Sherman R: Perspective in management of trauma to the spleen. J Trauma 20:1, 1980.
Singer DB: Post-splenectomy sepsis. Perspect Pediatr Pathol 1:3, 1973.

16.94 THE LYMPHATIC SYSTEM

The lymphatic system includes the free lymphocytes of the blood and lymph as well as organized lymphatic structures such as the lymph nodes, spleen, Peyer patches, appendix, and tonsils. The origin of lymphocytes is uncertain; some are believed to originate or be modified in the embryonic thymus, from which their progenitors migrated to populate other lymphatic tissues. Others may arise from the lymphoid areas of the gastrointestinal tract, tonsillar area, or appendix.

he lymph vessels start as small capillaries between the cells of all organs except the brain and heart. Small lymphatic capillaries join to form progressively larger channels that drain the extremities, trunk, and head. The largest of the lymphatic vessels is the thoracic duct, which discharges most of the central return of body lymph into the left subclavian vein.

The lymph channels are characteristically interrupted by lymph nodes. These structures are networks of dilated sinusoids lined by reticuloendothelial elements and surrounded by masses of actively proliferating lymphocytes. The lymph nodes are located in groups, through which the lymphatic drainage of well-defined anatomic areas passes. The lymph nodes function as protective barriers against the spread of infections. They also filter particulate antigens, and the lymphocytes and plasma cells within lymph nodes actively participate in antibody formation.

The superficial lymph nodes are evaluated by palpation. Small nodes can normally be felt in the neck, axillae, and groin. Roentgenograms of the chest assess enlargement of the mediastinal lymph nodes. Lymphangiography permits evaluation of the size and structure of the pelvic and retroperitoneal lymph nodes.

The lymph is a clear fluid. It has a protein content intermediate between that of interstitial fluid and plasma, and it contains a substantial number of small lymphocytes.

16.95 DISEASES OF THE LYMPH VESSELS

ACUTE LYMPHANGITIS

This is an inflammation of the lymphatics draining an area of acute infection, usually bacterial. It is manifested as red, painful streaks that radiate proximally from the infected site. Painful swelling of the regional nodes is also usually present. *S. aureus* and group A streptococci are common pathogens.

LYMPHEDEMA

Lymphedema is a diffuse, permanent, pitting edema resulting from obstruction of the lymph drainage of an area, usually an extremity. Congenital lymphedema occurs in those with Milroy disease and as part of the syndrome of gonadal dysgenesis. Acquired lymphedema may result from inflammatory processes or from surgical or radiologic obliteration of lymph nodes or lymph channels.

Hilliard RI, McKendry JBJ, Phillips MJ: Congenital abnormalities of the lymphatic system: A new clinical classification. Pediatrics 86:988, 1990.

16.96 DISEASES OF THE LYMPH NODES

Enlargement of the lymph nodes occurs in response to a wide variety of infectious, inflammatory, and neoplastic processes. Enlargement of a single node or group of nodes is most frequently caused by an infection in the area it drains. Generalized lymphadenopathy occurs in many acute infections, especially rubella, rubeola, typhoid, tularemia, and infectious mononucleosis. Leukemia, lymphoma, and reticuloendotheliosis are sometimes accompanied by striking degrees of lymph node enlargement. Malignant tumors such as neuroblastoma occasionally metastasize to lymph nodes, and large numbers of lipid-bearing histiocytes may be present in the lymph nodes of those with Gaucher disease or other lipidoses.

ACUTE LYMPHADENITIS

CLINICAL MANIFESTATIONS. As a result of cellulitis or other infections, bacteria and toxins and other by-products of acute inflammation are carried in the lymph to the regional lymph nodes, where an acute inflammatory process occurs. Bacteria may cause abscess formation. Acute cervical adenitis secondary to acute pharyngitis and inguinal lymphadenopathy resulting from infections of the lower extremity are common. The involved nodes become swollen and painful, and the overlying skin is hot and red. The primary infectious process is usually obvious, but the site of inoculation may not be apparent, as in cat-scratch disease. Mediastinal lymphadenitis secondary to pulmonary infections may produce obstructive symptoms and cough. Mesenteric lymphadenopathy may, on occasion, be associated with crampy abdominal pain simulating that of appendicitis.

TREATMENT. Antibiotic therapy that is appropriate for the primary infection benefits the lymphadenitis. When suppuration occurs, needle aspiration or surgical drainage is necessary.

CHRONIC LYMPHADENITIS

Chronic infection or inflammation is frequently associated with hyperplasia of the lymph nodes. Tuberculous infections regularly result in regional lymphadenopathy. Scrofula, or chronic cervical lymphadenopathy, may be secondary to infection of the nasopharynx with bovine tuberculosis. This organism is uncommon in the United States, where chronic lymphadenopathy is more often caused by infection by atypical acid-fast organisms. The organisms are trapped in the nodes, where granuloma and caseous necrosis occur. Affected nodes are hard, nontender, and frequently matted to adjacent tissues. Biopsy may be necessary to differentiate chronic infections from malignant processes.

JAMES A. STOCKMAN III

17

NEOPLASMS AND NEOPLASM-LIKE STRUCTURES

17.1 GENERAL CONSIDERATIONS

In the United States, cancer causes more deaths than any other disease of children between the ages of 1 and 15 yr. The incidence rate of malignant tumors in children under 15 yr of age is estimated to be 14/100,000/yr for the years 1986–1987 with a slight increase for acute lymphocytic leukemia and central nervous system (CNS) tumors during the previous 15 yr (Table 17–1). Mortality rates, however, for malignant neoplasms in children during this same period were only about one quarter the incidence rate, and each of the tumor types listed in Table 17–1 has shown a significant decrease in mortality during the same period. There are still, unfortunately, tumors such as disseminated neuroblastoma in the child over 1 yr that carry an extremely high mortality (80% or more). Some of the favorable rates reflect improvements in therapy and access to appropriate care over the past several decades. A child in whom possible cancer is diagnosed should be referred as soon as possible to a center where appropriate treatment is available. There is evidence that for most tumors prognosis improves if the patient is enrolled in a study protocol.

In most cases, the development of cancer probably involves environmental as well as host factors. In adults, of those cancers that occur primarily in organs exposed directly to the environment, from 60 to 90% are estimated to be caused by environmental carcinogens. Not all persons who work outdoors in strong sunlight will get skin cancer, however, nor will all those who smoke develop lung cancer; accordingly, even with these agents there are important host factors. Indeed, in tumors such as colon cancer, direct evidence indicates that cumulative changes in cells occur, including activation of proto-oncogenes, inactivation of suppressor genes, and gross chromosomal aberrations, and this supports the idea of multifactorial carcinogenesis. In children, in whom the common cancers tend to occur in tissues that are not exposed directly to the environment, such as hematopoietic, nervous, and supportive connective tissues, host factors may be more important.

ENVIRONMENTAL FACTORS

IONIZING RADIATION. Increases in the incidence of acute lymphocytic leukemia, acute myeloid leukemia, and chronic granulocytic leukemia followed exposure of children to the atomic bombs in Hiroshima and Nagasaki (Sec. 26.1). A linear relationship was found between the radiation dose and the frequency of leukemia. The type of leukemia and the rate at which it developed were related to the age of the individual at the time of exposure. The increases in acute lymphatic and chronic granulocytic leukemia were most dramatic in the younger children, whereas acute myelogenous leukemia was seen with increasing frequency among the older children. Leukemia developed after a relatively short incubation, with a peak rate of occurrence 5 years after exposure. There is also an increased incidence of breast cancer in middle aged women who were under 10 yr old at the time they were exposed. Thus, critical environmental events may cause cancers with long latency periods; these cancers under normal circumstances may be more difficult to discover than after an event such as massive exposure to atomic radiation.

The use of radiation therapy for nonmalignant conditions is now generally abandoned, because it is associated with the development of malignancy. An example is the increased incidence of thyroid cancer after external irradiation to the head and neck (once given for a variety of benign conditions, such as enlarged thymus, enlarged tonsils, or tinea capitis). Before 1955 significant doses of radiation were also administered during fluoroscopy in hospitals or physicians' offices, and even in shoe stores to measure children's feet. Such exposures are now sharply curtailed or eliminated. Either causally or coincidentally, leukemia mortality rates for children under the age of 5 yr dropped substantially during the early 1960s, before chemotherapy was producing the cures that it is today.

Exposure in utero of the fetus to diagnostic x-rays has been associated with a risk ratio of about 1.5 for development of a childhood tumor; but, although an as yet unexplained relationship exists, the fact that there was no increase in such cancer among children exposed in utero to the atomic bomb and that animal models do not indicate any supersensitivity of the fetus to radiation oncogenesis suggests that the relationship is probably not causal. Second malignancies also occur in patients who have received therapeutic radiation, for example, brain tumors in patients who have received cranial radiation for leukemia.

SOLAR RADIATION. Sunlight may cause cancer of the skin later in adult life when there is high exposure in childhood and adolescence. Children who have a genetic predisposition, such as xeroderma pigmentosum or another congenital defect in DNA repair, are also at increased risk of developing neoplasms.

ASBESTOS. Investigation of a cluster of cases of mesothelioma among adults in South Africa found that, although only a few worked with asbestos, most had as children lived near open pits where asbestos was mined and some had played on the refuse dumps. Moreover, asbestos carried home on the father's workclothes has been found to cause mesothelioma 3–4 decades later in the wife or children (Sec. 26.17). Children exposed to asbestos in their homes or neighborhoods may be especially susceptible to the carcinogenicity of cigarette smoking, because asbestos potentiates the capacity of cigarette smoking to cause lung cancer in adults. Mesotheliomas that occur in persons under 20 yr old, however, are apparently not due to asbestos and are histologically unlike those produced by this agent.

DRUGS. Intrauterine exposure to *diethylstilbestrol* (DES) carries an increased risk of clear cell adenocarcinoma of the vagina in daughters of women given this drug. In addition,

TABLE 17–1. Incidence and Mortality of Some Common Childhood Cancers: Summary of 15-Year Trends by Site*

Site	Incidence Average 1973–1974	Incidence Rate 1986–1987	% Change	Mortality Average 1973–1974	Mortality Rate 1986–1987	% Change
Acute lymphocytic leukemia	2.9	3.3	14.4†	1.4	0.7	−50.7†
Brain and nervous system	2.5	3.2	29.4†	1.0	0.8	−19.2†
Bone	0.7	0.8	12.5	0.3	0.2	−33.5†
Hodgkin disease	0.8	0.6	−17.5	0.1	0.0	−68.7†
Non-Hodgkin lymphoma	0.8	1.1	31.7	0.4	0.2	−50.2†
Kidney	0.7	0.8	7.5	0.2	0.1	−43.6†
Soft tissue	0.7	0.8	5.2	0.6	0.2	−68.1†
All sites	13.2	14.0	6.1†	5.5	3.6	−35.6†

*Cancer Statistics Review 1973–1987. The Surveillance Program Division of Cancer Prevention and Control. (Ries LAG, Hankey BF, Edwards BK [eds]) NIH Publication No. 90-2789, US Dept of Health and Human Services.

†The Estimated Annual Percent Change over the 15-yr interval is significantly different from O ($p<.05$).

Rates are per 100,000 whites, ages 0–14, and are age-adjusted to the 1970 US standard population.

The mortality rate for every major cancer in children has declined significantly since 1973.

The overall cancer mortality rate decreased 36% for children while the incidence rate increased by 6.1%. As expected with decreasing mortality and increasing incidence rates, the 5-yr relative survival rate has increased from 55.1% in 1974–1976 to 66.8% in 1981–1986.

exposed children of both sexes commonly have malformations of the genital tract (see also Sec. 18.54). DES is currently the only proven human transplacental carcinogen known, although two cases of neuroblastoma have been reported in infants with fetal *hydantoin* syndrome, and another has been reported in a child with fetal *alcohol* syndrome.

Immunosuppressive agents administered following renal or other transplantation have been associated with an increased incidence of malignancy (particularly non-Hodgkin lymphoma). Since the types of tumors that occur in immunosuppressed individuals do not have the same relative incidence as tumors that occur in other children, this effect cannot be merely a breakdown in immune surveillance against cancer; other mechanisms must be at work.

Treatment of aplastic anemia (especially of the Fanconi type) with *anabolic androgenic steroids* has led to various liver tumors: hepatocellular carcinoma, hepatoma, or hepatic adenoma. The underlying condition may enhance the induction of liver neoplasia by these drugs, because such neoplasms have not been reported in athletes who use these androgens to build up muscles; such athletes, however, may well be at risk (Sec. 10.12).

Chemotherapy for malignancy may result in second neoplasms, with a cumulative risk as high as 12% at 25 yr.

DIET. There is an unexplained association between high fat intake, obesity, and the development of cancers of breast, colon, and uterus in adults. Speculation is rife as to whether dietary manipulation may prevent the development of cancer in later life, with emphasis on the possible prevention of colon cancer through a diet high in vegetable fiber. No convincing clinical data support such ideas at present.

VIRUSES

RNA VIRUSES. There is convincing evidence for both vertical and horizontal transmission in animals of lymphatic leukemia and lymphoma associated with type c RNA viruses; retroviruses also cause leukemia/lymphoma in cats and cows, with horizontal transmission. A type of T cell leukemia in humans has been associated with a retrovirus (human T cell leukemia virus [HTLV 1]). This form of leukemia is endemic on two islands in southern Japan and also occurs in the Caribbean and sporadically elsewhere, including the United States and Israel. The youngest case reported to date was 17 yr old at the time of diagnosis; some cases are known to have had latency periods of over 20 yr.

DNA VIRUSES. The Epstein-Barr (EB) virus is implicated in the development of infectious mononucleosis as well as in African Burkitt lymphoma, lymphoepithelioma, and Hodgkin disease. In the United States, however, about 80% of cases of Burkitt lymphoma are not associated with EB virus. EB virus infection in vitro leads to "immortalization" of B cell lines. Uncontrolled proliferation of B cells that have been neoplastically transformed by EB virus may be an important factor in the development of Burkitt lymphoma, particularly in Africa. It is not clear how EB virus infection is related to the chromosomal changes in Burkitt lymphoma that are described below.

PAPOVA VIRUSES. This family of viruses is known to cause warts and papillomas in a variety of tissues. Subtypes of the virus appear to have strong tissue tropisms. Types 6 and 11 are found in the lesions of laryngeal papillomatosis as well as condyloma acuminata. Although these viral lesions rarely become spontaneously malignant, they can frequently be converted to squamous cell carcinomas by the action of a secondary carcinogen such as cigarette smoke or therapeutic irradiation. Subtypes 16 and 18 of the papova viruses seem to be the contributing etiologic agents in carcinoma of the uterine cervix.

GENETIC MECHANISMS

ONCOGENES AND MALIGNANCY. Oncogenes are DNA sequences that when applied to an appropriate target, such as the NIH 3T3 tissue culture cell line, will cause a transformed focus. Originally, oncogenes were identified as that portion of the genome of a retrovirus that led to malignant transformation, as distinct from the portion responsible for viral replication. The first oncogene studied was the *src* gene, which enables the Rous sarcoma virus to induce sarcomas in vivo and to transform chicken fibroblasts in monolayer culture. The *src* gene is now known to encode the structure of a tyrosine kinase. It is not a unique viral genome at all; instead, it stems from a closely related gene that is an integral part of the normal genome of the chicken. That is, the cellular genome contains a gene that can exhibit strong transforming properties when properly activated. This antecedent gene is called a *proto-oncogene.* Two dozen cellular proto-oncogenes have been discovered to date through the study of retrovirus and the use of gene transfer techniques.

Oncogenes may be important in pediatric tumors. In Burkitt lymphoma, a typical translocation occurs in which the proto-oncogene, c-*myc*, is translocated from chromosome 8 to the heavy chain locus on chromosome 14. In a small proportion of Burkitt lymphoma, a breakpoint is still present on chromosome 8, but the other breakpoint is in either the κ immunoglobulin light chain locus on chromosome 2 or the λ light chain locus on chromosome 22. In all these cases the c-*myc* oncogene comes to lie adjacent to immunoglobulin constant region sequences. These findings and others led to the conclusion that the proto-oncogene c-*myc* is in some way "activated" or abnormally expressed by this proximity and that this contributes to tumorigenesis. Because the level of c-*myc* messenger RNA in the cytoplasm is similar to that of other proliferating cells, the abnormality is not simply one of quantity but is likely to involve inappropriate expression. Other mechanisms may result in conversion of proto-oncogenes. N-*myc*, for example, is highly amplified in patients with widely disseminated neuroblastoma, whereas ganglioneuromas contain only one copy of the gene.

TUMOR SUPPRESSOR GENES. The second general mechanism by which a gene can promote cancer is to undergo a mutation that reduces or eliminates its function (rather than acquiring excessive activity or a different function). Knudson noted that familial retinoblastoma differed from sporadic retinoblastoma by occurring bilaterally or multifocally and at a younger age. He postulated that retinoblastoma requires two mutations (or two "hits"): in the familial form, the first mutation is inherited and the second is acquired, whereas in the sporadic form both are acquired. Recent laboratory data are consistent with this hypothesis. Some years ago certain patients with retinoblastoma and an associated syndrome of mental retardation and microcephaly were found to have a deletion of chromosome 13 (13q- syndrome). Since then, sensitive gene mapping techniques have related all forms of retinoblastoma to some abnormality of chromosome 13. The tumors studied have shown submicroscopic deletions in chromosome 13 even when the constitutional karyotype from the same patient is normal.

Antioncogene. The normal allele at the retinoblastoma locus acts to suppress cancer development when present in two copies (such as in normal persons) or even one copy, for example, in persons with one mutant retinoblastoma gene or a constitutional deletion of the normal allele, hence the term antioncogene. A retinoblastoma can occur clinically only when both copies of the antioncogene are lost, for example, through point mutation or mitotic recombination (i.e., only when there is loss of heterozygosity). Because osteosarcoma is a common second malignancy in patients with retinoblastoma, it is not surprising that some osteosarcomas have cytogenetic and molecular evidence of involvement of 13q14. Evidence is mounting for the similar action of other recessive mutant genes in the pathogenesis of Wilms' tumor and other pediatric and adult malignancies (Beckwith-Wiedemann syndrome of Wilms tumor, hepatoblastoma, and rhabdomyosarcoma; multiple endocrine neoplasia, type 2a; neurofibromatosis 1 and 2). The retinoblastoma gene was first identified and cloned in 1986. The gene product has also been characterized as a 110-kd nuclear phosphoprotein with DNA-binding activity. Because the gene has been cloned and characterized, mutations can be identified both in tumor and normal tissue from patients. This allows genetic definition with regard to whether the patient has constitutional or sporadic chromosome 13 deletions, facilitates distinguishing hereditary from nonhereditary retinoblastoma, and is useful in risk estimation and in genetic counseling.

Patients with soft tissue sarcomas often have primary relatives with brain tumors; breast cancer at a young age in the mother is also reported. This familial clustering of tumors, the *Li-Fraumeni syndrome*, is associated with deletion of another antioncogene, P53.

OTHER MECHANISMS. Although both oncogenes and antioncogenes have been described in pediatric tumors, additional syndromes associated with constitutional chromosomal abnormalities, such as Down syndrome, Fanconi anemia, and Bloom syndrome, are associated with an increased incidence of leukemia by mechanisms that are not yet understood. In addition, there appear to be certain families in which cancer is common. Hodgkin disease, brain tumors, and Ewing sarcoma have been reported in siblings more often than would likely occur by chance alone.

In the case of children with tumors, it is important to look for familial associations, either with malignancy or with any congenital syndrome or abnormality. Syndromes such as neurofibromatosis or hemihypertrophy may not become obvious until the patient is 5–10 yr old and may not be recognizable at the time the diagnosis of tumor is made in the child. Accordingly, in some situations it may be important to examine the parents as well as the child. Awareness of these associations may protect the parents as well; for example, one should make sure that the mother of a child with a soft tissue sarcoma knows how to perform breast self-examination.

There are as yet no rules that will help to prevent the development of cancer in children, but pediatricians can help to avoid cancers in adults. They should counsel patients about the avoidance of smoking, obesity, and excessive sun exposure, for example, and do Papanicolaou (Pap) smears regularly in teenage girls who are sexually active.

17.2 PRINCIPLES OF DIAGNOSIS

Because only about one child in 10,000 will develop cancer each year, it is unusual for a general physician in practice to encounter a child with cancer. Physicians must, therefore, be alert to the possible occurrence of a rare but important disease. The diagnosis of cancer is too frequently overlooked while studies for infection or collagen disease or both are pursued in detail. Atypical courses of what appear to be common childhood conditions, prolonged (over 3–4 wk) and unexplained pain or fever, or unexplained (and especially growing) masses, particularly when these are associated with weight loss, should initiate prompt and appropriate studies.

Delays in diagnosis are a particular problem in certain clinical situations. Tumors of the nasopharynx or middle ear may mimic infection; prolonged unexplained ear pain, nasal discharge, retropharyngeal swelling, or trismus should be investigated, therefore, as being possibly due to malignancy. Cervical lymph node enlargement is common in children with infection, but it is also common in children with Hodgkin and non-Hodgkin lymphoma. Persistent or progressively enlarging nodes, which are often nonpainful, can be the hallmark of lymphoma and should lead to consideration of biopsy. Osteosarcoma and Ewing sarcoma usually occur during the 2nd decade of life, a time associated with physical activity. The cardinal symptom is localized and persistent pain, which the patient often associates with an episode of trauma. Such persistent pain should be investigated radiologically. The early symptoms of leukemia may also be nonspecific: low grade fever, or bone or joint pain. Careful attention to blood counts in such patients, with particular sensitivity to the development of normocytic anemia or mild thrombocytopenia, may help to determine when bone marrow should be examined, even if leukemic blast forms are not seen in the blood smear. Malignancy may also occur in the neonate and should be considered in children with masses or "blueberry muffin" spots on the skin.

When a malignant neoplasm is suspected, the immediate goal is to determine its nature and extent. A tentative diagnosis can be inferred from such clinical features as the presenting symptoms, location of the tumor, and age of the child. Figure 17–1 shows the incidence of primary sites of tumor by age at the time of diagnosis. From this it can be seen, for example, that an abdominal mass is much more

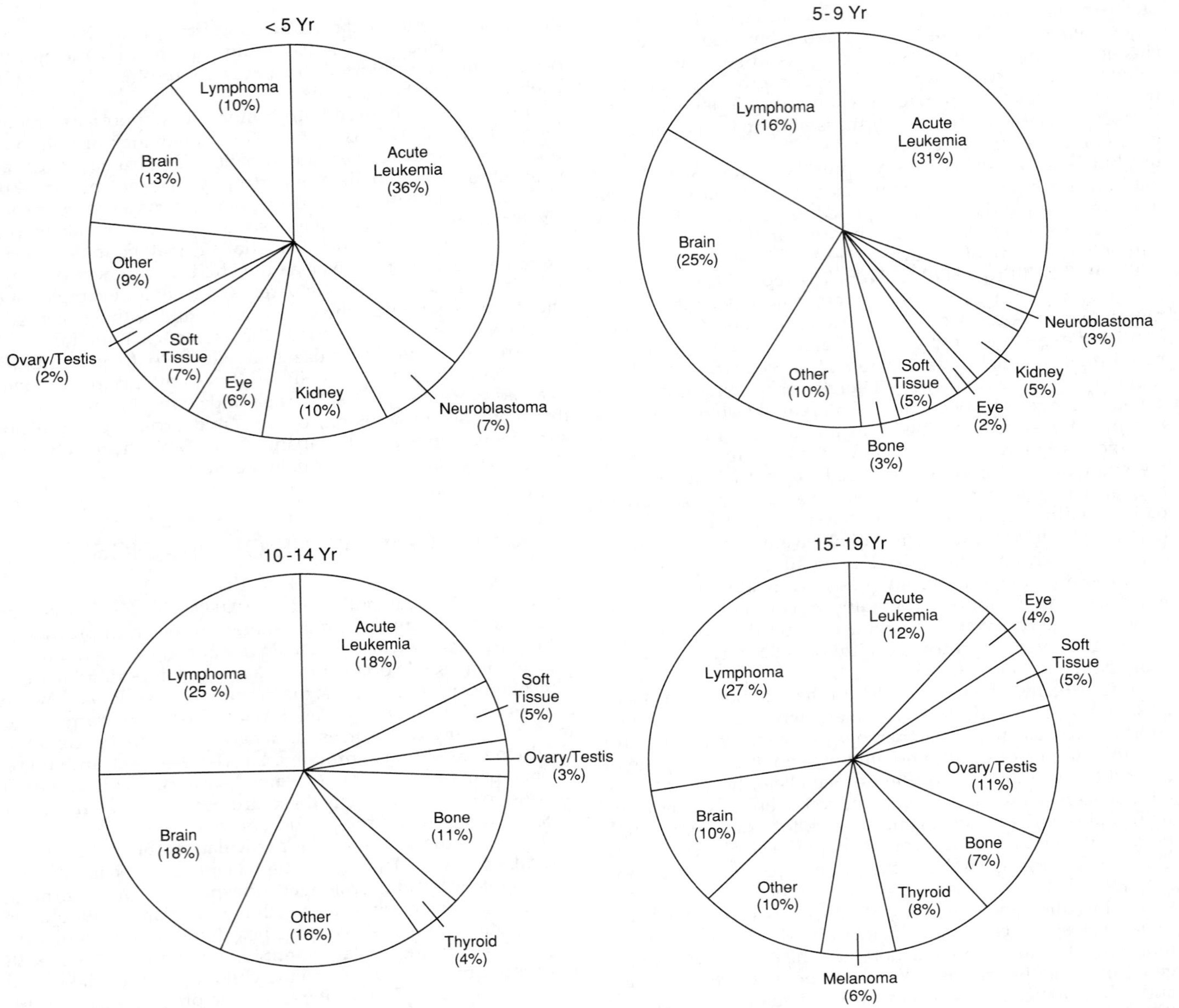

Figure 17–1. Percentage of primary tumors by site of origin at different ages at diagnosis. (Adapted from the National Cancer Institute Monograph No. 57. SEER Program.)

likely to be a neuroblastoma or Wilms tumor in a young child than in a child over the age of 10 yr.

It is usually appropriate to make a relatively thorough search for metastatic disease before obtaining a biopsy for confirmation of the diagnosis. If the surgeon knows the likelihood of disseminated disease, he or she can exercise better judgment in choosing between an attempt at complete resection and a more limited diagnostic biopsy. The studies appropriate for this preoperative review depend on the tentative diagnosis and are discussed for each specific tumor. A number of noninvasive techniques are useful in the search for metastases. The invasive procedure most often used before surgery is examination of bone marrow by aspiration or biopsy or both.

At the time of diagnosis, it is critical that the extent of disease be defined accurately; this delineation is called "staging." A system of staging must be designed for each tumor and will depend on the experience that has been gained in relating the extent of disease at the time of diagnosis to the subsequent clinical course. Staging helps to determine prognosis and treatment plan. Specific staging systems will be described for each tumor type, as appropriate.

At the core of the initial diagnostic studies of any tumor is the examination of its histologic character. The initial specimen of tumor tissue should be obtained under conditions that allow for the full range of pathologic studies that may be necessary to identify the tumor accurately; in some tumors, such as lymphoma, these studies may require fresh tissue for antigen marker or other studies such as electron microscopy. The results of these studies may take time to become available, and it is often impossible immediately after surgery to discuss diagnosis in detail with a family.

The surgeon must search carefully at biopsy, excision, or exploration for evidences of regional dissemination to lymph node groups or to adjacent organs. If an attempt is made to remove the whole tumor or the organ containing the tumor, the pathologist will need to examine carefully the margins of resection to make sure that no microscopic residual tumor remains. The planning for subsequent treatment of the patient rests on this cornerstone of initial diagnostic studies; the planning must be done by physicians trained and experienced in the care of children with cancer.

17.3 PRINCIPLES OF TREATMENT

GENERAL. Treatment of the child with cancer has two aspects: specific and supportive. For specific therapy the physician can offer surgical removal, irradiation, and chemotherapy. The majority of tumors in childhood have spread beyond the site of origin at the time of diagnosis and are not, therefore, amenable to complete surgical removal or to destruction by local irradiation alone. In most children with cancer, all three modalities will be necessary. The goal of all forms of treatment is the same: to remove or destroy as much tumor as possible, with the least damage to normal cells.

The patient's prognosis varies with the type of tumor and the extent of disease at the time of diagnosis as well as on the adequacy of treatment. The best chance for cure exists during the initial course of treatment, which should be optimized; accordingly, patients should be referred early to an appropriate specialized center. Major advances have been made in the treatment of childhood malignancy in the past 3 decades and at least half of patients diagnosed today will be cured. These advances have been made as a result of the participation by patients and their physicians in clinical research programs. Some of the discoveries, such as the importance of sanctuary therapy for the central nervous system in acute leukemia, have been made at individual institutions, whereas others, such as the curability of patients with stage I Wilms tumor through short-term chemotherapy without radiotherapy, have been made by collaborative groups of investigators. Not all patients and families may wish to participate in clinical experiments, but further progress will not be made without assessment of new treatments in a systematic fashion, and because there are such small numbers of patients with any single diagnosis, progress may well require that a patient be entered into a collaborative study directed by a protocol or treatment plan from one of the cooperative Clinical Cancer Research groups.

CHEMOTHERAPY. Drugs for treatment of cancer are selected from several classes of agents, including hormones, antimetabolites, antibiotics, plant alkaloids, and alkylating agents (Table 17–2). New agents with apparent antitumor activity can be identified in a number of ways. The effects of these agents are studied in animals for their efficacy in suppressing tumor growth and for toxicity. The few agents of promise are then studied in humans. The initial (phase I) studies are carried out to assess the toxicity of the new compounds. They are usually performed in adults with tumors for which there is no available therapy, who have given their informed consent to the procedure. The starting doses of a new drug to be tested are small, the dose increasing to the point of tolerance as the study progresses. With the maximum tolerated dose determined, the drug is then studied (phase II) in patients with a wide variety of tumors to determine its range of effectiveness. For those tumors found to be responsive to the drug, further trials are designed (phase III) in which the agent is incorporated into schedules with other active drugs and new and old regimens are compared for effectiveness.

BONE MARROW TRANSPLANTATION. Early experiments with marrow transplantation involved patients in florid relapse of leukemia, and the death rate after transplantation was high. Patients are now undergoing transplantation while in remission; the death rate from infection in the immediate post-transplantation period is much lower, and it appears that 40–60% of patients with selected diagnoses may show long-term survival. In general, the younger the patient, the more favorable the response may be. A number of centers now use or recommend transplantation of allogeneic or syngeneic bone marrow for patients with acute myeloblastic leukemia in first remission or for acute lymphoblastic leukemia in a second or subsequent remission.

There has as yet been no definitive comparison between the best available chemotherapy (which is continually improving) and marrow transplantation. The survival curves of groups of patients given chemotherapy alone take their origin from the day of first treatment and reflect the outcomes of patients who have failed to achieve remission or who have

TABLE 17–2. Cancer Chemotherapeutic Agents

Drug	Major Mode of Action	Important Toxicities
Methotrexate	Inhibits tetrahydrofolate synthesis	Marrow suppression, mucosal ulceration, liver damage, leukoencephalopathy*
6-mercaptopurine, 6-thioguanine	Inhibits purine biosynthesis	Marrow suppression, mucosal ulceration, liver damage
Cytosine arabinoside	Inhibits initiation of DNA synthesis	Marrow suppression, mucosal ulceration, febrile reaction, conjunctivitis, cerebellar toxicity with high dose*
Alkylating agents (all)	Alkylation of DNA	Marrow suppression, sterility in males
Cisplatin		Renal tubular damage, ototoxicity*
Cyclophosphamide		Hemorrhagic cystitis,* SIADH
Ifosfamide		Hemorrhagic cystitis,* nephrotoxicity, transient CNS toxicity
Bleomycin	DNA strand scission	Pulmonary fibrosis*
Epipodophyllotoxins (VP 16, VM 26)	DNA strand scission, topoisomerase inhibition	Myelosuppression, hypotension, anaphylaxis
Anthracyclines (doxorubicin, daunorubicin)	DNA intercalation, free radical formation	Marrow suppression, mucosal and gut ulceration, radiosensitization, myocardial damage*
Actinomycin D	Inhibits DNA-dependent RNA synthesis	Marrow suppression, gut ulceration, radiosensitization
Vinca alkaloids (vincristine, vinblastine)	Microtubule disruption with metaphase block	Marrow suppression, loss of deep tendon reflexes, constipation, cranial nerve palsies, SIADH
Asparaginase	Inhibits protein synthesis	Anaphylaxis, pancreatitis,* hyperglycemia, liver dysfunction

*Dose related, potentially irreversible.

died during introduction. On the other hand, the marrow transplant curves measure survival from the time of transplantation. To be eligible for marrow transplantation, a patient must already have achieved remission with induction chemotherapy. Such survival curves cannot, therefore, be directly compared.

Current methods of allogeneic bone marrow transplantation require an HLA-matched sibling as donor (see Sec. 6.39 and 6.42). As family size has tended to decrease, so has the proportion of patients for whom a match is available, since there is only one chance in four that any sibling will be appropriate. Studies are under way to determine whether minor degrees of HLA mismatch or better immunosuppression will allow the use of donors other than HLA-matched siblings.

Graft-versus-host disease (GVHD) and interstitial pneumonitis remain serious post-transplantation problems. GVHD occurs less often in younger patients, and newer agents such as cyclosporin are decreasing its incidence (see also Sec. 11.21). Chronic GVHD can remain a problem, however, and can lead to serious disfigurement (e.g., with a scleroderma-like skin picture as well as more debilitating conditions). Leukemic relapse also limits the proportion of patients achieving long-term disease control. Patients with GVHD appear to have a lesser likelihood of relapse (graft-versus-leukemia effect); accordingly, reducing the incidence and severity of GVHD may increase the likelihood of relapse. Another serious potentially fatal complication of marrow transplantation is veno-occlusive disease of the liver, thought to be related to the conditioning regimen.

A number of investigators are exploring the possibility of **autologous bone marrow transplantation.** After the patient's own bone marrow is harvested, doses of radiation or chemotherapy are administered that would usually be lethal owing to marrow toxicity. The autologous marrow is then reinfused so that the marrow can be repopulated. GVHD is generally not a problem in this situation, as long as meticulous care is taken to irradiate all blood products administered at the time of marrow harvest, as well as during the support period after marrow reinfusion. During this procedure the frozen marrow must be kept viable. The marrow is usually cryopreserved in dimethylsulfoxide (DMSO), which prevents ice crystals from forming, and DMSO will be reinfused with the marrow and excreted through the lungs (with a garlic odor), and may have toxicities of its own (specifically cataract formation). Veno-occlusive disease of the liver may occur and is more common in patients with abnormal liver function at the start of transplant. Moreover, there may be tumor cells in the harvested marrow that are reinfused after irradiation or drug therapy. A variety of techniques to circumvent this are under trial: first, the patient should be in remission at the time of harvest for autotransplantation; and second, cytoxan derivatives, which appear to kill tumor cells and spare marrow stem cells, have been used to purge bone marrow in vitro, as have specific monoclonal antibodies (e.g., against T cells). Another problem, which is shared with allogeneic transplantation, is that the intensive treatment, which sets the stage for autologous transplantation, may be insufficient to eradicate the disease.

Active investigation is under way in the use of autologous transplantation in acute myelogenous leukemia, non-Hodgkin lymphoma, neuroblastoma, Ewing sarcoma, and other solid tumors in which effective chemotherapy is available but hematopoietic toxicity may be dose-limiting. Unfortunately, when higher doses of antitumor agents are not restricted by hematopoietic toxicity, toxic effects on other organs are likely to appear. There has been some success in relapsed non-Hodgkin lymphoma with combination chemotherapy as preparation for autotransplantation. L-Phenylalanine mustard is a promising agent in both neuroblastoma and Ewing sarcoma.

COMPLICATIONS. Early complications of therapy include metabolic disorders, bone marrow suppression, and immunosuppression. Patients with a large tumor load may have been breaking down tumor cells for some time before the diagnosis is made. Their renal function may be impaired from tubular precipitates of uric acid crystals. Before initiating therapy, therefore, the serum levels of uric acid and creatinine should be measured in all patients, adequate hydration should be assured, and allopurinol (a xanthine oxidase inhibitor) should be given, if necessary, to bring the uric acid level to within the normal range. This problem arises particularly with hematopoietic tumors but may occur with other large tumors (e.g., neuroblastoma). If proper attention is not given and the metabolic *tumor lysis syndrome* ensues, phosphates and potassium will be released into the circulation in large quantities as further cell lysis takes place, and symptomatic hypocalcemia and hyperkalemia may develop.

All chemotherapeutic regimens are capable of producing *bone marrow suppression,* and tumors that invade and replace bone marrow can also result in pancytopenia. Anemia can be corrected by blood transfusions of packed red blood cells. Thrombocytopenia can be corrected by platelet infusions. Granulocytopenia poses a risk of serious bacterial infections when the granulocyte count is less than $500/mm^3$. Febrile granulocytopenic patients should have appropriate cultures obtained and receive intravenous antimicrobial therapy, usually with a penicillinase-resistant penicillin and an aminoglycoside to give broad antibacterial coverage until the granulocyte count rises. Granulocyte transfusions are toxic and are rarely used.

Immunosuppression of variable degree is a consequence of some tumors and of some treatment regimens. Viruses normally of low pathogenicity can then produce serious disease. Patients should not be given vaccines containing live virus. Patients on chemotherapy who are exposed to varicella should receive varicella zoster immunoglobulin and, if severe clinical disease develops, should be hospitalized and treated with acyclovir. An attenuated varicella vaccine is being developed that appears to be safe at present for use in patients with leukemia on chemotherapy. Fungal infections are common, particularly with *Candida* species. Opportunistic organisms such as *Pneumocystis carinii* can produce fatal disease. If severe degrees of immunosuppression are anticipated, prophylactic treatment against pneumonitis due to *P. carinii* should be given with trimethoprim/sulfamethoxazole. See also Sec. 14.58.

NUTRITION. It is not uncommon for patients undergoing cancer therapy to lose 10% or more of body weight. Malnutrition may become a particular problem in patients undergoing radiotherapy to the head and neck, or with intensive chemotherapy and total body irradiation for marrow transplantation. Such patients may require parenteral hyperalimentation. There is no evidence, however, that hyperalimentation improves a patient's chances of responding to therapy, and anxious parents should be reassured that they need not be concerned if the child's appetite is poor.

EMOTIONAL SUPPORT. A foremost consideration should be psychologic and emotional support for patient and family. An honest examination of the facts is the best policy in dealing with both child and parents. The child should be told all that he or she can understand and would find useful to know or wishes to know. Special problems, such as the need for amputation of a limb or of loss of hair during chemotherapy, must be anticipated and fully discussed. Explanations may have to be repeated several times before distraught family members feel that they really understand what is being said.

Whenever possible, the child should remain in school and with classmates. Because most treatment regimens are intensive, most of the patients will miss a considerable amount of schooling in the first year or two after diagnosis, even if they are eventually cured. Tutoring should be encouraged so that they do not fall behind academically. Parents, patients, siblings, and medical staff will need help in expressing feelings of anxiety, depression, guilt, and anger (Sec. 3.59).

LATE SEQUELAE. Late consequences of therapy may result in serious morbidity. Successful surgical removal of a tumor may require the sacrifice of important functional structures. Following the amputation of a leg for bone tumor, for example, careful attention must be given to rehabilitation with a functional prosthesis.

Irradiation may produce irreversible damage to organs, the symptoms and degree of limitation depending on the organ involved and the severity of injury (Sec. 26.1). These may not become fully obvious until the patient is fully grown, when it may be noted that irradiated and nonirradiated areas or extremities are markedly asymmetric. Irradiation of endocrine organs can cause abnormalities in function. Hypothyroidism and sterility commonly follow thyroid and gonadal irradiation, and neurologic dysfunction may follow cranial irradiation.

Chemotherapy also carries the risk of irreversible damage to organs. Of particular concern are the leukoencephalopathy that follows high-dose methotrexate therapy, sterility in the male after therapy with alkylating agents, myocardial damage with anthracyclines, pulmonary fibrosis after bleomycin, pancreatitis after asparaginase, and hearing loss with cisplatin. All of these may be dose-related and are poorly, if at all, reversible. Appropriate studies must be done before these medicines are administered, in order to ensure that dangerous damage to organs has not already occurred.

Another late effect is the occurrence of *second cancers* in patients successfully cured of a first. The risk appears to be cumulative at about 0.5%/yr, up to 12% for patients who are 25 yr beyond their treatment. Patients who have been treated for childhood cancer should be examined annually and should be carefully assessed for the late effects of therapy.

17.4 THE LEUKEMIAS

The leukemias are the most common form of childhood cancer. They account for about one third of new cases of cancer diagnosed each year. The acute lymphocytic leukemias make up about 76% of cases, with a peak in incidence around the age of 4 yr. Acute nonlymphocytic leukemia accounts for about another 20%, with incidence increasing with age into late adulthood. Chronic myelogenous leukemia and other leukemias difficult to classify account for the remainder. Chronic lymphocytic leukemia is essentially never seen in childhood.

Leukemia occurs in 42.1/million white and 24.3/million black children/yr. The difference is due mainly to the lower incidence of acute lymphocytic leukemia among black children. The acute lymphocytic leukemia (ALL) of childhood was the first form of disseminated cancer to respond completely to chemotherapy. It is, therefore, an important model on which concepts of chemotherapy in other malignancies have been developed.

The general clinical features of the leukemias are similar, since all involve a severe disruption of bone marrow function. Specific clinical and laboratory features differ, however, and there are considerable differences in the responses to therapy and prognosis.

17.5 ACUTE LYMPHOCYTIC LEUKEMIA

ALL occurs slightly more frequently in boys than in girls. Several reports of clusters of acute leukemia in children have suggested some common environmental factor in etiology, but careful statistical analyses have not supported this possibility. Lymphoid leukemias do occur more often than expected in patients with immunodeficiency, chromosomal abnormalities (e.g., Down syndrome), and ataxia-telangiectasia.

PATHOLOGY. Patients with ALL are subclassified according to the morphologic and immunologic features of their blast cells as well as by their clinical presentation. Definitive diagnosis must be made on examination of a bone marrow aspirate. The variability in cytologic appearance of the blast cells is so great, even within a single specimen, that no completely satisfactory system has yet been devised for differentiation of the various forms of ALL by cytologic appearance alone. A French-American-British (FAB) working group has devised a classification based on the appearance of bone marrow leukemia cells at the time of diagnosis. Three cytologic types are identified: L-1 lymphoblasts are predominantly small with little cytoplasm; L-2 cells tend to be larger and have greater amounts of cytoplasm, irregular nuclear membranes, and more prominent nucleoli; and L-3 cells have characteristic cytoplasmic vacuolization. L-3 morphology is uncommon and usually associated with blast cells having surface immunoglobulin (in B cell ALL).

The most useful classification of subtypes of ALL depends on *cell membrane markers*. It is first determined whether the cells represent a malignant proliferation of T (thymus-derived) lymphocytes, by using monoclonal antibody against pan T cell antigens (CD5, CD7). Within the subclass of T cells, monoclonal antibodies can be used further to determine whether the abnormal cell arises from early or late stages of T cell maturation. If the cells are not T cells, they are then screened with fluorescein-tagged anti-immunoglobulin reagents. If immunoglobulin is detected on the cell surface (sIg), the cell is considered a mature B (bone marrow–derived) cell. If immunoglobulin is found in the cytoplasm (cIg), the cell is considered a B cell precursor, or preB cell. The largest group of leukemic patients have lymphoblasts that do not react with any of the above reagents, but they generally represent an even earlier stage in B cell maturation than the preB cell. Almost all of them show immunoglobulin gene rearrangement, and the majority of them express the common ALL antigen (cALLa) and the immune-associated (Ia) antigen, both of which are lost with T cell maturation. Some leukemias in both the null and the preB class do not express cALLa. They represent a minority of the leukemias found in older children but virtually all the leukemias that have their onset before 6 mo of age. Some leukemias cannot be precisely classified because they demonstrate asynchronous antigen expression.

Chromosome translocations in the immunoglobulin forming region of DNA such as t8:14, or in the alpha T cell receptor gene (t11:14) can help define the subtype of leukemia. An overall increase in chromosome number (i.e., hyperdiploidy) is associated with a good outcome whereas the presence of the Philadelphia chromosome (Ph+) similar to that seen in adult chronic myelogenous leukemia carries a particularly ominous prognosis.

The subtypes of ALL with their relative incidences are shown in Table 17–3, along with certain clinical characteristics.

Another biologic marker with potential usefulness is the increased terminal desoxynucleotidyltransferase activity found in cells of null, preB, and T cell ALL. Because this enzyme is present only rarely in normal non-T lymphocytes, it may prove useful in identifying leukemic cells in difficult diagnostic situations; for example, it may help to distinguish early CNS relapse from aseptic meningitis.

Patients with leukemia almost always have disseminated disease at the time of diagnosis, with marrow involvement at all sites and with leukemic blast cells in blood. Spleen, liver, and lymph nodes are also usually involved. Accordingly,

TABLE 17–3. Incidence of the Subtypes of ALL in a Single Study, with Incidence of Some Clinical Features at the Time of Diagnosis*

Subtype	No. of Patients	%	Age (Median)	WBC × 10^3 (Median)	% Male	% Having a Mediastinal Mass	Common Chromosomal Abnormalities
T (T+)	44	14	7.4 yr	61.2	67.1	38.2	t (11:14)
B (sIg+)	2	0.6					t (8:14)
PreB (cIg+)	56	18	4.7 yr	12.2	54.8	1.2	t (1:19)
Early preB (T−, sIg−, cIg−)	209	67	4.4 yr	12.4	56.5	1.0	t (4:11)
Infant (Ia⁺, cAlla−)	33	NA	<1 yr	50.0	55	None	Breakpoints: 11 p 23–25; 9 p 21–22; 10 p 11–13

*Adapted from Pullen JD, Boyett JM, Crist WM, et al: Pediatric Oncology Group utilization of immunologic markers in the designation of acute lymphocytic leukemia subgroups: Influence on treatment response. Ann NY Acad Sci 428:26, 1983.

there is no staging system like those developed for solid tumors.

CLINICAL MANIFESTATIONS. Children with ALL present a fairly consistent clinical onset. About two thirds of them will have had signs and symptoms of their disease for less than 4 wk at the time of diagnosis. The first symptoms are usually nonspecific; there may be a history of a viral respiratory infection or exanthem from which the child has not appeared to recover fully. Frequent early manifestations are anorexia, irritability, and lethargy. Progressive failure of bone marrow function leads to pallor, bleeding, and fever, which are usually the features that precipitate diagnostic studies.

On initial examination most of the patients are pale, and about half have petechiae or mucous membrane bleeding. About a quarter have fever, which can sometimes be ascribed to a specific cause, such as respiratory infection. Lymphadenopathy is occasionally prominent, and splenomegaly (usually less than 6 cm below the costal margin) can be demonstrated in about two thirds of patients. Hepatomegaly is less common. Bone pain, probably secondary to marrow infarction and arthralgia, is an important presenting complaint in about one quarter of patients. About one third of patients will have bone tenderness, owing to periosteal invasion and subperiosteal hemorrhage. Rarely, signs of increasing intracranial pressure such as headache and vomiting may indicate leukemic meningeal involvement. Children with T cell ALL are likely to be older, are more often male, and more often have a mediastinal mass; these features do not distinguish between children with preB and those with null cell ALL (see Table 17–3).

DIAGNOSIS. On initial examination most patients will have anemia; only about 25% will have hemoglobin levels below 6 g/dL. Most patients will also have thrombocytopenia, but as many as 25% may have platelet counts greater than 100,000/mm³. A significant proportion of patients will have white blood cell counts less than 3,000/mm³, and about 20% will have counts greater than 50,000/mm³. The diagnosis of leukemia can be suspected on the finding of blast cells on blood smear, but the definitive study is examination of bone marrow, which in almost all patients will be found to be completely replaced by leukemic lymphoblasts. Occasionally, patients in whom an aspirated specimen is hypocellular will require a needle biopsy of the bone marrow to demonstrate the leukemic replacement.

A chest roentgenogram should be taken to determine if there is a mediastinal mass, as is frequently the case in patients with T cell ALL. Bone roentgenograms may show altered medullary trabeculae, cortical defects, or subepiphyseal bone resorption, but these findings have no clinical or prognostic significance. Cerebrospinal fluid should be examined for leukemic cells. Early CNS involvement has important prognostic implications. Uric acid level and renal function should be determined before treatment is started (see Sec. 17.3).

DIFFERENTIAL DIAGNOSIS. The diagnosis of ALL is usually easily made once the possibility of ALL has been considered, but thinking of the diagnosis may be delayed for a child who has been sick and febrile with adenopathy for several weeks. The diseases to be considered in the differential diagnosis are those also associated with bone marrow failure. Bone marrow infiltration by other malignant cells can occasionally produce pancytopenia. In children tumors capable of producing marrow replacement include neuroblastoma, rhabdomyosarcoma, Ewing sarcoma, and retinoblastoma. These tumors are usually found in clumps scattered throughout normal marrow tissue, but occasionally there may be complete replacement of marrow. In such patients there is usually evidence of a primary tumor in some other site.

The bone marrow failure of ALL needs to be distinguished from the nonmalignant marrow failure associated with aplastic anemia or myelofibrosis. Patients with ALL who have marked leukopenia sometimes have no evidence of blast cells either on a blood smear or in aspirated marrow, the hypoplastic marrow resembling that of aplastic anemia. Examination of an adequate bone marrow biopsy will usually resolve any uncertainty. Occasionally, a patient who presents with aplastic marrow will develop frank leukemia a few weeks later. When possible, chromosome studies should be done on such marrows to identify possible specific abnormalities associated with myelodysplastic and preleukemic syndromes

Infectious mononucleosis should rarely be confused with ALL despite their somewhat similar clinical pictures. Careful examination of the blood smear should permit identification of the typical cells of infectious mononucleosis. If doubt remains, a bone marrow aspirate will demonstrate a normal cell population.

TREATMENT. The treatment of ALL varies with the clinical risk features. A patient at standard risk at the time of diagnosis is more than 2 yr old and less than 10 yr old, has a white blood cell count under 100,000/mm³, a normal mediastinum on chest roentgenogram, no evidence of leukemic central nervous system involvement, and blast cells that do not have B or T cell features. The basic components of a treatment program for such an individual include initial induction therapy until the bone marrow no longer shows leukemic cells, prophylactic treatment to the CNS, and a continuation of systemic treatment for 2.5–3 yr. A sample plan is outlined in Table 17–4.

A combination of prednisone, vincristine, and asparaginase can be expected to produce remission in about 95% of children with standard-risk ALL. For almost all such patients remission is achieved within 4 wk. For the residual 5–10% of patients, another 2 wk of therapy should be given. Systemic continuation therapy should be given for 2.5–3 yr.

In more than 50% of patients who have not received prophylactic treatment of the CNS, this body system will be

TABLE 17–4. An Effective Treatment Regimen for Standard-Risk ALL

Remission induction (4–6 wk)	
Vincristine 1.5 mg/m² (max 2 mg) IV/wk	
Prednisone 40 mg/m² (max 60 mg) po/day	
Asparaginase (*E. coli*) 10,000 U/m²/day biweekly IM	
Intrathecal treatment	
Triple therapy:	Methotrexate* (MTX)
	Hydrocortisone* (HC)
	Cytosine arabinoside* (Ara C)
Wkly × 6 during induction, and then every 8 wk for 3 yr	
Systemic continuation treatment	
6-mercaptopurine 50 mg/m²/day po	
Methotrexate 20 mg/m²/wk po	
With reinforcement	
Vincristine 1.5 mg/m² (maximum 2 mg) IV every 8 wk	
Prednisone 40 mg/m²/day po × 28 days every 16 wk	

*The dose of intrathecal medication is age adjusted.

Age	MTX	HC	Ara C
≤ 1 yr	10 mg	10 mg	20 mg
2–8 yr	12.5 mg	12.5 mg	25 mg
≥9 yr	15 mg	15 mg	30 mg

the site of initial relapse. Evidence indicates that leukemic cells are present in the meninges at the time of diagnosis and that their survival is due to the lower drug concentrations achieved in the cerebrospinal fluid. Therapeutic attack on this sanctuary area was first achieved through cranial irradiation; this therapy has been found, however, to produce late effects on school performance and behavior, particularly in younger children. For the standard-risk patient, intrathecal chemotherapy alone, continued on a bimonthly basis throughout maintenance, is sufficient therapy for clinically inapparent CNS involvement.

The response of patients with T cell ALL is improving. A regimen similar to that for standard-risk ALL will often achieve an initial remission, but most patients with T cell ALL will relapse within 2 yr on such treatment. More intensive multidrug regimens are being explored by the Cooperative Treatment Groups with promising results and with 40% of patients achieving long-term remission. Investigators are trying to take advantage of characteristics of T cells that set them apart from other lymphocytes, in order to target specific therapy. The adenosine deaminase inhibitor deoxycoformycin may provide specific biochemical therapy for T cell disease. Acute myelogenous leukemia occurs as a late occurrence in 20% of patients with T cell leukemia treated with epipodophyllotoxin containing regimens. This has raised the possibility that both malignancies may arise from a common stem cell that has undergone clonal evolution.

The few patients with L-3 morphology and surface immunoglobulin have the worst prognosis. They are best treated according to regimens designed for B cell lymphoma and are considered candidates for early marrow transplantation.

In most centers, bone marrow is examined at regular intervals to determine whether remission is continuing. If bone marrow relapse occurs, particularly after the patient has completed continuation therapy, intensive retreatment with a combination such as cytosine arabinoside and the epipodophyllotoxin VM 26, will achieve cures in 15–20% of patients. Bone marrow transplantation should also be considered.

When relapse occurs in both standard and high-risk patients, it is often in an extramedullary site. The most important sites are the CNS and the testes. The common early manifestations of CNS leukemia are due to increasing intracranial pressure. Vomiting, headache, papilledema, and lethargy occur with increasing severity. These symptoms may also occur as part of a chemical meningitis secondary to intrathecal therapy, and this must be considered in the differential diagnosis. Convulsions and isolated cranial nerve palsies (such as of the 6th and 7th nerves) may also be manifestations of CNS leukemia but also of vincristine toxicity. Hypothalamic involvement is rare but must be suspected if excessive weight gain or behavioral disturbances occur. In almost all patients with leukemia involving the CNS, spinal fluid pressure is elevated and the fluid shows a pleocytosis due to leukemic cells. When the cell count is not increased, leukemic cells may be found in smears of spinal fluid specimens after centrifugation.

If CNS relapse occurs after preventive CNS therapy and during hematologic remission, the patient should be given intrathecal methotrexate weekly for 4–6 wk after the cells have disappeared. The dose of intrathecal methotrexate is age adjusted since cerebrospinal fluid volume is not proportional to body surface area (see Table 17–4). Craniospinal irradiation should then be given. In addition, the patient's systemic treatment should be intensified. Preventive CNS therapy should be repeated in all patients in whom relapses have occurred in the bone marrow or in other extramedullary sites.

Testicular size should be assessed as part of the routine examination of all patients with leukemia, to make sure the size is appropriate for age. Testicular relapse generally produces painless swelling of one or both testicles, of which the patient may not be aware. Diagnosis should be confirmed by biopsy. Treatment should include irradiation of the gonads (2,000 rad), but because a number of patients show involvement of retroperitoneal lymph nodes at the time of testicular relapse, systemic therapy should be reinforced, for patients still on treatment, or reinstituted for those off treatment. CNS preventive therapy should be repeated as well.

PROGNOSIS. Unfavorable prognostic features for patients with ALL include onset at age less than 2 yr or more than 10 yr of age, with a white cell count over 100,000/mm³, or with a mediastinal mass. The significance of these clinical signs was established before the subtypes of ALL were known; the latter now permit clearer delineation of prognosis.

Null cell ALL has the most favorable prognosis. Approximately 95% of affected patients will enter remission, and about 75% will still be in remission 5 yr after the start of therapy. A cure may be achieved in the majority of patients with this form of ALL. PreB cell ALL with t 1:19 has a somewhat less promising prognosis. About 95% of patients will achieve remission, but only about 60% will still be in remission after 5 yr. Patients whose cells lack cALLa may have a poor prognosis; almost all patients in whom ALL is diagnosed at less than 1 yr of age have cALLa-negative leukemia. T cell leukemia is curable in about half of the patients; B cell leukemia is rarely cured with current therapy.

TABLE 17–5. Subtypes of Nonlymphocytic Leukemia

Type	
Acute nonlymphocytic leukemia (ANLL)	*FAB classification*
Myeloblastic, no maturation	M1
Myeloblastic, some maturation	M2
Hypergranular promyelocytic	M3
Myelomonocytic	M4
Monocytic	M5
Erythroleukemia	M6
Megakaryocytic	M7
Chronic myelocytic leukemia (CML)	
Adult form	
Chronic phase	
Blast crisis	
Juvenile form	
Congenital leukemia	

17.6 ACUTE NONLYMPHOCYTIC LEUKEMIA

Acute nonlymphocytic leukemia (ANLL) accounts for about 20% of cases of leukemia in children. It is more common in older children and occurs with equal frequency in boys and girls. ANLL characteristically occurs in children having predisposing conditions, such as Fanconi anemia and Bloom syndrome, in which there is excessive chromosomal breakage, or as a second tumor after cancer chemotherapy.

PATHOLOGY. The subtypes of ANLL shown in Table 17–5 are distinguished in the FAB system by differences in cytomorphology in Wright-stained smears of blood and bone marrow. The degree to which the predominant cell resembles a normal cell of bone marrow provides the designation of type. In the most common type the leukemic cells resemble myeloblasts or myelomonoblasts. The proportion of cell types resembling myeloblasts or monoblasts in the admixture makes the distinction between these two subtypes, which account for 90% of all ANLL.

Although there are cytologic differences, the clinical presentations and responses to therapy are similar for subtypes, with one exception: when the predominant cell resembles a promyelocyte (M3), there is increased risk that bleeding associated with disseminated intravascular coagulation will occur during the course of an early response to therapy. This M3 subtype occurs in about 5% of patients with ANLL.

CLINICAL MANIFESTATIONS. The duration of symptoms and signs before the diagnosis is made in patients with ANLL is usually brief, 50% of patients having less than 6 wk of illness. In a few patients, however, the history may indicate a probable onset up to 12 mo before definitive presentation; in such patients the usual complaints are fatigue and recurrent infections. Worsening symptoms or signs during the 2 wk immediately before diagnosis are likely to include pallor, fever, active bleeding, bone pain, gastrointestinal distress, or severe infection. It is not possible to distinguish between ALL and ANLL on the basis of prediagnostic findings. A finding relatively specific for ANLL, however, is gingival swelling due to infiltration of leukemic cells.

The initial physical findings do not differ greatly from those in patients with ALL. The liver and spleen are enlarged in 60% of patients; marked hepatosplenomegaly occurs in only 10–15%. In 20% there may be marked lymphadenopathy. A few patients may initially have joint pain mimicking arthritis or a localized tumor mass (chloroma) that may produce such findings as proptosis or neurologic manifestations of CNS leukemia. In older girls menorrhagia may be prominent.

DIAGNOSIS. The variability of initial leukocyte and platelet counts is similar to that in patients with ALL. Initial hemoglobin levels range from markedly decreased to normal, most patients having levels from 5 to 10 g/dL. The suspected diagnosis is confirmed by examination of the blood smear and bone marrow. Since consistent chromosome abnormalities occur in ANLL, chromosome analysis of the marrow is indicated. In patients in whom the cytology is consistent with acute promyelocytic leukemia, coagulation studies must be done at the time of diagnosis to detect any acceleration of intravascular coagulation and to provide baseline values for evaluation of the subsequent clinical course.

The same considerations for differential diagnosis of ALL apply to ANLL. Additionally, there may be megaloblastic features in the bone marrow in ANLL that may superficially mimic those of folic acid or vitamin B_{12} deficiency. The experienced cytologist can easily distinguish ANLL by the more striking defects in maturation, the greater degree of atypical morphology, and the greater proportion of blast cells seen in this disease.

Sometimes children with ANLL have a long antecedent period of progressive marrow failure. In this early phase the proportion of blast cells may be so small that the diagnosis of leukemia cannot be confirmed. The diagnosis can sometimes be facilitated by the demonstration that there are clones of bone marrow cells having aneuploid karyotypes. In such patients the course of progressive marrow failure may be hastened rather than reversed by chemotherapy; accordingly, a period of observation is the best current management, there being no indication that early treatment is beneficial. Patients with therapy-linked leukemia or occupational exposure to potentially leukemogenic agents and those with myelodysplastic syndromes have an increased frequency of abnormalities involving chromosomes 5, 7, or both and a relatively poor response to therapy.

In most cases, standard Wright- or Giemsa-stained blood and bone marrow smears are adequate to differentiate between leukemias. Histochemical stains are also useful. The cells in ANLL are usually positive for peroxidase and Sudan B black stains; and when their cytoplasm is positive for the periodic acid-Schiff (PAS) stain, the reaction is diffuse rather than aggregated or clumped as in ALL. In monoblastic leukemia the cytoplasm will be positive with the nonspecific esterase stain.

Monoclonal antibodies are now being developed that detect membrane antigens associated with discrete phases of maturation of myeloid cells. These help to identify myeloid leukemia cells as being mature or less mature (i.e., as stem cell phenotypes). Monoclonal antibodies can be particularly helpful in patients in whom histologic diagnosis is confusing. Even with these aids there are a few patients whose leukemia cells show no definite markers and others who will be seen to have definite markers of two cell lines (e.g., myeloid surface antigens and immunoglobulin gene rearrangement). It is not clear at present how such patients should be treated.

TREATMENT. Treatment of ANLL is improving with the availability of new drugs and particularly with improvement in supportive care. Presumably because the myeloid leukemia cell closely resembles the normal myeloid stem cell, successful induction therapy seems to require a period of marrow aplasia. A regimen employing cytosine arabinoside 100 mg/m²/24 hr by continuous intravenous infusion for 7 days, with intravenous daunorubicin 45 mg/m² 24 hr for 3 days, should achieve remission in 70% or more of the patients. In patients with promyelocytic leukemia, heparin should be given during induction to prevent fatal hemorrhage from disseminated intravascular coagulation. Maintenance therapy is generally given with rotating combinations of several agents for a period of up to 2 yr. At least 50% of those who achieve remission will remain in remission when therapy is stopped. The CNS is an important site of relapse in ANLL, as in ALL. Following initial spinal taps for evaluation of CNS disease, prophylactic chemotherapy is administered in a fashion similar to that recommended for ALL. The use of bone marrow transplantation after the patient has achieved an initial remission is being studied. Children have longer remissions and survival than do adults, both with chemotherapy alone and after marrow transplantation; it is important, therefore, that experimental and control groups be matched for age.

PROGNOSIS. The prognosis for patients with ANLL has improved; 30–40% of children can be expected to be cured with chemotherapy alone. Studies done principally in adults, in whom the disease is more common, tend to show that patients with membrane markers consistent with "stem cell phenotype" will be less likely to do well than those with a mature cell phenotype. The immunologic phenotypes have not correlated well with histologic appearance.

17.7 CHRONIC MYELOCYTIC LEUKEMIA

Adult type chronic myelocytic leukemia (CML) is a clonal panmyelopathy involving all the hematopoietic cell lineages and at least some of the lymphoid. There is a specific cytogenetic marker, the Philadelphia (Ph^1) chromosome, a translocation (9;22) (q34;q11).

The adult type of CML accounts for only 3% of cases of leukemia in children. The age of maximal incidence in children is 10–12 yr. This condition has been seen with increased frequency in individuals exposed to radiation from the atomic bombs.

PATHOLOGY. In CML there are increased numbers of differentiating myeloid cells in blood and bone marrow. Splenomegaly is a prominent finding. Levels of vitamin B_{12} in serum and of fetal hemoglobin in erythrocytes will be elevated, whereas leukocyte alkaline phosphatase activity will be absent. If the pathognomonic Ph^1 chromosome is present, the diagnosis of CML is established; but some patients who have all the features of the clinical syndrome lack the Ph^1 chromosome (Ph^1-negative CML), and a few patients who have the clinical syndrome of ALL have the Ph^1 chromosome in their leukemic blast cells (Ph^1-positive ALL). In some patients a deletion in the break cluster region (bcr) will be equivalent to a Ph^1 chromosome.

CLINICAL FEATURES. The onset of symptoms is generally insidious. The diagnosis may not be suspected until splenomegaly or an abnormal blood count is found on routine examination. The spleen may become firm and enlarge as far as into the pelvis.

DIAGNOSIS. Laboratory abnormalities are usually confined initially to the white blood cell count, which may be greater than $100,000/mm^3$, with all forms of myeloid cells seen in the blood smear. There are no characteristic morphologic abnormalities of the cells, but eosinophilia and basophilia are usually present and may be striking. The bone marrow is hypercellular, with normal myeloid cells in all stages of differentiation, and megakaryocytes may be increased in number. Initially, the platelet count is usually normal or increased. Anemia may or may not be present, and nucleated red blood cells may be seen. Laboratory abnormalities are noted earlier. Examination of bone marrow, with chromosome studies, is essential for diagnosis.

TREATMENT. There is no treatment that will reverse the underlying disease process in CML, although intensive chemotherapy in adults has demonstrated that normal stem cells do exist in affected patients. Therapy should be aimed at preserving these stem cells in the hope that new treatments will be developed. The white blood cell count should probably be kept below $100,000/mm^3$, in order to avoid increased blood viscosity and cerebrovascular accidents. For this purpose, hydroxyurea (Litalir), which does not damage stem cells, is preferred to busulfan (Myleran), which does. Splenic radiation may be used if the enlarged spleen is causing severe discomfort. Allogenic bone marrow transplantation may be effective early in the disease, and some responses to interferon have been seen.

The terminal phase of this disease is characterized by a gradual increase in the number of myeloblasts in the blood (blast crisis) and by the development of anemia and thrombocytopenia. With the onset of a blast crisis, which may be myeloid or lymphoid, the treatment program is changed to that for acute leukemia. Median survival from the time of diagnosis is about 3 yr.

Juvenile chronic myelocytic leukemia is a term used to describe a rare disease, usually in patients under 2 yr. It is a clonal panmyelopathy associated with an elevated white blood cell count, prominent involvement of the monocytic series, splenomegaly, and cutaneous manifestations. Serum vitamin B_{12} is elevated, and leukocyte alkaline phosphatase is low, but Ph^1 chromosome is absent. This disorder is thought to represent abnormal sensitivity to growth factors.

17.8 CONGENITAL LEUKEMIA

True leukemia may occur in the neonatal period and is usually of myelocytic morphology. This disease often presents with cutaneous infiltration (blueberry muffin lesions), hemorrhage, and high white blood cell counts. It has a high fatality rate.

Sometimes an infant with an underlying chromosomal abnormality, and particularly 21-trisomy, may be born with hepatosplenomegaly, a high white blood cell count with immature myeloid forms, and thrombocytopenia. It is unclear whether this "**congenital leukemia**" represents a true leukemic process. Affected patients should be treated with supportive platelet transfusions only if needed for bleeding, or with single agent chemotherapy only if needed to control the white blood cell count, in order to see whether they will have spontaneous remission during the first few weeks of their disease.

LYMPHOMA

See Sec. 11.1–11.3 and 16.93 for related discussion of the immune and lymphatic systems.

Lymphoma, the third most common cancer in children in the United States, affects 13.2/million children/yr. The rates are similar for white and black children. The two broad categories of lymphoma, Hodgkin disease and non-Hodgkin lymphoma (NHL), have such different clinical manifestations, treatment, and prognosis that they will be considered separately.

17.9 HODGKIN DISEASE

INCIDENCE. This tumor rarely occurs before the age of 5 yr, the incidence increasing steadily thereafter to a peak at 15–34 yr of age; a second peak occurs after the age of 50. The condition is almost twice as common in boys as in girls. No definitive causal factors are known, but occurrence in like-sex siblings has suggested a virus of low virulence and infectivity. Hodgkin disease appears to arise in T-dependent areas of lymphoid tissue. The central histologic feature is the Reed-Sternberg cell (Fig. 17–2). This cell is thought to originate from an antigen-presenting cell of the mononuclear phagocyte-reticulum cell lineage, perhaps from the interdigitating reticulum cell. There is increasing evidence that EB virus may be involved in the pathogenesis.

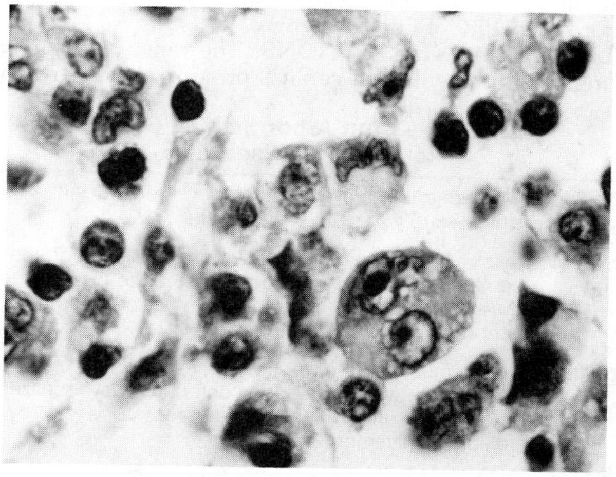

Figure 17–2. A Reed-Sternberg cell that contains 2 nuclei, each with a prominent nucleolus and distinct nuclear membrane. The cytoplasm of this cell is relatively abundant. Other cells present are lymphocytes, plasma cells, and tissue mononuclear cells. This appearance in a lymph node is diagnostic of Hodgkin disease.

PATHOLOGY. There are four histologic subtypes of Hodgkin disease, each with special clinical features and implications for prognosis. In the *lymphocytic predominant* variety, almost all of the cells appear to be mature lymphocytes or a mixture of lymphocytes and benign histiocytes, with only an occasional Reed-Sternberg cell. This type affects 10–20% of patients and has the best prognosis.

The *nodular sclerosing* variety, the most common form, affects about 50% of younger patients and 70% of adolescents. Broad bands of collagen divide the involved lymph node into nodular cellular areas. A special cytologic feature is clear spaces surrounding "lacunar cells," which are variants of the Reed-Sternberg cell. Because of the amount of collagen, the radiographic appearance of these lesions (particularly in the mediastinum) may be slow to return to normal, even when the patient is responding to therapy.

Hodgkin disease of *mixed cellularity* is the second most common form and affects 40–50% of patients. It is characterized by accumulations of lymphocytes, plasma cells, eosinophils, histiocytes, malignant reticular cells, and Reed-Sternberg cells. Foci of necrosis may be present. This form is more likely to involve extranodal areas at the time of diagnosis.

The least common and least favorable form of the disease is the *lymphocytic depletion* variety, which affects fewer than 10% of patients. Numerous bizarre malignant reticular cells are found, with Reed-Sternberg cells and relatively few lymphocytes. There may also be various degrees of partly hyalinized fibrosis with a paucity of cells, mostly of reticular and Reed-Sternberg types.

Hodgkin disease arises in lymph nodes in almost all cases; extranodal primary sites occur in fewer than 1% of patients. The manner of spread suggests direct anatomic extension. Adjacent lymph node areas are the first site of spread in most patients, presumably as the result of spread along adjacent lymphoid channels. These observations have provided the basis for radiotherapy regimens. When the disease is no longer confined to lymph nodes, the more common sites of extranodal involvement are spleen, liver, lung, bone, and bone marrow.

For determining prognosis and for planning treatment, anatomic staging should be done at the time of diagnosis (Table 17–6). This may involve exploratory laparotomy to establish the extent of intra-abdominal disease. In addition, patients should be assigned to an A or B category in accordance with the absence or presence, respectively, of systemic symptoms such as night sweats, fever, or recent weight loss of more than 10% of body weight.

CLINICAL MANIFESTATIONS. The most common presenting finding is enlarged cervical or supraclavicular lymph nodes. Occasionally, nodes of the axillary or inguinal areas may be the site of primary involvement. The enlargement is firm, nontender, and usually discrete, involving single or multiple lymph nodes. It is generally first noted by the patient or parents. Characteristically, no regional inflammation can be found to explain the lymphadenopathy. Mediastinal lymph node enlargement is common and may produce a cough, usually nonproductive, or symptoms of tracheal or bronchial compression. It may be found on a chest roentgenogram taken for an unrelated purpose. In younger children, mediastinal lymph node involvement may be difficult to distinguish from a large, normal thymus. Computed tomography (CT) or magnetic resonance imaging (MRI) of the mediastinum may reveal differences in texture from thymus.

The patient usually has few, if any, systemic manifestations at the time of diagnosis. Typical symptoms would include night sweats, unexplained fever, weight loss, lethargy, easy fatigability, and anorexia. Pruritus is an unusual early complaint; if pruritus occurs alone, it does not place the patient in a B category.

Extranodal involvement is unusual at the time of diagnosis, but may occur with progression of the disease. Lung involvement may be represented roentgenographically by diffuse fluffy exudates, difficult to distinguish from disseminated fungal infection. Fever and tachypnea are usual, and pulmonary insufficiency may develop. If pulmonary involvement is suspected, the lesions should be biopsied first, because establishment of this diagnosis will identify stage IV, and a staging laparotomy will not be required.

Liver involvement is associated early with signs of intrahepatic biliary obstructive disease. With progression, signs of hepatocellular disease may develop. Bone marrow involvement may result in neutropenia, thrombocytopenia, and anemia. Extradural tumor masses in the spinal canal can cause progressive cord compression. A variety of immune disorders may occur, such as immunohemolytic anemia, immunothrombocytopenia, or the nephrotic syndrome.

Cellular immunity is impaired in Hodgkin disease as a consequence both of the disease and of its treatment. Affected patients are at increased risk of the infections characteristic of immunosuppressed patients. Varicella-zoster infections occur in up to one third of the patients and should be treated with *acyclovir* if severe; fungal infections, such as cryptococcosis, histoplasmosis, and candidiasis, may also become disseminated. Once the spleen has been removed, sepsis with encapsulated bacteria (e.g., *Streptococcus pneumoniae* or *Haemophilus influenzae*) may be lethal.

DIAGNOSIS. Hodgkin disease should be suspected in the patient with persistent unexplained lymphadenopathy. The disease is more common in older children and adolescents, when infectious cervical lymphadenopathy is common. If a careful history and physical examination find no evidence that an underlying inflammatory process is responsible for the enlarged nodes and if the lymphadenopathy is persistent, then a biopsy is warranted. In a significant percentage of patients, there will be a history of relatively recent antecedent, serologically proven infectious mononucleosis; accordingly, enlarged nodes that fail to regress after infectious mononucleosis should also be considered for biopsy. Before a biopsy is done of a cervical node, a chest roentgenogram should explore the possibility of mediastinal involvement and examine the patency of the airway. The blood counts are generally not helpful; characteristic changes in the white blood cell count include a neutrophilic leukocytosis, lymphopenia, and sometimes eosinophilia and monocytosis. Anemia and thrombocytopenia occur only in patients with disseminated disease. Acute phase reactants, such as erythrocyte sedimentation rate, serum copper, and serum ferritin, may be elevated and may be useful, albeit nonspecific, markers of disease activity.

TABLE 17–6. Ann Arbor Staging System for Hodgkin Disease*

Stage I	Involvement of a single lymph node region or of a single extralymphatic organ or site
Stage II	Involvement of two or more lymphoid regions on the same side of the diaphragm; or localized involvement of an extralymphatic organ or site and of one or more lymph node regions on the same side of the diaphragm
Stage III	Involvement of lymph node regions on both sides of the diaphragm, which may be accompanied by localized involvement of an extralymphatic organ or site or by splenic involvement
Stage IV	Diffuse or disseminated involvement of one or more extralymphatic organs or tissues, with or without associated lymph node enlargement

*Patients are further categorized as A or B, based on the absence or presence, respectively, of systemic symptoms of fever and/or weight loss.

When the diagnosis is made, staging should be done in order to establish the extent of the disease. Most patients first present evidence of lymph node enlargement above the diaphragm. A roentgenogram and CT scan of the chest should be performed. Disease will sometimes be seen on the latter when the former appears normal. In addition, CT can evaluate the extent of pericardial and chest wall involvement, which may affect prognosis. Liver function tests are unreliable indicators of hepatic disease, and the size of the spleen correlates poorly with splenic involvement.

Lymphangiography is generally accurate in indicating lymph node involvement below the level of the second lumbar vertebra, but above that level involved lymph nodes may not be filled with contrast materials. This procedure is infrequently performed in children. CT or MRI of the abdomen may indicate node enlargement but not the nature of the underlying process. Accordingly, a staging laparotomy may be indicated to determine with certainty the presence or absence of infradiaphragmatic disease. At laparotomy the spleen is removed, the liver is biopsied, and samples are taken of nodes from all accessible areas. In addition, if radiotherapy to the pelvis is contemplated in a female, the ovaries should be moved to an area away from the radiation field, for example, tucked behind the uterus in the midline. Bone marrow biopsies may be done to determine possible marrow involvement. In about one third of affected children, the stage of disease assigned from clinical findings will be revised when the anatomic findings are known.

TREATMENT. Both radiation therapy and chemotherapy are highly effective in the treatment of Hodgkin disease. Many patients have a good chance of long-term disease control or of cure, and the goal of current treatment regimens is to achieve cure with as little morbidity and toxicity as possible. For localized (stage I or IIA) disease in patients who have achieved their full growth, radiation alone to standard fields with doses of 3,500–4,000 rad may be the treatment of choice. Up to 50% of such patients, however, will have recurrences and will require combination chemotherapy. Regimens of chemotherapy either with nitrogen mustard, vincristine (Oncovin), procarbazine, and prednisone (MOPP) or with doxorubicin (Adriamycin), bleomycin, vinblastine, and dacarbazine (ABVD) can produce long disease-free periods for patients with advanced Hodgkin disease. A usual course of therapy would consist of six cycles of either of these treatments and would take about 6 mo. Further treatment with low dose radiations (2,000–2,500 rad) to involved areas may be indicated. Questions such as which patients should be treated initially with chemotherapy, who should receive radiation and in what doses, and how toxic these treatments are to the growing child are still under investigation.

PROGNOSIS. With current treatment more than 90% of patients with Hodgkin disease achieve a complete initial clinical remission. The likelihood of prolonged remission or cure is related primarily to the stage at diagnosis. Most patients with disease in stages I and II will be cured, as will approximately 75% of those in stage III if treated with both chemotherapy and radiation, and at least 50% of those in stage IV if treated with intensive chemotherapy.

The longer survival of patients has created more concern about the complications of treatment. The complications of irradiation depend on the site. Irradiation of upper body node areas may lead to restriction of lung capacity, to cardiac involvement, or to late hypothyroidism. In the younger child the growth of the vertebral column, the clavicles, and the breast buds can be affected. Because of concerns about growth, standard dose radiation is rarely given to children. Irradiation of the ovaries in the female patient may induce sterility or premature menopause or both. With chemotherapy, there may also be late pulmonary (bleomycin) and cardiac (doxorubicin) toxicity. MOPP may produce sterility in the male.

One to two per cent of patients who have had splenectomy at staging laparotomy may develop overwhelming sepsis with *S. pneumoniae* or *H. influenzae*. These patients should be given pneumococcal vaccines around the time of laparotomy and should receive long-term prophylactic penicillin. Abdominal adhesions may follow laparotomy, particularly in patients whose abdomens have been irradiated. A second malignancy (most frequently acute leukemia in patients who have received chemotherapy) occurs with an incidence of about 0.5%/yr after treatment.

17.10 NON-HODGKIN LYMPHOMA (NHL)

NHL, which designates a heterogenous group of solid lymphoid tumors, is more common than Hodgkin disease in young children, and affects boys about three times as frequently as it does girls. Both congenital and acquired immunodeficiencies, including acquired immunodeficiency syndrome (AIDS), predispose to the development of this type of lymphoma. Children with infantile X-linked agammaglobulinemia or severe combined immunodeficiency have about a 5% incidence of malignancy, usually lymphoma, and children with Wiskott-Aldrich syndrome and ataxia-telangiectasia a 10% or greater incidence. The incidence of lymphomas is increased also in immunosuppressed patients after renal transplantation.

A form of lymphoma in American patients resembles the Burkitt lymphoma of African children; the cells carry surface immunoglobulins, are derived from B lymphocytes (e.g., in the African form of the disease), and show the chromosomal translocations described in Sec. 17–1. Unlike the African form, the American lymphoma does not have a nearly universal association with the EB virus.

PATHOLOGY. The classification of NHL is under continual revision. Children, more often than adults, tend to have the diffuse, more rapidly growing forms. A recent classification divides lymphomas into low, intermediate, and high grades. The majority of childhood lymphomas fall into the high-grade category.

As new techniques identify subpopulations of normal lymphocytes, NHL is being reclassified in accordance with the stage in differentiation of lymphocytes that each represents. There is a striking association between mediastinal primary site and T cell origin of the tumor, and between abdominal primary site and B cell origin. In general, immunologic type and histologic type are correlated; T cell tumors usually have lymphoblastic histology, whereas undifferentiated, Burkitt, and "histiocytic" lymphomas are of B cell origin. When it can be done, immunologic subtyping is important, because optimal therapies vary with subtype.

Since children tend to have the more high-grade tumors that do not spread in an orderly fashion and that disseminate readily, staging systems applicable to adults may not apply to children. A system devised for non-Hodgkin lymphoma in childhood is shown in Table 17–7.

CLINICAL MANIFESTATIONS. The clinical features of lymphoma depend on the site of primary tumor and the extent of local and distant disease. The tumor commonly presents in the head and neck region as a painless, unexplained swelling of cervical or supraclavicular lymph nodes. The growth may be rapid, significant increases occurring within 1–2 wk. There may also be periods of regression prior to therapy. The nodes are generally nontender and firm, discrete in the early phases of growth, but often confluent later. Other nodal areas such as axilla, ileocecal region, or groin may also be primary sites of tumor.

TABLE 17–7. A Staging System for Non-Hodgkin Lymphoma in Childhood*

Stage I
A single tumor (extranodal) or single anatomic area (nodal), with the exclusion of mediastinum or abdomen.

Stage II
A single tumor (extranodal) with regional node involvement.
Two or more nodal areas on the same side of the diaphragm.
Two single (extranodal) tumors with or without regional node involvement on the same side of the diaphragm.
A primary gastrointestinal tract tumor, usually in the ileocecal area, with or without involvement of associated mesenteric nodes only, which must be grossly (>90%) resected.

Stage III
Two single tumors (extranodal) on opposite sides of the diaphragm.
Two or more nodal areas above and below the diaphragm.
Any primary intrathoracic tumor (mediastinal, pleural, thymic).
Any extensive primary intra-abdominal disease.

Stage IV
Any of the above, with initial involvement of CNS and/or bone marrow at time of diagnosis.

*From Murphy SB: Classification, staging, and end results of treatment of childhood non-Hodgkin's lymphomas: Dissimilarities from lymphomas in adults. Semin Oncol 7:332–339, 1980.

Lymphoma of the chest generally arises in the anterior mediastinum, and the presenting feature may be cough or progressive dyspnea owing to compression of the airway or to pleural effusion, which may contain lymphoma cells. These patients should receive immediate attention. Obstruction of the superior vena cava may occur.

Abdominal lymphoma occurs most frequently in the ileocecal region, presenting possibly as an abdominal mass, as intestinal obstruction, or as intussusception. There may be associated ascites.

Lymphoma of bone produces local or diffuse bone pain and usually represents dissemination from some other primary site.

Along with findings related to the local tumor, there may be manifestations of systemic dissemination. Meningeal involvement may present signs of increased intracranial pressure, or there may be direct extension of tumor to involve cranial nerves or produce spinal cord compression. Bone marrow may be involved. If more than 25% of the marrow cells are lymphoblasts, the patient is classified arbitrarily as having leukemia. Systemic symptoms of fever and weight loss are not uncommon. Occasionally, particularly in patients with immunodeficiency, primary intracerebral lymphoma may present as a mass lesion.

TREATMENT. After biopsy, surgery has a role principally for the excision of localized lymphoma of the bowel. Because of the systemic nature of this tumor and its propensity for hematogenous dissemination, all patients require chemotherapy. Before therapy is started, renal function and serum uric acid levels should be determined (Sec. 17.3) and administration of allopurinol should be begun. Due to the extreme rapid progression of NHL, frequently with the threat of fulminant airway obstruction, acute renal failure and abrupt metabolic decompensation, expedient staging, and the start of specific therapy are medical emergencies. The airway should be evaluated by a CT scan prior to anesthesia. A tissue diagnosis should be obtained before any therapy is started. Steroids should not be given to decrease airway edema, because they may precipitate the tumor lysis syndrome.

Recommended therapy now depends on the site of origin of the tumor, as well as the degree of dissemination. For localized nodal disease, treatment similar to that for acute lymphoblastic leukemia (see Table 17–4), but lasting only 6 mo, currently represents the treatment of choice. For patients with a Burkitt lymphoma histology, regimens relying on high-dose methotrexate and cytoxan should be employed. In general, these tumors of B cell origin grow rapidly and recur quickly if they are going to do so. Thus, therapy is intensive but is usually not given for more than 1 yr.

For primary intrathoracic tumors, a more intensive, 10-drug regimen gives the best chance of cure. Particularly with lymphomas of T cell origin, some form of preventive CNS therapy (chemotherapy or irradiation or both) should be given, and maintenance should be continued for up to 1 yr.

PROGNOSIS. With current treatment, perhaps 90% of patients with stage I and II disease can expect to be cured, as can about 50% of those with stage III and IV disease. Once the tumor has spread to the bone marrow and undergone "leukemic conversion," the prognosis is worse. In patients who have had relapses, there has been some success in the use of intensive chemotherapy followed by autologous bone marrow reinfusion or identical-twin marrow transplantation.

17.11 HISTIOCYTOSES

A group of diseases characterized by proliferation of cells of the monocyte/macrophage line have been traditionally referred to as histiocytoses or reticuloendothelioses. Their nature is not known. Careful attention to clinical features and histologic characteristics permits sufficient definition to guide the treatment and to determine the prognosis. It should be remembered that "histiocytic lymphoma" is thought to represent malignant proliferation of B cells (Sec. 17.10). The majority of these disorders are now thought to represent benign processes (see Sec. 25.5).

NEOPLASMS OF NERVOUS TISSUE ORIGIN

Tumors of the central nervous system are discussed in Sec. 20.74. Other tumors arise from the primitive neural crest cells that form the adrenal medulla and sympathetic nervous system. In children, these tumors are represented almost exclusively by neuroblastoma and its benign variant, ganglioneuroma.

17.12 NEUROBLASTOMA

Neuroblastoma in children under the age of 15 yr occurs at a rate of about 1/100,000/yr. It is slightly more common in white children than in black and slightly more common in boys than in girls. The median age at the time of diagnosis is around 2 yr; about 75% of cases are diagnosed before the age of 5 yr. Occasionally, cases occur in older children or adults. Familial occurrence is known, including in identical twins, but this tumor seems generally to be sporadic. Deletions in chromosome 1 are commonly found in tumor tissue.

Neuroblastoma has a uniquely high rate of spontaneous regression. Microscopic clusters of neuroblasts are normally found in the adrenal glands of fetuses and in about 1/200 neonates at autopsy; this frequency is far above the incidence of clinical neuroblastoma. It is believed that most of these small tumors disappear spontaneously. Spontaneous regression of clinically apparent disease after birth also occurs, particularly in patients under the age of 1 yr who have stage I or stage IVS disease (see later and Table 17–8). Although the reasons for this spontaneous regression are unknown, proposed possibilities include an immunologic response to the tumor and the response to some normal growth factor as yet undefined. Some have questioned whether stage IVS

TABLE 17–8. Neuroblastoma Staging Systems

Evans Stages	Pediatric Oncology Group Stages
Stage I Tumor confined to organ or structure of origin.	***Stage A*** Complete gross resection of primary tumor with or without microscopic residual; intracavitary lymph nodes, not adherent to and removed with primary,* histologically free of tumor; if primary in abdomen or pelvis, liver histologically free of tumor.
Stage II Tumor extending in continuity beyond organ or structure of origin but not crossing the midline; regional nodes on homolateral side may be involved.	***Stage B*** Grossly unresected primary tumor; nodes and liver same as stage A.
Stage III Tumor extending in continuity beyond the midline; regional nodes may be involved bilaterally; bilateral extension of midline disease.	***Stage C*** Complete or incomplete resection of primary; intracavitary nodes not adherent to primary histologically positive for tumor; liver as in stage A.
Stage IV Remote disease involving skeleton, organs, soft tissue, distant nodes, and so on.	***Stage D*** Any dissemination of disease beyond intracavitary nodes—e.g., to extracavitary nodes, liver, skin, bone marrow, bone.
Stage IVS Patients who would otherwise be stage I or II, i.e., with small and/or resectable primary tumor; but who have remote disease confined only to one or more of the following sites: liver, skin, or bone marrow (not bone).	

*Nodes adherent to or within tumor resection may be positive for tumor without upstaging patient to stage C.

neuroblastoma in infancy represents a true malignancy, despite its dissemination. Hyperdiploid tumor cells of clonal origin have been reported in infants with stage IVS neuroblastoma, possibly indicating true malignancy rather than benign hyperplasia.

PATHOLOGY. Neuroblastoma is usually a firm, gray mass. Hemorrhage into this vascular neoplasm commonly imparts a variegated maroon color, often with necrosis and calcification. The degree of cell differentiation in neuroblastoma is variable. Most tumors consist of primitive neuroblastoma cells with little evidence of differentiation. Some tumors have admixtures of cells with larger amounts of cytoplasm, cytoplasmic processes, rosettes with central fibrillar material, and mature ganglion cells. Electron microscopy reveals distinctive features: peripheral dendritic processes containing longitudinally oriented microtubules; and small, spherical, membrane-bound granules with electron-dense cores, which represent cytoplasmic accumulation of catecholamines (neurosecretory granules). With treatment, serial biopsy specimens may contain increasing proportions of mature ganglion cells, and "maturation" of the tumor to a ganglioneuroma may take place at some sites; this does not, however, indicate an improved prognosis.

The tumor may arise in any site where neural crest cells are present. The sympathetic chain extends from the posterior cranial fossa to the coccyx. About 70% of the tumors arise in the abdomen, half of these in the adrenal gland. Another 20% arise in the thorax, usually in the posterior mediastinum, and the remainder arise elsewhere. In some children with widely disseminated tumor, the initial site cannot be defined.

Neuroblastoma may extend to surrounding tissue by local invasion or to regional lymph nodes via lymphatics. Extension of a paravertebral lesion into the spinal canal may produce spinal cord compression. Hematogenous spread most frequently involves liver, bone marrow, and skeleton. Metastases to the orbits not uncommonly result in proptosis; metastases to the dura, in signs of increasing intracranial pressure (including split sutures). Metastases to the brain are rare.

Two staging systems are currently in use for neuroblastoma (see Table 17–8). A special designation (stage IVS) is reserved for patients with small or unidentifiable primary tumors in whom remote involvement is confined to liver, skin, or bone marrow. Almost all such patients are under the age of 6 mo. Their skin nodules may have a firm, purplish blueberry muffin appearance. Patients with this form of neuroblastoma generally have a good prognosis with minimal or no therapy. Recent studies indicate that a normal DNA content of tumor cells compared with normal cells (DNA index) carries a poor prognosis, as does amplification of N-*myc* in the tumor.

CLINICAL MANIFESTATIONS. No tumor has such polymorphic symptoms as neuroblastoma, owing to the numerous sites for primary tumor, as well as to the patterns of widespread metastases. Moreover, some symptoms arise out of tumor-associated metabolic disturbances. The primary tumor is usually in the abdomen and presents as a firm, irregular, and nontender mass. Because the primary tumor is often in the adrenal, the mass is usually in the upper abdomen. Hemorrhage into the enlarging tumor is common and may produce pallor or even hypotension. With metastasis to the liver, hepatic enlargement and occasionally ascites occur. Severe ascites may result in respiratory embarrassment, and surgical decompression may be required. Bony metastases can produce pain and tenderness, generally manifested in the young child as extreme irritability.

Patients with primary tumors outside the abdomen are often not as sick at presentation. Thoracic masses are often discovered unexpectedly on the chest roentgenogram. Occasionally, a large upper thoracic mass will give rise to respiratory distress. Tumors in the head and neck may be palpable or may result in Horner syndrome. Tumors in the pelvis may produce problems in defecation or urination. A rectal examination should be performed at least once in any patient with such symptoms. Neuroblastoma can develop either intraspinally or extraspinally or can extend in dumb-bell fashion between intervertebral foramina to cause cord compression, with back tenderness, sphincter dysfunction, and gait disturbance. A primary tumor in the nasopharynx (esthesioneuroblastoma) usually presents unilateral epistaxis or occlusion of nasal passageways.

Other symptom complexes accompany neuroblastoma. An encephalopathy involving the cerebellum produces a syndrome *(opsomyoclonus)* characterized by progressive ataxia and titubation of the head, myoclonic jerks, and chaotic conjugate jerking movements of the eyes (opsoclonus), with progressive dementia. The cause of this syndrome is not known. Symptoms may disappear with the resection of the primary tumor. *Severe diarrhea* with atonic bowel and extreme loss of potassium may occur as an effect of overproduction of vasoactive intestinal peptide (VIP) and may disappear rapidly with resection of the primary tumor. *Hypertension* is relatively rare in patients with neuroblastoma; it is much more common in those with pheochromocytoma. Episodes of unexplained flushing and sweating are often reported, however, in patients with neuroblastoma and have even been reported in mothers of infants with the tumor in utero. The systemic syndromes occur in patients with all stages of disease and do not necessarily reflect disseminated disease or poor prognosis.

DIAGNOSIS. Initial studies are determined by the site of origin and the evidence of dissemination. For abdominal tumors, CT scans with oral and intravenous contrast are the most helpful studies. Conventional radiographic evaluation of adrenal neuroblastoma includes the abdominal roentgenogram, ultrasound, and excretory urography. Helpful findings include calcification, or displacement of the renal collecting system or of the ureter. The relationship of the tumor to adjacent retroperitoneal organs (particularly the great vessels) is usually inadequately assessed by these methods, however, and such determinations may be critical in deciding whether the tumor is resectable or not and in planning the initial surgical procedure. On the CT scan, neuroblastomas generally have mixed tissue density indicating both solid and cystic components. The cystic areas are either hemorrhage or necrotic tumor. Calcification, sometimes not appreciated on a plain x-ray film, is found on CT scan in as many as 80% of neuroblastomas. If there has been significant hemorrhage into the tumor, this calcification may have a ring configuration difficult to distinguish from that of traumatic adrenal hemorrhage. Metastases may also be appreciated on the CT scan of organs such as the liver or the skeleton. Posterior mediastinal or paraspinal tumors are usually revealed by chest roentgenography. Widening of intervertebral foramina may help in detection of intraspinal extension of tumor. Metrizamide myelography along with CT may be required to define fully the extent of intraspinal extension of disease.

Bone scan is also useful in detecting primary tumor and in defining the extent of metastatic disease. Sixty per cent of patients will show primary tumor uptake of technetium diphosphonate. Metastatic lesions are detected on bone scan, but they are sometimes difficult to identify because they often occur symmetrically at epiphyseal plates, for example, in the proximal humerus. Plain roentgenograms of symptomatic areas may help define the extent of metastatic disease.

Bone marrow aspiration or biopsy should be performed for staging in all patients. It may reveal infiltrating tumor cells in clumps (Fig. 17–3) or complete replacement of the marrow with sheets of tumor cells indistinguishable from those of acute lymphoblastic leukemia. Pancytopenia may result from marrow involvement.

A specific diagnostic feature is the elevated levels of catecholamines in urine. Increased amounts of dopa, dopamine, norepinephrine, normetanephrine, homovanillic acid (HVA), or vanillylmandelic acid (VMA) are found in about 90% of patients. The use of paper chromatography to identify VMA and HVA in 24-hr collections of urine may be confounded by medications or by dietary substances, such as bananas, nuts, chocolate, and vanilla. A method involving gas chromatography and mass spectrography ("mass fragmentography") has greater precision and sensitivity; is free of diet and drug interference; measures all end-products of metabolism of dopamine, norepinephrine, and epinephrine; and requires only a few milliliters of urine. Radiolabled metaiodobenzylguanidine (miBG) can be taken up by catecholamine producing tumors. This isotope can be used to identify neuroblastoma on nuclear medicine scans and in higher doses may represent potential therapy.

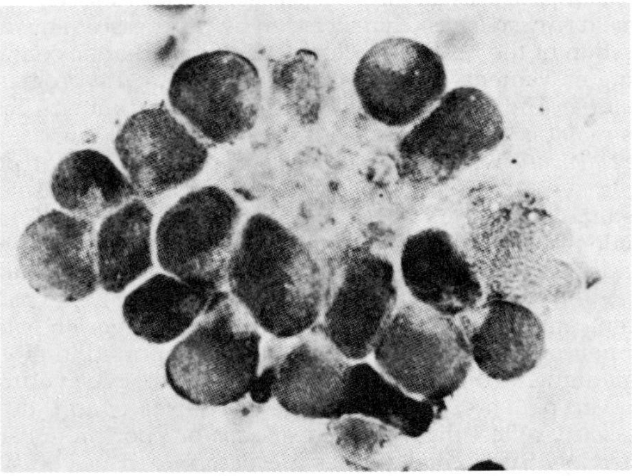

Figure 17–3. Neuroblastoma cells aspirated from the bone marrow. Clumps of cells often contain 3 cells or more without evidence of rosette formation. Rosettes of cells surrounding an inner mass of fibrillary material are characteristic of neuroblastoma.

Definitive diagnosis depends on the histologic characteristics of tumor obtained at excision or diagnostic biopsy. The aforementioned studies to demonstrate the site of primary tumor and the degree of dissemination should be done before surgery. For some patients with widely disseminated disease, a limited diagnostic biopsy of a superficial lesion or a bone marrow aspiration will be sufficient, particularly when accompanied by elevated catecholamine levels in the urine. When possible, material to determine ploidy and *n-myc* copy number should be obtained at biopsy.

TREATMENT. For localized tumor, complete surgical resection gives the best chance for cure. For unresectable regional disease, the surgeon should establish the degree and nature of the local extension. Biopsies of lymph nodes draining the tumor area should be obtained; and for tumors primarily in the abdomen, liver biopsy specimens should be examined for microscopic involvement. For cases in which metastatic disease has already occurred, the value of an attempt at resection of the primary tumor has not been established. For patients with disseminated disease who have shown a response to chemotherapy, attempts have been made later to resect the primary tumor; the value of this second look for therapy has not been established, but a significant percentage of patients thought to be tumor free by clinical restaging have been discovered at the time of such surgery to have residual disease and to require further therapy.

Most neuroblastomas are radiosensitive; irradiation may be used for local symptomatic relief of disseminated tumor or for reduction in size of tumor masses. The use of total body irradiation or extensive radiation alone to treat systemic disease has been generally disappointing.

Because disseminated disease is common at the time of diagnosis of this tumor, chemotherapy is the mainstay of treatment. A regimen incorporating cytoxan and doxorubicin has been shown to induce remission in about 50% of patients. The combination of cisplatinum and the epipodophyllotoxin VM 26 is also active. A number of other combinations have also been tried, with short-term responses. Bone marrow transplantation after preparation with melphalan and total body irradiation is now being assessed in patients with disseminated disease in first remission. Autologous marrow is reinfused after purging to remove possible contaminating tumor cells.

Patients whose tumors are identified as pure ganglioneuroma should not receive chemotherapy or radiation if the tumors have been resected and probably not even if total resection was impossible.

PROGNOSIS. The success of treatment in neuroblastoma depends greatly on age and stage. The older the patient and the more widespread the disease, the worse will be the prognosis. Patients whose tumors can be completely resected may do well with surgery alone. Local irradiation may be used if there are small amounts of residual tumor. Patients with stage III and IV disease generally receive chemotherapy. Patients under 1 yr of age may tolerate chemotherapy less well but are more likely than older patients to have a successful response to chemotherapy, particularly if their tumors are hyperdiploid. In Japan a mass screening program with urine VMA spot tests of 6-mo-old infants has been instituted for early detection of neuroblastoma.

Table 17–9 shows the results in a single institution of various regimens. The long-term survival of less than 10% for

TABLE 17–9. Neuroblastoma: Treatment Results by Stage and Age*

Evans Stage	Age at Diagnosis <1 yr	Age at Diagnosis >1 yr	2-Yr Survivors/Total (%)
I	5/5†	2/2	7/7 (100)
II	9/9	17/19	26/28 (93)
III	8/9	5/8	13/17 (76)
IV	9/10	4/46	13/56 (23)
IVS	6/7	3/3	9/10 (90)

*From Rosen EM, Cassady JR, Frantz CN, et al: Neuroblastoma: The Joint Center for Radiation Therapy/Dana Farber Cancer Institute Children's Hospital Experience. J Clin Oncol 2:719, 1984.

†Number of disease-free survivors at 2 yr/total number of patients in age group at given stage. Follow-up of 2–12 yr.

patients over the age of 1 yr with stage IV disease at the time of diagnosis illustrates the poor prognosis in this large group of patients. Marrow transplantation in remission may achieve closer to 25% long-term survival. The excellent prognosis of stage IVS patients is seen. Unless tumors in these patients seem likely to be lethal through interference with function of vital organs, they should probably not be treated but should rather be observed for the first few months after diagnosis to see whether spontaneous remission will occur.

NEOPLASMS OF THE KIDNEY

17.13 WILMS TUMOR

Wilms tumor accounts for almost all renal neoplasms in childhood. It occurs with approximately equal frequency in both sexes and in all races, with an annual incidence of 7.8/million children under the age of 15 yr.

An important feature of Wilms tumor is its association with congenital anomalies. The most common associations are with genitourinary anomalies (4.4%), hemihypertrophy (2.9%), and sporadic aniridia (1.1%). Wilms tumor has developed in children of parents with hemihypertrophy and in siblings of children with hemihypertrophy. Hemihypertrophy may often not become obvious until the time of the adolescent growth spurt; accordingly, a child with asymmetric growth following treatment for Wilms tumor may have hemihypertrophy rather than a complication of therapy.

A deletion in chromosome 11 was first noted in families of children with the aniridia-Wilms syndrome. It is consistently present at a submicroscopic level in cells of most Wilms tumors, even when the constitutional chromosomal composition is normal (see Sec. 17.1).

As with retinoblastoma (Sec. 17.21), the familial form of Wilms tumor is more likely to be bilateral than the sporadic form. Moreover, patients with bilateral or familial disease also have a higher incidence of congenital anomalies, and their tumor may develop at an earlier age. It is estimated that a child of a patient with bilateral or familial Wilms tumor has a 30% risk of developing the tumor.

PATHOLOGY. The classic Wilms tumor is a solitary growth that may occur in any part of either kidney. It is sharply demarcated and variably encapsulated. Small areas of hemorrhage are common. The tumors usually distort the renal outline, the residual normal kidney often being compressed into a thin rim around the tumor (Fig. 17–4*A* and *B*).

The microscopic appearance in patients with favorable histology generally includes both epithelial and stromal elements. There are three "unfavorable" histologic patterns; these are found in 10% of cases of Wilms tumor but are responsible for 60% of the deaths. *Anaplasia* involves marked variation in nuclear size with abnormal mitotic figures. It tends to occur in older patients. The *rhabdoid* tumor has cells with fibrillar eosinophilic inclusions; the presence of true striated muscle, however, excludes the diagnosis of rhabdoid Wilms tumor. This tumor type is found most often in very young patients. *Clear cell sarcoma* of the kidney is characterized by a spindle cell pattern with a striking vasocentric arrangement. This tumor is predominant in males and is most likely to metastasize to bone.

The staging system most frequently used is that of the

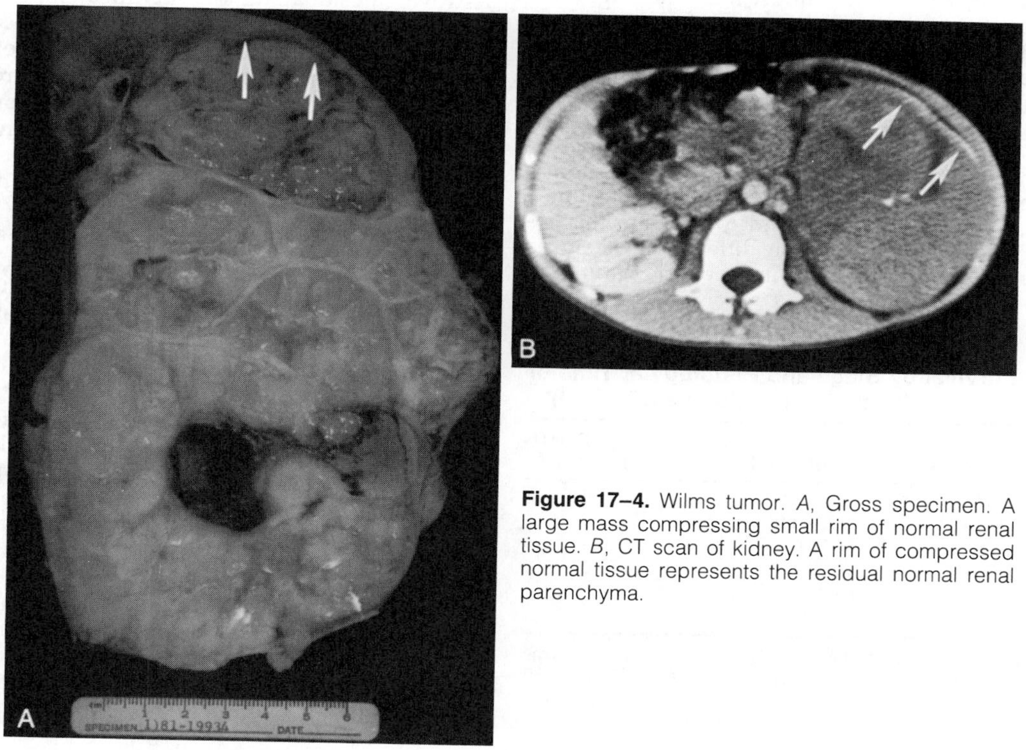

Figure 17–4. Wilms tumor. *A*, Gross specimen. A large mass compressing small rim of normal renal tissue. *B*, CT scan of kidney. A rim of compressed normal tissue represents the residual normal renal parenchyma.

National Wilms Tumor Study (NWTS) Group. Stage I tumors are limited to the kidney and can be completely excised with capsular surface intact. The stage II tumor extends beyond the kidney but can be completely excised. In stage III, there is residual nonhematogenous extension of tumor, confined to the abdomen following surgery. Stage IV indicates hematogenous metastases, which most frequently involve the lung. Five to ten per cent of Wilms tumors will be bilateral, and survival will be related to prognosis for the most severely involved kidney. (Stage V designates bilateral renal involvement, which is usually concordant in time). The relative incidence of stages I–IV and survival rates are shown in Table 17–10.

CLINICAL MANIFESTATIONS. The median age at time of diagnosis of Wilms tumor is about 3 yr. The most frequent sign is an abdominal mass, which is often asymptomatic. The mass is generally smooth and firm and rarely crosses the midline. Masses vary greatly in size at the time of discovery; mean diameter in one series of cases was 11 cm. Masses are often discovered on routine examination, or by parents. About half of affected children may have additional symptoms of abdominal pain or vomiting or both. In general, patients with Wilms tumor are slightly older and appear less ill than those whose abdominal mass will prove to be neuroblastoma.

Hypertension has been reported in as many as 60% of patients. Hypertension results from renal ischemia, usually owing to pressure of the tumor on the renal artery. It may be sufficiently severe and prolonged to produce congestive cardiac failure.

DIAGNOSIS. The diagnosis of Wilms tumor must be suspected in any young child with an abdominal mass. In 10–25% of patients, microscopic or gross hematuria may be an indication that the tumor is renal. Ultrasonography may indicate that the mass is intrarenal. The major differential diagnostic consideration may be neuroblastoma. CT is generally most helpful (see also Sec. 6.56). On CT studies without enhancement, the usual Wilms tumors arise from kidney as inhomogeneous masses with areas of low density indicating necrosis. Areas of hemorrhage and small focal calcifications are generally less common and less prominent than in neuroblastoma. After injection of a contrast medium, slight enhancement of tumors is noted. There is often a sharp demarcation between the tumor and normal parenchyma, correlated with a pseudocapsule, and persistent ellipsoid areas of increased attenuation corresponding to the compressed uninvolved renal parenchyma (see Fig. 17–4*B*). The primary clinical usefulness of CT in Wilms tumor is to establish the intrarenal origin of the tumor, which rules out neuroblastoma; to detect multiple masses; to determine the extent of tumor, including great vessel involvement; and to evaluate the opposite kidney. The major problems in differential diagnosis are hydronephrosis, renal cysts, and mesoblastic nephroma or other renal malignancies such as renal cell carcinoma, sarcoma, and lymphoma.

TABLE 17–10. Survival by Stage and Histology at Time of Diagnosis in National Wilms' Tumor Study 3 (NWTS 3)*

Stage	No. of Patients	% of Total	% Having 4-Yr RFS†
I	607	42.2	96.5
II	278	19.3	92.2
III	275	19.1	86.9
IV +UH	279	19.4	73.0
Total	1,439	100.0	

*Data from D'Angio GJ, Breslow N, Beckwith JB, et al: Treatment of Wilms' tumor: Results of the third national Wilms' tumor study. Cancer 64:349–360, 1989.

†RFS = relapse-free survival. UH = unfavorable histology.

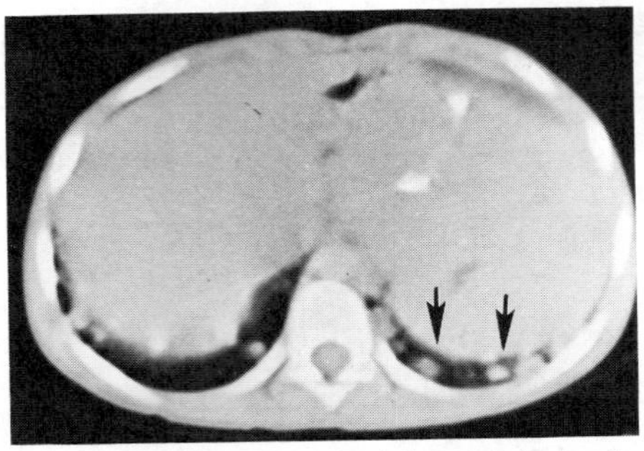

Figure 17–5. Wilms tumor. CT scan of the chest showing metastatic lesions below the dome of diaphragm, which would be difficult to visualize on plain radiograph.

Pulmonary metastases will be evident on roentgenograms in 10–15% of patients at the time of diagnosis, which is more common than in neuroblastoma. CT scan of the chest is useful, particularly to visualize the portions of the lung below the level of the dome of the diaphragm (Fig. 17–5). In a patient in whom hepatic metastases are suspected, radionuclide scan of the liver may be performed. Evaluation of bone and bone marrow should be done only after surgery and only if the patient has a tumor with unfavorable histology or has persistent pain.

Certain rare paraneoplastic syndromes may be associated with Wilms tumor. The neoplasm may produce erythropoietin, leading to polycythemia; and secondary hypercalcemia has been reported.

TREATMENT. The usual immediate treatment is surgical removal of the kidney containing the tumor even if pulmonary metastases are present. At the time of operation careful inspection should be made of the other kidney to exclude the possibility of bilateral tumor and of the liver for possible metastasis. The retroperitoneal lymph nodes and renal vein should be examined for involvement. Every attempt should be made to remove the tumor without spillage, but because postoperative chemotherapy and radiation are capable of destroying residual tumor, life-threatening attempts to remove every bit of tumor should not be undertaken.

Wilms tumor is sensitive both to chemotherapy and to radiotherapy. The logical and systematic treatment of this tumor has been greatly advanced by the formation in 1969 of the NWTS group of participating institutions. Prior to that time, virtually all patients received postoperative radiation and various single-agent chemotherapies. The NWTS group has shown that combination chemotherapy with vincristine and actinomycin is clearly superior to single-agent therapy in patients with localized disease, and that doxorubicin is a significant addition to the treatment of patients with advanced disease. In addition, the NWTS group has shown that postoperative radiotherapy is not necessary for patients with stage I disease, for whom a short postoperative course (6 mo or less) of combination chemotherapy appears to suffice. They are currently investigating the best dose and field for postoperative radiation in patients with stage II and III disease who also receive chemotherapy. For patients with stage IV disease, radiotherapy and combination chemotherapy with three or four drugs for 15 mo is recommended.

Preoperative therapy is not recommended for patients with unilateral disease, but it may be the treatment of choice for patients with bilateral disease so that shrinkage of primary tumors can allow partial nephrectomy with salvage of the greatest amount of residual normal kidney. For patients with bilateral disease, bilateral nephrectomy with secondary renal transplantation has usually not been effective.

PROGNOSIS. In general, prognosis is better in children diagnosed before the age of 2 yr and whose Wilms tumor weighs less than 250 g. The most significant prognostic variables, however, are histology and stage (see Table 17–10). Any recurrence of disease carries a poor prognosis.

Pulmonary involvement has not been studied systematically. Pulmonary lesions amenable to surgery at the time of recurrence should probably be resected.

17.14 OTHER RENAL NEOPLASMS

NEPHROBLASTOMATOSIS. One or more independent foci of malformation or benign neoplasia or both may accompany Wilms tumors in at least one third of patients. This condition is generally called the nephroblastomatosis complex; its pathologic features include the presence grossly of multicentric tumor-like lesions and microscopically of metanephric elements matured beyond the 36th wk of gestation. All patients with bilateral Wilms tumor have manifestations of nephroblastomatosis, and the finding of these blastomatous components in one kidney is an indication for careful inspection of the contralateral kidney. The incidence of development of an asynchronous second Wilms tumor in patients with unilateral and nephroblastomatous tumor was once thought to be as high as 60%, but it is declining, perhaps owing to a chemopreventive effect, since all patients now receive combination chemotherapy at the time of the diagnosis of the initial tumor. Patients with nephroblastomatosis should be followed carefully with CT scans.

MESOBLASTIC NEPHROMA. Congenital mesoblastic nephroma is a massive, firm, infiltrative, solitary renal mass, grossly and microscopically resembling a leiomyoma or a low-grade leiomyosarcoma with trapped nephrons. The infiltrative margins are difficult to delineate histologically from normal or dysplastic renal stroma. By electron microscopy, the cells are fibroblasts or myofibroblasts. This tumor accounts for the majority of congenital renal tumors. Male preponderance has been noted, as well as renin production. The tumor is generally thought to be benign, for which surgical removal represents adequate therapy. A patient may occasionally have a very cellular tumor that more closely resembles a clear cell sarcoma, and such patients may show local recurrence and even metastatic disease; they should receive chemotherapy and irradiation.

RENAL CELL CARCINOMA. This tumor is rare in the first decade of life, but occurs occasionally in teenagers. The initial findings are an abdominal mass and hematuria. The microscopic appearance and clinical course are similar to those found in adults with this neoplasm. Complete surgical resection may result in cure, but the prognosis is grim for patients with postoperative residual disease.

SOFT TISSUE SARCOMAS

Soft tissue sarcomas have an annual incidence of 8.4/million white children under the age of 15 yr and about half that incidence in black children. Rhabdomyosarcoma accounts for more than half of these tumors (Table 17–11).

17.15 RHABDOMYOSARCOMA

There appears to be a bimodal curve for incidence of rhabdomyosarcoma. An early peak occurs before 5 yr of age, with tumors of the neck, head, prostate, bladder, and vagina (in females) common; a later peak occurs around 15–19 yr of age, with involvement of the genitourinary tract (particularly of testes or paratesticular tissue in males). There is a slight predominance of male patients.

There appears to be a familial aggregation of rhabdomyosarcoma with other sarcomas. Rhabdomyosarcoma may complicate neurofibromatosis. In addition, patients with rhabdomyosarcoma are often found in "cancer families" with Li-Fraumeni syndrome (Sec. 17.1), in which there is a high incidence of brain tumors and breast cancer at an early age, particularly in parents.

PATHOLOGY. Rhabdomyosarcoma is thought to arise from the same embryonic mesenchyme as striated skeletal muscle. It can occur anywhere in the body. In general, rhabdomyosarcoma and the other soft tissue sarcomas belong to the group of tumors often called "small round cell tumors" on light microscopy; they include Ewing sarcoma, neuroblastoma, and lymphoma. Definitive diagnosis of a pathologic specimen may require additional studies such as antibodies to actin or electron microscopy to distinguish characteristic features. There are four recognized histologic subtypes of rhabdomyosarcoma. The *embryonal* type accounts for about 60% of the tumors. The *botryoid* type (also called **sarcoma botryoides**) is a variant of the embryonal form in which the tumor cells and an edematous stroma project into a body cavity like a bunch of grapes; it accounts for 6% of the total and is commonly seen in the vagina, uterus, bladder, nasopharynx, and middle ear. The *alveolar* type accounts for about 20% of cases. The tumor cells tend to grow in cores that often have cleft-like spaces resembling alveoli. It is found most often in trunk and extremities, primarily in older children, and carries the poorest prognosis. The *pleomorphic* type (adult form) is rare in childhood (1% of cases). About 20% of patients are considered to have *undifferentiated* tumor. New classification schemes that might have prognostic significance are under consideration by the Intergroup Rhabdomyosarcoma Study (IRS).

The most commonly used staging system is that of the IRS. Group I is localized disease, completely removable, with regional nodes not involved. Group II represents grossly resected tumor with regional nodes involved or microscopic residual disease. Group III indicates gross residual disease, and group IV distant metastatic disease at the time of diagnosis. The first IRS study found only 13% of patients in group I.

CLINICAL FEATURES. The most common presenting feature is a mass, which may be painful. Origin in the nasopharynx may be associated with nasal congestion, mouth breathing, epistaxis, and difficulty with swallowing and chewing. Regional extension into the cranium may produce cranial nerve paralysis, blindness, and signs of increasing intracranial pressure, with headache and vomiting. When the tumor develops in the face or cheek there may be swelling, pain, trismus, and, as extension occurs, paralysis of cranial nerves. In the neck region the original finding may be progressive swelling, with neurologic symptoms following regional extension. In the orbit there may be proptosis, periorbital edema, ptosis, change in visual acuity, and local pain. When the tumor arises in the middle ear, the early signs are usually pain, loss of hearing, chronic otorrhea, or a tumor mass in the ear canal; extensions of the tumor produce cranial nerve paralysis and signs of an intracranial mass on the involved side. With tumor of the larynx there may be an unremitting croupy cough and progressive stridor. Because most of these signs and symptoms are also associated with common problems of the head and neck area, the clinician must be alert to the possibility of tumor.

Rhabdomyosarcoma of the trunk or extremities appears as a tumor, not uncommonly first noticed after trauma and for a time regarded as a hematoma. When the tumor shows little change in size or even grows at a time when a hematoma should be resolving, the true diagnosis should be suspected. Involvement of the genitourinary tract may produce hema-

TABLE 17–11. Soft Tissue Sarcomas*

Tissue of Origin	Tumor	Natural History
Primitive Mesenchyme	Malignant mesenchymoma	May occur as a congenital tumor. Usually involves extremities or retroperitoneum. Characterized by rapid growth and frequent recurrence. Lung, brain, liver, and lymph nodes are the most frequent sites of metastases.
Connective Tissues		
Adipose	Liposarcoma	Rare in children. Generally develops in a previous lipoma, with rapid growth, occasionally with systemic symptoms (e.g., fever). Metastases relatively common in adults, less so in children. Outcome correlated with the degree of cellular differentiation.
Fibrous	Fibrosarcoma	May occur as a congenital tumor. Patients under 5 yr old (i.e., with infantile form) have a better survival rate (metastases in 7.5%) than patients over 15 yr old (metastases in 50%; local recurrence rate 40%). Extremities the most common site. Primary lesion related occasionally to prior irradiation.
	Dermatofibrosarcoma protuberans	Slow-growing tumor, especially likely on the trunk, scalp, or face. Usually progresses from skin nodule to pedunculated tumor over years, but (rarely) can grow rapidly. High frequency of local recurrence. Tumor spread is usually to subcutaneous tissue, muscle, and bone; metastasis predominantly to the lung and brain.
	Fibromatoses (fibrous hamartoma, fibrosis colli, infant and juvenile aponeurotic fibroma, congenital generalized fibromatosis, infantile digital fibroma)	Locally invasive; only rarely metastatic. An exception: congenital generalized fibromatosis (CGF), which usually has visceral involvement and a poor prognosis. Prognosis generally good for these tumors, but the local recurrence rate is high (90%).
	Malignant fibrous histiocytosis	Rare before the 4th decade; the most common soft tissue sarcoma of late adult life. Typically on the extremities (especially the thigh) and in the retroperitoneum, arising from deep fascia or muscle. Local recurrence rate is 44%. Prognosis is related to the size and the initial depth of the tumor (i.e., whether fascia or deeper structures are involved).
	Epithelioid sarcoma	Slow-growing, locally infiltrating tumor; usually presents as painful nodules on extremity (especially on forearm or hand or in popliteal area). The nodules frequently have ulcerated overlying skin. High rate of local recurrence. The most frequent metastases are to the lung, lymph nodes, and skin.
Vascular Tissue		
Lymphatic	Lymphangiosarcoma	Very rare tumor, presenting predominantly in the extremities, sometimes decades following congenital or acquired lymphedema. Rapidly progressive, with metastases to the chest wall or pleura.
Blood	Angiosarcoma	Rapidly progressive, highly fatal tumor, predominantly involving extremities, liver, and head and neck regions. Has been associated with exposure to Thorotrast and vinyl chloride. May occur in children 1 yr old. Metastasizes to the liver, bone, and adrenal gland.
	Hemangiopericytoma	May occur as a tumor. Most frequent primary sites are extremities and trunk. High rate of local recurrence (50%); metastases may occur late (10 yr), usually to lung, brain, and liver.
	Juvenile angiofibroma	The primary site is the nasopharynx. Does not metastasize but is locally invasive.
Supportive Tissue		
Synovium	Synovial cell sarcoma	Rare; occurs mainly between ages of 20 and 40 yr. Predominantly involves the extremities (80–90%), especially the knee, foot, and hand. Metastases common to lung, bone, and lymph nodes. Characterized by local recurrence and late relapse (even 10–15 yr after diagnosis).
Fascia	Alveolar soft part sarcoma	Generally slow-growing; most common primary site the thigh or abdominal wall. High rate of local recurrence and metastasis, generally late and especially to the lung, bone, and brain. Occurs in children as young as 3 yr old.
Mesothelioma	Malignant mesothelioma	Rare in children. Associated with exposure to asbestos in adults. The most common primary sites are the pleura and peritoneum. Rapidly progressive, with extensive local spread and metastases.
Muscle Tissue		
Aponeurotic	Desmoid	Rare in children: median age of onset 23 yr, most commonly in abdominal wall or shoulder girdle. Generally presents as a fixed, sometimes painful mass. Tumors may be exacerbated by estrogens or during the postpartum period.
Smooth	Leiomyosarcoma	Rare in children; has been observed in neonates. The gastrointestinal, genitourinary, and respiratory tracts represent the most common sites. Major sites of metastases: liver, regional nodes, lungs, peritoneum, and pancreas.
Striated	Rhabdomyosarcoma	See Sec. 17.15.

*Modified from Levine AS (ed): Cancer in the Young. New York, Masson Publishing, 1982, p 1330.

turia, obstruction of the lower urinary tract, recurrent urinary tract infections, incontinence, or a mass detectable on abdominal or rectal examination. Involvement of the paratesticular tissues usually presents a rapidly growing mass in the scrotum. Vaginal rhabdomyosarcoma may present as a grape-like mass of tumor tissue bulging through the vaginal orifice (sarcoma botryoides) and may cause symptoms relating to the urinary tract or to the large bowel. Vaginal bleeding or obstruction of the urethra or the rectum may occur. Similar findings may occur when the tumor arises in the uterus.

With tumors in any location there may be early dissemination, and the presenting symptoms can be bone pain or the respiratory distress of pulmonary metastases. Extensive bone involvement may produce symptomatic hypercalcemia. In patients with disseminated tumor, it is sometimes difficult to identify the primary lesions.

DIAGNOSIS. The early diagnosis of rhabdomyosarcoma requires an alert physician. Several months often elapse between first symptoms and biopsy.

Diagnostic procedures are determined mainly by the area of involvement. In the head and neck area, roentgenograms should be examined for evidence of the tumor mass and for indications of bony erosion. CT scans should be used as well to check for intracranial extension and to look for bony involvement at the base of skull, which is difficult to visualize roentgenographically. For abdominal tumors, ultrasound examinations and CT scanning with oral and intravenous contrast media can help delineate the tumor mass. Cystourethrograms are useful for tumors in the bladder. Before a patient has definitive surgery, a full skeletal metastatic survey should be done as well as radionuclide scans of the skeleton. A chest roentgenogram and CT should be obtained, and bone marrow should be examined. These studies should be evaluated before any surgical procedure so that the extent of proposed surgery can be defined. The most essential element of the diagnostic workup is the examination of tumor tissue.

TREATMENT. Rhabdomyosarcoma is rarely completely resectable. Tumor margins should be carefully defined, and an appropriate search for metastatic disease (e.g., to nodes or liver or both) should be made at the time of initial surgery, even if this is only a biopsy. The treatment program for each patient must be designed according to the location and stage of the tumor. Some patients are given chemotherapy prior to surgery in the hope that vital organs, particularly in the genitourinary tract, might be preserved and in order to reduce the amount of surgery required. In group I tumor, complete local excision is followed by chemotherapy to reduce the likelihood of subsequent metastatic disease. For groups II and III, surgery should be followed by a regimen involving local irradiation and systemic chemotherapy. The treatment of group IV rhabdomyosarcoma relies principally on systemic chemotherapy. Intrathecal therapy is generally given to patients with primary disease in parameningeal sites (nasopharynx, nasal cavity, paranasal sinuses, middle ear, mastoid, or pterygopalatine or infratemporal fossae).

PROGNOSIS. Of patients with resectable tumor, 80–90% have prolonged tumor-free survival. In addition, unresectable tumor localized at certain favorable sites (such as orbit) has a high likelihood of cure. About two thirds of patients with incompletely resected regional tumor will also achieve long-term disease-free survival. Patients with disseminated disease have a poor prognosis; only about half will achieve remission and less than half of these will be cured. Older children have a worse prognosis than younger ones and have a greater frequency of lesions of the extremities and of alveolar histology.

17.16 OTHER SOFT TISSUE SARCOMAS

Subtypes of soft tissue sarcoma can be identified with the normal tissues from which each appears to have arisen (see Table 17–11). Some grow aggressively, others grow relatively slowly. In most patients, the sarcomas appear as masses. Here again, it is critical to determine the extent of disease before surgery, particularly with respect to bony or pulmonary metastases. For a number of these tumors, radical surgical excision offers the only chance of cure. Perhaps for no other group of tumors is it so important to have the tissues reviewed carefully by an experienced pathologist, both for definition of the specific type of tumor and for an assessment of its malignant or benign nature. Postoperative chemotherapy is indicated for high-grade tumors with prominent mitotic activity, regardless of tumor size or resectability.

NEOPLASMS OF BONE

Bone tumors have an annual incidence in white children of 5.6/million and in black children 4.8/million. Osteosarcoma, the most common malignant bone tumor, is twice as common in white children as Ewing tumor. Ewing tumor almost never occurs among black children. Bone tumors tend to occur in adolescents, rather than in younger children. Rare bone tumors include chondrosarcomas and fibrosarcomas.

17.17 OSTEOSARCOMA

Bone growth and the occurrence of osteosarcoma seem to be correlated. Onset is most common during the adolescent growth spurt. The mean age at the time of diagnosis is 15 yr. During the first 13 yr of life, boys and girls have the same incidence of osteosarcoma, but older boys have an increasing rate whereas girls reach a plateau. One study found children with osteosarcoma to be taller at the time of diagnosis than control children with other cancers; it also found that osteosarcoma occurs more commonly in giant breeds of dogs (e.g., Great Danes). Osteosarcoma occurs most commonly in long bones at the metaphyseal ends, the points of most active growth and reconstruction. The most common primary site is the distal femur; the proximal humerus and proximal tibia are also common sites. Osteosarcoma can arise in any bone.

Children with bilateral retinoblastoma have an increased incidence of osteosarcoma. In past years osteosarcoma developed most often in the field of irradiation, but it is being increasingly reported in bones that were not included in the radiation portal and as multifocal disease. The gene associated with retinoblastoma predisposes to osteosarcoma as well (Sec. 17.1).

Certain diseases of bone, some genetically determined, may also predispose to osteosarcoma. These include multiple osteochondromatosis (Ollier disease), which may also be found with hemangiomas (Maffucci syndrome); multiple hereditary exostoses; osteogenesis imperfecta; and Paget disease. Osteosarcoma is occasionally familial. It occurs also as a secondary tumor in the treated bone of long-term survivors of Ewing tumor; latency period ranges from 4 to over 20 yr (Table 17–12).

PATHOLOGY. Osteosarcoma has been defined as a primary malignant bone tumor, the neoplastic cells of which produce osteoid. The classic osteosarcoma arises within the medullary canal of the shaft and may break through the cortex of the bone of origin to form a soft tissue mass which can achieve considerable size. The tumor may also extend along the medullary cavity. The tumor may have osteosarcomatous, chondrosarcomatous, and fibrosarcomatous differentiation within a single lesion. Osteosarcoma has some important subclassifications. *Parosteal* osteogenic sarcoma is a well-differentiated, extramedullary tumor of low metastatic potential. Surgical resection alone is often adequate therapy. In contrast,

TABLE 17–12. Comparison of Osteogenic and Ewing Sarcoma

	Osteogenic Sarcoma	Ewing Sarcoma
Age	> 10 yr	< 10 and >10 yr
Race	Both	White
Sex (M:F)	1.5:1	1.5:1
Cell	Spindle cell, osteoid	Nonosseous, small round cell
Predisposition	Retinoblastoma Radiotherapy Alkylating agents	None
Site	Metaphysis, epiphysis; distal femur > proximal tibia > proximal humerus	Diaphysis, medullary cavity, cortical bone, soft tissue; femur > pelvis > tibia > humerus
Presentation	Local pain	Pain, fever, increased ESR, FUO, weight loss
Roentgenogram	Lytic, sclerotic Sunburst pattern	Mottled, lytic Onion skin pattern
Differential diagnosis	Ewing sarcoma, osteomyelitis	Osteomyelitis, eosinophilic granuloma, lymphoma, neuroblastoma, rhabdomyosarcoma
Metastasis	Lung, bones Skip lesions in the same bone	Lung, bones
Treatment	Surgery, chemotherapy Limb salvage if resectable and the patient is near adult height	Surgery, radiotherapy Chemotherapy
Outcome	50–60% survival	60% survival without metastasis, 5–15% with metastasis, primary site dependent
Poor prognosis	Age < 10 yr, large tumor size (>15 cm), symptoms < 2 mo, metastasis	Pelvis, soft tissue tumor, increased LDH, metastasis, increased circulating PMN, decreased circulating lymphocytes

a similarly located lesion, *periosteal* osteogenic sarcoma, is histologically a much more pleomorphic lesion that behaves more aggressively clinically. *Telangiectatic* osteosarcoma is a bloody, cystic lesion that produces no new bone radiographically and may be confused with aneurysmal bone cyst. Prognosis may be poor.

Osteosarcoma may appear simultaneously in many sites, with a predominantly osteoblastic pattern (multifocal sclerosing osteosarcoma).

CLINICAL MANIFESTATIONS. The most common initial finding is pain at the site of the tumor. The patient and family usually ascribe this pain to trauma. Later, limitation of motion and a palpable or visible tumor may develop. With involvement of bones of the legs or pelvis, there may be limping or alterations of gait. Later manifestations are tenderness and local erythema and hyperthermia. The most common site of metastasis is the lungs; early pulmonary involvement is usually asymptomatic, but more extensive disease may produce respiratory embarrassment. Pleural effusion and pneumothorax can occur. Other sites of metastasis include other bones, hilar lymph nodes, and the CNS.

DIAGNOSIS. Persistent unexplained bone pain, particularly when associated with a palpable mass, requires roentgenographic examination of that bone. A typical lesion is shown in Fig. 17–6. Sclerosis of bone and periosteal new bone formation are common. Prior to initial surgery, minimal staging should include a radionuclide scan to look for metastatic bony lesions and a roentgenographic study (Fig. 17–7) and CT scan of the chest. CT scan of the chest will detect more lesions than will be seen on roentgenogram and is particularly important in the patient for whom the latter is negative. On the other hand, about half the additional nodules defined by CT scanning in a series of adult patients proved at thoracotomy to be benign granulomas or pleura-based lymph nodes.

CT scan with contrast enhancement of the affected extremity can help to define the extent of medullary involvement and will assist in surgical planning. If a limb salvage procedure is contemplated, arteriography will be performed to see whether it is possible to preserve function distal to the resected tumor. Serum alkaline phosphatase activity may be increased, and this may serve as a marker to follow the effect of therapy. Confirmation of the diagnosis must be made by histologic examination through open biopsy of the lesion.

TREATMENT. For the patient with no evident metastatic disease, the recommended treatment is radical surgery. This may consist of amputation of the affected extremity or wide local excision of a flat bone when feasible. Internal prostheses are now available for most sites, and amputation should be avoided when possible. Presurgical chemotherapy to improve resectability is being evaluated in experimental protocols. In the prechemotherapy era, amputation alone yielded a 5-yr survival rate of about 17%. The usual cause of death was pulmonary metastases, which developed within 2 yr in patients who had no obvious pulmonary metastases at the time of diagnosis. The thought that pulmonary micrometastases present at the time of diagnosis might account for this phenomenon has led to uncontrolled small studies with single agent chemotherapy. A randomized concurrent controlled trial by the Pediatric Oncology Group has compared a multiple chemotherapy regimen (high-dose methotrexate, cisplatin, doxorubicin, bleomycin, cytoxan, and dactinomycin) with surgery alone. The results indicate that complex, intensive chemotherapy is the postoperative treatment of choice for osteosarcoma with 80% disease-free survival compared to 20% for surgery alone. Osteosarcoma is not radiosensitive.

For patients with resectable pulmonary metastatic disease, surgery is recommended, since in this situation there is about a 20% disease-free survival rate with surgery alone. It is usual, however, that a patient in whom only a few lesions are seen on conventional roentgenograms will have more visible on CT scanning and even more seen at the time of surgery.

Careful rehabilitation must follow surgery. Patients are likely to experience postoperative phantom limb pain. Long-term psychologic support should be available.

PROGNOSIS. Prognosis is best with low-grade tumors, such as parosteal osteosarcoma. With surgery alone about 20% of patients with the classic form of osteosarcoma will have long-term survival. The survival rate after intensive chemotherapy is not yet known but will be at least 50%. Some cases of long-term survival have followed resection of metastatic pulmonary disease, but none have occurred in patients with diffuse pulmonary metastases or metastatic disease to bone.

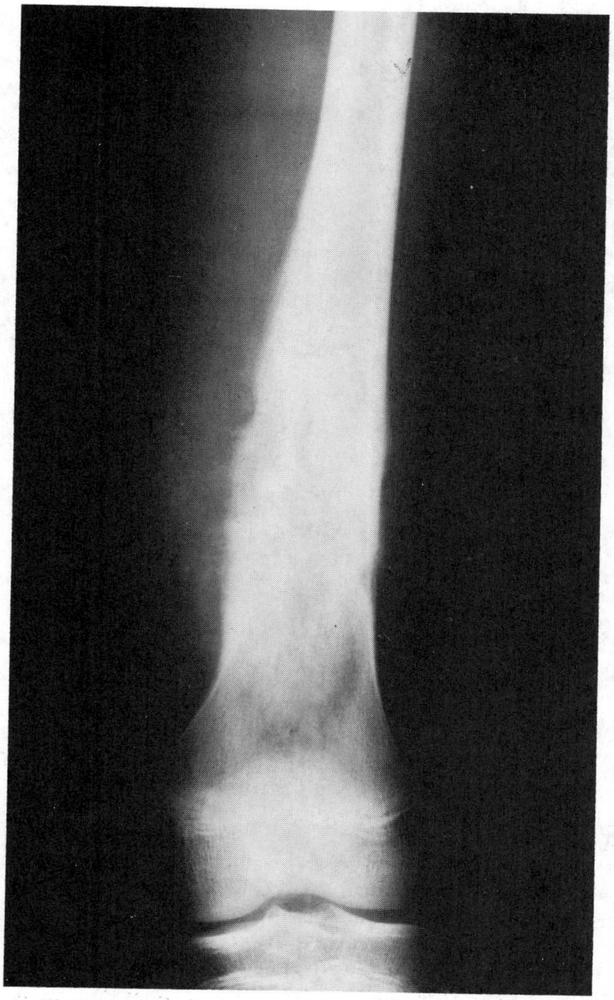

Figure 17–6. Osteosarcoma of the distal portion of the femur. The tumor has broken through the cortex; calcification of the tumor is seen in the surrounding soft tissues.

17.18 CHONDROSARCOMA

This tumor of bone is rare in children and is usually seen during the second decade. It occurs with equal frequency in boys and girls and is associated with Ollier disease and Maffucci syndrome (Sec. 24.48). Exposure to ionizing radiation is an etiologic factor in some patients.

The histologic picture is that of malignant formation of cartilage. The tumor may arise in any bone but is most common in the pelvis. It occurs in flat bones of the trunk as well as in long bones of the extremities. It can metastasize to lung and bone, but the usual form of spread is local extension to contiguous normal tissues, with recurrence following surgical removal.

Clinical features are local pain and tumor mass. Diagnosis can be suspected from the roentgenogram of the area; it must be confirmed by biopsy. Histologic examination requires care, because osteosarcoma can have a large chondrosarcomatous component. The prognosis for these two tumors is quite different as to likelihood of metastatic disease. Treatment is surgical removal of the tumor or amputation if an extremity is involved. Chondrosarcoma is relatively radioresistant. Owing to its rarity, the effect of chemotherapy has not been adequately evaluated.

17.19 EWING SARCOMA

Ewing sarcoma is a round-cell tumor of bone of later childhood and adolescence. It is more common in males than in females and is almost never seen in blacks either in the United States or in Africa. Familial cases have been described. There is no evidence that radiation exposure is important in the etiology.

PATHOLOGY. Histologically, Ewing tumor consists of uniform small round cells with scanty cytoplasm and little or no surrounding stroma. The presence of glycogen, as indicated by the periodic acid-Schiff reaction, helps to differentiate this tumor from neuroblastoma. The cell of origin for this tumor is uncertain.

The tumor may arise either in long bones of the extremities or in flat bones of the head and trunk. As with osteosarcoma, the most commonly involved long bone is the femur. The most commonly involved flat bone is the pelvis. Extraskeletal neoplasms histologically resembling Ewing sarcoma have been described, most frequently arising in the soft tissues of the lower extremity and paravertebral regions. Their relationship to Ewing sarcoma of bone is uncertain. Metastatic disease most frequently involves lungs and bone, occasionally bone marrow and CNS; and is present in up to one third of patients at the time of diagnosis.

CLINICAL MANIFESTATIONS. The primary symptom is pain, which may be accompanied by fever and tenderness. The degree of soft tissue involvement varies but may be massive. The two conditions most often mistaken clinically for Ewing sarcoma are eosinophilic granuloma and osteomyelitis. Occasionally, there may even be periods of improvement in symptoms of a Ewing sarcoma with antibiotic therapy. A clinician confronted with the diagnosis of osteomyelitis should always consider Ewing sarcoma when bacterial cultures are negative. Typical roentgenographic features are seen in Figure 17–8.

DIAGNOSIS. Ewing sarcoma may be suspected from clinical history and roentgenographic features; confirmation requires surgical biopsy. Differentiation from infection may be difficult unless pulmonary metastatic disease is present. This tumor may be difficult to distinguish on biopsy from the other

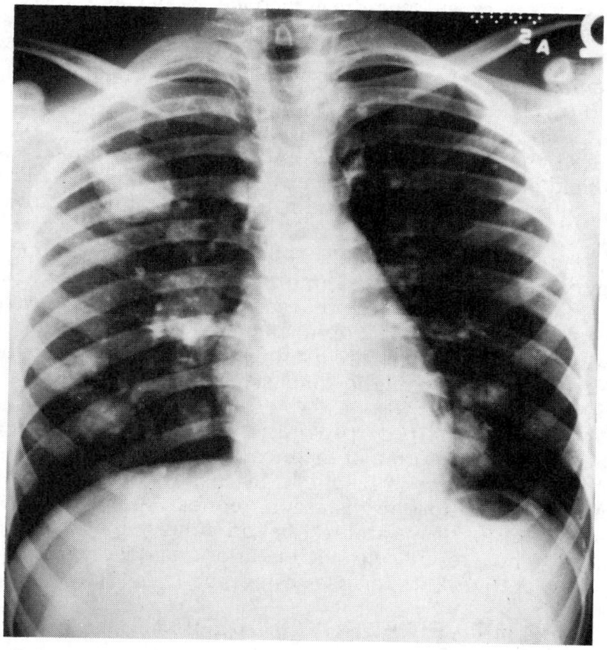

Figure 17–7. Multiple metastatic nodules of osteosarcoma.

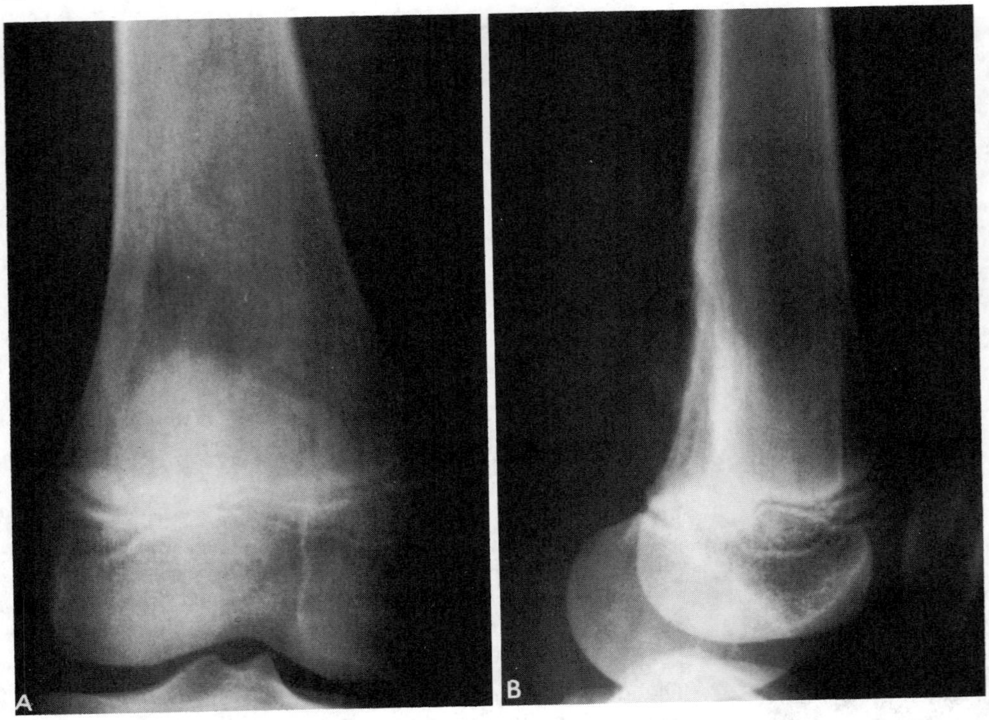

Figure 17–8. Anterior and lateral views of the distal femur of a patient with Ewing sarcoma. The lateral view shows the destruction of cortex, with growth of tumor into the surrounding soft tissues. With time, progressive calcification of periosteum lifted away from the bone may lead to a typical "sunburst" appearance.

small round-cell tumors of childhood. Evaluation by an experienced pathologist is critical.

Once the diagnosis is made, patients should be screened for metastases to the lung by roentgenography and CT scan, to the bones by radionuclide bone scan, and to the bone marrow by biopsy (so that an adequate tissue specimen is obtained). The extent of the primary lesion can be most precisely defined by CT scan, which will be helpful in following the response to therapy.

TREATMENT. In general, amputation is not recommended in patients with Ewing sarcoma, because the tumor is sensitive both to radiation and to chemotherapy. The possible contribution of excisional surgery to cure is being explored. Pathologic fracture may occur through bone, either as a result of tumor destruction or at a biopsy site. This may heal poorly during radiotherapy and chemotherapy and may cause pain. Patients should be warned against vigorous weight bearing on an involved bone during therapy.

High-dose irradiation of the primary tumor site and combination chemotherapy are recommended. The optimal dose and field of radiation are currently under investigation. Problems with high-dose radiation include failure of bone growth, fibrosis, and development of secondary osteosarcomas.

Ewing sarcoma that is clinically localized at the time of diagnosis develops into systemic disease with high frequency. All patients should, therefore, receive chemotherapy. Active agents are vincristine, cyclophosphamide, dactinomycin, and doxorubicin. It is probable that a four-drug regimen combining these agents will give the longest disease-free period after initiation of therapy.

PROGNOSIS. A poor prognosis is associated with metastatic disease at the time of diagnosis and a proximal primary site; primary tumors in pelvis, humerus, or rib carry a worse prognosis than those in distal long bones. Recent trials with combinations of drugs and irradiation indicate that 40–60% of patients who present without metastatic disease will be free of tumor at 3 yr. Late relapses can occur.

17.20 PRIMITIVE NEUROECTODERMAL TUMORS (PNET)

The term primitive neuroectodermal tumors (PNET) is widely used for a group of small round cell tumors that occur in peripheral sites, including soft tissue and bone, as well as in the CNS. There is disagreement among pathologists with regard to whether the PNET represents a midpoint on a spectrum of neural development from Ewing sarcoma to neuroblastoma.

PATHOLOGY. Although the criteria for a definitive diagnosis of PNET is not established, PNET is generally distinguished from soft tissue Ewing sarcoma by suggestive microscopic evidence of neural differentiation, including histochemical stains for neuron specific enolase or dense-core granules by electron microscopy.

TREATMENT AND PROGNOSIS. These tumors have been called *Askin tumor* when they arise in the chest wall and have been thought to have a less good prognosis than soft tissue Ewing sarcoma, although they have similar clinical presentation and are treated by similar protocols.

17.21 RETINOBLASTOMA

This tumor has an annual incidence of 3.4/million children, similar for black and white children. The average ages at time of diagnosis are 8 mo for bilateral tumors and 26 mo for unilateral tumors. About 30% of patients with retinoblastoma have bilateral involvement; they have a dominantly inherited predisposition to retinoblastoma. About 10–20% of patients with unilateral disease also have the genetic predisposition. The retinoblastoma locus was discovered to be on chromosome 13 when a group of patients with growth delay, mental retardation and a characteristic facies, and a deletion on the long arm of that chromosome (13q− syndrome) were found to have retinoblastoma as well. Genetic mapping techniques (Sec. 17.1) have shown that the cells of most retinoblastoma tumors have submicroscopic deletions of chromosome 13. The retinoblastoma gene also carries increased risk of other tumors; about 1% of the survivors of the hereditary form of retinoblastoma will develop osteosarcoma at around 10 yr of age. Such osteosarcomas may occur either at a site irradiated for treatment for retinoblastoma or at a nonirradiated site and are often multifocal. By 30 yr after cure of the ocular tumor, 30% of individuals with the hereditary form of the disease have developed a secondary malignancy. A "trilateral" retinoblastoma syndrome has been reported in patients who have shown bilateral ocular disease as well as pineal tumors.

PATHOLOGY. Retinoblastoma usually develops in the posterior portion of the retina. It consists of small, closely packed, round, malignant cells with scanty cytoplasm. Occasionally, rosette formation occurs, which is thought to be an abortive attempt at formation of rods and cones. Retinoblastoma may appear as a single tumor in the retina but typically arises in multiple foci. When it arises in the internal nuclear layers of the retina, it grows forward into the vitreous cavity. This endophytic growth is easily seen with the ophthalmoscope, whereas if the tumor is exophytic (arising in the external nuclear layer and growing into the subretinal space, with detachment of the retina), the diagnosis is more difficult, because the tumor is hidden. Tumor fragments may break off from endophytic tumors and float free in the vitreous to seed unaffected parts of the retina. These vitreous seeds are associated with large tumors (usually more than 5 disk diameters) and a poor prognosis. Extension of retinoblastoma into the choroid usually occurs with massive tumors and may indicate a propensity for hematogenous metastases. Extension of tumor through the lamina cribrosa and down the optic nerve may lead to involvement of the CNS.

Because these tumors rarely metastasize, the primary concern at the time of diagnosis is generally to preserve useful vision. Accordingly, staging of these tumors is in accord with the extent of disease within the eye (Table 17–13).

CLINICAL MANIFESTATIONS. This tumor usually presents with leukokoria, an asymptomatic patient being discovered to have a yellowish white reflex in the pupil due to tumor behind the lens. Other presenting findings can be loss of vision, sometimes reflected as a squint in the affected eye, or with more advanced tumor, complaints of pain, pupillary irregularity, or hyphema. With far advanced tumor, there may be proptosis, signs of increasing intracranial pressure, or bone pain associated with metastatic disease.

More than 80% of patients with the hereditary bilateral form have tumors involving both eyes at the time of diagnosis. Delay in involvement of the second eye rarely exceeds 18 mo. In many patients with the familial form of the disease, the retinoblastoma will be discovered on a routine funduscopic examination made under anesthesia, performed because a parent or sibling has had the disease.

DIAGNOSIS. The finding of leukokoria must be followed by a careful funduscopic examination, which will usually necessitate anesthesia in children. In about 75% of patients roentgenography will show calcification within the globe. CT scan of the orbits should be performed to evaluate the intraorbital extent of tumor and also to see whether optic nerve or bony structures are involved. Other causes of leukokoria include retinal detachment, persistent hyperplastic primary vitreous, nematode endophthalmitis (usually visceral larva migrans), bacterial panendophthalmitis, cataract, coloboma of the choroid, and the retinopathy of prematurity. These conditions can be differentiated by an experienced ophthalmologist.

Additional studies to search for metastatic disease should include a skeletal survey, radionuclide bone scan, CT scan of the head with contrast, and examination of the spinal fluid and bone marrow for tumor cells. Elevated plasma levels of carcinoembryonic antigen and α-fetoprotein are frequently found at the time of diagnosis; they fall to normal levels after removal of the tumor. Their subsequent rise may indicate recurrence of tumor.

TABLE 17–13. Staging for Retinoblastoma*

Group I
Solitary or multiple tumors, <4 disk diameters in size, at or behind the equator

Group II
Solitary or multiple tumors, 4–10 disk diameters in size, at or behind the equator

Group III
Any lesion anterior to the equator
Solitary tumors >10 disk diameters, behind the equator

Group IV
Multiple tumors; some >10 disk diameters, any lesion extending anterior to the ora serrata

Group V
Massive tumors involving over half the retina
Vitreous seeding

*After Ellsworth RM: The practical management of retinoblastoma. Trans Am Ophthalmol Soc 67:462, 1969.

TREATMENT. The standard treatment for unilateral disease is enucleation of the eye. If the tumors are so small that useful vision might be preserved after irradiation (e.g., group I, II, or III), then irradiation may be preferred. It is rare to see unilateral disease with tumors so small that useful vision can be preserved in the involved eye.

For patients with bilateral disease attempts should be made to salvage useful vision in at least one eye with radiotherapy. This can be administered bilaterally from the outset, because an eye that appears more involved may also have a more dramatic response. On the other hand, if an eye is so heavily involved that no useful vision remains, or if painful glaucoma has developed as a complication, then that eye should be enucleated. When enucleation is done, an attempt should be made to resect as much of the optic nerve as possible (10 mm or more). In addition, radiation therapy to the orbit should be considered if regional extraocular extension of the tumor has been found at the time of enucleation. Radiation therapy will require daily sedation of the patient and perhaps daily anesthesia.

There is no definite role for chemotherapy in patients whose tumor is localized to the globe. If there is gross or microscopic residual disease in the orbit after enucleation, then chemotherapy (probably with cytoxan and doxorubicin) should be considered along with radiotherapy. Widespread metastatic disease will respond to chemotherapy, but cure is most unlikely.

PROGNOSIS. In groups I–IV the survival rate is 100%. In group V survival is at least 85%. Less than 10% of patients have extraglobal extension of disease at the time of presentation. No cures have been reported in patients who have had massive orbital disease or extensive optic nerve involvement when first seen, because intracranial spread and distant metastases have already occurred. If microscopic examination finds tumor in the periglobal tissues of the optic nerve, there is about a 30% chance of long-term survival with irradiation and chemotherapy. This survival is from the primary tumor. Recent studies have indicated that overall survival of these patients in the third and fourth decade of life may be considerably lower because of their high incidence of second malignancies.

17.22 GASTROINTESTINAL NEOPLASMS

See also Sec. 13.68.

The incidence of tumors arising in the gastrointestinal tract is much lower in children than in adults. A malignant lesion in the oral cavity in the very young is likely to be sarcomatous.

SALIVARY GLAND TUMORS. Most enlargements of the salivary glands result from such benign causes as inflammation or the formation of mucocoeles. About two thirds of tumors involving the salivary glands are benign, such as hemangiomas, hamartomas, or the mixed tumor of salivary glands (pleomorphic adenoma).

Mixed tumors are rare during the first decade; they are seen occasionally during the second decade and are evenly distributed between boys and girls. The gland most often involved is the parotid, and the most frequent presenting manifestation is a mass in the area. The mass is usually hard, movable, and nontender. Facial nerve paralysis may occur. Treatment is excision of the tumor. The prognosis for control of the disease is excellent; recurrences may necessitate a second surgical procedure.

Mucoepidermoid carcinoma is the malignant tumor of salivary glands. It is found primarily during the second decade of life and most frequently involves the parotid gland, usually as a hard, nontender mass. Metastases to regional lymph nodes are unusual, but once they have occurred the prognosis is poor. Treatment is excision; if this is complete, the prognosis is excellent. Local recurrence may necessitate a second surgical procedure.

NASOPHARYNGEAL CARCINOMA (LYMPHOEPITHELIOMA). In adults this tumor is most common in the Far East and North Africa, where it occurs in familial clusters. There is high frequency of association with EB virus. In the United States it occurs in or after the second decade of life. Black children in the southern United States have 4 to 7 times the incidence of whites. Male predominance is observed in adults but not in children. The histologic appearance is that of undifferentiated carcinoma.

The most frequent early finding is cervical adenopathy, which is usually unilateral and frequently tender. Other early symptoms and signs are trismus, epistaxis, sore throat, and difficulty in swallowing. There may be weight loss due to dysphagia.

Diagnosis is made usually through biopsy of a cervical node. On careful examination, including CT scan, it is possible to find the primary tumor in the nasopharynx in the majority of affected children. If the tumor has not metastasized, multiple biopsies of the nasopharynx may be required to obtain appropriate tissue. Extension occurs locally to the base of the skull and to the soft tissues surrounding the nasopharynx. Regional lymph node metastases are common, and there may be hematogenous spread to bone (detectable on radionuclide scan) and to lung.

The primary therapy is irradiation of the involved areas of the nasopharynx. This will result in cure in up to 50% of patients. Experience with chemotherapy is limited; the tumor responds to cyclophosphamide, and doxorubicin, and continuous infusion of cisplatin/5-fluorouracil (5-FU) is being tried.

CARCINOMA OF THE STOMACH. This form of gastrointestinal cancer is rarely reported in children. The usual symptoms are caused by a mass; bleeding and gastric obstruction also occur.

Malignant lesions affecting the stomach are most often lymphomas or soft tissue sarcomas. If the lesion is a true carcinoma, resection is the treatment of choice.

PANCREATIC CARCINOMA. This tumor is rare in children. The usual site of origin is the head of the pancreas, and the initial clinical findings are those of upper abdominal mass, weight loss, and pain. Obstruction to the common bile duct may lead to obstructive jaundice. Treatment is resection when possible, and prognosis is poor.

Pancreatoblastoma is an exocrine tumor that behaves as a benign lesion located in the head of the pancreas. Because it is encapsulated and does not communicate with the pancreatic ducts, it can be removed without interfering with pancreatic function. The symptoms in these patients generally are those of an abdominal mass. The prognosis is favorable after resection of these tumors; it is important, therefore, that they be differentiated from pancreatic carcinoma.

β cell endocrine tumors are generally seen in the form of *nesidioblastosis* or diffuse islet cell malformation or dysplasia (Sec. 8.59 and 9.57). Diagnosis is based on the finding of hypoglycemia followed by the demonstration that there are high serum levels of insulin even at low glucose levels, confirming the autonomous behavior of islet cells. Pancreatectomy is the treatment of choice.

COLONIC POLYPS. The juvenile or retention polyp constitutes about 85% of all polypoid lesions found in the colon and rectum of children. Bright red rectal bleeding is the most common presenting sign or symptom, occurring in almost all cases. Polyps occur most commonly between 3 and 5 yr of age. Most can be removed through a sigmoidoscope. A new polyp will develop in about 25% of cases. This is not a premalignant lesion, but there is an entity of *multiple juvenile polyposis* that may not be benign. Adenomatous polyps may coexist with these lesions, but true adenomatous polyps of the colon in children are rare except as part of familial polyposis or Gardner syndrome.

ADENOCARCINOMA OF THE COLON AND RECTUM. Adenocarcinoma of the colon and rectum represents less than 1% of all the malignant tumors that occur in children but has occurred in a child as young as 9 mo of age. Affected patients may present bloody stools or melena. Abdominal pain (which may be colicky), anorexia, and weight loss are common. An abdominal mass may be found, and there may be liver enlargement owing to metastases. The diagnosis can be confirmed by barium enema or direct endoscopic examination or both. Radionuclide or CT scans of liver and spleen will help detect hepatic metastases. The tumor is rarely confined to the mucosa at the time of diagnosis; it has usually extended through the serosa with involvement of the regional lymph nodes. Other metastases can occur within the abdominal cavity, commonly to the liver. Late hematogenous dissemination may occur. Predisposing conditions are familial multiple polyposis, ulcerative colitis, regional enteritis, and the Peutz-Jeghers syndrome. For most patients with these conditions, regular endoscopic examination and occasionally prophylactic colectomy are recommended.

17.23 NEOPLASMS OF THE LIVER

Two kinds of primary liver cancer occur in children: hepatoblastoma and hepatocellular carcinoma (hepatoma).

EPIDEMIOLOGY. Hepatoblastoma is more common than hepatoma; it is seen almost exclusively in children under the age of 3 yr. Boys predominate in a ratio of 1.5:1. Hepatocellular carcinoma shows two age peaks, one before the age of 4 yr and the other between the ages of 12 and 15 yr. This tumor predominates in boys by a ratio of 1.3:1.

The congenital defects associated with hepatic malignancy are similar to those that occur in patients with Wilms tumor and adrenocortical neoplasms and include congenital hemihypertrophy and extensive hemangiomas. Hepatic tumor and Wilms tumor have occurred in the same patient, which indicates that similar mechanisms may be involved in the predisposition to all three neoplasms. Hepatoblastoma and hepatocellular carcinoma have been reported in siblings.

The occurrence of hepatic carcinoma with cirrhosis is much rarer in children than in adults; on the other hand, the cirrhosis of malnutrition and the biliary cirrhosis secondary to biliary atresia or giant cell hepatitis are associated with an increased incidence of primary malignant tumors of the liver. In addition, hepatic tumors develop in patients with Fanconi anemia who have been treated with androgens. Patients with the chronic form of hereditary tyrosinemia who survive beyond the age of 2 yr have about a 40% risk of developing hepatocellular carcinoma.

PATHOLOGY. Hepatoblastoma may consist entirely of cells with an epithelial appearance, or there may be an admixture of mesenchymal components. Gland-like structures may be seen. The individual cells are poorly differentiated. In the mixed type of tumor mesenchymal components and areas of primitive osteoid tissue may be seen. The hepatocellular carcinoma consists of well-differentiated large polygonal cells with highly eosinophilic cytoplasm. The cells form hepatic cord-like structures surrounded by sinusoidal vessels. Foci of extramedullary erythropoiesis are found in both tumors.

In both forms of hepatic cancer the right lobe is more commonly involved than the left. In about half the patients, however, the tumor involves both lobes or is multicentric. The most frequent site of metastasis is the lungs; local extension within the abdomen is also common. Less often, the CNS may be the site of metastasis.

CLINICAL MANIFESTATIONS. The most frequent finding is an upper abdominal mass with abdominal enlargement. Pain is present in only 15–20% of the patients at the time of diagnosis; anorexia and weight loss occur with the same frequency. Even less common initial complaints are vomiting and jaundice. Rarely, there may be virilization in affected boys, owing to production of gonadotropin by the tumor.

DIAGNOSIS. The major diagnostic problem is the differentiation of hepatic enlargement due to primary tumor from that caused by other diseases, benign or malignant. A careful search should be made for another primary site of tumor, which will most frequently be neuroblastoma. Infantile hemangioendotheliomas and cavernous hemangiomas can enlarge the liver, and a careful survey for other hemangiomas should be made. Metabolic storage diseases may also simulate hepatic tumor.

Results of laboratory studies of liver function are most often normal. About 20% of patients may have increases in bilirubin levels or in transaminase activities. Most patients will have increased serum levels of α-fetoprotein, and this is a useful marker to follow after surgery.

The roentgenogram of the abdomen will demonstrate hepatic enlargement; in about 30% of patients, calcification will be seen within the tumor. In about 10% of patients pulmonary metastases will be present at the time of diagnosis, and abdominal and chest CT are indicated for initial staging. Angiography is particularly valuable in providing the surgeon with an indication of the blood supply of the tumor, which will determine its resectability. Radionuclide scan of the liver will indicate tumor. Final diagnosis depends on histologic examination.

TREATMENT. The only effective treatment is surgical resection. In only about one third of patients are the size and location of the tumor at the time of diagnosis such that complete excision can be attempted. Rapid regeneration of the liver occurs within 4–6 wk after surgery, and it is at about this time that the postoperative baseline CT scan and liver scan should be obtained. The tumor is relatively radioresistant. Various chemotherapeutic agents have a temporarily beneficial effect in metastatic disease, but there is no definitive chemotherapy. Cisplatin, vincristine, and Adriamycin all appear active in hepatoblastoma. Liver transplantation is being evaluated and, currently, should be limited to children without extrahepatic tumor and combined with postoperative chemotherapy.

PROGNOSIS. The prognosis for patients with hepatic tumors is poor. Overall survival in hepatoblastoma is 35%; in hepatocellular carcinoma the overall survival is only 13%. The survivors are exclusively patients who have had complete surgical excision of the tumor. Less than complete excision is always associated with local recurrence and eventual death. Transplantation results have not been encouraging.

17.24 GONADAL AND GERM CELL NEOPLASMS

EPIDEMIOLOGY. Gonadal and germ cell tumors are uncommon in children, although sacrococcygeal teratoma is the most common solid tumor in newborns (1:40,000 live births). Most reports indicate a female preponderance. The age incidence for both ovarian and testicular tumors peaks before the age of 2 yr, with a second increase in rate beginning after the age of 6 yr for ovarian tumors and after the age of 14 yr for testicular tumors. Patients with cryptorchid testes have a 50 times greater risk of malignant testicular tumors. Of the tumors that occur in cryptorchid males, 20% arise in the descended testis. Gonadal dysgenesis is the consistent underlying clinical feature of patients who develop gonadoblastoma (Sec. 19.33).

PATHOLOGY. The germ cell tumors are an interrelated group of malignancies expressing the multipotential characteristics of differentiation of the cells from which they arise. These relationships are expressed graphically in Figure 17–9. The mixtures of different cell types that may occur in the same tumor confirms their interrelationship.

Germ cell tumors occur most commonly in the gonads but may appear in such sites as the retroperitoneum, mediastinum, sacrococcygeum, and CNS. These tumors in extragonadal sites are thought to represent aberrancies in the migration of germ cells from the yolk sac into the developing fetus.

Differentiation may occur in the direction of extra-embryonic tissues, resulting in choriocarcinoma or yolk sac carcinoma (endodermal sinus tumor).

Choriocarcinoma is a component of both gonadal and extragonadal germ cell neoplasms. It occurs after puberty in the testicle, but both before and after puberty in the ovary. Choriocarcinoma is not commonly the predominant pattern of the tumor. There is frequently hemorrhagic necrosis. Masses of cytotrophoblast are overlain by caps of syncytiotrophoblastic giant cells. Choriocarcinoma may also be gestational (arising in the placenta), and there are rare cases

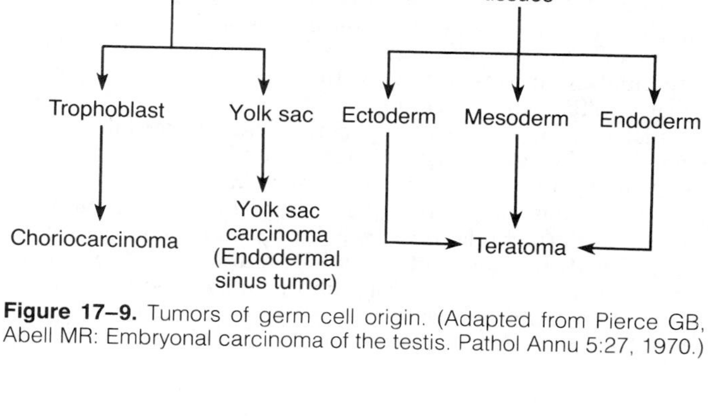

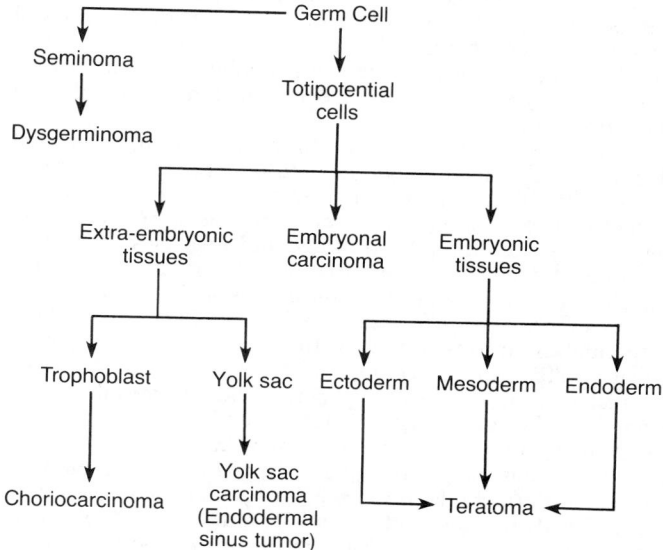

Figure 17–9. Tumors of germ cell origin. (Adapted from Pierce GB, Abell MR: Embryonal carcinoma of the testis. Pathol Annu 5:27, 1970.)

reported of infants developing widespread choriocarcinoma from maternal placental disease. The *yolk sac carcinoma (endodermal sinus tumor)* has histologic features resembling the endodermal sinuses of the placenta. A pattern of differentiation predominantly in the direction of embryonic tissues leads to *teratomas* or *teratocarcinomas*, which have elements of all three germ layers. The malignant component of a teratocarcinoma is usually an embryonal carcinoma.

Seminoma of the testicle occurs almost exclusively during the 2nd decade of life and later. The tissue is cellular, histologically, with clear cells aggregated in lobules and separated by fibrous stroma. *Dysgerminoma*, the ovarian counterpart, frequently occurs prior to puberty; the cells are morphologically and histochemically identical to primordial germ cells. These tumors metastasize to regional lymph nodes, with hematogenous dissemination to lung and bone. Metastasis from ovarian tumors may also be found within the peritoneal cavity, either by implantation, often with accompanying ascites, or by regional extension.

Just as the primary tumor may contain a mixture of histologic elements, metastatic tumor is generally also mixed; occasionally, a representation purely of one cell type may be found.

CLINICAL MANIFESTATIONS. During the 1st yr of life, the usual initial sign of a testicular tumor is a mass in the scrotum, sometimes found at birth. Delays in diagnosis arise when the mass is initially considered a hydrocele, and hydrocele may accompany these tumors. They are usually not painful at first, nor are there signs of inflammation. An initial finding of metastatic disease is uncommon. In older boys, a gradual swelling of the involved testicle is usually noted over some weeks, and pain and tenderness are found in more than half the cases. Clinical complications of metastasis to retroperitoneal lymph nodes or to lungs may be the initial findings in some patients. Gynecomastia may occur as an effect of chorionic gonadotropin. In a few patients the early clinical findings may be those of disseminated cancer, such as weight loss, anorexia, and lethargy.

With ovarian tumors the most common initial symptoms are pain, nausea, and vomiting. Some patients have no symptoms, an abdominal mass or abdominal fullness being noted incidentally. An acute onset of abdominal pain may occur in patients who have ovarian torsion; in such patients, the findings may simulate an inflammatory process, such as appendicitis. Germ cell tumors of the ovary seldom present with signs of metastatic disease. Of all ovarian germ cell tumors 95% are benign cystic teratomas, but an inverse relationship exists between age and likelihood of malignancy, with 84% of germ cell tumors being malignant in girls less than 10 yr old.

Sacrococcygeal teratoma or *teratocarcinoma* is usually detected during infancy and frequently at the time of birth. The most common finding is a mass in the area of the sacrum and buttocks. The incidence of malignancy is 10% in tumors diagnosed at less than 2 mo of age and increases to 50–70% for tumors diagnosed after this age. Additional symptoms and signs result if the growing mass causes obstruction of the rectum or urinary tract. Associated clinical features include congenital anomalies involving the lower vertebrae, genitourinary system, or anorectum.

Initial clinical features of patients with germ-cell tumors arising in other extragonadal sites depend on the location of the primary tumor. In the abdomen, tumors will usually present as masses. In the chest there may be respiratory symptoms. Intracranial tumors will present as mass lesions.

DIAGNOSIS. The chief diagnostic aid is careful examination. Testicular tumors are solid and usually opaque to transillumination (although they may be accompanied by hydrocele). Testicular size can be estimated via ultrasound or CT scan. Abdominal pain, nausea, and vomiting in a girl may be severe enough to warrant ultrasound evaluation of the ovaries.

A sacrococcygeal tumor in early infancy should immediately suggest teratoma. Other masses found in the same area include meningoceles, chordomas, duplications of the rectum, neurogenic tumors, lipoma, rhabdomyosarcoma, and hemangioma. Masses in the area may sometimes be confused with perirectal abscess. When the bulk of the tumor is intrapelvic, only constipation and anuria may ensue, as symptoms of obstruction. A rectal examination should always be done for an infant with such symptoms. Germ cell tumors in other extragonadal sites cannot in most cases be identified until excision or biopsy has been done and the histologic character established.

All patients suspected of having germ cell tumors should have roentgenograms and CT scans of the chest and radionuclide scans of bone to detect any metastatic disease. A CT scan of the abdomen in boys with testicular tumors may demonstrate retroperitoneal lymph node metastasis. Serum levels of α-fetoprotein and chorionic gonadotropin should be measured. The levels of these two biologic markers before treatment may be useful in the subsequent evaluation of the effectiveness of therapy.

TREATMENT. Therapy depends primarily on prompt recognition and surgical removal of the tumor. Dysgerminoma and seminoma are highly radiosensitive. Even when no metastatic disease is found, malignant germ cell tumors should receive combination chemotherapy, because it is likely that inapparent dissemination has already occurred. These tumors in adults are highly sensitive to chemotherapy. Cisplatin, bleomycin, and vinblastine (Velban) are most commonly used. Etoposide and ifosfamide are also active.

PROGNOSIS. This rests mainly on the extent of disease at the time of diagnosis. It is important, therefore, that germ cell tumors be suspected as early as possible. In general, the finding of extraembryonal elements in a germ cell tumor denotes a poor prognosis. It is difficult to assess results of treatment, because only a small number of patients have been treated in any consistent manner; treatment should be planned, however, with the assumption that early intervention and adjuvant chemotherapy provide reasonable expectation for long-term disease-free survival. Cures have been reported in adult patients even after recurrence.

OTHER TUMORS OF THE GONADS are uncommon in children. *Sertoli tumors* of the testicle are usually benign and arise from sustentacular cells originating from the primitive gonadal mesenchyme. Occasionally, endocrine activity can occur, with sexual precocity or gynecomastia. The tumor is most likely to occur during the 1st or 2nd yr of life. Treatment is surgical removal.

Almost half of ovarian tumors are *benign ovarian cysts*. These cysts may be found incidentally at laparotomy for other purposes or on physical examination of an otherwise well child. Occasionally, torsion of the involved ovary can cause acute abdominal pain, nausea, and vomiting. Other ovarian tumors are quite uncommon. The *granulosa-theca cell tumor* is thought to arise in cells of ovarian stromal origin; it is usually associated with precocious puberty and a mass in the lower abdomen. The tumor is only rarely malignant, and its removal alleviates the endocrine abnormality. *Cystadenocarcinoma* of the ovary is even more uncommon and cannot be differentiated by clinical manifestations from other malignant ovarian tumors. *Hemangiomas* may involve the ovary (Sec. 18.54). Occasionally, ovarian enlargement will be the first manifestation of *lymphoma*.

Gonadoblastomas are found exclusively in patients with gonadal dysgenesis. Of affected patients, 80% are phenotypic females, usually with evidence of virilization. The others are phenotypic males, usually with such abnormalities as cryptorchidism, hypospadias, or female internal or secondary sex organs. The gonadoblastoma is regarded as a cancer in situ from which germinomas may develop. The tumor may be bilateral; it presents as a growing mass with the additional features of virilization in some female patients. Histologic examination shows an intimate mixture of germ cells and elements resembling immature granulosa or Sertoli cells, with or without Leydig cells or lutein-type cells. The tumor should be removed along with the other normal gonad (and the uterus if one is present), because the other gonad may undergo malignant degeneration. Prolonged exogenous hormone administration may be required in such patients for development of secondary sexual characteristics, and secondary uterine cancer may occur under these circumstances.

17.25 MISCELLANEOUS CARCINOMAS

ADENOCARCINOMA OF THE VAGINA AND CERVIX

This tumor, once extremely rare, has become more common as the result of intrauterine exposure to diethylstilbestrol. Other genitourinary anomalies occur in affected patients (Sec. 18.54).

CARCINOMA OF THE THYROID

Thyroid cancer is discussed in Sec. 19.15. It occurs in increased incidence in patients who have had irradiation to the head and neck in childhood. Spontaneous thyroid cancer is more common in girls than in boys and is most likely to be papillary and to grow slowly. Medullary carcinoma of the thyroid may occur sporadically or in a familial pattern; in its familial form, it is associated with Marfan-like habitus, pheochromocytoma, hyperparathyroidism, and mucosal neuromas.

CARCINOMA OF THE ADRENAL GLAND

Adrenocortical carcinoma is quite rare. It may occur at any age during childhood but is more common during the first few years. The tumor may be associated with hemangiomas of the skin, hemihypertrophy, urinary tract anomalies, and astrocytomas. Girls predominate among patients with this tumor. The usual presenting symptoms are secondary to the endocrine function of the cancer. Affected children present signs of adrenal hyperfunction (Sec. 19.24), which may include Cushing syndrome (Sec. 19.23), virilization (Sec. 19.22), feminization (Sec. 19.25), or a combination of these.

CARCINOMA OF THE BREAST

See Sec 10.19 and 18.52.

CANCER OF THE SKIN

Cancer of the skin is rare in children (Sec. 23.33). *Malignant melanoma* may occur during the first two decades, with clinical behavior much like that in adults. It usually appears as a rapidly growing, easily traumatized, ulcerated lesion that is darkly pigmented or has changed in color. It may be found on any part of the body. Certain conditions such as *giant hairy cell nevus syndrome* or *dysplastic nevus syndrome* will predispose to the development of melanoma. Because malignant melanoma is rare in children, an excisional biopsy of a suspected lesion is indicated initially. If malignancy is found, then wide local resection is indicated, which may necessitate skin grafting. Regional lymph nodes should be examined carefully; if they are enlarged, then a lymph node dissection should also be done. For patients with metastatic disease, good clinical responses may be obtained with doxorubicin and cyclophosphamide.

Xeroderma pigmentosum is an autosomal recessive condition in which there is a defective mechanism for DNA repair. When the affected person is exposed to sunlight, the ultraviolet radiation produces breaks in DNA, which provides an opportunity for mutant malignant growth. The skin is the organ of primary involvement. Multiple skin cancers appear in the exposed areas. Surgical resection of the tumors is necessary, and affected children must be protected as much as possible from sunlight. The *nevoid basal cell carcinoma syndrome* (basal cell nevus syndrome) is discussed in Sec. 23.33.

MISCELLANEOUS BENIGN TUMORS

A variety of benign tumors in infants and children present problems in differential diagnosis; many will also require treatment. Some can be life-threatening, although they are histologically benign.

17.26 BENIGN TUMORS AND TUMOR-LIKE PROCESSES IN BONE

A number of benign processes in bone must be recognized by the clinician and distinguished from malignant tumors in order to avoid tragic consequences of overtreatment. Some of them may be reactions to trauma, but the putative trauma usually cannot be identified. Others appear to be hamartomas, or true overgrowths of normal tissue in situ. Still other lesions, less well understood, are considered to be benign neoplasia, with perhaps the potential for malignancy.

Osteoid osteoma occurs with moderate frequency in adolescents, especially in boys; it usually involves the femur or tibia, much less frequently the spine, humerus, or phalanges. The cardinal clinical feature is pain, which is dull at first and accentuated by weight-bearing, typically more severe at night, and relieved by aspirin. After weeks or months of increasing pain there may be localized tenderness, but signs of inflammation are unusual. The roentgenogram is diagnostic, disclosing a sharply demarcated radiolucent nidus of osteoid tissue surrounded by sclerotic bone. There may be calcification of the osteoid within the nidus. Treatment is surgical: the nidus must be removed completely to prevent recurrence. A related tumor is the *osteoblastoma*, which tends to be larger and to have little or no sclerosis. It involves the spine more commonly than does osteoid osteoma.

Fibrous (benign) cortical defects are eccentric in location and presumably arise from the periosteum to erode the cortex from without. They have been estimated to occur in as many as 53% of boys and 31% of girls, most commonly from 4–8 yr of age. They may persist into adolescence and even into early adult life. They are found always in the metaphyses of cylindrical bones, usually near the knees. The radiographic picture is characteristic. They are asymptomatic and heal spontaneously. Their recognition is important lest they be mistaken for malignant lesions.

Nonossifying fibroma or *fibroxanthoma* is most common in late childhood and early adolescence and may be related to the fibrous cortical defect. About half of all cases are found incidentally in roentgenograms made for other purposes. There are often no symptoms, but chronic bone pain may occur. A pathologic fracture may be the first sign. The ends of the shafts of the long bones of the lower limbs are most commonly involved. The roentgenographic picture of a rarefied scalloped lesion is so characteristic that biopsy for histologic confirmation may not be required. Treatment is often not required, spontaneous cure being expected after months or years. Curettage or other interventions may be required for weakened or fractured bones.

Osteochondroma (cartilaginous exostosis) is the solitary lesion that corresponds to those of osteochondromatosis (hereditary multiple exostoses, Sec. 24.48). Osteochondroma occurs in any bone formed in cartilage, most often near the ends of femur or tibia at the knee. Growth appears in childhood and early adolescence and ceases with closure of the neighboring epiphyseal plates, at which time ossification of its cartilaginous cap may occur. A mass may be present, or pain if there is a fracture. The roentgenographic features are characteristic; some lesions are pedunculated, others sessile. Reactivation of growth occurs spontaneously on rare occasions, sometimes after a fracture; such lesions should be considered malignant until proved otherwise by excisional biopsy. Lesions should be removed prophylactically when possible, particularly if there are symptoms.

Enchondroma is the solitary lesion that corresponds to those of multiple enchondromatosis (Ollier disease, Sec. 24.48). It is less common than osteochondroma and is most likely to involve metacarpals, metatarsals, and phalanges. Enchondromas appear as deforming masses or become apparent when they induce pathologic fractures. Roentgenograms show circumscribed areas of rarefied bone with thinning and often bulging of the cortex and stippled calcification. Lesions in the hands or feet are benign; those in the large long bones, in any diaphysis, or in membranous bone have malignant potential and may be difficult to separate histologically from malignant lesions. Treatment is curettage of clearly benign lesions or wide excision of doubtful ones.

Solitary (unicameral) cysts fall somewhere between dysplasias and true tumors. These common lesions begin close to the epiphyseal plate and appear to migrate toward the diaphysis with growth of bone. The cavity is unilocular or multilocular and contains fluid or blood. The origin of the cysts is unknown; they have been attributed to traumatic hematomas. Symptoms may be absent or scant; the cysts may first declare themselves because of pathologic fracture. The roentgenographic appearance consists of an area of rarefaction, often pseudoloculated, that does not cross the epiphyseal plate. These lesions may resolve spontaneously. Those in the upper extremity sometimes need no therapy; those of the lower extremity are at greater risk of fracture and should usually be treated with curettage or excision.

17.27 HEMANGIOMA

This tumor is among the most common neoplasms found in infants and children. Most occur in the skin and do not achieve great size (Sec. 23.8).

In a few children, large, rapidly growing hemangiomas can produce serious or life-threatening complications or grotesque deformity, especially in the area of the head and neck or on an extremity. Most such hemangiomas become evident before the age of 6 mo. They are evenly distributed between boys and girls. Their natural history is unpredictable. There is usually rapid growth during the 1st and 2nd yr of life, followed by slow regression. Hemangiomas in the head and neck area can be unsightly and may progressively distort normal structures. Growth of these tumors may produce airway obstruction, pressure necrosis of surrounding structures, difficult feeding, and obstruction of the ear canal. The tumors may become secondarily infected through the ulceration of overlying skin. If arteriovenous communications of sufficient size develop, congestive cardiac failure may ensue.

Treatment of large tumors by resection is frequently difficult because of extensive involvement, and complete removal may be impossible. In some patients the administration of prednisone may suppress tumor growth, and regression may occur. Stopping the treatment may be followed by regrowth of tumor.

Hemangioma of the liver most frequently becomes evident before the age of 6 mo. Histologically, hemangioendothelioma is more common than are cavernous hemangiomas. The initial symptoms may be jaundice, vomiting, or diarrhea, or, in some infants, increases in abdominal size without symptoms. The hemangioma is sometimes found when routine examination discloses an enlarged liver. Arteriovenous fistulas may lead to congestive cardiac failure. Roentgenograms of the abdomen show an enlarged liver and occasionally calcification in the tumor. Radionuclide and CT scans of liver and spleen will show the defect in hepatic tissue; hepatic angiograms will show an abnormal vascular pattern. Initial treatment with prednisone is recommended. If hemangioma of the liver is confined to a single lobe, surgical resection may be possible.

In some patients with large, cavernous hemangiomas, hemolysis and intralesional clotting may produce thrombocytopenia and hypofibrinogenemia with clinical symptoms. The anemia is not easily corrected by transfusion because of the ongoing red blood cell destruction, and a hemorrhagic diathesis may be impossible to correct by the transfusion of platelets and plasma clotting factors (Sec. 23.8).

17.28 LYMPHANGIOMA (CYSTIC HYGROMA)

Lymphangiomas are found in the head and neck region in about three fourths of cases. Like hemangiomas they appear early in life, with almost all evident by the age of 3 yr, and some have been diagnosed antenatally on maternal sonography. The embryonic origin of lymphangiomas is uncertain; it is not known whether they are malformations, benign neoplasms, or hamartomas. They may present as unilocular or multicystic masses, with thin, often-transparent walls. The contents of the cysts are straw colored. Histologically, the lining of the cystic areas is one or two cells thick, with varying amounts of intervening fibrous stroma.

Cystic hygroma is compressible and feels cystic. The tumors are not tender or painful. There may be some thinning of the overlying skin. There is no erythema unless the lesion becomes infected. Unlike hemangiomas, these lesions do not regress spontaneously, and they should be resected as soon as possible. Planning for surgery involves evaluation of the extent of disease. Roentgenograms and CT scans will demonstrate intrathoracic extension in at least 10% of patients, and the tumor as it grows may result in tracheal compression and respiratory embarrassment. The tongue may also be involved and enlarged in some patients. Complete surgical excision, which is required for cure, may involve extensive dissection, with reconstructive surgery if vital structures are involved.

17.29 THYMOMA

Thymoma is rare in children, occurring with equal frequency in boys and girls. This anterior mediastinal tumor may be found in an asymptomatic person on a routine chest roentgenogram. With growth of the tumor, there may be progressive compression of surrounding tissues, with the development of cough, dyspnea, dysphagia, and even superior vena cava compression.

A number of paraneoplastic syndromes have occurred with thymoma, including myasthenia gravis, hypogammaglobulinemia, and pure red blood cell aplasia. These disorders may arise as a result of imbalances in immune regulation (e.g., enhanced production of suppressor lymphocytes by the tumor). The tumor extends locally and rarely metastasizes outside the thorax.

The treatment of choice is complete surgical excision. The tumor is radiosensitive, and recurrent disease will respond to chemotherapy with agents such as doxorubicin, cyclophosphamide, and cisplatin.

17.30 SPLENIC CYSTS

Splenic cysts can produce an enlarged spleen, which may suggest a malignant neoplasm. Any such mass should be investigated by abdominal ultrasound or CT scan to establish its nature and exactly which organ is involved.

BRIGID G. LEVENTHAL

GENERAL CONSIDERATIONS

Doolittle RF, Hunkapiller MW, Hood LE, et al: Simian sarcoma virus *onc* gene, V-*sis*, is derived from the gene (or genes) encoding a platelet derived growth factor. Science 22KL:275, 1983.
Fearon E, Vogelstein B: A genetic model for colorectal tumorigenesis. Cell 61:759, 1990.
Knudson AG: Mutation and cancer: Statistical study of retinoblastoma. Proc Nat Acad Sci USA 68:820, 1971.
Land H, Parada LF, Weinberg RA: Cellular oncogenes and multistep carcinogenesis. Science 222:771, 1983.
Leder P, Battey J, Lenoir G, et al: Translocations among antibody genes in human cancer. Science 222:765, 1983.
Miller RW: Environmental causes of cancer in childhood. Adv Pediatr 25:97, 1978.
Skuse GR, Rowley PT: Tumor suppressor genes and inherited predisposition to malignancy. Semin Oncol 16:128, 1989.
Yandell DW, Campbell TA, Dayton SH, et al: Oncogenic point mutations in the human retinoblastoma gene: Their application to genetic counseling. N Engl J Med 321:1689, 1989.

BONE MARROW TRANSPLANTATION AS THERAPY

Begg CB, McGlave PB, Bennett JM, et al: A critical comparison of allogeneic bone marrow transplantation and conventional chemotherapy as treatment for acute nonlymphocytic leukemia. J Clin Oncol 2:369, 1984.
Fefer A, Cheever MA, Thomas ED, et al: Bone marrow transplantation for refractory acute leukemia in 34 patients with identical twins. Blood 57:421, 1981.
Johnson FL, Thomas ED, Clark BS, et al: A comparison of marrow transplantation with chemotherapy for children with acute lymphoblastic leukemia in second or subsequent remission. N Engl J Med 305:846, 1981.
Kersey JH, Weisdorf D, Nesbit ME, et al: Comparison of autologous and allogeneic bone marrow transplantation for treatment of high risk refractory acute lymphoblastic leukemia. N Engl J Med 317:461, 1987.
O'Reilly RJ: Allogeneic bone marrow transplantation: Current status and future directions. Blood 62:941, 1983.
Philip T, Bernard JL, Zucker JM, et al: High dose chemoradiotherapy with bone marrow transplantation as consolidation treatment in neuroblastoma: An unselected group of stage IV patients over 1 year of age. J Clin Oncol 5:266, 1987.
Yeager AM, Kaizer H, Santos G, et al: Autologous bone marrow transplantation in patients with acute nonlymphocytic leukemia using ex-vivo marrow treated with 4-hydroperoxycyclophosphamide. N Engl J Med 315:141, 1986.

ACUTE LYMPHOCYTIC LEUKEMIA (ALL)

Freeman AI, Weinberg V, Brecher ML, et al: Comparison of intermediate-dose methotrexate with cranial irradiation for the post-induction treatment of acute lymphocytic leukemia in children. N Engl J Med 308:477, 484, 1983.
Amylon M, Murphy S, Pullen J: Treatment of lymphoid malignancies according to immune phenotype: Preliminary results in T-cell disease. Proc ASCO 7:225, 1988.
Camitta B, Leventhal B, Lauer S, et al: Intermediate dose intravenous methotrexate and mercaptopurine therapy for non-T, non-B acute lymphocytic leukemia of childhood: A Pediatric Oncology Group Study. J Clin Oncol 7:1539, 1989.
Crist WM, Grosse CE, Pullen J, et al: Immunologic markers in childhood acute lymphocytic leukemia. Semin Oncol 12:105, 1985.
Hurwitz CA, Loken MR, Graham ML, et al: Asynchronous antigen expression in B lineage acute lymphoblastic leukemia. Blood 72:299, 1988.
Pui CH, Behm FG, Raimondi SC, et al: Secondary acute myeloid leukemia in children treated for acute lymphoid leukemia. N Engl J Med 321:136, 1989.
Rivera GK, Mauer AM: Controversies in the management of childhood acute lymphoblastic leukemia: Treatment intensification, CNS leukemia and prognostic factors. Semin Hematol 24:12, 1987.

ACUTE NONLYMPHOCYTIC LEUKEMIA (ANLL)

Lampkin BC, Woods W, Strauss R, et al: Current status of the end treatment of acute non lymphocytic leukemia in children (report of the ANLL strategy group of the Children's Cancer Study Group). Blood 61:215, 1983.
Steuber P, Ruymann F, Culbert S, et al: A Pediatric Oncology Group study: Comparison of two induction regimens for acute myelogenous leukemia. Blood 72:208A, 1983.
Weinstein HJ, Mayer RJ, Rosenthal DS, et al: Chemotherapy for acute myelogenous leukemia in children and adults: VAPA update. Blood 62:315, 1983.
Yates J, Glidewell O, Wiernik P, et al: Cytosine arabinoside plus daunorubicin or adriamycin for therapy of acute myelocytic leukemia: A CALGB study. Blood 60:454, 1982.

CHRONIC MYELOCYTIC LEUKEMIA (CML)

Altman AJ, Palmer CG, Baehner RL: Juvenile "chronic granulocytic" leukemia: A panmyelopathy with prominent monocytic involvement and circulating monocyte colony forming cells. Blood 43:341, 1974.
Kastan MB, Zehnbauer BA, Leventhal BG, et al: Philadelphia-chromosome positive essential thrombocythemia. Am J Ped Hem Onc 11:433, 1989.
Phillips GL, Herzig GP: Intensive chemotherapy, total body irradiation, and autologous marrow transplantation for chronic granulocytic leukemia: Blast phase. Report of four additional cases. J Clin Oncol 2:379, 1984.

HODGKIN DISEASE

Chilcote RR, Baehner RL, Hammond D: Septicemia and meningitis in children splenectomized for Hodgkin's disease. N Engl J Med 295:798, 1976.
DeVita VT Jr, Simon RM, Hubbard SM, et al: Curability of advanced Hodgkin's disease with chemotherapy. Long term follow up of MOPP treated patients at the National Cancer Institute. Ann Intern Med 92:57, 1980.
Donaldson SS, Whitaker SJ, Plowman PN, et al: Stage I-II pediatric Hodgkin's disease: long term follow up demonstrates equivalent survival following different management schemes. J Clin Oncol 8:1128, 1990.
Grufferman S, Delzell E: Epidemiology of Hodgkin's disease. Epidemiol Rev 6:76, 1984.
Kadin M: Possible origins of the Reed Sternberg cell from an interdigitating reticulum cell. Cancer Treat Rep 66:601, 1982.
Kaplan HS: Hodgkin's Disease. Cambridge, MA, Harvard University Press, 1980.
Russell KL, Donaldson SS, Cox RS, et al: Childhood Hodgkin's disease: Patterns of relapse. J Clin Oncol 2:80, 1984.
Santoro A, Bonadonna G, Bonfante V, et al: Alternating drug combinations in the treatment of advanced Hodgkin's disease. N Engl J Med 306:770, 1982.

NON-HODGKIN LYMPHOMA

Bernard A, Murphy SB, Melvin S, et al: Non-T, non-B lymphomas are rare in childhood and associated with cutaneous tumor. Blood 59:549, 1982.
Graham M: Non-Hodgkin's lymphomas. Pediatr Ann 17:192, 1988.
Jenkin RDT, Anderson JR, Chilcote R, et al: Pediatric non Hodgkin's lymphomas: The Children's Cancer Study Group experience—an interim report. *In:* Rosenberg S, Kaplan H (eds): Malignant lymphomas: etiology, immunology, pathology, treatment. New York, Academic Press, 1982, pp 591–601.
Link MP, Donaldson SS, Berard CW, et al: Results of treatment of childhood localized non-Hodgkins lymphoma with combination chemotherapy with or without radiotherapy. N Engl J Med 322:1169, 1990.
Murphy SB: Prognostic features and obstacles to cure of childhood non-Hodgkin's lymphoma. Semin Oncol 4:265, 1977.
Murphy SB, Melvin SL, Mauer AM: Correlation of tumor cell kinetic studies with surface marker results in childhood non-Hodgkin's lymphoma. Cancer Res 39:1534, 1979.
Stapleton FB, Strother DR, Roy S, et al: Acute renal failure at onset of therapy for advanced stage Burkitt lymphoma and B-cell acute lymphoblastic lymphoma. Pediatrics 82:863, 1988.

NEUROBLASTOMA

Brodeur GM, Seeger R: Gene amplification in human neuroblastomas: Basic mechanisms and clinical implications. Cancer Genet Cytogenet 19:101, 1986.
Look AT, Hayes FA, Nitschke R, et al: Cellular DNA content as a predictor of response to chemotherapy in infants with unresectable neuroblastoma. N Engl J Med 211:231, 1984.
Rosen EM, Cassady JR, Frantz DN, et al: Neuroblastoma: The Joint Center for Radiation Therapy/Dana Farber Cancer Institute Children's Hospital Experience. J Clin Oncol 2:719, 1984.
Sawada T, Sugimoto T, Tanaka T, et al: Number and cure rate of neuroblastoma cases detected by the mass screening program in Japan: Future aspects. Med Pediatr Oncol 15:14, 1987.
Shimada H, Chatten J, Newton WA Jr, et al: Histopathologic prognostic factors

in neuroblastic tumors: Definition of subtypes of ganglioneuroblastoma and an age-linked classification of neuroblastomas. J Nat Cancer Inst 73:405, 1984.

WILMS TUMOR

Beckwith JB, Palmer NF: Histopathology and prognosis of Wilms' tumor: Results from the First National Wilms' Tumor Study. Cancer 41:1937, 1978.
Bolande RP: Congenital mesoblastic nephroma. Arch Pathol Lab Med 98:357, 1974.
Bove KE, McAdams AJ: The nephroblastomatosis complex and relationship to Wilms' tumor; a clinico pathologic treatise. J Pediatr Pathol 3:185, 1976.
D'Angio GJ, Evans AE, Breslow N, et al: The treatment of Wilms' tumor: Results of the National Wilms' Tumor Study. Cancer 38:633, 1976.
D'Angio GJ, Evans AE, Breslow N, et al: The treatment of Wilms' tumor: Results of the Second National Wilms' Tumor Study. Cancer 47:2302, 1981.
Fishman EK, Hartmen DS, Goldman SM, et al: The CT appearance of Wilms' tumor. J Comput Assist Tomogr 7:659, 1983.

SOFT TISSUE SARCOMAS

Hays DM, Raney RB, Lawrence W Jr, et al: Bladder and prostatic tumors in the Intergroup Rhabdomyosarcoma Study (IRS-1). Cancer 50:1472, 1982.
Pizzo PA: Rhabdomyosarcoma and other soft tissue sarcomas. *In*: Levine AS (ed): Cancer in the Young. New York, Masson Publishing, 1982, pp 615–632.
Sarcomas of soft tissue and bone in childhood. NCI Monograph 56. United States Government Printing Office, 1981.

OSTEOSARCOMA

Dahlin DC, Unni KK: Osteosarcoma of bone and its important recognizable varieties. Am J Surg Pathol 1:61, 1977.
Goorin AM, Delorey MJ, Lack EE, et al: Prognostic significance of complete surgical resection of pulmonary metastases in patients with osteogenic sarcoma: Analysis of 32 patients. J Clin Oncol 2:425, 1984.
Link MP, Goorin AM, Miser AW, et al: The effect of adjuvant chemotherapy on relapse-free survival in patients with osteosarcoma of the extremity. N Engl J Med 314:1600, 1986.
Rosen G, Nienberg A: Preoperative chemotherapy for osteogenic sarcoma: Selection of postoperative adjuvant chemotherapy based on the response of primary tumor to preoperative chemotherapy. Cancer 49:1221, 1982.

EWING SARCOMA

Freeman CR, Geldhill R, Chevalier LM, et al: Osteogenic sarcoma following treatment with megavoltage radiation and chemotherapy for bone tumors in children. Med Pediatr Oncol 3:375, 1980.
Hayes FA, Thompson EI, Hustu HO, et al: The response of Ewing's sarcoma to sequential cyclophosphamide and adriamycin induction therapy. J Clin Oncol 1:45, 1983.
Rosen G, Caparros B, Nirenberg A, et al: Ewing's sarcoma: Ten years' experience with adjuvant chemotherapy. Cancer 47:2204, 1981.
Soule EH, Newton W Jr, Moon TE, et al: Extraskeletal Ewing's sarcoma: A preliminary study of 26 cases encountered in the Intergroup Rhabdomyosarcoma Study. Cancer 42:259, 1978.

PRIMITIVE NEUROECTODERMAL TUMORS

Askin FB, Rosai J, Sibley RK, et al: Malignant small cell tumor of the thoracopulmonary region in childhood: A distinctive clinicopathologic entity of uncertain histogenesis. Cancer 43:2438, 1979.
Dehner LP: Peripheral and central primitive neuroectodermal tumors: A nosologic concept seeking a consensus. Arch Pathol Lab Med 110:997, 1986.

GASTROINTESTINAL NEOPLASMS

Horie A, Yano Y, Kotto Y, et al: Morphogenesis of pancreatoblastoma, infantile carcinoma of the pancreas: Report of two cases. Cancer 39:247, 1977.
Krolls SO, Trodahl JN, Boyers RC: Salivary gland lesions in children—a survey of 430 cases. Cancer 30:459, 1972.
Pratt CB, Rivera G, Shanks E, et al: Colorectal carcinoma in adolescents: Implications regarding etiology. Cancer 40:2464, 1977.
Rich RH, Dehner LP, Okinaga K, et al: Surgical management of islet cell adenoma in infancy. Surgery 84:519, 1978.
Siegel SE, Hays DM, Romansky S, et al: Carcinoma of the stomach in childhood. Cancer 38:1781, 1976.
Taxy JB: Adenocarcinoma of the pancreas in childhood. Cancer 37:1508, 1976.
Toccalino H, Guastavino E, DePinni F, et al: Juvenile polyps of the rectum and colon. Acta Pediatr Scan 62:337, 1973.

NEOPLASMS OF THE LIVER

Evans AE, Land VJ, Newton WA, et al: Combination chemotherapy (vincristine, adriamycin, cyclophosphamide, and 5-fluorouracil) in the treatment of children with malignant hepatomas. Cancer 50:821, 1982.
Exelby PR, Filler RM, Grosfeld JL: Liver tumors in children in the particular reference to hepatoblastoma and hepatocellular carcinoma. American Academy of Pediatrics Surgical Survey—1974. J Pediatr Surg 10:329, 1975.
Vawter G: Hepatoblastoma: A clinical and pathologic study of 54 cases. Am J Surg Pathol 6:693, 1982.
Wineberg AG, Finegold MJ: Primary hepatic tumors of childhood. Hum Pathol 14:512, 1983.

GONADAL AND GERM CELL NEOPLASMS

Einhorn LH, Williams ST, Troner M, et al: The role of maintenance therapy in disseminated testicular cancer. N Engl J Med 305:727, 1981.
Hogan JM, Johnson DE: The etiology of testicular tumors. *In*: Johnson DE (ed): Testicular Tumors, 2nd ed. Flushing, NY, Medical Examination Publishing Co, 1976.
Witzleben CL, Bruninga G: Infantile choriocarcinoma: A characteristic syndrome. J Pediatr 73:378, 1968.
Woodruff JD, Protos P, Peterson WF: Ovarian teratomas: Relationship of histologic and oncogenic factors to prognosis. Am J Obstet Gynecol 102:702, 1968.

MISCELLANEOUS CARCINOMAS

Dudgeon DL: Lumps in the breast. Difficult diagnosis in pediatrics. Philadelphia, WB Saunders 391–400, 1990.
Hayes FA, Green AA: Malignant melanoma in childhood: Clinical cause and response to chemotherapy. J Clin Oncol 2:1229, 1984.
Herbst AL, Scully RE: Adenocarcinoma of the vagina in adolescence. Cancer 25:745, 1970.
Leape LL, Miller HH, Graze K, et al: Total thyroidectomy for occult familial medullary carcinoma of the thyroid in children. J Pediatr Surg 11:831, 1976.
Oberman HA, Stephens PJ: Carcinoma of the breast in childhood. Cancer 30:470, 1972.
Stewart DR, Jones PH, Jolleys A: Carcinoma of the adrenal gland in children. J Pediatr Surg 9:59, 1974.

18

THE URINARY SYSTEM AND PEDIATRIC GYNECOLOGY

NEPHROLOGIC DISEASES

18.1 ANATOMY OF THE GLOMERULUS

The kidneys lie in the retroperitoneal space slightly above the level of the umbilicus and range in length and weight, respectively, from approximately 6 cm and 24 g in the full-term newborn to 12 cm or more and 150 g in the adult. The kidney (Fig. 18–1) has an outer layer, the *cortex,* which contains the glomeruli, proximal and distal convoluted tubules, and collecting ducts, and an inner layer, the *medulla,* which contains the straight portions of the tubules, the loops of Henle, the vasa recta, and the terminal collecting ducts (Fig. 18–2).

The blood supply to each kidney usually consists of a main renal artery that arises from the aorta; multiple renal arteries are not uncommon. The main artery divides into segmental branches within the medulla and these into interlobar arteries that pass through the medulla to the junction of the cortex and medulla. At this point, the interlobar arteries branch to form the arcuate arteries, which run parallel to the surface of the kidney. Interlobular arteries originate from the arcuate arteries and give rise to the afferent arterioles of the glomeruli. Specialized muscle cells in the wall of the afferent arteriole, in combination with the lacis cells and that portion of the distal tubule (macula densa) that is adjacent to the glomerulus, form the juxtaglomerular apparatus that controls the secretion of renin. The afferent arteriole divides into the glomerular capillary network, which then merges into the efferent arteriole (Fig. 18–3). The efferent arterioles of glomeruli next to the medulla (juxtamedullary glomeruli) are larger than those in the outer cortex and provide the blood supply (vasa recta) to the tubules and medulla.

Each kidney contains approximately 1 million nephrons (glomeruli and associated tubules). In humans, formation of nephrons is complete at birth, but functional maturation does not occur until later. As no new nephrons can be formed after birth, progressive loss of nephrons may lead to renal insufficiency.

The glomerular network of specialized capillaries serves as the filtering mechanism of the kidney. The glomerular capillaries are lined by endothelial cells (Fig. 18–4) having very thin cytoplasm that contains many holes (fenestrations). The glomerular basement membrane (GBM) forms a continuous layer between the endothelial and mesangial cells on one side and the epithelial cells on the other. The membrane has three layers: (1) a central electron-dense lamina densa, (2) the lamina rara interna, which lies between the lamina densa and the endothelial cells, and (3) the lamina rara externa, which lies between the lamina densa and the epithelial cells. The visceral epithelial cells cover the capillary and project cytoplasmic

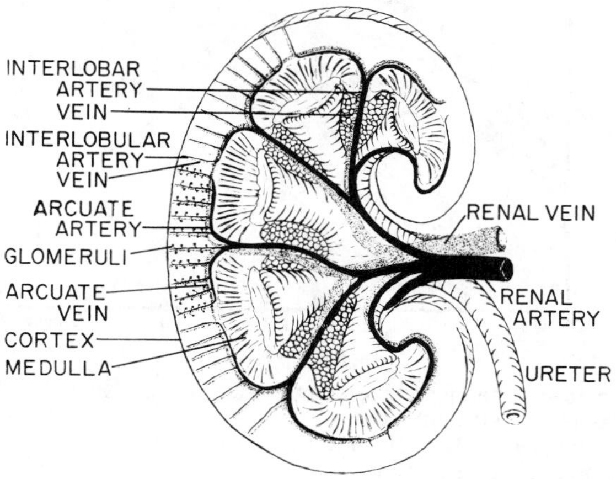

Figure 18–1. Gross morphology of the renal circulation. (From Pitts RF: Physiology of the Kidney and Body Fluids, 3rd ed. Chicago, Year Book Medical Publishers, 1974. Used by permission.)

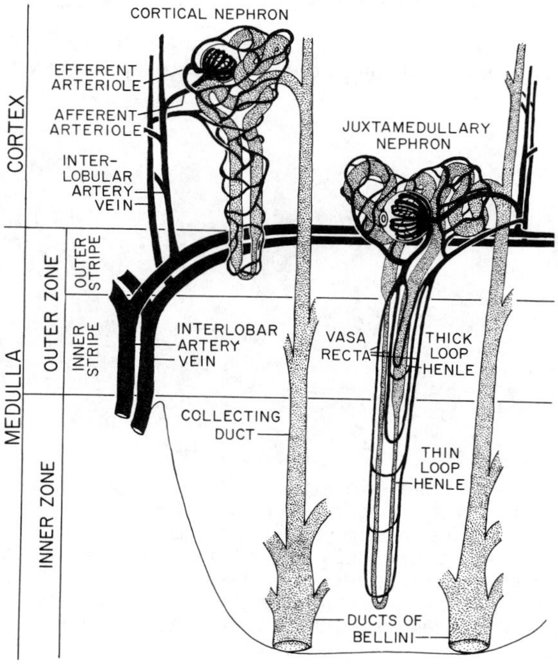

Figure 18–2. Comparison of the blood supplies of cortical and juxtamedullary nephrons. (From Pitts RF: Physiology of the Kidney and Body Fluids, 3rd ed. Chicago, Year Book Medical Publishers, 1974. Used by permission.)

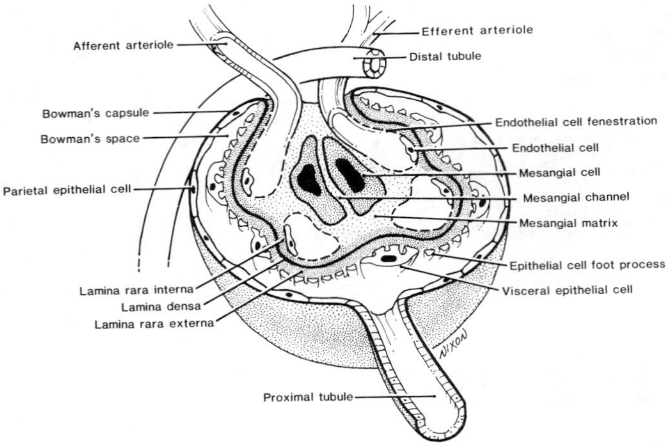

Figure 18–3. Schematic depiction of the glomerulus and surrounding structures.

"foot processes," which come in contact with the lamina rara externa. Between the foot processes are spaces or filtration slits. The mesangium (mesangial cells and matrix) lies between the glomerular capillaries on the endothelial cell side of the basement membrane and forms the medial part of the capillary wall. The mesangium may serve as a supporting structure for the glomerular capillaries and probably plays a role in the removal of macromolecules (such as immune complexes) from the glomerulus, either through intracellular phagocytosis or by transport through intercellular channels to the juxtaglomerular region. The Bowman capsule, which surrounds the glomerulus, is composed of (1) a basement membrane, which is continuous with the basement membranes of the glomerular capillaries and the proximal tubules, and (2) the parietal epithelial cells, which are continuous with the visceral epithelial cells.

18.2 GLOMERULAR FILTRATION

As the blood passes through the glomerular capillaries, the plasma is filtered through the glomerular capillary walls. The ultrafiltrate, which is cell-free, contains all the substances in the plasma (electrolytes, glucose, phosphate, urea, creatinine, peptides, low molecular weight proteins) except proteins (like albumin and the globulins) having a molecular weight exceeding 68,000. The filtrate is collected in Bowman space and enters the tubules, where its composition is modified in accordance with body needs until it leaves the kidney as urine.

Glomerular filtration is the net result of opposing forces across the capillary wall. The force for ultrafiltration (glomerular capillary hydrostatic pressure) stems from the systemic arterial pressure, as modified by the tone of the afferent and efferent arterioles. The major force opposing ultrafiltration is the glomerular capillary oncotic pressure, which is created by the gradient between the high concentration of plasma proteins within the capillary and the almost protein-free ultrafiltrate in Bowman space. Filtration may be modified by the rate of glomerular plasma flow, the hydrostatic pressure within Bowman space, and the permeability of the glomerular capillary wall. The permeability, as measured by the ultrafiltration coefficient (K_f), is the product of the water permeability of the membrane and the total glomerular capillary surface area available for filtration.

Although glomerular filtration begins around the 9th week of fetal life, kidney function does not appear necessary for normal intrauterine homeostasis, the placenta serving as the major excretory organ. Following birth, the rate of glomerular filtration increases until growth ceases toward the end of the 2nd decade of life. To facilitate the comparison of the glomerular filtration rates (GFR) of children and adults, the rate is standardized to the surface area (1.73 m^2) of a 70-kg adult. Even after correction for surface area, the GFR of the child does not approximate adult values until the 3rd year of life (Fig. 18–5).

The GFR may be estimated by measurement of the serum creatinine level (Fig. 18–6). Creatinine is derived from muscle metabolism. Its production is relatively constant, and its excretion is primarily through glomerular filtration (although tubular secretion may become important in renal insufficiency). In contrast to the concentration of blood urea nitrogen, the serum creatinine level is minimally influenced by factors (nitrogen balance, state of hydration) other than glomerular function. The serum creatinine is of value in estimating the GFR in the steady state only (e.g., a patient very

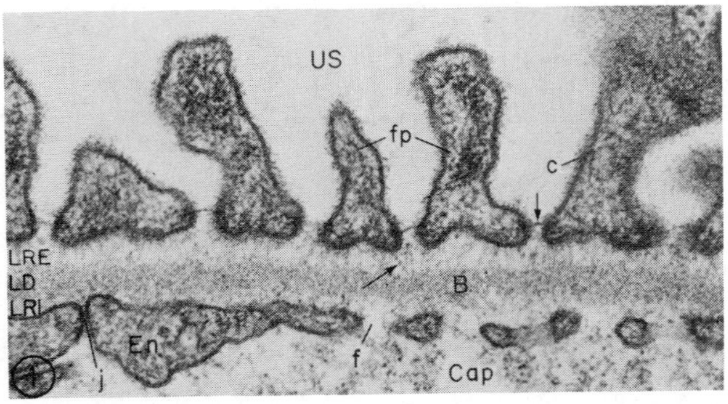

Figure 18–4. Electron micrograph of the normal glomerular capillary (Cap) wall demonstrating the endothelium (En) with its fenestrations (f), the glomerular basement membrane (B) with its central dense layer, the lamina densa (LD) and adjoining lamina rara interna (LRI) and externa (LRE; *long arrow*), and the epithelial cell foot processes (fp) with their thick cell coat (c). The glomerular filtrate passes through the endothelial fenestrae, crosses the basement membrane, and passes through the filtration slits *(short arrow)* between the epithelial cell foot processes to reach the urinary space (US). (× 60,000.) (From Farquhar MG, Kanwar YS: Functional organization of the glomerulus: State of the science in 1979. *In*: Cummings NB, Michael AF, Wilson CB [eds]: Immune Mechanisms in Renal Disease. New York, Plenum, 1982. Reprinted by permission.)

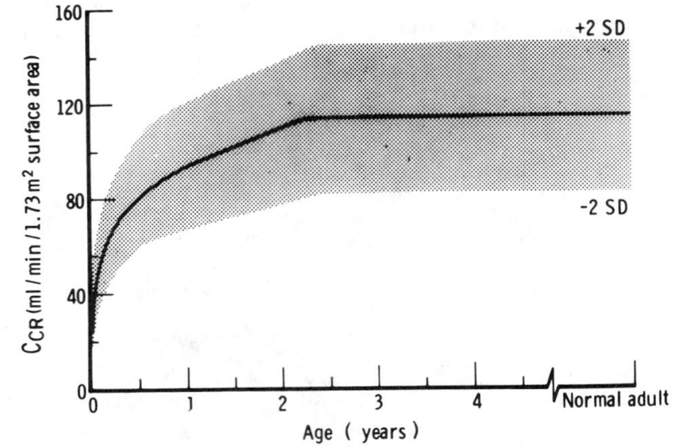

Figure 18–5. Changes in the normal value of the glomerular filtration rate, as measured by the creatinine clearance (C_{CR}), when standardized to mL/min/1.73 m^2 of body surface area. The *solid line* depicts the mean value, and the shaded area includes two standard deviations. (Reprinted by permission of the publishers from DEVELOPMENTAL NEPHROLOGY by Wallace McCrory. Cambridge, MA, Harvard University Press. Copyright © 1972 by the President and Fellows of Harvard College.)

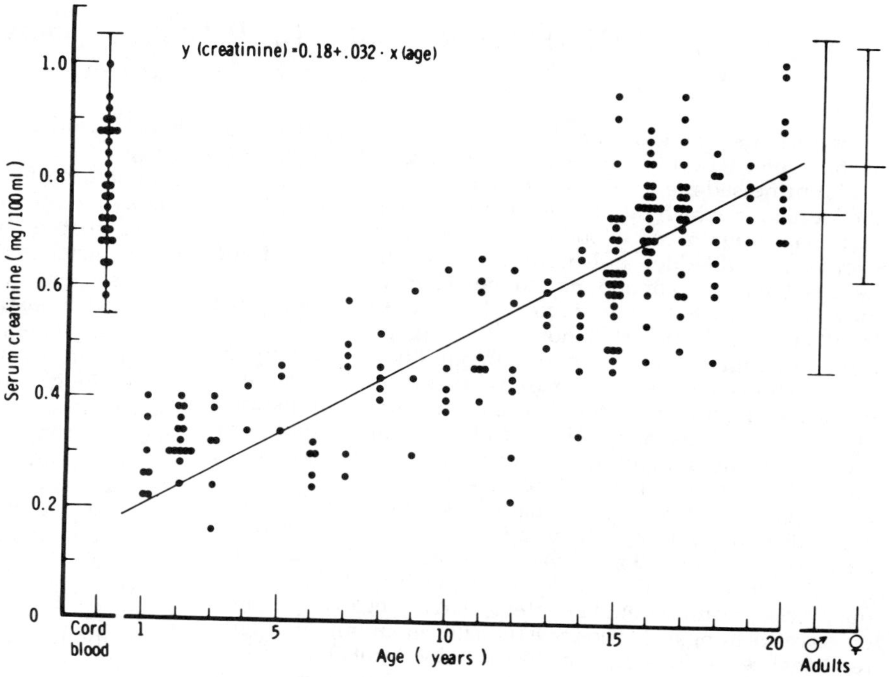

Figure 18–6. The serum creatinine in relation to age. (Reprinted by permission of the publishers from DEVELOPMENTAL NEPHROLOGY by Wallace McCrory. Cambridge, MA, Harvard University Press. Copyright © 1972 by the President and Fellows of Harvard College.)

shortly after the onset of acute renal failure and cessation of urine output may have a normal creatinine level but no effective renal function). The value of the serum creatinine is further compromised by the fact that its level does not rise above normal until the filtration rate falls below 70% of normal.

The precise measurement of the GFR is accomplished by quantitating the "clearance" of a substance that is freely filtered across the capillary wall and that is neither reabsorbed nor secreted by the tubules. The clearance (C_s) of such a substance(s) is that volume of plasma which, when completely "cleared" of the contained substance, would yield a quantity of that substance equal to that excreted in the urine over a specified time. The clearance is represented by the following formula:

$$C_s(\text{mL/min}) = \frac{U_s(\text{mg/mL})V(\text{mL/min})}{P_s(\text{mg/mL})}$$

where C_s equals the clearance of substance s, U_s reflects the urinary concentration of s, V represents the urinary flow rate, and P_s equals the plasma concentration of s. To correct the clearance for body surface area, the formula is:

$$\text{Corrected clearance} = C_s(\text{mL/min}) \times \frac{1.73}{\text{Patient's surface area (m}^2\text{)}}$$

The GFR is optimally measured by the clearance of inulin, a fructose polymer having a molecular weight of approximately 5,000. Because the inulin clearance technique is cumbersome, the GFR is commonly estimated by the clearance of endogenous creatinine. When the GFR is relatively normal, the creatinine clearance closely approximates the inulin clearance. However, as the GFR declines, an increasing proportion of the total creatinine in the urine is secreted by tubules, with the result that the creatinine clearance progressively overestimates the actual filtration rate. There is little merit, therefore, in measuring creatinine clearance when serum creatinine levels exceed 2.0 mg/dL (180 μmol/L); changes in renal function can then be monitored by the serum creatinine concentration.

The absence of plasma proteins larger than the size of albumin from the glomerular filtrate confirms the effectiveness of the glomerular capillary wall as a filtration barrier. Major factors restricting the filtration of these and other macromolecules include their size and their ionic charge.

Clearance studies of macromolecules in animals have shown no restriction to the filtration of molecules up to the size of inulin (molecular weight 5,000). As size increases further, filtration diminishes progressively, approaching zero for substances the size of albumin (molecular weight 68,000). Morphologic studies suggest that the size-selective filtration barrier resides within the GBM.

The endothelial cell, basement membrane, and epithelial cell of the glomerular capillary wall possess strong negative ionic charges. These anionic charges are a consequence of two negatively charged moieties: proteoglycans (heparan sulfate) and glycoproteins containing sialic acid. Proteins in the blood have a relatively low isoelectric point and carry a net negative charge. Consequently, they are repelled by the negatively charged sites in the glomerular capillary wall, thus restricting filtration.

Arant BS Jr: Postnatal development of renal function during the first year of life. Pediatr Nephrol 1:308, 1987.
Brenner BM, Bohrer MP, Baylis C, et al: Determinants of glomerular permselectivity: Insights derived from observations in vivo. Kidney Int 12:229, 1977.
Brenner BM, Hostetter TH, Humes HD: Glomerular permselectivity: Barrier function based on discrimination of molecular size and charge. Am J Physiol 234:F455, 1978.
Farquhar MG: The primary glomerular filtration barrier—basement membrane or epithelial slits? Kidney Int 8:197, 1975.
Michael AF, Keane WF, Raij L, et al: The glomerular mesangium. Kidney Int 17:141, 1980.
Renkin EM, Robinson RR: Glomerular filtration. N Engl J Med 290:785, 1974.
Venkatachalam MA, Rennke HG: The structural and molecular basis of glomerular filtration. Circ Res 43:337, 1978.

CONDITIONS PARTICULARLY ASSOCIATED WITH HEMATURIA

Hematuria may be gross (visible to the naked eye) or microscopic (detected only by dipstick or microscopic examination of the urine sediment). Gross hematuria may originate from the kidney, in which case it is generally brown or cola-colored and may contain red blood cell casts, or from the lower urinary tract (bladder and urethra), in which case the urine has a red to pink color and may contain clots. Gross hematuria may be associated with edema, hypertension, and renal insufficiency. This constellation of findings is typical of "the acute nephritic syndrome" and is frequently seen in patients with postinfectious (e.g., poststreptococcal) glomerulonephritis, systemic lupus erythematosus, membranoproliferative glomerulonephritis, anaphylactoid purpura, and rapidly progressive glomerulonephritis. The urine may be colored by pigments other than blood (Table 18–1).

In children, microscopic hematuria is most commonly discovered at periodic health examinations, by dipstick or by microscopic examination of the urine sediment. Because the quantitation of blood (actually hemoglobin) on dipsticks is not precise, results should be interpreted as negative (negative or trace readings) or positive (small, medium, and large readings). A positive dipstick test for blood calls for a urinalysis. Microscopic hematuria is defined as more than five red blood cells per high power field in the sediment from 10 mL of centrifuged freshly voided urine.

Asymptomatic microscopic hematuria is found in 0.5–2% of school-aged children, but whether screening for isolated microscopic hematuria can discover occult renal disease is unclear. Because of this uncertainty and its cost, screening urinalysis with microscopic examination of sediment for hematuria or pyuria seems unwarranted in asymptomatic children. On the other hand, a dipstick can detect blood or protein inexpensively, suggesting that this evaluation should be included in health maintenance routines.

Causes of hematuria are listed in Table 18–2. Children with gross hematuria should be hospitalized for evaluation because of the increased likelihood of finding hypertension and renal failure. Children having persistent microscopic hematuria (more than five red blood cells per high power field on three urinalyses at monthly intervals) should undergo further outpatient evaluation. The cost-effectiveness of such evaluation remains to be determined.

18.3 GLOMERULAR DISEASES

PATHOGENESIS. Glomerular injury may be the result of immunologic, inherited (presumably biochemical), or coagulation disorders. Immunologic injury is the most common cause and results in "glomerulonephritis," which is both a generic term for several diseases and a histopathologic term signifying inflammation of the glomerular capillaries. Evidence that glomerulonephritis is caused by immunologic injury includes (1) morphologic and immunopathologic similarities to experimental immune-mediated glomerulonephritis; (2) the demonstration of immune reactants (immunoglobulin and complement components) in glomeruli; and (3) abnormalities in serum complement and the finding of autoantibodies (e.g., anti–glomerular basement membrane [anti-GBM]) in some of these diseases. There appear to be two major mechanisms of immunologic injury: (1) localization of circulating antigen-antibody immune complexes; and (2) interaction of antibody with local antigen in situ. In the latter circumstance, the antigen may be a normal component of the glomerulus (e.g., the noncollagenous domain [NC-1] of type IV collagen, which is the putative antigen in human anti-GBM nephritis) or an antigen that has been planted in the glomerulus.

In immune complex–mediated diseases, antibody is produced against and combines with an antigen that is usually unrelated to the kidney. The immune complexes accumulate in glomeruli and activate the complement system, leading to immune injury. Experimental studies suggest that the complexes may be formed in the circulation and deposited in the kidney. Acute serum sickness in the rabbit is produced by a single intravenous injection of bovine albumin. Within 1 wk after injection, the rabbit produces antibody against bovine

TABLE 18–1. Urinary Hues

Dark Yellow
- Concentrated urine
- Bile pigments

Red
- Blood (red cells or hemoglobin)
- Myoglobin
- Porphyrins
- Beets
- Blackberries
- Red food coloring
- Phenolphthalein
- Urates
- Pyridium

Dark Brown or Black
- Blood
- Homogentisic acid

TABLE 18–2. Causes of Hematuria in Children

Glomerular Diseases
- Recurrent gross hematuria syndrome
  - IgA nephropathy
  - Idiopathic (benign familial) hematuria
  - Alport syndrome
- Acute poststreptococcal glomerulonephritis
- Membranous glomerulopathy
- Systemic lupus erythematosus
- Membranoproliferative glomerulonephritis
- Nephritis of chronic infection
- Rapidly progressive glomerulonephritis
- Goodpasture disease
- Anaphylactoid purpura
- Hemolytic-uremic syndrome

Infection
- Bacterial
- Tuberculosis
- Viral

Hematologic
- Coagulopathies
- Thrombocytopenia
- Sickle cell disease
- Renal vein thrombosis

Stones and Hypercalciuria

Anatomic Abnormalities
- Congenital anomalies
- Trauma
- Polycystic kidneys
- Vascular abnormalities
- Tumors

Exercise

Drugs

albumin, while the antigen remains in the blood in high concentration. As antibody enters the circulation, it forms immune complexes with antigen. While the amount of antigen in the circulation exceeds that of antibody (antigen excess), the complexes formed are small, remain soluble in the circulation, and are deposited in glomeruli. The processes involved in glomerular localization are not well understood but include attributes of the complex (concentration, charge, size), characteristics of the glomerulus (mesangial trapping, negatively charged capillary wall), hydrodynamic forces, and the influence of various mediators (angiotensin II, prostaglandins).

With deposition of immune complexes in glomeruli, rabbits develop an acute proliferative glomerulonephritis. Immunofluorescence microscopy demonstrates granular ("lumpy-bumpy") deposits containing immunoglobulin and complement in the glomerular capillary wall. Electron microscopic studies show these deposits to be on the epithelial side of the GBM and in the mesangium. Over the next few days, as additional antibody enters the circulation, the antigen is ultimately removed from the circulation and the glomerulonephritis subsides. In the rabbit, complement does not participate in the capillary injury, which is largely related to influx of macrophages. In other animal models, complement does play a role in capillary injury.

An example of in situ antigen-antibody interaction is anti-GBM antibody disease, in which antibody reacts with antigen(s) of the GBM. The antibody to GBM may be produced either in an animal species other than the one in which the disease will be produced (heterologous antibody) or in the host animal itself (autoantibodies) by immunization with GBM preparations. When rats are given an intravenous injection of anti-GBM antibody made in rabbits, the disease process evolves in two phases. In the initial or heterologous phase, rabbit antibody attaches to the rat GBM immediately after injection, fixing complement, and producing a mild glomerulonephritis with infiltration of polymorphonuclear leukocytes. The second or autologous phase begins a week later. This phase is due to the production by the host (rat) of antibody to the rabbit antibody fixed to the GBM. Fixation of host antibody to rabbit antibody also activates the complement and coagulation systems, producing a severe glomerulonephritis with crescent formation and infiltration of macrophages into the glomerulus. Immunopathologic studies reveal linear deposition of immunoglobulin and complement on the GBM, similar to that seen in Goodpasture disease and certain types of rapidly progressive glomerulonephritis. The severity of the second (autologous) phase can be markedly reduced if the animal is given anticoagulant therapy at the time of injection of the anti-GBM antibody.

The inflammatory reaction that follows immunologic injury results from activation of one or more biochemical mediation systems. Perhaps the most important of these is the complement system, which has two initiating sequences: (1) the classic pathway, which is activated by antigen-antibody immune complexes, and (2) the alternative or properdin pathway, which is activated by polysaccharides and endotoxin. These pathways converge at C3; from that point on, for both, the same sequence leads to lysis of cell membranes (see Fig. 11–1). The major noxious products of complement activation are produced after activation of C3 and include anaphylatoxin (which stimulates contractile proteins within vascular walls and increases vascular permeability) and chemotactic factors (C5a) that direct neutrophils and perhaps macrophages to the site of complement activation, where the cells release substances that damage vascular cells and basement membranes.

The coagulation system may be activated directly, following endothelial cell injury which bares the thrombogenic subendothelial layer (initiating the coagulation cascade), or indirectly, following complement activation. Fibrin deposits may occur within glomerular capillaries or within Bowman space in crescents. Activation of the coagulation process may activate the kinin system, which also produces chemotactic and anaphylatoxin-like factors.

PATHOLOGY. The glomerulus may be injured by several mechanisms but has only a limited number of histopathologic responses; accordingly, different disease states may produce similar microscopic changes.

Proliferation of glomerular cells occurs in most forms of glomerulonephritis and may be generalized, involving all glomeruli, or focal, involving only some glomeruli while sparing others. Within a single glomerulus, proliferation may be diffuse, involving all parts of the glomerulus, or segmental, involving only some areas but not others. Proliferation commonly involves the endothelial and mesangial cells and is frequently associated with an increase in the mesangial matrix. Immunofluorescent and electron microscopic studies indicate that mesangial proliferation may result from immune complex deposition within the mesangium. The resultant increase in cell size and number and in mesangial matrix may increase glomerular size and narrow the lumina of glomerular capillaries, leading to renal insufficiency.

Crescent formation in Bowman space (capsule) is a result of proliferation of parietal epithelial cells. Crescents develop in several forms of glomerulonephritis (termed "rapidly progressive") and are thought to be a response to fibrin deposited in Bowman space. New crescents contain fibrin, the proliferating epithelial cells of Bowman space, basement membrane-like material produced by these cells, and macrophages that may play a role in the genesis of glomerular injury. In days to weeks, the crescent is invaded by connective tissue (fibroepithelial crescent); this generally results in glomerular obsolescence. Crescent formation is frequently associated with glomerular cell death (necrosis). The necrotic glomerulus has a characteristic eosinophilic appearance with hematoxylin and eosin stain and usually contains nuclear remnants. Crescent formation is usually associated with generalized proliferation of the mesangial cells and with either immune complex or anti-GBM antibody deposition in the glomerular capillary wall.

In addition to proliferation, certain forms of acute glomerulonephritis show glomerular exudation of blood cells, most commonly neutrophils; eosinophils, basophils, and mononuclear cells may be seen in lesser numbers. The thickened appearance of GBM may result from a true increase in the width of the membrane (as seen in membranous glomerulopathy), from massive deposition of immune complexes which have staining characteristics similar to the membrane (as seen in systemic lupus erythematosus), or from the interposition of mesangial cells and matrix into the subendothelial space between the endothelial cells and the membrane. The latter may give the basement membrane a "split" appearance, as seen in type I membranoproliferative glomerulonephritis and other diseases.

Sclerosis refers to the presence of scar tissue within the glomerulus. Occasionally, pathologists will use this term to refer to an increase in mesangial matrix.

18.4 RECURRENT GROSS HEMATURIA OR PERSISTENT MICROSCOPIC HEMATURIA

In patients having a syndrome of recurrent gross hematuria (RGH), recurrent episodes of generally painless hematuria occur (mild flank pain may be felt). The gross hematuria usually develops 1–2 days after the onset of a presumably viral upper respiratory tract infection. This short latent period between the onset of infection and appearance of hematuria contrasts with the 7- to 14-day latent period seen in children

TABLE 18–3. Evaluation of the Child with Hematuria

Step 1: Studies Performed in All Patients
- Complete blood count
- Urine culture
- Serum creatinine level
- 24-hr urine collection for:
  - creatinine
  - protein
  - calcium
- Serum C3 level
- Ultrasound or intravenous pyelography

Step 2: Studies Performed in Selected Patients
- DNase B titer or streptozyme test if hematuria is of less than 6 mo duration
- Skin or throat cultures when appropriate
- ANA titer
- Urine erythrocyte morphology
- Coagulation studies/platelet count when suggested by history
- Sickle cell screen in all black patients
- Voiding cystourethrography with infection, or when a lower tract lesion is suspected

Step 3: Invasive Procedures

Renal biopsy indicated for:
1. Persistent high-grade microscopic hematuria
2. Microscopic hematuria plus any of the following:
   a. diminished renal function
   b. proteinuria exceeding 150 mg/24 hr (0.15 g/24 hr)
   c. hypertension
3. Second episode of gross hematuria

Cystoscopy indicated for:
pink to red hematuria, dysuria, and sterile urine culture

developing acute poststreptococcal glomerulonephritis. Patients with RGH do not usually have such manifestations of the acute nephritic syndrome as edema, hypertension, or renal insufficiency. Other patients have persistent microscopic hematuria without episodes of gross hematuria.

Patients having a first episode of gross hematuria are hospitalized and evaluated for other causes of hematuria (Table 18–3). In patients with RGH, routine radiographic and laboratory studies will fail to reveal a cause of hematuria. The gross hematuria resolves over 1–2 wk, but microscopic hematuria usually persists. Later, with another respiratory infection there is a recurrence of gross hematuria. Renal biopsy is indicated after the second episode, to determine the nature of any underlying disease, which will most frequently be IgA nephropathy, idiopathic hematuria, or familial nephritis (Alport syndrome).

IgA NEPHROPATHY (BERGER NEPHROPATHY). Patients with this disorder have glomerulonephritis with IgA as the predominant immunoglobulin in mesangial deposits, in the absence of any systemic disease such as systemic lupus erythematosus or anaphylactoid purpura.

Pathology and Pathogenesis. By light microscopy, most kidney biopsies reveal focal and segmental mesangial proliferation and increased matrix (Fig. 18–7). Some show generalized mesangial proliferation, occasionally associated with crescent formation and scarring. IgA is the predominant immunoglobulin deposited in the mesangium (Fig. 18–8), but lesser amounts of IgG, IgM, C3, and properdin are common. Electron microscopic studies confirm these findings.

Most evidence points to an immune complex etiology for IgA nephropathy. If the patient with IgA nephropathy has a kidney transplantation, the nephropathy commonly recurs in the transplanted kidney, indicating the systemic nature of this disorder.

Clinical and Laboratory Features. IgA nephropathy is more common in males than in females (2:1). Patients either present with an episode of gross hematuria or are found to have microscopic hematuria on routine examination. While the gross hematuria lasts, renal function usually remains relatively normal and proteinuria minimal (< 1 g/24 hr). Normal serum levels of C3 in IgA nephropathy help to distinguish this disorder from poststreptococcal glomerulonephritis.

Prognosis and Treatment. IgA nephropathy does not lead to significant kidney damage in most patients. Treatment is supportive and activity need not be restricted. Neither the number of episodes of gross hematuria nor the persistence of microscopic hematuria between episodes correlates with the likelihood of progressive disease. Progressive disease develops in 20% of patients, in whom a poor prognosis is associated with hypertension, diminished renal function, or proteinuria exceeding 1 g/24 hr between episodes of gross hematuria, or with histologic evidence of diffuse glomerulonephritis with crescents and scarring. Although controlled studies are lacking, immunosuppressive therapy may be beneficial in certain patients with progressive IgA nephropathy.

IDIOPATHIC HEMATURIA. Within the clinical spectrum of recurrent episodes of gross hematuria, *idiopathic* (benign familial) *hematuria* is defined histologically by normal findings on light and immunofluorescence microscopy. In some patients, electron microscopy demonstrates marked thinning of the GBM (thin basement membrane nephropathy), but the membrane width may be normal in others.

Idiopathic hematuria has an excellent prognosis, but long-term follow-up is required to exclude Alport syndrome. Both disorders may be familial and Alport syndrome may have minimal light microscopic changes, negative immunofluorescence, and thin basement membranes. In patients presumed to have idiopathic hematuria, the development of decreased renal function, proteinuria, or hypertension calls for a second renal biopsy.

ALPORT SYNDROME. This is the most common of several types of hereditary nephritis. There is marked variability in clinical presentation, natural history, histologic abnormalities, and genetic patterns.

Pathology. Kidney biopsies obtained during the first decade of life may show few changes by light microscopy. Later, the glomeruli may develop mesangial proliferation and capillary wall thickening, leading to progressive glomerular sclerosis. Tubular atrophy, interstitial inflammation and fibrosis, and foam cells (nonspecific lipid-laden tubular or interstitial cells) develop if the disease progresses. Immunopathologic studies are usually negative.

In most patients, electron microscopic studies have revealed thickening, thinning, splitting, and layering of the basement

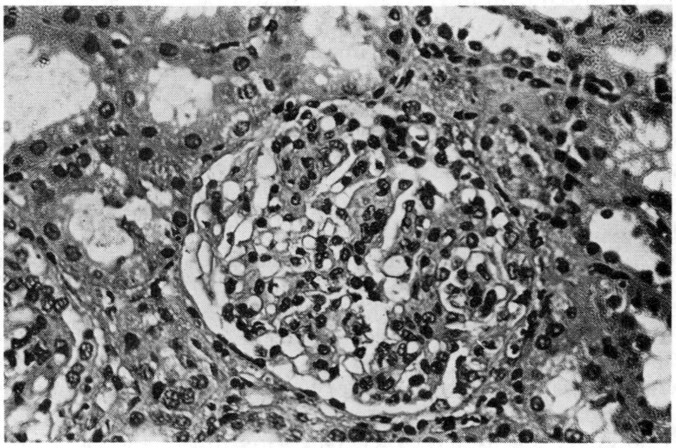

Figure 18–7. Light microscopy of IgA nephropathy demonstrating segmental mesangial proliferation and increased matrix. (× 180.)

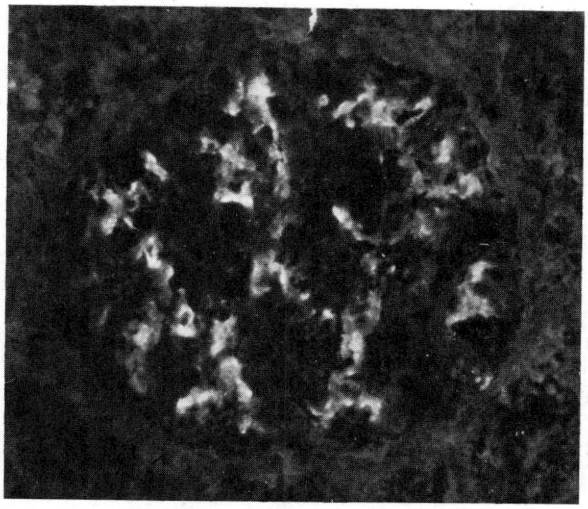

Figure 18–8. Immunofluorescence microscopy of the biopsy from a child having recurrent episodes of gross hematuria demonstrating mesangial deposition of IgA. (× 250.)

membranes of the glomeruli (Fig. 18–9) and tubules, but these lesions are not specific for Alport syndrome and may be absent in certain families that have the typical clinical manifestations of the syndrome.

Clinical Manifestations. Patients with Alport syndrome most commonly present with asymptomatic microscopic hematuria, but recurrent episodes of gross hematuria are not uncommon. In those with microscopic hematuria the development of proteinuria indicates the need for a kidney biopsy, which establishes the diagnosis.

Besides kidney involvement, a minority of patients have sensorineural hearing loss, which may begin in the high frequency range but progresses to involve the speech range and results in deafness. Approximately 10% of patients have eye abnormalities, the most frequent of which are cataracts, anterior lenticonus, and macular lesions.

Genetics. The inheritance of Alport syndrome best fits an X-linked dominant disorder. This explains the more severe clinical course in males than females. However, autosomal dominant transmission also has been described. Up to 20% of patients with Alport syndrome have no family history of renal disease; this suggests a high spontaneous mutation rate for the abnormal gene. The nature of the inherited defect is unknown; it may be related to the composition of membrane collagen.

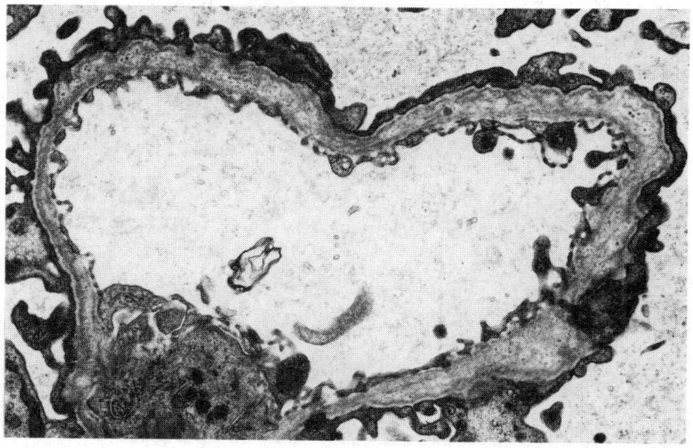

Figure 18–9. Electron micrograph of the biopsy from a child with Alport syndrome, depicting thickening, thinning, splitting, and layering of the glomerular basement membrane. (× 16,250.) (From Yum M, Bergstein JM: Basement membrane nephropathy. Hum Pathol 14:996, 1983. Used by permission.)

Complications. If renal function deteriorates, hypertension, urinary tract infections, and the manifestations of chronic renal failure may appear.

Prevention. Genetic counseling involving the entire family may limit propagation of the genetic abnormality.

Prognosis and Treatment. Males with Alport syndrome commonly develop end-stage renal failure in the 2nd or 3rd decade of life, occasionally in association with hearing loss. There is no specific therapy, but such patients are good candidates for dialysis and kidney transplantation. The development of anti-GBM nephritis in the transplanted kidneys of some patients with Alport syndrome suggests that the GBM of their native kidneys lacks a nephritogenic antigen. Females usually have a normal life span (for this reason, more mothers than fathers transmit the disease to their children) and only subclinical hearing loss.

IgA NEPHROPATHY

Andreoli SP, Bergstein JM: Treatment of severe IgA nephropathy in children. Pediatr Nephrol 3:248, 1989.

Andreoli SP, Yum MN, Bergstein JM: IgA nephropathy in children: Significance of glomerular basement membrane deposits of IgA. Am J Nephrol 6:28, 1986.

Levy M, Gonzalez-Burchard G, Broyer M, et al: Berger's disease in children. Medicine 64:157, 1985.

Wyatt RJ, Julian BA, Bhathena DB, et al: IgA nephropathy: Presentation, clinical course, and prognosis in children and adults. Am J Kidney Dis 4:192, 1984.

IDIOPATHIC HEMATURIA

Gauthier B, Trachtman H, Frank R, et al: Familial thin basement membrane nephropathy in children with asymptomatic microhematuria. Nephron 51:502, 1989.

Tiebosch ATMG, Frederik PM, Van Breda Vriesman PJC, et al: Thin-basement-membrane nephropathy in adults with persistent hematuria. N Engl J Med 320:14, 1989.

Yoshikawa N, White RHR, Cameron AH: Familial hematuria: Clinico-pathological correlations. Clin Nephrol 17:172, 1982.

Yum M, Bergstein JM: Basement membrane nephropathy: A new classification for Alport's syndrome and asymptomatic hematuria based on ultrastructural findings. Hum Pathol 14:996, 1983.

ALPORT SYNDROME

Bernstein J: The glomerular basement membrane abnormality in Alport's syndrome. Am J Kidney Dis 10:222, 1987.

Feingold J, Bois E: Genetics of Alport's syndrome. Pediatr Nephrol 1:436, 1987.

Grunfeld, J-P: The clinical spectrum of hereditary nephritis. Kidney Int 27:83, 1985.

Habib R, Gubler MC, Hinglais N, et al: Alport's syndrome: Experience at Hôpital Necker. Kidney Int 21:S-20, 1982.

Kashtan CE, Kleppel MM, Butkowski RJ, et al: Alport syndrome, basement membranes and collagen. Pediatr Nephrol 4:523, 1990.

18.5 ACUTE POSTSTREPTOCOCCAL GLOMERULONEPHRITIS

This disease is the classic example of the acute nephritic syndrome: the sudden onset of gross hematuria, edema, hypertension, and renal insufficiency. It was formerly the most common cause of gross hematuria in children, but its frequency has so declined during the last decade that IgA nephropathy now seems to be the most common cause of gross hematuria.

ETIOLOGY AND EPIDEMIOLOGY. Acute poststreptococcal glomerulonephritis follows infection of the throat or skin with certain "nephritogenic" strains of group A beta-hemolytic streptococci. The factors that allow only certain strains of streptococci to be "nephritogenic" remain unclear. During cold weather poststreptococcal glomerulonephritis commonly follows streptococcal pharyngitis, whereas during warm

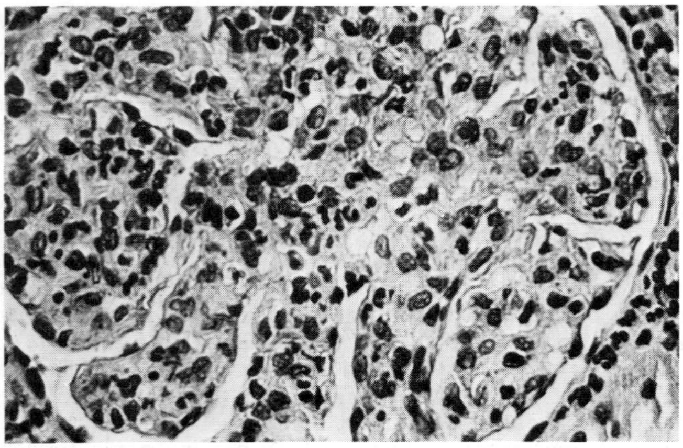

Figure 18–10. Glomerulus from a patient having poststreptococcal glomerulonephritis, appearing enlarged and relatively bloodless and showing mesangial proliferation and exudation of neutrophils. (× 400.)

weather the glomerulonephritis generally follows streptococcal skin infections or pyoderma. Epidemics of nephritis have been described in association with both throat (serotype 12) and skin (serotype 49) infections, but the disease is now most commonly sporadic.

PATHOLOGY. As in most forms of acute glomerulonephritis, the kidneys appear symmetrically enlarged. By light microscopy, all glomeruli appear enlarged and relatively bloodless and show diffuse mesangial cell proliferation with an increase in mesangial matrix (Fig. 18–10). Polymorphonuclear leukocytes are common in glomeruli during the early stage of the disease. Crescents and interstitial inflammation may be seen in severe cases. These changes are not specific for poststreptococcal glomerulonephritis.

Immunofluorescence microscopy reveals lumpy-bumpy deposits of immunoglobulin and complement on the GBMs and in the mesangium. By electron microscopy, electron-dense deposits, or "humps," are observed on the epithelial side of the GBM (Fig. 18–11).

PATHOGENESIS. Although morphologic studies and a depression in the serum complement (C3) level strongly suggest that poststreptococcal glomerulonephritis is mediated by immune complexes, the precise mechanisms whereby nephritogenic streptococci induce complex formation remain to be determined. Despite clinical and histologic similarities to acute serum sickness in the rabbit, the finding of circulating immune complexes in poststreptococcal glomerulonephritis is not uniform and complement activation is primarily through the alternative rather than the classic (immune complex–activated) pathway.

CLINICAL MANIFESTATIONS. Poststreptococcal glomerulonephritis is most common in children but rare before the age of 3 yr. The typical patient develops an acute nephritic syndrome 1–2 wk after an antecedent streptococcal infection. The severity of renal involvement may vary from asymptomatic microscopic hematuria with normal renal function to acute renal failure. Depending on the severity of renal involvement, patients may develop varying degrees of edema, hypertension, and oliguria. An encephalopathy or congestive heart failure or both may also develop. The edema is usually the result of salt and water retention, but a nephrotic syndrome may occur. Nonspecific symptoms such as malaise, lethargy, abdominal or flank pain, and fever are common. The acute phase generally resolves within 1 mo following onset, but urinary abnormalities may persist for more than 1 yr.

DIAGNOSIS. Urinalysis demonstrates red blood cells, frequently in association with red blood cell casts and proteinuria; polymorphonuclear leukocytes are not uncommon. A mild normochromic anemia may be present owing to hemodilution and low-grade hemolysis. The serum C3 level is usually reduced.

Confirmation of the diagnosis requires clear evidence of invasive streptococcal infection. Thus, positive throat cultures may support the diagnosis or may simply represent the carrier state. To document streptococcal infection properly, an elevated antibody titer to streptococcal antigen(s) should be confirmed. Although most commonly obtained, determination of the ASO titer may not be helpful because it rarely rises after streptococcal skin infections. The best single antibody titer to measure is that to the DNase B antigen. An alternative is the Streptozyme test (Wampole Laboratories, Stamford, CT), a slide agglutination procedure that detects antibodies to streptolysin O, DNase B, hyaluronidase, streptokinase, and NADase.

In the child with an acute nephritic syndrome, evidence of recent streptococcal infection, and a low C3 level, the clinical diagnosis of poststreptococcal glomerulonephritis is warranted and renal biopsy ordinarily is not indicated. It is important, however, to exclude systemic lupus erythematosus and an acute exacerbation of chronic glomerulonephritis. Considerations for renal biopsy would include the development of acute renal failure or nephrotic syndrome, the absence of evidence for streptococcal infection, the absence of hypocomplementemia, or the persistence of marked hematuria or proteinuria or both, diminished renal function, or a low C3 level for more than 3 mo after onset.

The differential diagnosis of poststreptococcal glomerulonephritis includes many of the causes of hematuria listed in Table 18–2. Acute glomerulonephritis may also follow infection with coagulase-positive and -negative staphylococci, *Streptococcus pneumoniae,* gram-negative bacteria, and certain fungal, rickettsial, and viral diseases.

COMPLICATIONS. The complications are those of acute

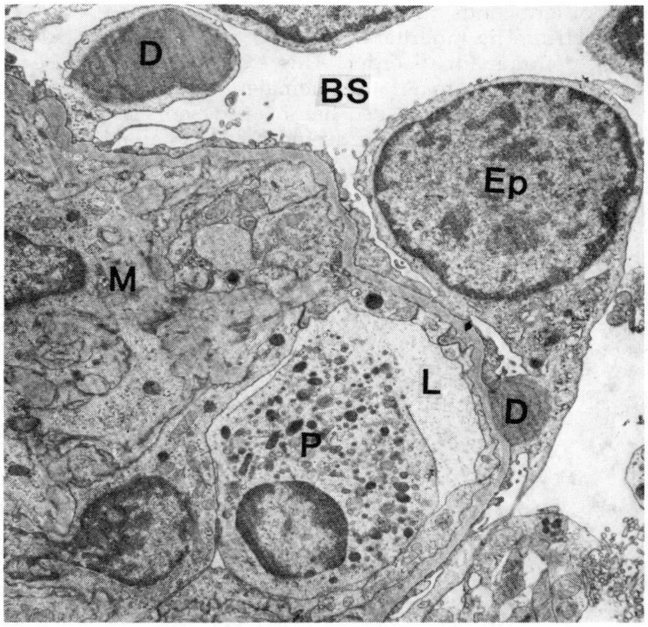

Figure 18–11. Electron micrograph in poststreptococcal glomerulonephritis, demonstrating electron-dense deposits (D) on the epithelial cell (EP) side of the glomerular basement membrane. A polymorphonuclear leukocyte (P) is present within the lumen (L) of the capillary. (BS = Bowman space; M = mesangium.)

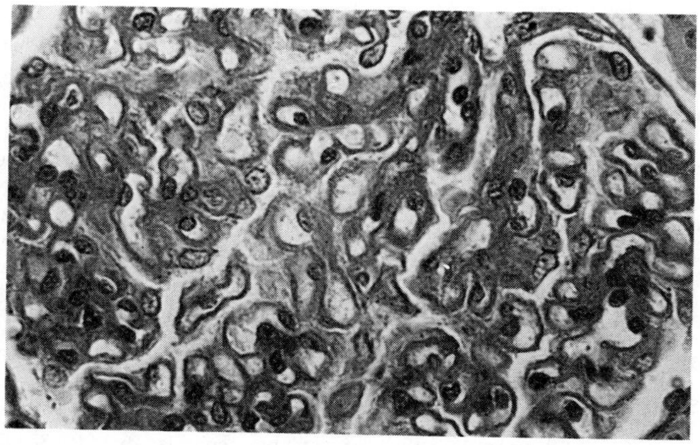

Figure 18–12. Glomerulus from a patient having membranous glomerulopathy, demonstrating diffuse thickening of the glomerular basement membrane in the absence of cellular proliferation. (× 400.)

renal failure and include volume overload, circulatory congestion, hypertension, hyperkalemia, hyperphosphatemia, hypocalcemia, acidosis, seizures, and uremia.

PREVENTION. Early systemic antibiotic therapy of streptococcal throat and skin infections will not eliminate the risk of glomerulonephritis. Family members of patients with acute glomerulonephritis should be cultured for group A beta-hemolytic streptococci and treated if culture-positive.

TREATMENT. As there is no specific therapy for acute poststreptococcal glomerulonephritis, the management is that of acute renal failure (see Sec. 18.35). Although a 10-day course of systemic antibiotic therapy, generally with penicillin, is recommended to limit the spread of the nephritogenic organisms, there is no evidence that antibiotic therapy affects the natural history of glomerulonephritis. Activity need not be restricted except during the acute phase of the disease when the complications of acute renal failure may be present, since activity has no detrimental effect on healing.

PROGNOSIS. Complete recovery occurs in more than 95% of children with acute poststreptococcal glomerulonephritis. There is no evidence that progression to chronic glomerulonephritis occurs. Infrequently, however, the acute phase may be very severe and lead to glomerular hyalinization and chronic renal insufficiency. Mortality in the acute stage can be avoided by appropriate management of the acute renal or cardiac failure. Recurrences are extremely rare.

Clark G, White RHR, Glasgow EF, et al: Poststreptococcal glomerulonephritis in children: Clinicopathological correlations and long-term prognosis. Pediatr Nephrol 2:381, 1988.

Heptinstall RH: Pathology of the Kidney. 3rd ed. Boston, Little, Brown, 1983.

Lange K, Seligson G, Cronin W: Evidence for the in situ origin of poststreptococcal glomerulonephritis: Glomerular localization of endostreptosin and the clinical significance of the subsequent antibody response. Clin Nephrol 19:3, 1983.

Vogl W, Renke M, Mayer-Eichberger D, et al: Long-term prognosis for endocapillary glomerulonephritis of poststreptococcal type in children and adults. Nephron 44:58, 1986.

18.6 MEMBRANOUS GLOMERULOPATHY (GLOMERULONEPHRITIS)

Membranous glomerulopathy is the most common cause of nephrotic syndrome in adults, but it is uncommon in childhood and a rare cause of hematuria.

PATHOLOGY. By light microscopy, the glomeruli show diffuse thickening of the GBM, without significant proliferative changes (Fig. 18–12). The thickening is presumably due to the production of membrane-like material by the visceral epithelial cells in response to immune complexes deposited on the epithelial side of the membrane. This new material may, in certain areas, appear as "spikes" on the epithelial side of the basement membrane. Immunofluorescent microscopy demonstrates granular deposits of IgG and C3, which electron microscopy shows to be located on the epithelial side of the membrane.

PATHOGENESIS. Morphologic studies suggest that membranous glomerulopathy is an immune complex–mediated disease, but the mechanism of complex formation and the nature of the antigen within the complexes remain unknown in most patients. Despite close clinical and histologic similarities to the experimental Heymann nephritis, attempts to demonstrate proximal tubular antigen in the deposits have been largely unsuccessful.

CLINICAL MANIFESTATIONS. In children, membranous glomerulopathy is most common in the 2nd decade of life. The disease usually presents as nephrotic syndrome. However, almost all patients have microscopic hematuria and occasional patients suffer gross hematuria. The blood pressure and C3 levels are normal.

DIAGNOSIS. The diagnosis is confirmed by kidney biopsy. The usual indications for biopsy include the presentation of nephrotic syndrome in a child over 8 yr of age or the presence of unexplained hematuria and proteinuria.

Membranous glomerulopathy may occasionally be seen in association with systemic lupus erythematosus, cancer, gold or penicillamine therapy, and syphilis and hepatitis B virus infections. These conditions should be considered in patients having membranous disease, since elimination of the presumed stimulus might lead to resolution of the glomerulopathy. Patients with membranous glomerulopathy are at increased risk of renal vein thrombosis.

TREATMENT. Fortunately, membranous glomerulopathy resolves spontaneously in the majority of children, although some may have persistent proteinuria. The nephrotic state is best controlled with salt restriction and diuretic agents. Studies in adults suggest that immunosuppressive therapy may retard the progressive renal insufficiency observed in some patients.

Cattran DC, Delmore T, Roscoe J, et al: A randomized controlled trial of prednisone in patients with idiopathic membranous nephropathy. N Engl J Med 320:210, 1989.

Kleinknecht C, Levy M, Gagnadoux MF, et al: Membranous glomerulonephritis with extra-renal disorders in children. Medicine 58:219, 1979.

Latham P, Poucell S, Koresaar A, et al: Idiopathic membranous glomerulopathy in Canadian children: A clinicopathologic study. J Pediatr 101:682, 1982.

Ponticelli C, Zucchelli P, Passerini P, et al: A randomized trial of methylprednisolone and chlorambucil in idiopathic membranous nephropathy. N Engl J Med 320:8, 1989.

Ramirez F, Brouhard BH, Travis LB, et al: Idiopathic membranous nephropathy in children. J Pediatr 101:677, 1982.

18.7 SYSTEMIC LUPUS ERYTHEMATOSUS

This systemic disease is characterized by fever, weight loss, rash, hematologic abnormalities, arthritis, and involvement of the heart, lungs, central nervous system, and kidneys. The nonrenal manifestations are discussed in Sec. 11.54. Kidney disease is one of the most common manifestations of lupus in childhood and may occasionally be the only manifestation.

PATHOGENESIS AND PATHOLOGY. Studies in a mouse (NZB/NZW) strain and in humans suggest that the clinical manifestations of lupus are mediated by immune complexes, which are formed in the circulation and deposited in various organs. Recent studies have revealed aberrations in both B-cell and T-cell function.

Of the several classifications of lupus nephritis, the one offered by the World Health Organization (WHO), which uses light, immunofluorescent, and electron microscopy, is most accepted. In patients with WHO class I nephritis, no histologic abnormalities are detected. In WHO class II (also called mesangial lupus nephritis), some glomeruli have mesangial deposits containing immunoglobulin and complement; light microscopy may be normal (class II-A) or show focal and segmental mesangial hypercellularity and increased matrix (class II-B).

WHO class III (also called focal proliferative lupus nephritis) shows mesangial deposits in almost all glomeruli, and subendothelial deposits (between the endothelial cells and GBM) in some. In addition to focal and segmental mesangial proliferation, occasional glomeruli show capillary wall necrosis and crescent formation.

WHO class IV (also called diffuse proliferative lupus nephritis) is the most common and most severe form of lupus nephritis. All glomeruli contain massive mesangial and subendothelial deposits of immunoglobulin and complement. By light microscopy, all glomeruli show mesangial proliferation. The capillary walls are frequently thickened (owing to subendothelial deposits), creating the "wire-loop" lesion, and commonly show necrosis, crescent formation, and scarring.

WHO class V (also called membranous lupus nephritis) is the least common form of lupus nephritis; it resembles idiopathic membranous glomerulopathy histologically, except for mild to moderate mesangial proliferation.

Transformation of the histologic lesion from one class to another (usually to a more severe class) is common, especially in inadequately treated patients.

CLINICAL MANIFESTATIONS. The large majority of children with systemic lupus are adolescent girls who present with evidence of systemic disease, leading to the ultimate diagnosis. The clinical findings in patients having the milder forms (all class II, some class III) of lupus nephritis include hematuria, normal renal function, and proteinuria of less than 1 g/24 hr. Some patients with class III and all with class IV nephritis have hematuria and proteinuria, with reduced renal function, nephrotic syndrome, or acute renal failure. In some patients with proliferative glomerulonephritis, the finding of normal urinary sediment obscures the renal involvement. Patients with class V nephritis commonly have a nephrotic syndrome.

DIAGNOSIS. The diagnosis of lupus is suggested by the detection of circulating antinuclear antibodies and is confirmed by demonstrating that these antibodies react with native (double-stranded) DNA. In most patients with active disease, C3 and C4 levels are depressed. In view of the lack of clear correlation between the clinical manifestations and the severity of the renal involvement, renal biopsy should be done in all patients with lupus. The findings will guide the selection of immunosuppressive therapy.

TREATMENT. Immunosuppressive therapy in lupus nephritis aims at clinical and serologic remission (normalization of the anti-DNA, C3, and C4 levels). Therapy is initiated in all patients with prednisone, 60 mg/m^2/day, divided into three or four doses. In patients having more severe forms of nephritis (some class III, all class IV), azathioprine is added in a once daily dosage of 2–3 mg/kg. When serologic remission is obtained after 1–2 mo, the dose of prednisone is reduced to 60 mg/m^2 taken every other day as a single morning dose, being certain that the serologic studies remain normal and renal function stable while the dose is reduced. After a varying period of time, the dose may then be further reduced by 5 mg decrements to 30 mg/m^2, so long as serologic studies remain normal and renal function stable. The dose of azathioprine may be reduced gradually while serology and renal function are monitored, and may be discontinued after 1 yr. Studies in adults suggest that monthly intravenous infusions of cyclophosphamide may also be effective in corticosteroid-unresponsive or -toxic patients.

PROGNOSIS. Aggressive immunosuppressive therapy has dramatically improved the prognosis of lupus in childhood; but the disease is controlled, not cured. The risk of relapse, as well as the side effects of chronic immunosuppressive therapy, persists; of special concern are the effects of corticosteroids in teenaged girls. Patients with lupus should be managed in conjunction with specialists in medical centers where both medical and psychologic support can be given to both patients and their families.

Appel GB, Cohen DJ, Pirani C, et al: Long-term follow-up of patients with lupus nephritis. Am J Med 83:877, 1987.
Balow JE, Austin HA, Muenz LR, et al: Effect of treatment on the evolution of renal abnormalities in lupus nephritis. N Engl J Med 311:491, 1984.
Cameron JS: The treatment of lupus nephritis. Pediatr Nephrol 3:350, 1989.
Laitman RS, Glicklich D, Sablay L, et al: Effect of long-term normalization of serum complement levels on the course of lupus nephritis. Am J Med 87:132, 1989.
McCune WJ, Golbus J, Zeldes W, et al: Clinical and immunologic effects of monthly administration of intravenous cyclophosphamide in severe systemic lupus erythematosus. N Engl J Med 318:1423, 1988.
Schwartz MM, Shu-ping L, Bonsib SM, et al: Clinical outcome of three discrete histologic patterns of injury in severe lupus glomerulonephritis. Am J Kidney Dis 13:273, 1989.
Steinberg AD: The treatment of lupus nephritis. Kidney Int 30:769, 1986.

18.8 MEMBRANOPROLIFERATIVE (MESANGIOCAPILLARY) GLOMERULONEPHRITIS

The term "chronic glomerulonephritis" implies continuing glomerular injury, such as frequently leads to glomerular destruction and end-stage renal failure. Membranoproliferative glomerulonephritis is the most common cause of chronic glomerulonephritis in older children and young adults.

PATHOLOGY AND PATHOGENESIS. Membranoproliferative glomerulonephritis was initially distinguished from other forms of chronic glomerulonephritis by the finding of hypocomplementemia, in some patients the result of an antibody (called C3 nephritic factor) that activates the alternative complement pathway. Not all patients have hypocomplementemia. Three histologic types are described.

Type I membranoproliferative glomerulonephritis is the most common form; the glomeruli reveal an accentuation of the lobular pattern, due to a generalized increase in mesangial cells and matrix (Fig. 18–13). The glomerular capillary walls appear thickened and, in some areas, duplicated or split, owing to interposition of mesangial cytoplasm and matrix between the endothelial cells and GBM. Crescents may be present; when detected in a high percentage of glomeruli, they indicate a poor prognosis. Immunofluorescent microscopy reveals C3 and lesser amounts of immunoglobulin in the mesangium and along the peripheral capillary walls in a lobular pattern (Fig. 18–14), and electron microscopy confirms the presence of immune complex–like deposits in the mesangial and subendothelial regions.

In type II disease, the mesangial changes are less prominent than in type I. The capillary walls demonstrate irregular ribbon-like thickening, owing to dense deposits. Splitting of the membrane is rare, but crescents are common. By electron microscopy, the dense deposits are seen as thickenings of GBM in the region of but distinct from the lamina densa. The deposits are also found in Bowman capsule, mesangium, and tubular basement membranes; their composition is unknown. Immunofluorescent studies show C3, usually with minimal immunoglobulin, along the margin of the dense deposit material.

In type III disease, the light and immunofluorescent microscopic findings resemble those found in type I disease. Electron microscopy reveals contiguous subepithelial and suben-

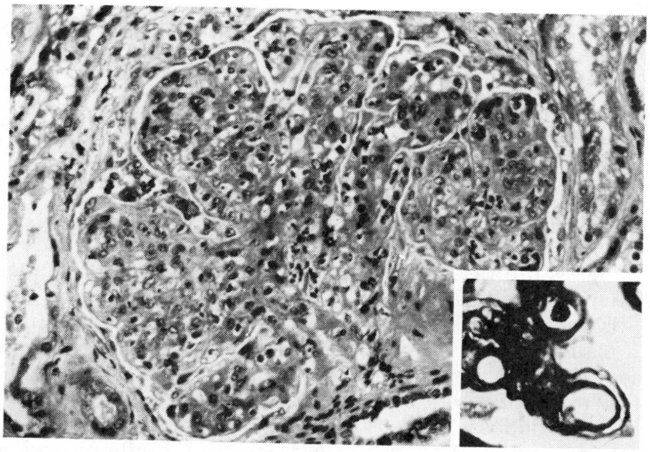

Figure 18–13. Glomerulus from a patient with type I membranoproliferative glomerulonephritis, demonstrating an accentuated lobular pattern, a generalized increase in mesangial cells and matrix, and "splitting" of the glomerular capillary wall *(inset).* (× 250.) (From Kim Y, Michael AF: Idiopathic membranoproliferative glomerulonephritis. Reproduced, with permission, from the Annual Review of Medicine, Vol 31. © 1980 by Annual Reviews, Inc.)

dothelial deposits, associated with disruption and layering of the lamina densa portion of the basement membrane.

CLINICAL MANIFESTATIONS. Membranoproliferative glomerulonephritis is most common in the second decade of life. The majority of patients present with mild nephrotic syndrome, others with gross hematuria or asymptomatic microscopic hematuria and proteinuria. Renal function may be normal to depressed. Hypertension is common. The serum C3 complement level may be decreased.

DIAGNOSIS AND DIFFERENTIAL DIAGNOSIS. The diagnosis of membranoproliferative glomerulonephritis is made by renal biopsy. Indications for biopsy include onset of nephrotic syndrome in a child more than 8 yr of age, or persistent microscopic hematuria and proteinuria.

Both membranoproliferative glomerulonephritis and poststreptococcal glomerulonephritis may present gross hematuria, low C3 levels, and elevated antistreptococcal antibody titers (coincidental in patients with membranoproliferative disease); their natural histories will distinguish between the two. Patients with poststreptococcal glomerulonephritis will improve dramatically within 2 mo of onset, whereas in children having membranoproliferative glomerulonephritis, persistent clinical manifestations will lead to kidney biopsy.

PROGNOSIS AND TREATMENT. The outlook for all types of membranoproliferative disease is poor. Complete recovery has been reported, but most patients with type II and many patients with types I and III progress to end-stage renal failure. Types I and II membranoproliferative glomerulonephritis have been found to recur in patients with kidney transplants, suggesting the presence of systemic disorder.

No definitive therapy exists, but stabilization of the clinical course has been reported in some patients receiving long-term alternate-day prednisone therapy and in others treated with inhibitors of platelet function.

Bennett WM, Fassett RG, Walker RG, et al: Mesangiocapillary glomerulonephritis type II (dense-deposit disease): Clinical features of progressive disease. Am J Kidney Dis 13:496, 1989.

Cameron JS, Turner DR, Heaton J, et al: Idiopathic mesangiocapillary glomerulonephritis. Am J Med 74:175, 1983.

Donadio JV Jr, Anderson CF, Mitchell JC, et al: Membranoproliferative glomerulonephritis. A prospective clinical trial of platelet-inhibitor therapy. N Engl J Med 310:1421, 1984.

Kim Y, Michael AF: Idiopathic membranoproliferative glomerulonephritis. Annu Rev Med 31:273, 1980.

Strife CF, Jackson EC, McAdams AJ: Type III membranoproliferative glomerulonephritis: Long-term clinical and morphologic evaluation. Clin Nephrol 21:323, 1984.

West CD: Childhood membranoproliferative glomerulonephritis: An approach to management. Kidney Int 29:1077, 1986.

18.9 GLOMERULONEPHRITIS OF CHRONIC INFECTION

Occurrence of glomerulonephritis has been recognized during the course of various chronic infections, including subacute bacterial endocarditis (*S. viridans* and other organisms), infected ventriculoatrial shunts for hydrocephalus *(Staphylococcus epidermidis)*, syphilis, hepatitis B, candidiasis, and malaria. In each condition, the infecting organism has low virulence, and the host is chronically seeded with foreign antigen. In the presence of high levels of circulating antigen, the host's antibody response leads to formation of immune complexes, which deposit in the kidneys and initiate the glomerulonephritis.

The histopathologic findings may resemble poststreptococcal, membranous, or membranoproliferative glomerulonephritis. The clinical manifestations are generally those of an acute nephritic or nephrotic syndrome. The C3 level is frequently depressed.

Eradication of the infection before severe glomerular injury occurs usually results in resolution of the glomerulonephritis. Progression to end-stage renal failure has been described.

Arze RS, Rashid H, Morley R, et al: Shunt nephritis: Report of two cases and review of the literature. Clin Nephrol 19:48, 1983.

Chesney RW, O'Regan S, Guyda HJ, et al: Candida endocrinopathy syndrome with membranoproliferative glomerulonephritis: Demonstration of glomerular candida antigen. Clin Nephrol 5:232, 1976.

Collins AB, Bhan AK, Dienstag JL, et al: Hepatitis B immune complex glomerulonephritis: Simultaneous glomerular deposition of hepatitis B surface and e antigens. Clin Immunol Immunopathol 26:137, 1983.

Hendrickse RG, Adeniyi A: Quartan malarial nephrotic syndrome in children. Kidney Int 16:64, 1979.

Neugarten J, Baldwin DS: Glomerulonephritis in bacterial endocarditis. Am J Med 77:297, 1984.

O'Regan S, Fong JSC, de Chadarevian JP, et al: Treponemal antigens in congenital and acquired syphilitic nephritis. Ann Intern Med 85:325, 1976.

18.10 RAPIDLY PROGRESSIVE (CRESCENTIC) GLOMERULONEPHRITIS

The term "rapidly progressive" describes the clinical course of several forms of glomerulonephritis whose unifying abnor-

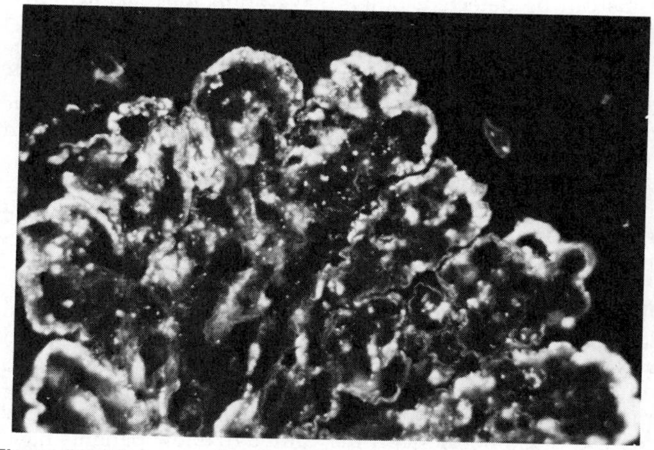

Figure 18–14. Immunofluorescence microscopy in type I membranoproliferative glomerulonephritis, demonstrating granular deposition of C3 along the glomerular basement membranes and in the mesangium. (× 610.) (From Kim Y, Michael AF: Idiopathic membranoproliferative glomerulonephritis. Reproduced, with permission, from the Annual Review of Medicine, Vol 31. © 1980 by Annual Reviews, Inc.)

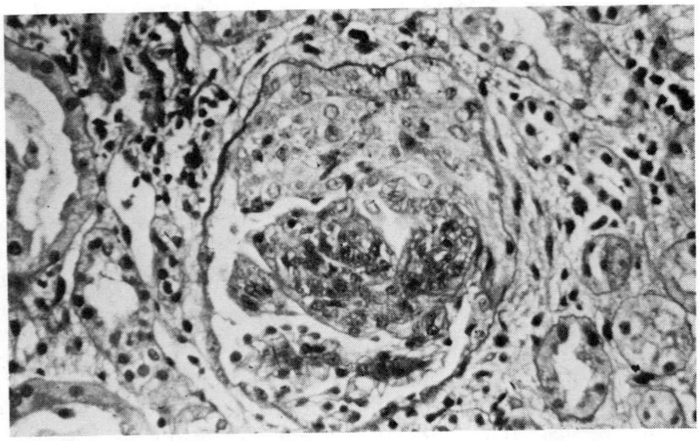

Figure 18–15. Light micrograph of a biopsy specimen from a child with anaphylactoid purpura glomerulonephritis, demonstrating a crescent overlying the glomerulus. (× 180.)

mality is the presence of crescents in the majority of glomeruli. The natural history in most forms is rapid progression to end-stage renal failure.

CLASSIFICATION. Crescents may be found in several well-defined types of glomerulonephritis, such as poststreptococcal, lupus, membranoproliferative, and the glomerulonephritides of Goodpasture disease or anaphylactoid purpura. In these diseases, the typical findings on light, immunofluorescent, and electron microscopic examinations are maintained despite crescent formation, and these histologic findings, in conjunction with appropriate laboratory studies, should reveal the underlying disease. After these recognized forms of glomerulonephritis are excluded, an idiopathic variety of rapidly progressive disease remains.

PATHOLOGY AND PATHOGENESIS. Crescents are found on the inside of Bowman capsule and are composed of the proliferating epithelial cells of the capsule, and of fibrin, basement membrane–like material, and macrophages (Fig. 18–15). The stimulus for crescent formation is presumed to be the deposition of fibrin in Bowman space, probably as a result of necrosis or disruption of the glomerular capillary wall.

In many patients having the idiopathic variety of rapidly progressive disease, no evidence for immunologic mechanisms can be detected; others have antibodies against GBM or deposits of immune complexes on capillary walls. The C3 level is normal.

CLINICAL MANIFESTATIONS. Most patients develop acute renal failure, often after an acute nephritic or nephrotic episode. Progression to end-stage renal failure follows within weeks to months after onset.

DIAGNOSIS AND DIFFERENTIAL DIAGNOSIS. Appropriate serologic studies (ANA, C3, anti-DNase B titers) should be obtained to search for defined types of glomerulonephritis. The diagnosis is confirmed by kidney biopsy.

PROGNOSIS AND TREATMENT. Children having rapidly progressive disease associated with poststreptococcal glomerulonephritis may recover spontaneously. We have had success in treating the rapidly progressive nephritis of lupus and of anaphylactoid purpura with prednisone and azathioprine. The prognosis is poor for the remaining types of rapidly progressive glomerulonephritis, although a few patients have been reported to improve with therapy combining immunosuppressive agents, anticoagulants, and plasmapheresis.

Couser WG: Rapidly progressive glomerulonephritis: Classification, pathogenic mechanisms, and therapy. Am J Kidney Dis 11:449, 1988.
Miller MN, Baumal R, Poucell S, et al: Incidence and prognostic importance of glomerular crescents in renal diseases of childhood. Am J Nephrol 4:244, 1984.
Salant DJ: Immunopathogenesis of crescentic glomerulonephritis and lung purpura. Kidney Int 32:408, 1987.
Southwest Pediatric Nephrology Study Group: A clinico-pathologic study of crescentic glomerulonephritis in 50 children. Kidney Int 27:450, 1985.

18.11 GOODPASTURE DISEASE

Goodpasture disease (pulmonary hemorrhage and glomerulonephritis associated with antibodies against lung and against GBM) should be distinguished from Goodpasture syndrome (a clinical picture of pulmonary hemorrhage and glomerulonephritis that may be seen with several disorders, including systemic lupus erythematosus, anaphylactoid purpura, polyarteritis nodosa, and Wegener granulomatosis). In some patients, anti-GBM nephritis occurs without pulmonary hemorrhage as one form of rapidly progressive glomerulonephritis.

PATHOLOGY. In most patients, the changes on light microscopy resemble those of rapidly progressive glomerulonephritis; immunofluorescent microscopy shows a continuous linear pattern of IgG along the GBM, typical of anti-GBM antibody (Fig. 18–16).

CLINICAL MANIFESTATIONS. Goodpasture disease is extremely rare in childhood. Hemoptysis is usually the presenting complaint, and pulmonary hemorrhage is a potential cause of death. In days to weeks, hematuria, proteinuria, and progressive renal failure develop. The C3 level is normal.

DIAGNOSIS. The diagnosis is suggested by kidney biopsy. Other diseases that may show linear GBM staining for IgG are excluded when serum is found to contain anti-GBM antibody.

PROGNOSIS AND TREATMENT. Patients who survive the pulmonary hemorrhage commonly progress to end-stage renal failure. No definitive therapy exists; some patients have improved following combined immunosuppression and plasmapheresis.

Briggs WA, Johnson JP, Teichman S, et al: Antiglomerular basement membrane antibody-mediated glomerulonephritis and Goodpasture's syndrome. Medicine 58:348, 1979.
Herman PG, Balikian JP, Seltzer SE, et al: The pulmonary-renal syndrome. Am J Roentgenol 130:1141, 1978.
Simpson IJ, Doak PB, Williams LC, et al: Plasma exchange in Goodpasture's syndrome. Am J Nephrol 2:301, 1982.

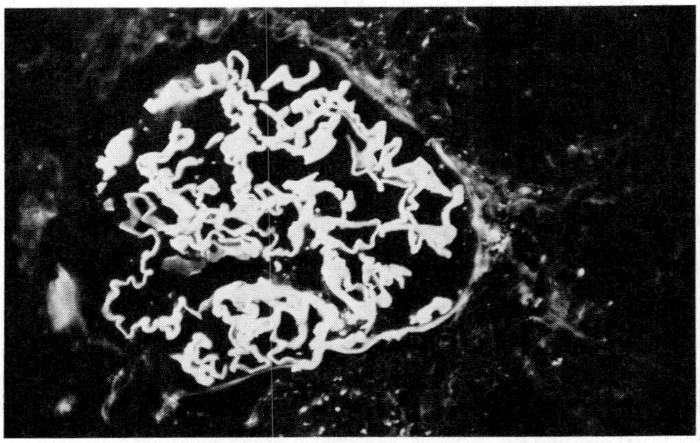

Figure 18–16. Immunofluorescence micrograph demonstrating the continuous linear staining of IgG along the glomerular basement membrane, as found in diseases mediated by antiglomerular basement membrane antibody. (× 250.)

18.12 ANAPHYLACTOID (HENOCH-SCHÖNLEIN) PURPURA GLOMERULONEPHRITIS

Anaphylactoid purpura is the most common form of systemic vasculitis in children. It is presumably an immune complex–mediated disease, but the precise etiology is unclear (see Sec. 11.56).

PATHOLOGY. Anaphylactoid purpura is a vasculitis of the smallest blood vessels. Perivascular accumulation of white blood cells may be seen in several organs, and in the majority of patients with renal involvement, there are focal and segmental increases in mesangial cells and matrix. A minority of patients show generalized mesangial changes, and rare patients will have diffuse necrotizing glomerulitis with crescent formation.

Immunofluorescent microscopy reveals mesangial deposits of IgA, frequently in association with IgG, C3, and fibrin. The predominant deposition of IgA suggests a relationship to IgA nephropathy. Electron microscopy confirms the presence of mesangial deposits and may also reveal deposits along the capillary wall in the subendothelial space.

CLINICAL MANIFESTATIONS. The typical patient presents with an urticarial and/or purpuric rash on the buttocks and lower extremities, arthritis or arthralgias, and abdominal pain. Intussusception or perforation of the bowel may occur. Evidence for renal involvement is usually detected within 1 mo of onset but may appear later.

Clinical evidence of kidney disease develops in approximately 50% of patients. A large majority have only mild renal involvement, characterized by hematuria, preserved renal function, and proteinuria of less than 2 g/24 hr. Patients with severe kidney involvement have diminished renal function and heavy proteinuria and frequently a nephrotic syndrome.

DIAGNOSIS. The disease is usually defined by the clinical constellation of the typical rash and abdominal and joint complaints, with normal platelet count and C3 level and absence of antinuclear antibodies in serum.

Renal involvement is usually mild and kidney biopsy rarely necessary. Indications for biopsy include diminished renal function, proteinuria exceeding 2 g/24 hr, or development of a nephrotic syndrome.

PROGNOSIS AND TREATMENT. In most patients, the clinical manifestations resolve completely over several months, although microscopic hematuria may persist for more than 1 yr. With severe renal involvement, especially when biopsy shows the morphologic picture of rapidly progressive glomerulonephritis, the ultimate prognosis is extremely poor. No form of therapy is reliably effective in patients having severe renal involvement, but dramatic improvement occurs in some such patients following treatment with prednisone and azathioprine.

Allen DM, Diamond LK, Howell DA: Anaphylactoid purpura in children (Schönlein-Henoch syndrome). Am J Dis Child 99:833, 1960.
Meadow SR: The prognosis of Henoch-Schönlein nephritis. Clin Nephrol 9:87, 1978.
Meadow SR, Glasgow EF, White RHR, et al: Schönlein-Henoch nephritis. Q J Med 4:241, 1972.
Sinniah R, Feng PH, Chen BTM: Henoch-Schönlein syndrome: A clinical and morphological study of renal biopsies. Clin Nephrol 9:219, 1978.

18.13 HEMOLYTIC-UREMIC SYNDROME

The hemolytic-uremic syndrome is the most common cause of acute renal failure in young children, and the incidence is increasing. It was initially believed to be a renal disorder with secondary hematologic manifestations, but recent studies indicate that the syndrome should be regarded as a systemic disease.

ETIOLOGY. The precise etiology of the disease is unknown. It has been associated with bacterial (*Shigella, Salmonella, E. coli [especially 0157:H7], S. pneumoniae), Bartonella,* and viral (coxsackie, ECHO, influenza, varicella, Epstein-Barr) infections and with endotoxemia. It has been reported also to follow use of oral contraceptives and pyran copolymer, an inducer of interferon. In addition, a hemolytic-uremic type of disorder has been reported to be associated with systemic lupus erythematosus, malignant hypertension, pre-eclampsia, postpartum renal failure, and radiation nephritis. There may be an absence of a plasma factor that stimulates endothelial cell prostacyclin production. There are several reports of occurrence in more than one member of a family, but the role of genetic factors in predisposition to the disease is unknown.

PATHOLOGY. The initial changes in the glomeruli include thickening of the capillary walls, narrowing of the capillary lumina, and widening of the mesangium. Electron microscopy shows these changes to be the result of subendothelial and mesangial deposition of a granular, amorphous material of unknown origin. Fibrin thrombi can be found in glomerular capillaries and arterioles and may lead to cortical necrosis.

Severely involved glomeruli progress to partial or total sclerosis; severe vascular involvement may render others obsolescent from ischemia. In these severely involved small arteries and arterioles, concentric intimal proliferation leads to vascular occlusion.

PATHOGENESIS. The primary event in pathogenesis of the syndrome appears to be endothelial cell injury. Capillary and arteriolar endothelial injury in the kidney leads to localized clotting. Evidence for disseminated intravascular coagulation is commonly lacking. The microangiopathic anemia results from mechanical damage to the red blood cells as they pass through the altered vasculature. Thrombocytopenia is due to intrarenal platelet adhesion or damage. Damaged red cells and platelets are removed from circulation by the liver and spleen.

CLINICAL MANIFESTATIONS. The syndrome is most common in children under the age of 4 yr. The onset is usually preceded by gastroenteritis (fever, vomiting, diarrhea, which is often bloody) or, less commonly, by an upper respiratory tract infection. This is followed in 5–10 days by the sudden onset of pallor, irritability, weakness, lethargy, and oliguria. Physical examination may reveal dehydration, edema, petechiae, hepatosplenomegaly, and marked irritability.

DIAGNOSIS AND DIFFERENTIAL DIAGNOSIS. The diagnosis of the syndrome is supported by the findings of a microangiopathic hemolytic anemia, thrombocytopenia, and acute renal failure. The hemoglobin is commonly in the range of 5–9 g/dL (50–90 g/L). The blood film reveals helmet cells, burr cells, and fragmented red blood cells (see Sec. 16.83). Plasma hemoglobin levels are elevated and plasma haptoglobin levels diminished. The reticulocyte count is moderately elevated; Coombs test is negative. The white blood cell count may rise to 30,000/mm^3 (30 × 10^9/L). Thrombocytopenia (20,000–100,000/mm^3; 10^9/L) occurs in more than 90% of patients. Findings on urinalysis are surprisingly mild and usually consist of low-grade microscopic hematuria and proteinuria. Partial thromboplastin time and prothrombin time are usually normal; their prolongation is more commonly due to vitamin K deficiency than to disseminated intravascular coagulation. The severity of the renal involvement, and the complications thereof, vary from mild renal insufficiency to acute renal failure requiring dialysis.

The sudden onset of acute renal failure in a child should always call this entity to mind. The typical history, clinical picture, and laboratory findings confirm the diagnosis in most patients. Other causes of acute renal failure, especially those that can be associated with a microangiopathic anemia (lupus, malignant hypertension), should be excluded. Except in the rare patient who suffers prolonged renal failure (more than 2 wk) or who fails to develop thrombocytopenia, a renal biopsy is rarely indicated; it cannot be performed in the thrombocytopenic patient.

Patients who have bilateral renal vein thrombosis (see Sec. 18.15) may be difficult to distinguish from those with the hemolytic-uremic syndrome. Both disorders may be preceded by gastroenteritis, and in both the children may present with dehydration, pallor, and evidence of microangiopathic hemolytic anemia, thrombocytopenia, and acute renal failure. The marked enlargement of kidneys of the child with renal vein thrombosis helps to distinguish the disorders, but angiography may be necessary in obscure cases.

COMPLICATIONS. Complications may include anemia, acidosis, hyperkalemia, fluid overload, congestive heart failure, hypertension, and uremia. In addition, extrarenal involvement may include central nervous system manifestations (irritability, seizures, coma), colitis (melena, perforation), diabetes mellitus, and rhabdomyolysis. The pathogenesis of these complications is unknown; they seem likely to be the result of intravascular thrombosis.

PROGNOSIS AND TREATMENT. With aggressive management of the acute renal failure, more than 90% of patients survive the acute phase and the majority of these recover normal renal function. It has been difficult to evaluate the results of therapy. Corticosteroids appear to have no value, and experience with platelet inhibitors is so far inconclusive. The treatment has mostly involved anticoagulants, primarily heparin. Analysis of the results fails to demonstrate beneficial effects in most patients, who in any case lack evidence of active hypercoagulation. Fibrinolytic therapy to dissolve intrarenal thrombi would have theoretical benefit, but the risks seem to outweigh the potential gains. Plasmapheresis or the administration of fresh-frozen plasma, or both, has been recommended in hopes of replacing a missing plasma stimulator of prostacyclin production, but results do not as yet permit interpretation.

Currently, we believe that careful medical management of the hematologic and renal manifestations, in conjunction with early and frequent peritoneal dialysis, offers the best chance of recovery from the acute phase. Long-term observation is necessary to watch for late development of hypertension or chronic kidney disease. Recurrence of the disease is quite rare.

Andreoli SP, Bergstein JM: Development of insulin-dependent diabetes mellitus during the hemolytic-uremic syndrome. J Pediatr 100:541, 1982.
Andreoli SP, Bergstein JM: Acute rhabdomyolysis associated with the hemolytic-uremic syndrome. J Pediatr 103:78, 1983.
Bergstein JM, Kuederli U, Bang NU: Plasma inhibitor of glomerular fibrinolysis in the hemolytic-uremic syndrome. Am J Med 73:322, 1982.
Goldstein MH, Churg J, Strauss L, et al: Hemolytic-uremic syndrome. Nephron 23:263, 1979.
Martin DL, MacDonald KL, White KE, et al: The epidemiology and chemical aspects of the hemolytic-uremic syndrome in Minnesota. N Engl J Med 323:1161, 1990.
Milford DV, White RHR, Taylor CM: Prognostic significance of proteinuria one year after onset of diarrhea-associated hemolytic-uremic syndrome. J Pediatr 118:191, 1991.
Remuzzi G, Misiani R, Marchesi D, et al: Treatment of the hemolytic uremic syndrome with plasma. Clin Nephrol 12:279, 1979.
Riella MC, George CRP, Hickman RO, et al: Renal microangiopathy of the hemolytic-uremic syndrome in childhood. Nephron 17:188, 1976.
Siegler RL: Management of hemolytic-uremic syndrome. J Pediatr 112:1014, 1988.
Siegler RL, Milligan MR, Burningham TH, et al: Long-term outcome and prognostic indicators in the hemolytic-uremic syndrome. J Pediatr 118:195, 1991.

18.14 INFECTION AS A CAUSE OF HEMATURIA

Gross or microscopic hematuria may be associated with bacterial, mycobacterial, or viral infections of the urinary tract (see Sec. 18.39). Why the same organism may cause hematuria in one patient with cystitis and not in another is unclear; the occurrence of hematuria may be related to the depth and severity of the inflammatory reaction within the bladder wall.

Urethritis may present gross or microscopic hematuria, usually in conjunction with urgency and urethral discomfort. Urinalysis reveals red blood cells and pyuria. Urine cultures occasionally reveal bacteria, *Ureaplasma*, or *Chlamydia*, but are usually negative. A history of trauma should be sought. The disorder frequently resolves spontaneously. Treatment can be considered with a 10-day course of tetracycline, with a urinary analgesic (phenazopyridine hydrochloride) given for relief of pain. If conservative management fails, cystoscopy may be required to determine the nature of any underlying abnormality.

18.15 HEMATOLOGIC DISEASES CAUSING HEMATURIA

COAGULOPATHIES AND THROMBOCYTOPENIA

Gross or microscopic hematuria may be associated with inherited or acquired disorders of coagulation (e.g., with hemophilias or with disseminated intravascular coagulation or with thrombocytopenia of any cause). In these cases, however, hematuria is almost never the presenting complaint but usually develops after other manifestations (see Sec. 16.63).

SICKLE CELL NEPHROPATHY

Gross or microscopic hematuria may be seen in children with sickle cell disease or trait. The hematuria presumably results from sickling in the relatively hypoxic, acidic, hypertonic renal medulla, with vascular stasis, diminished blood flow, ischemia, papillary necrosis, and interstitial fibrosis. Additional clinical manifestations of sickle cell nephropathy may include a urinary concentrating defect, renal tubular acidosis and, rarely, a nephrotic syndrome that morphologically resembles membranoproliferative glomerulonephritis. The hematuria resolves spontaneously in the majority of patients (see Sec. 16.19).

Buckalew VM, Someren A: Renal manifestations of sickle cell disease. Arch Intern Med 133:660, 1974.
DeJong PE, Statius Van Eps LW: Sickle cell nephropathy: New insights into its pathophysiology. Kidney Int 27:711, 1985.
Tejani A, Phadke K, Adamson O, et al: Renal lesions in sickle cell nephropathy in children. Nephron 39:352, 1985.

RENAL VEIN THROMBOSIS

EPIDEMIOLOGY. Renal vein thrombosis seems to occur in two distinct patterns. In newborns and infants, the disease is commonly associated with asphyxia, dehydration, shock, and sepsis; it occurs rarely in infants of diabetic mothers. After infancy, the disease is more commonly associated with the nephrotic syndrome (most frequently with membranous nephropathy), with cyanotic heart disease, and with the use of angiographic contrast agents.

PATHOGENESIS. The disease presumably begins in the intrarenal venous radicles, with both antegrade and retrograde spread. The main renal vein may escape involvement. Thrombus formation is presumably mediated by endothelial cell injury (by hypoxia, endotoxin, or contrast media) in conjunction with a hypercoagulable state (nephrotic syndrome) and diminished vascular blood flow, which may be due to hypovolemia (shock, sepsis, dehydration, or nephrotic syndrome) or to the intravascular sludging of blood that results from polycythemia.

CLINICAL MANIFESTATIONS. The development of renal vein thrombosis in infants is usually heralded by the sudden onset of gross hematuria and unilateral or bilateral flank masses. Older children commonly present with gross or microscopic hematuria and flank pain. The disease is more frequently unilateral than bilateral; bilateral involvement results in acute renal failure.

DIAGNOSIS. The diagnosis is suggested by the development of hematuria and flank masses in a patient with predisposing clinical factors. Most patients will also have a microangiopathic hemolytic anemia and thrombocytopenia. Ultrasonography will show marked enlargement, whereas radionuclide studies reveal little or no renal function in involved kidneys. Doppler flow studies or venacavography of the inferior vena cava may be necessary to confirm the diagnosis in occult cases, but contrast studies should generally be avoided in order to minimize the risk of further vascular damage.

DIFFERENTIAL DIAGNOSIS. The differential diagnosis includes other causes of hematuria (especially the hemolytic-uremic syndrome) or renal enlargement (hydronephrosis, cystic disease, Wilms tumor, abscess, hematoma).

TREATMENT. For unilateral renal vein thrombosis, treatment is supportive and involves correction of fluid and electrolyte abnormalities and treatment of infection. Prophylactic anticoagulation to prevent thrombosis in the remaining kidney is unwarranted, except perhaps in patients with disseminated intravascular coagulation.

Since bilateral renal vein thrombosis frequently leads to chronic renal failure, consideration should be given to use of such measures as thrombectomy or the systemic use of fibrinolytic agents.

PROGNOSIS. In infants, the thrombosed kidney undergoes progressive atrophy, ultimately leaving a small scarred kidney. Nephrectomy should not be performed in the acute phase, and later only if hypertension or chronic infection develops. In older children, the involved kidney may recover function, especially if the thrombosis was associated with nephrotic syndrome or cyanotic heart disease.

Arnell GC, MacDonald AM, Murphy AV, et al: Renal venous thrombosis. Clin Nephrol 1:119, 1973.
Baum NH, Moriel E, Carlton CE Jr: Renal vein thrombosis. J Urol 119:443, 1978.
Belman AB: Renal vein thrombosis in infancy and childhood. Clin Pediatr 15:1033, 1976.
Llach F, Papper S, Massry SG: The clinical spectrum of renal vein thrombosis: Acute and chronic. Am J Med 69:819, 1980.
Rowe JM, Rasmussen RL, Mader SL, et al: Successful thrombolytic therapy in two patients with renal vein thrombosis. Am J Med 77:111, 1984.

18.16 ANATOMIC ABNORMALITIES ASSOCIATED WITH HEMATURIA

CONGENITAL ANOMALIES

Gross or microscopic hematuria may be associated with almost any type of malformation of the urinary tract. The sudden onset of usually painless gross hematuria after minor trauma to the flank is frequently associated with ureteropelvic junction obstruction or cystic kidneys.

TRAUMA

Blunt or penetrating injury to the abdomen may injure the kidney. Gross or microscopic hematuria, flank pain, and abdominal rigidity may occur; associated injuries may be present. Urethral trauma may result from crushing-type injury, frequently associated with a fractured pelvis, or from direct injury by a foreign object. The injury is suspected when gross blood appears at the external meatus.

Lieu TA, Fleisher GR, Mahboubi S, et al: Hematuria and clinical findings as indications for intravenous pyelography in pediatric blunt renal trauma. Pediatrics 82:216, 1988.
Taylor GA, Eichelberger MR, Potter BM: Hematuria: A marker of abdominal injury in children after blunt trauma. Ann Surg 208:688, 1988.
Yale-Loehr AJ, Kramer SS, Quinlan DM, et al: CT of severe renal trauma in children: Evaluation and course of healing with conservative therapy. AJR 152:109, 1989.

18.17 INFANTILE POLYCYSTIC DISEASE

This rare autosomal recessive disorder may not be detected until after infancy. Besides cysts in the kidneys, cysts may be found also in the liver, with significant liver disease.

PATHOLOGY. Both kidneys are markedly enlarged and grossly show innumerable cysts throughout the cortex and medulla. Microscopic studies show the "cysts" to be dilatations of the collecting ducts. The interstitium and remainder of the tubules may be normal at birth, but development of interstitial fibrosis and tubular atrophy may lead to renal failure.

The majority of patients also have cysts in the liver. In severe cases, the cysts in the liver may be associated with cirrhosis, portal hypertension, and death from ruptured esophageal varices. When the severity of hepatic manifestations exceeds that of renal involvement, the disorder is called *congenital hepatic fibrosis*. Whether infantile polycystic disease and congenital hepatic fibrosis are the opposite ends of the spectrum of a single disorder or distinct autosomal recessive disorders with similar manifestations remains to be determined.

CLINICAL MANIFESTATIONS. The typical patient has bilateral flank masses at birth. The disorder may be associated with oligohydramnios, owing to inadequate formation of urine by the fetus. The oligohydramnios may produce Potter syndrome (flat nose, recessed chin, epicanthal folds, low-set abnormal ears, limb abnormalities), as a result of compression of the fetus, and pulmonary hypoplasia. The pulmonary hypoplasia may produce neonatal respiratory distress, with spontaneous pneumothorax. The association of developmental disorders of the lungs and kidneys is sufficiently frequent to warrant ultrasonic evaluation of the kidneys in all neonates who have spontaneous pneumothorax. Gross or microscopic hematuria and hypertension (which may be severe) are common. Renal function may be normal or diminished, depending on the severity of the renal malformation. Rarely, patients beyond infancy may first present with a nephrogenic diabetes insipidus–like state, renal insufficiency, or hypertension.

DIAGNOSIS. The diagnosis is suggested by the clinical manifestations. Since ultrasonic evaluation of the kidneys may fail to define the cysts, intravenous pyelography should be done. A satisfactory pyelogram will reveal opacification of the dilated collecting ducts. Because these ducts run from cortex to medulla, they will appear as radial streaks similar to the spokes of a wheel. But radiographic studies are rarely able to confirm the diagnosis; it is our practice, therefore, in questionable instances, to perform open surgical biopsy of the liver and right kidney toward the end of the 1st yr of life, to confirm the diagnosis and to permit genetic counseling.

The differential diagnosis includes other causes of bilateral renal enlargement, such as multicystic dysplasia, hydronephrosis, Wilms tumor, and renal vein thrombosis.

TREATMENT. The treatment is supportive, including careful management of the hypertension.

PROGNOSIS. Children with severe renal involvement may die in the neonatal period of pulmonary or renal insufficiency. Survivors may live for several years before developing renal insufficiency. During this period, the kidneys shrink in size and the hypertension becomes less severe. When renal failure develops, dialysis and kidney transplantation should be considered. In patients having hepatic fibrosis, cirrhosis may lead to portal hypertension, for which the prognosis is poor.

Cole BR, Conley SB, Stapleton FB: Polycystic kidney disease in the first year of life. J Pediatr 111:693, 1987.
Kaariainen H, Koskimes O, Norio R: Dominant and recessive polycystic kidney disease in children: Evaluation of clinical features and laboratory data. Pediatr Nephrol 2:296, 1988.
Kaplan BS, Fay J, Shah V, et al: Autosomal recessive polycystic disease. Pediatr Nephrol 3:43, 1989.
Zerres K: Genetics of cystic kidney diseases. Pediatr Nephrol 1:397, 1987.

Adult Polycystic Disease

This autosomal dominant disorder is a common cause of end-stage renal failure in adults but is rarely encountered in childhood. In most families the genetic defect seems to involve a locus on the short arm of chromosome 16. In affected adults, both kidneys are enlarged and show cortical and medullary cysts that are primarily dilated tubules. The disease commonly presents in the 4th or 5th decade of life with gross or microscopic hematuria, bilateral flank pain or masses, or both, and hypertension. Associated abnormalities may include hepatic cysts of no clinical significance and aneurysms of the cerebral circulation that may result in intracranial hemorrhage. Children with the disease may present with unilateral or bilateral flank masses. Hypertension may develop. The cysts are frequently demonstrable by ultrasonography, intravenous pyelography, or computed tomography (CT) scan. In conjunction with the clinical manifestations and family history, radiographic studies usually confirm the diagnosis. In occult cases, especially those lacking a family history of the disease (the disease has a high spontaneous mutation rate), open renal biopsy may be necessary to confirm the diagnosis. Treatment is supportive. End-stage renal failure frequently develops by the 6th or 7th decade.

Gabow PA: Autosomal dominant polycystic kidney disease—more than a renal disease. Am J Kidney Dis 16:403, 1990.
Kaplan BS, Rabin I, Nogrady MG, et al: Autosomal dominant polycystic renal disease in children. J Pediatr 90:782, 1977.
Kaye C, Lewy PR: Congenital appearance of adult-type (autosomal dominant) polycystic kidney disease. J Pediatr 85:807, 1974.
Sedman A, Bell P, Manco-Johnson M, et al: Autosomal dominant polycystic kidney disease in childhood: A longitudinal study. Kidney Int 31:1000, 1987.

18.18 KIDNEY STONES AND HYPERCALCIURIA

Kidney stones in children usually result from chronic infection or the excessive urinary excretion of calcium, uric acid, oxalate, or cystine. Presenting complaints may include abdominal or flank pain, gross or microscopic hematuria, or symptoms of urinary tract infection (see Sec. 18.48).

18.19 VASCULAR ABNORMALITIES

Hemangiomas and arteriovenous malformations of the kidneys and lower urinary tract are extremely rare causes of hematuria. They usually present with gross hematuria and the passage of blood clots. Renal colic may develop if the upper tract is involved. The diagnosis is confirmed by angiography.

18.20 TUMORS

Kidney tumors in children (Wilms tumor is most common) rarely have hematuria as the first sign; a flank mass is most common (see Sec. 17.13). Extrarenal tumors, such as the leukemias, lymphomas, or neuroblastoma, may cause hematuria, by direct infiltration of the kidney or by infiltration of the bone marrow, with resulting thrombocytopenia.

18.21 EXERCISE HEMATURIA

Gross or microscopic hematuria may follow vigorous exercise. Exercise hematuria is rare in females and can be associated with dysuria. The color of the urine may vary from red to black; myoglobinuria should be excluded. Blood clots may be present in the urine. Findings on urine culture, intravenous pyelography, voiding cystourethrography, and cystoscopy are normal in most patients. This seems to be a benign condition, and the hematuria generally resolves within 48 hr after cessation of exercise. The absence of red blood cell casts or of evidence of renal disease, and the presence of dysuria and blood clots in some patients, suggest that the source of bleeding lies in the lower urinary tract.

Bailey RR, Dann E, Gillies AHB, et al: What the urine contains following athletic competition. N Z Med J 83:309, 1976.
Fred HL, Natelson EA: Grossly bloody urine of runners. South Med J 70:1394, 1977.
Siegel AJ, Hennekens CH, Solomon HS, et al: Exercise-related hematuria. JAMA 241:391, 1979.

18.22 DRUGS

Gross or microscopic hematuria has been associated with use of various medications. Mechanisms include alterations in the coagulation system (heparin, warfarin, aspirin), tubular damage (penicillins, sulfonamides), and hemorrhagic cystitis (cyclophosphamide).

Northway JD: Hematuria in children. J Pediatr 78:381, 1971.

18.23 EVALUATION OF THE CHILD WITH HEMATURIA

A thorough history and physical examination may give clues to the etiology of hematuria. For example, a history of recent upper respiratory, skin, or gastrointestinal infection may suggest acute glomerulonephritis or the hemolytic-uremic syndrome. Frequency, dysuria, and unexplained fevers suggest urinary tract infection. A flank mass may indicate hydronephrosis, cystic disease, renal vein thrombosis, or tumor. Recurrent episodes of gross hematuria suggest IgA nephropathy, idiopathic hematuria, Alport syndrome, or hypercalciuria. Rash and joint pains point toward anaphylactoid purpura or lupus. A history of trauma, of bleeding difficulties, of drug usage, or of kidney disease or high blood pressure in other family members could be useful.

Laboratory evaluation of the child with hematuria is done in steps, beginning with the studies most likely to reveal the etiology (see Table 18–3). Depending on the results of the initial group of tests, additional studies may be indicated.

The finding of certain hematologic abnormalities may narrow the differential diagnosis. Anemia may be dilutional (the result of fluid overload in acute renal failure), hemolytic (hemolytic-uremic syndrome, systemic lupus erythematosus), or the result of blood loss (pulmonary hemorrhage in Goodpasture disease, melena in anaphylactoid purpura, hemolytic-uremic syndrome). Confirmation of a hemolytic state (elevated reticulocyte count and plasma hemoglobin level, with depressed plasma haptoglobin level) indicates additional studies. Observation of the blood film may reveal a microangiopathic process as seen in the hemolytic-uremic syndrome, renal vein thrombosis, vasculitis, and systemic lupus erythematosus. In the last, the presence of autoantibodies may result in a positive Coombs test, ANA, leukopenia, and multisystem disease. All black children with hematuria should be screened for sickle hemoglobin, even in the absence of anemia. Thrombocytopenia may result from decreased platelet production (malignancies) or increased platelet consumption (lupus, idiopathic thrombocytopenic purpura, hemolytic-uremic syndrome, renal vein thrombosis). Although red blood cell morphology may be normal with lower tract bleeding and dysmorphic from glomerular bleeding, cell morphology does not reliably correlate with the site of hematuria. The best screening test for a bleeding diathesis, however, is a good history; coagulation studies or platelet counts are not routinely obtained unless personal or family history suggests a bleeding tendency.

Urine culture evaluates the possibility of urinary tract infection. Optimally, a timed urine specimen is also collected to measure the creatinine clearance, and protein and calcium excretion. If this is not possible, then determination of the serum creatinine, urine protein by dipstick, and calcium-to-creatinine ratio in a random urine specimen are adequate.

The serum C3 level is determined in all patients, since a low level narrows the differential diagnosis to certain forms of glomerulonephritis: poststreptococcal, lupus, membranoproliferative, and chronic infection. When the hematuria is of less than 6 mo duration, serologic evidence for streptococcal infection should be sought. Throat or skin infections should be cultured for streptococci. An ANA titer should be obtained as a test for lupus.

If the above mentioned studies do not yield the diagnosis, ultrasound or intravenous pyelography should be carried out to exclude structural abnormalities. Cystography is done only in patients with infection or in patients in whom a lesion of the lower tract is suspected.

The studies in steps 1 and 2, as presented in Table 18–3, will frequently reveal the etiology of the hematuria. In some patients, however, results of all these studies will be normal and no cause for the hematuria will be found. In such patients, despite the lack of a diagnosis, no further studies need be performed. The parents should be reassured that the child does not at present have evidence of urinary tract disease. Because it remains possible, however, that significant renal disease (e.g., IgA nephropathy, Alport syndrome) may be present, the child with persistent microscopic hematuria should have long-term follow-up, with an annual re-evaluation consisting of history, physical examination, blood pressure determination, urinalysis, creatinine clearance, and determination of protein level in a 24-hr specimen.

Renal biopsy may not yield a definitive diagnosis in children with unexplained microscopic hematuria and no other laboratory abnormalities. The finding of normal histology can be reassuring to the family and physician, however, as it excludes the most serious kidney diseases and reduces the need for close surveillance of the child. Biopsy is indicated in children with persistent microscopic hematuria associated with decreased renal function, proteinuria, or hypertension; in those children having one or more episodes of unexplained gross hematuria; and in those with persistent high-grade microscopic hematuria.

Cystoscopy is not part of the routine evaluation of hematuria in children. We have found cystoscopy most helpful in patients having bright red hematuria, dysuria, and sterile urine cultures. In boys, cystoscopy frequently reveals a hemorrhagic lesion in the urethra, probably the result of local trauma. Although neoplasms of the lower urinary tract rarely present as asymptomatic gross hematuria in children, debate persists regarding the need for cystoscopy to exclude the remote possibility of a tumor.

18.24 CONDITIONS PARTICULARLY ASSOCIATED WITH PROTEINURIA

Protein may be found in the urine of healthy children. Estimates vary, but a reasonable upper limit of normal protein excretion in healthy children is 150 mg/24 hr (0.15 g/24 hr). Approximately half of this protein derives from the plasma, albumin representing the largest fraction (less than 30 mg/24 hr; 0.03 g/24 hr). The remainder of normal urinary protein is Tamm-Horsfall protein, a mucoprotein of unknown function produced in the distal tubule.

Proteinuria is commonly detected by the dipstick test and is reported as negative, trace, 1+ (closest to 30 mg/dL), 2+ (closest to 100 mg/dL), 3+ (closest to 300 mg/dL), and 4+ (greater than 2,000 mg/dL). Dipsticks detect primarily albuminuria and are less sensitive than (and may miss) other forms of proteinuria (e.g., low molecular weight proteins, Bence Jones protein, gamma globulins). The depth of color of the dipstick reaction increases in a semi-quantitative manner with increasing urinary protein concentrations. Owing to their high sensitivity, dipsticks may detect amounts of protein in the urine that are within normal limits. Because the dipstick reaction cannot accurately measure protein excretion, persistent proteinuria should be quantitated by a more precise method (sulfosalicylic acid) in a timed (preferably 24 hr) urine collection. False-positive test results for proteinuria may be found with both the dipstick test (highly concentrated urine, gross hematuria, contamination with chlorhexidine or benzalkonium, pH over 8.0, phenazopyridine therapy) and the sulfosalicylic acid method (radiographic contrast media, penicillin or cephalosporin therapy, tolbutamide, sulfonamides).

18.25 NONPATHOLOGIC PROTEINURIA

Proteinuria in excess of 150 mg/24 hr (0.15 g/24 hr) may be divided into two categories (Table 18–4). In the first category, nonpathologic proteinuria, the excessive protein excretion is apparently not the result of a disease state. The level of proteinuria in this category is generally less than 1,000 mg/24 hr (1.00 g/24 hr) and is never associated with edema.

POSTURAL (ORTHOSTATIC) PROTEINURIA

Children with this disorder excrete normal or slightly increased amounts of protein in the supine position. In the upright position, the amount of protein in the urine may increase 10-fold or more. The proteinuria is usually discovered at routine urinalysis; its etiology is unknown. Hematuria is absent, and the creatinine clearance and C3 complement level are normal. Renal biopsy (not part of the evaluation) is normal or shows mild nonspecific alterations.

In the child having asymptomatic low-grade proteinuria, a study for postural proteinuria should be performed. At bedtime, the child goes to bed without voiding. After 30 min supine, the child voids in this position. This urine is discarded but the time of voiding is recorded as the beginning of the supine collection. The child is then given a large glass of liquid and allowed to sleep. In the morning, the child again voids supine before rising; this ends the supine collection and begins the upright collection, which is terminated at bedtime.

TABLE 18–4. Classification of Proteinuria

Nonpathologic Proteinuria
- Postural (orthostatic)
- Febrile
- Exercise

Pathologic Proteinuria
- Tubular
  - *Hereditary*
    - Cystinosis
    - Wilson disease
    - Lowe syndrome
    - Proximal renal tubular acidosis
    - Galactosemia
  - *Acquired*
    - Analgesic abuse
    - Vitamin D intoxication
    - Hypokalemia
    - Antibiotics
    - Interstitial nephritis
    - Acute tubular necrosis
    - Sarcoidosis
    - Cystic diseases
    - Homograft rejection
    - Penicillamine
    - Heavy metal poisoning (mercury, gold, lead, bismuth, cadmium, chromium, copper)
- Glomerular
  - Persistent asymptomatic
  - Nephrotic syndrome
    - Idiopathic nephrotic syndrome
      - Minimal change
      - Mesangial proliferation
      - Focal sclerosis
    - Glomerulonephritis
    - Tumors
    - Drugs
    - Congenital

The child may have normal daily activities, avoiding the supine position. The protein excretion is measured in the two urine collections, and for each collection the result is calculated as mg of protein excreted per min. A finding of essentially normal protein excretion in the supine collection and increased protein excretion in the upright collection establishes the proteinuria as orthostatic.

Studies in adults suggest that postural proteinuria is a benign process, but similar data are not available for children. Accordingly, long-term follow-up of children is necessary (unless the proteinuria resolves) in order to monitor the patient for evidence of renal disease (hematuria, hypertension, diminished renal function, or proteinuria exceeding 1 g/24 hr).

Springberg PD, Garrett LE Jr, Thompson AL, et al: Fixed and reproducible orthostatic proteinuria: Results of a 20-year follow-up study. Ann Intern Med 97:516, 1982.

FEBRILE PROTEINURIA

Transient proteinuria may be found in patients having fever in excess of 38.3° C (101° F). The mechanism of proteinuria associated with fever is unknown. The proteinuria does not exceed +2 on the dipstick and may be considered benign if it resolves when the fever abates.

Jensen H, Henriksen K: Proteinuria in non-renal infectious disease. Acta Med Scand 196:75, 1974.
Marks MI, McLaine PN, Drummond KN: Proteinuria in children with febrile illnesses. Arch Dis Child 45:250, 1970.

EXERCISE PROTEINURIA

Proteinuria, like hematuria, may follow vigorous exercise. The level rarely exceeds +2 on the dipstick. The disorder can be considered benign if the proteinuria resolves after 48 hr of rest.

Campanacci L, Faccini L, Englaro E, et al: Exercise-induced proteinuria. Contr Nephrol 26:31, 1981.
Poortmans JR: Postexercise proteinuria in humans. JAMA 253:236, 1985.

18.26 PATHOLOGIC PROTEINURIA

The second category of proteinuria may result from glomerular or tubular disorders.

TUBULAR PROTEINURIA

Healthy individuals filter large amounts of proteins of lower molecular weight than albumin (e.g., lysozyme, light chains of immunoglobulin, β_2-microglobulin, insulin, growth hormone); these are normally reabsorbed in the proximal tubule. Injury to the proximal tubules results in diminished reabsorptive capacity and the loss of these low molecular weight proteins in the urine; such proteinuria rarely exceeds 1 g/24 hr; it is not associated with edema. Tubular proteinuria (see Table 18–4) may be seen in acquired and inherited disorders and may be associated with other defects of proximal tubular function, such as glucosuria, phosphaturia, bicarbonate wasting, and aminoaciduria. Tubular proteinuria rarely presents a diagnostic dilemma because the underlying disease is usually detected before the proteinuria. Asymptomatic patients having persistent proteinuria generally have glomerular rather than tubular proteinuria. In occult cases, glomerular and tubular proteinuria can be distinguished by electrophoresis of the urine. In tubular proteinuria, the low molecular weight proteins migrate primarily in the alpha and beta regions and little or no albumin is detected, whereas in glomerular proteinuria the major protein is albumin.

Alt JM, Von der Heyde D, Assel E, et al: Characteristics of protein excretion in glomerular and tubular disease. Contr Nephrol 24:115, 1981.
Maack T, Johnson V, Kau ST, et al: Renal filtration, transport, and metabolism of low-molecular-weight proteins: A review. Kidney Int 16:251, 1979.
Waller KV, Ward KM, Mahan JD, et al: Current concepts in proteinuria. Clin Chem 35:755, 1989.

GLOMERULAR PROTEINURIA

The most common cause of proteinuria is increased permeability of the glomerular capillary wall. The amount of glomerular proteinuria may range from less than 1 to more than 30 g/24 hr. Glomerular proteinuria may be termed selective (loss of plasma proteins of molecular weight up to and including albumin) or nonselective (loss of albumin and of larger molecular weight proteins such as IgG). Most forms of glomerulonephritis are accompanied by nonselective proteinuria. Selective proteinuria is seen primarily in minimal-change nephrosis and in that disease, the finding of selective proteinuria increases the likelihood of corticosteroid responsiveness. The determination of urinary protein selectivity is generally of little clinical value, owing to considerable overlap of selectivities among various forms of renal disease.

PERSISTENT ASYMPTOMATIC PROTEINURIA

Persistent asymptomatic proteinuria is defined as proteinuria in an apparently healthy child that occurs without hematuria and persists for 3 mo. The prevalence in school-aged children may be as high as 6%. The amount of proteinuria is usually less than 2 g/24 hr; it is never associated with edema. Causes include postural proteinuria, membranous and membranoproliferative glomerulonephritis, pyelonephritis, hereditary nephritis, developmental anomalies, and "benign" proteinuria.

Evaluation of the child having persistent asymptomatic proteinuria should include urine culture; measurement of creatinine clearance, 24-hr protein excretion, serum albumin, and C3 complement levels; and intravenous pyelography. In patients with low-grade proteinuria (150 to 1,000 mg/24 hr [0.15 to 1.00 g/24 hr]) in whom findings are normal, renal biopsy may not be indicated because evidence for a progressive disease is rarely found. Such patients should have an annual re-evaluation consisting of physical examination and blood pressure determination, urinalysis, creatinine clearance, and 24-hr protein excretion. Indications for renal biopsy include persistent asymptomatic proteinuria in excess of 1,000 mg/24 hr (1 g/24 hr) or the development of hematuria, hypertension, or diminished renal function.

Dodge WF, West EF, Smith EH, et al: Proteinuria and hematuria in school-age children: Epidemiology and early natural history. J Pediatr 88:327, 1976.
McLaine PN, Drummond KN: Benign persistent asymptomatic proteinuria in childhood. Pediatrics 46:548, 1970.
Vehaskari VM, Rapola J: Isolated proteinuria: Analysis of a school-age population. J Pediatr 101:661, 1982.
Yoshikawa N, Uehara S, Yamana K, et al: Clinicopathological correlations of persistent asymptomatic proteinuria in children. Nephron 25:127, 1980.

18.27 NEPHROTIC SYNDROME (NEPHROSIS)

The nephrotic syndrome is characterized by proteinuria, hypoproteinemia, edema, and hyperlipidemia.

ETIOLOGY. Most (90%) children with nephrosis have some form of the idiopathic nephrotic syndrome; minimal-change disease is found in approximately 85%, mesangial proliferation in 5%, and focal sclerosis in 10%. In the remaining 10% of children with nephrosis, the nephrotic syndrome is largely mediated by some form of glomerulonephritis, membranous and membranoproliferative being most common.

PATHOPHYSIOLOGY. The underlying pathogenetic abnormality in nephrosis is proteinuria, which results from an increase in glomerular capillary wall permeability. The mechanism of this increase in permeability is unknown but may be related, at least in part, to loss of negatively charged glycoproteins within the capillary wall. In the nephrotic state, the protein loss generally exceeds 2 g/24 hr and is composed primarily of albumin; the hypoproteinemia is fundamentally a "hypoalbuminemia." In general, edema appears when the serum albumin level falls below 2.5 g/dL (25 g/L).

The mechanism of edema formation in nephrosis is incompletely understood. It seems likely that the edema is initiated by the development of hypoalbuminemia, the result of urinary protein loss. The hypoalbuminemia leads to a decrease in the plasma oncotic pressure, which permits the transudation of fluid from the intravascular compartment to the interstitial space. The reduction in intravascular volume decreases renal perfusion pressure, activating the renin-angiotensin-aldosterone system, which stimulates distal tubular reabsorption of sodium. The reduced intravascular volume also stimulates the release of antidiuretic hormone, which enhances the reabsorption of water in the collecting duct. Because of the decreased plasma oncotic pressure, the reabsorbed sodium and water are lost into the interstitial space, exacerbating the edema. That other factors may also play a role in the formation of the edema is indicated by the observations that some patients with nephrotic syndrome have normal or increased intravascular volume and normal to diminished plasma levels of renin and aldosterone. Hypothetical explanations include an intrarenal defect in sodium and water excretion or the presence of a circulating agent that increases capillary wall permeability throughout the body, as well as in the kidneys.

In the nephrotic state, almost all serum lipid (cholesterol, triglycerides) and lipoprotein levels are elevated. Two factors offer at least partial explanation: (1) the hypoproteinemia stimulates generalized protein synthesis in the liver, including the lipoproteins; and (2) lipid catabolism is diminished, owing to reduced plasma levels of lipoprotein lipase, the major enzyme system that removes lipids from the plasma. Whether lipoprotein lipase is lost in the urine is unclear.

Dorhout Mees EJ, Geers AB, Koomans HA: Blood volume and sodium retention in the nephrotic syndrome: A controversial pathophysiological concept. Nephron 36:201, 1984.
Oetliker OH, Mordasini R, Lutschg J, et al: Lipoprotein metabolism in nephrotic syndrome in childhood. Pediatr Res 14:64, 1980.
Strauss J, Freundlich M, Zilleruelo G: Nephrotic edema: Etiopathogenic and therapeutic considerations. Nephron 38:78, 1984.
Tulassay T, Rascher W, Scharer K: Intra- and extrarenal factors of oedema formation in the nephrotic syndrome. Pediatr Nephrol 3:92, 1989.
Usberti M, Federico S, Meccariello S, et al: Role of plasma vasopressin in the impairment of water excretion in nephrotic syndrome. Kidney Int 25:422, 1984.
Wheeler DC, Varghese Z, Moorhead JF: Hyperlipidemia in nephrotic syndrome. Am J Nephrol 9:78, 1989.

IDIOPATHIC NEPHROTIC SYNDROME

This syndrome accounts for approximately 90% of nephrosis in childhood. Occasional reports that one of the three histologic types has been transformed into another type suggest that this syndrome may be a single disorder with varying histologic features. It seems more likely, however, that the syndrome represents several diseases having similar clinical manifestations. The resolution of this issue awaits the discovery of the pathogenetic factors. The syndrome has been reported in certain families with a frequency that appears to be increased over that expected, but it does not appear to be inherited.

ETIOLOGY. The cause of the syndrome remains unknown. Early success in controlling nephrosis with "immunosuppressive" drugs suggested that the disease was mediated by immunologic mechanisms, but evidence for classic mechanisms of immunologic injury has been lacking, and it now seems clear that "immunosuppressive" drugs have many effects other than suppression of antibody formation. A few patients have evidence supporting IgE mediation of the disease, but increasing evidence suggests that the syndrome may result from an abnormality in thymus-derived (T-cell) lymphocyte function, perhaps through the production of a factor that increases vascular permeability.

PATHOLOGY. Idiopathic nephrotic syndrome occurs in three morphologic patterns. In minimal-change disease (85%), the glomeruli appear normal or show a minimal increase in mesangial cells and matrix. Findings on immunofluorescent microscopic studies are typically negative. Electron microscopy reveals retraction of the epithelial cell foot processes. More than 95% of children with minimal-change disease respond to corticosteroid therapy.

The mesangial proliferative group (5%) is characterized by a diffuse increase in mesangial cells and matrix. The frequency of mesangial deposits containing IgM and C3 by immunofluorescence is not different from that observed in minimal change disease. Approximately 50–60% of patients with this histologic lesion will respond to corticosteroid therapy.

In biopsies from patients having the focal sclerosis lesion (10%), the majority of glomeruli appear normal or manifest

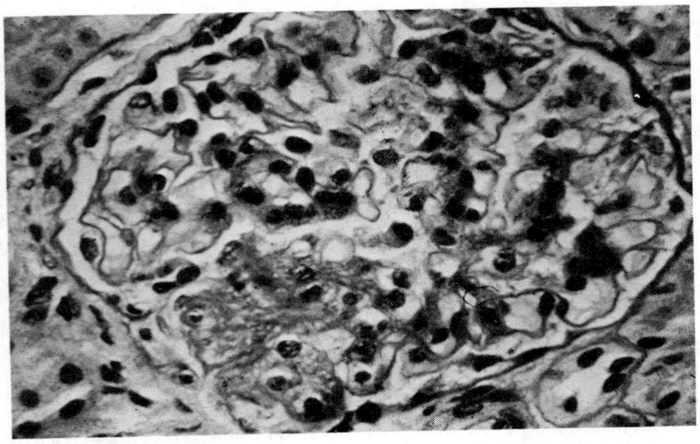

Figure 18–17. Glomerulus from a patient having corticosteroid-resistant nephrotic syndrome, showing mesangial hypercellularity and an area of sclerosis in the lower portion. (× 250.)

mesangial proliferation. Others, especially those close to the medulla (juxtamedullary), show segmental scarring in one or more lobules (Fig. 18–17). The disease is frequently progressive, ultimately involving all glomeruli, and leads to end-stage renal failure in most patients. Approximately 20% of such patients respond to prednisone or cytotoxic therapy or both. The disease may recur in a transplanted kidney.

CLINICAL MANIFESTATIONS. The idiopathic nephrotic syndrome is more common in boys than in girls (2:1) and most commonly appears between the ages of 2 and 6 yr. It has been reported as early as the last half of the 1st yr of life and is not uncommon in adults. The initial episode and subsequent relapses may follow an apparent viral upper respiratory tract infection. The disease usually presents as edema, which is initially noted around the eyes and in the lower extremities, where it is "pitting" in nature. With time, the edema becomes generalized and may be associated with weight gain, the development of ascites and/or pleural effusions, and declining urine output. The edema accumulates in dependent sites and appears to shift from the face and back to the abdomen, perineum, and legs as the day progresses. Anorexia, abdominal pain, and diarrhea are common; hypertension is uncommon.

DIAGNOSIS. Urinalysis reveals +3 or +4 proteinuria; microscopic hematuria may be present, but gross hematuria is rare. Renal function may be normal or reduced. The low creatinine clearance is due to diminished renal perfusion resulting from contraction of the intravascular volume and will return to normal when intravascular volume is restored. Protein excretion exceeds 2 g/24 hr. The serum cholesterol and triglyceride levels are elevated, the serum albumin level is generally less than 2 g/dL (20 g/L), and the total serum calcium level is diminished, owing to a reduction in the albumin-bound fraction. The C3 level is normal.

Children with onset of nephrotic syndrome between the ages of 1 and 8 yr are likely to have steroid-responsive minimal-change disease, and corticosteroid therapy should be initiated without renal biopsy. Minimal-change disease remains common in children above the age of 8 yr who present with nephrosis, but membranous and membranoproliferative glomerulonephritis become increasingly common; renal biopsy is recommended in this group to establish a firm diagnosis prior to considering therapy.

COMPLICATIONS. Infection is the major complication of nephrosis; it results from increased susceptibility to bacterial infections during relapse. Proposed explanations include decreased immunoglobulin levels, the edema fluid acting as a culture medium, protein deficiency, decreased bactericidal activity of the leukocytes, "immunosuppressive" therapy, decreased perfusion of the spleen due to hypovolemia, and loss in the urine of a complement factor (properdin factor B) that opsonizes certain bacteria. For reasons that are unclear, **peritonitis** is the most frequent type of infection; sepsis, pneumonia, cellulitis, and urinary tract infections may also be seen. *S. pneumoniae* is the most common organism causing peritonitis; gram-negative bacteria are also encountered. Fever and physical findings may be minimal in the presence of corticosteroid therapy. Accordingly, a high index of suspicion, prompt evaluation (including cultures of blood and peritoneal fluid), and the early initiation of therapy that covers both gram-positive and gram-negative organisms are critical to prevention of life-threatening illness. When in remission, all patients having nephrosis should receive a single injection of polyvalent pneumococcal vaccine.

Additional complications may include an increased tendency to arterial and venous thrombosis (owing at least in part to elevated plasma levels of certain coagulation factors and inhibitors of fibrinolysis, decreased plasma level of antithrombin III, and increased platelet aggregation), deficiencies of coagulation factors IX, XI, and XII, and reduced serum levels of vitamin D.

TREATMENT. The child may be hospitalized with the first episode of nephrosis for diagnostic, educational, and therapeutic purposes. When edema develops, sodium intake is reduced by the initiation of a "no added salt diet." The mother is advised to cook without salt, to hide the salt shaker, and to avoid serving obviously salty foods. Salt restriction is terminated when the edema resolves. Unless the edema is severe, fluid intake is not restricted but need not be encouraged. The child may attend school and participate in physical activities as tolerated. Until corticosteroid-induced diuresis begins, mild to moderate edema can be managed at home with chlorothiazide, 10–40 mg/kg/24 hr, in two divided doses. If hypokalemia develops, an oral potassium chloride supplement or spironolactone (3–5 mg/kg/24 hr divided into four doses) may be added. If the edema becomes severe, resulting in respiratory distress from massive pleural effusions and ascites or in severe scrotal edema, the child should be hospitalized. Sodium restriction should be continued, but further reduction in intake is rarely effective in controlling edema. The swollen scrotum is elevated with pillows to enhance the removal of fluid by gravity. In the past, severe edema was treated with intravenous administration of albumin, followed in some patients by an intravenous dose of furosemide. This type of therapy has now been supplanted by the oral administration of furosemide (1–2 mg/kg every 4 hr) in conjunction with metolazone (0.2–0.4 mg/kg/24 hr in two divided doses); metolazone may act in both proximal and distal tubules. When using this potent combination, electrolyte levels and renal function must be closely monitored. In some instances of severe edema, intravenous administration of 25% human albumin (1 g/kg/24 hr) may be necessary, but the effect is usually transient and volume overload with hypertension and heart failure must be avoided.

After the diagnosis is confirmed by the appropriate laboratory studies, the pathophysiology and treatment of nephrosis is reviewed with the family to enhance their understanding of the child's disease. Remission is then induced by administration of prednisone, the least expensive corticosteroid, at a dosage of 60 mg/m²/24 hr (maximum daily dose 60 mg), divided into three or four doses over the day. Divided-dose rather than single-dose therapy is used because some patients who fail to respond to a single daily dose will respond to divided doses. The time needed for response to prednisone averages about 2 wk, response being defined as the point at which urine becomes free of protein. If the child continues to have proteinuria (2+ or greater) after 1 mo of continuous, daily, divided-dose prednisone, the nephrosis is termed "steroid-resistant" and renal biopsy is indicated to determine the precise etiology of the disease.

Five days after the urine becomes free (negative, trace, or 1+ on the dipstick) of protein, the dose of prednisone is changed to 60 mg/m² (maximum dose 60 mg) taken every other day as a single dose with breakfast. This alternate-day regimen is continued for 3–6 mo. The purpose of alternate-day therapy is to maintain the remission using a relatively nontoxic dose of prednisone, thus avoiding frequent relapses of the disease and the cumulative toxicity of frequent courses of daily administration of corticosteroids. After such a period of alternate-day therapy, the prednisone may be discontinued abruptly. Adequate experience indicates that there has been sufficient recovery of pituitary-adrenal axis function that the patient is not at risk for adrenal insufficiency after abrupt withdrawal of the alternate-day prednisone. On the other hand, for up to 1 yr after completing corticosteroid therapy, the child will require corticosteroid supplementation for severe illness or surgery.

Each relapse of the nephrosis is treated in a similar manner. A relapse is defined as the recurrence of edema and not simply of proteinuria, as many children with this condition will have intermittent proteinuria that resolves spontaneously. A small number of patients who respond to daily, divided-dose therapy will have relapses shortly after switching to or after terminating alternate-day therapy. Such patients are termed "steroid-dependent."

If there are repeated relapses and especially if the child suffers severe corticosteroid toxicity (cushingoid appearance, hypertension, growth failure), then cyclophosphamide therapy should be considered. Cyclophosphamide has been shown to prolong the duration of remission and to prevent relapses in children with frequently relapsing nephrotic syndrome. The potential side effects of the drug (leukopenia, disseminated varicella infection, hemorrhagic cystitis, alopecia, sterility) should be reviewed with the family. A renal biopsy is recommended to confirm the diagnosis prior to initiating such therapy. The dose of cyclophosphamide is 3 mg/kg/24 hr as a single dose, for a total duration of 8 wk. Alternate-day prednisone therapy is often continued during the course of cyclophosphamide administration. During cyclophosphamide therapy, the white count must be monitored weekly and the drug withheld if the count falls below 5,000/mm³.

PROGNOSIS. The large majority of children with steroid-responsive nephrosis will have repeated relapses until the disease resolves itself spontaneously toward the end of the 2nd decade of life. It is important to indicate to the family that the child will have no residual renal dysfunction, that the disease is generally not hereditary, and that the child (in the absence of cyclophosphamide or chlorambucil therapy) will remain fertile. To minimize the psychologic effects of the nephrosis, we emphasize that when in remission, the child is normal and may have unrestricted diet and activity. While the child is in remission, it is generally unnecessary to test the urine for protein.

Arbeitsgemeinschaft für Pädiatrische Nephrologie: Short versus standard prednisone therapy for initial treatment of idiopathic nephrotic syndrome in children. Lancet 1:380, 1988.
Arbeitsgemeinschaft für Pädiatrische Nephrologie: Alternate-day prednisone is more effective than intermittent prednisone in frequently relapsing nephrotic syndrome. Eur J Pediatr 135:229, 1981.
Arbus GS, Poucell S, Bacheyie GS, et al: Focal segmental glomerulosclerosis with idiopathic nephrotic syndrome: Three types of clinical response. J Pediatr 101:40, 1982.
Arnold WC: Efficacy of metolazone and furosemide in children with furosemide-resistant edema. Pediatrics 74:872, 1984.
Berns JS, Gaudio KM, Krassner LS, et al: Steroid-responsive nephrotic syndrome of childhood: A long-term study of clinical course, histopathology, efficacy of cyclophosphamide therapy and effects on growth. Am J Kidney Dis 9:108, 1987.
Chiu J, McLaine PN, Drummond KN: A controlled prospective study of cyclophosphamide in relapsing, corticosteroid-responsive, minimal-lesion nephrotic syndrome in childhood. J Pediatr 82:607, 1973.
Churg J, Habib R, White RHR: Pathology of the nephrotic syndrome in children. Lancet 1:1299, 1970.
Freundlich M, Bourgoignie JJ, Zilleruelo G, et al: Calcium and vitamin D metabolism in children with nephrotic syndrome. J Pediatr 108:383, 1986.
Geary DF, Farine M, Thorner D, et al: Response to cyclophosphamide in steroid-resistant focal segmental glomerulosclerosis: A reappraisal. Clin Nephrol 22:109, 1984.
Gorensek MJ, Lebel MH, Nelson JD: Peritonitis in children with nephrotic syndrome. Pediatrics 81:849, 1988.
Habib R, Girardin E, Gagnadoux M-F, et al: Immunopathological findings in idiopathic nephrosis: Clinical significance of glomerular "immune deposits." Pediatr Nephrol 2:402, 1988.
International Study of Kidney Disease in Children: Minimal change nephrotic syndrome in children: Deaths during the first 5 to 15 years' observation. Pediatrics 73:497, 1984.
Krensky AM, Ingelfinger JR, Grupe WE: Peritonitis in childhood nephrotic syndrome. Am J Dis Child 136:732, 1982.
Llach F: Hypercoagulability, renal vein thrombosis, and other thrombotic complications of nephrotic syndrome. Kidney Int 28:429, 1985.
Schnaper HW: The immune system in minimal change nephrotic syndrome. Pediatr Nephrol 3:101, 1989.
Southwest Pediatric Nephrology Study Group: Focal segmental glomerulosclerosis in children with idiopathic nephrotic syndrome. Kidney Int 27:442, 1985.
Trompeter RS: Immunosuppressive therapy in the nephrotic syndrome in children. Pediatr Nephrol 3:194, 1989.
Trompeter RS, Lloyd BW, Hicks J, et al: Long-term outcome for children with minimal-change nephrotic syndrome. Lancet 1:368, 1985.
Williams SA, Makker SP, Ingelfinger JR, et al: Long-term evaluation of chlorambucil plus prednisone in the idiopathic nephrotic syndrome of childhood. N Engl J Med 302:929, 1980.

GLOMERULONEPHRITIS

Nephrotic syndrome may develop during the course of any type of glomerulonephritis but is most common in association with membranous, membranoproliferative, poststreptococcal, lupus, chronic infection (including malaria and schistosomiasis), and anaphylactoid purpura glomerulonephritis. Although the development of a secondary nephrotic syndrome may indicate severe glomerular disease, the nephrotic syndrome frequently resolves if the nephritis improves.

Andrade ZA, Rocha H: Schistosomal glomerulopathy. Kidney Int 16:23, 1979.
Hendrickse RG, Adeniyi A: Quartan malarial nephrotic syndrome in children. Kidney Int 16:64, 1979.
Sitprija V: Nephropathy in falciparum malaria. Kidney Int 34:867, 1988.

TUMORS

See also Sec. 17.9 and 17.10.

Nephrotic syndrome has been associated with several extrarenal neoplasms. In patients having solid tumors, such as carcinomas, the glomerular changes resemble membranous glomerulopathy. The renal involvement is presumably mediated by immune complexes composed of tumor antigens and tumor-specific antibodies. In lymphomas (especially Hodgkin disease), minimal-change disease is most commonly found; proliferative lesions have also been described. In patients having the minimal-change lesion, the nephrosis may develop before or after the malignancy is detected, may resolve as the tumor regresses, and may return if the tumor recurs. The mechanism of the nephrosis is unknown; it has been proposed that the tumor produces a lymphokine that increases glomerular capillary wall permeability.

Alpers CE, Cotran RS: Neoplasia and glomerular injury. Kidney Int 30:465, 1986.
Dabbs DJ, Striker L, Mignon F, et al: Glomerular lesions in lymphomas and leukemias. Am J Med 80:63, 1986.

DRUGS

Nephrotic syndrome has developed during therapy with several types of drugs and chemicals. The histologic picture may resemble membranous glomerulopathy (penicillamine, gold, mercury compounds), minimal-change disease (probenecid, ethosuximide, methimazole, lithium), or proliferative glomerulonephritis (procainamide, chlorpropamide, phenytoin, trimethadione, paramethadione).

CONGENITAL NEPHROTIC SYNDROME

Nephrotic syndrome is rare during the 1st yr of life. Causes of nephrosis developing during the first 6 mo of life include the congenital nephrotic syndrome, congenital infection (syphilis, toxoplasmosis, cytomegalovirus), and diffuse mesangial sclerosis of unknown etiology (**Drash syndrome**, consisting of nephropathy, Wilms tumor, and genital abnormalities). Nephrosis developing during the last half of the 1st yr is most commonly associated with the idiopathic nephrotic syndrome or drugs. Owing to the diversity of causes of development of nephrotic syndrome during the 1st year of life, all such patients should have kidney biopsy to determine the precise etiology and severity of the disease.

The congenital nephrotic syndrome (Finnish type) is an autosomal recessive disorder that is most common in populations of Scandinavian descent. The major pathologic feature in some patients is dilatation of the proximal convoluted tubules (microcystic disease), but this is variable even within the same kindred. The glomeruli show mesangial proliferation and sclerosis. The pathogenesis of the syndrome is unknown; a reduction in the number of heparan sulfate–rich anionic sites has been demonstrated in the glomerular basement membrane. Although proteinuria is present at birth, the nephrotic syndrome becomes apparent within the first 3 mo of life. Additional clinical features include prematurity, an enlarged placenta, respiratory distress, and separation of the cranial sutures. The clinical course is one of persistent edema and recurrent infections. Death due to infection or renal failure is likely by the age of 5 yr. Corticosteroid and immunosuppressive agents are of no value. Treatment is supportive, with the ultimate goal of kidney transplantation. In families at risk, antenatal diagnosis is possible by measuring α-fetoprotein level of the amniotic fluid prior to 20 wk of gestation.

Aula P, Rapola J, Karjalainen O, et al: Prenatal diagnosis of congenital nephrosis in 23 high-risk families. Am J Dis Child 132:984, 1978.

Eddy AA, Mauer SM: Pseudohermaphroditism, glomerulopathy, and Wilms tumor (Drash syndrome): Frequency in end-stage renal failure. J Pediatr 106:584, 1985.

Jadresic L, Leake J, Gordon I, et al: Clinicopathologic review of twelve children with nephropathy, Wilms tumor, and genital abnormalities (Drash syndrome). J Pediatr 117:717, 1990.

Mahan JD, Mauer SM, Sibley RK, et al: Congenital nephrotic syndrome: Evolution of medical management and results of renal transplantation. J Pediatr 105:549, 1984.

Rapola J: Congenital nephrotic syndrome. Pediatr Nephrol 1:441, 1987.

Shahin B, Papadopoulou ZL, Jenis EH: Congenital nephrotic syndrome associated with congenital toxoplasmosis. J Pediatr 85:366, 1974.

Sibley RK, Mahan J, Mauer SM, et al: A clinicopathologic study of forty-eight infants with nephrotic syndrome. Kidney Int 27:544, 1985.

Vernier RL, Klein DJ, Sisson SP, et al: Heparan sulfate-rich anionic sites in the human glomerular basement membrane. N Engl J Med 309:1001, 1983.

18.28 TUBULAR DISORDERS

TUBULAR FUNCTION

Except for reduced protein levels, the ultrafiltrate of blood that enters the proximal tubule is similar to plasma. Body homeostasis is maintained by tubular reabsorption of salts and water.

SODIUM. After the 1st year of life, the tubules have the reabsorptive capacity to lower the urinary sodium concentration to 1 mEq/L (1 mmol/L). Approximately 65% of filtered sodium is isotonically reabsorbed in the proximal tubule. Glucose and amino acids are also reabsorbed in the proximal tubule in conjunction with sodium transport. An additional 25% of filtered sodium is reabsorbed from the ascending limb of the loop of Henle in association with the active transport of chloride. The remainder of sodium reabsorption is accomplished in the distal tubule and collecting duct, mediated in part by aldosterone. Sodium excretion is closely related to the extracellular fluid volume and may be modified by factors that regulate the extracellular fluid volume.

POTASSIUM. Essentially all of the filtered potassium is reabsorbed, primarily in the proximal tubules. The potassium excreted is derived from distal tubular and collecting duct potassium secretion, as modified by the pH of the extracellular fluid, by aldosterone, and by the urinary flow rate and sodium concentration.

CALCIUM. Approximately 98% of filtered calcium is reabsorbed by the tubules. Proximal tubular reabsorption (65% of the filtered load) is linked to sodium reabsorption. Calcium reabsorption is enhanced by parathyroid hormone, thiazide diuretics, and reduction of the extracellular fluid volume. Calcium excretion is increased by saline infusion and furosemide.

PHOSPHATE. The majority of the filtered phosphate is reabsorbed in the proximal tubule. Reabsorption is inhibited by parathyroid hormone.

MAGNESIUM. About 25% of filtered magnesium is reabsorbed in the proximal tubule; the major site of magnesium reabsorption and the principal moderator of magnesium excretion is the thick ascending limb of Henle.

ACIDIFICATION AND CONCENTRATING MECHANISMS. These are discussed in the sections on renal tubular acidosis and nephrogenic diabetes insipidus (Sec. 18.29 and 18.30).

MATURATION OF TUBULAR FUNCTION. At birth and for several months thereafter, tubular functional capabilities are at less than adult levels. Tubular function is adequate for healthy infants, but limitations may contribute to fluid and electrolyte abnormalities in sick infants.

Maximal urinary concentrating capacity in the healthy full-term newborn is 600–700 mOsm/kg (mmol/kg) H_2O. This reduction in concentrating capacity in comparison with older children and adults (who can concentrate to more than 1,000 mOsm/kg (mmol/kg) H_2O) is related to reduced GFR, to tubular cell immaturity, to reduced nephron length, to reduced medullary solute gradient due to increased medullary blood flow and low urea production, and to diminished tubular responsiveness to antidiuretic hormone. Although the ability of newborn infants to dilute the urine is comparable to that of adults, their capacity to excrete a water load is diminished, owing to the reduced GFR. The capacity of the neonate to excrete sodium, potassium, hydrogen ion, and phosphate is also limited, owing in part to the low GFR and/or immaturity of tubular function.

Hogg RJ, Stapleton FB: Renal tubular function. *In*: Holliday MA, Barratt TM, Vernier RL (eds): Pediatric Nephrology. Baltimore, Williams & Wilkins, 1987, p 59.

McCrory WW: Developmental Nephrology. Cambridge, Harvard University Press, 1972.

TUBULAR DISEASES

18.29 RENAL TUBULAR ACIDOSIS

Renal tubular acidosis (RTA) is a clinical state of systemic hyperchloremic acidosis resulting from impaired urinary acidification. Three types exist: distal RTA (type I), proximal RTA (type II), and mineralocorticoid deficiency (type IV). A proposed type III has been found to be a variant of type I.

NORMAL URINARY ACIDIFICATION. After the first few months of life, approximately 85% of the filtered bicarbonate is reabsorbed in the proximal tubules, but in premature infants and neonates, such reabsorption of bicarbonate is transiently reduced, and bicarbonate wasting results when the serum bicarbonate level exceeds 20–22 mEq/L (mmol/L). The proximal tubular reabsorption of bicarbonate involves the secretion of hydrogen ion into the tubular lumen in exchange for sodium (see Sec. 6.8). The hydrogen ion combines with filtered bicarbonate to form carbonic acid, which, under the influence of carbonic anhydrase, dissociates into carbon dioxide and water. The carbon dioxide diffuses into the proximal tubular cells, where, under the influence of carbonic anhydrase, it is reconverted to carbonic acid. The carbonic acid dissociates to yield a hydrogen ion that is again secreted to absorb additional bicarbonate, and to yield also a bicarbonate ion that enters the peritubular capillary. The remaining 15% of filtered bicarbonate is reabsorbed in the distal tubule. The normal kidney reabsorbs all filtered bicarbonate, but this does not make the urine acid. Acidification of the urine is mediated by distal tubular secretion of hydrogen ion (which is in part mineralocorticoid-dependent) and of ammonia (which forms ammonium ion in an acidic urine).

Proximal Renal Tubular Acidosis

PATHOGENESIS. Proximal RTA results from reduced proximal tubular reabsorption of bicarbonate, presumably owing to deficient carbonic anhydrase production. Rather than reabsorbing the normal 85% of filtered bicarbonate, the proximal tubules in this condition may reabsorb only 60%, thus presenting the distal tubules with 40% rather than the usual 15% of the filtered load. Because the distal tubules can, at a maximum, reabsorb only 15% of the normal filtered load of bicarbonate, up to 25% may be lost in the urine. Proximal RTA is generally more severe than distal RTA, as complete loss of the distal bicarbonate recovery mechanism (which is rare) would waste only 15% of filtered bicarbonate. With urinary bicarbonate loss, the serum bicarbonate level falls until it reaches a level (bicarbonate threshold) at which bicarbonate wasting ceases. At this level (15–18 mEq/L [mmol/L]), the quantity of filtered bicarbonate is reduced to an amount that can be totally reabsorbed by the tubules. Because distal tubular acidification mechanisms remain intact, the urine may then be acidified (pH less than 5.5). Flooding the distal tubule with sodium bicarbonate stimulates sodium reabsorption in exchange for potassium, leading to hypokalemia. Contraction of the extracellular fluid volume (as a result of the loss of sodium bicarbonate) stimulates chloride reabsorption (resulting in hyperchloremia) and aldosterone secretion (enhancing potassium loss).

Proximal RTA (Table 18–5) may occur as an isolated disorder not associated with other diseases or with other abnormalities of proximal tubular function. Isolated proximal RTA may be transient or persistent, sporadic or inherited (usually autosomal dominant). Proximal RTA may also occur as part of a generalized defect in proximal tubular transport (Fanconi syndrome), characterized by glucosuria, phosphaturia, aminoaciduria, carnitinuria, and proximal RTA. A primary form of Fanconi syndrome, also not associated with other disease states, has been reported to show both autosomal dominant and recessive modes of inheritance. Secondary Fanconi syndrome may develop during the course of several inherited or acquired disease states.

INHERITED FORMS

Cystinosis (see Sec. 8.5). This autosomal recessive defect results from the accumulation of cystine within the lysosomes of the bone marrow, liver, spleen, lymph nodes, kidneys, fibroblasts, leukocytes, corneas, and conjunctivae. It may present either during the first 3 yr of life (nephropathic form) or later (juvenile form). In the nephropathic variety, initial clinical manifestations may include polyuria and polydipsia (concentrating defect), fever (dehydration), growth retardation, rickets, blond hair and fair skin (diminished pigmenta-

TABLE 18–5. Classification of Renal Tubular Acidosis

Proximal	Distal	Mineralocorticoid Deficiency*
Isolated	Isolated	Adrenal disorders (↓ A, ↑ R)
Sporadic	Sporadic	Addison disease
Hereditary	Hereditary	Congenital hyperplasia
Fanconi syndrome	Secondary	Primary hypoaldosteronism
Primary	Interstitial nephritis	Hyporeninemic hypoaldosteronism (↓ A, ↓ R)
Secondary	Obstructive	Obstruction
Inherited	Pyelonephritis	Pyelonephritis
Cystinosis	Transplant rejection	Interstitial nephritis
Lowe syndrome	Sickle cell nephropathy	Diabetes mellitus
Galactosemia	Lupus nephritis	Nephrosclerosis
Hereditary fructose intolerance	Ehlers-Danlos syndrome	Pseudohypoaldosteronism (↑ A, ↑ R)
Tyrosinemia	Nephrocalcinosis	
Wilson disease	Hepatic cirrhosis	
Medullary cystic disease	Elliptocytosis	
Acquired	Medullary sponge kidney	
Heavy metals	Toxins	
Outdated tetracycline	Amphotericin B	
Proteinuria	Lithium	
Interstitial nephritis	Toluene	
Hyperparathyroidism		
Vitamin D deficiency rickets		

*A = aldosterone; R = renin.

tion), and photophobia. The diagnosis is suggested when cystine crystals are observed in the corneas with use of the slit-lamp biomicroscope and is confirmed by demonstration of an elevated cystine content of leukocytes. Intracellular accumulation of cystine in the kidney leads to progressive renal damage, resulting in end-stage renal failure by the end of the first decade. No therapy is known to prevent intracellular cystine accumulation; a clinical trial with cysteamine is currently in progress. The juvenile form of the disease presents later in life; it has the same but less severe clinical manifestations but may also progress to renal failure.

Lowe Syndrome. This X-linked disorder is associated with mental retardation, hypotonia, cataracts, glaucoma, and generalized proximal tubular dysfunction. The underlying metabolic defect is unknown (see Sec. 24.73).

Galactosemia (see Sec. 8.37). The renal manifestations of this disorder result from prolonged galactose accumulation in the proximal tubules.

Hereditary Fructose Intolerance (see Sec. 8.37). This autosomal recessive deficiency of fructose 1-phosphate aldolase leads to proximal tubular dysfunction.

Tyrosinemia. Generalized proximal tubular dysfunction is common in hereditary tyrosinemia (see Sec. 8.3).

Wilson Disease. The clinical manifestations of this autosomal recessive disorder include proximal tubular dysfunction; it is discussed in Sec. 13.88 and 22.10.

Medullary Cystic Disease. This disorder is inherited as an autosomal dominant trait, whereas a similar disorder, juvenile nephronophthisis, is inherited as an autosomal recessive trait. Whether these are separate disorders or the same disorder with variable inheritance is uncertain. Children more commonly have the recessive form, whereas the dominant form is more common in adults. The major pathologic finding is cysts in the medulla. As the "cysts" seem to be dilatations of the distal tubules and collecting ducts, some may also be found in the renal cortex. Progressive interstitial inflammation and fibrosis lead to glomerular sclerosis, cortical atrophy, and renal insufficiency. Some children suffer no clinical problems until reaching end-stage renal failure. Others show manifestations of tubular dysfunction such as polyuria and polydipsia (concentrating defect), sodium wasting, and proximal RTA. Red or blond hair is common. Urinalysis may be normal or show minimal abnormalities. Radiographic studies show small, poorly functioning kidneys. The diagnosis is confirmed by biopsy or at nephrectomy, if either is warranted in preparation for transplantation.

CAUSES OF ACQUIRED FANCONI SYNDROME. These include tubular toxins such as heavy metals (lead, mercury, cadmium, uranium), outdated tetracycline, proteinuric states (myeloma, nephrotic syndrome), and interstitial nephritis. Excessive parathyroid hormone secretion (primary and secondary hyperparathyroidism, vitamin D deficient rickets) may also cause proximal RTA, presumably by inhibition of carbonic anhydrase.

Distal Renal Tubular Acidosis

PATHOGENESIS. The genesis of distal RTA is best explained as a deficiency of hydrogen ion secretion by the distal tubule and collecting duct, although other mechanisms may also be involved. The lack of secreted hydrogen ion reduces the formation of carbonic acid and then carbon dioxide in the tubular lumen. The loss of bicarbonate in the urine may be 5 to 15% of the filtered load. Owing to the nature of the defect, the pH of the urine cannot be reduced below 5.8 despite severe systemic acidosis. Loss of sodium bicarbonate results in hyperchloremia and hypokalemia. The hypokalemia is usually less severe than that found in proximal RTA because less bicarbonate is wasted. Nephrocalcinosis may be present.

Distal RTA may occur as an isolated condition not associated with any other disorder; as such it may be sporadic or inherited as an autosomal dominant or recessive trait. Secondary distal RTA may develop during the course of several diseases and intoxications involving the distal tubules and collecting ducts (see Table 18–5).

MEDULLARY SPONGE KIDNEY. This noninherited disorder is characterized by cystic dilatation of the terminal portions of the collecting ducts as they enter the renal pyramids. Although renal function and life span are typically normal, the disorder may be complicated by pyelonephritis, hypercalciuria, nephrocalcinosis, nephrolithiasis, impaired concentrating capacity, and distal RTA.

Mineralocorticoid Deficiency

PATHOGENESIS. This form of RTA results from inadequate production of or reduced distal tubular responsiveness to aldosterone. The lack of aldosterone effect impairs the establishment across the tubular cell membrane of an electrochemical gradient (with negative electrical potential in the tubular lumen) favorable to hydrogen ion secretion. In the absence of aldosterone-mediated sodium reabsorption, hyperkalemia develops. Hyperkalemia suppresses renal ammonia production, resulting in a reduction of ammonium ion excretion and, thus, net acid excretion. The net effect is a hyperkalemic, hyperchloremic acidosis. The systemic acidosis may render the urine pH acid (less than 5.5).

Mineralocorticoid-deficiency RTA may result from diseases of the adrenal gland (Addison disease, congenital adrenal hyperplasia, primary hypoaldosteronism) in which aldosterone production is deficient. In these disorders, renal function is normal, urinary sodium wasting is common, and the plasma renin level is elevated. Hyporeninemic hypoaldosteronism is a form of RTA that may result from kidney diseases associated with interstitial damage and destruction of the juxtaglomerular apparatus; it may also be observed with volume expansion and prostaglandin inhibition. In these conditions, plasma levels of renin and, as a result, of aldosterone are reduced; renal function may be compromised. Rarely, type IV RTA may be the result of distal tubular unresponsiveness to aldosterone (pseudohypoaldosteronism); plasma renin and aldosterone levels are elevated, renal function is usually normal, and salt wasting is the rule. In adults, this form of RTA may be observed in patients with medullary disease and renal insufficiency.

Clinical Management of Renal Tubular Acidosis

CLINICAL MANIFESTATIONS. Children having isolated forms of proximal or distal RTA commonly present with growth failure toward the end of the first year of life. Gastrointestinal symptoms are common. Children having secondary forms of proximal or distal RTA may present in a similar fashion or with complaints unique to their fundamental disease. Mineralocorticoid deficiency is usually found as an underlying feature of a primary kidney disease.

Distal RTA is complicated by hypercalciuria, which may lead to nephrocalcinosis, nephrolithiasis, and renal parenchymal destruction. The causes of the hypercalciuria are unknown; potential mechanisms include bone breakdown to release calcium carbonate (the carbonate to be converted to bicarbonate in an attempt to control the acidosis) and diminished levels of urinary citrate (which chelates calcium).

DIAGNOSIS. Before considering the diagnosis of RTA, other causes of systemic acidosis such as diarrhea, lactic acidosis, diabetes mellitus, and renal failure should be excluded. The biochemical features of proximal and distal RTA include low serum bicarbonate and potassium levels in association with hyperchloremia. In mineralocorticoid-deficiency RTA, systemic acidosis is associated with hyperkalemia. The anion gap in all forms of RTA is usually normal (see Sec. 6.8).

Patients suspected of having proximal or distal RTA should be evaluated by comparing the pH (by pH meter) of a first morning urine specimen (collected under mineral oil to prevent the loss of carbon dioxide) with simultaneous measurements of serum electrolytes. In patients who have substantial systemic acidosis (serum bicarbonate less than 16 mEq/L [mmol/L]), a urine pH of less than 5.5 supports the diagnosis of proximal RTA, whereas patients with distal RTA will have a urine pH of 5.8 or greater. In patients having mild acidosis (serum bicarbonate 17–20 mEq/L [mmol/L]), ammonium chloride loading may be required to distinguish between the two types. In occult cases, measurement of the fractional excretion of bicarbonate after raising the serum bicarbonate to normal by intravenous infusion of bicarbonate should be considered. If proximal RTA is detected, then other defects of proximal tubular function should be sought (glucosuria, phosphaturia, aminoaciduria). When any form of RTA is confirmed, potential underlying causes (see Table 18–5) should be investigated.

TREATMENT. The goals of therapy are correction of the acidosis and maintenance of normal serum bicarbonate and potassium levels. Most patients' conditions can be corrected with oral therapy; in infants having severe acidosis and hypokalemia, intravenous therapy may be required initially. The least expensive and easiest alkalinizing solution for oral use is Shohl solution (Bicitra, Willen Drug Company, Baltimore, MD) containing 1 mEq/mL of sodium as sodium citrate. For patients requiring potassium supplementation, potassium citrate can be added (Polycitra, Willen Drug Company, Baltimore, MD) to form a solution that contains 1 mEq/mL each of sodium and potassium and 2 mEq/mL of bicarbonate equivalent. Sodium bicarbonate tablets (325 and 650 mg) may be used in older patients. Patients having mineralocorticoid-deficiency RTA may also require diuretics and/or polystyrene sulfonate resin (Kayexalate, Winthrop Pharmaceuticals, New York, NY) to reduce the serum potassium level to normal. Carnitine supplements may be beneficial if serum levels are reduced.

PROGNOSIS. Isolated proximal RTA, although initially more severe than the distal variety, may resolve over the first decade of life. Isolated distal RTA seems to be a lifelong disease; in some instances, renal failure may develop; the prognosis is excellent, however, if the disease is recognized and therapy initiated prior to the development of nephrocalcinosis. A continuing need for alkali therapy and for lifelong monitoring of clinical status is the rule.

Mineralocorticoid-deficiency RTA most frequently results from obstructive uropathy and usually resolves within 12 mo after correction of the obstruction. In other secondary forms of RTA, the ultimate prognosis may depend on the severity of the primary disorder.

Burke JR, Inglis JA, Craswell PW, et al: Juvenile nephronophthisis and medullary cystic disease—the same disease (report of a large family with medullary cystic disease associated with gout and epilepsy). Clin Nephrol 18:1, 1982.

Chan JCM, Alon U: Tubular disorders of acid-base and phosphate metabolism. Nephron 40:257, 1985.

Chesney RW: Etiology and pathogenesis of the Fanconi syndrome. Mineral Electrolyte Metab 4:303, 1980.

Gahl WA: Cystinosis: Progress in a prototypic disease. Ann Intern Med 109:557, 1988.

Kurtzman NA: Acquired distal renal tubular acidosis. Kidney Int 24:807, 1983.

McSherry E, Morris RC Jr: Attainment and maintenance of normal stature with alkali therapy in infants and children with classic renal tubular acidosis. J Clin Invest 61:509, 1978.

O'Neil M, Breslau NA, Pak CYC: Metabolic evaluation of nephrolithiasis in patients with medullary sponge kidney. JAMA 245:1233, 1981.

Portale AA, Booth BE, Morris RC Jr: Renal tubular acidosis. *In*: Holliday MA, Barratt TM, Vernier RL (eds): Pediatric Nephrology. Baltimore, Williams & Wilkins, 1987, p 606.

Rodriguez-Soriano J, Vallo A, Castillo G, et al: Natural history of distal renal tubular acidosis treated since infancy. J Pediatr 101:669, 1982.

Sebastian A, Hulter HN, Kurtz I, et al: Disorders of distal nephron function. Am J Med 72:289, 1982.

Steele BT, Lirenman DS, Beattie CW: Nephronophthisis. Am J Med 68:531, 1980.

18.30 Nephrogenic Diabetes Insipidus

In this disorder, the kidney fails to respond to antidiuretic hormone despite elevated blood levels of antidiuretic hormone.

ETIOLOGY. Primary nephrogenic diabetes insipidus is a rare inherited (usually X-linked recessive) disease characterized by complete tubular unresponsiveness to antidiuretic hormone in males and partial unresponsiveness in females. Partial or complete nephrogenic diabetes insipidus (secondary) may also be associated with disorders that (1) result in loss of the medullary concentrating gradient (acute or chronic renal failure, obstructive and post-obstructive uropathy, vesicoureteral reflux, cystic diseases, interstitial nephritis, osmotic diuresis, nephrocalcinosis); or (2) diminish the effect of antidiuretic hormone on the tubules (hypokalemia, hypercalcemia, lithium, and demeclocycline therapy).

PATHOGENESIS. Concentration of the urine depends on the establishment of a hypertonic renal medulla and the permeability of the distal tubules and collecting ducts to water. The hypertonicity of the medulla is established by a countercurrent mechanism linked to reabsorption of sodium and urea. The permeability of the collecting ducts is regulated by antidiuretic hormone, release of which from the neurohypophysis is triggered primarily by osmosensitive neurons located in the hypothalamus and secondarily by monitors of intravascular volume that reside in the heart, large arteries, kidney, liver, and brain. In the kidney, the hormone acts to increase the permeability of the distal tubules and collecting ducts to water by means of a cyclic adenosine monophosphate–dependent mechanism. This permits water to flow by passive diffusion from the tubule into the hypertonic medullary interstitium of the kidney.

In primary nephrogenic diabetes insipidus, the distal tubule fails to respond normally to antidiuretic hormone, whether endogenous or exogenous. In secondary forms of nephrogenic diabetes insipidus, the hypertonic medullary gradient may be diminished owing to a solute diuresis or inability of tubules to reabsorb sodium chloride and urea. Alternatively, the secondary form may result from induced tubular unresponsiveness to the hormone.

CLINICAL MANIFESTATIONS. Males with primary nephrogenic diabetes insipidus have dramatic history of polyuria and polydipsia in infancy, often with episodes of hypernatremic dehydration. Females with the primary defect have milder symptoms that may not be detected until later in life. Patients having secondary forms of the disease present with hypernatremia during the course of their primary disorder.

DIAGNOSIS. The diagnosis of primary nephrogenic diabetes insipidus is suspected on clinical history, often with a positive family history in males. Laboratory findings include hypernatremia and dilute urine. If the serum osmolality at initial study exceeds 295 mOsm/kg (mmol/kg) H_2O and concurrent urine osmolality is less than this value, then a dehydration test to establish the diagnosis is unnecessary. The diagnosis is confirmed by administering an intramuscular injection of 0.1–0.2 unit/kg of aqueous vasopressin and measuring the serum and urine osmolality each hour for 4 hr. If the ratio of urine-to-plasma osmolality remains less than 1.0, the patient has nephrogenic diabetes insipidus. If the ratio becomes greater than 1.0, then central diabetes insipidus is suggested, but psychogenic polydipsia must be excluded. Patients with initial serum osmolality levels less than 295 mOsm/kg (mmol/kg) H_2O should be fasted (during the day rather than overnight) until serum osmolality exceeds 295 mOsm/kg (mmol/kg) H_2O; vasopressin is then given as before. The withholding of fluids should be terminated if body weight declines by as much as 3%. In patients suspected of primary nephrogenic diabetes insipidus, appropriate biochemical and radiographic studies should be done to exclude secondary causes.

COMPLICATIONS. As originally described, primary nephrogenic diabetes insipidus was associated with mental retardation. Retardation is more likely the result of repeated episodes of hypertonic dehydration than the consequence of the disease itself. Growth retardation is uniformly present in males with the primary disorder but is usually absent in females. Growth failure was originally thought to result from inadequate caloric intake due to excessive fluid intake, but it now seems that growth failure is intrinsic to the homozygous state. Dilatation of the urinary collecting system may result from excessive urine production. Accordingly, the anatomy of the urinary tract should be examined for evidence of hydronephrosis every few years by renal scan (intravenous pyelography may not visualize the collecting systems when there is rapid flow of large volumes of dilute urine).

TREATMENT. The keys to treatment include the provision of adequate fluid and caloric intake and reduction of the urinary solute load. These are accomplished by limiting the intake of a low sodium formula (SMA, Wyeth Laboratories, Philadelphia, PA; Similac PM 60/40, Ross Laboratories, Columbus, OH) to only that which is necessary to supply optimal caloric intake for growth. The remainder of the daily fluid requirement (as determined by the maintenance of a normal serum sodium level) is administered as water or fruit juice. The parents should be cautioned that until the child can obtain free access to water, fluids should be offered every 1–2 hr during the day and three times during the night. Once the child becomes old enough to obtain free access to water, the intact thirst mechanism will provide the appropriate stimulus for fluid intake.

In patients with the primary disorder, the urinary volume can be dramatically reduced by diuretic therapy. This paradoxical response results because sodium depletion seems to enhance proximal tubular reabsorption of sodium and water. Less water, therefore, is presented to the defective portion of the tubules. Chlorothiazide (20–40 mg/kg/24 hr in divided doses) in conjunction with moderate salt restriction may significantly reduce the need for fluid intake and the frequency of voiding. The patient should be monitored for the development of hypokalemia. Patients who fail to respond to a low-solute diet and diuretics may be candidates for treatment with inhibitors of prostaglandin synthesis (e.g., indomethacin). This type of therapy is of no value for secondary forms of the disease.

PROGNOSIS. Primary nephrogenic diabetes insipidus is a lifelong disease with a good prognosis if hypernatremic dehydration can be avoided. Genetic counseling should be provided for the family. The prognosis of secondary forms of the disease depend on the nature of the primary disorder. The syndrome may resolve after correction of obstructive lesions.

Gibbons MD, Koontz WW Jr: Obstructive uropathy and nephrogenic diabetes insipidus in infants. J Urol 122:556, 1979.
Hodjatilt S Jr: Polyuria in children: Clinical evaluation and differential diagnosis. J Urol 121:223, 1979.
Jamison RL, Oliver RE: Disorders of urinary concentration. Am J Med 72:308, 1982.
Libber SL, Harrison H, Spector D: Treatment of nephrogenic diabetes insipidus with prostaglandin synthesis inhibitors. J Pediatr 108:305, 1986.
Rascher W, Rosendahl W, Henrichs IA, et al: Congenital nephrogenic diabetes insipidus—vasopressin and prostaglandins in response to treatment with hydrochlorothiazide and indomethacin. Pediatr Nephrol 1:485, 1987.
Shapiro SR, Woerner S, Adelman RD, et al: Diabetes insipidus and hydronephrosis. J Urol 119:715, 1978.

18.31 BARTTER SYNDROME

This rare form of renal potassium wasting is characterized by hypokalemia, normal blood pressure, vascular insensitivity to pressor agents, and elevated plasma concentrations of renin and aldosterone. In certain families, the disorder may be inherited as an autosomal recessive trait.

PATHOLOGY. Generalized hyperplasia of the juxtaglomerular apparatus, the site of renin production, is observed in most patients with the syndrome. The renal parenchyma is otherwise normal in most patients; a few have shown nonspecific glomerular disease or interstitial disease or both.

PATHOGENESIS. The etiology is unknown. Currently, the disorder is best explained as a primary defect in chloride reabsorption in the ascending limb of the loop of Henle. The resultant decrease in sodium chloride reabsorption in this portion of the loop will reduce medullary hypertonicity, perhaps explaining the concentrating defect. The defect in chloride reabsorption presents extra sodium chloride to the distal tubule, where sodium is reabsorbed in exchange for potassium; the result is urinary potassium wasting. The induced hypokalemia stimulates the synthesis of prostaglandins (which may account for the vascular insensitivity to pressor agents and the defect in platelet aggregation); these, in turn, activate the renin-angiotensin-aldosterone system by increasing renin release and by stimulating aldosterone synthesis. The latter exacerbates renal potassium wasting.

CLINICAL MANIFESTATIONS. Young children typically present with growth failure, muscle weakness, constipation, polyuria, and dehydration due to urinary salt and water loss. Older children have muscle weakness or cramps and carpopedal spasms.

DIAGNOSIS. The diagnosis is suggested by the finding of hypokalemia; the serum potassium level is usually less than 2.5 mEq/L (mmol/L). Supportive findings include normal blood pressure; defective platelet aggregation; hypochloremia; metabolic alkalosis; elevated plasma levels of renin, aldosterone, and prostaglandin E_2; and high urinary levels of potassium and chloride. Some patients may also have hypercalciuria, hyperuricemia, hypomagnesemia, and urinary sodium-wasting. The diagnosis is confirmed by the histologic demonstration of hyperplasia of the juxtaglomerular apparatus, but this abnormality is not found in all patients and is most frequently absent in young children.

Bartter syndrome must be differentiated from licorice abuse, laxative or diuretic use, persistent vomiting or diarrhea, pyelonephritis, and diabetes insipidus. Several of these (laxative use, vomiting, diarrhea, diabetes insipidus) are associated with hypovolemia, which results in a low urinary chloride level; whereas Bartter syndrome is associated with an elevated level.

TREATMENT. The goals of therapy are to supply adequate nutrition and to maintain the serum potassium level above 3.5 mEq/L (mmol/L). Therapy is initiated with oral potassium chloride supplementation, increasing the dose until the serum potassium level reaches 3.5 mEq/L (mmol/L) or the dosage reaches 250 mEq/24 hr. A reasonably well-tolerated potassium preparation is K-Lyte/Cl (Mead Johnson Company, Evansville IN), flavored effervescent tablets containing 25 or 50 mEq of potassium chloride. Sodium chloride supplementation may also be required in small children. If the serum potassium level remains below 3.5 mEq/L (mmol/L) after reaching a dose

TABLE 18–6. Causes of Interstitial Nephritis

Acute	Chronic
Drugs	***Drugs***
Penicillin derivatives	Analgesics
Cephalosporins	Lithium
Sulfonamides	***Infections***
Co-trimoxazole	Pyelonephritis
Rifampin	***Disease-Associated***
Phenytoin	Vesicoureteral reflux
Thiazides	Nephrocalcinosis
Furosemide	Prolonged hypokalemia
Allopurinol	Oxalate nephropathy
Cimetidine	Heavy metals
Amphotericin B	Radiation
Nonsteroidal anti-inflammatory drugs	Obstructive uropathy
Infections	Medullary cystic disease
Streptococcal	
Pyelonephritis	
Toxoplasmosis	
Diphtheria	
Brucellosis	
Leptospirosis	
Mononucleosis	
Cytomegalovirus	
Disease-Associated	
Sarcoidosis	
Glomerulonephritis	
Transplant rejection	
Idiopathic	

of 250 mEq/24 hr of potassium chloride, then triamterene, 5–10 mg/kg/24 hr in divided doses, should be added. If this fails to resolve the hypokalemia, then indomethacin, 3–5 mg/kg/24 hr divided into three doses, should be given. The use of indomethacin is generally avoided or minimized because of gastrointestinal complications.

PROGNOSIS. The long-term prognosis of Bartter syndrome is uncertain. Many patients remain well, but some (especially those with glomerular or interstitial abnormalities) progress to renal insufficiency. Despite severe growth retardation in infancy, normal stature is ultimately obtained. The suggestion that mental retardation occurs in patients who have severe disease in the 1st yr of life remains to be confirmed.

Bartter FC: On the pathogenesis of Bartter's syndrome. Mineral Electrolyte Metab 3:61, 1980.
Chan JCM: Bartter's syndrome. Nephron 26:155, 1980.
Dunn MJ: Prostaglandins and Bartter's syndrome. Kidney Int 19:86, 1981.
Gill JR Jr: Bartter's syndrome. Annu Rev Med 31:405, 1980.
Robson WL, Arbus GS, Balfe JW: Bartter's syndrome. Am J Dis Child 133:636, 1979.
Simopoulos AP: Growth characteristics in patients with Bartter's syndrome. Nephron 23:130, 1979.
Stoff JS, Stemerman M, Steer M, et al: A defect in platelet aggregation in Bartter's syndrome. Am J Med 68:171, 1980.

18.32 INTERSTITIAL NEPHRITIS

Interstitial nephritis is a histopathologic term signifying inflammation between the glomeruli in the areas surrounding the tubules (the interstitium). Acute and chronic forms are recognized, depending on the nature of the inflammatory infiltrate and the presence or absence of edema and fibrosis. Tubular damage is generally present; glomerular changes may be minimal. Common causes of interstitial nephritis in children are listed in Table 18–6.

ACUTE INTERSTITIAL NEPHRITIS

PATHOLOGY. Whatever the cause of interstitial disease, the interstitial infiltrate is composed of lymphocytes, plasma cells, eosinophils, and occasional neutrophils (Fig. 18–18). The tubules are separated by edema and may show degeneration or frank necrosis. Unless the interstitial nephritis is associated with glomerulonephritis, the glomeruli are normal.

PATHOGENESIS. The genesis of acute interstitial nephritis is poorly understood. When it is due to drug ingestion, failure of the amount of drug administered to correlate with incidence of the syndrome suggests a hypersensitivity reaction. For methicillin, an immunologic mechanism has been suggested in several instances by the finding of anti–tubular basement membrane antibodies. Whether infections cause interstitial inflammation by direct invasion or by other mechanisms remains unclear. In certain forms of glomerulonephritis, tubular basement membrane deposition of immune complexes (lupus, membranoproliferative) or of anti–basement membrane antibodies (Goodpasture, membranous) may initiate the inflammatory reaction. In sarcoidosis and transplant rejection, cell-mediated mechanisms may play a role.

CLINICAL MANIFESTATIONS. In hospitalized patients, drugs are the most common cause of acute interstitial nephritis. After a week or so of drug therapy, patients typically present fever and a maculopapular skin rash. Urine output may be normal or diminished. Increased numbers of eosinophils may be detected in the blood or urine or both. Acute renal failure or generalized tubular dysfunction or both may result. Other forms of acute interstitial nephritis present a clinical picture resembling acute glomerulonephritis or acute renal failure, along with manifestations of the initiating disorder.

DIAGNOSIS. The diagnosis is confirmed by renal biopsy, although acute interstitial nephritis may not be suspected prior to the biopsy. The differential diagnosis includes other causes of acute nephritis or renal failure.

PREVENTION. The development of drug-related interstitial nephritis may be reduced by using alternative therapeutic agents when possible (e.g., the substitution of nafcillin for methicillin).

TREATMENT AND PROGNOSIS. Following appropriate management of the acute renal failure, withdrawal of possible inciting agents, and treatment of precipitating infection, the acute interstitial nephritis may resolve completely, but residual renal dysfunction is not uncommon. In patients suffering

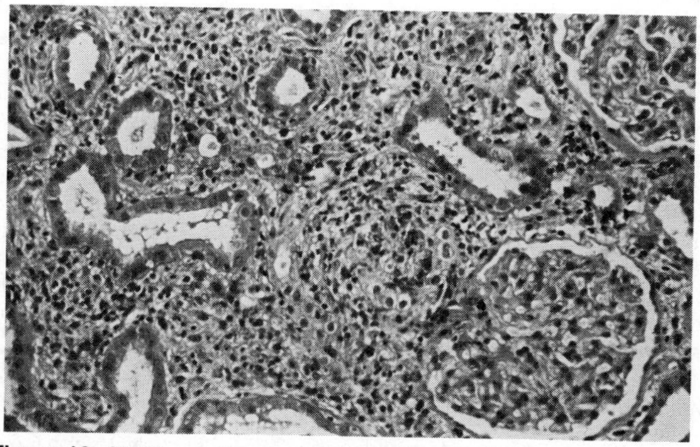

Figure 18–18. Biopsy from a patient having acute interstitial nephritis. The tubules are widely separated by edema and an intense inflammatory infiltrate containing lymphocytes, plasma cells, eosinophils, and neutrophils. The glomeruli are preserved. (× 80.)

severe histologic injury and renal failure, high-dose corticosteroid therapy may bring dramatic improvement.

CHRONIC INTERSTITIAL NEPHRITIS

PATHOLOGY. In chronic interstitial nephritis, the inflammatory infiltrate consists of lymphocytes and plasma cells. The edema of the acute form is replaced by interstitial fibrosis. Tubular dilatation and atrophy are widespread. The glomeruli show partial or total sclerosis, presumably as a result of ischemia.

CLINICAL MANIFESTATIONS. In children, chronic interstitial nephritis usually develops in association with an occult structural abnormality of the kidneys or lower urinary tract (cystic disease, obstruction, reflux). The presenting clinical manifestations may be those of chronic renal failure (nausea, vomiting, pallor, headache, fatigue, hypertension, growth failure) or manifestations of the underlying disorder (urinary tract infection, flank mass).

DIAGNOSIS. The diagnosis is suggested by the presence of chronic renal insufficiency in association with a known cause of the disorder; renal biopsy is not usually indicated.

TREATMENT AND PROGNOSIS. The natural history of chronic interstitial nephritis is progression to end-stage renal failure. Whether elimination of infection or correction of reflux or obstruction will alter this progression is unclear. In adults, avoidance of analgesics (phenacetin) and lithium prior to the development of end-stage renal failure may result in improvement in renal function.

Ellis D, Fried WA, Yunis EJ, et al: Acute interstitial nephritis in children: A report of 13 cases and review of the literature. Pediatrics 67:862, 1981.
Galpin JE, Shinaberger JH, Stanley TM, et al: Acute interstitial nephritis due to methicillin. Am J Med 65:756, 1978.
Kincaid-Smith P: Analgesic abuse and the kidney. Kidney Int 17:250, 1980.
Linton AL, Clark WF, Driedger AA, et al: Acute interstitial nephritis due to drugs. Ann Intern Med 93:735, 1980.
Neilson EG: Pathogenesis and therapy of interstitial nephritis. Kidney Int 35:1257, 1989.
Ten RM, Torres VE, Milliner DS, et al: Acute interstitial nephritis: Immunological and clinical aspects. Mayo Clin Proc 63:921, 1988.

18.33 TOXIC NEPHROPATHIES

Medications, diagnostic agents (iodinated radiographic contrast media), and chemicals may alter the kidneys directly (through reduction of renal blood flow, acute tubular necrosis, intratubular obstruction) or indirectly (through induction of an allergic or hypersensitivity reaction in the vessels or interstitium). Commonly nephrotoxic agents and their clinical manifestations are listed in Table 18–7. Nephrotoxicity is frequently reversible if the noxious agent is removed.

Useful agents should not be withheld because of potential nephrotoxicity, but preventive measures may reduce the risks of nephrotoxicity: (1) in patients with pre-existing renal disease, substitution of ultrasound or isotopic scans for studies using contrast media; (2) substitution of non-nephrotoxic agents for nephrotoxic agents if possible; (3) use of the lowest effective dose of the agent in conjunction with monitoring of the blood level; (4) reduction of the dose in patients with renal insufficiency; (5) avoidance of simultaneous use of several nephrotoxic agents.

Abraham PA, Keane WF: Glomerular and interstitial disease induced by nonsteroidal anti-inflammatory drugs. Am J Nephrol 4:1, 1984.
Bennett WM: Aminoglycoside nephrotoxicity. Mineral Electrolyte Metab 6:277, 1981.
Bennett WM: Lead nephropathy. Kidney Int 28:212, 1985.
Bennett WM, Plamp C, Porter CA: Drug-related syndromes in clinical nephrology. Ann Intern Med 87:582, 1977.
Fer MF, McKinney TD, Richardson RL, et al: Cancer and the kidney: Renal complications of neoplasms. Am J Med 71:704, 1981.
Mendoza SA: Nephrotoxic drugs. Pediatr Nephrol 2:466, 1988.
Murgo AJ: Thrombotic microangiopathy in the cancer patient including those induced by chemotherapeutic agents. Semin Hematol 24:161, 1987.
Porter GA, Bennett WM: Nephrotoxic acute renal failure due to common drugs. Am J Physiol 241:F1, 1981.
Roxe DM: Toxic nephropathy from diagnostic and therapeutic agents. Am J Med 69:759, 1980.
Safirstein R, Winston J, Goldstein M, et al: Cisplatin nephrotoxicity. Am J Kidney Dis 8:356, 1986.
Schwab SJ, Hlatky MA, Pieper KS, et al: Contrast nephrotoxicity: A randomized controlled trial of a nonionic and an ionic radiographic contrast agent. N Engl J Med 320:149, 1989.
Wedeen RP: Occupational renal disease. Am J Kidney Dis 3:241, 1984.

18.34 KIDNEY PROBLEMS IN THE NEWBORN INFANT

Almost all premature and full-term infants void within the first 24 hr after birth. If an infant has not voided by the end of the 1st day of life, a search should be initiated for underlying anatomic abnormalities.

The urine of the healthy neonate may have a pH from 5–7 and an osmolality of 60–600 mOsm/kg (mmol/kg) H_2O. It usually has many epithelial cells and may contain an occasional red blood cell. White blood cells should be absent, and the culture should be sterile. Trace amounts of glucose and protein may be found on dipstick testing.

RENAL DYSGENESIS

APLASIA (see Sec. 18.38).

HYPOPLASIA. This term signifies small kidneys having a reduction in the number of nephrons. Hypoplasia is not inherited; it may be unilateral or bilateral. When unilateral, the hypoplasia may involve the entire kidney or portions thereof. In the latter case (segmental hypoplasia or Ask-Upmark kidney), transverse scars may run from cortex to medulla. Unilateral hypoplasia of either type is one of the more common causes of hypertension in the first decade of life.

Bilateral hypoplasia usually presents with the manifestations of chronic renal failure and is a leading cause of end-stage renal failure during the first decade of life. A history of polyuria and polydipsia is common. Urinalysis may be normal. A rare form of bilateral hypoplasia is called *oligomeganephronia*, in which the number of nephrons is markedly reduced but those present are markedly hypertrophied.

DYSPLASIA. This term indicates altered structural differentiation of the fetal kidney such that it contains cysts, abnormal ducts, undifferentiated mesenchyme, or nonrenal elements (such as cartilage).

Dysplasia may result from *intrauterine obstruction* of the urinary tract (prune-belly syndrome, ureterocele, urethral valves, ureteropelvic junction, and so on). Such dysplasia is usually bilateral and frequently leads to end-stage renal failure.

Another form of the disorder is *multicystic dysplasia*. This may be unilateral or bilateral and is commonly associated with developmental anomalies of the lower tracts. In the unilateral form, the patient presents with a nonfunctioning flank mass that appears histologically to be a mass of cysts containing little or no identifiable renal tissue. The mass is usually removed if hypertension or infection develops. Bilateral multicystic dysplasia is associated with chronic renal failure; severe cases may show Potter syndrome.

Arant BS Jr, Sotelo-Avila C, Bernstein J: Segmental "hypoplasia" of the kidney (Ask-Upmark). J Pediatr 95:931, 1979.

TABLE 18–7. Nephrotoxic Compounds*

Nephrotic Syndrome
- Angiotensin converting enzyme inhibitors
- Gold salts
- Mercurial diuretics
- Mercury compounds
- Nonsteroidal anti-inflammatory drugs
- Paramethadione
- Penicillamine
- Perchlorate
- Probenecid
- Tolbutamide
- Trimethadione

Nephrogenic Diabetes Insipidus
- Amphotericin B
- Demeclocycline
- Lithium carbonate
- Methoxyflurane
- Propoxyphene

Fanconi Syndrome
- Aminoglycosides
- Cadmium
- Lead
- Lysol
- Mercury
- Nitrobenzene
- Outdated tetracycline
- Salicylate
- Uranium

Renal Tubular Acidosis
- Amphotericin B
- Lithium salts
- Toluene sniffing

Interstitial Nephritis with or without Papillary Necrosis
- Amidopyrine
- p-Aminosalicylate
- Bunamiodyl (papillary necrosis only)
- Penicillins (especially methicillin)
- Phenacetin
- Phenylbutazone
- Salicylate
- Sulfonamides
- Nonsteroidal anti-inflammatory agents

Renal Vasculitis with or without Glomerular Capillary Involvement
- Hydralazine
- Isoniazid
- Sulfonamides
- Any of the numerous other drugs that may cause a hypersensitivity reaction

Nephrocalcinosis or Nephrolithiasis
- Allopurinol
- Ethylene glycol
- Methoxyflurane
- Vitamin D

Miscellaneous Renal Manifestations Including Proteinuria, Hematuria, Oliguria, Tubular Necrosis, and Renal Failure
- Acyclovir
- Angiotensin converting enzyme inhibitors
- Arsenic
- Bacitracin
- Cadmium
- Carbon tetrachloride
- Cephaloridine
- Cephalothin
- Cisplatin
- Colistin
- Copper
- Cyclosporine
- Ethylene glycol
- Gentamicin
- Gold salts
- Indomethacin
- Iron
- Kanamycin
- Mercury salts
- Mitomycin C
- Neomycin
- Pentamidine
- Poisonous mushrooms
- Polymyxin B
- Radiocontrast agents
- Streptomycin
- Sulfonamides
- Tetrachlorethylene
- Vancomycin
- Viomycin

*The agents are grouped according to the principal site of injury or manifestations. (Dr. Sean O'Regan assisted in the preparation of this table.)

Ashkenazi S, Merlob P, Stark H, et al: Renal anomalies in neonates with spontaneous pneumothorax—incidence and evaluation. Int J Pediatr Nephrol 4:25, 1983.

Carter JE, Lirenman DS: Bilateral renal hypoplasia with oligomeganephronia. Am J Dis Child 120:537, 1970.

Clark DA: Times of first void and first stool in 500 newborns. Pediatrics 60:457, 1977.

Moore ES, Galvez MB: Delayed micturition in the newborn. J Pediatr 80:867, 1972.

Roodhooft AM, Birnholz JC, Holmes CB: Familial nature of congenital absence and severe dysgenesis of both kidneys. N Engl J Med 310:1341, 1984.

Thomas IT, Smith DW: Oligohydramnios, cause of the nonrenal features of Potter's syndrome, including pulmonary hypoplasia. J Pediatr 84:811, 1974.

Vinocur L, Slovis TL, Perlmutter AD, et al: Follow-up studies of multicystic dysplastic kidneys. Radiology 167:311, 1988.

CORTICAL NECROSIS

Renal cortical (and frequently medullary) necrosis seems to represent a final common result of several types of renal injury. It usually involves both kidneys and may be patchy or involve the entire cortex.

ETIOLOGY. In the newborn, cortical necrosis develops after dehydration, asphyxia, shock, disseminated intravascular coagulation, or renal vein thrombosis. After the newborn period, cortical necrosis most commonly develops with the hemolytic-uremic syndrome.

PATHOLOGY. Involved portions of the cortex show infarction, with congestion of the glomeruli, thrombosis of the arterioles, and necrosis of the tubules.

PATHOGENESIS. Cortical necrosis seems to develop when endothelial cell injury occurs in conjunction with diminished renal cortical blood flow. Toxins that presumably develop during shock, hemolytic-uremic syndrome, or sepsis (endotoxin) may injure the endothelial cells and initiate intrarenal coagulation, leading to thrombosis and cortical necrosis.

CLINICAL MANIFESTATIONS. Cortical necrosis commonly presents as acute renal failure developing in infants having the above-mentioned predisposing causes. The kidneys are frequently enlarged. Urine output is diminished and may show gross hematuria.

DIAGNOSIS. The diagnosis is supported by the detection on ultrasonography of enlarged, nonobstructed kidneys, which on isotopic renal scan show little or no renal blood flow or function. The differential diagnosis includes other causes of renal failure (Table 18–8).

TREATMENT AND PROGNOSIS. Therapy is supportive and involves correction of dehydration, asphyxia, and shock

TABLE 18–8. Causes of Acute Renal Failure in the Newborn

Renal dysgenesis	Hemorrhage
Obstructive uropathy	Sepsis
Renovascular accidents	Anoxia
Congenital heart disease	Shock
Dehydration	Renal vein thrombosis

and treatment of sepsis. The prognosis depends on the amount of surviving renal cortex.

Anand SK, Northway JD, Smith JA: Neonatal renal papillary and cortical necrosis. Am J Dis Child 131:773, 1977.
Chevalier RL, Campbell F, Brenbridge ANAG: Prognostic factors in neonatal acute renal failure. Pediatrics 74:265, 1984.
Dauber IM, Krauss AN, Symchych PS, et al: Renal failure following perinatal anoxia. J Pediatr 88:851, 1976.
Guignard JP, Torrado A, Mazouni SM, et al: Renal function in respiratory distress syndrome. J Pediatr 88:845, 1976.
Reimold EW, Don TD, Worthen HG: Renal failure during the first year of life. Pediatrics 59:987, 1977.
Rodriguez-Soriano J, Vallo A, Bilbao F, et al: Different functional characteristics of residual nephrons in infantile vs adult diffuse cortical necrosis. Int J Pediatr Nephrol 3:71, 1982.

URINARY TRACT INFECTION IN THE NEWBORN

This subject is reviewed in Sec. 9.66 and 18.39.

RENAL FAILURE

18.35 ACUTE RENAL FAILURE

Acute renal failure develops when renal function is diminished to the point at which body fluid homeostasis can no longer be maintained. Although oliguria (daily urine volume less than 400 mL/m^2) is common, the urine volume may approximate normal (nonoliguric renal failure) in certain types of acute renal failure (aminoglycoside nephrotoxicity). To monitor renal function, it is important to use biochemical studies (BUN, creatinine) as well as measurement of urine volume.

ETIOLOGY. The causes of acute failure are listed in Table 18–9. In the first category (prerenal), decreased perfusion of the kidney results in decreased renal function; the second category includes diseases of the kidney, while the third is composed primarily of obstructive disorders.

PATHOGENESIS. *Prerenal causes* of acute renal failure produce decreased renal perfusion through decreases in the total or "effective" circulating blood volume. Evidence of kidney damage is absent. Diminished intravascular volume leads to a fall in cardiac output, causing a decline in renal cortical blood flow and GFR. If, within a certain time, the underlying cause of the hypoperfusion is reversed, then renal function may return to normal. If hypoperfusion persists beyond this critical point, then renal parenchymal damage may develop.

Renal causes of acute renal failure include the rapidly progressive forms of several types of glomerulonephritis (see Table 18–9) that are common causes of acute renal failure in older children. Activation of the coagulation system within the kidney, resulting in small vessel thrombosis, may lead to acute renal failure. The hemolytic-uremic syndrome is the most common cause of acute renal failure in toddlers.

The term "acute tubular necrosis" originally described a syndrome of acute renal failure in the absence of arterial or glomerular lesions. The proposed mechanism of the renal failure was necrosis of the tubular cells. Certain agents (heavy metals, chemicals) may indeed cause renal failure by producing tubular cell necrosis, but significant histologic changes are absent in kidneys from patients having other forms of "acute tubular necrosis." The precise mechanism of renal failure in these patients is unknown. Proposed mechanisms include alterations in intrarenal hemodynamics, tubular obstruction, and passive backflow of the glomerular filtrate across injured tubular cells into the peritubular capillaries.

TABLE 18–9. Causes of Acute Renal Failure

Prerenal	Renal	Postrenal
Hypovolemia	Glomerulonephritis	Obstructive uropathy
Hemorrhage	Poststreptococcal	Ureteropelvic junction
Gastrointestinal losses	Lupus erythematosus	Ureterocele
Hypoproteinemia	Membranoproliferative	Urethral valves
Burns	Idiopathic rapid progressive	Tumor
Renal or adrenal disease with salt wasting	Anaphylactoid purpura	Vesicoureteral reflux
Hypotension	Localized intravascular coagulation	Acquired
Septicemia	Renal vein thrombosis	Stones
Disseminated intravascular coagulation	Cortical necrosis	Blood clot
Hypothermia	Hemolytic-uremic syndrome	
Hemorrhage	Acute tubular necrosis	
Heart failure	Heavy metals	
Hypoxia	Chemicals	
Pneumonia	Drugs	
Aortic clamping	Hemoglobin, myoglobin	
Respiratory distress syndrome	Shock	
	Ischemia	
	Acute interstitial nephritis	
	Infection	
	Drugs	
	Tumors	
	Renal parenchymal infiltration	
	Uric acid nephropathy	
	Developmental abnormalities	
	Cystic disease	
	Hypoplasia-dysplasia	
	Hereditary nephritis	

Acute interstitial nephritis is an increasingly common cause of acute renal failure and is usually the result of a hypersensitivity reaction to a therapeutic agent. Tumors may produce acute renal failure by infiltration of the kidney or by obstruction of the tubules by uric acid crystals (see Sec. 17.3 and 17.4).

Developmental abnormalities and hereditary nephritis may be associated with acute renal failure. Inability to conserve sodium and water is common in patients having these disorders, but losses are usually compensated by increased oral intake. If oral intake is compromised (vomiting) and/or extrarenal salt and water loss develops (diarrhea), then these, in conjunction with the obligate urinary salt and water losses, may lead to intravascular volume contraction and renal failure.

Postrenal causes of acute renal failure include obstructions of the urinary tract. With two functioning kidneys, ureteral obstruction must be bilateral to produce renal failure. It is important to recognize that dilatation of the upper collecting system may not occur until several days after acute ureteral obstruction.

CLINICAL MANIFESTATIONS. The presenting signs and symptoms may be dominated or modified by the precipitating disease. Clinical findings related to the renal failure include pallor (anemia), diminished urine output, edema (salt and water overload), hypertension, vomiting, and lethargy (uremic encephalopathy). Complications of acute renal failure include volume overload with congestive heart failure and pulmonary edema, arrhythmias, gastrointestinal bleeding due to stress ulcers or gastritis, seizures, coma, and behavioral changes.

DIAGNOSIS. A careful history may aid in defining the cause of renal failure. Vomiting, diarrhea, and fever suggest dehydration and prerenal azotemia, but these may also precede development of the hemolytic-uremic syndrome or renal vein thrombosis. Antecedent skin or throat infection suggests poststreptococcal glomerulonephritis. Rash may be found in systemic lupus erythematosus or anaphylactoid purpura. A history of exposure to chemicals and medications should be sought. Flank masses suggest renal vein thrombosis, tumors, cystic disease, or obstruction.

Laboratory abnormalities may include anemia (with the rare exception of blood loss, the anemia is usually dilutional or hemolytic, as seen in lupus, renal vein thrombosis, and the hemolytic-uremic syndrome); leukopenia (lupus); thrombocytopenia (lupus, renal vein thrombosis, hemolytic-uremic syndrome); hyponatremia (dilutional); hyperkalemia; acidosis; elevated serum concentrations of BUN, creatinine, uric acid, and phosphate (diminished renal function); and hypocalcemia (hyperphosphatemia). The serum C3 level may be depressed (poststreptococcal, lupus, or membranoproliferative glomerulonephritis), and antibodies may be detected in the serum to streptococcal (poststreptococcal glomerulonephritis), nuclear (lupus) or to basement membrane (Goodpasture disease) antigens. Chest roentgenography may reveal cardiomegaly and pulmonary congestion (fluid overload). In all patients presenting in acute renal failure, the possibility of obstruction (which, if detected, is quickly reversed by percutaneous nephrostomy) should be immediately assessed by obtaining a plain roentgenogram study of the abdomen, renal ultrasound, and a radionuclide scan; retrograde pyelography may occasionally be needed to detect occult obstructions. Renal biopsy may ultimately be required to determine the precise cause of renal failure.

TREATMENT. In children with *hypovolemia*, the need for volume replacement may be critical. The initial physical examination of the patient should include a careful assessment of the state of hydration. In some oliguric patients, it may be impossible to distinguish whether oliguria is due to hypoperfusion (hypovolemia) or impending acute tubular necrosis. Evaluation of the urine may prove helpful in this regard. In patients with hypovolemia, the urine is concentrated (urine osmolality exceeds 500 mOsm/kg [mmol/L] H_2O), its sodium content is usually less than 20 mEq/L (mmol/L), and the fractional excretion of sodium (urine/plasma sodium concentration divided by the urine/plasma creatinine concentration $\times$ 100) is usually less than 1%. By contrast, in patients with tubular necrosis, the urine is dilute (osmolality less than 350 mOsm/kg [mmol/L] H_2O), the sodium concentration usually exceeds 40 mEq/L (mmol/L), and the fractional excretion of sodium usually exceeds 1%.

If hypovolemia is detected, intravascular volume should be expanded by the intravenous administration of isotonic saline, 20 mL/kg, over 30 min. In the absence of blood loss or hypoproteinemia, colloid-containing solutions are not required for volume expansion. Following this infusion, the dehydrated patient will generally void within 2 hr. Failure to do so mandates a thorough re-evaluation of the patient. Catheterization of the bladder and determination of the central venous pressure may be helpful. If clinical and laboratory evaluations show that the patient is adequately hydrated, then aggressive diuretic therapy may be considered.

In patients with *impending renal failure* the value of diuretics in preventing development of anuria remains controversial. It seems clear that diuretics have no value in patients with established anuria. In some oliguric patients, furosemide or mannitol or both may increase the rate of urine production. These agents act by altering tubular function, but it should be recognized that the increase in urine flow does not represent an improvement in renal function nor will it affect the natural history of the disease that precipitated the renal failure. On the other hand, enhancement of urine output may be valuable in the management of hyperkalemia and fluid overload.

The pharmacodynamics of furosemide in renal failure are such that the urinary response (which is a function of the dose and blood level obtained) may be delayed for several hours. In the oliguric patient who lacks clinical and laboratory evidence of hypovolemia (and who may have already failed to respond to volume expansion), furosemide may be administered as a single intravenous dose of 2 mg/kg at the rate of 4 mg/per min (to avoid ototoxicity); if no response occurs, a second dose of 10 mg/kg may be given. Bumex may be given (0.1 mg/kg) as an alternative to Lasix. If no increase in urine production is obtained following this dose, then further furosemide therapy is contraindicated. A single intravenous dose of 0.5 g/kg of mannitol may be given over 30 min in addition to or in place of furosemide. Regardless of the response, no additional mannitol should be given, owing to the risk of toxicity. To increase renal cortical blood flow, dopamine (5 μg/kg/min) may be administered (in the absence of hypertension) in conjunction with diuretic therapy.

Fluid restriction is essential for the patient who fails to obtain adequate urine output following volume expansion or the administration of diuretics. The degree of fluid restriction depends upon the state of hydration. For the patient with oliguria or anuria having a relatively normal intravascular volume, fluid administration should be limited to 400 $mL/m^2/24$ hr (insensible losses) plus an amount of fluid equal to the urine output for that day. On the other hand, markedly hypervolemic patients may require almost total fluid restriction; omitting the replacement of insensible fluid losses and urine output will aid in diminishing the expanded intravascular volume. Access to the vascular space should be maintained; this is best obtained using an infusion pump at the slowest possible rate. In general, glucose-containing solutions (10–30%) without electrolytes are used as maintenance fluids.

The composition of the fluid may be modified in accordance with the state of electrolyte balance. Except in the overhydrated patient, extrarenal (blood, gastrointestinal tract) fluid losses should be replaced, milliliter for milliliter, with appropriate fluids.

In acute renal failure, rapid development of *hyperkalemia* (serum level greater than 6 mEq/L [mmol/L]) may lead to cardiac arrhythmia and death. *The patient should receive no potassium-containing fluid, foods, or medications until adequate renal function is re-established.* The earliest electrocardiographic change seen in patients with developing hyperkalemia is the appearance of tall, peaked T waves. This may be followed by ST-segment depression, prolongation of the P-R and widening of the QRS intervals, ventricular fibrillation, and cardiac arrest.

In children with acute renal failure, procedures to deplete body potassium are initiated when the serum potassium rises to 5.5 mEq/L (mmol/L). To minimize the rate at which the serum potassium rises, all solutions given to the patient should contain high concentrations of glucose. Sodium polystyrene sulfonate resin (Kayexalate), 1 g/kg, should be given orally or by retention enema. This material exchanges sodium for potassium. For best results, the resin should be given orally, suspended in 2 mL/kg of 70% sorbitol. Sorbitol produces an osmotic diarrhea, which will increase fluid and electrolyte losses (the usual patient in renal failure is hypervolemic with increased total body sodium and potassium levels), as well as enhance the movement of the resin through the gastrointestinal tract. Because 70% sorbitol is locally irritating to the rectum, the concentration should be reduced to 20% and the volume increased to 10 mL/kg when it is given by enema. Resin therapy may be repeated every 2 hr, the frequency being limited primarily by the risk of sodium overload.

If the serum potassium rises above 7 mEq/L (mmol/L), emergency measures in addition to Kayexalate must be initiated. The following agents should be given sequentially:

1. Calcium gluconate 10% solution, 0.5 mL/kg intravenously, over 10 min. The heart rate must be closely monitored during the infusion; a fall in rate of 20 beats/min requires stopping the infusion until the pulse returns to the preinfusion rate.
2. Sodium bicarbonate 7.5% solution, 3 mEq/kg intravenously. Possible complications include volume expansion, hypertension, and tetany.
3. Glucose 50% solution, 1 mL/kg, with regular insulin, 1 unit/5 g of glucose, given intravenously over 1 hr. The patient should be monitored closely for hypoglycemia.

Calcium gluconate does not lower the serum potassium but counteracts the potassium-induced increase in myocardial irritability. Bicarbonate lowers serum potassium; the mechanism is not clearly defined. The effect of glucose and insulin is to shift potassium from the extracellular to the intracellular compartment. β-Adrenergic receptor agonists given by aerosol also acutely lower potassium levels. The duration of action of these emergency measures is just a few hours. Persistent hyperkalemia, therefore, especially in patients requiring the emergency measures, should be managed by dialysis.

Moderate *acidosis* is common in renal failure as a result of inadequate excretion of hydrogen ion and ammonia but it rarely requires treatment. Severe acidosis (arterial pH less than 7.15, serum bicarbonate less than 8 mEq/L [mmol/kg]) may increase myocardial irritability and requires treatment. Because of the risks involved in the rapid infusion of alkali, the acidosis should be corrected only partially by the intravenous route, generally giving enough bicarbonate to raise the arterial pH to 7.20 (which approximates a serum bicarbonate level of 12 mEq/L [mmol/L]). The correction formula is:

$$\text{mEq NaHCO}_3\text{ required} = 0.3 \times \text{weight (kg)} \times (12 - \text{serum bicarbonate [mEq/L]}$$

The remainder of the correction, which should be accomplished only after normalization of the serum calcium and phosphorous, may be made by the oral administration of sodium bicarbonate tablets or sodium citrate solution.

In addition to the risks involved in administration of intravenous bicarbonate that have been noted, correction of acidosis with intravenous bicarbonate may precipitate tetany (see Sec. 6.27). In patients with renal failure, an inability to excrete phosphorus leads to hyperphosphatemia and a reciprocal hypocalcemia. Acidosis prevents the development of tetany by increasing the ionized fraction of the total calcium. Rapid correction of acidosis will reduce the ionized calcium concentration, resulting in tetany.

Hypocalcemia is treated by lowering the serum phosphorus. Unless tetany develops, calcium is not given intravenously, in order to avoid reaching a calcium × phosphorus product (mg/dL × mg/dL [mmol/L × mmol/L]) of 70 (6) in the serum, the point at which calcium salts are deposited in tissue. To lower the serum phosphorus, a phosphate-binding calcium carbonate antacid is given by mouth, increasing fecal phosphate excretion; common agents include Titralac Liquid (3M Company, St. Paul, MN; starting dose 5–15 mL/6 hr) and Os-Cal 500 tablets (Marion Laboratories, Kansas City, MO; starting dose 1–3 tablets/6 hr). The total daily dose should be gradually increased until the serum phosphorus level falls to normal.

Hyponatremia is commonly the result of administration of excessive amounts of hypotonic fluids to the oliguric-anuric patient. Correction may be accomplished by fluid restriction. Patients whose serum sodium levels fall below 120 mEq/L (mmol/L) are at increased risk for developing cerebral edema and central nervous system hemorrhage. In the absence of dehydration, water restriction is essential. When the serum sodium falls below 120 mEq/L (mmol/L), it may be elevated to 125 mEq/L (mmol/L) by the intravenous infusion of hypertonic (3%) sodium chloride, using the following formula:

$$\text{mEq NaCl required} = 0.6 \times \text{weight (kg)} \times (125 - \text{serum sodium [mEq/L]})$$

The risks of administration of hypertonic saline include volume expansion, hypertension, and congestive heart failure; if these occur, they may be treated by dialysis.

Gastrointestinal bleeding may be prevented with calcium carbonate antacids, which also serve to lower the serum phosphorus. Alternatively, intravenous Tagamet (Smith, Kline & French, Philadelphia, PA) may be administered at a dose of 5–10 mg/kg/12 hr.

Hypertension may result from the primary disease process or expansion of the extracellular fluid volume or both. In patients with renal failure and hypertension, salt and water restriction is critical.

In children with severe hypertension, a useful drug is diazoxide. This potent vasodilator must be given by rapid (less than 10 sec) intravenous injection at a dose of 5 mg/kg (maximum dose of 300 mg). A fall in blood pressure is usually seen within 10 to 20 min; if that following the first injection is insufficient, a second injection may be given 30 min later. Alternatively, nifedipine may be given acutely (0.25–0.5 mg/kg, sublingual). Sodium nitroprusside or labetalol as continuous intravenous infusion is indicated for hypertensive crises. For less severe hypertension, control of extracellular volume expansion (salt and water restriction, furosemide), and use of beta-blockers (e.g., propranolol) and vasodilators (e.g., apresoline) are generally effective.

Seizures may be the result of the primary disease process (e.g., systemic lupus erythematosus), hyponatremia (water intoxication), hypocalcemia (tetany), hypertension, or the uremic state itself. If possible, therapy should be directed toward the precipitating cause.

We have found that some of the usual anticonvulsant agents (paraldehyde, phenobarbital, phenytoin) are of limited effectiveness in uremia. Diazepam seems to be the most effective agent in controlling seizures. It should be remembered that its metabolic products are excreted in the urine and may accumulate in patients with renal insufficiency.

Except in the presence of hemolysis (e.g., hemolytic-uremic syndrome, lupus) or bleeding, the *anemia* of acute renal failure is generally mild (hemoglobin 9–10 g/dL [90–100 g/L]), is primarily the result of volume expansion (hemodilution), and does not require transfusion. Blood loss from active bleeding should be replaced appropriately.

In patients with hemolytic anemia or prolonged renal failure, if hemoglobin levels fall below 7 g/dL (70 g/L), blood should be given. In the hypervolemic patient, blood transfusion carries the risk of further volume expansion, which may produce hypertension, congestive heart failure, and pulmonary edema. Slow (4–6 hr) transfusion with fresh (to minimize the amount of potassium administered) packed red blood cells (10 mL/kg) will diminish the risk of hypervolemia. In the presence of severe hypervolemia, anemia should be corrected during dialysis.

The diet of most previously healthy and well-nourished children who suddenly develop acute renal failure should be restricted initially to fats and carbohydrates (gum drops and jelly beans), given the likelihood that the acute renal failure will resolve or respond to therapy within a reasonably brief period of time. Restrictions of sodium, potassium, and water administration have already been mentioned. If renal failure persists beyond 7 days, then an expanded oral diet for renal failure or parenteral hyperalimentation with essential amino acids should be considered.

Indications for *dialysis* in acute renal failure may comprise various combinations of the following factors: acidosis, electrolyte abnormalities (especially hyperkalemia), central nervous system disturbances, hypertension, fluid overload, and congestive heart failure. It appears that the early initiation of dialysis has significantly improved the survival in children with acute renal failure.

In certain patients with acute renal failure, careful medical management may minimize complications and delay the need for dialysis; other patients will eventually require dialysis for the uremic state itself. The life-threatening complications of uremia are hemorrhage, pericarditis, and central nervous system dysfunction; their precise causes are unknown. The risk of developing these complications correlates more closely with the level of BUN than with that of creatinine.

PROGNOSIS. The prognosis for recovery of renal function depends on the disorder that precipitated the renal failure. In general, recovery of function is likely following renal failure resulting from prerenal causes, the hemolytic-uremic syndrome, acute tubular necrosis, acute interstitial nephritis, or uric acid nephropathy. On the other hand, recovery of renal function is unusual when renal failure results from most types of rapidly progressive glomerulonephritis, bilateral renal vein thrombosis, or bilateral cortical necrosis.

Chesney RW, Kaplan BS, Freedom RM, et al: Acute renal failure: An important complication of cardiac surgery in infants. J Pediatr 87:381, 1975.
Diamond JR, Yoburn DC: Nonoliguric acute renal failure. Arch Intern Med 142:1882, 1982.
Feld LG, Springate JE, Fildes RD: Acute renal failure. I. Pathophysiology and diagnosis. J Pediatr 109:401, 1986.
Hodson EM, Kjellstrand CM, Mauer SM: Acute renal failure in infants and children: Outcome of 53 patients requiring hemodialysis treatment. J Pediatr 93:756, 1978.
Kjellstrand CM, Pru CE, Jahnke WK, et al: Acute renal failure. *In*: Drukker W, Parsons FM, Maher JF (eds): Replacement of Renal Function by Dialysis. Boston, Martinus Nijhoff, 1983, p 536.
Miller TR, Anderson RJ, Linas SL, et al: Urinary diagnostic indices in acute renal failure. Ann Intern Med 89:47, 1978.
Myers BD, Moran SM: Hemodynamically mediated acute renal failure. N Engl J Med 314:97, 1986.
Niaudet P, Haj-Ibrahim M, Gagnadoux M-F, et al: Outcome of children with acute renal failure. Kidney Int Suppl 17:148, 1985.
Steiner RW: Interpreting the fractional excretion of sodium. Am J Med 77:669, 1984.

18.36 CHRONIC RENAL FAILURE

ETIOLOGY. The etiology of chronic renal failure in childhood correlates closely with the age of the patient at the time when the renal failure is first detected. Chronic renal failure in children under 5 yr of age is commonly the result of anatomic abnormalities (hypoplasia, dysplasia, obstruction, malformations), whereas after 5 yr of age, acquired glomerular diseases (glomerulonephritis, hemolytic-uremic syndrome) or hereditary disorders (Alport syndrome, cystic disease) predominate.

PATHOGENESIS. Regardless of the cause of kidney damage, once a critical level of renal functional deterioration is reached, progression to end-stage renal failure is inevitable. The precise mechanisms resulting in progressive functional deterioration are unclear, but factors that may play important roles include ongoing immunologic injury; hemodynamically mediated hyperfiltration in surviving glomeruli; dietary protein and phosphorus intake; persistent proteinuria; and systemic hypertension.

Ongoing deposition of immune complexes or anti–GBM antibodies in the glomerulus may result in persistent glomerular inflammation that leads to eventual scarring.

Hyperfiltration injury may be an important final common pathway of ultimate glomerular destruction, independent of the initiating mechanism of renal injury. Once nephrons are lost for any reason, the remaining nephrons undergo structural and functional hypertrophy mediated, at least in part, by an increase in glomerular blood flow. The increased blood flow increases the driving force for glomerular filtration in the surviving nephrons. This beneficial "hyperfiltration" in surviving glomeruli, which serves to preserve renal function, may also damage these glomeruli by mechanisms that are not understood. Potential mechanisms of damage include the direct effect of the elevated hydrostatic pressure on the integrity of the capillary wall, the resultant increase in the passage of proteins across the capillary wall, or both. Ultimately, this leads to changes in the mesangium and epithelial cells with the development of glomerular sclerosis. As sclerosis advances, the remaining nephrons suffer an increasing excretory burden, resulting in a vicious cycle of increasing glomerular blood flow and hyperfiltration. Angiotensin converting enzyme inhibition reduces hyperfiltration and may slow the progression of renal failure.

Experimental models of chronic renal insufficiency have shown that a high-protein diet accelerates the development of renal failure, perhaps by means of afferent arteriolar dilatation and hyperperfusion injury. Conversely, a low-protein diet diminishes the rate of functional deterioration. Studies of humans confirm that in normal individuals the GFR correlates directly with protein intake and suggest that restriction of dietary protein may reduce the rate of functional deterioration in chronic renal insufficiency.

Some controversial studies in animal models suggest that dietary phosphorus restriction preserves renal function in chronic renal insufficiency. Whether this beneficial effect is due to the prevention of calcium-phosphate salt deposition in the blood vessels and tissues or to suppression of secretion of parathyroid hormone, a potential nephrotoxin, is unclear.

Persistent proteinuria or systemic hypertension from any cause may directly damage the glomerular capillary wall, leading to glomerular sclerosis and initiation of hyperfiltration injury.

As renal function begins to deteriorate, compensatory mechanisms develop in remaining nephrons to maintain a normal internal environment. When the GFR falls below 20% of normal, however, a complex constellation of clinical, biochemical, and metabolic abnormalities develop that together constitute the uremic state. The pathophysiologic manifestations of the uremic state are listed in Table 18–10.

CLINICAL MANIFESTATIONS. In patients developing chronic renal failure from glomerular or hereditary diseases, the renal disease is usually detected because of clinical manifestations apparent prior to the onset of renal insufficiency. The development of renal failure may be insidious, however, in patients having anatomic abnormalities, and their presenting complaints may be nonspecific (headache, fatigue, lethargy, anorexia, vomiting, polydipsia, polyuria, growth failure). Physical examination occasionally may be surprisingly unrewarding, but most patients with chronic renal failure appear pale and weak and have high blood pressure. Patients having anatomic abnormalities, in whom the renal failure has developed slowly over several years, may also have growth retardation and rickets.

TREATMENT. The management of the child having chronic renal failure requires close monitoring of the patient's clinical (physical examination and blood pressure) and laboratory status. Blood studies to be followed routinely include the hemoglobin (anemia), electrolytes (hyponatremia, hyperkalemia, acidosis), BUN and creatinine (nitrogen accumulation and level of renal function), calcium and phosphorus levels, and alkaline phosphatase activity (hypocalcemia, hyperphosphatemia, osteodystrophy). Periodic examination of parathyroid hormone levels and roentgenographic studies of bone may be of value in detecting early evidence of osteodystrophy. Chest roentgenography and echocardiography may be helpful in assessing cardiac function. Nutritional status may be monitored by periodic evaluation of the serum albumin, zinc, transferrin, folic acid, and iron levels. Optimally, the patient should be managed in conjunction with a medical center capable of supplying medical, nursing, social service, and nutritional support as the patient progresses to end-stage renal failure.

TABLE 18–10. Pathophysiology of Chronic Renal Failure

Manifestation	Mechanisms
Accumulation of nitrogenous waste products (azotemia)	Decline in glomerular filtration rate
Acidosis	Urinary bicarbonate wasting Decreased ammonia excretion Decreased acid excretion
Sodium wasting	Solute diuresis Tubular damage Functional tubular adaption for sodium excretion
Sodium retention	Nephrotic syndrome Congestive heart failure Anuria Excessive salt intake
Urinary concentrating defect	Nephron loss Solute diuresis Increased medullary blood flow
Hyperkalemia	Decline in glomerular filtration rate Acidosis Excessive potassium intake Hypoaldosteronism
Renal osteodystrophy	Decreased intestinal calcium absorption Impaired production of 1,25-dihydroxy-vitamin D by the kidneys Hypocalcemia and hyperphosphatemia Secondary hyperparathyroidism
Growth retardation	Protein-calorie deficiency Renal osteodystrophy Acidosis Anemia Unknown factors
Anemia	Decreased erythropoietin production Low grade hemolysis Bleeding Decreased erythrocyte survival Inadequate iron intake Inadequate folic acid intake Inhibitors of erythropoiesis
Bleeding tendency	Thrombocytopenia Defective platelet function
Infection	Defective granulocyte function Impaired cellular immune functions
Neurologic (fatigue, poor concentration, headache, drowsiness, loss of memory, slurred speech, muscle weakness and cramps, seizures, coma, peripheral neuropathy, asterixis)	Uremic factor(s) Aluminum toxicity
Gastrointestinal ulceration	Gastric acid hypersecretion
Hypertension	Sodium and water overload Excessive renin production
Hypertriglyceridemia	Diminished plasma lipoprotein lipase activity
Pericarditis and cardiomyopathy	Unknown
Glucose intolerance	Tissue insulin resistance

Diet in Chronic Renal Failure

In children with renal insufficiency, the growth rate diminishes when the GFR falls below 50% of normal. The precise cause of growth failure is unknown; a major factor is inadequate caloric intake (less than 70% of recommended dietary allowance). The optimal caloric intake in renal insufficiency is unknown, but an attempt should be made to equal or exceed (in patients with growth failure) the recommended daily caloric allowance for age. Caloric intake can be enhanced by adding to the diet unrestricted amounts of carbohydrate (sugar, jam, honey, glucose polymers: Polycose, Ross Laboratories, Columbus, OH) and fat (medium-chain triglycerides oil: MCT Oil, Mead Johnson and Company, Evansville, IN) as tolerated by the patient.

When BUN exceeds approximately 80 mg/dL (30 mmol/L of urea), patients may develop nausea, vomiting, and anorexia. These symptoms result from the accumulation of nitrogenous waste products and can be relieved by restricting dietary protein intake. Because children in renal failure continue to require adequate protein intake for growth, protein is provided at the level of 1.5 g/kg/24 hr and should consist of proteins of high biologic value that are metabolized primarily to usable amino acids rather than to nitrogenous wastes. The proteins of highest such biologic value are those of eggs and milk, followed by meat, fish, and fowl. Because cow's milk contains a high concentration of phosphate, moderate restriction or the use of a formula containing a reduced amount of phosphate (Similac PM 60/40, Ross Laboratories, Columbus, OH), sometimes in conjunction with an oral phosphate binder (see subsequent section on renal osteodystrophy), may be indicated.

Owing to inadequate intake or dialysis losses, children with renal insufficiency may become deficient in water-soluble vitamins. These should be routinely supplied, using preparations such as Nephrocaps (Fleming, Fenton, MO). Zinc and iron supplements should be added only after deficiencies are confirmed. Supplementation with fat-soluble vitamins A, E, and K is not required.

Water and Electrolyte Management in Chronic Renal Failure

Until the development of end-stage renal failure requires the initiation of dialysis, water restriction is rarely necessary in children with renal insufficiency, since water needs are regulated by the thirst center in the brain.

Most children with renal insufficiency will maintain normal sodium balance with the sodium intake derived from an appropriate diet. Some patients whose renal insufficiency is a consequence of anatomic abnormalities may waste sodium in the urine and require dietary salt supplementation. On the other hand, patients with high blood pressure, edema, or congestive heart failure may require sodium restriction, sometimes in conjunction with aggressive furosemide therapy (1–4 mg/kg/24 hr).

In most children with renal insufficiency, potassium balance will be maintained until renal function deteriorates to the level at which dialysis is initiated. Hyperkalemia may develop in patients having only moderate renal insufficiency, however, as a result of excessive dietary potassium intake, the development of severe acidosis, or aldosterone deficiency (destruction of the juxtaglomerular apparatus). The hyperkalemia may be controlled by reducing dietary potassium intake and adding oral alkalinizing agents and/or Kayexalate (Winthrop Pharmaceuticals, New York, NY), an oral resin that (in 1 g/kg/dose) binds to and removes potassium from the intestine.

Acidosis in Chronic Renal Failure

Acidosis develops in almost all children with renal insufficiency and need not be treated unless the serum bicarbonate falls below 20 mEq/L (mmol/L). Either Bicitra (1 mL equals 1 mEq of base) or sodium bicarbonate tablets (325 and 650 mg; 325 mg equals 4 mEq of base) may be used to raise the serum bicarbonate above 20 mEq/L (mmol/L).

Renal Osteodystrophy

Renal osteodystrophy commonly develops in association with hyperphosphatemia, hypocalcemia, and elevation of parathyroid hormone levels and serum alkaline phosphatase activity. In general, serum phosphorus levels rise when the GFR falls below 30% of normal. Hyperphosphatemia lowers the serum calcium level because of the reciprocal solubility relationship; secondary hyperparathyroidism results. Hyperphosphatemia may be controlled with a low phosphate formula (Similac PM 60/40) and by enhancing fecal excretion by using oral calcium carbonate, an antacid that coincidentally also binds phosphate in the intestinal tract. The usual dosage range is 1–4 tsp (Titralac, 3M Company, St. Paul, MN) or tablets (Os-Cal 500 Tablets, Marion Laboratories, Kansas City, MO) with each meal and before bed. Because aluminum may be absorbed from the gastrointestinal tract, especially in small children, and lead to aluminum poisoning (dementia, osteomalacia), aluminum antacids should be used rarely, if ever, with periodic monitoring of the serum aluminum level.

Hypocalcemia may result from hyperphosphatemia, inadequate dietary intake, and decreased intestinal calcium absorption caused by a deficiency in the active form (1,25-dihydroxycholecalciferol) of vitamin D. If the serum calcium remains low after correction of the serum phosphorus, then oral calcium supplements (Neo-Calglucon Syrup, Dorsey Pharmaceuticals, East Hanover, NJ; Os-Cal Tablets, Marion Laboratories, Kansas City, MO) at a dose of 500–1,000 mg/24 hr can be administered.

Vitamin D is converted to its active form (1,25-dihydroxycholecalciferol) by 1-hydroxylation in the kidney. With severe kidney destruction, insufficient conversion results in vitamin D deficiency. Vitamin D therapy is indicated (1) in patients having persistent hypocalcemia despite reduction of the serum phosphorus below 6 mg/dL (1.90 mmol/L) and the addition of oral calcium supplements; and (2) in patients with osteodystrophy, as indicated by elevated serum alkaline phosphatase activities and roentgenographic evidence of rickets. Therapy may be initiated with 1 capsule (0.25 μg) per day of the active form of dihydroxy vitamin D (Rocaltrol, Roche Laboratories, Nutley, NJ) or 0.05–0.20 mg/24 hr of dihydrotachysterol solution (DHT Oral Solution, Roxane Laboratories, Columbus, OH), which is metabolized to its active form in the liver. The dose of vitamin D is progressively increased until the serum calcium level and alkaline phosphatase activity are normal and roentgenographic healing of the rickets is seen. The dose of vitamin D should then be reduced to the initial level.

Anemia in Chronic Renal Failure

Anemia is common in chronic renal failure and is primarily the result of inadequate erythropoietin production by the failing kidneys, but inadequate dietary intake of iron and folic acid should not be overlooked. In most patients, the hemoglobin level will stabilize in the range of 6–9 g/dL (60–90 g/L); transfusion therapy is not indicated, as this would further suppress erythropoietin production. If the hemoglobin falls below 6 g/dL (60 g/L), 10 mL/kg of packed red blood cells should be administered cautiously (the small volume reduces the risk of circulatory overload). The problem of anemia may be alleviated with the introduction of recombinant human erythropoietin therapy.

Hypertension in Chronic Renal Failure

Hypertensive emergencies should be treated with sublingual nifedipine or intravenous administration of diazoxide (Hyperstat, Schering Corporation, Kenilworth, NJ). The dose of diazoxide is 5 mg/kg, up to a maximum of 300 mg; it is given within 10 sec by manual injection. When severe hypertension is associated with circulatory overload, 2–4 mg/kg of furosemide may also be administered at the rate of 4 mg/min. Sodium nitroprusside should be used with great caution in renal insufficiency, owing to the possible accumulation of toxic thiocyanate.

The treatment of sustained hypertension may include a combination of salt restriction (2–3 g/24 hr), furosemide (1–4 mg/kg/24 hr), propranolol (Inderal, Ayerst Laboratories, New York, NY; 1–4 mg/kg/24 hr), and hydralazine (Apresoline, CIBA Pharmaceutical Company, Summit, NJ; 1–5 mg/kg). Minoxidil and captopril should be used only in patients whose blood pressure is inadequately controlled with the above measures and should be administered with the guidance of a pediatric nephrologist. Captopril may produce hyperkalemia.

TABLE 18–11. Value of Continuous Ambulatory Peritoneal Dialysis (CAPD)

Advantages	Disadvantages
Rapid training	Catheter malfunction
Technical simplicity (no machines)	Infection
Greater mobility	Poor appetite
Minimal dietary restriction	Poor body image
Feel better than hemodialysis patients	Parental "burnout" (emotional exhaustion)
Steady state chemistries	Elevated serum lipids
Can live far from medical center	
Cheaper than hemodialysis	
Improved growth rate	
Fewer blood transfusions	

Drug Dosage in Chronic Renal Failure

As many drugs are excreted by the kidneys, their administration to patients with renal insufficiency must be altered to maximize effectiveness and minimize the risk of toxicity (see Sec. 6.55).

18.37 END-STAGE RENAL FAILURE

In the treatment of end-stage renal failure in children, the ultimate goal is a successful kidney transplant (see Sec. 6.44). Both cadaver and living-related donors have been used extensively as sources for the organ graft. In centers using predominantly living-related donors, when the patient's serum creatinine is progressively increasing and is in the range of 5–6 mg/dL (450–530 μmol/L), the patient and his or her family (parents and siblings over the age of 18 yr) are generally typed for histocompatibility antigens. At that point, the physicians, nurses, and social workers begin a thorough education program for the family regarding both dialysis and transplantation. If there is a willing, compatible potential donor in the family, the person undergoes a complete medical evaluation prior to confirmation as the donor.

Dialysis is generally initiated when the patient's creatinine level approaches 10 mg/dL (900 μmol/L), depending on the patient's clinical status, the results of other laboratory studies, and the availability of a kidney donor. If no family donor is available, after beginning dialysis, the patient is placed on a waiting list for a cadaver kidney. Children are usually hospitalized for initiation of dialysis. If, in preparation for transplantation, bilateral nephrectomies are required (for severe hypertension, vesicoureteral reflux, or chronic pyelonephritis), these may be done at this time.

Continuous ambulatory peritoneal dialysis (CAPD) is the standard technique for the majority of children requiring chronic dialysis. However, some require hemodialysis and the use of long-term indwelling subclavian vein catheters and arteriovenous fistulas created at the wrist.

In CAPD, dialysis across the peritoneal membrane removes excess body water through an osmotic gradient created by the glucose concentration in the dialysate; wastes are removed by diffusion from the periotoneal capillaries into the dialysate. CAPD is not as efficient as hemodialysis, but the fact that it is continuous around the clock (as contrasted with 12–18 hr/wk for hemodialysis) permits the maintenance of satisfactory levels of BUN and creatinine.

Access to the peritoneal cavity is achieved by inserting a soft Tenckhoff catheter through a midline infraumbilical incision; the catheter is brought out through the skin by means of a subcutaneous tunnel and connected to an extension tube that has a spike for insertion into the dialysis bag.

The parents (and patient, if more than 10–12 yr old) are then taught the techniques of spiking the bags of dialysate, allowing the dialysate to run in and dwell in the peritoneal cavity for the prescribed period of time, draining the dialysate back into the dialysate bag, and replacing the used bag of dialysate with a fresh one. Such "exchanges" are performed 3–5 times per day between arising and bedtime. Because the advantages of CAPD seem to far outweigh the risks (Table 18–11), CAPD is the optimal form of chronic dialysis for most children.

An alternative to CAPD is continuous cyclic peritoneal dialysis (CCPD). This procedure reverses the schedule of CAPD by providing the exchanges at night rather than during the day. The exchanges are performed automatically during sleep by a simple cycler machine. This permits an uninterrupted day of activities, a reduction in the number of connections and disconnections (which should decrease the risk of peritonitis), and a reduction in the time required by the patient and parent to perform dialysis, reducing the risk of fatigue and burn-out.

The success rate for kidney transplants in children over the age of 5 yr approximates that for adults, and successful grafts have been performed in children as small as 5 kg. Ongoing research into better and less toxic means to prevent graft rejection should improve these statistics. Psychologic aspects of care of these children are discussed in Sec. 3.56 and 3.57.

JERRY MICHAEL BERGSTEIN

Andreoli SP, Bergstein JM, Sherrard DJ: Aluminum intoxication for aluminum-containing phosphate binders in children with azotemia not undergoing dialysis. N Engl J Med 310:1079, 1984.

Baldwin DS, Neugarten J: Treatment of hypertension in renal disease. Am J Kidney Dis 5:A57, 1985.

Baum M, Powell D, Calvin S, et al: Continuous ambulatory peritoneal dialysis in children. N Engl J Med 307:1537, 1982.

Bennett WM, Aronoff GR, Morrison G, et al: Drug prescribing in renal failure: Dosing guidelines for adults. Am J Kidney Dis 3:155, 1983.

Eschbach JW: The anemia of chronic renal failure: Pathophysiology and the effects of recombinant erythropoietin. Kidney Int 35:134, 1989.

Fine LG: Preventing the progression of human renal disease: Have rational therapeutic principles emerged? Kidney Int 33:116, 1988.

Frasier CL, Arieff AI: Nervous system complications in uremia. Ann Intern Med 109:143, 1988.

French CB, Genel M: Pathophysiology of growth failure in chronic renal insufficiency. Kidney Int 30:S59, 1984.

Geary DF, Haka-Ikse K: Neurodevelopmental progress of young children with chronic renal disease. Pediatrics 84:68, 1989.

Hager SR: Insulin resistance of uremia. Am J Kidney Dis 14:272, 1989.

Hanna JD, Chan JCM, Gill JR Jr: Hypertension and the kidney. J Pediatr 118:327, 1991.

Hellerstein S, Holliday MA, Grupe WE, et al: Nutritional management of children with chronic renal failure. Pediatr Nephrol 1:195, 1987.

Jubelirer SJ: Hemostatic abnormalities in renal disease. Am J Kidney Dis 5:219, 1985.

Klahr S, Schreiner G, Ichikawa I: The progression of renal disease. N Engl J Med 318:1657, 1988.

Levey AS, Harrington JT: Continuous peritoneal dialysis for chronic renal failure. Medicine 61:330, 1982.

Mehls O, Salusky IB: Recent advances and controversies in childhood renal osteodystrophy. Pediatr Nephrol 1:212, 1987.

Mooradian AD, Morley JE: Endocrine dysfunction in chronic renal failure. Arch Intern Med 144:351, 1984.

Morrison G, Murray TG: Electrolyte, acid-base, and fluid homeostasis in chronic renal failure. Med Clin North Am 65:429, 1981.

Nevins TE, Kjellstrand CM: Hemodialysis for children—a review. Int J Pediatr Nephrol 4:155, 1983.

Novello AC, Fine RN: Renal transplantation in children—a review. Int J Pediatr Nephrol 3:87, 1982.

Olson JL, Heptinstall RH: Nonimmunologic mechanisms of glomerular injury. Lab Invest 59:564, 1988.

Polinsky MS, Kaiser BA, Stover JB, et al: Neurologic development of children with severe chronic renal failure from infancy. Pediatr Nephrol 1:157, 1987.

Suki WN: Pericarditis. Kidney Int 33:S10, 1988.

UROLOGIC DISORDERS IN INFANTS AND CHILDREN

18.38 CONGENITAL ANOMALIES OF THE KIDNEYS

RENAL AGENESIS. *Bilateral agenesis* is not compatible with extrauterine life. The stillborn fetus has the stigmata of severe prenatal renal failure and oligohydramnios; the facies is characteristic (Fig. 18–19). The eyes are widely separated and have epicanthic folds, the ears are low set, the nose is broad and flat, the chin is receding, and there are limb anomalies. The hypoplastic lungs preclude survival. The syndrome of bilateral renal agenesis occurs in 1/3,000 births and accounts for one fifth of newborns with the Potter phenotype. Other common causes of severe prenatal renal failure associated with the Potter phenotype include cystic renal dysplasia and obstructive uropathy. Less common causes are infantile polycystic kidney disease (autosomal recessive), renal hypoplasia, and medullary dysplasia. Agenesis should be distinguished from aplasia, an extreme form of dysplasia in which a nubbin of nonfunctioning tissue is seen capping a normal or abnormal ureter. Clinically this distinction may be difficult. Hereditary renal adysplasia should be differentiated from bilateral renal agenesis because of its genetic implications; this condition has an autosomal dominant inheritance pattern with a penetrance of 50–90% and variable expression. Associated anorectal, cardiovascular, and skeletal abnormalities are seen in both hereditary renal adysplasia and bilateral renal agenesis.

Bilateral renal agenesis should be suspected prenatally when maternal ultrasound demonstrates oligohydramnios, nonvisualization of the bladder, and absent kidneys in the second trimester. Death occurs in the first months of life from uremia or pulmonary insufficiency.

Unilateral renal agenesis is often discovered during the course of an evaluation for other congenital anomalies or for urinary tract symptoms. It should be suspected in newborns with a single umbilical artery. The ureter and the ipsilateral bladder hemitrigone are usually absent. The contralateral kidney undergoes compensatory hypertrophy after birth. Associated anomalies involve the genitourinary system in 40% of cases, the skeletal system in 30%, cardiovascular and gastrointestinal systems in 15% of cases each, and the central nervous and respiratory systems in 10% of cases each. Unilateral aplasia is seen in about 1/1000 live births; males are affected more than females, and the left kidney is usually absent. Notable among the genitourinary malformations are vaginal atresia or agenesis **(Mayer-Rokitansky syndrome)**, agenesis of the vas deferens, and seminal vesicle cysts. Individuals with solitary kidneys may be at risk for hypertension and proteinuria and should be followed appropriately.

ANOMALIES IN SHAPE AND POSITION. The normal process of ascent and rotation of the kidney may be incomplete, resulting in renal ectopia (usually in the pelvis) or nonrotation. The lower poles of the kidneys may fuse in the midline, resulting in a horseshoe kidney (Fig. 18–20). The fusion may be asymmetric, or one kidney may cross the midline resulting in crossed ectopia with or without fusion.

Horseshoe kidneys occur in 1:500 births but are seen in 7% of patients with Turner syndrome. Horseshoe kidney is one of the many renal anomalies that occur in one third of these patients. Wilms tumors are 2 to 8 times more frequent in

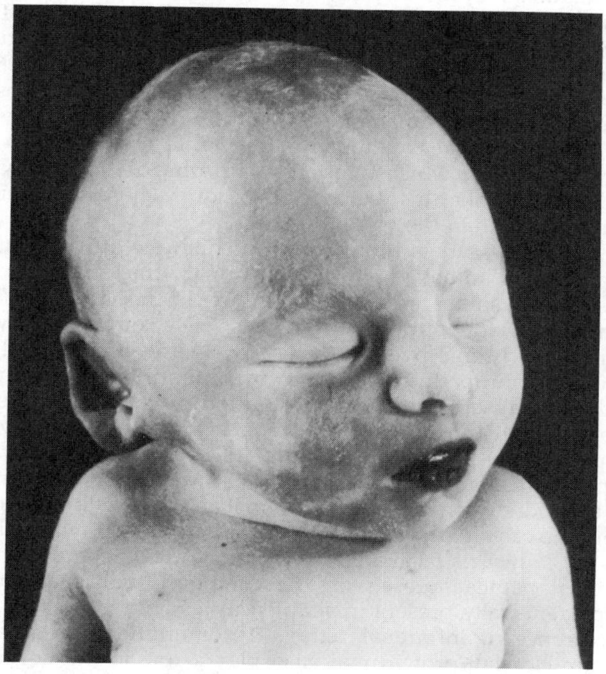

Figure 18–19. Stillborn with renal agenesis exhibiting the characteristic Potter facies. (Courtesy of Barbara Burke, M.D., Department of Laboratory Medicine and Pathology, University of Minnesota Hospital, Minnesota.)

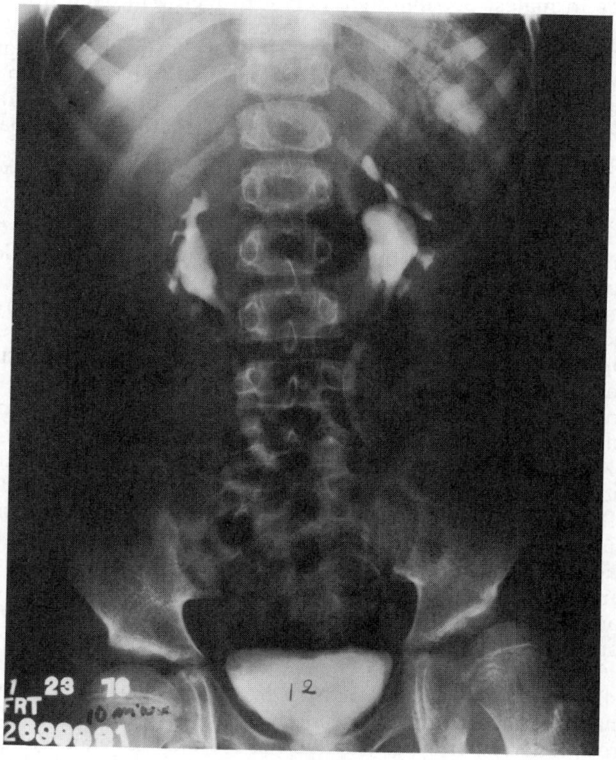

Figure 18–20. Excretory renogram showing classic characteristics of a horseshoe kidney. Notice the bilateral malrotation and the vertical axes of the kidneys. (Courtesy of Drs. S. Sane, L. Prewitt, K. Blumberg, and R. Patterson, Department of Radiology, Minneapolis Children's Medical Center, Minnesota.)

children with horseshoe kidneys than in the general population.

Kelalis PP: Anomalies of the urinary tract. *In*: Kelalis PP, King LR, Belman AB (eds): Clinical Pediatric Urology. Philadelphia, WB Saunders, 1985, pp 643–672.
McPherson E, Carey J, Kramer A, et al: Dominantly inherited renal adysplasia. Am J Med Genet 26:863, 1987.
Pitts WR, Muecke EC: Horseshoe kidneys: A 40 year experience. J Urol 113:743, 1975.
Tarry WF, Duckett JW, Stephens FD: The Mayer-Rokitansky syndrome: Pathogenesis, classification and management. J Urol 136:648, 1986.
Wilson RD, Baird PA: Renal agenesis in British Columbia. Am J Med Genet 21:153, 1985.

18.39 URINARY TRACT INFECTIONS

PREVALENCE AND ETIOLOGY. The prevalence of urinary infections varies markedly with sex and age. Symptomatic urinary tract infections occur in about 1.4/1,000 newborn infants, with a slight male preponderance. Reports indicate that urinary tract infections are more common in uncircumcised male infants. Thereafter, infections are much more common in females. Symptomatic and asymptomatic urinary tract infections occur in 1.2–1.9% of school-aged females and are most common in the 7- to 11-yr-old age group (2.5%). Infections are quite rare in males of similar age. Sexually active females are at increased risk for cystitis; both male and female sexually active adolescents may have urethritis.

Urinary tract infections are caused mainly by colonic bacteria. In females 75–90% of all infections are caused by *Escherichia coli*, followed by *Klebsiella* and *Proteus*. Some series report that in males over 1 yr of age, *Proteus* is as common as *E. coli*; others report a preponderance of gram-positive organisms in males. *S. saprophyticus* is a proven pathogen in both sexes. Viral infections may also occur.

PATHOGENESIS AND PATHOLOGY. In the neonatal period bacteria reach the urinary tract via the bloodstream or urethra, whereas later in life they ascend the urinary tract from below. Individual differences in susceptibility to urinary tract infections may be explained by such host factors as production of urethral and cervical antibodies (IgA) and other factors that influence bacterial adherence to the epithelium of the introitus and the urethra. Once the organisms gain entrance to the bladder, the severity of the infection may reflect the virulence of the bacteria and such anatomic factors as vesicoureteral reflux, obstruction, urinary stasis, and the presence of calculi. With urinary stasis, bacteria have increased opportunity to multiply, since urine is an excellent culture medium. In addition, vesical overdistention decreases the blood flow to the bladder wall and may decrease the bladder's natural resistance to infection.

Acute bacterial cystitis is characterized by mucosal congestion and edema, occasionally with petechiae and hemorrhage. The inflammatory reaction causes hyperactivity of the detrusor muscle and a decrease in the functional capacity of the bladder. These changes may precipitate vesicoureteral reflux, particularly when the vesicoureteral junction is already abnormally developed. Chronic or frequently recurrent infections may cause changes of *cystitis cystica* in the bladder wall, with characteristic endoscopic and histologic appearances.

Bacteria can reach the kidney from the bladder by way of established vesicoureteral reflux or through transient reflux precipitated by the inflammation of the bladder wall. Patients with the P1 blood group can develop ascending recurrent pyelonephritis in the absence of vesicoureteral reflux, because *E. coli* binds specifically to the P1 antigens on the epithelial cell surface. *Acute pyelonephritis* leads to enlargement of the kidney due to edema and acute inflammatory infiltrates in the medulla and pelvis. If untreated, these changes may lead to the formation of renal microabscesses, which may become confluent. Acute pyelonephritis is always more severe when obstruction is present. These changes may result in the development of renal scars, with the histologic findings commonly known as chronic pyelonephritis; however, prompt treatment of the infection can result in complete healing.

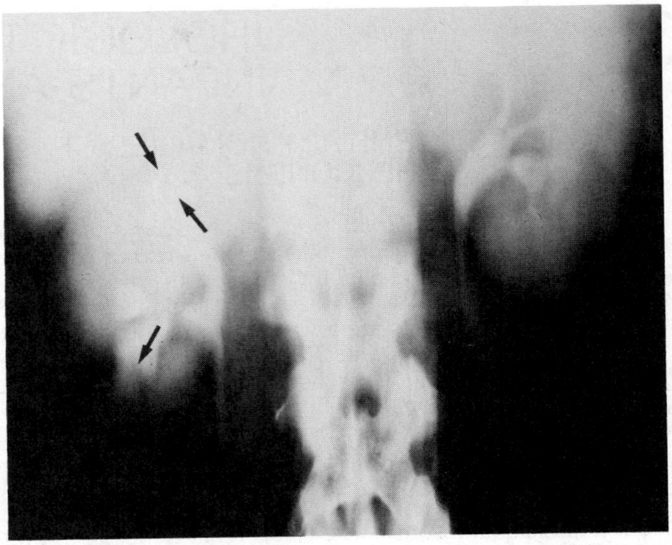

Figure 18–21. Chronic pyelonephritis. Tomographic cut made during intravenous urography, showing characteristic changes of chronic pyelonephritis on the right side. Note the smaller size of the right kidney, the clubbing of the calyces, particularly those of the upper and lower poles, and the marked thinning of the cortex in the poles of the kidney. The left kidney is normal.

Histologically, *chronic pyelonephritis* is often difficult to distinguish from other causes of end-stage renal scarring such as medullary cystic disease, ischemia, irradiation, analgesic abuse, and others. The scars can be focal or diffuse. The characteristic finding in chronic pyelonephritis is a cortical scar with an underlying calyceal deformity (Fig. 18–21). Microscopically, the lesions are patchy with glomerular fibrosis, interstitial chronic inflammation, and fibrosis and atrophy of the tubules. Local conditions of the renal medulla such as high osmolality, which interferes with phagocytic activity of leukocytes, make this region of the kidney more susceptible to infections than the cortex.

Such renal scars are found also in children with vesicoureteral reflux who have no history of urinary tract infection; for this reason some prefer the term "reflux nephropathy" to "chronic pyelonephritis." In any case, 90% of children with lesions of chronic pyelonephritis have vesicoureteral reflux. Reflux nephropathy or chronic pyelonephritis is the most common cause of arterial hypertension in children; some of the vascular and glomerular changes may be secondary to hypertension rather than to the inflammatory process. In experimental animals reflux nephropathy occurs only in areas of the kidney where the renal papillae allow reflux of urine from the calyx to the collecting tubules (intrarenal reflux) (Fig. 18–22), which is facilitated by the anatomic configuration of the flat papillae present in the compound calyces; conical papillae usually present in simple calyces help to prevent the occurrence of intrarenal reflux. Autoimmune responses to Tamm-Horsfall protein may also play a role in the development and progression of the pyelonephritic scar.

In addition to the inflammatory changes just described, infection by urea-splitting organisms such as *Proteus* can lead to stone formation. The ammonia derived from urea produces

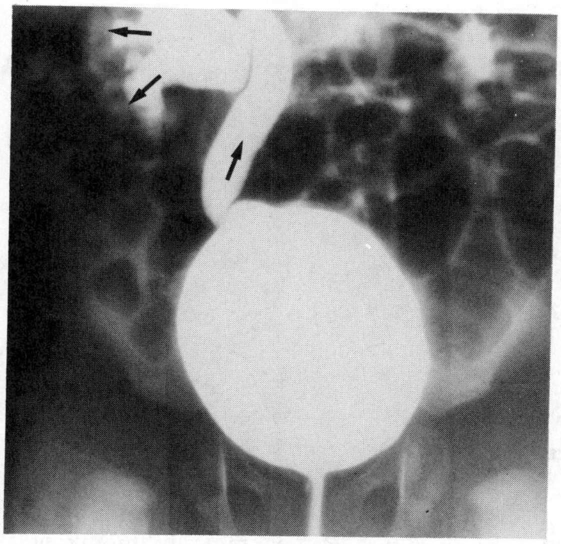

Figure 18–22. Intrarenal reflux. Retrograde cystogram in a young infant male with a past history of a urinary tract infection. Note the right vesicoureteral reflux with ureteral dilatation, with opacification of the renal parenchyma representing intrarenal reflux.

a strongly alkaline urine in which calcium phosphate and triple calcium, magnesium, and ammonium phosphate can precipitate. The calculi act as foreign bodies and help perpetuate the infection. With ureteral obstruction, renal infection can rapidly lead to septicemia, pyonephrosis, and the formation of renal and perirenal abscesses.

Xanthogranulomatous pyelonephritis is a distinct histologic type of renal infection characterized by granulomatous inflammation with giant cells and foamy histiocytes. It may present clinically as a renal mass or an acute or chronic infection. Renal calculi, obstruction, and infection with *Proteus* or *E. coli* contribute to the development of this rare lesion, which usually requires nephrectomy.

CLINICAL MANIFESTATIONS. Asymptomatic bacteriuria is common; in most cases either there have been symptoms suggestive of urinary tract infection or there will be. The clinical manifestations often fail to indicate clearly whether the infection is confined to the bladder or involves the kidneys as well. In infancy, fever, weight loss, failure to thrive, nausea, vomiting, diarrhea, and jaundice are common. In children with fever of unknown origin, cultures of urine should be obtained to exclude urinary tract infection. Later in childhood, urinary frequency, pain during micturition, urinary incontinence associated with urgency, bedwetting in a previously dry child, abdominal pain, and foul-smelling urine are common symptoms. Chronic or frequently recurrent cystitis is often responsible for daytime incontinence and other manifestations of bladder instability, which may persist even after the urine has become sterile (see Sec. 18.44).

Hematuria is occasionally observed as a sign of hemorrhagic cystitis caused by *E. coli*. In acute pyelonephritis, fever, chills, and flank or abdominal pain and tenderness are common. The kidney may be enlarged. Children with chronic pyelonephritis are often asymptomatic. Arterial hypertension is commonly associated with renal scars. Reflux nephropathy, commonly attributed to the combination of vesicoureteral reflux and infection, is responsible for up to 15% of cases of end-stage renal failure in children. Sepsis is common in infants and older children with infection and urinary tract obstruction. Hyperammonemia with central nervous system manifestations is a rare complication of urinary tract infections due to *Proteus* and is associated with urinary stasis or obstruction.

LABORATORY DATA. The diagnosis of urinary tract infections depends on the culture of bacteria from the urine. The finding of any bacteria in urine obtained from the bladder or renal pelvis is indicative of infection. An accurate diagnosis may be difficult to establish, owing to the frequent contamination of voided specimens or to prior treatment of the patient with antibiotics.

In toilet-trained children, a midstream urine culture obtained after cleansing the urethral meatus with a povidone-iodine solution and rinsing with sterile water or saline is usually satisfactory. In females the labia should be spread manually to avoid contamination of the urine or contact with the skin. In uncircumcised males the prepuce must be retracted; if the prepuce is not retractable, this method of urine collection is not reliable. Skillful nurses can help the child's parent to obtain these specimens. For midstream voided specimens the colony count is often used to differentiate between infected and contaminated specimens. Cultures indicating more than 10^5 colonies/mL of a single organism are more than 90% specific for urinary tract infections. It should be recognized, however, that lower colony counts in infected patients may be due to overhydration, to recent bladder emptying, or to antibiotic therapy; such counts do not rule out infection.

In infants and both male and female young children, the application of an adhesive, sealed, sterile collection bag after disinfection of the skin of the genitalia can be useful, particularly if a sterile culture results. The specificity of these cultures is much lower than that of a midstream specimen. When greater assurance as to the possiblity of infection is needed, a catheterized specimen must be obtained. Proper skin preparation and good technique of catheterization are important. The use of a No. 5 French polyethylene feeding tube in infants or of a No. 8 French tube with proper lubrication in older children minimizes the chance of urethral trauma and contamination. Catheterization shortly after spontaneous voiding produces a measure of the residual urine in the bladder and helps assess problems related to bladder emptying. In theory, the normal flora of the distal urethra may be a source of false-positive culture results, but in practice the finding of any colonies grown from bladder urine should be considered as indicative of infection.

The use of a suprapubic puncture of the full bladder with a 25- or 22-gauge needle yields reliable results. With the child properly hydrated (when the bladder can be percussed or palpated), the skin is disinfected and a puncture performed 1 finger-breadth above the pubis in the midline. A syringe is used to aspirate as the needle is inserted; 1 or 2 mL of urine is sufficient for culture. The urine specimen for bacterial culture should be kept refrigerated until the culture is plated to avoid bacterial overgrowth. False-negative findings on urine culture may result from unrecognized antibiotic treatment, dilution from overhydration, or contamination of the specimen with the antiseptic solution.

A urinalysis should be obtained from the same specimen as that cultured. Pyuria (leukocytes in the urine) suggests infection, but infection can occur in the absence of pyuria; accordingly, this finding is more confirmatory than diagnostic. Conversely, pyuria can be present without urinary tract infections. Microscopic hematuria is common in acute cystitis. Casts in the urinary sediment suggest renal involvement. *Proteus* infections consistently produce an alkaline pH.

With acute renal infection, leukocytosis and neutrophilia are common. Unfortunately, in children such tests to differentiate upper from lower urinary tract infections as the detection of antibody coated bacteria, response to single-dose antibiotic therapy, and other immunologic and biochemical tests are unreliable. Inability to concentrate the urine is a common but unreliable finding in acute and chronic pyelonephritis. In 30% of infants with renal infections the serum creatinine level is transiently elevated. Because sepsis is common in renal infections, particularly in infants and with obstruction, blood cultures should be obtained during febrile infections.

IMAGING STUDIES. During acute febrile infection, renal ultrasound should be obtained to rule out hydronephrosis and renal or perirenal abscesses; other indications for this study are when the response to antibiotic therapy is not prompt, when the child is severely ill and toxic, and when the serum creatinine level is elevated. Renal ultrasound is also very sensitive for detecting pyonephrosis, a condition that often demands prompt drainage of the collecting system by percutaneous nephrostomy.

When the diagnosis of acute pyelonephritis is uncertain, renal scanning with technetium labeled 2,3-dimercaptosuccinic acid (DMSA) or glucoheptanate is useful. The presence of a parenchymal filling defect on the renal scan supports the diagnosis of pyelonephritis but cannot differentiate an acute from a chronic process. Computerized axial tomography (CAT) is the definitive diagnostic test for acute pyelonephritis. However, a CT scan is seldom necessary to establish such diagnosis.

Approximately 3 wk after treatment of the acute infection all children should have voiding cystourethrography to assess reflux. Some physicians would restrict such studies to all males and to females under 5 yr of age who have an initial infection; older females would be studied at the time of a second infection. We prefer the former approach, since reflux will be found in 25% of all children under the age of 10 yr who have had symptomatic or asymptomatic bacteriuria; it is more frequently observed in children under 3 yr of age. If it is available, radioisotopic voiding cystourethrography can be used in females; this technique is sensitive and exposes the ovaries to 50- to 100-fold less radiation than would conventional voiding cystourethrography with intermittent fluoroscopic control. In males radiographic definition of the urethra is important; accordingly, radiographic voiding cystourethrography with fluoroscopic control is recommended for the initial work-up. Renal ultrasound may also be carried out as part of the initial work-up in order to exclude obstruction and to determine kidney size.

If vesicoureteral reflux is present, intravenous pyelography with nephrotomography should be obtained to evaluate kidney size and detect possible calyceal blunting, ureteral dilatation, and renal scarring. A better alternative to intravenous urography for detection of renal scars is radioisotopic renal scanning with DMSA or glucoheptanate. These diagnostic tests are more sensitive than urography and avoid the possible adverse reactions associated with an intravenously administered contrast medium. Renal scanning is particularly useful in infants and young children, in whom abdominal gas makes the interpretation of urography difficult (Fig. 18–23). Further evaluation of children with infections and reflux or obstructive uropathy will be discussed in other sections.

The frequently performed cystoscopies and measurements of urethral caliber advocated for girls in the past contribute nothing to the therapeutic decisions to be made in children with normal findings on radiographic study or with primary reflux. Narrowing of the female urethra was once postulated to be a contributing factor in the development of urinary tract infections, but the urethras of girls with recurrent urinary tract infections are not narrower than those of girls without infections.

DIFFERENTIAL DIAGNOSIS. Inflammations of the external genitalia, vulvitis, and vaginitis caused by yeast, pinworms, and other agents may be accompanied by symptoms mimicking cystitis. Viral and chemical cystitis must be distinguished from bacterial cystitis on the basis of history and

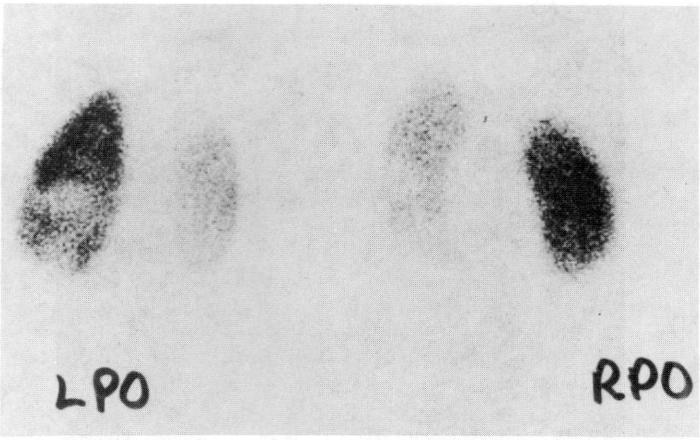

Figure 18–23. DMSA renal scan showing bilateral photopenic areas indicative of renal scarring.

results of urine culture. Radiographically, the hypoplastic or dysplastic kidney or a small kidney secondary to a vascular accident may appear similar to a kidney with chronic pyelonephritis. With the latter, however, vesicoureteral reflux is usually present.

Acute hemorrhagic cystitis is frequently caused by *E. coli;* it has been attributed also to adenovirus types 11 and 21. Adenovirus cystitis is more frequent in males; it is self-limiting, with hematuria lasting approximately 4 days. *Eosinophilic cystitis* is a rare form of cystitis of obscure origin that occasionally has been found in children. Usual symptoms are those of cystitis with hematuria, ureteral dilatation, and filling defects in the bladder caused by masses that consist histologically of inflammatory infiltrates with eosinophils.

TREATMENT. Acute cystitis should be treated promptly to prevent its possible progression to pyelonephritis. If the symptoms are severe, a specimen of bladder urine is obtained for culture and treatment is started immediately. If the symptoms are mild or the diagnosis doubtful, treatment can be delayed until the results of culture are known and the culture can be repeated if the results are uncertain. For example, if midstream culture grew between 10^4 and 10^5 colonies of a gram-negative organism, a second culture may be obtained by catheterization or suprapubic aspiration before treatment is initiated. If treatment is initiated before the results of a culture and sensitivities are available, a 7- to 10-day course of therapy with trimethoprim-sulfamethoxazole (see below) will be effective against most strains of *E. coli*. Nitrofurantoin (5–7 mg/kg/24 hr in 3–4 divided doses) is also very effective and has the advantage of being active against *Klebsiella-Enterobacter* organisms. Amoxicillin (50 mg/kg/24 hr) is also effective as initial treatment but has no clear advantages over the sulfonamides or nitrofurantoin.

In acute febrile infections suggestive of pyelonephritis, the use of broad-spectrum antibiotics capable of reaching significant tissue levels is preferable. If the child is acutely ill, parenteral treatment with cefotaxime (100 mg/kg/24 hr) or ampicillin (100 mg/kg/24 hr) with an aminoglycoside such as gentamicin (3 mg/kg/24 hr in 3 divided doses) is preferable. The potential ototoxicity and nephrotoxicity of aminoglycosides should be considered, and serum creatinine levels must be obtained prior to initiating treatment as well as daily thereafter so long as treatment continues. Treatment with aminoglycosides is particularly effective against *Pseudomonas*, and alkalinization of urine with sodium bicarbonate increases their effectiveness in the urinary tract. The combination of sulfamethoxazole and trimethoprim (Cotrim, Bactrim, Septra), either orally or intravenously, is effective against a variety of gram-negative organisms other than *Pseudomonas* and is considered by some authorities to be the treatment of choice for oral therapy. The oral dosage is 20 mg/kg/24 hr for sulfamethoxazole and 4 mg/kg/24 hr for trimethoprim, given in two divided doses. Ciprofloxacin is an alternative agent for resistant microorganisms in patients older than 18 yr.

A urine culture should be obtained a week after the termination of treatment of any urinary tract infection to assure that the urine remains sterile. Given the tendency of urinary tract infections to recur even in the absence of predisposing anatomic factors, follow-up urine cultures should be obtained at 3-mo intervals for 1–2 yr even when the child is asymptomatic. If recurrences are frequent, prophylaxis against reinfection, using either sulfamethoxazole-trimethoprim combination or nitrofurantoin at one third the normal therapeutic dose once a day, is often effective. It is important, however, to obtain periodic urine cultures if the child is receiving prolonged prophylactic treatment, in order to rule out asymptomatic infections caused by resistant organisms. Antibacterial prophylaxis is also indicated for as long as vesicoureteral reflux persists (see Sec. 18.40), or when recurrent cystitis causes such symptoms as incontinence, frequency, and urgency of urination, which are perpetuated by frequent reinfections. Other indications for long-term prophylaxis (neurogenic bladder, urinary tract stasis and obstruction, reflux, and calculi) are discussed in a later section. Because the probability of finding vesicoureteral reflux is 25% and the probability of a recurrent infection is 50% it is logical to continue antibacterial prophylaxis with low dose sulfamethoxazole-trimethoprim combinations or nitrofurantoin until completion of the radiologic evaluation. The prolonged use of any chemotherapeutic agent should be monitored for evidence of toxicity (anemia, leukopenia, and so on). Broad-spectrum antibiotics are usually ineffective for prophylaxis, since the colonic bacteria likely to be responsible for reinfections quickly become resistant to these agents.

The long-term prognosis for urinary tract infections is usually excellent, provided prompt and adequate treatment is instituted when the diagnosis is established. The prompt treatment of acute bacterial pyelonephritis in animals has prevented the development of renal scars. Notwithstanding this usually favorable long-term outcome, children with recurrent urinary tract infections often present difficult and frustrating problems in treatment and prophylaxis. The main consequences of chronic renal damage caused by pyelonephritis are arterial hypertension and renal insufficiency; when they are found they should be treated appropriately. Some children with urinary tract infections void infrequently and many also have severe constipation. Counseling of parents to try to establish more normal patterns of voiding and defecation may be helpful in controlling recurrences.

Children with renal or perirenal abscesses or with infections in obstructed urinary tracts require surgical or percutaneous drainage in addition to antibiotic therapy and other supportive measures.

18.40 VESICOURETERAL REFLUX

Reflux of urine from the bladder to the ureter and renal pelvis results from incompetence of the valvular mechanism at the ureterovesical junction that normally allows passage of urine only from the ureter to the bladder. Reflux can be harmful to the kidneys because (1) it exposes the renal pelvis (which has a normal pressure of less than 10 mm Hg) to the much higher vesical pressures produced during voiding, and (2) it facilitates the passage of bacteria from the bladder to the kidneys.

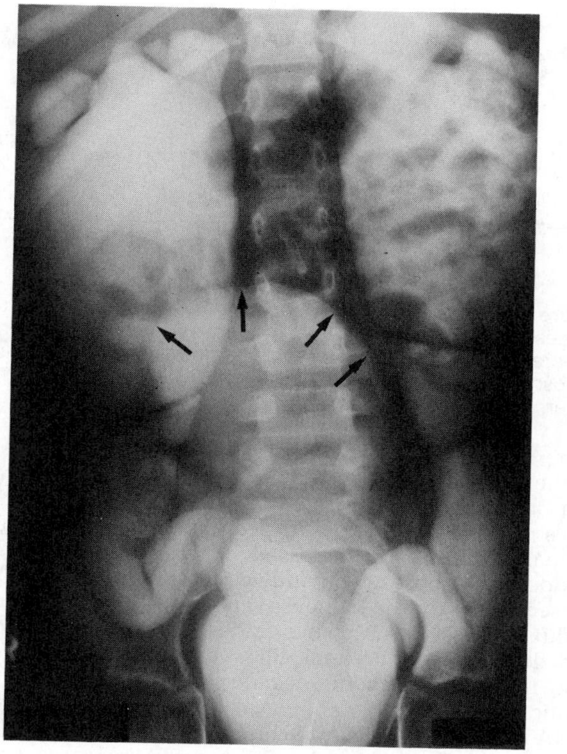

Figure 18–24. Excretory urogram in a male with megaureter-megacystic syndrome. Note the massive ureteral dilatation due to high-grade vesicoureteral reflux. The bladder is very distended, reaching the level of the third lumbar vertebra. There was no urethral obstruction or neurogenic dysfunction.

Accordingly, reflux can result in dilatation of the ureter and upper collecting systems as well as the development of renal scars, particularly in association with urinary tract infections. Reflux of urine from the intrarenal collecting system to the collecting tubules also plays an important role in the development of renal scars (see Sec. 18.39). Massive reflux into dilated ureters also prevents complete bladder emptying, inasmuch as urine "voided" into the upper collecting system rapidly returns to the bladder, with development of progressive bladder dilatation, as in the megaureter-megacystic syndrome (Fig. 18–24). Reflux nephropathy accounts for 15–20% of all end-stage renal failure in children and young adults and is an important cause of hypertension in children.

CLASSIFICATION. Primary vesicoureteral reflux results from a congenital anomaly of the ureterovesical junction in which the intramural ureteral tunnel is short, the ureteral orifice is placed in a lateral and cephalad direction, and the trigone is underdeveloped. This shortening of the intramural tunnel decreases the efficiency of the valvular mechanism. The degree of vesicoureteral reflux varies with the degree of malformation of the orifice (Fig. 18–25). A wide spectrum of anomalies may be associated (Table 18–12).

With duplication of the ureters and ureterocele, the ureterocele obstructs the upper collecting system, and there is often reflux to the ureter of the lower collecting system and occasionally to the contralateral side. In duplicated systems, reflux is more common in the lower ureter, which enters the bladder higher and more laterally and has a less competent valve. Reflux is always present when the ureter enters a diverticulum (Figs. 18–26 and 18–27).

In cases of congenital neurogenic bladder, such as myelomeningocele and sacral agenesis, reflux is present in one third

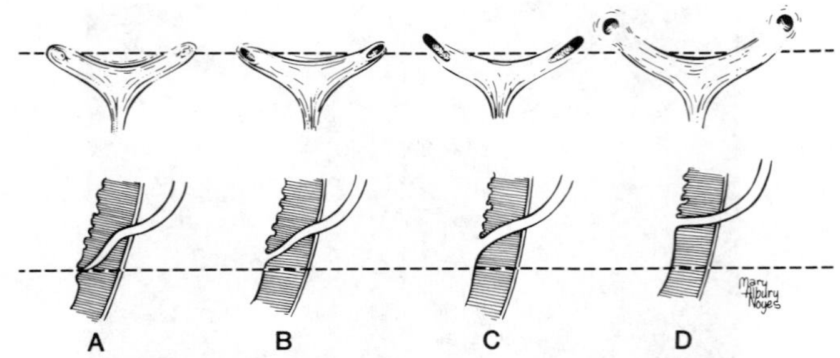

Figure 18–25. Normal and abnormal configuration of the ureteral orifices. Shown from left to right, progressive lateral displacement of the ureteral orifices and shortening of the intramural tunnels. *Top*, Endoscopic appearance. *Bottom*, Sagittal view through the intramural ureter.

of the cases at birth and develops eventually in more than half of affected children. Reflux is seen in more than half of cases of posterior urethral valves. Both clinically and experimentally, reflux with increased intravesical pressures (as in bladder outlet obstruction and vesical dysfunction) has severe consequences for the kidney, even in the absence of infection. Reflux is classified into five grades according to its severity and the degree of ureteral dilatation and calyceal deformity (Fig. 18–28). This grading of reflux has prognostic and therapeutic significance.

NATURAL HISTORY. In children with reflux the incidence of renal scarring or reflux nephropathy increases with the grade of reflux. Intrarenal reflux seems to increase the risk of scarring. In grades I and II reflux in patients who have no ureteral dilatation, the anatomy of the vesicoureteral region tends to be nearly normal, and in about 80% of cases reflux will cease spontaneously with maturation of the child. With greater degrees of ureteral dilatation and of abnormality of the vesicoureteral junction, the chances of spontaneous disappearance decrease. Reflux may be familial.

PRESENTATION. In the majority of children, reflux is discovered during an evaluation for urinary tract infection. In other children, voiding cystourethrography is part of an evaluation of voiding dysfunction, renal insufficiency, hypertension, or other suspected pathology of the urinary tract. It has become increasingly common to diagnose reflux in asymptomatic siblings of children with reflux.

TABLE 18–12. Classification of Vesicoureteral Reflux

Type	Cause
1. Primary	Congenital incompetence of the valvular mechanism of the vesicoureteral junction
2. Primary associated with other malformations of the ureterovesical junction	Ureteral duplication Ureterocele with duplication Ureteral ectopia Paraureteral diverticula
3. Secondary to increased intravesical pressure	Neurogenic bladder Non-neurogenic bladder dysfunction Bladder outlet obstruction
4. Secondary to inflammatory processes	Severe bacterial cystitis Foreign bodies Vesical calculi Clinical cystitis
5. Secondary to surgical procedures involving the ureterovesical junction	

DIFFERENTIAL DIAGNOSIS. The distinction between primary and secondary reflux is usually easy to make on the basis of history and radiographs. In the case of the child who has reflux, infection, and voiding dysfunction, it may be difficult to determine whether the voiding dysfunction is secondary to infection or the cause of reflux that predisposes to infection. Urodynamic studies of the lower urinary tract (see Sec. 18.44) may be necessary in such cases.

EVALUATION. Once reflux is diagnosed, graded, and determined to be primary, secondary to other malformations of the vesicoureteral junction, or secondary to inflammatory processes or increased intravesical pressure, it is important then to know the renal size and whether scars are present; ultrasound is indicated to evaluate renal size, and isotopic parenchymal renal scanning is helpful to rule out scars. Intravenous pyelography and tomography are also appropriate studies for these purposes. Blood pressure and baseline creatinine clearance should also be measured. In patients with primary reflux, the degree of abnormality of the intramural tunnel can be predicted from the grade of reflux. Accordingly, when anomalies of the urethra or bladder and associated anomalies of the vesicoureteral junction can be ruled out radiographically, cystoscopy is of doubtful value in determining the prognosis or choosing between surgical and medical treatment.

TREATMENT. The treatment of *primary reflux* and reflux associated with complete duplication of the ureters can be considered together. In grades I and II reflux the likelihood of spontaneous resolution is great, and a period of expectant treatment is warranted, during which the child must be protected from infection by administration of low doses of an antibacterial medication such as sulfamethoxazole-trimethroprim combination or nitrofurantoin (see Sec. 18.39). At the beginning of treatment, urine cultures are obtained at monthly intervals; when the efficacy of prophylaxis has been established, cultures can be obtained at 3-mo intervals.

Since asymptomatic bacteriuria and reflux can be harmful, it is important to culture the urine even in the absence of symptoms. Using a radionuclide, voiding cystourethrography is obtained at yearly intervals. A yearly renal ultrasound study is useful to evaluate renal growth. When a radiographic study indicates spontaneous cessation of the reflux, another study made in 3–6 mo should confirm this before antibacterial

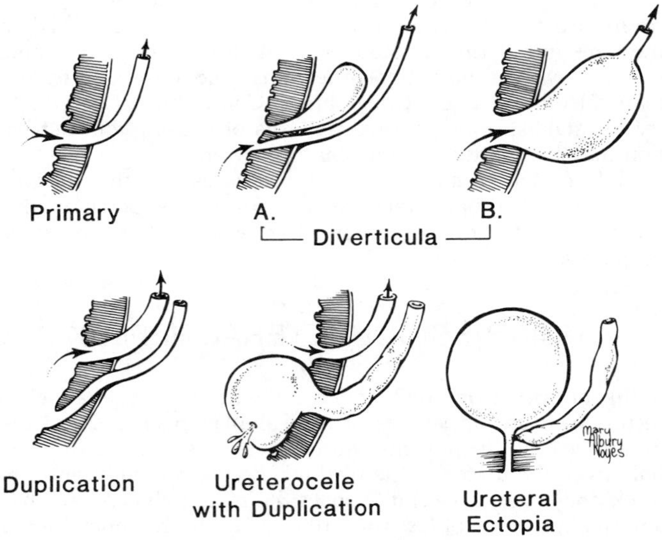

Figure 18–26. Various anatomic defects of the ureterovesical junction associated with vesicoureteral reflux.

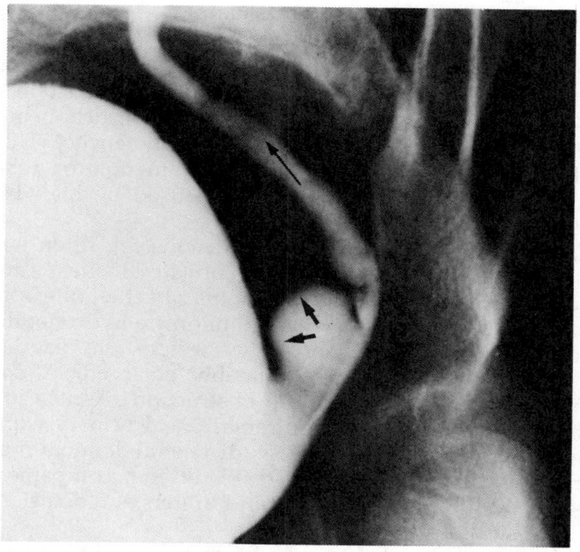

Figure 18–27. Reflux and bladder diverticulum. The voiding cystourethrogram demonstrates left vesicoureteral reflux and a paraureteral diverticulum.

therapy is discontinued, since reflux is occasionally intermittent. Grade II reflux seldom needs surgical correction, but if antibacterial prophylaxis fails to keep the urine consistently sterile, surgery is indicated.

In cases of grade III reflux, the follow-up is similar, but periodic parenchymal scans are useful if new scar formation is suspected. More than 50% of children with grade III reflux may ultimately need surgical treatment.

In grades IV and V reflux (reflux associated with significant ureteral dilatation and upper urinary tract changes), spontaneous cessation is unlikely and early surgical treatment is indicated after a brief period of prophylaxis and confirmation of the persistence of the reflux. Surgical treatment is particularly indicated for the infant and young child because the risk of renal scarring is higher in children less than 5 yr of age.

Secondary reflux associated with duplications can be treated exactly as primary reflux. When a periureteral diverticulum is present, spontaneous cessation of reflux is significantly less likely, and early surgical treatment is therefore indicated. For a large bladder diverticulum, surgical treatment is necessary to improve bladder emptying. Reflux secondary to severe cystitis, such as that which may accompany foreign bodies or chemical irritation, will usually cease once the primary cause of the cystitis is removed. Iatrogenic reflux usually requires surgical treatment. The treatment of reflux in cases of ureteroceles, posterior urethral valves, and neurogenic bladder is discussed in a later section.

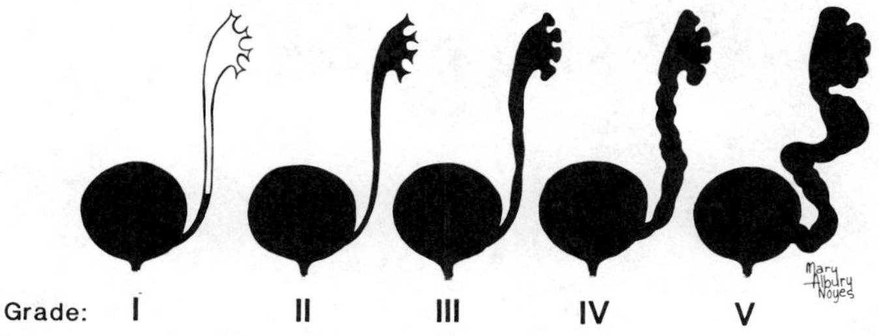

Figure 18–28. Grading of a vesicoureteral reflux. Grade I: reflux into a nondilated distal ureter. Grade II: reflux into the upper collecting system without dilatation. Grade III: reflux into dilated ureter and/or blunting of calyceal fornices. Grade IV: reflux into a grossly dilated ureter. Grade V: massive reflux, with ureteral dilatation and tortuosity and effacement of the calyceal details.

The results of surgical treatment of reflux are usually excellent. On the other hand, most past series reporting up to 95% or greater success included many cases of low grade reflux, which is now known seldom to need corrective surgery. Antireflux operations involving dilated ureters carry a lower success rate, but with one or more reoperations success is usually achieved.

Complications of antireflux surgery include persistence of reflux and obstruction of the distal ureter. Careful follow-up of patients after surgery is therefore required. When only unilateral reflux has been demonstrated, bilateral correction of reflux is usually unnecessary. Reflux may appear transiently on the opposite side after surgery, but it usually ceases spontaneously.

Endoscopic injection of polytetrafluoroethylene (Polytef) under the ureteral orifice has been effective in the short term to control reflux in some children. The safety of Polytef paste injection in the bladder wall remains questionable. Some are experimenting with the use of other substances. In the future, endoscopic techniques may become part of the surgical treatment of reflux in selected patients.

18.41 OBSTRUCTIONS OF THE URINARY TRACT

Obstructive lesions of the urinary tract occur at any level from the urethral meatus to the calyceal infundibula. In children, obstruction can be congenital (anatomic) or caused by trauma, neoplasia, calculi, inflammatory processes, or surgical procedures. The pathophysiologic effects of obstruction depend on its level, extent of involvement, age of onset, and acute or chronic nature. In childhood most obstructive lesions are congenital and may therefore be present during fetal life.

A partial list of obstructive lesions is given in Table 18–13. High-grade ureteral obstruction of early onset in fetal life results in renal dysplasia, ranging from the multicystic kidney, usually associated with ureteral or pelvic atresia (Fig. 18–29), to various degrees of histologic renal cortical dysplasia seen with less severe obstruction. Chronic ureteral obstruction in late fetal life or after birth results in hypertrophy and later dilatation of the ureter and upper collecting system, with alterations of renal parenchyma ranging from minimal tubular changes to dilatation of Bowman space, glomerular atrophy, and interstitial fibrosis. After birth, infections often complicate obstruction and may increase renal damage.

Urethral obstruction in the fetus can result in a patent urachus, which serves to decompress the bladder. More commonly there is urethral dilatation above the obstruction and hypertrophy of the detrusor muscle. The ureters are dilated because of impeded drainage into the obstructed bladder, owing to high intravesical pressure and to obstruction of the intramural portion of the ureter by the hypertrophied detrusor muscle. Vesicoureteral reflux commonly complicates congenital urethral obstruction. Urinary extravasation sometimes occurs in children with congenital obstruction when urine under pressure leaks out of the intrarenal collecting system, usually through ruptured calyceal fornices, into the subcapsular or perirenal spaces (urinomas) or into the peritoneal cavity (urinary ascites). Bilateral ureteral obstruction or urethral obstruction may cause oligohydramnios and pulmonary hypoplasia. The newborn may exhibit the facies and stigmata of severe prenatal renal failure (see Sec. 18.38). The immediate prognosis for newborns with severe obstruc-

TABLE 18–13. Types and Causes of Urinary Tract Obstruction

Location	Cause
Infundibula	Congenital Calculi Inflammatory (tuberculosis) Traumatic Postsurgical Neoplastic
Renal pelvis	Congenital (infundibulopelvic stenosis) Inflammatory (tuberculosis) Calculi Neoplasia (Wilms tumor, neuroblastoma)
Ureteropelvic junction	Congenital stenosis Calculi Neoplasia Inflammatory Postsurgical Traumatic
Ureter	Congenital obstructive megaureter Ureteral ectopia Ureterocele Retrocaval ureter Ureteral fibroepithelial polyps Ureteral valves Calculi Postsurgical Extrinsic compression Neoplasia (neuroblastoma, lymphoma, and other retroperitoneal or pelvic tumors) Inflammatory (Crohn disease, chronic granulomatous disease) Hematoma, urinoma Lymphocele Retroperitoneal fibrosis
Bladder outlet and urethra	Neurogenic bladder dysfunction (functional obstruction) Posterior urethral valves Anterior urethral valves Diverticula Urethral strictures (congenital, traumatic, or iatrogenic) Urethral atresia Ectopic ureterocele Meatal stenosis (males) Calculi Foreign bodies Phimosis Extrinsic compression by tumors Urogenital sinus anomalies

tive uropathy is often more closely related to the degree of pulmonary insufficiency than to the degree of renal damage.

In high-grade urethral obstruction or bilateral ureteral obstruction there is renal failure. The urinary output may be low, normal, or increased because of tubular dysfunction with decreased concentrating ability. Renal function usually recovers completely following relief of a brief acute obstruction. The potential for recovery of renal function in chronic (including all congenital) cases depends on the degree of dysplasia or irreversible renal damage. In renal failure with obstructive uropathy both the concentrating ability and the ability of the tubules to excrete hydrogen ions are decreased. Accordingly, infants with renal failure secondary to obstruction may, after relief of obstruction, continue to have polyuria, dilute urine, and chronic acidosis with normal serum creatinine levels.

Hypertrophy and dilatation in the bladder and collecting systems persist long after correction of the obstruction and are often irreversible. Following relief of obstruction in the uremic child, postobstructive diuresis may ensue. This is usually transient and due to the combination of tubular dysfunction and an osmotic diuresis caused by high blood levels of urea.

DIAGNOSIS. Urinary tract obstructions are often silent, and advanced lesions (particularly unilateral ones) can be found in children without symptoms. In the newborn a palpable abdominal mass is most commonly a hydronephrotic kidney. With infravesical obstructive lesions the bladder as well as the kidneys may be palpably enlarged. A patent urachus should suggest urethral obstruction. Ascites in the newborn may be caused by intraperitoneal urinary extravasation (see earlier). Prune-belly syndrome (abdominal muscle deficiency and undescended testes) is often accompanied by massive dilatation of the bladder and ureters and occasionally by infravesical obstruction.

Urinary tract obstruction may be diagnosed prenatally by ultrasonography. In such cases further ultrasound and, if indicated, a more complete evaluation should be undertaken in the neonatal period. Oligohydramnios and various degrees of pulmonary hypoplasia accompany the more severe cases of urethral or bilateral ureteral obstruction.

Infection and sepsis may be the first indications of an obstructive lesion of the urinary tract. The combination of infection and obstruction poses a serious threat to infants and children and usually requires parenteral administration of antibiotics and drainage of the obstructed kidney. For this reason renal ultrasound should be performed for all children during the acute stage of febrile urinary tract infections. Obstructive renal insufficiency can manifest itself by failure to thrive, vomiting, diarrhea, or other nonspecific signs and symptoms. In older children infravesical obstruction can be associated with overflow urinary incontinence or a poor urinary stream. Acute ureteral obstruction causes flank or abdominal pain, and there may be nausea and vomiting.

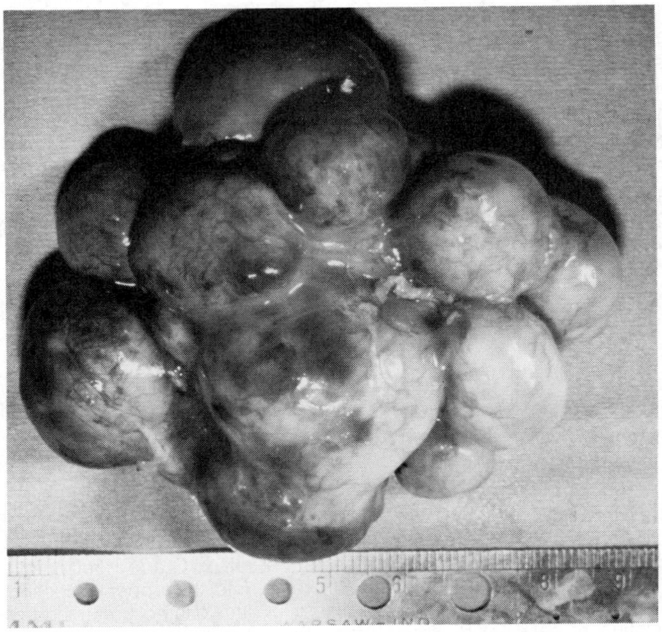

Figure 18–29. Surgical specimen of a multicystic dysplastic kidney associated with ureteral atresia.

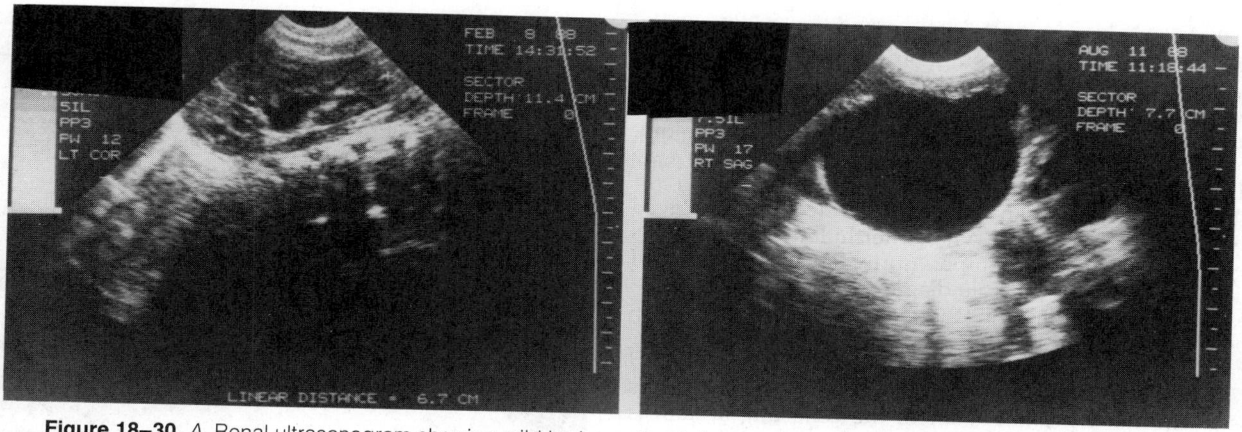

Figure 18–30. *A*, Renal ultrasonogram showing mild hydronephrosis in a newborn. Notice the minimal calyceal dilatation and well-preserved parenchyma. *B*, Renal ultrasonogram showing marked hydronephrosis in a newborn. Notice the massive dilatation and thinning of the renal parenchyma.

Chronic ureteral obstruction can be silent or cause vague abdominal or typical flank pain with increased fluid intake. Abdominal ultrasound should be the initial imaging study in all children with abdominal pain. If attention is focused initially on the gastrointestinal tract, the diagnosis of ureteral obstruction is often delayed unnecessarily.

IMAGING STUDIES. The common characteristic of obstruction is the presence of a dilated urinary tract. Dilatation is frequently an ultrasonographic finding (Fig. 18–30). However, dilatation is not always indicative of obstruction but may persist after surgical correction or spontaneous resolution of an obstructive lesion. Dilatation may result from vesicoureteral reflux, or it may be a manifestation of abnormal development of the urinary tract even when there is no obstruction. Renal ultrasound is, nonetheless, useful in the assessment of the presumably obstructed urinary tract, not only as a screening method but also to evaluate renal size and parenchymal thickness, to determine whether ureteral dilatation is present, and to evaluate the bladder. In acute or intermittent obstruction, the dilatation of the collecting system may be minimal and ultrasound may be misleading.

Radioisotopic renography using technetium labeled diethylenetriaminepentaacetic acid (DTPA) gives a gross estimate of differential renal function. In a normal renogram, the isotope is excreted spontaneously but when dilatation is present, it tends to remain in the renal pelvis. If furosemide is administered, the unobstructed system promptly excretes the isotope, whereas the obstructed urinary tract will excrete it slowly or not at all (Fig. 18–31). Because there are many cases of both false-negative interpretations and, more importantly, false-positive interpretations of this test, it should be interpreted cautiously. The furosemide renogram is probably even less reliable in the 1st yr of life. In the newborn and in cases of compromised renal function, even nonobstructed and nondilated kidneys may fail to respond to furosemide. Isotopic renography with iodine-labeled Hippuran is probably more accurate, but when obstruction is present, it exposes the kidneys to unreasonably high doses of radiation. Newly developed radiopharmaceuticals such as MAG3 (^{99m}Tc mercaptoacetylglycine) promise the accuracy of Hippuran and the safety of DTPA.

In older children, the intravenous urogram is still quite useful. The preliminary radiography of the abdomen should be inspected for calculi, spinal abnormalities, or an abnormal intestinal gas pattern. In infravesical obstruction, the bladder wall is irregular or trabeculated because of detrusor hypertrophy. A postvoiding film may show residual bladder urine. In ureteral obstruction there is dilatation of the collecting system

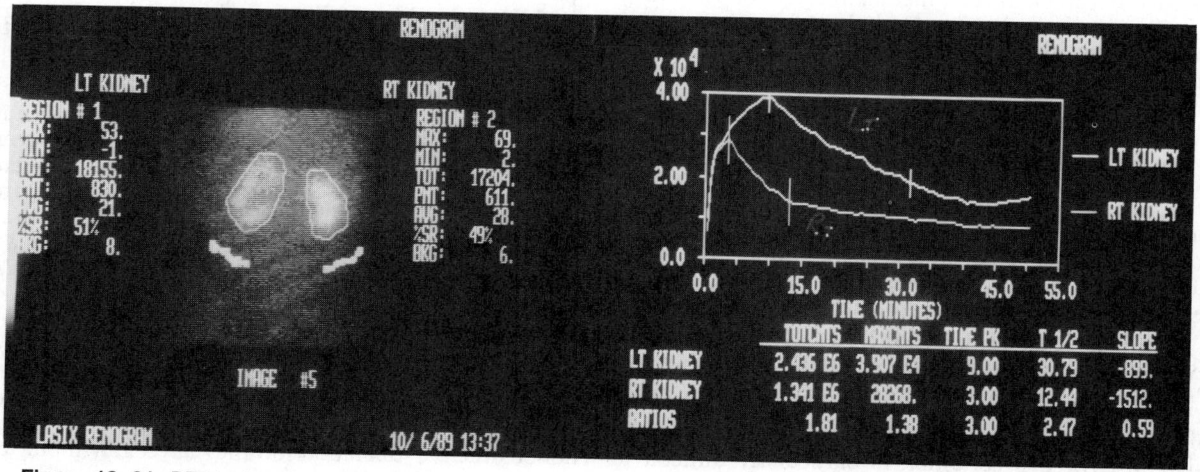

Figure 18–31. DTPA diuresis renogram in a child with left flank pain. The renal function is symmetric. The excretory curve on the right is normal. The kidney excretes the isotope before the injection of furosemide at the 10-min mark. The left kidney retains the isotope and excretes it slowly (T 1/2 30 min) after an injection of furosemide.

above the obstruction and blunting of the calyces. Concentration of the radiopaque medium on the obstructed side is decreased, and there may be delayed appearance of the dye in the collecting system with progressive increase in dye concentration at the point of obstruction when delayed radiographs are obtained. In high-grade obstruction the dye may remain in the collecting system after 24 hr.

Urinary extravasation can be detected in the early or delayed films of a urographic study. When intermittent obstruction is suspected, intravenous urography during an acute episode of pain is often the most valuable diagnostic study.

Pressure Flow Studies. Another way to establish the diagnosis of obstruction of the upper collecting systems in equivocal cases is by performing pressure flow studies, as described by Whitaker. With a No. 22-gauge needle, percutaneous access to the renal pelvis is gained; the collecting system is then perfused with radiopaque dye at a measured flow rate, usually 10 mL/min. The pressures in the renal pelvis and the bladder are monitored during this infusion, and pressure differences exceeding 20 cm of water indicate obstruction. This test usually requires general anesthesia for immobilization. Antegrade pyelography is obtained at the same time, which provides excellent delineation of the anatomy of the collecting system.

Voiding Cystourethrography. In all cases of ureteral dilatation, voiding cystourethrography should be obtained to rule out vesicoureteral reflux as a possible cause of the dilatation. The voiding cystourethrogram is also necessary to rule out urethral obstruction, particularly in cases of posterior urethral valves. In infravesical obstruction in infants the bladder may be palpable because of chronic distention and incomplete emptying. In older children the urinary flow rate can be measured in a simple noninvasive way with a urinary flow meter, and decreased flow in the presence of normal bladder contraction is diagnostic of infravesical obstruction. When the urethra cannot be catheterized to obtain a voiding cystourethrogram, one must suspect a urethral stricture or an obstructive urethral lesion other than valves. Retrograde urethrography with dye injected into the urethral meatus will help delineate the anatomy of the urethral obstruction.

SPECIFIC TYPES OF URINARY TRACT OBSTRUCTION

HYDROCALYCOSIS. This term refers to a localized dilatation of the calyx caused by obstruction of its infundibulum. Such obstruction can be developmental in origin or secondary to inflammatory processes (particularly tuberculosis, now rarely seen). In congenital obstructions due to stenosis or extrinsic vascular compressions, the presenting symptom is usually pain, which can be relieved by surgical correction of the obstruction. The diagnosis of infundibular obstruction is usually established by intravenous urography.

OBSTRUCTION OF THE URETEROPELVIC JUNCTION. This is the most common obstructive lesion in childhood and is caused most often by congenital stenosis of the ureteropelvic junction. Ureteral kinks, fibrous bands, and apparently aberrant vessels are usually secondary phenomena caused by dilatation of the pelvis above the obstruction. Ureteropelvic junction obstruction most commonly presents as: (1) maternal ultrasonography revealing fetal hydronephrosis; (2) a palpable renal mass in a newborn; (3) abdominal, flank, or back pain; (4) a febrile urinary tract infection; or (5) hematuria after minimal trauma. Twenty per cent of obstructions are bilateral.

The diagnosis of this condition is particularly difficult to establish in the asymptomatic infant in whom dilatation of the renal pelvis is found incidentally in a prenatal ultrasonogram. The recognition of unilateral hydronephrosis in the fetus with a normal contralateral kidney and normal volume of amniotic fluid is not an indication for prenatal intervention or early induction of labor. After birth the sonographic study is repeated to confirm the prenatal finding. If no dilatation is found after birth, the newborn may have had transient fetal hydronephrosis. However, renal ultrasonograms should be repeated at 3-mo intervals for the first year, since the dilatation may be minimal after birth but may become more evident later in life. If the kidney is hydronephrotic, a period of observation is usually advisable provided that the serum creatinine level and the other kidney are normal. In many infants, mild to moderate hydronephrosis improves with time and may not require treatment. However, the natural history of prenatally diagnosed hydronephrosis is incompletely understood and long-term follow-up may be indicated. If the degree of hydronephrosis is marked or if the renal parenchyma is thin, an isotopic renogram will give a gross estimation of the differential renal function. If the function is normal, the infant should be followed with serial ultrasonograms. If there is no improvement, a diuresis renogram and pressure flow studies after 6–12 mo may help to decide between continued observation or surgical repair. Early surgical repair is indicated in infants in whom the function of the involved kidney is decreased, in those with bilateral involvement or solitary kidneys, and when there is diminished overall renal function. Early repair should also be done when there is a palpable mass.

In older children who present with symptoms, diagnosis is established by intravenous urography (Fig. 18–32). When the kidneys function poorly and are not visualized on the delayed postinjection radiographs, renal ultrasonography will show hydronephrosis. Retrograde pyelography or percutaneous antegrade pyelography on the operating table will establish the point of obstruction. In the differential diagnosis the following entities should be considered: (1) megacalycosis, a congenital nonobstructive dilatation of the calyces without pelvic or ureteric dilatation; (2) vesicoureteral reflux with marked dilatation and kinking of the ureter (voiding cystourethrography should be done on all patients with suspected ureteropelvic

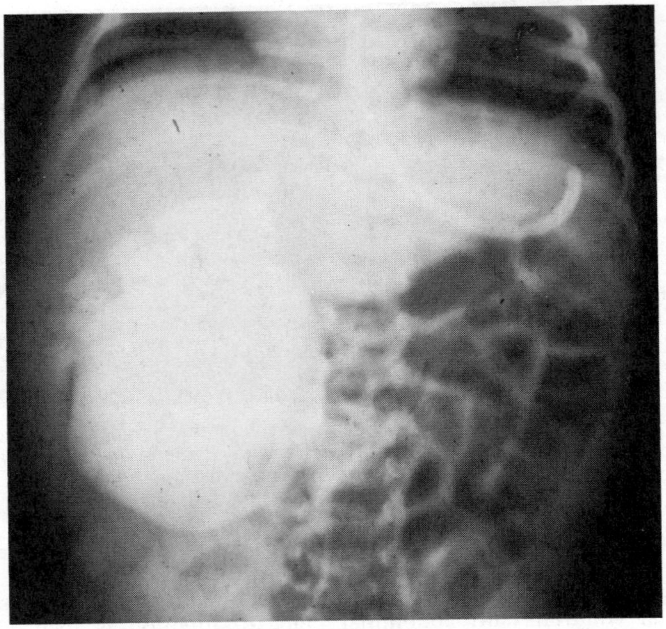

Figure 18–32. Ureteropelvic junction obstruction. Excretory urogram on a newborn, showing dilatation of the right renal pelvis and blunting of the calyces characteristic of a ureteropelvic junction obstruction.

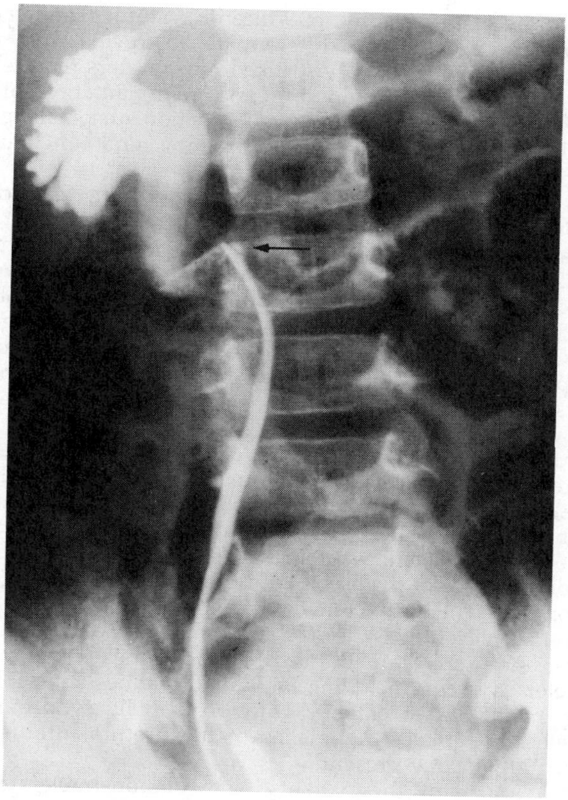

Figure 18–33. Circumcaval ureter. Retrograde pyelogram showing medial deviation of a dilated upper ureter to the level of the 3rd lumbar vertebra, characteristic of a circumcaval ureter.

junction obstruction); and (3) midureteral or distal ureteral obstructions when the ureter is not well visualized on the urogram.

In the neonate with a renal mass, ureteropelvic junction obstruction must be distinguished from multicystic renal dysplasia, solid renal tumors, and renal vein thrombosis. The clinical picture and imaging studies will help establish an accurate diagnosis. A multicystic dysplastic kidney may mimic a ureteropelvic junction obstruction on ultrasound but invariably shows no function on the radioisotopic renogram. Treatment consists of surgical excision of the obstructed ureteropelvic junction with reanastomosis of the ureter and renal pelvis. The success rate of pyeloplasties is high, but postoperative ultrasound and intravenous urography often show persistent dilatation of the calyces. Diuresis renography is useful for the longitudinal follow-up of these patients.

MIDURETERAL OBSTRUCTION. Congenital ureteral stenosis or ureteral valves can sometimes occur in the midureter. A retrocaval ureter can be partially obstructed; such *circumcaval ureters* are invariably on the right side and represent anomalous development of the vena cava, with persistence of the ventral infrarenal subcardinal veins. Excretory urography shows the right ureter to be medially deviated at the level of the 3rd lumbar vertebra (Fig. 18–33). Surgical treatment is needed only when obstruction is present. Retroperitoneal tumors, fibrosis caused by surgical procedures, inflammatory processes (as in chronic granulomatous disease), and radiation therapy can cause acquired midureteral obstruction.

URETERAL ECTOPIA. An ectopic ureteral orifice can be located anywhere along the path of migration of the mesonephric duct. The ectopic ureter may drain a single collecting system, but more commonly it belongs to the upper moiety of a duplicated collecting system. The ureteral orifice of the upper collecting system is always caudal to that of the lower collecting system. In males, ectopic ureters are usually single; they may enter the bladder neck, the urethra above the external sphincter, the seminal vesicle, or the vas deferens; ectopic ureters are commonly associated with high-grade obstruction and symptoms of urinary tract infection or epididymitis. When the contralateral side is normal, nephroureterectomy is usually indicated. When single ectopic ureters are bilateral, or in the rare unilateral cases when the function of the involved kidney is good, the ectopic ureter should be reimplanted.

In females, ureteral ectopia is usually associated with duplication. When the ureter of the upper collecting system enters the bladder neck or the urethra at or above the level of the sphincter there is obstruction, and treatment consists of an upper pole nephroureterectomy. When the ureter enters the vestibule, vagina, or uterus, the most common presenting complaint is urinary incontinence or vaginal discharge. In either case the diagnosis is established by careful inspection of the urogram, renal ultrasonography, and endoscopy. Although obstructed, the collecting system drained by a duplicated ectopic ureter may be very small and difficult to detect even after careful inspection of the intravenous urogram. A high degree of suspicion is always necessary to establish this diagnosis. In bilateral simple ectopic ureters in the female there is usually bladder hypoplasia in addition to ureteral obstruction; such cases are difficult to manage and may require bladder reconstruction, urinary diversion, or renal transplantation.

URETEROCELE. Ureterocele is a congenital cystic dilatation of the distal ureter that protrudes into the bladder and has a pinpoint ureteral orifice. Its embryogenesis remains uncertain. Ureteroceles are more common in females than in males. *Simple ureteroceles* are associated with nonduplicated collecting systems, and the orifice is in the expected location in the bladder. They are usually discovered during an investigation for a urinary tract infection. Intravenous pyelography reveals varying degrees of ureteral and calyceal dilatation, and there is a round filling defect in the bladder (Fig. 18–34). In delayed films the cystic dilatation of the ureter may be clearly visible and full of contrast material. Transurethral incision of the ureterocele effectively relieves the obstruction, but it may result in vesicoureteral reflux necessitating ureteral reimplantation later. Some prefer open excision of the ureterocele and reimplantation as the initial form of treatment. Small, simple ureteroceles incidentally discovered without upper tract dilatation may not require treatment. In questionable cases diuresis renography and pressure flow studies (see earlier) are useful.

More commonly, ureteroceles are associated with ureteral duplication. The ureter involved with the ureterocele drains the upper renal moiety, which frequently functions poorly or is dysplastic because of congenital obstruction. The more cephalad ureter drains the lower renal moiety and frequently refluxes. These *ectopic ureteroceles* may extend submucosally into the posterior urethra. Affected children also present with urinary tract infections. Rarely, large ectopic ureteroceles may cause bladder outlet obstruction and retention of urine; in females the ureterocele may prolapse from the urethral meatus. Reflux to the ipsilateral lower segment ureter is common. Contralateral reflux is usually present when the bladder neck is obstructed. Both simple and ectopic ureteroceles can be bilateral. Intravenous pyelography usually shows a large filling defect in the bladder corresponding to the ureterocele and characteristic findings of duplication of the collecting systems (poor or absent function of the upper collecting system and caudal displacement of the lower collecting system) (Fig. 18–35).

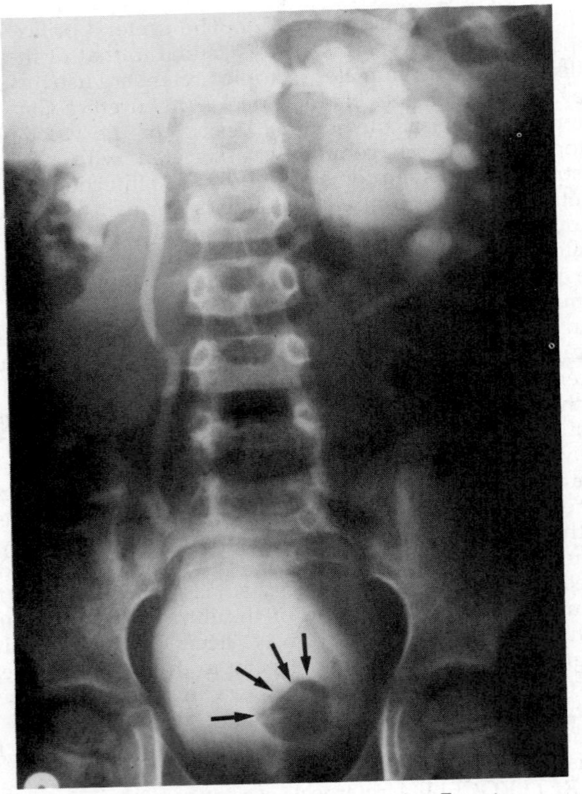

Figure 18–34. Simple intravesical ureterocele. Excretory urogram showing left hydronephrosis and a round filling defect on the left side of the bladder corresponding to a simple ureterocele causing left ureteral obstruction.

Treatment of ectopic ureteroceles is the excision of the upper collecting system, involving partial nephrectomy and ureterectomy. When the ectopic ureterocele is small and there is low grade or no reflux in the ipsilateral duplicated ureter, the decompressed ureterocele need not be excised and usually will cause no further problems. Large ureteroceles, however, or those with high-grade reflux to the ipsilateral lower ureter are best treated by excision of the ureterocele and reimplantation of the remaining ureter, plus partial upper moiety nephroureterectomy. This can usually be accomplished in a single operation. In the treatment of an acutely ill, septic infant with an obstructing ureterocele, drainage of the involved collecting system may be necessary, either transureterally or (preferably) by percutaneous nephrostomy of the upper collecting system.

MEGAURETER. This term refers generally to the dilated ureter. A classification of megaureters is given in Table 18–14. In this section, primary obstructed and nonrefluxing nonobstructed megaureters will be discussed. Megaureters are usually discovered through intravenous urography done for urinary tract infections, hematuria, or abdominal pain. A careful history, physical examination, and voiding cystourethrography will help to rule out causes of secondary megaureters and refluxing megaureters as well as the prune-belly syndrome. Primary obstructed megaureters and nonobstructed megaureters probably represent opposite extremes of a spectrum of the same anomaly.

Radiographically, the distal ureter is more dilated in its distal segment and tapers abruptly at or above the junction of the bladder (Fig. 18–36). The lesion may be unilateral or bilateral. Dilatation of the upper collecting system and calyceal blunting are suggestive of obstruction. In most cases, however, diuresis renography, pressure flow studies, and careful follow-up are needed to differentiate obstructed from nonobstructed megaureters. Obstructed megaureters require surgical treatment, with tapering and reimplantation of the ureter. The results of surgical reconstruction are usually good, but the prognosis depends on pre-existing renal function and whether complications develop.

PRUNE-BELLY SYNDROME. This syndrome, also called abdominal muscle deficiency syndrome or **Eagle-Barrett syndrome**, occurs in approximately 1/40,000 births. The characteristic association of deficient abdominal muscles, undescended testes, and urinary tract abnormalities probably results from severe urethral obstruction in fetal life (Fig. 18–37). Oligohydramnios and pulmonary hypoplasia are frequent complications in the perinatal period. Many affected infants are stillborn. Urinary tract abnormalities include massive dilatation of the ureters and upper tracts, and a very large bladder, with a patent urachus or a urachal diverticulum. There may be vesicoureteral reflux. The prostatic urethra is usually dilated and the prostate is hypoplastic. The anterior urethra may be dilated, resulting in a megalourethra. Rarely, there is urethral stenosis or atresia. The kidneys usually show various degrees of dysplasia, and the testes are usually intra-abdominal. There is often malrotation of the bowel with a universal mesentery. Cardiac abnormalities occur in 10% of cases, and more than 50% have abnormalities of the musculoskeletal system, including limb abnormalities and scoliosis. Only about 3% of patients with prune-belly syndrome are females. In females, anomalies of the urethra, uterus, and vagina are usually present.

One fourth of the patients have demonstrable urethral

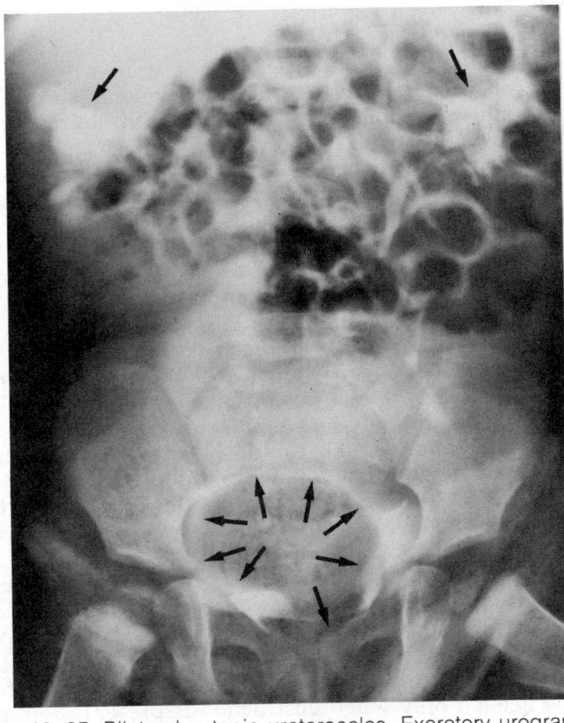

Figure 18–35. Bilateral ectopic ureteroceles. Excretory urogram of a 1-yr-old girl with a history of febrile urinary tract infections. The large filling defect in the bladder represents bilateral ectopic ureteroceles. The visualized portion of the upper urinary tracts reveals only the lower moiety of the duplicated kidneys, with characteristic drooping lily configuration. The upper moieties drained by the ureters involved in the ureteroceles function poorly and are not opacified. Most cases of ectopic ureteroceles are unilateral.

TABLE 18–14. International Classification of Megaureters*

	Primary	Secondary
Obstructed	Intrinsic ureteral obstruction	Associated with urethral obstruction or extrinsic lesions
Refluxing	Reflux is only abnormality	Associated with bladder outlet obstruction or neurogenic bladder
Nonrefluxing, nonobstructed	Idiopathic ureteral dilatation	Associated with polyuria (diabetes insipidus) or infection

*From King LR: Ureter and ureterovesical junction. *In*: Kelalis PP, King LR, Belman AB (eds): Clinical Pediatric Urology. Philadelphia, WB Saunders, 1985, p 486.

obstruction at the time of birth. When no obstruction is present, the goal of treatment is the prevention of urinary tract infection. When obstruction of the ureters or urethra can be demonstrated or suspected, temporary drainage procedures such as pyelostomies or vesicostomies may help to preserve renal function until the child is old enough for reconstructive surgery. Some children with prune-belly syndrome have been found to have classic or atypical posterior urethral valves. Urinary tract infections are frequent and should be treated promptly. Antibacterial prophylaxis is often necessary. Correction of the undescended testis by orchidopexy in these children can be quite difficult and is best accomplished in the 1st yr of life.

The prognosis ultimately depends on the degree of pulmonary and renal dysplasia. One third of children with prune-belly syndrome are stillborn or die in the first few months of life of pulmonary complications. Of the long-term survivors, one half develop chronic renal failure from dysplasia or complications of infection or reflux and eventually require renal transplantation. The results of renal transplantation in these patients are favorable.

BLADDER NECK OBSTRUCTION. Bladder neck obstruction is usually secondary to ectopic ureteroceles, bladder calculi, or tumors of the prostate (rhabdomyosarcoma). The manifestations include difficulty voiding, urinary retention, urinary tract infection, and bladder distention with overflow incontinence. Apparent bladder neck obstruction is common in cases of posterior urethral valves, but it seldom has any functional significance. Primary bladder neck obstruction is exceptional in males and, according to current thinking, probably never occurs in females. Functional bladder neck obstruction can also result from nonrelaxation of the bladder neck in neurogenic bladder dysfunction.

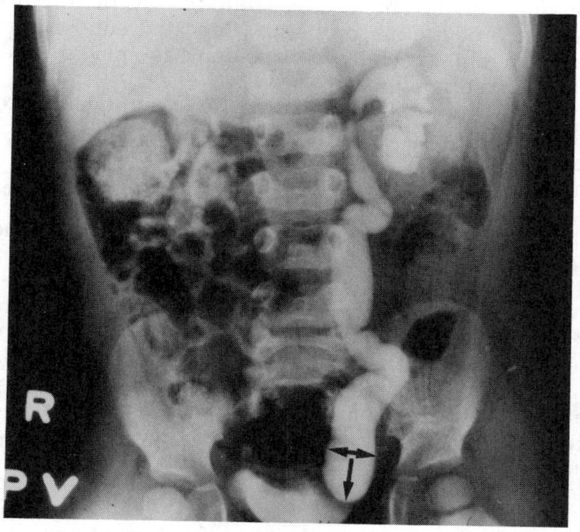

Figure 18–36. Obstructed megaureter. Excretory urogram in a girl with a history of a febrile urinary tract infection. The right side is normal. The left side reveals hydroureteronephrosis with predominant dilatation of the distal ureter. Note the characteristic appearance of the distal ureter. There was no vesicoureteral reflux. The diagnosis of obstruction was confirmed by pressure-flow studies.

POSTERIOR URETHRAL VALVES. The most common type of urethral valves are located in the posterior urethra. They are sail-shaped membranes that arise from the verumontanum in males and extend distally and attach to the anterolateral walls of the urethra. Valves are congenitally abnormal structures of unclear embryologic origin and cause varying degrees of obstruction. The prostatic urethra dilates and the detrusor muscle hypertrophies. There may be vesicoureteral reflux or distal ureteral obstruction resulting from a chronically distended bladder or bladder muscle hypertrophy. The renal changes range from mild hydronephrosis to severe dysplasia; their severity probably depends on the severity of the obstruction and the time of its onset in fetal life. As in other cases of obstruction or renal dysplasia, there may be oligohydramnios and pulmonary hypoplasia.

With increasing frequency, posterior urethral valves are being discovered prenatally when maternal ultrasonography reveals bilateral hydronephrosis, a dilated bladder and, if the obstruction is severe, oligohydramnios. Prenatal bladder decompression by percutaneous vesicoamniotic shunt or open fetal surgery has been reported. However, experimental and clinical evidence of the possible benefits of fetal intervention is lacking and these procedures should be considered experimental. In the male neonate posterior urethral valves are suspected when there is a palpably distended bladder and the urinary stream is weak. If the obstruction is severe and goes unrecognized during the neonatal period, infants will present later in life with failure to thrive due to uremia or sepsis caused by infection in the obstructed urinary tract. With lesser degrees of obstruction children present later in life with difficulty in maintaining urinary continence during the daytime or with urinary tract infections. The diagnosis is established by voiding cystourethrography (Fig. 18–38).

Vesicoureteral reflux is present in two thirds of cases and may be unilateral or bilateral. The prognosis for renal function is worse when reflux is present. Once the diagnosis is established, renal function and the anatomy of the upper urinary tract should be carefully evaluated. In the healthy neonate, a small polyethylene feeding tube (No. 5 French or No. 8 French) is inserted in the bladder and left indwelling for several days. If the serum creatinine level remains normal or returns to normal, treatment is by primary ablation of the valves through a transurethral approach or by temporary vesicostomy. If the urethral caliber is insufficient for transurethral ablation, temporary vesicostomy is preferred, to be followed by closure of the vesicostomy and transurethral ablation of the valves at a later date when the growth of the child permits use of urethral instrumentation.

If the serum creatinine level remains high or increases despite bladder drainage by a small catheter, secondary ureteral obstruction, irreversible renal damage, or renal dysplasia should be suspected. In such cases, upper tract drainage by cutaneous pyelostomy or high ureterostomy is necessary. If renal function does not improve, the child should have reconstructive surgery at a relatively early age to prevent infections and restore bladder function before the need for renal transplantation arises. If renal function improves between the ages of 6 mo and 1 yr, the ureters are re-evaluated by pressure flow studies. Distal obstruction caused by hyper-

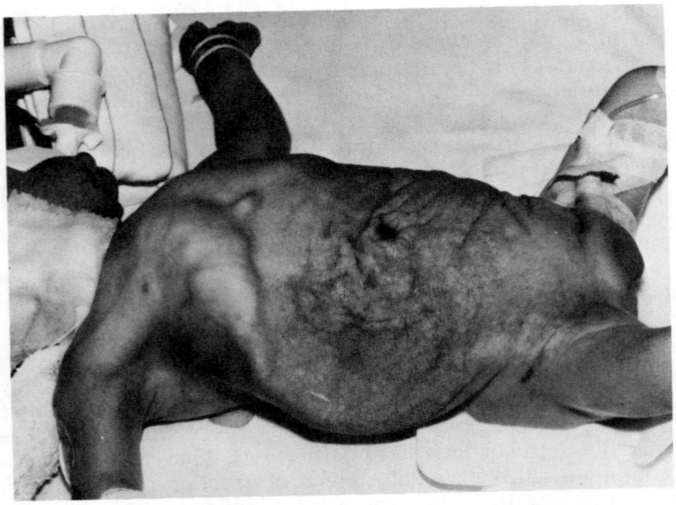

Figure 18–37. Eagle-Barrett syndrome. Photograph of a 1,600-g newborn with the prune-belly syndrome. Note the lack of tonicity of the abdominal wall and the wrinkled appearance of the skin.

trophy of the detrusor muscle may reverse spontaneously; if it persists, however, the child should have ablation of the valves, closure of the pyelostomies, and correction of the distal ureteral obstruction.

Infants presenting later in life with uremia without infection should be evaluated and treated following identical guidelines. In the septic and uremic infant, lifesaving measures must include prompt correction of the electrolyte imbalance and control of the infection by appropriate antibiotics. Drainage of the upper tracts by percutaneous nephrostomy and hemodialysis are frequently required. After the patient's condition becomes stable, step-by-step evaluation and treatment

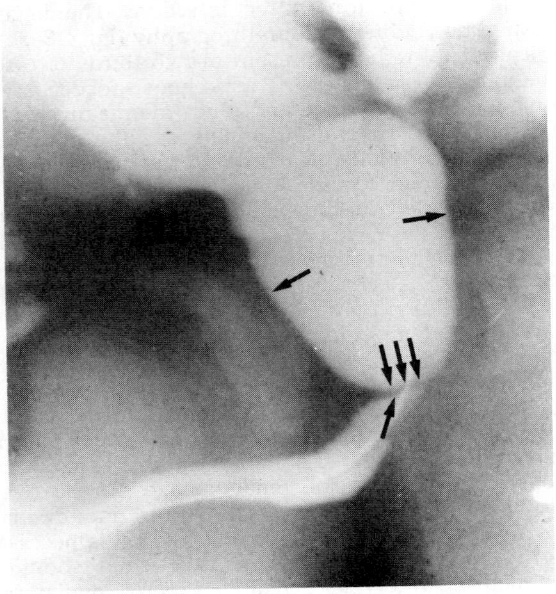

Figure 18–38. Posterior urethral valves. Voiding cystourethrogram in an infant with posterior urethral valves. Note the dilatation of the prostatic urethra and the transverse linear filling defect corresponding to the valves.

can be undertaken. Prolonged use of intubated nephrostomy drainage is inconvenient for the parents, introduces infection, and is generally detrimental to renal function.

Most children presenting with incontinence can be treated by primary valve ablation. When vesicoureteral reflux is present, expectant treatment and suppressive doses of antibacterial drugs are advisable; however, if reflux persists more than 1 yr after ablation of the valves and if the function of the involved kidney warrants it, surgical correction should be undertaken.

There is some degree of urinary incontinence in up to 50% of children after treatment of posterior urethral valves. Assuming there has been no surgical damage to the sphincter, the dilatation of the prostatic urethra, poor bladder compliance, and polyuria from renal damage are all important factors that contribute to incontinence. Urinary incontinence usually improves with age, particularly after puberty.

The prognosis in the newborn is related to the degree of pulmonary hypoplasia and potential for recovery of renal function. Severely affected infants are often stillborn. Of those who survive the neonatal period, approximately one third will retain some degree of renal insufficiency and many will eventually require renal transplantation. Renal transplantation in children with posterior urethral valves has a lower success rate than transplantation in children with normal bladders, presumably because of the adverse influence of altered bladder function on graft function and survival. Meticulous attention to bladder compliance, emptying, and infection may improve results in the future.

URETHRAL STRICTURES. Urethral strictures *in males* are rarely congenital. They usually result from urethral trauma, either iatrogenic (catheterization, endoscopic procedures, or previous urethral reconstruction) or accidental (straddling injuries or pelvic fractures). Because these lesions may develop gradually, the decrease in force of the urinary stream is seldom noticed by the child or his parents. More commonly, the obstruction causes symptoms of bladder instability, hematuria, or dysuria. Catheterization of the bladder is usually impossible. The diagnosis is made by a voiding film obtained during intravenous urography; retrograde urethrography and endoscopy are confirmatory. Endoscopic treatment of short strictures by dilatation or internal urethrotomy is usually successful. Longer strictures surrounded by periurethral fibrosis often require urethroplasty. Repeated endoscopic procedures should generally be avoided, as they may cause additional urethral damage.

In females true urethral strictures are exceptional, since the female urethra is protected from trauma, particularly in childhood. In the past it was thought that the urethral ring commonly caused obstruction of the female urethra and urinary tract infection and that affected girls benefited from urethral dilatation. The diagnosis was suspected when a "spinning top" deformity of the urethra was found in the voiding cystourethrogram and was confirmed by urethral calibration. Treatment for this condition invariably included antibiotic therapy, and adequately controlled studies were not done. Moreover, other studies have found no correlation between the radiologic appearance of the urethra in the voiding cystourethrogram and the urethral caliber and no significant difference in urethral caliber between females with recurrent cystitis and normal age-matched controls. This area remains somewhat controversial, but endoscopy and urethral dilatation are seldom justified solely by the radiologic appearance of the urethra or by a history of recurrent urinary tract infections. Likewise, there is no justification for performing urethral dilatation in girls with diurnal or nocturnal enuresis because there is no evidence that urethral obstruction plays a role in the pathogenesis of these symptoms. The evaluation and treatment of these conditions are discussed in Sec. 18.44.

ANTERIOR URETHRAL VALVES AND URETHRAL DIVERTICULA IN THE MALE. *Anterior urethral valves* are usually associated with congenital urethral diverticulum. They are considerably rarer than valves of the posterior urethra, but they may cause similar symptoms and have identical effects on the urinary tract. The diagnosis is established on voiding cystourethrography. *Urethral diverticula* are discovered on voiding cystourethrography, often during evaluation for hematuria or urinary tract infections. Many diverticula are believed to arise from dilatations of Cowper glands and ducts. Small diverticula require no treatment; larger ones are usually managed endoscopically.

Fusiform dilatation of the urethra or megalourethra may result from underdevelopment of the corpus spongiosum and support structures of the urethra. This is commonly associated with the prune-belly syndrome.

MALE URETHRAL MEATAL STENOSIS. Congenital stenosis of the urethral meatus in the male is rare. It has in the past probably been overdiagnosed, and unrelated conditions, such as nocturnal enuresis, have been blamed on presumed meatal stenosis. True urethral meatal stenosis (a meatus less than No. 8 French in boys under 4 yr old, or less than No. 10 French in prepubertal boys over the age of 10) usually results from inflammation associated with ammoniacal dermatitis of the glans following neonatal circumcision. Children with hypospadias rarely may have stenosis of the urethral meatus. The treatment of symptomatic urethral meatal stenosis is by a meatoplasty with careful follow-up to avoid reapproximation of the edges of the enlarged meatus. A more common abnormality is the development of a thin ventral membrane that partially covers the meatus and produces dorsal deflection of the urinary stream. Even though the actual meatus is often of normal caliber, these children may require meatoplasty to allow them to aim their urinary stream as desired.

18.42 OTHER DISORDERS AND ANOMALIES OF THE BLADDER

BLADDER EXSTROPHY

Exstrophy of the urinary bladder occurs about once in every 10,000–40,000 births. It is more common in boys than in girls. The severity ranges from a small cutaneous fistula in the abdominal wall or simple epispadias to complete exstrophy of the cloaca involving exposure of the entire hindgut and the bladder.

These anomalies result when the mesoderm fails to invade the cephalad extension of the cloacal membrane; the extent of this failure determines the degree of the anomaly. In classic bladder exstrophy (Fig. 18–39), the bladder protrudes from the abdominal wall and its mucosa is exposed. The umbilicus is displaced downward, the pubic rami are widely separated in the midline, and the recti muscles are separated. In males there is complete epispadias with a wide and shallow scrotum. Undescended testes and inguinal hernias are common. Females also have epispadias, with duplication of the clitoris and wide separation of the labia. The anus is displaced anteriorly in both sexes, and there may be rectal prolapse. The consequences of untreated bladder exstrophy are total urinary incontinence and increased incidence of bladder cancer, usually adenocarcinoma. The genital deformities produce sexual disability in both sexes, but particularly in the male. The wide separation of the pubic rami causes a characteristic broad-based gait but no significant disability.

Treatment for bladder exstrophy should start at birth. The bladder should be covered with a Silastic shield or another appropriate plastic dressing that will prevent desiccation of

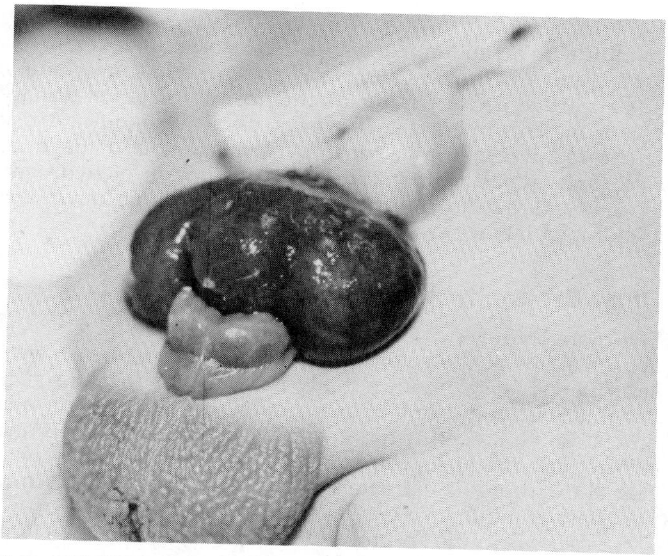

Figure 18–39. Classic bladder exstrophy. The bladder is exposed in the midline; the umbilical cord is displaced caudally; the penis is epispadiac; and the scrotum is broad.

the bladder mucosa but allow urinary drainage. Application of gauze or Vaseline-gauze to the bladder mucosa should be avoided. The infant should then be transferred promptly to a center equipped for the treatment of such anomalies.

Closure of the exstrophied bladder is the preferred treatment, ideally performed during the first 48 hr of life before permanent changes in the bladder wall are established. At this time the flexibility of the pelvic joints allows precise reconstruction of the bladder and prostatic urethra in the male, with approximation of the pubic rami and reconstruction of the abdominal wall without the iliac osteostomies that are often required in the older child. This treatment can be applied to more than three fourths of infants with classic bladder exstrophy. Treatment should be deferred in certain exceptional circumstances when surgery would be excessively risky or complex, such as when the bladder is extremely small or there are upper tract changes, or when there are complex genital anomalies such as complete duplication of the penis.

The purpose of the initial operation is the precise closure of the bladder and prostatic urethra in the male, elongation of the urethral plate and penis, and closure of the abdominal wall. Postoperatively, the infant's upper urinary tract is watched closely for the possible development of hydronephrosis and infection. The majority of such infants have vesicoureteral reflux and should receive antibiotics. When the child is between 1 and 2 yr old, the resulting epispadias is repaired, to create an anterior urethra and correct the malformation of the penis. At about 3 yr of age, most children will have total incontinence, and bladder neck reconstruction with bilateral ureteral reimplantation is undertaken.

This plan of treatment has yielded less than 15% deterioration of the upper urinary tract and over 70% continence in some centers. This continence rate reflects not only the successful reconstruction but also the quality and size of the bladder. It appears that children who have reconstructive surgery as newborns have a greater chance for obtaining a normally functioning bladder. Children whose sphincters cannot be successfully reconstructed should have artificial sphincters implanted. If the cause of incontinence is a small bladder capacity, an augmentation cystoplasty using a segment of the large bowel will help obtain continence. The exceptional children whose anomaly cannot be reconstructed can have a urinary diversion by means of a sigmoid urinary conduit with an abdominal stoma. Ureterosigmoidostomy has been popular in the past and is still employed in some centers; it is attractive because it avoids the need for external urinary diversion. This operation, however, carries a significant risk of chronic pyelonephritis, of upper urinary tract damage, of electrolyte imbalance resulting from absorption of hydrogen ion and chloride in the intestine, and of colonic carcinoma after a long latency period.

Other Exstrophy Anomalies

The more complex cases of *cloacal exstrophy* may have severe abnormalities of the colon and the rectum and often have a short bowel syndrome. Mortality in infancy is high for such patients, but some can undergo genital reconstruction and others can be helped with permanent urinary diversions and colostomies. Because genital reconstruction in males with cloacal exstrophy is extremely difficult, most authors recommend assigning female gender to such infants.

Epispadias is in the spectrum of exstrophy anomalies. Distal epispadias should be repaired by reconstructing the urethra and the penis. The more severe cases of epispadias also have separation of the pubic rami and urinary incontinence. Such children require surgical reconstructions analogous to those of the 2nd and 3rd stages of management of patients with classic bladder exstrophy.

BLADDER DIVERTICULA

Bladder diverticula usually occur at the ureterovesical junction and are associated with vesicoureteral reflux (see Fig. 18–26). Congenital diverticula in other locations also occur. Bladder diverticula are also commonly associated with distal urethral obstruction or neurogenic bladder dysfunction. Small diverticula require no treatment other than that of the primary disease, whereas large diverticula may contribute to inefficient voiding, residual urine, urinary stasis, and urinary tract infections and should be excised.

URACHAL ANOMALIES

Urachal abnormalities are more common in males than in females. A patent urachus can occur as an isolated anomaly, in which case it should be corrected surgically, or it may be associated with prune-belly syndrome. Other anomalies related to the urachus are cysts and bladder diverticula and umbilical sinus; these should be excised.

18.43 NEUROGENIC BLADDER

Neurogenic bladder dysfunction in children is often congenital and may result from myelomeningocele, lipomeningocele, sacral agenesis, or other spinal abnormalities. Acquired diseases and traumatic lesions of the spinal cord are less frequent. Cerebral palsy, central nervous system tumors and their treatment, and pelvic operations such as repair of imperforate anus or excision of a sacrococcygeal teratoma can result in abnormal innervation of the bladder and the sphincters. The two most important consequences of neurogenic bladder dysfunction are upper tract deterioration and urinary incontinence.

Renal damage is the result of lack of coordination between the contraction of the detrusor muscle and the relaxation of the sphincter, normally a function located in the brain stem. This dyssynergia results in functional obstruction of the bladder outlet leading to high intravesical pressures, bladder muscle hypertrophy and trabeculation, vesicoureteral reflux, and rapid deterioration of the upper tracts. Infection often compounds the problem. For example, vesicoureteral reflux is present in 30% of neonates with myelomeningocele and develops later in life in another 20%. Reflux secondary to neurogenic bladder has much more severe consequences than primary reflux. However, not all children with myelomeningocele (or any other neurologic anomaly) have similar patterns of lower tract dysfunction, so that its occurrence cannot be predicted accurately from the neurologic examination or radiographic appearance of the spine. Accordingly, accurate urodynamic studies (by cystometrography and sphincter electromyography) and radiologic evaluation of the urinary tract are required in every case. If the bladder is atonic or the sphincters are denervated, bladder pressure tends to be low, and vesicoureteral reflux is unlikely to develop even when bladder emptying is incomplete.

Urinary incontinence in the child with neurogenic bladder can result from total or partial denervation of the sphincter, from bladder hyper-reflexia or poor bladder compliance, from chronic urinary retention, or from a combination of factors. The treatment of children with neurogenic bladder aims at protecting the upper urinary tracts and eventually providing continence. Supravesical diversion, once commonly performed to achieve these goals, yielded unsatisfactory long-term results and is now seldom employed. The neonate with low intravesical pressures and no vesicoureteral reflux can be treated expectantly with follow-up renal ultrasound to detect possible development of hydronephrosis and radioisotopic cystography for the early detection of reflux. Occasionally, limited intravenous pyelography is needed as well. Recurrent urinary tract infections may require prolonged antibiotic prophylaxis (see Sec. 18.39). Urodynamic studies should be repeated at 6 mo of age to detect possible neurologic changes following repair of the myelomeningocele. The neurologic lesion in myelomeningocele can vary with time owing to tethering of the spinal cord or to development of secondary central changes.

When reflux is present or there are elevated intravesical pressures (indicative of high risk for developing reflux), treatment with antibacterial prophylaxis, intermittent catheterization, and often anticholinergic drugs (oxybutynin up to 0.4 mg/kg/24 hr in 2 divided doses) will cure the reflux in up to 40% of patients without ureteral dilation (grades I and II). Children with more severe reflux require corrective surgery followed by intermittent catheterization and anticholinergic drugs. When intermittent catheterization is impossible, as may be the case in male neonates and small infants, when there are urethral abnormalities that preclude catheterization, or when anticholinergics are not well tolerated, a temporary cutaneous vesicostomy provides effective, temporary bladder decompression. Failure of these methods to relieve intravesical pressures is an indication for augmentation enterocystoplasty and intermittent catheterization. Attempts to denervate the bladder to control bladder hypertonicity have yielded unsatisfactory long-term results.

The treatment of incontinence should be tailored to the individual case. If the sphincter tone is sufficient and the bladder has adequate compliance, intermittent catheterization every 4 hr is usually successful in keeping the child dry. Anticholinergic drugs are sometimes needed to relax the bladder and enhance continence. Most children 7–8 yr old who have adequate manual dexterity can learn the technique of intermittent self-catheterization. Bacteriuria is seen in up to 50% of children using intermittent self-catheterization, but it seldom causes symptoms. In the absence of reflux, there seems to be little cause for concern. Antibacterial prophylaxis can often be effective in keeping the urine sterile while intermittent catheterization is used.

When the bladder capacity and compliance are adequate

but the urethral resistance is low, implantation of an artificial sphincter is usually successful. This sphincter consists of an inflatable cuff that is placed around the bladder neck, a pressure-regulating balloon implanted in the extraperitoneal space, and a pumping mechanism that is implanted in the scrotum of males and in the labia of females. Sometimes bladder augmentation by enterocystoplasty alone or in combination with other means to increase outlet resistance is necessary, along with intermittent catheterization. With the treatment as outlined earlier and lifelong follow-up, urinary diversion can be avoided in most cases, children can reach a satisfactory degree of continence, and the chances of upper tract deterioration are low.

The more frequent application of *enterocystoplasty* for increasing bladder capacity—not only in children with neurogenic bladder but also in some patients with bladder exstrophy, posterior urethral valves, and other congenital and acquired bladder disorders that result in a small functional bladder capacity—requires that pediatricians be informed about some of the implications of these operations. The bowel segments used to enlarge the bladder are isolated from the right or left side of the colon and the ileum. Most children with augmented bladders require intermittent catheterization for emptying. The urine is usually colonized with gram-negative bacteria, and attempts to sterilize the urine for prolonged periods of time usually fail. Therefore only symptomatic urinary tract infections should be treated in these patients. Even when there is no reflux, the upper tracts may be colonized as well. However, there is no evidence that chronic bacteriuria in these patients is associated with renal damage. Nevertheless, long-term follow-up is necessary.

The enteric mucosal surface in contact with the urine absorbs chloride and hydrogen ions and losses of potassium. Hyperchloremic metabolic acidosis can result and may require medical treatment. This complication is more common in patients with compromised renal function. To overcome this limitation of enterocystoplasty in patients with chronic renal insufficiency, a gastric segment can be used instead of a segment of the small or large intestine. The stomach secretes chloride and hydrogen ions; thus, pre-existing metabolic acidosis will remain stable or improve.

Perforation of the augmented bladder and peritonitis is a serious complication that has occurred in up to 10% of patients in some series. Prompt diagnosis and treatment is lifesaving. Although the precise pathogenesis of these perforations remains unclear, meticulous adherence to the prescribed program of intermittent catheterization to avoid bladder overdistention is important.

The potential for malignancy secondary to enterocystoplasty is unknown but, based on past experience with ureterosigmoidostomy and some reported cases, it is prudent to advise yearly endoscopic examinations or urine cytology beginning in the 7th to 10th postoperative years.

18.44 VOIDING DYSFUNCTION

Nocturnal Enuresis (See also Sec. 3.28)

Enuresis is the occurrence of involuntary voiding at an age when volitional control of micturition is expected. *Nocturnal enuresis* without overt daytime voiding symptoms affects up to 20% of children at the age of 5 yr; it ceases spontaneously in approximately 15% of the involved children every year thereafter. Its frequency among adults is probably less than 1%. The cause of nocturnal enuresis is not precisely known but appears to involve delayed maturation of the cortical mechanisms that allow voluntary control of the micturition reflex. The disorder can be primary (when the child never has a period of night-time continence) or secondary (developing in a formerly "dry" child following some emotionally disruptive event). Nocturnal enuresis is 3 times more common in males than in females, and there is often a family history of bedwetting.

The child with nocturnal enuresis should be examined carefully for neurologic and spinal abnormalities. A careful history should be obtained especially with respect to fluid intake and urinary output. Children with diabetes insipidus, diabetes mellitus, and chronic renal disease may have high obligatory urinary output and a compensatory polydipsia. A complete examination should include palpation of the abdomen and rectal examination after voiding, to assess the possibility of a chronically distended bladder. If possible, the child should be watched during micturition to observe the force and quality of the urinary stream; measurement of the urinary flow rate helps rule out obstructive lesions. Bacteriuria has increased frequency in enuretic girls and, if found, should be investigated and treated (see Sec. 18.39), though this will not always lead to resolution of bedwetting. Urinalysis should be obtained after an overnight fast and evaluated for specific gravity or osmolality, or both, in order to exclude polyuria as a cause of frequency and incontinence and to ascertain that the concentrating ability is normal. The absence of glycosuria should be confirmed. Urine culture should be done routinely. If there are no daytime symptoms and if the physical examination, urinalysis, and culture are normal, then further evaluation for urinary tract pathology is not warranted, even in older children.

The best approach to treatment is to assure parents that the problem is self-limited and to eliminate punitive measures that may adversely affect the psychologic development of the child (see Sec. 3.28).

Unstable Bladder

Voiding dysfunction not related to neurologic abnormalities or dysfunction is common in children. The child with an unstable bladder usually exhibits urinary frequency, urgency, and episodes of diurnal urinary incontinence with or without bladder pain. Such symptoms are seen also in about 15% of children with nocturnal enuresis, but sometimes the daytime symptoms predominate and certainly always have greater psychosocial consequences, particularly in school-aged children. In females, a history of recurrent urinary tract infection is common, but incontinence may persist long after infections are brought under control. It is not clear in these cases if the voiding dysfunction is a sequel of the infections or if the voiding dysfunction disposes to recurrent infections. In other female cases and usually in male cases, there is no antecedent history of infection and the cause of uninhibited bladder is obscure. Many authors attribute it to a delayed maturation of the neurologic mechanisms that modulate the spinal micturition reflex. Bladder outlet obstructions result in detrusor hyper-reflexia and can also lead to uninhibited bladder contractions.

In the evaluation of affected children, a careful history helps rule out the possibility of previous urinary tract infections. Constipation is sometimes associated. Its treatment may lead to improvement of the urinary symptoms. The physical examination is directed at detecting neurologic abnormalities and residual urine after voiding. Urinalysis and urine culture rule out infection and causes of polyuria. Examination of the urinary flow rate by visual inspection of the urinary stream or, ideally, with a uroflowmeter helps rule out gross urethral obstruction. Abdominal ultrasound excludes hydronephrosis and gross bladder abnormalities and confirms the completeness of bladder emptying. In males, voiding cystourethrography is usually necessary to rule out bladder or urethral abnormalities. If the evaluation rules out significant urinary tract pathology, a therapeutic trial with oxybutynin or other anticholinergic drugs is warranted and often effective. The treatment is usually prolonged and should be interrupted periodically to determine its continued need. If there is a history of cystitis but no other abnormalities such as vesicoureteral reflux that require additional evaluation and treatment, prophylactic antibacterial agents help prevent recurrence of infection, which can exacerbate bladder instability. Children not responding to this simple treatment should be evaluated endoscopically and urodynamically to rule out other possible forms of bladder or sphincter dysfunction.

Non-neurogenic Neurogenic Bladder

This is a more serious but less common disorder involving failure of the external sphincter to relax during voiding, in children without neurologic abnormalities. Children with this syndrome, also called non-neurogenic detrusor/sphincter dyssynergia, exhibit daytime and night-time wetting. There is usually a history of urinary tract infections and constipation, with or without encopresis. Evaluation of affected children usually reveals vesicoureteral reflux, a trabeculated bladder, and decreased urinary flow rate with an intermittent pattern. The pathogenesis of this syndrome appears to involve problems during toilet training, since the syndrome is not seen in children before the age when voluntary micturition occurs. The urodynamic evaluation should be complemented with magnetic resonance imaging of the spine to rule out a neurologic cause for the bladder dysfunction. The treatment is usually difficult and requires appropriate treatment of the reflux with antibacterial prophylaxis. Behavioral modification and encouragement of relaxation during voiding are sometimes useful. Biofeedback has been used successfully in older children to teach relaxation of the external sphincter. Some investigators have recommended intermittent catheterization and anticholinergic drugs to decrease intravesical pressures; others have administered diazepam to facilitate relaxation of the external sphincter. The prognosis for this condition is poor, and many patients develop chronic renal failure. Therefore, aggressive treatment of the bladder dysfunction is often justified and may include antireflux surgery, intermittent catheterization, and bladder augmentation. These children require long-term treatment and careful follow-up.

Infrequent Voiding

Infrequent voiding is a common disorder of micturition usually associated with urinary tract infections. Affected children, usually girls, void only twice a day rather than the normal three to five times. With bladder overdistention and prolonged retention of urine, growth of bacteria leads to recurrent urinary tract infections. Some such children are constipated. There is sometimes a family history of infrequent voiding. Some of these children also have occasional episodes of incontinence due to overflow or urgency. The etiology of this disorder appears to be behavioral. When the children have urinary tract infections, the treatment is by antibacterial prophylaxis, and encouragement of frequent voiding and of complete emptying of the bladder by double voiding until a normal pattern of micturition is re-established.

Other Causes of Incontinence in Females

Table 18–15 lists other causes of urinary incontinence. *Ureteral ectopia*, usually associated with a duplicated collecting system in girls, can produce urinary incontinence characterized by constant dribbling of urine during day and night, in addition to a normal voiding pattern. Sometimes the urine production from the renal segment drained by the ectopic ureter is small and urinary drainage is confused with watery vaginal discharge. Children with a history of vaginal discharge or incontinence and an abnormal voiding pattern require careful study. The ectopic orifice is usually difficult to find. On intravenous urography, one may suspect duplication of the collecting system (Fig. 18–40), but the upper collecting system drained by the ectopic ureter usually has poor or very delayed function. Ultrasound and CT scan of the kidneys help rule out subtle duplication that may not be discovered on intravenous urography. Examination under anesthesia for an ectopic ureteral orifice in the vestibule or the vagina is often

TABLE 18–15. Urinary Incontinence in Childhood

With Complete Bladder Emptying	
Ectopic ureter and fistulas	
Sphincter failure (with total or partial incontinence)	Neurogenic Traumatic Iatrogenic
Urgency Incontinence	
Detrusor hyperactivity is caused by inflammation, neurogenic dysfunction, or detrusor instability secondary to functional or mechanical obstruction	Cystitis Unstable bladder Neurogenic bladder Hyperreflexia Bladder outlet obstruction Noncompliant bladder, neurogenic or non-neurogenic Detrusor sphincter dyssynergia, neurogenic or non-neurogenic
With Incomplete Bladder Emptying	
Overflow incontinence (incomplete bladder emptying may be due to decompensated obstruction or paralysis of the detrusor muscle)	Bladder outlet obstruction (e.g., posterior urethral valves) Neurogenic detrusor areflexia Detrusor sphincter dyssynergia, neurogenic or non-neurogenic Behavioral
Other	
Combination of above	Multiple factors

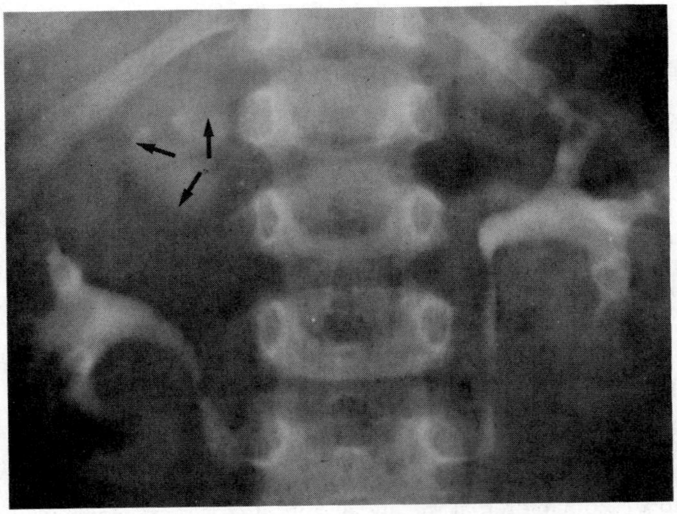

Figure 18–40. Duplication of the right collecting system with ectopic ureter. Excretory urogram in a female presenting with a normal voiding pattern and constant urinary dribbling. The left kidney is normal and the right side, well visualized, is the lower collecting system of a duplicated kidney. On the upper pole opposite the 1st and 2nd vertebral bodies, note the accumulation of contrast material corresponding with a poorly functioning upper pole drained by a ureter opening in the vestibule.

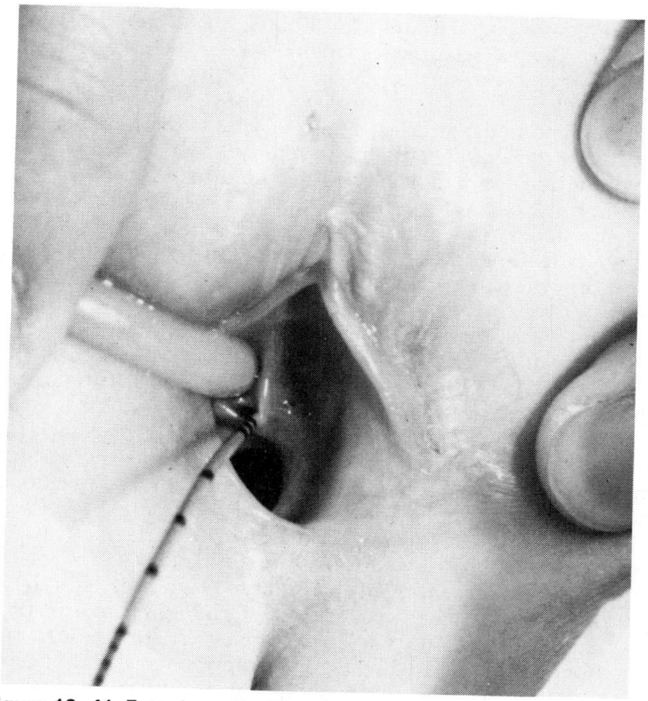

Figure 18–41. Ectopic ureter. The photograph shows an ectopic ureter entering the vestibule next to the urethral meatus. The thin ureteral catheter with transverse marks has been introduced into this ectopic ureter. This girl had a normal voiding pattern and constant urinary dribbling.

necessary (Fig. 18–41). The treatment in these cases is by partial nephroureterectomy, removing the involved segment of the duplicated kidney and the ureter down to the pelvic brim. A short, incompetent urethra may be associated with certain urogenital sinus malformations. The diagnosis of these malformations requires a high index of suspicion and a careful physical examination of all incontinent girls. In these cases, urethral and vaginal reconstruction can often restore continence.

18.45 OTHER DISEASES AND ANOMALIES OF THE PENIS AND URETHRA

HYPOSPADIAS. Hypospadias occurs in approximately 1 of 500 newborns. In the mildest cases the urethral meatus opens on the ventral aspect of the glans, there are various degrees of malformation of the glans, and the prepuce is defective ventrally with the appearance of a dorsal hood. With increasing degrees of severity the penis is curved ventrally (chordee) and the penile urethra is progressively shorter (Fig. 18–42), but the distance between the meatus and the glans may not increase significantly until the chordee is corrected. It is misleading, therefore, to classify hypospadias solely on the basis of the location of the meatus. In some cases, the meatus is at the penoscrotal junction; in extreme cases, the urethra opens in the perineum, the scrotum is bifid and sometimes extends to the dorsal base of the penis (scrotal transposition), and the chordee is extreme (Fig. 18–43). In such cases, there is usually a urethral diverticulum opening at the level of the verumontanum, representing a vestige of müllerian structures. In variant cases ventral curvature of the penis occurs without a hypospadiac urethral meatus. In these cases, the prepuce is usually hooded and the corpus spongiosum may be underdeveloped.

Testes are undescended in 10% of boys with hypospadias. Inguinal hernias are also common. In the newborn period the differential diagnosis of severe penoscrotal and perineal hypospadias with undescended testes should include other forms of ambiguous genitalia, particularly masculinization of females (congenital adrenal hyperplasia). A karyotype should be obtained in all patients with hypospadias and cryptorchidism (see Sec. 19.37). The incidence of other anomalies of the genitourinary tract in boys with hypospadias is low, and with the probable exception of the more severe cases of perineal hypospadias, radiographic studies of the urinary tract are not justified.

The treatment of hypospadias starts in the newborn period. Routine circumcisions should be avoided, as the foreskin is often essential for repair later in life. Mild cases of hypospadias are usually repaired for cosmetic reasons alone, but with increasing severity, repair becomes essential in order to allow the child to void standing, to allow future normal sexual function, and to avoid psychologic consequences of having malformed external genitalia. The ideal age for repair is somewhat controversial; the current trend is to operate before the age of 18 mo. Most of these anomalies can now be repaired in a single operation with minimal hospitalization; accordingly, emotional trauma is less likely or severe now than with the older techniques. We prefer to do these repairs before the child is toilet trained and, if possible, during the 1st yr of life. Repair of hypospadias is a technically demanding operation and should be performed by surgeons with extensive experience.

AGENESIS AND MICROPENIS. *Agenesis* of the penis is rare and usually associated with anorectal and renal anomalies. If the child is likely to survive the associated anomalies, rearing as a female is recommended, with later genital reconstruction.

The length of the normal newborn penis is 3.5 ± 0.7 cm. *Micropenis* results from primary or secondary testicular failure during fetal life after morphogenesis is complete. Secondary congenital testicular failure is seen in anencephaly, pituitary agenesis, and Kallmann, Noonan, Prader-Willi, and other syndromes. Other cases may be due to the presence of rudimentary testes, dwarfism, or maternal hormone administrations. Treatment options include a trial of hormonal stimulation, or rearing as female, with later genital reconstruc-

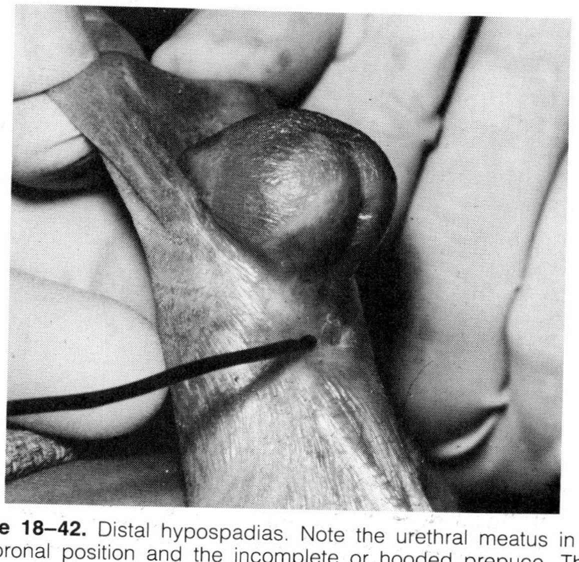

Figure 18–42. Distal hypospadias. Note the urethral meatus in the subcoronal position and the incomplete or hooded prepuce. There was no ventral curvature of the penis in this case.

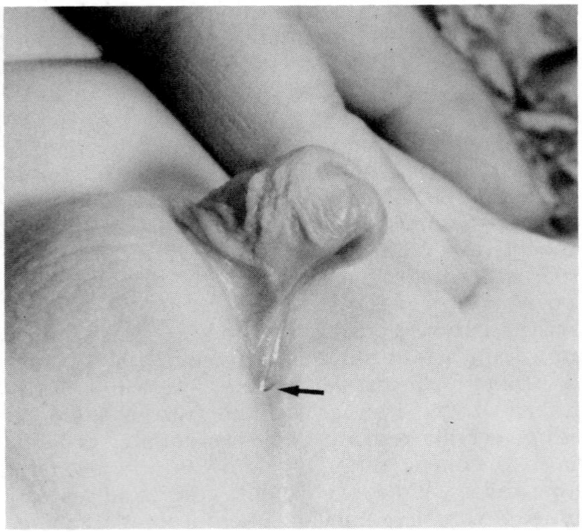

Figure 18–43. Severe perineoscrotal hypospadias. Note the ventral curvature and the underdeveloped ventral surface of the penis, the hooded prepuce, and the urethral meatus in the midline of the bifid scrotum. This child had palpable gonads and a normal chromosome pattern.

tion. Adjustment to the male gender role and sexual satisfaction is possible in some of these patients.

PHIMOSIS AND PARAPHIMOSIS. In 90% of uncircumcised males the prepuce becomes retractable by the age of 3 yr. Inability to retract the prepuce before this age is therefore not pathologic and not an indication for circumcision. *Phimosis* is the inability to retract the prepuce at an age when it should normally be retractable. Phimosis can be congenital or a sequel of inflammation. True phimosis usually requires surgical enlargement of the phimotic ring or circumcision. Accumulation of smegma under the infantile prepuce is not pathologic and does not require surgical treatment.

Paraphimosis occurs when a phimotic prepuce is retracted behind the coronal sulcus and this retraction cannot be reduced. This causes venous stasis distal to the corona, with edema leading to severe pain and inability to reduce the foreskin. If discovered early, the condition can be treated by reduction of the foreskin with appropriate lubrication, while the child is under heavy sedation or a short-acting general anesthetic. In some cases, circumcision is required.

CIRCUMCISION. In the United States, circumcision is usually performed for cultural reasons, or because it prevents phimosis, paraphimosis, and balanoposthitis, and decreases the incidence of cancer of the penis. A relationship between circumcision and a lower incidence of urinary tract infections in infancy has been established. Routine neonatal circumcision carries a very small but real risk of potentially serious complications, including sepsis, amputation of the distal part of the glans, removal of an excessive amount of foreskin, and the occurrence of urethrocutaneous fistulas.

URETHRAL PROLAPSE. Urethral prolapse is encountered predominantly in black females who exhibit vulvar bleeding (Fig. 18–44). Surgical excision and reapproximation of the mucosal edges is curative.

18.46 DISORDERS AND ANOMALIES OF THE SCROTAL CONTENTS

UNDESCENDED TESTES

UNDESCENDED AND ECTOPIC TESTES. Failure to find one or both testes in the scrotum may indicate any of a variety of congenital or acquired conditions, including true undescended testes, ectopic or maldescended testes, retractile testes, and absent testes.

True undescended testes and *maldescended or ectopic* testes can be differentiated from each other only by surgical exploration, and both conditions usually are referred to as cryptorchidism or hidden testes. The true undescended testis is found along the normal path of descent, and the processus vaginalis is usually patent. The ectopic testis has completed its descent through the inguinal canal but ends up in a subcutaneous location other than the scrotum, the most common being a point lateral to the external inguinal ring, below the subcutaneous fascia. Cryptorchidism is present in 0.7% of children after 1 yr of age and in adults. The incidence is high in full-term newborns (3.4%) and increases with prematurity (to 17% in infants with birthweights between 2,000 and 2,500 g and to 100% in those under 900 g). This reflects the fact that testicular descent from the inguinal canal into the scrotum takes place in the 7th mo of gestation. Spontaneous testicular descent does not occur after the age of 1 yr.

The consequences of cryptorchidism include infertility in adulthood, tumor development in the undescended testes, associated hernias, torsion of the cryptorchid testis, and the possible psychologic effects of an empty scrotum. Cryptorchidism is bilateral in up to 30% of cases. Infertility is the rule in adults with untreated bilateral cryptorchidism, and of those treated in childhood less than one third will be fertile. With unilateral undescended testis, the rate of infertility is similar to that in the general population.

The undescended testis is often histologically normal at birth, but *failure of development and atrophy* are detectable by the end of the 1st yr of life, and by the end of the 2nd yr the number of germ cells in the affected testis is severely reduced. Surgical correction at an early age results in a greater probability of fertility in adulthood. The patient with cryptorchidism has a 20–44% increase in risk of developing a *malignant testicular tumor* in the 3rd or 4th decade of life. Patients with untreated intra-abdominal cryptorchidism or those who underwent surgical correction during or after puberty are at greatest risk. Although surgical correction of the cryptorchidism does not change the overall risk of malignant transformation, very few cases of tumors have been reported in patients whose operations were performed before 8 yr of age. Carcinoma in situ is occasionally discovered when the testis

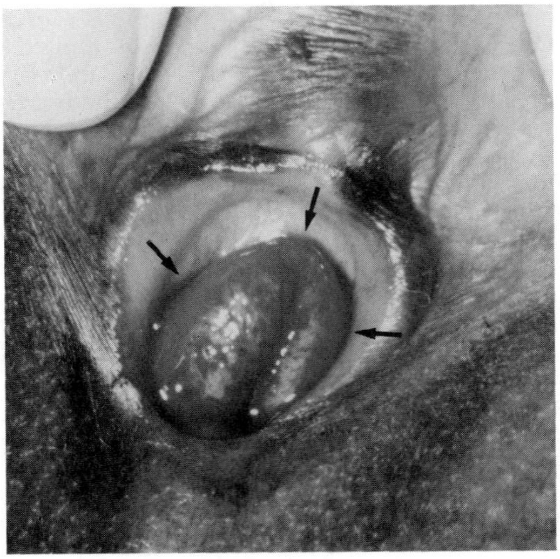

Figure 18–44. Urethral prolapse in a 4-yr-old black girl who had blood spotting on her underwear.

is biopsied at the time of orchiopexy or during evaluation for infertility later in life; its significance is unclear. The most common tumor developing in undescended testes is the seminoma (60%); in contrast, seminomas represent only 30% of tumors occurring in normally descended testes.

Indirect inguinal hernias always accompany true undescended testes and are common with ectopic testes. *Torsion and infarction* of the undescended testis can occur because of excessive mobility of such testes. The treatment of the unilateral cryptorchid testis is best undertaken early in the 2nd yr of life. Most testes located extra-abdominally can be brought down to the scrotum and the associated hernia corrected with an operation **(orchiopexy)**. This can often be performed without hospitalization. When the testis is not palpable, ultrasonography is used to determine its location. In the majority of cases, orchiopexy of the intra-abdominal testis located immediately inside the internal inguinal ring offers little difficulty, but orchiectomy should be considered in the more difficult cases or when the testis appears to be severely atrophied. Testicular prostheses are available for older children and adolescents when the absence of the gonad in the scrotum may have an undesirable psychologic effect.

Treatment of bilateral undescended testes is identical to the treatment of unilateral undescended testis when the testes are palpable. When testes are not palpable, however, differential diagnosis must be made from absent testes by measuring serum testosterone levels before and after stimulation with human chorionic gonadotropin (hCG). If the testosterone level rises, an abdominal exploration and orchiopexy should be undertaken. A negative response does not rule out the possible existence of intra-abdominal testicular tissue. An attempt is made to preserve these gonads for hormonal production after puberty; the likelihood of preserving fertility is very low.

Hormonal treatment with hCG or luteinizing hormone releasing hormone (LH-RH) has not replaced surgical treatment of cryptorchidism. Most agree that hormonal stimulation, which induces an early pseudopuberty, succeeds only in bringing down retractile testes (see later). Some believe that preoperative treatment with hCG facilitates surgery.

RETRACTILE TESTES. These testes retract into the inguinal canal in response to an exaggerated cremasteric reflex. The cremasteric reflex is weak or absent at birth. Consequently, when testes that were palpable at birth become nonpalpable later, retractile testes should be suspected. Retractile testes can be brought down by careful palpation when the child is relaxed in a warm room, and scrotal examination is facilitated if the child is in a squatting position. Often more than one examination is required to establish the diagnosis. The retractile testis usually adopts a permanent scrotal position during puberty and has none of the complications commonly associated with the true undescended or ectopic testis.

ABSENT TESTES. Approximately 20% of nonpalpable testes are absent. Congenital absence of the testis is possible, but it is quite rare and may be associated with some degree of feminization of the internal organs on the ipsilateral side. More commonly, the fetal testis disappears some time after the differentiation of the internal and external genitalia has occurred. This vanishing of the testis is usually attributed to a vascular accident that has taken place prenatally or after birth but was not recognized clinically. At exploration, the spermatic vessels and the vas deferens end blindly, usually somewhere in the inguinal region or in the scrotum. Because this condition is analogous to testicular torsion, some authors advocate fixation of the contralateral testis to prevent torsion from occurring in the remaining gonad. In these cases, placement of a testicular prosthesis can be considered as well.

TORSION OF THE TESTIS OR APPENDICES

Testicular torsion requires prompt diagnosis and treatment if the gonad is to survive. Testicular torsion accounts for approximately 40% of all cases of acute scrotal pain and swelling and for the majority of such cases in patients less than 6 yr old. It is caused by an abnormal fixation of the testis to the scrotal envelope. Under normal conditions, the testis is partially covered on its anterior portion by the tunica vaginalis, a serosal membrane derived from the processus vaginalis of the peritoneum. When the tunica vaginalis covers not only the testis but also the epididymis and the distal part of the spermatic cord, the testis is allowed to rotate freely within this serosal space and torsion can occur (bell clapper deformity). This abnormality of the tunica vaginalis is often bilateral.

Testicular torsion produces acute pain and swelling of the scrotum. On examination, the scrotum is swollen, very tender, and often difficult to examine. The cremasteric reflex is absent. The condition can be differentiated from an incarcerated hernia because swelling in the inguinal area is often absent. The differential diagnosis includes torsion of one of the testicular or epididymal appendices (embryologic vestiges), which usually causes less swelling and pain; occasionally a blue dot is observed above the testis and there is localized tenderness in this area. Often, however, differentiation can be made only at the time of surgical exploration. Torsion of the appendices is more common between the ages of 7 and 12 yr.

In children over 13 yr old, the differential diagnosis should include *epididymitis.* In epididymitis, the urinalysis is often abnormal, and there may be an antecedent history of sexual activity or urinary tract infection. Epididymitis is the most common cause of acute scrotal pain and swelling in patients over 18 yr of age. Nevertheless, in the prepubertal or adolescent boy with acute painful and swollen testes, testicular torsion should be considered present until proven otherwise. The accuracy of ultrasonography, Doppler examination, and isotopic scans in differentiating testicular torsion from other conditions is uncertain, and these diagnostic measures often delay unnecessarily a surgical procedure that can salvage the gonad.

The optimal treatment is prompt surgical exploration. If the testis is explored within 6 hr of torsion, up to 90% of the gonads will survive after detorsion and fixation to the scrotum. Survival decreases rapidly with a delay of more than 6 hr, and such cases usually require orchiectomy. It is probably unwise not to remove a necrotic testis if torsion is confirmed. The contralateral testis should be fixed to the scrotum to prevent future torsion. If torsion of the appendices or epididymis is found, surgical removal of the necrotic appendix will result in cure.

In cases of *neonatal torsion* the mechanism for torsion appears to be different, in that abnormal fixation of the testis to the scrotum is not necessarily present. These torsions are usually extravaginal, as the entire testis and tunica vaginalis rotate within the lax subcutaneous tissue of the scrotum. This type of torsion can occur in utero or be present at birth. Salvage of testes with neonatal torsion is extremely rare. Many authors recommend exploration to remove the necrotic testis and to fix the contralateral side, since there have been some reports of later torsion involving the remaining testis.

VARICOCELE

Dilatation of the pampiniform venous plexus results from valvular incompetence of the spermatic vein. Varicoceles occur predominantly on the left side, are bilateral in 10% of cases, and rarely involve the right side only. Rarely seen before the age of 10 yr, varicoceles are present in 15% of adult males. In some cases, varicoceles cause male subfertility with decreased sperm concentration or motility. Varicoceles are also associated with decrease in size of and characteristic testicular histologic changes in the involved testis.

A large varicocele can be painful, particularly during strenuous physical activity. In the standing position, venous varicosities can be palpated along the spermatic cord. This venous distention increases with the Valsalva maneuver and collapses with recumbency. A fixed varicocele is suggestive of a retroperitoneal tumor. Surgical treatment by ligation of the internal spermatic vein is sometimes required in adolescents to relieve pain or, when there is disparity in testicular size, to allow normal development of the testis. The effect of early surgical correction of varicoceles on future fertility is unknown. Improved testicular growth has been reported after surgery for varicocele in adolescents.

HYDROCELE

Hydrocele is an accumulation of fluid in the tunica vaginalis. When the amount of fluid varies with time, there is communication with the peritoneal cavity. Small hydroceles can disappear by the age of 1 yr, but larger ones often persist and require surgical treatment. Communicating hydroceles should be treated as indirect inguinal hernias.

EPIDIDYMITIS

Acute inflammation of the epididymis presents acute scrotal pain and swelling; it is rare before puberty and should raise the question of a congenital abnormality of the wolffian duct, such as an ectopic ureter entering the vas. After puberty, epididymitis becomes progressively more common and is the principal cause of acute painful scrotal swelling in young adults. Urinalysis usually reveals pyuria. Epididymitis can be bacterial (gonococcus, chlamydia), but often the organism remains undetermined. Treatment is by bed rest and antibiotics. Differentiation from torsion can be very difficult, and in children surgical exploration is usually required.

18.47 TRAUMA TO THE GENITOURINARY TRACT

Accidental injuries to the genitourinary tract in children are usually the result of blunt trauma from falls, athletic activities, or motor vehicle accidents. In childhood, genitourinary trauma is exceeded in frequency only by trauma to the skeleton and the central nervous system. In more than half of the cases there are also major injuries to the brain, spinal cord, skeleton, lungs, or other intraperitoneal organs. In cases of isolated renal injury, particularly following minor trauma, a pre-existent anomaly such as a horseshoe kidney, renal ectopia, hydronephrosis, or tumor should be suspected. Hematuria, bleeding through the urethral meatus, a flank mass, fractured lower ribs or lumbar transverse processes, or a perineal or scrotal hematoma suggests a major injury to the genitourinary tract in a child with trauma. In lesions involving the renal pedicle, hematuria is often absent.

Evaluation of the patient starts as soon as an adequate airway has been established and the patient is hemodynamically stable. The bladder should be catheterized in all cases except when there is bleeding from the urethral meatus, an indication of potential urethral injury. Straddling injuries are usually associated with trauma to the bulbous urethra. Rupture of the membranous urethra occurs in 3% of cases of pelvic fractures. Passing the catheter in the presence of a urethral injury may increase the extent of the damage and convert a partial tear to a total disruption. Instead, a retrograde urethrogram should be performed by injecting a radiopaque medium into the urethral meatus. Oblique radiographs will demonstrate the extent of the injury and whether urethral continuity is preserved or has been disrupted. Treatment is by suprapubic cystostomy drainage until the hematoma is reabsorbed, followed by urethroplasty when necessary to correct a resulting stricture. Erectile impotence, urethral stricture, and urinary incontinence are the major complications of rupture of the membranous urethra.

When the bladder can be catheterized, cystography is performed by infusing radiopaque medium through the catheter by gravity. If possible, flat and oblique views are obtained; a roentgenogram is also obtained after the bladder is drained. Bladder ruptures can be intraperitoneal or extraperitoneal. All intraperitoneal ruptures require surgical repair. Minor extraperitoneal near-ruptures might be treated by catheter drainage but generally require surgical treatment as well.

Intravenous urography is next done, to evaluate the kidneys. Complete absence of function of the one kidney without contralateral compensatory hypertrophy (indicative of congenital absence) should be regarded as an indication of major injury to the renal pedicle. Renal angiography should be done immediately before surgical exploration.

Renal injuries are usually classified as minor and major. *Minor renal injuries* include contusion of the renal parenchyma and shallow cortical lacerations not involving the collecting system. The majority of renal injuries fall into this category and can be treated nonoperatively with bed rest and supportive measures. *Major renal injuries* include deep lacerations involving the collecting system, the shattered kidney, and renal pedicle injuries. After the bladder is evaluated by cystography, intravenous pyelography is obtained; in some cases, this can be done intraoperatively when immediate surgical exploration is required for related life-threatening conditions. The observation of prompt function of both kidneys without extravasation usually excludes major renal injury. When findings on intravenous urography are not diagnostic, however, CT scanning is the ideal method for evaluating these lesions and has largely replaced angiography. CT scanning better defines the extent of injury and also allows evaluation of other intra-abdominal organs.

Major renal injuries may require surgical treatment either during the course of an exploration for other intra-abdominal injuries or as management of the renal injury per se to control bleeding or significant urinary extravasation. Besides loss of renal parenchyma, the main long-term complication of renal injury is arterial hypertension. Children who sustain renal injuries should have periodic measurement of the blood pressure for approximately 1 yr following injury. All penetrating injuries of the kidneys should be surgically explored.

Ureteral injuries are usually iatrogenic. Injuries of the ureter by blunt or penetrating trauma require immediate surgical attention.

Testicular injuries are relatively uncommon in children because of the small size of the testes and their great mobility. Such injuries usually result from athletic activities. Prompt surgical treatment of testicular injuries increases the testicular salvage rate.

18.48 URINARY LITHIASIS

Urinary lithiasis in children is very common in some parts of the world but rare in the United States. The wide geographic variations in the incidence of lithiasis in childhood appear related to climatic, dietary, and socioeconomic factors. These

TABLE 18–16. Laboratory Tests Suggested to Evaluate Urolithiasis

Serum
- Calcium
- Phosphorus
- Uric acid
- Electrolytes and acid-base balance
- Creatinine
- Alkaline phosphatase

Urine
- Urinalysis
- Urine culture
- Urinary pH
- Calcium/creatinine ratio
- Spot test for cystinuria
- 24-hr collection for:
  - creatinine clearance
  - calcium
  - phosphorus
  - oxalate
  - uric acid
  - dibasic amino acids (if cystine spot test is positive)

factors also influence the location of the calculi; primary bladder stones are common in developing countries, whereas upper tract stones predominate in the United States (except in children with pre-existing bladder diseases, such as neurologic dysfunction, obstruction, or previous surgical procedures).

Children with urolithiasis almost always have either gross or microscopic hematuria. In order of frequency, abdominal pain, flank or back pain, and symptoms of urinary tract infection follow. When the diagnosis of urolithiasis is suspected, a plain roentgenogram of the abdomen will detect radiopaque stones, mainly those containing calcium. Cystine stones and infectious stones (composed of struvite) may be faintly radiopaque. Radiolucent stones (uric acid, 2,8-dihydroxyadenine and xanthine calculi) can be detected by abdominal ultrasonography or as filling defects found in the upper collecting system or bladder on intravenous urography or on CT scanning of the abdomen. When lithiasis is diagnosed, a complete functional and radiographic evaluation of the urinary tract is made, to rule out stasis, obstruction, or infection as predisposing factors. One fourth of children with urinary calculi have vesicoureteral reflux. The best insight into the etiology of lithiasis in a particular patient is the complete chemical and crystallographic analysis of the stone (as obtained by spontaneous passage, or surgical or endoscopic extraction).

A metabolic evaluation for the most common predisposing factors should be undertaken as well, keeping in mind that structural, infectious, and metabolic factors often coexist. The basic laboratory studies required are listed in Table 18–16.

The causes of urolithiasis are multiple, and a complete listing is given in Table 18–17. Some of the more frequently encountered types of calculi are discussed here.

CALCIUM STONES. The most common urinary calculi in children in the United States are made of calcium oxalate. Cases in which no metabolic explanation for the stone formation is found are referred to as *idiopathic urolithiasis*. Hypercalciuria often leads to the formation of calcium oxalate stones and may be associated with hypercalcemia (due to hyperparathyroidism, sarcoidosis, immobilization, hypervitaminosis D, or idiopathic causes, and so on) but more often is an isolated phenomenon. Normocalcemic hypercalciuria may result from administration of furosemide (which often leads to stone formation in neonates), or from uncontrolled distal renal tubular acidosis, total parenteral alimentation, or alkalosis. In most cases, however, hypercalciuria leading to stone disease is idiopathic and may result from a renal tubular calcium "leak" which causes usually mild, secondary compensatory hyperparathyroidism and intestinal hyperabsorption of calcium. Another type of isolated hypercalciuria is related to *primary intestinal hyperabsorption* of calcium, which increases the filtered load of calcium and causes parathyroid inhibition.

The precise cause of these disorders remains unclear. Children with hypercalciuria sometimes have recurrent episodes of gross hematuria and flank pain years before the 1st stone is detected; accordingly, the work-up of children with recurrent gross hematuria should include the measurement of urinary calcium. Upper limits of normal are 4 mg/kg/24 hr or a urinary calcium/creatinine ratio greater than 0.25. A detailed metabolic work-up to differentiate the various types of hypercalciuria has been described by Pak. Despite careful evaluation, there remains a group of children who are stone-formers, in whom neither metabolic nor anatomic abnormalities can be detected. Calculi of calcium oxalate can also occur in children in whom small bowel disease and malabsorption lead to excessive reabsorption of oxalate in the colon (intestinal hyperoxaluria). Renal stone formation and nephrocalcinosis in primary hyperoxaluria (type 1 or 2) usually begins before the age of 4–5 yr and often runs a progressive course leading to renal failure.

TABLE 18–17. Classification of Urolithiasis*

Renal Tubular Syndromes
- Renal tubular acidosis
  - Distal defect, type I
- Carbonic anhydrase inhibitors
- Cystinuria
- Glycinuria

Enzyme Disorders
- Primary hyperoxaluria
  - Type I, glycolic aciduria
  - Type II, L-glyceric aciduria
- Xanthinuria
- Metabolic (enzymatic) hyperuricosuria
- 2,8-Dihydroxyadeninuria

Hypercalcemic States
- Primary hyperparathyroidism
- Sarcoidosis
- Hypervitaminosis D
- Milk-alkali syndrome
- Neoplasms
- Cushing syndrome
- Hyperthyroidism
- Idiopathic infantile hypercalcemia
- Immobilization

Uric Acid Lithiasis and Related Disorders
- Hereditary metabolic hyperuricosuria
- Hereditary renal hypouricemia
- 2,8-Dihydroxyadeninuria
- Myeloproliferative disorders
- Low urine output states

Nephrolithiasis and Intestinal Disease
- Acquired hyperoxaluria
- Uric acid lithiasis

Idiopathic Renal Lithiasis

Infected Urolithiasis and Urinary Stasis

Endemic Calculi

Nephrocalcinosis

*Modified from Malek RS: Urolithiasis. *In*: Kelalis PP, King LR, Belman AB (eds): Clinical Pediatric Urology. Philadelphia, WB Saunders, 1985.

CYSTINURIA. This inborn error of transport of the dibasic amino acids (cystine, ornithine, arginine, and lysine) results in excessive urinary excretion of these products. The only known complication of this familial disease is the formation of calculi, owing to the low solubility of cystine. The sulfur content of cystine gives these stones their faint radiopaque appearance.

STRUVITE STONES. Urinary tract infections caused by urea-splitting organisms (e.g., *Proteus* and occasionally *Klebsiella, E. coli, Pseudomonas,* and others) result in urinary alkalinization and excessive production of ammonia, which can lead to the precipitation of magnesium ammonium phosphate (struvite) and calcium phosphate. The stones act as foreign bodies, causing obstruction and perpetuating infection. Patients with struvite stones may also have metabolic abnormalities that predispose to stone formation.

URIC ACID STONES. Calculi containing uric acid represent less than 5% of all cases of lithiasis in children in this country but are more common in less developed areas of the world. Hyperuricosuria with or without hyperuricemia is the common underlying factor in most cases. The stones are radiolucent. The diagnosis should be suspected when there is a persistently acid urine and urate crystalluria. Hyperuricosuria may result from various inborn errors of purine metabolism that lead to overproduction of uric acid, the end product of purine metabolism in humans. Children with the Lesch-Nyhan syndrome and patients with glucose-6-phosphatase deficiency (G-6-PD) form urate calculi as well. In children with short bowel syndrome, and particularly in those with ileostomies, chronic dehydration and acidosis are sometimes complicated by uric acid lithiasis. One of the most common causes of uric acid lithiasis is the rapid turnover of purine with some tumors and myeloproliferative diseases. The risk of uric acid lithiasis is especially great when treatment of these diseases causes rapid breakdown of nucleoproteins. Uric acid calculi or "slush" can fill the entire upper collecting system and cause renal failure and even anuria. In addition, urates also are present within calcium-containing stones. In these cases more than one predisposing factor for stone formation may exist. A related disorder only recently recognized is *2,8-dihydroxyadenine lithiasis*, which results from a deficiency in adenine phosphoribosyltransferase. The stones are radiolucent and can be differentiated from uric acid calculi by mass spectrometry but not by routine chemical analysis. In contrast to uric acid, which is very soluble in alkaline urine, the solubility of 2,8-dihydroxyadenine changes little within physiologic pH ranges.

TREATMENT. The treatment of urinary lithiasis is approached from two perspectives. One aspect is the treatment of the underlying metabolic disorder, infections, or predisposing anatomic factors; the other is the treatment of complications associated with the stone itself, principally obstruction and infection. The simplest and most effective measure to prevent recurrence in all forms of lithiasis is to maintain an adequate state of hydration and diuresis 24 hr a day, in order to keep the urine dilute and to diminish the likelihood of precipitation of stone ingredients.

Alterations of the urine pH can also prevent recurrence of calculi. Cystine is much more soluble when the urinary pH is over 7.5, and alkalinization of urine with sodium bicarbonate or sodium citrate is effective. Recurrence of uric acid lithiasis may likewise be prevented by keeping the urinary pH above 7.5; indeed, hydration, urinary alkalinization, and measures directed at reducing uric acid excretion can cause dissolution of uric acid calculi. Acidification impairs the growth of struvite stones, but this cannot be achieved in practice so long as the stone or an infection by urea-splitting organisms is present.

Whenever possible, and if simple measures fail, specific therapy for any underlying metabolic disorder should be used. Thiazides appear to be effective in controlling primary renal hypercalciuria, but their effectiveness in the treatment of calcium oxalate stones caused by primary hypercalciuria remains debatable. Treatment of renal tubular acidosis controls recurrence of stone disease or nephrocalcinosis. Allopurinol is an inhibitor of xanthinoxidase and is effective in reducing the production both of uric acid and of 2,8-dihydroxyadenine, and can help control recurrence of both types of stones. Rarely, excessive urinary excretion of xanthine with stone formation has been reported during treatment with allopurinol. D-Penicillamine is a chelating agent that binds to cysteine or hemicystine, increasing the solubility of the product. Although poorly tolerated by many patients, it has been reported to be effective in dissolving cystine stones and in preventing recurrences when hydration and urinary alkalinization fail. *N*-acetylcysteine appears to have low toxicity and may be effective in controlling cystinuria, but long-term experience with it is lacking. Other specific therapies for lithiasis include the use of cellulose phosphate to bind calcium in the intestine in cases of primary absorptive hypercalciuria. Poor compliance with treatment and poor tolerance of the medication are significant drawbacks to its use. Pyridoxine has been used in some cases of hyperoxaluria. Salts of phosphate, citrate, magnesium, and other compounds directed at increasing the solubility of calcium oxalate and other stone ingredients in the urine are used in some centers, with varying success. Citrate is especially useful in the presence of hypocitraturia.

Surgical treatment of stone disease has been widespread in the past. Stones must be removed when they cause obstruction of the collecting system, pain, or bleeding, or if they are a factor in perpetuating infections. All struvite stones should be removed, because these carry a significant risk of renal parenchymal destruction and of renal or perirenal abscess formation. Newer modalities of stone removal, both endoscopically and by percutaneous access to the kidney, have been applied on a limited scale in children. The extracorporeal lithotriptor has made surgery for renal lithiasis unnecessary in most children.

RICARDO GONZALEZ

URINARY TRACT INFECTIONS

Burbige KA, Retik AB, Colodny AH, et al: Urinary tract infection in boys. J Urol 132:54, 1984.
Gillenwater YJ, Harrison RB, Kunin CM: Natural history of bacteriuria in school girls: A long term case control study. N Engl J Med 301:396, 1979.
Gonzalez R, Sheldon CA: Septic obstruction and uremia in the newborn. Urol Clin North Am 9:297, 1982.
Govan DE, Fair WR, Fredland GW: Management of children with UTI. Urology 6:275, 1975.
Kunin CM: Emergence of bacteriuria, proteinuria and symptomatic urinary tract infections among a population of school girls followed for 7 years. Pediatrics 41:968, 1968.
Mayrer AR, Miniter P, Andriole VT: Immunopathogenesis of chronic pyelonephritis. Am J Med 75:59, 1983.
Newcastle Asymptomatic Bacteriuria Research Group: Asymptomatic bacteriuria in school children in Newcastle upon Tyne. Arch Dis Child 50:90, 1975.
Sheldon CA, Gonzalez R: Differentiation of upper and lower urinary tract infections. How and when? Med Clin North Am 68:321, 1984.
Sinha B, Gonzalez R: Hyperammonemia in boys with obstructive ureterocele and Proteus infection. J Urol 131:1, 1984.
Stamey TA: Pathogenesis and Treatment of Urinary Tract Infections. Baltimore, Williams & Wilkins, 1980.
Wiswell TE, Roscelli JD: Corroborative evidence for the decreased incidence of urinary tract infections in circumcised male infants. Pediatrics 78:96, 1986.

VESICOURETERAL REFLUX

Bauer SB, Willscher MK, Ammuto PJ, et al: Longterm results of antireflux surgery in children. *In*: Hodson J, Kinkaid-Smith P (eds): Reflux Nephropathy. New York, Masson Publishing, 1979, chap 20.
Chantler C, Donckerwolcke RA, Brunner FP, et al: Combined report on regular

dialysis and transplantation in children in Europe, 1978. Proceedings of the European Dialysis and Transplant Association 16:76, 1979.
Edwards D, Normand ICS, Prescod N, et al: Disappearance of vesicoureteric reflux during longterm prophylaxis of urinary tract infection in children. Br Med J 2:285, 1977.
Jenkins GR, Noe N: Familial vesicoureteral reflux: A prospective study. J Urol 128:774, 1982.
Koff SA, Murtagh DS: Uninhibited bladder in children: Effect of treatment on recurrent urinary tract infection and on vesicoureteral reflux resolution. J Urol 130:1138, 1983.
Nasrallah PF, Nava S, Crawford J: Clinical application of nuclear cystography. J Urol 128:550, 1982.
Puri P, O'Donnell R: Endoscopic correction of grades IV and V primary vesicoureteral reflux: 6 to 30 months follow-up in 42 ureters. J Pediatr Surg 2:1087, 1987.
Rance CP, Arbus GS, Balfe JW, et al: Persistent systemic hypertension in infants and children. Pediatr Clin North Am 21:801, 1974.
Ransley PG: Intrarenal reflux: Anatomical, dynamic and radiological studies. Urol Res 5:61, 1977.
Report of the International Reflux Committee: Special article: Medical versus surgical treatment of primary vesicoureteral reflux. Pediatrics 67:392, 1981.

OBSTRUCTION

Churchill BM, Krueger RP, Fleischer MH, et al: Complications of posterior urethral valve surgery and their prevention. Urol Clin North Am 10:519, 1983.
Gonzalez R, Chiou RK: The diagnosis of upper urinary tract obstruction in children: Comparison of diuresis renography and pressure flow studies. J Urol 133:1, 1985.
Gonzalez R, Lapointe S, Sheldon CA, et al: Undiversion in children with chronic renal failure. J Pediatr Surg 19:632, 1984.
Harrison MR, Golbus MS, Filly RA: Congenital hydronephrosis. *In*: The Unborn Patient: Prenatal Diagnosis and Treatment. Orlando, FL, Grune & Stratton Inc., 1984, p 277.
Hendren WH: Posterior urethral valves in boys: A broad clinical spectrum. J Urol 106:298, 1971.
Homsy YL, Williot P, Danais S: Transitional neonatal hydronephrosis: Fact or fantasy? J Urol 136:339, 1986.
Immergut M, Notman GE: The urethral course of female children with recurrent urinary tract infection. J Urol 99:189, 1965.
Kaplan GW, Sammons TA, King LR: Blind comparison of dilatation urethrotomy and medication alone in the treatment of infection in girls. J Urol 109:917, 1973.
Keating MA, Escala J, Snyder HM, et al: Changing concepts in management of primary obstructive megaureter. J Urol 142:636, 1989.
Kelalis PP: Ureteropelvic junction. *In*: Kelalis PK, King LR, Belman AB (eds): Clinical Pediatric Urology. Philadelphia, WB Saunders, 1985, chap 16.
Kramer SA: Current status of fetal intervention for congenital hydronephrosis. J Urol 130:641, 1983.
Kroovand RL, Perlmutter AD: A one stage surgical approach to ectopic ureterocele. J Urol 122:367, 1979.
Lapointe S, Gonzalez R: Acute and chronic urinary tract obstruction: Pathophysiology, diagnosis and management. *In*: Mandel A (ed): Clinical Nephrology. Philadelphia, Lea & Febiger, 1988, p 380.
Lockhart JL, Singer AM, Glenn JF: Congenital megaureter. J Urol 122:310, 1979.
Manivel JC, Pettmato G, Reinberg Y, et al: Prune belly syndrome: Clinicopathological study of 28 cases. Pediatr Pathol 9:691, 1989.
Nguyen DH, Aliabadi H, Ercole CJ, et al: Nonintubated Anderson-Hines repair of ureteropelvic junction obstruction in 60 patients. J Urol 142:704, 1989.
Reinberg Y, Gonzalez R, Fryd D, et al: The outcome of renal transplantation in children with posterior urethral valves. J Urol 140:1491, 1988.
Sullivan M, Halpern L, Hodges CV: Extravesical ureteral ectopia. Urology 11:577, 1978.
Whitaker RH: Percutaneous upper urinary tract dynamics in equivocal obstruction. Urol Radiol 2:187, 1981.
Williams DI, Whitaker RH, Barratt TM, et al: Urethral valves. Br J Urol 45:200, 1973.
Woodhouse CRJ, Kellett JS, Williams DI: Minimal surgical interference in prune belly syndrome. Br J Urol 51:475, 1979.

OTHER DISEASES AND ANOMALIES OF THE BLADDER

Exstrophy

Arap S, Giron DM, Menezes de Goes G: Initial results of the complete reconstruction of bladder exstrophy. Urol Clin North Am 7:477, 1980.
Jeffs RD: Exstrophy and cloacal exstrophy. Urol Clin North Am 5:127, 1978.
Sheldon CA, McKinley R, Hartig P, et al: Carcinoma at the site of the ureterosigmoidostomy. J Dis Colon Rectum 26:55, 1983.

Bladder Diverticula

Johnston JH: Vesical diverticula without urinary obstruction in childhood. J Urol 84:535, 1960.

Urachal Anomalies

Bauer SB, Retik AB: Urachal and related umbilical disorders. Urol Clin North Am 5:195, 1978.

Neurogenic Bladder

Bauer SB: Urodynamic evaluation and neuromuscular dysfunction. *In*: Kelalis PK, King LR, Belman AB (eds): Clinical Pediatric Urology. Philadelphia, WB Saunders, 1985.
Gonzalez R, Aliabadi H: Sigmoid cystoplasty. *In*: King LR, Stone, AR, Webster GD (eds): Bladder Reconstruction and Continent Urinary Diversion. Chicago, Year Book Medical Publishers, 1991.
Gonzalez R, Nguyen D, Koleliat N, et al: The artificial sphincter AS800 in congenital urinary incontinence. J Urol 142:512, 1989.
Kaplan WE, Firlit CF: Management of reflux in myelodysplastic child. J Urol 129:1195, 1983.
Kass EJ, Koff SA, Biokno AC: Fate of vesicoureteral reflux in children with neuropathic bladders managed by intermittent catheterization. J Urol 125:63, 1981.
Lapides J, Diokno AC, Lowe BS: Follow-up on unsterile intermittent self catheterization. J Urol 111:184, 1974.
Reinberg Y, Shapiro E, Manivel JC, et al: Prune belly syndrome in females: A triad of abdominal wall musculature deficiency and anomalies of the urinary and genital systems. J Pediatr 118:395, 1991.
Sidi AA, Dykstra DD, Gonzalez R: The value of urodynamic testing in the management of neonates with myelodysplasia. A prospective study. J Urol 135:90, 1986.
Sidi AA, Peng W, Gonzalez R: Vesicoureteral reflux in children with myelodysplasia: Natural history and results of treatment. J Urol 136:329, 1986.

Enuresis and Voiding Dysfunction

Allen TD: The non-neurogenic neurogenic bladder. J Urol 117:232, 1977.
Bauer SB, Retik AB, Colodny AH, et al: The unstable bladder in childhood. Urol Clin North Am 7:321, 1980.
Fermandes E, Vernier R, Gonzalez R: Bladder instability in children. J Pediatr 118:399, 1991.
Mikkelsen EJ, Rappaport JL: Enuresis: Psychopathology, sleep stage and drug response. Urol Clin North Am 7:361, 1980.
Pedersen PS, Hejl M, Kjoller SS: Desamino-D-arginine vasopressin in childhood. Nocturnal enuresis. J Urol 133:65, 1985.
Perlmuter AD: Enuresis. *In*: Kelalis PP, King LR, Belman AB (eds): Clinical Pediatric Urology. Philadelphia, WB Saunders, 1985, p 311.

OTHER DISEASES AND ANOMALIES OF THE PENIS AND URETHRA

Hypospadias

American Academy of Pediatrics: Report of the task force on circumcision. Pediatrics 84:388, 1989.
Bauer SB, Retik AB, Colodny AH: Genetic aspects of hypospadias. Urol Clin North Am 8:559, 1981.
Johnston JH: Abnormalities of the penis. *In*: Williams DI, Johnston JH (eds): Paediatric Urology. London, Butterworth Scientific, 1982, p 435.
Kaplan GW: Complications of circumcision. Urol Clin North Am 10:543, 1983.
Reilly JM, Woodhouse CRJ: Small penis and the male sexual role. J Urol 142:569, 1989.
Rozenman J, Hertz M, Boichis H: Radiological findings of the urinary tract in hypospadias: A report of 770 cases. Clin Radiol 30:471, 1979.
Section on Urology, American Academy of Pediatrics: The timing of elective surgery on the genitalia of male children with particular reference to undescended testes and hypospadias. Pediatrics 56:479, 1975.
Wallerstein E: Circumcision: The uniquely American medical enigma. Urol Clin North Am 12:123, 1985.

DISEASES AND ANOMALIES OF THE SCROTAL CONTENTS

Bartsch G, Frank ST, Marberger H: Testicular torsion: Late results with special regard to fertility and endocrine function. J Urol 124:375, 1980.
Cendron M, Keating MH, Huff DS, et al: Cryptorchidism, orchiopexy and infertility: A critical long-term retrospective analysis. J Urol 142:559, 1989.
Farrington GH: The position and retractability of the normal testes in childhood with reference to the diagnosis and treatment of cryptorchidism. J Pediatr Surg 3:353, 1968.
Fonkalsrud EW, Menzel W (eds): The Undescended Testes. Chicago, Year Book Medical Publishers, 1981.
Gonzalez R: Outpatient orchidopexy in children. *In*: Kaye KW (ed): Outpatient Urologic Surgery. Philadelphia, Lea & Febiger, 1985.
Heinz HA, Voggenthaler J, Weissbach L: Histologic findings in testes with varicocele during childhood and their therapeutic consequences. Eur J Pediatr 133:139, 1980.
Martin DC: Malignancy on the cryptorchid testes. Urol Clin North Am 9:371, 1982.
Papadotos C, Moutsouris C: Bilateral testicular torsion in the newborn. J Pediatr Surg 71:249, 1967.

Sarer CG: The descent of the testes. Arch Dis Child 39:605, 1964.

TRAUMA

Brower P, Paul J, Brosman SA: Urinary tract abnormalities presenting as a result of shunt abdominal trauma. J Trauma 18:719, 1978.
Burrington JD: Childhood trauma. *In*: Holder TM, Ashcroft KLW (eds): Pediatric Surgery. Philadelphia, WB Saunders, 1980, p 149.
Cass AS: Blunt renal trauma in children. J Trauma 23:123, 1983.
Pinhas ML, Gonzales ET: Genitourinary trauma in children. Urol Clin North Am 12:53, 1985.

URINARY LITHIASIS

Churchill DN, Malone CM, Nolan MH, et al: Pediatric urolithiasis in the 1970s. J Urol 123:233, 1980.
Gearhart JP, Herzberg GZ, Jeffs RD: Childhood urolithiasis: Experiences and advances. Pediatrics 87:445, 1991.
Hulbert JC, Reddy PK, Gonzalez R, et al: Percutaneous nephrostolithotomy: An alternative approach to the management of pediatric calculous disease. Pediatrics 76:610, 1985.
Malek RS: Urolithiasis. *In*: Kelalis PP, King LR, Belman BA (eds): Clinical Pediatric Urology. Philadelphia, WB Saunders, 1985, p 1093.
Nijman RJM, Ackaer TK, Scholtneijer RJ, et al: Long-term results of extracorporeal shock wave lithotripsy in children. J Urol 142:609, 1989.
Noe HN, Stapleton FB, Roxy S III: Potential surgical implications of hematuria in children. J Urol 132:737, 1984.
Pak CYC: The spectrum and pathogenesis of hypercalciuria. Urol Clin North Am 8:245, 1981.
Sinno K, Boyce WH, Resnick MI: Childhood urolithiasis. J Urol 121:662, 1979.
Stapleton FB, Rog S, Noe HN, et al: Hypercalciuria in children with hematuria. N Engl J Med 310:1345, 1984.

18.49 GYNECOLOGIC PROBLEMS OF CHILDHOOD

18.50 HISTORY AND PHYSICAL EXAMINATION

The pediatric or adolescent patient undergoing her first gynecologic examination should be managed with particular care, as the initial encounter may well set the tone for all future gynecologic examinations. If the examination is painful or uncomfortable, or if there is a significant lack of rapport between the patient and the examiner, the child may suffer lasting psychologic consequences. A gentle, caring attitude by the physician will go far in helping the patient relax during all future gynecologic examinations.

The parent or guardian usually provides the medical history for the pediatric patient. However, the child should be encouraged to take part in the history-taking process, and specific time should be allotted for obtaining the medical history from the adolescent patient (see Sec. 6.1 and 10.22). The older child and adolescent should be assured that confidentiality will be maintained. Not uncommonly, the clinician must play the role of detective to ascertain why the patient is seeking consultation: for example, is sexual activity and desire for birth control disguised as a chief complaint of "vaginal discharge," or is she worried about being pregnant? When the general history is completed, the clinician should inquire, in a private conversation with a patient of appropriate age, whether the patient is sexually active and has a need for birth control information. Most adolescents are sexually active for 6 mo prior to requesting contraception. If the adolescent is not sexually active, it may be appropriate to discuss concepts such as "It's OK to say No" (to drugs and intercourse), as suggested by the American College of Obstetricians and Gynecologists and the American Academy of Pediatrics.

A questionnaire for identification of individual health care needs for which preventive counseling may be necessary has been suggested. Whether family members should be present during the gynecologic examination is a frequently asked question that has been addressed by Phillips et al; in a study of 1,358 patients, the presence of a family member was viewed as beneficial for the patient or the physician, or both, in 86% of the cases; the remaining 13% communicated no preference.

For all age groups, patients should be told what to expect during the pelvic examination. It is helpful to inquire of the adolescent patient whether tampons are used, offering the reassurance that the small Pederson speculum is no bigger than a tampon. Such reassurance will help establish a good rapport throughout the examination. A successful examination also depends on the availability of the proper equipment at the start: pediatric-sized vaginal specula, nasal specula, a good light source (gooseneck lamp or headlamp), and appropriate collection materials for culture and cytology. A bulb syringe with catheter may be helpful in obtaining a vaginal specimen for either culture or wetmount.

The most important principle to remember in conducting a pelvic examination is to allow the patient to be in control. Often, a well-meaning allied health professional will tell the patient what position she should be in, whether her buttocks are properly positioned, and so forth. A more appropriate and effective method is for the physician to conduct the examination while allowing the patient to be in charge of what she does with her body during it.

The most common positions for examination of the pediatric patient include the frog-legged position, knee-chest, and dorsal lithotomy. If the child is reluctant to be examined, it is sometimes helpful to have the mother lie on the examination table in the dorsal lithotomy position with the child on her abdomen, or have the parent sit in a chair with the child on his or her lap. Again, ideally the child should be "in command" of the examination, and the clinician should be aware of alternatives. For example, in the case of vulvovaginitis, the most common problem in the pediatric or adolescent gynecologic patient, visualization of only the lower third of the vagina may be all that is required for diagnosis.

Cavanaugh R: Obtaining a personal and confidential history from adolescents: An opportunity for prevention. J Adolesc Health Care 2:118, 1986.
Greydanus DE: Contraception. *In*: Sanfilippo JS, Lavery JP (eds): Pediatric and Adolescent Obstetrics and Gynecology. New York, Springer-Verlag, 1985, p 234.
Phillips S, Bohannon W, Heald F: Teenager's choices regarding the presence of family members during the examination of genitalia. J Adolesc Health Care 7:245, 1986.
Pokorny SF: Pediatric vulvovaginitis. *In* Kaufman R, Friedrich E, Gardner H (eds): Benign Diseases of the Vulva and Vagina. Chicago, Year Book Medical Publishers, 1989, p 55.
Talbot CW: The gynecologic examination of the pediatric patient. Pediatr Ann 15:501, 1986.

18.51 VULVOVAGINITIS

This is the most common childhood or adolescent gynecologic problem. Vulvovaginal irritation results from the lack of labial fat pads and pubic hair for protection of the external genitalia. The labia minora tend to open when the child squats; this in turn causes exposure of the more sensitive tissues within the hymenal ring. In addition, the close proximity of the anal orifice to the vagina allows transfer of fecal bacteria to the vulvovaginal area. Masturbation may also be a contributing factor.

The squamous epithelium of the vaginal mucosa is sensitive to steroid hormones. In the relatively low estrogenic environment, the thin atrophic epithelium becomes susceptible to bacterial invasion. Thus, recurrent vulvovaginitis usually ceases once a female child reaches puberty and the pH of the vagina becomes more acidic. In part, this is due to increased production of acetic and lactic acids, a phenomenon accompanied by an increase in superficial cell proliferation and glycogen as well as by enhancement of normal bacterial flora.

CLINICAL MANIFESTATIONS

PHYSIOLOGIC VAGINAL DISCHARGE. A normal physiologic increase in vaginal discharge occurs 6–12 mo prior to the onset of menarche. This discharge frequently presents as a yellow staining of the patient's underpants; there is no specific malodor, and the vulva is not inflamed. Microscopically, the discharge is composed of Döderlein's bacilli. The patient should simply be reassured that this is a normal occurrence.

PATHOLOGIC VAGINAL DISCHARGE. In the pediatric patient, vaginal discharge is a common presenting complaint. It is often the primary symptom of vulvitis, vaginitis, or vulvovaginitis. Pruritus, frequent urination, dysuria, or enuresis may be associated signs and symptoms. Vulvitis is manifested primarily by dysuria and pruritus, associated with erythema of the vulva. Vulvitis commonly has a more protracted course than vaginitis, which is characterized by discharge without associated dysuria, pruritus, or erythema of the vulva. Vulvovaginitis involves a combination of these manifestations. The color, odor, and duration of the discharge should be noted. Although there are a number of causes of vulvovaginitis in the pediatric patient, the more common ones include poor perineal hygiene, *Candida* infection, and foreign body.

NONSPECIFIC VULVOVAGINITIS. Patients with poor perineal hygiene often develop a condition known as nonspecific vulvovaginitis. The discharge is characteristically brown or green, has a fetid odor, and is associated with a vaginal pH of 4.7–6.5. In 68% of reported cases, this type of vaginitis is associated with coliform bacteria secondary to fecal contamination. The next most common bacterial organisms associated with nonspecific vulvovaginitis are β-hemolytic *Streptococcus* and coagulase positive *Staphylococcus*. These organisms are often transmitted manually from the nasopharynx. Clothing, chemicals, cosmetics, and soap products or detergents used for bathing or laundry may also cause irritation that leads to nonspecific vulvovaginitis. Tight-fitting clothing such as jeans or leotards and tights, as well as rubber pants or plastic coated paper diapers, have also been implicated.

Nonspecific vulvovaginitis occasionally can result in a state of "chronic infection," which may cause significant psychologic consequences for child and parent alike. The physician should stress the importance of avoiding "vaginal fixation," while encouraging proper perineal hygiene.

Successful treatment of nonspecific vulvovaginitis should include instruction in perineal hygiene, switching from tight fitting underwear, use of sitz baths with mild soap, and air drying the vulva. The patient should be instructed in appropriate bowel and bladder habits, emphasizing the necessity of wiping fecal material away from the vulvovaginal area. Recurrent vulvovaginitis should be treated with systemic antibiotics such as amoxicillin or cephalosporins. Topical estrogen cream or Polysporin ointment is often helpful.

SPECIFIC VULVOVAGINITIS. *Gardnerella vaginalis* is the most common organism cultured in the pediatric or adolescent patient with vulvovaginitis, followed by *Candida* and *Trichomonas*. Other identified organisms include enterococci and anaerobic bacteria such as *Peptococcus, Peptostreptococcus, Veillonella parvula, Eubacterium, Propionibacterium,* and *Bacteroides* species. Protozoa, helminths, and viruses should also be considered as etiologic agents. Vulvovaginal *Corynebacterium diphtheria* has been reported in a 7-yr-old female. Treatment will depend on the offending organism (Table 18–18).

MOLLUSCUM CONTAGIOSUM. This common infection of the skin is associated with the pox virus group. Molluscum contagiosum presents as an umbilicated, dome-shaped papule. The central umbilication usually is associated with a pulpy core. Vulvar lesions appear to result from autoinoculation or from close contact (sexual or nonsexual) with an infected individual. The incubation period is 2–7 wk. Diagnosis is confirmed by light microscopic visualization of viral inclusions (molluscum bodies) in the central core. Treatment requires elimination of the lesions, usually by application of silver nitrate after gentle curettage. Other methods of therapy include cryosurgery or electrocautery.

LICHEN SCLEROSUS. This is a chronic atrophic skin disease characterized by small, pink to ivory, flat topped papules that are several millimeters in diameter. The papules appear to coalesce into plaques that become wrinkled and atrophic. The anogenital lesions frequently resemble an hourglass or a "figure 8" (Fig. 18–45 [color plate section]). Vesicles and bullae may spread over the vulva with associated hemorrhage. A biopsy is often required for accurate diagnosis.

The onset of lichen sclerosus in most children usually occurs before 7 yr of age. The youngest reported patient was an infant only several weeks old. Onset of menarche often results in spontaneous improvement of the lesions, but the process usually continues. Patients are often "intermittently symptomatic," and there is no relationship between menarche and symptomatic improvement or resolution of the disease. Atrophy of the labia minora and clitoral phimosis as well as contracture of the introitus may occur.

The cause of lichen sclerosus is unknown, but it is believed to be related to an autoimmune disorder. Positive immunofluorescence for fibrin, serum complement (C'3), or immunoglobulin M (IgM) in involved areas has been demonstrated in 75% of patients.

Treatment is symptomatic: emollients and topical corticosteroids usually provide relief. Topical estrogens and androgens also have been used, but these agents may produce a vaginal discharge as well as other secondary problems such as breast development and clitoral enlargement. Secondary infection should be treated with antibiotics. Some affected individuals demonstrate what is known as the *Koebner phenomenon,* the precipitation of lesions secondary to trauma. For relief, these individuals should avoid tight clothing and genital trauma. Newer treatment modalities include laser vaporization to the level of the first surgical plane.

LICHEN PLANUS (see Sec. 23.16). Vulvar lichen planus is often associated with oral mucosal and subcutaneous lesions. The vulvar lesions are characterized by angular violaceous, flat-topped papules that may simulate leukoplakia. The oral lesion consists of minute white papules that form a lacy pattern, usually on the buccal mucosa. The lesions are intensely pruritic and may become excoriated and macerated; erosions and ulcerations may even occur in severe cases. Diagnosis requires biopsy. Exacerbation or recurrence of the lesions is common.

Treatment consists of topical intralesional corticosteroids and antihistamines to control pruritus. Squamous cell carcinoma may occur with longstanding, hypertrophic, vulvar lichen planus; therefore, long-term follow-up and the histologic examination of any changed or otherwise suspicious area is advisable.

TABLE 18–18. Specific Vulvovaginitis*

Organism	Presentation	Diagnosis	Treatment†
Calymmatobacterium granulomatis-Donovania (Granuloma inguinale)	Insidious onset mucosal lesions (oral, genital, perineal), painless ulcer with red friable base	Donovan bodies in intracytoplasmic cysts (Wright stain)	Tetracycline, 500 mg qid × 2 wk, *or* ampicillin, 500 mg qid × 2 wk
Cytomegalovirus	Jaundice, hepatosplenomegaly, purpura, thrombocytopenia, intrauterine infection	Positive cell culture or serologic tests	No specific treatment
Enterobiasis (Pinworms)	Perineal pruritus (nocturnal), variable GI symptoms, vulvovaginal contamination from feces	Adult worms in stool or eggs on perianal skin; Scotch tape test (perianal skin)	Pyrantel pamoate, 10 mg/kg orally; repeat in 2 and 4 wk
Entamoeba histolytica (Amebiasis)	Diarrhea, cramps, mucoid stools, vulvovaginal contamination from feces	Amebas in stool, serologic tests; Diloxanide furotate	Metronidazole, 750 mg tid × 10 day, *or* iodoquinol, 650 mg tid × 3 wk
Giardia lamblia (Giardiasis)	Asymptomatic fecal contaminant, vaginal discharge, diarrhea, malabsorption syndrome	Protozoal flagellate (cyst ortrophozoites) in feces	Metronidazole, 250 mg orally tid × 10 day, *or* tinazole, 2 g orally, *or* quinacrine, 100 mg orally tid × 1 wk
Hemophilus ducreyi (Chancroid)	Fever, chills, malaise, vesicle, pustule, painful soft ulcer with surrounding erythema, inguinal adenitis	Gram-negative bacillus on chocolate agar with 1% Isovitalex and Vancomycin or positive skin test	Tetracycline, 500 mg orally qid × 10 day, *or* erythromycin, 500 mg orally qid × 10 day, *or* trimethoprim-sulfamethoxazole, 2 Tab q 12 hr
Herpes genitalis (Type II)	Fever, malaise, anorexia, localized pain—paresthesias, leukorrhea, dysuria, vaginal bleeding, multiple shallow ulcerated vesicles with erythematous papules, painful inguinal adenopathy	Smear of lesions, multinucleated giant cells with inclusion bodies	5% Acyclovir ointment q 4 hr × 24 hr *and/or* acyclovir—oral or intravenous, dosage individualized
Lymphogranuloma venereum	Fever, arthritis, arthralgia, conjunctivitis, iritis, anorectal manifestations including proctitis, tenesmus, bloody discharge, obstipation, rectal stricture	*Chlamydia trachomatis* type L_1–L_3 Frei test (skin) Complement fixing antibody, immunofluorescent antibody test, false-positive VDRL	Tetracycline, 500 mg orally qid × 10 day, *or* minocycline, 100 mg orally bid × 10–20 day, *or* sulfadiazine, 1 g orally tid × 3 wk
Molluscum contagiosum	Vulvar lesions, nodules with umbilicated area—white core of curd-like material	Isolation of pox virus	Dermal curettage of papule
Phthirus pubis (Pediculosis pubis)	Pruritus, excoriation, sky blue macules—inner thigh or lower abdomen	Nits on hair shafts, lice—skin or clothing	Lindane lotion (Kwell) wash off medication in 12 hr; topical permethrin
Sarcoptes scabiei (Scabies)	Nocturnal pruritus, pruritic vesicles, pustules in runs	Mites—ova black dots of feces (microscopic)	1% Lindane applied overnight, discard infected clothing; topical permethrin
Shigella species (Shigellosis)	Fever, malaise, fecal contamination, diarrhea with blood and mucus, cramps, pus in stool	Stools—WBC and RBC, positive for *Shigella*	Trimethoprim and sulfamethoxazole, 1:5, *or* chloramphenicol, 50 mg/kg/24 hr, *or* tetracycline, 500 mg orally qid × 1 wk‡
Staphylococcus and *Streptococcus* species	Vaginal discharge to vulvovaginal area; spread from primary lesion	Positive culture for appropriate organism	Penicillin *or* cephalosporin—dose variable
Treponema pallidum (Syphilis)	Chancre (painless ulcer), regional lymphadenopathy, gummatous lesion, CNS-ocular syndromes	Positive VDRL, RPR, or treponemal antibody (FTA-ABS)	Penicillin, tetracycline, *or* erythromycin–dose variable depending on stage and patient's age
Trichomonas vaginalis and *Gardnerella vaginalis*—Vaginitis emphysematosa	Gas-filled bubbles in the vagina caused by concomitant infection by *G. vaginalis* and *T. vaginalis*	Vaginal blebs with identification of *G. vaginalis* and *T. vaginalis*	Metronidazole, 250 mg orally tid × 1 wk

*From Sanfilippo JO: Specific vulvovaginitis. Pediatr Ann 15:512, 1986.
†Dosages are given for a 70-kg female.
‡In adolescents.

LICHEN SIMPLEX CHRONICUS (NEURODERMATITIS). This is a chronic, lichenified plaque that causes pruritus. Scratching and inflammation may result, causing a vicious cycle. The condition is rare in children. Treatment with antihistamines and topical or intralesional corticosteroids is recommended.

SEBORRHEIC DERMATITIS (see Sec. 23.14). This presents as erythematous, oily, circumscribed patches that can be found on the face, scalp, and chest as well as on intertriginous areas of the body. There may also be fissures and associated secondary infection around the vulva. This secondary bacterial or candidal infection is quite common, causing pain, pruritus, dysuria, and vaginal bleeding. Acute episodes are best treated with sitz baths or topical aluminum acetate solution (Burow solution). Exacerbating factors such as tight clothing or rubber pants should be eliminated. Systemic antibiotics with appropriate topical antifungal medication should be administered for secondary infection.

ATOPIC DERMATITIS (see Sec. 23.14). This affects 3% of all children. Patients present with hay fever or asthma or both and generally have a family history positive for such allergies. The vulvar lesion is characterized as a chronic condition accompanied by intense pruritus, erythema, papules, and vesicles, with oozing and crusting of the involved areas. There may be associated circumscribed, lichenified scaly patches on the vulvar area. Pruritus often causes scratching, which results in excoriation of the lesions. Secondary bacterial or candidal infection is common.

Antihistamines are necessary for control of pruritus. Sitz baths with mild soap and lubricants are helpful. Topical corticosteroids such as 1% hydrocortisone are also effective. Secondary bacterial or candidal infections require specific treatment.

CONTACT DERMATITIS (see Sec. 23.14). In either allergic or irritant contact dermatitis, the vulva may be affected by edematous, erythematous, oozing lesions that are sometimes accompanied by vesicles or pustules. Chronic contact dermatitis is often associated with thickened and lichenified lesions. The clue for correct diagnosis of this condition is the limitation of the dermatitis to the area of contact with the etiologic agent. There may also be a secondary candidal or bacterial infection. Some common etiologic agents are soaps, powders, bubble baths, feminine hygiene spray, topical medications, toilet paper, rubber, and certain types of clothing. Treatment should include avoidance of the offending agents and sitz baths or compresses with topical aluminum acetate solution (Burow solution) during acute episodes. Mild topical corticosteroids such as 0.5–1% hydrocortisone cream applied several times daily may further aid healing and alleviate vulvar irritation. Recurrence can be prevented by removal of the offending etiologic agent.

VULVAR PSORIASIS (see Sec. 23.16). This is frequently associated with lesions of other parts of the body and is characterized by violaceous papules or plaques with a thick, adherent silvery scale (Fig. 18–46 [color plate section]). The intertriginous areas may show "inverse" psoriasis, a variation that does not occur on the extremities. Vulvar lesions usually are poorly demarcated and may present as scaly patches, most commonly on the mons pubis. The vulvar lesions are often resistant to therapy; therefore, a multifaceted approach is essential. A corticosteroid cream (e.g., 1% hydrocortisone) should be used in conjunction with control of secondary infection and pruritus.

ENTEROBIASIS (see Sec. 12.123). Pinworms *(Enterobias vermicularis)* are helminths that may carry colonic bacteria to the perineum, causing recurrent vulvovaginitis. The female pinworm emerges from the anus to deposit eggs. Vulvovaginitis develops in about 20% of girls infected with *E. vermicularis*. The "Scotch tape" test should be used to search for the organism if there is any suspicion or if there is undiagnosed recurrent vulvovaginitis. Victims typically have pruritus and nocturnal episodes of scratching. Treatment consists of pyrantel pamoate (Table 18–18).

SHIGELLOSIS (see Sec. 12.30). *Shigella flexneri* and *S. sonnei* cause various gastrointestinal symptoms in association with vaginitis. Forty seven per cent of patients present with a bloody vaginal discharge and 2%, with diarrhea. Systemic antibiotics are the treatment of choice (see Table 18–18). Bowel colonization with *Shigella* can result in subclinical gastrointestinal symptoms in 10% of household members.

VITILIGO. This presents as sharply demarcated pink to ivory patches that tend to spread and coalesce (Fig. 18–47 [color plate section]). The skin on the patch is smooth with no palpable changes. It may be differentiated from lichen sclerosus because the hyperpigmented patches are asymptomatic. No treatment is necessary unless cosmetic problems result.

LABIAL ADHESIONS. In this disorder, the labia minora have a central line of adherence from an area immediately inferior to the clitoris to the fourchette (Fig. 18–48 [color plate section]). Labial adhesions are commonly seen in patients under 6 yr of age, and the condition is often symptomatic. The lesions usually are associated with local inflammation in association with the hypoestrogenic state of the preadolescent. Pooling of urine in the vagina and recurrent vulvovaginitis appear to provide a continuous nidus for recurrent urinary tract infections. Recurrent urinary tract symptoms occur in 20–40% of patients and should be treated. If the patient is asymptomatic and the vaginal examination is normal, there is no need for treatment other than to reassure the patient and her parents. Once the vaginal pH becomes more acidic, as occurs with adolescence, the recurrent labial adhesions almost always disappear.

Topical estrogen cream applied each evening is the treatment of choice and is effective in over 90% of reported cases. Polysporin, Bacitracin, or Neosporin ointment may be applied each evening for 1 wk. Elimination of the lesions may require 2–8 wk of therapy. Cleansing followed by application of a bland ointment such as petrolatum should continue for 1–2 mo after the adhesions separate. Mechanical separation of the adhesions is advisable only if the lesions appear to separate easily and if it does not cause significant trauma. Once the adhesions are separated, the patient should be re-examined for any predisposing cause, such as the presence of a vaginal septum.

CLITORITIS. This is caused by the same organisms that may produce vulvovaginitis. Treatment is the same as for vulvitis. Synechiae also occur in association with the clitoral hood. The synechiae can cause pain when the child masturbates and may result in engorgement of the clitoris. Treatment consists of warm soaks and retraction of the clitoral hood. If chronic irritation is a problem, night-time application of an estrogen-containing cream for 2 wk is an excellent means of separating the adhesions.

FOREIGN BODIES. These are sometimes responsible for vaginal bleeding in the pediatric patient. The presence of a foul smelling discharge with vaginal bleeding should suggest the possibility of a foreign body. A plain roentgenogram or ultrasound of the abdomen is often helpful. Wadded toilet paper is the most common foreign body identified in the vagina. A vaginal foreign body was found in 18% of preadolescent girls with vaginal bleeding with or without discharge and in 50% of those with bleeding and no discharge.

Arsenault P, Gerbie A: Vulvovaginitis in the pre-adolescent girl. Pediatr Ann 15:577, 1986.
Bacon JL: Pediatric vulvovaginitis. Adolesc Pediatr Gynecol 2:86, 1989.

TABLE 18–19. How To Do Breast Self-Examination*

1. Lie down. Flatten your right breast by placing a pillow under your right shoulder. If your breasts are large, use your right hand to hold your right breast while you do the exam with your left hand.
2. Use the sensitive pads of the middle three fingers on your left hand. Feel for lumps using a rubbing motion.
3. Press firmly enough to feel different breast tissues.
4. Completely feel all of the breast and chest area to cover breast tissue that extends toward the shoulder. Allow enough time for a complete exam. Women with small breasts will need at least 2 minutes to examine each breast. Larger breasts will take longer.
5. Use the same pattern to feel every part of the breast tissue. Choose the method easiest for you. The diagrams show the three patterns preferred by women and their doctors: the circular, clock or oval pattern, the vertical strip, and the wedge.
6. After you have completely examined your right breast, then examine your left breast using the same method. Compare what you have felt in one breast with the other.
7. You may also want to examine your breasts while bathing, when your skin is wet and lumps may be easier to feel.
8. You can check your breasts in a mirror looking for any change in size or contour, dimpling of the skin, or spontaneous nipple discharge.

*Published with permission of The American Cancer Society, Kentucky Division.

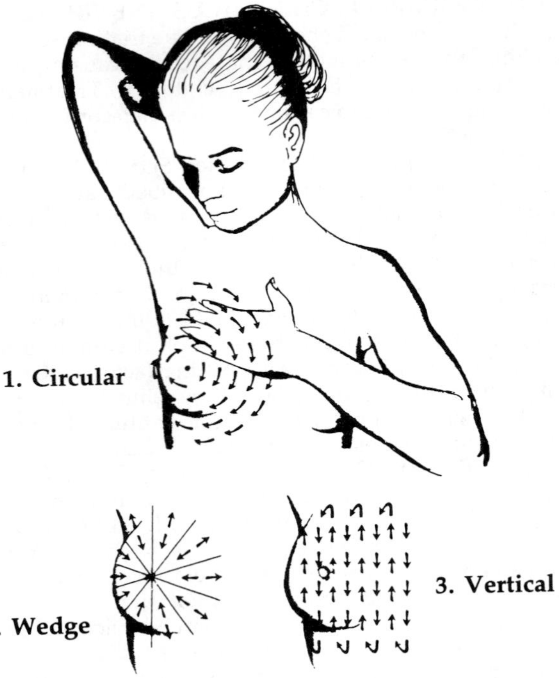

Charles V, Charles SX: A case of vulvo-vaginal diphtheria in a girl of seven years. Indian Pediatr 15:257, 1978.
Clark JA, Muller SA: Lichen sclerosus et atrophicus in children: A report of 24 cases. Arch Dermatol 95:476, 1967.
Davis AJ, Goldstein DP: Treatment of pediatric lichen sclerosus with the CO_2 laser. Adolesc Pediatr Gynecol 2:103, 1989.
Gerstner G, Grunberger W, Boschitsch E, et al: Vaginal organisms in prepubertal children with and without vulvovaginitis. Arch Gynecol 231:247, 1982.
Huffman J, Dewhurst J, Capraro V: The Gynecology of Childhood and Adolescence, 2nd ed. Philadelphia, WB Saunders, 1981.
Murphy T, Nelson J: Shigella vaginitis: Report of 38 patients and review of the literature. Pediatrics 63:511, 1979.
Paradise J, Willis E: Probability of vaginal body in girls with genital complaints. Am J Dis Child 139:472, 1985.
Redmond CA, Cowell CA, Krafchik BR: Genital lichen sclerosus in prepubertal girls. Adolesc Pediatr Gynecol 1:177, 1988.
Williams T, Callen J, Owen L: Vulvar disorders in the prepubertal female. Pediatr Ann 15:588, 1986.

18.52 BREAST DISORDERS

See Sec. 10.19.

The mammary glands are derived from the epidermal layer. Beginning at approximately 6 wk of gestation, epidermal cells migrate to the mesenchyme and form the mammary ridges. Breast buds, lactiferous ducts, and fully developed mammary glands eventually form. Breast development normally occurs in girls between the ages of 8 1/2–13 yr (see Sec. 3.9 and 10.19). The rate of breast growth varies, and development is often asymmetric. Complete development may not occur until a woman is in her early 20s.

BREAST SELF-EXAMINATION. Early diagnosis is central to improvement in health care for breast abnormalities including carcinoma. Instruction in breast self-examination should be given during the initial gynecologic evaluation of the adolescent with reinforcement during follow-up visits (Table 18–19).

CONGENITAL ANOMALIES. Complete absence of a breast, *amastia*, is rare; it is unilateral and often associated with other abnormalities, such as Poland syndrome (aplasia of the pectoralis muscles, rib deformities, webbed fingers, and radial nerve aplasia). Amastia can be iatrogenic, as a result of the inadvertent excision of a breast bud. *Athelia* is defined as absence of one or both nipples. This condition is also rare and may not be associated with absent breast tissue. Both abnormalities require surgical correction.

Supernumerary breasts (polymastia) and *supernumerary nipples* (polythelia) are relatively common (Fig. 18–49); they occur along the "milk lines" and are usually asymptomatic. There is an association between polythelia and anomalies of the urinary and cardiovascular systems. In general, surgical excision of accessory breasts or nipples is not necessary. However, if the aberrant breasts or nipples become symptomatic, excision may be indicated.

Hypoplasia of the breasts varies in degree from a nearly total absence of breast tissue to well-formed breasts that are considered by the patient to be too small. There are three general causes for poor or absent breast development. (1) The onset of breast development may be delayed, and the breast will develop slowly but be normal in all other respects. (2) There may be a family history of late breast development. (3) Ovarian function may have failed or been suppressed (see Sec. 19.34). Treatment depends on the underlying cause.

Breast atrophy is seen occasionally in adolescents and is almost uniformly secondary to dietary changes such as occur in anorexia nervosa. Correction of the underlying problem results in re-establishment of breast tissue.

NEONATAL BREAST ABNORMALITIES. Bilateral breast hypertrophy may occur as a result of elevated circulating endogenous steroid hormones in late gestation. It may be associated with discharge from the nipples known as "witches' milk." Repeated manipulation of the breasts can exacerbate the condition. On occasion, the hypertrophy is associated with mastitis caused by a staphylococcal infection; antibiotics should be administered.

MASTODYNIA. Painful breast engorgement (mastodynia) is usually associated with ovulatory cycles; this is uncommon in the adolescent until 18 mo following menarche. There is frequently a cyclical pattern to the breast discomfort. Analgesics such as nonsteroidal anti-inflammatory drugs (NSAIDs) such as naproxen sodium and ibuprofen, as well as the use

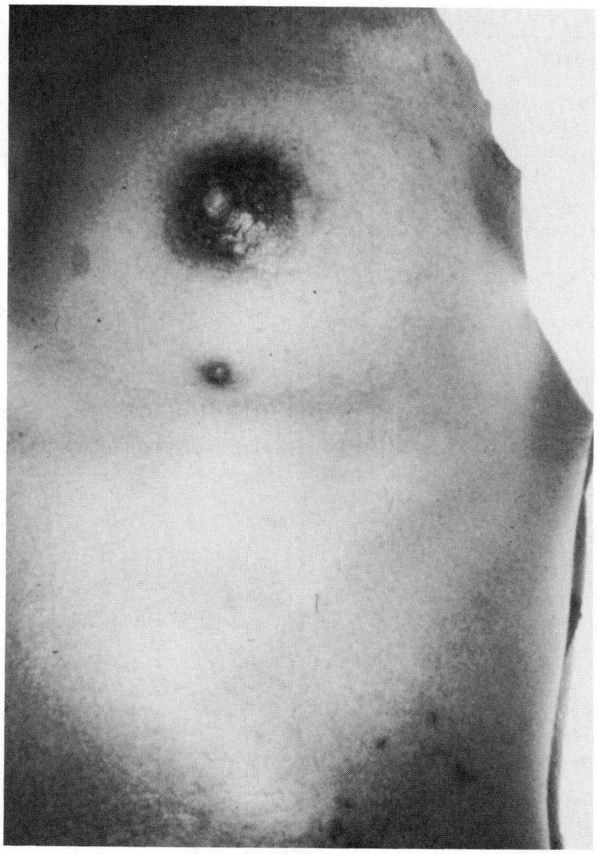

Figure 18–49. Polythelia.

of good support bras, are often helpful in alleviating discomfort.

BREAST MASSES. Retrospective reviews of breast disease in adolescent females reveal that about 54% have fibroadenomas and 13% have virginal hypertrophy. Fibrocystic or proliferative breast disease occurs in about 24%. Primary rhabdomyosarcoma, metastatic rhabdomyosarcoma, metastatic neuroblastoma, and non-Hodgkin lymphoma occur in 2–3% of all breast masses in this age group. Other diagnoses include polythelia, accessory breast tissue, mastitis, hemangioma, fat necrosis, and intramammary lymph nodes.

A thorough history and complete physical examination are mandatory for any pediatric or adolescent patient who has a breast mass. The clinical problem should be reviewed with a radiologist prior to rendering specific radiologic assessments. Needle aspiration and biopsy are often essential for evaluation of palpable breast abnormalities. Large breast tumors also occur in adolescents. Although malignancy is often suspected because of rapid growth of the mass and skin ulceration, breast tumors can have varied presentations. Giant fibroadenomas in adolescence may be treated by simple enucleation.

Malignant Tumors. Although rare, breast *cancer* does occur in the adolescent. Early menarche in association with anovulatory cycles is a risk factor. The estrogen-to-androgen ratio appears to be critical, with androgens having a protective effect.

Cystosarcoma phylloides, an uncommon breast tumor in adults, may occur in adolescents. It is characterized by asymmetric breast enlargement in association with a firm, mobile, circumscribed mass. Often the tumor increases rapidly in size and can become quite large. Fixation of the tumor to the skin or chest wall is rare. The majority of these tumors are benign, but malignant cystosarcoma phylloides with metastases has been reported. Excision is the preferred initial therapy in the adolescent patient, regardless of the histologic classification of the lesion. Malignant cystosarcoma is more likely to recur than is a benign lesion. Fatal metastatic cystosarcoma phylloides in an adolescent has been reported.

Breast tumors also may be the first manifestation of relapse (extramedullary) in *acute lymphoblastic leukemia.* Reports in the literature include a case of *radiation-induced sarcoma* of the breast in a female adolescent and a case of *liposarcoma* in a 17-yr-old black female who previously had a total mastectomy.

MACROMASTIA (VIRGINAL HYPERTROPHY). The etiology of massive breast enlargement during puberty and early adolescence is unknown but probably represents an end-organ increased sensitivity to circulating estrogens. It is bilateral, often occurs over a brief period, and most commonly affects girls from 13–17 yr old (see Sec. 19.33). Physical and psychologic problems may occur in the adolescent with macromastia. Posture problems and discomfort often result. Reduction mammoplasty is the treatment of choice but should be delayed until late adolescence to allow for complete breast development. Surgical intervention often necessitates relocation of the nipple, which may result in decreased sensation and altered lactation. In addition, strong emotional support should be provided.

MASTITIS AND ABSCESS. Mastitis and breast abscess may require antibiotic therapy as well as incision and drainage.

TRAUMA AND INFLAMMATION. Breast trauma in adolescent females is more common because of the increased number of young women participating in contact sports. The trauma usually takes the form of contusion or hematoma and often resolves without incident. Occasionally, fat necrosis occurs and results in either late cystic changes in the breast or fibrosis with retraction of skin or the nipple over the injured area. These late changes may mimic those associated with malignancy; biopsy may be the only means of differentiating between the two.

MAMMARY DYSPLASIA. This common lesion is characterized by changes associated with the menstrual cycle. The etiology may be related to hormonal imbalance, a relative excess of estrogen, and deficient corpus luteum activity. This imbalance produces exaggerated responses in the breast tissue, especially in the upper and outer quadrants during the premenstrual phase of the cycle. Mammography is helpful in establishing the diagnosis. The extent of treatment depends on the degree of symptomatology. Danazol, a synthetic androgen derived from ethisterone (Danocrine, Winthrop Laboratories, New York, NY) can be beneficial in the adolescent patient; daily doses range from 100–800 mg, depending on weight. In addition, methylxanthines (e.g., coffee, tea, carbonated drinks) and chocolate should be eliminated from the diet.

NIPPLE DISCHARGE. This must be carefully evaluated and a distinction made between the presence of galactorrhea (''spontaneous flow of milk'') and bloody discharge. Evaluation of galactorrhea in children is the same as for adults. Serum prolactin levels are obtained to rule out the presence of pituitary prolactinoma (see Sec. 19.5). If there is suspicion of a pituitary tumor or adenoma based on markedly elevated serum prolactin levels, with or without headaches, and bitemporal hemianopsia, appropriate radiologic (CT, MRI) assessment is necessary. Another cause of galactorrhea is hypothyroidism in association with elevated levels of thyroid releasing hormone, which also stimulates prolactin release. Treatment of galactorrhea consists primarily of dopamine agonists such as bromocriptine (Parlodel, Sandoz, East Hanover, NJ). Surgical intervention, usually in the form of trans-sphenoidal hypophysectomy, is rare. Galactorrhea secondary to chest wall surgery in an adolescent has also been reported. The galactorrhea occurred for 2 mo and was associated with transient amenorrhea.

Bloody nipple discharge can be indicative of *duct ectasia.* Cytologic assessment and surgical consultation are indicated. Nipple discharge in association with *Montgomery tubercles* also has been reported. These secretions can be episodic and vary in color from clear to brown, but they are usually not milky. This discharge evolves over a period of 3–5 wk and may be associated with "breast lumps." This is a benign, self-limited problem. *Intraductal breast papillomas* have also been reported in adolescents. *Areolar gland discharge* is a self-limited problem that does not require treatment.

PREMATURE THELARCHE (see Sec. 19.8).

Apter D, Vinko R: Early menarche, a risk factor for breast cancer, indicates early onset of ovulatory cycles. J Clin Endocrinol Metab 57:82, 1983.

Briggs R, Walters M, Rosenthal D: Cystosarcoma phylloides in adolescent female patients. Am J Surg 146:712, 1983.

Cromer B, Frankel M, Kader L: Compliance with breast self-examination and instruction in healthy adolescents. J Adolesc Health Care 10:105, 1989.

Diehl G, Kaplan D: Breast masses in adolescent females. J Adolesc Health Care 6:353, 1985.

Ellegaard J, Bendix-Hanson K, Boesen A, et al: Breast tumor as a first manifestation of extramedullary relapse in acute lymphoblastic leukemia. Scand J Haematol 33:288, 1984.

Heyman R, Rauh J: Areolar gland discharge in adolescent females appears to be benign. J Adolesc Health Care 4:285, 1983.

Letson G, Moore D: Galactorrhea secondary to chest wall surgery in an adolescent. J Adolesc Health Care 5:277, 1984.

Ngala Kenda J: Fatal metastatic cystosarcoma phylloides in a young woman: Report of a case. Arch Surg 118:871, 1983.

Onnis G, Chiarelli S, Dalla-Palma P: Intraductal breast papilloma in adolescents: Case report. Eur J Gynaecol Oncol 4:211, 1983.

Pietsch J: Breast disorders. *In:* Sanfilippo JS, Lavery JP (eds): Pediatric and Adolescent Obstetrics and Gynecology. New York, Springer-Verlag, 1985, p 96.

Raganoonan C, Fairbairn J, Williams S, et al: Giant breast tumors of adolescence. Aust NZ J Surg 57:243, 1987.

Simmons P, Wold L: Surgically treated breast disease in adolescent females: A retrospective review of 185 cases. Adolesc Pediatr Gynecol 2:95, 1989.

Squire R, Bianchi A, Jakate S: Radiation-induced sarcoma of the breast in a female adolescent: Case report with histologic and therapeutic considerations. Cancer 61:2444, 1988.

Watkind F, Giacomantonio M, Salisbury S: Nipple discharge and breast lump related to Montgomery's tubercles in adolescent females. J Pediatr Surg 23:718, 1988.

18.53 HIRSUTISM AND POLYCYSTIC OVARIAN SYNDROME

EXCESSIVE ANDROGEN PRODUCTION PRIOR TO PUBERTY. Hirsutism (excessive hair growth) must be distinguished from virilization, which involves increased body hair, acne, voice change, change in body habitus due to increased muscle mass, and clitoromegaly (see Sec. 19.41). Premature pubarche is defined as the appearance of genital hair or axillary hair, or both, before 8 yr of age (see Sec. 19.8). Adrenarche, the output of excess androgen from the adrenal gland, usually occurs between 12 and 18 yr of age and is discussed in Sec. 19.8.

HIRSUTISM IN THE ADOLESCENT. Table 18–20 lists the causes of hirsutism. *Androgen-producing tumors* of adrenal or gonadal origin should be considered when an adolescent presents with excessive hair growth. However, hirsutism is most often *idiopathic* with normal total circulating androgen levels. Sex hormone binding globulin (SHBG) levels may be decreased in hirsute patients, which allows a higher fraction of bioactive androgens despite normal total serum androgen levels. SHBG levels are affected by a number of factors. Androgens, specifically testosterone, cause a decrease in SHBG levels; estrogens and dexamethasone tend to increase SHBG. Furthermore, a decline in SHBG occurs with increasing age, especially from prepuberty to adolescence. Body weight has an inverse correlation with SHBG levels independent of androgen levels.

TABLE 18–20. Causes of Hirsutism*

Peripheral
- Idiopathic
- Partial androgen insensitivity (5-α-reductase deficiency)
- HAIR-AN syndrome (hirsutism, androgenization, insulin resistance, and acanthosis nigricans)
- Hyperprolactinemia

Gonadal
- Polycystic ovary syndrome (PCO, chronic anovulation)
- Ovarian neoplasm (Sertoli-Leydig cell, granulosa cell, thecoma, gynandroblastoma, lipoid cell, luteoma, hypernephroma, Brenner tumor)
- Gonadal dysgenesis (Turner mosaic with XY, or H-Y antigen positive)

Adrenal
- Cushing syndrome
- Adrenal hyperresponsiveness
- Congenital adrenal hyperplasia (classic, cryptic, adult onset)
  - 21-hydroxylase deficiency
  - 11-hydroxylase deficiency
  - 3-β-ol-dehydrogenase deficiency
  - 17-ol-dehydrogenase deficiency
- Adrenal neoplasm (adenoma, cortical carcinoma)

Exogenous
- Minoxidil
- Dilantin
- Cyclosporine
- Anabolic steroids
- Diamox
- Penicillamine
- Oral contraceptives (progestin dominant)
- Danazol
- Androgenic steroids
- Psoralens
- Diazoxide
- Phenothiazines

Congenital Anomalies
- 18-Trisomy (Edward syndrome)
- Cornelia de Lange syndrome
- Hurler syndrome
- Juvenile hypothyroidism

*From Bailey-Pridham DD, Sanfilippo JS: Hirsutism in the adolescent female. Pediatr Clin North Am 36:581, 1989; with permission. See also Chapter 19.

HAIR-AN syndrome is the acronym for the association of hirsutism, androgen excess, insulin resistance, and acanthosis nigricans. The pathogenesis of this syndrome is unknown. However, there is a defect in membrane insulin receptors. Elevated androgen levels contribute to the development of acanthosis.

Hyperprolactinemia, a central nervous system disorder, is an occasional cause of hyperandrogenemia (see Sec. 19.5). Approximately 40% of patients with hyperprolactinemia exhibit androgen abnormalities. Laboratory findings may include elevated free testosterone due to decreased SHBG levels and increased adrenal production of 17-hydroxyprogesterone and androstenedione following ACTH stimulation.

Polycystic ovary syndrome (PCO, chronic anovulation, Stein-Leventhal syndrome) is the most commonly diagnosed ovarian cause of hirsutism (see Sec. 19.36). The underlying biochemical cause of PCO is unknown, and controversy exists over whether the basic defect is central (hypothalamic or pituitary regulation of gonadotropins) or ovarian (defect in a peptide hormone, perhaps inhibin, with resultant abnormal feedback to the pituitary gland). The usual hormonal pattern of PCO begins with altered luteinizing hormone release (a luteinizing hormone-to-follicle stimulating hormone ratio of 2:1 or 3:1, shortened pulse frequency, slightly increased pulse amplitude of luteinizing hormone). Adolescents with hyperandrogenism display an exaggerated luteinizing hormone pulsatility similar to that found in adults with PCO syndrome.

Hirsutism in adolescents can also be due to a heterozygous form of 21-hydroxylase deficiency (see Sec. 19.23). This has been called adult onset congenital adrenal hyperplasia (AOCAH). Various forms of *congenital adrenal hyperplasia* and *congenital anomalies* are also associated with hirsutism. Clinically, it may be difficult to distinguish between PCO and AOCAH.

Ovarian hyperthecosis, which can be familial, may be a variant of PCO. Hyperthecosis is defined as isolated islands of luteinized cells within the ovary contributing to increased androgen production. Ovarian androgen production and peripheral effects are similar to those associated with PCO.

Medications, radiation, and chronic irritation (such as the placement of a cast) can also initiate localized, nonendocrinologic hair growth.

DIAGNOSIS AND TREATMENT OF THE HIRSUTE PATIENT. Cushing's syndrome or disease, androgen producing tumors, and congenital adrenal hyperplasia are discussed in Sec. 19.24, Sec. 19.39, and Sec. 19.23, respectively.

Treatment alternatives for idiopathic hirsutism and PCO are outlined in Table 18–21. Hirsutism secondary to hyperprolactinemia is best treated with bromocriptine. In patients with multicystic (polycystic) ovaries and primary hypothyroidism, the polycystic ovaries resolve rapidly with adequate doses of thyroid replacement therapy. If an exogenous cause such as a medication is producing hirsutism, it must be eliminated.

Even when the increased tissue androgen effect is reversed by appropriate treatment, hair follicles converted to terminal hair may still produce that type of hair. Electrolysis may then provide improved cosmetic appearance, with the assurance that if the underlying abnormality is controlled there should be no new growth of hair.

Apter D, Siegberg R, Laatikainen T: Pulsatile secretion of luteinizing hormone in adolescents with hyperandrogenism. Adolesc Pediatr Gynecol 1:104, 1988.
Belgorosky A, Rivarola M: Progressive increase in non-sex hormone binding globulin-bound testosterone and estradiol from infancy to late pre-puberty in girls. J Clin Endocrinol Metab 67:234, 1988.
Ferriman D, Gallwey J: Clinical assessment of body hair growth in women. J Clin Endocrinol Metab 21:1440, 1961.
Judd H, Scully R, Herbst A, et al: Familial hyperthecosis: Comparison of endocrinologic and histologic findings with polycystic ovarian disease. Am J Obstet Gynecol 117:976, 1973.
Kamilaris T, DeBold C, Manolus K, et al: Testosterone secreting adrenal adenoma in a peripubertal patient. JAMA 258:2558, 1987.
Leng J, Greenblatt R: Hirsutism in adolescent girls. Pediatr Clin North Am 19:681, 1972.
Lindsay A, Voorhess M, MacGillivray M: Multicystic ovaries in primary hypothyroidism. Obstet Gynecol 61:433, 1983.
Mathur R, Moody L, Langriebe S, et al: Sex hormone binding globulin in clinically hyperandrogenic women: Association of plasma concentration with body weight. Fertil Steril 38:207, 1982.
Parker L, Sack J, Fisher D, et al: The adrenarche: Prolactin, gonadotropins, adrenal androgens and cortisol. J Clin Endocrinol Metab 60:409, 1985.
Rosen G, Kaplan B, Lobo R: Menstrual function and hirsutism in patients with gonadal dysgenesis. Obstet Gynecol 71:677, 1988.
Speroff L, Glass RH, Kase NG: Hirsutism. *In:* Speroff L, Glass RH, Kase NG (eds): Clinical Gynecologic Endocrinology and Infertility, 4th ed. Baltimore, Williams & Wilkins, 1989, p 233.
Zumogg B, Freeman R, Coupa S, et al: A chronobiologic abnormality of luteinizing hormone secretion in teenage girls with the polycystic ovary syndrome. N Engl J Med 309:1206, 1983.

18.54 NEOPLASMS

The most common gynecologic neoplasm found in children is of ovarian origin and usually presents as an abdominal mass. The vagina or vulva, or both, may also be the site of benign or malignant lesions in children (see Sec. 17.24); cervical dysplasias may occur in adolescents (see Sec. 17.25). Breast masses are discussed in Sec. 18.52.

OVARIES. Ovarian tumors are the most frequent type of pelvic tumors found in patients under 18 yr of age; paraovarian tumors are next in frequency, followed by uterine neoplasms. The most common clinical presentation is abdominal pain or a mass, or both. In the adolescent, the most common ovarian tumor is the *teratoma*. It is usually benign, but malignant teratomas may occur. Calcification on abdominal roentgenogram is often a hallmark of a benign teratoma. During surgery the opposite ovary should be palpated. If there is any question about the possibility of a neoplasm, a biopsy of the opposite ovary should be taken. Ovarian adenomas are the second most common benign ovarian tumor.

The majority of these tumors are of the *germ cell* type, the most common of which includes dysgerminomas, followed in incidence by malignant teratomas, endodermal sinus tumors, embryonal carcinomas, mixed cell neoplasms, and gonadoblastomas. Germ cell neoplasms of more aggressive malignancy than dysgerminomas (e.g., immature teratomas, endodermal sinus tumors) occur in a significantly higher proportion of younger females (under 10 yr of age). In this age group, 10-yr survival rates determined by life table analyses were 73% for epithelial carcinomas, 44% for sex cord stromal tumors, 73% for dysgerminomas, 33% for malignant teratomas, 39% for endodermal sinus tumors, 25% for embryonal carcinomas, 30% for other germ cell neoplasms, and 100% for gonadoblastomas. Dysgerminomas usually are associated with XY gonadal dysgenesis, and Y-DNA probes are becoming increasingly important in their diagnosis. The role

TABLE 18–21. Treatment of Hirsutism: Idiopathic and Polycystic Ovary Syndrome*

Medication	Dose†	Comments
Oral contraceptives (estrogen dominant)	35 μg	Decrease in plasma testosterone, androstenedione, and DHEA-S
Spironolactone	100 mg bid	Decreased androgen production and androgen receptor competition
Medroxyprogesterone acetate-depo (Depo-Provera)	150–250 mg q 2–4 wk	Decreased testosterone production and 17-ketosteroid levels
Cyproterone acetate	Diane, 2 mg Androcur, 100 mg	Decreased plasma testosterone, androstenedione, SHBG, induces "insulinemia"
Dexamethasone	0.25–0.5 mg	Dose adequate if plasma-free testosterone < 15 pg/mL
Cimetidine	200–300 mg tid–qid	Decreased serum testosterone, increased serum estradiol
GnRH agonist (Nafarelin)	1,000 μg	Decreased testosterone and androstenedione

*From Bailey-Pridham DD, Sanfilippo JS: Hirsutism in the adolescent female. Pediatr Clin North Am 36:581, 1989; with permission.
†Dosage for 70-kg female. Daily dosage unless otherwise specified.

of tumor markers such as α-fetoprotein, carcinoembryonic antigen, and cancer antigen (CA)-125 are also used to assess ovarian malignancies.

Surgical excision followed by postoperative chemotherapy and radiotherapy is often necessary. Staging at the beginning of therapy is of the utmost importance. In many cases, a second-look procedure can assist further in the treatment of these neoplasms.

Ovarian follicular cysts, which occur from birth to puberty, usually disappear spontaneously within 3–32 wk. By ultrasound the cyst usually presents as a nonecogenic area, frequently larger than 20 mm at its greatest diameter; diffuse swelling of the ovarian parenchyma and follicular enlargement of the cortical zone are also seen. Torsion of an ovarian cyst is a complication that must always be considered, and prompt surgical intervention is necessary. Torsion of an adnexa often presents with intermittent sharp abdominal pain that, in many cases, radiates down the ipsilateral extremity. Bilateral ovarian torsion may occur in infancy and should be considered in the differential diagnosis of abdominal pain in the pediatric female patient. When unilateral torsion is diagnosed, pexing or plication of the contralateral adnexa is recommended.

Autoamputation of the ovary, presenting as a small calcified free-floating mass associated with an absent adnexa, has been described. The child may be asymptomatic, and ultrasound is often helpful in establishing the diagnosis. It has been hypothesized that antenatal or subclinical ovarian torsion leads to necrosis, calcification, and separation of the adnexa from its blood supply.

Sex cord stromal tumors comprise 5% of ovarian neoplasms, of which the *granulosa cell tumor* is the most common. Isosexual precocity and occasionally virilization may be observed in the juvenile variety. The characteristic histologic features include nodular architecture, follicle formation, microcysts, cell necrosis, and high mitotic activity.

CERVIX. Cervical intraepithelial neoplasia (CIN), diagnosed in sexually active teenagers and young adults, is associated with abnormal cytology in 2–3% of patients. The prevalence of dysplasia and carcinoma in situ is 18.8/1,000 for ages 15–19 yr. Biopsy proven cases of all grades of CIN in the teenage population have a prevalence of 13.3/1,000. Sexually transmitted diseases are well correlated with CIN. In a case-controlled study, human papilloma virus infection and altered vaginal flora were consistent findings in patients with CIN. Abnormal Papanicolaou (Pap) smears in adolescents also correlate with significant CIN; abnormal Pap smears should be evaluated and a tissue diagnosis should be obtained. Colposcopic examination is essential when CIN is diagnosed in the adolescent. Other pathologic abnormalities of the cervix include cervical polyps and mixed mesodermal tumor of the uterine cervix. The latter may represent a mixed, heterologous, or homologous sarcoma of the uterine cervix.

BENIGN AND MALIGNANT TUMORS OF THE UTERINE CORPUS. *Adenocarcinoma* of the corpus is rare in children and adolescents. Vaginal bleeding that is not associated with sexual precocity in the pediatric patient is a frequent sign at presentation. The treatment of malignant tumors consists of hysterectomy, ideally with removal of the ovaries, followed by adjunctive radiotherapy or chemotherapy, or both, depending on the operative findings. Mixed *mesodermal tumors* of the uterus also have been noted. *Leiomyomata* have been described in this age group and should be included in the differential diagnosis of an adolescent presenting with a pelvic mass. Leiomyosarcoma has also been reported in an adolescent; the presentation is variable, but usually abnormal vaginal bleeding is present.

VAGINA. One of the more common vaginal wall abnormalities is the *Gartner duct (mesonephric) cyst.* Usually, these findings are incidental and require no specific therapy. In the sexually active patient, excision may be necessary if there is associated dyspareunia. *Paramesonephric (müllerian) duct cysts* often become symptomatic at menarche when the cavity fills with menstrual blood. Women who were exposed to diethylstilbestrol (DES) in utero have a high incidence of *adenosis* of the vagina and cervix (see Sec. 17.1). These patients have a host of potential reproductive abnormalities including infertility, habitual abortion, and tubal and uterine cavity abnormalities. *Clear cell adenocarcinoma* of the vagina and cervix is a rare sequela of DES exposure in utero.

Sarcoma botryoides, a vaginal carcinoma that occurs primarily in the pediatric patient, is best treated by surgical excision. A combination of vincristine, actinomycin-D, and cyclophosphamide is usually given postoperatively (see Sec. 17.16).

Any questionable vulvar lesion should be submitted for histologic examination. *Liposarcoma* of the vulva has been reported in a 15-yr-old girl. Malignant melanoma of the vulva has been described in a 14-yr-old patient.

Barber HR: Ovarian cancers in childhood. Int J Radiat Oncol Biol Phys 8:1427, 1982.

Berenson A, Pokorny S, Dutton R: The autoamputated ovary: A rare cause of abdominal calcification. Adolesc Pediatr Gynecol 2:99, 1989.

Biscotti C, Hart W: Juvenile granulosa cell tumors of the ovary. Arch Pathol Lab Med 113:40, 1989.

Brooks J, LiVolsi V: Liposarcoma presenting on the vulva. Am J Obstet Gynecol 156:73, 1987.

Copeland LJ, Gershenson DM, Saul PB, et al: Sarcoma botryoides of the female genital tract. Obstet Gynecol 66:262, 1985.

Freedman R, Kopf A, Jones W: Malignant melanoma in association with lichen sclerosus on the vulva of a 14-year-old. Am J Dermatopathol 6:253, 1984.

Graif M, Itzchak Y: Sonographic evaluation of ovarian torsion in childhood and adolescence. AJR 150:647, 1988.

Guijon F, Paraskevas M, Brunham R: The association of sexually transmitted diseases with cervical intraepithelial neoplasia: A case-controlled study. Am J Obstet Gynecol 151:185, 1985.

Jones DED, Russo JF, Dombroski RA, et al: Cervical intraepithelial neoplasia in adolescence. J Adolesc Health Care 5:243, 1984.

Lavecchia C, Morris H, Draper G: Malignant ovarian tumors in childhood in Britain 1962–78. Br J Cancer 48:363, 1983.

Liapi C, Evain-Biron D: Diagnosis of ovarian follicular cyst from birth to puberty: A report of 20 cases. Acta Paediatr Scand 76:91, 1987.

de Rooy TC, Wiegerinck M: A 15-year-old girl with an expansively growing tumor. Eur J Obstet Gynecol Reprod Biol 22:373, 1986.

Rosenfeld WD, Kleinhaus S, Kutcher R, et al: Leiomyoma in a 15-year-old girl. Adolesc Pediatr Gynecol 1:109, 1988.

Sadeghi S, Hsieh E, Gonn S: Prevalence of cervical intraepithelial neoplasia in sexually active teenagers and young adults: Results of data analysis of mass Papanicolaou screening of 796,337 women in the United States in 1981. Am J Obstet Gynecol 148:726, 1984.

Sanfilippo JS, Pokorny SF, Reindollar R: Pediatric and Adolescent Gynecology. (Curr Probl Obstet Gynecol Fertil Vol 13, No 5.) St Louis, Mosby/Year Book, 1990.

Starceski P, Lee P, Siever W: Bilateral ovarian pathology and torsion in infancy: Assessment of pubertal and gonadal function. Adolesc Pediatr Gynecol 1:199, 1988.

DYSMENORRHEA AND PREMENSTRUAL SYNDROME

(See Sec. 10.18)

18.55 PREMATURE OVARIAN FAILURE

Premature ovarian failure may occur in adolescent females as a result of gonadal dysgenesis, gonadotropin resistant ovary syndrome, ovarian tumors, and extirpation of the ovaries secondary to surgery, radiation, or chemotherapy. The adolescent presents with secondary amenorrhea and hypogonadism. Although it is not often indicated, a biopsy of the ovary would reveal premature ovarian failure, characterized by absence of or rare presence of oocytes. Gonadotropin-resistant ovary syndrome is characterized by a normal complement of primordial follicles but an inability to respond to gonadotropin stimulation. Autoimmune oophoritis presents with lymphocytic and plasma cell infiltration around developing ovarian follicles but not adjacent to the follicles.

Hormone replacement therapy is prescribed in the form of exogenous estrogens, usually given at physiologic dosages (conjugated estrogens [Premarin], 0.625 mg/24 hr for 25 days/mo; micronized estradiol [Estrace], 1 mg/24 hr; or estradiol patches [Estraderm], 0.05 mg). Progestins should be added to the estrogen regimen either in the form of medroxyprogesterone acetate, 10 mg/24 hr during the last 13 days of the cycle, or norethindrone acetate (Norlutate) 2.5–5 mg/24 hr for the last 13 days of the cycle.

Coulam C: Premature gonadal failure. Fertil Steril 38:645, 1982.
Coulam C, Kempers R, Randall R: Premature ovarian failure: Evidence for the autoimmune mechanism. Fertil Steril 36:238, 1981.
Elder M, MacLaren N, Riley W: Gonadal autoantibodies in patients with hypogonadism and/or Addison's disease. J Clin Endocrinol Metab 52:1137, 1981.

18.56 CONSTITUTIONAL TALL STATURE

See also Sec. 19.5.

Defined as height greater than the 97th percentile (more than 2 standard deviations above the mean of the population), constitutional tall stature affects 3% of the female population. Treatment should be considered only for girls whose expected maximum height is projected to be over 180–183 cm (5 ft, 11 in–6 ft). Bone age can be used as an accurate predictor of final adult height. Any decisions regarding treatment should be individualized and should take into consideration the psychologic, social, and philosophical issues involved.

Referral for psychologic counseling is appropriate, but treatment with hormones is rarely indicated. Regimens for hormonal therapy vary: for example, conjugated estrogen tablets (1.25 mg each) are given to a total dose of 7.5 mg/24 hr. In general, the mean duration of treatment is 18 mo and includes monitoring of bone age and somatomedin C levels. Somatomedin C levels fall as circulating levels of estrogen increase. Alternatively estradiol valerate is injected intramuscularly, 10 mg weekly for 3 wk, followed by an injection of 125 mg of medroxyprogesterone caproate; or conjugated estrogens can be given in 5–10 mg/24 hr oral doses. Care must be taken to prevent unopposed estrogen producing endometrial hyperplasia with associated breakthrough bleeding, which may be a precancerous condition. Ethinyl estradiol is another commonly used estrogen in a dose of 0.1–0.5 mg/24 hr, with a progestin added during the last 13 days of the cycle (medroxyprogesterone acetate, 10 mg/24 hr). Opinions vary as to when therapy should begin. Bierich has initiated treatment at 170 cm, whereas other researchers begin to reduce height when the adolescent is 5–6 in less than the predicted final height. Side effects associated with this therapy are summarized in Table 18–22.

TABLE 18–22. Effects of Estrogen Treatment*

Desirable
Rapid slowing and cessation of linear growth
Accelerated epiphyseal closure: 2 yr maturation per calendar year
Accelerated development of secondary sexual characteristics
Amelioration of adolescent acne
Improved self-image
Undesirable
Nuisances
Morning sickness
Pigmentation
Night cramps
Leukorrhea
Obesity
Hypertension
Migraine
Menometrorrhagia
Urticaria due to progesterone
Gonadotropin suppression
Potential major hazards
Intractable anxiety
Neoplasms of the genital tract, breast, and liver
Sterility
Thromboembolism
Vascular catastrophe
Precipitation of diabetes, cholelithiasis, or atherosclerosis

*Reproduced by permission of Pediatrics 62:1189, 1978.

Bailey J, Hark E, Cowell C: Estrogen treatment of girls with constitutional tall stature. Pediatr Clin North Am 28:501, 1981.
Bierich J: Estrogen treatment of girls with constitutional tall stature. Pediatrics 62:1196, 1978.
Crawford J: Treatment of tall girls with estrogen. Pediatrics 62:1189, 1978.
Schoenle E, Theintz G, Torresani T: Lack of bromocriptine-induced reduction of predicted height in tall adolescents. J Clin Endocrinol Metab 65:355, 1987.

18.57 DEVELOPMENTAL ANOMALIES

EMBRYOLOGY. The *uterus* is formed by fusion of the cordal elements of the müllerian ducts, a process that occurs at 8 wk of gestation. The fusion begins from the cordal end (Müller tubercle) and is completed at the upper level of the fundus. A median septum is present until the end of the 1st trimester of gestation.

The *vagina* is formed from the terminal portion of the uterovaginal canal (müllerian origin), which is met by the posterior aspect of the urogenital sinus (terminal portion of Müller tubercle). Further thickening occurs in the portion of the posterior wall of the urogenital sinus that is in contact with Müller tubercle. The tissue is of combined urogenital and müllerian duct origin and is known as the vaginal epithelial plate. Bilateral evaginations of the vaginal epithelial plate encircle the caudal aspect and form the uterine canal. Canalization of the vaginal plate occurs and proceeds in a caudal direction to form the vagina. The process elongates

TABLE 18–23. Common Müllerian Anomalies

Hydrocolpos	Accumulation of mucus or nonsanguineous fluid in the vagina
Hemihematometra	Atretic segment of vagina with menstrual fluid accumulation
Hydrosalpinx	Accumulation of serous fluid in the fallopian tube, often an end result of pyosalpinx
Didelphic uterus	Two cervices each associated with one uterine horn
Bicornuate uterus	One cervix associated with two uterine horns
Unicornuate uterus	Result of failure of one müllerian duct to descend

the vaginal structure, leaving the cranial two thirds of müllerian origin and the caudal one third of urogenital origin.

Common müllerian duct anomalies are defined in Tables 18–23 and 18–24.

CONGENITAL ABSENCE OF THE VAGINA (MAYER-ROKITANSKY-KUSTER-HAUSER SYNDROME). This anomaly is often discovered in adolescents who present with primary amenorrhea. Absence of the vagina has significant anatomic, physiologic, and psychologic implications for the patient and family. Vaginal agenesis is characterized by primary amenorrhea with absence of the vagina and presence of a normal vulva, a duplication anomaly of the uterus, attenuated fallopian tubes, normal ovaries, normal female karyotype, normal female phenotype, and associated anomalies (most frequently renal and skeletal).

INCOMPLETE VERTICAL FUSION OF THE VAGINA. Transverse and longitudinal vaginal septa represent failure of completion of canalization of the vagina. Not uncommonly, the patient presents with amenorrhea and with cyclical pain, which is a result of cryptomenorrhea. Müllerian agenesis must be differentiated from androgen insensitivity (testicular feminization). A serum testosterone level will usually distinguish whether the levels are in the male range, as occurs in androgen insensitivity syndrome. Müllerian agenesis is associated with renal anomalies in 34% and skeletal anomalies in 12% of patients. Unilateral renal agenesis (15%) is the most common abnormality followed by skeletal anomalies, the most frequent of which are vertebral abnormalities. Klippel-Feil syndrome has been reported in association with müllerian agenesis. Müllerian agenesis, with a reported incidence of 1/5,000 to 1/20,000, is more common than androgen insensitivity and second in frequency to gonadal dysgenesis as a cause of primary amenorrhea. There is usually a normal female karyotype of 46 XX, but autosomal translocation of chromosomes 12q and 14q occurs. Affected siblings have been reported, as well as families with variable expression of defects in müllerian, renal, and skeletal systems.

An intravenous pyelogram (IVP) is indicated to determine the presence and extent of associated renal anomalies. Skeletal anomalies should also be ruled out. Karyotype determination will help in ruling out other diagnoses, such as androgen insensitivity (46XY). A pelvic ultrasound is helpful in defining the anomaly, and CT scanning and MRI provide increased refinement in detail. Laparoscopy is usually reserved for evaluation of a pelvic mass and associated abnormalities.

Vaginoplasty is best deferred until the patient has matured and should be supported by counseling for both patient and family. The MacIndoe procedure, the usual treatment of choice, involves the use of a skin graft, usually from the buttocks, to create a vagina after appropriate dissection of the vulvovaginal area. Other procedures have included the use of human amniotic membrane as an allograft and the use of fasciocutaneous flaps for vaginal reconstruction. The artificial vaginal epithelium changes cytologically to an almost normal-appearing vaginal mucosa. Various dilatation procedures result in an increased vaginal size, which ultimately permits intercourse. Squamous cell carcinoma of the reconstructed vagina has been reported and appears to be related to the type of tissue transplanted. Radiotherapy is probably the primary method of treatment for this particular squamous cell carcinoma.

TRANSVERSE VAGINAL SEPTA. The incidence of transverse vaginal septa is approximately 1/80,000 females. The patient presents with amenorrhea, which may be associated with cyclical pelvic pain, and often a pelvic mass as well as *cryptomenorrhea*. The problem is usually asymptomatic until puberty, although it may present in pediatric patients as *hydrometrocolpos*. It may be associated with other congenital anomalies, although this occurs less often than with müllerian agenesis. The most common site of the septum is between the middle and upper thirds of the vagina. These patients have a functional uterus, although their fertility is often compromised; 47% of affected females in one retrospective series had spontaneous abortions. The prognosis is worse for higher obstructions. There is also an increased incidence of endometriosis secondary to retrograde menstruation.

Evaluation of transverse vaginal septa includes careful pelvic examination and often pelvic imaging to delineate the anatomic abnormalities. Treatment is surgical resection of the obstruction from below. Anastomosis of the upper and lower segments should be attempted, if at all possible, to prevent stenosis. A skin graft may be necessary. Often a lucite form is placed in the vagina to maintain patency.

DISORDERS OF LATERAL FUSION. These include a number of anatomic variations of nonobstructive longitudinal septum as well as the obstructed hemivagina (Fig. 18–50). The latter may be associated with a didelphic uterus and often

TABLE 18–24. Heritable Disorders Associated with Müllerian Anomalies*

Mode of Inheritance	Disorder	Associated Müllerian Defect
Autosomal dominant	Camptobrachydactyly	Longitudinal vaginal septa
	Hand-foot-genital	Incomplete müllerian fusion
Autosomal recessive	Kaufman-McCusick	Transverse vaginal septa
	Johanson-Blizzard	Longitudinal vaginal septa
	Renal-genital-middle ear anomalies	Vaginal atresia
	Fraser syndrome	Incomplete müllerian fusion
	?Uterine hernia syndrome	Persistent müllerian duct derivatives
Polygenic/Multifactorial	Mayer-Rokitansky-Kuster-Hauser syndrome	Müllerian aplasia
X-linked	?Uterine hernia syndrome	Persistent müllerian duct derivatives

*From Shulman P, Elias S: Developmental abnormalities of the female reproductive tract: Pathogenesis and nosology. Adolesc Pediatr Gynecol 1:232, 1988.

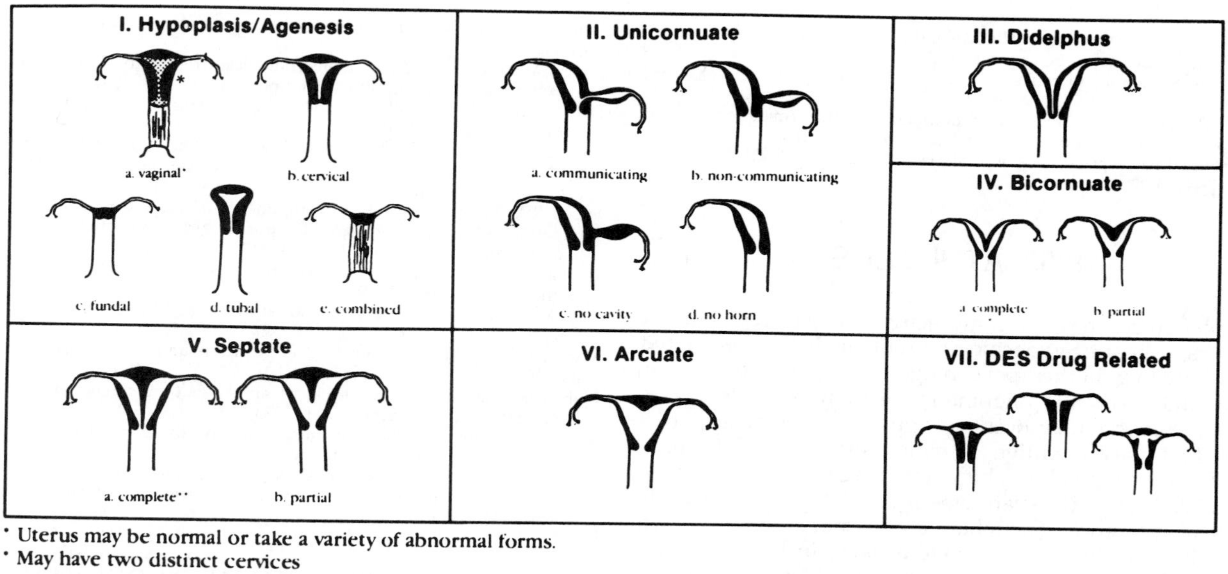

Figure 18–50. The American Fertility Society Classification of Müllerian Anomalies. (Reprinted with permission of the publishers, The American Fertility Society.)

with a pelvic mass, which represents retrograde menstruation associated with the occluded hemivagina. The patient presents with menses that are often cyclical, representing an unobstructed outflow tract from one of the uterine horns.

The incidence of uterine anomalies ranges from 1/100 to 1/1,000. Anomalous development of the uterine cavity may have a host of clinical presentations. The patient may present with primary amenorrhea or with irregular or even regular menses. There may be an asymptomatic pelvic mass or dysmenorrhea. In the adult, pregnancy wastage and infertility may cause the first suspicion of a uterine anomaly. Evaluation should include a pelvic ultrasound, IVP, and skeletal inspection for anomalies. Karyotyping and diagnostic laparoscopy may be necessary, depending on the presentation and laboratory assessment. A hysterosalpingogram may be helpful in further delineating the uterine anomaly.

Treatment depends on the specific anomaly and must be individualized accordingly. Traditionally, surgical repair of uterine malformations have included Strassman metroplasty, Jones "wedge" metroplasty, and Tompkins metroplasty. The obstructions to the outflow tract must also be relieved; this may necessitate creation of a vaginal window or excision of a hemivagina. Careful determination of retrograde menstruation in a uterine horn must also be considered and appropriate surgical correction provided.

CONGENITAL ATRESIA OF THE UTERINE CERVIX. The patient often presents at puberty with cryptomenorrhea, amenorrhea, and pelvic pain. This problem is extremely rare and is associated with significant renal anomalies in 5–10% of patients. On examination, there is complete absence of a cervix but the presence of a palpable uterus. Pelvic imaging is helpful in defining the abnormality. Treatment may include laparotomy to create a uterovaginal fistula. If this is impossible, a hysterectomy may be necessary. Other anomalies include mesonephric cysts, which are remnants of the wolffian duct. Incomplete reduplication of internal genitalia and unilateral renal aplasia also have been reported. Each of these patients had a didelphic uterus, in which one uterus emptied into a normally developed vagina and the other into a blind pouch (hemihematometra) or into an atretic vagina (hemihematocolpos). In addition, gastrointestinal (42.9%), respiratory (47.6%), central nervous system (28.6%), cardiovascular (38.1%), and musculoskeletal abnormalities (33.3%) also may be associated.

COMPLETE VULVAR DUPLICATION. This rare congenital anomaly presents in infancy and consists of two vulvas, vaginas, and bladders, a didelphic uterus, a single rectum and anus, and two renal systems.

LABIAL HYPERTROPHY. Elongation of the labia minora can be present at birth. Usually this is of no consequence. Surgical revision may be necessary if the problem is symptomatic.

CLITORAL ABNORMALITIES. Agenesis of the clitoris is rare. Clitoral duplication has been reported and is often associated with pelvic organ abnormalities, including agenesis of other genital structures as well as associated bladder exstrophy.

CLITORAL HYPERTROPHY IN ASSOCIATION WITH AMBIGUOUS GENITALIA. See Sec. 19.38.

HYMENAL ABNORMALITIES. An imperforate hymen can be present in the pediatric patient and is often associated with mucocolpos; it can also be associated with hydrometrocolpos. Other hymenal abnormalities include cribriform or stenotic hymen.

UROGYNECOLOGIC PROBLEMS AND SEXUALLY TRANSMITTED DISEASES

See Sec. 10.17 and 18.51.

Bergh P, Breen J, Gregori C: Congenital absence of the vagina—the Mayer-Rokitansky-Kuster-Hauser syndrome. Adolesc Pediatr Gynecol 2:73, 1989.
Freedman M: Uterine anomalies. Semin Reprod Endocrinol 4:39, 1986.
Hopkins M, Marley G: Squamous cell carcinoma of the neovagina. Obstet Gynecol 69:525, 1987.
Horejsi JA: Incomplete reduplication of internal genitalia and unilateral renal aplasia syndrome. Adolesc Pediatr Gynecol 1:42, 1988.
Jeffcoat T: Principles in Gynecology. London, Butterworth, 1957, p 153.
Joshi N, Sotrel G: Diagnostic laparoscopy in apparent uterine agenesis. J Adolesc Health Care 9:403, 1988.
Kucheria K, Taneja N, Kinra G: Autosomal translocation of chromosomes 12q and 14q in müllerian duct failure. Indian J Med Res 87:290, 1988.
Lewis V, Money J: Gender-identify/role. Par A:XY (androgen insensitivity) syndrome and XX (Rokitansky) syndrome, vaginal atresia compared. *In*: Dennerstein L, Burroughs G (eds): Handbook of Psychosomatic Obstetrics and Gynecology. New York, Elsevier Biomedical Press, 1983, p 61.

Morton K, Davies D, Dewhurst J: The use of the fasciocutaneous flap in vaginal reconstruction. Br J Obstet Gynaecol 93:970, 1986.
Rock J, Azziz R: Genital anomalies in childhood. Clin Obstet Gynecol 30:682, 1987.
Shulman LP, Elias S: Developmental abnormalities of the female reproductive tract: Pathogenesis and nosology. Adolesc Pediatr Gynecol 1:230, 1987.
Sorenson S: Estimated prevalence of müllerian anomalies. Acta Obstet Gynecol Scand 67:441, 1988.

18.58 ATHLETICS

As more females have become actively engaged in athletic endeavors, a host of gynecologic problems have been noted. It is unknown whether psychologic stress per se is a key factor in amenorrhea or oligomenorrhea among athletic girls.

Delayed menarche may occur in young women who participate in highly competitive activities such as ballet, figure skating, and gymnastics. The average age of onset of menarche is 12.23 yr, but for athletes it is 13.58 yr, a statistically significant difference. This change does not occur for swimmers. Ballet dancers tend to have a delay in both thelarche and menarche, but pubarche and adrenarche are not affected. The role of a threshold level of body fat in determining the onset of menarche and maintenance of regular ovulatory cycles is controversial.

Menstrual irregularity may be associated with intensity of exercise. The incidence of amenorrhea has varied widely (5–100%) depending on the population studied. Dale and associates noted that oligomenorrhea or amenorrhea occurred in 4% of control women versus 23% of joggers (5–30 miles/wk) and 34% of "runners" (>30 miles/wk). Decreased spontaneous luteinizing hormone pulse frequency may be associated with the onset of secondary amenorrhea in long-distance runners. Ballet dancers frequently experience oligomenorrhea with the onset of increased training without significant weight change. Secondary amenorrhea is defined as the cessation of menstruation for at least 6 mo or 3 menstrual cycles after the patient has attained menarche. The diagnosis of secondary amenorrhea due to athletic endeavors is a "diagnosis of exclusion." The clinician should approach any menstrual aberration in the athlete in a manner similar to that in a nonathlete (see Sec. 10.18). Pregnancy tests should always be obtained, as well as serum prolactin and gonadotropin levels (follicle stimulating hormone and luteinizing hormone).

It has been reported that women have less *premenstrual tension* when they actively exercise. This may be attributable to a reduction in antidiuretic hormone levels or an increase in the output of β-endorphins.

Other *endocrinologic changes* associated with athletic activity include hypoestrogenism and an altered follicle stimulating hormone–to–luteinizing hormone ratio, as well as acute elevation of serum testosterone, prolactin, catecholamines, and opioids. *Premature bone loss* has also been reported.

Breast injuries are uncommon in most sports. However, mastodynia and nipple irritation do occur. A proper fitting bra that is not too tight often prevents this discomfort. Adhesive strip bandages or nursing pads tend to alleviate the problems of nipple abrasion. The American College of Obstetricians and Gynecologists (ACOG) has issued safety guidelines for women in sports that may be helpful to patients experiencing problems.

American College of Obstetricians and Gynecologists: Women and Exercise. Washington, D.C., Technical Bulletin No. 87, Sept. 1985.
Beldhuis J, Evans W, Demer L, et al: Altered neuroendocrine regulation of gonadotropin secretion in women distance runners. J Clin Endocrinol Metab 61:557, 1985.
Bonen A, Keizer H: Athletic menstrual cycle irregularity: Endocrine response to exercise and training. Physician Sports Med 12:78, 1984.
Dale E, Gerlach D, Wilhite A: Menstrual dysfunction in distance runners. Obstet Gynecol 54:47, 1979.
Emans SJ: The athletic adolescent with amenorrhea. Pediatr Ann 13:605, 1984.
Falk RJ: Ovarian malfunction: When is it exercise induced? Contemp Obstet Gynecol 9:187, 1984.
Frisch RE, Revelle R, Cook S: Components of weight at menarche and the initiation of the adolescent growth spurt in girls: Estimated total water, lean body weight and fat. Hum Biol 45:469, 1973.
Gonzalez E: Premature bone loss found in some nonmenstruating sports women. JAMA 248:513, 1982.
Hale R: Exercise, sports, and menstrual function. Clin Obstet Gynecol 26:728, 1983.
Malina RM: Menarche in athletes: A synthesis and hypothesis. Ann Human Biol 10:1, 1983.
Malina R, Harper A, Avent H, et al: Age at menarche in athletes and nonathletes. Med Sci Sports 5:11, 1973.
Scott E, Johnston F: Critical fat, menarche, and the maintenance of menstrual cycles: A critical review. J Adolesc Health Care 2:249, 1982.
Shangold M, Gatz M, Thysen B: Acute effects of exercise on plasma concentrations of prolactin and testosterone in recreational women runners. Fertil Steril 35:699, 1981.

18.59 CHILDREN WITH SPECIAL NEEDS

Gynecologic care for the mentally handicapped pediatric or adolescent patient is a challenging task. When the mentally handicapped adolescent presents to the clinician with the problem of "perineal hygiene," an adequate gynecologic examination is required. Outpatient sedation with oral ketamine (Ketalar) and midazolam (Versed) markedly decreases the need for examination under anesthesia. Once an adequate examination, including a Pap smear, is obtained, the various alternative treatments should be discussed.

A number of medical approaches have been proposed to suppress the menses, for example, depomedroxyprogesterone acetate, usually prescribed at a dose of 125 mg/60 kg, injected intramuscularly every 6–12 wk. Other alternatives are the use of oral contraceptives, which will not produce amenorrhea but will result in marked decrease in the quantity of menstrual flow, resulting in a more manageable condition. Before the clinician considers a surgical approach such as hysterectomy, there should be a thorough discussion with parents or custodians after a trial of medical treatment that has not been successful.

An ethics advisory committee should be consulted to aid in decisions to sterilize mentally handicapped patients (see also Sec. 2.4).

SEXUAL ABUSE (See Sec. 3.53)

TEENAGE PREGNANCY (See Sec. 10.15)

JOSEPH S. SANFILIPPO

Braham D: House of Lords upholds decision to sterilise 17-year-old mentally handicapped girl. Lancet 1:1099, 1987.
Elkins T, Hoyle D, Darnton T, et al: The use of a societally based ethics class advisory committee to aid in decisions to sterilize mentally handicapped patients. Adolesc Pediatr Gynecol 1:190, 1988.
Elkins T, McNeeley S, Rosen D, et al: A clinical observation of a program to accomplish pelvic exams in difficult-to-manage patients with mental retardation. Adolesc Pediatr Gynecol 1:195, 1988.

19

THE ENDOCRINE SYSTEM

19.1 DISORDERS OF THE HYPOTHALAMUS AND PITUITARY GLAND

The anterior pituitary originates from the Rathke pouch as an invagination of the oral endoderm. It then detaches from the oral epithelium and becomes an individual structure of rapidly proliferating cells. Persistent postnatal fetal rests of the original connection of the Rathke pouch with the oral cavity often develop into craniopharyngiomas, the most common tumor arising in this area. There are five clearly distinguishable cell types in the anterior pituitary. They are growth hormone (GH)–secreting somatotropes, prolactin-secreting lactotropes, thyrotropin-secreting thyrotropes, corticotropes that secrete corticotropin and other pro-opiomelanocortin–derived peptides, and gonadotropes that synthesize follicle-stimulating and luteinizing hormones. However, pituitary adenomas are often plurihormonal, producing two hormones or more, the most frequent combination being GH and prolactin.

FUNCTION. ***Anterior Lobe*.** The anterior pituitary secretes a variety of protein hormones. These hormones act either on other endocrine glands or directly on certain body cells to affect almost every organ. The pituitary gland itself is under the control of hypothalamic secretions, each of which regulates specific pituitary cells. Many conditions formerly classified as of pituitary origin in fact have a hypothalamic origin, and availability of the major pituitary-releasing hormones now permits more precise delineation of these endocrinologic conditions. The endings of some hypothalamic fibers liberate their hormones into the capillaries of the median eminence, from which they are carried by portal veins to the pituitary gland. Accordingly, the median eminence is the final common pathway of all the hypothalamic hormones.

GH is a protein with 191 amino acids; its gene (hGH-N) is one of a cluster of five closely related genes on the long arm of chromosome 17 (q22-24). The four other genes have 90% homology with the GH gene; they consist of two coexpressed chorionic somatomammotropin genes (hCS-A and -B) and a related gene (hCS-L), and a GH variant gene (hGH-V), which encodes a protein detectable in the placenta, suggesting a role in the fetomaternal unit. The secretion of GH is controlled mainly by two hypothalamic hormones, the *growth hormone–releasing hormone* (GHRH), which consists of three molecular species (37, 40, and 44 amino acids), and *somatostatin*, a 14-amino acid cyclic peptide, which inhibits the secretion of GH. Somatostatin also acts as a neurohormone and a neurotransmitter via autocrine and paracrine mechanisms, especially in the gastrointestinal tract. Thus, it also inhibits secretion of insulin, glucagon, secretin, gastrin, and vasoactive intestinal peptide as well as thyrotropin. In the pancreatic islets it is localized to the D cells; somatostatin-secreting pancreatic tumors *(somatostatinoma)* have been reported in adults. A potent long-acting somatostatin analog, *octreotide*, which inhibits GH preferentially over insulin, is now available to treat patients with GH-secreting tumors; it is also useful in managing patients with gastrinomas, insulinomas, glucagonomas, vipomas, and carcinoids (see Sec. 8.59 and 13.68). ^{123}I-labeled octreotide also appears to be useful in localizing these somatostatin receptor–positive tumors and their metastases. The alternating secretion of GHRH and somatostatin accounts for the rhythmic secretion of GH.

Growth hormone circulates bound predominantly to a specific high-affinity 150-dalton protein, which is a fragment of the GH receptor. The mitogenic actions of GH are mediated through synthesis of *insulin-like growth factor-1* (IGF-1), formerly named somatomedin C, a single-chain peptide with 70 amino acids coded for by a gene on the long arm of chromosome 12. IGF-1 has considerable homology to insulin. Circulating IGF-1 is synthesized primarily in the liver, but it is also formed locally in mesodermal and ectodermal cells, particularly in the growth plate of children, where its effect is exerted by paracrine or autocrine mechanisms. Circulating levels of IGF-1 are related to blood levels of GH to a large extent, except in the fetus and during the neonatal period. IGF-1 circulates bound to several different binding proteins; the major one is a 150-dalton complex (SmBP), which is decreased in GH-deficient children but is in the normal range in non–GH-deficient short children. Human recombinant IGF-1 is currently being used experimentally to determine its therapeutic potential. IGF-2 is a single-chain protein with 67 amino acids that is coded for by a gene on the short arm of chromosome 11; it has homology to IGF-1, but much less is known about its physiologic roles, although it appears to be an important mitogen in bone cells, where it occurs in a concentration many times higher than IGF-1.

Disorders of growth owing to deficiencies of GHRH, GH, or IGF-1 are known. At the molecular level, one form of GH deficiency and one form of GH-receptor abnormality have been delineated.

When plasma levels of GH are measured by standard radioimmunoassay (RIA), its secretion appears to be pulsatile, but when measured by an ultrasensitive immunoradiometric assay (IRMA), which can measure GH in the previously undetectable range, it is observed to be secreted in a rhythmic fashion with a dominant 2-hr periodicity. The highest levels of GH are achieved during sleep when measured by either RIA or IRMA.

Prolactin is composed of 199 amino acids, and its gene is located on chromosome 6. The identity of the prolactin-releasing factor (PRF) is still unknown, but recent evidence suggests that it is localized almost exclusively in the intermediate lobe of the pituitary rather than in the hypothalamus. The major prolactin-inhibiting factor (PIF) is dopamine, and medications that disrupt hypothalamic dopaminergic pathways result in increased serum levels of prolactin. Serum levels of prolactin are increased after administration of thyrotropin-releasing hormone (TRH), in states of primary hypothyroidism, and after disruption of the pituitary stalk, as may occur in children with craniopharyngioma.

The main established role for prolactin is the initiation and maintenance of lactation. Concentrations in amniotic fluid are 10–100 times the levels in maternal or fetal serum; the major source of amniotic prolactin appears to be the decidua. Mean serum levels in children and in fasting adults of both sexes are about 5–20 ng/mL, but levels in the fetus and in neonates during the 1st wk of life are usually over 200 ng/mL.

Thyrotropin (TSH) consists of two glycoprotein chains linked by hydrogen bonding. The α chain is identical to that found in follicle-stimulating hormone (FSH), luteinizing hormone (LH), and chorionic gonadotropin (hCG). The β chain is unique in each of these hormones and confers specificity. The gene for the α chain has been mapped on chromosome 6, that for the β chain of TSH on chromosome 1, and those for the β chains for LH and hCG on chromosome 19. TSH increases iodine uptake, iodide clearance from the plasma, iodotyrosine and iodothyronine formation, thyroglobulin proteolysis, and release of thyroxine and triiodothyronine from the thyroid. Most of the effects of TSH are mediated by cyclic adenosine monophosphate (cAMP). Deficiency results in inactivity and atrophy of the thyroid, and excess results in hypertrophy and hyperplasia.

TSH-releasing hormone (TRH) was the first hypothalamic hormone to be isolated, characterized, and synthesized; it is a tripeptide ([pyro] Glu-His-Pro-NH_2). Thyroxine (T_4) and triiodothyronine (T_3) inhibit TSH secretion by blocking the action of TRH on the pituitary cell. TRH also stimulates the release of prolactin, in males as well as in females. Synthetic TRH is useful for testing pituitary reserves of TSH and prolactin.

Corticotropin (ACTH) is derived by proteolytic cleavage from a large precursor glycoprotein product of the pituitary gland called *pro-opiomelanocortin* (POMC). Cleavage of POMC yields both ACTH (a single, unbranched glycoprotein chain of 39 amino acids) and β-lipotropin (β-LPH) (a 91-amino acid glycoprotein). Further cleavage of ACTH and β-LPH in the pituitary yields yet other hormonal products. Thus, α-melanocyte–stimulating hormone (α-MSH) is identical to the first 13 amino acids of ACTH but has no corticotropin activity; cleavage of β-LPH results in neurotropic peptides with morphinomimetic activity (fragment 61–91 is β-endorphin); and β-melanocyte–stimulating hormone (β-MSH) consists of a 17-amino acid fragment of β-LPH.

Corticotropin acts primarily on the adrenal gland; it produces changes in structure, chemical composition, enzymatic activity, and release of corticosteroid hormones. ACTH release has a diurnal rhythm; it is lowest between 10 P.M. and 2 A.M. with peak levels reached about 8 A.M. Levels of β-LPH and of β-endorphin are elevated in patients with endocrine disorders with increased ACTH. It appears that ACTH rather than MSH is the principal pigmentary hormone in humans.

Pro-opiomelanocortin peptides are also produced in nonpituitary tissues; in the testis some peptides act as autocrine regulators of androgen-secreting Leydig cells, whereas others may either potentiate or oppose the action of FSH on Sertoli cells.

Secretion of ACTH, of β-endorphin, and of other pro-opiomelanocortin-related peptides is regulated by corticotropin-releasing hormone (CRH). CRH is a 41-amino acid peptide found predominantly in the median eminence but also in other areas of the brain and in tissues outside the brain, particularly the placenta. During pregnancy, levels of CRH rise several hundred-fold, increase further during labor and delivery, and then fall to nonpregnant levels within 24 hr; its source is probably the placenta, which contains the peptide and its gene. Both synthetic ovine (oCRH) and human CRH (hCRH) have been used clinically; oCRH is the clinical agent of choice because responses to it are greater and longer lasting than with hCRH. It is particularly useful in differentiating different forms of Cushing syndrome.

Gonadotropic hormones include two glycoproteins: LH (luteinizing hormone or lutropin) and FSH (follicle-stimulating hormone or follitropin). Each has an α subunit and a β subunit. The α subunits of these two hormones and of TSH are identical; specificity of hormone action resides in the β subunit, which is different for each of the three. Receptors for FSH on the ovarian granulosa cells and on testicular Sertoli cells mediate FSH stimulation of follicular development in the ovary and of gametogenesis in the testis. On binding to specific receptors on ovarian theca cells and testicular Leydig cells, LH promotes luteinization of the ovary and Leydig cell function of the testis. Both LH and FSH activate adenyl cyclase by way of a guanine nucleotide–regulatory protein.

Hypothalamic control of gonadotropic hormones has long been known, and separate releasing hormones for FSH and LH were once anticipated. Luteinizing hormone–releasing hormone (LHRH), a decapeptide, has been isolated, synthesized, and widely used in clinical studies. Since it leads to the release of both LH and FSH, it is now proposed that there may be only one gonadotropin-releasing hormone.

Secretion of LH is inhibited by androgens and estrogens, whereas secretion of FSH is suppressed by gonadal production of *inhibin*, a 31-kD glycoprotein, produced by the Sertoli cells. Inhibin consists of α and β subunits joined by disulfide bonds. The β-β dimer *(activin)* also occurs, but its biologic effect is to stimulate FSH secretion. The biology of these new hormones is only now being delineated. In addition to its endocrine effect, activin has paracrine effects in the testis; it facilitates LH-induced testosterone production, indicating a direct effect of Sertoli cells on Leydig cells analogous to the interaction of these cells through the paracrine effects of pro-opiomelanocortin.

Posterior Lobe. The posterior lobe of the pituitary is part of a functional unit (the neurohypophysis) that consists of (1) the neurons of the supraoptic and paraventricular nuclei of the hypothalamus; (2) neuronal axons, which form the pituitary stalk; and (3) neuronal terminals, either in the median eminence or in the posterior lobe.

The neurohypophysis is the source of *arginine vasopressin* (AVP, the antidiuretic hormone) and of *oxytocin;* both are octapeptides, differing in only two amino acids. These hormones are produced by neurosecretion in the hypothalamic nuclei. Vasopressin derives its name from early observations of its pressor and its antidiuretic activities; however, the latter is its physiologically important function. At levels 50–1,000 times those found in blood, it affects blood pressure, intestinal contractibility, hepatic glycogenolysis, platelet aggregation, and release of factor VIII. Vasopressin and oxytocin are secreted by separate cells of the supraoptic and paraventricular nuclei. Secreted concurrently in equimolar amounts with these hormones are vasopressin neurophysin (neurophysin II) and oxytocin neurophysin (neurophysin I). Each hormone binds to its respective neurophysin and is transported to the nerve terminals in the posterior pituitary, where it is secreted in the free form. Radioimmunoassays of the neurophysins provide a direct index of vasopressin and oxytocin levels in plasma. The concentration of arginine vasopressin in umbilical cord plasma appears to be a sensitive indicator of fetal stress.

Vasopressin has a short half-life and responds very quickly to changes in hydration. It changes the permeability of the renal tubular cell membrane via cAMP. A synthetic analog, desmopressin, is resistant to peptidases and has a prolonged half-life. Small amounts administered intranasally are effective in therapy of patients with diabetes insipidus.

19.2 HYPOPITUITARISM

This section discusses only those hypopituitary states associated with deficiency of growth hormone (Table 19–1). Affected

TABLE 19–1. Etiologic Classification of Hypopituitarism: Pituitary and/or Hypothalamic Dysfunction

- Developmental defects
  - Anencephaly
  - Holoprosencephaly (cyclopia, cebocephaly, orbital hypotelorism)
  - Midfacial anomalies (e.g., hypertelorism)
  - Basal encephalocele
  - Septo-optic dysplasia (de Morsier syndrome)
  - Cleft lip and palate
  - Solitary maxillary central incisor
  - Hall-Pallister syndrome (hypothalamic hamartoblastoma, imperforate anus, polydactyly)
  - Rieger syndrome
  - Fanconi syndrome
- Genetic defects of GH or GHRH
  - Isolated GH deficiency
    - Autosomal recessive—type I
      - Type IA—deletion of gene for GH
      - Type IB
    - Autosomal dominant–type II
    - X-linked—type III
  - Multiple pituitary deficiencies
    - Autosomal recessive–type I
    - X-linked—type III
- Destructive lesions
  - Trauma
    - Perinatal (trauma, anoxia, hemorrhagic infarction)
    - Basal skull fractures
    - Child abuse
  - Infiltrative lesions
    - Tumors
      - Histocytosis X
      - Craniopharyngioma
      - Hypothalamic tumors
      - Germinoma
      - Optic glioma
      - Pituitary adenomas
      - Sarcoidosis
      - Hemochromatosis
      - Tuberculosis
      - Toxoplasmosis
      - Irradiation (central nervous system, eyes, middle ears)
      - Surgery
      - Removal of pharyngeal pituitary
      - Surgery for craniopharyngioma and other tumors
  - Vascular
    - Infarctions (e.g., hemoglobinopathy)
    - Aneurysm
- Autoimmune hypophysitis
- Unresponsiveness to growth hormone
  - Insulin-like growth factor deficiency
    - Laron syndrome (GH receptor gene deletion or mutations)
    - African pygmy (GH receptor deficiency)
    - Little women of Loja
  - Bioinactive growth hormone
- Other functional deficiency
  - Hypothyroidism
  - Psychosocial deprivation

children have usually been referred to as pituitary dwarfs, a designation best avoided. Isolated deficiencies of thyrotropin, corticotropin, and gonadotropin are discussed later.

ETIOLOGY. Congenital Defects. Aplasia or hypoplasia of the pituitary is rare. Developmental abnormalities of the pituitary are associated with such defects as anencephaly, holoprosencephaly (cyclopia, cebocephaly, orbital hypotelorism), and septo-optic dysplasia (de Morsier syndrome). In *Hall-Pallister syndrome* absence of the pituitary gland is associated with hypothalamic hamartoblastoma, postaxial polydactyly, nail dysplasia, bifid epiglottis, imperforate anus, and anomalies of the heart, lungs, and kidneys; most patients die neonatally, but in at least one case neonatal hypopituitarism was recognized, computed tomography (CT) scan revealed the hypothalamic tumor, and surgical removal was successful at 1 yr of age. In the neonate, symptoms of hypopituitarism with postaxial polydactyly and bifid epiglottis should suggest this diagnosis. Hypoplasia of the pituitary with anencephaly has long been known, but recent observations reveal a large residuum of normal pituitary function and suggest that hypoplasia may be secondary to the hypothalamic defect. With hypothalamic-releasing hormones it is possible to determine whether defects in pituitary function reside in the pituitary or in the hypothalamus. Many of these conditions are lethal early in life, but partial defects may occur in siblings. A child has been reported with isolated deficiency of growth hormone and mild hypotelorism who had two siblings with holoprosencephaly with hypopituitarism. Deficiency of growth hormone occurs in 4% of all patients with *cleft lip* or *cleft palate* and in 32% of those who also have short stature. Midfacial anomalies or the finding of a *solitary maxillary central incisor* indicates a high likelihood of growth hormone deficiency.

Optic nerve hypoplasia, bilateral or unilateral, is often associated with hypopituitarism. When it is also associated with absence of the septum pellucidum, the condition is known as *septo-optic dysplasia*. The fundus exhibits hypoplastic disks with typical double rims and sparse retinal vessels. Endocrine abnormalities are extremely variable. Hormonal deficiency most often involves GH alone, but multiple pituitary deficiencies, including diabetes insipidus, may occur. The defect resides primarily in the hypothalamus. Delay in linear growth may begin as early as 3 mo of age or may not be observed before 3–4 yr of age. Affected newborns often have apnea, hypotonia and seizures, prolonged jaundice, hypoglycemia without hyperinsulinism, and (in males) microphallus. The condition is usually sporadic but has been reported in first cousins. The cause is unknown but young maternal age and nulliparity are strongly associated.

Aplasia of the pituitary without abnormalities of the brain or skull is very rare, but affected infants are being increasingly recognized because hypoglycemia occurs early and in males there is microphallus. Some infants have shown evidence of the neonatal hepatitis syndrome, but the relationship of hypopituitarism is obscure. The condition has been reported in siblings of both sexes, and consanguinity has been noted in two families; autosomal recessive inheritance is suggested. Studies in some children have placed the defect in the hypothalamus. This may be a heterogeneous group of disorders.

In *empty-sella syndrome* a deficient sellar diaphragm leads to herniation of the suprasellar subarachnoid space into the sella turcica, with remodeling of the sella and flattening of the pituitary gland. It may follow surgery or radiation therapy or be idiopathic. Of 17 cases reported in children, significant hypopituitarism was present in 5. Empty-sella with an enlarged sella and hypopituitarism has been observed in siblings.

Hypogammaglobulinemia has been associated with isolated GH deficiency in two families as an X-linked trait. The relationship between the two disorders is not clear.

Other syndromes in which short stature is a prominent feature may be associated with deficiency of GH; for example, occasionally patients with Turner, Fanconi, Russell-Silver, Rieger, Williams, or the CHARGE syndrome have been found to have hypopituitarism.

Destructive Lesions. Any lesion that damages the anterior pituitary or hypothalamus may cause cessation of growth. Since such lesions are not selective, multiple hormonal deficiencies are usually observed. The most common lesion is the craniopharyngioma; central nervous system germinoma, eosinophilic granuloma and other hypothalamic tumors, tuberculosis, sarcoidosis, toxoplasmosis, and aneurysms may also cause hypothalamic-hypophyseal destruction. These lesions are frequently associated with roentgenographic changes in the skull. Besides diabetes insipidus, deficiency of GH and other pituitary hormones may occur in children with histiocytosis, especially if treated with cranial irradiation. Enlargement of the sella or deformation or destruction of the clinoid processes usually indicates a tumor. Intrasellar or suprasellar calcifications usually indicate a craniopharyngioma. Trauma, including child abuse, traction at delivery, anoxia, and hemorrhagic infarction, may also damage the pituitary, its stalk, or the hypothalamus.

Improved survival of children who receive radiotherapy for malignancies of the central nervous system or other cranial structures has resulted in a substantial group of patients with deficiency of growth hormone. Children with acute lymphocytic leukemia who have received prophylactic cranial irradiation also belong in this group. Deceleration of growth usually appears slowly during the years after cancer therapy. The dose of irradiation and the fractionation schedule used are important determinants of the incidence of hypopituitarism. Growth hormone deficiency is almost universal 5 yr after therapy when the dose is 35–45 Gy; harmful radiation dose is probably close to 18–20 Gy. Deficiency of GH is usually the only defect, but deficiencies of TSH, ACTH, and gonadotropins may also occur.

Idiopathic Hypopituitarism. In most patients with hypopituitarism, there is no demonstrable lesion of the pituitary or hypothalamus; and in most, the functional defect is hypothalamic rather than pituitary. The deficiency may be of GH only or of multiple hormones. The condition is most often sporadic. Association with breech birth, forceps delivery, and intrapartum and maternal bleeding suggests that birth trauma and anoxia may be pathogenic factors in some instances.

In 5–10% of cases, the deficiency is familial. Patients with isolated GH deficiency (IGHD) are classified on the basis of mode of inheritance—autosomal recessive (type I), autosomal dominant (type II), or X-linked (type III). Patients with type I IGHD are subdivided into two subtypes, those with deletion of the GH gene (type IA) and those with no gene deletion (type IB). Likewise, patients with multiple pituitary deficiencies are classified into autosomal recessive (type I) and X-linked (type II).

Approximately 38 patients with type IA IGHD and gene deletion have been reported from 15 countries. Patients often have onset of growth retardation before 6 mo of age and by early childhood have heights greater than 5 standard deviations (SD) below the mean. Plasma levels of GH, both spontaneous secretion and after provocative stimulation, are virtually absent. There is no response to stimulation with GHRH. Initially, there is a response to treatment with hGH, but most patients become refractory to treatment. These patients develop high titers of anti-hGH antibodies, presumably because it acts as a foreign protein in a patient who has never been exposed to endogenous hGH. Other patients have good long-term growth despite high antibody titers. The gene cluster has been examined in a large number of patients with type IA and in most a 6.7-kb deletion has been found. Since the hGH gene is part of a cluster of five very similar genes, it appears that the highly homologous DNA sequences are predisposed to unequal recombination, leading to deletion of the gene.

Patients with type IB isolated growth hormone deficiency produce small amounts of GH to provocative stimuli and respond well to exogenous hGH. These patients respond to stimulation with GHRH, suggesting that the defect is a genetic deficiency in GHRH.

Growth Hormone–Receptor Defects. Children with *Laron syndrome* have all the clinical findings of those with hypopituitarism, but they have elevated plasma levels of biologically active growth hormone, whereas levels of IGF-1 are very low, and they fail to respond to exogenous hGH. One of the high-affinity GH-binding proteins present in the plasma of normal children is absent in patients with Laron syndrome; this protein is derived from the extracellular domain of the GH receptor. Sephardic Jews have been found to have deletions of a large portion of the GH-binding receptor gene; in other families, the defect appears to be a point mutation of the receptor gene. The condition is recessively inherited and, although originally reported in 14 Oriental Jewish families, it has also been reported in other ethnic groups. A normal spontaneous pregnancy in an affected woman indicates that IGF-1 is not obligatory for fertility. Acute administration of biosynthetic IGF-1 to affected children results in the expected biologic effects and suggests that its long-term administration may prove effective in enhancing growth.

African pygmies in the rain forest of Equatorial Africa have normal levels of GH and low levels of IGF-1. Affected children are usually below the 20th percentile in height until 10 yr of age, when growth stops. This growth pattern differs from that seen in children with Laron syndrome. Levels of the specific GH-binding protein are relatively normal in early childhood but fail to increase with increasing age as they do in normal individuals. This suggests that the defect is a failure of receptors to increase in a normal manner rather than a structural defect in the GH-receptor gene.

The *little women of Loja* is a newly reported syndrome of high plasma levels of GH associated with very low levels of IGF-1. The condition has been found in a small, highly inbred Spanish community in Loja, Ecuador. It is distinctive from Laron syndrome in that only females are affected. The condition is thought to be lethal for males in early fetal life. The nature of the presumed receptor defect is unknown.

CLINICAL MANIFESTATIONS. In Patients without Demonstrable Lesions of the Pituitary. The child with hypopituitarism is usually of normal size and weight at birth. In about half of affected children the retardation of growth is noticed by 1 yr of age. In others there may be regular but slow growth in height, with the increments always below normal percentiles, or periods of lack of growth may alternate with short spurts of growth. Delayed closure of the epiphyses permits growth beyond the age when normal persons cease to grow.

Infants with congenital defects of the pituitary or hypothalamus usually present such neonatal emergencies as apnea, cyanosis, or severe hypoglycemia. Microphallus in the male is an important diagnostic clue. Deficiency of growth hormone may be accompanied by hypoadrenalism and hypothyroidism, and clinical manifestations of hypopituitarism evolve more rapidly than in the usual hypopituitary child.

The head is round and the face short and broad. The frontal bone is prominent and the bridge of the nose depressed and saddle-shaped. The nose is small, and the nasolabial folds are well developed. The eyes are somewhat bulging. The mandible and the chin are underdeveloped and infantile, and the teeth, which erupt late, are frequently crowded. The neck is short and the larynx small. The voice is high-pitched and remains high after puberty. The extremities are well proportioned, with small hands and feet. The genitalia are usually underdeveloped for the child's age, and sexual maturation may be delayed or absent. Facial, axillary, and pubic hair is usually absent; the hair of the scalp is fine. Symptomatic hypoglycemia, usually after fasting, occurs in 10–15% of children with panhypopituitarism as well as with isolated growth hormone deficiency. Intelligence is usually normal. Affected children may become shy and retiring.

Patients with Demonstrable Lesions of the Pituitary. The child is normal initially, and manifestations similar to those seen in idiopathic pituitary growth failure gradually appear and progress. When complete or almost complete destruction of the pituitary gland occurs, severe manifestations of pituitary insufficiency are present. Atrophy of the adrenal cortex, thyroid, and gonads results in loss of weight, asthenia, sensitivity to cold, mental torpor, and absence of sweating. Sexual maturation fails to take place or regresses if already present. Thus, there may be atrophy of the gonads and genital tract with amenorrhea and loss of pubic and axillary hair. There is a tendency to hypoglycemia and coma. Growth ceases. Diabetes insipidus may be present early but tends to improve spontaneously as the anterior pituitary is progressively destroyed.

If the lesion is an expanding tumor, symptoms such as headache, vomiting, visual disturbances, pathologic sleep, decreased school performance, seizures, polyuria, and growth failure may be present. Growth failure frequently antedates the neurologic signs and symptoms, especially in patients with craniopharyngiomas, but symptoms of hormonal deficit account for only 10% of presenting complaints. In other patients the neurologic manifestations may precede the endocrinologic, or evidence of pituitary insufficiency may first appear after surgical intervention. In children with craniopharyngiomas, visual field defects, optic atrophy, papilledema, and cranial nerve palsy are common.

LABORATORY DATA. The diagnosis of classic growth hormone deficiency, with or without an organic lesion of the hypothalamus or pituitary, rests upon demonstration of absent or low levels of GH in response to stimulation. GH appears to be secreted episodically because plasma levels are often below the level of detectability on assay; its plasma concentration fluctuates over a wide range with major secretory pulses occurring during early nocturnal slow-wave sleep. A variety of provocative tests have been devised that rapidly increase the level of growth hormone in normal children. These include a 20-min period of strenuous exercise or administration of L-dopa, insulin, arginine, clonidine, or glucagon. Because administration of each of these agents can result in false-negative responses, two tests or more are usually performed. Peak levels of GH below 7 ng/mL strongly suggest GH deficiency.

During the 3 decades when hGH was obtained by extraction from human pituitary glands culled at autopsy, its supply was sharply limited, and only patients with classic GH deficiency were treated. With the advent of an unlimited supply of recombinant GH, there has been a marked interest in redefining the criteria for GH deficiency in order to include children with lesser degrees of deficiency. In recent years it has become popular to evaluate the spontaneous secretion of GH by measuring its level every 20 min during a 24- or 12-hr (8 P.M.–8 A.M.) period; this mode of evaluation appears to offer advantages over the traditional provocative tests. Some short children with normal levels of GH when studied by provocative tests have been found to have a marked deficiency of pulsatile secretion when levels are measured every 30 min; such children are thought to have GH *neurosecretory dysfunction*. With the collection of more normative data, it is now clear that frequent GH sampling offers little diagnostic advantage in most short children because of the wide range of secretory patterns in children with normal heights; marked variations have been observed in the same child on consecutive nights, and GH levels in normal children may even overlap those in children with classic GH deficiency. Although the laboratory criteria for GH deficiency in patients with severe (classic) hypopituitarism are well established, diagnostic criteria are unsettled for short children with lesser degrees of GH deficiency.

Levels of IGF-1 (somatomedin C) reflect those of GH and are often used to indicate GH deficiency. Diagnostic use of IGF-1 levels requires comparison with age- and sex-matched controls. In healthy children, levels of IGF-1 gradually increase from birth to a peak at puberty; in girls, peak levels occur 2 yr earlier than in boys. In classic GH-deficient children, levels of IGF-1 are low but usually rise significantly within 16–28 hr of hGH administration. Before 10 yr of age, a single measurement of IGF-1 level cannot usually discriminate between children with and those without GH deficiency.

In addition to establishing the diagnosis of GH deficiency, it is necessary to examine other pituitary functions. Levels of TSH and T_4, ACTH, cortisol, dehydroepiandrosterone sulfate (DHEAS), gonadotropins, and gonadal steroids may provide evidence of other pituitary hormonal deficiencies. The defect can be localized to the hypothalamus if there is a normal response to the administration of hypothalamic-releasing hormones for GH, TSH, ACTH, or gonadotropins. Thus, when there is a deficiency of TSH, serum levels of T_4 and TSH are low. A normal rise in TSH and prolactin following stimulation with thyrotropin-releasing hormone places the defect in the hypothalamus, whereas absence of such a response localizes the defect to the pituitary. An elevated level of plasma prolactin taken at random in the patient with hypopituitarism is also strong evidence that the defect is in the hypothalamus rather than in the pituitary. Some children with craniopharyngioma have elevated prolactin levels before surgery but after surgery prolactin deficiency occurs owing to pituitary damage. Antidiuretic hormone deficiency may be established by appropriate studies.

ROENTGENOGRAPHIC EXAMINATION. The long bones are slender and poor in minerals, the centers of ossification appear late, and the epiphyseal clefts remain open. The fontanels may remain open beyond the 2nd yr, and intersutural wormian bones may be found. The sella turcica may be abnormally small, but a normal sellar volume does not exclude the diagnosis. Occasionally the sella turcica may be partially or completely filled with cerebrospinal fluid; it is then known as an *empty sella*. In one study only 2 of 32 children with GH deficiency had an empty sella. Roentgenograms of the skull are most helpful when there is a destructive or space-occupying lesion causing hypopituitarism. In patients with nausea, vomiting, loss of vision, headache, or increase in circumference of the head, evidence of increased intracranial pressure may be found. Enlargement of the sella, especially ballooning with erosion and calcifications within or above the sella, may be detected. CT scan or magnetic resonance imaging (MRI) is indicated in all patients with hypopituitarism.

DIFFERENTIAL DIAGNOSIS. The causes of growth disorders are legion; systemic conditions such as inflammatory bowel disease, occult renal disease, and Turner syndrome must always be considered.

A small number of children with decreased growth velocity have normal levels of immunoreactive GH but deficient levels by radioreceptor assay and an abnormal ratio of the two levels. Levels of IGF-1 may be low or normal. Treatment with GH may result in normalization of growth rate and in increase in somatomedin levels. In one such patient the circulating GH was an abnormal polymer with low bioactivity. Many other theoretical defects of GH structure resulting in *bioinactive GH* are possible; this cause of hypopituitarism may be more frequent than previously recognized.

A small number of otherwise normal children are short (more than 3 SD below the mean for age) and grow 5 cm/yr or less but have normal levels of GH in response to provocative tests as well as normal spontaneous episodic secretion. A significant percentage of such children have increased rates of growth when treated with GH in doses comparable to those used to treat children with hypopituitarism. Plasma levels of IGF-1 in these patients may be normal or low. No long-term results are available, and it is not known whether the final heights in this group of patients will be improved. There are no methods that predict reliably which of these children will respond to GH. Treatment of otherwise normal short children without proven hypopituitarism is still undergoing experimental trials.

Constitutional growth delay is one of the frequent variants of normal growth encountered by the pediatrician. Length and weight of affected children are normal at birth, and growth is normal for the first 4–12 mo of life. Growth then decelerates to near or below the 3rd percentile for height and weight. By 2–3 yr of age, growth resumes at a normal rate of 5 cm/yr or more. Studies of GH secretion and other studies are within normal limits. Osseous maturation is consistent with height age rather than with chronologic age. Detailed questioning will reveal other family members (frequently one or both of the parents) with histories of short stature in childhood, delayed puberty, and eventual normal stature. The prognosis for these children to achieve normal adult height is excellent. Boys with unusual degrees of delayed puberty may occasionally require a short course of testosterone therapy to initiate puberty. The cause of this variant of normal growth is thought to be persistence of the relatively hypogonadotropic state of childhood (see Sec. 19.31). Constitutional growth delay can be differentiated from *genetic short stature* by the level of skeletal maturation, which is consistent with chronologic age in the latter condition. Genetic short stature is usually found in other family members. Results of studies of growth, however, are normal.

Primary hypothyroidism is usually easily distinguished on clinical grounds. Responses to GH provocative tests may be subnormal, however, and enlargement of the sella may be present. Elevated levels of TSH clearly establish the diagnosis, and these secondary changes disappear following treatment with thyroid hormone. Since thyroid hormone is a necessary prerequisite for normal GH synthesis, its levels must always be assessed prior to GH studies. Hypothyroidism produces decreased levels of GH in the pituitary and serum and an attenuated response to GHRH.

Emotional deprivation is an important cause of retardation of growth and mimics hypopituitarism. The condition is known as psychosocial dwarfism, deprivation dwarfism, or reversible hyposomatotropism. The mechanisms by which sensory and emotional deprivation interfere with growth are not fully understood. Functional hypopituitarism is indicated by low levels of IGF-1, by inadequate responses of GH to provocative stimuli, and perhaps by delayed puberty. Appropriate history and careful observations reveal disturbed mother-child or family relations and provide clues to diagnosis. Proof may be difficult to establish because the adults responsible often hide from professionals the true situation in the family, and the children rarely divulge their plight. Emotionally deprived children frequently have perverted or voracious appetities, enuresis, encopresis, insomnia, crying spasms, and sudden tantrums. They may be excessively passive or aggressive and are borderline or dull-normal in intelligence. When child-rearing practices are altered or when the child is removed from the domicile of abuse, the rate of growth improves significantly. During this period of catch-up growth, separation of the cranial sutures and other evidence of pseudotumor cerebri may occur; these should not be mistaken for signs of a mass lesion.

The *Silver-Russell syndrome* is characterized by short stature, frontal bossing, small triangular facies, sparse subcutaneous tissue, shortened and incurved 5th fingers, and, in many cases, asymmetry (hemihypertrophy). Affected children have low birthweights for gestational age. Recent studies have revealed some degree of GH secretory deficiency in very short children with intrauterine growth retardation, whether or not they have Silver-Russell syndrome. Short-term treatment with GH often results in increased rates of growth, but its long-term benefits are unknown.

TREATMENT. In patients with demonstrable organic lesions treatment should be directed to the underlying disease process. Evaluation of pituitary function is indicated after surgery or irradiation.

Treatment of children with classic GH deficiency should begin as early as possible; younger children respond better than older ones, and long-term expectations are better. The recommended dose of hGH is 0.18–0.3 mg/kg/wk; it is administered subcutaneously in 6 or 7 divided doses. Therapy should be continuous until there is no further response, a point usually concomitant with closure of the epiphyses. If the effect of therapy wanes, the dose should be increased. Some patients treated with growth hormone have subsequently developed leukemia; the risk for leukemia in treated patients may be double that in the general population, but this is still under investigation.

Maximal response to GH occurs in the 1st yr of treatment; with each successive year of treatment, the response tends to decrease. Occasional patients receiving GH develop reversible hypothyroidism owing to enhanced conversion of T_4 to T_3 and decreased levels of TSH. Periodic evaluation of thyroid function is indicated in all patients treated with GH. GHRH is just as effective as GH in the treatment of children with hypopituitarism with a deficiency of GHRH, but multiple daily subcutaneous injections are required. When a depot form becomes available, it may provide a practical form of treatment for this group of children. Recombinant IGF-1 may prove useful in the treatment of children with Laron syndrome and possibly those with gene deletions and high titers of antibodies.

The doses of GH used to treat children with classic GH deficiency usually enhance growth of many non–GH-deficient children as well. Therefore, intensive investigation is in progress to determine the full spectrum of short children who may benefit from treatment with GH. Children with intrauterine growth retardation, chronic renal failure, Noonan syndrome, Turner syndrome, and others experience short-term increased growth velocity when treated with GH. Girls with Turner syndrome treated with GH appear to have a final height several centimeters greater than that seen in untreated girls. For children with all other causes of short stature it is unknown whether GH treatment increases their final height, and treatment of such patients should be confined to prospective clinical trials until further data establish the validity of this expensive, chronic form of therapy.

Replacement should also be directed at other hormonal deficiencies when present. In TSH-deficient subjects, thyroid hormone is given in full replacement doses; in corticotropin-deficient patients the dose of hydrocortisone should not exceed 10–15 mg/m^2/24 hr, and therapy can often be deferred until growth has been completed if the deficiency is partial. In patients with a deficiency of gonadotropins, gonadal steroids are given when the bone age reaches the age when puberty usually takes place. For infants with microphallus one or two 3-mo courses of monthly intramuscular injections of 25 mg of testosterone enanthate may bring the penis to normal size without inordinate effect on osseous maturation.

Older GH-deficient patients treated with cadaver pituitary extracts are at risk for Creutzfeldt-Jakob disease for at least 10–15 yr after therapy. Recombinant growth hormone (r-hGH) has eliminated this risk.

19.3 DIABETES INSIPIDUS (DI)
(Arginine Vasopressin Deficiency)

Diabetes insipidus, characterized by polyuria and polydipsia, results from lack of the antidiuretic hormone, arginine vasopressin (AVP). Destruction of the supraoptic and paraventricular nuclei or division of the supraoptic-hypophyseal tract above the median eminence results in permanent diabetes insipidus. Transection of the tract below the median eminence or removal of just the posterior lobe may result in transitory polyuria, but in this case arginine vasopressin released into the median eminence prevents occurrence of diabetes insipidus. Vasopressin acts directly on the distal tubules and collecting ducts of the kidney by binding to V_2 receptors, which are coupled to cAMP. Vasopressin deficiency may be total or partial with varying degrees of polydipsia and polyuria.

ETIOLOGY. Any lesion that damages the neurohypophyseal unit may result in diabetes insipidus. Tumors of the suprasellar and chiasmatic regions, particularly craniopharyngiomas (Fig. 19–1), optic gliomas, and germinomas, are common causes; the symptoms of increased intracranial pressure may accompany those of diabetes insipidus or may follow years later. Approximately 25% of patients with histiocytosis develop diabetes insipidus as a consequence of histiocytic infiltration of the hypothalamus and pituitary. DI is seldom present when histiocytosis is diagnosed but almost always occurs within 4–5 yr. It occurs most often in children with multisystem disease and in those with proptosis. About half of these patients have cytoplasmic antibodies to vasopressin (VP)–producing cells, suggesting an autoimmune response to histiocytic cell invasion of the hypothalamus. Encephalitis, sarcoidosis, tuberculosis, actinomycosis, and leukemia are occasional causes. Injuries to the head, especially basal skull fractures, may produce diabetes insipidus immediately or after a delay of several months. Operative procedures near the pituitary or hypothalamus may result in transitory or permanent diabetes insipidus.

In a few cases diabetes insipidus is hereditary. An autosomal dominant form is characterized by variable onset, from birth to several years of age, and variable severity within a family and in individuals over time. Symptoms decrease in the 3rd–5th decades. Levels of AVP may be absent (<0.5 pg/mL) or variably decreased. DNA studies have localized the defect to the preprovasopressin-neurophysin II-glycoprotein complex (AVP-NP II gene) on chromosome 20, but the precise molecular defect remains unknown. An even rarer X-linked familial form of AVP deficiency is known.

DI is associated with insulin-dependent diabetes mellitus (IDDM), optic atrophy, deafness, and neurogenic bladder in *Wolfram syndrome*, also known by the acronym DIDMOAD. IDDM usually occurs first, and an autosomal recessive mode of inheritance appears likely. Absence of islet cell antibodies and of the usual HLA haplotypes associated with classic IDDM clearly differentiates the cause of diabetes mellitus in this condition from that of the usual type 1 autoimmune diabetes mellitus. Pathologic studies suggest a degenerative process involving the β cells, the supraoptic and paraventricular nuclei, the optic nerve, and cranial nerve VIII.

Diabetes insipidus occasionally accompanies *septo-optic dysplasia*.

Diabetes insipidus has been reported in the newborn infant following asphyxia, intraventricular hemorrhage, intravascular coagulopathy, *Listeria monocytogenes* sepsis, and group B β-hemolytic streptococcal meningitis.

In many instances, the cause of diabetes insipidus cannot be found initially, but disease in only about 20% of affected patients will eventually be classified as idiopathic. In over half of all patients with intracranial tumors clinical or neuroradiologic signs (or both) are not manifest until 1 yr after diabetes insipidus has been diagnosed, and in 25% the delay is as long as 4 yr. Periodic re-evaluation is required for at least 4 yr before the entity can be called idiopathic. About one third of patients with idiopathic diabetes insipidus have antibodies to vasopressin-producing cells suggesting an autoimmune basis for the condition; this idea is further supported by the frequent occurrence in this subgroup of patients of other autoimmune endocrine disorders, especially autoimmune thyroid disease; these autoimmune disorders are particularly evident in adults. Diabetes insipidus is being increasingly recognized as a terminal event in brain dead individuals.

CLINICAL MANIFESTATIONS. Polydipsia and polyuria are the outstanding symptoms of diabetes insipidus. In families with the hereditary disorder the polyuria is often noted in early infancy. The infant cries excessively and is not satisfied with additional milk but is quieted with water.

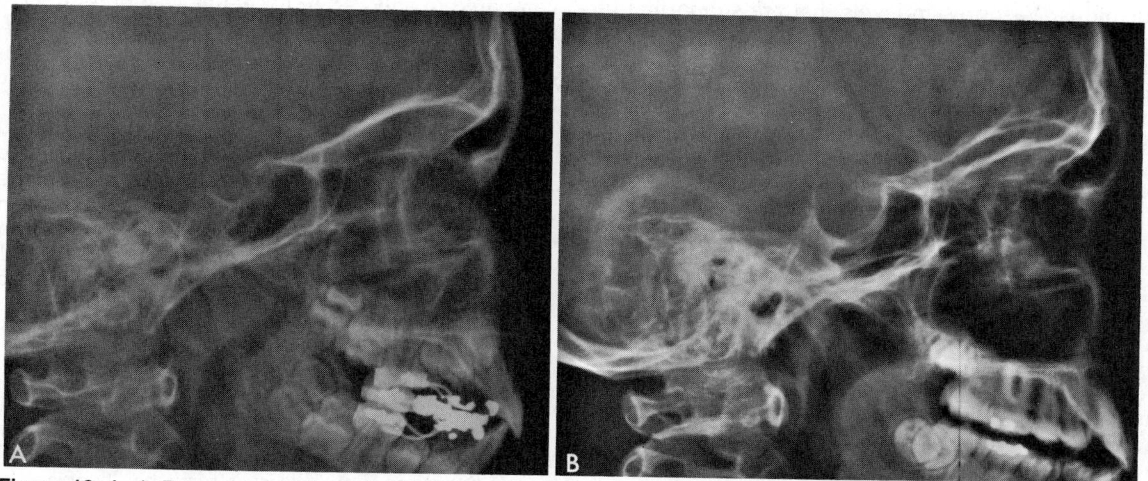

Figure 19–1. *A*, Roentgenograph of the skull of a 9-yr-old boy with polydipsia, polyuria, nocturia, and enuresis. Urine specific gravity was 1.010 after water deprivation. Growth was normal, and the sella turcica was considered roentgenographically to be at the upper limit of normal but was probably enlarged. Over the ensuing 6 mo, the symptoms of diabetes insipidus abated. *B*, The patient returned at 14 yr of age because of growth failure and delay in sexual maturation. Studies revealed a deficiency of growth hormone, gonadotropins, corticotropin, and thyrotropin. Note the enlargement and the thinning of the sella turcica but also the absence of intrasellar or suprasellar calcification. The neurologic and ophthalmologic examinations were normal. There was exacerbation of diabetes insipidus with the administration of hydrocortisone and thyroxine. At surgery, a large craniopharyngioma was found.

Hyperthermia, rapid loss of weight, and collapse are common in infancy. Vomiting, constipation, and growth failure may be observed. Dehydration in early infancy may result in brain damage and mental impairment. In children with vasopressin deficiency there is wide variability in manifestations. Severity tends to increase with age, some affected children being asymptomatic until adolescence. Many affected families accept polydipsia and polyuria as a family habit and do not seek medical attention or may even prefer the symptoms to therapy.

In a child who has acquired bladder control, enuresis may be the first symptom. The excessive thirst is disturbing and interferes with play, learning, and sleep. Children with diabetes insipidus do not perspire; their skin is dry and pale. Anorexia is common; there is a preference for carbohydrates.

Other signs and symptoms depend on the primary lesion; for example, patients with tumors in the region of the hypothalamus may have disturbance of growth, progressive cachexia or obesity, hyperpyrexia, sleep disturbance, sexual precocity, or emotional disorders. Lesions initially causing diabetes insipidus may eventually destroy the anterior pituitary; in such instances the diabetes insipidus tends to become milder or disappear completely.

LABORATORY DATA. The daily volume of urine may be 4–10 or more liters. The urine is pale or colorless; the specific gravity varies from 1.001 to 1.005, with a corresponding osmolality of 50–200 mOsm/kg water. During periods of severe dehydration the specific gravity may rise to 1.010 and the osmolality to 300. Other renal function studies are normal. Serum osmolality is normal with adequate hydration. During water deprivation tests patients must be closely observed to prevent surreptitious intake of water on the one hand and to avoid severe and rapid development of dehydration on the other. In patients with severe deficiency a 3-hr period of dehydration leads to elevation of plasma osmolality while urine osmolality characteristically remains below plasma levels. Administration of desmopressin or vasopressin quickly raises urine osmolality. When polyuria is mild and the deficiency is incomplete, urine osmolality may exceed that of plasma, and the response to vasopressin is attenuated.

Radioimmunoassay for vasopressin is available; plasma levels consistently below 0.5 pg/mL indicate severe neurogenic diabetes insipidus. Vasopressin levels that are subnormal for the concomitant hyperosmolality indicate partial neurogenic diabetes insipidus. The assay is particularly useful in distinguishing partial diabetes insipidus from primary polydipsia.

Roentgenograms of the skull may reveal evidence of an intracranial tumor such as calcifications, enlargement of the sella turcica, erosion of the clinoid processes, or increased width of the suture lines. Roentgenograms of the skull or other bones in patients with reticuloendothelioses may reveal areas of rarefaction. CT scan or MRI of the head is indicated in such cases.

DIFFERENTIAL DIAGNOSIS. Polydipsia, polyuria, and impaired concentration are common in patients with hypercalcemia or potassium deficiency. In the male infant nephrogenic diabetes insipidus must be differentiated from inherited or acquired vasopressin deficiency; failure of response to exogenous vasopressin or desmopressin is a critical differential criterion (see Sec. 18.30).

Defects in urinary concentrations also occur in a variety of chronic renal disorders. Familial nephronophthisis, in particular, can mimic diabetes insipidus. Elevated plasma levels of urea and creatinine, anemia, and isotonic rather than hypotonic urine are characteristics of primary renal disease.

Compulsive water drinking *(psychogenic polydipsia)* is rare but may easily be confused with diabetes insipidus. Affected persons are usually able to produce a concentrated urine when fluids are withheld. Occasionally, however, diagnosis is difficult because prolonged polydipsia lowers the maximal urinary concentrations achievable following dehydration or even following infusion of hypertonic saline solution. As a rule, a urine osmolality greater after dehydration than after administration of vasopressin alone indicates the ability to secrete vasopressin. On the other hand, if administration of vasopressin produces a urinary osmolality that is substantially higher than that with dehydration alone, vasopressin secretion is deficient. This rule seems to apply no matter how low or how high the urinary concentration may be.

Adipsia or hypodipsia, as an isolated defect of the thirst center, is extremely rare. Since the osmoreceptors for thirst and vasopressin occupy contiguous areas of the anterior hypothalamus, hypodipsic hypernatremia is usually associated with defects in antidiuretic function. This most often occurs in patients with hypothalamic tumors, especially germinomas, gliomas, histiocytosis, congenital malformations, and microcephaly. Adipsia seriously complicates the management of problems of water balance.

PROGNOSIS. When diabetes insipidus is diagnosed the underlying process must be determined. Diabetes insipidus itself rarely threatens life, but it may signify a serious underlying condition. It may be only transitory following trauma or surgical intervention in the region of the hypothalamus or pituitary. In some patients with reticuloendothelioses spontaneous remission occurs, whereas in others diabetes insipidus may be the only residuum long after remission of the primary condition. Amelioration of clinical diabetes insipidus may herald development of anterior pituitary insufficiency. The prognosis of patients with brain tumors depends upon the site of the lesion and the type of neoplastic cell.

TREATMENT. The causative factor deserves first consideration in the treatment. Patients with uncomplicated diabetes insipidus may live untreated for years with only the inconvenience of polyuria and polydipsia so long as they have an intact thirst mechanism and are allowed free access to water.

The drug of choice is desmopressin (1-desamino-8-D-arginine vasopressin; dDAVP), a highly effective analog of vasopressin. This analog is more resistant to degradation by peptidases than native vasopressin. The antidiuretic activity of desmopressin is 2,000 to 3,000 times greater than its pressor activity, and 1 μg produces an antidiuresis that lasts 8–10 hr compared to only 2–3 hr for native vasopressin. Desmopressin is given by a nasal tube delivery system that delivers precise amounts to the nasal mucosa. The usual dose ranges from 5 to 15 μg given either as a single dose or divided into two doses. Children under 2 yr of age require smaller doses (0.15–0.5 μg/kg/24 hr). The dose must be individualized, and it is important that the dosage schedule be adjusted to allow patients to revert to mild polyuria before the next dose is given. For patients requiring over 10 μg/dose, a nasal spray preparation is also available. A parenteral preparation of desmopressin (0.03–0.15 μg/kg) is available and is useful postoperatively, particularly after transsphenoidal surgery, when nasal packing precludes nasal insufflation.

Great care must be taken in patients with diabetes insipidus who are comatose, undergoing surgery, or receiving intravenous fluids for any reason. Regardless of the form of therapy, any effective dose should be repeated only after its effect has worn off and polyuria recurs. Postoperative diabetes insipidus is often transient; daily reassessment of the need for antidiuretic hormone is necessary after it has been initiated.

Desmopressin also has an effect on V_2-like extrarenal receptors, resulting in release of factor VIII and von Willebrand factor. Selected patients with mild or moderate hemophilia A or von Willebrand disease can be successfully treated with doses of dDAVP 15 times higher than the dose used for antidiuresis. Desmopressin is being increasingly used in the management of children with enuresis. Some of these children appear to have an unexplained nocturnal deficiency of vasopressin secretion. The dose required is slightly higher (20–40 μg) than that used to treat neurogenic diabetes insipidus. It is given as a nasal spray before bedtime.

Nephrogenic Diabetes Insipidus
(Vasopressin-Insensitive Diabetes Insipidus)

See Sec. 18.30.

19.4 INAPPROPRIATE SECRETION OF ANTIDIURETIC HORMONE
(Hypersecretion of Vasopressin)

The syndrome of inappropriate secretion of antidiuretic hormone (SIADH) is now recognized as one of the most common aberrations of arginine vasopressin (AVP) secretion. In this condition plasma levels of AVP are inappropriately high for the concurrent osmolality of the blood and are not suppressed by further dilution of body fluids.

ETIOLOGY. The syndrome is being recognized in an increasing number of clinical conditions, particularly those involving the central nervous system, including meningitis, encephalitis, brain tumor and abscesses, subarachnoid hemorrhage, Guillain-Barré syndrome, head trauma, and after transsphenoidal surgery for pituitary tumors. Pneumonia, tuberculosis, acute intermittent porphyria, cystic fibrosis, infant botulism, perinatal asphyxia, use of positive-pressure respirators, and certain drugs such as vincristine and vinblastine also produce the syndrome. The mechanism of the disturbed regulation of vasopressin in these conditions is not fully understood, but in many instances there is direct involvement of the hypothalamus. The syndrome has been observed in patients with Ewing sarcoma; with malignant tumors of the pancreas, duodenum, or thymus; and particularly with oat cell carcinoma of the lung. In these instances the tumor presumably synthesizes and secretes vasopressin, the syndrome disappearing when the tumor is removed. In rare cases no cause for the syndrome has been found.

The syndrome has occurred during chlorpropamide therapy for diabetes mellitus, presumably because this drug potentiates vasopressin. Patients with diabetes insipidus treated with various antidiuretic preparations readily develop the syndrome during periods of excessive ingestion of fluids or during intravenous fluid therapy.

CLINICAL MANIFESTATIONS. The syndrome is probably most often latent and asymptomatic and forms the basis for the long known observation that serum sodium levels may be unexpectedly low in conditions such as pneumonia, tuberculosis, and meningitis. Careful attention to fluid replacement in patients with conditions known to be associated with the syndrome may prevent the development of symptoms.

The clinical manifestations are attributable to hypotonicity of body fluids and are those of water intoxication. If the serum sodium is not below 120 mEq/L, there may be no symptoms. Early, there is loss of appetite followed by nausea and sometimes vomiting. Irritability and personality changes, including hostility and confusion, may occur. When the serum sodium falls below 110 mEq/L, neurologic abnormalities or stupor is common, and convulsive seizures may occur. Skin turgor and blood pressure are normal, and there is no evidence of dehydration.

Serum sodium and chloride concentrations are low, whereas serum bicarbonate usually remains normal. Despite low serum sodium there is continued renal excretion of sodium. The serum is hypo-osmolar, but the urine is less than maximally dilute, and its osmolality is greater than appropriate for the tonicity of the serum. Hypouricemia is often present, probably owing to increased urate clearance secondary to volume expansion. Concurrence of hypouricemia with hyponatremia is a clue to the diagnosis of SIADH and is especially helpful in the neonate. Renal and adrenal functions are normal.

TREATMENT. Successful treatment of the underlying disorder (meningitis, pneumonia) is followed by spontaneous remission. Immediate management of the hyponatremia consists simply of *restriction of fluids*. Sodium should be made available to replace the soidum loss; hypertonic saline solution is usually of little benefit, however, since even large sodium loads are excreted in the urine. In cases of severe water intoxication, with convulsions or coma, administration of hypertonic saline solution will increase osmolality and control the central nervous system manifestations. In such emergencies administration of furosemide with 300 mL/m^2 of 1.5% sodium chloride will cause both a rise in sodium levels and a diuresis. Demeclocycline interferes with the action of AVP on the renal tubule. Experience in adults with SIADH indicates that this agent may be useful, but its role in the treatment of children is not established. An 8-yr-old child with chronic SIADH has been successfully treated with single daily doses of furosemide.

19.5 HYPERPITUITARISM

Hypersecretion of pituitary hormones is an expected finding in conditions in which deficiency of a target organ gives decreased hormonal feedback, as in primary hypogonadism or hypoadrenalism. In primary hypothyroidism pituitary hyperfunction and hyperplasia can enlarge and erode the sella and on rare occasions increase intracranial pressure. Such changes are not to be confused with primary pituitary tumors; they disappear when the underlying thyroid condition is treated. Pituitary hyperplasia also occurs in response to stimulation by ectopic production of releasing hormones such as that seen occasionally in patients with Cushing syndrome, secondary to CRH, or in children with acromegaly, which is secondary to GHRH produced by a variety of systemic tumors.

Primary hypersecretion of pituitary hormones by a suspected or proved adenoma is rare in childhood. The most commonly encountered pituitary tumors are those that secrete corticotropin, prolactin, or GH. With very rare exceptions, pituitary adenomas that secrete gonadotropins or thyrotropin occur primarily in adults. Hypothalamic hamartomas that secrete gonadotropin-releasing hormone are known to cause precocious puberty. It is suspected that some pituitary tumors may result from stimulation with hypothalamic-releasing hormones. Any pituitary tumor may also cause various hormonal deficiencies by compressing pituitary tissue.

Pituitary Gigantism and Acromegaly

In young persons with open epiphyses, overproduction of GH results in gigantism; in persons with closed epiphyses, the result is acromegaly. Often some acromegalic features are seen with gigantism, even in children and adolescents; after closure of the epiphyses, the acromegalic features become more prominent.

ETIOLOGY. Pituitary gigantism is rare. The cause is most often a pituitary adenoma, but gigantism has been observed in a 2.5-yr-old boy with a hypothalamic tumor that presumably secreted GHRH. Other tumors, particularly in the pancreas, have also produced acromegaly owing to secretion of large amounts of GHRH with resultant hyperplasia of the somatotrophs; GHRH was first isolated from two such pancreatic tumors. Growth hormone–secreting adenomas are also associated with McCune-Albright syndrome (see Sec. 19.7). The usual manifestations consist of rapid linear growth, coarse facial features, and enlarging hands and feet. In young children rapid growth of the head may precede linear growth. Some patients have behavioral and visual problems.

CLINICAL MANIFESTATIONS. In most of the recorded cases the abnormal growth became evident at puberty, but the condition has been established as early as the newborn period in one child and at 21 mo of age in another. Giants may grow to a height of 8 ft or more. Acromegaly consists chiefly of enlargement of the distal parts of the body, but manifestations of abnormal growth actually involve all portions. The circumference of the skull increases, the nose becomes broad, and the tongue is often enlarged, with coarsening of the facial features. The mandible grows excessively, and the teeth become separated. The fingers and toes grow chiefly in thickness. There may be dorsal kyphosis. Fatigue and lassitude are early symptoms. Delayed sexual maturation or hypogonadism may occur. Signs of increased intracranial pressure appear later; visual loss may be demonstrable only on careful examination of visual fields.

LABORATORY DATA. Growth hormone levels are elevated and may occasionally reach 400 ng/mL. The episodic pattern of secretion and the nocturnal surge may be preserved in some patients. There is usually no suppression of growth hormone levels by the hyperglycemia of a glucose tolerance test. There may be no response, normal responses, or paradoxic responses to various other stimuli. For example, L-dopa may paradoxically decrease GH levels. Administration of thyrotropin-releasing hormone results in increased GH levels in some acromegalics, and in a 5-yr-old giant it resulted in a 3-fold increase in levels of GH. IGF-1 levels are consistently elevated in acromegaly, in one study ranging from 2.6–21.7 U/mL; normal levels are 0.31–1.4 U/mL. Most patients also have marked hyperprolactinemia.

Adenomas may compromise other anterior pituitary function through growth or cystic degeneration. Secretion of gonadotropins, thyrotropin (TSH), or ACTH may be impaired.

Roentgenograms of the skull may reveal enlargement of the sella turcica and of the paranasal sinuses; CT scans or magnetic resonance imaging (MRI) delineates the tumor. Tufting of the phalanges and increased heel pad thickness are common. Osseous maturation is normal.

DIFFERENTIAL DIAGNOSIS. In the differential diagnosis hereditary tall stature must be considered; in this condition there is usually abnormal height in one or both parents or in close relatives. Such tall persons are well proportioned and free of signs of increased intracranial pressure. Excessive growth during preadolescence in obese children is a temporary state; though such children may become tall, they do not attain the height of giants. Children with precocious puberty are often unusually tall but do not develop into giants because their epiphyses close early and growth ceases prematurely. Patients with tall stature associated with hypogonadism or Marfan syndrome are easily distinguished clinically and have normal levels of growth hormone. Gigantism and increased growth hormone levels may occur in some patients with lipodystrophy, but absence of subcutaneous fat is a characteristic finding; there is increasing evidence of disordered hypothalamic function in this condition. Cerebral gigantism, which is more common than pituitary gigantism, can usually be differentiated on clinical grounds (see later).

TREATMENT. Modalities include surgery, irradiation, and medical therapy; there are advantages and disadvantages of each. Bromocriptine, a dopamine agonist that binds to pituitary dopamine receptors, is helpful in some patients as primary therapy or when surgery or irradiation has not been successful. More recently, octreotide, a long-acting somatostatin analog, has been found to be more effective than bromocriptine in lowering levels of GH and in shrinking the size of the tumor. However, since octreotide must be given subcutaneously every 8 hr and is expensive, bromocriptine should be tried first when medical treatment is indicated.

Sotos Syndrome
(Cerebral Gigantism)

This disorder is characterized by rapid growth, but there is no evidence that it is an endocrine disorder. A hypothalamic defect has been suggested as a cause, but none has been demonstrated functionally or at necropsy. Birthweight and length are above the 90th percentile in most affected infants, and macrocrania may be noted. Growth is rapid, and by 1 yr of age affected infants are over the 97th percentile in height. Accelerated growth continues for the first 4–5 yr, and then returns to a normal rate. Puberty usually occurs at the normal time but may occur slightly early. The hands and feet are large, with thickened subcutaneous tissue. The head is large and dolichocephalic, the jaw prominent; there is hypertelorism, and the eyes have an antimongoloid slant. Clumsiness and awkward gait are characteristic, and affected children have great difficulty in sports, in learning to ride a bicycle, and in other tasks requiring coordination. Some degree of mental retardation is present in most patients; in some children, perceptual deficiencies may predominate (Fig. 19–2).

Roentgenograms reveal a large skull, a high orbital roof, a sella of normal size but slightly posterior inclination, and an increased interorbital distance. Osseous maturation is compatible with the patient's height. GH levels and results of other endocrine studies are usually normal; there are no

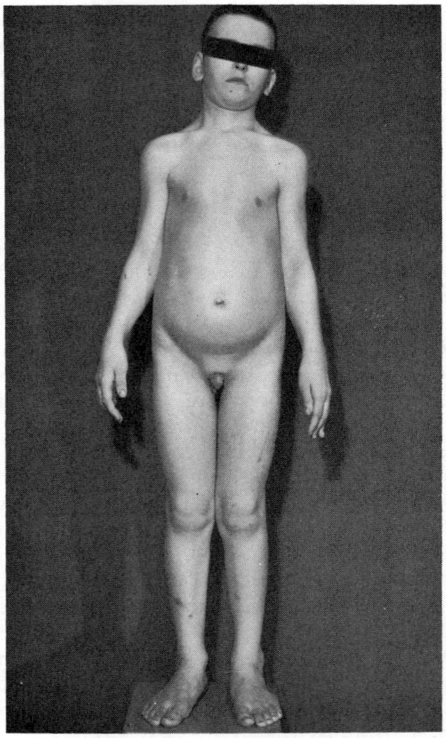

Figure 19–2. Cerebral gigantism in an 8-yr-old boy. The height age was 12 yr; the bone age was 12 yr; IQ was 60; the electroencephalogram had abnormal findings. Note the prominence of the forehead and the jaw and also the large hands and feet. Sexual development was consistent with chronologic age. Hormone studies were normal. The adult height was 208 cm (6 ft 10 in); his sexual development was normal. He wears size 18 shoes.

distinctive laboratory markers for the syndrome. Abnormal electroencephalograms are common; other studies frequently reveal a dilated ventricular system.

The cause of the disorder is unknown, nor is it clear whether all patients with this syndrome have the same defect. Most cases are sporadic. Familial cases are usually consistent with autosomal dominant inheritance, occasionally with autosomal recessive inheritance. Affected patients may be at increased risk for neoplasia; hepatic carcinoma and Wilms, ovarian, and parotid tumors have been reported.

Prolactinoma

Prolactin-secreting pituitary adenomas are the most common tumor of the pituitary in adults, and more than 50 cases have been reported in children and adolescents. With the advent of MRI more of these adenomas are being detected. In some kindreds with type I multiple endocrine neoplasia, prolactinomas are the presenting features during adolescence. Presenting features in children and adolescents include headache, decreased growth rate and delayed puberty, primary or secondary amenorrhea, gynecomastia, galactorrhea, and advanced puberty either singly or in various combinations. Prolactin levels may be moderately or markedly elevated (as high as 5,000 ng/mL) and are not appropriately increased by TRH stimulation. Most prolactinomas thus far recognized in children have been large (macroadenomas), have caused the sella to enlarge, and in some cases have caused visual field defects. The mechanism causing pubertal delay is probably multifactorial, possible mechanisms being decreased secretion of growth hormone, gonadotropic hormones, or luteinizing hormone–releasing hormone (LHRH) as well as direct inhibition of the gonads by prolactin.

Prolactinomas should not be confused with the hyperprolactinemia and pituitary hyperplasia that may occur in patients with primary hypothyroidism, which is readily treated with thyroid hormone (see Sec. 19.12). Moderate elevations (<200 ng/mL) of prolactin are also associated with a variety of medications, with pituitary stalk dysfunction such as may occur with craniopharyngioma, and with other benign conditions. Treatment for most children has been surgical resection by transfrontal or transsphenoidal approach. Bromocriptine is highly effective in reducing levels of prolactin and in decreasing tumor size by 50% or more in two thirds of adults. Experience in adults indicates that microadenomas usually do not become macroadenomas and that spontaneous remission of clinical manifestations is common. The management of microadenomas is becoming increasingly conservative.

19.6 PUBERTY

PHYSIOLOGY OF PUBERTY. The hypothalamus, pituitary, and gonads are active and interacting for years before the secondary sex characteristics associated with puberty appear. However, after the first years of life, plasma levels of FSH, LH, estradiol, and testosterone are very low or below the limited sensitivity of conventional radioimmunoassays. Evidence of hypothalamic-pituitary-gonadal interaction prior to puberty resides in the fact that young children with Turner syndrome or anorchia have levels of gonadotropins higher than those of normal children of the same age. In the prepubertal child, very small amounts of gonadal steroids are able to suppress the activity of the hypothalamus and pituitary. One to two years before the clinical onset of puberty becomes evident, low plasma levels of LH during sleep become demonstrable. This sleep-entrained LH secretion occurs in a pulsatile fashion and probably reflects endogenous episodic discharge of hypothalamic LHRH. After the onset of nocturnal LH pulses, one can predict that clinical onset of puberty will occur within the next year or two.

Nocturnal pulses of LH continue to increase in frequency and amplitude as clinical puberty approaches. By midpuberty, LH pulses become evident even before sleep and occur at about 90- to 120-min intervals. It is the pulsatile secretion of gonadotropins that is the initial stimulation for gonadal maturation. The major drive to the pituitary is LHRH from the hypothalamic neurons and their associated afferent inputs; this neurosecretory unit is known as the LHRH pulse generator, but the factors that normally activate or restrain it are unknown. Pulsed administration of LHRH can induce puberty in the infantile monkey that will disappear when treatment is discontinued and subsequently reappear spontaneously at the appropriate age. Likewise, chronic pulsatile administration of LHRH intravenously to patients with idiopathic hypogonadotropic hypogonadism leads to the initiation and progression of pubertal development.

The situation is complicated by the heterogeneity of pituitary gonadotropins. The bioactive to immunoreactive ratio of LH increases during puberty, indicating qualitative as well as quantitative changes. Furthermore, FSH and LH act synergistically to promote changes in the gonad at puberty.

A second critical event occurs in middle or late adolescence, at least in girls, in whom cyclicity and ovulation occur. A positive feedback mechanism develops whereby rising levels of estrogen in midcycle cause a distinct increase (rather than decrease) of LH. Prior to midadolescence this ability of estrogen to release LH is not found.

Adrenal cortical androgens also play a role in pubertal maturation (adrenarche). Levels of dehydroepiandrosterone (DHEA) and its sulfate (DHEAS) begin to rise before the earliest physical changes of puberty are apparent. This increase occurs before those of gonadotropins, testosterone, or estradiol at about 6 yr of age; the rise is more rapid in girls than in boys. DHEAS is the most abundant adrenal C-19 steroid in blood, but its function is unknown. It has been postulated that an adrenal androgen-stimulating factor other than ACTH initiates adrenarche.

Age of onset of puberty varies and is more closely correlated with osseous maturation than with chronologic age (see Sec. 3.9). In girls the breast bud is usually the first sign of puberty (10–11 yr), and the interval to menarche is usually 2–2.5 yr but may be as long as 6 yr. In the United States about 95% of girls have at least one sign of puberty by 12 yr, and the mean age of menarche is about 12½ yr. Peak height velocity always precedes menarche and is attained about 2 yr earlier in girls than in boys. There are, however, wide variations in the sequence of changes involving growth spurt, breast bud, pubic hair, and genital development.

Genetic and environmental factors also affect onset of puberty. The drop in menarchal age in the past century is probably due to better nutrition and improved general health. Black girls are significantly more advanced in development of secondary sex characteristics than white girls. Ballet dancers, gymnasts, swimmers, runners, and other girl athletes in whom leanness and strenous physical activity have coexisted from early childhood frequently exhibit a marked delay in puberty or menarche. This observation supports the thesis that there may be a growth tracking device (somatometer) that is responsible for synchronizing somatic development with LHRH and initiating puberty (Sec. 18.58).

In boys, growth of the testes is the first sign of puberty (prepubertal testicular volume is 1–3 mL). This is followed by pigmentation and thinning of the scrotum and growth of the penis (Sec. 3.9). Pubic hair then appears. Appearance of axillary hair usually marks the midpoint of puberty. In boys, unlike girls, acceleration of growth begins after puberty is well under way and is maximal from 14–16 yr of age; growth may continue well beyond 18 yr of age.

Precocious puberty is difficult to define because of the marked variation in the age at which puberty begins normally. Onset of secondary sexual characteristics before 8 yr of age in girls and 9 yr in boys may be considered precocious, but these are arbitrary guidelines.

19.7 DISORDERS OF PUBERTAL DEVELOPMENT

Precocious pubertal development may be classified as true precocious puberty or precocious pseudopuberty (Table 19–2). True precocious puberty is always isosexual and involves hypothalamic-pituitary-gonadal activation; the precocity involves not only secondary sexual characteristics but also an increase in the size and activity of the gonads. In precocious pseudopuberty some of the secondary sex characteristics appear, but the gonads do not mature and there is no activation of normal hypothalamic-pituitary-gonadal interplay. In this latter group the sex characteristics may be isosexual or heterosexual (see Sec. 19.23, 19.32, and 19.39).

TABLE 19–2. Conditions Causing Precocious Puberty

True precocious puberty (gonadotropin-dependent)
Idiopathic (constitutional, functional)
Central nervous system lesion
Hypothalamic hamartoma, brain tumors, hydrocephalus, postencephalitic scars, and so on
Prolonged untreated primary hypothyroidism
Therapy of congenital adrenal hyperplasia
McCune-Albright syndrome—late
Administration of gonadotropins
Precocious pseudopuberty (gonadotropin-independent)
Females
Isosexual (feminization)
Ovarian tumors
Granulosa–theca cell tumor
Associated with Ollier disease
Teratoma, chorionepithelioma
Sex-cord tumor with annular tubules (associated with Peutz-Jeghers syndrome)
Autonomous functional cyst of ovary
McCune-Albright syndrome
Adrenocortical tumor
Exogenous estrogen
Heterosexual (virilization)
Congenital adrenal hyperplasia
Adrenocortical tumor
Testosterone-secreting tumor
Androblastoma (arrhenoblastoma)
Androgen-producing teratoma
Exogenous androgen
Males
Isosexual (masculinization)
Male-limited autosomal dominant
Congenital adrenal hyperplasia
Adrenocortical tumor
Leydig cell tumor
Teratoma (containing adenocortical tissue)
hCG-secreting tumor
CNS tumor
Hepatoblastoma
Mediastinal tumor
Associated with Klinefelter syndrome
Exogenous androgen
Heterosexual (feminization)
Adrenocortical tumor
Exogenous estrogen
Sertoli cell tumor
Sex-cord tumor with annular tubules (associated with Peutz-Jeghers syndrome)
Partial precocious puberty
Premature adrenarche
Premature thelarche
Premature menarche

True Precocious Puberty

PRECOCIOUS PUBERTY WITHOUT OTHER PATHOLOGIC FINDINGS (CONSTITUTIONAL)

In the past, no causative factor could be found to account for precocious puberty in about 80–90% of girls and 50% of boys. CT scans and MRI have lowered the percentages of children in this category. The condition occurs far more frequently in girls and is usually sporadic.

CLINICAL MANIFESTATIONS. The clinical course is extremely variable. Affected children may complete sexual maturation rapidly or slowly; manifestations may remain stationary or even regress, only to resume development later. Sexual development may begin at any age. In girls the first sign is development of the breasts; pubic hair may appear simultaneously but more often appears later. Development of the external genitalia, the appearance of axillary hair, and the onset of menstruation follow. The early menstrual cycles may be more irregular than they are with normal puberty. The initial cycles are usually anovulatory, but pregnancy has been reported as early as 5.5 yr of age (Fig. 19–3).

In boys enlargement of the penis and testes, appearance of pubic hair, acne, and frequent erections occur. The voice deepens, and linear growth is accelerated. Spermatogenesis has been observed as early as 5–6 yr of age, and nocturnal emissions may occur. Testicular biopsies have shown stimulation of all elements of the testes. If the precocity is complete, various degrees of spermatogenesis are present; even if it is incomplete, the interstitial cells are present.

In both girls and boys height, weight, and osseous maturation are advanced. The increased rate of ossification results in early closure of epiphyses so that ultimate stature is less than it would have been otherwise. Without treatment, approximately one third of patients do not achieve a height of 152 cm (5 ft) as adults. Dental age and mental development are usually compatible with chronologic age.

LABORATORY DATA. Levels of plasma FSH and LH may be elevated for the age of the patient. In as many as 50% of patients, however, these levels overlap those seen in normal children of the same age. Serial determinations often reveal well-defined pulsatile secretion of gonadotropins, especially during sleep, with LH secretion predominating. After administration of LHRH, a brisk response occurs, similar in degree to that seen in normal puberty. Markedly elevated LH levels should suggest the presence of a human chorionic gonadotropin (hCG)–secreting tumor because most assays for LH cross-react with hCG.

Plasma testosterone (in boys) and estradiol (in girls) are usually elevated to levels consistent with the stage of puberty and osseous maturation. Like normal pubertal girls, girls with idiopathic precocious puberty may have wide fluctuations in levels of estrogens. Osseous maturation is advanced and consistent with the stage of pubertal development. Ultrasound examination of the ovaries reveals enlargement to pubertal size. CT scan or MRI is indicated to rule out intracranial lesions.

DIFFERENTIAL DIAGNOSIS. Gonadotropin-independent causes of precocious puberty must be considered in the differential diagnosis (see Table 19–2). In girls, these include tumors of the ovaries, autonomously functioning luteinized ovarian cysts, feminizing adrenal tumors, McCune-Albright syndrome, and exogenous sources of estrogens. In boys, congenital adrenal hyperplasia, adrenal tumors, Leydig cell tumors, gonadotropin-producing hepatoma, and familial male

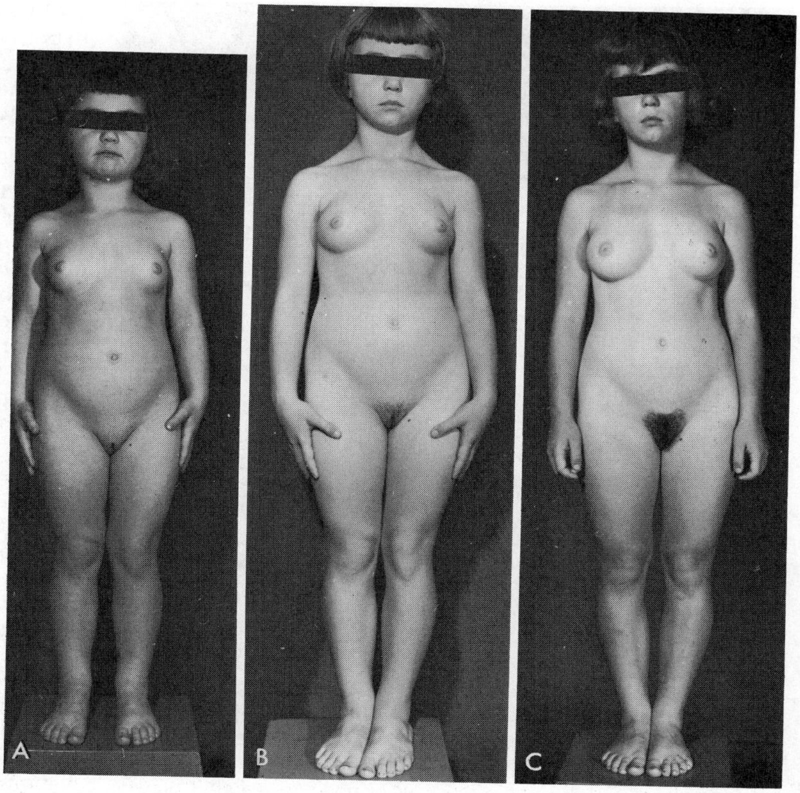

Figure 19–3. Idiopathic precocious puberty. Patient *(A)* at 3 11/12, *(B)* at 5 8/12, and *(C)* at 8 1/2 yr of age. Breast development and vaginal bleeding began at 2 1/2 yr of age. Osseous age was 7 1/2 yr at 3 11/12 and 14 yr at 8 yr of age. Repeated estrogen assays varied between normal prepubertal and adult female levels. Urinary gonadotropins were not demonstrable until the child was 5 yr of age. Intelligence and dental age were normal for chronologic age. Growth was completed at 10 yr; ultimate height was 142 cm (56 in).

precocious puberty should be considered. In children with gonadotropin-dependent precocious puberty, cerebral lesions should be ruled out by CT or MRI scans.

TREATMENT. Treatment consists of administration of an analog of LHRH that is more potent, has a longer duration of action than native LHRH, and suppresses pulsatile discharge of gonadotropins, because to maintain sustained release of gonadotropin pituitary gonadotropic cells require intermittent periods of absence of stimulation by LHRH.

A variety of analogs have been used to treat several hundred children with gonadotropin-dependent precocious puberty. Gonadotropins in children who have been treated longest (6 yr) have remained continuously suppressed, and no serious adverse effects have been noted. Breast development regresses or does not advance. Growth returns to normal rates, osseous maturation decreases, and predicted height is enhanced. LHRH-stimulated peak levels of gonadotropin and sex steroid levels remain suppressed. Discontinuation of therapy results in resumption of puberty.

In the past, treatment required daily subcutaneous or multiple (t.i.d.) intranasal administrations of the LHRH analog. The recent advent of a long-acting depot analog has markedly simplified therapy. The available preparation, luprolide acetate (Lupron Depot), is given in a dose of 0.2–0.3 mg/kg (maximum 7.5 mg) intramuscularly once every 4 wk. Gonadotropin suppression is comparable with that achieved with preparations administered daily.

Precocious Puberty Resulting from Organic Brain Lesions

ETIOLOGY. A wide variety of lesions of the central nervous system have been associated with gonadotropin-dependent sexual precocity. Postencephalitic scars, tuberculous meningoencephalitis, hydrocephalus, tuberous sclerosis, and severe head trauma have each, on occasion, been etiologic factors. Optic gliomas, astrocytomas, ependymomas, and neurofibromas may cause sexual precocity. How these lesions activate hypothalamic mechanisms that initiate puberty is unknown, but they usually involve the hypothalamus by scarring, invasion, or pressure.

With the advent of CT scan and MRI, *hypothalamic hamartoma* is being increasingly recognized as a cause of true precocious puberty (Fig. 19–4). These congenital malformations consist of ectopically located neural tissue resembling nerve cells of the tuber cinereum. These lesions are small, grow slowly or remain static in size, and are occasionally connected to the tuber cinereum by a stalk. Some of these hamartomas have been found to contain LHRH and, in at least one instance, other hypothalamic peptides such as ACTH.

About half of the tumors in the pineal region are *germinomas* or *astrocytomas;* the remainder consist of a wide variety of histologically distinct tumor types. These tumors cause precocious puberty in boys by secreting hCG, which stimulates the Leydig cells of the testes. Intracranial hCG-secreting germinomas usually do not produce precocious puberty in girls, presumably because complete ovarian function cannot occur without FSH priming; precocious puberty in one such girl without measurable estrogen has been attributed to a direct effect of hCG and/or the associated hyperprolactinemia on the breast.

CLINICAL MANIFESTATIONS. Some of these tumors grow slowly and produce no signs other than precocious puberty. Neuroendocrine manifestations may be present for 1–2 yr before tumors can be detected radiologically. Other hypothalamic signs or symptoms such as diabetes insipidus, adipsia, hyperthermia, obesity, and cachexia should suggest the possibility of an intracranial lesion. Unnatural crying or laughing (gelastic seizures) may occur in children with hypothalamic hamartomas.

The sexual precocity is always isosexual, and the endocrine patterns are those found in children without demonstrable

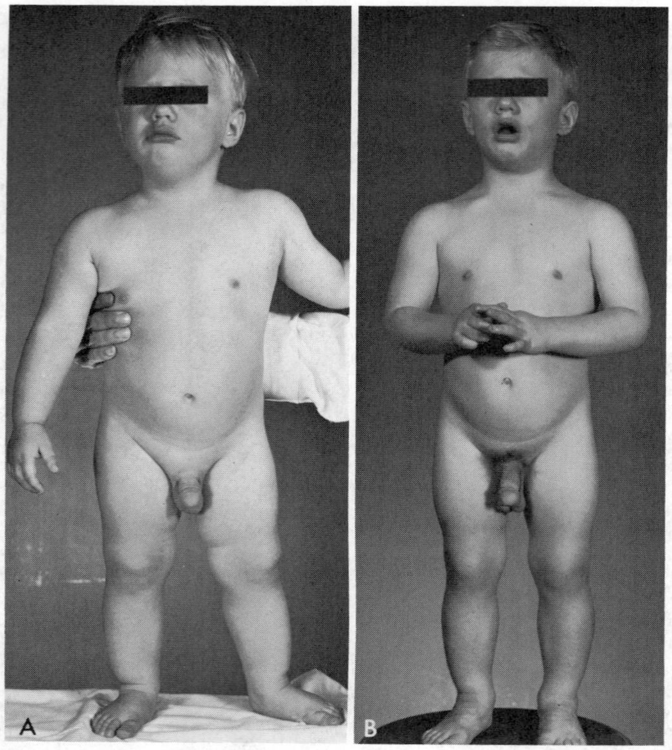

Figure 19–4. Precocious puberty with central nervous system lesion. Photographs at *(A)* 1.5 and *(B)* 2.5 yr of age. Accelerated growth, muscular development, osseous maturation, and testicular development were consistent with the degree of secondary sexual maturation. Urinary gonadotropins were repeatedly negative, 17-ketosteroids usually 2–3 mg/24 hr. In early infancy he began having frequent spells of rapid, purposeless motion; later in life he had episodes of uncontrollable laughing with ocular movements. At 7 yr he exhibited emotional lability, aggressive behavior, and destructive tendencies. Although a hypothalamic hamartoma had been suspected, it was not established until computed tomographic scanning became available, when the patient was 23 yr of age. Epiphyses fused at 9 yr of age; final height was 142 cm (56 inches). At 24 yr of age, he developed an embryonal cell carcinoma of the retroperitoneum.

organic lesions. About 40% of boys but only 10% of girls with true precocious puberty have an intracranial tumor; accordingly, the diagnosis of idiopathic precocious puberty can be made with less confidence in boys than in girls. Rapidly progressive sexual precocity in very young children suggests the likelihood of a hamartoma of the tuber cinereum. CT scan or MRI is indicated in all children with true precocious puberty. Serum hormone levels are essentially the same as those occurring in children with idiopathic gonadotropin-dependent precocious puberty. Very high levels of LH should suggest a chorionic gonadotropin–secreting tumor because LH and hCG cross-react in radioimmunoassays.

TREATMENT. Therapy depends on the nature and location of the lesion. Hypothalamic hamartomas that are pedunculated may be surgically removed; otherwise, their effects are best treated with an LHRH analog, as described for true precocious puberty without organic lesions. Other untreatable lesions, such as trauma, may also be treated in this fashion.

SYNDROME OF PRECOCIOUS PUBERTY AND HYPOTHYROIDISM

In children with untreated hypothyroidism, onset of puberty is usually delayed until epiphyseal maturation has reached 12–13 yr of age. Precocious puberty in a child with untreated hypothyroidism and a prepubertal bone age presents, therefore, a striking appearance and an unphysiologic association. The phenomenon appears to be not uncommon. Among 54 carefully studied children with primary hypothyroidism, half had varying degrees of isosexual development prior to osseous maturation.

Affected patients have usually had severe hypothyroidism of long duration, with the usual manifestations including retardation of growth and of osseous maturation. The causes of the hypothyroidism include lymphocytic thyroiditis, thyroidectomy, and overtreatment with antithyroid drugs.

A preponderance of the reported instances have involved girls, probably reflecting the higher incidence of hypothyroidism in females. A significant number have also had Down syndrome; this observation probably relates to the delay in recognition of hypothyroidism in children with Down syndrome. Sexual development in girls consists primarily of breast enlargement or menstrual bleeding, even in girls with minimal breast enlargement. Boys have testicular enlargement without signs of virilization. Enlargement of the sella and suprasellar extension of the pituitary may occur and are best demonstrated by MRI. Plasma levels of TSH are markedly elevated (often over 1,000 mIU/mL). Plasma levels of prolactin, FSH, and LH are elevated, but there is preferential secretion of FSH over LH. As a consequence, unlike true precocious puberty in boys, testicular enlargement occurs without Leydig cell stimulation, and in girls ovarian estrogen production occurs without a concomitant increase in androgens. Thus, the precocious puberty associated with hypothyroidism is an incomplete form of gonadotropin-dependent puberty. Since TSH and gonadotropins have similar α chains, it is believed that in patients in whom TSH is markedly elevated for prolonged periods, the specificity of TRH spills over to involve the gonadotropins. Whatever the mechanism, treatment of the hypothyroidism results in rapid return to normal of the biochemical and clinical manifestations.

GONADOTROPIN-SECRETING TUMORS

HEPATIC TUMORS. About 30 patients with isosexual precocious puberty associated with hepatoblastoma have been recorded. All have been males, the age of onset varying from 4 mo–8 yr, the average being 2 yr. An enlarged liver or mass in the upper quadrant should suggest the diagnosis. Testicular histology reveals interstitial cell hyperplasia and absence of spermatogenesis. The tumor cells produce chorionic gonadotropin (hCG), which stimulates precocious maturation of the testes. Plasma levels of hCG and α-fetoprotein are usually markedly elevated; they serve as useful markers for following the effects of therapy. Plasma levels of testosterone are elevated, FSH levels are low, and LH levels are high because it cross-reacts with hCG on radioimmunoassay. Treatment for these tumors is the same as that for other carcinomas of the liver; survival is usually less than 1 yr from the time of diagnosis. One patient has survived disease free for over 7 yr.

OTHER TUMORS. Chorionic gonadotropin–secreting choriocarcinomas, teratocarcinomas, or teratomas (also called ectopic pinealomas or atypical teratomas) may also cause precocious puberty. These tumors may be located in the central nervous system, mediastinum, or gonads. They are much more common in boys with precocious puberty (21/100) than in girls (1/100). About a dozen boys with mediastinal tumors and precocious puberty had small testes leading to the diagnosis of Klinefelter syndrome. Why extragonadal tumors (particularly mediastinal) occur more frequently than gonadal tumors in patients with Klinefelter syndrome is not known. Affected patients often have very marked elevation of hCG and α-fetoprotein. FSH is suppressed, but LH levels appear elevated because of cross-reactivity with hCG assay.

PRECOCIOUS PSEUDOPUBERTY

The adrenal causes of pseudopuberty are discussed in Sec. 19.23 and the gonadal causes in Sec. 19.32 and 19.37.

McCune-Albright Syndrome

(Precocious Puberty with Polyostotic Fibrous Dysplasia, and Abnormal Pigmentation)

This is a syndrome of endocrine dysfunction associated with patchy cutaneous pigmentation and fibrous dysplasia of the skeletal system. In the first 4 decades after Albright's description of this entity, sexual precocity in girls was the major recognized endocrinopathy. During the past decade, associated pituitary, thyroid, and adrenal aberrations have been increasingly recognized. For many years the disorder was presumed to originate in the hypothalamus, but now it appears that the disorders in this syndrome result from autonomous hyperfunction of the involved glands.

Precocious puberty has been described predominantly in girls (Fig. 19–5). The average age at onset in affected girls is about 3 yr, but vaginal bleeding has occurred as early as 4 mo of age and secondary sex characteristics as early as 6 mo. Young girls have suppressed levels of LH and FSH, and there is no response to LHRH stimulation. Estradiol levels vary from normal to markedly elevated (>900 pg/mL) and may be cyclic. Ovarian cysts are often found by ultrasound, and levels of estradiol may correlate with the size of the cyst. Sexual precocity appears to be caused by functioning leuteinized follicle cysts of the ovary independent of gonadotropins and is resistant to treatment with long-acting agonists of LHRH. Gonadotropin-independent ovarian function is seen primarily in young girls. When the bone age reaches the usual pubertal age range, gonadotropin secretion begins, and response to LHRH is normal. Thus, true precocious puberty (gonadotropin-dependent) may supersede the antecedent precocious pseudopuberty (gonadotropin-independent). Menses become regular, and fertility has been documented.

The hyperthyroidism that occurs in this condition differs from that characteristic of Graves disease. There is an equal distribution in males and females, and the goiters tend to be multinodular. Clinical hyperthyroidism is uncommon in children, but goiters, mildly elevated T_3 levels, suppressed TSH levels, and abnormalities on ultrasound have been reported.

In patients with associated Cushing syndrome, bilateral nodular adrenocortical hyperplasia has occurred in early infancy, antedating the sexual precocity. ACTH levels are low, and adrenal function is not suppressed by large doses of dexamethasone.

Seventeen patients with McCune-Albright syndrome are known who have increased secretion of growth hormone. This increase is manifested clinically by gigantism or acromegaly or by increased rates of growth even in the absence of precocious puberty. Girls and boys are equally affected. Levels of growth hormone are elevated and increase during sleep; they are augmented by TRH and poorly inhibited by oral glucose. Serum levels of prolactin are increased in most patients, suggesting a plurihormonal-secreting adenoma, but fewer than half of the patients have a demonstrable pituitary tumor.

All patients must be thoroughly investigated. Functioning ovarian cysts often disappear spontaneously; aspiration or surgical excision of cysts is rarely indicated. For girls with persistent estradiol secretion, limited experience with testolactone, an aromatase inhibitor that interferes with the final step of estrogen biosynthesis, is encouraging. Cushing syndrome requires adrenalectomy. Octreotide, a long-acting somatostatin inhibitor, has been used to treat the hypersomatotropism. Prognosis is favorable for longevity, but deformity and repeated fractures may result from the bony lesions.

FAMILIAL MALE GONADOTROPIN-INDEPENDENT PRECOCIOUS PUBERTY

Male-limited autosomal dominant sexual precocity had been assumed to be gonadotropin dependent but is now established to be gonadotropin independent. In the dozen or so described pedigrees, the disorder has been transmitted through affected males and unaffected female carriers of the gene. Signs of puberty appear by 2–3 yr of age. The testes are only slightly enlarged. Testicular biopsies show Leydig cell maturation and, in some instances, marked hyperplasia. Maturation of seminiferous tubules may be present. Testosterone levels are markedly elevated to the same range seen in boys with true precocious puberty; however, baseline levels of LH are prepubertal, pulsatile secretion of LH is absent, and LH does not respond to stimulation with LHRH. The cause for activation of Leydig cells independent of gonadotropin stimulation is unknown. Osseous maturation may be markedly advanced; when it reaches around 13 yr of age, normal gonadotropin secretion intervenes because maturation of the hypothalamus is enhanced owing to exposure to abnormal levels of androgens. Precocious puberty then becomes gonadotropin dependent. This situation is analogous to that occurring in children with McCune-Albright syndrome or in those with congenital adrenal hyperplasia, in whom sexual precocity is initially gonadotropin independent but becomes gonadotropin dependent when maturation of the hypothalamus initiates normal gonadotropin secretion.

Treatment. Young boys have been successfully treated with ketoconazole (600 mg/24 hr in 8-hr divided doses), an antifungal drug that inhibits C-17,20 lyase and testosterone synthesis. However, older boys whose LHRH pulse generator has matured become resistant to treatment. LHRH agonists may then be used. Other investigators have successfully used a combination of spironolactone (to block androgen action) and testolactone (a competitive inhibitor of aromatase). Further experience is necessary to assess these forms of therapy.

19.8 INCOMPLETE (PARTIAL) PRECOCIOUS DEVELOPMENT

Isolated manifestations of precocity without development of other signs of puberty are not unusual; development of the breasts and growth of sexual hair are the two most common forms.

PREMATURE THELARCHE. This term applies to a transient condition of isolated breast development that most often appears in the first 2 yr of life; in some infants breast development is present at birth and persists. Breast development may be unilateral or asymmetric and often fluctuates in degree. Growth and osseous maturation are normal or slightly advanced. The genitalia show no evidence of estrogenic stimulation. The condition is usually sporadic and is rarely familial. Breast development may regress after 2 yr, often persists for 3–5 yr, and is rarely progressive. Menarche occurs at the expected age, and reproduction is normal. Plasma levels of LH and estradiol are below the limits of the assays, but basal levels of FSH and their responses to LHRH stimulation are greater than those seen in normal controls. In contrast, children with true precocious puberty secrete predominantly LH. Ultrasound examination of the ovaries reveals

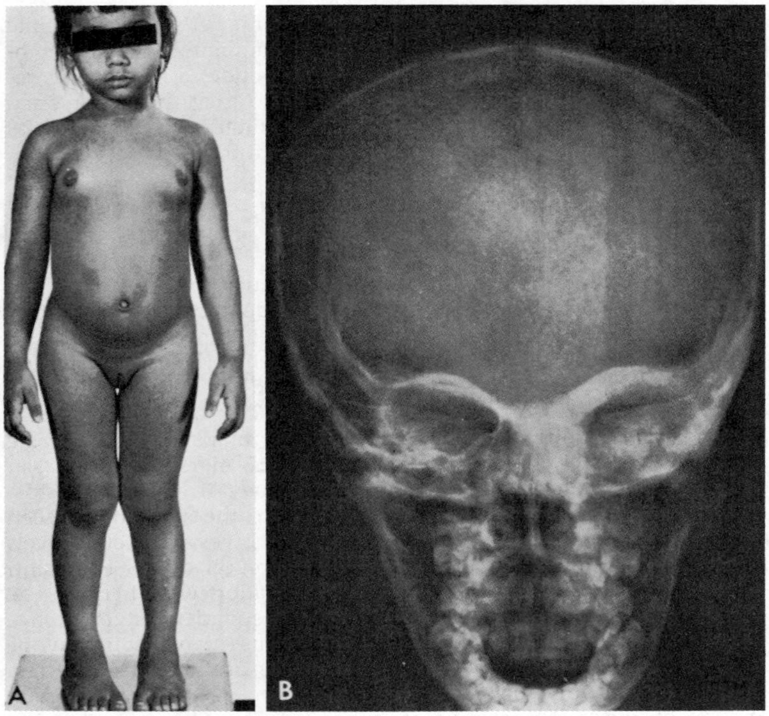

Figure 19–5. Precocious puberty associated with polyostotic fibrous dysplasia (McCune-Albright syndrome) in a girl 4.5 yr of age; at this time her height age and osseous age were normal. Menarche occurred at 4 yr of age. *A*, Note the bilateral breast development, hyperpigmented spots on the abdomen, and the prominence of the left side of the face. *B*, Roentgenograms revealed fibrous dysplasia in the distal end of the left ulna and the thickening of the bones about the left orbit and the maxillary portion of the frontal bones shown here.

normal size, but there may be a few small cysts, usually not larger than 9 mm. The condition is thought to arise from a maturational aberration of the hypothalamic-pituitary-gonadal axis resulting in an imbalance in the ratio of LH-FSH secretion.

Premature thelarche is a benign condition but may be the first sign of true or pseudoprecocious puberty, or it may be caused by exogenous exposure to estrogens. In addition to a detailed history, plasma levels of FSH, LH, and estradiol should be obtained. Pelvic ultrasound examination is rarely indicated. Continued observation is important because the condition cannot be readily distinguished from true precocious puberty. Regression and recurrence suggest functioning follicular cysts. Occurrence of thelarche in children older than 2 yr of age most often is caused by a condition other than benign precocious thelarche.

PREMATURE ADRENARCHE. This term applies to the appearance of sexual hair before the age of 8 yr in girls or 9 yr in boys without other evidence of maturation. It is much more frequent in girls than in boys and may occur more frequently in black girls than in others. Hair appears first on the labia majora; in young children it progresses slowly to the pubic region and finally appears in the axilla. Adult-type axillary odor is common. Affected children are slightly advanced in height and osseous maturation.

Basal and ACTH-stimulated levels of DHEAS, androstenedione, 17-hydroxyprogesterone, and 17-hydroxypregnenolone are often higher than the levels seen in age-matched controls. This may lead to an erroneous diagnosis of an enzymatic defect in adrenal steroidogenesis due to nonclassic forms of adrenal hyperplasia. However, the levels of these steroids are usually found to be in the normal range when they are compared with those of children in the early stages of normal puberty. Thus, it appears that premature adrenarche is simply an early maturational event of adrenal androgen production. A non-ACTH factor is believed to initiate the adrenarche. This event coincides with maturation of the zona reticularis, an associated decrease in 3β-hydroxysteroid-dehydrogenase activity, and an increase in C-17,20 lyase activity (see Fig. 19–12).

Premature adrenarche is a benign condition. When it is associated with clitoral enlargement, cystic acne, or advanced bone age (>3 SD above the mean for age), an ACTH stimulation test with measurement of adrenal steroids is indicated.

PREMATURE MENARCHE. Isolated menses without other evidence of sexual development occurs less frequently than premature thelarche or premature adrenarche. The majority of affected girls have only 1–3 episodes of bleeding; puberty occurs at the usual time and menstrual cycles are normal. Plasma levels of gonadotropins are normal, but estradiol levels may be elevated, probably owing to bursts of ovarian activity. Occasional patients are found to have ovarian follicular cysts on ultrasound. Vaginal causes of bleeding such as vulvovaginitis, foreign body, urethral prolapse, and sarcoma botryoides must be ruled out by careful physical examination.

19.9 MEDICATIONAL PRECOCITY

A variety of medicaments can induce the appearance of secondary sexual characteristics that may be confused with precocious puberty. A careful history focused on exploring the possibility of accidental exposure to or ingestion of sex hormones is important. Precocious pseudopuberty has occurred in both boys and girls from the accidental ingestion of estrogens (including contraceptive pills) and from the administration of anabolic steroids. Estrogens in cosmetics, hair creams, and breast augmentation creams have caused breast development in girls and gynecomastia in boys; estrogens are readily absorbed through the skin. Contamination of vitamin tablets by sex hormones has been reported to cause precocious pseudopuberty. A recent "epidemic" of premature thelarche and precocious pseudopuberty in Puerto Rico has been attributed to contamination of meats, particularly chicken, with estrogens used in animal husbandry but has not been proved. Exogenous estrogens may produce an intense, dark brown color in the areola of the breasts that is not usually seen in endogenous types of precocity. The precocious changes disappear after cessation of exposure to the hormones.

GENERAL

Kaplan SA: Clinical Pediatric Endocrinology. Philadelphia, WB Saunders, 1990.

HYPOPITUITARISM

Allen DB, Fost NC: Growth hormone therapy for short stature: Panacea or Pandora's box. J Pediatr 117:16, 1990.

Amselem S, Duquesnoy P, Goossens M: Molecular basis of Laron dwarfism. Trends in Endocrinol Metab 2:35, 1991.

Asa SL, Bilbao JM, Kovacs K, et al: Lymphocytic hypophysitis of pregnancy resulting in hypopituitarism: A distinct clinicopathologic entity. Ann Intern Med 95:166, 1981.

Bala RM, Lopatka J, Leung A, et al: Serum immunoreactive somatomedin levels in normal adults, pregnant women at term, children at various ages, and children with constitutionally delayed growth. J Clin Endocrinol Metab 52:508, 1981.

Baumann G, Shaw MA, Merimee T: Low levels of high-affinity growth hormone-binding protein in African pygmies. N Engl J Med 320:1705, 1989.

Blethen SL, Welden VV: Hypopituitarism and septo-optic "dysplasia" in first cousins. Am J Med Genet 21:123, 1985.

Brown RS, Vijayalakshmi B, Hayes E: An apparent cluster of congenital hypopituitarism in central Massachusetts: Magnetic resonance imaging and hormonal studies. J Clin Endocrinol Metab 72:11, 1991.

Clayton PE, Shalet SM: Dose dependency of time of onset of radiation-induced growth hormone deficiency. J Pediatr 118:226, 1991.

Costin G, Murphree AL: Hypothalamic-pituitary function in children with optic nerve hypoplasia. Am J Dis Child 139:249, 1985.

Dean HJ, Bishop A, Winter JSD: Growth hormone deficiency in patients with histiocytosis. J Pediatr 109:615, 1986.

Donaldson DL, Hallowell JG, Pan E, et al: Growth hormone secretory profiles: Variation on consecutive nights. J Pediatr 115:51, 1989.

Ellyin F, Khatir AH, Singh SP: Hypothalamic-pituitary functions in patients with transsphenoidal encephalocele and midfacial anomalies. J Clin Endocrinol Metab 51:854, 1980.

Fleisher TA, White RM, Broder S, et al: X-linked hypogammaglobulinemia and isolated growth hormone deficiency. N Engl J Med 302:1429, 1980.

Frasier SD: Human pituitary growth hormone (hGH) therapy in growth hormone deficiency. Endocrinol Rev 4:155, 1983.

Gertner JM, Genel M, Gianfredi SP, et al: Prospective clinical trial of human growth hormone in short children without growth hormone deficiency. J Pediatr 104:172, 1984.

Godowski PJ, Leung DW, Meacham LR, et al: Characterization of the human growth hormone receptor gene and demonstration of a partial gene deletion in two patients with Laron-type dwarfism. Proc Natl Acad Sci USA 86:8083, 1989.

Hall JG, Pallister PD, Carren SK, et al: Congenital hypothalamic hamartoblastoma, hypopituitarism, imperforate anus, and postaxial polydactyly—a new syndrome? Part 1: Clinical, causal and pathogenetic considerations. Am J Med Genet 7:47, 1980.

Hanna CE, Krainz PL, Skeels MR, et al: Detection of congenital hypopituitary hypothyroidism: Ten year experience in The Northwest Regional Screening Program. J Pediatr 109:959, 1986.

Herman SP, Baggenstoss AM, Clothier MD: Liver dysfunction and histiologic abnormalities in neonatal hypopituitarism. J Pediatr 87:892, 1975.

Kamijo T, Phillips JA III, Ogawa M, et al: Screening for growth hormone gene deletions in patients with isolated growth hormone deficiency. J Pediatr 118:245, 1991.

Lippe B, Frasier D: How should we test for growth hormone deficiency, and whom should we treat. J Pediatr 115:585, 1989.

Littley MD, Shalet SM, Beardwell CG, et al: Radiation-induced hypopituitarism is dose-dependent. Clin Endocrinol 31:363, 1989.

Lovinger RD, Kaplan SL, Grumbach MM: Congenital hypopituitarism associated with neonatal hypoglycemia and microphallus: Four cases secondary to hypothalamic hormone deficiencies. J Pediatr 87:1171, 1975.

Margalith D, Tze WJ, Jan JE: Congenital optic nerve hypoplasia with hypothalamic-pituitary dysplasia. Am J Dis Child 139:361, 1985.

Miller WL, Kaplan SL, Grumbach MM: Child abuse as a cause of post-traumatic hypopituitarism. N Engl J Med 302:724, 1980.

Money J: The syndrome of abuse dwarfism (psychosocial) or reversible hyposomatotropism. Am J Dis Child 131:508, 1977.

Nishi Y, Aihara K, Usui T, et al: Isolated growth hormone deficiency type 1 A in a Japanese family. J Pediatr 104:885, 1984.

Rapaport EB, Ulstrom RA, Gorlin RJ, et al: Solitary maxillary central incisor and short stature. J Pediatr 91:924, 1977.

Rappaport R, Brauner R: Growth and endocrine disorders secondary to cranial irradiation. Pediatr Res 25:561, 1989.

Rivarola MA, Phillips JA III, Migeon CJ, et al: Phenotypic heterogeneity in familial isolated growth hormone deficiency Type 1-A. J Clin Endocrinol Metab 59:34, 1984.

Rogol AD, Blizzard RM, Foley TP, et al: Growth hormone releasing hormone and growth hormone: Genetic studies in familial growth hormone deficiency. Pediatr Res 19:489, 1985.

Rose SR, Ross JL, Uriarte M, et al: The advantage of measuring stimulated as compared with spontaneous growth hormone levels in the diagnosis of growth hormone deficiency. N Engl J Med 319:201, 1988.

Rosenbloom AL, Aquirre JG, Rosenfeld RG, et al: The little women of Loja—growth hormone-receptor deficiency in an inbred population of southern Ecuador. N Engl J Med 323:1367, 1990.

Rudman D, Davis GT, Priest JH, et al: Prevalence of growth hormone deficiency in children with cleft lip or palate. J Pediatr 93:378, 1978.

Schriock EA, Lustig RH, Rosenthal SM, et al: Effect of growth hormone (GR)-releasing hormone (GRH) on plasma GH in relation to magnitude and duration of GH deficiency in 26 children and adults with isolated GH deficiency or multiple pituitary hormone deficiencies: Evidence for hypothalamic GRH deficiency. J Clin Endocrinol Metab 58:1083, 1984.

Sklar CA, Grumbach MM, Kaplan SL, Conte FA: Hormonal and metabolic abnormalities associated with central nervous system germinoma in children and adolescents and effect of therapy: Report of 10 patients. J Clin Endocrinol Metab 52:9, 1981.

Tanner JM, Lejarraga H, Cameron N: The natural history of the Silver-Russell syndrome: A longitudinal study of thirty-nine cases. Pediatr Res 9:611, 1975.

Taylor AL, Fishman LM: Corticotropin-releasing hormone. N Engl J Med 319:213, 1988.

Thomasett MJ, Conte FA, Kaplan SL, Grumbach MM: Endocrine and neurologic outcome in childhood craniopharyngioma: Review of effect of treatment in 42 patients. J Pediatr 97:728, 1980.

Tsu-Hui L, Kirkland RT, Sheman BM, et al: Growth hormone testing in short children and their responses to growth hormone therapy. J Pediatr 115:57, 1989.

Valenta LJ, Siegel MB, Lesniak MA, et al: Pituitary dwarfism in a patient with circulating abnormal growth hormone polymers. N Engl J Med 312:214, 1985.

Vnencak-Jones CL, Phillips JA III, De-Fen W: Use of polymerase chain reaction in detection of growth hormone gene deletions. J Clin Endocrinol Metab 70:1550, 1990.

White MC, Chahal P, Banks L, et al: Familial hypopituitarism associated with an enlarged pituitary fossa and an empty sella. Clin Endocrinol 24:63, 1986.

Wilkinson IA, Duck SC, Gager WE, et al: Empty-sella syndrome. Occurrence in childhood. Am J Dis Child 136:245, 1982.

HYPERPITUITARISM

Bale AE, Drum A, Perry DM, et al: Familial Sotos syndrome (cerebral gigantism): Craniofacial and psychological characteristics. Am J Med Genet 20:613, 1985.

Costin G, Fefferman RA, Kogut MD: Hypothalamic gigantism. J Pediatr 83:419, 1973.

Cutler L, Jackson JA, Uz-zafar S, et al: Hypersecretion of growth hormone and prolactin in McCune-Albright syndrome. J Clin Endocrinol Metab 68:1148, 1989.

Dodge PR, Holmes SJ, Sotos JF: Cerebral gigantism. Devel Med Child Neurol 25:248, 1983.

Guyda H, Robert F, Colle E, et al: Histologic, ultrastructural and hormonal characterization of a pituitary tumor secreting both HGH and prolactin. J Clin Endocrinol Metab 36:531, 1973.

Lightner ES, Winter JSD: Treatment of juvenile acromegaly with bromocriptine. J Pediatr 98:494, 1981.

Liuzzi A, Dellabonzana D, Oppizzi G, et al: Low doses of dopamine agonists in the long-term treatment of macroprolactinomas. N Engl J Med 313:656, 1985.

Melmed S: Acromegaly. N Engl J Med 322:966, 1990.

Moran A, Asa SL, Kovacs K, et al: Gigantism due to pituitary mammosomatotroph hyperplasia. N Engl J Med 323:322, 1990.

Patton ML, Woolf PD: Hyperprolactinemia and delayed puberty: A report of three cases and their response to therapy. Pediatrics 71:572, 1983.

Sack J, Friedman E, Tadmor R, et al: Growth and puberty arrest due to prolactinoma. Acta Paediatr Scand 73:863, 1984.

Sadeghi-Nejad A, Wolfsdorf JI, Biller BJ, et al: Hyperprolactinemia causing primary amenorrhea. J Pediatr 99:802, 1981.

Spense JH, Trias EP, Raiti S: Acromegaly in a 9½ year old boy. Am J Dis Child 123:504, 1972.

Whitaker MD, Scheithaver BW, Hayles AB, et al: The hypothalamus and pituitary in cerebral gigantism. A clinico-pathologic and immunocytochemical study. Am J Dis Child 139:679, 1985.

DIABETES INSIPIDUS

Adams JM, Kenny JD, Rudolph AJ: Central diabetes insipidus following intraventricular hemorrhage. J Pediatr 88:292, 1976.

Assadi FK, John EG: Hypouricemia in neonates with syndrome of inappropriate secretion of antidiuretic hormone. Pediatr Res 19:424, 1985.

Bode HH, Harley BM, Crawford JD: Restoration of normal drinking behavior by chlorpropamide in patients with hypodipsia and diabetes insipidus. Am J Med 51:304, 1971.

Czernichow P, Pomerade R, Basmaciogullari A, et al: Diabetes insipidus in children. III. Anterior pituitary dysfunction in idiopathic types. J Pediatr 106:41, 1985.

Dunger DB, Broadbent V, Yeoman E, et al: The frequency and natural history of diabetes insipidus in children with Langerhans-cell histiocytosis. N Engl J Med 321:1157, 1989.

Friedman AL, Segar WE: Antidiuretic hormone excess. J Pediatr 94:521, 1979.

Hammond DN, Moll GW, Robertson GL, et al: Hypodipsic hypernatremia with normal osmoregulation of vasopressin. N Engl J Med 315:433, 1986.

Hays RM: Antidiuretic hormone. N Engl J Med 295:659, 1976.
Hendricks SA, Lippe B, Kaplan SA, et al: Differential diagnosis of diabetes insipidus: Use of DDAVP to terminate the seven-hour water deprivation test. J Pediatr 98:244, 1981.
Khare SK: Neurohypophyseal dysfunction following perinatal asphyxia. J Pediatr 90:628, 1977.
Kohn B, Norman ME, Feldman H, et al: Hysterical polydipsia (compulsive water drinking). Am J Dis Child 130:210, 1976.
Lee WP, Lippe B, LaFranchi SH, et al: Vasopressin analogue DDAVP in the treatment of diabetes insipidus. Am J Dis Child 130:166, 1976.
Miller M, Moses AM: Urinary antidiuretic hormone in polyuric disorders and in appropriate ADH syndrome. Ann Intern Med 77:715, 1972.
Richardson DW, Robinson AG: Desmopressin. Ann Intern Med 103:228, 1985.
Richman RA, Post EM, Notman DD, et al: Simplifying the diagnosis of diabetes insipidus in children. Am J Dis Child 135:839, 1981.
Scherbaum WA, Wass JAH, Besser GM, et al: Autoimmune cranial diabetes insipidus: Its association with other endocrine diseases and with histiocytosis X. Clin Endocrinol 25:411, 1986.
Sklar C, Fertig A, David R: Chronic syndrome of inappropriate secretion of antidiuretic hormone in childhood. Am J Dis Child 139:733, 1985.
Toth EL, Bowen PA, Crockford PM: Hereditary central diabetes insipidus: Plasma levels of antidiuretic hormone in a family with a possible osomoreceptor defect. Canad Med Assoc J 131:1237, 1984.
Zerbe RL, Robertson GL: A comparison of plasma vasopressin with a standard direct test in the differential diagnosis of polyuria. N Engl J Med 305:1539, 1981.

PRECOCIOUS PUBERTY

Barnes ND, Hayles AB, Ryan RJ: Sexual maturation in juvenile hypothyroidism. Mayo Clin Proc 48:849, 1973.
Comite F, Pescovitz OH, Rieth KG, et al: Luteinizing hormone-releasing hormone analog treatment of boys with hypothalamic hamartoma and true precocious puberty. J Clin Endocrinol Metab 59:888, 1984.
Comite F, Shawker TH, Pescovitz OH, et al: Cyclical ovarian function resistant to treatment with an analogue of luteinizing hormone releasing hormone in McCune-Albright syndrome. N Engl J Med 311:1032, 1984.
Conn PM, Crowley WR Jr: Gonadotropin-releasing hormone and its analogues. N Engl J Med 324:93, 1991.
Danon M, Robboy SJ, Sully R, et al: Cushing syndrome, sexual precocity and polyostotic fibrous dysplasia in infancy. J Pediatr 87:817, 1975.
DiGeorge AM: Albright syndrome: Is it coming of age? J Pediatr 87:1018, 1975.
Dunkel L, Alfthan H, Stenman UH, et al: Gonadal control of pulsatile secretion of luteinizing hormone and follicle-stimulating hormone in prepubertal boys by ultrasensitive time-resolved immunofluorometric assays. J Clin Endocrinol Metab 70:107, 1990.
Feuillan P, Foster CM, Pescovitz OH, et al: Treatment of precocious puberty in the McCune Albright syndrome with the aromatase inhibitor testolactone. N Engl J Med 315:115, 1986.
Foster CM, Ross JR, Shawker T, et al: Absence of pubertal gonadotropin secretion in girls with McCune-Albright syndrome. J Clin Endocrinol Metab 58:1161, 1984.
Hardy M, O'Connell J, Gilbertson N, et al: Precocious puberty associated with hyperprolactinemia in a male patient. J Pediatr 113:508, 1988.
Harlan WR, Grillo GP, Cornoni-Huntley J, Leaverton PE: Secondary sex characteristics of boys 12–17 years of age. J Pediatr 95:293, 1979.
Harlan WR, Harlan EA, Grillo GP: Secondary sex characteristics of girls 12 to 17 years of age: The US Health Examination Survey. J Pediatr 96:1074, 1980.
Hertz R: Accidental ingestion of estrogens by children. Pediatrics 21:203, 1958.
Holland FS, Kirsch SE, Selby R: Gonadotropin-independent precocious puberty ("testotoxosis"): Influence of maturational status of response to ketoconazole. J Clin Endocrinol Metab 64:328, 1987.
Ilicke A, Prager Lewin R, Kauli R, et al: Premature thelarche—Natural history and sex hormone secretion in 68 girls. Acta Paediatr Scand 73:756, 1984.
Jenner MR, Kelch KP, Kaplan SL, et al: Plasma estradiol in prepubertal children, pubertal females, and in precocious puberty, premature thelarche, hypogonadism, and in a child with a feminizing ovarian tumor. J Clin Endocrinol 34:521, 1972.
Kaplan SL, Grumbach MM: Pathophysiology and treatment of sexual precocity. J Clin Endocrinol Metab 71:785, 1990.
Lave L, Kenisberg D, Peskovitz O, et al: Treatment of familial male precocious puberty with spironolactone and testolactone. N Engl J Med 320:496, 1989.
Lee PA, Xenakis T, Winer J, et al: Puberty in girls: Correlation of serum levels of gonadotropins, prolactin, androgens, estrogens, and progestins with physical changes. J Clin Endocrinol Metab 42:775, 1976.
Lightner ES, Penny R, Frasier SD: Pituitary adenoma in McCune-Albright syndrome: Follow-up information. J Pediatr 89:159, 1976.
Lin TH, LePage ME, Henzl M, et al: Intranasal nafarelin: An LH-RH analogue treatment of gonadotropin-dependent precocious puberty. J Pediatr 109:954, 1986.
Lucky AW, Rich BH, Rosenfield RL, et al: LH bioactivity increases more than immunoactivity during puberty. J Pediatr 97:205, 1980.
Mills JL, Stolley PD, Davies J, et al: Premature thelarche. Natural history and etiologic investigation. Am J Dis Child 135:743, 1981.
Morris AH, Reiter EO, Geffner ME, et al: Absence of nonclassical congenital adrenal hyperplasia in patients with precocious adrenarche. J Clin Endocrinol Metab 69:709, 1989.
Nakagawara A, Ikeda K, Tsuneyoshi M, et al: Hepatoblastoma producing alpha-fetoprotein and human chorionic gonadotropin. Cancer 56:1636, 1985.
Oberfield SE, Mayes DM, Levine LS: Adrenal steroidogenic function in a black and Hispanic population with precocious puberty. J Clin Endocrinol Metab 76:76, 1990.
Pescovitz OH, Comite F, Hench K, et al: The NIH experience with precocious puberty: Diagnostic subgroups and response to short-term luteinizing hormone releasing hormone analogue therapy. J Pediatr 108:47, 1986.
Price RA, Lee PA, Albright AL, et al: Treatment of sexual precocity by removal of a luteinizing hormone-releasing hormone secreting hamartoma. JAMA 251:2247, 1984.
Rieter EO, Fuldauer VG, Root AW: Secretion of the adrenal androgen dehydroepiandrosterone sulfate, during normal infancy, childhood and adolescence in sick infants, and in children with endocrinologic abnormalities. J Pediatr 90:766, 1977.
Romshe CA, Sotos JF: Intracranial human chorionic gonadotropin-secreting tumor with precocious puberty. J Pediatr 86:250, 1975.
Rosenfeld RG, Reitz RE, King AB, et al: Familial precocious puberty associated with isolated elevation of luteinizing hormone. N Engl J Med 303:859, 1980.
Schimke RN, Madigan CM, Silver BJ, et al: Choriocarcinoma, thyrotoxicosis, and the Klinefelter syndrome. Cancer Genet Cytogenet 9:1, 1983.
Shaul PW, Towbin RB, Chernausek SD: Precocious puberty following severe head trauma. Am J Dis Child 139:467, 1985.
Stanhope R, Abdulwahid NA, Adams J, et al: Studies of gonadotropin pulsatility and pelvic ultrasound examination distinguish between isolated premature thelarche and central precocious puberty. Eur J Pediatr 145:190, 1986.
Stanhope R, Adams J, Brook CGD: The treatment of central precocious puberty using an intranasal LHRH analogue (Buserlin). Clin Endocrinol 22:795, 1985.
Starceski PJ, Lee PA, Albright AL, et al: Hypothalamic hamartomas and sexual precocity. Am J Dis Child 144:225, 1990.
Styne DM, Harris DA, Egli CA, et al: Treatment of true precocious puberty with a potent luteinizing hormone-releasing factor agonist: Effect on growth, pelvic sonography and hypothalamic-pituitary gonadal axis. J Clin Endocrinol Metab 61:142, 1985.
Wu FCW, Butler GE, Kelnar CJH, et al: Patterns of pulsatile luteinizing hormone secretion before and during the onset of puberty in boys: A study using an immunoradiometric assay. J Clin Endocrinol Metab 70:629, 1990.

19.10 DISORDERS OF THE THYROID GLAND

The main function of the thyroid gland is to synthesize thyroxine (T_4) and 3,5,3′-triiodothyronine (T_3). The only known physiologic role of iodine is in the synthesis of these hormones; the recommended dietary allowance of iodine is 40–50 μg/24 hr for infants, 70–120 μg/24 hr for children, and 150 μg/24 hr for adolescents and adults. The daily intake in North America varies from 240 to more than 700 μg. Whatever the chemical form ingested, iodine eventually reaches the thyroid gland as iodide. Thyroid tissue has an avidity for iodine and is able to trap (with a gradient of 100–1), transport, and concentrate it in the follicular lumen for synthesis of thyroid hormone.

Before trapped iodide can react with tyrosine, it must be oxidized; this reaction is catalyzed by thyroidal peroxidase. The thyroid cells also elaborate a specific thyroprotein, a globulin with approximately 120 tyrosine units. Iodination of tyrosine forms monoiodotyrosine and diiodotyrosine; two molecules of diiodotyrosine then couple to form one molecule of T_4, or one molecule of diiodotyrosine and one of monoiodotyrosine to form T_3. Once formed, hormones are stored as thyroglobulin in the lumen of the follicle (colloid) until ready to be delivered to the body cells. Thyroglobulin (Tg) is a large globular glycoprotein with a molecular weight of about 660,000 and under normal conditions is detectable in the blood of most individuals at nanogram levels. T_4 and T_3 are liberated from thyroglobulin by activation of proteases and peptidases.

The metabolic potency of T_3 is 3–4 times that of T_4. Only

20% of circulating T_3 is secreted by the thyroid; the remainder is produced by deiodination of T_4 in the liver, kidney, and other peripheral tissues by type I 5′-deiodinase. In the pituitary and brain approximately 80% of required T_3 is produced in situ from T_4 by a different enzyme, type II 5′-deiodinase. In the fetal rat, although plasma levels of T_3 are very low, cerebral concentrations increase to almost adult levels. T_3 carries out most of the physiologic actions of the thyroid hormones. T_4 is more abundant, but it binds weakly to nuclear receptors, and most of its physiologic effects occur via conversion to T_3. The level of T_3 in blood is 1/50 that of T_4. The thyroid hormones increase oxygen consumption, stimulate protein synthesis, influence growth and differentiation, and affect carbohydrate, lipid, and vitamin metabolism. The free hormones enter cells, bind to cytosol receptors specific for T_3 or T_4, and are transported to the nucleus, where they participate in activating transcription. The protein products of the *c-erb* A proto-oncogene have been identified as nuclear thyroid hormone receptors.

About 70% of the circulating thyroid hormones are firmly bound to *thyroxine-binding globulin* (TBG). Less important carriers are thyroxine-binding prealbumin, now named *transthyretin* (TTR), and albumin. Only 0.03% of T_4 in serum is not bound and comprises free thyroxine (FT_4). Because concentration of TBG is altered in many clinical circumstances, its status must be considered when interpreting T_4 or T_3 levels.

The thyroid is regulated by thyroid-stimulating hormone (TSH), a glycoprotein produced and secreted by the anterior pituitary. This hormone activates adenylate cyclase in the thyroid gland to effect release of thyroid hormones. TSH is composed of two noncovalently bound subunits (chains): α and β (hTSH-β). The α subunit is common to LH, FSH, and hCG; the specificity of each hormone is conferred by their β subunit. TSH synthesis and release are stimulated by TSH-releasing hormone (TRH), which is synthesized in the hypothalamus and secreted into the pituitary. TRH is found in other parts of the brain besides the hypothalamus and in many other organs; aside from its endocrine function, it seems to serve as a neurotransmitter. TRH, a simple tripeptide, was the first neuropeptide to be identified, synthesized, and utilized in clinical medicine. In states of decreased production of thyroid hormone, TSH and TRH are increased. An excess of TRH or of TSH results in hypertrophy and hyperplasia of thyroid cells, increased trapping of iodine, and increased synthesis of thyroid hormones. Exogenous thyroid hormone or increased thyroid hormone synthesis inhibits TSH and TRH production. Except in the neonate, levels of TRH in serum are very low.

Further control of the level of circulating thyroid hormones occurs in the periphery. In many nonthyroidal illnesses extrathyroidal production of T_3 decreases; factors that inhibit thyroxine-5′-deiodinase include fasting, chronic malnutrition, acute illness, and certain drugs. Levels of T_3 may be significantly decreased while levels of T_4 and TSH remain normal. Presumably, the decreased levels of T_3 result in decreased rates of oxygen production, of substrate utilization, and of other catabolic processes.

19.11 THYROID HORMONE STUDIES

SERUM THYROID HORMONES. Methods are available to measure all of the thyroid hormones in sera. These include T_4, free T_4, T_3, free T_3, and the diiodothyronines. A metabolically inert T_3 (3,5′,3′-triiodothyronine), called reverse T_3, is also present in sera. Age must be considered in interpreting results, particularly in the neonate (see later).

Thyroglobulin (Tg) is a glycoprotein dimer that is secreted through the apical surface of the thyrocyte into the colloid. Small amounts escape into the circulation and are measurable in serum. Levels increase with TSH stimulation and decrease with TSH suppression. Levels are increased in the neonate, in patients with Graves disease, and in those with endemic goiter. The most marked elevations of Tg occur in patients with differentiated carcinoma of the thyroid. Athyreotic infants may have no measurable Tg in serum.

Thyrotropin (TSH) levels in serum are an extremely sensitive indicator of primary hypothyroidism. RIA methods for the measurement of serum levels of TSH have been replaced by immunometric assay methods, which are capable of quantitating the lower limits of normal as well as elevated levels. A 3rd generation of assays (chemiluminescent assays) that can measure complete suppression of TSH is now available.

After the neonatal period, normal levels of TSH are below 6 μU/mL. TSH secretion can be stimulated by intravenous administration (7 μg/kg) of thyrotropin-releasing hormone (TRH). In normal subjects TRH administration increases baseline levels of TSH within 30 min. In hyperthyroidism there is no rise in serum levels of TSH in response to TRH because the elevated levels of thyroid hormones block the effect of TRH on the pituitary. On the other hand, in patients with even very mild degrees of thyroid failure, administration of TRH results in an exaggerated TSH response. Patients with pituitary or hypothalamic failure have low basal levels of TSH; a normal response to TRH localizes the defect in the hypothalamus.

FETAL AND NEWBORN THYROID. The fetal hypothalamic-pituitary-thyroid system develops independently of maternal influence. By 10–12 wk of gestation the fetal thyroid is able to concentrate iodine and to synthesize iodothyronines. By the same time the fetal pituitary contains TSH. Fetal serum T_4 increases progressively from midgestation to approximately 11.5 μg/dL at term. Fetal levels of T_3 are below measurable levels before 30 wk and then gradually rise to about 50 ng/dL at term. Reverse T_3 levels, however, are very high in the fetus (250 ng/dL at 30 wk) and fall to 150 ng/dL at term. Serum levels of TSH peak in the fetus at 20–24 wk to about 15 μU/mL and then gradually decrease to 10 μU/mL at term.

At birth there is an acute release of TSH; peak serum concentrations reach 70 μU/mL in 30 min in full-term infants. A rapid decline occurs in the ensuing 24 hr and a more gradual decline within the next 2 days to below 10 μU/mL. The acute increase in TSH produces a dramatic rise in levels of T_3 to approximately 300 ng/dL in about 4 hr. This T_3 seems largely derived from increased peripheral conversion of T_4 to T_3. T_3 levels then decline during the 1st wk of life to levels under 200 ng/mL. Reverse T_3 levels are maintained for 2 wk (200 ng/dL) and fall by 4 wk to around 50 ng/dL. Small amounts of T_4 cross the placenta but are not sufficient to interfere with a diagnosis of congenital hypothyroidism in the neonate.

SERUM THYROXINE-BINDING GLOBULIN (TBG). The thyroid hormones are transported in plasma bound to TBG, a glycoprotein synthesized in the liver. Estimation of TBG levels is occasionally necessary because TBG is increased or decreased in a variety of clinical situations, with effects on the level of thyroxine. TBG binds about 75% of T_4 and 70% of T_3. TBG levels increase in pregnancy and in the newborn period, and with administration of estrogens (oral contraceptives), perphenazine, and heroin and decrease with androgens, anabolic steroids, glucocorticoids, and L-asparaginase. These effects are the results of modulation of hepatic synthesis of TBG. Phenytoin (diphenylhydantoin) is another cause of drug-induced abnormality of thyroid function tests. Phenytoin, an inducer of hepatic enzymes, stimulates hepatic degradation of T_4 and accelerates transport of T_4 into tissues. Phenobarbital has a similar effect. Some drugs, particularly phenytoin, also inhibit binding of T_4 and T_3 to TBG. Decreased or increased levels of TBG also occur as genetic traits (see later).

The most commonly used measures of TBG or TBG-binding capacity are variations of the resin triiodothyronine uptake test, RT_3U, a screening test with which to interpret T_4 results; it should never be used as an autonomous test of thyroid function. The product of the serum T_4 concentration and T_3 uptake (thyroxine-resin T_3 index or T_4-RT_3U index) correlates closely with free T_4 concentration in serum. This index increases in hyperthyroidism, decreases in hypothyroidism, and is normal in euthyroid patients with abnormalities in the concentration of TBG. Normal values for the index vary among laboratories since T_4 levels and T_3 uptakes are often determined by a variety of kit methods and calculations and expressions of the index vary also among laboratories. A radioimmunoassay method for TBG is available.

IN VIVO RADIONUCLIDE STUDIES. Markedly improved direct tests of thyroid function have made radioiodine uptake studies less useful. The iodine-trapping or concentrating mechanism of the thyroid can be evaluated by the radioactive isotope ^{123}I (half-life of 13 hr). Present technology allows doses of radioiodine (0.1–0.5 μCi) that are only a fraction of those formerly used. Technetium (^{99m}Tc) is a particularly useful radioisotope for children because, in contrast to iodine, it is trapped but not organified by the thyroid and has a half-life of only 6 hr. Thyroid scanning may be indicated to detect ectopic thyroid tissue, to evaluate thyroid nodules, or to assess the presence of thyroid tissue in questions of thyroid agenesis. These studies should be performed with ^{99m}Tc as pertechnetate because it has the advantages of lower radiation exposure and high-quality scintigrams. Use of ^{131}I in children should be limited to those known to have thyroid cancer.

DEFECTS OF THYROXINE-BINDING GLOBULIN

Abnormalities in levels of TBG are not associated with clinical disease and do not require treatment. They are usually uncovered by a chance finding of abnormally low or high levels of T_4 and may be sources of confusion in the diagnosis of hypo- or hyperthyroidism.

TBG deficiency occurs as an X-linked dominant disorder. Congenital TBG deficiency is most often discovered through screening programs for neonatal hypothyroidism that utilize levels of T_4 as the primary screen. Affected patients have low levels of T_4, but levels of free T_4 and TSH are normal. The diagnosis is confirmed by the finding of absent or low levels of TBG by RIA. The disorder is more readily recognized in males because it is caused by a gene on the short arm of the X chromosome. TBG deficiency occurs in 1 in 2,800 newborn males, of whom 36% have TBG levels below 1 mg/L. Complete TBG deficiency (<5 μg/L) occurs much less frequently. Three of eight families with complete TBG deficiency have been found to have a codon mutation (leucine to proline); other patients with reduced affinity of TBG for T_4 have had other point mutations that affect the tertiary structure of the protein.

Elevated TBG is also a harmless X-linked dominant anomaly, occurring in about 1 in 2,500 persons. It has been recognized primarily in adults, but neonatal screening programs are now uncovering the condition in the neonate. The level of T_4 is elevated, T_3 is variably elevated, TSH and free T_4 are normal, and RT_3U is decreased. The elevated levels of TBG and normal levels of free T_4 confirm the diagnosis. In neonates, levels of T_4 as high as 95 μg/dL have been found, which decrease to 20–30 μg/dL after 2–3 wk. Such high levels of T_4 are thought to be related in part to the normally elevated levels of TBG in neonates during the 1st mo of life, presumably as an effect of maternal estrogens. Affected patients are euthyroid. Family studies may be indicated to alert other affected individuals. Acquired elevations of TBG occur with pregnancy, estrogen treatment, and hepatitis.

Familial dysalbuminemic hyperthyroxinemia is an autosomal dominant disorder that may be confused with hyperthyroidism. Markedly increased binding of T_4 to an abnormal albumin variant leads to increased serum concentrations of T_4. However, the levels of free T_4, free T_3, and TSH are normal. Levels of T_3 are normal or only slightly elevated. Affected patients are euthyroid.

19.12 HYPOTHYROIDISM

Hypothyroidism results from deficient production of thyroid hormone or a defect in its receptor (Table 19–3). The disorder may be manifest very early in life. When symptoms appear after a period of apparently normal thyroid function, the disorder may be either truly "acquired" or may only appear so as a result of one of a variety of congenital defects in which the manifestation of the deficiency is delayed. The term

TABLE 19–3. Etiologic Classification of Hypothyroidism

Deficiency of thyrotropin-releasing hormone (TRH)
- Isolated?
- Multiple hypothalamic deficiencies (e.g., idiopathic hypopituitarism)

Deficiency of thyrotropin (TSH*)
- Isolated
  - Autosomal recessive (point mutation in β chain)
- Multiple pituitary deficiencies (e.g., craniopharyngioma)

Deficiency of thyroid hormone
- Fetal thyroid developmental defects
  - Aplasia, ectopia (dysgenesis)
- Defective synthesis (goitrous hypothyroidism)
  - Iodide-trapping defect
  - Iodide-organification defect (thyroid peroxidase deficiency)
    - Pendred syndrome
  - Iodotyrosine deiodination defect
  - Thyroglobulin synthesis defect
- Iodine deficiency (endemic cretinism)
  - Neurologic type
  - Myxedematous type
- Maternal medications or antibiodies
  - Radioiodine
  - Propylthiouracil, methimazole
  - Iodide
  - Amiodarone
  - TSH-inhibiting antibody (TBIAb)
  - Thyroid growth-blocking antibody
- Autoimmune
  - Hashimoto thyroiditis
  - Idiopathic hypothyroidism
  - TSH-blocking antibody
- Iatrogenic
  - Propylthiouracil, methimazole, lithium, amiodarone, iodides
  - Thyroidectomy
  - Neck or whole body irradiation
- Systemic disease
  - Cystinosis

Receptor defects
- TSH unresponsiveness
  - Defective G unit (e.g., type 1a pseudohypoparathyroidism)
- Thyroid hormone unresponsiveness
  - Generalized
    - Complete
    - Partial
  - Limited to pituitary gland

*TSH = thyroid-stimulating hormone.

cretinism is often used synonymously with congenital hypothyroidism but should be avoided.

CONGENITAL HYPOTHYROIDISM

Congenital causes of hypothyroidism may be sporadic or familial, goitrous or nongoitrous. In many cases the deficiency of thyroid hormone is severe, and symptoms develop in the early weeks of life. In others, lesser degrees of deficiency occur, and manifestations may be delayed for months or years.

ETIOLOGY. Thyroid Dysgenesis. Since the establishment of nationwide programs for neonatal screening for congenital hypothyroidism, many millions of neonates have been screened. The prevalence of congenital hypothyroidism has been found to be 1 in 4,000 infants worldwide, lower in Japan (1 in 5,500) and in African-Americans (1 in 32,000). Developmental defects (thyroid dysgenesis) account for 90% of infants in whom hypothyroidism is detected; in about one third even sensitive radionuclide scans can find no remnants of thyroid tissue *(aplasia)*. In most of the other infants, rudiments of thyroid tissue are found in an ectopic location anywhere from the base of the tongue *(lingual thyroid)* to the normal position in the neck. Most infants with congenital hypothyroidism are asymptomatic at birth even when there is complete agenesis of the thyroid gland. This situation is attributed to the transplacental passage of moderate amounts of maternal T_4, which provide fetal levels that are 25–50% of normal at birth. These low serum levels of T_4, and concomitantly elevated levels of TSH, make it possible to screen and detect most hypothyroid neonates.

Little is known about the factors that interfere with the normal migration and development of the thyroid gland. Thyroid dysgenesis occurs sporadically, but familial cases have occasionally been reported. Twice as many females as males are affected. The frequent finding of thyroid dysgenesis confined to only one of a pair of monozygotic twins suggests the operation of a deleterious factor during intrauterine life. For years it had been proposed that maternal antithyroid antibodies might be that factor, especially because antibodies in patients with autoimmune thyroid disease belong predominantly to the IgG class and can cross the placenta. Although thyroid antimicrosomal antibodies have been detected in some mother-infant pairs, there is little evidence of their pathogenicity. The recent demonstration of thyroid growth-blocking and cytotoxic antibodies in some infants with thyroid dysgenesis and in their mothers suggests a more likely pathogenetic mechanism. Maternal TSH-binding antibodies as a cause of transient congenital hypothyroidism and of neonatal Graves disease are well established (see later).

Ectopic thyroid tissue (lingual, sublingual, subhyoid) may provide adequate amounts of thyroid hormone for many years or may fail in early childhood. Affected children come to clinical attention because of a growing mass at the base of the tongue or in the midline of the neck, usually at the level of the hyoid. Occasionally, ectopia is associated with thyroglossal duct cysts. It may occur in siblings. Surgical removal of ectopic thyroid tissue from a euthyroid individual usually results in hypothyroidism because most such patients have no other thyroid tissue. Newborn screening programs detect most of these patients and obviate delayed diagnosis.

TSH-Binding Inhibitory Antibody (TBIAb). An unusual cause of transitory congenital hypothyroidism is the transplacental passage of maternal antibodies that inhibit binding of TSH to its receptor in the neonate. The frequency of this occurrence is unknown, but it should be suspected whenever there is a history of maternal autoimmune thyroid disease, including Hashimoto thyroiditis, Graves disease, or hypothyroidism on replacement therapy. In these situations, maternal levels of TBIAb should be measured during pregnancy. Affected infants and their mothers often also have TSH-stimulating and antimicrosomal antibodies. Technetium pertechnetate and ^{125}I scans may fail to detect any thyroid tissue, mimicking thyroid agenesis, but after the condition remits, a normal thyroid gland is demonstrable after discontinuation of replacement treatment. The half-life of the antibody is 7½ days, and remission of the hypothyroidism occurs in about 2 mo. Correct diagnosis of this cause of congenital hypothyroidism prevents protracted unnecessary treatment, alerts the clinician to possible recurrences in future pregnancies, and allows him to offer a favorable prognosis to the parents.

Radioiodine. Hypothyroidism has been reported as a result of inadvertent administration of radioiodine during pregnancy for treatment of cancer of the thyroid or of hyperthyroidism. Although only a few affected infants have been reported, a 1976 mail survey of endocrinologists uncovered 237 women who had inadvertently received therapeutic doses of ^{125}I during the 1st trimester of pregnancy. The fetal thyroid is capable of trapping iodide by 70–75 days. Whenever radioiodine is administered to a woman of child-bearing age, a pregnancy test must be made before a therapeutic dose of ^{131}I is given, regardless of the menstrual history or putative history of contraception. Administration of radioactive iodine to lactating women is also contraindicated because it is readily excreted in milk.

Thyrotropin Deficiency. Deficiency of TSH and hypothyroidism may occur in any of the conditions associated with developmental defects of the pituitary or hypothalamus (Sec. 19.2). More often in these conditions the deficiency of TSH is secondary to a deficiency of TRH. TSH-deficient hypothyroidism is found in 1 in 30,000–50,000 infants, but only 30–40% of these are detected by neonatal thyroid screening. The majority of affected infants have multiple pituitary deficiencies and present with hypoglycemia, persistent jaundice, and micropenis in association with septo-optic dysplasia, midline cleft lip, midface hypoplasia, and other midline facial anomalies.

Isolated deficiency of TSH is a rare autosomal recessive disorder that has been reported in five sibships. DNA studies in two Japanese children and in three children in two related Greek families have revealed different point mutations in the TSH β-subunit gene.

Thyrotropin Hormone Unresponsiveness. Mild congenital hypothyroidism has been detected in newborn infants who subsequently proved to have type Ia pseudohypoparathyroidism. The molecular cause of resistance to TSH in these patients is the generalized impairment of cAMP activation caused by genetic deficiency of the α subunit of the guanine nucleotide regulatory protein (αG_s) (Sec. 19.19).

Only a few other instances of isolated TSH unresponsiveness have been detected. Serum levels of T_4 were low, those of TSH by both RIA and bioassay were elevated, and there was no response to exogenous TSH administration. The defect appears to be located somewhere in the TSH receptor–G protein cAMP system.

Defective Synthesis of Thyroxine. A variety of defects in the biosynthesis of thyroid hormone may result in congenital hypothyroidism; when the defect is incomplete, compensation occurs, and onset of hypothyroidism may be delayed for years. A goiter is almost always present, and the defect is detected in 1 in 30,000–50,000 live births in neonatal screening programs. These defects are genetically determined and are transmitted in an autosomal recessive manner.

DEFECT OF IODIDE TRANSPORT. This rare defect has been reported in nine related infants of the Hutterite sect, and about half the cases are from Japan. Consanguinity has been present in about one third of the families. In the past, clinical hypothyroidism with or without a goiter often developed in the first few months of life, but in recent years the condition has been detected in neonatal screening programs. In Japan, however, untreated patients develop goiter and hypothyroidism after 10 yr of age, perhaps because of the very high iodine content (often 19 mg/24 hr) of the Japanese diet.

The energy-dependent mechanisms for concentrating iodide are defective not only in the thyroid but also in the salivary glands. In contrast to other defects of thyroid hormone synthesis, uptake of both radioiodine and pertechnetate is low; a saliva-serum ratio of ^{123}I may be required to establish the diagnosis. This condition responds to treatment with large doses of potassium iodide, but treatment with thyroxine is preferable.

Defects of Organification. After iodide is trapped by the thyroid, it is rapidly oxidized to reactive iodine, which is then incorporated into tyrosine units. This process requires generation of H_2O_2, thyroid peroxidase, and hematin (an enzyme cofactor); defects are now known that involve each of these components. Hence, there is considerable clinical as well as biochemical heterogeneity. In the Dutch neonatal screening program 23 infants have been found with a complete organification defect (1 in 60,000), but its prevalence in other areas is unknown. A characteristic finding in all patients with this defect is a marked decrease in thyroid radioactivity when perchlorate or thiocyanate is administered 2 hr after administration of a test dose of radioiodine. In these patients perchlorate discharges 40–90% of radioiodine compared to less than 10% in normal individuals. Patients with **Pendred syndrome**, a disorder comprising sensorineural deafness and goiter, also have a positive perchlorate discharge, but the precise biochemical defect in these people is unknown (Sec. 19.14).

Defects of Thyroglobulin Synthesis. This is a heterogeneous group of disorders characterized by goiter, elevated TSH, low T_4 levels, and absent or low levels of thyroglobulin (Tg); patients with normal levels of Tg have qualitative defects in the protein. Studies in animal models with congenital goiter have disclosed a nonsense mutation of the gene for Tg in Afrikander cattle, and a point mutation in Dutch goitrous goats. Delineation of a variety of analogous molecular defects in humans is anticipated.

Defects in Deiodination. Monoiodotyrosine and deiodotyrosine released from thyroglobulin are normally deiodinated within the thyroid or in peripheral tissues by a deiodinase. The liberated iodine is reused in the synthesis of thyroglobulin. Patients with a deficiency of this enzyme develop severe iodine loss from the constant urinary excretion of nondeiodinated tyrosines, leading to hormonal deficiency and goiter. The deiodination defect may be limited to thyroid tissue only or to peripheral tissue only, or it may be universal.

Thyroid Hormone Unresponsiveness. An increasing number of patients are being found who have resistance to the actions of endogenous and exogenous T_4 and T_3. Most patients have a goiter, and levels of T_4, T_3, free T_4, and free T_3 are elevated. These findings have often led to the erroneous diagnosis of Graves disease, although most affected patients are clinically euthyroid. It is presumed that these patients have incomplete resistance to thyroid hormone. TSH levels are diagnostic in that they are not suppressed as in Graves disease but instead are moderately elevated or normal but inappropriate for the levels of T_4 and T_3 when measured by a sensitive TSH assay. A TSH response to TRH occurs in these patients, unlike the situation in Graves disease. The failure of TSH suppression indicates that the resistance is generalized and affects the pituitary gland as well as peripheral tissues. The disorder is most often inherited in an autosomal dominant fashion. Several distinct point mutations in the hormone binding domain of the β-thyroid receptor have been identified. Elevated levels of T_4 on neonatal thyroid screening should suggest the possibility of this diagnosis. No treatment is usually required.

Two infants of consanguineous matings are known to have an autosomal recessive form of thyroid resistance. These infants had manifestations of hypothyroidism early in life, and DNA studies revealed a major deletion of the β-thyroid receptor in one individual. The resistance appears to be more severe in this form of the entity.

On rare occasions, resistance to thyroid hormone may selectively affect the pituitary gland. Because the peripheral tissues are not resistant to thyroid hormones, the patient presents with a goiter and manifestations of hyperthyroidism. The laboratory findings are the same as those seen with generalized thyroid hormone resistance. This condition must be differentiated from a pituitary TSH-secreting tumor. At least one young child has been successfully treated with D-thyroxine therapy.

Other Causes of Hypothyroidism. Congenital hypothyroidism may result from fetal exposure to excessive iodides or antithyroid drugs. This condition is transitory and must not be mistaken for the other forms of hypothyroidism described. The usual sources of iodides are proprietary preparations used to treat asthma. In a few instances, the cause of hypothyroidism was amiodarone, an antiarrhythmic drug with a high iodine content. In most of these instances a goiter is present (Sec. 19.14). In the neonate, topical iodine-containing antiseptics utilized in nurseries and by surgeons can also cause transient congenital hypothyroidism, especially in low-birthweight infants, and can lead to abnormal results on neonatal screening tests.

CLINICAL MANIFESTATIONS. The clinician is becoming increasingly dependent on neonatal screening tests for diagnosis of congenital hypothyroidism. Laboratory errors occur, however, and awareness of early symptoms must be maintained. Congenital hypothyroidism is twice as common in girls as in boys. Prior to neonatal screening programs congenital hypothyroidism was rarely recognized in the newborn since the signs and symptoms are usually not sufficiently developed. It can be suspected and the diagnosis established during the early weeks of life if the initial but less characteristic manifestations are recognized. Hypothyroid infants may be significantly heavier at birth than normal newborn infants, but there is little diagnostic value to this observation. Prolongation of physiologic icterus, owing to delayed maturation of glucuronide conjugation, may be the earliest sign. Feeding difficulties, especially sluggishness, lack of interest, somnolence, and choking spells during nursing, are often present during the 1st mo of life. Respiratory difficulties, due in part to the large tongue, include apneic episodes, noisy respirations, and nasal obstruction. Typical respiratory distress syndrome may also occur. Affected infants cry little, sleep much, have poor appetites, and are generally sluggish. There may be constipation that does not usually respond to treatment. The abdomen is large, and an umbilical hernia is usually present. The temperature is subnormal, often below 35° C (95° F), and the skin, particularly of the extremities, may be cold and mottled. Edema of the genitals and extremities may be present. The pulse is slow; heart murmurs and cardiomegaly are common. Anemia is often present and is refractory to treatment with hematinics. Since symptoms appear gradually, the diagnosis is often delayed.

These manifestations progress; retardation of physical and mental development becomes greater during the following months, and by 3–6 mo of age the clinical picture is fully developed (Fig. 19–6). When there is only a partial deficiency of thyroid hormone, the symptoms may be milder, the syndrome incomplete, and the onset delayed. Although breast milk contains significant amounts of thyroid hormones, par-

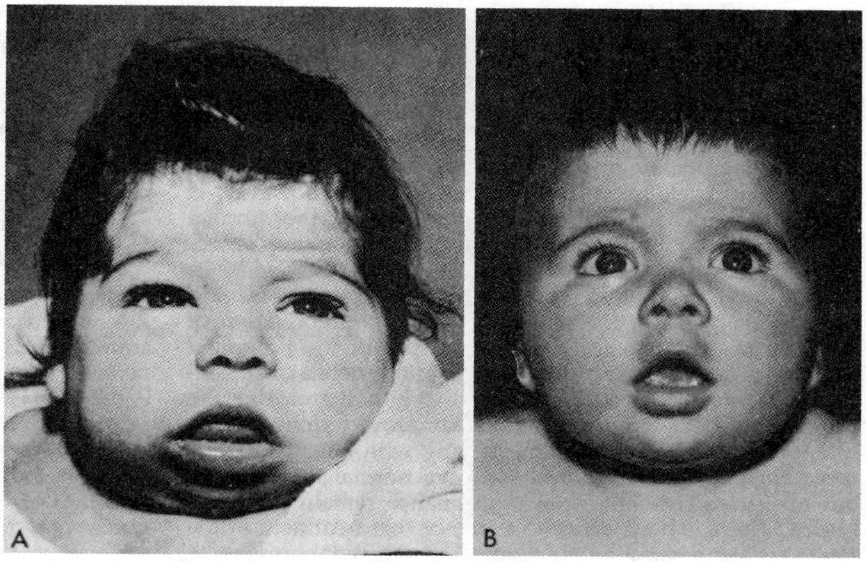

Figure 19–6. Congenital hypothyroidism in an infant 6 mo of age. The infant fed poorly in the neonatal period and was constipated. She had a persistent nasal discharge and a large tongue; she was very lethargic; and she had no social smile and no head control. *A*, Note the puffy face, dull expression, and hirsute forehead. Negligible uptake of radioiodine. Osseous development was that of a newborn. *B*, Four mo after treatment. Note the decreased puffiness of the face, decreased hirsutism of the forehead, and the alert appearance.

ticularly T_3, it is inadequate to protect the breast-fed infant with congenital hypothyroidism, and it has no effect on neonatal thyroid screening tests.

The child is stunted in growth, the extremities short, with head size normal or even increased. The anterior and posterior fontanels are widely open; observation of this sign at birth may serve as an initial clue to the early recognition of congenital hypothyroidism. Only 3% of normal newborn infants have a posterior fontanel larger than 0.5 cm. The eyes appear far apart, and the bridge of the broad nose is depressed. The palpebral fissures are narrow and the eyelids swollen. The mouth is kept open, and the thick and broad tongue protrudes from it. Dentition is delayed. The neck is short and thick, and there may be deposits of fat above the clavicles and between the neck and shoulders. The hands are broad and the fingers short. The skin is dry and scaly, and there is little perspiration. Myxedema is manifest, particularly in the skin of the eyelids, of the back of the hands, and of the external genitalia. Carotenemia may cause a yellow discoloration of the skin, but the scleras remain white. The scalp is thickened, and the hair is coarse, brittle, and scanty. The hairline reaches far down on the forehead, which usually appears wrinkled, especially when the infant cries.

Development is usually retarded. Hypothyroid infants appear lethargic and are late in learning to sit and stand. The voice is hoarse, and they do not learn to talk. The degree of physical and mental retardation increases with age. Sexual maturation may be delayed or may not take place at all.

The muscles are usually hypotonic, but in rare instances generalized muscular hypertrophy occurs *(Kocher-Debré-Sémélaigne syndrome)*. Affected children may have an athletic appearance due to pseudohypertrophy, particularly in the calf muscles. Its pathogenesis is unknown; nonspecific histochemical and ultrastructural changes seen on muscle biopsy return to normal with treatment. Boys are more prone to develop the syndrome, which has been observed in siblings born to a consanguineous mating. Affected patients have hypothyroidism of longer duration and severity.

LABORATORY DATA. Most newborn screening programs in North America measure levels of T_4, supplemented by measurement of TSH when T_4 is low. This approach identifies infants with low TBG and some infants with low TSH and can be used to identify infants with hyperthyroxinemia. European and Japanese neonatal screening programs are based on a primary measurement of TSH; this approach misses infants with hyperthyroxinemia, low TBG, and hypothalamic or pituitary hypothyroidism. With any of these assays, special care should be given to the normal range of values for age of the patient, particularly in the first weeks of life. Regardless of the approach used for screening, some infants escape detection because of technical or human errors; clinicians must maintain their vigilance for clinical manifestations of hypothyroidism.

Serum levels of T_4 and T_3 are low or borderline. If the defect is primarily in the thyroid, levels of TSH are elevated, often to above 100 μU/mL. Serum levels of prolactin are elevated, correlating with those of TSH. Serum levels of Tg are usually low in infants with thyroid dysgenesis or defects of Tg synthesis or secretion. Undetectable levels of Tg usually indicate thyroid aplasia.

Special attention should be paid to monoamniotic twins because in at least four cases neonatal screening failed to detect the discordant twin with hypothyroidism, and diagnosis was not made until the infants were 4–5 mo of age. Apparently transfusion of euthyroid blood from the unaffected twin normalized the serum level of T_4 and TSH in the affected twin at the initial screening.

Retardation of osseous development can be shown roentgenographically at birth in about 60% of congenitally hypothyroid infants and indicates some deprivation of thyroid hormone during intrauterine life. For example, the distal femoral epiphysis, normally present at birth, is often absent (Fig. 19–7*A*). In untreated patients the discrepancy between chronologic age and osseous development increases. The epiphyses often have multiple foci of ossification (epiphyseal dysgenesis, Fig. 19–7*B*); deformity ("beaking") of the 12th thoracic or 1st or 2nd lumbar vertebra is common. Roentgenograms of the skull show large fontanels and wide sutures; intersutural (wormian) bones are common. The sella turcica is often enlarged and round; in rare instances there may be erosion and thinning. Delays in formation and eruption of teeth may occur. Cardiac enlargement or pericardial effusion may be present.

Scintigraphy is indicated in infants with congenital hypothyroidism, but treatment should not be unduly delayed for this study. ^{125}I sodium iodide is superior to the ^{99m}Tc sodium

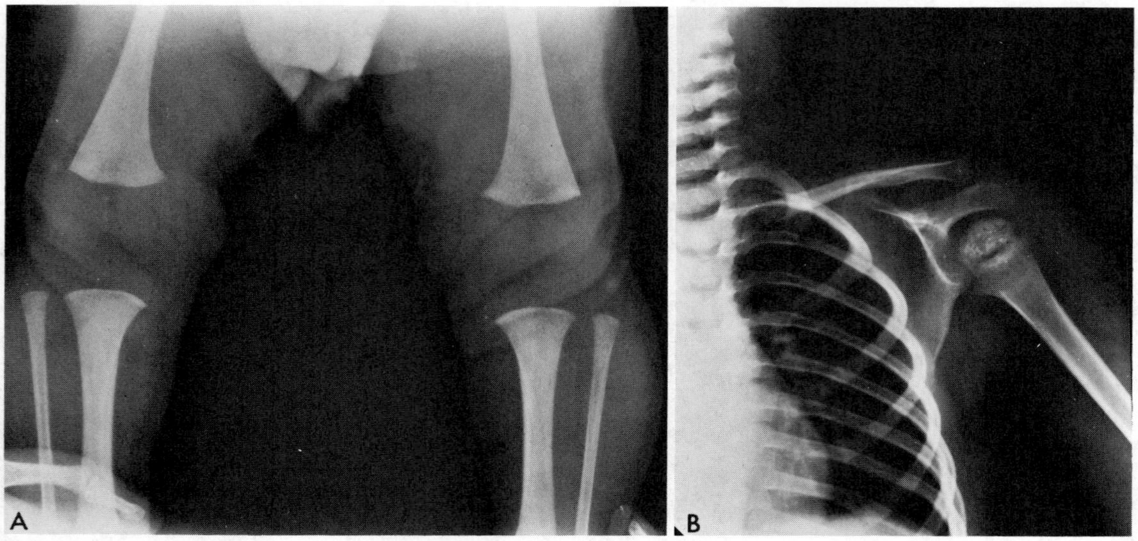

Figure 19–7. Congenital hypothyroidism. *A*, Absence of distal femoral epiphysis in a 3-mo-old infant who was born at term. This is evidence for the onset of the hypothyroid state during fetal life. *B*, Epiphyseal dysgenesis in the head of the humerus in a 9-yr-old girl who had been inadequately treated with thyroid hormone.

pertechnetate for this purpose. Neither thyroid ultrasound examination nor serum levels of Tg are reliable alternatives to radionuclide scanning. Demonstration of ectopic thyroid tissue is diagnostic of thyroid dysgenesis and establishes the need for lifelong treatment with T_4. Failure to demonstrate any thyroid tissue suggests thyroid aplasia but also occurs in neonates with TSH-binding inhibitory immunoglobulin and in infants with the iodide-trapping defect. A normally situated thyroid gland with a normal or avid uptake of radionuclide indicates a defect in thyroid hormone biosynthesis. Patients with goitrous hypothyroidism may require extensive evaluation, including radioiodine studies, perchlorate discharge tests, kinetic studies, chromatography, and studies of thyroid tissue if the biochemical nature of the defect is to be determined.

The electrocardiogram may show low-voltage P and T waves with diminished amplitude of QRS complexes. The electroencephalogram frequently shows low voltage. In children over 2 yr of age the serum cholesterol level is usually elevated.

PROGNOSIS. With the advent of neonatal screening programs for detection of congenital hypothyroidism, the prognosis for affected infants has improved dramatically. Early diagnosis and adequate treatment from the first weeks of life result in normal linear growth and intelligence comparable with that of unaffected siblings. No specific learning problems unrelated to intelligence have been detected in a carefully followed treated group of children through the first 10 yr of life. Without treatment, affected infants become mentally deficient dwarfs. Thyroid hormone is critical for normal cerebral development in the early postnatal months; biochemical diagnosis must be made soon after birth, and effective treatment must be initiated promptly to prevent irreversible brain damage. Delay in diagnosis, inadequate treatment, and poor compliance result in variable degrees of brain damage. When onset of hypothyroidism occurs after 2 yr of age, the outlook for normal development is much better even when diagnosis and treatment have been delayed, indicating how much more important thyroid hormone is to the rapidly growing brain of the infant.

TREATMENT. Sodium-L-thyroxine given orally is the treatment of choice. Because 80% of circulating T_3 is formed by monodeiodination of T_4, serum levels of both T_4 and T_3 in treated infants return to normal. This is also true in the brain, where 80% of required T_3 is produced locally from T_4. In neonates, the dose is 10–15 μg/kg (37.5 *or* 50 μg/24 hr). Levels of both T_4 and TSH should be monitored and maintained in the normal range. Children with hypothyroidism require about 4 μg/kg/24 hr, whereas adults require only 2 μg/kg/24 hr.

Later, confirmation of diagnosis may be necessary in some infants to rule out the possibility of transient hypothyroidism. This is not necessary in infants with proven thyroid ectopia or in those who manifest elevated levels of TSH after 6–12 mo of therapy owing to poor compliance or an inadequate dose of T_4. Discontinuation of therapy at about 3 yr of age for 3–4 wk results in a marked increase in TSH levels in hypothyroid children.

The only untoward effects of sodium-L-thyroxine are related to its dose. An occasional older child (8–13 yr) with acquired hypothyroidism may develop pseudotumor cerebri within the first 4 mo of treatment. In older children, after catch-up growth is complete, the growth rate provides an excellent index of the adequacy of therapy. Parents should be forewarned about changes in behavior and activity expected with therapy, and special attention must be given to any developmental or neurologic deficits.

JUVENILE HYPOTHYROIDISM
(Acquired Hypothyroidism)

ETIOLOGY. The most common cause of acquired hypothyroidism is lymphocytic thyroiditis (Sec. 19.13). Some patients with congenital thyroid dysgenesis or with incomplete genetic defects in thyroid hormone synthesis may not develop clinical manifestations until childhood and therefore appear to have acquired hypothyroidism; most patients with these conditions are now detected in newborn screening programs. Subtotal thyroidectomy for thyrotoxicosis or cancer may result in hypothyroidism, as may removal of ectopic thyroid tissue. For example, *lingual thyroid, subhyoid median thyroid*, or thyroid tissue in a *thyroglossal duct cyst* usually constitutes the only source of thyroid hormone, and excision results in hypothyroidism. Because subhyoid glands usually mimic thyroglossal duct cysts, a radionuclide scan before surgery is indicated in these patients.

Children with *nephropathic cystinosis*, a disorder characterized by intralysosomal storage of cystine in body tissues, develop impaired thyroid function. Hypothyroidism may be overt, but compensated forms are more common, and periodic assessment of TSH levels is indicated. By 13 yr of age, two thirds of these patients require thyroxine replacement.

Irradiation to the area of the thyroid that is incidental to the treatment of Hodgkin disease or other malignancies or that is given prior to bone marrow transplantation often results in thyroid damage. About one third of such children develop elevated TSH levels within a year following therapy, and 15–20% progress to hypothyroidism within 5–7 yr. Some clinicians recommend periodic TSH measurements, but others recommend treatment of all exposed patients with doses of T_4 to suppress TSH (Sec. 19.16).

Protracted ingestion of medications containing iodides can cause hypothyroidism, usually accompanied by a goiter (see Sec. 19.14). Amiodarone, a drug used for cardiac arrhythmias, consisting of 37% by weight of iodine, causes hypothyroidism in about 20% of treated children. It affects thyroid function directly by its high iodine content as well as by inhibition of 5′-deiodinase, which converts T_4 to T_3. Children treated with this drug should have serial measurements of T_4, T_3, and TSH.

CLINICAL MANIFESTATIONS. Deceleration of growth is usually the first clinical manifestation, but this sign often goes unrecognized (Fig. 19–8). Myxedematous changes of the skin, constipation, cold intolerance, decreased energy, and increased need for sleep develop insidiously. Surprisingly, school work and grades usually do not suffer even in severely hypothyroid children. Osseous maturation is delayed, often strikingly, which is an indication of the duration of the hypothyroidism.

Some children present with headaches, visual problems, precocious puberty, or galactorrhea. These children usually have hyperplastic enlargement of the pituitary gland, often with suprasellar extension, after longstanding hypothyroidism; this condition may be mistaken for a pituitary tumor (see Sec. 19.6).

All of these changes return to normal with adequate replacement of thyroxine, but in children with longstanding hypothyroidism, catch-up growth may be incomplete. During the first 18 mo of treatment, skeletal maturation often exceeds expected linear growth, resulting in a loss of about 7 cm of predicted adult height. The cause for this is not known.

Diagnostic studies and treatment are the same as those described for congenital hypothyroidism. During the 1st yr of treatment deterioration of school work, poor sleeping habits, restlessness, short attention span, and behavioral problems may ensue, but these are transient; forewarning families about these manifestations enhances appropriate management.

19.13 THYROIDITIS

LYMPHOCYTIC THYROIDITIS

(Hashimoto Thyroiditis; Autoimmune Thyroiditis)

Lymphocytic thyroiditis is the most common cause of thyroid disease in children and adolescents and accounts for many of the enlarged thyroids formerly designated "adolescent" or "simple" goiter. It is also the most common cause of juvenile hypothyroidism, with or without goiter. Its incidence may be as high as 1% in school children.

ETIOLOGY. This is a typical organ-specific autoimmune disease. The condition is characterized histologically by lymphocytic infiltration of the thyroid. Early in the course of the disease there may be only hyperplasia; this is followed by infiltration of lymphocytes and plasma cells between the follicles and by atrophy of the follicles. Lymphoid follicle formation with germinal centers is almost always present; the degree of atrophy and of fibrosis of the follicles varies from mild to moderate.

Intrathyroidal lymphocyte subsets differ from those in blood. About 60% of infiltrating lymphoid cells are T cells, and about 30% express B cell markers; the T cell population is represented by both helper (CD4+) and cytotoxic (CD8+) cells. Participation of cellular events in the pathogenesis is clear, but much remains to be discovered about the disturbance in immunoregulation and how it interacts with genetic predisposition and environmental factors in the pathogenesis of autoimmune thyroid disease.

A variety of different thyroid antigen autoantibodies are also involved in the process. Thyroid antimicrosomal antibodies (MicAb) are demonstrable in the sera of 90% of children with lymphocytic thyroiditis and in many patients with

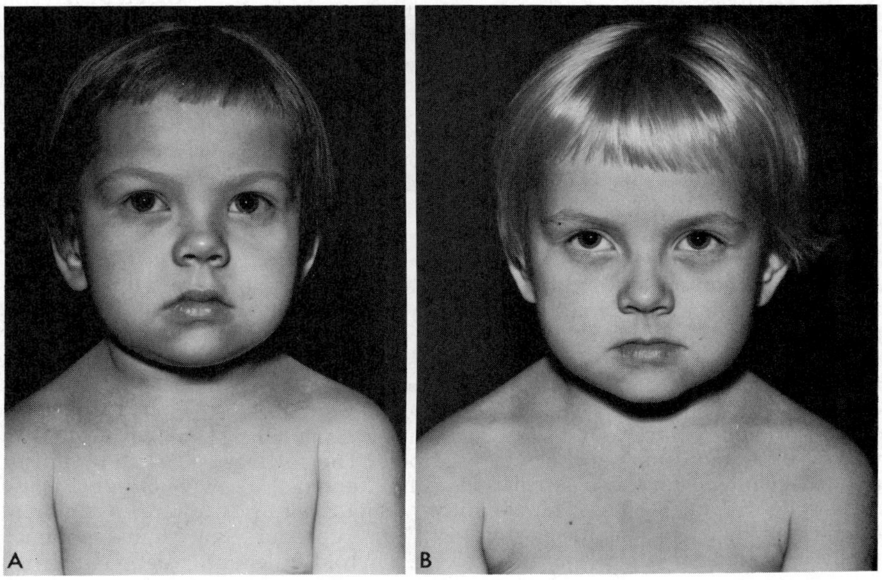

Figure 19–8. *A*, Acquired hypothyroidism in a girl 6 yr of age. She was treated with a wide variety of hematinics for refractory anemia for 3 yr. She had almost complete cessation of growth, constipation, and sluggishness of 3 yr duration. The height age was 3 yr; the bone age was 4 yr. She had a sallow complexion and immature facies with a poorly developed nasal bridge. Serum cholesterol, 501 mg/dL; radioiodine uptake, 7% at 24 hr; PBI, 2.8 μg/dL. *B*, After therapy for 18 mo. Note the nasal development, the increased luster and decreased pigmentation of hair, and maturation of face. The height age was 5.5 yr; the bone age was 7 yr. There was a decided improvement in her general condition. Menarche occurred at 14 yr. The ultimate height was 155 cm (61 in). She graduated from high school. She was well controlled with sodium-L-thyroxine daily.

Graves disease. This antibody has now been identified as thyroid peroxidase (TPO), an enzyme that catalyzes the iodination of tyrosine residues on thyroglobulin. For many years MicAb has been considered nonpathogenic, but now that it is known to be TPO its pathogenetic role is being reconsidered. With the molecular cloning of the TPO gene, a new generation of ultrasensitive tests for the measurement of these antibodies is under development.

Antithyroglobulin antibodies occur in only a small percentage of affected children but are much more common in adults. Blocking TSH antibodies, thought to be rare until recently, are frequently present, especially in patients with hypothyroidism, and it is now believed they are related to the development of hypothyroidism and thyroid atrophy in patients with autoimmune thyroiditis.

CLINICAL MANIFESTATIONS. The disorder is 4–7 times more frequent in girls than in boys. It may occur during the first 3 yr of life but becomes sharply more common after 6 yr of age and reaches a peak incidence during adolescence. The goiter may appear insidiously and may vary in size from slight to marked. In most patients the thyroid is diffusely enlarged, firm, and nontender. In about a third of the patients the gland is lobular and may seem to be nodular. Most of the affected children are clinically euthyroid and asymptomatic; some may have symptoms of pressure in the neck. Some children have clinical signs of hypothyroidism, while others who appear clinically euthyroid have laboratory evidence of hypothyroidism. A few children have manifestations suggestive of hyperthyroidism, such as nervousness, irritability, increased sweating, or hyperactivity, but results of laboratory studies are not those of hyperthyroidism. Occasionally, the disorder may coexist with Graves disease. Ophthalmopathy may occur in lymphocytic thyroiditis in the absence of Graves disease.

The clinical course is variable. The goiter may become smaller or may disappear spontaneously, or it may persist unchanged for years while the patient remains euthyroid. A significant percentage of patients who are euthyroid initially exhibit hypothyroidism gradually within months or years; thyroiditis is the cause of most cases of nongoitrous juvenile hypothyroidism. Lymphocytic thyroiditis may also occur without symptoms, and in many children persists for many years.

Familial clusters of lymphocytic thyroiditis are common; the incidence in siblings or parents of affected children may be as high as 25%. Autoantibodies to Tg and human thyroid peroxidase (hTPO) (see later) in these families appear to be inherited in an autosomal dominant fashion with reduced penetrance in males. The concurrence within families of patients with lymphocytic thyroiditis, "idiopathic" hypothyroidism, and Graves disease provides cogent evidence for a basic relationship among these three conditions. The disorder has been associated with many of the other autoimmune disorders more often than would be expected by chance alone. The association of Addison disease with insulin-dependent diabetes mellitus or autoimmune thyroid disease or both is known as *Schmidt syndrome* or *type II polyglandular autoimmune disease.* Autoimmune thyroid disease also tends to be associated with pernicious anemia, vitiligo, or alopecia. Thyroid microsomal antibodies are found in approximately 20% of white and 4% of black children with diabetes mellitus. Autoimmune thyroid disease has an increased incidence in children with congenital rubella. Lymphocytic thyroiditis is also associated with certain chromosomal aberrations, particularly Turner syndrome and Down syndrome. The pathogenetic mechanisms for these associations is not known.

LABORATORY DATA. The definitive diagnosis can be established by biopsy of the thyroid, but this procedure is rarely indicated for clinical purposes alone. Thyroid function tests are often normal, though the level of TSH may be slightly or even moderately elevated in some euthyroid individuals. With progressive thyroid failure a decrease in the levels of T_4 is followed by a decrease in levels of T_3 and progressive increases in levels of TSH. The fact that many patients with lymphocytic thyroiditis do not have elevated levels of TSH indicates that the goiter may be caused by the lymphocytic infiltrations or by thyroid growth–stimulating immunoglobulins. In 50% of patients thyroid scans reveal irregular and patchy distribution of the radioisotope, and in about 60% or more the administration of perchlorate results in a greater than 10% discharge of iodide from the thyroid gland. The majority of patients with lymphocytic thyroiditis have serum antibody titers to thyroid microsomal antigens, whereas the antithyroglobulin test for thyroid antibodies is positive in fewer than 50%. When both tests are used, approximately 95% of patients with thyroid autoimmunity will be detected. In general, levels in children and adolescents are lower than those in adults with lymphocytic thyroiditis, and repeated measurements are indicated in questionable instances because titers may increase later in the course of the disease.

Antithyroid antibodies may be found also in almost half the siblings of affected patients and in a significant percentage of the mothers of children with Down syndrome or Turner syndrome without demonstrable thyroid disease. They are also found in 20% of children with diabetes mellitus and in 23% of children with the congenital rubella syndrome.

TREATMENT. If there is evidence of hypothyroidism, replacement treatment with sodium-L-thyroxine (50–150 μg daily) is indicated. The goiter usually shows some decrease in size but may persist for years. Antibody levels fluctuate in both treated and untreated patients and persist for years. Since the disease may be self-limited in some instances, the need for continued therapy requires periodic re-evaluation. Untreated patients should also be periodically checked. Prominent nodules that persist despite suppressive therapy should be examined histologically because thyroid cancer has occurred in patients with lymphocytic thyroiditis.

OTHER CAUSES OF THYROIDITIS

Specific conditions such as tuberculosis, sarcoidosis, mumps, and cat-scratch disease are rare causes of thyroiditis.

Acute suppurative thyroiditis is uncommon; it is usually preceded by a respiratory infection. The left lower lobe is affected predominantly. Abscess formation may occur. Anaerobic organisms, with or without aerobes, are the most common organisms; *Eikenella corrodens* has been reported. Recurrent episodes or the detection of a mixed bacterial flora suggests that the infection arises from a thyroglossal duct remnant or, more often, from a pyriform sinus fistula. Exquisite tenderness of the gland, swelling, erythema, dysphagia, and limitation of head motion are characteristic findings. Systemic manifestations are often but not invariably absent and leukocytosis is present. Scintigrams of the thyroid often reveal decreased uptake in the affected areas and ultrasonography may show a complex echogenic mass. Thyroid function is usually normal, but thyrotoxicosis due to escape of thyroid hormone has been encountered in a child with suppurative thyroiditis resulting from *Aspergillus.* When suppuration occurs, incision and drainage and administration of antibiotics are indicated. After infection subsides, a barium esophagram is indicated to search for a fistula tract; if found, exteriorization is indicated.

Subacute nonsuppurative thyroiditis (deQuervain disease) is rare in children. It is thought to have a viral etiology and remits spontaneously. The disorder becomes manifest by a vague tenderness over the thyroid and low-grade fever or by

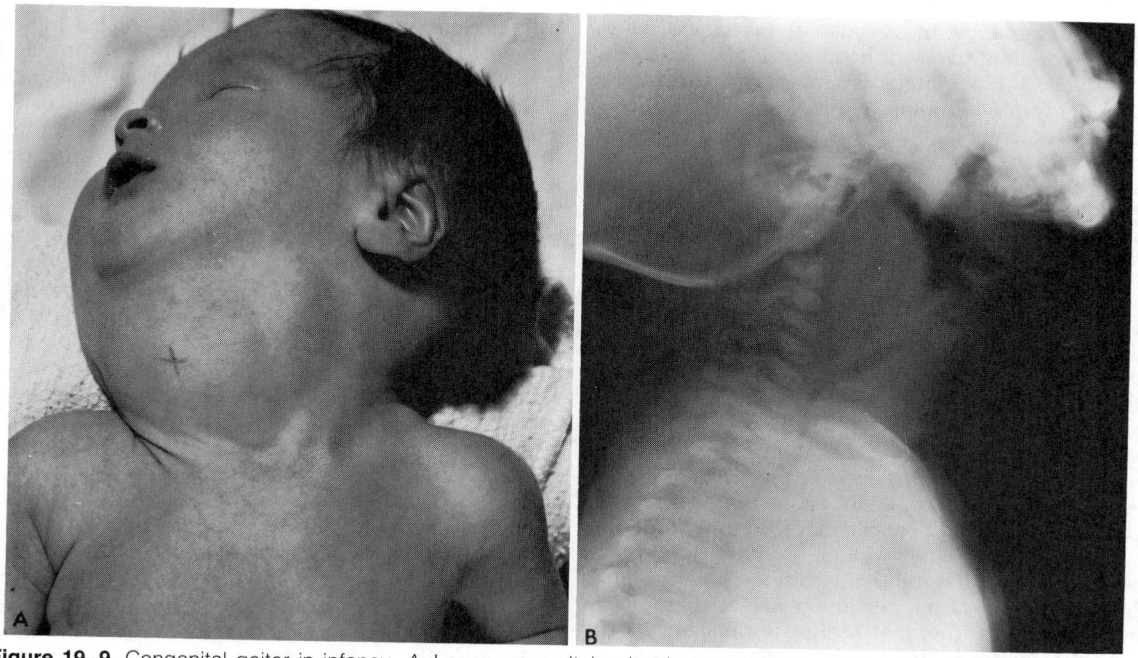

Figure 19–9. Congenital goiter in infancy. *A*, Large congenital goiter in an infant born to a mother with thyrotoxicosis who had been treated with iodides and methimazole during pregnancy. *B*, A 6-wk-old infant with increasing respiratory distress and cervical mass since birth. The operation revealed a large goiter that almost completely encircled the trachea. Note the anterior deviation and posterior compression of the trachea. Partial thyroidectomy completely relieved the symptoms. The cause for the goiter was not found. It is apparent why a tracheostomy is not adequate treatment for these infants.

severe pain in the region of the thyroid and systemic manifestations with chills and high fever. Serum levels of T_4 and T_3 are elevated, and mild symptoms of hyperthyroidism may be present, but radioiodine uptake is depressed. The erythrocyte sedimentation rate is increased. The course is variable, and remission usually occurs in several months. Occasionally, this condition is superimposed on lymphocytic thyroiditis.

19.14 GOITER

A goiter is an enlargement of the thyroid gland. Persons with enlarged thyroids may have normal function of the gland *(euthyroidism)*, thyroid deficiency *(hypothyroidism)*, or overproduction of the hormones *(hyperthyroidism)*. Goiter may be congenital or acquired, endemic or sporadic.

The goiter often results from increased pituitary secretion of thyrotropic hormone in response to decreased circulating levels of thyroid hormones. Thyroid enlargement may also result from infiltrative processes that may be inflammatory or neoplastic. Goiter in patients with thyrotoxicosis is caused by TSH-stimulating antibodies (TSAb).

CONGENITAL GOITER

Congenital goiter is usually sporadic and may result from the administration of antithyroid drugs or iodides during pregnancy for the treatment of thyrotoxicosis. The concomitant administration of thyroid hormone with the goitrogen does not prevent this effect. Iodides are included in many proprietary preparations used to treat asthma; these preparations must be avoided during pregnancy because they have often been a cause of unexpected congenital goiter. Amiodarone, an antiarrhythmic drug with a 37% iodine content, has also caused congenital goiter with hypothyroidism. Goitrogenic drugs and iodides cross the placenta and at high doses may interfere with synthesis of thyroid hormone, resulting in goiter and hypothyroidism in the fetus. Even when the infant is clinically euthyroid, there may be retardation of osseous maturation, low levels of T_4, and elevated levels of TSH. Since these effects can occur when the mother takes only 100–200 mg of propylthiouracil/24 hr, all such infants should undergo thyroid studies at birth. Administration of thyroid hormone to affected infants may be indicated to treat clinical hypothyroidism, to hasten the disappearance of the goiter, and to prevent brain damage. Since the condition is rarely permanent, thyroid hormone may be safely discontinued after several months.

Enlargement of the thyroid at birth may occasionally be sufficient to cause respiratory distress that interferes with nursing and may even cause death. The head may be maintained in extreme hyperextension. When respiratory obstruction is severe, partial thyroidectomy rather than tracheostomy is indicated (Fig. 19–9).

Goiter is almost always present in the congenitally hyperthyroid infant. These goiters are usually not large; the infant manifests clinical symptoms of hyperthyroidism, and the mother often has a history of Graves disease (Sec. 19.15).

When no causative factor is identifiable, a defect in synthesis of thyroid hormone should be suspected. One in 30,000–50,000 live births is found in neonatal screening programs to have such a defect. Study of this group of infants is complex. If the infant is hypothyroid, it is advisable to treat immediately with thyroid hormone and to postpone more detailed studies for later in life. Since these defects are transmitted by recessive genes, precise diagnosis is important for sound counseling. Monitoring subsequent pregnancies with ultrasound can be useful in detecting fetal goiters.

Iodine deficiency as a cause of congenital goiters has become rare but persists in isolated endemic areas (see later). More important is the recent recognition that severe iodine deficiency early in pregnancy may cause neurologic damage during fetal development even in the absence of goiter.

When the "goiter" is lobulated, asymmetric, firm, or large to an unusual degree, a teratoma within or in the vicinity of the thyroid must be considered in the differential diagnosis (Sec. 17.24).

ENDEMIC GOITER AND CRETINISM

The association between dietary deficiency of iodine and the prevalence of goiter or cretinism has been recognized for over half a century. If there is a moderate deficiency of iodine, the demand can be satisfied by increased efficiency in synthesis of thyroid hormone. Iodine liberated in the tissues is returned rapidly to the gland, which resynthesizes the hormone at a higher rate than normal. This increased activity is achieved by compensatory hypertrophy and hyperplasia, which satisfy the demands of the tissues for thyroid hormone. In geographic areas where deficiency of iodine is severe, decompensation and hypothyroidism may result. It is estimated that 800 million people in Third World countries live in areas of iodine deficiency.

Sea water is rich in iodine, and the iodine content of fish and shellfish is also high. Endemic goiter is rare therefore in populations living along the sea. Iodine is deficient in the water and native foods in the Pacific West and the Great Lakes areas of the United States. Deficiency of dietary iodine is even greater in certain Alpine valleys, the Himalayas, the Andes, the Congo, and the Highlands of Papua New Guinea. In areas such as the United States, where iodine is provided in foods from other areas and in iodized salt, endemic goiter has disappeared. Iodized salt in the United States contains potassium iodide (100 μg/g) and provides excellent prophylaxis. Further iodine intake in the United States is contributed by iodates used in baking, iodine-containing coloring agents, and iodine-containing disinfectants used in the dairy industry. The recommended daily allowance of iodine for infants is 40–50 μg/24 hr; this amount is exceeded 4-fold in breast-fed infants and 10-fold in cowmilk-fed infants in the United States.

CLINICAL MANIFESTATIONS. If the deficiency of iodine is mild, thyroid enlargement does not become noticeable except when there is increased demand for the hormone during periods of rapid growth, as in adolescence and during pregnancy. In regions of moderate iodine deficiency, goiter observed in school children may disappear with maturity and reappear during pregnancy or lactation. Iodine-deficient goiters are more common in girls than in boys. Where iodine deficiency is severe, as in the hyperendemic Highlands of Papua New Guinea, nearly half the population have large goiters, and endemic cretinism is common.

Serum thyroxine levels are often low in people with endemic goiter, though clinical hypothyroidism is rare. This is true in New Guinea, the Congo, the Himalayas, and South America. Despite low serum levels of thyroid hormone, serum TSH concentrations are often only moderately increased. In such patients circulating levels of T_3 are elevated. Moreover, T_3 levels are also elevated in those patients with normal T_4 levels, indicating a preferential secretion of T_3 by the thyroid in this disease.

Endemic cretinism, the most serious consequence of iodine deficiency, has been recognized for centuries; it occurs only in geographic association with endemic goiter. The term endemic cretinism includes two different but overlapping syndromes, a neurologic type and a myxedematous type. The frequency of the two types varies among different populations; in Papua, New Guinea, the "nervous" type occurs almost exclusively, whereas in Zaire the myxedematous type predominates. Both types are found in all endemic areas, and some individuals have intermediate or mixed features.

The neurologic syndrome is characterized by mental retardation, deaf-mutism, disturbances in standing and gait, and pyramidal signs such as clonus of the foot, Babinski sign, and patellar hyperreflexia. Affected individuals are goitrous but euthyroid, have normal pubertal development and adult stature, and have little or no impaired thyroid function. Individuals with the myxedematous syndrome also are mentally retarded and deaf and have neurologic symptoms, but in addition they have delayed sexual development and growth, myxedema, and absence of goiter; serum T_4 levels are low, and TSH levels are markedly elevated. Delayed skeletal maturation may extend into the 3rd decade or later. Ultrasound examination shows thyroid atrophy.

The pathogenesis of the neurologic syndrome has been attributed to iodine deficiency and hypothyroxinemia during pregnancy leading to fetal and postnatal hypothyroidism. Although some investigators have attributed brain damage to a direct effect of elemental iodine deficiency in the fetus, others believe the neurologic symptoms are caused by the hypothyroxinemia. There is evidence that the human fetal brain has receptors for thyroid hormone before development of the fetal thyroid, and there is also evidence of some transplacental passage of thyroid hormone into the fetus. The pathogenesis of the myxedematous syndrome leading to thyroid atrophy is more bewildering. Searches for additional environmental factors that may provoke continuing postnatal hypothyroidism have led to incrimination of selenium deficiency, goitrogenic foods, thiocyanates, and *Yersinia*. Studies from Western China suggest that thyroid autoimmunity may play a role. Myxedematous cretins with thyroid atrophy, but not euthyroid cretins, were found to have thyroid growth-blocking immunoglobulins of the kind found in infants with sporadic congenital hypothyroidism. No other types of antibodies were found. The precipitants of the thyroid autoimmune process are unknown.

In many areas of the Third World administration of a single intramuscular injection of iodinated poppy seed oil to women prevents iodine deficiency during future pregnancies for about 5 yr. This form of therapy given to children under 4 yr of age with myxedematous cretinism results in a euthyroid state in 5 mo. However, older children respond poorly and adults not at all to iodized oil injections, indicating an inability of the thyroid gland to synthesize hormone; these patients require treatment with thyroxine.

SPORADIC GOITER

The term sporadic goiter encompasses goiters developing from a variety of causes; patients are usually euthyroid but may be hypothyroid. The most common cause of sporadic goiter is lymphocytic thyroiditis (see Sec. 19.13). Intrinsic biochemical defects in the synthesis of thyroid hormone are almost always associated with goiter (see earlier); the occurrence of the disorder in siblings, onset in early life, and possible association with hypothyroidism (goitrous hypothyroidism) are important clues to the diagnosis.

IODIDE GOITER. A small percentage of patients treated with iodide preparations for prolonged periods develop goiters. Iodides are commonly included for their expectorant effect in cough medicines and in proprietary mixtures for asthma. Goiters resulting from iodide administration are firm and diffusely enlarged, and in some instances hypothyroidism may develop. In normal subjects acute administration of large doses of iodine inhibits the organification of iodine and the synthesis of thyroid hormone (Wolff-Chaikoff effect). This effect is short-lived and does not lead to hypothyroidism.

When iodide administration continues, an autoregulatory mechanism in normal persons limits iodine trapping and thus permits the level of iodide in the thyroid to fall and organification to proceed normally. In patients with iodide-induced goiter this escape does not occur because of an underlying abnormality of biosynthesis of thyroid hormone. Subjects most susceptible to the development of iodide goiter are those with lymphocytic thyroiditis or with a subclinical inborn error in thyroid hormone synthesis as well as those who have had partial thyroidectomy.

Lithium carbonate also causes goiters; it is currently widely used as a psychotropic drug. Lithium competes with iodide; the mechanism producing the goiter or hypothyroidism is similar to that described earlier for iodide goiter. Lithium and iodide also act synergistically to produce goiter; their combined use should be avoided.

Amiodarone, a drug used to treat cardiac arrhythmias, can cause thyroid dysfunction with goiter because it is rich in iodine. It is also a potent inhibitor of 5′-deiodinase, preventing conversion of T_4 to T_3. It can cause hypothyroidism, particularly in patients with underlying autoimmune disease; in other patients, it may cause hyperthyroidism.

SIMPLE GOITER (COLLOID GOITER). A few children with euthyroid nontoxic goiters have simple goiters, a condition of unknown etiology not associated with hypothyroidism or hyperthyroidism and not caused by inflammation or neoplasia. The condition predominates in girls and has a peak incidence before and during the pubertal years. Histologic examination of the thyroid either is normal or reveals variable follicular size, dense colloid, and flattened epithelium. The goiter may be small or large. It is firm in consistency in half the patients and is occasionally asymmetric or nodular. Levels of TSH are normal or low; scintiscans are normal; thyroid antibodies are absent. Differentiation from lymphocytic thyroiditis may not be possible without a biopsy, but biopsy is ordinarily not indicated. Therapy with thyroid hormone may be indicated to avoid progression to a large multinodular goiter. Untreated patients should be re-evaluated periodically. This condition must be differentiated from lymphocytic thyroiditis (see Sec. 19.13).

MULTINODULAR GOITER. Rarely, a firm goiter with a lobulated surface and single or multiple palpable nodules is encountered. Areas of cystic change, hemorrhage, and fibrosis may be present. The incidence of this condition has decreased markedly with the use of iodine-enriched salt. A mild goitrogenic stimulus, acting over a long time, is thought to be the cause. Ultrasound examination may reveal multiple echo-free and echogenic lesions that are nonfunctioning on scintiscans. Thyroid studies are usually normal, but TSH may be elevated and thyroid antibodies may be present. The condition occurs in children with McCune-Albright syndrome and has been described in three children (including two siblings) with digital anomalies and cystic renal disease. If the nodules are not suppressed with replacement therapy with thyroxine, surgery is indicated because malignancy cannot readily be ruled out.

PENDRED SYNDROME
(Goiter and Congenital Deafness)

This syndrome of congenital deafness and goiter is transmitted in an autosomal recessive fashion and is not to be confused with the deaf-mutism seen in people with endemic cretinism or with the minor impairment of hearing that may be found in severely hypothyroid persons. It must also be differentiated from the lymphocytic thyroiditis that may be associated with congenital rubella. The hearing loss is usually severe and is present at birth, although it may not be recognized until later. It is most pronounced in the higher frequencies, is of the perceptive type, and exhibits recruitment. The goiter generally appears at puberty or later but may be present in early childhood; it may be barely detectable or pronounced. Initially, the goiter is soft and diffuse; it tends to become nodular in adult life. Most affected persons are clinically euthyroid, but hypothyroidism may ensue even during childhood. Affected persons are otherwise normal.

Administration of perchlorate causes a significant discharge of iodide from the thyroid gland, indicating a defect in organification. The biochemical defect is not known. There does not appear to be a deficiency in iodide peroxidase or iodotyrosine synthesis or any defect in binding to apoenzyme. Lifelong treatment with thyroid hormone is indicated to prevent development or progression of the goiter.

INTRATRACHEAL GOITER

One of the many ectopic locations of thyroid tissue is within the trachea. The intraluminal thyroid lies beneath the tracheal mucosa and is frequently continuous with the normally situated extratracheal thyroid. The thyroid tissue is susceptible to goitrous enlargement, which involves the normally situated as well as the ectopic thyroid. When there is obstruction of the airway associated with a goiter, it must be ascertained whether the obstruction is extratracheal or endotracheal. If obstructive manifestations are mild, administration of sodium-L-thyroxine usually causes the goiter to decrease in size. When symptoms are severe, surgical removal of the endotracheal goiter is indicated.

19.15 HYPERTHYROIDISM

Hyperthyroidism results from excessive secretion of thyroid hormone and, with few exceptions, is due to diffuse toxic goiter (Graves disease) during childhood. Other rare causes of hyperthyroidism that have been observed in children include toxic uninodular goiter (Plummer disease), hyperfunctioning thyroid carcinoma, thyrotoxicosis factitia, and acute suppurative thyroiditis. Hyperthyroidism occurs in some patients with McCune-Albright syndrome; suppression of plasma TSH indicates that the hyperthyroidism is not hypothalamic in origin. Hyperthyroidism due to excess thyrotropin secretion is rare and in most cases is caused by pituitary unresponsiveness to thyroid hormone. TSH-secreting pituitary tumors have been reported only in adults. In infants born to mothers with Graves disease hyperthyroidism may occur as a transitory phenomenon or as classic Graves disease during the neonatal period. Choriocarcinoma, hydatidiform mole, and struma ovarii have caused hyperthyroidism in adults but have not yet been recognized as causes in children.

GRAVES DISEASE

ETIOLOGY. Enlargement of the thymus, splenomegaly, lymphadenopathy, infiltration of the thyroid gland and of retro-orbital tissues with lymphocytes and plasma cells, and peripheral lymphocytosis are well-established findings in Graves disease. In the thyroid gland T helper cells (CD4+) tend to predominate in dense lymphoid aggregates; in areas of lower cell density, cytotoxic T cells (CD8+) predominate. The percentage of activated B lymphocytes infiltrating the thyroid is higher than in peripheral blood; these B cells appear to be the source of the antithyroid antibodies that occur in Graves disease. The most characteristic antibody produced is an immunoglobulin that binds to the receptor for TSH and stimulates cAMP, analogous to TSH itself. In addition to TSAb, TSH-inhibiting antibodies (TBIAb) may also be produced, and the clinical course of the disease usually correlates with the ratio between the two antibodies.

The ophthalmopathy occurring in Graves disease is caused by antibodies that bind to the extraocular muscles and orbital fibroblasts, stimulate the synthesis of glycosaminoglycans by orbital fibroblasts, and produce cytotoxic effects on muscle cells.

In whites Graves disease is associated with HLA-B8 and HLA-DR3, especially the latter. Therefore, it is not surprising that Graves disease is also associated with other HLA-D3–related disorders such as Addison disease, insulin-dependent diabetes mellitus, myasthenia gravis, and celiac disease. In family clusters, the most frequent association with Graves disease is lymphocytic thyroiditis, autoimmune hypothyroidism, and neonatal hyperthyroidism.

CLINICAL MANIFESTATIONS. About 5% of all patients with hyperthyroidism are under 15 yr of age; the peak incidence occurs during adolescence. Graves disease has begun between 6 wk and 2 yr of age in children born to mothers without a history of hyperthyroidism. The incidence is about 5 times higher in girls than in boys.

The clinical course in children is highly variable but is in general not so fulminant as in many adults. Symptoms develop gradually; the usual interval between onset and diagnosis is 6–12 mo. The earliest signs in children may be emotional disturbances accompanied by motor hyperactivity. The children become irritable, excitable, and cry easily. Their school work suffers, and their restlessness, which may resemble that of chorea, causes conflicts. Tremor of the fingers can be noticed if the arm is extended. There may be a voracious appetite combined with loss of or no increase in weight. The size of the thyroid is variable. It may be enlarged, or it may be so little enlarged that it escapes detection. Exophthalmos is noticeable in the majority of patients but is rarely severe. Lagging of the upper eyelid as the eye looks downward, impairment of convergence, and retraction of the upper eyelid and infrequent blinking may be present. The skin is smooth and flushed, with excessive sweating. Muscular weakness is uncommon but may be severe enough to result in falling spells. Tachycardia, palpitations, dyspnea, and cardiac enlargement and insufficiency cause discomfort and may endanger the patient's life. Atrial fibrillation is a rare complication. Mitral regurgitation, probably resulting from papillary muscle dysfunction, is the cause of the apical systolic murmur present in some patients. The systolic blood pressure and the pulse pressure are increased. Many of the findings in Graves disease are due to hyperactivity of the sympathetic nervous system.

Thyroid "crisis" or "storm" is a form of hyperthyroidism manifested by an acute onset, hyperthermia, and severe tachycardia and restlessness. There may be rapid progression to delirium, coma, and death. "Apathetic" or "masked" hyperthyroidism is another variety of hyperthyroidism characterized by extreme listlessness, apathy, and cachexia. A combination of both forms may also occur. These symptom complexes are rare in children.

LABORATORY DATA. Serum levels of T_4, T_3, free T_4, and free T_3 are elevated. In some patients levels of T_3 may be more elevated than those of T_4. Levels of TSH measured by a sensitive assay are suppressed below normal levels. Antimicrosomal antibodies are often present. Most patients with newly diagnosed Graves disease have measurable TSH receptor–stimulating antibodies, and their disappearance predicts remission of the disease. Assays of TSH-receptor antibodies are rarely necessary for diagnosis or management of Graves disease. Radioiodine is rapidly and diffusely concentrated in the thyroid, but this study is rarely necessary. Very young children with Graves disease often have advanced skeletal maturation and craniostenosis.

DIFFERENTIAL DIAGNOSIS. Diagnosis is rarely difficult once it has been considered. Elevated levels of T_4 and free T_4 in association with suppressed levels of TSH are usually diagnostic. The presence of TSAb establishes the cause as Graves disease.

Most other causes of hyperthyroxinemia are rare but may result in erroneous diagnosis. Patients with elevated TBG or familial dysalbuminemic hyperthyroxinemia have normal levels of free T_4 and TSH. If a thyroid nodule is palpable, or if T_3 is preferentially elevated, a functional thyroid nodule must be considered; radionuclide study is diagnostic. If precocious puberty, polyostotic fibrous dysplasia, or café-au-lait pigmentation is present, the autonomous thyroid disorder of McCune-Albright syndrome is likely. Patients with generalized thyroid hormone unresponsiveness have elevated levels of free T_4, but levels of TSH are inappropriately elevated. Patients with pituitary unresponsiveness to thyroid hormone also have clinical hyperthyroidism, but their levels of TSH are elevated, and they must be differentiated from patients with TSH-secreting pituitary tumors.

When hyperthyroxinemia is caused by exogenous thyroid hormone, levels of free T_4 and TSH are the same as those seen in Graves disease, but the level of thyroglobulin is very low, whereas in patients with Graves disease it is elevated.

TREATMENT. Most pediatric endocrinologists recommend medical therapy rather than subtotal thyroidectomy or radioiodine. The two thionamide drugs in widest use are propylthiouracil (PTU) and methimazole (Tapazole). Both compounds inhibit incorporation of trapped inorganic iodide into organic compounds, and they may also suppress levels of TSH-receptor antibody by directly affecting intrathyroidal autoimmunity. But there are important differences between the two drugs. Methimazole is at least 10 times more potent than propylthiouracil and has a much longer serum half-life (6–8 hr versus 1/2 hr); PTU must be administered 3 times daily, whereas methimazole can be given once daily. Unlike methimazole, PTU is heavily protein-bound and has a lesser ability to cross the placenta and to pass into milk; theoretically, PTU is the preferred drug during pregnancy and for nursing mothers. PTU, but not methimazole, inhibits extrathyroidal conversion of T_4 to T_3; this may be advantageous in the treatment of neonatal thyrotoxicosis.

Toxic reactions occur with both drugs; most are mild, but some are life-threatening. They are unpredictable and can occur after therapy of any duration. There is increasing evidence that these reactions may be fewer in patients treated with methimazole. Transient leukopenia ($<4,000/mm^3$) is common; it is asymptomatic and not a harbinger of agranulocytosis, and usually is not a reason to discontinue treatment. Transient urticarial rashes are common. The most severe reactions are hypersensitive in nature and include agranulocytosis, hepatitis, hepatic failure, a lupus-like syndrome, and a vasculitis involving the skin and other organs. Although rare, these reactions have been reported with both drugs, and it is probably best to treat unusually hypersensitive patients with thyroidectomy. Cases of congenital skin defects (aplasia cutis) have been seen in infants exposed in fetal life to methimazole, but this association does not appear to be a strong one.

The initial dose of PTU is 100–150 mg 3 times daily, and that of methimazole is 30 mg once daily. Smaller initial doses should be used in early childhood. Careful surveillance is required after treatment is initiated. Raising serum levels of TSH above normal indicates overtreatment and leads to increased size of the goiter. Clinical response becomes apparent in 2–3 wk, and adequate control is evident in 1–3 mo. The dose is decreased to the minimal level required to maintain a euthyroid state.

Drug therapy may be continued for 6 yr or longer because

there appears to be a remission rate of about 25% every 2 yr. If a relapse occurs, it will usually appear within 3 mo and almost always within 6 mo after therapy has been discontinued. Therapy may be resumed in case of a relapse. Patients over 13 yr of age, boys, and those with small goiters and modestly elevated T_3 levels appear to have earlier remissions.

A β-adrenergic blocking agent such as propranolol is a useful supplement in management of severely toxic patients. Thyroid hormones potentiate the actions of catecholamines, which include tachycardia, tremor, excessive sweating, lid lag, and stare. These symptoms abate with use of propranolol, which does not, however, alter thyroid function or exophthalmos.

Operation is indicated when adequate cooperation for medical management is not possible or when adequate trial of medical management has failed to result in permanent remission. Subtotal thyroidectomy, a rather safe procedure, is performed only after the patient has been brought to a euthyroid state. This may be accomplished with propylthiouracil or methimazole over 2–3 mo. After a euthyroid state has been attained, 5 drops of a saturated solution of potassium iodide/24 hr are added to the regimen for 2 wk before operation in order to decrease the vascularity of the gland. Complications of surgical treatment are rare and include hypoparathyroidism (transient or permanent) and paralysis of the vocal cords. The incidence of residual or recurrent hyperthyroidism or of hypothyroidism depends on the extent of the surgery. With extensive thyroidectomy the incidence of recurrence may be low, but that of hypothyroidism may exceed 50%.

The ophthalmopathy remits gradually and usually independently of the hyperthyroidism. Severe ophthalmopathy may require treatment with prednisone.

CONGENITAL HYPERTHYROIDISM

Onset of neonatal hyperthyroidism usually occurs a few days after birth; occasionally, onset may be delayed for several weeks or more. The mothers of these infants have active Graves disease, Graves disease in remission, or, on rare occasions, hypothyroidism and a history of lymphocytic thyroiditis. The condition is caused by transplacental passage of TSAb, but the clinical onset, severity, and course may be modified by the concurrent presence of TBIAb and by the transplacental passage of antithyroid drugs taken by the mother. Very high levels of TSAb usually result in classic neonatal hyperthyroidism, but if the infant has been exposed to the antithyroid drugs, onset of symptoms is delayed 3–4 days to allow degradation of the maternally derived antithyroid drug. If TBIAb is also present, onset of hyperthyroid symptoms may be delayed for several weeks.

Neonatal hyperthyroidism occurs in only about 1% of infants born to mothers with a history of Graves disease. The finding of very high levels of TSAb in these mothers usually predicts the occurrence of an affected infant. Unlike Graves disease at all other ages, neonatal hyperthyroidism affects males as often as females. The disorder usually remits spontaneously within 6–12 wk but may persist longer depending on the levels of TSAb. Mild asymptomatic hyperthyroxinemia also occurs. Occasionally, classic neonatal Graves disease does not remit but persists for several years or longer. These patients have impressive family histories of Graves disease. In these infants TSAb transfer from the mother apparently blends with the infantile onset of autonomous Graves disease.

Many of the infants are premature; the majority, but not all, have goiters. The infant is extremely restless, irritable, and hyperactive and appears anxious and unusually alert. The eyes are widely opened and appear exophthalmic. There may be extreme tachycardia and tachypnea, and the temperature is elevated. In severely affected infants there is progression of symptoms; weight loss occurs despite a ravenous appetite, hepatomegaly increases, and jaundice may become manifest. Cardiac decompensation is common, and severe hypertension may occur. The infant may die if therapy is not instituted promptly. The serum level of T_4 is markedly elevated. Advanced bone age, frontal bossing, and cranial synostosis are common, especially in those infants with persistent clinical manifestations of hyperthyroidism. Prognosis for intellectual development is guarded for infants with craniostenosis.

Treatment consists of oral administration of Lugol solution (1 drop every 8 hr) and propylthiouracil (10 mg every 8 hr). If the thyrotoxic state is severe, parenteral fluid therapy, digitalization, and propranolol (2 mg/kg/24 hr po given in 3 divided doses) may be indicated. When propranolol is used during pregnancy to treat thyrotoxicosis, it crosses the placenta and may cause respiratory depression in the newborn infant.

19.16 CARCINOMA OF THE THYROID

Carcinoma of the thyroid is rare in children; only 37 new cases/1 million people are found annually, and about 7% of these occur in children under 18 yr of age. Unlike other malignancies in childhood, thyroid cancer usually has a very indolent course even after pulmonary metastases have developed.

The thyroid gland of children is unusually sensitive to exposure to external radiation. There probably is no threshold dose; even 7 rads increases the incidence of cancer. In the past, about 80% of children with cancer of the thyroid were found to have received irradiation of the neck and adjacent areas during infancy for such benign conditions as "enlarged" thymus, hypertrophied tonsils and adenoids, hemangiomas, nevi, eczema, tinea capitis, and "cervical adenitis." With the disuse of irradiation for benign conditions, this cause of thyroid cancer has vanished. However, the increasing long-term survival of children who have received therapeutic irradiation to areas of the neck for neoplastic disease has now made this cause of thyroid cancer and nodules increasingly prevalent; increased dose, younger age at time of treatment, and female sex are factors that increase the risk of developing thyroid cancer. Long-term risk data for cancer are sparse, but 15–50% of children who have received irradiation and chemotherapy for Hodgkin disease, leukemia, and other malignancies of the head and neck develop elevated levels of TSH within the 1st yr of therapy, and 5–20% progress to hypothyroidism during the next 5–7 yr. Most large groups of treated patients have a 10–30% incidence of benign thyroid nodules and an increased incidence of thyroid cancer. Thyroid cancer begins to appear within 3–5 yr after irradiation treatment and reaches a peak in 15–25 yr. It is unknown whether there is a period after which no more tumors develop.

Histologically, the carcinomas are papillary, follicular, or mixed differentiated tumors. These are usually slow-growing tumors and may remain dormant for years. The type of tumor and the natural course of disease in irradiated and nonirradiated patients are the same except that multicentricity is more frequent in irradiation-induced cancer. In about 4% of patients with papillary cancer, another family relative is affected. Undifferentiated thyroid neoplasms are very rare in children and usually have a rapidly fatal course.

Girls are affected twice as often as boys. The average age at diagnosis is 9 yr, but the onset may be as early as the 1st yr of life. A painless nodule in the thyroid or in the neck is the usual first evidence of disease. Cervical lymph node involvement is often present at the time of initial diagnosis. Any unexplained cervical lymph node enlargement requires examination of the thyroid, which occasionally has a primary tumor too small to be felt, the diagnosis being made on biopsy of the lymph node. The lungs are the most common site of metastases beyond the neck. There may be no clinical manifestations referable to them; roentgenographically, they appear as diffuse miliary or nodular infiltrations, principally in the basal portions. They may be mistaken for tuberculosis, histoplasmosis, or sarcoidosis. Other sites of metastases include the mediastinum, long bones, skull, and axilla. On rare occasions the carcinoma may be functional and produce symptoms of hyperthyroidism.

A thyroid scan should be performed whenever a thyroid nodule is found. ^{123}I or ^{99m}Tc pertechnetate is the preferred scanning agent. Most malignant lesions show decreased concentration of radioisotope (are "cold"), but some cold lesions are benign. Serum levels of Tg are often elevated and return to normal after surgical removal of differentiated tumors; this test also permits early detection of metastases. Tg levels do not correlate with any histologic characteristics or with malignancy or benignity of thyroid tumors. Other tests of thyroid function are normal, but Hashimoto thyroiditis has been associated on a number of occasions with thyroid cancer.

Because differentiated thyroid carcinoma is a chronic disease with a long survival, optimal therapy is still evolving. There is increasing evidence that papillary carcinoma, the least aggressive type, is effectively treated by subtotal thyroidectomy and suppressive doses of thyroid hormone. Total thyroidectomy and treatment with ^{131}I do not appear to improve prognosis. Many patients with cervical or pulmonary metastases have survived for many years. Pure follicular and mixed papillary and follicular cancers are more aggressive; affected patients may require total thyroidectomy and neck dissection. For any form of therapy, survival or recurrence does not appear to be different for patients with or without involvement of the cervical nodes. Even patients with cervical or pulmonary metastases have survived for many years.

More than 95% of patients are alive 25 yr after initial treatment if the tumor is intrathyroid, less than 2 cm in size, and classified as grade 1. Greater tumor size, distant spread, and greater atypia are associated with increased cumulative mortality.

After surgery all patients should be treated with sodium-L-thyroxine in doses sufficient to suppress TSH. Periodic determinations of Tg levels should also be performed, since Tg is an excellent marker for tumor recurrence in patients taking T_4.

SOLITARY THYROID NODULE

Solitary nodules of the thyroid are uncommon in children. In the past it was estimated that as many as half were carcinomas, but more recent studies indicate that there is about a 15% incidence of malignancy, perhaps because of decreasing exposure of children to irradiation. Children exposed to irradiation have a high incidence of benign adenoma as well as of carcinoma of the thyroid.

Benign disorders that may present as solitary thyroid nodules include benign adenomas (follicular, embryonal, Hürthle cell), lymphocytic thyroiditis, thyroglossal duct cyst, ectopically located normal thyroid tissue, a single median thyroid, agenesis of one of the lateral thyroid lobes with hypertrophy of the contralateral lobe, thyroid cysts, and abscess. Sudden appearance of or rapidly enlarging thyroid mass may indicate hemorrhage into a benign adenoma. In most cases the child is euthyroid and thyroid function studies are normal. A ^{99m}Tc scan is usually indicated. Ultrasound is particularly useful in detecting cystic lesions. When lymphocytic thyroiditis is the cause of the nodule, T_4 may be low, TSH may be elevated, and thyroid antibodies are usually present. The scan may reveal a moth-eaten appearance. Rarely, lymphocytic thyroiditis may be associated with carcinoma of the thyroid.

Some nodules are "cold" on ^{99m}Tc scan, as is the case with carcinoma, but other lesions, such as developmental defects of the thyroid, are usually "hot." In questionable cases one may use suppressive therapy with 0.1–0.2 mg daily of sodium-L-thyroxine. Cold nodules that continue to grow over 4–6 mo or that do not reduce in size by 50% in 1 yr should be surgically explored. Surgery without delay is indicated when the nodule is hard or has grown rapidly, when there is evidence of tracheal or vocal cord involvement, or when there is enlargement of adjacent lymph nodes. All persons with a history of head or neck irradiation should have careful examinations of the thyroid at least every 2 yr, indefinitely.

Very rarely, thyroid nodules may be functional, producing hyperthyroidism (Plummer disease). The uptake of radionuclide is concentrated in the nodule ("hot" or "warm" nodule), and thyroid function studies indicate that the nodule is functioning autonomously. Such nodules are usually benign, but a few instances of carcinoma in such cases have been reported. T_4 levels are usually normal, whereas T_3 levels are elevated (T_3 toxicosis), and TSH levels are suppressed. Treatment consists of surgical removal of the nodule.

A suppressible functioning nodule in a euthyroid child has been reported only once.

MEDULLARY CARCINOMA

This carcinoma of the thyroid arises from the parafollicular cells (C cells) of the thyroid and accounts for about 10% of thyroid malignancies. The tumor is pleomorphic, with sheets of spindle or small cells with eosinophilic granular cytoplasm. Amyloid is invariably deposited in the stroma, and calcification is common. The most common symptom is goiter or a palpable thyroid nodule. Roentgenograms may reveal dense, conglomerate, homogeneous calcification in the thyroid. Metastases to the regional lymph nodes and to the liver are common, and these too may calcify. Death may result, but long survivals are not uncommon.

The tumors occur sporadically and as components of two distinct autosomal dominant syndromes (see later). When the tumor occurs sporadically, it is usually unicentric, whereas in the familial form it is usually multicentric, and it begins as hyperplasia of parafollicular cells. The tumors are often too small to be found by palpation, scintigraphy, or ultrasound examination in at-risk patients in these families. Diagnosis of medullary carcinoma should lead to a careful search for associated tumors, particularly pheochromocytoma. No clinically recognizable manifestations result from the elevated serum levels of calcitonin or from the calcitonin gene-related peptide and the carboxy-terminal flanking peptide (katacalcin) that are associated.

MULTIPLE ENDOCRINE NEOPLASIA (MEN), TYPE IIa. When hyperplasia or carcinoma of C cells is associated with adrenal medullary hyperplasia or pheochromocytoma and parathyroid hyperplasia, it is known as MEN-IIa. The gene locus is on chromosome 10 next to the centromere. DNA testing that can identify family members with the mutant gene is now possible, thus narrowing the number of family members requiring endocrine studies. C cell hyperplasia or tumors usually appear earlier than pheochromocytoma. Pheochromocytomas are frequently bilateral and may be multiple. Adrenal medullary hyperplasia is known to precede pheochromocytoma, but the detectable latent period is short.

Hypercalcemia is a late manifestation and indicates hyperparathyroidism. The parathyroids may reveal chief-cell hyperplasia or only hypercellularity. A primary defect of the neural crest can account for all the findings in the syndrome. Since basal levels of calcitonin are often normal in affected individuals, provocative tests using infusions of pentagastrin or calcium or both may be required to detect C cell hyperplasia. Other biochemical markers frequently found in serum include histaminidase and dopa decarboxylase. Ectopic secretion of ACTH or vasoactive intestinal peptide accounts for the occasional association with Cushing syndrome or watery diarrhea.

MULTIPLE ENDOCRINE NEOPLASIA (MEN), TYPE IIb. The distinguishing feature of MEN-IIb, also called the *mucosal neuroma syndrome*, is the occurrence of multiple neuromas and a characteristic phenotype associated with medullary carcinoma and pheochromocytoma. The genes for MEN-IIa and MEN-IIb seem to be allelic.

The neuromas most often occur on the tongue, buccal mucosa, lips, and conjunctivae. Peripheral neurofibromas and café-au-lait patches may be present, and intestinal ganglioneuromatosis is common. Diffuse proliferation of nerves and ganglion cells is found in mucosal, submucosal, myenteric, and subserosal plexuses involving the small and large bowel as well as the esophagus. The patients may be tall, with arachnodactyly and a Marfan-like appearance. Scoliosis, pectus excavatum, pes cavus, and muscular hypotonia are common. The eyelids may be thickened and everted, the lips patulous and blubbery, the jaw prognathic. Feeding difficulties, poor sucking, diarrhea, constipation, and failure to thrive may begin in infancy or early childhood many years before the appearance of neuromas or endocrine symptoms.

TREATMENT. Total thyroidectomy is indicated for all children with medullary carcinoma of the thyroid, even for those in whom C cell hyperplasia is demonstrable only by calcitonin stimulation tests. Recognition of familial forms of this tumor is critical to early diagnosis in patients at risk. Evidence suggests that thyroidectomy must be done very early because medullary carcinoma has been seen in a 6-mo-old child with MEN-IIb and in a 3-yr-old child with MEN-IIa. Monitoring the levels of calcitonin is useful in detecting metastatic lesions and for following the course of the disease after operation.

HYPOTHYROIDISM

American Academy of Pediatrics and American Thyroid Association: Newborn screening for congenital hypothyroidism: Recommended guidelines. Report. Pediatrics 80:745, 1987.

Bachrach LK, Daneman D, Daneman A, et al: Use of ultrasound in childhood thyroid disorders. J Pediatr 103:547, 1983.

Bogner U, Gruters A, Sigle B, et al: Cytotoxic antibodies in congenital hypothyroidism. J Clin Endocrinol Metab 68:671, 1989.

Burrow GN, Dussault JH (eds): Neonatal Thyroid Screening. New York, Raven Press, 1980.

Codaocioni JL, Cargyon P, Miche-Bechet M, et al: Congenital hypothyroidism associated with thyrotropin unresponsiveness and thyroid cell membrane alterations. J Clin Endocrinol Metab 50:932, 1980.

Connors MA, Styne DM: Transient neonatal "athyreosis" resulting from thyrotropin-binding inhibiting immunoglobulins. Pediatrics 78:287, 1986.

Cosman BC, Schullmger JN, Bell JJ, et al: Hypothyroidism caused by topical povidone-iodine in a newborn with omphalocele. J Pediatr Surg 23:356, 1988.

Costigan DC, Holland FJ, Daneman D, et al: Amiodarone therapy effects on childhood thyroid function. Pediatrics 77:703, 1986.

Cutler AT, Benezra-Obeiter R, Brink SJ: Thyroid function in young children with Down syndrome. Am J Dis Child 140:479, 1986.

Dacou-Voutetakis C, Felquate DM, Drakopoulou M, et al: Familial hypothyroidism by a nonsense mutation in the thyroid-stimulating hormone β-subunit gene. Am J Hum Genet 46:988, 1990.

Dussault JH, Letarte J, Guyda H, et al: Lack of influence of thyroid antibodies on thyroid function in the newborn infant and on a mass screening program for congenital hypothyroidism. J Pediatr 96:385, 1980.

Fisher DA: Management of congenital hypothyroidism. J Clin Endocrinol Metab 72:523, 1991.

Fisher DA, Foley BL: Early treatment of congenital hypothyroidism. Pediatrics 83:785, 1989.

Fisher DA, Klein AH: Thyroid development and disorders of thyroid function in the newborn. N Engl J Med 304:702, 1981.

Francis G, Riley W: Congenital familial transient hypothyroidism secondary to transplacental thyrotropin-blocking antibodies. Am J Dis Child 141:1061, 1987.

Gushurst CA, Muehler JA, Green JA, et al: Breast milk iodide: Reassessment in the 1980's. Pediatrics 73:354, 1984.

Hann CE, Krainz PL, Skeels MR, et al: Detection of congenital hypopituitary hypothyroidism: Ten-year experience in The Northwest Regional Screening Program. J Pediatr 109:959, 1986.

Hopwood NJ, Sauder SE, Shapiro B, et al: Familial partial peripheral and pituitary resistance to thyroid hormone: A frequently missed diagnosis. Pediatrics 78:1114, 1986.

Kleinhaus N, Faber J, Kahana L, et al: Euthyroid hyperthyroxinemia due to a generalized 5'-deiodinase defect. J Clin Endocrinol Metab 66:684, 1988.

Levine MA, Jap TS, Hung W: Infantile hypothyroidism in two sibs: An unusual presentation of pseudohypoparathyroidism type Ia. J Pediatr 107:919, 1985.

Menezes-Fereira MM, Eil C, Wortsman J, et al: Decreased nuclear uptake of (^{123}I)triiodo-L-thyronine in fibroblasts from patients with peripheral thyroid hormone resistance. J Clin Endocrinol Metab 59:1081, 1984.

Muir A, Daneman D, Daneman A, et al: Thyroid scanning, ultrasound, and serum thyroglobulin in determining the origin of congenital hypothyroidism. Am J Dis Child 142:214, 1988.

Najjar SS: Muscular hypertrophy in hypothyroid children. The Kocher-Debré-Sémélaigne syndrome. J Pediatr 85:236, 1974.

New England Congenital Hypothyroidism Collaborative: Elementary school performance of children with congenital hypothyroidism. J Pediatr 111:17, 1990.

New England Congenital Hypothyroidism Collaborative: Neonatal hypothyroidism screening: Status of patients at 6 years of age. J Pediatr 107:915, 1985.

Refetoff S, DeGroot LJ, Barsano CP: Defective thyroid hormone feedback regulation in the syndrome of peripheral resistance to thyroid hormone. J Clin Endocrinol Metab 51:41, 1980.

Rezvani I, DiGeorge AM: Reassessment of the daily dose of oral thyroxine for replacement therapy in hypothyroid children. J Pediatr 90:291, 1977.

Rivkees SA, Bode HH, Crawford JD: Long-term growth in juvenile acquired hypothyroidism: The failure to achieve normal adult stature. N Engl J Med 318:519, 1988.

Sklar CA, Qazi R, David R: Juvenile autoimmune thyroiditis. Hormonal status at presentation and after long-term follow-up. Am J Dis Child 140:877, 1986.

Smith DW, Klein AM, Henderson JR, et al: Congenital hypothyroidism—signs and symptoms in the newborn period. J Pediatr 87:958, 1975.

Thorpe-Beeston JG, Nicolaides KH, Fetton CV, et al: Maturation of the secretion of thyroid hormone and thyroid-stimulating hormone in the fetus. N Engl J Med 324:532, 1991.

Usala SJ, Menke JB, Watson TL, et al: A new point mutation in the 3,5,3'-triiodothyronine-binding domain of the c-erbAβ thyroid hormone receptor is tightly linked to generalized thyroid hormone receptor resistance. J Clin Endocrinol Metab 72:32, 1991.

van der Gaag RD, Drexhage HA, Dussault JH: Role of maternal immunoglobulin blocking TSH-induced thyroid growth in sporadic forms of congenital hypothyroidism. Lancet 1:246, 1985.

VanDop C, Conte FA, Koch TK, et al: Pseudotumor cerebri associated with initiation of levothyroxine therapy for juvenile hypothyroidism. N Engl J Med 308:1076, 1983.

Vulsma T, Gons MH, deVijlder JJM: Maternal-fetal transfer of thyroxine in congenital hypothyroidism due to a total organification defect or thyroid agenesis. N Engl J Med 321:13, 1989.

GOITROUS CRETINISM

Boyages SC, Halpern JP, Maberly GF, et al: A comparative study of neurological and myxedematous endemic cretinism in Western China. J Clin Endocrinol Metab 67:1262, 1988.

Boyages SC, Halpern JP, Maberly GF, et al: Supplementary iodine fails to reverse hypothyroidism in adolescents and adults with endemic cretinism. J Clin Endocrinol Metab 70:336, 1990.

Boyages SC, Halper JP, Maberly GF, et al: Endemic cretinism: Possible role for thyroid autoimmunity. Lancet 2:529, 1989.

Burrow GN, Spaulding SW, Alexander NM, et al: Normal peroxidase activity in Pendred's syndrome. J Clin Endocrinol Metab 36:522, 1973.

Couch RM, Dean HJ, Winter JSD: Congenital hypothyroidism caused by defective iodide transport. J Pediatr 106:950, 1985.

Gattereau A, Bernard B, Bellabarba D, et al: Congenital goiter in four euthyroid siblings with glandular and circulating iodoproteins and defective iodothyronine synthesis. J Clin Endocrinol Metab 37:118, 1973.

Goslings BM, et al: Hypothyroidism in an area of endemic goiter and cretinism in central Java, Indonesia. J Clin Endocrinol Metab 44:481, 1977.

Illum P, Kiaer HW, Hvidberg-Hansen J, et al: Fifteen cases of Pendred's syndrome. Congenital deafness and sporadic goiter. Arch Otolaryngol 96:297, 1972.

Silva JE, Santelices R, Kishihara M, Schneider A: Low molecular weight thyroglobulin leading to a goiter in a 12-year-old girl. J Clin Endocrinol Metab 58:526, 1984.

Vanderpas JB, Rivera-Vanderpas MT, Bourdoux P, et al: Reversibility of severe hypothyroidism with supplementary iodine in patients with endemic cretinism. J Clin Endocrinol Metab 315:791, 1986.

GOITER

Daneman D, Davy T, Mancer K, et al: Association of multinodular goiter, cystic renal disease, and digital anomalies. J Pediatr 107:270, 1985.
Davidson KM, Richards DS, Schatz DA, et al: Successful in utero treatment of fetal goiter and hypothyroidism. N Engl J Med 324:543, 1991.
DeLuca G, Chaussain JL, Job JC: Hyperfunctioning thyroid nodules in children and adolescents. Acta Paediatr Scand 75:118, 1986.
Feuillan PP, Shawker T, Rose SR, et al: Thyroid abnormalities in the McCune-Albright syndrome. Ultrasonography and hormonal studies. J Clin Endocrinol Metab 71:1596, 1990.
Hay ID: Thyroiditis: A clinical update. Mayo Clin Proc 60:836, 1985.
Patel YC, Pharoah POD, Hornabrook RW, et al: Serum triiodothyronine, thyroxine and thyroid-stimulating hormone in endemic goiter: A comparison of goitrous and non-goitrous subjects in New Guinea. J Clin Endocrinol Metab 7:783, 1973.
Pharoah POD, Buttfield IH, Hetzel BS: Neurological damage to the foetus resulting from severe iodine deficiency during pregnancy. Lancet 1:308, 1971.
Queen JS, Clegg HW, Council JC, et al: Acute suppurative thyroiditis caused by *Eikenella corrodens*. J Pediatr Surg 23:359, 1988.
Randolph J, Grunt JA, Vawter GF: The medical and surgical aspects of intratracheal goiter. N Engl J Med 268:457, 1963.
Rich EJ, Mendelman PM: Acute suppurative thyroiditis in pediatric patients. Pediatr Infect Dis J 6:936, 1987.

HYPERTHYROIDISM

Cheron RG, Kaplan MM, Larsen PR, et al: Neonatal thyroid function after propylthiouracil therapy for maternal Graves' disease. N Engl J Med 304:525, 1981.
Collen RJ, Landaw EM, Kaplan SA, et al: Remission rates of children and adolescents with thyrotoxicosis treated with antithyroid drugs. Pediatrics 65:550, 1980.
Cooper DS: Which anti-thyroid drug. Am J Med 80:1165, 1986.
Daneman D, Howard NJ: Neonatal thyrotoxicosis: Intellectual impairment and craniosynostosis in later years. J Pediatr 97:257, 1980.
Darby CP: Three episodes of spontaneous thyroid storm occurring in a nine year-old child. Pediatrics 30:927, 1962.
Foley TP, White C, New A: Juvenile Graves disease: Usefulness and limitations of thyrotropin receptor antibody determinations. J Pediatr 110:378, 1987.
Lightner ES, Allen HD, Laughlin G: Neonatal hyperthyroidism and heart failure. Am J Dis Child 131:68, 1977.
Lippe BM, Landow EM, Kaplan SA: Hyperthyroidism in children treated with long-term medical therapy: Twenty-five percent remission rate every two years. J Clin Endocrinol Metab 64:1241, 1987.
McGregor AM, Peterson MM, McLachlan SM, et al: Carbimazole and the autoimmune response in Graves' disease. N Engl J Med 303:302, 1980.
McKenzie JM, Zakarija M: The clinical use of thyrotropin receptor antibody measurements. J Clin Endocrinol Metab 68:1093, 1989.
Mihailovic V, Feller MS, Kourides IA, et al: Hyperthyroidism due to excess thyrotropin secretion: Follow-up studies. J Clin Endocrinol Metab 50:1135, 1980.
Milham S Jr: Scalp defects in infants of mothers treated for hyperthyroidism with methimazole or carbimazole during pregnancy. Teratology 32:321, 1985.
Pompa BH, Cloutier MD, Hayles AB: Thyroid nodule producing T_3 toxicosis in a child. Mayo Clin Proc 48:273, 1973.
Riggs W Jr, Wilroy RS Jr, Etteldorf JN: Neonatal hyperthyroidism with accelerated skeletal maturation, craniosynostosis, and brachydactyly. Radiology 105:621, 1972.
Roti E, Gardini E, Minelli R, et al: Methimazole and serum thyroid hormone concentrations in hyperthyroid patients: Effects of single and multiple daily doses. Ann Intern Med 111:181, 1989.
Samuel S, Gilman S, Maurer HS, et al: Hyperthyroidism in an infant with McCune-Albright syndrome: Report of a case with myeloid dysplasia. J Pediatr 80:275, 1972.
Smith CS, Howard NJ: Propranolol in treatment of neonatal thyrotoxicosis. J Pediatr 83:1046, 1973.
Stenszky V, Kozma L, Balazs C, et al: The genetics of Graves disease: HLA and disease susceptibility. J Clin Endocrinol Metab 61:835, 1985.
Totterman TH, Karlsson FA, Bengstsson M, et al: Induction of circulating activated suppressor-like T cells by methimazole therapy for Graves disease. N Engl J Med 316:15, 1987.
Viscardi RM, Shea M, Sriwantanakul K, et al: Hyperthyroxinemia in newborns due to excess thyroxine-binding globulin. N Engl J Med 309:897, 1983.
Volpe R, Ehrlich R, Steiner G, et al: Graves' disease in pregnancy years after hypothyroidism with recurrent passive-transfer neonatal Graves' disease in offspring. Therapeutic considerations. Am J Med 77:572, 1984.
Zakarija M, McKenzie JM: Pregnancy-associated changes in the thyroid-stimulating antibody of Graves' disease and the relationship to neonatal hyperthyroidism. J Clin Endocrinol Metab 57:1036, 1983.

LYMPHOCYTIC THYROIDITIS

Boyages SC, Halpern JP, Maeberly GF, et al: Possible role for thyroid autoimmunity. Lancet 2:529, 1989.
Chiovato L, Vitti P, Santini F, et al: Incidence of antibodies blocking thyrotropin effect in vitro in patients with euthyroid or hypothyroid autoimmune thyroiditis. J Clin Endocrinol Metab 71:40, 1990.
Doniach D, Nilsson LR, Roitt IM: Autoimmune thyroiditis in children and adolescents. Acta Pediatr 54:260, 1965.
Hung W, Chandra R, August GP, et al: Clinical, laboratory and histologic observations in euthyroid children and adolescents with goiters. J Pediatr 82:10, 1973.
Lautenschlager I, Maenpaa J, Nyberg M, et al: Thyroid infiltrating cells in juvenile autoimmune thyroiditis: A follow-up of 1 year. Clin Immunol Immunopathol 49:143, 1988.
Loeb PB, Drash AL, Kenny FM: Prevalence of low titer and "negative" antithyroglobulin antibodies in biopsy-proven juvenile Hashimoto's thyroiditis. J Pediatr 82:17, 1973.
Phillips D, McLachlan S, Stephenson A, et al: Autosomal dominant transmission of autoantibodies to thyroglobulin and thyroid peroxidase. J Clin Endocrinol Metab 70:742, 1990.
Rallison ML, Dobyns BM, Keating FR, et al: Occurrence and natural history of chronic lymphocytic thyroiditis in childhood. J Pediatr 86:675, 1975.
Riley WJ, Maclaren NK, Lezotte DC, et al: Thyroid autoimmunity in insulin-dependent diabetes mellitus. The case for routine screening. J Pediatr 98:350, 1981.
Yokoyama N, Taurog A, Klee GG: Thyroid peroxidase and thyroid microsomal antibodies. J Clin Endocrinol Metab 68:766, 1989.

CARCINOMA OF THE THYROID

Ashcroft NW, Van Herle AJ: The comparative value of serum thyroglobulin measurements and iodine ^{131}I total body scans in the follow-up of patients treated with differentiated thyroid cancer. Am J Med 71:806, 1981.
Black EG, Cassoni A, Gimlette TMD, et al: Serum thyroglobulin in thyroid cancer. Lancet 2:443, 1981.
Carney JA, Go VLW, Sizemore GW, et al: Alimentary tract ganglioneuromatosis. A major component of the syndrome of multiple endocrine neoplasia, type 2b. N Engl J Med 295:1287, 1976.
Crile Y Jr, Antunex AR, Esselstyn CB, et al: The advantages of subtotal thyroidectomy and suppression of TSH in the primary treatment of papillary carcinoma of the thyroid. Cancer 55:2691, 1985.
DeGroot LJ: Diagnostic approach and management of patients exposed to irradiation of the thyroid. J Clin Endocrinol Metab 69:925, 1989.
Fisher DA: Thyroid nodules in children and their management. J Pediatr 89:866, 1976.
Fleming ID, Black TL, Thompson EI, et al: Thyroid dysfunction and neoplasia in children receiving neck irradiation for cancer. Cancer 55:1190, 1985.
Gagel RF: The impact of gene mapping techniques on the management of multiple endocrine neoplasia type 2. Trends in Endocrinol Metab 2:19, 1991.
Griffiths AM, Mack DR, Byard RW, et al: Multiple endocrine neoplasia IIb: An unusual cause of chronic constipation. J Pediatr 116:285, 1990.
Gutjahr P, Spranger J: Thyroidectomy in type IIb multiple-endocrine-neoplasia syndrome. Lancet 1:1149, 1977.
Hempelmann LH, Hall WJ, Phillips M, et al: Neoplasms in persons treated with x-rays in infancy: Fourth survey in 20 years. J Natl Cancer Inst 55:519, 1975.
Jones BA, Sisson JC: Early diagnosis and thyroidectomy in multiple endocrine neoplasia, type 2b. J Pediatr 102:219, 1983.
Keiser HR, Beaven MA, Doppham J, et al: Sipple's syndrome: Medullary thyroid carcinoma, pheochromocytoma and parathyroid disease. Ann Intern Med 78:561, 1973.
Kirkland RT, Kirkland JL, Rosenberg HS, et al: Solitary thyroid nodules in 30 children and report of a child with a thyroid abscess. Pediatrics 51:85, 1973.
Razack MS, Sako K, Shimaoka K, et al: Radiation-associated thyroid carcinoma. J Surg Oncol 14:287, 1980.
Rojeski MT, Gharib H: Nodular thyroid disease. Evaluation and management. N Engl J Med 313:428, 1985.
Samaan NA, Schultz PN, Ordunez NG, et al: A comparison of thyroid carcinoma in those who have and have not had head and neck irradiation in childhood. J Clin Endocrinol Metab 64:219, 1987.
Sazmaan NA, Maheshwari YK, Nader S, et al: Impact of therapy for differentiated carcinoma of the thyroid: An analysis of 706 cases. J Clin Endocrinol Metab 56:1131, 1983.
Scott MD, Crawford JD: Solitary thyroid nodules in childhood: Is the incidence of thyroid carcinoma declining? Pediatrics 58:521, 1976.
Stjernholm MR, Freudenborrg JC, Mooney HS, et al: Medullary carcinoma of the thyroid before age 2 years. J Clin Endocrinol Metab 51:252, 1980.
Sussman L, Librik L, Clayton GW: Hyperthyroidism attributable to a hyperfunctioning thyroid carcinoma. J Pediatr 72:208, 1968.
Vane D, King DR, Boles ET Jr: Secondary thyroid neoplasma in pediatric cancer patients: Increased risk with improved survival. J Pediatr Surg 19:855, 1984.

19.17 DISORDERS OF THE PARATHYROID GLANDS

Parathyroid hormone (PTH), vitamin D, and calcitonin are the principal regulators of calcium homeostasis.

PARATHYROID HORMONE. PTH is an 84-amino acid chain (9,500 dalton), but its biologic activity resides in the first 34 residues. In the parathyroid gland a proparathyroid hormone (90-amino acid chain) and a pre-pro-PTH (115-amino acid chain) are synthesized. Pre-pro-PTH is converted to pro-PTH in the endoplasmic reticulum and pro-PTH to PTH in the Golgi apparatus. PTH (1–84) is the major secretory product of the gland, but it is rapidly cleaved in the liver and kidney into smaller COOH-terminal, midregion, and NH_2-terminal fragments.

The occurrence of these fragments has complicated the reliable measurement of PTH in serum and has led to the development of a variety of assays. The 1–34 amino-terminal (N-terminal) fragments possess biologic activity but are present in very low amounts in the circulation; assay of these fragments is most useful for detecting acute secretory changes. The carboxy-terminal (C-terminal) and midregion fragments, although biologically inert, are cleared more slowly from the circulation and represent 80% of plasma immunoreactive PTH; values of the C-terminal fragment are 50–500 times the level of the active hormone. The C-terminal assays are very effective in detecting patients with hyperparathyroidism, but, since C-terminal fragments are removed from the circulation by glomerular filtration, these assays are less useful for evaluating the secondary hyperparathyroidism characteristic of renal disease. Only certain sensitive radioimmunoassays for PTH can distinguish the subnormal concentrations that occur in hypoparathyroidism from normal levels. No RIA satisfactorily distinguishes between the hypercalcemia of malignancy and that of primary hyperparathyroidism. These assays are being replaced by immunometric assays that measure intact PTH with greater sensitivity, specificity, and precision; a shortened incubation period also allows their intraoperative use to provide the surgeon with useful information.

When serum levels of calcium fall, secretion of PTH increases. PTH stimulates activity of 1α-hydroxylase in the kidney, enhancing production of 1,25-dihydroxycholecalciferol (1,25-$(OH)_2D_3$). The increased level of 1,25-$(OH)_2D_3$ induces synthesis of a calcium-binding protein *(calbindin-D)* in the intestinal mucosa with resultant absorption of calcium. PTH also mobilizes calcium by directly enhancing bone resorption, an effect that requires 1,25-$(OH)_2D_3$. The effects of PTH on bone and kidney are mediated through binding to specific receptors on the membranes of target cells and through activation of the adenylate cyclase system.

PTH-RELATED PEPTIDE (PTHrP). This recently isolated protein is homologous to PTH only in the first 13 amino acids of its amino terminus, 8 of which are identical to PTH. Its gene is on the short arm of chromosome 12, whereas that of PTH is on the short arm of chromosome 11. PTHrP, like PTH, activates PTH receptors in kidney and bone, increases urinary cAMP and renal production of 1,25-$(OH)_2D$, induces bone resorption, increases serum levels of calcium, and increases phosphate excretion. Although its physiologic role is unknown, PTHrP is widely distributed in normal tissues and cells such as placenta, lactating mammary tissue, gastric cells, and keratinocytes, as well as in fetal tissues, suggesting a physiologic role at these sites. The humoral hypercalcemia syndrome of malignancy is caused by elevated concentrations of PTHrP. Breast milk and pasteurized bovine milk have levels of PTHrP that are 10,000 times higher than those of normal plasma.

VITAMIN D. See Sec. 4.7 and 24.59.

CALCITONIN (CT). CT is a 32-amino acid polypeptide. Its gene is on chromosome 11p and is tightly linked to that of PTH. The CT gene encodes three peptides: CT, a 21-amino acid carboxy-terminal flanking peptide (katacalcin), and a CT gene-related peptide. Katacalcin and CT are cosecreted in equimolar amounts by the parafollicular cells (C cells) of the thyroid gland. Although CT was discovered through its hypocalcemic effect, patients with medullary carcinoma of the thyroid (a tumor arising from the C cells) usually have normal plasma levels of calcium. Patients with thyroid aplasia or those who have been thyroidectomized have little discernible disturbance in calcium metabolism; basal calcitonin levels are normal, but secretory response after calcium infusion is impaired.

Its action appears to be independent of PTH and of vitamin D. Its main biologic effect appears to be the inhibition of bone resorption by decreasing the number and activity of bone-resorbing osteoclasts. This action of CT is the rationale behind its use in treatment of Paget disease. Calcitonin is synthesized also in other organs, such as the gastrointestinal tract, pancreas, brain, and pituitary. In these organs CT is believed to behave as a neurotransmitter to impose a local inhibitory effect on cell function.

The physiologic role of calcitonin remains uncertain. Its mean circulating basal levels are higher in children than in adults and are four times higher in men than in women.

19.18 HYPOPARATHYROIDISM

ETIOLOGY (Table 19–4). The normal level of PTH in cord blood is low; it doubles by the 6th day to reach a level nearly that of normal infants and children. Hypocalcemia is common from 12–72 hr of life, especially in premature infants, in infants with asphyxia at birth, and in infants of diabetic mothers *(early neonatal hypocalcemia)* (see also Sec. 6.6). After the 2nd–3rd day and during the 1st wk of life, the type of feeding is also a determinant of the level of serum calcium *(late neonatal hypocalcemia)*. The role played by the parathyroids in these hypocalcemic infants remains to be clarified, although functional immaturity of the parathyroids has often been invoked as a pathogenetic factor. In a group of infants with *transient idiopathic hypocalcemia* (1–8 wk of age) serum levels of PTH were significantly lower than in normal infants. It is possible that the functional immaturity is a manifestation of a delay in development of the enzymes that convert glandular PTH to secreted PTH; other mechanisms are possible.

Hyperparathyroidism during pregnancy may result in transient hypocalcemia of the newborn infant. It appears that the hypocalcemia in such infants results from suppression of the fetal parathyroids by exposure to elevated levels of calcium in maternal serum. Tetany usually develops within 3 wk but may be delayed 1 mo or more if the infant is breast-fed. Hypocalcemia may persist for weeks or months. When the cause of hypocalcemia in young infants is unknown, their mothers should have measurements of calcium, phosphorus,

TABLE 19–4. Etiologic Classification of Hypocalcemia

- Parathyroid hormone (PTH) deficiency
  - Transient hypofunction
    - Early neonatal hypocalcemia
    - Late neonatal hypocalcemia
    - Maternal hyperparathyroidism
    - Other
  - Congenital aplasia or hypoplasia of parathyroids
    - With thymic and other III–IV arch defects (DiGeorge syndrome)
    - With Zellweger, Vater, CHARGE syndromes
    - With chromosomal abnormalities (especially 22p−)
    - With maternal diabetes mellitus, alcoholism, or retinoic acid treatment
    - With congenital hypothyroidism due to maternal ^{131}I
  - Familial hypoparathyroidism
    - X-linked
    - Autosomal dominant
  - Idiopathic hypoparathyroidism
    - Autoimmune hypoparathyroiditis
      - Isolated
      - With Addison disease or mucocutaneous candidiasis (type I autoimmune polyendocrinopathy)
- Surgical removal or damage to parathyroids
- Hemosiderosis (treatment of thalassemia)
- Copper deposition (Wilson disease)
- Parathyroid hormone unresponsiveness (pseudohypoparathyroidism)
  - Type Ia—reduced cellular αG_S (G unit)
  - Type Ib—normal G unit
  - Type II—normal cAMP response
- Vitamin D deficiency
  - Inadequate irradiation (clothing, housing, smog, climate)
  - Dietary deficiency
  - Malabsorption
    - Deficiency of bile salts (liver disease)
    - Deficiency of calcium-binding protein (gluten-sensitive enteropathy)
    - Intestinal bypass operations
  - Depletion (bile fistulas)
  - Altered metabolism (chronic therapy with phenytoin [diphenylhydantoin] or phenobarbital)
  - Impaired synthesis of 25-(OH)D_3 (severe hepatic disease)
  - Impaired synthesis of 1,25-$(OH)_2D_3$
    - Renal failure
    - Renal tubular disease?
    - Genetic deficiency of 1α-hydroxylase (vitamin D–dependent rickets, type I)
    - Hypoparathyroidism
  - End-organ resistance to 1,25-$(OH)_2D_3$ (vitamin D–dependent rickets, type II)
    - With alopecia
    - Without alopecia
- Magnesium deficiency
  - Familial hypomagnesemia
  - Other malabsorption syndromes
- Inorganic phosphate excess
  - Poisoning
  - Initial therapy of leukemia

and parathyroid hormone. Most affected mothers are asymptomatic, and the etiology of their hypoparathyroidism is usually a parathyroid adenoma.

Aplasia of the parathyroid glands is often associated with other developmental defects arising from the 3rd and 4th pharyngeal pouches *(DiGeorge syndrome)* (Fig. 19–10 and Sec. 11.13). The most common associations are aplasia or hypoplasia of the thymus and congenital heart defects (especially those involving the aorta, such as truncus arteriosus and interruption of the aortic arch). The disorder is usually sporadic, but autosomal dominant and autosomal recessive inheritance have been reported. In other instances, deletions of the short arm of chromosome 22 have been associated. The syndrome has occurred in infants of diabetic mothers, in association with the fetal alcohol and CHARGE syndromes, and in infants born to mothers who were inadvertently treated with retinoic acid for acne early in pregnancy. Tetany may be transient, may remit and recur later, or may appear initially during childhood. *Hypoplasia of the parathyroid glands* probably occurs more often than aplasia. The thymic deficiency may be likewise attenuated.

Administration of ^{131}I during pregnancy has resulted in hypoparathyroidism as well as in hypothyroidism.

Familial Congenital Hypoparathyroidism. In two large pedigrees this disorder appears to be transmitted by an X-linked recessive gene. Onset of afebrile seizures characteristically occurs in infants from 2 wk–6 mo of age. Familial hypoparathyroidism that has been observed also in both sexes in successive generations suggests autosomal dominant inheritance. The age of onset ranges from infancy to young adulthood. Absence of any parathyroid tissue after detailed examination at autopsy in a boy with the X-linked form of the condition suggests that it is a defect of embryogenesis. Hypocalcemia, hyperphosphatemia, and low levels of immunoreactive PTH occur. Parathyroid antibodies are absent in both genetic types.

Removal or damage of the parathyroid glands may complicate thyroidectomy *(surgical hypoparathyroidism)*. Hypoparathyroidism has developed even when the parathyroid glands have been identified and left undisturbed at the time of operation. This presumably is the result of interference with the blood supply or of postoperative edema and fibrosis. Symptoms of tetany may occur abruptly postoperatively and be temporary or permanent. In some instances symptoms may develop insidiously and go undetected until months after thyroidectomy. Occasionally, the first evidence of surgical hypoparathyroidism may be the development of cataracts. The status of parathyroid function should be carefully monitored in all patients subjected to thyroidectomy.

Deposition in the parathyroid glands of iron pigment (e.g., in thalassemia) or of copper (e.g., in Wilson disease) may produce hypoparathyroidism.

Idiopathic Hypoparathyroidism. The term idiopathic should be reserved for the small residuum of children with hypoparathyroidism for which no etiologic mechanism can be defined. The majority of children in whom onset of hypoparathyroidism occurs after the first few years of life have an autoimmune condition. A much smaller percentage have incomplete forms of DiGeorge syndrome or the autosomal dominant type of familial hypoparathyroidism.

Autoimmune Hypoparathyroidism. An autoimmune mechanism for hypoparathyroidism is strongly suggested by the finding of parathyroid antibodies and by the frequent association with other autoimmune disorders or organ-specific antibodies. Autoimmune hypoparathyroidism is usually associated with Addison disease and chronic mucocutaneous candidiasis. The association of at least two of these three conditions has been tentatively classified as *polyglandular autoimmune disease, type I.* One third of patients with this syndrome have all three components; two thirds have only two of three conditions. The candidiasis almost always precedes the other disorders (70% of cases occur in children under 5 yr of age); the hypoparathyroidism (90% after 3 yr of age) usually occurs before Addison disease (90% after 6 yr of age). In addition, a variety of other disorders occur at variable times; these include alopecia areata or totalis, malabsorption disorder, pernicious anemia, gonadal failure, chronic active hepatitis, autoimmune thyroid disease, and vitiligo. These associations may occur in 10–25% of patients; insulin-independent diabetes and IgA deficiency are much less frequent concomitants.

Affected siblings may have the same or different constellations of disorders (e.g., hypoparathyroidism and Addison

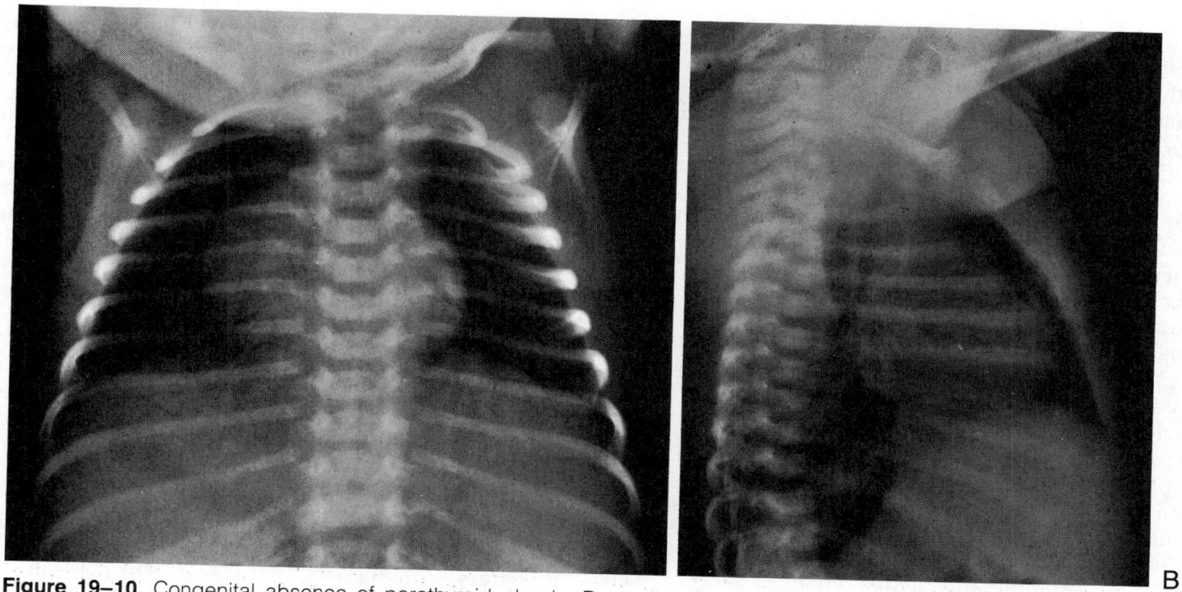

A B

Figure 19–10. Congenital absence of parathyroid glands. Roentgenograms of the chest exposed at 6 days of age reveal no evidence of thymus. *A*, The mediasinum is narrow; *B*, the substernal area is radiolucent. (From Kirkpatrick JA Jr, DiGeorge AM: Am J Roentgenol 103:32, 1968.)

disease). No HLA type has been found in excess in these patients. There is a slight predominance of affected females (4:3), but the disorder is thought to have an autosomal recessive mode of inheritance.

Siblings have been observed with nephrosis, nerve deafness, and hypoparathyroidism, a constellation also likely to have an autoimmune basis.

CLINICAL MANIFESTATIONS. There is a spectrum of parathyroid deficiencies with clinical manifestations varying from no symptoms to those of complete and longstanding deficiency. Mild deficiency may be revealed only by appropriate laboratory studies. Muscular pain and cramps are early manifestations; they progress to numbness, stiffness, and tingling of the hands and feet. There may be only a positive Chvostek or Trousseau sign or laryngeal and carpopedal spasms. Convulsions with loss of consciousness may occur at intervals of days, weeks, or months. These may begin with abdominal pain, followed by tonic rigidity, retraction of the head, and cyanosis. Hypoparathyroidism is frequently mistaken for epilepsy. Headache, vomiting, increased intracranial pressure, and papilledema may be associated with convulsions and may suggest a brain tumor.

The teeth erupt late and irregularly. Enamel formation is irregular, and the teeth may be unusually soft. The skin may be dry and scaly, and the nails of the fingers and toes may have horizontal lines. Manifestations of a wide variety of other disorders that are not direct consequences of PTH deficiency may also be seen. Mucocutaneous candidiasis, when present, antedates the development of hypoparathyroidism; the candidal infection most often involves the nails, the oral mucosa, the angles of the mouth, and, less often, the skin.

Cataracts in patients with longstanding untreated disease are a direct consequence of hypoparathyroidism; other autoimmune ocular disorders such as keratoconjunctivitis may also occur. Manifestations of Addison disease, lymphocytic thyroiditis, pernicious anemia, alopecia areata or totalis, hepatitis, and primary gonadal insufficiency may also be associated with those of hypoparathyroidism.

Permanent physical and mental deterioration occur if initiation of treatment is long delayed.

LABORATORY DATA. The serum calcium level is low (5–7 mg/dL) and the phosphorus elevated (7–12 mg/dL). Blood levels of ionized calcium (approximately 45% of the total) more nearly reflect physiologic adequacy. The serum level of alkaline phosphatase is normal or low, and the level of 1,25-$(OH)_2D_3$ is usually low, but high levels have been found in some children with severe hypocalcemia. The level of magnesium is normal but should always be checked in hypocalcemic patients (see later). By immunometric assay serum levels of PTH are low. Administration of the synthetic 1–34 fragment of human PTH (teriparatide acetate) results in increased urinary levels of cAMP and phosphate. This response differentiates hypoparathyroidism from pseudohypoparathyroidism. With the advent of very sensitive PTH assays, this test may no longer be necessary. Roentgenograms of the bones occasionally reveal an increased density limited to the metaphyses, suggestive of heavy metal poisoning, or an increased density of the lamina dura. Roentgenograms or computed tomography of the skull may reveal calcifications in the basal ganglia. There is a prolongation of the Q-T interval on the electrocardiogram, which disappears when the hypocalcemia is corrected. The electroencephalogram usually reveals widespread slow activity; the tracing returns to normal after the serum calcium has been within the normal range for a few weeks unless irreversible brain damage has occurred or unless the parathyroid insufficiency is associated with epilepsy. When hypoparathyroidism occurs concurrently with Addison disease, the serum level of calcium may be normal, but hypocalcemia appears after effective treatment of the adrenal insufficiency.

TREATMENT. Emergency treatment for neonatal tetany consists of intravenous injections of 5–10 mL of a 10% solution of calcium gluconate at the rate of 0.5–1 mL/min. Additionally, 1,25-dihydroxycholecalciferol (calcitriol) should be given. The initial dose is 0.25 μg/24 hr; the maintenance dose ranges from 0.01 to 0.10 μg/kg/24 hr up to a maximum of 1–2 μg/24 hr. Calcitriol has a short half-life and should be given in two equal divided doses; it has the advantages of rapid onset of effect (1–4 days) and rapid reversal of hypercalcemia after discontinuation in the event of overdosage (calcium begins to fall in 3–4 days).

Once normocalcemia has been achieved, one may wish to continue therapy with vitamin D_2 because it is considerably less costly than calcitriol. The usual doses are 0.1–0.5 mg/24 hr in infants and young children. One mg of vitamin D_2 has a biologic activity of 40,000 IU. Older children require 1.25–2.00 mg (50,000–100,000 IU) once daily. Vitamin D_2 has a slow onset of effect, and reversal of hypercalcemia after discontinuation of treatment is markedly delayed; its main advantage is its low cost.

An adequate intake of calcium should be ensured. Supplemental calcium can be given in the form of calcium gluconate or calcium glubionate (Neo-Calglucon) to provide 800 mg of elemental calcium daily, but it is rarely essential. Foods with a high phosphorus content such as milk, eggs, and cheese should be reduced in the diet.

Clinical evaluation of the patient and frequent determinations of the serum calcium levels are indicated in the early stages of treatment to determine the requirement for calcitriol or vitamin D_2. If hypercalcemia occurs, therapy should be discontinued and resumed at a lower dose after the serum calcium level has returned to normal. In cases of long standing, repair of cerebral and dental changes is not likely. Pigmentation, lowering of the blood pressure, or weight loss may indicate adrenal insufficiency, which requires specific treatment.

DIFFERENTIAL DIAGNOSIS. *Magnesium deficiency* must be considered in patients with unexplained hypocalcemia. Concentrations of magnesium in serum below 1.5 mg/dL (1.2 mEq/L) are usually abnormal. *Familial hypomagnesemia* with secondary hypocalcemia has been reported in 32 patients, most of whom developed tetany and seizures from 2–4 wk of age. Administration of calcium is ineffective, but administration of magnesium promptly corrects both calcium and magnesium levels. Oral supplements of magnesium are necessary to maintain levels of magnesium in the normal range. The profoundly low levels of magnesium result from a specific defect in intestinal absorption. The disorder has been most frequently diagnosed in boys, but it appears to be caused by an autosomal recessive gene (see also Sec. 9.54 for treatment).

Hypomagnesemia also occurs in malabsorption syndromes and has been noted in granulomatous colitis and cystic fibrosis. Therapy with aminoglycosides causes hypomagnesemia by increasing urinary losses. Patients with autoimmune hypoparathyroidism may have concurrent steatorrhea and low magnesium levels.

It is not clear how low levels of magnesium lead to hypocalcemia. Current evidence suggests that hypomagnesemia impairs release of PTH and induces resistance to the effects of the hormone, but other mechanisms also may be operative.

Poisoning with inorganic phosphate leads to hypocalcemia and tetany. Infants administered large doses of inorganic phosphates, either as laxatives or as sodium phosphate enemas, have had sudden onset of tetany, with serum calcium levels below 5 mg/dL and markedly elevated levels of phosphate. Symptoms are quickly relieved by intravenous administration of calcium. The mechanism of the hypocalcemia is not clear.

Hypocalcemia may occur early in the course of treatment of *acute lymphoblastic leukemia*. It is usually associated with hyperphosphatemia (resulting from destruction of lymphoblasts), which is probably the primary cause of hypocalcemia.

Episodic symptomatic hypocalcemia occurs in the *Kenny-Caffey syndrome*, which is characterized by medullary stenosis of the long bones, short stature, and high hyperopia, with onset ranging from the neonatal period to the 4th decade. Recent evidence suggests heterogeneity of the syndrome; idiopathic hypoparathyroidism and abnormal PTH have both been found.

19.19 PSEUDOHYPOPARATHYROIDISM
(Albright Hereditary Osteodystrophy)

In this syndrome, in contrast to the situation in idiopathic hypoparathyroidism, the parathyroid glands are normal or hyperplastic histologically, and they can synthesize and secrete parathyroid hormone. Serum levels of immunoreactive PTH are elevated when the patient is hypocalcemic. Neither endogenous nor administered PTH raises the serum levels of calcium or lowers the levels of phosphorus. The genetic defects in the hormone receptor–adenylate cyclase system are classified into various types depending on the phenotypic and biochemical findings.

TYPE Ia. This type accounts for 50% of patients with pseudohypoparathyroidism (PHP). Affected patients have a genetic defect of the α subunit of the guanine nucleotide–binding protein ($G_s\alpha$). This coupling factor is required for the hormone-bound receptor to activate cAMP. In four unrelated individuals, four distinct mutations of the $G_s\alpha$ gene have been documented. Deficiency of the G unit is a generalized cellular defect and accounts for the association of other endocrine disorders with type Ia PHP. The defect is inherited as an autosomal dominant trait, and the paucity of father-to-son transmissions is thought to be due to decreased fertility in males.

Tetany is often the presenting sign. Affected children have a short, stocky build and a round face. Brachydactyly with dimpling of the dorsum of the hand is usually present. The 2nd metacarpal is the least often involved. As a result, the index finger may occasionally be longer than the middle finger. Likewise, the 2nd metatarsal is only rarely affected. There may be other skeletal abnormalities such as short and wide phalanges, bowing, exostoses, and thickening of the calvaria. These patients frequently have calcium deposits and metaplastic bone formation subcutaneously. Moderate degrees of mental retardation, calcification of the basal ganglia, and lenticular cataracts are common in patients who are diagnosed late.

Some members of affected kindreds may have the usual anatomic stigmata of PHP, but serum levels of calcium and phosphorus are normal despite reduced $G_s\alpha$ activity and mutations in its gene. This variant of PHP type Ia is called *pseudopseudohypoparathyroidism*. Transition from the normocalcemic to the hypocalcemic form has been observed; however, it is not known what other factors cause clinically overt hypocalcemia.

In addition to resistance to PTH, resistance to the metabolic effects of TSH, gonadotropins, and glucagon may be detected in patients with type Ia PHP. Clinical hypothyroidism is uncommon, but basal levels of TSH are elevated, and TRH-stimulated TSH responses are exaggerated. Moderately decreased levels of thyroxine and increased levels of TSH have been detected in newborn thyroid screening programs, leading to the detection of type Ia PHP in infancy. In adults, gonadal dysfunction is common, as manifested by sexual immaturity, amenorrhea, oligomenorrhea, and infertility. Each of these abnormalities can be related to deficient synthesis of cAMP secondary to a deficiency of $G_s\alpha$, but it is not clear why resistance to other G protein–dependent hormones (e.g., ACTH, vasopressin) is much less affected.

Serum levels of calcium is low, and those of phosphorus and alkaline phosphatase are elevated. Levels of both immunoreactive and bioactive PTH are elevated. Definitive diagnosis rests on the demonstration of a markedly attenuated response in urinary phosphate and cAMP after intravenous infusion of the synthetic 1–34 fragment of human PTH (teriparatide acetate).

TYPE Ib. Affected patients have normal levels of G protein activity and a normal phenotypic appearance. These patients have resistance to PTH but not to other hormones. Serum levels of calcium, phosphorus, and immunoreactive PTH are the same as those in patients with type Ia PHP; however, bioactive PTH is not increased. The pathophysiology of the disorder in this group of patients is uncertain. Proposed explanations include production of a defective, biologically inactive hormone, presence of inhibitory PTH peptides, and a defect in the PTH receptor or in the catalytic subunit of adenyl cyclase. It is likely that the cause of the abnormality in this group is heterogeneous.

TYPE II. This type of pseudohypoparathyroidism has been detected in only a few patients and differs from type I in that the urinary excretion of cAMP is elevated both in the basal state and after stimulation with PTH, but phosphaturia does not increase. It appears that cAMP is normally activated, but the cell is unable to respond to the signal.

19.20 HYPERPARATHYROIDISM

Excessive production of PTH may result from a primary defect of the parathyroid glands such as an adenoma or idiopathic hyperplasia *(primary hyperparathyroidism)*.

More often, the increased production of PTH is compensatory, usually aimed at correcting hypocalcemic states of diverse origins *(secondary hyperparathyroidism)*. In vitamin D–deficient rickets and in the malabsorption syndromes, intestinal absorption of calcium is deficient, but hypocalcemia and tetany may be averted by increased activity of the parathyroid glands. In chronic renal disease, hyperphosphatemia and the consequent hypocalcemia result in compensatory hyperparathyroidism with marked increases in serum levels of PTH. In some instances, if stimulation of the parathyroids has been sufficiently intense and protracted, the glands may continue to secrete increased levels of PTH for months or years after renal transplantation, with resulting hypercalcemia (Table 19–5). This situation, in which there may be some autonomy of the parathyroids, has been called *tertiary hyperparathyroidism*.

ETIOLOGY. *Primary hyperparathyroidism* is rare in children. When its onset occurs in the neonatal period, it is always caused by generalized hyperplasia of the parathyroid glands, whereas onset during childhood is usually due to a single benign adenoma.

Neonatal primary hyperparathyroidism has been reported in 31 infants. Symptoms develop shortly after birth and consist of anorexia, irritability, lethargy, constipation, and failure to thrive. Roentgenograms reveal subperiosteal bone resorption, osteoporosis, and pathologic fractures. Symptoms may be mild, resolving without treatment, or may have a rapidly fatal course if diagnosis and treatment are delayed. Histologically, the parathyroid glands consist of diffuse hyperplasia with light chief cells. Affected siblings have been observed in three kindreds, and parental consanguinity has been reported in four kindreds.

About half the affected infants have been in kindreds with the clinical and biochemical features of *familial hypocalciuric hypercalcemia* (FHH) (see below). It is not clear why newborn infants born into families with this autosomal dominant cause of benign hypercalcemia exhibit the clinical manifestations of hyperparathyroidism only on rare occasions. It appears that the generalized insensitivity to calcium ion, which is a characteristic of FHH, may be more profound in some neonates carrying the gene. Infants who inherit the gene from the father may recognize the mother's normal calcium as low and develop hyperplasia of the parathyroids. Another possible explanation for the condition (though rare) is homozygosity for the gene.

TABLE 19–5. Etiologic Classification of Hypercalcemia

Parathyroid hormone (PTH) excess
Primary hyperparathyroidism
Adenoma
Sporadic
Autosomal dominant
Hyperplasia or adenoma
Multiple endocrine neoplasia type I–autosomal dominant
Multiple endocrine neoplasia type II–autosomal dominant
Parathyroid hyperplasia of infancy
With familial hypocalciuric hypercalcemia
Sporadic?
Secondary hyperparathyroidism
Chronic renal failure, postrenal transplant, rickets, malabsorption, pseudohypoparathyroidism
Transient neonatal hyperparathyroidism
Maternal hypoparathyroidism
Ectopic PTH production
Nonendocrine malignancies
Parathyroid hormone–related peptide (PTHrP) excess
Nonendocrine malignancies
Vitamin D excess
Poisoning, iatrogenic
Ectopic production
Granulomatous disease
Sarcoidosis, tuberculosis
Subcutaneous fat necrosis
Vitamin D sensitivity
Idiopathic hypercalcemia of infancy
Insensitivity to calcium ion
Familial hypocalciuric hypercalcemia (FHH)
Miscellaneous
Hypervitaminosis A
Hypophosphatasia
Thyrotoxicosis
Prolonged immobilization

Childhood hyperparathyroidism usually becomes manifest after 10 yr of age and is most frequently due to a single adenoma. There have been many kindreds in which three or more members have hyperparathyroidism. In such cases of autosomal dominant hyperparathyroidism, most of the affected family members are adults, but children have been involved in about a third of the pedigrees. Some affected patients in these families are asymptomatic and are detected only by careful study. In some kindreds, hyperparathyroidism also occurs as part of the constellation known as the MEN syndromes.

MEN type I is a disorder characterized by hyperplasia or adenomas of the pancreatic islets (which secrete gastrin, insulin, pancreatic polypeptide, or occasionally glucagon), the anterior pituitary (which usually secretes prolactin), and the parathyroids. In most kindreds hyperparathyroidism is usually the presenting manifestation, with a prevalence approaching 100% by 50 yr of age but occurring only rarely in children under 18 yr of age. In the past, once an affected family was identified, it was necessary to perform repeated metabolic screening for many years to detect other affected family members. With appropriate DNA probes, it is now possible to detect carriers of the gene with 95% accuracy as early as birth.

The gene for MEN type I has been localized to the pericentric region of the long arm of chromosome 11 (q11.13). The gene appears to function as a recessive oncogene (antioncogene). The 1st mutation (germinal) is inherited and is recessive to the dominant allele; this does not result in tumor formation. A 2nd mutation (somatic) is required to eliminate the normal allele, which then leads to tumor formation.

MEN type II is also associated with hyperparathyroidism (see Sec. 19.16).

Ectopic PTH production had been suggested in the past as an explanation for the hypercalcemia that occurs with various nonendocrine tumors. However, it is now established that in most instances the hypercalcemic hormone produced by these tumors is a PTHrP rather than PTH (see Sec. 19.17). The usual RIAs for PTH frequently do not distinguish this condition from primary hyperparathyroidism, but with immunometric assays, levels of PTH are found to be suppressed.

Transient neonatal hyperparathyroidism has occurred in a few infants born to mothers with hypoparathyroidism (idiopathic or surgical) or with pseudohypoparathyroidism. In each case the maternal disorder had been undiagnosed or inadequately treated during pregnancy. The cause of the condition is chronic intrauterine exposure to hypocalcemia with resultant hyperplasia of the fetal parathyroid glands. In the newborn, manifestations involve the bones primarily, and healing occurs between 4 and 7 mo.

CLINICAL MANIFESTATIONS. At all ages the clinical manifestations of hypercalcemia of any cause include muscular weakness, anorexia, nausea, vomiting, constipation, polydipsia, polyuria, loss of weight, and fever. Calcium may be deposited in the renal parenchyma (nephrocalcinosis), with progressively diminished renal function. Renal calculi are common and may produce renal colic and hematuria. Osseous changes may produce pain in the back or extremities, disturbances of gait, genu valgum, fractures, and tumors. Height may decrease from compression of vertebrae; the patient may become bedridden. Completely asymptomatic patients are now being detected with the increasing use of automated serum calcium determinations.

Abdominal pain is occasionally prominent and may be associated with acute pancreatitis. Parathyroid crisis may occur, manifested by serum calcium levels greater than 15 mg/dL and progressive oliguria, azotemia, stupor, and coma. In infants, failure to thrive, poor feeding, and hypotonia are common. Mental retardation, convulsions, and blindness may occur as sequelae.

LABORATORY DATA. The serum calcium level is elevated; 39 of 45 children with adenomas had levels over 12 mg/dL. The hypercalcemia is more severe in infants with parathyroid hyperplasia; concentrations ranging from 15 to 20 mg/dL are common, and values as high as 30 mg/dL have been reported. Ionized (Ca^{2+}) calcium levels are often elevated even when total serum calcium is borderline or only slightly elevated. The serum phosphorus level is reduced to about 3 mg/dL or less, and the level of serum magnesium is low. The urine may have a low and fixed specific gravity, and serum levels of nonprotein nitrogen and uric acid may be elevated. In patients with adenomas who have skeletal involvement serum phosphatase is elevated, whereas in infants with hyperplasia the levels of alkaline phosphatase may be normal even when there is extensive involvement of bone.

Serum levels of PTH, as measured by carboxy-terminal antisera, are elevated, especially in relation to the level of calcium. Results may vary markedly from one laboratory to another, depending on the antibody used. Calcitonin levels are normal. Acute hypercalcemia can stimulate calcitonin release, but with prolonged hypercalcemia, hypercalcitoninemia does not occur.

The most consistent and characteristic roentgenographic findings are resorption of subperiosteal bone, best seen along the margins of the phalanges of the hands. In the skull there may be gross trabeculation or a granular appearance resulting from focal rarefaction; the lamina dura may be absent. In more advanced disease there may be generalized rarefaction, cysts, tumors, fractures, and deformities. About 10% of patients have roentgenographic signs of rickets. Roentgenograms of the abdomen may reveal renal calculi or nephrocalcinosis.

DIFFERENTIAL DIAGNOSIS. *Hypercalcemia* of any origin results in a similar clinical pattern; other causes must be differentiated from hyperparathyroidism (see Table 19–5). A low serum phosphorus level with hypercalcemia is characteristic of primary hyperparathyroidism; elevated levels of PTH are also diagnostic. With hypercalcemia of any cause except hyperparathyroidism and familial hypocalciuric hypercalcemia, PTH levels are suppressed. Pharmacologic doses of corticosteroids lower the serum calcium level to normal in patients with hypercalcemia from other causes but generally do not affect the calcium level in patients with hyperparathyroidism.

TREATMENT. Surgical exploration is indicated in all instances. All glands should be carefully inspected; if an adenoma is discovered, it should be removed; only two instances of carcinoma are known in children. Neonates with severe hypercalcemia require total parathyroidectomy. A portion of a parathyroid gland may be autografted into the forearm; four infants treated in this fashion were able to maintain normocalcemia without supplementary treatment, but no long-term outcome has yet been reported. The patient should be carefully observed postoperatively for the development of hypocalcemia and tetany; intravenous administration of calcium gluconate may be required for a few days. The serum calcium level then gradually returns to normal, and, under ordinary circumstances, a diet high in calcium and phosphorus needs to be maintained for only several months after operation.

Arteriography and selective venous sampling with radioimmunoassay of PTH for preoperative localization and for differentiation of a single adenoma from hyperplasia have been replaced by imaging methods. Computed tomography, real-time ultrasound, and subtraction scintigraphy using ^{99m}Tc pertechnetate and ^{201}Tl have each proved effective in 50–90% of adults. These procedures are rarely required by the expert parathyroid surgeon but may be advisable before re-exploration in cases of persistent or recurrent hyperparathyroidism.

PROGNOSIS. The prognosis is good if the disease is recognized early and there is appropriate surgical treatment. When extensive osseous lesions are present, deformities may be permanent; with renal disease the prognosis is less hopeful. A search for other affected family members is indicated.

Other Causes of Hypercalcemia

FAMILIAL HYPOCALCIURIC HYPERCALCEMIA (FAMILIAL BENIGN HYPERCALCEMIA). Children with this disorder are usually asymptomatic, and the hypercalcemia comes to light by chance during routine investigation for other conditions. The parathyroid glands are normal, PTH levels are not elevated, and subtotal parathyroidectomy does not correct the hypercalcemia. Serum levels of magnesium are high normal or mildly elevated. The rate of calcium to creatinine clearance is usually decreased despite hypercalcemia. The disorder is inherited in an autosomal dominant manner. Detection of other affected family members is important to avoid inappropriate parathyroid surgery. The basic defect in the condition is unknown; the insensitivity of the kidneys and parathyroid glands to hypercalcemia suggests generalized insensitivity to calcium ion. On rare occasions, an infant born to an affected parent may have severe neonatal hypercalcemia associated with generalized hyperplasia of the parathyroid glands and require total parathyroidectomy (see earlier).

GRANULOMATOUS DISEASES. Hypercalcemia occurs in 30–50% of children with sarcoidosis and less often in patients with other granulomatous diseases such as tuberculosis. Levels of PTH are suppressed, and levels of 1,25-$(OH)_2D_3$ are elevated. The source of the ectopic 1,25-$(OH)_2D_3$ is the activated macrophage, through stimulation by interferon α from T lymphocytes, which are present in abundance in granulomatous lesions. Unlike renal tubular cells, the 1α-hydroxylase in macrophages is unresponsive to homeostatic regulation. Oral administration of prednisone (2 mg/kg/24 hr) lowers serum levels of 1,25-$(OH)_2D_3$ to normal and corrects the hypercalcemia.

HYPERCALCEMIA OF MALIGNANCY. Hypercalcemia frequently occurs in adults with a wide variety of solid tumors but is identified much less often in children. It has been reported in 14 infants with malignant rhabdoid tumors of the kidney or congenital mesoblastic nephroma and in a few children with neuroblastoma, medulloblastoma, leukemia, Burkitt lymphoma, and rhabdomyosarcoma. Serum levels of PTH are rarely elevated. In most patients the hypercalcemia associated with malignancy is caused by elevated levels of PTHrP. An assay to measure plasma levels of PTHrP is now available. Very rarely, tumors produce 1,25-$(OH)_2D_3$ or PTH ectopically.

MISCELLANEOUS CAUSES OF HYPERCALCEMIA. Hypercalcemia may occur in infants with *subcutaneous fat necrosis*. Levels of PTH are normal. In one infant the level of 1,25-$(OH)_2D$ was elevated, and biopsy of the skin lesion revealed granulomatous infiltration, suggesting that the mechanism of the hypercalcemia was akin to that seen in patients with other granulomatous disease. Treatment with prednisone is effective.

Hypophosphatasia, especially the severe infantile form, is usually associated with mild to moderate hypercalcemia. Serum levels of phosphorus are normal, and those of alkaline phosphatase are subnormal. The bones exhibit rachitic-like lesions on roentgenograms. Urinary levels of phosphoethanolamine, inorganic pyrophosphate, and pyridoxal 5′-phosphate are elevated; each is a natural substrate to a tissue-nonspecific (liver, bone, kidney) alkaline phosphatase enzyme. Point mutations of the gene appear to result in an inactive enzyme in this autosomal recessive disorder.

Idiopathic hypercalcemia of infancy is manifested by failure to thrive and hypercalcemia during the 1st yr of life followed by spontaneous remission. Serum levels of phosphorus and PTH are normal. The hypercalcemia results from increased absorption of calcium. Vitamin D may be involved in the pathogenesis. Both normal and elevated levels of 1,25-$(OH)_2D$ have been reported. An excessive rise in the level of 1,25-$(OH)_2D$ in response to PTH administration years after the hypercalcemic phase suggests that vitamin D has a role in the pathogenesis. A blunted calcitonin response to intravenous calcium has also been reported. A phenotype consisting of elfin face, supravalvular aortic stenosis or other cardiac defects, mental retardation, and other abnormalities is known as **Williams syndrome**. This syndrome is frequently, but not always, associated with neonatal hypercalcemia. Heterogeneity of these entities remains a strong possibility. Hypercalcemia has been successfully controlled with either prednisone or calcitonin.

When hypercalcemia is caused by *vitamin D intoxication*, levels of 25-OHD are markedly elevated (Sec. 4.31). Total parenteral nutrition in the neonate may induce *phosphate depletion*, leading in turn to hypercalcemia.

Barakat AY, D'Albora JB, Martin MM, et al: Familial nephrosis, nerve deafness and hypoparathyroidism. J Pediatr 91:61, 1977.
Berliner BC, Shenker IR, Weinstock MS: Hypercalcemia associated with hypertension due to prolonged immobilization. (An unusual complication of extensive burns.) Pediatrics 49:92, 1972.
Broadus AE, Mangin M, Ikeda K, et al: Humoral hypercalcemia of cancer: Identification of a novel parathyroid hormone-like peptide. N Engl J Med 319:556, 1988.
Bronsky D, Kiamko RT, Moncado R, et al: Intrauterine hyperparathyroidism secondary to maternal hypoparathyroidism. Pediatrics 42:606, 1968.
Burtis WJ, Brady TG, Orloff JJ, et al: Immunochemical characterization of circulating parathyroid hormone-related protein in patients with hormonal hypercalcemia of cancer. N Engl J Med 322:1106, 1990.
Chesney RW: Requirements and upper limits of vitamin D intake in the term neonate, infant, and older child. J Pediatr 116:159, 1990.
Cooper L, Wertheimer J, Levey R, et al: Severe primary hyperparathyroidism in a neonate with two hypercalcemic parents: Management with parathyroidectomy and heterotopic autotransplantation. Pediatrics 78:263, 1986.
Culler FL, Jones KL, Deltos LJ: Impaired calcitonin secretion in patients with Williams syndrome. J Pediatr 107:720, 1985.
Daum F, Rosen JF, Boley SJ: Parathyroid adenoma, parathyroid crisis and acute pancreatitis in an adolescent. J Pediatr 83:275, 1973.
Davis RF, Eichner JM, Bleyer WA, et al: Hypocalcemia, hyperphosphatemia, and dehydration following a single hypertonic phosphate enema. J Pediatr 90:484, 1977.
DiGeorge AM: Congenital absence of the thymus and its immunologic consequences, concurrence with congenital hypoparathyroidism. *In*: Bergsma D, Good RA (eds): Birth Defects. Original Article Series, No. 1, Vol. IV. New York, The National Foundation, 1968.
Fanconi S, Fischer JA, Wieland P, et al: Kenny syndrome: Evidence for idiopathic hypoparathyroidism in two patients and for abnormal parathyroid in one. J Pediatr 109:469, 1986.
Fairney A, Jackson D, Clayton BE: Measurement of serum parathyroid hormone, with particular reference to some infants with hypocalcemia. Arch Dis Child 48:419, 1973.
Finne PH, Sanderud J, Aksnes L, et al: Hypercalcemia with increased and unregulated 1,25-dihydroxyvitamin D production in a neonate with subcutaneous fat necrosis. J Pediatr 112:792, 1988.
Fisher G, Skillern PG: Hypercalcemia due to hypervitaminosis A. JAMA 227:1413, 1974.
Fitch N: Albright's hereditary osteodystrophy: A review. Am J Med Genet 11:11, 1982.
Goodyer PR, Frank A, Kaplan BS: Observations on the evolution and treatment of idiopathic infantile hypercalcemia. J Pediatr 105:771, 1984.
Green CG, Doershuk CF, Stern RC: Symptomatic hypomagnesemia in cystic fibrosis. J Pediatr 107:425, 1985.
Hanukoglu A, Chalew S, Kowarski AA: Late-onset hypocalcemia, rickets and hypoparathyroidism in an infant of a mother with hyperparathyroidism. J Pediatr 112:751, 1988.
Jayabose S, Igbal K, Newman L, et al: Hypercalcemia in childhood renal tumors. Cancer 61:788, 1988.
Key LL, Thorne M, Pitzer B, et al: Management of neonatal hyperparathyroidism with parathyroidectomy and autotransplantation. J Pediatr 116:923, 1990.
Khosla S, Johansen KL, Ory SJ, et al: Parathyroid hormone-related peptide in lactation and in umbilical cord blood. Mayo Clin Proc 65:1408, 1990.
Law WM Jr, Bollman S, Kumar R, et al: Vitamin D metabolism in familial benign hypercalcemia (hypocalciuric hypercalcemia) differs from that in primary hyperparathyroidism. J Clin Endocrinol Metab 58:744, 1984.
Leblanc A, Caillaud JM, Hartmann O, et al: Hypercalcemia preferentially occurs in unusual forms of childhood non-Hodgkin's lymphoma, rhabdomyosarcoma, and Wilms' tumor. Cancer 54:2132, 1984.
Levine MA, Downs RW Jr, Moses AM, et al: Resistance to multiple hormones in patients with pseudohypoparathyroidism. Association with deficient activity of guanine nucleotide regulatory protein. Am J Med 74:545, 1983.
Levitt M, Gessert C, Finberg L: Inorganic phosphate (laxative) poisoning resulting in tetany in an infant. J Pediatr 82:479, 1973.
Lund B, Sorensen OH, Lund B, et al: Vitamin D metabolism in hypoparathyroidism. J Clin Endocrinol Metab 51:606, 1980.
Mallette LE: Synthetic human parathyroid hormone 1–34 fragment for diagnostic testing. Ann Intern Med 109:800, 1988.
Markowitz ME, Rosen JF, Smith C, et al: 1,25-Dihydroxyvitamin D_3-treated hypoparathyroidism: 35 patient years in 10 children. J Clin Endocrinol Metab 55:727, 1982.
Martin TJ, Suva LJ: Parathyroid hormone–related protein in hypercalcaemia of malignancy. Clin Endocrinol 31:631, 1989.
Marx SJ, Fraser D, Rapoport A: Familial hypocalciuric hypercalcemia. Mild expression of the gene in heterozygotes and severe expression in homozygotes. Am J Med 78:15, 1985.
Miller RR, Menke JA, Mentser MI: Hypercalcemia associated with phosphate depletion in the neonate. J Pediatr 105:814, 1984.
Morris CA, Demsey SA, Leonard CD, et al: Natural history of Williams syndrome: Physical characteristics. J Pediatr 113:318, 1988.
Patten JL, Johns DR, Valle D, et al: Mutation in the gene encoding the stimulating G protein of adenylate cyclase in Albright's hereditary osteodystrophy. N Engl J Med 322:1412, 1990.
Pronicka E, Kulczcka H, Lorenc R: Increased serum level of 1,25-dihydroxyvitamin D_3 after parathyroid hormone in the normocalcemic phase of idiopathic hypercalcemia. J Pediatr 112:930, 1988.
Radeke HH, Auf'mkolk B, Juppner H, et al: Multiple pre- and postreceptor defects in pseudohypoparathyroidism (a multicenter study with twenty-four patients). J Clin Endocrinol Metab 62:393, 1986.
Rapaport D, Rubin ZM, Huminer D, et al: Primary hyperparathyroidism in children. J Pediatr Surg 21:395, 1986.

Reichel H, Koeffler HP, Norman AW: The role of the vitamin D endocrine system in health and disease. N Engl J Med 320:980, 1989.
Ross AJ III, Cooper A, Attie MF, et al: Primary hyperparathyroidism in infancy. J Pediatr Surg 21:493, 1986.
Silue C, Santora A, Breslav N, et al: Selective resistance to parathyroid hormone in cultured skin fibroblasts from patients with pseudohypoparathyroidism type Ib. J Clin Endocrinol Metab 62:640, 1986.
Sobel H, Narod SA, Nakamura Y, et al: Screening for multiple endocrine neoplasia type 2a with DNA-polymorphism analyses. N Engl J Med 321:996, 1989.
Stewart AF, Broadus A: Parathyroid hormone-related proteins: Coming of age in the 1990's. J Clin Endocrinol Metab 71:1410, 1990.
Stromme JH, Steen-Johnson J, Harnaes K, et al: Familial hypomagnesemia—a follow-up examination of three patients after 9 to 12 years of treatment. Pediatr Res 15:1134, 1981.
Taylor AB, Stern PH, Bell NH: Abnormal regulation of circulating 25-hydroxyvitamin D in the Williams syndrome. N Engl J Med 306:972, 1982.
Thakker RV, Bouloux P, Wooding C, et al: Association of parathyroid tumors in multiple endocrine neoplasia type 1 with loss of alleles in chromosome 11. N Engl J Med 321:218, 1989.
Tsang RC, Venkatararaman P, Ho M, et al: The development of pseudohypoparathyroidism. Involvement of progressively increasing serum parathyroid hormone concentrations, increased 1,25-dihydroxyvitamin D concentrations, and "migratory" subcutaneous calcifications. Am J Dis Child 138:654, 1984.
Van Dop C, Bourne HR, Neer RM: Father to son transmission of decreased N activity in pseudohypoparathyroidism Type Ia. J Clin Endocrinol Metab 59:825, 1984.
Whyte MP, Weldon VV: Idiopathic hypoparathyroidism presenting with seizures during infancy: X-linked recessive inheritance in a large Missouri kindred. J Pediatr 99:608, 1981.
Winter WE, Silverstein JH, MacLaren NK, et al: Autosomal dominant hypoparathyroidism with variable, age-dependent severity. J Pediatr 103:387, 1983.
Wu J, Carson NL, Myers S, et al: The genetic defect in multiple endocrine neoplasia type 2A maps next to the centromere on chromosome 10. Am J Hum Genet 46:624, 1990.
Young TO, Satzstein EC, Boman DA: Parathyroid carcinoma in a child: Unusual presentation with seizures. J Pediatr Surg 19:194, 1984.

19.21 DISORDERS OF THE ADRENAL GLANDS

The adrenal gland is composed of two endocrine systems, the medullary and the cortical systems. Mesodermal cells contribute to the development of the adrenal cortex, the gonads, and the liver; these three tissues are active in steroid metabolism in the fetus. Adrenals and gonads have in common certain enzymes involved in steroid synthesis, and an inborn defect in one tissue may also involve the other.

At about the 7th wk of gestation the primordium of the adrenal cortex is invaded by sympathetic neural elements. About 1 wk later these cells begin to differentiate into the chromaffin cells capable of synthesizing and storing catecholamines; the methyl transferase, which converts norepinephrine to epinephrine, develops later.

In a fetus of 2 mo the adrenals are larger than the kidneys, but from the 4th mo the kidneys grow rapidly, becoming about twice as large as the adrenals by the end of the 6th mo. In the full-term infant the adrenal gland is one third the size of the kidney, and the combined weight of both glands is 7–9 g.

The adrenal cortex in the fetus and the newborn infant has two histologically distinct components: an outer portion, the true cortex, and a more central portion, the "fetal cortex." At birth the fetal cortex makes up about 80% of the gland. Within a few days it begins to involute, undergoing a 50% reduction by 2 wk of age and disappearing completely by about 6 mo of age. The major steroids produced by the fetal cortex are DHEA and its sulfurylated derivative (DHEAS).

The true cortex consists of three zones. In the zona glomerulosa, situated beneath the capsule, there is an alveolar arrangement of the cells; in the broader zona fasciculata the columns of cells are radially arranged; in the zona reticularis the cells form a network next to the medulla.

FETOPLACENTAL UNIT. Until near the end of gestation the fetal adrenal does not possess the 3β-hydroxysteroid dehydrogenase necessary to form progesterone; it utilizes placental pregnenolone to synthesize cortisol, aldosterone, and particularly DHEAS. The placenta in turn utilizes the fetal DHEAS to produce estrone and estriol. Estriol is the major estrogen found in maternal urine in pregnancy, especially in the late stages. In instances of fetal adrenal hypoplasia, maternal urinary estriol levels are markedly reduced.

ADRENAL CORTEX. The adrenal cortex secretes various steroid compounds essential to life. Studies indicate that the zona fasciculata and zona glomerulosa behave as two separate glands: ACTH primarily stimulates the zona fasciculata to secrete cortisol and androgens; the zona glomerulosa is involved primarily in synthesis of aldosterone.

Glucocorticoids have a 21-carbon structure and are produced by the zona fasciculata; they are also referred to as 17-hydroxycorticosteroids or simply as corticosteroids. The principal one is cortisol, also known as compound F or hydrocortisone. Cortisol can be interconverted to cortisone by the enzyme 11β-hydroxysteroid dehyrogenase (11β-OHSD) in peripheral tissues; surprisingly, a deficiency of this enzyme results in heritable forms of apparent mineralocorticoid excess (see Sec. 19.25).

Glucocorticoids affect the metabolism of most tissues. They attach to specific intracellular receptor proteins, which then bind to the cell nucleus to influence RNA and protein synthesis. In many tissues glucocorticoids have a catabolic effect, resulting in increased degradation of protein; primarily affected are muscles, skin, and connective, adipose, and lymphoid tissues. On the other hand, glucocorticoids are anabolic in the liver, where they stimulate a number of enzymes, increase protein and glycogen content, and enhance its capacity for gluconeogenesis. Patients with cortisol excess (e.g., Cushing syndrome) have increased glucose production, whereas those with deficiency of cortisol (Addison disease) have decreased gluconeogenesis, with hypoglycemia. The effects of insulin and androgens are antagonistic to those of glucocorticoids. Glucocorticoids have effects on the immune and nervous systems. As with all steroid hormones, the receptors are cytosolic proteins. The receptor for glucocorticoids and mineralocorticoids is the same. It appears that mineralocorticoid-responsive tissues (e.g., kidney), by converting cortisol to cortisone, exclude the glucocorticoid from the receptor. Thus, specificity is dependent on prereceptor enzyme activity.

The 17-hydroxycorticosteroids are excreted in urine; cortisol itself is also excreted in urine in amounts less than 1% of the adrenal production. Levels of cortisol and of its precursors and metabolites can be measured by radioimmunoassay and by high-performance liquid chromatography (HPLC) in biologic fluids and tumor tissues. Levels of cortisol in plasma vary with the time of day; after the first few years of life a circadian rhythm follows that of corticotropin.

Glucocorticoid synthesis is regulated primarily by ACTH, with cortisol exerting negative feedback on ACTH secretion. One of the major regulators of ACTH is corticotropin-releasing hormone (CRH).

Many synthetic analogs of cortisone and hydrocortisone are available. Derivatives with an additional double bond in ring A are known as prednisone and prednisolone. They are 4 times as potent in anti-inflammatory and carbohydrate activity as the natural steroids but have less effect on salt and water retention. Halogenated derivatives have different effects; 9α-fluorohydrocortisone has approximately 15 times more anti-inflammatory activity than hydrocortisone but is more than 20 times as active in salt and water retention. Betamethasone and dexamethasone are approximately 25 times as potent as cortisol and have little effect on the retention of water and electrolytes. These analogs are usually used in pharmacologic doses for their anti-inflammatory or immunosuppressive properties.

Aldosterone, a potent mineralocorticoid, is the 18-aldehyde of corticosterone and is produced primarily in the zona glomerulosa. Its secretion is regulated by activation of the renin-angiotensin system. Renin produced by the juxtaglomerular apparatus of the kidney reacts with renin substrate, an α_2-globulin produced by the liver, to yield the inactive decapeptide, angiotensin. A converting enzyme rapidly changes angiotensin I to the biologically active octapeptide, angiotensin II. Angiotensin II is a pressor agent 50 times more potent than norepinephrine. One of its main functions is to act directly on the adrenal cortex to stimulate the secretion of aldosterone.

In good health and on a normal dietary intake, ACTH plays a minor role in the regulation of aldosterone secretion, but under some conditions, as in anephric man, it may have a more significant effect. On the other hand, potassium may be equally important in the regulation of aldosterone secretion as the renin-angiotensin system. In studies of aldosterone secretion, dietary potassium and sodium must be rigidly controlled. Aldosterone and renin activity in plasma can be measured by radioimmunoassay.

Sodium deprivation is a potent stimulus to secretion of aldosterone. Changes in intake of sodium result in small changes in blood volume, arterial pressure, and renal blood flow. These changes are sensitively monitored by the juxtaglomerular cells on the renal afferent arterioles, which form the receptor site or volume receptor. Activation of the juxtaglomerular apparatus results in increased output of renin, followed by increased secretion of aldosterone.

The principal action of aldosterone is the maintenance of electrolyte equilibrium, which in turn contributes to the stabilization of blood volume and blood pressure. Aldosterone controls sodium reabsorption (and hence water reabsorption) in the distal tubule of the kidney.

Androgens are produced mainly by the zona fasciculata. They are capable of increasing retention of nitrogen, potassium, phosphorus, and sulfate. They promote growth and have androgenic effects, which are most conspicuous when adrenal hyperplasia or adrenal tumors induce precocious growth and development of male secondary sex characteristics. The adrenal androgens seem to be partly responsible for the development of axillary and pubic hair in the female.

DHEAS is the most abundant adrenal androgen in the circulation. It is derived either from adrenal secretion or from peripheral sulfation of DHEA secreted by the adrenal. DHEAS levels are low during childhood but begin to rise before the other hormonal changes of puberty take place in a process called adrenarche. The zona reticularis is probably the major source of these adrenarcheal changes. Aside from a relationship of these hormones to the growth of sexual hair, their function remains unknown; they do not appear to be an initiator of puberty. Levels are low in patients with Addison disease as well as in those with adrenal insufficiency secondary to ACTH deficiency. However, administration of ACTH does not acutely increase DHEAS levels, indicating that it is not the corticotropic hormone that initiates adrenarche. For many years, a separate adrenal cortical androgen–stimulating hormone (CASH) has been proposed but has not yet been identified. Marked elevations of DHEAS occur in patients with virilizing adrenal cortical tumors, lesser elevations occur in patients with congenital adrenal hyperplasia, and modest elevations occur in children with isolated precocious adrenarche.

ADRENAL MEDULLA. The principal hormones of the adrenal medulla are the physiologically active catecholamines: dopamine, norepinephrine, and epinephrine. The sequence of their biosynthetic reactions is shown in Figure 19–11. Catecholamine synthesis occurs also in the brain, in sympathetic nerve endings, and in chromaffin tissue outside the adrenal medulla. Metabolites of catecholamines are excreted in the urine. The principal ones are 3-methoxy-4-hydroxymandelic acid (VMA), metanephrine, and normetanephrine. Measurement of metanephrines and catecholamines is used to detect functioning tumors of the adrenal medulla.

The proportions of epinephrine and norepinephrine in the adrenal vary with age. In early fetal stages there is practically no epinephrine, and even at birth norepinephrine is predominant. In adults norepinephrine makes up only 10–30% of the pressor amines in the medulla. Both epinephrine and norepinephrine raise the mean arterial blood pressure, norepinephrine without changing the cardiac output. By increasing peripheral vascular resistance, norepinephrine increases systolic and diastolic blood pressures with only a slight reduction in the pulse rate. Epinephrine increases the pulse rate and, by decreasing the peripheral vascular resistance, decreases the diastolic pressure. The hyperglycemic and calorigenic effects of norepinephrine are much less pronounced than those of epinephrine.

19.22 ADRENOCORTICAL INSUFFICIENCY

Deficient production of cortisol or aldosterone may result from a wide variety of congenital or acquired lesions of the hypothalamus, pituitary, or adrenal cortex (Table 19–6). Depending upon the pathologic lesions, symptoms may be severe or mild, appear abruptly or insidiously, begin in infancy or later, and be permanent or temporary.

ETIOLOGY. Corticotropin Deficiency. Congenital hypoplasia or aplasia of the pituitary is almost always associated with secondary hypoplasia of the adrenals as well as with other hormonal deficiencies. These congenital defects are usually associated with abnormalities of the skull and brain such as anencephaly and holoprosencephaly. Such infants have a considerable residuum of pituitary function, and the hypoplasia of the pituitary is probably secondary to a hypothalamic deficiency of CRH. Isolated deficiency of corticotropin has been reported in eight children including two sets of siblings. Idiopathic hypopituitarism and destructive lesions in the area of the pituitary, such as craniopharyngioma, are the most common causes of corticotropin deficiency; the defect is in the hypothalamus in many patients. Isolated deficiency of CRH has been documented in an Arabic kindred as an autosomal recessive trait. In rare instances, autoimmune hypophysitis has been the cause of corticotropin deficiency.

Primary Adrenal Aplasia or Hypoplasia. Aplasia and hypoplasia have been noted in the same patient or in siblings. The disorder appears to be a defect of organogenesis. Corticotropin is present, and the adrenal defect involves both cortisol and aldosterone. The condition occurs predominantly in males and has been observed in half-brothers with different fathers, establishing X-linked inheritance. In most patients with the X-linked form histologic examination of hypoplastic adrenal cortex reveals disorganization and cytomegaly, findings not present in the adrenals from corticotropin-deficient infants.

In several dozen infants X-linked congenital adrenal hypoplasia has occurred in association with glycerol kinase defi-

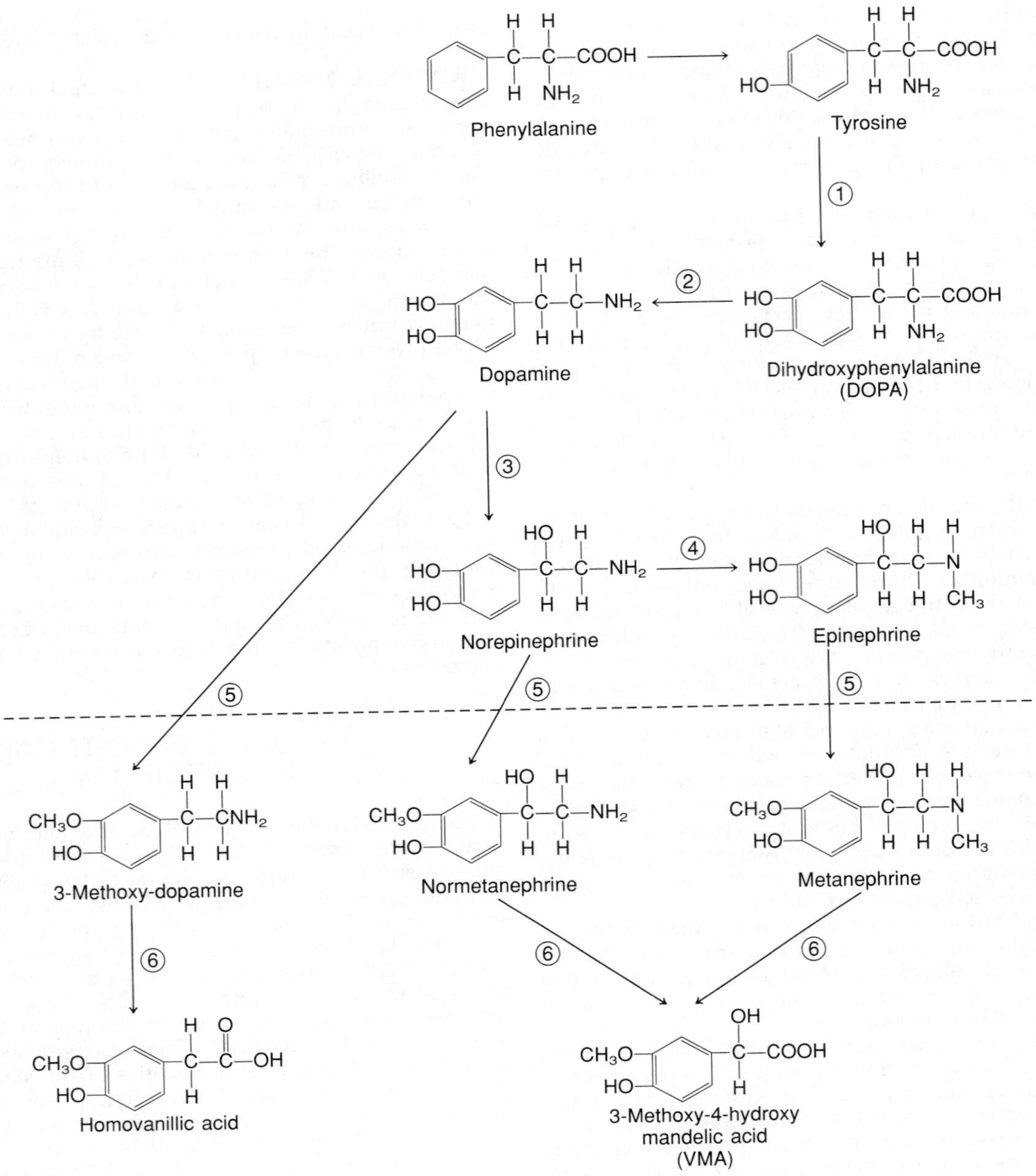

Figure 19–11. Biosynthesis (above dashed line) and metabolism (below dashed line) of the catecholamines: norepinephrine and epinephrine.

1. Tyrosine hydroxylase
2. Dopa decarboxylase
3. Dopamine β-oxidase
4. Phenylethanolamine-*N*-methyl transferase
5. Catechol-o-methyltransferase
6. Monocrine oxidase

ciency and/or Duchenne muscular dystrophy. Most of these boys are mentally retarded. High resolution of chromosome bands discloses a microdeletion in the Xp21 region. DNA probe analysis reveals a deletion in the genome of affected patients and their mothers.

Most boys with isolated congenital adrenal hyperplasia have failed to undergo puberty because of hypogonadotropic hypogonadism. The cause is not known, but an associated X-linked gene disorder is likely. Little is known about pubertal development in boys with the glycerol kinase complex because they usually die early in life of muscular dystrophy. In one boy with X-linked congenital adrenal hypoplasia and Becker muscular dystrophy who was studied by the author, pubertal development was normal.

Familial Glucocorticoid Deficiency. This form of chronic adrenal insufficiency is characterized by isolated deficiency of glucocorticoids, elevated levels of corticotropin, and normal aldosterone production. The salt-losing manifestations of most other forms of adrenal insufficiency do not occur; instead, patients present primarily with hypoglycemia, seizures, and pigmentation during the 1st decade of life. The disorder affects both sexes equally and is inherited in an autosomal recessive

TABLE 19–6. Etiologic Classification of Adrenocortical Hypofunction

- Corticotropin-releasing hormone deficiency
  - Isolated deficiency
  - Multiple deficiencies
    - Congenital defects (e.g., anencephaly, septo-optic dysplasia)
    - Destructive lesions (e.g., tumor)
    - Idiopathic (e.g., idiopathic hypopituitarism)
- Corticotropin deficiency
  - Isolated
  - Autosomal recessive
  - Multiple deficiencies
    - Pituitary hypoplasia or aplasia
    - Destructive lesions (e.g., craniopharyngioma)
    - Autoimmune hypophysitis
- Primary adrenal hypoplasia or aplasia
  - X-linked
    - With hypogonadotropic hypogonadism and/or Duchenne muscular dystrophy (Xp21 deletion)
    - With glycerol kinase deficiency
- Familial glucocorticoid deficiency
  - With autonomic dysfunction (alacrima, achalasia)
  - Without autonomic dysfunction
- Defects of steroid biosynthesis (adrenal hyperplasia)
  - Lipoid adrenal hyperplasia (P_{450}scc deficiency)
    - Severe
    - Mild
  - 3β-Hydroxysteroid dehydrogenase deficiency
    - Severe
    - Mild
  - 21-Hydroxylase (P_{450}c21) deficiency
    - Classic
      - Salt-loser
      - Non–salt-loser
    - Nonclassic
  - Isolated aldosterone deficiency
    - P_{450}c11 deficiency
  - Aldosterone unresponsiveness—pseudohypoaldosteronism
  - Adrenoleukodystrophy (lignnoceroyl-CoA deficiency)
    - With neurologic involvement
    - Isolated adrenal involvement
  - Lysosomal acid lipase deficiency (Wolman syndrome)
- Destructive lesions of adrenal cortex
  - Granulomatous lesions (e.g., tuberculosis)
- Autoimmune adrenalitis (idiopathic Addison disease)
  - Isolated
    - Associated with hypoparathyroidism and/or mucocutaneous candidiasis (Type I autoimmune polyglandular syndrome)
    - Associated with autoimmune thyroid disease and insulin-requiring diabetes (Type II autoimmune polyglandular syndrome)
- Neonatal hemorrhage
- Acute infection (Waterhouse-Friderichsen syndrome)
- Iatrogenic
  - Abrupt cessation of exogenous corticosteroids or corticotropin
  - Removal of functioning adrenal tumor
  - Adrenalectomy for Cushing disease
  - Drugs
    - Aminoglutethimide
    - Mitotane (o,p′-DDD)
    - Metyrapone
    - Ketoconazole
- Fetal adrenal suppression—maternal hypercortisolism
  - Endogenous
  - Therapeutic

manner. Histologically, there is marked adrenocortical atrophy with relative sparing of the zona glomerulosa. It has been suggested that the unresponsiveness of the adrenal cortex may be due to a failure of membrane attachment or to failure of activation of adenyl cyclase by corticotropin. Absence of ACTH binding to peripheral blood mononuclear leukocytes has been reported in one child. The syndrome may be heterogeneous. Most patients exhibit achalasia of the cardia, deficient tear production, and other autonomic dysfunctions. How these manifestations are related to the adrenal disorder is not clear.

Inborn Defects of Steroidogenesis. The most common causes of adrenocortical insufficiency in infancy are the salt-losing forms of congenital adrenal hyperplasia (Sec. 19.23). About half the infants with the 21-hydroxylase defect, all infants with lipoid adrenal hyperplasia, and most infants with a deficiency of 3β-hydroxysteroid dehydrogenase manifest salt-losing symptoms in the newborn period. In these defects there is a deficiency in the synthesis of both cortisol and aldosterone, and elevated levels of steroids are precursors to the enzymatic defect.

Isolated Deficiency of Aldosterone. This rare disorder is caused by impaired conversion of 18-hydroxycorticosterone (18-OHB) to aldosterone. The enzyme involved is P_{450}c11; this single enzyme mediates the 11β-hydroxylation of 11-deoxycortisol to cortisol as well as the three final steps in the synthesis of aldosterone. It is speculated that a point mutation affects 18-oxidase activity while sparing 11β- and 18-hydroxylase activities (Fig. 19–12).

Affected infants fail to thrive and become dehydrated in the newborn period. Hyponatremia, hyperkalemia, metabolic acidosis, and hyperreninemia occur and may be severe. Levels of aldosterone are low, and those of its precursor, 18-hydroxycorticosterone, are elevated. Specific diagnosis depends on the measurement of the ratio of 18-OHB to aldosterone in plasma; a markedly elevated ratio has been found even on the 1st day of life in an infected infant.

Treatment consists of administration of enough salt or 9α-fluorocortisol (0.05 mg twice a day) to return plasma renin to normal. With increasing age, the salt-losing manifestations improve, and it appears that therapy may be discontinued; however, levels of plasma renin rise and growth decelerates, indicating chronic salt depletion. The biosynthetic defect persists and can be demonstrated in adults. This autosomal recessive defect is especially frequent in Iranian Jews. Carrier detection and prenatal diagnosis are possible.

Pseudohypoaldosteronism. This salt-losing syndrome also presents in the neonate; however, levels of aldosterone in plasma and urine are markedly elevated. Levels of plasma renin activity are elevated, indicating hyperactivity of the renin-angiotensin system. The defect is target-organ unresponsiveness to aldosterone. Administration of mineralocorticoids is ineffective; the condition is treated by supplementary dietary salt, which may be discontinued as the condition improves, usually by 2 yr of age. The syndrome appears to be heterogeneous. In some patients salt loss involves only the renal tubules, whereas in others the salivary and sweat glands may be involved, and occasionally the colonic mucosal cells may be affected. In the 70 reported patients, both autosomal dominant and autosomal recessive forms have been identified.

Addison Disease. Destruction of the adrenal cortex during childhood is one of the more common causes of adrenal insufficiency. Tuberculosis, a common cause of adrenal destruction in the past, has virtually vanished as a cause. Now the most common cause is autoimmune destruction of the glands. The glands may be so small that they are not visible at autopsy, and only remnants of tissue are found in microscopic sections. Usually, the medulla is not destroyed, and there is marked lymphocytic infiltration in the area of the former cortex. In advanced disease, all adrenal cortical function is lost, but early in the clinical course isolated cortisol deficiency may antedate aldosterone deficiency and salt-losing manifestations. Most patients have antiadrenal cytoplasmic antibodies in their plasma. About 75% of affected patients have immunoglobulins that block the growth and steroido-

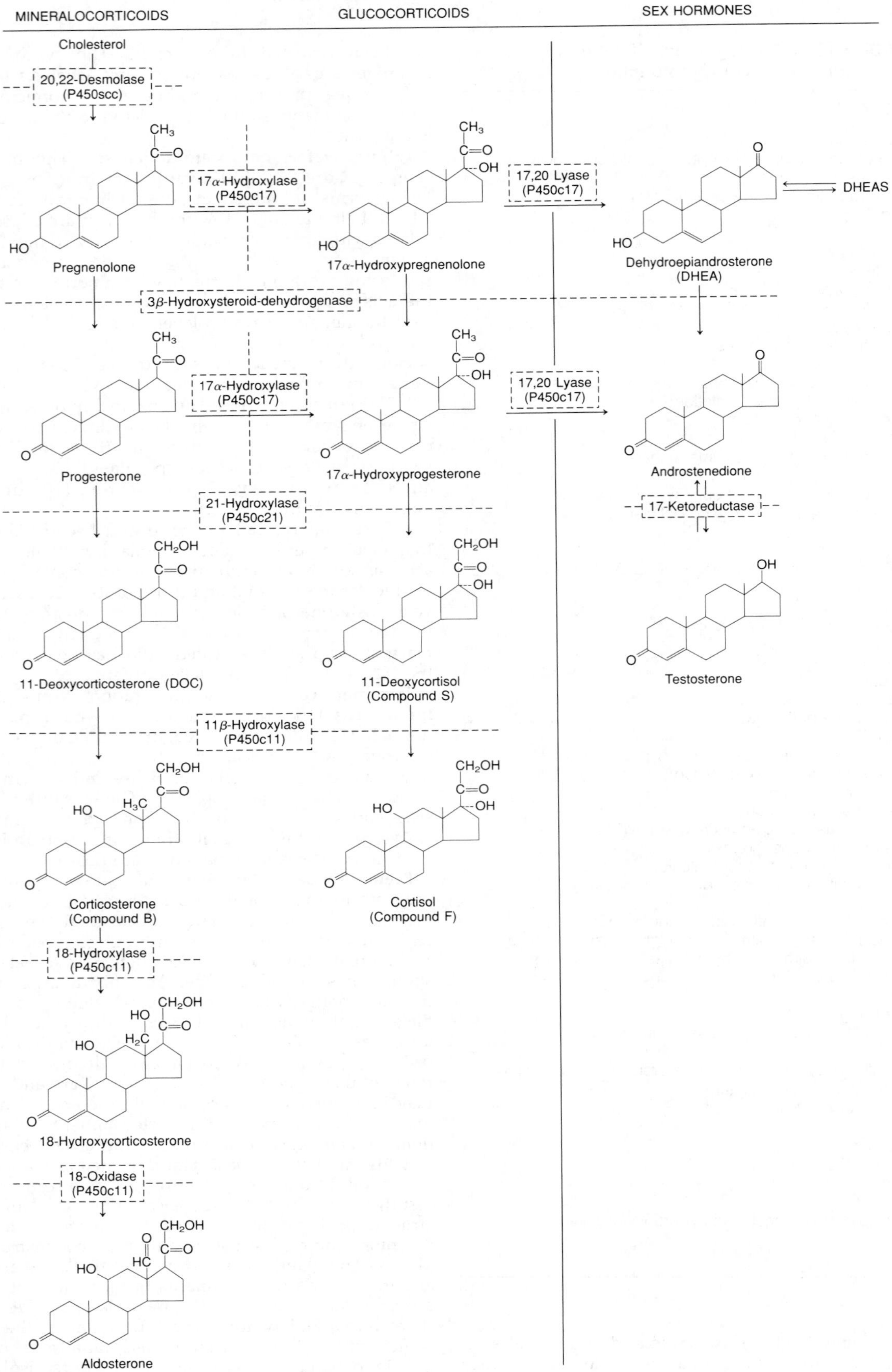

Figure 19–12. The synthesis of cortisol and aldosterone is shown to the left of the vertical line. To the right of the solid vertical line are the predominant adrenal androgens that lead to conversion to testosterone. Note that a single polypeptide, $P_{450}c17$, catalyzes both 17α-hydroxylase and 17,20-lyase activities. Likewise, polypeptide $P_{450}c11$ mediates the last step in cortisol synthesis as well as the last three steps in aldosterone synthesis.

genic effects of ACTH. How the various antibodies act in concert with cell-mediated processes to cause disease is unknown.

Addison disease often occurs as a component of two syndromes, each consisting of a constellation of autoimmune disorders. *Type I autoimmune polyendocrinopathy* is also known as *autoimmune polyendocrinopathy-candidiasis-ectodermal dystrophy* (APECED). Chronic mucocutaneous candidiasis is most often the first manifestation, followed by hypoparathyroidism and then by Addison disease. Other closely associated autoimmune disorders include gonadal failure, alopecia, vitiligo, keratopathy, enamel hypoplasia, nail dystrophy, intestinal malabsorption, and chronic active hepatitis. Hypothyroidism and type I diabetes mellitus occur in fewer than 10% of affected patients. The disorder is inherited as an autosomal recessive disorder. Some components of the syndrome continue to develop as late as the 5th decade. The presence of antiadrenal antibodies and steroidal-cell antibodies in these patients usually indicates a high likelihood of developing Addison disease or, in females, ovarian failure.

Type II autoimmune polyendocrinopathy consists of Addison disease associated with autoimmune thyroid disease or insulin-dependent diabetes. HLA-D3 and HLA-D4 predominate in these patients.

Adrenoleukodystrophy (see Sec. 8.17 and 20.61). About one third of patients with this disorder develop adrenal insufficiency, usually after 4 yr of age. Boys with adrenocortical failure due to adrenoleukodystrophy have been identified who have no evidence of neurologic involvement after 8 yr. It is unknown whether isolated adrenal involvement may be the only manifestation of this disorder or if these patients will eventually develop adrenomyeloneuropathy.

Hemorrhage into Adrenal Glands. This may occur in the neonatal period as a consequence of difficult labor or of asphyxia. The hemorrhage may be sufficiently extensive to result in death from exsanguination or from hypoadrenalism. Often the hemorrhage is asymptomatic initially and is identified by later calcification of the adrenal. On rare occasions, gradual impairment in function resulting from progressive fibrosis or cystic changes may culminate in adrenocortical insufficiency in infancy or childhood. Another cause of hemorrhage into the adrenal glands is the *Waterhouse-Friderichsen syndrome*, the characteristic state of shock resulting from meningococcemia (Sec. 12.23).

Abrupt Cessation of Administration of Corticotropin or a Corticosteroid. This condition may result in adrenal insufficiency. Symptoms are most likely to occur if these substances have been given in large doses for a long time to patients who are subsequently subjected to stressful situations such as severe infections or surgical procedures.

Drugs. Ketoconazole, an antifungal drug, can cause adrenal insufficiency by inhibiting adrenal enzymes. Rifampicin and anticonvulsive drugs such as phenytoin and phenobarbital reduce the effectiveness and bioavailability of corticosteroid replacement therapy by inducing steroid-metabolizing enzymes in the liver.

CLINICAL MANIFESTATIONS. The age at onset of symptoms and the clinical manifestations depend on the specific etiologic factor involved. In patients with adrenal hypoplasia, defects in steroidogenesis, or pseudohypoaldosteronism, symptoms and signs begin shortly after birth and are those characteristic of salt loss. Failure to thrive, vomiting, lethargy, anorexia, and dehydration occur; circulatory collapse may be fatal.

In older children with Addison disease the onset is usually more gradual and is characterized by muscular weakness, lassitude, anorexia, loss of weight, general wasting, and low blood pressure. Abdominal pain may simulate an acute abdominal process, and there may be an intense craving for salt. If the condition is not recognized and treated, *adrenal crisis* may supervene. The patient suddenly becomes cyanotic, the skin cold, and the pulse weak and rapid. The blood pressure falls, and respirations are rapid and labored. In the absence of immediate and intensive therapy, the course is rapidly fatal. In patients with inadequately treated chronic adrenal insufficiency, crises may be precipitated by infection, trauma, excessive fatigue, or drugs such as morphine, barbiturates, laxatives, thyroid hormone, or insulin.

Increased pigmentation of the skin should always alert the clinician to the possibility of adrenocortical insufficiency. This manifestation occurs in those conditions in which there are a deficiency of cortisol and excessive secretion of corticotropin, as in primary adrenal hypoplasia, familial glucocorticoid deficiency, adrenoleukodystrophy, and Addison disease. Pigmentation may be first apparent on the face and hands and is most intense around the genitalia, umbilicus, axillae, nipples, and joints. Scars and freckles may be especially pigmented. Areas of depigmentation (vitiligo) may be interspersed with dark areas. The exposed areas of the skin are the most intensely affected, and failure of a suntan to disappear may be the first clue to the condition. In the buccal mucosa the pigmentation is usually bluish brown.

The presenting manifestations may be those of hypoglycemia, particularly in the neonate with congenital adrenal hypoplasia. Patients with adrenocortical insufficiency are deficient in gluconeogenic substrates; the hypoglycemia may therefore be associated with ketosis and confused with ketotic hypoglycemia (see Sec. 8.59).

In young children with familial glucocorticoid deficiency, salt-losing manifestations do not occur, and the symptoms consist primarily of increased pigmentation and hypoglycemia. Symptoms may begin shortly after birth and almost always appear by 5 yr of age. Many affected children have received other treatment for seizures before the hypoglycemic cause was recognized.

In patients with a deficiency of corticotropin, pigmentation does not occur. Hypoglycemia is the usual presenting manifestation, but salt-losing is uncommon, presumably because of residual ability of the adrenal to secrete aldosterone.

In those conditions known to have a genetic basis it is important to evaluate fully the adrenocortical function of siblings.

LABORATORY DATA. When salt-losing manifestations are present, the levels of sodium and chloride in the serum are usually low and that of potassium elevated, with increased plasma renin activity. Urinary excretion of sodium and chloride is increased and that of potassium decreased. The nonprotein nitrogen level in plasma is elevated if dehydration is present. Hypoglycemia may be striking or may become manifest only after prolonged fasting. The blood eosinophils may be increased in number. When hemorrhage, adrenal cysts, or tuberculosis has been a causative factor, roentgenograms of the abdomen may reveal calcifications in the area of the adrenals. Ultrasound and computed tomography may also be helpful. A small and narrow roentgenographic shadow of the heart reflects hypovolemia. Electrocardiographic changes reflect potassium levels.

The most definitive test is measurement of the plasma levels of cortisol before and after administration of corticotropin; resting levels are low, and no increase occurs after administration of corticotropin. Occasionally, normal resting levels that do not increase after administration of corticotropin indicate an absence of adrenocortical reserve. A low initial level followed by a significant response to corticotropin may indicate adrenal insufficiency secondary to endogenous insufficiency of corticotropin. Levels of corticotropin are elevated in disorders of primary cortisol deficiency and are low when the adrenal insufficiency is secondary to a hypothalamic or pituitary disorder. Testing with CRH may be helpful in localizing the defect.

Measurement of plasma levels of cortisol precursors is necessary in infants in whom congenital adrenal hyperplasia is suspected. Aldosterone secretion may be low in patients with salt-losing congenital adrenal hyperplasia, adrenal hypoplasia, or Addison disease. Measurement of aldosterone is necessary in infants suspected of having isolated defects of aldosterone synthesis (in whom it is low) and in those suspected of having pseudohypoaldosteronism (in whom it is usually elevated). In patients with familial glucocorticoid deficiency aldosterone levels are normal and rise appropriately with salt deprivation.

TREATMENT. Treatment for acute adrenal insufficiency or for adrenal crises must be immediate and vigorous. If the cause of adrenal insufficiency has not been established, a blood sample should be obtained prior to therapy for determination of levels of cortisol, 17-hydroxyprogesterone, and adrenal androgens. Intravenous administration of 5% glucose in 0.9% saline solution should be given to correct the hypoglycemia and the sodium loss. Concomitantly, a water-soluble form of hydrocortisone, such as hydrocortisone hemisuccinate, should be given intravenously. High levels are achieved instantaneously, and large doses can be used safely. As much as 25 mg for infants and 75 mg for older children should be given intravenously at 6-hr intervals for the first 24 hr. These doses may be reduced during the next 24 hr if progress is satisfactory. A salt-retaining hormone should be added to maintain electrolyte balance; desoxycorticosterone acetate (DOCA) in oil may be used in doses of 1–5 mg/24 hr intramuscularly. After the first 48 hr, if oral intake is satisfactory, intravenous fluids may be discontinued and the corticosteroid given orally as cortisol in doses of 5–20 mg at 8-hr intervals. Further reduction can then be accomplished until maintenance levels and a stable clinical situation are achieved. Daily administration of DOCA is continued throughout this period of treatment.

Once the acute manifestations are under control, most patients require chronic replacement therapy for their aldosterone and cortisol deficiencies. The cortisol may be given orally in daily doses of 5 mg twice daily for infants, and 15 mg twice daily for adolescents. During situations of stress, such as periods of infection or operative procedures, the dose of hydrocortisone should be increased. The daily injections of DOCA can be replaced by fluorohydrocortisone, administered orally in doses of 0.05–0.1 mg/24 hr. Measurements of serum renin activity are useful in monitoring adequacy of mineralocorticoid replacement.

Overdosage with DOCA or fluorohydrocortisone results in hypertension and may lead to cardiac enlargement and edema because of excessive retention of sodium chloride and water; excessive loss of potassium may produce weakness or paralysis.

Patients with primary corticotropin deficiency or with familial glucocorticoid deficiency do not require a salt-retaining hormone because their ability to secrete aldosterone is intact. On the other hand, patients with primary defects in aldosterone synthesis do not require cortisol; a salt-retaining hormone may be required, but in milder forms the addition of salt to the diet is adequate to maintain homeostasis. In patients with pseudohypoaldosteronism administration of salt-retaining hormones does not correct the urinary sodium loss; therapy must consist of supplementation with sodium chloride. In newborn infants with adrenal hemorrhage vitamins K and C and transfusions with whole blood may be indicated.

Patients with apparent Addison disease must be differentiated from those with familial glucocorticoid deficiency and adrenoleukodystrophy (Sec. 8.17); absence of salt-losing manifestations and presence of alacrima suggest the former, and elevated levels of very long chain fatty acids are diagnostic for the latter. The presence of antiadrenal antibodies suggests an autoimmune pathogenesis; these patients must be closely observed for the development of other associated autoimmune disorders. Infants with congenital adrenal hypoplasia should undergo chromosomal analysis to search for a deletion of the Xp21 region; elevated levels of creatine phosphokinase indicate an association with Duchenne muscular dystrophy, and elevated levels of triglycerides suggest glycerol kinase deficiency. DNA probe analysis for the gene defect, glycerol kinase enzyme assay, and negative dystrophin staining of muscle tissue permit confirmation of the components of this complex.

ADRENOCORTICAL HYPERFUNCTION

Four syndromes are attributable to hyperadrenocorticism: the *adrenogenital syndrome, Cushing syndrome, hyperaldosteronism,* and *feminization* (Table 19–7).

19.23 ADRENOGENITAL SYNDROME

The adrenogenital syndrome is produced by congenital adrenal hyperplasia and by virilizing adrenocortical tumors.

Congenital Adrenal Hyperplasia

PATHOGENESIS. When the adrenogenital syndrome is associated with congenital adrenal hyperplasia, it is caused

TABLE 19–7. Etiologic Classification of Adrenocortical Hyperfunction

- Excess androgen (adrenal hyperplasia)
  - Congenital adrenal hyperplasia
    - 21-Hydroxylase ($P_{450}c21$) deficiency
    - 11β-Hydroxylase ($P_{450}c11$) deficiency
    - 3β-Hydroxysteroid dehydrogenase defect (females)
  - Tumor
    - Carcinoma
  - Adenoma—isolated testosterone secretion
- Excess cortisol (Cushing syndrome)
  - Bilateral adrenal hyperplasia
    - Hypersecretion of corticotropin (Cushing disease)
    - Ectopic secretion of corticotropin
    - Exogenous corticotropin
  - Tumor
    - Carcinoma
    - Adenoma
      - Adrenocortical nodular dysplasia
      - Pigmented nodular adrenocortisol disease (Carney complex)
- Excess mineralocorticoid (hypertensive hypokalemic syndrome)
  - Primary hyperaldosteronism
    - Aldosterone-secreting adenoma
    - Bilateral micronodular adrenocortical hyperplasia
    - Glucocorticoid-suppressible aldosteronism
  - Tumor
    - Adenoma
    - Carcinoma
- Desoxycorticosterone excess
  - Adrenal hyperplasia
    - 11β-Hydroxylase ($P_{450}c11$) deficiency
    - 17α-Hydroxylase ($P_{450}c17$) deficiency
  - Tumor—carcinoma
- Apparent mineralocorticoid excess
  - 11β-hydroxysteroid dehydrogenase deficiency
- Excess estrogen (adrenal feminization syndrome)
  - Carcinoma
  - Adenoma
- Mixed hypercorticism—tumor

by a family of autosomal recessive disorders of adrenal steroidogenesis leading to a deficiency of cortisol (see Fig. 19–12). The deficiency of cortisol results in increased secretion of corticotropin, which leads in turn to adrenocortical hyperplasia and overproduction of intermediary metabolites. Each defect has severe and mild forms, presumably because of allelic variants.

Deficiency of 21-hydroxylase accounts for 95% of affected patients. This P_{450} enzyme (P_{450}c21) hydroxylates progesterone and 17-hydroxyprogesterone (17-OHP) to yield 11-deoxycorticosterone and 11-deoxycortisol (see Fig. 19–12). There are two steroid 21-hydroxylase genes (CYP21A and CYP21B), which alternate in tandem with two genes for the 4th component of complement (C4A and C4B) on the short arm of chromosome 6 between the HLA-B and HLA-DR loci. The CYP21B gene is the active gene; the CYP21A gene is 98% homologous to the CYP21B gene but is a pseudogene. The majority of mutations causing 21-hydroxylase deficiency are recombinations (deletions or gene conversions) between the active CYP21B gene and the adjacent CYP21A pseudogene.

Newborn screening programs, utilizing capillary heel blood on filter paper disks, have been developed to detect 21-hydroxylase deficiency. Data on more than 2 million neonates screened thus far indicate that the disorder occurs in 1 in 20,000 population in Japan, 1 in 10,000–16,000 in Europe and North America, and 1 in 300 in Yupik Eskimos of Alaska. About 75% of affected infants have the salt-losing, virilizing form and 25% have the simple virilizing form of the disorder.

Deficiency of 11β-hydroxylase accounts for a very low percentage of cases of adrenal hyperplasia. This P_{450}c11 enzyme mediates the 11β-hydroxylation of 11-deoxycortisol to cortisol as well as the final steps in the synthesis of aldosterone from 11-deoxycorticosterone (DOC). This deficit occurs relatively frequently in Israeli Jews of North African origin; in this ethnic group a point mutation (Arg448 to His) has been found in the CYP11B1 gene encoded on chromosome 8q22.

Hypertension is a distinctive clinical feature of the disorder but is absent in the first few years of life. Virilization occurs as in 21-hydroxylase deficiency. The plasma characteristically contains large amounts of both 11-deoxycortisol and DOC. The elevated levels of DOC are thought to cause the hypertension and prevent symptoms of salt-losing. Prenatal diagnosis is possible by measuring levels of 11-deoxycortisol in maternal urine during pregnancy or in amniotic fluid, and by DNA probes.

Deficiency of 3β-hydroxysteroid dehydrogenase (3β-HSD) occurs in fewer than 5% of patients with adrenal hyperplasia. This enzyme is required for conversion of Δ^5 steroids (pregnenolone, 17-hydroxypregnenolone, DHEA) to Δ^4 steroids (progesterone, 17-hydroxyprogesterone, and androstenedione). Deficiency of the enzyme results in decreased synthesis of cortisol, aldosterone, and androgens (see Fig. 19–12). The 3β-HSD enzymatic system is present in adrenal and gonadal tissue, but regulatory control in the two tissues differs. In the classic form of the disease, salt-wasting is present in the neonate, boys are incompletely virilized and have hypospadias, and girls are only mildly virilized. In milder forms of the condition, the genitalia are normal, and salt-losing is absent. Incomplete forms in which onset occurs after puberty are manifested by hirsutism, menstrual disorders, and often polycystic ovaries. The hallmark of this disorder is the marked elevation of the Δ^5 steroids preceding the block. Patients may also have elevated levels of 17-hydroxyprogesterone and may be readily mistaken for patients with 21-hydroxylase deficiency because of the extra-adrenal 3β-HSD activity that occurs in peripheral tissues.

Lipoid adrenal hyperplasia has been reported in 32 patients, 18 of whom were Japanese. Failure of cleavage of the side chain of cholesterol results in marked accumulation of cholesterol and lipids in the adrenal cortex, and in failure of synthesis of any adrenal steroids. A single protein termed P_{450}SCC is responsible for all three steps in the conversion of cholesterol to pregnenolone (formerly termed 20,22 desmolase); the gene is encoded on chromosome 15. The same enzymatic defect is present in the testes, preventing synthesis of testicular hormones. As a consequence, genetic males are phenotypically female and females exhibit no genital abnormality. Salt-losing manifestations are usual, and most infants have died in early infancy. Because adrenal steroid levels are not elevated in this form of adrenal hyperplasia, affected infants are apt to be confused with those with adrenal hypoplasia.

17α-Hydroxylase deficiency has been described in more than 50 patients. A single polypeptide, P_{450}17, catalyzes two distinct reactions: 17α-hydroxylation of pregnenolone and progesterone, and the 17,20 lyase reaction mediating conversion of 17α-pregnenolone to C-19 steroid precursors of testosterone and estrogen (see Fig. 19–12). The enzyme is encoded on chromosome 10, and the gene is expressed in both the adrenal cortex and the gonads. The deficiency results in overproduction of DOC, leading to hypertension, hypokalemia, and suppression of renin and aldosterone. In addition, there is an inability to synthesize normal amounts of sex hormones. Affected males are unvirilized and present as phenotypic females or with sexual ambiguity (male pseudohermaphroditism). Affected females usually present with failure of sexual development at the expected time of puberty. Patients have been described with complete or partial combined 17α-hydroxylase–17,20 lyase deficiencies as well as with deficiencies of only one of these activities. The gene has been cloned; a deletion of more than one base pair in three patients and a duplication of more than one pair in another have been reported thus far. This defect must be considered in the differential diagnosis of male pseudohermaphroditism or of testicular feminization. 17-Hydroxylase deficiency in females must be considered in the differential diagnosis of primary hypogonadism (see Sec. 19.35).

CLINICAL MANIFESTATIONS. Most patients with congenital adrenal hyperplasia have the defect in 21-hydroxylation and exhibit the classic form of the disease. In newborn screening programs, about 75% of infants in whom this condition is detected are salt-losers, whereas without screening only about 50% of clinically diagnosed infants are salt-losers, presumably because of undiagnosed neonatal deaths.

Patients without Salt-Losing. In the *male* the main clinical manifestations are those of premature isosexual development. The infant usually appears normal at birth, but signs of sexual and somatic precocity may appear within the first 6 mo of life or develop more gradually, becoming evident at 4–5 yr of age or later. Enlargement of the penis, scrotum, and prostate, appearance of pubic hair, and development of acne and a deep voice are noted. Muscles are well developed, and bone age is advanced for chronologic age. Premature closure of the epiphyses causes growth to stop relatively early, and adult stature is stunted (Fig. 19–13).

The testes are prepubertal in size so that they appear relatively small in contrast to the enlarged penis. Occasionally, ectopic adrenocortical cells in the testes of patients with adrenal hyperplasia become hyperplastic just as the adrenal glands do, producing enlargement of the testes (Sec. 19.32). Mental development is usually normal, but the abnormal physical development may result in behavioral problems.

In the *female* congenital adrenal hyperplasia results in female pseudohermaphroditism (Fig. 19–14). Since the disorder of steroidogenesis begins early in fetal life, there is almost always evidence of some degree of masculinization at birth. It is manifested by enlargement of the clitoris and varying degrees of labial fusion. The vagina has a common opening with the

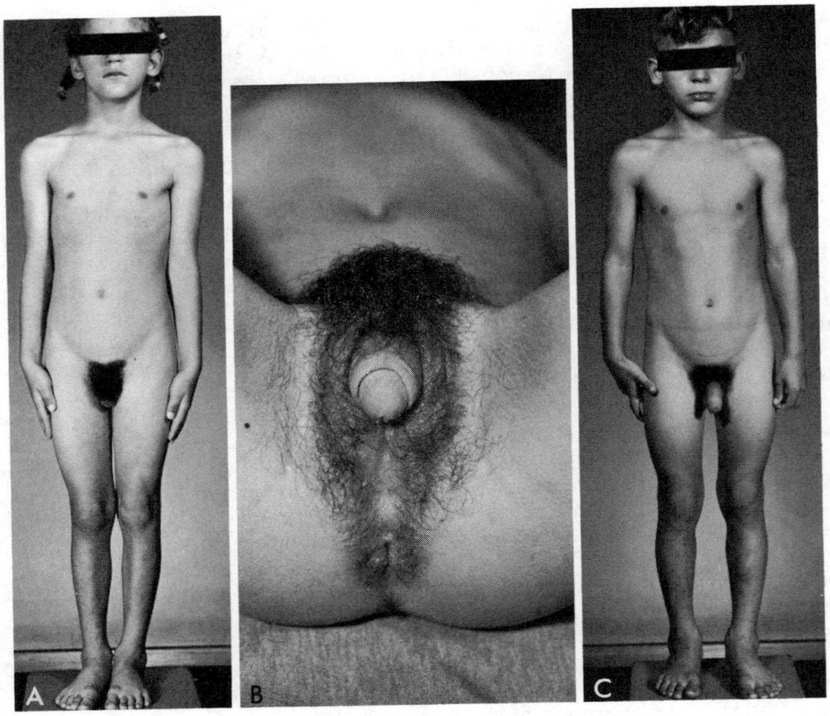

Figure 19–13. *A*, A 6-yr-old girl with congenital virilizing adrenal hyperplasia. The height age was 8.5 yr; the bone age was 13 yr; and urinary 17-ketosteroids were 50 mg/24 hr. *B*, Note the clitoral enlargement and labial fusion. *C*, Five-yr-old brother of girl in *A* was not considered to be abnormal by the parents. The height age was 8 yr; the bone age was 12.5 yr; and the urinary 17-ketosteroids were 36 mg/24 hr.

urethra (urogenital sinus). The clitoris may be so enlarged that it resembles a penis, and, since the urethra opens below this organ, a mistaken diagnosis of hypospadias and cryptorchidism is often made. About 2% of females have a male phenotype; there is complete labial fusion, a phallic urethra, and an external meatus at the tip of the penis. The severity of the virilization is in general greater in infants who are salt-losers than in those who are not. The internal genital organs are those of a normal female.

After birth the masculinization progresses. Pubic and axillary hair develop prematurely, acne appears, and the voice assumes a masculine quality. Affected girls are tall for their age, and ossification is advanced; they show good muscular development and, in general, have the body build of a boy (see Fig. 19–13). Although the internal genitalia are female, breast development and menstruation do not occur unless the excessive production of androgens is suppressed by adequate treatment.

A number of such virilized female pseudohermaphrodites whose condition was not diagnosed until adult life have been erroneously reared as males. These patients have behaved in every way as males, including having sexual intercourse; some have had satisfactory (albeit infertile) marriages.

With the *11-hydroxylase defect* salt-losing manifestations do not occur. Most patients are hypertensive, but several have been normotensive or have had intermittent hypertension only. The disorder has been diagnosed only rarely in early life, but hypertension was not present. Several prepubertal children with this defect presented with gynecomastia. Virilization occurs in all patients and is as severe as with the 21-hydroxylase defect.

Patients with Salt-Losing. In patients with the salt-losing variant, symptoms begin shortly after birth with failure to regain birthweight, progressive weight loss, and dehydration. Vomiting is prominent, with anorexia. Disturbances in cardiac rate and rhythm may occur, with cyanosis and dyspnea. Without treatment, collapse and death may occur within a few weeks.

In females virilization of the external genitalia in an infant with the above manifestations directs attention to the correct diagnosis. In the male, on the other hand, the genitalia appear normal, and clinical manifestations are apt to be confused with those of pyloric stenosis, intestinal obstruction, heart disease, cow milk intolerance, or other causes of failure to thrive.

Familial homogeneity of defect is usually observed for the salt-losing and non–salt-losing forms. Under conditions of stress or sodium deprivation, salt-losing may be provoked in compensated patients.

Patients with the *3β-hydroxysteroid dehydrogenase* defect are usually salt-losers but are less virilized. In the female, labial fusion and enlargement of the clitoris may be so mild as to escape detection; rarely, the genitalia are normal. In the male, varying degrees of hypospadias may occur, with or without bifid scrotum or cryptorchidism. Most patients with *lipoid adrenal hyperplasia* are salt-losers, and their phenotype is female with normal genitalia.

Nonclassic 21-Hydroxylase Deficiency. In this attenuated form, affected females have normal genitalia at birth and are usually asymptomatic before puberty. Then they develop hirsutism, acne, menstrual disorders, and infertility later in life. Some females and all males are completely asymptomatic. About 75% of patients are HLA-B14,DR1. The genetic defect is allelic with classic 21-hydroxylase; a mutation in codon 281 appears to be a marker for the disorder. It is estimated that 1% of North American whites have this disorder with the highest frequency occurring in Ashkenazic Jews.

LABORATORY DATA. Salt-losers may have low serum concentrations of sodium and chloride and elevated levels of potassium and nonprotein nitrogen. Plasma levels of renin are elevated. In classic 21-hydroxylase deficiency, plasma levels of 17-hydroxyprogesterone (17-OHP) are markedly elevated and are especially helpful in diagnosis, but they are normally high during the first 2–3 days of life and may range as high as levels found in affected patients; by the 3rd day, however, levels in normal infants fall and those in affected infants rise to clearly diagnostic levels. Blood levels of cortisol are usually low in patients with the salt-losing type but are

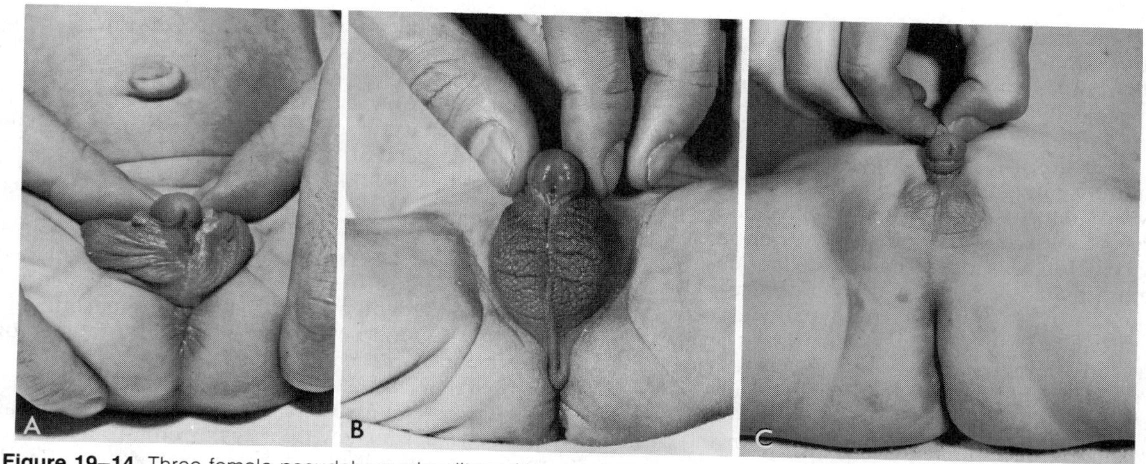

Figure 19–14. Three female pseudohemaphrodites with untreated congenital adrenal hyperplasia. All were erroneously assigned male sex at birth, and each had normal female sex-chromosome complement. Infants *A* and *B* were salt-losers and were diagnosed in early infancy. Infant *C* was referred at 1 yr of age because of bilateral cryptorchidism. Note the completely penile urethra; such complete degrees of masculinization in females with adrenal hyperplasia are rare; most of these infants are salt-losers.

normal in those with the simple virilizing type. A large part of the virilization is caused by increased levels of testosterone; the excess 17-OHP is partially diverted to androstenedione, which is converted to testosterone in the periphery (see Fig. 19–12). Levels of urinary 17-ketosteroids and pregnanetriol are elevated; 24-hr urine collections are often unnecessary, however, since radioimmunoassay permits measurement in plasma of the levels of the steroids involved in all forms of congenital adrenal hyperplasia.

In the late-onset variant of congenital adrenal hyperplasia, basal plasma levels of 17-OHP are not as high as in the classic form and may even be normal. There is, however, a diagnostic rise in level 60 min following an intravenous bolus of 0.25 mg of ACTH (1–24).

In patients with the 11-hydroxylase defect, plasma levels of DOC and 11-deoxycortisol (compound S) are elevated.

The 3β-hydroxysteroid dehydrogenase defect is characterized by markedly elevated Δ^5 steroids such as 17-hydroxypregnenolone. 17-OHP levels are also elevated, however, and the condition may be confused with the 21-hydroxylase defect. It is necessary to determine the ratios of Δ^5 to Δ^4 steroids in plasma or urine for definitive diagnosis.

Affected females have an XX karyotype; males have a normal XY chromosome constitution. Injection of contrast medium into the urogenital sinus of female pseudohermaphrodites usually demonstrates a vagina and uterus. Ultrasonography is also helpful.

DIAGNOSIS. Congenital adrenal hyperplasia in an infant or child should always alert one to the diagnosis in later siblings. The salt-losing form of the disorder must be suspected in any infant who fails to thrive and especially in female infants with ambiguous external genitalia. When virilization occurs postnatally, in either male or female, a virilizing adrenocortical tumor must be considered in the differential diagnosis.

An adrenal tumor may be palpable or suggested on pyelography by displacement of the adjacent kidney. Ultrasound or CT scans may be necessary if hormonal studies have ruled out congenital adrenal hyperplasia. Urinary 17-ketosteroid excretion and plasma levels of DHEAS are elevated with congenital hyperplasia and with cortical tumors, but very high values favor the diagnosis of neoplasm. Administration of hydrocortisone quickly reduces these and other elevated steroid levels to normal in patients with congenital adrenal hyperplasia but does not do so in those with a virilizing tumor. Corticosteroids, by inhibiting secretion of corticotropin, reduce the excessive stimulation of the adrenals in patients with hyperplasia, whereas adrenocortical tumors are not subject to pituitary regulation.

In males with adrenal hyperplasia the testes are small for the degree of virilization, whereas in those with true precocious puberty or with Leydig cell tumors, the testes are enlarged for age.

Females with this condition must be differentiated from those with other causes of ambiguous external genitalia. Only in this condition are adrenal cortical steroid levels elevated. Males with the 3β-hydroxysteroid dehydrogenase defect may be confused with female pseudohermaphrodites because they lack normal virilization of the external genitalia. These male patients are 46XY and also have elevated adrenal cortical steroids.

Detection of the heterozygous carrier is possible by measuring the ratio of 17-OHP to 11-deoxycorticosterone 60 min after an intravenous bolus injection of 0.25 mg of ACTH (1–24). In families in which there is an affected individual with 21-hydroxylase deficiency, HLA genotyping provides a reliable basis for counseling. Molecular DNA techniques are now also available.

Prenatal Diagnosis and Treatment. Prenatal diagnosis of 21-hydroxylase is possible in the 1st trimester by performing biopsy of the chorionic villi followed by HLA typing or DNA analysis. In the 2nd trimester, the diagnosis can be established by measuring 17-OHP in amniotic fluid as well as by HLA typing and DNA analysis of amniotic fluid cells. Prenatal treatment of 17 affected infants has resulted in limited success in mitigating the genital abnormality; possible reasons include late onset of treatment and inadequate suppressive doses of the therapeutic drug. Current recommendations for pregnancies at risk consist of administration of dexamethasone, a steroid that readily crosses the placenta, by the 5th wk of pregnancy in an amount of 1.5 mg/24 hr in 2 or 3 divided doses. First-trimester chorionic villus biopsy is then done to determine the sex and genotype of the fetus; therapy is continued only if the fetus is an affected female. It is unknown whether or to what degree such a regimen will be effective.

TREATMENT. Administration of glucocorticoids inhibits excessive production of androgens and stems virilization. A variety of glucocorticoids and dosage schedules have been used for this purpose. We recommend hydrocortisone (20–25 mg/m²/24 hr) administered orally in 2 divided doses. Infants usually require 5 mg twice daily and pubertal children 10–15 mg twice daily. Doses are individualized by monitoring growth and hormonal levels. Patients with disturbances of electrolyte regulation (salt-losers) and elevated plasma renin activity require a mineralocorticoid in addition to the glucocorticoid. Maintenance therapy with 0.05–0.10 mg, once daily, of 9α-fluorocortisol is usually sufficient to normalize plasma renin activity. Non–salt-losers may also manifest elevated plasma renin activity and require a mineralocorticoid.

The optimal way to monitor these patients varies with personal preference. Measurements of urinary levels of 17-ketosteroids and pregnanetriol are no longer necessary. Plasma levels of 17-OHP, androstenedione, testosterone, and renin, measured preferably at 9:00 A.M., usually provide adequate indices of control. Monitoring of growth and osseous maturation is equally important.

The administration of hydrocortisone must be continued indefinitely in *all* patients. Increased doses are indicated during periods of stress such as infection or surgery or during periods of decreased salt intake for both salt-losers and non–salt-losers, including those with the 11-hydroxylase defect because they all have defective adrenal reserve.

The enlarged clitoris of female infants usually requires surgical correction; a good age for this elective surgery is 6–12 mo. Recession of the clitoris is preferred rather than its removal; the clitoris is freed and repositioned beneath the pubis with preservation of the glans, corporal components, and all neural and vascular elements. Parents should be reassured that complete sexual gratification, including orgasm, can be achieved. The menarche occurs at the appropriate age in most girls in whom good control has been achieved. It is not exceptional for adolescents past the age of 16 not to have begun menstruating; such delay is probably related to suboptimal control.

Non–salt-losers, particularly males, are frequently not diagnosed until 3–7 yr of age, at which time osseous maturation may be 5 yr or more in advance of chronologic age. Institution of treatment slows growth and osseous maturation to more nearly normal rates in some children; in others, especially if the bone age is 12 yr or more, spontaneous gonadotropin-dependent puberty may occur, therapy with hydrocortisone having suppressed production of adrenal androgens and permitted release of pituitary gonadotropins if the appropriate level of hypothalamic maturation is present. This form of superimposed true precocious puberty may now be effectively treated with a luteinizing hormone–releasing hormone analog.

Males who have had inadequate corticosteroid therapy may develop bilateral testicular tumors, which may or may not regress with increased dosage. The tumors are thought to arise from adrenal rest cells present in the testes (Sec. 19.32). Prolonged inadequate adrenal suppression may also result in adenomatous changes in the adrenal gland.

Virilizing Adrenocortical Tumors

Tumors of the adrenal cortex may result in masculinization in girls and precocious pseudopuberty in boys. Hypertension is common, and manifestations of Cushing syndrome may accompany virilization because these tumors frequently secrete excessive cortisol and mineralocorticoids in addition to androgens.

In males the symptoms are usually the same as those occurring with non–salt-losing congenital adrenal hyperplasia. It is virtually impossible to differentiate the two conditions on clinical grounds. *In females* virilizing tumors of the adrenal cause masculinization of a previously normal female, whereas congenital hyperplasia is almost always associated with genital abnormalities at birth. However, virilization in congenital adrenal hyperplasia may have its onset during childhood, and an adrenal adenoma is known to have caused intrauterine clitoral enlargement and mild labial fusion. Fourteen instances of an adrenal cortical carcinoma arising in the newborn period are known.

Tumors of the adrenal (with or without Cushing syndrome) may be associated with hemihypertrophy, usually during the first few years of life. These tumors are also associated with Beckwith-Wiedemann syndrome and other congenital defects, particularly genitourinary tract and central nervous system abnormalities and hamartomatous defects.

Urinary 17-ketosteroids and serum levels of DHEA, DHEAS, and androstenedione are usually elevated, often markedly. Serum levels of testosterone are also usually increased as a result of peripheral conversion of androstenedione, but infants who have had predominantly testosterone-secreting adenomas are known. Many adrenocortical tumors have 11β-hydroxylase deficiency and secrete increased amounts of deoxycorticosterone; these patients are hypertensive, and the tumor is usually malignant. Ultrasound and CT scans are indicated and can detect masses as small as 1.3 cm. Carcinomas are three times more common than adenomas. Differentiation between benign and malignant tumors by histologic criteria is often not possible.

The treatment is surgical; a transperitoneal approach is usually recommended. Some of these neoplasms are highly malignant and metastasize widely, but cure with regression of the masculinizing features may follow removal of less malignant encapsulated tumors.

A neoplasm of one adrenal may produce atrophy of the other as excessive production of cortical hormones by the tumor suppresses ACTH stimulation of the normal gland. Consequently, adrenal insufficiency may follow surgical removal of the tumor. This situation can be avoided by giving 10–25 mg of hydrocortisone every 6 hr, starting on the day of operation and continuing for 3–4 days postoperatively. It may also be necessary to give corticotropin concurrently with cortisol to reactivate the atrophied gland. Adequate quantities of water, sodium chloride, and glucose must also be provided. On rare occasions, the tumors are bilateral, and in at least five instances the contralateral adrenal was absent; in such instances replacement therapy must be continued indefinitely.

Patients with tumors that are easily resected and weigh less than 150 g have a good prognosis. If the tumor is large or incompletely removed, prognosis is guarded. Radiotherapy is not generally helpful. Adrenal androgen levels should be measured at monthly intervals to detect recurrences early. Adjuvant therapy with mitotane (o,p′-DDD), an isomer of DDD, is indicated for inoperable tumors and for recurrences. This agent can induce regression of abnormal steroid production in most patients and tumor regression in some patients; only a few long-term survivals are known. In at least eight patients a second primary tumor has developed, the central nervous system being the most frequent site.

19.24 CUSHING SYNDROME

Cushing syndrome, a characteristic pattern of obesity with associated hypertension, is the result of maintenance of abnormally high blood levels of cortisol by hyperfunction of the adrenal cortex. The syndrome is caused by either ACTH-dependent or ACTH-independent tumors.

ETIOLOGY. In infants, Cushing syndrome is most often caused by a *functioning adrenocortical tumor,* usually a malignant carcinoma but occasionally a benign adenoma. Over 50%

of cortical tumors occur in children 3 yr of age or younger and 85% occur in children 7 yr or younger. Patients with cortical tumors often exhibit a mixed form of hypercortisolism owing to overproduction of such other steroids as androgens, estrogens, and aldosterone.

Primary pigmented nodular adrenocortical disease is a distinctive form of ACTH-independent Cushing disease in infants and children. The adrenal glands are small and have characteristic multiple small (less than 4 mm in diameter), pigmented (black) nodules containing large cells with cytoplasm and lipofuscin; between the nodules there is cortical atrophy. Recent evidence suggests that the condition is caused by circulating immunoglobulins directed toward the ACTH receptor with ensuing stimulation of adrenal steroidogenesis. This adrenal disorder occurs as a component of the **Carney complex**, an autosomal dominant disorder consisting of centrofacial lentigines, cardiac and cutaneous myxomas, sexual precocity in boys with testicular tumors, functioning pituitary tumors, and pigmented melanotic schwannomas.

In children over 7 yr of age *bilateral adrenal hyperplasia,* an ACTH-dependent form of Cushing syndrome, is usually found. This entity is due to a basophilic adenoma of the pituitary in about 20% of affected children. On the other hand, covert pituitary adenomas (microadenomas) are present in most instances of Cushing disease, and resection of these tumors results in correction of the hypercorticism. In some children the pituitary tumors become overt after adrenalectomy *(Nelson syndrome)*; these consist principally of chromophobe cells and produce increased levels of β-lipotropin and β-endorphin as well as of ACTH. There are only two reports of ACTH-secreting tumors in infants with Cushing syndrome.

Bilateral hyperplasia of the adrenals may also result from *ectopic production of ACTH.* Cushing syndrome has been associated with an islet cell carcinoma of the pancreas in four children, with neuroblastoma or ganglioneuroblastoma in several children, with a hemangiopericytoma arising from the cerebral tentorium in a 7-yr-old boy, with Wilms tumors in two children, and with thymic carcinoid in a 10-yr-old girl.

Prolonged exogenous administration of corticotropin or hydrocortisone or its analogs results in a clinical pattern identical to the spontaneous disorder and is frequently referred to as *cushingoid syndrome.*

CLINICAL MANIFESTATIONS. Symptoms may begin in the neonatal period and have been recognized in infants under 1 yr of age on at least 35 occasions. Early in life girls outnumber boys 3:1, and adrenocortical tumors (carcinoma, adenoma, and nodular hyperplasia) are the usual causative lesions. The disorder appears to be more severe and the clinical findings more flagrant in infants than when the onset occurs in older children. The face is rounded, with prominent cheeks and a flushed appearance (moon facies). The chin is doubled, there is a buffalo hump, and generalized obesity is common. Signs of abnormal masculinization due to the androgen production of tumors occur frequently; accordingly, there may be hypertrichosis on the face and trunk, pubic hair, acne, deepening of the voice, and, in girls, enlargement of the clitoris. Growth is impaired, length falling below the 3rd percentile, except when significant virilization produces normal or even accelerated growth. Hypertension is common and may lead to heart failure. An increased susceptibility to infection may lead to fatal sepsis. Infants with Cushing syndrome, despite a robust appearance, are generally very fragile. Occasionally, the condition is associated with hemihypertrophy or other congenital defects.

In older children bilateral hyperplasia of the adrenals is the most common lesion, and the sex incidence is equal. In addition to obesity, short stature is a common presenting feature. Gradual onset of obesity and deceleration or cessation of growth may be the only early manifestations. Purplish striae on the hips, abdomen, and thighs are common. Pubertal development may be delayed, or amenorrhea may occur in girls past menarche. Weakness, headache, deterioration in school work, and emotional lability may be prominent. Hypertension is usual. Renal stones have occurred both in older children and in infants.

LABORATORY DATA. Polycythemia, lymphopenia, and eosinopenia are common. The glucose tolerance test may be diabetic despite elevated levels of insulin. Levels of serum electrolytes are usually normal, but potassium may be decreased.

Cortisol levels in blood are normally elevated at 8:00 A.M. and decrease to less than 50% by 8:00 P.M. except in children under 3 yr of age, in whom a diurnal rhythm is not always established. In patients with Cushing syndrome this diurnal rhythm is lost, and cortisol levels at 8:00 P.M. are usually elevated. Urinary excretion of free cortisol is almost always increased; normal values are 20–90 μg/24 hr. Urinary excretion of 17-hydroxycorticosteroids is usually increased (>5 $mg/m^2/24$ hr). In questionable cases a single-dose dexamethasone suppression test may be helpful; a dose of 0.3 mg/m^2 given at 11:00 P.M. will result in a plasma cortisol level of less than 5 μg/dL at 8:00 A.M. the next morning in normal children.

After the diagnosis of Cushing syndrome has been established, it is necessary to determine whether it is ACTH-dependent or -independent. ACTH concentrations alone usually are not helpful in the differential diagnosis because of the large range of normal basal levels. The ovine corticotropin-releasing hormone (oCRH) stimulation test is still experimental but seems promising. After an intravenous bolus of oCRH (1 μg/kg), patients with ACTH-dependent Cushing syndrome have an exaggerated ACTH and cortisol response, whereas those with adrenal tumors show no increase in ACTH and cortisol. Another test consists of administration of dexamethasone, 30 and 120 μg/kg/24 hr, divided into 4 doses and given for 2 consecutive days each. In children with ACTH-dependent Cushing syndrome, the larger dose will suppress urinary free cortisol or 17-hydroxycorticosteroids to less than 50% of baseline, and serum levels of cortisol will decrease to less than 7 μg/dL. Occasional parodoxic results have been reported.

Osseous maturation is usually moderately retarded but may be normal; in virilized children the bone age is apt to be advanced. Osteoporosis is common and is most evident in roentgenograms of the spine. Pathologic fractures may be noted. Levels of growth hormone, both secreted spontaneously and stimulated, are suppressed but return to normal when the hypercortisolism is corrected. Diminution of muscle mass and increased deposition of adipose tissue may be noted in roentgenograms of the extremities. The thymic shadow is absent because excessive cortisol produces involution. CT scanning detects virtually all adrenal tumors over 1.5 cm in diameter. Adrenal scintigraphy with radiocholesterol is rarely indicated except for patients with pigmented micronodular adrenal hyperplasia, in whom it may be more accurate than CT scan. MRI is the screening method of choice to detect ACTH-secreting pituitary adenomas; the addition of gadolinium contrast increases the sensitivity of detection. Bilateral inferior petrosal blood sampling to measure concentrations of ACTH may be required when a pituitary adenoma is not visualized.

DIFFERENTIAL DIAGNOSIS. Cushing syndrome is frequently suspected in children with obesity, particularly when striae and hypertension are present. Differential diagnosis is complicated by the fact that elevated urinary concentrations of corticosteroids are frequently secondary to obesity itself. Children with simple obesity are usually tall, whereas those with Cushing syndrome are short or have a decelerating growth rate. The excretion of urinary corticosteroids is rapidly suppressed by oral administration of low doses of dexamethasone in persons with uncomplicated obesity. Elevated levels of cortisol and ACTH without clinical evidence of Cushing syndrome occur in patients with *cortisol resistance*. This genetic disorder is caused by a defect in glucocorticoid receptor function. The condition is usually asymptomatic, but mild elevations of ACTH have resulted in increased adrenal androgens and precocious pseudopuberty.

TREATMENT. If the lesion is a benign cortical adenoma, unilateral adrenalectomy is indicated. Such adenomas are occasionally bilateral; then the treatment of choice is subtotal adrenalectomy. In either instance an excellent therapeutic result is achieved by removing the tumor. Adrenocortical carcinomas, on the other hand, frequently metastasize, especially to the liver and lungs, and the prognosis may be unfavorable in spite of removal of the primary lesion. Rarely, the tumors are bilateral and require total adrenalectomy. It is often impossible to differentiate between benign and malignant tumors by histologic appearance alone.

Management of Cushing syndrome is still unsettled. Total adrenalectomy has fallen into disfavor because about 30% of patients develop an expanding pituitary tumor postoperatively. Intense melanosis, markedly elevated serum levels of ACTH (often >1,000 pg/mL), and enlargement of the sella turcica occur *(Nelson syndrome)*. To circumvent this problem, current treatment is directed at the pituitary. External irradiation of the pituitary is advocated by some, but remission is slow and sequelae include hypopituitarism and behavioral changes. The most frequently recommended approach is transsphenoidal pituitary microsurgery. In the hands of an experienced neurosurgeon, selective adenoma resection has produced low morbidity and a good remission rate.

Cyproheptadine, a centrally acting serotonin antagonist that blocks ACTH release, has been used to treat Cushing disease in adults; remissions are usually not sustained after discontinuation of therapy. A child with Cushing disease treated with this agent has had a 3-yr remission after cessation of therapy; further therapeutic trials are needed.

Management of patients undergoing adrenalectomy requires adequate preoperative and postoperative replacement therapy with a corticosteroid. Tumors that produce corticosteroids usually lead to atrophy of the normal adrenal tissue, and replacement with both cortisol and corticotropin may be required. Postoperative complications have included sepsis, pancreatitis, thrombosis, poor wound healing, and sudden collapse, particularly in infants with Cushing syndrome. Substantial catch-up growth occurs, but adult height is often compromised.

19.25 EXCESS MINERALOCORTICOID SECRETION

The principal mineralocorticoid secreted by the adrenal is aldosterone. Increased secretion may result from a primary defect of the adrenal (primary hyperaldosteronism) or from factors that activate the renin-angiotensin system (secondary hyperaldosteronism). Patients with primary hyperaldosteronism usually have hypertension or hypokalemia; those with secondary hyperaldosteronism do not.

Desoxycorticosterone is a precursor of aldosterone, with only about one thirtieth the sodium-retaining potency of aldosterone (see Fig. 19–12). Overproduction of desoxycorticosterone occurs with two distinct defects of adrenal steroidogenesis: the first defect involves 11-hydroxylation, which also leads to androgen excess and presents clinically as the hypertensive form of congenital adrenal hyperplasia (see Sec. 19.23); the second defect involves 17-hydroxylation, producing hypogonadism in the female and male pseudohermaphroditism in the male because the synthesis of androgens and estrogens as well as of cortisol is impaired.

ETIOLOGY. Primary aldosteronism encompasses disorders characterized by excessive aldosterone secretion independent of the renin-angiotensin system. These disorders, rare in children, are characterized by hypertension, hypokalemia, and suppression of the renin-angiotensin system.

Aldosterone-secreting adenomas are unilateral and have been reported in about 12 children as young as 3½ yr of age; they mainly affect girls.

Bilateral micronodular adrenocortical hyperplasia tends to occur in older children. There is increasing evidence that the adrenal is being stimulated by a circulating glycoprotein that appears to originate in the pituitary.

Glucocorticoid-suppressible aldosteronism is characterized by bilateral adrenal hyperplasia and a dramatic response to treatment with glucocorticoids. Two new adrenal corticosteroid hormones have been identified in the urine of patients with this disorder, 18-hydroxycortisol and 18-oxocortisol. Because these hybrid steroids have characteristics of both the zona glomerulosa and the zona fasciculata, they appear to arise from the transitional zona of the adrenal. Aldosterone secretion in these patients is regulated by ACTH, which explains the prompt suppression with corticosteroids. This is an autosomal dominant disorder; at-risk family members of affected patients should be investigated for this easily treated cause of hypertension.

CLINICAL MANIFESTATIONS. Some affected children have no symptoms, the diagnosis being established after incidental discovery of moderate hypertension. Others have severe hypertension (up to 240/150 mm Hg), with headache, dizziness, and visual disturbances. Chronic hypokalemia may lead to "clear cell nephrosis," polyuria, nocturia, enuresis, and polydipsia. Muscle weakness and discomfort, tetany, intermittent paralysis, fatigue, and growth failure have been noted.

LABORATORY STUDIES. Hypertension, hypokalemia, and suppressed plasma renin activity are the hallmarks of hyperaldosteronism. The serum pH, carbon dioxide content, and sodium concentrations may be elevated and the serum chloride and magnesium levels decreased. Serum levels of calcium are normal, even in children who manifest tetany. The urine is neutral or alkaline. Plasma and urine levels of aldosterone are increased, and plasma levels of renin are persistently low. In patients with glucocorticoid-suppressible aldosteronism, urinary and plasma levels of 18-oxocortisol and 18-hydroxycortisol are markedly increased.

DIFFERENTIAL DIAGNOSIS. After establishing the diagnosis of primary aldosteronism, it is necessary to determine the etiology. All children should have a therapeutic trial with dexamethasone before invasive studies are done. Daily administration of 0.25 mg every 6 hr results in marked suppression of aldosterone and disappearance of hypertension in those patients with the glucocorticoid-suppressible variant of hyperaldosteronism. If there is no response to dexamethasone, computed tomography may help to detect an adrenal adenoma, but the tumors are often quite small. If CT scans are normal, adrenal vein catheterization is indicated. High concentrations of aldosterone are found in only one adrenal vein when an adenoma is present and in both when bilateral hyperplasia is the cause. If adrenal vein catheterization is not successful, exploratory laparotomy may be required to establish the diagnosis.

Hyperaldosteronism occurs in many other conditions in which it is a normal homeostatic response. In such *secondary hyperaldosteronism*, serum renin activity is high or rises with a low-salt diet, whereas in primary hyperaldosteronism the renin-angiotensin system is suppressed. Increased aldosterone secretion occurs in edematous disorders with reduced effective volume, such as nephrotic syndrome, congestive cardiac failure, and cirrhosis of the liver. Increased secretion of aldosterone also occurs in conditions in which compromise of renal perfusion results in increased secretion of renin, such as in stenosis of the renal artery. Wilms tumor and juxtaglomerular cell tumors may also secrete renin and cause secondary hyperaldosteronism.

In *pseudohypoaldosteronism* the increased levels of aldosterone are due to a deficiency or abnormality of aldosterone receptors, with ensuing activation of the renin-angiotensin system (Sec. 19.22).

Bartter syndrome is also characterized by hypokalemic alkalosis, hypochloremia, and hyperaldosteronism, but the blood pressure is normal, and secretion of renin is increased. Growth failure is the usual presenting complaint. The primary defect appears to be deficient reabsorption in the ascending limb of the loop of Henle. Renal biopsy reveals hyperplasia of the juxtaglomerular apparatus. Urinary excretion of prostaglandin $F_1\alpha$ has been demonstrated, and it has been suggested that this mediates the hyperreninemia (Sec. 18.31).

11β-hydroxysteroid dehydrogenase deficiency (11β-OHSD) has been reported in 18 children. Onset occurs in early childhood with failure to thrive, polyuria and polydipsia secondary to the effects of hypokalemia, and severe hypertension. Strokes have occurred in young children. The disorder has been reported in siblings and appears to have a genetic basis. Although clinically the disorder mimics that seen in patients with elevated aldosterone levels, renin and aldosterone levels are low *(low renin hypertension)*. For several decades the condition was thought to be caused by production of an undetected mineralocorticoid and was named the *syndrome of apparent mineralocorticoid excess*. It is now clear that the disorder is caused by a deficiency of the enzyme that converts cortisol to cortisone. Plasma levels of cortisol are normal, but those of cortisone are low, and the ratio of the urinary tetrahydro products of cortisol to cortisone is characteristically elevated.

How this glucocorticoid defect can cause such profound mineralocorticoid effects has only recently been elucidated. Type I mineralocorticoid receptors (kidney, parotid glands, colon) have equal affinity for aldosterone and cortisol. Under normal conditions, 11β-OHSD acts as a paracrine protector for the mineralocorticoid receptor in the proximal tubules of the kidney; by converting cortisol to cortisone at this site, it can no longer bind to the receptor. In the absence of this enzyme, and with failure of conversion of cortisol to cortisone, cortisol binds to the mineralocorticoid receptor and elicits effects similar to those of aldosterone. Another name suggested for this condition is *pseudohyperaldosteronism*. The well-known hypertensive effect of glycorrhetinic acid, a constituent of licorice, is now known to be caused by its inhibition of renal 11β-OHSD.

TREATMENT. Glucocorticoid-suppressible hyperaldosteronism is managed by daily administration of dexamethasone. Bilateral adrenal hyperplasia that does not respond to this therapy requires bilateral adrenalectomy; the results are excellent, but adrenal replacement therapy is required. Removal of an aldosterone-secreting adenoma results in a cure.

Treatment of secondary hyperaldosteronism is directed to the specific causative disorder.

19.26 FEMINIZING ADRENAL TUMORS

Adrenocortical tumors have been associated in nine boys with excessive production of estrogens and heterosexual precocious puberty. Gynecomastia was the initial manifestation, appearing from 6 mo–7 yr of age. Growth and development were otherwise normal, or concomitant virilization was sometimes evidenced by acne, deep voice, phallic enlargement, and advanced osseous maturation. The testes were not enlarged. Hypertension is common in affected adults but has not been observed in children. Levels of estrogens and often of androgens in plasma and urine are markedly elevated. Tumors may be either carcinomas or benign adenomas and may be calcified on roentgenography. Gynecomastia regresses after removal of the tumor, and hormone values return to normal.

Estrogen-secreting adrenocortical tumors have been reported in 12 girls ranging in age from 6 mo–10 yr. The majority of the tumors were adenomas, some of which also elaborated androgens (with virilization) or mineralocorticoids (with hypertension). In addition to elevated plasma and urinary levels of estrogens, there were usually elevated levels of 17-ketosteroids in urine and of Δ^5 adrenal steroids (DHEA and DHEAS) in plasma. Plasma gonadotropin levels are suppressed and GNRH stimulation does not elicit a response. Computed tomography usually localizes the tumor.

19.27 EXCESSIVE SECRETION OF CATECHOLAMINES

PHEOCHROMOCYTOMA

The pheochromocytoma, a catecholamine-secreting tumor, arises from the chromaffin cells. The most common site of origin is the adrenal medulla; tumors may develop, however, anywhere along the abdominal sympathetic chain and are particularly apt to be located near the aorta at the level of the inferior mesenteric artery or at its bifurcation. They also appear in the periadrenal area, the urinary bladder or ureteral walls, the thoracic cavity, and the cervical region. Fewer than 5% of reported instances have occurred in children. Tumors vary from about 1–10 cm in diameter; they are found more often on the right side than on the left. In 20% of affected children the adrenal tumors are bilateral, and in 30% tumors are found in both the adrenal and extra-adrenal areas or only in an extra-adrenal area.

Pheochromocytoma is frequently inherited as an autosomal dominant trait. In affected families the ages of patients at the time of diagnosis have varied from the 1st to 5th decades of life; more than half the patients have had multiple tumors.

Pheochromocytoma is frequently associated with other syndromes or tumors. Approximately 5% of patients with pheochromocytoma have neurofibromatosis. Sporadic as well as familial instances of pheochromocytoma have been noted in patients with von Hippel–Lindau disease. Kinships have been reported in which some affected members also have asymptomatic islet cell adenomas, and some people with pheochromocytoma are asymptomatic despite elevated urinary concentrations of catecholamines.

Pheochromocytoma is a component of MEN, types IIa and IIb; medullary carcinoma of the thyroid usually appears at an earlier age than pheochromocytoma (see Sec. 19.16). These syndromes are inherited in an autosomal dominant fashion.

CLINICAL MANIFESTATIONS. These result from excessive secretion of epinephrine and norepinephrine; the clinical picture varies with quantitative variations in their secretion. All patients have hypertension at some time. The hypertension is usually sustained, but it may often be *paroxysmal*. Paroxysms should particularly suggest pheochromocytoma as a diagnostic possibility. When there are paroxysms of hypertension, the attacks are usually infrequent at first but become more frequent and eventually give way to a continuous hypertensive state. Between attacks of hypertension the patient may be free of symptoms. During attacks the patient complains of headache and palpitations, and pallor, vomiting, and sweating also occur. Convulsions and other manifestations of hypertensive encephalopathy may occur. In severe cases precordial pains radiate into the arms, and pulmonary edema and cardiac and hepatic enlargement may develop. The child has a good appetite but because of hypermetabolism does not gain weight, and severe cachexia may develop. Polyuria and polydipsia can be sufficiently severe to suggest diabetes insipidus. Growth failure may be striking. The blood pressure may range from 180–260 systolic and 120–210 diastolic, and the heart may be enlarged. Ophthalmoscopic examination may reveal papilledema, hemorrhages, exudate, and arterial constriction.

LABORATORY DATA. The urine contains protein, a few casts, and occasionally glucose. Gross hematuria suggests that the tumor is in the bladder wall. Polycythemia is occasionally noted. The diagnosis is established by demonstration of elevated plasma or urinary levels of catecholamines and their metabolites.

Pheochromocytomas produce both norepinephrine and epinephrine; norepinephrine in plasma is derived, however, from both the adrenal gland and adrenergic nerve endings, whereas epinephrine is derived primarily from the adrenal. In contrast to adults, the predominant catecholamine in children is norepinephrine, and total urinary catecholamine excretion usually exceeds 300 μg/24 hr. The concentrations of catecholamines in urine are directly related to those in the tumor. Urinary excretion of vanillylmandelic acid (VMA, 3-methoxy-4-hydroxymandelic acid), the major metabolite of epinephrine and norepinephrine, and of metanephrine (see Fig. 19–11) are also increased. Catecholamine levels can be measured by RIA and high-pressure liquid chromatography methods. Excretion of catecholamine metabolites may be similar in children with neuroblastoma and with pheochromocytoma, but levels are usually higher in those with pheochromocytoma. Daily urinary excretion of these compounds by unaffected children increases with age; and vanilla-containing foods and fruits can produce falsely elevated levels of VMA. Certain drugs interfere with fluorometric determinations of catecholamines.

Most tumors in the area of the adrenal are readily localized by CT scans; their frequent bilateral occurrence must not be forgotten. Extra-adrenal tumors, anywhere from the neck to the bladder, may be difficult to detect. ^{131}I-metaiodobenzylguanidine is taken up by chromaffin tissue anywhere in the body and is useful for localizing small tumors. Venous catheterization with sampling of blood at different levels for catecholamine determinations is now only rarely necessary for localizing the tumor.

DIFFERENTIAL DIAGNOSIS. The various causes of hypertension in children must be considered, such as renal or renovascular disease, coarctation of the aorta, acrodynia, thallium intoxication, hyperthyroidism, Cushing syndrome, 11β-hydroxylase, 17-hydroxylase, and 11β-hydroxysteroid dehydrogenase deficiency, primary aldosteronism, adrenal cortical tumors, and essential hypertension. A nonfunctioning kidney may result from compression of a ureter or of a renal artery by a pheochromocytoma. Paroxysmal hypertension may be associated with familial dysautonomia. Urinary excretion of VMA is low in familial dysautonomia because of a defect in release rather than in synthesis of catecholamines. Cerebral disorders, diabetes insipidus, diabetes mellitus, and hyperthyroidism must also be considered in the differential diagnosis. Hypertension in patients with neurofibromatosis may be caused by renal vascular involvement as well as by concurrent pheochromocytoma.

Neuroblastoma, ganglioneuroblastoma, and ganglioneuroma frequently produce catecholamines. Secreting neurogenic tumors commonly produce hypertension, excessive sweating, flushing, pallor, rash, polyuria, and polydipsia. Diarrhea also may be associated with these tumors, particularly with ganglioneuroma, and at times may be sufficiently persistent to suggest the "celiac syndrome."

TREATMENT. Removal of these tumors results in cure, but the operation is not without danger. Careful preoperative, intraoperative, and postoperative management is essential. Preoperative α- and β-adrenergic blockade is required. Since these tumors are often multiple in children, a thorough transabdominal exploration of all the usual sites offers the best chance of finding all of them. Appropriate choice of anesthesia and expansion of blood volume with appropriate fluids during surgery are critical to avoid a precipitious drop in blood pressure during operation or within 48 hr postoperatively. Manipulation and excision of these tumors result in marked increases in catecholamine secretion that cause rises in blood pressure and heart rate. Surveillance must continue postoperatively.

Although these tumors often appear malignant histologically, only rarely has malignancy been established unequivocally in a child by the appearance of metastases. Prolonged follow-up is indicated because functioning tumors at other sites may become manifest many years after the initial operation. Examination of relatives of affected patients may reveal other persons harboring unsuspected tumors. In one family with 10 affected individuals the highest blood pressures and urinary concentrations of catecholamines were found in the children, whereas some of the affected adults were normotensive and had only moderately elevated urinary concentrations of catecholamines and VMA.

OTHER CATECHOLAMINE-SECRETING NEURAL TUMORS

See Sec. 13.68 and 17.12.

19.28 CALCIFICATION WITHIN THE ADRENAL

Calcification within the adrenal glands may occur in a wide variety of situations, some serious and others of no obvious consequence. Adrenal calcifications are often detected as incidental findings in roentgenographic studies of the abdomen in infants and children. One may elicit a history of anoxia or trauma at birth. Hemorrhage into the adrenal at or immediately after birth is probably the common factor that leads to subsequent calcification. Though it is advisable to assess the adrenocortical reserve of such patients, there is rarely any functional disorder.

Neuroblastomas, ganglioneuromas, cortical carcinomas, pheochromocytomas, and cysts of the adrenal gland may be responsible for calcifications, particularly if hemorrhage has occurred within the tumor. Calcification in such lesions is almost always unilateral.

In the past tuberculosis was a common cause of calcification within the adrenals and of Addison disease. Calcifications may also develop in the adrenal glands of children who recover from the Waterhouse-Friderichsen syndrome; such patients are usually asymptomatic.

Infants with *Wolman syndrome*, a rare lipid disorder due to deficiency of lysosomal acid lipase, have extensive bilateral calcifications of the adrenal glands (see Sec. 8.18).

ADRENAL CORTICAL INSUFFICIENCY

Ahonen P, Miettinen A, Perheentupa J: Adrenal and steroidal cell antibodies in patients with autoimmune polygandular disease type I and risk of adrenocortical and ovarian failure. J Clin Endocrinol Metab 64:494, 1987.

Ahonen P, Myllarniemi S, Spila I, et al: Clinical variation of autoimmune polyendocrinopathy-candidiasis-ectodermal dystrophy (APECED) in a series of 68 patients. N Engl J Med 322:1824, 1990.

Armanini D, Kuhnle U, Strasser T, et al: Aldosterone-receptor deficiency in pseudohypoaldosteronism. N Engl J Med 313:1178, 1985.

Aubourg P, Blanche S, Jambaque T, et al: Reversal of early neurologic and neuroradiologic manifestations of X-linked adrenoleukodystrophy by bone marrow transplantation. N Engl J Med 322:1860, 1990.
Carey DE: Isolated ACTH deficiency in childhood: Lack of response to corticotropin-releasing hormone alone and in combination with arginine vasopressin. J Pediatr 107:925, 1985.
Carney JA, Hruska LS, Beauchamp GD, et al: Dominant inheritance of the complex of myxomas, spotty pigmentation, and endocrine overactivity. Mayo Clinic Proc 61:165, 1986.
Globerman H, Rosler A, Theodor R, et al: An inherited defect in aldosterone biosynthesis caused by a mutation in or near the gene for steroid 11-hydroxylase. N Engl J Med 319:1193, 1988.
Hay ID: Pubertal failure in congenital adrenocortical hypoplasia. Lancet 2:1035, 1977.
Kelch RP, Kaplan SL, Biglieri EG, et al: Hereditary adrenocortical unresponsiveness to adrenocorticotropic hormone. J Pediatr 81:726, 1972.
Kirkland RT, Kirkland JL, Johnson CM, et al: Congenital lipoid adrenal hyperplasia in an eight-year-old phenotypic female. J Clin Endocrinol Metab 36:488, 1973.
Kruse K, Sippell WG, Schnakenburg KV: Hypogonadism in congenital adrenal hypoplasia: Evidence for a hypothalamic origin. J Clin Endocrinol Metab 58:12, 1984.
Kuhnle U, Nielsen MD, Tietze U, et al: Pseudohypoaldosteronism in eight families: Different forms of inheritance are evidence for various genetic defects. J Clin Endocrinol Metab 70:638, 1990.
Lee PDK, Patterson BD, Hintz RL, et al: Biochemical diagnosis and management of corticosterone methyloxidase type II deficiency. J Clin Endocrinol Metab 62:225, 1986.
Linder BL, Esteban NV, Yergey AL, et al: Cortisol production rate in childhood and adolesence. J Pediatr 117:892, 1990.
Matsumoto T, Kondoh T, Yoshimoto M, et al: Complex glycerol kinase deficiency: Molecular genetic, cytogenetic and clinical studies of five Japanese patients. Am J Med Genet 31:603, 1988.
McCabe ERB, Towbin J, Chamberlain J, et al: Complementary DNA probes for the muscular dystrophy locus demonstrate a previously undetectable deletion in a patient with dystrophic myopathy, glycerol kinase deficiency, and congenital adrenal hyperplasia. J Clin Invest 83:95, 1989.
Moser HW, Moser AE, Singh J, et al: Adrenoleukodystrophy: Survey of 303 cases: Biochemistry, diagnosis, and therapy. Ann Neurol 16:628, 1984.
Sadegji-Nejad A, Senior B: Adrenomyeloneuropathy as Addison's disease in childhood. N Engl J Med 322:13, 1990.
Sauler NP, Tons R, McLaughlin CE, et al: Isolated adrenocorticotropin deficiency associated with an antibody to a corticotroph antigen that is not adrenocorticotropin or other pro-opiomelanocortin-derived peptides. J Clin Endocrinol Metab 70:1391, 1990.
Smith EM, Brosnan P, Meyer WH III, et al: An ACTH receptor on human mononuclear leukocytes. Relation to adrenal ACTH-receptor activity. N Engl J Med 317:1266, 1987.
Wolffraat NM, Drexhage HA, Bottazzo GF, et al: Immunoglobulins of patients with idiopathic Addison's disease block the in vitro action of adrenocorticotropin. J Clin Endocrinol Metab 69:231, 1989.

ADRENAL CORTICAL HYPERFUNCTION

Bitton RN, Cobbs R, Schneider BS: Development of Nelson syndrome in a patient with recurrent Cushing disease: Analysis of secretory behavior of the pituitary tumor. Am J Med 84:319, 1988.
Bryer-Ash M, Wilson DM, Tune BM, et al: Hypertension caused by an aldosterone-secreting adenoma. Occurrence in a 7-year-old child. Am J Dis Child 138:673, 1984.
Burr IM, Sullivan J, Graham T, et al: A testosterone-secreting tumour of the adrenal producing virilization in a female infant. Lancet 2:643, 1973.
Cara JF, Moshang T Jr, Bongiovanni AM, et al: Elevated 17-hydroxyprogesterone and testosterone in a newborn with 3-beta-hydroxysteroid dehydrogenase deficiency. N Engl J Med 313:618, 1985.
Carey RM, Sen S, Dolan LM, et al: Idiopathic hyperaldosteronism. A possible role for aldosterone-stimulating factor. N Engl J Med 313:94, 1984.
Chan-Cua S, Freidenberg G, Jones KL: Occurrence of male phenotype in genotypic females with congenital virilizing adrenal hyperplasia. Am J Med Genet 34:406, 1989.
Clark RV, Albertson BD, Munabi A, et al: Steroidogenic enzyme activities, morphology, and receptor studies of a testicular adrenal rest in a patient with congenital adrenal hyperplasia. J Clin Endocrinol Metab 70:1408, 1990.
Comite F, Schiebinger RJ, Alertson BD, et al: Isosexual precocious pseudopuberty secondary to a feminizing adrenal tumor. J Clin Endocrinol Metab 58:435, 1984.
Couch RM, Smail PJ, Dean HJ, et al: Prolonged remission of Cushing disease with cyproheptadine. J Pediatr 104:906, 1984.
Cutler GB Jr, Lave L: Congenital adrenal hyperplasia due to 21-hydroxylase deficiency. N Engl J Med 323:1806, 1990.
Duck SC: Acceptable linear growth in congenital adrenal hyperplasia. J Pediatr 97:93, 1980.
Edwards CRW, Stewart PM, Burt D, et al: Localization of 11-β-hydroxysteroid dehydrogenase: Tissue specific protector of the mineralocorticoid receptor. Lancet 2:986, 1988.
Eldar-Geva T, Hurwitz A, Velsei P, et al: Secondary biosynthetic defects in women with late-onset congenital adrenal hyperplasia. N Engl J Med 323:855, 1990.
Fraumeni JF Jr, Miller RW: Adrenocortical neoplasms with hemihypertrophy, brain tumors, and other disorders. J Pediatr 70:129, 1967.
Ganguly A, Grim CE, Bergstein J, et al: Genetic and pathophysiologic studies of a new kindred with glucocorticoid-suppressible hyperaldosteronism manifest in three generations. J Clin Endocrinol Metab 53:1040, 1981.
Grim CE, McBryde AC, Glenn JF, et al: Childhood primary aldosteronism with bilateral adrenocortical hyperplasia. Plasma renin activity as an aid to diagnosis. J Pediatr 71:377, 1967.
Gomez MT, Malazowski S, Winterer J, et al: Urinary free cortisol values in children and adolescents. J Pediatr 118:256, 1991.
Gomez-Sanchez CE, Gill JR Jr, Ganguly A, et al: Glucocoid-suppressible aldosteronism: A disorder of the adrenal transitional zona. J Clin Endocrinol Metab 67:444, 1988.
Holler W, Scholz S, Knon D, et al: Genetic differences between the salt-wasting simple virilizing and nonclassical types of congenital adrenal hyperplasia. J Clin Endocrinol Metab 60:757, 1985.
Howard CP, Takahashi H, Hayles AB: Feminizing adrenal adenoma in a boy. Case report and literature review. Mayo Clin Proc 52:354, 1977.
Kaye TB, Crapo L: The Cushing syndrome: An update on diagnostic tests. Am J Intern Med 112:434, 1990.
Lee PDK, Winter RJ, Green OC: Virilizing adrenocortical tumors in childhood: Eight cases and a review of the literature. Pediatrics 76:437, 1985.
LeFevre M, Gerard-Marchant R, Gubler JP, et al: Adrenal cortical carcinoma in children: 42 patients treated from 1958 to 1980 at Villejuif. Cancer Treat Res 17:265, 1983.
Levy SR, Val Wynne C Jr, Lorentz WB Jr: Cushing's syndrome in infancy secondary to pituitary adenoma. Am J Dis Child 136:605, 1982.
Luton LP, Cerdas S, Billaud L, et al: Clinical features of adrenocortical carcinoma, prognostic factors, and the effect of mitotane therapy. N Engl J Med 322:1195, 1990.
McArthur RG, Bahn RC, Hayles AB: Primary adrenocortical nodular dysplasia as a cause of Cushing's syndrome in infants and children. Mayo Clin Proc 57:58, 1982.
Malchoff CD, Javier EC, Malchoff DM, et al: Primary cortisol resistance presenting as isosexual precocity. J Clin Endocrinol Metab 70:503, 1990.
Mampalam TJ, Tyrell JB, Wilson CB: Transsphenoidal microsurgery for Cushing disease. Ann Intern Med 109:487, 1988.
Miller WL: Gene conversions, deletions, and polymorphisms in congenital adrenal hyperplasia. Am J Hum Genet 42:4, 1988.
Miller WL: Molecular biology of steroid hormone synthesis. Endocrine Rev 9:295, 1988.
Muguruza MTG, Chrousos GP: Periodic Cushing syndrome in a short boy: Usefulness of the ovine corticotropin-releasing hormone test. J Pediatr 115:270, 1990.
New MI, Lorenzen F, Lerner AJ, et al: Genotyping steroid 21-hydroxylase deficiency: Hormonal reference data. J Clin Endocrinol Metab 57:320, 1983.
Pang S, Levine LS, Stoner E, et al: Nonsalt-losing congenital adrenal hyperplasia due to 3β-hydroxysteroid dehydrogenase deficiency with normal glomerulosa function. J Clin Endocrinol Metab 56:808, 1983.
Pang S, Pollack MS, Marshall RN, et al: Prenatal treatment of congenital adrenal hyperplasia due to 21-hydroxylase deficiency. N Engl J Med 322:111, 1990.
Pescovitz OH, Comite F, Cassorla F, et al: True precocious puberty complicating congenital adrenal hyperplasia: Treatment with a luteinizing hormone-releasing hormone analog. J Clin Endocrinol Metab 58:857, 1984.
Rescoria FJ, Vane DW, Fitzgerald JF, et al: Vasoactive intestinal polypeptide-secreting ganglioneuromatosis affecting the entire colon and rectum. J Pediatr Surg 23:635, 1988.
Schackleton CHL, Rodriquez J, Arteago E, et al: Congenital 11β-hydroxysteroid dehydrogenase deficiency associated with juvenile hypertension: Corticosteroid metabolite profiles of four patients and their families. Clin Endocrinol 22:701, 1985.
Speiser PW, Agdere L, Ueshiba H, et al: Aldosterone synthesis in salt-wasting congenital adrenal hyperplasia with complete absence of adrenal 21-hydroxylase. N Engl J Med 324:145, 1991.
Speiser PW, New MI, White PC: Molecular genetic analysis of nonclassic steroid 11-hydroxylase deficiency associated with HLA-B14,DR1. N Engl J Med 319:19, 1988.
Stewart PM, Edwards CRW: Specificity of the mineralocorticoid receptor. Crucial role of 11β-hydroxysteroid dehydrogenase. Trends Endocrinol Metab 1:225, 1990.
Strachan T: Molecular pathology of congenital adrenal hyperplasia. Clin Endocrinol 32:373, 1990.
Streetan DHP, Faas FH, Elders MJ, et al: Hypercortisolism in childhood: Shortcomings of conventional diagnostic criteria. Pediatrics 56:797, 1975.
Sultan C, Descomps B, Garandeau P, et al: Pubertal gynecomastia due to an estrogen-producing adrenal adenoma. J Pediatr 95:744, 1979.
Styne DM, Grumbach MM, Kaplan SL, et al: Treatment of Cushing's disease in childhood and adolescence by transsphenoidal microadenomectomy. N Engl J Med 310:889, 1984.
Styne DM, Isaac R, Miller WL, et al: Endocrine, histological and biochemical studies of adrenocorticotropin-producing islet cell carcinoma of the pancreas in childhood with characterization of propiomelanocortin. J Clin Endocrinol Metab 57:723, 1983.

Urabe K, Kimura A, Harada F, et al: Gene conversions in steroid 21-hydroxylase genes. Am J Hum Genet 46:1178, 1990.
Wolffraat NM, Drexhage HA, Wiersinga WM, et al: Immunoglobulins of patients with Cushing's syndrome due to pigmented adrenocortical micronodular dysplasia stimulate in vitro steroidogenesis. J Clin Endocrin Metab 66:301, 1988.
Yane T, Sanders D, Shibata A, et al: Combined 17α-hydroxylase/17,20-lyase deficiency due to a 7-base pair duplication in the N-terminal region of the cytochrome $P_{450}17\alpha$-(CYP 17) gene. J Clin Endocrinol Metab 70:1325, 1990.
Zachman M, Tassinari D, Prader A: Clinical and biochemical variability of congenital adrenal hyperplasia due to 11β-hydroxylase deficiency. A study of 25 patients. J Clin Endocrinol Metab 56:222, 1983.

PHEOCHROMOCYTOMA AND OTHER NEURAL TUMORS

El Shafie M, Samuel D, Klippel CH, et al: Intractable diarrhea in children with VIP-secreting ganglioneuroblastoma. J Pediatr Surg 18:34, 1983.
Gitlow SE, Bertani LM, Greenwood SM, et al: Benign pheochromocytoma associated with elevated excretion of homovanillic acid. J Pediatr 81:1112, 1972.
Kaufman BH, Telander RL, VanHeerden JA, et al: Pheochromocytoma in the pediatric age group: Current status. J Pediatr Surg 18:879, 1983.
Keiser HR, Beauen MA, Doppman J, et al: Sipple's syndrome: Medullary thyroid carcinoma, pheochromocytoma, and parathyroid disease. Ann Intern Med 78:561, 1973.
Kogut MD, Kaplan SA: Systemic manifestations of neurogenic tumors. J Pediatr 60:697, 1962.
Phillips AF, McMurty RJ, Taubman J: Malignant pheochromocytoma in childhood. Am J Dis Child 130:1252, 1976.
Sawada T, Hirayama M, Nakata T, et al: Mass screening for neuroblastoma in infants in Japan. Interim report of a mass screening study group. Lancet 2:271, 1984.
Schimke RN, Hartman WH, Prout TE, et al: Syndrome of bilateral pheochromocytoma, medullary thyroid carcinoma and multiple neuromas. A possible regulatory defect in the differentiation of chromaffin tissue. N Engl J Med 279:1, 1968.
Stackpole RH, Melicow MM, Uson AC: Pheochromocytoma in children. Report of 9 cases and review of the first 100 published cases with follow-up studies. J Pediatr 63:315, 1963.
Voorhess ML: Urinary catecholamine excretion by healthy children. I: Daily excretion of dopamine, norepinephrine, epinephrine and 3-methoxy-4-hydroxymandelic acid. Pediatrics 39:252, 1967.
Voorhess ML: Neuroblastoma-pheochromocytoma: Products and pathogenesis. Ann NY Acad Sci 230:187, 1974.
Wise KS, Gibson JA: Von Hippel–Lindau's disease and pheochromocytoma. Br Med J 1:441, 1971.

ADRENAL CALCIFICATION

Crocker AC, Vawter GF, Neuhauser EBO, et al: Wolman's disease: Three new patients with recently described lipidosis. Pediatrics 35:627, 1965.
Hill EE, Williams JA: Massive adrenal haemorrhage in the newborn. Arch Dis Child 34:178, 1959.
Jarvis JL, Seaman WB: Idiopathic adrenal calcification in infants and children. Am J Roentgenol 82:510, 1959.
Stevenson J, MacGregor AM, Connelly P: Calcification of the adrenal glands in young children: A report of three cases with a review of the literature. Arch Dis Child 36:316, 1961.

19.29 DISORDERS OF THE GONADS

FUNCTION OF THE TESTES. Testosterone. In the 1st trimester of pregnancy, levels of placental chorionic gonadotropin peak (8–12 wk) and stimulate the fetal Leydig cells to secrete testosterone, the main hormonal product of the testis. This period (8–12 wk) is critical for normal virilization of the XY fetus. Defects in this process of fetal masculinization lead to different forms of male pseudohermaphroditism (see Sec. 19.42). After masculinization occurs, fetal levels of testosterone decrease but are maintained at low levels in the latter half of pregnancy by LH secreted by the fetal pituitary; this is required for continued penile growth.

Shortly after birth a transient increase of gonadotropins, especially LH, occurs, leading to a sharp increase in serum levels of testosterone, which peak at about 1–3 mo of age (80–400 ng/dL). Thereafter, levels of gonadotropins subside, and by 6 mo of age levels of testosterone decrease to the low prepubertal levels (10–20 ng/mL) that persist until the beginning of puberty. The significance of this "mini-puberty" in the neonate is not known. Neonates with testicular torsion and atrophy have very low levels of testosterone and markedly elevated levels of FSH and LH. Development of nocturnal pulsatile secretion of LH marks the advent of puberty (see Sec. 19.6).

Within specific target cells, about 6–8% of testosterone is converted by 5α-reductase to dehydrotestosterone, another potent androgen (see Fig. 19–18), and about 0.3% is acted on by aromatase to produce estradiol (Fig. 19–15). Approximately half of circulating testosterone is bound to *sex hormone–binding globulin* (SHBG) and half to albumin; only 2% circulates in the free form. Plasma levels of SHBG are low at birth, rise rapidly during the first 10 days of life, and then remain stable until the onset of puberty. Thyroid hormone may play a role in this physiologic increase because neonates with athyreosis have very low levels of SHBG.

Müllerian-inhibiting factor (MIF), also termed antimüllerian hormone (AMH), is a glycoprotein hormone secreted by the Sertoli cells of the fetal testes. It causes involution of the embryologic precursors of the cervix, uterus, and fallopian tubes (müllerian ducts) during sexual differentiation. Recent studies indicate that MIF persists after birth; levels remain elevated until about 2 yr of age, diminishing thereafter but remaining measurable until just before puberty. Its function after involution of the müllerian ducts is unknown.

Inhibin is another glycoprotein hormone secreted by the Sertoli cells of the testes. This recently characterized hormone consists of α and β subunits and appears to have an important regulatory role in the secretion of FSH. In the 1st yr of life, levels are elevated; then they decrease and rise again during puberty, correlating with those of FSH. Since current RIAs measure dimeric inhibin as well as inhibin proteins, the precise role of this hormone has yet to be elucidated.

The functional integrity of the pituitary-testicular axis in the neonate can be assessed by the measurement of FSH, LH, and testosterone levels. In the near future, measurements of MIF and inhibin levels may also become clinically useful. After the neonatal period, the ability of the quiescent prepubertal testes to secrete testosterone can be assessed by admin-

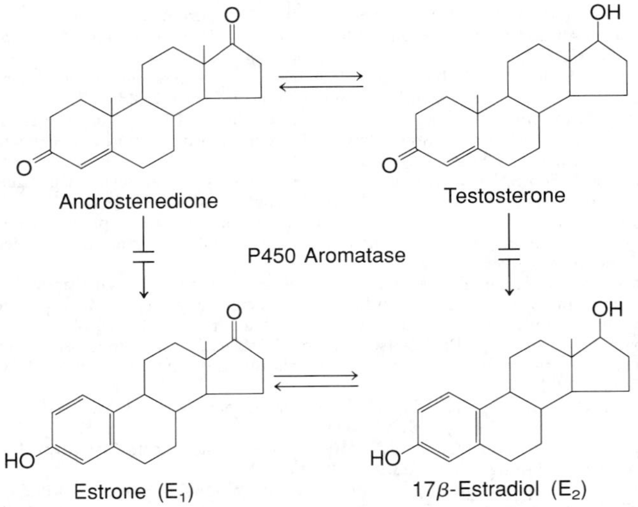

Figure 19–15. Conversion of androgens to estrogens. Aromatase activity results in loss of the C-19 methyl group and the formation of an aromatic A ring.

istering chorionic gonadotropin (hCG), which stimulates the Leydig cells in a manner analogous to LH. Many different dosage schedules have been devised; a common regimen is intramuscular administration of 3,000 units/m^2 once daily for 3–5 days.

Clinical patterns of pubertal changes vary widely (see Sec. 3.9 and 9.6). In 95% of boys enlargement of the genitalia begins between 9½ and 13½ yr, reaching maturity from 13 to 17 yr. In a small minority of normal boys puberty begins after 15 yr of age. In 50% of boys pubic hair is present by 11 yr of age, and by 13–17½ yr it is equivalent in amount to that of normal adult females. In some boys pubertal development is completed in less than 2 yr, whereas in others it may take longer than 4½ yr. The adolescent growth spurt occurs later in boys than in girls at corresponding levels of sexual maturation; for example, the peak velocity of change in height is not attained in boys until the genitalia are well developed, whereas in girls the growth rate is usually at its maximum when the nipple and areola have developed but before there is any other significant breast development.

The median age of sperm production (*spermarche*) is 14 yr. This event occurs in midpuberty as judged by pubic hair, testes size, evidence of growth spurt, and testosterone levels. Night-time levels of FSH are in the adult male range at the time of spermarche; the first conscious ejaculation occurs at about the same time.

FUNCTION OF THE OVARIES. The most important estrogens produced by the ovary are estradiol-17β (E_2) and estrone (E_1); estriol is a metabolic product of these two, and all three estrogens may be found in the urine of mature females. Estrogens also arise from androgens, both in the adrenal and in the testis; the pathway for this conversion is shown in Figure 19–15. This conversion explains why in certain types of male pseudohermaphroditism feminization occurs at puberty; in 17-ketosteroid reductase deficiency, for example, the enzymatic block results in markedly increased secretion of androstenedione, which is converted in the peripheral tissues to estradiol and estrone; these estrogens, in addition to those directly secreted by the testis, result in gynecomastia. The ovary also synthesizes progesterone, a progestational steroid; adrenal cortex and testis also synthesize progesterone as a precursor for other adrenal and testicular hormones.

Plasma levels of estradiol increase slowly but steadily with advancing sexual maturation and correlate well with clinical evaluation of pubertal development, skeletal age, and rising levels of FSH. Levels of LH do not rise until secondary sexual characteristics are well developed. Estrogens, like androgens, inhibit secretion of both LH and FSH (negative feedback). In females estrogens also provoke the surge of LH secretion that occurs in the midmenstrual cycle. The capacity for this positive feedback is another maturational milestone of puberty. The average age at menarche in American girls is 12½–13 yr, but the range of "normal" is wide, and 1–2% of "normal" girls have not menstruated by 16 yr of age. Menarche generally correlates closely with skeletal age (see Sec. 3.9 and 9.6).

DIAGNOSTIC AIDS. Rapid advances in understanding the hypothalamic-pituitary-gonadal interactions involved with puberty and in the clinical diagnosis of aberrations of pubertal development have been made possible by markedly improved assays for pituitary and gonadal hormones that can be measured in small amounts of blood. With LHRH it is also possible to differentiate between primary pituitary and hypothalamic defects in hypogonadotropic patients.

THERAPEUTIC AIDS. Naturally occurring estrogens administered orally are rapidly destroyed by gastrointestinal and liver enzymes; accordingly, they are usually given as conjugates or esters. The most widely used oral preparations are equine conjugated estrogens (e.g., Premarin) and ethinyl estradiol. Androgens are generally injected as long-acting esters (enanthate, cyclopentylpropionate, or phenylacetate) because of their potency and steady response. Oral preparations, such as methyltestosterone or fluoxymesterone, do not produce as potent an androgenic response.

HYPOFUNCTION OF THE TESTES

Testicular hypofunction may be primary in the testis (primary hypogonadism) or secondary to deficiency of pituitary gonadotropic hormones (secondary hypogonadism). Patients with primary hypogonadism have elevated levels of gonadotropin (hypergonadotropic); those with secondary hypogonadism have low or absent levels (hypogonadotropic).

19.30 HYPERGONADOTROPIC HYPOGONADISM IN THE MALE

(Primary Hypogonadism)

Defects of androgen production involving the fetal testis and resulting in male pseudohermaphroditism are discussed in Sec. 19.42.

ETIOLOGY. *Congenital anorchia* occurs in 0.6% of boys with nonpalpable testes (1 in 20,000 males). These boys have normal external genitalia, indicating that a noxious factor damaged the fetal testes of the genetic male fetus sometime after sexual differentiation had taken place (14th wk of fetal life). The condition has been reported in monozygotic twins. Low levels of testosterone (<10 ng/dL) and markedly elevated levels of LH and FSH are found in the early postnatal months; thereafter, levels of gonadotropins tend to decrease even in agonadal children, rising to castrate levels as the pubertal years approach. Stimulation with hCG fails to evoke an increase in the levels of testosterone.

A syndrome of *rudimentary testes* has been described in which the testes are exceedingly small; this appears to be inherited as an autosomal or X-linked recessive trait. The etiology is unknown. *Atrophy* of the testes may follow damage to the vascular supply as a result of unskillful manipulation of the testes during surgical procedures for correction of cryptorchidism or as a result of bilateral torsion of the testes. *Acute orchitis* in pubertal or adult males with mumps may also damage the testes; usually, only the reproductive function of the testes is impaired. The routine immunization of all prepubertal males with mumps vaccine should prevent this complication.

Testicular damage is a frequent sequela of *chemotherapy* and of *radiotherapy* for cancer. The frequency and extent of damage depend on the agent used, total dosage, duration of therapy, and post-therapy interval of observation. Another important variable is age at therapy; germ cells are less vulnerable in prepubertal than in intrapubertal and postpubertal boys. On the other hand, nitrosourea administered before the age of 16 yr almost always causes permanent damage to the germinal epithelium with a high likelihood of infertility. Because of these variables, reports of the frequency and degree of testicular damage are often conflicting. Testicular function should be carefully evaluated in adolescents who have prolonged survival after multimodal treatment for cancer in childhood. Replacement therapy with testosterone or counseling concerning fertility may be indicated.

In *germinal cell aplasia (Del Castillo syndrome)* sexual maturation occurs normally, Leydig cells are normal, and testosterone secretion is normal. The testes are small, however, and the seminiferous tubules are small and devoid of germ cells. Azoospermia and infertility are the rule. The disorder has affected brothers, but the mode of transmission is not clear. FSH levels are elevated, LH levels normal. These findings are readily explained by the absence of inhibin, the specific Sertoli cell inhibitor of FSH.

The term hypogonadism has been widely used to describe aspects of children with a variety of syndromes of multiple malformations. The term often refers simply to cryptorchidism, a small phallus, or a scrotal anomaly. In many of these syndromes little is known about the function of the testes; hyper- or hypogonadotropic hypogonadism has been proved in some instances.

Varying degrees of hypogonadism also occur in a significant percentage of patients with chromosomal aberrations such as Klinefelter syndrome or XX males (see later).

CLINICAL MANIFESTATIONS. Primary hypogonadism may be suspected at birth if the testes and penis are abnormally small. The condition often is not noted until puberty is expected and secondary sex characteristics fail to develop. Facial, pubic, and axillary hair is scant or absent; there is neither acne nor regression of scalp hair, and the voice remains high pitched. The penis and scrotum remain infantile and may be almost obscured by pubic fat; the testes are small or absent. Fat accumulates in the region of the hips and buttocks and sometimes also in the breasts and on the abdomen. The epiphyses close late in life; therefore, extremities are long. The span is several inches longer than the height, and the distance from the symphysis pubis to the soles of the feet is much greater than from the symphysis to the vertex. This clinical state is also known as *eunuchism,* and the proportions of the body are described as eunuchoid. Many individuals with milder degrees of hypogonadism may be detected only by appropriate studies of the pituitary-gonadal axis.

DIAGNOSIS. Levels of serum FSH and, to a lesser extent, of LH are elevated above age-specific normal values. These elevated levels indicate that even in the prepubertal child there is an active hypothalamic-gonadal feedback relationship. After the age of 11 yr FSH and LH levels rise significantly, reaching the postmenopausal range. Plasma testosterone levels are ordinarily low in normal prepubertal children, rising during puberty to attain adult levels. During puberty these levels correlate better with testicular size and stage of sexual maturity than with age. In patients with primary hypogonadism, testosterone levels remain low at all ages, and there is an attenuated rise or no rise following administration of hCG, whereas in normal males at any stage of development hCG produces a significant rise in plasma testosterone.

Noonan Syndrome

The term Noonan syndrome has been applied to phenotypic males and females who have certain anomalies that occur also in females with Turner syndrome. These boys and girls have normal karyotypes. The disorder is usually sporadic, but affected siblings of the same and of different genders have been reported. Total or partial expression is present in 20% of relatives. Reports of male-to-male transmission suggest an autosomal dominant gene with variable expressivity.

The most common abnormalities are short stature, webbing of the neck, pectus carinatum or pectus excavatum, cubitum valgum, congenital heart disease, and a characteristic facies. Hypertelorism, epicanthus, an antimongoloid palpebral slant, ptosis, micrognathia, and ear abnormalities are common. Other abnormalities such as clinodactyly, hernias, and vertebral anomalies occur less frequently. Moderate mental retardation occurs in 25% of patients. The cardiac defect is most often pulmonary valvular stenosis or atrial septal defect. Recent reports of a number of children with the Noonan phenotype associated with *neurofibromatosis* suggest a separate disorder. Males frequently have cryptorchidism and small testes; they may be hypogonadal or normal. Puberty is delayed 2 yr on average; adult height is achieved by the end of the 2nd decade and usually reaches the lowest limit of the normal population. Premature ovarian failure has been noted in at least one teenage girl.

Klinefelter Syndrome

ETIOLOGY. Approximately 1 in 1,000 newborn males has a 47,XXY chromosome complement. The incidence approximates 1% among the mentally retarded, clustering among patients with IQs above 50 and among children admitted to psychiatric hospitals or referred to psychiatric clinics. The chromosomal aberration most often results from meiotic nondisjunction of an X chromosome during parental gametogenesis; the extra X chromosome is maternal in origin in 67% and paternal in origin in 33% of patients. Increased maternal age predisposes to meiotic nondisjunction and to this syndrome, but in most instances maternal age is not advanced.

The 47,XXY complement is the most common chromosomal pattern in persons with Klinefelter syndrome; some have mosaic patterns: 46,XY/47,XXY; 46,XY/48,XXYY; 45,X/46,XY/46,XXY; or 46,XX/47,XXY. Rarely, occurrence of more than two X chromosomes may result in Klinefelter variants: 48,XXXY; 49,XXXYY; 49,XXXXY; 50,XXXXYY; 47,XXY/48,XXXY; 47,XXY/49,XXXXY; or 48,XXYY karyotype. Even with as many as four X chromosomes, the Y chromosome determines a male phenotype.

CLINICAL MANIFESTATIONS. The diagnosis is rarely made prior to puberty because of the paucity or subtleness of clinical manifestations in childhood. Since behavioral or psychiatric disorders may often be apparent long before defects in sexual development, the condition should be considered in all boys with mental retardation as well as in children with psychosocial, learning, or school adjustment problems. Affected children may be anxious, immature, excessively shy, or aggressive; they may engage in antisocial acts. Fire-setting behavior has been noted in some of these children. Problems often first become apparent after the child begins school. The patients tend to be tall, slim, and underweight and to have relatively long legs, but body habitus can vary markedly. The testes tend to be small for age, but this sign may become substantially apparent only after puberty, when normal testicular growth fails to occur. The phallus tends to be smaller than average, and cryptorchidism or hypospadias may occur in a few patients.

Pubertal development may be delayed. Some degree of androgen deficiency is usually noted, though some patients may undergo almost normal masculinization. About 80% of adults have gynecomastia; they have sparser facial hair, most shaving less than daily. Azoospermia and infertility are usual, though rare instances of fertility are known. Height tends to be increased. There is also an increased incidence of pulmonary disease, varicose veins, cancer of the breast, and extragonadal germ cell neoplasms, particularly within the mediastinum and brain.

In a prospective study a group of children with 47,XXY karyotypes identified at birth exhibited relatively mild deviations from normal during the first 5 yr of life. None had major physical, intellectual, or emotional disabilities; some were inactive, with poorly organized motor function and mild delay in language acquisition.

In adults with XY/XXY *mosaicism* the features of Klinefelter syndrome are decreased in severity and frequency. Little is known of children with mosaicism, but they have a better prognosis for virilization, fertility, and psychosocial adjustment. The XXYY *male* phenotype is not distinctively different from that of the XXY patient except that XXYY adults tend to be taller than the average XXY patient.

Klinefelter Variants. When the number of X chromosomes exceeds two, the clinical manifestations, including mental retardation and impairment of virilization, are more severe. The 49,XXXXY variant has been reported in more than 100 patients and is sufficiently distinctive to be detected in childhood. The disorder arises from sequential nondisjunction in meiosis. Affected patients are severely retarded, and many have large malformed ears, a short neck, and a typical facies with wide-set eyes that have a mild mongoloid slant; epicanthus, strabismus, a wide, flat upturned nose, and a large open mouth may also be present. The testes are small and may be undescended, the scrotum is hypoplastic, and the penis is very small. Defects suggestive of Down syndrome (such as short incurved terminal 5th phalanges, single palmar creases, and hypotonia) and other skeletal abnormalities (including defects in the carrying angle of the elbows and restricted supination) are common. The most frequent radiographic abnormalities are radioulnar synostosis or dislocation, elongated radius, pseudoepiphyses, scoliosis or kyphosis, coxa valga, and retarded osseous age. Most patients with such extensive changes have a 49,XXXXY chromosome karyotype; the following mosaic patterns have also been observed: 48,XXXY/49,XXXXY (Fig. 19–16); 48,XXXY/49,XXXXY/-50,XXXXXY; and 48,XXXY/49,XXXXY/50,XXXXYY.

LABORATORY DATA. The chromosomes should be examined in all patients suspected of Klinefelter syndrome, particularly those attending child guidance, psychiatric, and mental retardation clinics. Prior to 10 yr of age boys with 47,XXY Klinefelter syndrome have normal basal plasma levels of FSH and LH. Responses to gonadotropin-stimulating hormone and to hCG are also normal. The testes show normal growth early in puberty, but by midpuberty testicular growth stops, gonadotropins become elevated, and testosterone levels are slightly low. Elevated levels of estradiol resulting in a high estradiol:testosterone ratio account for the development of gynecomastia during puberty.

Testicular biopsy before puberty may reveal only a deficiency or absence of germinal cells. After puberty the seminiferous tubular membranes are hyalinized, and there is adenomatous clumping of Leydig cells. Azoospermia is characteristic, and infertility is the rule.

TREATMENT. Replacement therapy with a long-acting testosterone preparation should begin at 11–12 yr of age. The enanthate ester may be used in a starting dose of 50 mg injected intramuscularly every 3 wk with 50-mg increments every 6–9 mo until a maintenance dose for adults (200–250 mg every 3–4 wk) is achieved. For older boys larger initial doses and increments can achieve more rapid virilization.

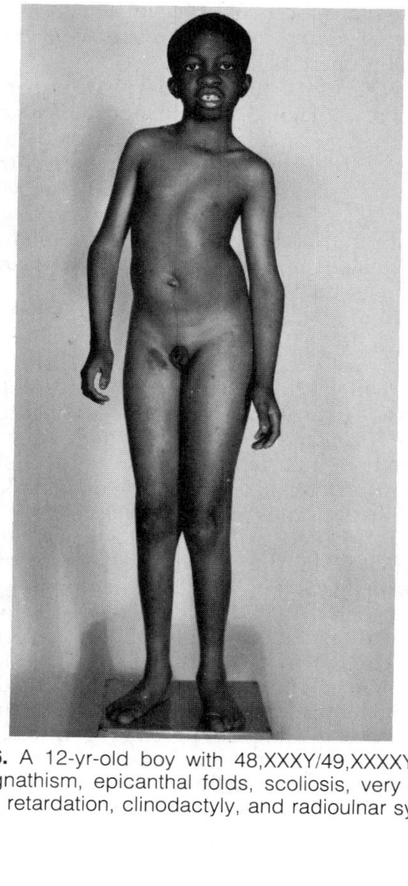

Figure 19–16. A 12-yr-old boy with 48,XXXY/49,XXXXY mosaicism, who has prognathism, epicanthal folds, scoliosis, very small testes, severe mental retardation, clinodactyly, and radioulnar synostoses.

XX Males

Approximately 140 males with 46,XX chromosome constitution have been identified; the disorder is thought to occur in 1 in 25,000 newborn males. Affected individuals have a male phenotype, small testes, a small phallus, and no evidence of ovarian or müllerian duct tissue; they appear, therefore, to be distinct from the XX true hermaphrodite (Sec. 19.43). This disorder resembles Klinefelter syndrome, but stature is greater in the latter. The histologic features of the testes are essentially the same in the two conditions. Only about 20% of reported patients have been prepubertal; patients with the condition usually come to medical attention in adult life because of hypogonadism or gynecomastia. About 50% of those detected as children have had hypospadias or chordee. Hypergonadotropic hypogonadism occurs secondary to testicular failure.

For 2 decades it has been theorized that male-determining genes have been translocated from the Y chromosome to the X chromosome. It is now established that one of the X chromosomes carries the testis-determining factor (TDF). This gene has been designated SRY (sex-determining region of the Y). The exchange from the Y to the X chromosome occurs during paternal meiosis, when the short arms of the Y and X chromosomes pair. Thus, XX males inherit one maternal X chromosome and one paternal X chromosome containing the translocated male-determining gene. Such exchanges occur because of the proximity of TDF to the pseudoautosomal region where recombination between X and Y chromosomes normally occurs in meiosis. Probes are now available to determine the amount of the Y material transferred to the X chromosome of XX males (see Sec. 19.40).

XYY Males

The 47,XYY male does not have hypogonadism; his condition is discussed here for easy comparison with the XXY and the XX male syndromes.

Approximately 1 in 1,000 newborn males has an XYY chromosome pattern. When this disorder was first discovered in adults, studies of XYY individuals in mental or penal institutions created a stereotype of affected individuals as having deviant behavior marked by physical aggressiveness and violence. It now appears that the rate at which XYY males are found in mental or penal settings may be as high as 20 times the rate at which they are born. Adults with this karyotype may be relatively impulsive, antisocial, and likely to break the law, but they are not especially aggressive. Unselected 47,XXY boys detected in screening programs tend to exhibit attention deficits, impulsive behavior, inadequate poor interactions, and poor self-image. Patients with 48,XXYY and 48,XYYY karyotypes also tend to have similar deviant behavior.

The XYY adult has few phenotypic manifestations. He tends

to be tall and to have severe nodulocystic acne. In affected persons genital abnormalities have been noted, but cryptic mosaicism, such as X/XYY, is a possibility in these instances. Prolonged P-R intervals on electrocardiography and radioulnar synostosis appear to occur more often than in the general population. No clear-cut endocrine abnormalities have been found. This condition poses a serious dilemma for counseling of parents of infants or children discovered to have this sex chromosome complement. The risks for some developmental disability may not be trivial, but neither do they appear to be as dire as earlier thought.

19.31 HYPOGONADOTROPIC HYPOGONADISM IN THE MALE
(Secondary Hypogonadism)

In hypogonadotropic hypogonadism there is deficiency of FSH or LH. The primary defect may lie in the anterior pituitary or in the hypothalamus as a deficiency of gonadotropin-releasing hormone. The testes are normal but remain in the prepubertal state because stimulation by gonadotropins is lacking.

ETIOLOGY. Hypopituitarism. Most causes of hypopituitarism may be associated with deficiency of gonadotropins and hypogonadotropic hypogonadism (see Sec. 19.2). In patients with organic lesions in or near the pituitary (e.g., craniopharyngioma), the gonadotropin deficiency is pituitary in origin. On the other hand, in many patients with "idiopathic" or "familial" hypopituitarism, the defect resides in the hypothalamus and is caused by a deficiency of LHRH. Microphallus (<2.5 cm) in the newborn male with growth hormone deficiency suggests the likelihood of gonadotropin deficiency, and diagnostic confirmation is feasible; after 6 mo of age gonadotropin deficiency cannot be established with certainty until the teenage years.

Isolated Deficiency of Gonadotropin. Usually this disorder involves the hypothalamus rather than the pituitary. It affects about 1 in 10,000 males and 1 in 50,000 females and encompasses a heterogeneous group of entities. LHRH deficiency may be complete or partial; it may occur sporadically or as a component of the **Kallmann syndrome**, a disorder characterized by anosmia and LHRH deficiency. The LHRH-secreting neurons arise within the nasal placode, the precursor of the nose, and migrate into the hypothalamus during fetal life, thus explaining the association of LHRH deficiency with agenesis of the olfactory lobes.

The disorder has been transmitted in an autosomal dominant, autosomal recessive, or X-linked fashion. In the X-linked form of the disease, the gene has been localized to the Xp 22.3 region. Some kindreds contain anosmic individuals with and without hypogonadism; others include hypogonadal individuals who are euosmic. Cleft palate, hypotelorism, median facial clefts, and other findings occur in some affected families.

In some patients more complex phenotypes have been described, including association of the Kallmann syndrome with steroid sulfatase deficiency, a cause of *X-linked ichthyosis*. Since the Xp 22.3 region contains contiguous genes for the Kallmann syndrome, steroid sulfatase, chondrodysplasia punctata (Conradi syndrome), and others, associations of these conditions have occurred as a result of varying X chromosome deletions. Several families have been reported with X-linked ichthyosis and hypogonadism without anosmia, whereas in another kindred of 10 males in four generations hypogonadotropic hypogonadism was associated with anosmia, ichthyosis, and mild mental retardation.

Hypogonadotropic hypogonadism is associated with the X-linked form of *congenital adrenal hypoplasia* (Sec. 19.22) and has been observed in two young men with *polyglandular autoimmune syndrome*. A variety of other syndromes such as Bardet-Biedl, Prader-Willi, multiple lentigines, and several syndromes of ataxia have been reported in association with hypogonadism. Many of these have not been evaluated by current techniques, and the sites of the defects are unknown. It is not known whether or not these patients had markedly delayed puberty that eventually resolved spontaneously.

DIAGNOSIS. Levels of gonadotropins and gonadal steroids remain in the prepubertal range, and nocturnal pulsatile secretion of LH does not occur. The gonadotropin response to the standard LHRH stimulation test is markedly blunted. All of these findings are also consistent with those observed in normal adolescents with the variant known as *constitutional delayed puberty*; a variety of tests proposed in the past to separate these two conditions have proved inadequate. Recently, preliminary data suggest that a single test dose of a potent LHRH agonist will evoke a greater release of LH in patients with constitutional growth delay than in those with deficiency of LH; further evaluation of this test is necessary.

Gonadotropin deficiency is likely if the patient has other evidence of pituitary deficiency, such as a deficiency of growth hormone, particularly if it is associated with ACTH deficiency. The presence of anosmia usually indicates permanent gonadotropin deficiency, but occasional instances of markedly delayed puberty (18–20 yr of age) have been observed in anosmic individuals. Although anosmia may be present in the family or in the patient from early childhood, its existence is rarely volunteered, and direct questioning is necessary in all patients with delayed puberty. Prolactinomas are being increasingly recognized as a cause of delayed puberty and should be ruled out by determination of serum levels of prolactin.

Probes are available to establish the diagnosis in heterozygotes and newborn infants with the X-linked form of Kallmann syndrome. During the first 3–4 mo of life unaffected infants demonstrate the usual physiologic rise in gonadotropins and gonadal steroids, and the response to LHRH exceeds that seen in prepubertal children.

TREATMENT. Constitutional delayed puberty must be ruled out before a diagnosis of isolated deficiency of LHRH can be established. Testicular volume of less than 4 mL by 14 yr of age occurs in about 3% of boys, whereas true hypogonadotropic hypogonadism is a rare condition. Even relatively moderate delays in sexual development and growth may result in significant psychologic distress and require attention. Initially, an explanation of the variations characteristic of puberty and reassurance suffice for the majority of boys. If by 15 yr of age there is no clinical evidence of puberty beginning and the testosterone level is less than 50 ng/dL, a brief course of testosterone is indicated. Testosterone enanthate, 100–200 mg intramuscularly once monthly for 4 mo, usually initiates puberty and differentiates constitutional delay in puberty from isolated gonadotropin deficiency. Only rarely is a second course indicated if puberty is not sustained.

Patients with established deficiency of gonadotropins can be treated with the same program of repository testosterone as that used for those with primary testicular deficiency (see Sec. 19.30). With this therapy the testes will remain small. Treatment with hCG, given subcutaneously or intramuscularly in doses of 500–1,000 IU, 3 times weekly, will stimulate growth of the testes and spermatogenesis. If after 6–12 mo of therapy sufficient growth of the testes has not occurred, human menopausal gonadotropin may be added in doses of 37.5–150 IU, 3 times weekly. It may require up to 2 yr of treatment to achieve adequate spermatogenesis in adults.

A more physiologic but cumbersome form of treatment consists of episodic administration (subcutaneously or intravenously) of LHRH. Long-term therapy has been utilized with a programmable peristalic infusion pump. Most patients require about 2 yr of treatment to maximize testicular growth and to achieve spermatogenesis.

19.32 PSEUDOPRECOCITY RESULTING FROM TUMORS OF THE TESTES

Leydig cell tumors of the testis are rare causes of precocious pseudopuberty. Leydig cells are sparse before puberty; tumors derived from them are more common in the adult. About 50 cases have been reported in children, including one member in each of two pairs of identical twins. These tumors are usually unilateral and benign. Reinke crystalloids are a characteristic microscopic feature but are present in fewer than 50% of Leydig cell tumors.

The clinical manifestations are those of puberty in the male; onset occurs usually from 5 to 9 yr of age. Gynecomastia has occurred in five patients. The tumor of the testis can usually be readily felt; the contralateral unaffected testis is normal in size for the age of the patient.

Plasma levels of testosterone are markedly elevated. FSH and LH levels are suppressed, and there is no response to LHRH. Ultrasound may aid in the detection of small nonpalpable tumors. Treatment consists of surgical removal of the affected testis. Progression of virilization ceases, and partial reversal of the signs of precocity may occur.

Testicular adrenal rests may develop into tumors that mimic Leydig cell tumors; in the absence of Reinke crystals these two tumors cannot be differentiated histologically. Adrenal rest tumors are usually bilateral and occur in patients with congenital adrenal hyperplasia, usually salt-losers, during adolescence or young adult life. The stimulus for the growth of the adrenal rests is inadequate corticosteroid suppressive therapy, and treatment with adequate doses almost always results in their regression. Definite evidence of the origin of these tumors has been achieved by demonstrating their 21-hydroxylase activity. The misdiagnosis of these tumors in patients with congenital adrenal hyperplasia has led to unnecessary orchidectomy. Successful pregnancy after treatment of adrenal rest tumors by conservative steroid replacement therapy has been reported.

The *fragile X syndrome* is another cause of testicular enlargement (macro-orchidism). Volumes of more than 3 mL are found in 15–40% of affected prepubertal boys, and the condition has been recognized in a child as young as 5 mo of age; after puberty, 80% of these patients have testicular enlargement, which usually reaches 40–50 mL. The testes are bilaterally enlarged and are not nodular. There is no evidence of precocious puberty. Hormonal studies and testicular histology are normal. Males with this condition have a constriction near the end of the X chromosome at position Xp 27.3 and are mentally retarded (see Sec. 7.30). Identification of affected boys requires genetic screening of their families.

In boys with *unilateral cryptorchidism* the contralateral testis is about 25% larger than normal for age.

19.33 GYNECOMASTIA

Gynecomastia, or the occurrence of mammary tissue in the male, is a common condition. It is almost always a sign of estrogen-androgen imbalance, but its cause is often obscure. It occurs in most newborn males as a result of stimulation by maternal hormones. The effect disappears in a few weeks.

During midpuberty approximately two thirds of boys develop varying degrees of subareolar hyperplasia of the breasts. *Physiologic pubertal gynecomastia* may involve only one breast, and it is not unusual for both breasts to enlarge at disproportionate rates or at different times. Tenderness of the breast is common but transitory. Spontaneous regression may occur within a few mo; it rarely persists longer than 2 yr. Mean concentrations of FSH, LH, prolactin, testosterone, estrone, and estradiol are the same as in boys without gynecomastia. When, however, levels are correlated with stage of puberty, a decreased ratio of testosterone to estradiol is found in boys with gynecomastia. Treatment usually consists of reassurance of the boy and his family of the physiologic and transient nature of the phenomenon. Surgical removal of the breast is rarely indicated; when enlargement is striking and persistent and causes serious emotional disturbance to the patient, removal may be justified.

Occasionally, breast development may mimic female breast development (to Tanner stages 3–5) and fails to regress. *Familial gynecomastia* has occurred in several kindreds as an X-linked or autosomal dominant sex-limited trait. Levels of gonadotropins, testosterone, prolactin, and steroid-binding globulins are normal. Increased peripheral conversion of C_{19}-steroids to estrogens (increased aromatization) has been found in both familial and sporadic cases of gynecomastia and may explain some instances of this condition (see Fig. 19–15).

In young children with gynecomastia an exogenous source of estrogens must be sought. Either accidental or therapeutic exposure to small amounts of estrogens by inhalation, percutaneous absorption, or ingestion may cause gynecomastia. Increased pigmentation of the nipple and areola should suggest this cause. Gynecomastia may also be caused by exogenously administered androgens.

A number of other pathologic conditions may cause gynecomastia. It has been noted in four reports of children with the 11β-hydroxylase–deficient form of congenital virilizing adrenal hyperplasia. It may be associated with Leydig cell tumors of the testis or with feminizing tumors of the adrenal. Four young boys with the *Peutz-Jeghers syndrome* and gynecomastia had *sex-cord tumors with annular tubules* of the testes. The testis may not be enlarged; the tumor is usually multifocal and bilateral. Extensive study of one tumor established excessive aromatase production to account for the gynecomastia. Gynecomastia occurs in patients with Klinefelter syndrome and with other types of testicular failure (hypergonadotropic states). It is a common finding in boys with certain types of male pseudohermaphroditism, particularly Reifenstein syndrome, the testicular feminization syndrome, and in patients with the 17-ketosteroid reductase defect. When gynecomastia is associated with galactorrhea, a prolactinoma should be considered. In adults gynecomastia occurs with liver cirrhosis, with digitalis therapy for congestive heart failure, with bronchogenic carcinoma, with administration of various nonsteroidal therapeutic agents, and with heavy marijuana smoking. Ketoconazole, an antifungal drug, causes gynecomastia by directly inhibiting testosterone synthesis. In a pubertal boy with fibrolamellar carcinoma of the liver, the associated gynecomastia and elevated estrogen level were attributed to increased aromatization of circulating androgens by the tumor.

HYPOFUNCTION OF THE OVARIES

Hypofunction of the ovaries may be due to congenital failure of development, to postnatal destruction (primary or hypergonadotropic hypogonadism), or to lack of stimulation by the pituitary (secondary or hypogonadotropic hypogonadism). Many chronic diseases may result in the latter type.

19.34 HYPERGONADOTROPIC HYPOGONADISM IN THE FEMALE
(Primary Hypogonadism)

Diagnosis of hypergonadotropic hypogonadism prior to puberty is possible. Except in the case of Turner syndrome, most affected patients have no prepubertal clinical manifestations.

Turner Syndrome

In 1938 Turner described a syndrome consisting of sexual infantilism, webbed neck, and cubitum valgum in adult females. Such women have elevated levels of urinary gonadotropins and their gonads consist of rudimentary elongated streaks containing no germinal elements but whorls of connective tissue suggestive of ovarian stroma.

PATHOGENESIS. In 1959 it was demonstrated that patients with Turner syndrome have a single X chromosome (45,X). In about 30% of patients with the Turner phenotype, the chromosomal constitution consists of mosaics or nonmosaic partial deletion of one of the X chromosomes. Deletions of the short arm of the X chromosome do not affect ovarian function but do result in short stature and the Turner phenotype. On the other hand, deletions of the long arm of one of the X chromosomes in the q13–q27 band lead to failure of ovarian development.

Turner syndrome occurs in about 1 in 3,000 live-born females. The frequency of the 45,X karyotype at conception is about 1.5%, but 95% of these are spontaneously aborted, accounting for 5–10% of all abortuses. Mosaicism (45,X/46,XX) occurs in about 25% of patients with Turner syndrome, a proportion higher than that seen with any other aneuploid state, whereas the mosaic Turner constitution is rare among the abortuses; these findings indicate preferential survival for mosaic forms.

The normal fetal ovary contains about 7 million oocytes, but these begin to disappear rapidly at about 5 mo of gestation. At birth there are only 3 million, by menarche there are 400,000, and at menopause 10,000 remain. In the absence of one X chromosome, this process is accelerated, and nearly all oocytes are gone by 2 yr of age. In aborted 45,X fetuses, the number of primordial germ cells in the gonadal ridge appears to be normal, suggesting that the normal process is accelerated in patients with Turner syndrome. Eventually, the ovaries are described as "streaks" and consist only of connective tissue, but a few germ cells may persist.

CLINICAL MANIFESTATIONS. In the past the diagnosis was generally first suspected in childhood or at puberty when sexual maturation failed to occur. Now many patients with Turner syndrome are recognizable at birth because of a characteristic edema of the dorsa of the hands and feet and loose skinfolds at the nape of the neck. Significantly low birthweight and decreased length are common. Clinical manifestations in childhood include webbing of the neck, a low posterior hairline, small mandible, prominent ears, epicanthic folds, high arched palate, a broad chest presenting the illusion of widely spaced nipples, cubitum valgum, and hyperconvex fingernails.

Short stature, the cardinal finding in all girls with Turner syndrome, may be present with minimal other clinical manifestations. During the first 3 yr of life the rate of growth is normal, albeit in the lower percentiles; thereafter, it begins to decelerate and results in significant short stature. Sexual maturation fails to occur at the expected age. The mean adult height is 143 cm (132–155 cm) (Fig. 19–17). Pigmented nevi become more prominent with increasing age.

Associated covert defects are common. Complete cardiologic evaluation, including echocardiography, reveals isolated nonstenotic bicuspid aortic valves in about one third of

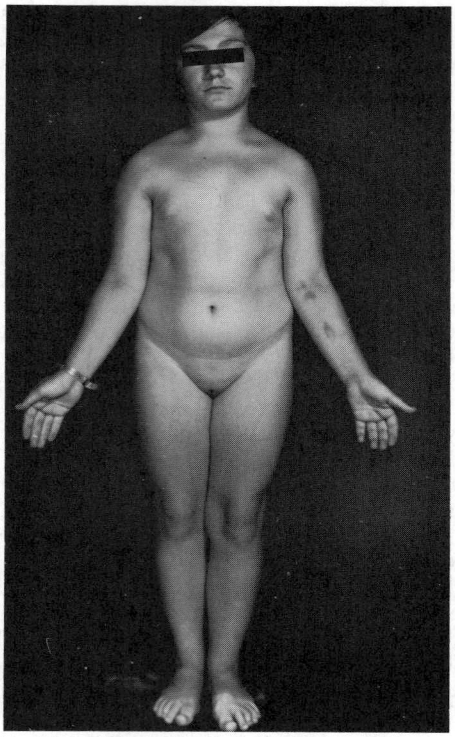

Figure 19–17. Turner syndrome in a 15-yr-old girl exhibiting failure of sexual maturation, short stature, cubitus valgus, and a goiter. There is no webbing of the neck. Karyotype revealed 45,X/46,XX chromosome complement, and urinary gonadotropin was over 96 mouse units/24 hr. T_4 was 2.2 μg/dL. Biopsy of the thyroid revealed lymphocytic thyroiditis.

patients. Less frequent but more serious defects include aortic stenosis, aortic coarctation, and anomalous pulmonary venous drainage. Approximately one third of patients have renal malformations on ultrasound examination. The more serious defects include pelvic kidney, horseshoe kidney, double collecting system, complete absence of one kidney, and ureteropelvic junction obstruction.

When the ovaries are examined by ultrasound, small but nonstreak ovaries are found in half the patients in the first 4 yr of life; between 4 and 10 yr of age the ovaries appear as streaks in 90% of patients. Sexual maturation usually fails to occur, but 10–20% of girls have spontaneous breast development, and an occasional girl may even have some menstrual periods. Fertility has been reported in about 12 45,X patients.

Recurrent bilateral otitis media occurs in about 75% of patients. Sensorineural hearing deficits are common and frequency increases with age. Increased problems with gross and fine motor-sensory integration, failure to walk before 15 mo of age, and early language dysfunction often raise questions about developmental delay, but intelligence is normal. In adults, deficits in perceptual spatial skills are more common than they are in the general population.

The presence of a goiter should suggest lymphocytic thyroiditis. Abdominal pain, tenesmus, or bloody diarrhea may represent inflammatory bowel disease; and recurrent gastrointestinal bleeding may indicate gastrointestinal telangiectasia.

In patients with 45,X/46,XX mosaicism the abnormalities are attenuated and fewer; short stature is as frequent as it is in the 45,X patient and may be the only manifestation of the condition other than ovarian failure (see Fig. 19–17).

LABORATORY DATA. Chromosomal analysis must be considered in all short girls. If a chromosomal fragment is present that cannot be clearly identified cytogenetically, DNA probe analysis is indicated to rule out the presence of a Y chromosome (see later discussion of mixed gonadal dysgenesis). Ultrasound of the heart, kidneys, and ovaries is indicated once the diagnosis is established. The most common skeletal abnormalities are shortening of the 4th metatarsal and metacarpal bones, epiphyseal dysgenesis in the joints of the knees and elbows, Madelung deformity, scoliosis, and, in older patients, inadequate osseous mineralization.

Plasma levels of gonadotropins, particularly FSH, are markedly elevated above those of age-matched controls during infancy; at about 2–3 yr of age a progressive decrease in levels occurs until they reach a nadir at 6–8 yr of age, and by 10–11 yr they rise to adult castrate levels.

Antimicrosomal thyroid antibodies should be checked periodically, and, if positive, levels of T_4 and TSH should be obtained. Extensive studies have failed to establish that growth hormone deficiency plays a primary role in the pathogenesis of the growth disorder. Mild carbohydrate intolerance in young girls tends to improve with puberty.

TREATMENT. Current data indicate that treatment with recombinant human growth hormone alone or in combination with an anabolic steroid increases height velocity. Although data on the final height of girls being treated in a large multicenter study are not complete, many girls may achieve heights of 150 cm or more.

Replacement therapy with estrogens is indicated, but there is little consensus about the optimal age at which to initiate treatment. The psychologic preparedness of the patient to accept therapy must be taken into account. In the past there has been a tendency to delay replacement therapy with estrogens in order to achieve maximal height. The improved growth achieved by girls treated with GH permits initiation of estrogen replacement at 12–13 yr. Premarin, 0.3–0.625 mg given daily for 3–6 mo, is usually effective in inducing puberty. The estrogen then is cycled (taken on days 1–23), and Provera, a progestin, is added (taken on days 10–23) in a dose of 5–10 mg daily. In the remainder of the calendar month, during which no treatment is given, withdrawal bleeding usually occurs. Other estrogen preparations and regimens of treatment are also in current use.

Psychosocial support for these girls is an integral component of treatment. The Turner Syndrome Society, which has local chapters in the United States, and similar groups in Canada and other countries provide a valuable support system for these patients and their families in addition to that given by the physician.

Pregnancy is now possible by means of ovum donation and in vitro fertilization.

XX Gonadal Dysgenesis

Some phenotypically and genetically normal females have gonadal lesions identical to those in 45,X patients but without somatic features of Turner syndrome; their condition is termed "pure" gonadal dysgenesis or *pure ovarian dysgenesis.* Here we discuss only those with the XX chromosome constitution. XY gonadal dysgenesis, also termed *Swyer syndrome,* is discussed later in the section on male pseudohermaphroditism. These two conditions are quite distinct entities; in no instance have XX and XY gonadal dysgenesis been reported in the same family.

The disorder is rarely recognized in children because the external genitalia are normal, no other abnormalities are visible, and growth is normal. At pubertal age sexual maturation fails to take place. Plasma gonadotropin levels are elevated. Delay of epiphyseal fusion results in a eunuchoid habitus. Pelvic ultrasound reveals streak ovaries.

Affected siblings, parental consanguinity, and failure to uncover mosaicism (even in the streak gonads) all point to autosomal recessive inheritance. It appears that autosomal genes have an important role in the differentiation of normal ovaries. In five families XX gonadal dysgenesis has been associated with sensorineural deafness *(Perrault syndrome).* There may be distinct genetic forms of this disorder. Tumors of the gonads have not been reported in these patients. Treatment consists of replacement therapy with estrogens.

45,X/46,XY Gonadal Dysgenesis

This condition, *mixed gonadal dysgenesis,* has extreme variability, which may extend from a Turner-like syndrome to a male phenotype with a penile urethra; it is possible to delineate three major clinical phenotypes. Short stature is a major finding in all affected patients.

Some patients have no evidence of masculinization; they have a female phenotype and often the somatic signs of Turner syndrome. The condition is discovered prepubertally when chromosomal studies are made in short girls, or later, when chromosomal studies are made because of failure of sexual maturation. Fallopian tubes and uterus are present. The gonads consist of intra-abdominal undifferentiated streaks; chromosome study of the streak often reveals an XY cell line. The streak gonad differs somewhat from that in girls with Turner syndrome; in addition to wavy connective tissue there are often tubular or cord-like structures, occasional clumps of granulosa cells, and frequently mesonephric or hilar cells.

Some patients have mild virilization manifested only by prepubertal clitorimegaly. Normal müllerian structures are present, but at puberty virilization occurs. These patients usually have an intra-abdominal testis, a contralateral streak gonad, and bilateral fallopian tubes.

Many patients present with frank ambiguity of the genitalia; this is the most frequent phenotype encountered in infants. A testis and vas deferens are found on one side in the labioscrotal fold, and a streak gonad on the contralateral side. Despite the presence of a testis, fallopian tubes are often present bilaterally. An infantile or rudimentary uterus is almost always present.

Other genotypes and phenotypes have been described. About 25% of the more than 200 reported patients have a dicentric Y chromosome (45,X/46,X,dic Y). In some patients the Y chromosome may be represented by only a fragment (45,X/45,X +fra); application of Y-specific probes can establish the origin of the fragment. It is not clear why the same genotype (45,X/46,XY) can result in such diverse phenotypes.

Patients with a female phenotype present no problem in gender of rearing. Patients who are only slightly virilized are usually assigned a female gender of rearing before a diagnosis is established. Patients with ambiguity of the genitalia are readily confused with various types of male pseudohermaphrodites. In most instances these patients are best reared as females; the short stature, the ease of genital reconstruction, and the predisposition of the gonad to develop malignancy favor this choice. In some patients followed to adulthood the putative normal testis proved to be dysgenetic with eventual loss of Leydig and Sertoli cell function.

Gonadal tumors, usually gonadoblastomas, occur in about 25% of these patients, particularly in those with the more female phenotypes. These germ cell tumors are preceded by the changes of carcinoma in situ. Accordingly, both gonads should be removed in all patients reared as girls, and the undifferentiated gonad should be removed in the few patients reared as males.

In the past, all patients came to clinical attention because of their abnormal phenotypes. However, 45,X/46,XY mosaicism is found in about 7% of fetuses with true chromosome mosaicism encountered prenatally. Of 76 infants with 45,X/46,XY mosaicism diagnosed prenatally, 72 had a normal male phenotype, 1 had a female phenotype, and only 3 males had hypospadias. Of 12 males whose gonads were examined, only 3 were abnormal. These data must be taken into account when counseling a family in which a 45,X/46,XY infant is discovered prenatally.

XXX, XXXX, and XXXXX Females

XXX FEMALES. The 47,XXX chromosomal constitution is the most frequent X chromosomal abnormality in females, occurring in almost 1 in 1,000 live-born females. This condition is most often caused by maternal meiotic nondisjunction, whereas the majority of 45,X and half of the 47,XXY constitutions are caused by paternal sex chromosome errors. The phenotype is that of a normal female; affected infants and children are not recognized.

Sexual development and menarche are normal. Most pregnancies have resulted in normal infants. However, prospective studies of infants diagnosed at birth and followed to young adult life have provided new information about these patients. By 2 yr of age, delays in speech and language become evident, and lack of coordination, poor academic performance, and immature behavior are seen. These girls tend to be tall and gangly, manifest behavior disorders, and are placed in special education classes. There is marked variability within the syndrome, and a small proportion of affected girls are well coordinated, socially outgoing, and academically superior.

XXXX AND XXXXX FEMALES. About 36 females with four X and 6 with five X chromosomes have been described. All have been mentally retarded except for one of the 48,XXXX girls. Commonly associated defects are epicanthal folds, hypertelorism, clinodactyly, simian crease, radioulnar synostosis, and congenital heart disease. Sexual maturation is often incomplete and may not occur at all. Nevertheless, one woman with the tetra-X syndrome gave birth to three normal children.

Noonan Syndrome

Girls with Noonan syndrome show certain anomalies that also occur in girls with 45,X Turner syndrome, but they have normal 46,XX chromosomes. The most common abnormalities are the same as those described for males with Noonan syndrome (see Sec. 19.30). The phenotype differs from Turner syndrome in the following respects: (1) Mental retardation is often present; (2) the cardiac defect is most often pulmonary valvular stenosis or an atrial septal defect rather than an aortic defect; and (3) gonadal defects may be present, but normal sexual maturation usually occurs.

Other Ovarian Defects

An increasing number of other young women with no chromosomal abnormality are being found to have streak gonads that may contain only occasional germ cells, if any. Gonadotropins are increased. *Cytotoxic drugs* and exposure of the ovaries to radiation for the treatment of malignancy are increasingly frequent causes of ovarian failure. A study of young women with Hodgkin disease found that combination chemotherapy and pelvic irradiation may be more deleterious than either therapy alone. Teenagers are more likely than older women to retain or recover ovarian function after either irradiation or combined chemotherapy; normal pregnancies have occurred after such treatment. Current treatment regimens may result in some ovarian damage in the majority of girls treated for cancer. The LD_{50} for the human oocyte has been estimated to be about 4 Gy.

Autoimmune ovarian failure occurs in 60% of patients over 13 yr of age with *type 1 autoimmune polyendocrinopathy* (Addison disease, hypoparathyroidism, candidiasis). Affected girls may not develop sexually, or secondary amenorrhea may occur in young women. The ovaries may have lymphocytic infiltration or appear simply as streaks. The majority of affected patients have circulating steroid cell antibodies.

The condition also occurs in young women as an isolated event or in association with other autoimmune disorders, leading to secondary amenorrhea *(premature menopause)*. About 70% of sera from affected adult patients contains antibodies against the ovaries and oocytes. Some adults treated with immunosuppressive doses of glucocorticoids resume menses and become pregnant; in one case, fertility returned spontaneously 7 yr after onset of autoimmune ovarian failure.

Galactosemia, particularly the classic form of the disease, almost always results in ovarian damage, beginning during intrauterine life. Levels of FSH and LH are elevated early in life. Ovarian damage had been thought to be caused by fetal accumulation of galactose-1-phosphate, but more recent evidence suggests that deficient UDP-galactose may be the basis for the defect (see Sec. 8.36).

Ataxia-telangiectasia may be associated with ovarian hypoplasia and elevated gonadotropins; the cause is not known. Gonadoblastomas and dysgerminomas have occurred in a few girls.

19.35 HYPOGONADOTROPIC HYPOGONADISM IN THE FEMALE
(Secondary Hypogonadism)

Hypofunction of the ovaries can result from failure to secrete normal levels of gonadotropins. The defect may lie in the anterior pituitary, but, as in the male, there is increasing evidence of a hypothalamic defect in most such hypogonadal females.

ETIOLOGY. Hypopituitarism. Destructive lesions in or near the pituitary almost always result in impaired secretion of gonadotropins as well as of other pituitary hormones. In patients with idiopathic hypopituitarism, however, the defect is usually found in the hypothalamus. In these patients administration of LHRH results in increased plasma levels of FSH and LH, establishing the integrity of the pituitary gland.

Isolated Deficiency of Gonadotropins. This heterogeneous group of disorders is only now being sorted out with the help of the LHRH test. Isolated pituitary deficiency of FSH has been documented, but in most patients the pituitary is normal, the defect residing in the hypothalamus.

Several sporadic instances of anosmia with hypogonadotropic hypogonadism have been reported. Anosmic hypogonadal females have also been reported in kindreds with Kallmann syndrome, but hypogonadism more frequently affects the males in these families.

Some autosomal recessive disorders such as the Laurence-Moon-Biedl, multiple lentigines, and Carpenter syndromes also appear in some instances to include gonadotropic hormone deficiency. Girls with severe thalassemia may have gonadotropin deficiency owing to pituitary damage caused by chronic iron overload secondary to multiple transfusions.

DIAGNOSIS. The diagnosis is not difficult in patients with other deficiencies of pituitary tropic hormones. On the other hand, it is difficult to differentiate isolated hypogonadotropic hypogonadism from physiologic delay of puberty. Repeated measurements of FSH and LH, particularly during sleep, may reveal the rising levels that herald the onset of puberty.

19.36 POLYCYSTIC OVARIES
(Stein-Leventhal Syndrome)

The classic polycystic ovaries syndrome (PCOS) is characterized by obesity, hirsutism, and secondary amenorrhea, with bilaterally enlarged polycystic ovaries, but these manifestations may not all be present. Onset often occurs at puberty or shortly thereafter; menstrual irregularities and hirsutism are the most frequent complaints. In the reproductive years, the condition is the most common cause of anovulatory infertility. The enlarged ovaries can often be felt on combined rectal and abdominal palpation, and are always demonstrable by ultrasound.

The cause of the disorder in most patients is unsettled despite intensive investigation. PCOS is a heterogeneous condition that may be associated with several distinct entities, such as late-onset 21-hydroxylase deficiency, partial deficiency of 3β-hydroxysteroid dehydrogenase, or Cushing syndrome; it also has been caused by ovarian 17-ketoreductase deficiency, the enzyme that converts androstenedione to testosterone and estrone to estradiol. However, in most patients with PCOS the elevated plasma level of free testosterone or androstenedione is not suppressed by dexamethasone, thus ruling out an adrenal cause of the disorder. About 75% of patients have an increased ratio of LH to FSH levels, an increased amplitude and frequency of plasma LH levels, and an exaggerated response to LHRH. Premenarcheal girls may have an early morning rise in LH rather than the characteristic nocturnal one. These perturbances of LH secretion are believed to bring about hyperplasia of theca cells, arrested follicular development, and impaired estradiol production. These effects lead to hyperandrogenemia and irregular cycles or amenorrhea.

Insulin-resistant hyperinsulinemia and *acanthosis nigricans* are associated with PCOS, especially in obese patients. The role of hyperinsulinemia in the etiology is not known; some investigators believe it is primary in this syndrome because suppression of androgen levels does not improve insulin resistance.

In the differential diagnosis, adrenal disorders must be ruled out. Basal levels of adrenal steroids may be normal; an ACTH (1–24) stimulation test is necessary to reveal these defects. A deficiency of 17-ketoreductase is suggested when there are affected brothers or when the estrone-estradiol and androstenedione-testosterone ratios are increased.

The optimal method of treatment is still evolving but usually consists of ovarian suppression by the contraceptive pill. Further suppression can be achieved with testolactone, a compound with antiandrogen and weak progestin properties. Attention to the obesity is important because its correction often leads to correction of the insulin resistance.

19.37 PSEUDOPRECOCITY OWING TO LESIONS OF THE OVARY

Functioning lesions of the ovary consist of benign cysts or malignant tumors. The majority synthesize estrogens; a few synthesize androgens (see also Sec. 17.24).

19.38 ESTROGENIC LESIONS OF THE OVARY

These lesions cause isosexual precocious sexual development but account for only a small percentage of all cases of precocity.

Juvenile Granulosa-Cell Tumor

In childhood the most common neoplasm of the ovary with estrogenic manifestations is the granulosa-cell tumor, although it comprises only 9% of all ovarian tumors. These tumors have distinctive histologic features that differ from those encountered in older women (adult granulosa-cell tumor). Follicles are often irregular, Call-Exner bodies are rare, and luteinization is frequent. The tumor may be solid, cystic, or both. In at least six instances this tumor has been associated with multiple enchondromas *(Ollier disease)* and in two of these cases with multiple subcutaneous hemangiomas *(Maffucci syndrome)* as well.

CLINICAL MANIFESTATIONS. The tumor has been observed in a newborn infant, and in 36 known instances sexual precocity occurred at 2 yr of age or younger; about half of these tumors have occurred before 10 yr of age. They are almost always unilateral. The breasts become enlarged, rounded, and firm and the nipples prominent. The external genitalia resemble those of a normal girl at puberty, and the uterus is enlarged. A white vaginal discharge is followed by irregular or cyclic menstruation. Ovulation, however, does not occur. The presenting manifestation may be abdominal pain or swelling. Pubic hair is usually absent unless there is mild virilization.

A mass is readily palpable in the lower portion of the abdomen in most patients by the time sexual precocity is evident. The tumor may be small, however, and escape detection even on careful rectal and abdominal examination; such tumors are usually detectable by ultrasound.

Plasma estradiol levels are markedly elevated; a 9-yr-old girl with a granulosa-cell tumor had a level of 413 pg/dL, whereas levels in fully mature women or in children with idiopathic precocious puberty are under 100 pg/dL. Plasma levels of gonadotropins are suppressed and do not respond to LHRH stimulation. α-Fetoprotein levels may be elevated. Osseous development is moderately advanced.

The tumor should be removed as soon as the diagnosis is established. Prognosis is excellent because fewer than 5% of these tumors in children are malignant. Vaginal bleeding immediately after removal of the tumor is common. Signs of precocious puberty abate and may disappear within a few months after operation. The secretion of estrogens returns to normal.

Sex-cord tumor with annular tubules is a distinctive tumor, thought to arise from granulosa cells, that occurs primarily in patients with Peutz-Jeghers syndrome. In three girls (two siblings) with Peutz-Jeghers syndrome, precocious puberty developed in association with this tumor.

Chorionepithelioma has been reported in only about 20 girls. This very malignant tumor is thought to arise from a preexisting teratoma. The usually unilateral tumor produces large amounts of chorionic gonadotropin (hCG), which stimulates the contralateral ovary to secrete estrogens and progesterone. Elevated levels of hCG are diagnostic.

Follicular Cyst

Small ovarian cysts (< 0.7 cm in diameter) are common in prepubertal children. At puberty and in girls with true isosexual precocious puberty, larger cysts (1–6 cm) are often seen; these are secondary to stimulation by gonadotropins. However, similar larger cysts occur occasionally in young girls with precocious puberty in the absence of LH and FSH. Since surgical removal or spontaneous involution of these cysts results in regression of pubertal changes, there is little doubt that they are its cause. The mechanism of production of these autonomously functioning cysts is not known. Such cysts may form only once, or they may disappear and recur, resulting in waxing and waning of the signs of precocious puberty. They may be unilateral or bilateral. The sexual precocity that occurs in young girls with McCune-Albright syndrome is usually caused by such autonomous follicular cysts (Sec. 19.7). Gonadotropins are suppressed, and estradiol levels are often markedly elevated, but they may fluctuate widely and even return to normal. LHRH stimulation fails to evoke an increase in gonadotropins. Because gonadotropins are suppressed in these patients, the mechanism of ovarian stimulation is unknown. In one girl with such a functioning cyst immunoglobulins stimulated FSH action, suggesting an autoimmune mechanism as a pathogenesis. Ultrasound is the method of choice for the detection and monitoring of such cysts. A short period of observation to ascertain a lack of spontaneous resolution is advisable before cyst aspiration or cystectomy is considered. Cystic neoplasms must be considered in the differential diagnosis.

19.39 ANDROGENIC LESIONS OF THE OVARY

Virilizing ovarian tumors are rare at all ages but particularly so in prepubertal girls. The *arrhenoblastoma* has been reported as early as 14 days of age, but fewer than 2 dozen cases have been reported in girls under 16 yr of age.

The *gonadoblastoma* occurs exclusively in dysgenetic gonads, particularly in phenotypic females who have a Y chromosome in their phenotype (46,XY; 45,X/46,XY; 45,X/46,X fra). The tumor may be bilateral. Virilization occurs with some but not all tumors. The clinical features are the same as those seen in patients with virilizing adrenal tumors and include accelerated growth, acne, clitoral enlargement, and growth of sexual hair. A palpable abdominal mass is found only in about 50% of patients. Plasma levels of testosterone and androstenedione are elevated, and those of gonadotropins are suppressed. Ultrasound and CT scans usually localize the lesion. The dysgenetic gonad of phenotypic females with a Y chromosome should be removed prophylactically. When a unilateral tumor is removed, the contralateral dysgenetic gonad should also be removed.

Virilizing manifestations occur occasionally in girls with *juvenile granulosa-cell tumors*.

19.40 HERMAPHRODITISM
(Intersexuality)

Hermaphroditism implies a discrepancy between the morphology of the gonads and that of the external genitalia. Many chromosomal aberrations resulting in ambiguity of the external genitalia have been discussed earlier in this section. Here those conditions of aberrant sexual differentiation that are imposed on the XX or XY genotype (female and male pseudohermaphrodites) are discussed (Table 19–8). An increasing number of such conditions are now understood through advances in the understanding of normal sexual differentiation. The category known as true hermaphroditism, with few exceptions, is still a poorly understood heterogeneous group of disorders.

TABLE 19–8. Etiologic Classification of Hermaphroditism

- Female pseudohermaphroditism
  - Androgen exposure
    - Fetal source
      - Congenital adrenal hyperplasia
        - 21-Hydroxylase (P_{450}c21) deficiency
        - 11β-Hydroxylase (P_{450}c11) deficiency
        - 3β-Hydroxysteroid dehydrogenase deficiency
      - Adrenal tumor?
    - Maternal source
      - Virilizing tumor
        - Ovary
        - Adrenal
      - Androgenic drugs
      - Progestational drugs
      - Placental aromatase deficiency
  - Undetermined origin
    - Usually associated with other defects (skeleton, urinary and gastrointestinal tracts)
- Male pseudohermaphroditism
  - Defect in testicular differentiation
    - Deletion of short arm of Y chromosome
    - XY pure gonadal dysgenesis (Swyer syndrome)
    - XY gonadal agenesis syndrome
    - XY antigen deficiency with camptomelic dysplasia
  - Defect in testicular hormones
    - Leydig cell aplasia—abnormality of hCG-LH receptor?
    - Inborn errors of testosterone synthesis
      - Lipoid adrenal hyperplasia (P_{450}scc) deficiency
      - 3β-Hydroxysteroid dehydrogenase deficiency
      - 17α-Hydroxylase (P_{450}c17) deficiency
      - 17,20-Lyase deficiency
      - 17-Ketosteroid reductase/17,20-lyase (P_{450}17α) deficiency
    - Defect in antimüllerian hormone action (uterine hernia syndrome)
      - Defective synthesis
      - Defective receptor
  - Defect in androgen action
    - Defect in conversion of testosterone to dihydrotestosterone—5α-reductase deficiency
    - Testicular feminization syndrome
      - Cytosol receptor defect
      - Postreceptor defect
    - Incomplete testicular feminization
    - Reifenstein syndrome
      - Decreased cytoplasmic receptor
      - Normal cytoplasmic receptor
  - Undetermined—male pseudohermaphroditism
    - With aniridia and/or Wilms tumor
    - With nephropathy and/or Wilms tumor
- True hermaphroditism
  - XX
  - XY
  - XX/XY chimeras
  - Familial

EMBRYONIC SEXUAL DIFFERENTIATION. In normal differentiation, the final form of all sexual structures is consistent with normal sex chromosomes (either XX or XY). A 46,XX complement of chromosomes is necessary for the development of normal ovaries. Both the long and the short arms of X chromosomes bear genes for normal ovarian development. An autosomal gene also appears to play a role in normal ovarian organogenesis (see XX gonadal dysgenesis, earlier). A deletion affecting the short arm of the X chromosome produces the typical somatic anomalies of Turner syndrome.

Development of the male phenotype is more complex. Maleness requires a Y chromosome, but only the short arm of the Y chromosome is critical for sex determination; a testicular-determining factor (TDF) at this site has been proposed, the gene for which has been localized. During male meiosis the Y chromosome must segregate from the X chromosome so that both X and Y chromosomes do not occur in the same spermatozoa. The major portion of the Y chromosome is composed of Y-specific sequences that do not pair with the X chromosome. However, a minor portion of the Y chromosome shares sequences with the X chromosome, and pairing does occur in this region. Since the genes and sequences in this area recombine between the sex chromosomes, they behave like autosomal genes; the term *pseudoautosomal* is used to describe the genetic behavior of these genes. The gene for TDF has now been localized adjacent to this pairing and exchange (pseudoautosomal) region of the Y chromosome and has been designated SRY (sex-determining region of the Y). This TDF gene appears to be present in most XX males and accounts for their phenotype.

TDF in some unknown way induces the indifferent genital ridge to develop into a testis. The first hormone produced by the fetal testis (6–7 wk) is müllerian-inhibiting factor (MIF), a high molecular weight glycoprotein produced by the Sertoli cells. MIF causes the müllerian ducts to regress; in its absence, they persist. By about 8 fetal wk the Leydig cells of the testis begin to produce testosterone. During this critical period of male differentiation, testosterone secretion is stimulated by placental hCG, which peaks at 8–12 wk. In the latter half of pregnancy, lower levels of testosterone are maintained by LH secreted by the fetal pituitary. Testosterone initiates virilization of the wolffian duct into the epididymis, vas deferens, and seminal vesicle. Development of the external genitalia also requires dihydrotestosterone (DHT), an active metabolite of testosterone. DHT is necessary to fuse the genital folds to form the penis and scrotum. A functional androgen receptor, controlled by an X-linked gene, is required for testosterone to effect these masculinizing changes.

In the XX fetus, the bipotential gonad does not develop into an ovary until about the 12th wk. This occurs only in the absence of testosterone and müllerian-inhibiting factor. Thus, the female phenotype develops independently of the fetal gonads, whereas maleness is imposed upon a basically female potential by the hormones of the fetal testes.

19.41 FEMALE PSEUDOHERMAPHRODITISM

In the female pseudohermaphrodite the genotype is XX and the gonads are ovaries, but the external genitalia are virilized. Since there is no müllerian-inhibiting factor, uterus, tubes, and ovaries develop. The mechanisms involved in normal female differentiation are considerably less complex than those required for male differentiation, and the varieties and causes of female pseudohermaphroditism are fewer. Most instances result from exposure of the female fetus to excessive androgens during intrauterine life; and the changes consist principally of virilization of the external genitalia (clitoral hypertrophy and labioscrotal fusion).

CONGENITAL ADRENAL HYPERPLASIA. This is the most common cause of the condition. Females with the 21-hydroxylase and 11-hydroxylase defects are the most highly virilized, though minimal virilization also occurs with the 3β-hydroxysteroid dehydrogenase defect. Salt-losers tend to have greater degrees of virilization than non–salt-losers. Masculinization may be so intense that a complete penile urethra results, and the condition may mimic a male with cryptorchidism (Sec. 19.23).

PLACENTAL AROMATASE DEFICIENCY. A single instance of a highly virilized 46,XX girl born to a mother with progressive virilization during pregnancy has been reported. Maternal serum and urinary levels of estrogen were very low, and serum levels of androgens were high. Cord serum levels of estrogen were also extremely low, whereas those of androgens were elevated. The fetal adrenal cortex normally synthesizes large quantities of DHEAS, which are metabolized to potent androgens and subsequently converted to estrogens by aromatase produced in the placenta. In vitro studies of the placenta documenting very low aromatizing activity explains this new cause of female pseudohermaphroditism (see Sec. 19.21 and Fig. 19–15).

MASCULINIZING MATERNAL TUMORS. In 18 instances the female fetus has been virilized during fetal life by a maternal androgen-producing tumor. In five cases the lesion was a benign adrenal adenoma, but all others were ovarian tumors, particularly androblastomas, luteomas, and Krukenberg tumors. Maternal virilization may be manifested by enlargement of the clitoris, acne, deepening of the voice, decreased lactation, hirsutism, and elevated levels of androgens. In the infant there is enlargement of the clitoris of varying degrees, often with labial fusion. Mothers of children with unexplained female pseudohermaphroditism should undergo measurements of their own levels of plasma testosterone and DHEAS.

ADMINISTRATION OF ANDROGENIC DRUGS TO WOMEN DURING PREGNANCY. Testosterone and 17-methyltestosterone have been reported to cause female pseudohermaphroditism in some instances. The greatest number of cases, however, have resulted from the use of certain progestational compounds for the treatment of threatened abortion. In recent years most of these progestins have been replaced by nonvirilizing ones.

Infants with female pseudohermaphroditism have been reported for whom no masculinizing agent could be identified. In such instances the disorder is usually associated with other congenital defects, particularly of the urinary and gastrointestinal tracts. No etiologic factors are known.

19.42 MALE PSEUDOHERMAPHRODITISM

In the male pseudohermaphrodite the genotype is XY, but the external genitalia are incompletely virilized, ambiguous, or completely female. When gonads can be found, they are invariably testes; their development may range from rudimentary to normal. Because the process of normal virilization in the fetus is so complex, it is not surprising that there are many varieties of male hermaphroditism.

Defects in Testicular Differentiation

The first step in male differentiation is conversion of the indifferent gonad to a testis. If in the XY fetus there is a deletion of the *short arm of the Y chromosome* or deletion of the male-determining genes, male differentiation does not occur. The phenotype is female; müllerian ducts are well developed, but gonads consist of undifferentiated streaks. By contrast, even extreme deletions of the *long arm of the Y chromosome* (Yq–) have been found in normally developed males, most of whom are azoospermic and have short stature, indicating that the long arm of the Y chromosome normally has genes that prevent these manifestations. In other syndromes in which the testes fail to differentiate, Y chromosomes are morphologically normal.

CAMPTOMELIC SYNDROME. This form of short-limbed dysplasia is probably inherited as an autosomal trait (Sec. 24.36). Many of the affected phenotypic females have an XY karyotype and exhibit sex reversal. Uterus and fallopian tubes are present. The gonads appear grossly to be ovaries; histologically, some resemble dysgenetic testicular tissue, and others more closely resemble the ovaries of the newborn. The pathogenesis of sex reversal in this condition is unknown.

XY PURE GONADAL DYSGENESIS (SWYER SYNDROME). The designation "pure" distinguishes this condition from forms of gonadal dysgenesis that are of chromosomal origin and associated with somatic anomalies. Affected patients have normal stature and a female phenotype, including vagina, uterus, and fallopian tubes, but at pubertal age breast development and menarche fail to occur. None of the defects associated with 45,X patients are present. Patients present at puberty with hypergonadotropic primary amenorrhea. Familial cases suggest either an X-linked or a sex-limited dominant autosomal transmission. Y-specific probes have detected instances in which there were normal and deleted segments of the short arm of the Y chromosome. Mutations of the gene for TDF, biologically inactive TDF, or defects of the TDF receptors are possible explanations of the condition. In any case, the gonads consist of almost totally undifferentiated streaks despite the presence of a cytogenetically normal Y chromosome. The primitive gonad cannot accomplish any testicular function, including suppression of müllerian ducts. There may be hilar cells in the gonad capable of producing some androgens; accordingly, some virilization, such as clitoral enlargement, may occur at the age of puberty. The streak gonads may undergo neoplastic changes, such as gonadoblastomas and dysgerminomas, and should, therefore, be removed shortly after ascertainment, regardless of age.

Pure gonadal dysgenesis also occurs in XX individuals (Sec. 19.34).

XY GONADAL AGENESIS SYNDROME (EMBRYONIC TESTICULAR REGRESSION SYNDROME). In this rare syndrome the external genitalia are slightly ambiguous but more nearly female. Hypoplasia of the labia, some degree of labioscrotal fusion, a small clitoris-like phallus, and a perineal urethral opening are present. No uterus, no gonadal tissue, and usually no vagina can be found. At the age of puberty no sexual development occurs, and gonadotropins are elevated. Most patients have been reared as females. In several patients with XY gonadal agenesis in whom no gonads could be found on exploration, significant rises in testosterone followed stimulation with hCG, indicating Leydig cell function somewhere. Siblings with the disorder are known.

In this condition it is presumed that testicular tissue was active long enough during fetal life for MIF to inhibit development of müllerian ducts but not long enough for testosterone production to result in virilization. Testicular degeneration seems to occur between the 8th and 12th fetal wk. Regression of the testis before the 8th fetal wk results in Swyer syndrome (see earlier), between the 14th and 20th wk of gestation the rudimentary testis syndrome, and after the 20th wk anorchia (see later).

In *bilateral anorchia* testes are absent, but the male phenotype is complete; it is presumed that tissue with fetal testicular function was active during the critical period of genital differentiation but that sometime later it was damaged. Bilateral anorchia in identical twins and unilateral anorchia both in identical twins and in siblings suggest a genetic predisposition. Coexistence of anorchia and the gonadal agenesis syndrome in a sibship is evidence for a relationship between the disorders.

Defects in Testicular Hormones

Five genetic defects have been delineated in the enzymatic synthesis of testosterone by fetal testis, and a defect in Leydig cell differentiation has been described. These defects produce male pseudohermaphroditism through inadequate masculinization of the XY fetus (Fig. 19–18). Since levels of testosterone are normally low prior to puberty, a chorionic gonadotropin stimulation test must be used in children to assess the ability of the testes to synthesize testosterone.

LEYDIG CELL APLASIA. Ten patients with aplasia or hypoplasia of the Leydig cells have been described. The phenotype is usually female, but there may be mild virilization. Testes, epididymis, and vas are present; uterus and fallopian tubes are absent. There are no secondary sexual changes at puberty; pubic hair may be normal. Plasma levels of testosterone are low and do not respond to hCG; gonadotropins are elevated. The Leydig cells of the testes are absent or markedly deficient. The defect may involve lack of receptors that permit hCG or LH to bind to Leydig cells. In children, hCG stimulation is necessary to differentiate the condition from testicular feminization. Male-limited autosomal recessive inheritance is suggested.

20,22-DESMOLASE DEFICIENCY. This enzyme, now designated P_{450}SCC, is required to cleave the cholesterol side chain early in the biosynthesis of all steroid hormones (Sec. 19.23). In its absence, the adrenal is unable to synthesize any steroid. There is marked accumulation of lipids in the adrenal (lipoid adrenal hyperplasia). Affected males have a female phenotype but male genital ducts. Salt-losing manifestations and early adrenal crisis are the presenting manifestations in both genetic males and females. Partial defects with partially virilized males and delayed onset of salt loss have been described.

3β-HYDROXYSTEROID DEHYDROGENASE DEFICIENCY. Males with this form of congenital adrenal hyperplasia (Sec. 19.23) have varying degrees of hypospadias, with or without bifid scrotum and cryptorchidism. Affected infants usually develop salt-losing manifestations shortly after birth. Incomplete defects have been reported, and normal pubertal changes have occurred in some boys.

DEFICIENCY OF 17-HYDROXYLASE/17,20 LYASE. A single peptide, P_{450}C17, has both 17-hydroxylase and 17,20 lyase activities in adrenal and gonadal tissues (Sec. 19.23). Four allelic variants of P_{450}C17 deficiency have been described leading to different phenotypes. Genetic males usually present with a complete female phenotype or, less often, with varying degrees of virilization from labioscrotal fusion to perineal hypospadias and cryptorchidism; both 17-hydroxylase and 17,20-lyase activities are deficient. The rare patient with isolated deficiency of 17-hydroxylase and normal gonadal 17,20 lyase activity has a similar phenotype.

In the classic disorder there is decreased synthesis of cortisol by the adrenal and of sex steroids by the adrenal and gonads (see Figs. 19–12 and 19–18). Levels of deoxycorticosterone and corticosterone are markedly increased and lead to the hypertension and hypokalemia characteristic of this form of male pseudohermaphroditism. Although levels of cortisol are low, the elevated ACTH and corticosterone levels maintain a eucorticoid state, and the renin-aldosterone axis is suppressed. Virilization does not occur at puberty; levels of testosterone are low and those of gonadotropins are increased. Since fetal production of MIF is normal, no müllerian duct remnants are present. In phenotypic females, gonadectomy and replacement therapy with hydrocortisone and sex steroids are indicated.

The gene is on chromosome 10, and the defect follows autosomal recessive inheritance. Affected females are usually not detected until young adult life, when they fail to experience normal pubertal changes and are found to have hypertension and hypokalemia. The gene has been cloned, and gene deletions have been reported. Of the 50 or so reported patients, 16 have been Japanese.

DEFICIENCY OF 17-KETOSTEROID REDUCTASE. This enzyme is necessary for the conversion of androstenedione to testosterone, DHEA to androstenediol, and estrone to estradiol in gonadal and adrenal tissue. Affected genetic males have a female phenotype or sufficiently severe ambiguity of the external genitalia to be reared as females. Synthesis of MIF is normal, hence, müllerian ducts are absent. A shallow vagina is present. At puberty, gonadotropic stimulation of the testis results in very high levels of DHEA and androstenedione; levels of testosterone may be near normal as a result of transformation in peripheral tissues. Virilization occurs, and some patients reared as females have spontaneously adopted a male gender role; about half develop gynecomastia.

The defect is inherited in an autosomal recessive fashion

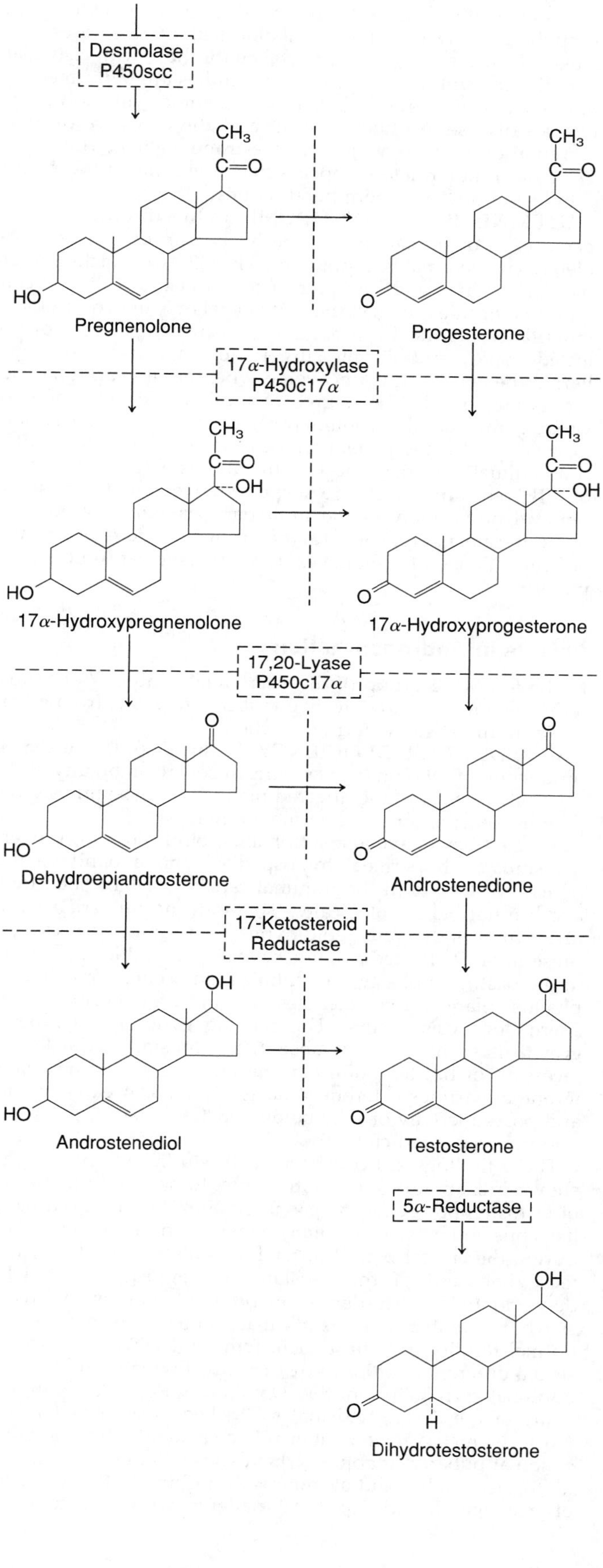

Figure 19–18. Biosynthesis of androgens. The *dotted lines* indicate enzymatic defects associated with male pseudohermaphroditism. The *vertical dotted line* indicates a defect in 3β-hydroxysteroid dehydrogenase. Note that a single polypeptide, $P_{450}c17$, catalyzes both 17α-hydroxylase and 17,20-lyase activities.

and has been identified in 52 patients, including 25 from a highly inbred Arab kindred. Diagnosis is established by measurement of the ratio of testosterone to androstenedione; in prepubertal children prior stimulation with hCG is necessary. Affected children are readily mistaken for those with testicular feminization unless the appropriate studies are performed. A few females with this defect have presented with polycystic ovarian disease at puberty because of the excessive ovarian secretion of androstenedione and estrone. Genetic control of 17-ketosteroid reductase appears to be the same in testes and ovaries but differs in peripheral tissues.

UTERINE HERNIA SYNDROME. In this disorder there is persistence of müllerian duct derivatives in otherwise completely virilized males. Approximately 142 cases, including 11 pairs of siblings and one pair of identical twins, have been reported. Studies suggest that autosomal or X-linked recessive inheritance occurs. Cryptorchidism is present in 80% of affected males, and during surgery for this or for inguinal hernia the condition is uncovered when a fallopian tube and uterus are found. The degree of müllerian development is variable and may be asymmetric. Testicular function is normal. Some of these patients have isolated deficiency of MIF; codon mutations are suspected. In patients with normal levels of MIF, receptor defects are suspected. Treatment consists of removal of as many of the müllerian structures as possible without causing damage to the testis, epididymis, or vas deferens. Some affected males develop testicular tumors after puberty.

Defects in Androgen Action

In the following group of disorders fetal synthesis of testosterone is normal, and defective virilization results from inherited abnormalities in androgen action.

5α-REDUCTASE DEFICIENCY. In this disorder decreased production of DHT in utero results in severe ambiguity of the external genitalia of the affected male fetus. Biosynthesis and peripheral action of testosterone are normal.

Affected boys have a small phallus, bifid scrotum, urogenital sinus with perineal hypospadias, and a blind vaginal pouch. Testes are in the inguinal canals or labioscrotal folds and are normal histologically. There are no müllerian structures; the vas deferens, epididymis, and seminal vesicles are present. Most affected patients have been identified as females in the past. At puberty, masculinization occurs normally; the phallus enlarges, the testes descend and grow normally, and spermatogenesis occurs. There is no gynecomastia. Beard growth is scanty, acne is absent, the prostate is small, and recession of the temporal hairline fails to occur. The testosterone-dihydrotestosterone ratio is elevated in early infancy and postpubertally or may be demonstrable by hCG stimulation in prepubertal children.

These findings are consistent with studies in animals that show virilization of the wolffian duct to be due to the action of testosterone itself, whereas masculinization of the urogenital sinus and external genitalia depends on the action of DHT during the critical period of fetal masculinization. Growth of facial hair and of the prostate also appears to be DHT dependent. The disorder is inherited as an autosomal recessive but is limited to males; normal homozygous females with normal fertility indicate that in females DHT has no role in sexual differentiation or in ovarian function later in life. In 23 interrelated families in the Dominican Republic, although many of the 38 affected males had been reared as females, most assumed a male gender role coincident with masculinization at puberty. It appears that exposures to testosterone in utero, neonatally, and at puberty contribute to the formation of male gender identity. All patients with this condition should be considered boys and reared accordingly. Treatment of an affected male infant with DHT resulted in phallic enlargement.

TESTICULAR FEMINIZATION SYNDROME. In this extreme form of failure of virilization genetic males appear female at birth and are invariably reared accordingly. The external genitalia are female; the vagina ends blindly in a pouch, and the uterus is absent. In about one third of patients unilateral or bilateral fallopian tube remnants are found. The testes are usually intra-abdominal but may descend into the inguinal canal; they consist largely of seminiferous tubules. At puberty there is normal development of breasts and the habitus is female, but menstruation does not occur and sexual hair is absent. Adult heights of these women are commensurate with those of normal males despite profound congenital deficiency of androgenic effects. Psychosexual orientation of such persons is entirely female.

The testes of affected adult patients produce normal male levels of testosterone and DHT. Failure of normal male differentiation during fetal life reflects defective response to androgens at that time, whereas the absence of müllerian ducts indicates normal fetal testicular production of MIF. The absence of androgenic effects is due to a striking resistance to the action of endogenous or exogenous testosterone at the cellular level. In many patients receptor binding for androgen is undetectable (receptor-negative androgen resistance). In other clinically identical patients, receptor binding is quantitatively normal (receptor-positive androgen resistance), and the defect is presumed to be postreceptor.

The disorder follows X-linked recessive inheritance, and the gene encoding the androgen receptor has been localized to Xq11–12. Female heterozygotes are normal, but about 20% have delayed menarche. Availability of DNA probes for the androgen receptor has revealed a variety of defects in patients with receptor-negative androgen resistance. Gross alterations of the locus are unusual; more commonly, exonic point mutations that seriously impair androgen-receptor binding activity are found.

Prepubertal children with this disorder are often detected when inguinal masses prove to be a testis or when a testis is unexpectedly found during herniorrhaphy in a phenotypic female. About 1–2% of girls with an inguinal hernia will prove to have this disorder. In adults, amenorrhea is the usual presenting symptom. Affected patients should always be reared as females. In prepubertal children the condition must be differentiated from other types of XY male pseudohermaphroditism in which there is complete feminization. These include XY gonadal dysgenesis (Swyer syndrome), true agonadism, Leydig cell aplasia, and 17-ketosteroid reductase deficiency; all of these conditions are characterized by low levels of testosterone as neonates and during adult life and by failure to respond to hCG during the prepubertal years.

The testes should be removed as soon as they are discovered. In one third of patients, malignant tumors, usually seminomas, develop by 50 yr of age. Several 14-yr-old girls have developed seminomas, and a 2-mo-old infant was found to have a carcinoma in situ. Replacement therapy with estrogens is indicated at the age of puberty.

Affected girls who have not had their testes removed by the age of puberty will develop normal breasts. In these individuals elevated production of estradiol by the testes results from defective androgen feedback at the hypothalamic-pituitary level, leading to enhanced secretion of LH. The absence of androgenic activity also contributes to the feminization of these women.

INCOMPLETE TESTICULAR FEMINIZATION. In this disorder patients exhibit some degree of masculinization and at birth may have enlargement of the phallus and labioscrotal fusion. The vagina ends blindly, and the uterus is absent.

Testes are present in the inguinal canal or in the labioscrotal folds. At puberty, breast development occurs as well as axillary and pubic hair. These patients have lesser degrees of insensitivity to androgen than those with the complete syndrome. The disorder may be due to a deficient level of normal androgen receptor activity (receptor-deficient), to qualitative defects, such as acceleration of dissociation of androgen-receptor complex (receptor-positive), or to postreceptor defects. Several patients with qualitative abnormalities of androgen receptor binding have had point mutations of the androgen receptor gene. The pattern of inheritance is compatible with X-linkage; the "complete" and "incomplete" forms have not been reported in the same family.

REIFENSTEIN SYNDROME. This syndrome and other syndromes of defective virilization are caused by decreased end-organ responsiveness to androgens and are best described as *partial androgen insensitivity*. Androgen receptor studies in skin fibroblasts have revealed a variety of quantitative and qualitative abnormalities. Treatment with large doses of depot testosterone may increase phallic growth and virilization, particularly in patients with partial receptor resistance. Inheritance is X-linked recessive. These patients differ from those in the previous section; the phenotype is more male than female. There are marked phenotypic differences in various affected individuals, even within affected families. Severely affected children have perineal hypospadias, a small phallus, and cryptorchidism. Most patients are sufficiently virilized, however, to be considered male at birth. Mildly affected individuals may manifest only microphallus and a bifid scrotum. After puberty there is inadequate masculinization. There is lack of both facial hair and voice change. Female escutcheon, azoospermia, and infertility are usual. The disorder is being increasingly recognized in adults with relatively normal male phenotype who have a small phallus, small testes, and azoospermia.

In adults, plasma levels of testosterone and of DHT are normal or elevated. Levels of LH, and often of FSH, are also elevated. Diagnosis is also possible in the neonatal period when plasma levels of testosterone and LH are elevated.

Undetermined Causes

Other XY male pseudohermaphrodites display much variability of the external and internal genitalia and varying degrees of phallic and müllerian development. Testes may be histologically normal or rudimentary, or there may only be one. Even the newer techniques may find no recognized cause of pseudohermaphroditism in as many as one third of patients. Some ambiguity of genitalia is associated with a wide variety of chromosomal aberrations, which must always be considered in the differential, the most common being the 45,X/46,XY syndrome (Sec. 19.34). It may be necessary to examine several tissues in order to establish mosaicism. Other complex genetic syndromes, many resulting from single gene mutations, are associated with varying degrees of ambiguity of the genitalia, particularly in the male. For example, XY males with the Smith-Lemli-Opitz syndrome may have external genitalia that are normal, markedly ambiguous, or completely female. These entities must be identified on the basis of the associated extragenital malformations.

Drash syndrome, consisting of nephropathy associated with genital abnormalities or Wilms tumor, has been reported in 60 children. Most patients are 46,XY; the phenotype may be female or may be ambiguous with penoscrotal hypospadias and cryptorchidism. Müllerian ducts are often present, indicating a global deficiency of fetal testicular function. Proteinuria, commonly with the nephrotic syndrome, begins when the infant is less than 1 yr of age and progresses to end-stage renal failure by 2 yr of age. Wilms tumor most often develops in patients under 2 yr of age and is frequently bilateral. Gonadoblastomas occur in some instances. All cases have been sporadic, and the etiology is thought to be defective embryogenesis of the urogenital ridge. Treatment by early bilateral nephrectomy, dialysis, and renal transplantation has been proposed; management of the pseudohermaphroditism follows the same principles as those used for this condition due to other causes.

Sporadic aniridia in genetic males is usually associated with ambiguous genitalia and mental retardation. Cryptorchidism and severe deficiency of virilization has in some instances resulted in incorrect gender assignment. Wilms tumor occurs in about 30% of affected children, usually at about 2 yr of age. Gonadoblastoma has arisen from the dysgenetic gonads in at least five cases. The syndrome also occurs in XX females, in whom the genitalia are always normal. The complex has also been termed the Wilms tumor-aniridia-genitourinary-mental retardation (WAGR) syndrome. Affected patients have an 11p13 deletion, which is often cytogenetically demonstrable. The pathogenesis of male pseudohermaphroditism is unknown. All newly born infants with sporadic aniridia require chromosomal studies and careful prospective evaluation.

19.43 TRUE HERMAPHRODITISM

In true hermaphroditism both ovarian and testicular tissues are present, either in the same or in opposite gonads. The clinical features may include any of those described for the other types of hermaphroditism. The phenotype may be male or female; usually, the external genitalia are ambiguous.

Patients with 46,XX/46,XY mosaicism are the best understood of those with true hemaphroditism. Of 25 reported cases, derivation from more than one zygote was documented in about half; they were chimeras (chi 46,XX/46,XY). The presence of both paternal alleles for some blood groups and of both maternal alleles for other blood groups is clear evidence of chimerism. Various mechanisms are possible.

More than 500 cases of true hermaphroditism have been reported, 80% of which have a 46,XX karyotype. These patients must not be confused with 46,XX males with small testes and testicular-determining genes (Sec. 19.30). Examination of a number of 46,XX true hermaphrodites with X-specific probes has failed to detect any Y-specific sequences. Etiology of true hermaphroditism remains enigmatic. The condition is usually sporadic, but familial occurrence has been reported. An unusually high prevalence has been reported in the black population of South Africa.

The most frequently encountered gonad in true hermaphroditism is an ovotestis; a testis is the rarest. In ovotestes the ovarian and testicular portions are often arranged end-to-end, permitting clear differentiation. The testicular tissue is often defective in secretion of androgens and of antimüllerian hormone. The majority of true hermaphrodites are best reared as females, with selective removal of testicular tissue. Many pregnancies with living offspring have been reported in true hermaphrodites reared as females.

Diagnosis and Management

In the neonate ambiguity of the genitalia requires emergency medical attention to settle the sex of rearing as early in life as possible. While awaiting the results of chromosomal analysis, pelvic ultrasound examination is indicated to determine the presence of a uterus and ovaries. Presence of a uterus and absence of palpable gonads usually suggests a virilized XX female. Search for the source of virilization should be undertaken; this includes studies of adrenal hormones to rule out varieties of congenital adrenal hyperplasia. Female pseudohermaphrodites should be reared as females even when highly virilized.

The absence of a uterus, with or without palpable gonads, almost always indicates male pseudohermaphroditism and an XY karyotype. Measurements of levels of gonadotropins, testosterone, and DHT are necessary to determine whether testicular production of androgen is normal. Male pseudohermaphrodites who are totally feminized must be reared as females. However, certain significantly feminized infants, such as those with 5α-reductase deficiency, should be reared as males because these children virilize normally at puberty. On the other hand, an infant with a comparable degree of feminization resulting from an androgen-receptor defect is best reared as a female. It is more feasible to reconstruct the external genitalia to create a functional female, particularly when a vagina is present, than to create a functional male phallus. Infants with 45,X/46,XY whose phenotype varies from almost completely male to completely female are usually reared as females because they are generally short in stature and have a uterus, and they will require gonadectomy.

When receptor disorders are suspected in the XY male with a small phallus (micropenis), a course of 3 monthly intramuscular injections of testosterone enanthate (25–50 mg) may assist in the differential diagnosis as well as in treatment.

The management of the potential psychologic upheaval that these disorders can generate in the patient or the family is of paramount importance and requires physicians with sensitivity, training, and experience in this field. Once the appropriate sex of rearing has been established, parents should be left with no ambiguity in their minds as to the gender of the child.

In some mammals the female exposed to androgens prenatally or in early postnatal life will exhibit aberrant sexual behavior in adult life. Girls who have undergone fetal masculinization from congenital adrenal hyperplasia or from maternal progestin therapy have no such problems in sexual identity, although during childhood they may appear to prefer male playmates and activities over female playmates and feminine play with dolls in mothering roles.

ANGELO M. DIGEORGE

HYPOFUNCTION OF TESTES

Barkam AL, Kelch RP, Marshall JC: Isolated gonadotrope failure in the polyglandular autoimmune failure. N Engl J Med 312:1535, 1985.
Borgaonkar DS, Mules E, Char F: Do the 48 XXYY males have a characteristic phenotype? Clin Genet 1:272, 1970.
Borghgraef M, Fryns JP, Smeets E, et al: The 49,XXXXY syndrome. Clinical and psychological follow-up data. Clin Genet 33:429, 1988.
Burger HG, McLachlan RI, Bangah M, et al: Serum inhibin concentrations rise through normal male and female puberty. J Clin Endocrinol Metab 67:689, 1988.
Burger HG, Yamada Y, Bangah ML, et al: Serum gonadotropin, sex steroid, and immunoreactive inhibin levels in the first two years of life. J Clin Endocrinol Metab 72:682, 1991.
Chaussain JL, Lemerle J, Roger M, et al: Klinefelter syndrome, tumor and sexual precocity. J Pediatr 97:607, 1980.
Clayton PE, Shalet SM, Price DA, et al: Testicular damage after chemotherapy for childhood brain tumors. J Pediatr 112:922, 1988.
Crowne EC, Shalet SM: Management of constitutional delay in growth and puberty. Trends Endocrinol Metab 1:239, 1990.
Dunkel L, Perheentupa J, Tapanainen J, et al: Hypergonadotropic hypogonadism in newborn males with primary testicular failure. Acta Pediatr Scand 73:740, 1984.
Dunkel L, Perheentupa J, Virtanen M, et al: Gonadotropin-releasing hormone test and human chorionic gonadotropin test in the diagnosis of gonadotropin deficiency in prepubertal boys. J Pediatr 107:388, 1985.
Ehrmann DA, Rosenfield RL, Cuttler L, et al: A new test of combined pituitary-testicular function using the gonadotropin-releasing hormone agonist Nafarelin in the differentiation of gonadotropin deficiency from delayed puberty: Pilot studies. J Clin Endocrinol Metab 69:963, 1989.
Evain-Brion D, Gendred D, Bozzola M, et al: Diagnosis of Kallmann's syndrome in early infancy. Acta Paediatr 71:937, 1982.
Finkel DM, Phillips JL, Snyder PJ: Stimulation of spermatogenesis by gonadotropins in men with hypogonadotropic hypogonadism. N Engl J Med 313:651, 1985.
Kaplowitz PB: Diagnostic value of testosterone therapy in boys with delayed puberty. Am J Dis Child 143:116, 1989.
Kulin HE, Frontera A, Demers LM, et al: The onset of sperm production in pubertal boys. Relationship to gonadotropin excretion. Am J Dis Child 143:190, 1989.
Lieblich JM, Rogol AD, White BJ, et al: Syndrome of anosmia with hypogonadotropic hypogonadism (Kallmann syndrome). Clinical and laboratory studies in 23 cases. Am J Med 73:506, 1982.
Matus-Ridley M, Nicosia SV, Meadows AT: Gonadal effects of cancer therapy in boys. Cancer 55:2353, 1985.
Meisner LF, Inhorn SL: Normal male development with Y chromosome long arm deletion (Yq-). J Med Genet 9:373, 1972.
Meitinger T, Heye B, Petit C, et al: Definitive localization of X-linked Kallmann syndrome (hypogonadotropic hypogonadism and anosmia) to Xp22.3. Close linkage to the hypervariable repeat sequence CR1-S232. Am J Hum Genet 47:664, 1990.
Melman A, Leiter E, Perez JM, et al: The influence of neonatal orchiopexy upon the testis in persistent müllerian duct syndrome. J Urol 125:856, 1981.
Money J, Franzke A, Borgaonkar DS: XYY syndrome, stigmatization, social class, and aggression. South Med J 68:1536, 1975.
Najjar SS, Takla RJ, Nassar VH: The syndrome of rudimentary testes: Occurrence in five siblings. J Pediatr 84:119, 1974.
Philip J, Lundsteen C, Owen D, et al: The frequency of chromosome aberrations in tall men with special reference to 47,XYY and 47,XXY. Am J Hum Genet 28:404, 1976.
Pike MG, Hammerton M, Edge J, et al: A family with X-linked ichthyosis and hypogonadism. Eur J Pediatr 148:442, 1989.
Ranke MB, Heidemann P, Knupter C, et al: Noonan syndrome: Growth and clinical manifestations in 144 cases. Eur J Pediatr 148:220, 1988.
Rose SR, Cassorla F, Sherins RJ: Normal neonatal surge of gonadotropins and sex steroids in infants of men with isolated hypogonadotropic hypogonadism. Clin Endocrinol 29:577, 1988.
Rosenfeld RL: Diagnosis and management of delayed puberty. J Clin Endocrinol Metab 70:559, 1990.
Salbenblatt JA, Bender BG, Puck MH, et al: Development of eight pubertal males with 47,XXY karyotype. Clin Genet 20:141, 1981.
Salbenblatt JA, Bender BG, Puck MH, et al: Pituitary-gonadal function in Klinefelter syndrome before and during puberty. Pediatr Res 19:82, 1985.
Saunder SE, Corley KP, Hopwood NJ, Kelch RP: Subnormal gonadotropin responses for gonadotropin-releasing hormone persist into puberty in children with isolated growth hormone deficiency. J Clin Endocrinol Metab 53:1186, 1981.
Seyler LE, Arulananthan K, O'Connor CF: Hypergonadotropic-hypogonadism in the Prader-Labhart-Willi syndrome. J Pediatr 94:435, 1979.
Shalet SM, Hann IM, Lendon M, et al: Testicular function after combination chemotherapy in childhood for acute lymphoblastic leukaemia. Arch Dis Child 56:275, 1981.
Sherins RJ, Olweny CLM, Ziegler JL: Gynecomastia and gonadal dysfunction in adolescent boys treated with combination chemotherapy for Hodgkin's disease. N Engl J Med 299:12, 1978.
Spratt DI, Carr DB, Merriam GR, et al: The spectrum of abnormal patterns of gonadotropin-releasing hormone secretion in men with idiopathic hypogonadotropic hypogonadism: Clinical and laboratory correlations. J Clin Endocrinol Metab 64:283, 1987.
Stanhope R, Brook CGD, Pringle PJ, et al: Induction of puberty by pulsatile gonadotropin-releasing hormone. Lancet 2:552, 1987.
VanDop C, Burstein S, Conte FA, et al: Isolated gonadotropin deficiency in boys: Clinical characteristics and growth. J Pediatr 111:684, 1987.
White BJ, Rogol AD, Brown KS, et al: The syndrome of anosmia with hypogonadotropic hypogonadism: A genetic study of 18 new families and a review. Am J Med Genet 15:417, 1983.
Witkin HA, Mednick SA, Schulsinger F, et al: Criminality in XYY and XXY men. Science 193:547, 1976.

TUMORS OF THE TESTES

Carmi R, Meryash DL, Wood J, et al: Fragile-X syndrome ascertained by the presence of macro-orchidism in a 5 month-old infant. Pediatrics 74:883, 1984.
Clark RV, Albertson BD, Monabi A, et al: Steroidogenic enzyme activities, morphology and receptor studies of a testicular rest in a patient with congenital adrenal hyperplasia. J Clin Endocrinol Metab 70:1408, 1990.
Coen P, Kulin H, Ballantine T, et al: An aromatase-producing sex-cord tumor resulting in prepubertal gynecomastia. N Engl J Med 324:317, 1991.
Cunnah D, Perry L, Dacie JA, et al: Bilateral testicular tumors in congenital adrenal hyperplasia: A continuing diagnostic and therapeutic dilemma. Clin Endocrinol 30:141, 1989.
Nisula BC, Loriaux DL, Sherins RJ, et al: Benign bilateral testicular enlargement. J Clin Endocrinol Metab 38:440, 1974.
Rosenberg T, Gilboay, Golik A, et al: Pseudoprecocious puberty in a young boy due to interstitial cell adenomas of the testis. Helv Paediatr Acta 39:79, 1984.

Turner G, Daniel A, Frost M: X-linked mental retardation, macro-orchidism, and the Xq 27 fragile site. J Pediatr 96:837, 1980.

Turner WR, Derrick FC, Wohltmann W: Leydig cell tumor in identical twin. Urology 7:194, 1976.

GYNECOMASTIA

August GP, Chandra R, Hung W: Prepubertal male gynecomastia. J Pediatr 80:259, 1972.

Berkovitz GD, Guerami A, Brown TR, et al: Familial gynecomastia with increased extraglandular aromatization of plasma carbon$_{19}$-steroids. J Clin Invest 75:1763, 1985.

Bulard J, Mowszowicz I, Schaison G: Increased aromatase in pubic skin fibroblasts from patients with isolated gynecomastia. J Clin Endocrinol Metab 64:618, 1987.

Hochberg Z, Even L, Zadik Z: Mineralocorticoid in the mechanism of gynecomastia in adrenal hyperplasia caused by 11 β-hydroxylase deficiency. J Pediatr 118:258, 1991.

Lee PA: The relationship of concentrations of serum hormones to pubertal gynecomastia. J Pediatr 86:212, 1975.

Maclaren NK, Migeon CJ, Raiti S: Gynecomastia with congenital virilizing adrenal hyperplasia (11β-hydroxylase deficiency). J Pediatr 86:579, 1975.

Nydick M, Bustos J, Dale JH Jr, et al: Gynecomastia in adolescent boys. JAMA 178:449, 1961.

Van Meter QL, Gareis FJ, Hayes JW, et al: Galactorrhea in a 12-year-old boy with a chromophobe adenoma. J Pediatr 90:756, 1977.

HYPOFUNCTION OF THE OVARIES

Ahonen P, Myllarnjemi S, Sipila I, et al: Clinical variation of autoimmune polyendocrinopathy-candidiasis-ectodermal dystrophy (APECED) in a series of 68 patients. N Engl J Med 322:1829, 1990.

Allanson JE, Hall JG, VanAllen MI: Noonan phenotype associated with neurofibromatosis. Am J Med Genet 21:457, 1985.

Arulanantham K, Kramer MS, Gryboski J: The association of inflammatory bowel disease and X chromosomal abnormality. Pediatrics 66:63, 1980.

Barnes R, Rosenfield RL: The polycystic ovary syndrome: Pathogenesis and treatment. Ann Intern Med 110:386, 1989.

Bender B, Puck M, Salbenblatt J, et al: Cognitive development of unselected girls with complete and partial X monosomy. Pediatrics 73:175, 1984.

Chang HJ, Clark RD, Bachman H: The phenotype of 45,X/46,XY mosaicism: An analysis of 92 prenatally diagnosed cases. Am J Hum Genet 46:156, 1990.

Franks S: Polycystic ovary syndrome. Trends Endocrinol Metab 1:60, 1990.

Fryns JP, Kleczkowska A, Petit P, et al: X-chromosome polysomy in the female: Personal experience and review of the literature. Clin Genet 23:341, 1983.

Horning SJ, Hoppe RT, Kaplan HS, et al: Female reproductive potential after treatment for Hodgkin's disease. N Engl J Med 304:1377, 1981.

Kaufman FR, Kogut MD, Donnell GH, et al: Hypergonadotropic hypogonadism in female patients with galactosemia. N Engl J Med 304:994, 1981.

Krasna IH, Lee M, Sciorre L, et al: The importance of surgical evaluation of patients with "Turner-like" sex chromosomal abnormalities. J Pediatr Surg 20:61, 1985.

Krauss CM, Turksoy N, Atkins L, et al: Familial premature ovarian failure due to an interstitial deletion of the long arm of the X chromosome. N Engl J Med 317:125, 1987.

Luborsky JL, Visintin I, Boyers, et al: Ovarian antibodies detected by immobilized antigen immunoassay in patients with premature ovarian failure. J Clin Endocrinol Metab 70:69, 1990.

Magenis RE, Tochen ML, Holalan KP, et al: Turner syndrome resulting from partial deletion of Y chromosome short arm: Localization of male determinants. J Pediatr 105:916, 1984.

Massarano AA, Adams JA, Preece MA, et al: Ovarian ultrasound appearances in Turner syndrome. J Pediatr 114:568, 1989.

May KM, Jacobs PA, Lee M, et al: The parental origin of the extra X chromosome in 47,XXX females. Am J Hum Genet 46:754, 1990.

McDonough PG, Thi Tho P: The spectrum of 45,X/46,XY gonadal dysgenesis and its implications (a study of 19 patients). Pediatr Adoles Gynecol 1:1, 1973.

Muller J, Shakkeback NE, Ritzen M, et al: Carcinoma in situ of the testis in children with 45,X/46,XY gonadal dysgenesis. J Pediatr 106:431, 1985.

Nicosia SV, Matus-Ridley M, Meadows AT: Gonadal effects of cancer therapy in girls. Cancer 55:2364, 1985.

Rosenfeld RG: Update on growth hormone therapy for Turner syndrome. Acta Paediatr Scand (Suppl) 356:103, 1989.

Rosenfeld RG, Grumbach MM (ed): Turner Syndrome. New York, Marcel Dekker, 1989.

Toscano V, Bolducci R, Bianchi P, et al: Ovarian 17-ketoreductase deficiency as a possible cause of polycystic ovarian disease. J Clin Endocrinol Metab 71:288, 1990.

Yeh J, Rebar RW, Liu JH, et al: Pituitary function in isolated gonadotropin deficiency. Clin Endocrinol 31:375, 1989.

TUMORS OF THE OVARY

Dewhurst J, Pryse-Davies J, Helm W, et al: Diagnosis and management of granulosa/theca cell tumors of childhood. Pediatr Adolesc Gynecol 3:131, 1985.

Lack EE, Perez-Atayde AR, Murthy AS, et al: Granulosa theca cell tumors in premenarchal girls: A clinical and pathologic study of ten cases. Cancer 48:1846, 1981.

Solh HM, Azoury RS, Najjar SS: Peutz-Jeghers syndrome associated with precocious puberty. J Pediatr 103:593, 1983.

Stokns-Brantsma WH, von Weissenbruch MM, Schoemaker WH, et al: Sexual precocity induced by ovarian follicular cysts. Is autoimmunity involved? Clin Endocrinol 32:603, 1990.

Tucci JR, Zäh W, Kalderon AE: Endocrine studies in arrhenoblastoma responsive to dexamethasone, ACTH and human chorionic gonadotropin. Am J Med 55:681, 1973.

Young RH, Dickersin GR, Scully RE: Juvenile granulosa cell tumor of the ovary. A clinicopathologic analysis of 125 cases. Am J Surg Pathol 8:575, 1984.

Zaloudek C, Norris JH: Granulosa cell tumors of the ovary in children: A clinical and pathological study of 32 cases. Am J Surg Pathol 6:513, 1982.

HERMAPHRODITISM

Amrhein JA, Jones Klingensmith G, Walsh PC, et al: Partial androgen in sensitivity. The Reinfenstein syndrome revisited. N Engl J Med 297:350, 1977.

Avruskin TW, Imperato-McGinley J, O'Shaughnessy PJ, et al: Steroid patterns and in vitro testicular enzyme studies in male pseudohermaphroditism due to 17-ketosteroid reductase deficiency. J Pediatr Endocrinol 3:135, 1989.

Berkovitz GD, Lee PA, Brown TR, et al: Etiologic evaluation of male pseudohermaphroditism in infancy and childhood. Am J Dis Child 138:755, 1984.

Bernstein R, Koo GC, Wachtel SS: Abnormality of the X chromosome in human 46,XY female siblings with dysgenetic ovaries. Science 207:768, 1980.

Burstein S, Grumbach MM, Kaplan SL: Early determination of androgen-responsiveness is important in the management of microphallus. Lancet 2:983, 1979.

Carpenter TO, Imperato-McGinley J, Boulware SD, et al: Variable expression of 5α-reductase deficiency: Presentation with male phenotype in a child of Greek origin. J Clin Endocrinol Metab 71:318, 1990.

David R, Yoon DJ, Landin L, et al: A syndrome of gonadotropin resistance possibly due to luteinizing hormone receptor defect. J Clin Endocrinol Metab 59:156, 1984.

Dean HJ, Shackleton CHL, Winter JSD: Diagnosis and natural history of 17-hydroxylase deficiency in a newborn male. J Clin Endocrinol Metab 59:513, 1984.

Eil C, Austin RM, Sesterhenn I, et al: Leydig cell hypoplasia causing male pseudohermaphroditism: Diagnosis 13 years after prepubertal castration. J Clin Endocrinol Metab 58:441, 1984.

Fitch N, Richer CL, Pinsky L, et al: Deletion of the long arm of the Y chromosome and review of Y chromosome abnormalities. Am J Med Genet 20:31, 1985.

Fitzgerald PH, Donald RA, Kirk RL: A true hermaphrodite dispermic chimera with 46,XX and 46,XY karyotypes. Clin Genet 15:89, 1979.

Greene C, Pitts W, Rosenfeld R, et al: Smith-Lemli-Opitz syndrome in two 46,XY infants with female external genitalia. Clin Genet 25:366, 1984.

Griffin JE, Wilson JD: The syndromes of androgen resistance. N Engl J Med 302:198, 1980.

Guerami A, Griffin JE, Kovacs WJ, et al: Estrogen and androgen production rates in two brothers with Reifenstein syndrome. J Clin Endocrinol Metab 71:247, 1990.

Guerrier D, Tran D, Vanderwinden JM, et al: The persistent müllerian duct syndrome: A molecular approach. J Clin Endocrinol Metab 68:46, 1989.

Imperato-McGinley J, Gautier T, Pichardo M, et al: The diagnosis of 5-α-reductase deficiency in infancy. J Clin Endocrinol Metab 63:1313, 1986.

Imperato-McGinley J, Peterson RE, Gautier T, et al: Androgens and the evolution of male gender identity among male pseudohermaphrodites with 5α-reductase deficiency. N Engl J Med 300:1233, 1979.

Jadresic L, Leake J, Gordon I, et al: Clinicopathologic review of twelve children with nephropathy, Wilms tumor, and genital abnormalities (Drash syndrome). J Pediatr 117:717, 1990.

Jensen JC, Ehrlich RM, Hanna MK, et al: A report of 4 patients with the Drash syndrome and a review of the literature. J Urol 141:1174, 1989.

Josso N, Briard ML: Embryonic testicular regression syndrome: Variable phenotypic expression in siblings. J Pediatr 97:200, 1980.

Kaufman FR, Costin G, Goebelsmann U, et al: Male pseudohermaphroditism due to 17,20-desmolase deficiency. J Clin Endocrinol Metab 57:32, 1983.

Kirk JMW, Perry LA, Shand WS, et al: Female pseudohermaphroditism due to maternal adrenocortical tumor. J Clin Endocrinol Metab 70:1280, 1990.

McLaren A: What makes a man a man? Nature 346:216, 1990.

Marcelli M, Tilley WD, Wilson CM, et al: A single nucleotide substitution introduces a premature termination codon in the androgen receptor gene of a patient with receptor-negative androgen resistance. J Clin Invest 85:1522, 1990.

Medina M, Chavez B, Perez-Palacios G: Defective androgen action at the cellular level in the androgen resistance syndromes. I: Differences between the complete and incomplete testicular feminization syndromes. J Clin Endocrinol Metab 53:1243, 1981.

Migeon CJ, Brown TR, Lanes R, et al: A clinical syndrome of mild androgen insensitivity. J Clin Endocrinol Metab 59:672, 1984.

Nagel RA, Lippe BM, Griffin JE: Androgen resistance in the neonate: Use of hormones of hypothalamic-pituitary-gonadal axis for diagnosis. J Pediatr 109:486, 1986.

Nihoul-Fékété C, Lorat-Jacob S, Cachin O, et al: Preservation of gonadal function in true hermaphroditism. J Pediatr Surg 19:50, 1984.
Ramsay M, Bernstein R, Zwane E, et al: XX True hermaphroditism in Southern African blacks: An enigma of primary sexual differentiation. Am J Hum Genet 43:4, 1988.
Rockhill TA, Schmidt CL: Male pseudohermaphroditism secondary to early fetal testicular regression. Pediatr Adoles Gynecol 3:15, 1985.
Rohmer V, Barbot N, Bertrand P, et al: A case of male pseudohermaphroditism due to 17α-hydroxylase deficiency and hormonal profiles in the nuclear family. J Clin Endocrinol Metab 71:523, 1990.
Saenger P: Abnormal sexual differentiation. J Pediatr 104:1, 1984.
Sai T, Seino S, Chang C, et al: An exonic point mutation of the androgen receptor gene in a family with complete androgen insensitivity. Am J Hum Genet 6:1095, 1990.
Savage MD, Low DG: Gonadal neoplasia and abnormal sexual differentiation. Clin Endocrinol 32:519, 1990.
Shanfield I, Young RB, Hume DM: True hermaphroditism with XX/XY mosaicism: Report of a case. J Pediatr 83:471, 1973.
Shozu M, Akasofu K, Harda T, Kubota Y: A new cause of female pseudohermaphroditism: placental aromatase deficiency. J Clin Endocrinol Metab 72:560, 1991.
Siiteri PK, Wilson JD: Testosterone formation and metabolism during male sexual differentiation in the human embryo. J Clin Endocrinol Metab 38:113, 1974.
Turleau C, de Grouchy J, Dufier JL, et al: Aniridia, male pseudohermaphroditism, gonadoblastoma, mental retardation, and del 11 p13. Hum Genet 57:300, 1981.
Ulloa-Aquirre A, Bassal S, Poo J, et al: Endocrine and biochemical studies in a 46,XY phenotypically male infant with 17-ketoreductase deficiency. J Clin Endocrinol Metab 60:639, 1985.
Weckworth PF, Johnson HW, Pantzar JT, et al: Dicentric Y chromosome and mixed dysgenesis. J Urol 139:91, 1988.
Wenstrup RJ, Pagon RA: Female pseudohermaphroditism with anorectal, Müllerian duct and urinary tract malformations: Report of four cases. J Pediatr 107:751, 1985.
Wu RH, Boyer RM, Knight R, et al: Endocrine studies in a phenotypic girl with XY gonadal agenesis. J Clin Endocrinol Metab 43:506, 1976.
Yanase T, Simpson ER, Waterman MR: 17α-Hydroxylase/17,20-lyase deficiency: From clinical investigation to molecular definition. Endocrine Rev 12:91, 1991.

20

THE NERVOUS SYSTEM

20.1 NEUROLOGIC EVALUATION

The neurologic evaluation seeks to assess the integrity of the central nervous system (CNS) by means of a thorough history and physical examination and thus to determine the location (and causes) of abnormal function. This section highlights those features of the history and neurologic examination that are peculiar to the infant and provides the framework for the history and neurologic examination in the premature, infant, and child.

HISTORY

The history is the most important component of the evaluation of a child with a neurologic problem. The history should carefully document in chronologic order the onset of symptoms and a thorough description of their frequency, duration, and associated characteristics. Most children beyond the age of 3–4 yr are capable of contributing to their history, particularly concerning facts relating to the present illness. It is essential to obtain a comprehensive review of the function and interaction of all organ systems, because abnormalities of the CNS may initially present with clinical manifestations (e.g., vomiting, pain, constipation, or urinary tract disorders) implicating other systems. A detailed history might suggest that the child's vomiting is due to increased intracranial pressure, that the pain behind the eye may be caused by migraine headaches or multiple sclerosis, and that the constipation and urinary dribbling may be due to a spinal cord tumor.

It is important to start with a concise description of the chief complaint within its developmental context. For example, parents may be concerned that their child cannot talk. The seriousness of this problem depends on many factors, including the age of the patient, the normal range of language development for age, the parent/child interaction, function of the auditory system, and the intellectual level of the child. A comprehensive understanding of developmental milestones is essential in order to ascertain the relative importance of the parents' observations (Sec. 3.10–3.12). There is no particular order to the neurologic history; each physician should utilize the method that is personally most comfortable and familiar, but the history should be comprehensive.

Following the chief complaint and history of present illness, a review of the pregnancy, labor, and delivery is indicated, particularly if a congenital disorder is suspected (Sec. 9.2–9.3). Was the mother exposed to a viral illness during the pregnancy and what is the mother's rubella immune status? The history should also include information about the quantity of cigarette and alcohol consumption and drug use (legal and illicit) that are known to have an adverse effect on fetal development. Decreased or absent fetal activity may be associated with the congenital myopathies and other neuromuscular disorders. Seizures in utero occasionally occur and suggest placental insufficiency or rare inborn errors of metabolism, such as pyridoxine dependency. Seizure activity in utero is difficult to evaluate, particularly in the primigravida. The fact that seizures occurred during pregnancy is often made retrospectively after the mother has had an opportunity to observe her infant's seizures. The mother's postpartum health may provide a clue as to the cause of her infant's neurologic problem; for example, maternal fever, drug dependence, cervical or vaginal vesicles (e.g., herpes simplex), hemorrhage, petechiae, or the presence of an abnormal placenta.

The history of the birthweight, length, and head circumference are particularly important. It may be necessary to obtain the infant's hospital records to determine the head circumference, particularly if congenital microcephaly is a consideration, and the Apgar score, for suspected asphyxia. There are, however, several indicators of neurologic dysfunction during the newborn period that can reliably be obtained from the history. The fact that a full-term infant was unable to breathe spontaneously and required ventilatory assistance may suggest a CNS abnormality. A poor, uncoordinated suck or a full-term infant that requires an inordinate amount of time to feed suggests a neurologic disorder requiring careful evaluation. If such an infant requires gavage feeding, there is almost certainly a significant problem. All of the aforementioned abnormalities may be common to the premature infant, particularly the very low birthweight infant, and do not necessarily signify a poor neurologic outcome. Additional important information in the newborn period includes the presence of jaundice, its degree, and management. The physician should also attempt to assess the activity, sleep patterns, the nature of the cry, and the general well-being of the newborn infant from the history.

The most important component of a neurologic history is the child's developmental assessment (see Sec. 3.11). A careful evaluation of a child's developmental milestones usually determines the presence of a global delay in language, gross and fine motor or social skills, or a delay in a particular subset of development. An abnormality in development from birth suggests an intrauterine or perinatal cause. A slowing of the rate of acquisition of skills later in infancy or childhood may imply an acquired abnormality of the nervous system. A loss of skills over time strongly suggests an underlying degenerative disease of the CNS. The ability of parents to precisely recall the timing of their child's developmental milestones is extremely variable. Some are very reliable and others are uncertain, particularly if the patient in question has a significant neurodevelopmental problem. Table 20–1 provides some guidelines with regard to the upper range of normal skills that are usually recalled by the parents and that, if not present, should alert the physician. It is often helpful to request photographs taken at an earlier age or to review the family's baby book, because milestones for a child may have been dutifully recorded. Parents (particularly mothers) are usually aware when their child has a developmental problem, and the physician should show appropriate concern.

The family history is extremely important in the neurologic evaluation of the child. Parents are sometimes unwilling to discuss or may be unaware of family members with debilitat-

TABLE 20–1. Screening Scheme for Developmental Delay

Age (Months)	Gross Motor	Fine Motor	Social Skills	Language
3	Supports weight on forearms	Opens hands spontaneously	Smiles appropriately	Coos, laughs
6	Sits momentarily	Transfers objects	Shows likes and dislikes	Babbles
9	Pulls to stand	Pincer grasp	Plays patty-cake, peek-a-boo	Imitates sounds
12	Walks with one hand held	Releases an object on command	Comes when called	1–2 meaningful words
18	Walks upstairs with assistance	Feeds from a spoon	Mimics actions of others	At least six words
24	Runs	Builds a tower of six blocks	Plays with others	2–3 word sentences

ing neurologic disorders, particularly if they are institutionalized. However, most parents are extremely cooperative in securing medical information concerning family members, particularly if it may have relevance for their child. The history should document the ages and well-being of all close relatives and the presence of neurologic disease, including epilepsy, migraine, cerebrovascular accidents, and heredofamilial disorders. The sex and age at death of miscarriages or live-born siblings, including the results of post mortem examinations, should be obtained because this information may have a direct bearing on the patient's condition. It should also be determined whether the parents are related, because the incidence of metabolic and degenerative disorders affecting the CNS is increased significantly in children of consanguineous marriages.

Finally, an attempt should be made to learn about the patient as a person. The child's performance in school, both academically and socially, may shed light on the diagnosis, particularly if there has been an abrupt change. A description of the child's personality before and after the onset of symptoms may provide a clue with regard to the cause of the disorder. Discussions with the day-care worker, kindergarten, or school teacher may provide useful information that is not available from the parent.

NEUROLOGIC EXAMINATION

The neurologic examination of a child begins at the outset of the interview. Observation during interaction with the parents, while playing, or during the time when little attention is directed to the child can provide useful information. It may be obvious that the child has characteristic facies, an unusual posture, an abnormality of motor function manifested by a gait disturbance or hemiparesis. Furthermore, much can be learned from observing the child's behavior during the interview. The normally inquisitive child or toddler may play independently but soon wishes to become involved with the interview process. The child with an attention disorder may display inappropriate behaviors in the examining room, whereas the neurologically abnormal child may appear lethargic or disinterested or may show a complete lack of awareness of the environment. The degree of interaction between the parent and the child should be noted. As the neurologic examination of a newborn or premature infant requires a somewhat modified approach from the older child, the differences in the examination will be highlighted for both age groups (see also Sec. 6.1 and 9.3).

The examination should be conducted in a setting that is nonthreatening and enjoyable for the child. The more it seems like a game, the greater will be the degree of cooperation. The child may be most comfortable on a parent's lap or interacting on the floor of the examination room. It is unwise to force the child to sit on the examining table or to demand that all clothes be removed at the beginning of the procedure. Cooperation is essential for a comprehensive neurologic examination; as a child's confidence increases, so too does the level of participation. Several methods may be used to assess *mental status, cognitive function,* and the level of *alertness,* depending on the age of the child. Simple puzzles may be useful. A child's ability to tell a story or to draw a picture is often a powerful method for assessing cognitive function or for determining the developmental level. The manner in which a child plays with toys or explores the function of a new object or game is an excellent indicator of intellectual curiosity. The level of alertness of a newborn infant depends on many factors, including the time of the last feeding, the room temperature, and the gestational age. Prematures less than 28 wk of gestation do not consistently demonstrate periods of alertness, whereas gentle physical stimulation applied to a slightly older infant arouses the child from sleep and results in a brief period of alertness. Sleep and waking patterns are well developed at term.

The examiner must take advantage of the opportunities provided by the patient; if the circumstances permit, evaluation of muscle power and tone or cerebellar function might precede the cranial nerve examination. However, if a hearing assessment is considered to be important from the historical information, attention should be directed initially to that portion of the examination so that full cooperation can be achieved before the interest and curiosity of the child is lost.

THE HEAD. The *size* and *shape* of the head should be documented carefully. The tower-head or oxycephalic skull suggests premature closure of sutures and is associated with various forms of inherited craniosynostosis (see Sec. 20.16). A broad forehead may indicate hydrocephalus and a small head microcephaly. The observation of a square or a "box-shaped" skull should suggest chronic subdural hematomas, because the longstanding presence of fluid in the subdural space causes enlargement of the middle fossa. Inspection of the scalp should include observation of the venous pattern, because increased intracranial pressure and thrombosis of the superior sagittal sinus can produce marked venous distention.

The infant has two *fontanels* at birth; a diamond-shaped open anterior fontanel that is situated in the midline at the junction of the coronal and sagittal sutures and a posterior fontanel placed between the intersection of the occipital and parietal bones that may be closed at birth or, at the most, admit the tip of a finger. The posterior fontanel is usually closed and nonpalpable beyond the first 6–8 wk of life; its persistence suggests underlying hydrocephalus or the possibility of congenital hypothyroidism. The anterior fontanel varies greatly in size, but the usual measurement approximates 2 × 2 cm. The average time of closure is 18 mo, but the fontanel may normally close as early as 9–12 mo. A very small or absent anterior fontanel at birth may indicate premature fusion of the sutures of microcephaly, whereas a very large fontanel could signify a variety of problems (see Table 9–2). *The fontanel is normally slightly depressed and pulsatile and is best evaluated when the infant is held upright and asleep or feeding.* A bulging fontanel is a reliable indicator of increased intracranial pressure, but vigorous crying can cause a protuberant fontanel in a normal infant.

Palpation of the newborn's skull characteristically shows overriding of the cranial sutures for the first several days of life due to the pressures exerted on the skull during its descent through the pelvis. Marked overriding of the sutures beyond a few days is cause for alarm and suggests the possibility of an underlying abnormality of the brain. Palpation may uncover cranial defects or **craniotabes,** a peculiar softening of the parietal bone so that gentle pressure produces a sensation similar to indenting a ping-pong ball. Craniotabes is often associated with prematurity.

Auscultation of the skull is an important adjunct to the neurologic examination. **Cranial bruits** are most prominent over the anterior fontanel, temporal region, or the orbits and are best heard by the diaphragm of the stethoscope. Soft symmetric bruits may be discovered in normal children less than 4 yr of age or in association with a febrile illness. Arteriovenous malformations of the middle cerebral artery or vein of Galen may produce a loud bruit. Murmurs arising from the heart or great vessels frequently are transmitted to the cranium. The child with severe anemia is often found to have a skull bruit that disappears when the anemia is corrected. Increased intracranial pressure resulting from hydrocephalus, tumor, subdural effusions, or purulent meningitis frequently produce significant intracranial bruits. *The demonstration of a loud or localized bruit is usually significant and warrants further investigation.*

Transillumination of the cranium is an important diagnostic screening procedure that should be performed on any child 2 yr of age and under who is suspected of having a neurologic disorder. The child should be examined in a dark room with a bright flashlight (with a molded rubber adapter) or with a commercially available transilluminator with a high-intensity light source. The degree of transillumination varies with the patient's age, the area of the skull, and the thickness of the cortical mantle. The newborn or premature infant has a very thin skull, particularly in the frontal region, resulting in greater transillumination. Generally, asymmetric, localized, or diffuse transillumination suggests an underlying pathologic process. Increased transillumination is typically observed in hydranencephaly or marked hydrocephalus with a thin cortical mantle. Porencephalic or arachnoid cysts as well as the Dandy-Walker syndrome are frequently demonstrated by this technique. The result of transillumination is often positive in children with subdural effusions complicating meningitis, and the procedure offers a quick, reliable, and noninvasive method of following their size and dissolution. In contrast, acute subdural hematomas may reveal a decreased area of transillumination due to the viscidity of fresh blood.

The correct *measurement of the head circumference* is important. It should be performed on every patient, at every visit, and should be recorded on a suitable head growth chart. A nondistensible plastic measuring tape should be utilized. The tape is placed over the midforehead and is extended circumferentially to include the most prominent portion of the occiput so that the greatest volume of the cranium is measured. The head circumferences of the parents and siblings should also be recorded if the patient is found to have an abnormally sized skull. Errors in the accurate measurement of a newborn skull are frequent and result from scalp edema, overriding of the sutures, intravenous fluid infiltration, and the presence of a cephalohematoma. The average rate of head growth in a healthy premature infant is 0.5 cm in the first 2 wk, 0.75 cm during the 3rd wk, and 1.0 cm in the 4th wk and thereafter until the 40th wk of development. The head circumference of the term infant at birth measures 34–35 cm, 44 cm by 6 mo, and 47 cm by 1 yr of age (see Sec. 3.3).

CRANIAL NERVES. Olfactory Nerve (1). Anosmia, loss of smell, is most commonly found in association with an upper respiratory tract infection in children and, therefore, is a transient abnormality. A fracture of the base of the skull and cribriform plate as well as a frontal lobe tumor also may produce anosmia. Occasionally, a child who recovers from purulent meningitis or who develops hydrocephalus will have a diminished sense of smell. Rarely, anosmia is congenital. Although not a routine component of the examination, smell can be tested reliably as early as the 32nd wk of gestation. Care should be taken to use appropriate stimuli, such as coffee, peppermint, and peanut butter, that are familiar to the child, and strongly aromatic substances should be avoided.

Optic Nerve (2). Examination of the optic disk and retina is an important component of the neurologic examination. In order to visualize a good portion of the retina, dilation of the pupil is necessary. One drop of a combination of 1% cyclopentolate hydrochloride, 2.5% phenylephrine hydrochloride, and 1% tropicamide repeated every 15 min on three occasions effectively produces mydriasis. Mydriatics should not be used if a patient's pupil reaction is necessary to follow the level of consciousness or if a cataract is present. Examination of the retina in an infant is enhanced by providing a nipple or soother and by placing the head on one side. The physician gently strokes the patient to maintain arousal, while examining the closest eye. The older child should be placed in the parent's lap and should be distracted by bright objects or toys that are presented during the ophthalmologic examination. The optic nerve is a salmon-pink color in the child but is a gray-white color in the newborn, particularly in a blond infant. This normal finding may cause confusion and may lead to the improper diagnosis of optic atrophy.

Papilledema rarely occurs in infancy because the skull sutures are capable of separating to accommodate the expanding brain. Papilledema in the older child may be recognized by the following changes in the optic nerve and surrounding retina (Fig. 20–1):

1. The optic nerve becomes hyperemic.
2. The small capillaries that normally transverse the optic nerve are no longer visualized as they become constricted.
3. The larger veins become dilated, and the accompanying arterioles become constricted.

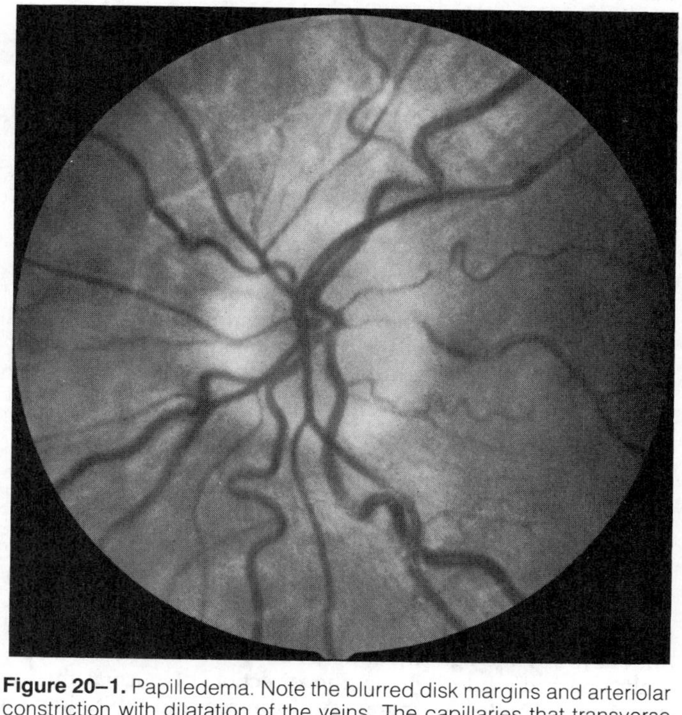

Figure 20–1. Papilledema. Note the blurred disk margins and arteriolar constriction with dilatation of the veins. The capillaries that transverse the optic nerve are difficult to identify.

4. The border of the optic nerve becomes indistinct from the surrounding retina, particularly along the temporal edge.

5. Subhyaloid, flame-shaped hemorrhages appear in the retina surrounding the optic nerve.

6. In some cases, a macular star develops due to retinal edema in the region of the macula. Visual activity and color vision remain intact in acute papilledema as contrasted with optic neuritis, but the blind spot is increased in both.

Retinal hemorrhages occur in 30–40% of all full-term newborn infants. The hemorrhages are more common after vaginal delivery compared with infants delivered by cesarean section and are not associated with birth injury or with neurologic complications. They disappear spontaneously by 1–2 wk of age.

Vision (see also Sec. 22.4). The normal 28-wk-old premature infant blinks when a bright light is directed to the eyes, and by 32 wk the infant maintains eye closure until the light source is removed. At 37 wk, the normal premature turns the head and the eyes to a soft light, and by term, visual fixation and the ability to follow a brilliant target is present. During a period of alertness, optokinetic nystagmus can be demonstrated in the newborn. The visual acuity in the term infant approximates 20/150 and reaches the adult level of 20/20 by about 6 mo of age. Children who are too young to read the standard letters on the Snellen Eye Chart may learn the "E game" by pointing a finger in the direction that the "E" is oriented. Children as young as 2½ or 3 yr of age with normal vision will identify the objects on the Allen Chart at a distance of 15 or 20 ft. Peripheral vision may be tested in an infant by bringing an object from behind the patient into the peripheral field of vision that normally produces a visual recognition response. The examiner should be assured that the object rather than a sound produces the visual response.

The *pupil* is difficult to examine in the premature due to the poorly pigmented iris and the resistance to lid opening. The pupil reacts to light by the 29th–32nd wk of gestation. The equality of the pupils, their size, and reaction to light may be affected by drugs, a space occupying lesion, metabolic disorders, and abnormalities of the midbrain and optic nerves. **Horner syndrome** is characterized by miosis, ptosis, enophthalmos, and ipsilateral anhidrosis of the face. It may be congenital or may result from a lesion involving the sympathetic nervous system in the brain stem, cervical spinal cord, or the sympathetic plexus in juxtaposition to the carotid artery. Localization of the lesion within the sympathetic nervous system is aided by the pupillary response to a series of topical drugs, including cocaine, epinephrine, hydroxyamphetamine, and phenylephrine.

Oculomotor (3), Trochlear (4), and Abducens Nerves (6). The eye is moved by the extraocular muscles that are innervated by the oculomotor, trochlear, and abducens nerves. The oculomotor nerve innervates the superior, inferior, and medial rectus as well as the inferior oblique and the levator palpebra superioris muscle. Complete paralysis of the oculomotor nerve causes ptosis, dilation of the pupil, displacement of the eye outward and downward, and impairment of adduction and elevation. The trochlear nerve supplies the superior oblique muscle, and isolated paralysis causes the eye to deviate upward and outward, often with an associated head tilt. The abducens nerve innervates the lateral rectus muscle so that its paralysis causes medial deviation of the eye and the inability to abduct beyond the midline. In the older child, the **red glass test** is used to assess extraocular palsies. A red glass is placed over one eye, and the patient is requested to follow a white light in all fields of direction. The child sees only one red/white light in the direction of normal muscle function but notes a separation of the red and white images that is greatest in the plane of action of the affected muscle. *Internuclear ophthalmoplegia* results from a lesion in the brain stem and consists of paralysis of medial rectus function of the adducting eye and nystagmus confined to the abducting eye. *Internal ophthalmoplegia* refers to a dilated pupil that is unreactive to light and accommodation but has normal extraocular function, and *external ophthalmoplegia* is associated with ptosis and paralysis of all eye muscles with preservation of the pupillary response. *Nystagmus* is an involuntary rapid movement of the eye that may be horizontal, vertical, rotatory, pendular, or mixed. Jerk nystagmus is used to describe a fast and slow phase. Horizontal nystagmus occurs with an abnormality of the peripheral labyrinth or with a lesion of the vestibular system in the brain stem or cerebellum. Vertical nystagmus is indicative of brain stem dysfunction.

Complete ocular movement may be demonstrated as early as 25 wk of gestation utilizing the **doll's eye maneuver**. This technique is used to examine horizontal and vertical eye movements in the infant, the uncooperative, or the comatose patient. If the head is suddenly turned to the right, the eyes look to the left in a symmetric fashion. Horizontal eye movements in the opposite direction may then be evaluated if the head is turned to the left. Vertical movements may be assessed in a similar fashion by rapid flexion and extension of the head. The normal infant and child will follow a toy or interesting object in all directions. The examiner observes the completeness and flow of the eye movements and determines the presence or absence and the direction of nystagmus, diplopia, opsoclonus, ocular bobbing, or other abnormal eye positions. Premature infants tend to have slightly dysconjugate eyes at rest with one eye horizontally displaced from the other by 1 or 2 mm. Skew deviation of the eyes (vertical displacement) is always abnormal and requires investigation. Strabismus is discussed in Sec. 22.6.

Trigeminal Nerve (5). The sensory distribution of the face is divided into three areas: the ophthalmic area, the maxillary area, and the mandibular area. Each region may be tested by light touch and by pinprick and may be compared with the opposite side. The corneal response is elicited by touching the cornea with a small pledget of cotton and by observing the eye closure response. Trigeminal nerve function in the premature is best documented by facial grimacing from a pinprick (away from the eye) or by stimulating the nostril with a cotton tip. Motor function may be tested by examination of the masseters, pterygoid, and temporalis muscles during mastication as well as by evaluation of the jaw jerk.

Facial Nerve (7). Decreased voluntary movement of the lower face with flattening of the nasolabial angle on the ipsilateral side indicates an upper motor neuron or supranuclear corticospinal lesion. A lower motor neuron lesion tends to equally involve upper and lower facial muscles. Facial nerve paralysis may be congenital or secondary to trauma, infection, intracranial tumor, hypertension, toxins, or myasthenia gravis. Taste may be tested in the cooperative child by placing a solution of saline or glucose on one side of the extended tongue. The normal child can identify the substance with little difficulty.

Auditory Nerve (8). Screening for hearing loss is an important component of the neurologic examination, because a hearing deficit is not readily recognized by parents (see Sec. 22.19). A normal newborn will pause briefly during sucking when a bell is presented, but after several stimuli the pauses will cease as habituation occurs. The neurologically abnormal infant will not habituate. The normal hearing infant will turn its head toward a bell, rattle, or crumpled paper and by 3 mo of age will look at the direction of the sound source. The normally intelligent, hard-of-hearing toddler is visually alert and responds appropriately to physical stimuli. Temper tantrums and abnormal speech are common symptoms in a hard-of-hearing child. Audiometry or brain stem–evoked potential testing is mandatory for any child suspected of a hearing loss (Sec. 22.19). The risk factors that indicate a need for testing during the first few months of life include a family history of deafness, prematurity, severe asphyxia, use of ototoxic drugs in the newborn period, hyperbilirubinemia, congenital anomalies of the head or neck, bacterial meningitis, and congenital infections due to rubella, toxoplasmosis, herpes, and cytomegalovirus.

Vestibular function may be evaluated by the **caloric test**. In the obtunded or comatose patient, approximately 5 mL of ice water is delivered by syringe into the external auditory canal with the patient's head elevated 30 degrees from the horizontal position. A much smaller quantity of ice water (0.5 mL) is used in the alert, awake subject. In the normal subject, introduction of ice water produces nystagmus with the quick component in the opposite direction to the stimulated labyrinth. No response implies severe dysfunction of the brain stem and medial longitudinal fasciculus. If the otoscopic examination reveals a ruptured tympanic membrane, the test should not be performed in that ear.

Glossopharyngeal Nerve (9). This nerve supplies innervation to the stylopharyngeus muscle. An isolated lesion of the ninth cranial nerve is rare. The nerve is tested by observing the gag response to tactile stimulation of the posterior pharyngeal wall. Taste for the posterior one third of the tongue is provided by the sensory portion of the glossopharyngeal nerve.

Vagus Nerve (10). A unilateral injury of the vagus nerve produces weakness and asymmetry of the ipsilateral soft palate and a hoarse voice due to paralysis of a vocal cord. Bilateral lesions may produce respiratory distress as a result of vocal cord paralysis as well as nasal regurgitation of fluids, pooling of secretions, and an immobile, low-lying soft palate. Isolated lesions of the vagus nerve may occur postoperatively following a thoracotomy due to separation of the recurrent laryngeal nerve, and these lesions are not uncommon during the neonatal period in children with the type II Chiari malformation. If a lesion involving the vagus nerve is suspected, visualization of the vocal cords is necessary.

Accessory Nerve (11). Paralysis and atrophy of the sternomastoid and trapezius muscles result from lesions of the accessory nerve. The sternomastoid muscle has two origins; sternal and clavicular, and is tested by forceful rotation of the head and neck against the examiner's hand. Motor neuron disease, myotonic dystrophy, and myasthenia gravis are the most common conditions producing weakness and atrophy of these muscles.

Hypoglossal Nerve (12). The hypoglossal nerve innervates the tongue. Examination of the tongue includes an assessment of its motility, size, and shape and the presence of atrophy or fasciculations. Malfunction of the hypoglossal nucleus or nerve produces wasting, weakness, and fasciculations of the tongue. If the injury is bilateral, tongue protrusion is not possible and dysphagia may be present. Werdnig-Hoffmann disease (infantile spinal muscular atrophy) and congenital anomalies in the region of the foramen magnum are the principle causes of hypoglossal nerve involvement.

MOTOR EXAMINATION. The motor examination includes an assessment of the integrity of the musculoskeletal system and the search for abnormal movements that may indicate an abnormality of the peripheral nervous system or the CNS. The components of the motor examination include testing of power, muscle bulk, tone, posture, locomotion and motility, deep tendon reflexes, and the presence of primitive reflexes, when applicable.

Power. The testing of muscle power is relatively straightforward in the cooperative child. It may begin by requesting that the child squeeze the examiner's fingers, flex and extend the wrist and elbow, and adduct and abduct the shoulder against resistance. Shoulder girdle muscle strength may be evaluated in the newborn or infant by supporting the child by the axillae. The patient with weakness will be unable to support body weight and will "slip through" the examiner's hands. Distal power can be tested in the infant by evaluating the palmar grasp; the child with weakness will not adequately grasp or will show abnormalities in the manipulation of objects. A normal 3- to 4-yr-old child will cooperate in the testing of the extension or flexion of the muscles of the foot, knee, and hip. Examination of the pelvic girdle and proximal lower extremity muscles is also performed by observing the child climb steps or stand up from a prone position. Weakness in these muscles causes the child to use the hands to "climb up" the legs in order to assume an upright position, a maneuver called **Gowers' sign** (Fig. 20–2). The infant with diminished power in the lower extremities tends to have decreased spontaneous activity in the legs and refuses to support body weight when suspended by the axillae. It is important not only to assess individual muscle groups but also to carefully compare muscle power between the upper and lower extremities as well as the opposite extremities. Muscle power in a cooperative child is graded by a scale of 0–5 as follows: 0 = no movement, 1 = movement with gravity eliminated, 2 = full range against gravity, 3 = movement against slight resistance, 4 = movement against moderate resistance, and 5 = normal strength. Examination of muscle power should include the muscles of respiration. Observation of the action of the intercostal muscles, diaphragmatic movement, and the use of accessory muscles of respiration should be documented. Finally, the evaluation of power should include an assessment of muscle bulk and nutrition. Weakness may be associated with muscle atrophy and fasciculations. Because most infants have an excess of body fat, muscle fasciculations and atrophy are most commonly demonstrated in the denervated tongue in this age group.

Tone. Muscle tone is tested by assessing the degree of resistance when an individual joint is moved passively. Tone undergoes considerable change and assumes different forms depending on age. The premature or newborn infant is relatively hypotonic compared with the child. Tone in this age group is tested by a variety of maneuvers (see Sec. 9.17 and Fig. 9–9). When the upper extremity of the normal term infant is pulled gently across the chest, the elbow normally does not quite reach the mid-sternum **(scarf sign)**. The elbow of the hypotonic infant extends beyond the midline with ease. Measurement of the popliteal angle is a useful method to document tone in the legs of the newborn. The examiner flexes the child's lower extremity on the abdomen and extends the knee. The normal term infant allows extension of the knee to approximately 80 degrees. Abnormalities of tone consists of spasticity, rigidity, and hypotonia.

Spasticity is characterized by an initial resistance to passive movement, followed by a sudden release called the **clasp-knife** phenomenon. Spasticity is most apparent in the upper extremity flexors and lower extremity extensor muscles. It is associated with brisk tendon reflexes and an extensor plantar reflex, clonus, diminished active movements, and disuse atrophy. **Clonus** may be demonstrated in the lower extremity by sudden dorsiflexion of the foot with the knee partially flexed. Whereas sustained clonus is always abnormal, 5–10 beats in the newborn is a normal finding unless the clonus is asymmetric. Spasticity results from a lesion that involves upper motor neuron tracts and may be unilateral or bilateral. *Rigidity*, the result of a basal ganglia lesion, is characterized by a constant resistance to passive movement of both extensor and flexor muscles. As the extremity is undergoing passive movement, a typical **cogwheel** sensation may be evident. The rigidity persists with repetitive passive extension and flexion of a joint and does not "give away" or release, such as with

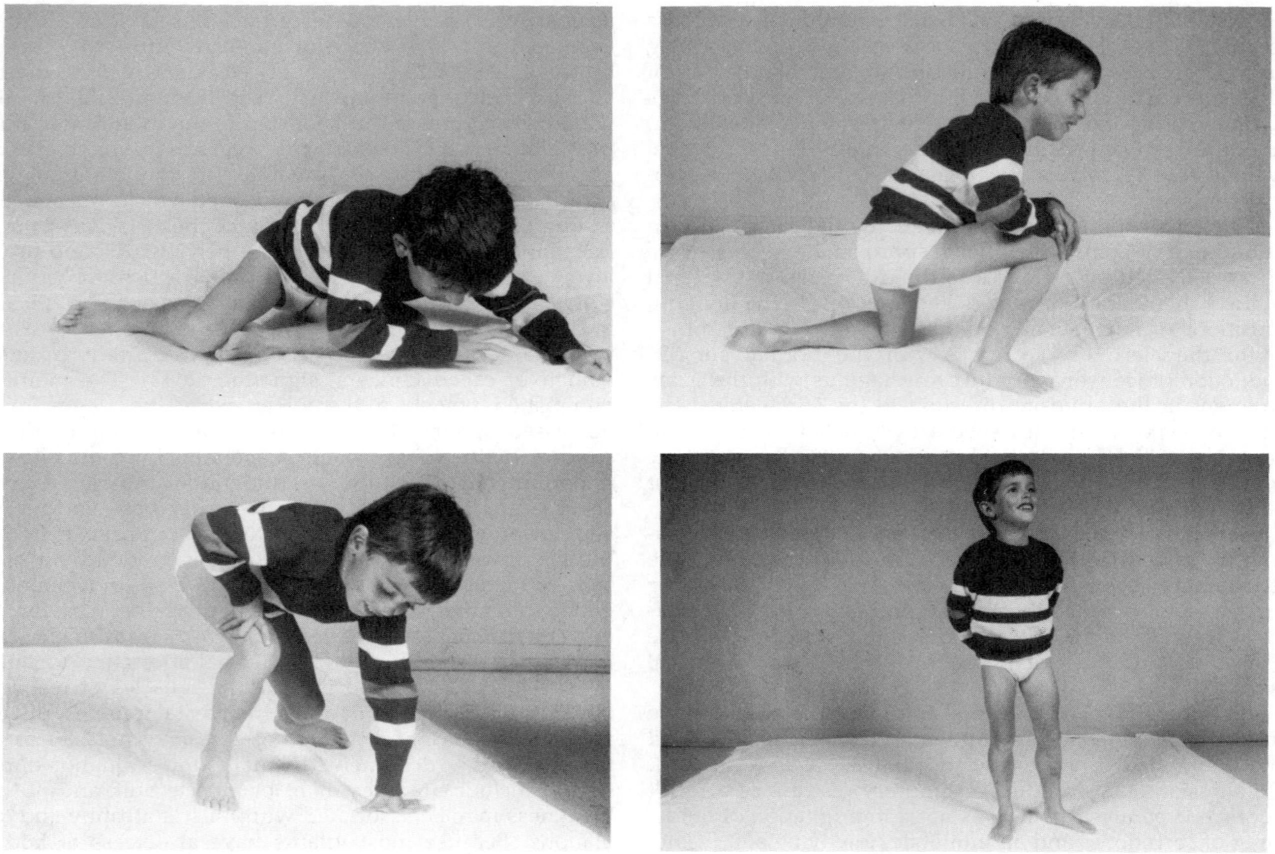

Figure 20–2. Gowers' sign. A boy with hip girdle weakness due to Duchenne muscular dystrophy.

spasticity. The child with spastic lower extremities will drag the legs while crawling or will walk on tip-toes. The patient with marked spasticity or rigidity will develop a posture of opisthotonus in which the head and the heels are bent backward and the body bowed forward (Fig. 20–3). *Hypotonia* refers to abnormally diminished tone and is the most common abnormality of tone in the neurologically compromised premature neonate. The demonstration of hypotonia may reflect pathology of the cerebral hemispheres, cerebellum, spinal cord, anterior horn cell, peripheral nerve, myoneural junction, or muscle. An unusual position or posture by an infant is a reflection of abnormal tone. The hypotonic infant is **floppy** and may have difficulty in maintaining head support or a straight back while sitting. Such infants may assume a **frog-leg** posture in the supine position. The premature infant of 28 wk of gestation tends to extend all extremities at rest, but by 32 wk there is evidence of flexion, particularly in the lower extremities. The normal full-term infant's posture is characterized by flexion of all extremities.

Motility and Locomotion. The premature of less than 32 wk of gestation displays random slow writhing movements interspersed with rapid, myoclonic-like activity of the extremities. Beyond 32 wk, the motor activity is primarily flexor. Observation of crawling, cruising, walking, or running may uncover movement disorders, most of which are most likely to be apparent during motion and to disappear with rest or sleep. *Ataxia* refers to incoordination of movement or a disturbance of balance. It may be primarily truncal or may be limited to the extremities. Truncal ataxia is characterized by unsteadiness during sitting or standing and results primarily from involvement of the cerebellar vermis. Abnormalities of the cerebellar hemispheres characteristically cause intention tremor unaffected by visual attention. Ataxia may be demonstrated by the finger-to-nose and heel-to-shin tests, heel-to-toe or tandem walking, and, in the infant, by observation of reaching for or playing with toys. Additional abnormalities associated with cerebellar lesions include dysmetria (errors in measuring distances), rebound (inability to inhibit a muscular action, such as when the examiner suddenly releases the flexed arm and the patient inadvertently strikes the face), and dysdiadochokinesia (diminished performance of rapid alternating movements). Hypotonia, dysarthria, nystagmus, and decreased deep tendon reflexes are common features of cer-

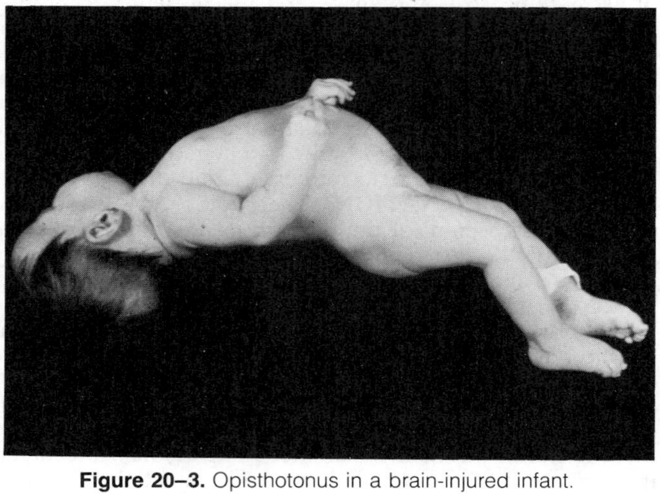

Figure 20–3. Opisthotonus in a brain-injured infant.

ebellar abnormalities. Sensory ataxia is found with diseases of the spinal cord and peripheral nerves. In these disorders, the **Romberg sign** (patient is unsteady with eyes closed but not open) is positive, and there are often related sensory findings including abnormalities in joint position and vibration sense.

Chorea is characterized by involuntary movements of the major joints, trunk, and the face that are rapid and jerky. The child is incapable of extending the arms without producing abnormal movements. There is a tendency to pronate the arms when held above the head. The hand grip contracts and relaxes **(milk-maid sign)**, the speech is explosive and inarticulate, the deep tendon reflexes of the knee are "hung up," and the patient may have difficulty in maintaining protrusion of the tongue. *Athetosis* is a slow, writhing movement that is often associated with abnormalities of muscle tone. It is most prominent in the distal extremities and is enhanced by voluntary activity or emotional upset. Speech and swallowing may be affected. Chorea and athetosis are the result of basal ganglia lesions and are difficult to separate clinically. They may both be prominent in the same patient. *Dystonia* is an involuntary, slow, twisting movement that primarily involves the proximal muscles of the extremities, trunk, and neck.

Deep Tendon Reflexes and the Plantar Response. The deep tendon reflexes are readily elicited in most infants and children. In the premature and term infant, the biceps, knee, and ankle jerks are the most reliable deep tendon reflexes. The ankle reflex is difficult to obtain by percussing the Achilles tendon in this age group. Gentle dorsiflexion of the foot and tapping the plantar surface with the reflex hammer will usually elicit a response. The knee jerk in the infant may produce a crossed adductor response (tapping the patellar tendon in one leg causes contraction in the opposite extremity), which does not become abnormal until 6–7 mo of age. The deep tendon reflexes are absent or decreased in primary disorders of the muscle (myopathy), nerve (neuropathy), myoneural junction, and abnormalities of the cerebellum. They are characteristically increased in upper motor neuron lesions. Asymmetry of deep tendon reflexes suggests a lateralizing lesion. The plantar response is obtained by stimulation of the external portion of the sole of the foot, beginning at the heel and extending to the base of the toes. Firm pressure from the examiner's thumb is a useful method for eliciting the response. The **Babinski reflex** is characterized by extension of the great toe and by fanning of the remaining toes. Too vigorous stimulation may produce withdrawal, which may be misinterpreted as a Babinski response. Most newborn infants show an initial flexion of the great toe upon plantar stimulation. As with adults, asymmetry of the plantar response between extremities is a useful lateralizing sign in infants and children.

Primitive Reflexes. Primitive reflexes appear and disappear in sequence during specific periods of development. Their absence or persistence beyond a given time frame signifies dysfunction of the CNS. Some primitive reflexes, such as the snout or **rooting reflex**, reappear during old age or with specific degenerative diseases involving the cerebral cortex. Although many primitive reflexes have been described, the Moro, grasp, tonic neck, and parachute reflexes are the most important. The **Moro reflex** is obtained by placing the infant in a semi-upright position. The head is momentarily allowed to fall backward with immediate resupport by the examiner's hand. The child will symmetrically abduct and extend the arms, flex the thumbs, followed by flexion and adduction of the upper extremities. An asymmetric response may signify a fractured clavicle, brachial plexus injury, or a hemiparesis. Absence of the Moro reflex in the term newborn is ominous, suggesting a significant dysfunction of the CNS. The **grasp** response is elicited by placing a finger or object in the open palm of each hand. The normal infant will grasp the object and with attempted removal, the grip is reinforced. The **tonic neck** reflex is produced by manually turning the head to one side while supine. Extension of the arm occurs on that side of the body corresponding to the direction of the face, while flexion develops in the contralateral extremities. An obligatory tonic neck response, by which the infant remains "locked" in the fencer's position, is always abnormal and implies a disorder of the CNS. The **parachute reflex** is demonstrated by suspending the child by the trunk and by suddenly producing forward flexion as if the child were to fall. The child spontaneously extends the upper extremities as a protective mechanism. The parachute reflex appears before the onset of walking.

SENSORY EXAMINATION. The sensory examination is difficult to interpret in the infant or uncooperative child. Furthermore, the understanding child soon tires of the examination because it requires considerable attention to repetitious and uninteresting tasks. The more this part of the neurologic examination can be made to simulate a game, the greater will be the likelihood that the child will cooperate. Fortunately, disorders involving the sensory system are less common in the pediatric population than among adults, so that this component of the neurologic assessment is less important for infants and children than for the adolescent and adult. While the infant is distracted by a parent or an interesting toy, the examiner touches the patient with a piece of cotton or a sterile pin. The normal child indicates an awareness of the stimulus by pausing during play, withdrawing the extremity, crying, or looking at and touching the stimulated area. Unfortunately, the child quickly loses patience and soon begins to disregard the examiner. It is critical, therefore, that the area in question is tested efficiently and, if necessary, re-examined at an appropriate time.

The identification of a sensory level in association with a *spinal cord lesion* can be very difficult in the infant. Observation may suggest a difference in color, temperature, or perspiration, with the skin cooler and dry below the spinal cord level. Touching the skin lightly above the level evokes a response that is usually in the form of a squirming movement or physical withdrawal. The superficial abdominal reflexes may be absent. A child with a spinal cord lesion may have evidence of rectal sphincter incontinence that is manifested by a patulous anus, by the absence of contraction of the sphincter when the skin in the anal region is stimulated with a sharp object (anal wink), and by a lack of contraction of the anal sphincter during the rectal examination. Children 4–5 yr of age are capable of detailed sensory testing, including joint position, vibration, temperature, stereognosis, two-point discrimination, double simultaneous extinction, light touch, and pain. The success of the sensory examination depends on the ingenuity and the patience of the examiner.

GAIT AND STATION. Observation of a child's gait is an important aspect of the neurologic examination. The *spastic gait* is characterized by stiffness and by a "tin-soldier"-like steppage appearance. The spastic child may walk on tip toes because of tightness or contractures of the Achilles tendons. *Hemiparesis* is associated with a decreased arm swing on the affected side and a lateral circular motion of the leg **(circumduction gait)**. Extrapyramidal movements, such as dystonia or chorea, may become apparent while the child is walking or running. Cerebellar ataxia produces a broad-based unsteady gait and, if severe, the child requires support to prevent falling. Heel-to-toe or tandem walking is performed poorly in patients with abnormalities of the cerebellum. A **waddling gait** results from weakness of the proximal hip girdle. These children often develop a compensatory lordosis and have difficulty in climbing stairs. Weakness or hypotonia of the lower extremities may result in genu recurvatum and flat feet, which causes a clumsy, tentative gait. *Scoliosis* may cause an abnormal gait and can result from disorders of muscle and spinal cord.

SOFT NEUROLOGIC SIGNS. These signs should be interpreted cautiously because they are present in normal children during various stages of neurodevelopment. A soft neurologic sign may be defined as a particular form of deviant performance on a motor or sensory test in the neurologic examination that is abnormal for a particular age. Testing for the presence of soft neurologic signs involves the observation of a series of timed motor tasks and a comparison of the quality and the precision of the patient's movement with normal controls of similar age and sex. The tests include repetitive and successive finger movements, hand pats, arm pronation-supination movements, foot-taps, hopping, and tandem walking. There is considerable variation in the expression of these signs, depending on age, sex, and maturation of the nervous system. For example, minimal choreoathetoid movements in the fingers of the extended arms are normal at 4 yr of age but disappear by 7 or 8 yr of age. The neurodevelopment of girls is more accelerated than that of boys for many motor tasks, including hopping, skipping, and fine balance maneuvers. Although intellectually normal children may demonstrate a soft neurologic sign, the finding of two or more persistent soft signs correlates significantly with neurologic dysfunction, including attention deficit disorder, learning disorders, and cerebral palsy. Because specific soft signs lack association with a particular disability and can occur in the normal child, it is unwise to label a child who manifests several soft neurologic signs. It is more appropriate to monitor such a patient closely and to ensure that a developmental disability has been excluded.

SPECIAL DIAGNOSTIC PROCEDURES

LUMBAR PUNCTURE AND CEREBROSPINAL FLUID EXAMINATION. An examination of the cerebrospinal fluid (CSF) is essential in confirming the diagnosis of meningitis, encephalitis, and subarachnoid hemorrhage and is often helpful in the evaluation of demyelinating, degenerative, and collagen vascular diseases and the presence of tumor cells within the subarachnoid space. Preparation of the patient is important in order to successfully complete the procedure. The skin is thoroughly prepared with a cleansing agent, and the patient is placed in the lateral recumbent position. The physician should be gowned and gloved; drapes are optional. The neck and legs of the patient are flexed by an assistant to enlarge the intervertebral spaces. The ideal interspace for lumbar puncture (LP) is L3–L4 or L4–L5, which is found by drawing an imaginary horizontal line from the anterior superior spine of the ilium. The skin and underlying tissue are anesthetized with a local anesthetic. A No. 18- to 22-gauge, 1- to 2-inch sharp, beveled spinal needle with a properly fitting stylet is introduced into the midsagittal plane directed slightly in the cephalad direction. The stylet is removed frequently as the needle is slowly advanced to determine whether CSF is present. A "pop" is felt as the needle penetrates the dura and enters the subarachnoid space. A manometer and a three-way stopcock may be attached to obtain an opening pressure. The opening pressure in the recumbent position should be less than 160 mm of water. The most common cause of an elevated opening pressure is a crying, uncooperative, and struggling patient. The pressure is recorded most reliably with the child positioned comfortably with the head and the legs extended. Newborns and neonates should be placed in the upright position for a spinal tap, because decreased ventilation and perfusion abnormalities leading to respiratory arrest are more common in the recumbent position in this age group.

The *contraindications* for performing an LP include: (1) raised intracranial pressure owing to a suspected mass lesion of the brain or spinal cord, which may develop transtentorial herniation or herniation of the cerebellar tonsils following the procedure. Inspection of the eyegrounds for the presence of papilledema is mandatory before proceeding with an LP; (2) A skin infection at the site of the LP. If examination of the CSF is urgent in such a patient, a ventricular or cisterna magna tap performed by a skilled physician is indicated; (3) Thrombocytopenia, with a platelet count less than 20×10^9/L may cause uncontrolled bleeding in the subarachnoid or subdural space; and (4) on *rare occasions*, an LP is temporarily withheld from a critically ill moribund patient because the procedure may produce cardiorespiratory arrest. In this situation, blood cultures are drawn; antibiotics and supportive care are administered; and when the patient is stabilized, the LP may be accomplished safely under more controlled circumstances.

Normal CSF is the color of water. Cloudy CSF results from an elevated white blood cell (WBC) or red blood cell (RBC) count. The normal CSF contains up to five lymphocytes, and the newborn may have as many as 15 per mm^3. Polymorphonuclear (PMN) cells are always abnormal in the child, but 1–2 per mm^3 may be present in the normal neonate. The presence of PMN cells raises suspicion of a pathologic process. An elevated PMN count suggests bacterial meningitis or the early phase of an aseptic meningitis (Sec. 12.6). CSF lymphocytosis indicates aseptic, tuberculous, or fungal meningitis; demyelinating diseases; brain or spinal cord tumor; immunologic disorders including collagen vascular diseases; and chemical irritation (e.g., postmyelogram, intrathecal methotrexate). A Gram stain of the CSF is essential in the investigation of suspected bacterial meningitis; an acid-fast stain or India ink preparation is used if tuberculous or fungal meningitis is a possibility. The fluid is placed on appropriate culture media based on the clinical findings and on the CSF analysis. There are no RBCs in normal CSF. The presence of RBCs indicates a traumatic tap or a subarachnoid hemorrhage. Bloody CSF should be centrifuged immediately. The supernatant of a bloody tap will be clear, but it will be xanthochromic in the presence of a subarachnoid hemorrhage. Progressive clearing of bloody CSF is noted during the collection of the fluid in the case of a traumatic tap. The presence of crenated RBCs does not differentiate a traumatic tap from a subarachnoid hemorrhage. In addition to a subarachnoid hemorrhage, xanthochromia may result from hyperbilirubinemia, carotenemia, and a markedly elevated CSF protein.

The normal *CSF protein* ranges from 10–40 mg/dL in the child and as high as 120 mg/dL in the neonate. The CSF protein falls to the normal childhood range by 3 mo of age. The CSF protein may be elevated in multiple processes, including infectious, immunologic, vascular, and degenerative diseases as well as tumors of the brain and spinal cord. The CSF protein is increased following a bloody tap by approximately 1 mg/dL for every 1,000 RBC/mm^3. Elevation of CSF immunoglobulin G (IgG), which normally represents approximately 10% of the total protein, is observed in subacute sclerosing panencephalitis, postinfectious encephalomyelitis, and in some cases of multiple sclerosis.

The *CSF glucose* content is about 60% of the blood glucose in the healthy child. In order to prevent a spuriously elevated blood/CSF glucose ratio in a case of suspected meningitis, it is advisable to collect the blood glucose prior to the LP when the child is relatively calm. Hypoglycorrhachia is found in association with diffuse meningeal disease, particularly bacterial and tuberculous meningitis. In addition, widespread neoplastic involvement of the meninges, subarachnoid hemorrhage, fungal meningitis, and, on occasion, aseptic meningitis can produce a low CSF glucose.

The CSF may also be examined for specific *antigens* (e.g., latex agglutination for suspected meningitis) and the investigation of a series of metabolic diseases (e.g., lactate, endolase determination).

SUBDURAL TAP. This procedure may be indicated to establish the diagnosis of a subdural effusion or hematoma. A blunt, short-beveled No. 20 gauge needle and stylet are used for the procedure. The subdural space is approached at the lateral border of the anterior fontanel or along the upper margin of the coronal suture at least 2–3 cm from the midline to prevent injury to the underlying sagittal sinus. Following adequate cleansing and preparation of the skull, including shaving of the hair from the operative site, the patient is placed in the supine position and is firmly held by an attendant. The needle and stylet are slowly advanced through the skin and underlying tissue with a z-like movement until the dura is entered with a sudden "popping" sensation. Considerable care is taken to prevent advancement of the needle into the cerebral cortex, which in the infant is approximately 1.5 cm from the skin surface. The attachment of a hemostat approximately 5–7 mm from the beveled end of the needle should provide an adequate safeguard. The subdural fluid, which may squirt out under pressure, is collected and is sent for protein analysis, cell count, and culture. The color of the fluid may be xanthochromic, bright red, or an oily brown (depending on the age of the subdural collections). Bilateral subdural taps may be indicated, because subdural collections are bilateral in most cases. The amount of fluid removed with each tap should be limited to a total of 15–20 mL from each side in order to prevent rebleeding from a sudden shift of the intracranial contents. At the termination of the procedure, a sterile dressing is applied, and the child is placed in a sitting position that tends to prevent leakage of fluid from the puncture site. (See Sec. 12.15 for a discussion of subdural fluid associated with meningitis.)

VENTRICULAR TAP. A ventricular tap is used for the removal of CSF in the management of life-threatening increased intracranial pressure when conservative measures have failed. The procedure should not be undertaken by a pediatrician except when the patient's life is in jeopardy and a neurosurgeon is not available. For the infant, the procedure is similar to a subdural tap. A No. 20 gauge ventricular needle with a stylet is placed in the lateral border of the anterior fontanel and is directed toward the inner canthus of the ipsilateral eye. The needle is advanced slowly, and the stylet is removed frequently to determine the presence of CSF. The ventricle is usually encountered about 4 cm from the skin surface.

NEURORADIOLOGIC PROCEDURES (see also Sec. 6.56). The *skull roentgenogram* remains a useful diagnostic procedure but unfortunately is frequently overlooked in the era of computed tomography (CT) scanning and magnetic resonance imaging (MRI). It may demonstrate fractures, intracranial calcification, craniosynostosis, congenital anomalies, or bony defects and evidence of increased intracranial pressure. Acute increased intracranial pressure is characterized by separation of the sutures, whereas erosion of the posterior clinoid processes, enlargement of the sella turcica, and an increase in convolutional markings indicate long-standing intracranial hypertension. *CT scanning* has revolutionized the neuroradiologic examination of children, obviating pneumoencephalography, and has greatly reduced the requirement for cerebral angiography. CT scanning is a noninvasive procedure that utilizes conventional x-ray techniques (Sec. 6.56). Sedation is usually required for infants and young children, because a lack of head movement is essential during the study. Pentobarbital, 4 mg/kg intramuscularly (IM), 30 min before the CT scan with a supplementary dose of 2 mg/kg IM, 1–1½ hr later if necessary, is usually effective. Chloral hydrate, 50–75 mg/kg PO 45 min before the procedure is an alternate method of sedation. CT scanning is useful in demonstrating congenital malformations of the brain, including hydrocephalus and porencephalic cysts, subdural collections, cerebral atrophy, intracranial calcification, intracerebral hematoma, brain tumors and areas of cerebral edema, infarction, and demyelination. The intravenous injection of radiographic contrast medium enhances areas of increased vascular permeability due to abnormalities of the blood-brain barrier and highlights abnormal collections of blood vessels in an arteriovenous malformation. *MRI* is a noninvasive procedure that does not utilize ionizing radiation. It is especially well suited for the study of neoplasms, cerebral edema, degenerative diseases, and congenital anomalies, particularly of the posterior fossa and spinal cord. MRI is capable of detecting small plaques in patients with multiple sclerosis and areas of localized gliosis in children with uncontrolled seizures. Intracerebral calcifications are not detected by MRI. *Radionuclide brain scan* utilizes a radioactive material such as ^{99}Tc, which concentrates in regions where the blood-brain barrier has been disrupted. It is useful in the investigation of herpes encephalitis and cerebral abscess. *Cerebral angiography* is reserved for the study of vascular disorders. The procedure requires a general anesthetic in most children. Cerebral angiography, utilizing subtraction techniques, is particularly useful for the delineation of arteriovenous malformations, aneurysms, arterial occlusions, and venous thrombosis. In most cases, a four-vessel study (internal carotids and vertebral arteries) is accomplished. *Cranial ultrasound*, for the detection of intracranial hemorrhage, hydrocephalus, and intracranial tumors, is limited to the infant with a patent fontanel. The procedure is utilized intraoperatively in older children for the placement of shunts, for the location of small tumors, and for the direction of needle biopsies. *Myelography* was used in the past for the demonstration of congenital anomalies, tumors, and vascular malformations of the spinal cord. MRI is superior in most cases to contrast myelography and is not associated with arachnoiditis, which occasionally complicates the injection of contrast material into the subarachnoid space.

ELECTROENCEPHALOGRAPHY. The *electroencephalogram* (EEG) provides a continuous recording of electrical activity between reference electrodes placed on the scalp. Although the genesis of the electrical activity is not certain, it likely originates from postsynaptic potentials in the dendrites of cortical neurons. Even with amplification of the electrical activity, not all potentials are recorded due to the buffering effect of the scalp, muscles, bone, vessels, and subarachnoid fluid. The EEG waves are classified according to their frequency as delta (1–3/sec), theta (4–7/sec), alpha (8–12/sec), and beta (13–20/sec). These waves are altered by many factors, including age, state of alertness, eye closure, drugs, and disease states. The maturational changes between the neonate and childhood are evident in Figure 20–4. High-voltage slow and sharp waves (K complexes) and sleep spindles (regular 12–14/sec waves) confined to the central regions occur during sleep in the normal EEG. Abnormalities of waveform include spikes and slow waves. Spikes are characteristically paroxysmal, sharp, and of high voltage followed by a slow wave. Spike and slow waves are associated with epilepsy, but some normal patients may have this EEG finding. Focal spikes are often associated with irritative lesions, including cysts, slow-growing tumors, and glial scar tissue. Epileptiform activity may be enhanced by activation procedures, including hyperventilation, photic stimulation, and sleep deprivation. Slow waves may be focal, in which case a circumscribed lesion such as a hematoma, tumor, infarction, or a localized infectious process may be considered; generalized slow waves suggest a metabolic, inflammatory, or more widespread process.

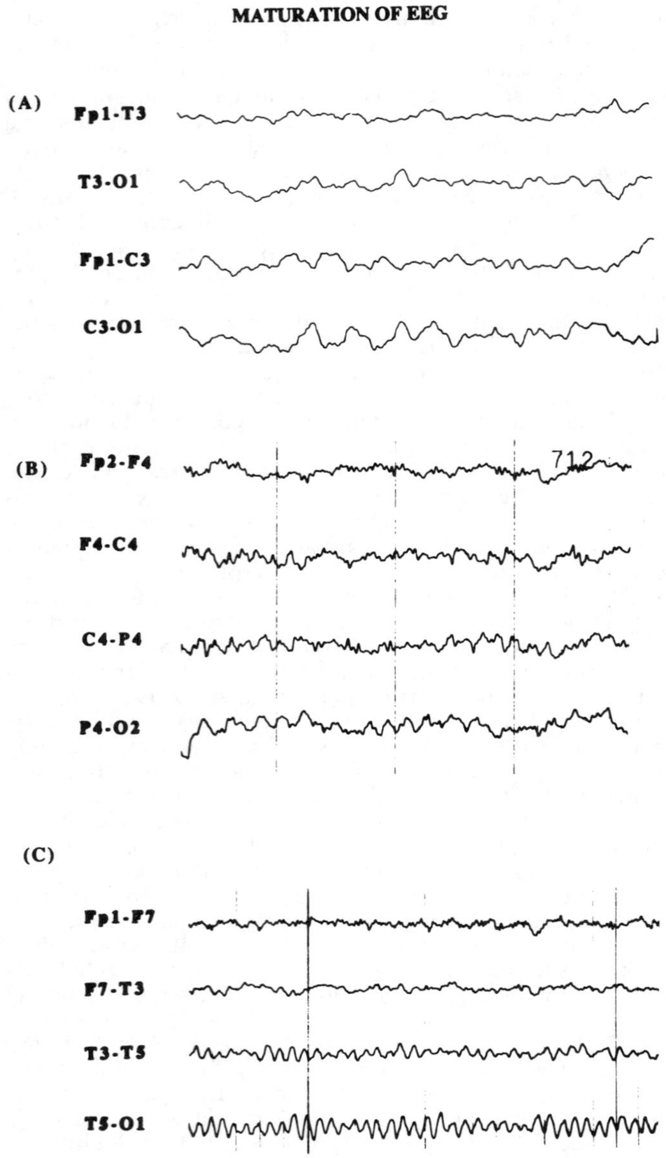

Figure 20–4. *A*, Normal waking record in a term infant. The background rhythm consists of low-amplitude 3- to 4-Hz activity. *B*, An 8-mo-old infant with occipital θ (5 Hz) and superimposed frontal β waves. *C*, Normal 9 yr old. Note the regular α rhythm in the occipital region.

EEG/polygraphic/video monitoring provides precise characterization of seizure types, which allows for specific medical or surgical management. In addition, the physician is more accurately able to differentiate epileptic seizures from paroxysmal events that mimic epilepsy, including pseudoseizures. EEG/polygraphic/video monitoring provides for the quantification of seizure discharges and for the study of the efficacy of various therapeutic regimens. Finally, polygraphic/EEG with video monitoring simultaneously records physiologic and EEG changes, which is particularly useful in the neonate, in whom the characterization of seizures is difficult.

EVOKED POTENTIALS. An evoked potential is an electrical response that follows stimulation of the CNS by a specific stimulus of the visual, auditory, or sensory system. The clinical application of evoked potentials in infants and children has increased dramatically during the last decade. Stimulation of the visual system by a flash or patterned stimulus, such as a black and white checkerboard, produces *visual evoked potentials* (VEPs), which are recorded over the occiput and averaged in a computer. Abnormal VEPs result from lesions involving the visual system from the retina to the visual cortex. Neurodegenerative diseases, such as Tay-Sachs, Krabbe, Pelizaeus-Merzbacher disease, and neuronal ceroid lipofuscinoses, show characteristic VEP abnormalities. Lesions of the optic nerve and chiasm also produce abnormalities in the VEP response. The VEP, using patterned stimuli, is useful particularly in the assessment of visual function in the at-risk neonate. *Brain stem auditory evoked potentials* (BAEPs) may be used to objectively measure hearing acuity, particularly in the neonate or uncooperative child when routine hearing assessment techniques have failed. The BAEP is abnormal in many neurodegenerative diseases in children and is an important tool in the evaluation of patients with suspected tumors of the cerebellopontine angle. BAEPs are helpful in the assessment of brain stem function in the comatose patient, because the waveforms are unaffected by drugs or by the level of consciousness. They are less accurate in predicting neurologic recovery and outcome. *Somatosensory evoked potentials* (SSEPs) are obtained by stimulating a peripheral nerve (peroneal, median) and by recording the electrical response over the cervical region and contralateral parietal somatosensory cortex. The SSEP determines the functional integrity of the dorsal column–medial-lemniscal system and is useful in monitoring spinal cord function during operative procedures, such as scoliosis, the repair of coarctation of the aorta, and myelomeningocele. SSEPs are abnormal in many neurodegenerative disorders in children and are the most accurate evoked potential in the assessment of neurologic outcome following a severe CNS insult.

Backman DS, Hodges FJ, Freeman JM: Computerized axial tomography in neurologic disorders of children. Pediatrics 59:352, 1977.

Fagan ER, Taylor MJ, Logan WJ: Somatosensory evoked potentials. Part II: A review of the clinical applications in pediatric neurology. Pediatr Neurol 3:249, 1987.

Gooding CA, Brasch RC, Lallemand DP, et al: Nuclear magnetic resonance imaging of the brain in children. J Pediatr 104:509, 1984.

Mizrahi EM: Electroencephalographic/polygraphic/video monitoring in childhood epilepsy. J Pediatr 105:1, 1984.

Packer RJ, Zimmerman RA, Sutton LN, et al: Magnetic resonance imaging of spinal cord disease of childhood. Pediatrics 78:251, 1986.

Portnoy JM, Olson LC: Normal cerebrospinal fluid values in children: Another look. Pediatrics 75:484, 1985.

CONGENITAL ANOMALIES OF THE CENTRAL NERVOUS SYSTEM

20.2 NEURAL TUBE DEFECTS (DYSRAPHISM)

Neural tube defects account for most congenital anomalies of the CNS and result from the failure of the neural tube to close spontaneously between the 3rd and 4th wk of in utero development. Although the precise cause of neural tube defects remains unknown, there is evidence that many factors, including radiation, drugs, malnutrition, chemicals, and genetic determinates, may adversely affect the normal development of the CNS from the time of conception. In some cases, an abnormal maternal nutritional state or exposure to radiation prior to conception may increase the likelihood of a CNS congenital malformation. The major neural tube defects include spina bifida occulta, meningocele, myelomeningocele, encephalocele, anencephaly, dermal sinus, tethered cord, syringomyelia, diastematomyelia, and lipoma involving the conus medullaris.

The human nervous system originates from the primitive ectoderm that also develops into the epidermis. The ectoderm, endoderm, and mesoderm form the three primary germ layers that are developed by the 3rd week. The endoderm, particularly the notochordal plate and the intraembryonic mesoderm, induces the overlying ectoderm to develop the neural plate during the 3rd week of development (Fig. 20–5*A*). Failure of normal induction is responsible for most of the neural tube defects. Rapid growth of cells within the neural plate causes further invagination of the neural groove and the differentiation of a conglomerate of cells, the neural crest, which migrate laterally on the surface of the neural tube (see Fig. 20–5*B*). The notochordal plate becomes the centrally placed notochord, which acts as a foundation around which the vertebral column ultimately develops. With the formation of the vertebral column, the notochord undergoes involution and becomes the nucleus pulposus of the intervertebral disks. The neural crest cells differentiate to form the peripheral nervous system, including the spinal and autonomic ganglia as well as the ganglia of cranial nerves V, VII, IX, and X. In addition, the neural crest forms the leptomeninges, including the dura, as well as Schwann cells, which are responsible for myelinization of the peripheral nervous system.

During the 3rd week of embryonic development, invagination of the neural groove is completed and the neural tube is formed by separation from the overlying surface ectoderm (see Fig. 20–5*C*). The initial closure of the neural tube is accomplished in the area corresponding to the future junction of the spinal cord and medulla and moves rapidly both caudally and rostrally. For a brief period the neural tube is open at both ends, and the neural canal communicates freely with the amniotic cavity (see Fig. 20–5*D*). Failure of closure of the neural tube allows the excretion of fetal substances (e.g., α-fetoprotein, acetylcholine) into the amniotic fluid, serving as biochemical markers for a neural tube defect. Normally, the rostral end of the neural tube closes on the 25th day, and the caudal neuropore closes by the 27th day of development, prior to the time that many women realize they are pregnant.

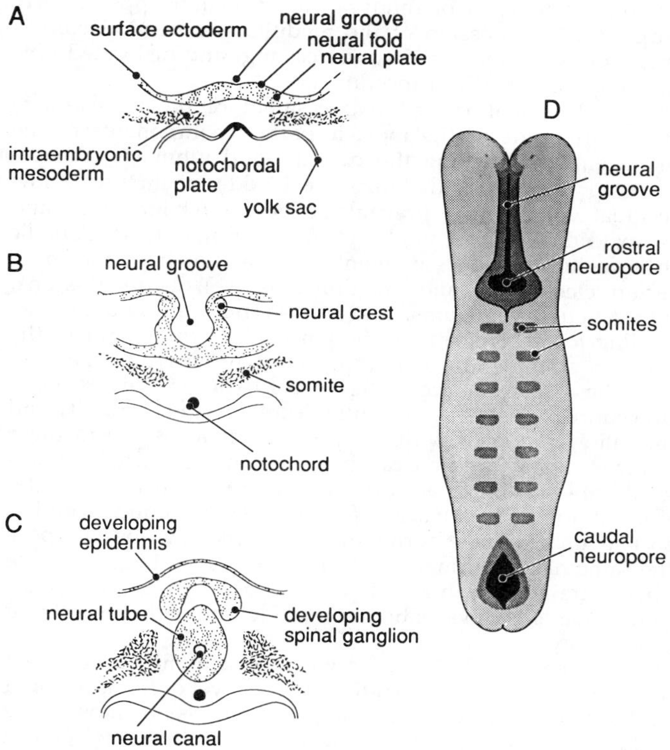

Figure 20–5. Diagrammatic illustration of the developing nervous system. *A*, Transverse sections of the neural plate during the 3rd week. *B*, Formation of the neural groove and the neural crest. *C*, The neural tube is developed. *D*, Longitudinal drawing showing the initial closure of the neural tube in the central region.

20.3 SPINA BIFIDA OCCULTA

This common anomaly represents the most benign form of dysraphism. Most individuals are asymptomatic and lack neurologic signs, and the condition is usually of no consequence. In some cases patches of hair, a lipoma, discoloration of the skin, or a dermal sinus in the midline of the low back signifies an underlying spina bifida occulta. A spine roentgenogram shows a defect in the closure of the posterior vertebral arches and laminae, typically involving L5 and S1. There is no abnormality of the meninges, spinal cord, or nerve roots. Spina bifida occulta is occasionally associated with more significant developmental abnormalities of the spinal cord, including syringomyelia, diastematomyelia, and a tethered cord (see Sec. 20.78, 20.79, and 20.80).

20.4 MENINGOCELE

A meningocele is formed when the meninges herniate through a defect in the posterior vertebral arches. A fluctuant midline mass that may transilluminate occurs along the vertebral column, usually in the low back. Most meningoceles are well covered with skin and pose no threat to the patient. A careful neurologic examination is mandatory. Asymptomatic children with a normal neurologic examination and full-thickness skin covering the meningocele may have surgery delayed. Prior to surgical correction of the defect, the patient must be thoroughly examined with the use of plain roentgenograms, ultrasound, and CT scanning with metrizamide or MRI to determine the extent of neural tissue involvement and associated anomalies, including diastematomyelia, tethered spinal cord, and lipoma. Those patients with leaking CSF or a thin skin covering should undergo immediate surgical treatment to prevent meningitis. A CT scan of the head is recommended for children with a meningocele because of the association with hydrocephalus in some cases. An anterior meningocele projects into the pelvis through a defect in the sacrum. Symptoms of constipation and bladder dysfunction develop owing to the increasing size of the lesion. Female patients may have associated anomalies of the genital tract, including a rectovaginal fistula and vaginal septa. Plain roentgenograms demonstrate a defect in the sacrum and CT scanning or MRI outline the extent of the meningocele.

20.5 MYELOMENINGOCELE

Myelomeningocele represents the most severe form of dysraphism involving the vertebral column and occurs with an incidence of approximately 1/1,000 live births.

ETIOLOGY. The cause of myelomeningocele is unknown, but as with all neural tube closure defects, a genetic predisposition exists; the risk of recurrence after one affected child rises to 3–4% and increases to approximately 10% with two previous abnormal pregnancies. Nutritional and environmental factors undoubtedly play a role in the etiology of myelomeningocele. During the last decade, studies have suggested that preconceptual vitamins and folic acid supplements greatly reduce the incidence of neural tube defects in pregnancies at risk. Unfortunately, the interpretation of the impact of vitamin supplementation is difficult owing to the lack of a randomized trial. Certain drugs are known to increase the risk of myelomeningocele. Valproic acid, an effective anticonvulsant, causes neural tube defects in approximately 1–2% of pregnancies if the drug is administered during pregnancy. Pregnant animals exposed to hyperthermia or vitamin A produce offspring with defects in neural tube closure. Recent studies have suggested that dysraphism might result from specific biochemical abnormalities of the basement membrane, particularly hyaluronate, which plays a role in cell division and the shape of the primitive neuroepithelium.

CLINICAL MANIFESTATIONS. The condition produces dysfunction of many organs and structures, including the skeleton, skin, and genitourinary tract in addition to the peripheral nervous system and the CNS. A myelomeningocele may be located anywhere along the neuraxis, but the lumbosacral region accounts for at least 75% of the cases. The extent and degree of the neurologic deficit depends on the location of the myelomeningocele. A lesion in the low sacral region causes bowel and bladder incontinence associated with anesthesia in the perineal area but with no impairment of motor function. The newborn with a defect in the mid-lumbar region typically has a sac-like cystic structure covered by a thin layer of partially epitheliolized tissue (Fig. 20–6). Remnants of neural tissue are visible beneath the membrane, which may occasionally rupture and leak CSF. An examination of the infant shows a flaccid paralysis of the lower extremities, an absence of deep tendon reflexes, a lack of response to touch and pain, and a high incidence of postural abnormalities of the lower extremities (including club feet and subluxation of the hips). Constant urinary dribbling and a relaxed anal sphincter may be evident. Thus, a myelomeningocele in the mid-lumbar region tends to produce lower motor neuron signs due to abnormalities and disruption of the conus medullaris. Infants with myelomeningocele typically have an increasing neurologic deficit as the myelomeningocele goes higher into the thoracic region. However, patients with a myelomeningocele in the upper thoracic or the cervical region usually have a very minimal neurologic deficit and in most cases do not have hydrocephalus.

Hydrocephalus in association with a type II Chiari defect develops in at least 80% of patients with myelomeningocele. Generally, the lower the deformity in the neuraxis (e.g., sacrum), the less likely will be the risk of hydrocephalus. Ventricular enlargement may be indolent and slow-growing or it may be rapid, causing a bulging anterior fontanel, dilated scalp veins, "setting-sun" appearance of the eyes, irritability, and vomiting associated with an increased head circumference. Not infrequently, infants with hydrocephalus and the Chiari II malformation develop symptoms of hindbrain dysfunction, including difficulty feeding, choking, stridor, apnea, vocal cord paralysis, pooling of secretions, and spasticity of the upper extremities, which, if untreated, can lead to death.

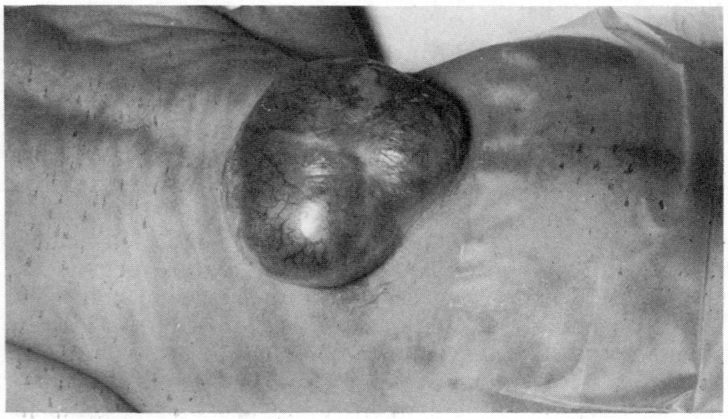

Figure 20–6. A lumbar myelomeningocele is covered by a thin layer of skin.

TREATMENT. The management and supervision of a child and family with a myelomeningocele requires a *multidisciplinary team approach*, including surgeons, physicians, and therapists, with one individual (often a pediatrician) acting as the advocate and coordinator of the treatment program. The news that a newborn child has a devastating condition such as myelomeningocele causes considerable grief and anger in the parents. They need time to learn about the handicap and the associated complications and to reflect on the various procedures and treatment plans. The parents must be given the facts by a knowledgeable individual in an unhurried and nonthreatening setting. If possible, discussions with other parents of children with neural tube defects are helpful in resolving important questions and issues.

In the past, it was advocated that the myelomeningocele should be repaired as soon as possible after birth to preserve neurologic function and to prevent further deterioration. Recent studies indicate similar long-term results with a delay in *surgery* for several days (with the exception of a CSF leak), which allows the parents to begin to adjust to the shock and to prepare for the multiple procedures and inevitable problems that lay ahead. Some centers have attempted to develop criteria for determining which infants will be treated aggressively and which will receive only supportive care. The most quoted exclusion criteria, developed in the United Kingdom, consist of the following: marked paralysis of the legs, thoracolumbar or thoracolumbosacral lesions, kyphosis or scoliosis, associated birth injury, other congenital defects of the heart, brain, or gastrointestinal tract, and a grossly enlarged head. More recent information suggests that such selective criteria have little prognostic value, and as a result most pediatric centers aggressively treat the majority of infants with myelomeningocele. After the repair of the myelomeningocele, most infants require a shunting procedure for hydrocephalus. If symptoms or signs of hindbrain dysfunction appear, early surgical decompression of the medulla and cervical cord is indicated. Club feet may require casting, and dislocated hips may require operative procedures.

Careful evaluation and reassessment of the *genitourinary system* are some of the most important components of the management. Teaching the parents, and ultimately the patient, to regularly catheterize the bladder maintains a low residual volume that prevents urinary tract infections and reflux leading to pyelonephritis and hydronephrosis. Periodic urine cultures and assessment of renal function, including serum electrolytes and creatinine as well as renal scans, intravenous pyelograms, and ultrasounds, are obtained according to the progress of the patient and the results of the physical examination. This approach to urinary tract management has greatly reduced the need for surgical diversionary procedures and has significantly decreased the morbidity and mortality associated with progressive renal disease in these patients. Some children can become continent with the surgical implantation of an artificial urinary sphincter at a later age. Although *incontinence of fecal matter* is common and is socially unacceptable during the school years, it does not pose the same risks as urinary incontinence. Many children can be "bowel-trained" with a regimen of timed enemas or suppositories that allow evacuation at a predetermined time once or twice a day.

Functional *ambulation* is the wish of each child and parent and may be possible depending on the level of the lesion and on the intact function of the iliopsoas muscles. Almost every child with a sacral or lumbosacral lesion obtains functional ambulation; approximately one half of the children with higher defects will ambulate with the use of braces and canes.

PROGNOSIS. For the child born with a myelomeningocele who is treated aggressively, the mortality rate is approximately 10–15%, and most deaths occur before 4 yr of age. At least 70% of survivors have normal intelligence, but learning problems and seizure disorders are more common than in the general population. Previous episodes of meningitis or ventriculitis adversely affect the ultimate intelligence quotient. Because myelomeningocele is a chronic handicapping condition, periodic multidisciplinary follow-up is required for life.

20.6 ENCEPHALOCELE

There are two major forms of dysraphism affecting the skull, resulting in protrusion of tissue through a bony midline defect, called **cranium bifidum**. A *cranial meningocele* consists of a CSF-filled meningeal sac only, and a *cranial encephalocele* contains the sac plus cerebral cortex, cerebellum, or portions of the brain stem. Microscopic examination of the neural tissue within an encephalocele is often abnormal. The cranial defect occurs most commonly in the occipital region at or below the inion, but in certain parts of the world frontal or nasofrontal encephaloceles are more prominent. These abnormalities are one tenth as common as neural tube closure defects involving the spine. The etiology is presumed to be similar to that for anencephaly and myelomeningocele, because examples of each have been reported in the same family.

Infants with a cranial encephalocele are at increased risk for developing hydrocephalus due to aqueduct stenosis or a Chiari malformation and the Dandy-Walker syndrome. Examination may show a small sac with a pedunculated stalk or a large cyst-like structure that may exceed the size of the cranium. The lesion may be completely covered with skin, but areas of denuded skin can occur and require urgent surgical management. Transillumination of the sac may indicate the presence of neural tissue. A plain roentgenogram of the skull and cervical spine is indicated to define the anatomy of the vertebra. An ultrasound is most helpful in determining the contents of the sac, obviating the need for a CT scan in most cases. Children with a cranial meningocele generally have a good prognosis, whereas patients with an encephalocele are at risk for visual problems, microcephaly, mental retardation, and seizures. Generally, children with neural tissue within the sac and associated hydrocephalus have the poorest prognosis. **Meckel-Grüber syndrome** is a rare autosomal recessive condition that is characterized by an occipital encephalocele, cleft lip or palate, microcephaly, abnormal genitalia, congenital nephrosis, and polydactyly. Encephaloceles may be diagnosed in utero by the determination of α-fetoprotein levels and ultrasound measurement of the biparietal diameter.

20.7 ANENCEPHALY

The anencephalic infant presents a distinctive appearance with a large defect of the calvarium, meninges, and scalp associated with a rudimentary brain, which results from a failure of closure of the rostral neuropore. The primitive brain consists of portions of connective tissue, vessels, and neuroglia. The cerebral hemispheres and cerebellum are usually absent, and only a residue of the brain stem can be identified. The pituitary gland is hypoplastic, and the spinal cord pyramidal tracts are missing due to the absence of the cerebral cortex. Additional anomalies include folding of the ears, cleft palate, and congenital heart defects in 10–20% of cases. Most anencephalic infants die within several days of birth. The incidence of anencephaly approximates 1/1,000 live births, and the greatest frequency is in Ireland and Wales. The recurrence risk is approximately 4% and increases to 10% if a couple has had two previously affected pregnancies. Many factors have been implicated as the cause of anencephaly (in addition to a genetic basis), including low socioeconomic status and poverty, nutritional and vitamin deficiencies, and a large number of environmental and toxic factors. It is very likely that several noxious stimuli interact on a genetically susceptible host to produce anencephaly. Fortunately, the frequency of anencephaly has been decreasing during the last 2 decades. Approximately 50% of anencephalic pregnancies are associated with polyhydramnios. Couples who have had an anencephalic infant should have successive pregnancies monitored, including amniocentesis, determination of α-fetoprotein levels, and an ultrasound examination between the 14th–16th week of gestation.

Charney EB, Weller SC, Sutton LN, et al: Management of the newborn with myelomeningocele: Time for a decision-making process. Pediatrics 75:58, 1985.
Copp AJ, Bernfield M: Accumulation of basement membrane-associated hyaluronate is reduced in the posterior neuropore region of mutant (curly tail) mouse embryo developing spinal neural tube defects. Devel Biol 130:583, 1988.
Hannigan KF: Teaching intermittent self-catheterization to young children with myelodysplasia. Dev Med Child Neurol 21:365, 1979.
Lemire RJ, Beckwith JB, Warkany J: Anencephaly. New York, Raven Press, 1978.
Lorber J, Salfiedl S: Results of selective treatment of spina bifida cystica. Arch Dis Child 56:822, 1981.
McLone DG: Results of treatment of children born with a myelomeningocele. Clin Neurosurg 30:407, 1983.
McLone DG, Czyzewski D, Raimondi AJ, et al: Central nervous system infections as a limiting factor in the intelligence of children with myelomeningocele. Pediatrics 70:338, 1982.
Milunsky A, Alpert E: The value of alpha-fetoprotein in the prenatal diagnosis of neural tube defects. J Pediatr 84:889, 1974.
Moore KL: The Developing Human, 4th ed. Philadelphia, WB Saunders, 1988.
Norman D, Brant-Zawadski M, Yeates A, et al: Magnetic resonance imaging of the spinal cord and canal: Potentials and limitations. AJNR 5:9, 1985.
Opitz JM, Howe JJ: The Meckel syndrome. Birth Defects 5:167, 1969.
Robert E, Guibaud P: Maternal valproic acid and congenital neural tube defects. Lancet 2:937, 1982.
Smithells RW, Sheppard S, Schorah CJ: Possible prevention of neural tube defects by periconceptional vitamin supplementation. Lancet 1:339, 1980.

20.8 DISORDERS OF CELL MIGRATION

Disorders of cell migration may result in minor abnormalities with little or no clinical consequence (e.g., small heterotopia of neurons) or devastating abnormalities of the CNS (e.g., mental retardation, lissencephaly, schizencephaly). One of the most important mechanisms in the control of neuronal migration is the radial glial fiber system that guides neurons to their proper site. The severity and the extent of the disorder are related to numerous factors including the timing of a particular insult and a host of environmental and genetic factors. Although abnormalities of lamination of the six layers of the cerebral cortex account for some important neurologic conditions related to cell migration, a brief description of the formation of the spinal cord will highlight the potential for errors in migration.

The embryonic neural tube consists of three zones: ependymal (ventricular), mantle (intermediate), and marginal (Fig. 20–7). The ependymal layer consists of a pluripotential pseudostratified columnar neuroepithelium. Specific neuroepithelial cells differentiate into primitive neurons or neuroblasts that form the mantle layer. The marginal zone is formed from cells in the outer layer of the neuroepithelium, which ultimately becomes the white matter. Glioblasts, which act as the primitive supportive cells of the CNS, also arise from the neuroepithelial cells in the ependymal zone. They migrate to the mantle and marginal zones and become future astrocytes and oligodendrocytes. It is likely that microglia originate from mesenchymal cells at a later stage of fetal development when blood vessels begin to penetrate the developing nervous system. A brief description of selected examples of disordered cell migration follows.

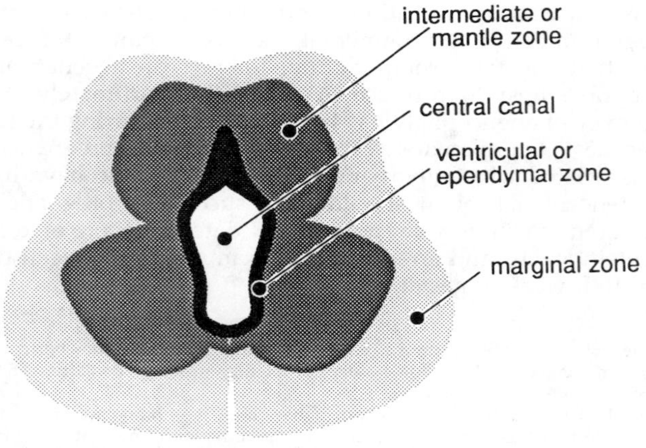

Figure 20–7. A cross-sectional drawing of the embryonic neural tube.

20.9 Lissencephaly

Lissencephaly or agyria refers to a rare disorder that is characterized by the absence of cerebral convolutions and a poorly formed sylvian fissure, giving the appearance of a 3–4 mo fetal brain. The condition is probably the result of faulty neuroblast migration during early embryonic life and is usually associated with enlarged lateral ventricles and heterotopias in the white matter. Clinically, these infants present with failure to thrive, microcephaly, marked developmental delay, and a severe seizure disorder. Ocular abnormalities are common, including hypoplasia of the optic nerve and microphthalmia. The facies are distinctive in some patients and include a prominent occiput, a broad forehead, and anteverted nostrils. The CT scan typically shows a smooth brain with an absence of sulci (Fig. 20–8).

20.10 Schizencephaly

Schizencephaly refers to the presence of unilateral or bilateral clefts within the cerebral hemispheres due to an abnormality of morphogenesis. The cleft may be fused or unfused and, if unilateral and large, may be confused with a porencephalic cyst. Not infrequently, the borders of the cleft are surrounded by abnormal brain, particularly microgyria. The CT scan is diagnostic and clearly demonstrates the size and extent of the cleft. Many patients are severely mentally retarded with seizures that are difficult to control and microcephalic with spastic quadriparesis when the clefts are bilateral.

20.11 Porencephaly

Porencephaly refers to the presence of cysts or cavities within the brain that result from developmental defects or acquired lesions, including infarction of tissue. *True porencephalic cysts* are most frequently located in the region of the sylvian fissure and typically communicate with the subarachnoid space, the ventricular system, or both. They represent developmental abnormalities of cell migration and are often associated with other malformations of the brain, including microcephaly, pachygyria, and encephalocele. These infants tend to have multiple problems, including mental retardation, spastic quadriparesis, optic atrophy, and seizures. *Pseudoporencephalic cysts* characteristically develop during the perinatal or postnatal period and result from abnormalities of arterial or venous circulation. These cysts tend to be unilateral; they do not communicate with a fluid-filled cavity; and they are not associated with abnormalities of cell migration or CNS malformations. Infants with pseudoporencephalic cysts present with hemiparesis and focal seizures during the 1st year of life.

20.12 AGENESIS OF THE CORPUS CALLOSUM

Agenesis of the corpus callosum consists of a heterogeneous group of disorders that vary in expression from severe intellectual and neurologic abnormalities to the asymptomatic and normally intelligent individual. The corpus callosum develops from the commissural plate that lies in proximity to the anterior neuropore. An insult to the commissural plate during early embryogenesis causes agenesis of the corpus callosum. When agenesis of the corpus callosum is an isolated phenomenon the patient may be normal, whereas individuals with neurologic symptoms including mental retardation, microcephaly, hemiparesis, diplegia, and seizures have associated brain anomalies due to cell migration defects, such as heterotopias, microgyria, and pachygyria (broad, wide gyri) in addition to the absence of the corpus callosum. The anatomic features are best depicted on a CT scan or by MRI and show widely separated frontal horns with an abnormally highly positioned third ventricle between the lateral ventricles. The MRI precisely outlines the extent of the corpus callosum defect. An absence of the corpus callosum may be inherited as an X-linked recessive trait or as an autosomal dominant trait. The condition may be associated with specific chromosomal disorders, particularly 8-trisomy and 18-trisomy. The **Aicardi syndrome** represents a complex disorder that affects many systems and is typically associated with agenesis of the corpus callosum. These patients are exclusively female, suggesting a genetic abnormality of the X chromosome. Seizures become evident during the first few months and are typically resistant to anticonvulsants. The EEG shows independent activity recorded from both hemispheres as a result of the absent corpus callosum. All patients are severely mentally retarded and may have abnormal vertebrae that may be fused or only partially developed (e.g., hemivertebra).

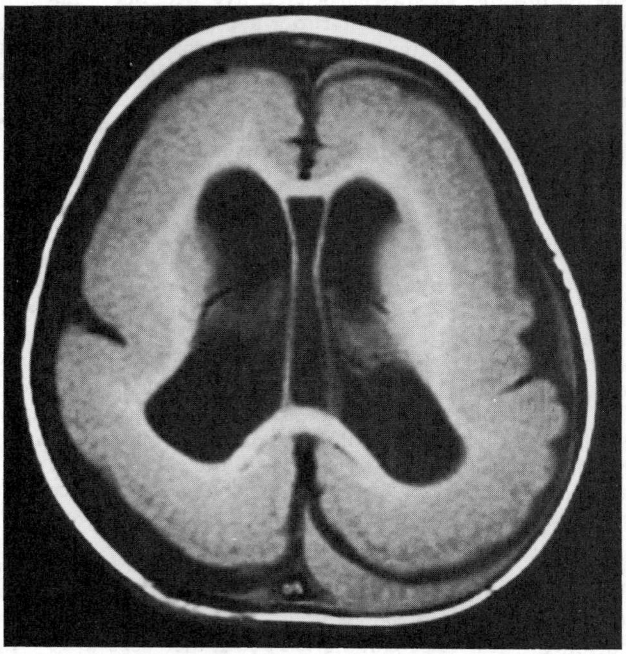

Figure 20–8. MRI of an infant with lissencephaly. Note the absence of cerebral sulci and the maldeveloped sylvian fissures associated with enlarged ventricles.

Abnormalities of the retina, including circumscribed pits or lacunae and coloboma of the optic disk, are the most characteristic findings of the Aicardi syndrome.

20.13 AGENESIS OF THE CRANIAL NERVES

Absence of the cranial nerves or the corresponding central nuclei have been described in several conditions and include the optic nerve, congenital ptosis, the Marcus Gunn phenomenon, the trigeminal and auditory nerves, and cranial nerves IX, X, XI, and XII. **Möbius syndrome** is characterized by bilateral facial weakness, which is often associated with abducens nerve paralysis. Hypoplasia or agenesis of brain stem nuclei as well as absent or decreased numbers of muscle fibers have been reported. These infants present in the newborn period with facial weakness, causing feeding difficulties due to a poor suck. The immobile, dull facies may give the incorrect impression of mental retardation; the prognosis for normal development is excellent in most cases.

20.14 MICROCEPHALY

Microcephaly is defined as a head circumference that measures more than three standard deviations below the mean for age and sex. This condition is relatively common, particularly among the mentally retarded population. Although there are many causes of microcephaly, abnormalities in neuronal migration during fetal development, including heterotopias of neuronal cells and cytoarchitectural derangements, are found in many brains. Microcephaly may be subdivided into two main groups: primary (genetic) microcephaly and secondary (nongenetic) microcephaly. A precise diagnosis is important for genetic counseling and for prediction for future pregnancies.

ETIOLOGY. Primary microcephaly refers to a group of conditions that usually have no other malformations and follow a mendelian pattern of inheritance or are associated with a specific genetic syndrome. These infants are usually identified at birth because of a small head circumference. The more common types include familial and autosomal dominant microcephaly and a series of chromosomal syndromes that are summarized in Table 20–2. Secondary microcephaly results from a large number of noxious agents that may affect the fetus in utero or the infant during periods of rapid brain growth, particularly the first 2 yr of life.

CLINICAL MANIFESTATIONS. A thorough family history should be taken seeking additional cases of microcephaly or disorders affecting the nervous system. It is important to obtain the patient's head circumference at birth. A very small head circumference implies a process that began early in embryonic or fetal development. An insult to the brain that occurs later in life, particularly beyond the age of 2 yr, is less likely to produce severe microcephaly. Serial head circumference measurements are more meaningful than a single determination, particularly when the abnormality is minimal. In addition, the head circumference of each parent and sibling should be recorded.

The laboratory investigation of the microcephalic child is determined by the history and physical examination. If the cause of the microcephaly is unknown, the mother's serum phenylalanine level should be determined. High phenylalanine serum levels in an asymptomatic mother can produce marked brain damage in the otherwise normal nonphenylketonuric infant. A karyotype is obtained if a chromosomal syndrome is suspected or if the child has abnormal facies, short stature, and additional congenital anomalies. Skull roentgenograms, CT scanning, or MRI may be useful in identifying structural abnormalities of the brain or intracerebral calcification. Additional studies include a fasting plasma and urine amino acid analysis, serum ammonium, *t*oxoplasmosis, *r*ubella, *c*ytomegalovirus, and *h*erpes simplex (TORCH) titers of the mother and child, and a urine sample for the culture of cytomegalovirus.

TREATMENT. Once the cause of the microcephaly has been established, the physician must provide accurate and supportive genetic and family counseling. Because many children with microcephaly will also be mentally retarded, the physician must assist with placement in an appropriate program that will provide the maximum development of the child (Sec. 3.57).

Barth PG: Disorders of neuronal migration. Can J Neurol Sci 14:1, 1987.
Bertoni JM, Von Loh S, Allen RJ: The Aicardi syndrome: Report of 4 cases and review of the literature. Ann Neurol 5:475, 1979.
Dobyns WB, Stratton RF, Greenberg F: Syndromes with lissencephaly. 1: Miller-Dieker and Norman-Roberts syndromes and isolated lissencephaly. Am J Med Genet 18:509, 1984.
Harwood-Nash DC: Congenital craniocerebral abnormalities and computed tomography. Semin Roentgenol 12:39, 1977.
Haslam RHA: Microcephaly. *In*: Vinken PJ, Bruyn G, Klawans HL (eds): Handbook of Clinical Neurology. Amsterdam, Elsevier Science Publishers, 1987, pp 267–284.
Miller GM, Stears JC, Guggenheim MA, et al: Schizencephaly: A clinical and CT study. Neurology 34:997, 1984.
Molina JA, Mateos F, Merino M, et al: Aicardi syndrome in two sisters. J Pediatr 115:282, 1989.
Naeff RW: Clinical features of porencephaly. Arch Neurol Psychiatry 80:133, 1958.
Nerdich JA, Nussbaum RL, Packer TCJ, et al: Heterogeneity of clinical severity and molecular lesions in Aicardi syndrome. J Pediatr 116:911, 1990.
Parrish ML, Roessmann U, Levinsohn MW: Agenesis of the corpus collosum: A study of the frequency of associated malformations. Ann Neurol 6:349, 1979.
Qazi QH, Reed TE: A possible major contribution to mental retardation in the general population by the gene for microcephaly. Clin Genet 7:85, 1975.
Sudarshan A, Goldie WD: The spectrum of congenital facial diplegia (Moebius syndrome). Pediatr Neurol 1:180, 1985.

20.15 HYDROCEPHALUS

Hydrocephalus is not a specific disease, rather it represents a diverse group of conditions, which result from impaired circulation and absorption of CSF or, in the rare circumstance, from increased production by a choroid plexus papilloma.

PHYSIOLOGY. The CSF is formed primarily in the ventricular system by the choroid plexus which occupies the lateral, third, and fourth ventricles. Although the majority of CSF is produced in the lateral ventricles, approximately 25% originates from extrachoroidal sources, including the capillary endothelium within the brain parenchyma. There is active neurogenic control of CSF formation as the choroid plexus is innervated by adrenergic and cholinergic nerves. Stimulation of the adrenergic system diminishes CSF production, whereas excitation of the cholinergic nerve may double the normal CSF production rate. In the normal child, approximately 20 mL of CSF is produced per hour. The total volume of CSF approximates 50 mL in an infant and 150 mL in an adult. CSF is formed by the choroid plexus in several stages; through a series of intricate steps a plasma ultrafiltrate is ultimately processed into a secretion, the CSF.

CSF movement results from the hydrostatic gradient that exists between the ventricular system and venous channels. The intraventricular pressure may be as high as 180 mm of water in the normal state, whereas the pressure in the superior sagittal sinus is in the range of 90 mm of water. Normally, CSF flows from the lateral ventricles through the foramina of Monro into the third ventricle. It then traverses the narrow aqueduct of Sylvius, which is approximately 3 mm in length and 2 mm in diameter in the child, to enter the fourth ventricle. The CSF exits the fourth ventricle through the paired lateral foramina of Luschka and the midline foramen of

TABLE 20–2. Causes of Microcephaly

Causes	Characteristic Findings
Primary (Genetic)	
1. Familial (autosomal recessive)	• Incidence 1/40,000 births • Typical appearance with slanted forehead, prominent nose and ears; severely mentally retarded and prominent seizures; surface convolutional markings of the brain poorly differentiated and disorganized cytoarchitecture
2. Autosomal dominant	• Nondistinctive facies, upslanting palpebral fissures, mild forehead slanting, and prominent ears • Normal linear growth, seizures readily controlled, and mild or borderline mental retardation
3. Syndromes	
Down (21-trisomy)	• Incidence 1/800 • Abnormal rounding of occipital and frontal lobes and a small cerebellum; narrow superior temporal gyrus, propensity for Alzheimer neurofibrillary alterations, and ultrastructure abnormalities of cerebral cortex
Edward (18-trisomy)	• Incidence 1/6,500 • Low birthweight, microstomia, micrognathia, low-set malformed ears, prominent occiput, rocker-bottom feet, flexion deformities of fingers, congenital heart disease, increased gyri, heterotopias of neurons
Cri-du-chat (5 p-)	• Incidence 1/50,000 • Round facies, prominent epicanthic folds, low-set ears, hypertelorism, and characteristic cry • No specific neuropathology
Cornelia de Lange	• Prenatal and postnatal growth delay, synophrys, thin down-turning upper lip • Proximally placed thumb
Rubinstein-Taybi	• Beaked-nose, downward slanting of palpebral fissures, epicanthic folds, short stature with broad thumbs and toes
Smith-Lemli-Opitz	• Ptosis, scaphocephaly, inner-epicanthic folds, anteverted nostrils • Low birthweight, marked feeding problems
Secondary (Nongenetic)	
1. Radiation	• Microcephaly and mental retardation most severe if exposure prior to 15 wk of gestation
2. Congenital infections	
Cytomegalovirus	• Small for dates, petechial rash, hepatosplenomegaly, chorioretinitis, deafness, mental retardation, and seizures • CNS calcification and microgyria
Rubella	• Growth retardation, purpura, thrombocytopenia, hepatosplenomegaly, congenital heart disease, chorioretinitis, cataracts, and deafness • Perivascular necrotic areas, polymicrogyria, heterotopias, subependymal cavitations
Toxoplasmosis	• Purpura, hepatosplenomegaly, jaundice, convulsions, hydrocephalus, chorioretinitis, and cerebral calcification
3. Drugs	
Fetal alcohol	• Growth retardation, ptosis, absent philtrum and hypoplastic upper lip, congenital heart disease, feeding problems, neuroglial heterotopia, and disorganization of neurons
Fetal hydantoin	• Growth delay, hypoplasia of distal phalanges, inner epicanthic folds, broad nasal ridge, and anteverted nostrils
4. Meningitis/encephalitis	• Cerebral infarcts, cystic cavitation, diffuse loss of neurons
5. Malnutrition	• Controversial cause of microcephaly
6. Metabolic	• Maternal diabetes mellitus and maternal hyperphenylalaninemia
7. Hyperthermia	• Significant fever during 1st 4–6 wk has been reported to cause microcephaly, seizures, and facial anomalies • Pathologic studies show neuronal heterotopias • Further studies showed no abnormalities with maternal fever
8. Hypoxic-ischemic encephalopathy	• Initially diffuse cerebral edema; late stages characterized by cerebral atrophy

Magendie into the cisterns at the base of the brain. Hydrocephalus resulting from obstruction within the ventricular system is called *obstructive or noncommunicating hydrocephalus*. The CSF circulates from the basal cisterns posteriorly over the cerebellum and cerebral cortex and anteriorly through the cistern system and over the convexities of the cerebral hemispheres. CSF is absorbed primarily by the arachnoid villi through tight junctions of their endothelium by hydrostatic forces that were noted earlier. CSF is absorbed to a much lesser extent by the lymphatic channels directed to the paranasal sinuses, along nerve root sleeves, and by the choroid plexus itself. Hydrocephalus resulting from obliteration of the subarachnoid cisterns or malfunction of the arachnoid villi is called *nonobstructive or communicating hydrocephalus*.

PATHOPHYSIOLOGY AND ETIOLOGY. Obstructive or noncommunicating hydrocephalus develops most commonly in children because of an abnormality of the aqueduct or a lesion in the fourth ventricle. *Aqueductal stenosis* results from an abnormally narrow aqueduct of Sylvius that is often associated with branching or forking. In a small percentage of cases, aqueductal stenosis is inherited as a sex-linked recessive trait. These patients occasionally have minor neural tube closure defects, including spina bifida occulta. Rarely, aqueductal stenosis is associated with neurofibromatosis. *Aqueductal gliosis* may also give rise to hydrocephalus. As a result of neonatal meningitis or a subarachnoid hemorrhage in a premature infant, the ependymal lining of the aqueduct is interrupted and a brisk glial response results in complete obstruction. Intrauterine viral infections may also produce aqueductal stenosis followed by hydrocephalus, and mumps meningoencephalitis has been reported as a cause in a child. A vein of Galen malformation can expand to a large size and, because of its midline position, obstruct the flow of CSF. Lesions of the fourth ventricle are prominent causes of hydrocephalus, including posterior fossa brain tumors, the Chiari malformation, and the Dandy-Walker syndrome.

Nonobstructive or communicating hydrocephalus most commonly follows a subarachnoid hemorrhage, which is usually the result of intraventricular hemorrhage in the premature infant. Blood in the subarachnoid spaces may cause obliteration of the cisterns or arachnoid villi and obstruction of CSF flow. Pneumococcal and tuberculous meningitis have a propensity to produce a thick, tenacious exudate that obstructs the basal cisterns, and intrauterine infections may also destroy the CSF pathways. Finally, leukemic infiltrates may seed the subarachnoid space and produce communicating hydrocephalus.

CLINICAL MANIFESTATIONS. The clinical presentation of hydrocephalus is variable and depends on many factors including the age of onset, the nature of the lesion causing obstruction, and the duration and rate of rise of the intracranial pressure. In the infant, an accelerated rate of enlargement of the head is the most prominent sign. In addition, the anterior fontanel is wide open and bulging, and the scalp veins are dilated. The forehead is broad and the eyes may deviate downward because of the impingement of the dilated suprapineal recess on the tectum, producing the "setting sun" eye sign. Long tract signs including brisk tendon reflexes, spasticity, clonus, and Babinski sign are common, particularly in the lower extremities, owing to stretching and disruption of the corticospinal fibers originating from the leg region of the motor cortex. In the older child, the cranial sutures are partially closed so that the signs of hydrocephalus may be more subtle. Irritability, lethargy, poor appetite, and vomiting are common to both age groups, and headache is a prominent symptom in the older age patient. A gradual change in personality and a deterioration in academic productivity suggests a slowly progressive form of hydrocephalus. Serial measurements of the head circumference indicate an increased velocity of growth. Percussion of the skull may produce a "cracked-pot" or **Macewen sign** indicating separation of the sutures. A foreshortened occiput suggests the Chiari malformation, and a prominent occiput suggests the Dandy-Walker malformation. Papilledema, abducens nerve palsy, and pyramidal tract signs, which are most evident in the lower extremities, are apparent in most cases.

The *Chiari malformation* consists of two major subgroups. Type I typically produces symptoms during adolescence or adult life and is usually not associated with hydrocephalus. These patients complain of recurrent headache, neck pain, urinary frequency, and progressive lower extremity spasticity. The deformity consists of displacement of the cerebellar tonsils into the cervical canal. Although the pathogenesis is unknown, the prevailing theory suggests that obstruction of the caudal portion of the fourth ventricle during fetal development is responsible. The type II Chiari malformation is characterized by progressive hydrocephalus and a myelomeningocele. This lesion represents an anomaly of the hindbrain, probably due to a failure of pontine flexure during embryogenesis, and results in elongation of the fourth ventricle, kinking of the brain stem, with displacement of the inferior vermis, pons, and medulla into the cervical canal. Approximately 10% of type II malformations produce symptoms during infancy consisting of stridor, weak cry, and apnea, which may be relieved by shunting or by posterior fossa decompression. A more indolent form consists of abnormalities of gait, spasticity, and increasing incoordination during childhood. Plain skull radiographs show a small posterior fossa and a widened cervical canal. CT scanning with contrast and MRI display the cerebellar tonsils protruding downward into the cervical canal and the hindbrain abnormalities. The anomaly is treated by surgical decompression.

The *Dandy-Walker malformation* consists of a cystic expansion of the fourth ventricle in the posterior fossa, which results from a developmental failure of the roof of the 4th ventricle during embryogenesis. Approximately 90% of patients have hydrocephalus, and a significant number of children have associated anomalies, including agenesis of the posterior cerebellar vermis and corpus callosum. Infants present with a rapid increase in head size and a prominent occiput. Transillumination of the skull may be positive. Most children have evidence of long-tract signs, cerebellar ataxia, and delayed motor and cognitive milestones, probably owing to the associated structural anomalies. The Dandy-Walker malformation is managed by shunting the cystic cavity and the ventricles in the presence of hydrocephalus.

DIAGNOSIS AND DIFFERENTIAL DIAGNOSIS. The investigation of a child with hydrocephalus begins with the history. Familial cases suggest X-linked hydrocephalus secondary to aqueductal stenosis. A past history of prematurity with intracranial hemorrhage, meningitis, or mumps encephalitis is important to ascertain. Multiple café-au-lait spots and other clinical features of neurofibromatosis point to aqueductal stenosis as the cause of hydrocephalus. Examination includes careful inspection, palpation, and auscultation of the skull and spine. The occipitofrontal head circumference is recorded and compared with previous measurements. The size and configuration of the anterior fontanel is noted, and the back is inspected for abnormal midline skin lesions including tufts of hair, lipoma, or angioma that might suggest spinal dysraphism. The presence of a prominent forehead or abnormalities in the shape of the occiput may suggest the pathogenesis of the hydrocephalus. A cranial bruit is audible in association with many cases of vein of Galen arteriovenous malformation. Transillumination of the skull is positive with massive dilatation of the ventricular system or in the Dandy-Walker syndrome. Inspection of the eyegrounds is mandatory, because the finding of chorioretinitis suggests an intrauterine infection such as toxoplasmosis as a cause of the hydrocephalus. Papilledema is observed in older children but is rarely present in infants because the cranial sutures separate as a result of the increased pressure. Plain skull films typically show separation of the sutures, erosion of the posterior clinoids in the older child, and an increase in convolutional markings ("beaten-silver appearance") with longstanding increased intracranial pressure. The CT scan or MRI along with ultrasound in the infant are the most important studies to identify the specific cause of hydrocephalus.

The head may appear enlarged secondary to a thickened cranium resulting from chronic anemia, rickets, osteogenesis imperfecta, and epiphyseal dysplasia. Chronic subdural collections can produce bilateral parietal bone prominence. Various metabolic and degenerative disorders of the CNS produce megalencephaly due to abnormal storage of substances within the brain parenchyma. These disorders include lysosomal diseases (e.g., Tay-Sachs, gangliosidosis, and the mucopolysaccharidoses), the aminoacidurias (e.g., maple syrup urine disease [MSUD]), and the leukodystrophies (e.g., metachromatic, Alexander disease, and Canavan disease). In addition, cerebral gigantism and neurofibromatosis are characterized by increased brain mass. Familial megalencephaly is inherited as an autosomal dominant and is characterized by delayed motor milestones and hypotonia but normal or near-normal intelligence. Measurement of the parent's head circumference is necessary to establish the diagnosis. *Hydranencephaly* may be confused with hydrocephalus. The cerebral hemispheres are absent or represented by membranous sacs with remnants of frontal, temporal, or occipital cortex dispersed over the membrane. The midbrain and brain stem are relatively intact (Fig. 20–9). The cause of hydranencephaly is unknown, but bilateral occlusion of the internal carotid arteries during early fetal development would explain most of the pathologic abnormalities. The infant may have a normal or enlarged head circumference at birth that grows at an excessive rate postnatally. Transillumination shows an absence of the cerebral hemispheres. The child is irritable, feeds poorly, develops seizures and spastic quadriparesis, and has little or no cognitive development. A ventriculoperitoneal shunt prevents massive enlargement of the cranium.

TREATMENT. Therapy for hydrocephalus depends on the cause. Medical management, including the use of acetazolamide and furosemide, may provide temporary relief by reducing the rate of CSF production, but long-term results have been disappointing. Most cases of hydrocephalus require extracranial shunts, particularly a ventriculoperitoneal shunt. The major complication of shunts is bacterial infection, usually due to *Staphylococcus* epidermidis (Sec. 12.19). With meticulous preparation, the shunt infection rate can be reduced to 0–2%. The results of intrauterine surgical management of fetal hydrocephalus have been poor, possibly because of the high rate of associated cerebral malformations in addition to the hydrocephalus.

PROGNOSIS. This depends on the cause of the dilated ventricles and not on the size of the cortical mantle at the time of operative intervention. Hydrocephalic children are at increased risk for a variety of developmental disabilities. The mean intelligence quotient is reduced compared with the general population, particularly for performance tasks as contrasted to verbal abilities. Most children have abnormalities in memory function. Visual problems are common, including strabismus, visuospatial abnormalities, visual field defects, and optic atrophy with decreased acuity secondary to increased intracranial pressure. The visual-evoked potential latencies are delayed and take some time to recover following correction of the hydrocephalus. Although most hydrocephalic children are pleasant and mild mannered, some children show aggressive and delinquent behavior. It is imperative that the hydrocephalic child receive long-term follow-up in a multidisciplinary setting.

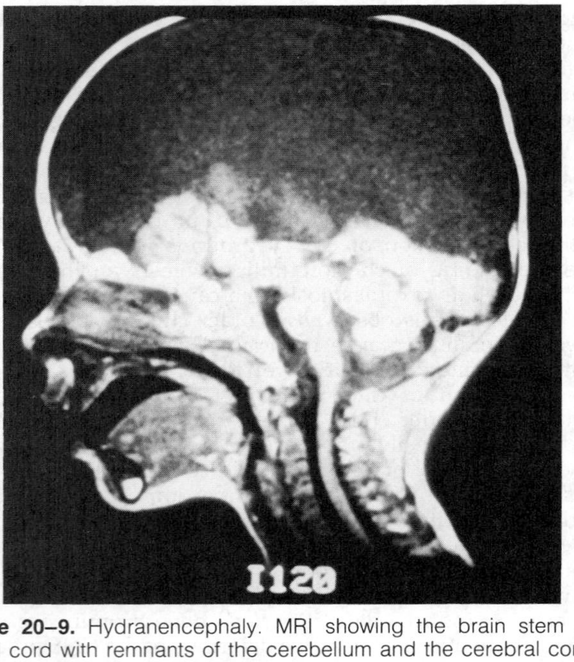

Figure 20–9. Hydranencephaly. MRI showing the brain stem and spinal cord with remnants of the cerebellum and the cerebral cortex. The remainder of the cranium is filled with CSF.

Cochrane DD, Myles ST, Nimrod C, et al: Intrauterine hydrocephalus and ventriculomegaly: Associated abnormalities and fetal outcome. Can J Neurol Sci 12:51, 1985.

Cull C, Wyke MA: Memory function of children with spina bifida and shunted hydrocephalus. Dev Med Child Neurol 26:177, 1984.

De Myer W: Megalencephaly in children. Neurology 22:634, 1972.

Dennis M, Fitz CR, Netley CT, et al: The intelligence of hydrocephalic children. Arch Neurol 38:607, 1981.

Fitzsimmons JS: Laryngeal stridor and respiratory obstruction association with myelomeningocele. Dev Med Child Neurol 15:533, 1973.

Greene M, Benaceraf B, Crawford J: Hydranencephaly: Ultrasound appearance in utero evolution. Radiology 156:779, 1985.

Hirsch JF, Pierre-Kahn A, Renier D, et al: The Dandy-Walker malformation. J Neurosurg 61:515, 1984.

Hoffman HJ, Hendrick EB, Humphreys RP: Manifestations and management of Arnold-Chiari malformations in patients with myelomeningocele. Childs Brain 1:255, 1975.

Jackson JC, Blumhagen JD: Congenital hydrocephalus due to prenatal intracranial hemorrhage. Pediatrics 72:344, 1983.

Johnson RT, Johnson KP, Edmonds CJ: Virus-induced hydrocephalus: Development of aqueductal stenosis in hamsters after mumps infection. Science 157:1066, 1967.

Satz A, Felgenhaueur K: Development of the blood-CSF barrier. Dev Med Child Neurol 25:152, 1983.

20.16 CRANIOSYNOSTOSIS

Craniosynostosis is defined as premature closure of the cranial sutures and is classified as primary or secondary. *Primary craniosynostosis* refers to the closure of one or more sutures due to abnormalities of skull development, whereas *secondary craniosynostosis* results from failure of brain growth and expansion and will not be discussed further. The incidence of primary craniosynostosis approximates 1 per 2,000 births. The cause is unknown in the majority of children; however, genetic syndromes account for 10–20% of cases.

DEVELOPMENT AND ETIOLOGY. A review of skull development is helpful in understanding the genesis of craniosynostosis. During early development, the brain is enveloped by a film of mesenchyme. By the 2nd mo, osseous tissue is evident in that portion of the mesenchyme corresponding to the cranium, and cartilaginous tissue is formed at the base of the skull. The bones of the cranium are well developed by the 5th mo of gestation (frontal, parietal, temporal, and occipital) and are separated by sutures and fontanels. The brain grows rapidly during the first several years of life and is normally not impeded because of equivalent growth along the suture lines. The etiology of craniosynostosis is unknown, but the prevailing hypothesis suggests that abnormal development of the base of the skull creates exaggerated forces on the dura that act to disrupt normal cranial suture development. Dysfunctional osteoblasts or osteoclasts are not responsible for craniosynostosis.

CLINICAL MANIFESTATIONS AND TREATMENT. Most cases of craniosynostosis are evident at birth and are characterized by a skull deformity that is the direct result of premature suture fusion. Palpation of the suture reveals a prominent bony ridge, and fusion of the suture may be confirmed by plain skull roentgenograms or bone scan in ambiguous cases. Premature closure of the sagittal suture produces a long and narrow skull or *scaphocephaly*, the most common form of craniosynostosis. Scaphocephaly is associated with a prominent occiput and a broad forehead and a small or absent anterior fontanel. The condition is sporadic and more common in males and often causes difficulties during labor because of cephalopelvic disproportion. Scaphocephaly does not produce increased intracranial pressure or hydrocephalus and the neurological examination of affected patients is normal. *Frontal plagiocephaly* is the next most common form of craniosynostosis and is characterized by unilateral flattening of the forehead, elevation of the ipsilateral orbit and eyebrow, and a prominent ear on the corresponding side. The condition is more common in females and is the result of premature fusion of a coronal and sphenofrontal suture. Surgical intervention produces a cosmetically pleasing result. *Occipital plagiocephaly* is most often the result of positioning during infancy and is more common in an immobile or handicapped child, but fusion or sclerosis of the lambdoid suture can cause unilateral occipital flattening and bulging of the ipsilateral frontal bone. *Trigonocephaly* is a rare cause of craniosynostosis due to premature fusion of the metopic suture. These children have a keel-shaped forehead and hypotelorism and are at risk for associated developmental abnormalities of the forebrain. *Turricephaly* refers to a conical-shaped head due to premature fusion of the coronal and often sphenofrontal and frontoethmoidal sutures. The *kleeblattschädel deformity* is a peculiarly shaped skull that resembles a cloverleaf. These children have very prominent temporal bones, and the remainder of the cranium is constricted. Hydrocephalus is a common complication. Premature fusion of only one suture rarely causes a neurologic deficit. In this situation, the sole indication for surgery is to enhance the cosmetic appearance of the child, and the prognosis depends on the suture involved and on the degree of disfigurement. Neurologic complications, including hydrocephalus and increased intracranial pressure, are more likely to occur when two or more sutures are prematurely fused, in which case operative intervention is essential.

The most prevalent genetic disorders associated with craniosynostosis include Crouzon, Apert, Carpenter, Chotzen, and Pfeiffer syndromes. **Crouzon syndrome** is characterized by premature craniosynostosis and is inherited as an autosomal dominant trait. The shape of the head depends on the timing and order of suture fusion but most often produces a compressed back-to-front diameter or brachycephalic skull due to bilateral closure of the coronal sutures. The orbits are underdeveloped, and ocular proptosis is prominent. Hypoplasia of the maxilla and orbital hypertelorism are typical facial features.

Apert syndrome has many features in common with Crouzon syndrome. However, Apert syndrome is usually a sporadic condition, although autosomal dominant inheritance may occur. It is associated with premature fusion of multiple sutures, including the coronal, sagittal, squamosal, and lambdoid sutures. The facies tend to be asymmetric, and the eyes are less proptotic compared with Crouzon syndrome. Apert syndrome is characterized by syndactyly of the 2nd, 3rd, and 4th fingers, which may be joined to the thumb and the 5th finger. Similar abnormalities often occur in the feet. All patients have progressive calcification and fusion of the bones of the hands, feet, and cervical spine.

Carpenter syndrome is inherited as an autosomal recessive condition, and the multiple fusion of sutures tends to produce the kleeblattschädel skull deformity. Soft-tissue syndactyly of the hands and feet are always present, and mental retardation is common. Additional but less common abnormalities include congenital heart disease, corneal opacities, coxa valga, and genu valgum.

Chotzen syndrome is characterized by asymmetric craniosynostosis and plagiocephaly. The condition is the most prevalent of the genetic syndromes and is inherited as an autosomal dominant trait. It is associated with facial asymmetry, ptosis of the eyelids, shortened fingers, and soft-tissue syndactyly of the 2nd and 3rd fingers.

Pfeiffer syndrome is most often associated with turricephaly. The eyes are prominent and widely spaced, and the thumbs and great toes are short and broad. Partial soft-tissue syndactyly may be evident. Most cases appear to be sporadic, but autosomal dominant inheritance has been reported.

Each of the genetic syndromes are at risk for additional anomalies, including hydrocephalus, increased intracranial pressure, papilledema, optic atrophy due to abnormalities of the optic foramina, respiratory problems secondary to a deviated nasal septum or choanal atresia, and disorders of speech and deafness. Craniectomy is mandatory for the management of increased intracranial pressure, and a multidisciplinary craniofacial team is essential for the long-term follow-up of affected children.

Cohen MM: Craniofacial disorders. *In*: Emery AEH, Rimoin DL (eds): Principles and Practice of Medical Genetics. Edinburgh, Churchill Livingstone, 1983, pp 576–621.

David DJ, Poswillo D, Simpson D: The Craniosynostoses: Causes, Natural History and Management. Berlin, Springer Verlag, 1982.

Shillito J, Matson BD: Craniosynostosis: A review of 519 surgical patients. Pediatrics 41:829, 1968.

20.17 SEIZURES IN CHILDHOOD

Seizures are a common neurologic disorder in the pediatric age group and occur with a frequency of 4–6 cases/1,000 children. They are the most common cause for referral to a pediatric neurology practice. The presence of a seizure disorder does not constitute a diagnosis but is a symptom of an underlying CNS disorder that requires a thorough investigation and management plan. In most children an etiology for the seizure cannot be determined, and a diagnosis of idiopathic epilepsy is made. Although the outcome for most uncomplicated seizures in children is good, a small number have persistent seizures refractory to drugs, and these pose a diagnostic and management challenge. The terms "seizure" and "convulsion" may be incorrectly used interchangeably with "epilepsy." A *seizure* (convulsion) is defined as a paroxysmal involuntary disturbance of brain function that may be manifested as an impairment or loss of consciousness, abnormal motor activity, behavioral abnormalities, sensory disturbances, or autonomic dysfunction. Some seizures are characterized by abnormal movements without loss or impairment of consciousness. *Epilepsy* is defined as recurrent seizures unrelated to fever or to an acute cerebral insult.

EVALUATION. The *history* should attempt to define factors that may have promoted the convulsion and provide a detailed description of the seizure and the child's postictal state. Children who have a propensity to develop epilepsy may experience the first convulsion in association with a viral illness or a low-grade fever. Seizures that occur during the early morning hours or with drowsiness, particularly during the initial phase of sleep, are common in childhood epilepsy. In retrospect, irritability, mood swings, headache, and subtle personality changes may precede a seizure by several days. Some parents can accurately predict the timing of the next seizure based on changes in the child's disposition.

Most parents vividly recall their child's initial convulsion and can describe it in detail. The first step in an evaluation is to determine whether the seizure has a focal onset or is generalized. Focal seizures may be characterized by motor or sensory symptoms and include forceful turning of the head and eyes to one side, unilateral clonic movements beginning in the face or extremities, or a sensory disturbance such as paresthesias or pain localized to a specific area. Focal seizures in the adult usually indicate a localized lesion, but the investigation of focal seizures during childhood is frequently negative. Motor seizures may be focal or generalized and tonic-clonic, tonic, clonic, myoclonic or atonic. Tonic seizures are characterized by increased tone or rigidity, and atonic seizures are characterized by flaccidity or by lack of movement during a convulsion. Clonic seizures consist of rhythmic muscle contraction and relaxation, and myoclonus is most accurately described as shock-like contractions of a muscle. The duration of the seizure and state of consciousness (retained or impaired) should be documented. The history should determine whether an aura preceded the convulsion and the behavior of the child immediately preceding the seizure. The posture of the patient, presence and distribution of cyanosis, vocalizations, loss of sphincter control (particularly of the urinary bladder), and postictal state (including sleep and headache) should be noted.

Some parents can precisely act out or recreate a seizure. The physical portrayal by the parent or caregiver is often surprisingly similar to the actual convulsion and is much more accurate than the verbal description. Aside from the description of the seizure pattern, the frequency, time of day, precipitating factors, and alteration in the type of convulsive disorder are important. Although generalized tonic-clonic seizures are readily documented, the frequency of absence seizures is often underestimated by the parent. A prolonged personality change or intellectual deterioration may suggest a degenerative disease of the CNS, whereas constitutional symptoms, including vomiting and failure to thrive, might indicate a primary metabolic disorder or a structural lesion. It is essential to obtain details of prior anticonvulsant medication, the child's response to the regimen, and to determine whether drugs that may potentiate seizures, including chlorpromazine or methylphenidate, were prescribed.

The *examination* of a child with a seizure disorder should be geared toward the search for an organic cause. The blood pressure is recorded, and the child's head circumference, length, and weight are plotted on a growth chart and compared with previous measurements. The finding of unusual facial features or associated physical findings such as hepatosplenomegaly point to an underlying metabolic or storage disease as the cause of the neurologic disorder. A search for vitiliginous lesions of tuberous sclerosis utilizing an ultraviolet light source, examination for adenoma sebaceum, shagreen patch, multiple café-au-lait spots, or a nevus flammeus and the presence of retinal phakoma would indicate a neurocutaneous disorder as the cause of the seizure. Localizing neurologic signs such as a subtle hemiparesis with hyperreflexia, an equivocal Babinski, and a downward drifting arm with eyes closed might suggest a contralateral hemispheric structural lesion such as a slow-growing temporal lobe glioma as the cause of the seizure disorder. A unilateral growth arrest of the thumbnail, hand, or extremity in a child with a focal seizure disorder suggests a chronic condition such as porencephalic cyst, arteriovenous malformation, or cortical atrophy in the opposite hemisphere. The eyegrounds must be examined for the presence of papilledema, retinal hemorrhages, chorioretinitis, coloboma, and macular changes as well as retinal phakoma. Hyperventilation for a 3- or 4-min period produces an immediate seizure in virtually all children with absence epilepsy.

CLASSIFICATION OF SEIZURES

It is important to classify the type of seizure for several reasons. First, the seizure type may provide a clue to the cause of the seizure disorder. In addition, precise delineation of the seizure may allow a firm basis for making a prognosis. The child with generalized tonic-clonic epilepsy is usually readily controlled with anticonvulsants, whereas the patient with partial seizures may fare less well. The infant with benign myoclonic epilepsy has a more favorable outlook than a patient with infantile spasms. Similarly, the school-aged child who has benign partial epilepsy with centrotemporal spikes (rolandic epilepsy) has an excellent prognosis and is unlikely to require a prolonged course of anticonvulsants. The clinical classification of seizures may be difficult because the manifestations of different seizure types may be similar. For example, the clinical features of a child with absence seizures may be almost identical to that of another patient with complex partial epilepsy. The EEG is a useful adjunct to the classification of epilepsy because of the variability of seizure expressivity in this age group. A classification useful in delineating childhood epilepsy is shown in Table 20–3.

20.18 Partial Seizures

Partial seizures account for a large proportion of childhood seizures, up to 40% in some series. Partial seizures may be classified as *simple* or *complex;* consciousness is maintained with simple seizures and is impaired in patients with complex seizures.

SIMPLE PARTIAL SEIZURES (SPS). Motor activity is the most common symptom of SPS. The movements are characterized by asynchronous clonic or tonic movements, and they tend to involve the face, neck, and extremities. *Versive seizures* consisting of head turning and conjugate eye movements are particularly common in SPS. Automatisms do not occur with SPS, but some patients complain of aura (e.g., chest discomfort and headache), which may be the only manifestation of a seizure. Unfortunately, children have difficulty in describing aura and often refer to them as "feeling funny" or "something crawling inside me." The average seizure persists for 10–20 sec. SPS may be confused with tics; however, *tics* are characterized by shoulder shrugging, eye blinking, and facial grimacing and primarily involve the face and shoulders. Tics can be briefly suppressed, but partial seizures cannot be controlled. The EEG may show spikes or sharp waves unilaterally or bilaterally or a multifocal spike pattern in patients with SPS.

TABLE 20–3. International Classification of Epileptic Seizures

Partial Seizures
Simple partial (consciousness retained)
Motor
Sensory
Autonomic
Psychic
Complex partial (consciousness impaired)
Simple partial, followed by impaired consciousness
Consciousness impaired at onset
Partial seizures with secondary generalization
Generalized Seizures
Absences
Typical
Atypical
Generalized tonic-clonic
Tonic
Clonic
Myoclonic
Atonic
Infantile spasms
Unclassified Seizures

COMPLEX PARTIAL SEIZURES (CPS). A CPS may begin with a simple partial seizure with or without an aura, followed by impaired consciousness, or, conversely, the onset of the CPS may coincide with an altered state of consciousness. An *aura* consisting of vague, unpleasant feelings is present in approximately one third of children with SPS and CPS. As partial seizures are difficult to document in the infant and child, the frequency of their association with CPS may be underestimated. Impaired consciousness in the infant and child is difficult to appreciate. There may be a brief blank stare or a sudden cessation or pause in activity that is frequently overlooked by the parent. Furthermore, the child is unable to communicate or to describe the periods of impaired consciousness in most cases. Finally, the periods of altered consciousness may be brief and infrequent, and only an experienced observer or an EEG may be able to identify the abnormal event.

Automatisms are a common feature of CPS in infants and children, occurring in approximately 50–75% of cases; the older the child, the greater will be the frequency of automatisms. Automatisms develop following the loss of consciousness and may persist into the postictal phase, but they are not recalled by the child. The automatic behavior observed in infants is characterized by alimentary automatisms, including lip smacking, chewing, swallowing, and excessive salivation. These movements can represent normal infant behavior and are difficult to distinguish from the automatisms of CPS. Prolonged and repetitive alimentary automatisms associated with a blank stare or with a lack of responsiveness almost always indicate CPS in an infant. Automatic behavior in older children consists of semipurposeful, incoordinated, and unplanned gestural automatisms, including picking and pulling at clothing or the bed sheets, rubbing or caressing objects, and walking or running in a nondirective, repetitive, and often fearful fashion.

Spreading of the epileptiform discharge during CPS can result in secondary generalization with a tonic-clonic convulsion. During the spread of the ictal discharge throughout the hemisphere, contralateral versive turning of the head, dystonic posturing, and tonic or clonic movements of the extremities and face including eye blinking may be noted. The average duration of a CPS is 1–2 min, which is considerably longer than an SPS.

CPS are associated with interictal *EEG* anterior temporal lobe sharp waves or focal spikes, and multifocal spikes are a frequent finding. Approximately 20% of infants and children with CPS have a normal routine interictal EEG. In these patients, a sleep-deprived EEG study, zygomatic leads during EEG, prolonged EEG recording, or study of the hospitalized patient weaned from anticonvulsants are techniques that can be utilized to increase the identification of spikes and sharp waves (Fig. 20–10*A*). In addition, some children with CPS have interictal sharp waves or spikes originating from the frontal, parietal, or occipital lobes. Radiographic studies including CT scanning and MRI are most likely to identify an abnormality in the temporal lobe in a child with CPS. These lesions include mesial temporal sclerosis, hamartoma, postencephalitic gliosis, subarachnoid cysts, infarction, arteriovenous malformations, and a slow-growing glioma.

BENIGN PARTIAL EPILEPSY WITH CENTROTEMPORAL SPIKES (BPEC). BPEC is a common type of partial epilepsy in childhood and has an excellent prognosis. The clinical features, EEG findings, and lack of a neuropathologic lesion are characteristic and readily separate BPEC from CPS. BPEC occurs between the ages of 2 and 14 and has a peak age of onset of 9–10 yr. The disorder occurs in normal children with an unremarkable past history and a normal neurologic examination. There is often a positive family history of epilepsy. The seizures are usually partial, and motor signs and somatosensory symptoms are often confined to the face. Oropharyngeal symptoms include tonic contractions and paresthesias of the tongue, unilateral numbness of the cheek (particularly along the gum), guttural noises, dysphagia, and excessive salivation. Frequently, unilateral tonic-clonic contractures of the lower face accompany the oropharyngeal symptoms as do clonic movements or paresthesias of the ipsilateral extremities. Consciousness may be intact or impaired, and the partial seizure may proceed to secondary generalization. Approximately 20% of children experience only one seizure, the majority have infrequent seizures, and about one quarter have repeated clusters of seizures. BPEC occurs during sleep in 75% of patients, whereas CPS tends to be observed during the waking hours. The EEG pattern is diagnostic for BPEC and is characterized by a repetitive spike focus localized in the centrotemporal or rolandic area with a normal background activity (see Fig. 20–10*A*). Anticonvulsants are necessary for patients who have frequent seizures but should not be prescribed automatically after the initial convulsion. Carbamazepine is the preferred drug, which is continued until 14–16 yr of age when spontaneous remission of BPEC usually occurs.

20.19 Generalized Seizures

ABSENCE SEIZURES. Simple absence (petit mal) seizures are characterized by a sudden cessation of motor activity or speech with a blank facial expression and flickering of the eyelids. These seizures, which are uncommon prior to the age of 5 yr, are more prevalent in girls; they are never associated with an aura; they rarely persist longer than 30 sec; and they are not associated with a postictal state. These features tend to differentiate absence seizures from complex partial seizures. The patient does not lose body tone, but the head may fall forward slightly. Immediately after the seizure, the patient resumes preseizure activity with no indication of postictal impairment. Automatic behavior frequently accompanies simple absence seizures. Hyperventilation for 3–4 min routinely produces an absence seizure. The EEG shows a typical 3/sec spike and generalized wave discharge (see Fig. 20–10*B*). Complex absence seizures have associated motor components consisting of myoclonic movements of the face, fingers, or extremities and, on occasion, loss of body tone. These seizures produce atypical EEG spike and wave discharges at 2–2.5/sec.

GENERALIZED TONIC-CLONIC SEIZURES. These seizures are extremely common and may follow a partial seizure with a focal onset (secondary generalization) or occur de novo. They may be associated with an aura suggesting a focal origin of the epileptiform discharge. It is important to inquire about the presence of an aura, because its presence and site of origin may indicate the area of pathology. The patient suddenly loses consciousness and in some cases emits a shrill, piercing cry. The eyes roll back, the entire body musculature undergoes tonic contractions, and the child rapidly becomes cyanotic in association with apnea. The clonic phase of the seizure is heralded by rhythmic clonic contractions alternating with relaxation of all muscle groups. The clonic phase slows toward the end of the seizure, which usually persists for a few minutes, and the patient often sighs as the seizure comes to an abrupt stop. During the seizure the child may bite the tongue but rarely vomits. Loss of sphincter control, particularly the bladder, is common during a generalized tonic-clonic seizure.

Tight clothing and jewelry around the neck should be loosened, the patient should be placed on one side, and the neck and jaw should be gently hyperextended to enhance breathing. The mouth should not be opened forcibly by an

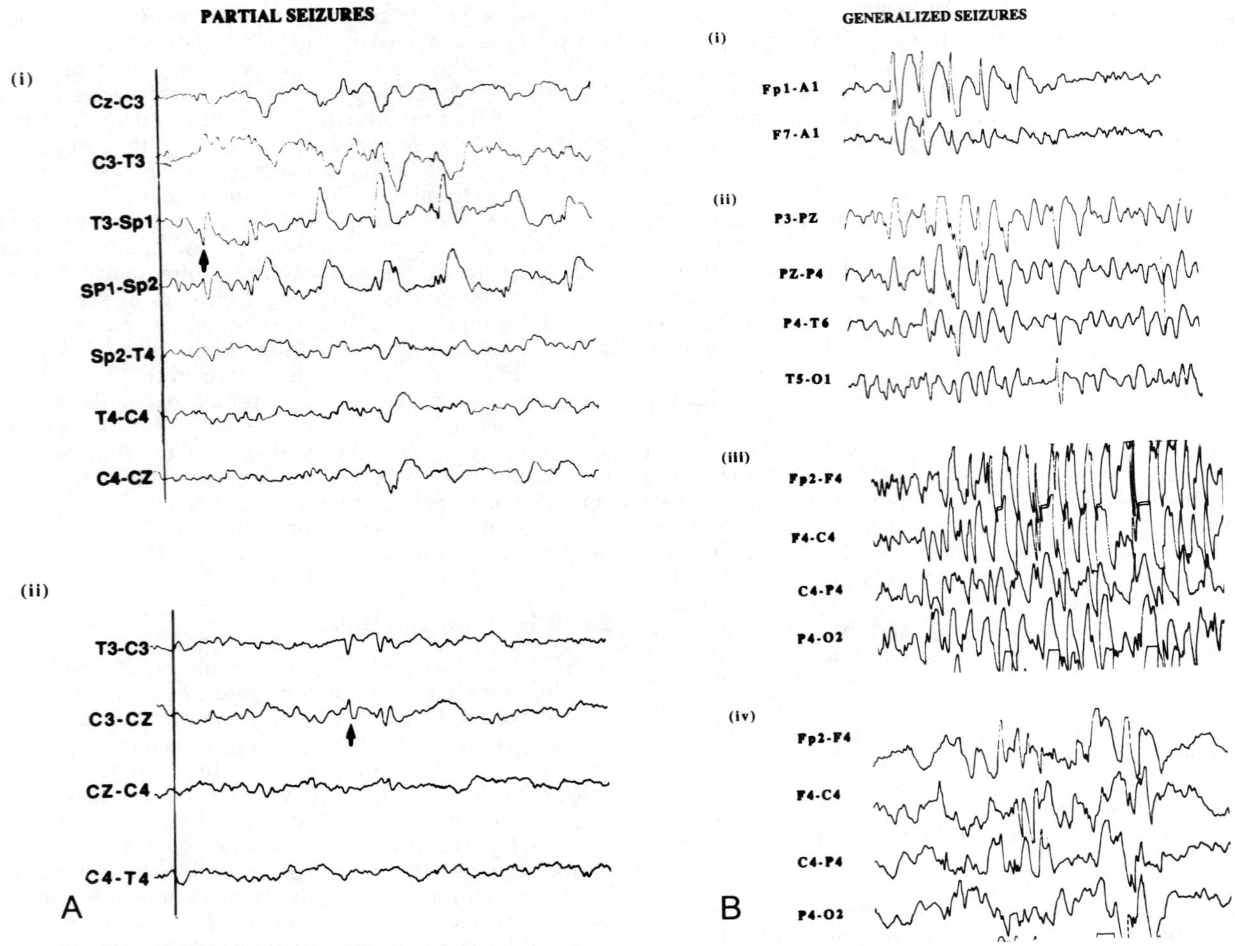

Figure 20–10. *A*, An EEG of partial seizures: (i) spike discharges from the left temporal lobe *(arrow)* in a patient with CPS, (ii) left parietal central spikes *(arrow)* characteristic of BPEC. *B*, Representative EEGs of generalized seizures: (i) 3/sec spike and wave discharge of absence seizures with normal background activity, (ii) complex myoclonic epilepsy (Lennox-Gastaut syndrome) with interictal slow spike waves, (iii) juvenile myoclonic epilepsy showing 6/sec spike and waves enhanced by photic stimulation, and (iv) hypsarrhythmia with an irregular high-voltage spike and wave activity.

object or by a finger because the patient's teeth may be dislodged and aspirated or significant injury to the oropharyngeal cavity may result. Postictally the child will initially be semicomatose and typically remains in a deep sleep from 30 min to 2 hr. If the patient is examined during the seizure or immediately postictally, he or she may demonstrate truncal ataxia, hyperactive deep tendon reflexes, clonus, and a Babinski reflex. The postictal phase is often associated with vomiting and an intense bifrontal headache. An *idiopathic seizure* is a term applied when the cause of a generalized seizure cannot be ascertained. Many factors are known to precipitate generalized tonic-clonic seizures in children including low-grade fever associated with infections, excessive fatigue or emotional stress, and various drugs including psychotropic medications, theophylline, and methylphenidate.

MYOCLONIC EPILEPSIES OF CHILDHOOD. This disorder is characterized by repetitive seizures consisting of brief, often symmetric muscular contractions with loss of body tone and falling or slumping foward, which has a tendency to cause injuries to the face and the mouth. Myoclonic epilepsies include a heterogeneous group of conditions with multiple causes and variable outcomes. However, at least four distinct subgroupings can be identified that represent the broad spectrum of myoclonic epilepsies in the pediatric population.

Benign Myoclonus of Infancy. Benign myoclonus begins during infancy and consists of clusters of myoclonic movements confined to the neck, trunk, and extremities. The myoclonic activity may be confused with infantile spasms; however, the EEG is normal in patients with benign myoclonus. The prognosis is good with normal development and the cessation of myoclonus by 2 yr of age. An anticonvulsant is not indicated.

Typical Myoclonic Epilepsy of Early Childhood. Children who develop typical myoclonic epilepsy are near normal prior to the onset of seizures with an unremarkable pregnancy, labor, and delivery and intact developmental milestones. The mean age of onset is approximately 2½ yr, but the range spreads from 6 mo–4 yr. The frequency of myoclonic seizures varies; they may occur several times daily or children may be seizure-free for weeks. A few patients have febrile convulsions or generalized tonic-clonic afebrile seizures that precede the onset of myoclonic epilepsy. Approximately one half of the patients occasionally have tonic-clonic seizures in addition to the myoclonic epilepsy. The EEG shows fast spike wave complexes of ≥2.5 Hz and a normal background rhythm in most cases. At least one third of the children have a positive family history of epilepsy, which suggests a genetic etiology in some cases. The long-term outcome is relatively favorable. Mental retardation develops in the minority, and more than 50% are seizure-free several years later. However, learning and language problems and emotional and behavioral disorders occur in a significant number of these children and require prolonged follow-up by a multidisciplinary team.

Complex Myoclonic Epilepsies. These consist of a heterogeneous group of disorders with a uniformly poor prognosis. Typically, focal or generalized tonic-clonic seizures beginning during the 1st year of life antedate the onset of myoclonic epilepsy. The generalized seizure is often associated with an upper respiratory tract infection and a low-grade fever and frequently develops into status epilepticus. Approximately one third of these patients have evidence of delayed developmental milestones. A history of hypoxic-ischemic encephalopathy in the perinatal period and the finding of generalized upper motor neuron and extrapyramidal signs with microcephaly constitute a common pattern among these children. A family history of epilepsy is much less prominent in this group compared with typical myoclonic epilepsy. Some children display a combination of frequent myoclonic and tonic seizures, and when interictal slow spike waves are evident in the EEG, the seizure disorder is classified as the **Lennox-Gastaut syndrome.** Patients with complex myoclonic epilepsy routinely have interictal slow spike waves and are refractory to anticonvulsants (see Fig. 20–10*B*). The seizures are persistent, and the frequency of mental retardation and behavioral problems is approximately 75% of all patients.

Juvenile Myoclonic Epilepsy. Juvenile myoclonic epilepsy usually begins between the ages of 12 and 16 yr and accounts for approximately 5% of the epilepsies. Patients note frequent myoclonic jerks upon awakening, which makes hair-combing and tooth-brushing difficult. As the myoclonus tends to abate later in the morning, most patients do not seek medical advice at this stage and some deny the episodes. A few years later, early morning generalized tonic-clonic seizures develop in association with the myoclonus. The EEG shows a 4–6/sec irregular spike and wave pattern, which is enhanced by photic stimulation (see Fig. 20–10*B*). The neurologic examination is normal, and the majority respond dramatically to valproate, which is required lifelong. Discontinuance of the drug causes a high rate of recurrence of seizures.

INFANTILE SPASMS. Infantile spasms usually begin between the ages of 4–8 mo and are characterized by brief symmetric contractions of the neck, trunk, and extremities. There are at least three types of infantile spasms: flexor, extensor, and mixed. *Flexor spasms* occur in clusters or volleys and consist of sudden flexion of the neck, arms, and legs onto the trunk, whereas *extensor spasms* produce extension of the trunk and extremities and are the least common form of infantile spasms. *Mixed infantile spasms*, consisting of flexion in some volleys and extension in others, is the most common type of infantile spasm. Clusters or volleys of seizures may persist for minutes with brief intervals between each spasm. A cry may precede or follow an infantile spasm, accounting for the confusion with colic in a few cases. The spasms occur during sleep and arousal but have a tendency to develop while drowsy or immediately upon awakening. The EEG that is most commonly associated with infantile spasms is referred to as hypsarrhythmia, which consists of a chaotic pattern of high-voltage, bilaterally asynchronous, slow-wave activity (see Fig. 20–10*B*), or a modified hypsarrhythmia pattern.

Infantile spasms are typically classified into two groups: *cryptogenic* and *symptomatic*. The child with cryptogenic infantile spasms has an uneventful pregnancy and birth history as well as normal developmental milestones prior to the onset of seizures. The neurologic examination and the CT scan of the head are normal, and there are no associated risk factors. Approximately 10–20% of infantile spasms are classified as cryptogenic, and the remainder are classified as symptomatic. Symptomatic infantile spasms are related directly to several prenatal, perinatal, and postnatal factors. Prenatal and perinatal factors include hypoxic-ischemic encephalopathy with periventricular leukomalacia, congenital infections, inborn errors of metabolism, neurocutaneous syndromes such as tuberous sclerosis, cytoarchitectural abnormalities including lissencephaly and schizencephaly, and prematurity. Postnatal conditions include CNS infections, head trauma (especially subdural hematoma and intraventricular hemorrhage), and hypoxic-ischemic encephalopathy. In the past, immunization, particularly with the pertussis antigen, had been implicated as a cause of infantile spasms. The fact that infantile spasms and immunizations often occur simultaneously around 6 mo of age has now been shown to be a coincidence of timing rather than a cause and effect. Infants with cryptogenic infantile spasms have a good prognosis whereas those with the symptomatic type have an 80–90% risk of mental retardation. The underlying CNS disorder plays the major role in the neurologic outcome. Several theories have been advanced with regard to the pathogenesis of infantile spasms, including dysfunction of the monoaminergic neurotransmitter system in the brain stem, derangement of neuronal structures in the brain stem, and an abnormality of the immune system. The therapy of infantile spasms follows in the treatment section.

20.20 Febrile Seizures

Febrile convulsions rarely develop into epilepsy, and they spontaneously remit without specific therapy. They are the most common seizure disorder during childhood with a uniformly excellent prognosis. However, a febrile convulsion may signify a serious underlying acute infectious disease such as sepsis or bacterial meningitis so that each child must be carefully examined and appropriately investigated for the cause of the associated fever (Sec. 12.4). Febrile seizures are age dependent and are rare prior to 9 mo and after 5 yr of age. The peak age of onset is approximately 14–18 mo of age, and the incidence approaches 3–4% of young children. There is a strong family history of febrile convulsions in siblings and parents, suggesting a genetic predisposition. Animal studies suggest that arginine vasopressin may be an important mediator in the pathogenesis of hyperthermia-induced seizures.

CLINICAL MANIFESTATIONS. The convulsion is associated with a rapidly rising temperature and usually develops when the core temperature reaches 39° C or greater. The seizure is typically generalized, tonic-clonic of a few seconds to 10-min duration, followed by a brief postictal period of drowsiness. Febrile seizures persisting longer than 15 min suggest an organic cause such as an infectious or toxic process and require a thorough investigation. As the seizure is no longer present by the time that the child reaches the hospital, the physician's most important responsibility is to determine the cause of the fever and to rule out meningitis. *If any doubt exists with regard to the possibility of meningitis, a lumbar puncture with examination of the CSF is indicated.* Viral infections of the upper respiratory tract, roseola, and acute otitis media are most frequently the causes of febrile convulsions.

An EEG is not warranted following a simple febrile seizure because the recording will prove nonepileptiform or normal and that finding will not alter the management. An EEG is indicated for atypical febrile seizures or for the child at risk for developing epilepsy. Atypical febrile seizures include a seizure persisting for more than 15 min, repeated convulsions for several hours or days, and a focal seizure. Approximately 50% of children have recurrent febrile seizures, and a small minority have multiple recurrent seizures. The risk factors for the development of epilepsy as a complication of febrile seizures include a positive family history of epilepsy, initial febrile seizure prior to 9 mo of age, a prolonged or atypical febrile seizure, delayed developmental milestones, and an abnormal neurologic examination. The incidence of epilepsy is approximately 9% when several risk factors are present compared with an incidence of 1% in children who have febrile convulsions and no risk factors.

TREATMENT. The routine management of the normal infant who has simple febrile convulsions includes a careful search for the cause of the fever, active measures to control the fever including the use of antipyretics, and reassurance of the parents. Short-term anticonvulsant prophylaxis is not indicated. Prolonged anticonvulsant prophylaxis for the prevention of recurrent febrile convulsions is controversial and no longer recommended. Antiepileptics such as phenytoin and carbamazepine have no effect on febrile seizures. Phenobarbital has been ineffective in preventing recurrent febrile seizures and may decrease cognitive function in treated children compared with untreated children. Sodium valproate is effective in the management of febrile seizures, but the potential risks of the drug do not justify its use in a disorder with an excellent prognosis irrespective of treatment. Rectal diazepam or lorazepam is the drug of choice for the acute management of prolonged febrile seizures. Parents can be taught to administer the drug safely to children with recurrent seizures.

MECHANISMS OF SEIZURES

Although the precise mechanisms of seizures are unknown, there is considerable knowledge concerning the influence of anatomic lesions, developmental and genetic factors, pharmacologic agents, and cellular function that enhances the understanding of the origin of seizures. For example, it is well known that lesions in the temporal lobe (including slow-growing gliomas, hamartomas, gliosis, and arteriovenous malformations) cause seizures, and when the abnormal tissue is removed surgically, the seizures are likely to cease. Seizures may be produced in animals by the phenomenon of *kindling*. In this model, repeated subconvulsive stimulation of the brain (e.g., amygdala) leads ultimately to a generalized convulsion. In humans, it has been proposed that recurrent seizure activity from an abnormal temporal lobe may produce seizures in the contralateral normal temporal lobe by transmission of the stimulus via the corpus callosum. Seizures are more common in the infant and in the immature experimental animal. Certain seizures in the pediatric population are age specific (e.g., infantile spasms), which suggests that the underdeveloped brain is more susceptible to specific seizures than the older child or adult. It has also been shown that the substantia nigra plays an integral role in the development of generalized seizures. Electrographic seizure activity spreads from within the substantia nigra, causing an increase in uptake of 2-deoxyglucose in adult animals, but there is little or no metabolic activity within the substantia nigra when immature animals have a convulsion. It has been proposed that the functional immaturity of the substantia nigra may play a role in the increased seizure susceptibility of the immature brain. Additionally, the γ-aminobutyric acid (GABA)–sensitive substantia nigra pars reticulata (SNR) neurons play a role in preventing seizures. Recent evidence suggests that excitatory amino acid neurotransmitters (glutamate, aspartate) may play a role in producing neuronal excitation by acting on specific cell receptors.

DIAGNOSIS OF SEIZURES

The investigation of a seizure depends on many factors, including the age of the patient, the type and frequency of the seizure, and the presence or absence of neurologic findings and constitutional symptoms. The minimum work-up for the first afebrile seizure in an otherwise healthy child includes a fasting glucose, calcium, magnesium, serum electrolytes, and a routine *EEG*. The demonstration of paroxysmal discharges on the EEG during a clinical seizure is diagnostic of epilepsy, but seizures rarely occur in the EEG laboratory. A normal EEG does not exclude the diagnosis of epilepsy, because the interictal recording is normal in approximately 40% of patients. Activation procedures including hyperventilation, eye-closure, photic stimulation, and, when indicated, sleep deprivation and special electrode placement (e.g., zygomatic leads) substantially increase the positive yield. Seizure discharges are more likely to be recorded in the infant and child than in the adolescent or adult.

Prolonged EEG monitoring with simultaneous closed-circuit video recording is reserved for the complicated patient with protracted and unresponsive seizures. It provides an invaluable method for the recording of ictal seizure events that are rarely obtained during routine EEG studies. This technique is extremely helpful in the classification of seizures because it can accurately determine the location and frequency of seizure discharges while recording alterations in the level of consciousness and the presence of clinical signs. Patients with pseudoseizures can be readily distinguished from those with true epilepsy, and the seizure type (e.g., complex partial versus generalized) can be more precisely identified, which is critical in the investigation of a child who may be a candidate for epilepsy surgery.

The role of *CT scanning or MRI* in the investigation of seizures is controversial. The yield in the routine use of these procedures in the patient with a first afebrile seizure and a normal neurologic examination is negligible. In studies of children with chronic seizure disorders, the results are similar. Although approximately 30% of these children show a structural abnormality (e.g., focal cortical atrophy or dilated ventricles), only a small minority benefit from active intervention as a result of CT scanning. Thus, CT scanning or MRI should be reserved for patients in whom an intracranial lesion is suspected on the basis of the history or an abnormal neurologic examination. Prolonged partial seizures, intractability to anticonvulsant therapy, a focal neurologic deficit, and evidence of increased intracranial pressure are indications for neuroimaging studies.

Examination of the CSF is indicated if the seizure is potentially related to an infectious process, subarachnoid hemorrhage, or a demyelinating disorder. Specific metabolic tests are outlined in the sections on neonatal seizures and status epilepticus.

20.21 TREATMENT OF EPILEPSY

The first step in the management of epilepsy is to ensure that the patient has a seizure disorder and not a condition that mimics epilepsy (see later). It is sometimes difficult to be certain about the etiology of a paroxysmal event in a normal child. A negative result on a neurologic examination and EEG usually supports the approach of watchful waiting rather than the administration of an anticonvulsant. The true cause of the paroxysmal disorder eventually becomes apparent. Although there is not uniform agreement, most would concur that antiepileptics should be withheld from a previously healthy child with the first afebrile convulsion if there is a negative family history, a normal examination and EEG, and a cooperative and compliant family. Approximately 70% of these children will not experience another convulsion. A recurrent seizure, particularly if it occurs in close proximity to the first seizure, is an indication to begin an anticonvulsant. Table 20–4 suggests an approach to a child with a suspected seizure disorder.

TABLE 20–4. An Approach to the Child with a Suspected Convulsive Disorder

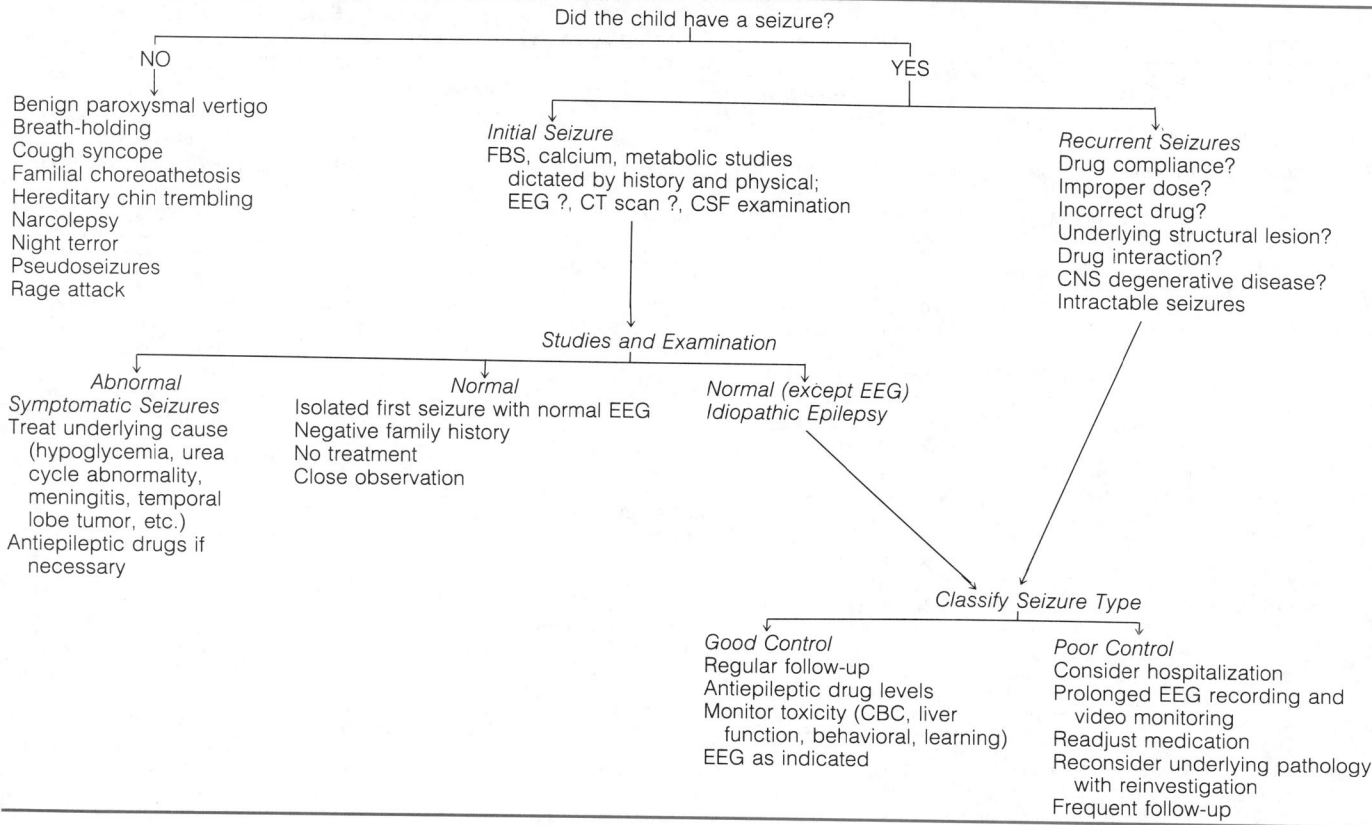

Did the child have a seizure?

- NO
  - Benign paroxysmal vertigo
  - Breath-holding
  - Cough syncope
  - Familial choreoathetosis
  - Hereditary chin trembling
  - Narcolepsy
  - Night terror
  - Pseudoseizures
  - Rage attack
- YES
  - *Initial Seizure*
    - FBS, calcium, metabolic studies dictated by history and physical; EEG ?, CT scan ?, CSF examination
    - → *Studies and Examination*
      - *Abnormal Symptomatic Seizures*
        - Treat underlying cause (hypoglycemia, urea cycle abnormality, meningitis, temporal lobe tumor, etc.)
        - Antiepileptic drugs if necessary
      - *Normal*
        - Isolated first seizure with normal EEG
        - Negative family history
        - No treatment
        - Close observation
      - *Normal (except EEG) Idiopathic Epilepsy* → *Classify Seizure Type*
  - *Recurrent Seizures*
    - Drug compliance?
    - Improper dose?
    - Incorrect drug?
    - Underlying structural lesion?
    - Drug interaction?
    - CNS degenerative disease?
    - Intractable seizures
    - → *Classify Seizure Type*

Classify Seizure Type

- *Good Control*
  - Regular follow-up
  - Antiepileptic drug levels
  - Monitor toxicity (CBC, liver function, behavioral, learning)
  - EEG as indicated
- *Poor Control*
  - Consider hospitalization
  - Prolonged EEG recording and video monitoring
  - Readjust medication
  - Reconsider underlying pathology with reinvestigation
  - Frequent follow-up

The second step involves the choice of an anticonvulsant. The drug of choice depends on the classification of the seizure, determined by the history and EEG findings. The goal for every patient should be the use of only one drug with the fewest possible side effects for the control of seizures. The drug is increased slowly until seizure control is accomplished or until undesirable side effects develop. The child's serum anticonvulsant level should be monitored during this stage, and the dosage should be altered accordingly. Table 20–5 summarizes the common antiepileptic drugs used in childhood epilepsy and highlights the recommended daily dosage, therapeutic serum levels, and common side effects. A suggested loading dose is indicated for drugs that are useful for the treatment of status epilepticus. The physician should be familiar with the pharmacokinetics of the anticonvulsant and its toxic actions and should monitor the child on a regular basis to gauge the seizure control while watching for unwanted side effects.

Anticonvulsants that are introduced during childhood may be required during adolescence and the child-bearing years. Unfortunately, some anticonvulsants including phenytoin, valproic acid, carbamazepine, and primidone are associated with the occurrence of specific birth defects, including facial and limb anomalies and spinal dysraphism. A debate continues with regard to whether the teratogenic effect is secondary to the mother's epilepsy or the anticonvulsant medication. Meanwhile, the pediatrician should counsel the family about the possible relationship and should avoid prescribing an anticonvulsant to a pregnant patient unless it is absolutely necessary.

If complete seizure control is accomplished by an anticonvulsant, a minimum of two seizure-free years is an adequate and safe period of treatment in a patient with no risk factors. Prominent risk factors include neurologic dysfunction (motor handicap or mental retardation), focal seizures, and a long duration of epilepsy prior to control. In the child with complete seizure control for a minimum of 2 yr and low risk factors, the chance of recurrence is approximately 20–25%, particularly during the first 6 mo after the discontinuation of the anticonvulsant. When the decision is made to discontinue the drug, the weaning process should occur for 3–6 mo, because abrupt withdrawal may cause status epilepticus.

CARBAMAZEPINE. This drug is effective for the management of generalized tonic-clonic and partial seizures. Significant leukopenia (<1,000 neutrophils/mL^3) and hepatotoxicity may rarely develop, particularly during the initial 3–4 mo of therapy. Therefore, a complete blood count (CBC) and differential and a SGOT and SGPT should be obtained on a monthly basis during this period, although serious idiosyncratic drug reactions may develop despite normal liver function tests and routine bloodwork. Subsequent laboratory testing is determined by the presence of adverse symptoms or signs. The parents should be informed of untoward drug effects and instructed to report them immediately to the physician. Erythromycin should not be prescribed with carbamazepine because the two drugs compete for metabolism by the liver. The plasma concentration of carbamazepine is lowered by phenytoin, phenobarbital, and valproate. Carbamazepine 10, 11 epoxide, which is an active metabolite of carbamazepine, may produce toxicity despite therapeutic carbamazepine levels, particularly when sodium valproate is added to the drug regimen. Carbamazepine is supplied in 100- and 200-mg tablets and in a controlled release (CR) form, 200- and 400-mg tablets. The half-life is 8–20 hr, and the drug should be given two or three times daily.

PHENOBARBITAL AND PRIMIDONE. These are rela-

TABLE 20–5. Common Anticonvulsant Drugs

Drug	Seizure Type	Oral Dose	Loading Dose (IV)	Therapeutic Serum Level (μg/mL)	Side Effects and Toxicity
Carbamazepine	Generalized tonic-clonic Partial	Begin 10 mg/kg/24 hr Increase to 20 mg/kg/24 hr	—	8–12	Dizziness, drowsiness, diplopia, liver dysfunction, anemia, leukopenia
Clonazepam	Absence Myoclonic Infantile spasms Partial	Begin 0.05 mg/kg/24 hr Increase 0.05 mg/kg/wk Maximum 0.2 mg/kg/24 hr	—	>0.013	Drowsiness, irritability, behavioral abnormalities, depression, excessive salivation
Ethosuximide	Absence Myoclonic	Begin 20 mg/kg/24 hr Increase to maximum of 40 mg/kg/24 hr or 1.5 g/24 hr whichever is less	—	40–100	Abdominal discomfort, skin rash, liver dysfunction, leukopenia
Nitrazepam	Absence Myoclonic Infantile spasms	Begin 0.2 mg/kg/24 hr Increase slowly to 1 mg/kg/24 hr	—		Similar to clonazepam
Paraldehyde	Generalized status epilepticus	Make a 5% solution by adding 1.75 mL of paraldehyde to D_5W with total volume of 35 mL	150–200 mg/kg Maintenance, 20 mg/kg/hr	10–40	
Phenobarbital	Generalized tonic-clonic Partial	3–5 mg/kg/24 hr	10–20 mg/kg 20–30 mg/kg in the neonate	15–40	Hyperactivity, irritability, short attention span, temper tantrums, altered sleep pattern, Stevens-Johnson syndrome, depression of cognitive function
Phenytoin	Generalized tonic-clonic Partial	5 mg/kg/24 hr	10–20 mg/kg	10–20	Hirsutism, gum hypertrophy, ataxia, skin rash, Stevens-Johnson syndrome
Primidone	Generalized tonic-clonic Partial	Begin 50 mg/24 hr in two divided doses Gradually increase to 150–500 mg/24 hr given in three divided doses	—	5–12	Aggressive behavior, personality changes, similar to phenobarbital
Sodium valproate	Generalized tonic-clonic Absence Myoclonic Partial	Begin 10 mg/kg/24 hr Increase by 5–10 mg/kg/wk Usual dose, 30–40 mg/kg/24 hr	—	50–100	Weight gain, alopecia, hepatotoxicity

tively safe anticonvulsants that are particularly useful for generalized tonic-clonic seizures. Unfortunately, approximately 25% of children undergo severe behavioral changes on these drugs. Neurologically abnormal children are at greater risk. Furthermore, there is evidence that phenobarbital may adversely effect the cognitive performance of children treated for febrile seizures. Sodium valproate interferes with the metabolism of phenobarbital, causing elevated phenobarbital plasma levels and toxicity despite the usual daily doses. Phenobarbital is supplied in an elixir (4 mg/mL) and in 15-, 30-, 60-, and 100-mg tablets. Primidone is prepared in a suspension, 50 mg/mL, and in 125- and 250-mg tablets. Phenobarbital is prescribed twice daily, and primidone is prescribed three times a day. Routine bloodwork is not indicated for these anticonvulsants.

PHENYTOIN. This drug may be used interchangeably with carbamazepine. Because of the long list of side effects including rashes, Stevens-Johnson syndrome, lymphadenopathy, a lupus-like disease, gum hyperplasia, hirsutism, megaloblastic anemia, polyneuropathy, and rickets (especially with polytherapy), the drug has become less popular in the treatment of children. Phenytoin is supplied in 50-mg tablets, 30- and 100-mg capsules, and a suspension. The latter is not recommended, because phenytoin is immiscible in liquid and is more likely to produce erratic serum levels and toxicity.

SODIUM VALPROATE. This drug is useful for the management of many seizure types, including generalized tonic-clonic, absence, atypical absence, and myoclonic seizures. It rarely induces behavioral changes but is associated with mild gastrointestinal disturbances, alopecia, tremor, and hyperphagia. There are two rare, but serious side effects of valproate: a Reye-like syndrome and irreversible hepatotoxicity. A small number of children develop progressive lethargy and coma with elevated serum ammonia and decreased levels of serum carnitine. Valproate may block the metabolism of carnitine, producing the altered state of consciousness in these patients. Discontinuation of valproate leads to recovery over several days. Another small group of patients, particularly children less than 2 yr of age with specific neurologic syndromes, who are managed with several anticonvulsants simultaneously, may develop an idiosyncratic hepatotoxic syndrome characterized by abdominal pain, anorexia, weight loss, and retching within a few weeks to months of beginning valproate therapy. These patients have normal liver function studies during the initial stages so that significant and persistent gastrointestinal symptoms are cause for alarm during the initial few months of valproate therapy. If reduction in the valproate dose does not provide immediate relief, the physician should discontinue the drug. These serious and sometimes lethal side effects do not tend to occur after several months of symptom-free therapy. Sodium valproate is available in a syrup, 50 mg/mL, 250- and 500-mg capsules, and 125-, 250-, and 500-mg tablets.

ADRENOCORTICOTROPIC HORMONE (ACTH). This is the preferred drug for the management of infantile spasms, although there is nonuniformity with regard to the dose and duration of therapy. Prednisone is equally effective. A common schedule includes ACTH 20 units IM daily for 2 wk, and if no response occurs, the dose is increased to 30 and then 40 units IM daily for an additional 4 wk. Unless there is complete seizure control, the ACTH is replaced with oral prednisone, 2 mg/kg/24 hr for 2 wk. If the seizures persist, prednisone is given for an additional 4 wk. The side effects of ACTH include hyperglycemia, hypertension, electrolyte abnormalities, gastrointestinal disturbances, and transient brain shrinkage observed by CT scanning. ACTH and prednisone are equally effective for the treatment of cryptogenic and symptomatic seizures, and control can be expected in approximately 70% of patients. There is no relationship between the ease or degree of seizure control and ultimate neurologic and cognitive outcome. The response to medication is usually apparent within a few weeks of therapy, but one third of patients who respond will relapse when the ACTH or prednisone is discontinued.

KETOGENIC DIET. This treatment should be considered for the management of recalcitrant seizures, particularly for children with complex myoclonic epilepsy with associated tonic-clonic convulsions. The diet restricts the quantity of carbohydrate and protein, and most calories are provided as fat. Most children beyond the age of 2–3 yr will not tolerate this fatty unpalatable diet. Because the diet demands precise weighing of foodstuffs and is time-consuming to prepare, it is not tolerated by all families. Some children respond to a liberalized ketogenic diet that substitutes medium-chain triglycerides for the high-fat content of the former diet. Although the mechanism of action of the ketogenic diet is unknown, there is some evidence that it has an effect on increasing the inhibitory neurotransmitter GABA.

SURGERY FOR EPILEPSY. Surgery should be considered for children with intractable seizures unresponsive to anticonvulsants. Until recently, surgery was reserved for adults with longstanding seizures with a focal onset. Studies have now shown that certain children, particularly those with focal seizures, are also candidates for surgery. Although the history and neurologic examination may suggest a focal onset of seizure activity, the EEG is critical in documenting the localization and extent of the epileptogenic discharges. Prolonged EEG recording with video monitoring, frequently necessary on more than one occasion, is essential for the precise localization of the epileptogenic area. It is often helpful to decrease or discontinue the anticonvulsant in the hospitalized patient to increase the probability of recording ictal and interictal epileptogenic activity. In those rare cases when the EEG with the use of sphenoidal or nasopharyngeal electrodes does not adequately localize the focus, the placement of subdural electrodes may provide invaluable information. The EEG studies are complemented by neuropsychologic testing, the WADA (intracarotid injection of amobarbital to establish the dominant hemisphere) test, single photon emission computed tomography (SPECT) or positron emission tomography (PET) scanning, and neuroimaging procedures including CT scanning and MRI. The results of surgery in children with a well-defined focus of epileptogenic activity supported by an identical structural lesion on CT scanning or MRI are extremely favorable and are comparable with the adult with similar pathology. Further refinement in electrophysiologic testing and neuroimaging will undoubtedly lead to even better surgical results in children with anticonvulsant-unresponsive epilepsy.

COUNSELING THE PARENTS. Most parents are initially frightened by the diagnosis of epilepsy and require support and accurate information. The physician should anticipate questions, including inquiries about the duration of the seizure disorder, side effects of medication and convulsions, etiology, social and academic repercussions, and parental guilt. Parents usually wish to know if restrictions should be placed on the child and whether the teacher should be informed. Others inquire about the genetic implications, including the risks for future children. The parents should be encouraged to treat the child as normally as possible. For most children with epilepsy, restriction of physical activity is unnecessary except that the child must be attended by a responsible adult while the child is bathing and swimming. The mechanism of the seizure and what epilepsy means should be explained, and the purpose and side effects of the specific anticonvulsant should be reviewed. Parents who understand the fundamental action and purpose of anticonvulsants and the need for a specific drug regimen are generally very compliant. Counseling should include first-aid measures to be used if the seizure recurs. Fortunately, most parents and children readily adapt to the seizure disorder and to the requirement for long-term anticonvulsants. Most children with epilepsy are well controlled on medication, have normal intelligence, and can be expected to lead normal lives. Cooperation and understanding among the parent, physician, teacher, and child enhance the outlook for the patient with epilepsy.

Annegers JF, Hauser WA, Shirts SB, et al: Factors prognostic of unprovoked seizures after febrile convulsions. N Engl J Med 316:493, 1987.
Backman DS, Hodges FJ, Freeman JM: Computed axial tomography in chronic seizure disorders of childhood. Pediatrics 58:828, 1976.
Clemens B, Ohah R: Sleep studies in benign epilepsy of childhood with rolandic spikes. 1: Sleep pathology. Epilepsia 28:20, 1987.
Commission on Classification and Terminology of the International League Against Epilepsy: Proposal for revised clinical and electroencephalographic classification of epileptic seizures. Epilepsia 22:489, 1981.
Delgado-Escueta AV, Bacsal FE, Treiman DM: Complex partial seizures on closed-circuit television and EEG: A study of 691 attacks in 79 patients. Ann Neurol 11:292, 1982.
Delgado-Escueta AV, Enrile-Bacsal FE: Juvenile myoclonic epilepsy of Janz. Neurology 34:285, 1984.
Dravet C, Bureau M, Roger J: Benign myoclonic epilepsy of infants. *In:* Roger J, Dravet C, Bureau M, et al (eds): Epileptic Syndromes in Infancy, Childhood and Adolescence. London, John Libbey, 1985, pp 68–72.
Duchowny MS: Complex partial seizures of infancy. Arch Neurol 44:911, 1987.
Engel JE Jr (ed): Surgical Treatment of the Epilepsies. New York, Raven Press, 1987.
Erba G, Browne TR: Atypical absence, myoclonic, atonic and tonic seizures and the "Lennox-Gastaut syndrome." *In:* Browne TR, Feldman RG (eds): Epilepsy, Diagnosis and Management. Boston, Little Brown, 1983.
Farwell JR, Lee YJ, Hirtz DG, et al: Phenobarbital for febrile seizures: Effects on intelligence and on seizure recurrence. N Engl J Med 322:364, 1990.
Holmes GL: Partial seizures in children. Pediatrics 77:725, 1986.
Hrachovy RA, Frost JD Jr, Kellaway P, et al: Double-blind study of ACTH vs prednisone therapy in infantile spasms. J Pediatr 103:641, 1983.
Jabbari B, Gunderson CH, Wippold F, et al: Magnetic resonance imaging in partial complex epilepsy. Arch Neurol 43:869, 1986.
Jeavons PM, Bower BD: The natural history of infantile spasms. Arch Dis Child 36:17, 1961.
Lombroso CT: A prospective study of infantile spasms. Epilepsia 24:135, 1983.
Nelson KB, Ellenberg JH: Predictors of epilepsy in children who have experienced febrile seizures. N Engl J Med 295:1029, 1976.
Sato S, Dreifuss FE, Penry JK: Prognostic factors in absence seizures. Neurology 26:788, 1976.
Thompson PJ, Trimble MR: Anti-convulsant drugs and cognitive functions. Epilepsia 23:531, 1982.
Thurston JH, Thurston DL, Hixon BB, et al: Prognosis in childhood epilepsy: Additional follow-up of 148 children 15–23 years after withdrawal of anticonvulsant therapy. N Engl J Med 306:831, 1982.

20.22 NEONATAL SEIZURES

The neonate is at particular risk for the development of seizures, because metabolic, toxic, structural, and infectious diseases are more likely to become manifest during this time than at any other period of life. Neonatal seizures are dissimilar from those in a child or adult because generalized tonic-clonic convulsions tend not to occur during the 1st mo of life. The arborization of axons and dendritic processes as well as myelination is incomplete in the neonatal brain. A seizure discharge therefore cannot readily be propagated throughout the neonatal brain to produce a generalized seizure. There are at least five seizure types that are recognizable in the newborn infant.

CLINICAL MANIFESTATIONS AND CLASSIFICATION. *Focal seizures* consist of rhythmic twitching of muscle groups, particularly the extremities and face. These seizures are often associated with localized structural lesions as well as with infections and subarachnoid hemorrhage. *Multifocal clonic* convulsions are similar to focal clonic seizures but differ in that multiple muscle groups are involved, frequently several simultaneously. *Tonic seizures* are characterized by rigid posturing of the extremities and trunk and are sometimes associated with fixed deviation of the eyes. *Myoclonic seizures* are brief focal or generalized jerks of the extremities or body that tend to involve distal muscle groups. *Subtle seizures* consist of chewing motions, excessive salivation, alterations in the respiratory rate including apnea, blinking, nystagmus, bicycling or pedaling movements, and changes in color.

Neonatal seizures may be difficult to recognize clinically, and some behaviors in the newborn that were considered previously to be convulsions are not substantiated by the EEG recording. Nonetheless, there are several clinical features that distinguish seizures from nonepileptic activity in the neonate. Autonomic changes such as tachycardia and elevation of the blood pressure are common with seizures but do not occur with nonepileptic events. Nonepileptic movements are suppressed by gentle restraint, but true seizures are not. Nonepileptic phenomena are enhanced by sensory stimuli that have no influence on seizures. Correct classification of neonatal seizures is important for the appropriate selection of anticonvulsant therapy. Recent studies utilizing polygraphic EEG recording with video monitoring have greatly enhanced the characterization of neonatal seizures and their medical management.

EEG CLASSIFICATION OF NEONATAL SEIZURES. Clinical Seizure with a Consistent EEG Event. In this category, a clinical seizure occurs in relationship to seizure activity recorded on the EEG and includes focal clonic, focal tonic, and some myoclonic seizures. These seizures are clearly epileptic and are likely to respond to an anticonvulsant.

Clinical Seizures with Inconsistent EEG Events. A neonate may have a clinical seizure without a corresponding seizure discharge. This is observed with all generalized tonic seizures and subtle seizures and with some myoclonic seizures. These infants tend to be neurologically depressed or comatose as a result of hypoxic-ischemic encephalopathy. Seizures in this category are likely to be of nonepileptic origin and may not require or respond to antiepileptics.

Electrical Seizures with Absent Clinical Seizures. Electrical seizures associated with a markedly abnormal background EEG may develop in the comatose infant who is not on anticonvulsants. Conversely, electrical seizures may persist in patients with focal tonic or clonic seizures without clinical signs following the introduction of an anticonvulsant.

ETIOLOGIC DIAGNOSIS. The most common cause of neonatal seizures, hypoxic-ischemic encephalopathy, is discussed in Sec. 9.28. There are many additional disorders that are likely to cause seizures, including metabolic, infectious, traumatic, structural, and maternal disturbances. Because seizures in the neonate may indicate a serious life-threatening and potentially reversible disease, it is imperative that a timely and organized approach to the investigation of neonatal seizures occur.

A careful neurologic examination of the infant may uncover the cause of the seizure disorder. An examination of the retina may show the presence of chorioretinitis, suggesting a congenital infection in which case TORCH titers of mother and infant are indicated. The Aicardi syndrome, which occurs exclusively in female infants, is associated with coloboma of the iris and retinal lacunae, refractory seizures, and absence of the corpus callosum. Inspection of the skin may show hypopigmented lesions characteristic of tuberous sclerosis or the typical crusted vesicular lesions of incontinentia pigmenti; both neurocutaneous syndromes are associated with generalized myoclonic seizures beginning early in life. An unusual body odor suggests an inborn error of metabolism.

Blood should be obtained for glucose, calcium, magnesium, electrolytes, and BUN. If hypoglycemia is a possibility, a serum Dextrostix is indicated so that treatment can be initiated immediately. See Sec. 9.57 for discussion of the diagnosis and treatment of hypoglycemia. Hypocalcemia may occur in isolation or in association with hypomagnesemia. A lowered serum calcium is often associated with birth trauma or a CNS insult in the perinatal period. Additional causes include maternal diabetes, prematurity, the DiGeorge syndrome, and high phosphate feedings. See Sec. 6.28 and 9.54 for full discussion. Hypomagnesemia (<1.5 mg/dL) is often associated with hypocalcemia and occurs particularly in infants of malnourished mothers. In this situation, the seizures are resistant to calcium therapy but respond to intramuscular magnesium, 0.2 mL/kg of a 50% solution of $MgSO_4$. See Sec. 9.54 for diagnosis and treatment of hypomagnesemia. The serum electrolytes may indicate significant hyponatremia (serum sodium <135 mEq/L) or hypernatremia (serum sodium >150 mEq/L) as a cause of the seizure disorder.

A *lumbar puncture* is indicated in virtually all neonates with seizures, unless the cause is obviously related to a metabolic disorder such as hypoglycemia or hypocalcemia secondary to feeding of high concentrations of phosphate. These latter infants are normally alert interictally and usually respond promptly to appropriate therapy. The CSF findings may indicate a bacterial meningitis or aseptic encephalitis (Sec. 9.63). Prompt diagnosis and appropriate therapy improves the outcome for these infants. A bloody CSF indicates a traumatic tap or a subarachnoid/intraventricular bleed. Immediate centrifugation of the specimen may assist in the differentiation of the two disorders. A clear supernatant suggests a traumatic tap, and a xanthochromic color suggests a subarachnoid bleed. However, the mildly jaundiced normal infant may have a yellowish discoloration of the CSF that makes inspection of the supernatant less reliable in the newborn period.

Many *inborn errors of metabolism* cause generalized convulsions in the newborn period. As these conditions are often inherited in an autosomal recessive or X-linked recessive fashion, it is imperative that a careful family history be obtained to determine if siblings or close relatives developed seizures or expired at an early age. A serum ammonia is useful for the screening of suspected urea cycle abnormalities, such as ornithine transcarbamylase, arginosuccinic lysate, and carbamylphosphate synthetase deficiencies. Other than generalized clonic seizures, these infants present during the first few days of life with increasing lethargy progressing to coma, anorexia and vomiting, and a bulging fontanel. If the blood gases show an anion gap and a metabolic acidosis with hyperammonemia, urine organic acids should be immediately determined to investigate the possibility of methylmalonic or propionic acidemia. MSUD should be suspected when a metabolic acidosis occurs in association with generalized clonic seizures, vomiting, and muscle rigidity during the 1st wk of life. The result of a rapid screening test utilizing 2, 4-dinitrophenylhydrazine that identifies ketoderivatives in the urine is positive in MSUD. Additional metabolic causes of neonatal seizures include nonketotic hyperglycemia, a lethal condition characterized by markedly elevated plasma and CSF glycine levels, persistent generalized seizures, and lethargy rapidly leading to coma; ketotic hyperglycinemia in which seizures are associated with vomiting, fluid and electrolyte disturbances, and a metabolic acidosis; and Leigh disease suggested by elevated levels of serum and CSF lactate or an increased lactate/pyruvate ratio. A comprehensive description of the diagnosis and management of these metabolic diseases is discussed in Chapter 8.

The unintentional *injection of a local anesthetic* into the fetus during labor can produce intense tonic seizures. These infants are often thought to have had a traumatic delivery because they are flaccid at birth, they have abnormal brain stem reflexes, and they show signs of respiratory depression that sometimes requires ventilation. Examination may show a needle puncture of the skin or a perforation or laceration of the scalp. An elevated serum anesthetic level confirms the diagnosis. The treatment consists of supportive measures and promotion of urine output by IV fluids with appropriate monitoring to prevent fluid overload.

Pyridoxine dependency, a rare disorder, must be considered when generalized clonic seizures begin shortly after birth with signs of fetal distress in utero. These seizures are particularly resistant to conventional anticonvulsants, such as phenobarbital or phenytoin. The history may suggest that similar seizures occurred in utero. Some cases of pyridoxine dependency are reported to begin later in infancy or in early childhood. This condition is inherited as an autosomal recessive. Although the precise biochemical defect is unknown, pyridoxine is essential for the synthesis of glutamic acid decarboxylase, which in turn is required for the synthesis of GABA. In these infants, large amounts of pyridoxine are required to maintain adequate production of GABA. When pyridoxine dependent seizures are suspected, 100- to 200-mg of pyridoxine should be immediately administered IV. The seizures will abruptly cease, and the EEG will normalize during the next few hours. In the future, measurement of CSF and plasma pyridoxal-5-phosphate may prove to be the more precise method of confirming the diagnosis of pyridoxine dependency. These children require lifelong supplementation of oral pyridoxine, 10 mg/day. Generally, the earlier the diagnosis and therapy with pyridoxine, the more favorable will be the outcome. Untreated children have persistent seizures and are uniformly severely mentally retarded (see also Sec. 4.26).

Drug withdrawal seizures can present in the newborn nursery but may take several weeks to develop because of prolonged excretion of the drug by the neonate. The incriminated drugs include barbiturates, benzodiazepines, heroin, and cocaine. The infant may be jittery, irritable, and lethargic and may show myoclonus or frank clonic seizures. Mother may deny the use of drugs; a serum analysis may identify the responsible agent (see Sec. 9.54).

Infants with severe *cytoarchitectural abnormalities* of the brain including lissencephaly, schizencephaly, neonatal adrenoleukodystrophy, and chromosome abnormalities are susceptible to severe seizures. The investigation of these infants may include a karyotype, CT scanning, MRI, and a long-chain fatty acid determination.

TREATMENT. Anticonvulsants should be utilized in the management of infants with seizures secondary to hypoxic-ischemic encephalopathy (Sec. 9.28) or an acute intracranial bleed (Sec. 9.23). The dose and administration of phenobarbital, diazepam, phenytoin, and paraldehyde for the treatment of neonatal seizures is included in Table 20–5. The greater use of EEG recording in the infant with subtle seizures has identified a number of patients with abnormal movements unrelated to seizure discharges; anticonvulsants are not indicated for this group of neonates.

PROGNOSIS. This depends mainly on the primary cause of the disorder or the severity of the insult. In the case of the hypoglycemic infant of the diabetic mother or hypocalcemia associated with excessive phosphate feedings, the prognosis is excellent. Conversely, the child with intractable seizures due to severe hypoxic-ischemic encephalopathy or a cytoarchitectural abnormality of the brain will usually not respond to anticonvulsants and is susceptible to status epilepticus and early death. The challenge for the physician is to identify patients who will recover with prompt treatment and to avoid delays in diagnosis that could lead to severe irreversible neurologic damage.

Donn S, Grasela T, Goldstein G: Safety of a higher loading dose of phenobarbital in the term newborn. Pediatrics 75:1061, 1985.
Gilman JT, Gal P, Duchowny MS, et al: Rapid sequential phenobarbital treatment of neonatal seizures. Pediatrics 83:674, 1989.
Herzlinger RA, Krandall SR, Vaughan HG: Neonatal seizures associated with narcotic withdrawal. J Pediatr 91:683, 1977.
Hillman L, Hillman R, Dodson WE: Diagnosis, treatment and follow-up of neonatal mepivacaine intoxication secondary to paracervical and pudendal blocks during labor. J Pediatr 95:472, 1979.
Hunt AD, Stokes J, McCrory WW, et al: Pyridoxine dependency: Report of a case of intractable convulsions in an infant controlled by pyridoxine. Pediatrics 13:140, 1964.
Kellaway P, Mizrahi EM: Neonatal seizures. *In*: Luders H, Lesser RP (eds): Epilepsy, Electroclinical Syndromes. New York, Springer-Verlag, 1987, pp 13–47.
Koren G, Warwicke B, Rajchgot R, et al: Intravenous paraldehyde for seizure control in newborn infants. Neurology 36:108, 1986.
Mizrahi E, Kellaway P: Characterizations and classification of neonatal seizures. Neurology 37:1837, 1987.
Painter MJ, Pippenger C, Wasterlain C, et al: Phenobarbital and phenytoin in neonatal seizures: Metabolism and tissue distribution. Neurology 31:1107, 1981.
Shin YS, Rasshofer R, Endres W: Pyridoxal-5-phosphate concentration: Marker for vitamin B_6-dependent seizures in the newborn. Lancet 2:870, 1984.
Van Orman CB, Darwish HZ: Efficacy of phenobarbital in neonatal seizures. Can J Neurol Sci 12:95, 1985.
Volpe JJ: Neonatal seizures: Current concepts and revised classification. Pediatrics 84:422, 1989.

20.23 STATUS EPILEPTICUS

Status epilepticus is defined as a convulsion lasting greater than 30 min or the occurrence of serial convulsions between which there is no return of consciousness. Status epilepticus may be classified as generalized (tonic-clonic, absence) or partial (simple, complex, or with secondary generalization). Generalized tonic-clonic seizures predominate in cases of status epilepticus. Status epilepticus is a medical emergency that requires an organized and skillful approach in order to minimize the associated mortality and morbidity.

ETIOLOGY. There are three major subtypes of status epilepticus in children: prolonged *febrile seizures*, *idiopathic status epilepticus* in which a seizure develops in the absence of an underlying CNS lesion or insult, and *symptomatic status epilepticus* when the seizure occurs in association with a longstanding neurologic disorder or a metabolic abnormality. A febrile seizure lasting for more than 30 min, particularly in a child less than 3 yr of age, is the most common cause of status epilepticus. The idiopathic group includes epileptic patients who have had sudden withdrawal of anticonvulsants followed by status epilepticus. Children who are given anticonvulsants on an irregular basis or who are noncompliant are more likely to develop status epilecticus. Status epilepticus may also be the initial presentation of epilepsy. Sleep deprivation and an intercurrent infection tend to render epileptic patients more susceptible to status epilepticus. The mortality and morbidity among patients with prolonged febrile seizures and idiopathic status epilepticus are low. Symptomatic status epilepticus has a much higher mortality. The cause of death is usually directly attributable to the underlying abnormality. Unlike those with idiopathic status epilepticus, many of these children have not previously had a convulsion. Severe anoxic encephalopathy presents with seizures during the first few days of life, and the ultimate prognosis relates partly to the ease in controlling the seizures. A prolonged convulsion may be the initial manifestation of encephalitis, and epilepsy may be a long-term complication of meningitis. Infants with congenital malformations of the brain (e.g., lissencephaly or schizencephaly) may have recurrent episodes of status epilepticus that are frequently refractory to anticonvulsants. Metabolic inborn errors of metabolism may present with status epilepticus in the newborn. These infants often have a progressive loss of consciousness associated with failure to thrive and excessive vomiting. Electrolyte abnormalities, hypocalcemia, hypoglycemia, drug intoxication, Reye syndrome, lead intoxication, extreme hyperpyrexia, and brain tumors, particularly in the frontal lobe, are additional causes of status epilepticus.

PATHOPHYSIOLOGY. The relationship between the neurologic outcome and the duration of status epilepticus is unknown in children and adults. There is some evidence that the period of status epilepticus that produces neuronal injury in a child is less than that for an adult. In the primate, pathologic changes can occur in the brain of the ventilated animal after 60 min of constant seizure activity when metabolic homeostasis is maintained. Thus, cell death may result from excessively increased metabolic demands by continually discharging neurons. The most vulnerable areas of the brain include the hippocampus, amygdala, cerebellum, middle cortical areas, and the thalamus. Characteristic acute pathologic changes consist of venous congestion, small petechial hemorrhages, and edema. Ischemic cellular changes are the earliest histologic finding, followed by neuronophagia, microglial proliferation, cell loss, and increased numbers of reactive astrocytes. Prolonged seizures are associated with lactic acidosis, an alteration in the blood-brain barrier, and elevation of intracranial pressure. A series of complex, poorly understood hormonal and biochemical changes ensues. Circulating levels of prolactin, adrenocorticotropic hormone, cortisol, glucagon, growth hormone, insulin, epinephrine, and cyclic nucleotides are elevated during status epilepticus in the animal. Neuronal concentrations of calcium, arachidonic acid, and prostaglandins rise and may promote cell death. Initially, the animal may be hyperglycemic, but ultimately hypoglycemia occurs. Inevitably, dysfunction of the autonomic nervous system develops, which may lead to hypotension and shock. Constant tonic-clonic muscle activity during a seizure may produce myoglobinuria and lower nephron nephrosis.

Several investigations have shown significant increases in cerebral blood flow and metabolic rate during status epilepticus. In the animal, approximately 20 min of status epilepticus produces regional oxygen insufficiency, which promotes cell damage and necrosis. These studies have led to the concept of a critical period during status epilepticus when irreversible neuronal changes may develop. This *transitional period* varies between 20 and 60 min in the animal during constant seizure activity. Management of the child should be directed to supporting vital functions and to controlling the convulsions as expeditiously as possible, because the precise transitional period in humans is unknown.

TREATMENT. The *initial management* of the patient begins with an assessment of the respiratory and cardiovascular systems. The child should be transferred to an intensive care unit if possible. The oral airway is inspected for patency, and the pulse, temperature, respirations, and blood pressure are recorded. Excessive oral secretions are removed by gentle suction, and a proper fitting face mask attached to oxygen is applied. If the patient does not respond to oxygen by mask or is difficult to ventilate by an Ambu Bag, consideration should be given to intubation and assisted ventilation. An IV catheter is immediately inserted. If hypoglycemia is confirmed by Dextrostix, a rapid infusion of 5 mL/kg of 10% dextrose is provided. Blood is obtained for a CBC, electrolytes, glucose, creatinine, and anticonvulsant levels, if indicated. Blood and urine may be obtained for toxicology, keeping in mind that some drugs potentiate or precipitate status epilepticus (e.g., amphetamines, phenothiazines, and the tricyclic antidepressants). Arterial blood gases should be determined, and it is wise to maintain an arterial line for repeated examinations. If the seizures are refractory to anticonvulsants, or the patient is paralyzed and is on a respirator, continuous EEG monitoring is important to follow the frequency of seizure discharges, their location, and the response to anticonvulsant therapy. A physical and neurologic examination should be carried out concurrently to assess evidence of trauma; papilledema, a bulging anterior fontanel, or lateralizing neurologic signs suggesting increased intracranial pressure; manifestations of sepsis or meningitis; retinal hemorrhages that may indicate a subdural hematoma; Kussmaul breathing and dehydration suggestive of metabolic acidosis or irregular respirations signifying brain stem dysfunction; evidence of failure to thrive, a peculiar body odor, or abnormal hair pigmentation that suggests an inborn error of metabolism; and constriction or dilatation of pupils suggesting a toxin or drugs as the cause of the status epilepticus. A comprehensive examination should be undertaken once the seizures are under control. Further investigation of the patient including neuroradiologic studies depends on the physical and neurologic findings and on a precise history of the seizure type and frequency.

Drugs should always be delivered IV in the management of status epilepticus; the IM route is unreliable because some drugs are bound by muscle. One of the major drawbacks in the management of status epilepticus is the inappropriate use of anticonvulsants. Too often an unsuitably low drug dose is given, and with lack of response, another antiepileptic is introduced immediately. Care should be given with regard to how the anticonvulsant is delivered. Phenytoin forms a precipitate in glucose solutions and is rendered ineffective. Other drugs interact with plastic containers or are altered by sunlight (e.g., paraldehyde). It is essential to have resuscitation equipment at the bedside and the ability to intubate and ventilate the patient immediately if respiratory depression should supervene.

Either **diazepam** or **lorazepam** may be used initially, because they are effective for the immediate control of prolonged tonic-clonic seizures in most children. Diazepam should be given IV directly into the vein (not the tubing) with a dose of 0.3 mg/kg and with a maximum dose of 10 mg at a rate no greater than 1 mg/min. Respiratory depression and hypotension can occur, especially if administered with a barbiturate. Diazepam is effective in the management of tonic-clonic status, but the drug has a short half-life so that the seizures will recur unless a longer acting anticonvulsant is administered simultaneously. Lorazepam is an equally effective short-term anticonvulsant, with a greater duration of action and decreased likelihood of producing hypotension and respiratory arrest. The recommended dose is 0.05–0.1 mg/kg administered slowly, IV. If an IV line cannot be established or the child is some distance from a medical center, rectal diazepam or lorazepam can be used safely. Undiluted diazepam is placed into the rectum by a syringe and a flexible tube at a dose of 0.3–0.5 mg/kg. The effective dose of rectal lorazepam is 0.05–0.1 mg/kg. Therapeutic serum levels occur within 5–

10 min. Sublingual lorazepam may be used to treat children with serial seizures that tend to develop into status epilepticus while the children are at home. The dose of sublingual lorazepam is 0.05–0.1 mg/kg. The tablet is placed under the patient's tongue and dissolves in a few seconds.

Following the administration of diazepam or lorazepam, several options are available for further management. If the convulsive activity ceases after diazepam or lorazepam therapy or if the seizures persist, **phenytoin** is given immediately. The loading dose of phenytoin is 15–20 mg/kg IV at the rate of 1 mg/kg/min. Phenytoin may be safely added to half-normal or normal saline; the undiluted drug can cause pain, irritation, and phlebitis of the vein. If the seizures do not recur, a maintenance dose of 5–8 mg/kg divided into two equal doses daily is begun 12–24 hr later. Serum phenytoin levels should be monitored as the maintenance dose varies considerably with age. Phenytoin is not always effective in controlling tonic-clonic status epilepticus, in which case an alternative drug is necessary. In some centers, **phenobarbital** is initiated before phenytoin. It is given in a loading dose of 10–15 mg/kg or in the neonate 20 mg/kg IV during 10–30 min. With control of the seizures, the maintenance dose is 3–5 mg/kg/24 hr divided into two equal doses.

If the status epilepticus is not controlled by the preceding strategy, the physician must make some important therapeutic decisions, because it is likely the *transitional period* has been surpassed. The choices for further drug management include paraldehyde, a diazepam drip, lidocaine, or general anesthesia. By this stage the patient is usually sedated and may show signs of respiratory depression, necessitating elective intubation and assisted ventilation.

Paraldehyde is an excellent anticonvulsant and is relatively safe for administration to children. A 5% solution of paraldehyde is prepared by adding 1.75 mL of paraldehyde (1 g/mL) to D_5W to a total volume of 35 mL. The loading dose is 150–200 mg/kg IV slowly for 15–20 min, and then seizure control is maintained with an infusion of 20 mg/kg/hr in a 5% concentration in a glass bottle, because the drug is incompatible with plastic. The IV drip rate may be lowered as the seizures and EEG improve. The drug should be freshly opened, because outdated paraldehyde can deteriorate to acetylaldehyde and acetic acid. Paraldehyde administered rectally or IM can produce tissue damage and sloughing, thus these routes should be reserved for exceptional circumstances.

A **diazepam constant infusion** may be considered rather than paraldehyde, particularly if the initial loading dose of diazepam briefly controlled the seizures. Diazepam is soluble in sterile water, normal saline, and Ringer lactate. A dilution of 0.04 mg/mL offers the greatest assurance of redissolution of diazepam and 24-hr stability. The suggested flow rate is 2 to 3 mg/hr, but the dose should be titrated against the patient's response and side effects.

If the status epilepticus persists following diazepam or lorazepam, and a trial of phenytoin, phenobarbital, and paraldehyde, serious consideration should be given to the induction of **pentobarbital coma.** In an intensive care setting, the patient is placed on a ventilator and a continuous EEG monitor. The initial IV loading dose of pentobarbital is 3–5 mg/kg followed by 2–3 mg/kg/hr to maintain the serum pentobarbital level between 25 and 40 μg/mL. A burst-suppression EEG pattern is maintained for a minimum of 48 hr, followed by cessation of the pentobarbital until the serum level falls to the therapeutic range. Pentobarbital coma requires careful monitoring by an experienced physician, because hypotension requiring pressor agents and electrolyte abnormalities are likely to occur.

General anesthesia is an alternative adjunct to the management of status epilepticus if conventional drug therapy is not effective or if pentobarbital coma is not an option. Several agents have been used successfully, including halothane and isoflurane. General anesthesia probably acts by reversing cerebral anoxia and the concomitant metabolic abnormalities, allowing the previously administered anticonvulsants to exert their effect. The major disadvantage of general anesthesia is that it must be administered in an operating room with anesthetic gas scavenging equipment for prolonged periods.

Sodium valproate has been an effective anticonvulsant in the management of several types of seizures. Because sodium valproate is not available parenterally, it must be given orally or rectally in patients with status epilepticus. Because vomiting or paralytic ileus are common in children with recurrent seizures, sodium valproate should be administered rectally during status epilepticus in order to achieve maximal absorption. Sodium valproate syrup (50 mg/mL) is diluted 1:1 with tap water and is given as a retention enema in a loading dose of 20 mg/kg. It may be considered in the management of status epilepticus in patients who do not respond to the conventional anticonvulsants and pentobarbital coma.

The use of anticonvulsant therapy following status epilepticus is controversial. There is little question that a long-term antiepileptic should be maintained in the child with a progressive neurologic disorder or with a history of recurrent seizures before the onset of status epilepticus. However, it is unlikely that a lengthy period of anticonvulsant treatment is necessary following an initial attack of idiopathic status epilepticus, particularly when a prolonged febrile seizure was the cause. Anticonvulsant therapy is maintained arbitrarily for 3 mo in this case and is discontinued if the child remains asymptomatic.

PROGNOSIS. The neurologic outcome following status epilepticus has improved significantly since the advent of modern pediatric intensive care units and the aggressive management of prolonged seizures. The mortality rate of status epilepticus is approximately 5% in most series. Most deaths occur in the symptomatic group, most of whom have a serious and life-threatening CNS disorder known before the onset of status epilepticus. In the absence of a progressive neurologic insult or metabolic disorder, the morbidity from status epilepticus is low. The fact that long-term sequelae such as hemiplegia, extrapyramidal syndromes, mental retardation, and epilepsy are more common in children less than 1 yr of age following status epilepticus is related to the fact that this group is more likely to have a premorbid underlying CNS disorder than the older child.

Aicardi J, Chevrie JJ: Consequences of status epilepticus in infants and children. Adv Neurol 34:115, 1983.

Aicardi J, Chevrie JJ: Convulsive status epilepticus in infants and children: A study of 239 cases. Epilepsia 11:187, 1970.

Cranford RE, Leppik IE, Patrick B, et al: Intravenous phenytoin in acute treatment of seizures. Neurology 29:1474, 1979.

Curless RG, Holzman BH, Ramsay RE: Paraldehyde therapy in childhood status epilepticus. Arch Neurol 40:477, 1983.

Delgado-Escueta AV, Bajorek JG: Status epilepticus: Mechanisms of brain damage and rational management. Epilepsia 23:S29, 1982.

Delgado-Escueta AV, Wasterlain CG, Treiman DM, et al: Management of status epilepticus. N Engl J Med 306:1337, 1982.

Dulac O, Aicardi J, Rey E, et al: Blood levels of diazepam after single rectal administration in infants and children. J Pediatr 93:1039, 1978.

Hauser AW: Status epilepticus, frequency, etiology and neurological sequelae. *In*: Delgado-Escueta AV, Wasterlain CG, Treiman DM, et al (eds): Status Epilepticus, Advances in Neurology, Vol 34. New York, Raven Press, 1983, pp 3–14.

Kreisman NR, Rosenthal M, LaManna JC, et al: Cerebral oxygenation during recurrent seizures. Adv Neurol 34:231, 1983.

Maytal J, Shinnar S, Moshe SL, et al: Low morbidity and mortality of status epilepticus in children. Pediatrics 83:323, 1989.

Walker JE, Homan RW, Vasko MR, et al: Lorazepam in status epilepticus. Ann Neurol 6:207, 1979.

Yager JY, Seshia SS: Sublingual lorazepam in childhood serial seizures. Am J Dis Child 142:931, 1988.

Young RSK, Ropper AH, Hawkes D, et al: Pentobarbital in refractory status epilepticus. Pediatr Pharmacol 3:63, 1983.

CONDITIONS THAT MIMIC EPILEPSY

Several conditions share features in common with epilepsy. Because these disorders may be associated with altered levels of consciousness, tonic or clonic movements, or cyanosis, they are often confused with epilepsy. These patients may be inappropriately placed on multiple anticonvulsants with no response and some risk; conditions that mimic epilepsy are refractory to antiepileptic drugs. The management of these children differs significantly from that of epilepsy.

20.24 Benign Paroxysmal Vertigo

Benign paroxysmal vertigo (BPV) typically develops in the toddler and is relatively rare beyond 3 yr of age. The attacks develop suddenly and are associated with ataxia, causing the child to fall or refuse to walk or sit. Horizontal nystagmus may be evident during the duration of the attack. The child appears frightened and pale. Nausea and vomiting may be prominent. Consciousness and the ability to verbalize are not disturbed, and there is a lack of lethargy or drowsiness at the completion of the episode. The attacks vary in duration (seconds to minutes), frequency (daily to monthly), and intensity. A rotational sensation (vertigo) is verbalized by the older child with BPV. These children are susceptible to motion sickness and may develop migraine headaches several years later, suggesting a relationship between BPV and migraine. The neurologic evaluation characteristically has negative results, except for the finding of abnormal vestibular function detected by ice water caloric testing. Patients with clusters of attacks usually respond to dimenhydrinate 5 mg/kg/24 hr with a maximum of 300 mg/24 hr PO, IM, IV, or per rectum.

20.25 Night Terrors

Night terrors are common, particularly in boys between 5 and 7 yr of age (see Sec. 3.30). They occur in 1–3% of children and are usually short-lived. A night terror has a sudden onset between midnight and 2.00 A.M. during stage 3 or 4 of slow-wave sleep. The child screams and appears frightened, with dilated pupils, tachycardia, and hyperventilation. There is little or no verbalization; the child may thrash violently, cannot be consoled, and is unaware of parents or surroundings. Sleep follows in a few minutes, and there is total amnesia the following morning. Approximately one third of children with night terrors experience somnambulism. An underlying emotional disorder should be explored in children with persistent and prolonged night terrors. A short course of diazepam or imipramine may be considered for treatment of protracted night terrors while the family dynamics are under investigation.

20.26 Breath-Holding Spells

A breath-holding spell can be a frightening experience for the parent because the infant becomes lifeless and unresponsive owing to cerebral anoxia at the height of the attack. There are two major types of breath-holding spells: the more common cyanotic form and the pallid form.

CYANOTIC SPELLS. A cyanotic breath-holding spell is usually predictable and is always provoked by upsetting or scolding an infant. The episode is heralded by a brief, shrill cry followed by forced expiration and apnea. There is rapid onset of generalized cyanosis and a loss of consciousness that may be associated with repeated generalized clonic jerks, opisthotonus, and bradycardia. The interictal EEG is normal. A breath-holding spell can occur repeatedly within a few hours or it can recur sporadically, but it is always stereotyped. Breath-holding spells are rare prior to 6 mo of age; they peak at about 2 yr of age, and they abate by 5 yr of age. The management of breath-holding spells concentrates on the support and reassurance of the parents. Some parents feel that, whatever the physician recommends, they must splash cold water on the face, turn the child upside down, or initiate mouth-to-mouth resuscitation and even cardiopulmonary resuscitation. A thorough examination followed by an explanation of the mechanism of breath-holding spells is reassuring for most parents. The counseling session should emphasize the need for both parents to be consistent and not reinforce the child's behavior after the child recovers from the spell. This may be accomplished by placing the child safely in bed and by refusing to cuddle, play, or hold the child for a given period of time when recovery is complete.

PALLID SPELLS. These spells are much less common than cyanotic breath-holding spells, but they share several characteristics. Pallid spells are typically initiated by a painful experience, such as falling and striking the head or a sudden startle. The child stops breathing, rapidly loses consciousness, becomes pale and hypotonic, and may have a tonic seizure. Bradycardia with periods of asystole of longer than 2 sec may be recorded. The interictal EEG is normal. Pallid spells can in some cases be induced spontaneously in the laboratory by ocular compression that produces the oculocardiac reflex by afferent stimulation of the trigeminal nerve and by efferent inhibition of the heart by way of the vagus nerve. This procedure should not be attempted by an inexperienced physician, and appropriate resuscitation equipment should be readily available. Most children respond to conservative measures as outlined for cyanotic spells, but a trial of an anticholinergic, oral atropine sulfate 0.01 mg/kg/24 hr in divided doses with a maximum daily dose of 0.4 mg, which increases the heart rate by blocking the vagus nerve, may be considered in refractory cases. Atropine should not be prescribed during very hot weather as an episode of hyperpyrexia may be initiated.

20.27 Syncope

SIMPLE SYNCOPE. Syncope follows an alteration in brain metabolism, the consequence of decreased cerebral blood flow, usually secondary to systemic hypotension. The brain depends on a constant blood flow, and autoregulation protective mechanisms maintain cerebral circulation and oxygenation despite wide fluctuations in the systemic blood pressure. Decreased blood flow causes loss of consciousness, and the concomitant ischemia influences the higher cortical centers to release their inhibiting influence on the reticular formation within the brain stem. Neuronal discharges from the reticular formation then produce brief tonic contractions of the muscles of the face, trunk, and extremities in approximately 50% of patients with syncope. During a syncopal episode, the child may have fixed upward deviation of the eyes that can be confused with epilepsy. Simple syncope results from vasovagal stimulation and is precipitated by pain, fear, excitement, and extended periods of standing still, particularly in a warm environment. The EEG shows transient slowing during the attack but no seizure discharges. Simple syncope is uncommon prior to 10-12 yr of age but is quite prevalent in adolescent females.

COUGH SYNCOPE. This is most common in asthmatic children. It often occurs shortly after the onset of sleep, and the coughing paroxysm abruptly awakens the child. The patient's face becomes plethoric, and the child perspires, becomes agitated, and frightened. Loss of consciousness is associated with generalized muscle flaccidity, vertical upward gaze, and clonic muscle contractions lasting for several seconds. Urinary incontinence is frequent. Recovery begins within seconds, and consciousness is usually restored a few minutes later. The child has no recollection of the attack except for the events surrounding the paroxysm of coughing. Coughing produces a marked increase in intrapleural pressure followed by a lowered venous return to the right side of the heart and an associated decrease in right ventricular output. Reduction of left ventricular filling follows, and a rapidly diminished cardiac output results in altered cerebral blood flow, cerebral hypoxia, and a loss of consciousness. The cornerstone of management for asthmatic children with cough syncope is an aggressive approach to the prevention of bronchoconstriction.

20.28 Familial Paroxysmal Choreoathetosis

This rare autosomal dominant disorder is characterized by a sudden onset of choreoathetosis and is precipitated by movement, particularly after awakening and during the first few steps. The patient may fall and lose consciousness, which persists for a few seconds to several minutes. The child is normal between attacks, and although familial paroxysmal athetosis is not a seizure disorder, clonazepam is often successful in preventing the episodes.

20.29 Shuddering Attacks

Shuddering attacks have their onset at 4–6 mo of age and may persist to 6–7 yr of age. They produce an interesting posture with sudden flexion of the head and trunk and shuddering or shivering movements similar to what must occur if ice-cold water is poured down the back of an unsuspecting individual. These children may have 100 attacks/day followed by several symptom-free weeks. Shuddering attacks may be the childhood precursor of benign essential tremor, because examination of parents and relatives reveals a high incidence of that common condition.

20.30 Benign Paroxysmal Torticollis of Infancy

Infants with benign paroxysmal torticollis have recurrent attacks of head tilt associated with pallor, agitation, and vomiting with an onset between 2 and 8 mo of age. During the attack, the child resists passive head movement. There is no loss of consciousness, and spontaneous remission occurs by 2–3 yr of age. As with benign paroxsymal vertigo, abnormalities in vestibular function have been documented in these patients. Children with persistent torticollis should be investigated for abnormalities of the cervical vertebra, including dislocation or fracture or a tumor located in the posterior fossa. Some infants with benign paroxysmal torticollis develop migraine headaches later in childhood.

20.31 Hereditary Chin Trembling

Hereditary chin trembling may be confused with epilepsy due to repeated episodes of rapid 3/sec chin trembling movements. These brief attacks are precipitated by stress, anger, and frustration and are inherited as an autosomal dominant trait. The findings on the neurologic examination and EEG are normal.

20.32 Narcolepsy and Cataplexy

See also Sec. 3.30 and 10.13. Narcolepsy is a disorder that rarely begins before adolescence and is characterized by paroxysmal attacks of irrepressible sleep, which is sometimes associated with transient loss of muscle tone (cataplexy). An EEG shows that the recurrent sleep attacks consist of rapid eye movement (REM) sleep. Patients with narcolepsy are easily aroused and become spontaneously alert, whereas a convulsion is followed by a deep sleep, postictal drowsiness, lethargy, and often a headache. Cataplexy is also occasionally confused with epilepsy. These patients experience sudden loss of muscle tone and fall to the floor because of laughter, stress, or frightening experiences. The cataplectic patient does not lose consciousness but lies without moving for a few minutes until normal body tone returns. Treatment consists of scheduled naps, amphetamines, methylphenidate, tricyclic antidepressants, and counseling with respect to occupational safety and driving.

20.33 Rage Attacks or Episodic Dyscontrol Syndrome

The *episodic dyscontrol syndrome,* a nonepileptic condition, can be confused with complex partial seizures. These patients develop sudden and recurrent attacks of violent physical behavior with minimal provocation. The attacks consist of kicking, scratching, biting, and shouting (including abusive and profane language). The child or adolescent cannot seem to control the behavior and may seem momentarily psychotic throughout the attack. The episode is followed by fatigue, amnesia, and sincere remorse. The routine EEG may show nonspecific abnormalities in patients with the rage syndrome. The EEG in such patients during the attack remains normal, which distinguishes this condition from complex partial seizures that always show an abnormal EEG during an attack.

20.34 Pseudoseizures

The diagnosis of a pseudoseizure should be made only after a thorough history and physical examination and exclusion of "true" seizures by prolonged EEG recording when indicated. Pseudoseizures occur typically between 10 and 18 yr of age and are more frequent among female patients. Pseudoseizures occur in many patients with a past history of epilepsy and in some with ongoing "true" seizures. A pseudoseizure may be quite realistic but frequently it is bizarre, with unusual postures, verbalizations, and uncharacteristic tonic or clonic movements. There are several distinguishing features of a pseudoseizure, including lack of cyanosis, normal reaction of the pupil to light, no loss of sphincter control, normal plantar responses, and the absence of tongue biting or injury during the attack. Many patients moan or cry during a pseudoseizure, and some patients can be persuaded to have an attack on request by the physician. Patients with pseudoseizures are likely to have a neurotic personality documented by formal psychologic testing. It is not unusual to find a patient on three or four anticonvulsants which, of course, have no effect. The most reliable method of differentiating epilepsy from suspected pseudoseizures is to record an attack. The EEG shows an excess of muscle artifact during the pseudoseizure, but a normal background rhythm devoid of seizure discharges. Following true epileptic seizure there is a significant increase in serum prolactin, whereas there is no change from the baseline at the termination of a pseudoseizure.

Basser LS: Benign paroxysmal vertigo of childhood. Brain 87:141, 1964.
Grossman BJ: Trembling of the chin—an inheritable dominant character. Pediatrics 19:453, 1957.
Haslam RHA, Freigang B: Cough syncope mimicking epilepsy in asthmatic children. Can J Neurol Sci 12:45, 1985.
Koenigsberger MR, Chutorian AM, Gold AP, et al: Benign paroxysmal vertigo of childhood. Neurology 20:1108, 1970.

Lombroso CT, Lerman P: Breath-holding spells (cyanotic and pallid infantile syncope). Pediatrics 39:563, 1967.
Mount LA, Reback S: Familial paroxysmal choreoathetosis. Arch Neurol Psychiatr 44:841, 1940.
Pritchard PB, Wannamaker BB, Sagel J, et al: Serum prolactin and cortisol levels in evaluation of pseudoepileptic seizures. Ann Neurol 18:87, 1985.
Schneider S, Rice DR: Neurologic manifestations of childhood hysteria. J Pediatr 94:153, 1979.
Snyder CH: Paroxysmal torticollis in infancy. Am J Dis Child 117:458, 1969.
Vanasse M, Bedard P, Andermann F: Shuddering attacks in children: An early clinical manifestation of essential tremor. Neurology 26:1027, 1976.
Yoss R, Daly D: Nacrolepsy in children. Pediatrics 25:1025, 1960.
Zarcone V: Narcolepsy. N Engl J Med 288:1156, 1973.

20.35 HEADACHES

Headache is a common problem in pediatrics. The effect that headaches have on a child's academic performance, memory, personality, and interpersonal relationships as well as school attendance depends on their etiology, frequency, and intensity. A headache may occasionally indicate a severe underlying disorder (e.g., a brain tumor) and thus careful evaluation of children with recurrent, severe, or unconventional headaches is mandatory. Infants and children respond to a headache in unpredictable fashions. Most toddlers cannot communicate the characteristics of a headache, but rather they may become irritable and cranky, vomit, prefer a darkened room because of photophobia, or repeatedly rub their eyes and head. Children are poor historians when describing a headache and its associated symptoms. The most important causes of headache in children include migraine, increased intracranial pressure, and psychogenic or stress headaches. Refractive errors, strabismus, sinusitis, and malocclusion of the teeth are much less common causes of significant headaches in children.

20.36 MIGRAINE

Migraine is defined as a recurrent headache with symptom-free intervals and at least three of the following symptoms or associated findings: abdominal pain, nausea or vomiting, throbbing headache, unilateral location, associated aura (visual, sensory, motor), relief following sleep, and a positive family history. It is the most important and frequent type of headache in the pediatric population. Most migraine headaches are not severe and are readily managed by conservative measures without requiring medical attention. The youngest child reported to develop migraine was 1 yr of age. The incidence of migraine among school-aged children between 7 and 15 yr of age was 4% in a comprehensive Swedish study. Girls are more likely to develop a migraine as adolescents, whereas males are in the slight majority among children under 10 yr old with migraine headaches. More than one half undergo spontaneous prolonged remission following the 10th birthday. The etiology of migraine headaches is unknown, but an inherited predisposition to vasomotor instability appears to be an important underlying factor. Hormonal changes, food allergies, personality traits characterized by high achievement, stress, bright flashing lights, and excessive sound have all been implicated. Increased levels of circulating serotonin and substance P, a vasodilating polypeptide, may act directly on the extracranial and intracranial vessels.

CLINICAL MANIFESTATIONS AND CLASSIFICATION. Migraine may be classified into subgroups, including common and classic migraine, migraine variants, cluster headaches, and complicated migraine. As cluster headaches rarely occur in children, they are not discussed here.

Common Migraine. This migraine is not associated with an aura and is the most prevalent type of migraine in children. The headache is throbbing or pounding and tends to be located in the bifrontal or temporal regions. It is often not hemicranial in children and is less intense compared with the migraine in an adult. The headache usually persists for 1–3 hr, although the pain may last for as long as 24 hr. A characteristic feature of childhood migraine is intense nausea and vomiting, which may be more bothersome than the headache. The vomiting may be associated with abdominal pain and fever, thus conditions such as appendicitis and a systemic infection may be erroneously confused with the primary diagnosis. Additional symptoms include photophobia, light-headedness, and paresthesias of the hands and feet. A family history, particularly on the maternal side, is present in approximately 90% of children with common migraine. Thus, considerable caution should be exercised when making the diagnosis of a common migraine in the absence of a positive family history.

Classic Migraine. In this disorder an aura precedes the onset of the headache. Visual aura are rarely present in children with migraine, but when they occur they may take the form of blurred vision, scotoma (an area of depressed vision within the visual field), photopsia (flashes of light), fortification spectra (brilliant white zig-zag lines), or irregular distortion of objects. Some patients also have vertigo and light-headedness during this stage of the headache. Sensory symptoms include perioral paresthesias and numbness of the hands and feet. Distortions of body image may predominate as a prelude to a classic migraine headache. A graphic description of visual misinterpretation was recorded by Lewis Carroll, a migraine sufferer, in his *Alice's Adventures in Wonderland*, where Alice is addressing the caterpillar: "I can't remember things as I used—and I don't keep the same size for ten minutes together." Following the aura, a patient with classic migraine develops typical symptoms of a common migraine as described earlier.

Migraine Variants. These variants include cyclic vomiting, acute confusional states, and benign paroxysmal vertigo. The last condition is discussed in Sec. 20.24. *Cyclic vomiting* is characterized by recurrent, sometimes monthly bouts of severe vomiting that may be so intense that dehydration and electrolyte abnormalities occur, particularly in an infant. Initially, systemic symptoms such as fever, abdominal pain, and diarrhea are absent, but they may become prominent in association with excessive fluid losses secondary to vomiting. The vomiting may be protracted and persist for several days. The child may appear pale and frightened but does not lose consciousness. After a period of deep sleep, the child awakens and resumes normal play and eating habits as if the vomiting had not existed. Most children with cyclic vomiting have a positive family history of migraine, and, as they grow older and become verbal, they describe a typical migraine headache that leaves little doubt about the diagnosis and the association of the cyclic vomiting with the condition. Cyclic vomiting is treated with rectally administered antiemetics such as dimenhydrinate 5 mg/kg/24 hr in four divided doses (maximum of 300 mg/24 hr) and careful attention to fluid replacement if the vomiting is excessive.

Acute confusional states may be a manifestation of migraine. Migraine may present in a bizarre fashion, particularly in children, characterized by confusion, hyperactivity, disorientation, unresponsiveness, memory disturbances, vomiting, and lethargy. The neurologic examination shows defects of the sensorium, delayed responses to stimuli including touch and pain, and occasionally plantar extensor responses. The differential diagnosis includes toxic encephalopathy (particularly in an adolescent), encephalitis, acute psychosis, postictal state, petit mal (absence) status epilepticus, head trauma, and sepsis. The episode of acute confusion may persist for several hours and characteristically clears spontaneously following sleep; the patient has no recall of the confusional state. The diagnosis is usually made in retrospect as the patient or family recalls the onset of a severe headache or visual symptoms preceding the acute attack of confusion, and a family history of migraine is established. Acute confusional states as a component of migraine probably result from localized cerebral edema due to increased vascular permeability during the headache. The EEG shows regional areas of slowing (2–4 cps) during and shortly after the attack but routinely returns to normal within a few days.

Complicated Migraine. Complicated migraine refers to the development of neurologic signs during a headache that persist following the termination of the headache. The presence of neurologic signs in association with a headache suggests the possibility of an underlying structural lesion and requires a thorough investigation. There are three subsets of complicated migraine.

Brain stem signs predominate in patients with *basilar migraine*, owing to vasoconstriction of the basilar and posterior cerebral arteries. The major symptoms include vertigo, tinnitus, diplopia, blurred vision, scotoma, ataxia, and an occipital headache. The pupils may be dilated, and ptosis may be evident. Alterations in consciousness followed by a generalized seizure may result. After the attack there is a complete resolution of the neurologic symptoms and signs. There is a strongly positive family history for migraine in most of the children. Many develop classic migraine as adolescents or adults. Relatively minor head trauma may precipitate an episode of basilar migraine. The condition has been described in children of both sexes, with girls less than 4 yr of age at particular risk.

Ophthalmoplegic migraine is relatively rare in children. These patients develop a third-nerve palsy ipsilateral to the headache during the attack, owing to altered blood supply to the oculomotor nerve. The major differential diagnosis is a congenital aneursym compressing the oculomotor nerve.

Hemiplegic migraine refers to the onset of unilateral sensory or motor signs during an episode of migraine. Hemisyndromes are more common in children than in adults and may be characterized by numbness of the face, arm, and leg, unilateral weakness, and aphasia. More than one attack is uncommon in the pediatric age group. The neurologic signs may be transient or may persist for days. It is unusual for a child to develop a completed stroke following a single episode. Hemiplegic migraine in the older child or adolescent has a relatively good prognosis, and often a positive family history of similar hemiplegic events is elicited. On the other hand, some children with migraine develop the syndrome of alternating hemiplegia, which has its onset during infancy. Acute hemiplegia may be the initial manifestation of migraine and may recur affecting one side and then the other. Frequent episodes of vasoconstriction associated with ischemia may result in irreversible cerebral injury leading to mental retardation and epilepsy in this subgroup of children.

DIAGNOSIS AND DIFFERENTIAL DIAGNOSIS. A thorough history and physical examination suffice to establish the diagnosis in most cases. Basilar migraine may be confused with several conditions, including congenital malformations of the skull and cervical vertebrae, posterior fossa tumors, toxins and drugs, and metabolic abnormalities including Leigh disease and pyruvate decarboxylase deficiency. In children with hemiplegic migraine, an arteriovenous malformation, cerebral tumor, Todd paralysis, clotting disorders, hemoglobinopathies such as sickle cell disease, and metabolic conditions including homocystinuria should be considered. A lipid profile should be obtained in children with migraine and a positive family history of premature myocardial infarction or cerebrovascular accident. The organization of laboratory tests and radiologic studies depends on the constellation of symptoms and findings during the neurologic examination. A CT scan or MRI is indicated if the headache is associated with an unusual constellation of symptoms or signs or when increased intracranial pressure is suspected (Table 20–6).

TABLE 20–6. Indications for Neuroimaging a Child with Headaches*

Abnormal neurologic signs
Recent school failure, behavioral change, fall-off in linear growth rate
Headache awakens child during sleep; early morning headache, with increase in frequency and severity
Periodic headaches and seizures coincide, especially if seizure has a focal onset
Migraine and seizure occur in the same episode, and vascular symptoms precede the seizure (20–50% risk of tumor or arteriovenous malformation)
Cluster headaches in child; any child <5 or 6 years whose principal complaint is a headache
Focal neurologic symptoms or signs developing during a headache (i.e., complicated migraine)
Focal neurologic symptoms or signs (except classic visual symptoms of migraine) develop during the aura, with fixed laterality; focal signs of the aura persisting or recurring in the headache phase
Visual graying out occurring at the peak of a headache instead of the aura
Brief cough headache in a child or adolescent

*Modified from Barlow CF: Headaches and Migraine in Childhood. Philadelphia, JB Lippincott, 1984, p 205.

TREATMENT. Migraine may be prevented or ameliorated by *avoiding certain initiating stimuli*. A few children can identify specific factors that uniformly result in a headache. The most common precipitator of migraine headaches is stress and anxiety. The child may be under undue stress because of difficulties at home or school, particularly when unrealistic pressures or demands are placed on the patient. Children who experience recurrent migraine headaches during the school year may have a learning disability or may have been placed in a too highly competitive classroom. Reassessment of the child's school placement and academic abilities may be the most important step in the management of the headache disorder. Some studies implicate certain foods as a cause of migraine, particularly nuts, chocolate, cola drinks, hot dogs, spicy meats, kippers, and Chinese food (monosodium glutamate). Elimination of the incriminating foodstuff is indicated if the history suggests a relationship between the ingestion of a particular food and the onset of headache. Avoidance of bright flashing lights, sun exposure, excessive physical exertion, mild head trauma, loud noises, hunger, fatigue, motion sickness, and drugs (including alcohol and oral contraceptives) are indicated when the history suggests a direct relationship. It is important to note that the frequency and severity of migraine headaches is reduced significantly in at least 50% of pediatric patients who undergo a careful history and neurologic examination followed by reassurance from the physician.

Management of an acute attack of migraine should include the use of *analgesics and antiemetics*. Most migraine headaches in children can be treated by the judicious use of **acetaminophen**, particularly if the headaches are mild, infrequent, and of short duration. The **ergotamine preparations** (ergotamine tartrate) should be considered for children with severe, classic migraine headaches and are most efficacious during the early stages of the migraine attack. The usual dose is 1 mg, which may be administered orally, subcutaneously, or per rectum in the form of a suppository. A repeat dose may be given 30 min later. Ergotamine should not be prescribed for patients with hemiplegic episodes. The ergotamines are frequently ineffective in children because they must be used early in the evolution of the headache. Most children are either unaware of an aura or fail to communicate the onset of the headache to their parents. An antiemetic such as **dimenhydrinate** 5 mg/kg/24 hr in four divided doses is the mainstay of treatment when vomiting is the major symptom. The child usually prefers to rest in a quiet darkened room and typically awakens, refreshed and headache-free, several hours later after a deep sleep.

The decision to use *continuous daily medication* is based on the severity and frequency of the headaches and on the impact of the migraine on the child's daily activities, including school attendance and performance as well as participation in recreation. The use of prophylactic drugs should be considered if the child experiences more than 2–4 severe episodes monthly or is unable to attend school regularly (Table 20–7). Although few drugs have been subjected to well-designed clinical trials in children, propranolol, a β-adrenergic blocker, is the drug of choice in most centers. If a drug is effective, it is usually maintained for 1 yr, particularly during the school term.

Behavior management is an effective method for the treatment of migraine in some children and adolescents. Biofeedback and self-hypnosis are replacing pharmacologic treatment in some centers because of the undesirable side effects of drugs and the concern that some may produce chemical dependency. Biofeedback can be mastered by most children over 8 yr of age and has been effective in many clinical trials. Several studies of migrainous children show a significant decrease in frequency and no change in intensity of headaches in those treated by self-hypnosis compared with those taking the placebo or propranolol.

20.3 ORGANIC HEADACHES

A headache may be the earliest symptom of increased intracranial pressure. The headache results from tension or traction of the cerebral blood vessels and dura and occurs initially in a sporadic fashion, primarily in the early hours in the morning or shortly after the patient arises. The headache is diffuse and generalized and is more prominent over the frontal and occipital regions. Its onset may be insidious, and the pain is enhanced by any activity that raises the intracranial pressure (e.g., coughing, sneezing, or straining during a bowel movement). As the intracranial pressure increases, the child becomes lethargic and irritable, and the headache becomes constant. Early morning vomiting is often associated with increased intracranial pressure. Causes of organic headaches in children include brain tumors, particularly those located in the posterior fossa, hydrocephalus, meningitis and encephalitis, cerebral abscess, subdural hematoma, chronic lead poisoning, and pseudotumor cerebri. Additional causes of organic headaches in children that may not be associated with increased intracranial pressure include arteriovenous malformations, berry aneurysm, collagen vascular diseases affecting the CNS, hypertensive encephalopathy, acute subarachnoid hemorrhage, and stroke. The management of organic headaches depends on the cause. The initial step includes a thorough history and physical examination, including recording of the blood pressure and inspection of the eyegrounds. Ordering of laboratory tests and neuroradiologic procedures depends on the clues provided by the history and physical examination.

20.38 PSYCHOGENIC OR STRESS HEADACHES

Psychogenic, stress, or tension headaches, are relatively uncommon in the pediatric age group particularly before puberty and are often difficult to differentiate from migraine headaches. The two are often associated in the same patient. Psychogenic headaches infrequently appear in the morning hours but are most apparent during the school day, particularly coinciding with a test or similarly anxiety provoking circumstance. Although these headaches can be continuous and persist for weeks, they tend to wax and wane and build in intensity during the day. The headache is described as hurting or aching but is rarely perceived as throbbing. Most psychogenic headaches in children are distributed in the frontal region, but they may localize over the vertex or the occipital area. Unlike migraine or headaches associated with increased intracranial pressure, psychogenic headaches are not, as a rule, associated with nausea and vomiting.

The *diagnosis* of psychogenic headache is made by exclusion at the completion of the history and physical examination. Studies such as an EEG or a CT scan are rarely necessary. Management consists of a search for possible underlying emotional or stressful factors. Most children have considerable insight into the origin of psychogenic headaches and, when given the opportunity, will share concerns and conflicts. A poor self-image, fear of school failure, and lack of self-confidence are common factors. Occasionally, a depressed child presents with severe headaches. These patients may also complain of sudden mood changes, weight loss, anorexia, disturbed sleep, fatigue, and withdrawal from social activities.

TABLE 20–7. Drugs for Migraine Prophylaxis

Drug	Dose	Side Effects	Contraindications
Propranolol	Children: begin 10 mg bid or tid, max 20 mg tid; adolescents: begin 10–20 mg tid, max 80 mg tid	Nausea, insomnia, fatigue, bradycardia, hypertension	Asthma, cardiac arrhythmias, depression, diabetes
Phenytoin	3–5 mg/kg/24 hr; adjust to maintain serum levels at 40–80 μmol/L	Hirsutism, gingival hyperplasia, ataxia, skin reaction, rarely hepatotoxicity	
Phenobarbital	2–5 mg/kg/24 hr; do not exceed serum level of 130 μmol/L	Hyperactivity, short attention span in 20% of children	Probable side effects in hyperactive or developmentally delayed child
Amitriptyline	Not approved for children; adolescents: 25–50 mg/24 hr	Dizziness, fatigue, urinary retention, constipation, weight gain, dry mouth	
Cyproheptadine	Children: 0.2–0.4 mg/kg/24 hr in 2–3 divided doses; adolescents: 4–10 mg/24 hr	Impaired learning, drowsiness, increased appetite, and weight gain	
Methysergide	Not recommended for children under 10 yr old; adolescents: 2 mg/bid or tid after meals. Do not use longer than 3 mo	Nausea, dizziness, drowsiness, retroperitoneal fibrosis with prolonged use	Restricted to patients with severe headache when other drug regimens have failed

The *treatment* of psychogenic headaches begins with reassurance and an explanation with regard to how stress may cause a headache. Anxiety and stress may unconsciously produce constant isometric contraction of the temporalis, masseter, or trapezius muscles, which leads to the characteristic dull, aching headache. Steps should be introduced to remove obvious anxiety-provoking situations. Acetaminophen and other mild analgesics are often all that is required to treat a psychogenic headache. Sedatives and antidepressants are rarely necessary. Children with severe psychogenic headaches may benefit from a brief hospitalization, particularly if an underlying depressive illness is under consideration. In the hospital setting, the child's interaction with other patients, nursing and medical staff, and family is observed while a plan is formulated for counseling or psychiatric intervention. In most cases, the child's headaches are considerably relieved during the period of observation. As with migraine headaches, biofeedback and self-hypnosis exercises are effective in the management of some patients with psychogenic headaches.

Barlow CF: Headaches and Migraine in Childhood. Philadelphia, JB Lippincott, 1984.
Billie B: Migraine in school children. Acta Paediatr Scand (Suppl 136) 51:1, 1962.
Carroll L: Alice's Adventures in Wonderland and Through the Looking Glass. New York, New American Library, 1960.
Forsythe WI, Gillies D, Sills MA: Propranolol in the treatment of childhood migraine. Dev Med Child Neurol 26:737, 1984.
Gascon G, Barlow C: Juvenile migraine, presenting as an acute confusional state. Pediatrics 45:628, 1970.
Glueck CJ, Bates SR: Migraine in children: Association with primary and familial dyslipoproteinemias. Pediatrics 77:316, 1986.
Ling W, Oftedal G, Weinberg W: Depressive illness in childhood presenting as severe headache. Am J Dis Child 120:122, 1970.
Olness H, MacDonald JT, Uden DL: Comparison of self-hypnosis and propranolol in the treatment of juvenile classic migraine. Pediatrics 79:593, 1987.
Presnky AL, Sommer D: Diagnosis and treatment of migraine in children. Neurology 29:506, 1979.
Verret S, Steel JC: Alternating hemiplegia of childhood: A report of eight patients with complicated migraine beginning in infancy. Pediatrics 47:675, 1971.

NEUROCUTANEOUS SYNDROMES

The neurocutaneous syndromes include a heterogeneous group of disorders characterized by abnormalities of both the integument and CNS. Although the etiology is unknown, most disorders are familial and believed to arise from a defect in the differentiation of the primitive ectoderm. Disorders classified as neurocutaneous syndromes include neurofibromatosis, tuberous sclerosis, Sturge-Weber disease, von Hippel-Lindau disease, ataxia telangiectasia (discussed in section on Movement Disorders), linear nevus syndrome, and incontinentia pigmenti.

20.39 NEUROFIBROMATOSIS

Neurofibromatosis (NF) (von Recklinghausen disease) is a common autosomal dominant disorder affecting approximately 1 in 4000 of the population. The condition is protean, as virtually every system and organ may be affected, and progressive in that distinctive features may be present at birth but the development of complications is delayed for decades. Neurofibromatosis is the consequence of an abnormality of neural crest differentiation and migration during the early stages of embryogenesis, possibly related to the influence of nerve or glial growth factor (see also Sec. 23. 11).

CLINICAL MANIFESTATIONS AND DIAGNOSIS. There are two distinct forms of neurofibromatosis. NF-1 is the most prevalent type of neurofibromatosis and is diagnosed if any two of the following signs are present: (1) *At least five café-au-lait spots over 5 mm in greatest diameter in prepubertal patients or at least six café-au-lait spots over 15 mm in postpubertal patients.* Café-au-lait spots are the hallmark of neurofibromatosis and are present in almost 100% of patients. They are present at birth but increase in size, number, and pigmentation, especially during the first few years of life. The spots are scattered throughout the body surface with predilection for the trunk and extremities and sparing of the face. (2) *Axillary or inguinal freckling* consists of multiple hyperpigmented areas of 2–3 mm in diameter. (3) *Two or more iris Lisch nodules.* Lisch nodules are hamartomas located within the iris and are best identified with a slit lamp examination. They are present in more than 90% of patients with NF-1 but are not a component of NF-2. (4) *Two or more neurofibromas or one plexiform neurofibroma.* Neurofibromas typically involve the skin, but they may be situated along peripheral nerves, blood vessels, and within viscera including the gastrointestinal tract. The cutaneous lesions appear characteristically during adolescence or pregnancy, suggesting a hormonal influence. They are usually small, rubbery lesions with a slight purplish discoloration of the overlying skin. Plexiform neurofibromas are usually evident at birth and result from diffuse thickening of nerve trunks that are frequently located in the orbital or temporal region of the face. The skin overlying a plexiform neurofibroma may be hyperpigmented to a greater degree than a café-au-lait spot. Plexiform neurofibromas may produce overgrowth of an extremity and a deformity of the corresponding bone. (5) *A distinctive osseous lesion.* Abnormalities of the skeleton are a common feature of neurofibromatosis. Kyphoscoliosis is reported in approximately 40% of patients. Dysplasia of the sphenoid wing causes a pulsating exophthalmos, whereas bowing of the tibula and fibula are often associated with pathologic fractures that have a propensity to develop pseudoarthroses. (6) *Optic gliomas* are present in approximately 15% of patients with NF-1. These relatively benign tumors consist of glial cells and a mucinous material. Most patients with optic gliomas are asymptomatic and have normal or near-normal vision, but approximately 20% have visual disturbances or evidence of precocious sexual development secondary to tumor invasion of the hypothalamus. Children rarely are aware of unilateral visual loss, thus diagnosis may be delayed. Patients with a unilateral optic glioma typically display an afferent pupillary defect. To test for this, each eye is alternatively stimulated by a bright light source (swinging flashlight test). The affected pupil dilates rather than constricts, whereas light in the unaffected eye causes both pupils to constrict equally. Patients with NF-1 and a plexiform neuroma of the eyelid have a high association with an ipsilateral optic glioma. The CT findings of an optic glioma include diffuse thickening, localized enlargement, or a distinct focal mass originating from the optic nerve or chiasm. (7) *A first-degree relative with NF-1 whose diagnosis was based on the aforementioned criteria.* The NF-1 gene is located on chromosome 17.

Children with NF-1 are susceptible to *neurologic complications.* MRI studies in selected children have shown abnormal signals in the globus pallidus, thalamus, and internal capsule, which probably represent low-grade glioma or hamartoma that are not detected by CT scanning. These findings may account for the high incidence of learning disabilities, attention deficit disorders, and abnormalities of speech among affected children. Complex partial and generalized tonic-clonic seizures are a frequent complication. Hydrocephalus is a rare manifestation secondary to aqueductal stenosis, whereas macrocephaly with normal-sized ventricles is a common finding. The cerebral vessels may be occluded owing to the neurofibromatosis, resulting in hemiparesis and intellectual deficits. Not surprisingly, *psychologic disturbances* are prevalent owing to the seriousness and uncertainty of the disease. *Malignant neoplasms* are also a significant problem in patients with NF-1. A neurofibroma occasionally differentiates into a neurofibrosarcoma or malignant schwannoma. The incidence of pheochromocytoma, rhabdomyosarcoma, leukemia, and Wilms tumor is higher than the general population. However, tumors of the CNS (including optic gliomas, meningiomas of the brain and spinal cord, neurofibromas, astrocytomas, and neurilemmomas) account for significant morbidity and mortality because of their increased frequency in patients with NF-1.

NF-2 accounts for 10% of all cases of neurofibromatosis and may be diagnosed when one of the following is present: (1) *bilateral eighth nerve masses* consistent with acoustic neuromas as demonstrated by CT scanning or MRI. (2) A *parent, sibling, or child with NF-2* and either unilateral eighth nerve masses or any two of the following: neurofibroma, meningioma, glioma, schwannoma, or juvenile posterior subcapsular lenticular opacities. **Bilateral acoustic neuromas** are the most distinctive feature of NF-2. Symptoms of hearing loss, facial weakness, headache, or unsteadiness may appear during childhood, although signs of a cerebellopontine angle mass are more commonly present in the 2nd and 3rd decades of life. Although café-au-lait spots and skin neurofibromas are classic findings in NF-1, they are much less common in NF-2. Posterior subcapsular lens opacities are identified in approximately 50% of patients with NF-2. As with NF-1, CNS tumors including schwann-cell and glial tumors, and meningiomas are common in patients with NF-2. Linkage analysis has shown that the gene for NF-2 is located near the center of the long arm of chromosome 22.

TREATMENT. As there is no specific treatment for neurofibromatosis, the management includes genetic counseling and early detection of treatable conditions or complications. The evaluation of a child with neurofibromatosis should include several baseline studies, such as an audiogram, auditory brain stem and visual evoked potentials, an EEG, psychologic testing (including studies predictive for learning disorders), a roentgenographic skeletal survey, and CT scanning or MRI of the brain and optic nerves. The asymptomatic patient should be re-examined annually with a neurologic assessment including blood pressure, auditory and visual screening, and a thorough search for the complications of neurofibromatosis. A parent with neurofibromatosis has a 50% chance of transmitting the disease with each pregnancy. The type of neurofibromatosis (NF-1 and NF-2) "breeds true" for successive generations. Because approximately one half of all cases of neurofibromatosis result from fresh mutations, each parent should be carefully examined (including a search for Lisch nodules) before counseling for the risk of affected future pregnancies. Prenatal diagnosis is not available.

20.40 TUBEROUS SCLEROSIS

Tuberous sclerosis (TS) is inherited as an autosomal dominant trait with an estimated frequency of 1/30,000. The TS gene is located on chromosome 9, but at least one half of the cases are sporadic owing to new mutations. TS is an extremely heterogeneous disease with a wide clinical spectrum. The disease varies from severe mental retardation and incapacitating seizures to normal intelligence and a lack of seizures, often within the same family. As a rule, the younger the patient presents with symptoms and signs of TS, the greater will be the likelihood of mental retardation. The disease affects many organ systems other than the skin and brain, including the heart, kidney, eyes, lung, and bone.

PATHOLOGY. The characteristic brain lesions consist of tubers. Tubers are located in the convolutions of the cerebral hemispheres and are typically present in the subependymal region, where they undergo calcification and project into the ventricular cavity producing a "candle-dripping" appearance. Tubers in the region of the foramen of Monro may cause obstruction of CSF flow and hydrocephalus. The microscopic appearance of the tuber consists of decreased numbers of neurons and a proliferation of astrocytes and the presence of oddly shaped multinucleated giant neurons. MRI is useful for identification of the lesions. Generally, the greater the number of tubers, the more neurologically impaired will be the patient.

CLINICAL MANIFESTATIONS. TS may present during infancy with infantile spasms and a hypsarrhythmic EEG pattern. Careful examination of the skin on the trunk and extremities shows the typical hypopigmented skin lesions that have been likened to an "ash leaf" in more than 90% of cases in this age group. The visualization of the hypopigmented lesions is enhanced by the use of a Wood's ultraviolet lamp (Sec. 23.12). The CT scan typically shows calcified tubers in the periventricular area, but these may not be apparent until 3–4 yr of age. The seizures may be difficult to control, and at a later age they may develop into myoclonic epilepsy. There is a high incidence of mental retardation in young patients with TS and infantile spasms.

During childhood, TS presents most often with a generalized seizure disorder and pathognomonic skin lesions. Sebaceous adenomas develop between 4 and 6 yr of age; they appear as tiny red nodules over the nose and cheeks and are sometimes confused with acne. Later, they enlarge, coalesce, and assume a fleshy appearance. A **shagreen patch** is also characteristic of TS and consists of a roughened, raised lesion with an orange-peel consistency located primarily in the lumbosacral region. Subungual or periungual fibromas arise from the stratum lucidum of the finger and toe in many patients with TS during adolescence. Retinal lesions consist of two types: mulberry tumors that arise from the nerve head or round and flat gray-colored lesions (phakoma) in the region of the disk (Fig. 20–11). Brain tumors are much less common in TS compared with neurofibromatosis, but occasionally a tuber differentiates into a malignant astrocytoma. Approximately 50% of children with TS have rhabdomyomas of the

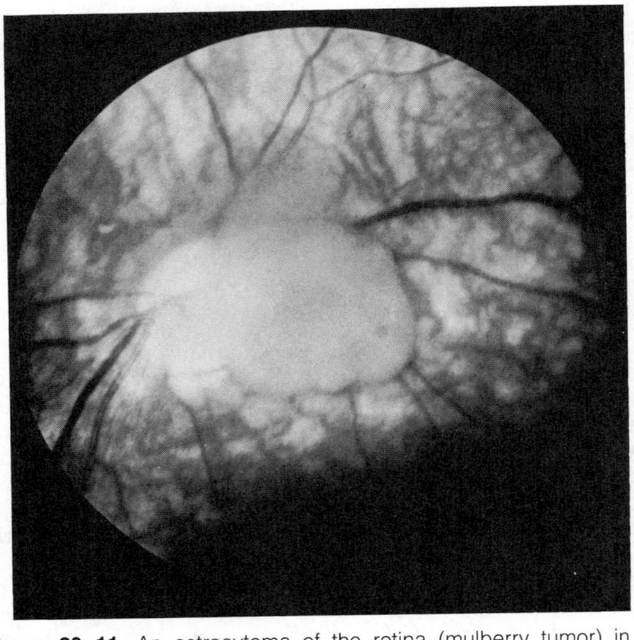

Figure 20–11. An astrocytoma of the retina (mulberry tumor) in a patient with tuberous sclerosis.

heart, which may be detected in the fetus at risk by an echocardiogram. The rhabdomyomas may be multiple or located at the apex of the left ventricle and, although they can cause congestive heart failure and arrhythmias, they tend to slowly resolve spontaneously. The kidney is involved in most patients by hamartomas or polycystic disease resulting in hematuria, pain, and, in some cases, renal failure. Angiomyolipomas may produce generalized cystic or fibrous pulmonary changes in the lung and lead to spontaneous pneumothorax.

DIAGNOSIS. The diagnosis of TS relies on a high index of suspicion when assessing a child with infantile spasms. A careful search for the typical skin and retinal lesions should be completed in all patients with a seizure disorder. The head CT scan or MRI confirms the diagnosis in most cases.

TREATMENT. The management consists of seizure control and baseline studies including renal ultrasound, an echocardiogram, and a chest roentgenogram with follow-up as indicated. Symptoms and signs of increased intracranial pressure suggest obstruction of the foramen of Monro by a tuber, or malignant transformation of a tuber, and warrant immediate investigation and surgical intervention.

20.41 STURGE-WEBER DISEASE

Sturge-Weber disease consists of a constellation of symptoms and signs including a facial nevus (port-wine stain), seizures, hemiparesis, intracranial calcifications, and in many cases, mental retardation. It occurs sporadically with a frequency of approximately 1/50,000.

ETIOLOGY. The condition is thought to result from the anomalous development of the primordial vascular bed during the early stages of cerebral vascularization. At this stage the blood supply to the brain, meninges, and face is undergoing reorganization, while the primitive ectoderm in the region differentiates into the skin of the upper face and the occipital lobe of the cerebrum. The overlying leptomeninges are richly vascularized and the brain beneath becomes atrophic and calcified, particularly in the molecular layer of the cortex, in patients with Sturge-Weber disease.

CLINICAL MANIFESTATIONS. The facial nevus is present at birth and tends to be unilateral and always involves the upper face and eyelid. The nevus may also be evident over the lower face, trunk, and in the mucosa of the mouth and pharynx. Not all children with facial nevi have Sturge-Weber disease (see Sec. 23.8). Buphthalmos and glaucoma of the ipsilateral eye are a common complication. Seizures develop in most patients during the 1st year of life. They are typically focal tonic-clonic and contralateral to the side of the facial nevus. The seizures tend to become refractory to anticonvulsants and are associated with a slowly progressive hemiparesis in many cases. Although neurodevelopment appears to be normal during the 1st year of life, mental retardation or severe learning disabilities are present in at least 50% during later childhood, probably the result of prolonged generalized seizures and increasing cerebral atrophy secondary to hypoxia and multiple anticonvulsants.

DIAGNOSIS. The skull radiograph shows intracranial calcification in the occipitoparietal region in most patients. This characteristically assumes a serpentine or "railroad-track" appearance. The CT scan highlights the extent of the calcification that is usually associated with unilateral cortical atrophy and ipsilateral dilatation of the lateral ventricle (Fig. 20–12).

TREATMENT. The management of Sturge-Weber disease is multifaceted and somewhat controversial. Seizure frequency and the significant risk for mental retardation influence the treatment plan. For patients with well-controlled seizures and normal or near-normal development, the management is straightforward and conservative. However, there is increasing evidence that a hemispherectomy or lobectomy may prevent the development of mental retardation in the patient with recalcitrant seizures, particularly if the surgery is accomplished during the 1st year of life. Because of the risk of glaucoma, regular measurements of intraocular pressure with a tenonometer is indicated. The facial nevus is often a target for ridicule by classmates, leading to psychologic trauma. Flashlamp-pulsed laser therapy holds considerable promise for clearing of the port-wine stain. Finally, because of the high frequency of developmental disabilities, special educational facilities are frequently required.

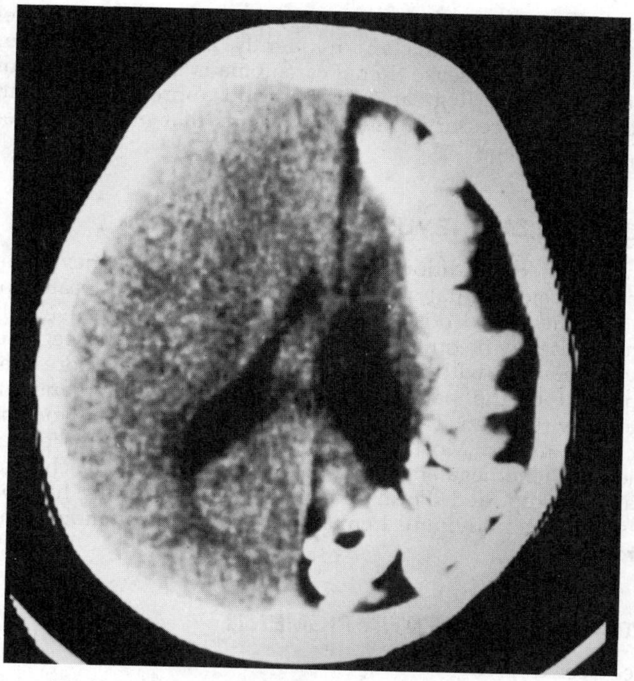

Figure 20–12. A CT scan of a patient with Sturge-Weber syndrome, showing unilateral calcification and atrophy of a cerebral hemisphere.

20.42 VON HIPPEL-LINDAU DISEASE

As with most of the neurocutaneous syndromes, von Hippel-Lindau disease affects multiple organs, including the cerebellum, spinal cord, medulla, retina, kidney, pancreas, and epididymis. Von Hippel-Lindau disease is inherited as an autosomal dominant trait with variable penetrance and delayed expression. The major neurologic features of the condition include cerebellar hemangioblastomas and retinal angiomata. Patients with cerebellar hemangioblastoma present in early adult life or beyond with symptoms and signs of increased intracranial pressure. A smaller number of patients have hemangioblastoma of the spinal cord, producing abnormalities of proprioception and disturbances of gait and bladder dysfunction. The CT scan typically shows a cystic lesion with a vascular mural nodule. Total surgical removal of the tumor is curative. Approximately 25% of patients with cerebellar hemangioblastoma have retinal angiomata.

Retinal angiomata are characterized by small masses of thin-walled capillaries that are fed by large and tortuous arterioles and venules. They are usually located in the peripheral retina so that vision is unaffected. However, exudation in the region of the angiomata may lead to retinal detachment and visual loss. Retinal angiomata are treated with photocoagulation and cryocoagulation with good results. Cystic lesions of the kidney, pancreas, liver, and epididymis as well as pheochromocytoma are frequently associated with von Hippel-Lindau disease. Renal carcinoma is the most common cause of death. Regular follow-up and appropriate imaging studies are necessary to identify lesions that may be treated at an early stage.

20.43 LINEAR NEVUS SYNDROME

This sporadic condition is characterized by a facial nevus and neurodevelopmental abnormalities. The nevus is located on the forehead and nose and tends to be midline in its distribution. It may be quite faint during infancy but later becomes hyperkeratotic with a yellow-brown appearance. More than one half of the patients have a seizure disorder and are mentally retarded. The seizures may be generalized myoclonic or focal motor. Most patients have normal CT studies, although hemimegalencephaly with hamartomatous changes has been reported. Focal neurologic signs including hemiparesis and homonymous hemianopia are more common in this group.

20.44 INCONTINENTIA PIGMENTI

See Sec. 23.11.

Alexander GL, Norman RM: The Sturge-Weber Syndrome. Bristol, John Wright, 1960.
Barker D, Wright E, Nguyen K, et al: Gene for von Recklinghausen neurofibromatosis is in the pericentromeric region of chromosome 17. Science 236:1100, 1987.
Gomez MR: Tuberous Sclerosis, 2nd ed. New York, Raven Press, 1988.
Hoffman HJ, Hendrick EB, Dennis M, et al: Hemispherectomy for Sturge-Weber syndrome. Childs Brain 5:233, 1979.
Horton WA, Wong V, Eldridge R: Von Hippel-Lindau disease: Clinical and pathological manifestations in nine families with 50 affected members. Arch Intern Med 136:769, 1976.
Hurst RW, Newman SA, Cail WS: Multifocal intracranial MR abnormalities in neurofibromatosis. AJNR 9:293, 1988.
Listernick R, Charrow J: Neurofibromatosis type 1 in childhood. J Pediatr 116:845, 1990.
Listernick R, Charrow J, Greenwald MJ, et al: Optic gliomas in children with neurofibromatosis type 1. J Pediatr 114:788, 1989.
Lovejoy FH, Boyle LE: Linear nevus sebaceous syndrome: Report of two cases and a review of the literature. Pediatrics 52:382, 1973.
Martuza RL, Eldridge R: Neurofibromatosis 2 (Bilateral acoustic neurofibromatosis). N Engl J Med 318:684, 1988.
Riccardi VM: Neurofibromatosis. Curr Probl Cancer 7:1, 1982.
Riccardi VM: Von Recklinghausen neurofibromatosis. N Engl J Med 305:1617, 1981.
Roach ES, Williams MD, Laster MD: Magnetic resonance imaging in tuberous sclerosis. Arch Neurol 44:301, 1987.
Seizinger BR, Martuza RL, Gusella JF: Loss of genes on chromosome 22 in tumorigenesis of human acoustic neuroma. Nature 322:644, 1986.
Tan OT, Sherwood K, Gilchrest BA: Treatment of children with port-wine stains using the flashlamp-pulsed tunable dye laser. N Engl J Med 320:416, 1989.

MOVEMENT DISORDERS

Abnormalities of movement in children constitute a wide range of conditions with multiple causes. The type of movement disorder assists in the localization of the pathologic process, whereas the onset, age, and degree of the abnormal motor activity and associated neurologic findings help to classify the disorder and organize the investigation. Movement disorders are rarely limited to one form such as ataxia; the examination usually demonstrates additional abnormal movements such as tremor or chorea. This section highlights the major movement disorders in children and classifies the conditions based on the predominant motor disturbance.

20.45 ATAXIAS

Congenital anomalies of the posterior fossa, including the Dandy-Walker syndrome, the Chiari malformation, and encephalocele, are prominently associated with ataxia because of their destruction or replacement of the cerebellum (see Sec. 20.2–20.14). **Agenesis of the cerebellar vermis** presents in infancy with generalized hypotonia and decreased deep tendon reflexes. Delayed motor milestones and truncal ataxia are typical. A familial variety is inherited as an autosomal recessive trait. These patients typically have abnormalities of respiration during infancy, characterized by alternating periods of hyperpnea and apnea. In addition to ataxia, mental retardation and abnormal eye movements have been described. MRI is the method of choice for investigating congenital abnormalities of the cerebellum, vermis, and related structures.

The major *infectious causes of ataxia* include cerebellar abscess, acute labyrinthitis, and acute cerebellar ataxia. **Acute cerebellar ataxia** occurs primarily in children 1–3 yr of age and is a diagnosis by exclusion. The condition often follows a viral illness, such as varicella, coxsackie, or echovirus infection by 2–3 wk and is thought to represent an autoimmune response to the viral agent affecting the cerebellum (see Sec. 12.80). The onset is sudden, and the truncal ataxia can be so severe that the child is unable to stand or sit. Vomiting may be present initially, but fever and nuchal rigidity are absent. Horizontal nystagmus is evident in approximately 50% of cases and, if the child is able to speak, dysarthria may be impressive. Examination of the CSF is typically normal at the onset of ataxia; however, a slight pleocytosis of lymphocytes (10–30 mm^3) is not unusual. Later in the course, the CSF protein undergoes a moderate elevation. The ataxia begins to improve in a few weeks but may persist for as long as 2 mo. The prognosis for complete recovery is excellent; however, a small number have long-term sequelae, including behavioral and speech disorders as well as ataxia and incoordination. **Acute labyrinthitis** may be difficult to differentiate from acute cerebellar ataxia in the toddler. The condition is associated with middle-ear infections and intense vertigo, vomiting, and abnormalities in labyrinthine function, particularly ice water caloric testing.

Toxic causes of ataxia include alcohol, thallium (which is used occasionally in the home as a pesticide), and the anticonvulsants, particularly phenytoin when serum levels reach or exceed 30 μg/mL (120 μmol/L).

Brain tumors including tumors of the cerebellum and frontal lobe as well as neuroblastoma may present with ataxia. Frontal lobe tumors may cause ataxia owing to the destruction of the association fibers connecting the frontal lobe with the cerebellum. Neuroblastoma may be associated with an encephalopathy characterized by progressive ataxia, myoclonic jerks, and opsoclonus (nonrhythmic horizontal and vertical oscillations of the eyes).

Several *metabolic disorders* are characterized by ataxia, including abetalipoproteinemia, arginosuccinic aciduria, and Hartnup disease. **Abetalipoproteinemia** (Bassen-Kornzweig disease) begins in childhood with steatorrhea and failure to thrive (Sec. 8.34). A blood smear shows acanthocytosis and decreased serum levels of cholesterol and triglycerides, and the serum β-lipoproteins are absent. Neurologic signs become evident by late childhood and consist of ataxia, retinitis pigmentosa, peripheral neuritis, abnormalities in position and vibration sense, muscle weakness, and mental retardation.

Degenerative diseases of the CNS represent an important group of ataxic disorders of childhood because of the genetic consequences and poor prognosis. **Ataxia telangiectasia,** an autosomal recessive condition, is the most common of the degenerative ataxias and is heralded by ataxia beginning at about 2 yr of age and progressing to loss of ambulation by adolescence (Sec. 11.19). Oculomotor apraxia, defined as having difficulty fixating smoothly on an object and therefore overshooting the target with lateral movement of the head followed by "re-fixating" the eyes, is a frequent finding, as is horizontal nystagmus. The telangiectasia becomes evident by mid-childhood and is found on the bulbar conjunctiva, over the bridge of the nose, and on the ears and exposed surfaces of the extremities. Examination of the skin shows a loss of elasticity. Abnormalities of immunologic function that lead to frequent sinopulmonary infections include decreased serum and secretory IgA as well as diminished IgG_2, IgG_4, and IgE levels in more than 50% of patients. Children with ataxia telangiectasia have a 50- to 100-fold greater chance of developing lymphoreticular tumors (lymphoma, leukemia, and Hodgkin disease) as well as brain tumors, compared with the normal population. Additional laboratory abnormalities include an increased incidence of chromosome breaks, particularly of chromosome 14, and elevated levels of α-fetoprotein. Death results from infection or tumor dissemination.

Friedreich ataxia is inherited as an autosomal recessive or dominant trait. The onset of ataxia is somewhat later than in ataxia telangiectasia but occurs usually prior to 10 yr of age. The ataxia is slowly progressive and involves the lower extremities to a greater degree than the upper extremities. The Romberg test is positive; the deep tendon reflexes are absent (particularly the Achilles); and the plantar response is extensor. Patients develop a characteristic explosive, dysarthric speech, and nystagmus is present in most children. Although the patient may appear apathetic, the intelligence is preserved. There may be significant weakness of the distal musculature of the hands and feet. Typically, there is a marked loss of vibration and position sense owing to degeneration of the posterior columns and indistinct sensory changes in the distal extremities. Friedreich ataxia is also characterized by skeletal abnormalities, including high-arched feet (pes cavus) and hammer toes as well as progressive kyphoscoliosis. Electrophysiologic studies including visual, auditory brain stem, and somatosensory evoked potentials are often abnormal. Hypertrophic cardiomyopathy with progression to intractable congestive heart failure is the cause of death for most patients. Several forms of *spinocerebellar ataxia* are similar to Friedreich ataxia. **Roussy-Levy disease** has, in addition, atrophy of the muscles of the lower extremity and the **Ramsay Hunt syndrome,** myoclonic epilepsy.

The **olivopontocerebellar atrophies** (OPCA) include at least five subtypes and usually have the onset of ataxia, cranial nerve palsies, and abnormal sensory findings in the 2nd or 3rd decade. However, some cases have been described in children, particularly of Finnish ancestry, with rapidly progressive ataxia, nystagmus, dysarthria, and seizures.

Rare forms of progressive cerebellar ataxia have been described in association with **vitamin E deficiency.** Additional degenerative ataxias include **Pelizaeus-Merzbacher disease,** neuronal ceroid lipofuscinoses, and late onset GM_2 gangliosidosis (see Sec. 20.59–20.60).

20.46 CHOREA

Sydenham chorea is the most common acquired chorea of childhood and is the sole neurologic manifestation of rheumatic fever (Sec. 11.74). With the resurgence of rheumatic fever during the last few years, it is likely that greater numbers of children with Sydenham chorea will be identified. The three major features of Sydenham chorea include chorea, hypotonia, and emotional lability. The chorea is usually symmetric, although children may have the choreic movements limited to one side of the body. The movements, which are rapid and jerky, are prominent in the face, trunk, and distal extremities and dart from one muscle group to another, are increased by stress, and disappear during sleep. The onset may be abrupt, but typically the chorea has a slowly progressive course. Hypotonia may be a prominent sign and when combined with severe chorea the child may be incapable of feeding, dressing, or walking. The speech is often involved and is sometimes unintelligible. Periods of uncontrollable crying and extreme mood swings are characteristic, perhaps in part as the result of the motor handicap and feeling of helplessness. Several typical signs are associated with Sydenham chorea, including the "milkmaid's grip" (relaxing and tightening hand shake), the "choreic hand" (spooning of the extended hand by flexion at the wrist and extension of the fingers), "the darting tongue" (the tongue cannot be protruded for longer than a few seconds), and the "pronator sign" (the arms and palms turn outward when held above the head). Sydenham chorea may persist for several months and as long as 1–2 yr. Cases with minimal signs are treated conservatively with avoidance of stress as much as possible. Incapacitating chorea is managed with a trial of diazepam followed by phenothiazines or haloperidol if the former is unsuccessful. Although the phenothiazines and haloperidol are effective drugs in the treatment of Sydenham chorea, long-term use may be complicated by the development of another movement disorder, **tardive dyskinesia.** As patients with Sydenham chorea are at risk for the development of rheumatic carditis, particularly mitral stenosis, a regimen of daily penicillin prophylaxis should be instituted and maintained until adulthood. A much rarer cause of chorea during childhood, *familial paroxysmal choreoathetosis* is discussed in Sec. 20.28.

Huntington disease is a progressive degenerative disorder of the CNS of unknown etiology, inherited as an autosomal dominant trait. The gene is located on the tip of the long arm of chromosome 4. The onset of symptoms of progressive chorea and presenile dementia occurs most typically between 35 and 55 yr of age. The disease is rare in the pediatric population; less than 1% of cases have the onset of symptoms prior to 10 yr of age. Rigidity and dystonia are the most common neurologic findings in the childhood patient. Chorea tends to involve proximal muscles, and the abnormal movements are often incorporated into semipurposeful acts in an attempt to mask the abnormality. Mental deterioration and behavioral problems are prominent in children. Generalized tonic-clonic seizures are common and are typically resistant to anticonvulsants. Cerebellar signs are present in 50%, and oculomotor apraxia occurs in approximately 20% of the cases. The course of the disease is more rapid in children, with an average duration of 8 yr until death compared with 14 yr in the adult. CT scanning, although nondiagnostic, shows the mean bifrontal to bicaudate ratio is decreased, indicating atrophy of the caudate nucleus and putamen. There is no specific therapy for Huntington disease, but once the diagnosis is confirmed, the pediatrician should provide genetic counseling to the family so that risks for additional cases in future generations are understood and the opportunity for molecular diagnosis is advanced.

20.47 DYSTONIAS

Dystonia is a slow, intermittent twisting motion that produces exaggerated turning and posture of the extremities and trunk. The principal causes of dystonia include perinatal asphyxia (see Sec. 9.10 and 9.28), dystonia musculorum deformans, drugs, Wilson disease (hepatolenticular degeneration), and Hallervorden-Spatz disease.

Dystonia musculorum deformans (DMD) is a slowly progressive disorder that typically begins during childhood. The etiology is unknown, but an abnormality of catecholamine metabolism within the CNS has been proposed. There are at least two varieties of DMD, an autosomal dominant and an autosomal recessive form, the latter being more common among Ashkenazi Jews. The initial manifestation of the disease during childhood is often unilateral posturing of the lower extremity, particularly the foot, which assumes an extended and rotated position causing tip-toe walking. Because the dystonic movement is initially intermittent and is aggravated by stress, patients are often labeled as hysterical. Ultimately, all four extremities and the axial musculature are affected as well as the muscles of the face and tongue so that speech and swallowing become impaired. Patients with generalized dystonia including those with involvement of the muscles of swallowing may respond to large doses of trihexphenidyl (artane). The initial dose is 2 mg/24 hr and the drug is slowly increased to 60–80 mg/24 hr or until untoward side effects (urinary retention, mental confusion, or blurred vision) occur. Additional drugs that have been effective include carbamazepine, levodopa, bromocriptine, and diazepam. Segmental dystonia, including writer's cramp, blepharospasm, and buccomandibular dystonia, are more common in the adult and tend to be limited to a specific group of muscles. Adults with segmental dystonia, particularly blepharospasm, may respond to local injections of botulism toxin, which holds promise for some children with generalized DMD. Cryothalamectomy with the placement of a lesion in the ventrolateral thalamus is reserved primarily for patients with extremity involvement.

Certain *drugs* are capable of producing an acute dystonic reaction in children. Therapeutic doses of phenytoin or carbamazepine may rarely cause progressive dystonia in children with epilepsy, particularly in those who have an underlying structural abnormality of the brain. Children may have an idiosyncratic reaction to the phenothiazines, characterized by acute dystonic posturing that is sometimes confused with encephalitis. IV diphenhydramine, 1–2 mg/kg/dose, may rapidly reverse the drug-related dystonia.

Wilson disease is a rare autosomal recessive inborn error of copper metabolism characterized by cirrhosis of the liver and degenerative changes in the CNS, particularly the basal ganglia (see Sec. 13.88). The gene for Wilson disease is located on chromosome 13 close to esterase D and the retinoblastoma locus. The precise etiology is unknown, but the basic mechanism relates to decreased excretion of biliary copper, owing partly to a lysosomal defect of the liver cells. The initial symptoms and signs in children under the age of 10 yr relate to acute or subacute hepatic failure that is frequently misinterpreted as infectious hepatitis. The neurologic manifestations of Wilson disease rarely appear before 10 yr of age, and the initial sign is often progressive dystonia. Tremors of the extremities develop, unilaterally at first, but eventually they become coarse, generalized, and incapacitating (the so-called "wing-beating" tremor). Signs of progressive basal ganglia destruction include drooling, a "fixed smile" owing to retraction of the upper lip, dysarthria, dysphonia, rigidity, contractures, dystonia, and choreoathetosis. The Kayser-Fleischer ring, which is best seen with the slit lamp, is pathognomonic and results from deposition of copper in Descemet membrane. In the untreated state, the patient typically becomes bedridden and demented and dies in coma within a few years from the onset of the disease. The MRI or CT scan shows ventricular dilatation in advanced cases with atrophy of the cerebrum and lesions in the thalamus and basal ganglia (Fig. 20–13). The treatment of Wilson disease is discussed in Sec. 13.88.

Hallervorden-Spatz disease is a rare degenerative disorder inherited as an autosomal recessive trait. The condition begins usually during childhood and is characterized by progressive dystonia, rigidity, and choreoathetosis. Spasticity, extensor plantar responses, dysarthria, and intellectual deterioration become evident during adolescence, and death usually occurs by early adulthood. The CT scan shows lesions of the globus pallidus, and neuropathologic examination indicates an excessive accumulation of iron-containing pigments in the globus pallidus and substantia nigra.

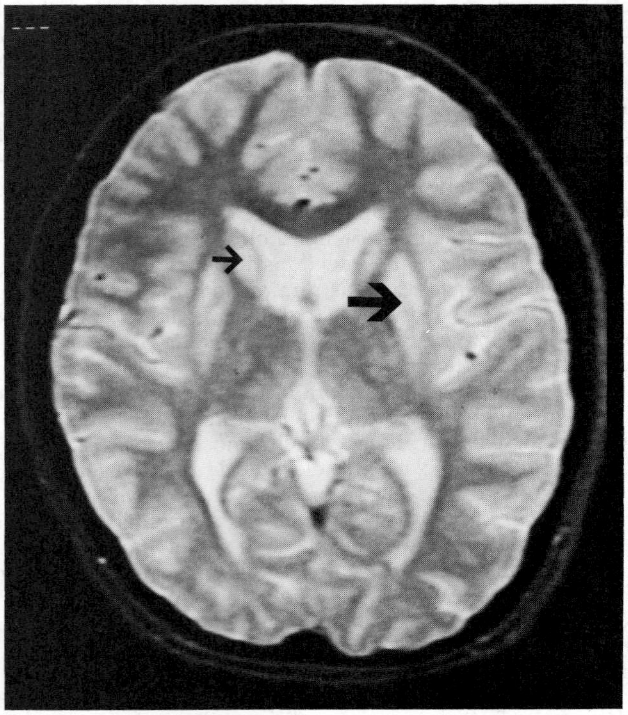

Figure 20–13. Wilson disease. MRI, T_2 image showing increased density of the caudate *(small arrow)* and the putamen *(large arrow)*.

Athetosis is most commonly associated with *perinatal brain insults* and is occasionally the major movement disorder of *phenothiazine toxicity*. Rigidity is associated with progressive destructive or neurodegenerative conditions, including Krabbe disease.

20.48 TICS

Tics are spasmodic, repetitive, stereotyped movements that are nonrhythmic and are often exacerbated by stress. Tics can be classified into three groups: transient tics of childhood, chronic tics, and Gilles de la Tourette syndrome. The *transient tic disorder* is the most common movement abnormality of childhood (see Sec. 3.31). The tics are more prevalent in boys, and there is often a positive family history. They consist of eyeblinking or facial movements and occasional throat-clearing noises. The disorder persists from weeks to less than 1 yr and does not require drug therapy. The *chronic motor tic disorder* occurs in children and adults beyond the age of 40 yr. The tics characteristically involve up to three muscle groups simultaneously and may occur throughout life. There is no clear-cut family history or sex prevalence.

Gilles de la Tourette syndrome is a lifelong condition that has its onset between 2 and 15 yr of age and is associated with numerous fluctuating tics of the face, eyes, neck, and shoulders. Ultimately the tics are accompanied by vocalizations, including throat clearing, sniffling, coughing, barking, coprolalia (obscene words), echolalia (repetition of words addressed to the patient), palilalia (repetition of one's own words), and

TABLE 20–8. Classification of Cerebral Palsy*

Physiologic	Topographic	Etiologic	Functional
Spastic	Monoplegia	Prenatal (e.g., infection, metabolic, anoxia, toxic, genetic)	Class I—no limitation of activity
Athetoid	Paraplegia		
Rigid	Hemiplegia		Class II—slight to moderate limitation
Ataxic	Triplegia		
Tremor	Quadriplegia	Perinatal (e.g., anoxia)	Class III—moderate to great limitation
Atonic	Diplegia		
Mixed	Double hemiplegia	Postnatal (e.g., toxins, trauma, infection)	Class IV—no useful physical activity
Unclassified			

*Adapted from Minear WL: A classification of cerebral palsy. Pediatrics 18:841, 1956.

echokinesis (imitation of movement of others). The vocalizations are uncontrollable and frequently jeopardize the patient's social interaction with other children. Compulsive behavior including touching, licking, repetitive thoughts and motor actions, and a greater than 50% incidence of attention deficit disorder are common to Gilles de la Tourette syndrome. Medication should be considered when the tics or vocalizations interfere significantly with the child's social and academic interactions, although behavior management and biofeedback programs have been successful for some patients. Haloperidol, a dopamine-blocking agent, is effective in the management of approximately 50% of children. The initial dose is 0.25 mg/24 hr, and the drug is increased weekly by 0.25 mg to the usual dose range of 2–6 mg/24 hr, although some children can tolerate larger doses. Side effects include cognitive impairment, lethargy, fatigue, depression, restlessness, extrapyramidal movements, and tardive dyskinesia. Additional drugs that may prove useful include penfluridol, pimozide, and clonidine. Because Gilles de la Tourette syndrome is a chronic disorder associated with multiple social, behavioral, and learning problems, the pediatrician can play an important role in the multidisciplinary management as an advocate for the child.

Aron AM, Freeman JM, Carter S: The natural history of Sydenham's chorea. Am J Med 38:83, 1965.
Boder E, Sedgwick RP: Ataxia-telangiectasia: A familial syndrome of progressive cerebellar ataxia, oculocutaneous telangiectasia and frequent pulmonary infection. Pediatrics 21:526, 1958.
Bray PF: Coincidence of neuroblastoma and acute cerebellar encephalopathy. J Pediatr 75:983, 1969.
Eldridge R: The torsion dystonia: Literature review and genetic and clinical studies. Neurology 20:1, 1970.
Fahn S: High dose anticholinergic therapy in dystonia. Neurology 33:1255, 1983.
Golden GS: Tics and Tourette's: A continuum of symptoms? Ann Neurol 4:145, 1978.
Hansotia P, Cleeland CS, Chun RWM: Juvenile Huntington's chorea. Neurology 18:217, 1968.
Harding AE: Friedreich's ataxia: A clinical and genetic study of 90 families with an analysis of early diagnostic criteria and intrafamilial clustering of clinical features. Brain 104:589, 1981.
Joubert M, Eisenring JJ, Robb JP, et al: Familial agenesis of the cerebellar vermis. Neurology 19:813, 1969.
Konigsmark BW, Weiner LP: The olivopontocerebellar atrophies: A review. Medicine 49:227, 1970.
Myers RH: Factors related to onset age of Huntington's disease. Am J Hum Genet 34:481, 1982.
Shapiro AK, Shapiro E, Wayne H, et al: Gilles de la Tourette Syndrome. New York, Raven Press, 1978.
Singer HS: Dopaminergic dysfunction in Tourette syndrome. Ann Neurol 12:361, 1982.
Vakili S: Hallervorden-Spatz syndrome. Arch Neurol 34:729, 1977.
Van Caillie-Bertrand M, Degenhart HJ, Visso HKA, et al: Oral zinc sulphate for Wilson's disease. Arch Dis Child 60:656, 1985.
Walshe JM: Wilson's disease: The presenting symptoms. Arch Dis Child 37:253, 1962.
Weiss S, Carter S: Course and prognosis of acute cerebellar ataxia in children. Neurology 9:711, 1959.

ENCEPHALOPATHIES

Encephalopathy is a term used to describe a generalized disorder of cerebral function which may be acute or chronic, progressive or static. The etiology of the encephalopathies in children includes infectious, toxic, metabolic, and ischemic causes. Hypoxic-ischemic encephalopathy is discussed in Sec. 9.28.

20.49 CEREBRAL PALSY

See also Sec. 3.56–3.58.

Cerebral palsy (CP) is a static encephalopathy that may be defined as a nonprogressive disorder of posture and movement, often associated with epilepsy and abnormalities of speech, vision, and intellect resulting from a defect or lesion of the developing brain. CP is a common disorder with an estimated prevalence of 2/1,000 population. The condition was first described almost 150 yr ago by Little, an orthopedic surgeon. He suggested that the primary causes included birth trauma and asphyxia as well as prematurity and that improved obstetrical care would significantly reduce the incidence of CP. During the last 2–3 decades, there have been considerable advances in obstetric and neonatal care, but, unfortunately, there has been virtually no change in the incidence of CP.

EPIDEMIOLOGY AND ETIOLOGY. The Collaborative Perinatal Project, in which approximately 45,000 children were regularly followed from pregnancy to the age of 7 yr, reported the prevalence rate of CP to be 4/1,000 live births. Birth asphyxia was an uncommon cause of CP; moreover, most high-risk pregnancies resulted in neurologically normal children. Although a cause for CP could not be identified in most cases, a substantial number of children with CP had congenital anomalies external to the CNS, which may have placed them at increased risk for developing asphyxia during the perinatal period. An Australian study comparing children with spastic CP with a group of matched controls had similar findings. Less than 10% of children with CP had evidence of intrapartum asphyxia. Although the increased survival of premature infants resulted in more children with CP, the rate did not increase (see Sec. 9.15–9.17). These studies suggest that future developments aimed at enhancing perinatal care will have minimal impact on the incidence of CP and that research might be directed more profitably to the field of developmental biology in order to understand the pathogenesis of CP.

CLINICAL MANIFESTATIONS. CP may be classified by a description of the motor handicap in terms of physiologic, topographic, and etiologic categories and functional capacity (Table 20–8). The physiologic classification identifies the major motor abnormality, whereas the topographic taxonomy indicates the involved extremities. CP is also commonly associated with a spectrum of developmental disabilities, including mental retardation, epilepsy, and visual, hearing, speech, cognitive, and behavioral abnormalities. The motor handicap may be the least of the child's problems.

Infants with *spastic hemiplegia* have decreased spontaneous movements on the affected side and show hand preference at a very early age. The arm is often more involved than the leg, and difficulty in hand manipulation is obvious by 1 yr of age. Walking is usually delayed until 18–24 mo, and a circumductive gait is apparent. Examination of the extremities may show growth arrest particularly in the hand and thumbnail, especially if the contralateral parietal lobe is abnormal, because extremity growth is influenced by this area of the brain. Spasticity is apparent in the affected extremities, particularly the ankle, causing an equinovarus deformity of the foot. The child often walks on tiptoes because of the increased tone, and the affected upper extremity assumes a dystonic posture when the child runs. Ankle clonus and a Babinski sign may be present; the deep tendon reflexes are increased; and weakness of the hand and foot dorsiflexors is evident. About one third of patients with spastic hemiplegia have a seizure disorder that usually develops during the first year or two, and approximately 25% have cognitive abnormalities including mental retardation. A CT scan characteristically shows an atrophic cerebral hemisphere with a dilated lateral ventricle contralateral to the side of the affected extremities.

Spastic diplegia refers to bilateral spasticity of the legs. The first indication of spastic diplegia is often noted when the infant begins to crawl. The child uses the arms in a normal reciprocal fashion but tends to drag the legs behind more as a rudder rather than using the normal four-stance crawling movement. If the spasticity is severe, the application of a diaper is difficult owing to excessive adduction of the hips. Examination of the child reveals spasticity in the legs with brisk reflexes, ankle clonus, and a bilateral Babinski sign. When suspended by the axillae, a scissoring posture of the lower extremities is maintained. Walking is significantly delayed; the feet are held in a position of equinovarus; and the child walks on tiptoes. Severe spastic diplegia is characterized by disuse atrophy and impaired growth of the lower extremities and by disproportionate growth with normal development of the upper torso. The prognosis for normal intellectual development is excellent for these patients, and the likelihood of seizures is minimal. The most common neuropathologic finding is periventricular leukomalacia, particularly in the area where fibers innervating the legs course through the internal capsule.

Spastic quadriplegia is the most severe form of CP because of marked motor impairment of all extremities and the high association with mental retardation and seizures. Swallowing difficulties are common owing to supranuclear bulbar palsies and often lead to aspiration pneumonia. At autopsy, the central white matter is disrupted by areas of necrotic degeneration that may coalesce into cystic cavities. Neurologic examination shows increased tone and spasticity in all extremities, decreased spontaneous movements, brisk reflexes, and plantar extensor responses. Flexion contractures of the knees and elbows are often present by late childhood. Associated developmental disabilities, including speech and visual abnormalities, are particularly prevalent in this group of children. Children with spastic quadriparesis often have evidence of athetosis and may be classified as mixed CP.

Athetoid CP is relatively rare, especially since the advent of aggressive management of hyperbilirubinemia and the prevention of kernicterus. These infants are characteristically hypotonic and have poor head control and marked head lag. Feeding may be difficult, and tongue thrust and drooling may be prominent. The athetoid movements may not become evident until 1 yr of age and tend to coincide with hypermyelination of the basal ganglia, a phenomenon called **status marmoratus.** Speech is typically affected owing to involvement of the oropharyngeal muscles. Sentences are slurred, and voice modulation is impaired. Generally, upper motor neuron signs are not present; seizures are uncommon; and intellect is preserved in most patients.

DIAGNOSIS. A thorough history and physical examination should eliminate a progressive disorder of the CNS, including degenerative diseases, spinal cord tumor, or muscular dystrophy. Depending on the severity and the nature of the neurologic abnormalities, a baseline EEG and CT scan may be indicated to determine the location and extent of structural lesions or associated congenital malformations. Additional studies may include tests of hearing and visual function. As CP is usually associated with a wide spectrum of developmental disorders, a multidisciplinary approach is most helpful in the assessment and management of such children.

TREATMENT. A team of physicians from various specialties as well as the occupational and physical therapists, speech pathologist, social worker, educator, and developmental psychologist provide important contributions to the management of the child. Parents should be taught how to handle their child in daily activities such as feeding, carrying, dressing, bathing, and playing in ways that will limit the effects of abnormal muscle tone. They also need to be instructed in the supervision of a series of exercises designed to prevent the development of contractures, especially a tight Achilles tendon. There is no proof that physical or occupational therapy will prevent the development of CP in the infant at risk or that it will correct the neurologic deficit, but there is ample evidence that therapy optimizes the development of the abnormal child. The child with spastic diplegia is treated initially with the assistance of adaptive equipment, such as walkers, poles, and standing frames. If the patient has marked spasticity of the lower extremities or if there is evidence of hip dislocation, consideration should be given to performing surgical soft-tissue procedures that reduce muscle spasm around the hip girdle, including an adductor tenotomy or psoas transfer and release. A rhizotomy procedure where the roots of the spinal nerves are divided has produced considerable improvement in selected patients with severe spastic diplegia. A tight heel cord in a child with spastic hemiplegia may be treated surgically by tenotomy of the Achilles tendon. The quadriplegic patient is managed with motorized wheelchairs, special feeding devices, modified typewriters, and customized seating arrangements. Communication skills may be enhanced by the use of Bliss symbols, talking typewriters, and specially adapted computers including artificial intelligence computers to augment motor and language function. Significant behavior problems may substantially interfere with the development of a child with CP; their early identification and management is important, and the assistance of the psychologist or psychiatrist may be necessary. Learning and attention deficit disorders and mental retardation are assessed and managed by a psychologist and educator. Strabismus, nystagmus, and optic atrophy are common in children with CP, thus an ophthalmologist should be included in the initial assessment. Several drugs have been utilized to treat spasticity, including dantrolene sodium, the benzodiazepines, and baclofen. These medications are generally ineffective but should be considered if severe spasticity is not controlled by other measures. Occasionally, patients with incapacitating athetosis will respond to levodopa, and children with dystonia may benefit from carbamazepine or trihexyphenidyl.

20.50 ACQUIRED IMMUNODEFICIENCY SYNDROME (AIDS) ENCEPHALOPATHY

Encephalopathy is an unfortunate and common manifestation of infants and children with human immunodeficiency virus

(HIV) infection (see Sec. 12.82). Neurologic signs in the congenitally infected patient may appear during early infancy or may be delayed to as late as 5 yr of age. The encephalopathy may have an acute onset with a relentless progressive course, but in some cases the process is either static or is characterized by insidious deterioration. The primary features of AIDS encephalopathy include an arrest in brain growth, evidence of developmental delay, and the evolution of neurologic signs.

20.51 MITOCHONDRIAL ENCEPHALOMYOPATHIES

At least three associated disorders are characterized by cerebral disease and mitochondrial myopathy and are included in this section devoted to the encephalopathies. Leigh disease and Reye syndrome are discussed here because they result from disorders of mitochrondrial function, and Zellweger syndrome is included as an abnormality of peroxisomal function. Further discussion may be found in Sec. 8.16, 13.96, and 21.25.

MITOCHONDRIAL MYOPATHY, ENCEPHALOPATHY, LACTIC ACIDOSIS, AND STROKE (MELAS). Patients with MELAS are normal for the first several years, but gradually they display delayed motor and cognitive developmental milestones. These children develop short stature and either a focal or generalized seizure disorder. Ultimately, the patient presents with an acute hemiparesis that can alternate from side to side. CT studies show basal ganglia calcification in some patients and lucent areas that do not correspond to specific cerebral vessels. Serum lactate levels during an acute episode are elevated. Muscle biopsies typically show ragged-red fibers, suggesting an abnormality of the electron transport system. MELAS is a progressive disorder that has been reported in siblings. It is punctuated with episodes of hemiparesis, hemianopia, cortical blindness, and dementia. The location of the lucent lesions noted on the CT scan is compatible with the acute neurologic deficit. Post mortem studies have demonstrated focal encephalomalacia and cortical microcystic liquefaction. There is no therapy for the prevention of the neurologic complications of MELAS disease.

MYOCLONUS EPILEPSY AND RAGGED-RED FIBERS (MERRF). Patients with MERRF are also normal during the early years of development. However, all patients ultimately develop myoclonic epilepsy and progressive ataxia associated with dysarthria and nystagmus, and a few have optic atrophy. Because some patients have abnormalities of deep sensation and pes cavus, the condition may be confused with Friedreich ataxia. Intellectual deterioration is slowly progressive in patients with MERRF. As with MELAS, a significant number of patients have a positive family history and short stature. Pathologic findings include elevated serum lactate levels, ragged-red fibers in muscle biopsies, marked loss and degeneration of neurons in the dentate nuclei, and degeneration of the subcortical cerebellar white matter.

KEARNS-SAYRE SYNDROME. This is characterized by ophthalmoplegia, retinal degeneration, and ataxia. More than 50% of patients have short stature and a sensorineural hearing loss, but seizures and a positive family history are rare. Many patients have heart block, diabetes mellitus, and significantly elevated CSF protein. Ragged-red fibers are also found in the muscle biopsies of patients with the Kearns-Sayre syndrome.

Studies of the muscle mitochondrial electron transport system in most cases of MELAS, MERRF, and Kearns-Sayre syndrome show reduced activities of complex I (NADH-CoQ reductase) and/or complex IV (cytochrome oxidase). There is good evidence that the mitochondria proliferating in ragged-red fibers are abnormal because of a defect in mitochondrial DNA. The fact that the mitochondrial DNA defect is heteroplasmic in each of these diseases means that the deleterious effect of the mutation on the assembly of electron transport complexes is manifest only in tissues where these abnormal mitochondria are proliferating, muscle and brain. Early development is normal presumably because there are few abnormal mitochondria in infancy.

LEIGH DISEASE (SUBACUTE NECROTIZING ENCEPHALOMYELOPATHY). There are at least three known genetically determined causes of Leigh disease: deficiency of the pyruvate dehydrogenase complex, deficiency of complex I, and deficiency of complex IV of the respiratory chain (see also Sec. 8.39). Unlike the defects present in the MELAS, MERRF, and Kearns-Sayre group of patients that are either sporadic or have strong elements of maternal inheritance, these defects are autosomally recessively inherited. Most patients present during infancy with feeding and swallowing problems, vomiting, and failure to thrive. Delayed motor and language milestones may be evident, and generalized seizures, weakness, hypotonia, ataxia, and nystagmus are prominent findings. Intermittent respirations with associated sighing or sobbing is characteristic and suggests brain stem dysfunction. Some patients have external ophthalmoplegia and decreased visual acuity. The primary pathologic changes are confined to the basal ganglia, tegmental gray matter, and periventricular and periaqueductal regions and consist of scattered foci of necrosis and capillary proliferation not unlike the lesions found in Wernicke encephalopathy. Abnormal results on CT scans consisting of bilaterally symmetric areas of low attenuation in the basal ganglia have been described in some patients. Elevated serum lactate levels are the hallmark of Leigh disease. Leigh disease has been treated with thiamine that may be associated with temporary improvement in some cases. Most children die within 6 mo of the onset of symptoms, but a few patients experience prolonged periods of remission.

REYE SYNDROME. This encephalopathy is associated with fatty degeneration of the viscera and a disorder of mitochondrial function (see Sec. 13.96).

ZELLWEGER SYNDROME (CEREBROHEPATORENAL SYNDROME [CHRS]). This rare, lethal disorder is inherited as an autosomal recessive trait. It represents the prototype of a group of peroxisomal disorders that have overlapping symptoms, signs, and biochemical abnormalities (see Sec. 8.16). Infants with Zellweger syndrome have dysmorphic facies consisting of frontal bossing and a large anterior fontanel. The occiput is flattened, and the external ears are abnormal. A high-arched palate, excessive skin folds of the neck, severe hypotonia, and areflexia are usually evident. Examination of the eyes reveals searching nystagmoid movements, bilateral cataracts, and optic atrophy. Generalized seizures become evident early in life, associated with severe global developmental delay and a significant bilateral hearing loss. Hepatomegaly is a prominent finding shortly after birth, often associated with a history of prolonged neonatal jaundice. Patients with Zellweger syndrome rarely survive beyond 1 yr of age.

LEAD ENCEPHALOPATHY

See Sec. 26.16.

20.52 BURN ENCEPHALOPATHY

An encephalopathy develops in approximately 5% of children with significant burns during the first several weeks of hospitalization (see also Sec. 6.37). There is no single cause of burn encephalopathy but rather a combination of factors that include anoxia (smoke inhalation, carbon monoxide poisoning, laryngospasm), electrolyte abnormalities, bacteremia and sepsis, cortical vein thrombosis, a concomitant head injury, cerebral edema, drug reactions, and emotional distress. Seizures are the most common clinical manifestation of burn encephalopathy, but altered states of consciousness, hallucinations, and coma may also occur. The management of burn encephalopathy is directed to a search for the underlying cause and treatment of hypoxemia, seizures, specific electrolyte abnormalities, or cerebral edema. The prognosis for complete neurologic recovery is generally excellent, particularly if seizures are the primary abnormality.

20.53 HYPERTENSIVE ENCEPHALOPATHY

Hypertensive encephalopathy is most commonly associated with renal disease in children including acute glomerulonephritis, chronic pyelonephritis, and end-stage renal disease (see Sec. 6.37). In some cases, hypertensive encephalopathy is the initial manifestation of underlying renal disease. Marked systemic hypertension produces vasoconstriction of the cerebral vessels, which leads to vascular permeability causing areas of focal cerebral edema and hemorrhage. The onset may be acute with seizures and coma or more indolent with headache, drowsiness and lethargy, nausea and vomiting, blurred vision, transient cortical blindness, and hemiparesis. Examination of the eyegrounds may be normal in children, but papilledema and retinal hemorrhages may occur. Treatment is directed to the restoration of a normotensive state and control of seizures with appropriate anticonvulsants.

20.54 RADIATION ENCEPHALOPATHY

Although techniques for administering radiation therapy to the brain have improved considerably and the incidence of serious side effects has decreased significantly, radiation encephalopathy remains an important complication. *Acute radiation encephalopathy* is most likely to develop in young patients who have received large daily doses. The excessive radiation injures vessel endothelium, resulting in enhanced vascular permeability, cerebral edema, and multiple hemorrhages. The child may suddenly become irritable, lethargic, complain of headache, or present with focal neurologic signs and seizures. The patient occasionally develops hemiparesis due to an infarct secondary to vascular occlusion of the cerebral vessels. Steroids are often beneficial in reducing the cerebral edema and reversing the neurologic signs. *Late radiation encephalopathy* develops months to years after the completion of therapy. It is rare in children. The condition is characterized by headaches and slowly progressive focal neurologic signs, including hemiparesis and seizures. Although the cause of late radiation encephalopathy is unknown, the CT scan shows cerebral atrophy and low-density lesions. Some children with acute lymphatic leukemia who are treated with a combination of intrathecal methotrexate and cranial irradiation develop neurologic signs months or years later, consisting of increasing lethargy, loss of cognitive abilities, dementia, and focal neurologic signs and seizures (see Sec. 17.4). The CT scan shows calcifications in the white matter, and the post mortem examination demonstrates a necrotizing encephalopathy. This devastating complication of the treatment of leukemia has prompted a re-evaluation of the use of cranial radiation in the management of these children.

Belman AL, Diamond G, Dickson D, et al: Pediatric acquired immunodeficiency syndrome: Neurologic syndromes. Am J Dis Child 142:29, 1988.
Blair E, Stanley FJ: Intrapartum asphyxia: A rare cause of cerebral palsy. J Pediatr 112:515, 1988.
Fukuhara N, Tokiguchi S, Shirakawa K, et al: Myoclonus epilepsy associated with ragged-red fibres (mitochondrial abnormalities): Disease entity or a syndrome? J Neurol Sci 47:117, 1980.
Goto Y, Itami N, Kajii N, et al: Renal tubular involvement mimicking Barter syndrome in a patient with Kearns-Sayre syndrome. J Pediatr 116:904, 1990.
Karpati G, Carpenter S, Larbrisseau A, et al: The Kearns-Shy syndrome: A multisystem disease with mitochondrial abnormality demonstrated in skeletal muscle and skin. J Neurol Sci 19:133, 1973.
Levitt S: Treatment of Cerebral Palsy and Motor Delay, 2nd ed. Boston, Blackwell, 1982.
Lovejoy FH, Smith AL, Bresnan MJ, et al: Clinical staging in Reye syndrome. Am J Dis Child 128:36, 1974.
Mohnot D, Snead OC, Benton JW: Burn encephalopathy in children. Ann Neurol 12:42, 1982.
Monnens L, Heymans H: Peroxisomal disorders: Clinical characterization. J Inher Metab Dis 10 (Suppl 1):23, 1987.
Nelson KB, Ellenberg JH: Antecedents of cerebral palsy: Multivariate analysis of risk. N Engl J Med 315:81, 1986.
Pavlakis SG, Phillips PC, Di Mauro S, et al: Mitochondrial myopathy, encephalopathy, lactic acidosis, and strokelike episodes: A distinctive clinical syndrome. Ann Neurol 16:481, 1984.
Peacock WJ, Arens LT, Berman B: Cerebral palsy spasticity: Selective posterior rhizotomy. Pediatr Neurosci 13:61, 1987.
Robinson BH, Taylor J, Sherwood WG: The genetic heterogeneity of lactic acidosis: Occurrence of recognizable inborn errors of metabolism in a pediatric population with lactic acidosis. Pediatr Res 14:956, 1980.
Sheline GE: Irradiation injury of the human brain: A review of clinical experience. *In:* Gilbert HA, Kagan AR (eds): Radiation Damage to the Nervous System. New York, Raven Press, 1980.
Still JL, Cottom D: Severe hypertension in childhood. Arch Dis Child 42:34, 1967.

20.55 COMA IN THE PEDIATRIC PATIENT

Coma is defined as a state of unconsciousness from which the child cannot be aroused by ordinary verbal, sensory, or physical stimuli. Coma is a medical emergency (see Sec. 6.33–6.35). Prompt diagnosis and appropriate management may be lifesaving. Treatment often precedes a thorough physical examination. The patient's airway and cardiorespiratory system must be examined immediately, and the vital signs must be recorded. If the patient is in shock or has had a cardiorespiratory arrest, the immediate management is directed to resuscitation and to the establishment of life support systems. Generally, a child with a Glasgow Coma Scale of seven or less should be intubated and placed on a respirator (see later). On the other hand, if the patient's vital signs and cardiovascular system are intact, attention may be directed to the history and physical examination.

The history may indicate the cause, but frequently the parent is unavailable or was not present at the onset of the coma. It is important to determine whether there has been a gradual change in personality and behavior or an abrupt loss of consciousness. The amount, type, and time of the last dose of insulin in the diabetic child is important to document. Because intoxication is a prominent cause of coma in the toddler and adolescent patient, a careful review of medications and their location at home should be completed. Furthermore, the discovery of the child in close proximity to the medicine cabinet or storage area or the finding of pills and empty medication containers is overwhelming evidence of drug-induced coma. If there is any doubt about the history, or if the clinical and laboratory findings do not support the history, a home visit may be invaluable. An altered state of consciousness in the newborn period associated with vomiting, failure to thrive, and seizures suggests an inborn error of metabolism. The patient in a postictal state following an initial seizure and the child with a history of chronic renal disease associated with hypertensive encephalopathy may present with coma. A child with severe pulmonary or heart disease or profound anemia may develop coma as a consequence of cerebral anoxia and ischemia. Rarely, brain tumors or cerebral abscess, particularly if there is rupture into the ventricular system, may produce sudden coma. These children may have a history of headache, vomiting, change in personality, or congenital heart disease. Acute subarachnoid hemorrhage secondary to a bleed from an arteriovenous malformation causes a sudden alteration in consciousness.

The child's level of consciousness and the response to stimuli should be carefully documented. A modification of the *Glasgow Coma Scale* in Table 6–25 is a useful tool for the grading of the degree of coma and the severity of the insult in infants and children. It is important to remember that the assessment of the verbal response is much different from that of the adult, and the child's developmental level must be kept in mind during the evaluation. A coma score of less than five is associated with a grave prognosis, whereas a score of five to eight may indicate a better prognosis in the child than in the adult.

The *physical examination* is helpful in distinguishing between a metabolic cause and structural cause for the coma. A slow, irregular pulse combined with systemic hypertension indicates increased intracranial pressure or hypertensive encephalopathy. The rate and rhythm of the respiratory pattern provide useful information about the etiology of the coma. Regular and deep hyperventilation (Kussmaul breathing) indicates metabolic acidosis; subdued and slow breathing suggests respiratory depression or sedation; and irregular, ataxic respiration suggests cerebellar herniation. Cherry red discoloration of the face and cheeks is associated with carbon monoxide poisoning. A fruity breath is typical of diabetic ketoacidosis; a putrid odor indicates hepatic coma; and a sweet-smelling urine suggests MSUD.

The examination should include a careful search for trauma and should test for the presence of nuchal rigidity. CSF rhinorrhea, hematotympanum, and **Battle sign** (bruising over the mastoid) are suggestive of a basilar skull fracture. Nuchal rigidity may indicate meningitis, encephalitis, subarachnoid bleed, or herniation of the cerebellar tonsils. Pin-point *pupils* are associated with narcotics, barbiturate toxicity, organophosphates, and phencyclidine. Small and irregular pupils suggest a lesion in the pons, and dilated and unresponsive pupils are seen in the postictal state, with botulism, and with certain drugs including glutethimide, amphetamine, atropine, cocaine, ethyl alcohol, and mydriatics. A unilaterally dilated and unresponsive pupil in the comatose child indicates herniation of the uncus of the ipsilateral temporal lobe. Check to ensure that a mydriatic was not the cause of the abnormal pupil. The integrity of the extraocular muscles may be tested by the doll's eye maneuver. The fundi must be examined for the presence of papilledema and retinal hemorrhages.

Brain stem function may be evaluated by *ice water* caloric testing (unless the tympanic membrane is ruptured) (see Sec. 20.1). The comatose child with an intact brain stem shows a fixed deviation of the eyes to the side of the stimulus, and the patient with irreversible coma has no response.

Focal neurologic signs may be difficult to elicit in the comatose patient. *Hemiparesis* may be demonstrated by passively flexing the legs and hips. The examiner suddenly releases the extremities. The hemiparetic leg will rapidly fall to an externally rotated position, whereas the normal limb will slowly slide back to the original posture. This maneuver should be carried out with the patient supine and on a flat surface. The quadriceps may be flattened, and the foot of the affected extremity is externally rotated owing to a decrease in muscle tone. Finally, the hemiparetic extremities may have altered reflexes, changes in muscle tone, and an extensor plantar reflex.

During the initial evaluation an *IV line* is established and blood is obtained for a complete blood count, electrolytes, calcium, phosphorus, glucose, creatinine, blood gases, liver function studies, prothrombin and partial thromboplastin, ammonium level, and a toxic screen. It is important to collect and store an additional 5 mL of heparinized blood that can be utilized later if a specific metabolic disease becomes apparent. Table 20–9 provides a framework to differentiate the various common causes of metabolic coma. If the initial Dextrostix suggests hypoglycemia, 2 mL/kg of 25% dextrose should be given IV. A *urinary catheter* is inserted; the urine volume is noted; and a sample is examined for glucose, ketones, and further studies as indicated. A *nasogastric tube* is placed in position, and the stomach is emptied with care to prevent aspiration, particularly if a toxin is suspected. The stomach contents may be analyzed in the laboratory for specific toxins. Structural causes of coma include concussion, contusion, subdural and epidural hematoma, cerebral edema, brain tumors, and cerebral abscess. The diagnosis and management of these conditions is discussed elsewhere in this chapter.

The principles of *treatment* include maintenance of the respiratory status, normalization of cardiovascular function, and correction of acid-base, fluid, and electrolyte abnormalities. Seizures, increased intracranial pressure, and hyperthermia (or hypothermia) are managed appropriately. The primary goal of treatment is to identify the specific cause of the coma and to correct the problem in a safe and controlled fashion.

The use of **invasive intracranial pressure monitoring** should be considered for any infant or child with nontraumatic coma and suspected increase in intracranial pressure to assess cerebral perfusion and to anticipate shifts in brain tissue. Cerebral perfusion is calculated as the difference between the mean arterial blood pressure and the mean intracranial pressure. Neurologic outcome is improved if the intracranial pressure can be reduced and maintained at 15 mm Hg or less and if the cerebral perfusion pressure is above 50 mm Hg. Poor neurologic outcome or death is associated with intracranial pressures above 50 mm Hg or cerebral perfusion pressures of less than 40 mm Hg. Intracranial pressure in the child may be monitored by the use of a subarachnoid screw, a subdural pressure transducer, or a fluid-filled intraventricular catheter. Raised intracranial pressure may be lowered by paralysis and sedation with pancuronium, phenobarbital, morphine, or diazepam, mechanical hyperventilation ($Pa{CO_2}$ lowered to 30–35 mm Hg), osmotherapy with IV mannitol or furosemide, or drainage of CSF through the ventricular catheter. A decrease in cerebral perfusion pressure associated with a low systemic arterial pressure may be enhanced by infusions of colloid or dopamine.

The induction of pentobarbital coma and the use of steroids does not appear to influence the neurologic *prognosis* in the comatose child. The prediction of coma outcome during the acute illness depends in part on the etiology of the condition; diabetic ketoacidosis has a more favorable outlook than Reye syndrome. However, certain physical signs provide some indication of outcome before inducing paralysis and placement on the respirator. These signs include severity of the coma (i.e., modified Glasgow score), eye movement, pupil reaction, level of blood pressure, temperature, motor patterns, and the seizure type. The EEG is also useful to estimate the potential for neurologic recovery. For example, the reappearance of normal sleep spindles is an encouraging finding even if associated with high-voltage slow waves that have no predictive value. EEG patterns associated with a poor prognosis include burst suppression, α-like activity, very low amplitude activity for age, and electrocerebral silence. Neurophysiologic studies have also been used to make a prognosis about comatose children, including brain stem auditory, visual, and somatosensory evoked potentials. Generally, the absence of all wave forms in these three modalities is associated with death or severe neurologic residua. Somatosensory evoked potentials are the most sensitive and reliable method for the evaluation of neurologic outcome in the comatose child.

TABLE 20–9. Coma in the Pediatric Population: Metabolic Coma

Etiology	Symptoms and Signs	Diagnosis
Intoxication		
Salicylism	Hyperventilation, dehydration, seizures	Metabolic acidosis, ketonuria, urine ferric chloride (burgundy color), increased serum salicylate
Barbiturates	Hypoventilation, decreased blood pressure, pin-point pupils	Increased serum phenobarbital level (>30 μg/mL)
Alcohol	Respiratory failure, seizures	Serum alcohol: coma = 300–500 mg/dL, >500 mg/dL may be lethal
Hyperglycemia		
Diabetes mellitus	Hyperventilation, fruity odor	Glycosuria, ketonuria, ketonemia, metabolic acidosis
Head injury	External evidence of trauma or focal signs	Glycosuria, no ketonemia or ketonuria
Hypoglycemia		
Insulin excess	Perspiration, pallor, seizures	Blood glucose <30 mg/dL (<20 mg/dL in premature)
Salicylism	As above	—
Alcohol	As above	—
Inborn Errors	Vomiting, changes in tone, seizures	Metabolic acidosis, positive 2, 4 dinitrophenyl-hydrazine, increased organic acids, increased amino acids, increased serum lactate
Electrolyte Abnormalities	Hypernatremia, hyponatremia, hypocalcemia, hypokalemia	Serum electrolytes, calcium and magnesium
Meningo-encephalitis	Fever, nuchal rigidity, seizures	Examination of CSF; brain scan, EEG, and CT scan if herpes suspected
Encephalopathy		
Anoxic	Cardiac arrest, severe anemia/pulmonary disease	Pulseless, ECG, Hb, chest radiograph
Reye syndrome	Hyperpnea, apneic breathing, decerebrate posture, dilated pupils, seizures	Increased serum ammonia, SGOT, SGPT, and prolonged PT hyperaminoacidemia (lysine and glutamine), characteristic liver biopsy
Hypertensive	Renal disease, coarctation of the aorta, collagen vascular disease, pheochromocytoma	Increased blood pressure, retinal changes, decreased femoral pulses, neurofibromatosis?
Hemorrhagic shock (HSES)	Malaise, fever, vomiting and diarrhea, seizures, cyanosis	Metabolic acidosis, acute renal failure, increased liver enzymes, anemia, and DIC
Hemolytic-uremic syndrome (HUS)	Irritability, pallor, purpura, oliguria, seizures	Decreased Hb, decreased platelets, fragmented red blood cells, hematuria, renal failure, verotoxin producing *Escherichia coli*
Lead	Vomiting, abdominal pain, ataxia, seizures	Blood lead greater than 100 μg/dL
Post-seizure	Dilated pupils, Babinski, rapid return of consciousness	Medicalert bracelet?

20.56 BRAIN DEATH

See also Sec. 2.6.

The President's commission commented that "Death is defined as irreversible cessation of circulatory and respiratory functions or irreversible cessation of all functions of the entire brain, including the brain stem. A determination of death must be made in accordance with accepted medical standards." The criteria for establishing brain death are similar for adults and children; however, the period of observation may be longer in the latter. The diagnosis of brain death is established when the cause of coma is determined; the possibility for recovery of any brain function is excluded; and the cessation of all brain functions are documented for an appropriate period of observation or trial of therapy. The diagnosis of brain death is made primarily by clinical methods, irrespective of the age of the patient. The physical examination criteria are as follows: (1) the patient must be comatose, apneic, normothermic, and normotensive with absence of vocalization and volitional movement. Apnea is defined as an absence of spontaneous respirations despite an adequate carbon dioxide stimulus (i.e., 45–60 mm Hg). During apnea testing the patient is maintained on continuous positive airway pressure ventilation and is oxygenated with 100% oxygen. The confirmation of apnea is achieved when the patient fails to breathe spontaneously after 15 min or until the P_{CO_2} rises to 60 mm Hg. Apnea testing is reserved until the physical examination is completed and the diagnosis of brain death appears to be certain. (2) All brain stem responses must be absent. The pupils are midposition or fully dilated, and there is no direct or consensual pupillary response to a bright light. There is absence of spontaneous eye movements, including lack of a blink or eye movement to a loud noise (auriculo-ocular response), no response to ice water caloric stimulation (vestibulo-ocular), and no lateral eye movement with head turning (doll's eye maneuver). There is no corneal response, rooting reflex, gag, cough, or sucking reflexes. (3) Spontaneous movements (with the exception of spinal cord reflex withdrawal and myoclonus) must be absent and there is generalized flaccidity. Laboratory studies are also performed to establish the cause of the coma and to specifically exclude a remedial condition, such as a toxic, metabolic, paralytic, or sedative cause.

Because the period of asphyxia or cause of coma may be unknown in the premature infant or newborn, a longer period of observation is required than in the older child or adult before a diagnosis of brain death is established. The diagnosis of brain death in these patients as well as in older children may be substantiated by an EEG, showing a period of electrocerebral silence utilizing standard techniques, or by the absence of carotid circulation at the base of the skull and intracranial arterial circulation utilizing a cerebral radionuclide angiogram. Unfortunately, the correlation among the physical examination, EEG, and cerebral radionuclide angiogram is not absolute. Until more precise laboratory or imaging studies are developed, the diagnosis of brain death for all ages continues to be made on the basis of a careful physical examination with an appropriate period of observation to ensure that all the criteria discussed earlier have been met.

Ashwal S, Schneider S: Brain death in the newborn: Pediatrics 84:429, 1989.
Drake B, Ashwal S, Schneider S: Determination of cerebral death in the pediatric intensive care unit. Pediatrics 78:107, 1986.
Fois A, Malandrini F: Electroencephalographic findings in pediatric cases of coma. Clin Electroenceph 14:207, 1983.
Guidelines for the determination of brain death: Report of the medical consultants on the diagnosis of death to the President's Commission for the Study of Ethical Problems in Medicine and Biomedical and Behavioral Research. Neurology 32:395, 1982.
Johnston B, Seshia SS: Prediction of outcome in non-traumatic coma in childhood. Acta Neurol Scand 69:417, 1984.
Plum F, Posner JB: Diagnosis of Stupor and Coma, 3rd ed. Philadelphia, FA Davis, 1980.
Reilly PL, Simpson DA, Sprod R, et al: Assessing the conscious level in infants and young children: A paediatric version of the Glasgow Coma Scale. Childs Nerv Syst 4:30, 1988.
Tasker RC, Matthew DJ, Helms P, et al: Monitoring in non-traumatic coma. 1: Invasive intracranial measurements. Arch Dis Child 63:888, 1988.

20.57 HEAD INJURIES

Accidents are the major cause of morbidity and mortality in children beyond 1 yr of age, and head trauma is the injury most responsible for death (Sec. 6.31). It is estimated that 100,000 children are hospitalized annually in the United States because of head injury, and 5–10% have long-term mental or physical handicaps as a result. Most head injuries involve an automobile; however, auto-bicycle and motorcycle accidents, falls, and nonaccidental trauma (i.e., child abuse) account for a significant number of head injuries in children. Injuries of males outnumber those of females by a ratio of 2:1. The degree of brain trauma depends on many variables, including age, velocity of the fall, whether the injury was a closed or open wound, and the use of protective head gear. It requires greater physical force to produce unconsciousness and brain trauma when the head is maintained in a fixed position compared with a freely moving skull at impact, which strongly supports the use of infant car seats and appropriate automobile seat belts and shoulder restraints.

SKULL FRACTURES. A skull fracture in association with head trauma does not necessarily imply injury to the underlying brain. Approximately one third of all children with a history of a head injury have radiologic evidence of a skull fracture, but most of these children are intact neurologically at the time of examination and remain free of sequelae. Conversely, approximately 50% of children who die of an acute brain injury have no evidence of a skull fracture. Furthermore, subdural hematoma occur in twice as many injured children without a fracture compared with those with a skull fracture. Epidural hematoma is associated with a skull fracture in approximately 50% of cases. Finally, the location and type of skull fracture are rarely correlated with symptoms and physical findings. Thus, careful clinical appraisal and observation are more valuable in determining the extent of brain injury and the presence of neurologic complications than the finding of a skull fracture.

The most common skull fracture is *linear and nondepressed*. It does not, as a rule, interfere with the function and integrity of the brain and, thus, the outcome in most cases is excellent. Serious consequences may result if the fracture traverses the groove of the meningeal vessels, the sagittal sinus, or the lamboid suture. A **leptomeningeal cyst** is a rare and late complication of a linear skull fracture and is characterized by a slowly expanding pulsatile mass on the surface of the skull. The cyst is caused by the protrusion of the leptomeninges and traumatized brain through the interrupted dura and skull fracture and expansion by the propulsion of CSF into the cyst by the pulsating brain.

Basilar skull fractures are difficult to demonstrate by radiologic examination. Most frequently, the temporal bone is fractured producing a bloody discharge from the middle ear (hematotympanum) or Battle sign, a few days later (Fig. 20–14). Cranial nerve palsies may occur, particularly injury to the facial and auditory cranial nerves. Bilateral ecchymosis and swelling of the upper eyelids **(raccoon's eye sign)** suggests a basal anterior fossa fracture. Fracture of the sphenoid bone may damage the oculomotor, trochlear, and abducens nerves. CSF otorrhea or rhinorrhea may complicate a basilar skull fracture. Although CSF otorrhea usually does not persist beyond 24–48 hr, CSF rhinorrhea is less likely to arrest spontaneously. It may be difficult to distinguish CSF rhinorrhea from excessive nasal secretions. The fluid is clear in the former, tends to be profuse (particularly upon sitting), and tests positive for glucose using Dextrostix. If the rhinorrhea persists longer than 14 days, surgical repair of the defect is usually necessary. Bacterial meningitis, particularly *Streptococcus pneumoniae*, may complicate a basilar skull fracture because of the open defect between the nasopharynx or middle ear and the brain. The use of prophylactic antibiotics is controversial, but they are rarely used during the first week of CSF rhinorrhea because of the likelihood of spontaneous closure of the defect. *Depressed skull fractures* must be treated surgically

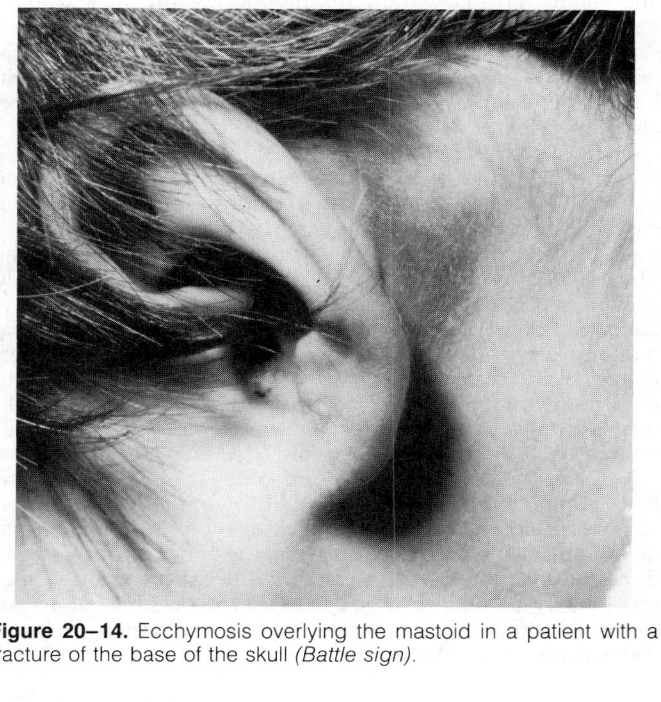

Figure 20–14. Ecchymosis overlying the mastoid in a patient with a fracture of the base of the skull *(Battle sign)*.

if a neurologic deficit results or a compound wound is present. Surgical treatment is necessary if the depression is greater than 3–5 mm.

There is no consensus about the guidelines for obtaining skull roentgenograms in the investigation of a pediatric head injury. National guidelines recommend that all children less than 5 yr of age with a history of head trauma undergo roentgenographic examination because of the unreliability of the history and neurologic examination in this age group. Unfortunately, the roentgenogram is usually ordered in a defensive, medicolegal-oriented atmosphere, and the negative results may add a false sense of security. A skull roentgenogram is indicated for a child with a cephalohematoma, prolonged unconsciousness, a penetrating scalp wound, palpable bony defects, focal neurologic signs including irregular pupils and hemiparesis, discharge from the nose or ear, a discolored tympanic membrane, blackened eyes, and symptoms and signs of increased intracranial pressure.

CONCUSSION. This is defined as a brief but variable and reversible alteration in the level of consciousness associated with transient paralysis of reflexes and amnesia for the events immediately surrounding the injury. The duration of retrograde and post-traumatic amnesia is a good indicator of the severity of the trauma. During the acute phase of concussion there is loss of tone, flaccidity and areflexia, dilatation of the pupils, and brief apnea. Cortical blindness may follow a concussion, probably as the result of localized cerebral edema in the region of the calcarine fissure. The child may appear irritable and restless, and the older child may deny blindness. The period of blindness is transient, and full recovery usually occurs within hours. The recovery phase of concussion is characterized by tachycardia, vomiting, pallor, lethargy, and confusion. Several mechanisms for the pathogenesis of concussion have been proposed, including shearing or stretching of the fibers within the white matter, temporary paralysis of nerve function, an alteration in neurotransmitter elaboration, and temporary changes in cerebral blood flow and oxygen consumption. Although the outcome for children with concussion is uniformly excellent, it is sometimes difficult to determine which patients should be hospitalized for observation at the time of the accident. The following clinical manifestations are indicators for concern following concussion and justify hospitalization for monitoring and a period of frequent observation: (1) deterioration in the level of consciousness, (2) persistence of confusion and lethargy, (3) excessive and copious vomiting, (4) unwitnessed or uncertain history of trauma, (5) focal neurologic signs, (6) a seizure, and (7) any child with a confirmed skull fracture.

SUBDURAL HEMATOMA. A subdural hematoma is a collection of bloody fluid between the dura and cerebral mantle. It occurs as a consequence of the rupture of bridging cortical veins that drain the cerebral cortex. Although any form of head trauma may produce subdural hematoma, the physically abused infant who is repeatedly and forcedly shaken is particularly susceptible to this type of head injury. Large collections of blood that may be unilateral or bilateral interfere with normal cerebral function and may cause herniation of the brain. Inevitably, there is a degree of trauma to the underlying brain as a direct result of the initial injury. In the physically abused child there are often additional sites of trauma, including rib and extremity fractures.

Acutely, the subdural hematoma consists of dark red blood that changes to a straw-colored fluid owing to disintegration of the red blood cells. Within 1 wk of the injury, a subdural membrane begins to develop from the inner surface of the dura and eventually encapsulates the hematoma. The hematoma may gradually enlarge owing to the presence of a high concentration of albumin which, by osmotic pressure, draws water across the subdural membrane. Repeated trauma can produce fresh bleeding into a chronic subdural hematoma. Infantile subdural hematoma presents during the first 6 mo of life, often with a focal or generalized convulsion. In addition, there is typically a history of poor feeding, failure to thrive, irritability, lethargy, vomiting, and fever. These common constitutional symptoms may have been present for some time and may have been overlooked. The examination may show a tense and bulging anterior fontanel and an enlarged head circumference. Frequently there is evidence of cerebral injury, because the infant is irritable with a shrill, high-pitched cry. The eyes may show a "setting-sun" position owing to increased intracranial pressure. Examination of the eyegrounds is critical because more than 50% show retinal or subhyaloid hemorrhages. The CT scan or MRI is invaluable in confirming the diagnosis (Fig. 20–15). Acute subdural hematomas produce a hyperdense image that may be indistinguishable from the surrounding bone, whereas chronic subdurals are hypodense and readily identified by the CT scan. A prothrombin and partial thromboplastin time are important to rule out the remote possibility of a coagulation disorder. An infant who is a suspected victim of physical abuse should be admitted to hospital and should be evaluated thoroughly for evidence of additional injuries while the social and environmental factors are carefully investigated. Acute subdural hematomas may be associated with severe underlying brain injuries, including contusion and intracerebral hemorrhage. The prognosis for recovery is poor because of the cerebral insult rather than the presence of blood in the subdural space.

Chronic subdural hematomas are typically observed in the infant and the elderly adult, because these patients have a discrepancy between the size of the brain and the skull. The lesions tend to be bilateral in younger children and are characterized by increasing head circumference, headache, dullness, personality change, a focal convulsion, sudden loss of consciousness, and signs of increased intracranial pressure.

EPIDURAL HEMATOMA. An epidural hematoma results from bleeding into the extradural space from rupture of the middle meningeal artery or a tear in the dural veins owing to direct trauma to the region of the temporal bone. The hematoma enlarges rapidly because of arterial bleeding or more

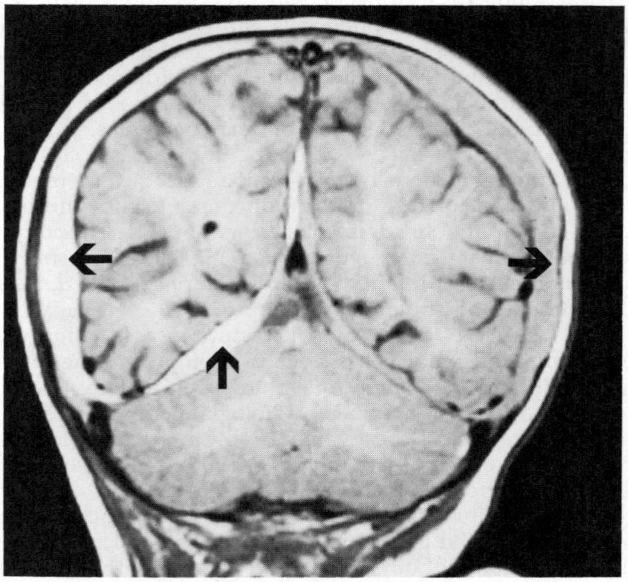

Figure 20–15. MRI of bilateral subdural hematoma *(arrows)* with suboccipital extension. Compare the color (age) of the hematomas between the right and left sides.

gradually if venous bleeding occurs; each is capable of causing compression of the temporal lobe and ultimately herniation of the uncus, which is life-threatening and demands immediate surgical intervention. After the injury, the child typically experiences a brief period of unconsciousness followed by a variable lucid interval from minutes to days, depending on the source of bleeding. As the hematoma impinges on the temporal lobe, the child undergoes progressive loss of consciousness associated with vomiting, a severe headache, and focal neurologic signs, including ipsilateral dilatation of the pupil followed by a complete third-nerve paresis, contralateral hemiparesis, and papilledema in approximately 20%. The CT scan is the diagnostic test of choice, because a skull fracture is present in only one half of the cases. An epidural hematoma typically assumes a hyperdense biconcave image on the CT scan (Fig. 20–16). The prognosis for an epidural hematoma is excellent if the diagnosis is made early with prompt surgical evacuation, but there is significant mortality and morbidity in those cases in which treatment is delayed or when severe underlying brain injury accompanies the epidural hematoma.

SEVERE HEAD INJURIES. Major insults to the brain may result from contusion, particularly to the frontal lobes or inferolateral portion of the temporal lobes, a penetrating injury, the presence of an intracerebral hemorrhage, and diffuse axonal injury due to cerebral edema. The clinical findings depend on the site and nature of the injury and on the degree of cerebral edema. The development of additional neurologic signs following admission to hospital implies increased cerebral edema; an expanding intracerebral, subdural, or epidural hematoma; or compromised cerebral blood flow secondary to vasospasm. Initial signs associated with a poor prognosis include fixed and dilated pupils, apneic breathing, decorticate posturing, and a Glasgow Coma Scale revised for children of less than 5 yr of age.

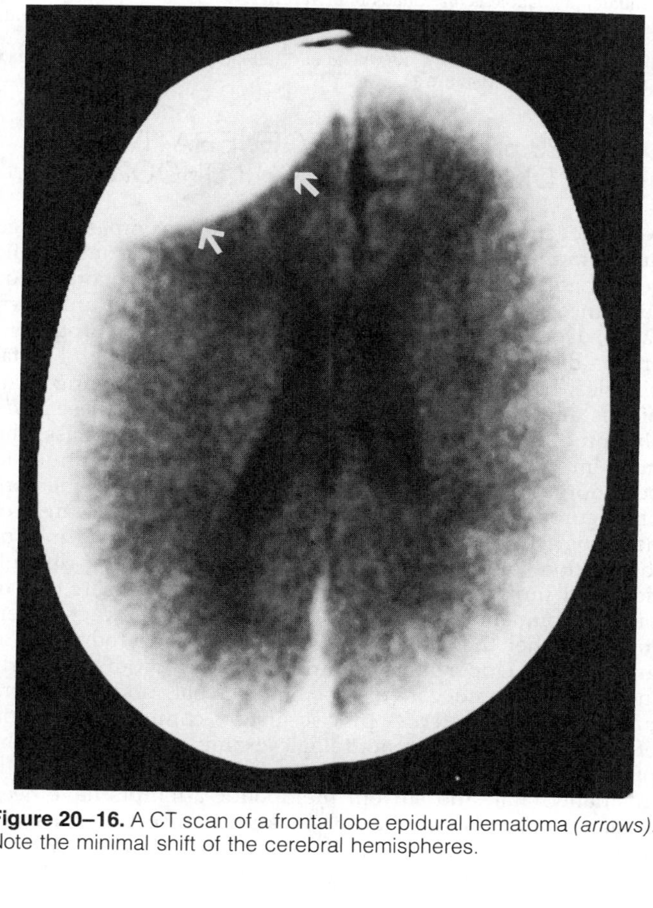

Figure 20–16. A CT scan of a frontal lobe epidural hematoma *(arrows)*. Note the minimal shift of the cerebral hemispheres.

TREATMENT. A head-injured child requires identification and treatment of all injuries, including fractures and trauma to the pelvis, abdomen, and chest. The vital signs should be monitored and serial examination should be performed including palpation of the scalp, inspection of the tympanic membranes, and a detailed neurologic evaluation (including pupillary reaction, eye movements, funduscopic examination, and a search for localizing signs). The Glasgow Coma Scale revised for children should be utilized to repeatedly document the level of consciousness in an accurate and reproducible fashion, avoiding ambiguous statements concerning the neurologic state and alerting the management team to deterioration in neurologic function. A minor head injury is sometimes difficult to distinguish from serious trauma, so that hospitalization and frequent observation for 24–48 hr may be necessary (see Concussion).

In the child with a major head injury, immediate attention must be directed to the cardiovascular and respiratory systems. Adequate oxygenation is essential to prevent further tissue damage. Endotracheal intubation is indicated when the respiratory effort is compromised, and ventilatory assistance is provided to maintain adequate exchange. A tracheostomy is required if ventilation is necessary for longer than a 10- to 14-day period. The circulatory system should be examined, and hypovolemic shock should be corrected. An infant may lose sufficient quantities of blood into the cranial cavity that may cause severe anemia or shock without evidence of external bleeding. The cervical spine should be stabilized because there is an association between head trauma and neck injuries. When convenient and early in the course of management, a portable lateral neck roentgenogram should be obtained. Additional radiologic studies depend on the findings of the physical examination. A CT scan may readily identify correctable lesions, including subdural, epidural, and intracerebral hematomas as well as localized areas of cerebral edema and penetrating bony injuries. MRI is more reliable than a CT scan in the detection of posterior fossa hematomas.

Cerebral edema is a major complication of head trauma and is the most common cause of death in the first few days after an accident. The management of cerebral edema and the concomitant increased intracranial pressure include adequate oxygenation, elevation of the head of the bed to 30 degrees, and the judicious use of IV fluids. Inappropriate secretion of antidiuretic hormone may complicate acute head injury, in which case excessive fluid administration enhances the cerebral edema. Monitoring of the intracranial pressure is an important method of documenting the effectiveness of therapy (see Sec. 20.55). Since an elevated P_{CO_2} causes vasodilation of the cerebral vessels and increases intracranial pressure, the patient is hyperventilated to maintain a P_{CO_2} in the region of 25–30 mm Hg. The use of hyperosmolar agents such as mannitol may be effective in controlling cerebral edema. Mannitol is given IV in a 20% solution at a dose of 1–1.5 g/kg. Subsequent pulses of mannitol of 0.25–0.5 g/kg are determined by the clinical state, intracranial pressure, and serum osmolarity, which should not be allowed to exceed 320 mOsmol/L. Glucocorticoids, which are thought to "stabilize" the blood-brain barrier, may be useful but have a delayed action of approximately 24 hr. The most widely utilized steroid is dexamethasone, with a loading dose of 0.1 mg/kg IV followed by 0.05 mg/kg IV every 6 hr. Hypothermia also should be considered for the management of serious head injuries in children. Aside from reducing the metabolic demand of the brain, hypothermia acts to decrease acute cerebral edema. The child is cooled by ice packs or a cooling blanket to a core temperature of 32–33° C for 2–3 days, at which time the cerebral edema usually begins to subside spontaneously.

The surgical management of head injuries includes the repair of depressed skull fractures, debridement of bony fragments within the cerebrum, evacuation of intracerebral hematomas producing a mass effect, removal of an epidural hematoma, and control of dural bleeding. Subdural hematomas of infancy may initially require percutaneous subdural taps if they are large or symptomatic. After bilateral subdural taps relieve the increased intracranial pressure, the child may be followed with repeated fontanel assessment, skull transillumination, head circumference measurements, and occasional CT scan to monitor the spontaneous resorption of the subdural hematoma over a period of weeks to months. Some children require repeated removal of the subdural collections because of recurrent symptoms and signs of increased intracranial pressure. Repeated subdural taps on alternate sides for several days may resolve the reaccumulation of subdural fluid and ameliorate the increased intracranial pressure. Rarely, a more aggressive surgical approach including stripping of the membranes and the placement of a subdural-peritoneal shunt is necessary to control subdural collections.

Seizures may complicate a head injury and can occur following relatively minor trauma. Seizures that develop within minutes or a few hours of head trauma are frequently brief and result from transient mechanical and neurochemical changes within the CNS. Most of these children will not have additional seizures and do not require anticonvulsants. Convulsions that develop within 24–48 hr of the injury are classified as early post-traumatic seizures and result from cerebral edema, petechial and hemorrhagic lesions, or a penetrating wound. Status epilepticus, which demands prompt management, may ensue. IV phenytoin is recommended with a loading dose of 15–20 mg/kg followed by maintenance doses of 5–10 mg/kg/24 hr. Phenytoin is desirable in the acute stages of management, because it does not alter the level of consciousness in a neurologically compromised patient.

PROGNOSIS. The most important determinant of neurologic and intellectual recovery in the head-injured child is the duration of coma. If the child survives the immediate consequences of the head injury and recovers from coma within 14 days, the likelihood of normal or near-normal cognitive and neuromotor function is extremely favorable. The reasons for optimism in the child compared with the adult is the contention that the former's brain is more "plastic" than the adult's and generally recovers more completely in a shorter time. However, infants less than 2 yr of age with major brain trauma have a uniformly poor prognosis compared with older children, perhaps as the result of immature autoregulation of the cerebral blood vessels, the greater susceptibility of the incompletely myelinated brain to irreversible injury, and the fact that open cranial sutures permit greater distortion among the meninges, cerebral vessels, and the underlying brain.

Late post-traumatic seizures tend to develop within 2 yr of the initial insult. Post-traumatic epilepsy is more likely to occur if the original trauma to the brain was severe and the dura disrupted. Anticonvulsant prophylaxis is not warranted for every head-injured child because the majority will not develop seizures. For patients who develop a seizure during hospitalization (excluding those with a brief seizure within a few hours of the accident), an anticonvulsant is prescribed for 2–3 mo. If the seizures recur, the drug is reinstituted for a more prolonged period. Post-traumatic seizures that result from localized glial scars may be unresponsive to anticonvulsants and require surgical extirpation in order to control the seizures.

With severe head injuries, a variety of persistent neurologic deficits may result including hemiparesis, aphasia, cognitive disturbances, and behavioral disorders. Many studies have noted that children with personality disorders following serious head trauma had unusual behavioral traits prior to the injury that seemed to be enhanced by the accident. Abnormalities of short-term memory, specifically storage and retrieval of important information, is the most common cognitive sequela of significant head injury in children and adolescents. Children may show gradual recovery of neuropsychologic function up to 5 yr after an accident. Cognitive deficits may not be readily apparent during hospitalization. Neuropsychologic evaluation of the severely injured child, or the patient with an apparently mild injury who copes poorly at school following the accident, is an important method of identifying specific language, memory, or cognitive deficits that may be responsive to special education techniques.

The **post-traumatic syndrome** may occur in children following relatively minor head trauma. The essential features include hyperactivity, decreased attention span, temper outbursts, sleep disturbances, moodiness, and discipline problems. Occasionally, dizziness and headaches are also present. Treatment of the post-traumatic syndrome should include a thorough evaluation of the child to eliminate other causes, followed by reassurance and support; the condition improves spontaneously without specific intervention in most children.

Black P, Jeffries JJ, Blumer D, et al: The post-traumatic syndrome in children. *In*: Walker AE, Caveness WF, Critchley M (eds): The Late Effects of Head Injury. Springfield, IL, Charles C Thomas, 1969.

Bruce DA, Schut L, Bruno LA, et al: Outcome following severe head injuries in children. J Neurosurg 48:679, 1978.

Dershewitz RA, Kaye BA, Swisher CN: Treatment of children with post-traumatic transient loss of consciousness. Pediatrics 72:602, 1983.

Hendrick EB, Harwood-Nash DC, Hudson AR: Head injuries in children: A survey of 4,465 consecutive cases at the Hospital for Sick Children, Toronto, Canada. Clin Neurosurg 11:46, 1963.

Klonoff H, Low MD, Clark C: Head injuries in children: A prospective 5 year follow-up. J Neurol Neurosurg Psychiatry 40:1211, 1977.

Kraus JF, Fife D, Conroy C: Pediatric brain injuries: The nature, clinical course and early outcomes in a defined United States population. Pediatrics 79:501, 1987.

Leonidas JC, Ting W, Binkiewicz A, et al: Mild head trauma in children: When is a roentgenogram necessary? Pediatrics 69:139, 1982.

Levin HS, Eisenberg HM: Neuropsychological outcome of head injury in children and adolescents. Childs Brain 5:281, 1979.

Mahoney WJ, D'Souza BJ, Haller JA, et al: Long-term outcome of children with severe head trauma and prolonged coma. Pediatrics 71:756, 1983.

Masters SJ, McClean PM, Arcarese JS, et al: Skull x-ray examinations after head trauma. N Engl J Med 316:84, 1987.

20.58 NEURODEGENERATIVE DISORDERS OF CHILDHOOD

Neurodegenerative disorders of childhood encompass a large number of heterogeneous diseases, which result from specific genetic and biochemical defects, chronic viral infections, toxic substances, and a significant group of conditions of unknown cause. Until recently, children with suspected neurodegenerative disorders were routinely subjected to brain and rectal biopsies, but with the advent of modern neuroimaging techniques and specific biochemical diagnostic tests, these invasive procedures are now rarely necessary. Nevertheless, the most important component of the investigation continues to be a thorough history and physical examination. The hallmark of a neurodegenerative disease is progressive deterioration of neurologic function with loss of speech, vision, hearing, or locomotion, often associated with seizures, feeding difficulties, and impairment of intellect. The age of onset, rate of progression, and the principal neurological findings determine whether the disease is primarily affecting the white or gray matter. Upper motor neuron signs are prominent early in the former and convulsions, intellectual, and visual impairment in the latter. A precise history confirms regression of milestones, and the neurologic examination localizes the process within the nervous system. Although the outcome is invariably fatal, and current therapeutic attempts have been unsuccessful, it is important to make the correct diagnosis so that genetic counseling may be offered and prevention strat-

TABLE 20–10. Heredity and Biochemical Defects in the Neurodegenerative Disorders

Neuro-degenerative Disorder	Mode of Inheritance	Biochemical Defect	Specimen for Analysis
Sphingolipidosis			
GM_1 gangliosidosis	AR*	β-Galactosidase	Serum, leukocytes, skin fibroblasts
GM_2 gangliosidosis			
Tay-Sachs	AR	Hexosaminidase A	Serum, leukocytes, skin fibroblasts
Sandhoff	AR	Hexosaminidase A and B	Serum, leukocytes, skin fibroblasts
Krabbe disease	AR	Galacto-cerebrosidase	Leukocytes and skin fibroblasts
Metachromatic leukodystrophy	AR	Arylsulfatase A	Leukocytes and skin fibroblasts
Neuronal Ceroid Lipofuscinoses	AR	?	EM† of skin biopsy
Adrenoleuko-dystrophy	XLR‡	VLCFA§ oxidation	Plasma, skin fibroblasts
Sialidosis	AR	Neuraminidase	Skin fibroblasts

*AR = autosomal recessive.
†EM = electron microscopy.
‡XLR = x-linked recessive.
§VLCFA = very long chain fatty acids.

egies can be implemented. For all conditions in which the specific enzyme defect is known, prevention by prenatal diagnosis (chorionic villus sampling or amniocentesis) is possible. Carrier detection is also often possible by enzyme assay. Table 20–10 summarizes the heredity, biochemical defects, and specific diagnostic abnormality in the inherited neurodegerative disorders.

The inherited neurodegenerative disorders include the sphingolipidoses, neuronal ceroid lipofuscinoses, adrenoleukodystrophy, and sialidosis. The sphingolipidoses are characterized by the intracellular storage of a normal lipid component of the cell membrane owing to a defect in the catabolism of the compound. The sphingolipidoses are subclassified into six categories: Niemann-Pick disease, Gaucher disease, GM_1 gangliosidosis, GM_2 gangliosidosis, Krabbe disease, and metachromatic leukodystrophy. Niemann-Pick disease and Gaucher disease are discussed in Sec. 8.18. The spinocerebellar degenerative diseases (Friedreich ataxia, ataxia telangiectasia, olivopontocerebellar atrophy, and abetalipoproteinemia) and degenerative disorders of the basal ganglia (Huntington disease, dystonia musculorum deformans, Wilson disease, and Hallervorden-Spatz disease) are included in Sec. 20.45–20.46. Finally, a miscellaneous group of degenerative diseases are discussed in this section, including multiple sclerosis, Pelizaeus-Merzbacher disease, Alexander disease, Canavan spongy degeneration, kinky hair disease, Rett syndrome, and subacute sclerosing panencephalitis.

SPHINGOLIPIDOSES

20.59 GANGLIOSIDOSES

See also Sec. 8.18.

Gangliosides are glycosphingolipids, normal constituents of the neuronal and synaptic membranes. The basic structure of GM_1 ganglioside consists of an oligosaccharide chain attached to a hydroxyl group of ceramide and sialic acid bound to galactose. The gangliosides are catabolized by sequential cleavage of the sugar molecules by specific exoglycosidases. Abnormalities in catabolism result in accumulation of the ganglioside within the cell. Defects in ganglioside degradation can be classified into two groups, the GM_1 gangliosidoses and the GM_2 gangliosidoses.

GM_1 GANGLIOSIDOSES. The three subtypes of GM_1 gangliosidoses are classified according to age of presentation: infantile (type 1), juvenile (type 2), and adult (type 3). The condition is inherited as an autosomal recessive trait and results from a marked deficiency of acid β-galactosidase. This enzyme may be assayed in leukocytes and cultured fibroblasts. Prenatal diagnosis is possible by the measurement of acid β-galactosidase in cultured amniotic cells. *Infantile GM_1 gangliosidosis* presents at birth or during the neonatal period with anorexia, poor suck, and inadequate weight gain. Development is globally retarded, and generalized seizures are prominent. The phenotype is striking and shares many characteristics with Hurler syndrome. The facial features are coarse; the forehead is prominent; the nasal bridge is depressed; the tongue is large (macroglossia); and the gums are hypertrophied. Hepatosplenomegaly is present early in the course owing to accumulation of foamy histiocytes, and kyphoscoliosis is evident owing to anterior beaking of the vertebral bodies. The neurologic examination is dominated by apathy, progressive blindness, deafness, spastic quadriplegia, and decerebrate rigidity. A cherry red spot in the macular region is visualized in approximately 50% of cases. The **cherry-red spot** is characterized by an opaque ring (sphingolipid-laden retinal ganglion cells) encircling the normal red-colored fovea (Fig. 20–17). Children rarely survive beyond 2–3 yr of age, and death is due to aspiration pneumonia. *Juvenile GM_1 gangliosidosis* has a delayed onset beginning about 1 yr of age. The initial symptoms consist of incoordination, weakness, ataxia, and regression of language. Thereafter convulsions, spasticity, decerebrate rigidity, and blindness are the major findings. Unlike the infantile type, coarse facial features and hepatosplenomegaly are usually absent. Radiographic examination of the lumbar vertebra may show minor beaking. Children rarely survive beyond 10 yr of age. *Adult GM_1*

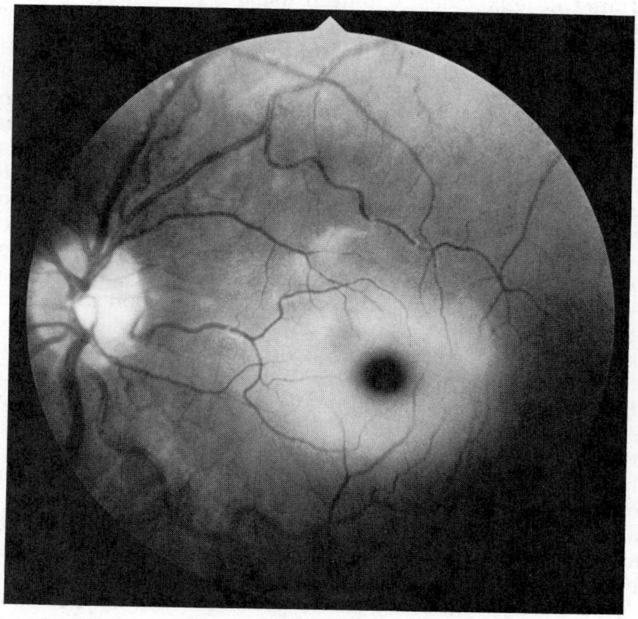

Figure 20–17. A cherry red spot in a patient with GM_1 gangliosidosis. Note the whitish ring of sphingolipid-laden ganglion cells surrounding the fovea.

gangliosidosis is a slowly progressive disease consisting of spasticity, ataxia, dysarthria, and a gradual loss of cognitive function.

GM_2 GANGLIOSIDOSES. The GM_2 gangliosidoses are a heterogeneous group of autosomal recessive inherited disorders that consist of several subtypes, including Tay-Sachs disease (TSD), Sandhoff disease, juvenile GM_2 gangliosidosis, and adult GM_2 gangliosidosis. *TSD* is most prevalent in the Ashkenazi Jewish population and has a carrier rate of approximately 1/30. Affected infants appear normal until approximately 6 mo of age, except for a marked "startle" reaction to noise that is evident soon after birth. The affected child then begins to lag in developmental milestones, and by 1 yr of age the child loses the ability to stand, sit, and vocalize. Early hypotonia develops into progressive spasticity, and relentless deterioration follows with convulsions, blindness, deafness, and cherry red spots in almost all patients (see Fig. 20–17). Macrocephaly becomes apparent by 1 yr of age and results from the 200- to 300-times normal content of GM_2 ganglioside deposited within the brain. Few children live beyond 3–4 yr of age, and death is usually associated with bronchopneumonia. A deficiency of the isoenzyme hexosaminidase A is found in tissues of patients with TSD. Mass screening for the prenatal diagnosis of TSD is a reliable and cost-effective method of prevention because the condition occurs in a defined population (Ashkenazi Jews). An accurate and inexpensive carrier detection test is available (serum or leukocyte hexosaminidase A), and the disease can be reliably diagnosed by chorionic villus sampling during the 1st trimester of pregnancy in couples at risk (heterozygote parents).

Sandhoff disease is very similar to TSD in the mode of presentation, including progressive loss of motor and language milestones beginning at 6 mo of age. Seizures, cherry red spots, macrocephaly, and doll-like facies are present in most patients; however, children with Sandhoff disease may also have splenomegaly. The visual-evoked responses (VEP) are normal early in the course of Sandhoff disease and TSD but become abnormal or absent as the disease progresses. The auditory brain stem responses (ABR) show prolonged latencies. The diagnosis of Sandhoff disease is established by the finding of deficient levels of hexosaminidase A and B in serum and leukocytes. Children usually succumb by 3 yr of age.

Juvenile GM_2 gangliosidosis develops in mid-childhood, initially with clumsiness followed by ataxia. Signs of spasticity, athetosis, loss of language, and seizures gradually develop. Progressive visual loss is associated with optic atrophy, but cherry red spots rarely occur in juvenile GM_2 gangliosidosis. A deficiency of hexosaminidase is variable (total deficiency to near-normal) in these patients. Death occurs around 15 yr of age. *Adult GM_2 gangliosidosis* is characterized by a myriad of neurologic signs, including slowly progressive gait ataxia, spasticity, dystonia, proximal muscle atrophy, and dysarthria. Generally, visual acuity and intellectual function are unimpaired. Hexosaminidase A or A and B activity is reduced significantly in the serum and leukocytes.

KRABBE DISEASE (GLOBOID CELL LEUKODYSTROPHY). Krabbe disease (KD) is a rare autosomal recessive neurodegenerative disorder characterized by severe myelin loss and the presence of globoid bodies in the white matter. The disease results from a marked deficiency of the lysosomal enzyme galactocerebroside β-galactosidase, which cleaves a galactose moiety from the ceramide portion of galactocerebroside. KD is a disorder of myelin destruction rather than abnormal myelin formation. Normally, myelination begins during the 3rd trimester, corresponding with a rapid rise of galactocerebroside β-galactosidase activity in the brain. In patients with Krabbe disease, galactocerebroside cannot be metabolized during the normal turnover of myelin because of the deficiency of galactocerebroside β-galactosidase. When galactocerebroside is injected into the brains of experimental animals, a globoid cell reaction ensues. It has been postulated that a similar phenomenon occurs in humans; nonmetabolized galactocerebroside stimulates the formation of globoid cells that reflect the destruction of oligodendroglia cells. Because oligodendroglia are responsible for the elaboration of myelin, their loss results in myelin breakdown, thus producing additional galactocerebroside and causing a vicious cycle of myelin destruction.

The symptoms of KD become evident during the first few months of life and include excessive irritability and crying, unexplained episodes of hyperpyrexia, feeding problems, vomiting, and failure to thrive. During the initial stages of KD, children are often treated for colic or "milk allergy" with frequent formula changes. Generalized seizures may appear early in the course of the disease. Alterations in body tone with rigidity and opisthotonus and visual inattentiveness owing to optic atrophy become apparent as the disease progresses. During the later stages of the illness, blindness, deafness, absent deep tendon reflexes, and decerebrate rigidity constitute the major physical findings. Most patients expire by 2 yr of age.

A *late onset KD* has been described beginning in childhood or during adolescence. These patients present with optic atrophy and cortical blindness and are often confused with the adrenoleukodystrophies. Slowly progressive gait disturbances, including spasticity and ataxia, are prominent. As with classic KD, globoid cells are abundant in the white matter and a deficiency in galactocerebroside β-galactosidase is present in leukocytes. An examination of the CSF shows an elevated protein content, and the nerve conduction velocities are markedly delayed owing to segmental demyelination of the peripheral nerves. The VEPs decrease gradually in amplitude with no response in the late stages of the disease, and the ABRs are characterized by the presence of only waves I and II. CT scans and MRI studies highlight the marked decrease in white matter, especially of the cerebellum and centrum semiovale, with sparing of the subcortical u fibers. Prenatal diagnosis is possible by the assay of galactocerebroside β-galactosidase activity in chorionic villi or in cultured amniotic fluid cells.

METACHROMATIC LEUKODYSTROPHY (MLD). This disorder of myelin metabolism is inherited as an autosomal recessive trait and characterized by a deficiency of arylsulfatase A activity. The absence or deficiency of arylsulfatase A leads to the accumulation of cerebroside sulfate within the myelin sheath of the CNS and peripheral nervous system, owing to the inability to cleave sulfate from galactosyl-3-sulfate ceramide. The excessive cerebroside sulfate is thought to cause myelin breakdown and destruction of oligodendroglia. The prenatal diagnosis of MLD is made by the assay of arylsulfatase A in chorionic villi or cultured amniotic fluid cells. Cresyl violet applied to tissue specimens produces metachromatic staining of the sulfatide granules, giving the disease its name. Six disorders are included in the MLD group of diseases, classified by the age of onset and enzyme deficiency. Three conditions are briefly discussed: the classic or late infantile, juvenile, and adult leukodystrophy.

Late infantile MLD begins with the insidious onset of gait disturbance between 1 and 2 yr of age. Initially the child appears awkward and frequently falls, but gradually locomotion is impaired significantly and support is required in order to walk. The extremities are hypotonic, and the deep tendon reflexes are absent or diminished. During the next several months the child can no longer stand, and a deterioration in intellectual function becomes apparent. The speech is slurred and dysarthric, and the child appears dull and apathetic. Visual fixation is diminished; nystagmus is present;

and examination of the retina shows optic atrophy. Within 1 year from the onset of the disease the child is unable to sit unsupported, and progressive decorticate postures develop. Feeding and swallowing are impaired owing to pseudobulbar palsies, and a feeding gastrostomy is required. The patient ultimately becomes stuporous and dies of bronchopneumonia by 5–6 yr of age. Neurophysiologic evaluation shows progressive changes in the VEPs, ABRs, and the somatosensory evoked potentials (SSEP), and the nerve conduction velocities (NCVs) of the peripheral nerves are significantly reduced. CT images of the brain indicate diffuse symmetric attenuation of the cerebellar and cerebral white matter, and examination of the CSF shows an elevated protein content. *Juvenile MLD* shares many features in common with late infantile MLD, but the onset of symptoms is delayed to 5–10 yr of age. Deterioration in school performance and alterations in personality may herald the onset of the disease. This is followed by incoordination of gait, urinary incontinence, and dysarthria. Muscle tone becomes increased, and ataxia, dystonia, or tremor may be present. During the terminal stages, generalized tonic-clonic convulsions are prominent and are difficult to control. The child rarely lives beyond midadolescence. *Adult MLD* occurs from the 2nd to 6th decade. Abnormalities in memory, psychiatric disturbances, and personality changes are prominent features. Slowly progressive neurologic signs, including spasticity, dystonia, optic atrophy, and generalized convulsions, lead eventually to a bedridden state characterized by decorticate postures and unresponsiveness.

20.60 NEURONAL CEROID LIPOFUSCINOSES

These are the most common class of neurodegenerative diseases in children and consist of three disorders inherited as autosomal recessive traits. They are characterized by the storage of an autofluorescent substance within neurons and other tissues. *Infantile type (Haltia-Santavuori)* begins toward the end of the 1st year of life with myoclonic seizures, intellectual deterioration, and blindness. Optic atrophy and brownish discoloration of the macula is evident upon examination of the retina, and cerebellar ataxia is prominent. The electroretinogram (ERG) typically shows small amplitude or absent wave forms. Death occurs at approximately 10 yr of age. *Late infantile (Jansky-Bielschowsky)* is the most common type of neuronal ceroid lipofuscinosis. It presents with myoclonic seizures between 2 and 4 yr of age in a previously normal child. Dementia and ataxia are combined with a progressive loss of visual acuity and microcephaly. An examination of the retina shows marked attenuation of vessels, peripheral black "bone spicule" pigmentary abnormalities, optic atrophy, and a subtle brown pigment in the macular region. The ERG is abnormal early in the course due to the deposition of the abnormal storage substance within the rod and cone area of the retina. The VER is characteristic and consists of markedly enlarged responses followed by absent wave forms with progression of the disease. The autofluorescent material is deposited in neurons, fibroblasts, and secretory cells. Electron microscopic examination of the storage material in skin or conjunctival biopsies typically shows curvilinear bodies or "fingerprint profiles." *Juvenile type (Spielmeyer-Vogt)* is characterized by progressive visual loss and intellectual impairment beginning between 5 and 10 yr of age. The funduscopic changes are similar to those for the late infantile type. The ERG is also abnormal early in the course of the disease, but in the juvenile type, the VER typically consists of small amplitude waves followed by absent wave forms as the disease progresses. Myoclonic seizures are not as prominent as in the late infantile type of neuronal ceroid lipofuscinosis, but dystonic posturing is marked during the late stages of the disease. Elevated urine dolichol levels are a nonspecific finding. Ultrastructural abnormalities of skin biopsies are present in most cases.

20.61 ADRENOLEUKODYSTROPHY

(See Sec. 8.17)

The adrenoleukodystrophies consist of a group of CNS degenerative disorders that are often associated with adrenal cortical insufficiency and are inherited by X-linked recessive transmission. *Classic adrenoleukodystrophy* becomes symptomatic between 5 and 15 yr of age with evidence of academic deterioration, behavioral disturbances, and gait abnormalities. Generalized seizures are common in the early stages. Upper motor neuron signs include spastic quadriparesis and contractures, ataxia, and marked swallowing disturbances secondary to pseudobulbar palsy. These dominate the terminal stages of the illness. Hypoadrenalism is present in approximately 50% of cases, and adrenal insufficiency characterized by abnormal skin pigmentation may precede the onset of neurologic symptoms. CT scans and MRI studies of patients indicate periventricular demyelination beginning posteriorly, which advances progressively to the anterior regions of the cerebral white matter. ABR, VER, and SSEP may be normal initially but ultimately show prolonged latencies and abnormal wave forms. Death supervenes within 10 yr of the onset of the neurologic signs. *Adrenomyeloneuropathy* begins with a slowly progressive spastic paraparesis, urinary incontinence, and impotence during the 3rd or 4th decade despite the fact that adrenal insufficiency may have been present since childhood. Cases of typical adrenoleukodystrophy have occurred in families in whom the propositus presented with adrenomyeloneuropathy. *Neonatal adrenoleukodystrophy* is characterized by marked hypotonia, severe psychomotor retardation, and the early onset of seizures. It is inherited as an autosomal recessive condition. Visual inattention is secondary to optic atrophy. Adrenal function tests are normal, but adrenal atrophy is evident at post mortem. Correction of adrenal insufficiency is ineffective in halting neurologic deterioration.

20.62 SIALIDOSIS

Sialidosis is inherited as an autosomal recessive trait and results from the accumulation of a sialic acid-oligosaccharide complex secondary to a deficiency in the lysosomal enzyme neuraminidase. The urinary excretion of sialic acid–containing oligosaccharides is increased significantly in affected patients. *Sialidosis type I*, coined the cherry red spot–myoclonus syndrome (CRSM), usually presents during the 2nd decade with complaints of visual deterioration. Inspection of the retina shows a cherry red spot, but, unlike patients with Tay-Sachs disease, visual acuity declines slowly in individuals with CRSM. Myoclonus of the extremities is gradually progressive, often debilitating, and eventually renders the patient nonambulatory. The myoclonus is triggered by voluntary movement, touch, and sound and is not controlled with anticonvulsants. Generalized convulsions responsive to antiepileptics have been reported in most patients. *Sialidosis type II* may be subdivided into an infantile and juvenile form, depending on the age of presentation. In addition to cherry red spots and myoclonus, these patients have somatic involvement including coarse facial features, corneal clouding in a few, and dysostosis multiplex, producing anterior beaking of the lumbar vertebrae. An examination of lymphocytes shows vacuoles in the cytoplasm; biopsy of the liver demonstrates cytoplasmic vacuoles in Kupffer cells; and membrane-bound vacuoles are found in Schwann cell cytoplasm, all attesting to the multiorgan nature of sialidosis type II. There are no distinctive neuroimaging findings or abnormalities in electrophysiologic studies in this group of disorders. Patients with sialidosis have been reported to live beyond the 5th decade.

MISCELLANEOUS CAUSES OF NEURODEGENERATIVE DISORDERS

20.63 MULTIPLE SCLEROSIS

Multiple sclerosis (MS) is a chronic and remitting disorder characterized by white matter lesions in the CNS disseminated in time and space. The condition is rare in the pediatric population, and onset prior to 10 yr of age is 0.2–2% of all cases. There is a greater incidence of MS in females in the pediatric age group compared with adults. The etiology of MS is unknown, but interactive genetic, immunologic, and infectious factors are probably responsible. The most frequent presenting symptom is unilateral weakness or ataxia. Headache is an important early component of the disease and is often severe, prolonged, and generalized. Ill-defined paresthesias involving the lower extremities, distal portions of the hands and feet, and the face are common. Visual symptoms including diplopia, blurred vision, or sudden visual loss secondary to optic neuritis are also important early manifestations of MS. Vertigo, dysarthria, and sphincter disturbances are relatively uncommon. *Neuromyelitis optica (Devic disease)* is a variant of classic MS and consists of optic neuritis and transverse myelitis, which occur conjointly.

The pathology of MS consists of demyelination with the formation of plaques. There is no reliable laboratory test that unequivocally confirms the diagnosis of MS, except for an autopsy. MRI is the neuroimaging technique of choice; small plaques of 3–4 mm can be identified, particularly those located in the brain stem and spinal cord.

The treatment of MS is supportive, and particular attention is given to the management of a neurogenic bladder. There is no evidence that corticosteroids alter the long-term course of the disease, but they may expedite recovery following an acute attack. The prognosis for childhood MS is similar to that in adults; recovery is often complete, and the progression of the disease tends to be slow with long periods of remission in most cases.

20.64 PELIZAEUS-MERZBACHER DISEASE

This disease consists of a group of disorders that is characterized by nystagmus and abnormalities of myelin. The classic form is inherited as an X-linked recessive trait and is recognized by nystagmus and roving eye movements with head-nodding during infancy. The child's developmental milestones are delayed, and ultimately ataxia, choreoathetosis, and spasticity develop. Optic atrophy and dysarthria are associated findings, and death occurs in the 2nd or 3rd decade. The major pathologic finding is a loss of myelin with intact axons, suggesting a defect in the function of oligodendroglia. Studies point to a genetic defect in the biosynthesis of proteolipid apoprotein, a protein that is concerned with the differentiation and maintenance of oligodendrocytes. The CT scan is normal or, in the late stages, shows ventricular dilatation. Multimodal evoked potential studies demonstrate an interesting pattern early in the course, consisting of loss of waves III–V on the ABR. This finding is useful in the investigation of nystagmus in the male infant. VEPs show prolonged latencies, and SSEPs show absent cortical responses or delayed latencies.

20.65 ALEXANDER DISEASE

Alexander disease is a rare disorder that causes progressive macrocephaly during the 1st year of life. Pathologic examination of the brain features the deposition of eosinophilic hyaline bodies in a perivascular distribution throughout the brain and beneath the pia mater. Degeneration of white matter is most prominent in the frontal lobes, and a CT scan during this stage shows corresponding attenuation of the cerebral white matter. The child develops progressive loss of intellect, spasticity, and unresponsive seizures causing death by 5 yr of age.

CANAVAN SPONGY DEGENERATION

See Sec. 8.14.

20.66 KINKY HAIR DISEASE

Kinky hair disease (Menkes' disease) is a progressive neurodegenerative condition inherited as a sex-linked recessive trait. Symptoms begin during the first few months of life and include hypothermia, hypotonia, and generalized myoclonic seizures. The facies are distinctive with chubby, rosy cheeks and kinky, colorless, friable hair. Microscopic examination of the hair shows several abnormalities, including trichorrhexis nodosa (fractures along the hair shaft) and pili torti (twisted hair). Feeding difficulties are prominent and lead to failure to thrive. Severe mental retardation and optic atrophy are constant features of the disease. Low serum copper and ceruloplasmin levels have been found consistently in patients with kinky hair disease, and a defect in copper absorption and transport across the gut has been postulated as the cause of the condition. Neuropathologic changes include tortuous cerebral vessels secondary to defects in the intima, focal degeneration of the gray matter, and marked changes in the cerebellum with loss of the internal granule cell layer and necrosis of the Purkinje cells. Although the use of parenteral copper has been reported to give inconsistent results, a course of IV cupric acetate (550–800 μg/kg/24 hr) until the serum copper and ceruloplasmin return to normal, followed by a dose of 190–220 μg/kg IV twice a week, is recommended. The copper infusions are maintained indefinitely as long as neurodevelopment proceeds but are discontinued if the degenerative process cannot be controlled. More recently, subcutaneous copper histidinate (250–600 μg/24 hr) has been used with encouraging results, particularly if therapy is begun during the neonatal period. The copper histidinate compound is probably permeable across the blood-brain barrier and will likely replace IV cupric acetate as the treatment of choice.

20.67 RETT SYNDROME

This is a neurodegenerative disorder of unknown etiology that occurs exclusively in female children and has an incidence of 1/15,000. Development proceeds normally until 1 yr of age when regression of language and motor milestones and acquired microcephaly become apparent. An ataxic gait or fine tremor of hand movements is an early neurologic finding. Most children develop peculiar sighing respirations with intermittent periods of apnea that may be associated with cyanosis. The hallmark of Rett syndrome is repetitive hand-wringing movements and a loss of purposeful and spontaneous use of the hands, which may not appear until 2–3 yr of age. Autistic behavior is a typical finding in all patients.

Generalized tonic-clonic convulsions occur in the majority and are usually well controlled by anticonvulsants. Feeding disorders and poor weight gain are common. Several studies have shown elevated CSF levels of endorphins in Rett syndrome. Trials of opiate receptor–blocking agents (e.g., naltrexone) have improved the apnea and behavior abnormalities in some patients. After the initial period of neurologic regression, the disease process appears to plateau, with a persistence of the autistic behavior.

20.68 SUBACUTE SCLEROSING PANENCEPHALITIS

Subacute sclerosing panencephalitis (SSPE) is a rare, progressive slow-virus infection of the CNS caused by a measles-like virus (Sec. 12.83). The number of reported cases has decreased dramatically to 0.06 cases/million population, paralleling the decline in reported measles cases. The initial clinical manifestations include personality changes, aggressive behavior, and impairment of cognitive function. Myoclonic seizures soon dominate the clinical picture. Later, generalized tonic-clonic convulsions, hypertonia, and choreoathetosis become evident followed by progressive bulbar palsy, hyperthermia, and decerebrate postures. Funduscopic examination early in the course of the disease reveals papilledema in approximately 20% of the cases. Optic atrophy, chorioretinitis, and macular pigmentation are observed in most patients. The *diagnosis* is established by the typical clinical course and one of the following: (1) measles antibody detected in the CSF, (2) a characteristic EEG consisting of bursts of high-voltage slow waves interspersed with a normal background in the early stages, and (3) typical histologic findings in the brain biopsy or post mortem specimen. *Treatment* with a series of antiviral agents has been attempted without success. Death occurs usually within 1–2 yr from the onset of symptoms.

Banker BQ, Robertson JT, Victor M: Spongy degenerations of the central nervous system in infancy. Neurology 14:981, 1964.
Baram TZ, Goldman AM, Percy AK: Krabbe disease: Specific MRI and CT findings. Neurology 36:111, 1986.
Boustany RMN, Alroy J, Kolodny EH: Clinical classification of neuronal ceroid-lipofuscinosis subtypes. Am J Med Genet 5(Suppl):47, 1988.
Centerick C, Martin J-J: Diagnostic role of skin or conjunctival biopsies in neurological disorders: An update. J Neurol Sci 65:179, 1984.
Danks DM, Campbell PE, Stevens BJ, et al: Menkes' kinky hair syndrome: An inherited defect in copper absorption with widespread effects. Pediatrics 50:188, 1972.
De Meirleir LJ, Taylor MJ, Logan WJ: Multimodal evoked potential studies in leukodystrophies of children. Can J Neurol Sci 15:26, 1988.
Duquette P, Murray TJ, Pleines J, et al: Multiple sclerosis in childhood: Clinical profile in 125 patients. J Pediatr 111:359, 1987.
Dyken PR, Cunningham SC, Ward LC: Changing character of subacute sclerosing panencephalitis in the United States. Pediatr Neurol 5:339, 1989.
Ebers GC, Bulman DE, Sadovnick AD, et al: A population-based study of multiple sclerosis in twins. N Engl J Med 315:1638, 1986.
Farrell DF, Swedberg K: Clinical and biochemical heterogeneity of globoid cell leukodystrophy. Ann Neurol 10:364, 1981.
Farrell K, Chuang S, Becker LE: Computed tomography in Alexander's disease. Ann Neurol 15:605, 1984.
Ferriero D, Koch TK: Computed tomography in white matter diseases. Ann Neurol 17:314, 1985.
Grover WD, Scrutton MC: Copper infusion therapy in trichopoliodystrophy. J Pediatr 86:216, 1975.
Hagberg B, Aicardi J, Dias K, et al: A progressive syndrome of autism, dementia, ataxia and loss of purposeful hand use in girls: Rett's syndrome: Report of 35 cases. Ann Neurol 14:471, 1983.
Hartter DE, Barnea A: Brain tissue accumulates ^{6}F copper by two-ligand-dependent saturable processes. J Biol Chem 263:799, 1988.
Johnson WG: The clinical spectrum of hexosaminidase deficiency disease. Neurology 31:1453, 1981.
Kelley RI, Datta NS, Dobyns WB, et al: Neonatal adrenoleukodystrophy: New cases, biochemical studies and differentiation from Zellweger and related peroxisomal polydystrophy syndromes. Am J Med Genet 23:869, 1986.
Koeppen AH, Ronca NA, Greenfield EA, et al: Defective biosynthesis of proteolipid protein in Pelizaeus-Merzbacher disease. Ann Neurol 21:159, 1987.
Lowden JA, O'Brien JS: Sialidosis: A review of human neuraminidase deficiency. Am J Hum Genet 31:1, 1979.
MacFaul R, Cavanagh N, Lake BD, et al: Metachromatic leukodystrophy: Review of 38 cases. Arch Dis Child 57:168, 1982.
McKhann GM: Metachromatic leukodystrophy: Clinical and enzymatic parameters. Neuropediatrics 15(Suppl):4, 1984.
Mobley WC, White CL, Tennekoon G, et al: Neonatal adrenoleukodystrophy. Ann Neurol 12:204, 1982.
Moser HW, Moser AE, Singh I, et al: Adrenoleukodystrophy: Survey of 303 cases: Biochemistry, diagnosis, and therapy. Ann Neurol 16:628, 1984.
O'Brien JS: Beta-galactosidase deficiency; ganglioside sialidase deficiency. *In:* Scriver CR, Beaudet AL, Shy WS, Valle D (eds): The Metabolic Basis of Inherited Disease, 6th ed. New York, McGraw-Hill, 1989.
Percy AK: The inherited neurodegenerative disorders of childhood: Clinical assessment. J Child Neurol 2:82, 1987.
Rapin I, Goldfischer S, Katzman R, et al: The cherry-red spot myoclonus syndrome. Ann Neurol 3:234, 1978.
Suzuki K, Suzuki Y: Globoid cell leukodystrophy (Krabbe's disease): Deficiency of galactocerebroside β-galactosidase. Proc Natl Acad Sci (USA) 66:302, 1970.
Tyler HR: Pelizaeus-Merzbacher disease. Arch Neurol Psychiatr 80:162, 1958.
Zeman W, Dyken P: Neuronal ceroid-lipofuscinosis (Batten's disease): Relationship to amaurotic family idiocy? Pediatrics 44:570, 1969.

VASCULAR DISORDERS

Hemiplegia secondary to vascular disorders occurs in children with an incidence of 3–8/100,000. The pediatric causes of *stroke* are distinctive compared with the adult. They include arterial and venous thrombosis, intracranial hemorrhage, embolism, and various miscellaneous conditions. The cause of a stroke in children is established in approximately 50% of cases. As the mode of presentation of acute stroke syndromes is not uniform, a brief description of the most prevalent causes follows.

20.69 ARTERIAL THROMBOSIS

Thrombosis of the internal carotid artery may result from blunt trauma due to a fall on a pencil or popsicle stick in the child's mouth. The injury produces a tear in the intima of the vessel wall, which may lead to the formation of a dissecting aneurysm. Cerebral symptoms result from the shedding of emboli from the thrombus. The onset of symptoms may be delayed up to 24 hours following the accident, with a stuttering but progressive flaccid hemiplegia, lethargy, and aphasia if the dominant hemisphere is involved. Focal motor seizures are a common complication. A *retropharyngeal abscess* may produce an identical clinical picture, but in this case the arterial thrombosis results from inflammation of the intima. A cerebral angiogram typically demonstrates occlusion of the internal carotid artery, and the CT scan shows a hypodense lesion representing the area of infarction. *Cyanotic congenital heart disease* in children less than 2 yr of age may cause thrombosis of the middle cerebral artery. These patients are particularly vulnerable when the oxygen saturation is significantly decreased together with a viral illness or state of dehydration. The *collagen vascular diseases*, particularly lupus erythematosus and polyarteritis nodosa, frequently produce cerebral symptoms and signs including hemiparesis owing to arterial thrombosis. A series of occlusive vascular disorders, some of which are unique in children, are prominent causes of acute hemiplegia. *Basal arterial occlusion without telangiectasia* results from narrowing of the supraclinoid portion of the internal carotid artery or the proximal segments of the anterior and middle cerebral arteries. As these lesions tend to be congenital and collateral vessels develop, the prognosis for recovery is usually excellent.

Basal arterial occlusion with telangiectasia or *Moyamoya disease* has a characteristic angiogram (Fig. 20–18). The condition is more common in girls and often presents with severe headache and bilateral upper motor neuron signs. It may present with chorea. The prognosis for recovery is poor, with inter-

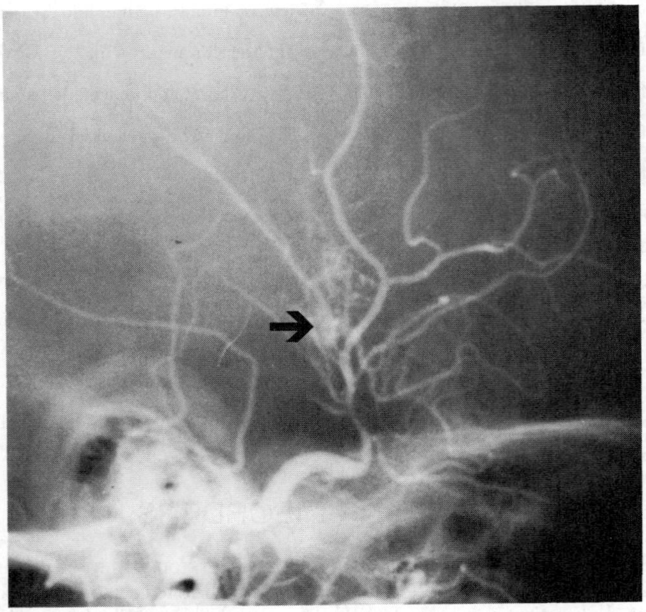

Figure 20–18. Cerebral angiogram showing idiopathic supraclinoid-internal carotid arteriopathy with classical Moyamoya collaterals *(arrow)*.

mittent episodes of transient ischemic attacks coupled with progressive neurologic signs and severe disability. Surgical procedures have been designed to enhance cerebral blood flow (superficial temporal artery to middle cerebral artery shunt and laying the superficial temporal artery on the arachnoid membrane) with variable results. *Occlusion of distal arteries* is associated with diabetes mellitus, neurofibromatosis, sickle cell disease, and IV drug abuse. The patient presents with unilateral neurological signs, and recovery is often complete owing to the small area of infarction. Patients with *thrombosis of small arteries*, including the perforating striate vessels, due to polyarteritis nodosa and homocystinuria, have a progressive debilitating course characterized by bilateral signs and a high mortality.

20.70 VENOUS THROMBOSIS/EMBOLISM

Hemiplegia is a relatively common complication of *bacterial meningitis* due to thrombosis of the superficial cortical and deep penetrating veins. Additional infectious causes of stroke in children include *otitis media* and *mastoiditis* with involvement of the dural vessels, and retrograde orbital infections producing *cavernous sinus thrombosis*. *Severe dehydration* during infancy may cause thrombosis of the superior sagittal sinus and the superficial cortical veins due to hyperviscosity and sludging of blood. Conditions causing hypercoagulopathy, cyanotic congenital heart disease, and leukemic infiltrates of cerebral veins are additional causes of acute hemiplegia of childhood. *Embolization* of cerebral vessels, although rare in children, may also produce acute hemiparesis. Cardiac causes include arrhythmias (particularly atrial fibrillation), myxoma, and bacterial endocarditis that results in a mycotic aneurysm. Air emboli may complicate surgery, and fat emboli occur with fracture of long bones. Septic emboli may seed in the cerebral vessels and evolve into an area of cerebritis leading to a cerebral abscess.

20.71 INTRACRANIAL HEMORRHAGE

Arteriovenous malformations result as a consequence of the failure of normal capillary bed development between arteries and veins during embryogenesis. The arteriovenous malformation produces abnormal shunting of blood, causing an expansion of vessels and a space-occupying effect or rupture of a vein and intracerebral bleeding. Arteriovenous malformations are typically located in the cerebral hemispheres, but they may be situated in the cerebellum, brain stem, or spinal cord. Although the malformation may remain asymptomatic throughout life, rupture and bleeding can occur at any age. Children with arteriovenous malformations frequently have a history of migraine-like headaches. Typical migraine alternates from one side of the head to the other, whereas headaches associated with an arteriovenous malformation classically remain on the same side. Auscultation of the skull is positive for a high-pitched bruit in approximately 50% of cases. Rupture of an arteriovenous malformation causes a severe headache, vomiting, nuchal rigidity due to subarachnoid bleeding, progressive hemiparesis, and a focal or generalized seizure. An **arteriovenous malformation of the vein of Galen** during infancy can cause high-output congestive heart failure secondary to shunting of large volumes of blood or progressive hydrocephalus and increased intracranial pressure due to obstruction of the CSF pathways.

Cerebral aneurysms producing symptoms in children are relatively rare. In contrast to adults, aneurysms in children tend to be large and are located at the carotid bifurcation or on the anterior and posterior cerebral arteries rather than the circle of Willis. The aneurysmal dilatation results from a congenital weakness of the vessel, and in some cases a deficiency of type III collagen has been demonstrated. In children, there is an association between cerebral aneurysms and coarctation of the aorta and bilateral polycystic kidney disease. Although most ruptured aneurysms bleed into the subarachnoid space causing an intense headache, nuchal rigidity, and coma, intracerebral hemorrhage and progressive hemiparesis also occur. Additional causes of intracerebral hematoma include hematologic disorders, particularly thrombocytopenic purpura and hemophilia. Finally, trauma can produce hemiparesis due to intracerebral bleeding or a subdural or epidural hematoma. A contrast CT scan is useful for the identification of large arteriovenous malformations; however, four-vessel cerebral angiography is the study of choice for the investigation of arteriovenous malformations and cerebral aneurysm.

20.72 BRAIN ABSCESS

A brain abscess may be a complication of embolization due to congenital heart disease with right to left shunts in children over 2 yr of age, meningitis, penetrating head injuries, and direct extension from mastoiditis, otitis, sinusitis, or soft tissue infection of the face, orbit, or scalp. The responsible bacteria include *S. aureus*, microaerophilic streptococci, and a large group of ubiquitous aerobic and anaerobic organisms, fungi, and parasites. Mixed organisms are cultured in approximately 25% of the cases. Abscesses associated with a penetrating wound tend to be single, whereas those caused by septic emboli or congenital heart disease are often multiple. The early stages of cerebritis and abscess formation are associated with nonspecific findings including a low-grade fever, headache, and lethargy. An antibiotic is often inappropriately prescribed (for an upper respiratory infection or otitis media), and the symptoms are briefly relieved during the course of therapy. The white blood count is characteristically normal, and an examination of the CSF may show a few white blood cells and an elevated protein content count. As the abscess enlarges, signs of increased intracranial pressure, including papilledema and progressive hemiparesis, become evident. If the abscess ruptures into the ventricular cavity, overwhelming shock and death usually ensue. The EEG shows corresponding focal slowing; the brain scan shows an area of enhancement due to disruption of the blood-brain barrier; and the CT scan shows the typical abscess cavity. The management of a cerebral abscess includes prompt diagnosis and the institution of broad-spectrum antibiotics, such as the combination of IV penicillin and chloramphenicol. The antibiotics are adjusted according to the results of the blood and abscess culture and sensitivity. Although some children with cerebral abscess may be managed conservatively with appropriate antibiotics and frequent CT scans, most require a combination of surgical drainage or excision of the abscess cavity and antibiotic therapy for a minimum of 6 wk. Mortality is 10–30%; 40–65% have neurologic sequellae.

20.73 MISCELLANEOUS CAUSES OF STROKE

Alternating hemiplegia complicating migraine (Sec. 20.36), which begins during infancy and early childhood, has a poor prognosis. There is often a strong maternal family history of classic migraine. These attacks have an abrupt onset and recovery typically begins within a few hours. Residual neurologic deficits that result from prolonged vasospasm and ischemia during the migraine attack are common and consist of permanent hemiparesis, mental retardation, focal seizures, and movement disorders. *Todd paralysis* may be confused initially with a stroke. The hemiparesis follows a focal seizure, but the weakness and neurologic signs disappear completely within 24 hr of the convulsion. Although the cause of Todd paralysis remains unknown, the hemiparesis probably results from an inhibitory phenomenon, possibly related to neurotransmitter dysfunction. Additional causes of hemiparesis include *cerebral tumor, encephalitis* (particularly herpes), *focal postviral encephalitis,* and *status epilepticus.* In some pediatric series of unexplained stroke, *lipid abnormalities* including elevated triglycerides and low levels of high-density lipoprotein cholesterol have been found in approximately 20% of the cases. The family histories of these children reveal an increased incidence of premature coronary heart disease and early ischemic cerebrovascular diseases. Screening of at-risk families will identify children who may benefit from long-term dietary management.

Investigation of Strokes

The most critical component of the investigation is a thorough history and physical examination, searching for an underlying disease process; evidence of trauma; an infectious, metabolic, or hematologic disorder; neurocutaneous syndrome; increased intracranial pressure; or hydrocephalus. Appropriate tests for infectious diseases, metabolic disorders, and hematologic disorders are based on the results of the history and physical examination. An EEG may be helpful in localizing the disease process but will rarely establish the diagnosis. A brain scan is extremely useful in cases of focal encephalitis, cerebritis, cerebral abscess, and infarction. A CT scan or MRI is mandatory in the investigation of children with acute hemiparesis. A cerebral angiogram is essential for those children in whom a CT scan or MRI is nondiagnostic. In these cases, a four-vessel cerebral angiogram should be planned. Electrocardiography and echocardiography may help to exclude intrinsic cardiac diseases or an arrhythmia as a cause of the stroke. Finally, a search for a lipid disorder is indicated in those cases of stroke with an unknown cause, particularly when a family history of premature cardiac or cerebrovascular disease is elicited.

Banker BQ: Cerebral vascular disease in infancy and childhood: Occlusive vascular diseases. J Neuropathol Exp Neurol 20:127, 1961.
Fischer EG, McLennan JE, Suzuki Y: Cerebral abscess in children. Am J Dis Child 135:746, 1981.
Glueck CJ, Daniels SR, Bates S, et al: Pediatric victims of unexplained stroke and their families: Familial lipid and lipoprotein abnormalities. Pediatrics 69:308, 1982.
Harwood-Nash DC, McDonald P, Argent W: Cerebral arterial disease in children: An angiographic study of 40 cases. Am J Roentgenol Radium Ther Nucl Med 111:672, 1971.
Kelly JJ, Mellinger JF, Sundt TM: Intracranial arteriovenous malformations in childhood. Ann Neurol 3:338, 1978.
Pitner SE: Carotid thrombosis due to intraoral trauma. N Engl J Med 274:764, 1966.
Schoenberg BS, Mellinger JF, Schoenberg DG: Cerebrovascular disease in infants and children: A study of incidence, clinical features and survival. Neurology 28:763, 1978.
Seeler RA, Royal JE, Powe L, et al: Moya-moya in children with sickle cell anemia and cerebrovascular occlusion. J Pediatr 93:808, 1978.
Shillito J Jr: Carotid arteritis: A cause of hemiplegia in childhood. J Neurosurg 21:540, 1964.
Thompson JR, Harwood-Nash DC, Fitz CR: Cerebral aneurysms in children. Am J Roentgenol 188:163, 1973.
Tomsick TA, Lukin RR, Chambers AA, et al: Neurofibromatosis and intracranial arterial occlusive disease. Neuroradiology 11:229, 1976.
Tyler HR, Clark DB: Cerebrovascular accidents in patients with congenital heart disease. Arch Neurol Psychiatry 77:483, 1957.
Watanabe K, Negoro T, Maehara M, et al: Moyamoya disease presenting with chorea. Pediatr Neurol 6:40, 1990.
Wisoff HS, Rothballer AB: Cerebral arterial thrombosis in children. Arch Neurol 4:258, 1961.

20.74 BRAIN TUMORS IN CHILDREN

(See also Sec. 17.1)

Brain tumors are second only to leukemia as the most prevalent malignancy in childhood, and they account for the most common solid tumors in this age group. Brain tumors can present at any age, but each tends to have a peak age incidence. Metastatic brain tumors are common in the adult but are relatively rare in the child.

EPIDEMIOLOGY. Generally, infratentorial tumors (located in the posterior fossa) are more prevalent in the pediatric age group, except for infants less than 2 yr of age and adolescents, where the frequency of supratentorial tumors is equivalent to those located in the posterior fossa. Approximately two thirds of all intracranial tumors between the ages of 2 and 12 are infratentorial in location. Supratentorial tumors predominate in the adult.

PATHOLOGY AND PATHOGENESIS. There are two major histologic types of brain tumors in children, glial cell tumors and those of primitive neuroectodermal cell origin. Glial cell tumors are the most common and consist of a variety of cell types with variable prognoses including the astrocytoma, ependymoma, and glioblastoma multiforme. Neuroectodermal tumors probably arise from a primitive, undifferentiated cell line and are prominent throughout the CNS, involving the cerebellum (medulloblastoma), cerebrum, spinal cord, and pineal gland (pineoblastoma) (see Sec. 17.20). Some tumors are unique because they originate from embryonic remnants such as the craniopharyngioma, which arises from Rathke pouch, dermoid and epidermoid tumors from the invagination of epithelial cells during the closure of the neural tube, and the chordoma that develops from traces of the embryonic notochord. The pathogenesis of brain tumors is complex because there appear to be many factors at play in their development. Certain diseases associated with immunologic dysfunction (e.g., ataxia telangiectasia and AIDS) render the host susceptible to brain tumors, particularly lymphomas. Conditions that result from abnormalities of neural crest development have a high association with tumors of the CNS. Patients with neurofibromatosis have a greater chance than the general population of developing optic

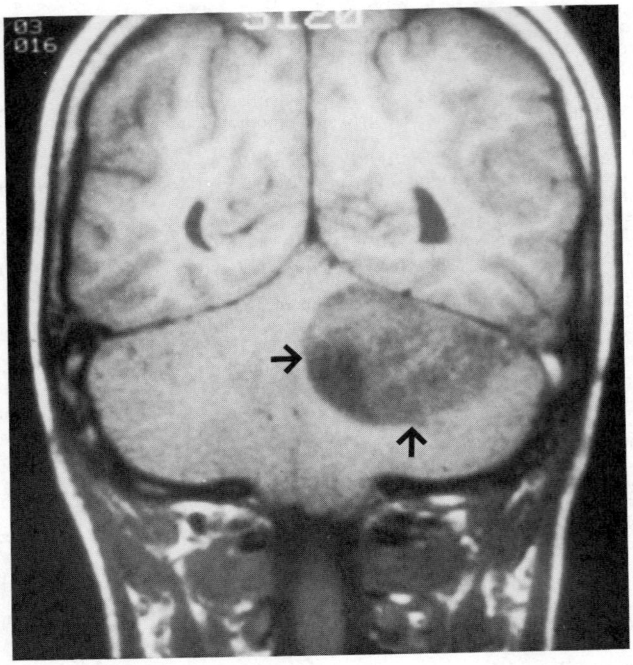

Figure 20–19. A coronal MRI of a large, primarily solid, cerebellar astrocytoma *(arrows)*.

glioma, acoustic neuroma, meningioma, or tumors involving the spinal cord. Some patients who received radiation for scalp disorders during childhood develop cranial tumors years later and, occasionally, second brain tumors develop after radiation for the treatment of a primary brain tumor. Growth factors are known to be important for the development of the nervous system, and they may operate in the neoplastic transformation of neural cells. The role of oncogenes in the pathogenesis of CNS tumors is unquestionably important, and with the application of molecular genetics to the study of tumor formation and control, critical information about the mechanisms of malignant cell transformation should be forthcoming.

CLINICAL MANIFESTATIONS. Brain tumors present in many ways depending on the location, type, and rate of growth of the tumor and the age of the child. Generally, there are two distinct patterns of presentation: symptoms and signs of increased intracranial pressure or focal neurologic signs. Tumors located within the posterior fossa primarily produce symptoms and signs of increased intracranial pressure due to obstruction of CSF pathways and the development of hydrocephalus. Supratentorial tumors are more likely to be associated with focal abnormalities including long-tract signs and seizures.

Alterations in personality are often the first symptoms of a brain tumor, irrespective of its location. The child, for weeks or months prior to the discovery of the tumor, may have become lethargic, irritable, hyperactive, forgetful, and performed poorly academically. It is not certain as to whether the behavioral changes result from increased intracranial pressure, the site of the lesion, or both. After the tumor has been removed and amelioration of the increased intracranial pressure occurs, there is usually a significant reversal of the behavioral problems.

Increased intracranial pressure is characterized by headache, vomiting, diplopia, and papilledema and in the infant a bulging fontanel and increasing head size (macrocrania) develop. Initially, the *headache* tends to occur in the morning and improves with standing as venous flow away from the head is enhanced in the upright position. The headache is described as dull, generalized, and steady and may be intermittent, worsened by coughing, sneezing, or during defecation. The headache is typically associated with *vomiting,* which often relieves the headache. Tumors that occupy the fourth ventricle are often associated with pernicious vomiting. Children who present with vomiting as the initial symptom of a brain tumor are frequently subjected to a series of gastrointestinal investigations. A thorough history and neurologic examination would obviate those tests in many cases. *Diplopia* is a common symptom of posterior fossa tumors. Children do not usually complain of double vision, because they seem to readily suppress the image of the affected eye. Examination of the eye movements shows strabismus owing to involvement of the abducens, oculomotor nerve or, rarely, the trochlear nerve. Some children with diplopia compensate by tilting the head in an attempt to align the two images. *Head tilting and nuchal rigidity* may also indicate herniation of the cerebellar tonsils. In this situation, a lumbar puncture may enhance the herniation and result in death. *Nystagmus* is a prominent sign associated with posterior fossa tumors. Unilateral cerebellar tumors cause horizontal nystagmus, which is exaggerated upon looking to the side of the lesion. Tumors located in the posterior cerebellar vermis or fourth ventricle produce nystagmus in all directions of gaze. Brain stem tumors may result in horizontal, vertical, and rotatory nystagmus. *Papilledema* is the cardinal finding of increased intracranial pressure, but it is important to remember that the infant may decompress the contents of the skull by separation of the cranial sutures and bulging of the anterior fontanel. The head may continue to accelerate in size without associated symptoms and signs of increased intracranial pressure. In this case, papilledema may be conspicuous by its absence. A rapid rise or prolonged increase in intracranial pressure may result in coma with alterations in the vital signs. Bradycardia, an irregular pulse, and systemic hypertension occur associated with alterations in the respiratory pattern. Initially, hyperventilation is noted which, without intervention, progresses to ataxic and irregular breathing followed by respiratory arrest.

Supratentorial tumors may also be associated with symptoms and signs of increased intracranial pressure. However, focal neurologic signs including hemiparesis and complex partial seizures predominate, particularly with a temporal lobe tumor. The greatest oversight in the examination of a child with headache and vomiting is failure to examine the retina and optic nerve. *Obscurations of vision* characterized by blurring is a serious symptom that indicates marked vasoconstriction of cerebral vessels and impending cerebellar herniation.

Ataxia is often associated with posterior fossa tumors, although it is interesting that some large tumors cause absolutely no abnormality of movement. Tumors of the cerebellar vermis characteristically cause truncal ataxia that is enhanced with sitting or standing, and involvement of the anterior cerebellum results in marked gait disturbances that are typically broad-based. Tumors of a cerebellar hemisphere produce ipsilateral extremity ataxia and dysdiadochokinesia. The following sections highlight the pathology, management, and prognosis of the major brain tumors in the pediatric age group.

INFRATENTORIAL TUMORS. The *cerebellar astrocytoma* is the most common posterior fossa tumor of childhood and has the best prognosis. These tumors tend to be cystic and have a mural nodule of solid tumor; however, conversely, they can be solid with little or no cystic cavitation. Those tumors with cystic cavities are filled with a thickened xanthochromic fluid. Cerebellar astrocytomas may be midline involving the vermis or confined to a hemisphere, and, although usually low-grade, they are capable of invading the cerebellar peduncles

(Fig. 20–19). The tumor causes hydrocephalus and symptoms and signs of increased intracranial pressure by obstructing the aqueduct of Sylvius or fourth ventricle. Histologically, the astrocytoma is characterized by protoplasmic and fibrillary astrocytes arranged in a radial fashion interspersed with Rosenthal fibers. The treatment is surgical resection, and the 5-yr survival approaches 90%. Radiation therapy is reserved for patients with high-grade astrocytomas or in whom postoperative tumor progression is evident by clinical and radiologic investigation.

The *medulloblastoma* is the next most common posterior fossa tumor in the pediatric age group and is the most prevalent brain tumor in children less than 7 yr of age. Although the site of origin of the medulloblastoma is unknown, in some cases it starts from the roof of the fourth ventricle and grows rapidly to fill the contents of the fourth ventricle or invade the adjacent cerebellar hemisphere. This tumor may spread over the cerebral convexities or along the spinal cord and is capable of metastasizing to extracranial sites. Microscopically, the tumor is vascular and cellular and is characterized by deeply staining nuclei with scant cytoplasm arranged in pseudorosettes. The prognosis and treatment depends on the age of the child and the size and dissemination of the tumor. Children less than 4 yr of age have a poorer prognosis than older patients. All patients are treated with surgical extirpation and irradiation, particularly those with small tumors and no evidence of dissemination, for whom the expected 5-yr survival rate is 70%. Irradiation is directed to the entire neuroaxis because of the propensity for medulloblastomas to seed to remote sites. In children with large tumors (with or without evidence of dissemination), chemotherapy in addition to surgery and irradiation improve the survival to approximately 45% compared with no survival without chemotherapy. Chemotherapeutic agents used for the treatment of medulloblastoma by the Children's Cancer Study Group include vincristine, lomustine, and prednisone. In the very young patient, most centers follow surgery with chemotherapy and withhold radiation therapy to a later age when the brain is more tolerant to the effects of radiation.

Brain stem gliomas are the third most frequent posterior fossa tumor in children. These tumors are of two types: those that produce diffuse infiltration in the pons extending throughout the brain stem, which at post mortem examination are found to be anaplastic astrocytomas, and low-grade focal tumors in the midbrain and medulla (Fig. 20–20). The symptoms and signs result from invasion and destruction of cranial nerve nuclei and the pyramidal tracts. The most common cranial nerve symptoms include diplopia and facial weakness due to abducens and facial nerve involvement. Later, dysarthria, dysphagia, and dysphonia may result owing to infiltration of the cranial nuclei in the medulla. Pyramidal tract symptoms are manifest by gait disturbances and the presence of generalized upper motor neuron signs. Changes in personality are particularly common with brain stem gliomas and include lethargy, irritability, and aggressive behavior.

Clinical manifestations of increased intracranial pressure including papilledema occur late (if at all) in the course, because the CSF pathways remain patent in most cases until the tumor has grown to a massive size. The surgical treatment of brain stem gliomas is controversial. With newer radioimaging techniques, particularly MRI, the diagnosis is usually apparent and biopsy is unnecessary. However, if the tumor assumes an irregular shape or there is a suggestion of nasopharyngeal origin, biopsy and debulking of the tumor are indicated. The primary treatment is irradiation and, although some brain stem gliomas are radiosensitive, the mean 5-yr survival is approximately 20%. Because the prognosis is so poor, studies are underway to investigate the outcome of high doses (7,000 rad) of hyperfractionated radiation therapy that involves administering radiotherapy at more frequent intervals so that a greater total dose of radiation can be given. Chemotherapy has not proven efficacious for the management of brain stem gliomas. Low-grade focal tumors of the midbrain or medulla have an excellent prognosis following radical excision. The patient is observed, and radiotherapy is withheld unless the residual tumor shows evidence of regrowth.

Ependymomas account for approximately 10% of childhood posterior fossa tumors. These lesions arise from within the fourth ventricle and cause hydrocephalus and signs of increased intracranial pressure due to obstruction of the CSF pathways. Aside from vomiting, headache, and diplopia, nuchal rigidity and torticollis may result owing to herniation of the cerebellar tonsils. Ataxia and focal neurologic signs are usually absent; however, papilledema is a consistent finding in the symptomatic child. The histologic picture consists of rosettes of ependymal cells with cilia protruding into the central cavity. Treatment includes surgical removal and radiation therapy to the tumor region, with a 5-yr survival approximating 50%. If the tumor histology reveals an aggressive anaplastic ependymoma, radiation should be delivered to the entire craniospinal region, because these tumors readily disseminate and are associated with a much less favorable prognosis. Additional tumors that have a proclivity for the posterior fossa include several benign tumors, such as dermoids, epidermoids, chordomas, and teratomas. Although generally nonmalignant, these lesions are capable of producing significant morbidity and death due to their location, size, and possibility of obstructing the normal flow of CSF.

SUPRATENTORIAL TUMORS. The *craniopharyngioma* is the most common supratentorial tumor in children. The tumor may be confined to the sella turcica or it can extend through the diaphragma sella and compress the optic nerve system, pons, or third ventricle, producing hydrocephalus. The tumor consists of solid and cystic areas that have a tendency to calcify. Approximately 90% of craniopharyngiomas show calcification on the plain skull roentgenogram or CT scan. Many children with craniopharyngioma are referred to endocrine clinics because of short stature due to pituitary-hypothalamic involvement. Pressure or injury to the optic chiasm typically produces bitemporal visual field defects, although most chil-

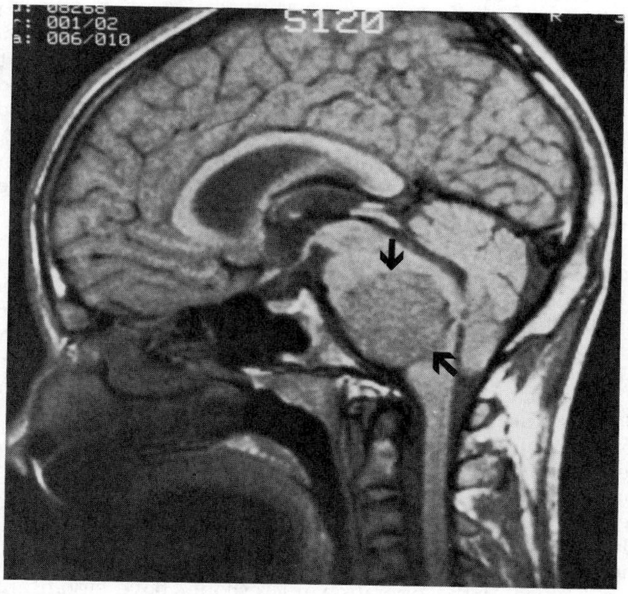

Figure 20–20. MRI of a solid brain stem glioma, an anaplastic astrocytoma *(arrows)*.

dren are unaware of peripheral visual loss until the time of testing. Papilledema and symptoms of increased intracranial pressure are evident when hydrocephalus is prominent. The treatment is a craniotomy using a subfrontal approach. With complete or near-total removal, 75% of patients experience no further recurrence. The role of radiation therapy is still debated, but many centers favor radiation to the sellar region postoperatively only in those cases in which tumor removal is incomplete. Endocrine disorders including diabetes insipidus, hypothyroidism, growth hormone, and adrenocortical deficiency may develop postoperatively and warrant close follow-up. There is no effective chemotherapeutic agent.

Optic nerve gliomas present with decreased visual acuity and pallor of the disks. These tumors are primarily low-grade astrocytomas, and approximately 25% of patients have associated neurofibromatosis (Sec. 20.39). Because optic nerve gliomas may be very slow growing and their response to radiation and chemotherapy is uncertain, most centers follow these patients and resort to surgery, radiation, or chemotherapy when progression of the tumor is documented. The glioma may invade the optic chiasm and hypothalamus, producing visual field defects or the **diencephalic syndrome**. These children are anorectic and emaciated and have little or no subcutaneous tissue but normal linear growth. Their behavior is not in keeping with the nutritional state, because they are often hyperalert and euphoric. Approximately 25% have a coarse horizontal nystagmus. Conversely, tumor invasion of the hypothalamus can result in an insatiable appetite, obesity, diabetes insipidus, and hypogonadism. Resection of the optic glioma confined to an optic nerve produces blindness but prevents recurrence or extension through the chiasm, which may be the preferred therapy if the eye is already blind from tumor invasion. Optic chiasm gliomas with hypothalamic involvement may be treated with chemotherapy (actinomycin D and vincristine) in children less than 3 yr of age, and this may delay the requirement for radiation therapy. Radiotherapy in older patients with chiasmatic/hypothalamic gliomas results in an excellent prognosis, with 10-yr survival rates of almost 90%.

Astrocytoma and related glial tumors (ependymoma and oligodendrogliomas) have a less favorable prognosis when located in the cerebral hemisphere compared with the cerebellum. These patients may have a chronic history of complex partial epilepsy, particularly if the tumor is located within the temporal lobe. Neurologic examination frequently exhibits subtle upper motor neuron signs or a contralateral growth arrest of the extremities. Surgical excision of a low-grade astrocytoma results in a 50–80% 5-yr survival. High-grade astrocytomas have a much greater mortality, with only a 30% survival following surgery and radiation therapy. Recent studies utilizing chemotherapeutic regimens have improved the 5-yr survival rate to approximately 50%.

There are a series of *tumors peculiar to children that arise in the region of the pineal gland*, including varieties of germ cell tumors, pinealomas, pineoblastomas, and teratomas. These tumors are remarkably different in degrees of malignancy and invasion of surrounding structures. They may cause obstruction of the CSF pathways, resulting in macrocrania and hydrocephalus. Pressure by the tumor on the quadrigeminal plate produces **Parinaud syndrome**, consisting of paralysis of conjugate upward movement of the eyes and poorly reactive pupils. There is no uniform agreement with regard to the management of pineal area tumors, because of the heterogeneity of the tumors and the variable response to radiotherapy. Most would concur that a tissue diagnosis is preferable before the initiation of therapy. Modern surgical techniques, including the use of the operating microscope, have significantly decreased the morbidity and mortality and have allowed total resection of some tumors in the pineal region. The radiosensitive germinoma has a 5-yr survival greater than 75%. Some tumors (e.g., pinealomas) are resistant to radiation and are more likely to respond to chemotherapy, whereas others such as mature teratomas may be treated exclusively by surgery.

The *choroid plexus papilloma* produces slowly progressive hydrocephalus owing to excessive production of CSF. The most common location is the lateral ventricle, followed by the third and fourth ventricles. These tumors arise from the choroid plexus epithelium and protrude into the ventricular cavity. The prognosis is excellent following surgical removal. A small number fragment and spread through the CNS by way of the CSF pathways.

Leukemia may invade the leptomeninges, causing increased intracranial pressure due to infiltration of the pacchionian granulations, or may involve the brain parenchyma and, in combination with an acute hemorrhage, result in a mass lesion. Finally, cranial nerves, particularly the facial, or peripheral nerves, such as the peroneal and sciatic nerves, may be invaded by leukemic infiltrates resulting in weakness, pain, and sensory phenomenon.

LABORATORY FINDINGS. The MRI is the best test for the delineation of brain tumors in children. Aside from the lack of ionizing radiation, the MRI provides a superior image of the posterior fossa structures compared with a CT scan. Furthermore, the fine detail of MRI has identified cerebral tumors that are not visible with a CT scan. In addition, MRI is more accurate in defining the extent of an infiltrating tumor. Metastases to the spinal cord can be identified by the noninvasive MRI and the contrast agent gadolinium; however, contrast myelography remains the study of choice for small metastatic lesions in that region. Children with tumors of the sella turcica should undergo a series of baseline endocrine studies, including measurement of growth hormone, thyroid-stimulating hormone, ACTH, luteinizing hormone, follicle stimulating hormone, antidiuretic hormone, and prolactin, as these hormones may require replacement if they are deficient. Germ cell tumors in the pineal gland are associated with elevated CSF human chorionic gonadotropin and α-fetoprotein levels. CSF monoclonal antibodies are proving helpful in differentiating medulloblastoma and CNS lymphoma antigens. CSF tumor cells may be examined at the time of surgery or as a component of routine follow-up. Positive CSF cytology postoperatively is common, but the interpretation of the finding is not certain, because seeding and new growth may not occur.

PROGNOSIS. Neuropsychologic deficits, including changes in cognitive behavior, verbal performance, perceptual-motor function, and academic achievement, have been reported as frequent complications of cranial radiation therapy. Neurophysiologic abnormalities consisting of generalized slowing of the EEG and increased evoked potential latencies have also been noted. Following radiation, CT scanning and MRI have shown a variety of lesions involving the cortex and myelin, including calcification, ventricular dilatation, white matter hypodensities, and cortical atrophy. Generally, the younger the patient, the greater will be the disability. However, there is little correlation between the site of the pathology as identified by imaging studies and the cognitive disorder. Abnormalities in linear growth and related endocrine disorders (particularly thyroid dysfunction) are common after radiation therapy, secondary to growth hormone dysfunction. Baseline endocrine studies should be carried out on all newly diagnosed patients before the initiation of therapy. Second malignancies are rare after treatment of a primary brain tumor in children. Prospective studies by the age of the child and specific therapeutic regimens are required to better understand the consequences of cranial radiation therapy.

New therapeutic modalities, such as implantation of radiated pellets and hyperfractionated radiotherapy, add promise for the treatment of brain tumors in children. Bone marrow transplantation may potentially allow the use of higher concentrations of chemotherapeutic agents. Molecular biologic studies are also likely to define the mechanisms of tumor behavior and provide a method for more effective therapy in the future.

20.75 PSEUDOTUMOR CEREBRI

Pseudotumor cerebri is a clinical syndrome that mimics brain tumors and is characterized by increased intracranial pressure with a normal CSF cell count and protein content and normal ventricular size, anatomy, and position.

ETIOLOGY. There are many explanations for the development of pseudotumor cerebri, including alterations in CSF absorption and production, cerebral edema, abnormalities in vasomotor control and cerebral blood flow, and venous obstruction. The causes of pseudotumor are multiple and include *metabolic disorders* (galactosemia, hypoparathyroidism, pseudohypoparathyroidism, hypophosphatasia, prolonged corticosteroid therapy, hypervitaminosis A, vitamin A deficiency, Addison disease, obesity, menarche, oral contraceptives, and pregnancy), *infections* (roseola infantum, Guillain-Barré syndrome), *drugs* (nalidixic acid, tetracycline), *hematologic disorders* (polycythemia, hemolytic and iron-deficiency anemia, Wiskott-Aldrich syndrome), and *obstruction of intracranial venous drainage* (lateral sinus, posterior sagittal sinus, head injury, and obstruction of the superior vena cava).

CLINICAL MANIFESTATIONS. The most frequent symptom is headache, and although vomiting is present, it is rarely as persistent and pernicious as that associated with a posterior fossa tumor. Diplopia secondary to paralysis of the abducens nerve is a frequent complaint. Most patients are alert and lack constitutional symptoms. An examination of the infant is characterized by a bulging fontanel and a positive "crack-pot" or Macewen sign (percussion of the skull produces a resonant sound) due to separation of the cranial sutures. Papilledema with an enlarged blind spot is the most consistent sign in the child beyond infancy. An inferior nasal defect may be detected on formal tangent screen testing. The presence of focal neurologic signs indicates a process other than pseudotumor cerebri.

TREATMENT. The prime goal in management should be directed toward the discovery and treatment of the underlying cause. Pseudotumor cerebri is mainly a self-limited condition, but optic atrophy and blindness are the most significant complications. For many patients, repeated follow-up and determination of the visual acuity are all that is required. Serial VEPs are useful, if the visual acuity cannot be reliably documented. For others, the initial lumbar tap that follows a CT scan is diagnostic and therapeutic. The spinal needle produces a small rent in the dura that allows CSF to escape the subarachnoid space and reduce the intracranial pressure. Occasionally, several additional lumbar taps and the removal of sufficient CSF to reduce the opening pressure by 50% lead to resolution of the process. Acetazolamide, 10–30 mg/kg/24 hr, and corticosteroids have been effective for some patients. Rarely, a lumboperitoneal shunt or subtemporal decompression is necessary, if the aforementioned approaches are unsuccessful and optic atrophy supervenes. Finally, any patient who proves to be refractory to treatment warrants consideration for repeat neuroradiologic studies. A slow-growing tumor or obstruction of a venous sinus may become evident at the time of reinvestigation.

Amacher AL: Craniopharyngioma: The controversy regarding radiotherapy. Childs Nerv Syst 6:57, 1980.
Bloom HJG: Medulloblastoma in children: Increasing survival rates and further prospects. Int J Radiat Oncol Biol Phys 8:2023, 1982.
Cohen ME, Duffner PK (eds): Brain Tumors in Children. New York, Raven Press, 1984.
Dowell RD Jr, Copeland DR: Cerebral pathology and neuropsychological effects. Am J Pediatr Hematol Oncol 9:68, 1987.
Duffner PK, Cohen ME, Myers MH, et al: Survival of children with brain tumors: SEER Program, 1973–1980. Neurology 36:597, 1986.
Edwards MSB, Hudgins RJ, Wilson CB, et al: Pineal region tumors in children. J Neurosurg 68:689, 1988.
Epstein F, McCleary EL: Intrinsic brain-stem tumors of childhood: Surgical indications. J Neurosurg 64:11, 1986.
Finlay JL, Uteg R, Giese WL: Brain tumors in children. II: Advances in neurosurgery and radiation oncology. Am J Pediatr Hematol Oncol 9:256, 1987.
Hoffman JH: Benign brain stem gliomas in children. Prog Exp Tumor Res 30:154, 1987.
Horowitz ME, Mulhern RK, Kun LE, et al: Brain tumors in the very young child. Cancer 61:428, 1988.
Huckman MS: Computed tomography in the diagnosis of pseudotumor cerebri. Radiology 119:593, 1976.
Johnston I, Paterson A: Benign intracranial hypertension: Diagnosis and prognosis. Brain 97:289, 1974.
Kadota RP, Allen JB, Hartman GA, et al: Brain tumors in children. J Pediatr 114:511, 1989.
Marsh WR, Laws ER Jr: Intracranial ependymomas. Progr Exp Tumor Res 30:175, 1987.
Packer RJ, Batnitzky S, Cohen ME: Magnetic resonance imaging in the evaluation of intracranial tumors of childhood. Cancer 56:1767, 1985.
Packer RJ, Sutton LN, Bilaniuk LT, et al: Treatment of chiasmatic/hypothalamic gliomas of childhood with chemotherapy: An update. Ann Neurol 23:79, 1988.
Phillips PC, Kremzner LT, DeVivo DC: Cerebrospinal fluid polyamines: Biochemical markers of malignant childhood brain tumors. Ann Neurol 19:360, 1986.
Rush JA: Pseudotumor cerebri. Mayo Clin Proc 55:541, 1980.
Schmidek HH: The molecular genetics of nervous system tumors. J Neurosurg 67:1, 1987.
Sutton LN: Current management of low-grade astrocytomas of childhood. Pediatr Neurosci 13:98, 1987.
Tomita T, McLone DG, Naidich TP: Brain stem gliomas in childhood. J Neurooncol 2:117, 1984.

20.76 SPINAL CORD DISORDERS IN CHILDREN

SPINAL CORD TUMORS

In children, spinal cord tumors account for approximately 20% of neuraxial tumors and are classified according to anatomic position (Fig. 20–21). *Intramedullary tumors* arise within the substance of the cord and grow slowly by infiltration, usually in the cervical region. The most common intramedullary tumor is a low-grade astrocytoma, followed by an ependymoma. *Extramedullary, intradural tumors* tend to be benign and arise from neural crest tissue. Tumors in this area include neurofibroma, ganglioneuroma, and meningioma. *Extramedullary, extradural tumors* characteristically consist of metastatic lesions, particularly neuroblastoma, sarcoma, and leukemia.

CLINICAL MANIFESTATIONS. Most spinal cord tumors in children present with a combination of gait disturbance and back pain, depending on the locale of the tumor. Intramedullary gliomas are slow growing. Progressive difficulties in locomotion and sphincter disturbances are the earliest symptoms. Glial tumors in the cervical cord produce lower motor neuron signs in the upper extremities and upper motor neuron signs in the legs. Denervation of the intercostal muscles decreases chest wall movement and results in a weak cough. Loss of pain, temperature, and light touch sensation are evident in the lower extremities, and a cord level can be documented with the starch-iodine test or somatosensory evoked potentials. Extramedullary tumors often present with back pain. The child has difficulty in sleeping because of pain and maintains a tripod posture while attempting to assume the supine position. If the tumor is attached to a nerve root,

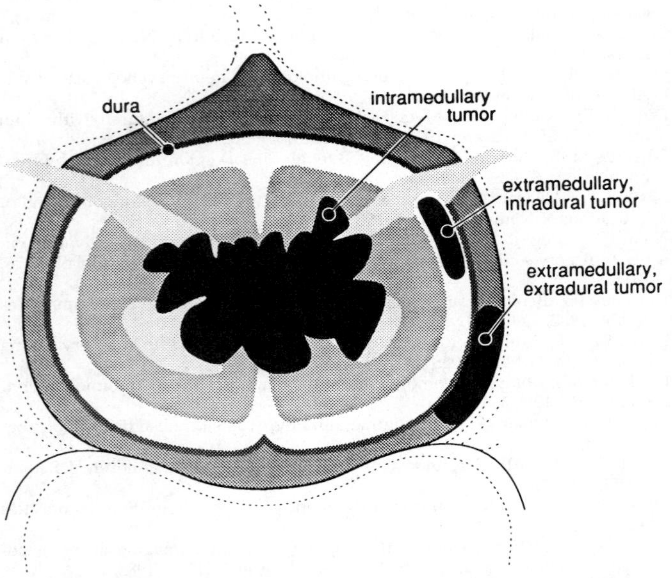

Figure 20–21. Diagram of the location of spinal cord tumors in children.

segmental pain, paresthesia, and weakness will be evident. Extramedullary, extradural tumors have a propensity to cause an acute block of the CSF pathways due to rapid growth within a confined space. Such children present with a flaccid paraplegia, urinary retention, and a patulous anus. Some extramedullary tumors produce the **Brown-Sequard syndrome** that consists of homolateral weakness, spasticity, and ataxia, and contralateral loss of pain and temperature sensation. Papilledema is observed in a few patients, usually in association with markedly elevated CSF protein levels that presumably interfere with normal CSF flow dynamics.

DIAGNOSIS. It is important to establish the diagnosis of a spinal cord tumor as early as possible, because the surgical management will be facilitated and irreversible damage to the cord will be prevented. In approximately 40% of the cases, routine roentgenograms show abnormalities including widening of the interpediculate distance, destruction or sclerosis of the adjacent vertebral bodies or pedicles, and widening of a vertebral foramina on an oblique view in the case of a neurofibroma or ganglioneuroma. MRI is the most important diagnostic test to establish the diagnosis. Intramedullary tumors produce a fusiform swelling of the cord, often with a complete block of the CSF. Neurofibroma tend to create a circular indentation of the cord, and extramedullary tumors show various degrees of blockage.

TREATMENT. With modern surgical techniques, many tumors can be totally and safely resected. Surgical removal of benign extramedullary tumors is associated with a good prognosis. For children with a primary neuroblastoma who present with a sudden onset of paraplegia secondary to metastases in the extradural space, immediate radiation therapy may circumvent the need for a laminectomy.

20.77 SPINAL CORD TRAUMA

See also Sec. 6.35 and 9.24.

Acute spinal cord injuries in children may result from indirect trauma due to hyperflexion, hyperextension, or vertical compression accidents; however, fracture dislocation of the vertebral column or epidural bleeding may also compromise spinal cord integrity secondary to a mass effect. As with the brain, the degree of injury to the spinal cord is variable and includes concussion, contusion, laceration, and transection. Recovery depends on the extent of the trauma as well as on the immediate and long-term management. Common causes of spinal cord injury include traumatic breech deliveries, extensive shaking of the physically abused child, automobile and diving accidents, falls from playground equipment, and congenital defects such as the underlying vertebral abnormality in Down syndrome. Because individuals with Down syndrome are susceptible to dislocation of the atlantoaxial joint because of lax ligaments, a roentgenogram of the cervical spine should be obtained in each patient. Those with an abnormality of the atlantoaxial joint should be counseled to refrain from exercises that are likely to cause excessive flexion/extension of the neck (tumbling/diving). Those with abnormal radiographs should be followed regularly for the development of neurologic signs that might require surgical stabilization of the cervical spine.

A *severe cord injury* presents with **spinal shock**, consisting of flaccidity, areflexia, and loss of sensation. This may persist for up to 4 wk and results from dysfunction of synaptic activity in the pathways caudal to the injury. Ultimately, reflex flexor movements develop, followed by extensor reflex activity associated with hyperactive deep tendon reflexes, spasticity, and an automatic bladder. *Fracture dislocations at the C5–C6 level* are the most common acute cause of spinal cord injuries and are characterized by a flaccid quadriparesis, loss of sphincter function, and a sensory level corresponding to the upper sternum. A transverse injury in the high cervical cord level (C1–C2) causes respiratory arrest and death in the absence of ventilatory support. Fractures in the low thoracic (T12–L1) region may produce the **conus medullaris syndrome** that includes a loss of urinary and rectal sphincter control, flaccid weakness, and sensory disturbances of the legs. A **central cord lesion** may result as a consequence of contusion and hemorrhage and typically involves the upper extremities to a greater degree than the legs. There are lower motor neuron signs in the upper extremities and upper motor neuron signs in the legs, bladder dysfunction, and loss of sensation caudal to the lesion. There may be considerable recovery, particularly in the lower extremities.

Spinal cord injuries should be managed by stabilization and immobilization of the spine at the accident site using a cervical collar or sandbags. An adequate airway should be maintained, respiratory support should be provided, and shock should be treated with appropriate volume expanders. Following transportation, roentgenograms of the spine, including oblique views, should be obtained. Approximately 50% of children with severe cord injuries show no abnormality of the spine roentgenogram. Fracture dislocations are treated with traction, immobilization, and, if unstable, by vertebral fusion. Laminectomy and inspection of the cord are reserved for the patient with progression of neurologic signs and a CT scan or MRI that suggests an epidural or intraspinal hemorrhage. Additional therapeutic measures include management of bladder and gastrointestinal disturbances, nutritional and skin care, and a rigorous multidisciplinary rehabilitation program.

20.78 TETHERED CORD

During fetal development the spinal cord occupies the entire length of the vertebral column, but due to differential growth, the conus medullaris in the child ultimately assumes a position at the level of L1. Normal regression of the distal embryonic spinal cord produces a slender, thread-like filum terminale that is attached to the coccyx. A tethered cord results when a thickened rope-like filum terminale persists and anchors the conus at or below the L2 level. Neurologic signs may develop due to abnormal tension on the spinal cord, compromising blood supply, particularly during flexion and extension movements. Diastematomyelia may coexist with a tethered cord. Inspection of the back shows a midline skin lesion in approximately 70% of cases, including a lipoma, cutaneous hemangioma, tuft of hair, hyperpigmentation, or a dermal pit. The clinical presentation varies, and signs may be evident at birth or may be delayed until adulthood. Infants may have asymmetric growth in a foot or leg associated with talipes cavus deformities and muscle wasting due to prolonged denervation. Abnormalities in bladder function with overflow incontinence, progressive scoliosis, and diffuse pain in the lower extremities are more common findings in the child. Plain roentgenograms of the lumbosacral spine demonstrate spina bifida in most cases. A CT scan with a small amount of metrizamide or MRI precisely outlines the level of the conus medullaris and the filum terminale. Surgical transection of the thickened filum terminale tends to halt the progression of neurological signs and prevent the development of dysfunction in the asymptomatic patient.

20.79 DIASTEMATOMYELIA

Diastematomyelia refers to the division of the spinal cord into two halves by the projection of a fibrocartilaginous or bony septum originating from the posterior vertebral body and extending posteriorly. It represents a disorder of neural tube fusion with the persistence of mesodermal tissue from the primitive neurenteric canal acting as the septum. The defect involves the lumbar vertebrae (L1–L3) in approximately 50% of cases and tends to be associated with abnormalities of the vertebral bodies including fusion defects, hemivertebra, hypoplasia, kyphoscoliosis, spina bifida, and myelomeningocele. A midline abnormality of the skin, including a cutaneous hemangioma, provides a clue to the possibility of an underlying abnormality. The neurologic signs are thought to result from flexion and extension movements of the cord, which produce traction and additional trauma by the impaling septum. The clinical presentation of diastematomyelia varies, and in some cases the patient may remain asymptomatic. Most often, unilateral foot abnormalities, including talipes equinovarus, claw toes, atrophy of the gastrocnemius, and loss of pain and temperature sensation, are apparent in the preschool child. A more progressive course may ensue, characterized by bilateral weakness and muscle atrophy in the lower extremities, absent ankle jerks, urinary incontinence, and low back pain. Plain roentgenograms of the vertebra may not detect the septum due to lack of calcification, so that CT scanning or MRI is the study of choice. The treatment of symptomatic patients is excision of the bony spur or septum and lysis of the adjacent adhesions.

20.80 SYRINGOMYELIA

Syringomyelia may be defined as a cystic cavity within the spinal cord, which may communicate with the CSF pathways or remain localized and noncommunicating. *Syringobulbia* exists when the cystic cavity extends into the medulla. Although the pathogenesis of communicating syringomyelia is unknown, the prevailing hypothesis suggests a constriction of the central canal at the level of the foramen magnum during embryogenesis. CSF may pass caudad through the narrowed canal, especially during periods of increased intracranial pressure (e.g., sneezing, coughing), and produce dilatation of the central canal. Because of the constriction, CSF is prevented from flowing in a cephalad direction. Communicating syringomyelia is frequently associated with the Chiari type I malformation, whereas the noncommunicating syrinx is complicated by cord tumors, vascular accidents, trauma, and arachnoiditis. Due to its slow evolution, syringomyelia rarely produces symptoms during childhood.

Interruption of the anterior white commissure at the level of the cervical cord disrupts the lateral spinothalamic tracts, causing an asymmetric loss of pain and temperature sensation in the upper extremities, with preservation of light touch (dissociation of sensation). Progressive enlargement of the cavity impinges on the anterior horn cells and corticospinal tracts, resulting in muscle wasting of the hands, absent deep tendon reflexes in the upper extremities, and upper motor neuron signs in the lower extremities. A rapidly progressive scoliosis may be the initial manifestation of syringomyelia. Trophic ulcers associated with vasomotor disturbances of the hands and arms indicate the loss of appreciation of pain. CT scanning with the intrathecal injection of metrizamide outline an enlarged spinal cord in the region of the syrinx, and a delayed scan displays the contrast medium within the cavity. The MRI is the study of choice. The management is surgical and depends on the site and etiology of the syringomyelia. Decompression of the foramen magnum and the upper cervical vertebrae is recommended when the syrinx is associated with a Chiari type I anomaly. Additional procedures include insertion of a tissue plug in the open end of the central canal, draining the cystic cavity into the subarachnoid space, and the percutaneous aspiration of the syrinx which may result in marked improvement in neurologic function for prolonged periods.

20.81 TRANSVERSE MYELITIS

Transverse myelitis is characterized by the abrupt onset of progressive weakness and sensory disturbances in the lower extremities. A history of a preceding viral infection accompanied by fever and malaise is documented in most cases. Several viruses have been implicated including the Epstein-Barr virus, herpes, influenza, rubella, mumps, and varicella virus. At least three hypotheses have been proposed to explain the pathogenesis of transverse myelitis: cell-mediated autoimmune response, direct viral invasion of the spinal cord, and an autoimmune vasculitis. Pathologic examination of the cord shows marked softening and perivascular cuffing by lymphocytes, supporting an immunologic basis for the disorder.

Low back or abdominal pain and paresthesias of the legs are prominent symptoms in the early stages. The legs are weak and flaccid, and a sensory level is present usually in the midthoracic region. Pain, temperature, and light touch sensation are affected, but joint position and vibration sense may be preserved. Sphincter disturbances are common, in which case catheterization of the bladder is necessary. Fever and nuchal rigidity are present early in most cases. The neurologic deficit evolves for 2–3 days and then plateaus, with flaccidity gradually changing to spasticity and with the concomitant development of upper motor neuron signs in the lower extremities. An examination of the CSF shows moderate lymphocyte pleocytosis and a normal or slightly elevated protein. CT scanning or MRI reveals mild fusiform swelling in the affected region. Spontaneous recovery occurs for a period of weeks or months and is complete in approximately 60% of cases. Residual deficits include bowel and bladder dysfunction and weakness in the lower extremities. Management is directed to bladder care and physiotherapy. There is no evidence that steroids influence the course or the outcome of transverse myelitis. The differential diagnosis includes meningitis, infectious polyneuropathy (Guillain-Barré syndrome), poliomyelitis, neuromyelitis optica (Devic disease), spinal cord neoplasm, epidural abscess, and a vascular malformation.

20.82 ARTERIOVENOUS MALFORMATION

An arteriovenous malformation of the spinal cord consists of a collection of tortuous dilated veins that are usually located on the dorsal aspect of the thoracic cord. The malformation may cause neurologic symptoms by its mass effect on the cord or by the "steal" phenomenon by which blood is shunted through the abnormal veins, bypassing the spinal cord, which produces transient and in some cases progressive loss of neurologic function. Occasionally, the patient presents with acute paraparesis and a sensory deficit due to a subarachnoid bleed from the malformation. More commonly, a gradual onset of gait abnormalities, low back pain, and bowel and bladder dysfunction is noted. The deep tendon reflexes are absent or reduced in the lower extremities, and the Babinski reflex is present. In approximately one third of cases, a midline cutaneous angioma overlies the arteriovenous malformation, and occasionally a spinal bruit may be auscultated. Roentgenograms of the spine may show erosion of the pedicles; however, contrast myelography and selective spinal angiography are required to delineate the blood supply and the extent of the malformation. The malformation is removed by surgical excision with the use of an operating microscope or is obliterated by embolization.

ROBERT H. A. HASLAM

Cahan LD, Bentson JR: Considerations in the diagnosis and treatment of syringomyelia and Chiari malformation. J Neurosurg 57:24, 1982.
De La Torre JC: Spinal cord injury: Review of basic and applied research. Spine 6:315, 1981.
Haft H, Ransohoff J, Carter S: Spinal cord tumors in children. Pediatrics 23:1152, 1959.
Hendrick EB, Hoffman HJ, Humphreys RP: The tethered spinal cord. Clin Neurosurg 30:457, 1982.
Hilal S, Marton D, Pollack E: Diastematomyelia in children. Radiology 112:609, 1974.
Newman PK, Terenty TR, Foster JB: Some observations on the pathogenesis of syringomyelia. J Neurol Neurosurg Psychiatry 44:964, 1981.
Paine RS, Byers RK: Transverse myelopathy in childhood. Am J Dis Child 85:151, 1953.
Pueschel SM, Findley TW, Furia J, et al: Atlantoaxial instability in Down syndrome: Roentgenographic, neurologic and somatosensory evoked potential studies. J Pediatr 110:515, 1987.
Riche MC, Modenesi-Freitas J, Djindjian M, et al: Arteriovenous malformations (AVM) of the spinal cord in children: Review of 38 cases. Neuroradiology 22:171, 1982.
Scotti G, Musgrave MA, Harwood-Nash DC, et al: Diastematomyelia in children: Metrizamide and CT metrizamide myelography. AJR 135:1225, 1980.
Sheptak PE, Susen AF: Diastematomyelia. Am J Dis Child 113:210, 1967.

21

NEUROMUSCULAR DISORDERS

The term *neuromuscular disease* refers to disorders of the motor unit and specifically excludes suprasegmental disorders, such as cerebral palsy, even though muscle tone, strength, function, and reflexes are influenced by cerebral disease. The *motor unit* consists of four components: (1) a motor neuron in the brain stem or ventral horn of the spinal cord; (2) its axon that, together with other axons, forms the peripheral nerve; (3) the neuromuscular junction; and (4) all muscle fibers innervated by a single motor neuron. The size of the motor unit varies among different muscles and with the precision of muscular function required. In large muscles, such as the glutei and quadriceps femoris, hundreds of muscle fibers are innvervated by a single motor neuron; in small, finely tuned muscles, such as the stapedius or the extraocular muscles, a 1:1 ratio may prevail. The motor unit is influenced by suprasegmental or upper motor neuron control that alters properties of muscle tone, precision of movement, reciprocal inhibition of antagonistic muscles during movement, and sequencing of muscle contractions to achieve smooth, coordinated movements. Suprasegmental impulses also augment or inhibit the monosynaptic stretch reflex.

Diseases of the motor unit are common in children. These neuromuscular diseases may be genetically determined or nonhereditary, congenital or acquired, acute or chronic, and progressive or static. Because specific therapy is available for many diseases and because of genetic and prognostic implications, precise diagnosis is important; laboratory confirmation is required for most diseases because of overlapping clinical manifestations.

21.1 EVALUATION AND INVESTIGATION

CLINICAL MANIFESTATIONS. Examination of the neuromuscular system should always include an assessment of muscle bulk, tone, and strength. Hypotonia may be associated with normal strength or with weakness; enlarged muscles may be weak or strong; thin, wasted muscles may be weak or have unexpectedly normal strength. The distribution of these components is of diagnostic importance. In general, myopathies follow a proximal distribution of weakness and muscle wasting (with the notable exception of myotonic muscular dystrophy); neuropathies, by contrast, are generally distal in distribution (with the notable exception of juvenile spinal muscular atrophy). Involvement of the face, tongue, palate, and extraocular muscles provides an important distinction in the differential diagnosis. Tendon stretch reflexes are generally lost in neuropathies and in motor neuron diseases and are diminished but preserved in myopathies. A few specific clinical features are important in the diagnosis of some neuromuscular diseases. Fasciculations of muscle, which are often best seen in the tongue, are a sign of denervation. Sensory abnormalities indicate neuropathy. Fatigable weakness is characteristic of neuromuscular junctional disorders. Myotonia is specific for a few myopathies.

Some features do not distinguish myopathy from neuropathy. Muscle pain or myalgias are associated with acute disease of either myopathic or neurogenic origin. Acute dermatomyositis and acute polyneuropathy (Guillain-Barré syndrome) are both characterized by myalgias. Muscular dystrophies and spinal muscular atrophies are not associated with muscle pain. Myalgias also occur in several metabolic diseases of muscle and in ischemic myopathy. Contractures of muscles, whether present at birth or developing later in the course of an illness, occur in both myopathic and neurogenic diseases.

Male infants who are weak in late fetal life and in the neonatal period often have undescended testicles. The testicles are actively pulled into the scrotum from the anterior abdominal wall by a pair of cords that consist of smooth and striated muscle called the *gubernaculum*. The gubernaculum is weakened in many congenital neuromuscular diseases, including spinal muscular atrophy, myotonic muscular dystrophy, and many congenital myopathies.

The thorax of infants with congenital neuromuscular disease often has a funnel shape, and the ribs are thin and radiolucent due to intercostal muscle weakness during intrauterine growth. This phenomenon is found characteristically in infantile spinal muscular atropy but also occurs in myotubular myopathy, neonatal myotonic dystrophy, and other disorders. Because of the small muscle mass, birth weight may be low for gestational age.

Generalized hypotonia and developmental delay are the most common presenting manifestations of neuromuscular disease in infants and young children. These features may also be expressions of neurologic disease, endocrine and systemic metabolic diseases, and Down syndrome, or they may be nonspecific neuromuscular expressions of malnutrition or chronic systemic illness. A prenatal history of decreased fetal movements and intrauterine growth retardation are often found in patients who are symptomatic at birth.

LABORATORY FINDINGS. Serum Enzymes. Several lysosomal enzymes are released by damaged or degenerating muscle fibers and may be measured in serum. The most useful of these is the creatine phosphokinase (CPK or CK), which is found in only three organs and may be separated into corresponding isozymes: MM for skeletal muscle; MB for cardiac muscle; and BB for brain. The serum CK is by no means a universal screening test for neuromuscular disease, because many diseases of the motor unit may not be associated with elevated enzymes. However, the CK is characteristically elevated in certain diseases, such as Duchenne muscular dystrophy, and the magnitude of increase is characteristic for particular diseases.

Nerve Conduction Velocity (NCV). Motor and sensory nerve conduction may be measured electrophysiologically by using surface electrodes. Neuropathies of various types are detected by decreased conduction. The site of a traumatic nerve injury may also be localized. The nerve conduction at birth is about half of the mature value achieved by 2 yr of age. Tables are available for normal values at various ages in infancy, including for preterm infants. Because the NCV study measures only the fastest conducting fibers in a nerve, 80% of the total nerve fibers must be involved before slowing in conduction becomes evident.

Electromyography (EMG). EMG is less useful in pediatrics than in adult medicine, in part because of technical difficulties in recording young children and in part because the best results require patient cooperation for full relaxation and maximal voluntary contraction of a muscle. Most children are too frightened to provide such cooperation. EMG requires the insertion of a needle into the belly of a muscle and recording the electrical potentials in various states of contraction. Characteristic patterns distinguish denervation from myopathic involvement. The specific type of myopathy is not usually definitively diagnosed, but certain specialized myopathic conditions, such as myotonia, may be demonstrated.

EMG combined with repetitive electrical stimulation of a motor nerve supplying a muscle to produce tetany is useful in demonstrating myasthenic decremental responses. Small muscles, such as the abductor digiti quinti of the hypothenar eminence, are used for such studies.

Muscle Biopsy. The muscle biopsy is the most important and specific diagnostic study of muscle. Not only are neurogenic and myopathic processes distinguished, but also the type of myopathy and specific enzymatic deficiencies may be determined. The vastus lateralis (quadriceps femoris) is the muscle that is most commonly sampled. The deltoid muscle should be avoided in most cases, because it normally has an 80% predominance of type I fibers, so thus the distribution patterns of fiber types are difficult to recognize. Muscle biopsy is a simple outpatient procedure that may be performed under local anesthesia with or without femoral nerve block. Needle biopsies, advocated by some authors, require an incision in the skin similar to open biopsy, and numerous samples must be taken to do an adequate examination of the tissue; needle biopsies are as traumatic as open biopsies and provide inferior specimens.

Histochemical studies of frozen sections of the muscle are obligatory in all pediatric muscle biopsies, because many congenital and metabolic myopathies cannot be diagnosed from paraffin sections using conventional histologic stains. Immunofluorescence is a useful supplement in some cases. A portion of the biopsy should be fixed for potential electron microscopy, but ultrastructure has additional diagnostic value only in selected cases. Muscle biopsy interpretation is complex and should be done by an experienced pathologist.

Nerve Biopsy. The most commonly sampled nerve is the sural nerve, which is a pure sensory nerve that supplies a small area of skin on the lateral surface of the foot. Whole or fascicular biopsies of this nerve may be taken. When the sural nerve is severed behind the lateral malleolus of the ankle, regeneration of the nerve occurs in more than 90% of cases, so that permanent sensory loss is not experienced. The sural nerve is often involved in many neuropathies that are clinically predominantly motor.

Electron microscopy should be performed on all nerve biopsies, because the most important morphologic alterations cannot be appreciated at the resolution of the light microscope. Teased fiber preparations are sometimes useful in demonstrating segmental demyelination, axonal swellings, and other specific abnormalities, but this time-consuming procedure is not done routinely.

Electrocardiography (ECG). Cardiac evaluation is important if myopathy is suspected, because of involvement of the heart in muscular dystrophies and in inflammatory and metabolic myopathies. The ECG often detects early cardiomyopathy or conduction defects that are clinically asymptomatic. Serial **pulmonary function tests** should be performed in muscular dystrophies and in other chronic or progressive diseases of the motor unit.

DEVELOPMENTAL DISORDERS OF MUSCLE

A heterogeneous group of congenital neuromuscular disorders is sometimes known as the *congenital myopathies,* but in many of these disorders, the assumption that the pathogenesis is primarily myopathic is unjustified. Most congenital myopathies are nonprogressive conditions, but some patients show slow clinical deterioration accompanied by additional changes in their muscle biopsy. Some of the diseases in the category of congenital myopathies are hereditary; others are sporadic. Although clinical features, including phenotype, may raise a strong suspicion of a congenital myopathy, the definitive diagnosis is determined by the histopathologic findings in the muscle biopsy. These morphologic and histochemical abnormalities differ considerably from those of the muscular dystrophies, spinal muscular atrophies, and neuropathies. Many are reminiscent of stages in the embryologic development of muscle and may represent aberrations of ontogenesis.

21.2 MYOTUBULAR MYOPATHY

The term myotubular myopathy implies a maturational arrest of fetal muscle during the myotubular stage of development at 8–15 wk of gestation. It is based on the morphologic appearance of myofibers: A row of central nuclei lie within a core of cytoplasm; contractile myofibrils form a cylinder around this core (Fig. 21–1). Many challenge this interpretation and use the more neutral term *centronuclear myopathy* when referring to this myopathy. But this term is too nonspecific because internal nuclei occur in many unrelated myopathies.

PATHOGENESIS. Although the pathogenesis may be neurogenic, spinal motor neurons are normal in number and morphology. Peripheral nerves also usually have normal ultrastructure and conduction velocity. Persistently high fetal concentrations of vimentin and desmin are demonstrated in myofibers of infants with myotubular myopathy. These intermediate filament proteins serve as cytoskeletal elements in fetal myotubes, attaching nuclei and mitochondria to the sarcolemmal membranes to preserve their central positions. As intracellular organization changes with maturation, the nuclei move to the periphery and mitochondria are redistributed between myofibrils. At the same time, vimentin and desmin diminish. Vimentin disappears altogether by term and desmin remains only in trace amounts. Persistent fetal vimentin and desmin in muscle fibers may be the mechanism of "maturational arrest."

CLINICAL MANIFESTATIONS. Decreased fetal movements are perceived in late gestation. At birth, affected infants have a thin muscle mass involving axial, limb-girdle, and distal muscles; severe generalized hypotonia; and diffuse weakness. Respiratory efforts may be ineffective, requiring ventilatory support. Gavage feeding may be required because of weakness of the muscles of suck and deglutition. The testicles are often undescended. Facial muscles may be weak, but infants do not have the characteristic facies of myotonic dystrophy. Ophthalmoplegia is observed in a few cases. The palate may be high. The tongue is thin, but fasciculations are not seen. Tendon stretch reflexes are weak or absent. Myotubular myopathy is not associated with cardiomyopathy; mature cardiac muscle fibers normally have central nuclei. Congenital anomalies of the central nervous system or of other systems are not associated.

The original case described as "myotubular myopathy" in 1966 was an adolescent boy with mild weakness. Many subsequent cases of older children and adults with centronuclear myopathy and variable weakness have been reported, but their relation to the severe neonatal disease is uncertain.

LABORATORY FINDINGS. Serum CK is normal. The EMG does not show evidence of denervation and is usually normal or shows minimal nonspecific myopathic features in early infancy. Nerve conduction velocity may be slow but is

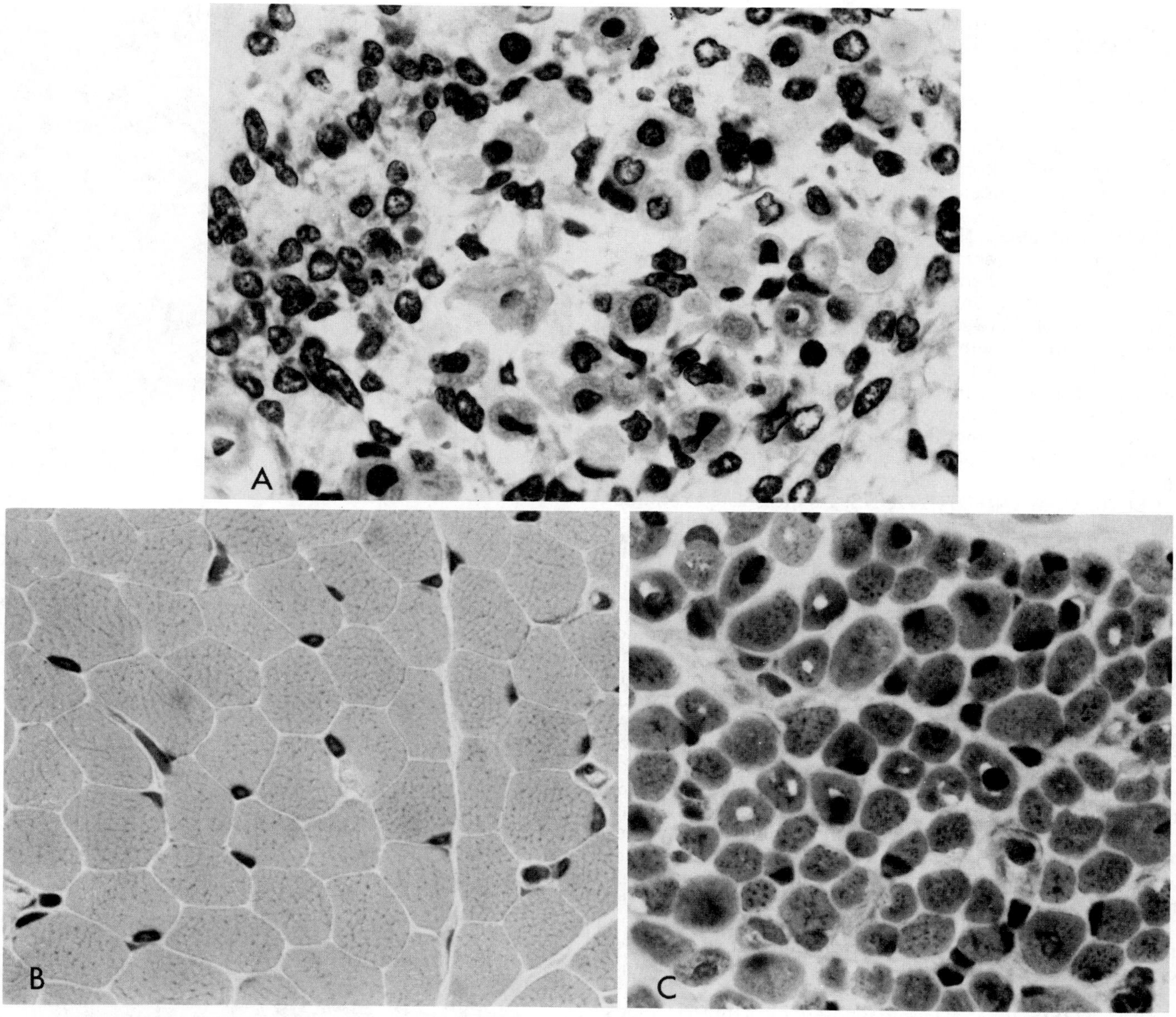

Figure 21–1. *A*, Cross-section of muscle from a 14-wk-old human fetus; *B*, normal full-term neonate; and *C*, term neonate with X-linked recessive myotubular myopathy. Myofibers have large central nuclei in the fetus and in myotubular myopathy, and nuclei are at the periphery of the muscle fiber in the term neonate as in the adult. (Hematoxylin & eosin, ×500.)

usually normal. The ECG is normal. Roentgenograms of the chest show no cardiomegaly, but the ribs may be thin.

DIAGNOSIS. The muscle biopsy is diagnostic at birth, even in premature infants. More than 90% of muscle fibers are small and have centrally placed, large vesicular nuclei in a single row. Spaces between nuclei are filled with sarcoplasm containing mitochondria. Histochemical stains for oxidative enzymatic activity and glycogen reveal a central distribution as in fetal myotubes. The cylinder of myofibrils shows mature histochemical differentiation with adenosine triphosphatase (ATPase) stains, however. The connective tissue of muscle, spindles, blood vessels, intramuscular nerves, and motor endplates are mature. Ultrastructural features in neonatal myotubular myopathy, other than those that define the disease, are also mature. Vimentin and desmin show strong immunoreactivity in muscle fibers in myotubular myopathy and no demonstrable activity in normal term neonatal muscle.

GENETICS. X-linked recessive inheritance is the most common trait, therefore most patients are boys. The mothers of affected infants are clinically asymptomatic, but their muscle biopsy shows scattered small centronuclear fibers with increased vimentin and desmin. Autosomal dominant and autosomal recessive forms are also reported but are rarer.

Genetic linkage on the X chromosome has been localized to the Xq28 site, a different locus than the Xp21 gene of Duchenne and Becker muscular dystrophies. If persistent vimentin and desmin are primary defects, the genetics of this disease is probably complex, because synthesis of human vimentin is controlled by chromosome 10 (10p13), and synthesis of desmin is controlled by chromosome 2 (2q35).

PROGNOSIS. About 75% of severely affected neonates die within the first few weeks or months of life. Survivors do not experience a progressive course but have major physical handicaps, rarely walk, and remain severely hypotonic.

21.3 CONGENITAL MUSCLE FIBER-TYPE DISPROPORTION (CMFTD)

This condition occurs as an isolated "congenital myopathy" but also develops in associated with a variety of unrelated disorders that include nemaline rod disease, Krabbe's disease (globoid cell leukodystrophy), cerebellar hypoplasia and certain other brain malformations (see later), fetal alcohol syndrome, some glycogenoses, and some cases of myotonic muscular dystrophy.

PATHOGENESIS. The association of CMFTD with cerebellar hypoplasia (see later) suggests that the pathogenesis may be an abnormal suprasegmental influence on the developing motor unit during the stage of histochemical differentiation of muscle between 20 and 28 wk of gestation. Muscle fiber types and growth are determined by innervation and are mutable even in the adult. Although CMFTD does not actually correspond with any normal stage of development, it appears to be an embryologic disturbance of fiber type differentiation and growth. From an evolutionary perspective, CMFTD is the normal physiologic condition in small mammals such as rodents.

CLINICAL MANIFESTATIONS. As an isolated condition not associated with others diseases, CMFTD is a nonprogressive disorder present at birth. There is generalized hypotonia and weakness, but the weakness is usually not severe and respiratory distress and dysphagia are rare. Mild congenital contractures are often present. Poor head control and developmental delay for gross motor skills are common in infancy. Walking is usually delayed until 18–24 mo but is eventually achieved. Because of the hypotonia, subluxation of the hips may occur. Muscle bulk is reduced. The muscle wasting and hypotonia are proportionately greater than the weakness, and the child may be stronger than expected during examination.

The facies of children with CMFTD often raise the suspicion, especially if the child is referred for assessment of developmental delay and hypotonia. The head is dolichocephalic and facial weakness is present. The palate is usually high-arched. Thin muscles of the trunk and extremities give a thin, wasted appearance to the body habitus. Patients do not complain of myalgias. The clinical course is benign and nonprogressive.

LABORATORY FINDINGS. Serum CK, ECG, EMG, and nerve conduction velocity are all normal in simple CMFTD. If other diseases are associated, the laboratory investigation of those conditions will disclose the specific features.

DIAGNOSIS. CMFTD is diagnosed by a muscle biopsy that shows a disproportion in both size and relative ratios of histochemical fiber types: type I fibers are uniformly small and type II fibers are hypertrophic; type I fibers are more numerous than those of type II. Degeneration of myofibers and other primary myopathic features are absent. The biopsy is diagnostic at birth.

GENETICS. Most cases of simple CMFTD are sporadic, although autosomal recessive inheritance is often suspected. A few autosomal dominantly transmitted cases have been described. CMFTD may also be associated with cerebellar hypoplasia.

TREATMENT. No drug therapy is available. Physiotherapy may be helpful for some patients in strengthening muscles that do not receive sufficient exercise in daily activities. Mild congenital contractures often respond well to gentle range of motion exercises and rarely require plaster casting or surgery.

21.4 NEMALINE ROD DISEASE

Nemaline rods (derived from the Greek *nema,* meaning thread) are rod-shaped inclusion-like abnormal structures within muscle fibers. In histologic sections of muscle, they are difficult to demonstrate with conventional hematoxylin-eosin stain but are easily seen with special stains. They are not foreign inclusion bodies but rather consist of excessive Z-band material with a similar ultrastructure (Fig. 21–2). Nemaline rod formation may be an unusual reaction of muscle fibers to injury, because these rod structures have been found uncommonly in a variety of diseases. They are most abundant in the congenital myopathy known as nemaline rod disease.

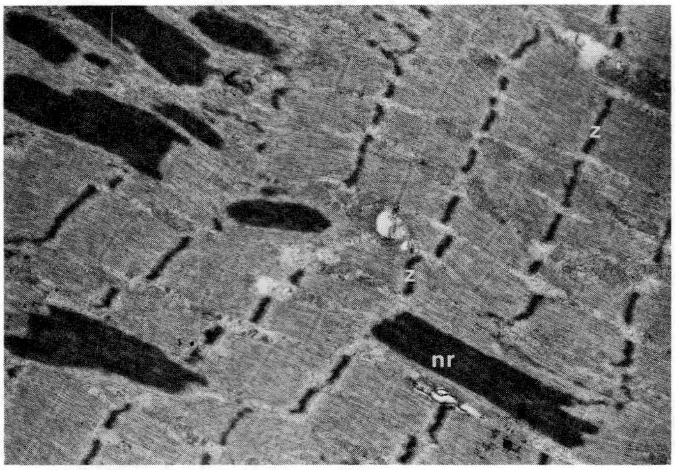

Figure 21–2. Electron micrograph of the muscle from a patient shown in Figure 21–4. Nemaline rods (nr) are seen within many myofibrils. They are identical in composition to the normal Z-bands (z) (×6000).

CLINICAL MANIFESTATIONS. Severe infantile and juvenile forms of the disease are known. Patients resemble those with CMFTD, except that they are more severely affected. Generalized hypotonia, weakness including bulbar-innervated and respiratory muscles, and a very thin muscle mass are characteristic (Fig. 21–3). The head is dolichocephalic, and the palate high-arched or even cleft. Muscles of the jaw may be too weak to hold it closed (Fig. 21–4). Infants may be severely weak at birth, and some die in the neonatal

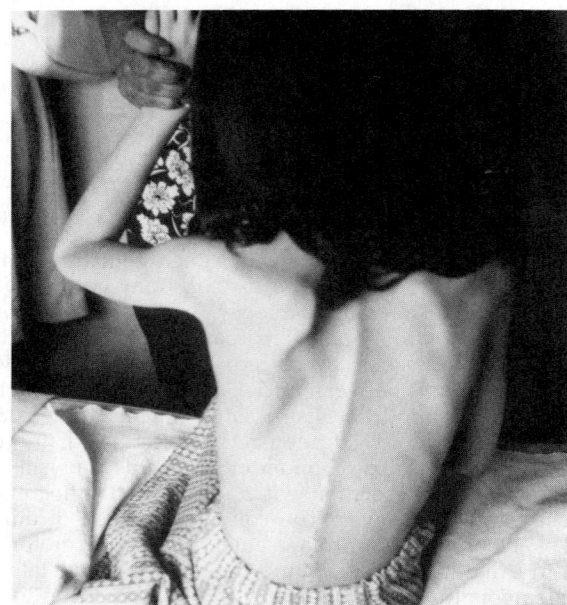

Figure 21–3. Back of 13-yr-old girl with the juvenile form of nemaline rod disease. The paraspinal muscles are very thin, and winging of the scapulae is evident. The muscle mass of the extremities is also greatly reduced both proximally and distally.

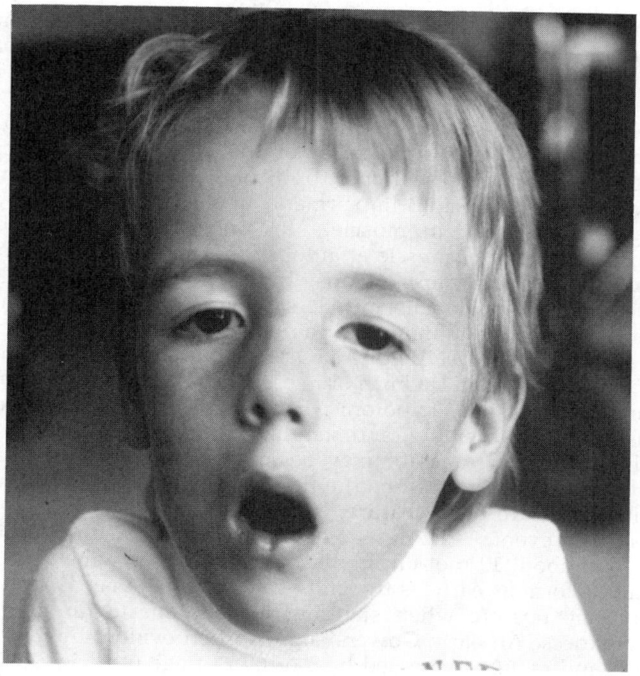

Figure 21–4. Infantile form of nemaline rod disease in a 6-yr-old boy. Facial weakness and generalized muscle wasting are severe. The head is dolichocephalic. The mouth is usually open because the masseters are too weak to lift the mandible against gravity for more than a few seconds.

period. Survivors are confined to an electric wheelchair and are usually unable to overcome gravity. Both proximal and distal muscles are involved. Gastrostomy may be needed for chronic dysphagia. In the juvenile form, patients are ambulatory and are able to perform most tasks of daily living. Weakness is not usually progressive, but some patients have more difficulty over time or enter a phase of progressive weakness. Cardiomyopathy is an uncommon complication.

LABORATORY FINDINGS. Serum CK is normal. The muscle biopsy shows CMFTD or at least fiber type I predominance in addition to the nemaline rods. In some patients, uniform type I fibers are seen with few or no type II fibers. Focal myofibrillar degeneration and an increase in lysosomal enzymes have been found in a few severe cases associated with progressive symptoms.

GENETIC ASPECTS. Autosomal dominant and autosomal recessive forms of nemaline rod disease are well documented, and an X-linked dominant form in girls may occur.

21.5 CENTRAL CORE DISEASE

This autosomal dominant disease is characterized pathologically by central cores within muscle fibers in which only amorphous, granular cytoplasm is found with an absence of myofibrils and organelles. Histochemical stains show a lack of enzymatic activities of all types within these cores. Clinically, infantile hypotonia, proximal weakness, muscle wasting, and involvement of facial muscles and neck flexors are the typical features. The course is nonprogressive, and the weakness is not usually severely disabling. Congenital dislocated hips and skeletal deformities are common.

Central core disease is consistently associated with malignant hyperthermia, and all patients should have special precautions before an anesthetic agent is administered. The serum CK is normal in central core disease, except during crises of malignant hyperthermia.

Variants of central cores, called minicores and multicores, are described in some families. Some children with Prader-Willi syndrome have focal loss of myofilaments resembling early central cores.

21.6 BRAIN MALFORMATIONS AND MUSCLE DEVELOPMENT

Infants with *cerebellar hypoplasia* are hypotonic and developmentally delayed. Muscle biopsy is sometimes performed to exclude a congenital myopathy. Such biopsies may show delayed maturation of muscle, fiber-type predominance, or CMFTD. Other malformations of the brain may also be associated with abnormal histochemical patterns, but supratentorial lesions are less likely than brain stem or cerebellar lesions to alter muscle development. Abnormal descending impulses along bulbospinal pathways probably alter discharge patterns of lower motor neurons that determine the histochemical differentiation of muscle. The corticospinal tract does not participate because it is not yet functional during this period of fetal life.

21.7 AMYOPLASIA

Congenital absence of individual muscles is common and is often asymmetric. One of the most common is the *palmaris longus* muscle of the ventral forearm, which is absent in one third of normal subjects and is compensated fully by other flexors of the wrist. Unilateral *absence of a sternocleidomastoid* muscle (SCM) is one cause of congenital torticollis. Absence of one *pectoralis major* muscle is part of the ***Poland anomalad.***

When innervation does not develop, such as in the lower limbs in severe cases of *myelomeningocele,* muscles may fail to develop. In *sacral agenesis,* the abnormal somites that fail to form bony vertebrae may also fail to form muscles from the same defective mesodermal plate. Skeletal muscles of the extremities fail to differentiate from embryonic myomeres if the long bones do not form. Absence of one long bone, such as the radius, is associated with variable aplasia or hypoplasia of associated muscles, such as the *carpi flexor radialis.*

21.8 BENIGN CONGENITAL HYPOTONIA

Benign congenital hypotonia is not a disease but is a descriptive term for infants or children with nonprogressive hypotonia of unknown origin. The hypotonia is not usually associated with weakness or developmental delay, although some children acquire gross motor skills more slowly than normal. Tendon stretch reflexes are normal or hypoactive. There are no cranial nerve abnormalities. Intelligence is normal.

The diagnosis is one of exclusion, after laboratory studies including muscle biopsy and imaging of the brain with special attention to the cerebellum are normal.

The *prognosis* is generally good, and no specific therapy is required. Contractures do not develop. Hypotonia persists into adult life. The disorder is not always as "benign" as its name implies, because a common complication is recurrent dislocation of joints, especially the shoulders. Excessive motility of the spine may result in stretch injury, compression, or vascular compromise of nerve roots or of the spinal cord. These are particular hazards for patients who perform gymnastics or who become circus performers, because of agility of joints without weakness or pain.

21.9 ARTHROGRYPOSIS

See Sec. 24.58.

Arthrogryposis multiplex congenita is not a disease but is a descriptive term that signifies multiple congenital contractures. The etiologies encompass both neurogenic and primary myopathic diseases, but most cases, and indeed the most severe cases, are not due to neuromuscular disease. Myopathies that have a high incidence of either minor congenital contractures or extensive arthrogryposis include myotonic muscular dystrophy, many congenital myopathies, and intrauterine viral myositis. Neurogenic diseases causing arthrogryposis include infantile spinal muscular atrophy and the Pena-Shokeir and Marden-Walker syndromes (see later).

21.10 TORTICOLLIS

Torticollis is a tilt and rotation of the head to one side and restricted rotation to the other (see also Sec. 20.30 and 24.23). The most common cause is a stretch injury of one SCM muscle during delivery. A fibrotic mass may be palpable within the muscle. The lesion may entrap a branch of the accessory nerve that passes through the sternal head to supply the clavicular head, denervating this portion of the muscle. Rarer causes of torticollis include congenital absence of one SCM, accessory nerve palsy, bony anomalies of the cervical spine, vestibular and ocular disturbances, and dystonia. Infants who consistently lie on one side may develop torticollis. Treatment depends on the cause, but physiotherapy may be a major benefit. Surgical release of a fibrotic SCM is sometimes required.

MUSCULAR DYSTROPHIES

The term *dystrophy* means abnormal growth and is derived from the Greek *trophe* meaning nourishment. Muscular dystrophy, a term coined by Erb in 1891, implies much more than simply aberrant growth or nutrition of muscle fibers, however. A *muscular dystrophy* is distinguished from all other neuromuscular diseases by four obligatory criteria: (1) It is a primary myopathy; (2) There is a genetic basis for the disorder; (3) The course is progressive; (4) Degeneration and death of muscle fibers occur at some stage in the disease. This definition excludes neurogenic diseases such as spinal muscular atrophy, nonhereditary myopathies such as dermatomyositis, nonprogressive and non-necrotizing congenital myopathies such as CMFTD, and nonprogressive inherited metabolic myopathies. Some metabolic myopathies may fulfill the definition of a progressive muscular dystrophy but are not traditionally classified as dystrophies. An example is muscle carnitine deficiency. Conversely, all muscular dystrophies might be reclassified eventually as metabolic myopathies once the biochemical defects are better defined.

Muscular dystrophies are a group of unrelated diseases, each transmitted by a different genetic trait and each differing in its clinical course and expression. Some are severe diseases at birth or lead to early death; others follow very slowly progressive courses over many decades, may be compatible with normal longevity, or may not even become symptomatic until late adult life. Some categories of dystrophies, such as limb-girdle muscular dystrophy, are probably not homogeneous diseases but rather syndromes encompassing several unrelated myopathies. Relationships between the various muscular dystrophies will be resolved by molecular genetics rather than by similarities or differences in clinical and histopathologic features.

21.11 DUCHENNE MUSCULAR DYSTROPHY

Duchenne muscular dystrophy is the most common hereditary neuromuscular disease, affecting all races and ethnic groups. Its incidence is 1:3,600 liveborn male infants. This disease is inherited as an X-linked recessive trait. The abnormal gene is on the X-chromosome at the Xp21 locus and is one of the largest yet identified.

Duchenne provided the first detailed description in 1861, in which he recognized most of the characteristic clinical features of the disease: hypertrophy of the calves, progressive weakness, intellectual impairment, and the proliferation of connective tissue in muscle. Not only did he study the histopathology of muscle at autopsy, but he also conceptualized the modern muscle biopsy by designing a harpoon-like biopsy needle to obtain muscle samples from living patients and a technique to minimize pain and bleeding.

CLINICAL MANIFESTATIONS. Male infants are only rarely symptomatic at birth or in early infancy, although some are already mildly hypotonic. Early gross motor skills, such as rolling over, sitting, and standing, are usually achieved at the appropriate ages or may be mildly delayed. Poor head control in infancy may be the first sign of weakness. Distinctive facies are not a feature, because facial muscle weakness is a late event. Walking is often accomplished at the normal age of about 12 mo, but hip girdle weakness may be seen in subtle form as early as the 2nd year. Toddlers may assume a lordotic posture when standing to compensate for gluteal weakness. An early **Gowers' sign** is often evident by 3 yr of age and is fully expressed by 5 or 6 yr of age (see Fig. 20–2). A **Trendelenberg gait,** or hip waddle, appears at this time.

The length of time that a patient remains ambulatory varies greatly. Some patients are confined to a wheelchair by 7 yr of age; most patients continue to walk with increasing difficulty until 10 yr of age without orthopedic intervention. With orthotic bracing, physiotherapy, and sometimes minor surgery (e.g., Achilles tendon lengthening), most boys with Duchenne dystrophy are able to walk until 12 yr of age. Ambulation is important not only for postponing the psychological depression that accompanies the loss of an aspect of personal independence but also because scoliosis usually does not become a major complication as long as a patient remains ambulatory even for as little as 1 hr/day; scoliosis becomes rapidly progressive after confinement to the wheelchair.

The relentless progression of weakness continues in the 2nd decade. The function of distal muscles is usually relatively well enough preserved, allowing the child to continue to use eating utensils, a pencil, and a computer keyboard. Respiratory muscle involvement is expressed as a weak and ineffective cough, frequent pulmonary infections, and decreasing respiratory reserve. Pharyngeal weakness may lead to episodes of aspiration, nasal regurgitation of liquids, and an airy or nasal voice quality. The function of the extraocular muscles remains well preserved. Incontinence due to anal and urethral sphincter weakness is an uncommon and very late event.

Contractures most often involve the ankles, knees, hips, and elbows. Scoliosis is common. The thoracic deformity further compromises pulmonary capacity and compresses the heart. Scoliosis is also uncomfortable or painful at times.

Enlargement of the calves (**pseudohypertrophy**) and wasting of thigh muscles is a classic feature. The enlargement is due to hypertrophy of some muscle fibers, infiltration of muscle by fat, and proliferation of collagen. After the calves, the next most common site of muscular hypertrophy is the tongue, followed by muscles of the forearm. Fasciculations of the tongue do not occur.

Unless ankle contractures are severe, ankle jerks remain well preserved until terminal stages. The knee jerks may be present until about 6 yr of age but are less brisk than the ankle jerks and are eventually lost. In the upper extremities, the brachioradialis reflex is usually stronger than the biceps or triceps brachii jerks.

Cardiomyopathy is a constant feature of this disease. The

severity of cardiac involvement does not necessarily correlate with the degree of skeletal muscle weakness. Some patients die early of severe cardiomyopathy while still ambulatory; others in terminal stages of the disease have well compensated cardiac function.

Intellectual impairment occurs in all patients, although only 20–30% have an intelligence quotient (IQ) less than 70. The majority have learning disabilities that still allow them to function in a regular classroom, particularly if remedial help is available. A few patients are profoundly mentally retarded, but there is no correlation with the severity of the myopathy. Epilepsy is slightly more common than in the general pediatric population.

The degenerative changes and fibrosis of muscle constitute a painless process. Myalgias and muscle spasms do not occur. Calcinosis of muscle is rare.

Death occurs usually at about 18 yr of age. The causes of death are respiratory failure in sleep, intractable congestive heart failure, pneumonia, or occasionally aspiration and airway obstruction.

LABORATORY FINDINGS. The serum CK is consistently greatly elevated in Duchenne muscular dystrophy, even in presymptomatic stages including at birth. The usual serum concentration is 15,000–35,000 IU/L (normal <160 IU/L). A normal serum CK is incompatible with the diagnosis of Duchenne dystrophy, although in terminal stages of the disease the serum CK may be considerably lower than it was a few years earlier, because there is less muscle to degenerate. Other lysosomal enzymes present in muscle, such as aldolase and AST, are also increased but are less specific.

Cardiac assessment by ECG and chest roentgenogram are essential and should be repeated periodically. After the diagnosis is established, the patient should be referred to a pediatric cardiologist for long-term cardiac care.

EMG shows characteristic myopathic features but is not specific for Duchenne muscular dystrophy. No evidence of denervation is found. Motor and sensory nerve conduction velocities are normal.

DIAGNOSIS. The muscle biopsy is diagnostic and shows characteristic changes (Fig. 21–5). Myopathic changes include endomysial connective tissue proliferation, scattered degenerating and regenerating myofibers, foci of mononuclear inflammatory cell infiltrates as a reaction to muscle fiber necrosis, mild architectural changes in still functional muscle fibers, and many dense fibers. These hypercontracted fibers probably result from segmental necrosis at another level, allowing calcium to enter the site of breakdown of the sarcolemmal membrane and trigger a contraction of the whole length of the muscle fiber.

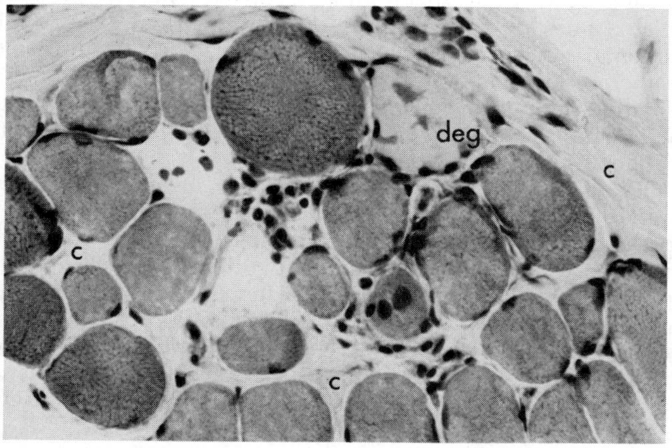

Figure 21–5. Muscle biopsy of 4-yr-old boy with Duchenne muscular dystrophy. Both atrophic and hypertrophic muscle fibers are seen, and some fibers are degenerating *(deg)*. Connective tissue (c) between muscle fibers is increased. Compare with the normal muscle shown in Figure 21–1*B*. (Hematoxylin & eosin, ×400.)

The decision of whether muscle biopsy should be performed to establish the diagnosis sometimes presents problems. If there is a family history of the disease, particularly in the case of an involved brother whose diagnosis has been confirmed, a patient with typical clinical features of Duchenne muscular dystrophy and high concentrations of serum CK probably does not need to undergo biopsy. A first case in a family, even if the clinical features are typical, should have the diagnosis confirmed to ensure that another myopathy is not masquerading as Duchenne dystrophy. The most common muscles sampled are the vastus lateralis (quadriceps femoris) and the gastrocnemius.

Newer molecular genetic studies using DNA probes may eventually become the routine and most specific method of accurate diagnosis.

GENETIC ETIOLOGY AND PATHOGENESIS. Despite the X-linked recessive inheritance in Duchenne muscular dystrophy, about 30% of patients are new mutations and the mother is not a carrier. The female carrier state usually shows no muscle weakness or any clinical expression of the disease, but affected girls are occasionally encountered, usually having much milder weakness than boys. These symptomatic girls are explained by the Lyon hypothesis in which the normal X chromosome becomes inactivated and the one with the gene deletion is active (Sec. 7.24). The full clinical picture of Duchenne dystrophy has occurred in several girls with Turner syndrome in whom the single X chromosome must have had the Xp21 gene deletion.

The asymptomatic carrier state is associated with elevated serum CK in 80% of cases. The level of increase is usually in the magnitude of hundreds or a few thousand but does not have the extreme values seen in affected males. Prepubertal girls who are Duchenne carriers also have increased serum CK, with highest levels at 8–12 yr of age. Approximately 20% of Duchenne carriers have normal serum CK. If the mother of an affected boy has a normal CK, it is unlikely that her daughter can be identified as a carrier by measuring CK. Muscle biopsy of suspected female carriers may detect an additional 10% in whom serum CK is not elevated.

Detection of the carrier state by serum CK or muscle biopsy will probably become obsolete because of recent discoveries in the molecular genetics of Duchenne muscular dystrophy. The Xp21 site of the Duchenne gene was previously recognized from translocations. The gene has more than 2,000 kilobases (kb) (2 million base pairs), but Duchenne DNA encompasses only 14 kb; less than 1% of the total genomic DNA is eventually transcribed into protein. Cloning of the breakpoint of the Xp21 gene has subsequently been accomplished, and the entire sequence of the gene has been mapped. The deletion at the breakpoint of the Xp21 gene in Duchenne muscular dystrophy is the DNA that encodes for a protein of sarcolemmal membranes called *dystrophin.* Dystrophin mRNA normally is detected in cardiac and smooth muscle as well as in skeletal muscle and brain. All of these tissues show various degrees of clinical involvement. The exact function of dystrophin is not yet completely elucidated, but a deficiency of dystrophin probably results in functional abnormalities in stretch-activated cation channels, allowing an influx of Ca^{2+} that causes muscle degeneration.

The isolation and cloning of the Duchenne gene and the discovery of dystrophin as the encoded protein that is deficient in Duchenne muscular dystrophy provides a new and precise method of molecular genetic diagnosis not only for confirming suspected cases but also for accurate carrier detection and for precise prenatal diagnosis. It also provides a potential future opportunity for cure by gene splicing and by replacement of the genetic deletion.

TREATMENT. There is presently no medical cure for this disease or method of slowing its progression. Nevertheless, much can be done to treat complications and to improve the quality of life of affected children. *Cardiac decompensation* often responds well to digoxin, at least in early stages. *Pulmonary infections* should be promptly treated. Patients should avoid contact with children who have obvious respiratory or other contagious illnesses.

Preservation of a good *nutritional state* is important. Duchenne muscular dystrophy is not a vitamin deficiency disease, and excessive doses of vitamins should be avoided. Adequate calcium intake is important to minimize osteoporosis in boys confined to the wheelchair, and fluoride supplements may also be given, particularly if the local drinking water is not fluoridated. Because sedentary children burn fewer calories than active children and because of depression as an additional factor, these children tend to eat excessively and gain weight. Obesity makes a patient with myopathy even less functional because part of the limited reserve muscle strength is dissipated in lifting the weight of excess subcutaneous adipose tissue. Dietary restrictions with supervision may be needed.

Physiotherapy delays but does not always prevent contractures. At times, contractures may actually be useful to functional rehabilitation. For example, if contractures prevent extension of the elbow beyond 90 degrees and the muscles of the upper limb no longer are strong enough to overcome gravity, the elbow contractures are functionally beneficial in fixing an otherwise flail arm and in allowing the patient to eat and write. The surgical correction of the elbow contracture may be technically feasible, but the result may be deleterious. Physiotherapy contributes little to muscle strengthening because the patient usually is already using his or her entire reserve for daily function, and exercise cannot further strengthen involved muscles. Excessive exercise may actually accelerate the process of muscle fiber degeneration.

Steroid hormones, either natural hydrocortisone or synthetic analogs such as prednisone, have no place in the conventional treatment of Duchenne muscular dystrophy. The complications of steroids including steroid-induced myopathy may actually worsen the clinical course.

Myoblast transfer is a new experimental approach to treatment. It involves the in vitro culture of myoblasts obtained from the mature normal muscle of a close but unaffected relative, usually the father. Satellite cells are embryonic presumptive myoblasts that lie dormant in mature muscle but are capable of mitotic proliferation, and differentiation into muscle cells as a regenerative or repair process when muscle is injured. The myoblast culture is then injected into dystrophic muscles of the patient with the theoretical expectation that they will replace degenerating muscle fibers with healthy ones that do not lack dystrophin. The patient must first be immunosuppressed to prevent rejection, as with any organ transplantation. The success of myoblast transfer therapy is not yet established.

21.12 BECKER MUSCULAR DYSTROPHY

This disease is the same as Duchenne muscular dystrophy but follows a slower, more protracted course. In classical Duchenne dystrophy boys almost never remain ambulatory beyond 12 yr of age; in Becker dystrophy they are ambulatory until age 16 yr or later. Intermediate cases also occur. Calf hypertrophy, cardiomyopathy, learning disabilities, greatly elevated serum CK, and muscle biopsy changes are similar in Becker and Duchenne dystrophies. The onset of weakness is later in Becker dystrophy than in Duchenne dystrophy. Death often occurs in the mid- or late 20s. Fewer than half of the patients are still alive by 40 yr of age, and these survivors are severely disabled.

Becker muscular dystrophy is transmitted by X-linked recessive inheritance, and the mutation of the Xp21 gene is identical to that of Duchenne muscular dystrophy. However, there is no correlation between the size and the position of a deletion in the dystrophin gene and clinical expression as the Duchenne or Becker type. Several molecular genetic hypotheses have been proposed to explain the difference between these clinical forms, but none has been verified.

21.13 EMERY-DREIFUSS MUSCULAR DYSTROPHY

Emery-Dreifuss muscular dystrophy, also known as *scapuloperoneal* or *scapulohumeral muscular dystrophy,* is another X-linked recessive dystrophy, but the gene has not been isolated. Unlike Duchenne and Becker muscular dystrophies, it is rare.

Clinical manifestations begin in middle childhood, but many patients survive to late adult life because of the slow progression of its course. Hypertrophy of muscles does not occur. Contractures of elbows and ankles develop early, and muscle becomes wasted in a scapulohumeroperoneal distribution. Facial weakness does not occur, distinguishing this disease clinically from autosomal dominant scapulohumeral and scapuloperoneal syndromes of neurogenic origin. Myotonia is absent. Intellectual function is normal. Cardiomyopathy is severe and is often the cause of death. The serum CK is only mildly elevated, further distinguishing this disease from other X-linked recessive muscular dystrophies.

Nonspecific myofiber necrosis and endomysial fibrosis are seen in the muscle biopsy. Many centronuclear fibers and selective histochemical type I muscle fiber atrophy may cause confusion with myotonic dystrophy. Treatment should be supportive.

21.14 MYOTONIC MUSCULAR DYSTROPHY

Myotonic dystrophy (**Steinert's disease**) is the second most common muscular dystrophy in North America, Europe, and Australia, having an incidence of 1:30,000 general population. It is inherited as an autosomal dominant trait.

Myotonic dystrophy is an example of a genetic defect causing dysfunction in multiple organ systems. Not only is striated muscle severely affected, but smooth muscle of the alimentary tract and uterus is also involved; cardiac function is altered; and patients have multiple and variable endocrinopathies, immunologic deficiencies, cataracts, dysmorphic facies, intellectual impairment, and other neurologic abnormalities.

CLINICAL MANIFESTATIONS. In the usual clinical course, excluding the severe neonatal form, infants may appear almost normal at birth, or facial wasting and hypotonia may already be early expressions of the disease. The facial appearance is characteristic, consisting of an inverted V-shaped upper lip, thin cheeks, and scalloped, concave temporalis muscles (Fig. 21–6). The head may be narrow, and the palate is high and arched because the weak temporal and pterygoid muscles in late fetal life do not exert sufficient lateral forces on the developing head and face.

Weakness is mild in the first few years. Progressive wasting of distal muscles becomes increasingly evident, particularly involving intrinsic muscles of the hands. The thenar and hypothenar eminences are flattened, and the atrophic dorsal interossei leave deep grooves between the fingers. The dorsal

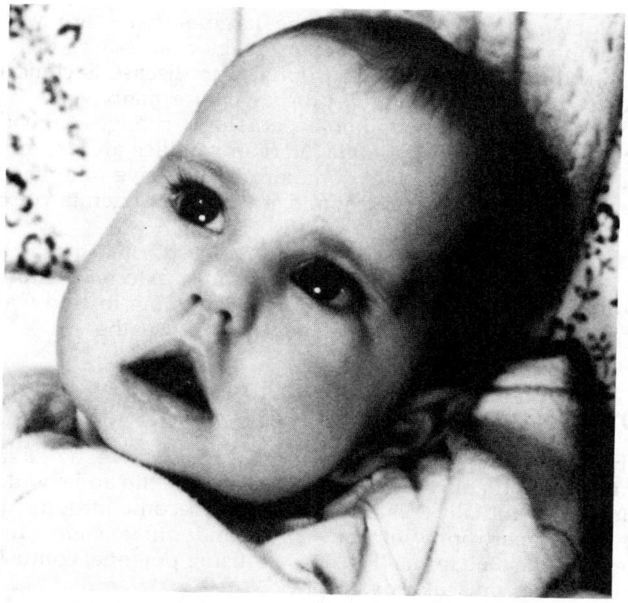

Figure 21–6. Facial weakness, inverted V-shaped upper lip, and loss of muscle mass in the temporal fossae are characteristic of myotonic muscular dystrophy even in infancy, as seen in this 8-mo-old girl.

forearm muscles and anterior compartment muscles of the lower legs also become wasted. The tongue is thin and atrophic. Wasting of the sternocleidomastoids gives the neck a long, thin, cylindrical contour. Eventually, proximal muscles also undergo atrophy, and scapular winging appears. Difficulty with climbing stairs and Gowers' sign are progressive. Tendon stretch reflexes are usually preserved.

The distal distribution of muscle wasting in myotonic dystrophy is an exception to the general rule of myopathies having proximal and neuropathies distal distribution patterns. The muscular atrophy and weakness in myotonic dystrophy are slowly progressive throughout childhood and adolescence and continue into adulthood. It is rare for patients with myotonic dystrophy to lose the ability to walk, however, even in late adult life, although splints or bracing may be required to stabilize the ankles.

Myotonia, a characteristic feature shared by few other myopathies, does not occur in infancy and is usually not clinically or even electromyographically evident until about 5 yr of age. Exceptional patients develop it as early as 3 yr of age. Myotonia is a very slow relaxation of muscle after contraction, regardless of whether that contraction was voluntary or was induced by a stretch reflex or electrical stimulation. During the physical examination, myotonia may be demonstrated by asking the patient to make tight fists and then to quickly open the hands. It may be induced by striking the thenar eminence with a rubber percussion hammer, and it may be detected by watching the involuntary drawing of the thumb across the palm. Myotonia may also be demonstrated in the tongue by pressing the edge of a wooden tongue blade against its dorsal surface and by observing a deep furrow that disappears slowly.

The severity of myotonia does not necessarily parallel the degree of weakness, and the weakest muscles often have only minimal myotonia. Myotonia is not a painful muscle spasm. Myalgias do not occur in myotonic dystrophy.

The speech of patients with myotonic dystrophy is often articulated poorly and is slurred because of the involvement of the muscles of the face, tongue, and pharynx. Difficulties with swallowing sometimes occur. Aspiration is a risk in severely involved children. Incomplete external ophthalmoplegia may sometimes result from extraocular muscle weakness.

Smooth muscle involvement of the gastrointestinal tract results in slow gastric emptying, poor peristalsis, and constipation. Some patients have encopresis associated with anal sphincter weakness. Women with myotonic dystrophy may have ineffective or abnormal uterine contractions during labor and delivery.

Cardiac involvement usually manifests as blocks in the Purkinje conduction system and arrhythmias rather than as cardiomyopathy, unlike most other muscular dystrophies.

Endocrine abnormalities may involve many glands and appear at any time during the course of the disease, so that re-evaluation of endocrine status must be done annually in the first few years and every several years after that. Hypothyroidism is commonly associated; hyperthyroidism may occur rarely. Adrenocortical insufficiency may lead to an Addisonian crisis, even in infancy. Diabetes mellitus is common in patients with myotonic deficiency; some children have a disorder of insulin release rather than defective insulin production by islet cells of the pancreas. Onset of puberty may be precocious or, more commonly, delayed. Testicular atrophy and testosterone deficiency are common in adults and are responsible for a high incidence of male infertility. A corresponding ovarian atrophy is rare. Frontal baldness is also characteristic in males and often begins in adolescence.

Immunologic deficiencies are common in myotonic dystrophy. The plasma IgG is often low.

Cataracts occur frequently in myotonic dystrophy. They may be congenital or they may begin at any time during childhood or adult life. Early cataracts are detected only by slit lamp examination, and periodic examination by an ophthalmologist is recommended. Visual evoked potentials are often abnormal in children with myotonic dystrophy and are unrelated to cataracts. They are not usually accompanied by visual impairment, however.

About half of the patients with myotonic dystrophy are intellectually impaired, but severe mental retardation is unusual. The remainder are of average or occasionally above average intelligence. Epilepsy is not common.

A **severe neonatal form of myotonic dystrophy** appears in a minority of involved infants born to mothers with myotonic dystrophy. Clubfoot deformities alone or more extensive congenital contractures of multiple joints may involve all extremities and even the cervical spine. Generalized hypotonia and weakness are present at birth. Some infants require gavage feeding or even ventilator support for respiratory muscle weakness or apnea. One or both leaves of the diaphragm may be nonfunctional. The abdomen becomes distended with gas in the stomach and intestine because of poor peristalsis due to smooth muscle weakness. The distention further compromises respiration. Inability to empty the rectum may compound the problem. About 75% of severely affected neonates die within the 1st year.

LABORATORY FINDINGS. The classic myotonic EMG is not found in infancy but may appear in toddlers or during the early school years. The serum CK and other serum enzymes from muscle may be normal or only mildly elevated in the hundreds (never the thousands).

An ECG should be performed annually in early childhood.

Ultrasonic imaging of the abdomen may be indicated in affected infants to determine diaphragmatic function. Roentgenograms of the chest and abdomen and contrast studies of gastrointestinal motility may be needed.

Endocrine assessment should be undertaken to determine thyroid and adrenal cortical function and to verify carbohydrate metabolism (e.g., glucose tolerance test with serum insulin levels).

Immunoglobulins should be examined, and more extensive immunologic studies should be performed if needed.

DIAGNOSIS. The muscle biopsy often shows many muscle fibers with central nuclei and selective atrophy of histochemical type I fibers, but degenerating fibers are usually few and widely scattered, and there is little or no fibrosis of muscle. Intrafusal fibers of muscle spindles are also abnormal. In young children with the common form of the disease, the biopsy may even appear normal or may at least not show myofiber necroses, which is a striking contrast with Duchenne muscular dystrophy. In the severe neonatal form of myotonic dystrophy, the muscle biopsy reveals maturational arrest in various stages of development. It is likely that the sarcolemmal membrane of muscle fibers not only has abnormal properties of electrical polarization but is also incapable of responding to trophic influences of the motor neuron. Muscle biopsy is not usually required for diagnosis, which in typical cases can be based on the clinical manifestations. It is recommended in severe neonatal cases because the biopsy may be of prognostic as well as of diagnostic value. Experimental studies in mice indicate that there is a factor in the serum of mothers with myotonic dystrophy that impairs fetal muscle maturation.

GENETICS. The defective gene has been localized to chromosome 19, although the gene is not yet isolated. The clinical expressivity varies, even among affected siblings. The genetic aspect is more complex than it appears because the mother transmits the disease in 94% of cases, a fact that cannot be explained by the increased incidence of male infertility alone. Myotonic dystrophy often exhibits a pattern of *anticipation,* in which each successive generation has a tendency to be more severely involved than the previous generation.

TREATMENT. There is no specific medical treatment, but the cardiac, endocrine, gastrointestinal, and ocular complications can often be treated. Physiotherapy and orthopedic treatment of contractures in the neonatal form of the disease may be beneficial.

Myotonia may be diminished and function may be restored by drugs that raise the depolarization threshold of muscle membranes, such as phenytoin (PHT), carbamazepine (CBZ), procainamide, and quinidine sulfate. These drugs also have cardiotropic effects, thus cardiac evaluation is important before prescribing them. PHT and CBZ are used in doses similar to their use as anticonvulsants (Sec. 20.21); serum concentrations of 40–80 μmol/L for PHT and 35–50 μmol/L for CBZ should be maintained. If the patient's disability is due mainly to weakness rather than to myotonia, these drugs will be of no value.

21.15 OTHER MYOTONIC SYNDROMES

Most patients with myotonia have myotonic dystrophy. However, myotonia is not specific for this disease and occurs in several rarer conditions.

Myotonic chondrodystrophy **(Schwartz-Jampel disease)** is a rare congenital disease characterized by generalized muscular hypertrophy and weakness. Dysmorphic phenotypical features and the roentgenographic appearance of long bones are reminiscent of Morquio's disease (Sec. 8.19), but abnormal mucopolysaccharides are not found. Dwarfism, joint abnormalities, and blepharophimosis are present. Several patients have been the products of consanguinity, suggesting autosomal recessive inheritance.

EMG reveals continuous electrical activity in muscle fibers closely resembling or identical to myotonia. Muscle biopsy reveals nonspecific myopathic features, which are minimal in some cases and pronounced in others. The sarcotubular system is dilated.

Myotonia congenita **(Thomsen's disease)** was first described by Thomsen in 1876 in his own family. It is characterized by generalized muscular hypertrophy, so that affected children resemble body builders, but the large muscles are weak. Myotonia is prominent and may develop at 2–3 yr of age, earlier than in myotonic dystrophy. The disease is clinically stable and is apparently not progressive for many years. The muscle biopsy shows minimal pathologic changes, and the EMG demonstrates myotonia. Various families are described showing either autosomal dominant or recessive inheritance. Rarely, myotonic dystrophy and myotonia congenita coexist in the same family.

Paramyotonia is a temperature-related myotonia that is aggravated by cold and alleviated by warm external temperatures. Patients have difficulty when swimming in cold water or if they are dressed inadequately in cold weather.

21.16 LIMB-GIRDLE MUSCULAR DYSTROPHY

This term encompasses a group of progressive hereditary myopathies that mainly affect muscles of the hip and shoulder girdles. Eventually, distal muscles also become atrophic and weak. Hypertrophy of the calves and ankle contractures develop in some forms (Fig. 21–7) causing potential confusion with Becker muscular dystrophy.

The initial symptoms and signs rarely appear before middle or late childhood or may be deferred until early adult life. Low back pain may be a presenting complaint because of the lordotic posture resulting from gluteal muscle weakness. Confinement to a wheelchair does not usually become obligatory until about 30 yr of age. The rate of progression varies from one pedigree to another but is uniform within a kindred. Although weakness of neck flexors and extensors is universal, facial, lingual, and other bulbar-innervated muscles rarely are clinically involved. As weakness and muscle wasting progresses, tendon stretch reflexes become diminished. Cardiac involvement is unusual. Intellectual function is generally normal. The clinical differential diagnosis of limb-girdle muscular dystrophy includes juvenile spinal muscular atrophy (**Kugelberg-Welander disease**), myasthenia gravis, and metabolic myopathies.

Most cases of limb-girdle muscular dystrophy are of autosomal recessive inheritance, but some families express an

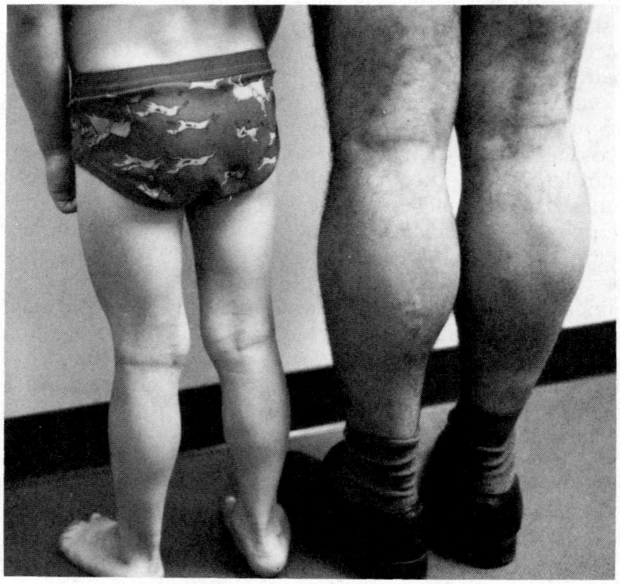

Figure 21–7. Posterior aspect of the legs of a father and his 6-yr-old son with a rare autosomal dominant muscular dystrophy. Hypertrophy of the calves resembles Duchenne muscular dystrophy, but the clinical course is benign and causes little disability throughout life.

autosomal dominant trait. The latter often follows a benign course with little functional impairment (see Fig. 21–7).

The EMG and muscle biopsy show confirmatory evidence of muscular dystrophy, but none of the findings are specific enough to make the definitive diagnosis without additional clinical criteria. Increased serum CK is usual, but the magnitude of elevation varies among families. The ECG is usually unaltered.

21.17 FACIOSCAPULOHUMERAL MUSCULAR DYSTROPHY

Facioscapulohumeral (FSH) muscular dystrophy, also known as **Landouzy-Déjerine disease,** is probably not a single disease entity but a group of diseases with similar clinical manifestations. Autosomal dominance is the rule, and the phenomenon of *anticipation* is often seen within several generations of a family, the succeeding more severely involved at an earlier age than the preceding.

CLINICAL MANIFESTATIONS. As the name implies, FSH dystrophy shows the earliest and most severe weakness in facial and shoulder girdle muscles. The facial weakness differs from that of myotonic dystrophy; rather than an inverted V-shaped upper lip, the mouth in FSH dystrophy is rounded and appears puckered because the upper and lower lips protrude. Inability to close the eyes completely in sleep is a common expression of upper facial weakness, and some patients have extraocular muscle weakness, although ophthalmoplegia is rarely complete. FSH dystrophy has been reported in association with Möbius syndrome on rare occasions. Pharyngeal and tongue weakness may be absent and are never as severe as the facial involvement.

Scapular winging is prominent, often even in infants. Flattening or even concavity of the deltoid contour is seen, and the biceps and triceps brachii muscles are wasted and weak. Muscles of the hip girdles and thighs also eventually lose strength and undergo atrophy, and Gowers' sign and a Trendelberg gait appear. Contractures are rare, however. Occasionally, finger and wrist weakness is the first symptom recognized by the patient with FSH muscular dystrophy. Weakness of the anterior tibial and peroneal muscles may lead to foot drop, but this complication usually occurs only in advanced cases with severe proximal weakness. Lumbar lordosis and kyphoscoliosis are common complications of axial muscle involvement. Calf hypertrophy is not a feature.

FSH muscular dystrophy may be a mild disease causing minimal disability in some cases. At times, clinical manifestations may not even be expressed in childhood and are delayed into middle adult life. Unlike most other muscular dystrophies, asymmetry of weakness is common.

LABORATORY FINDINGS. Serum CK and other enzymes vary greatly, ranging from normal or near-normal to elevations of several thousand. ECG should be performed, although the anticipated findings are usually normal. EMG reveals nonspecific myopathic muscle potentials.

DIAGNOSIS AND DIFFERENTIAL DIAGNOSIS. The muscle biopsy distinguishes more than one form of FSH, consistent with clinical evidence that several distinct diseases are embraced by the term FSH dystrophy. Muscle biopsy and EMG also distinguish the primary myopathy from a neurogenic disease with a similar distribution of muscular involvement. The general histopathologic findings in the muscle biopsy are extensive proliferation of connective tissue between muscle fibers, extreme variation in fiber size with many hypertrophic as well as atrophic myofibers, and scattered degenerating and regenerating fibers. An "inflammatory" type FSH muscular dystrophy is also distinguished, characterized by extensive lymphocytic infiltrates within muscle fascicles. Despite the resemblance of this form to true inflammatory myopathies, such as polymyositis, there is no evidence of autoimmune disease and steroids and immunosuppressive drugs do not alter the clinical course. A precise histopathologic diagnosis, therefore, has important therapeutic implications. Mononuclear cell "inflammation" in a muscle biopsy of infants less than 2 yr of age is usually FSH dystrophy.

TREATMENT. Physiotherapy is of no value in regaining strength or in retarding progressive weakness or muscle wasting. Foot drop and scoliosis may be treated by orthopedic measures. Cosmetic improvement of the facial muscles of expression may be achieved by reconstructive surgery, which grafts a fascia lata to the zygomatic muscle and to the zygomatic head of the *quadratus labiae superioris* muscle.

21.18 CONGENITAL MUSCULAR DYSTROPHY

The term "*congenital*" muscular dystrophy is misleading because all muscular dystrophies are genetically determined, hence congenital, diseases. It is used to encompass several distinct diseases with a common characteristic of severe involvement at birth but which ironically usually follow a benign clinical course. Autosomal recessive inheritance is the rule in each.

CLINICAL MANIFESTATIONS. Infants often have contractures or arthrogryposis at birth and are diffusely hypotonic. The muscle mass is thin in the trunk and extremities. Head control is poor. Facial muscles may be mildly involved, but ophthalmoplegia, pharyngeal weakness, and a weak suck are not common. Tendon stretch reflexes may be hypoactive or absent. Arthrogryposis is common in all forms of congenital muscular dystrophy (Sec. 24.58).

One form of congenital muscular dystrophy, the **Fukuyama type,** is the 2nd most common muscular dystrophy in Japan (following Duchenne dystrophy), but this disease has also been reported in children of Dutch, German, Scandinavian, and Turkish ethnic backgrounds and therefore is not limited to the Japanese. In the Fukuyama variety, severe cardiomyopathy and malformations of the brain usually accompany the skeletal muscle involvement. Signs and symptoms related to these organs are prominent: cardiomegaly and congestive failure, mental retardation, seizures, microcephaly, and failure to thrive.

Neurologic disease may accompany forms of congenital muscular dystrophy other than Fukuyama disease. Mental and neurologic status are the most variable features, and an apparently normal brain and normal intelligence do not preclude the diagnosis if other manifestations indicate this myopathy. The cerebral malformations that occur are not consistently of one type and vary from severe dysplasias (e.g., holoprosencephaly or lissencephaly) to milder conditions (e.g., agenesis of the corpus callosum, focal heterotopia of the cerebral cortex and subcortical white matter, and cerebellar hypoplasia).

LABORATORY FINDINGS. Serum CK is usually moderately elevated from several hundred to many thousand IU/L, but only marginal increases are sometimes found. EMG shows nonspecific myopathic features. Investigation of all forms of congenital muscular dystrophy should include cardiac assessment and an imaging study of the brain.

DIAGNOSIS. The muscle biopsy is diagnostic in the neonatal period or thereafter. An extensive proliferation of endomysial collagen envelops individual muscle fibers even at birth, also causing them to be rounded in cross-sectional contour by acting as a rigid sleeve, especially during contraction. The perimysial connective tissue and fat are also increased, and the fascicular organization of the muscle may be disrupted by the fibrosis. Tissue cultures of intramuscular fibroblasts exhibit increased collagen synthesis, but the structure of the collagen is normal. Muscle fibers vary in diameter, and many show central nuclei, myofibrillar splitting, and other cytoarchitectural alterations. Scattered degenerating and regenerating fibers are seen. No inflammation or abnormal inclusions are found.

ENDOCRINE AND METABOLIC MYOPATHIES

21.19 THYROID MYOPATHIES

See also Sec. 19.10.

Thyrotoxicosis causes proximal weakness and wasting accompanied by myopathic EMG changes. Thyroxine binds to myofibrils, and an excess impairs contractile function. Hyperthyroidism may also induce myasthenia gravis and hypokalemic periodic paralysis (see later).

Hypothyroidism, whether congenital or acquired, consistently produces hypotonia and a proximal distribution of weakness. Although muscle wasting is most characteristic, one form of cretinism, the **Kocher-Debré-Sémélaigne syndrome** is characterized by hypertrophy of weak muscles. The serum CK is elevated in hypothyroid myopathy and returns to normal after thyroid replacement therapy. The muscle biopsy reveals myopathic changes, including myofiber necrosis and sometimes central cores.

Both the clinical and pathologic features of hyperthyroid myopathy and hypothyroid myopathy resolve after appropriate treatment of the thyroid disorder.

21.20 HYPERPARATHYROIDISM

See also Sec. 19.20.

Most patients with primary hyperparathyroidism develop weakness, fatigability, and muscle wasting that are reversible after the removal of the parathyroid adenoma.

21.21 STEROID-INDUCED MYOPATHY

Both natural **Cushing's disease** and the iatrogenic **Cushing syndrome** from exogenous corticosteroid administration may cause progressive proximal weakness, increased serum CK, and a myopathic EMG and muscle biopsy (Sec. 19.24). Myosin filaments may be selectively lost. Fluorinated steroids, such as dexamethasone, are the most likely to produce *steroid myopathy*. In patients with dermatomyositis or other myopathies treated with steroids, it is sometimes difficult to distinguish refractoriness of the disease from steroid-induced weakness, especially after the chronic administration of these drugs.

Hyperaldosteronism (Conn's syndrome) is accompanied by episodic and reversible weakness similar to that of periodic paralysis (see later). The proximal myopathy may become irreversible in chronic cases. Elevated CK and even myoglobinuria sometimes occur during acute attacks.

21.22 POTASSIUM-RELATED PERIODIC PARALYSIS

Episodic weakness or paralysis known as *periodic paralysis* is associated with transient alterations in serum potassium, usually hypokalemia but occasionally hyperkalemia and sometimes even biphasic in the same patient. The disorder is inherited as an autosomal dominant trait. It is precipitated in some patients by hyperaldosteronism or hyperthyroidism, by amphotericin B, or by ingestion of licorice.

In childhood, periodic paralysis often occurs as an episodic event, the patient being unable to move after awakening and gradually recovering muscle strength during the new few minutes or hours. Muscles that remain active in sleep, such as the diaphragm and cardiac muscle, are not affected. Patients are normal between attacks, but in adult life the attacks become more frequent and the disorder causes progressive myopathy with permanent weakness even between attacks.

Alterations in serum potassium are seen only during acute episodes and are accompanied by T wave changes in the ECG. The CK may be mildly elevated at those times. The muscle biopsy is often normal between attacks, but during an attack a vacuolar myopathy is demonstrated. The vacuoles are dilated sarcoplasmic reticulum and invaginations of the extracellular space into the cytoplasm, and they are filled with glycogen. Hypoglycemia does not occur.

21.23 MALIGNANT HYPERTHERMIA

See also Sec. 6.51.

This syndrome is usually inherited as an autosomal dominant trait. It occurs in all patients with central core disease but is not limited to that particular myopathy. It occurs rarely in Duchenne and other muscular dystrophies, in a variety of other myopathies, and in an isolated syndrome not associated with other muscle disease. Affected children sometimes have peculiar facies. All ages are affected, including even a premature infant whose mother underwent general anesthesia for cesarean section.

Acute episodes are precipitated by exposure to general anesthetics and occasionally even to local anesthetic drugs. The patient suddenly develops extreme fever, rigidity of muscles, and the serum CK rises to as high as 35,000 IU/L. Myoglobinuria may result in tubular necrosis and acute renal failure.

The muscle biopsy during an episode of malignant hyperthermia or shortly afterward shows widely scattered necrosis of muscle fibers, known as *rhabdomyolysis*. Between attacks, the muscle biopsy is normal unless there is an underlying chronic myopathy.

It is important to recognize patients at risk for malignant hyperthermia because the attacks may be prevented by administering dantrolene sodium before an anesthetic is given. Identification of patients at risk, such as siblings of those who have experienced an episode, is done by the caffeine contracture test: a portion of fresh muscle biopsy tissue in a saline bath is attached to a strain gauge and exposed to caffeine and other drugs; an abnormal spasm is diagnostic.

21.24 GLYCOGENOSES

See also Sec. 8.40 and 20.58.

Glycogenosis I **(von Gierke's disease)** is not a true myopathy because the deficient liver enzyme, glucose-6-phosphatase, is not normally present in muscle. Nevertheless, children with this disease are hypotonic and mildly weak for uncertain reasons.

Glycogenosis II **(Pompe's disease)** is an autosomal recessively inherited deficiency of the glycolytic lysosomal enzyme acid maltase. Two forms are described. The infantile form is a severe generalized myopathy and cardiomyopathy. Cardiomegaly and hepatomegaly are present, and patients are diffusely hypotonic and weak. The serum CK is greatly elevated. Muscle biopsy reveals a vacuolar myopathy with abnormal lysosomal enzymatic activity (Fig. 21–8). Death in infancy or early childhood is usual.

The late childhood or adult form of acid maltase deficiency is a much milder myopathy without cardiac or hepatic enlarge-

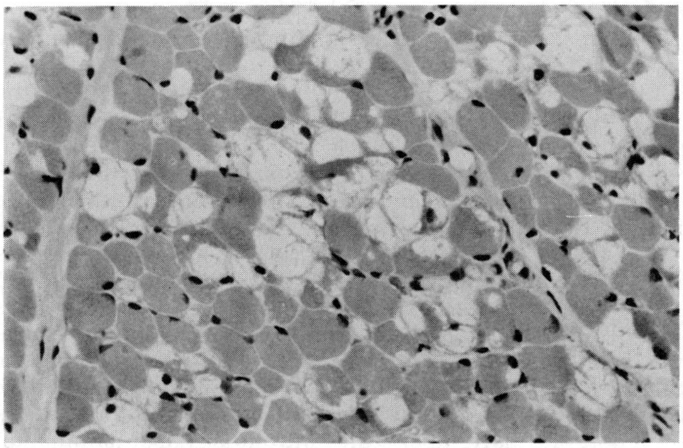

Figure 21–8. Muscle biopsy of 2-yr-old boy with glycogenosis II (Pompe's disease; acid maltase deficiency). More than half of the myofibers have large vacuoles replacing contractile myofibrils and cytoplasmic organelles. Special stains show glycogen storage and abnormally strong activity of lysosomal enzymes. (Hematoxylin & eosin, ×250.)

ment. It does not become clinically expressed until later childhood or early adult life, but the serum CK is greatly elevated and the muscle biopsy is diagnostic even in the presymptomatic stage.

The diagnosis of glycogenosis II is confirmed by quantitative assay of acid maltase activity in muscle or liver biopsy tissue.

Glycogenosis III **(Cori-Forbes disease),** deficiency of debrancher enzyme (amylo-1,6-glucosidase), is the most common of the glycogenoses, but also the least severe clinically. Hypotonia, weakness, hepatomegaly, and fasting hypoglycemia in infancy are common, but these features often resolve spontaneously, and patients become asymptomatic in childhood and adult life. Others experience slowly progressive distal muscle wasting, hepatic cirrhosis, and heart failure. Minor myopathic findings including vacuolation of muscle fibers are found in the muscle biopsy.

Glycogenosis IV **(Andersen's disease)** is a deficiency of brancher enzyme, resulting in the formation of an abnormal glycogen molecule, amylopectin, in the liver, reticuloendothelial cells, and skeletal and cardiac muscle. Hypotonia, generalized weakness, muscle wasting, and contractures are the usual signs of myopathic involvement. Most patients die before 4 yr of age because of hepatic or cardiac failure. A few children are described without neuromuscular manifestations.

Glycogenosis V **(McArdle's disease)** is due to muscle phosphorylase deficiency, inherited as an autosomal recessive trait. Exercise intolerance is the cardinal clinical feature. Physical exertion results in cramps, weakness, and myoglobinuria, but strength is normal between attacks. The serum CK is elevated only during exercise. A characteristic clinical feature is lack of the normal rise in serum lactate during ischemic exercise, because of inability to convert pyruvate to lactate under anaerobic conditions in vivo. Myophosphorylase activity or its deficiency may be demonstrated histochemically and biochemically in the muscle biopsy.

A rare *neonatal form* of myophosphorylase deficiency causes feeding difficulties in early infancy, may be severe enough to result in neonatal death, or may follow a course of slowly progressive weakness resembling a muscular dystrophy.

The long-term prognosis is good. Patients must learn to moderate their physical activities, but they do not develop severe chronic myopathic handicaps or cardiac involvement.

Glycogenosis VII **(Tarui's disease)** is muscle phosphofructokinase deficiency. Although rarer than glycogenosis V, the symptoms of exercise intolerance, clinical course, and inability to convert pyruvate to lactate are identical. The distinction is made by biochemical study of the muscle biopsy.

21.25 MITOCHONDRIAL MYOPATHIES

See also Sec. 20.51.

Several diseases involving muscle, brain, and other organs are associated with structural and functional abnormalities of mitochondria, producing defects in aerobic cellular metabolism, the electron transport chain, and the Krebs cycle. The structural aberrations are best demonstrated by electron microscopy of the muscle biopsy, revealing abnormally shaped cristae and fusion of cristae to form *paracrystalline inclusions*. Histochemical study of sections of muscle biopsy reveal abnormal clumping of oxidative enzymatic activity, sometimes increased neutral lipids because of impaired lipid metabolism, and "ragged-red" muscle fibers with accumulations of membranous material beneath the muscle fiber membrane, best demonstrated by special stains. Several distinct mitochondrial diseases are identified.

The *Kearns-Sayre syndrome* is characterized by the triad of progressive external ophthalmoplegia, pigmentary degeneration of the retina, and onset before 20 yr of age. Heart block, cerebellar deficits, and high cerebrospinal fluid protein content are often associated. Visual evoked potentials are abnormal. Patients usually do not experience weakness of the trunk or extremities or dysphagia. Most cases are sporadic.

Chronic progressive external ophthalmoplegia may be isolated or accompanied by limb muscle weakness, dysphagia, and dysarthria. A few patients described as **ophthalmoplegia plus** have additional central nervous system (CNS) involvement. Autosomal dominant inheritance is found in some pedigrees, but most cases are sporadic.

Myoclonic epilepsy and ragged-red fibers (MERRF) and the *MELAS syndrome,* an acronym for *m*itochondrial myopathy, *e*ncephalopathy, *l*actic *a*cidosis, and *s*troke-like episodes, are other mitochondrial disorders affecting children. The latter is characterized by stunted growth, episodic vomiting, seizures, and recurrent cerebral insults causing hemiparesis, hemianopia or even cortical blindness, and dementia. The disease behaves as a degenerative disorder and children die within a few years.

Other "degenerative" diseases of the CNS that also involve myopathy with mitochondrial abnormalities include *Leigh's subacute necrotizing encephalopathy* (Sec. 20.58) and *cerebrohepatorenal* **(Zellweger)** disease (Sec. 8.16). Another recognized mitochondrial myopathy is *cytochrome-c-oxidase deficiency. Oculopharyngeal muscular dystrophy* also is fundamentally a mitochondrial myopathy. Many other rare diseases with only a few case reports are suspected of being mitochondrial disorders.

The genetics of mitochondrial disease may involve mitochondrial DNA, which is distinct from the DNA of the cell nucleus and is inherited exclusively from the mother; mitochondria are present in the cytoplasm of the ovum but not in the sperm. The rate of mutation of mitochondrial DNA is 10 times higher than that of nuclear DNA.

21.26 LIPID MYOPATHIES

See Sec. 8.15.

Considered as a metabolic organ, the skeletal muscle is the most important site in the body for long-chain fatty acid metabolism because of its large mass and its rich density of mitochondria, where fatty acids are metabolized. Hereditary disorders of lipid metabolism that cause progressive myopathy are an important, relatively common, and often treatable group of muscle diseases.

Muscle carnitine deficiency (Sec. 8.15) is an autosomal recessive disease involving deficient transport of dietary carnitine across the intestinal mucosa. Carnitine, acquired from dietary sources and also synthesized in the liver and kidney from lysine and methionine, is the obligatory carrier of long- and medium-chain fatty acids into muscle mitochondria.

The clinical course is that of a progressive muscular dystrophy with generalized proximal myopathy and sometimes facial, pharyngeal, and cardiac involvement. Symptoms usually begin in late childhood or adolescence, or may be delayed until adult life. Progression is slow but may end in death.

Serum CK is mildly elevated. Muscle biopsy shows vacuoles filled with lipid within muscle fibers, in addition to nonspecific changes suggestive of a muscular dystrophy. Mitochondria may appear normal or abnormal. Carnitine measured in muscle biopsy tissue is reduced, but serum carnitine is normal.

Treatment stops the progression of the disease and may even restore lost strength if the disease is not too advanced. It consists of special diets low in long-chain fatty acids. Steroids may enhance fatty acid transport. Specific therapy with L-carnitine taken by mouth in large doses overcomes the intestinal barrier in some patients. Some patients also improve with supplementary riboflavin, and other patients seem to improve with propranolol.

Systemic carnitine deficiency (Sec. 8.15) is a disease of impaired renal and hepatic synthesis of carnitine rather than a primary myopathy. Patients with this autosomal recessive disease experience progressive proximal myopathy and show muscle biopsy changes similar to muscle carnitine deficiency. But the onset of weakness is earlier and may be evident at birth. Endocardial fibroelastosis also may occur. Episodes of acute hepatic encephalopathy resembling Reye's syndrome may occur. Hypoglycemia and metabolic acidosis complicate acute episodes.

The concentration of carnitine is reduced in serum as well as in muscle and liver. A similar clinical syndrome may be a complication of the renal *Fanconi syndrome,* because of excessive urinary loss of carnitine or during chronic hemodialysis.

Treatment with L-carnitine improves the maintenance of blood glucose and serum carnitine levels but does not reverse the ketosis or acidosis or improve exercise capacity.

Muscle carnitine palmityltransferase (CPT) deficiency presents as episodes of rhabdomyolysis, coma, and elevated serum CK that may be indistinguishable from Reye's syndrome. CPT transfers long-chain fatty acid-acyl-CoA residues to carnitine on the outer mitochondrial membrane for transport into the mitochondria. Exercise intolerance and myoglobinuria resemble glycogenoses V and VII (see earlier). Fasting hypoglycemia may also occur. Genetic transmission is autosomal recessive in some cases and autosomal dominant in others.

21.27 VITAMIN E DEFICIENCY MYOPATHY

Deficiency of vitamin E in experimental animals produces a progressive myopathy closely resembling a muscular dystrophy. Myopathy and neuropathy are recognized in humans who lack adequate intake of this antioxidant. Patients with malabsorption, on chronic dialysis, and premature infants who do not receive vitamin E supplements are particularly vulnerable.

INFLAMMATORY MYOPATHIES

21.28 DERMATOMYOSITIS

Juvenile dermatomyositis is a nonhereditary multisystem disease that commonly produces progressive weakness and may be life-threatening but is treatable. This discussion focuses on the manifestations in muscle as the disorder is primarily presented in Sec. 11.61.

CLINICAL MANIFESTATIONS. Four criteria define the myopathy in both adults and children: (1) predominantly or exclusively proximal, symmetric muscle weakness that progresses for weeks or months; myalgias and muscle tenderness to palpation are often present but are not an obligatory criterion; dermatologic lesions may or may not be evident early in the course; (2) serum CK and other muscle enzymes are elevated, although the magnitude of increase varies with the acuity of the process and other factors, and sometimes the CK is only mildly increased or even normal; (3) multifocal EMG changes of primary myopathy; and (4) characteristic alterations in the muscle biopsy that may include evidence of vasculopathy and ischemic myopathy, degeneration and regeneration of muscle fibers, and intramuscular inflammation with lymphocytes. The diagnosis is most likely if all four criteria are present, but the first and at least two of the last three are required.

The proximal myopathy shows typical features of limb-girdle weakness: Gowers' sign, Trendelenberg gait, difficulty with lifting the arms above the head, inability to sit up from the supine position, and weakness of neck flexors. As the disease progresses, more distal muscles of the extremities become involved. Dysphagia and respiratory muscle weakness are serious complications that may be life-threatening. Facial weakness is mild if it occurs. Extraocular muscles are rarely symptomatic. Sphincters do not become involved, but at least half of the children with dermatomyositis have impaired esophageal motility.

Calcinosis is a serious chronic complication of dermatomyositis and may progress despite improved strength with drug therapy. Dermal and subdermal calcifications occur in 20–50% of children with this disease, a much higher incidence than in adults. The calcium deposits may sometimes be palpated as subcutaneous nodules or may be demonstrated roentgenographically. They rarely occur within the muscle itself. Periarticular sites around the knees, elbows, and wrists are most usual. They also commonly involve the gluteal region and the groin. Children with a slowly progressive course of chronic myopathy are the most susceptible. Calcium deposits may cause contractures and focal atrophy of muscle. They may break through the skin to cause ulcerations that heal poorly.

LABORATORY FINDINGS. Serum CK should be determined before and periodically during the course of treatment. It may be greatly elevated to several thousand, mildly elevated in the hundreds, or normal in mild or early cases. The erythrocyte sedimentation rate and rheumatoid factor are almost always normal.

The EMG shows a myopathic pattern of small, short duration polyphasic motor unit potentials with or without increased insertional activity. Spontaneous potentials of denervation (fibrillations) are also occasionally seen, which result from a zone of segmental necrosis along a muscle fiber, isolating the distal segment from its nerve supply. Motor and sensory nerve conduction velocities remain normal.

The ECG may show evidence of cardiomyopathy in either mild or severe cases of skeletal myositis, but the heart is not commonly involved.

DIAGNOSIS. The muscle biopsy is the most specific test to confirm the diagnosis and to distinguish dermatomyositis from other myopathies. Muscle biopsy should be performed in all suspected cases before committing a child to a protracted course of therapy with steroids and immunosuppressive drugs and their attendant toxicity. About one fourth of patients with dermatomyositis fail to show lymphocytic inflammation in the muscle biopsy, perhaps due to sampling bias. Except in the earliest stages of the disease, a pattern of *perifascicular atrophy* is seen, in which peripheral fibers of muscle fascicles are atrophic and show cytoarchitectural alterations, degeneration and regeneration; fibers in the interior of fascicles are much less altered or even appear normal. Perifascicular atrophy results from progressive ischemia due to decreased perfusion through small vessels. Inflammatory cells infiltrate the muscle fascicles or cuff larger vessels in the perimysium.

Electron microscopy of muscle reveals severe changes in capillary endothelial cells: swelling of cytoplasm that narrows or occludes the lumen; reduced numbers of pinocytotic vesicles; thickening or duplication of the basement membrane surrounding the endothelium; degeneration of membranous organelles; and inclusion-like deposits of antigen-antibody complexes known as *tubuloreticular aggregates*. The latter structures in intramuscular endothelial cells are only found in one other disease: lupus erythematosis with myopathic involvement. Electron microscopy is therefore obligatory in the muscle biopsy examination of suspected cases of dermatomyositis.

It is not necessary to sample more than one muscle for diagnostic purposes. Repeat muscle biopsy at a later date is usually not required, but in some cases it may be useful to determine whether the disease is still active and to plan further treatment.

If calcinosis is suspected, roentgenograms using a radiographic technique for soft tissues rather than for bone are useful in demonstrating subcutaneous calcifications.

TREATMENT. See Sec. 11.61.

21.29 POLYMYOSITIS

It has been debated for decades whether polymyositis is a separate disease or whether it is simply dermatomyositis without the cutaneous lesions. The debate remains unresolved, but from the perspective of laboratory investigation, treatment, and prognosis, there is no difference.

Inclusion body myositis is a rare inflammatory disease resembling polymyositis, but granular inclusions are seen within the nuclei and sarcoplasm of muscle fibers, in addition to the less specific changes of myositis.

21.30 FOCAL MYOSITIS

A focal inflammatory myopathy may appear as a pseudotumor in any muscle, presenting as a local firm swelling of muscle that is often tender to palpation and may or may not be adherent to the overlying skin. The skin is not erythematous or abnormally warm. Contractures of nearby joints may develop because of traction of the involved muscle. Focal myositis tends to involve proximal muscles, such as the periscapular muscles, pectoralis major, deltoid, glutei, or quadriceps femoris, but distal muscles such as the gastrocnemius or intrinsic muscles of the foot may be the site of the lesion. It generally does not involve more than one muscle. All ages may be affected by this subacute process, but it is rare in infancy. The etiology is unknown. A history of preceding trauma to the region can sometimes be elicited, but its significance is speculative.

The serum CK is usually elevated in the hundreds or thousands. No laboratory evidence of infection, systemic disease, or cardiomyopathy is found. Biopsy of the lesion is essential to confirm the *diagnosis* and to distinguish it from the principal differential diagnoses, rhabdomyosarcoma, and intramuscular abscess. The biopsy reveals severe acute and chronic changes of inflammatory myopathy, fibrosis, and distorted muscle fiber architecture, but there are no neoplastic changes or evidence of infection. If other muscles are simultaneously biopsied, they are normal.

Treatment consists of corticosteroids, usually prednisone, 1 mg/kg 24 hr, administered systemically for a minimum period of 3 mo while tapering the dosage. The mass should slowly shrink in size and become nontender, and the serum CK should fall to normal values. Surgical lysis of adhesions to surrounding tendons and soft tissues may be needed to release contractures or correct anatomical distortions. Azathioprine is reserved for cases resistant to steroids alone.

Recurrence is rare, and the prognosis is excellent.

21.31 VIRAL MYOSITIS

Myalgias are common in transient systemic viral infections but whether they represent a true viral myositis is uncertain. Some viruses, particularly Coxsackie A2 and influenza viruses, produce an intense inflammatory reaction in the muscles of chick and mouse embryos, causing necrosis and fibrosis of muscle and severe arthrogryposis at birth. These viruses have been isolated from muscles of human infants with congenital myositis and from older children with chronic myopathy. There is no treatment.

21.32 MYOSITIS IN OTHER DISEASES

Polymyositis may be one component of more generalized collagen vascular diseases, such as systemic lupus erythematosis. In systemic vasculitis, such as periarteritis nodosa, the inflammation around intramuscular blood vessels consists of eosinophils and plasma cells in addition to lymphocytes, unlike dermatomyositis in which the inflammatory cell is almost exclusively the lymphocyte. In juvenile rheumatoid arthritis, muscle adjacent to affected joints may show mild lymphocytic infiltrates and the serum CK may be mildly increased. Scleroderma and psoriasis may have inflammatory myopathic components. Granulomatous myopathy is rare in children and is usually due to a foreign body in the muscle.

21.33 PARASITIC MYOSITIS

Trichinosis is an intramuscular infiltration by the larval nematode *Trichinella spiralis,* acquired from eating improperly cooked infected pork (see Sec. 12.127). The diaphragm, the tongue, and the gastrocnemius are the muscles most affected. The host muscle secretes a hyaline capsule around the worms, but in cardiac muscle the worms undergo necrosis without encapsulation. Muscles are acutely painful and tender, serum CK is increased only in acute stages, and eosinophilia is seen in peripheral blood. The ECG may indicate cardiac muscle involvement. Toxoplasmosis, schistosomiasis, and sarcocyst may also infiltrate muscle.

DISORDERS OF NEUROMUSCULAR TRANSMISSION

21.34 MYASTHENIA GRAVIS

Myasthenia gravis is a disease caused by neuromuscular blockade. The release of acetylcholine (ACh) into the synaptic cleft by the axonal terminal is normal, but the postsynaptic muscle membrane or *motor end-plate* is less responsive than normal. A decreased number of available ACh receptors is due to circulating receptor-binding antibodies. In most cases the disease is nonhereditary and is in the category of an autoimmune disorder. A rare familial myasthenia gravis is probably an autosomal recessive trait. Infants born to myasthenic mothers may have a transient neonatal myasthenic syndrome secondary to placentally transferred anti-ACh receptor antibodies.

CLINICAL MANIFESTATIONS. Ptosis and some degree of extraocular muscle weakness are the earliest and most constant signs in myasthenia gravis. Older children may complain of diplopia, and young children may hold open their eyes with their fingers or thumbs if the ptosis is severe enough to obstruct vision. The pupillary responses to light are preserved. Dysphagia and facial weakness are also common, and in early infancy feeding difficulties are often the cardinal sign of myasthenia. Poor head control due to weakness of the neck flexors also is prominent. Involvement may be limited to bulbar-innervated muscles, but the disease is systemic and weakness involves limb-girdle muscles and distal muscles of the hands in most cases. Fasciculations of muscle, myalgias, and sensory symptoms do not occur. Tendon stretch reflexes may be diminished but rarely are lost.

Rapid fatigue of muscles is a characteristic feature of myasthenia gravis that distinguishes it from most other neuromuscular diseases. Ptosis increases progressively as the patient is asked to sustain upward gaze for 30–90 sec. Holding the head up from the surface of the examining table while lying supine is very difficult, and gravity cannot be overcome for more than a few seconds. Repetitive opening and closing of the fists produces rapid fatigue of hand muscles, and the patient cannot elevate the arms for more than 1–2 min because of fatigue of the deltoids. A careful history also discloses that the patient is more symptomatic late in the day or when tired. Dysphagia may interfere with eating, and the muscles of the jaw soon tire when the child chews.

If untreated, myasthenia gravis is usually progressive and may become life-threatening because of respiratory muscle involvement and the risk of aspiration. Familial myasthenia gravis is usually not progressive.

Infants born to myasthenic mothers may have respiratory insufficiency, inability to suck or swallow, generalized hypotonia and weakness, and show little spontaneous motor activity for several days. Some require ventilatory support and feeding by gavage during this period. After the abnormal antibodies disappear, the infants have normal strength and are not at increased risk for developing myasthenia gravis in later childhood. The syndrome of **transient neonatal myasthenia gravis** is to be distinguished from a rare and often hereditary *congenital myasthenia gravis* not related to maternal myasthenia, that is often permanent.

Myasthenia gravis is occasionally secondary to hypothyroidism, usually *Hashimoto's thyroiditis.* Other collagen vascular diseases may also be associated. Thymomas are not found in myasthenia gravis in children as they are in adults, nor are oat cell carcinomas of the lung that produce a myasthenic syndrome in adults.

LABORATORY FINDINGS AND DIAGNOSIS. Myasthenia gravis is one of the few neuromuscular diseases in which the *EMG* is more specifically diagnostic than the muscle biopsy. A decremental response is seen in response to repetitive nerve stimulation; the muscle potentials diminish rapidly in amplitude until the muscle becomes refractory to further stimulation. Motor nerve conduction velocity remains normal. This unique EMG pattern is the electrophysiologic correlate of the fatigable weakness observed clinically and is reversed after a cholinesterase inhibitor is administered. A myasthenic decrement may be absent or difficult to demonstrate in muscles that are not involved clinically. This feature may be confusing in early cases or in patients showing only weakness of extraocular muscles.

Anti-ACh antibodies should be assayed in the serum but are not always demonstrated. Other serologic tests of autoimmune disease, such as antinuclear antibodies and abnormal immune complexes, should also be sought. A thyroid profile should always be examined. The serum CK is normal.

The heart is not involved, and the ECG remains normal. Roentgenograms of the chest often reveal an enlarged thymus, but the hypertrophy is not a *thymoma.* It may be further defined by tomography or by computed imaging of the anterior mediastinum.

The role of *muscle biopsy* in myasthenia gravis is controversial. It is not required in most cases, but about 17% of patients show inflammatory changes sometimes called **lymphorrhages** that are interpreted by some authors as a mixed myasthenia-polymyositis immune disorder. The muscle biopsy in myasthenia gravis shows nonspecific type II muscle fiber atrophy, similar to that seen with disuse atrophy, steroid effects on muscle, polymyalgia rheumatica, and many other conditions. The ultrastructure of motor end-plates shows simplification of the membrane folds.

A *clinical test for myasthenia gravis* is the administration of a short-acting cholinesterase inhibitor, usually edrophonium chloride. A small test dose is given intravenously (IV) initially to ensure that the patient is not allergic; if tolerated, the full dose of 0.2 mg/kg (maximum dose 10 mg) is given IV a few minutes later. Children weighing less than 30 kg should be given only 1–2 mg total dose. Within a few seconds, the ptosis and ophthalmoplegia improve, and fatigability of other muscles is greatly decreased. The effects only last 1–2 min, however. Edrophonium should not be given to young infants because cardiac arrhythmias may result. An alternative with fewer cardiogenic side effects is intramuscular (IM) neostigmine. If the initial test of 0.04 mg/kg is negative, the infant may be retested 4 hr later with 0.08 mg/kg. A maximal effect is seen in 20–40 min. Because of muscarinic side effects, such as abdominal distention, diarrhea, and profuse tracheal secretions, 0.01 mg/kg of atropine may be given just before the neostigmine.

TREATMENT. Some patients with mild myasthenia gravis require no treatment. *Cholinesterase-inhibiting drugs* are the primary therapeutic agents. Neostigmine methylsulfate (0.04 mg/kg) may be given IM every 4–6 hr, but most patients tolerate oral neostigmine bromide, 0.4 mg/kg every 4–6 hr. If dysphagia is a major problem, the drug should be given about 30 min before meals to improve swallowing. Pyridostigmine is an alternative; the dosage required is about four times greater than neostigmine, but it may be slightly longer acting. Overdoses of cholinesterase inhibitors produce cholinergic crises; atropine blocks the muscarinic effects but does not block the nicotinic effects that produce additional skeletal muscle weakness.

Because of the autoimmune basis of the disease, long-term *steroid treatment* with prednisone is often effective. *Thymectomy* should be considered and may provide a cure. Thymectomy is ineffective in congenital and familial forms of myasthenia gravis, however. Treatment of hypothyroidism usually abolishes an associated myasthenia.

Plasmapheresis is effective treatment in some children, particularly those who do not respond to steroids, but plasma exchange therapy may provide only temporary remission.

Neonates with transient maternally transmitted myasthenia gravis require cholinesterase inhibitors for only a few days or occasionally for a few weeks, especially to allow feeding. No other treatment is usually necessary.

COMPLICATIONS. Children with myasthenia gravis tolerate neuromuscular blocking drugs, such as succinylcholine and pancuronium, very poorly and may be paralyzed for weeks after a single dose. An anesthesiologist should carefully review myasthenic patients who require a surgical anesthetic. Also, certain antibiotics may potentiate myasthenia and should be avoided; these include kanamycin and streptomycin in particular.

PROGNOSIS. This is difficult to predict. Some patients undergo spontaneous remission after a period of months or years; others have a permanent disease extending into adult life. Immunosuppression, thymectomy, and treatment of associated hypothyroidism may provide a cure.

21.35 OTHER CAUSES OF NEUROMUSCULAR BLOCKADE

Organophosphate chemicals, commonly used as insecticides, may cause a myasthenia-like syndrome in children exposed to these toxins (Sec. 26.4).

Botulism results from ingestion of food containing the toxin of *Clostridium botulinum,* a gram-positive, spore-bearing, anaerobic bacillus (Sec. 12.39). Honey is a common source of contamination. The incubation period is short, only a few hours, and symptoms begin with nausea, vomiting, and diarrhea. Cranial nerve involvement soon follows, with diplopia, dysphagia, weak suck, facial weakness, and absent gag reflex. Generalized hypotonia and weakness then develop and may progress to respiratory failure. Neuromuscular blockade is documented by EMG with repetitive nerve stimulation. Respiratory support may be required for days or weeks, until the toxin is cleared from the body. There is no specific antitoxin available. Guanidine, 35 mg/kg/24 hr, may be effective for extraocular and limb muscle weakness but not for respiratory muscle involvement.

Tick paralysis is a disorder of ACh release from axonal terminals due to a neurotoxin that blocks depolarization. It also affects large myelinated motor and sensory nerve fibers. This toxin is produced by the wood tick or dog tick, insects common in the Appalachian and Rocky Mountains of North America. The tick embeds its head into the skin, usually the scalp, and neurotoxin production is maximal about 5–6 days later. Motor symptoms include weakness, loss of coordination, and sometimes an ascending paralysis resembling the Guillain-Barré syndrome. Tendon reflexes are lost. Sensory symptoms of tingling paresthesias may occur in the face and extremities. The diagnosis is confirmed by EMG and nerve conduction studies and by identifying the tick. The tick must be removed completely, and the buried head not left beneath the skin of the scalp. The patient then recovers completely within hours or days.

21.36 SPINAL MUSCULAR ATROPHIES

Spinal muscular atrophies (SMA) are degenerative diseases of motor neurons that begin in fetal life and continue to be progressive in infancy and childhood. The progressive denervation of muscle is compensated in part by reinnervation from an adjacent motor unit, but giant motor units are thus created with subsequent atrophy of muscle fibers when the reinnervating motor neuron eventually becomes involved. Upper motor neurons remain normal.

SMA is classified into a severe infantile form, also known as **Werdnig-Hoffmann disease** or SMA type I; a late infantile and more slowly progressive form, SMA type 2; and a more chronic or juvenile form, also called **Kugelberg-Welander disease** of SMA type 3. A variant of SMA, **Fazio-Londe disease,** is a progressive bulbar palsy resulting from motor neuron degeneration more in the brain stem than the spinal cord. Whether these clinical variants are identical in terms of genetic deletions is not yet known.

ETIOLOGY. Apart from the modes of genetic transmission (see later), the etiology of SMA is unknown. One hypothesis is that the disease or diseases are a pathologic continuation of a process of programmed cell death that is normal in embryonic life. A surplus of motor neuroblasts and of other neurons is generated from primitive neuroectoderm, but only about half survive and mature to become neurons; the excess cells have a limited life cycle and degenerate. If the process that arrests physiologic cell death fails to intervene by a certain stage, neuronal death may continue in late fetal life and postnatally. A defect in the transcription of neuronal RNA is suggested by some evidence and is compatible with progressive neuronal loss. Other evidence points to a disorder of ganglioside metabolism. None of these data are conclusive.

CLINICAL MANIFESTATIONS. Severe hypotonia, generalized weakness, thin muscle mass, absent tendon stretch reflexes, involvement of the tongue, face, and jaw muscles, and sparing of extraocular muscles and sphincters are the cardinal features of SMA type I. Infants who are symptomatic at birth may have respiratory distress and are unable to feed. Congenital contractures occur in about 10% of severely involved neonates. Infants lie flaccid with little movement, unable to overcome gravity. They lack head control. More than two thirds die by 2 yr of age, many early in infancy.

In type II SMA the infants are usually able to suck and swallow, and respiration is adequate in early infancy. They show progressive weakness, but many survive into the school years or beyond, though confined to an electric wheelchair and severely handicapped. Nasal speech and problems with deglutition develop later. Scoliosis becomes a major complication in many patients with long survival.

Kugelberg-Welander disease is the mildest SMA (type III), and patients may appear normal in infancy. The progressive weakness is proximal in distribution, particularly involving shoulder girdle muscles. Patients are ambulatory. Symptoms of bulbar muscle weakness are rare. Longevity may extend well into middle adult life.

Fasciculations are a specific clinical sign of denervation of muscle. In thin children, they may be seen in the deltoid, biceps brachii, and occasionally the quadriceps femoris, but the continuous involuntary worm-like movements may be masked by a thick pad of subcutaneous fat. Fasciculations are best observed in the tongue, where almost no subcutaneous connective tissue separates the muscular layer from the epithelium. If the intrinsic lingual muscles are contracted, such as in crying or when the tongue protrudes, fasciculations are more difficult to see than when the tongue is relaxed.

The outstretched fingers of children with SMA often show a characteristic tremor due to fasciculations and weakness. It should not be confused with a cerebellar tremor. Myalgias are not a feature of SMA.

The heart is not involved in SMA. Intelligence is normal, and children often appear brighter than their normal peers because the effort they cannot put into physical activities is redirected to intellectual development, and they are often exposed to adult speech more than to juvenile language because of the social repercussions of the disease.

LABORATORY FINDINGS. The serum CK may be normal, but more commonly is mildly elevated in the hundreds. Occasionally, a CK of several thousand is demonstrated. Motor nerve conduction studies are normal, an important feature distinguishing SMA from peripheral neuropathy. The EMG shows fibrillation potentials and other signs of denervation of muscle.

DIAGNOSIS. The muscle biopsy in SMA reveals a characteristic pattern of perinatal denervation that is unlike that of mature muscle. Groups of giant type I fibers are mixed with fascicles of severely atrophic fibers of both histochemical types (Fig. 21–9). In juvenile SMA, the pattern may be more similar to adult muscle that has undergone many cycles of denervation and reinnervation.

Sural nerve biopsy sometimes shows mild sensory neuropathic changes, and sensory nerve conduction velocity may be slowed. At autopsy, mild degenerative changes are seen in sensory neurons of dorsal root ganglia and in somatosensory nuclei of the thalamus, but these alterations are not perceived clinically as sensory loss or paresthesias. The most

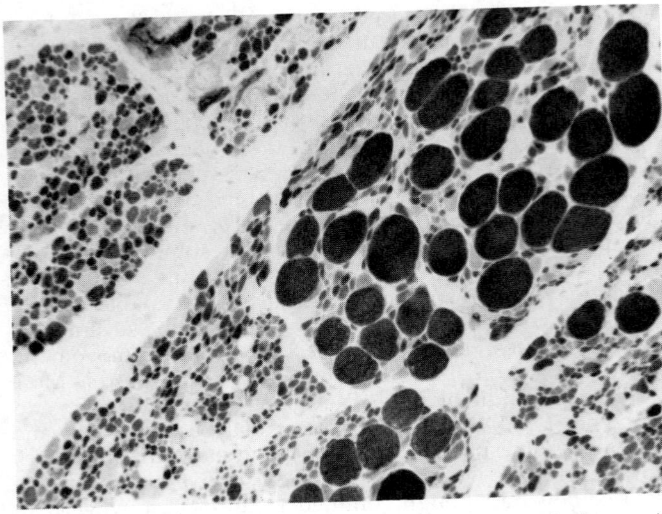

Figure 21–9. Muscle biopsy of neonate with infantile spinal muscular atrophy. Groups of giant type I (darkly stained) fibers are seen within muscle fascicles of severely atrophic fibers of both histochemical types. This is the characteristic pattern of perinatal denervation of muscle. Myofibrillar ATPase, preincubated at pH 4.6. (×400.)

pronounced neuropathologic lesions are the extensive neuronal degeneration and gliosis in the ventral horns of the spinal cord and brain stem motor nuclei, especially the hypoglossal nucleus.

GENETICS. Most cases are inherited as an autosomal recessive trait, and the incidence of SMA is 1:25,000, affecting all ethnic groups. It is the second most common neuromuscular disease, following Duchenne muscular dystrophy. The defective gene in SMA is on chromosome 5. A few families are described with autosomal dominant inheritance.

TREATMENT. There is no medical treatment to delay the progression. Supportive therapy includes orthopedic care with particular attention to scoliosis and joint contractures, mild physiotherapy, and mechanical aids for assisting the child to eat and to be as functionally independent as possible. Most children learn to use a computer keyboard with great skill but cannot use a pencil easily.

21.37 OTHER MOTOR NEURON DISEASES

Motor neuron diseases other than SMA are rare in children.

Poliomyelitis used to be a major cause of chronic disability, but since the routine use of polio vaccine, this viral infection has now become rare (Sec. 12.80). Other enteroviruses, such as Coxsackie and ECHO viruses, may also cause an acute infection of motor neurons with symptoms and signs similar to poliomyelitis, although usually milder. Serologic tests for specific antibodies and viral cultures of CSF are diagnostic.

A juvenile form of *amyotrophic lateral sclerosis* is rare. Upper motor neuron loss as well as lower motor neuron loss is evident clinically, unlike SMA. The course is progressive and is ultimately fatal.

The **Pena-Shokeir** and **Marden-Walker syndromes** are progressive motor neuron degenerations associated with severe arthrogryposis and congenital anomalies of many organ systems.

Motor neurons become involved in several metabolic diseases of the nervous system, such as gangliosidosis (Tay-Sachs disease), ceroid-lipofuscinosis (Batten's disease), and glycogenosis II (Pompe's disease), but the signs of denervation may be minor or obscured by the more prominent involvement of other parts of the CNS or of muscle.

21.38 HEREDITARY MOTOR-SENSORY NEUROPATHIES

The hereditary motor-sensory neuropathies (HMSN) are a group of progressive diseases of peripheral nerves. Motor components generally dominate the clinical picture, but sensory and autonomic involvement become expressed later.

21.39 PERONEAL MUSCULAR ATROPHY (CHARCOT-MARIE-TOOTH DISEASE; HMSN TYPE I)

This disease is the most common genetically determined neuropathy and has an overall prevalence of 3.8:100,000. It is transmitted as an autosomal dominant trait with 83% expressivity.

CLINICAL MANIFESTATIONS. Most patients are asymptomatic until late childhood or early adolescence, but young children sometimes show signs of gait disturbance as early as the 2nd year. The peroneal and tibial nerves are the earliest and most severely affected. The child is often described as being clumsy, falling easily, or tripping over her or his own feet. The onset of symptoms may be delayed until after the 5th decade.

Muscles of the anterior compartment of the lower legs become wasted, and the legs have a characteristic "stork-like" contour. The muscular atrophy is accompanied by progressive weakness of dorsiflexion of the ankle and eventual foot drop. The process is bilateral but may be slightly asymmetric. Pes cavus deformities may develop because of denervation of intrinsic foot muscles, further destabilizing the gait. Atrophy of muscles of the forearms and hands is usually not as severe as that of the lower extremities, but in advanced cases contractures of the wrists and fingers produce a "claw hand." Proximal muscle weakness is a late manifestation and is usually mild. Axial muscles are not involved.

The disease is slowly progressive throughout life, but patients occasionally show accelerated deterioration of function over a few years. Most patients remain ambulatory and have a normal longevity, although orthotic appliances are required to stabilize the ankles.

Sensory involvement mainly affects large myelinated nerve fibers that convey proprioceptive information and vibratory sense, but the threshold for pain and temperature may also increase. Some children complain of tingling or burning sensations of the feet, but pain is rare. Because the muscle mass is reduced, the nerves are more vulnerable to trauma or compression. Autonomic manifestations may be expressed as poor vasomotor control with blotching or pallor of the skin of the feet and inappropriately cold feet.

Nerves often become palpably enlarged. Tendon stretch reflexes are lost distally. Cranial nerves are not clinically affected. Sphincter control remains well preserved. Autonomic neuropathy does not affect the heart, gastrointestinal tract, or bladder. Intelligence is normal.

The **Davidenkow syndrome** is a variant of HMSN type I with a scapuloperoneal distribution.

LABORATORY FINDINGS AND DIAGNOSIS. Motor and sensory nerve conduction velocities are greatly reduced, sometimes as slow as 20% of normal conduction time. EMG and muscle biopsy are not usually required for diagnosis, but they show evidence of many cycles of denervation and reinnervation. Serum CK is normal. CSF protein may be elevated, but no cells appear in the CSF.

In uncertain cases, and particularly if the family history is negative, sural nerve biopsy is diagnostic. Large- and medium-sized myelinated fibers are reduced in number, collagen is increased, and characteristic *onion-bulb formations* of proliferated Schwann cell cytoplasm surround axons. This pathologic finding is called *interstitial hypertrophic neuropathy.* Extensive segmental demyelination and remyelination also occur.

TREATMENT. Stabilization of the ankle is a primary concern. In early stages, stiff boots that extend to midcalf often suffice, particularly for when the patient walks on uneven surfaces such as ice and snow or stones. As the dorsiflexors of the ankles further weaken, lightweight plastic splints may be custom-made to extend beneath the foot and around the back of the ankle. They are worn inside the socks and are not visible, reducing self-consciousness. External short leg braces may be required when foot drop becomes complete. Surgical fusion of the ankle may be considered in some cases.

The leg should be protected from traumatic injury. Compression neuropathy during sleep may be prevented by soft pillows beneath or between the lower legs in advanced cases. Burning paresthesias of the feet are not common but are often abolished by phenytoin or carbamazepine. No medical treatment is available to arrest or slow the progression.

In new cases, without a family history, both parents should be examined and nerve conduction studies should be performed.

21.40 PERONEAL MUSCULAR ATROPHY, AXONAL TYPE (HMSN TYPE II)

This disease is genetically and clinically similar to HMSN type I, but the rate of progression is slower and the disability is less. EMG shows denervation of muscle. Sural nerve biopsy reveals axonal degeneration rather than demyelination and whorls of Schwann cell processes.

21.41 DÉJERINE-SOTTAS DISEASE (HMSN TYPE III)

This interstitial hypertrophic neuropathy of autosomal dominant transmission is similar to HMSN type I but is more severe. Symptoms develop in early infancy and are rapidly progressive. Pupillary abnormalities such as lack of reaction to light or **Argyll-Robertson pupil** are common. Kyphoscoliosis and pes cavus deformities complicate about 35% of patients. Nerves become palpably enlarged at an early age.

The onion bulb formations seen in the sural nerve biopsy are more pronounced. Hypomyelination also occurs.

21.42 ROUSSY-LÉVY SYNDROME

This syndrome is defined as a combination of HMSN type I and Friedreich's ataxia.

21.43 REFSUM'S DISEASE

See Sec. 8.16.

This rare disease is due to an enzymatic block in α-oxidation of phytanic acid to pristanic acid. Phytanic acid is a branched-chain fatty acid that is derived mainly from dietary sources: spinach, nuts, and coffee. Phytanic acid is greatly elevated in plasma, CSF, and in brain tissue.

Clinical onset is usually between 4 and 7 yr of age, with intermittent motor and sensory neuropathy. Ataxia, progressive neurosensory hearing loss, retinitis pigmentosa and loss of night vision, ichthyosis, and liver dysfunction also develop in varying degrees. Motor and sensory nerve conduction velocities are delayed. Treatment is by dietary management and periodic plasma exchange.

21.44 GIANT AXONAL NEUROPATHY

This rare autosomal recessive disease with onset in early childhood is a progressive mixed peripheral neuropathy. Ataxia and nystagmus also usually develop. Most affected children have been noted to have peculiar curly reddish hair. Focal axonal enlargements are seen in both peripheral nervous system and the CNS, but the myelin sheath is intact. The disease is thought to be a disorder of neurofilament synthesis or organization.

21.45 LEUKODYSTROPHIES

Several hereditary degenerative diseases of white matter of the CNS also cause peripheral neuropathy. The most important are *Krabbe's disease* (globoid cell leukodystrophy) and *metachromatic leukodystrophy* (see Sec. 20.58).

NEUROFIBROMATOSIS

See Sec. 20.39.

21.46 TOXIC NEUROPATHIES

Many chemicals, toxins, and drugs are capable of causing peripheral neuropathy. *Heavy metals* are well-known neurotoxins. Lead poisoning, especially if chronic, causes mainly a motor neuropathy involving selective large nerves, such as the common peroneal, radial, or median nerves, a condition known as **mononeuritis multiplex** (Sec. 26.16). Arsenic produces painful burning paresthesias as well as motor polyneuropathy.

Antimetabolic drugs, especially vincristine, produce polyneuropathies as complications of chemotherapy for neoplasms.

Chronic uremia is associated with toxic neuropathy and myopathy. The neuropathy is due to excessive levels of circulating parathormone. Reduction in serum parathyroid hormone is accompanied by clinical improvement and a return to normal of nerve conduction velocity.

AUTONOMIC NEUROPATHIES

21.47 FAMILIAL DYSAUTONOMIA

Familial dysautonomia (**Riley-Day syndrome**) is an autosomal recessive disorder that is common in eastern European Jews, among whom the incidence is 1:10,000–20,000 and the carrier state is estimated to be 1%. It is rare in other ethnic groups.

PATHOLOGY. This disease of the peripheral nervous system is characterized pathologically, by a reduced number of small unmyelinated nerve fibers that carry pain, temperature, and taste sensations and that mediate autonomic functions. Large myelinated afferent nerve fibers that relay impulses from muscle spindles and Golgi tendon organs are also deficient. The degree of demonstrable anatomic change in peripheral and especially autonomic nerves is variable. Fungiform papillae of the tongue (taste buds) are absent or reduced in number.

CLINICAL MANIFESTATIONS. The disease is expressed in infancy by poor sucking and swallowing. Aspiration pneumonia may occur. Feeding difficulties remain a major symptom throughout childhood. Vomiting crises may occur. Excessive sweating and blotchy erythema of the skin are common, especially at mealtime or when the child is excited. Breath-holding spells followed by syncope are common in the first 5 yr. As the child becomes older, insensitivity to pain becomes evident and traumatic injuries are frequent. Corneal ulcerations are common. Newly erupting teeth cause tongue ulcerations. Walking is delayed, clumsy, or appears ataxic because of poor sensory feedback from muscle spindles. The "ataxia" is probably related more to deficient muscle spindle feedback and to vestibular nerve dysfunction than to cerebellar involvement. Tendon stretch reflexes are absent. Overflow tearing when crying does not normally develop until 2–3 mo of age but fails to develop after that time or is severely reduced in children with familial dysautonomia.

About 40% of patients have generalized major motor seizures, some of which are associated with acute hypoxia during breath-holding, some with extreme fevers, but most without an apparent precipitating event. Intellectual function is usually impaired but is unrelated to epilepsy. Puberty is often delayed, especially in girls. Body temperature is poorly controlled, and hypothermia and extreme fevers both occur. Speech is often slurred or nasal.

After 3 yr of age, **autonomic crises** begin, usually with attacks of cyclic vomiting lasting 24–72 hr or even several days. Retching and vomiting occur every 15–20 min associated with hypertension, profuse sweating, blotching of the skin, apprehension, and irritability. Prominent gastric distention may occur, causing abdominal pain and even respiratory distress. Hematemesis may complicate pernicious vomiting.

LABORATORY FINDINGS. Chest roentgenograms show atelectasis and pulmonary changes resembling cystic fibrosis. Urinary VMA is decreased, and HVA is increased. Sural nerve biopsy shows a decreased number of unmyelinated fibers. The EEG is useful for evaluating seizures.

DIAGNOSIS. A slow IV infusion of norepinephrine produces an exaggerated pressor response. The hypotensive response to infusion of methacholine is increased. Intradermal injection of 1:1000 histamine phosphate fails to produce a normal axon flare, and local pain is absent or diminished. Because normal infant skin reacts more intensely to histamine, a 1:10,000 dilution should be used. The instillation of 2.5% methacholine into the conjunctival sac produces miosis in patients with familial dysautonomia and no detectable effect on the normal pupil; this is a nonspecific sign of parasympathetic denervation from any cause, however. The methacholine is applied to only one eye in this test, the other eye serving as a control; the pupils are compared at 5-min intervals for 20 min.

TREATMENT. Symptomatic treatment includes special attention to the respiratory and gastrointestinal systems, methylcellulose eye drops or topical ocular lubricants to replace tears and prevent corneal ulceration, orthopedic management of scoliosis and joint problems, and appropriate anticonvulsants for epilepsy. Chlorpromazine is an effective antiemetic and may be given as rectal suppositories during autonomic crises. It also reduces apprehension and lowers the blood pressure. Dehydration and electrolyte disturbances should be anticipated. Bethanechol may be an alternative drug for cyclic vomiting. It is also useful for enuresis, another common complication, and augments tear production. Protection from injuries is important because of the lack of pain as a protective mechanism.

PROGNOSIS. This is poor. Most patients die in childhood, usually of chronic pulmonary failure or aspiration.

21.48 MYENTERIC PLEXUS NEUROPATHIES

Aganglionic megacolon (Hirschsprung disease) is a failure of embryonic development of parasympathetic neurons in the submucosal and myenteric plexuses of segments of the colon and rectum. Nerves between the longitudinal and circular layers of smooth muscle of the gut wall are hypertrophic; ganglion cells are absent (see Sec. 13.32). *Pyloric stenosis* is due to hypertrophy of the smooth muscle of the pylorus at the distal end of the stomach (see Sec. 13.27).

21.49 CONGENITAL INSENSITIVITY TO PAIN AND ANHIDROSIS

This hereditary disorder of uncertain genetic transmission affects boys much more frequently than girls and presents in early infancy. Patients have episodes of high fever related to warm environmental temperatures because they do not perspire. Frequent burns and traumatic injuries result from apparent lack of pain perception. Intelligence is normal. Nerve biopsy reveals an almost total absence of unmyelinated nerve fibers that convey impulses of pain, temperature, and autonomic functions.

21.50 GUILLAIN-BARRÉ SYNDROME

The Guillain-Barré syndrome is a postinfectious polyneuropathy that causes demyelination in mainly motor but sometimes also sensory nerves. This syndrome affects people of all ages and is not hereditary. The disorder closely resembles experimental allergic polyneuritis in animals.

CLINICAL MANIFESTATIONS. The paralysis usually follows a nonspecific viral infection by about 10 days. The original infection may have caused only gastrointestinal or upper respiratory tract symptoms. Weakness begins usually in the lower extremities and progressively involves the trunk, the upper limbs, and finally the bulbar muscles, a pattern formerly known as *Landry's ascending paralysis.* Proximal and distal muscles are involved relatively symmetrically, but asymmetry is found in 9% of patients. The onset is gradual and progresses over days or weeks. Particularly in cases with an abrupt onset, tenderness to palpation and pain in muscles is common in the initial stages. The child is irritable. Weakness may progress to inability or refusal to walk and later to flaccid tetraplegia. Paresthesias occur in some cases.

Bulbar involvement occurs in about half of the cases. Respiratory insufficiency may result. Dysphagia and facial weakness are often impending signs of respiratory failure. They interfere with eating and increase the risk of aspiration. Extraocular muscle involvement is rare, but in an uncommon variant, oculomotor and other cranial neuropathies are severe early in the course. The **Miller-Fisher syndrome** consists of acute external ophthalmoplegia, ataxia, and areflexia. Papilledema is found in some cases, although visual impairment is not clinically evident. Urinary incontinence or retention of urine is a complication in about 20% of cases but is usually transient.

Tendon reflexes are lost, usually early in the course, but are sometimes preserved until later, and this finding may be misleading in arriving at an early diagnosis.

The clinical course is usually benign, and spontaneous recovery begins with 2–3 wk. Most patients regain full muscular strength, although some are left with residual weakness. The tendon reflexes are usually the last function to recover. Improvement usually follows a gradient inverse to the direction of involvement, with recovery of bulbar function first and lower extremity weakness resolving last. Bulbar and respiratory muscle involvement may lead to death if the syndrome is not recognized and treated.

The autonomic nervous system may also be involved in some cases. Lability of blood pressure and cardiac rate, postural hypotension, episodes of profound bradycardia, and occasional asystole occur. Cardiovascular monitoring is important. A few patients require the insertion of a temporary venous cardiac pacemaker.

Occasional cases of acute Guillain-Barré syndrome are associated with *Mycoplasma pneumoniae* or *Campylobacter* sp. infections of the respiratory system.

Chronic relapsing polyradiculoneuropathy and *chronic unremit-*

ting polyradiculoneuropathy are chronic forms of Guillain-Barré syndrome that recur intermittently or do not improve for a period of months and years. About 7% of children with Guillain-Barré syndrome experience relapses. Patients are usually severely weak and may have a flaccid tetraplegia with or without bulbar and respiratory muscle involvement.

LABORATORY FINDINGS AND DIAGNOSIS. CSF studies are essential for diagnosis. The CSF protein is elevated to more than twice the upper limit of normal, glucose is normal, and there is no pleocytosis. Fewer than 10 white cells/mm^3 are found. The results of bacterial cultures are negative, and viral cultures rarely isolate specific viruses. The dissociation between high CSF protein and a lack of cellular response in a patient with an acute or subacute polyneuropathy is diagnostic of the Guillain-Barré syndrome.

Motor nerve conduction velocities are greatly reduced, and sensory nerve conduction time also is often slow. The EMG shows evidence of acute denervation of muscle. Serum CK may be mildly elevated or normal. Muscle biopsy is not usually required for diagnosis; it is normal in early stages and shows evidence of denervation atrophy in chronic stages. Sural nerve biopsy shows segmental demyelination, focal inflammation, and wallerian degeneration but also is usually not required for diagnosis.

TREATMENT. Patients in early stages of this *acute* disease should be admitted to the hospital for observation, because the ascending paralysis may rapidly involve respiratory muscles during the next 24 hr. Patients with slow progression may simply be observed for stabilization and spontaneous remission without treatment. Rapidly progressive ascending paralysis is treated with plasma exchange therapy or with steroids and immunosuppressive drugs. Plasmapheresis may be the most effective treatment. Supportive care, such as respiratory support, prevention of decubiti in children with flaccid tetraplegia, and treatment of secondary bacterial infections are important.

Chronic relapsing polyradiculoneuropathy or unremitting chronic neuropathy is treated with plasma exchange, sometimes requiring as many as 10 exchanges daily. Remission in these cases may be sustained, but relapses may occur within days, weeks, or even after many months; relapses usually respond to another course of plasmapheresis. Steroid and immunosuppressive drugs are an alternative, but their effectiveness is less predictable. High-dose "pulsed" methylprednisolone given IV is successful in some cases. The prognosis in chronic forms of the Guillain-Barré syndrome is more guarded than in the acute form, and many patients are left with major residual handicaps.

21.51 BELL'S PALSY

Bell's palsy is an acute unilateral facial nerve palsy that is not associated with other cranial neuropathies or brain stem dysfunction. It is a common disorder at all ages from infancy through adolescence and usually develops abruptly about 2 wk after a systemic viral infection. The preceding infection is due to the Epstein-Barr virus in about 20% of cases; Lyme disease (Sec. 12.57), herpes virus, and mumps virus are identified in many others. The disease is believed to be a postinfectious allergic or immune demyelinating facial neuritis rather than an active viral invasion of the nerve or of its motor neurons or origin.

CLINICAL MANIFESTATIONS. The upper and lower face is paretic, and the corner of the mouth droops. The patient is unable to close the eye on the involved side, and the patient may develop an exposure keratitis at night. Taste on the anterior two thirds of the tongue is lost on the involved side in about half of the cases, which helps to establish the anatomic limits of the lesion proximal or distal to the chorda tympani branch of the facial nerve. Numbness and paresthesias do not occur.

TREATMENT. Protection of the cornea with methylcellulose eye drops or an ocular lubricant is especially important at night. Steroids do not induce remission and are not recommended. Surgical decompression of the facial canal, theoretically to provide more space for the swollen facial nerve, has not proved to be of value.

PROGNOSIS. The prognosis is excellent. More than 85% of cases recover spontaneously with no residual facial weakness; another 10% have mild facial weakness as a sequel; only 5% are left with permanent severe facial weakness. In chronic cases that do not recover within a few weeks, electrophysiologic examination of the facial nerve helps to determine the degree of neuropathy and regeneration. In chronic cases, other causes of facial neuropathy should be considered, including facial nerve tumors such as schwannomas and neurofibromas, infiltration of the facial nerve by leukemic cells or by a rhabdomyosarcoma of the middle ear, brain stem infarcts or tumors, and traumatic injury of the facial nerve.

FACIAL PALSY AT BIRTH. This is usually a compression neuropathy from forceps application during delivery and recovers spontaneously in a few days or weeks in most cases. Congenital Bell's palsy should not be diagnosed. *Congenital absence of the depressor angularis oris muscle* causes facial asymmetry, especially when the infant cries. It is not a facial nerve lesion but is a cosmetic defect that does not interfere with feeding.

HARVEY B. SARNAT

GENERAL NEUROMUSCULAR

Brooke MH: A Clinician's View of Neuromuscular Disease, 2nd ed. Baltimore, Williams & Wilkins, 1986.
Dubowitz V: Color Atlas of Muscle Disorders in Childhood. Chicago, Year Book Med Publ, 1989.
Dubowitz V: The Floppy Infant, 2nd ed. Philadelphia, JB Lippincott, 1980.
Mastaglia FL, Walton J (eds): Skeletal Muscle Pathology, 2nd ed. Edinburgh, Churchill Livingstone, 1990.
Sarnat HB: Muscle Pathology and Histochemistry. Chicago, Am Soc Clin Pathol Press, 1983.
Walton J: Disorders of Voluntary Muscle, 4th ed. Edinburgh, Churchill Livingstone, 1981.

EMBRYOLOGY AND DEVELOPMENTAL DISORDERS OF MUSCLE

Barth PG, van Wijngaarden GK, Bethlem J: X-linked myotubular myopathy with fatal neonatal asphyxia. Neurology 25:531, 1975.
Fardeau M: Congenital myopathies. *In:* Mastaglia FL, Walton J (eds): Skeletal Muscle Pathology, 2nd ed. Edinburgh, Churchill Livingstone, 1991.
Martinez BA, Lake BD: Childhood nemaline myopathy: A review of clinical presentation in relation to prognosis. Dev Med Child Neurol 29:815, 1987.
Nonaka I, Ishiura S, Arahata K, et al: Progression in nemaline myopathy. Acta Neuropathol 78:484, 1989.
Sarnat HB: Cerebral dysgeneses and their influence on fetal muscle development. Brain Dev 8:495, 1986.
Sarnat HB: Myotubular myopathy: arrest in morphogenesis of myofibers associated with persistent fetal vimentin and desmin. Can J Neurol Sci 17:109, 1990.
Sarnat HB: Ontogenesis of striated muscle. *In:* Polin RA, Fox WW (eds): Neonatal and Fetal Medicine: Physiology and Pathophysiology. Orlando, Florida, WB Saunders, 1991.
Shimomura C, Nonaka I: Nemaline myopathy: Comparative muscle histochemistry in the severe neonatal, moderate congenital, and adult-onset forms. Pediatr Neurol 5:25, 1989.

MUSCULAR DYSTROPHIES

Dubowitz V: The Duchenne dystrophy story: From phenotype to gene and potential treatment. J Child Neurol 4:240, 1989.
Duncan CJ: Dystrophin and the integrity of the sarcolemma in Duchenne muscular dystrophy. Experientia 45:175, 1989.
Egger J, Kendall BE, Erdohazi M, et al: Involvement of the central nervous system in congenital muscular dystrophies. Dev Med Child Neurol 25:32, 1983.
Fukuyama Y, Osawa M, Suzuki H: Congenital progressive muscular dystrophy

of the Fukuyama type: Clinical, genetic and pathological considerations. Brain Dev 3:1, 1981.

Greenberg CR, Rohringer M, Jacobs HK, et al: Gene studies in newborn males with Duchenne muscular dystrophy detected by neonatal screening. Lancet 2:425, 1988.

Höweler CJ, Busch HFM, Bernini LF, et al: Dystonia myotonica and myotonia congenita occurring in one family. Brain 103:513, 1980.

Höweler CJ, Busch HFM, Geraedts JPM, et al: Anticipation in myotonic dystrophy: Fact or fiction? Brain 112:779, 1989.

Kunkel LM: Analysis of deletions in DNA from patients with Becker and Duchenne muscular dystrophy. Nature 322:73, 1986.

Sarnat HB, O'Connor T, Byrne PA: Clinical effects of myotonic dystrophy on pregnancy and the neonate. Arch Neurol 33:459, 1976.

Sarnat HB, Silbert SW: Maturational arrest of fetal muscle in neonatal myotonic dystrophy. Arch Neurol 33:466, 1976.

Siegel IM: Early signs of Landouzy-Déjerine disease: Wrist and finger weakness. JAMA 221:302, 1972.

Witkowski JA: Dystrophin-related muscular dystrophies. J Child Neurol 4:251, 1989.

METABOLIC AND ENDOCRINE MYOPATHIES

DiMauro S, Bonilla E, Zeviani M, et al: Mitochondrial myopathies. J Inher Metab Dis 10:(Suppl 1), 113, 1987.

Dimauro S, Hartlage PL: Fatal infantile form of muscle phosphorylase deficiency. Neurology 28:1124, 1978.

Lestienne P, Ponsot G: Kearns-Sayre syndrome with muscle mitochondrial DNA deletion. Lancet 1:885, 1988.

Lombes A, Bonilla E, DiMauro S: Mitochondrial encephalomyopathies. Rev Neurol 145:671, 1989.

Mastaglia FL, Ojeda VJ, Sarnat HB, et al: Myopathies associated with hypothyroidism. Aust NZ J Med 18:799, 1988.

Najjar SS: Muscular hypertrophy in hypothyroid children: The Kocher-Debré-Sémélaigne syndrome: A review of 23 cases. J Pediatr 85:236, 1974.

Sarnat HB, Machin G, Darwish HZ, et al: Mitochondrial myopathy of cerebro-hepato-renal (Zellweger) syndrome. Can J Neurol Sci 10:170, 1983.

INFLAMMATORY MYOPATHIES

Heffner RR Jr: Focal inflammatory diseases of muscle. *In:* Heffner RR Jr (ed): Muscle Pathology. New York, Churchill Livingstone, 1983, p 171.

Mastaglia FL, Ojeda VJ: Inflammatory myopathies. Ann Neurol 17:215, 1985.

Sarnat HB: Juvenile dermatomyositis. *In:* Mastaglia FL (ed): Inflammatory Diseases of Muscle. Oxford, Blackwell Scientific Publications, 1988, p 71.

Silver RM, Maricq HR: Childhood dermatomyositis: Serial microvascular studies. Pediatrics 83:278, 1989.

DISORDERS OF NEUROMUSCULAR TRANSMISSION

Engel AG, Lambert EH, Mulder DM, et al: Recently recognized congenital myasthenic syndrome. Ann NY Acad Sci 377:614, 1981.

Grob D (ed): Myasthenia gravis: Pathophysiology and management. Ann NY Acad Sci v:377, 1981.

Pickett J, Berg B, Chaplin E, et al: Syndrome of botulism in infancy: Clinical and electrophysiologic studies. N Engl J Med 295:770, 1976.

SPINAL MUSCULAR ATROPHIES

Gamstorp I, Sarnat HB (eds): Progressive Spinal Muscular Atrophies. New York, Raven Press, 1984.

Hageman G, Willemse J, van Ketel BA, et al: The heterogeneity of the Pena-Shokeir syndrome. Neuropediatrics 18:45, 1987.

Pearn JH, Gardner-Medwin D, Wilson J: A clinical study of chronic childhood spinal muscular atrophy: A review of 141 cases. J Neurol Sci 38:23, 1978.

Russman BS, Melchreit R, Drennan JC: Spinal muscular atrophy: The natural course of disease. Muscle Nerve 6:179, 1983.

Sees JN Jr, Towfighi J, Ladda RP: Marden-Walker syndrome: Neuropathologic findings. Pediatr Pathol, 1991.

HEREDITARY MOTOR-SENSORY NEUROPATHIES

Buchtal F, Behse F: Peroneal muscular atrophy (PMA) and related disorders. I: Clinical manifestations as related to biopsy findings, nerve conduction, and electromyography. Brain 100:41, 1977.

Carpenter S, Karpati G, Andermann F: Giant axonal neuropathy: A clinically and morphologically distinct neurological disease. Arch Neurol 31:312, 1974.

Dyck PJ, Lambert EH: Lower motor and primary sensory neuron diseases with peroneal muscular atrophy. I: Neurologic, genetic, and electrophysiologic findings in various neuronal degenerations. Arch Neurol 18:619, 1968.

Pena SD: Giant axonal neuropathy: An inborn error of organization of intermediate filaments. Muscle Nerve 5:166, 1982.

Ronen GM, Lowry N, Wedge JH, et al: Hereditary motor-sensory neuropathy type I presenting as scapuloperoneal atrophy (Davidenkow syndrome): Electrophysiological and pathological studies. Can J Neurol Sci 13:264, 1986.

AUTONOMIC NEUROPATHIES

Axelrod FB, Gouge TH, Ginsburg HB, et al: Fundoplication and gastrostomy in familial dysautonomia. J Pediatr 118:388, 1991.

Axelrod FB, Nachtigal R, Dancis J: Familial dysautonomia: Diagnosis, pathogenesis and management. Adv Pediatr 21:75, 1974.

Goebel HH, Veit S, Dyck PJ: Confirmation of virtual unmyelinated fiber absence in hereditary sensory neuropathy type IV. J Neuropathol Exp Neurol 39:670, 1980.

GUILLAIN-BARRÉ SYNDROME

D'Cruz OF, Shapiro ED, Spiegelman KN: Acute inflammatory demyelinating polyradiculoneuropathy (Guillain-Barré syndrome) after immunization with *Haemophilus influenzae* type b conjugate vaccine. J Pediatr 115:743, 1989.

Maytal J, Eviatar L, Brunson SC: Use of demand pacemaker in children with Guillain-Barré syndrome and cardiac arrhythmias. Pediatr Neurol 5:303, 1989.

McKhann GM, Griffin JN, Cornblath DR, et al: Plasmapheresis and Guillain-Barré syndrome: Analysis of prognostic factors and the effects of plasmapheresis. Ann Neurol 23:347, 1988.

Shuaib A, Becker WJ: Variants of Guillain-Barré syndrome: Miller-Fisher syndrome, facial diplegia and multiple cranial nerve palsies. Can J Neurol Sci 14:611, 1987.

Thomas PK, Lascelles RG, Hallpike JF, et al: Recurrent and chronic relapsing Guillain-Barré polyneuritis. Brain 29:589, 1969.

22

DISORDERS OF THE EYE AND EAR

PEDIATRIC OPHTHALMOLOGY

22.1 GROWTH AND DEVELOPMENT

At birth the eye of the normal full-term infant is approximately two thirds of adult size. Postnatal growth is maximal during the 1st yr, proceeds at a rapid but decelerating rate until the 3rd yr, and continues at a slower rate thereafter until puberty, after which little change occurs. In general, the anterior structures of the eye are relatively large at birth and thereafter grow proportionately less than the posterior structures. This growth pattern results in a progressive change in the shape of the globe; it becomes more nearly spherical.

In the infant the *sclera* is thin and translucent, with a bluish tinge. The *cornea* is relatively large in the newborn (averaging 10 mm) and attains adult size (nearly 12 mm) by the age of 2 yr or earlier. Its curvature tends to flatten with age, with progressive change in the refractive properties of the eye. The normal cornea is perfectly clear. In infants born prematurely there may be a transient opalescent haze. The anterior chamber in the newborn appears shallow, and the angle structures, so important to the maintenance of normal intraocular pressure, must undergo further differentiation after birth. The *iris*, typically light blue or gray at birth in Caucasians, undergoes progressive change of color as the pigmentation of the stroma increases in the 1st 6 mo of life. The pupils of the newborn infant tend to be small and are often difficult to dilate. Often remnants of the pupillary membrane (anterior vascular capsule) are evident on ophthalmoscopic examination as cobweb-like lines crossing the pupillary aperture, especially in preterm infants.

The *lens* of the newborn infant is more nearly spherical than that of the adult; its greater refractive power helps to compensate for the relative shortness of the young eye. The lens continues to grow throughout life; new fibers added to the periphery continually push older fibers toward the center of the lens. With age, the lens becomes progressively more dense and more resistant to change of shape during accommodation.

The *fundus* of the newborn eye is less pigmented than that of the adult; the choroidal vascular pattern is highly visible, and the retinal pigmentary pattern often has a fine "peppery" or mottled appearance. In some darkly pigmented infants, however, the fundus has a gray or opalescent sheen. In the newborn the macular landmarks, particularly the foveal light reflex, are less well defined and may not be readily apparent to ophthalmoscopic examination. The peripheral retina appears pale or grayish, and the peripheral retinal vasculature is immature, especially in the premature infant. The optic nervehead color varies from pink to slightly pale, sometimes grayish. Within 4–6 mo the appearance of the fundus more nearly approximates that of the mature eye.

Superficial retinal hemorrhages may be observed in many newborn infants. These are usually absorbed promptly and rarely leave any permanent effect. Conjunctival hemorrhages also may occur at birth and are resorbed spontaneously without consequence.

Remnants of the primitive hyaloid vascular system may also be seen as small tufts or worm-like structures projecting from the disk (Bergmeister papilla) or as a fine strand traversing the vitreous; in some cases only a small dot (Mittendorf dot) remains on the posterior aspect of the lens capsule.

As a rule, the infant eye is somewhat hyperopic (farsighted), but the refractive state at any time in life depends on the net effect of many factors, the principal ones being the size of the eye, the state of the lens, and the curvature of the cornea.

Newborn infants tend to keep their eyes closed much of the time, but the normal newborn can see, responds to changes in illumination, and can fixate points of contrast. The *visual acuity* in the newborn is estimated to be in the range of 20/400. One of the earliest responses to a formed visual stimulus is the infant's regard for the mother's face, evident especially during feeding. By 2 wk of age the infant shows more sustained interest in large objects, and by 8–10 wk of age the normal infant can follow an object through an arc of 180°. The acuity improves rapidly and may reach 20/30–20/20 by the age of 2–3 yr.

In many normal infants there may be imperfect coordination of the *eye movements* and *alignment* during the early days and weeks, but proper coordination should be achieved by 3–6 mo, usually sooner. Persistent deviation of an eye in an infant requires evaluation.

Tears often are not present with crying until after 1–3 mo.

Gordon RA, Donzis PB: Refractive development of the human eye. Arch Ophthalmol 103:785, 1985.

Greenwald MJ: Visual development in infancy and childhood. Pediatr Clin North Am 30:977, 1983.

Hendrickson AE, Youdelis C: The morphological development of the human fovea. Ophthalmology 91:603, 1984.

Khodadoust AA, Ziai M, Biggs SL: Optic disc in normal newborns. Am J Ophthalmol 66:502, 1968.

Krishnamohan VK, Wheeler MB, Testa MA, et al: Correlation of postnatal regression of the anterior vascular capsule of the lens to gestational age. J Pediatr Ophthalmol Strab 19:28, 1982.

Roarty JD, Keltner JL: Normal pupil size and anisocoria in newborn infants. Arch Ophthalmol 108:94, 1990.

Robb RM: Increase in retinal surface area during infancy and childhood. J Pediatr Ophthalmol Strab 19:16, 1982.

Roth AM: Retinal vascular development in premature infants. Am J Ophthalmol 84:636, 1977.

Spieres A, Isenberg SJ, Inkelis SH: Characteristics of the iris in 100 neonates. J Pediatr Ophthalmol Strab 26:28, 1989.

22.2 EXAMINATION OF THE EYE

Examination of the eye should be a routine part of the periodic pediatric assessment beginning in the newborn period. Screening in schools and community programs can also be effective in detecting problems early. The child should be examined by an ophthalmologist whenever a significant ocular abnormality or vision defect is noted or even suspected. Ideally, every child should have a thorough ophthalmologic examination sometime in early childhood, preferably by the age of 3–4 yr; these are the crucial years for the detection and treatment of amblyopia, strabismus, high refractive errors, and many other significant disorders.

Basic examination, whether done by the pediatrician or ophthalmologist, must include evaluation of visual acuity and the visual fields, assessment of the pupils, ocular motility and alignment, a general external examination, and an ophthalmoscopic examination of the media and fundi. When indicated, biomicroscopy (slit lamp examination), cycloplegic refraction, and tonometry are performed by the ophthalmologist. In some cases special diagnostic procedures, such as ultrasonic examination, fluorescein angiography, electroretinography (ERG), or visual evoked response (VER) testing, are also indicated.

VISUAL ACUITY. This is best measured by the standard Snellen chart (Fig. 22–1), and this method should be used as early as the child's ability to name, copy, or match letters or numbers allows. The "E" chart, consisting of rows of the letter E in various sizes and directions, can also be used; children are asked to indicate the direction of the selected E by pointing their hand or fingers (or a matching cardboard E) up, down, right, or left. For the very young child or the retarded, shy, or frightened child, a calibrated picture test can be used to elicit a verbal or picture matching response.

It is often best to start with both of the child's eyes open. This allows time for the child to become familiar with the test in a relaxed manner. Each eye can then be tested individually. It is essential to prevent peaking. The examiner should hold the occluder in place and observe the child throughout the test. It is equally important to ensure that the child does not memorize portions of the chart, nor should the child be allowed to squint to pass the test. The child should be reassured and encouraged throughout the test, because many children are intimidated by the procedure and fear a "bad grade" or punishment for errors. For young children or for those with concentration problems, testing at 10 or 15 ft using charts calibrated for the reduced distance may be more productive than testing at 20 ft. Also, testing near vision with a standardized reading card at 15 in may often yield useful information.

In infants and toddlers, in the very retarded, and in the psychiatrically disturbed youngster, vision can be estimated by the response to toys and familiar objects of various sizes, particularly food items, recording the distance at which the response is elicited.

Optokinetic nystagmus (the response to a sequence of moving targets; "railroad" nystagmus), can also be used to assess vision; this can be calibrated by various-sized targets (stripes or dots) or a rotating drum at specified distances. The VER, an electrophysiologic method of evaluating the response to light and special visual stimuli, such as calibrated stripes or a checkerboard pattern, can also be used to study visual function in selected cases. Preferential looking tests are also used for the evaluation of vision in infants and children who cannot respond to standard acuity tests. This is a behavioral technique based on the observation that, given a choice, an infant prefers to look at patterned rather than unpatterned stimuli.

Subnormal vision in one or both eyes warrants further evaluation. For the child who can be tested with a standard chart, acuity of less than 20/30, or an acuity difference of more than one line between the two eyes, is reason for referral. In the infant or very young child, lack of age-appropriate responses to interesting visual stimuli or a consistent difference in behavior when one or the other eye is covered is reason for referral.

VISUAL FIELD ASSESSMENT. Like visual acuity testing, visual field assessment must be geared to the child's age and abilities. Formal visual field examination (perimetry and scotometry) can often be accomplished in the school-aged child. Often, however, the examiner must rely on confrontation techniques and finger counting in quadrants of the visual field. In many children only testing by attraction can be accomplished; the examiner observes the child's response to familiar objects brought into each of the four quadrants of the visual field of each eye in turn. The child's bottle, a favorite toy, and lollipops are particularly effective attention-getting items. Even such gross methods can often detect diagnostically significant field changes such as the bitemporal hemianopsia of a chiasmal lesion or the homonymous hemianopsia of a cerebral lesion.

COLOR VISION TESTING. This can be accomplished whenever the child is able to name or trace the test symbols; these may either be numbers or Xs, Os, triangles, or other symbols. Color vision testing is not frequently necessary in young children, but parents sometimes request it, particularly if the child seems to be slow in learning colors. Defective color vision is not uncommon in males but is rare in females. Occasionally, there is achromatopsia, a total color vision defect with subnormal visual acuity, nystagmus, and photophobia. A change in color discrimination can be a sign of optic nerve or retinal disease.

PUPILLARY EXAMINATION. This includes evaluation of both the direct and consensual reactions to light, the reaction on near gaze, and the response to reduced illumination, noting the size and symmetry of the pupils under all conditions. Special care must be taken to differentiate the reaction to light from the reaction to near gaze; the natural tendency

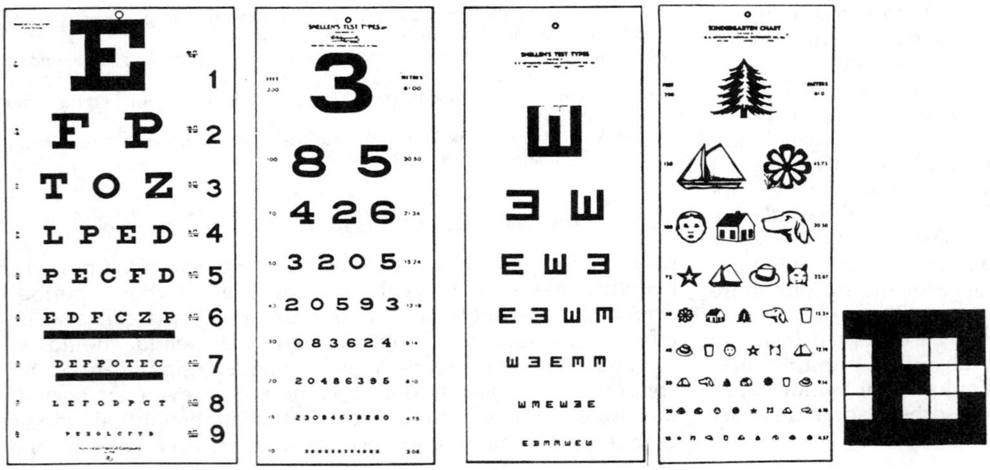

Figure 22–1. Various types of visual acuity charts. As illustrated by the Snellen E, each optotype is designed to subtend 5 min of arc and each component 1 min of arc.

of a child is to look directly at the approaching light, inducing the near gaze reflex when one is attempting to test only the reaction to light; accordingly, every effort must be made to control fixation. The swinging flashlight test is especially useful for detecting unilateral or asymmetric prechiasmatic afferent defects in children (see Marcus Gunn pupil, Sec. 22.5).

OCULAR MOTILITY. This is tested by having the child follow an object into the various positions of gaze. Movements of each eye individually (ductions) and of the two eyes together (versions, conjugate movements, and convergence) are assessed. Alignment is judged by the symmetry of the corneal light reflexes and by the response to alternate occlusion of each eye (see *cover tests for strabismus*, Sec. 22.6).

EXTERNAL EXAMINATION. This begins with general inspection in good illumination, noting size, shape, and symmetry of the orbits, position and movement of the lids, and the position and symmetry of the globes. Viewing the eyes and lids from above aids in detection of orbital asymmetry, lid masses, proptosis (exophthalmos), and abnormal pulsations. Palpation is also important in detection of orbital and lid masses.

The lacrimal apparatus is assessed by looking for evidence of tear deficiency, overflow of tears (epiphora), and erythema and swelling in the region of the tear sac or gland. The sac is massaged to check for reflux when obstruction is suspected. The presence and position of the puncta are also checked.

The lids and conjunctiva are specifically examined for focal lesions, foreign bodies, and inflammatory signs; loss and maldirection of lashes should also be noted. When necessary, the lids can be everted in the following manner: (1) instruct the patient to look down; (2) grasp the lashes of the patient's upper lid between the thumb and index finger of one hand; (3) place a probe, a cotton-tipped applicator, or the thumb of the other hand at the upper margin of the tarsal plate; and (4) pulling the lid down and outward, evert it over the probe, using the instrument as a fulcrum. Skill at eversion of the lid should be acquired. Foreign bodies commonly lodge in the concavity just above the lid margin and are exposed only by fully everting the lid.

The anterior segment of the eye is then evaluated with oblique focal illumination, noting luster and clarity of the cornea, depth and clarity of the anterior chamber, and features of the iris. Transillumination of the anterior segment aids in detecting opacities and in demonstrating atrophy or hypopigmentation of the iris; these latter signs are important when ocular albinism is suspected. When necessary, fluorescein dye can be used to aid in the diagnosis of abrasions, ulcerations, and foreign bodies.

BIOMICROSCOPY (SLIT LAMP EXAMINATION). This provides a highly magnified view of the various structures of the eye and an optical section through the media of the eye—that is, the cornea, aqueous humor, lens, and vitreous. Lesions can be not only identified but also localized as to their depth within the eye, and the resolution is sufficient to allow detection even of individual inflammatory cells in the aqueous and vitreous. With the addition of special lenses and prisms, the angle of the anterior chamber and regions of the fundus also can be examined with the slit lamp. Biomicroscopy is often crucial in trauma and in examining for iritis. It is also helpful in the diagnosis of many metabolic diseases of childhood.

FUNDUS EXAMINATION (OPHTHALMOSCOPY). This is best done with the pupil dilated unless there are neurologic or other contraindications. Tropicamide (Mydriacyl), 0.5–1%, and phenylephrine (Neo-Synephrine), 2.5%, are recommended as mydriatics of short duration. These are safe for most children, but the possibility of adverse systemic effects must be recognized. For very small infants more dilute preparations may be advisable. Beginning with posterior landmarks, the disk and the macula, the four quadrants are systematically examined by following each of the major vessel groups to the periphery. More of the fundus can be seen if the child is directed to look up, down, right, and left. Even with care, only a limited amount of the fundus can be seen with the direct or handheld ophthalmoscope. For examination of the far periphery the indirect ophthalmoscope is used, and full dilation of the pupil is essential.

It should be noted that, before the retina is examined, the ophthalmoscope is used to examine the clarity of the media. With a high plus lens (+8 or +10) in place, the ophthalmoscope can also be used for examination of external lesions and foreign bodies, because it provides magnification and good illumination.

REFRACTION. This determines the refractive state of the eye—that is, the degree of nearsightedness, farsightedness, or astigmatism. Retinoscopy provides an objective determination of the amount of correction needed and can be done at any age. In young children it is best done with cycloplegia. Subjective refinement of refraction involves asking the patient for preferences in the strength and axis of corrective lenses; it can be accomplished in many school-aged children. Refraction and determination of visual acuity with appropriate corrective lenses in place are essential steps in deciding whether or not the patient has a visual defect or amblyopia.

TONOMETRY. This measures intraocular pressure; it is usually done by the indentation method with the Schiotz gauge or by the applanation method with the slit lamp. Alternative methods are pneumatic and electronic tonometry. When accurate measurement of the pressure is necessary in a child who cannot cooperate, it may be done with sedation or general anesthesia. A gross estimate of pressure can be made by palpating the globe with the index fingers placed side by side on the upper lid above the tarsal plate.

Hoyt CS: The clinical usefulness of the visual evoked response. J Pediatr Ophthalmol Strab 21:231, 1984.
Isenberg S, Everett S, Parelhoff E: A comparison of mydriatic eyedrops in low-weight infants. Ophthalmology 91:278, 1984.
Isenberg SJ: Clinical application of the pupil examination in neonates. J Pediatr 118:650, 1991.
Linksz A: Color vision tests in clinical practice. Trans Am Acad Ophthalmol Otolaryngol 75:1078, 1971.
Marsh WR, Rawlings SC, Mumma JV: Evaluation of clinical stereoacuity tests. Ophthalmology 87:1265, 1980.
Sokol S, Hansen VC, Moskowitz A, et al: Evoked potentials and preferential looking estimates of visual acuity in pediatric patients. Ophthalmology 90:552, 1983.
Sturner RA, Green JA, Funk S, et al: A developmental approach to preschool vision screening. J Pediatr Ophthalmol Strab 18:61, 1981.
Teller DY, McDonald MA, Preston KI, et al: Assessment of visual acuity in infants and children: The acuity card procedure. Dev Med Child Neurol 28:779, 1986.

22.3 ABNORMALITIES OF REFRACTION AND ACCOMMODATION

When parallel rays of light come to focus on the retina with the eye in a state of rest (nonaccommodating), emmetropia exists. Such an ideal optical state is not uncommon, but more often the opposite condition, ametropia, exists. Three principal types occur: hyperopia (farsightedness), myopia (nearsightedness), and astigmatism. The majority of children are physiologically hyperopic at birth, but a significant number, especially those born prematurely, are myopic, and there is often some degree of astigmatism. With growth, the refractive state tends to change and should be evaluated periodically.

Measurement of the refractive state of the eye (refraction) can be accomplished objectively and subjectively. The objective method involves focusing a beam of light from a retinoscope onto the patient's retina through lenses of various powers placed in front of the eye. This method is precise and can be carried out at any age, because it requires no response from the patient. In infants and children it is best done after the instillation of eye drops that produce *mydriasis* (dilatation of the pupil) and *cycloplegia* (relaxation of accommodation); those used most commonly are tropicamide (Mydriacyl), cyclopentolate (Cyclogyl), homatropine hydrobromide, and atropine sulfate. The subjective method involves placing various lenses in front of the eye and having the patient report which lenses provide the clearest image of the letters on the chart. This method depends on the patient's ability to discriminate and communicate, but it can be used for some children and can be helpful in determining the best refractive correction for many youngsters who are developmentally capable of these tasks.

HYPEROPIA

If parallel rays of light come to focus posterior to the retina with the eye in a state of rest (nonaccommodating), hyperopia or farsightedness exists. This may result because the anteroposterior diameter of the eye is too short, because the refractive power of the cornea or lens is less than normal, or because the lens is dislocated posteriorly.

In hyperopia, accommodation is used to bring objects into focus for both far and near gaze. If the accommodative effort required is not too great, the child has clear vision and is comfortable for both distant and close work. In high degrees of hyperopia requiring greater accommodative effort, vision may be blurred, and the child may complain of "eye strain," headaches, or fatigue. Squinting, eye rubbing, lid inflammation, and lack of interest in reading are also frequent manifestations. There may be associated esotropia (convergent strabismus, accommodative esotropia, Sec. 22.6). Convex lenses (spectacles or contact lenses) of sufficient strength to provide clear vision and comfort are prescribed when indicated.

MYOPIA

In myopia parallel rays of light come to focus anterior to the retina. This may result because the anteroposterior diameter of the eye is too long, because the refractive power of the cornea or lens is greater than normal, or because the lens is dislocated forward. The principal symptom is blurred vision for distant objects. The far point of clear vision varies inversely with the degree of myopia; as the myopia increases, the far point of clear vision comes closer. With myopia of 1 diopter, for example, the far point of clear focus is 1 m from the eye; with myopia of 3 diopters, the far point of clear vision is only 1/3 m from the eye. Thus, myopic children tend to hold objects and reading matter close, prefer to be close to the blackboard, and may be uninterested in distant activities. Frowning and squinting are common, because the visual acuity is improved when the lid aperture is reduced; the effect is similar to that achieved by closing or "stopping down" the aperture of the diaphragm of a camera.

Myopia is infrequent in infants and preschool children. It is more common in preterm infants and in infants with retinopathy of prematurity. Also, there is a hereditary tendency to myopia, and children of myopic parents should be examined at an early age. The incidence of myopia increases during the school years, especially during the preteen and teen years. The degree of myopia also tends to increase with age during the growing years.

Concave lenses (spectacles or contact lenses) of appropriate strength to provide clear vision and comfort are prescribed. Changes are usually needed periodically, sometimes in 1–2 yr, sometimes every few months. Some practitioners advocate the use of cycloplegic agents and bifocals in an effort to retard the progression of myopia, but the value of such treatment is controversial.

In most cases myopia is not a result of pathologic alteration of the eye and is referred to as simple or physiologic myopia. Some children, however, may have pathologic myopia, a rare condition caused by a pathologically abnormal axial length of the eye; this is usually associated with thinning of the sclera, choroid, and retina, and often with some degree of uncorrectable visual impairment. Myopia may also occur as the result of other ocular abnormalities, such as keratoconus, ectopia lentis, and glaucoma, and is also a major feature of Stickler syndrome.

ASTIGMATISM

In astigmatism there is a difference in the refractive power of the various meridians of the eye. Most cases are caused by irregularity in the curvature of the cornea; some astigmatism results from changes in the lens. Mild degrees of astigmatism are very common and may produce no symptoms. With greater degrees there may be distortion of vision. In an effort to achieve a clearer image, the person with astigmatism uses accommodation or frowns or squints to obtain a pinhole effect. Symptoms include "eye strain," headache, and fatigue. Eye rubbing and lid hyperemia, indifference to schoolwork, and holding reading matter close are common manifestations in childhood. Cylindric or spherocylindric lenses are used to provide optical correction when indicated. Glasses may be needed constantly or only part time, depending on the degree of astigmatism and the severity of the attendant symptoms. In some cases, contact lenses are used.

Infants and children with corneal irregularity resulting from injury, periorbital and eyelid hemangiomas, and ptosis are at increased risk for astigmatism and attendant amblyopia.

ANISOMETROPIA

When the refractive state of one eye is significantly different from the refractive state of the other eye, anisometropia exists. Uncorrected, this may lead to amblyopia, or "lazy eye." Early detection and correction are essential if normal visual development in both eyes is to be achieved.

ACCOMMODATION

During accommodation the ciliary muscle contracts, the suspensory fibers of the lens relax, and the lens assumes a more rounded shape to bring rays of light into focus on the retina. The amplitude of accommodation is greatest during childhood and gradually diminishes with age. The physiologic decrease in accommodative ability that occurs with age is called presbyopia.

Disorders of accommodation in children are relatively rare. Premature presbyopia is occasionally seen in youngsters. The most common cause of paralysis of accommodation in children is the intentional or inadvertent use of cycloplegic substances, topically or systemically; included are all the anticholinergic drugs and poisons, as well as plants and plant substances having these effects. Neurogenic causes of accommodative paralysis include lesions affecting the oculomotor nerve (3rd cranial nerve) in any part of its course. Differential diagnosis includes tumors, degenerative diseases, vascular lesions, trauma, and infectious diseases. Impairment of accommodation may occur in botulism, diphtheria, Wilson disease, diabetes mellitus, and syphilis, and after some viral illnesses.

Rarely, inability to accommodate is caused by a congenital defect of the ciliary muscle. An apparent defect in accommodation may be psychogenic in origin; it is not uncommon for a child to feign inability to read when it can be demonstrated that visual acuity and ability to focus are normal.

Brodstein RS, Brodstein DE, Olson RJ, et al: The treatment of myopia with atropine and bifocals: A long-term prospective study. Ophthalmology 91:1373, 1984.
Curran RE, Hedges TR, Boger WP: Loss of accommodation and the near response in Wilson's disease. J Pediatr Ophthalmol Strab 19:157, 1982.
Curtin BJ: Physiologic vs pathologic myopia: Genetics vs environment. Ophthalmology 86:681, 1979.
Fulton AB, Dobson V, Salem D, et al: Cycloplegic refractions in infants and young children. Am J Ophthalmol 90:239, 1980.
Gordon RA, Donzia PB: Refractive development of the human eye. Arch Ophthalmol 103:785, 1985.
Mäntyjärvi MI: Changes in refraction in schoolchildren. Arch Ophthalmol 103:790, 1985.
Slataper FJ: Age norms of refraction and vision. Arch Ophthalmol 43:466, 1950.

22.4 DISORDERS OF VISION

AMBLYOPIA

Amblyopia is subnormal visual acuity in one or both eyes despite correction of any significant refractive error. The term may embrace various vision defects of organic or nonorganic origin (e.g., organic amblyopia designates vision loss directly attributable to trauma or to an organic lesion or disease of the eye or visual pathways), but the term is preferentially used to denote a specific developmental disorder of visual function arising from sensory stimulation deprivation or abnormal binocular interaction (i.e., malalignment or strabismus). In the latter sense amblyopia is familiarly known as "lazy eye."

Under normal conditions the development of visual acuity proceeds rapidly in infancy and early childhood. Anything that interferes with the formation of a clear retinal image during this early developmental period can produce *sensory deprivation amblyopia*. For example, during a critical developmental period in early life, a cataract can interfere with retinal stimulation to such a degree that even after the cataract is successfully removed and the aphakic refractive error is corrected with glasses or a contact lens that provides a clear retinal image, vision may be relatively poor. Similarly, uncorrected anisometropia in the young child can lead to amblyopia; in this condition the eye with the more normal refractive state and clearer retinal image is used for definitive seeing and the eye with the greater refractive error and blurred retinal image becomes amblyopic from sensory deprivation or disuse. Even the child with an abnormally high refractive error in both eyes may develop some degree of bilateral amblyopia because of retinal blur during the critical period of development.

In children with strabismus there is a tendency to suppress or "tune out" the image of the deviating eye as a sensory adaptation to avoid diplopia. If allowed to persist untreated in the young child, such suppression can result in amblyopia.

Susceptibility to amblyopia is greatest within the 1st 2–3 yr of life and especially in the 1st months of life, but risk of amblyopia lasts until full visual potential and stability have been achieved, generally by the age of 5–6 yr (sometimes later).

The key to the successful treatment of amblyopia is early detection and prompt intervention. In an infant amblyopia can often be reversed in a matter of days or weeks. In an older child with longstanding amblyopia, months or years of treatment may be required.

Treatment of amblyopia involves the following: (1) providing the clearest possible retinal image (e.g., by correction of refractive error, removal of cataract); and (2) stimulation or forced use of the amblyopic eye. The latter is accomplished by occlusion therapy, often referred to as "patching"; the better eye is covered to force use of the amblyopic eye. In many cases best results are achieved with complete and constant occlusion throughout the waking hours by the use of adhesive eye "patches"; in some cases part-time occlusion is sufficient or preferred. Occluders placed on spectacles allow peeking, and the adjustable headband type of cloth or plastic occluder is too easily removed by the child. In selected cases an opaque contact lens or a contact lens of sufficiently high power to blur the vision in the better eye is used. In certain cases cycloplegic drops are used to blur the image in the better eye. Most children and their families tolerate occlusion therapy well. In some cases the child resists therapy because of the severity of the vision defect, the cosmetic blemish of the patching, or related psychologic disturbances. The goals of treatment must be thoroughly understood and the treatment carefully supervised. Close monitoring of occlusion therapy is essential, especially in the very young, to avoid deprivation amblyopia in the occluded eye. Also, many families need reassurance and support throughout the trying course of treatment.

AMAUROSIS

The term "amaurosis" refers to partial or total loss of vision; it is usually reserved for profound impairment, blindness, or near blindness. When amaurosis exists from birth, primary consideration in differential diagnosis must be given to developmental malformations, damage consequent to gestational or perinatal infection, anoxia or hypoxia, perinatal trauma, and the genetically determined diseases that can affect the eye itself or the visual pathways. In certain cases the reason for the amaurosis can be readily determined by objective ophthalmic examination; examples are severe microphthalmia, corneal opacification, dense cataracts, chorioretinal scars, macular defects, retinal dysplasia, and severe optic nerve hypoplasia. In some cases there is intrinsic retinal disease that may not be apparent on initial ophthalmoscopic examination; an example is Leber congenital retinal amaurosis. In this retinal dystrophy the fundus may appear normal or near normal for some time before ophthalmoscopically appreciable signs of retinal degeneration (e.g., pigmentary deposits, arteriolar attenuation, optic disk pallor) develop; in such cases electroretinography is important in diagnosis, because the electroretinographic response in this condition is markedly reduced or absent. In many cases of amaurosis the defect lies not in the eye or optic nerve but in the brain, requiring neurologic and neuroradiologic evaluation, including computed tomography or magnetic resonance imaging.

Amaurosis that develops in a child who once had useful vision has different implications. In the absence of obvious ocular disease (e.g., cataract, chorioretinitis, retinoblastoma, retinitis pigmentosa) consideration must be given to many neurologic and systemic disorders that can affect the visual pathways. Amaurosis of rather rapid onset may indicate an encephalopathy (such as might occur with hypertension), infectious or parainfectious processes, vasculitis, migraine, leukemia, toxins, or trauma. It may be caused by acute demyelinating disease affecting the optic nerves, chiasm, or cerebrum. In some cases precipitous loss of vision is the result of increased intracranial pressure, a rapidly progressive hydrocephalus, or dysfunction of a shunt. More slowly progressive visual loss suggests tumor or neurodegenerative disease. Gliomas of the optic nerve and chiasm and craniopharyngiomas are primary diagnostic considerations in children who show progressive loss of vision.

Manifestations of impairment of vision vary with the age

and abilities of the child, the mode of onset, and the laterality and severity of the deficit. The 1st clue to amaurosis in an infant may be nystagmus or strabismus, the vision defect itself passing undetected for some time. Timidity, clumsiness, or behavioral change may be the initial clues in the very young. Deterioration in school progress and indifference to school activities are common signs in the older child. School-aged children often try to hide their disability and, in the case of very slowly progressive disorders, may not themselves realize the severity of the problem; some detect and promptly report small changes in their vision.

Any evidence of loss of vision requires prompt and thorough ophthalmic evaluation. More often than not, the complete delineation of childhood amaurosis and its etiology requires extensive investigation involving neurologic evaluation, electrophysiologic tests, neuroradiologic procedures, and sometimes metabolic and genetic studies. Furthermore, there may be attendant special educational, social, and emotional needs to be met.

NYCTALOPIA

Nyctalopia or "night blindness" refers to vision that is defective in reduced illumination. It generally implies impairment in function of the rods, particularly in dark adaptation time and perceptual threshold. *Stationary congenital night blindness* may occur as an autosomal dominant, autosomal recessive, or X-linked recessive condition. It may be associated with myopia and disk anomaly. *Progressive night blindness* usually indicates primary or secondary retinal, choroidal, or vitrioretinal degeneration (Sec. 22.13); it occurs also in vitamin A deficiency or as the result of retinotoxic drugs such as quinine.

DIPLOPIA

Diplopia or "double vision" is most frequently the result of malalignment of the visual axes—that is, displacement or deviation of the eye. It is common in heterophoria, in heterotropia of recent onset (particularly when caused by acquired nerve palsy), and in proptosis. Because in such cases occluding one eye relieves the diplopia, affected children commonly squint, cover one eye with a hand, or assume abnormal head postures (a face turn or head tilt) to alleviate the bothersome sensation. These mannerisms, especially in preverbal children, are important clues to diplopia. The onset of diplopia in any child warrants prompt evaluation; it may signal the onset of a serious problem such as increased intracranial pressure, a brain tumor, an orbital mass, or myasthenia gravis.

Monocular diplopia results from dislocation of the lens or some defect in the media or macula.

PSYCHOGENIC DISTURBANCES

Vision problems of psychogenic origin are not uncommon in school-aged children. Both conversion reactions and willful feigning are encountered. The usual manifestation is a report of reduced visual acuity in one or both eyes. Another common manifestation is constriction of the visual field. In some cases the symptom is diplopia or polyopia.

Important clues to the diagnosis are inappropriate affect, excessive grimacing, inconsistency in performance, and suggestibility. Thorough ophthalmologic examination is essential to differentiate organic from functional visual disorders.

As a rule, affected children do well with reassurance and positive suggestion. In some cases psychiatric care is indicated. In all cases the approach must be supportive and nonpunitive.

DYSLEXIA

The term "dyslexia" is used to describe a specific reading disability that is attributable to a primary or developmental defect in the higher cortical processing of graphic symbols. It is to be differentiated from reading retardation that may be secondary to other causes (e.g., intellectual impairment, maturational delay, cultural or educational deprivation, emotional disturbances, organic brain disease, or sensory defects) and from acquired word blindness (alexia) occurring as the result of a lesion in the dominant cerebral hemisphere.

Neither dyslexia nor the often associated symptoms such as letter or word reversal and so-called mirror writing are caused by any defect in the eye or visual acuity per se, nor are they attributable to a defect in ocular motility or binocular alignment, but ophthalmologic evaluation of the child with a reading problem is recommended for several reasons: (1) such assessment is of value in differential diagnosis; (2) correction of any concurrent ocular problems such as a refractive error, amblyopia, or strabismus ensures the best possible visual function for the child's education; and (3) the ophthalmologist can be of help in counseling patient and family.

The approach to treatment is remedial instruction. Treatment directed to the eyes themselves cannot be expected to correct developmental dyslexia.

Barnet AB, Manson JI, Wilmer E: Acute cerebral blindness in childhood. Six cases studied clinically and electrophysiologically. Neurology 30:1147, 1970.
Catalano RA, Simon JW, Krohel GB, et al: Functional visual loss in children. Ophthalmology 93:385, 1986.
Duffy FH, Burchfield JL, Snodgrass SR: The pharmacology of amblyopia. Ophthalmology 86:489, 1978.
Francois J: Diagnosis of blindness in the infant. Ann Ophthalmol 2:533, 1970.
Flynn JT, Cassady JC: Current trends in amblyopia therapy. Ophthalmology 85:428, 1978.
Hittner HM, Borda RP, Justice J Jr: X-linked recessive congenital stationary night blindness, myopia, and tilted discs. J Pediatr Ophthalmol 18:15, 1981.
Jastrzebski GR, Hoyt CS, Marg E: Stimulus deprivation amblyopia in children: Sensitivity, plasticity, and elasticity (SPE). Arch Ophthalmol 102:1030, 1984.
Kushner BJ: Functional amblyopia associated with organic ocular lesions. Am J Ophthalmol 91:39, 1981.
Mäntyjärvi MI: The amblyopic schoolgirl syndrome. J Pediatr Ophthalmol Strab 18:30, 1981.
Mellor DH, Fields AR: Dissociated visual development: Electrodiagnostic studies in infants who are "slow to see." Dev Med Child Neurol 22:327, 1980.
Stager DR: Amblyopia and the pediatrician. Pediatr Ann 8(2):91, 1977.
Tongue AC: Low vision examination in children with visual impairment. J Pediatr Ophthalmol Strab 17:175, 1980.
Von Noorden GK, Milane JB: Penalization in the treatment of amblyopia. Am J Ophthalmol 88:511, 1979.

22.5 ABNORMALITIES OF PUPIL AND IRIS

ANIRIDIA

This developmental anomaly is characterized by marked hypoplasia of the iris. Usually only a narrow rim of rudimentary iris tissue is present peripherally at the base or root. The pupil is abnormally large, often irregular, and unreactive. In addition to the iris defect, there is usually some degree of hypoplasia of the macula and optic nerve. Also frequently associated are cataracts, ectopia lentis, glaucoma, and progressive corneal degeneration. Most patients have some degree of vision impairment, nystagmus, and photophobia. High refractive errors and strabismus are also common.

At least two distinct types of aniridia have been delineated. Type I is transmitted in an autosomal dominant manner; the involved gene appears to be on chromosome 2. It is characterized by variable expressivity. Autosomal recessive cases of aniridia have also been described, sometimes in association with cerebellar ataxia and retardation. Type II usually occurs sporadically and is caused by an interstitial deletion on the short arm of chromosome 11. Patients with type II often have associated genitourinary anomalies and mental retardation, the AGR triad. In patients with AGR and the chromosome 11 defect there is marked predisposition for the development of Wilms' tumor, the WAGR or Wilms' tumor–aniridia association (see also Sec. 17.13).

COLOBOMA OF THE IRIS

Coloboma is a developmental defect that may take the form of a defect in a sector of the iris, a hole in the substance of the iris, or a notch in the pupillary margin. Simple colobomata are frequently transmitted as an autosomal dominant characteristic, and may occur alone or be associated with other anomalies. An iris coloboma may be part of an extensive coloboma involving the fundus and optic nerve as a result of malclosure of the embryonic fissure (Sec. 22.13).

MICROCORIA

Absence or malformation of the dilator pupillae muscle may result in an abnormally small pupil that is difficult to dilate, a condition referred to as congenital miosis, or microcoria. Both sporadic and hereditary cases (autosomal dominant and autosomal recessive) occur. They may be associated with other anomalies of the anterior segment.

CONGENITAL MYDRIASIS

In this disorder the pupils appear dilated, do not constrict significantly to light or near gaze, and respond minimally to miotic agents. The iris is otherwise normal and the affected child is usually healthy. The basis for the abnormality is not clear, though a defect of the iris musculature must be considered. There is evidence for autosomal dominant and possibly X-linked dominant transmission.

This congenital condition should be differentiated from aniridia or other structural abnormalities of the iris, from the fixed dilated pupil of neurologic disease, and from pharmacologic mydriasis.

DYSCORIA AND CORECTOPIA

Dyscoria is abnormal shape of the pupil, and corectopia is abnormal pupillary position. They may occur together or independently as congenital anomalies. Corectopia may be associated with dislocation of the lens. Distortion and displacement of the pupil are frequently the result of trauma and are important signs of prolapse of the iris in perforating injuries of the eye; they may also be seen with tears of the iris, with segmental iridoplegia, and with synechiae (adhesions of iris to lens or cornea).

ANISOCORIA

This is inequality of the pupils. As a general rule, if the inequality is more pronounced in the presence of bright focal illumination or on near gaze, the larger pupil is abnormal, whereas if the anisocoria is worse in reduced illumination, the smaller pupil is abnormal. Neurologic causes of anisocoria (parasympathetic or sympathetic lesions) must be differentiated from local causes such as synechiae (adhesions), congenital iris defects (colobomata, aniridia), and pharmacologic effects. Simple central anisocoria may occur in otherwise healthy individuals.

DILATED FIXED PUPIL

Differential diagnosis of the dilated unreactive pupil includes internal ophthalmoplegia caused by a central or peripheral lesion, the Hutchinson pupil of transtentorial herniation, tonic pupil, pharmacologic blockade, and iridoplegia secondary to ocular trauma.

The most common cause of a dilated unreactive pupil is the purposeful or accidental instillation of a cycloplegic agent, particularly atropine and related substances. Internal ophthalmoplegia may occur with central lesions, and in children the possibility of pinealoma must be considered. The "blown pupil" of transtentorial herniation, as occurs with subdural hematoma and increasing intracranial pressure, is generally unilateral, and usually the patient is obviously ill. The pilocarpine test can help differentiate neurologic iridoplegia from pharmacologic blockade. In the case of neurologic iridoplegia the dilated pupil constricts within minutes after the instillation of 1 or 2 drops of 0.5–1% pilocarpine; if the pupil has been dilated with atropine, the pilocarpine has no effect. Because pilocarpine is a long-acting drug, this test is not to be used in acute situations in which pupillary signs must be carefully monitored.

TONIC PUPIL

This is typically a large pupil that reacts poorly to light (the reaction may be very slow or essentially nil), reacts poorly and slowly to accommodation, and redilates in a slow, tonic manner. The features of tonic pupil are explained by cholinergic supersensitivity of the sphincter following peripheral (postganglionic) denervation and imperfect reinnervation. A distinctive feature of the tonic pupil is its sensitivity to dilute cholinergic agents, such as 0.125% pilocarpine. The condition is usually unilateral.

Tonic pupil may develop after the acute stage of a partial or complete iridoplegia. It can be seen after trauma to the eye or orbit, and may occur in association with toxic or infectious conditions. In those in the pediatric age group, tonic pupil is uncommon. Infectious processes (primarily viral syndromes) and trauma are the primary causes. Features of tonic pupil may also be seen in infants and children with familial dysautonomia (Riley-Day syndrome), although the significance of these findings has been questioned. Tonic pupil has also been reported in young children with Charcot-Marie-Tooth disease. The occurrence of tonic pupil in association with decreased deep tendon reflexes in young women is referred to as *Adie syndrome*.

MARCUS GUNN PUPIL

The Marcus Gunn pupil sign indicates an asymmetric, prechiasmatic, afferent conduction defect. It is best demonstrated by the swinging flashlight test; this allows comparison of the direct and consensual pupillary responses in both eyes. With the patient fixing on a distant target (to control accommodation) a bright focal light is directed alternately into each eye in turn. In the presence of an afferent lesion, both the direct response to light in the affected eye and the consensual response in the fellow eye are subnormal. Swinging the light to the better or normal eye causes both pupils to react (constrict) normally. Swinging the light back to the affected eye causes both pupils to redilate to some degree, reflecting the defective conduction. This is a very sensitive and useful test for detecting and confirming optic nerve and retinal disease. A relative afferent defect may be found in some children with amblyopia.

HORNER SYNDROME

The principal signs of oculosympathetic paresis (Horner syndrome) are homolateral miosis, mild ptosis, and apparent enophthalmos with slight elevation of the lower lid. There may also be decrease in facial sweating, increased amplitude of accommodation, and transient decrease in intraocular pressure. If paralysis of the ocular sympathetic fibers occurs before the age of 2 yr, there may be heterochromia iridis with hypopigmentation of the iris on the affected side.

Oculosympathetic paralysis may be caused by a lesion in the midbrain, brain stem, upper spinal cord, neck, middle fossa, or orbit. Congenital oculosympathetic paresis resulting from birth trauma, often as part of Klumke brachial palsy, is common, although the ocular signs, particularly the anisocoria, may pass undetected for years. Horner syndrome is also seen in some children following thoracic surgery, as for congenital heart disease. Congenital Horner syndrome may occur in association with vertebral anomalies and with enterogenous cysts. In some infants and children, Horner syndrome is the presenting sign of tumor in the mediastinal or cervical region, particularly neuroblastoma. Rare causes of Horner syndrome, such as vascular lesions, also occur in the pediatric age group. In some cases, no etiology for the Horner syndrome can be identified. Occasionally, the condition is familial.

When the etiology of Horner syndrome is in question, investigative procedures should be implemented, including chest radiography, computed tomography, magnetic resonance imaging of the head and neck, and 24-hr urinary catecholamine assay. Sometimes examining old photographs and old records can be helpful in establishing the age of onset of the Horner syndrome.

The cocaine test is useful in the diagnosis of oculosympathetic paralysis; a normal pupil dilates within 20–45 min after instillation of 1 or 2 drops of 4% cocaine, whereas the miotic pupil of an oculosympathetic paresis dilates poorly, if at all, to cocaine. In some cases there is denervation supersensitivity to dilute phenylephrine; 1 or 2 drops of a 1% solution dilates the affected but not the normal pupil. Furthermore, the instillation of 1% hydroxyamphetamine hydrobromide dilates the pupil only if the postganglionic sympathetic neuron is intact.

PARADOXIC PUPIL REACTION

Some children exhibit paradoxic constriction of the pupils to darkness. There is an initial brisk constriction of the pupils when the light is turned off, followed by slow redilation of the pupils. The response to direct light stimulation and the near response are normal. The mechanism is not clear, but paradoxic constriction of the pupils in reduced light can be a sign of retinal or optic nerve abnormalities. The phenomenon has been observed in children with congenital stationary night blindness, albinism, retinitis pigmentosa, Leber congenital retinal amaurosis, and Best disease. It has also been observed in those with optic nerve anomalies, optic neuritis, optic atrophy, and possibly amblyopia.

PERSISTENT PUPILLARY MEMBRANE

Involution of the pupillary membrane and anterior vascular capsule of the lens is usually completed prior to birth. It is not uncommon, however, to see some remnants of the pupillary membrane in newborns, particularly in premature infants. These fine, web-like strands or vascular arcades are arranged in a radiating or spoke-like pattern in the pupil and can be visualized with the ophthalmoscope. The remnants tend to atrophy in time and usually present no problem. In some cases, however, significant remnants remain, sometimes forming a dense band that traverses and distorts the pupil, a broad sheath of tissue that may be firmly attached to the anterior lens capsule, or an opaque hyperplastic membrane that obscures the pupil and interferes with vision. Rarely, there is patency of the vascular elements; hyphema resulting from rupture of persistent vessels may occur.

Intervention must be considered to minimize amblyopia in infants with extensive persistent pupillary membrane of sufficient degree to interfere with vision in the early months of life. In some cases mydriatics and occlusion therapy may be effective, but in others surgery may be needed to provide an adequate pupillary aperture.

HETEROCHROMIA

In heterochromia the two irides are of different color (heterochromia iridum), or a portion of an iris differs in color from the remainder (heterochromia iridis). Simple heterochromia may occur as an autosomal dominant characteristic. Congenital heterochromia is also a feature of Waardenburg syndrome, an autosomal dominant condition characterized principally by lateral displacement of the inner canthi and puncta, pigmentary disturbances (usually a median white forelock and patches of hypopigmentation of the skin), and defective hearing. Change in the color of the iris may occur as the result of trauma, hemorrhage, intraocular inflammation (iridocyclitis, uveitis), intraocular tumor (especially retinoblastoma), intraocular foreign body, glaucoma, iris atrophy, oculosympathetic palsy (Horner syndrome), or melanosis oculi.

OTHER IRIS LESIONS

Discrete nodules of the iris, referred to as Lisch nodules, may be seen in patients with neurofibromatosis. The lesions vary from slightly elevated pigmented areas to distinct ball-like excrescences. Slit lamp examination may aid in the diagnosis of neurofibromatosis.

In leukemia there may be infiltration of the iris, sometimes with hypopyon, an accumulation of white cells in the anterior chamber, which may herald relapse or involvement of the central nervous system.

The lesion of juvenile xanthogranuloma (nevoxanthoendothelioma) may occur in the eye as a yellowish fleshy mass or plaque of the iris. Spontaneous hyphema (blood in the anterior chamber), glaucoma, or a red eye with signs of uveitis may be associated. A search for the skin lesions of xanthogranuloma (see also Sec. 23.33) should be made in any infant or young child with spontaneous hyphema. In many cases the ocular lesion responds to topical corticosteroid therapy.

LEUKOCORIA

This term describes any white pupillary reflex, or so-called cat's eye reflex. Primary diagnostic considerations in any child with leukocoria are cataract, persistent hyperplastic primary vitreous, cicatricial retinopathy of prematurity, retinal detachment and retinoschisis, larval granulomatosis, and retinoblas-

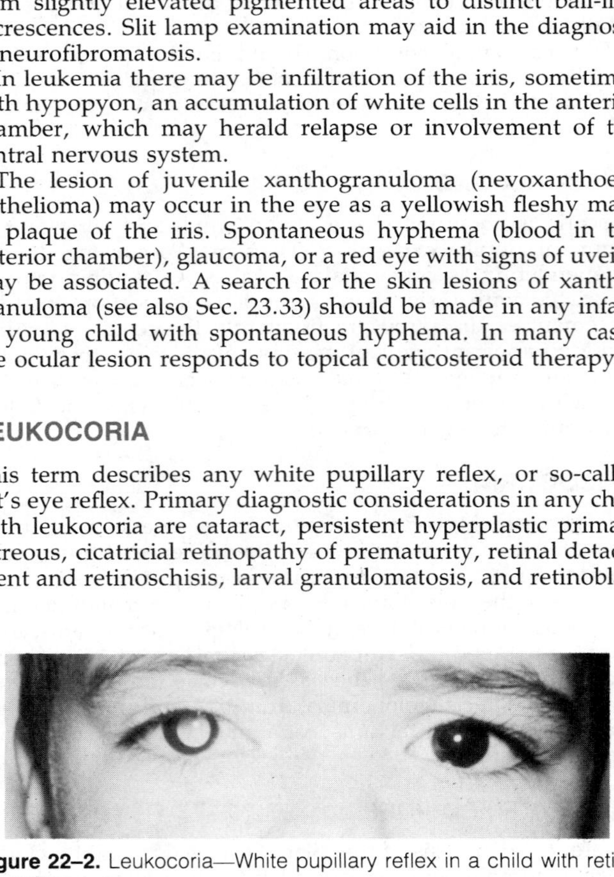

Figure 22–2. Leukocoria—White pupillary reflex in a child with retinoblastoma.

toma (Fig. 22–2). Also to be considered are endophthalmitis, organized vitreous hemorrhage, leukemic ophthalmopathy, exudative retinopathy (as in Coats disease), and a few rare conditions such as medulloepithelioma, massive retinal gliosis, the retinal pseudotumor of Norrie disease, the so-called pseudoglioma of the Bloch-Sulzberger syndrome, retinal dysplasia, and the retinal lesions of the phakomatoses. A white reflex may also be seen with fundus coloboma, large atrophic chorioretinal scars, and ectopic medullation of retinal nerve fibers. Leukocoria is an indication for prompt and thorough evaluation.

Often the diagnosis can be made by direct examination of the eye by ophthalmoscopy and biomicroscopy. Ultrasonographic and radiologic examinations are often helpful. In some cases the final diagnosis rests with the pathologist.

DiGeorge AM, Harley RD: The association of aniridia, Wilms' tumor, and genital abnormalities. Arch Ophthalmol 75:796, 1966.

Francois J: Differential diagnosis of leukokoria in children. Ann Ophthalmol 10:1375, 1978.

Frank JW, Kushner BJ, France TD: Paradoxic pupillary phenomenon: A review of patients with pupillary constriction to darkness. Arch Ophthalmol 106:1564, 1988.

Grant WM, Walton DS: Progressive changes in the angle in congenital aniridia with development of glaucoma. Am J Ophthalmol 78:842, 1974.

Greenwald MJ, Folk ER: Afferent pupillary defects in amblyopia. J Pediatr Ophthalmol Strab 20:63, 1983.

Hersh JH, Douglas C, Houston J, et al: Familial iridoplagia. J Pediatr Ophthalmol Strab 24:49, 1982.

Jaffe N, Cassady JR, Filler RM, et al: Heterochromia and Horner syndrome associated with cervical and mediastinal neuroblastoma. J Pediatr 87:75, 1975.

Krishnamohan VK, Wheeler MD, Testa MA, et al: Correlation of postnatal regression of the anterior vesicular capsule of the lens to gestational age. J Pediatr Ophthalmol Strab 19:28, 1982.

Layman PR, Andersen DR, Flynn JT: Frequent occurrence of hypoplastic discs in patients with aniridia. Am J Ophthalmol 77:513, 1974.

Lewis RA, Riccardi VM: Von Recklinghausen neurofibromatosis: Incidence of iris hamartomata. Ophthalmology 88:348, 1981.

Lowenfeld IE: "Simple, central" anisocoria: A common condition seldom recognized. Trans Am Acad Ophthalmol Otolaryngol 83:832, 1977.

Mackman G, Brightbill FS, Opitz JM: Corneal changes in aniridia. Am J Ophthalmol 87:497, 1979.

Margo C: Congenital aniridia: A histopathologic study of the anterior segment in children. J Pediatr Ophthalmol Strab 20:192, 1983.

Maloney WF, Younge BR, Moyer NJ: Evaluation of the causes and accuracy of pharmacologic localization in Horner's syndrome. Am J Ophthalmol 90:394, 1980.

Miller RW, Fraumeni JF, Manning MD: Association of Wilms' tumor with aniridia, hemihypertrophy and other congenital malformations. N Engl J Med 270:922, 1964.

Schachat AP, Jabs DA, Graham ML, et al: Leukemic iris infiltration. J Pediatr Ophthalmol Strabismus 25:135, 1988.

Thompson HS: Segmental palsy of the iris sphincter in Adie's syndrome. Arch Ophthalmol 96:1615, 1978.

Thompson HS, Newsome DA, Loewenfeld IE: The fixed dilated pupil: Sudden iridoplegia or mydriatic drops? A simple diagnostic test. Arch Ophthalmol 86:21, 1971.

Woodruff G, Buncic JR, Morin JD: Horner syndrome in children. J Pediatr Ophthalmol Strab 25:40, 1988.

22.6 DISORDERS OF EYE MOVEMENT AND ALIGNMENT

STRABISMUS

(Squint, Cast; Tropia, Phoria; Cross-Eye, Walleye)

The development of normal vision in each eye, the maintenance of proper alignment of the visual axes (orthophoria), and the ability to integrate the images from the two eyes into a single visual perception are essential to normal depth perception, or stereopsis. Any variation from normal sensorimotor development in early life may result in lifelong patterns of defective vision or abnormal ocular alignment. Early detection and treatment of strabismus in children is of primary importance, and proper assessment and management require knowledge of the various types of strabismus, the methods of detection, and the principles of treatment.

CLINICAL TYPES OF STRABISMUS: CLASSIFICATION AND TERMINOLOGY. The two principal types of deviation or malalignment of the eyes are heterophoria and heterotropia. *Heterophoria* is a latent tendency to malalignment; the eye deviates only under certain conditions (e.g., fatigue, illness, stress, or dissociative testing) that interfere with maintenance of normal fusion. Phorias are common and may give rise to bothersome symptoms such as transient diplopia, asthenopia ("eye strain"), or headaches. When the deviation exceeds the amplitude of fusion and becomes manifest, the malalignment is termed *heterotropia* or simply tropia. The condition may be monocular or alternating, depending on the vision and fixation pattern. In *alternating strabismus* the patient uses either eye for fixation or definitive seeing while the other eye deviates; because each eye is being used in turn, vision develops more or less equally in both. The patient in effect learns to suppress the image in the deviating (nonfixating) eye. When only one eye is used (or preferred) for fixation and the fellow eye consistently deviates, the deviation may be referred to as monocular or as right or left strabismus; in this situation the child is prone to amblyopia or defective central vision in the deviating eye as the result of disuse or misuse.

Strabismus is further described according to the direction of the deviation. Convergent deviation, a crossing or turning in of the eyes, is designated by the prefix *eso-* (thus esotropia, esophoria), whereas a divergent deviation or turning outward of the eyes (commonly referred to as wall-eye) is designated by the prefix *exo-*. Vertical deviations are indicated by the prefixes *hyper-* and *hypo-*. These may occur singly or in various combinations. In addition, torsional or cyclovertical deviations may occur.

The etiologic classification of strabismus is complex and knowledge of the causative factors and mechanisms incomplete. Certain major types must be distinguished; these are paralytic (noncomitant), nonparalytic (comitant), accommodative, and nonaccommodative.

Paralytic strabismus is caused by weakness or paralysis of one or more of the extraocular muscles. The deviation characteristically worsens on gaze into the field of action of the affected muscle. Hence, in the case of a right abducent paresis, the eyes appear crossed on looking to the right but appear straight (orthotropic) on looking to the left. The subjective manifestation is diplopia; to avoid this bothersome sensation, the child may turn the head to compensate for the paretic muscle or may close or cover one eye to eliminate the double image. Such mannerisms are important clues to the presence of an extraocular muscle palsy. With few exceptions, acquired extraocular muscle palsies are ominous signs of a serious pathologic process; the development of a noncomitant strabismus may be the first sign of an intracranial tumor, an infectious or parainfectious process (e.g., meningitis, encephalitis, neuritis), a demyelinizing or neurodegenerative disease, myasthenia gravis, or a progressive myopathy. A notable exception is benign 6th nerve palsy (see later). Congenital paralytic strabismus is more commonly a result of developmental defects of the cranial nerve nuclei or fibers, muscle anomalies, congenital infection syndromes, or birth trauma.

Nonparalytic strabismus is the more common type. There is no defect in the action of the individual extraocular muscles, and the amount of deviation is constant or relatively constant in all directions of gaze. Most congenital or infantile esotropias are of the nonparalytic or comitant type; this type is best treated surgically, but successful treatment must also involve treatment of any concurrent amblyopia.

Some cases of nonparalytic strabismus are caused by underlying ocular or visual defects, such as may occur with cataracts, lesions of the optic nerve or macula, high refractive errors, or asymmetric refractive errors (anisometropia). When possible, the underlying ocular condition is corrected first; in selected cases surgery may then be offered to "straighten" the eyes.

A special type of nonparalytic strabismus is *accommodative esotropia* (Fig. 22–3). This type depends on the relationship between the accommodation and convergence reflexes. In certain individuals activation of accommodation results in overconvergence or crossing of the eyes; also, in some cases, the amount of crossing with near gaze is greater than that with gaze into the distance. This type of deviation most commonly appears at 2–3 yr of age, with a range of onset from approximately 6 mo–7 or 8 yr. Most affected children have some degree of hyperopia (farsightedness). In most cases the crossing can be controlled with glasses that correct the hyperopia; some children require the use of bifocal lenses to control fully the excessive convergence for near gaze. Some respond to topical miotics such as phospholine iodide, but these must be used with great care because they are long-acting cholinesterase inhibitors. With early treatment of accommodative esotropia good vision should be maintained in both eyes; when amblyopia occurs, it is necessary to use occlusion therapy as well as glasses. A few children with accommodative esotropia require surgery for a residual amount of crossing that cannot be controlled with glasses alone.

True strabismus must be differentiated from the false impression of deviation created by certain anatomic variations. Children with prominent epicanthal folds and broad, flat nasal bridges often appear cross-eyed when they are in fact orthotropic; this is *pseudoesotropia*. Similarly, an orthotropic child may appear to have a divergent strabismus because of an increased interpupillary distance or a slight disparity between the position of the corneal light reflex and the pupillary axis; this is *pseudoexotropia*. Various types of facial asymmetry can also contribute to the false impression of vertical malalignment of the eyes.

ASSESSMENT. Two relatively simple and reliable techniques for assessing the alignment of the eyes in children are the Hirschberg or corneal light reflex test and the cover, uncover, and cross-cover tests. The *Hirschberg test* involves simply observing the position of the corneal reflexes (reflections) when a small focal light is directed toward the patient's eyes. If the light reflex is well centered in each eye or falls symmetrically on corresponding points of both pupils simultaneously, the eyes are properly aligned. If the light reflex in one eye is well centered but the light reflex in the other eye falls nasally or temporally, superiorly or inferiorly, a deviation exists. The amount of prism needed to recenter the light reflex in the deviating eye provides an accurate measurement of the degree of strabismus.

In the *cover, uncover,* and *cross-cover tests* the eyes are observed for compensatory or adjustive refixation movements. With the patient focusing on a distant target, the examiner alternately covers each eye in turn with an occluder. If no movement of either eye occurs as the occluder is moved back and forth from one eye to the other, alignment is normal (orthotropic). If there is esotropia, the deviating eye is seen to move outward to focus on the target as the fixating eye is occluded; if there is exotropia, the deviating eye moves inward to focus on the target as the fixating eye is occluded. In the case of a phoria or latent deviation it is the occluded eye that tends to deviate because of the temporary disruption of binocular fusion; the adjustive or refixation movement is seen at the moment of uncovering, as the eye once again focuses on the target. The tests should be performed both for distance and for near gaze to ensure detection of any accommodative component or any abnormality of the distance-near relationship; the tests should also be done in the cardinal positions of gaze to ensure detection of any incomitancy. In addition, the extraocular muscle functions of each eye should be tested individually. Simple toys, particularly those that create a pleasing noise, are especially useful in attracting the attention of young children for these tests, but detailed targets such as letters, numbers, and pictures are better for eliciting accommodative deviations.

Before proceeding with the light reflex and cover testing it is advisable to take time simply to observe the child at a nonthreatening distance in quiet, pleasant surroundings while the child plays or sits comfortably with a parent, particularly when the child is very young, shy, fearful, or retarded.

PRINCIPLES OF TREATMENT. The 1st goal of treatment is to achieve the best possible vision in each eye and, if possible, equal or nearly equal vision in both eyes. Any correctable underlying defect such as a cataract must be dealt with, contributing refractive errors must be corrected with lenses, and any amblyopia must be vigorously treated with occlusion therapy.

The 2nd goal is to achieve the best possible ocular alignment, especially for the primary or forward gaze position and for the reading or eyes-down position. In many cases surgery is required. Surgical treatment is particularly important in congenital strabismus, and it should be carried out at the earliest possible time to give the child the best possible opportunity to develop normal sensorimotor patterns. The longer the deviation persists untreated, the less chance there is for development of good or reasonably good function. Surgery is also required in some children with accommodative or partially accommodative esotropia when there is some degree of residual crossing that cannot be controlled with glasses and/or miotics. Surgical correction of a deviation is also an option in selected cases for cosmetic reasons, particularly when there is an underlying ocular defect such as an optic nerve or macular lesion or a dense amblyopia that cannot be corrected. In some cases multiple surgical procedures are required for strabismus, but most uncomplicated cases can be corrected with only one or two procedures.

In addition or alternative to surgery some patients have been successfully treated with an injection of botulinum toxin

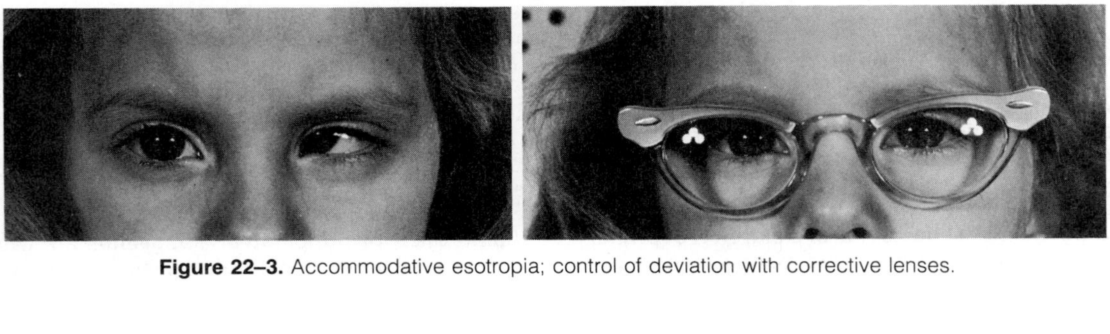

Figure 22–3. Accommodative esotropia; control of deviation with corrective lenses.

into the opposing (unaffected) muscle, producing chemodenervation and allowing the weakened muscle to realign.

The ultimate goal of treatment is to develop fusion (binocular function) and depth perception. In some cases the ophthalmologist and the patient must be satisfied with less than an ideal functional result.

DUANE SYNDROME

This congenital disorder of ocular motility is characterized by retraction of the globe on adduction. This is attributed to anomalous innervation, which results in cocontraction of the medial and lateral rectus muscles on attempted adduction of the affected eye. Within the spectrum of Duane syndrome patients may exhibit impairment of abduction, impairment of adduction, or upshoot or downshoot of the involved eye on adduction. They may have esotropia, exotropia, or relatively straight eyes. Many exhibit compensatory posturing for the defect in horizontal eye movement. Some develop amblyopia. Surgery to improve ocular motility and alignment can be helpful in selected cases.

Duane syndrome usually occurs sporadically. Sometimes it is inherited as an autosomal dominant condition. It usually occurs as an isolated condition but may occur in association with various other ocular and systemic anomalies.

MÖBIUS SYNDROME

The distinctive features of Möbius syndrome are congenital facial paresis and abduction weakness. The facial palsy is commonly bilateral, frequently asymmetric, and often incomplete, tending to spare the lower face and platysma. Ectropion, epiphora, and exposure keratopathy may develop. The abduction defect may be unilateral or bilateral. It is usually complete, and esotropia is common. The etiology is unknown. Whether the primary defect is maldevelopment of cranial nerve nuclei, hypoplasia of the muscles, or a combination of central and peripheral factors is unclear. Gestational factors such as trauma, illness, and intake of various drugs, particularly thalidomide, have been implicated. Some familial cases have been reported. Associated developmental defects may include ptosis, palatal and lingual palsy, hearing loss, pectoral and lingual muscle defects, micrognathia, syndactyly, supernumerary digits, or the absence of hands, feet, fingers, or toes. Surgical correction of the esotropia is indicated in selected cases, and any attendant amblyopia should be treated.

GRADENIGO SYNDROME

This is an acquired abducens palsy with pain in the distribution of the homolateral trigeminal nerve, indicating involvement of the petrous portion of the 6th cranial nerve and the adjacent gasserian ganglion. The usual causes are otitis media or mastoiditis with inflammation extending into the petrous bone, its meninges, and the inferior petrosal sinus. Tumor is rarely the cause. Principal signs and symptoms are weakness of the lateral rectus, diplopia, ocular and facial pain, photophobia, lacrimation, and sometimes corneal hypesthesia. There may also be involvement of the 7th nerve, with facial palsy.

BENIGN 6TH NERVE PALSY

This is a painless acquired abducens palsy that resolves spontaneously, usually without residua. The palsy typically develops 1–3 wk after a nonspecific febrile illness or upper respiratory infection; in some cases the palsy precedes other symptoms of infection or occurs during the prodrome of an exanthem. Improvement usually begins within 3–6 wk after onset, and recovery is usually complete within 10–12 wk. Episodes may be recurrent. The paresis is thought to be a neurotropic effect of a viral infection. Except for benign 6th nerve palsy, the development of a cranial nerve palsy in a child is usually a sign of a serious pathologic process, such as intracranial tumor, increased intracranial pressure, meningitis, or demyelinating disease.

BROWN SYNDROME

In this syndrome elevation of the eye in the adducted position is restricted or absent. Often, there is an associated downward deviation of the affected eye in adduction. There may be a compensatory tilt of the head. Various causes have been described. Some cases have been attributed to structural abnormalities such as a tight superior oblique tendon, congenital shortening or thickening of the superior oblique tendon sheath, or connective tissue trabeculae between the superior oblique tendon and the trochlea. Sometimes no anatomic abnormality is found.

Acquired Brown syndrome may follow trauma to the orbit involving the region of the trochlea or sinus surgery. It may also occur with inflammatory processes, particularly sinusitis and juvenile rheumatoid arthritis.

Acquired inflammatory Brown syndrome may respond to treatment with steroids. Surgery may be helpful for children with true congenital Brown syndrome.

PARINAUD SYNDROME

This eponym designates a palsy of vertical gaze, isolated or associated with pupillary or nuclear oculomotor (cranial nerve III) paresis. It indicates a lesion affecting the mesencephalic tegmentum. The ophthalmic signs of midbrain disease include vertical gaze palsy, dissociation of the pupillary responses to light and to near focus, general pupillomotor paralysis, corectopia, dyscoria, accommodative disturbances, pathologic lid retraction, ptosis, extraocular muscle paresis, and convergence paralysis. In some cases there are spasms of convergence, convergent retraction nystagmus, and vertical nystagmus, particularly on attempted vertical gaze. Combinations of these signs are referred to as the Koerber-Salus-Elschnig or sylvian aqueduct syndrome.

A principal cause of vertical gaze palsy and associated mesencephalic signs in children is tumor of the pineal gland or 3rd ventricle. Differential diagnosis includes trauma and demyelinating disease. In children with hydrocephalus, impairment of vertical gaze and pathologic lid retraction are referred to as the *setting sun sign*. A transient supranuclear disorder of gaze is sometimes seen in healthy neonates.

CONGENITAL OCULAR MOTOR APRAXIA

This congenital disorder of conjugate gaze is characterized by a defect in voluntary horizontal gaze, compensatory jerking movement of the head, and retention of slow pursuit and reflexive eye movements. Additional features are absence of the fast (refixation) phase of optokinetic nystagmus and obligate contraversive deviation of the eyes on rotation of the body. Typically, the affected child is unable to look quickly to either side voluntarily in response to command or in response to an eccentrically presented object but may, however, be able to follow a slowly moving target to either side. To compensate for the defect in purposive lateral eye movements, the child jerks the head to bring the eyes into the desired position and may also blink repetitively in an attempt to change fixation. The signs tend to become less conspicuous with age.

The pathogenesis of congenital ocular motor apraxia is unknown. It may be a result of delayed myelination of the ocular motor pathways. Structural abnormalities of the CNS have been found in a few patients, including agenesis of the corpus callosum and cerebellar vermis, porencephaly, hamartoma of the foramen of Monro, and macrocephaly. Many children with congenital ocular motor apraxia show delayed motor and cognitive development.

A disorder of eye movement resembling congenital ocular motor apraxia may occur in patients with certain metabolic neurodegenerative diseases (particularly Gaucher disease) or with ataxia-telangiectasia, or as a sign of brain tumor.

NYSTAGMUS

Nystagmus (rhythmic oscillations of one or both eyes) may be caused by an abnormality in any one of the three basic mechanisms that regulate position and movement of the eyes: the fixation, conjugate gaze, or vestibular mechanisms. In addition, physiologic nystagmus may be elicited by appropriate stimuli.

Congenital pendular nystagmus is commonly associated with ocular and visual defects; it typically occurs with albinism, aniridia, achromatopsia, congenital cataracts, congenital macular lesions, congenital optic atrophy, and high refractive errors. In some instances pendular nystagmus occurs as a dominant or X-linked characteristic without obvious ocular abnormalities. There may be associated rhythmic movements of the head.

Congenital jerky nystagmus is characterized by horizontal jerky oscillations with gaze preponderance; the nystagmus is coarser in one direction of gaze than in the other, with the jerk toward the direction of gaze. There is usually a point of reversal or a null point in which the nystagmus lessens and in which position vision is best; compensatory posturing, turning of the head to bring the eyes into the position of least nystagmus, is characteristic. The cause of congenital jerky nystagmus is unknown; in some instances it is familial.

Acquired nystagmus requires prompt and thorough evaluation. Worrisome pathologic types are the gaze-paretic or gaze-evoked oscillations of cerebellar, brain stem, or cerebral disease.

Nystagmus retractorius or *convergent nystagmus* is repetitive jerking of the eyes into the orbit or toward each other. It is usually seen with vertical gaze palsy as a feature of the Parinaud or Koerber-Salus-Elschnig (sylvian aqueduct) syndrome. The causal condition may be neoplastic, vascular, or inflammatory. In children nystagmus retractorius suggests particularly the presence of pinealoma or hydrocephalus.

Spasmus nutans is a special type of acquired nystagmus in childhood (see also Sec. 20.30). In its complete form it is characterized by the triad of pendular nystagmus, head nodding, and torticollis. The nystagmus is characteristically very fine, very rapid, horizontal, and pendular; it is often asymmetric, sometimes unilateral. Signs usually develop within the 1st year or two of life. Components of the triad may develop at varying times. In many cases the condition is benign and self-limited, usually lasting a few months, sometimes years. The cause of this classic type of spasmus nutans, which resolves spontaneously, is unknown. Many children exhibiting signs resembling those of spasmus nutans have underlying brain tumors, particularly hypothalamic and chiasmal optic gliomas. Appropriate neurologic and neuroradiologic evaluation and careful monitoring of infants and children with nystagmus is therefore recommended.

OTHER ABNORMAL EYE MOVEMENTS

To be differentiated from true nystagmus are certain special types of abnormal eye movements, particularly opsoclonus, ocular dysmetria, and flutter.

Opsoclonus

Opsoclonus and ataxic conjugate movements are terms that describe spontaneous, nonrhythmic, multidirectional, chaotic movements of the eyes. The eyes appear to be in agitation, with bursts of conjugate movement of varying amplitude in varying directions. Opsoclonus is most often associated with encephalitis. It may be the first sign of neuroblastoma.

Ocular Motor Dysmetria

This is analogous to dysmetria of the limbs. There is lack of precision in performing movements of refixation, characterized by an overshoot (or undershoot) of the eyes with several corrective to-and-fro oscillations on looking from one point to another. Ocular motor dysmetria is a sign of cerebellar or cerebellar pathway disease.

Flutter-Like Oscillations

These intermittent to-and-fro horizontal oscillations of the eyes may occur spontaneously or on change of fixation. They are characteristic of cerebellar disease.

Anthony JH, Ouvrier RA, Wise G: Spasmus nutans: A mistaken identity. Arch Neurol 37:373, 1980.

Baker JD, Parks MM: Early-onset accommodative esotropia. Am J Ophthalmol 90:11, 1980.

Bixenman WW, von Noorden GK: Benign recurrent VI nerve palsy in childhood. J Pediatr Ophthalmol Strab 18:29, 1981.

Chan CC, Sogg RL, Steinman L: Isolated oculomotor palsy after measles immunization. Am J Ophthalmol 89:446, 1980.

Cogan DG: Heredity of congenital ocular motor apraxia. Trans Am Acad Ophthalmol Otolaryngol 76:60, 1972.

Harley RD: Paralytic strabismus in children: Etiologic incidence and management of the third, fourth and sixth nerve palsies. Ophthalmology 87:24, 1980.

Harley RD, Rodrigues MM, Crawford JS: Congenital fibrosis of the extraocular muscles. J Pediatr Ophthalmol Strab 15:346, 1978.

Hiatt RL: Medical management of accommodative esotropia. J Pediatr Ophthalmol Strab 20:199, 1983.

Hoyt CS, Mousel DK, Weber AA: Transient supranuclear disturbance of gaze in healthy neonates. Am J Ophthalmol 89:708, 1980.

Ing M: Early surgical alignment for congenital esotropia. Ophthalmology 90:132, 1983.

Kalpakian B, Choy AE, Sparkes RS: Duane syndrome associated with features of the cat-eye syndrome and mosaicism for a supernumerary chromosome probably derived from number 22. J Pediatr Ophthalmol Strab 25:293, 1988.

Katz NNK, Whitmore PV, Beauchamp GR: Brown's syndrome in twins. J Pediatr Ophthalmol Strab 18:32, 1981.

Kornder LD, Nursey JN, Pratt-Johnson JA, et al: Detection of manifest strabismus in young children: 1. A prospective study. Am J Ophthalmol 77:209, 1974.

Kornder LD, Nursey JN, Pratt-Johnson JA, et al: Detection of manifest strabismus in young children. 2. A retrospective study. Am J Ophthalmol 77:211, 1974.

Kushner BJ: Ocular causes of abnormal head postures. Ophthalmology 86:2115, 1979.

Lavery MA, O'Neill JF, Chau FC, et al: Acquired nystagmus in early childhood: A presenting sign of intracranial tumor. Ophthalmology 91:425, 1984.

Magoon EH: Botulinum toxin chemo-denervation for strabismus in infants and children. J Pediatr Ophthalmol Strab 21:110, 1984.

Miller MT, Ray V, Owens P, et al: Möbius and Möbius-like syndromes (TTV-OFM, OMLH). J Pediatr Ophthalmol Strab 26:176, 1989.

Miller NR: Solitary oculomotor nerve palsy in children. Am J Ophthalmol 83:106, 1977.

Mohindra I, Zwann J, Held R, et al: Development of acuity and stereopsis in infants with esotropia. Ophthalmology 92:691, 1985.

Morre RT, Morin JD: Bilateral acquired inflammatory Brown's syndrome. J Pediatr Ophthalmol Strab 22:26, 1985.

Norton EWD, Cogan DG: Spasmus nutans: A clinical study of twenty cases followed two years or more since onset. Arch Ophthalmol 52:442, 1954.

O'Malley ER, Helveston EM, Ellis FD: Duane's retraction syndrome—plus. J Pediatr Ophthalmol Strab 19:161, 1982.

Parks MM, Eisenbaum AM: Duane's syndrome: What to do and what to expect. Am Orthoptic J 37:28, 1987.

Rappaport L, Urlon D, Strand K, et al: Concurrence of congenital oculomotor apraxia and other motor problems: An expanded syndrome. Dev Med Child Neurol 29:85, 1987.

Richard JM, Parks M: Intermittent exotropia: Surgical results in different age groups. Ophthalmology 90:1172, 1983.

Saunders RA, Stratas BA, Gordon RA, et al: Acute-onset Brown's syndrome associated with pansinusitis. Arch Ophthalmol 108:58, 1980.
Scott WE, Kraft SP: Surgical treatment of compensatory head position in congenital nystagmus. J Pediatr Ophthalmol Strab 21:85, 1984.
Shetty T, Rosman NP: Opsoclonus in hydrocephalus. Arch Ophthalmol 88:585, 1972.
Smith JL, Walsh FB: Opsoclonus—ataxic conjugate movements of the eye. Arch Ophthalmol 64:244, 1960.
Smith JL, Ziepes I, Gay AJ, et al: Nystagmus retractorius. Arch Ophthalmol 62:864, 1959.
Summers CG, MacDonald JT, Wirtschafter JD: Oculomotor apraxia associated with intracranial lipoma. J Pediatr Ophthalmol Strab 24:267, 1987.
Utrata J: Gradenigo's syndrome—bilateral occurrence. The Eye, Ear, Nose and Throat Monthly 52:54, 1973.
Wang FM, Wertenbaker C, Behrens MM, et al: Acquired Brown's syndrome in children with juvenile rheumatoid arthritis. Ophthalmology 91:23, 1984.
Zaret CR, Behrens MM, Eggers HM: Congenital ocular motor apraxia and brain stem tumor. Arch Ophthalmol 98:328, 1980.

22.7 ABNORMALITIES OF THE LIDS

PTOSIS

Blepharoptosis exists when the upper eyelid droops below its normal level. Congenital ptosis is usually a result of faulty development of the levator muscle or its innervating branch of the 3rd nerve. There may be associated involvement of the superior rectus muscle and attendant impairment in elevation of the eye. The condition may be familial, transmitted as a dominant trait. Congenital ptosis can be corrected surgically; the age at which surgery is done depends on its degree, its cosmetic and functional severity, the presence or absence of compensatory posturing, the wishes of the parents, and the discretion of the surgeon. Ptosis of sufficient degree to interfere with visual development requires early correction to prevent amblyopia. Correction of mild ptosis for purely cosmetic reasons is often deferred until age 3–4 yr. Children with ptosis may have associated anisometropia and/or strabismus, which may lead to amblyopia. Early evaluation and treatment of these problems are indicated in all children with ptosis.

Congenital ptosis occurs with a large number of syndromes. In the Marcus Gunn jaw winking syndrome of aberrant innervation, there is abnormal synkinesis of lid and jaw movements; paradoxic elevation of the ptotic lid occurs as the child sucks, chews, or cries. In the congenital fibrosis syndrome, a hereditary condition, ptosis is associated with paralysis or "fibrosis" of other extraocular muscles. Minimal ptosis occurs in the Horner syndrome (oculosympathetic palsy). In the Sturge-Weber syndrome, ptosis is often secondary to hemangiomatous involvement of the upper lid, and in von Recklinghausen syndrome there may be ptosis resulting from plexiform neuroma of the upper lid.

Differential diagnosis of acquired ptosis in childhood includes myasthenia gravis, botulism, progressive external ophthalmoplegia, progressive intracranial lesions affecting the 3rd nerve, and inflammation or tumors affecting the levator, the orbit, or lid. Ptosis may also result from trauma. Aberrant regeneration of injured 3rd nerve fibers may produce paradoxic lid and eye movements.

EPICANTHAL FOLDS

These vertical or oblique folds of skin extend on either side of the bridge of the nose from the brow or lid area, covering the inner canthal region. They are present to some degree in most young children and become less apparent with age. The folds may be sufficiently broad to cover the medial aspect of the eye, making the eyes appear crossed (pseudoesotropia).

Epicanthal folds are a common feature of many syndromes, including chromosomal aberrations (particularly the trisomies) or disorders of single genes.

LAGOPHTHALMOS

This exists when complete closure of the lids over the globe is difficult or impossible. It may be paralytic, because of a facial palsy involving the orbicularis muscle, or spastic, as in thyrotoxicosis. It may be structural when retraction or shortening of the lids results from scarring or atrophy consequent to injury (e.g., burns) or disease. Infants with collodion membrane may have temporary lagophthalmos caused by the restrictive effect of the membrane on the lids. Lagophthalmos may accompany proptosis or buphthalmos when the lids, although normal, cannot effectively cover the enlarged or protuberant eye. A degree of physiologic lagophthalmos may occur normally during sleep, but functional lagophthalmos in the unconscious or debilitated patient can be a problem.

When lagophthalmos exists, exposure of the eye may lead to drying, infection, corneal ulceration, or perforation of the cornea; the result may be loss of vision, even loss of the eye. In lagophthalmos protection of the eye by artificial tear preparations, ophthalmic ointment, or moisture chambers is essential. Gauze pads are to be avoided, because the gauze may abrade the cornea. In some cases surgical closure of the lids (tarsorrhaphy) may be necessary for long-term protection of the eye.

LID RETRACTION

Pathologic retraction of the lid may be myogenic or neurogenic. Myogenic retraction of the upper lid occurs in thyrotoxicosis, in which it is associated with three classic signs: a staring appearance (Dalrymple sign), infrequent blinking (Stellwag sign), and lag of the upper lid on downward gaze (von Graefe sign).

Neurogenic retraction of the lids may occur in conditions affecting the anterior mesencephalon. Lid retraction is a feature of the syndrome of the sylvian aqueduct. In children it is commonly a sign of hydrocephalus. It may occur with meningitis.

Paradoxic retraction of the lid is a feature of the Marcus Gunn jaw winking syndrome. Paradoxic lid retraction may also occur during recovery from a 3rd nerve palsy as a result of aberrant regeneration or misdirection of oculomotor fibers.

To be differentiated from pathologic lid retractions are simple staring and the physiologic or reflexive lid retraction ("eye popping") that occurs in infants in response to a sudden reduction in illumination or as a startle reaction.

ENTROPION AND ECTROPION

Entropion is inversion of the lid margin, which may cause discomfort and corneal damage because of the inward turning of the lashes (trichiasis). A principal cause is scarring secondary to inflammation such as occurs in trachoma or as a sequela of Stevens-Johnson syndrome. There is also a rare congenital form. Surgical correction is effective in many cases.

Ectropion is eversion of the lid margin; it may lead to overflow of tears (epiphora) and subsequent maceration of the skin of the lid, to inflammation of exposed conjunctiva, or to superficial exposure keratopathy. Common causes are scarring consequent to inflammation, burns, or trauma, or weakness of the orbicularis muscle as a result of facial palsy; these forms may be corrected surgically. Protection of the cornea is essential. Eversion of the lids may occur during delivery; this can resolve with conservative management.

Ectropion is also seen in certain children who have faulty development of the lateral canthal ligament; this may occur in Down syndrome.

BLEPHAROSPASM

This spastic or repetitive closure of the lids may be caused by irritative disease of the cornea, conjunctiva, or facial nerve, fatigue or uncorrected refractive error, or common tic. Thorough ophthalmic examination for pathologic causes such as trichiasis, keratitis, conjunctivitis, or foreign body is indicated. Local injection of botulinum toxin may give relief.

BLEPHARITIS

This inflammation of the lid margins is characterized by erythema and crusting or scaling; the usual symptoms are irritation, burning, and itching. The condition is commonly bilateral and chronic or recurrent. There are two main types, staphylococcal and seborrheic. In *staphylococcal blepharitis* ulceration of the lid margin is common, the lashes tend to fall out, and there is often associated conjunctivitis and superficial keratitis. In *seborrheic blepharitis* the scales tend to be greasy, the lid margins are less red, and ulceration usually does not occur. The blepharitis is often of mixed type.

Thorough daily cleansing of the lid margins with a cloth or moistened cotton applicator to remove scales and crusts is important in the treatment of both forms of blepharitis. Staphylococcal blepharitis is treated with antistaphylococcal antibiotic or sulfonamide ophthalmic ointment applied directly to the lid margins daily at bedtime. When seborrhea exists, concurrent treatment of the scalp is important.

Pediculosis of the eyelashes may produce the clinical picture of blepharitis. The lice can be smothered with opthalmic-grade petrolatum ointment applied to the lid margin and lashes. Nits should be mechanically removed from the lashes.

HORDEOLUM

Infection of the glands of the lid may be acute or subacute; there is tender focal swelling and redness. The usual agent is *Staphylococcus aureus*.

When the meibomian glands are involved the lesion is referred to as an *internal hordeolum*; the abscess tends to be large and may point through either the skin or conjunctival surface. When the infection involves the glands of Zeis or Moll the abscess tends to be smaller and more superficial and points at the lid margin; it is then referred to as an *external hordeolum* or *stye*.

As with abscesses elsewhere, treatment is frequent, warm compresses and, if necessary, surgical incision and drainage. In addition, topical antibiotic or sulfonamide preparations are often used. Untreated, the infection may progress to cellulitis of the lid or orbit, requiring the use of systemic antibiotics. Recurrence is common, possibly by reinfection through contaminated hands. Itching resulting from an underlying allergy is a common contributory factor. Recurrent styes in children may also signal an immunologic defect.

CHALAZION

Chalazion is granulomatous inflammation of a meibomian gland characterized by a firm, nontender nodule in the upper or lower lid. This lesion tends to be chronic and differs from internal hordeolum in the absence of acute inflammatory signs. When a chalazion is large enough to distort vision (it may cause astigmatism by exerting pressure on the globe) or to be a cosmetic blemish, excision is advised. In some cases chalazion subsides spontaneously.

COLOBOMA OF THE EYELID

This cleft-like deformity may vary from a small indentation or notch of the free margin of the lid to a large defect involving almost the entire lid. If the gap is extensive, xerosis, ulceration, and corneal opacities may result from exposure. Early surgical correction of the lid defect is recommended. Other deformities frequently associated with lid colobomata include dermoid cysts or dermolipomata on the globe; often, they occur in a position corresponding to the site of the lid defect. Lid colobomata may also be associated with extensive facial malformation, as in mandibulofacial dysostosis (Franceschetti or Treacher Collins syndrome).

TUMORS OF THE LID

A number of lid tumors arise from surface structures (the epithelium and sebaceous glands). Nevi may appear in early childhood; most are junctional. Compound nevi tend to develop in the prepubertal years, dermal nevi at puberty. Malignant epithelial tumors (basal cell carcinoma and squamous cell carcinoma) are rare in children, but the basal cell nevus syndrome and the malignant lesions of xeroderma pigmentosum and of the Rothmund-Thomson syndrome may develop in childhood. Adenoma sebaceum (vascular fibroma) may also occur in the lid, sometimes forming extensive masses. The small yellowish papules of juvenile xanthogranuloma may occur on the lids, with or without cutaneous lesions elsewhere; these usually appear in infancy and regress spontaneously by the age of 1–2 yr.

Other lid tumors arise from deeper structures (the neural, vascular, and connective tissues). Hemangiomas are especially common. Most tend to regress spontaneously, although they may show alarmingly rapid growth in infancy. In many cases the best management of such hemangiomas is patient observation, allowing spontaneous regression to occur (Sec. 23.8). In the case of a rapidly expanding lesion that threatens to obstruct vision and produce sensory deprivation amblyopia, corticosteroid treatment should be considered.

Nevus flammeus (port wine stain), a noninvoluting hemangioma, occurs as an isolated lesion or in association with other signs of Sturge-Weber syndrome. Affected patients should be examined for glaucoma.

Lymphangiomas of the lid appear as firm masses at or soon after birth and tend to enlarge slowly during the growing years. Associated conjunctival involvement, appearing as a clear, cystic, sinuous conjunctival mass, may provide a clue to the diagnosis. In some cases there is also orbital involvement. The treatment is surgical excision.

Plexiform neuromas of the lids occur in children with neurofibromatosis, often with ptosis as the first sign.

The lids may also be involved by other tumors, such as retinoblastoma, neuroblastoma, and rhabdomyosarcoma of the orbit; these conditions are discussed elsewhere.

Crawford JS: Congenital eyelid anomalies in children. J Pediatr Ophthalmol Strab 21:140, 1984.
Crawford JS, Iliff CE, Stasier OG: Symposium on congenital ptosis. J Pediatr Ophthalmol Strab 19:245, 1982.
Johnson CC: Epicanthus and epiblepharon. Arch Ophthalmol 96:1030, 1978.
Kushner BJ: Intralesional corticosteroid injection for infantile adnexal hemangioma. Am J Ophthalmol 93:496, 1982.
Masaki S: Congenital bilateral facial paralysis. Arch Otolaryngol 94:260, 1971.
McCully JP, Dougherty JM, Deneau DG: Classification of chronic blepharitis. Ophthalmology 89:1173, 1982.
Merriam WW, Ellis FD, Helveston EM: Congenital blepharoptosis, anisometropia, and amblyopia. Am J Ophthalmol 89:401, 1980.
Moainie R, Kopelowitz N, Rosenfeld W, et al: Congenital eversion of the eyelids: A report of two cases treated with conservative management. J Pediatr Ophthalmol Strab 19:326, 1982.
Picó G: Congenital ectropion and distichiasis. Etiologic and hereditary factors. A report of cases and review of the literature. Am J Ophthalmol 47:363, 1959.
Pratt SG, Beyer CK, Johnson CC: The Marcus Gunn phenomenon: A review of 71 cases. Ophthalmology 91:27, 1984.
Stigmar G, Crawford JS, Ward CM, et al: Ophthalmic sequelae of infantile hemangiomas of the eyelid and orbit. Am J Ophthalmol 85:806, 1978.

Zak TA: Congenital primary upper eyelid entropion. J Pediatr Ophthalmol Strab 21:69, 1984.

22.8 DISORDERS OF THE LACRIMAL SYSTEM

DACRYOSTENOSIS AND DACRYOCYSTITIS

Normally, tears produced by the lacrimal gland and the secretions produced by the accessory glands of the lid and conjunctiva drain medially into the punctal openings of the lid margins and flow through the canaliculi into the lacrimal sac, and then through the nasolacrimal duct into the nose. When partial or complete obstruction to the drainage system occurs, the condition is commonly referred to as dacryostenosis; in many cases more specific terms are applicable.

In infants and children the problem is usually congenital, resulting from maldevelopment or incomplete canalization of some portion of the drainage system. In most cases there is a congenital narrowing, a membranous or valve-like obstruction of the nasolacrimal duct, more often involving the distal or nasal segment than the proximal portion. In some cases there is involvement of the puncta, the canaliculi, the opening into the sac, or the sac itself. Rarely, there may be a more complex anomaly or atresia of some portion of the system.

Signs may appear days or weeks after birth, and are often aggravated by upper respiratory infection or by exposure to cold or wind. The usual manifestations of nasolacrimal obstruction are "tearing," ranging in degree from a "wetness" of the eye (an increase in the tear lake, "pooling," or "puddling") to frank overflow of tears (epiphora), accumulation of mucoid or mucopurulent discharge (often described by the parents as "matter"), and crusting. There may be erythema or maceration of the skin because of irritation and rubbing produced by dripping of tears and discharge. In many cases reflux of clear fluid or mucopurulent discharge can be elicited by massaging the nasolacrimal sac, proving obstruction to outflow.

Infants with obstruction may have acute infection and inflammation of the nasolacrimal sac (dacryocystitis), inflammation of the surrounding tissues (pericystitis), or even periobital cellulitis. With dacryocystitis the sac area is swollen, red, and tender, and there may be systemic signs of infection such as fever and irritability.

Rarely, nasolacrymal obstruction leads to distention of the nasolacrimal sac, producing a tense, bluish mass (nasolacrimal mucocele, amniotocele or amniocele) that sometimes transilluminates.

The primary treatment of uncomplicated nasolacrimal obstruction is a regimen of nasolacrimal massage, usually two to three times a day, often accompanied by cleansing of the lids with warm water and instillation of an antibacterial drop. In most cases, the problem resolves with conservative management by the age of 1 yr, if not earlier. In persistent or severe cases, dilatation, probing, and irrigation of the nasolacrimal system may be indicated. In more complicated cases, placement of tubes or more extensive reconstructive surgery (such as dacryocystorhinostomy) may be required to provide adequate drainage.

Acute dacryocystitis or cellulitis requires prompt treatment with antibiotics. In such cases some form of definitive surgical intervention is usually indicated.

Although nasolacrimal obstruction in children is most often congenital, lacrimal problems may develop later in life as the result of acquired infection, inflammation, or trauma.

It should be noted that not all tearing in infants and children is caused by nasolacrimal obstruction. Tearing may also be a sign of glaucoma, intraocular inflammation, or external irritation, such as that from a corneal abrasion or foreign body.

DACRYOADENITIS

Dacryoadenitis, or inflammation of the lacrimal gland, is uncommon in childhood. It may occur with mumps (in which case it is usually acute and bilateral, subsiding in a few days or weeks), or with infectious mononucleosis. Chronic dacryoadenitis is associated with certain systemic diseases, particularly sarcoidosis, tuberculosis, and syphilis. Some systemic diseases may produce enlargement of the lacrimal and salivary glands (Mikulicz syndrome).

ALACRIMA AND "DRY EYE"

Marked deficiency of tears may occur as an isolated unilateral or bilateral congenital defect or in association with other nervous system anomalies, such as aplasia of cranial nerve nuclei. It occurs congenitally in familial dysautonomia (Riley-Day syndrome) and in the anhidrotic type of ectodermal dysplasia; it may occur with glucocorticoid deficiency, sometimes in association with swallowing dysfunction. Tear deficiency may be a sign of Sjögren syndrome, in which it is sometimes associated with salivary gland enlargement and with arthritis. Deficiency of tears may also follow inflammation; it is not uncommon after Stevens-Johnson syndrome. Drying of the eye, corneal ulceration, and scarring may result. Preventive care includes the frequent instillation of an artificial tear preparation. In some cases occlusion of the lacrimal puncta is helpful. In severe cases tarsorrhaphy may be necessary to protect the cornea.

Caccamise WC, Townes PL: Congenital absence of the lacrymal puncta associated with alacrima and aptyalism. Am J Ophthalmol 89:62, 1980.
Geffner ME, Lippe BM, Kaplan SA, et al: Selective ACTH insensitivity, achalasia, and alacrima: A multisystem disorder presenting in childhood. Pediatr Res 17:532, 1983.
Goldberg MF, Payne JW, Brunt PW: Ophthalmologic studies of familial dysautonomia. Arch Ophthalmol 80:732, 1966.
Kushner BJ: Congenital nasolacrymal system obstruction. Arch Ophthalmol 100:597, 1982.
Mondino BJ, Brown SI: Hereditary congenital alacrima. Arch Ophthalmol 94:1478, 1976.
Paul TO: Medical management of congenital nasolacrymal duct obstruction. J Pediatr Ophthalmol Strab 22:68, 1985.
Pinsky L, DiGeorge AM: Congenital familial sensory neuropathy with anhidrosis. J Pediatr 68:1, 1966.
Sevel D: Developmental and congenital abnormalities of the nasolacrymal apparatus. J Pediatr Ophthalmol Strab 18:13, 1981.
Weinstein GS, Biglan AW, Patterson JH: Congenital lacrimal sac mucoceles. Am J Ophthalmol 94:106, 1982.
Welham RAN, Hughes SM: Lacrimal surgery in children. Am J Ophthalmol 99:27, 1985.

22.9 DISORDERS OF THE CONJUNCTIVA

CONJUNCTIVITIS

The conjunctiva reacts to a wide range of bacterial and viral agents, allergens, irritants, toxins, and systemic diseases. Conjunctivitis is common in childhood and may be infectious or noninfectious.

Acute Purulent Conjunctivitis

This is characterized by more or less generalized conjunctival hyperemia, edema, mucopurulent exudate, and various degrees of ocular discomfort. It is usually a result of bacterial infection. The most frequent causes are staphylococci, pneumococci, *Haemophilus influenzae*, and streptococci. Conjunctival smear and culture are helpful in differentiating specific types. These common forms of acute purulent conjunctivitis usually respond well to warm compresses and frequent topical instillation of antibiotic drops. Brazilian purpuric fever due to *Haemophilis aegyptius* manifests conjunctivitis and sepsis. Unfortunately, however, *Neisseria gonorrhoeae* and *Chlamydia* are emerging as common causes of acute purulent conjunctivitis in children beyond the newborn period, especially in adolescents. These infections require specific testing and treatment (Sec. 12.24 and 12.59).

Ophthalmia neonatorum is acute conjunctivitis in the newborn infant. Any of the common bacterial conjunctivitides can occur in the newborn period, but emphasis in differential diagnosis must be given to recognition of gonococcal and chlamydial infections (see Sec. 9.61). To be differentiated from the infectious types of ophthalmia neonatorum is the chemical conjunctivitis caused by the prophylactic use of silver nitrate. This usually develops 12–24 hr after instillation and lasts only 24–48 hr; no treatment is needed.

Viral Conjunctivitis

This is generally characterized by a watery discharge. Often, there are follicular changes (small aggregates of lymphocytes) in the palpebral conjunctiva. Conjunctivitis resulting from adenovirus infection is relatively common, sometimes with corneal involvement (see later). Outbreaks of conjunctivitis caused by enterovirus are also seen; this type may be hemorrhagic.

Conjunctivitides are commonly associated with such systemic viral infections as the childhood exanthems, particularly measles. These are self-limited.

Epidemic Keratoconjunctivitis

This is caused by adenovirus type 8 and is transmitted by direct contact. Initially there is a sensation of a foreign body beneath the lids with itching and burning. Edema and photophobia develop rapidly, and large oval follicles appear within the conjunctiva. Preauricular adenopathy and a pseudomembrane on the conjunctival surface occur frequently. Subepithelial corneal infiltrates may develop and may cause blurring of vision; these usually disappear but may reduce visual acuity permanently. Corneal complications are less common in children than in adults. Children may have associated upper respiratory infection. No specific therapy is available. Emphasis must be placed on prevention of spread of the disease.

Membranous and Pseudomembranous Conjunctivitis

These types can be seen in a number of diseases. The classic membranous conjunctivitis is that of diphtheria, accompanied by a fibrin-rich exudate that forms on the conjunctival surface and permeates the epithelium; the membrane is removed with difficulty and leaves raw bleeding areas. In pseudomembranous conjunctivitis the layer of fibrin-rich exudate is superficial and can often be stripped easily, leaving the surface smooth. This type occurs with many bacterial and viral infections, including staphylococcal, pneumococcal, streptococcal, or chlamydial conjunctivitis, and in epidemic keratoconjunctivitis. It is seen also in vernal conjunctivitis and in Stevens-Johnson disease.

Allergic Conjunctivitis

This is usually accompanied by intense itching, tearing, and conjunctival edema. It is commonly seasonal. Cold compresses and decongestant drops give symptomatic relief. Topical cromalyn sodium also may help. In selected cases, topical corticosteroids are used under ophthalmic supervision.

Vernal Conjunctivitis

This usually begins in the prepubertal years and may recur for many years. Atopy appears to play a role in its origin, but the pathogenesis is uncertain. Extreme itching and tearing are the usual complaints. Large, flattened, cobblestone-like papillary lesions of the palpebral conjunctivae are characteristic. A stringy exudate and a milky conjunctival pseudomembrane are frequently present. There may be small elevated lesions of the bulbar conjunctiva adjacent to the limbus (limbal form). Smear of the conjunctival exudate reveals many eosinophils. Topical corticosteroid therapy and cold compresses afford some relief. Cromolyn sodium drops may help.

Chemical Conjunctivitis

This can result when an irritating substance enters the conjunctival sac (as in the acute but benign conjunctivitis caused by silver nitrate in the newborn). Other common offenders are household cleaning substances, sprays, smoke, smog, and industrial pollutants.

Alkalis tend to linger in the conjunctival tissues and continue to inflict damage over a period of hours or days. Acids precipitate the proteins in tissues and so produce their effect immediately. In either case prompt, thorough, and copious irrigation is crucial. Extensive tissue damage, even loss of the eye, can result, especially if the offending agent is an alkali.

OTHER CONJUNCTIVAL DISORDERS

Subconjunctival hemorrhage is manifested by bright or dark red patches in the bulbar conjunctiva and may result from injury or inflammation. It may occasionally result from severe sneezing or coughing or be a manifestation of a blood dyscrasia.

Pingueculum is a yellowish-white, slightly elevated mass on the bulbar conjunctiva, usually in the interpalpebral region. It represents elastic and hyaline degenerative changes of the conjunctiva. No treatment is required except for cosmetic reasons, in which case simple excision suffices.

Pterygium is a fleshy triangular conjunctival lesion that may encroach on the cornea. It typically occurs in the nasal interpalpebral region. The pathologic findings are similar to those of a pingueculum. Irritation such as exposure to dust or wind is thought to aggravate the lesion. Removal is suggested when the lesion encroaches far onto the cornea.

Dermoid cyst and *dermolipoma* are benign lesions, clinically similar in appearance. They are smooth, elevated, round to oval lesions of various sizes. The color varies from yellowish-white to a fleshy pink. The most frequent site is the upper outer quadrant of the globe; they also commonly occur near or straddle the limbus. The dermolipoma is composed of adipose and connective tissue. Dermoid cysts may also contain glandular tissue, hair follicles, and hair shafts. Excision for cosmetic reasons is feasible.

Conjunctival nevus is a small, slightly elevated lesion that may vary in pigmentation from pale salmon to dark brown. It is usually benign, but careful observation for progressive growth or changes suggestive of malignancy is advised.

Symblepharon is a cicatricial adhesion between the conjunctiva of the lid and the globe; the lower lid is usually affected. It follows operation or injuries, especially burns from lye, acids, or molten metals. It is a serious complication of Stevens-Johnson syndrome. It may interfere with motion of the eyeball and cause diplopia. The adhesions should be separated and the raw surfaces kept from uniting during healing. Grafts of oral mucous membrane may be necessary.

Arstikaitis MJ: Ocular aftermath of Stevens-Johnson syndrome. Arch Ophthalmol 90:376, 1973.
Brook I: Anaerobic and aerobic bacterial flora of acute conjunctivitis in children. Arch Ophthalmol 98:833, 1980.
Clark SW, Culbertson WW, Forster RK: Clinical findings and results of treatment in an outbreak of acute hemorrhagic conjunctivitis in southern Florida. Am J Ophthalmol 99:45, 1983.
Cohen KL, McCarthy LR: *Haemophilus influenzae* ophthalmia neonatorum. Arch Ophthalmol 98:1214, 1980.
Fischer MC: Conjunctivitis in children. Pediatr Clin North Am 34:1447, 1987.
Forster RK, Dawson CR, Schachter J: Late followup of patients with neonatal inclusion conjunctivitis. Am J Ophthalmol 69:467, 1970.
Gigliotti F, Williams WT, Hayden FG, et al: Etiology of acute conjunctivitis in children. J Pediatr 98:531, 1981.
Howard GM: The Stevens-Johnson syndrome. Am J Ophthalmol 55:893, 1963.
Isenberg SJ, Apt L, Yoshimora R, et al: Bacterial flora of the conjunctiva at birth. J Pediatr Ophthalmol Strab 23:284, 1986.
Knopf HLS, Hierholzer JC: Clinical and immunologic responses in patients with viral keratoconjunctivitis. Am J Ophthalmol 80:661, 1975.
Matobu A: Ocular viral infections. Pediatr Infect Dis 3:358, 1984.

22.10 ABNORMALITIES OF THE CORNEA

MEGALOCORNEA

This denotes a developmental anomaly in which the diameter of the cornea is greater than 13 mm. The condition is nonprogressive and produces no ill effects, although there is often a high refractive error. Megalocornea is often familial and may be associated with other developmental abnormalities.

Pathologic corneal enlargement caused by glaucoma is to be differentiated from this anomaly. Any progressive increase in the size of the cornea, especially when accompanied by photophobia, lacrimation, or haziness of the cornea, requires prompt opthalmologic evaluation.

MICROCORNEA

Microcornea, or anterior microphthalmia, describes an abnormally small cornea in an otherwise relatively normal eye. It may be familial, transmission being dominant more often than recessive. More commonly, a small cornea is just one feature of an otherwise developmentally abnormal or microphthalmic eye; associated defects include colobomata, microphakia, congenital cataract, and glaucoma.

KERATOCONUS

Keratoconus, or conical cornea, is characterized by ectasia and increased curvature of the central or axial portion of the cornea. It commonly appears in adolescence and with increased frequency in Down syndrome. It may occur as a late complication of congenital rubella. The etiology is obscure. There is usually considerable impairment of vision resulting from a high degree of astigmatism, although vision can often be improved with contact lenses. In some cases acute ectasia and corneal edema (hydrops) develop. In selected cases perforating keratoplasty (corneal transplant) is done.

Keratoconus is to be differentiated from keratoglobus, a globular configuration of the cornea present at or soon after birth. Both anomalies can be associated with other developmental abnormalities, including blue sclera, hearing impairment, abnormal teeth, and hyperextensible joints.

SCLEROCORNEA

Also known as scleralization of the cornea, this is a congenital malformation in which part or all of the cornea is opaque, having the appearance of sclera. This anomaly may be sporadic or familial, and may be associated with other developmental defects of the eye, with defects of other systems, or with chromosomal abnormalities. In generalized sclerocornea, early keratoplasty should be considered in an effort to provide vision.

DENDRITIC KERATITIS

Infection of the eye with the virus of herpes simplex produces a characteristic lesion of the corneal epithelium, referred to as a dendrite; it has a branching tree-like pattern that can be demonstrated by fluorescein staining. The acute episode is accompanied by pain, photophobia, tearing, blepharospasm, and conjunctival injection. Specific treatment is 5-iodo-2'-deoxyuridine (IDU) in the form of drops or ointment, or topical vidarabine or trifluridine. In addition, a cycloplegic agent is used, preferably atropine. Recurrent infection and deep stromal involvement can lead to corneal scarring.

It has been clearly demonstrated that the topical use of corticosteroids causes exacerbation of superficial herpetic disease of the eye; eyedrops combining steroids and antibiotics are, therefore, to be avoided in treatment of "red eye" unless there are clear-cut indications for their use and close supervision during therapy.

Infants born to mothers infected with herpes simplex should be examined carefully for signs of ocular involvement.

CORNEAL ULCERS

In corneal ulcers, the usual signs and symptoms are focal or diffuse corneal haze, hyperemia, lid edema, pain, photophobia, tearing, and blepharospasm. Often, there is hypopyon (pus in the anterior chamber).

Corneal ulcers require prompt treatment. They result most frequently from traumatic lesions that become secondarily infected. Many organisms are capable of infecting the cornea. One of the most troublesome is *Pseudomonas aeruginosa;* it can rapidly destroy stromal tissue and lead to corneal perforation. *N. gonorrhoeae* also is particularly damaging to the cornea. Indolent ulcers may be caused by fungi, often in association with the use of contact lenses. In each case scrapings of the cornea must be studied in an effort to identify the infectious agent and to determine the best therapy. Generally, both systemic and local treatment are needed to save the eye. Perforation or scarring resulting from corneal ulceration is an important cause of blindness throughout the world and is estimated to be responsible for 10% of blindness in the United States.

Unexplained corneal ulcers in infants and young children should raise the question of a sensory defect, as in Riley-Day or Goldenhar-Gorlin syndrome, or of a metabolic disorder such as tyrosinemia.

PHLYCTENULES

These are small, yellowish, slightly elevated lesions usually located at the corneal limbus; they may encroach on the cornea and extend centrally. Often, there is a small corneal ulcer at the head of the advancing lesion, with a fascicle of blood vessels behind the head of the lesion. Phlyctenular keratoconjunctivitis was once thought to represent hypersensitivity to tuberculin proteins, but the cause is not really known. Staphylococcal infections may be associated with phlyctenular changes. There is strong evidence for an immunologic factor. The condition usually responds to topical corticosteroid therapy, sometimes leaving superficial stromal pannus and scarring.

INTERSTITIAL KERATITIS

This denotes inflammation of the corneal stroma. The most common cause is syphilis, interstitial keratitis being one of the characteristic late manifestations of congenital syphilis. The deep inflammation produces pain, photophobia, tearing, circumcorneal injection, and corneal haze. Corneal vascularization and opacities develop and generally remain as permanent stigmata of the disease.

Cogan syndrome is a nonluetic interstitial keratitis associated with hearing loss and vestibular symptoms. Both the corneal changes and the auditory involvement may respond to corticosteroids.

Less frequently, interstitial keratitis is caused by other infectious diseases, such as tuberculosis or leprosy.

PETERS ANOMALY

In this condition maldevelopment of the anterior segment of the eye may affect the cornea, anterior chamber angle, and iris. The terms "mesodermal dysgenesis," "anterior cleavage syndrome," and others describe these defects and various combinations thereof.

Peters anomaly consists of a congenital corneal opacity (leukoma) with corresponding defects in the posterior corneal stroma, Descemet membrane, and endothelium, often with associated iridocorneal or lenticulocorneal adhesions. The condition is usually bilateral. It is generally sporadic, but recessive and dominant inheritances have been suggested.

Other anomalies within the spectrum of anterior chamber cleavage syndrome are abnormalities of the peripheral cornea and angle, including a prominent, anteriorly displaced ring of Schwalbe, Axenfeld anomaly (fine iris strands that cross the chamber to the displaced ring of Schwalbe), or Rieger anomaly. There may be associated glaucoma or lens abnormalities.

CORNEAL MANIFESTATIONS OF SYSTEMIC DISEASE

Several metabolic diseases produce distinctive corneal changes in childhood. Refractile polychromatic crystals are deposited throughout the cornea in cystinosis. Corneal deposits producing various degrees of corneal haze also occur in certain of the mucopolysaccharidoses, particularly MPS IH (Hurler), MPS IS (Scheie), MPS I H/S (Hurler-Scheie compound), MPS IV (Morquio), MPS VI (Maroteaux-Lamy), and sometimes MPS VII (Sly). Corneal deposits may develop in patients with GM_1 (generalized) gangliosidosis. In Fabry disease fine opacities radiating in a whorl or fan-like pattern occur, and corneal changes can be important in identifying the carrier state. A spray-like pattern of corneal opacities may also be seen in the Bloch-Sulzberger syndrome. In Wilson disease the distinctive corneal sign is the Kayser-Fleischer ring, a golden brown ring in the peripheral cornea resulting from changes in Descemet membrane. Pigmented corneal rings may develop in neonates with cholestatic liver disease. Corneal changes may occur in autoimmune hypoparathyroidism, and band keratopathy in patients with hypercalcemia. Transient keratitis may occur with rubeola, sometimes with rubella.

Beauchamp GR, Gillette TE, Friendly DS: Phlyctenular keratoconjunctivitis. J Pediatr Ophthalmol Strab 18:22, 1981.

Biglan AW, Brown SI, Johnson BL: Keratoglobus and blue sclera. Am J Ophthalmol 83:225, 1977.

Boger WP III, Peterson RA, Robb RM: Keratoconus and acute hydrops in mentally retarded patients with congenital rubella syndrome. Am J Ophthalmol 91:231, 1981.

Burns RB: Soluble tyrosine aminotransferase deficiency: An unusual cause of corneal ulcers. Am J Ophthalmol 73:400, 1972.

Cobo LM, Haynes BF: Early corneal findings in Cogan's syndrome. Ophthalmology 91:903, 1984.

Deckard PS, Bergstrom TJ: Rubeola keratitis. Ophthalmology 88:810, 1981.

Dunn LL, Annable WL, Kliegman RM: Pigmented corneal rings in neonates with liver disease. J Pediatr 110:771, 1987.

Elliott JH, Feman SS, O'Day DM, et al: Hereditary sclerocornea. Arch Ophthalmol 103:676, 1985.

Goldberg MF: A review of selected inherited corneal dystrophies associated with systemic disease. Birth Defects: Original Article Series VII:13, 1971.

Goldberg MF, Payne JW, Brunt PW: Ophthalmologic studies of familial dysautonomia. Arch Ophthalmol 80:732, 1966.

Hutchison DS, Smith RE, Haughton PB: Congenital herpetic keratitis. Arch Ophthalmol 93:70, 1975.

Kraft SP, Judisch GF, Grayson DM: Megalocornea: A clinical and echographic study of an autosomal dominant pedigree. J Pediatr Ophthalmol Strab 21:190, 1984.

Mohandessan MM, Romano PE: Neuroparalytic keratitis in Goldenhar-Gorlin syndrome. Am J Ophthalmol 85:111, 1978.

Schanzlin DJ, Goldberg DB, Brown SI: Transplantation of congenitally opaque corneas. Ophthalmology 87:1253, 1980.

Stieglitz LM, Kind HP, Kazden JJ, et al: Keratitis with hypoparathyroidism. Am J Ophthalmol 84:467, 1972.

Stone DL, Kenyon KR, Green WR, et al: Congenital central corneal leukoma (Peters' anomaly). Am J Ophthalmol 81:173, 1976.

Tso MOM, Fine BS, Thorpe HE: Kayser-Fleischer ring and associated cataract in Wilson's disease. Am J Ophthalmol 79:479, 1975.

22.11 ABNORMALITIES OF THE LENS

CATARACTS

A cataract is any opacity of the lens. Some are clinically insignificant, others significantly affect visual function, and many signify associated ocular or systemic disease.

DIFFERENTIAL DIAGNOSIS. The differential diagnosis of cataracts in infants and children includes a wide range of developmental disorders, infectious and inflammatory processes, metabolic diseases, and toxic and traumatic insults. Cataracts may also develop secondary to intraocular processes, such as retinopathy of prematurity, persistent hyperplastic primary vitreous, retinal detachment, retinitis pigmentosa, and uveitis.

Developmental Variants. Early developmental processes may lead to various congenital lens opacities. Not uncommon are discrete dots or white plaque-like opacities of the lens capsule, sometimes with involvement of the contiguous subcapsular region. Small opacities of the posterior capsule may be associated with persistent remnants of the primitive hyaloid vascular system (the common Mittendorf dot), whereas those of the anterior capsule may be associated with persistent strands of the pupillary membrane or vascular sheath of the lens. Congenital cataracts of this type are usually stationary and rarely interfere with vision; in some cases, however, progression occurs.

Prematurity. A special type of lens change seen in some preterm newborns is the so-called cataract of prematurity. The appearance is of a cluster of tiny vacuoles in the distribution of the Y sutures of the lens. They can be visualized with the ophthalmoscope and are best seen with the pupil well dilated. The pathogenesis is unclear. In most cases the opacities disappear spontaneously, often within a few weeks.

Mendelian Inheritance. Many cataracts are hereditary, unassociated with other disease. The most common mode of inheritance is autosomal dominant. Penetrance and expressivity vary. Autosomal recessive inheritance occurs less frequently; it is sometimes found in populations with high rates of consanguinity. X-linked inheritance of cataracts unassociated with disease is relatively rare, whereas cataracts occurring in association with X-linked disease, such as Lowe syndrome, Alport syndrome, and Fabry disease, are not uncommon.

Congenital Infection Syndrome. Frequently, cataracts in infants and children are the result of prenatal infection. Lens opacity may occur in any of the major congenital infection syndromes (e.g., toxoplasmosis, cytomegalovirus infection, syphilis, rubella, perinatal herpes simplex virus infection). Cataracts attributed to other maternal infections, including measles, poliomyelitis, influenza, varicella-zoster and vaccinia, have also been reported.

Metabolic Disorders. Cataracts are a prominent manifestation of many metabolic diseases, particularly certain disorders of carbohydrate, amino acid, calcium, and copper metabolism. A primary consideration in any infant with cataracts is the possibility of galactosemia (Sec. 8.36). In classic infantile galactosemia, galactose-1-phosphate uridyl transferase deficiency, the cataract is typically of the zonular type, with haziness or opacification of one or more of the perinuclear layers of the lens; often, haziness or clouding of the nucleus also occurs. In its early stages the cataract generally has a distinctive "oil droplet" appearance and is best detected with the pupil fully dilated. There may be progression to complete opacification of the lens within weeks. With early treatment (galactose-free diet) the lens changes may be reversible.

In galactokinase deficiency, cataracts may be the sole or presenting clinical manifestation. The cataracts are usually zonular and may appear in the 1st months or years of life, or later in childhood.

In children with juvenile-onset diabetes mellitus, lens changes are uncommon. Some, however, develop snowflake-like white opacities and vacuoles of the lens. Others develop cataracts that may progress and mature rapidly, sometimes in a matter of hours or days, especially during adolescence. An antecedent event may be the sudden development of myopia caused by changes in the optical density of the lens.

Congenital lens opacities may be seen in children of diabetic and prediabetic mothers. Hypoglycemia in the neonate can also be associated with early development of cataracts. Another disorder of carbohydrate metabolism associated with the development of cataracts is ketotic hypoglycemia of childhood.

An association between cataracts and hypocalcemia is well established. Various lens opacities may be seen in patients with hypoparathyroidism.

A metabolic disorder of major importance in the differential diagnosis of cataracts in infants and children is the oculocerebral renal syndrome of Lowe. Affected male children frequently have dense bilateral cataracts at birth, often in association with glaucoma and miotic pupils. Punctate lens opacities are frequently present in heterozygous females.

The distinctive sunflower cataract of Wilson disease is not commonly seen in children. Various lens opacities may be seen in children with certain of the sphingolipidoses, mucopolysaccharidoses and mucolipidoses, particularly Niemann-Pick disease, mucosulfatidosis, Fabry disease, and aspartylglycosaminuria.

Miscellaneous Disorders. The list of multisystem syndromes and diseases associated with lens opacities of various types is long. The clinical features of some of the major disorders are presented in Table 22–1.

Chromosomal Defects. Lens opacities of various types may occur in association with chromosomal defects, including 13-, 18-, and 21-trisomy, Turner syndrome and a number of deletion (e.g., 11p13, 18p, 18q), and duplication syndromes (e.g., 3q, 20p, 10q).

Drugs, Toxic Agents, and Trauma. Of the various drugs and toxic agents that may produce cataracts, corticosteroids are of major importance in the pediatric age group. Steroid-related cataracts characteristically are posterior subcapsular lens opacities. The incidence and severity vary. The relative significance of dose, duration of treatment, and individual susceptibility is controversial, and the pathogenesis of steroid-induced cataracts is unclear. The effect on vision depends on the extent and density of the opacity. In many cases, the acuity is only minimally or moderately impaired. Reversibility of steroid-induced cataracts may occur in some cases. All children being treated with long-term steroids should have periodic eye examinations.

Trauma to the eye is a major cause of cataracts in children. Opacification of the lens may result from contusion or penetrating injury. Cataracts are an important manifestation of child abuse. Other physical agents, such as radiation, can also damage the lens and produce cataracts.

MANAGEMENT PRINCIPLES. The treatment of cataracts that significantly interfere with vision includes the following: (1) surgical removal of lens material to provide an optically clear visual axis; (2) correction of the resultant aphakic refractive error with spectacles, contact lenses or, in selected cases, intraocular lens implantation or refractive corneal surgery; and (3) correction of any associated sensory deprivation amblyopia. Treatment of the amblyopia may be the most demanding and difficult step in the visual rehabilitation of infants or children with cataracts.

PROGNOSIS. Prognosis depends on many factors, including the nature of the cataract, age of onset, age of intervention, duration and severity of any attendant amblyopia, and presence of any associated ocular abnormalities (e.g., microphthalmia, retinal lesions, optic atrophy, glaucoma, nystagmus, strabismus). In addition, secondary conditions and complications may develop in children who have had cataract surgery, including inflammatory sequelae, secondary membranes, glaucoma, retinal detachment, and changes in the axial length of the eye. All these factors and possibilities should be considered in planning treatment. The ultimate management decision should rest jointly with the ophthalmologist, pediatrician, and family.

ECTOPIA LENTIS

Normally, the lens is suspended in place behind the iris diaphragm by the zonular fibers of the ciliary body. Abnormalities of the suspensory system resulting from a developmental defect, disease, or trauma may result in instability or displacement of the lens. Displacement of the lens is classified as luxation (dislocation—complete displacement of the lens) or as subluxation (partial displacement—shifting or tilting of the lens). Symptoms include blurring of vision, which is often the result of refractive changes such as myopia, astigmatism, or aphakic hyperopia. Some patients experience diplopia. An important sign of displacement is iridodenesis, a tremulousness of the iris caused by the loss of its usual support. Also, the anterior chamber may appear deeper than normal. Sometimes the equatorial region ("edge") of the displaced lens may be visible in the pupillary aperture. On ophthalmoscopy this may appear as a black cresent. Also, the difference between the phakic and aphakic portions can be appreciated when focusing on the fundus.

DIFFERENTIAL DIAGNOSIS. A major cause of lens displacement is trauma. Displacement may occur as the result of ocular disease, such as uveitis, intraocular tumor, congenital glaucoma, high myopia, megalocornea, or aniridia, or in association with cataract. Also important in the differential diagnosis of lens displacement in children are the hereditable forms of ectopia lentis and those associated with systemic disease.

Displacement of the lens occurring as a hereditable ocular condition unassociated with systemic abnormalities is referred to as simple ectopia lentis. Usually simple ectopia lentis is transmitted as an autosomal dominant condition. The lens is generally displaced upward and temporally. The ectopia may be present at birth or appear later in life.

Text continued on page 1586

TABLE 22–1. Clinical Features of Ocular Changes in Developmental Pediatric Syndromes

- CNS anomalies
  - Anencephaly (see Sec. 20.17)
    - Optic nerve aplasia or hypoplasia
  - Holoprosencephaly (see Sec. 20.8)
    - Hypotelorism; in extreme form, cyclopia; in some cases, iris coloboma
  - Cyclopia
    - A single eye of variable complexity, usually accompanied by a proboscis-like structure on the forehead; often associated with holoprosencephaly; sometimes fusion of both eyes with duplication of lenses, corneas, and other structures; rosette formation in the retina; optic nerve rudimentary or absent; orbit diamond-shaped
  - Arnold-Chiari malformation (see Sec. 20.2)
    - Nystagmus, usually vertical, often downbeat; ocular motor palsies with diplopia; sometimes skew deviation
  - Dandy-Walker syndrome (see Sec. 20.15)
    - Ophthalmic manifestations of increased intracranial pressure
  - Septo-optic dysplasia (deMorsier syndrome)
    - Malformation of anterior midline structures (agenesis of septum pellucidium, primitive optic ventricle, with hypoplasia of optic nerves, chiasm, and infundibulum); sometimes associated endocrine abnormalities; vision defects, strabismus, nystagmus; in some cases, other anomalies of eyes
- Craniostenosis syndromes (see Sec. 20.16)
  - Apert syndrome (acrocephalosyndactyly)
    - Orbits shallow, eyes protuberant (proptosis) and widely spaced; antimongoloid slant of palpebral fissures; ocular motor abnormalities (strabismus, partial ophthalmoplegia, nystagmus); papilledema; optic atrophy; cataracts; sometimes dislocated lenses; occasionally iris and fundus colobomata
  - Carpenter syndrome (acrocephalopolysyndactyly)
    - Orbits shallow; lateral displacement of medial canthi; epicanthus; antimongoloid slant of palpebral fissures; optic atrophy; microcornea and corneal opacities in some cases
  - Crouzon syndrome (dysostosis craniofacialis)
    - Eyes protuberant (proptosis) and widely spaced; luxation of globe may occur; antimongoloid slant of palpebral fissures; strabismus; papilledema; optic atrophy; vision loss; cataracts in some patients
  - Kleeblattschädel syndrome (cloverleaf skull)
    - Shallow orbits with proptosis; high risk of corneal ulceration
- Miscellaneous craniofacial defects and syndromes
  - Frontonasal dysplasia (median cleft-face syndrome)
    - Hypertelorism (radiographic interobital distance 2 SD above normal for age); in some cases, anophthalmia, microphthalmia, epibulbar dermoids, lid colobomata, congenital cataracts
  - Opitz syndrome
    - Hypertelorism, particularly associated with hypospadias; antimongoloid slant of palpebral fissures; epicanthus; strabismus
  - Waardenburg syndrome
    - Lateral displacement of medial canthi and inferior puncta; heterochromia iridis, total or partial; in some cases both irides completely blue (isochromia); fundus pigmentary changes in some cases
  - Oculodentodigital dysplasia (Meyer-Schwickerath syndrome)
    - Hypotelorism, microphthalmos, microcornea, dental anomalies and enamel hypoplasia, camptodactyly, syndactyly, and other skeletal defects; persistent pupillary membrane; glaucoma
  - Hallermann-Streiff syndrome (dyscephalia oculomandibulofacialis)
    - Microphthalmos, cataract, sparse eyebrows and lashes, blue sclerae, nystagmus
  - Pierre Robin syndrome
    - Congenital glaucoma; retinal detachment; strabismus
  - Treacher Collins syndrome (mandibulofacial dysostosis; Franceschetti-Klein syndrome)
    - Antimongoloid slant of palpebral fissures; underdevelopment of supraorbital ridges, coloboma of lower eyelids and in some cases of iris or choroid
  - Goldenhar syndrome (oculoauriculovertebral dysplasia)
    - Antimongoloid slant of palpebral fissures; colobomata of eyelid, upper lid more commonly involved than lower; hypoplasia or coloboma of iris; hypertelorism; sometimes microphthalmos
- Chromosomal abnormalities
  - 21-Trisomy (Down syndrome; see Sec. 7.14)
    - Mongoloid slant of palpebral fissures; epicanthus; dacryostenosis; blepharitis; Brushfield spots of iris; peripheral thinning of iris stroma; keratoconus and corneal hydrops; cataracts; high refractive errors; strabismus; nystagmus; increased vessels at disk
  - 18-Trisomy (Edwards syndrome; see Sec. 7.15)
    - Ptosis; short palpebral fissures; epicanthus; hypoplastic supraorbital ridges; microphthalmia; corneal opacities; anisocoria; cataracts; fundus and disk colobomata; retinal hypopigmentation
  - 13-Trisomy (Patau syndrome; see Sec. 7.16)
    - Microphthalmos; anophthalmos; cyclopia in some cases; dysgenesis of anterior segment (iris hypoplasia, iris adhesions, chamber angle abnormalities); corneal opacities; congenital glaucoma; cataracts; persistent hyperplastic primary vitreous; retinal dysplasia; colobomata of iris, ciliary body, fundus; intraocular cartilage, optic nerve hypoplasia
  - 9-Trisomy
    - Antimongoloid slant of palpebral fissures; deeply set eyes; corectopia; strabismus
  - 8-Trisomy
    - Dysmorphic skull; strabismus
  - Syndrome 45X (Turner, and mosaic variants; see Sec. 7.25 and 19.34)
    - Ptosis; epicanthus; blue sclerae; defective color vision; cataracts; strabismus; nystagmus
  - 47,XXY; 48,XXXY; 49,XXXXY (Klinefelter) syndromes (see Sec. 7.26 and 19.30)
    - Hypertelorism; epicanthus; Brushfield spots of iris; myopia; strabismus
  - Partial deletion short arm chromosome 4 (4p −) (see Sec. 7.21)
    - Ptosis; hypertelorism; epicanthus; colobomata

TABLE 22–1. Clinical Features of Ocular Changes in Developmental Pediatric Syndromes *Continued*

Chromosomal abnormalities *Continued*
  Partial deletion short arm chromosome 5 (5p −) (cri-du-chat syndrome; see Sec. 7.21)
    Antimongoloid slant of palpebral fissures; hypertelorism; epicanthus; strabismus
  Partial deletion short arm chromosome 9 (9p −) (see Sec. 7.21)
    Mongoloid slant of palpebral fissures; epicanthus; arched brows
  Partial deletion long arm chromosome 13 (13q −)
    Ptosis; epicanthus; hypertelorism; microphthalmos; colobomata; retinoblastoma
  Partial deletion long arm chromosome 18 (18q −) (see Sec. 7.21)
    Horizontal palpebral fissures; epicanthus; deeply set eyes; optic disk pallor; tapetoretinal degeneration; nystagmus
  Partial deletion, long arm chromosome 21 (21q −)
    Downward slanting palpebral fissures
  Partial deletion long arm chromosome 22 (22q −)
    Ptosis; epicanthus
  Extrachromosomal material (cat-eye syndrome)
    Antimongoloid slant of palpebral fissures; epicanthus; hypertelorism; microphthalmos; colobomata of iris, fundus, optic nerve; macular defects; pale disks; cataracts; strabismus; nystagmus

Disorders of amino acid metabolism
  Albinism*
    Defect in the formation of melanin; several forms:
    (1) *Oculocutaneous albinism, tyrosinase negative;* generalized hypopigmentation; iris blue or gray; generalized hypopigmentation of eye; typical pink or orange reflex; fundus bright, with increased choroidal vascular pattern; macula/fovea poorly defined (hypoplastic); photophobia; nystagmus; subnormal vision; often high refractive error
    (2) *Oculocutaneous albinism, tyrosinase positive;* pigmentation may increase with age; iris blue, yellow, or brownish; color increasing with age; photophobia; nystagmus; subnormal vision, which may improve with age
    (3) *Amish* or *yellow* mutant; generalized albinism in which a yellowish pigment is produced instead of melanin, providing some skin and hair color
    (4) *Hermansky-Pudlak syndrome;* tyrosine negative albinism associated with a hemorrhagic diathesis; iris blue-gray to brown; photophobia; nystagmus; slight to moderate vision defect
    (5) *Cross syndrome,* tyrosine positive; a syndrome of hypopigmentation, gingival fibromatosis, spasticity, athetoid movements, and microphthalmos; iris blue-gray; microphthalmos; cataracts; severe vision defect; nystagmus
    (6) *Ocular albinism;* pigment deficiency limited to the eye; generalized ocular hypopigmentation; macular hypoplasia; nystagmus (in blacks, fundus tessellated)
  Alcaptonuria (see Sec. 8.6)
    Black discoloration of sclera, most noticeable at insertion of extraocular muscles
  Tyrosinemia (Richner-Hanhart syndrome; see Sec. 8.3)
    Corneal ulceration, "herpetiform"
  Cystinosis (see Sec. 8.5)
    Accumulation of refractile crystals in cornea (best seen with slit lamp, but corneal haze may be detected grossly); photophobia; pigmentary retinopathy; fundi generally hypopigmented, with fine to coarse spotty pigmentation, most marked peripherally; vision usually normal to nearly normal
  Homocystinemia, type I (see Sec. 8.4)
    Ectopia lentis; cataract; secondary glaucoma; peripheral cystic degeneration of retina
  Sulfite oxidase deficiency (see Sec. 8.6)
    Subluxation of lens; spherophakia; strabismus
  Hartnup disease (see Sec. 8.6)
    Photophobia; nystagmus; strabismus
  Maple syrup urine disease (see Sec. 8.7)
    Strabismus, varying with condition of child

The mucopolysaccharidoses (MPS)
  Hurler syndrome (MPS IH; α-L-iduronidase deficiency; see Sec. 8.43)
    Hypertelorism, prominent eyes; puffy lids; heavy brows; deposition of MPS and attendant cellular changes throughout most regions of eye, particularly the conjuctiva, cornea, sclera, iris, ciliary body, retina, and optic nerve; characteristic corneal clouding, clinically evident early in life, and progressing to dense milky "ground-glass" haze, often with associated photophobia; progressive retinal degeneration with pigmentary dispersion and clumping, arteriolar attentuation and disk pallor, and reduced ERG; optic atrophy; vision loss, principally because of corneal, retinal, and optic nerve changes; hydrocephalus and cerebral changes; glaucoma in some cases
  Scheie syndrome (MPS IS; α-L-iduronidase deficiency; see Sec. 8.43)
    Progressive corneal clouding, diffuse but sometimes more dense peripherally than centrally; progressive retinal degeneration; visual symptoms, field loss, and night blindness often commencing in 2nd or 3rd decade; glaucoma in some cases
  Hurler-Scheie Compound (MPS IH/S; α-L-iduronidase deficiency; see Sec. 8.43)
    Corneal clouding, diffuse and progressive; glaucoma in some cases; vision loss because of corneal clouding or optic nerve effects of arachnoid cysts
  Hunter syndrome (MPS II; iduronosulfate sulfatase deficiency)
    Phenotypically similar to MPS IH; both mild and severe forms occur; progressive retinal degeneration with pigmentary changes, arteriolar attenuation, optic atrophy, vision, loss, reduced ERG; corneas macroscopically (clinically) clear, but microscopic corneal changes documented; papilledema secondary to hydrocephalus in some cases
  Sanfillippo syndrome (MPS III; type A [heparin sulfate sulfatase deficiency], B [*N*-acetyl-α-D-glucosaminidase deficiency], and C [acetyl-Co A:α-glucosaminide *N*-acetyl transferase deficiency])
    Retinal changes in some patients—arteriolar narrowing; reduced ERG; corneas clinically clear but some microscopic changes reported
  Morquio syndrome (MPS IV; galactosamine-6-sulfate sulfatase deficiency in classic form; β-galactosidase deficiency reported in variants; see Sec. 8.43)

*To be differentiated from these forms of albinism is the Chédiak-Higashi syndrome in which the defect is in the morphology of the melanosomes, not in the formation of melanin. Ocular signs include hypopigmentation of iris and fundus, photophobia, nystagmus, and papilledema with lymphocytic infiltration of optic nerve.

Table continued on following page

TABLE 22–1. Clinical Features of Ocular Changes in Developmental Pediatric Syndromes *Continued*

- The mucopolysaccharidoses (MPS) *Continued*
    - Fine corneal clouding in many patients; slowly, progressive; often not clinically apparent for several years
  - Maroteaux-Lamy syndrome (MPS VI; arylsulfatase-B deficiency; see Sec. 8.43)
    - Diffuse corneal clouding, usually evident within 1st few yr of life; tortuosity of retinal vessels in some patients; papilledema and 6th nerve paresis in some patients with hydrocephalus
  - Sly syndrome (MPS VII; β-D-glucuronidase deficiency)
    - Some diversity of phenotype; corneas clear or cloudy; corneal haze of either fine or coarse type
  - Di Ferrenti syndrome (MPS VIII: *N*-acetylglucosamine-6-sulfate sulfatase deficiency)
    - Short stature; mild dysostosis multiplex; odontoid hypoplasia; hepatosplenomegaly; mental retardation; ophthalmologic abnormalities not yet described
- The sphingolipidoses
  - Generalized gangliosidosis (GM_1 gangliosidosis type 1; β-galactosidase deficiency; see Sec. 8.18)
    - Diffuse corneal clouding (MPS accumulation); macular cherry red spot of retinal ganglioside accumulation; retinal vascular tortuosity and retinal hemorrhages; optic atrophy; vision loss, nystagmus, strabismus
  - Juvenile GM_1 gangliosidosis (GM_1 gangliosidosis type 2; β-galactosidase deficiency; see Sec. 8.18)
    - Corneas clinically clear; histologic changes of retinal ganglioside storage without clinically obvious signs; optic atrophy and vision loss; nystagmus and strabismus
  - Tay-Sachs disease (GM_2 gangliosidosis type 1; hexosaminidase A deficiency; see Sec. 8.18)
    - Macular cherry red spot; optic atrophy (demyelination and degeneration of optic nerves, chiasm, and tracts); progressive loss of vision, caused by ocular and cerebral abnormalities; sequential deterioration of eye movements
  - Sandhoff variant (GM_2 gangliosidosis type 2; hexosaminidase A and B deficiency; see Sec. 8.18)
    - Macular cherry red spot; optic atrophy and progressive loss of vision; corneas clinically clear or slightly opalescent; histologic evidence of storage cytosomes in cornea
  - Juvenile GM_2 gangliosidosis (GM_2 gangliosidosis type 3; partial deficiency of hexosaminidase; see Sec. 8.8)
    - Retinal pigmentary degeneration; macular changes (cherry red spot type) in some cases; optic atrophy; blindness later in course of disease
  - Krabbe globoid cell leukodystrophy (galactosyl ceramide lipidosis; galactosylceramide β-galactosidase deficiency)
    - Cortical blindness and optic atrophy caused by degenerative changes in brain and visual pathways; nystagmus; strabismus
  - Gaucher disease (glycosyl ceramide lipidosis; glucosyl ceramide β-glucosidase deficiency; see Sec. 8.18)
    - Paralytic strabismus caused by brain stem and cranial nerve involvement in neuronopathic forms; nystagmus; macular changes (grayness) in some cases; retinal hemorrhages secondary to anemia, thrombocytopenia; discrete white spots in or on retina reported in juvenile form; pingueculae (wedge-shaped conjunctival lesions) in chronic non-neuronopathic form; possibly corneal clouding
  - Niemann-Pick disease (sphingomyelin lipidoses; sphingomyelinase deficiency; see Sec. 8.18)
    - Grayish macular haze in classic infantile neuronopathic form (type A), and in subacute neurovisceral or juvenile form (type C); corneal clouding, lens opacities in some cases (type A); vertical gaze palsy in some patients
  - Fabry disease (glycosphingolipid lipidosis; α-galactosidase A deficiency; see Sec. 8.18)
    - Corneal dystrophy related to epithelial lipid deposits (radiating lines/whorls in affected males and in carrier females); aneurysmal dilatation and tortuosity of conjunctival and retinal vessels; renovascular signs of renal hypertension; papilledema; orbital and lid edema; cataracts (spoke-like posterior cortical lens opacities—anterior lens opacities in some cases)
  - Farber disease (ceramide lipidosis; ceramidase deficiency; see Sec. 8.18)
    - Cherry red-like spot; grayish posterior pole; retinal pigmentary mottling; granulomata in and around eye
- Ceroid lipofuscinoses (see also Sec. 8.18 and 20.60)
  - Infantile (Finnish variant; unsaturated fatty acid lipidosis)
    - Microcephaly; marked atrophy of brain; loss of vision; granular inclusions; ataxia; myoclonus; profound dementia, decorticate state; onset 1–2 yr; death by 10 yr
  - Late infantile (Jansky-Bielschowsky)
    - Intellectual deterioration, seizures, ataxia; pigmentary retinal degeneration, in some cases, predominantly macular; ERG abnormal; optic atrophy; inclusions of curvilinear type; onset 2–4 yr; death by 10 yr
  - Juvenile (Batten-Mayou-Spielmeyer-Vogt)
    - Intellectual deterioration, seizures, ataxis, progressive loss of motor function; pigmentary retinal degeneration, resembling retinitis pigmentosa, with progressive loss of vision; in some cases predominantly macular degeneration; ERG abnormal; optic atrophy as a late manifestation; mixed inclusion bodies including curvilinear and fingerprint types, and lipofuscin in brain; onset 5–8 yr, sometimes later; death in teens or 20s
  - Late juvenile or adult (Kufs)
    - Behavior disturbances and intellectual impairment; ataxia, spasticity, myoclonic seizures; vision and fundi usually normal; macular degeneration in some cases; mostly lipofuscin in brain; onset in childhood, adolescence, or early adult life
  - Cherry red spot myoclonus syndrome
    - Macular cherry red spot; vision loss; intention myoclonus; variable inclusions in brain; light inclusions in hepatocytes and Kupffer cells; onset in childhood; survival to adulthood
- Leukodystrophies (see also Sec. 8.17 and 20.61)
  - Metachromatic leukodystrophy (arylsulfatase A deficiency)
    - Retinal degeneration resembling retinitis pigmentosa; in some cases, early macular involvement (macular grayness with accentuation of central red spot); optic atrophy; vision loss; strabismus and nystagmus
  - Pelizaeus-Merzbacher syndrome
    - "Eye-rolling" (rhythmic eye movements) noted soon after birth, sometimes with rotary movements of the head; optic atrophy as a late manifestation
  - Canavan disease
    - Vacuolization of ganglion cell layer of retina reportedly detectable with slit lamp; retinal pigmentary changes; optic atrophy; blindness early in course; ERG normal; VER reduced; strabismus, roving eye movements, and nystagmus
- Demyelinating scleroses (see Sec. 20.63)
  - Schilder disease (encephalitis periaxialis diffusa)
    - Involvement of visual pathways, producing retrobulbar neuritis, optic atrophy, central scotomas, chiasmal syndromes, homonymous field defects; disorders of cortical gaze functions; nystagmus

TABLE 22–1. Clinical Features of Ocular Changes in Developmental Pediatric Syndromes *Continued*

Demyelinating scleroses *Continued*
- Multiple sclerosis
  - Optic neuritis (episodic loss of vision, typically a central scotoma, unilateral more often than bilateral, often with retrobulbar pain); other visual pathway lesions (various field defects); internuclear ophthalmoplegia; supranuclear gaze palsies; nystagmus; sheathing of peripheral retinal vessels in some cases
- Neuromyelitis optica (Devick disease)
  - Optic neuritis (usually papillitis with visible disc edema), with resultant optic atrophy; other visual pathway lesions (various visual field defects); in some cases extraocular muscle palsies, conjugate gaze palsies, nystagmus, pupil abnormalities

Hamartomatoses and phakomatoses
- Tuberous sclerosis (Bourneville disease; see Sec. 20.40 and 23.12)
  - Retinal phakomata (glial hamartomas, ranging from small flat or slightly elevated white or yellowish lesions to large elevated refractile yellowish multinodular or cystic masses often likened to an unripe mulberry); fibroangioma of the lids; in some, papilledema or optic atrophy, vision defects, pupil or ocular motor signs related to CNS changes (tumors, hydrocephalus); occasionally iris or pigmentary changes.
- Neurofibromatosis (von Recklinghausen syndrome; see Sec. 20.39 and 23.11)
  - Plexiform neuromas of eyelids, often producing ptosis; episcleral and conjunctival neurofibromas; prominent corneal nerves; Lisch iris nodules; uveal hypercellularity; glaucoma (related to angle anomalies, uveal hypercellularity, neovascularization, or synechiae); hamartomas (phakomata) of disk and retina; fundus pigmentary changes likened to café-au-lait spots; optic gliomas and vision loss (presenting with proptosis, strabismus, nystagmus if intraorbital—with signs of increased intracranial pressure, hydrocephalus, or diencephalic syndrome when intracranial); orbital asymmetry; orbital wall defects; pulsatile exophthalmos, intraorbital neurofibromas, with proptosis
- Angiomatosis of the retina and cerebellum (von Hippel-Lindau disease; see Sec. 20.42)
  - Retinal hemangioblastoma (reddish or yellowish globular mass with paired vessels coursing to and from the lesion, sometimes likened to a toy balloon in the fundus); may lead to hemorrhage, exudates, retinal detachment
- Encephalofacial angiomatosis (Sturge-Weber syndrome; see Sec. 20.41)
  - Lid and conjunctival involvement of facial nevus flammeus; choroidal hemangioma; dilated and tortuous retinal vessels; glaucoma, congenital or later in infancy or childhood (related to possible angle anomalies, vascular lesion, or hypersecretion); visual field defects associated with CNS lesions; hemianopsia in some cases
- Angiomatosis of mid-brain and retina (Wyburn-Mason syndrome)
  - Extensive vascular malformations involving principally the midbrain and eye; angiomatosis of the retina; vessels dilated and tortuous; angiomatosis affecting optic nerve and orbit

Neurocutaneous syndromes
- Ataxia-telangiectasia (Louis-Bar syndrome; see Sec. 11.19)
  - Telangiectasias of bulbar conjunctivae, usually by the age of 4–6 yr; apraxic disorder of conjugate eye movements; horizontal and vertical gaze performed in halting dyssynergic fashion; difficulty in maintaining eccentric gaze; sometimes convergence defect; nystagmus
- Sjögren-Larsson syndrome (see Sec. 23.17)
  - Chorioretinal lesions; discrete defects in retinal pigment epithelium of unknown etiology; circumscribed symmetric lesions of varying size in and about the macula in approximately 25% of cases
- Incontinentia pigmenti (Bloch-Sulzberger syndrome; see Sec. 23.11)
  - Intraocular retrolental masses ("pseudogliomas") and membranes, apparently secondary to an underlying retinal vascular disorder characterized by aneurysmal dilatation, abnormal arteriovenous connections, and vasoproliferative changes; sometimes intraocular hemorrhage and inflammation; microphthalmos; corneal opacities; cataracts; optic atrophy
- Linear nevus sebaceus of Jadassohn (see Sec. 23.10)
  - Coloboma of the eyelids, iris, and fundus; corectopia; epibulbar lipodermoids; orbital teratomas; proptosis; aberrant lacrimal gland; corneal vascularization; ocular motor palsies; nystagmus; defective vision
- Xerodermic idiocy of de Sanctis and Cacchione (see Sec. 23.15)
  - Atrophy of eyelids; loss of cilia, ectropion, entropion, symblepharon, ankyloblepharon; drying and infection of conjunctiva; ulceration of cornea; iritis; photophobia
- Klippel-Trenaunay-Weber syndrome (see Sec. 23.8)
  - Conjunctival telangiectasia; choroidal hemangioma; iris coloboma; heterochromia; glaucoma; strabismus

Special neurobiothrophies
- Subacute sclerosing panencephalitis (Dawson disease; Van Bogaert disease; see Sec. 12.85)
  - Focal retinitis (edema, hemorrhage, pigmentary changes), with chorioretinal scarring (usually macular or paramacular, usually bilateral)—may precede other neurologic manifestations; papilledema; optic atrophy; visual symptoms of retinal and optic nerve involvement; field defects of cerebral involvement; nystagmus; extraocular muscle palsies; ptosis
- Subacute necrotizing encephalomyopathy (Leigh disease; see see Sec. 8.39 and 18.29)
  - Abnormal eye movements (bizarre rolling eye movements, disconjugate eye movements, horizontal and vertical nystagmus, saccadic ocular movements); extraocular muscle palsies (sometimes complete external ophthalmoplegia); blepharoptosis; progressive optic atrophy and vision loss; sometimes retinal changes (diminished macular reflex); afferent and efferent pupil defects
- Hepatolenticular degeneration (Wilson disease; see Sec. 13.88)
  - Kayser-Fleischer ring of cornea (copper deposition in periphery of Descemet membrane, particularly in deepest zone adjacent to endothelium, seen as granules of golden, greenish, grayish, or brown hue); Sonnenblumenkatarakt ("sunflower" cataract); occasionally ocular motor abnormalities (jerky oscillations of eyes, involuntary upward deviation of eyes, or paresis of upward gaze); accommodation sometimes affected; in some cases, optic neuritis secondary to penicillamine therapy
- Trichopoliodystrophy (Menkes disease; kinky hair disease; see Sec. 20.65)
  - Decrease in retinal ganglion cells, thinning of retinal nerve fiber layer, and partial atrophy of optic nerve; progressive vision loss; abnormal ERG; microcysts of pigment epithelium of iris
- Abetalipoproteinemia (acanthocytosis; Bassen-Kornzweig disease; see Sec. 8.34)
  - Pigmentary retinal degeneration with progressive impairment of visual function (pigment dispersion, arteriolar attenuation, disk pallor, impaired dark adaptation); cataracts, ptosis, and ocular motor abnormalities; in some cases, progressive exotropia, paresis of medial recti, and dissociated nystagmus on lateral gaze

Table continued on following page

TABLE 22–1. Clinical Features of Ocular Changes in Developmental Pediatric Syndromes *Continued*

- Special neurobiothrophies *Continued*
  - Heredopathia atactica polyneuritiformis (Refsum syndrome; phytanic acid α-hydrolase deficiency; see Sec. 8.16 and 21.43)
    - Pigmentary retinal degeneration (pigmentary clumping, arteriolar attenuation, optic atrophy, progressive impairment of night vision and visual field); ERG abnormal; sometimes vitreous opacities, cataracts, cornea guttata, miosis; ophthalmoparesis; nystagmus
  - Familial dysautonomia (Riley-Day syndrome; see Sec. 21.47)
    - Depressed or absent corneal sensation, with corneal ulceration and scarring common; defective lacrimation; tortuosity of retinal vessels; tonic pupil in some cases; myopia and exotropia common
  - Congenital familial sensory neuropathy with anhidrosis (Pinsky-DiGeorge syndrome; see Sec. 21.49)
    - Defective corneal sensation, with defective lacrimation; corneal ulceration and scarring may result
- Disorders of connective tissues, bones, and joints
  - Arachnodactyly (Marfan syndrome; see Sec. 24.56)
    - Ectopia lentis (lens dislocation, usually upward) and iridodonesis (tremulous iris); microphakia, spherophakia; cataract; myopia; glaucoma; retinal changes: degeneration, detachment
  - Cutis hyperelastica (Ehlers-Danlos syndrome; see Sec. 23.18)
    - Epicanthus; blue sclera; keratoconus; subluxation of lens; retinal detachment
  - Pseudoxanthoma elasticum (see Sec. 23.18)
    - Angioid streaks (breaks in Bruch membrane appearing as dark lines in the fundus radiating from the disk); tendency to retinal hemorrhage
  - Osteogenesis imperfecta (see Sec. 24.50)
    - Blue sclera; prominent eyes; in some cases, megalocornea, keratoconus, corneal opacities
  - Polyostotic fibrous dysplasia (McCune-Albright syndrome; see Sec. 19.7)
    - Thickening of bones of orbit
  - Osteopetrosis (Albers-Schönberg disease; "marble bones"; see Sec. 24.49)
    - Vision loss and extraocular muscle palsies, caused by bony overgrowth of cranial foramina; in some cases, retinal degeneration, optic atrophy
  - Chondrodystrophia calcificans congenita (Conradi syndrome; see Sec. 24.46)
    - Cataract; optic atrophy; hypertelorism
  - Spondyloepiphyseal dysplasia congenita (see Sec. 24.37)
    - Myopia; retinal detachment; cataract; buphthalmos
  - Spondyloepiphyseal dysplasia variants (see Sec. 24.37)
    - Punctate corneal dystrophy without impairment of vision
  - Hereditary onchyo-osteodysplasia (nail-patella syndrome)
    - Dark "cloverleaf" pigmentation of iris; cataract; microphakia; microcornea; keratoconus; ptosis
  - Progressive arthro-ophthalmopathy (Stickler syndrome)
    - Pain and stiffness of joints with bony enlargement; kyphosis; cleft palate; Pierre Robin anomaly; deafness; progressive myopia; retinal detachment; glaucoma
- Dermatologic disorders
  - Focal dermal hypoplasia (Goltz syndrome; see Sec. 23.6)
    - Nystagmus; strabismus; microphthalmos; coloboma
  - Hypohidrotic (anhidrotic) ectodermal dysplasia (see Sec. 23.7)
    - Deficiency of tears, leading to keratopathy, photophobia; stenosis of the lacrimal puncta; cataracts; lashes and brows sparse
  - Dyskeratosis congenita (see Sec. 23.6)
    - Bullous conjunctivitis, with minimal scarring of cornea; chronic blepharitis, loss of lashes and ectropion; keratinization of lacrimal puncta
  - Ichthyosis (see Sec. 23.17)
    - Conjunctivitis, ectropion, and corneal erosions in lamellar and sex-linked forms; cataracts in congenital and vulgaris forms
  - Basal cell nevus syndrome (see Sec. 23.33)
    - Prominent supraorbital ridges; hypertelorism or dystopia canthorum; cataracts; coloboma; vision defects; strabismus
  - Juvenile xanthogranuloma (nevoxanthoendothelioma; see Sec. 23.33)
    - Xanthogranuloma in ocular tissues, as infiltrates in orbit, iris, episclera, ciliary body; presenting signs may be proptosis, heterochromia, spontaneous hyphema, uveitis, glaucoma
  - Poikiloderma congenitale (Rothmund-Thomson syndrome; see Sec. 23.15)
    - Sparse eyebrows and eyelashes; cataracts (onset 2–7 yr); corneal dystrophy
  - Bloom syndrome (see Sec. 23.15)
    - Conjunctivitis; conjunctival telangiectasias; drusen at posterior pole of fundus
- Syndromes of multiple developmental abnormalities
  - Cornelia de Lange syndrome
    - Microbrachycephaly, short neck, low hair line, anteverted nares, micrognathism, and low-set ears; physical and mental retardation; limb defects including micromelia, phocomelia, oligodactyly, polydactyly; cardiac and urogenital anomalies; synophrys (confluent eyebrows) and long curly eyelashes; ptosis; epicanthus; microphthalmos with eccentric pupils; corneal opacities; optic atrophy; strabismus
  - Fraser syndrome
    - Facial, genitourinary, skeletal anomalies (including lateral cleft of nostril, ear deformity, renal agenesis, hydronephrosis, hypospadias, cryptorchidism, syndactyly); cerebral defects, meningoencephalocele; cryptophthalmos (eye hidden, fused lids—absence of palpebral fissure), sometimes with symblepharon (adhesion of lid to globe); microphthalmos in some cases; flat supraorbital ridge
  - Rieger syndrome
    - Various dental and limb anomalies; occasionally intellectual retardation, muscular dystrophy, and myotonic dystrophy; dysplasia of anterior segment of the eye; posterior embryotoxon (prominence and anterior displacement of Schwalbe line), often with bands of iris tissue attached (Axenfeld syndrome); iris hypoplasia; glaucoma; cataracts; ectopia lentis; colobomata; micro- or megalocornea; strabismus; ptosis; optic atrophy
  - Peter syndrome
    - Skeletal anomalies; developmental defects of the gastrointestinal tract and central nervous system; hydrocephalus and mental retardation; central defect of Descemet membrane, with central corneal leukoma, shallow anterior chamber, peripheral anterior synechia; cataracts

TABLE 22–1. Clinical Features of Ocular Changes in Developmental Pediatric Syndromes *Continued*

Syndromes of multiple developmental abnormalities *Continued*

- Lenz syndrome
  - Microcephaly, mental retardation; short stature, digital anomalies, and dental defects; colobomatous microphthalmos; blepharoptosis; nystagmus; strabismus
- Meckel syndrome (Meckel-Gruber syndrome)
  - Microcephaly, occipital encephalocele, or anencephaly; polycystic kidneys; polydactyly; congenital heart disease; genital abnormalities; microphthalmos, anophthalmos, cryptophthalmos; sclerocornea; partial aniridia; cataract; retinal dysplasia; optic nerve hypoplasia
- Otopalatodigital syndrome (Rubinstein-Taybi syndrome)
  - Intellectual and growth retardation; abnormally broad thumbs and broad great toes; characteristic facies with hypoplasia of maxilla and mandible, beaked nose, posterior rotation of ears; hypertrichosis; cryptorchidism; cardiac and renal anomalies; hypertelorism, with epicanthus, ptosis, and antimongoloid slant of palpebral fissures; cataract; colobomata; strabismus
- Seckel syndrome
  - Growth retardation, with small head circumference and characteristic face, narrow with beak-like nose ("bird head"); micrognathia and apparent prominence of maxilla; sometimes musculoskeletal and genitourinary anomalies; hypertelorism, with antimongoloid slant of palpebral fissures, prominent eyes; strabismus
- Freeman-Sheldon syndrome
  - Syndrome characterized by mask-like face with small pursed mouth, "whistling face"; ulnar deviation of the hand and fingers; talipes equinovarus; deep-set eyes; epicanthus, blepharophimosis, ptosis; strabismus
- Aicardi syndrome
  - Agenesis of the corpus callosum, with cortical heterotopia; seizures; mental retardation; costovertebral anomalies; multiple discrete chorioretinal defects of varying size; sometimes microphthalmos
- Wildervanck syndrome
  - Association of the Klippel-Feil malformation with congenital deafness and *Duane syndrome*, unilateral or bilateral (congenital defect in abduction with retraction of the globe or attempted adduction of the affected eye); epibulbar dermoid cysts
- Falls-Kertesz syndrome
  - Pterygium colli; later onset of lymphedema of lower extremities; distichiasis of all four lids; partial ectropion of lower lids
- Kartagener syndrome (see Sec. 14.53)
  - Pigmentary retinal disorder; cataracts

Miscellaneous multisystem disorders

- Oculocerebrorenal syndrome (Lowe syndrome; see Sec. 18.39)
  - Congenital cataracts in affected males; fine lens opacities in carrier females; glaucoma; rarely, microphthalmos
- Cerebrohepatorenal syndrome (Zellweger syndrome) (congenital adrenoleukodystrophy)
  - Profound hypotonia, growth retardation, and failure to thrive; hepatomegaly, jaundice, hypoprothrombinemia; renal cortical cysts; characteristic facies, flat profile; accumulation of iron in various organs; mild hypertelorism, flat supraorbital ridges, and epicanthal folds, cataracts; glaucoma (also, nonglaucomatous corneal haze); vitreous opacities; optic nerve hypoplasia; retinal pigmentary disorder (fundi generally hypopigmented, with fine to coarse spotty pigmentation, most marked peripherally)
- Laurence-Moon-Biedl syndrome (see Sec. 19.31)
  - Pleomorphic pigmentary retinal degeneration (retinitis pigmentosa type, with prominent macular involvement in some cases), with progressive vision impairment
- Prader-Willi syndrome
  - Hypotonia, hypomentia, hypogonadism, and obesity, with tendency to diabetes mellitus; strabismus
- Cockayne syndrome (see Sec. 23.15)
  - Pigmentary retinal degeneration; optic atrophy; cataracts; photophobia
- Werner syndrome
  - Syndrome of premature aging; in the 2nd decade, with cessation of growth, graying of the hair, alopecia, scleroderma-like changes of the skin, atherosclerosis, and diabetes mellitus; hypogonadism; increased risk of neoplasia; cataracts, juvenile onset; pigmentary retinal degeneration ("retinitis pigmentosa"); macular degeneration; glaucoma
- Asphyxiating thoracic dysplasia (Jeune syndrome; see Sec. 14.98)
  - Pigmentary retinal degeneration, with progressive vision impairment in some cases
- Alstrom disease
  - Nerve deafness, diabetes mellitus, and obesity in childhood; pigmentary retinal degeneration; cataracts
- Renal-retinal dystrophy
  - Interstitial nephritis; progressive pigmentary retinal degeneration, with attenuation of arterioles, reduced ERG, optic atrophy, and loss of vision
- Usher syndrome
  - Nerve deafness; mental retardation; epilepsy; pigmentary retinal degeneration ("retinitis pigmentosa"); cataracts
- Norrie disease
  - A syndrome of retinal malformation, mental retardation, and deafness; congenital retinal pseudoglioma; persistent hyperplastic primary vitreous, with vision loss; degenerative changes with phthisis bulbi; corneal opacities; cataracts

Congenital infection syndromes

- Congenital rubella (see Sec. 9.73)
  - Ophthalmic sequelae, both teratogenic and inflammatory; bilateral or unilateral effects; persistence of virus in the eye for months or years; microphthalmia; cataract (usually a dense pearly nuclear opacity with relatively clearer cortical rim); iris hypoplasia, atrophy synechiae (pupils often difficult to dilate); congenital glaucoma; transient nonglaucomatous corneal clouding in the newborn; retinopathy (pigmentary mottling "salt and pepper," focal or generalized, without loss of function); acute maculopathy (submacular neovascularization) as a delayed complication later in childhood in some cases, with attendant vision impairment; optic atrophy; vision defects and ocular motor abnormalities (nystagmus, strabismus) related not only to ocular involvement but also to effects of encephalomyelitis
- Congenital cytomegalovirus infection (see Sec. 9.69)
  - Chorioretinitis (single or multifocal atrophic and pigmented fundus lesions, more often peripheral than macular—sometimes perivascular retinal exudates and hemorrhages); anterior uveitis, conjunctivitis, and corneal clouding; optic atrophy; optic nerve hypoplasia; coloboma; microphthalmos; vision defects with strabismus, nystagmus
- Congenital toxoplasmosis (see Sec. 12.117)

Table continued on following page

TABLE 22–1. Clinical Features of Ocular Changes in Developmental Pediatric Syndromes *Continued*

Congenital infection syndromes *Continued*
Retinochoroiditis (retinitis, with secondary choroiditis, often with exudate into vitreous in early stages, resulting in single or multifocal atrophic and pigmented scars); often large macular lesions; satellite lesions and recurrent inflammation common in later years caused by persistence of organism in eye; vision loss, optic atrophy, retinal detachment, cataract, and glaucoma common; attendant oculomotor abnormalities (strabismus, nystagmus) attributed to ocular and/or CNS involvement; congenital anomalies of eye (e.g., microphthalmos)
Congenital syphilis (see Sec. 12.50)
Perivascular infiltration by *T. pallidum*, with inflammation in the cornea, uvea, retina, and optic nerve; persistence of the organism in the eye for years; interstitial keratitis, usually appearing after age 5 or 6 yr (iridocyclitis and intense photophobia in acute phase, vascularization and corneal opacification later, with decreased vision); retinopathy ("salt and pepper" pigmentary changes, frequently with arteriolar attenuation and disk pallor); retinal periphlebitis, sometimes with vascular occlusion; exudative uveitis in some cases; phthisis may result; disk edema; optic atrophy

Another form of hereditable dislocation is ectopia lentis et pupillae. In this condition there is displacement of both the lens and pupil, usually in opposite directions. This condition is generally bilateral, with one eye being almost a mirror image of the other. Ectopia lentis et pupillae is a recessive condition, although variable expression with some intermingling with simple ectopia lentis has been reported.

Systemic disorders associated with displacement of the lens include Marfan syndrome, homocystinuria, Weill-Marchesani syndrome, and sulfite oxidase deficiency. Ectopia lentis occurs in approximately 80% of patients with Marfan syndrome, and in about 50% of patients the ectopia is evident by the age of 5 yr. In most cases the lens is displaced superiorly and temporally; it is almost always bilateral and relatively symmetric. In homocystinuria the lens is usually displaced inferiorly and somewhat nasally. It occurs early in life, and is often evident by 5 yr of age. In Weill-Marchesani syndrome the displacement of the lens is often downward and forward and the lens tends to be small and round.

Ectopia lentis is also associated occasionally with other conditions, including Ehlers-Danlos, Sturge-Weber, Crouzon, or Klippel-Feil syndrome, oxycephaly, and mandibulofacial dysostosis. A syndrome of dominantly inherited blepharoptosis, high myopia, and ectopia lentis has also been described.

TREATMENT AND PROGNOSIS. Displacement of the lens often results only in optical problems; in other cases, however, more serious complications may develop, such as glaucoma, uveitis, retinal detachment, or cataract. Management must be individualized according to the type of displacement, its etiology, and the presence of any complicating ocular or systemic conditions. For many patients optical correction by spectacles or contact lenses can be provided. Sometimes manipulation of the iris diaphragm with mydriatic or myotic drops may help improve vision. In selected cases the best treatment is surgical removal of the lens. In many children treatment of any associated amblyopia must be instituted early. In addition, for the child with ectopia lentis, safety precautions should be taken to prevent injury to the eye.

MICROSPHEROPHAKIA

The term "microspherophakia" refers to a small, round lens that may occur as an isolated anomaly (probably autosomal recessive) or in association with other ocular abnormalities, such as ectopia lentis, myopia, or retinal detachment (possibly autosomal dominant). Microspherophakia may also occur in association with various systemic disorders, including Marfan syndrome, Marchesani syndrome, Alport syndrome, mandibulofacial dysostosis, and Klinefelter syndrome.

POSTERIOR LENTICONUS

This unusual anomaly is characterized by a circumscribed round or oval bulge of the posterior lens capsule and cortex, restricted to the 2- to 7-mm central (axial) region. It occurs in infants and young children and it tends to increase with age, often with cataractous changes in the lens cortex of the cone. Lenticonus usually occurs as an isolated ocular anomaly. It is generally unilateral but may be bilateral. It is believed to be sporadic, although autosomal dominant heredity has been suggested in some cases. Occasionally, it is a feature of a systemic disorder such as Alport syndrome. The infant or child with lenticonus may require lens surgery for progressive cataract, optical correction, amblyopia treatment, and care of secondary conditions, such as strabismus.

Alden ER, Kalina RE, Hodson WA: Transient cataracts in low-birth-weight infants. J Pediatr 82:314, 1973.

Bateman JB, Spence MA, Marazita ML, et al: Genetic linkage analysis of autosomal dominant congenital cataracts. Am J Ophthalmol 101:218, 1986.

Birch EE, Stager DR: Prevalence of good visual acuity following surgery for congenital unilateral cataract. Arch Ophthalmol 106:40, 1988.

Casper DS, Simon JW, Nelson LB, et al: Familial simple ectopia lentis. A case study. J Pediatr Ophthalmol Strab 22:227, 1985.

Chrousos GA, Parks MM, O'Neill JF: Incidence of chronic glaucoma, retinal detachment and secondary membrane surgery in pediatric aphakic patients. Ophthalmology 91:1238, 1984.

Cotlier E: Congenital varicella cataract. Am J Ophthalmol 86:627, 1978.

Cross HE: Ectopia lentis et pupillae. Am J Ophthalmol 88:381, 1979.

Cross HE, Jensen AD: Ocular manifestations in the Marfan syndrome and homocystinuria. Am J Ophthalmol 75:405, 1973.

Forman AR, Loreto JA, Tina LU: Reversibility of corticosteroid-associated cataracts in children with the nephrotic syndrome. Am J Ophthalmol 84:75, 1977.

Francois J: Late results of congenital cataract surgery. Ophthalmology 86:1586, 1979.

Gelbart SS, Hoyt CS, Jastrebski G, et al: Long-term visual results in bilateral congenital cataracts. Am J Ophthalmol 93:615, 1982.

Gillum WN, Anderson RL: Dominantly inherited blepharoptosis, high myopia, and ectopia lentis. Arch Ophthalmol 100:282, 1982.

Goldberg MF: Clinical manifestations of ectopia lentis et pupillae in 16 patients. Ophthalmology 95:1080, 1988.

Hiles DA: Intraocular lens implantation in children with monocular cataracts, 1974–1983. Ophthalmology 91:1231, 1984.

Jaafar MS, Robb RM: Congenital anterior polar cataract: A review of 63 cases. Ophthalmology 91:249, 1984.

Jensen AD, Cross HE, Paton D: Ocular complications in the Weill-Marchesani syndrome. Am J Ophthalmol 77:261, 1975.

Khalil M, Saheb N: Posterior lenticonus. Ophthalmology 91:1429, 1984.

Kirkam TH: Mandibulofacial dysostosis with ectopia lentis. Am J Ophthalmol 70:947, 1979.

Kohn BA: The differential diagnosis of cataracts in infancy and childhood. Am J Dis Child 130:184, 1976.

Levin AV, Edmonds SA, Nelson LB, et al: Extended-wear contact lenses for the treatment of pediatric aphakia. Ophthalmology 95:1107, 1988.

Maumenee IH: Classification of hereditary cataracts in children by linkage analysis. Ophthalmology 86:1554, 1979.

Morgan KS, McDonald MB, Hiles DA, et al: The nationwide study of epikeratophakia for aphakia in older children. Ophthalmology 95:526, 1988.

Morgan KS, McDonald MB, Hiles DA, et al: The nationwide study of epikeratophakia for aphakia in children. Am J Ophthalmol 103:366, 1989.

Nelson LB, Calhoun JH, Simon JW, et al: Progression of congenital anterior polar cataracts in childhood. Arch Ophthalmol 103:1842, 1985.

Parks MM: Visual results in aphakic children. Am J Ophthalmol 94:441, 1982.

Rasoby R, Ben Ezra D: Congenital and traumatic cataracts: The effect on ocular axial length. Arch Ophthalmol 106:1066, 1988.

Schimke RN, McKusick VA, Huang T, et al: Homocystinuria: Studies of 28 families with 38 affected members. JAMA 193:87, 1965.

Seetner AA, Crawford JS: Surgical correction of lens dislocation in children. Am J Ophthalmol 91:106, 1981.
Smith T, Holland MG, Woody NC: Ocular manifestations of familial hyperlysinemia. Trans Am Acad Ophthalmo Otolaryngol 75:355, 1971.
Townes PL: Ectopia lentis et pupillae. Arch Ophthalmol 94:1126, 1976.
Wets B, Milot JA, Polomeno RC, et al: Cataracts and ketotic hypoglycemia. Ophthalmology 89:999, 1982.

22.12 DISORDERS OF THE UVEAL TRACT

UVEITIS
(Iritis, Cyclitis, Chorioretinitis)

The uveal tract (the inner vascular coat of the eye, consisting of the iris, ciliary body, and choroid) is subject to inflammatory involvement in a number of systemic diseases, both infectious and noninfectious, and in response to exogenous factors, including trauma and toxic agents. Inflammation may affect any one portion of the uveal tract preferentially or all parts together.

Iritis may occur alone or in conjunction with inflammation of the ciliary body as iridocyclitis or in association with pars planitis. Pain, photophobia, and lacrimation are the characteristic symptoms of acute anterior uveitis, but the inflammation may develop insidiously without disturbing symptoms. Signs of anterior uveitis include conjunctival hyperemia, particularly in the perilimbal region (ciliary flush), cells and protein ("flare") in the aqueous humor, inflammatory deposits on the posterior surface of the cornea (keratic precipitates, or "KP"), congestion of the iris, and sometimes neovascularization of the iris. In more chronic cases there may be degenerative changes of the cornea (band keratopathy), lenticular opacities (cataract), and impairment of vision. The etiology of anterior uveitis is often obscure; primary considerations in children are rheumatoid disease, particularly pauciarticular rheumatoid arthritis, Kawasaki disease, and sarcoidosis. Iritis may be secondary to corneal disease, such as herpetic keratitis or a bacterial or fungal corneal ulcer, or to a corneal abrasion or foreign body. Traumatic iritis and iridocyclitis are especially common in children.

Choroiditis, inflammation of the posterior portion of the uveal tract, invariably also involves the retina; when both are obviously affected, the term "chorioretinitis" is used (Fig. 22–4). The causes of posterior uveitis are numerous; the more common are toxoplasmosis, histoplasmosis, cytomegalic inclusion disease, sarcoidosis, syphilis, tuberculosis, and toxocariasis. Depending on the etiology, the inflammatory signs may be diffuse or focal. Often there is vitreous reaction as well. With many types the result is atrophic chorioretinal scarring demarcated by pigmentation, often with visual impairment. Secondary complications include retinal detachment, glaucoma, or phthisis.

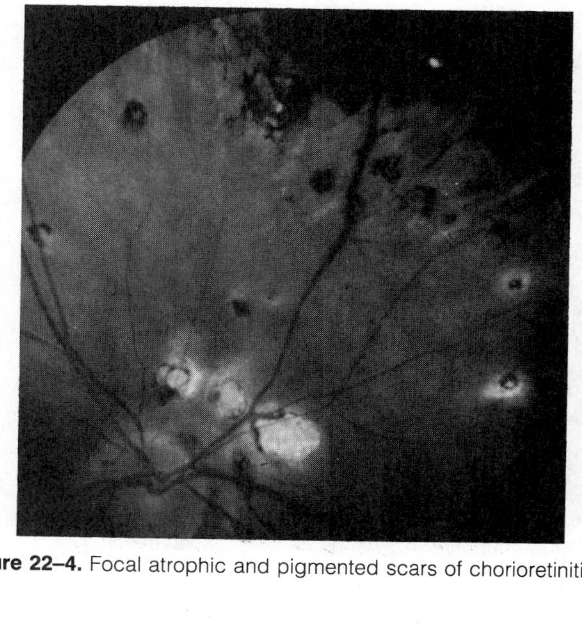

Figure 22–4. Focal atrophic and pigmented scars of chorioretinitis.

Panophthalmitis is inflammation involving all parts of the eye. It is frequently suppurative, most often as a result of a perforating injury or of septicemia. It produces severe pain, marked congestion of the eye, inflammation of the adjacent orbital tissues and eyelids, and loss of vision. In many cases the eye is lost despite intensive treatment of the infection and inflammation. Enucleation of the eye or evisceration of the orbit may be necessary.

Sympathetic ophthalmia is a rare type of inflammatory response that affects both eyes following perforating injury of one eye. It may occur weeks or even months after the injury. A hypersensitivity phenomenon is the most probable cause. Loss of vision may result.

TREATMENT. The various forms of intraocular inflammation are treated according to their etiologic factors. When infection is proven or suspected, appropriate antimicrobial therapy is used. Often, systemic and ocular treatment are required. In some cases subconjunctival or intravitreal injection of antibiotics is indicated. Prevention or reduction of inflammatory sequelae is also important in the treatment of these conditions; in selected cases, topical or systemic corticosteroids are used. Cycloplegic agents, particularly atropine, are also used to reduce inflammation and to prevent adhesion of the iris to the lens, especially in anterior uveitis.

Burke MJ, Rennebohm RM: Eye involvement in Kawasaki disease. J Pediatr Ophthalmol Strab 18:7, 1981.
Contreras F, Pereda J: Congenital syphilis of the eye with lens involvement. Arch Ophthalmol 96:1052, 1978.
Hart WM, Reed AB, Freedman HL, et al: Cytomegalovirus in juvenile iridocyclitis. Am J Ophthalmol 86:329, 1978.
Kanski JJ: Anterior uveitis in juvenile rheumatoid arthritis. Arch Ophthalmol 96:1794, 1977.
Kimura SJ: Uveitis in children: Analysis of 274 cases. Trans Am Ophthalmol Soc 62:171, 1964.
Lonn LL: Neonatal cytomegalic inclusion disease chorioretinitis. Arch Ophthalmol 88:434, 1972.
Lou P, Kazdan J, Basu PK: Ocular toxoplasmosis in three consecutive siblings. Arch Ophthalmol 96:613, 1978.
Makkey TA, Azar A: Sympathetic ophthalmia: A long-term follow-up. Arch Ophthalmol 96:257, 1978.
Molk R: Ocular toxocariasis: A review of the literature. Ann Ophthalmol 15:216, 1983.
Ryan SJ, Hardy PH, Hardy JM, et al: Persistence of virulent *Treponema pallidum* despite penicillin therapy in congenital syphilis. Am J Ophthalmol 73:258, 1972.
Smith ME, Zimmerman LE, Harley RD: Ocular involvement in congenital cytomegalic inclusion disease. Arch Ophthalmol 76:696, 1966.
Stern GA, Romano PE: Congenital ocular toxoplasmosis: Possible occurrence in siblings. Arch Ophthalmol 96:615, 1978.
Wilkinson CP, Welch RB: Intraocular toxocara. Am J Ophthalmol 71:921, 1971.

22.13 DISORDERS OF THE RETINA AND VITREOUS

RETINOPATHY OF PREMATURITY

This retinal angiopathy occurs primarily but not exclusively in preterm infants (see also Sec. 9.32). It may be active (early stages) or chronic (late stages). Clinical manifestations range from mild or transient changes of the peripheral retina to severe progressive vasoproliferation, cicatrization, and potentially blinding retinal detachment. Retinopathy of prematurity (ROP) refers to all stages of the disease and its sequelae.

Retrolental fibroplasia (RLF), the term previously used for this disease, described only the cicatricial stages.

PATHOGENESIS. Beginning at 16 wk of gestation, retinal angiogenesis normally proceeds from the disk to the periphery, reaching the outer rim of the retina (ora serrata) nasally at about 36 wk and temporally by approximately 40 wk. Injury to the process can result in various pathologic and clinical changes. The 1st observation in the acute or active phase is cessation of vasculogenesis. Rather than a gradual transition from vascularized to avascular retina there is an abrupt termination of the vessels, marked by a line in the retina. The line may then grow into a ridge composed of mesenchymal and endothelial cells. Cell division and differentiation may later resume, and vascularization of the retina may proceed. Alternatively, there may be progression to an abnormal proliferation of vessels out of the plane of the retina, into the vitreous, and over the surface of the retina, the ciliary body, and the equator of the lens. Cicatrization and traction on the retina may follow, leading to detachment.

The factors that cause ROP and determine its outcome are not fully known, but prematurity and the degree of retinal immaturity at birth are major factors. Hyperoxia is also a major factor, but other problems such as respiratory distress, apnea, bradycardia, heart disease, infection, hypoxia, hypercarbia, acidosis, anemia, and the need for transfusion may be contributory factors. Generally, the lower the birth weight and the sicker the infant, the greater the risk for ROP.

CLASSIFICATION. The currently used international classification of ROP (ICROP) describes the location, extent, and severity of the disease. To delineate location the retina is divided into three concentric zones, centered on the optic disk. Zone I, the posterior or inner zone, extends twice the disk-macular distance, or 30 degrees in all directions from the optic disk. Zone II, the middle zone, extends from the outer edge of zone I to the ora serrata nasally and to the anatomic equator temporally. Zone III, the outer zone, is the residual crescent that extends from the outer border of zone II to the ora serrata temporally; this area of the retina is vascularized last and is most frequently involved with ROP.

The extent of involvement is described by the number of circumferential clock hours involved. In the right eye 3 o'clock is nasal and 9 o'clock is temporal, whereas in the left eye 3 o'clock is temporal and 9 o'clock is nasal.

The phases and severity of the disease process are classified into five stages. Stage 1 is characterized by a demarcation line that separates vascularized from avascular retina (Fig. 22–5*A*). This line lies within the plane of the retina and appears relatively flat and white. There is often abnormal branching or arcading of the retinal vessels that lead into the line. Stage 2 is characterized by a ridge—the demarcation line has grown, acquiring height, width, and volume and extending up and out of the plane of the retina. It may change from white to pink. Vessels may leave the plane of the retina to enter the ridge. Stage 3 is characterized by the presence of a ridge and by the development of extraretinal fibrovascular tissue. Stage 4 is characterized by subtotal retinal detachment caused by traction from the proliferating tissue in the vitreous or on the retina. Stage 4 is subdivided into two phases: (1) subtotal retinal detachment not involving the macula; and (2) subtotal retinal detachment involving the macula. Stage 5 is total retinal detachment.

When signs of vascular decompensation accompany the active stages of ROP, the term "plus" disease is used. These signs include dilatation and tortuosity of the retinal vessels, engorgement of the iris, pupillary rigidity, and vitreous haze.

CLINICAL COURSE AND PROGNOSIS. In more than 90% of infants the course is one of spontaneous arrest and regression of the usually asymmetric disease process, with little or no residual effects or visual disability. In less than 10% of infants there is progression toward severe disease, with significant extraretinal vasoproliferation, cicatrization, detachment of the retina, and impairment of vision.

Some children with arrested or regressed ROP are left with demarcation lines, undervascularization of the peripheral retina, or abnormal branching, tortuosity, or straightening of the retinal vessels. Some are left with retinal pigmentary changes, dragging of the retina (so-called "dragged disk"), ectopia of the macula, retinal folds, or retinal breaks (Fig. 22–5*B*). Others proceed to total retinal detachment, which commonly assumes a funnel-like configuration. The clinical picture is often that of a retrolental membrane, producing leukocoria (a white or cat's eye reflex in the pupil). Some patients develop cataract, glaucoma, and signs of inflammation. The end stage is often a painful blind eye or a degenerated phthisical eye. The spectrum of ROP also includes myopia, which is often progressive and of significant degree in infancy. There may also be an increased incidence of anisometropia, strabismus, amblyopia, and nystagmus.

DIAGNOSIS. Systematic ophthalmologic examination of infants at risk is recommended. Guidelines vary and are

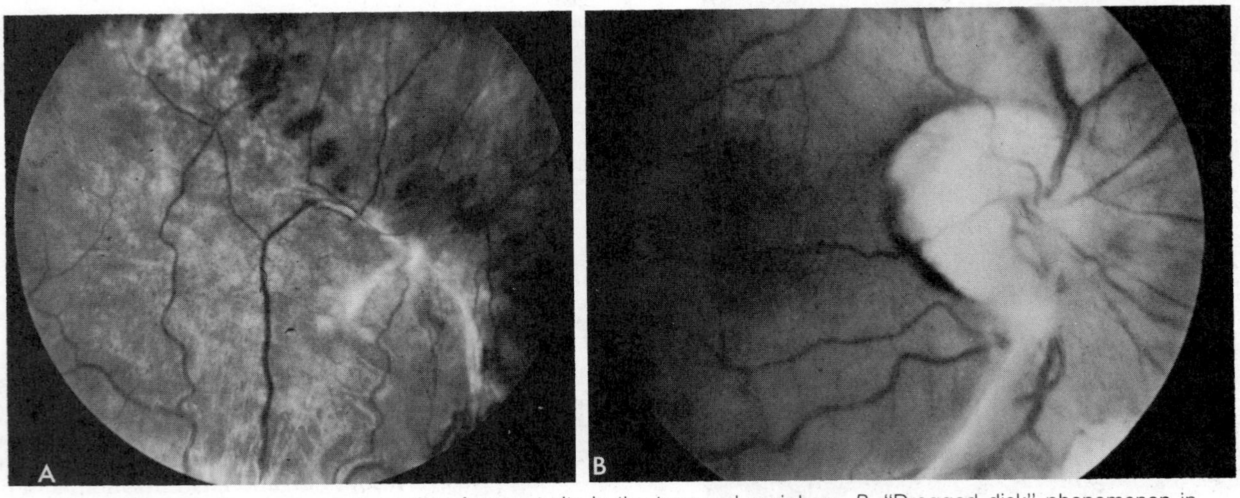

Figure 22–5. *A*, Developing retinopathy of prematurity in the temporal periphery. *B*, "Dragged disk" phenomenon in cicatricial retinopathy of prematurity.

changing but generally include infants weighing less than 2,000 g at birth, especially those weighing less than 1,500 g, those born before 33 wk gestational age, and those requiring supplemental oxygen. Some studies suggest that the optimal time for initial examination is from 7–9 wk, whereas others suggest 4–7 wk. ROP is diagnosed most often at 32–44 wk postconception. The examination can be stressful to the fragile preterm infant and the dilating drops can have untoward side effects, so discretion must be used in timing the eye examination and the infant must be carefully monitored during and after the examination. Follow-up is based on the initial findings and risk factors.

TREATMENT. In selected cases, cryotherapy to the avascular retina has been shown to reduce the more severe complications of progressive ROP to some extent. Also, advances in vitreoretinal surgical techniques have led to some success in reattaching the retina in infants with total retinal detachment (stage 5 ROP), but the visual results are often disappointing.

PREVENTION. Prevention of ROP ultimately depends on the prevention of premature birth and its attendant problems. Despite advances in technology and the meticulous care given to high-risk infants in modern nurseries, ROP continues to occur. Oxygen alone is neither sufficient nor necessary to produce ROP, and no safe level of oxygen has yet been determined. Each infant must be treated with whatever is necessary to sustain life and neurologic function. Some investigators have suggested the use of supplemental vitamin E for its antioxidant properties in infants at risk for ROP. Its efficacy has not been proven, however, and at certain dosage levels it may produce untoward side effects (see Sec. 9.32), but maintaining a sufficient vitamin E level is prudent.

PERSISTENT HYPERPLASTIC PRIMARY VITREOUS

Persistent hyperplastic primary vitreous (PHPV) refers to a spectrum of manifestations caused by the persistence of various portions of the fetal hyaloid vascular system and associated fibrovascular tissue.

During development of the eye, the hyaloid artery extends from the optic disk to the posterior aspect of the lens; it sends branches into the vitreous (vasa hyaloidea propria) and ramifies to form the posterior portion of the vascular capsule of the lens (tunica vasculosa lentis). The posterior portion of the hyaloid system normally regresses by the 7th fetal mo and the anterior portion by the 8th fetal mo. Small remnants of the system, such as a tuft of tissue at the disk (Bergmeister papilla) or a tag of tissue on the posterior capsule of the lens (Mittendorf dot) are common findings in healthy persons. More extensive remnants and associated complications constitute PHPV. Two major forms are described, anterior PHPV and posterior PHPV. Variability is great, and mixed or intermediate forms occur.

The usual manifestation of anterior PHPV is the presence of a vascularized plaque of tissue on the back surface of the lens in an eye that is microphthalmic or slightly smaller than normal. The condition is usually unilateral and may occur in infants with no other abnormalities and no history of prematurity. The fibrovascular tissue tends to undergo gradual contracture. The ciliary processes characteristically become elongated and the anterior chamber may become shallow. The lens usually is smaller than normal. The lens may be clear, but often it becomes cataractous and may swell or absorb fluid. Large or anomalous vessels of the iris may be present. There may be abnormalities of the anterior chamber angle. In time, the cornea may become cloudy.

Anterior PHPV is usually noted in the 1st weeks or months of life. The most frequent presenting signs are leukocoria (white or cat's eye reflex), strabismus, or nystagmus. The course is usually progressive and ill fated. Major complications are spontaneous intraocular hemorrhage, swelling of the lens caused by rupture of the posterior capsule, and glaucoma. The eye may eventually deteriorate. In selected cases, surgery can be done in an effort to prevent complications, to preserve the eye and a reasonably good cosmetic appearance and, in some cases, to salvage vision. Surgical treatment usually involves aspirating the lens and excising the abnormal tissue. If useful vision is to be attained, refractive correction and aggressive amblyopia therapy are required, but the visual results tend to be disappointing.

In some cases the affected eye is enucleated, because the differential diagnosis between this white mass and that of retinoblastoma can be difficult. Ultrasound and computed tomography are valuable aids in the differential diagnosis.

The spectrum of posterior PHPV includes fibroglial veils around the disk and macula, vitreous membranes and stalks containing hyaloid artery remnants projecting from the disk, and meridional retinal folds. Traction detachment of the retina may occur. Vision may be impaired, but the eye is usually retained.

RETINOBLASTOMA

Retinoblastoma (Fig. 22–6) is the most common primary malignant intraocular tumor of childhood (see also Sec. 17.21). The most frequent 1st sign is leukocoria, a white or cat's eye reflex in the pupil. Another frequent sign is strabismus, secondary to impairment of vision. Some children present with ocular inflammation, intraocular hemorrhage, glaucoma, or heterochromia iridis. On examination the tumor appears as a white mass, sometimes small and relatively flat, sometimes large and protuberant. It may appear nodular. Vitreous haze or tumor seeding may be evident.

RETINITIS PIGMENTOSA

This progressive retinal degeneration is characterized by pigmentary changes, arteriolar attenuation, usually some degree of optic atrophy, and progressive impairment of visual function. Dispersion and aggregation of the retinal pigment produce various ophthalmoscopically visible changes, ranging from granularity or mottling of the retinal pigment pattern to distinctive focal pigment aggregates with the configuration of bone spicules (Fig. 22–7).

Impairment of night vision or dark adaptation is often the 1st symptom. Progressive loss of peripheral vision, often in the form of an expanding ring scotoma or concentric contraction of the field, is usual. There may be loss of central vision. Retinal function, as measured by electroretinography (ERG), is characteristically reduced. Manifestations commonly begin in childhood. The disorder may be autosomal recessive, autosomal dominant, or sex-linked.

A special form of retinitis pigmentosa is Leber congenital retinal amaurosis, in which the retinal changes tend to be pleomorphic, with varying degrees of pigment disorder, arteriolar attenuation, and optic atrophy. Vision impairment is usually evident soon after birth, and the ERG is abnormal early.

To be differentiated from retinitis pigmentosa are clinically similar, secondary, pigmentary retinal degenerations that occur in a wide variety of metabolic diseases, neurodegenerative processes, and multifaceted syndromes. Examples include the progressive retinal changes of the mucopolysaccharidoses (particularly the syndromes of Hurler, Hunter, Scheie, and Sanfilippo) and certain of the late-onset gangliosidoses (the

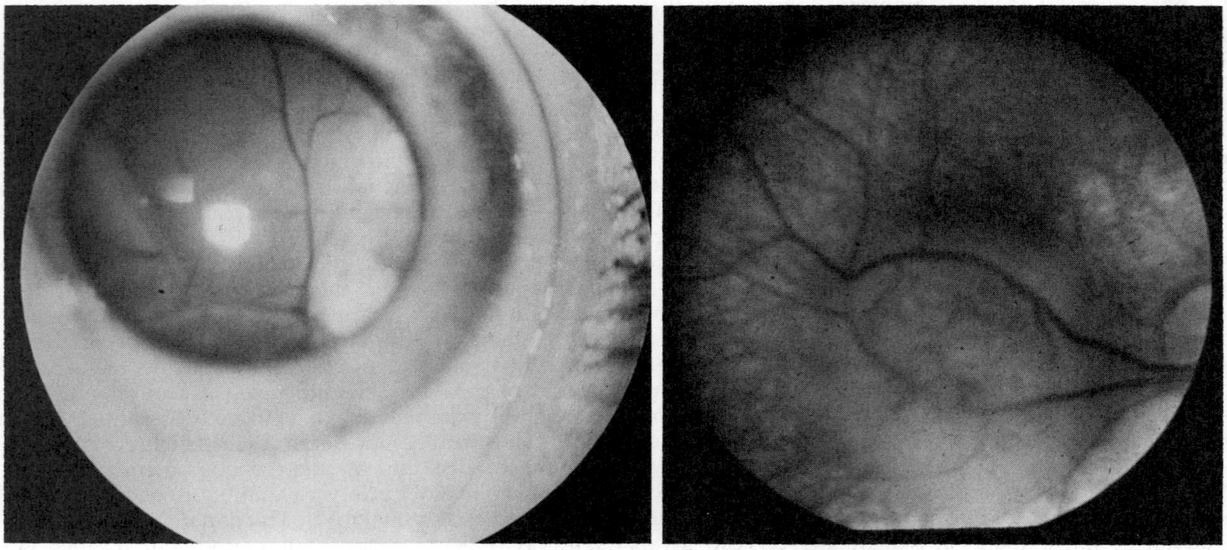

Figure 22–6. Retinoblastoma.

syndromes of Batten-Mayou, Spielmeyer-Vogt, and Jansky-Bielschowsky), the retinal manifestations of abetalipoproteinemia (Bassen-Kornzweig syndrome), the progressive retinal degeneration that is associated with progressive external ophthalmoplegia (Kearns-Sayre syndrome), and the retinitis pigmentosa-like changes in the Laurence-Moon-Biedl syndrome. There is also a high association of retinitis pigmentosa and hearing loss, as in Usher syndrome.

STARGARDT DISEASE
(Fundus Flavimaculatus)

This autosomal recessive retinal disorder is characterized by slowly progressive bilateral macular degeneration and vision impairment. It usually appears at 8–14 yr of age. The foveal reflex becomes obtunded or appears grayish, pigment spots develop in the macular area, and eventually macular depigmentation and chorioretinal atrophy occur. Macular hemorrhages also may develop. In some patients there are also white or yellow spots beyond the macula or pigmentary changes in the periphery; for such patients the term "fundus flavimaculatus" is used. Central visual acuity is reduced, often to 20/200, but total loss of vision does not occur. ERG findings vary. The condition is not associated with CNS abnormalities and is to be differentiated from the macular changes of many progressive metabolic neurodegenerative diseases.

BEST VITELLIFORM DEGENERATION

This macular dystrophy is characterized by a distinctive yellow or orange discoid subretinal lesion in the macula, resembling the intact yolk of a fried egg. Diagnosis is usually made at 5–15 yr of age; vision is usually normal at this stage. The condition may be progressive; the yolk-like lesion may eventually degenerate ("scramble") and result in pigmentation, chorioretinal atrophy, and vision impairment. There is no association with systemic abnormalities. Inheritance is usually autosomal dominant.

In vitelliform macular degeneration the electroretinographic response is normal. The electro-oculogram, however, is abnormal in affected patients and carriers and is therefore a useful test in diagnosis and in genetic counseling.

CHERRY RED SPOT

Because of the special histologic features of the macula, certain pathologic processes affecting the retina produce an ophthalmoscopically visible sign referred to as a cherry red spot, a bright to dull red spot at the center of the macula surrounded and accentuated by a grayish-white or yellowish halo. The halo is the result of loss of transparency of the multilayered ganglion cell ring as a result of edema, lipid accumulation, or both. The sign occurs typically in certain sphingolipidoses, principally in Tay-Sachs disease (GM_2 type 1), in the Sandhoff variant (GM_2 type 2), and in generalized gangliosidosis (GM_1 type 1). Similar but less distinctive macular changes occur in some cases of metachromatic leukodystrophy (sulfatide lipidosis), in some forms of neuronopathic Niemann-Pick disease, and in certain mucolipidoses. To be differentiated from the cherry red spot of neurodegenerative disease is the cherry red spot that characteristically occurs as the result of retinal ischemia secondary to vasospasm, ocular contusion, or occlusion of the central retinal artery.

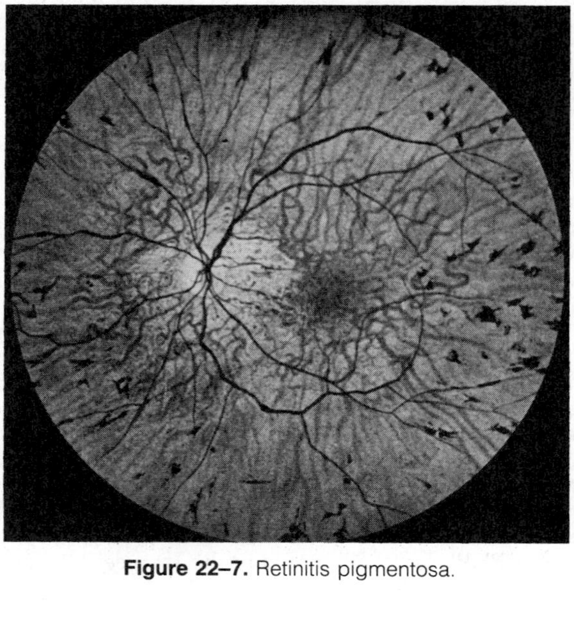

Figure 22–7. Retinitis pigmentosa.

PHAKOMATA

These are the herald lesions of the hamartomatous disorders. In Bourneville disease (tuberous sclerosis) the distinctive ocular lesion is a refractile, yellowish, multinodular cystic lesion arising from the disk or retina; the appearance of this typical lesion is often compared to that of an unripe mulberry (Fig. 22–8). Equally characteristic and more common in tuberous sclerosis are flatter, yellow to whitish retinal lesions, varying in size from minute dots to large lesions approaching the size of the disk. These lesions are benign astrocytic proliferations. Rarely, similar retinal phakomata occur in von Recklinghausen disease (neurofibromatosis). In von Hippel-Lindau disease (angiomatosis of the retina and cerebellum) the distinctive fundus lesion is a hemangioblastoma; this vascular lesion usually appears as a reddish globular mass with large paired arteries and veins passing to and from the lesion. In Sturge-Weber syndrome (encephalofacial angiomatosis) the fundus abnormality is a choroidal hemangioma; the hemangioma may impart a dark color to the affected area of the fundus, but the lesion is best seen with fluorescein angiography.

RETINOSCHISIS

Congenital hereditary retinoschisis, also referred to as *juvenile X-linked retinoschisis,* is a bilateral vitreoretinal dystrophy that appears early in life, often in infancy. It is characterized by a splitting of the retina into inner and outer layers. The usual ophthalmoscopic finding in affected males is an elevation of the inner layer of the retina, most commonly in the inferotemporal quadrant of the fundus, often with round or oval holes visible in the inner layer. There are often associated cystoid macular changes. In some cases frank retinal detachment or vitreous hemorrhage occurs.

Vision impairment varies from mild to severe; visual acuity may worsen with age, but good vision is often retained.

Carrier females are asymptomatic, but linkage studies may be useful to help detect carriers.

RETINAL DETACHMENT

Retinal detachment refers to separation of the neuroretina from the underlying retinal pigment epithelium. It may result from the development of a tear or hole in the retina (rhegmatogenous detachment) with the accumulation of fluid beneath the neuroretina, from the accumulation of fluid because of inflammatory processes (exudative detachment), subretinal hemorrhage, or neoplastic processes; or from the pull of vitreal or retinal scar tissue, membranes, or adhesions (traction detachment).

Most retinal detachments in the pediatric population are nonrhegmatogenous and occur in association with other ocular abnormalities or disease processes, such as retinopathy of prematurity, persistent hyperplastic primary vitreous, Coats' disease, retinoblastoma, toxocariasis, and certain anomalies of the optic nerve head (e.g., coloboma, pit, and morning glory disk anomaly). High myopia, ectopia lentis, and aphakia also predispose to retinal detachment. Rhegmatogenous detachments occur in children primarily as a result of trauma. Retinal detachment is also a feature of a number of systemic syndromes, particularly the Pierre Robin sequence.

The presenting sign of retinal detachment in an infant or child may be loss of vision, secondary strabismus and/or nystagmus, or leukocoria (white pupillary reflex). In addition to direct examination of the eye, special diagnostic studies such as ultrasonography and neuroimaging (CT, MRI) may be necessary to establish the etiology of the detachment and the appropriate treatment. Prompt care is essential if vision is to be salvaged.

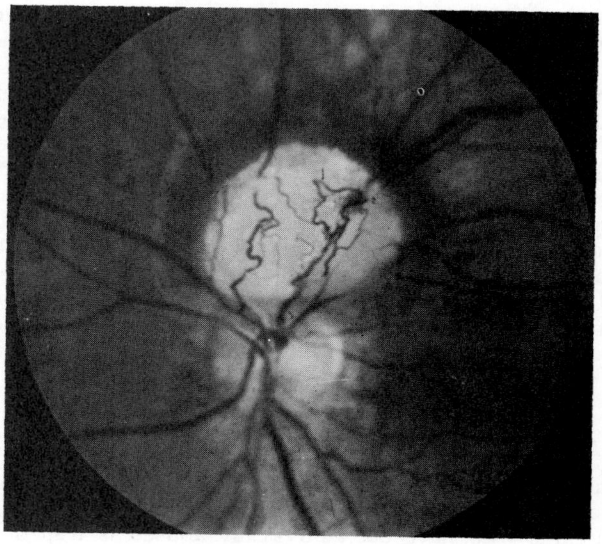

Figure 22–8. Retinal phakoma of tuberous sclerosis.

COATS' DISEASE

This exudative retinopathy of obscure etiology is characterized by telangiectasis of retinal vessels with leakage of plasma to form intraretinal and subretinal exudates, and by retinal hemorrhages and detachment. The condition is usually unilateral. It affects predominantly boys, usually appearing in the 1st decade. The condition is nonfamilial and for the most part occurs in otherwise healthy children. The most frequent presenting signs are blurring of vision, leukocoria, and strabismus. Rubeosis of the iris, glaucoma, and cataract may develop. Treatment with photocoagulation or cryotherapy may be helpful.

FAMILIAL EXUDATIVE VITREORETINOPATHY

This progressive retinovascular disorder is of unknown etiology, but clinical and angiographic findings suggest an aberration of vascular development. A significant finding in most cases is avascularity of the peripheral temporal retina, with abrupt cessation of the retinal capillary network in the region of the equator. The avascular zone often has a wedge- or V-shaped pattern in the temporal meridian. There may be glial proliferation or well-marked retinochoroidal atrophy in the avascular zone. Excessive branching of retinal arteries and veins, dilatation of the capillaries, arteriovenous shunt formation, neovascularization, and leakage from retinal vessels of the farthest vascularized retina occur. Vitreoretinal adhesions are usually present at the peripheral margin of the vascularized retina. Traction, retinal dragging and temporal displacement of the macula, falciform retinal folds, and retinal detachment are common. Intraretinal or subretinal exudation, retinal hemorrhage, and recurrent vitreous hemorrhages may develop. Patients may also develop cataracts and glaucoma. Vision impairment of varying severity occurs. The condition is usually bilateral. Familial exudative retinopathy (FEV) is an autosomal dominant condition; sporadic cases have been reported.

The findings in FEV may resemble those of retinopathy of prematurity in the cicatricial stages but, unlike ROP, the neovascularization of FEV seems to develop years after birth and in most patients with FEV there is no history of prematurity, oxygen therapy, prenatal or postnatal injury or infection, or developmental abnormalities.

FEV is also to be differentiated from Coats' disease, angiomatosis of retina, peripheral uveitis, and other disorders of the posterior segment.

HYPERTENSIVE RETINOPATHY

In the early stages of hypertension there may be no observable retinal changes. Generalized constriction and irregular narrowing of the arterioles are usually the 1st signs in the fundus. Other alterations include retinal edema, flame-shaped hemorrhages, "cotton-wool patches," and papilledema (Fig. 22–9). These changes are reversible if the disease can be controlled in the early stages, but in hypertension of longstanding, irreversible changes may occur. Thickening of the vessel wall may produce a silver- or copper-wire appearance.

Hypertensive retinal changes in the child should alert the physician to renal disease, pheochromocytoma, collagen disease, and cardiovascular disorders, particularly coarctation of the aorta.

DIABETIC RETINOPATHY

The retinal changes of diabetes mellitus are classified as simple or nonproliferative (early) or proliferative (more advanced).

Nonproliferative diabetic retinopathy is characterized by retinal microaneurysms, venous dilatation, and retinal hemorrhages and exudates. The microaneurysms appear as tiny red dots. The hemorrhages may be of both the dot and blot type, representing deep intraretinal bleeding, and the splinter or flame-shaped type, involving the superficial nerve fiber layer. The exudates tend to be deep and to appear waxy. There may also be superficial nerve fiber infarcts called cytoid bodies or cotton-wool spots, and retinal edema. These signs may wax and wane. They are seen primarily in the posterior pole, around the disc and macula, well within the range of direct ophthalmoscopy.

Proliferative retinopathy, the more serious form, is characterized by neovascularization and proliferation of fibrovascular tissue on the retina, extending into the vitreous. The vision-threatening complications of proliferative diabetic retinopathy are retinal and vitreous hemorrhages, cicatrization, traction, and retinal detachment. Rubeosis of the iris and secondary glaucoma may develop.

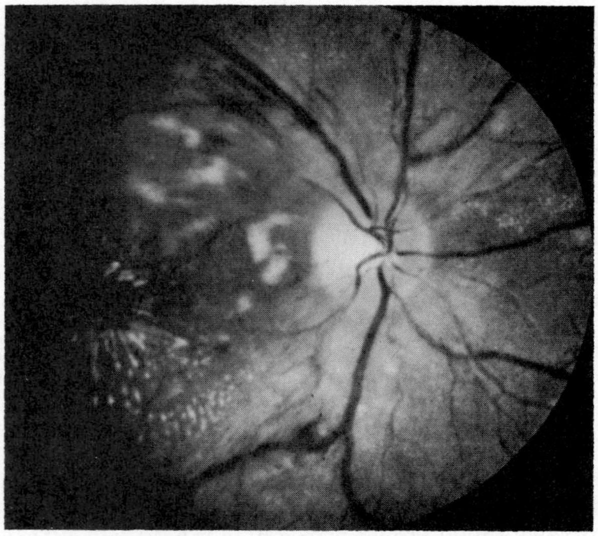

Figure 22–9. Hypertensive retinopathy.

Diabetic retinopathy involves the alteration and nonperfusion of retinal capillaries, retinal ischemia, and neovascularization, but its pathogenesis is not yet completely understood, either as to location of the primary pathogenetic mechanism (retinal vessels versus surrounding neuronal or glial tissue) or to the specific biochemical factors involved. The precise relationship between control of blood glucose and the genesis or progression of retinopathy remains unsettled, but data suggest that the better the degree of long-term metabolic control, the lower the risk of diabetic retinopathy.

Clinically, the prevalence and course of retinopathy relate to the patient's age and to duration of disease. Detectable microvascular changes are rare in prepubertal children, with the prevalence of retinopathy increasing significantly after puberty, especially after the age of 15 yr. The incidence of retinopathy is low during the 1st 5 yr of disease and increases progressively thereafter, with the incidence of proliferative retinopathy becoming substantial after 10 yr and with increased risk of visual impairment after 15 yr or more. Periodic ophthalmologic evaluation is recommended for all patients with diabetes mellitus.

In addition to retinopathy, patients with juvenile-onset diabetes may develop optic neuropathy, characterized by swelling of the disk and blurring of vision. Patients with diabetes may also develop cataracts, even at an early age, sometimes with rapid progression.

It is also prudent to check the color vision of children and their caregivers who must interpret the results of color-dependent glucose strip tests.

Advances in ocular therapy, such as retinal photocoagulation and vitrectomy, offer hope in reducing visual morbidity in some patients with diabetes. The value of technologic advances such as insulin infusion pumps and pancreatic transplants in the prevention of ocular complications is under investigation (Sec. 8.53).

SUBACUTE BACTERIAL ENDOCARDITIS

At some time during the course of the disease, retinopathy is present in approximately 40% of cases of subacute bacterial endocarditis. The lesions include hemorrhages, hemorrhages with white centers (Roth spots), papilledema and, rarely, embolic occlusion of the central retinal artery.

BLOOD DISORDERS

In primary and secondary anemias, retinopathy in the form of hemorrhages and cotton-wool patches may occur. Vision can be affected if hemorrhage occurs in the macular area. The hemorrhages may be light and feathery or dense and preretinal. In polycythemia vera, the retinal veins are dark, dilated, and tortuous. Retinal hemorrhages, retinal edema, and papilledema may be observed. In leukemia the veins are characteristically dilated, with sausage-shaped constrictions; hemorrhages, particularly white-centered hemorrhages and exudates, are common during the acute stage. In the sickling disorders, fundus changes include vascular tortuosity, arterial and venous occlusions, "salmon patches," refractile deposits, pigmented lesions, arteriolar-venous anastomoses, and neovascularization (with "sea-fan" formations), sometimes leading to vitreous hemorrhage and retinal detachment.

TRAUMA-RELATED RETINOPATHY

Retinal changes may occur in patients who suffer trauma to other parts of the body. The occurrence of retinal hemorrhages in infants who have been physically abused is well documented (Sec. 3.52). Retinal, subretinal, subhyaloid, and vitreous hemorrhages have been described. Often there are no signs of direct trauma to the eye, periocular region, or head. Such cases may result from violent shaking of the infant, and permanent retinal damage may result.

Retinal, subhyaloid, and vitreous hemorrhages are common in patients with traumatic and nontraumatic subarachnoid hemorrhage, an association referred to as Terson syndrome.

In patients with head or chest trauma, a traumatic retinal angiopathy known as Purtscher retinopathy may occur. This is characterized by retinal hemorrhage, cotton-wool spots, sometimes disk swelling, and decreased vision. The pathogenesis is unclear, but there is evidence for arteriolar obstruction in this condition.

Retinal hemorrhages and cotton-wool spots may also be seen after bone fractures or pelvic surgery, probably as the result of fat embolism.

MEDULLATED NERVE FIBERS

Myelination of the optic nerve fibers normally terminates at the level of the disk, but in some individuals ectopic medullation extends to nerve fibers of the retina. The condition is most commonly seen adjacent to the disk, although more peripheral areas of the retina may be involved. The characteristic ophthalmoscopic picture is a focal white patch with a feathered edge or brush-stroke appearance. Vision is generally not affected, but there may be relative or absolute visual field defects corresponding to areas of ectopic medullation. The eye is usually otherwise normal, but various abnormalities have been associated with ectopic medullation, including coloboma, cranial anomalies (oxycephaly), neurofibromatosis, basal cell nevus syndrome, anisometropic myopia, strabismus, and amblyopia, which may respond to treatment.

COLOBOMA OF THE FUNDUS

The term "coloboma" describes a defect such as a gap, notch, fissure, or hole. The typical fundus coloboma is a result of malclosure of the embryonic fissure, which leaves a gap in the retina, retinal pigment epithelium, and choroid, thus baring the underlying sclera. The defect may be extensive, involving the ciliary body, iris, and even lens, or it may be localized to one or more portions of the fissure. The usual appearance is of a well-circumscribed, wedge-shaped white area extending inferonasally below the disk, sometimes involving or engulfing the disk. In some cases there is ectasia or cyst formation in the area of the defect. Less extensive colobomatous defects may appear as only single or multiple focal "punched-out" chorioretinal defects or anomalous pigmentation of the fundus in the line of the embryonic fissure. Colobomata may occur in one or both eyes. Usually a visual field defect corresponds to the chorioretinal defect. Visual acuity may be impaired, particularly if the defect involves the disk or macula.

Fundus colobomata may occur in isolation as sporadic defects or inherited as a dominant or recessive condition, or may be associated with such abnormalities as microphthalmia, glioneuroma of the eye, cyclopia, or an encephaly. They occur in children with various chromosomal disorders, including 13-trisomy, 18-trisomy, triploidy, cat-eye syndrome, and 4p−. Ocular colobomata also occur in many multisystem disorders, including the CHARGE* association, Joubert, Aicardi, Meckel, Warburg, and Rubinstein-Taybi, linear sebaceous nevus, Goldenhar, Lenz microphthalmia syndromes, and Goltz focal dermal hypoplasia. Colobomata of the optic nerve in particular may be associated with basal encephalocele and serous detachment of the retina. Ocular colobomata have also been associated with congenital infection, including cytomegalovirus infection, and with the maternal use of thalidomide and lysergic acid diethylamide (LSD).

*C = coloboma; H = heart disease; A = atresia choanae; R = retarded growth and development and/or CNS anomalies; G = genetic anomalies and/or hypogonadism; E = ear anomalies and/or deafness.

Aaby AA, Kushner BJ: Acquired and progressive myelinated nerve fibers. Arch Ophthalmol 103:542, 1985.

Abramson DH, Ellsworth RM, Kitchin FD, et al: Second nonocular tumors in retinoblastoma survivors: Are they radiation-induced? Ophthalmology 91:1351, 1984.

Barr CC, Glaser JS, Blankenship G: Acute disc swelling in juvenile diabetes: Clinical profile and natural history of 12 cases. Arch Ophthalmol 98:2185, 1980.

Bateman JB, Riedner E, Levin LS, et al: Heterogeneity of retinal degeneration and hearing impairment syndromes. Am J Ophthalmol 90:755, 1980.

Berson EL, Rosner B, Siminoff E: Risk factors for genetic typing and detection in retinitis pigmentosa. Am J Ophthalmol 89:763, 1980.

Biglan AW, Brown DR, Reynolds JD, et al: Risk factors associated with retrolental fibroplasia. Ophthalmology 91:1504, 1984.

Boldrey EE, Egbert P, Gass DM, et al: The histopathology of familial exudative vitreoretinopathy: A report of two cases. Arch Ophthalmol 103:238, 1985.

Burns RP, Lourien EW, Cibis AB: Juvenile sex-linked retinoschisis: Clinical and genetic studies. Trans Am Acad Ophthalmol Otolaryngol 75:1011, 1971.

Chang M, McLean IW, Merritt JC: Coats' disease: A study of 62 histologically confirmed cases. J Pediatr Ophthalmol Strab 21:163, 1984.

Cotlier E: Café-au-lait spots of the fundus in neurofibromatosis. Arch Ophthalmol 95:1990, 1977.

CRYD-ROP group: Multicenter trial of cryotherapy for retinopathy of prematurity: three month outcome. Arch Ophthalmol 108:195, 1990.

Doft BH, Kingsley LA, Orchard TJ, et al: The association between long-term diabetic control and early retinopathy. Ophthalmology 91:763, 1984.

Dryja TP, Cavena W, White R, et al: Homozygosity of chromosome 13 in retinoblastoma. N Engl J Med 319:550, 1984.

Duane TD, Osher RH, Green WR: White-centered hemorrhages: Their significance. Ophthalmology 87:66, 1980.

Eagle RC, Lucier AC, Bernardino VB Jr, et al: Retinal pigment epithelial abnormalities in fundus flavimaculatus. Ophthalmology 87:1189, 1980.

Fishman GA: Retinitis pigmentosa: Genetic percentages. Arch Ophthalmol 96:822, 1978.

Foos RY: Chronic retinopathy of prematurity. Ophthalmology 92:563, 1985.

Frank RN: On the pathogenesis of diabetic retinopathy. Ophthalmology 91:626, 1984.

Frank RN, Hoffman WH, Podgor MJ, et al: Retinopathy in juvenile-onset diabetes of short duration. Ophthalmology 87:1, 1980.

Gallie BL, Phillips RA: Retinoblastoma: A model of oncogenesis. Ophthalmology 91:666, 1984.

Goldberg MF, Mafee M: Computed tomography for diagnosis of persistent hyperplastic primary vitreous (PHPV). Ophthalmology 90:442, 1983.

Hardwig P, Robertson DM: Von Hippel-Lindau disease: A familial, often lethal, multi-system phakomatosis. Ophthalmology 91:263, 1984.

Hittner HM, Rudolph AJ, Kretzer FL: Suppression of severe retinopathy of prematurity with vitamin E supplementation: Ultrastructural mechanism of clinical efficacy. Ophthalmology 91:1512, 1984.

Jackson RL, Ide CH, Guthrie RA, et al: Retinopathy in adolescents and young adults with onset of insulin-dependent diabetes in childhood. Ophthalmology 89:7, 1982.

Juan Verdaguer T: Juvenile retinal detachment. Am J Ophthalmol 93:145, 1982.

Kline R, Klein BEK, Moss SE, et al: The Wisconsin epidemiologic study of diabetic retinopathy: II. Prevalence and risk of diabetic retinopathy when age at diagnosis is less than 30 years. Arch Ophthalmol 102:520, 1984.

Knobloch WH, Layer JM: Clefting syndromes associated with retinal detachment. Am J Ophthalmol 73:517, 1972.

Kushner BJ: Strabismus and amblyopia associated with regressed retinopathy of prematurity. Arch Ophthalmol 100:256, 1982.

Kushner BJ, Essner D, Cohen IJ, et al: Retrolental fibroplasia. II: Pathologic correlation. Arch Ophthalmol 95:29, 1977.

Kushner BJ, Sondheimer S: Medical treatment of glaucoma associated with cicatricial retinopathy of prematurity. Am J Ophthalmol 94:313, 1982.

Laverda AM, Saia OS, Drigo P, et al: Chorioretinal coloboma and Joubert syndrome: A nonrandom association. J Pediatr 105:282, 1984.

Mann E, Kut LJ, Lee CB: Rheumatogenous retinal detachment in infancy. Arch Ophthalmol 95:1774, 1971.

Matthews JD, Weiter JJ, Kolodny EH: Macular halos associated with Niemann-Pick type B disease. Ophthalmology 93:933, 1986.

Margo C, Hidayat A, Kopelman J, et al: Retinocytoma: A benign variant of retinoblastoma. Arch Ophthalmol 101:1519, 1983.

Miyakulo H, Hashimoto K, Miyakulo S: Retinal vascular pattern in familial exudative vitreoretinopathy. Ophthalmology 91:1524, 1984.

Mohler CW, Fine SL: Long-term evaluation of patients with Best's vitelliform dystrophy. Ophthalmology 88:688, 1981.

Noble KG, Carr RE: Leber's congenital amaurosis: A retrospective study of 33

cases and a histopathological study of one case. Arch Ophthalmol 96:818, 1978.
Noble KG, Carr RE: Stargardt's disease and fundus flavimaculatus. Arch Ophthalmol 97:1281, 1979.
Nyboer JH, Robertson DM, Gomez MR: Retinal lesions in tuberous sclerosis. Arch Ophthalmol 94:1277, 1976.
Pagon RA: Ocular coloboma. Survey Ophthalmol 25:223, 1981.
Pagon RA, Graham JM, Zonana J, et al: Coloboma, congenital heart disease, and choanal atresia with multiple anomalies: CHARGE association. J Pediatr 99:223, 1981.
Palmer EA: Optimal timing of examination for acute retrolental fibroplasia. Ophthalmology 88:662, 1981.
Pruett RC, Schepens CI: Posterior hyperplastic primary vitreous. Am J Ophthalmol 69:535, 1970.
Ridgeway EW, Jaffe N, Walton DS: Leukemic ophthalmopathy in children. Cancer 38:1744, 1976.
Ridley ME, Shields JA, Brown GC, et al: Coats' disease: Evaluation of management. Ophthalmology 89:1381, 1982.
Riley FC, Campbell RJ: Double phakomatosis. Arch Ophthalmology 97:518, 1979.
Romayananda N, Goldberg MF, Green WR: Histopathology of sickle cell retinopathy. Ophthalmology 77:652, 1973.
Rosenthal AR: Ocular manifestations of leukemia. Ophthalmology 90:899, 1983.
Salazar FG, Lamiell JM: Early identification of retinal angiomas in a large kindred with von Hippel-Lindau disease. Am J Ophthalmol 89:540, 1980.
Shields JA, Augsburger JJ: Current approaches to the diagnosis and management of retinoblastoma. Surv Ophthalmol 25:347, 1981.
Stark WJ, Lindsey PS, Fagadau WR, et al: Persistent hyperplastic primary vitreous: Surgical treatment. Ophthalmology 90:452, 1983.
Stein MR, Gay AJ: Acute chorioretinal infarction in sickle cell trait. Arch Ophthalmol 84:485, 1970.
Straatsma BR, Foos RY, Heckenlively JR, et al: Myelinated retinal nerve fibers. Am J Ophthalmol 91:25, 1981.
Tasman W: Late complications of retrolental fibroplasia. Ophthalmology 86:1724, 1979.
The Committee for the Classification of Retinopathy of Prematurity: An international classification of retinopathy of prematurity. Arch Ophthalmol 102:1130, 1984.
The International Committee for the Classification of the Late Stages of Retinopathy of Prematurity: An international classification of retinopathy of prematurity. II: The classification of retinal detachment. Arch Ophthalmol 105:906, 1987.
Topilow HW, Ackerman AL, Wang FM: The treatment of advanced retinopathy of prematurity by cryotherapy and scleral buckling surgery. Ophthalmology 92:379, 1985.
Trese MT: Surgical results of stage V retrolental fibroplasia and timing of surgical repair. Ophthalmology 91:461, 1984.
Tso MOM, Jampol LM: Pathophysiology of hypertensive retinopathy. Ophthalmology 89:1132, 1982.
Walsh JB: Hypertensive retinopathy: Description, classification and prognosis. Ophthalmology 89:1127, 1982.
Yassur Y, Nissenkorn I, Ben-Sira I, et al: Autosomal dominant inheritance of retinoschisis. Am J Ophthalmol 94:338, 1982.
Zimmerman LE, Buras RP, Wankum G, et al: Trilateral retinoblastoma: Ectopic intracranial retinoblastoma associated with bilateral retinoblastoma. J Pediatr Ophthalmol Strab 19:320, 1982.

22.14 ABNORMALITIES OF THE OPTIC NERVE

OPTIC NERVE HYPOPLASIA

This developmental deficiency of optic nerve fibers has been attributed to primary failure in the differentiation of retinal ganglion cells or their axons. Alternatively, it may result from prenatal degeneration of the ganglion cell axons. In typical cases the nerve head is small and pale, with a pale or pigmented peripapillary halo or "double ring sign." This anomaly is associated with defects of vision and of visual fields of varying severity, ranging from blindness to normal or near-normal vision in the affected eye. Hypoplasia may be unilateral or bilateral, with clinical findings varying with the severity and laterality of the condition. Unilateral or asymmetric hypoplasia commonly presents as deviation (heterotropia, strabismus) of the more severely affected eye; the deviation usually develops early in life, but often the underlying visual defect is not suspected or detected until a later age. When there is bilateral hypoplasia of relatively severe degree, the defect in vision is usually appreciated early, and there is often obvious strabismus or secondary nystagmus. Mild hypoplasia may be unrecognized for years.

Optic nerve hypoplasia may occur alone or with other developmental abnormalities, including microphthalmia, anencephaly, hydrocephalus, and encephalocele. Optic nerve hypoplasia is a principal feature of septo-optic dysplasia of de Morsier, a developmental disorder characterized by the association of anomalies of the midline structures of the brain with hypoplasia of the optic nerves, optic chiasm, and optic tracts; typically, there is agenesis of the septum pellucidum, partial or complete agenesis of the corpus callosum, and malformation of the fornix, with a large chiasmatic cistern. There may be hypothalamic abnormalities and endocrine defects, ranging from panhypopituitarism to isolated deficiency of growth hormone, hypothyroidism, diabetes insipidus, or diabetes mellitus. Neonatal hypoglycemia and seizures are important presenting signs in affected infants. The condition does not appear to be familial, although it has occurred in siblings. There is no regularly associated chromosomal defect, although it may be present in infants with chromosomal aberrations such as 13-trisomy. Optic nerve hypoplasia is common in patients with albinism and aniridia. It may occur with somewhat increased frequency in infants of diabetic mothers. Optic nerve hypoplasia has been associated with the maternal use of dilantin, quinine, LSD, and alcohol during pregnancy.

OPTIC NERVE APLASIA

This very rare congenital anomaly is characterized by the absence of the optic nerves, retinal ganglion cells, and retinal blood vessels, with attendant blindness and absence of the pupillary reaction to light in the affected eye. It may occur as an isolated anomaly or in association with gross maldevelopment of the globe, malformation of the brain, or other developmental defects.

MORNING GLORY DISK ANOMALY

This term describes a congenital malformation of the optic nerve characterized by an enlarged, excavated, funnel-shaped disk with an elevated rim, resembling the flower for which it is named. There often is whitish tissue in the funnel, the abnormal vessel pattern involves multiple branches emerging radially, and there is usually pigmentary mottling of the peripapillary region. One or both eyes may be affected. There may be other developmental defects of the affected or fellow eye. Vision is usually impaired, and strabismus may be the 1st sign. Detachment of the retina may occur. The anomaly may be associated with developmental midline defects, including cleft lip and palate, agenesis of the corpus callosum, hypertelorism, and encephalocele.

TILTED DISK

In this congenital anomaly the vertical axis of the optic disk is directed obliquely, so a that the upper temporal portion of the nerve head is more prominent and anterior to the lower nasal portion of the disk, and the retinal vessels emerge from the upper temporal portion of the disk rather than from the nasal side. Often there is a peripapillary crescent or conus. There may be associated visual field defects and myopic astigmatism. Clinical recognition of the tilted disk syndrome is important to avoid confusion of its disk and visual field signs with those of papilledema and intracranial tumor.

DRUSEN OF THE OPTIC NERVE

These globular, acellular bodies are thought to arise from axoplasmic derivatives of disintegrating nerve fibers. Drusen may be buried within the optic nerve, producing elevation of the optic nerve head (which can be confused with papilledema), or they may be partially or completely exposed, appearing as refractile bodies at the surface of the disk. Visual field defects and spontaneous peripapillary nerve fiber layer hemorrhages may occur in association with drusen. Drusen may occur as an autosomal dominant condition. They have also been observed in children with various neurologic disorders, including primary megalencephaly, seizures, learning disorders, mental retardation, schizophrenia, tuberous sclerosis, and intracranial tumors.

PAPILLEDEMA

The term papilledema ("choked disk") can be applied to swelling of the nerve head of diverse etiologies, but it preferentially denotes the disk changes of increased intracranial pressure, including edematous blurring of the disk margins, fullness or elevation of the nervehead, partial or complete obliteration of the disk cup, capillary congestion and hyperemia of the nerve head, generalized engorgement of the veins, loss of spontaneous venous pulsation, nerve fiber layer hemorrhages around the disk, and peripapillary exudates. In some cases there may be edema extending into the macula, producing a fan- or star-shaped figure. In addition, there may be concentric peripapillary retinal wrinkling. There may be transient obscuration of vision, lasting seconds. Normally, when the intracranial pressure is relieved, the papilledema resolves and the disk returns to a normal or nearly normal appearance within 6–8 wk. Sustained chronic papilledema or longstanding unrelieved increased intracranial pressure may, however, lead to permanent nerve fiber damage, atrophic changes of the disk, macular scarring, and impairment of vision. In cases of impending or progressive vision loss caused by papilledema in patients with benign intracranial hypertension, decompression of the optic nerve by slitting the sheath may preserve vision.

The sequence of events as increased intracranial pressure leads to papilledema is probably as follows: elevation of intracranial subarachnoid cerebrospinal fluid pressure, elevation of cerebrospinal fluid pressure in the sheath of the optic nerve, elevation of tissue pressure in the optic nerve, stasis of axoplasmic flow and swelling of the nerve fibers in the optic nervehead, and secondary vascular changes and the characteristic ophthalmoscopic signs of venous stasis. Associated neurophthalmic signs of increased intracranial pressure in infants and children include abducent palsy and attendant esotropia, lid retraction, paresis of upward gaze, tonic downward deviation of the eyes, and convergent nystagmus.

The common causes of increased intracranial pressure and choked disk in childhood are intracranial tumors and obstructive hydrocephalus, intracranial hemorrhage, the cerebral edema of trauma, meningoencephalitis and toxic encephalopathy, and certain metabolic diseases. Whatever the etiology, the disk signs of increased intracranial pressure in early childhood may be modified by the distensibility of the young skull. In the absence of conditions associated with early closure of sutures and early obliteration of the fontanel (craniosynostosis, Crouzon, and Apert syndromes), infants with increased intracranial pressure usually do not develop papilledema.

To be differentiated from true papilledema are certain structural changes of the disk ("pseudopapilledema," "pseudoneuritis," drusen, and medullated fibers), with which it may be confused, and the disk swelling of hypertension and diabetes mellitus.

OPTIC NEURITIS

This term is used to describe any inflammation, demyelinization, or degeneration of the optic nerve with attendant impairment of function. The process is usually acute, with rapidly progressive loss of vision. It may be unilateral or bilateral. Pain on movement of the globe or pain on palpation of the globe may precede or accompany the onset of visual symptoms.

When the retrobulbar portion of the nerve is affected without ophthalmoscopically visible signs of inflammation at the disk, the term "retrobulbar neuritis" is applied. When there is ophthalmoscopically visible evidence of inflammation of the nervehead, the term "papillitis" or "intraocular optic neuritis" is used. When there is involvement of both the retina and papilla, the term "optic neuroretinitis" is used.

In childhood, optic neuritis rarely occurs as an isolated condition but is usually a manifestation of a neurologic or systemic disease. It may occur with bacterial meningitis or with viral infection (often accompanying encephalomyelitis following an exanthem). It may signify one of the many demyelinizing diseases of childhood. It may be the first manifestation of disseminated sclerosis. Alternatively, the cause may be an exogenous toxin or drug; optic neuritis may develop, for example, with lead poisoning or as a complication of long-term, high-dose treatment with chloramphenicol or vincristine therapy. Extensive pediatric neurologic and ophthalmic investigation, including neuroradiologic and electrophysiologic studies, is usually required.

In most cases of acute optic neuritis there is some improvement in vision beginning within 1–4 wk after onset, and vision may improve to normal or near normal within weeks or months. In some cases there is permanent impairment of vision. The course varies with etiology. Treatment of optic neuritis with high doses of systemic corticosteroids may sometimes be helpful in reducing inflammation and improving vision.

LEBER OPTIC NEUROPATHY

This maternally (mitochondrial DNA) inherited disorder may manifest in childhood, and affects males and females. Early signs include peripapillary telangiectatic microangiopathy, disk swelling, and sudden or gradual decrease in vision. One eye is usually affected before the other. In time there is usually progressive optic atrophy and vision loss. There may be associated electrocardiographic abnormalities.

OPTIC ATROPHY

This denotes degeneration of optic nerve axons, with attendant loss of function. The ophthalmoscopic signs of optic atrophy are pallor of the disk and loss of substance of the nerve head, sometimes with enlargement of the disk cup. The associated vision defect varies with the nature and site of the primary disease or lesion.

Optic atrophy is the common expression of a wide variety of congenital or acquired pathologic processes. The cause may be traumatic, inflammatory, degenerative, neoplastic, or vascular; intracranial tumors and hydrocephalus are principal causes of optic atrophy in children. In some cases, progressive optic atrophy is hereditary. Dominantly inherited infantile optic atrophy is a relatively mild heredodegenerative type that tends to progress through childhood and adolescence. Autosomal recessively inherited congenital optic atrophy is a rare condition that is evident at birth or develops at a very early age; the visual defect is usually profound. Behr optic atrophy is a hereditary type associated with hypertonia of the extremities, increased deep tendon reflexes, mild cerebellar ataxia, some degree of mental deficiency, and possibly external ophthalmoplegia. This disorder afflicts principally males from 3–11 yr of age. Some forms of heredodegenerative optic atrophy are associated with sensorineural hearing loss, as may occur in some children with juvenile-onset (insulin-dependent) diabetes mellitus. In the absence of an obvious cause, optic atrophy in an infant or child warrants extensive etiologic investigation.

OPTIC GLIOMA

The most frequent tumor of the optic nerve in childhood is optic glioma. This neuroglial tumor may develop in the intraorbital, intracanalicular, or intracranial portion of the nerve; often the chiasm is involved.

Histologically, optic glioma is usually a benign lesion; its deleterious effects vary with its location and growth pattern. Rarely, it may show malignant characteristics. The principal manifestations of intraorbital optic glioma are unilateral loss of vision, proptosis, and deviation of the eye; there may be optic atrophy or congestion of the optic nerve head. With chiasmal gliomas there may be defects of vision and visual fields (often bitemporal hemianopsia), increased intracranial pressure, papilledema or optic atrophy, hypothalamic dysfunction, pituitary dysfunction, and, sometimes, nystagmus, and/or strabismus.

Optic glioma occurs with increased frequency in patients with neurofibromatosis.

The natural clinical course of optic glioma often involves relatively slow, often self-limited progression; there may, however, be relentless progression to death. In some cases the course is rapidly progressive to death.

Management of optic glioma is controversial. When the tumor is confined to the intraorbital, intracanalicular, or prechiasmal portion of the nerve, resection is often done, especially when there is unsightly proptosis with complete or nearly complete loss of vision of the affected eye. When the chiasm is involved, surgery is not advocated, although surgical intervention to control secondary hydrocephalus and increased intracranial pressure, or to obtain biopsy material, may be necessary. Radiation may alter growth of the tumor. Chemotherapy is under trial.

Barr CC, Glaser JS, Blankenship G: Acute disc swelling in juvenile diabetes: Clinical profile and natural history of 12 cases. Arch Ophthalmol 98:2185, 1980.
Beck RW: The neuritis treatment trial. Arch Ophthalmol 106:1051, 1988.
Costin G, Murgpree AL: Hypothalamic-pituitary function in children with optic nerve hypoplasia. AJDC 139:249, 1985.
Danoff BF, Kramer S, Thompson N: The radiotherapeutic management of optic nerve gliomas in children. J Radiation Oncol Biol Phys 6:45, 1980.
Flickinger JC, Torres C, Deutsch M: Management of low-grade gliomas of the optic nerve and chiasm. Cancer 61:635, 1988.
Haik BG, Greenstein SH, Smith ME, et al: Retinal detachment in the morning glory anomaly. Ophthalmology 91:1638, 1984.
Hayreh SS: Optic disc edema in raised intracranial pressure: V. Pathogenesis. Arch Ophthalmol 95:1553, 1977.
Hayreh SS: Optic disc edema in raised intracranial pressure: VI. Associated visual disturbances and their pathogenesis. Arch Ophthalmol 95:1566, 1977.
Hoover DL, Robb RM, Petersen RA: Optic disc drusen and primary megalencephaly in children. J Pediatr Ophthalmol Strab 26:81, 1989.
Hotchkiss ML, Green WR: Optic nerve aplasia and hypoplasia. J Pediatr Ophthalmol Strab 16:225, 1979.
Hoyt CS: Autosomal dominant optic atrophy: A spectrum of disability. Ophthalmology 87:245, 1980.
Imes RK, Hoyt WF: Childhood chiasmal gliomas: Update on the fate of patients in the 1969 San Francisco study. Br J Ophthalmol 70:179, 1986.
Kazarian EL, Gager WE: Optic neuritis complicating measles, mumps and rubella vaccination. Am J Ophthalmol 86:544, 1978.
Kennedy C, Carter S: Relation of optic neuritis to multiple sclerosis in children. Pediatrics 28:377, 1961.
Kim RY, Hoyt WF, Lessell S, et al: Superior segmental optic hypoplasia: A sign of maternal diabetes. Arch Ophthalmol 107:1312, 1989.
Koenig SB, Naidich TP, Lissner G: The morning glory syndrome associated with sphenoidal encephalocele. Ophthalmology 89:1368, 1982.
Layman PR, Anderson DR, Flynn JT: Frequent occurrence of hypoplastic optic discs in patients with aniridia. Am J Ophthalmol 77:513, 1974.
Lessell S, Rosman P: Juvenile diabetes mellitus and optic atrophy. Arch Neurol 34:759, 1977.
Lewis RA, Gerson LP, Axelson KA, et al: Von Recklinghausen neurofibromatosis: II. Incidence of optic gliomata. Ophthalmology 91:929, 1984.
Margalith D, Jan JE, McCormick AQ, et al: Clinical spectrum of congenital optic nerve hypoplasia: Review of 51 patients. Dev Med Child Neurol 26:311, 1984.
Margalith D, Tse WJ, Jan JE: Congenital optic nerve hypoplasia with hypothalamic-pituitary dysplasia: A review of 16 cases. Am J Dis Child 139:361, 1985.
McLeod AR: Acute blindness in childhood optic glioma caused by hematoma. J Pediatr Ophthalmol Strab 20:31, 1983.
Nikoskelainen EK, Savontaus M-L, Wanne OP, et al: Leber's hereditary optic neuropathy, a maternally inherited disease: A genealogic study in four pedigrees. Arch Ophthalmol 105:665, 1987.
O'Dwyer JA, Newton TH, Hoyt WF: Radiologic features of septo-optic dysplasia: deMorsier syndrome. AJNR 1:443, 1980.
Packer RJ, Savino PJ, Bilaniuk LT, et al: Chiasmatic gliomas of childhood: A reappraisal of natural history and effectiveness of cranial irradiation. Child's Brain 10:393, 1983.
Petersen RA, Walton DS: Optic nerve hypoplasia with good visual acuity and visual field defects: A study of children of diabetic mothers. Arch Ophthalmol 95:254, 1977.
Repka MX, Miller NR: Optic atrophy in children. Am J Ophthalmol 106:191, 1988.
Rosenberg MA, Savino PJ, Glaser JS: A clinical analysis of pseudopapilledema. I: Population, laterality, acuity, refractive error, ophthalmoscopic characteristics, and coincident disease. Arch Ophthalmol 97:65, 1979.
Rosenstock JG, Packer RJ, Bilaniuk L, et al: Chiasmatic optic glioma treated with chemotherapy: A preliminary report. J Neurosurg 63:862, 1985.
Rush JA, Younge BR, Campbell RJ, et al: Optic glioma: Long-term follow-up of 85 histopathologically verified cases. Ophthalmology 89:1213, 1982.
Schwartz JF, Chutorian AM, Evans RA, et al: Optic atrophy in childhood. Pediatrics 34:670, 1964.
Selbst RG, Selhorst JB, Harbison JW, et al: Parainfectious optic neuritis: Report and review following varicella. Arch Neurol 40:347, 1983.
Sergott RC, Savino PJ, Bosley TM: Modified optic nerve sheath decompression provides long-term visual improvement for pseudotumor cerebri. Arch Ophthalmol 106:1384, 1988.
Skarf B, Hoyt CS: Optic nerve hypoplasia in children: Association with anomalies of the endocrine and CNS. Arch Ophthalmol 102:62, 1984.
Traboulsi EI, O'Neill JE: The spectrum in the morphology of the so-called "morning glory disc anomaly." J Pediatr Ophthalmol Strab 25:93, 1988.
Weiss AH, Beck RW: Neuroretinitis in childhood. J Pediatr Ophthalmol Strb 26:198, 1989.
Weiter JJ, McClean IW, Zimmerman IE: Aplasia of the optic nerve and disc. Am J Ophthalmol 83:569, 1977.

22.15 DISORDERS OF OCULAR PRESSURE

GLAUCOMA

Glaucoma refers to the abnormal elevation of the intraocular pressure of sufficient degree and duration to cause damage to the eye and changes in visual function. In infants and young children, the principal clinical manifestations of glaucoma are tearing, photophobia, blepharospasm, corneal clouding (edema), and progressive enlargement of the eye (buphthalmos). Optic atrophy, excavation (cupping) of the nerve head, and loss of visual acuity or visual field may result.

Glaucoma in infants and children is usually caused by a developmental abnormality of the filtration angle of the anterior chamber; commonly, there is residual mesodermal tissue that impedes drainage of the aqueous humor through the trabecular meshwork and canal of Schlemn. Primary or simple congenital glaucoma, long thought to be a recessive condition, is most probably inherited in a multifactorial fashion. Glaucoma associated with dominantly inherited goniodysgenesis has also been described.

In some infants and children with early-onset glaucoma there is more extensive maldevelopment of the anterior segment of the eye. Mesodermal dysgenesis, anterior cleavage syndrome, or various eponyms are used to describe these defects. One type, Peters anomaly, is characterized by the presence of a central corneal opacity (leukoma) with corresponding defects in the posterior corneal stroma, Descemet membrane, and endothelium, often with associated iridocorneal or lenticulocorneal adhesions. The condition is usually bilateral, although often asymmetric. It is generally sporadic, but recessive and dominant inheritance patterns have been suggested. Other anomalies within the spectrum of anterior chamber cleavage syndromes are anterior embryotoxon (prominent anteriorly displaced ring of Schwalbe), Axenfeld anomaly (presence of fine iris strands crossing the anterior chamber, attaching to the displaced ring of Schwalbe), and Rieger anomaly (anteriorly displaced ring of Schwalbe and iris adhesions, iris hypoplasia, and dyscoria). Within the spectrum there may be associated cataracts and various other abnormalities. Chromosomal defects have been found in some patients.

Other ocular anomalies that may be associated with glaucoma in infants and children are aniridia, cataract, spherophakia, and ectopia lentis. Glaucoma may also develop secondary to persistent hyperplastic primary vitreous (PHPV) or retinopathy of prematurity (ROP).

Trauma, intraocular hemorrhage, ocular inflammatory disease, and intraocular tumor are also important causes of glaucoma in the pediatric population.

Systemic disorders associated with glaucoma in infants and children are Sturge-Weber syndrome, von Recklinghausen disease, Lowe syndrome, Marfan syndrome, congenital rubella, a number of chromosomal syndromes, and juvenile xanthogranuloma.

TREATMENT. The treatment of congenital and infantile glaucoma is primarily surgical; surgery should be performed as early as the child's general medical condition allows. Procedures used to reduce and control ocular tension are goniotomy, goniopuncture, trabeculotomy, trabeculectomy and, in some cases, cyclocryotherapy. Frequently, multiple surgical procedures are required. In many cases, even after surgery, long-term medical therapy is also required. The prognosis for vision depends on normalization of intraocular pressure and prevention of optic nerve damage. In addition to control of ocular pressure, attention must be directed to the correction of associated refractive errors and the treatment of amblyopia. In some children there are also complicating factors such as cataracts, corneal opacities, and retinal and optic nerve abnormalities that affect visual outcome.

HYPOTONY

Abnormally low intraocular pressure may result from perforating ocular injury, or from ocular inflammation (cyclitis/uveitis) that impairs aqueous secretion. Acute hypotony occurs in infants or children with moderate to severe dehydration.

Barsoum-Homsy M, Chevrette L: Incidence and prognosis of childhood glaucoma: A study of 63 cases. Ophthalmology 93:1323, 1986.
Bardelli AM, Hadjistilianou T: Congenital glaucoma associated with other abnormalities in 150 cases. Glaucoma 9:10, 1987.
Boger WP III, Walton DS: Timolol in uncontrolled childhood glaucomas. Ophthalmology 88:253, 1981.
Cibis GW, Tripathi RC, Tripathi BJ: Glaucoma in Sturge-Weber syndrome. Ophthalmology 91:1061, 1984.
Cohen SMZ, Brown FR, Martyn L, et al: Ocular histopathologic and biochemical studies of the cerebrohepatorenal syndrome (Zellweger's syndrome) and its relationship to neonatal adrenoleukodystophy. Am J Ophthalmol 96:488, 1983.
Ginsberg J, Bove KE, Fogelson MH: Pathological features of the eye in the oculocerebrorenal (Lowe) syndrome. J Pediatr Ophthalmol Strabism 18:16, 1981.
Heckenlively JR, Isenberg SJ, Fox LE: The Reiger syndrome: A heritable disorder associated with glaucoma. Genet Clin Johns Hopkins Hosp 151:351, 1982.
Kivlin JD, Fineman RM, Crandall AS, et al: Peter's anomaly as a consequence of genetic and nongenetic syndromes. Arch Ophthalmol 104:61, 1986.
Kushner BJ, Sondheiner S: Medical treatment of glaucoma associated with cicatricial retinopathy of prematurity. Am J Ophthalmol 94:313, 1982.
McMahon CD, Hetherington J Jr, Hoskins HD, et al: Timolol and pediatric glaucomas. Ophthalmology 88(3):249, 1981.
McPherson SD Jr, Berry DP: Goniotomy vs external trabeculotomy for developmental glaucoma. Am J Ophthalmol 95:427, 1983.
Quigley HA: Childhood glaucoma: Results with trabeculotomy and study of reversible cupping. Ophthalmology 89:219, 1982.
Robin AL, Quigley HA, Pollack IP, et al: An analysis of visual acuity, visual fields, and disc cupping in childhood glaucoma. Am J Ophthalmol 88:847, 1979.
Zimmerman L: Ocular lesions of juvenile xanthogranuloma (nevoxanthoendothelioma). Trans Am Acad Ophthalmol Otolaryngol 69:412, 1965.

22.16 ORBITAL ABNORMALITIES

HYPERTELORISM AND HYPOTELORISM

Hypertelorism refers to wide separation of the eyes or an increased interorbital distance, which may occur as a morphogenetic variant, a primary deformity, or a secondary phenomenon in association with developmental abnormalities, such as frontal meningocele or encephalocele or the persistence of a facial cleft. There is often associated strabismus, generally exotropia, and sometimes optic atrophy.

Hypotelorism refers to narrowness of the interorbital distance, which may occur as a morphogenetic variant alone or in association with other anomalies, such as epicanthus, holoprosencephaly, or secondary to a cranial dystrophy, such as scaphocephaly.

EXOPHTHALMUS AND ENOPHTHALMUS

Protrusion of the eye is referred to as exophthalmos or proptosis. It may be caused by shallowness of the orbits, as in many craniofacial malformations, or by increased tissue mass within the orbit, as with neoplastic, vascular, and inflammatory disorders. Ocular complications include exposure keratopathy, ocular motor disturbances, and optic atrophy with loss of vision.

Posterior displacement or sinking of the eye back into the orbit is referred to as enophthalmos. This may occur with orbital fracture or with atrophy of orbital tissue. It is a feature of Horner syndrome.

ORBITAL CELLULITIS

Orbital cellulitis refers to a condition involving inflammation of the tissues of the orbit, with proptosis, limitation of movement of the eye, edema of the conjunctiva (chemosis), and inflammation and swelling of the eyelids. There is often some discomfort, usually with general symptoms of toxicity, fever, and leukocytosis (see also Sec. 14.31).

In general, orbital cellulitis may follow direct infection of the orbit from a wound, metastatic deposition of organisms during bacteremia, or direct extension or venous spread of infection from contiguous sites such as the lids, conjunctiva, globe, lacrimal gland, nasolacrimal sac, or paranasal sinuses. In some cases primary or metastatic tumor in the orbit can produce the clinical picture of orbital cellulitis.

The most common cause of orbital cellulitis in children is paranasal sinusitis, with the most frequent pathogenic organisms being *H. influenzae*, *S. aureus*, group A beta-hemolytic streptococci, and *S. pneumoniae*.

The orbital inflammatory manifestations of paranasal sinusitis vary with the location and extent of involvement. Stage 1 is swelling of the lids—the edema of impaired venous drainage or the reactive inflammation of underlying periostitis; in this stage the infection is still confined to the sinus. The 2nd stage is subperiosteal abscess, a collection of pus between the periosteum and the wall of the orbit, often with localized tenderness, displacement of the globe, and some limitation of eye movement. The 3rd stage is true orbital cellulitis, diffuse inflammation of the tissues within the orbit, with proptosis and impairment of ocular motility. The 4th stage is orbital abscess, resulting from localization of infection in the orbit or from extension of a subperiosteal abscess through the periosteum.

The potential for complications is great. Involvement of the optic nerve may result in loss of vision. Extension of infection from the orbit into the cranial cavity may lead to cavernous sinus thrombosis or meningitis or to epidural, subdural, or brain abscess.

Orbital cellulitis must be recognized promptly and treated aggressively. Hospitalization and systemic antibiotic therapy are usually indicated. In some cases surgical intervention is necessary to drain infected sinuses or a subperiosteal or orbital abscess.

PERIORBITAL CELLULITIS

Inflammation of the lids and periorbital tissues without signs of true orbital involvement (such as proptosis or limitation of eye movement) is generally referred to as periorbital or preseptal cellulitis. This is common in young children and may be caused by trauma, or by an infected wound, or by abscess of the lid or periorbital region (e.g., pyoderma, hordeolum, conjunctivitis, dacryocystitis, insect bite). It may be associated with respiratory infection or bacteremia, often with *H. influenzae,* streptococcus, or pneumococcus. What initially appears to be periorbital or preseptal cellulitis may be the 1st sign of sinusitis that may progress to true orbital cellulitis. Prompt antibiotic therapy and careful monitoring for signs of progression are essential.

TUMORS OF THE ORBIT

Various tumors occur in and about the orbit in childhood. Among benign tumors, the most common are vascular lesions (principally hemangiomas) and dermoids. Among malignant neoplasms, rhabdomyosarcoma, lymphosarcoma, and metastatic neuroblastoma are the most frequent. Optic gliomata and retinoblastomas that extend into the orbit also occur.

The effects of orbital tumors vary with their locations and growth patterns. The principal signs are proptosis, resistance to retroplacement of the eye, and impairment of eye movement. There may be a palpable mass. Other significant signs are ptosis, optic nerve head congestion, optic atrophy, and loss of vision. Bruit and visible pulsation of the globe are important clues to vascular lesions.

The differential diagnosis of orbital tumors is difficult; ultrasonography, magnetic resonance imaging, and computed tomography may be particularly helpful. Pseudotumor of the orbit also must be considered in children with signs of a mass lesion.

Haik BG, Jakobiec FA, Ellsworth RM, et al: Capillary hemangioma of the lids and orbit: An analysis of the clinical features and therapeutic results in 101 cases. Ophthalmology 86:760, 1979.

Hawkins DB, Clark RW: Orbital involvement in acute sinusitis: Lessons from 24 childhood patients. Clin Pediatr 16:464, 1977.

Mottow LS, Jakobiec FA: Idiopathic inflammatory orbital pseudotumor in childhood. Arch Ophthalmol 96:1410, 1978.

Pollard ZF, Calhoun J: Deep orbital dermoid with draining sinus. Am J Ophthalmol 79:310, 1975.

Porterfield JF: Orbital tumors in children: A report of 214 cases. Int Ophthalmol Clin 2:319, 1962.

Shields JA, Bakewell B, Augsberger JJ, et al: Classification and incidence of space-occupying lesions of the orbit: A survey of 645 biopsies. Arch Ophthalmol 102:1606, 1984.

Smith TF, O'Day D, Wright PF: Clinical implications of preseptal (periorbital) cellulitis in childhood. Pediatrics 62:1006, 1978.

Weiss A, Friendly D, Eglin K, et al: Bacterial periorbital cellulitis in childhood. Ophthalmology 90:195, 1983.

22.17 INJURIES TO THE EYE

About one third of all blindness in children results from trauma, usually avoidable. Injuries are caused by air rifles, arrows, darts, stones and missile-throwing toys, sticks, sharp tools, explosives, and strong chemicals. Many injuries cause acute pain, photophobia, tearing, blepharospasm, redness, or bleeding, prompting immediate consultation with a physician; unfortunately, some injuries do not produce such signs and symptoms and are often ignored.

ECCHYMOSES AND SWELLING OF THE EYELIDS

These are common after blunt trauma. Hemorrhage into the lids and periorbital region (the "black eye" or "shiner") is usually of no consequence and absorbs spontaneously, but it should prompt careful examination of the eye for deeper, more serious injury, such as intraocular hemorrhage or rupture of the globe.

LACERATIONS OF THE EYELIDS

These require careful management. Horizontal laceration of the upper lid may involve the levator, the tarsal plate, or the orbital septum. Faulty repair can result in ptosis, distortion of the lid, or herniation of orbital fat. Lacerations involving the lid margins require meticulous surgical apposition to prevent notching, eversion, or inversion of the margin or misdirection of the lashes that might lead to epiphora (tear overflow) and chronic irritation. Lacerations situated near the medial canthus may involve the punctum, canaliculi, or nasolacrimal duct and require the attention of an experienced ophthalmic surgeon. In all cases of lid laceration, examination of the globe for perforating injury is mandatory.

SUPERFICIAL ABRASIONS OF THE CORNEA

These usually produce pain or a foreign body sensation, sensitivity to light, tearing, redness, blepharospasm, and sometimes blurring of vision. The diagnosis is facilitated by fluorescein staining. Sterile paper strips impregnated with fluorescein dye are moistened and applied to the conjunctiva. The yellow dye diffuses in the tear film and "stains" any epithelial defect; the stain is best seen with the aid of a blue light.

Most superficial corneal abrasions heal promptly without complication. The injury is best treated initially by instillation of an antibiotic eye drop or ophthalmic ointment to prevent infection and application of a firm bandage (eye pad) to reduce eyelid movement and promote healing. The eye should then be examined within a day, preferably by an ophthalmologist, to determine the progress of healing and the need for further treatment (such as removal of a foreign body). In some cases attendant iritis requires the topical use of a cycloplegic agent or corticosteroid.

FOREIGN BODY ON OR IN THE CORNEA OR CONJUNCTIVA

This usually produces acute discomfort, lacrimation, and inflammation. Most foreign bodies can be detected by examination in good light with the aid of magnification; the direct ophthalmoscope set on a high plus lens (+10 or +12) is helpful. In many cases slit lamp examination is necessary, especially if the particle is deep or metallic. Some conjunctival foreign bodies tend to lodge under the upper eyelid, producing the sensation of corneal foreign body as they come into contact with the globe on eyelid movement; eversion of the lid may be necessary to detect such foreign particles (Sec. 22.2). If a foreign body is suspected but not found, further examination is indicated. If the history suggests injury with a high-velocity particle, roentgenographic examination of the eye may be needed to explore the possibility of intraocular foreign body.

Removal of a foreign body can be facilitated by the instillation of a drop of topical anesthetic. Many foreign bodies can be removed by irrigating or by gently wiping them away with a moistened cotton-tipped applicator. Embedded foreign bodies should be handled by an ophthalmologist. Removal of corneal foreign bodies may leave epithelial defects, which are treated as corneal abrasions. Metallic foreign bodies may cause rust to form in the corneal tissues; examination by an ophthalmologist a day or two after removal of a foreign body is recommended, because a rust ring would require further treatment (curettage).

LACERATIONS AND PERFORATING WOUNDS OF THE CORNEA OR SCLERA

These require immediate referral to an ophthalmologist and prompt surgical repair if the eye and vision are to be saved. Important clues to perforating injury of the eye are collapse of the anterior chamber, distortion and displacement of the pupil, and protrusion of dark tissue (uvea) into the wound. Emergency treatment consists of protecting the injured eye from further damage by applying a sterile bandage and a rigid eye shield. If these medical supplies are not on hand, an adequate eye shield can be fashioned from a plastic or styrofoam cup or from a piece of cardboard bent into a box or cone shape. Manipulation should be kept to a minimum, and no medication should be instilled except under the direction of an ophthalmologist.

HYPHEMA

This is the presence of blood in the anterior chamber of the eye. It may occur with either a blunt or perforating injury. Hyphema appears as a bright or dark red fluid level between the cornea and iris or as a diffuse murkiness of the aqueous humor. The treatment of hyphema usually includes bed rest, with the head elevated 30–45 degrees to promote settling and resorption of the blood. In some cases topical mydriatics, miotics, steroids, or oral aminocaproic acid are used. In some cases secondary bleeding occurs 3–5 days after the initial hemorrhage, increasing the risk of sequelae. The blood in the anterior chamber may produce elevation of intraocular pressure and blood staining of the cornea. These complications may affect vision. In such cases surgical evacuation of the clot and irrigation of the anterior chamber may be necessary.

OTHER INJURIES

Chemical Injuries

These require immediate, thorough, and copious irrigation. Whereas acids do their damage on contact, caustic alkalis may continue to penetrate and damage the tissue long after the initial contact, and require long-term ophthalmic care. In some cases reparative surgery is necessary for resultant corneal and conjunctival scarring.

Fracture of the Orbit

This is a common result of blunt trauma. Routine roentgenograms may fail to show the fracture; tomography is frequently necessary. Any portion of the orbital rim or any wall may be involved, but fracture of the floor of the orbit ("blow-out" fracture) is of special concern. Possible complications are entrapment of the extraocular muscles (resulting in restriction of movement of the eye and diplopia) and herniation of orbital fat or of the eye itself (resulting in enophthalmos). Such cases require surgical repair.

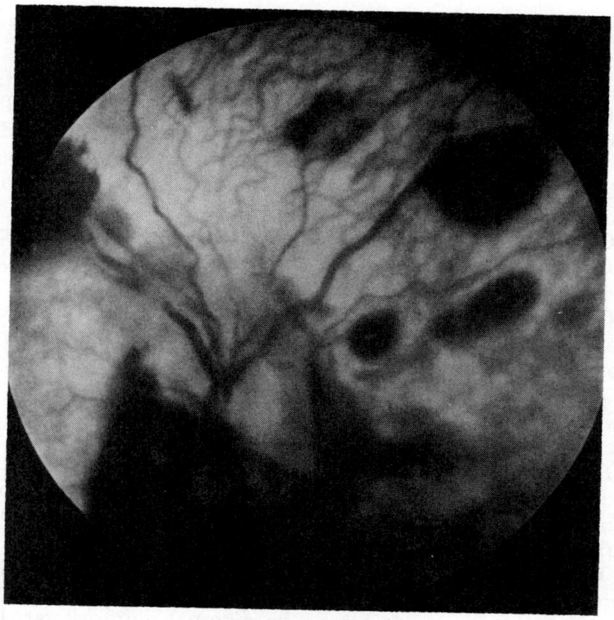

Figure 22–10. Retinal hemorrhages in the abused child with subdural hematoma.

Penetrating Wounds of The Orbit

These demand careful evaluation for possible damage to the eye, the optic nerve, or the brain. Examination should include investigation for retained foreign body. Orbital hemorrhage and infection are common with penetrating wounds of the orbit; such injuries must be treated as emergencies.

Child Abuse

This is a major cause of injuries to the eye and orbital region. The manifestations are numerous and may play a prominent role in the recognition of this syndrome. The possibility of nonaccidental trauma must be considered in any child with ecchymosis or laceration of the lids, hemorrhage in or about the eye, cataract or dislocated lens, retinal detachment, or fracture of the orbit (Fig. 22–10).

LOIS J. MARTYN

Emery JM, von Noorden GK, Schlernitzauer DA: Orbital floor fractures: Long-term follow-up of cases with and without surgical repair. Trans Am Acad Ophthalmol Otolaryngol 75:802, 1971.

Friendly DS: Ocular manifestations of physical child abuse. Trans Am Acad Ophthalmol Otolaryngol 75:318, 1971.

Hofman RF, Paul TO, Pentelei-Molner J: The management of corneal birth trauma. J Pediatr Ophthalmol Strab 18;45, 1981.

Pfister RR: Chemical injuries of the eye. Ophthalmology 90:1246, 1983.

Vinger PF: Sports eye injuries: A preventable disease. Ophthalmology 88:108, 1981.

Wilson FM: Traumatic hyphema: Pathogenesis and management. Ophthalmology 87:910, 1980.

22.18 THE EAR

Diseases and disorders of the ear are among the most frequently encountered morbid conditions of childhood. The ability to recognize their presence, the adequate knowledge of the most efficacious treatment, and the skills to prevent complications and sequelae are imperative for every physician caring for children.

CLINICAL MANIFESTATIONS. Eight prominent signs and symptoms are associated primarily with diseases of the ear and temporal bone:

Otalgia. This is most commonly associated with inflammation of the external and middle ear, but it may also arise from involvement of the temporomandibular joint, teeth, or pharynx. In young infants, pulling at the ear or general irritability, especially when either is associated with fever, may be the only sign of ear pain.

Purulent Otorrhea. This is a sign of otitis externa, otitis media with perforation of the tympanic membrane, or both. Bloody discharge may be associated with acute or chronic inflammation, trauma, neoplasm, or blood dyscrasias. Clear drainage suggests either a perforation of the drum with a serous middle ear effusion or a cerebrospinal fluid otorrhea draining through a defect in the external auditory canal or through the tympanic membrane from the middle ear.

Hearing Loss. This results from disease of either the external or middle ear (conductive hearing loss) or from pathology in the inner ear, retrocochlea, or central auditory pathways (sensorineural hearing loss).

Swelling. Swelling about the ear is most commonly the result of inflammation (e.g., external otitis, perichondritis, mastoiditis), trauma (hematoma) or, on rare occasions, neoplasm.

Vertigo. This is not a common complaint in children, but may sometimes be present. *Vertigo,* a specific type of dizziness, is defined as any hallucination or illusion of motion; *dizziness* refers to any altered orientation in space. The most frequent cause is eustachian tube–middle-ear disease, but vertigo may also be caused by labyrinthitis, perilymphatic fistula between the inner and middle ear from a congenital defect, trauma, or cholesteatoma, vestibular neuronitis, benign paroxysmal positional vertigo, Meniere disease, or disease of the central nervous system. Older children may describe a feeling of spinning or turning, whereas younger children may manifest the disequilibrium only by falling, stumbling, or clumsiness.

Nystagmus. Unidirectional, horizontal, or jerk nystagmus, usually associated with vertigo, is vestibular in origin.

Tinnitus. Although infrequently described by children, tinnitus is common, especially in patients with eustachian tube–middle-ear disease or with conductive or sensorineural hearing loss.

Facial Paralysis. This is an infrequent but frightening condition for both child and parents. When resulting from disease within the temporal bone in children, it most commonly occurs as a complication of acute or chronic otitis media, but it may also be idiopathic (Bell palsy) or be the result of temporal bone fracture or neoplasm; on rare occasions it may be caused by herpes zoster oticus. Other conditions associated with ear disease may also be present (e.g., symptoms of upper respiratory allergy associated with otitis media).

DIAGNOSIS. Adequately examining the entire child, paying special attention to the head and neck, can reveal a condition that may predispose to or be associated with ear disease. The facial appearance and the character of speech may be important clues to an abnormality of the ear. Many of the craniofacial anomalies, such as mandibulofacial dysostosis (Treacher Collins syndrome) and 21-trisomy (Down syndrome), are associated with disorders of the ear. Mouth breathing and hyponasality may indicate intranasal or postnasal obstruction; hypernasality is a sign of velopharyngeal insufficiency. Examining the oropharyngeal cavity may uncover an overt cleft palate or a submucous cleft, both of which predispose to otitis media with effusion. A bifid uvula may also be associated with middle-ear disease. Examination may reveal posterior nasal or pharyngeal inflammation and discharge. Polyposis, severe deviation of the nasal septum, or a nasopharyngeal tumor may be associated with otitis media.

The position of the patient for examination of the ear, nose, and throat depends on the patient's age, ability to cooperate, clinical setting, and preference of the examiner. The evaluation of an infant is best performed on an examining table. The presence of a parent or assistant is necessary to restrain the baby, because undue movement usually prevents an adequate evaluation (Fig. 22–11). Some clinicians prefer to place the infant prone on the table, whereas others prefer the patient to be supine. Use of the examining table is also desirable for older infants who are uncooperative or when a tympanocentesis or myringotomy is performed without general anesthesia. Infants and young children who are only apprehensive and not struggling actively can be evaluated adequately while sitting on the parent's lap. When necessary, the child may be restrained firmly on an adult's lap if the parent holds the child's wrists over the abdomen with one hand and holds the patient's head against the adult's chest with the other hand. If necessary, the child's legs can be held between the adult's thighs. Some infants can be examined by placing the child's head on the parent's knee. Cooperative children sitting in a chair or on the edge of an examination table can usually be evaluated successfully. The examiner should hold the otoscope with the hand or finger placed firmly against the child's head or face, so that the otoscope moves with the head rather than cause trauma (pain) to the ear canal if the child moves suddenly. Pulling up and out on the pinna usually straightens the ear canal enough to allow exposure of the tympanic membrane. In the young infant, the tragus must be moved forward and out of the way.

Examining the ear itself is the most critical assessment. The auricle and external auditory meatus should be examined first, because the presence or absence of signs of infection in

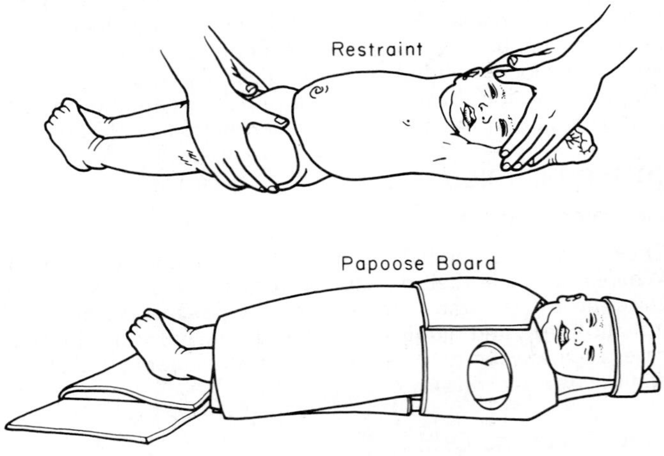

Figure 22–11. Methods of restraining an infant for examination and for procedures such as tympanocentesis or myringotomy. (From Bluestone CD, Klein JO: Otitis Media in Infants and Children. Philadelphia, WB Saunders, 1988.)

these areas may aid later in the differential diagnosis or evaluation of complications of otitis media. For instance, eczematoid external otitis may result from acute otitis media with discharge, or inflammation of the postauricular area may indicate a periosteitis or subperiosteal abscess extending from the mastoid air cells.

Next, the otoscopic examination, the most important part of physical assessment, is undertaken. However, before adequate visualization of the external canal and tympanic membrane is possible, obstructing cerumen must be removed from the canal. Removal of cerumen can usually be accomplished by use of an otoscope with a surgical head and a wire loop or a blunt cerumen curette, or by irrigating the ear canal *gently* with warm water. Instillation of hydrogen peroxide (3% solution) in the ear canal for 2–3 min softens cerumen and may facilitate removal with subsequent irrigation. Use of some commercial preparations (e.g., triethanolamine polypeptide oleate-condensate [Cerumenex]) may cause dermatitis of the external canal. These materials may be of value, however, if used infrequently and under the physician's supervision. The absence of cerumen and inflammation of the ear canal indicate external otitis. The external canal of the newborn is filled with vernix caseosa, which disappears shortly after birth.

The tympanic membrane and its mobility are properly assessed by using the pneumatic otoscope; assessing the light reflex is of limited value. The normal tympanic membrane is in the neutral position; a drum that is bulging is a condition that may be caused by increased middle-ear air pressure, by an effusion within the middle ear, or by both; the visualization of the malleus handle and short process is obscured by a bulging drum. Retraction of the tympanic membrane usually indicates the presence of middle-ear negative pressure, but it may also result from previous disease and subsequent fixation of the ossicles and ligaments. When retraction is present, the short process of the malleus is prominent and the long process is foreshortened.

The normal tympanic membrane has a "ground-glass" appearance; a blue or yellow color usually indicates a middle-ear effusion. A red membrane alone may not indicate pathology, because the blood vessels of the drum head may be engorged as the result of crying, sneezing, or blowing the nose. The normal tympanic membrane is also translucent, allowing the observer to look through it to visualize the middle-ear landmarks—incudostapedial joint, promontory, round window niche, and frequently the chorda tympani nerve. If a middle-ear effusion is present medial to a translucent drum, an air-fluid level or bubbles of air mixed with the fluid may be visible. Inability to visualize the middle-ear structures indicates opacification of the drum, usually caused by thickening of the tympanic membrane, to a middle-ear effusion, or to both.

Normal and abnormal middle-ear pressure are reflected in the pattern of tympanic membrane mobility when positive and then negative pressure are applied to the external canal using a pneumatic otoscope with a rubber ring around the tip of the end of the ear speculum to obtain a better seal in the external auditory canal. Normal middle-ear pressure is reflected by the neutral position of the tympanic membrane as well as by its response to both positive and negative pressures.

The eardrum may be retracted, usually because negative middle-ear pressure is present. The compliant membrane is maximally retracted by even moderate negative middle-ear pressure and hence cannot visibly be deflected inward farther with applied positive pressure in the ear canal. Negative pressure produced by releasing the rubber bulb of the pneumatic otoscope, however, causes a return of the eardrum toward the neutral position if a negative pressure equivalent to that in the middle ear can be created by releasing the rubber bulb, a condition that occurs when air, with or without an effusion, is present in the middle ear. When the middle ear pressure is even lower, there may be only slight outward mobility of the tympanic membrane because of the limited negative pressure that can be exerted through the otoscopes that are currently available. When assessing the mobility of the tympanic membrane in which a negative pressure is present within the middle ear, return of the tympanic membrane to the resting retracted position after the application of applied negative external canal pressure should not be confused with movement to applied positive pressure. This "rebound" of the eardrum after applied negative pressure may lead the examiner to conclude erroneously that the tympanic membrane is mobile to both positive and negative pressures and that, therefore, the middle-ear pressure is ambient. If the eardrum is severely retracted with extremely high negative middle-ear pressure or in the presence of a middle-ear effusion or both, the examiner is not able to produce significant outward movement.

The tympanic membrane that exhibits fullness moves to applied positive pressure but not to applied negative pressure if the pressure within the middle ear is positive and air, with or without an effusion, is present. In such an instance, the tympanic membrane is stretched laterally to the point of maximal compliance and does not visibly move outward any farther to the applied negative pressure but moves inward to applied positive pressure as long as some air is present within the middle ear-mastoid air cell system. A full tympanic membrane and positive middle-ear pressure without a middle-ear effusion are frequently seen in neonates and in young infants who are crying during the otoscopic examination; in older infants and children, the same situation may be encountered after the patient has sneezed, blown the nose, or swallowed when the nose was obstructed. However, in the initial stage of acute otitis media, the tympanic membrane may be full, with the characteristic findings of pneumatic otoscopy described before, because air is usually present within the middle ear. When the middle ear–mastoid air cell system is filled with an effusion and little or no air is present, the mobility of the bulging tympanic membrane is severely decreased or absent to both applied positive and negative pressures.

Aspiration of the middle ear is the definitive method of verifying the presence and type of a middle-ear effusion. Diagnostic tympanocentesis is performed by inserting, through the inferior portion of the tympanic membrane, an 18-gauge spinal needle attached to a syringe or a collection trap (Fig. 22–12). Alcohol cleansing and culturing of the ear canal should precede tympanocentesis and culture of the middle-ear aspirate. The canal culture helps to determine whether cultured organisms are contaminants from the external canal or pathogens from the middle ear.

Roentgenographic assessment of the ear and temporal bone is frequently helpful. When the tympanic membrane is not intact (as a result of perforation or insertion of a tympanostomy tube), *assessment of the ventilatory function of the eustachian tube* by pressure-flow studies may be an additional diagnostic aid. *Assessment of labyrinthine function* is essential in the evaluation of a child with a vestibular disorder (Sec. 20.24).

22.19 HEARING LOSS

INCIDENCE AND PREVALENCE. Although estimates vary because of differences in criteria for defining hearing impairment, the age group surveyed, and the methods of testing employed, from 0.5–1 newborn/1,000 live births has permanent, moderate to severe, bilateral sensorineural hearing loss. In addition, onset of hearing loss can occur at any time throughout childhood, for various reasons (see later). Thus, it is estimated that the prevalence of permanent, bilateral hearing loss of moderate to severe degree increases to 1.5–2/1,000 children under the age of 6 yr. When considering hearing loss of less severity or the transient or fluctuating hearing loss that accompanies middle-ear disease, so common in young children, the number of children with hearing loss at any given point in time increases substantially.

TYPES. Hearing loss can be peripheral or central in origin. Peripheral hearing loss is commonly caused by dysfunction in the transmission of sound through the external or middle ear or by the transduction of sound energy into neural activity at the inner ear and the 8th nerve. It can be conductive, sensorineural, or mixed. Conductive hearing loss occurs when sound transmission through the external or middle ear, or both, is physically impeded. Conditions such as impacted cerumen or foreign bodies in the external ear canal, an atretic or stenotic ear canal, interruption or fixation of the ossicular chain, perforation of the tympanic membrane, otitis media with effusion, otosclerosis, and cholesteatoma can cause conductive hearing loss. Damage to or maldevelopment of structures in the inner ear, such as destruction of hair cells because of noise, disease, or ototoxic agents, cochlear agenesis, perilymphatic fistula of the round or oval window membrane, and lesions of the 8th nerve are some conditions that cause sensorineural hearing loss. A combined conductive and sensorineural hearing loss is considered a mixed hearing loss.

Auditory deficits originating along the central auditory nervous system pathways, from the proximal 8th nerve to the cortex, are generally considered central hearing losses. Tumors, demyelinating disease, seizures, and various syndromes (e.g., Landau syndrome), can cause hearing deficits in the presence of normal outer, middle, and inner ears. Other forms of central auditory deficits, known as central auditory processing disorders, include those that make it difficult for normal hearing children to listen selectively in noise, to combine information from the two ears properly, to process speech when it is slightly degraded, and to integrate auditory information that is delivered faster than at a slow rate. Often no organic cause can be identified for such problems, but they can be quantified. They often manifest as poor attention or academic achievement, or as behavior problems in school. Strategies for coping with such disorders are available, and identification and documentation of the central auditory processing disorder is often valuable because parents and teachers are made aware of a valid reason for the child's poor attention or behavior, so adjustments can be made.

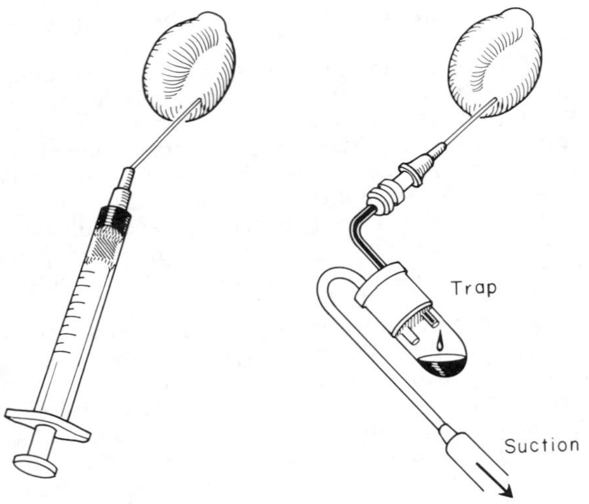

Figure 22–12. Tympanocentesis can be performed by employing a needle attached to a tuberculin syringe *(left)* or by using an Alden-Senturia collection trap (Storz Instrument Co., St. Louis). (From Bluestone CD, Klein JO: Otitis Media in Infants and Children. Philadelphia, WB Saunders, 1988.)

ETIOLOGY. The etiology of hearing impairment can be divided into four categories. Hearing impairment can be caused prior to or during birth (congenital), can occur at some time after birth (postnatal), can be caused by genetic factors, or may be acquired in another, nongenetic fashion. It is estimated that about 50% of cases of childhood hearing impairment of moderate to profound degree are genetically determined.

Genetic–Congenital Hearing Impairment. These disorders may be associated with other abnormalities or may be part of a syndrome. Hearing impairment occurs along with abnormalities of the external ear and eye and with disorders of the metabolic, musculoskeletal, integumentary, renal, and nervous systems. Pendred, Usher, and Waardenburg syndromes account for a large proportion of the sensorineural hearing impairments in this category. Chromosomal abnormalities such as 13–15-trisomy, 18-trisomy, and 21-trisomy can also be accompanied by hearing impairment. Agenesis or malformation of cochlear structures, including the Scheibe, Bing-Siebermann, Mondini, and Michel anomalies, are also genetic causes of congenital sensorineural hearing impairment.

Conductive hearing loss can also be genetically determined. Conditions, diseases, or syndromes that include craniofacial abnormalities are often associated with conductive hearing loss, and possibly also with sensorineural hearing loss. Pierre Robin, Treacher Collins, Klippel-Feil, and Crouzon syndromes and osteogenesis imperfecta are often associated with hearing loss. Congenital anomalies causing conductive hearing loss include malformations of the middle-ear structures and atresia of the external auditory canal.

A child with a parent having familial deafness is at risk for hearing impairment. Familial deafness can be dominant, recessive, or X-linked. Familial hearing impairment of the autosomal recessive type accounts for 70–80% of genetic-congenital sensorineural hearing impairment; X-linked disorders account for 1–3%. Whereas children with an easily identified syndrome or with anomalies of the outer ear may be identified as being at risk for hearing loss and monitored adequately, deafness of autosomal recessive genetic origin is often difficult to identify.

Genetic-Postnatal. Some genetically determined causes of hearing impairment do not express themselves until after birth. Familial hearing impairment can be of late onset with no other signs. Alport, Alstrom, and von Recklinghausen diseases and Hunter-Hurler syndrome are genetically determined hearing impairments with late onset in childhood.

Nongenetic-Congenital. Early in pregnancy the embryo is vulnerable to the effects of toxic modalities and substances. In the 1st trimester, ototoxic drugs (e.g., streptomycin, quinine, thalidomide), radiation, and infection (e.g., rubella, cytomegalovirus [CMV]) can damage the developing ear. Table 22–2 lists factors that place a newborn at risk for hearing impairment, including the genetic factors described in the

TABLE 22–2. Risk Factors That Identify Neonates At-risk for Sensorineural Hearing Impairment*

Family history of congenital or delayed onset childhood sensorineural impairment
Congenital infection known or suspected to be associated with sensorineural hearing impairment, such as toxoplasmosis, syphilis, rubella, cytomegalovirus, and herpes
Craniofacial anomalies including morphologic abnormalities of the pinna and ear canal, absent philtrum, low hairline
Birth weight less than 1,500 g (~3.3 lb)
Hyperbilirubinemia at a level exceeding indication for exchange transfusion
Ototoxic medications including but not limited to the aminoglycosides used for more than 5 days (e.g., gentamicin, tobramycin, kanamycin, streptomycin) and loop diuretics used in combination with aminoglycosides
Bacterial meningitis
Severe depression at birth, which may include infants with Apgar scores of 0–3 at 5 minutes or those who fail to initiate spontaneous respiration by 10 minutes or those with hypotonia persisting to 2 hours of age
Prolonged mechanical ventilation for a duration equal to or greater than 10 days (e.g., persistent pulmonary hypertension)
Stigmata or other findings associated with a syndrome known to include sensorineural hearing loss (e.g., Waardenburg syndrome or Usher syndrome)

*From the Joint Committee on Infant Hearing (1991) and Position Statement. ASHA 33:3, 1990.

previous section. Congenital CMV warrants special attention because it is associated with hearing loss in its symptomatic and asymptomatic forms, and the hearing loss may be progressive. Some children with congenital CMV have lost residual hearing suddenly at 4–5 yr of age. Persistent pulmonary hypertension of the newborn (PPHN) may also place newborns at risk for hearing impairment. All these factors account for about 50% of cases of moderate to profound sensorineural hearing impairment in neonates.

Nongenetic-Postnatal. Many of the risk factors mentioned in the preceding section (and in Table 22–2) can also affect the child after birth. Viral and bacterial infections can damage the inner ear. Some infections in children that are associated with sudden deafness include cryptococcal meningitis, measles, and mumps. Bacterial meningitis (especially pneumococcus and *H. influenzae*) is a major cause of childhood acquired hearing impairment (see also Sec. 12.15). Hearing loss in childhood can also be caused by ototoxic medications (e.g., aminoglycosides, platinum), noise exposure, head trauma, otitis media, vascular insults, lesions of the cranium, and various toxic substances.

EFFECTS OF HEARING IMPAIRMENT. These depend on the nature and degree of the hearing loss and on the individual characteristics of the child. Hearing loss may be unilateral or bilateral, conductive, sensorineural, or mixed, mild, moderate, severe, or profound, of sudden or gradual onset, stable, progressive, or fluctuating, and selective in the region of the acoustic spectrum affected (or it can affect most of the audible spectrum). Factors such as intelligence, medical or physical condition (including accompanying syndromes), family support, age at onset, age at time of identification, and promptness of intervention also affect the impact of hearing loss on a child.

Most hearing-impaired children have some usable hearing—only 6% of those in the hearing-impaired population have profound hearing loss. In general, hearing loss very early in life can affect the development of speech and language, social and emotional development, behavior, attention, and academic achievement. Some hearing-impaired children are misdiagnosed because they have sufficient hearing to respond to environmental sounds, can learn some language, and have some speech but, when challenged in the classroom, cannot perform to full potential.

Even a mild or unilateral hearing loss may have a detrimental effect on the development of a young child and on school performance. Children with such hearing impairments have greater difficulty when listening conditions are unfavorable (e.g., when there is background noise and poor acoustics), such as may occur in the classroom. Unfortunately, the fact that schools are auditory-verbal environments is not appreciated by those who minimize the impact of hearing impairment on learning. Hearing loss should be considered in any child with below-par performance, poor behavior, or inattention in school (Table 22–3).

Children with moderate, severe, or profound hearing impairment and/or those with other handicapping conditions are often educated in classes or schools for exceptional children. The auditory management and choices regarding modes of communication and education for children with hearing handicaps must be individualized, because these children are not a homogeneous group. A team approach to individual case management is essential, because each child and family unit represents unique needs and abilities.

HEARING SCREENING. Because hearing impairment can have a major impact on the development of a child, and because the earlier the impairment is identified the better the prognosis, early identification through screening programs is widely advocated. Many medical centers have such programs. Some use the high-risk register criteria (see Table 22–2) to decide which infants to screen, some screen all infants who require intensive care, and some do both. Screening methods include observing behavioral responses to uncalibrated noisemakers, using automated systems such as the Crib-o-gram or the auditory response cradle (in which movement of the infant in response to sound is recorded by motion sensors), and carrying out evoked potentials testing. The auditory brain stem response (ABR) test, an auditory evoked electrophysiologic response that correlates highly with hearing, also has been used successfully and cost-effectively to screen newborns.

Many children who are congenitally hearing impaired are not identified by the high-risk register or do not spend time in intensive care units. Such infants are not routinely screened at birth, although some centers advocate screening of all newborns. Furthermore, many children become hearing impaired after the neonatal period (see earlier). It is not until children are in school (or possibly in preschool) that formal hearing screening efforts are made. Consequently, the primary care physician or pediatrician should be alert to the signs and symptoms of childhood hearing impairment, so that those with hearing impairment who are not screened formally can be identified as early as possible.

Identification of Hearing Impairment. The impact of hearing impairment is greatest on the infant who has yet to develop language; therefore, identification, diagnosis, description, and habilitation should be done as soon as possible. In general, infants with a prenatal or perinatal history that puts them at risk (see Table 22–2) or those who have failed a formal hearing screening, should be followed closely by a clinical audiologist experienced in the evaluation and management of hearing-impaired children until a reliable assessment of auditory function has been obtained. The pediatrician and family physician are important in encouraging families to cooperate with the follow-up plan. Infants born at risk but who have not been screened as neonates should have a

TABLE 22–3. Hearing Handicap as a Function of Average Hearing Threshold Level of the Better Ear*

Average Threshold Level (dB) at 500–2,000) Hz (ANSI)†	Description	Common Causes	What Can Be Heard Without Amplification	Degree of Handicap (if not treated in 1st yr of life)	Probable Needs
0–15	Normal range		All speech sounds	None	None
16–25	Slight hearing loss	Serous otitis, perforation, monomeric membrane, sensorineural loss, tympanosclerosis	Vowel sounds heard clearly, may miss unvoiced consonant sounds	Possible mild or transitory auditory dysfunction Difficulty in perceiving some speech sounds	Consideration of need for hearing aid Lip reading Auditory training Speech therapy Preferential seating Appropriate surgery
26–40	Mild	Serous otitis, perforation, tympanosclerosis, monomeric membrane, sensorineural loss	Hears only some of speech sounds, the louder voiced sounds	Auditory learning dysfunction Mild language retardation Mild speech problems Inattention	Hearing aid Lip reading Auditory training Speech therapy Appropriate surgery
41–65	Moderate hearing loss	Chronic otitis, middle ear anomaly, sensorineural loss	Misses most speech sounds at normal conversational level	Speech problems Language retardation Learning dysfunction Inattention	All of the above, plus consideration of special classroom situation
66–95	Severe hearing loss	Sensorineural loss or mixed loss, caused by sensorineural loss plus middle ear disease	Hears no speech sound of normal converations	Severe speech problems Language retardation Learning dysfunction Inattention	All of the above; probable assignment to special classes
96+	Profound hearing loss	Sensorineural loss or mixed	Hears no speech or other sounds	Severe speech problems Language retardation Learning dysfunction Inattention	All of the above; probable assignment to special classes

*From Northern JL, Downs MP: Hearing in Children, 3rd ed. © 1984, The Williams & Wilkins Co., Baltimore.
†ANSI = American National Standards Institute.

hearing screening by 6 mo of age, carried out by a pediatric audiologist. Most infants, however, are born at facilities that do not have hearing screening programs.

Hearing-impaired infants who are born at risk and/or screened for hearing loss in a neonatal hearing screening program comprise only a portion of those in the pediatric hearing-impaired population. Those who are congenitally deaf because of autosomal recessive inheritance or silent TORCH infection are often not identified until the 2nd or 3rd year of life. Usually, the more severe the hearing loss, the earlier the age at identification, but, identification occurs later than the age necessary for an optimal outcome. Normal hearing children have developed a great deal of language by 3 yr of age. Parental concern regarding hearing and any delayed development of speech and language should alert the practitioner; often, parental concern precedes formal identification and diagnosis of hearing impairment by 6 mo–1 yr. Primary care physicians are uniquely able to respond to the concerns of parents and to monitor the development of speech and language. Table 22–4 presents guidelines for screening language development in young children and Table 22–5 provides guidelines for identifying children with abnormal auditory behavior. Failure to fulfill these criteria should be reason for referral for an audiologic evaluation.

Clinical Audiologic Evaluation. The importance of identification and diagnosis of hearing loss is widely understood, but what is not so well understood is the ability of a pediatric audiologist to obtain information on the hearing of infants and young children in a diagnostic setting. Even the youngest infants can be evaluated for auditory function. When hearing impairment is suspected in the young child, reliable and valid estimates of auditory function can be obtained. Successful management strategies for hearing-impaired children rely on prompt identification and ongoing assessment to define the dimensions of auditory function. Cooperation among the pediatrician and those specializing in such areas as audiology, speech and language pathology, education, and child development is necessary to optimize auditory-verbal development. Management of the hearing-impaired child includes the consideration (and often fitting) of an amplification device; the

TABLE 22–4. Criteria for Referral for Audiologic Assessment*

Age (mo)	Referral Guidelines for Children with "Speech" Delay
12	No differentiated babbling or vocal imitation
18	No use of single words
24	Single-word vocabulary of ≤10 words
30	Fewer than 100 words; no evidence of two-word combinations; unintelligible
36	Fewer than 200 words; no use of telegraphic sentences, clarity <50%
48	Fewer than 600 words; no use of simple sentences; clarity ≤80%

*From Matkin ND: Early recognition and referral of hearing-impaired children. Pediatr Rev 6:151, 1984. Reproduced by permission of Pediatrics.

TABLE 22–5. Guidelines for Referral of Children Suspected of Hearing Loss*

Age (mo)	Normal Development
0–4	Should startle to loud sounds, quiet to mother's voice, momentarily cease activity when sound is presented at a conversational level
5–6	Should correctly localize to sound presented in a horizontal plane, begin to imitate sounds in own speech repertoire or at least reciprocally vocalize with an adult
7–12	Should correctly localize to sound presented in any plane Should respond to name, even when spoken quietly
13–15	Should point toward an unexpected sound or to familiar objects or persons when asked
16–18	Should follow simple directions without gestural or other visual cues; can be trained to reach toward an interesting toy at midline when a sound is presented
19–24	Should point to body parts when asked; by 21–24 mo, can be trained to perform play audiometry

*From Matkin ND: Early recognition and referral of hearing-impaired children. Pediatr Rev 6:151, 1984. Reproduced by permission of Pediatrics.

monitoring hearing and auditory skills, counseling parents and families, advising teachers, and dealing with public agencies.

Audiometry. The goal of the audiologic evaluation can vary as a function of the age or developmental level of the child, the reason for the evaluation, and the child's otologic condition and/or history. The audiogram provides the fundamental description of hearing sensitivity (Fig. 22–13). Hearing thresholds are assessed as a function of frequency using pure tones (sine waves) at octave intervals from 250–8,000 Hz. Typically, earphones are used and hearing is assessed independently for each ear. Air-conducted signals are presented through earphones (or loudspeakers) and are used to provide information regarding the sensitivity of the auditory system. To begin the differential diagnosis of hearing loss, these same test sounds can be delivered to the ear through an oscillator that is placed on the head, usually on the mastoid. Such signals are considered bone-conducted signals, because the bones of the skull are vibrated and sound energy is transmitted directly to the inner ear, essentially bypassing the outer and middle ears. In the normal ear, the air and bone conduction thresholds are the same; they are also the same in those with sensorineural hearing loss. In those with conductive hearing loss, however, there is a difference between the air and bone conduction thresholds. This is called the air-borne gap; it indicates the amount of hearing loss attributable to dysfunction in the outer and/or middle ear. When there is mixed hearing loss, both the bone and air conduction thresholds are abnormal, and there is an air-bone gap.

Speech Recognition Threshold. Another measure useful for describing auditory function is the speech recognition threshold (SRT), which is the lowest intensity level at which a score of approximately 50% correct is obtained on a task of recognizing spondee words. Spondee words are two-syllable words or phrases that have equal stress on each syllable (e.g., baseball, hot dog, pancake). The listener must be familiar with all the words in order for a valid test result to be obtained. The SRT should correspond with the average of pure-tone thresholds at 500, 1,000, and 2,000 Hz, the pure-tone average (PTA). The SRT is relevant because much of the rationale for assessing hearing in children involves determining the adequacy for development and use of speech and language. It also serves to check the validity of the evaluation, because children with nonorganic hearing loss (i.e., malingerers) often have a large discrepancy between the PTA and SRT. Audiometric configuration, however, can also affect the SRT-PTA relationship and should be considered before assessing the possibility of malingering.

The basic battery of hearing tests concludes with an assessment of the child's ability to understand monosyllabic words when presented at a comfortable listening level. Performance on such word intelligibility tests assists in the differential diagnosis of hearing impairment, and also provides a measure of how well a child performs when speech is presented at loudness levels similar to those encountered in the environment.

Play Audiometry. For children at or above the developmental level of a 5- or 6-yr-old, conventional test methods can be used. For children from 2½–5 yr old, a technique called play audiometry can be used. Responses in play audiometry are usually conditioned motor activities associated with a game, such as dropping blocks in a bucket, placing rings on a peg, stringing beads, or completing a puzzle. The technique can be used to obtain a reliable audiogram of the preschool child. For those who will not or cannot repeat words clearly for the SRT and word intelligibility tasks, pictures can be used with a pointing response.

Visual Reinforcement Audiometry. For those between the ages of about 5–6 mo and 2½ yr, visual reinforcement audiometry (VRA) is commonly used. The technique incorporates a head-turning response with the activation of an animated (mechanical) toy reinforcer. If infants are properly conditioned, VRA can provide reliable estimates of hearing sensitivity for tones and speech sounds. In most applications of VRA sounds are presented by loudspeaker(s) in a sound field, so no ear-specific information is obtained. Often, how-

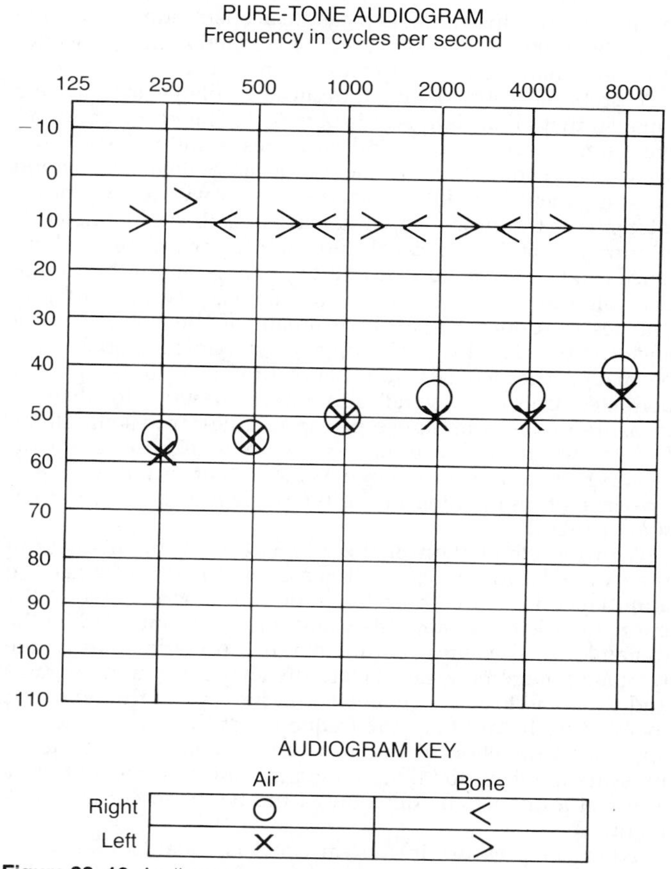

Figure 22–13. Audiogram demonstrating a bilateral conductive hearing loss.

ever, assessment of the infant is designed to rule out hearing loss that would affect the development of speech and language. Normal sound field response levels of infants indicate sufficient hearing for this purpose in spite of the possibility of different hearing levels in the two ears.

Behavioral Observation Audiometry. For those below 5 mo of age, behavioral hearing assessment is limited to unconditioned, reflexive responses to complex (i.e., not frequency-specific) test sounds, such as noise, speech, or music presented using calibrated signals from a loudspeaker or uncalibrated noisemakers. Response levels can vary widely within and across infants, and usually do not represent a good estimate of sensitivity. Behavioral observation audiometry (BOA), as this technique is called, is used primarily as a screening device.

Assessment of a child with suspected hearing loss is not complete until pure-tone hearing thresholds and SRTs have been obtained in each ear (i.e., until a reliable audiogram has been obtained). Estimates of hearing responsivity obtained using BOA or VRA in a sound field (loudspeakers) cannot be used satisfactorily to describe hearing in both ears.

Acoustic Immittance Testing. This is a standard part of the clinical audiologic test battery and includes tympanometry. Acoustic immittance testing is a useful, objective assessment technique that provides information about the status of the middle ear. It is helpful in the diagnosis and management of otitis media with effusion, one of the leading causes of mild to moderate hearing loss in young children. Tympanometry may also be performed by physicians.

Tympanometry. This technique provides a graph of the ability of the middle ear to transmit sound energy (admittance, or compliance) or impede sound energy (impedance) as a function of air pressure in the external ear canal. Because most immittance test instruments measure acoustic admittance, the term "admittance" is used here. In general, the principles apply to whatever units of measure are used.

A probe is inserted into the entrance of the external ear canal so that an airtight seal is obtained. The probe varies air pressure, presents a tone, and measures sound pressure level in the ear canal through the probe assembly. The sound pressure measured in the ear canal relative to the known intensity of the probe signal is used to estimate the acoustic admittance of the ear canal and middle-ear system. Admittance can be expressed in a unit called a millimho (mmho) or as a volume of air (in mL) with equivalent acoustic admittance. The test is done so that an estimate of the volume of air enclosed between the probe tip and tympanic membrane can be made. The acoustic admittance of this volume of air is deducted from the overall admittance measure to obtain a measure of the admittance of the middle-ear system alone. Estimating ear canal volume also has some diagnostic benefit, because an abnormally large value is consistent with the presence of an opening in the tympanic membrane (perforation or tube).

With the elimination of the admittance of the air mass in the external auditory canal, it is assumed that the remaining admittance measure accurately reflects the admittance of the entire middle-ear system. Its value is largely controlled by the dynamics of the tympanic membrane. Abnormalities of the tympanic membrane can dictate the shape of tympanograms and thus obscure abnormalities that lie beyond the tympanic membrane. In addition, the frequency of the probe tone, the speed and direction of the air pressure change, and the air pressure at which the tympanogram is initiated are all factors that can influence the outcome of the tympanometric assessment.

When air pressure in the ear canal is equal to that in the middle ear, the middle-ear system is functioning optimally. Therefore, the ear canal pressure at which there is the greatest

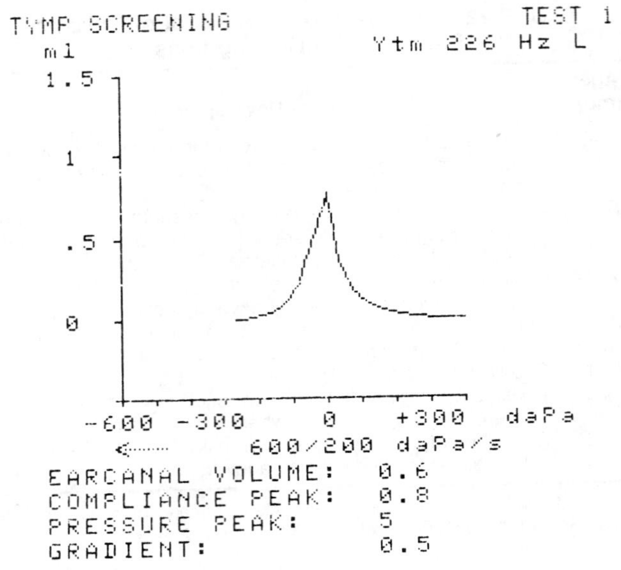

Figure 22–14. Admittance tympanogram of a normal ear of a 7-yr-old child. Ear canal volume, compliance peak (i.e., peak admittance in mL using the y-axis scale), and tympanometric peak pressure and gradient are all within normal limits. For this instrument, the gradient can range from 0 to 1.0, and the sharpest peaks get the highest values.

flow of energy (admittance) should be a reasonable estimate of the air pressure in the middle-ear space. This pressure is determined by finding the admittance maximum (peak) on the tympanogram and obtaining its value on the x axis. The value on the y axis at the tympanogram peak is an estimate of peak admittance. This peak measure is sometimes referred to as static acoustic admittance, even though it is estimated from a dynamic measure (Fig. 22–14). Table 22–6 presents the norms for peak admittance based on admittance tympanometry for normal adults and children.

Acoustic Reflex Test. This is also part of the immittance test battery. With a properly functioning middle-ear system, admittance at the tympanic membrane changes on activation of the stapedius and tensor tympani muscles. In healthy ears, the stapedial reflex occurs following exposure to loud sounds. Admittance instruments are designed to present reflex activating signals (pure tones of various frequencies or noise), either to the same or the contralateral ear, while monitoring admittance. Very small admittance changes that are time-locked to presentations of the signal are considered to be a result of middle-ear muscle reflexes. Absence of admittance

TABLE 22–6. Norms for Peak (Static) Admittance (in mL) Using a 226-Hz Probe Tone for Children and Adults*

		Speed of Air Pressure Sweep	
		≤50 da/Pa/sec†	200 da/Pa/sec‡
Children (3–5 yr)	Lower limit	0.30	0.36
	Median	0.55	0.61
	Upper limit	0.90	1.06
Adults	Lower limit	0.56	0.27
	Median	0.85	0.72
	Upper limit	1.36	1.38

*Adapted from Margolis RH, Shanks JE: Tympanometry: Basic principles of clinical application. *In* Rintelman WS (ed): Hearing Assessment, 2nd ed. Austin, TX, PRO-ED, 1991, pp 179–245.

†Ear canal volume measurement based on admittance at lowest tail of tympanogram.

‡Ear canal measurement based on admittance at lowest tail of tympanogram for children and at +200 da/Pa for adults.

changes can occur when the hearing loss is sufficient to prevent the signal from reaching the loudness level necessary to elicit the reflex, or if there is a middle-ear condition present that affects the ability to monitor a small admittance change. Reflexes cannot usually be measured in those with conductive hearing loss because of the examiner's inability to measure any change in admittance in an ear with an abnormal transfer system. As a result, the acoustic reflex test is useful in the differential diagnosis of hearing impairment. The acoustic reflex also has applications to the assessment of sensorineural hearing loss and the integrity of the neurologic components of the reflex arc, including cranial nerves VII and VIII.

Tympanometry in Otitis Media with Effusion. Often, children with otitis media have high negative tympanometric peak pressure (Fig. 22–15) and/or reduced peak admittance values. However, in regard to the diagnosis of middle-ear effusion, the tympanometric measure that has the greatest sensitivity and specificity is the tympanogram shape, rather than its peak pressure (poor predictive value) or peak admittance (fair predictive value). This shape is sometimes referred to as the tympanometric gradient or tympanometric width; it quantifies the degree of roundness or "peakedness" of the tympanogram. Generally, the more rounded the peak (or, ultimately, an absent peak), the higher the probability that an effusion is present (Fig. 22–16). Some instruments compute gradient automatically, whereas others do not. Various ways to compute this gradient can be used so, until the measure becomes standardized, the individual characteristics of the instrument used must be known and applied accordingly.

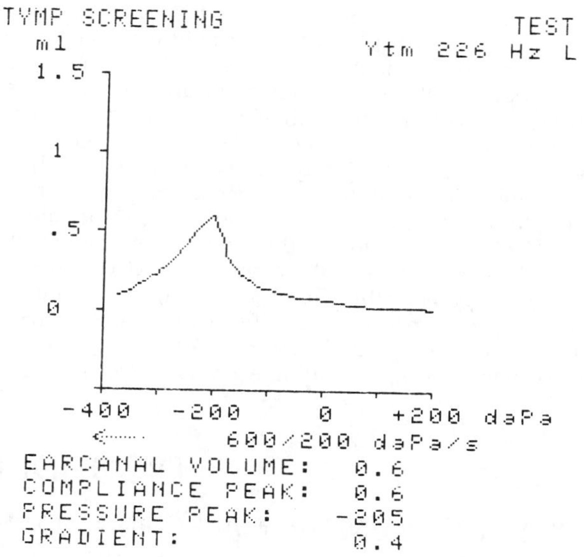

Figure 22–15. Admittance tympanogram of the same ear as that shown in Figure 22–14, only 2 wk earlier. On this occasion, tympanometric peak pressure is abnormal. Whereas the other variables are in the normal range, peak admittance and gradient are both slightly reduced relative to the values shown in Figure 22–14.

Auditory Brain Stem Response. The ABR test is used for neonatal newborn hearing screening, and it is also important in the diagnosis of auditory dysfunction and of disorders of the auditory nervous system. The ABR is a far-field recording of minute electrical discharges from multiple neurons. The stimulus, therefore, must be able to cause the simultaneous discharge of the large numbers of neurons involved. Stimuli with very rapid onset, such as clicks or tone bursts, must be used. Unfortunately, the rapid onset required to create a measurable ABR also causes energy to be spread in the frequency domain, reducing the frequency-specificity of the response.

The ABR is not affected by sedation or general anesthesia. Infants and children from about 6 mo–6 yr of age are routinely sedated to avoid problems related to the electrical interference caused by muscle activity during testing. Also, ABR testing can be done in the operating room when a child is anesthetized for another procedure.

The ABR is recorded as five to seven waves. Waves I, III, and V can be obtained consistently in all age groups. Waves II and IV appear less consistently, between and within subjects. The latency of each wave (i.e., time of occurrence of the wave peak following stimulus onset) increases with reductions in stimulus intensity or loudness. There is developmental change in the latency of the various waves; latency decreases with increasing age, with the earliest waves reaching mature latency values earlier in life than the later waves.

The ABR commonly has two major uses in the pediatric setting: (1) it is used as an audiometric test, providing information regarding the ability of the peripheral auditory system to transmit information to the auditory nerve and beyond; (2) it is used in the differential diagnosis or monitoring of central nervous system pathology. For the audiometric approach, a search is conducted for the minimum stimulus intensity that yields an observable ABR. Plotting latency versus intensity for various waves also aids in the differential diagnosis of hearing impairment. A major advantage of auditory assessment using the ABR is that ear-specific threshold estimates on infants or otherwise difficult-to-test patients can be obtained. ABR thresholds using click stimuli are correlated best with behavioral hearing thresholds in the higher frequencies (1,000–4,000 Hz). Measurement of the responsivity of the peripheral auditory system to low-frequency stimuli requires different stimuli (tone bursts or filtered clicks) or the use of masking, neither of which isolates the low-frequency region of the cochlea in all cases. ABR responses for low frequencies should be interpreted by those knowledgeable and experienced in ABR testing.

The ABR test does not assess "hearing." It reflects auditory neuronal electric responses that can be correlated to behavioral hearing thresholds, but a normal ABR only suggests that the

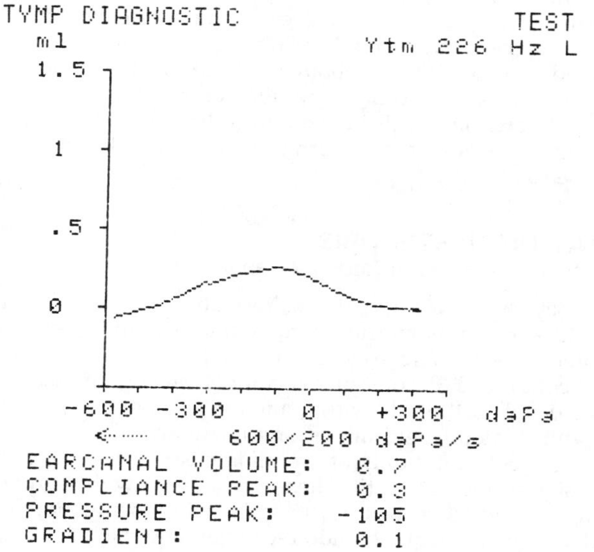

Figure 22–16. Admittance tympanogram of the left ear of a 4-yr-old child with middle-ear effusion. Note that the peak admittance and gradient are both very low, whereas the tympanometric peak pressure is grossly within normal limits.

auditory system, up to the level of the midbrain, is responsive to the stimulus used. Conversely, a failure to elicit an ABR indicates an impairment of the system's synchronous response, but does not necessarily mean that there is no "hearing." Sometimes the behavioral response to sound is normal but no ABR can be elicited (e.g., neurologic demyelinating disease). The ABR may be used to infer whether and at what level of the auditory system an impairment exists. Hearing losses that are sudden, progressive, or unilateral are indications for ABR testing. Although it is commonly believed that the different waves of the ABR reflect activity in increasingly rostral levels of the auditory system, the neural generators of the response have not been determined precisely. Each ABR wave beyond the earliest waves is probably the result of neural firing at multiple levels of the system, and each level of the system probably contributes to multiple ABR waves.

For the neurologic application, typically high intensity click stimuli are used. The morphology of the response and wave and interwave latencies are examined in respect to age appropriate forms. Delayed or missing waves in the ABR often have diagnostic significance.

The ABR and other electrical responses are extremely complex and difficult to interpret. A number of factors, including instrumentation design and settings, environment, degree and configuration of hearing loss, and patient characteristics may influence the quality of the recording. Therefore, testing and interpretation of electrophysiologic activity should be done by trained professionals to avoid the risk that unreliable and/or erroneous conclusions will affect patient care.

DISORDERS OF THE EAR

22.20 CONGENITAL MALFORMATIONS

The external and middle ears, which are derived from the 1st and 2nd branchial arches and grooves, continue to grow throughout puberty, but the inner ear, which develops from the otocyst, reaches adult size and shape by the middle of fetal development. Malformed external and middle ears may be associated with serious renal anomalies, mandibulofacial dysostosis, and many other craniofacial malformations. Severely deformed external and middle ears may also be associated with malformations of the inner ear.

MINOR DEFORMITIES

Severe malformations of the external ear are rare, but minor deformities are common. A pit-like cutaneous depression just in front of the helix and above the tragus may represent a cyst or an epidermis-lined fistulous tract; these are common but do not require surgical removal unless they become recurrently infected. Accessory skin tags on narrow pedicles may be removed by ligation but, if the pedicle is broad-based or contains cartilage, the defect should be corrected surgically. The unusually prominent or "lop" ear results from lack of bending of the cartilage that creates the antihelix; it may be improved cosmetically by otoplasty after the auricle has developed sufficiently (at about the age of 5 yr). Microtia includes cases of rudimentary auricles that, in addition to being abnormally small in size, are often more anterior and inferior in placement than normal auricles. Rarely, the auricle may be totally absent (anotia).

CONGENITAL STENOSIS

(Atresia of the External Auditory Canal)

This may be associated with malformation of the auricle and middle ear. Audiometric, tympanometric, and roentgenographic assessments are essential in diagnosing and managing these conditions. Reconstructive middle-ear surgery for atresia is restricted to the following patients: (1) above 5 yr of age; (2) with bilateral deformities or unilateral lesions in which there is a deformity only of the middle-ear ossicles, resulting in a significant conductive hearing loss; (3) with significant bilateral conductive hearing loss; (4) with roentgenographic evidence of an adequate middle-ear cleft and mastoid; and (5) with a normally positioned facial nerve. A congenital perilymphatic fistula of the oval or round window membrane may present as a rapid-onset, fluctuating, or progressive sensorineural hearing loss with or without vertigo and should be repaired to prevent possible spread of infection from the middle ear to the labyrinth, hearing loss, or both. Computed tomography can be helpful in detecting congenital fistula.

Congenital malformations of the inner ear are rare but usually result in severe sensorineural hearing loss. The bony deformities are frequently associated with central nervous system malformations.

CONGENITAL CHOLESTEATOMA

This is a congenital rest of epithelial tissue that may appear as a white, cyst-like structure medial to or within an intact tympanic membrane. It is unrelated to infections of the middle ear and should be promptly removed because it invariably enlarges, causing irreversible structural change.

INFLAMMATORY DISEASES

22.21 EXTERNAL OTITIS

In the infant, the outer two thirds of the ear canal is cartilaginous and the inner third is bony, whereas in the older child and adult only the outer third is cartilaginous. The highly viscid secretions of the sebaceous glands and the watery, pigmented secretions of the apocrine glands in the outer portion of the canal combine with exfoliated surface cells of the skin to form a protective, waxy, water-repellent coating. The normal flora of the external canal consists of *Staphylococcus epidermidis*, *Corynebacterium* (diphtheroids), *Micrococcus* sp., and occasionally *S. aureus* and *Streptococcus viridans*. Excessive wetness (swimming, bathing, or increased environmental humidity) or dryness (previous infection, dermatoses, or insufficient cerumen) and trauma (digital or foreign body) make the skin of the canal vulnerable to infection by endogenous bacteria or virulent exogenous bacteria.

ETIOLOGY. External otitis is most commonly caused by *Pseudomonas aeruginosa*, *Enterobacter aerogenes*, *Proteus mirabilis*, *Klebsiella pneumoniae*, streptococci, and *S. epidermidis*, and fungi such as *Candida* and *Aspergillus*. The condition known as "swimmer's ear" results from the loss of protective cerumen and chronic irritation and maceration from excessive moisture in the canal; *Pseudomonas* sp. is the most commonly isolated bacterium. Herpesvirus hominis and varicella-zoster may also cause external otitis.

CLINICAL MANIFESTATIONS. The predominant symptom is ear pain, accentuated by manipulation of the pinna and especially by pressure on the tragus. The severity of the pain and tenderness may be disproportionate to the degree of inflammation, because the skin of the external ear canal is attached to the perichondrium and periosteum. Itching is a frequent precursor of pain and is usually characteristic of chronic inflammation of the canal. Conductive hearing loss may occur as a result of edema of the skin and tympanic membrane, serous or purulent secretions, or the progressive meatal skin thickening associated with longstanding external otitis. Edema of the canal, erythema, and greenish otorrhea are prominent signs of the acute disease.

Frequently, the canal is so tender and swollen that the entire ear canal and tympanic membrane cannot be adequately visualized, in which instance complete otoscopic examination should be delayed until the acute swelling subsides. If the tympanic membrane can be visualized, it may be either normal or opaque in appearance and the mobility of the drum may be normal or, when the drum is thickened, reduced in response to positive and negative pressure.

Periauricular edema and fever often result from a combined infection with *Pseudomonas* sp. and *Streptococcus pyogenes* or from *S. aureus*. When there is such secondary infection, lymphadenitis, with tender nodes anterior to the tragus or in the postauricular region, may also occur.

DIFFERENTIAL DIAGNOSIS. Diffuse external otitis may be confused with furunculosis, otitis media, and mastoiditis. A furuncle usually causes a localized swelling of the canal limited to one quadrant, whereas external otitis is associated with concentric swelling. In otitis media the eardrum may be perforated, severely retracted, or bulging and immobile, and hearing is usually impaired. Pain on manipulation of the auricle and lymphadenitis are not features of middle-ear disease. In some patients with external otitis, the periauricular edema is so extensive that the auricle is pushed forward, creating a condition that may be confused with acute mastoiditis and a subperiosteal abscess; however, in mastoiditis the postauricular fold is obliterated, whereas in external otitis the fold is maintained. When the edema over the mastoid process is a result of mastoiditis, there is also usually a history of otitis media and hearing loss, and tenderness is noted over the mastoid antrum or tip and not on movement of the auricle as in external otitis. Sagging of the posterior external canal wall may also occur with acute mastoiditis.

TREATMENT. Topical otic preparations containing neomycin (active against gram-positive organisms and also against some gram-negative organisms, notably *Proteus* sp.) with either colistin or polymyxin (active against gram-negative bacilli, notably *Pseudomonas* sp.) and corticosteroids are effective in treating most forms of acute diffuse external otitis. If canal edema is marked, a cotton or selvedged-gauze wick should be inserted into the outer third of the ear canal and the medication applied to the wick as frequently as possible for 24–48 hr; the wick can be removed after these applications and the otic medication instilled 3–4 times a day. Acetic acid preparations (2%), with or without corticosteroids, or half-strength Burow solution (aluminum acetate, 1:20) are probably equally effective. When the pain is severe, analgesics (e.g., salicylates, codeine) and dry heat may be necessary.

As the inflammatory process subsides, cleaning the canal with cotton-tipped applicators or, more effectively, irrigating with 2% acetic acid to remove the debris enhances the effectiveness of the topical medications. In subacute and chronic infections, periodic cleansing of the canal is essential. In severe, acute, diffuse external otitis associated with fever and lymphadenitis from which bacteria have been cultured, oral and, on occasion, parenteral antibiotics are indicated; the choice of drug depends on the antibiotic susceptibility of the organism. A fungal infection (otomycosis) of the external auditory canal may be treated by applying metacresol acetate. Preventing external otitis may be necessary for individuals susceptible to recurrences, especially children who swim frequently. The most effective prophylaxis is instillation of dilute alcohol or acetic acid immediately following swimming or bathing.

Furunculosis. This is caused by *S. aureus* and is seen only in the hair-containing outer third of the ear canal. It is treated with incision and drainage and systemic penicillin or one of the penicillinase-resistant penicillins, depending on the antibiotic susceptibility of the organism.

Acute Cellulitis. Acute cellulitis of the auricle and external auditory canal is usually caused by *S. pyogenes*, occasionally by *S. aureus*. The skin is red, hot, and indurated, without a sharply defined border. Fever may be present with little or no exudate in the canal. Parenteral administration of penicillin G or a penicillinase-resistant penicillin is the therapy of choice.

Dermatoses. Various dermatoses (e.g., seborrheic, contact, infectious eczematoid, atopic, or neurodermatoid) are common causes of inflammation of the external canal and can be precursors of acute diffuse external otitis caused by scratching and the introduction of infecting organisms.

Seborrheic dermatitis is characterized by greasy scales that flake and crumble as they are detached from the epidermis; associated changes in the scalp, forehead, cheeks, brow, postauricular areas, and the concha are usual.

Contact dermatitis may be caused by topical otic medications such as neomycin, polymyxin, and colistin, which may produce erythema, vesiculation, edema, and weeping. Poison ivy, oak, and sumac may also produce contact dermatitis.

Infectious eczematoid dermatitis is caused by a purulent infection of the external canal, middle ear, or mastoid; the purulent drainage infects the skin of the canal, auricle, or both. The lesion is weeping, erythematous, or crusted.

Atopic dermatitis occurs in children with familial or personal histories of allergy; the auricle, particularly the postauricular fold, becomes thickened, scaly, and excoriated.

Neurodermatitis is recognized by the intense itching and erythematous, thickened epidermis localized to the concha and orifice of the meatus. Treatment of these dermatoses depends on the type but should include application of the aural medication described for external otitis, elimination of the source of infection or contactant when identified, and management of any underlying dermatologic problem.

Herpes Simplex. This may appear as vesicles on the auricle and lips, which eventually become encrusted and dry up, and may be confused with impetigo. Topical application of a 10% solution of carbamide peroxide in anhydrous glycerol is symptomatically helpful.

Herpes Zoster Oticus (Ramsay Hunt Syndrome). This is a vesicular eruption on the posterior canal wall accompanied by facial paralysis. Spontaneous recovery is usual.

Bullous Myringitis. This is commonly associated with an acute upper respiratory infection. The ear is very painful, and there are hemorrhagic or serous blebs on the membrane. The disease is difficult to differentiate from acute otitis media, because early in the course of acute otitis the drum may appear to have bullae. The organisms involved are probably the same as those causing acute otitis media. Treatment consists of antibiotic therapy of the type generally used for acute otitis media. Incision of the bullae, although not necessary, promptly relieves the pain.

22.22 OTITIS MEDIA

Inflammation of the middle ear, otitis media, is the most prevalent disease of childhood after respiratory tract infections. The complications and sequelae of acute otitis media and otitis media with effusion represent significant health hazards for children. Acute otitis media is usually suppurative or purulent, but serous effusions may also have an acute onset. There are many terms for otitis media with effusion, including serous, secretory, catarrhal, mucoid, nonsuppurative, and allergic otitis media.

EPIDEMIOLOGY. Infants and young children are at highest risk for otitis media; incidence rates are 15–20%, with peaks occurring from 6–36 mo and 4–6 yr of age. Children who develop otitis media in the 1st year of life have an increased risk of recurrent acute or chronic disease. A study of 2,565 children followed during their 1st 3 years found that only 29% of infants failed to develop at least one attack of otitis media, whereas about 33% had three or more episodes. In addition, after the 1st episode, 40% of children had a middle-ear effusion that persisted for 4 wk and 10% had an effusion that was still present at 3 mo. The incidence of the disease tends to decrease as a function of age after the age of 6 yr. The incidence is high in males, lower socioeconomic groups, Alaskan natives, native Americans, and children with cleft palate and other craniofacial anomalies, and is higher in whites than in blacks. The incidence is also increased in winter and early spring.

PATHOGENESIS. The eustachian tube protects the middle ear from nasopharyngeal secretions, provides drainage into the nasopharynx of secretions produced within the middle ear, and permits equilibration of air pressure with atmospheric pressure in the middle ear. Mechanical or functional obstruction of the eustachian tube can result in middle-ear effusion. Intrinsic mechanical obstruction can result from infection or allergy and extrinsic obstruction from obstructive adenoids or nasopharyngeal tumors. Persistent collapse of the eustachian tube during swallowing can result in functional obstruction related to decreased tubal stiffness, an inefficient active opening mechanism, or both. Functional obstruction is common in infants and younger children because the amount and stiffness of the cartilage support of the tube are less than that in older children and adults. All infants with unrepaired palatal clefts have chronic otitis media with effusion because of the functional obstruction of the eustachian tube.

Eustachian tube obstruction results in negative middle-ear pressure and, if persistent, in a sterile transudative middle-ear effusion. Drainage of the effusion is inhibited by impaired mucociliary transport and by sustained negative pressure. When the eustachian tube is not totally obstructed mechanically, contamination of the middle-ear space from nasopharyngeal secretions may occur by reflux (especially when the tympanic membrane has a perforation or when a tympanostomy tube is present), by aspiration (from high negative middle-ear pressure), or by insufflation during crying, nose blowing, sneezing, and swallowing when the nose is obstructed. Rapid alterations in ambient pressure or barotrauma during deep water diving or flying can also result in acute middle-ear effusion that may be hemorrhagic. Infants and young children have a shorter eustachian tube than older children and adults, which makes them more susceptible to reflux of nasopharyngeal secretions into the middle-ear space and to the development of acute otitis media.

Acute Otitis Media

CLINICAL MANIFESTATIONS. In the usual course, a child suffering an upper respiratory infection for several days suddenly develops otalgia, fever, and hearing loss. Examination with the pneumatic otoscope reveals a hyperemic, opaque, bulging tympanic membrane of poor mobility; purulent otorrhea may be present, but earache and fever are not invariably present. Children with diminished or absent mobility and opacification of the tympanic membrane should be suspected of having bacterial otitis media with effusion. Any child with a "fever of undetermined origin" must also be evaluated for a middle-ear infection (Sec. 12.2 and 12.3).

DIAGNOSIS. When the diagnosis of acute otitis media is doubtful or identification of the causative agent is desirable, aspiration of the middle ear should be performed. Tympanocentesis should also be considered in the following: for seriously ill children or those who appear toxic; for children who respond unsatisfactorily to antibiotic therapy; for an onset of otitis media in a patient receiving antibiotic agents; for patients who develop suppurative intratemporal or intracranial complications; and for otitis in the newborn, the very young infant, or the immunologically deficient patient, in each of whom unusual organisms may cause infection.

TREATMENT. Therapy depends on the bacterial cause of the disease (Fig. 22–17) and on the results of susceptibility testing (Table 22–7). *Streptococcus pneumoniae* is the most common causative agent of acute otitis media with effusion in all age groups: in neonates, approximately 20% of effusions may contain gram-negative enteric bacilli. The causative organism is rarely known before therapy begins, so oral amoxicillin, 40 mg/kg/24 hr tid for 10 days, is recommended, because it is usually effective against the most commonly encountered bacteria (see Table 22–7). An increasing percentage of *H. influenzae* and *Moraxalla catarrhalis* strains have now become β-lactamase producing and, therefore, ampicillin-resistant. When a resistant organism is cultured from a middle-ear aspirate or from otorrhea, or when the patient fails to improve clinically after initial amoxicillin treatment (probably because of an ampicillin-resistant bacterium) and if a tympanocentesis or myringotomy is not performed, the initial antimicrobial agent should be changed. Appropriate choices may be erythromycin (50 mg/kg/24 hr) combined with a sulfonamide (100 mg/kg/24 hr of triple sulfonamides or 150 mg/kg/24 hr of sulfisoxazole) qid, trimethoprim-sulfamethoxazole (8 and 40 mg/kg/24 hr) bid, cefaclor (40 mg/kg/24) tid, amoxicillin-clavulanate (40 mg/kg/24) tid, cefuroxime axetil (125–250 mg/24 hr) bid, or cefixime (8 mg/kg/24 hr) once daily or bid. If the patient is allergic to the penicillins, the combination of oral erythromycin and triple sulfonamides or sulfisoxazole is an alternative. Combined trimethoprim-sulfamethoxazole can also be given initially to penicillin-sensitive individuals, but its effectiveness in treating acute otitis media caused by *Staphlococcus pyogenes* is uncertain. Sulfonamide combinations have a high rate of adverse side effects, which on rare occasion have been serious and even fatal. The administration of cefaclor has been associated with a serum sickness-type reaction.

Additional supportive therapy, including analgesics, antipyretics, and local heat, is usually helpful. Meperidine hydrochloride may also be required for sedation. An oral decongestant (e.g., pseudoephedrine hydrochloride) may relieve some nasal congestion and antihistamines may help patients with known or suspected nasal allergy. The efficacy of antihistamines and decongestants in the treatment of acute otitis media, however, is not established.

In patients with unusually severe earache, myringotomy may be performed initially to provide immediate relief. When therapeutic drainage is required, a myringotomy knife should be used and the incision made large enough to allow for adequate drainage of the middle ear.

If the patient's clinical manifestations of acute infection increase during the 1st 24 hr despite antimicrobial therapy a concurrent infection such as meningitis or a suppurative complication of otitis media should be suspected. The child should be re-examined and tympanocentesis and myringotomy performed. Similarly, if the patient continues to have appreciable pain, fever, or both after 24–48 hr, tympanocentesis and myringotomy should be performed as diagnostic and therapeutic procedures; identification of the organism(s)

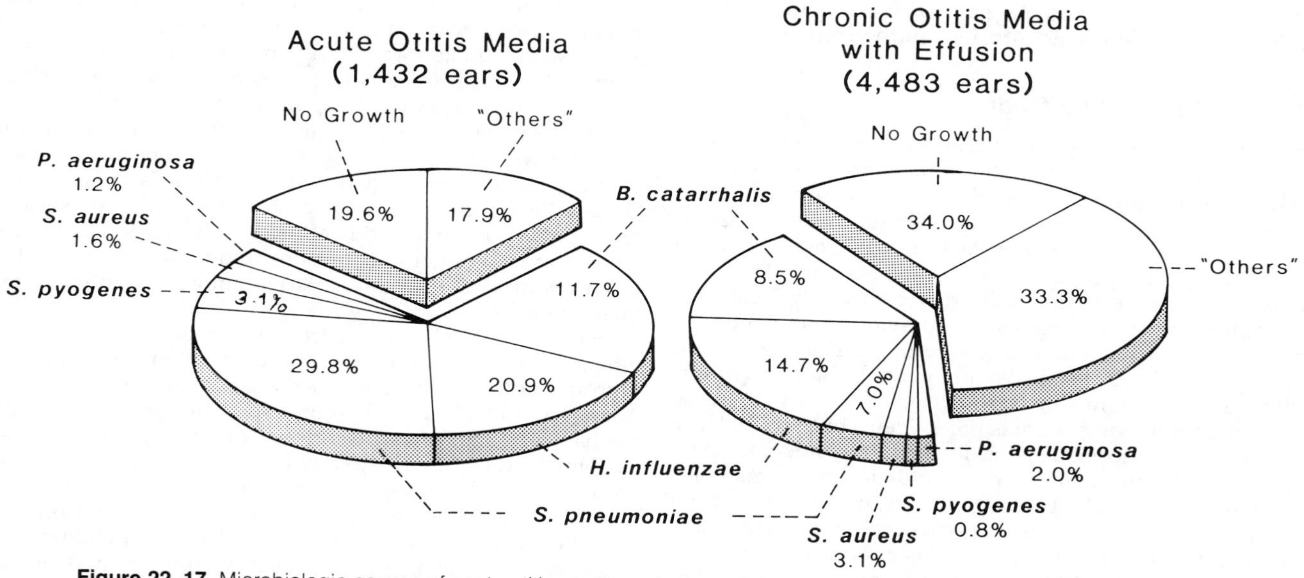

Figure 22–17. Microbiologic causes of acute otitis media and chronic otitis media with effusion from the Pittsburgh Otitis Media Research Center 1980–1985. (From Bluestone CD, Klein JO: Otitis Media in Infants and Children. Philadelphia, WB Saunders, 1988.) *Branhamella catarrhalis* has been renamed *Moraxella catarrhalis*.

is recommended at this stage but, when a diagnostic aspiration is not performed, antimicrobials effective against resistant organisms prevalent in the community should be administered.

All patients should be re-evaluated approximately 2 wk after the institution of treatment, at which time there should be some otoscopic evidence of resolution, such as a decrease in inflammation and return of mobility of the tympanic membrane. Periodic follow-up is indicated for patients who have had recurrent episodes. If the middle-ear fluid is persistent, the patient should be treated as described in the next section.

Persistent Middle-Ear Effusion

If the middle-ear effusion persists after the initial 10–14 days of antimicrobial therapy for acute otitis media, one or more of the following options may help resolve it during the next, subacute phase: (1) a course of an antimicrobial different from the initial agent (the new antimicrobial agent may be effective against an organism resistant to the previous one); (2) a topical or systemic nasal decongestant, antihistamine, or combination of these drugs; (3) systemic corticosteroids; and (4) eustachian tube–middle-ear inflation. None of these have been demonstrated to be effective in randomized, controlled trials. Many clinicians do not treat children who have asymptomatic (except for hearing loss) middle-ear effusion still present after 2 wk, but rather re-examine the child 6 wk later—that is, 2 mo after the initial visit—at which time most patients are effusion-free. Treatment with another antimicrobial, such cefaclor, trimethoprim-sulfamethoxazole, erythromycin-sulfisoxazole, amoxicillin-clavulanate, cefuroxime axetil, or cefixime, which are effective against resistant bacteria, may be indicated if the child has any signs or symptoms of

TABLE 22–7. Comparative Efficacy of Selected Oral Antimicrobial Agents for Common Pathogens in Acute Otitis Media*

	Pathogen†							
	Streptococcus pneumoniae (30%)‡	*Haemophilus influenzae* (25%)		*Moraxella catarrhalis* (13%)		*Streptococcus pyogenes* (3%)	*Staphylococcus aureus* (2%)	
		β-Lactamase		β-Lactamase			β-Lactamase	
Antimicrobial Agent		Negative	Positive	Negative	Positive		Negative	Positive
Amoxicillin	+§	+	−	+	−	+	+	−
Amoxicillin-clavulanate	+	+	+	+	+	+	+	+
Cefaclor	+	+	+	+	−	+	+	+
Cefuroxime axetil¶	+	+	+	+	+	+	+	+
Cefixime	+	+	+	+	+	+	−	−
Erythromycin-sulfisoxazole	+	+	+	+	+	+	+	+
Trimethoprim-sulfamethoxazole	+	+	+	+	+	−	+	+

*Based on available data from clinical trials and laboratory studies.
†+ = effective; − = not effective.
‡Refers to percentage of bacterium found in middle-ear aspirates of acute otitis media.
§Resistant strains have been isolated on rare occasion (Pittsburgh Otits Media Research Center: Unpublished data).
¶Not available in liquid formulation.

persistent infection, such as otalgia, or if such organisms have been isolated from subacute effusions in the community.

Recurrent Acute Otitis Media

Some children develop recurrent acute episodes of otitis media with almost every respiratory tract infection, have more or less dramatic symptoms, respond well to therapy, and have fewer episodes with advancing age. Others have persistent middle-ear effusion and suffer recurrent episodes of acute otitis media superimposed on the chronic disorder. The child with recurrent acute otitis media that completely clears between episodes may be managed as previously outlined, but if the bouts are frequent and close together, further evaluation similar to that described below for patients having chronic otitis media with effusion is indicated. In many of these children the underlying cause is not evident, but prophylactic antibiotics (a daily dose of amoxicillin or sulfonamides) appear to be effective. Myringotomy and ventilating tubes may also be effective but should be reserved for patients in whom antimicrobial prophylaxis fails to prevent recurrent acute otitis media or in whom chemoprophylaxis is not desirable because of allergy to the penicillins or the sulfonamides. The preventive efficacies of antimicrobial chemoprophylaxis and myringotomy with tympanotomy tube insertion have been demonstrated in clinical trials. Adenoidectomy is of uncertain benefit for the prevention of recurrent acute otitis media. However, immunization with the polyvalent pneumococcal vaccine may be effective when administered to patients above 2 yr of age.

OTITIS MEDIA WITH EFFUSION

Otitis media with effusion is a middle-ear effusion lacking the clinical manifestations of acute infection, such as otalgia and fever. The duration (not the severity) of the effusion can be divided into acute (less than 3 wk), subacute (3 wk–3 mo), and chronic (greater than 3 mo). The effusions may be serous (thin), mucoid (thick), and purulent.

CLINICAL MANIFESTATIONS. Frequently, either a retracted or convex tympanic membrane is seen. The membrane is usually opaque but, when it is translucent, an air-fluid level or air bubbles may be seen and an amber or sometimes bluish fluid may be apparent in the middle ear. The mobility of the eardrum is almost always impaired. Occasionally, even when there is little effusion, the tympanic membrane is retracted and its mobility impaired, usually because of negative middle-ear air pressure; when extreme, this is termed "atelectasis of the tympanic membrane." The auditory acuity is usually decreased and, although systemic symptoms are generally absent, there may be behavioral disturbances resulting from the child's inability to communicate adequately. A feeling of fullness in the ear, tinnitus, and even vertigo may be present. Some patients, even with thick middle-ear effusions, can hear fairly well; tympanometry is more reliable than audiometry.

TREATMENT. Treatment may not be indicated, because little is known about the possible complications and sequelae associated with this condition, and because most of these effusions resolve spontaneously. However, although the significance of hearing loss is uncertain, such a loss may impair cognitive and language development and result in disturbances in psychosocial adjustment. Because of these uncertainties, some clinicians believe treatment is indicated under certain conditions. For example, treatment may be indicated for a child with bilateral chronic middle-ear effusions and a marked hearing loss, although treatment may not be necessary for a child having a unilateral, asymptomatic otitis media with effusion and only a mild hearing loss, without serious secondary changes in the tympanic membrane. In addition to conductive or sensorineural hearing loss, other conditions to be considered include the following: (1) occurrence of otitis media with effusion in young infants who are unable to communicate about their symptoms and may have suppurative disease; (2) an associated purulent upper respiratory tract infection; (3) vertigo; (4) alterations of the tympanic membrane such as severe atelectasis, especially a deep retraction pocket in the posterosuperior quadrant, the pars flaccida, or both; (5) middle-ear changes such as adhesive otitis or ossicular involvement; (6) when the effusion persists for 2–3 mo or longer; and (7) when the episodes frequently recur, resulting in an accumulation of an excessive amount of effusion over many months.

One of the most popular treatments for otitis media with effusion, an orally administered combination of a decongestant and antihistamine, has been shown to be ineffective in infants and children with acute, subacute and chronic otitis media with effusion. The efficacy of topical intranasal and systemic corticosteroid therapy is unproven, and the risks of corticosteroid therapy generally outweigh the possible benefits. However, even though the efficacy of immunotherapy and allergy control has not been established for children with evidence of upper respiratory allergy, this method of management seems reasonable for those who have frequent recurrent otitis media with effusion. Inflation of the eustachian tube, using the method of Politzer or employing the Valsalva maneuver, is also ineffective in children with chronic otitis media with effusion.

A trial of antibiotics is currently the most appropriate treatment for those children who have not recently received antibiotics. Because bacteria similar to those found in acute otitis media have been isolated from a significant proportion of middle-ear aspirates in children with otitis media with effusion, the antibiotic chosen and duration of treatment should be the same as that recommended for acute otitis media. In clinical trials, both amoxicillin and amoxicillin-clavulanate have been shown to be significantly more effective than placebo; recommended treatment is for 10–30 days in therapeutic doses. The efficacy of other antimicrobial agents for the treatment of this stage of otitis media has not been demonstrated adequately in clinical trials.

If the effusion persists for 3 mo or longer, or if there have been frequent recurrences of episodes of acute otitis media, the patient requires further evaluation for respiratory allergy, adenoid tissue obstructing the nose and nasopharynx, an immunologic disorder (if other organs are involved), or abnormalities such as submucous cleft palate or a tumor of the nasopharynx.

If nonsurgical methods of management fail, surgical intervention should be considered. Myringotomy with aspiration of the middle-ear effusion is appropriate in those children in whom the procedure can be performed without the aid of a general anesthetic. A second myringotomy with or without the insertion of a tympanostomy tube may be indicated if the effusion is still present soon after the myringotomy incision heals (i.e., if the disease is persistent). It is desirable to avoid the risk of administering a 2nd general anesthetic; if a myringotomy is elected and general anesthesia is required, a tympanostomy or ventilation tube should be inserted at the time of the initial myringotomy to preclude, if possible, the necessity of performing a 2nd procedure under general anesthesia should a tube later be required. Myringotomy and the insertion of ventilation tubes may also be helpful in patients with atelectasis of the tympanic membrane when pain, hearing loss, vertigo, or tinnitus is present. Ventilation tubes may prevent permanent structural damage and cholesteatoma if a deep retraction pocket develops in the posterosuperior quadrant or in the attic (pars flaccida) portion of the tympanic membrane. The efficacy of ventilation tubes in these various circumstances, however, is not proven. Furthermore, troublesome otorrhea occasionally develops after the insertion of tubes and can usually be treated successfully with ear drops containing neomycin, polymyxin, or colistin with hydrocortisone. Because these medications may be ototoxic, some physicians use systemic antibiotics without the aural drops.

Adenoidectomy for chronic otitis media with effusion can benefit some children, but others spontaneously improve, and still other patients have persistent disease despite adenoid or tonsil surgery. Because the effectiveness of adenoidectomy for chronic otitis media with effusion apparently is not related to adenoid size, the selection of children who might benefit from adenoidectomy at present must be related to the potential benefits weighed against the costs and potential risks. For children who have recurrent or chronic otitis media with effusion and who had had one or more myringotomy and tympanostomy tube operations in the past, adenoidectomy is a reasonable option. The presence of upper airway obstruction, recurrent acute or chronic adenoiditis, or both conditions are also more compelling indications in the consideration of adenoidectomy for children who have chronic otitis media with effusion.

ATELECTASIS OF THE TYMPANIC MEMBRANE-MIDDLE EAR AND HIGH NEGATIVE PRESSURE

Atelectasis of the tympanic membrane may be acute or chronic, generalized or localized, and mild or severe. The tympanic membrane may be retracted or collapsed. High negative pressure may be present or absent. When middle-ear effusion is also present the clinical picture is the same as when acute or chronic otitis media is present. In such cases it is not unusual to visualize a severely retracted malleus through the otoscope in association with a tympanic membrane that is full or even bulging in the posterior portion. The malleus is retracted by concurrent high negative middle-ear pressure, chronic inflammation of the tensor tympani muscle or the malleolar ligaments, or both, whereas the hydrostatic pressure of the effusion (not completely filling the middle ear–mastoid air cell system) results in bulging of the most compliant (floppy) portion of the pars tensa, the posterosuperior and posteroinferior quadrants. Frequently an effusion is evident by the presence of an air-fluid level or bubbles behind a severely retracted tympanic membrane.

There may not be specific otologic symptoms with or without effusion. The child may have a severely retracted translucent tympanic membrane with evidence of high negative pressure by pneumatic otoscopy (immobile to applied positive pressure and decreased or absent mobility to applied negative pressure) or a high negative middle-ear pressure tracing on the tympanogram. The otoscopist can look through the tympanic membrane and see that there is no effusion present. Some children with such an otoscopic (and tympanometric) examination may not have any complaint, whereas others may have a feeling of fullness in the ear, otalgia, tinnitus, hearing loss, and even vertigo. The condition may be self-limited and in some it may be physiologic because of temporary eustachian tube obstruction. In others, however, especially those with symptoms, the condition is pathologic and should be managed in a manner similar to that employed when an effusion is present.

When there is localized atelectasis or a retraction pocket, especially in the pars flaccida or posterosuperior portion of the pars tensa of the tympanic membrane, the condition may be more serious than when only generalized atelectasis is present. The child may be totally asymptomatic but the retraction pocket may be associated with a significant conductive hearing loss, especially if there is erosion of one or more of the ossicles.

The evaluation of children with atelectasis caused by high negative pressure is similar to that described for those with chronic otitis media with effusion. Management is also similar and ranges from watchful waiting to tympanostomy tube insertion, depending on the duration, frequency, and severity of the problem. If a chronic retraction pocket has developed tympanoplasty may be necessary to correct the defect, because a cholesteatoma can develop at the site of a retraction pocket.

Complications and Sequelae

The intracranial suppurative complications of otitis media are relatively uncommon except in neglected cases. However, complications occurring within the aural cavity and adjacent structures of the temporal bone are more common.

HEARING LOSS

This is the most prevalent complication, and morbid outcome of otitis media, and may be caused by one or more of the intratemporal complications. To a varying degree, fluctuating or persistent loss of hearing is usually associated with acute or chronic middle-ear effusions or, in the absence of an effusion, with high negative pressure within the middle ear. The audiogram usually reveals a mild to moderate conductive loss. However, there may be a sensorineural component, generally attributed to the effect of increased tension and stiffness of the round window membrane. This hearing loss is usually reversible with resolution of the effusion, but permanent conductive hearing loss can result from irreversible changes secondary to recurrent acute or chronic inflammation (e.g., adhesive otitis, tympanosclerosis, ossicular discontinuity). Irreparable sensorineural loss may also occur, presumably as the result of spread of infection through the round or oval window membrane.

Persistent or episodic conductive hearing loss in children may impair their cognitive, language, and emotional development, but the degree and duration of the hearing loss required to produce such deficits are unknown. The accumulated results of the over 60 reported studies suggest that children do suffer such long-term effects from otitis media early in life. The scientific evidence, however, remains incomplete. Some experts are skeptical about the available data and have concluded that no causal link can be established between early, recurrent, middle-ear effusion and language delay or learning problems. Several studies, however, have shown an association between early otitis media and later deficits. Prolonged durations of middle-ear effusions, which are associated with significant loss of hearing, may be detrimental to the child's ability to develop speech and language optimally when the otitis media occurs early in life.

PERFORATION

Perforation of the tympanic membrane most frequently occurs when the central portion of the eardrum spontaneously ruptures during an episode of acute otitis media. In addition, a large numbers of temporary perforations are created by the surgical treatment of otitis media with tympanostomy tubes. Approximately 1 million tympanostomy tubes are inserted annually for the treatment of recurrent acute otitis media and otitis media with effusion, and approximately two thirds of these children develop otorrhea once or more while the tubes are in place and patent. The organisms most frequently cultured from the aural discharge, which occurs through a perforation by tympanostomy tube when acute otitis media is present, are the same as those cultured from acute middle-ear effusions when a tympanocentesis was performed (e.g., *S. pneumoniae*, *H. influenzae* and *B. catarrhalis*). *S. pyogenes*, when present and untreated, has been associated with acute, spontaneous perforation of the tympanic membrane.

Antimicrobial therapy for patients with acute perforation of the eardrum is the same as that for acute otitis media when a perforation is not present. When an aural discharge is present, however, it may be desirable to culture the drainage. The antimicrobial regimen can then be adjusted according to the results of the Gram stain, culture, and antibiotic susceptibility testing. The patient may also benefit from otic drops instilled into the external canal. Ototopical medication is usually beneficial when infectious eczmatoid external otitis is present. The application of an antibiotic-cortisone otic medication whenever a discharge is present has been advocated by many clinicians, despite the possibility of ototoxicity, because the topical medication may treat or prevent an external canal infection and hasten the resolution of the middle-ear infection. In addition, the ototopical drops may prevent bacteria in the external canal (e.g., staphylococci and *Pseudomonas* SPG) from entering the middle ear and causing a chronic infection. Healing of the tympanic membrane frequently follows cessation of the suppurative process in the middle ear, but, the perforated tympanic membrane may remain open after an episode of acute otitis media. When the perforation is present with no signs of healing and there are no signs of otitis media for several months, the perforation is considered to be chronic and possibly permanent.

The management of noninfected chronic perforations in children is difficult and controversial. The perforation provides ventilation and drainage of the middle ear, but the physiologic protective function of the eustachian tube and middle-ear system is impaired. The middle ear and mastoid air cells no longer have an air cushion to prevent nasopharyngeal secretions from entering the ear, which can result in reflux otitis media. In addition, the middle ear may be infected from the external canal, especially when swimming and bathing. Many infants and young children may benefit by the open tympanic membrane but, for patients over 5 yr of age, the perforation should be evaluated for repair (i.e., tympanoplasty) to restore the eustachian tube–middle-ear air cushion.

If otorrhea persists despite adequate antimicrobial therapy, or if the drainage seems to be coming from an apparent posterosuperior or attic (pars flaccida) defect, a cholestratoma should be suspected. Aural polyps, which appear as red, friable masses, may protrude through one of these defects, indicating the presence of a cholesteatoma.

CHRONIC SUPPURATIVE OTITIS MEDIA WITH MASTOIDITIS

In this stage of ear disease there is chronic infection of the middle ear and mastoid (mastoiditis), a nonintact tympanic membrane (because of perforation or tympanostomy tube), and discharge (otorrhea). It develops from a chronic bacterial infection, but the bacteria that caused the initial episode of acute otitis media with perforation are usually not those that are isolated from the chronic discharge. The most common bacterial species isolated are *P. aeruginosa* and *S. aureus*. The most common anaerobic species isolated are *Bacteroides, Peptostreptococcus*, and *Peptococcus*. Thus, the antimicrobial therapy recommended for acute otitis media is not effective for most cases of chronic suppurative otitis media. Tympanomastoid surgery is indicated when cholesteatoma is present.

The medical treatment of chronic suppurative otitis media without cholesteatoma is directed toward eliminating the infection from the middle ear and mastoid. Antimicrobial agents should be selected for effectiveness against the cultured organisms. Because of the high prevalence of *P. aeruginosa*, suspensions that contain polymyxin B, neomycin, and hydrocortisone (Cortisporin), or neomycin, polymyxin E, and hydrocortisone (ColyMycin), have been recommended, but their potential ototoxicity limits their usefulness. In children, orally administered antibiotics are usually not effective unless an organism is seen on Gram stain or is cultured from the discharge that is susceptible to a specific antibiotic, such as *S. aureus*, pneumococcus, or *H. influenzae*. Ciprofloxacin, a new oral antimicrobial agent with activity against most organisms that cause chronic suppurative disease (including *Pseudomonas*), may be effective, but this drug is *not* indicated for patients below the age of 17 yr.

Because of concern over the toxicity of the ototopical agents, patients and parents should be informed of their potential danger if they are used. If a topical antibiotic medication is used, the patient should return to the outpatient facility daily so that the discharge can be thoroughly aspirated. The discharge rapidly improves with this type of treatment, usually within 1–2 wk.

As an alternative, it is recommended that children be hospitalized and given a parenteral β-lactam antipseudomonal drug, such as ticarcillin. The middle ear is aspirated daily. In most children, the middle ear is free of discharge and the signs of otitis media greatly improved or absent within 7–10 days.

When the discharge fails to respond to intensive medical therapy, surgery on the middle ear and mastoid is indicated. In a study of 36 pediatric patients with chronic suppurative otitis media, in which all received parenteral antimicrobial therapy and daily aural cleansing, 32 children (89%) had their initial infection resolved with medical therapy alone and 4 (11%) required tympanomastoidectomy.

If the infection is eliminated using these methods, prevention of recurrence is usually achieved by the following: (1) prophylactic antimicrobial therapy; (2) removal of the tympanostomy tube; or (3) surgical repair of the tympanic membrane defect. The appropriate choice depends on the age of the patient and the function of the eustachian tube.

ACQUIRED CHOLESTEATOMA

This sac-like structure within the middle ear is lined by keratinized, stratified, squamous epithelium and contains desquamated epithelium or keratin. White, shiny, greasy debris accompanied by a foul-smelling discharge may be observed. Tympanomastoid surgery is indicated but if it is delayed, the disease can invade and destroy other structures of the temporal bone and spread to the intracranial cavity. A retraction pocket is a deformity of the tympanic membrane that is usually caused by persistent or fluctuating high negative middle-ear pressure, and can progress into cholesteatoma.

MASTOIDITIS

Mastoiditis is classified into acute and chronic forms. Acute mastoiditis is further subdivided into pathologic stages, which are the basis for management. In almost every child with acute otitis media the mastoid air cells are also inflamed; thus, acute mastoiditis is a natural extension and part of the pathologic process of the acute middle-ear infection. No specific signs or symptoms of the mastoid infection are present in this most common stage of acute mastoiditis. The hearing loss, otalgia, and fever are primarily the result of the acute infection within the middle ear. CT scans of the mastoid area are usually interpreted as "cloudy mastoids," which is indicative of the general inflammation. No mastoid osteitis is evident on the CT scan. The process is usually reversible because the middle-ear–mastoid effusion resolves, either as a natural process or as a result of treatment of the acute infection. If resolution of the infection does not occur at this stage, one or more of the following conditions may develop: (1) acute mastoiditis with periosteitis; (2) acute mastoid osteitis (with or without a subperiosteal abscess); or (3) chronic mastoiditis.

ACUTE MASTOIDITIS WITH PERIOSTEITIS

This occurs when the infection within the mastoid air cells spreads to the periosteum covering the mastoid process, causing periosteitis. The condition should not be confused with the presence of a subperiosteal abscess, because the management of the latter condition requires incision and drainage of the abscess and a complete simple (cortical) mastoidectomy; the former, however, usually responds to immediate but less aggressive surgical intervention.

When acute mastoiditis with periosteitis occurs in the absence of roentgenographic evidence of osteitis of the mastoid, management consists of hospitalization, immediate tympanocentesis (for aspiration and microbiologic assessment of the middle-ear–mastoid effusion), and myringotomy for drainage of the system. The insertion of a tympanostomy tube is desirable and enhances drainage over a longer period than myringotomy alone. Parenteral antimicrobial agents should be administered as described in the section on acute mastoid osteitis (see later).

Resolution of the periosteal involvement should occur within 24–48 hr after the tympanic membrane has been opened for drainage and appropriate antimicrobial therapy has begun. Surgical drainage of the mastoid—complete simple mastoidectomy—should be performed if the symptoms of the acute infection, such as fever and otalgia, persist, if the postauricular involvement does not progressively improve, or if a subperiosteal abscess develops.

Failure to institute immediate treatment at this stage may result in the development of acute mastoid osteitis with or without a subperiosteal abscess or, more dangerous to the child, a suppurative intratemporal or intracranial complication such as lateral sinus thrombosis, extradural abscess, or meningitis.

ACUTE MASTOID OSTEITIS
(Acute Coalescent Mastoiditis, Acute Surgical Mastoiditis)

This occurs when the infection within the mastoid progresses, causing destruction of the bony trabeculae that separate the mastoid cells and coalescence of the cells. A mastoid empyema is present. The primary clinical manifestations include swelling, redness, and tenderness to touch over the mastoid bone. The pinna is displaced outward and downward, and swelling or sagging of the posterosuperior canal wall may also be present. A purulent discharge may issue through a perforation in the tympanic membrane. Ear drainage may be persistent and the ear canal filled with pus and debris. Alternatively, there may be a nipple-like protrusion at the site of the tympanic membrane perforation. A fluctuant subperiosteal abscess or even a drainage fistula from the mastoid to the postauricular area may be present. The patient may be toxic and febrile, with systemic signs of acute illness. In the subacute disease, fever may be prolonged and low grade, with occasional temperature spikes. When no clinical signs of extension of pus from the mastoid are evident, CT scans of the mastoids must be obtained to rule out the presence of an acute mastoid osteitis. Any infant or child with a fever of unknown origin also should have CT scans of the mastoids to eliminate the possibility that the fever is caused by acute mastoid osteitis (without otitis media).

The diagnosis should be suspected on the basis of clinical signs. CT scans of the mastoid area may reveal one or more of the following: (1) haziness, distortion, or destruction of the mastoid outline; (2) fuzziness of the shadows of cellular walls as a result of demineralization, atrophy, and/or ischemia of the bony septa; (3) a decrease in the density and cloudiness of the areas of pneumatization because of inflammatory swelling of the air cells; and (4) in longstanding cases, a chronic osteoblastic inflammatory reaction that may obliterate the cellular structure. Small abscess cavities in sclerotic bone may be confused with pneumatic cells. CT scans may also be helpful in ruling out the coexistence of other suppurative intratemporal or intracranial complications of otitis media.

Antimicrobial agents are the mainstay of treatment of acute disease. If the case is otherwise uncomplicated (i.e., there was no prior infection), *S. pneumoniae* or *H. influenzae* is probably responsible, and a 2nd- or 3rd-generation cephalosporin should be used (see Sec. 12.21 and 12.22). A complete, simple ("cortical") mastoidectomy should also be performed, especially when the mastoid empyema has extended outside the mastoid bone. The procedure should be considered an emergency, but the timing of the operation must depend on the status of the child. Failure to control infection during the acute stage of mastoid osteitis may lead to a chronic infection within the mastoid bone or to a suppurative complication.

CHRONIC MASTOIDITIS

Chronic mastoiditis is invariably associated with chronic suppurative otitis media. The mastoid may be poorly pneumatized or sclerotic. The chronic infection should be controlled by medical treatment, but when extensive granulation tissue and osteitis in the mastoid are present, mastoidectomy is usually necessary to eliminate the chronic mastoid osteitis, especially if a cholesteatoma is present.

PETROSITIS

This may result from acute or chronic infections of the pneumatized apical and perilabyrinthine cells of the temporal bone. The triad of otitis media, paralysis of the external rectus muscle, and pain in the homolateral orbit or retro-orbital area with headache constitutes petrous apicitis, i.e., Gradenigo syndrome.

ADHESIVE OTITIS

This is the result of healing following chronic inflammation of the middle ear. The mucous membrane is thickened by proliferation of fibrous tissue, which frequently impairs the movement of the ossicles and results in an irreversible conductive hearing loss.

TYMPANOSCLEROSIS

This is a complication of chronic middle-ear inflammation characterized by whitish plaques in the tympanic membrane and nodular deposits in the submucosal layers of the middle ear. There is hyalinization with deposition of calcium and phosphate crystals and conductive hearing loss may result from the ossicles embedding in the deposits. Prevention is the only successful means of controlling this disease and adhesive otitis media.

OSSICULAR DISCONTINUITY

This is the result of rarefying osteitis secondary to chronic middle-ear inflammation. The long process of the incus is commonly involved, but the crural arch of the stapes, the body of the incus, or the manubrium of the malleus may also be eroded. The conductive hearing loss that frequently results can be corrected surgically.

FACIAL PARALYSIS

This may occur during an episode of acute otitis media because of exposure of the facial nerve from a congenital bony dehiscence within the middle ear. When it occurs as an isolated complication, a myringotomy should be performed and parenteral antibiotics administered. The paralysis usually improves rapidly without further surgery (i.e., facial nerve decompression). Mastoidectomy is not indicated unless mastoid osteitis is present. However, immediate surgical intervention is indicated when a facial paralysis develops in a child who has chronic suppurative otitis media with or without cholesteatoma.

SUPPURATIVE LABYRINTHITIS

This may occur during an episode of acute otitis media from the direct invasion of bacteria through the round or oval windows. When chronic otitis media is present the infection may penetrate the windows or enter through a fistula of the bony horizontal semicircular canal. There may be vertigo, nystagmus, tinnitus, hearing loss, nausea, and vomiting. Treatment consists of intensive parenteral antibiotic therapy, but labyrinthectomy may be indicated to prevent spread to the intracranial cavity.

CHOLESTEROL GRANULOMA

Cholesterol granuloma is a sequela of chronic otitis media with effusion. It has been described as "idiopathic hemotympanum," because the tympanic membrane appears to be dark blue. The treatment of choice is middle-ear and mastoid surgery.

INFECTIOUS ECZEMATOID DERMATITIS

This may be associated with an infection of the external auditory canal (Sec. 22.21), or may occur secondary to a discharge from the middle ear and mastoid. Management should be directed toward resolving the middle ear-mastoid infection (see Sec. 23.14).

INTRACRANIAL SUPPURATIVE COMPLICATIONS

The incidence of suppurative intracranial complications of otitis media has declined because of the use of antimicrobial agents. They now occur most often in association with chronic suppurative otitis media and mastoiditis, with or without cholesteatoma. The middle-ear and mastoid air cells are adjacent to important structures, including the dura of the posterior and middle cranial fossa, the sigmoid venous sinus of the brain, and the inner ear. Suppuration in the middle ear or mastoid, or both, may spread to these structures through progressive thromboplebitis, bony erosion, or direct extension, resulting in meningitis, extradural abscess, subdural empyema, focal encephalitis, brain abscess, lateral (sigmoid) sinus thrombosis, and otic hydrocephalus. Multiple complications frequently depend on the route of infection. For example, a patient may have meningitis, lateral sinus thrombosis, and a cerebellar abscess.

Any child with acute or chronic otitis media who develops one or more of the following signs or symptoms, especially while receiving medical treatment, should be suspected of having a suppurative intracranial complication: persistent headache, lethargy, malaise, irritability, change in personality, severe otalgia, persistent or recurrent fever, nausea, and vomiting. Fever is rarely present in children with chronic suppurative otitis media; when present, it should suggest an impending intracranial complication. The following are definitive clinical manifestations requiring an intensive search for an intracranial complication: stiff neck, focal seizures, ataxia, blurred vision, papilledema, diplopia, hemiplegia, aphasia, dysdiadochokinesia, intention tremor, dysmetria, and hemianopsia. Conversely, children with intracranial infection, such as meningitis or a brain abscess, should have middle-ear–mastoid disease ruled out as the origin of, or concomitant with, the central nervous system disease.

The diagnosis of intracranial complications is greatly improved by the use of CT scanning, but, when unavailable, arteriography should be used. Magnetic resonance imaging (MRI) also provides excellent resolution of intracranial suppuration and its consequences (e.g., edema, thrombosis, hydrocephalus).

MENINGITIS

Meningitis may occur because of the following: (1) direct invasion, in which a suppurative focus in the middle ear or mastoid spreads through the dura and extends to the pia-arachnoid, causing generalized meningitis; (2) suppuration in an adjacent area, such as a subdural abscess, brain abscess, or lateral sinus thrombophlebitis, which causes the meninges to become inflamed, and (3) concurrent infection, in which otitis media arises by contiguous spread from an infectious focus in the upper respiratory tract, and meningitis results from invasion of the blood from the upper respiratory focus. The latter is the most common route. The infections are simultaneous, but meningitis does not arise from the middle-ear infection. See Sec. 12.15 for a more detailed discussion of meningitis.

EXTRADURAL ABSCESS

Extradural (epidural) abscess usually results from the destruction of bone adjacent to dura by cholesteatoma, infection, or both. This occurs when granulation tissue and purulent material collect between the lateral aspect of the dura and adjacent temporal bone. Dural granulation tissue within a bony defect is more common than an actual accumulation of pus. When an abscess is present a dural sinus thrombosis or, less commonly, a subdural or brain abscess may also be present. If extensive bony destruction has occurred because of acute mastoid osteitis (acute coalescent mastoiditis), an extradural abscess may develop in the area of the sigmoid dural sinus.

Clinical manifestations may include severe earache, low-grade fever, and headache in the temporal region with deep local throbbing pain; usually, however, there are no signs or symptoms. Frequently, an asymptomatic extradural abscess is found in patients undergoing elective mastoidectomy for cholesteatoma. When otorrhea occurs, it is characteristically profuse, creamy, and pulsatile. Compression of the ipsilateral jugular vein may increase the rate of discharge and the degree of pulsation. Usually, there is no accompanying fever (but malaise and anorexia may be observed), no neurologic signs, the intracranial pressure is normal, and it is difficult to detect any displacement of the brain. The cerebrospinal fluid cell count and pressure are normal unless meningitis is also present. CT scanning may reveal a large extradural abscess.

The treatment of extradural abscess consists of surgical drainage. A mastoidectomy is performed, enough bone is removed so that the dura of the middle and posterior fossae may be inspected directly, the extradural abscess is identified and removed (and sometimes a drain is also inserted), and the otologic procedure that can provide optimal exteriorization of the diseased area is completed by removing all the granulation tissue until normal dura is found.

SUBDURAL EMPYEMA

A subdural empyema is a collection of purulent material within the potential space between the dura externally and arachnoid membrane internally. It may develop as a direct extension of infection or, more rarely, by thrombophlebitis through venous channels. It is a rare complication of otitis media and mastoiditis (see also Sec. 12.15).

Children with subdural empyema are extremely toxic and febrile. There are usually the signs and symptoms of a locally expanding intracranial mass. Severe headache in the temporoparietal area is usually present. Central nervous system findings may include seizures, hemiplegia, dysmetria, belligerent behavior, somnolence, stupor, deviation of the eyes, dysphagia, sensory deficits, stiff neck, and a positive Kernig sign. Hemiplegia and jacksonian epilepsy in a child with suppurative disease of the middle ear and mastoid usually indicate a subdural empyema. CT scanning is often diagnostic. The peripheral white blood cell count is high and there is a predominance of polymorphonuclear leukocytes. The cerebrospinal fluid glucose concentration is normal and no microorganisms are seen on smear or culture of the cerebrospinal fluid.

Treatment of subdural empyema includes intensive intravenous antimicrobial therapy, anticonvulsants, and neurosurgical drainage of the empyema through burr holes or craniectomy. Corticosteroids are occasionally needed to diminish severe edema. Mastoid surgery to locate and drain the source of infection is usually delayed until after neurosurgical intervention has yielded some improvement in neurologic status. The condition has a high mortality rate, and more than 50% of children who recover have some residual neurologic deficit.

FOCAL OTITIC ENCEPHALITIS

Edematous and inflamed focal areas of brain may occur as a complication of acute or chronic otitis media or of the other suppurative complications of these disorders. The signs and symptoms of this focal otic encephalitis may be similar to those of a brain abscess or subdural empyema, except that the suppuration within the brain is absent. Ataxia, nystagmus, vomiting, and giddiness suggest a possible focus within the cerebellum, whereas drowsiness, disorientation, restlessness, seizures, and coma suggest a cerebral focus. At both sites, headache may be present. CT and/or needle aspiration may be necessary to eliminate the presence of an abscess. If an abscess is not present, the focal encephalitis should be treated by administering antimicrobial agents and by carrying out an appropriate otologic surgical procedure to remove the source of infection as soon as possible. Failure to control the source of the infection within the temporal bone, as well as the focal encephalitis, may result in the development of a brain abscess. Anticonvulsive medication is given when there is cerebral involvement.

OTOGENIC BRAIN ABSCESS

Otogenic abscess of the brain may result directly from acute or chronic middle-ear and mastoid infection (with or without cholesteatoma) or may follow the development of an adjacent infection, such as lateral sinus thrombophlebitis, petrositis, or meningitis. The dura overlying the infected mastoid is invaded along vascular pathways or by adherence of the dura to underlying infected bone. Chronic otitis media or mastoiditis (with or without cholesteatoma) may lead to erosion of the tegmen tympani by pressure necrosis and perforation of the bone, with resultant inflammation of the dura and invasion by pathogenic organisms. An extradural abscess occurs with subsequent infiltration of the dura and spreads to the subdural space. A localized subdural abscess or leptomeningitis ensues. Invasion of brain tissue follows. The abscess is located closest to the primary source of infection. Thus, temporal lobe abscesses occur following invasion through the tegmen tympani or petrous bone. Cerebellar abscesses occur when the infectious focus is the posterior surface of the petrous bone or thrombophlebitis of the lateral sinus. The former occurs more frequently than the latter, and multiple abscesses are not uncommon.

Signs and symptoms of invasion of the central nervous system usually occur about 1 mo after an episode of acute otitis media or an acute exacerbation of chronic otitis media. Most children are febrile, although systemic signs, including fever and chills, vary and may be absent. Signs of a generalized central nervous system infection include severe headache, vomiting, drowsiness, seizures, irritability, personality change, altered levels of consciousness, anorexia and weight loss, and meningismus. Temporal lobe abscesses are associated with seizures in some children, may be associated with visual field deficits (e.g., optic radiation involvement), or may be silent. Cerebellar abscesses cause vertigo, nystagmus, ataxia, dysmetria, and symptoms of hydrocephalus. There may be persistent purulent ear drainage, suggesting the primary site of infection.

LATERAL SINUS THROMBOSIS

Lateral and sigmoid sinus thrombosis or thrombophlebitis arises from inflammation in the adjacent mastoid. The superior and petrosal dural sinuses are also intimately associated with the temporal bone, but are rarely affected. The mastoid infection in contact with the sinus walls produces inflammation of the adventitia followed by penetration of the venous wall. Formation of a thrombus occurs after the infection has spread to the intima. The mural thrombus may become infected and propagate, occluding the lumen. Embolization of septic thrombi or extension of infection into the tributary vessels may cause further disease. This complication is still common in children, and can be caused by both acute and chronic otitis media and mastoiditis.

The clinical signs of lateral sinus thrombosis include the following: (1) general—fever, headache, and malaise (with the formation of the infectious mural thrombus, the patient may have spiking fever and chills); (2) central nervous system—headache, papilledema, signs of increased intracranial pressure, altered states of consciousness, and seizures; (3) metastatic disease caused by infected thrombi and septic infarcts—pneumonia, septic infarcts, empyema, bone and joint infection, and, less commonly, thyroiditis, endocarditis, ophthalmitis, and abscess of the kidney; (4) spread to skin and soft tissues—cellulitis or abscess; and (5) signs of intracranial complications, including meningitis, cavernous sinus thrombosis, and brain abscess.

CT and MRI are invaluable in making the diagnosis, and their use should precede a lumbar puncture. Variations in cerebrospinal fluid pressure can occur, so demonstration by the Queckenstedt test is contraindicated because of the risk of herniation. In some cases, there is leakage of red cells and subsequent xanthochromia may occur.

Treatment includes the use of antimicrobial agents and surgery. The administration of anticoagulant medication is controversal because of the risks of releasing septic emboli or causing uncontrollable hemorrhage in the mastoid. The sinus should be uncovered and any perisinuous abscesses drained. The lateral sinus should be opened and the thrombus removed if there is septic thrombophlebitis.

OTITIC HYDROCEPHALUS

Otic hydrocephalus is a syndrome of increased intracranial pressure without other abnormalities of the cerebrospinal fluid, complicating acute otitis media. The pathogenesis is unknown, but, because the ventricles are not dilated, the term "benign intracranial hypertension" may also be appropriate. The disease is frequently associated with lateral sinus thrombosis. Symptoms include a headache that is often intractable, blurring of vision, nausea, vomiting, and diplopia. Signs include a draining ear, abducens paralysis of one or both lateral rectus muscles, and papilledema.

CT should be performed prior to lumbar puncture to prevent brain herniation. The cerebrospinal fluid pressure is sometimes above 300 mm H_2O, and the ventricles are of normal or small size. Although usually benign, otic hydrocephalus may proceed to loss of vision secondary to optic atrophy (see Sec. 20.15).

Treatment includes the use of antimicrobial agents mastoidectomy, normalization of intracranial pressure by medications (e.g., acetazolamide, furosemide), repeated lumbar punctures, or a lumboperitoneal shunt. An aggressive approach is warranted because of the possibility of optic atrophy.

INNER EAR

The inner ear may be affected by viral or bacterial infections. Congenital rubella, cytomegalovirus, and mumps are causes of severe sensorineural deafness. Labyrinthitis may be a complication of acute or chronic otitis media and mastoiditis but may also follow bacterial meningitis as a result of organisms entering the labyrinth through the internal auditory meatus, endolymphatic duct, vascular channel, or perilymphatic duct.

22.23 TRAUMATIC INJURIES OF THE EAR AND TEMPORAL BONE

AURICLE AND EXTERNAL AUDITORY CANAL

Hematoma, or accumulation of blood between the perichondrium and the cartilage, may follow trauma to the pinna. Immediate needle aspiration or, when the hematoma is extensive, incision and drainage and a pressure dressing are necessary to prevent perichondritis, which can result in a cauliflower ear deformity.

Frostbite of the auricle should be managed by rapidly rewarming the exposed pinna with warm irrigation or warm compresses.

Foreign bodies in the external canal are common in childhood. These can usually be removed without general anesthesia if the child is informed of the procedure (if old enough to understand it), if the child is properly restrained, when an adequate headlight or surgical head otoscope is used for visualizing the object, and when an alligator forceps, wire loop, or blunt cerumen curet is used, depending on the shape of the object. Irrigation is sometimes helpful. General anesthesia and the otomicroscope are necessary for the removal of more difficult foreign bodies, especially those deeply embedded in the canal just lateral to the tympanic membrane. Following removal of the external canal foreign body, the tympanic membrane should be carefully inspected for possible traumatic perforation or for a pre-existing middle-ear effusion. If the foreign body has resulted in acute inflammation of the canal, treatment as described for acute diffuse external otitis should be instituted.

TYMPANIC MEMBRANE AND MIDDLE EAR

Traumatic perforation of the tympanic membrane usually occurs as the result of a sudden external compression (e.g., a slap) or penetration by a foreign object (e.g., a stick or cotton-tipped applicator). The perforation may be linear or stellate and is most frequently in the anterior portion of the pars tensa when it is caused by compression; it may be in any quadrant of the tympanic membrane when caused by a foreign object. Spontaneous healing usually occurs but, if the drum does not heal within 2–3 mo, tympanoplastic surgery is indicated. Systemic antibiotics and topical otic medications are not required unless suppurative otorrhea is present. However, otorrhea may occur at any time during periods of upper respiratory tract infection, because the middle-ear air cushion is lost, permitting reflux of nasopharyngeal secretions into the middle-ear cavity. Perforations resulting from penetrating foreign bodies are less likely to heal than those caused by compression. Implantation of epithelium from a traumatic perforation can result in a cholesteatoma. Immediate surgical exploration is indicated if the injury is accompanied by one or more of the following: vertigo, nystagmus, severe tinnitus, moderate to severe hearing loss, or cerebrospinal fluid otorrhea. Exploratory tympanotomy is necessary to inspect the ossicles, especially the stapes, that may have been dislocated.

Perilymphatic fistula may occur following sudden barotrauma or increase in cerebrospinal fluid pressure. This condition is probably more common than generally appreciated and should always be suspected in a child who develops a sudden or fluctuating sensorineural hearing loss, vertigo, or both, following physical exertion, deep water diving, flying in an airplane, playing a wind instrument, or any other activity that suddenly increases the pressures within the middle ear or the intracranial-labyrinthine system. Characteristically, the leak is at the oval or the round window, which may be congenitally abnormal; immediate repair of the fistula is essential, because the hearing loss may become irreversible.

TEMPORAL BONE FRACTURES

Children are particularly prone to basilar skull fractures, which usually involve the temporal bone. Most temporal bone fractures are longitudinal and are commonly manifested by the following: bleeding from a laceration of the external canal and tympanic membrane or, if the drum is intact, a hemotympanum; conductive hearing loss resulting from the laceration of the tympanic membrane, hemotympanum, or ossicular injury; delayed onset of facial paralysis (which usually improves spontaneously); and temporary cerebrospinal fluid otorrhea. Transverse fractures of the temporal bone have a graver prognosis than longitudinal fractures and are associated with the following: immediate facial paralysis, which may not improve without surgical intervention; severe sensorineural hearing loss, vertigo, nystagmus, tinnitus, nausea, and vomiting associated with complete loss of cochlear and vestibular function; hemotympanum and, rarely, external canal bleeding; and cerebrospinal otorrhea, seen either in the external auditory canal or behind the tympanic membrane, which may come through the nose via the eustachian tube.

Vigorous removal of external auditory canal blood clots, tympanocentesis, and application of otic preparations are not indicated, but prophylactic parenteral administration of antibiotics when cerebrospinal otorrhea is present has been advocated. Surgical intervention is reserved for children who require tympanoplastic repair of the perforated tympanic membrane (that fails to heal spontaneously), who have suffered dislocation of the ossicular chain, or who need decompression of the facial nerve. Sensorineural hearing loss can also occur following a blow to the head without an obvious fracture of the temporal bone (labyrinthine concussion).

ACOUSTIC TRAUMA

This results from exposure to high-intensity sound (e.g., fireworks, gunfire, rock music) and is manifested by a depression at 4,000 Hz on the audiometric examination. The loss is usually temporary but may become permanent if the noise exposure is chronic. Avoiding chronic exposure to loud noise and protecting the ear against unavoidable exposure are preventive measures.

22.24 TUMORS OF THE EAR AND TEMPORAL BONE

Benign tumors of the external canal include osteoma and monostotic and polyostotic fibrous dysplasia. Osteomas present as bony masses in the canal and require removal only if hearing is impaired or external otitis results.

Eosinophilic granuloma of the middle ear should be suspected when there are otalgia, otorrhea, hearing loss, and roentgenographic findings of a sharply delineated destructive lesion of the temporal bone.

Rhabdomyosarcoma originating in the middle ear should be considered when there is bleeding from the ear or otorrhea associated with paralysis of the facial nerve.

Reticulum cell sarcoma and leukemia may also present in the middle ear. Although primary neoplasms of the middle ear are relatively uncommon, the initial signs and symptoms of the more common nasopharyngeal neoplasms (e.g., angiofibroma, rhabdomyosarcoma, epidermoid carcinoma) may be associated with the insidious onset of a chronic otitis media with effusion (see Chapter 17).

22.25 DISEASES OF THE BONY LABYRINTH

Otosclerosis, an autosomal dominant disease, can cause a fixation of the stapes, resulting in progressive hearing loss in older children and teenagers. A hearing aid may be necessary. Corrective surgery is more successful and permanent in adults than in children.

Osteogenesis imperfecta may involve both the middle and inner ears. If the hearing loss is severe enough, a hearing aid is a preferable alternative to surgical correction of the fixed stapes, because the disease is progressive.

Osteoporosis may involve the middle ear, resulting in a moderate to severe hearing loss. A hearing aid may be necessary for rehabilitation.

CHARLES D. BLUESTONE
ROBERT J. NOZZA

GENERAL REFERENCES

American Academy of Otolaryngology—Head and Neck Surgery Subcommittee on cochlear implants. Status of cochlear implantation in children. J Pediatr 118:1, 1991.

American Academy of Pediatrics: Joint committee on infant hearing [Position statement 1982]. Pediatrics 70:496, 1982.

Arola M, Ziegler T, Ruuskanen O: Respiratory virus infection as a cause of prolonged symptoms in acute otitis media. J Pediatr 116:697, 1990.

Bergstrom L: Infectious agents that deafen. *In*: Bess FH (ed): Hearing Impairment in Children. Parkton, MD, York Press, 1988.

Bess FH (ed): Hearing Impairment in Children. Parkton, MD, York Press, 1988.

Bluestone CD, Klein JO: Otitis Media in Infants and Children. Philadelphia, WB Saunders, 1988, pp 249–257.

Bluestone CD, Klein JO: Intracranial suppurative complications of otitis media and mastoiditis. *In*: Bluestone CD, Stool SE (eds): Pediatric Otolaryngology, 2nd ed. Philadelphia, WB Saunders, 1990, pp 537–546.

Bluestone CD, Klein JO: Intratemporal complications and sequelae of otitis media. *In*: Bluestone CD, Stool SE (eds): Pediatric Otolaryngology, 2nd ed. Philadelphia, WB Saunders, 1990, pp 487–536.

Bluestone CD, Klein JO: Methods of examination: Clinical examination. *In*: Bluestone CD, Stool SE (eds): Pediatric Otolaryngology, 2nd ed. Philadelphia, WB Saunders, 1990, pp 111–124.

Bluestone CD, Klein JO: Otitis media, atelectasis, and eustachian tube dysfunction. *In*: Bluestone CD, Stool SE (eds): Pediatric Otolaryngology, 2nd ed. Philadelphia, WB Saunders, 1990, pp 320–486.

Brookhouser PE, Moeller MP: Choosing the appropriate habilitative track for the newly identified hearing-impaired child. Ann Oto Rhinol Laryngol 95:51, 1986.

Carlin SA, Marchant CD, Shurin PA, et al: Host factors and early therapeutic response in acute otitis media. J Pediatr 118:178, 1991.

Catlin FI: Etiology and pathology of hearing loss in children. *In*: Martin FN (ed): Pediatric Audiology. Englewood Cliffs, NJ, Prentice-Hall, 1978, pp 3–34.

De Jonge R: Normal tympanometric gradient: A comparison of three methods. Audiology 25:299, 1986.

Glasscock ME, McKennan KX, Levine SC: Differential diagnosis of sensorineural hearing loss in children. *In*: Bess FH (ed): Hearing Impairment in Children. Parkton, MD, York Press, 1988, pp 1–14.

Koebsell KA, Margolis RH: Tympanometric gradient measured from normal preschool children. Audiology 25:149, 1986.

Konigsmark BW, Gorlin RJ: Genetic and Metabolic Deafness. Philadelphia, WB Saunders, 1976.

Mancuso AA, Hanafee WN: Computed Tomography and Magnetic Resonance Imaging of the Head and Neck, 2nd ed. Baltimore, Williams & Wilkins, 1985.

Margolis RH, Heller JW: Screening tympanometry: Criteria for medical referral. Audiology 25:197, 1987.

Matkin ND: Early recognition and referral of hearing-impaired children. Pediatr Rev 6:151, 1984.

Matkin ND: Re-evaluating our approach to evaluation: Demographics are changing—are we? *In*: Bess FH (ed): Hearing Impairment in Children. Parkton, MD: York Press, 1988, pp 101–11.

Northern JL, Downs MP: Hearing in Children, 3rd ed. Baltimore, Williams & Wilkins, 1984.

Nozza RJ, Fria TJ: The assessment of hearing and middle ear function in children. *In*: Bluestone CD, Stool SE (eds): Pediatric Otolaryngology, 2nd ed. Philadelphia, WB Saunders, 1990, pp 125–153.

Ruben RJ, Rapin I: Management of hearing-impaired deaf infant and child. *In*: Alberti P, Ruben RJ (eds): Otological Medicine and Surgery. New York, Churchill Livingston, 1988.

Shapiro GG, Virant FS, Furukawa CT, et al: Immunologic defects in patients with refractory sinusitis. Pediatrics 87:311, 1991.

Shaver KA. Genetic causes of childhood deafness. *In*: Bess FH (ed): Hearing impairment in children. Parkton, MD, York Press. 1988, pp 15–32.

Van Camp KJ, Margolis RH, Wilson RH, et al: Normative static acoustic immittance. Principles of tympanometry. ASHA Monogr, 24, 1986.

Vignaud J, Jardin C, Rosen L: The Ear—Diagnostic Imaging. New York, Masson Publishing USA, 1986.

SPECIAL REFERENCES

Bluestone CD: Otitis media and congenital perilymphatic fistula as a cause of sensorineural hearing loss in children. Pediatr Infect Dis J 7:S141, 1988.

Casselbrant ML, Brostoff LM, Cantekin EI, et al: Otitis media with effusion in preschool children. Laryngoscope 95:428, 1985.

Chan KH, Bluestone CD: Lack of efficacy of middle-ear inflation: Treatment of otitis media with effusion in children. Otolaryngol Head Neck Surg 100:317, 1989.

Chan KH, Mandel EM, Rockette HE, et al: A comparative study of amoxicillin-clavulanate and amoxicillin. Arch Otolaryngol 114:142, 1988.

Fria TJ, Cantekin EI, Eichler JA: Hearing acuity of children with otitis media with effusion. Arch Otolaryngol 111:10, 1985.

Gates GA, Avery CA, Prihoda TJ, et al: Effectiveness of adenoidectomy and tympanostomy tubes in the treatment of chronic otitis media with effusion. N Engl J Med 317:1444, 1987.

Harrison CJ, Marks MI, Welch PF: Microbiology of recently treated acute otitis media compared with previously untreated acute otitis media. Pediatr Infect Dis 4:641, 1985.

Hayden GF, Schwartz RH: Characteristics of earache among children with acute otitis media. Am J Dis Child 139:721, 1985.

Hough JVD, Stuart WD: Middle ear injuries in skull trauma. Laryngoscope 78:899, 1968.

Kaleida PH, Bluestone CD, Rockette HE, et al: Amoxicillin-clavulanate potassium comparison with cefaclor for acute otitis media in infants and children. Pediatr Infect Dis J 6:265, 1987.

Kaleida PH, Casselbrant ML, Rockette HE, et al: Amoxicillin or myringotomy or both for acute otitis media: results of a randomized clinical trial. Pediatrics 87:466, 1991.

Kenna M, Bluestone CD, Reilly J: Medical management of chronic suppurative otitis media without cholesteatoma in children. Laryngoscope 96:146, 1986.

Kenna MA, Bluestone CD, Fall P, et al: Cefixime vs. cefaclor in the treatment of acute otitis media in infants and children. Pediatr Infect Dis J 6:992, 1987.

Levine LR: Quantitative comparison of adverse reactions to cefaclor vs. amoxicillin in a surveillance study. Pediatr Infect Dis 4:358, 1985.

Mandel EM, Rockette HE, Bluestone CD, et al: Efficacy of amoxicillin with and without decongestant-antihistamine for otitis media with effusion in children. N Engl J Med 316:432, 1987.

Mandel EM, Rockette HE, Bluestone CD, et al: Myringotomy with and without tympanostomy tubes for chronic otitis media with effusion. Arch Otolaryngol Head Neck Surg 115:1217, 1989.

Odio CM, Kusmiesz H, Shelton S, et al: Comparative treatment trial of augmentin versus cefaclor for acute otitis media with effusion. Pediatrics 75:819, 1985.

Paradise JL, Bluestone CD, Rogers KD, et al: Efficacy of adenoidectomy for recurrent otitis media: Results from parallel random and nonrandom trials. Pediatr Res 21:286A, 1987.

Pukander JS, Karma PH: Persistence of middle-ear effusion and its risk factors after an acute attack of otitis media with effusion. *In*: Lim DJ, Bluestone CD, Klein JO, et al, (eds): Proceedings of the Fourth International Symposium on Recent Advances in Otitis Media. Toronto, BC Decker, 1988, pp 8–11.

Pukander JS, Sipila M, Karma P: Occurrence of and risk factors in acute otitis media. *In*: Lim DJ, Bluestone CD, Klein JO, et al (eds): Recent Advances in Otitis Media with Effusion. Philadelphia, BC Decker, 1984, pp 9–13.

Samuel J, Fernandes CMC, Steinberg JL: Intracranial otogenic complications: A persisting problem. Laryngoscope 96:272, 1986.

Teele DW, Klein JO, Rosner BA: Otitis media with effusion during the first three years of life and development of speech and language. Pediatrics 74:282, 1984.

Teele DW, Klein JO, Rosner BA, et al: Epidemiology of otitis media during the first seven years of life in children in greater Boston: A prospective, cohort study. J Infect Dis 160:83, 1989.

23

THE SKIN

23.1 MORPHOLOGY OF THE SKIN

EPIDERMIS. The mature epidermis, a stratified epithelial tissue, is constantly renewed by mitotic division of the cells of the basal layer. In addition to the squamous cells or keratinocytes, the epidermis contains melanocytes (the pigment-forming cells) and Langerhans cells (dendritic cells of the mononuclear phagocyte system).

The continuous renewal of the surface cells of the epidermis normally proceeds in an orderly fashion as the cells of the basal cell layer move upward to the stratum corneum. The transit time of the epidermal cell is relatively fixed; the total life span is approximately 28 days. In hyperproliferative diseases the movement of the cells is more rapid, so that the newly arrived epidermal cells in the stratum corneum, being immature, form a defective barrier; this may alter permeability.

Keratinocytes are joined together by attachment plaques, the desmosomes. Cytoplasmic tonofibrils project to the desmosome and aid in cell attachment. Autoantibodies to various desmosomal glycoproteins cause acantholysis (detachment of joined keratinocytes with bullae formation).

Epidermal melanocytes are derived from the neural crest and migrate to the skin during embryonic life. They reside in the interfollicular epidermis and in the hair follicles and multiply by mitosis to repopulate the epidermis. Melanocytes are responsible for skin color as they produce the melanosomes containing melanin that are ingested by the keratinocytes; the melanin is shed with the stratum corneum cells.

The Langerhans cells have a dendritic form like that of melanocytes, but rather than melanosomes, they contain a specific organelle, the Birbeck granule. These cells are derived from bone marrow and participate in immune reactions in the skin, playing an active role in antigen presentation and processing.

DERMIS. The dermis, or corium, forms a tough, pliable, fibrous supporting structure between the epidermis and the subcutaneous fat. It consists of collagen and elastic and reticulin fibers embedded in an amorphous ground substance; it contains blood vessels, lymphatics, neural structures, eccrine and apocrine sweat glands, hair follicles, sebaceous glands, and smooth muscle. Morphologically, the dermis can be divided into two layers, the superficial papillary layer that interdigitates with the rete ridges of the epidermis and the deeper reticular layer that lies beneath the papillary dermis. The papillary layer is less dense and more cellular, whereas the reticular layer appears more compact because of the coarse network of interlaced collagen and elastic fibers.

The dermoepidermal junction includes the basal cell membrane of the epidermal basal cell. Half desmosomes containing tonofilaments appear above the bullous pemphigoid antigen layer at this junction. Other macromolecules, such as laminin, proteoglycan, type IV collagen, KF-1 antigen, and anchoring fibril antigens (AF1, AF2), are present and aid in the diagnosis of various cutaneous diseases affecting the dermoepidermal junction (e.g., bullous, pemphigoid, epidermolysis bullosa).

The predominant cell is a spindle-shaped fibroblast that is responsible for the synthesis of collagen, elastic fibers, and mucopolysaccharides. Phagocytic histiocytes, mast cells, and motile leukocytes are also present. The gelatinous ground substance serves as a supporting medium for the fibrillar and cellular components as well as a storage place for a substantial portion of body water. Nutrients are supplied to both epidermis and dermis via the dermal blood vessels.

SUBCUTANEOUS TISSUE. Panniculus, or subcutaneous tissue, consists of fat cells, which form and store lipid, and of fibrous septa that divide it into lobules and anchor it to the underlying fascia and periosteum. Blood vessels and nerves are also present in this layer, which serves as a storage depot for lipid, an insulator to conserve body heat, and a protective cushion against trauma.

APPENDAGEAL STRUCTURES. These structures are derived from aggregates of epidermal cells that become specialized during early embryonic development. Small buds (primary epithelial germs) appear during the 3rd fetal mo and give rise to hair follicles, sebaceous and apocrine glands, and the attachment bulges for the arrector pili muscles. Eccrine sweat glands are derived from separate epidermal downgrowths that arise during the 2nd fetal mo and are completely formed by the 5th mo. Formation of nails is initiated during the 3rd intrauterine mo.

HAIR FOLLICLES. The hair follicle is the most prominent structure in the pilary complex, which includes the sebaceous gland, the arrector pili muscle, and in areas such as the axillae, an apocrine gland. Hair follicles are distributed throughout the skin, except in the palms, soles, lips, and glans penis; if destroyed, they cannot regenerate. Individual follicles extend from the surface of the epidermis to the deep dermis, where the matrix cells with the dermal papilla form a bulbous hair root. The growing hair consists of a bulb and a matrix from which the keratinized hair shaft is generated; the shaft consists of an inner medulla, a cortex, and an outer cuticular layer.

Human hair growth is cyclical, with alternate periods of growth (anagen) and rest (telogen). The length of the anagen phase varies from months to years. At birth, all hairs are in the anagen phase. Subsequent generative activity lacks synchrony, so that an overall random pattern of growth and shedding prevails. Scalp hair usually grows about 0.35 mm/24 hr.

The types of hair are fetal lanugo, terminal, and vellus. *Lanugo* hair is thin and short; this hair is shed prior to term and is replaced by vellus hair by 36–40 wk of gestation. *Terminal* hair is long and coarse and is found on the scalp, beard, eyebrows, eyelashes, axillary, and pubic areas. *Vellus* hair is short, soft, and frequently unpigmented and is distributed over the rest of the body. During puberty, androgenic hormone stimulation causes pubic, axillary, and beard hair to change from vellus hair to terminal hair.

SEBACEOUS GLANDS. These glands occur in all areas except the palms, soles, and dorsa of the feet, but they are most numerous on the face, upper chest, and back. Their ducts open into the hair follicles except on the lips, prepuce, and labia minora, where they emerge directly onto the mucosal surface. These holocrine glands are saccular structures that are often branched and lobulated and consist of a proliferative basal layer of small flat cells peripheral to the central mass of lipidized cells. The latter cells disintegrate as they move toward the duct and form the lipid secretion known as sebum, which consists of cellular debris, triglycerides, phospholipids, and cholesterol esters.

Sebaceous glands depend on hormonal stimulation and are activated by androgens at puberty. Fetal sebaceous glands are stimulated by maternal androgens, and their lipid secretion, together with desquamated stratum corneum cells, comprise the vernix caseosa.

APROCRINE GLANDS. The apocrine glands are located in the axillae, areolae, perianal and genital areas, and the periumbilical region. These large, coiled, tubular structures continuously secrete an odorless milky fluid that is discharged in response to adrenergic stimuli, usually the result of emotional stress. Bacterial decomposition of apocrine sweat accounts for the unpleasant odor associated with perspiration.

Apocrine glands remain dormant until puberty, when they enlarge and secretion begins in response to androgenic activity. The secretory coil of the gland consists of a single layer of cells enclosed by a layer of contractile myoepithelial cells. The duct is lined with a double layer of cuboidal cells and opens into the pilosebaceous complex. Although apocrine glands do not function in thermoregulation, they are involved in certain disease processes.

ECCRINE SWEAT GLANDS. These glands are distributed over the entire body surface including the palms and soles, where they are most abundant. Those on the hairy skin respond to thermal stimuli and serve to regulate the body temperature by delivering water to the skin surface for evaporation; in contrast, sweat glands on the palms and soles respond mainly to psychophysiologic stimuli.

Each eccrine gland consists of a secretory coil located in the reticular dermis or subcutaneous fat and a secretory duct that opens onto the skin surface. Sweat pores can be identified on the epidermal ridges of the palm and fingers with a magnifying lens but are not readily visualized elsewhere.

Two types of cells compose the single-layered secretory coil: small dark cells and large clear cells; these rest on a layer of contractile myoepithelial cells and a basement membrane. The glands are supplied by sympathetic nerve fibers, but the pharmacologic mediator of sweating is acetylcholine rather than epinephrine. Sweat consists of H_2O, Na, K, Ca, Cl, P, lactate, and small quantities of Fe, glucose, and protein. The composition varies with the rate of sweating but is always hypotonic in normal children.

NAILS. Nails are specialized protective epidermal structures that form convex, translucent, tight-fitting plates on the distal dorsal surfaces of the fingers and toes. The nail plate, which is derived from a metabolically active matrix of multiplying cells situated beneath the posterior nail fold, grows forward at the rate of approximately 0.1 mm/24 hr. The nail plate is bounded by the lateral and posterior nail folds; a thin eponychium (the cuticle) protrudes from the posterior fold over a crescent-shaped white area called the lunula. The pink color above it reflects the underlying vascular bed.

23.2 EXAMINATION OF THE PATIENT

Although many skin disorders are recognized easily by simple inspection, a painstaking history and physical examination are often necessary for accurate assessment. In all cases the entire body surface, the mucous membranes, the conjunctiva, the hair, and nails should be examined thoroughly under adequate illumination. The color, turgor, texture, temperature, and moisture of the skin and the growth, texture, caliber, and luster of the hair and nails should be noted. Skin lesions should be palpated as well as inspected and should be classified on the bases of morphology, size, color, texture, firmness, configuration, location, and distribution. One must also decide whether the changes are those of the primary lesion itself or whether the clinical pattern has been altered by a secondary factor such as infection, trauma, or therapy.

Primary lesions are classified as macules, papules, nodules, tumors, vesicles, bullae, pustules, wheals, and cysts. A *macule* represents an alteration in skin color but cannot be felt. When larger than 1 cm, the term *patch* is used. *Papules* are palpable solid lesions smaller than 0.5–1 cm, whereas *nodules* are larger in diameter. *Tumors* are usually larger than nodules and vary considerably in mobility and consistency. *Vesicles* are raised, fluid-filled lesions less than 0.5 cm in diameter; when larger, they are called *bullae*. *Pustules* contain purulent material. *Wheals* are flat-topped, palpable lesions of variable size and configuration that represent dermal collections of edema fluid. *Cysts* are circumscribed, thick-walled lesions that are located deep in the skin, are covered by a normal epidermis, and contain fluid or semisolid material. Aggregations of papules and pustules are referred to as *plaques*.

Secondary lesions include scales, ulcers, excoriations, fissures, crusts, and scars. *Scales* consist of compressed layers of stratum corneum cells that are retained on the skin surface. *Ulcers* are excavations of necrotic or traumatized tissue. Ulcerated lesions inflicted by scratching are often linear or angular in configuration and are called *excoriations*. *Fissures* are caused by splitting or cracking; they occur usually in diseased skin. *Crusts* consist of matted, retained accumulations of blood, serum, pus, and epithelial debris on the surface of a weeping lesion. *Scars* are end-stage lesions that can be thin, depressed and atrophic, raised and hypertrophic, or flat and pliable; they are composed of fibrous connective tissue. *Lichenification* is a thickening of skin with accentuation of normal skin due to chronic irritation (rubbing, scratching) or inflammation.

If the diagnosis is not clear after a thorough examination, one or more diagnostic procedures may be indicated. Besides those discussed later, others are identified in appropriate subsections (e.g., scrapings of scabies lesions and smears and cultures of vesicles and pustules for detection of virus or bacteria).

BIOPSY OF SKIN. Biopsy of skin by excision is rarely required for diagnosis in children. *Punch biopsy* is a simple, relatively painless procedure and usually provides adequate tissue for examination. A fresh but well-developed lesion should be selected for removal. Xylocaine, 1 or 2%, with or without epinephrine, should be injected intradermally with a 27- or 30-gauge needle following cleansing of the site. A punch, 3 or 4 mm in diameter, is pressed firmly against the skin and rotated until it sinks to the proper depth. All three layers (epidermis, dermis, and subcutis) should be contained in the plug. The plug should be lifted gently with forceps or extracted with a needle and separated from the underlying tissue with an iris scissors. Bleeding abates with firm pressure; suturing is optional. The biopsy specimen should be placed in 10% formalin for appropriate processing.

WOOD LAMP. The Wood lamp transmits ultraviolet light mainly in a wavelength of 365 nm. The examination, which is performed in a darkened room, is useful mainly in certain superficial fungal infections of the scalp. Blue-green fluorescence is detectable at the base of each infected hair shaft in ectothrix and in some endothrix infections. Scales and crusts may appear pale yellow, but this is not evidence of a fungal infection. Dermatophyte lesions of the skin (tinea corporis) do not fluoresce; macules of tinea versicolor, however, have

TABLE 23–1. Immunofluorescent Findings in Immune-Mediated Cutaneous Diseases

Disease	Involved Skin	Uninvolved Skin	Direct IF	Indirect IF	Other Antibodies
Dermatitis herpetiformis	Negative	Positive	Granular IgA ± C* in papillary dermis	None	IgA antireticulum in 20–70%. Antigliadin antibodies with celiac disease
Bullous pemphigoid	Positive	Positive	Linear IgG and C band in BMZ,† occasionally IgM, IgA, IgE	IgG to BMZ in 70%	None
Pemphigus (all variants)	Positive	Positive	IgG in intercellular spaces of epidermis between keratinocytes	IgG to intercellular space	None
Pemphigus foliaceus	Positive	Positive	IgG to desmosomal glycoprotein, desmoglein	Same as direct IF	None
Herpes gestationis	Positive	Positive	C3 at BMZ, occasionally IgG	IgG anti-BMZ	None
Linear IgA bullous dermatosis (chronic bullous dermatosis of childhood)	Positive	Positive	Linear IgA at BMZ, occasionally C	Low titer, rare IgA, anti-BMZ	None
Discoid lupus erythematosus	Positive	Negative	Linear IgG, IgM, IgA, and C3 at BMZ (lupus band)	None	Antinuclear antibody negative
Systemic lupus erythematosus	Positive	Variable: exposed to sun, 30–50%; nonexposed, 10–30%	Linear IgG, IgM, C3 at BMZ (lupus band)	None	ANA Anti Ro (SSA) Anti-RNP Anti-DNA Anti-Sm
Henoch-Schönlein purpura	Positive	Negative	IgA around vessel walls	None	IgA rheumatoid factor, occasionally

*C = complement.
†BMZ = basement membrane zone at the dermoepidermal junction.

a golden fluorescence under the Wood lamp. *Erythrasma*, an intertriginous infection due to *Corynebacterium minutissimum* may fluoresce pink-orange, whereas *Pseudomonas aeruginosa* has a yellow-green color under a Wood lamp.

Discrete areas of altered pigment can often be visualized more clearly by use of a Wood lamp, particularly if the pigmentary change is epidermal. Hyperpigmented lesions appear darker and hypopigmented lesions lighter than the surrounding skin.

KOH PREPARATION. The KOH preparation provides a rapid and reliable method for the detection of fungal elements of both yeasts and dermatophytes. Scaly lesions should be scraped at the active border for optimal recovery of mycelia and spores. Vesicles should be unroofed, and the blister top should be clipped and placed on a slide for examination. In tinea capitis, infected hairs must be plucked from the follicle; scales from the scalp usually will not contain mycelia. A few drops of 20% potassium hydroxide are added to the specimen, which is then gently heated over an alcohol lamp until it begins to bubble. The preparation is examined under low-intensity light for fungal elements.

TZANCK SMEAR. A Tzanck smear is useful in the diagnosis of some viral infections (herpes simplex, varicella, herpes zoster, and eczema herpeticum) as well as for detection of acantholytic cells in pemphigus. An intact, fresh blister should be ruptured and drained of fluid. The base of the blister is then vigorously scraped with a dull-edged instrument; the material is smeared on a clear glass slide and air-dried. Staining with Giemsa stain is preferable, but Wright stain is acceptable. Balloon cells and multinucleated giant cells are diagnostic of herpesvirus infection; acantholytic epidermal cells are characteristic of pemphigus.

IMMUNOFLUORESCENCE STUDIES. Immunofluorescence studies of skin can be used to detect tissue-fixed antibodies to skin components and complement; characteristic staining patterns are specific for certain skin disorders. Serum can be used for the identification of circulating antibodies. Skin biopsies for direct immunofluorescence preparations should be obtained from involved sites except in those diseases for which paralesional skin or uninvolved skin is required (Table 23–1). A punch biopsy is obtained, and the tissue is placed in a special transport medium or *immediately* frozen in liquid nitrogen for transport or storage. Thin cryostat sections of the specimen are incubated with fluorescein-conjugated goat or rabbit antihuman globulin or complement.

Serum of patients can be examined by indirect immunofluorescence techniques using sections of normal human skin, guinea pig lip, or monkey esophagus as substrate. A substrate is incubated with fresh or thawed frozen serum and then with fluorescein-conjugated antihuman globulin. If the serum contains antibody to epithelial components, its specific staining pattern can be seen on fluorescence microscopy. By serial dilutions, the titer of circulating antibody can be estimated.

23.3 PRINCIPLES OF THERAPY

Dermatologic therapy is a mixture of art and science in which the nuances often determine the success of management. Competent skin care requires a specific diagnosis and knowledge of the natural course of the disease as well as an appreciation of primary versus secondary lesions. If the diagnosis is uncertain, it is better to err on the side of less rather than more aggressive treatment. Even when the diagnosis is clear, an acute dermatitis may require gentle and bland therapy initially.

In the use of topical medication, consideration of vehicle is as important as the specific therapeutic agent. Acute weeping lesions respond best to wet compresses, followed by lotions or creams. For dry, thickened, scaly skin, an ointment base is more effective. Gels and solutions are most useful for the scalp and other hairy areas. The site of involvement is of considerable importance because the most desirable vehicle may not be cosmetically or functionally appropriate, such as an ointment on the face or hands. The patient's preference should also play a role in the choice of vehicle, because compliance is poor if the medication is not acceptable to the patient.

Lotions are a suspension of water and insoluble powder; as the water evaporates, cooling the skin, a thin film of powder covers the skin. *Ointments* have oils and a small amount of water; they feel greasy, lubricate dry skin, trap water, and may be occlusive if there is a high water content. *Creams* are emulsions of oil and water (more water than in ointments); as the water evaporates, the small amount of oil covers the skin.

Therapy should be kept as simple as possible, and specific written instructions with regard to the frequency and duration of application should be provided. Drug combinations in a single vehicle may exacerbate a dermatitis and cause diagnostic confusion. The physician should become familiar with one or two preparations in each category and should learn to use them appropriately. The careless prescribing of nonspecific proprietary medications that often contain sensitizing agents is not to be condoned. Certain preparations such as topical antihistamines and sensitizing anesthetics are never indicated.

WET DRESSINGS. These dressings will alleviate pruritus, burning, and stinging sensations; they are indicated for any acutely inflamed moist or oozing dermatitis. Although a variety of astringent and antiseptic substances may be added to the solution, tap water compresses are just as effective.

OPEN WET DRESSINGS. These dressings cool and dry the skin by evaporation and cleanse by removal of crusts and exudates that cause further irritation if permitted to remain. The solution should be cool or tepid and consist of tap water, isotonic saline, or aluminum acetate (Burow solution) in a 1:20 or 1:40 dilution. Potassium permanganate is messy and offers no advantage. Boric acid can be toxic if absorbed and should *never* be used for compresses. Dressings of multiple layers of Kerlix, gauze, or soft cotton material should be saturated with the solution and remoistened as often as necessary. Compresses should be applied for 10–20 min at least every 4 hr and should be continued usually for 24–48 hr.

CLOSED WET DRESSINGS. These dressings are indicated for abscesses and cellulitis. The solution should be warm, and the dressings should be covered with plastic to prevent evaporation. Closed wet dressings, if prolonged, cause maceration, because they prevent evaporation and heat loss.

BATH OILS, COLLOIDS, SOAPS. *Bath oil* may be added to the bath or to compressing solutions when the skin is dry. Bath oils, which are highly dispersible and have surfactant activity, may be obtained scented or unscented for the allergic patient. These preparations leave a fine film of oil on the skin for lubrication; parents should be cautioned that the child and the tub will be slippery. Alpha Keri oil, Lubath, and Domol are examples of commercial preparations. Bath oils containing tar (Balnetar, Zetar) can be prescribed for psoriasis and atopic dermatitis.

Colloids such as starch powder or Aveeno are soothing and antipruritic for some patients when added to the bath water. Oilated Aveeno contains mineral oil and lanolin derivatives for lubrication if the skin is dry.

Ordinary toilet *soaps* may be irritating and drying if patients have dry skin or dermatitis. Examples of soaps that are usually not harmful to skin are Dove, Lowila, Aveeno, Neutrogena, Basis, Alpha Keri, and Oilatum. When skin is acutely inflamed, avoidance of soap is advised. Some patients find the use of lipid-free cleansers (Cetaphil) soothing.

LUBRICANTS. Lubricants, such as lotions, creams, and ointments, can be used as emollients for dry skin and as vehicles for topical agents such as corticosteroids and keratolytics. In general, ointments are the most effective emollients. Numerous commercial preparations are available in addition to standard U.S.P. items, such as petrolatum, cold cream, stearin-lanolin cream, and hydrophilic ointment. Some patients do not tolerate ointments, and some may be sensitized to a component of the lubricant; some preservatives of creams (most commonly parabens) are sensitizers.

Useful lubricating lotions include Lubriderm, Shepard's lotion, Nutraderm, and Nivea. Creams include Eucerin, Neutrogena, Nutraderm, Purpose, Vanicream, and Complex 15. Aquaphor is a cosmetically acceptable alternative to petrolatum. These preparations can be applied several times a day if necessary. Maximal effect is achieved when they are applied *immediately* following a bath or shower. Sarna lotion contains menthol and camphor in an emollient vehicle for control of pruritus as well as dryness.

SHAMPOOS. Special shampoos containing sulfur, salicylic acid, antiseptics, and selenium sulfide (Selsun, Exsel) are useful for conditions in which there is scaling of the scalp. Most shampoos also contain surfactants and detergents. Shampoos with sulfur or salicylic acid include Ionil, Sebulex, Fostex, and Vanseb. Those with only antiseptic agents include DHS-zinc, Danex, and Head and Shoulders. Tar-containing shampoos such as T-gel, Ionil-T, Sebutone, and Polytar are useful for psoriasis and severe seborrheic dermatitis. In general, they can be used as frequently as necessary to control scaling, but use must be limited to avoid irritation. Patients should be instructed to leave the lathered shampoo in contact with the scalp for 5–10 min.

SHAKE LOTIONS. These lotions are useful antipruritic agents; they consist of a suspension of powder in a liquid vehicle. A water-dispersible oil may be added for lubrication. Calamine lotion is acceptable but tends to cake on the skin. A prototype lotion is zinc oxide 20 g, talc 20 g, glycerine 20 g, Alpha Keri 5 g, and water to make 120 g. These preparations can be used effectively in combination with wet dressings for exudative dermatitis. Cooling occurs as the lotion evaporates and moisture is absorbed by the powder deposited on the skin.

POWDERS. Powders are hygroscopic and serve as effective absorptive agents in areas of excessive moisture. They are most useful in the intertriginous areas and between the toes, where maceration and abrasion may result from friction on movement. Coarse powders may cake; therefore, they should be of fine particle size and inert unless medication has been incorporated in the formulation. Zeasorb is a bland, finely milled, general purpose powder that can be applied to any area of the body.

PASTES. Pastes contain a fine powder in an ointment vehicle and are not often prescribed in current dermatologic therapy; in certain situations, however, they can be used effectively to protect vulnerable or damaged skin. For example, a stiff zinc oxide paste is bland and inert and can be applied to the diaper area to avert irritant diaper dermatitis. Zinc paste should be applied in a thick layer completely obscuring the skin and is removed more easily with mineral oil than with soap and water.

KERATOLYTIC AGENTS. *Urea*-containing agents are hydrophilic; they hydrate the stratum corneum and make the skin more pliable. In addition, because urea dissolves hydrogen bonds and epidermal keratin, it is effective in treatment of scaling disorders. Concentrations of 10–25% are available in several commercial lotions and creams (Carmol 20, Carmol 10, Nutraplus, Ultra Mide, Aquacare HP), which can be applied once or twice daily as tolerated.

Salicylic acid is an effective keratolytic agent and can be incorporated into a variety of vehicles in concentrations up to 6% to be applied 2–3 times daily. Salicylic acid preparations should not be used in the treatment of small infants or on large surface areas or denuded skin; percutaneous absorption may result in salicylism.

The α-hydroxy acids, particularly *lactic acid* and *glycolic acid*, are available in commercial preparations (Lacticare, Lac-Hydrin, Aqua Glycolic) or can be incorporated in an ointment vehicle such as petrolatum or Aquaphor in concentrations up to 5%. These preparations are useful for the treatment of keratinizing disorders and may be applied once or twice daily. Some patients complain of burning; in this case, the frequency of application should be decreased. A useful keratolytic agent for the scalp is P&S Plus.

TAR COMPOUNDS. Tars are obtained from bituminous coal, shales, petrolatum (coal tars), and wood. They are antipruritic and astringent and appear to promote normal keratinization. They are particularly useful for chronic eczema and psoriasis, and their efficacy may be increased if the affected area is exposed to ultraviolet light. (The tar should be removed prior to exposure to light; otherwise a phototoxic dermatitis may ensue.) Tars *should not be used* in acute inflammatory lesions.

Tars may be incorporated into shampoos, bath oils, lotions, and ointments. A useful preparation for pediatric patients is liquor carbonis detergens (LCD) 2–5% in a cream or ointment vehicle. Tar gels (Psorigel, Estargel, Aquatar) and tar in a light body oil (T-Derm) are relatively pleasant cosmetic preparations that cause minimum staining of skin and fabrics. Tars can also be incorporated into a vehicle with a topical corticosteroid. The frequency of application varies from 1 to 3 times daily according to tolerance.

ANTIFUNGAL AGENTS. These agents are now available as powders, lotions, creams, and ointments for the treatment of dermatophyte and yeast infections. Nystatin and amphotericin B (Fungizone) are specific for *Candida* and are ineffective in other fungal disorders. Tolnaftate (Tinactin) is effective against the dermatophytes and is somewhat effective in the treatment of tinea versicolor. The spectrum for haloprogin (Halotex) includes the dermatophytes, *Pityrosporon orbiculare* and *Candida albicans*. The imidazoles, miconazole (Monistat-Derm), clotrimazole (Lotrimin), econazole (Spectazole), and ketoconazole (Nizoral) have a spectrum similar to haloprogin. They should be applied 2–3 times a day for most fungal infections. All these agents have low sensitizing potential; however, additives such as preservatives and stabilizers in the vehicles may cause allergic contact dermatitis. Whitfield ointment (6% benzoic acid and 3% salicylic acid) is a potent keratolytic agent that has also been used for the treatment of dermatophyte infections. Irritant reactions are common.

TOPICAL ANTIBIOTICS. Topical antibiotics have been used to treat local cutaneous infections for many years, although their efficacy has been questioned. Ointments are the preferable vehicle, and combinations with other topical agents, such as corticosteroids, are in general inadvisable. Whenever possible, the etiologic agent should be identified and treated specifically. Antibiotics in wide use as systemic preparations should be avoided because of the risk of sensitization. The sensitizing potential of certain other antibiotics (e.g., neomycin, Furacin) should be kept in mind. Polysporin and bacitracin are useful preparations for pyoderma; however, mupirocin appears to be the most effective topical agent currently available.

TOPICAL CORTICOSTEROIDS. Topical corticosteroids are potent anti-inflammatory agents and effective antipruritic agents. Successful therapeutic results have been achieved in a wide variety of skin conditions. In general, corticosteroids fall into two classes: nonfluorinated preparations, such as hydrocortisone (Hytone), desonide (Tridesilon, Des Owen), hydrocortisone butyrate (Locoid), and mometasone furoate (Elocon), and fluorinated compounds including triamcinolone (Kenalog, Aristocort), flurandrenolone (Cordran), fluocinolone (Synalar), betamethasone (Valisone, Benisone, Flurobate), and amcinonide (Cyclocort). The nonfluorinated steroids are of lesser potency but also cause fewer local and systemic side effects, whereas fluorinated steroids are potentially more harmful, particularly with long-term use. Other fluorinated compounds, for example, fluoronide (Lidex), halcinonide (Halog), betamethasone dipropionate (Diprolene), and clobetasol propionate (Temovate), are extremely potent and should be prescribed with care. Some of these compounds are formulated in several strengths based on their clinical efficacy and vasoconstrictive ability.

Virtually all of the corticosteroids can be obtained in a variety of vehicles, including creams, ointments, solutions, gels, and aerosols. Absorption is enhanced by an ointment or gel vehicle, but the selection of the vehicle should be based on the type of disorder and the site of involvement. Frequency of application should be determined by the potency of the preparation and the severity of the eruption. In general, the application of a *thin film* 2 times daily will suffice. Adverse local effects include cutaneous atrophy, striae, telangiectasia, hypopigmentation, and increased hair growth.

Percutaneous absorption of corticosteroids can be enhanced up to 100-fold by the use of occlusive pliable plastic wraps (Handi-Wrap, Saran Wrap). The steroid is applied in a thin film and tightly covered with a strip of plastic that is taped to the skin. Plastic bags may be used for the feet, and disposable plastic gloves can be used for the hands. Occlusion should be carried out for no more than 8–10 hr, because prolonged occlusion may produce undesirable side effects such as pyoderma, folliculitis, miliaria, and malodor from maceration and bacterial overgrowth. This procedure is appropriate in chronic recalcitrant disorders such as lichen simplex chronicus, dyshidrotic eczema, and psoriasis. The possibility of systemic absorption and adrenal suppression must be considered if large areas are occluded. Fluorinated corticosteroids with or without occlusion are seldom indicated in infancy.

In selected circumstances, corticosteroids may be administered by intralesional injection (for acne cysts, keloids, psoriatic plaques, alopecia areata, and persistent insect bite reactions). This method of administration should be used only by physicians who are experienced in techniques of dermatologic therapy.

SUNSCREENS. Sunscreens are of two general types: those that reflect all wavelengths of the ultraviolet (UV) and visible spectrums, such as zinc oxide and titanium dioxide; and a heterogeneous group of chemicals that selectively absorb energy of various wavelengths within the ultraviolet spectrum. Some sunscreens permit tanning without burning; others prevent both. In addition to the spectrum of light that is blocked, other factors to be considered include cosmetic acceptance, sensitizing potential, retention on skin while swimming or sweating, required frequency of application, and cost. Effective opaque total barrier agents are A-Fil, zinc oxide ointment, Covermark, Dermablend, and RVPaque. Para-aminobenzoic acid–ethanol (Pabanol, PreSun) and cinnamate-benzophenone combinations (Maxafil, Solbar, Uval) effectively prevent transmission of ultraviolet B (UVB) and at least some ultraviolet A (UVA) wavelengths. Para-aminobenzoic acid (PABA) esters (Eclipse, Pabafilm, Sundown) afford partial protection. Lip protectants that absorb in the UVB range (Sunstick, RVPaba lipstick, Blistik, PreSun) are also available for patients with photo-induced lip disorders such as recurrent herpesvirus infections. Sunscreens are now designated by sun protection factor (SPF) values ranging from 2 (minimal protection) to 15 and above (maximal protection) and are so labeled on the container. Examples of sunscreens offering maximal protection are Supershade, Photoplex, and Total Eclipse. The efficacy of these agents depends on careful attention to instructions for use. PABA-containing sunscreens should be applied at least 30 min before sun exposure to permit penetration of the epidermis. Most patients with photosensitivity eruptions require protection by agents that absorb UVB wavelengths; patients with porphyria, phototoxic eruptions, and some types of solar urticaria require agents with a broader spectrum of prevention.

DISEASES OF THE SKIN

23.4 TRANSIENT LESIONS OF THE NEONATE

Minor evanescent lesions of the newborn infant, particularly when florid, may cause undue concern. Most of the entities described in this section are relatively common, benign, and transient; they do not require therapy.

SEBACEOUS HYPERPLASIA. Minute profuse yellow-white papules are frequently found on the forehead, nose, upper lip, and cheeks of the term infant; they represent hyperplastic sebaceous glands. These tiny papules diminish gradually in size and disappear entirely within the first few weeks of life.

MILIA. The milium is a superficial epidermal inclusion cyst that contains laminated keratinized material. The lesion is a firm papule, 1–2 mm in diameter and pearly, opalescent white in color. Milia may occur at any age but in the neonate are most frequently scattered over the face and gingivae and on the midline of the palate, where they are called *Epstein pearls.* Milia exfoliate spontaneously in most infants and may be ignored; those that appear in scars or sites of trauma in older children may be gently unroofed and "shelled out" with a fine-gauge needle.

SUCKING BLISTERS. Solitary or scattered superficial bullae on the upper limbs of infants at birth are presumed to be induced by vigorous sucking on the affected part in utero. Common sites are the radial aspect of the forearm, the thumb, and the index finger. These bullae resolve rapidly without sequelae. These lesions should be distinguished from sucking pads (calluses), which are found on the lips in the first few months and represent combined intracellular edema and hyperkeratosis. The diagnosis can be confirmed by observing the neonate suck the affected area.

CUTIS MARMORATA. When the newborn infant is exposed to low environmental temperatures, an evanescent, lacy, reticulated red or blue cutaneous vascular pattern appears over most of the body surface. This vascular change represents an accentuated physiologic vasomotor response that disappears with increasing age, although it is sometimes discernible even in older children. Persistent and pronounced cutis marmorata occurs in the Cornelia de Lange, Down, and 18-trisomy syndromes. Cutis marmorata telangiectatica congenita is clinically similar, but the lesions are more intense and are persistent.

HARLEQUIN COLOR CHANGE. This rare but dramatic vascular event occurs in the immediate newborn period and is most common in infants of low birthweight. It probably reflects an imbalance in the autonomic vascular regulatory mechanism. When the infant is placed on his or her side, the body is bisected longitudinally into a pale upper half and a deep red dependent half. The color change lasts only for a few minutes and occasionally affects only a portion of the trunk or face. The pattern may be reversed by changing the infant's position. Muscular activity will cause generalized flushing and will obliterate the color differential. Multiple episodes may occur but do not indicate permanent autonomic imbalance.

SALMON PATCH (NEVUS SIMPLEX). Salmon patches are small, pale pink, ill-defined, flat vascular lesions that occur most commonly on the glabella, eyelids, upper lip, and nuchal area of 30–50% of normal newborn infants. These lesions, which represent localized plaques of vascular ectasia, persist for several months and may become more visible during crying or changes in environmental temperature. The lesions on the face eventually fade and disappear completely, but those on the posterior neck and occipital area often persist. When they become covered with hair, they are not noticeable. The facial lesions should not be confused with a port-wine stain, which is a permanent lesion.

MONGOLIAN SPOTS. These blue or slate-gray macular lesions have variably defined margins; they occur most commonly in the presacral area but may be found over the posterior thighs, legs, back, and shoulders. They may be solitary or multiple and often involve large areas. More than 80% of black, oriental, and East Indian infants have these lesions, whereas the incidence in white infants is less than 10%. The peculiar hue of these macules is due to the dermal location of melanin-containing melanocytes that are presumed to have been arrested in their migration from neural crest to epidermis. Mongolian spots usually fade during the first few years of life, but occasionally persist. Malignant degeneration does not occur. Widespread multiple lesions, particularly those in unusual sites, are unlikely to disappear. The characteristic appearance and congenital onset distinguish these spots from the bruises of child abuse.

ERYTHEMA TOXICUM. This benign, self-limited, evanescent eruption occurs in approximately 50% of full-term infants; preterm infants are affected less commonly. The lesions are firm, yellow-white, 1- to 2-mm papules or pustules with a surrounding erythematous flare (Fig. 23–1 [color plate section]). At times, splotchy erythema is the only manifestation. Lesions may be sparse or numerous and clustered in several sites or widely dispersed over much of the body surface. Palms and soles are usually spared. Peak incidence occurs on the 2nd day of life, but new lesions may erupt during the 1st few days as the rash waxes and wanes.

The pustules form below the stratum corneum or deeper in the epidermis and represent collections of eosinophils that also accumulate around the upper portion of the pilosebaceous follicle. The eosinophils can be demonstrated in Wright-stained smears of the intralesional contents. Cultures are sterile.

The cause of erythema toxicum is unknown. The lesions can mimic pyoderma, candidosis, herpes simplex, transient neonatal pustular melanosis, and miliaria but can be differentiated by the characteristic infiltrate of eosinophils and the absence of organisms on a stained smear. The course is brief, and no therapy is required. Incontinentia pigmenti and eosinophilic pustular folliculitis also have eosinophilic infiltration but can be distinguished by their distribution, histology, and chronicity.

TRANSIENT NEONATAL PUSTULAR MELANOSIS. Pustular melanosis, which is more common in black than in white infants, is a transient, benign, self-limited dermatosis of unknown cause that is characterized by three types of lesions: (1) evanescent superficial pustules; (2) ruptured pustules with a collarette of fine scale, at times with a central hyperpigmented macule; and (3) hyperpigmented macules (Fig. 23–2). The lesions are present at birth, and one or all types of lesions may be found in a profuse or sparse distribution. The pustules represent the early phase of the disorder, the macules, the late phase. Sites of predilection are the anterior neck, forehead, and lower back, although the scalp, trunk, limbs, palms, and soles may be affected.

Biopsies of tissue during the active phase show an intracorneal or subcorneal pustule filled with polymorphonuclear leukocytes, debris, and an occasional eosinophil. The macules are characterized only by increased melanization of epidermal cells. Cultures and smears can be used to distinguish these pustules from those of erythema toxicum and pyoderma because they do not contain bacteria or dense aggregates of eosinophils.

The pustular phase rarely lasts more than 2–3 days; hyperpigmented macules may persist for as long as 3 mo. No therapy is required.

23.5 DEVELOPMENTAL DEFECTS

23.6 CUTANEOUS DEFECTS

SKIN DIMPLES. Deep dimpling over bony prominences and in the sacral area, at times associated with pits and creases, may occur in normal children as well as in association with some dysmorphologic syndromes, such as those of congenital rubella, deletion of the long arm of chromosome 18, Bloom, and the cerebrohepatorenal syndromes.

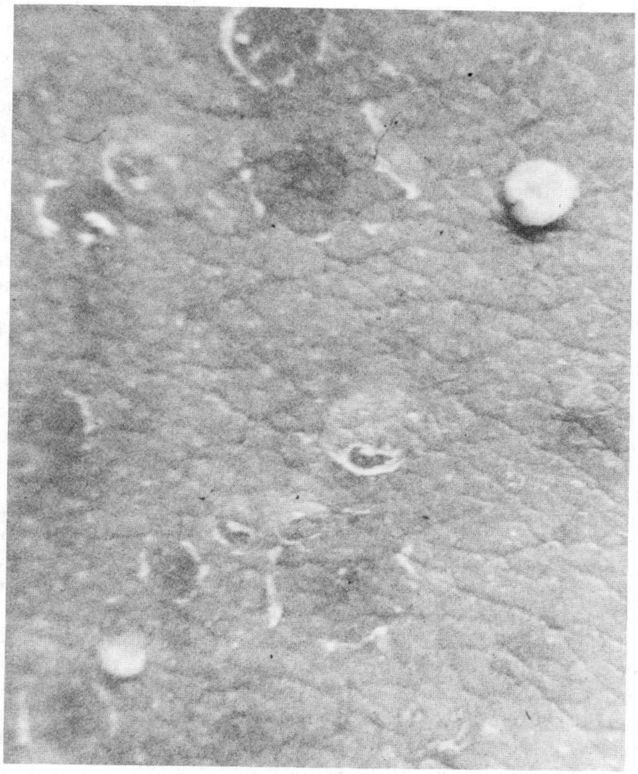

Figure 23–2. Transient neonatal pustular melanosis showing pustules, rings of scales, and hyperpigmented macules.

REDUNDANT SKIN. Loose folds of skin must be differentiated from cutis laxa, a congenital defect of elastic tissue. Redundant skin over the posterior neck is common in the Turner and Down syndromes; more generalized folds of the skin occur in infants with 18-trisomy, with combined immunodeficiency disease, and with short-limbed dwarfism.

AMNIOTIC CONSTRICTION BANDS. Partial or complete constriction bands that produce defects in extremities and digits are found occasionally in otherwise normal infants. Associated abnormalities include craniofacial anomalies and thoracic or abdominal wall defects. Bands are thought to result from intrauterine rupture of amnion with formation of fibrous strands that encircle the fetal parts and cause permanent depression of the underlying tissue. Alternatively, they may represent a reparative process following vascular compromise. Rarely, amputation of one or more digits may result. Constriction bands on the limbs may be removed by plastic procedures.

PREAURICULAR SINUSES AND PITS. Pits and sinus tracts anterior to the pinna may be the result of imperfect fusion of the tubercles of the 1st and 2nd branchial arches, from which the tragus and pinna are derived. These anomalies may be unilateral or bilateral, may be familial, are more common in females and blacks, and at times are associated with other anomalies of the ears and face. When the tracts become chronically infected, retention cysts may form and drain intermittently; such lesions may require excision.

ACCESSORY TRAGI. Multiple or single, unilateral or bilateral, sessile or pedunculated, soft or cartilaginous skin tags may occur in the preauricular area or on the neck anterior to the sternocleidomastoid muscle. They may occur as isolated defects or in syndromes that include anomalies of the ears and face, such as Goldenhar syndrome. Surgical excision is appropriate. Infants should be screened for deafness.

BRANCHIAL CLEFT AND THYROGLOSSAL CYSTS AND SINUSES. Cysts and sinuses in the neck may be formed along the course of the 1st and 2nd branchial clefts as a result of improper closure during embryonic life. The lesions may be unilateral or bilateral and may open onto the cutaneous surface or drain into the pharynx. Secondary infection is an indication for systemic antibiotic therapy. These anomalies may be inherited as autosomal dominant traits.

Thyroglossal cysts and fistulas are similar defects located in or near the midline of the neck; they may extend to the base of the tongue. These cysts occasionally contain aberrant thyroid tissue as well as the usual mucinous material. Surgical excision is the appropriate treatment, but care must be taken to preserve thyroid tissue (Sec. 19.10).

SUPERNUMERARY NIPPLES. Solitary or multiple accessory nipples may occur in a unilateral or bilateral distribution along a line from the midaxilla to the inguinal area. The accessory nipples may or may not have areolae and may be mistaken for congenital nevi. They may be excised for cosmetic reasons. Rarely, they undergo malignant change. Urinary tract anomalies may occur in children with this finding.

APLASIA CUTIS CONGENITA (CONGENITAL ABSENCE OF SKIN). Developmental absence of skin is usually noted on the scalp as multiple or solitary (70%), noninflammatory, well demarcated, oval or circular 1- to 2-cm ulcers. The majority occur at the vertex just lateral to the midline, but similar defects may also occur on the face, trunk, and limbs, where they are often symmetric. The depth of the ulcer varies; it may involve only the epidermis and upper dermis, or it may extend to the deep dermis, subcutaneous tissue, and, rarely, to the periosteum, skull, and dura. The defects are covered occasionally by a tough membrane and simulate a bulla. Although sporadic, in some cases, multiple family members have been afflicted; both autosomal recessive and dominant patterns of inheritance have been observed. Defects of the limbs (syndactyly, polydactyly) and trunk (umbilical hernia, omphalocele), usually symmetric, have been associated with intrauterine events such as placental infarcts and monozygotic twinning with fetus papyraceus. The etiology is unknown.

The major complications are massive hemorrhage, secondary local infection, and meningitis. Associated developmental defects are rare; they include cleft lip and palate, hamartomas, vascular malformations, congenital heart disease, limb anomalies, and defects of the central nervous system. Aplasia cutis is also associated with malformation syndromes such as 13-trisomy, 4p-, Johanson-Blizzard syndrome, focal dermal hypoplasia, ectodermal dysplasias, and amniotic band disruption complex. Congenital localized defects of skin, generalized recurrent blisters of skin and mucous membranes, and nail defects inherited as an autosomal dominant trait are known as Bart syndrome, which is probably a rare form of epidermolysis bullosa. The differential diagnosis includes injury from amniocentesis and the congenital hairless nevus sebaceus of Jadassohn.

If the defect is small, recovery is uneventful with gradual epithelialization and formation of a hairless atrophic scar over a period of several weeks (Fig. 23–3). Small bony defects usually close spontaneously during the 1st yr of life. Large or multiple scalp defects may require excision and primary closure, if feasible, rotation of a flap to fill the defect, or the use of tissue expanders. Truncal and limb defects, despite large size, usually epithelialize and form atrophic scars, which can later be revised, if necessary.

FOCAL FACIAL DERMAL DYSPLASIA (*Bitemporal aplasia cutis congenita*; ectodermal dysplasia of the face). This rare disorder is characterized by congenital atrophic depressed lesions on the temples and a spectrum of associated facial anomalies including frontal bossing, upward slanting eyebrows, absence of or multiple rows of eyelashes, and a prominent chin with a median ridge. The pattern of inheritance is not established, but both autosomal dominant and autosomal recessive inheritance have been documented in affected kindreds.

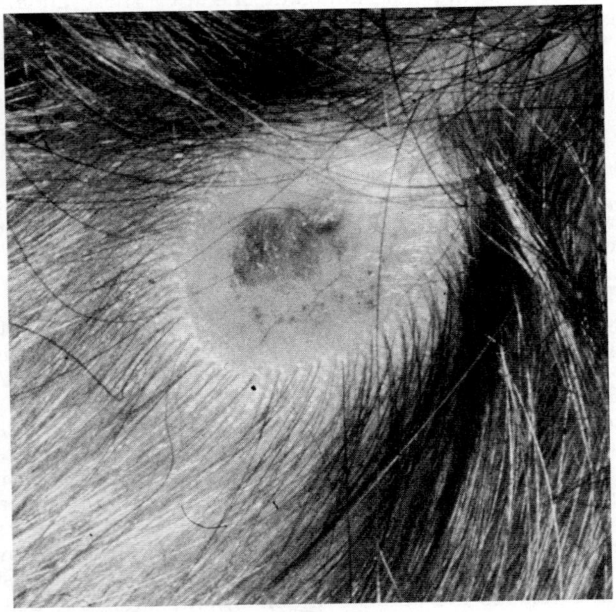

Figure 23–3. Healing solitary lesion of aplasia cutis.

FOCAL DERMAL HYPOPLASIA (GOLTZ SYNDROME). This rare congenital mesoectodermal disorder is characterized by herniations of fat through thinned, partially deficient dermis that are responsible for multiple soft, tan-colored papillomas. Other types of skin changes include linear cribriform atrophic lesions, reticulated hypopigmentation and hyperpigmentation, telangiectasia, congenital absence of skin, angiofibromas presenting as verrucous excrescences, and papillomas of the lips, tongue, circumoral region, vulva, anus, and the inguinal, axillary, and periumbilical areas. Partial alopecia, sweating disorders, and dystrophic nails are additional less common ectodermal anomalies.

The most frequent skeletal defects include syndactyly, clinodactyly and polydactyly, and scoliosis and other spinal anomalies. Ocular abnormalities are legion, but the most common are colobomas, strabismus, nystagmus, and microphthalmia. Small stature, dental defects, soft-tissue anomalies, and peculiar dermatoglyphic patterns are also common. Mental deficiency occurs occasionally.

This familial disorder occurs principally in girls. It has been postulated that an X-linked dominant gene, lethal in males, may account for the sex distribution. Affected males may be mosaic or may have a less severe mutation. This disorder is often confused with incontinentia pigmenti because it shares a sex predilection for females and has some similar skin manifestations and mesodermal anomalies. The cutaneous lesions may also superficially resemble epidermal nevi. Treatment should be directed at amelioration of specific anomalies; genetic counseling is advisable.

CONGENITAL DYSKERATOSIS (ZINSSER-ENGMAN-COLE SYNDROME). This rare familial syndrome usually affects males and is inherited most often in an X-linked fashion. However, autosomal recessive or dominant inheritance may occur. The onset occurs during childhood; nail dystrophy is the usual initial manifestation. The nails become ridged and atrophic, and there is considerable loss of the nail plate. The skin changes resemble a poikiloderma consisting of reticulated gray-brown pigmentation, atrophy, and telangiectasia, especially on the neck, face, and chest. Hyperhidrosis and hyperkeratosis of the palms and soles, acrocyanosis, and occasional bullae on the hands and feet are also characteristic. Blepharitis, ectropion, and excessive tearing due to atresia of the lacrimal ducts are occasional manifestations. Vesiculobullous lesions may occur on the oral mucous membranes and result in ulceration, formation of epithelial tags, atrophic changes of the tongue, and premalignant oral leukokeratosis. Similar changes have been noted in the urethral and anal mucosa. The scalp hair, eyebrows, and lashes may become sparse. Hypoplastic anemia, at times of the Fanconi variety, is a common late complication; T and B lymphocyte abnormalities have been noted.

The differential diagnosis includes the ectodermal dysplasias, pachyonychia congenita, poikilodermas, epidermolysis bullosa, keratoderma of the palms and soles, and lichen sclerosus et atrophicus. The abnormalities noted in skin biopsies are those of poikiloderma. Congenital dyskeratosis is progressive and may be complicated by squamous cell carcinoma of the mouth or anus as well as by the potentially lethal pancytopenia. Management includes biopsy of leukoplakic sites to identify malignancies and corticosteroids, androgens, or bone marrow transplantation for aplastic anemia.

CUTIS VERTICIS GYRATA. This bizarre alteration of the scalp, which is more common in males, may be present from birth or develop during adolescence. The scalp is characterized by convoluted elevated folds, 1–2 cm in thickness, usually in the fronto-occipital axis. Unlike the lax skin of other disorders, the convolutions cannot be flattened by traction.

Primary cutis gyrata is often associated with mental retardation, ocular defects, abnormal size and shape of the head, seizures, and spasticity. Secondary cutis gyrata may be due to chronic inflammatory diseases, tumors, nevi, acromegaly, and pachydermoperiostosis, a syndrome characterized by hypertrophy of the skin and bones.

23.7 ECTODERMAL DYSPLASIAS

The term ectodermal dysplasia is used to designate a group of disorders characterized by a constellation of defects involving the teeth, skin, and appendageal structures, including hair, nails, and eccrine and sebaceous glands. Disturbances in tissue derived from embryologic layers other than ectoderm are not uncommon. Many of the syndromes have overlapping features and are distinguished by the presence or absence of a single defect.

HYPOHIDROTIC (ANHIDROTIC) ECTODERMAL DYSPLASIA. This syndrome is manifested by a triad of defects: hypohidrosis, anomalous dentition, and hypotrichosis. It is usually inherited as an X-linked recessive trait, with full expression only in males; however, an autosomal recessive mode of inheritance may be operative in some families. Heterozygotic females may have some clinical manifestations.

Affected children unable to sweat may experience episodes of high fever in warm environments and may be mistakenly considered to have fever of unknown origin. This is particularly the case in infancy when the facial changes are not easily appreciated. The typical facies is characterized by frontal bossing, malar hypoplasia, a flattened nasal bridge, recessed columella, thick, everted lips, wrinkled, hyperpigmented periorbital skin, and prominent, low set ears (Fig. 23–4). The skin over the entire body is dry and hypopigmented, often with a prominent venous pattern. The hair is sparse, unruly, and lightly pigmented, and eyebrows and lashes are sparse or absent. Anodontia or hypodontia with widely spaced, peg-shaped teeth is a consistent feature (see Fig. 23–4). Less commonly, stenotic lacrimal puncta, corneal dysplasia, cataracts, hypoplastic or absent mammary glands, and conductive hearing loss have been observed. The incidence of atopic diseases in these children is relatively high.

The sweating deficit is a reflection of hypoplasia or absence of the eccrine glands; this may be confirmed by skin biopsy. The palmar skin is an appropriate site for biopsy. Reduction or absence of sweating can be documented by pilocarpine iontophoresis or by topical application of *o*-phthalaldehyde to the palmar skin. Sweat pores are not visible in the palmar ridges in affected children and are decreased in number in carrier females. Diminished lacrimation and atrophic rhinitis are due to maldevelopment of the secretory glands, which predisposes to purulent rhinitis. These glands are also deficient in the tracheobronchial mucosa, the esophagus, and the duodenum; recurrent pulmonary infections, hoarseness, and dysphonia are the clinical manifestations.

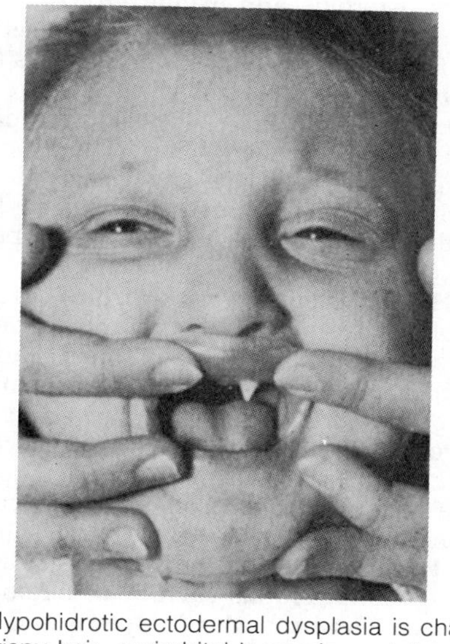

Figure 23–4. Hypohidrotic ectodermal dysplasia is characterized by pointed ears, wispy hair, periorbital hyperpigmentation, midfacial hypoplasia, and pegged teeth.

Children with hypohidrotic ectodermal dysplasia must be protected from exposure to high ambient temperatures. Early dental evaluation is necessary so that prostheses can be provided for cosmetic reasons and for adequate nutrition. The use of artificial tears will prevent damage to the cornea in patients with defective lacrimation. Alopecia may necessitate the wearing of a wig to improve the appearance.

HIDROTIC ECTODERMAL DYSPLASIA (CLOUSTON TYPE). Dystrophic, hypoplastic, or absent nails, sparse hair, and hyperkeratosis of the palms and soles are the salient features of this autosomal dominant disorder. The dentition is usually normal, although small teeth and rampant caries are occasionally associated. Sweating is always normal. Absence of eyebrows and lashes and hyperpigmentation over the knees, elbows, and knuckles have been noted in some affected individuals.

EEC SYNDROME. Ectrodactyly, ectodermal dysplasia, and cleft lip and palate compose the EEC syndrome, which is probably inherited as an autosomal dominant trait of low penetrance and variable expressivity. The ectodermal dysplasia consists of a dry, poorly pigmented integument, light-colored, wispy, sparse scalp hair and eyebrows, and absence of lashes. Decreased numbers of hair follicles and sebaceous glands have been demonstrated by biopsy.

Associated defects include anomalies of the hands and feet, nail hypoplasia, granulomatous perlèche frequently complicated by candidosis, defective dentition, ocular abnormalities such as blepharophimosis, atretic or absent lacrimal puncta, strabismus, and abnormalities of the urinary tract.

RAPP-HODGKIN ECTODERMAL DYSPLASIA. This disorder is inherited as an autosomal dominant trait and consists of hypohidrosis with reduced numbers of sweat pores, anomalous dentition, ocular abnormalities, sparse hair, dysplastic nails, oral clefts, variable growth deficiency, and hypospadias.

ROBINSON-TYPE ECTODERMAL DYSPLASIA. This autosomal dominant disorder combines sensorineural deafness, nail dystrophy, and peg-shaped teeth with partial anodontia.

23.8 VASCULAR LESIONS

Developmental vascular anomalies may occur as isolated defects or as part of a syndrome. They can be separated into two major categories: hemangiomas and malformations. Hemangiomas are proliferative lesions of vascular endothelium that predictably spontaneously involute. Malformations are derived from capillaries, veins, arteries, or lymphatics or any combination thereof, are relatively static, and do not regress.

NEVUS FLAMMEUS (PORT-WINE NEVUS, PORT-WINE STAIN). Port-wine nevi are always present at birth; they consist of mature dilated dermal capillaries and represent a permanent developmental defect. The lesions are macular, sharply circumscribed, pink to purple in color (or occasionally black in deeply pigmented infants), and tremendously varied in size, occasionally involving up to one half of the body surface (Fig. 23–5). The posterior surface of the neck is a common site (Unna nevus). The face is also a site of predilection; distribution is often unilateral, and the mucous membranes can be involved. With maturation, the port-wine nevus may become slightly raised and pebbly in consistency; alternatively, the paler lesions may fade somewhat.

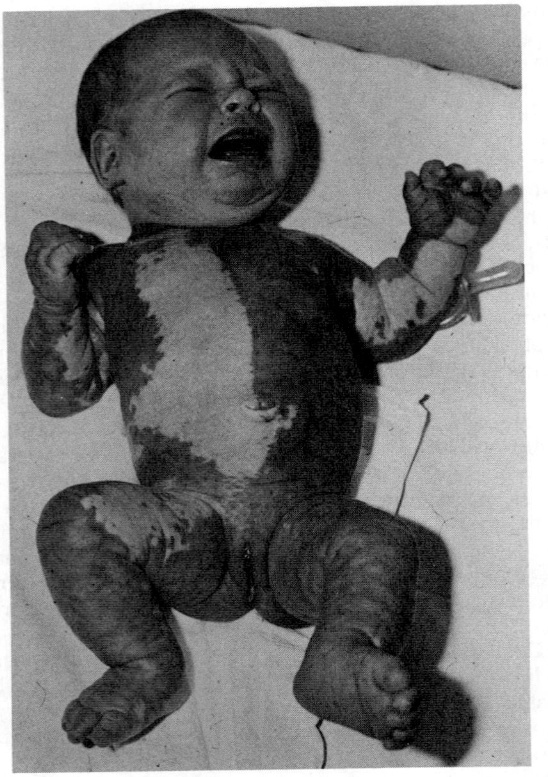

Figure 23–5. Widespread nevus flammeus in an infant with Klippel-Trenaunay-Weber syndrome.

True nevus flammeus should be distinguished from the common salmon patch of the neonate, which is, in contrast, a relatively transient lesion. When the nevus is localized to the trigeminal area of the face, the diagnosis of *Sturge-Weber syndrome* (leptomeningeal venous angioma, seizures, hemiparesis contralateral to the facial lesion, and intracranial calcification) must be considered (Sec. 20.41). Rarely, Sturge-Weber syndrome is associated with a bilateral facial lesion or with a nevus flammeus elsewhere on the body surface. Nevus flammeus also occurs as a component of Klippel-Trenaunay-Weber syndrome and with moderate frequency in other syndromes, including the Rubinstein-Taybi, Cobb (spinal arteriovenous malformation and nevus flammeus), Beckwith-Wiedemann, and 13-trisomy syndromes. In the absence of associated anomalies, the morbidities from these lesions may include a poor self-image, hypertrophy of underlying structures, and traumatic bleeding.

Several types of therapy including masking with cosmetics (e.g., Covermark, Dermablend), cryosurgery, excision and grafting, and tattooing have been utilized in the management of this defect in the past; however, laser therapy has become the modality of choice.

Although the argon and CO_2 lasers have been used with moderate success in adolescents and adults, the best results in infants and children have been with the flash-lamp–pulsed dye laser. This therapy is targeted at the lesion and avoids thermal injury to the surrounding normal tissue. After such treatment, the texture and pigmentation of the skin is generally normal and without scarring.

HEMANGIOMAS. Hemangiomas are the most common tumor of infancy and, with rare exception, they occur sporadically and without a genetic basis. Cutaneous hemangiomas are superficial (capillary) in approximately 60% of cases and are deep (cavernous) in 15% of cases; they have both a superficial and a deep component (mixed) in approximately 20%.

CAPILLARY HEMANGIOMA (STRAWBERRY NEVUS). So-called strawberry hemangiomas are bright red, protuberant, compressible, sharply demarcated lesions that may occur on any area of the body. Although sometimes present at birth, more often they appear within the first 2 mo, heralded by an erythematous mark or by an area of pallor, which subsequently develops a fine telangiectatic pattern prior to the phase of expansion. Girls are affected more often than boys. Favored sites are the face, scalp, back, and anterior chest; lesions may be solitary or multiple.

Most superficial hemangiomas undergo a phase of rapid expansion followed by a stationary period and finally by spontaneous involution. Regression may be anticipated when the lesion develops blanched or pale gray areas that are indicative of fibrosis. The course of a particular lesion is unpredictable, but approximately 60% of these lesions have involuted completely by the age of 5 yr, and 90–95% have involuted by the age of 9 yr. Spontaneous involution cannot be correlated with size or site of involvement, but lip lesions seem to persist most often. Complications include ulceration, secondary infection, and, rarely, hemorrhage. The location of a lesion may interfere with a vital function (e.g., eyelid with vision, urethra with urination). Respiratory symptoms should suggest a tracheobronchial lesion.

In the usual patient who has no serious complications or extensive overgrowth that results in tissue destruction and severe disfigurement, a course of expectant observation should be followed. Because almost all of these lesions resolve spontaneously, interference is rarely indicated and may, in fact, cause further harm. Parents require repeated reassurance and support. After spontaneous resolution, approximately 10% of patients are left with small cosmetic defects, such as puckering or discoloration of skin. These defects can be eliminated or minimized by judicious plastic repair if it is desired.

In the rare case in which intervention is required, excision may be advisable; the extent of scarring anticipated should influence the final decision. Radiation can be hazardous and should be considered only in life-threatening situations, such as the Kasabach-Merritt syndrome. Elastic bandages may reduce the amount of tissue distortion resulting from rapid growth, but they are appropriate only in selected patients with large hemangiomas. Systemic or intralesional administration of corticosteroids and α-interferon may be indicated for infants at risk for serious sequelae from exceptionally large or rapidly growing hemangiomas in vital areas (see later).

CAVERNOUS HEMANGIOMAS. These are more deeply situated lesions and, therefore, appear more diffuse and ill-defined than capillary hemangiomas. The lesions are cystic, firm, or compressible, and the overlying skin may appear normal in color or have a bluish hue. Mixed hemangiomas consist of a deep component with a superimposed capillary hemangioma (Fig. 23–6).

Cavernous hemangiomas progress from a growth phase to a stationary phase to a period of involution. These lesions are likely to regress as capillary hemangiomas, and the outcome cannot be predicted from size or site of involvement. A course of expectant observation should be followed in most cases. If involvement of underlying structures is suspected, appropriate radiologic studies should be performed for elucidation. Rarely, these lesions impinge on vital structures, interfere with functions such as vision or feeding, cause grotesque disfigurement because of rapid growth, or are associated with life-threatening complications such as thrombocytopenia and hemorrhage (see Kasabach-Merritt syndrome). If it becomes necessary to intervene, a course of prednisone (2–4 mg/kg/24 hr) has proved effective in some infants. Termination of

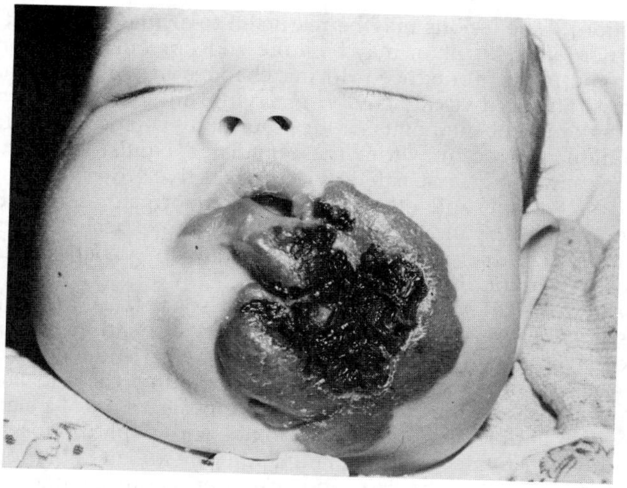

Figure 23–6. Large mixed capillary and cavernous hemangioma with central crusted ulcer.

growth and sometimes regression may be evident after approximately 4 wk of therapy. When a response is obtained, the dosage should be decreased gradually. Alternate day corticosteroid therapy has also been administered with success. Intralesional corticosteroid injection with the patient anesthetized can also induce rapid involution of a localized hemangioma. This technique has been useful particularly in patients with eyelid hemangiomas, which have a high incidence of complications including amblyopia, strabismus, and refractive errors. Alpha-interferon therapy may also be effective.

Cavernous hemangiomas are associated with macrocephaly and pseudopapilledema in a rare autosomal dominant syndrome and occur with variable frequency in I cell disease and in Gorham disease (cavernous hemangiomas and disappearing bones).

KASABACH-MERRITT SYNDROME. This syndrome is a combination of a rapidly enlarging hemangioma, thrombocytopenia, and an acute or chronic consumption coagulopathy. It is usually clinically evident during early infancy, but occasionally the onset is later. The hemangiomas are often present at birth and characteristically are solitary and large, although multiple and small hemangiomas have also been associated with this complication. The vascular lesions are usually cutaneous and are only rarely located in viscera. The associated platelet defect may lead to precipitous hemorrhage accompanied by ecchymoses, petechiae, and a rapid increase in size of the hemangioma. Severe anemia due to hemorrhage or microangiopathic hemolysis may ensue. The platelet count is depressed, but the bone marrow contains increased numbers of normal or immature megakaryocytes. The thrombocytopenia has been attributed to sequestration or increased destruction of platelets within the hemangioma. Hypofibrinogenemia and decreased levels of consumable clotting factors are relatively common (Sec. 16.75–16.77).

Therapy includes the management of thrombocytopenia, anemia, and consumptive coagulopathy by administering platelets and by transfusion of red blood cells and fresh frozen plasma. Heparinization is controversial but has benefitted some patients when combined with transfusions. Arteriovenous shunts in large lesions may produce high-output heart failure requiring digitalization. Treatment of the lesion includes systemic steroids, embolization, radiation therapy, aminocaproic acid (inhibits fibrinolysis), and recombinant α-interferon, which may inhibit proliferation of endothelial and smooth muscle cells. The mortality rate is 20–30%.

DISSEMINATED HEMANGIOMATOSIS. This is a serious condition in which multiple hemangiomas are widely distributed cutaneously and internally; on the skin there are usually numerous small, red, or purple papular hemangiomas, but infrequently they may be sparse or absent. The internal hemangiomas may involve any of the viscera; the liver, gastrointestinal tract, central nervous system, and lung are the most common sites. Ultrasound and CT scanning are indicated to determine the extent of visceral or neural involvement. The disorder is often fatal because of high-output cardiac failure, visceral hemorrhage, obstruction of the respiratory tract, or compression of central neural tissue. In some cases, systemic corticosteroid therapy alone or in combination with surgery or irradiation has apparently been lifesaving. Myriads of cutaneous hemangiomas may occur in the absence of visceral involvement (benign neonatal hemangiomatosis); spontaneous regression of the lesions without complications is probable in such cases.

Multiple hemangiomas may also occur in several rare syndromes, such as macrocephaly combined with pseudopapilledema or with lipomas.

BLUE RUBBER BLEB NEVUS. This syndrome consists of multiple cavernous hemangiomas of the skin, mucous membranes, and gastrointestinal tract. Typical lesions are blue-purple in color and rubbery in consistency; they vary in size from a few millimeters to a few centimeters in diameter. They are sometimes painful or tender. Large disfiguring hemangiomas and irregular blue marks may also occur. The lesions, which can rarely be located in the liver, spleen, and central nervous system in addition to the skin and gastrointestinal tract, do not involute spontaneously. Recurrent gastrointestinal hemorrhage may lead to severe anemia. Palliation can be achieved by excision of involved bowel. Cutaneous angiomas have been removed successfully by laser therapy.

MAFFUCCI SYNDROME. The association of cavernous hemangiomas, phlebectasias, lymphangiomas, and lymphangiectasias with nodular echondromas in the metaphyseal or diaphyseal portion of long bones is known as the Maffucci syndrome. Onset occurs during childhood. Bone lesions may produce limb deformities and pathologic fractures. Chondrosarcoma or angiosarcoma may become complications.

KLIPPEL-TRENAUNAY-WEBER SYNDROME. A macular vascular nevus (port-wine nevus) in combination with bony and soft-tissue hypertrophy and venous varicosities constitutes the triad of defects of this nonheritable disorder. The anomaly is present at birth and usually involves a lower limb but may involve more than one as well as portions of the trunk or face (see Fig. 23–5). Enlargement of the soft tissues may be gradual and may involve the entire extremity, a portion of it, or selected digits. In addition to venous varicosities, arteriovenous fistulas can develop, and bruits are audible in the affected part. This disorder can be confused with Maffucci syndrome or, if the surface hemangioma is minimal, with Milroy disease. Pain, limb swelling, and cellulitis may occur. Thrombophlebitis, dislocations of joints, gangrene of the affected extremity, congestive heart failure, hematuria secondary to urinary tract hemangiomas, rectal bleeding from lesions of the gastrointestinal tract, pulmonary lesions, and malformations of the lymphatic vessels are infrequent complications. Arteriograms and venograms may delineate the extent of the anomaly, but surgical correction or palliation is often difficult. The indications for radiologic studies of viscera and bones are best determined by clinical evaluation. Supportive care includes compression bandages for varicosities; surgical treatment may help carefully selected patients. Leg length differences should be treated with orthotic devices to prevent the development of spinal deformities. Eventually, corrective bone surgery may be needed to treat significant leg length discrepancy.

HEREDITARY HEMORRHAGIC TELANGIECTASIA (OSLER-WEBER-RENDU DISEASE). This disorder is inherited as an autosomal dominant trait. Affected children may experience recurrent epistaxis prior to detection of the characteristic skin and mucous membrane lesions. The mucocutaneous lesions, which usually develop at puberty, are 1–4 mm, sharply demarcated, red to purple macules, papules, or spider-like projections, each composed of a tightly woven mat of tortuous telangiectatic vessels. The nasal mucosa, lips, and tongue are usually involved; less commonly, cutaneous lesions occur on the face, ears, palms, and nail beds. Vascular ectasias may also arise in the conjunctivae, larynx, pharynx, gastrointestinal tract, bladder, vagina, bronchi, brain, and liver.

Massive hemorrhage is the most serious complication and may result in severe anemia. Bleeding may occur from the nose, mouth, gastrointestinal tract, genitourinary tract, and lungs. Persons with hereditary hemorrhagic telangiectasia have normal levels of clotting factors and an intact clotting mechanism. In the absence of serious complications, life span is normal. Local lesions may be ablated temporarily with chemical cautery or electrocoagulation. More drastic surgical measures may be required for lesions in critical sites such as the lung or gastrointestinal tract. Anemia should be treated with iron.

SPIDER ANGIOMAS. The vascular spider (nevus araneus) consists of a central feeder artery with multiple dilated radiating vessels and a surrounding erythematous flush, varying from a few millimeters to several centimeters in diameter. Pressure over the central vessel will cause blanching; pulsations visible in larger nevi are evidence for the arterial source of the lesion. Spider angiomas are associated with conditions in which there are increased levels of circulating estrogens, such as cirrhosis and pregnancy, but they also occur in up to 15% of normal preschool-aged children and 45% of school-aged ones. Sites of predilection in children are the dorsum of the hand, forearm, face, and ears. Angiomas can be obliterated by application of liquid nitrogen, by electrocoagulation, or by pulsed dye laser; they may also regress spontaneously.

GENERALIZED ESSENTIAL TELANGIECTASIA. A rare and presumably nevoid anomaly of unknown etiology, essential telangiectasia may have its onset in childhood or adulthood. Mild expression consists of patchy retiform telangiectases, particularly on the limbs, with occasional progression to involve large areas of the body surface. The condition must be distinguished from the secondary telangiectasia of connective tissue diseases, xeroderma pigmentosum, poikiloderma, and ataxia-telangiectasia. There is no treatment; however, patients can be reassured that their health will not be affected by the cutaneous disorder.

UNILATERAL NEVOID TELANGIECTASIA. This unusual entity is characterized by the appearance of telangiectasia in a unilateral distribution, particularly in females at onset of menses or during pregnancy. The appearance of these lesions usually coincides with elevated levels of circulating estrogens, whatever the cause. When initiated by pregnancy, the telangiectasia may fade or disappear postpartum.

HEREDITARY BENIGN TELANGIECTASIA. This rare disorder is inherited as an autosomal dominant trait and develops during childhood. The face, upper trunk, and arms are the areas of predilection. The condition is progressive but remains limited to the skin.

CUTIS MARMORATA TELANGIECTATICA CONGENITA (CONGENITAL GENERALIZED PHLEBECTASIA). This benign vascular anomaly represents dilatation of superficial capillaries and veins and is apparent at birth. Involved areas of skin have a reticulated pattern of a red or purple hue that resembles physiologic cutis marmorata but is more pronounced and relatively unvarying (Fig. 23–7 [color plate section]). The lesions may be restricted to a single limb and a portion of the trunk or may be more widespread. The lesions become more pronounced during changes in environmental temperature, physical activity, or crying. In some cases, the underlying subcutaneous tissue is underdeveloped, and ulceration may occur within the reticulated bands. Port-wine stain may also be associated. Rarely, defective growth of bone and soft tissue and other congenital abnormalities may be present. No specific therapy is indicated; the expected course is one of gradual steady improvement, with partial or complete resolution by adolescence.

ATAXIA-TELANGIECTASIA (see also Sec. 11.19). This disorder *(Louis-Bar syndrome)* is transmitted as an autosomal recessive trait. The characteristic telangiectasia develops at about 3 yr of age, first on the bulbar conjunctivae and later on the nasal bridge, malar areas, external ears, hard palate, upper anterior chest, and antecubital and popliteal fossae. Additional cutaneous stigmata include café-au-lait spots, premature graying of the hair, and sclerodermatous changes.

ANGIOKERATOMAS. Several forms of angiokeratomas have been described, but some do not occur during childhood or adolescence. Angiokeratomas are flat hemangiomas with a verrucous irregular surface. *Angiokeratoma of Mibelli*, probably transmitted in an autosomal dominant pattern, is characterized by 1- to 8-mm red, purple, or black scaly, verrucous, occasionally crusted papules and nodules that appear on the dorsum of the fingers and toes and on the knees and the elbows. Less commonly, palms, soles, and ears may be affected. In many patients, onset has followed frostbite or chilblains. These nodules bleed freely following injury and may involute in response to trauma or may be effectively eradicated by cryotherapy or fulguration. *Angiokeratoma circumscriptum* is a rare solitary lesion that presents as a plaque of blue-red papules or nodules with a verrucous surface. These usually develop during infancy and early childhood, and they may increase in size at adolescence. The lower limb is the site of predilection. Excision is the treatment of choice.

ANGIOKERATOMA CORPORIS DIFFUSUM (FABRY DISEASE) (see Sec. 8.18). This inborn error of glycolipid metabolism is an X-linked recessive disorder that is fully penetrant in males and is of variable penetrance in carrier females. The skin lesions have their onset prior to puberty and occur in profusion over the genitalia, hips, buttocks, thighs, and in the umbilical and inguinal regions. They consist of 0.1- to 3-mm red to blue-black papules that may have a hyperkeratotic surface. Telangiectasias are seen in mucosa and in the conjunctivae. On light microscopy these angiokeratomas appear as blood-filled, dilated, endothelial-lined vascular spaces. Granular lipid deposits are demonstrable in dermal macrophages, fibrocytes, and endothelial cells.

Additional clinical features include recurrent episodes of fever and agonizing limb pain, cyanosis and flushing of the acral areas, paresthesias of the hands and feet, corneal opacities detectable by slit-lamp examination, and hypohidrosis. Renal and cardiac involvement are the usual causes of death. The biochemical defect is a deficiency of the lysosomal enzyme α-galactosidase, with accumulation of ceramide trihexoside in tissues and excretion in urine. There is no specific therapy.

Similar cutaneous lesions have also been described in another lysosomal enzyme disorder, α-L-fucosidase deficiency, and in sialidosis, a storage disease with neuraminidase deficiency.

NEVUS ANEMICUS. Although nevus anemicus is present at birth, it may not be detectable until early childhood. The nevus consists of solitary or multiple, sharply delineated, pale macules that are most often on the trunk but may also occur on the neck or limbs. These nevi may simulate plaques of vitiligo, leukoderma, or nevoid pigmentary defects, but they can be readily distinguished by their response to firm stroking.

Stroking will evoke an erythematous line and flare in areas of pigment loss, but the skin of a nevus anemicus fails to redden. Although the cutaneous vasculature appears normal histologically, the blood vessels within the nevus do not respond to injection of vasodilators. It has been postulated that the persistent pallor may represent a sustained localized adrenergic vasoconstriction.

LYMPHANGIOMAS

See Sec. 17.28.

23.9 CUTANEOUS NEVI

The term *nevus* often causes semantic confusion because the precise definition of the word has been blurred by common usage. In this section it is used to designate skin lesions that histologically are characterized by collections of well-differentiated cell types normally found in the skin. Not all nevi, however, are discussed in this section; the most notable exceptions are vascular nevi (hemangiomas), which are described in the preceding section.

ACQUIRED PIGMENTED NEVI. Common pigmented nevi or moles are also called *nevocytic* or *nevocellular nevi* to distinguish them from the pigmented lesions arising from mature melanocytes. Nevus cells are related closely to melanocytes and may be derived from a common stem cell *(nevoblast)*. An alternative theory is that nevus cells are of dual origin, with superficially located cells arising from melanocytes *(melanocytic nevus)* and cells in the deeper layers arising from Schwann cells *(neuroid nevus)*.

Nevocellular nevi have a well-defined life history. Nevi are classified as junctional, compound, or dermal in accordance with the location of the nevus cells in the skin. Early lesions are usually junctional in type. Although some nevi remain junctional throughout life, most become compound or intradermal and change morphologically as well as histologically.

Junctional nevi may be present at birth but appear most often in early childhood or during adolescence. The lesions appear in varying shades of brown; they are relatively small, discrete, flat, and variable in shape. They may appear anywhere on the body; those on the palms, soles, and genitalia usually remain junctional throughout life. The melanized nevus cells are cuboidal or epithelioid in configuration and occur in nests on the epidermal side of the basement membrane.

With maturation *compound* and *intradermal nevi* may become raised, dome-shaped, verrucous, or pedunculated. Slightly elevated lesions are usually compound (i.e., the nevus cells inhabit both the epidermis and the dermis). Distinctly elevated lesions are usually intradermal. The amount of melanin in a lesion may vary greatly, or there may be none.

Acquired pigmented nevi are benign lesions and need be removed only to improve appearance or to avoid chronic irritation and infection if they are subject to repeated trauma. A very small percentage of nevi undergo malignant transformation; there is no way, however, to determine which are potentially dangerous, and random excision is neither feasible nor rational. Suspicious changes such as rapid increase in size, development of satellite lesions, variegation of color (particularly shades of red, gray, and blue), pigmentary incontinence, notched borders, regional lymphadenopathy, induration, itching, or pain are indications for excision and histologic evaluation. Most of these changes will be due to irritation, infection, or maturation; darkening and gradual increase in size and elevation normally occur during adolescence and should not be cause for concern. Nevertheless, if there is doubt about the benign nature of a nevus, excision is a safe and simple outpatient procedure that may be justified to allay anxiety.

DYSPLASTIC NEVI. Dysplastic nevocellular nevi occur in both a familial melanoma-prone setting (dysplastic nevus syndrome: autosomal dominant) and as a sporadic event. The morphologic features include large size (5–15 mm), round to oval shape, irregular margins, variegated color, and elevation of a portion of the lesion. These nevi are most common on the posterior trunk but may occur in sun-protected areas, such as the breasts, buttocks, and scalp. Dysplastic nevi do not usually develop until puberty, although scalp lesions may be present earlier. It is important to obtain histologic documentation of dysplastic change by biopsy in order to identify these individuals. Dysplastic nevi demonstrate disordered proliferation of atypical intraepidermal melanocytes.

All affected children should have frequent complete examinations of the integument. Melanoma can develop in any dysplastic nevus. Patients from melanoma-prone families should be examined every 6 mo, because their risk of developing malignant melanoma is 150-fold greater than that found in the general population. In nonfamilial cases, the lifetime risk of melanoma associated with dysplastic nevi is 5–10%; this risk is almost 100% in familial cases.

CONGENITAL PIGMENTED NEVI. Nevocellular nevi are present in approximately 1% of newborn infants. They are viewed with more concern than are acquired nevocellular nevi because they pose an increased risk over a lifetime for development of malignant melanoma.

Sites of predilection are the lower trunk, upper back and shoulders, chest, and proximal limbs. The lesions may be flat, elevated, verrucous, or nodular; they may appear in various shades of brown, blue, or black and may develop numerous coarse hairs or remain hairless and leathery in texture. The term giant congenital pigmented nevus is used for nevi measuring more than 20 cm (Fig. 23–8). Numerous smaller satellite nevi may be scattered elsewhere. The lesions, if significantly disfiguring, may cause severe emotional problems.

Some congenital nevi have the histologic features of ordinary junctional, compound, or intradermal nevi, but others

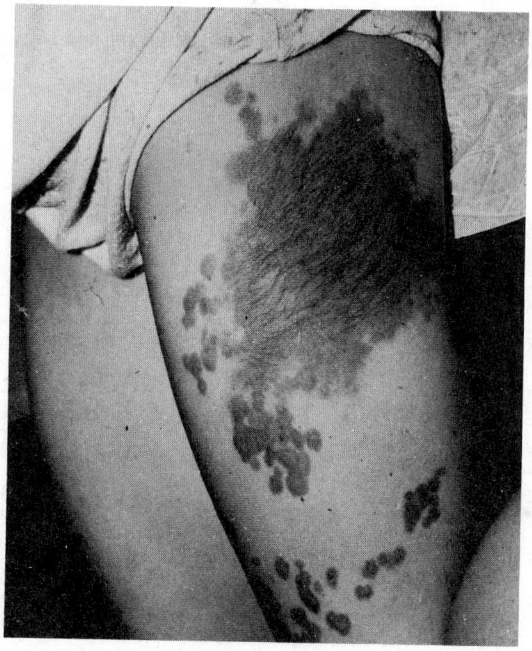

Figure 23–8. Congenital pigmented nevocytic nevus on the thigh.

are characterized by nevus cells dispersed between the collagen bundles of the lower two thirds of the dermis with occasional extension into the underlying tissues and infiltration of nevus cells into the cutaneous nerves, vessels, and appendages. Less commonly, the histologic pattern is that of a neural nevus, blue nevus, or spindle and epithelioid cell nevus.

Giant congenital pigmented nevi (1:500,000 births) are of special significance for 2 reasons: (1) the association of leptomeningeal melanocytosis and (2) the predisposition for development of malignant melanoma. Leptomeningeal involvement may cause hydrocephalus, seizures, retardation, and motor deficits and may result in melanoma. Malignancy can be identified by careful cytologic examination of the cerebrospinal fluid for melanin-containing cells. The incidence of malignant melanoma arising in giant congenital nevi is estimated to be approximately 6–10%; melanoma develops by age 5 in about 50%. Affected patients usually succumb despite palliative measures. Early total excision and repair aided by tissue expanders or grafting is the treatment of choice. Extensive spotty involvement of peripheral skin with small nevi often limits the use of the patient's skin for grafting. If excision is delayed, frequent examinations and biopsy of enlarging nodules or suspicious areas are mandatory. Although there is agreement concerning the management of giant congenital nevi (larger than 20 cm), there is considerable controversy concerning the appropriate approach to medium-sized (1.5–20 cm) and small (smaller than 1.5 cm) congenital nevi. Although there are no definitive data on the incidence of melanomas arising in these lesions, it has been estimated that the risk is 0.8–4.9% until 60 yr of age. It is now the prevailing, but not universal, opinion that these nevi should be excised prior to adolescence. Benign-appearing macular lesions of uniform color may be observed expectantly until late childhood, when they can be removed under local anesthesia. In the neonate, all pigmented macules are not congenital nevi; the differential diagnosis includes mongolian spots, café-au-lait spots, smooth muscle hamartoma, and dermal melanocytosis (nevi of Ota and Ito).

HALO NEVUS (LEUKODERMA ACQUISITUM CENTRIFUGUM). Occasionally, the common pigmented nevus develops a peripheral zone of depigmentation up to 5 mm in width (Fig. 23–9). In tissue biopsy there is a dense inflammatory infiltrate of lymphocytes and histiocytes in addition to the nevus cells. The pale halo reflects disappearance of the melanocytes. This phenomenon has also been associated with blue nevi, neurofibromas, and primary and secondary malignant melanoma. Patients with certain organ-specific autoimmune disorders and vitiligo have an increased incidence of halo nevi.

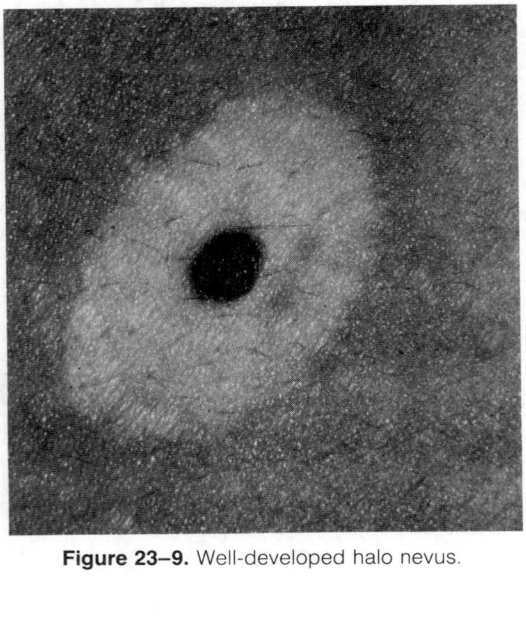

Figure 23–9. Well-developed halo nevus.

These lesions occur primarily in children and young adults; development of the halo may coincide with puberty or pregnancy. Frequently, several pigmented nevi will develop halos simultaneously. Subsequent disappearance of the central nevus is the usual outcome, and the depigmented area may or may not be repigmented. Excision and histopathologic examination of the lesion is indicated only when the nature of the central lesion is in question.

SPINDLE AND EPITHELIOID CELL NEVUS (SPITZ NEVUS). This type is commonly referred to as a *juvenile melanoma*; however, because it is always benign, the anxiety-provoking term melanoma should be avoided. Spindle and epithelioid cell nevi are pink to red, smooth, dome-shaped, firm, hairless nodules, which appear suddenly, grow rapidly, and are most often situated on the face, shoulder, or upper limb. They achieve a maximal size of about 1.5 cm. Rarely, they occur as multiple grouped lesions. Visually similar lesions include pyogenic granuloma, hemangioma, nevocellular nevus, juvenile xanthogranuloma, and basal cell carcinoma, but histologically these entities are distinguishable. The spindle and epithelioid cell nevus, a variant of the compound nevus, presents epidermal changes, vascular ectasias, and dermal and epidermal collections of pleomorphic, fusiform, and polygonal nevus cells, giant cells, and multinucleated giant cells. Although the histologic pattern may appear ominous to the inexperienced observer, the benign nature of the lesion permits conservative excision with little likelihood of reappearance or spread.

ZOSTERIFORM LENTIGINOUS NEVUS. This nevus is a unilateral, linear, band-like lesion composed of multiple small brown or black macules on the face, trunk, or limbs. The lesions may be present at birth or they may develop during childhood; they represent collections of melanin-containing nevus cells at the tips of the dermal papillae.

NEVUS SPILUS (SPECKLED LENTIGINOUS NEVUS). This nevus is a flat, brown patch, within which are darker brown macules. These nevi vary considerably in size and can occur anywhere on the body. The darker macules usually develop gradually and represent nevus cells in a junctional or dermal location. These nevocellular nevi are benign and need not be excised.

NEVUS OF OTA. This nevus consists of a permanent, blue-gray, macular, facial stain caused by aggregates of melanocytes in the dermis. The macular nevi resemble mongolian spots in color and occur unilaterally in the areas supplied by the 1st and 2nd divisions of the trigeminal nerve. They are sometimes present at birth, and in other cases may arise during the 1st or 2nd decade of life. Patchy involvement of the sclera and other ocular tissues and of the nasal and buccal mucosa occurs in some patients. Nevus of Ota is more common in females and in oriental and black patients.

Nevus of Ito is localized to the shoulder, supraclavicular area, lateral neck, and upper arm. It can also be regarded as a persistent mongolian spot. The only available treatment is masking with cosmetics.

BLUE NEVI. These nevi are solitary lesions that may be present at birth or develop during childhood, most frequently on the face, neck, arms, buttocks, hands, and feet; they are more common in females. Typical lesions are smooth, dome-shaped, hairless, blue or black nodules that rarely exceed 1 cm in diameter. Microscopically, they are characterized by groups of intensely pigmented, spindle-shaped melanocytes in the dermis and around appendicular structures.

Cellular blue nevi, which differ somewhat histologically, are larger and occur most frequently on the buttocks and in the sacrococcygeal area. They have a low but definite incidence of malignant transformation, and therefore excision is the treatment of choice.

ACHROMIC NEVI (NEVUS DEPIGMENTOSUS). These nevi are usually present at birth; they are localized macular hypopigmented patches or streaks, often with bizarre, irregular borders. They can resemble hypomelanosis of Ito clinically, except that they are more localized, and often unilateral. Small lesions may also resemble the white leaf macules of tuberous sclerosis. They appear to represent a focal defect in melanin production.

EPIDERMAL NEVI. These nevi may be visible at birth or may develop within the first months or years of life. They affect both sexes equally and only occur very rarely in more than one family member. The epidermal nevus may appear initially as a discolored, slightly scaly patch that, with maturation, becomes more thickened, verrucous, and hyperpigmented. Several morphologic types include pigmented papillomas, often in a linear distribution; unilateral hyperkeratotic streaks (nevus unius lateris) involving a limb and perhaps a portion of the trunk; velvety hyperpigmented plaques; and feathered, whorled, or marbled hyperkeratotic lesions in localized plaques (Fig. 23–10) or over extensive areas of the body. An inflammatory linear verrucous variant is markedly pruritic and may become eczematized.

The histologic pattern evolves as the lesion matures; but epidermal hyperplasia of some degree is apparent in all stages of development. One or another dermal appendage may predominate in a particular lesion. The diagnosis can be confirmed by biopsy. These nevi must be distinguished from lichen striatus, lymphangioma circumscriptum, shagreen patch of tuberous sclerosis, congenital hairy nevi, and nevus sebaceus (Jadassohn). Keratolytic agents such as retinoic acid or salicylic acid may be moderately effective in reducing scaling and controlling pruritus, but definitive treatment requires full-thickness excision; recurrence is usual if more superficial removal is attempted. Alternatively, the nevus may be left intact.

With some frequency, epidermal nevi are associated with abnormalities of other organs; this combination has been designated as the *epidermal nevus syndrome*. The additional defects include localized soft tissue hypertrophy, hemangiomas, pigmentary changes, skeletal anomalies of various sorts, ocular defects, and neurologic abnormalities, such as developmental delay, seizures, motor deficits, and cerebrovascular malformations. Associated malignancies such as Wilms tumor and astrocytoma, although rare, have been reported.

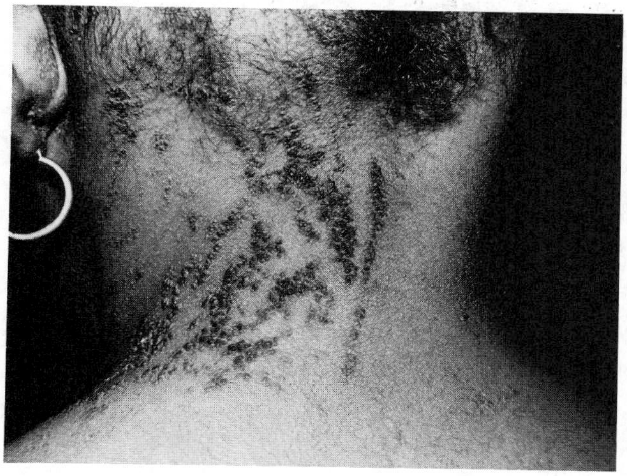

Figure 23–10. Verrucous streaky epidermal nevus on the neck.

NEVUS SEBACEUS (JADASSOHN). This type is a relatively small, sharply demarcated, oval or linear, yellow-orange, elevated plaque that is usually devoid of hair and occurs on the head and neck of infants. Although characterized histologically by an abundance of sebaceous glands, all elements of the skin are represented. With maturity, usually during adolescence, the lesions become verrucous and studded with large rubbery nodules. The changing clinical appearance reflects the histologic pattern, which is characterized by a variable degree of hyperkeratosis, hyperplasia of the epidermis, malformed hair follicles, and often a profusion of sebaceous and apocrine glands. During adulthood, these nevi are frequently complicated by secondary malignancies and benign adnexal tumors, most commonly basal cell carcinoma or syringocystadenoma papilliferum. The diagnosis can be established by biopsy; the treatment of choice is total excision prior to adolescence. Sebaceous nevi associated with central nervous system, skeletal, and ocular defects probably represent variants of the epidermal nevus syndrome.

BECKER NEVUS. This lesion, also called Becker melanosis, is a form of epidermal nevus. It occurs predominantly in males, usually becoming apparent during childhood or adolescence. Macular pigmentation is followed by hypertrichosis, which is limited to the area of hyperpigmentation. The most common sites are the upper torso and the upper arm. The nevus is benign, has no risk for malignant change, and is very rarely associated with other anomalies.

NEVUS COMEDONICUS. This type is an uncommon form of epidermal nevus that consists of linear plaques of plugged follicles that simulate comedones; they may be present at birth or appear during childhood. The horny plugs represent keratinous debris within dilated, malformed pilosebaceous follicles. The lesions are most often unilateral and may develop at any site. They are not associated with other congenital malformations. Although often asymptomatic, some individuals experience recurrent inflammatory lesions resulting in cyst formation, fistulas, and scarring. There is no effective treatment except full-thickness excision; palliation of larger lesions may be achieved by regular applications of a retinoic acid preparation.

CONNECTIVE TISSUE NEVUS. This type may occur as a solitary defect or as a manifestation of an associated disorder. These nevi may occur at any site but are most common on the trunk. They are skin-colored, ivory, or yellow plaques, 2–15 cm in diameter, composed of multiple tiny papules or grouped nodules that are frequently difficult to appreciate visually because of the subtle color changes. The plaques have a rubbery or cobblestone consistency on palpation. Biopsy findings are variable and include increased amounts of dermal elastic tissue or a predominance of thickened collagen bundles. Similar lesions occurring with tuberous sclerosis are called shagreen patches. The association of multiple small papular connective tissue nevi with osteopoikilosis is called *dermatofibrosis lenticularis disseminata* (Buschke-Ollendorf syndrome).

SMOOTH MUSCLE HAMARTOMA. This uncommon lesion is a developmental anomaly resulting in hyperplasia of the smooth muscle (arrector pili) associated with the hair follicles. It is usually evident at birth or shortly thereafter as a flesh-colored or lightly pigmented plaque with overlying hypertrichosis on the trunk or limbs. Transient elevation or a rippling movement of the lesion can sometimes be elicited by stroking the surface because of contraction of the muscle bundles. Smooth muscle hamartoma can be mistaken for congenital pigmented nevus, but the distinction is important because it has no risk for malignant melanoma. These lesions need not be removed.

23.10 DISORDERS OF PIGMENT

Alterations in skin color may be generalized or localized and may result from a variety of defects ranging from absence of melanocytes and defective melanization of melanosomes to overproduction of melanin and increased numbers of melanocytic cells. Some of these aberrations are induced by hormones (hyperpigmentation of Addison disease); others represent focal developmental defects (white spots of tuberous sclerosis); still others may be nonspecific and the result of cutaneous inflammation (postinflammatory hypopigmentation or hyperpigmentation).

TABLE 23–2. Disorders with Café-au-Lait Spots

Neurofibromatosis
McCune-Albright syndrome
Russell-Silver syndrome
Multiple lentigenes
Ataxia telangiectasia
Fanconi anemia
Tuberous sclerosis
Bloom syndrome
Epidermal nevus syndrome
Gaucher disease
Chédiak-Higashi syndrome

23.11 HYPERPIGMENTED LESIONS

EPHELIDES OR FRECKLES. These are light or dark brown macules that occur in sun-exposed areas, such as the face, upper back, arms, and hands. They are induced by exposure to sun, particularly during the summer, and may fade or disappear during the winter. They are more common in fair-haired individuals, appear first during the preschool years, and are probably genetically determined. Histologically, they are marked by increased melanin pigment in the epidermal basal layer with no increase in the number of melanocytes. Actually the freckle contains fewer but larger melanocytes than the surrounding paler skin.

LENTIGINES. Lentigines, often mistaken for freckles or pigmented nevi, are small (1–3 cm), round, dark brown macules that can appear anywhere on the body, are unrelated to sun exposure, and remain permanently. They differ from other hyperpigmented macules histologically in that they have elongated, club-shaped, epidermal rete ridges with increased numbers of melanocytes and dense epidermal deposits of melanin. The lesions are benign and, when few, may be viewed as a normal occurrence. Some juvenile lentigines may be precursors of nevocellular nevi (pigmented moles). The *multiple lentigines (LEOPARD) syndrome* is an autosomal dominant entity consisting of a generalized, symmetric distribution of Lentigines in association with Electrocardiogram abnormalities, Ocular hypertelorism, Pulmonary stenosis, Abnormal genitalia (cryptochidism, hypogonadism), growth Retardation, and sensoneural Deafness. Other features include hypertrophic obstructive cardiomyopathy and pectus excavatum or carinatum.

The *Peutz-Jeghers syndrome* is characterized by melanotic macules on the lips and mucous membranes and by polyposis of the small intestine. It is inherited as an autosomal dominant trait. Onset is noted during early childhood when pigmented macules appear on the lips, buccal mucosa, and gingivae and occasionally on the nose, hands, and feet. Polyposis usually involves the small intestine but may also occur in the stomach and large intestine. Episodic abdominal pain, melena, and intussusception are frequent complications. Malignant degeneration has been reported, but the risk of malignancy is small, and a normal life span is usual. Peutz-Jeghers syndrome must be differentiated from other syndromes associated with multiple lentigines, from ordinary freckling, from *Gardner syndrome*, and from *Cronkhite-Canada syndrome* (a disorder characterized by gastrointestinal polyposis, alopecia, onychodystrophy, and skin pigmentation).

CAFÉ-AU-LAIT SPOTS. Café-au-lait spots are uniformly hyperpigmented, sharply demarcated, macular lesions, the hues of which vary with the normal depth of pigmentation of the individual: they are tan or light brown in white individuals and may be dark brown in black children. Café-au-lait spots vary tremendously in size and may be quite large, covering a significant portion of the trunk or limb. Generally, the borders are smooth, but some have an exceedingly irregular border. The lesions are characterized by increased numbers of melanocytes and melanin in the epidermis but lack the clubbed rete ridges that typify lentigines. One to three café-au-lait spots are common in normal children. They may be present at birth or develop during childhood.

Large, often unilateral café-au-lait spots with irregular borders are characteristic of patients with *McCune-Albright syndrome* (Sec. 19.7), a disorder that includes polyostotic bone dysplasia, precocious puberty, and multiple endocrine dysfunctions. The macular hyperpigmentation may be present at birth or develop late in childhood; if segmentally localized, it suggests an embryonic developmental defect.

Neurofibromatosis-1 (von Recklinghausen disease). The café-au-lait spot is the most familiar cutaneous hallmark of this autosomal dominant neurocutaneous syndrome (see Sec. 20.39). These lesions also occur with certain other disorders, including other types of neurofibromatosis (Table 23–2). These lesions are soft, skin-colored, sessile or pedunculated nodules (Fig. 23–11) that may grow to considerable size and occasionally undergo sarcomatous change. Subcutaneous nodules may also occur along the course of nerve trunks. Deforming plexiform neurofibromas that often have overlying hyperpigmentation are another cutaneous feature. The histologic features of these lesions are diagnostic.

INCONTINENTIA PIGMENTI (BLOCH-SULZBERGER DISEASE). This disease is a rare, heritable, multisystem disorder that is thought to be transmitted as an X-linked

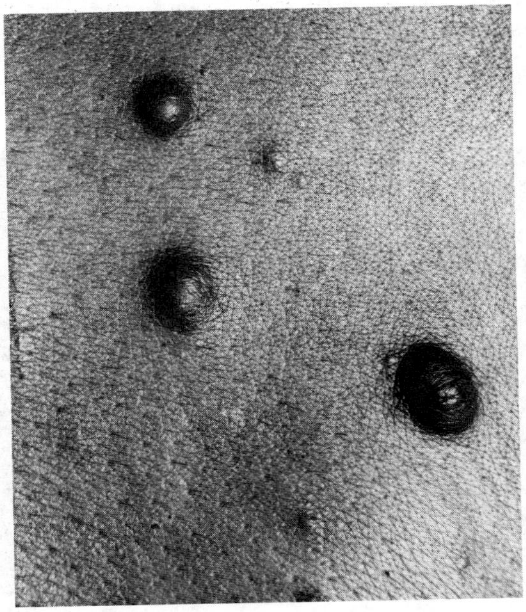

Figure 23–11. Multiple sessile neurofibromas.

dominant trait and is lethal in males. The paucity of affected males and the high frequency of spontaneous abortions in carrier females lend credence to this supposition.

The cutaneous manifestations can be divided into four phases, all of which may not occur in a given patient:

1. The 1st phase is evident at birth or shortly thereafter and consists of erythematous, linear streaks and plaques of vesicles that are most pronounced on the limbs (Fig. 23–12*A*). The lesions may be confused with those of herpes simplex, bullous impetigo, or mastocytosis, but the linear configuration is unique. They demonstrate eosinophils. Blood eosinophilia up to 65% is common but disappears after 4–5 mo of age.
2. The vesicular phase is followed by an intermediate verrucous stage, which may persist for several months. These lesions eventually involute, at times leaving atrophic or depigmented areas.
3. The 3rd or pigmentary stage is variable in time of onset; it may overlap the earlier phases and may even be evident at birth or, more commonly, within the 1st few weeks of life; sites of involvement are not necessarily those of the preceding vesicular and warty lesions. The pigment is distributed in macular whorls, reticulated patches, flecks, splashes, and linear streaks and, once present, persists throughout childhood (see Fig. 23–12*B*).
4. Hypopigmented streaks that are also hairless and anhidrotic are considered a late manifestation of incontinentia pigmenti and develop mainly on the flexor aspect of the legs and less often on the arms and trunk.

Histologically, an early vesicular lesion is characterized by epidermal edema and an intraepidermal vesicle filled with eosinophils. Epidermal hyperplasia, hyperkeratosis, and papillomatosis are characteristic of the 2nd phase. The 3rd stage pigmentary lesion typically shows vacuolar degeneration of the epidermal basal cells and melanin in melanophages of the upper dermis. The name of the disease is derived from the latter histologic feature.

Although the skin lesions may constitute the only manifestation, approximately 80% of affected children have other defects. Alopecia, which may be scarring and patchy or diffuse, occurs in up to 40% of patients; dental anomalies, present in over half the children, consist of late dentition, conical teeth, and partial anodontia. Central nervous system manifestations, including developmental retardation, seizures, microcephaly, spasticity, and paralysis, are found in up to a third of affected children; ocular anomalies, such as strabismus, optic nerve atrophy, cataracts, or retrolenticular masses, which may result in severe impairment of vision or blindness occur in over 30% of children. Less common abnormalities include dystrophy of nails and skeletal defects. The choice of investigative studies and the plan of management depend on the occurrence of particular noncutaneous abnormalities because skin lesions are benign and often become less evident during adulthood. The high incidence of associated major anomalies warrants genetic counseling.

POSTINFLAMMATORY PIGMENTARY CHANGES. Either hyperpigmentation or hypopigmentation can occur as a result of cutaneous inflammation. Alteration in pigmentation usually follows a severe inflammatory reaction but may result from mild dermatitis. Dark-skinned children are more likely to show these changes than fair-skinned ones. Although altered pigmentation may persist for weeks to months, patients can be reassured that these lesions are usually temporary. These changes must be distinguished from nevoid lesions and diseases manifested by pigmentary alterations such as vitiligo.

23.12 HYPOPIGMENTED LESIONS

ALBINISM. Several types of congenital oculocutaneous albinism have been defined, each of which is inherited in an autosomal recessive fashion. The various forms of albinism may be distinguished by clinical manifestations, morphology of the melanosomes, and the hair bulb incubation test, which determines whether tyrosinase is present. Examples of some well-defined types of oculocutaneous albinism follow (see also Sec. 8.3).

Tyrosinase-negative albinism is characterized by a lack of visible pigment in hair, skin, and eyes that results in photophobia, nystagmus, defective visual acuity, white hair, and white skin. The irides are blue-gray in oblique light and pink in reflected light.

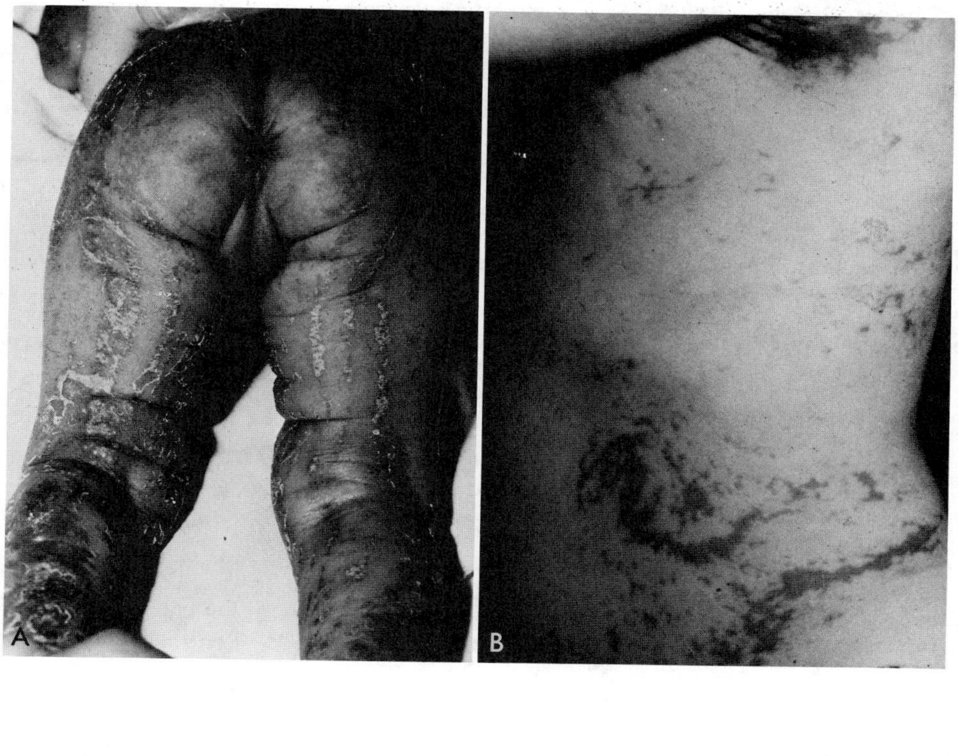

Figure 23–12. *A*, Vesicular and verrucous linear lesions on buttocks and legs of an infant girl with incontinentia pigmenti. *B*, Whorled macular hyperpigmentation of incontinentia pigmenti.

Tyrosinase-positive albinism may resemble the aforementioned pattern, except that the hair may be straw colored or light brown. With aging, the irides may accumulate some brown pigment, and thus there is some improvement in visual acuity. The skin color is cream or pink.

In *tyrosinase-variable albinism* (yellow mutant), the infant has white hair, pink skin, and gray eyes at birth but develops bright yellow hair, light tanning of skin on sun exposure, and some pigment in the iris. Photophobia and nystagmus are present but mild.

The *Hermansky-Pudlak syndrome* is albinism with platelet storage-pool deficiency and a hemorrhagic diathesis. Pigmentation is extremely variable. Associated features are accumulation of ceroid in the tissue, pulmonary fibrosis, and granulomatous colitis.

The *Cross-McKusick-Breen syndrome* consists of tyrosinase-positive albinism with microphthalmia, retardation, spasticity, and athetosis.

Because of the absence of normal protection by adequate amounts of epidermal melanin, persons with albinism are predisposed to develop actinic keratoses and cutaneous carcinoma secondary to skin damage by ultraviolet light. Protection with a broad-spectrum sunscreen preparation (Sec. 23.15) should be provided during exposure to sunlight.

PARTIAL ALBINISM (PIEBALDISM). This autosomal dominant disorder is characterized by amelanotic plaques; they occur most frequently on the forehead, anterior scalp (producing a white forelock), thorax, elbows, and knees. Although sharply demarcated from normally pigmented skin, islands of normal pigmentation may be present within the amelanotic areas. The plaques are the result of localized absence or reduction in the number of melanocytes; the defect is permanent. Piebaldism must be differentiated from vitiligo, which is progressive and is not usually congenital; achromic nevus; and Waardenburg syndrome.

WAARDENBURG SYNDROME. This syndrome is characterized by a white forelock, heterochromic irides, broad nasal root, dystopia canthorum, congenital deafness, defects in fundus pigment, and cutaneous hypopigmentation; it is inherited as an autosomal dominant trait.

CHÉDIAK-HIGASHI SYNDROME (see Sec. 11.31).

TUBEROUS SCLEROSIS (see Sec. 20.40). This disorder, as well as many of the neurocutaneous syndromes, is a multisystemic disorder affecting primarily tissues derived from ectoderm but also involving organs of mesodermal and endodermal origin. The most reliable early cutaneous sign is the *white leaf macule,* which is present but not always easily detectable at birth. They are sharply demarcated, pale, 0.5- to 3-cm lesions that often assume the shape of a mountain ash leaflet. Single or multiple lesions are most often found on the trunk (Fig. 23–13*A*) but also occur on the face and limbs. Small, confetti-like hypopigmented macules are also present in some instances, reflecting inadequate melanization of the melanosomes of the pigment-generating cells.

Adenoma sebaceum is the most commonly recognized cutaneous marker of tuberous sclerosis; the lesions appear on the face during mid to late childhood or adolescence in approximately 80% of patients. These pink or flesh-colored papulonodular growths may erupt in profusion on the cheeks, nose, forehead, and chin but often spare the upper lip (see Fig. 23–13*B*). The term adenoma sebaceum is a misnomer because these growths are angiofibromas rather than tumors of the sebaceous glands. Similar fibromatous nodules may be scattered on the forehead, trunk, and limbs. Large, skin-colored, raised or flat collagenous plaques with an orange peel or cobblestone texture *(shagreen patches)* occur with some frequency in the lumbosacral area. At puberty, distinctive, clove-like, periungual fibromas (see Fig. 23–13*C*) appear on the fingers and toes of some children; gingival fibromas may also occur, unassociated with the administration of anticonvulsant medications. Café-au-lait spots occur with increased frequency but are not as numerous as in neurofibromatosis.

HYPOMELANOSIS OF ITO (INCONTINENTIA PIGMENTI ACHROMIANS). This congenital skin disorder affects children of both sexes and is frequently associated with defects in several organ systems. There is no evidence for genetic transmission, but chromosomal mosaicism has been demonstrated in some of these patients. The skin lesions consist of bizarre, patterned, hypopigmented macules arranged in sharply demarcated whorls, streaks, and patches over the body surface (Fig. 23–14). The hypopigmentation remains unchanged throughout childhood but is said to fade during adulthood. Neither inflammatory nor vesicular lesions precede the development of the pigmentary changes as in Bloch-Sulzberger incontinentia pigmenti. Histologic changes in affected skin are nonspecific. Commonly associated abnormalities include seizures, developmental retardation, scoliosis, limb asymmetry, and ophthalmologic defects, but there is no consistent pattern of anomalies. The differential diagnosis includes nevus depigmentosus or achromicus.

VITILIGO. This acquired pigmentary defect may occur at any age in persons of any skin color. The lesions are depigmented macules, sharply circumscribed, often with a hyperpigmented border; they vary in size and shape. Preferred sites are the face, particularly around the eyes or mouth (Fig. 23–15), the genitalia, hands and feet, elbows, knees, and upper chest. When the scalp or brow is affected, the hair may also lose its pigment.

Although no clearcut pattern of genetic transmission is established, vitiligo is known to occur with increased frequency in some families. It is also more prevalent in patients with hyperthyroidism, adrenal insufficiency, pernicious anemia, and diabetes mellitus; some patients have detectable circulating antibodies to thyroid, adrenal, and other tissues.

The cause is unknown, but trauma appears to play a role in induction of the lesions. An autoimmune mechanism has been suggested. Melanocytes are absent from involved sites and repopulate the epidermis from the hair follicle epithelium when repigmentation occurs. Although the diagnosis is usually made clinically, the disappearance of melanocytes can be confirmed by DOPA stains or electron microscopy of specimens obtained from depigmented skin. The course of vitiligo varies; some lesions may remit spontaneously while others are developing, but relentlessly progressive depigmentation may occur. Treatment is difficult and usually involves administration of oral or topical psoralen compounds (8-methoxypsoralen or trimethylpsoralen [Trisoralen]) in conjunction with exposure to sunlight or an ultraviolet light (UVA) source twice weekly. Repigmentation may be partial or complete, but many months of therapy may be required and should be carefully monitored by physicians experienced in the use of photosensitizing drugs. High-potency topical steroids are sometimes effective in repigmenting small areas of vitiligo or early lesions in areas not amenable to phototherapy such as the lips. Small lesions may be camouflaged by application of a specially prepared makeup (Covermark; Dermablend). Because of the absence of melanin, vitiliginous skin will burn readily on sun exposure and should be protected at all times by the use of an appropriate sunscreen agent.

23.13 VESICOBULLOUS DISORDERS

Many diseases are characterized by vesicobullous lesions; they vary considerably in etiology, in age of occurrence, and in the pattern of the lesions. Some of them (e.g., varicella) are discussed in other chapters; some are described in other

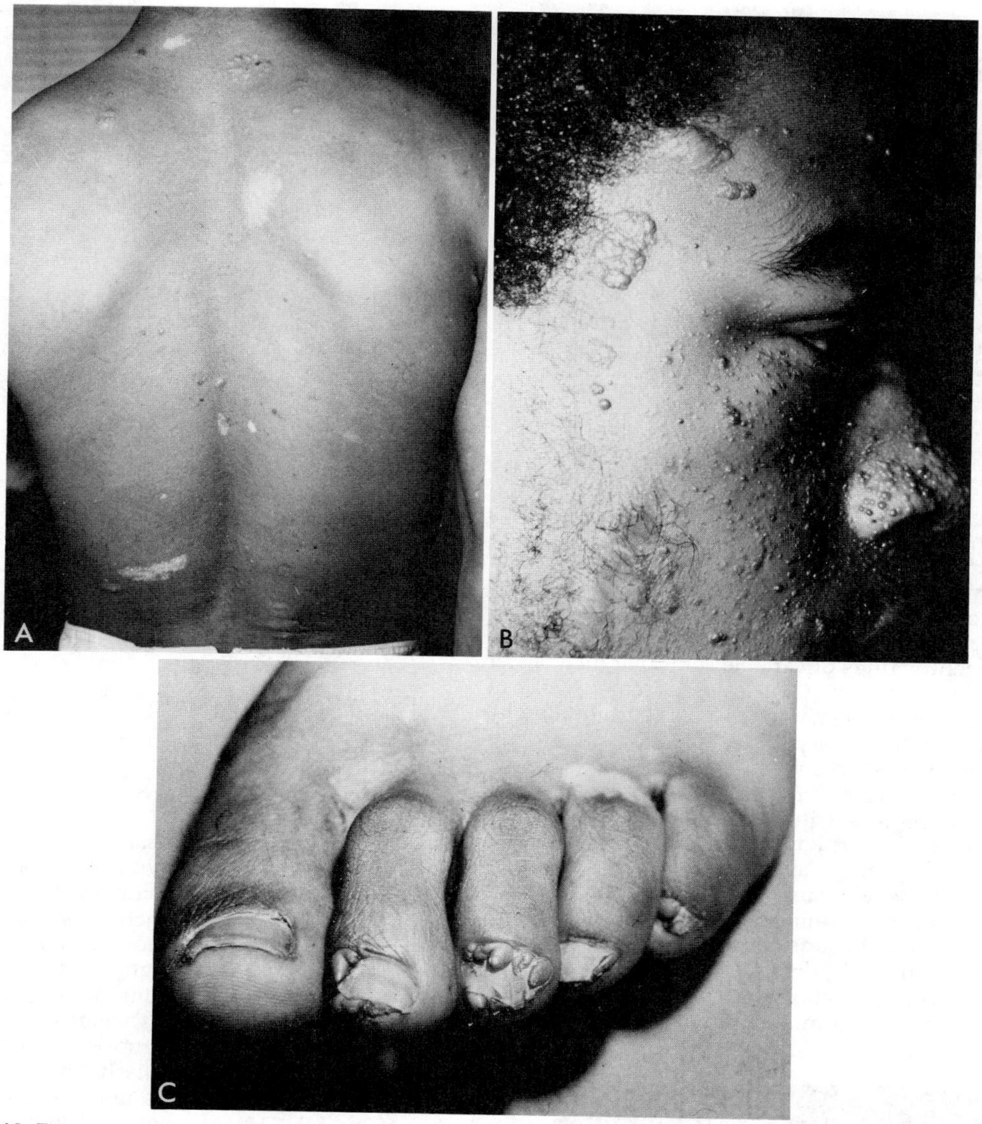

Figure 23–13. Tuberous sclerosis. *A*, Multiple white leaf macules, small papular fibromas, and shagreen patch on lower back. *B*, Adenoma sebaceum and angiofibromatous plaques on the temple. *C*, Periungual fibromas.

sections of this chapter because the vesicobullous lesions represent only a transient stage of the disease (e.g., incontinentia pigmenti and mastocytosis). The morphology of the blister often provides a visual clue to the location of the lesion within the skin. Blisters localized to the epidermal layers are thin-walled and relatively flaccid and tend to rupture easily. Subepidermal blisters are tense, thick-walled, and more durable. Biopsies of blisters can be diagnostic because the level of cleavage within the skin is constant and characteristic for a particular disorder. Blister cleavage sites are depicted schematically in Figure 23–16.

The freshest intact blister should be selected for biopsy because partial healing may obscure the true cleavage plane. The differential diagnosis of the disease process can often be narrowed by histologic examination in consideration with other diagnostic procedures (Table 23–3).

ERYTHEMA MULTIFORME. This is an acute, sometimes recurrent, inflammatory disease of the skin and mucous membranes. It occurs at any age, but it is more common during childhood and more frequent in males than in females. The pathogenesis is unknown, but the disorder is generally regarded as a hypersensitivity reaction triggered by drugs, infections, and exposure to toxic substances (Table 23–4).

Clinical Manifestations. There are two forms of the disease. In *erythema multiforme minor,* the most common type, the diverse morphology of the skin lesions is the prominent manifestation. This form of erythema multiforme may represent an immune-mediated response to herpes simplex virus present in epidermis despite absence of clinically apparent infection. The *Stevens-Johnson syndrome* (erythema multiforme major) is a serious systemic disorder in which at least two mucous membranes as well as skin are involved.

The cutaneous lesions of erythema multiforme minor are usually symmetric, appear in crops, and show a predilection for the extensor surfaces of the hands, arms, feet, legs, palms, and soles. The eruption appears 1–2 wk after a prodromal nonspecific upper respiratory illness, varies considerably in extent and severity, and may involve the entire body except the scalp. Lesions begin as macules or wheals and evolve into papules or plaques. The center of the lesion may be vesicular, purpuric, or necrotic. "Multiforme" refers to this changing pattern of a fixed lesion over several days. Vesicobullous

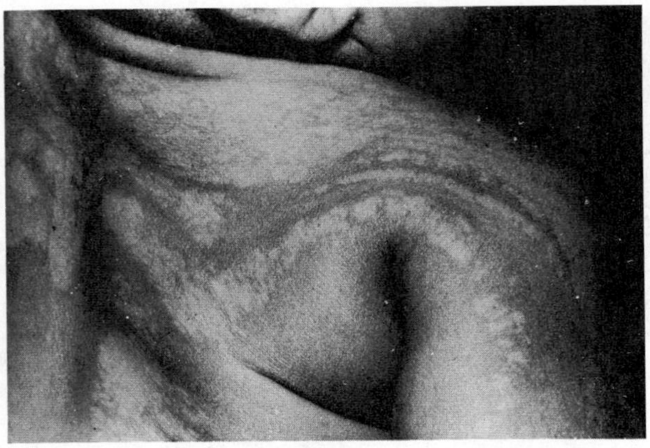

Figure 23–14. Marbled hypopigmented streaks of hypomelanosis of Ito (incontinentia pigmenti achromians).

lesions arise centrally within pre-existent lesions; urticarial lesions may fuse to form annular polycyclic plaques of bizarre outline. Intradermal hemorrhage is common and may be florid or may consist only of petechiae. Iris or target lesions, pathognomonic for erythema multiforme, have dusky centers and develop concentric rings of variable color that may blister when the reaction is intense. Oral lesions occur in 25% of patients and consist of erythematous macules surmounted by vesicobullae that rapidly form painful necrotic ulcers, often with a pseudomembranous surface.

Skin lesions in erythema multiforme minor appear abruptly, evolve over 1 wk, regress within 2–4 wk, and heal with hypopigmentation or hyperpigmentation but without scarring. Pruritus is minimal to absent. The rash sometimes develops more extensively in sun-exposed areas and in areas of prior trauma (the isomorphic or Koebner phenomenon). The differential diagnosis includes bullous pemphigoid, pemphigus, linear IgA dermatosis, urticaria, viral infections, Reiter disease, Kawasaki disease, Behçet disease, allergic vasculitis, erythema annulare centrifugum, and periarteritis nodosa.

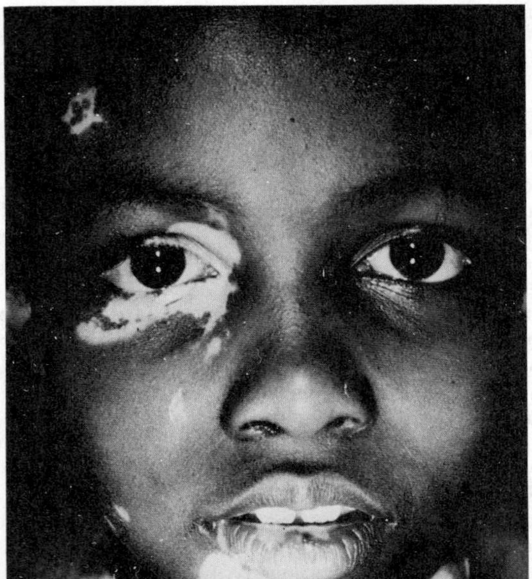

Figure 23–15. Multiple, sharply demarcated, depigmented areas of vitiligo.

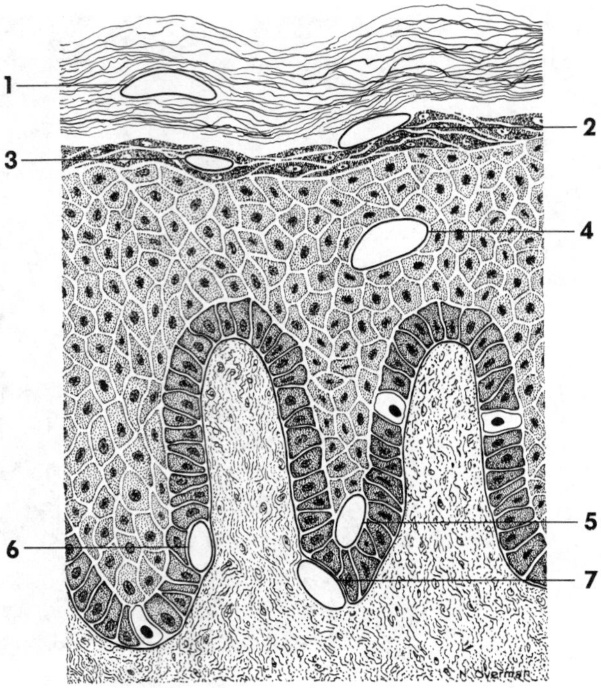

Figure 23–16. Blister cleavage sites in the skin: (1) intracorneal, (2) subcorneal, (3) granular layer, (4) intraepidermal, (5) suprabasal, (6) junctional (between basal cell membrane and basement membrane), and (7) subepidermal.

The cutaneous and mucosal lesions in erythema multiforme major (Stevens-Johnson syndrome) have an abrupt onset following a prodromal respiratory illness. Bullae involve the lips, the mouth, and conjunctiva. A purulent conjunctivitis is usual, as is uveitis; cutaneous lesions rupture and the denuded skin may result in significant fluid losses. New lesions erupt for 1–4 wk, and healing occurs during the following 6 wk. Fever, chills, malaise, weakness, neutropenia, and anemia are common. The diagnosis can usually be made from the clinical features, particularly when iris lesions are apparent. When the diagnosis is uncertain, a skin biopsy should be performed. The differential diagnosis of Stevens-Johnson syndrome includes toxic epidermal necrolysis, benign mucous membrane pemphigoid, phemphigus, graft-versus-host disease, gingivostomatitis, bullous drug reactions, Behçet syndrome, and Reiter disease. The histologic changes vary with the severity of the lesions. There is intraepidermal edema with vesicular alteration in the epidermal basal layer and necrosis of individual epidermal cells. The dermis is edematous, with lymphocytic infiltration around the vessels and at the dermoepidermal junction. When the changes are severe, red blood cells may be extravasated into the dermis, subepidermal bullae may form, and the epidermis may become necrotic. Eosinophils and neutrophils are sparse.

This treatment is local and symptomatic. Ophthalmologic consultation is mandatory because ocular sequelae can lead to loss of vision. Oral lesions should be managed with mouthwashes, glycerin swabs, and chlorhexidine rinses. Topical anesthetics (Benadryl, dyclonine, and viscous Xylocaine) may provide relief from pain, particularly when applied before eating. Denuded skin lesions can be cleansed with saline or Burow solution compresses. Antibiotic therapy is appropriate for secondary bacterial infection. Frequent recurrences of herpes-associated erythema multiforme may warrant prophylactic acyclovir. Treatment of erythema multiforme major (Stevens-Johnson syndrome) includes intensive care admis-

TABLE 23–3. Sites of Blister Formation and Diagnostic Studies for the Vesicobullous Disorders

Disorder	Blister Cleavage Site	Cutaneous Diagnostic Studies
Acrodermatitis enteropathica	IE	—
Bullous impetigo	GL	Smear, culture
Bullous pemphigoid	SE (junctional)	Direct and indirect immunofluorescence studies
Candidosis	SC	KOH preparation, culture
Chronic bullous dermatosis of childhood	SE	Direct immunofluorescence studies
Dermatitis herpetiformis	SE	Direct immunofluorescence studies
Dermatophytosis	IE	KOH preparation, culture
Dyshidrotic eczema	IE	—
Epidermolysis bullosa (EB) simplex	IE	Electron microscopy; immunofluorescence mapping
Hands and feet	IE	Electron microscopy; immunofluorescence mapping
Junctional EB (Letalis)	SE (junctional)	Electron microscopy; immunofluorescence mapping
Recessive dystrophic EB	SE	Electron microscopy; immunofluorescence mapping
Dominant dystrophic EB	SE	Electron microscopy; immunofluorescence mapping
Epidermolytic hyperkeratosis	IE	—
Erythema multiforme	SE	—
Erythema toxicum	SC, IE	Smear for eosinophils
Incontinentia pigmenti	IE	Smear for eosinophils
Insect bites	IE	—
Mastocytosis	SE	Smear for mast cells
Miliaria crystallina	IC	—
Pachyonychia congenita	IC	—
Pemphigus foliaceus	GL	Direct and indirect immunofluorescence studies Tzanck smear
Pemphigus vulgaris	SB	Direct and indirect immunofluorescence studies Tzanck smear
Pseudomonas infection	IE, SE	Smear, culture
Scabies	IE	Scraping
Staphylococcal scalded skin syndrome	GL	Frozen section biopsy
Syphilis	SE	Darkfield preparation
Toxic epidermal necrolysis (Lyell)	SE	Frozen section biopsy
Transient neonatal pustular melanosis	SC, IE	Smear for cells
Viral blisters	IE	Tzanck smear for herpesvirus infections

GL = granular layer; IC = intracorneal; IE = intraepidermal; SB = suprabasal; SC = subcorneal; SE = subepidermal.

sion, intravenous fluids, nutritional support, sheepskin or air-fluid bedding, topical antibiotics (2% mupirocin to the skin and nose, chloramphenicol or erythromycin to the eyes), daily saline or Burow solution compresses, paraffin gauze or hydrogel dressing to denuded areas, saline compresses to the eyelids, lips, or nose, analgesics, and urinary catheterization (when needed). A daily examination for infection and ocular lesions, which constitute the major cause of long-term morbidity, is essential. Systemic antibiotics are indicated for urinary or cutaneous infections and for suspected bacteremia, because infection is the leading cause of death. Prophylactic systemic antibiotics, systemic steroids, and extensive debridement are not necessary.

TOXIC EPIDERMAL NECROLYSIS. This appears to be a hypersensitivity phenomenon triggered by many of the same factors that are responsible for erythema multiforme: drugs, infections, vaccination, radiotherapy, and malignancies. It may represent the most devastating form of erythema multiforme; widespread epidermal necrosis rapidly follows blister formation at the dermoepidermal junction.

The prodrome consists of fever, malaise, and localized skin tenderness and diffuse erythema. Flaccid bullae develop, and full-thickness epidermis is lost in large sheets. *Nikolsky sign* (denudation of the skin with gentle pressure) is positive, but only in the areas of erythema. Conjunctivitis and oral lesions are common but are usually not as severe as in Stevens-Johnson syndrome. The course may be relentlessly progressive, complicated by severe dehydration, electrolyte imbalance, shock, and secondary localized infection and septicemia.

The differential diagnosis includes the staphylococcal scalded skin syndrome, in which the blister cleavage plane is intraepidermal, graft-versus-host disease, chemical burns, drug eruptions, and pemphigus. Appreciation of the specific etiologic factor is crucial, particularly when the disorder is drug-induced. Management is similar to that for severe burns: strict reverse isolation, appropriately calculated fluid and electrolyte therapy, use of an air-fluid bed, and daily cultures.

TABLE 23–4. Potential Etiologies of Erythema Multiforme

Infectious Agents	Antibiotics
Herpes simplex 1,2*	Penicillin
Mycoplasma pneumoniae†	Sulfonamides†
Tuberculosis	INH
Group A streptococcus	Tetracyclines
Hepatitis B vaccine	***Anticonvulsants***
BCG vaccine	Phenytoin†
Yersinia	Phenobarbital†
Enteroviruses	Carbamazepine†
Histoplasmosis	Other drugs
Coccidioidomycosis	Phenylbutazone
Chemicals	Captopril
Terpenes	Etopside
Perfumes	Aspirin
Nitrobenzene	***Other***
Specific Diseases	Radiation therapy
Leukemia	
Lymphoma	

*Recurrent erythema multiforme.

†Erythema multiforme major (Stevens-Johnson syndrome: toxic epidermal necrolysis).

Drug reactions occur 1–3 wk after exposure.

Systemic antibiotic therapy is indicated when secondary infection is evident or suspected. Skin care consists of cleansing with isotonic saline or Burow solution, aluminum acetate, and applications of mupirocin ointment. Biologic or hydrogel dressings alleviate pain and reduce fluid loss. Narcotics are often required for pain relief. Mouth and eye care may be necessary, such as for erythema multiforme major. The fatality rate is approximately 25%.

EPIDERMOLYSIS BULLOSA. The diseases categorized under this general term are a heterogeneous group of congenital, hereditary blistering disorders. They differ in severity and prognosis, clinical and histologic features, and inheritance patterns (Table 23–5). The disorders can be categorized under three major headings: epidermolytic epidermolysis bullosa (EB), junctional EB, and dermolytic EB. The pathogenesis is poorly understood in all types; some involve structural defects and others apparent enzymatic abnormalities. Because mechanical trauma and high environmental temperatures are provocative factors in all of the types, affected children should be protected to the extent warranted by the severity of their disease. Parents usually become quite knowledgeable about what their child will tolerate. Metal closures on clothing, tape of any kind, rough or tight clothing, and sharp-edged toys should be avoided. Hot baths may also initiate new lesions. Blisters should be drained by puncturing, but the blister tops should be left intact to protect the underlying skin. Management must be individualized to permit maximum safe participation in childhood activities. Genetic counseling should be offered to families of affected children; therefore, early diagnosis is desirable whenever possible. Immunofluorescence mapping with monoclonal antibodies to identify the location of type IV collagen, bullous pemphigoid antigen, and laminin, and electron microscopy of skin are helpful in establishing a diagnosis of the specific type of disease by determining the depth of the blister formation (see Table 23–5).

Epidermolytic EB. *Epidermolysis bullosa simplex* is a nonscarring, autosomal dominant disorder. Blisters are usually present at birth or during the neonatal period. The bullae are intraepidermal and result from disintegration of the basal cells. Sites of predilection are the hands, feet, elbows, knees, legs, and scalp; intraoral lesions are minimal, and nails rarely become dystrophic and may be shed but usually regrow. The infants are usually vigorous. Secondary infection is the only serious complication. The propensity to blister decreases with age, and the long-term prognosis is good.

Epidermolysis bullosa of hands and feet (Weber-Cockayne type) is also an autosomal dominant disorder. This nonscarring variant begins some time after the 1st yr of life. Bullae are usually restricted to the hands and feet, including the palms and soles; rarely, they occur elsewhere. The intraepidermal blisters involve the cells of the suprabasal and granular layers, which may be dyskeratotic with clumped tonofilaments. The disorder is only mildly incapacitating.

In a less common variant, *EB herpetiformis Dowling-Meara*, affected children are not heat-sensitive. Grouped blisters, intense inflammation and milia formation, later development of hyperkeratosis of palms and soles, and distinctive electron microscopic findings are characteristic.

Junctional EB. *Epidermolysis bullosa letalis (Herlitz type)*, although basically a nonscarring condition, is life-threatening, and the complications are such that serious morbidity and disfigurement can be predicted. The infant is usually blistered at birth or develops lesions during the neonatal period, particularly on the perioral area, scalp, legs, diaper area, and thorax. Large, moist, erosive plaques may provide a portal of entry for bacteria, and septicemia is a frequent cause of death. Healing is delayed, and vegetating granulomas may persist for a long time. Mucous membrane involvement may be severe and ulceration of the respiratory, gastrointestinal, and genitourinary epithelium has been documented in many affected children. Defective dentition with early loss of teeth due to rampant caries is characteristic. In contrast to other variants of epidermolysis bullosa, sparing of the hands and feet is striking, with the exception of the distal digits and the nail plates; these are dystrophic or permanently lost. Growth retardation and recalcitrant anemia are almost invariable. A subepidermal blister is found on light microscopic examination, and electron microscopy demonstrates a cleavage plane between the plasma membranes of the basal cells and the basement membrane. Hypoplasia or absence of hemidesmosomes in the basal cell layer as seen by electron microscopy is diagnostic.

Therapy is supportive; an adequate caloric diet and iron should be provided. Infections should be treated promptly with antibiotics. Transfusions of packed red blood cells may be required. In addition to infection, cachexia and circulatory failure are common causes of death. This disorder is an autosomal recessive disease; genetic counseling should be offered to the family.

Generalized atrophic benign EB, a milder autosomal recessive variant, is also nonscarring and is characterized by identical histologic changes. The course is compatible with normal growth and life span.

Dermolytic EB. *Dominant dystrophic epidermolysis bullosa* appears to occur sporadically in many cases, although an autosomal dominant mode of transmission has been documented

TABLE 23–5. Characteristics of Epidermolysis Bullosa

Type	Predominant Inheritance	Level of Blister Formation	Features
Simplex (epidermolytic)	Autosomal dominant	Superficial; basal cell layer; above hemidesmosomes	7 Variants; usually congenital onset; hands and feet involved; minimal mucosal lesions; no scarring
Junctional (letalis)	Autosomal recessive	Lamina lucida, between bullous pemphigoid antigen and laminin; absence or rare hemidesmosomes	6 Variants; localized or progressive; congenital; heals with scarring; pyloric atresia; mucosal lesions; dysplastic teeth; loss of nails
Recessive dystrophic (dermolytic)	Autosomal recessive	Deep in dermis below the lamina densa; excessive production of abnormal dermal collagenase; absent anchoring fibrils	2 congenital variants; mitten scarring of the hands and feet; marked deformities; mucosal lesions produce esophageal stricture or gastrointestinal perforation; varied clinical course; risk for aggressive squamous cell cancer of the skin, tongue, esophagus
Dominant dystrophic (dermolytic)	Autosomal dominant	Deep in dermis below the lamina densa, below type IV collagen layer; sparse anchoring fibrils	2 Variants; hyperkeratotic lesions; variable severity; risk for squamous cell cancer

in some families. Blisters may be present at birth and are often limited to the hands, feet, and sacrum. The lesions heal promptly with the formation of soft, wrinkled scars, milia, and alterations in pigmentation. The general health is unimpaired, and in many cases the blistering process is rather mild, causing little restriction of activity and unimpaired growth and development. Mucous membrane involvement tends to be minimal, but nail loss is common. The *Cockayne-Touraine* variant of dominant dystrophic EB is milder than the *Pasini* form, in which blistering is more widespread and flesh-colored papules called albopapuloid lesions develop on the trunk at adolescence. The blister is subepidermal in both variants, with separation beneath the basement membrane. On electron microscopy anchoring fibrils are abnormal and decreased in number over the entire skin in the Pasini type but only in areas of blister predilection in the Cockayne-Touraine variant.

Recessive dystrophic epidermolysis bullosa is probably the most incapacitating form of the disorder. Extensive erosions and blister formation may occur at birth and seriously impede the care and feeding of the infant. Mucous membrane lesions are common and may cause severe nutritional deprivation, even in older children, whose growth may be retarded. During childhood, esophageal erosions and strictures, scarring of the buccal mucosa, flexion contractures of joints secondary to scarring of the integument, and the development of the digital fusion (Fig. 23–17) significantly limit the quality of life. The subepidermal bullae are located beneath the basement membrane, and there is an absence of anchoring fibrils. Excessive amounts of an aberrant collagenase are produced by dermal fibroblasts.

Although the skin becomes less sensitive to trauma with aging, the progressive and permanent deformities complicate management tremendously, and the overall prognosis is poor. If esophageal scarring develops, a semiliquid diet and esophageal dilatations may be required. Endoscopy and bougie dilatation may cause perforation; alternatively, stricture excision or colonic interposition may be needed to relieve esophageal obstruction. In infants, severe oropharyngeal involvement may necessitate the use of special feeding devices. Continuous iron therapy for anemia, intermittent antibiotic therapy for secondary infections, which are a common cause of death, and periodic plastic procedures for release of digits may reduce morbidity. Phenytoin may reduce blister formation in the recessive dystrophic type and corticosteroids occasionally reduce dysphagia due to esophageal stricture.

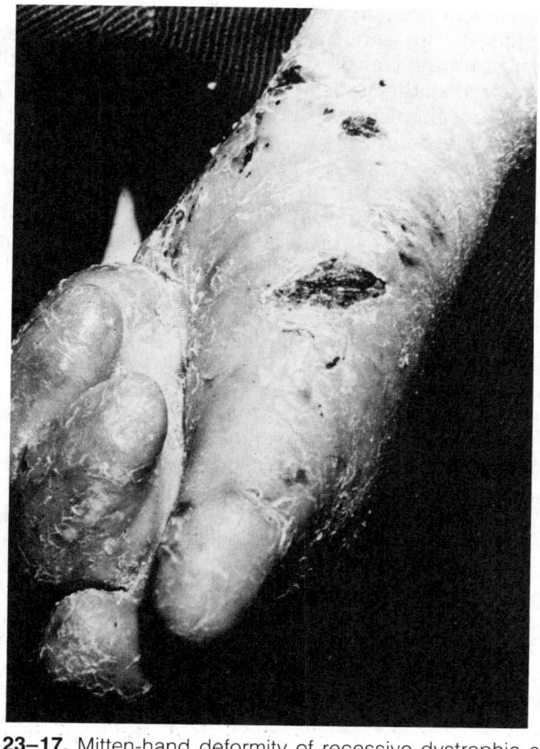

Figure 23–17. Mitten-hand deformity of recessive dystrophic epidermolysis bullosa.

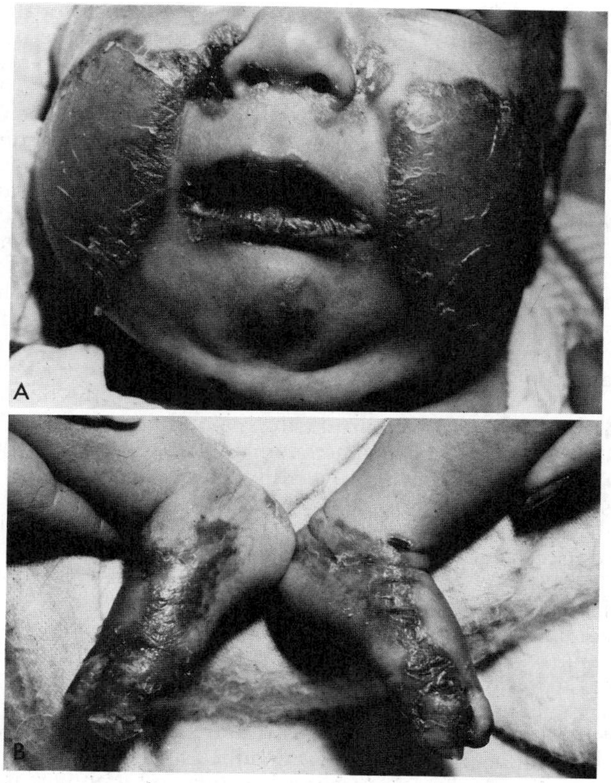

Figure 23–18. *A*, Psoriasiform facial lesions of zinc deficiency dermatitis. *B*, Similar lesions on the feet with secondary nail dystrophy.

ACRODERMATITIS ENTEROPATHICA. This is a rare, autosomal recessive disorder of zinc deficiency. The onset is insidious, occurring usually during the 1st yr of life. Initial symptoms are often noted following weaning from breast milk to cow's milk. The cutaneous eruption consists of vesicobullous, eczematous, and psoriasiform skin lesions symmetrically distributed in the perioral, acral, and perineal areas as well as on the cheeks, knees, and elbows. Initially these lesions are intensely erythematous and erosive, but with chronicity they become dry, hyperkeratotic, and psoriasiform in appearance (Fig. 23–18*A* and *B*). The hair often has a peculiar reddish tint, and alopecia of some degree is characteristic. Ocular manifestations include photophobia, conjunctivitis, blepharitis, and corneal dystrophy, detectable by slit-lamp examination. Associated manifestations include chronic diarrhea, stomatitis, glossitis, paronychia, nail dystrophy, growth retardation, personality changes, intercurrent bacterial infections, and superinfection with *Candida albicans*. The course without treatment is chronic and intermittent but often relentlessly progressive, terminating in severe marasmus and death. When the disease is less severe, only growth retardation and delayed development may be apparent.

The diagnosis is established by the constellation of clinical findings and by low concentrations of plasma zinc and of alkaline phosphatase, a zinc-dependent enzyme. Histopathologic changes in the skin and gastrointestinal tract are nonspecific, except that a cytoplasmic inclusion body has been noted in the Paneth cells. The basic metabolic defect in the disease relates to reduced intestinal absorption of zinc. A possible deficiency in amount or function of a zinc-binding ligand has been suggested as a pathogenetic factor.

For many years, acrodermatitis enteropathica was treated empirically, but often successfully, with diiodohydroxyquin and breast milk; however, the possibility of serious untoward effects of the drug, particularly optic atrophy, was a hazard. Oral therapy with zinc compounds has replaced diiodohydroxyquin as the treatment of choice. Optimal doses range from 50 mg of zinc sulfate, acetate, or gluconate daily for infants up to 150 mg/day for children; plasma zinc levels should be monitored, however, to individualize the dosage. Zinc therapy rapidly abolishes the manifestations of the disease. A few patients with acrodermatitis enteropathica without hypozincemia have recovered when given pharmacologic doses of zinc. A syndrome resembling acrodermatitis enteropathica has been observed in patients of all ages receiving total parenteral nutrition without supplemental zinc.

PEMPHIGUS. This occurs during childhood as pemphigus vulgaris or as pemphigus foliaceus.

Pemphigus Vulgaris. This type usually first appears as painful oral ulcers, which may be the only evidence of the disease for weeks or months. Subsequently, large, flaccid bullae emerge on nonerythematous skin, most commonly on the head and trunk. The lesions rupture and enlarge peripherally, producing painful, raw, denuded areas that have little tendency to heal. Malodorous verrucous and granulomatous lesions may develop at sites of ruptured bullae. Nikolsky sign (avulsion of epidermis on gentle pressure) is always present.

Histologically, the lesion is a suprabasal (intraepidermal) blister containing loose, acantholytic epidermal cells. IgG antibody to epidermal intercellular substance produces a characteristic pattern on direct immunofluorescence preparations (see Table 23–1). Serum antibody titers to the epidermal intercellular substance usually correlate with the clinical course; thus, serial determinations may have predictive value.

The disease can be confused with erythema multiforme, bullous pemphigoid, Stevens-Johnson syndrome, and toxic epidermal necrolysis. Since the course may rapidly lead to debility, malnutrition, and death, prompt diagnosis is essential. The disease is best controlled initially with high-dose systemic corticosteroid therapy. Azathioprine, cyclophosphamide, methotrexate, and gold therapy have all been useful in maintenance regimens.

Pemphigus Foliaceus. This type is also characterized by intraepidermal blisters; the site of cleavage, however, is high in the epidermis rather than suprabasal. The blisters are very superficial, rupture quickly, and may be missed on examination. Crusting and scaling are typical manifestations. When generalized, the eruption may resemble exfoliative dermatitis or any of the chronic blistering disorders, but localized erythematous plaques simulate seborrheic dermatitis, psoriasis, impetigo, eczema, or lupus erythematosus. Focal lesions are usually localized to the scalp, face, neck, and upper trunk. Mucous membrane lesions are minimal or absent. Pruritus, pain, and a burning sensation are frequent complaints.

An intraepidermal acantholytic bulla high in the epidermis is diagnostic; it is imperative, however, to select an early lesion for biopsy. Tissue-bound and circulating intercellular epidermal antibodies to a desmosomal glycoprotein, desmoglein, may be found (see Table 23–1). The course varies but is generally more benign than that of pemphigus vulgaris. Long-term remission is usual following suppression of the disease by systemic corticosteroid therapy. A topical corticosteroid preparation is occasionally sufficient.

BULLOUS PEMPHIGOID. This lesion rarely occurs in children, but it must be considered in the differential diagnosis of any chronic blistering disorder. Typically, the blisters arise in crops on a normal, erythematous, or urticarial base. Individual lesions vary greatly in size and are tense and filled with serous fluid, which may become hemorrhagic or turbid. Oral lesions are common. Pruritus and a burning sensation may accompany the eruption, but constitutional symptoms are not prominent.

A subepidermal bulla can be identified by histologic examination. In sections of a blister or paralesional skin, a band of immunoglobulin (usually IgG) and C3 can be demonstrated in the basement membrane zone by means of immunofluorescence preparations (see Table 23–1). Indirect immunofluorescence studies of serum are usually positive for IgG antibodies to the basement membrane zone; the titers, however, do not correlate well with the clinical course.

The differential diagnosis includes bullous erythema multiforme, pemphigus, linear IgA dermatosis, bullous drug eruption, dermatitis herpetiformis, and bullous impetigo, which can be differentiated by histologic examination, immunofluorescence studies, and cultures. The cause of bullous pemphigoid is unknown, and the course is chronic and intermittent. Nevertheless, the disease can be successfully suppressed with systemic corticosteroid therapy alone or in combination with azathioprine, and ultimately it usually remits permanently. Local skin care consists of compresses and a drying lotion.

DERMATITIS HERPETIFORMIS. This disorder is characterized by grouped, small, tense, erythematous, stinging, pruritic papules and vesicles. The eruption tends to be symmetrically distributed; the sites of predilection are the knees, elbows, shoulders, buttocks, and scalp; mucous membranes are usually spared. When pruritus is severe, excoriations may be the only visible sign.

The cause is unknown; however, an association with gluten-sensitive enteropathy is found with some frequency (Sec. 13.49). Subepidermal blisters are found on skin biopsy, and IgA and C3 can be detected in the dermal papillae of paralesional skin by immunofluorescence studies. The frequent finding of immune complexes and autoimmune antibodies in serum, as well as the association with HLA B8 or D3 suggests an immune mechanism.

Dermatitis herpetiformis may mimic other chronic blistering diseases and may also resemble scabies, papular urticaria, insect bites, contact dermatitis, and papular eczema. The most effective treatment is oral administration of sulfapyridine or dapsone. These drugs provide immediate relief from the intense pruritus but must be used with caution because of possible serious side effects. Local antipruritic measures may also be useful. Jejunal biopsy is indicated to diagnose celiac disease, because cutaneous manifestations may precede malabsorption. The enteropathy will respond to a gluten-free diet more rapidly than the skin lesions will.

LINEAR IgA DERMATOSIS (CHRONIC BULLOUS DERMATOSIS OF CHILDHOOD). This disorder is most common in the 1st decade of life, with a peak incidence during the preschool years. The eruption consists of multiple large, tense bullae filled with clear or hemorrhagic fluid that develop on a normal or erythematous base. Areas of predilection are the trunk, genitalia, and legs, as well as the face, scalp, and dorsum of the feet. In the smaller lesions sausage-shaped bullae may be arranged in an annular or rosette-like fashion around a central crust (Fig. 23–19). Erythematous plaques with gyrate margins bordered by intact bullae may develop over larger areas. Pruritus may be absent or very intense.

The cause of the eruption is unknown. Histologic examination discloses a subepidermal bulla infiltrated with a mixture of inflammatory cells. Direct immunofluorescence studies

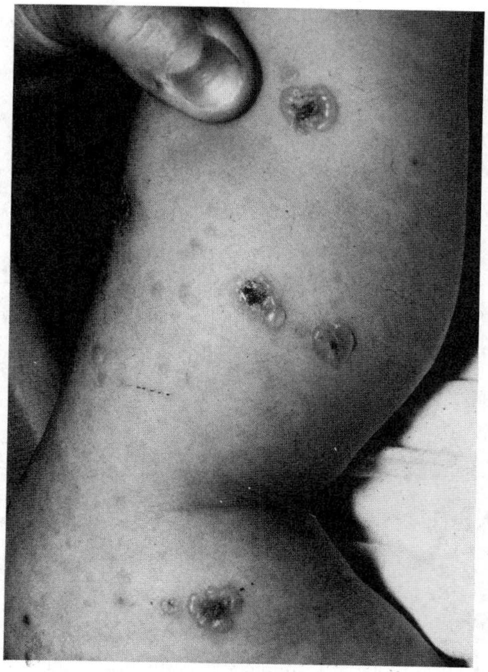

Figure 23–19. Rosette-like blisters around a central crust typical of linear IgA dermatosis (chronic bullous dermatosis of childhood).

demonstrate linear deposition of IgA and sometimes C3 at the dermoepidermal junction (see Table 23–1). Indirect immunofluorescence studies are sometimes positive for circulating antibodies. These studies serve to differentiate this eruption from pemphigus, bullous pemphigoid, dermatitis herpetiformis, and erythema multiforme, with which it may be confused. Gram stain and culture will exclude the diagnosis of bullous impetigo. The lack of bullous formation in response to trauma differentiates epidermolysis bullosa.

Many patients respond favorably to oral sulfapyridine or dapsone. During therapy with sulfapyridine, attention should be paid to urinary output and alkalinization of the urine to avoid crystal formation within the renal parenchyma. Hematologic and biochemical studies must be obtained at regular intervals during treatment with either drug to avoid serious side effects. Children who do not respond to either of these drugs may benefit from oral therapy with a corticosteroid or a combination of these drugs. The usual course is 2–4 yr, although some children have persistent or recurrent disease; there are no long-term sequelae.

INFANTILE ACROPUSTULOSIS. This disorder has its onset between 2 and 10 mo of age; lesions are occasionally noted at birth. Black males have a predisposition for this eruption, but infants of both sexes and all races may be affected. The cause is unknown.

The lesions are initially discrete, erythematous papules that become vesiculopustular within 24 hr and subsequently crust prior to healing. They are intensely pruritic, and a fresh outbreak is usually accompanied by extreme fretfulness. Preferred sites are the palms and soles, where the lesions may develop in profusion. A less dense eruption may be found on the dorsum of the hands and feet, the ankles, and the wrists. Pustules may occasionally occur elsewhere on the body. Each episode lasts for 7–10 days, during which time pustules continue to appear in crops. After a 2- to 3-wk remission, a new outbreak follows. This cyclical pattern continues for about 2 yr; permanent resolution is often preceded by longer intervals of remission between periods of activity. Infants with acropustulosis are otherwise well, and there are no constitutional findings.

The white blood count and differential are normal. Wright-stained smears of intralesional contents show masses of neutrophils or, occasionally, a predominance of eosinophils. Cultures for all types of organisms are negative. Histologically the pustules are well circumscribed, subcorneal in location, and filled with polymorphonuclear leukocytes, with or without eosinophils.

The differential diagnosis in the neonate includes transient neonatal pustular melanosis, erythema toxicum, cutaneous candidosis, and staphylococcal pustulosis. In the older infant and toddler additional diagnostic considerations include scabies, dyshidrotic eczema, pustular psoriasis, subcorneal pustular dermatosis, and hand, foot, and mouth disease.

Therapy is directed at minimizing discomfort; however, infantile acropustulosis is relatively unresponsive to topical corticosteroid preparations or oral antihistamines. Dapsone has been used effectively orally but has potentially serious side effects and should be used only with great caution.

23.14 ECZEMA

Eczema is a generic term used to designate a particular type of reaction pattern in the skin, which includes exudation, lichenification, and pruritus. Acute eczematous lesions are characterized by erythema, weeping, oozing, and the formation of microvesicles within the epidermis. Chronic lesions are generally thickened, dry, and scaly with coarse skin markings (lichenification) and altered pigmentation. Many types of eczema occur in children, of which the most common is atopic dermatitis (Sec. 11.42); however, seborrheic dermatitis, allergic and irritant contact dermatitis, nummular eczema, and dyshidrosis are also relatively common childhood eczemas. Pyoderma may become eczematized from scratching as may insect bites, papular urticaria, dermatophytosis, and a variety of dermatoses. Atopic skin is sensitive to many factors that increase pruritus, such as soap, wool, cool air, and food allergens.

Once the diagnosis of eczema has been established, it is important to classify the eruption more specifically for proper management. Pertinent historical data will often provide the clue. In some instances the subsequent course and character of the eruption permit classification. Histologic changes are relatively nonspecific, but all types of eczematous dermatitis are characterized by intraepidermal edema known as spongiosis.

CONTACT DERMATITIS. This form of eczema can be subdivided into irritant dermatitis, resulting from nonspecific injury to the skin, and allergic contact dermatitis, in which the mechanism is a delayed hypersensitivity reaction. Of the two, irritant dermatitis is more frequent in children, particularly during the early years of life.

Irritant contact dermatitis can result from prolonged or repetitive contact with a variety of substances that include saliva, citrus juices, bubble bath, detergents, abrasive materials, strong soaps, and proprietary medications. Saliva is probably one of the most common offenders; it may cause dermatitis on the face and in the neck folds of the drooling infant or retarded child. The older child who habitually licks his or her lips because of dryness may develop a striking, sharply demarcated perioral rash (Fig. 23–20*A*). Among the exogenous irritants, citrus juices, proprietary medications, and bubble bath preparations are relatively common; bubble bath dermatitis is a cause of severe pruritus. Excessive accumulation of sweat and moisture as a result of wearing occlusive shoes may also be responsible for irritant dermatitis.

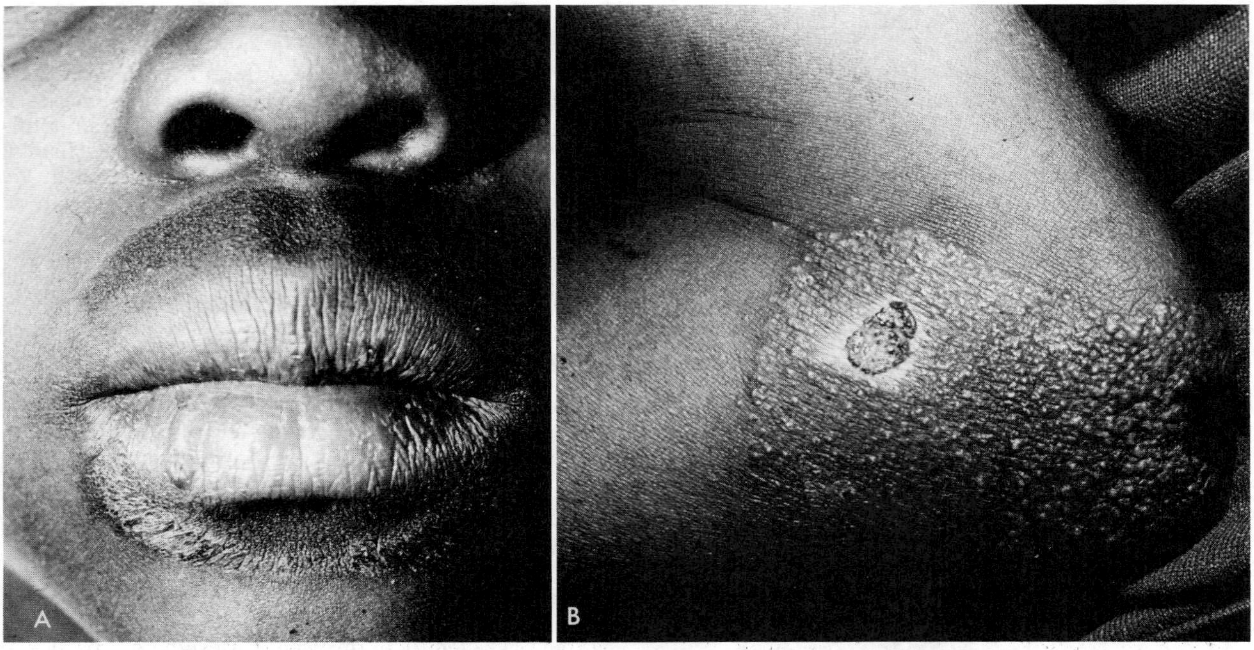

Figure 23–20. *A*, Perioral irritant contact dermatitis from lip-licking. *B*, Allergic contact dermatitis to Merthiolate spray. Note the sharp angular border of vesicular eruption.

Clinically, irritant contact dermatitis may be indistinguishable from atopic dermatitis or allergic contact dermatitis. A detailed history and consideration of the sites of involvement, the age of the child, and contactants usually provide clues to the etiology. The propensity to develop irritant dermatitis varies considerably among children, and some may respond to minimal injury in this fashion. In general, all irritant contact dermatitis will clear after removal of the stimulus and after temporary treatment with a topical corticosteroid preparation. Education of patient and parents as to the causes of contact dermatitis is crucial to successful therapy.

Diaper dermatitis can be regarded as the prototype of irritant contact dermatitis. As a reaction to overhydration of the skin, friction, maceration, and prolonged contact with urine and feces, retained diaper soaps, and topical preparations, the skin of the diaper area may become erythematous and scaly, often with papulovesicular or bullous lesions, fissures, and erosions. The eruption can be patchy or confluent, but the genitocrural folds are often spared. Chronic hypertrophic, flat-topped papules, and infiltrative nodules may simulate syphilitic lesions. Secondary infection with bacteria and yeasts is common; discomfort may be marked because of intense inflammation. Such conditions as allergic contact dermatitis, seborrheic dermatitis, candidosis, atopic dermatitis, and rare disorders such as histiocytosis X and acrodermatitis enteropathica should be considered when the eruption is persistent or recalcitrant to simple therapeutic measures.

Diaper dermatitis often responds to simple measures; however, some infants seem predisposed to diaper dermatitis, and management may prove difficult. The damaging effects of overhydration of the skin and prolonged contact with feces and ammoniacal urine can be obviated by frequent changing of diapers and meticulous washing of the genitalia with warm water and mild soap. Disposable diapers containing a superabsorbent material may help to maintain a relatively dry environment. Frequent applications of a bland protective topical agent (petrolatum or zinc oxide paste) following thorough gentle cleansing may suffice to prevent dermatitis.

When the aforementioned measures are not sufficient to promote healing, a light application of 0.5–1% topical hydrocortisone ointment after each diaper change for a limited time is often effective. Prior to initiation of such therapy, the possibility of candidal infection should be excluded by a KOH preparation or culture. For infants requiring additional protection, zinc oxide paste can be applied, after the steroid, as a thick covering. Secondary complications can result from prolonged use of corticosteroids, especially fluorinated compounds.

Juvenile plantar dermatosis is a common form of irritant contact dermatitis occurring mainly in prepubertal children. The dermatitis characteristically involves the weight-bearing surfaces, is painful rather than pruritic, and causes a glazed appearance of the plantar skin. Fissuring may become extensive, producing considerable discomfort. The dermatitis results from alternating excessive hydration and rapid moisture loss, which causes chapping of the skin and cracking of the stratum corneum. Affected children often have hyperhidrosis, wear occlusive synthetic footwear, and subject their feet to rapid drying without moisturization. Immediate application of a thick emollient when socks and shoes are removed or immediately after swimming will usually prevent this condition.

Allergic contact dermatitis is a T cell–mediated hypersensitivity reaction that is provoked by application of an antigen to the skin surface. The antigen penetrates the skin, where it is conjugated with a cutaneous protein, and the hapten-protein complex is transported to the regional lymph nodes. A primary immunologic response occurs locally in the nodes and becomes generalized, presumably because of dissemination of sensitized T cells. Sensitization requires several days and, when followed by a fresh antigenic challenge, becomes manifest as allergic contact dermatitis. Generalized distribution may also occur if enough antigen finds its way into the circulation. Once sensitization has occurred, each new antigenic challenge may provoke an inflammatory reaction within 8–12 hr; sensitization to a particular antigen usually persists for many years.

Acute allergic contact dermatitis is an erythematous, intensely pruritic, eczematous dermatitis, which, if severe, may be edematous and vesicobullous. Chronic contact dermatitis has the features of a longstanding eczema: lichenification, scaling, fissuring, and pigmentary change. The distribution of the eruption often provides a clue to the diagnosis. Volatile sensitizers usually affect exposed areas, such as face and arms. Jewelry, topical agents, shoes, clothing, and plants cause dermatitis at points of contact.

Rhus dermatitis (poison ivy, poison sumac, or poison oak) is often vesicobullous, and may be distinguished by linear streaks of vesicles where the plant leaves have brushed against the skin. Contrary to popular opinion, fluid from ruptured vesicles does not spread the eruption; however, antigen retained on the skin, under the fingernails, and on clothing will initiate new plaques of dermatitis if they are not removed by washing with soap and water. Antigen may also be carried by animals on their fur. The sap-like allergen (olecresin) is present on live or dead leaves, and sensitization to one plant produces cross reactions with the others.

Nickel dermatitis usually develops from contact with jewelry or metal closures on clothing and is seen most frequently on the ear lobes, such as when nickel-containing posts rather than nonmetallic materials or stainless steel are used to keep a pierced tract open. Some children are exquisitely sensitive to nickel, with even the traces found in gold jewelry provoking eruptions.

Shoe dermatitis typically affects the dorsum of the feet and toes, sparing the interdigital spaces; it is usually symmetric. Allergic contact dermatitis, in contrast to irritant dermatitis, rarely involves the palms and soles. Common allergens are the antioxidants and accelerators in shoe rubber and the chromium salts in tanned leather or shoe dyes. These substances are often leached out by excessive sweating.

Wearing apparel contains a number of sensitizers, including dyes, mordants, fabric finishes, fibers, resins, and cleaning solutions. Dye may be poorly fixed to clothing and leached out with sweating, as are the partially cured formaldehyde resins. The elastic in garments is also a frequent cause of clothing dermatitis.

Topical medications and cosmetics may be unsuspected as allergens, particularly if the medication is being used for a pre-existing dermatitis. The most common offenders are neomycin, thimerosal (Merthiolate) (see Fig. 23–20*B*), topical antihistamines (e.g., Caladryl), anesthetics (e.g., Nupercaine and Surfacaine), preservatives (e.g., parabens), and ethylenediamine, a stabilizer present in many medications. All types of cosmetics can cause facial dermatitis; involvement of the eyelids is characteristic for nail polish sensitivity.

Contact dermatitis can be confused with other types of eczema, dermatophytosis, and vesicobullous diseases. Patch testing may clarify the situation but should be performed only by an experienced person. The essential principle in treatment is elimination of contact with the allergen. Acute dermatitis responds to cool compresses and a corticosteroid agent applied several times daily. Chronic dermatitis often requires a more potent fluorinated steroid ointment with protective covering at night. An antihistamine may be used orally for its sedative effect. Massive acute bullous reactions such as those of poison ivy are best treated by a short course of oral corticosteroid therapy. If secondary infection has occurred, appropriate systemic antibiotic therapy should be given. Desensitization therapy is rarely indicated.

NUMMULAR ECZEMA. This disorder is unusual in children and unrelated to other types of eczema. The eczematous plaques are more or less coin-shaped. Common sites are the extensor surfaces of the extremities (Fig. 23–21), the buttocks, and the shoulders. The plaques are relatively discrete, boggy, vesicular, severely pruritic, and exudative; when chronic, they often become thickened and lichenified. The cause is unknown. Most frequently, these lesions are mistaken for tinea corporis, but plaques of nummular eczema are distinguished by the lack of a raised, sharply circumscribed border, and they often weep or bleed when scraped. A KOH study can be helpful in differentiation. Secondary infection is common. Control of pruritus is usually achieved with a fluorinated corticosteroid preparation with or without occlusion with a polyethylene wrap. Sedation with an antihistamine is helpful, particularly at night. Antibiotics are indicated for secondary infection.

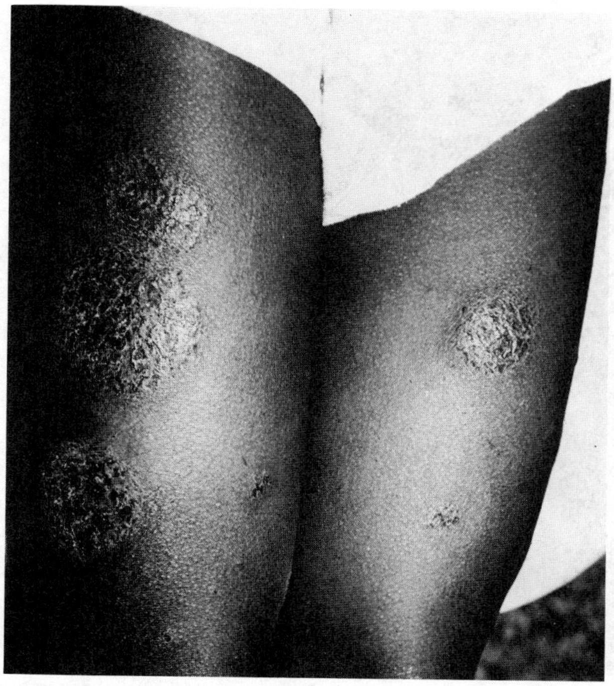

Figure 23–21. Multiple hyperpigmented scaly plaques of nummular eczema.

PITYRIASIS ALBA. This occurs mainly in children; the lesions are hypopigmented, round or oval, macular or slightly elevated patches with fine adherent scales (Fig. 23–22 [color plate section]). They may be mildly erythematous and relatively well defined, but lack a sharply marginated border. Lesions occur on the face, neck, upper trunk, and proximal arms. Itching is minimal or absent.

The etiology is unknown, but the eruption appears to be exacerbated by dryness and is often regarded as a mild form of eczema. Pityriasis alba is frequently misdiagnosed as tinea versicolor or tinea corporis, each of which can be readily excluded by performing a KOH examination of surface scales. The lesions wax and wane but eventually disappear. Application of a lubricant may ameliorate the condition; if pruritus is troublesome, a topical 1% hydrocortisone preparation applied 3–4 times daily may be more effective. Normal pigmentation returns in weeks to months.

LICHEN SIMPLEX CHRONICUS. This lesion is characterized by a chronic pruritic, eczematous, circumscribed, solitary plaque that is usually lichenified and hyperpigmented. The most common sites are the posterior neck, dorsum of the feet, wrists, and ankles. Trauma from rubbing and scratching accounts for persistence of the plaque, although the initiating event may be a transient lesion, such as an insect bite. Pruritus must be controlled to permit healing. A topical fluorinated corticosteroid preparation is often helpful, but constant irritation to the skin must be avoided. A covering to prevent scratching may be necessary.

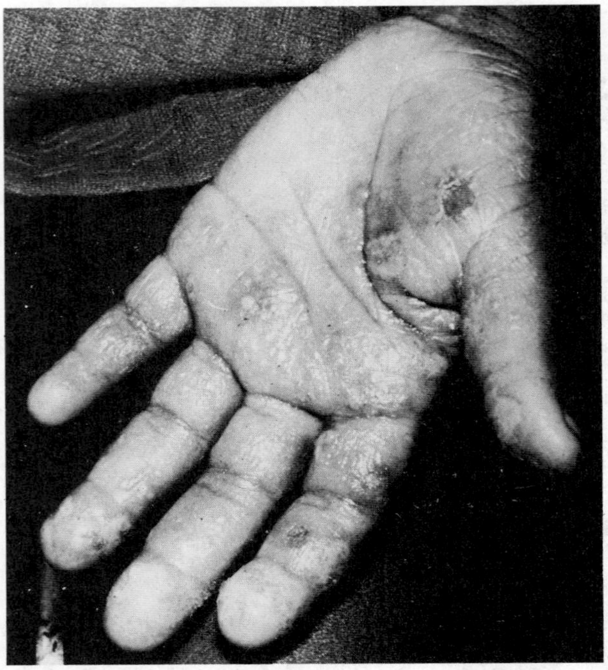

Figure 23–23. Vesicular palmar lesions of dyshidrotic eczema that have become secondarily infected.

DYSHIDROTIC ECZEMA (DYSHIDROSIS, POMPHOLYX). This is a recurrent, sometimes seasonal, blistering disorder of the hands and feet; it occurs in all age groups but is uncommon in infancy. The pathogenesis is not known; there does not appear to be a genetic factor, although an increased incidence of atopy has been recorded in patients and their relatives.

The disease is characterized by recurrent crops of intensely pruritic, small vesicles on the hands and feet. Sites of predilection are the palms, soles, and lateral aspects of the fingers and toes. Primary lesions are noninflammatory and filled with clear fluid, which, unlike sweat, has a physiologic pH and contains protein. Larger vesicobullae may occur, and maceration and secondary infection are frequent because of scratching (Fig. 23–23). The chronic phase is characterized by thickened, fissured plaques that may cause considerable discomfort. Hyperhidrosis is common in many patients, but the association may be fortuitous.

The diagnosis is made clinically. The disorder may be confused with allergic contact dermatitis, which usually affects the dorsal rather than the volar surfaces, and with dermatophytosis, which can be distinguished by a KOH preparation of the roof of a vesicle and by appropriate cultures.

Dyshidrotic eczema responds to wet dressings, followed by a topical corticosteroid preparation during the acute phase. Control of the chronic stage is difficult; lubricants containing mild keratolytic agents in conjunction with a potent topical fluorinated corticosteroid preparation and occlusion with a polyethylene wrap may be indicated. Secondary bacterial infection should be treated systemically with an appropriate antibiotic. Patients should be told to expect recurrence and should protect their hands and feet from the damaging effects of excessive sweating, chemicals, harsh soaps, and adverse weather.

SEBORRHEIC DERMATITIS. This is a chronic inflammatory disease that occurs at all ages; in the pediatric age group, it is most common during infancy and adolescence. The cause is unknown, as is the role of the sebaceous gland in this disease. A generalized eruption with features of seborrheic dermatitis is extremely common in HIV-infected children and adolescents.

The disorder may begin within the 1st mo of life and may be most troublesome during the 1st yr. Diffuse or focal scaling and crusting of the scalp, sometimes called *cradle cap,* may be the initial and at times the only manifestation. A greasy, scaly, erythematous papular dermatitis, which is usually nonpruritic, may involve the face, neck, retroauricular areas, axillae, and diaper area. The dermatitis may be patchy and focal or may spread to involve almost the entire body (Fig. 23–24). Postinflammatory pigmentary changes are common, particularly in black infants. When the scaling becomes pronounced, the condition may resemble psoriasis and at times can be distinguished only with difficulty. The possibility of coexistent atopic dermatitis must be considered when there is an acute weeping dermatitis with pruritus. An intractable seborrhea-like dermatitis with chronic diarrhea and failure to thrive (Leiner disease) may reflect dysfunction of the immune system. A chronic seborrhea-like pattern, which responds poorly to treatment, may also result from cutaneous histiocytic infiltrates in infants with histiocytosis X. Seborrheic dermatitis is a common cutaneous manifestation of acquired immunodeficiency syndrome (AIDS) among young adults and is characterized by thick, greasy scalp scales and large hyperkeratotic erythematous plaques on the face, chest, and genitalia.

During adolescence, seborrheic dermatitis is more localized and may be confined to the scalp and intertriginous areas. There may also be marginal blepharitis and involvement of the external auditory canal. Scalp changes may vary from diffuse, brawny scaling to focal areas of thick, oily, yellow crusts with underlying erythema. Loss of hair is not uncommon, and pruritus may be absent to marked. When the dermatitis is severe, erythema and scaling may occur at the frontal hairline, at the medial aspects of the eyebrows, and in the nasolabial and retroauricular folds. Red, scaly plaques may appear in the axillae, inguinal region, gluteal cleft, and umbilicus. On the extremities seborrheic plaques may be more eczematous and less erythematous and demarcated.

Seborrheic dermatitis is a condition that is reactivated in some patients by stressful situations, poor hygiene, and excessive perspiration. *Pityrosporum ovale (M. furfur)* has also been implicated as a causative agent. The differential diagnosis includes psoriasis, atopic dermatitis, dermatophytosis, and candidosis. Secondary bacterial infections and superimposed candidosis are not uncommon.

Scalp lesions should be controlled with an antiseborrheic shampoo (selenium sulfide, sulfur, salicylic acid, zinc pyri-

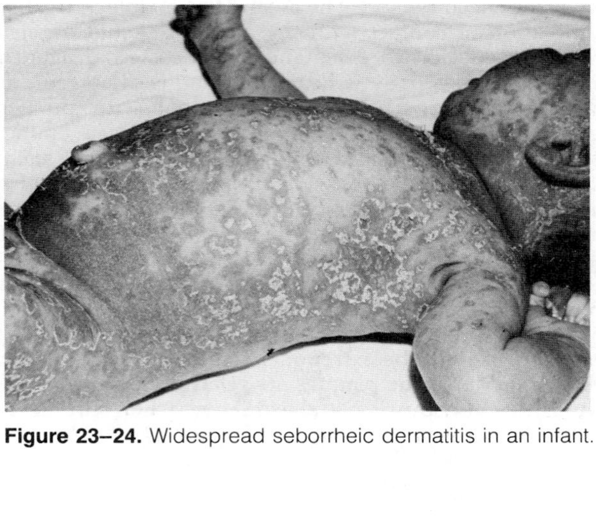

Figure 23–24. Widespread seborrheic dermatitis in an infant.

thion, tar), used daily if necessary. Inflamed lesions usually respond promptly to topical corticosteroid therapy given 2–4 times daily. A 3% sulfur ointment in a washable base is an alternative means of therapy. Topical antifungal agents effective against *Pityrosporum* have also been advocated as therapy. Wet compresses should be applied to the moist or fissured lesions prior to application of the steroid ointment. Many patients require the continued use of an antiseborrheic shampoo for control. Response to therapy is usually rapid unless there are complicating factors or the diagnosis is in error.

23.15 PHOTOSENSITIVITY

Photosensitivity denotes a qualitatively or quantitatively abnormal cutaneous reaction to sunlight or, less commonly, to artificial light. The adverse effects of sunlight are due principally to wavelengths of light ranging from 250 to 800 nm, a range that includes both ultraviolet and visible light. Host factors play an important role, particularly natural skin pigmentation, because melanin serves to reflect, absorb, and scatter light.

ACUTE SUNBURN REACTION. This is the most common light-induced effect seen in children; it is caused mainly by UVB radiation (290–320 nm wavelength). UVA radiation (320–400 nm) is more abundant but must be encountered in large quantities to produce sunburn. Children vary in susceptibility to ultraviolet radiation depending on their skin type (amount of pigment) (Table 23–6). Erythema appears 6–12 hr after initial exposure and reaches a peak in 24 hr when intense redness, exquisite tenderness, pain, edema, and blistering may occur. Additional effects of sun exposure include increase in thickness of the stratum corneum and increased formation and melanization of melanosomes, resulting in deepening of the skin color (tanning). Acute severe sunburn should be managed with cool tap water compresses, shake lotions, and, if necessary, a mild oral analgesic. Topical corticosteroids, judiciously chosen, may diminish inflammation and pain. Proprietary preparations containing topical anesthetics are relatively ineffective and potentially hazardous because of their propensity to cause contact dermatitis. A bland emollient is effective in the desquamative phase.

Although the long-term sequelae of chronic and intense sun exposure are not often seen in children, pediatricians should advise patients, children, and adolescents regarding the harmful effects, potential malignancy risks, and irreversible skin damage that results from unduly prolonged exposure to the sun and tanning lights. Premature aging, senile elastosis, actinic keratoses, squamous and basal cell carcinomas, and melanomas all occur with greater frequency in sun-damaged skin. Blistering sunburns in childhood and adolescence significantly increase the risk for later development of malignant melanoma. Adequate protection is readily provided by a wide variety of sunscreen agents. Physical opaque sunscreens (zinc oxide, titanium dioxide) block ultraviolet light, whereas chemical sunscreens (e.g., PABA, PABA esters, benzophenones, cinnamates) absorb damaging radiation. Children with skin types I–III (see Table 23–6) require sunscreens with SPF of at least 15. Protective clothing (hats) and avoidance of sun exposure between 10.00 AM–2.00 PM are additional prudent practices.

TABLE 23–6. Sun Reactive Skin Types

Type	Demographics	Sunburn, Tanning History
I	Red hair, freckles, Celtic origin	Always burns easily; no tanning
II	Fair skin, fair-haired, blue-eyed, Caucasian	Always burns easily; minimal tanning
III	Darker skinned Caucasians	Moderate burns, gradual light brown tan
IV	Mediterranean background	Minimal burn, tans well
V	Middle eastern Caucasians, Mexican	Rarely burns, tans profusely dark brown
VI	Blacks	Never burns, pigmented black

PHOTOTOXICITY AND PHOTOALLERGY. *Exogenous photosensitizers* in combination with a particular wavelength of light cause dermatitis that can be classified as a phototoxic or a photoallergic reaction.

Phototoxic reactions occur in all individuals who accumulate adequate amounts of a photosensitizing drug or chemical within the skin. The eruption is confined to light-exposed areas and often resembles an exaggerated sunburn, but it may be urticarial or bullous, and it results in hyperpigmentation.

Photoallergic reactions, in contrast, occur only in a small percentage of persons exposed to photosensitizers and light and require a time interval for sensitization to take place. A photoallergic dermatitis is a T cell–mediated delayed hypersensitivity reaction in which the drug, acting as a hapten, combines with a skin protein to form the antigenic substance. Photoallergic reactions vary in morphology and may occur on partially covered as well as on light-exposed skin. Some of the important classes of drugs and chemicals responsible for photosensitivity reactions are listed in Table 23–7.

Although photodermatitis due to drugs or chemicals may be diagnosed by photopatch testing, facilities for this diagnostic procedure are not widely available. A high index of suspicion combined with an appreciation of the distribution pattern of the eruption (sparing of eyelids, areas beneath the nose and chin, wrists, and antecubital fossae) and a history of application or ingestion of a known photosensitizing agent are all that is required to make a diagnosis. Discontinuation of the offending medication or avoidance of sun exposure, oral administration of an antihistamine, and application of a topical corticosteroid preparation to alleviate pruritus are appropriate therapeutic measures. Severe reactions may necessitate systemic corticosteroid therapy for a brief time.

THE PORPHYRIAS. These are acquired or inborn abnormalities of specific enzymes in the heme biosynthetic pathway; they are quite diverse in their clinical manifestations (Sec. 8.49). Two in particular occur in children and have photosensitivity as a consistent feature. Signs and symptoms may be negligible during the winter, when sun exposure is minimal.

Congenital erythropoietic porphyria (Gunther) is a rare autosomal recessive disorder. Affected persons are exquisitely sensitive to light, which may induce repeated severe bullous eruptions that result in mutilating scars. Hyperpigmentation, hyperkeratosis, vesiculation, and fragility of skin in light-exposed areas are a consequence of permanent skin damage. Hirsutism, red urine, erythrodontia, hemolytic anemia, splenomegaly, and increased amounts of uroporphyrin I in urine, plasma, and erythrocytes and of coproporphyrin I in feces are additional characteristic manifestations.

Erythropoietic protoporphyria is inherited as an autosomal dominant trait; photosensitivity becomes apparent in early childhood and is manifested by pain, pruritus, and a sensation of burning within 30 min of sun exposure, followed by erythema, edema, urticaria, vesicles, and, rarely, bullae on light-exposed areas. Nail changes consist of opacification of the nail plate, onycholysis, pain, and tenderness. Mild systemic symptoms of malaise, chills, and fever may accompany the acute skin reaction. Recurrent sun exposure produces a chronic eczematous dermatitis with thickened, lichenified

TABLE 23–7. Cutaneous Reactions to Sunlight

Sunburn
Photo-induced drug eruptions
  Systemic drugs include tetracyclines (Declomycin), psoralens, chlorthiazides, sulfonamides, barbiturates, griseofulvin, phenothiazines
  Topical agents include coal tar derivatives, furocoumarins (plants), psoralens, halogenated salicylanilides (soaps), perfume oils (e.g., oil of bergamot)
Genetic disorder with photosensitivity
  Xeroderma pigmentosum
  Bloom syndrome
  Cockayne syndrome
  Rothmund-Thomson syndrome
Disorders involving immune mechanisms
  Lupus erythematosus
  Dermatomyositis
  Scleroderma
  Solar urticaria
  Polymorphous light eruptions (?)
  Hydroa aestivale and vacciniforme (?)
Inborn errors of metabolism
  Porphyrias
  Hartnup disease
  Pellagra
Infectious diseases associated with photosensitivity
  Recurrent herpes simplex infection
  Lymphogranuloma venereum
  Viral exanthems (accentuated photodistribution)
Skin disease exacerbated or precipitated by light
  Lichen planus
  Darier disease
  Granuloma annulare
  Psoriasis
  Erythema multiforme
  Sarcoid
  Atopic dermatitis
Deficient protection due to lack of pigment
  Vitiligo
  Oculocutaneous albinism
  Partial albinism
  Phenylketonuria
  Chédiak-Higashi syndrome

skin, especially over the finger joints, and persistent violaceous erythema, ulcers, and pitted or vermicular atrophic scars on the face and rims of the ears. Protoporphyrin is elevated in the red blood cells, plasma, and feces.

The *porphyrias* may be confused with other diseases characterized by photosensitivity. Biopsies of lesions from patients with porphyria have shown deposits of a lipomucopolysaccharide-protein complex in perivascular areas and the papillary dermis.

The wavelengths of light mainly responsible for eliciting cutaneous reactions in porphyria are in the region of 400 nm. Window glass, which transmits wavelengths greater than 320 nm, is not protective. Patients must avoid direct sunlight, wear protective clothing, and use a sunscreen agent that effectively blocks wavelengths in the region of 400 nm. The administration of β-carotene (Solatene) quenches the fluorescence of the porphyrin molecule by imparting a yellow color to the skin; it effectively reduces the photosensitivity in patients with protoporphyria.

COLLOID MILIUM. This is a rare childhood disorder that occurs on the face and dorsum of the hands as a profuse eruption of ivory to yellow, firm, tiny, grouped papules. Although the translucent quality of the lesions suggests vesiculation, no fluid is obtained by puncture. The eruption is asymptomatic and usually remits spontaneously after puberty.

HYDROA AESTIVALE (summer prurigo; juvenile polymorphous light eruption). This is a controversial entity thought by some to be a variant of polymorphous light eruption and by others a mild form of hydroa vacciniforme. It occurs more frequently in girls with onset in the 1st decade. Papulovesicular lesions occur primarily, but not exclusively, on light-exposed areas: the ears, the face, the upper chest, and the dorsa of the hands and forearms. Itching and burning may precede the onset of visible lesions. Peak incidence occurs in the spring and early summer, before the time when ultraviolet light exposure is at a maximum. The pathogenesis is unknown, and no biochemical abnormalities have been identified. Phototesting appears to be of no value diagnostically. Sunscreens provide only partial relief.

HYDROA VACCINIFORME. This vesicobullous disorder is more common in boys than girls. The peak incidence is in the spring and summer. Symmetric crops of vesicles appear over the ears, the nose, the lips, the cheeks, and the dorsa of the hands and forearms. Itching and burning precede and accompany the lesions; occasionally, fever and malaise are also noted. Severe lesions of hydroa vacciniforme resemble the vesicles of chickenpox; they become ulcerated and crusted and heal with pitted scars. The pathogenesis is unknown, but typical lesions have been reproduced with repeated doses of UVA light. Hydroa vacciniforme begins in early childhood but may remit at puberty. It should be distinguished from erythropoietic protoporphyria. A topical corticosteroid may be useful for the inflammatory phase of the eruption. Sunscreens offer relatively little protection. β-Carotene taken orally and antimalarial agents are sometimes beneficial.

ACTINIC PRURIGO. This lesion was previously regarded as a subtype of polymorphous light eruption but is now defined as a distinct disorder. It is a chronic familial photodermatitis inherited as an autosomal dominant trait that occurs with some frequency among the Indians of North and South America, but it also occurs in European populations. The onset is in early childhood. Characteristic lesions follow sun exposure by several hours to 2 days and are intensely pruritic erythematous papules that merge to form eczematous plaques that lichenify and may become secondarily infected. Associated features that distinguish this disorder from other photoeruptions include cheilitis, conjunctivitis with pterygium, and traumatic alopecia of the outer half of the eyebrows. Actinic prurigo is a chronic condition that persists into adult life. Topical corticosteroids palliate the pruritus and inflammation. Sunscreens, antimalarials, and β-carotene all afford little to no protection. Thalidomide has been found to be an effective treatment in the American Indian population.

COCKAYNE SYNDROME. This disorder is inherited as an autosomal recessive trait and is characterized by normal appearance at birth, photosensitivity, loss of adipose tissue, dwarfism, mental retardation, and thin, atrophic, hyperpigmented skin, particularly over the face. The ears are large and protuberant, the nose is pinched, the teeth are carious, the hands and feet are cool and sometimes cyanotic. An unsteady gait with tremor, limitation of joint mobility, partial deafness, cataracts, retinal pigmentary abnormalities, optic atrophy, decreased sweating and tearing, and premature graying of the hair are additional features. The syndrome is distinguished from progeria (Sec. 25.4) by photosensitivity and the ocular abnormalities.

ROTHMUND-THOMSON SYNDROME. This is also known as poikiloderma congenitale because of the striking skin changes; it is thought to be inherited as an autosomal recessive trait, although a preponderance of affected females has been reported. Skin changes are noted in infancy as early as the 3rd mo. Plaques of erythema and edema appear on the cheeks, buttocks, hands, and feet and are replaced gradually by reticulated, atrophic, hyperpigmented, telangiectatic plaques. Exposure to the sun may provoke formation of bullae. Short stature, small hands and feet, sparse eyebrows and eyelashes, sparse, prematurely gray hair or alopecia, dystrophic nails, defective dentition, bony defects, hypogenitalism, and mental retardation are common. Cataracts commonly become apparent at 2–7 yr of age.

HARTNUP DISEASE (Sec. 8.6). This is a rare inborn error of metabolism with autosomal recessive inheritance; renal aminoaciduria and intestinal malabsorption of tryptophan is associated with a photo-induced, pellagra-like eruption. Approximately 20% of patients are mentally retarded, and others evidence emotional instability and episodic cerebellar ataxia. The initial cutaneous manifestations are detectable during the early months of life when an eczematous, occasionally vesicobullous, eruption is noted on the face and on the extremities in a glove and stocking pattern. Hyperpigmentation and hyperkeratosis may supervene and are intensified by further exposure to sunlight. Episodic flares may be precipitated by febrile illness, sun exposure, emotional stress, and poor nutrition. Administration of nicotinamide and protection from sunlight result in improvement of both cutaneous and neurologic manifestations.

BLOOM SYNDROME. This is characterized by erythema and telangiectasia in a butterfly distribution on the face, photosensitivity, and dwarfism of prenatal onset; inheritance is autosomal recessive. The facial erythema develops during infancy following exposure to sunlight. A bullous eruption may appear on the lips and telangiectatic erythema on the hands and forearms. Café-au-lait spots, ichthyosis, acanthosis nigricans, and hypertrichosis are less constant cutaneous manifestations. Defective dentition, prominent ears, pilonidal cysts, sacral dimples, syndactyly, polydactyly, clinodactyly of the 5th fingers, shortened lower extremities, and club feet are additional inconstant features. Intellect is normal. Chromosomal breaks and rearrangements are common, and affected children have an unusual tendency to develop lymphoreticular malignancies.

XERODERMA PIGMENTOSUM. This is a rare autosomal recessive genetic disorder in which skin changes are first noted during infancy or early childhood. Affected children, who are unable to repair DNA damaged by ultraviolet light, develop extensive changes in exposed skin. Sun-exposed areas such as the face, neck, hands, and arms are most severely involved, but lesions may occur at other sites including the scalp. The skin lesions consist of erythema, scaling, bullae, crusting, ephelides, telangiectasia, keratoses, basal and squamous cell carcinomas, and malignant melanomas. Ocular manifestations include photophobia, lacrimation, blepharitis, symblepharon, keratitis, corneal opacities, tumors of the lids, and possible eventual blindness. Neurologic abnormalities such as mental deterioration and sensorineural deafness may develop in some patients. The association of xeroderma pigmentosum with microcephaly, mental retardation, dwarfism, and hypogonadism is known as *De Sanctis–Cacchione syndrome.*

This disease is a serious, mutilating disorder, and the life span is often quite brief. Affected families should have genetic counseling. The defect is detectable in cells cultured from amniotic fluid. Affected children should be totally protected from sun exposure; protective clothing, eyeglasses, and opaque broad-spectrum sunscreens should be employed even for mildly affected children. Light from unshielded fluorescent bulbs and sunlight passing through glass windows are also harmful. Early detection and removal of malignancies is mandatory. Grafting of skin from non–light-exposed areas may be helpful, as is the use of topical antimitotic agents such as 5-fluorouracil.

23.16 DISEASES OF THE EPIDERMIS

PSORIASIS. This common, chronic skin disorder is first evident in approximately one third of affected individuals within the first 2 decades of life. When the onset occurs during childhood about 50% have a positive family history of the disease, and girls are more frequently affected. The mode of transmission is unknown; a multifactorial type of inheritance has been proposed. There is an association with HLA BW17, B13, B16, and BW37, but the most significant association is with CW6. These HLA types are not associated with the pustular form of the disease. The pathogenesis is also unknown; epidermal turnover time, however, is distinctly accelerated compared with that of normal epidermis.

Clinical Manifestations. The lesions consist of erythematous papules which coalesce to form plaques with sharply demarcated, irregular borders. If they are unaltered by treatment, a thick silvery or yellow-white scale (resembling mica) develops; removal of it may result in pinpoint bleeding (Auspitz sign). The Koebner, or isomorphic, response in which new lesions appear at sites of trauma is a valuable diagnostic feature. Lesions may occur anywhere, but preferred sites are the scalp, knees (Fig. 23–25*A*), elbows, umbilicus, and genitalia. Scalp lesions may be confused with seborrheic dermatitis or tinea capitis. Small, raindrop-like lesions on the face are moderately common. Nail involvement, a valuable diagnostic sign, is characterized by pitting of the nail plate (see Fig. 23–25*B*), detachment of the plate (onycholysis), and accumulation of subungual debris.

Age is an important factor in determining the clinical pattern. Psoriasis is rare in the neonate but may be severe, recalcitrant, and pose a diagnostic problem. The initial lesions may involve the diaper area and mimic seborrheic dermatitis, eczematous diaper dermatitis, perianal streptococcal disease, or candidosis. Biopsy or prolonged observation may be required for definitive diagnosis. Other rare forms include psoriatic erythroderma, localized or generalized pustular psoriasis, and linear psoriasis. Hospitalization may be required for severe forms of the disease.

Guttate psoriasis, a variant that occurs predominantly in children is characterized by an explosive eruption of profuse, small, oval or round lesions that morphologically are identical to the larger plaques of psoriasis (see Fig. 23–25*C*). Sites of predilection are the trunk, face, and proximal portions of the limbs. The onset frequently follows a recent streptococcal respiratory infection; a culture of the throat and serologic titers should be obtained. Guttate psoriasis has also been observed following perianal streptococcal infection, viral infections, sunburn, and withdrawal of systemic corticosteroid therapy. The lesions may be confused with viral exanthems and guttate parapsoriasis (see later).

Diagnosis. The differential diagnosis includes Reiter syndrome, which in contrast to psoriasis involves mucous membranes and pityriasis rubra pilaris.

Treatment. The therapeutic approach varies with the age of the child, the type of psoriasis, the sites of involvement, and the extent of the disease. Therapy is mainly palliative and should not be overly aggressive. Physical and chemical trauma to the skin should be avoided as much as possible (see the Koebner response, earlier).

Tar preparations may be used in the form of an emulsion added to the daily bath, gel preparations, or ointments such as crude coal tar (1–5%) and liquor carbonis detergens (5–15%) in petrolatum alone or in conjunction with ultraviolet light (UVB) or natural sunlight. Occasionally, sunlight has an adverse rather than a beneficial effect, and the use of tar preparations may have to be decreased during the summer

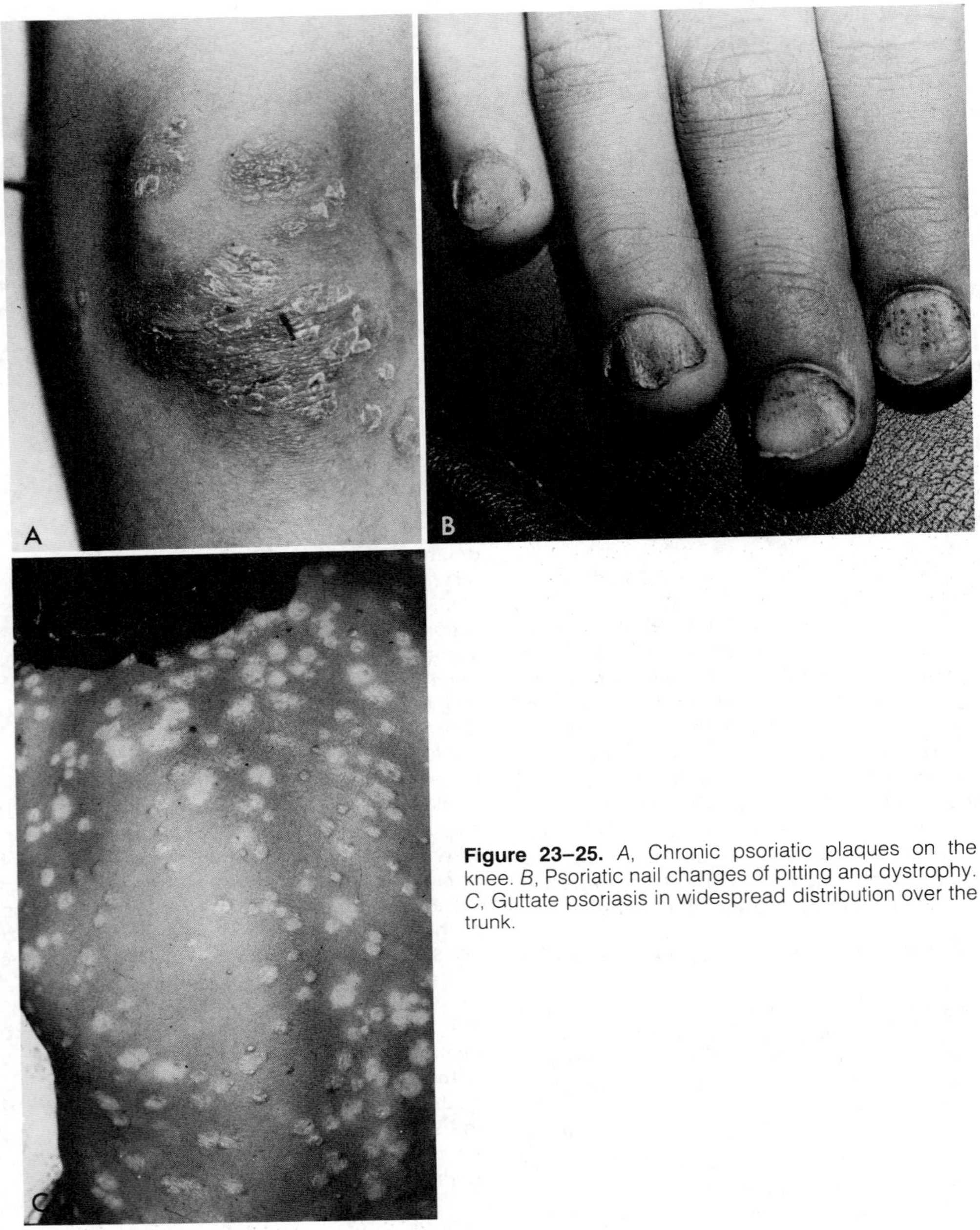

Figure 23–25. *A*, Chronic psoriatic plaques on the knee. *B*, Psoriatic nail changes of pitting and dystrophy. *C*, Guttate psoriasis in widespread distribution over the trunk.

to avoid phototoxic reactions. Salicylic acid ointment (1–3%) may provide an alternative for removal of scale, but extensive application may result in toxicity, particularly in small children. Topical corticosteroid preparations are extremely effective, but they must be used with caution; fluorinated compounds produce cutaneous atrophy if applied excessively or if occluded with polyethylene film for prolonged periods of time. The least potent effective preparation should be applied 1–2 times daily. For scalp lesions, applications of a phenol and saline solution (Baker P & S) followed by a tar shampoo are effective in the removal of scales. A corticosteroid in a lotion or gel base may be applied when the scaling is diminished. Rarely, the more severe forms of psoriasis may require systemic therapy; such management should be under the direction of an experienced physician.

The use of psoralens and ultraviolet light (PUVA) is effective in severe psoriasis in adults, but the safety of PUVA has not been established for children. Methotrexate and oral retinoids (in combination with PUVA) are utilized for the rare severe and generalized forms of psoriasis. The retinoid etretinate is useful in severe disorders, has a half-life of several years, and may have serious side effects; dermatologic consultation is essential when its use is being considered. Psoriasis in infants and acute guttate psoriasis may flare with vigorous treatment and should be managed conservatively. Nail lesions are usually recalcitrant to therapy.

Prognosis. This is best for children with limited disease. Psoriasis is characterized by remissions and exacerbations, and, if present during adolescence, it is a lifelong disease. Arthritis may be an extracutaneous complication.

KERATOSIS PILARIS. This moderately common papular eruption may vary in extent from sparse lesions over the extensor aspects of the limbs to involvement of most of the body surface. The lesions may resemble gooseflesh; they are

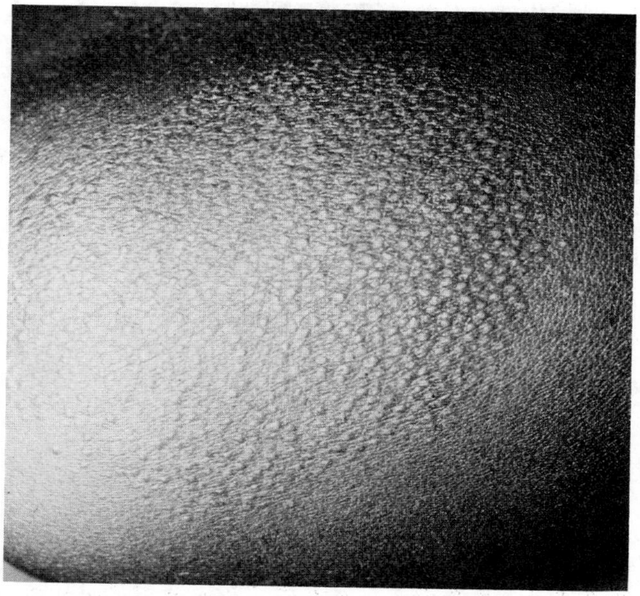

Figure 23–26. Sharply circumscribed plaque of follicular papules characteristic of lichen spinulosus.

noninflammatory, scaly, follicular papules that do not coalesce. Irritation of the follicular plugs occasionally causes folliculitis. Because the lesions are associated with and accentuated by dry skin, they are often more prominent during the winter. They are more frequent in patients with atopic dermatitis and are most common during childhood and early adulthood, tending to subside during the 3rd decade of life. Mild or localized eruptions respond to lubrication with a bland emollient; more pronounced or widespread lesions require regular applications of a 10–25% urea cream, an α-hydroxy acid preparation such as lactic acid in an emollient, or topical retinoic acid.

LICHEN SPINULOSUS. This uncommon disorder occurs principally in children and more frequently in boys. The cause is unknown. The lesions consist of sharply circumscribed irregular plaques of spiny, keratinous projections that protrude from the orifices of the pilosebaceous canals (Fig. 23–26). Plaques may occur anywhere on the body and are often distributed symmetrically on the trunk, elbows, knees, and extensor surfaces of the limbs. Although sometimes erythematous, the lesions are usually skin-colored. They are readily palpable and represent keratotic follicular plugs.

Lichen spinulosus is easily differentiated from keratosis pilaris because the latter lesions are never grouped to form plaques. More commonly, it is confused with papular eczema.

Treatment is usually unnecessary. For patients who regard the eruption as a cosmetic defect, keratolytic agents such as salicylic acid ointment (3–7%), urea-containing lubricants (10–25%), and retinoic acid preparations are often effective in flattening the projections. The plaques usually disappear spontaneously after several months or years.

PITYRIASIS ROSEA. This benign, common eruption occurs most frequently in children and young adults. Although a prodrome of fever, malaise, arthralgia, and pharyngitis may precede the eruption, children rarely complain of such symptoms. A *herald patch*, a solitary, round or oval lesion that may occur anywhere on the body and is often but not always identifiable by its large size, usually precedes the generalized eruption. Herald patches vary from 1 to 10 cm in diameter; they are annular in configuration; and they have a raised border with fine, adherent scales. Approximately 5–10 days after the appearance of the herald patch, a widespread, symmetric eruption becomes evident involving mainly the trunk and proximal limbs (Fig. 23–27). When the disease is extensive, the face, scalp, and distal limbs may be involved, or, in the inverse form of pityriasis rosea, only those sites may be affected. Lesions may appear in crops for several days. Typical lesions are oval or round, less than 1 cm in diameter, slightly raised, and pink to brown in color. The developed lesion is covered by a fine scale that gives the skin a crinkly appearance; some lesions clear centrally, producing a collarette of scale that is attached only at the periphery. Papular, vesicular, urticarial, hemorrhagic, and large, annular lesions are unusual variants. The long axis of each lesion is usually aligned with the cutaneous cleavage lines, a feature that creates the so-called "Christmas tree" pattern on the back. Actually, conformation to skin lines is often more discernible in the anterior and posterior axillary folds and supraclavicular areas. Duration of the eruption varies from 2 to 12 wk. The lesions may be asymptomatic or mildly to severely pruritic. The cause of pityriasis rosea is unknown; a viral agent has been sought.

The diagnosis is clinical. The herald patch may be mistaken for tinea corporis, a pitfall that can be avoided if a KOH preparation is obtained. The generalized eruption resembles a number of other diseases; of these, secondary syphilis is the most important. Drug eruptions, viral exanthems, guttate psoriasis, pityriasis lichenoides chronica, and eczema can also be confused with pityriasis rosea.

Treatment is unnecessary for the asymptomatic patient. If scaling is prominent, a bland emollient may suffice. Pruritus may be suppressed by a lubricating lotion containing menthol and camphor or by an oral antihistamine for sedation, particularly at night, when itching may be troublesome. Occasionally, a nonfluorinated topical corticosteroid preparation may be necessary to alleviate pruritus. After the eruption has resolved, postinflammatory hypopigmentation or hyperpigmentation may be pronounced, particularly in black patients; these changes disappear during subsequent weeks.

PITYRIASIS RUBRA PILARIS. This rare chronic dermatosis often has an insidious onset with diffuse scaling and erythema of the scalp, indistinguishable from seborrheic dermatitis, and with thick hyperkeratosis of the palms and soles. The characteristic primary lesion is a firm, dome-shaped, tiny,

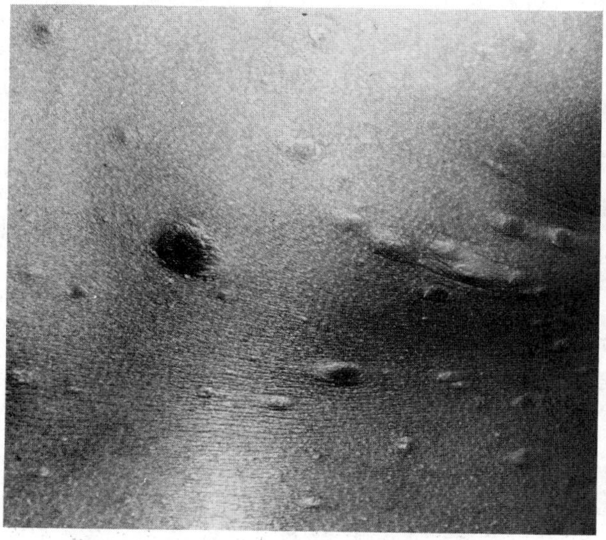

Figure 23–27. Ovoid, maculopapular lesions of pityriasis rosea. Note the distribution along the skin lines and the herald patch on the chest.

acuminate papule, which is pink to red in color and has a central keratotic plug pierced by a vellus hair. Masses of these papules coalesce to form large, erythematous, sharply demarcated plaques, within which islands of normal skin can be distinguished, creating a bizarre effect. Typical papules on the dorsum of the proximal phalanges are readily palpated. Gray plaques or papules resembling lichen planus may be found in the oral cavity. Dystrophic changes in the nails may occur and mimic those of psoriasis. In advanced stages, marked hyperkeratosis of the scalp and face may cause alopecia and ectropion. Differential diagnosis includes ichthyosis, seborrheic dermatitis, keratoderma of the palms and soles, and psoriasis.

The etiology is unknown. A genetic form with autosomal dominant transmission may account for some cases in childhood, but most appear to be sporadic. Attempts to link the disease with a defect in vitamin A metabolism have not been definitive. Skin biopsy may help to differentiate this condition from psoriasis and seborrheic dermatitis, which it resembles most closely.

The numerous therapeutic regimens recommended are difficult to evaluate because the disease has a capricious course with exacerbations and remissions. Oral and topical retinoids as well as vitamin A have been used most frequently. When vitamin A or synthetic retinoids are administered orally, the child should be observed carefully for signs of toxicity (see Psoriasis, Treatment). In childhood the prognosis for eventual resolution is relatively good.

DARIER DISEASE (KERATOSIS FOLLICULARIS). This rare genetic disorder is inherited as an autosomal dominant trait. Onset occurs usually during late childhood. Typical lesions are small, firm, skin-colored papules that are not always follicular in location. Eventually, the lesions acquire yellow, malodorous crusts; coalesce to form large, gray-brown, vegetative plaques; and usually involve the face, neck, shoulders, chest, back, and limb flexures in a symmetric distribution. Papules, fissures, crusts, and ulcers may appear on the mucous membranes of the lips, tongue, buccal mucosa, pharynx, larynx, and vulva. Hyperkeratosis of the palms and soles and nail dystrophy with subungual hyperkeratosis are variable features. Severe pruritus, secondary infection, offensive odor and aggravation of the dermatosis on exposure to sunlight may occur.

Darier disease is most likely to be confused with seborrheic dermatitis or juvenile flat warts. Histologic changes are diagnostic; hyperkeratosis, intraepidermal separation with formation of suprabasal clefts, and dyskeratotic epidermal cells are characteristic features.

Therapy is nonspecific. Some patients have responded to large oral doses of vitamin A or to topical retinoic acid, with or without occlusive dressings. Secondary infection may require local cleansing and systemically administered antibiotics. Affected individuals usually suffer more during the summer.

LICHEN NITIDUS. This chronic, benign, papular eruption is characterized by minute (1–2 mm), flat-topped, shiny, firm papules of uniform size, which are most often skin-colored but may be pink or red and, in black individuals, are usually hypopigmented. Sites of predilection are the genitalia, abdomen, chest, forearms, wrists, and inner aspects of the thighs. The lesions may be sparse or numerous and form large plaques; careful examination usually discloses linear papules in a line of scratch (Koebner phenomenon), a valuable clue to the diagnosis because it occurs in only a few diseases (Fig. 23–28).

Lichen nitidus occurs in all age groups. The cause is unknown. Patients are usually asymptomatic and constitutionally well. The lesions may be confused with and rarely coexist with those of lichen planus. Widespread keratosis

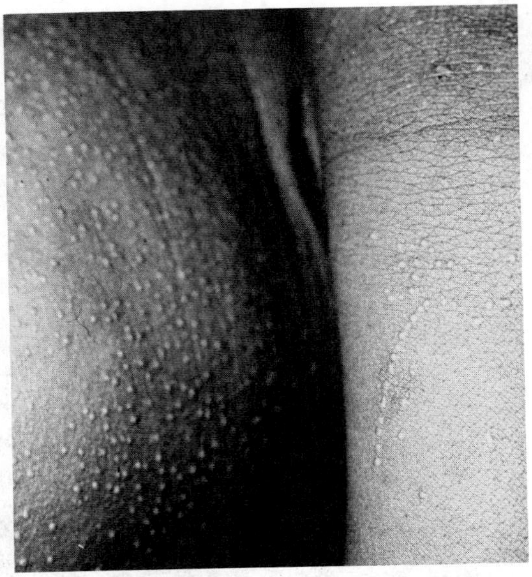

Figure 23–28. Tiny flat-topped papules of lichen nitidus on the arm and trunk. Note the Koebner response on the arm (papules in a line of scratch).

pilaris can also be confused with lichen nitidus, but the follicular localization of the papules and the absence of the Koebner phenomenon in keratosis pilaris will distinguish them. Verruca plana (flat warts), if small and uniform in size, may occasionally resemble lichen nitidus. Although the diagnosis can be made clinically, a biopsy is occasionally indicated. Histopathologically, the lichen nitidus papule consists of sharply circumscribed nests of lymphocytes and histiocytes in the upper dermis enclosed by claw-like epidermal rete ridges. The course of lichen nitidus takes months to years, but the lesions eventually involute completely. There is no effective therapy.

LICHEN STRIATUS. This benign, self-limited eruption consists of a continuous or discontinuous linear band of papules in a zosteriform distribution. The primary lesion is a flat-topped red to violaceous papule covered with a fine scale. Aggregates of these papules form multiple bands or plaques (Fig. 23–29). In black patients, the lesions may be hypopigmented.

The etiology and explanation for the linear distribution are unknown. The eruption evolves over a period of days or weeks in an otherwise healthy child, remains stationary for weeks to months, and finally remits without sequelae. Symptoms are usually absent; some children complain of itching. Nail dystrophy may occur when the eruption involves the posterior nail fold and matrix.

Lichen striatus is confused occasionally with other disorders. The initial plaque may resemble papular eczema or lichen nitidus until the linear configuration becomes apparent. Linear lichen planus and linear psoriasis are often associated with typical individual lesions elsewhere on the body. Linear epidermal nevi are permanent lesions that often become more hyperkeratotic and hyperpigmented than those of lichen striatus. A lubricating lotion containing menthol and camphor or a mild corticosteroid preparation provides sufficient relief when pruritus is a problem.

LICHEN PLANUS. This is a rare disorder in the young child and uncommon in the older one. The primary lesion is a violaceous, sharply demarcated, polygonal papule with fine lines or thin white scales on the surface; papules may coalesce to form large plaques. The papules are intensely pruritic, and additional ones are often induced by scratching (Koebner

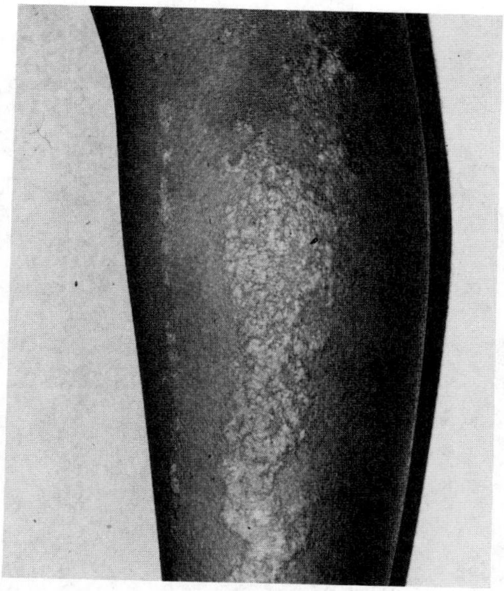

Figure 23–29. Multiple linear plaques and streaks of lichen striatus.

phenomenon) so that lines of them are often detected (Fig. 23–30). Sites of predilection are the flexor surfaces of the wrists, the forearms, and the inner aspects of the thighs. Characteristic lesions of the mucous membrane consist of pinhead-sized, white papules that coalesce to form reticulated and lacy patterns on the oral mucosa and sometimes on the lips and tongue.

Acute eruptive lichen planus is probably the most common form in children. The lesions erupt in an explosive fashion, much like a viral exanthem, and spread to involve most of the body surface. Hypertrophic, linear, bullous, atrophic, annular, follicular, erosive, and ulcerative forms of lichen planus may also occur. Nail involvement may develop in the chronic forms but is rarely evident in children (twenty nail dystrophy, Sec. 23.23). The disorder may persist for months to years, but the acute eruptive form is most likely to involute permanently. Frequently, intense hyperpigmentation persists for a long time following the resolution of lesions. The pathology of lichen planus is quite specific, and a biopsy is indicated if the diagnosis is unclear.

Treatment is directed at alleviation of the intense pruritus as well as amelioration of the skin lesions. Oral antihistamines and/or tranquilizers are often helpful. The skin lesions respond best to regular applications of a topical corticosteroid preparation. Rarely, systemic corticosteroid therapy is necessary to gain control of widespread, intractable lesions.

POROKERATOSIS. This rare, chronic, progressive disease is inherited as an autosomal dominant trait. Several forms have been delineated: solitary plaques, linear porokeratosis, hyperkeratotic lesions of the palms and soles, disseminated eruptive lesions, and superficial actinic porokeratosis. The last form, probably induced by excessive sun exposure, occurs more commonly in adult females. Other types of porokeratosis are more common in males and begin during childhood. Sites of predilection are the limbs, face, neck, and genitalia. The primary lesion is a small, keratotic papule that enlarges peripherally so that the center becomes depressed, the edge forming an elevated wall or collar. The configuration of the plaque may be round, oval, or gyrate; its elevated border is split by a thin groove from which minute cornified projections protrude. The enclosed central area is yellow, gray, or tan, sclerotic, smooth, and dry, whereas the hyperkeratotic border is a darker gray, brown, or black.

The differential diagnosis includes warts, epidermal nevi, lichen planus, granuloma annulare, and elastosis perforans serpiginosa. A skin biopsy discloses the characteristic cornoid lamella (plug of stratum corneum cells with retained nuclei), which is responsible for the invariable linear ridge of the lesion.

The disease is slowly progressive but relatively asymptomatic. Lesions are sometimes responsive to applications of liquid nitrogen or occasionally may be surgically excised. Topical agents such as retinoic acid and 5-fluorouracil may be effective in some patients.

PAPULAR ACRODERMATITIS OF CHILDHOOD (GIANOTTI-CROSTI SYNDROME). This distinctive eruption is associated with malaise and low-grade fever but few other constitutional symptoms. The incidence peaks in early childhood. Occurrences are usually sporadic, but epidemics have been recorded.

The skin lesion is a monomorphous, usually nonpruritic, dusky or coppery red, flat-topped, firm papule ranging in size from 1 to 5 mm. The papules appear in crops and may become profuse but remain discrete forming a symmetric eruption on the face, buttocks, and limbs including the palms and soles. The papules sometimes become hemorrhagic. Lines of papules (Koebner phenomenon) may be noted on the extremities. The trunk is relatively spared, as are the scalp and mucous membranes. Generalized lymphadenopathy and hepatomegaly (in those with hepatitis B viremia) constitute the only other abnormal physical findings. The eruption resolves spontaneously in about 3 wk. Lymphadenopathy and hepatomegaly may persist for several months.

This eruption in Italy is most often associated with primary liver infection by hepatitis B virus and hepatitis B surface antigenemia. Elevation of serum transaminase and alkaline phosphatase values without concomitant hyperbilirubinemia is usual. Skin biopsy is characterized by a perivascular mononuclear cell infiltrate and capillary endothelial swelling.

Generally the disease is benign, self-limited, and does not recur. The hepatitis usually resolves in 2–3 mo but, occasionally, may progress to chronic hepatitis with persistent antigenemia and elevated transaminase activity. The surface an-

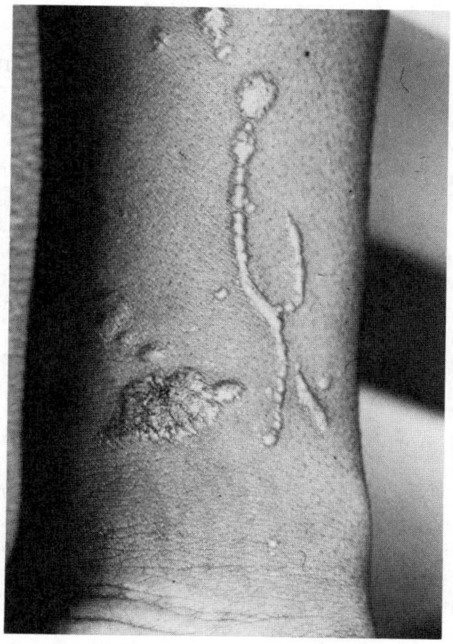

Figure 23–30. Violaceous polygonal papules of lichen planus. Note the striking Koebner response.

tibody of the hepatitis B virus is not detected during the phase of dermatitis, appearing approximately 6–12 mo later in patients who become HB_sAg negative.

A similar cutaneous eruption has also been observed in patients in the United States infected with Epstein-Barr virus, coxsackievirus A16, and parainfluenza virus and undoubtedly accompanies other viral infections. Papular acrodermatitis can be confused with lichen planus, erythema multiforme, histiocytosis X, and Henoch-Schönlein purpura.

23.17 ICHTHYOSIS

Ichthyosis is a primary group of inherited keratinizing disorders characterized by visible scaling in distinctive patterns of distribution. They are usually distinguishable on the basis of inheritance patterns, clinical features, associated defects, and histologic changes. Because some of these conditions cause disfigurement and considerable mental anguish, early diagnosis is helpful in order to predict probable course and prognosis and to provide supportive management for the patient and family.

HARLEQUIN FETUS. This very rare keratinizing disorder is inherited as an autosomal recessive trait. Some infants have an abnormality of keratinization, and others have a disorder of epidermal lipid metabolism, therefore, harlequin fetus may represent a phenotype for several different genotypes. Affected infants are extremely grotesque. Markedly thickened, ridged, and cracked skin forms horny plates over the entire body, disfiguring the facial features and constricting the digits. Severe ectropion and chemosis obscure the orbits; the nose and ears are flattened, and the lips are everted and gaping. Nails and hair may be absent. Joint mobility is restricted, and the hands and feet appear fixed and ischemic. The infants have respiratory difficulty and suck poorly. Most succumb within the 1st wk of life, but infants occasionally survive and are afflicted with severe ichthyosis. Initial therapy includes a high fluid intake to avoid dehydration from transepidermal water loss, use of a humidified heated incubator, emulsifying ointments, antiseptic solutions, paraffin, and oral retinoids such as etretinate. Ectropion and eclabion resolve and the cracked, horny plated skin is replaced by large, thin scales with surrounding erythema. Prenatal diagnosis has been accomplished by fetoscopy and fetal skin biopsy.

COLLODION BABY. These infants are covered at birth by a thick, taut membrane resembling oiled parchment or collodion, which is subsequently shed. The condition is usually a primary manifestation of one of the ichthyoses, most often of the autosomal recessive, lamellar variety; like harlequin fetus, the collodion baby appears to be a phenotype for several genotypes. Infrequently an affected infant has normal skin after the membrane is shed. There is ectropion, flattening of the ears and nose, and fixation of the lips in an O-shaped configuration (Fig. 23–31). Hair may be absent or may perforate the horny covering. The membrane cracks with initial respiratory efforts and, shortly after birth, begins to desquamate in large sheets. Complete shedding may take several weeks, and occasionally a new membrane may form in localized areas.

Neonatal morbidity and mortality may be due to cutaneous infection, aspiration pneumonia (squamous material), or hypernatremic dehydration from excessive transcutaneous fluid losses due to increased skin permeability. The outcome is uncertain, and accurate prognosis is impossible with respect to the subsequent development of ichthyosis. Maintenance in a high-humidity environment and application of nonocclusive lubricants may facilitate shedding of the membrane.

ICHTHYOSIS VULGARIS. This most common type of ichthyosis is transmitted as an autosomal dominant trait. Onset occurs sometime after the 1st yr of life. Scaling is most prominent on the extensor aspects of the extremities and back. The flexural surfaces are spared, and the abdomen and face are relatively uninvolved. Accentuated markings and creases are apparent on palms and soles. Atopy is relatively common. Scaling is most pronounced during the winter months and may abate completely during warm weather. The condition may improve and even disappear with age.

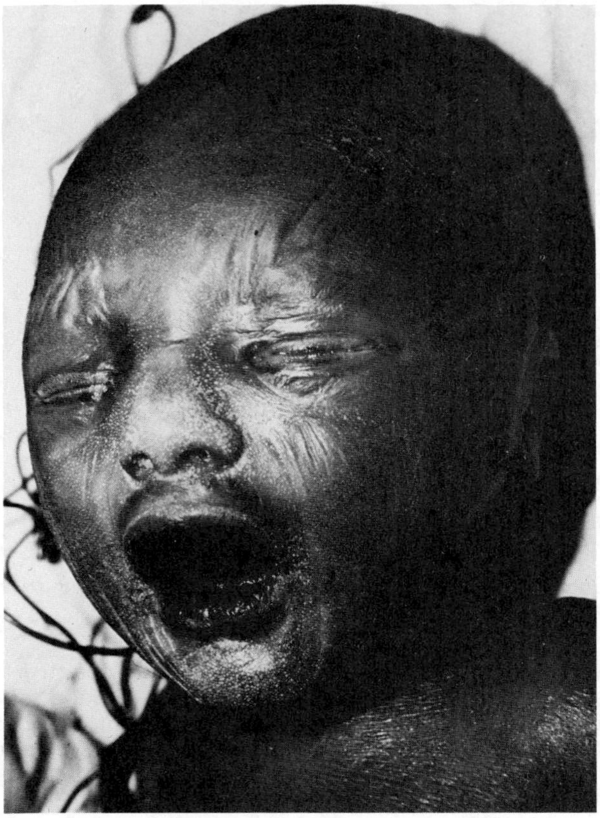

Figure 23–31. Typical facial appearance of a collodion baby.

The histologic changes differ from those of other types of ichthyosis in that the hyperkeratosis is associated with a decreased or absent granular layer. Abnormally small and crumbly keratohyalin granules are found in epidermal cells on electron microscopy.

Scaling may be diminished by use of a bath oil and by daily applications of an emollient or a lubricant containing urea or an α-hydroxy acid, such as lactic acid.

X-LINKED ICHTHYOSIS. This disorder is limited to males and is often present at birth. Scaling is most pronounced on the scalp, neck, sides of the face, anterior trunk, and limbs. The face, palms, and soles are usually spared. The distribution pattern of scaling differs from that of ichthyosis vulgaris, but biopsy may be required to distinguish the two conditions. Histologic changes in X-linked ichthyosis include hyperkeratosis of the stratum corneum, a well-developed granular layer, a hyperplastic epidermis, and a mononuclear, perivascular dermal infiltrate. Epidermal transit time is normal.

The inherited biochemical defect in X-linked ichthyosis is a deficiency of steroid sulfatase. This defect can be demonstrated in the fibroblasts, leukocytes, epidermal cells and scales from affected males. Steroid sulfatase hydrolyzes cholesterol sulfate and other sulfated steroids; cholesterol sulfate accumulates in the stratum corneum and plasma in X-linked ichthyosis. The increase in plasma cholesterol sulfate can be detected by serum lipoprotein electrophoresis or by direct measurement. Carrier mothers demonstrate a placental steroid sulfatase deficiency reflected by low urinary and serum estriol values, prolonged labors, and insensitivity of the uterus to oxytocin and prostaglandins. The role that these enzymes have in the keratinization process is as yet unknown. The gene for steroid sulfatase is located on the short arm of the X chromosome, closely linked with the Xg^2 blood group locus.

Deep corneal opacities that do not interfere with vision develop during late childhood or adolescence and are a useful marker for the disease because they may also be present in carrier females. Cryptorchidism occurs in approximately 25% of affected males. Although the disease does not represent a serious keratinizing defect, affected boys are usually embarrassed by the disfigurement and request treatment. Hydration by bathing with bath oil and daily application of emollients and a urea-containing lubricant are usually effective. Glycolic or lactic acid (5%) in an emollient base and propylene glycol 40–60% in water with occlusion overnight are alternative forms of therapy.

LAMELLAR ICHTHYOSIS/CONGENITAL ICHTHYOSIFORM ERYTHRODERMA. This is either an autosomal recessive disorder with two distinct clinical variants or two separate entities. The clinical manifestations are evident at birth, often as a collodion membrane. Once the membrane is shed, a generalized erythroderma becomes apparent. Scaling is often pronounced and involves the entire body surface, including flexural surfaces, palms, and soles (Fig. 23–32). In phenotypic lamellar ichthyosis, the scales are large, dark, and adherent; a moderate to marked degree of ectropion is present as is keratoderma of the palms and soles. In congenital ichthyosiform erythroderma (CIE), the scales are fine and white and the other features, such as erythroderma, ectropion, and palmoplantar keratoderma, are more variable.

Pruritus may be severe and responds minimally to antipruritic therapy. Hair growth may be curtailed, and patients may suffer in hot weather because of an inability to sweat freely through plugged sweat ducts. Mild growth retardation may also occur in children with severe CIE. The unattractive appearance of the child and the malodor from bacterial colonization of macerated scales may create serious psychologic problems.

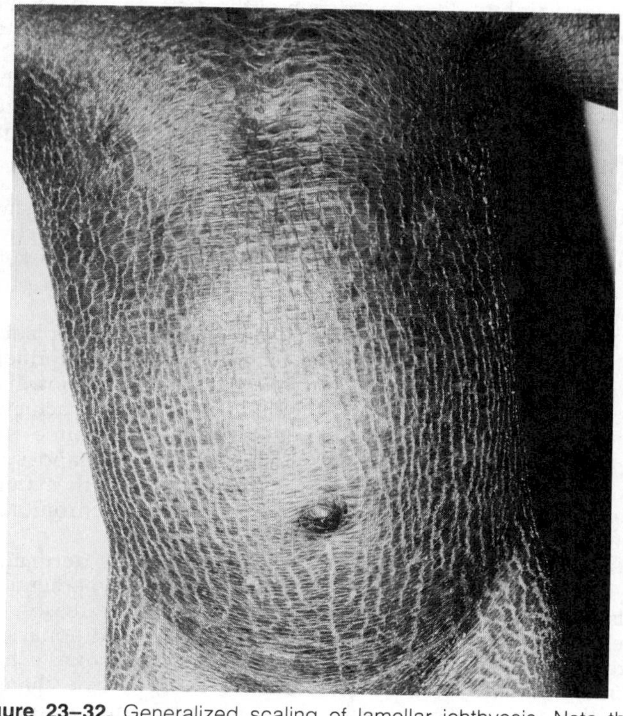

Figure 23–32. Generalized scaling of lamellar ichthyosis. Note the involvement of the axillary areas.

Skin biopsy shows hyperkeratosis, a well-developed granular layer, epidermal hyperplasia, and a mononuclear, perivascular dermal infiltrate. Epidermal transit time is decreased in CIE but is normal in lamellar ichthyosis. *N*-alkanes accumulate in scales from patients with CIE, suggesting an inborn error of lipid metabolism.

Effective treatment includes prolonged baths with bath oil to remove excessive scales. The restriction of bathing, on the erroneous premise that accentuation of dryness will occur, only promotes malodor and accumulation of keratinous debris and contributes to pruritus and discomfort. A high-humidity environment in winter and air conditioning in summer will reduce discomfort. Generous and frequent applications of emollients as well as keratolytic agents such as lactic or glycolic acid (5%), urea (10–25%), and retinoic acid (0.1% cream) may lessen the scaling to some extent. Oral synthetic retinoids have a beneficial effect in these conditions but do not alter the underlying defect and, therefore, must be administered indefinitely. The long-term risks of these compounds (e.g., teratogenic effects and toxicity to bone) limit their usefulness. Ectropion requires ophthalmologic care and, at times, plastic procedures. Genetic counseling should be provided.

EPIDERMOLYTIC HYPERKERATOSIS (BULLOUS CONGENITAL ICHTHYOSIFORM ERYTHRODERMA). This autosomal dominant keratinizing disorder is characterized by onset at birth, generalized erythroderma, and severe hyperkeratosis with accentuation in the flexural areas. The scales are small, hard, and verrucous and in many areas assume a columnar configuration, thus differing from those of other forms of ichthyosis. Recurrent bullae, which are characteristic during childhood and are usually localized to the lower limbs, may be widespread in the neonate and may cause diagnostic confusion with other blistering disorders. Secondary bacterial infection is common and requires appropriate antibiotic therapy.

The histologic pattern is pathognomonic and consists of hyperkeratosis and vacuolization of the cells of the granular layer and midepidermis with abnormally large clumped keratohyaline granules. Epidermal transit time is decreased. Localized forms of the disease may resemble epidermal nevi (ichthyosis hystrix) or keratoderma of the palms and soles but share the distinctive histologic changes of epidermolytic hyperkeratosis.

Epidermolytic hyperkeratosis is difficult to treat. Bacterial colonization of macerated scales produces a distinctive malodor that can be controlled somewhat by use of an antibacterial cleanser. Keratolytic agents may be prescribed with caution but are often poorly tolerated. Genetic counseling should be provided. Prenatal diagnosis has been accomplished by fetoscopy and fetal skin biopsy.

ICHTHYOSIS LINEARIS CIRCUMFLEXA. This rare autosomal recessive disorder is characterized by migratory hyperkeratotic lesions, hyperkeratosis of the flexures, and hyperhidrosis of the palms and soles. The skin is diffusely red and scaly at birth. Superimposed serpiginous scaly plaques, bordered by a distinctive double-edged scale, appear at various sites on the trunk and limbs. This type of ichthyosis is characteristic of patients with the Netherton syndrome (see later).

ERYTHROKERATODERMA VARIABILIS. This is characterized by two types of lesions: sharply demarcated hyperkeratotic plaques with bizarre borders and discrete areas of macular erythema that disappear or migrate but may eventually become hyperkeratotic and fixed. Sites of predilection are the face, buttocks, and extensor surfaces of the limbs. The palms and soles may be thickened, but hair, teeth, and nails are normal. The disorder is inherited as an autosomal dominant trait. Histologic changes include lamination of the stratum corneum, focal parakeratosis, papillomatosis, and irregular hyperplasia of the epidermis. The epidermal transit time is normal.

ICHTHYOSIFORM DERMATOSES

Several syndromes that include ichthyosis as a constant feature have been established as rare but distinct entities.

Sjögren-Larsson syndrome, an autosomal recessive disorder, has three major and constant components: ichthyosis of the lamellar type, mental deficiency, and spastic diplegia. A degenerative defect of retinal pigment epithelium has been detected in 20–30% of affected individuals. Glistening dots in the foveal area, although easily overlooked, are believed to be a cardinal ophthalmologic sign (see also Table 22–1). Some patients may walk with the aid of braces, but most are confined to a wheelchair. The primary defect appears to be an abnormality of fatty alcohol metabolism due to a deficiency of nicotinamide adenine dinucleotide oxidoreductase activity.

Rud syndrome consists of mental retardation, epilepsy, ichthyosis (type uncertain), and sexual infantilism. Associated defects of the skeleton, eyes, dentition, and hearing have also been reported.

Netherton syndrome is characterized by ichthyosis (usually ichthyosis linearis circumflexa but occasionally the lamellar type), trichorrhexis invaginata and other hair shaft anomalies, and atopic diathesis. The ichthyosis is present at birth. Scalp hair is sparse and fractures easily; eyebrows, eyelashes, and body hair are also abnormal. The most frequent allergic manifestations are urticaria, angioedema, and asthma. Some patients are mentally retarded. Although the disease is believed to be inherited in an autosomal recessive fashion, a preponderance of females has been reported.

Refsum syndrome (see also Sec. 8.16), a multisystem disorder, is inherited as an autosomal recessive trait and becomes symptomatic during the 1st or 2nd decade of life. The ichthyosis is relatively mild and is not clinically distinctive but resembles ichthyosis vulgaris. Chronic polyneuritis with progressive paralysis and ataxia, atypical retinitis pigmentosa, anosmia, deafness, bony abnormalities, and ECG changes are the most characteristic features. Affected patients have a deficiency of the enzyme phytanic oxidase, and cannot degrade phytanic acid which accumulates in the serum and tissues. Dietary avoidance of chlorophyll (phytanic acid) containing foods is all that is available therapeutically.

Chondrodysplasia punctata (see also Sec. 24.36) includes several genetically heterogeneous disorders: *Conradi-Hunermann syndrome*, inherited as an autosomal dominant trait; *rhizomelic dwarfism*, transmitted as an autosomal recessive trait; and an *X-linked dominant* form affecting females only. Approximately 25% of patients with the recessive or dominant type have cutaneous lesions, ranging from severe, generalized erythema and scaling to mild hyperkeratosis. Patients with the X-linked dominant form have a distinctive ichthyosiform eruption at birth. Thick, yellow, tightly adherent keratinized plaques are distributed in a whorled pattern over the entire body, which may be intensely erythematous. The histologic changes include hyperkeratosis that penetrates to the depths of the hair follicles. The eruption disappears completely during the first few weeks of life and may be superseded by a follicular atrophoderma. Patchy alopecia may be associated.

Additional features in all variants include cataracts with or without optic atrophy, an abnormal facies with saddle nose and hypertelorism, and cardiovascular and central nervous system abnormalities. The pathognomonic defect, which also disappears with age, is stippled epiphyses in the cartilaginous skeleton. Other bony abnormalities consist of shortened femora and humeri, flexion contractures of joints, dysplasia of the hips, and asymmetric deformities of the limbs. A similar clinical syndrome without ichthyosis has been described in association with maternal warfarin ingestion.

A number of other rare syndromes with ichthyosis as a consistent feature include the following: *ichthyosis with keratitis and deafness (KID syndrome); ichthyosis with defective hair having a banded pattern under polarized light and a low sulfur content (trichothiodystrophy) and mental and growth retardation (Tay syndrome); multiple sulfatase deficiency; neutral lipid storage disease with ichthyosis (Chanarin-Dorfman syndrome); CHILD syndrome (congenital hemidysplasia with ichthyosiform erythroderma and limb defects).*

KERATODERMA OF PALMS AND SOLES (KERATOSIS PALMARIS ET PLANTARIS). This is due to excessive accumulation of stratum corneum and may occur as a manifestation of a focal or generalized congenital hereditary skin disorder or may result from such chronic skin diseases as psoriasis, eczema, or pityriasis rubra pilaris.

Although strict classification is difficult, the hereditary types of keratoderma may be categorized as follows:

Diffuse hyperkeratosis of palms and soles (tylosis) is an autosomal dominant disorder characterized by sharply demarcated areas of scaling. Striate and punctate forms have also been described.

Localized epidermolytic hyperkeratosis of palms and soles is an autosomal dominant defect with characteristic histologic changes.

Mal de Meleda is a rare, progressive autosomal recessive condition characterized by erythema and thick scales on the palms, soles, and dorsal surfaces of the limbs, hyperhidrosis, EEG abnormalities, and mental retardation.

Keratoma hereditaria mutilans (progressive dystrophic hyperkeratosis) is a progressive autosomal dominant disease with honeycombed hyperkeratosis of palms and soles, starfish-like linear and annular keratoses on the dorsum of the hands and feet, and ainhum-like constriction of the digits that sometimes leads to autoamputation. This disorder may be associated with scarring, alopecia, and deafness.

Papillon-Lefèvre syndrome is an autosomal recessive erythematous hyperkeratosis of the palms and soles characterized by periodontal inflammation and early shedding of teeth, nail dystrophy, and ectopic calcification of the dura.

Keratoderma of palms and soles also occurs in association with corneal dystrophy and with carcinoma of the esophagus as an autosomal dominant trait and as a feature of pachyonychia congenita, ichthyosis, ectodermal dysplasia, dyskeratosis congenita, and tyrosinemia as well as of several other conditions.

Patients with hyperhidrosis may develop macerated plaques that become secondarily infected and malodorous. Morbidity is lessened if the hyperkeratosis can be controlled; however, treatment is difficult, and only mild palliation is achieved with applications of lubricants, keratolytic agents (urea, salicylic acid, lactic acid), and retinoic acid. Excision and split-skin grafting have been successful in patients with extreme hyperkeratosis and painful fissuring that cause chronic disability.

ACANTHOSIS NIGRICANS. This symmetric dermatosis is characterized by hyperpigmented, velvety, hyperkeratotic plaques that are most often localized to flexural creases, the neck, groin, axillae, and inframammary areas. Additional sites are the elbows, knees, and knuckles where the plaques exhibit a more verrucous or pebbly surface. The histologic changes are those of papillomatosis and scaling rather than acanthosis and excessive pigment formation.

Acanthosis nigricans has classically been associated with obesity, endocrinopathies, metabolic diseases, and malignancies; occasionally it may be familial. The skin lesions are a manifestation of insulin resistance. The clinical syndromes are classified into two types. Type A results from insulin receptor or postreceptor defects. Type B is associated with autoantibodies to the insulin receptor. Conditions characterized by acanthosis nigricans and insulin resistance include lipoatrophic diabetes, partial lipodystrophy, leprechaunism, hyperandrogenic syndromes, hypogonadal syndromes, Cushing syndrome, and acromegaly. Obesity is a common cause of acanthosis nigricans, which is reversible when the excess weight is lost. Malignant neoplasms, which may secrete an insulin-like polypeptide, are often associated with acanthosis nigricans in adults, but in children the association is rare.

This skin disorder is extremely difficult to treat but may be improved by palliation of the underlying disorder and by reduction of insulin resistance.

PACHYONYCHIA CONGENITA. This heritable disorder is transmitted as an autosomal dominant trait with variable expressivity. Several clinical variants have been described. The nail dystrophy is common to all types. Additional features include keratoderma of the palms and soles, follicular hyperkeratosis, hyperhidrosis, and oral leukokeratosis. Less common findings include epidermal cysts, corneal dystrophy, natal teeth, and abnormalities of the hair. The nail dystrophy is the most striking feature and may be present at birth or develop early in life. The nails are thickened and tubular, projecting upward at the free edge to form a conical roof over a mass of subungual keratotic debris. Repeated paronychial inflammation may result in shedding of the nails.

Treatment is relatively ineffective, although keratolytic agents may be of some benefit.

ESSENTIAL FATTY ACID DEFICIENCY. This deficiency may be responsible for generalized, scaly dermatitis that resembles congenital ichthyosis. The eruption has also been observed in patients sustained on fat-free diets or fat-free parenteral alimentation and is caused by a deficiency of linoleic and arachidonic acids. Additional manifestations of essential fatty acid deficiency include alopecia, thrombocytopenia, increased susceptibility to bacterial infections, and failure to thrive. Daily application of sunflower seed oil, which contains linoleic acid, may ameliorate the clinical and biochemical manifestations, but it does not readily replenish tissue stores of linoleic acid. Intravenous lipid emulsion is preventive as well as the treatment of choice for essential fatty acid deficiency. This condition should be distinguished from ichthyosis since it is amenable to therapy.

23.18 DISEASES OF THE DERMIS

GRANULOMA ANNULARE. This common dermatosis occurs predominantly in children; it can be polymorphous. Typical lesions begin as erythematous, firm, flat-topped papulonodules; they gradually enlarge to form ring-shaped plaques with a normal, slightly atrophic or discolored central area (Fig. 23–33) up to several cm in size. Lesions occur most frequently on the dorsum of the hands and feet but can also develop on the scalp, trunk, arms, and legs. *Annular lesions* are often mistaken for tinea corporis because of the elevated advancing border; they differ in that they are never scaly. *Papular lesions,* another variant, may simulate rheumatoid nodules, particularly when grouped on the fingers and elbows. The generalized papular form is rare in children. *Subcutaneous granuloma annulare,* a less common form, may appear on the scalp, and limbs, particularly in the pretibial area. These lesions are firm, usually nontender, skin-colored

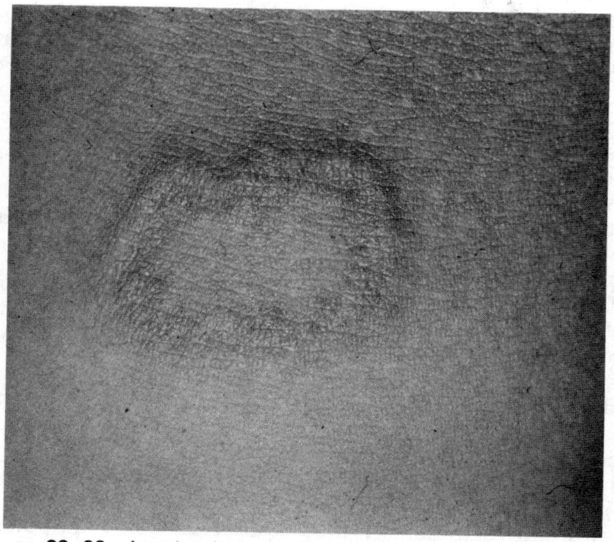

Figure 23–33. Annular lesion with a raised papular border and depressed center, characteristic of granuloma annulare.

nodules. They may be confused with other nodular and cystic lesions; identification of typical annular lesions elsewhere on the body, if present, will resolve the diagnostic dilemma.

A biopsy is occasionally required for diagnosis. The lesions consist of a granuloma with a central area of necrotic collagen, mucin deposition, and a peripheral palisading infiltrate of lymphocytes, histiocytes, and foreign body giant cells. The pattern resembles that of necrobiosis lipoidica and rheumatoid nodule, but subtle histologic differences usually permit differentiation. The cause of granuloma annulare is unknown. Affected children are usually healthy. The eruption persists for months to years, but spontaneous resolution without residual change is usual. Application of a potent topical corticosteroid preparation or intralesional injections of corticosteroid may hasten involution, but nonintervention is acceptable.

LICHEN SCLEROSUS ET ATROPHICUS. This dermatosis of unknown etiology rarely occurs in children. Initial lesions consist of ivory-colored, shiny, indurated papules, often with violaceous halos. These coalesce to form irregular atrophic plaques of variable size, which may develop hemorrhagic bullae in their margins. Sites of predilection are the anogenital skin, buttocks, upper back, chest, forearms, and face. In boys, the prepuce and glans penis are often involved. In girls, extensive involvement of the anogenital area may produce a sclerotic, atrophic plaque of hourglass configuration. Severe itching and burning are common.

In children, this disorder is most frequently confused with focal scleroderma (morphea). In the genital area, it may be mistakenly attributed to sexual abuse. Biopsy is diagnostic. The lesions may involute spontaneously and, in children, resolve without residua. Resolution has sometimes coincided with menarche. Corticosteroid creams provide relief from pruritus. Topical estrogen and androgen preparations have been used for genital lesions. None has been invariably curative; the risks of side effects must be weighed against the benefits of therapy.

MACULAR ATROPHIES (ANETODERMA). This disorder may occur in the absence of inflammation (primary macular atrophy) or as a sequel of an inflammatory process (secondary macular atrophy). Lesions vary from 0.5 to 1 cm in diameter and, if inflammatory, may initially be erythematous but subsequently become thinned, wrinkled, and blue-white in color or hypopigmented. The lesions often protrude as small outpouchings that, on palpation, may be readily indented into the subcutaneous tissue because of the dermal atrophy. Secondary macular atrophy may follow cutaneous lesions of lupus erythematosus, sarcoidosis, and certain other dermatoses.

All types of macular atrophy show loss of elastic tissue on histopathologic examination, a change that is not recognizable unless special stains are used. These lesions occasionally resemble morphea, lichen sclerosus et atrophicus, or end-stage lesions of chronic bullous dermatoses. There is no effective therapy.

NECROBIOSIS LIPOIDICA. This disorder is rare in children and is often associated with diabetes mellitus. The lesions begin as erythematous papules and evolve into irregularly shaped, yellow, sclerotic plaques with central telangiectasia and a violaceous border. Scaling, crusting, and ulceration are frequent. Necrobiosis must be differentiated clinically from xanthomas, morphea, and pretibial myxedema. The lesions persist despite good control of the diabetes but may improve minimally after applications of high-potency topical steroids or local injection of a corticosteroid.

KELOID. This sharply demarcated benign growth of connective tissue is found in the dermis; it consists of whorled and interlaced hyalinized collagen fibers. The lesions are firm, raised, pink, and rubbery; they may be tender or extremely pruritic. Sites of predilection are the face, ears, sternum, and extremities. Keloids are usually induced by trauma and commonly follow ear piercing, burns, scalds, and surgical procedures. Certain individuals, especially blacks, seem predisposed to keloid formation. Keloids may enlarge to form grotesque excrescences with numerous claw-like projections, and, on the ear lobe, where they tend to be round, may hang in a pendulous fashion.

Keloids should be differentiated from hypertrophic scars, which remain confined to the site of injury and gradually involute over time. Young keloids may diminish in size if injected intralesionally at 4-wk intervals with triamcinolone suspension (10 mg/mL). At times a more concentrated suspension is required. Large or old keloids may require surgical excision followed by intralesional injections of corticosteroid. The risk of recurrence at the same site argues against surgical excision alone.

STRIAE DISTENSAE. These thinned, depressed, erythematous bands of atrophic skin eventually become silvery, opalescent, and smooth in consistency. They occur most frequently in areas that have been subject to distention, such as the lower back, buttocks, thighs, breasts, abdomen, and shoulders. The most frequent causes are rapid growth, pregnancy, obesity, Cushing disease, or prolonged corticosteroid therapy. The lesions result from rupture, retraction, and disintegration of the dermal elastic fibers.

SCLEREDEMA (SCLEREDEMA ADULTORUM, SCLEREDEMA OF BUSCHKE). This occurs in children as well as in adults. The onset is sudden with brawny edema of the face and neck that spreads rapidly to involve the thorax and arms but usually spares the abdomen, hands, and feet. The face acquires a waxy, mask-like appearance; the involved areas feel indurated and woody and are nonpitting. The overlying skin cannot be wrinkled, but it is normal in color and there are no atrophic changes. Systemic involvement, which is uncommon, is marked by thickening of the tongue, dysarthria, dysphagia, restriction of eye movements, and pleural, pericardial, and peritoneal effusions. Electrocardiographic changes may also be observed.

The disease often follows an infection such as tonsillitis, influenza, or scarlet fever after an interval of days or weeks, but its cause remains obscure. Onset may be heralded by a prodrome of fever, arthralgia, myalgia, and malaise. Laboratory data are not helpful. Skin biopsy demonstrates an increase in dermal thickness due to swelling and homogenization of the collagen bundles, which are separated by large interfibrous spaces. Increased amounts of mucopolysaccharides in the dermis can be identified by special stains.

The active phase of the disease persists for 2–8 wk; spontaneous and complete resolution usually occurs in 6 mo–2 yr. Recurrent attacks are unusual. The disorder must be differentiated from scleroderma, myxedema, trichinosis, dermatomyositis, and other conditions causing widespread edema. There is no specific therapy.

LIPOID PROTEINOSIS. This autosomal recessive disorder may be initially noted in early infancy as hoarseness. Skin lesions appear during childhood and consist of yellowish papules and nodules that may coalesce to form plaques on the face, forearms, neck, genitalia, dorsum of the fingers, and scalp, where they result in patchy alopecia. Similar deposits are found on the lips, tongue, fauces, uvula, epiglottis, and vocal cords. Translucent nodules along the margins of the eyelids are the most characteristic clinical manifestation. Hypertrophic, hyperkeratotic nodules occur at sites of friction such as the elbows and knees; the palms may be diffusely thickened. The distinctive histologic pattern includes extreme dilatation of the dermal blood vessels and infiltration of the dermis with extracellular hyaline material, which is also deposited in the vessel walls. Calcification of the hippocampal gyri, identifiable roentgenographically, is pathognomonic but is not always present. The biochemical defect is unknown; the infiltrates appear to contain both lipid and mucopolysaccharide substances. There is no specific treatment.

CUTIS LAXA (DERMATOMEGALY, GENERALIZED ELASTOLYSIS). This congenital disorder is inherited as an autosomal recessive or autosomal dominant trait. A newborn infant may appear prematurely aged. When onset appears to occur during childhood or adulthood, usually after a febrile illness or a course of drug therapy (e.g., D-penicillamine), the disorder is designated as *acquired cutis laxa;* such clinical expression may, however, represent the variable expressivity of the congenital types.

In all forms of cutis laxa, the skin hangs in pendulous folds. Characteristic facial features include an aged appearance with sagging jowls ("bloodhound" appearance), a hooked nose with everted nostrils, a short columella, a long upper lip, and everted lower eyelids. The skin is lax elsewhere on the body as well and may resemble an ill-fitting suit (Fig. 23–34). Hyperelasticity and hypermobility of the joints are not present as they are in the Ehlers-Danlos syndrome. Many infants

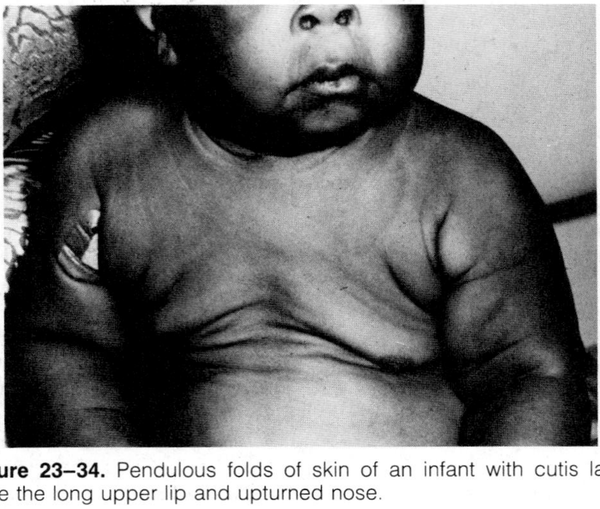

Figure 23–34. Pendulous folds of skin of an infant with cutis laxa. Note the long upper lip and upturned nose.

have a hoarse cry, probably due to laxity of the vocal cords. Tensile strength of the skin is normal. Histologically, elastic tissue is reduced throughout the dermis, with fragmentation, distention, and clumping of the elastic fibers.

The dominant form of cutis laxa is generally benign and mainly of cosmetic significance; a few affected individuals have had mild cardiovascular or pulmonary manifestations. In contrast, the more common recessive form of the disease is susceptible to severe complications, such as multiple hernias, diaphragmatic atony, diverticula of the gastrointestinal and genitourinary tracts, and cardiopulmonary disease with emphysema, pneumothoraces, peripheral pulmonary artery stenosis, and aortic dilatation. Such patients often have a shortened life span. Skeletal anomalies, growth retardation, and developmental delay also occur. Another rare recessive form of cutis laxa is associated with growth retardation, lax joints, and hip dislocations as well as hernias, emphysema, and diverticulae of the gastrointestinal and urinary tracts. Plastic surgery procedures may be helpful in ameliorating the cutaneous defect.

EHLERS-DANLOS SYNDROME. This is a genetically heterogeneous connective tissue disorder whose severity varies because of mild or incomplete forms of the disease. Affected children appear normal at birth. The most striking feature is the hyperelasticity, fragility, and bruisability of the skin. It has been classified into 10 distinct clinical forms:

I. *Gravis type*, autosomal dominant, is characterized by skin hyperelasticity and fragility, easy bruising, generalized and severe joint hypermobility, and preterm birth from premature rupture of the fetal membranes.

II. *Mitis type*, autosomal dominant, is characterized by mild skin and joint manifestations, the latter limited to hands and feet.

III. *Benign, hypermobile type*, autosomal dominant, has generalized severe joint hypermobility and minimal skin manifestations.

IV. *Ecchymotic (Sack) type*, autosomal dominant and autosomal recessive, is characterized by joint hypermobility limited to digits, minimal skin hyperextensibility, severe bruisability with prominent venous network, extensive ecchymoses from trauma, high incidence of keloids and contractures, and rupture of bowel and great vessels. Type III collagen is absent.

V. *X-linked type*, has minimal joint hypermobility, extensive hyperelasticity, moderate bruising, fragility, and scarring. Lysyl oxidase is deficient in some but not all affected individuals.

VI. *Ocular type*, autosomal recessive, has fragile cornea, sclera, deformed cornea, joint hyperextensibility, skin hyperelasticity, fragile bones and lysyl hydroxylase deficiency.

VII. *Arthrochalasis multiplex congenita*, A type, autosomal recessive, is characterized by short stature, marked joint hyperextensibility and dislocation, moderate hyperelasticity and bruisability of skin, and procollagen-n-peptidase deficiency; B type, possibly autosomal dominant, is characterized by hyperelasticity, marked hypermobility, and structural mutation of pro-α 2 (I) chain.

VIII. *Periodontitis type*, autosomal dominant, has mild skin hyperelasticity, joint hypermobility and bruisability, moderate cutaneous fragility, and severe periodontitis leading to premature loss of teeth and alveolar bone.

IX. *X-linked recessive skeletal type* is characterized by occipital exostoses, widening and bowing of long bones at tendinous and ligamentous insertion sites, deformed clavicles, mild skin hyperelasticity, low serum copper and ceruloplasm, dimished lysyl oxidase activity, and defective collagen cross-linking.

X. *Dysfibronectinemic type*, autosomal recessive, has fibronectin-correctable failure of platelet aggregation, easy bruisability, joint hypermobility, and skin hyperextensibility.

Ehlers-Danlos syndrome has been confused with cutis laxa, but the features of the two disorders differ considerably. The skin in Ehlers-Danlos syndrome is hyperextensible and snaps back into place when stretched. Because of its marked fragility, minor trauma results in ecchymoses, bleeding, and poor healing with atrophic cigarette-paper scars, which are most prominent on the forehead and lower legs and over pressure points. Surgical procedures are fraught with risk; dehiscence of wounds is common. Additional cutaneous manifestations include molluscoid pseudotumors over pressure points, small, subcutaneous, lipid-containing cysts that often calcify, and redundant skin on the palms and soles. Joint hypermobility with skeletal deformity, mitral valve prolapse, ocular defects, and ruptures of the bowel, great vessels, and lung are the major complications. Hernias and gastrointestinal diverticula may also occur.

All types of Ehlers-Danlos syndrome have been attributed to a defect of collagen; specific procollagen defects have been identified in types IV, VI, and VII disease.

There is no specific treatment for these disorders and, although death may occur secondary to the internal manifestations of the disease, life expectancy is usually normal. Orthopedic management with braces and physical therapy may improve musculoskeletal function; surgical intervention may be indicated to correct vascular or bleeding abnormalities.

PSEUDOXANTHOMA ELASTICUM. This rare, heritable disorder of elastic tissue involves the skin, eyes, cardiovascular system, and gastrointestinal tract. Of four distinct forms of the disease, two are transmitted in an autosomal dominant and two in an autosomal recessive fashion.

Onset of skin manifestations often occurs during childhood, but the changes produced by early lesions are subtle and may not be recognized. The characteristic "plucked chicken skin" cutaneous lesions are asymptomatic; 1- to 2-mm yellow papules are arranged in a linear or reticulated pattern or in confluent plaques. Preferred sites are the neck, axillary and inguinal folds, umbilicus, and antecubital and popliteal fossae. As the lesions become more pronounced, the skin acquires a velvety texture and droops in lax, inelastic folds. Mucous membrane lesions may involve the lips, buccal cavity, rectum, and vagina. Additional manifestations include visual disturbances, angioid streaks and other chorioretinal changes, intermittent claudication, cerebral and coronary occlusion, hypertension, and hemorrhage from the gastrointestinal tract and uterus.

The four forms of the disorder can be distinguished by pedigree data and the clinical patterns. Most of the features described earlier occur in each of the two autosomal dominant forms of the disease; they differ principally in the incidence of vascular and ophthalmologic complications. Patients with the type 1 disorder tend to have extensive disease with numerous complications, whereas those with type 2 have a less prominent macular skin eruption and low incidences of vascular involvement and of debilitating ophthalmologic disease. Patients with the recessive type 1 form have the classic flexural skin changes, but vascular changes are minimal, and the degenerative retinopathy is localized. In the recessive type 2 form there is elastic tissue degeneration of the entire integument, in contrast to the flexural accentuation in the other forms of the disease, and systemic involvement does not occur.

The basic defect is unknown. Pathologic and clinical manifestations are related to deposition of calcium and to degenerative changes in the elastic fibers of the skin and blood vessels. Because of the serious nature of the systemic complications, even suggestive skin changes are an indication for skin biopsy. There is no effective therapy.

ELASTOSIS PERFORANS SERPIGINOSA. This is an unusual skin disorder in which 1- to 3-mm, skin-colored, keratotic, firm papules tend to cluster in arcuate and annular patterns on the posterolateral neck and limbs and occasionally on the face and trunk. Onset occurs usually during childhood or adolescence. The etiology is unknown, but it occurs frequently with osteogenesis imperfecta, Marfan syndrome, pseudoxanthoma elasticum, Ehlers-Danlos syndrome, Rothmund-Thomson syndrome, and Down syndrome. It has also occurred in association with D-penicillamine therapy.

Proliferation, thickening, and branching of dermal elastic fibers that perforate the epidermis and stimulate a reactive epidermal hyperplasia and inflammatory response are diagnostic. Differential diagnosis includes tinea corporis, granuloma annulare, lichen planus, creeping eruption, and porokeratosis of Mibelli. Treatment is ineffective; however, the lesions are asymptomatic and disappear spontaneously.

XANTHOMAS (see Sec. 8.23–8.32).

FARBER DISEASE (LIPOGRANULOMATOSIS) (see Sec. 8.18).

MUCOPOLYSACCHARIDOSES (MPS). MPS are distinguished by differences in clinical and genetic patterns and specific enzymatic defects (Sec. 8.43). In several of these disorders, thick, inelastic, rough skin, particularly on the extremities, and generalized hirsutism are characteristic but nonspecific features. Telangiectases on the face, forearms, trunk, and legs have been observed in the Scheie and Morquio syndromes. In some patients with Hunter syndrome, distinctive skin lesions occur; they are ivory-colored, firm papulonodules that have a corrugated surface texture and aggregate to form plaques on the upper trunk, arms, and thighs. Onset of these unusual lesions occurs during the 1st decade, and spontaneous disappearance has been noted.

Biopsies of affected skin and nodular lesions demonstrate thickening of the dermis with swelling and separation of the collagen bundles and deposition of metachromatic material. The epidermal cells may be vacuolated, and large mononuclear "gargoyle" cells, which also contain metachromatic material, may be identified in the upper dermis.

MASTOCYTOSIS. *Mastocytosis* encompasses a spectrum of disorders that range from solitary cutaneous nodules to diffuse infiltration of skin associated with involvement of other organs. All the disorders are characterized by aggregates of tissue mast cells in the dermis; the local and systemic manifestations of the disease are due to the release of histamine and heparin from mast cell granules. Biopsy of involved skin is diagnostic.

Affected children may have intense pruritus. Systemic signs of histamine release, such as episodic flushing, tachycardia, respiratory distress, headache, colic, diarrhea, hypotension, and syncope, occur most frequently in the more severe types of mastocytosis. Flushing can be precipitated by excessively hot baths, by vigorous rubbing of the skin, and by certain drugs, such as codeine, aspirin, morphine, atropine, alcohol, *d*-tubocurarine, and polymyxin B. Avoidance of these triggering factors will reduce discomfort considerably. For patients who are symptomatic, oral antihistamines may be palliative. H_1 receptor antagonists are the initial drugs of choice for systemic signs of histamine release. If H_1 antagonists are unsucessful, H_2 receptor antagonists (e.g., ranitidine) may be helpful in controlling pruritus or gastric hypersecretion. Oral mast cell stabilizing agents, such as disodium cromoglycate or ketotifen, may also be effective. Avoidance of factors known to precipitate histamine release, such as cold or hot stimuli, drugs, or trauma, is advisable.

The cause is unknown. Most cases are sporadic; rarely, other family members have been affected.

Mastocytomas are solitary lesions that constitute approximately 10% of childhood cases of mastocytosis. Lesions may be present at birth or arise during early infancy; they can occur at any site, although the wrist, neck, and trunk are sites of predilection. Initially the lesions may present as recurrent, evanescent wheals or bullae; however, in time, an infiltrated, rubbery, pink, yellow, or tan plaque develops at the site of whealing or blistering (Fig. 23–35*A*). The surface acquires a pebbly, orange-peel–like texture, and hyperpigmentation may become prominent. Stroking or trauma to the nodule may result in urtication (Darier sign); rarely, systemic signs of histamine release become apparent. The differential diagnosis includes recurrent bullous impetigo, nevi, and juvenile xanthogranuloma. Mastocytomas usually involute spontaneously during early childhood; troublesome lesions can be excised and do not recur. Only rarely do multiple cutaneous lesions develop.

Urticaria pigmentosa is the most common form of mastocytosis and occurs primarily in infants and children; onset occurs before the 2nd year. Lesions may be present at birth but more often erupt in crops over a period of several months. In some cases, early lesions are bullous or urticarial and fade repeatedly only to recur at the same site until they become fixed and hyperpigmented; in others, the initial lesions are hyperpigmented. Vesiculation usually abates by 2 yr of age. Individual lesions range in size from a few millimeters to several centimeters and may be macular, papular, or nodular; they range in color from yellow-tan to chocolate brown and often have ill-defined borders (see Fig. 23–35*B*). Larger nodular lesions, like mastocytomas, may have a characteristic orange-peel texture (see Fig. 23–35*C*).

Lesions of urticaria pigmentosa may be sparse or numerous and are often symmetrically distributed. Palms, soles, and face are sometimes spared, as are the mucous membranes. The rapid appearance of erythema and whealing in response to vigorous stroking of a lesion (Darier sign) can usually be elicited; dermographism of intervening normal skin is also common. Urticaria pigmentosa can be confused with drug eruptions, postinflammatory pigmentary change, juvenile xanthogranuloma, pigmented nevi, ephelides, xanthomas, chronic urticaria, insect bites, and bullous impetigo.

The prognosis is good; spontaneous involution occurs in about 50% of patients by puberty; another 25% will have partial resolution by adulthood.

Diffuse cutaneous mastocytosis is characterized by diffuse involvement of the skin rather than discrete hyperpigmented lesions. Rarely, there are no discernible skin changes, but usually the skin appears thickened and pink to yellow in color; it may also have a doughy feel and a texture resembling orange peel. Surface changes are accentuated in the flexural areas. Recurrent bullae, intractable pruritus, and flushing attacks are common, as is systemic involvement.

Telangiectasia macularis eruptiva perstans is another variant that consists of telangiectatic hyperpigmented macules that are usually localized to the trunk. These lesions do not urticate when stroked. This form of the disease is seen in adolescents and adults primarily.

Systemic mastocytosis occurs in approximately 5–10% of patients with mastocytosis and is more common in adults than in children. Bone lesions may be silent but are detectable radiologically as osteoporotic or osteosclerotic areas, principally in the axial skeleton. Gastrointestinal tract involvement may produce diarrhea and steatorrhea. Mucosal infiltrates may be detectable by barium studies or by small bowel biopsy. Peptic ulcers also occur. Hepatosplenomegaly due to mast cell infiltrates and fibrosis has been described, as well as mast cell proliferation in lymph nodes, kidneys, periadrenal fat, bone marrow, and peripheral blood. The prognosis is guarded.

The need for laboratory studies is determined by the symptoms and physical findings. Urinary excretion of free histamine and its metabolites is increased. Prostaglandin D_2 metabolites may be elevated in the urine of patients with systemic mastocytosis. Coagulation abnormalities are rare.

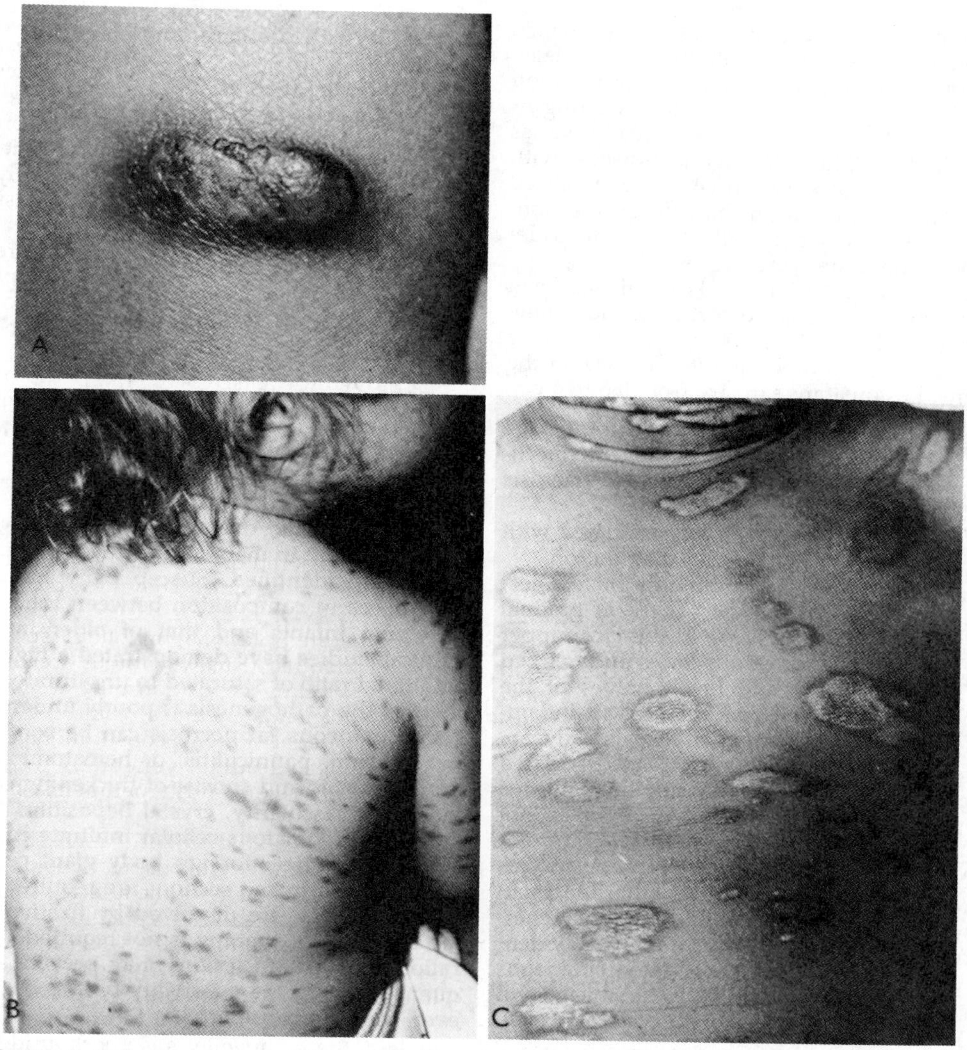

Figure 23–35. *A*, Solitary mastocytoma that is partially blistered. *B*, Hyperpigmented papular lesions of urticaria pigmentosa, some of which exhibit a surrounding flare. *C*, Infiltrated plaques of urticaria pigmentosa.

EPIDERMAL INCLUSION CYSTS. These cysts are sharply circumscribed, firm, freely movable, skin-colored nodules, often with a central dimple or dilated pore. They form most frequently on the face, neck, or trunk and may periodically become inflamed and secondarily infected. The wall of the cyst consists of stratified epithelium that surrounds a mass of layered keratinized material that may have a cheesy consistency. Epidermal cysts may be confused with dermatofibromas, branchial cleft cysts, and small lipomas. Excision of the cysts with removal of the entire sac and its contents is the appropriate procedure.

23.19 DISORDERS OF SUBCUTANEOUS TISSUE

Diseases involving the subcutis are usually characterized histologically by necrosis or inflammation; they may occur either as a primary event or as a secondary response to a variety of stimuli or disease processes. Unfortunately, these disorders are not all separable on the basis of the histologic changes; the histologic pattern may merely reflect the stage of the lesion at biopsy. The principal diagnostic criteria the clinician must rely on are the appearance and distribution of the lesions, associated symptoms, laboratory studies, and an appreciation of the exogenous provocative factors.

CORTICOSTEROID ATROPHY. The injection of a corticosteroid intradermally can produce deep atrophy accompanied by surface pigmentary changes and telangiectasia. These changes occur approximately 2 wk after injection and may last for months. The deltoid area is most susceptible to this complication; lesions also occur on the buttocks and thighs.

PANNICULITIS. This inflammation of fibrofatty subcutaneous tissue may occur as an idiopathic process with or without vasculitis. It may also be precipitated by various factors including infections, trauma, systemic lupus erythematosus, α_1-antitrypsin deficiency, diabetes, thyroid disease, pancreatic disease, malignancy, steroid withdrawal, and nutritional deficiencies.

Lobar panniculitis primarily affects the fat lobule. It occurs in the systemic, nonvasculitic nodular paniculitis of Weber-Christian disease (Sec. 11.68). Physical-induced lobar panniculitis is also a common response to cold in young children (see later). In contrast, septal panniculitis involving inflammation of the septal structures of the subcutaneous tissue occurs in erythema nodosum.

The skin lesions consist of erythematous or skin-colored,

tender, firm to fluctuant nodules usually measuring from 0.5–3 cm. These lesions develop in crops, most often on the legs, but also elsewhere on the body. Ulceration and suppuration may occur, and healing may be accompanied by scarring or by lipoatrophy. The clinical spectrum of the panniculitis varies from benign, self-limited conditions to relentless disease with an unfavorable outcome. Death may occur in generalized systemic disease and is most often attributable to infection, hemorrhage or thrombosis, or hepatic failure. Treatment depends on the nature of the underlying process.

POSTCORTICOSTEROID PANNICULITIS. This has been observed in children who have received corticosteroids orally for relatively short periods of time. Within 1–2 wk after discontinuation of the drug, multiple nodules appear on the face, trunk, and arms. Lesions range in size from 0.5 to 4 cm; they are erythematous or skin-colored and may be pruritic. The mechanism of the inflammatory reaction in the fat is unknown. Treatment is unnecessary, because the lesions remit spontaneously without scarring.

COLD PANNICULITIS. Cold panniculitis may result in localized lesions in infants after prolonged cold exposure, especially on the cheeks, or after prolonged application of a cold object such as an ice cube, ice bag, or Popsicle to any area of the skin. Erythematous, indurated lesions arise within hours of exposure, persist for 2–3 wk, and heal without residua. It may be confused with facial cellulitis due to *Haemophilus influenzae* type B. The pathogenic mechanism may be similar to that of subcutaneous fat necrosis (later and Sec. 15.78).

WEBER-CHRISTIAN PANNICULITIS. This type is discussed in Sec. 11.68.

LIPODYSTROPHY. Several rare conditions are associated with loss of fatty tissue in a partial or generalized distribution.

Partial lipodystrophy occurs more commonly in females than in males, often with the onset during the 1st decade. There is gradual symmetric loss of subcutaneous tissue over the face, upper trunk, and arms, resulting in a cadaverous facies and marked disproportion between the upper and lower halves of the body. Loss of adipose tissue is not preceded by an inflammatory phase, and histologic examination reveals only absence of subcutaneous fat. Some patients have had associated renal disease, disordered glucose metabolism, or abnormal serum lipid profiles. The etiology of the disorder is not understood, and there is no effective treatment.

Congenital generalized lipodystrophy (Seip-Lawrence syndrome) is a progressive multisystem disorder inherited as an autosomal recessive trait. The earliest manifestation is generalized loss of subcutaneous and visceral fat; it may be evident at birth or may occur during early infancy. Associated cutaneous changes include prominent superficial veins, hirsutism, and skin pigmentation with acanthosis nigricans. Accelerated skeletal and muscle growth and advanced bone age are seen. Abnormalities of carbohydrate homeostasis, insulin production, and growth hormone appear to be age-dependent. Hyperlipidemia, hyperinsulinism, and insulin-resistant nonketotic diabetes mellitus develop gradually and are reflected by increasing hepatomegaly due to fatty infiltration and cirrhosis. Serum levels of growth hormone may be normal, but its secretion in response to stimuli may be disturbed. Hypothalamic releasing factors that are not ordinarily found in plasma have been identified in affected patients and suggest a lack of hypothalamic regulation. There is no treatment.

SCLEREMA NEONATORUM. This is an uncommon disorder of adipose tissue that occurs primarily in preterm, sick, or debilitated infants. There is abrupt onset of a diffuse and generalized hardening of the skin, which becomes stony in consistency, cold, and nonpitting. Joint mobility may be compromised, and the face assumes a mask-like expression owing to inflexibility of the skin.

Sclerematous change is nonspecific and is almost always associated with serious illness, such as sepsis, gastroenteritis, pneumonia, or multiple congenital anomalies. The appearance of sclerema in a sick infant should be regarded as an ominous prognostic sign. The outcome depends on the response to treatment of the underlying disorder. When recovery is imminent, sclerema tends to disappear rapidly.

The histologic changes in sclerema consist only of edema and thickening of the connective tissue septa. Early and extensive subcutaneous fat necrosis may resemble sclerema, but the evolution of the process usually permits differentiation. Edema of the newborn is localized to dependent parts, pits easily with pressure, and should not be confused with sclerema.

SCLERODERMA (see Sec. 11.62).

SUBCUTANEOUS FAT NECROSIS. This inflammatory disorder of adipose tissue occurs primarily in the newborn infant. Sites of predilection are the buttocks, thighs, back, upper arms, and face. Lesions may be focal or extensive and may be preceded by a brawny edema of the affected skin. Typical well-developed lesions are firm, irregular nodules that may be skin-colored or have a red or violaceous hue (Fig. 23–36 [color plate section]). They are tender during the acute phase.

Uncomplicated lesions involute spontaneously within weeks to months, usually without scarring or atrophy. Occasionally, calcium deposition may occur within areas of fat necrosis and may sometimes result in rupture and drainage of liquid material. Rarely, constitutional symptoms such as hypotonia, poor feeding, vomiting, and fever are complications. Hypercalcemia and hyperlipemia have also been associated.

Fat necrosis in the infant has been attributed to birth trauma, asphyxia, overexposure to cold, and prolonged hypothermia, but in many of the affected infants no provocative factors are identified. Susceptibility has been attributed to differences in composition between the subcutaneous tissue of young infants and that of older infants and children. Clinical studies have demonstrated a high melting point and an altered ratio of saturated to unsaturated fatty acids. Nevertheless, the pathogenesis is poorly understood.

Subcutaneous fat necrosis can be confused with sclerema neonatorum, panniculitis, or hematoma. Histologic changes are diagnostic and consist of thickening of the fibrous septa, increased vascularity, crystal deposition within the fat cells, and a granulomatous cellular infiltrate composed of lymphocytes, histiocytes, foreign body giant cells, and fibroblasts. Lipid-stained frozen sections are required to demonstrate the crystals, which are dissolved by fixatives. Because the lesions are self-limited, therapy is not required. Careful needle aspiration of fluctuant lesions may prevent rupture and subsequent scarring; the possibility of introducing infection, however, may be a contraindication.

23.20 DISEASES OF THE SWEAT GLANDS

MILIARIA. *Miliaria*, or *prickly heat*, results from retention of sweat in ducts and pores of the eccrine sweat glands when they are occluded by keratinous plugs. Retrograde pressure may result in rupture of the duct and leakage of sweat into the dermis, where an inflammatory response is evoked. The eruption is most often induced by hot, humid weather, but it may also be caused by high fever. Infants who are kept too warmly dressed indoors may develop this eruption even during the winter.

In *miliaria crystallina* the lesions are very superficial and

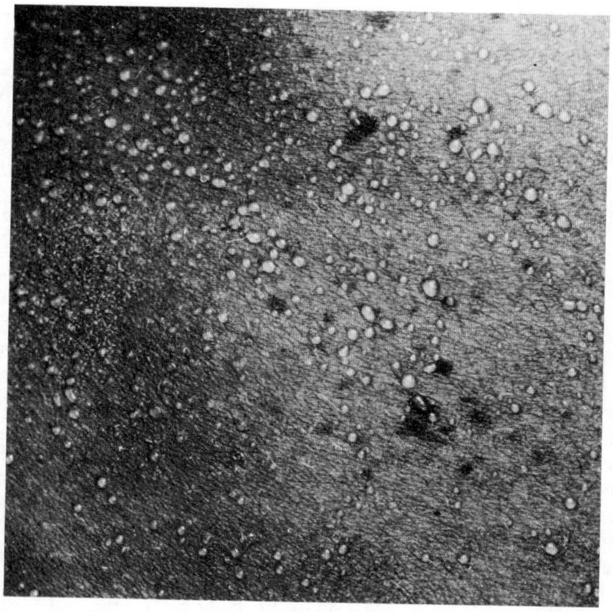

Figure 23–37. Superficial clear vesicles of miliaria crystallina in a patient with hyperpyrexia and lymphoma.

noninflammatory. The tiny clear vesicles rupture readily with gentle pressure. They can erupt suddenly and occur in profusion over large areas of the body surface (Fig. 23–37). The clarity of the fluid, the extreme superficiality of the vesicles, and the absence of inflammation permit differentiation from other blistering disorders. This type of miliaria occurs most frequently in newborn infants and in older patients with hyperpyrexia. *Miliaria rubra* is a less superficial eruption and is characterized by papulovesicles with intense erythema. The lesions are usually localized to sites of occlusion or to flexural areas where the skin may become macerated and eroded. This lesion may be confused with or superimposed on other diaper area eruptions, including candidosis and folliculitis. *Pustular miliaria,* unusual in children, is often a consequence of sweat retention associated with an underlying dermatitis.

All forms of miliaria respond dramatically to cooling the patient by regulation of environmental temperatures and by removal of excessive clothing and, in patients with fever, to administration of antipyretics. Topical agents are usually ineffective and may exacerbate the eruption. A cool bath is often helpful in alleviating pruritus.

HIDRADENITIS SUPPURATIVA. This inflammatory suppurative disease of the apocrine glands is a chronic, indolent disorder that involves the axillae and genitocrural area and, rarely, the scalp and mammary and umbilical skin. The onset usually occurs during puberty or early adulthood. The disease is probably initiated by plugging of apocrine gland ducts with keratinous debris. Progressive dilatation below the obstruction leads to rupture of the duct, inflammation, and often to secondary bacterial infection. Healing is by fibrosis and scarring. Clinically, affected patients have solitary or multiple painful, erythematous nodules, deep abscesses, and contracted scars, sharply confined to areas of skin containing apocrine glands. When the disease is severe and chronic, sinus tracts, ulcers, and fistulas develop.

Early lesions are often mistaken for infected epidermal cysts or for furuncles (abscesses of the hair follicles), but the sharp localization to particular areas of the body should suggest hidradenitis.

Systemic antibiotics chosen on the basis of bacterial culture (usually staphylococcal and streptococcal pathogens) and sensitivity tests should be administered in the acute phase even though such therapy is not always effective. Warm compresses will encourage spontaneous rupture of abscesses; those that are "pointing" should be incised and drained. The addition of a limited course of prednisone (40–60 mg/24 hr) to the regimen of patients who respond poorly to antibiotics may decrease fibrosis and scarring. Axillary shaving and the use of deodorants should be avoided. Ultimately, surgical measures are required for control or cure. Solitary lesions can be excised and closed by primary intention, and sinus tracts and fistulas should be exteriorized and excised. Extensive involvement may require the removal of all diseased tissue and the placement of skin grafts. Surgical management should not be withheld in the mistaken belief that such an approach is radical.

23.21 DISORDERS OF HAIR

Disorders of hair in infants and children may be due to intrinsic disturbances of hair growth, to structural anomalies of the hair shafts, or to underlying biochemical or metabolic defects. Excessive and abnormal hair growth is referred to as hypertrichosis or hirsutism. Hypertrichosis is excessive hair growth at inappropriate locations; hirsutism is noted in women who have a male pattern of hair growth and distribution. Deficient hair growth is known as hypotrichosis, and hair loss, partial or complete, is called alopecia. Alopecia may be classified as nonscarring or scarring; the latter type is rare in children and, if present, is most often due to prolonged or untreated inflammatory conditions such as pyoderma or tinea capitis.

HYPERTRICHOSIS

Hypertrichosis is rare in children and may be localized or generalized, permanent or transient. Localized hypertrichosis is most often due to a heritable condition or to a nevoid defect. Generalized hypertrichosis has many causes; some are listed in Table 23–8.

TABLE 23–8. Causes of and Conditions Associated with Hypertrichosis

1. *Intrinsic factors*
   - Racial and familial forms such as hairy ears, hairy elbows, intraphalangeal hair, or generalized hirsutism
2. *Extrinsic factors*
   - Local trauma or casts
   - Drugs
     - Diazoxide, phenytoin, corticosteroids, corticotropin, cyclosporine, androgens, anabolic agents, hexachlorobenzene, minoxidil
3. *Hamartomas or nevi*
   - Congenital pigmented nevocytic nevus, nevus pilosus, Becker nevus, congenital smooth muscle hamartoma
4. *Endocrine disorders*
   - Virilizing ovarian tumors, Cushing syndrome, acromegaly, congenital adrenal hyperplasia, adrenal tumors, gonadal dysgenesis, male pseudohermaphroditism, nonendocrine hormone–secreting tumors
5. *Congenital and genetic disorders*
   - Hypertrichosis lanuginosa, mucopolysaccharidoses, leprechaunism, congenital generalized lipodystrophy, Cornelia de Lange syndrome, craniofacial dysostosis, 18-trisomy, Rubinstein-Taybi syndrome, Bloom syndrome, congenital hemihypertrophy, gingival fibromatosis with hypertrichosis, porphyrias

HYPOTRICHOSIS AND ALOPECIA

Some of the disorders associated with hypotrichosis and alopecia are listed in Table 23–9. True alopecia is only rarely congenital; it is more often related to infections, an inflammatory dermatosis, drug ingestion, or mechanical factors. Hair loss as well as alterations in texture and quality are associated with some of the endocrinopathies that involve the ovary, thyroid, parathyroid, adrenal, or pituitary glands. Bacterial, viral, and fungal infections of the scalp may also cause focal or diffuse hair loss. Metabolic disturbances, such as protein deprivation, celiac disease, hypervitaminosis A, and hypozincemia are additional causes. Any inflammatory condition of the scalp, such as atopic dermatitis or seborrheic dermatitis, if severe enough, may result in partial alopecia. In all these disorders, hair growth will return to normal if the underlying condition is treated successfully unless there has been permanent damage to the hair follicle.

TELOGEN EFFLUVIUM. This loss of scalp hair, because of premature conversion of growing hairs to the resting phase, accounts for the loss of hair by infants during the first few months of life, for postpartum loss, and for that lost 2–4 mo after an acute febrile illness. Telogen effluvium may also occur after the discontinuation of oral contraceptives. There is no inflammatory reaction; the hair follicles remain intact, and telogen bulbs can be demonstrated microscopically on shed hairs. Because more than 50% of the scalp hair is rarely lost, alopecia is usually not severe; the sudden loss of large amounts of hair with brushing, combing, and washing of hair, however, can generate considerable anxiety. Parents should be reassured that normal hair growth will return shortly and that alopecia will not be permanent.

TRACTION ALOPECIA (MARGINAL OR TRAUMATIC ALOPECIA). This results in follicular damage and may be caused by tight braiding or "ponytails," headbands, rubber bands, curlers, and rollers (Fig. 23–38*A*). Associated folliculitis in the parietal areas, if severe, may cause scarring and regional lymphadenopathy. The alopecia is usually reversible; children and parents must be encouraged to avoid these devices and, if necessary, to alter the hair style. Otherwise, irreparable damage to hair follicles may occur.

TOXIC ALOPECIA. This is the side effect of radiation and certain drugs. Cancer chemotherapeutic agents, such as antimetabolites, alkylating agents, and mitotic inhibitors, inhibit synthesis of hair in growing (anagen) follicles. Hairs become dystrophic, and the hair shaft breaks at the narrowed segment. Loss is diffuse, rapid (1–3 wk after treatment), and temporary; regrowth occurs when administration of the drug(s) is discontinued. Thallium, heparin, and the coumarins induce shedding of the hair by converting it from the growing (anagen) to the resting (telogen) phase. Hair loss is diffuse and temporary.

TABLE 23–9. Disorders Associated with Alopecia and Hypotrichosis

1. Congenital universal alopecia, atrichia with papular lesions
2. Localized congenital alopecia: aplasia cutis, alopecia triangularis
3. Ectodermal dysplasias
4. Heritable syndromes: Marie-Unna hypotrichosis, Cockayne, progeria, Rothmund-Thomson, dyskeratosis congenita, Seckel, cartilage-hair hypoplasia, Conradi, trichorhinophalangeal, pachyonychia congenita, Hallerman-Streiff, Treacher Collins, popliteal web, oculodentodigital, orofaciodigital, incontinentia pigmenti, focal dermal hypoplasia, keratosis follicularis spinulosa decalvans
5. Metabolic defects: homocystinuria, acrodermatitis enteropathica, biotin deficiency
6. Hamartomas of the scalp and the hair follicles

TRICHOTILLOMANIA. This compulsive pulling, twisting, and breaking of hair is responsible for irregular areas of incomplete hair loss. These are most often located on the crown and in the occipital and parietal areas of the scalp (see Fig. 23–38*B*), but occasionally eyebrows, eyelashes, and body hair are traumatized. Some plaques of alopecia may have a linear outline. The hairs remaining within the areas of loss are of varying lengths and are typically blunt-tipped because of breakage. The scalp is normal in appearance.

The diagnosis of trichotillomania is often difficult and may require biopsy confirmation. Histologic changes include coexistent normal and damaged follicles, parafollicular hemorrhages, atrophy of some follicles, and catagen transformation of hair. Tinea capitis and alopecia areata must be considered in the differential diagnosis. Parents often acknowledge that the child frequently plucks or twists the hair. Amelioration of the condition requires the patient's cooperation. Denial on the part of both patient and parents complicates management, and occasionally psychiatric counseling is required. Long-term repeated trauma may result in irreversible damage and permanent alopecia.

ALOPECIA AREATA. This idiopathic disorder is characterized by rapid and complete loss of hair in round or oval patches on the scalp (see Fig. 23–38*C*) as well as on other body sites. In *alopecia totalis* all the scalp hair is lost; in *alopecia universalis* body hair as well as scalp hair is nonexistent. Peripheral spread and confluence of plaques of alopecia areata often result in bizarre patterns. At the margin of active plaques, the hairs can often be extracted with gentle traction and, on examination, demonstrate an attenuated or catagen bulb at the termination of a tapered, poorly pigmented shaft. The skin within the plaques of hair loss is normal in appearance. In patients with severe alopecia, dystrophy of the nails is common.

The cause of alopecia areata is unknown. A perifollicular infiltrate of inflammatory round cells is found in biopsy specimens from affected areas. Emotional factors and stress have been suggested as triggering factors, but supportive evidence is tenuous. About 20% of patients have a family history of alopecia areata. The infrequent but striking association with autoimmune diseases, such as Hashimoto thyroiditis, Addison disease, pernicious anemia, collagen vascular diseases, and vitiligo, has suggested an autoimmune pathogenesis. Some patients have serum antibodies to thyroglobulin, parietal cells, and adrenal gland. An increased incidence of alopecia areata has been reported in patients with Down syndrome.

The differential diagnosis includes tinea capitis, seborrheic dermatitis, trichotillomania, traumatic alopecia, and lupus erythematosus. The course is unpredictable because spontaneous resolution is usual, but recurrences are common. In general, onset at a young age and extensive or prolonged hair loss are poor prognostic signs. Alopecia universalis and totalis as well as *ophiasis*, a type of alopecia areata in which hair loss is circumferential, are less likely to resolve permanently.

Treatment is difficult to evaluate because the course is erratic and unpredictable. The use of high-potency topical, fluorinated corticosteroids with occlusion at night is thought to be effective in some patients. Intradermal injections of steroid may also stimulate hair growth locally, but this mode of treatment is impractical in young children or in those with extensive hair loss. Systemic corticosteroid therapy has, on occasion, been associated with good results; however, the permanence of cure is questionable, and the side effects are a serious deterrent. Additional therapies that are sometimes effective include short-contact anthralin, topical minoxidil, and applications of contact allergens (squaric acid dibutylester). In general, parents and patients can be reassured that spontaneous remission will usually occur. New hair growth

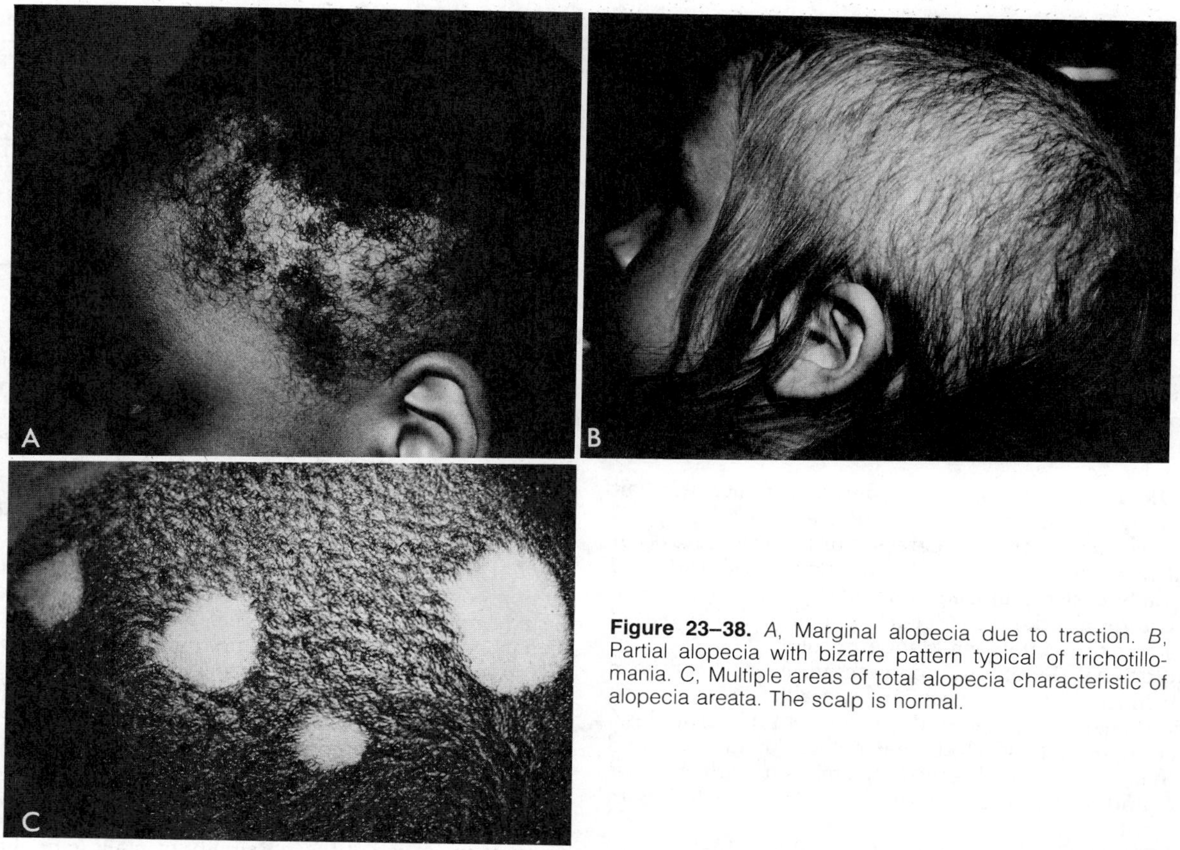

Figure 23–38. *A*, Marginal alopecia due to traction. *B*, Partial alopecia with bizarre pattern typical of trichotillomania. *C*, Multiple areas of total alopecia characteristic of alopecia areata. The scalp is normal.

may initially be of finer caliber and lighter color, but replacement by normal terminal hair can be expected.

23.22 STRUCTURAL DEFECTS OF HAIR

Structural defects of the hair shaft can be congenital or acquired. Some reflect known biochemical aberrations; others are of unknown cause; and one, at least, appears to be related to damaging grooming practices. All the defects can be demonstrated by microscopic examination of affected hairs. Scanning and transmission electron microscopy has contributed greatly to an understanding of the structural abnormalities.

TRICHORRHEXIS NODOSA. This is the most common of the structural defects. Clinically, the defect appears as a node or swelling on the hair shaft. Microscopically, it has the appearance of two interlocking brushes. The defect is due to a fracture of the hair shaft with derangement of the cells in the cortex. Weakness at the nodal points accounts for the fragility of the shaft, resulting in broken stubs and partial alopecia. Trichorrhexis nodosa has been noted as a congenital defect in some families and has also been observed in some infants with argininosuccinic aciduria.

Acquired trichorrhexis nodosa, the most common cause of hair breakage, occurs in two forms. *Proximal defects* are found most frequently in black children, whose complaint is not of alopecia but of the failure of their hair to grow. The hair is short, often in brush-stroke patches; easy breakage is demonstrated by gentle traction on the hair shafts. A history of other affected family members may be obtained. The problem is thought to be caused by a combination of genetic predisposition and the cumulative mechanical trauma of rough combing and brushing, hair straightening procedures, and "permanents." The longitudinal splits, knots, and nodal defects can be demonstrated in hair mounts. The patient must be cautioned to avoid damaging grooming techniques. A soft, natural-bristle brush and a wide-toothed comb should be used. The condition is self-limited with resolution in 2–4 yr if the patient avoids damaging practices.

Distal trichorrhexis nodosa is seen more frequently in white and oriental children; it is also traumatic in origin. The distal portions of the hair shafts are thinned, ragged, and faded and may have white specks (sometimes mistaken for nits) along the shaft. Hair mounts reveal the paint-brush defect and the sites of excessive fragility and breakage. Avoidance of diverse insults, including saltwater soaking and traumatic grooming, as well as regular trimming of affected ends and the use of cream rinses to lessen tangling will ameliorate the condition.

MONILETHRIX. This rare defect of the hair shaft is inherited as an autosomal dominant trait. The hair appears dry, lusterless, and brittle, and it fractures spontaneously or with mild trauma. Eyebrows, lashes, and body and sexual hair as well as scalp hair may be affected. Keratosis pilaris is always present, and, less commonly, there are other ectodermal defects. Microscopically, a distinctive, regular beading pattern of the hair shafts is evident; the narrowed internodal portions of the shaft lack a medulla and are the sites of fracture. The etiology is unknown; treatment is ineffective. Spontaneous improvement may occur at puberty.

TRICHORRHEXIS INVAGINATA (BAMBOO HAIR). This is a distinguishing feature of the Netherton syndrome. Dry, fragile hair without apparent growth is characteristic. The nodal defects of the shaft have the appearance of a ball and socket joint in which the distal portion has been invaginated into the cup-like proximal portion. The abnormality is thought to result from a transient defect in keratinization.

The defects may be identified in body hair as well as in scalp hair and seem to decrease in frequency as the child matures. Hair growth may improve significantly at puberty.

TRICHOSCHISIS. This refers to a defect that has the appearance of a clean fracture perpendicular to the hair shaft. Affected children have brittle hair (trichothiodystrophy). Under the light microscope, the hair resembles a flat ribbon and folds back on itself at intervals along the hair shaft. On scanning electron microscopy, near absence of the cuticular hair cells can be demonstrated along with ridging and fluting of the shaft. A zebra-striped pattern of alternating bright and dark bands is characteristic on polarizing microscopy. There is decreased hair sulfur content.

These changes have also been described in association with other abnormalities, including ichthyosis; intellectual impairment; short stature; defects of the teeth, nails, and eyes; and photosensitivity. Several different syndromes have trichothiodystrophy.

PILI TORTI. This is a structural defect in which the hair shaft is grooved and flattened at irregular intervals and is twisted on its axis in varying degrees. Minor twists that occur in normal hair should not be misconstrued as pili torti. Pili torti is usually first recognized at about 2–3 yr of age, when the hair acquires a striking spangled appearance and increased fragility. The hair is often ash-blonde in color.

Both autosomal dominant and recessive forms have been described; most cases, however, are sporadic. Pili torti has, on occasion, been associated with sensorineural hearing loss, mental retardation, and ectodermal defects of the hair and teeth. It has also been observed in children with Menkes syndrome and citrullinemia and in children treated with retinoid agents.

PILI ANNULATI. This consists of ringed hair that is characterized by hair shafts banded with bright rings when viewed in reflected light. The bands are caused by reflection of light from focal aggregates of abnormal air-filled cavities within the hair shafts. The hair is not fragile. The defect may be familial or sporadic.

Pseudo-pili annulati is a variant of normal blond hair; an optical effect caused by the refraction and reflection of light from the flattened and twisted shaft creates the phenomenon of banding.

WOOLY HAIR DISEASE. This disease presents peculiarly tight, curly, abnormal hair at birth. Three types have been recognized: (1) an autosomal dominant form in which other ectodermal structures and hair color are normal; (2) an autosomal recessive type in which the scalp hair has a bleached appearance and body hair is short and pale; and (3) wooly hair nevus, a sporadic form in which only a portion of the scalp hair is fine and light-colored and grows poorly.

23.23 DISEASES OF THE NAILS

Nail abnormalities in children may be manifestations of generalized skin disease or of systemic disease. They may also be due to trauma, localized bacterial and fungal infections, or skin diseases involving the nail fold. Nail changes occur in psoriasis, Reiter disease, Norwegian scabies, lichen planus, lichen striatus, Darier disease, alopecia areata, hypoparathyroidism, and acrodermatitis enteropathica. Nail anomalies are also common in certain congenital disorders (Table 23–10).

Anonychia is absence of the nail plate, usually the result of a congenital disorder or trauma. *Koilonychia* is flattening and concavity of the nail plate with loss of normal contour. *Macronychia* is an abnormally large nail; *micronychia* is an unusually small one. *Leukonychia* is a white opacity of the nail plate that may involve the entire plate or may be punctate or striate; the nail plate, however, remains smooth and undamaged. Leukonychia can be traumatic; associated with infection, dermatosis, malnutrition, anemia, and heavy metal poisoning; or may be a benign hereditary defect. *Onychogryphosis* is an acquired defect characterized by a thickened, overgrown, distorted nail plate. *Onycholysis* indicates separation of the nail plate from the nail bed. Common causes are trauma, psoriasis, fungal infection (distal onycholysis), contact dermatitis, porphyria, drugs (bleomycin, vincristine, retinoid agents), and drug-induced phototoxicity. *Beau lines* are transverse grooves in the nail plate that represent an inability of the nail matrix to produce a nail plate of normal thickness. Beau lines are usually indicative of periodic trauma or episodic shutdown of the nail matrix secondary to a systemic disease.

TABLE 23–10. Congenital Disease with Nail Defects

Large nails:	Pachyonychia congenita, Rubinstein-Taybi syndrome, hemihypertrophy
Small or absent nails:	Syndromes: the ectodermal dysplasias, nail-patella, dyskeratosis congenita, focal dermal hypoplasia, cartilage-hair hypoplasia, Ellis–van Creveld, Larsen, epidermolysis bullosa, incontinentia pigmenti, Rothmund-Thomson, Turner, popliteal web, 13-trisomy, 18-trisomy, Apert, Gorlin-Pindborg, long arm 21 deletion, otopalatodigital, fetal alcohol, fetal hydantoin, and elfin facies

Pigmentation of an entire nail plate or linear bands of pigmentation are common in black individuals. The pigment is produced by melanocytes in the nail matrix and nail bed and is of no consequence. Pigmentation may also be due to nevus cells in the nail matrix (junctional nevus). Extension or alteration in pigment in the latter lesion should be evaluated by biopsy because of the possibility of malignant change.

Paronychial inflammation is often responsible for dystrophies of the nail plate that are due to damage to the nail matrix; the lesions include bacterial infections, candidosis, eczema, psoriasis, and lichen striatus. Tumors in the paronychial area include pyogenic granulomas, mucous cysts, and junctional nevi. Periungual fibromas that appear during late childhood should suggest a diagnosis of tuberous sclerosis.

Twenty nail dystrophy is characterized by longitudinal ridging, fragility, distal notching, and opalescent discoloration of all the nails. The onset is insidious; there are no associated skin or systemic diseases and no other ectodermal defects. It has been suggested that nail dystrophy is due to lichen planus, but the typical skin lesions of lichen planus are never associated. The disorder must be differentiated from fungal infections, psoriasis, nail changes of alopecia areata, and nail dystrophy secondary to eczema. Eczema and fungal infections rarely produce changes of all the nails simultaneously. The disorder is self-limited and eventually remits; treatment is ineffective.

23.24 DISEASES OF THE MUCOUS MEMBRANES

The mucous membranes may be involved in developmental disorders, infections, acute and chronic skin diseases, genodermatoses, and benign and malignant tumors. A discussion of a few of the more common diseases specific to mucous membranes follows.

FORDYCE DISEASE. This disease is characterized by multiple, yellow-white papules located on the mucosa of the lips and the buccal surface. They are aberrant sebaceous glands and may be found in otherwise normal individuals. They are asymptomatic and require no therapy.

GEOGRAPHIC TONGUE. Geographic tongue, or glossitis

areata migrans, is seen most often in children and young adults. The lesions consist of sharply demarcated, irregular, smooth red plaques, often with elevated, gray margins. The erythematous areas are due to a loss of the normal papillae other than the fungiform ones. The cause is unknown. Symptoms of mild burning or irritation are occasionally bothersome. The onset is rapid, and individual lesions may persist for months. These lesions should not be confused with mucous patches of secondary syphilis. No therapy other than reassurance is necessary.

CHEILITIS. This inflammation of the lips and angles of the mouth (angular cheilitis) may be due to a variety of causes. In children it is commonly due to dryness, chapping, and constant lip-licking; excessive salivation and drooling, particularly in children with neurologic deficits, may also cause chronic irritation. The lesions of oral thrush may occasionally extend to the angles of the mouth. Protection can be provided by frequent applications of a bland ointment such as petrolatum. Candidosis should be treated with an appropriate antifungal agent, and contact dermatitis of the perioral skin should be treated with a topical corticosteroid preparation and a lubricant for protection.

LIP PITS AND FISTULAS. These are usually located symmetrically in the vermilion of the lower lip; they represent the mucosa-lined sinus tracts from underlying minor salivary glands. They may occasionally exude a mucous secretion and should be excised for cosmetic reasons.

MUCOCELES. These mucous retention cysts usually form as a result of trauma to the lips or buccal mucosa. Severance of the duct of a mucous gland leads to retention of mucous secretion within the interrupted duct lumen and subsequent cystic dilatation. Lesions are common on the lips, tongue, palate, and buccal mucosa. Those on the floor of the mouth are known as *ranulas* when the submaxillary or sublingual salivary ducts are involved. Fluctuations in size are usual, and the lesions may disappear temporarily after traumatic rupture. Mucoceles must be excised to prevent recurrence.

APHTHOUS STOMATITIS (CANKER SORES) (see Sec. 13.9). This recurrent painful ulceration of the oral mucous membranes is a common condition in which several factors probably play a role. Solitary or multiple lesions occur on the labial, buccal, and lingual mucosa as well as on the sublingual, palatal, and gingival mucosa. Initial lesions are erythematous and indurated papules that erode rapidly to form sharply circumscribed, necrotic ulcers with a gray fibrinous exudate and an erythematous halo. The lesions heal spontaneously in 10–14 days. A more severe form of this disorder in which there are larger, more debilitating lesions is called *periadenitis aphthae*.

Aphthous stomatitis is often cyclical in occurrence. It has been attributed to a variety of causes that include food hypersensitivity, allergic or toxic drug reactions, infectious agents, endocrine factors, emotional stress, and trauma. Immunologic studies have demonstrated lymphocytotoxicity for oral epithelial cells, suggesting a cell-mediated pathogenesis. It is a common misconception that aphthous stomatitis is a manifestation of herpes simplex. Recurrent herpes infections remain localized to the lips and rarely cross the mucocutaneous junction; involvement of the oral mucosa occurs only in primary infections.

Treatment of aphthous stomatitis is extremely difficult and is palliative at best. Relief of pain, particularly before eating, may be achieved by use of a topical anesthetic such as viscous Xylocaine or an oral rinse with 1 teaspoonful of elixir of Benadryl. A topical corticosteroid in a mucosal adhering agent (0.1% triamcinolone in Orabase) may be helpful if applied 2–3 times daily. Alternatively, Gelusil used as a rinse may provide some relief.

23.25 VASCULITIS

Cutaneous vasculitis can occur as a variable feature of a large number of disorders including connective tissue diseases, infections, and hypersensitivity reactions. Although the morphology of the skin lesions may vary considerably in these diseases, palpable purpura can be regarded as pathognomonic of vasculitis, reflecting the intense inflammatory process in the dermal vessels (Sec. 11.56 and Table 23–11).

PITYRIASIS LICHENOIDES ET VARIOLIFORMIS ACUTA (PLEVA, MUCHA-HABERMANN DISEASE). This disorder can occur at any age and is sometimes classified as a form of parapsoriasis but is, in fact, a type of vasculitis. The eruption is polymorphous; small, red-brown, scaly papules and varicelliform vesicles appear in crops and evolve as papulonecrotic, crusted, hemorrhagic lesions that heal as pitted scars. The anterior trunk and proximal limbs are preferred sites; the palms, soles, and mucous membranes are spared. There are no constitutional signs, and mild itching is often the only symptom. The general health is unimpaired, and the process eventually resolves spontaneously.

The disease must be differentiated from varicella, other

TABLE 23–11. Types of Vasculitis and Associated Skin Lesions*

Type of Vasculitis	Blood Vessels Involved	Type of Skin Lesion
Leukocytoclastic or hypersensitivity angiitis: Henoch-Schönlein purpura, cryoglobulinemia, hypocomplementemic vasculitis	Dermal capillaries, venules, and occasional small muscular arteries in internal organs	Purpuric papules, hemorrhagic bullae, cutaneous infarcts
Rheumatic vasculitis: systemic lupus erythematosus; rheumatoid vasculitis	Dermal capillaries, venules, and small muscular arteries in internal organs	Purpuric papules; ulcerative nodules; splinter hemorrhages; periungual telangiectasia and infarcts
Granulomatous vasculitis		
Churg and Strauss allergic granulomatous angiitis	Dermal small and larger muscular arteries and medium muscular arteries in subcutaneous tissue and other organs	Erythematous, purpuric, and ulcerated nodules, plaques, and purpura
Wegener granulomatosis	Small venules, arterioles of dermis, and small muscular arteries	Ulcerative nodules, peripheral gangrene
Periarteritis: classic type limited to skin and muscle	Small and medium muscular arteries in deep dermis, subcutaneous tissue, and muscle	Deep subcutaneous nodules with ulceration; livedo reticularis; ecchymoses
Giant cell arteritis: temporal arteritis, polymyalgia rheumatica, Takayasu disease	Medium muscular arteries and larger arteries	Skin necrosis over scalp

*From Wyngaarden JB, Smith LH (eds): Cecil Textbook of Medicine, 18th ed. Philadelphia, WB Saunders, 1988.

viral exanthems, papular urticaria, drug eruptions, and other vasculitides. The protracted episodic course of weeks to months (or even years) serves to exclude some of these disorders. The histologic changes are lymphocytic vasculitis, invasion of the epidermis by lymphocytes and erythrocytes, edema, necrosis, and vesicle formation. Cultures of intact lesions are always negative.

Oral administration of erythromycin can often control the eruption, but the response is slow. The medication must be given for several months, and the dose is reduced gradually when the disease appears to be quiescent. Ultraviolet light treatments are often effective.

PITYRIASIS LICHENOIDES CHRONICA (GUTTATE PARAPSORIASIS, PLC). This is the chronic form of PLEVA. The eruption can be polymorphous, but typical lesions are small (1–5 mm), superficial, erythematous papules covered by a fine, white scale. Occasional lesions may become infiltrated, vesicular, hemorrhagic, and crusted. Prolonged postinflammatory pigmentary loss is usual and may be prominent in darker-skinned children. There is a predilection for involvement of the trunk, but all body sites may be affected except the nails and mucous membranes. An individual lesion may persist for 2–6 wk, but exacerbations and remissions persist for months to years.

Despite the prolonged course, PLC is benign and unassociated with systemic manifestations. The lesions may be asymptomatic or may cause minimal pruritus. The diagnosis is entirely clinical. Differential diagnosis includes guttate psoriasis, pityriasis rosea, drug eruptions, secondary syphilis, viral exanthems, and lichen planus. Because the pathologic changes are specific in some of these disorders, a skin biopsy may be indicated to exclude them. The chronicity of pityriasis lichenoides helps to exclude pityriasis rosea, viral exanthems, and some drug eruptions.

Some patients show remarkable improvement following intense sun exposure. Topical corticosteroid-tar preparations and ultraviolet light have been used with variable success. A lubricant to remove excessive scaling may be all that is necessary if the patient is asymptomatic. Parents should be reassured that the child will remain well.

23.26 CUTANEOUS BACTERIAL INFECTIONS

IMPETIGO CONTAGIOSA. This superficial form of pyoderma occurs most commonly in children and is most prevalent during the hot, humid summer months.

Clinical Manifestations. The infection is characterized by erythematous macules that very rapidly evolve into thin-walled vesicles and pustules (Fig. 23–39*A*). The vesicopustular stage is also brief, and, following rupture, sticky, heaped-up, honey-colored crusts are formed (see Fig. 23–39*B*). Removal of crusts leaves a moist, red base over which a fresh exudate quickly accumulates. The lesions often spread peripherally and clear centrally to form circinate plaques and gyrate patterns. The infection may be spread to other parts of the body by the fingers, clothing, and towels. The sites usually involved are exposed areas such as the face, neck, and limbs, but lesions may develop anywhere on the body. Insect bites, scabies, cutaneous injuries, and preceding dermatitis serve as portals of entry for the organism, which does not penetrate intact skin. Regional lymphadenopathy is frequently associated.

Etiology. Nonbullous impetigo has classically been regarded as an infection with group A β hemolytic streptococcus, which first colonizes normal skin. Secondary invasion by staphylococci can occur, and both organisms may be recovered on culture. *S. aureus* alone may also cause this type of impetigo (as well as bullous impetigo) and may be the prevalent agent in some areas. An appreciation of the primary agent is especially important in choosing the appropriate antibiotic.

Epidemiology. The strains of streptococci that colonize the skin and cause impetigo are different from the strains that are usually responsible for pharyngeal infection. Skin strains elaborate streptolysin, hyaluronidase, and DNase B, but ASO and antihyaluronidase titers are not consistently elevated; anti-DNase B titers are more frequently elevated. The white blood cell and differential counts and erythrocyte sedimentation rate are usually normal.

Type specificity and virulence of streptococci are associated with their M protein, and only certain types are associated with the development of poststreptococcal acute glomerulonephritis. The incidence of nephritis following streptococcal impetigo varies considerably in epidemiologic studies and is higher in areas where cutaneous infection is endemic (Sec. 18.5). Rheumatic fever has not been associated with impetigo.

Treatment. Impetigo is an indolent but self-limited disease. It should, however, be treated to decrease morbidity and prevent spread to other children. Local measures should include improvement of personal hygiene, compresses with Burow solution applied 4 times a day to remove crusts, and washing with an antibacterial soap. Topical therapy with mupirocin alone is often effective for impetigo owing to *S. aureus* and streptococci and has minimal adverse effects. Alternative therapy with penicillin, erythromycin, or dicloxacillin is also effective depending on the etiologic agent and its antibiotic sensitivities. It is important to be aware of the patterns of resistance for organisms prevalent in a particular community. Early treatment of impetigo caused by nephritogenic strains of streptococci does not appear to lessen the occurrence of acute glomerulonephritis.

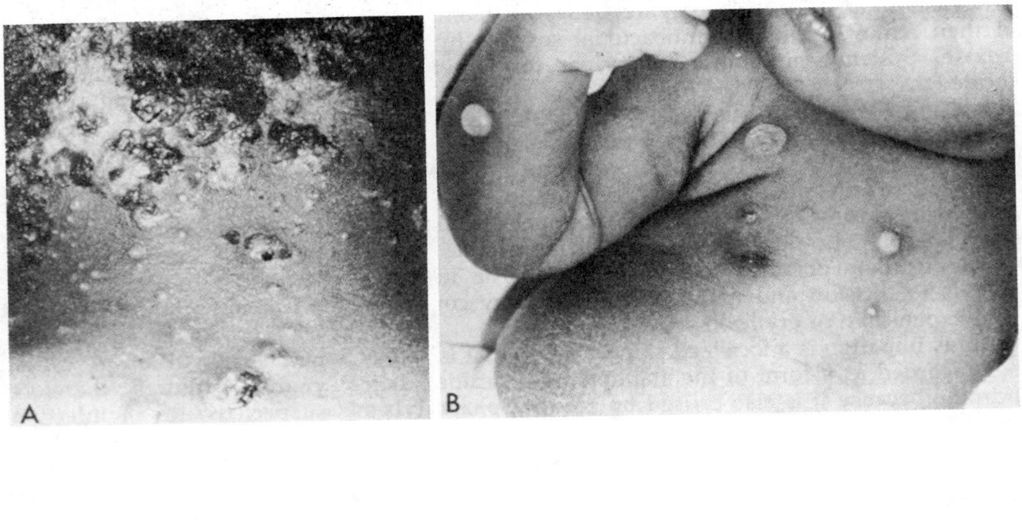

Figure 23–39. *A*, Multiple crusted and oozing lesions of streptococcal impetigo. *B*, Multiple tense and flaccid blisters of bullous impetigo on the trunk and arm of an infant.

BULLOUS IMPETIGO. This is a localized skin infection that is sometimes regarded as a form of the staphylococcal scalded skin syndrome because it is also caused by group 2 phage types of *S. aureus*. It is mainly an infection of infants and young children. Neonatal bullous impetigo begins in the diaper area. Typical bullae arise on normal skin or have a narrow, erythematous halo; they are filled with a clear, pale to dark yellow fluid that may become turbid if the bullae remain intact. The blisters are relatively superficial and rupture easily, leaving a moist denuded base that is rapidly covered with a thin crust. There is no intradermal separation of adjacent skin (positive Nikolsky sign). The lesions occasionally become widespread, particularly in young infants, but rarely cause systemic manifestations.

The differential diagnosis in the neonate includes epidermolysis bullosa, bullous mastocytosis, herpetic infection, and early scalded skin syndrome. In older children, erythema multiforme, chronic bullous dermatosis of childhood, pemphigus, and pemphigoid must be considered, particularly if the lesions fail to respond to therapy. Examination of smears of blister fluid disclose polymorphonuclear leukocytes and clusters of gram-positive cocci. Cultures of fluid from an intact blister should yield the causative agent; when the patient appears ill, blood cultures should be obtained.

Bullae will rupture and dry rapidly with frequent application of wet compresses followed by gentle cleansing. Localized lesions can be treated topically with an antibiotic such as mupirocin 3 times daily. Patients with widespread lesions and small infants should receive a 5- to 7-day course of oral therapy with a penicillinase-resistant penicillin, cephalexin, or erythromycin in the case of the penicillin-allergic patient.

ECTHYMA. Ecthyma resembles impetigo in onset and appearance but gradually evolves into a deeper, more chronic infection. The initial lesion is a vesicle or vesicopustule with an erythematous base that erodes through the epidermis into the dermis to form an ulcer with elevated margins. The ulcer becomes obscured by a dry, heaped-up, tightly adherent crust that contributes to the persistence of the infection and to scar formation. Lesions vary in size and may be as large as 4 cm. Sites of predilection are the legs, where trauma probably plays a major role. Pruritic lesions, such as insect bites, scabies, or pediculosis, which are subject to frequent scratching, act as a focus for the infection.

The causative agent is usually a β-hemolytic streptococcus; the lesions are infectious and may be spread by autoinoculation. Crusts should be softened by frequent warm compresses and should then be removed with an antibacterial soap or hydrogen peroxide. Systemic antibiotic therapy, as for impetigo, is indicated.

Ecthyma gangrenosa is a necrotic ulcer covered with a gray-black eschar and is due to *P. aeruginosa* sepsis, usually occurring in immunosuppressed patients. Therapy with an antipseudomonal penicillin and an aminoglycoside is effective.

BLISTERING DISTAL DACTYLITIS. This is a β-hemolytic streptococcal infection of the fingertips. The superficial bullae are located over the volar fat pad on the distal portion of the fingers or thumb. If left untreated, they may continue to enlarge and extend to the paronychial area. Polymorphonuclear leukocytes and chains of gram-positive cocci are demonstrable in the purulent exudate obtained from the blister. The infection responds to incision and drainage and a 10-day course of systemic penicillin or erythromycin therapy.

PERIANAL STREPTOCOCCAL DERMATITIS. This type is characterized by an erythematous, confluent, moist, pruritic eruption associated with painful defecation and blood-streaked stools. The diagnosis is made by culture of the perianal area. A positive pharyngeal culture for group A β-hemolytic streptococcus is often found as well. The differential diagnosis includes psoriasis, seborrheic dermatitis, candidiasis, pinworm infestation, and sexual abuse. Treatment with oral penicillin or erythromycin should be followed by repeat culture because recrudescence requiring retreatment is not uncommon.

ERYSIPELAS. See Sec. 12.18.

STAPHYLOCOCCAL SCALDED SKIN SYNDROME. This disorder is, almost without exception, a disease of infants and children under 10 yr of age. In most cases it is caused by a group 2 phage type *S. aureus*; rarely, group 1 phage types are isolated.

Etiology and Pathogenesis. The clinical manifestations are due to the elaboration of an exfoliative (epidermolytic) toxin by the infecting strain of bacteria. This extracellular toxin is distinct from other staphylococcal toxins. The toxin has reproduced the disease in both animal models and human volunteers. There may be two distinct epidermolytic toxins: ETA is heat stabile and is encoded by chromosomal genes, and ETB is heat labile and is encoded on a 37.5-kb plasmid. Scalded skin syndrome is due to the presence of one or both toxins, which produce lysis of intracellular connections in the epidermal granular cell layer.

Clinical Manifestations. The onset of the rash may be preceded by a prodrome of malaise, fever, and irritability associated with exquisite tenderness of the skin, or the appearance of generalized erythema may be abrupt without preceding symptoms. Initially, the eruption is macular and involves the face, neck, axilla, and groin; rapid extension is usual, and the brightly erythematous skin may acquire a wrinkled appearance due to the formation of ill-defined flaccid bullae filled with clear fluid. At this stage, areas of epidermis may separate in response to gentle stroking (Nikolsky sign). Facial edema and perioral crusting are usual and result in a typically lugubrious facies. Crusting around the eyes, mouth, and nose produce a characteristic "sunburst" radial pattern. The child is irritable and lies motionless due to pain. As large sheets of epidermis peel away, moist, glistening, denuded areas become apparent, initially in the flexures and subsequently over much of the body surface (Fig. 23–40 [color plate section]). These areas dry quickly and heal by postinflammatory desquamation, which begins within 2–3 days. There may be pharyngitis, conjunctivitis, and superficial erosions of the lips. Although some patients appear desperately ill, many are reasonably comfortable except for the marked skin tenderness. Once the desquamative phase has started, healing proceeds at a rapid rate and is complete in 10–14 days.

A presumed abortive form of the disease (resembling *scarlet fever*) is less dramatic in presentation. The facial appearance in staphylococcal scarlet fever is similar to that of the classic scalded skin syndrome, but the generalized scarlatiniform eruption, which may be accentuated in the flexural areas, does not progress to blister formation. In these patients the Nikolsky sign may be absent.

Diagnosis. The portal of entry for the toxin-producing staphylococcus may be a preceding impetiginous skin eruption, conjunctivitis, gastroenteritis, or pharyngitis that may be unobserved or subclinical. Cultures, therefore, should be obtained from all suspected sites of infection and from the blood, although septicemia is a rare complication. Intact bullae are consistently sterile, unlike those of bullous impetigo; the organism, however, may be cultured from other cutaneous sites.

In staphylococcal scalded skin syndrome the site of blister cleavage is the granular layer, the feature that accounts for the rapid healing of denuded areas of skin. Scattered acantholytic cells are evident in the cleft-like bullae; mild edema and vascular ectasia are present in the dermis, but the absence of inflammatory infiltrate is striking. Ultrastructural studies have consistently demonstrated separation of the two halves of the desmosome without preceding cytolysis or demonstrable removal of the cellular surface.

The differential diagnosis varies with the presentation and age of the child. Incipient scalded skin syndrome in infants may be mistaken for bullous impetigo, epidermolysis bullosa, epidermolytic hyperkeratosis (a type of ichthyosis), sunburn, acrodynia, *Arcanobacterium haemolyticum* pharyngitis, toxic shock syndrome, or boric acid poisoning. Florid lesions of the scalded skin syndrome in older children may mimic erythema multiforme, drug-induced toxic epidermal necrolysis, pemphigus, and other blistering disorders. Toxic epidermal necrolysis can often be distinguished by a history of drug ingestion, presence of the Nikolsky sign only at the site of erythema, absence of perioral crusting, and a deeper blister cleavage plane. A frozen biopsy specimen of exfoliated epidermis provides a rapid method to distinguish the scalded skin syndrome from toxic epidermal necrolysis because the entire thickness of epidermis will be exfoliated only in the latter. The scarlatiniform variety of scalded skin syndrome is most frequently mistaken for streptococcal scarlet fever, but it lacks the palatal enanthem, strawberry tongue, and perioral pallor of scarlet fever. Drug eruptions and other hypersensitivity reactions must also be considered in the differential diagnosis.

Treatment. Systemic therapy, either orally or parenterally, with a semisynthetic penicillinase-resistant penicillin should be prescribed because the staphylococci are usually penicillin-resistant. The skin should be gently moistened and cleansed with Burow solution, isotonic saline, or 0.25% silver nitrate compresses. During the desquamative phase, applications of a bland nonocclusive emollient will provide lubrication and will decrease itching. Topical antibiotics are unnecessary. Recovery is usually rapid, but occasionally complicating factors such as excessive fluid loss, electrolyte imbalance, faulty temperature regulation, pneumonia, septicemia, and cellulitis cause increased morbidity. Uncomplicated skin lesions should heal without scarring.

FOLLICULITIS. This superficial infection of the hair follicle is most often caused by *S. aureus*. The lesions are typically small, dome-shaped pustules with an erythematous base; they are located at the mouth of the pilosebaceous canals. Hair growth is unimpaired. Favored sites include the scalp, buttocks, extremities, and perioral and paranasal areas. Poor hygiene, maceration, and drainage from wounds and abscesses can be provocative factors. Folliculitis can also occur as a result of tar therapy or occlusive wraps; the moist environment encourages bacterial proliferation. The causative organism can be identified by Gram stain and culture of the pus.

Treatment includes frequent cleansing; the use of an antibacterial soap may be helpful. Local antibiotic therapy is usually all that is required. In chronic recurrent folliculitis, daily application of a benzoyl peroxide lotion or gel may facilitate resolution.

Hot tub folliculitis is attributable to *Pseudomonas aeruginosa* (serotype O-11). The lesions are pruritic papules and pustules or deeply erythematous nodules that develop 8–48 hr after exposure and are most dense in areas covered by a bathing suit. They may resolve spontaneously but sometimes require topical antipseudomonal agents.

FURUNCLES AND CARBUNCLES. These follicular lesions may originate from a preceding folliculitis or may arise initially as a deep-seated, tender, erythematous nodule. Although lesions are initially indurated, central necrosis and suppuration follow and lead to rupture and discharge of a central core of necrotic tissue. Pain may be intense if the lesion is situated in an area where the skin is relatively fixed, such as in the external auditory canal or over the nasal cartilages. Sites of predilection are the face, neck, buttocks, and axillae. Confluent furuncles with multiple drainage points are called carbuncles. Furuncles may become chronic and recurrent, particularly in obese individuals and in those with poor hygiene and hyperhidrosis. Patients with furuncles usually have no constitutional symptoms, whereas carbuncles may be accompanied by fever, leukocytosis, and bacteremia.

The causative agent is almost always *S. aureus*, but other bacteria or fungi may be responsible, and Gram stain and culture of the pus are indicated.

Initial treatment should consist of frequent applications of hot, moist compresses to encourage localization and drainage. Large lesions may be drained by a small incision or by repeated needle aspirations but should not be tampered with until fluctuant. Lesions in the paranasal area should not be incised because of the danger of extension to the cavernous sinus. Carbuncles and large or multiple furuncles should be treated with systemic antibiotics. Because penicillinase-producing staphylococci are frequently involved, a penicillinase-resistant penicillin (e.g., cloxacillin orally or oxacillin parenterally) should be used. The penicillin-allergic patient can be treated with a cephalosporin or clindamycin.

Treatment of chronic furunculosis is often difficult. Attention to personal hygiene, use of an antibacterial soap, low dose oral antistaphylococcal penicillin or clindamycin and frequent hand washing may be beneficial.

PITTED KERATOLYSIS. This problem arises in chronically moist and macerated skin and is most often attributable to the wearing of occlusive footgear or to frequent swimming. The lesions consist of plaques of irregularly shaped, superficial erosions of the horny layer that produce crateriform defects on the soles. Occasionally they become secondarily infected. Although usually mild and asymptomatic, the lesions may be quite painful.

The etiologic agent is thought to be a species of keratinophilic diphtheroid. A KOH preparation of scrapings from the lesion demonstrates filamentous coccobacilli. Of the various therapeutic regimens that have been tried, 20% formalin solution in Aquaphor applied topically, with avoidance of maceration, has been the most effective. Topical antibiotics and imidazoles are also acceptable therapeutic agents.

ERYTHRASMA. This benign chronic superficial infection occurs on the skin in adolescents, particularly if they are obese, and occurs more commonly in warmer climates. It is caused by the filamentous diphtheroid, *Corynebacterium minutissimum*. The most frequently affected sites are moist intertriginous areas, such as the groin, axillae, and toe webs. Sharply demarcated, brownish-red, slightly scaly patches are characteristic of the disease. Mild pruritus is the only constant symptom.

The diagnosis is readily made with a Wood lamp; the lesions fluoresce a brilliant coral-red color under ultraviolet light. The gram-positive pleomorphic coccobacilli can be cultured on routine laboratory media. Erythrasma can be differentiated from dermatophyte infections and from tinea versicolor by the Wood lamp examination.

A 10- to 14-day course of oral use of erythromycin therapy is usually curative. Recurrence may be inhibited by frequent use of an antibacterial soap.

TUBERCULOSIS OF THE SKIN (see also Sec. 12.47). ***Primary cutaneous tuberculosis*** is rare in the United States but occurs with the greatest frequency in infants and children. Primary lesions result when *Mycobacterium tuberculosis* is inoculated at a site of injury on the skin or mucous membranes. Sites of predilection are the chin, lips, nose, limbs, and genitalia. The initial lesion, referred to as a *tuberculous chancre*, develops 2–3 wk after introduction of the organism into the damaged tissue. A red-brown papule gradually enlarges and ulcerates, forming an indolent, firm, sharply demarcated ulcer. Some lesions acquire a crust resembling impetigo, and others become heaped-up and verrucous at the margins. Regional adenopathy with or without lymphangitis appears at approximately 3–4 wk.

The primary lesion is a tuberculoid granuloma with caseation necrosis. *M. tuberculosis* is demonstrable in the skin lesion and local lymph nodes. Clinically, the lesions can resemble syphilitic chancres or deep fungal infections. Spontaneous healing coincides with acquisition of immunity, at which time the skin lesions and infected nodes may become calcified. Antituberculous therapy is indicated (Sec. 12.47).

Direct cutaneous inoculation of a previously infected individual with the tubercle bacillus produces a verrucous plaque known as *tuberculosis verrucosa cutis*. These children have a markedly positive response to a tuberculin skin test. The lesions heal gradually with antituberculous therapy.

Miliary tuberculosis may rarely be manifested cutaneously. The skin lesions result from bloodstream invasion by massive numbers of mycobacteria. The eruption consists of symmetrically distributed, erythematous papules that ulcerate and crust and may become purpuric. Subcutaneous gummatous nodules are often associated. Tubercle bacilli are readily identified in an active lesion. A fulminant course should be anticipated, and aggressive antituberculous therapy is indicated.

Lupus vulgaris is, fortunately, relatively rare today and represents reinfection tuberculosis in children with immunity induced by previous infection. Infection follows traumatic cutaneous inoculation of mycobacteria, direct extension from underlying joints or nodes, or lymphatic or hematogenous spread. Typical lesions consist of tiny red papules that evolve into small nodules. When examined by diascopy, these lesions are sharply marginated, yellow-brown macules. Relentless progression occurs by peripheral spread and coalescence of nodules to form irregular plaques of varying sizes, often with central spontaneous healing. These lesions usually ulcerate and cause extreme disfigurement with eventual formation of atrophic and hypertrophic scars.

Lupus vulgaris occurs most frequently on the head and neck, but no site is exempt. Lesions involving the nasal, buccal, and conjunctival mucosa may cause extensive facial deformity. Chronicity is characteristic, and persistence of plaques for many years is not uncommon. The histopathologic changes are those of a tuberculoid granuloma without caseation; organisms are extremely difficult to demonstrate. Small lesions can be excised; antituberculous drug therapy will usually halt further spread and induce involution.

Scrofuloderma is caused by infection of the skin from caseous tuberculous cervical lymph nodes. The infection is initiated in the larynx and is believed to be caused most often by the ingestion of milk containing *M. tuberculosis*. The lymph nodes become enlarged and fluctuant, stretching the overlying skin, which may slough, forming ulcerations and multiple draining sinuses. Healing results in cord-like cicatrices.

Caseous tubercles can be demonstrated in the deep dermis and subcutaneous tissue. Tubercle bacilli are readily identified.

Scrofuloderma may occasionally resemble actinomycosis, sporotrichosis, or pyogenic lymphadenitis. The course is predictably indolent, but constitutional symptoms are typically absent. Antituberculous therapy is usually effective.

Tuberculids represent a variety of noninfectious cutaneous lesions and have been ascribed to hypersensitivity to the tubercle bacillus. The most commonly observed reaction pattern is the *papulonecrotic tuberculid*; lesions appear in crops of symmetrically distributed, sterile papules that undergo central ulceration and eventually heal, leaving sharply delineated, circular, depressed scars. Preferred sites are the extensor aspects of the limbs and the dorsum of the hand and foot. Histologically, nonspecific inflammation, tubercles, and minimal caseation coexist with an obliterative vasculitis of the deep dermis. The duration of the eruption is variable, but disappearance usually follows eradication of the primary infection.

Lichen scrofulosorum, another form of tuberculid, is characterized by grouped, pinhead-sized, pink or red papules that form large plaques, mainly on the trunk. Clinically and histologically, the eruption can simulate sarcoidosis; in such cases, hypersensitivity to tuberculin is supportive evidence of tuberculous disease. Healing occurs without scarring.

Atypical mycobacterial infection (swimming pool granuloma) may be responsible for cutaneous lesions in children; *M. marinum*, an organism found in saltwater fish, tropical fish tanks, dolphin bites, and swimming pools, is responsible for most of the infections. Swimming pool granulomas are usually initiated by traumatic abrasion of the skin, which serves as a portal of entry for the organism; the knees and elbows are most often affected. Approximately 3 wk after inoculation with the organism, single or multiple reddish papules develop and enlarge slowly to form violaceous nodules. The lesions occasionally break down and become covered with adherent brown crusts. Systemic signs and symptoms, including regional lymphadenopathy, are absent.

M. marinum granulomas may mimic sporotrichosis or pyoderma. A biopsy specimen of a fully developed lesion will demonstrate a granulomatous infiltrate with tuberculoid architecture and caseation necrosis; intracellular organisms can be identified within the histiocytes with appropriate stains. Cultures of material obtained from the granuloma must be incubated at 30–33° C, since *M. marinum* does not grow at 37° C. This organism is a photochromogen, that is, colonies will change color (white to yellow) on exposure to daylight. The purified protein derivative skin test demonstrates 5–15 mm of induration.

There is no specific treatment, because these organisms are resistant to antituberculous drugs. Tetracycline, minocycline, and trimethoprim-sulfamethoxazole for 1–2 mo after resolution have been effective in some cases. Surgical excision may be curative for small lesions; however, recurrences are not uncommon. Spontaneous healing can be expected within a period of several years.

23.27 CUTANEOUS FUNGAL INFECTIONS

TINEA VERSICOLOR. This is a rather common, innocuous, chronic fungal infection caused by the dimorphic yeast *Pityrosporon orbiculare (Malassezia furfur)*. The lesions vary widely in color; in whites they are typically reddish-brown, whereas in blacks they may be either hypopigmented or hyperpigmented. The characteristic macules are covered with a fine scale; they often begin in a perifollicular location, enlarge, and merge to form confluent patches, most commonly on the neck, upper chest, back, and upper arms (Fig. 23–41*A*). Facial lesions are not unusual in adolescents, and lesions occasionally appear on the forearms, the dorsum of the hands, and the pubis. There may be little or no pruritus. Involved areas do not tan following sun exposure.

P. orbiculare is part of the normal flora, predominantly in the yeast form, but proliferation of filamentous forms occurs in the disease state. Predisposing factors include excessive sweating, high plasma cortisol levels, debilitating diseases, and genetically determined susceptibility. The disease is most prevalent in adolescents and young adults.

Examination with a Wood lamp will disclose a deep gold fluorescence. A KOH preparation of scrapings is diagnostic, demonstrating groups of thick-walled spores and myriads of short, thick, angular hyphae (see Fig. 23–41*B*).

Tinea versicolor must be distinguished from dermatophyte infections and scaling disorders such as seborrheic dermatitis and pityriasis alba. Nonscaling pigmentary disorders, such as

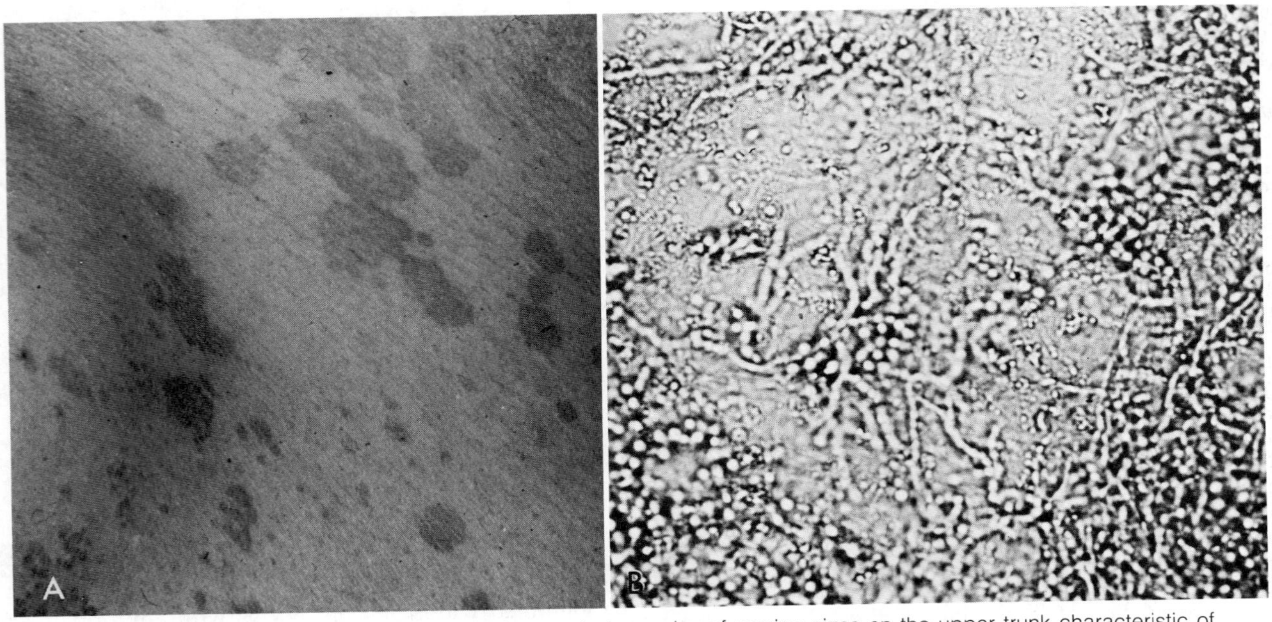

Figure 23–41. *A*, Hyperpigmented, sharply demarcated macules of varying sizes on the upper trunk characteristic of tinea versicolor. *B*, KOH preparation of *Pityrosporon orbiculare* demonstrating short, thick hyphae and clusters of spores.

postinflammatory pigmentary change, may be mimicked if the patient has removed the scales by scrubbing.

Many therapeutic agents can be used to treat this disease successfully; however, it must be appreciated that the causative agent is a normal human saprophyte, and the disorder will recur in predisposed individuals. Appropriate therapy may include one of the following: a selenium sulfide suspension applied for 4 consecutive evenings and repeated the following week; 25% sodium hyposulfite or thiosulfate lotion applied twice daily for 2–4 wk; lotions, ointments, or creams containing 3–6% salicylic acid twice daily for 2–4 wk; haloprogin, miconazole, clotrimazole or ketoconazole twice daily for 2–4 wk. Recurrent episodes continue to respond promptly to the above agents.

23.28 THE DERMATOPHYTOSES

DERMATOPHYTOSES (RINGWORM). These disorders are caused by a group of closely related filamentous fungi with a propensity for invading the stratum corneum, hair, and nails. The three principal genera responsible for dermatophyte infections are *Trichophyton, Microsporum*, and *Epidermophyton*. The *Trichophyton* species cause lesions of all keratinized tissue, including skin, nails, and hair; the *Microsporum* species principally invade the hair; and the *Epidermophyton* species invade the intertriginous skin. The dermatophytic infections are designated by the word tinea followed by the Latin word for the anatomic site of involvement. The dermatophytes are also classified according to source and natural habitat. Fungi acquired from the soil are called *geophilic*, those from animals, *zoophilic*; dermatophytes acquired from humans are referred to as *anthropophilic*. *Epidermophyton* infections are transmitted only by humans, but various species of *Trichophyton* and *Microsporum* can be acquired from both human and nonhuman sources.

Anthropophilic dermatophytes apparently elicit delayed-type hypersensitivity in the infected host; some dermatophytes, most notably the zoophilic species, tend to elicit a more severe, suppurative inflammation in humans. Some degree of resistance to reinfection apparently is acquired by most infected persons and may be associated with a positive delayed hypersensitivity response. Humoral immunity to dermatophytes can be detected by serologic techniques, but no relationship between antibody and resistance to infection has been demonstrated.

Occasionally, a secondary skin eruption referred to as a **dermatophytid** or **"id" reaction** appears in sensitized individuals and has been attributed to circulating fungal antigens derived from the primary infection. The eruption occurs most frequently on the fingers, hands, and arms and is characterized by grouped papules and vesicles and occasionally by sterile pustules. Symmetric urticarial lesions and a more generalized maculopapular eruption can also occur. Id reactions are most often associated with tinea pedis but also occur with tinea capitis and, in the latter case, most often appear as a generalized papulovesicular follicular eruption.

The important diagnostic procedures for the various dermatophyte diseases include examination of infected hairs with a Wood lamp, microscopic examination of potassium hydroxide (KOH) preparations of infected material, and cultural identification of the etiologic agent. Hairs infected with common *Microsporum* species fluoresce a bright blue-green color; most *Trichophyton*-infected hairs do not fluoresce.

Tinea capitis is a dermatophyte infection of the scalp most often caused by the species *Microsporum canis* or *Trichophyton tonsurans* and much less commonly by other microsporum and trichophyton species. In microsporum and some trichophyton infections, the spores are distributed in a sheath-like fashion around the hair shaft (ectothrix infection), whereas *T. tonsurans* produces an infection within the hair shaft (endothrix).

The clinical presentation of tinea capitis varies with the infecting organism. The pattern produced by *M. audouini* is characterized initially by a small papule at the base of a hair follicle. The infection spreads peripherally, forming an erythematous and scaly circular plaque within which the infected hairs become brittle and broken. Multiple, confluent patches of alopecia develop, and the patient may complain of severe pruritus. Although *M. audouini* infection was formerly the most common type of scalp ringworm, this organism is no longer ubiquitous. Endothrix infections such as those caused by *T. tonsurans* create a pattern known as "black-dot ring-

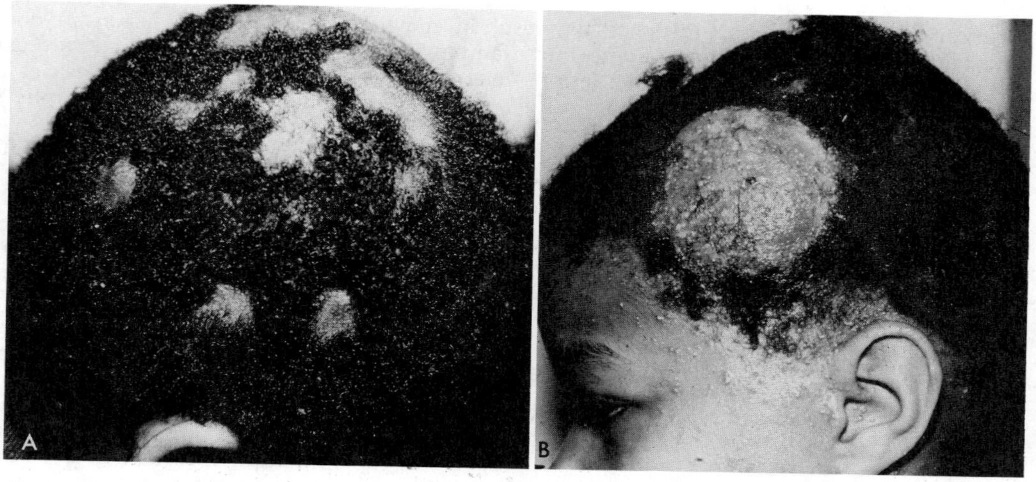

Figure 23–42. *A*, Patchy alopecia associated with tinea capitis. *B*, Elevated, boggy granuloma with multiple pustules (kerion) due to inflammatory tinea capitis.

worm"; it is characterized initially by multiple, small, circular patches with only a few hairs involved; they are broken off close to the hair follicle and create a polka-dot appearance. Diffuse scaling with minimal hair loss secondary to traction is another clinical variant and strongly resembles seborrheic dermatitis. This organism may also produce a chronic and more diffuse alopecia (Fig. 23–42*A*). A severe inflammatory response will produce elevated, boggy granulomatous masses *(kerions)*, which are often studded with sterile pustules (see Fig. 23–42*B*). Permanent scarring and alopecia may result. *Favus*, a form of tinea capitis that is rare in the United States, is caused by the fungus *T. schoenleini*; it is characterized by development of scaly, erythematous patches with yellow, honeycomb-like crust and a dull green fluorescence under the Wood lamp.

M. audouini and *T. tonsurans* are anthropophilic species acquired most often by contact with infected hairs and epithelial cells that are on such surfaces as theater seats, hats, and combs. Dermatophyte spores may also be airborne within the immediate environment, and high carriage rates have been demonstrated in noninfected schoolmates. *M. canis* is a zoophilic species whose preferred hosts are cats and dogs; children acquire it from them.

In microsporum-infected lesions a characteristic bright green fluorescence is seen at the base of each hair on examination with the Wood lamp, whereas lesions caused by *T. tonsurans* fail to fluoresce. Microscopic examination of a KOH preparation of infected hair from the active border of a lesion discloses tiny spores surrounding the hair shaft in microsporum infections and chains of spores within the hair shaft in *T. tonsurans* infections. Fungal elements are usually not seen in scales. A specific etiologic diagnosis of tinea capitis may be obtained by planting broken off infected hairs on Sabouraud medium or Mycosel agar; such identification may require 2 wk or more.

Tinea capitis can be confused with seborrheic dermatitis, psoriasis, alopecia areata, trichotillomania, and certain dystrophic hair disorders. When inflammation is pronounced, as in kerion, primary or secondary bacterial infection must also be considered. In adolescents, the patchy, motheaten type of alopecia associated with secondary syphilis may resemble tinea capitis.

Oral administration of griseofulvin microcrystalline (15 mg/kg/24 hr) is recommended for all forms of tinea capitis. Treatment may be necessary for 8–12 wk and should be terminated only after examination by the Wood lamp or KOH preparation is negative. Adverse reactions to griseofulvin are rare but include nausea, vomiting, headache, blood dyscrasias, phototoxicity, and hepatotoxicity. Oral ketoconazole is an effective alternative medication.

Topical therapy alone is ineffective; it may be an important adjunct because it may decrease the shedding of spores. For this purpose vigorous shampooing with a 2.5% selenium sulfide or zinc pyrithione preparation is helpful. It is not necessary to shave the scalp.

Tinea corporis, or dermatophytic infection of the skin of the face, trunk, and extremities, can be caused by most of the dermatophyte species, although *T. rubrum* and *T. mentagrophytes* are the most prevalent etiologic organisms. In children, infections with *M. canis* are also frequent.

The most typical clinical lesion begins as a dry, mildly erythematous, elevated, scaly papule or plaque and spreads centrifugally as it clears centrally to form the characteristic annular lesion responsible for the designation "ringworm" (Fig. 23–43). At times plaques with advancing borders may spread over large areas. Grouped pustules are another variant. Most lesions clear spontaneously within several months, but some may become chronic. Central clearing does not always

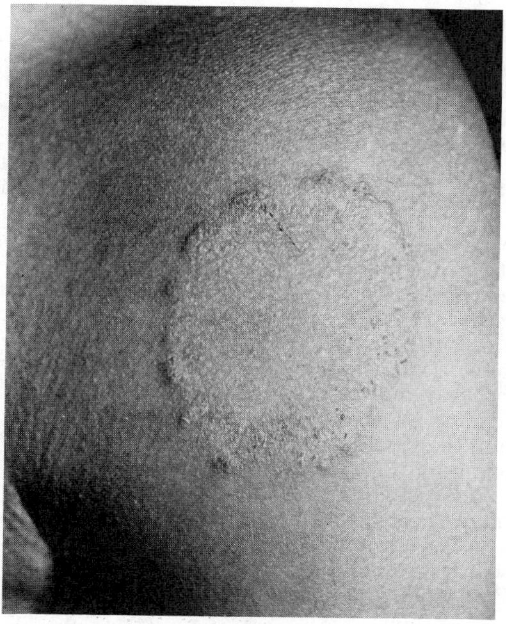

Figure 23–43. Circinate lesion of tinea corporis on the shoulder. Note the active papular border, scaling, and relative clearing centrally.

occur, and differences in host response may result in tremendous variability in the clinical appearance, for example, granulomatous lesions and the kerion-like lesions referred to as **tinea profunda**.

Tinea corporis can be acquired by direct contact with infected persons or by contact with infected scales or hairs deposited on environmental surfaces. *M. canis* infections are usually acquired from infected pets. Not infrequently, a single dermatophyte lesion is responsible for dissemination.

Many skin lesions, both infectious and noninfectious, must be differentiated from the lesions of tinea corporis. Those most frequently confused are granuloma annulare, nummular eczema, pityriasis rosea, psoriasis, seborrheic dermatitis, erythema chronicum migrans, and tinea versicolor. Microscopic examination of KOH wet mount preparations or cultures should always be obtained when fungal infection is considered. Tinea corporis usually does not fluoresce with a Wood lamp.

Tinea corporis will usually respond to treatment with one of the topical antifungal agents (haloprogin, miconazole, clotrimazole, econazole) twice daily for 2–4 wk. In unusually severe or extensive disease, a course of therapy with oral griseofulvin microcrystalline may be required for several weeks.

Tinea cruris, or dermatophyte infection of the groin, occurs most often in adolescent males and is usually caused by the anthropophilic species, *Epidermophyton floccosum* or *T. rubrum*, but occasionally by the zoophilic species *T. mentagrophytes*.

The initial lesion is a small, raised, scaly, erythematous patch on the inner aspect of the thigh that spreads peripherally, often developing multiple tiny vesicles at the advancing margin. It eventually forms bilateral, irregular, sharply bordered patches with hyperpigmented, scaly centers. In some cases, particularly in infections of *T. mentagrophytes*, the inflammatory reaction is more intense, and the infection may spread beyond the crural region. Pruritus may be severe initially but abates as the inflammatory reaction subsides. Bacterial superinfection may alter the clinical appearance, and erythrasma or candidosis may coexist with the dermatophytosis. Tinea cruris is more prevalent in obese persons and in those who perspire excessively and wear tight-fitting clothing.

The diagnosis is confirmed by culture and by demonstrating septate hyphae on a KOH preparation of epidermal scrapings. Tinea cruris must be differentiated from intertrigo, allergic contact dermatitis, candidosis, and erythrasma. Bacterial superinfection must be excluded when there is a severe inflammatory reaction.

The patient should be advised to use a bland absorbent powder and to wear loose cotton underwear. Topical therapy with an imidazole is recommended for severe infection, especially because these agents are effective in mixed candidal-dermatophytic infections. Pure dermatophytic infection may also be treated with haloprogin or tolnaftate.

Tinea pedis (athlete's foot), a dermatophyte infection of the toe webs and soles of the feet, is uncommon in young children but occurs with some frequency in preadolescent and adolescent males. The usual etiologic agents are *T. rubrum*, *T. mentagrophytes*, and *E. floccosum*.

Most commonly the toe webs in the 3rd and 4th interdigital spaces and the subdigital crevice are fissured with maceration and peeling of the surrounding skin. Severe tenderness, itching, and a persistent, foul odor are characteristic. These lesions may become chronic, but they can usually be treated effectively. Less commonly, a chronic, diffuse hyperkeratosis of the sole of the foot occurs with only mild erythema. This type of infection is more refractory to treatment and tends to recur.

An inflammatory, vesicular type of reaction may occur with *T. mentagrophytes* infection; this type is most common in young children. These lesions involve any area of the foot, including the dorsal surface, and are usually circumscribed. The initial papules progress to vesicles and bullae which may become pustular (Fig. 23–44). A number of factors, such as occlusive footwear and warm, humid weather, predispose to infection. The disease may be transmitted in shower facilities and swimming pool areas. Despite its severity, the infection tends to resolve spontaneously.

Tinea pedis must be differentiated from simple maceration and peeling of the interdigital spaces, which is common in children. Infection with *C. albicans* and with a variety of bacterial organisms (erythrasma) may cause confusion or may coexist with primary tinea pedis. Contact dermatitis, dyshidrotic eczema, and atopic dermatitis also simulate tinea pedis. Fungal mycelia can be seen on microscopic examination of a KOH preparation or by culture; the 4th toe web provides a high yield of infected scales; a blister top can also be used.

Simple measures such as avoidance of occlusive footwear, careful drying between the toes after bathing, and the use of an absorbent antifungal powder such as zinc undecylenate may suffice for milder infections. Topical therapy with clotrimazole, miconazole, or econazole is curative in most cases; each of these agents is also effective against candidal infection. Haloprogin and tolnaftate can be used in uncomplicated dermatophyte infections. Several weeks of therapy may be necessary, and low-grade, chronic infections, particularly those caused by *T. rubrum*, may be refractory. In such patients, oral griseofulvin therapy may effect a cure, but recurrences are common.

Tinea unguium is a dermatophyte infection of the nail plate; it occurs most often in patients with tinea pedis, but it may occur as a primary infection. It can be caused by a number of dermatophytes, of which *T. rubrum* and *T. mentagrophytes* are the most common.

The most superficial form of tinea unguium is often due to *T. mentagrophytes*; it is manifested by irregular, single, or multiple white patches on the surface of the nail unassociated with paronychial inflammation or deep infection. *T. rubrum* generally causes a more invasive, subungual infection that is initiated at the lateral distal margins of the nail and is often preceded by mild paronychia. The middle and ventral layers of the nail plate, and perhaps the nail bed, are the sites of

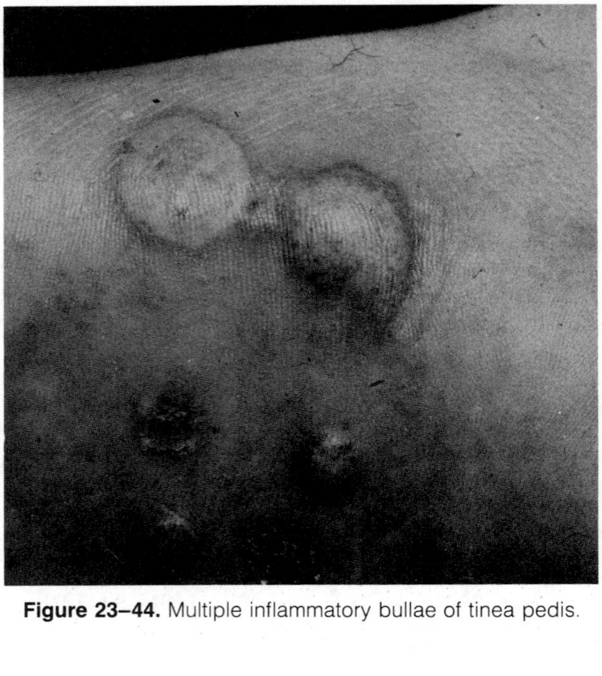

Figure 23–44. Multiple inflammatory bullae of tinea pedis.

infection. The nail initially develops a yellowish discoloration and slowly becomes thickened, brittle, and loosened from the nail bed. In advanced infection the nail may turn dark brown to black and may crack or break off.

Tinea unguium must be differentiated from a variety of dystrophic nail disorders. Changes due to trauma, psoriasis, lichen planus, and eczema can all be confused with tinea unguium. Nails infected with *C. albicans* have several distinguishing features, most prominently the presence of pronounced paronychial swelling. Thin shavings taken from the infected nail, preferably from the deeper areas, should be examined microscopically with KOH and cultured. Repeated attempts may be required to demonstrate the fungus.

Therapy of tinea unguium is frequently disappointing. Prolonged therapy with griseofulvin and the application of topical fungistatic agents to the nail bed may be effective in some cases. Griseofulvin therapy may be required for more than 1 yr and should be reserved for especially severe disease in patients who are motivated to obtain a cure.

Tinea nigra palmaris is a rare but distinctive superficial fungal infection that occurs principally in children and adolescents. It is caused by the dimorphic fungus *Cladosporium wernecki*, which imparts a gray-black color to the affected palm. The characteristic lesion is a well-defined hyperpigmented macule; scaling and erythema are rare, and the lesions are asymptomatic. Tinea nigra is often mistaken for a junctional nevus, melanoma, or staining of the skin by contactants. Treatment with Whitfield ointment, undecylenic acid ointment, or tincture of iodine is most successful.

23.29 CANDIDAL INFECTIONS
(Candidosis, Candidiasis, or Moniliasis)

The dimorphic yeasts of the genus *Candida* are ubiquitous in the environment, but *Candida albicans* is the one that usually causes candidosis in children. This yeast is not a member of the normal skin flora, but it is a frequent transient on skin and may colonize the human alimentary tract and the vagina as a saprophytic organism. Certain environmental conditions, notably elevated temperature and humidity, are associated with an increased frequency of isolation of *C. albicans* from the skin. Many bacterial species inhibit the growth of *C. albicans*, and alteration of normal flora by the use of antibiotics may promote overgrowth of the yeast.

Candidal infections in infants and children may be acute or chronic and localized or generalized; widespread lesions may occur in the newborn infant, in children with an immunodeficiency or with a serious disease of any etiology, and in patients with a multiple endocrinopathy syndrome (Sec. 12.13 and 19.18). Infants and older children with AIDS often present with mucocutaneous candidiasis, which is often difficult to treat with topical agents. In addition to the mucocutaneous lesions, candidosis may occur as a granulomatous process (candidal granuloma).

ORAL CANDIDOSIS (THRUSH) See Sec. 9.75 and 12.13.

VAGINAL CANDIDOSIS (see Sec. 18.51). *C. albicans* is an inhabitant of the adult female vagina in at least 5–10% of women, and vaginal candidosis is not uncommon in adolescent girls. A number of factors can predispose to this infection, including antibiotic therapy, corticosteroid therapy, diabetes mellitus, pregnancy, and the use of oral contraceptives. The infection is manifested by cheesy white plaques on an erythematous vaginal mucosa and by a thick white-yellow discharge. The disease may be relatively mild or may produce pronounced inflammation and scaling of the external genitalia and surrounding skin with progression to vesiculation and ulceration. Patients often complain of severe itching and burning in the vaginal area. The infection may be eradicated by insertion of nystatin or imidazole vaginal tablets, suppositories, creams, or foam. If these products are ineffective, the addition of oral nystatin tablets, 1–2 tablets 3 times daily for 14 days, may eliminate or decrease the candidal population in the gastrointestinal tract.

CONGENITAL CUTANEOUS CANDIDOSIS. See Sec. 9.75.

CANDIDAL DIAPER DERMATITIS. This is a ubiquitous problem in infants and, although relatively benign, is often frustrating because of its tendency to recur. Predisposed infants usually carry *C. albicans* in their intestinal tract, and the warm, moist, occluded skin of the diaper area provides optimal environment for its growth. Usually a seborrheic, atopic, or primary irritant contact dermatitis provides a portal of entry for the yeast.

The primary *clinical manifestation* consists of an intensely erythematous, confluent plaque with a scalloped border and a sharply demarcated edge. It is formed by the confluence of numerous papules and vesicopustules; satellite pustules, those that stud the contiguous skin, are a hallmark of localized candidal infections. Usually the perianal skin, inguinal folds, perineum, and lower abdomen are involved (Fig. 23–45 [color plate section]). In males the entire scrotum and penis may be involved with an erosive balanitis of the perimeatal skin; in females the lesions may be found on the vaginal mucosa as well as on the labia. In some infants the process is generalized, with erythematous lesions distant from the diaper area; in some cases the generalized process may represent a fungal id (hypersensitivity) reaction.

The differential *diagnosis* includes other eruptions of the diaper area that may coexist with candidal infection. For this reason, it is important to establish a diagnosis by a KOH preparation or culture.

Treatment consists of applications of an anticandidal agent (nystatin, miconazole, clotrimazole, ketoconazole) with each diaper change or 4 times daily. Ointments are better tolerated than creams; lotions and creams may cause a burning sensation when applied to irritated skin, and powder may cake and cause erosion from friction during movement. The combination of a corticosteroid and antifungal agent is justified if inflammation is severe but may confuse the situation if the diagnosis is not firmly established. Protection of the diaper area by an application of thick zinc oxide paste overlying the anticandidal preparation may be helpful; the paste is more easily removed with mineral oil than with soap and water. **Fungal id reactions** will gradually abate with successful treatment of the diaper dermatitis or may be treated with a mild corticosteroid preparation. When recurrences of diaper candidosis are frequent, it may be helpful to prescribe a course of oral anticandidal therapy to decrease the yeast population in the gastrointestinal tract. Some infants seem to be receptive hosts for *C. albicans* and may reacquire the organism from a colonized adult.

INTERTRIGINOUS CANDIDOSIS. This occurs most often in the axillae and the groin, under the breasts, under pendulous abdominal fat folds, in the umbilicus, and in the gluteal cleft. Typical lesions are large, confluent areas of moist, denuded, erythematous skin with an irregular, macerated, scaly border. Satellite lesions are characteristic and consist of small vesicles or pustules on an erythematous base. With time, intertriginous candidal lesions may become lichenified, dry, scaly plaques. The lesions develop on skin subjected to irritation and maceration. Candidal superinfection is more likely to occur under conditions that lead to excessive perspiration, especially in obese children and in those with underlying disorders, such as diabetes mellitus.

A similar condition, *interdigital candidosis*, commonly occurs in individuals whose hands are constantly immersed in water; fissures occur between the fingers and have red, denuded centers, with an overhanging, white epithelial fringe. Similar lesions between the toes may be secondary to occlusive footgear.

Treatment is the same as for other candidal infections.

PERIANAL CANDIDOSIS. Perianal dermatitis is caused by irritation of the skin from occlusion, constant moisture, poor hygiene, anal fissures, and pruritus due to pinworm infestation. It may become superinfected with *C. albicans*, especially in children who are receiving oral antibiotic or corticosteroid medication. The involved skin becomes erythematous, macerated, and excoriated, and the lesions are identical to those of candidal intertrigo or candidal diaper rash. Application of a topical antifungal agent in conjunction with improved hygiene is usually effective. Underlying disorders such as pinworm infection must also be treated.

CANDIDAL PARONYCHIA AND ONYCHIA. These disorders are characterized by tender, erythematous swellings at the base of the nails (posterior nail fold) that occasionally discharge purulent material. If the lesion becomes chronic, the nail is secondarily invaded and becomes brittle and thickened, initially in the proximal portion but subsequently over the entire nail plate. The nail may develop a brownish discoloration and prominent transverse ridges or grooves, or it may be completely destroyed. Associated infection with *Pseudomonas* imparts a green color to the nail plate, particularly at the lateral margins.

This type of onychia is more common on the fingers, particularly in thumb-sucking children and in those whose hands are frequently immersed in water. The candidal paronychia is often mistaken for a dermatophyte infection, which is rare in children and has different clinical characteristics. It may also be confused with bacterial paronychia. *C. albicans* can usually be cultured from the posterior nail fold and can often be identified on a KOH preparation of nail scrapings or a Gram stain of exudate. Effective management necessitates keeping the finger as dry as possible and applying nystatin, miconazole, or clotrimazole 3 times daily for weeks to months, until the nail plate grows out normally.

CANDIDAL GRANULOMA. This is a rare response to an invasive candidal infection of skin. Clinically the lesions appear as crusted, verrucous plaques and horn-like projections on the scalp, face, and distal limbs. Affected patients may have single or multiple defects in immune mechanisms and are often refractory to topical therapy. When topical antifungal agents prove ineffective, a systemic anticandidal agent may be required for palliation or eradication of the infection.

23.30 CUTANEOUS VIRAL INFECTIONS

WARTS (VERRUCAE). All types of warts are caused by DNA viruses in the papillomavirus group; those that infect humans are not readily transmissible to animals. Warts can affect the skin and the mucous membranes, including the larynx (laryngeal papillomas). Histologically, the various types of verrucae differ in minor ways, but the basic changes consist of hyperplasia of the epidermal cells and vacuolization of the spinous keratinocytes, which may contain basophilic intranuclear inclusions (viral particles). Parakeratosis (retained stratum corneum cell nuclei), papillomatosis, and eosinophilic cytoplasmic inclusions thought to represent altered keratohyalin are additional variable histologic changes.

The incidence of all types of warts is highest in children and adolescents. The warts are probably transferred by direct contact, although transmission by contaminated fomites is possible. Incubation periods range from 1 to 8 mo. Once acquired, warts are spread by autoinoculation. Antibodies occur in response to infection but appear to have little protective effect.

Clinical Manifestations. *Common warts (verruca vulgaris)* occur most frequently on the fingers, dorsum of the hands, paronychial areas, face, knees, and elbows. They are well-circumscribed papules with a roughened, keratotic, irregular surface. When the surface is pared away, multiple black dots representing thrombosed dermal capillary loops are often visible. Periungual warts are less sharply circumscribed and often painful and may spread beneath the nail plate, separating it from the nail bed.

Filiform warts are frequently located on the face or neck; the lesion is a single projection of several millimeters that has a sharply circumscribed base. The digitate wart is a related morphologic type of verruca that is often found on the scalp and neck. It has multiple projections from a sessile base.

Plantar warts, although essentially similar to the common wart, are usually flush with the surface of the sole because of the constant pressure from weight bearing. Similar lesions (palmar) can also occur on the palms. They are sharply demarcated, often with a ring of thick callus. The surface keratotic material must sometimes be removed before the boundaries of the wart can be appreciated; in contrast to calluses, warts obliterate normal skin markings. Several contiguous warts may fuse to form a large plaque, the so-called mosaic wart. Plantar warts may be exceedingly painful.

Juvenile flat warts (verruca plana) are slightly elevated, minimally hyperkeratotic papules that usually remain less than 3 mm in size and vary in color from pink to brown. They may occur in profusion on the face, arms, dorsum of the hands, and knees. The distribution of multiple lesions along a line of scratch is a helpful diagnostic feature. Lesions may be disseminated in the beard area by shaving and from the hairline onto the scalp by combing the hair.

Condylomata acuminata (mucous membrane warts) are moist, fleshy, papillomatous lesions that occur on the perianal mucosa (Fig. 23–46), the labia, vaginal introitus, and perineal raphe and on the shaft, corona, and glans penis. They may occasionally obstruct the urethral meatus or the vaginal introitus. Because they are located in intertriginous areas, they may become moist and friable. When untreated, condylomata proliferate and become confluent, at times forming large cauliflower-like masses. Condylomata acuminata can be transmitted with or without sexual contact and are often referred to as venereal warts. These lesions in prepubertal children

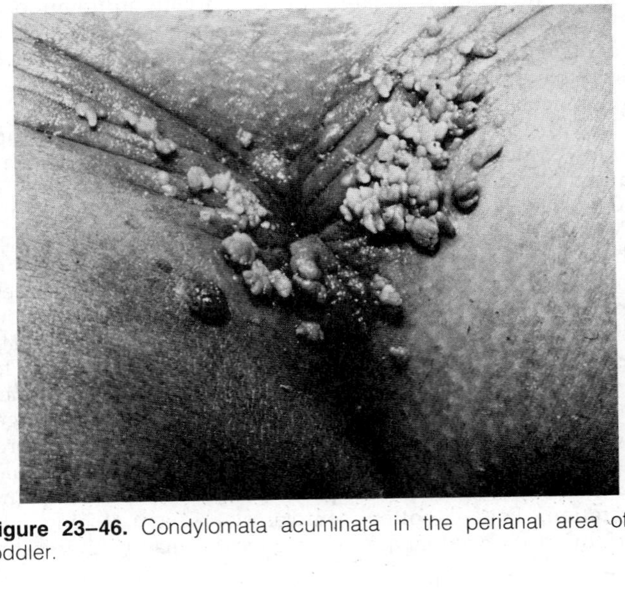

Figure 23–46. Condylomata acuminata in the perianal area of a toddler.

suggest sexual abuse. Lesions can also occur on the lips, gingivae, and tongue. Cervical infections with these viruses may become latent and are associated with cervical cancer.

Differential Diagnosis. Common warts are most often confused with molluscum contagiosum. Plantar and palmar warts may be difficult to distinguish from punctate keratoses, corns, and calluses. Juvenile flat warts mimic lichen planus, lichen nitidus, adenoma sebaceum, syringomas, milia, and acne papules. Condylomata acuminata may resemble condylomata lata of secondary syphilis.

Treatment. A variety of therapeutic measures are effective in the treatment of warts. More than 50% of warts will disappear spontaneously within 2 yr, but failure to treat incurs the risk of spread to other sites. Warts are epidermal lesions and do not produce scarring unless they are managed surgically or treated in an overly aggressive fashion. Hyperkeratotic lesions (common, plantar, and palmar warts) are more responsive to therapy if the excess keratotic debris is gently pared with a scalpel only until thrombosed capillaries are apparent; further paring will induce bleeding.

Common warts can be destroyed by light electrodesiccation and curettage or by applications of liquid nitrogen or cantharidin. Daily applications of 10–17% lactic acid and 10–17% salicylic acid in flexible collodion is a slow but painless method of removal. Filiform, digitate, and periungual warts respond best to liquid nitrogen. Plantar and palmar warts may be treated with cantharidin, liquid nitrogen, salicylic and lactic acids in collodion, or 40% salicylic acid plasters. After prolonged soaking keratotic debris can be removed by an emery board or pumice stone. Occlusive taping for several days may also be effective. Condylomata respond best to weekly applications of 25% podophyllin in tincture of benzoin; the medication should be left on the warts for 4–6 hr and then removed by bathing. Condylomata localized to keratinized sites (e.g., buttocks) may not respond to podophyllin. Resistant lesions can usually be eradicated by weekly freezing with liquid nitrogen or by treatment with a CO_2 laser. Although intralesion injection of 1 million units of α- or β-interferon, 3 times/wk for 3–4 wk, appears to be effective against condylomata, the Centers for Disease Control does not recommend it because of a low incidence of effectiveness, high toxicity rate, and high cost. With all types of therapy, extreme care should be taken to protect the surrounding normal skin from irritation.

MOLLUSCUM CONTAGIOSUM. This common cutaneous viral infection is caused by a DNA virus, the largest member of the poxvirus group and the largest true virus that infects humans. The disease is acquired by direct contact with an infected person or from fomites and is spread by autoinoculation. The incubation period is estimated to be 2–8 wk.

Clinical Manifestations. The lesions are discrete, pearly, skin-colored, dome-shaped papules varying in size from 1 to 5 mm; typically they have central umbilication from which a plug of cheesy material can be expressed (Fig. 23–47). The papules may occur anywhere on the body, but the face, eyelids, neck, axillae, and thighs are sites of predilection. They may be found in clusters on the genitalia or in the groin of adolescents and may be associated with other venereal diseases in sexually active individuals. Mucosal lesions occur occasionally. An eczematous dermatitis may obscure the molluscum papules.

Diagnosis. Although biopsy is not indicated, an appreciation of the histologic pattern of the lesions is helpful diagnostically. The molluscum papule consists of a lobulated adhesive mass of virus-infected epidermal cells that degenerate gradually as they move upward from basal layer to stratum corneum. The eosinophilic viral inclusions become more prominent as the cells reach the surface and pack the cytoplasm. The central plug of material that represents these virus-laden cells (molluscum bodies) may be shelled out from a lesion (see later) and examined under the microscope with 10% KOH or with Wright or Giemsa stain. The rounded, cup-shaped mass of homogeneous cells, often with identifiable lobules, is diagnostic.

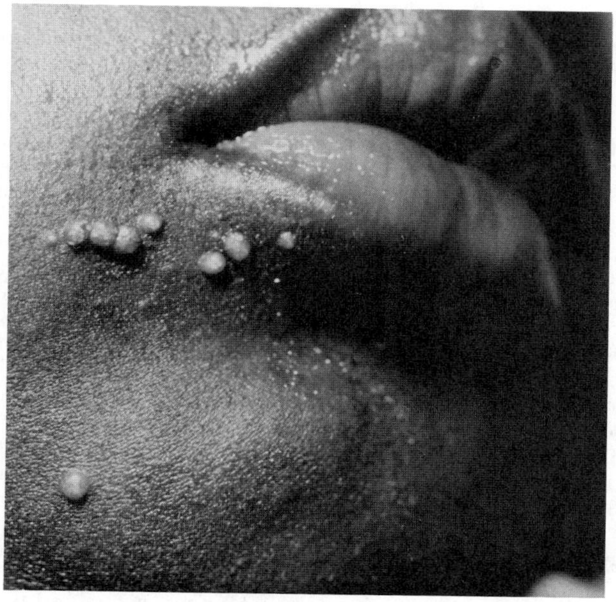

Figure 23–47. Grouped papules of molluscum contagiosum on the face.

Treatment. Molluscum contagiosum is a self-limited disease, but lesions can persist for months to years, can be spread to distant sites, and may be transmitted to others. It is therefore advisable to eradicate the lesions in all infected children. It is mandatory to treat children who also have atopic dermatitis or an immunodeficiency because the infection may spread rapidly and produce hundreds of lesions. The papules can be destroyed by expressing the plug with a needle, a sharp curette, a comedo extractor, or a curved forceps; the base of the lesion can be touched with iodine. Brief application of liquid nitrogen is also very effective. Cantharidin 0.9% may be applied to each lesion without occlusion and frequently causes enough inflammation to facilitate spontaneous extrusion of the plug. Molluscum is an epidermal disease and should not be overtreated so that scarring results.

23.31 INSECT BITES AND PARASITIC INFESTATIONS

INSECT BITES

Insect bites are a common affliction of children and usually pose no problem in diagnosis. Occasionally, the patient is unaware of the source of the lesions or denies being bitten; in these cases, precise interpretation of the eruption may be difficult. Insect bites may occur as solitary, multiple, or profuse lesions but, when numerous, are usually grouped because of the tendency of a single insect to inflict several bites in a localized area.

Clinical Manifestations. The type of reaction that occurs depends on the species of insect and the age group and reactivity of the human host. Infants often display no reaction, young children manifest only a delayed hypersensitivity reaction, and older children experience both an immediate and a delayed reaction. By adolescence or adulthood, the delayed component of the insect bite reaction is lost, and the host responds only with an immediate reaction, which is characterized by an evanescent, erythematous wheal. A central punctum is usually visible, but the punctum may disappear as the lesion ages, and, if edema is marked, the wheal may be surmounted by a tiny vesicle. Certain beetles produce bullous lesions through the action of cantharidin, and hemorrhagic lesions may be caused by a variety of insects including beetles and spiders. Delayed hypersensitivity reactions to insect bites are characterized by firm persistent papules that may become hyperpigmented and are often excoriated and crusted. Pruritus may be mild or severe, transient or persistent. The reaction is a response to introduction of insect toxins and antigens into the tissues. Severe hypersensitivity reactions that result from certain types of bites and stings are discussed in Chapters 11 and 26.

Treatment. Acute local reactions may be ameliorated by cool water compresses followed by application of a soothing shake lotion such as calamine, to which 0.25% menthol and 0.5% phenol can be added. Topical corticosteroids can also be helpful for control of pruritus. If lesions are extensive and extremely pruritic, an oral antihistamine may provide some relief. Topical antihistamines are potent sensitizers and have no role in the treatment of insect bite reactions or other skin diseases. Insect repellents containing diethyl-meta-toluamide (DEET) or ethyl hexanediol may afford moderate protection against mosquitoes, fleas, flies, chiggers, and ticks but are relatively ineffective against wasps, bees, and spiders.

PAPULAR URTICARIA. This is a persistent, annoying eruption that occurs principally in the 1st decade of life and appears to represent a delayed hypersensitivity reaction to the bites of insects, the most common of which are species of fleas and mites, bedbugs, gnats, mosquitoes, and animal lice. The disorder is most prevalent during the warmer months.

Typical lesions are firm, hyperpigmented, intensely pruritic, discrete papules which cluster mainly on the trunk and extensor surfaces of the extremities (Fig. 23–48). The initial and acute lesion may be an urticarial wheal that in turn is replaced by a papule. When new lesions are acquired, quiescent papules may flare and become erythematous and edematous. A central punctum is visible initially; however, when the lesions become severely excoriated, central crusting or a secondary pyoderma can obscure the typical morphologic aspects.

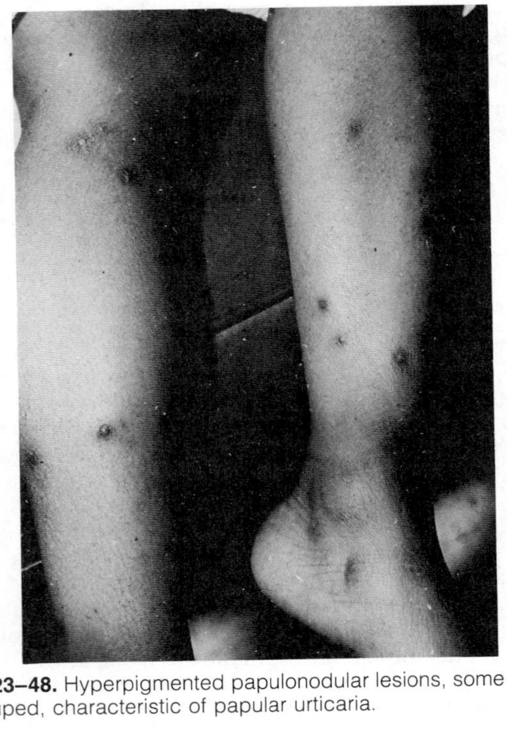

Figure 23–48. Hyperpigmented papulonodular lesions, some of which are grouped, characteristic of papular urticaria.

It is important to *identify the etiologic agent*. The nature of the eruption may not be suspected because older family members are usually not afflicted. When it is appreciated that papular urticaria represents a delayed hypersensitivity reaction to insect bites and that this phenomenon is age related, the sparing of others in the household becomes explicable.

Papular urticaria can be confused with papular exanthems, varicella, and scabies. The histologic changes are relatively nonspecific; they consist of dermal edema and a mixed inflammatory perivascular infiltrate. At times, however, the dermal cellular infiltrate is so dense that a lymphoma or foreign body reaction may be suspected.

Treatment is directed at alleviation of pruritus by oral antihistamines, cool compresses, soothing lotions, and topical corticosteroid creams or lotions for the more annoying lesions. An effort should be made to identify and eradicate the etiologic agent: pets should be carefully inspected; crawl spaces, eaves, and other sites of the house or outbuildings frequented by animals and birds should be decontaminated because insects such as fleas can survive for many months without feeding; baseboard crevices, mattresses, rugs, furniture, and animal sleeping quarters should also be sprayed with insecticide.

PARASITIC INFESTATIONS

SCABIES. This infection is caused by the itch mite *Sarcoptes scabiei* var. *hominis*. Scabies is transmitted by direct contact with infected persons and only rarely by fomites because the isolated mite dies within 2–3 days.

Clinical Manifestations. The intensely pruritic eruption consists of wheals, papules, vesicles, thread-like burrows, and a superimposed eczematous dermatitis. In older children and adolescents the clinical pattern is similar to that in adults; preferred sites are the interdigital spaces, wrists, elbows, ankles, buttocks, umbilicus, groin, genitalia, areolae, and axillae (Fig. 23–49*A*). The head, neck, palms and soles are generally spared. In infants, bullae and pustules are relatively common; burrows may be absent, and the palms, soles (see Fig. 23–49*B*), face, and scalp are often affected. Red-brown nodules, most often located in the axillae and groin and on the genitalia, are a less common variant. All lesions are extremely pruritic, particularly at night; scratching inevitably results in eczematization, excoriation, and secondary pyoderma, which may mask the true nature of the disorder.

Etiology and Pathogenesis. The adult female mite measures approximately 0.4 mm in length and has four sets of legs and a hemispherical body marked by transverse corrugations and brown spines and bristles on the dorsal surface. The male mite is approximately half her size and is similar in configuration. After fertilization on the skin surface, the gravid female burrows into the stratum corneum and gradually extends this tract as she deposits 1–3 oval eggs daily and numerous brown fecal pellets (scybala). When egg-laying is completed in 4–5 wk, she dies within the burrow. The eggs hatch in 3–5 days, releasing larvae that grow and molt into nymphs on the skin surface. Maturity is achieved in about 2–3 wk. Mating occurs, and the gravid female invades the skin to complete the life cycle.

Diagnosis. This is made by microscopic identification of mites (see Fig. 23–49C), ova, and scybala in epithelial debris.

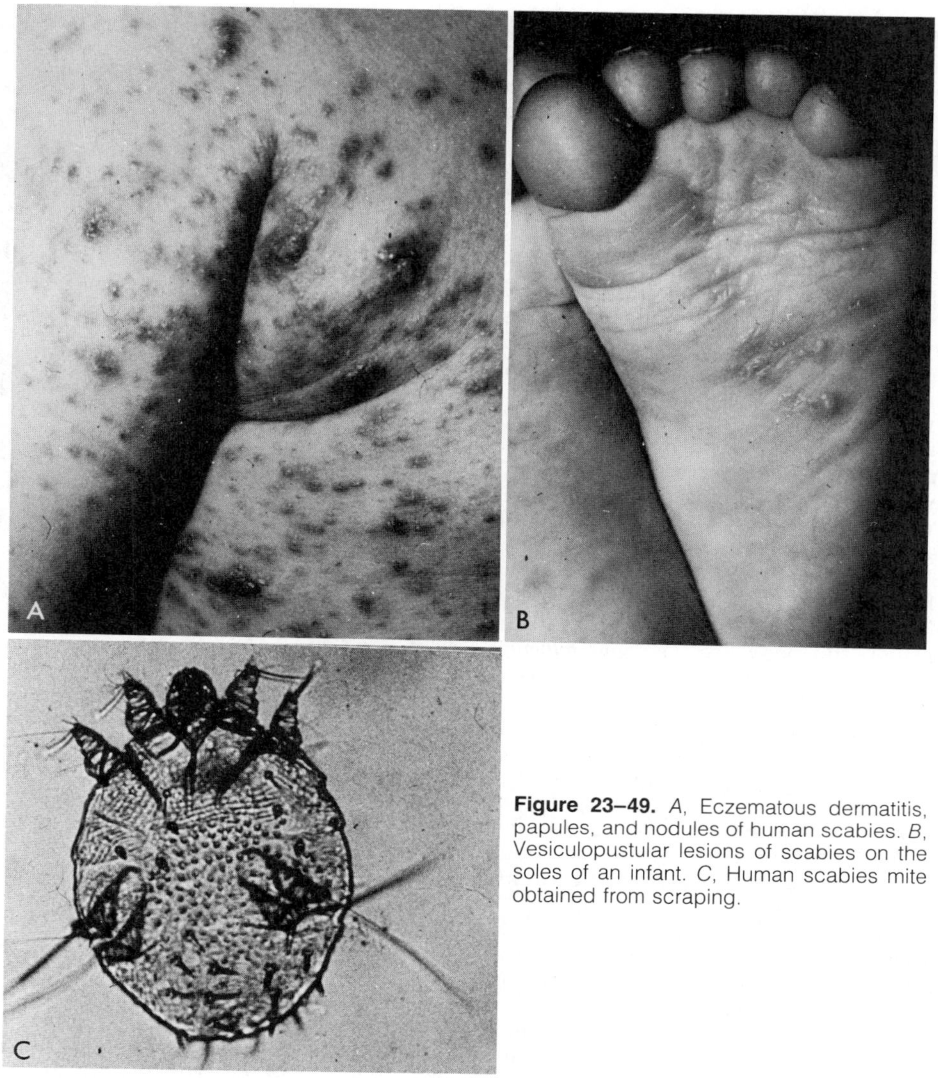

Figure 23–49. *A*, Eczematous dermatitis, papules, and nodules of human scabies. *B*, Vesiculopustular lesions of scabies on the soles of an infant. *C*, Human scabies mite obtained from scraping.

Scrapings are most often positive when obtained from burrows, eczematous lesions, or fresh papules. The most reliable method is application of a drop of mineral oil on the selected lesion, vigorous scraping of it with a dull-edged instrument, and transfer of the oil and scrapings to a glass slide. The mite can be detected microscopically by its movement.

The *differential diagnosis* depends on the types of lesions present. Burrows are virtually pathognomonic for human scabies. Papulovesicular lesions are confused with papular urticaria, canine scabies, chickenpox, viral exanthems, drug eruptions, dermatitis herpetiformis, and folliculitis. Eczematous lesions may mimic atopic dermatitis and seborrheic dermatitis, and the less common bullous disorders of childhood may be suspected in the infant with predominantly bullous lesions. Nodular scabies is frequently misdiagnosed as urticaria pigmentosa, histiocytosis X, and insect bite granuloma.

Treatment. Application of 1% gamma benzene hexachloride cream or lotion to the entire body from the neck down, with particular attention to intensely involved areas, has been standard therapy. The medication is left on the skin for 8–12 hr, and if necessary it may be reapplied in 1 wk for another 8–12 hr period. The vulnerability of small infants to percutaneous absorption of this potentially neurotoxic substance should dictate extreme caution in prescribing it for them. A shorter application time (6–8 hr) is less hazardous for infants under 1 yr of age. Permethrin 5% cream (Elimite) is an equally effective scabicide now widely available for use in children over 2 mo of age. It is poorly absorbed, rapidly metabolized by tissue esterases and, therefore, of very low toxicity. For infants less than 6 mo, as well as older individuals, alternative therapy includes 10% crotamiton cream or lotion applied daily for 5 consecutive days or 6% sulfur in petrolatum applied for three consecutive 24 hr periods. Pruritus, which is due to hypersensitivity to mite antigens, may persist for a number of days and may be alleviated by a topical corticosteroid preparation. Nodules are extremely resistant to treatment and may take several months to resolve. Persistent pruritus may not reflect inadequate treatment because the hypersensitivity reaction to the mite may outlast the presence of live parasites. The entire family should be treated as well as caretakers of the infested child. A latent period of approximately 1 mo follows infestation, so that itching may be absent and lesions relatively inapparent in contacts who are asymptomatic carriers. Clothing, bed linens, and towels should be thoroughly laundered.

Norwegian scabies, a variant of human scabies, is highly contagious and occurs mainly in institutions among mentally and physically debilitated patients. Affected individuals are infested by myriads of mites which inhabit the crusts and exfoliating scales of the skin and scalp lesions. The nails may become thickened and dystrophic and are densely populated by mites. Management is extremely difficult; it requires scrupulous isolation measures and repeated but careful applications of antiscabetic preparations.

Canine scabies is caused by *Sarcoptes scabiei* var. *canis*, the dog mite that is associated with mange. The eruption in the human, which is most frequently acquired by cuddling an infested puppy, consists of tiny papules, vesicles, wheals, and excoriated eczematous plaques. Burrows are not present because the mite infrequently inhabits human stratum corneum. The rash is pruritic and has a predilection for the arms, chest, and abdomen, the usual sites of contact. Onset is sudden and usually follows exposure by 1–10 days, possibly resulting from development of a hypersensitivity reaction to mite antigens. Recovery of mites or ova from scrapings of human skin is rare. The disease is self-limited in humans, but removal or treatment of the infested animal is necessary. Symptomatic therapy for itching is helpful. In the rare cases in which mites are demonstrated in scrapings from the affected child, they can be eradicated by the same measures applicable to human scabies.

PEDICULOSIS. Three types of lice are obligate parasites of the human host: pubic or crab lice *(Phthirus pubis)*, head lice *(Pediculus humanus capitis)*, and body lice *(Pediculus humanus corporis)*. Only the body louse is a vector for pathogens of human disease (typhus, trench fever, relapsing fever). Body and head lice are related and have similar physical characteristics; they are about 2–4 mm in length, whereas pubic lice have a striking crab-like anatomy and are only 1–2 mm in length. Female lice live for approximately 1 mo and deposit up to 10 eggs daily on the human host. Ova hatch in 1 wk and require another week to mature. Both nymphs and adult lice feed on human blood, injecting their salivary juices into the host and depositing their fecal matter on the skin.

Pediculosis pubis is usually encountered in adolescents, although small children may acquire pubic lice on the eyelashes by close contact with an infested individual. Patients experience moderate to severe pruritus and may develop a secondary pyoderma from scratching. Maculae caeruleae (blue spots) may appear in the pubic area and on the abdomen and thighs; they are thought to represent altered blood pigments or excretion from the salivary gland of the louse. Oval, translucent nits, which are firmly attached to the hair shafts, may be visible to the naked eye or may be readily identified by a hand lens or by microscopic examination (Fig. 23–50). Adult lice are occasionally detected.

Because the pubic louse may occasionally wander or be transferred to other sites on fomites, terminal hair on the trunk, thighs, axillary region, beard area, and eyelashes should be examined for nits. The patient also should be checked for manifestations of other venereal diseases.

Infestation may be effectively treated by a 10 min application of a pyrethrin preparation. Retreatment may be required in 7–10 days. Nits can be removed with a fine-tooth comb. The shampoo form of lindane, which requires a 5-min application time, is an alternative choice. Lindane cream and lotion are no longer recommended for treatment of pubic lice. Infestation of eyelashes is eradicated by petrolatum applied 3–5 times/day for 8–10 days. A less safe but effective alternative is 0.25% physostigmine ophthalmic ointment applied twice daily for 8–10 days. Pubic lice survive for only a short time when separated from the host; nevertheless, clothing, towels, and bed linens may be contaminated with nit-bearing hairs and should be thoroughly laundered or dry-cleaned.

Pediculosis corporis is rare in children except under conditions of poor hygiene, because the parasite is transmitted mainly on contaminated clothing or bedding. The lesions consist of papules, wheals, excoriations, secondary eczematization, and pyoderma; itching is intense in all stages. Lice are found on the skin only when they are feeding; at other times they inhabit the seams of clothing, which are also a repository for nits. Therapy consists of improved hygiene and laundering or boiling all infested clothing and bedding. Gamma benzene hexachloride or permethrin can be used to eradicate nits on body hair.

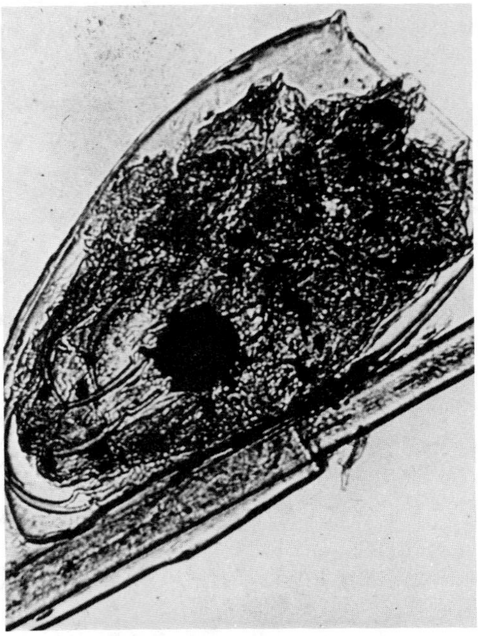

Figure 23–50. Intact nit on a human hair.

Pediculosis capitis is responsible for intense pruritus, and the infestation may be complicated by secondary pyoderma and lymphadenopathy. Pediculi are not always visible, but nits are detectable on the hairs, most commonly in the occipital region and above the ears. Dermatitis may also be noted on the neck and pinnae. Head lice can be transmitted on infested clothing, combs, brushes, and furniture or by direct human contact.

The treatment of choice is permethrin 1% cream rinse applied for 10 min with a repeat application in 10–14 days. Alternative treatments include natural pyrethrin shampoos and 1% gamma benzene hexachloride for 4 min with a repeat application in 10–14 days. All household members should be treated at the same time. Nits can be removed with a fine-tooth comb after a 1:1 vinegar-water rinse or, if tenacious, following application of a creme rinse containing 8% formic acid (stept 2), which dissolves the chitin attaching the nits to the hair shafts. Clothing and bed linens should be laundered in very hot water or dry-cleaned; brushes and combs should be discarded or coated with a pediculicide for 15 min and then thoroughly cleaned in boiling water.

CREEPING ERUPTION. See Sec. 12.126.

23.32 ACNE

ACNE VULGARIS. The appearance of this type of acne is often regarded as a physiologic event because it occurs almost universally during adolescence and frequently persists into adulthood. It is a self-limited inflammatory process of the pilosebaceous unit, and is somewhat more common in males. For girls the incidence peaks between 14 and 17 yr of age, for boys between 16 and 19 yr. Genetic factors probably play some role, but no clear-cut patterns of transmission are evident.

Pathology. The lesions of acne vulgaris develop in sebaceous follicles; these appendicular structures have a large, multilobular sebaceous gland and a wide follicular canal containing a rudimentary hair. The primary histologic alteration appears to be abnormal keratinization of the epithelium in the duct with impaction of the keratinized cells within the lumen. The initial lesions are *comedones,* which are impactions of lamellated keratinous material containing lipid and bacteria. Two types are recognized: open comedones, known as blackheads, and closed comedones, called whiteheads. A patulous pilosebaceous orifice permits visualization of the plug (open comedo). Open comedones are presumed to be mature lesions because they less commonly become inflammatory. The closed comedo has only a pinpoint opening and represents a follicular sac filled with densely aggregated keratinous material, lipids, and bacteria.

Inflammatory papules and nodules develop from comedones in which the follicular epithelium has ruptured and extruded the follicular contents into the subjacent dermis, where a neutrophilic inflammatory response is induced. Suppuration and an occasional giant cell reaction to the keratin and hair are the cause of nodulocystic lesions; these are not true cysts but liquefied masses of inflammatory debris.

Etiology and Pathogenesis. The cause of acne vulgaris is not fully known, but certain aspects of the pathogenesis are understood. A functionally mature sebaceous gland is fundamental. At puberty, the sebaceous gland enlarges and sebum production increases in response to the increased activities of testicular, ovarian, and adrenal androgens. Adolescents with extensive acne usually have increased sebum production. There may also be a local tissue abnormality of testosterone metabolism.

Freshly formed sebum consists of a mixture of lipids with a predominance of triglycerides. Normal follicular bacteria convert sebum triglycerides to free fatty acids, and those of medium chain length (C8–C14) may be one of the minor provocative factors in initiating an inflammatory reaction. There is also evidence that free fatty acids may stimulate formation of comedones.

The sebaceous follicles are colonized by organisms of three types: an anaerobic diphtheroid, *Propionibacterium acnes*; coagulase-negative *S. epidermidis*; and a dimorphic yeast, *Pityrosporon ovale*. Each of these organisms possesses lipolytic enzymes; however, *P. acnes* appears to be largely responsible for the formation of free fatty acids. It is probable that bacterial proteases, hyaluronidases, chemotactic factors, and hydrolytic enzymes released from neutrophils play significant roles in eliciting an inflammatory reaction.

Clinical Manifestations. Acne vulgaris is characterized by four basic types of lesions: open and closed comedones, papules, pustules, and nodulocystic lesions. The last may be firm and indolent, resembling true cysts, or fluctuant or draining, resembling furuncles. Pitted, atrophic or hypertrophic scars may be interspersed, depending on the severity and chronicity of the process. One or more types of lesions may predominate whether acne is mild or severe. Lesions may be confined to the face or may also involve the chest, upper back, and deltoid areas. A predominance of lesions on the forehead, particularly closed comedones, is often attributable to prolonged use of greasy hair preparations (pomade acne). Marked involvement on the trunk is most often seen in males. The diagnosis is rarely difficult, although flat warts, folliculitis, and other types of acne may be confused with acne vulgaris.

Treatment. There is no evidence that early treatment will prevent the emergence of acne lesions; however, acne can be controlled and severe scarring prevented by judicious therapy maintained until the disease process has spontaneously abated.

It is important to establish rapport with the adolescent patient and to explain the basic pathogenetic events in clear language. Parents should be included in discussions because their misconceptions about acne may lead to needless harassment of the afflicted adolescent.

General Measures. Diet plays *no* significant role in the pathogenesis of the usual case of acne. There is little evidence that ingestion of particular foods can trigger acne flares. When a patient is convinced that certain dietary items exacerbate acne, it is permissible to omit those foods; it is unnecessary, however, to impose unwarranted restrictions on most teenagers. A balanced diet should be encouraged for reasons of general health.

Climate appears to influence acne in that improvement frequently occurs during the summer months, and flares are more common during the wintertime. Remission during summer may relate, in part, to the relative absence of stress. Emotional tension and fatigue seem to exacerbate acne in many individuals.

Additional factors that should be discussed are cleansing, cosmetics, hair preparations, and facial manipulation. Cleansing with soap and water removes surface lipid and renders the skin less oily in appearance, but there is no evidence that surface lipid is harmful in acne. Only minimal drying and peeling are achieved by cleansing; repetitive cleansing can be harmful because it irritates and chaps the skin. Greasy cosmetic and hair preparations must be discontinued because they will exacerbate pre-existing acne and cause further plugging of follicular pores. Manipulation and squeezing of facial lesions will serve only to rupture intact lesions and provoke localized inflammatory reactions.

Topical Therapy. Cleansing agents that contain keratolytic agents, such as sulfur, salicylic acid, and benzoyl peroxide, may exert a mild drying and peeling effect and are acceptable if tolerated. Cleansers containing abrasives probably provide little additional help and may be excessively drying and irritating. There is no evidence that preparations containing alcohol or hexachlorophene decrease acne, because surface bacteria are not involved in the pathogenesis.

Topical lotions, creams, and gels containing sulfur, salicylic acid, and resorcinol may be added for additional mild keratolytic effect. Tinted preparations intended to replace cosmetics often mismatch normal skin color and highlight rather than mask the lesions.

The most effective topical preparations, particularly for comedones and papulopustular acne, include the benzoyl peroxide gels and retinoic acid. Benzoyl peroxide is an organic peroxide and oxidizing agent that dries and peels the skin and suppresses growth of *P. acnes*. Preparations are available in concentration of 2½%, 5%, and 10% (e.g., Desquam-X, Benzac, PanOxyl) and may be applied as a thin film once or twice daily as tolerated. Water-based gels are less irritating than alcohol-based gels for patients with sensitive skin. Retinoic acid (Retin-A) affects keratinization in the sebaceous follicle by increasing turnover of epidermal cells and by decreasing the cohesiveness of the squamous cells; it thus aids in elimination of the keratinous plug. Some erythema and peeling may be expected, and pustular flares due to rupture of microcomedones are common. Retinoic acid may be applied once daily, 30 min after washing, in the form best tolerated (0.025% gel; 0.01% gel; 0.1% cream; 0.05% cream, 0.025% cream, in decreasing order of potency). Increased sensitivity to sunlight may occur, and a sunscreen should be provided until partial tanning has occurred.

Topical antibiotics in a vehicle appropriate for use in patients with acne include clindamycin (Cleocin-T) or erythromycin (T-Stat, ATS) and may be applied once or twice daily.

Although not as effective as orally administered antibiotics, they serve as a useful therapeutic adjunct.

All topical preparations require several weeks for a demonstrable positive effect. They may be used alone or together in selected patients, for example, benzoyl peroxide gel in the morning and retinoic acid at night.

Systemic Therapy. Certain antibiotics, especially tetracycline and erythromycin, have been used in the treatment of papulopustular and nodulocystic acne. These drugs appear to act by suppressing the normal follicular flora, mainly *P. acnes*, and by decreasing the inflammatory reaction. For most patients, initiation of therapy with 1 g/day for 4 wk and gradual decrease in dosage to a maintenance dose of 500 mg/day will be effective. The drugs should always be administered in combination with topical therapy. Patients should be instructed to take the drug between meals and should be forewarned of such side effects as secondary candidal vaginitis and transient nausea. Tetracycline is contraindicated in pregnant adolescents.

Estrogen therapy is appropriate only for young women with premenstrual flares of acne; it is sometimes effective in such circumstances. The hazards of side effects must be considered.

Physical Therapy. Ultraviolet light appears to be beneficial in some patients who tan easily, possibly because of the peeling effect of tanning. It is best provided by natural sunlight. Periodic applications of CO_2 snow or slush for a peeling effect may be therapeutic for some patients. Radiation therapy is contraindicated.

Surgical Therapy. Extraction of open and closed comedones, needle aspiration of nodulocystic lesions, and injection of corticosteroid into acne cysts are additional helpful measures in selected patients. Planing of the skin by dermabrasion to minimize scarring is indicated only after the active process is quiescent. Not all patients, however, will be improved by dermabrasion, and some risks accompany it.

STEROID ACNE. Pubertal and postpubertal patients who are receiving systemic corticosteroid therapy or potent topical steroids are predisposed to steroid-induced acne, a monomorphous folliculitis that occurs on the face, neck, chest (Fig. 23–51*A*), shoulders, upper back, arms, and, rarely, the scalp. Onset follows the initiation of steroid therapy by 2 wk. The lesions are small, erythematous papules or pustules that may erupt in profusion and are all in the same stage of development. Comedones may occur subsequently, but nodulocystic lesions and scarring are rare. Pruritus is occasional. The steroid appears to induce focal degeneration of the follicular epithelium with a localized neutrophilic inflammatory response. Although steroid acne is relatively refractory if there is continued use of the drug, the eruption may respond to use of retinoic acid and a benzoyl peroxide gel.

Endogenous steroid (androgen) production may produce acne in children with congenital adrenal hyperplasia, of which severe acne in adolescence may be the only clinical manifestation. Studies of adrenal function are indicated in appropriate patients (Sec. 19.23).

HALOGEN ACNE. Administration of medications containing iodides or bromides or, rarely, ingestion of massive amounts of vitamin-mineral preparations or iodine-containing "health foods" such as kelp may induce halogen acne. The lesions are often very inflammatory. Discontinuation of the provocative agent and appropriate topical preparations will usually achieve reasonable therapeutic results.

INFANTILE ACNE. Acne vulgaris may occur in infants, principally in males; it has been attributed to a hypersensitive end-organ response to hormones, but the etiology is unknown. Onset may occur within the 1st mo of life, and lesions are confined to the face (see Fig. 23–51*B*). Papules, pustules, and open and closed comedones are usual, but only occasionally do nodulocystic lesions develop; pitted scarring is rare. The course may be relatively brief, or the lesions may persist for many months. Rarely, an unusual exposure to an occlusive ointment, a halogenated compound, or a topical fluorinated corticosteroid may cause the acneiform eruption, and appropriate history should be sought. The use of a mild acne lotion or a benzoyl peroxide gel will usually clear the eruption within a few weeks. There is often a history of severe acne in one or both parents, and the child may be predisposed to more severe acne in adolescence.

TROPICAL ACNE. A severe form of acne occurs in tropical climates and is believed to be due to the intense heat and humidity. Lesions occur mainly on the back, chest, and buttocks, with a predominance of suppurating nodulocystic lesions. Secondary infection with *S. aureus* may be a complication. The eruption is refractory to acne therapy if the environmental factors are not eliminated.

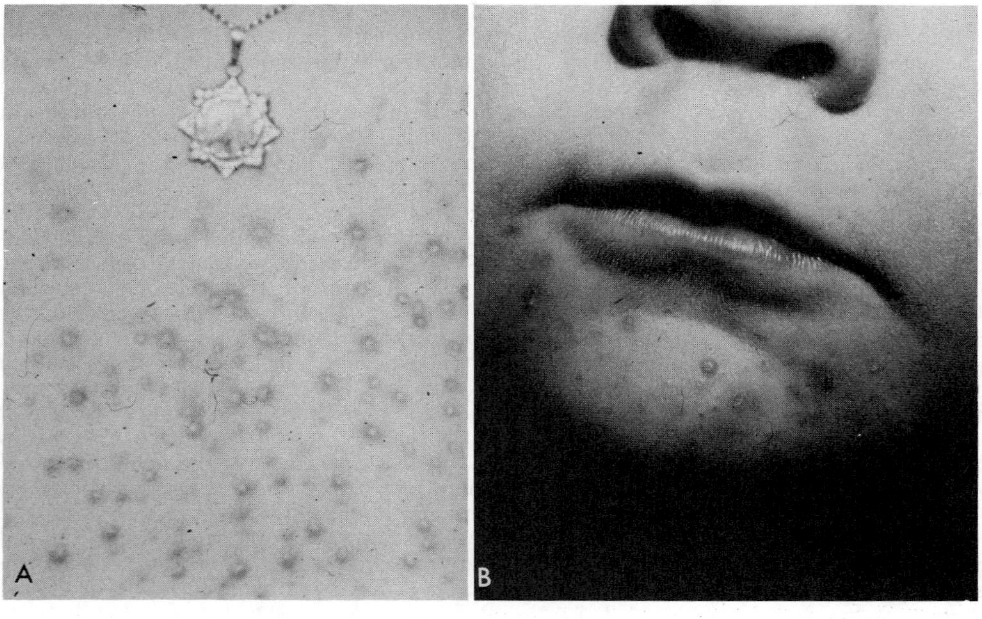

Figure 23–51. *A*, Monomorphous papular eruption of steroid acne. *B*, Acne in a male infant.

ACNE CONGLOBATA. This disorder is a chronic, progressive inflammatory disease that occurs mainly in adult males but may begin during adolescence. Papules, pustules, nodules, cysts, abscesses, sinus tracts, and severe scarring are characteristic. The face is relatively spared, but, in addition to the back and chest, the buttocks, abdomen, arms, and thighs may be involved. Constitutional symptoms and anemia may accompany the inflammatory process. Acne conglobata has been related to hidradenitis suppurativa and may occur coincidentally. Routine acne therapy is generally ineffective. Systemic therapy with a corticosteroid or sulfones may be required to suppress the intense inflammatory activity. Isotretinoin (Accutane) appears to be the most effective form of therapy for most of these patients. It is mandatory that physicians prescribing this drug be familiar with its side effects, including teratogenicity in pregnancy.

23.33 TUMORS OF THE SKIN

See also Sec. 17.25.

PYOGENIC GRANULOMA (TELANGIECTATIC GRANULOMA). This small, red, moist, sessile or pedunculated growth often has a discernible epithelial collarette (Fig. 23–52). The surface may be weeping and crusted, or completely epithelialized. Pyogenic granulomas initially grow rapidly and bleed easily when traumatized because they consist of exuberant granulation tissue. They are relatively common in children, particularly on the face, arms, and hands. Generally they arise at sites of injury, but often a history of trauma cannot be elicited. Clinically, they resemble and are often indistinguishable from small hemangiomas.

Microscopically, the lesions consist of a dense proliferation of capillaries and fibroblastic stroma. Masses of polymorphonuclear leukocytes that infiltrate the stroma account for the name pyogenic granuloma. These lesions are benign but a nuisance, because they bleed easily with trauma and may recur if incompletely removed. Small lesions may regress after cauterization with silver nitrate; larger lesions require excision and electrodesiccation of the base of the granuloma.

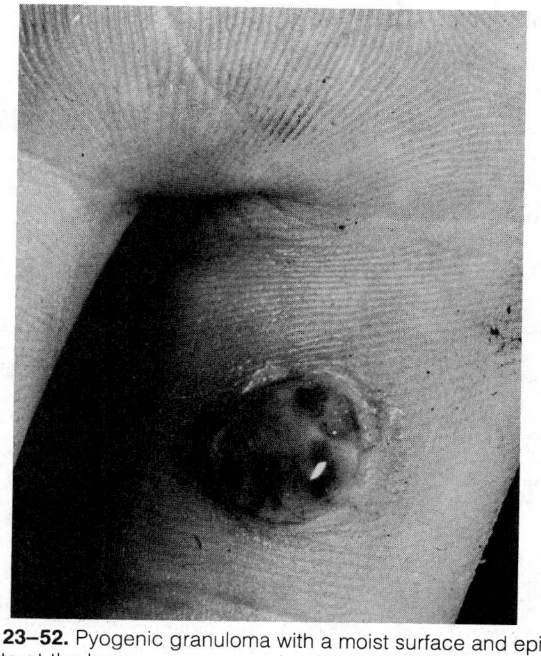

Figure 23–52. Pyogenic granuloma with a moist surface and epithelial collarette at the base.

INFANTILE DIGITAL FIBROMATOSIS. These are benign but destructive tumors identifiable as firm, smooth, erythematous or skin-colored nodules on the dorsal or lateral surfaces of the distal phalanges of the fingers and toes. More than 80% of reported tumors have been in infants less than 1 yr of age. Lesions may be solitary or multiple. Generally, they are asymptomatic, but flexion deformity of the digits may occur.

Clinically, the lesions resemble fibromas, leiomyomas, angiofibromas, and mucous cysts. The diagnosis is confirmed by finding characteristic pyroninophilic intracellular inclusion bodies within the proliferating fibroblasts on biopsy. A viral etiology has been postulated. Local recurrence following simple excision of this tumor has been reported in 60% of patients. Because the tumor does not metastasize and may occasionally regress spontaneously, a course of expectant observation is advised. If functional impairment or flexion deformity of the digit becomes apparent, prompt full excision of the tumor is indicated.

DERMATOFIBROMAS (HISTIOCYTOMAS, SCLEROSING HEMANGIOMAS). These benign dermal tumors rarely exceed 1 cm and arise most frequently on the limbs. They may be nodular, flat, or pedunculated and are usually firm and well circumscribed but occasionally feel soft on palpation. The overlying skin is usually hyperpigmented. The differential diagnosis includes epidermal inclusion cyst, juvenile xanthogranuloma, hypertrophic scar, and neurofibroma. Dermatofibromas may be excised or left intact according to the patient's preference. They represent collections of histiocytes, fibroblasts, and small capillaries in the dermis.

BASAL CELL EPITHELIOMA (BASAL CELL CARCINOMA). This is rare in children in the absence of a predisposing condition, such as nevoid basal cell carcinoma syndrome, xeroderma pigmentosum, nevus sebaceus of Jadassohn, or prior exposure to irradiation. Isolated lesions have been reported in children as young as 7 yr of age. Sites of predilection are the face, scalp, and upper back; the lesions are yellow to pink, smooth, crusted or verrucous papulonodules that enlarge slowly and may bleed occasionally or become chronically irritated. The differential diagnosis includes pyogenic granuloma, nevocellular nevus, epidermal inclusion cyst, closed comedo, dermatofibroma, and the various adnexal tumors. Simple excision is usually curative; occasional recurrences have been reported.

NEVOID BASAL CELL CARCINOMA SYNDROME. This syndrome includes a wide spectrum of defects involving the skin, eyes, central nervous system, bones, and endocrine system. The typical facies of this autosomal dominant syndrome is characterized by temporoparietal bossing, prominent supraorbital ridges, a broad nasal root, ocular hypertelorism or dystopia canthorum, and prognathism. Appearing in early childhood, basal cell carcinomas erupt in crops and vary in size, color, and number, mimicking numerous other types of skin lesions. Sites of predilection are the periorbital skin, nose, malar areas, and upper lip, but the lesions can develop on the trunk and limbs and are not restricted to sun-exposed areas. Ulceration, bleeding, and crusting can occur, with considerable destruction of surrounding tissue if the lesions are not removed. Small milia, epidermal cysts, pigmented lesions, hirsutism, and palmar and plantar pits are additional cutaneous findings.

Cysts in the maxilla and mandible occur in 65–75% of these patients; they may result in maldevelopment of the teeth and cause pain, fever, swelling of the jaw, facial deformity, bone erosion, pathologic fractures, and suppurating sinus tracts. Osseous defects such as anomalous rib development, spina bifida, kyphoscoliosis, and brachymetacarpalism occur in two thirds of patients, and ocular abnormalities including cataracts, coloboma, strabismus, and blindness in approximately one third. Neurologic manifestations include calcification of the falx, seizures, mental retardation, partial agenesis of the corpus callosum, hydrocephalus, and nerve deafness. There is increased incidence of medulloblastoma and ovarian fibroma.

The management of these patients requires participation of various specialists according to individual clinical problems. Genetic counseling is also indicated.

SYRINGOMAS. These benign tumors are more frequent in females and occasionally are inherited in an autosomal dominant fashion. They develop during childhood or adolescence. The tumors are soft, small, skin-colored, red, or brown papules that erupt in profusion on the face, particularly in the periorbital regions, and on the neck, upper chest, lower abdomen, and pubic area. Syringomas are derived from the sweat gland ducts and are readily distinguishable from other adnexal tumors by their histologic pattern. They are of cosmetic significance only. Sparse lesions may be excised, but they are often too numerous to remove.

TRICHOEPITHELIOMAS (EPITHELIOMA ADENOIDES CYSTICUM). These benign nevoid tumors are derived from the hair follicles; inheritance is autosomal dominant. Trichoepitheliomas occur on the face in a symmetric distribution but may also appear on the scalp, ears, neck, upper trunk, arms, and thighs. They arise during childhood and adolescence as firm, pink, yellow, or skin-colored papules that enlarge gradually, reaching a final size of 0.5–2 cm. They may be distinguished from other adnexal tumors, basal cell epitheliomas, syringomas, and adenoma sebaceum by biopsy. Surgical excision is the only available therapy.

LIPOMAS. These benign collections of fatty tissue appear on the trunk, neck, and proximal limbs. They are soft, compressible, lobulated growths that form skin-colored subcutaneous masses. They reach their maximal size and thereafter persist indefinitely. Occasionally, multiple lesions may occur. Atrophy, calcification, liquefaction, or xanthomatous change may sometimes complicate their course. They represent a cosmetic defect and may be surgically excised, or subjected to biopsy if diagnosis is in doubt.

JUVENILE XANTHOGRANULOMAS (NEVOXANTHOENDOTHELIOMA). These lesions may be present at birth or develop within the first several months of life. They are firm, dome-shaped, yellow, pink, or orange papules or nodules, varying in size from a few millimeters to approximately 4 cm in diameter. Rarely, they are macular, annular, or reticulated. Sites of predilection are the scalp (Fig. 23–53), face, and upper trunk, where they may erupt in profusion or remain as solitary lesions. Affected infants are otherwise normal, and blood lipid values are never elevated, as they are with xanthomas of hyperlipoproteinemic disorders.

The lesions may resemble papulonodular urticaria pigmentosa, dermatofibromas, or xanthomas of hyperlipoproteinemia. Biopsy is helpful diagnostically; mature lesions are characterized by a dermal infiltrate of lipid-laden histiocytes, admixed inflammatory cells, and Touton giant cells (multinucleated vacuolated cells with a wreath of nuclei and a peripheral rim of foamy cytoplasm) that are pathognomonic.

There is no need to remove these lesions because most of them regress spontaneously during the first few years.

Rare cases of similar lesions in the lung, testes, and pericardium have been reported. More commonly, juvenile xanthogranulomas occur in the ocular tissues, presenting as infiltrates in the orbit, iris, episclera, or ciliary body or as glaucoma, hyphema, uveitis, heterochromia iridum, iritis, or sudden proptosis (see Chapter 22). There appears to be an association among juvenile xanthogranuloma, neurofibromatosis, and childhood leukemia, most frequently juvenile chronic myelogenous leukemia.

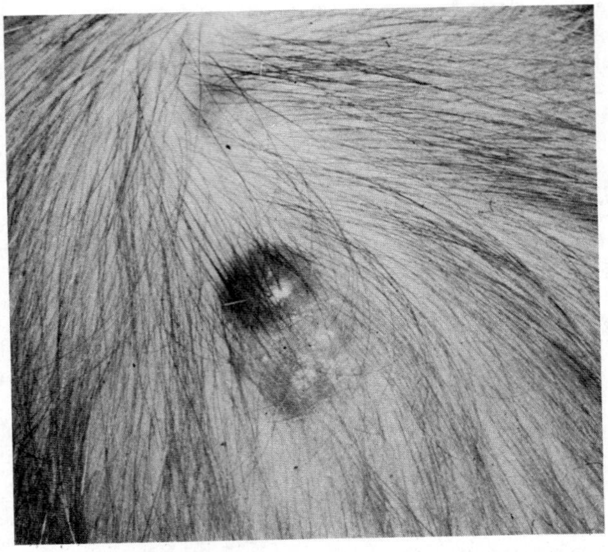

Figure 23–53. Multiple papulonodular juvenile xanthogranulomas on the scalp.

MUCOSAL NEUROMA SYNDROME (SIPPLE SYNDROME). This syndrome is inherited as an autosomal dominant trait and is easily recognized by characteristic physical features. An asthenic or marfanoid habitus is accompanied by scoliosis, pectus excavatum, pes cavus, and muscular hypotonia. There are thick, patulous lips and soft tissue prognathism simulating acromegaly. Multiple mucosal neuromas or neurofibromas appear as pink, pedunculated, or sessile nodules on the anterior third of the tongue, at the commissures of the lips, and on the buccal mucosa and palpebral conjunctiva. A variety of ophthalmologic defects and intestinal ganglioneuromatosis with recurrent diarrhea are additional common findings.

Of major concern in these patients is the high incidence of medullary thyroid carcinoma associated with high calcitonin levels, pheochromocytoma, and hyperparathyroidism, probably a compensatory response to the high levels of circulating calcitonin. Rarely, these patients are mistakenly diagnosed as having neurofibromatosis. Periodic screening tests for the associated malignant tumors are mandatory.

NANCY B. ESTERLY

GENERAL

Alper JC (ed): The genodermatoses. Dermatol Clin 5(1), 1987.
Arndt KA: Manual of Dermatologic Therapeutics, 3rd ed. Boston, Little, Brown, 1983.
Hurwitz S (ed): Pediatric Dermatology. Dermatol Clin 4(1), 1986.
Moschella SL, Hurley HM: Dermatology, 2nd ed. Vols I and II. Philadelphia, WB Saunders, 1985.
Rasmussen JE (ed): Pediatric dermatology. Pediatr Clin North Am 30(3) and 30(4), 1983.
Schachner LA, Hansen RC: Pediatric Dermatology, Vols I and II. New York, Churchill Livingstone, 1988.
Solomon LM, Esterly NB, Loeffel ED: Adolescent Dermatology. Philadelphia, WB Saunders, 1978.
Weston WL: Practical Pediatric Dermatology, 2nd ed. Boston, Little, Brown, 1985.

SPECIFIC DISEASES

Arons MS, Hurwitz S: Congenital nevocellular nevus: A review of the treatment controversy and a report of 46 cases. Plast Reconstr Surg 72:355, 1983.
Aronson IK, Zeitz HJ, Variakojis D: Panniculitis in childhood. Pediatr Dermatol 5:216, 1988.

Baley J, Silverman R: Systemic candidiasis: Cutaneous manifestations in low birth weight infants. Pediatrics 82:211, 1988.
Barton LL, Friedman AD: Impetigo: A reassessment of etiology and therapy. Pediatr Dermatol 4:185, 1987.
Beckett IH, Jacobs AH: Recurring digital fibrous tumors of childhood. Pediatrics 59:401, 1977.
Bigby M, Stern RS: Adverse reactions to isotretinoin. J Am Acad Dermatol 18:543, 1988.
Blumer JL, Lemon E, O'Horo J, et al: Changing therapy for skin and soft tissue infections in chidren: Have we come full circle? Pediatr Infect Dis J 6:117, 1987.
Carney RG Jr: Incontinentia pigmenti: A world statistical analysis. Arch Dermatol 112:535, 1976.
Castillo G: Chronic bullous disease of childhood: Linear IgA dermatosis of childhood. Dermatol Clin 1(2):231, 1983.
Cooper PH, Frierson HF, Kayne AL, et al: Association of juvenile xanthogranuloma with juvenile myeloid leukemia. Arch Dermatol 120:371, 1984.
Council on Scientific Affairs: Harmful effects of ultraviolet radiation. JAMA 262:380, 1989.
DEBRA workshop participants: Pathogenesis, clinical features and management of non-dermatologic complications of epidermolysis bullosa. Arch Dermatol 124:705, 1988.
Dicken CH: Retinoids: A review. J Am Acad Dermatol 11:541, 1984.
Duvic M: Erythema multiforme. Dermatol Clin 1:217, 1983.
Elias PM, Fritsch P, Epstein J: Staphylococcal scalded skin syndrome. Arch Dermatol 113:207, 1977.
Esterly NB: Cutaneous hemangiomas, vascular stains and associated syndromes. Curr Probl Pediatr 17:1, 1987.
Farber EM, Muller RH, Jacobs AH, et al: Infantile psoriasis: A follow-up study. Pediatr Dermatol 3:237, 1986.
Fergusson DM, Horwood J, Shannon FT: Early solid feeding and recurrent childhood eczema: a 10-year longitudinal study. Pediatrics 86:541, 1990.
Fine JD: Epidermolysis bullosa. Clinical aspects, pathology, and recent advances in research. Int J Dermatol 25:143, 1986.
Friedman A: Superficial bacterial and fungal infections of the skin. Adv Pediatr Infect Dis 5:205, 1990.
Frieden I: Aplasia cutis congenita: A clinical review and proposal for classification. J Am Acad Dermatol 14:646, 1986.
Frieden I: Blisters and pustules in the newborn. Curr Probl Pediatr 19:551, 1989.
Freire-Maia N, Pinheiro M: Ectodermal Dysplasias: A Clinical and Genetic Study. New York, Alan R Liss, 1984.
Ginsburg CM: Stevens-Johnson syndrome in children. Pediatr Infect Dis J 1:155, 1982.
Glover M, Brett EM, Atherton DJ: Hypomelanosis of Ito: Spectrum of the disease. J Pediatr 115:75, 1989.
Golitz LE, Weston WL, Lane AT: Bullous mastocytosis: Diffuse cutaneous mastocytosis with extensive blisters mimicking scalded skin syndrome or erythema multiforme. Pediatr Dermatol 1:288, 1984.
Green MS: Epidemiology of scabies. Epidemiol Rev 11:126, 1989.
Greene MH, Clark WH, Tucker MA, et al: Acquired precursors of cutaneous malignant melanoma. (The familial dysplastic nevus syndrome). N Engl J Med 312:91, 1985.
Gurevitch AW: Scabies and lice. Pediatr Clin North Am 32:987, 1985.
Halebian PH, Corder VJ, Madden MR, et al: Improved burn center survival of patients with toxic epidermal necrolysis managed without corticosteroids. Ann Surg 204:503, 1986.
Hazelrigg DE, Duncan C, Jarrett M: Twenty-nail dystrophy of childhood. Arch Dermatol 113:73, 1977.
Illig L, Weidner F, Hundeiker M, et al: Congenital nevi <10cm as precursors to melanoma: 52 cases, a review and a new conception. Arch Dermatol 12:1274, 1985.
Jacobs AH, Walton RG: The incidence of birthmarks in the neonate. Pediatrics 58:281, 1976.
Kaplan EN: The risk of malignancy in large congenital nevi. Plast Reconstr Surg 53:421, 1974.
Kousseff BG: Collodion baby, Sign of Tay syndrome. Pediatrics 87:571, 1991.
Kraemer KW, Slor H: Xeroderma pigmentosum. Clin Dermatol 3:33, 1985.
Krieger I, Evans GW: Acrodermatitis enteropathica without hypozincemia: Therapeutic effect of a pancreatic enzyme preparation due to a zinc-binding ligand. J Pediatr 96:32, 1980.
Krowchuk DP, Lucky AW, Primmer SI, et al: Current status of the identification and management of tinea capitis. Pediatrics 72:625, 1983.
Lin A, Carter D: Epidermolysis bullosa: When the skin falls apart. J Pediatr 114:349, 1989.
Lyell A: The staphylococcal scalded skin syndrome in historical perspective: Emergence of dermopathic strains of *Staphylococcus aureus* and discovery of the epidermolytic toxin. J Am Acad Dermatol 9:285, 1983.
Maddox JS, Ware JC, Dillon DC: The natural history of streptococcal skin infection: Prevention with topical antibiotics. J Am Acad Dermatol 13:207, 1985.
McMurdo SK, Moore SG, Brant-Zawadski M, et al: MR imaging in intracranial tuberous sclerosis. AJNR 8:77, 1987.
Milstone EG, Helwig EB: Basal carcinoma in children. Arch Dermatol 108:523, 1973.
Monoghan HP, Krafchik BP, MacGregor DL, et al: Tuberous sclerosis complex in children. Am J Dis Child 135:912, 1981.
Mulbauer JE: Granuloma annulare. J Am Acad Dermatol 3:217, 1980.
Neldner KH, Hambidge KM: Zinc deficiency of acrodermatitis enteropathica. N Engl J Med 292:879, 1975.
Nelson LB, Melick JE, Harley RD: Intralesional corticosteroid injections for infantile hemangiomas of the eyelids. Pediatrics 74:241, 1984.
NIH Consensus Development Conference. Neurofibromatosis. Arch Neurol 45:575, 1988.
Nordlund JJ (ed): Pigmentation disorders. Dermatol Clin 6(2), 1988.
Oranje AP, van Joost TH, van Reede EC: Infantile seborrheic dermatitis: Morphological and immunopathological study. Dermatologica 172:191, 1986.
Picascia DD, Esterly NB: Cutis marmorata telangectatica congenita: A report of 22 cases. J Am Acad Dermatol 20:1098, 1989.
Podmore P, Burrows D, Eady DJ, et al: Seborrheic eczema—a disease entity or a clinical variant of atopic eczema? Br J Dermatol 115:341, 1986.
Poh-Fitzpatrick MB, Ramsay CA, Frain-Bell W, et al: Photodermatoses in infants and children. Pediatr Dermatol 5:189, 1988.
Prendiville J, Hebert A, Greenwald M, et al: Management of Stevens-Johnson syndrome and toxic epidermal necrolysis in children. J Pediatr 115:881, 1989.
Prockop DJ, Kivirikko KI: Heritable diseases of collagen. N Engl J Med 311:376, 1984.
Prose NS, Mendez H, Menikoff H, et al: Pediatrics human immunodeficiency virus infection and its cutaneous manifestations. Ped Dermatol 4:67, 1987.
Revuz J, Penso D, Roujeau J-C, et al: Toxic epidermal necrolysis: Clinical findings and prognosis factors in 87 patients. Arch Dermatol 123:1160, 1987.
Revuz J, Roujeau J-C, Guillaume J-C, et al: Treatment of toxic epidermal necrolysis: Creteil experience. Arch Dermatol 123:1156, 1987.
Rhodes AR: Congenital nevi: should these be excised? JAMA 262:1696, 1989.
Rizzo WB, Dammaum AL, Craft DA, et al: Sjögren-Larsson Syndrome: Inherited defect in the fatty alcohol cycle. J Pediatr 115:228, 1989.
Rogers M, McCrossin I: Epidermal nevi and the epidermal nevus syndrome. J Am Acad Dermatol 20:476, 1989.
Schmidt H, Knitker G, Thomson K, et al: Erythropoietic protoporphyria: A clinical study based on 29 cases in 14 families. Arch Dermatol 110:58, 1974.
Schwartz MF Jr, Esterly NB, Fretzin DF, et al: Hypomelanosis of Ito (incontinentia pigmenti achromians): A neurocutaneous syndrome. J Pediatr 90:236, 1977.
Spear KL, Winkelmann, RK: Gianotti-Crosti syndrome: A review of 10 cases not associated with hepatitis B. Arch Dermatol 120:891, 1984.
Staka BF, Whitaker DL, Morrison SH, et al: Cutaneous manifestations of the acquired immunodeficiency syndrome in children. J Am Acad Dermatol 18:1089, 1988.
Stroud JB: Hair shaft anomalies. Dermatol Clin 5:581, 1987.
Swenen RJ: Management of congenital nevocytic nevi: A survey of current practices. J Am Acad Dermatol 11:629, 1984.
Tallman B, Tan OT, Morelli JG, et al: Location of port-wine stains and the likelihood of ophthalmic and/or central nervous system complications. Pediatrics 87:323, 1991.
Tan O, Sherwood K, Gilchrest B: Treatment of children with port-wine stains using the flashlamp pulsed tunable dye laser. N Engl J Med 320:416, 1989.
Teelman K: Retinoids: Toxicity and teratogenicity to date. Pharmac Ther 40:29, 1989.
Thiers BH, Bergfeld WF, Fiedler-Weiss VC, et al: Alopecia areata symposium. Pediatr Dermatol 4:136, 1987.
Truhan AP, Herbert AA, Esterly NB: Pityriasis lichenoides in children: Therapeutic response to erythromycin. J Am Acad Dermatol 15:66, 1986.
Tucker MA, Clarke WH, Fraser MC, et al: Dysplastic nevi on the scalp of prepubertal children from melanoma-prone families. J Pediatr 103:65, 1983.
Walter SD, Marrett LF, Hertzman C, et al: The association of cutaneous malignant melanoma with the use of sunbeds and sunlamps. Am J Epidemiol 131:232, 1990.
White CW, Wolf SJ, Korones DN, et al: Treatment of childhood angiomatous diseases with recombinant interferon alpha-2a. J Pediatr 118:59, 1991.
Williams ML: A new look at the ichthyoses: Disorders of lipid metabolism. Pediatr Dermatol 3:476, 1986.

24

THE BONES AND JOINTS

ORTHOPEDIC PROBLEMS

Musculoskeletal diseases constitute about 10% of problems of childhood. The majority of these problems can be managed safely and effectively by the pediatrician who has the understanding and skill necessary to establish an accurate diagnosis, to understand the natural history of the condition, and to employ appropriate management. Musculoskeletal diseases may be congenital or acquired, primary bone, muscle, tendon, or articular pathology, or secondary to a more generalized systemic inflammatory, metabolic, or neuromuscular disorder (Table 24–1). Musculoskeletal illness may be acute or chronic, manifesting with pain, limitation of movement or strength, gait disturbance (Table 24–2), abnormal posture or positioning, deformity, and signs of inflammation (warmth, erythema, swelling, tenderness, and limited range of motion). This chapter provides basic information relevant to these problems and emphasizes the importance of the pediatrician's role in making a diagnosis. A glossary of common orthopedic terminology is provided in Table 24–3. Neoplasms and infections of bone are discussed in Chapters 12 and 17.

24.1 EVALUATION

A careful history, thorough physical examination, appropriate imaging, and laboratory studies usually lead to the diagnosis. The birth and developmental history of the child are important. The neonatal history may reveal breech presentation, which is commonly noted among patients with congenital hip dislocation, neuromuscular disease, and hypotonia; birth trauma; or abnormal mechanical forces leading to fetal constraint or compression with resultant deformations. The latter includes craniofacial (scaphocephaly, plagiocephaly, mandibular asymmetry, torticollis, crumpled ear, craniostenosis), extremity (dislocated hips, metatarsus adductus, foot equinovarus, hyperflexed hips, hyperextended knees, joint contractures), or other (scoliosis, pulmonary hypoplasia) mechanical deformations. The neonatal history may reveal components of a malformation anomalad such as *v*ertebral defects, imperforate *a*nus, *t*racheo*e*sophageal fistula, and *ra*dial and *r*enal dysplasia (VATER) syndrome, which is associated with hemivertebra and congenital scoliosis. In-toeing associated with a history of delayed walking suggests a diagnosis of cerebral palsy. The significance of an acute history of injury should be carefully assessed. Injury is a common event in the life of a child. The diagnosis of a serious problem such as a neoplasm or infection may be inappropriately delayed if the symptoms are attributed to an injury. The parents' concerns should be seriously considered. Intuition may be surprisingly accurate; a mother often senses that something is wrong with her infant before the physician diagnoses conditions, such as cerebral palsy.

Disorders that cause pain in the older child may present only as altered function (e.g., pseudoparalysis) in the infant or toddler. Diskitis in toddlers, for example, often presents as refusal to walk, whereas in older children the constitutional features of an infection predominate. Diskitis during adolescence may manifest with back pain as the major complaint. The child with a "toddler's fracture" (undisplaced tibial fracture) simply limps. The infant with such a fracture often shows pseudoparalysis, which may be confused with a neurologic problem.

PHYSICAL EXAMINATION. Be thorough and start with a screening examination that includes observation of posture, gait, and positioning. This requires the removal of the outer

TABLE 24–1. Mechanisms of Common Pediatric Orthopedic Problems*

Category	Mechanism	Example
Congenital		
Malformation	Teratogenesis prior to 12th wk of gestation	Polydactyly, spina bifida
Disruption	Amniotic band constriction	Extremity amputation
	Fetal varicella infection	Limb scar/atrophy
Deformation	Leg compression	Clubfoot
	Neck compression	Torticollis
Dysplasia	Abnormal cell growth or metabolism	Osteogenesis imperfecta
		Dwarf syndromes
		Mucopolysaccharidosis
Acquired		
Infection	Pyogenic bacterial hematogenous spread	Osteomyelitis, septic arthritis
Inflammation	Antigen-antibody reaction, immune mediated	JRA, SLE, Reiter syndrome
Trauma	Mechanical forces, overuse, foreign body	Child abuse, sports injuries, accidents, birth injury, fractures, dislocations, tendinitis
Tumor	Primary bone tumor	Osteosarcoma, Ewing sarcoma
	Metastasis to bone from other site	Neuroblastoma
	Bone marrow tumor	Leukemia, lymphoma

*Modified from Allen B: Common orthopedic problems of children. *In:* Behrman R, Kliegman R: Nelson Essentials of Pediatrics. Philadelphia, WB Saunders, 1990.

TABLE 24–2. Mechanisms of Gait Disturbances*

Mechanical
- Trauma, fracture, sprain
- Sports injury, overuse injury
- Child abuse
- Dysplastic lesions
- Short leg

Osseous
- Legg-Perthes disease
- Slipped capital epiphysis
- Osteomyelitis
- Diskitis
- Osteoid osteoma
- Osgood-Schlatter

Articular
- Congenital hip dislocation
- Septic arthritis
- Toxic synovitis
- Rheumatic disease (JRA, SLE)
- Hemophilia
- Ankylosis of a joint

Neurologic
- Guillain-Barré syndrome (other peripheral neuropathies)
- Intoxication
- Cerebellar ataxia
- Brain tumor
- Lesion occupying spinal cord space
- Posterior spinal column disorders
- Myopathy
- Hemiplegia
- Sympathetic reflex dystrophy
- Cerebral palsy

Hematologic
- Sickle cell pain crisis
- Leukemia, lymphoma
- Metastatic tumor
- Primary bone tumor
- Histiocytosis

Other
- Soft-tissue infection
- Kawasaki disease
- Conversion reaction
- Gaucher disease
- Phlebitis
- Scurvy
- Rickets
- Peritonitis

*Modified from Allen B: Common orthopedic problems of children. *In:* Behrman R, Kliegman R: Nelson Essentials of Pediatrics, 13th ed. Philadelphia, WB Saunders, 1990.

clothing while honoring the child's modesty. It may be best to examine the infant or young child on a parent's lap, where the child feels more secure and is less likely to cry or struggle. First, observe the whole child and make a judgment about whether the child appears ill. This is one factor differentiating toxic synovitis from septic arthritis. Lack of spontaneous movement (pseudoparalysis) of a lower extremity is the most consistent finding in septic arthritis of the hip in the infant. The physician should look for asymmetry or other deformities (Fig. 24–1). Unusual posturing, such as an externally rotated leg in the older child or adolescent, is a classic feature of slipped capital femoral epiphysis.

The general physical examination should look for clues to systemic diseases affecting the musculoskeletal system. Dysmorphic signs should suggest a congenital, genetic, malformation anomalad or metabolic disorder. Inborn errors of connective tissue (Marfan disease, Ehlers-Danlos syndrome, homocystinuria, osteogenesis imperfecta) should be suspected in the presence of ocular (ectopic lens, severe myopia, blue sclera) abnormalities, high-arched palate, hypermobile joints, cardiovascular disease (dilated aorta, mitral valve prolapse), or multiple fractures. Ocular manifestations of conjunctivitis (Reiter syndrome), episcleritis-scleritis (systemic lupus erythematosus [SLE], rheumatoid arthritis), uveitis (juvenile rheumatoid arthritis [JRA], Kawasaki syndrome), or retinal hemorrhages (child abuse) suggest a generalized process. Cutaneous signs of facial butterfly rash (SLE), erythema nodosum (tuberculosis, inflammatory bowel disease), café-au-lait spots (neurofibromatosis, polyostotic fibrous dysplasia), erythema marginatum (rheumatic fever), livedo reticularis (SLE), and bruising, burns, or unexplained marks (child abuse) also suggest systemic problems.

The more detailed musculoskeletal examination tests for deformity, stiffness, strength, symmetry, tenderness, joint clicking, gait disturbances, contractures, and range of motion. Limitation of active and passive (gently to avoid pain) range of motion is assessed in degrees of movement from a zero degree or neutral position. Movement may be flexion-extension (most joints, spine), dorsiflexion-plantar (palmar) flexion (ankle, toe, wrist, finger), abduction (away from the midline)-adduction (shoulder, hip, finger, toe), inversion-eversion (subtalar, midtarsal-foot), internal-external rotation (hip, shoulder), pronation-supination (forearm), or rotation (neck, spine). Each joint should be examined individually because disease may be subclinical. Joint laxity is commonly associated with other orthopedic problems, such as flexible flatfeet, congenital hip dysplasia, and dislocating patella.

The *Trendelenburg test* identifies the pathology between the femur and the pelvis. The normal response to standing on one leg is that the opposite pelvis rises due to normal gluteus medius stabilizing action. Additional testing in infants involves the Ortolani and Barlow tests (see Sec. 24.8) for congenital dislocated hips, whereas in preadolescents and adolescents the examiner views the upright back for waist crease and asymmetry and the 70-degree forward bend position for paravertebral asymmetry (scoliosis) or a midline thoracic hump (kyphosis) (see Sec. 24.15 and 24.18).

Tenderness over the spine suggests trauma, fracture, infection (diskitis, osteomyelitis, epidural abscess, tuberculosis), Reiter syndrome, inflammatory bowel disease, ankylosing spondylitis, spondylolisthesis, spondylolysis, and, rarely, metastatic or primary tumor.

If feasible, the child should be observed both walking and running. Gait disturbances result from a variety of orthopedic problems and should prompt additional evaluation (see Table 24–2). The most common limp is described as the **antalgic** (painful) **gait**. The antalgic position is the one that attempts to limit pain. Because of pain, the stance phase on the effective side is shortened, producing an asymmetric gait. The second most common gait abnormality is the **abductor lurch** in which the upper trunk shifts to the affected side. This abnormality is common in dysplasia and in painful conditions of the hip. The **equine gait**, usually secondary to a contracture of the heel cord, causes a loss of the normal sequence of foot contact with the ground. The toe, rather than the heel, strikes the ground first.

Unless the condition is bilateral or involves the spine, a comparison of the two sides is often helpful. Usually, asymmetry arises from normal variability or from the effect of the intrauterine position, such as with tibial torsion. Asymmetry sometimes results from more serious problems, such as hip dysplasia or hemiparesis secondary to cerebral palsy. Atrophy should be distinguished from hemihypertrophy.

If a child has pain, the suspected site of the pain should be examined last. The physician should be gentle but thorough

TABLE 24–3. Glossary of Orthopedic Terminology*

Acheiria (achiria)	Absence of hand
Acheiriopodia	Absence of hands and feet
Acro-	End
Acromelia	Shortening of the hand
Adactylia or adactyly	Absence of all fingers or toes
Agenesis	Absence or no development
Amelia	Absence of limb
Amputation	Absence of a distal part of a limb
Anteversion	Anterior twist or angulation of the femoral head away from the frontal plane
Aplasia	Absence of a specific bone or bones
Apodia	Absence of foot
Apophysis	Bone growth center that is not a growth plate and that has a strong muscle insertion (e.g., greater trochanter of femur)
Arachnodactyly	Long, slender digits
Arthroplasty	Surgical reconstruction of a joint
Arthrotomy	Surgical incision into a joint
Brachy-	Short
Brachydactyly	Short fingers
Brachymegalodactyly	Short, broad digit
Calcaneus	Dorsiflexion of hindfoot
Camptodactyly	Curvature of finger in plane of flexion
Cavovarus	High longitudinal and medial arch of foot with medial rotation of forefoot and hindfoot
Cavus	High longitudinal arch of the foot
Central defect	(Cleft or lobster claw hand) Absence of one or more central rays of hand, the second, third, or fourth or any combination
Clinodactyly	Deviation of a finger in the plane of the hand
Coalition	Union of two foot bones
Compartment syndrome	Increased pressure from trauma, inflammation, or hemorrhage in a tightly encased (by fascia) muscle group, with the potential for ischemic damage to nerve, muscle, or blood vessels
Dactylia	With reference to digit
Dislocation	Complete loss of contact between two joint surfaces
Dys-	Deformed
Ectro-	Absence
Ectrodactyly	Total or partial absence of fingers or hand
Ectromelia	Total or partial absence of fingers or hand
Equinus	Plantar flexion of the forefoot, hindfoot, or entire foot
Fractures	
Longitudinal	Parallel to bone axis
Transverse	Perpendicular to bone axis
Oblique	Angulated to bone axis
Spiral	Curvilinear course around axis
Impacted	Bone ends crushed together
Comminuted	More than two separated bone fragments
Bowing	Bone bends without fracture
Greenstick	Fracture of one side with plastic deformity on the other side
Torus	Buckle and bending without fracture
Hemimelia	Absence of part of a limb
Hyper-	Above or increased
Hyperphalangia	Presence of more than the normal number of phalanges in the transverse direction
Hypo-	Below or decreased
Hypodactyly	Fewer than the normal number of fingers
Hypoplasia	Incomplete development
Macro-	Excessive size
Melia	Referring to the limb
Mero	Part or partial
Meromelia	Partial absence of the limb
Meso-	Middle
Micro	Small size
Oligo-	Few or little
Oligodactyly	Absence of some of the fingers
Pero-	Deformed or defective
Perodactyly	Deformed fingers
Pes	Foot deformity
Phoco-	Flipper-like
Phocomelia	In complete form, the hands and feet sprout directly from the trunk—the arm and forearm are absent in the upper limb, and the thigh and leg are absent in the lower limb; the deficiency may be proximal (arms and thighs missing) or distal (forearms and legs missing)
Pod-	Related to the foot
Poikilodactyly	Irregular or varied digit
Poly-	Many or increased number
Polydactyly	More than the normal number of digits
Postaxial	Pertaining to the ulnar side of the upper limb, fibular side of the lower limb
Preaxial	Pertaining to the radial side of the upper limb or thumb, the tibial side of the lower thumb
Spondylolisthesis	Forward slippage of a vertebral body over the underlying vertebral body
Spondylolysis	Defect in the pars interarticularis
Subluxation	Incomplete loss of contact between two joint surfaces
Syn-	Fusion
Syndactyly	Fusion of adjacent digits; may be complete or incomplete with reference to cutaneous involvement, simple or complex with reference to bony involvement
Synostosis	Bony fusion
Talipes	Congenital foot deformity
Tele-	Distant or end
Transverse deficiency	Absence of part of a limb (across the width of the limb)
Valgum	Angulation of a bone distal to a joint or of part of a bone away from the midline. Genu valgum results in knock-knee as angulation distal to the knee is away from the midline
Varum	Angulation of a bone or within a bone toward the midline. Genu varum results in bowleg

*Modified from Tachdjian M: Pediatric Orthopedics, 2nd ed. Philadelphia, WB Saunders, 1990.

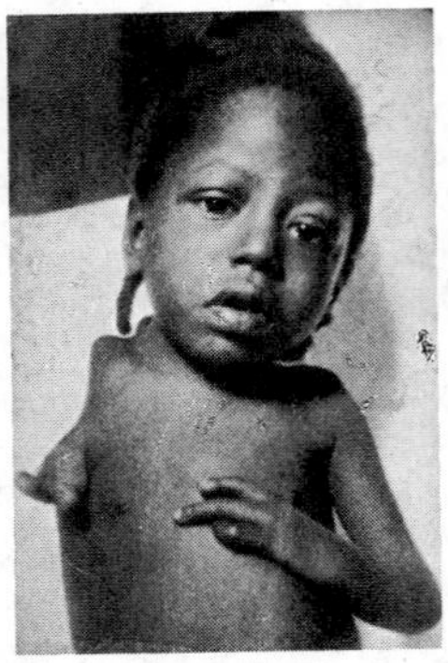

Figure 24–1. Phocomelia and partial adactyly in a girl 3.5 yr of age.

and should look for evidence of swelling, erythema, or discoloration. He or she should palpate for warmth, swelling, and tenderness. Localization of tenderness is one of the most helpful steps in the physical examination. The physician should palpate gently while watching the child's face for signs of discomfort in order to localize precisely the site of the tenderness, because this area may provide the diagnosis. For example, tenderness of the tibial tubercle is a typical finding in Osgood-Schlatter disease, whereas tenderness just anterior to the distal fibula is a classic finding in the common ankle sprain. Focal or point tenderness in patients with osteomyelitis suggests that the infection is confined to a metaphyseal abscess, whereas more diffuse tenderness is noted following rupture to the periosteal space.

HEMATOLOGIC STUDIES. The erythrocyte sedimentation rate (ESR) is a useful screening study to differentiate infections and rheumatologic disorders from benign inflammatory or traumatic (mechanical) problems. The ESR is usually elevated in septic arthritis but is normal or minimally increased in toxic synovitis of the hip. Tenderness over the upper tibial metaphysis should be supplemented by an ESR to aid in differentiating an early infection from a stress fracture. The ESR may be elevated in an infection but is normal with a stress fracture. A complete blood count (CBC) is often helpful to identify anemia due to chronic disease (JRA, renal failure, inflammatory bowel disease), hemolysis, (SLE, sickle cell anemia), bone marrow displacement (leukemia, neuroblastoma), leukocytosis (JRA, bacterial infection, rheumatic fever, Kawasaki syndrome), leukopenia (leukemia, neuroblastoma, SLE), and thrombocytopenia (leukemia, neuroblastoma). A normal CBC does not exclude serious primary or secondary musculoskeletal disorders, whereas abnormal findings may be present in the patient with multiple skeletal trauma (e.g., hemorrhage and anemia).

IMAGING STUDIES (see Sec. 6.56). Roentgenography remains the principle method of evaluation and should not be bypassed for other imaging techniques. The decision about which studies are needed should be based on the history and physical examination. An anteroposterior (AP) roentgenogram is adequate for an initial evaluation of hip dysplasia. If a slipped capital femoral epiphysis is suspected, a lateral roentgenogram of the hip is essential. The physical examination also aids in evaluating the roentgenogram. The differentiation of normal variations in ossification from a fracture is much easier if one knows whether tenderness is present over the site in question. Fractures are tender; ossicles are not. Finally, routine ordering of comparative roentgenograms of the opposite limb is not appropriate.

Bone scanning is very useful in screening for subtle fractures due to child abuse, evaluating the limping child, determining the site of pain about the pelvis or spine, identification of osteomyelitis before signs appear on plain roentgenograms, or staging a malignant tumor. If a lesion is seen in the roentgenogram, scanning is usually unnecessary. If septic arthritis is suspected, a diagnostic joint aspiration should not be delayed to obtain a bone scan. Delay may jeopardize the success of treatment, whereas the aspiration seldom affects the scan (see Sec. 12.16–12.17). Positive findings on bone scans depict increased metabolism and vascularity; thus, uptake of radionuclides (hot spot) is present in many pathologic conditions. In contrast, a cold spot is present in avascular necrosis (osteonecrosis).

Magnetic resonance imaging (MRI) studies are very important when evaluating the spinal cord and soft-tissue lesions, such as sarcomas of extremities. MRI is also useful to visualize meniscal injury in the knee. The use of the MRI in childhood is limited by problems of immobilization of the infant or young child for the study. Although MRI is helpful for soft-tissue lesions, computed tomography (CT) scanning is useful for bone lesions (anomalies, trauma, neoplasms, infections, foreign bodies).

Ultrasound studies are becoming increasingly valuable, particularly in screening for hip dysplasia, when performed and interpreted by an experienced ultrasonographer. Normal variability and age-related changes complicate the interpretation of all imaging studies. Ultrasound differentiates cystic lesions from solid lesions. Doppler flow studies can identify the vascular integrity of an extremity, the vascular supply of an arteriovenous malformation, and the presence of deep venous thrombosis.

DIAGNOSIS. Establishing a definitive diagnosis should be the priority for the pediatrician. The most common drawback in management is to initiate treatment before the diagnosis is clear. Common examples of ineffective treatment and waste of valuable time include the use of triple diapers when hip dysplasia is suspected, "corrective shoes" for gait abnormalities, or exercises for scoliosis. The delay in starting appropriate treatment is sometimes dangerous. Therapy with anti-inflammatory agents for undiagnosed bone pain or unwitnessed suspected trauma may mask infectious or neoplastic processes.

NATURAL HISTORY. After determining an accurate diagnosis, it is essential to understand the "natural history" of the condition, the outcome of the condition without interventions, before deciding on management. Most minor musculoskeletal problems of childhood resolve spontaneously and are simply normal variations, such as flexible flatfeet, bowlegs, knock-knees, and rotational problems. Most sports-related problems in children are overuse syndromes that heal with rest and time. Scoliosis uncommonly progresses to a level of severity that requires treatment. One of the greatest challenges for the primary care provider is to distinguish between self-resolving problems and uncommon problems that have the potential for disability and require treatment.

TALKING WITH PARENTS. Providing effective reassurance for concerned parents is a challenge. Because most problems are normal variations that resolve with time, only observation is often indicated. Active treatment is indicated only when the condition has the potential to produce disability and the treatment is effective in altering the natural history. Unnecessary treatment is expensive and often uncomfortable for the child.

Several steps are helpful in providing effective reassurance. The diagnosis should be accurate; the family should be given information regarding the natural history; and a follow-up evaluation should be provided to be certain that the condition resolves as expected. If the family seems unconvinced, an orthopedic consultation is needed. The need for reassurance should be communicated to the orthopedist.

Finally, not all physiologic conditions resolve. Normal variability includes "outlyers" that are on the edge of the normal curve. For example, tibial or femoral torsion may persist into late childhood, producing disability and requiring operative correction. The likelihood of such problems persisting is less than 1 in 1,000, but this fact should be included in discussions regarding the outcome. The longer a problem persists, the greater will be the chance that the problem is an outlyer. If similar problems exist in the adult members of the family, there are increased reasons for concern.

DRAWBACKS IN MANAGEMENT. Hidden among the many common musculoskeletal conditions that resolve without intervention are serious problems. These uncommon problems, such as congenital hip dislocations, septic arthritis, and tumors, require early treatment to avoid serious sequelae. Therefore, the differential diagnosis should include a broad spectrum of disorders. Screening laboratory and imaging studies should be performed if there is any doubt about the diagnosis.

REGIONAL PROBLEMS

24.2 FOOT AND TOES

FLATFEET. The flatfoot (pes planovalgus) is characterized by a lack of the longitudinal arch, producing an increased area of ground contact with weight bearing. Most flatfeet are flexible and are simply a variation of normal. Such feet are typical of the infant, common in the child (Fig. 24–2), and occur in approximately 15% of adults. The arch normally develops during childhood, eliminating the flatfoot appearance of the toddler. Flexible flatfoot is divided into three increasingly severe degrees based on the defect of the longitudinal arch (Fig. 24–3). If the patient stands on tiptoes, this will reveal the longitudinal arch in most cases.

The flexible flatfoot is usually asymptomatic. Pain is unusual and should suggest another process, such as contracture of the triceps surae muscle, trauma, rheumatologic diseases, foreign body, neoplasia, or tarsal coalition. Flexible flatfoot may be familial or, less often, part of a generalized syndrome (21-trisomy, Ehlers-Danlos syndrome, Marfan syndrome, osteogenesis imperfecta, cerebral palsy, muscular dystrophy, myelodysplasia).

Flexible flatfoot requires no therapy. The child can go barefoot or use sneakers or regular shoes.

Pathologic flatfeet show some degree of stiffness or rigidity detected by a physical examination. This stiffness may be due to a loss of the normal subtalar motion of inversion and eversion or to a tightness of the heelcord. Heelcord contracture is present if the ankle cannot be dorsiflexed to 10 degrees above neutral when the knee is extended. Three common causes of stiff flatfeet may occur in otherwise normal children and constitute serious problems that require referral to an orthopedist.

The **vertical talus** (congenital convex pes valgus) is the most severe and serious type of flatfoot. This deformity is a dorsal and lateral dislocation of the talocalcaneonavicular joint and produces not only flattening but also an actual convexity to the sole of the foot. The talus lies in a vertical position with the head of the talus projecting into the plantar aspects of the foot. The condition may be isolated or associated with central nervous or musculoskeletal system abnormalities, such as arthrogryposis multiplex congenita, congenital dislocated hips, neurofibromatosis, cerebral palsy, and autosomal trisomies (13-trisomy, 18-trisomy). The diagnosis is confirmed by a lateral roentgenogram of the foot showing the vertical orientation of the talus. Differentiation from flexible flatfoot is performed by demonstrating rigidity and persistence of the "rocker-bottom" deformity when not bearing weight. Correction requires soft-tissue lengthening and surgical repositioning of the talus. The procedure is best performed at about 6 mo of age.

Tarsal coalitions are fusions among two or more tarsal bones that restrict motion, producing a rigid planovalgus foot and loss of inversion motion. The altered mechanics produce arthritis with secondary peroneal spasm and a flatfoot. The condition is asymptomatic in early childhood but eventually produces pain and becomes symptomatic in later childhood or early adolescence. This condition occurs in approximately 0.5–1% of the population. The lesion may be isolated (usually bilateral, but may be unilateral in 50% of some types), may be inherited as an autosomal dominant trait with variable

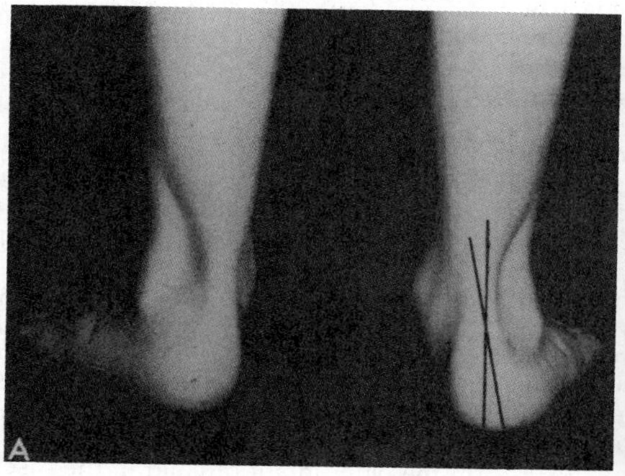

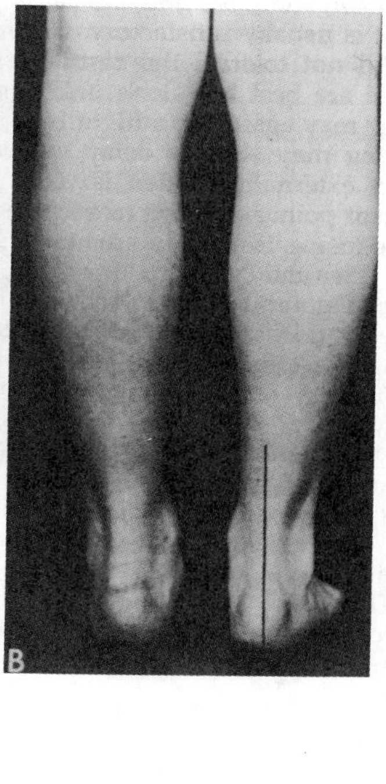

Figure 24–2. *A*, The heel in valgus. *B*, Normal heel.

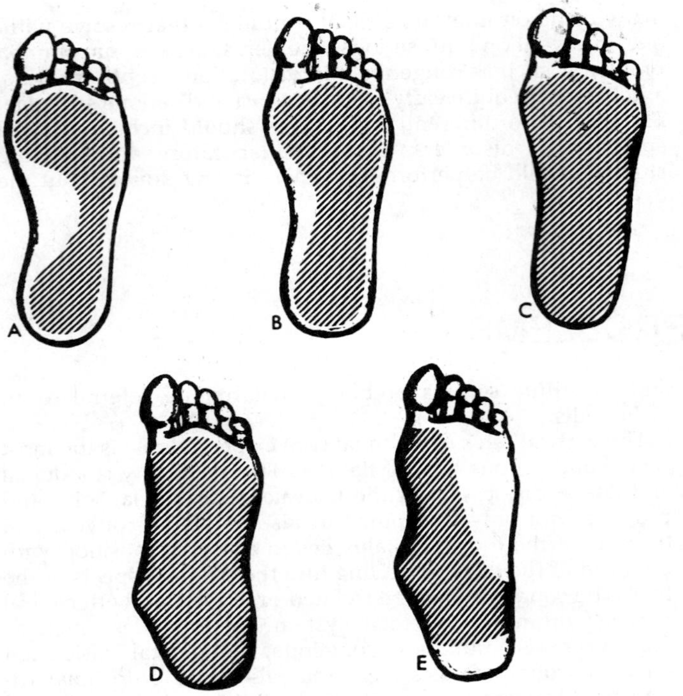

Figure 24–3. Footprints of varying degrees of flatfoot. *A*, Normal. *B*, Mild or 1st-degree—the longitudinal arch is low but still visible. *C*, Moderate or 2nd-degree—the longitudinal arch is absent. *D*, Severe or third degree—the longitudinal arch is absent and the medial border of the foot is convex with the head of the talus pressing on the plantar aspect of the foot. *E*, "Rocker-bottom" deformity in congenital convex pes valgus—the heel is in the equinus position; the forefoot is dorsiflexed and everted; and the head of the talus is prominent on the sole. The deformity is rigid; it does not disappear when not weight bearing. (From Tachdjian M: Pediatric Orthopedics, 2nd ed. Philadelphia, WB Saunders, 1990.)

penetrance, associated with fusion of other bones (carpus, phalanges), and less often part of complex malformations (Alport syndrome, Nievergelt-Pearlman syndrome) or major limb anomalies (absent toes, fibular hemimelia, phocomelia, proximal focal femoral deficiency).

The most common coalitions are between the calcaneus and the navicular and between the talus and the calcaneus. The coalition may be completely osseous (synostosis) or divided by fissures in cartilage (synchondrosis) or fibrous tissue (syndesmosis). Coalition produces pain in adolescence and occurs in the subtalar or midtarsal area. Spasms of the peroneal tendon (peroneal spasm flatfoot) may complicate coalition, are painful, and increase the valgus foot deformity. Peroneal spastic flatfoot also may be produced by other lesions that limit the motion of the talocalcaneonavicular joint (e.g., pauciarticular rheumatoid arthritis, osteoid osteoma).

Calcaneonavicular coalitions are diagnosed by an oblique roentgenogram of the foot. Talocalcaneal coalitions are best imaged by CT scanning. Symptomatic coalitions (pain, spasm, deformity) are best treated by operative resection of the connecting bar to allow free motion of the foot. Patients with minor symptoms may be managed with heel orthosis, anti-inflammatory agents, or special shoes.

The combination of **heelcord contracture and joint hypermobility** produces a painful flatfoot. The diagnosis is suspected by demonstrating a loss of dorsiflexion of the foot with the knee extended. The extended knee tightens the gastrocnemius and allows demonstration of the contracture. This combination results in an "obligatory" heel valgus, alters the mechanics of the foot, and results in increased joint wear and pain. Treatment includes lengthening of the heelcord and a hindfoot-stabilizing procedure.

CAVUS FOOT (PES CAVUS). This disorder is characterized by a high arch and is at the other end of the spectrum of flatfoot. The patient or parent often considers this high arch to be desirable, although a high arch is more likely to be pathologic and symptomatic than a flatfoot. Pain is common, because the body load is concentrated on the metatarsal heads and heel. The congenitally cavus foot may be part of the spectrum of normal arch patterns. Pathologic cavus feet, however, are frequently acquired and are due to some neuromuscular abnormality. The lesion may be a myopathy (muscular dystrophy) or peripheral neuropathy (Charcot-Marie-Tooth disease, hypertrophic neuritis, polyneuritis) or may be localized to the spinal nerve roots; anterior horn cell; spinal cord; or pyramidal, extrapyramidal, or spinocerebellar (Friedreich ataxia) tract. Without obvious associated neuromuscular signs, some cases of pes cavus are familial. Nonetheless, pes cavus must be considered to be due to neuromuscular disease unless proved otherwise. A thorough evaluation is needed to detect spinal dysraphisms and peripheral neuropathies. This includes a detailed family history, careful muscle and peripheral nerve examination, imaging of the spine and electromyography with nerve conduction studies. Unless the cavus foot is physiologic rather than pathologic, referral to an orthopedist or neurologist is indicated.

The *diagnosis* and severity of pes cavus are assessed with weight-bearing AP and lateral roentgenograms. *Treatment* can be conservative in mild cases, with a support insole to protect the metatarsals during weight bearing. Surgical correction is indicated for a severe, disabling deformity.

CLUBFOOT (CONGENITAL TALIPES EQUINOVARUS). This common congenital foot deformity includes features of equine, adductus, varus, and medial rotation (Fig. 24–4). Neuromuscular imbalance, uterine compression, or primary germ cell defects may produce in utero displacement and malalignment of the talocalcaneal navicular and calcaneocuboid joints, which are fixed by capsular, ligamentous, and musculotendinous contractures. Mild cases may be due to in utero postural-induced compression *(positional deformation)*, whereas more severe cases may be due to a developmental malformation. Postural clubfoot may be differentiated from talipes equinovarus by the presence of a normal-sized heel, a mild and flexible deformity rather than a marked and rigid deformity, the ability to be corrected to a neutral position by passive manipulation, normal position of the lateral malleolus, a forefoot in the varus position but not in the equinus position, and minimal or no calf atrophy in the postural deformation.

Involvement is bilateral in 50% of patients. The male to female ratio is approximately 2:1; the incidence varies from 1/1,000 live births in whites to 6.8/1,000 in Polynesian infants. Inheritance may be polygenic; associated disorders include congenital hip dysplasia, amniotic band syndrome, arthrogryposis, spina bifida, myotonic dystrophy, diastrophic dwarfism, craniocarpotarsal dysplasia, and Larsen, Möbius, and other syndromes. Acquired clubfoot may be seen in myelomeningocele, spinal tumors, poliomyelitis, myopathies, cerebral palsy, Guillain-Barré syndrome, or diastematomyelia.

The foot is stiff and smaller than normal. The diagnosis is seldom difficult because the clinical appearance is characteristic; early referral is indicated. Roentgenograms may be useful in the older infant or child in the case of talipes equinovarus in order to define the anatomy and to assess the degree of subluxation of the talocalcaneonavicular joint and the severity of the deformity and also to demonstrate improvement during closed nonoperative casting. Cast treatment should be started within the 1st wk of life. The more flexible clubfoot may be treated by serial casting; however, severe talipes equinovarus

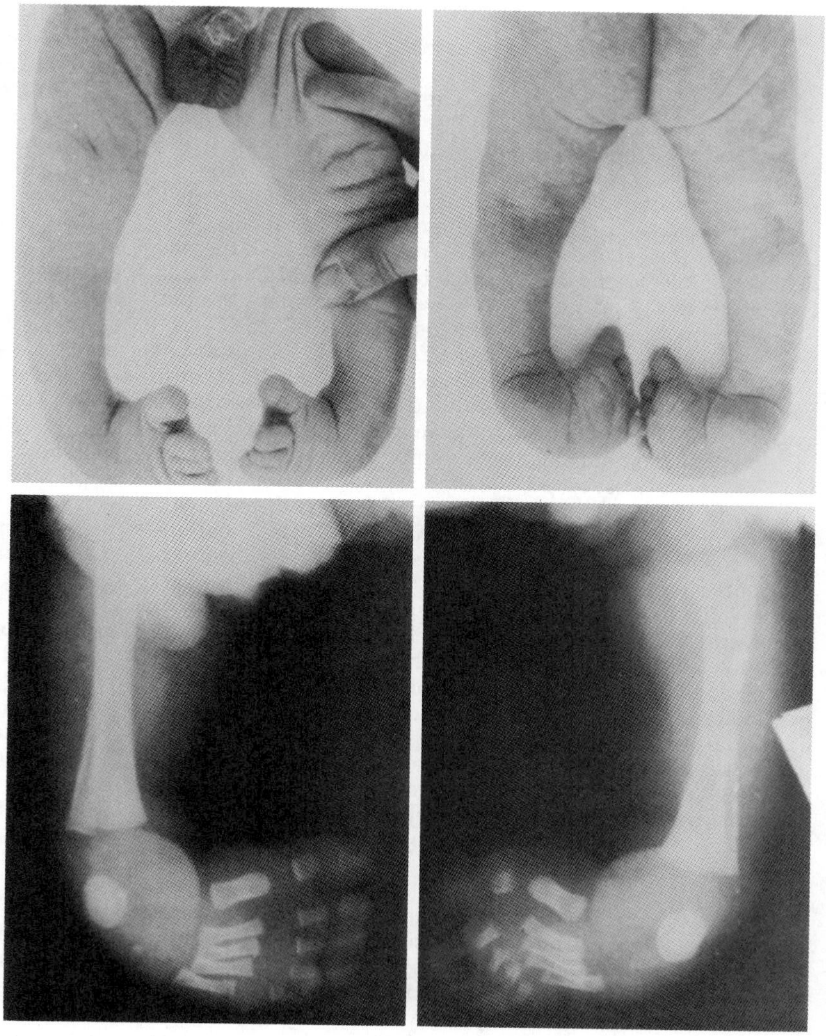

Figure 24–4. Bilateral talipes equinovarus in a newborn infant. (From Tachdjian M: Pediatric Orthopedics, 2nd ed. Philadelphia, WB Saunders, 1990.)

requires some operative correction, usually recommended between 4 and 12 mo of age.

METATARSUS ADDUCTUS. This is the most common congenital foot deformity and is thought to be secondary to intrauterine position deformity. An initial hip screening examination is most important because hip dysplasia occurs in approximately 2% of cases. **Metatarsus varus** (Fig. 24–5) involves medial subluxation of the tarsometatarsal joints and adduction and inversion of each metatarsal bone, with the hindfoot in a neutral or slight valgus position. Metatarsus adductus, which is the positional deformity, should be differentiated from metatarsus varus, which is an in utero subluxation that does not improve after birth. In metatarsus adductus, the forefoot can be brought to the neutral position because the varus position is flexible, whereas in metatarsus varus the posture is fixed. Some authors do not distinguish between the two anomalies. In both conditions, involvement may be bilateral or unilateral.

The adductus resolves spontaneously in 90% of deformational cases. The unresolved form is most likely to be stiff and severe and to show little improvement during the first months of infancy. This problem should be referred to an orthopedist if the foot is stiff or the problem persists after 6 mo of age.

If the condition persists, cast correction is indicated and is effective during infancy and early childhood. Operative correction of simple metatarsus adductus is not appropriate because no long-term disability occurs.

TOE PROBLEMS. *Polydactyly* or supernumerary toes are common and occur more frequently in blacks and females. They are often inherited in an autosomal dominant trait; they

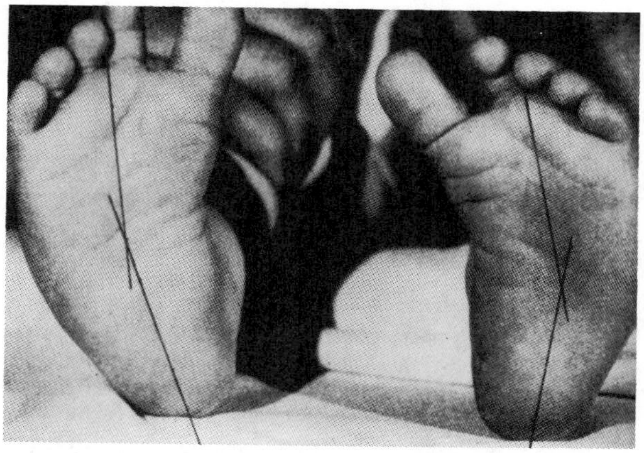

Figure 24–5. Metatarsus varus: A line bisecting the hindpart of the foot should pass through the 2nd toe or between the 2nd and 3rd toes.

are occasionally sporadic; and they often present on the lateral aspect of the foot. There may be associated hand polydactyly, absence or hypoplasia of the tibia, and various syndromes (Carpenter syndrome, Ellis-Van Creveld syndrome, Meckel-Gruber syndrome, polysyndactyly). Surgical removal is necessary and is planned before the child walks, between 9 and 12 mo of age. *Syndactyly*, congenital webbing of the toes, is most common between the 2nd and 3rd toes, is usually partial, and rarely causes disability or interferes with function (see Sec. 24.24). Associated syndromes include Apert, Carpenter, deLange, Holt-Oram, polysyndactyly, Laurence-Moon-Biedl, Fanconi pancytopenia, and 13-, 18-, and 21-trisomies. Surgery often requires skin grafting and is usually not indicated.

Congenital split or cleft foot (lobster claw), a rare deformity, is a form of ectrodactyly with 2–3 absent central digital rays (Fig. 24–6). Bilateral anomalies (hand anomalies may also be present) are usually autosomal dominant traits with incomplete penetrance, whereas less common unilateral lesions are not inherited. Associated anomalies include cleft lip and palate, deafness, triphalangeal thumb, and syndactyly. Surgical correction is indicated between 1 and 2 yr of age and includes alignment of deformed toes and syndactylization of the split forefoot and toes.

Congenital curly (varus) or overlapping toes are common, manifesting with one toe or more bent plantarward, deviated medially, and rotated laterally at the distal interphalangeal joint. The tip of the affected toe impinges on and curls under the adjacent toes, developing a callus. Congenital curly toes are familial and symmetric and are usually bilateral. Symptoms are unusual with mild deformities that require no therapy; taping and stretching does not improve the position. Children with the familial deformity of cocked-up, overlapping 5th toe *(congenital digitus minimus varus)* have difficulty with shoe-fitting and may require surgical syndactylism of the 4th and 5th digits or tendon-release surgery. Curly toes must be distinguished from *brachymetatarsia* (congenital short metatarsal), which manifests with curly (varus) deformity of the affected toes. Treatment of congenital short metatarsals includes the use of a metatarsal pad to redistribute body weight or lengthening of the metatarsals if the upriding toes cause pain from shoe pressure. Additional toe problems include *macrodactylism* due to neurofibromatosis or congenital lymphatic and adipose tissue hyperplasia and *microdactylism*, which is idiopathic or associated with amniotic bands.

Bunions in late childhood and adolescence are usually associated with *metatarsus primus varus*. This developmental deformity is hereditary, usually bilateral, seen predominantly in females, and is often unrecognized in young children. It is characterized by an increase in the angle between the 1st and 2nd metatarsals greater than 10 degrees, with medial deviation of the 1st metatarsal. The great toe deviates laterally at the metatarsophalangeal joint in compensation, and the head of the metatarsal becomes prominent, producing the bunion. The same condition may occur laterally, producing a prominence of the 5th metatarsal head, which is referred to as a "bunionette."

Bunions often become painful and may eventually require operative correction in adulthood. Otherwise, it is preferable to delay the correction until after growth has been completed; recurrence is frequent after early correction. The operation consists of an osteotomy of the metatarsal, correction of the malalignment, and excision of the prominence. If detected in infancy, stretching and casting may prevent bunion formation.

Ingrown toe nails are common in childhood; they usually involve the great toe and can be prevented by proper trimming of the toe nail. Excessively tight shoes and trimming the nail too short so that the edge digs into the nail bed have been implicated as causes of ingrown toe nails. Mild inflammation is managed best by a gentle packing of a cotton pledget under the edge of the nail to elevate the nail from the matrix beyond the skin edge. Prevention includes cutting the nail square and permitting it to extend beyond the end of the skin.

PAINFUL FOOT. The painful foot is usually relatively easily assessed by the history (trauma, fever, rash, athletic activity) and by the physical examination. The diagnosis is often suggested by the presence or absence of signs of a generalized system illness and by localizing the exact site of tenderness, which is facilitated by the paucity of obscuring muscle over the foot (Table 24–4). For example, tenderness over the calcaneus in late childhood suggests an overuse syndrome with inflammation at the insertion of the heelcord into the calcaneus. Tenderness over the tarsal navicula in late childhood is often associated with avascular necrosis or an accessory navicula. If the physician finds the site of tenderness, this guides in ordering and evaluating roentgenograms. Therapy depends on the specific disease, which is often age related and due to congenital, inflammatory (infections, rheumatologic illness), overuse, or neoplastic lesions (see Table 24–4).

SHOES. Clothing is worn for comfort, to enhance appearance, and for protection. Shoes should be selected on the same basis. They are not "corrective," and it is no more appropriate to place a child's foot in a stiff shoe than a hand in a stiff glove. The foot does not need "support," but rather it requires mobility and freedom. Barefooted people have better feet than those who wear shoes. The best shoes for children are those that simulate the bare foot. Shoes for children should be flexible, flat, and nonconstricting and should be made of material that "breathes." Shoes do not have to be expensive.

Because various overuse foot syndromes are common, especially in the athletic adolescent, shock-absorbing shoes are a good choice. A thick, cushioned sole absorbs some of the shock of impact and increases comfort.

Shoe modifications are sometimes appropriate for specific problems. Lifts may be prescribed if the limb is short. Shoe inserts may be helpful for the stiff and deformed foot or to distribute the weight load more evenly over the sole.

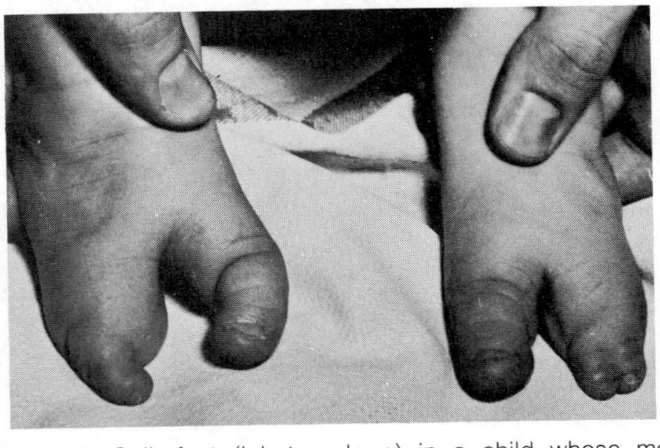

Figure 24–6. Split feet (lobster claws) in a child whose mother, maternal aunt, and maternal grandfather had similar malformations.

24.3 ROTATIONAL (TORSIONAL) PROBLEMS

In-toeing and out-toeing are common in infancy and early childhood. These problems are a subject of concern for the parents and are the reason for consulting a physician. Torsion (rotational deformity) is the twisting of a bone along its longitudinal axis. Rotation may be lateral (lateral tibial torsion: out-toeing) or medial (medial tibial torsion: in-toeing); ante-

TABLE 24–4. Differential Diagnosis of Foot Pain*

Age (Yr)		
0–6	*6–12*	*12–20*
Poor-fitting shoes	Poor-fitting shoes	Poor-fitting shoes
Foreign body		Stress fracture
Fracture	Enthesopathy (JRA)	Foreign body
Osteomyelitis†	Foreign body	Ingrown toe nail Bunion
Juvenile rheumatoid arthritis (JRA)	Accessory navicular Pes cavus	Metatarsalgia Pes cavus Ganglion
Leukemia	Tarsal coalition	Plantar fasciitis
Drawing of blood	Hypermobile flatfoot Trauma (sprains)	Avascular necrosis of metatarsal (Freiberg infarction) or navicular bone (Köhler disease) Severe disease Achilles tendinitis Trauma (sprains) Plantar warts
Tumor‡	Tumor Osteomyelitis	Tumor‡

*Modified from Allen B: Common orthopedic problems of children. *In:* Behrman R, Kliegman R: Nelson Essentials of Pediatrics, 13th ed. Philadelphia, WB Saunders, 1990.

†Osteomyelitis may be hematogenous or secondary to a puncture wound.

‡Soft-tissue mass, osteoid osteoma, synovial sarcoma, lipoma, digital fibroma, hemangioma, subungual exostosis, Ewing sarcoma.

torsion of the femoral neck axis produces medial femoral torsion and in-toeing, whereas femoral retrotorsion produces out-toeing. Almost all cases can be managed by the pediatrician. Rotational problems usually resolve spontaneously (Table 24–5). The resolution is not affected by shoe modifications or inserts, and daytime bracing is inappropriate. Rarely, these problems persist into late childhood with sufficient severity to warrant operative correction.

In the normal course of fetal growth and development, the lower limbs undergo changes in rotation. In utero the hips are laterally rotated and flexed, producing both the lateral rotation and flexion of the hip (with medially rotated and adducted feet) characteristic of early infancy. Many of the deformities of the foot and tibia in early infancy result from this intrauterine position. The foot may be medially rotated, producing *metatarsus adductus* or *medial tibial torsion*. The foot may be dorsiflexed, producing the *calcaneovalgus foot* deformity. This process is often asymmetric, and metatarsus adductus, when unilateral, is more common on the left side. With growth, postnatal alterations of ligament and muscle forces, and walking, both the hip flexion and lateral rotation contractures gradually resolve. This normal pattern accounts for the clinical presentation of rotational problems seen in infancy and childhood.

Evaluation of the infant with a rotational problem should include a history of the birth and motor development (to rule out neurologic problems), a screening examination, a hip examination (abduction, symmetry, instability) to exclude dysplasia, and an assessment of the rotational status.

The rotational status of the child is first evaluated by observing the gait, to determine the degree of in-toeing or out-toeing. Rotational deviation may result from malalignment of the femur, tibia, or foot (see Table 24–5). Therefore, the child is then examined in the prone position to determine the rotational status of each segment of the lower limb. The shape of the foot may reveal a convexity of its lateral border, indicating a metatarsus adductus. With the knee and ankle flexed to a right angle, the relationship of the axis of the foot and thigh should be observed from above. This is known as the ***thigh-foot axis*** (Figs. 24–7 and 24–8). The foot is usually laterally rotated in relation to the thigh. If the foot is turned in more than 10–20 degrees, medial tibial torsion is present. If the foot is laterally rotated more than 30 degrees, lateral tibial torsion is present. The thigh-foot angle has the greatest normal variability between 1 and 2 yr of age.

TABLE 24–5. Etiology of Toeing-In and Toeing-Out in Children*

Level of Affliction	Toe-In	Toe-Out
Feet-ankles	Pronated feet (protective toeing-in) Metatarsus varus Talipes varus and equinovarus	Pes valgus due to contracture of the triceps surae muscle Talipes calcaneovalgus Congenital convex pes planovalgus
Leg-knee	Tibia vara (Blount disease) and developmental genu varum Abnormal medial tibial torsion Genu valgum—developmental (protective toeing-in to shift body center of gravity medially) Congenital or acquired hypoplasia of the tibia with relative overgrowth of the fibula	Lateral tibial torsion Congenital absence or hypoplasia of the fibula
Femur-hip	Abnormal femoral antetorsion Spasticity of medial rotators of hip (cerebral palsy)	Abnormal femoral retroversion Flaccid paralysis of medial rotators of hip
Acetabulum	Maldirected—facing anteriorly	Maldirected—facing posteriorly

*From Tachdjian M: Pediatric Orthopedics, 2nd ed. Philadelphia, WB Saunders, 1990.

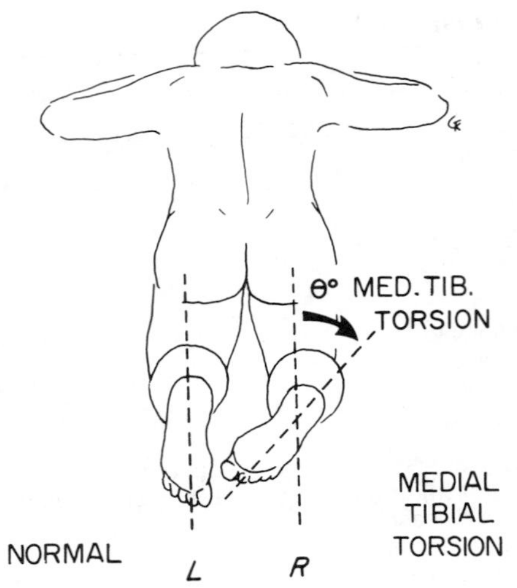

Figure 24–7. With the patient lying prone and the knees flexed 90 degrees, the position of the foot is examined for medial tibial torsion. The left foot is normal; the right foot is in medial torsion.

The hips should then be rotated medially and laterally (Fig. 24–9; see also Fig. 24–8). Medial rotation is normal to 70 degrees; if the rotation is greater, the child shows medial femoral torsion. This angle tends to be greater in the female than in the male at any age and has its greatest normal variability between 1 and 2 yr of age. The **foot progression angle** is that between the longitudinal axis of the foot and the forward line of progression, which is a neutral angle (0 degrees). The line is drawn by observing the child's gait in the office and by estimating the angle, which is negative with toeing-in and positive with toeing-out. The normal angle is approximately 10 degrees (see Fig. 24–8).

OUT-TOEING IN INFANCY. The examination usually shows more lateral than medial hip rotation, a normal pattern. Spontaneous resolution is expected during the first year or two when the child starts walking.

IN-TURNED FEET (PIGEON-TOED) IN THE FIRST YEAR. This condition is often caused by metatarsus varus or adductus (see Sec. 24.2). It is usually due to an intrauterine position and resolves spontaneously.

IN-TOEING IN THE SECOND YEAR. This is usually caused by *medial tibial torsion.* Medial tibial torsion is usually bilateral; may be associated with congenital metatarsus adductus, genu varum, or femoral antetorsion; and becomes most evident when the child begins to walk. The natural history is an improvement of the lateral rotation with increasing age. On examination, the medial malleolus is posterior to the lateral malleolus, the toes on standing point inward at angles of 15–35 degrees, and the center of gravity falls lateral to the usual 2nd metatarsal. The thigh-foot axis demonstrates a medially deviated foot (see Figs. 24–7 and 24–8). The differential diagnosis is noted in Table 24–5.

Only observation is indicated. If the condition is severe, some orthopedists recommend a splint to hold the feet laterally rotated at night. This may hasten the resolution but probably produces no more ultimate improvement than would occur spontaneously with time. Familial medial tibial torsion is least likely to resolve spontaneously and persists into adolescence (see later).

IN-TOEING IN EARLY CHILDHOOD. In-toeing with a later onset is usually due to *medial femoral torsion.* The excessive femoral torsion is present at birth but becomes most apparent with increasing age. Girls are affected more than boys (2:1); there is often a familial pattern. The child's gait is clumsy, pigeon-toed, with the thighs, knees, and patellae rotated inward. The appearance of the lower extremities is unattractive, while athletic activity is awkward. Compensatory lateral tibial tension develops with increasing age and results in a high quadriceps angle (Q angle) and subsequent patellar chondromalacia due to this torsional malalignment at the patellofemoral joint with the patella moving in and out of the intercondylar sulcus. The Q angle is a line drawn through the tibial tubercle to the midpatella, extending to the anterior superior iliac spine; angles above 15 degrees are associated with patellar instability. The child sits in the "W" (reverse tailor) position, shows limited lateral hip rotation, and medial hip rotation of more than 70 degrees, and in-toes when walking or running.

The condition usually peaks between 3 and 6 yr of age and then resolves spontaneously in most cases by 7–8 yr of age. Resolution may be due to weight bearing, muscle and ligamentous tension, gravitational forces, and growth of the femur. Shoe modifications, night splinting, and twister cables are ineffective and should be avoided. Rarely, femoral torsion persists into late childhood, producing disability and requiring operative correction.

IN-TOEING OR OUT-TOEING IN LATE CHILDHOOD AND ADOLESCENCE. Occasionally, rotational problems fail to resolve. In this rare situation, operative correction may be necessary but is best delayed until after 8–10 yr of age. Correction is indicated for medial femoral torsion (derotation osteotomy). If medial rotation is about 90 degrees, the femoral antetorsion measures 45 degrees by CT scan or MRI, the hip cannot be rotated laterally beyond the neutral position, lateral tibial torsion does not exceed 35 degrees, and the child shows a clear disability. Surgery should not be delayed beyond adolescence because the compensatory lateral tibial torsion may increase and become fixed. Medial rotation osteotomy may be needed for compensatory lateral excessive tibial torsion. There is no evidence to suggest that uncorrected medial femoral torsion produces degenerative arthritis of the hip or knee in adults.

24.4 ANGULAR DEFORMITIES: BOWLEGS AND KNOCK-KNEES

Bowlegs and knock-knees are physiologic variations in the shape of the lower limb. This variability is seen in the "frontal plane" in contrast to "transverse" or "coronal" plane problems discussed in Sec. 24.3. These two planes should be considered separately when evaluating children. Pathologic deformities of extremities in the frontal plan are referred to as genu varum (bowlegs) and valgum (knock-knees).

NORMAL DEVELOPMENT. During the 1st yr, lateral bowing of the tibia is common; during the 2nd yr, bowing of the entire limb is common (Fig. 24–10). The latter involves both the femur and tibia and is centered over the knee. During the 3rd and 4th yr, the physiologic knock-knee pattern emerges and usually peaks. The knock-knees spontaneously improve between 4 and 10 yr of age. Knock-knees seem to be more prominent in the obese, older child; however, in the normal individual, a slight case of knock-knee remains throughout life as the normal shape of the leg.

BOWLEGS (GENU VARUM). This becomes most evident when a child begins to stand and walk (Fig. 24–11). There is a wide space between the knees, a rolling gait, and in-toeing (owing to commonly present medial tibial torsion). This gait and appearance are accentuated when the child is tired or has recently been walking a long distance. The history should include information about the height of family members (short stature noted in rickets, achondroplasia), presence of similar problems in relatives, unusual dietary habits, trauma, the first

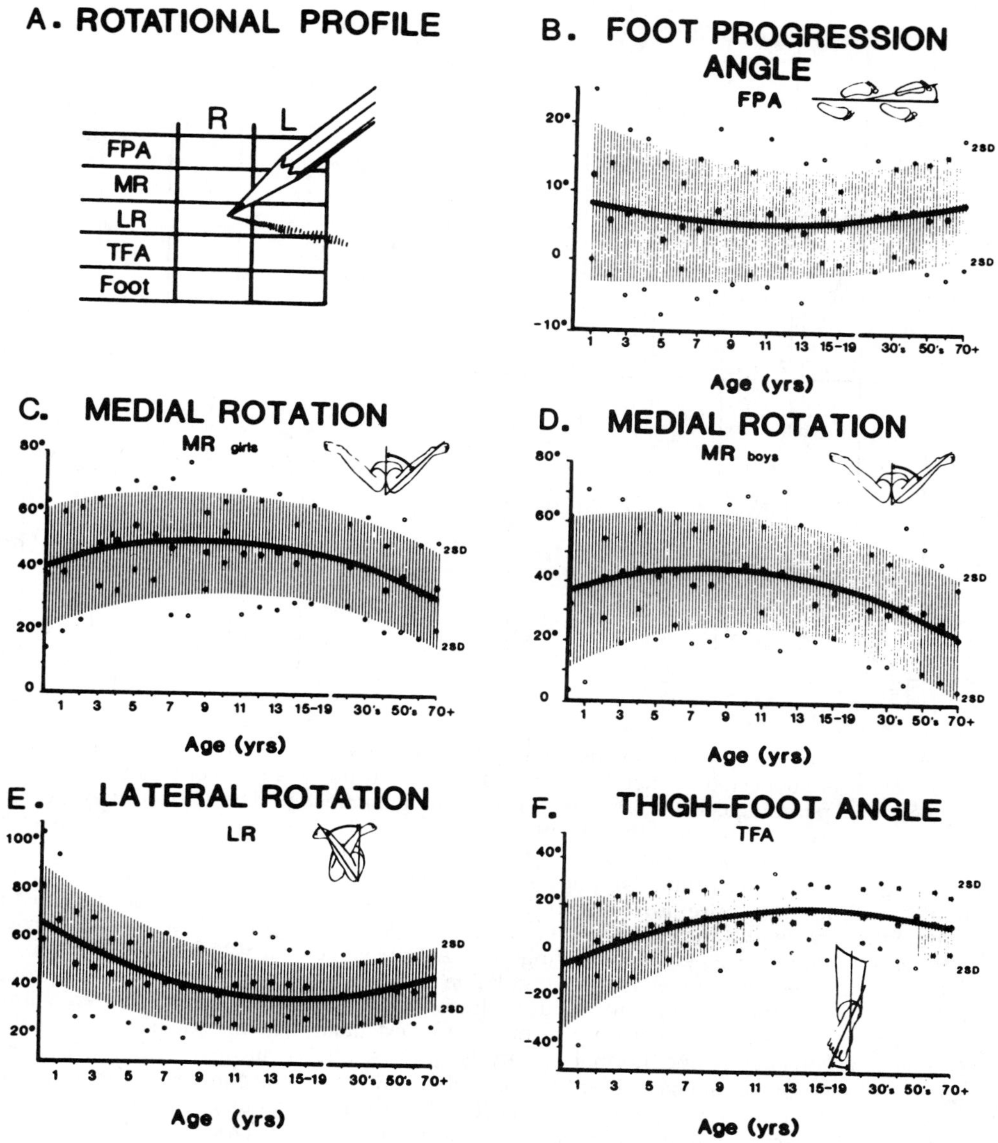

Figure 24–8. Range of normal values by age and sex with positions to determine specific angles. *A*, Rotational profile. *B*, Foot progression angle to determine the degree of in-toeing and out-toeing. *C* and *D*, Medial rotation normally < 70 degrees to determine the degree of femoral (medial femoral torsion) antetorsion (anteversion). *E*, Lateral rotation is limited in femoral antetorsion. *F*, Thigh-foot angle to determine the degree of tibial rotation. Medial torsion is present if the angle is more than 20–30 degrees. (From Staheli L: Torsional deformity. Pediatr Clin North Am 33:1373, 1986.)

time the deformity was noted, and the progression of the abnormality. Rapid progression suggests a pathologic process rather than a normal developmental process.

Diagnosis. *Physical examination* should determine the alignment of the lower limbs during stance and gait. With the patella facing forward and the medial malleoli touching, the degree of genu varum is assessed by determining the distance between the medial femoral condyles. The examination should look for signs of systemic, genetic, or metabolic process associated with pathologic genu varum. These diseases include vitamin D deficiency (nutritional, resistant rickets), hypophosphatasia, trauma, infection, tumor, metaphyseal dysplasia, camptomelic dwarfism, achondroplasia, enchondromatosis, fluorosis, congenital longitudinal deficiency of the tibia (with overgrowth of the fibula), congenital tibia vara, and Blount disease (tibia vara). Blount disease (see later) is the most common form of pathologic bowlegs and is distinguished from physiologic genu varum, as the former is often asymmetric, either unilateral or bilateral, has a short angulation at the proximal tibial metaphysis (rather than a gentle curve at the junction of the tibial proximal and middle third), has a normal contoured femur (rather than bowed), demonstrates a lateral thrust during the stance phase of gait, and demonstrates irregular rarefaction (fragmentation) of the medial upper tibial metaphysis, a medially sloping upper tibial epiphysis, a medially narrowing and laterally widening upper tibial physis, when compared with the normal roentgenographic findings in physiologic genu varum (Fig. 24–12).

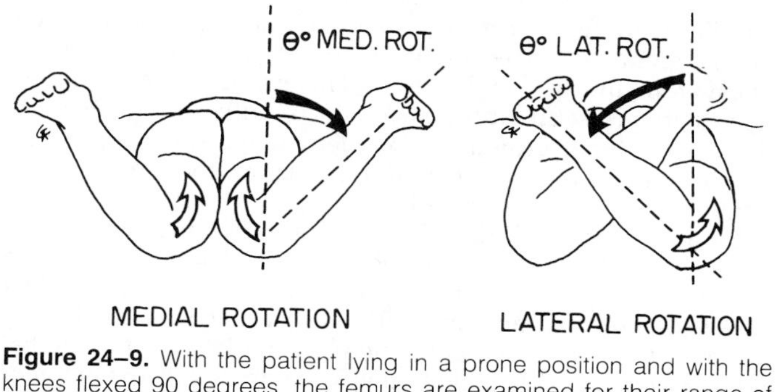

Figure 24–9. With the patient lying in a prone position and with the knees flexed 90 degrees, the femurs are examined for their range of motion at the hips in extension.

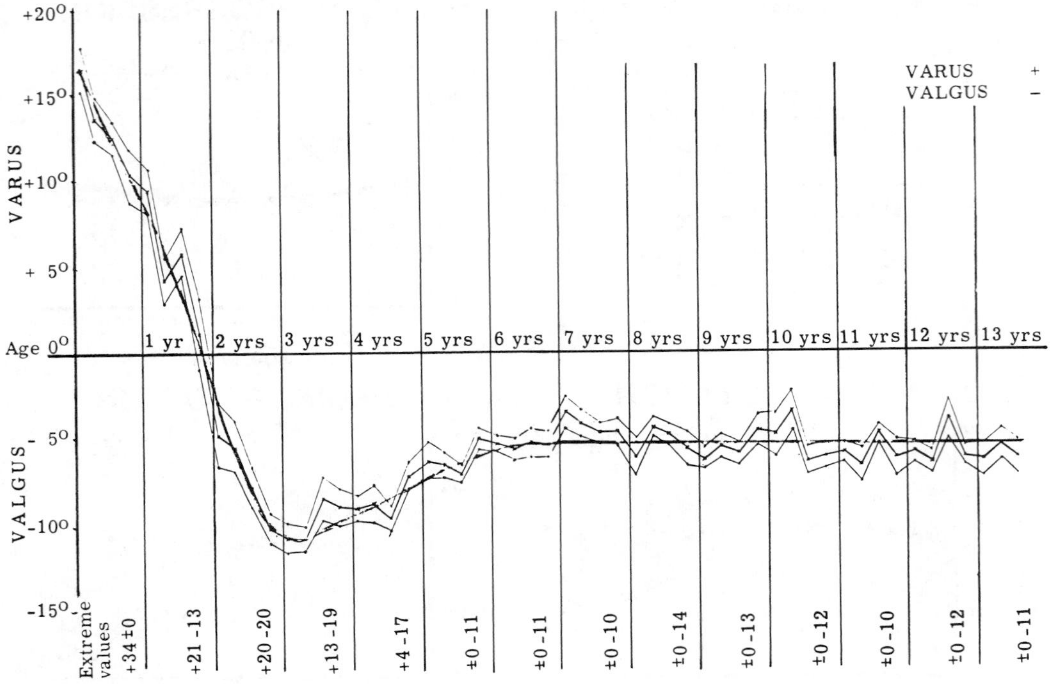

Figure 24–10. Development of the tibiofemoral angle. (From Salenius P, Vankka E: The development of the tibial femoral angle in children. J Bone Joint Surg 57A:259, 1975.)

Roentgenograms are not usually needed unless pathologic genu varum is suspected (rickets, Blount disease). Features suggesting a pathologic basis include (1) a positive family history; (2) stature below the 5th percentile; (3) severe deformity; (4) asymmetric pattern; and (5) a course that deviates from the normal developmental pattern. Roentgenograms should include the entire lower limb to demonstrate the alignment of the femur and tibia (see Fig. 24–11). Physiologic genu varum demonstrates medial tilting of the transverse planes of the knee and ankle, medial angulation of the tibia at the junction of the proximal and middle third, thickening and sclerosis of the medial cortices of the femur and tibia, symmetric involvement, and normal epiphysis, physis, and metaphysis (see later). Signs of Blount disease (tibia vara) (see Fig. 24–12), rickets (see Sec. 24.60), trauma, epiphyseal dysplasias, and infection should be identified. Metaphyseal-diaphyseal angles greater than 11 degrees suggest Blount disease. Pathologic variations warrant a referral to an orthopedist.

Treatment. The management of physiologic bowlegs is observation. The family should be reassured that this normal variant will correct itself spontaneously with time and that shoe wedges or other modifications, braces, or special diets are not helpful. The severity of the condition should be documented, and the child should be followed at 3- to 6-mo intervals to demonstrate resolution. If the deformity persists and is severe (e.g., in some congenital familial forms of tibia vara), operative correction may be indicated by a ***hemiepiphysiodesis*** in early adolescence. This produces an asymmetric growth arrest about the knee which, with growth, corrects the deformity. If growth is complete at the time of referral, an osteotomy of the tibia and fibula at the apex of the angulation can be performed.

Blount Disease (Tibia Vara). Formerly and incorrectly called osteochondrosis deformans tibia, Blount disease is a growth disorder of the medial aspect of the proximal tibial physis, epiphysis, and metaphysis (see Fig. 24–12). Blount disease demonstrates acute medial angulation and medial rotation of the tibia below the knee in the proximal metaphyseal region. Early (infantile)-onset deformity is noted before 3 yr of age, whereas juvenile onset (4–10 yr) and adolescent forms (>11 yr) occur later.

The *etiology* may be related to repeated stress, associated with severe physiologic bowlegs and differential growth of the leg. Obesity, early walking, female sex, and West Indian or West African black race are predisposing factors. Bilateral involvement is present in 50–75%. Tibia vara can be distinguished from physiologic bowlegs by the features discussed in the section on genu varum and by the progressive worsening rather than improvement, which is noted with increasing age in children with genu varum. Roentgenograms are diagnostic (see earlier). The *differential diagnosis* includes genu varum, rickets, Ollier multiple enchondromatosis, fracture, osteomyelitis (tibia vara is painless), and focal fibrocartilaginous dysplasia.

Treatment of tibia vara is indicated for progressive varus angulation and includes orthotic devices to relieve the stress of weight bearing. The knee-ankle-foot orthosis is a typical brace used in 24- to 36-mo-old children with a tibiofemoral angle greater than 15 degrees. Operative treatment is reserved for greater deformity in children (≥4 yr of age) and includes an osteotomy, which usually requires pin placement for stability.

DEVELOPMENTAL GENU VALGUM. Knock-knees is a physiologic developmental finding that is most evident at 2–6 yr of age (see Fig. 24–10). Valgus is present if the distance between the ankles exceeds 10 cm when the knees are approximated. Marked genu valgum results in an awkward gait with the knees rubbing, the feet kept apart, and a leg-swinging gait to avoid knee-to-knee contact. The child pronates and in-toes to shift the center of gravity. If there is contracture of the iliotibial band and triceps surae muscle, the child will out-toe. Calf and anterior thigh pain plus patellar subluxation are present in severe deformity.

The *differential diagnosis* includes pathologic genu valgum, especially if there is short stature (suggests epiphyseal dysplasia or endocrinopathy), asymmetric or unilateral disease, a family history of genu valgum, or a distance greater than 10 cm between the medial malleoli. Disease processes include primary tibia valgum (opposite to Blount disease), osteochon-

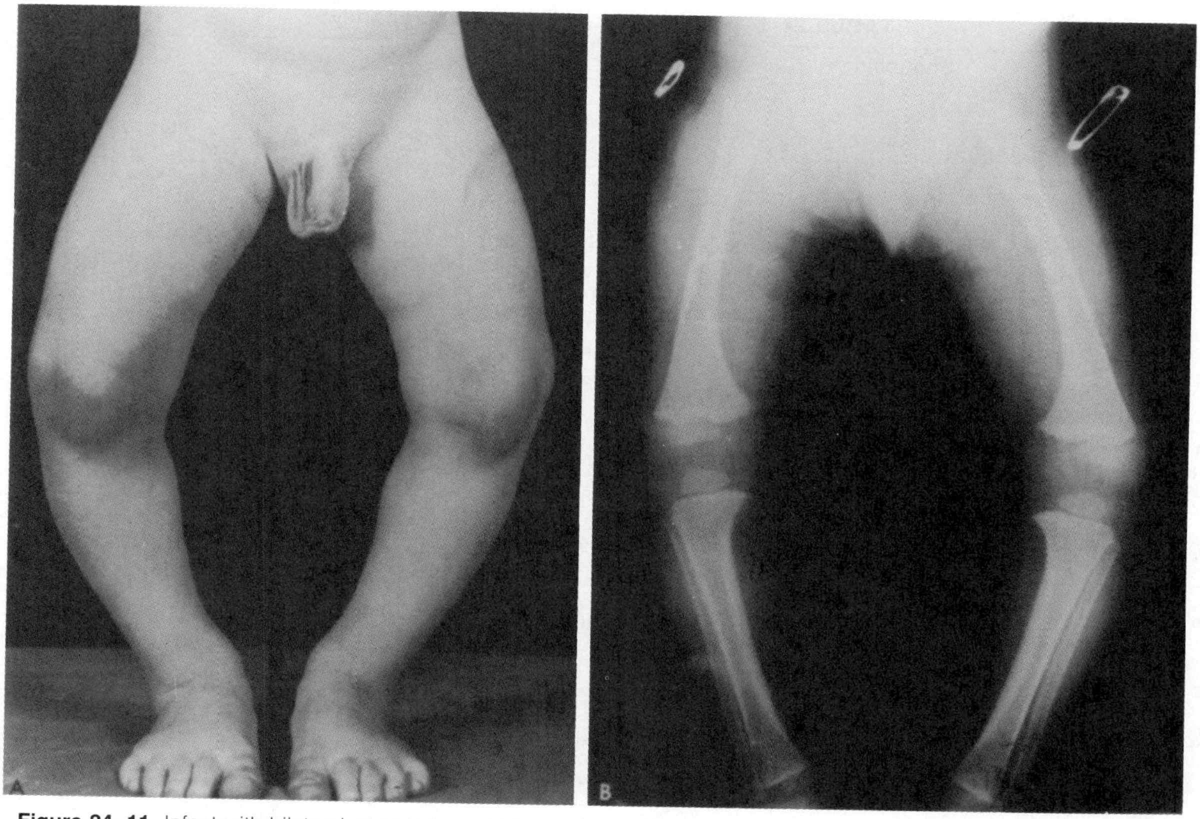

Figure 24–11. Infant with bilateral genu varum at 18 mo of age. This resolved spontaneously before 7 yr of age. (From Tachdjian M: Pediatric Orthopedics, 2nd ed. Philadelphia, WB Saunders, 1990.)

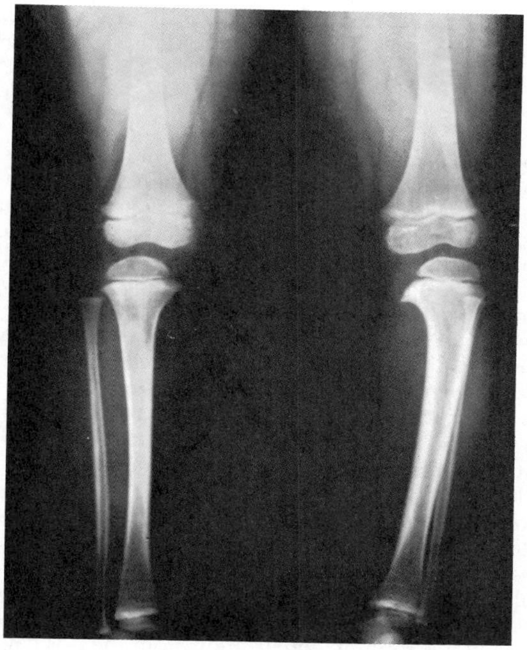

Figure 24–12. Blount disease. The medial aspect of the proximal end of the left tibia is irregular and "beaked." There is also minimal involvement of medial aspects of the proximal tibial epiphyseal center. As a consequence of the proximal tibial deformity, there was abnormal weight bearing, which in turn was responsible for the thickening shown in the medial cortex of the left tibia. The right tibia is normal.

droma, exostosis, enchondromatosis, subacute osteomyelitis, renal osteodystrophy, congenital longitudinal deficiency of the fibula, trauma, and contracture of the iliotibial band due to neuromuscular paralytic problems (myelomeningocele). Roentgenograms are indicated to determine the presence of such pathologic processes that produce excessive genu valgum.

Treatment of physiologic genu valgum of the 2- to 6-yr-old child consists of observation, because most will correct spontaneously. Surgical therapy is indicated if the intermalleolar distance exceeds 7.5 cm at 11–12 yr of age. A medial physeal retardation procedure is indicated in all except the skeletally mature patient for whom medial osteotomy is indicated.

24.5 LEG LENGTH DISCREPANCY

Leg length difference, discrepancy, or inequality, *anisomelia*, is defined as a difference of 1 cm or more. Differences less than 1 cm are considered to be a normal variation owing to nonpathologic asymmetry between the right and left sides of the body. Anisomelia may be real or apparent. Apparent or functional anisomelia is due to a tilting of the pelvis, which in turn is usually due to contracture of the adductor muscles. This contracture hikes the pelvis on the same side and creates an apparent shortening of the ipsilateral limb.

Leg length discrepancy may be due to shortening or overgrowth of one or more bones in a limb. Pathologic conditions may cause a difference in length without a change in growth rate (healed fracture with overlapping fragments) or first produce a change in growth rate without an initial leg length discrepancy (osteomyelitis). The etiology of leg length discrepancy must be determined to decide about the medical and surgical management of the patient (Table 24–6).

TABLE 24–6. Etiology of Leg Length Discrepancy*

Shortening	Lengthening
Congenital	***Congenital***
Hemiatrophy	Hemihypertrophy
Skeletal dysplasias	Local vascular malformation
Short femur	
Proximal focal femoral deficiency	
Fibular, tibial hemimelia	
Congenital dislocation of the hip	
Tumor—Developmental	***Tumor—Developmental***
Neurofibromatosis	Neurofibromatosis
Multiple exostosis	Soft-tissue hemangioma
Enchondromatosis (Ollier disease)	Arteriovenous malformation
Osteochondromatosis	Hemihypertrophy with Wilms tumor
Fibrous dysplasia (Albright syndrome)	Aneurysm
Punctate epiphyseal dysplasia	
Dysplasia epiphysealis hemimelia (Trevor disease)	
Radiation therapy prior to skeletal maturity (physeal arrest)	
Resection of benign or malignant neoplasm	
Infection	***Infection—Inflammation***
Osteomyelitis	Metaphyseal osteomyelitis
Septic arthritis	Rheumatoid arthritis
Tuberculosis	Hemarthrosis (hemophilia)
Trauma	***Trauma***
Physeal injury	Metaphyseal, diaphyseal fracture
Failed joint replacement	Diaphyseal operations (bone grafts, osteotomy, osteosynthesis, periosteal stripping)
Atrophic nonunion	
Overlapping, malposition of fracture fragments	
Burns	
Neuromuscular Disease	
Poliomyelitis	
Cerebral palsy	
Myelomeningocele	
Peripheral neuropathy	
Focal cerebral lesions (hemiplegia)	
Other	
Legg-Perthes disease	
Slipped capital femoral epiphysis	

*Adapted from Moseley C: Leg-length discrepancy. Pediatr Clin North Am 33:1385, 1986; and Tachdjian M: Pediatric Orthopedics, 2nd ed. Philadelphia, WB Saunders, 1990.

Leg length discrepancy produces a limp with a vaulting movement over the long leg. To compensate, the patient may walk on the toes of the short leg, flex the knee of the long leg, or tilt the pelvis with resultant functional scoliosis. The gait is not energy efficient, and the up-and-down motion is unattractive. Patients may use shoe lifts or corrective shoes. They may develop equinus contracture of the ankle and develop hip degenerative arthritis as adults.

DIAGNOSIS. After performing a general history and physical examination to identify disease processes noted in Table 24–6, the child should be observed from behind, with the fingers placed on the posterior iliac crests. Any difference in pelvic height should be noted. If the pelvis is not level, place a lift (e.g., a book) under the short side and adjust the thickness until the pelvis is level. The width of the lift will approximate the difference in leg length. In addition to pelvic obliquity, the patient should be observed for the vertical nature of the spine, position and size of the feet, configuration of the trunk, and relative levels of the knees.

Roentgenographic methods are essential to diagnose and assess leg length discrepancy because clinical measurements are inaccurate. CT scanning is the most accurate method, but orthoroentgenography is also helpful and involves a single exposure of the entire extremity (hips to ankles) on a long x-ray film.

TREATMENT. Treatment options of lower limb length discrepancy are based on the knowledge of patterns of skeletal growth, including past growth, potential future growth, growth rate, skeletal maturity, and ultimate growth prediction based partly on the parents' growth status. Charts are available to predict the remaining growth of specific bones for boys and girls and to predict eventual adult height.

Anticipated future or actual leg length differences of less than 2–2.5 cm should usually be left untreated. Anisomelia does not cause true structural scoliosis (a common misconception). Lifts are necessary only to improve the child's gait. Lifts are heavy, make the shoe less stable, and may place a cosmetic and social burden on the child.

Treatment varies with the age of the patient and the degree of leg length discrepancy and includes procedures to reduce the growth (epiphysiodesis, epiphyseal stapling), to shorten (osteotomy) the long leg, or to increase the length of the short leg (distraction, stimulation of physeal growth, vascular or avascular autologous fibular bone graft, cadaveric allografts).

Epiphysiodesis produces permanent growth arrest of the long limb and allows for limb equalization from the normal growth of the short leg. The procedure involves fusion across the growth plate of the long extremity. Indications include a projected limb discrepancy of 2–5 cm, an acceptable total height, and remaining growth potential for correction of the limb length difference. Referral at 8 yr of age is preferable in order to accumulate sequential growth studies and to determine the appropriate age of surgery, which is critical to avoid overcorrection or undercorrection. Epiphysiodesis is the preferred method. However, if the patient has already achieved skeletal maturity, tibial or femoral shortening of the longer leg may be indicated. Resection of a segment of bone is more difficult and has a higher complication rate than epiphysiodesis.

Lengthening procedures have a significant morbidity but are indicated for an unsatisfactory predicted final adult height and limb differences greater than 5 cm. Limb lengthening can be performed by osteotomy of the short limb with gradual distraction and (1) lengthening of diaphyseal bone with bone grafts and plating of the distraction gap (Wagner method); (2) lengthening of metaphyseal bone with corticotomy, gradual lengthening but no grafts (Ilizarov and DeBustiani methods of callotasis—callus distraction); and (3) cortical allografting of the distraction gap using a flexible intramedullary nail. In general, these procedures produce an osteotomy with preservation of the periosteum, endosteum, intramedullary circulation, and marrow. New bone growth (callus formulation) begins during the repair phase and slow (1 mm/24 hr) dynamic axial distraction (with an external fixator placed across the osteotomy) separates the margin of the osteotomy with resultant new longitudinal bone growth. Gradual application of longitudinal forces with weight bearing increases the strength and modeling of the new bone.

Complications of these procedures include postoperative wound infection, compartment syndrome, neurovascular injury, nonunion, osteomyelitis, and stress fractures.

24.6 KNEE

Knee disorders become more common during the 2nd decade, when the body grows to nearly an adult size and overuse problems become common.

HYPEREXTENSION OR KNEE DISLOCATION. Congenital knee dislocation and subluxation are deformities in which the tibia is displaced anteriorly onto the femur. Hyperextension of the knee need not be associated with true dislocation. Females are affected more than males; the disease is bilateral in 35%.

The *etiology* may be due to abnormal fetal position (e.g., breech). In addition there is fibrosis and contracture of the quadriceps muscle, which may be the cause or possibly the result of a hyperextended knee. These deformities are often associated with clubfeet, hip and elbow dislocations, familial Larsen syndrome (dislocation of hip, knee, elbow, ankles; hypertelorism; prominent forehead), 21-trisomy, spina bifida, and arthrogryposis.

The severity varies and determines the necessary treatment. Grade I (minimal subluxation) is characterized by a knee in a 15- to 20-degree hyperextension, which can be moved to 45–90 degrees of flexion. Grade II (moderate displacement) demonstrates some contact between the femoral and tibial articular surfaces despite the tibia being displaced onto the femur; the knee is held in 25- to 45-degree hyperextension and can be flexed into the neutral position. Grade III is characterized by total displacement of the tibial epiphysis in front of the femoral condyles with no contact between articular surfaces.

The *clinical manifestations* are distinctive with the knee in severe hyperextension, hips in hyperflexion, and prominent femoral condyles evident in the popliteal fossa. Dislocation should be distinguished from simple **genu recurvatum**, which is noted with breech presentation and ligamentous laxity but does not demonstrate tibial displacement over the femur. Roentgenograms demonstrate partial or complete anterior displacement of the tibia on the femur. *Treatment* consists of serial cast correction started in early infancy. If manipulation does not reduce the subluxation, traction may be needed. If correction to 60 degrees is not achieved by 3–4 mo of casting, operative open reduction is indicated. This involves lengthening of the quadriceps and correction of the intra-articular problems when necessary.

Physiologic hyperextension is seen in individuals with joint laxity. If hyperextension is greater than 10–15 degrees, evaluation for a collagen disorder such as Ehlers-Danlos syndrome and its variants may be indicated.

KNEE FLEXION CONTRACTURE. This may be due to many conditions. It may be congenital, as seen in arthrogryposis (Sec. 24.58). It is common in neuromuscular disorders, such as myelomeningocele or cerebral palsy (see Sec. 20.49). Inflammatory or traumatic disorders may also produce a contracture. *Management* involves determining the cause and treating the underlying condition when possible. Fixed flexion deformities, in patients with spina bifida, may require splinting in extension, proper posturing, exercises, and, if severe (limiting ambulation), surgical release procedures that permit extension of the knee joint. Hamstring lengthening may be indicated in some patients with cerebral palsy.

PATELLOFEMORAL DISORDERS. These disorders are due to altered function of the quadriceps mechanism. The patella may be congenitally dislocated and may produce a progressive flexion and valgus deformity unless it is corrected. Patellar *subluxation* and *dislocation* may also occur during childhood. Recurrent subluxation is common (noted predominantly in females), has a familial tendency, is associated with physical activity, and results from instability of the patellofemoral joints, permitting the patella to partially dislocate out of the intercondylar groove. Subluxation, as with the less common dislocation, occurs when the knee is flexed and the quadriceps muscle contracts. After subluxation, the patella snaps back to its normal position. Patients complain of a popping sensation or retropatellar pain, or that the knee gives out or buckles during subluxation. Chondromalacia may develop after repeated episodes; occasionally, there is an effusion. Subluxation may resemble a torn meniscus or lax ligaments.

Complete acute patellar dislocation is uncommon and dramatic and is characterized by a flexed knee with the patella visible on the lateral aspect of the joint. Concavity is present where the patella normally sits; an effusion may be present; and if the vastus medialis is torn, there will be medial tenderness. Acutely there is knee pain and the patient falls down; with chronic dislocation, pain and disability diminish. The so-called **habitual dislocation** is usually painless and results from a contracture of the vastus lateralis and tearing or stretching of the vastus medialis tendon. Whenever the knee is flexed, the patella subluxates or dislocates laterally. This process often occurs with walking and results in a loss of the lateral femoral condyle.

The etiologies associated with subluxation/dislocation of the patella include ligamentous laxity of the medial knee capsule in normal individuals or in patients with Ehlers-Danlos syndrome or related syndromes, contracture of lateral patellar soft tissues (vastus lateralis) and abnormal attachments of the iliotibial fascial band, muscle imbalance (weak vastus medialis, stronger vastus lateralis), femoral antetorsion, genu valgum, high-riding patella (patella alta), and trauma.

Recurrent subluxation-dislocation may produce degeneration of the patellofemoral joint, especially of the medial side of the patella, which may progress to osteoarthritis of the entire femorotibial joint.

Chondromalacia patellae, an overuse syndrome occurring in susceptible persons during adolescence, is the most common patellofemoral disorder. Most patients show some mild degree of patellofemoral malalignment. The principal symptom is anterior knee pain and a grating sensation aggravated by activities involving knee flexion (e.g., climbing stairs or running). The undersurface of the medial side of the patella may be tender and demonstrate crepitance, and the result of the **patellar inhibition test** is usually positive. This test is carried out by asking the patient to actively extend the knee while the examiner compresses the patella against the femoral condyles. The patient refuses to extend the leg, which necessitates contracting the quadriceps muscles, thus aggravating patellar instability. The chronic knee pain often results in disuse atrophy of the quadriceps.

Recurrent dislocation of the patella during adolescence is commonly associated with physical activity. Dislocation may occur spontaneously or may be initiated by some injury. If traumatic, dislocations may be associated with an articular fracture. If the injury is severe, arthroscopic evaluation may be indicated.

Most recurrent dislocations occur in individuals with **dysplastic knees.** The elements of this dysplasia may include one or more features. Bony malalignment may be present as a genu valgum or as a rotational problem. Medial femoral and lateral tibial torsion and a valgus knee align the tibial tubercle more laterally than normal, making dislocation easier. The quadriceps may be abnormal. Hypoplasia of the vastus medialis results in an absence of the normal fullness just superior medial to the patella. Shortening or tightness of the vastus lateralis results in a tethering of the patella laterally. The joint itself may be abnormal with the patella high-riding and the lateral femoral condyle deficient. Tracking of the patella is often abnormal. With the patient sitting and slowly extending the knee, normally the patella remains midline throughout extension. In patients with subluxation/dislocation, the patella often tracks laterally during the last 10–20 degrees of extension.

The physical examination should include a search for the dysplastic elements and should elicit the **patellar apprehension sign.** The latter is demonstrated by applying lateral pressure to the patella with the knee extended 30 degrees and the quadriceps relaxed. The patient, sensing that the patella may be about to dislocate, becomes fearful at the point of maximal displacement. The patient stops the examiner's hand while extending the knee to relocate the patella to a normal position.

Roentgenograms are indicated in the subluxable patella, especially after reduction of an acute dislocation, to demonstrate the presence of fractures, bone fragments, genu valgum, patellar position, hypoplasia of the femoral condyles, or changes in degenerative arthritis.

Treatment of subluxation or moderate chondromalacia includes an active isometric progressive resistance exercise program to strengthen the quadriceps. During the acute painful period, the use of nonsteroidal anti-inflammatory agents, rest, and temporary avoidance of activities that exacerbate the condition are indicated. Arthroscopy may be indicated to remove bone or cartilaginous fragments, to shave the underside of a patella with chrondromalacia, or to release lateral retinacular tethering structures. Arthroscopy may identify other pathology, such as meniscal tears.

Patellar subluxation with excessive lateral pressure, which does not respond to an exercise program, requires operative correction. This may include arthroscopic or surgical lateral patellar retinacular release or procedures to realign the quadriceps. Lateral release may be accompanied by transfer of the proximal tibial tubercle in a distal and medial direction to realign the quadriceps.

Reduction of acute dislocation may occur spontaneously or by gently straightening the knee to reduce quadriceps tension, thus permitting the patella to slide over the lateral femoral condyle.

INTRA-ARTICULAR DISORDERS. Meniscal problems are uncommon in children. Tears of the meniscus seldom occur during the 1st decade. ***Meniscus injuries*** occur in adolescents during weight bearing, with the knee in moderate flexion while exposed to twisting or bending forces. *Clinical manifestations* during the acute injury include a painful, audible snap, a popping sensation, knee buckling, limp, limitation of knee motion, and, if there is associated soft-tissue trauma, swelling and hemarthrosis. Chronic manifestations include a "clunk," popping, or snapping sensation if the meniscus is displaced between the articular surfaces. Impingement on articular surfaces may produce future arthritis and should be removed. The knee may also lock or give way with meniscal injuries and other knee disorders (subluxation or dislocation of the patella). There may be accompanying joint effusion, atrophy of the quadriceps, and localized tenderness at the joint line near the tear. A *diagnosis* is made by arthroscopy and arthrography. *Treatment* includes arthroscopic repair or partial resection of meniscal tissue impinging on articular surfaces. Total meniscectomy in childhood leads to premature degenerative arthritis and should be avoided.

Most meniscal abnormalities in childhood are due to a ***lateral diskoid meniscus.*** This is a congenitally malshaped meniscus, often with abnormal attachments and increased mobility. The child may be asymptomatic before 6–8 yr of age and may then develop a snapping (click) of the knee, catching or giving way, and a loss of full extension. Physical examination reveals an audible clunk during knee extension and a palpable fullness in the parapatellar joint line of the flexed knee. The *differential diagnosis* of a snapping-catching knee includes meniscal injury or cyst, congenital tibiofemoral joint subluxation, abnormal popliteus tendon motion, normal snapping of knee tendons, and patellofemoral or proximal tibiofibular joint subluxation/dislocation. *Diagnosis* of diskoid lateral meniscus is visualized by arthrography, arthroscopy, and MRI. *Treatment* is nonoperative in the absence of pain or functional disability. Open or arthroscopic, partial, or, less optimally, complete resection is indicated for frequent knee-locking episodes and severe pain and disability.

Osteochondritis dissecans (OD) is a condition characterized by subchondral bone necrosis and sometimes by complete or partial separation of articular fragments. The etiology may involve repeated trauma to a segment of bone with tenuous vascularity. Although usually unilateral and sporadic, there may be familial incidence. Multiple joints may be involved (e.g., knee, elbow, ankle, hip, shoulder); there is a preponderance of males (3:1) and two involved age groups (younger than 12 yr of age and young adults). The most common site is the lateral aspect of the medial femoral condyle. It may also occur in the patella and the lateral condyle.

Clinical manifestations include episodic knee pain, aching after exercises, stiffness, clicking, muscle atrophy, mild joint swelling, and occasionally locking. Localized tenderness is palpable by deep pressure over the lesion. The demarcated fragment of subchondral bone is best demonstrated roentgenographically by a "notch view" of the knee. This shows the femoral condyles and the radiolucent fragment. Ossification variations (irregular-ragged epiphysis) about the knee are often mistaken for OD. These may be differentiated from OD because they are often bilateral; they occur in locations that are uncommon for OD; and they are not tender. CT scanning and MRI are also helpful methods to visualize the anatomy.

The *treatment* of OD in the patient with open growth plates is conservative. Isometric quadriceps exercises, limitation of activities, and the passage of time lead to resolution of most lesions. Open arthrotomy or arthroscopic correction is appropriate for large lesions (>1 cm) when there is a history of joint locking or the persistence of symptoms for more than 6 mo. Arthroscopic procedures include multiple drilling of the transarticular cartilage for intact lesions; in situ pinning for early separated lesions; removal and replacement with pinning of partially detached lesions; curetting the crater and fragment-pinning of the salvageable loose body; and spongialization of the crater and removal of the fragment with an unsalvageable loose body. All attempts are made to preserve the articular weight-bearing surface to avoid future osteoarthritis.

OSGOOD-SCHLATTER DISEASE. This traction apophysitis of the tibial tubercle results from microtrauma. It is not avascular necrosis or an inflammatory process but is an overuse syndrome that occurs commonly in physically active males around puberty. Athletic activity combined with a recent growth spurt results in detachment of cartilage fragments from the tibial tuberosity. The disease is bilateral in 25–50% of cases.

Localized tenderness and swelling are present over the tibial tubercle. Pain is demonstrated by running, jumping, going up or down stairs, and kneeling. The tibial tuberosity is enlarged, but there is no synovial effusion or thickening of the knee joint.

A single roentgenogram is indicated to rule out other lesions. The tibial tubercle in adolescents is normally irregular but Osgood-Schlatter disease is associated with soft-tissue swelling and a thickened ligamentum patellae. More severe disease is characterized by free particles of bone anterior and superior to the tibial tuberosity. Fragments of the epiphysis are not typical of Osgood-Schlatter disease.

Treatment is focused on a reduction of activity; this should be negotiated with the patient to avoid over-restriction. The process is usually self-limited and remits when the tibial tubercle fuses to the diaphysis. A contracted quadriceps should be stretched. The use of a knee immobilizer splint may sometimes be helpful. Resolution occurs over a period of months, but in 5–10% of patients the condition becomes chronic (unresolved Osgood-Schlatter disease) with persistent tenderness, swelling, and an ossicle demonstrated by a lateral roentgenogram. Excision of the ossicle may be required. There are few indications for local corticosteroid injections, because such treatment is not indicated for a self-limited disease and may weaken the tendon and produce local cutaneous thinning and depigmentation.

POPLITEAL CYST. Popliteal or Baker cysts are lesions arising from the capsule or tendon sheaths. In contrast to adults, cysts in children seldom communicate with the joint and are not associated with intra-articular abnormalities. The parents often notice a nonpulsatile, painless swelling on the posterior and medial aspects of the knee that becomes most prominent on knee extension. The child occasionally has local pain, stiffness, and mild discomfort. The diagnosis may be confirmed by translumination of the hard, firm cyst or by aspiration of clear viscous fluid. In most cases, the cyst recurs following aspiration. Ultrasound may be used to differentiate a solid and cystic lesion. The differential diagnosis includes a lipoma, aneurysm, varices, thrombophlebitis, neuroma, pigmented villonodular synovitis, and, rarely, tumors (synovial and other sarcomas, histiocytoma) occurring in older patients and in the lateral aspect rather than the medial (typical for Baker cyst) aspect of the popliteal fossa. The lateral position and solid components are indications for further evaluation and excision. Because most cysts resolve in 1–2 yr, only observation is necessary. Excision is usually not necessary but is indicated for large, painful, and persisting cysts or when the diagnosis is uncertain.

24.7 HIP

Hip disorders have great potential to cause disability; many hip problems in adults originate in childhood. For most diseases, early detection and subsequent successful management prevent permanent joint damage.

The hip is vulnerable for many reasons. Because of upright posture, the body weight is shifted forward in the acetabulum, reducing the weight-bearing area and making the hip at risk for arthritis. The vascularity of the femoral head is precarious and is subject to reduced perfusion (with or without increased intra-articular pressure), making avascular necrosis (osteonecrosis) a common problem.

Hip disease may be congenital or acquired and manifests as deformity, disability, limp, stiffness, and hip or referred knee, buttock, or thigh pain, with or without signs of inflammation or systemic generalized illness (rheumatic fever, sepsis, sickle cell anemia). Traumatic injury is usually obvious, whereas acute or chronic nontraumatic hip pain due to intra-articular disease in childhood creates an important differential diagnosis.

The diagnosis of hip problems is difficult because of the hip's deep location and pattern of innervation. The obdurator nerve has a dual sensory distribution that includes the hip joint and the skin above the knee. Referred knee pain may therefore lead to mistakes in diagnosis and delays in treatment.

The orthopedic examination should evaluate the patient's stance and posture to identify asymmetry (short leg in congenital hip dysplasia, Legg-Calvé-Perthes disease, slipped capital femoral epiphysis), unilateral externally rotated foot (possible slipped capital femoral epiphysis), or a prominent femoral greater trochanter (dislocated hip). The walking and running gaits, squatting, and single leg standing should be evaluated to look for limp, instability, or demonstration of pain. Inspection may reveal signs of trauma, external rotation of the leg (e.g., in slipped capital femoral epiphysis), or flexion, abduction, and external rotation (e.g., in septic hip arthritis). Palpation should look for point localized tenderness and warmth over the femoral head (anterior groin) and should identify the pathology of the pelvis, abdomen, and spine. Range of motion should be performed gently to avoid pain, and measurements of the thigh should be made to identify swelling or disuse atrophy.

Screening laboratory tests include a CBC, ESR, and plain hip roentgenograms, bone scan, or ultrasound.

24.8 Developmental (Congenital) Dislocation of the Hip

Developmental dislocation of the hip (DDH) encompasses the severity spectrum from mild acetabular dysplasia to frank dislocation. *Subluxation* is present when the femoral head remains in the joint space but is not concentric with the acetabulum at rest. A *dislocatable* hip is similar to subluxation, except that the entire femoral head leaves the acetabulum with manipulation but remains in normal position at rest. An unstable hip in a neonate is usually subluxable or dislocatable. Such simple hip instability often stabilizes and improves spontaneously 1–3 mo after birth. *Developmental dislocation* is demonstrated by the femoral head riding superolaterally outside the acetabulum at rest but which is reducible during the neonatal period. DDH may not be clinically evident by examination at birth but demonstrates roentgenographic evidence of an acetabulum that is steeper and shallower than normal. Dysplasia may be associated with coxa valga antetorsion and delayed ossification of the femoral head. *Teratologic* DDH is associated with other serious malformations (arthrogryposis, lumbosacral agenesis, chromosomal disorder, spina bifida), develops early in gestation, is complicated by soft-tissue contractures and significant displacement of the femoral head, and is not reducible at birth.

If left untreated, DDH produces a functional disability with a limp in young children and continued disability with pain in adults. Unresolved degrees of DDH eventually produce degenerative hip arthritis.

EPIDEMIOLOGY AND ETIOLOGY. The incidence of DDH is 0.5–2% of live-born infants. The incidence of true dislocation is 1.5 in 1,000 live births. Ten to 20% of patients with hip dysplasia have a family history. DDH is associated with oligohydramnios, first-born infants, females, breech presentation, positive family history in 1st-degree relatives, white race, congenital scoliosis or torticollis, metatarsus adductus, hyperextension of the hip or knee, calcaneovalgus foot deformity, plagiocephaly, intrauterine crowding (twins, triplets), Larsen syndrome, spina bifida, and cerebral palsy. The left side is involved in 60% of cases; the right side is involved in 20%; and 20% are bilateral. The incidence is higher if screening is performed immediately after birth because 85–95% of unstable hips in neonates resolve by 2–3 mo of age.

The etiology of congenital DDH may be related to intrauterine malposition (breech) and associated abnormal mechanical forces, ligamentous laxity, or collagen disorders. Most cases of DDH are secondary to mechanical factors (positional deformation) rather than primary dysplasia of the acetabulum. Postnatal factors include abnormal anatomic alignment of the hip, positioning the infant with extended and adducted hips, and muscle contractures owing to neuromuscular disorders (cerebral palsy). Increased ligamentous laxity, due in part to placental passage of maternal estrogens, may explain some cases of subluxation or dislocatable hips that resolve spontaneously after birth.

The familial occurrence of DDH suggests that some genetic factors contribute to the etiology. These variables may include a predisposition to ligamentous laxity or to dysplastic development of the acetabulum. The concordance rate is 42% in monozygotic twins and 2.8% in dizygotic twins. The risk of recurrence is 6% with a normal parent and one affected sibling; 12% with an affected parent; and 36% with an affected parent and sibling.

PATHOPHYSIOLOGY. At birth, hips have four ultrasonographic characteristics: (1) normal well-formed bony acetabular roof, deep acetabular cavity, normal position of femoral head, small amounts of hyaline cartilage at the lateral margin of the acetabulum, and the labrum extending from the acetabulum and encompassing the femoral head, representing 60% of neonatal examinations; (2) physiologic immature appearance (30–40%) with a shallower bony acetabulum, rounded bony ridge, and wider and larger cartilaginous component; (3) the labrum is displaced laterally, and the bony acetabulum is very shallow with no covering of the femoral head; and (4) there is displacement with no contact of the labrum and femoral head.

Initial joint laxity (from whatever cause) produces hip instability. With established dislocation, the muscles about the hip shorten; the iliopsoas tendon becomes positioned between the femoral head and the acetabulum; the joint capsule constricts; fat fills the joint; the labrum inverts; the proximal femur becomes anteverted; and the femoral head becomes less spherical. These processes occur with advancing postnatal age and can be prevented by early diagnosis and management with prompt reduction and positioning until the acetabulum is normal.

CLINICAL MANIFESTATION AND DIAGNOSIS. In the newborn period, the diagnosis is made clinically by demonstrating hip instability using the Ortolani (passive reduction–re-entry of a dislocated femoral head) and Barlow (passive manipulation–provoked dislocation) maneuvers. Very gently, without applying force in a calm, relaxed infant while supine on an examining table, the physician should examine each hip independently, placing the knees and hips in flexion and manipulating the infant's hip to displace (Barlow) or reduce (Ortolani) the femoral head over the posterior rim of the acetabulum (Fig. 24–13). The femoral head is reduced by passive motion as the hip is abducted, and the examiner's middle finger applies gentle inward and upward pressure

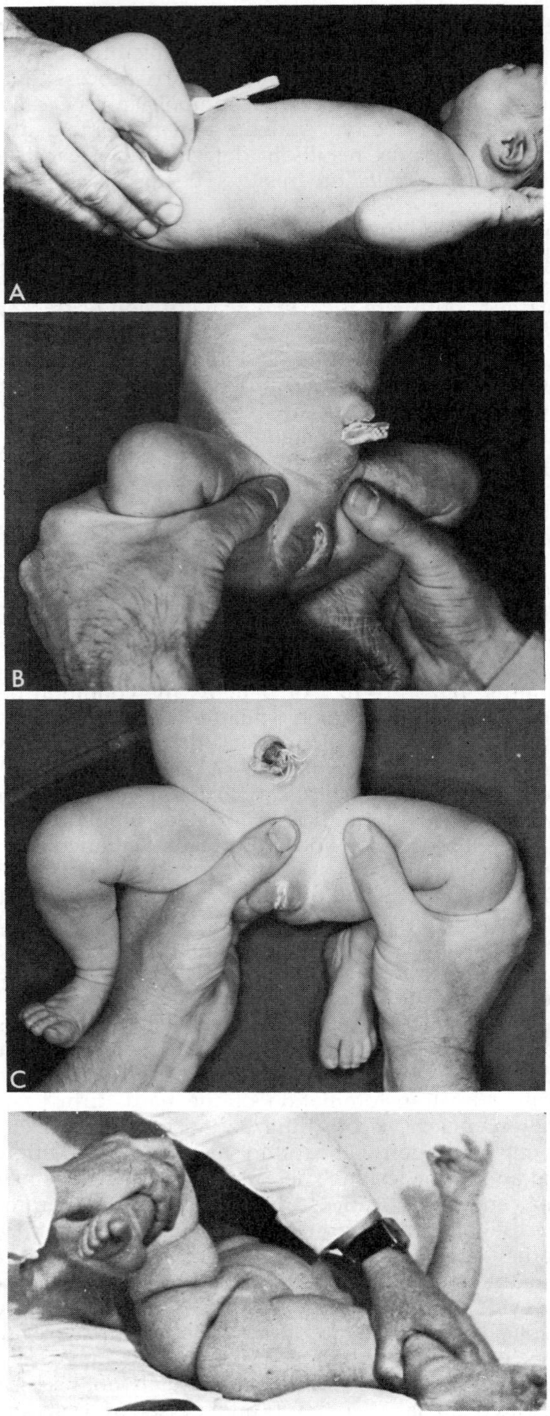

Figure 24–13. *A*, The newborn child is laid on her back with the hips and knees flexed, and the middle finger of each hand is placed over each greater trochanter. *B*, The thumb of each hand is applied to the inner side of the thigh opposite the lesser trochanter. *C*, In a doubtful case the pelvis may be steadied between a thumb over the pubis and fingers under the sacrum while the hip is tested with the other hand. *D*, Limitation of abduction is an early sign of congenital dislocation of the hip. Note the restriction in abduction of the right leg.

over the greater trochanter; the femoral head is gently dislocated as the hip is adducted with outward and backward pressure applied over the inner thigh with the examiner's thumb. The positive finding is a palpable clunk of entry or exit of the femoral head over the acetabular rim. This sensation is *not* an audible click that is caused by nonpathologic processes. Hip clicks are audible high-pitched sounds due to ligamentous snapping, normal joint space vacuum phenomena, patellar subluxation, or diskoid lateral meniscus but *not* DDH.

The Ortolani and Barlow tests detect most, but not all, cases of DDH; some cases of developmental hip dysplasia are not identified by clinical examination of the neonate but may be demonstrated by ultrasound, which is indicated in patients with a family history of DDH and no physical findings. The Ortolani and Barlow maneuvers are not definitive and should be "backed up" by repeated examination in later infancy. Because these provoked manipulations are less useful in infants older than 3–4 mo of age and because the diagnostic signs of DDH change with age, other manifestations must be demonstrated. With time, hip instability becomes less apparent owing to muscle contracture, whereas limited abduction, limb shortening, asymmetric perineal inguinal (thigh) folds (while in the frog-leg position), palpable nonreducible malposition of the femoral head, telescoping or a piston-like motion of the femur over the pelvis, and pelvic obliquity become more prominent. Children who are at the age when they should walk, instead limp. They have contralateral pelvis tilt and lateral spine deviation to the affected hip, and they demonstrate an abductor lurch as the shoulders sway laterally to the affected side. The result of the Trendelenburg test is positive. Bilateral disease is characterized by external lordosis, a wide pelvis, flat buttocks, and a "duck-like" waddle.

Roentgenography is unreliable and may be normal in the neonatal period because the pelvis is cartilaginous, the femoral head is unossified, and its relationship to the acetabulum is difficult to define. After 2–3 mo of age, conventional anteroposterior roentgenograms adequately visualize DDH (Fig. 24–14). Static nonstressed and dynamic *ultrasound* are valuable methods capable of identifying and monitoring DDH from birth throughout infancy. The static technique visualizes the iliac bone, triradiate cartilage, roof, wall, and cartilage of the acetabulum, labrum, intertrochanteric fossa, cartilaginous femoral head and growth plate, and the ossified femoral metaphysis. The dynamic stress method employs coronal and axial planes with real-time ultrasonographic observation of the motion of the femoral head. Ultrasound may detect dysplasia in the absence of clinical findings and may have a role in screening programs. Ultrasound allows grading of severity (see Pathophysiology) and permits monitoring of treatment.

TREATMENT. In infancy, the principles of treatment include a reduction of the dislocated hip and maintenance of the reduction with the use of a harness (splint) to position the hip in flexion and abduction. The infant younger than 6 mo of age with a dislocated hip should be treated with a **Pavlik harness** (Fig. 24–15). Double or triple diapers are rarely effective except in the case of minimally unstable hips and often delay definitive therapy. The Pavlik harness consists of Velcro closures, a shoulder harness with shoulder straps, lower limb stirrup straps, and open booties, which allow for active hip motion and gentle passive hip abduction to maintain reduction of the femoral head.

If the hip is dislocatable, the harness is used for 22 hr each day (for at least 3 wk) until the hip is stable. Thereafter, the harness is weaned by 4, 6, or 8 hr each day on a weekly or biweekly schedule. If the hip is dislocated but reducible the infant uses the harness all day for 3–4 wk. The hip usually becomes stable (not dislocatable) and roentgenographically demonstrated to be concentrically in the acetabulum by 4–6 wk of treatment; thereafter, the harness is weaned. *Complications* include aseptic (avascular) necrosis (osteonecrosis) of

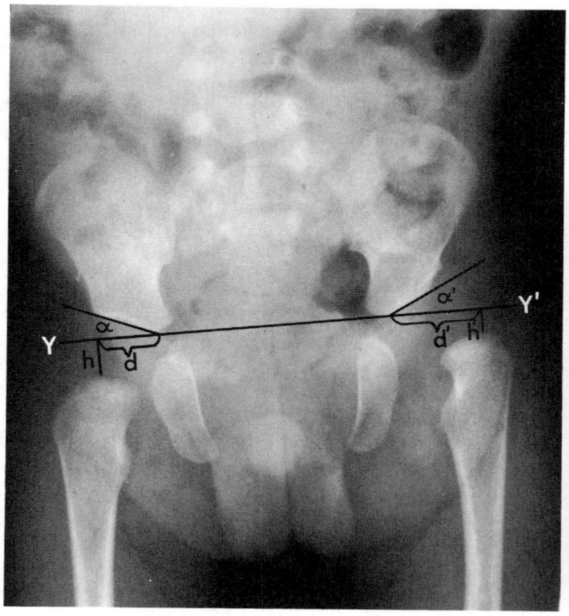

A

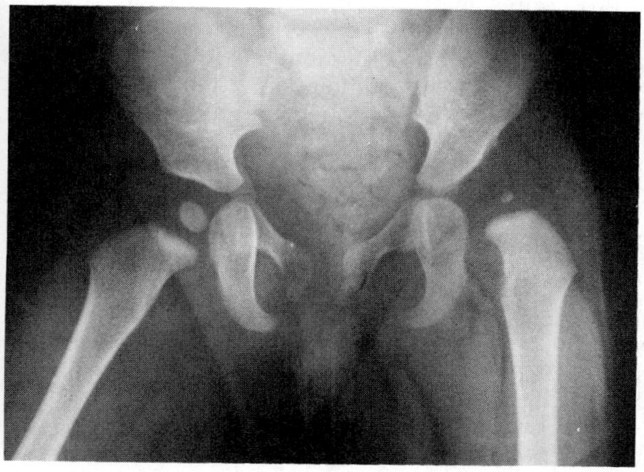

B

Figure 24–14. *A*, The Hilgenreiner method for identification of dysplasia of the hip prior to ossification of the capital femoral epiphysis: α' is greater than α, indicating greater obliquity of the acetabular roof. d' is greater than d, indicating lateral displacement of the femur. h is greater than h', indicating cephalic displacement of the femur. These relations indicate dysplasia of the patient's left hip. *B*, Congenital dislocation of the left hip. The bony roof of the left acetabulum is quite oblique, and there is the beginning of a false acetabulum above its most lateral aspect. The left femur is displaced laterally and superiorly. The left femoral capital epiphyseal center is smaller than the right.

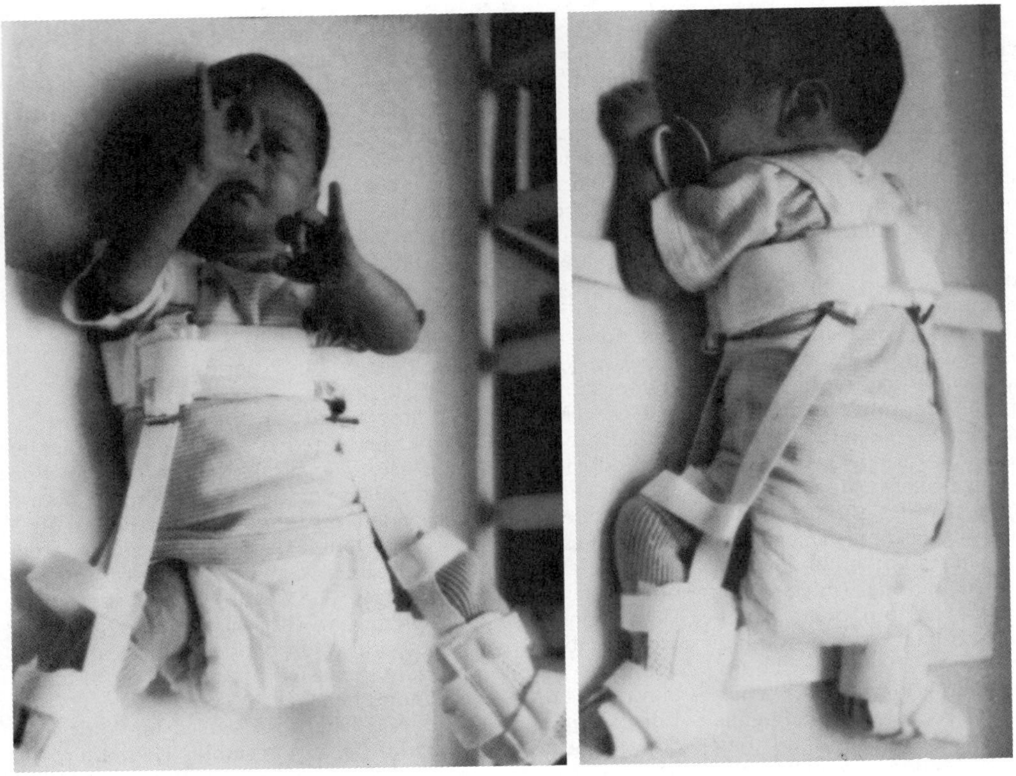

Figure 24–15. Pavlik harness. The hips become flexed and subsequently fall out passively into abduction. This adjustable harness is easy to apply and permits active lower extremity motion. (From Tachdjian M: Pediatric Orthopedics, 2nd ed. Philadelphia, WB Saunders, 1990.)

the proximal femur noted more often in dislocated than dislocatable or subluxed hips, inferior subluxation or dislocation, failure to achieve concentric reduction, anterior dislocation, failure to stretch taut hip adductors, femoral nerve palsy (entrapment syndrome), and medial knee joint instability. Other splints or harnesses include the von Rosen (Malmo), Craig (Ilfeldt), and Frejka.

If splint/harness treatment fails or the diagnosis is delayed until after 6 mo, treatment consists of preliminary traction followed by closed or open reduction under anesthesia and bilateral spica cast immobilization to retain the reduction. If treatment is delayed until walking age, management becomes complicated and prolonged and has a lower likelihood of full correction. Procedures in older children may include open reduction, acetabuloplasty, osteotomy, bone grafts, plate and pin placement, and correction of femoral antetorsion.

Early detection by frequent examination of the hips at birth and before 4 mo of age with subsequent closed reduction and harness therapy will prevent the significant morbidity associated with untreated DDH of the older child and adolescent.

24.9 LEGG-CALVÉ-PERTHES DISEASE

(Perthes Disease)

Perthes disease is a juvenile idiopathic avascular necrosis of the femoral head. The *etiology* is unknown although trauma, transient synovitis, venous congestion, hyperviscosity, coagulation abnormalities, and other mechanisms have been suggested. Repeated rather than one episode of infarction may best explain the pathology and long-term outcome.

Males are affected more often than females (4–5:1); 20% of cases are familial. The incidence is 1:1,000 to 1:5,000 in the general population but 1:35 in affected families. The familial occurrence of Perthes disease, especially with bilateral involvement, has been challenged as such cases may be skeletal dysplasias. The disease is associated with poor socioeconomic status, whites rather than blacks, a history of low birthweight, hernias, undescended testis, constitutional delayed growth, 4–8 yr of age, and delayed bone age. In 10% of cases the disease is bilateral.

The natural history includes four stages. The initial or **synovitic** stage demonstrates joint stiffness, an occasional effusion, and negative results on roentgenograms. The patients are seldom seen during this stage. The 2nd stage is that of **necrosis.** Early in this phase a subchondral lucency is often seen on the lateral radiogram and demonstrates the extent of the necrosis (Fig. 24–16). The bone undergoes progressive collapse during this phase. The 3rd phase is **fragmentation.** This is a reparative phase in which new bone replaces the necrotic dead bone. The final phase is that of **reconstitution** with restoration of normal bone structure. Remodeling is often incomplete, and the head remains large and nonspherical.

The *clinical manifestations* include an insidious onset (weeks-months), antalgic limp, stiffness, and mild pain in the groin, hip, thigh, or knee. Pain is aggravated by activity and relieved by rest. The condition is often present for months before medical care is sought. The physical findings include stiffness, thigh atrophy, tenderness with acute synovitis, and loss of motion, especially abduction and medial rotation.

Roentgenography is definitive except during the first weeks of the disease. In this early avascular stage, the bone scan shows decreased uptake (Fig. 24–17) (in the later revascularization stages there is increased uptake), and the MRI demonstrates necrosis. Plain roentgenograms in the early stage (1–3 wk) may demonstrate a wide articular cartilage space. A homogeneous increased radioopacity of the femoral head is noted in the avascular necrosis stage (months-years). The regenerative or fragmentation stage may reveal rarefaction and fragmentation due to bone resorption, ingrowth of fibrous tissue, and immature uncalcified bone. The reconstitution or residual stage demonstrates a spherical or flattened femoral head.

The *differential diagnosis* includes acute transient toxic syn-

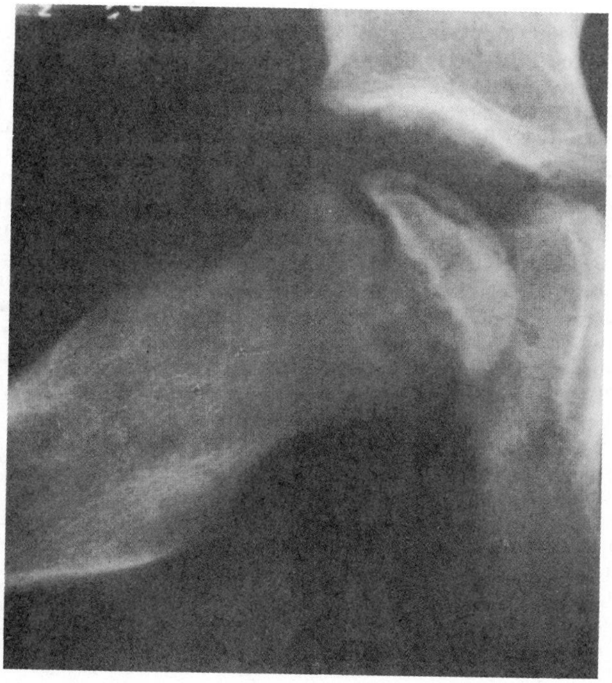

Figure 24–16. Legg-Calvé-Perthes disease. The lateral roentgenogram of the right hip reveals that the epiphyseal line is irregularly widened. The femoral capital epiphyseal center is flattened; there is a lucent defect in the anterior aspect of the center. Relative to the femoral neck, the secondary center is opaque.

ovitis (acute rather than chronic manifestation; normal to slightly increased rather than decreased bone scan uptake), sickle cell anemia, pyogenic or tuberculous arthritis, JRA, rheumatic fever, Gaucher disease, corticosteroid-induced osteonecrosis, bony dysplasias, tumors, and hypothyroidism.

The objective of *treatment* of Perthes disease is the maintenance of full joint mobility and a spherical femoral head, thus preventing progressive deformity and later degenerative hip arthritis. The 1st therapeutic step is rest to reduce synovitis. The 2nd step is containment, to position the hip so that the epiphysis is encompassed by the uninvolved acetabulum to prevent extrusion of the softened head. This is provided by abduction bracing or operative procedures to direct the femoral head into the acetabulum.

Perthes disease is difficult to manage owing to the necessity for long-term treatment and the need to limit activities. The psychologic status of the child should be monitored continually to avoid overwhelming the child or the family. A "balanced" approach is often necessary to compromise between the psychologic and orthopedic aspects of the problem. Braces and casting may require 1–2 yr of therapy, whereas surgery permits the child to return to normal activity in 4–6 mo.

The *prognosis* for Perthes disease is fair. Most patients do well until late middle adult life, when about half of the severe cases require some joint replacement procedure. The prognosis is poorest when the patient is older at the onset, the femoral head is completely involved, and treatment is inadequate. Additional high-risk situations ("head at risk") include a loss of hip motion, increased hip adduction contracture, rarefaction of the lateral epiphysis and metaphysis, calcification lateral to the epiphysis, lateral extrusion of the femoral head, and physeal growth disturbance.

24.10 TOXIC SYNOVITIS
(Irritable Hip)

This is an idiopathic, transient, nonspecific, common, unilateral (5% bilateral) inflammatory arthritis involving the hip joint, which occurs in children under 10 yr of age (typically 3–6 yr of age). It is the most common cause of limp with hip pain in this age group. The male to female ratio is 3–5:1. The condition is usually self-limited; however, 2–5% may develop Perthes disease, possibly owing to increased intra-articular pressure.

The child is usually seen with mild symptoms of a few days' duration. There may be a history of a preceding upper respiratory tract infection. Hip rotation is guarded, and there is an antalgic limp and loss of medial hip rotation and abduction. Pain may be present in the hip, anteromedial aspect of the thigh, and the knee. Constitutional findings, if present, are usually mild. Occasionally, a low-grade fever (100–101° F) and a mild elevation of the sedimentation rate are noted. Aspirated joint fluid is clear and sterile. *Roentgenography* demonstrates normal hips; however, an increased space between the medial acetabulum and the ossified femoral head may be evident. The bones are normal, thus reducing the likelihood of aseptic necrosis, osteomyelitis, and tumor. *Ultrasound* demonstrates the joint effusion. Radionuclide scans demonstrate normal to slightly increased uptake.

The *differential diagnosis* includes osteomyelitis, septic arthritis, Perthes disease, slipped capital femoral epiphysis, trauma, idiopathic hip chondrolysis, osteoid osteoma, rheumatologic disease, neuroblastoma, Gaucher disease, leukemia, Ewing sarcoma, and osteogenic sarcoma.

The objective of *treatment* is to differentiate toxic synovitis from septic arthritis (Fig. 24–18). This differentiation is usually possible because septic arthritis-osteomyelitis demonstrates higher fever, malaise, more pronounced spasm, guarding and fixed positioning, and a sedimentation rate greater than 25 mm/hr. Roentgenography is seldom helpful, whereas a bone scan may reveal marked uptake in bacterial arthritis-osteomyelitis. If the diagnosis is uncertain, synovial fluid should be examined and cultured following joint aspiration (see Sec. 12.17). Purulent fluid establishes the diagnosis of septic arthritis, and open joint draining is essential. If the diagnosis

Figure 24–17. Legg-Calvé-Perthes disease. The radionuclide scan of the pelvis and hips reveals an area of decreased uptake in the head of the right femur. This is best seen in the isolated image on the right and can be compared with the normal left hip.

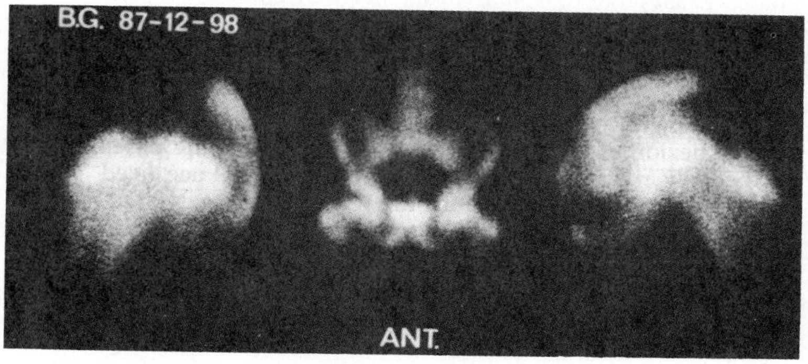

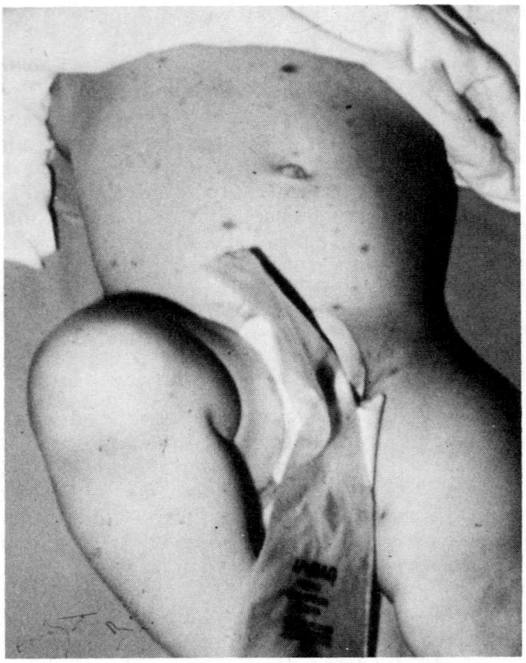

Figure 24–18. An infant with a bacterial infection of the hip holds the joint flexed, abducted, and laterally rotated.

of toxic synovitis is made but the clinical manifestations persist for more than 7–10 days or recur, the patient probably has Perthes disease in the synovitis phase (see Sec. 24.9).

Toxic synovitis resolves with bed rest at home, usually within 7–10 days. Nonsteroidal anti-inflammatory agents may be beneficial. Antibiotics and corticosteroids are not indicated.

24.11 SLIPPED CAPITAL FEMORAL EPIPHYSIS

Slipped capital femoral epiphysis (SCFE) represents a displacement of the femoral head from the femoral neck due to a stress fracture through the femoral capital epiphyseal growth plate (Fig. 24–19). SCFE occurs before the epiphyseal plate closes, usually before and during the maximal pubertal growth spurt (13–15 yr in males; 11–13 yr in females) with a male to female ratio of 2–5:1. This sporadic condition is the most common adolescent hip disorder and has an incidence of 1–4/100,000. Blacks are affected more often than whites. The disease is usually unilateral; simultaneous symptomatic bilateral disease is present in 10%.

Acute SCFE may result from a significant shear force applied to the epiphyseal plate with subsequent separation of the femoral head. Predisposing factors include severe trauma, motor vehicle accidents, falls from heights, child abuse, or obstetric accidents.

Chronic or *gradual SCFE* is more common and is associated with abnormal shear forces exerted over a long period. Such high mechanical forces can separate a normal epiphyseal plate, whereas normal forces may separate an abnormal epiphyseal plate. Chronic SCFE is often associated with obesity and deficient gonadal development. Growth hormone or chorionic gonadotropin administration, hypothyroidism (before or during treatment), pseudohypoparathyroidism, acromegaly, hypopituitarism, hyperparathyroidism, Klinefelter syndrome, and tall, thin, actively growing adolescents are additional potential, less frequent predisposing factors.

CLINICAL MANIFESTATIONS. Clinical manifestations are classified into four groups. *Preslip* or *minimal slip* is characterized by mild discomfort and slight limitation of medial rotation, abduction, and flexion. The growth plate is wide, but no slip has occurred. *Acute SCFE* demonstrates no symptoms or mild short-lived (< 3 wk) prior symptoms (pain, limp) before the sudden onset of severe pain, resulting in an inability to bear weight by the affected leg. There may or may not be a history of obvious trauma. The hip is tender, and range of motion is greatly reduced owing to spasm and guarding. The affected limb is shortened and is held in lateral rotation. The epiphyseal separation with associated synovitis produces pain that is often referred to the thigh or knee. Patients with acute SCFE should not be forced into range of motion exercises or to demonstrate walking because such movement may exacerbate the lesion and further displace the femoral head.

Acute on chronic SCFE develops with a sudden onset of severe pain and an inability to bear weight in a patient who has had a limp or hip, thigh, or knee pain for the past few weeks or months. The acute epiphyseal slippage may or may not be associated with trauma and occurs on an existing chronic SCFE.

Chronic SCFE is the presentation noted in 80% of cases and manifests with groin pain referred to the anteromedial aspect of the thigh and knee. The pain is either continuous or intermittent, dull, or vague and is exacerbated by activity. The onset of pain may be hard to determine because symptoms are present for months. The gait demonstrates an antalgic limp; the limb is held in lateral rotation; and there is local tenderness over the hip joint while the limitation of motion relates to the severity of the slip. There is a loss of internal rotation, accentuated external rotation, and occasionally limitation of flexion and abduction. Disuse atrophy and limb shortening are common with chronic SCFE. Shortening is due to posterior and inferior displacement of the femoral head.

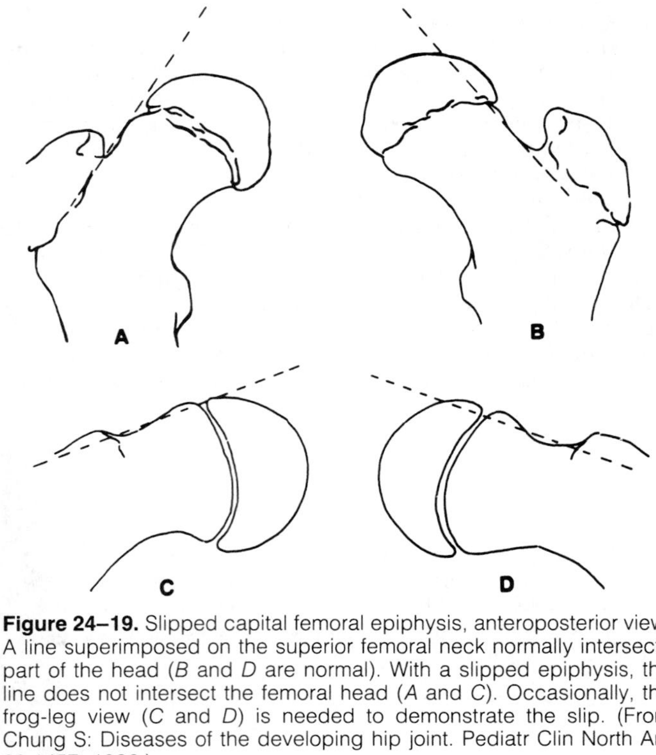

Figure 24–19. Slipped capital femoral epiphysis, anteroposterior view. A line superimposed on the superior femoral neck normally intersects part of the head (*B* and *D* are normal). With a slipped epiphysis, the line does not intersect the femoral head (*A* and *C*). Occasionally, the frog-leg view (*C* and *D*) is needed to demonstrate the slip. (From Chung S: Diseases of the developing hip joint. Pediatr Clin North Am 33:1457, 1986.)

Roentgenography using the anteroposterior and lateral frog-leg views is usually diagnostic and demonstrates medial displacement of the epiphysis and a bare upper portion of the femoral neck adjacent to the physis. There is widening of the growth plate and irregularity of the metaphysis. The capital femoral epiphysis remains in the acetabulum, but the femoral neck slips superiorly and posteriorly. The degree of separation of the epiphysis and femoral neck may be mild (0–33%), moderate (34–50%), or severe (> 50%). Radionuclide bone scan demonstrates increased uptake in the epiphyseal area. The other asymptomatic hip may demonstrate evidence of a *preslip* and should be included in the roentgenogram.

The *differential diagnosis* includes toxic synovitis, avascular (aseptic) necrosis, osteochondritis dissecans, idiopathic chondrolysis, rheumatologic disorders, and, rarely, chronic low-grade infective arthritis.

TREATMENT. SCFE is an emergency because immediate hospitalization and operative fixation are indicated. Stabilization of the SCFE is essential to prevent acute or gradual slipping. The management and outcome depend on the degree of displacement. *Pinning or external fixation,* a common therapy, locks the epiphysis in place and enhances physeal closure in 3–6 mo and is indicated for preslip, mild to moderate chronic SCFE, acute SCFE, and acute on chronic SCFE. *Open bone graft epiphysiodesis* is used for severe chronic SCFE and promotes epiphyseal closure. Spica hip casting is needed to decrease the risk of femoral neck fracture and to protect the epiphysis for 6–8 wk after the epiphysiodesis. In severe chronic poorly aligned SCFE, osteotomies are required to realign and stabilize the capital femoral epiphysis.

Problems associated with SCFE and its treatment include chondrolysis of the femoral head and acetabulum (associated with black race, females, pins penetrating into the joint space, prolonged immobilization) presenting with joint stiffness and loss of motion in all planes; avascular necrosis (osteonecrosis) presenting with persistent postoperative pain; and fracture after removal of the pin.

24.12 SPINE

Congenital and developmental spinal deformity are common and potentially serious nontraumatic musculoskeletal problems in children and adolescents. Deformity may involve the spine curvature (lateral or AP), appearing as a frontal plane curvature-scoliosis and as sagittal plane curves of lordosis and kyphosis. Deformities may be static, whereas some progress with time and require therapy.

The normal spine demonstrates cervical lordosis (convex anterior curve), thoracic kyphosis (concave anterior curve), lumbar lordosis, and sacrococcygeal kyphosis. Young children usually have less cervical lordosis and an exaggerated lumbar lordosis compared with adolescents. The major (larger) and minor (smaller) curves are named relative to the degree of angulation. Spinal curvatures may be idiopathic and primary or functional secondary to other disorders (e.g., leg length discrepancy; neuromuscular, metabolic, or collagen diseases, such as Marfan syndrome).

The physical examination should include a general assessment of the patient with specific attention to the lower extremity (for leg length discrepancy) and inspection of the back (Fig. 24–20). The general contour of the back should be observed for asymmetry or deformity. Because scoliosis is a rotational problem there may be rib deformity and unilateral prominence of lumbar musculature. The *forward bend test* permits observation from behind the patient and may demonstrate asymmetry; observation from the side will demonstrate kyphotic curves. Forward bending permits assessment of spine flexibility; spine stiffness suggests bone deformity, infection, inflammation, or neoplastic lesions. Joint stiffness should also be sought in other sites to determine the presence of a rheumatologic illness, although lumbosacral stiffness and pain may be the only sign of rheumatologic or other systemic illnesses. Back pain is unusual in children and warrants a diagnostic evaluation (Table 24–7).

Midline defects should be identified and include dimpling (dermal sinuses), hypertrichosis (hair patches), hemangiomata, cutaneous nevi, skin tags, and soft-tissue masses. These masses are often associated with underlying spinal abnormalities, such as spina bifida, diastematomyelia, lipomyelocele, lipoma, or teratoma.

Roentgenography in the AP and lateral positions will permit an assessment of curvature, rotation, vertebral bodies and spaces, skeletal maturity, and soft tissues.

24.13 CONGENITAL SPINE ANOMALIES

Anomalous vertebral development may produce simple, benign lesions (spina bifida occulta) or severe functional and deforming anomalies (congenital scoliosis, myelomeningocele, lumbosacral agenesis), which affect the cervical, thoracic, lumbar, or sacral vertebrae and which may be evident at birth or present in childhood or adolescence. Defective *unilateral segmentation* (fused, nonseparated vertebra along lateral aspect) produces congenital scoliosis (see Sec. 24.14), defective

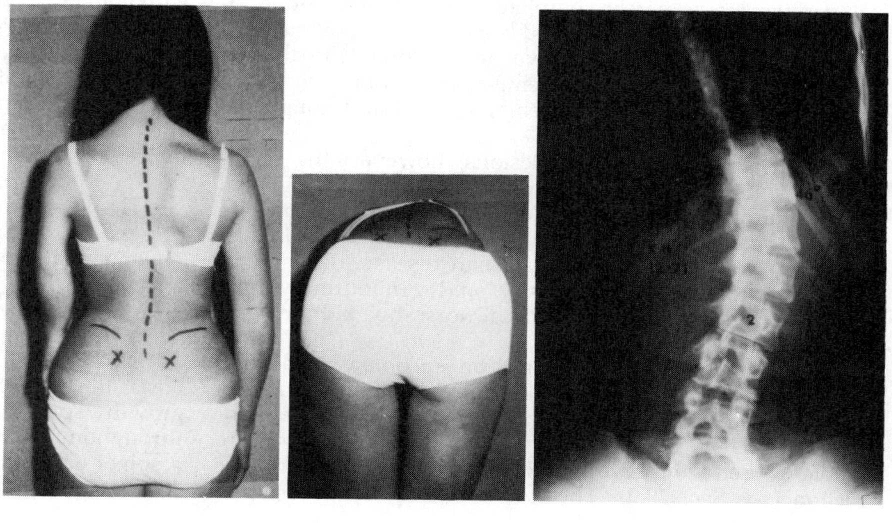

Figure 24–20. Scoliosis. The spine rotates as it curves, with the spinous processes moving toward the concavity. The severe curve of 46 degrees seen by roentgenogram on the right is only partly recognizable when the patient stands upright. However, an examination with the child's spine flexed shows the rotation on the right that indicates a structural scoliosis.

TABLE 24–7. Differential Diagnosis of Back Pain*

Inflammatory Diseases
Diskitis (common before 6 yr)
Vertebral osteomyelitis (pyogenic, tuberculosis)
Spinal epidural abscess
Pyelonephritis
Pancreatitis
Rheumatologic Diseases
Pauciarticular juvenile rheumatoid arthritis
Reiter syndrome
Ankylosing spondylitis
Psoriatic arthritis
Ulcerative colitis—regional enteritis
Developmental Diseases
Spondylolysis (common in adolescence)
Spondylolisthesis (common in adolescence)
Scheuermann syndrome (common in adolescence)
Scoliosis
Mechanical Trauma and Abnormalities
Hip/pelvic anomalies
Herniated disk
Overuse syndromes (common with athletic training and in gymnasts and dancers)
Vertebral stress fractures
Lumbosacral sprain
Neoplastic Diseases
Primary vertebral tumors (e.g., osteogenic sarcoma, Ewing sarcoma)
Metastatic tumor (e.g., neuroblastoma)
Primary spinal tumor (e.g., neuroblastoma, lipoma, cysts)
Malignancy of bone marrow (e.g., ALL, lymphoma)
Benign tumors (e.g., eosinophilic granuloma, osteoid osteoma)
Other
Disk space calcification
Conversion reaction
Sickle cell anemia
Hematocolpos

*Modified from Allen B: *In:* Behrman R, Kliegman R (eds): Nelson Essentials of Pediatrics, 13th ed. Philadelphia, WB Saunders, 1990.

anterior segmentation (fusion) produces congenital kyphosis (see Sec. 24.17), defective *posterior segmentation (fusion)* produces fixed congenital lordosis, *bilateral circumferential failure of segmentation* (bloc vertebra) affects vertical vertebral growth and motion (Klippel-Feil syndrome), whereas intraspinal abnormalities (tethered cord, diastematomyelia, diplomyelia, syringomyelia, teratoma) as determined by MRI are also associated with congenital spine deformities (scoliosis, kyphosis). *Vertebral formation defects* may be complete or partial (hemivertebra). Hemivertebrae may be segmented (separate), semisegmented, and nonsegmented (fused above and below). Unbalanced segmented hemivertebrae and semisegmented hemivertebrae may result in asymmetric vertebral growth and congenital scoliosis.

Hemivertebrae are sporadic lesions; however, the recurrence rate in siblings of patients with multiple congenital vertebral anomalies is 5–10%. Associated anomalies include posterior or anterior rib fusion, *spinal dysraphism*, Sprengel deformity, cleft palate, congenital heart disease, digit anomalies (supernumerary, hypoplasia), and genitourinary tract anomalies (renal hypoplasia, aplasia, horseshoe kidney, atresia of the vagina or uterus).

SPINAL DYSRAPHISM. This term encompasses a wide range of congenital anomalies of the spinal cord neural axis and bony vertebrae. Most visible and severe are myelomeningoceles, whereas other defects are not as obvious but are capable of producing severe deformity and loss of neurologic function (see Sec. 20.2). These latter lesions include diplomyelia, diastematomyelia, tight filum terminale, hamartoma, lipoma, lipomyelomeningocele, dermal and epidermal cysts, neurenteric canals, dermal sinus, and angiomas. **Diastematomyelia** is a sagittal division of the spinal cord due to an osseous or fibrous anterior projection from one vertebra or more. Tethered cord, thickened filum terminale, and scoliosis are associated lesions (see Sec. 20.2).

Cutaneous lesions over the spine are often clues to an underlying spinal dysraphism and include a soft-tissue mass, localized hypertrichosis–hair tuft, hemangioma, and midline high sacral–low lumbar (usually not in gluteal folds) sinus tracts or dimpling. The location of the cutaneous lesion does not always correspond with the spinal defect.

Musculoskeletal deformities associated with spinal dysraphism include unilateral small ilium, talipes equinovarus, congenital convex pes valgus, cavus or equinus, unilateral atrophy of the lower extremity, scoliosis, kyphosis, or congenital dislocated hips. *Neurologic* deficits appear by the 2nd yr of life and include difficulty with walking due to weakness or spasticity; one foot, calf, or thigh being smaller than the other; loss of sensation (position, temperature, touch, vibration) manifest as skin ulcerations of the lower extremity; and bladder dysfunction (incontinence, dribbling, enuresis, repeated urinary tract infections). Some patients are asymptomatic.

A **tethered (fixed) cord** is usually caused by a lipomyelomeningocele, repair of a myelomeningocele, a lipoma of the filum terminale, anomalous fibrous bands, and anomalous spinal nerve roots. Limitation of movement during flexion and extension stretches the cord. The resultant tension produces ischemic spinal cord injury and a variety of symptoms. Manifestations of a tethered cord include orthopedic foot deformities (see earlier), atrophy, pain radiating to the legs, lordosis, hamstring spasm, and bowel or bladder dysfunction. Some patients are asymptomatic.

24.14 CONGENITAL SCOLIOSIS

Anomalies of vertebral segmentation or formation (hemivertebrae) may result in structural spinal deformities which, with postnatal growth of the structurally abnormal curve or of the compensatory curve, produce spinal deviation. In utero malposture (positional deformation) does not produce congenital scoliosis. Thoracic curves with multiple unbalanced anomalies have the worst prognosis. Unilateral unsegmented bars and the presence of one or two hemivertebrae on the same side (unbalanced) produce marked curves that may demonstrate severe progression (> 30 degrees). Overall, 20% of patients with congenital scoliosis show no progression; 40–50% demonstrate moderate progression (5–30 degrees); and 30–40% have severe progression of the spinal curve after birth. Cervicothoracic, lumbar, and balanced curves are less progressive than thoracic curves. Cervicothoracic curves produce head and neck tilt, asymmetric neckline, and asymmetry and depression of the involved shoulder. Lumbar curves may produce pelvic obliquity, whereas thoracic curves produce lateral spinal deformity and occasionally kyphosis, which, if present, has a poor prognosis.

Congenital scoliosis may be associated with genitourinary tract anomalies, congenital heart disease, and various syndromes (Klippel-Feil syndrome, VATER syndrome, Goldenhar syndrome, spinal dysraphism).

TREATMENT. Congenital scoliosis, like idiopathic scoliosis, tends to progress most rapidly during the adolescent growth spurt. Slower progression, nonetheless, occurs throughout infancy and childhood. *Nonoperative therapy* with a spinal orthosis (Milwaukee brace) is indicated for long (8–10 vertebrae), flexible (50% correction with bending or traction) curves; short, rigid curves require surgical intervention. *Surgical therapy* is usually required and includes in situ fusion and resection of associated intradural lesions, tethered cord, or spurs to prevent progression of neurologic defects.

24.15 IDIOPATHIC SCOLIOSIS

Scoliosis is a lateral curvature of the spine associated with a rotational deformity. This deformity involves the frontal, sagittal, and transverse planes, and with progression, scoliosis produces the recognizable asymmetric back hump owing to the rotational deformity of the rib cage.

Postural scoliosis is unusual, is not rotational, disappears on recumbency, and is not progressive. *Functional scoliosis* is due to leg length discrepancy, is nonstructural, has the convexity of the curve toward the depressed side of the pelvis (shorter leg), has little rotational deformity, disappears with recumbency or with a leg lift, and resolves with correction of leg length discrepancy (see Sec. 24.5). *Nonstructural scoliosis* is often noted in infants with pelvic obliquity owing to intrauterine positional deformation and usually resolves with passive stretching exercises to relieve hip contractures. *Hysterical scoliosis* is associated with a long C curve and no rotation and may not disappear on recumbency. This type of scoliosis has varying degrees of deformity from day to day and requires psychotherapy. Osteoid osteoma or spinal tumor must be considered in the differential diagnosis of hysterical scoliosis.

Neuromuscular scoliosis is associated with imbalance of paraspinal muscles or other processes and is noted with progressive (spinal muscular atrophy, Friedreich ataxia, hereditary motor and sensory neuropathies, syringomyelia, neurofibromatosis) or static (cerebral palsy, spinal cord injury, poliomyelitis, arthrogryposis) neuropathic disorders and progressive (muscular dystrophy) and static (fiber-type disproportions, arthrogryposis) myopathic disorders (see Sec. 24.14). Miscellaneous conditions associated with scoliosis include prior radiation, vertebral or spinal cord tumors, and Marfan or Ehlers-Danlos syndrome.

Idiopathic scoliosis is familial and has a female to male ratio of 1:1 for small curves (< 10 degrees), 1.4:1 for curves of 11–20 degrees, 5.4:1 for curves greater than 20 degrees, and 7:1 for curves progressing to require treatment. The prevalence of small curves is 3–5% of school-aged children; the prevalence decreases with increasing severity of the curve. The etiology of idiopathic scoliosis is unknown but is associated with possibly abnormal proprioception and vibratory perception, collagen abnormalities, or asymmetric and abnormal growth of the vertebral column.

Idiopathic scoliosis may begin at three chronologic ages: infantile (from birth to 3 yr of age), juvenile (4 yr of age to the onset of puberty), and, the most common, adolescent (immediately before and during the onset of puberty but before closure of physes). *Idiopathic infantile scoliosis* represents fewer than 1% of scoliosis cases. This type is more common in boys, is not associated with vertebral anomalies, and usually has a left thoracic curve that spontaneously resolves in 85% without treatment. The disorder is more common in Europe than America and is associated with postnatal head molding (plagiocephaly). Factors associated with the 15% who demonstrate progressive scoliosis include later age of onset (> 1 yr), curves greater than 35 degrees, secondary curves, developmental anomalies, and a significant rib–vertebral angle difference. *Idiopathic juvenile scoliosis* is more common in girls, represents fewer than 10% of scoliosis cases, usually demonstrates a right thoracic curve, and requires treatment if the severity exceeds 25–30 degrees.

CLINICAL MANIFESTATIONS AND DIAGNOSIS. Symptoms and signs of idiopathic scoliosis are often subtle and are usually unnoticed by the patient or parents. Shirts may fit poorly, and even hemlines are difficult to level. As the curvature progresses there may be asymmetry noted in the standing position as determined by shifted flank, waist, or trunk creases; a high shoulder; a prominent shoulder blade, breast, or hip; asymmetric paravertebral musculature; and the spinal curvature. More subtle abnormalities are detected by observing the patient from the back with the most common screening examination, *the forward bend test.* Bending forward from the waist demonstrates the thoracic rotational deformity (rib hump) as the involved vertebral bodies rotate toward the convexity of the curve, posteriorly displacing the ribs and paraspinal muscles on the convex side (see Fig. 24–20). The degree of mild truncal prominence owing to rotation can be measured with a scoliometer (inclinometer) or by measuring the height of the paravertebral prominence. School-aged screening using the forward bend test identifies spinal asymmetry in 3–10% but identifies curves greater than 20 degrees in 0.5%. Cosmetic deformity is associated with the curvature degree and the location of the apex, because higher thoracic curves have the poorest appearance for a specific degree of curvature.

Back pain is not usually a feature of idiopathic scoliosis in children or adolescents and should raise the suspicion of another disorder that warrants a more detailed evaluation, even in the presence of a spinal curve (see Table 24–7).

Severe untreated scoliosis produces unacceptable cosmetic appearance and physiologic cardiopulmonary impairment in patients with curves greater than 60 degrees. Pulmonary abnormalities include reduced work capacity, reduced vital capacity, ventilation-perfusion mismatch, hypoxia, pulmonary hypertension, and cor pulmonale. Once present, these cardiopulmonary sequelae are not improved by surgery. Degenerative arthritis and nerve root impingement occur, but spinal cord compression is rare. Treatment of scoliosis before the curvature progresses is required to prevent these sequelae.

Roentgenography of the entire spine determines the location, number, and severity of the curves, compensatory or secondary curves, the presence of pelvic tilt, the direction of the curve's apex, anomalies of vertebral bodies, primary vertebral lesions (tumors), skeletal maturity, and the presence of associated kyphosis, lordosis, or spondylolisthesis. Various roentgenographic methods are used to determine the curvature angle and the degree of rotation (Fig. 24–21). The location of the apical vertebra defines the site: cervical (C1–C6); cervicothoracic (C7–T1); thoracic (T2–T11); thoracolumbar (T12–L1); lumbar (L2–L4); and lumbosacral (L5–S1). The direction of the curvature is determined by its convexity; an apex at T6 with a right convexity is a *right thoracic scoliosis.* The major or primary larger curve may be compensated by a secondary or minor curve or may be uncompensated (which appears cosmetically unattractive). Most major curves are thoracic and convex to the right. The direction and location do not change with age; however, the degree of curvature may remain stable or progress.

NATURAL HISTORY. The natural history of idiopathic scoliosis varies. Progression is defined by a sustained increase of 5 degrees or more of the Cobb angle. A progressive curve is usually greater than 30 degrees, and if left untreated the curve increases in adult life. Progression commonly occurs during periods of rapid growth (e.g., Tanner stage 2). Factors associated with an increased risk of progression include premenarchal appearance of a curve, younger age of diagnosis, larger curve at initial detection, higher (thoracic) curves, double thoracic curves, female sex, and excessive rotation of thoracic curves. Curves greater than 30 degrees in preadolescents with a bone age less than 12 yr generally progress, whereas curves less than 20 degrees in skeletally mature adolescents rarely progress. After skeletal growth is complete,

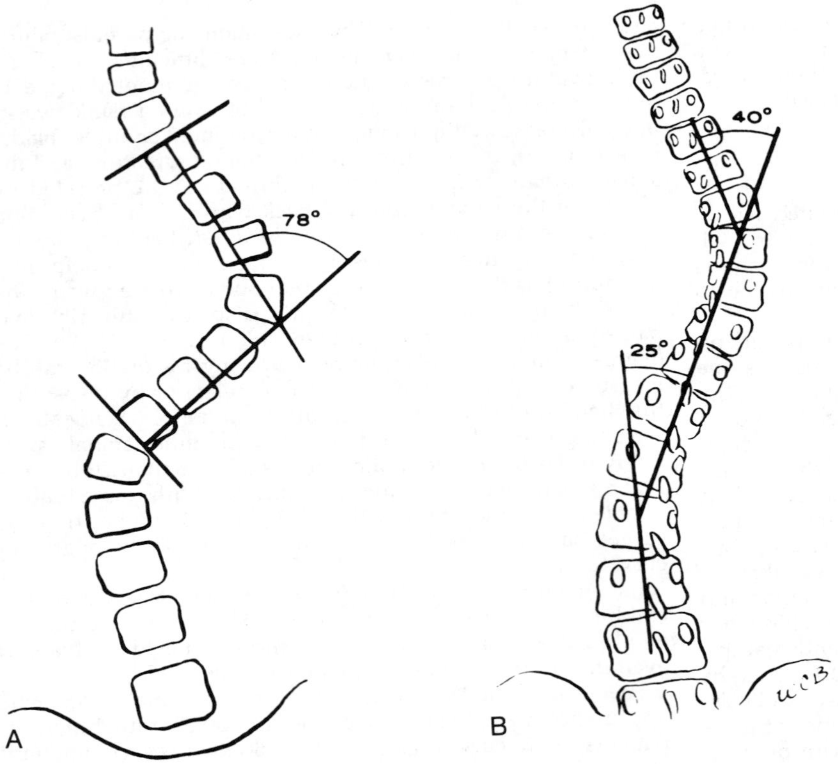

Figure 24–21. Methods to measure curvature angle in scoliosis. *A*, Cobb method. *B*, Ferguson method. The Cobb method is usually used to determine the curvature angle. (From Tachdjian M: Pediatric Orthopedics, 2nd ed. Philadelphia, WB Saunders, 1990.)

curves less than 30 degrees seldom progress, whereas those greater than 50–60 degrees at maturity may progress during adult life and produce significant morbidity.

TREATMENT. Options for therapy include nonoperative (observation, orthosis) and surgical methods. The goals of therapy are to avoid overtreatment of nonprogressing curves, to avoid iatrogenic loss of lumbar flexibility, and to have a cosmetically acceptable, stable, and balanced curve once the patient has reached skeletal maturity. Such a curve is unlikely to progress in adult life. Curves less than 30 degrees in a skeletally mature patient with no signs of spinal dysraphism may be observed. Curves less than 20 degrees in preadolescents may also be observed. Follow-up roentgenography or scoliometer and physical examination should be performed every 6–12 mo in young children with mild curves and every 3–6 mo in adolescents with larger curves.

The active *treatment of choice* for curves greater than 25–30 degrees in skeletally immature patients is *orthotic therapy*. The goal of orthotic therapy is to prevent further curve progression. Brace therapy may not improve the cosmetic appearance or rib deformity. Contraindications to orthotic treatment include a curve greater than 45 degrees. Flexible curves of 40 degrees may be treated if there is only 1 yr of growth remaining. Flexible curves of 40 degrees in young patients may require orthosis to improve growth prior to spinal fusion in a patient who does not emotionally accept the brace, or for thoracic hypokyphosis, skeletal maturity, and a high thoracic and cervicodorsal curve.

The **Milwaukee brace** is a common orthosis consisting of a pelvic girdle, a suprastructure of one anterior and two posterior upright supports, a cervical ring with a throat mold and occipital piece, and lateral pads that apply pressure on the apical vertebrae. This brace exerts passive and active forces on the longitudinal and transverse spinal planes. The patient wears the brace 23 hr each day until full skeletal growth is achieved. Thereafter, weaning over a 6- to 9-mo period is begun. The Milwaukee brace has a compliance rate of 75%, controls the progression of curvature in skeletally immature patients in 80%, and achieves permanent 5-yr correction in the coronal plane in 8%.

Thoracolumbosacral orthoses (TLSO) are prefabricated shells with prebuilt sites for corrective forces determined on a mold of a normal torso. The **Boston brace** is a prototype that applies derotational forces and may be combined with the Milwaukee suprastructure. The Boston brace fits under the patient's arms, envelops the torso, is more acceptable to patients than the Milwaukee brace, and is effective for low thoracic lumbar curves.

Complications of the orthosis include pressure sores, orofacial deformity (Milwaukee), nerve compression, esophageal reflux, sodium retention, thoracic cage compression (TLSO), and psychologic disturbances (poor self-esteem, body image) leading to noncompliance.

Surgical treatment can potentially correct the deformity, providing internal fixation (Harrington rod or C-D instrumentation) and arthrodesis (posterior spinal fusion) of the involved segments. Surgery is indicated in patients with progressive deformity who are not candidates for orthosis treatment and for curves exceeding the accepted maximal limits for adult life. Such curves exceed 50 degrees and have a high risk for continued progression during adult life. Other surgical indications include a cosmetically unacceptable deformity with truncal asymmetry and spinal decompensation in an adolescent or postadolescent, a progressive curve in a growing child that fails conservative treatment, and persistent backache in adults.

24.16 KYPHOSIS

Kyphosis is a sagittal plane deformity caused by an accentuation of the normal dorsal curve as seen on lateral examination and roentgenogram of the spine (Fig. 24–22). Normally, a dorsal curve of 20–50 degrees is observed on a standing lateral roentgenogram of the spine in childhood. If the value is less than 20 degrees, *hypokyphosis* or *flat back* is present, whereas if the angle is above 45–50 degrees hyperkyphosis or simply

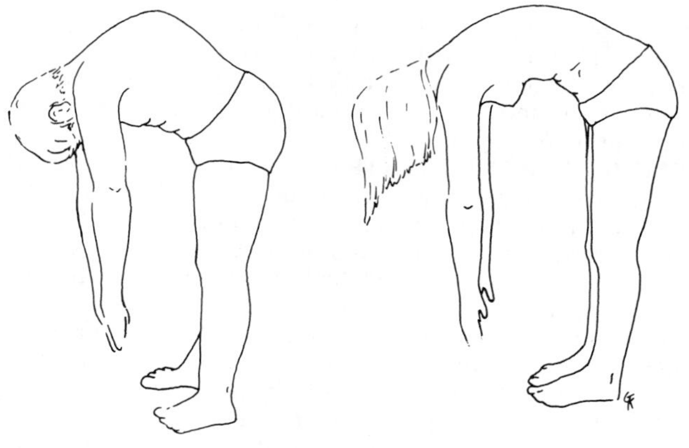

Figure 24–22. Note the sharp break in contour in the child with abnormal kyphosis *(A)* compared with the contour in the normal child *(B)*.

kyphosis is present. The etiology of kyphosis, like scoliosis, may be due to congenital structural vertebral anomalies, neuromuscular disorders, or idiopathic causes (see Sec. 24.15).

24.17 CONGENITAL KYPHOSIS

Failure of formation of all or part of the anterior vertebrae and failure of anterior segmentation of adjacent vertebrae produce congenital kyphosis. One, two, or three vertebrae may be affected. Congenital kyphosis must be differentiated from developmental kyphosis occurring in bone dysplasias (mucopolysaccharidosis).

Progression of congenital kyphosis is associated with growth spurts and mechanical forces, which may also erode vertebra and produce arching of the spinal cord across the apex with subsequent cord compression and paresis.

CLINICAL MANIFESTATIONS AND DIAGNOSIS. Kyphosis occurs usually between the 10th thoracic vertebra and the 2nd lumbar vertebra. The deformity is noted in infancy but becomes more evident when the child begins to stand and walk. There is no localized pain or paravertebral muscle spasm in young children. Paraplegia may develop with increased deformity. Compensatory hyperlordosis of the lumbar spine may be present and may produce back pain at that site. Extravertebral anomalies may be present as noted with congenital scoliosis (see Sec. 24.14).

Congenital kyphosis due to failure of vertebral formation progresses and is often associated with neurologic sequelae, whereas that due to failure of segmentation results in mild to moderate deformity, is less progressive, and is not associated with neurologic signs. Roentgenography confirms the diagnosis and underlying spinal defects; MRI demonstrates associated cord compression. The *differential diagnosis* includes spinal cord tumor, tuberculous spondylitis, postirradiation kyphosis, and mucopolysaccharidosis.

TREATMENT. Nonoperative management is ineffective, and surgical therapy includes arthrodesis before the deformity progresses. In situ simple, local spinal fusion of the posterior vertebra is indicated for a mild-to-moderate deformity owing to an anterior unsegmented bar. A severe deformity requires anterior and posterior fusion. Early fusion prevents progressive deformity and associated paraplegia.

24.18 IDIOPATHIC KYPHOSIS
(Scheuermann Juvenile Kyphosis)

Kyphosis developing in adolescents and young adults is associated with a wedge-shaped deformity of one or more vertebrae. This roentgenographic appearance is characteristic and demonstrates kyphosis involving at least three adjacent vertebrae with wedging of each vertebra of at least 5 degrees. Scheuermann kyphosis may be thoracic (familial, progressive, usually painless) or dorsolumbar (painful, predominantly found in males, progressive and secondary to repeated trauma). It is present in 5–8% of the adolescent population. The etiology is unknown but may include a familial predisposition and possibly a local osteochondritis.

CLINICAL MANIFESTATIONS. Symptoms become evident around puberty. Patients may have been thought to have poor posture or round back; the diagnosis of Scheuermann disease may be delayed because the roentgenographic appearance is not present before 10 yr of age. Therefore, all patients with "poor posture" must be followed beyond this age.

The patient may have fatigue and pain and localized tenderness at the site of the kyphotic curve, which is demonstrated best with the *forward bend test* by visualizing the patient from the side (see Fig. 24–22). There may be compensatory lumbar lordosis, a protuberant abdomen, and contracted taut hamstring and iliopsoas muscles. Deformity is usually mild-to-moderate, neurologic compromise is unusual, and the cosmetic appearance is usually acceptable.

Roentgenography demonstrates the characteristic wedging in addition to discrete irregular erosions of the vertebral endplate and disk protrusion into the vertebral spongiosa (Schmorl nodes).

The *differential diagnosis* includes **postural round back deformity** that consists of a smooth and mobile convexity rather than the rigid, fixed, and acutely angulated posterior spinal convexity noted with kyphosis. Roentgenography differentiates postural round back from Scheuermann disease. Kyphosis may also be congenital or may be due to bone dysplasias, traumatic compression vertebral fractures, infectious spondylitis, ankylosing spondylitis, tumors, and postirradiation.

The *natural history* of Scheuermann disease includes an active stage between 12 and 18 yr of age with fixation of kyphosis and the presence of backache at the kyphotic site. Adult sequelae include narrowing of disks, development of osteophytes, and sometimes back pain owing to low lumbar disk degeneration.

TREATMENT. Therapy depends on the degree of the deformity and on the patient's age. The goals are to relieve pain, correct the kyphosis, improve the cosmetic appearance, and prevent further progression. Therapy with the Milwaukee brace is usually successful in a skeletally immature patient (see Sec. 24.15). Surgical fusion with Harrington instrumentation is rarely indicated.

24.19 LORDOSIS

Lordosis is a sagittal plane deformity caused by an accentuation of the normal lumbar curve. The lumbar curve develops in early infancy to accommodate an upright position. *Hyperlordosis* may be caused by a compensation for a hip flexion contracture, is flexible and, therefore, is functional. Fixed hyperlordosis is manifest by a failure of the normal lumbar curve to reverse on forward flexion. A loss of the normal flexibility may occur from fixed deformity but arises more commonly from some painful spine condition owing to trauma, inflammation, or neoplasm. This finding requires careful evaluation.

The most common clinical presentation of lordosis is the benign juvenile form. The mother notices that her prepubescent child's buttock is prominent. The examination demonstrates only a mild prominence, an entirely normal physical examination with no pain, normal mobility, and no hip flexion contracture. The condition resolves with time. It is best documented by a lateral roentgenogram and is then managed by observation.

Lordosis is less commonly associated with kyphosis, poliomyelitis, muscular dystrophy, and myelomeningocele.

24.20 SPONDYLOLISTHESIS

The pars interarticularis is a segment of the posterior vertebral arch, usually L5, which, if narrower than normal, may undergo a stress fracture during childhood. This fracture may occur during normal activity or less often from an injury. A simple fracture without displacement of the vertebral body is *spondylolysis;* forward slippage of the vertebra is spondylolisthesis (hollow back) (Fig. 24–23).

Spondylolisthesis in childhood may be classified into four types: type I *(dysplastic spondylolisthesis)* is due to congenital dysplasia of the 5th lumbar vertebra and upper sacrum, produces a severe slip with potential for neurologic injury, and is more common in girls; type II *(isthmic ["true"] spondylolisthesis)* is the most common type, is due to a break of the pars interarticularis or less often due to its elongation, and is initiated by a stress fracture; type III *(traumatic)* is due to an acute fracture of the pedicle, lamina, or facet, with an intact pars interarticularis; and type IV *(pathologic)* is rare and associated with underlying bone disease (osteogenesis imperfecta, neoplasm, neurofibromatosis).

CLINICAL MANIFESTATIONS. Isthmic or true spondylolisthesis is associated with upright posture, lumbar lordosis (increased lordosis increases its incidence), and forces of rotation, flexion overload, and other unbalanced stresses. The incidence is 4–5%; spondylolisthesis is more common in males, Eskimos, and white Americans. There is a familial pattern, especially for the dysplastic type. Pars interarticularis defects are rare before 5 yr of age and often appear by 7–10 yr of age; its incidence increases until adult life. Slippage occurs before 20 yr of age. The degree of anterior displacement is graded as I (< 25% displacement), II (25–50%), III (50–75%), or IV (> 75%).

Forward displacement may be asymptomatic and identified as an incidental finding on roentgenography. There is usually back pain, stiffness, and limited straight leg raising owing to hamstring spasm or tautness. In children younger than 10 yr of age, there may be no symptoms other than poor posture and lumbar lordosis. During the adolescent growth spurt,

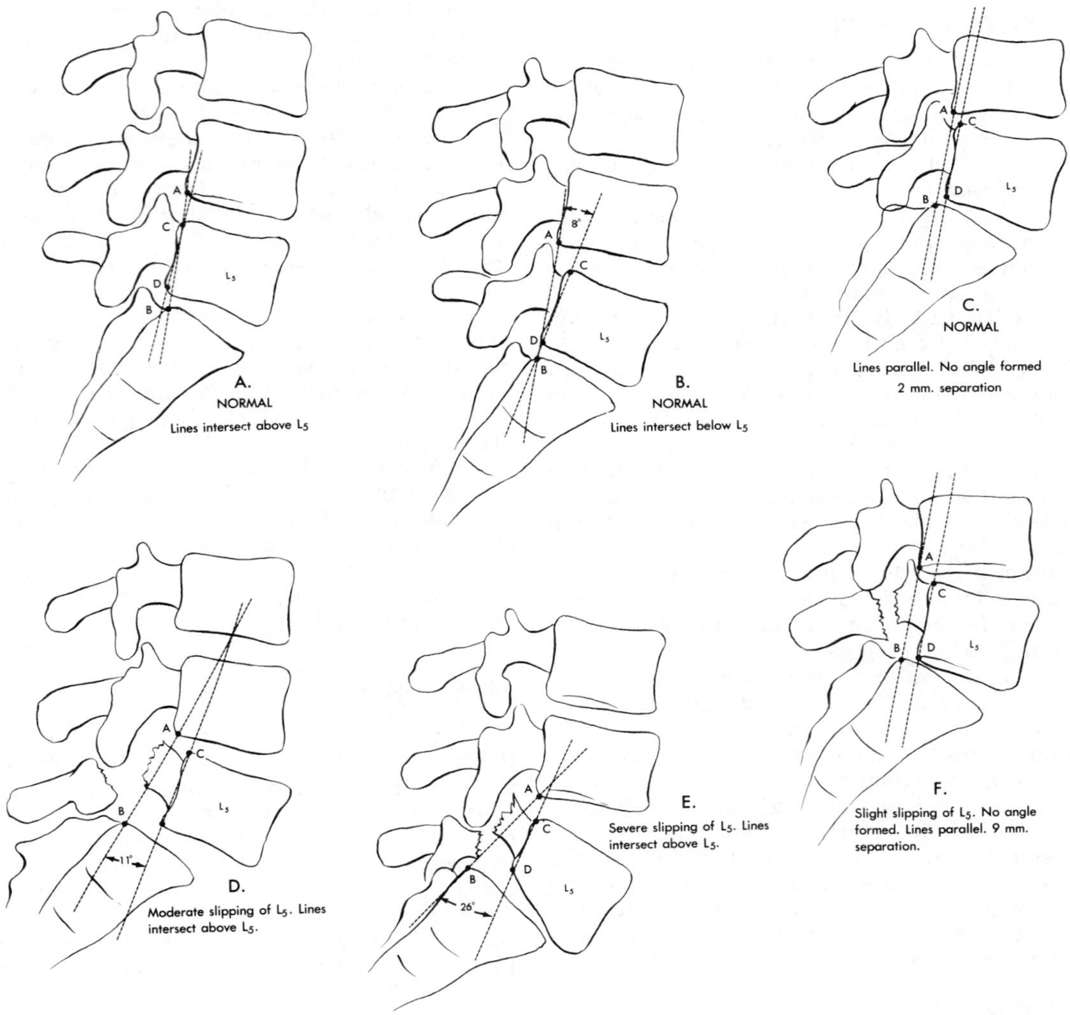

Figure 24–23. The Meschan method to measure the degree of spondylolisthesis. *A* to *C*, The three general normal variants of the lumbosacral spine. *Note*: The position of the apex of the angles made by intersecting lines is at L5 in *A* or below L5 in *B*. *D* to *F* *Note*: The arrangement of the lines in spondylolisthesis. (From Tachdjian M: Pediatric Orthopedics, 2nd ed. Philadelphia, WB Saunders, 1990.)

manifestations become more evident and include localized tenderness at L5–S1, dull low backache that is relieved with rest, pain radiating to the buttocks and posterior thighs, and radicular pain radiating along the sciatic nerve course. In severe cases the spine appears telescoped into the pelvis, and the sacrum is prominent and vertical.

Roentgenography confirms the diagnosis on a standing lateral roentgenogram of the lumbosacral spine. An oblique view may be needed to visualize the pars interarticularis. A bone scan will detect spondylolysis before it is evident on a plain roentgenogram. MRI is helpful to visualize the spinal cord if there is neurologic dysfunction.

TREATMENT. Therapy is predicated on the potential for progressive deformity. Risks for progressive displacement and disability include the age of onset younger than 10 yr, being female, ligamentous laxity (21-trisomy, Marfan syndrome), dysplastic-type lesion, 50% displacement, symptomatic disease, and instability or mobility of the defect.

Asymptomatic spondylolysis usually requires no therapy. Exaggerated lumbar lordosis is managed with pelvic tilt and other exercises. Repeat examination is indicated in 3–6 mo. Symptomatic spondylolysis is treated with a supportive brace, rest, or a plaster of Paris body cast to promote fracture healing and to prevent anterior displacement. Stress fractures heal within 6 mo. The patient should avoid sports that may further injure the spine (contact sports, weight lifting). Spinal fusion is indicated for spondylolysis that does not respond to nonoperative therapy.

Asymptomatic spondylolisthesis may be managed with conservative therapy if the slippage is less than 50%. Symptomatic lesions with a slip less than 25% may be treated with a brace. Operative therapy is indicated for persistent back pain and disability that interferes with activities of daily living, slip greater than 50%, progression of the slip to 25–50% with instability, neurologic deficits that do not improve with bracing, and persistent unresponsive sciatic scoliosis. The goals of surgery are stabilization to prevent progressive slippage, relief of nerve root compression, and improvement of posture, gait, and hamstring tautness. Posterolateral fusion of the alar transverse process of L5 to the sacrum is usually definitive and effective and rarely results in complications.

24.21 DISKITIS

Diskitis is an acute inflammatory process of the disk space that commonly occurs during infancy and early childhood (between 2 and 7 yr of age). The upper lumbar and lower thoracic intervertebral spaces are often affected and demonstrate narrowing of the disk space with minimal or no primary vertebral bone involvement. Diskitis is not vertebral osteomyelitis but is a relatively benign, self-limited inflammation of the intervertebral disk space. The *etiology* is often due to an acute bacterial *(Staphylococcus aureus)* disk infection but may also be due to a viral infection or an undefined inflammatory process.

Clinical manifestations vary with age. Young infants are irritable, refuse to sit, walk, or stand, and assume an exaggerated lumbar lordotic posture. There may be a mild fever (100–101° F), vague back pain and stiffness, paravertebral spasm, abdominal pain, an elevated ESR, sterile blood cultures, and minimal or no elevation of the peripheral leukocyte count. Back pain may be demonstrated with flexion, and the child may rise from sitting with a Gowers sign (see Sec. 21.11). Symptoms are usually present for less than 10 days. There is no neurologic deficit.

Roentgenography demonstrates a narrowed disk space 10–14 days after onset. A bone scan demonstrates increased uptake early in the course of the disease (before plain roentgenograms), whereas MRI demonstrates inflammatory swelling of the disk space.

The *differential diagnosis* includes vertebral osteomyelitis (*S. aureus,* brucellosis, salmonella), tuberculous spondylitis, epidural abscess, Scheuermann disease, tumor, appendicitis, pyelonephritis, Kawasaki disease, and trauma.

Treatment includes immobilization, rest, and nonsteroidal anti-inflammatory agents. Antistaphylococcal antibiotics are given for 4–6 wk when infection is suspected (fever, high ESR, leukocytosis, positive result of a blood culture) or when there is a positive disk space aspirate or progression of the disease despite immobilization. Immobilization may be achieved with bed rest or by casting (plaster of Paris jacket, fiberglass panty spica cast). Treatment is continued until the back pain and spasm are relieved; the ESR, leukocyte count, and temperature return to normal; and roentgenograms demonstrate healing as evident by sclerosis.

24.22 INTERVERTEBRAL DISK CALCIFICATION

Intervertebral disk calcification is of unknown etiology and is more common in males. Manifestations are acute and often follow mild trauma or an upper respiratory infection and include neck pain, limited neck motion, muscle spasm, torticollis, local tenderness, and inflammation (fever, elevated ESR, and leukocyte count). They usually appear at approximately 7 yr of age. In contrast to cervical spine disease, calcified thoracic or lumbar disks are often asymptomatic. Roentgenography confirms the diagnosis. Treatment includes analgesics, cervical collar, and neck traction. The prognosis is excellent because symptoms last for 1–2 mo, whereas calcifications resolve in some patients within 2–3 mo. In the remaining cases, the calcification is permanent.

24.23 CERVICAL SPINE, NECK, AND SHOULDERS

Congenital anomalies of the cervical spine may be asymptomatic or produce cosmetic, mechanical, or neurologic problems evident at birth or developing with the growth of the patient.

Platybasia is a flattening of the angle between the plane of the anterior fossa and the clivus. Alone, platybasia may be asymptomatic; however there may be signs of atlanto-occipital motion and spinal cord or hindbrain compression.

Congenital fusion of the 1st cervical vertebra and occiput (os odontoideum, occipitalization) is a partial or complete synostosis between the atlas and the base of the occiput. The patient may be asymptomatic, have symptoms following mild trauma, or manifest weakness, ataxia, numbness, head and neck pain, and papilledema from blocked cerebrospinal fluid at the foramen magnum. Symptoms resemble multiple sclerosis and involve long tracts. Physical examination reveals limited neck motion, a low hair line, and, occasionally, torticollis and high scapula. Roentgenography confirms the diagnosis. Treatment includes orthotics and surgery.

Congenital absence of cervical spine pedicles and facets becomes manifest in young adults with a history of mild trauma and resultant neck stiffness and pain, which may be radicular. Roentgenography demonstrates the lesion. CT scanning and MRI may be needed to exclude erosive lesions (neurofibromatosis, neoplasm). Treatment is generally conservative; surgical fusion is usually unnecessary.

KLIPPEL-FEIL SYNDROME. This rare malformation is due to a congenital fusion of two or more cervical vertebrae (congenital synostosis) and is also called brevicollis (short neck). There is a low hair line, limited neck motion, a short neck, and other anomalies of the urinary (agenesis, horseshoe kidney), genital (absent vagina, ovarian agenesis), cardiovascular (ventricular septal defect, patent ductus arteriosus, coarctation of aorta), pulmonary, and nervous systems (synkinesis, deafness, spinal cord compression, ptosis, 7th nerve palsy). Other common problems include scoliosis or kyphosis, torticollis (due to bone anomalies or sternocleidomastoid contractures), pterygium colli (webbing of each side of the neck), Sprengel deformity, cervical ribs, short trachea, syndactyly, hypoplastic thumbs, supernumerary digits, and unilateral hypoplasia of the pectoralis major muscle. The latter is *Poland anomaly* if it is associated with syndactyly and hypoplasia of the nipple and areola.

Roentgenography confirms the *diagnosis* and identifies other lesions, such as hemivertebrae, cervical ribs, and platybasia. The *differential diagnosis* includes bilateral Sprengel deformity, occipitalization of C1, and acquired postinflammatory (diskitis, rheumatoid arthritis) or post-traumatic fusion. *Treatment* is by observation.

SPRENGEL DEFORMITY (CONGENITAL HIGH SCAPULA). This uncommon congenital anomaly is due to failure of the normal descent of the scapula from its embryonic position to its normal location. This etiology is unknown; most cases are sporadic, whereas some families demonstrate an autosomal dominant inheritance. The female to male ratio is 3:1. Associated anomalies include Klippel-Feil syndrome, congenital scoliosis (hemivertebra), cervical spina bifida, congenital kyphosis, syringomyelia, platybasia, situs inversus, mandibulofacial dysostosis, ipsilateral shortened humerus and clavicular anomalies, and, rarely, renal anomalies. The scapula may be hypoplastic.

Clinical manifestations include shoulder asymmetry (best visualized from the back), usually left sided and less often bilateral. The neck appears full and short, and the cervicospinal line is less evident. There may be an associated torticollis owing to sternocleidomastoid contracture. Roentgenography confirms the *diagnosis*. *Treatment* by surgical correction is indicated for moderate or severe deformity.

ATLANTOAXIAL INSTABILITY. Atlantoaxial or atlanto-occipital dislocation may be due to congenital anomalies or trauma or may occur spontaneously in association with inflammatory processes of the retropharyngeal, neck, or pharyngeal spaces or with rheumatoid arthritis of the joint space. Instability may produce anteroposterior or rotary displacement (subluxation).

Congenital anomalies of the odontoid process include aplasia, hypoplasia (occasionally familial), and a separate odontoid process. The latter may also be post-traumatic (see Sec. 24.25). There may be localized pain, limited motion, transient neurologic manifestations, or quadriplegia owing to cord compression. Children with *21-trisomy* have atlantoaxial instability owing to laxity of the transverse ligament and abnormal odontoid process development (dysplasia, hypoplasia). Odontoid hypoplasia is also noted in children with skeletal dysplasias (osteochondrodystrophies). The latter inborn errors of metabolism include mucopolysaccharidosis (particularly Morquio disease), spondyloepiphyseal dysplasias, achondroplasia, pseudoachondroplasia, and multiple epiphyseal dysplasia.

Clinical manifestations of cord compression may not be evident during infancy but may occur spontaneously between 5 and 15 yr of age or after episodes of minor trauma. The older child complains of paresthesias of the upper extremities and manifests sleep apnea, neck pain, torticollis, distal muscle weakness, gait disturbances, and, later, bowel or bladder dysfunction, spasticity, or quadriplegia.

Roentgenography using neutral and then, if determined to be safe, flexion and extension lateral positions confirms the *diagnosis* and identifies the distance of displacement of the anterior arch of the atlas (C1) from the odontoid process of the axis (C2) and anomalies of the odontoid itself. The distance between the posterior margin of the atlas anterior arch and the front of the vertical odontoid process (atlanto-odontoid interval) is less than 4.5 mm in children and 2.5 mm in adults. The distance between the posterior margin of the axis (C2) body and the posterior atlas arch (AP canal diameter) helps to determine the risk for cord compression, which is unusual if the distance is more than 18 mm. Open-mouth AP roentgenograms may be needed to visualize rotary displacement. CT scanning and MRI may delineate bone abnormalities and cord involvement, respectively.

Treatment of an unstable atlantoaxial joint may require a posterior fusion of the upper cervical spine. Inflammatory related subluxation may be managed with reduction under general anesthesia and cast fixation or reduction with dorsally directed traction. Halo brace reduction and immobilization for approximately 3 mo may permit healing. If this method is unsuccessful, fusion is indicated.

TORTICOLLIS. Also known as *wryneck*, torticollis is characterized by head-tilting and rotation. The disorder may be congenital, acquired, acute and transient, or chronic and associated with deformity. The etiologies and differential diagnosis are noted in Table 24–8. The most common type of persistent torticollis is infantile congenital muscular torticollis; upper respiratory infections, trauma, unusual body positioning, and drug reactions are more often seen in older children.

TABLE 24–8. Differential Diagnosis of Torticollis

Congenital
Muscular torticollis
Positional deformation
Hemivertebra (cervicosuperior dorsal spine)
Unilateral atlanto-occipital fusion
Klippel-Feil syndrome
Unilateral absence of sternocleidomastoid
Pterygium colli

Trauma
Muscular injury (cervical muscles)
Atlanto-occipital subluxation
Atlantoaxial subluxation
C2–C3 subluxation
Rotary subluxation
Fractures

Inflammation
Cervical lymphadenitis
Retropharyngeal abscess
Cervical vertebral osteomyelitis
Rheumatoid arthritis
Spontaneous (hyperemia, edema) subluxation with adjacent head and neck infection (rotary subluxation syndrome)
Upper lobe pneumonia

Neurologic
Visual disturbances (nystagmus, superior oblique paresis)
Dystonic drug reactions (phenothiazines, haloperidol, metoclopramide)
Cervical cord tumor
Posterior fossa brain tumor
Syringomyelia
Wilson disease
Dystonia musculorum deformans
Spasmus nutans

Other
Acute cervical disk calcification
Sandifer syndrome (gastroesophageal reflux, hiatal hernia)
Benign paroxysmal torticollis
Bone tumors (eosinophilic granuloma)
Soft-tissue tumor
Hysteria

Congenital muscular torticollis is due to a sporadic, unilateral fibrosis and cord-like contracture of the sternocleidomastoid muscle, and it is associated with breech and forceps delivery, congenital dislocated hip, and female sex. The lesion is usually right sided, resulting in an asymmetric head and neck deformity with the head tilted toward the affected side and the chin tilted in the opposite direction. The etiology is unknown, and a biopsy of the "tumor" in the body of the sternocleidomastoid muscle reveals dense fibrous tissue (fibroma) but not a hematoma.

Clinical manifestations are present at birth or become evident in the 1st mo of life and include head tilt, chin rotation, and a hard fusiform nontender tumorous swelling of the muscle bed. The fibrous mass is not fixed to the skin and resolves by 2–6 mo of age. If a mass is not noted before this age, cervical spine anomalies should be suspected and spine roentgenograms should be obtained. If the contracture does not resolve (spontaneously or with treatment), secondary face and hand deformities appear and include plagiocephaly, facial asymmetry owing to alterations of the levels of the eyes and ears, cervical upper dorsal scoliosis, and further ipsilateral soft-tissue shortening with facial contractures. Eye strain may be present.

The differential diagnosis is noted in Table 24–8. **Postural torticollis** is due to an in utero positional deformation, has no tumor, is less severe, responds quickly to stretching, and often resolves spontaneously. Roentgenography is helpful to identify disorders of the spine and disk spaces.

Congenital muscular torticollis resolves spontaneously in most patients. The value of passive stretching is controversial. Operative correction is indicated for persisting deformity over age 2 yr. During the postoperative period, the head is held in the corrected position by a cast or brace to prevent a recurrence.

Acquired torticollis in the older child may be associated with trauma, inflammation, neurologic disorder, or other processes (see Table 24–8). *Benign paroxysmal torticollis* is of unknown etiology and manifests periodic recurrent episodes of head tilt with or without emesis, agitation, ataxia, and malaise. Episodes begin in the 1st yr of life and resolve by 5 yr of age. These episodes may be familial and may last for several hours to days. Patients may later develop benign paroxysmal vertigo or migraines.

Nontraumatic subluxation of the atlantoaxial spine may be due to inflammatory processes in (rheumatoid arthritis) or surrounding (head and neck infection) the spine. Edema and hyperemia may cause laxity of supporting ligaments with resultant spontaneous subluxation and secondary torticollis. Subluxation may be rotatory and may also follow mild trauma. Roentgenography by visualization of the excessive rotation of C1 or C2 confirms the diagnosis (see atlantoaxial subluxation). Treatment may require analgesics, muscle-relaxant drugs (Valium), a cervical collar, and traction.

Drug-induced dystonic spasmodic torticollis may be associated with other extrapyramidal signs (opisthotonos, trismus, dystonias, dysarthria, oculogyric crisis [spasmodic conjugate eye deviation]). Diphenhydramine (Benadryl) is the treatment of choice for such reactions.

PSEUDOARTHROSIS OF THE CLAVICLE. This disease is of unknown origin, occurs in the middle third of the clavicle, and must be distinguished from fracture, neurofibromatosis, and cleidocranial dysostosis. *Clinical manifestations* include unilateral nontender swelling noted usually on the right side, at or soon after birth in a patient with no birth trauma. In contrast to a fractured clavicle, there is no callus formation or spontaneous healing, and pain, arm pseudoparalysis, and limited motion are not present. The deformity grows during infancy and childhood, demonstrates a lump and mobility between the ends of the clavicle, and develops thin, atrophic skin over the lesion. Roentgenography confirms the *diagnosis* and excludes cleidocranial synostoses and fracture. *Treatment* includes internal fixation and grafting by 3–4 yr of age.

24.24 UPPER LIMB

Upper extremity problems may be congenital or acquired secondary to trauma, inflammation, neoplasm, and developmental (dysplasia, inborn errors of metabolism) disorders. Upper extremity problems are less frequent than those of the lower limbs and appear to be better tolerated, partly because of the nonweight-bearing nature of the upper limbs.

The general physical examination should identify manifestations of systemic or generalized skeletal disorders in addition to anomalies of the spine and lower extremity. The physician should view the alignment of the upper extremities in the anatomic position, and should look for asymmetry, deformity, length differences, and carrying angle. Each joint should be examined and moved through a passive range of motion to determine stiffness, pain, erythema, contractures, swelling, and limited motion. Associated muscle atrophy and neurologic signs should be assessed.

CONGENITAL UPPER LIMB ANOMALIES. *Congenital synostosis of the elbow* is a rare disorder that may be associated with other lesions of the upper extremity (absence of ulna, carpals, metacarpals, or phalanges). The lesion may be unilateral, occurring with other defects, or bilateral and isolated without other defects. In young children there may be cartilaginous synostosis that is not detected by roentgenography. Surgical osteotomy or arthroplasty is indicated.

Congenital radioulnar synostosis is an uncommon disorder that fixes the forearm in pronation. The lesion is bilateral in 60%, and there is familial, possibly autosomal dominant, inheritance. Functional disability depends upon the position in rotation. Surgical osteotomy rather than separation of synostosis is the preferred therapy when position is unacceptable.

Congenital dislocation of the head of the radius is rare and is unilateral or bilateral. Manifestations include a click or stiffness of the elbow and a bowed ulna; however, patients may be asymptomatic. The radial head may become prominent with growth, and excision of the radial head may be necessary after completion of growth. Traumatic dislocation must be distinguished from the congenital types. The latter demonstrate underdevelopment of the capitellum of the humerus and an ovoid radial head (see Sec. 24.25).

Congenital longitudinal deficiencies of the radius are of unknown origin, are bilateral in 50% of cases, have a male to female ratio of 1.5:1, and have an incidence of 1/100,000 live births. The lesion occurs sporadically except when part of specific syndromes, such as the autosomal recessive Fanconi pancytopenia (thumb hypoplasia-aplasia), the autosomal recessive thrombocytopenia with absent radius (TAR syndrome, thumb present), and the autosomal dominant Holt-Oram syndrome (atrial septal defect, finger-like triphalangeal or absent thumb). Associated problems include extremity (syndactyly, polydactyly, carpal coalition), spine (congenital and idiopathic scoliosis, Klippel-Feil syndrome, sacral agenesis), skeletal (clubfoot, congenital dislocated hips, pectus excavatum or carinatum, radioulnar synostosis), cardiac (atrial septal defect, ventricular septal defect, coarctation of the aorta, tetralogy of Fallot), genitourinary (renal agenesis or hypoplasia, hydronephrosis, horseshoe kidney), gastrointestinal (tracheoesophageal fistula, esophageal atresia, imperforate anus), and craniofacial (cleft lip and palate, craniosynostosis, ear) anomalies. The radial defect may be complete absence (seen in 50%), partial absence, or hypoplasia. In addition to bony anomalies, there are abnormalities of the associated muscles and neurovascular structures.

Clinical manifestations include a radially deviated hand and a short, radially bowed forearm with the prominent ulnar styloid process at its lower end. Functional disability is greatest with bilateral involvement.

Treatment of the hypoplastic radius includes correction of contractures with casting and radius-lengthening procedures. Therapy of the total or partial absent radius includes attempts to align the deviated hand over the ulna, to avoid further contractures with passive exercises, and casting begun in the neonatal period. By 6 mo of age surgery provides stabilization (centralization of the ulna) and correction of the deformity.

Ulnar dimelia (minor hand) has absence of the radial ray (radius, scaphoid, trapezium, 1st metacarpal, thumb) with duplication of the ulnar side, resulting in a hand with 7–8 fingers. The anomaly is unilateral, is not familial, and associated anomalies may be present in the lower extremity (absent tibia, duplicated fibula or foot). Treatment includes pollicization of the most normal preaxial (radial side) digit and release of flexion-radial deviation contractures.

Madelung deformity is a congenital lesion that retards the development of the ulnar and volar aspects of the distal radial physis, with resultant displacement and bowing of the distal radius that becomes shortened. The etiology is unknown, but the asymmetric growth is analogous to Blount disease (see Sec. 24.4). The deformity is inherited as an autosomal dominant trait, is bilateral, and is more common in females. Clinical manifestations become evident between 8 and 12 yr of age, and there is a visible prominence on the dorsal and ulnar side of the wrist. There is limited range of motion, joint instability, and pain. Roentgenograms confirm the diagnosis. The differential diagnosis includes bony dysplasias, rickets, trauma, infection, and rheumatoid arthritis. Treatment includes relief of pain and poor function with conservative therapy. Surgery is not needed for all patients, is delayed until 11–13 yr of age, and includes shortening of the ulna, correction of radial bowing, and fusion of the distal radial physis to prevent recurrent asymmetric growth.

Syndactyly, the most common hand congenital anomaly, is fusion or webbing of two digits (Fig. 24–24; see also Sec. 24.2). Occurring in 1:2,200 births, syndactyly is symmetric and bilateral in 50% of cases, affects males more than females, is usually sporadic (10–40% are familial), and occurs most often (55–60%) between the long and the ring fingers. Complete syndactyly extends to the tips of the involved fingers; in incomplete syndactyly, the web ends proximal to the tip. Simple syndactyly involves skin and soft tissue, whereas complex syndactyly includes various degrees of osseous fusion. Oligosyndactyly is fusion of digits on a hand with fewer than five possible digits. Treatment is indicated to separate the web in order to improve hand function and appearance. Early (6–12 mo of life) separation is needed if fingers of unequal length are involved (thumb-index or little-ring fingers) to avoid lateral deviation and flexion contractures and to permit unimpeded growth.

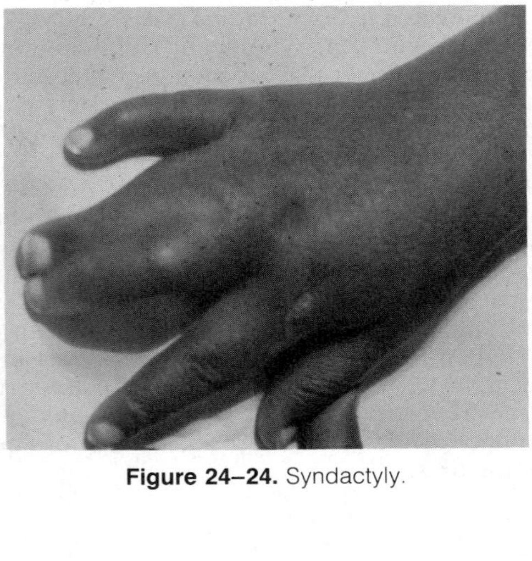

Figure 24–24. Syndactyly.

Polydactyly is digits in excess of 5, is the 2nd most common hand anomaly, and is more common in males and blacks (1:300, usually involving the little finger) than in whites (1:3,000, usually involving the thumb). Postaxial polydactyly (little finger side) occurs as an isolated lesion in blacks, inherited as an autosomal dominant trait, but in whites may be associated with other anomalies and syndromes. The extra digit may be just soft tissue (type I), a duplicated digit with normal finger bones and joints but an enlarged or bifid metacarpal (type II), or a rarer variant with duplication of the finger and metacarpals (type III). Other anomalies associated with postaxial polydactyly include syndactyly, triphalangeal thumb, absent thumb, carpal coalition, toe polydactyly, hemivertebra, and rarely genitourinary tract defects. Preaxial polydactyly with extra thumbs is common in whites; is usually sporadic and unilateral, unless associated with triphalangeal thumbs when the lesion may be familial; and is associated with vertebral anomalies, absent tibia, cleft palate, imperforate anus, 21-trisomy, acrocephalosyndactyly (Carpenter syndrome), Fanconi anemia, and Holt-Oram and Bloom syndromes.

Treatment of type I postaxial polydactyly with a rudimentary digit attached by a narrow pedicle involves ligation or electrocautery. More complicated polydactyly requires ablation surgery. Surgery for preaxial polydactyly attempts to preserve the size, stability, strength, and function of the dominant thumb.

Congenital longitudinal deficiency of the thumb demonstrates a hypoplastic or absent thumb. Hand function (grasp, prehension) is impaired. **Floating thumb** is also hypoplastic and is associated with hypoplasia or absence of the metacarpals and extrinsic tendons. Treatment of both lesions includes pollicization of the index finger and ablation for the functionless floating thumb. Surgery is performed between 6 and 12 mo of age. Transplantation of a toe to the thumb position is a new technique used by some orthopedic surgeons.

Congenital clasped thumb is a marked flexion of the metacarpophalangeal joint with thumb adduction into the palm. There is a male predominance, bilateral involvement, and familial occurrence. The etiology is an imbalance of the thumb flexor-extensor mechanisms. Treatment includes splinting, tendon transfer, soft-tissue release, or arthrodesis in unstable joints.

Trigger thumb is a stenosing tendovaginitis of the flexor pollicis longus, resulting in a thickened, constricted tendon sheath. There is stiffness, fixation of the thumb in flexion, snapping, and a nontender nodule over the tendon sheath. Congenital onset is bilateral in 50%, represents 25% of all cases, and resolves spontaneously in 30% of affected children by 1 yr of age. Childhood onset begins between 6 and 30 mo of age, is bilateral in 25%, and spontaneously resolves in 10%. Treatment includes passive stretching exercises, splinting, and, if needed, operative release of the fibrosed tendon sheath. Steroid injections are of no benefit.

24.25 TRAUMA

Trauma is the leading cause of death and disability in children between 1 and 18 yr of age (see Sec. 6.31). Trauma in children is usually blunt rather than penetrating and is the result of a motor vehicle accident or falls. Trauma in children may be localized to one anatomic area, but more often trauma produces multiple injuries. External signs of trauma may be absent in the presence of significant intracranial, intrathoracic, or intra-abdominal injury. Musculoskeletal injuries are difficult to diagnose in children due to lack of cooperation during the examination and variations of ossification of the less mature skeleton.

EVALUATION AND INITIAL STABILIZATION (see Sec. 6.31–6.35). The goals of trauma therapy are prioritized into the assessment and management during the primary survey. Musculoskeletal injury is assessed and treated as part of the secondary survey. A *primary survey* of the patient is performed to identify and treat life-threatening injuries, to initiate resuscitation, to determine the extent of injury, and to prepare for definitive therapy. Initial resuscitation of shock is provided in this phase, and all patients with signs of trauma above the clavicles, alteration of levels of consciousness, or neurologic signs should be considered at risk for cervical spine injury and should be managed with a rigid cervical collar and immobilization.

The *secondary survey* includes a head to toe assessment of the patient, including identification and initial management of musculoskeletal trauma. Even if one injury is detected, the secondary survey should continue to systematically evaluate the patient for other injuries.

Cranial fracture is suggested by the presence of a scalp hematoma, a soft mass, scalp (skull) depression, focal neurologic signs, cerebrospinal fluid leak (ears, nose), blood in the middle ear, the Battle sign (blood behind ears), and raccoon eyes.

Spinal cord accidents should be suspected in patients involved in motor vehicle accidents, falls, and, less often, sporting events (e.g., diving into shallow water). The most common site is the cervical spine followed by the thoracolumbar junction. In unconscious patients, spinal cord injury should be suspected in the presence of hypotension and bradycardia, flaccid paralysis, diaphragmatic breathing, priapism, malalignment of the spine (rotational deformity, widened interspinous spaces), urine retention, and apnea. In conscious patients these signs will be present in addition to neck pain, tenderness, and neurologic dysfunction such as the Beevor sign (upward motion of the umbilicus with contraction of the abdominal muscles), indicating a lesion below T10, and various cord syndromes. The **central cord syndrome** has predominant arm weakness; the **anterior cord syndrome** (flexion-rotation injuries) demonstrates lower extremity weakness and impaired pain and temperature sensation; the **posterior cord syndrome** (hyperextension injuries) has loss of vibration and proprioception, whereas hemisection of the cord **(Brown-Séquard syndrome)** produces ipsilateral weakness and contralateral loss of pain and temperature sensation.

The initial management of suspected spinal cord injury includes immobilization in a neck collar, roentgenographic evaluation of the spine (including all 7 cervical vertebrae), and the initiation of methylprednisolone (30 mg/kg followed by 5.4 mg/kg/hr × 23 hr) as soon as possible (preferably within 8 hr of injury). Lateral roentgenograms may demonstrate vertebral fractures or displacement and widened interspinous or prevertebral (secondary to hematoma) spaces. The retropharyngeal space (C2) should not exceed 6 mm, whereas the retrotracheal space (C6) should not exceed 22 mm in adults and 14 mm in children. Open-mouth and AP views may be needed to visualize rotary subluxation (see Sec. 24.23). In children, cervical spinal cord trauma may be present in the absence of cervical vertebral dislocation, subluxation, fracture, instability, or rotation; thus, a normal cervical spine roentgenogram does not exclude spinal cord injury.

The *extremities* should be examined to determine color, warmth, distal pulses, loss of distal sensation or motion, swelling (circumference differences), contusion, laceration (may indicate an open fracture), pseudoparalysis (fracture-related pain), asymmetry, abnormal interfragment (nonarticular) mobility, angular or rotational deformity, crepitus, instability, or shortening. Range of motion should not be determined if a fracture is evident. If a fracture is present, an immobilization splint should be placed prior to transfer or roentgenographic assessment. Splinting may reduce further damage and possibly prevent fat emboli.

Extremity trauma includes soft-tissue injuries, fractures, and dislocation or subluxation of the appendicular skeleton. *Life-threatening* extremity injuries include amputation, associated vascular injuries, disrupted pelvic fractures, open fractures with hemorrhage, multiple long bone fractures, and extensive crush injuries. *Limb-threatening* injuries include vascular injury, joint dislocations, crush injury, open fractures, nerve injury, and **compartment syndromes.** The latter are more common in forearm or lower leg trauma, can occur with open fractures, and produce ischemic injury secondary to swelling (hemorrhage or edema) within a tight nonyielding fascial compartment. The manifestations of a compartment syndrome include increased swelling and pain despite immobilization; altered sensation in a nerve passing through the compartment; tense and tender muscles; pain on muscle stretching; and normal, reduced, or absent distal pulses. If signs of a compartment syndrome are present, all constricting devices must be removed (bandages, casts, splints) and, if there is no improvement, a fasciotomy must be performed. If a deformity is present that produces distal ischemia (e.g., supracondylar fracture of the elbow), the initial management includes gentle traction with closed reduction to restore rotation and alignment in an attempt to improve distal perfusion.

Hemorrhage from multiple fractures may produce hypovolemic shock; however, other sources of bleeding should be determined. Significant hemorrhage is more common in pelvic fractures followed by femur, tibia, and humerus fractures. Blood loss is more common in open fractures.

The goals of management of open fractures are to avoid infection and to improve the chance of bone union. Initial treatment includes excision of devitalized tissue, meticulous wound cleansing and exploration, generous irrigation, fasciotomy if needed, and use of external skeletal fixation if the fracture is unstable.

If there are no signs of cervical spine injury, the patient may be rolled onto the side to *examine the back* to determine tenderness, deformity, contusion, laceration, malalignment, spasm, and increased intervertebral space distance.

FRACTURES. For all fractures a valuable finding is the demonstration of the exact location of maximal tenderness. This aids in the selection and interpretation of the appropriate roentgenographic studies. A growth plate or accessory ossicle may be confused with a fracture; if the site is nontender, it is not a fracture.

ROENTGENOGRAPHY. A fracture produces either an interruption in the cortex or an unexpected change in the contour of bone (Fig. 24–25). The fracture may involve the physis, epiphysis, metaphysis, or diaphysis. Diaphyseal (shaft) fractures of long bones may be complete, greenstick, torus (buckle), or bowed. Transverse fractures follow an angulation force; oblique fractures follow an axial overload, whereas spiral fractures follow a twisting force. The diagnosis is suspected clinically and is confirmed by demonstrating these roentgenographic changes that coincide with the site of tenderness on physical examination. Lateral, AP, and, rarely, oblique views are needed to identify fractures.

GROWTH PLATE FRACTURES. These are common in childhood and are classified into five types (Fig. 24–26). *Type I* usually occurs in infants, follows a shearing or avulsion force, or is pathologic owing to scurvy, rickets, or osteomyelitis. Reduction is not necessary, and growth remains undisturbed unless there is aseptic necrosis or premature closure

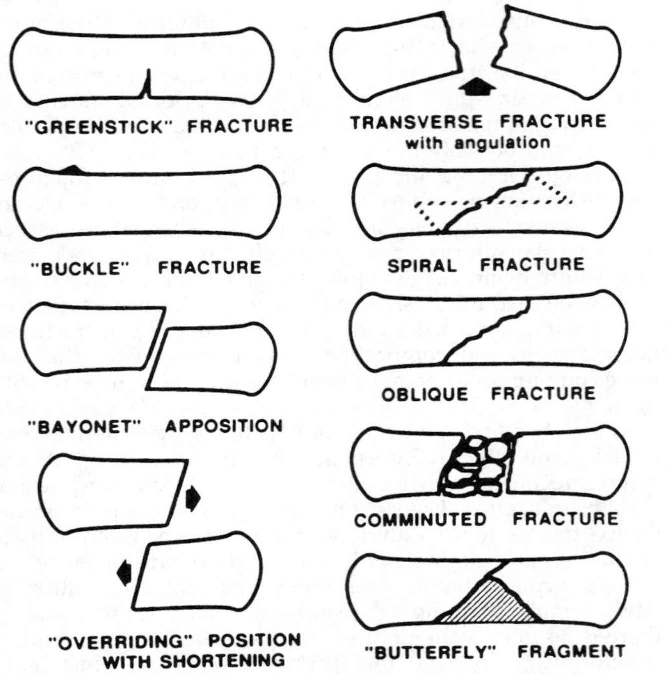

Figure 24–25. Fracture patterns. Not demonstrated is the avulsion fracture from a bony tuberosity by excessive tractional forces of a tendinous muscular insertion. (From Conrad E, Rang M: Fractures and sprains. Pediatr Clin North Am 33:1523, 1986.)

of the physis. *Type II* is the most common injury, usually occurs in children over 10 yr of age, and is due to shearing or avulsion forces. Reduction is easy to achieve and maintain; growth is unimpaired. *Type III* is a rare injury occurring after intra-articular shearing forces. Anatomic reduction is required. *Type IV* may produce osseous bridging of a joint or irregular articular surfaces if perfect anatomic reduction is not achieved. Internal fixation is needed to prevent future growth disturbances. *Type V* is a rare crush injury due to compression forces through the epiphysis to the physis. Displacement is minimal; however, severe growth impairment due to premature growth arrest is highly likely. Treatment of type V injuries includes a supporting cast and avoiding weight bearing for 3–4 wk.

DIFFERENTIAL DIAGNOSIS. In addition to trauma, fractures may be pathologic or due to child abuse. *Pathologic fractures* occur in the presence of pre-existing bone pathology, following a force that usually does not produce a fracture in normal bone. The most common lesion in a previously healthy child is a fracture through a unicameral bone cyst, occurring in the metaphysis (usually of the humerus). A nonossifying fibroma is another common lesion that produces a pathologic fracture in an otherwise healthy child. Less common causes of pathologic fractures include metastatic neuroblastoma, Ewing sarcoma, osteogenic sarcoma, Caffey disease, osteogenesis imperfecta, hyperparathyroidism, rickets, copper deficiency, osteomyelitis, and the child with spina bifida, cerebral palsy, or who is immobilized.

Child abuse or nonaccidental injury is a potentially lethal problem. See Sec. 3.51–3.54 for full discussion. Common patterns of skeletal injury owing to child abuse include spiral, oblique, or transverse fractures of long bones in children younger than 1 yr of age; a metaphyseal-epiphyseal "corner fracture" (bucket handle), which is a planar transmetaphyseal fracture with disk-like bone fragmentation and calcified cartilage; multiple posterior rib fractures at the costovertebral junction; physeal injuries; periosteal new bone reaction initiated by diaphyseal-periosteal separation and hemorrhage; avulsion fractures of the end of the clavicle and acromion process of the scapula; linear skull fractures; and vertebral body fractures. Rib fractures in children are not produced by falls or cardiopulmonary resuscitation but are caused by violent compression forces of the thorax. Common bones involved are the humerus > femur > tibia > skull > ribs > radius > ulna > other; 50% of children have only one fracture.

Multiple fractures in different stages of healing are specific for child abuse. Dating of the fracture is possible as soft-tissue swelling resolves by 4–10 days; new periosteal bone is formed by 7–14 days; fracture line definition is lost by 14–21 days, and a soft callus (10–21 days) and a hard callus (14–42 days) then form. Remodeling occurs within the 1st yr of the injury. Soft-tissue bruises can also be dated by the change in color of the hematoma; red-blue (1–2 days), blue-purple (3–5 days), green (6–7 days), and yellow-brown (8–10 days). Plain roentgenography with or without bone scans will reveal the site(s) and age of the fracture(s). The differential diagnosis of the skeletal injury owing to child abuse is similar to that listed for pathologic fractures. Child protective services should be notified of all cases of child abuse.

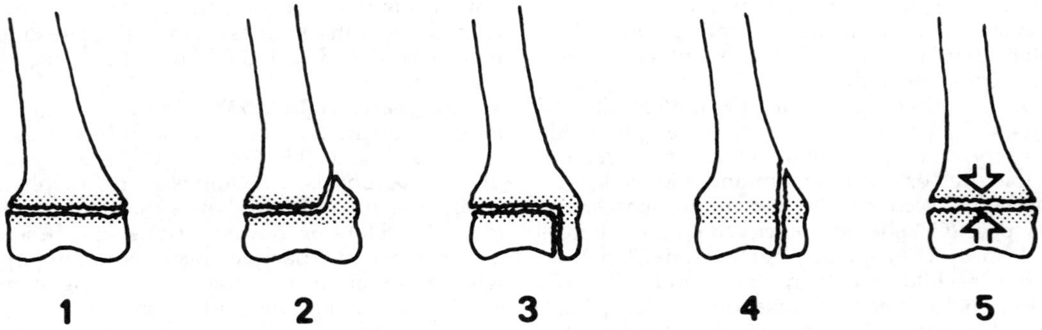

Figure 24–26. Salter-Harris classification of epiphyseal fractures. (1) The epiphysis separates from the metaphysis. The germinal cells remain with the epiphysis, usually uninjured. Healing is rapid and growth is seldom arrested. (2) Similar to type 1, except that a small piece of metaphysis breaks free to remain with the epiphysis. Healing is rapid and growth is usually normal. Types 1 and 2 are the most common. (3) Separation passes a variable distance along the growth plate, then enters the joint. Accurate reduction of the intra-articular fracture is necessary to prevent later traumatic arthritis. Open reduction may be needed. Growth disturbances are not usually a problem. (4) The fracture extends from the joint, across the growth plate, and into the metaphysis. This usually requires open reduction to prevent unilateral growth arrest and traumatic arthritis from malposition. (5) This is a crushing injury that leads to death of the germinal cells of the epiphyseal cartilage and arrest of growth. This type is rare.

PRINCIPLES OF PEDIATRIC FRACTURE MANAGEMENT. Fractures in children may differ from those in adults because the growth plates may dissipate force in comminuted fractures; the strong, thick periosteum has active osteogenic potential; the bone is more pliable, resulting in greenstick or buckle fractures; and healing is rapid but nonunion is very unusual. Angulation deformity is unusual owing to active remodeling during growth. If reduction of a deformity is needed, closed reduction is usually successful. Indications for open reduction (with internal fixation or pins) include failed closed reduction (older child with displaced femur, forearm, or tibial fracture), displaced intra-articular fractures of the distal femur, lateral humeral condyle, and distal tibia, displaced type III or IV growth plate fractures, and multiple injuries in some patients. Growth disturbances may result from physeal injuries, whereas bone overgrowth following diaphyseal metaphyseal long bone fractures may produce bone overgrowth.

Common drawbacks of pediatric fracture management include (1) Salter I fractures that are often not demonstrated by roentgenography. Tenderness over the growth plate may be the only sign. Therapy includes cast immobilization for 3 wk; (2) fractures (tender) may be confused with ossification centers (nontender), especially at the proximal aspect of the 5th metatarsal or the malleoli; and (3) fractures may "drift" in a cast. Such displacement indicates an unstable pattern that will be detected in the 1-wk follow-up roentgenogram; (4) some fractures are not apparent on the initial roentgenogram. Confirmation of point tenderness on the physical examination may be obtained by doing a bone scan or following 10–14 days of immobilization with a repeat roentgenogram. Multiple roentgenographic projections may be needed to visualize a fracture.

24.26 COMMON FRACTURES

CLAVICLE. A *fractured clavicle* may be due to birth trauma or, more often, may follow a fall onto a shoulder or the outstretched arm used to break the fall. There is pain, limited motion, marked callus formation, crepitance, and a lowered ipsilateral shoulder, and the arm is held against the body with the opposite hand supporting the ipsilateral elbow. Treatment in children is provided by a sling to rest the arm.

Acromioclavicular sprain and dislocation are common in athletic adolescents and manifest with pain on motion of the shoulder, local tenderness, and a palpable lateral end of the clavicle (with displacement). Treatment includes strapping and a sling for sprain, strapping and a plaster jacket for subluxation, and open repair for dislocation.

HUMERUS. *Upper epiphyseal fractures* occur in 11- to 15-yr-old patients after indirect trauma, usually with the arm adducted, extended, and laterally rotated. Injury may also result from direct trauma to the lateral aspect of the shoulder. Both mechanisms produce type I or II growth plate fractures. There is marked swelling, tenderness, and limited range of motion. Complete displacement demonstrates a short arm held in abduction and extension, with a prominence in the anterior axilla representing the distal fragment. Treatment includes Velpeau bandage immobilization (no displacement) and closed reduction for more angulated displaced lesions. Open reduction is rarely needed.

Fracture of the humeral shaft is less common in children than adults and follows direct trauma producing comminuted fractures, transverse fractures with or without displacement, and occasionally open fractures. Indirect trauma following falls on an elbow or an outstretched hand produce oblique spiral fractures. Pathologic oblique spiral fractures may follow muscular action (e.g., throwing a ball) (see Sec. 24.28). There is local pain, swelling, and potential for neurovascular injury with radial nerve damage producing anesthesia over the dorsum of the 1st and 2nd metacarpal regions and weakness of the thumb, finger, and wrist extensors. Treatment includes reduction of markedly displaced ends and immobilization for 4–6 wk with a modified Velpeau bandage or a hanging cast.

Supracondylar fracture is the most common elbow fracture and occurs at the metaphysis of the distal humerus in children between 5 and 8 yr of age. The injury is more common in males and usually results from falling on an outstretched arm that is hyperextended at the elbow. There is lateral and medial tenderness over the supracondylar area; deformity is present when there is displacement. Neurovascular injury may be present and manifest as distal pain, pallor, pain on passive finger extension, cyanosis, absent pulse, cool skin, paresthesias, and paralysis. These problems suggest the development of **Volkmann ischemia or contracture**, which, if left untreated, leads to paralysis and contracture due to ischemic necrosis of the forearm muscle. The arterial insufficiency may be due to direct arterial obstruction or injury (contusion) from the fracture, compression by tight bandages, or swelling associated with a compartment syndrome.

Treatment is an emergency and includes initial splinting in slight flexion, casting for undisplaced fractures, and closed reduction and percutaneous pinning for displaced fractures. Open reduction is indicated for acute vascular injury. Complications include malunion-induced deformity (cubitus varus or valgus), changes in the carrying angle, and Volkmann contracture.

Lateral condylar humeral fractures are common, occur in 6- to 10-yr-old children, and represent a type IV physeal injury following indirect trauma to the outstretched hand with elbow extension and forearm abduction. Tenderness, pain, swelling, and ecchymosis are present over the lateral aspect of the elbow. The fracture may be subtle on roentgenography and may be missed in young children owing to the small ossification center. Treatment of undisplaced fractures includes either immobilization in an above-elbow cast for 6 wk, with repeated roentgenograms to check for displacement or percutaneous pinning to prevent displacement. Displaced fractures are treated with open reduction and internal (pin) fixation. Delayed therapy may result in malunion, cubitus valgus deformity, and ulnar nerve palsy.

Medial epicondylar fractures of the humerus occur between 7 and 15 yr of age and may be associated with dislocation of the elbow and incarceration of fragments into the joint space. Local tenderness is present over the medial aspect of the joint; there is pain on motion; the elbow is held in partial flexion; and ulnar nerve injury is possible. Treatment includes casting for minimally displaced lesions and open reduction with fixation for more severely displaced fractures.

ELBOW. *Dislocation* is uncommon, occurs in children between 11 and 15 yr of age, and usually results in posterior, with some lateral, displacement following a fall on the outstretched hand when the forearm is supinated and the elbow is extended or partially flexed. There is pain, swelling, and refusal to move the elbow, which is held in partial flexion. The ulna is displaced posteriorly, and its semilunar notch may be palpated in this position. There may be associated neurovascular damage. Treatment with closed reduction and subsequent cast immobilization are effective. Reduction is performed with the patient prone on a table and with the arm hanging over the edge. An assistant applies gentle traction to the forearm, and the examiner's fingers encircle the arm and push the olecranon downward and forward with the examiner's thumbs.

Fractures of the proximal radial physis and radial neck occur in children between 5 and 13 yr of age and are caused by a fall on the outstretched hand with elbow extension and a supinated forearm. The elbow is held in flexion and is supported by the opposite hand. Treatment varies with the degree of angulation and includes an above-elbow cast for undisplaced or minimally displaced fractures, closed reduction for moderate displaced fractures, and open reduction for more severe injuries.

Nursemaid's elbow (subluxation of the radial head) or pulled elbow is common and is noted in children younger than 4 yr of age after sudden longitudinal traction on the hand with the elbow extended and the forearm pronated. The lesion may represent a tear of the annular ligament with entrapment of synovium (or ligament) in the radiohumeral joint. The child cries immediately after being pulled and refuses to move the elbow, which is partially flexed with the forearm pronated. The person who pulled the child may have heard or felt a click. Flexion and extension are usually normal, whereas supination is limited. Roentgenograms are normal. Closed reduction may occur during roentgenographic examination by the technician. Treatment consists of gentle supination with the arm in 90-degree flexion. A click may be felt or heard, and pain is immediately relieved with successful reduction. Immobilization is not necessary.

FOREARM. *Fractures of the shaft of the radius and ulna* may occur at the proximal, middle, or more often, distal (75% of fractures) third of one or both bones and may be greenstick or undisplaced, minimally or markedly displaced complete fractures. Indirect trauma from a fall on an outstretched hand or direct trauma ("both-bone") results in the fracture(s). Care must be taken to determine if there is an associated radial head dislocation. Treatment includes closed reduction, use of an appropriately fitted, usually above-elbow cast to avoid loss of reduction with redisplacement, and, rarely in some adolescents, open reduction.

The *torus or buckle fracture* of the distal radial and ulnar metaphysis is the most common childhood lower forearm fracture. Treatment includes a cast below the elbow or a volar splint for 3 wk.

Fracture separation of the distal radial physis (type II) is the most common physeal injury occurring in children between 6 and 10 yr of age after a fall on an outstretched hand. There is local pain, swelling, and roentgenographic confirmation in the lateral view. Treatment includes closed reduction and an above-elbow cast for 3–4 wk. The prognosis is good.

LOWER LIMB. *Fractures of the femoral neck* are uncommon and result from motor vehicle accidents or falls. There is often associated pelvic, skull, and soft-tissue injury. Treatment includes spica cast immobilization for undisplaced fractures and open reduction and internal fixation for displaced lesions.

Fractures of the femoral shaft are common owing to motor vehicle accidents, falls from heights, child abuse (especially in children younger than 1–3 yr of age), or sometimes after relatively minor injuries. There is pain, swelling, pseudoparalysis, shortening, deformity, lateral rolling of the distal leg, and crepitus. Treatment includes immobilization at the accident site. Infants require immobilization in a spica cast. Children between 2 and 10 yr of age are treated with a spica cast, if initial shortening is less than 2 cm. Skin traction is indicated if shortening exceeds 2 cm. Complications include leg overgrowth and angular deformity.

Fractures of the shaft of the tibia in infants and young children are spiral and are produced by torsional forces applied from a fall or by twisting against resistance if the foot is caught in a fixed position. The fibula is intact. This "toddler fracture" is manifest with refusal to walk or bear weight, antalgic limp, and local tibial tenderness. Roentgenography may demonstrate a hairline fracture; periosteal new bone formation will be evident, and may suggest the diagnosis of osteomyelitis or leukemia. Treatment includes an above-knee cast for 3 wk.

STRESS FRACTURES. See Sec. 24.27.

24.27 SPORTS MEDICINE

Participation in sports is important for normal development because it fosters physical fitness and overall health, provides opportunities for psychosocial development (team work, peer relations), improves decision-making abilities, and promotes self-confidence. Sports activity also provides the child with an enjoyable experience as well as an opportunity to learn some skills that can be continued throughout life. Play is sometimes referred to as the "occupation" of the child. The role of physicians is to provide health services, counseling, instruction, and rehabilitation. Physicians need to avoid unnecessary restriction of a child's play and sports activities, while trying to prevent injury. Restrictions of activity should be made: (1) when the need is definite; (2) for only the shortest necessary period; and (3) tailored to the child's specific requirements. Alternatives are often appropriate. For example, swimming is often a good substitute for contact sports. The most stressful activities are those that involve competition or body contact and are supervised or promoted by adults. It is prudent to tell parents that children should be allowed normal activity when parents impose restrictions that are too stringent and confining. Alternately, parents and coaches may push the child too far (see Overuse Injuries).

PREPARTICIPATION HEALTH EXAMINATION. The goal of this evaluation is to determine specific conditions that place the child at risk for injury or death during participation in sports. In addition, residual abnormalities of earlier athletic activity may become evident. Furthermore, as the preparticipation examination may be the only contact an adolescent athlete has with the health care provider, it provides an opportunity to perform a general health evaluation. The preparticipation examination should be performed every 3–4 yr or with changes in the level of competition (change to high school or college).

Areas of concern include *orthopedic* (knee or ankle injury, subluxing patella, chondromalacia patella, cervical spine disease, scoliosis), *cardiovascular* (heart murmur, hypertension, arrhythmia, current or repaired congenital heart disease), *pulmonary* (chronic versus exercise-induced asthma, obstructive lung disease), *anatomic* (organomegaly, absence of one of paired organs; e.g., eye, kidney, testis), *ocular* (poor vision, anisocoria), *hematologic* (sickle cell or other anemias, hemorrhagic disease), *cutaneous* (contagious infection including staphylococcal, streptococcal, herpes simplex), and *neurologic* (mental retardation, repeated head injury and concussions, seizures, syncope) problems.

Sudden death during sports may occur owing to cardiac disease such as hypertrophic or other cardiomyopathies, coronary artery disease (single or anomalous vessels, atherosclerosis), congenital heart disease (aortic stenosis), and ruptured aorta in Marfan syndrome. In many cases the underlying heart disease is not suspected, and sudden death is the first sign of heart disease. A chest roentgenogram, electrocardiogram, and echocardiogram are not recommended for screening but are indicated if there is concern about heart disease on the basis of history and physical examination. The screening orthopedic examination is noted in Table 24–9. Laboratory tests (hemoglobin, urinalysis, drug testing) are not routine screening procedures.

Disqualifications and limitations for sports participation among various medical conditions are noted in Table 24–10. Classification of sports activities is further delineated in Table 24–11. Students have a legal right to participate in a sport, despite a disqualifying condition. Physicians must, nonetheless, provide complete information about the risks associated with participation in sports.

The *psychologic assessment* should determine attitudes and behaviors that would suggest the risk for burnout and overuse

TABLE 24–9. 90-Second Orthopedic Screening Examination*

Instructions to Athlete	Observation
Stand facing examiner	Acromioclavicular joints; general habitus
Look at ceiling, floor, over both shoulders; touch ears to shoulders	Cervical spine motion
Shrug shoulders (examiner resists)	Trapezius strength
Abduct shoulders 90 degrees (examiner resists at 90 degrees)	Deltoid strength
Full external rotation of arms	Shoulder motion
Flex and extend elbows	Elbow motion
Arms at sides, elbows 90 degrees flexed; pronate and supinate wrists	Elbow and wrist motion
Spread fingers; make fist	Hand or finger motion and deformities
Tighten (contract) quadriceps; relax quadriceps	Symmetry and knee effusion; ankle effusion
"Duck walk" four steps (away from examiner with buttocks on heels)	Hip, knee, and ankle motion
Back to examiner	Shoulder symmetry; scoliosis
Knees straight, touch toes	Scoliosis, hip motion, hamstring tightness
Raise up on toes, raise heels	Calf symmetry, leg strength

*From American Academy of Pediatrics, Committee on Sports Medicine: Sports Medicine: Health Care for Young Athletes. Evanston, IL, American Academy of Pediatrics, 1983; Harris S, Runyan D: The Preparticipation Exam. *In:* Reider B (ed): Sports Medicine: The School Age Athlete. Philadelphia, WB Saunders, 1991.

injuries. Burnout may be prevented by keeping sports fun, by having a proper perspective with regard to winning and losing, and by taking time out from practice and competition. Pain is often reduced by rest, rehabilitation, and avoiding coming back to participation too soon.

Atlantoaxial instability (and the risk for subluxation) in patients with 21-trisomy has been thought to be a disqualifying condition for participation in some events of the Special Olympics. Cervical roentgenograms should be obtained because as many as 10–20% of these children have atlantoaxial instability.

OVERUSE INJURIES. Highly driven athletes, but more usually parents or coaches, place the child at risk for overuse injuries. Attitudes such as "no pain no gain," "giving 110%," "never miss a practice or competition," and other perfectionist behavior (especially when tied closely to the need for love and approval from parents or coaches) place the young athlete at risk for overuse injuries.

Overuse injuries are common in immature patients and are usually noted in the 2nd decade. Repeated trauma produces chronic irritation, inflammation, microtearing, or microfractures. Tennis or Little League elbow, chondromalacia patellae, shin splints, Achilles tendinitis, swimmer's shoulder, and stress fractures are examples of overuse injuries that may be exacerbated by poor technique, minor-to-moderate anatomic imbalance, and poor equipment. The diagnosis is determined by identifying high-risk attitudes or behaviors and by examination of the point of maximal tenderness of a specific anatomic site.

STRESS FRACTURES. Stress (fatigue) fractures are caused by chronic repetitive muscular action on a bony insertion site or by repeated direct trauma (march fracture), usually occurring in poorly trained patients engaged in physical activities. This common overuse syndrome produces local dissolution of bone and should be distinguished from conditions in which a physiologic force acts on a site with abnormal elastic resistance (osteogenesis imperfecta, osteopetrosis, rickets, scurvy, Cushing syndrome, hyperparathyroidism, disuse, immobilization, inflammatory lesions).

Stress fractures occur in typical locations associated with specific activities: 1st metacarpal sesamoid—standing; metatarsal shaft—marching, running, ballet; tarsal navicular—running, high-impact aerobics; distal fibula and proximal diaphysis of the tibia—running; patella—hurdling; neck and shaft of the femur—ballet, gymnastics, running; pelvic ischial pubic rami—bowling, gymnastics; lumbar vertebral pars interarticularis—ballet, weight lifting; ribs—coughing, golf; and coronoid ulnar process and distal humerus—throwing a ball.

Clinical manifestations include limp, gradual onset of pain that is increased with activity and relieved with rest, point tenderness, distal atrophy, and local swelling. There is no fever or abnormality of the CBC or erythrocyte sedimentation rate. Roentgenographic findings may be normal or demonstrate a radiolucent zone without periosteal reaction, focal sclerosis, and callus formation. Bone scans may be needed to identify the lesion if the results of plain roentgenograms are negative. The *differential diagnosis* includes osteoid osteoma, acute or chronic osteomyelitis, bone tumors, leukemia, and rickets.

Treatment includes rest, casting for complete fractures, and subsequent rehabilitation to correct muscle imbalance or anatomic variations.

SOFT-TISSUE INJURIES. Most sports-related injuries are not skeletal injuries but rather are injuries of the ligaments (sprains) and muscle-tendon units (strains). Additional injuries include muscle contusions and lacerations.

Musculotendinous strains also known as pulls, tears, or ruptures are an indirect injury due to excessive stretch from an antagonistic muscle group, external objects, gravity, or active muscle contraction. Muscle strains may occur rapidly with a single contraction and are classified as grade I (mild, microscopic muscle tear, intact fascia, local tenderness, minimal swelling, or ecchymosis), grade II (moderate, larger number of muscle fibers torn, fascia involved, a "pop" felt by athlete, small defect palpated), or grade III (severe, complete rupture, a palpable defect, severe pain, marked ecchymosis or hematoma formation, loss of function). The greater the size of the disruption (palpable defect) and the greater the ecchymosis, the more likely it is to be a grade III strain. Grade III tendon injuries do not bleed (tendons are relatively avascular), but a palpable defect is present before the onset of edema and swelling. Avulsion fractures from the point of bony tendinous insertion may occur instead of a muscle strain. Such lesions are common in muscles originating at the pelvis or femur and include rectus femoris, gluteus, sartorius, iliopsoas, adductor longus, and hamstrings.

Treatment of muscle strains includes ice and compression immediately after the injury, nonsteroidal anti-inflammatory agents for pain, very short periods of immobilization (1–2 days' rest), and subsequent strengthening (passive range of motion and active stretching exercises during rehabilitation). To avoid reinjury the child should not return to active partic-

TABLE 24–10. Recommendations for Participation in Competitive Sports*

			Noncontact		
Indications	**Contact/ Collision**	**Limited Contact/Impact**	***Strenuous***	***Moderately Strenuous***	***Nonstrenuous***
Atlantoaxial instability	No	No	Yes	Yes	Yes
*Swimming: no butterfly, breast stroke, or diving starts					
Acute illnesses	*	*	*	*	*
**Needs individual assessment (e.g., contagiousness to others, risk of worsening illness)*					
Cardiovascular					
Carditis	No	No	No	No	No
Hypertension					
Mild	Yes	Yes	Yes	Yes	Yes
Moderate	*	*	*	*	*
Severe	*	*	*	*	*
Congenital heart disease	†	†	†	†	†
**Needs individual assessment*					
†Patients with mild forms can be allowed a full range of physical activities; patients with moderate or severe forms, or who are postoperative, should be evaluated by a cardiologist before athletic participation					
Eyes					
Absence or loss of function of one eye	*	*	*	*	*
Detached retina	†	†	†	†	†
**Availability of American Society for Testing and Materials (ASTM)–approved eye guards may allow competitor to participate in most sports, but this must be judged on an individual basis*					
†Consult ophthalmologist					
Inguinal hernia	Yes	Yes	Yes	Yes	Yes
Kidney: absence of one	No	Yes	Yes	Yes	Yes
Liver: enlarged	No	No	Yes	Yes	Yes
Musculoskeletal disorders	*	*	*	*	*
**Needs individual assessment*					
Neurologic					
History of serious head or spine trauma, repeated concussions, or craniotomy	*	*	Yes	Yes	Yes†
Convulsive disorder					
Well controlled	Yes	Yes	Yes	Yes	Yes
Poorly controlled	No	No	Yes†	Yes	Yes†
**Needs individual assessment*					
†No swimming or weight lifting					
†No archery or riflery					
Ovary: absence of one	Yes	Yes	Yes	Yes	Yes
Respiratory					
Pulmonary insufficiency	*	*	*	*	Yes
Asthma	Yes	Yes	Yes	Yes	Yes
**May be allowed to compete if oxygenation remains satisfactory during a graded stress test*					
Sickle cell trait	Yes	Yes	Yes	Yes	Yes
Skin: boils, herpes, impetigo, scabies	*	*	Yes	Yes	Yes
**No gymnastics with mats, martial arts, wrestling, or contact sports until not contagious*					
Spleen: enlarged	No	No	No	Yes	Yes
Testicle: absence or undescended	Yes*	Yes*	Yes	Yes	Yes
**Certain sports may require protective cup*					

*From American Academy of Pediatrics, Committee on Sports Medicine: Sports Medicine: Health Care for Young Athletes. Evanston, IL, American Academy of Pediatrics, 1983; †Harris S, Runyan D: The Preparticipation Exam. *In:* Reider B (ed): Sports Medicine: The School Age Athlete. Philadelphia, WB Saunders, 1991.

ipation in sports until strength training returns the muscle to normal function. Prevention of strains may be possible by warming up and stretching.

Ligamentous sprains are likely to occur in forceful activities, such as football or wrestling. Sites include the knee, ankle, wrist, shoulder, or elbow. Sprains are graded on the basis of loss of stability: grade I demonstrates overstretching, microscopic tearing without instability; grade II involves partial tearing and instability; grade III includes marked ligamentous laxity, maximal instability, and discontinuous ligaments. Grade III (severe sprains) is associated with pain, a snapping or popping sound, hemorrhage, markedly diffuse swelling that develops rapidly, immediate disability, and loss of function. The patient often has instability. Fractures or dislocations usually produce more immediate pain than a sprain; however, the nature of the pain does not always distinguish a fracture from a sprain. Treatment of sprains includes immediate anti-inflammatory therapy (see strains), protection from tension-producing injuries during the healing phase, and occasionally casting or surgery (arthroscopic or open) for grade III sprains.

Muscle contusions are common in contact sports. There is local pain, disability, swelling, hematoma formation, and potential for subsequent connective tissue scar formation. The quadriceps muscle is the most common site of contusion that is graded as grade I (mild, local tenderness, normal gait, knee range of motion greater than 90 degrees); grade II (moderate, more tenderness and swelling, limp, inability to do deep leg bends, range of motion less than 90 degrees); and grade III (severe, cannot walk unassisted, marked swelling and tenderness, range of motion less than 45 degrees).

Treatment includes ice, elevation, compression, and nonsteroidal anti-inflammatory agents during the acute phase, followed by range of motion, stretching, and strengthening exercises. Massage is not recommended, and the serious nature of the injury should not be made trivial, because **myositis ossificans** is a common sequela to grade II–III contusions. The ossification of the intramuscular hematoma occurs mainly in adolescent patients, appears 2–4 wk after the injury, increases in size until 6 mo later, and manifests as continued pain and stiffness. Surgical excision is usually not indicated unless pain persists for more than 1 yr.

HEAD AND NECK INJURIES. High-risk sports for head and neck injuries include football, ice hockey, rugby, lacrosse, snowmobiling, diving, boxing, sledding, gymnastics, and horseback riding. Most injuries to the head and neck are self-limited and are not reported to the physician or coach.

Head injuries may be diffuse or focal, severe (contusion, intracranial hemorrhage, epidural or subdural hematoma, diffuse axonal injury), or mild-grade I–IV concussion and result in no or significant sequelae. Concussion, an immediate, transient (a few sec to 24 hr), post-traumatic alteration in level of consciousness, with or without retrograde or post-traumatic amnesia, is the most common head injury and is usually mild. There may be associated loss of or impaired vision and equilibrium. Grade I concussion manifests minimal symptoms such as transient confusion (5–15 min), being dazed; grade II (mild) concussion includes confusion, post-traumatic amnesia (loss of memory after the event), a sense of being "dinged" or having "bells rung," and the risk of developing the **postconcussion syndrome** consisting of difficulty concentrating, irritability, and headaches lasting for several weeks to months; grade III (moderate) concussion includes all the symptoms of grade II plus retrograde amnesia (no record of events before the injury) and the risk of the postconcussion syndrome; and grade IV (severe) concussion includes all the findings of grade III plus loss of consciousness and paralytic coma, a gradual return to consciousness (after several seconds to minutes) through the stages of stupor, confusion, automatic behavior, and lucid recovery and requires an examination by a physician and hospital observation if the loss of consciousness exceeds 5 min. Post-traumatic amnesia may be tested by asking "Who helped you to stand?", "How did you get to the bench?", while retrograde amnesia may be tested by asking the names of the coach, players, plays, opponents, and so forth.

Severe life-threatening concussion may be associated with cervical spine injury and is designated as grade V concussion if there is flaccid coma for 5 min, with or without cardiopulmonary arrest, or grade VI concussion if there is coma, cardiopulmonary arrest, and death. Grades V and VI concussion require cardiopulmonary resuscitation, cervical spine immobilization, and rapid transfer to a hospital for evaluation of serious intracranial (CT screening) and spine (lateral roentgenogram) injuries. Immediate and delayed sequelae of concussions include reduced mental capacity and post-traumatic migraine or seizures.

Athletes with grade I concussion may return to competition that day if symptoms resolve but must be observed for dizziness, headache, nausea, or photophobia; patients with grades II and III concussion should not return to competition for 1 wk if symptoms resolve; those with grade IV concussion should not play for 1 mo; and those with grade V concussion should be recommended to find an alternate sport and not to return to competition for a season.

Cervical spine fractures (see Sec. 24.23 and 24.25) are divided into the more common C1, C2 (diving, water skiing, surfing, trampolines) injuries and C3–C7 (football) fractures. Fractures may be immediately symptomatic, requiring neck immobilization and roentgenographic assessment or may present as persistent post-traumatic neck pain. Neurologic deficit (quadriplegia, paraplegia) may be immediate, associated with minimal neck pain, or delayed (for minutes or, rarely, days). *Neck*

TABLE 24–11. Classification of Sports*

Contact/Collision	Limited Contact/Impact	Noncontact: *Strenuous*	Noncontact: *Moderately Strenuous*	Noncontact: *Nonstrenuous*
Boxing	Baseball	Aerobic dancing	Badminton	Archery
Field hockey	Basketball	Crew	Curling	Golf
Football	Bicycling	Fencing	Table tennis	Riflery
Ice hockey	Diving	Field		
Lacrosse	Field	Discus		
Martial arts	High jump	Javelin		
Rodeo	Pole vault	Shot-put		
Soccer	Gymnastics	Running		
Wrestling	Horseback riding	Swimming		
	Skating	Tennis		
	Ice	Track		
	Roller	Weight lifting		
	Skiing			
	Cross-country			
	Downhill			
	Water			
	Softball			
	Squash			
	Handball			
	Volleyball			

*From American Academy of Pediatrics, Committee on Sports Medicine: Sports Medicine: Health Care for Young Athletes. Evanston, IL, American Academy of Pediatrics, 1983; Harris S, Runyan D: The Preparticipation Exam. *In:* Reider B (ed): Sports Medicine: The School Age Athlete. Philadelphia, WB Saunders, 1991.

sprain is a common football injury. This sprain is painful and produces local spasm with limited motion. The pain is not radicular, and there are no neurologic signs. If pain persists, there may be an associated small fracture or subluxation.

Cervical cord neurapraxia is a cervical cord syndrome but without obvious fracture, subluxation, or neck pain. The injury results from hyperextension, hyperflexion, or axial loading and may be caused by spinal stenosis, congenital fusion, cervical instability, or disk disease, with resultant reduced AP spinal canal diameter and spinal cord trauma (concussion, contusion). Manifestations may be present in the arms, hands, legs, or all sites and include numbness, tingling, burning pain, complete loss of sensation, or motor symptoms (quadriplegia). Neurapraxia lasts 10–15 min and resolves without sequelae. Evaluations include lateral spine roentgenography, CT scanning, and MRI. If there is no cervical spine instability or disk disease, the risk of permanent neurologic damage is low; however, many experts recommend avoiding participation in further contact sports.

24.28 SPECIFIC SPORTS AND ASSOCIATED INJURIES

GYMNASTICS. Competitive female gymnasts often begin the sport at 6 yr of age, achieve high-level competition at 16 yr of age, and retire at 18–20 yr of age. A similar activity pattern occurs in males at 9, 22, and 24–26 yr of age. In addition to mechanical or traumatic injuries, female gymnasts have delayed menarche and often have eating disorders.

Common problems include traumatic and overuse injuries, such as ankle sprain and wrist and spine injuries. The incidence of injury increases with the level of skill and is most common in the floor exercise. *Wrist pain* may be due to chronic upper extremity weight bearing with distal radial physeal trauma. *Ligamentous laxity* may predispose to elbow or shoulder dislocation and ankle sprains. *Spine problems* include acute traumatic or overuse injuries such as pars interarticularis injury, resulting in spondylolysis and spondylolisthesis. Therapy includes rest, immobilization, nonsteroidal anti-inflammatory agents, and, if pain persists, MRI or arthroscopic examination to rule out intra-articular tears, loose bodies, or ligamentous instability. Prevention includes wrist strengthening, flexibility exercises, and an ulnar variance brace.

SWIMMING. Shoulder injury is the most common overuse injury of competitive swimmers. *Swimmer's shoulder* is rotation cuff tendinitis of the supraspinatus or biceps and manifests as shoulder pain and tenderness of the supraspinatus tendon. The onset may be insidious. Supraspinatus tendinitis produces pain with active abduction between 60 and 100 degrees, whereas biceps tendinitis is demonstrated by resisting flexion of a straight supinated arm. Treatment includes ice, modification of stroke technique, rest, stretching, muscle strengthening, physiotherapy, and nonsteroidal anti-inflammatory agents. Prevention includes avoiding overwork, proper technique, and strengthening and stretching exercises.

BASEBALL. Throwing injuries of the elbow and shoulder (especially among pitchers) are the most common baseball injuries. *Shoulder pain syndromes* are due to a combination of some degree of shoulder instability and overuse injury. Supraspinatus, biceps, or subscapularis tendinitis, anterior capsule ligament or sternoclavicular sprain, acromioclavicular dysfunction, impingement syndromes, bursal inflammation, and labrum tears produce anterior or lateral shoulder pain, whereas posterior capsule injuries and intraspinatus tendinitis produce posterior shoulder pain. Treatment includes rest, oral nonsteroidal anti-inflammatory agents, intrabursal steroids for bursitis, and arthroscopy for persistent pain.

Elbow pain may be seen with flexion contractures, capsule inflammation, lateral epicondylitis, medial olecranon chondromalacia, flexor pronator tendinitis, medial collateral ligament sprains, and ulnar neuritis. Osteochondritis dissecans (OD) of the capitellum causes gradual onset of pain in children who have been pitching for 3–5 yr. There is pain over the lateral and anterior elbow, limited pronation and supination, and a flexion contracture (see Sec. 24.6). Surgery is indicated for a loose body causing mechanical problems and for a large defect causing grinding and catching of the elbow.

BALLET. This very demanding activity is associated with delayed menarche and eating disorders in female dancers. *Foot problems* include metatarsal stress fractures, subungual hematomas, callus, sesamoiditis, bunion formation, proximal phalangeal epiphysitis, and accessory navicular pain syndrome. *Ankle problems* include inversion sprains, anterior and posterior impingement syndromes, and OD of the talus. *Leg problems* include shin splints, tibial or fibular stress fracture, and compartment syndromes (see Running). *Knee* problems include Osgood-Schlatter disease, excessive recurvatum owing to lax ligaments (pseudo-genu varum), OD, and patellar malalignment (subluxation dislocation) owing to lax ligaments (see Sec. 24.6). *Hip* problems include the medial **snapping hip syndrome** due to iliopsoas tendon riding over the anterior hip capsule, tendinitis (pyriformis, iliopsoas, rectus femoris), and subclinical slipped capital femoral epiphysis, usually seen in male dancers (see Sec. 24.11). *Spine problems* include associated Scheuermann disease in males, idiopathic scoliosis in females, and purposeful excessive lumbar lordosis (see Sec. 24.15, 24.18, and 24.19).

WRESTLING. Wrestlers have great fluctuations in weight to meet weight-matched competition standards. Such fluctuations are associated with fasting, dehydration, and then binging.

Wrestling holds may produce injury by various torques or forces applied to the extremities and spine; wrestling throws with subsequent falls may produce concussions, neck strain, or spinal cord injury (see Sec. 24.27). "Stingers" and "burners" are neurogenic pain syndromes seen with traumatic stretching or pinching of the bracheal plexus (see Football). Severe electric-like pain starts with impact and radiates from the shoulders to the fingertips. There is numbness, weakness (predominantly of the abductor deltoid muscles), and tenderness over the paraspinous and trapezius muscles, lasting a few seconds to 5 min. Treatment includes ice, nonsteroidal anti-inflammatory agents, strengthening exercises, and, if severe, oral steroids, cervical collar for 24–48 hr, and transcutaneous electrical nerve stimulation (TENS).

Shoulder subluxation is common but does not usually present with only pain and weakness. Patients are usually aware of their shoulders slipping in and out. *Hand injuries* are usually not severe and include recurrent metacarpophalangeal and proximal interphalangeal sprains. Treatment of hand injuries includes splinting and taping.

Knee injuries are common, potentially serious, and include prepatellar bursitis, medial and lateral sprains, and medial and lateral meniscus tears. Prepatellar bursitis is the most common knee problem, is caused by a traumatic forceful impact to the mat or chronic trauma, demonstrates swelling over the knee and no limitation of motion except full flexion. Treatment includes protective neoprene knee sleeves, nonsteroidal anti-inflammatory agents, steroid application, aspiration of effusions, and bursectomy after the 3rd recurrence.

Dermatologic problems include herpes simplex (herpes gladiatorum), impetigo, staphylococcus furunculosis or folliculitis, superficial fungal infections, and contact dermatitis (see Sec. 23.14).

FOOTBALL. Football injuries are common, in part owing to the popularity of the sport. Fortunately, most injuries are minor because the incidence of serious injuries has been reduced by prohibition of clipping blocks and "spearing" or head-butting tackling, improvement of techniques, equipment (pads, shoes with wider, more, shorter cleats, helmet), preseason conditioning (strength and flexibility training), ankle taping, proper rehabilitation of injuries, and playing on grass rather than artificial surfaces.

Head and neck football injuries include concussion, neck sprain, and brachial plexus trauma ("stinger," "burner," see Wrestling) and often are unreported because athletes expect these problems. "Burners" represent a brachial plexus neurapraxia, possibly owing to lateral neck bending, manifesting without neck pain but with painful arm dysesthesia and deltoid muscle weakness. They are usually transient with immediate recovery. Cervical collars (neck rolls) may reduce the risks of this injury.

Lumbar spine injury manifest as low back pain probably represents spondylolysis. *Shoulder trauma* includes instability, rotator cuff, and tendinitis injury to the proximal humerus, shaft, and clavicular articulation. Rest, immobilization, and nonsteroidal anti-inflammatory agents may be effective therapies for mild shoulder injuries. Repeated shoulder subluxation requires strengthening exercises, bracing, and possible surgical stabilization in the off-season.

Contusions to the arm and thigh muscles are common, may produce knee effusions, and are at risk for the development of **myositis ossificans** (see Sec. 24.27).

Knee injuries are common reasons why a player seeks medical attention and include anterior cruciate (ACL), posterior cruciate (PCL), and collateral ligament tears. ACL injuries are common, debilitating, and reduce the chance of future competition. Functional hinged knee bracing for ACL injuries reduces the number of "giving-out" episodes and may improve performance. PCL injuries are usually isolated and respond to routine rehabilitation, whereas medial collateral ligament sprains are common, cause temporary disability, and may be rehabilitated with a brace.

Ankle sprains are frequent problems among football players and may be prevented by ankle taping or by reusable straps and supports. **Turf toe**, an injury to the 1st metatarsophalangeal joint (usually of the great toe), is caused by forceful dorsiflexion while playing on artificial turf in soft light-weight, flexible shoes. Treatment of turf toe includes ice, nonsteroidal anti-inflammatory agents, compression, and rest. Corticosteroid injections are not beneficial.

HOCKEY. Hockey is a collision sport associated with injuries caused by the puck and the stick, producing contusions, lacerations, or concussions or by the players' bodies, the ice, and the boards, producing fractures, sprains, or concussions. The risk for injury is reduced by proper equipment (helmets with face masks) and rules regarding dangerous body contact (checking from behind, high sticking).

Specific hockey injuries include *ankle sprains* (dorsiflexion, eversion, and external rotation in contrast to usual sprain of inversion in other sports), *hip adductor strain*, and various *shoulder injuries* from body contact. The latter include acromioclavicular sprain, dislocation, and clavicular fractures.

BASKETBALL AND VOLLEYBALL. Common physical activities of these two sports include shooting, jumping, pivoting, running, and sudden stopping that increase the risks for ankle, knee, and finger injury.

Knee overuse injuries include patellar tendinitis ("jumper knee"), traction apophysitis (Osgood-Schlatter disease), physeal fractures of the distal femur and proximal tibia, fracture of the patella, and ligament sprains (medial collateral with or without anterior cruciate ligaments).

Ankle sprain is the most common injury and is usually caused by inversion with plantar flexion placing the lateral ligaments at high tension. An avulsion fracture of the base of the 5th metatarsal at the insertion of the peroneus brevis tendon is another sequela of inversion ankle injuries. **Achilles tendinitis** is overuse injury, which may be exacerbated by rubbing of the tendon over high-top shoes. *Foot pain* may be due to retrocalcaneal bursitis, posterior tibial tendinitis, accessory tarsal navicular, calcaneal periostitis, plantar fasciitis, stress fracture of the tarsal navicular, Jones stress fracture of the 5th metatarsal, sesamoiditis, blisters, subungual hematoma, and paronychia.

RUNNING. Running problems are either due to *overuse* (chronic repetitive motion) injury exacerbated by muscle imbalance, minor skeletal deformity, or poor flexibility or to *overload* trauma from repeated poorly absorbed foot impact that ranges from 3–8 times the child's body weight. Most problems are seen as the child increases the distance or intensity of training. Minor variations (e.g., malalignment) in anatomy, which do not cause problems at rest, predispose to injury at specific sites (patellofemoral stress, overpronation). Muscle fatigue, environmental temperature, and running surface (grass versus unyielding concrete) also contribute to injuries. Prevention of injuries is possible by using good-quality running shoes without excessive sole wear, stretching, muscle-strengthening exercises, varying the running surface, cross-training (bicycling, swimming), and rest.

Iliac crest apophysitis produces pelvic pain and is probably caused by repeated microscopic stress fractures. *Stress fractures* may occur on the femoral neck, inferior pubic rami, subtrochanteric area, proximal femoral shaft, proximal tibia, fibula, navicular, metatarsal, sesamoid, and calcaneal apophysitis.

Muscle strains frequently affect the hamstrings followed by the quadriceps, adductors, soleus, and gastrocnemius muscles. *Tendinitis* involving the tendon and its sheath is commonly seen in the Achilles tendon followed by the posterior tibial, peroneal, iliopsoas, and proximal hamstring tendons. *Achilles tendinitis* develops chronically, initially may get better during a run, manifests tenderness, crepitance if acute, nodularity if chronic, and must be distinguished from a retrocalcaneal bursitis. Treatment includes temporary abstinence from running (begin cross-training), a ½-in heel lift, heelcord stretching, and nonsteroidal anti-inflammatory agents. Steroid injection is not needed.

Anterior knee pain is usually due to patellofemoral stress syndrome (runners' knee), which results from excessive dynamic, usually lateral, motion of the patellar tendon in relationship to the femoral intracondylar groove. Chondromalacia patellae may develop. Treatment includes stretching, quadriceps-strengthening exercises, and foot orthotics. *Posterior knee pain* is caused by gastrocnemius strain, whereas *posteromedial pain* is due to proximal tibial stress fractures or semimembranosus tendinitis and *lateral knee pain* may be due to iliotibial band syndrome and popliteus tendinitis. **Iliotibial band syndrome** may be a combination of a bursitis and tendinitis, owing to mechanical friction of the band (an extension of the tensor fasciae latae) and the lateral femoral epicondyle.

Shin splints is a descriptive term for pain over the anterior tibia and should be distinguished from tibial stress fractures and chronic compartment syndromes. Shin splints may be due to chronic fatigue tearing of collagenous fibers that connect muscle to bone. Bone scans may show diffuse uptake compared with the more focal area noted with stress fractures. Shin splints have diffuse areas of tibial tenderness involving bone and muscle, whereas stress fractures demonstrate point tenderness. Shin splints usually occur in new runners with overpronation. Treatment includes running on soft surfaces, shoe orthotics, nonsteroidal anti-inflammatory agents, and rest (or cross-training).

Compartment syndromes involving the anterior, lateral, deep posterior, or superficial posterior may be induced by running and produce local pain confined to the muscle (not to the bone). During exercise muscles gradually expand and if entrapped in unyielding fascia will result eventually in increased intracompartment pressure. Pain usually prevents further training, thus limiting the risk of permanent nerve damage.

Plantar fasciitis is an inflammation of the supporting structure of the longitudinal arch owing to repetitive cyclic loading with foot strike. Pain increases with running and is located on the medial aspect of the heel. Treatment is similar to that for shin splints.

SOCCER. Injuries in soccer include abrasions, contusions, muscle strains, and ligament sprains (ankle, knee) owing partly to body-to-body contact, falls, running, and the kicking or heading motion.

Hip problems include the "hip pointer" (iliac crest contusion), iliac crest apophysitis, and chronic groin pain (muscle strain, hernia, osteitis pubis). Femoral neck stress fractures, slipped femoral capital epiphysis, and avulsion fractures of the pelvis or femur may also cause hip pain.

Knee problems include injuries to the medial collateral ligament, anterior collateral ligament, and the menisci. Additional problems are similar to those in the section on running.

TENNIS. Common areas of injury in tennis include muscle and tendon problems of the elbow, shoulder, back, and abdomen. The risk for injury is increased by personal physical deficiencies (muscle imbalance, malalignment), prior injury, and poor technique. Acute injuries include ankle sprains, abdominal or leg muscle strains, and knee problems (patellofemoral syndrome, menisci); overuse injuries include tendinitis (shoulder, elbow, patellar, Achilles, plantar fascia) and apophysitis (elbow, knee, or calcis).

Shoulder tendinitis is caused by rotation cuff and biceps tendon inflammation. Subluxation of the glenohumeral joint may also be present.

Lateral tennis elbow tendinitis produces pain on backhand shots and tenderness over the extensor brevis origin. *Medial elbow tendinitis* manifests pain at the medial epicondyle with wrist flexion and forearm pronation. Medial epicondylar apophysitis is noted in young tennis players and may be associated with ulnar nerve dysfunction if there is an avulsion fracture. *Olecranon apophysitis* is similar to Osgood-Schlatter disease and manifests pain at the olecranon with elbow extension.

Wrist problems include dorsal ganglion, radiocarpal joint capsular (impingement) synovitis, and degenerative attrition (tears) of the triangular fibrocartilage.

Basic treatment includes rest, nonsteroidal anti-inflammatory agents, ice, compression (acute phase), rehabilitation, learning proper mechanics, protective counterforce bracing (elbow, wrist), strengthening exercises, and gradual return to tennis. Surgery is rarely needed but is indicated for rotator cuff tendinitis (subluxation), patellofemoral or meniscal injury, and capitellar osteochondritis.

SKIING. Injuries are related to falls (contusion, lacerations) and ski-specific mechanisms. Overall injuries have declined owing partly to better equipment (boots, bindings, poles) and slope conditions.

Thumb injuries resulting from falls with the thumb in abduction and hyperextension produce a sprain of the ulnar collateral ligament (skier thumb). Complete tears with a 45-degree joint opening require surgical intervention, whereas smaller degrees may be treated with a thumb spica cast for 4 wk. A Salter Harris type III fracture may also be present, and if the epiphyseal fracture is displaced it requires open reduction and internal fixation (see Sec. 24.25).

Lower extremity injuries include ankle sprains (less common in good boots), fractures (often spiral) of the tibia ("boot top") and ankle, and ACL sprains with or without tibial eminence fracture. Hemarthrosis is present in severe ACL sprain. Treatment of ACL sprains includes bracing, intra-articular reconstruction, and closed or open anatomic reduction of a tibial eminence fracture fragment.

LYNN T. STAHELI

GENERAL

Asher MA: Screening for congenital dislocation of the hip, scoliosis, and other abnormalities affecting the musculoskeletal system. Pediatr Clin North Am 33:1335, 1986.
Choban S, Killian J: Evaluation of acute gait abnormalities in preschool children. J Pediatr Orthop 10:74, 1990.
Conway JJ: Radionuclide bone scintigraphy in pediatric orthopedics. Pediatr Clin North Am 33:1313, 1986.
Dunne KB, Sterling KC: The origin of prenatal and postnatal deformities. Pediatr Clin North Am 33:1277, 1986.
Hensinger RN: Limp. Pediatr Clin North Am 33:1355, 1986.
Peterson H: Growing pains. Pediatr Clin North Am 33:1365, 1986.
Shapiro F: Epiphyseal disorders. N Engl J Med 317:1702, 1987.
Staheli LT: Philosophy of care. Pediatr Clin North Am 33:1269, 1986.
Tachdjian M: Pediatric Orthopedics, 2nd ed. Philadelphia, WB Saunders, 1990.
Wilkinson R: Imaging. Pediatr Clin North Am 33:1299, 1986.

FOOT-TOES

Bensahel H, Catterall A, Dimeglio A: Practical applications in idiopathic clubfoot: A retrospective multicentric study in EPOS. J Pediatr Orthop 10:186, 1990.
Berg EE: A reappraisal of metatarsus adductus and skew foot. J Bone Joint Surg 68A:1185, 1986.
Gross RF: Foot pain in children. Pediatr Clin North Am 33:1395, 1986.
Hamanishi C: Congenital vertical talus: Classification with 69 cases in a new measurement system. J Pediatr Orthop 4:318, 1984.
Phelps DA, Grogan DP: Polydactyly of the foot. J Pediatr Orthop 5:446, 1985.
Scranton PE Jr, Zuckerman JD: Bunion surgery in adolescence: Results of surgical treatment. J Pediatr Orthop 4:39, 1984.
Smith M: Flat feet in children. Br Med J 300:942, 1990.
Swiontkowski MF, Scranton PE, Hansen F: Tarsal coalition—long-term results of surgical treatment. J Pediatr Orthop 3:287, 1983.
Wenger DR, Leach J: Foot deformities in infants and children. Pediatr Clin North Am 33:1411, 1986.
Wenger DR, Mauldin D, Speck G, et al: Corrective shoes and inserts as treatment for flexible flatfoot in infants and children. J Bone Joint Surg 71A:800, 1989.

KNEE-LEG

Dinham JM: Popliteal cysts in children: The case against surgery. J Bone Joint Surg 57B:69, 1975.
Hensinger RN (ed): The pediatric lower extremity. Ortho Clin North Am Vol 18, 1987.
Kalamchi A, Cowell HR, Kim KI: Congenital deficiency in the femur. J Pediatr Orthop 5:129, 1985.
Krause BL, Williams JPR, Catterall A: Natural history of Osgood-Schlatter disease. J Pediatr Orthop 10:65, 1990.
Langenskiold A, Riska EB: Tibia vara (osteochondrosis deformans tibiae). J Bone Joint Surg 46A:1405, 1964.
Mosely CF: Leg-length discrepancy. Pediatr Clin North Am 33:1385, 1986.
Pappas AM: Congenital abnormalities of the femur and related lower extremity malformation: Classification and treatment. J Pediatr Orthop 3:45, 1983.
Salenius P, Wankka E: The development of the tibiofemoral angle in children. J Bone Joint Surg 57A:259, 1975.
Schonecker PL, Meade WC, Pierron RL, et al: Blount's disease: A retrospective review and recommendations for treatment. J Pediatr Orthop 5:181, 1985.
Smith JB: Knee problems in children. Pediatr Clin North Am 33:1439, 1986.
Staheli LT: Lower-extremity rotational problems in children: Normal values to guide management. J Bone Joint Surg 67A:39, 1985.
Staheli LT: Lower positional deformity in infants and children: A review. J Pediatr Orthop 10:559, 1990.
Staheli LT: Torsional deformity. Pediatr Clin North Am 33:1373, 1986.
Trueta J: The normal vascular anatomy of the human femoral head during growth. J Bone Joint Surg 39B:358, 1957.
Weinstein JN, Kuo KN, Millar EA: Congenital coxa vara: A retrospective review. J Pediatr Orthop 4:70, 1984.
Wenger DR, Mickelson M, Maynard JA: The evolution and histopathology of adolescent tibia vara. J Pediatr Orthop 4:78, 1984.
Wilkins KE: Bowlegs. Pediatr Clin North Am 33:1429, 1986.

HIP

Ando M, Gotoh E: Significance of inguinal folds for diagnosis of congenital dislocation of the hip in infants aged three to four months. J Pediatr Orthop 10:331, 1990.
Berman L, Klenerman L: Ultrasound screening for hip abnormalities: Preliminary findings in 1001 neonates. Br Med J 293:719, 1986.

Bialik V, Fishman J, Katzir J, et al: Clinical assessment of hip instability in the newborn by an orthopaedic surgeon and a pediatrician. J Pediatr Orthop 6:703, 1986.
Bower GD, Sprague P, Geijsel H, et al: Isotope bone scans in the assessment of children with hip pain or limp. Pediatr Radiol 15:319, 1985.
Burger BJ, Burger JD, Bos CFA, et al: Neonatal screening and staggered early treatment for congenital dislocation or dysplasia of the hip. Lancet 336:1549, 1990.
Chung SMK: Diseases of the developing hip joint. Pediatr Clin North Am 33:1457, 1986.
Cooperman DR, Emory H, Keller C: Factors relating to hip joint arthritis following three childhood diseases—juvenile rheumatoid arthritis, Perthes disease, and post-reduction avascular necrosis in congenital hip dislocation. J Pediatr Orthop 6:706, 1986.
Dunn PM, Evans RE, Thearle MN, et al: Congenital dislocation of the hip: Early and late diagnosis and management compared. Arch Dis Child 60:407, 1985.
Gardiner HM, Dunn PM: Controlled trial of immediate splinting versus ultrasonographic surveillance in congenitally dislocatable hips. Lancet 336:1553, 1990.
Haggaund G, Bylander B, Hansson LI, et al: Longitudinal growth of the distal fibula in children with slipped capital femoral epiphysis. J Pediatr Orthop 6:274, 1986.
Haueisen DC, Weiner DS, Weinder SD: The characterization of "transient synovitis of the hip" in children. J Pediatr Orthop 6:11, 1986.
Henderson R, Renner J, Sturdivant M, et al: Evaluation of magnetic resonance imaging in Legg-Perthes disease: A prospective, blinded study. J Pediatr Orthop 10:289, 1990.
Ippolito E, Tudisco C, Farsetti P: Long-term prognosis of Legg-Calvé-Perthes disease developing during adolescence. J Pediatr Orthop 5:652, 1985.
Kennedy J, Weiner D: Results of slipped capital femoral epiphysis in the black population. J Pediatr Orthop 10:224, 1990.
McGoldrick F, Bourke T, Blake N, et al: Accuracy of sonography in transient synovitis. J Pediatr Orthop 10:501, 1990.
Mukherjee A, Orth D, Fabry G: Evaluation of the prognostic indices in Legg-Calvé-Perthes disease: Statistical analysis of 116 hips. J Pediatr Orthop 10:153, 1990.
Nguyen D, Morrissy R: Slipped capital femoral epiphysis: Rationale for the technique of percutaneous in situ fixation. J Pediatr Orthop 10:341, 1990.
O'Brien T, Millis MB, Griffin PP: The early identification and classification of growth disturbances of the proximal end of the femur. J Bone Joint Surg 68A:970, 1986.
Prasad V, Greig F, Bastian W, et al: Slipped capital femoral epiphysis during treatment with recombinant growth hormone for isolated, partial growth hormone deficiency. J Pediatr 116, 3:397, 1990.
Salter RB, Dubos JP: The first fifteen years' personal experience with innominate osteotomy in the treatment of congenital dislocation and subluxation of the hip. Clin Orthop 98:72, 1974.
Staheli LT: Torsional deformity. Pediatr Clin North Am 33:1373, 1986.
Stone MJ, Clarke NMP, Campbell MJ, et al: Comparison of audible sound transmission with ultrasound in screening for congenital dislocation of the hip. Lancet 336:421, 1990.
Tonnis D, Storch K, Ulbrich H: Results of newborn screening for CDH with and without sonography and correlation of risk factors. J Pediatr Orthop 10:145, 1990.
Vila-Verde VMR, Gomes-Peres JFS, Kosta BAA: Value of the head at risk concept in assessing the prognosis in Legg-Calvé-Perthes disease. J Pediatr Orthop 5:422, 1985.
Yngve D, Gross R: Late diagnosis of hip dislocation in infants. J Pediatr Orthop 10:777, 1990.

SPINE

Bradford DS, Heithoff KB, Cohen M: Intraspinal abnormalities and congenital spine deformities: A radiographic and MRI study. J Pediatr Orthop 11:35, 1991.
Bunnell WP: Spinal deformity. Pediatr Clin North Am 33:1475, 1986.
Green NE: Part-time bracing of adolescent idiopathic scoliosis. J Bone Joint Surg 68A:738, 1986.
King HA: Evaluating the child with back pain. Pediatr Clin North Am 33:1489, 1986.
Letts M, Smallman T, Afanasiev R, et al: Fracture of the pars interarticularis in adolescent athletes: A clinical-biomedical analysis. J Pediatr Orthop 6:40, 1986.
McMaster MJ, David CV: Hemivertebra as a cause of scoliosis: A study of 104 patients. J Bone Joint Surg 68B:588, 1986.
Montgomery F, Willner S, Appelgren G: Long-term follow-up of patients with adolescent idiopathic scoliosis treated conservatively: An analysis of the clinical value of progression. J Pediatr Orthop 10:48, 1990.
Morin B, Poitras B, Duhaime M, et al: Congenital kyphosis by segmentation defect: Etiologic and pathogenic studies. J Pediatr Orthop 5:309, 1985.
Warren MP, Brooks-Gunn J, Hamilton L, et al: Scoliosis and fracture in young ballet dancers: Relation to delayed menarche and secondary amenorrhea. N Engl J Med 314(21):1348, 1986.
Winter RB, Moe JH, Eilers VE: Congenital scoliosis: A study of 234 patients treated and untreated. J Bone Joint Surg 50A:25, 1968.
Winter RB, Moe JH, Wang JF: Congenital kyphosis: Its natural history and treatment as observed in a study of 130 patients. J Bone Joint Surg 55A:223, 1973.

TRAUMA

Almquist EE: Hand injuries in children. Pediatr Clin North Am 33:1511, 1986.
Bracken MB, Shepard MJ, Collins WE, et al: A randomized, controlled trial of methylprednisolone or naloxone in the treatment of acute spinal-cord injury: Results of the Second National Acute Spinal Cord Injury Study. N Engl J Med 322:1405, 1990.
Conrad EU, Rang MC: Fractures and sprains. Pediatr Clin North Am 33:1523, 1986.
Dalton HJ, Slovis T, Helfer RE, et al: Undiagnosed abuse in children younger than 3 years with femoral fracture. Am J Dis Child 144:875, 1990.
Driscoll P, Skinner D: Initial assessment and management. I: Primary survey. Br Med J 300:1265, 1990.
Driscoll P, Skinner D: Initial assessment and management. II: Secondary survey. Br Med J 300:1329, 1990.
Hernandez J Jr, Peterson HA: Fracture of the distal radial physis complicated by compartment syndrome and premature physeal closure. J Pediatr Orthop 6:627, 1986.
Hobbs CJ: ABC of child abuse: Fractures. Br Med J 298:1015, 1989.
Lally KP, Senac M, Hardin WD Jr, et al: Utility of the cervical spine radiograph in pediatric trauma. Am J Surg 158:540, 1989.
Lloyd-Thomas AR, Anderson I: Paediatric trauma: Secondary survey. Br Med J 301:433, 1990.
Mann DC, Rajmaira S: Distribution of physeal and nonphyseal fracture in 2650 long-bone fracture in children aged 0–16 years. J Pediatr Orthop 10:713, 1990.
McCarty DL, Surpure JS: Pediatric trauma: Initial evaluation and stabilization. Pediatr Ann 19:584, 1990.
Merten D, Carpenter B: Radiologic imaging of inflicted injury in the child abuse syndrome. Pediatr Clin North Am 37:815, 1990.
Roberge RJ, Wears RC, Kelly M, et al: Selective application of cervical spine radiography in alert victims of blunt trauma: A prospective study. J Trauma 28:784, 1988.
Swain A, Dove J, Baker H: Trauma of the spine and spinal cord, Vol 1. Br Med J 301:34, 1990.
Swain A, Dove J, Baker H: Trauma of the spine and spinal cord, Vol 2. Br Med J 301:110, 1990.
Willett KM, Dorrell H, Kelly P: Management of limb injuries. Br Med J 301:229, 1990.

OTHER

Garrick JG: Sports medicine. Pediatr Clin North Am 33:1451, 1986.
Garrick JG, Smith NJ: Preparticipation sports assessment. Pediatrics 66:803, 1980.
Hensinger RN: Orthopedic problems of the shoulder and neck. Pediatr Clin North Am 33:1495, 1986.
Minamitani K, Inoue A, Tetsuko O: Results of surgical treatment of muscular torticollis for patients >6 years of age. J Pediatr Orthop 10:754, 1990.
Satku K, Ganesh B: Ganglia in children. J Pediatr Orthop 5:513, 1985.
Smith R, Lipke R: Treatment of congenital deformities of the hand and forearm. N Engl J Med 300:344, 402, 1979.
Williams PF: The management of arthrogryposis. Orthop Clin North Am 9:67, 1978.

24.29 GENETIC SKELETAL DYSPLASIAS

Developmental defects affecting the skeleton, although individually rare, contribute a major portion of the burden of short stature and skeletal deformity at all ages. They include dysplasias (disorders of growth), dysostoses (malformations of the bone), idiopathic osteolyses (pathologic resorption of bone), chromosomal aberrations with skeletal malformations, and metabolic disorders affecting the skeleton.

NOMENCLATURE. The term "dwarfism" has been re-

TABLE 24–12. Skeletal Dysplasias Associated with Immune Deficiency

	McKusick No.*
Metaphyseal chondrodysplasia, McKusick type	250,250
Metaphyseal chondrodysplasia with thymolymphopenia	200,900
Metaphyseal dysplasia with severe combined immunodeficiency (adenosine deaminase deficiency)	102,700
Metaphyseal dysplasia with pancreatic insufficiency and neutropenia (Shwachman)	260,400†
Metaphyseal dysplasia with short ribs, neutropenia, and pancreatic insufficiency	260,400†

*From McKusick VA: Mendelian Inheritance in Man, 9th ed. Baltimore, Johns Hopkins University Press, 1990.
†Probably two distinct syndromes.

placed by "dysplasia." The nomenclature of the skeletal dysplasias reflects clinical, genetic, or roentgenographic features. The name may describe the skeletal region involved or some characteristic feature of the disorder, or it may be an eponym. Disorders with short stature are divided into short-trunk or short-limb conditions; the latter are divided into rhizomelic (shortening involving mainly the proximal segment of the limbs), mesomelic (shortening of the middle segments), and acromelic (shortening of the distal segments). In acromesomelic dysplasia both middle and distal segments are involved. Other names of skeletal dysplasias describe unique roentgenographic features (e.g., chondrodysplasia punctata) or the pattern of involvement of skeletal elements (e.g., epiphyseal, metaphyseal, or diaphyseal). With primary involvement of skull the prefix cranio- may be used; with significant involvement of the spine, spondylo- may be used.

DIAGNOSIS AND ASSESSMENT. Most skeletal dysplasias show disproportionate lengths of limbs and trunk. Usually, it is the limbs that are relatively short, even in conditions such as spondyloepiphyseal dysplasia congenita and metatropic dysplasia, in which, as the child grows, disproportion becomes manifestly greater in the shortened trunk than in the limbs. When the disproportion between limbs and trunk is not obvious, the disproportionately large head size may suggest dysplasia (e.g., with hypochondroplasia). Associated abnormalities aid in diagnosis. Cleft palate occurs with high frequency in Kneist dysplasia, in spondyloepiphyseal dysplasia (SED) congenita, and in Stickler arthro-ophthalmopathy; polydactyly is often associated with chondroectodermal dysplasia (Ellis-van Creveld syndrome), asphyxiating thoracic dysplasia, and other short rib–polydactyly syndromes.

In infants with the short rib–polydactyly syndromes, thanatophoric dysplasia, and lethal perinatal osteogenesis imperfecta, respiratory distress owing to a short, small thorax is largely responsible for neonatal death.

Skeletal dysplasias vary in the ages at which they become apparent. When patients present beyond the newborn period, the most frequent reason for referral is disproportionate short stature, due either to relatively short limbs or to a short trunk with kyphosis or scoliosis. Asymmetric growth of the limbs also occurs, such as in chondrodysplasia punctata (Conradi-Hünermann), hemimelic epiphyseal dysplasia (Trevor), and multiple cartilaginous exostoses. Symptoms may arise from decreased density of the skeleton, such as in osteogenesis imperfecta syndromes, or from increased density with hematologic or neurologic complications, such as in osteopetrosis.

Whatever the presentation, the approach to these disorders of skeletal development is the same. Prenatal, perinatal, and postnatal growth history should be reviewed, and the family history should be taken. Physical examination should assess the symmetry and proportions of the patient, with a search for associated skeletal or extraskeletal malformations. Measurements should include height, length of upper segment (US) and lower segment (LS), span, head circumference, and chest circumference; these measurements should be made periodically and plotted on appropriate growth charts. Specific growth charts exist for patients with achondroplasia, diastrophic dysplasia, spondyloepiphyseal dysplasia, and pseudoachondroplasia. The upper segment/lower segment (US/LS) ratio and span/length ratio may aid in diagnosis. For example, a high US/LS ratio is characteristic of short-limb dysplasias (in which span is also usually less than height), whereas a decrease in US/LS ratio is found in short-trunk conditions, such as spondyloepiphyseal dysplasia.

Roentgenographic studies are required for the diagnostic differentiation of skeletal dysplasias; serial examinations are necessary for delineation of some conditions and for assessment of complications specific to each dysplasia.

At the first consultation a full series of skeletal views is usually required. These views include AP, lateral, and Towne views of the skull, AP and lateral views of the spine, and AP views of the pelvis and extremities, with separate views of hands and feet. Lateral views of the foot are particularly helpful in identifying punctate calcification of the calcaneus and in detecting absence or hypoplasia of the calcaneus and talus in the epiphyseal dysplasias.

In certain disorders radiologic features are diagnostic; others may require serial studies and consultation. Registries of skeletal dysplasias may be helpful.

PATHOLOGIC STUDIES. Specific histologic or ultrastructural changes are found in many dysplasias, especially in the lethal neonatal disorders. When affected infants die, autopsy should be obtained whenever possible, with specimens of costochondral junction and of growth plates of iliac crest and of long bones, such as femur, tibia, or fibula, preserved for study. During life a trephine biopsy of the iliac crest or a rib biopsy may be helpful. Appropriate studies may differentiate closely related conditions, but some dysplasias show only nonspecific histopathologic changes; in such cases, pathologic examination is useful in excluding other diagnoses.

BIOCHEMICAL STUDIES. Patients with severe congenital hypophosphatasia have a distinct pattern of abnormalities (Sec. 8.47 and 24.67), and patients with lysosomal storage disease have deficiencies of specific lysosomal enzymes (Sec. 8.18). Type I collagen abnormalities can be detected in most cases of osteogenesis imperfecta. On the other hand, the underlying biochemical defect in most cases of skeletal dysplasia is unknown.

Certain skeletal dysplasias, however, are characterized by disordered immune (Table 24–12), renal (Table 24–13), neurologic, cardiovascular, ophthalmologic, or hearing and speech functions (Table 24–14). These complications should

TABLE 24–13. Skeletal Dysplasias Frequently Associated with Renal Complications

	McKusick No.*
Lethal to newborn	
Short rib–polydactyly syndrome I (Saldino-Noonan)	263,530
Short rib–polydactyly syndrome II (Majewski)	263,520
Usually nonlethal	
Asphyxiating thoracic dysplasia	208,500
Acrodysplasia with retinitis pigmentosa and nephropathy (Saldino-Mainzer)	266,920

*From McKusick VA: Mendelian Inheritance in Man, 9th ed. Baltimore, Johns Hopkins University Press, 1990.

TABLE 24–14. Skeletal Dysplasias Associated with Hearing Impairment

	McKusick No.*
Predominantly sensorineural	
Congenital	
Spondyloepiphyseal dysplasia congenita	183,900
Kneist dysplasia	156,550
Diastrophic dysplasia	222,600
Otopalatodigital syndrome	311,300
Stickler syndrome	108,300
Due to progressive 8th nerve encroachment	
Osteopetrosis	166,600
Craniodiaphyseal dysplasia	218,300
Craniometaphyseal dysplasia	123,000 and 218,400
Endosteal hyperostosis (van Buchem)	239,100
Sclerosteosis	269,500
Hyperphosphatasia	239,000
Frontometaphyseal dysplasia	305,620
Predominantly conductive	
Achondroplasia†	100,800
Hypochondroplasia‡	146,000
Osteogenesis imperfecta (A.D.)	166,200
Metaphyseal dysplasia and mental retardation	250,420

*From McKusick VA: Mendelian Inheritance in Man, 9th ed. Baltimore, Johns Hopkins University Press, 1990.
†Recurrent and chronic serous otitis media.
‡Infrequent.

be sought at the time of diagnosis and with periodic screening throughout life.

MANAGEMENT. Effective management requires (1) precise diagnosis, (2) prompt recognition of specific skeletal and nonskeletal complications, (3) appropriate orthopedic and rehabilitative care, (4) emotional support and psychosocial counseling, and (5) genetic counseling. There is no specific cure for any of these conditions. Use of growth hormone is not presently indicated for short stature owing to skeletal dysplasia. Use of androgenic hormones has limited value in most patients, but oxandrolone has been used in closely supervised situations for growth promotion in selected patients.

Orthopedic management aims at maximizing mobility and correcting deformity; if deformities in the lower limbs are left uncorrected beyond puberty, early onset of osteoarthritis may lead to mechanically unsound joints. Recognition of spinal deformity and its early treatment with bracing or minimal surgical intervention may reduce morbidity (e.g., from scoliosis) in adult life.

The need for educational and emotional support and counseling is often intense and chronic. Several lay organizations (see references) may help to provide emotional support and an environment in which short persons can learn together to adjust to a world of taller people.

24.30 DEFECTS OF THE GROWTH OF TUBULAR BONES AND/OR SPINE

24.31 ACHONDROPLASIA

Achondroplasia, which occurs in about 1 in 25,000 births, is inherited as an autosomal dominant trait (Fig. 24–27). About 50% of cases represent new mutations. The pathogenesis is unknown. Disordered growth mainly involves a reduced rate of qualitatively normal endochondral bone formation and a marked disturbance in craniofacial growth.

CLINICAL MANIFESTATIONS. Rhizomelic shortening of the limbs can be recognized at birth, when most achondroplastic infants will already have large head size, frontal bossing, depression of the nasal bridge, and short stature. The limbs are covered with fatty folds of skin in infancy and early childhood. The hands are short and broad, with an appearance resembling a trident consisting of the thumb, the 2nd and 3rd digits, and the 4th and 5th digits, a wedge-shaped gap separating the 3rd and 4th fingers. The trident appearance is usually lost in late childhood or adolescence, the hand remaining short and broad. The elbows may be limited in extension and pronation. A lumbar gibbus is common in infancy, but after the 1st year this almost always disappears and is replaced frequently by a straight back, invariably with a prominent lumbar lordosis.

Achondroplastic infants are often hypotonic with delayed motor development. Normal neuromuscular tone is usually gained by 2–3 yr of age. Joint laxity, particularly in the interphalangeal joints, may persist throughout childhood. In the absence of hydrocephalus, mental and motor development are usually normal. A Denver developmental profile has been compiled for monitoring developmental progress in achondroplasia.

The head is large throughout life, with prominent frontal bossing, hypoplasia of the maxilla, and relative mandibular prognathism. The mean head circumference in achondroplasia follows a growth curve above the 97th percentile for normal individuals. Specific growth curves for achondroplasia have been developed, which are particularly valuable in monitoring the rapid growth in head size in infancy since hydrocephalus may complicate achondroplasia.

Dental malocclusion with anterior open bite is common and should be managed by an orthodontist who is familiar with the problem of achondroplasia. High frequencies of recurrent otitis media and chronic serous otitis media are found in these children and lead to a high incidence of conductive hearing loss in adulthood if not recognized and treated in childhood. Sleep apnea owing to obstructive or central apnea should be

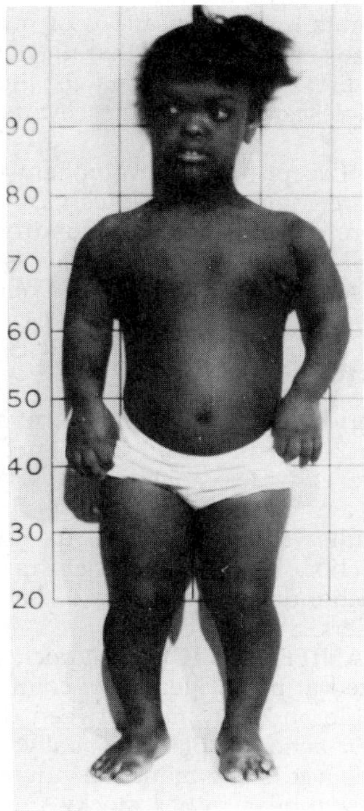

Figure 24–27. Achondroplasia demonstrating predominantly proximal (rhizomelic) limb shortening.

sought for, investigated, and treated if present. Sudden infant death is uncommon in achondroplastic infants.

ROENTGENOGRAPHIC MANIFESTATIONS. Roentgenograms show a short pelvis with broad iliac wings, horizontal acetabular roofs, and narrow, deep sacrosciatic notches. The vertebral interpedicular distance diminishes from L1 to L5, in contrast to the normal caudal widening; this is a distinctive feature of achondroplasia, although it may not be apparent in the newborn. The disk spaces are increased at the expense of the vertebral bodies, and the spinal canal is narrowed. There may be anterior tonguing and wedging of a lower thoracic or upper lumbar vertebra. There is posterior scalloping of the lumbar vertebrae; the pedicles appear short on lateral view. The base of the skull is shortened, and the foramen magnum is small and irregular. The cranium is large relative to the face, with frontal prominence and maxillary hypoplasia. The long bones are decreased in length, particularly in proximal limb segments, and appear rather wide and squat. The metaphyses have some flaring and may appear V-shaped (circumflex sign). There is relative overgrowth of the fibulas. The short tubular bones of the hands and feet are shorter and wider than normal; the shortening is greatest in the phalanges. The chest has a decreased AP diameter, with anterior cupping of the ribs.

TREATMENT. Achondroplasia may be complicated by *hydrocephalus* (see earlier and Sec. 20.15), which results from obstruction of the foramen magnum, and by lumbar cord and nerve root compression syndromes, dental malocclusion, hearing impairment from repeated otitis media, and strabismus (resulting from craniofacial dysmorphism). *Bowing of the legs* and persistent *kyphosis* may also require attention. Besides the prompt recognition and appropriate treatment of these problems, management during childhood will be concerned mainly with the social and psychologic effects of severe short stature and unusual appearance and with genetic counseling. Prompt and appropriate therapy is particularly necessary for each episode of *acute otitis media*. Hydrocephalus is not common but must be recognized as early as possible. There is some evidence that physiotherapy and bracing during childhood can ameliorate the complications of prolonged infantile kyphosis or of the severe lordosis that may aggravate lumbar stenosis in adult life. Osteotomies may be indicated just prior to or during adolescence to correct severe progressive leg bowing.

PROGNOSIS. Except for the rare patient with hydrocephalus or with severe complications of cervical or lumbar spinal cord compression, the life span in achondroplasia is normal. The mean adult height in achondroplasia is about 131.5 cm (51.8 in) in men and 125 cm (49.2 in) in women.

24.32 HYPOCHONDROPLASIA

This form of short-limbed (rhizomelic) short stature is usually recognized from 2–3 yr of age. It is distinct from achondroplasia, but there is wide variability in severity and much overlap in appearance with persons with achondroplasia. Morphologic studies of chondro-osseous tissue show qualitatively normal chondro-osseous transformation. Achondroplasia and hypochondroplasia appear to be allelic autosomal dominant disorders.

CLINICAL MANIFESTATIONS. Hypochondroplasia is not usually recognized at birth. Head size commonly falls above the 50th percentile and may fall between the normal range and the range for achondroplasia. Usually, the nasal bridge is not depressed, nor is the mandible unusually prominent. Affected persons appear rather stocky and muscular. The hands and feet are short and broad but not trident, and the legs are usually straight, but mild genu varum may develop. There may be a mild lumbar lordosis, pelvic tilt, and mild limitation of extension at the elbows, features that are always prominent in achondroplasia.

ROENTGENOGRAPHIC MANIFESTATIONS. These resemble those in achondroplasia but may be very mild. Features include prominent deltoid tubercles, relatively short ulnae with prominent radial styloids, relatively long fibulas, and narrowing or constancy of the interpedicular distance between L1 and L5.

COMPLICATIONS. Hypochondroplasia causes little morbidity apart from short stature.

TREATMENT. The condition may require orthopedic management of problems such as leg bowing or lumbar spinal cord claudication.

24.33 THANATOPHORIC DYSPLASIA

Thanatophoric dysplasia is probably the most frequent lethal congenital skeletal dysplasia. Most cases have been sporadic. An instance of familial occurrence of thanatophoric dysplasia with clover-leaf skull deformity (Kleeblattschädel) has been reported.

Infants with thanatophoric dysplasia are shorter at birth than those with achondroplasia. They have a prominent forehead, depressed nasal bridge, and bulging eyes (Fig. 24–28). The limbs are extremely short and held extended from the body. The chest is small and pear-shaped. Affected infants are hypotonic and lack primitive reflexes. Roentgenograms show marked rhizomelic shortening of the long bones, bowing of the femora, metaphyseal flaring, marginal spicules, and cupping. The changes in lumbar vertebrae are characteristic: inverted-U-shaped appearance in the AP view and marked flattening of vertebrae with central narrowing in the lateral view. The pelvis resembles that of achondroplasia with short, flat acetabula and small sacrosciatic notches, but spicules of bone protrude from both acetabula and ischia. The cranium is large and has a constricted base and a small foramen magnum. Clover-leaf skull deformity is found in some babies with thanatophoric dysplasia, all of whom have had hydrocephalus at autopsy (Fig. 24–29).

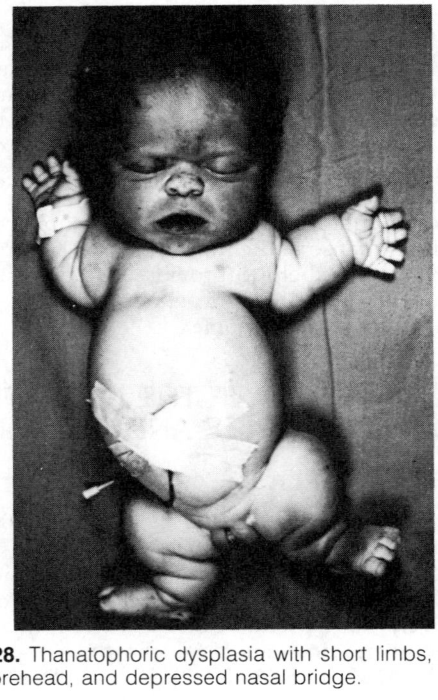

Figure 24–28. Thanatophoric dysplasia with short limbs, large head, prominent forehead, and depressed nasal bridge.

24.34 ACHONDROGENESIS I (PARENTI-FRACCARO) AND ACHONDROGENESIS II (LANGER-SALDINO)

These rare lethal autosomal recessive conditions have clinical features in common and are distinguished by roentgenographic findings. Infants with achondrogenesis I have heads that appear large relative to the trunk, and the skull is extremely soft, with multiple small bone islands palpable in a membranous calvarium. The neck is very short, and the arms are extremely short and stubby. The thorax is small and barrel-shaped rather than pear-shaped. Roentgenograms show no ossification in any vertebral body, although ossification of the pedicles and neural arches is present down to the midsacrum. The ribs are thin and may contain multiple fractures; there are usually no fractures of the long bones. The femora appear short and square with prominent bony projections at the border of the metaphyses.

Infants with achondrogenesis II have severe short limb stature, but the head is more proportionate to the body. The neck is short and hidden in skinfolds; the trunk is short, and the abdomen is distended. The roentgenographic features differ from those of achondrogenesis I or of thanatophoric dysplasia. The skull is poorly mineralized but not as defective as in achondrogenesis I. The ribs are short but relatively normal in diameter. There is often a lack of ossification of the vertebral bodies, but some infants show some ossification of the lower thoracic and upper lumbar vertebral centers. The ilia are small, with concave medial and inferior margins; ossification of the ischium and pubis is usually absent. The long bones are very short with metaphyseal flaring, spicules of ossification at both lateral and medial borders of the growth plate, and marked cupping.

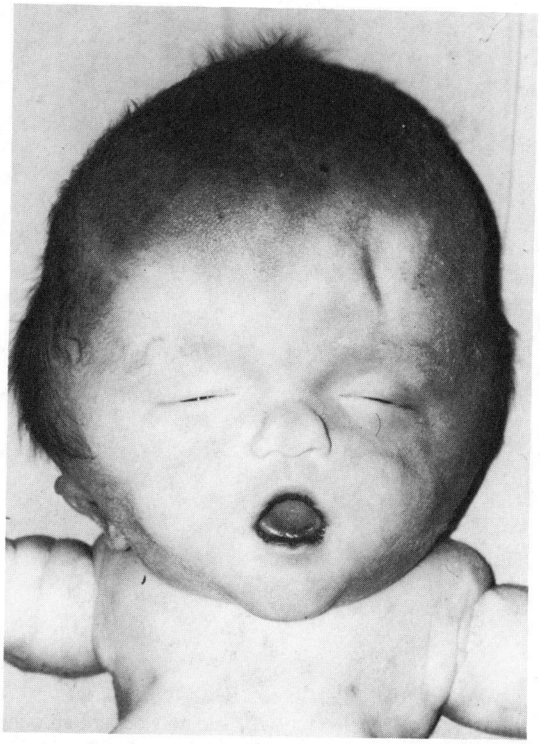

Figure 24–29. Clover-leaf skull deformity in association with thanatophoric dysplasia.

24.35 SHORT RIB–POLYDACTYLY SYNDROMES

Short rib–polydactyly (SRP) syndromes include lethal newborn skeletal dysplasias (Fig. 24–30), SRP I (Saldino-Noonan), SRP II (Majewski), and SRP III (Verma-Naumoff), and the usually nonlethal disorders, asphyxiating thoracic dysplasia (ATD) and chondroectodermal dysplasia (Ellis-van Creveld). All are inherited as autosomal recessive conditions. They have in common respiratory distress owing to pulmonary hypoplasia within a narrow dysplastic thorax with extremely short ribs. Polydactyly is almost always found in patients having short rib–polydactyly syndromes and chondroectodermal dysplasia, but not as often in those having ATD.

SRP I is characterized by relatively high frequencies of cloacal abnormalities (anal atresia, urogenital sinus) and of postaxial polydactyly, whereas *SRP II* has high frequencies of associated cleft upper lip or palate, multiple internal anomalies including hypoplastic epiglottis, cardiovascular defects, and preaxial as well as postaxial polydactyly. Roentgenographically, both show extremely short horizontal ribs. The pelvis is small and hypoplastic in SRP I, with an irregular acetabular margin, whereas in SRP II the pelvis is normal. In some cases of SRP I long bones are hypoplastic, with poor corticomedullary demarcation; other cases have longitudinal spurs at the margins of the metaphyses, with a convex central metaphysis. In SRP II long bones appear relatively normal apart from disproportionately short tibias.

In the newborn it may be difficult to distinguish between ATD and *chondroectodermal dysplasia*. Both have short limbs and polydactyly and respiratory distress owing to thoracic dysplasia. There is considerable clinical and roentgenographic variation in both. Roentgenograms may show short, horizontally oriented ribs and small pelvic bones with marked spurlike projections at the medial and lateral margins of the acetabula. Many patients survive the newborn period. Respiratory symptoms decrease with age.

In ATD, polydactyly may be absent or limited to the hands. Cardiac defects are uncommon. Many surviving patients develop a progressive renal disease that has glomerular, cystic, and interstitial elements.

Patients having *chondroectodermal dysplasia* often also have congenital cardiac anomalies (usually atrial septal defects) and ectodermal abnormalities, including hypoplastic nails, natal teeth, multiple frenula of the upper lip, cleft lip and palate, and epispadias.

Short ribs are found with other dysplasias besides the SRP syndromes (e.g., in thanatophoric dysplasia, sometimes in spondyloepiphyseal dysplasia congenita, in chondrodysplasia punctata, and in a syndrome of metaphyseal dysplasia associated with neutropenia), but polydactyly is associated with none of these conditions.

The respiratory distress of infants with SRP syndromes is not remediable. Some infants with ATD or severe chondroectodermal dysplasia who have severe respiratory distress show spontaneous improvement in respiratory function. In ATD, surgical enlargement of the thoracic cage with prolonged respirator management has permitted survival beyond the newborn period. Survivors have a high incidence of chronic renal failure leading to death in infancy.

24.36 CAMPOMELIC DYSPLASIAS

Campomelic dysplasia is characterized by short-limbed short stature and bowing or bending of the long bones, particularly in the lower limbs; pretibial skin dimples at the site of the bowing; and associated anomalies. It is inherited as an autosomal recessive trait. The majority of reported cases are in phenotypic females, some of whom have 46,XY karyotypes; cases with intersex have been reported. The relationship between sex reversal and skeletal dysplasia is not understood.

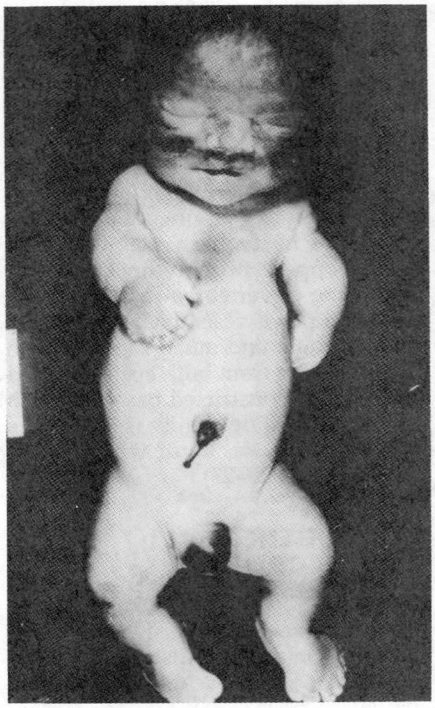

Figure 24–30. Short-rib polydactyly I (Saldino-Noonan) showing small thorax, postaxial hexadactyly in the fingers, and both preaxial and postaxial heptadactyly of the feet.

The classic finding in campomelic dysplasia is that the long bones are long and slender and usually bent at their midpoint. Cutaneous dimples may overlie the points of maximal curvature in the tibia or fibula. Severe respiratory distress usually leads to early death, presumably owing to small thoracic cage, narrow larynx, and hypoplasia of tracheal rings. Many other congenital abnormalities have been associated.

Roentgenograms show an enlarged dolichocephalic skull with narrow shallow orbits. The ribs usually number 11 and are often narrow. The cervical vertebral bodies may be hypoplastic and the lumbar interpedicular distance increased. The pelvis is usually tall, narrow, and hypoplastic.

Campomelia (bent limbs) is observed in the campomelic dysplasias, in osteogenesis imperfecta (at least four varieties), and in hypophosphatasia (dominant and recessive varieties). Bowing or angulation of the limbs is found also with other skeletal dysplasias and malformations.

24.37 CHONDRODYSPLASIA PUNCTATA
(Punctate Epiphyseal Dysplasia)

Chondrodysplasia punctata (CDP) comprises several dysplasias in which roentgenograms of the epiphyses, periarticular tissues, and growth plate zones show stippled calcification. At least three defined genetic skeletal dysplasias showing this finding have been referred to as Conradi disease, chondrodystrophia calcificans congenita, punctate epiphyseal dysplasia, stippled epiphyses, or other names. These defined syndromes include a severe autosomal recessive rhizomelic form, an autosomal dominant form (Conradi-Hünermann), and a milder X-linked form. Laryngomalacia with stippling of the laryngeal cartilages occurs in some patients who may have significant respiratory distress from upper airway obstruction during inspiration. Asymmetry of the length of the lower limbs is characteristic of the Conradi-Hünermann form. An abnormality in peroxisomal metabolism has been found in the rhizomelic type of CDP. The metabolic abnormality is similar but distinct from that in the cerebrohepatorenal syndrome (Zellweger), which also shows punctate stippling in the epiphyses.

24.38 EPIPHYSEAL DYSPLASIAS

These are characterized by flattened, fragmented, or irregular epiphyses. The earliest feature may be delay in the development of certain epiphyses. The epiphyseal dysplasias can be divided broadly into those with spinal involvement (the spondyloepiphyseal dysplasias) and those without spinal involvement (the multiple epiphyseal or polyepiphyseal dysplasias). Many patients cannot be precisely classified.

SPONDYLOEPIPHYSEAL DYSPLASIAS (SED). These are characterized by flattening and irregularity of the vertebrae and delay in ossification of the vertebral bodies. These changes are not pathognomonic of SED since vertebral irregularity, including an increased incidence of Schmorl nodes, also occurs in adults with multiple epiphyseal dysplasias. Accurate diagnosis can be made only from serial roentgenographic assessments of the vertebrae at various ages. In some spondyloepiphyseal dysplasias, skeletal dysplasia is evident at birth (SED congenita); in others, short stature develops during infancy or childhood (SED tarda). SED congenita has autosomal dominant inheritance with variable expressivity; SED tarda appears in both X-linked recessive and autosomal dominant forms.

Newborn infants with **SED congenita** have rhizomelic shortening of the limbs, but these appear long relative to the trunk. Hands and feet are of normal size so that the fingers appear excessively long. Clubfeet are common. The head is also normal in size, but the neck is extremely short with limited flexion. Odontoid hypoplasia is common and may lead to atlanto-occipital dislocation with cervical cord and root compression. Exaggerated dorsal kyphosis contributes to a broad barrel chest, and scoliosis commonly develops during childhood or adolescence. Marked lumbar lordosis, often with genu valgum or varum, leads to a waddling gait. Cleft palate is common. More than 50% of patients have severe myopia predisposing to retinal detachment.

Roentgenographically, SED congenita is characterized by platyspondyly and epiphyseal dysplasia. In the newborn, ossification of the epiphyseal centers is retarded, especially at the ankles, knees, and hips. Epiphyseal ossification centers ultimately appear but are irregular, fragmented, and flattened. The proximal femoral epiphysis is severely affected; severe coxa vara results. The long bones appear shortened, especially the humerus and femur, but the hands are normal or show only minor abnormalities. In childhood the vertebrae are ovoid but later become flat and irregular with narrowed disk spaces. Odontoid hypoplasia may be found with subluxation of C1 on C2.

Some patients with SED congenita later show atypical features or have a relatively mild disorder, suggesting genetic heterogeneity.

Short stature in **SED tarda** (X-linked recessive type) is recognized from 5 to 10 yr of age, when spinal growth appears to be slowed and the shoulders assume a humped appearance. Mild to severe kyphoscoliosis may develop, and US/LS ratio is reduced. As adults, affected men have mild short stature, with short trunk, large chest capacity, and relatively normal limb length. The hands, head, and feet appear normal. During late childhood or adolescence vague back pain may occur; in early adulthood painful osteoarthritis with limited mobility of the back and hips is usually present. Symptoms may also affect the shoulders and, less commonly, the knees and ankles.

Roentgenograms in SED tarda reveal diagnostic changes in the lumbar vertebrae by childhood or adolescence. Vertebral bodies show generalized mild flattening, with a hump-shaped build-up of bones in the central and posterior portions of the superior and inferior plates. Ossification of the ring epiphyses is delayed. Disk spaces appear narrowed and may appear to be calcified, but the calcification is part of the vertebral body itself. Premature disk degeneration occurs, and osteospondylotic changes develop in early childhood. The acetabula are deep, and the femoral neck is short. Mild dysplastic changes are seen in all large joints, especially the hips.

Differential Diagnosis. A dominantly inherited form of SED tarda has variable onset of manifestations after infancy, with distinctive roentgenographic features. Several conditions having metaphyseal as well as epiphyseal changes are called spondyloepimetaphyseal dysplasia or spondylometepiphyseal dysplasia, depending on the relative severity of metaphyseal or epiphyseal lesions (Fig. 24–31). *Stickler syndrome* (hereditary arthro-ophthalmopathy) is characterized by tall stature, myopia, and premature osteoarthritis. In the *Schwartz-Jampel* syndrome (myotonic chondrodysplasia) myotonia is associated with skeletal abnormalities. *Kneist dysplasia* is described below. Heterogeneity is marked among the spondyloepiphyseal dysplasias, many patients being unclassifiable.

KNEIST DYSPLASIA. In this autosomal dominant condition there is a marked delay in epiphyseal ossification at the hips, short-trunk short stature, progressive kyphoscoliosis, and progressive joint limitation. The joint deformity and limitation are most marked at the knee and the small joints of the hands. The face is round and flat. Myopia and cleft palate are common. Roentgenographic features include coronal clefts in the vertebrae, hypoplastic iliac bones having wide and irregular acetabular margins, dysplastic femoral heads that are very delayed in appearance, and short, thin tubular bones having flared metaphyses. Epiphyseal ossification is irregular and punctate, and a peculiar stippling occurs at the epiphyses and adjacent metaphyses as the patient becomes older.

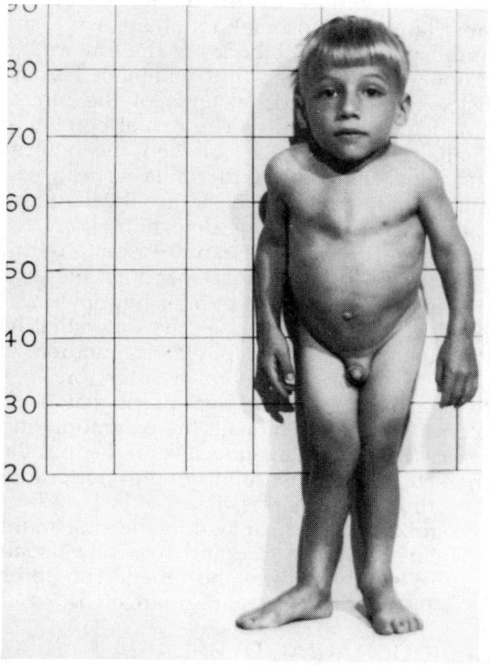

Figure 24–31. Spondylometepiphyseal dysplasia showing predominant shortening of the trunk characteristic of the spondylodysplasias.

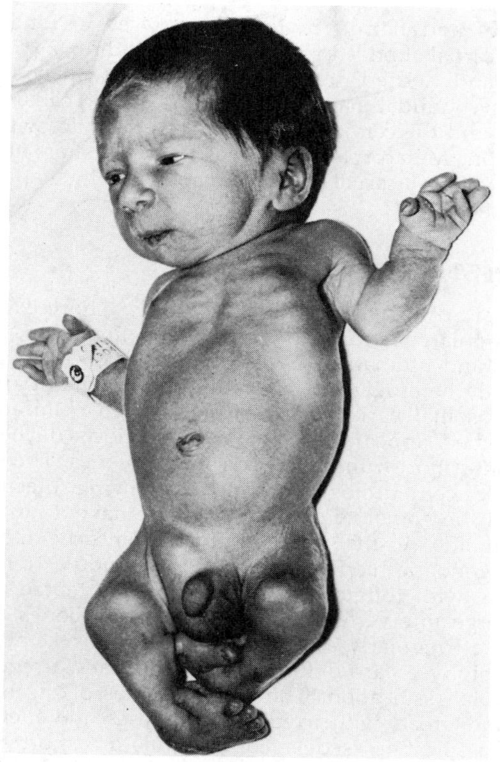

Figure 24–32. Diastrophic dysplasia showing fixed deformities of the knees and elbows, and hitchhiker thumbs (and halluces).

Kneist syndrome must be differentiated both from *Rolland-Desbuquois syndrome*, an autosomal recessive condition having many features in common with Kneist dysplasia but showing more severe vertebral segmentation defects, and from *dyssegmental dysplasia*, a lethal skeletal dysplasia of newborns that shows similar yet more severe vertebral malsegmentation and occipital encephalocele.

24.39 DIASTROPHIC DYSPLASIA

In this autosomal recessive disorder the dysplastic changes occur in auricular, tracheal, articular, and ligamentous tissues as well as in chondro-osseous tissues. Affected persons have short-limb (rhizomelic) short stature, severe clubfeet, joint contractures, and deformity of the hands with a proximally placed hypermobile (hitchhiker) thumb (Fig. 24–32). In about 85% of children the pinnae of the ears become acutely inflamed and swollen during the first 2–5 wk of life and remain thickened, firm, and irregular (cauliflower ear). With time, the ear lesions calcify and may ossify. The palate is broad and high arched; cleft palate occurs in approximately 25% of cases. Laryngomalacia may lead to respiratory distress. Midline frontal hemangiomas are common. The hips are normal at birth, but hip and knee dislocations frequently develop on weight bearing. Both stiff joints and loose joints may occur in the same patient, with subluxations and dislocations as well as contractures. Progressive scoliosis may develop during the 1st year of life. Kyphosis may begin at adolescence and lead to respiratory difficulty in adults. The head and skull are normal. Some cases involving milder features of diastrophic dysplasia have been termed "diastrophic variant."

Roentgenographic manifestations include hypoplasia of the

epiphyses and flaring of the metaphyses in long tubular bones, carpal bone irregularities (including extra carpal bones), and twisted or fused metatarsals with equinovarus deformity. Caudal narrowing of the spinal canal may be present, and the cervical spine may be kyphotic, with C2–C3 dislocation. Metacarpals and phalanges are short and wide, and the 1st metacarpal is oval or triangular in shape and set low on the carpus.

24.40 METATROPIC DYSPLASIA

Metatropic dysplasia is characterized by short extremities, bulbous enlargement of the joints, joint limitation, and progressive and ultimately severe kyphoscoliosis. It is probably genetically heterogeneous, having both dominant and recessive autosomal varieties. At birth, affected children have a short-limbed appearance, but kyphoscoliosis develops rapidly, and a short-trunk appearance supervenes. The kyphosis may produce neurologic complications owing to acute angulation of the spinal cord. Some patients have a peculiar tail-like skinfold over the sacrum. Some patients die in infancy.

Roentgenographic findings at birth include extreme platyspondyly with tongue-like flattening of vertebrae and relatively large intervertebral spaces. The long bones are short and have irregularly expanded metaphyses resembling barbells. Epiphyses are deformed, flattened and irregular, and delayed in ossification. The tubular bones of the hands are short and broad with irregular epiphyses and metaphyses. Carpal ossification is delayed. The ribs are short and have flared and cupped costochondral junctions. Marked flaring of the iliac crests produces a "battle-axe" (halberd) appearance.

The kyphoscoliosis requires bracing and surgical treatment at an early stage to prevent progression to severe disability.

24.41 MESOMELIC DYSPLASIAS

This heterogeneous group of skeletal dysplasias is characterized predominantly by shortening in the mesomelic segments

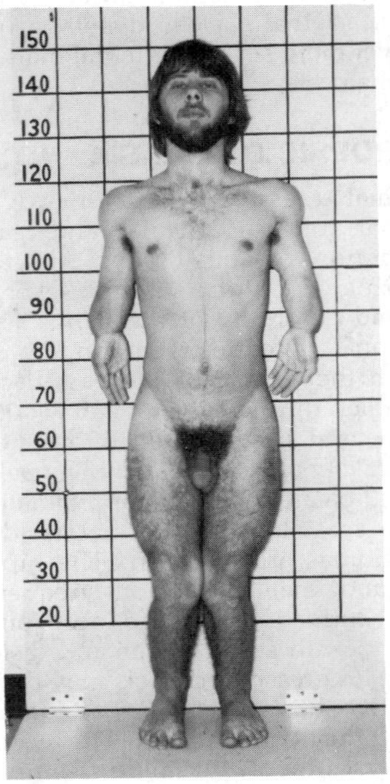

Figure 24–33. Mesomelic dysplasia with predominantly middle (mesomelic) limb shortening.

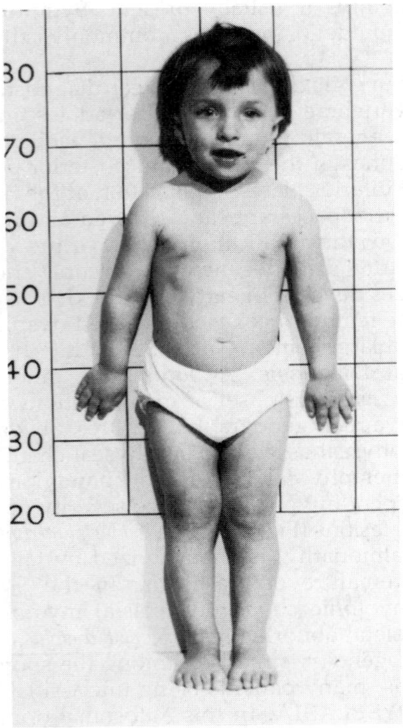

Figure 24–34. Peripheral dysostosis with disproportionate (acromelic) shortening of the fingers.

of the limbs (Fig. 24–33). Modes of inheritance vary. Five syndromes manifest at birth are clearly delineated: the Nievergelt, Langer, Robinow, Rheinhardt, and Werner mesomelic dysplasias. The most common mesomelic dysplasia, dyschondrosteosis, is not manifest until late childhood. A number of other conditions with mesomelia, short stature, and other congenital abnormalities do not fit into these categories.

Dyschondrosteosis (Léri-Weill syndrome) results in mild mesomelic short stature with Madelung deformity at the wrist (Sec. 24.24). Inheritance is autosomal dominant, with variable penetrance and expression. The bones of the forearm and leg are disproportionately shortened and widened. Hypoplasia and dorsal dislocation of the distal ends of the ulnae result in bilateral Madelung deformity. The carpal bones are wedged into a small triangular space between the deformed distal radius and ulna. The tibia and fibula appear widened. In some family members of normal stature the diagnosis is made solely on the basis of Madelung deformity.

Robinow mesomelic dysplasia is an autosomal dominant condition recognizable by the flat facial profile, mesomelic shortening, and high frequency of genital hypoplasia. The distal ulna is hypoplastic; in some cases there is radial head dislocation. Prominent forehead, hypoplastic mandible and hypertelorism, down-slanting palpebral fissures, and a short, flat nose are characteristic. Genital hypoplasia may occur, with or without cryptorchidism. The nails are commonly hypoplastic.

Acromesomelic dysplasias include several distinct skeletal dysplasias characterized by disproportionate shortening, predominantly affecting the forearms, hands, feet, and legs, which can be recognized at birth or within the first months of life (Fig. 24–34). In these the face and head are usually normal and the trunk is only slightly shortened. The epiphyses and metaphyses of the long bones are unaffected.

24.42 CLEIDOCRANIAL DYSPLASIA

The disorder is characterized by varying degrees of hypoplasia of membranous bones. Inheritance is autosomal dominant, with variable expressivity. Hypoplasia of the anterior ends of the clavicles and sacral rami, delayed closure of the anterior fontanel, and multiple wormian bones are characteristic. The hypoplasia of the clavicles leads to abnormally low positioning of the shoulders, which can commonly be apposed anteriorly. Frontal bossing, joint hyperlaxity leading to genu valgum, and dental anomalies are common. The primary dentition appears late and is frequently incomplete. The secondary dentition is similarly delayed and frequently malaligned, malformed, or hypoplastic. Proportionate short stature may occur.

Roentgenographically, there are variable degrees of hypoplasia of clavicles and scapulas, marked delay in ossification of the pubis and ischiopubic segments, and widening of the symphysis pubis in childhood. Normalization of skeletal elements occurs with age, and some affected adults have normal clavicles.

24.43 LARSEN SYNDROME

This is a genetically heterogeneous group of disorders characterized by marked hyperlaxity and multiple dislocations, especially of the hips, knees, and elbows. Skin hyperlaxity and dermatorrhexis are not features. Autosomal dominant and, rarely, autosomal recessive transmissions occur. Affected patients characteristically have a prominent forehead, low nasal bridge, hypertelorism, a flattened face, disproportionate short stature, and, in approximately 50% of cases, cleft uvula or palate.

Roentgenographically, joint dislocations with secondary epiphyseal deformities are seen. Supernumerary carpal and tarsal ossification centers develop, and the 1st–4th metacarpals are short and broad. There may be premature fusion of the epiphysis and shaft of the 1st distal phalanx.

Larsen syndrome must be distinguished from Ehlers-Danlos syndrome, types III (benign hypermobility) and VII (arthrochalasis multiplex congenita), in which associated skeletal abnormalities and craniofacial disproportion are not present. Multiple joint dislocations occur also in the otopalatodigital syndrome.

24.44 OTOPALATODIGITAL SYNDROME

This disorder is characterized by a distinct facies, abnormalities of the hands and feet, proportionate short stature, and, sometimes, mental retardation. Inheritance is X-linked dominant, with complete expression in males and milder features in carrier females. The facies has prominent supraorbital ridges, a broad nasal root, flattening of the midface, and a small jaw. The thumbs and distal segments of the other fingers are short and broad. Dislocation of the radial heads or hips may be present. Midline cleft palate and conductive deafness are commonly associated.

24.45 METAPHYSEAL DYSPLASIAS

The metaphyseal dysplasias (formerly called *metaphyseal dysostoses*) are a heterogeneous group of disorders predominantly involving the metaphyses, with relatively normal epiphyses and spine. They should always be considered in the differential diagnosis of vitamin D resistant rickets. Four principal types are the Jansen type (autosomal dominant), the Schmidt type (autosomal dominant), the Spahr type (autosomal recessive), and the McKusick type (autosomal recessive), which is also called cartilage-hair hypoplasia.

The *Jansen type* produces the most severe short stature (adult height about 125 cm) and can be recognized in the newborn period or early infancy by the predominantly rhizomelic short stature, severe bowing of the legs, and mandibular hypoplasia. Joints are large, with contractures, and because the legs are more severely affected than the arms, the arms appear to hang down around the knees. Roentgenographically, all metaphyses, including those of hands and feet, are severely involved, appearing markedly enlarged, wide, irregular, and cystic. Epiphyses and spine appear relatively normal. The long bones are broad and short, and bowing is evident. Deafness has been associated with hyperostosis of the calvarium. Serum calcium levels are elevated in some patients. Serum alkaline phosphatase activity is slightly elevated. New mutations account for most cases.

The *Schmid type* of metaphyseal dysplasia is characterized by mild to moderate short stature (adult height of 130–160 cm), bowing of the legs, and a waddling gait. It is usually recognized when the infant commences walking. Enlarged wrists and flaring of the rib cage are usually present. Roentgenographically, the metaphyseal changes are much less severe than those of the Jansen type. The metaphyses are flared and irregular and may be fragmented, with radiolucent streaks. Changes are most prominent in the hips, shoulders, knees, ankles, and wrists. In contrast to the McKusick variety, involvement of the femoral neck may be quite severe and result in marked coxa vara. This disorder has been frequently confused with vitamin D resistant rickets, but calcium and phosphorus metabolism appear to be normal.

The *Spahr type* is similar to the Schmid type but with autosomal recessive inheritance.

In the *McKusick type* of metaphyseal dysplasia (cartilage-hair hypoplasia) severe growth deficiency of postnatal onset, bowing deformities of the limbs, and particularly short, broad hands with loose joints are characteristic. Affected individuals also have an ectodermal dysplasia manifested by fine, light sparse hair and a light complexion. Increased susceptibility to severe viral infection, including varicella, in some patients reflects a deficiency in cellular immunity. Serum immunoglobulins may be abnormal in some families, and neutropenia may occur. Aganglionic megacolon may be associated.

Roentgenographically, cartilage-hair hypoplasia is characterized by multiple metaphyseal lesions in the long and short tubular bones, and a normal skull, spine, and epiphyses. Lesions especially involve the knees, and, in contrast to the Schmid type, the proximal femoral metaphyses are very mildly involved. The affected metaphyses are wide and irregular with sclerotic radiolucent cystic areas and linear streaks. The fibula is long relative to the tibia, producing an unstable ankle joint. Genu valgum is prominent. The ribs are short, with anterior cupping.

The *combination of metaphyseal abnormalities and immune deficiency* is found in at least three other autosomal recessive syndromes: (1) the Shwachman syndrome, in which skeletal lesions are associated with pancreatic exocrine insufficiency and chronic neutropenia; (2) metaphyseal chondrodysplasia-thymic alymphopenia syndrome; and (3) combined immunodeficiency owing to adenosine deaminase deficiency, in which growth failure with metaphyseal irregularities and flaring of the ribs may occur.

24.46 SPONDYLOMETAPHYSEAL DYSPLASIAS

In these conditions abnormalities primarily involve the vertebrae and metaphyses.

Spondylometaphyseal dysplasia (SMD) Kozlowski is an autosomal dominant condition. Growth retardation is not usually apparent until 1–2 yr of age, when short-trunk short stature and waddling gait develop. There is mild pectus carinatum, kyphoscoliosis, and precocious osteoarthritis in some patients. Affected children frequently have limb pains that are aggravated by exercise and relieved by rest; these may be misdiagnosed as "growing pains." Skeletal roentgenograms show generalized metaphyseal irregularities in the tubular bones, with normal or small and irregular epiphyses and platyspondyly. On an AP view the vertebral bodies appear flat and broad, with prominent articular facets and spinal processes contributing to an "open staircase" appearance.

SMDs other than the Kozlowski type have been described, some with other modes of inheritance.

24.47 PSEUDOACHONDROPLASIA

The pseudoachondroplasias are a group of disorders producing short-limb short stature with moderately severe reduction of trunk height and normal face. Both dominant and autosomal recessive forms have been described, although recessive inheritance is very uncommon. Growth retardation is usually not apparent until 2–3 yr of age, with considerable variability in its severity. In some patients shortening is predominantly rhizomelic; in others, shortening is predominantly mesomelic.

There is an exaggerated lumbar lordosis. Hypolaxity of the joint in the periphery may lead to valgus or varus deformities at the knees. Deformities of the legs lead to a waddling gait. The hands and feet are short and broad, ligamentous laxity permitting telescoping of the fingers similar to that seen in cartilage-hair hypoplasia. Dislocations may be troublesome, particularly at the knees. Contractures may also occur at the hips and knees, and there may be limitation of extension at the elbow. Ulnar deviation at the wrist is characteristic. The major complication is precocious osteoarthritis.

Roentgenographically, the epiphyses and metaphyses of the tubular bones are involved, with platyspondyly and irregularity of the vertebrae. The vertebrae have irregular endplates; anterior tonguing of the vertebral bodies is common in infancy.

24.48 TRICHORHINOPHALANGEAL SYNDROME

Trichorhinophalangeal (TRP) syndrome is characterized by mild disproportionate short stature involving deformities of the fingers, and a typical facies including sparse hair, pear-shaped nose, and medial accentuation of the eyebrows. Inheritance is autosomal dominant. The main roentgenographic features are numerous phalangeal cone-shaped epiphyses of the hands (PhCSEH), often associated with brachymetacarpism and brachymetatarsism. Legg-Perthes–like changes may occur occasionally in the hips. It is sometimes designated TRP type I in contradistinction to the Langer-Giedion syndrome, in which additional anomalies occur (see Sec. 24.49).

24.49 OSTEOCHONDRODYSPLASIAS WITH ANARCHIC DEVELOPMENT OF CARTILAGINOUS OR FIBROUS TISSUE

These form a group of disorders in which development of abnormally placed cartilage or fibrous elements leads to skeletal deformity during growth, with relative hyperplasia or hypoplasia of skeletal elements. Two subgroups can be distinguished according to whether the anarchic proliferation involves cartilage or fibrous tissue: those involving cartilage include dysplasia epiphysealis hemimelica, multiple cartilaginous exostoses, Langer-Giedion syndrome (multiple cartilaginous exostoses–peripheral dysplasia), multiple enchondromatosis (Ollier), enchondromatosis with hemangioma (Maffucci), and metachondromatosis. Those involving fibrous tissue include fibrous dysplasia (Jaffe-Lichtenstein), fibrous dysplasia with skin pigmentation and precocious puberty (McCune-Albright), cherubism, and neurofibromatosis.

Abnormally situated growths of osteocartilaginous tissue may be localized to the epiphyses, the metaphyses, or the diaphyses of the long bones. Dysplasia epiphysealis hemimelica or tarsomegaly affects the skeleton of only one portion of the lower extremity. Cartilage may develop within bone (i.e., as an enchondroma) or on the surface of bone, commonly at the edge of the metaphyses (i.e., as exostosis or enchondroma).

In **dysplasia epiphysealis hemimelica (Trevor disease)** there is asymmetric overgrowth of the epiphyses, tarsal centers, and, rarely, carpal centers. All cases have been sporadic, and there is a male predominance. Because there may be involvement of an entire epiphysis rather than half, the term "unilateral epiphyseal dysplasia" has been suggested as an alternative name.

This condition is usually recognized in the first years of life because of foot or knee deformity, a limp, or a painful gait. Usually, there is a medial or lateral firm swelling at the knee or tibiotarsal joint with minimal loss of length in the involved leg. Roentgenographically, fragmentation and excessive growth of the involved epiphysis are seen, which commonly involves only one part of the epiphysis. Simultaneous involvement of several epiphyses is common, especially of the foot and the knee. The talus, distal femoral, and distal tibial epiphyses are the most common sites of disease. Lesions of the upper extremities are rare.

Multiple cartilaginous exostoses (MCE) are bony projections found near the ends of the tubular bones and ribs, the vertebral bodies, the scapulas, and the iliac crest. Roentgenographically, these tumors appear to originate at the borders of metaphyses and sometimes along the shafts (diaphyses) of the long bones. They are distinct from enchondromata (chondromata), which arise within the metaphyses and sometimes the diaphyses and which appear to be expanding within the metaphyses into the epiphyses. Inheritance is autosomal dominant with high penetrance but widely variable expression. It is generally believed that the pathogenesis involves proliferation of normal cartilage at the borders of the metaphyses, along the diaphyses, or alongside the cartilaginous borders of the vertebrae and scapulas. Because regular endochondral ossification occurs within these cartilaginous tumors, the center of the tumor becomes ossified. The medullary cavity of this central ossified area may communicate with the marrow space of the shaft of the affected bone.

The tumors may undergo rapid growth during infancy but are rarely detected roentgenographically prior to 3 yr of age, when they appear as bony projections from the affected bones, which have a normal pattern of ossification. Exostoses at the ends of the long bones point away from the epiphyses. Involvement of metacarpals and phalanges frequently occurs, but the exostoses are small and rarely deform the fingers. Exostoses of the shaft of the humerus characteristically occur at the junction of the upper and middle thirds on the medial surface. The exostoses are not only unsightly but disturbing to the growth of long bones, producing deformation and sometimes compression of nerves and blood vessels. Severe deformity of the distal ulna is often associated with an asymmetric growth disturbance, dislocation of the radial head, and ulnar deviation of the hand. Involvement of the lower limbs may lead to coxa valga, genu valgum, or obliquity of the distal tibial epiphyses and limb length discrepancy. Final adult height tends to be in the normal range, but mild skeletal disproportion may occur because limb involvement (often asymmetric) is much greater than spinal involvement. Malignant degeneration may occur, but rarely, if ever, in childhood.

Surgical treatment is indicated for cosmetically deforming

lesions or those producing neurovascular complications. Wherever possible, surgery should be delayed until the end of growth because of the high chance of regression of the lesions.

MCE—peripheral dysplasia (Langer-Giedion syndrome), also known as trichorhinophalangeal syndrome type II, is characterized by predominantly acromelic or acromesomelic short stature of postnatal onset, facial appearance similar to that in the trichorhinophalangeal syndrome (see earlier), mild microcephaly of postnatal onset, and multiple cartilaginous exostoses. All reported cases have been sporadic. The characteristic facies includes large, poorly developed, laterally protruding ears, sparse scalp hair with thick eyebrows, a large bulbous nose with a thick prominent septum, a simple prominent elongated philtrum, and a relatively recessed chin. Redundant or loose skinfolds and hyperextensibility of skin and ligaments in infancy may lead to confusion with the Ehlers-Danlos syndromes.

Roentgenographically, two types of lesions are apparent: (1) multiple exostoses with all the possibilities for skeletal deformity produced by MCE alone, and (2) abnormalities in metacarpal and proximal phalanges consisting of cone-shaped epiphyses (see TRP syndrome), widening with lack of normal funnelization, and a hook-like, often asymmetric, projection of the metaphyses. Cytogenetic studies commonly show a deletion involving band 8q 24.

Enchondromata arise within bone, usually within areas of endochondral ossification. Single enchondromata of bone are not uncommon and may be incidentally detected. They may, on the other hand, produce local pain due to intramedullary expansion. *Multiple enchondromata* (Ollier disease) have widespread involvement of the skeleton, involving the hands; they are detected because of bone pain or deformity. Virtually all cases have been sporadic. Roentgenographically, the lesions may be detectable in early infancy as clear, homogeneous, oval lesions with axes parallel to the longitudinal axis of the bone.

Patients present because of growth disturbance, which may be asymmetric, leading to limp, or because of swelling of the fingers and toes in infancy. The tumors may produce visible or palpable swelling, particularly in the hands or the growing ends of the long bones; they are somewhat elastic and may limit mobility of neighboring joints. Phalangeal chondromas may lead to severe deformation of the fingers.

The effect of enchondromata on growth is usually much more serious than that of exostoses, and the prognosis is more serious than in MCE. Asymmetric growth disturbance is more severe. Involvement of distal ulna and radius may produce a severe deformation at the wrist leading to ulnar deviation of the hand. Malignant change is uncommon in childhood but has a higher frequency in adults. Pain and rapid growth in size or radiologic evidence of endosteal erosion may indicate malignant change.

Surgical intervention is indicated for lesions causing local symptoms or for growth plate deformation leading to marked limb asymmetry. Radionuclide scanning may be useful in investigating large enchondromata at risk of malignant change.

In **enchondromatosis with hemangiomatosis** *(Maffucci syndrome)* multiple enchondromata and hemangiomata of bone and overlying skin develop during childhood. The majority of affected persons are normal at birth; the lesions develop during infancy. All reported cases have been sporadic. The cutaneous lesions are usually cavernous or capillary hemangiomas, with or without lymphangiomas. Their distribution in skin appears to be independent of skeletal lesions; they may be found also in mucous membranes and intra-abdominal viscera. The skeletal lesions are typical enchondromata, involving metaphyses throughout the body; in some cases unilateral deformity predominates.

Maffucci syndrome produces a severe, cosmetically unsightly and often painful deformation of the skeleton. Neither the hemangiomata nor the enchondromata are amenable to surgical intervention except for palliation. The lesions lead to short stature or, if predominantly unilateral, to leg length discrepancy and scoliosis. The most serious complication is the development of malignancy, which has a higher incidence than malignant change in MCE. Chondrosarcomatous transformation of one or more enchondromata may occur; sarcomatous degeneration of hemangiomas and lymphangiomas has been reported.

Metachondromatosis is a condition in which typical multiple cartilaginous exostoses and multiple enchondromata are found in the same patient. Inheritance is autosomal dominant. Affected patients are normal at birth; in infancy they acquire lesions in digits and long bones. Short stature may occur, although most patients have normal stature.

24.50 ABNORMALITIES OF DENSITY OR MODELING OF THE SKELETON AND COLLAGENOUS TISSUE

This group of genetic skeletal dysplasias includes heritable conditions associated with osteoporosis (diminished or fragile bone), osteopetrosis, and hyperostosis or hyperplasia of bone producing abnormal modeling of the skull, long bones, or axial skeleton.

24.51 INHERITED OSTEOPOROSES

Osteopenia (insufficiency of bone) is a roentgenographic feature of many inherited or acquired disorders of childhood; it results from reduced production or increased breakdown of bone, or both. Osteoporosis (the clinical syndrome resulting from osteopenia) is characterized by susceptibility to fractures and particularly to crush fractures of vertebrae. Osteogenesis imperfecta is the most prevalent of the osteoporosis syndromes in childhood and is characterized by fractures and skeletal deformities. Some of the affected die in the newborn period with extreme fragility of bone and numerous fractures (osteogenesis imperfecta congenita); others manifest bone fragility in life and live a normal life span (osteogenesis imperfecta tarda). At least four genetic syndromes account for variability in osteogenesis imperfecta. Serum alkaline phosphatase activity is normal or elevated in all forms.

OSTEOGENESIS IMPERFECTA TYPE I (OI TYPE I). This is characterized by osteoporosis and excessive bone fragility, distinctly blue sclerae, and presenile conductive hearing loss in adolescents and adults. Inheritance is autosomal dominant. This most common variety of osteogenesis imperfecta has an incidence of about 1/30,000 live births.

The sclerae are generally of a deep blue-black hue. Fractures result from minimal trauma, but not all accidental trauma produces fractures. About 10% of affected infants have a few fractures at birth. Occurrence of neonatal fractures does not predict more deformity, more handicap, or a greater number of fractures than in other patients who have their first fractures after 1 yr of age. Deformities of the limbs in OI type I are largely the result of fractures, but bowing, particularly of the lower limbs, is common. Other deformities such as genu valgum and flat feet with metatarsus varus are also common. About 20% of affected adults have progressive kyphoscoliosis, which may be severe. Kyphosis alone is common in older adults but is rarely seen in children. There is usually excessive hyperlaxity of ligaments, particularly at the small joints of the hands, feet, and knees, but this feature is less marked in adults. There is usually mild short stature; body proportions depend on the relative involvement of limbs or spine. During adolescence there is a marked spontaneous reduction in the frequency of fractures.

Hearing impairment affects most patients by the 5th decade; it is rare, however, before the end of the 1st decade.

Hereditary opalescent dentin (dentinogenesis imperfecta) is observed in some families with this trait. It produces distinctively yellow (or sometimes gray-blue) transparent teeth, which are frequently prematurely eroded or broken. These teeth have short roots and constricted coronoradicular junctions. Opalescent dentin distinguishes a subgroup of patients with OI type I from a subgroup with normal teeth.

Roentgenographic studies in OI type I show generalized osteopenia, evidence of previous fractures, and normal callus formation at the site of recent fractures. Deformities are usually the result of angulation at the site of previous fractures, but bowing of the femora and tibia and fibula occurs as well as deformity in the bones of the feet, particularly metatarsus varus. Severe osteoporosis of the spine and codfish vertebrae are occasionally seen; kyphoscoliosis is not usually observed in childhood.

Studies of collagen synthesized by cultured skin fibroblasts show a reduction in type I collagen synthesis. However the collagen chains are usually structurally normal.

OSTEOGENESIS IMPERFECTA TYPE II (OI TYPE II). This lethal syndrome is characterized by low birthweight and length and typical roentgenographic findings of crumpled long bones and beaded ribs. Autosomal recessive inheritance occurs in a small proportion of cases, with the majority of instances representing fresh autosomal dominant mutations. The condition affects about 1 infant in 60,000 live births.

Approximately 50% are stillborn, and the remainder die soon after birth of respiratory insufficiency owing to a defective thoracic cage. The skull is soft, and there are multiple palpable bone islands. The face may show beaking of the nose and apparent hypotelorism, and the limbs are extremely short, bent, and deformed. The thighs are broad and fixed at right angles to the trunk (Fig. 24–35). The skin is thin and fragile and may be torn during delivery.

Roentgenograms show multiple fractures of the ribs, which

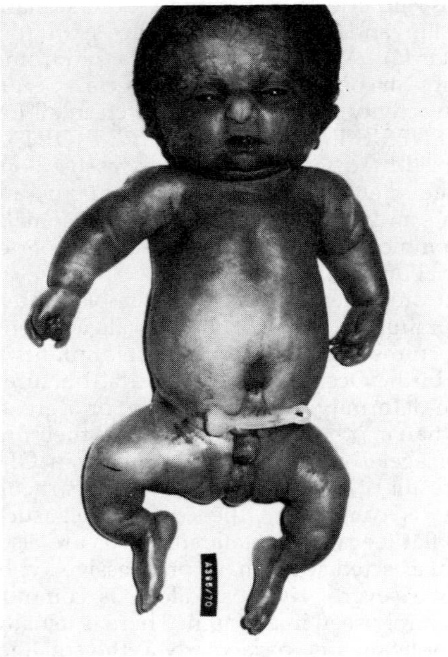

Figure 24–35. Osteogenesis imperfecta type II (lethal crumpled bone variety) with broad thighs and angulation deformities of the limbs.

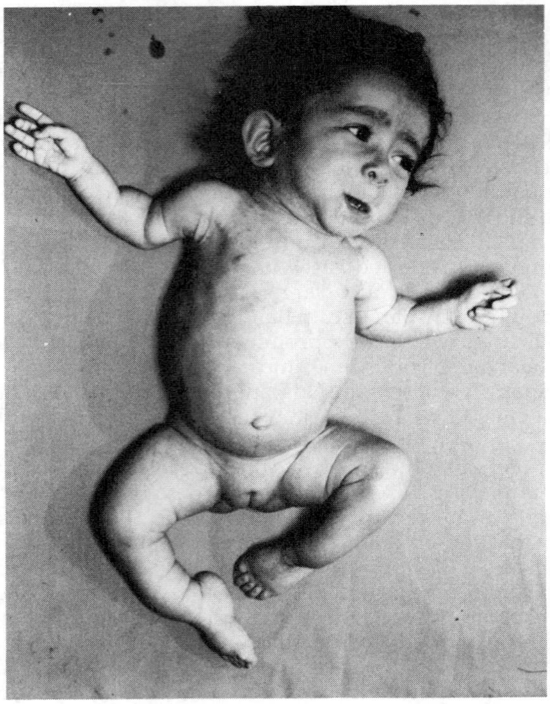

Figure 24–36. Osteogenesis imperfecta type III showing less shortening of the limbs but angulation deformities of the legs.

are often continuously beaded, and a crumpled (accordion-like) appearance of the long bones (especially the femora). There is diffuse osteopenia in the face and skull and multiple bone islands in the vault.

A number of distinct biochemical defects have been discovered predominantly in the α_1(I) chains of type I collagen that have the common effect of a marked reduction in the synthesis of type I collagen, the principal collagen of bone. These are mainly point mutations leading to substitution of an amino acid such as cysteine or arginine for glycine with disruption of triple helix formation.

OSTEOGENESIS IMPERFECTA TYPE III (OI TYPE III). This syndrome is characteristically manifested in the newborn or young infant by severe bone fragility and multiple fractures, which lead to progressive skeletal deformity (Fig. 24–36). The sclerae may be blue at birth and become less blue with age. Inheritance is autosomal recessive; clinical variability suggests genetic heterogeneity.

Very few patients with OI type III reach adult life. Infants generally have normal birthweight and often normal birth length, but the latter may be reduced by deformities of the lower limbs. Fractures are present in most cases at birth and occur frequently during childhood. Kyphoscoliosis develops during childhood and progresses into adolescence. Skull deformity is severe with temporal bulging contributing to the triangular appearance of the head. Final stature is very short. Hearing impairment has not been reported. A considerable proportion of patients succumb to cardiorespiratory complications in infancy or childhood.

Skeletal roentgenograms in OI type III show generalized osteopenia and multiple fractures, without the beading of the ribs or crumpling of long bones seen in OI type II. Osteopenia appears to be progressive, with platyspondyly and codfish vertebrae. The skull shows osteopenia and multiple wormian bones.

Collagen gene and protein biochemical studies in one case showed the α_2(I) chain of type I collagen could not be incorporated into the normal helix. Bone contained α_1(I) trimers.

OSTEOGENESIS IMPERFECTA TYPE IV (OI TYPE IV). This syndrome is characterized by osteoporosis leading to bone fragility without other features of classic OI type I. Inheritance is autosomal dominant. The sclerae in OI type IV may be bluish at birth but may become less blue as the patient matures. Hearing impairment is less common, but opalescent dentin has been observed in some families, suggesting heterogeneity within this group.

Patients with OI type IV have variable ages of onset of fractures, ranging from birth to adult life, and variable deformity of long bones and spine. Significant bowing of the lower limbs at birth may be the only feature of this syndrome, and progressive deformity of the long bones and spine has been reported without fractures. In several patients bowing has lessened with age. Like those with OI type I, patients with OI type IV show spontaneous improvement with puberty, few fractures showing up in adolescents and adults. Most patients, however, have short stature. Roentgenographically, there is generalized osteopenia. Multiple fractures may be observed at birth and occur throughout life, but these patients have less osteopenia and fewer fractures than infants with recessive varieties of osteogenesis imperfecta.

MANAGEMENT OF OSTEOGENESIS IMPERFECTA. For OI type II, no therapeutic intervention is effective. For other forms of OI careful nursing of the newborn on a firm mattress or pillows may prevent excessive fractures. Beyond the newborn period the mainstay of management is an aggressive orthopedic regimen aimed at prompt splinting of fractures and correction of deformities arising from fractures and from the progressive bowing or bending of the skeleton. Therapeutic regimens including supplements of calcium or fluoride, of vitamin C, or magnesium oxide, and calcitonin therapy have shown no clear benefit. Genetic counseling for affected families should aim at primary prevention. Reliable prenatal diagnosis is not available for all types of osteogenesis imperfecta, but some severely affected fetuses with OI type II may be confidently recognized prenatally through a combination of ultrasound, roentgenographic, and biochemical studies.

OSTEOPOROSIS WITH PSEUDOGLIOMATOUS BLINDNESS. This rare autosomal recessive syndrome is characterized by generalized osteoporosis leading to fractures and deformities of long bones and spine. Ocular pseudogliomas, which may be mistaken for retinoblastoma, develop in infancy. Mild mental retardation has been observed in several of those affected but may be unrelated.

24.52 OSTEOPETROSIS, PYKNODYSOSTOSIS, AND DYSOSTEOSCLEROSIS

These conditions are characterized by generalized increase in skeletal density. Individually, they are distinguished by their mode of inheritance, age of onset, and pattern of skeletal involvement. Several forms of **osteopetrosis** ("marble bone disease") have been described with overlapping spectra of clinical and roentgenographic features. A form with manifestations in the newborn and a progressive course leading to death at an early age is called *osteopetrosis with precocious manifestations.* A usually milder disorder with delayed manifestations is known as *osteopetrosis tarda* or *Albers-Schönberg disease.* Intermediate forms occur and include a type of osteopetrosis with renal tubular acidosis and cerebral calcification.

OSTEOPETROSIS WITH PRECOCIOUS MANIFESTATIONS. This form is most frequently discovered during the first months of life; it may appear as failure to thrive, malignant hypocalcemia, anemia with thrombocytopenia, or severe, perhaps overwhelming infection. Inheritance is generally autosomal recessive, but some cases may show autosomal dominant inheritance.

Rarely, fractures lead to medical attention. Hyperostosis may crowd the marrow cavity, with anemia and extramedullary hematopoiesis, hepatosplenomegaly, and thrombocytopenia. Anemia results from excessive hemolysis. A defect in macrophage killing of bacteria may account for recurrent and sometimes overwhelming infection. Bony encroachment on the optic foramina may lead to optic atrophy and blindness, in some cases detectable at birth. Hypocalcemia is not uncommon, and serum phosphorus may be low. Serum alkaline phosphatase activity is elevated. Roentgenographically, the diagnostic findings are a generalized increase in bone density, with defective metaphyseal modeling and a "bone in bone" appearance most marked in the vertebral bodies. Diffuse hyperostosis leads to loss of demarcation between the cortex and the medullary cavity. Irregular condensation of bone at the metaphyses may produce the appearance of parallel plates of dense bone at the ends of the long bones. The base of the skull is dense, having normal to increased density of the vault and markedly increased density in the orbital margins.

Treatment is aimed at decreasing or arresting progressive hyperostosis, correcting anemia and thrombocytopenia, and treating infections promptly and vigorously; a regimen of oral cellulose phosphate, prednisone, and low-calcium diet has been reported effective in some but not all patients. The prednisone arrests the progress of anemia and thrombocytopenia. Neurosurgical unroofing of the optic foramina is useful in selected cases. Bone marrow transplantation with appropriately HLA-matched donor marrow has been curative in several patients. Generally, the prognosis for survival is poor, and death in the first few months or years from anemia, bleeding, or overwhelming infection is not uncommon.

OSTEOPETROSIS WITH RENAL TUBULAR ACIDOSIS. This important entity is usually recognized because of failure to thrive in the 1st yr of life. Electrolyte investigation shows a metabolic acidosis. Intracerebral calcification may be found on a roentgenogram. Inheritance is autosomal recessive, and a defect in the enzyme carbonic anhydrase II can be shown in red blood cells.

OSTEOPETROSIS TARDA (ALBERS-SCHÖNBERG DISEASE). This condition presents in childhood, adolescence, or young adult life because of fractures (about 10% of patients), mild craniofacial disproportion, mild anemia, complications arising from neurologic involvement, or osteitis with osteonecrosis (usually of the mandible). Increased bone density may be discovered incidentally on a roentgenographic study made for some other problem. Most cases represent autosomal dominant inheritance, a few autosomal recessive.

Skeletal roentgenograms show generalized increase in density of cortical bone, with a club-shaped appearance of the long bones due to defective metaphyseal modeling. More than 50% of patients have longitudinal and transverse dense striations at the ends of the long bones. The vertebrae show alternating lucent and dense bands. The base of the skull is dense and thickened, but the face and vault are less affected.

Management should be directed at recognition and treatment of complications, with frequent testing of visual fields and acuity and periodic roentgenograms of the optic foramina. Transfusion may be required for anemia, and splenectomy may be useful in some patients.

PYKNODYSOSTOSIS. This autosomal recessive disorder is characterized by postnatal onset of short-limbed short stature and generalized hyperostosis. A disproportionately large skull, frontal and occipital bossing, and a wide anterior fontanelle may bring the patient to the physician's attention. The hands and feet are short and broad, and the nails may be deformed and brittle. The sclerae are often blue; this evidence combined with a tendency to fractures may lead to confusion with osteogenesis imperfecta.

Roentgenographically, there is a generalized increase in bone density without metaphyseal striation. The distal phalanges are characteristically hypoplastic or aplastic. The skull has wide sutures and wormian bones; the face has a small mandible with an obtuse mandibular angle.

DYSOSTEOSCLEROSIS. This rare autosomal recessive disorder is characterized by generalized increase in bone density and short stature of postnatal onset. Dysosteosclerosis differs from osteopetrosis and pyknodysostosis in showing platyspondyly with superior and inferior irregularity of vertebral ossification. Developmental defects of the teeth are common, with delayed eruption of primary dentition, severe hypodontia, and early loss of the teeth. Secondary dentition may fail to erupt. Other complications (fractures, visual and hearing loss, and recurrent infections of mandible and paranasal sinuses) are similar to those of osteopetrosis.

24.53 OSTEOPOIKILOSIS, OSTEOPATHIA STRIATA, AND MELORHEOSTOSIS

These three conditions are usually asymptomatic and encountered incidentally through roentgenographic studies. Some patients have several types of lesions.

In *osteopoikilosis,* numerous small osteodense round or oval foci are seen in the skeleton, most commonly in the epiphyses and carpal and tarsal centers. Joint pain is associated in about 20% of cases, and skin lesions occur in some patients. The latter are slightly elevated whitish-yellow fibrocollagenous infiltrations (dermatofibrosis lenticularis disseminata). The incidence of keloid formation is increased. Inheritance is autosomal dominant.

In *osteopathia striata,* linear regular bands of increased density radiate from the metaphyses throughout the skeleton, with a fan-like array in the iliac wings. Inheritance is possibly autosomal dominant. The lesions should be differentiated from those of osteopetrosis, which are associated with modeling defects and transverse bands of osteodensity at the metaphyses. Osteopathia occurs with focal dermal hypoplasia (Goltz syndrome), in which linear lesions of dermal hypoplasia and herniation of the adipose tissue are associated with skeletal defects (hypoplasia or aplasia of limbs or syndactyly).

In *melorheostosis,* irregular linear osteodense lesions are seen along the axes of the tubular bones in single or multiple areas of the skeleton. No hereditary basis has been established. The osteodense lesions have been likened to wax flowing down the side of a candle. Since the pattern of lesions may follow the sensory sclerotomes, it has been suggested that melorheostosis may result from lesions of the sensory nerve supply to skeletal elements. The lesions may be associated with shortening of certain bones, with contractures of the joints or palmar and plantar fasciae, and with intermittently painful swelling of joints.

24.54 CRANIOTUBULAR REMODELING DISORDERS

A distinction has been drawn between craniotubular dysplasias, for example, craniodiaphyseal dysplasia, in which modeling abnormalities are present, and craniotubular hyperostoses, for example, endosteal hyperostosis (van Buchem), in which deformity is due to overgrowth of osseous tissue rather than to defective bone modeling. The distinction may be arbitrary since these disorders must be the result of bone resorption and bone deposition, albeit with different patterns of skeletal involvement. In all of them there is generally minimal involvement of the spine, compared with osteopetrosis, pyknodysostosis, and dysosteoclerosis.

In diaphyseal dysplasia (Camurati-Engelmann), craniodiaphyseal dysplasia, the craniometaphyseal dysplasias, frontometaphyseal dysplasia, and pachydermoperiostosis, sclerosis in the region of optic foramina may lead to visual impairment, papilledema, and optic atrophy. Sclerosis of internal acoustic formina and the middle ear may also lead to conductive or sensorineural hearing loss. Encroachment on the facial nerve foramina may lead to facial paresis and encroachment on the foramen magnum, to long tract signs, hyperreflexia, weakness, and even sudden death or paraplegia.

DIAPHYSEAL DYSPLASIA (CAMURATI-ENGELMANN). This rare disorder, also known as progressive hereditary diaphyseal dysplasia, is associated with significant neuromuscular involvement. Inheritance is autosomal dominant, having variable penetrance and expression. Signs, symptoms, and severity vary among affected individuals within the same family. Symptoms usually begin at 4–10 yr of age but have occurred as early as 3 mo of age and as late as the 6th decade. Failure to thrive or gain weight, easy tiring, and abnormal gait are common presenting manifestations. Increasing leg pain may occur. The gait is waddling, with reduced muscle mass and poor muscle tone. Flexion contractures may develop at the elbows and knees. Bowleg or knock-knees may be seen; the feet may be flat and pronated. Deep tendon reflexes may be hypoactive or hyperactive, occasionally with ankle clonus. Lumbar lordosis, scoliosis, and back pain may occur. Symptoms and signs of encroachment on cranial nerves may be present. Exophthalmos is found in more than half of those affected.

The roentgenographic features include symmetric fusiform enlargement of the diaphyses of the long bones (especially the femur), with normal epiphyses and metaphyses. Diaphyseal cortex is enlarged by accretion of mottled endosteal and periosteal new bone. The lesions are often first noted in the centers of long bones, then gradual involvement of adjacent proximal and distal bone occurs. The skull may show sclerosis of frontal areas and base. Blood chemical findings are characteristically normal. There may be loss of individual muscle fibers and replacement by adipose tissue, atrophic muscle fibers, and slightly pyknotic sarcolemmal cell nuclei, with hyalinization and decreased prominence of cross-striations.

Management should aim for maximal mobility of the patient. Orthopedic correction of deformity of the lower limbs by appropriate osteotomy may help. A symptomatic response to low-dose corticosteroid therapy has been reported.

CRANIODIAPHYSEAL DYSPLASIA. This rare disorder is characterized by massive hyperostosis and sclerosis of the skull and facial bones and by hyperostosis and defective modeling of the shafts of the tubular bones. Inheritance is autosomal recessive. The early respiratory symptoms may be due to narrowing of the nasal passages. Flattening of the nasal root may be noted at birth, and symptoms may occur as early as 3 mo of age. Progressive hyperostosis of the cranial and facial bones usually leads to prominence of nasal and adjacent maxillary bones by 1–2 yr of age. Symptoms and signs produced by encroachment on cranial foramina are marked. Affected patients are often of normal to tall stature. Serum alkaline phosphatase activity is greatly decreased or increased.

Roentgenograms show massive hyperostosis of the cranial bones, which develops rapidly during infancy and completely obscures structural detail. The spine, ribs, clavicles, and scapulas appear hypermineralized but normal in shape. The metaphyses of the long bones show loss of normal funnelization and tubulation, which causes the long bones to appear broad and undermodeled.

No medical or surgical treatment can prevent progressive hyperostosis and sclerosis or their complications. Special attention should be given to amelioration of hearing and visual impairment and to psychosocial and genetic counseling.

ENDOSTEAL HYPEROSTOSIS AND SCLEROSTEOSIS. These form a group of disorders characterized by marked accretion of osseous tissue at the endosteal (inner) surface of bone leading to narrowing of the medullary canal or obliteration of the medullary space.

A rare, dominantly inherited variety of *endosteal hyperostosis* (Worth type) is frequently associated with torus palatinus. A recessively inherited variety *(van Buchem disease)* is characterized by progressive mandibular enlargement from childhood; in adult life signs and symptoms result from sclerotic encroachment on optic and acoustic foramina. Serum alkaline phosphatase activity is markedly elevated. Roentgenographically, there is marked thickening of the skull, from base to vault, and increased density of the mandible after puberty. Cortices of tubular bones show increased density, with narrowing of the marrow cavity.

Sclerosteosis, an autosomal recessive trait, is clinically and roentgenographically almost indistinguishable from van Buchem disease, of which it may be a variant. It is differentiated by a high incidence of hyperostosis in nasal and facial bones, which produces a broad, flat nasal bridge and hypertelorism, and by minor hand malformations consisting of cutaneous syndactyly, radial deviation of the 2nd and 3rd fingers, and absent or hypoplastic nails.

TUBULAR STENOSIS (CAFFEY-KENNY). This autosomal dominant syndrome is characterized by narrowing of the medullary canal. Features include delayed closure of the anterior fontanel, tetanic seizures secondary to hypocalcemia, and myopia. Roentgenographically, the medullary cavity is reduced, often markedly, with normal or increased cortical thickness. The diploic space may be absent.

FRONTOMETAPHYSEAL DYSPLASIA. This X-linked dominant condition produces a clinically striking facial appearance: a pronounced supraorbital ridge resulting from a torus-like bony overgrowth of the supraorbital ridges of the frontal bones. Changes are more severe in males. Affected patients show hirsutism, conductive deafness, and wasting of the muscles of arms and legs and particularly of the hypothenar and interosseous muscles of the hands. The prominent supraorbital ridge extending across the entire frontal bone is associated with poor development of frontal and other paranasal sinuses and with mandibular hypoplasia. The metaphyses of all the long and short tubular bones are undermodeled.

CRANIOMETAPHYSEAL DYSPLASIAS. These conditions manifest severe progressive cranial hyperostosis and undermodeling of the metaphyses. Both autosomal dominant and recessive transmissions are reported. The time of onset of symptoms and signs shows wide variability in families with dominant inheritance; some cases are recognized in infancy. Clinically, both dominant and recessively inherited forms show progressive facial dysmorphology, consisting of broad osseous prominence of the nasal root extending across the zygoma. Difficulty in breathing owing to encroachment on the nasal passages may be recognized in early infancy. The severity of sclerotic encroachment on cranial foramina is variable.

The essential roentgenographic features are hyperostosis of the skull; of the nasal and maxillary bones, extending bilaterally across the zygoma, with failure of pneumatization of the paranasal sinuses and mastoids; and of the mandible. The long bones show flaring and decreased density of the metaphyses (Erlenmeyer flask deformity). Hyperostosis and sclerosis of the mandible are less severe than in craniodiaphyseal dysplasia.

24.55 OSTEODYSPLASTY
(Melnick-Needles)

This disorder or group of disorders is characterized by "abnormally shaped" bones. The majority of familial cases have shown autosomal dominant inheritance, but an autosomal recessive variant is reported. The age at diagnosis is variable, and affected children are usually first evaluated because of an abnormal gait and bowing of the extremities, occasionally because of dislocation of hips or delayed closure of the anterior fontanel. On the whole, these patients do not have short stature, and psychomotor development and adult height are normal. Facial appearance is somewhat typical, consisting of slight exophthalmos, protruding cheeks, a high, narrow forehead, prominent orbital rims, micrognathia, and malaligned teeth. The lower thorax is narrow. Distal segments of the thumbs are incurved.

Roentgenographically, there is uneven thickening of the cortices of the long bones, in which irregular contours and multiple constrictions produce a wavy border. The diaphyses are slightly curved and show metaphyseal modeling defects.

Coxa valga and dislocation of the hips are common. The ribs are wavy in appearance. The supra-acetabular iliac wings appear narrowed.

HYPERPHOSPHATASIA WITH OSTEOECTASIA

See Sec. 24.70.

24.56 INFANTILE CORTICAL HYPEROSTOSIS
(Caffey Disease)

This condition of unknown cause must be differentiated from hyperphosphatasia with osteoectasia (Sec. 24.70). The disorder is usually recognized in the first 3 mo of life. The course is febrile, with marked swelling of soft tissues over the face and jaws and progressive cortical thickening of long bones and flat bones. Alkaline phosphatase activity is usually mildly increased. The condition has exacerbations and remissions with spontaneous regression after several years. Corticosteroids can relieve symptoms during exacerbations.

HYPOPHOSPHATASIA

See Sec. 24.61.

DAVID O. SILLENCE

GENERAL

Akeson WH, Bornstein P, Glimcher MJ: American Academy of Orthopaedic Surgeons Symposium on Heritable Disorders of Connective Tissue. St. Louis, CV Mosby, 1982.

Beighton P: Inherited Disorders of the Skeleton. Edinburgh, Churchill Livingstone, 1978.

Beighton P, Cremin B: Sclerosing Bone Dysplasias. New York, Springer Verlag, 1980.

Beighton P, Cremin B, Fauré C, et al: International nomenclature of constitutional diseases of bone. Ann Radiol 26:457, 1983.

McKusick VA: Heritable Disorders of Connective Tissues. St. Louis, CV Mosby, 1972.

McKusick VA: Mendelian Inheritance in Man, 8th ed. Baltimore, The Johns Hopkins Press, 1988.

Monaghan BA, Kaplan FS, August CS, et al: Transient infantile osteopetrosis. J Pediatr 118:252, 1991.

Rimoin DL (ed): Skeletal dysplasias. Clin Orthop 114:2, 1976.

Rimoin DL, Horton WA: Short stature, Parts I and II. J Pediatr 92:523, 93:697, 1978.

Shohat M, Gruber HE, Pagan RA, et al: Geleophysic dysplasia: A storage disorder affecting the skin, bone, liver, heart, and trachea. J Pediatr 117:227, 1990.

Sillence DO, Lachman R, Rimoin DL: Neonatal dwarfism. Pediatr Clin North Am 25:453, 1978.

Temtamy SA, McKusick VA: The genetics of hand malformations. Birth Defects, Original Article Series 14(3), 1978.

GROWTH CHARTS

Saul RA, Stevenson RE, Curtis Rogers R, et al: Growth references from conception to adulthood. Proc Greenwood Genetic Center Suppl No 1, 1988.

RADIOLOGY

Lachman R: Radiology of pediatric syndromes. Curr Probl Pediatr 9(4):52, 1979.
Spranger JW, Langer LO, Wiedemann HR: Bone Dysplasias: An Atlas of Constitutional Disorders of Skeletal Development. Philadelphia, WB Saunders, 1974.

CHONDRO-OSSEOUS MORPHOLOGY AND BIOCHEMICAL INVESTIGATION

Cetta G, Ramirez F, Tsipouras P: Third international conference on osteogenesis imperfecta. Ann NY Acad Sci 543:1, 1988.
Horton WA (ed): Biological basis of the human chondrodysplasias. Pathol Immunopathol Res 7:1, 1988.
Sillence DO, Horton WA, Rimoin DL: Morphologic studies in skeletal dysplasias. Ann J Pathol 96:813, 1979.
Stanescu V, Stanescu R, Maroteaux P: Pathogenetic mechanisms in osteochondrodysplasias. J Bone Joint Surg 66A:817, 1984.

MANAGEMENT

Coccia PF, Krivit W, Cervenka J, et al: Successful bone-marrow transplantation for infantile malignant osteopetrosis. N Engl J Med 302:701, 1980.
Goldberg MJ: Orthopedic aspects of bone dysplasia. Orthop Clin North Am 7:445, 1976.
Kopits SE: Orthopedic complications of dwarfism. Clin Orthop Rel Research 114:153, 1979.

NONPROFESSIONAL ORGANIZATIONS OF AND FOR PATIENTS WITH SKELETAL SHORT STATURE

American Brittle Bone Society, National Headquarters, Suite LL-3, Cherry Hill Plaza, 1415 East Marlton Pike, Cherry Hill, NJ 08034.
Human Growth Foundation, 11740 East 5th Street, Tulsa, OK 74128.
Little People of America, Inc, PO Box 633, San Bruno, CA 94066.
Osteogenesis Imperfecta Foundation, Inc, PO Box 14807, Clearwater, FL 34629-4807.

TABLE 24–15. Features of Marfan Syndrome

Skeletal	**Ocular**
Arachnodactyly	Ectopia lentis*
Tall stature	Flat cornea
Dolichostenomelia	Severe myopia
Pectus excavatum/carinatum	Retinal detachment
Scoliosis	Blue sclera
Thoracic lordosis	Iridodonesis
High-arched palate	**Cutaneous**
Dental crowding	Striae atrophicae
Congenital flexion contractures	Hernias (inguinal, incisional, umbilical)
Hypermobility, ligamentous laxity	
Pes planus	**Cardiovascular**
Central Nervous System	Dilatation of aortic root*
Dural ectasia*	Aortic dissection*
Learning disability	Aortic regurgitation
Hyperactivity	Mitral valve prolapse and regurgitation*
Other	
Pneumothorax	
Apical pulmonary blebs	
Family history	

*More specific major manifestations.
Diagnosis in the absence of a positive family history requires skeletal manifestations, two other systems and one major.
Diagnosis in the presence of an affected 1st-degree relative requires involvement of two systems with preferably one major.
Exclusion of homocystinuria, isolated mitral valve prolapse, isolated cystic medial necrosis/annuloaortic ectasia (Erdheim disease), pseudoxanthoma elasticum, congenital contractural arachnodactyly, and Stickler syndrome (autosomal dominant arthro-ophthalmopathy: flat facies, myopia, spondyloepiphyseal dysplasia, deafness, adult-onset arthritis) is necessary.

24.57 MARFAN SYNDROME
(Arachnodactyly)

Marfan syndrome is an autosomal dominant (sporadic in 15–30%) disorder with complete penetrance but variable expressivity and an incidence of 1 in 10,000 people. It is diagnosed on the basis of clinical features, some of which are growth dependent. The pathogenesis was once thought to be related to defective collagen synthesis or cross-linking. In some patients, there is an abnormality of dermal microfibrils, which may be caused by defective synthesis of fibrillin (a large glycoprotein component of microfibrils). The defective gene may be on chromosome 15.

CLINICAL MANIFESTATIONS. The diagnosis of Marfan syndrome is made on the overall pattern of malformation (typically skeletal, cardiovascular, and ocular; Table 24–15); in isolation these features are nonspecific. Tallness and slimness of stature are often present at birth and persist postnatally. Diminished subcutaneous fat may suggest failure to thrive. Hypotonia and ligamentous laxity may suggest developmental delays, but cognitive performance is usually normal.

Infantile (congenital) Marfan syndrome, often confused with congenital contractural arachnodactyly, manifests as joint laxity and dislocations, arachnodactyly, flexion contractures, dolichocephaly, large floppy ears, narrow maxilla, pectus deformity, iridodonesis, micrognathia, ectopia lentis, myopia, megalocornea, mitral valve prolapse with regurgitation, and aortic root dilatation.

Most affected older individuals have a long, thin face with a narrow maxilla and dental crowding. *Ocular abnormalities* reflect the connective tissue defect and include ectopia lentis, blue sclerae, and severe myopia. Slit lamp examination as early as infancy may disclose lens dislocation, which may be congenital. Iridodonesis (iris tremor) is a helpful clinical sign; suspected cases of Marfan syndrome should have ophthalmologic evaluations that include slit lamp examinations.

A wide range of *skeletal malformations* has been reported in some patients (Fig. 24–37). The limbs are long and thin (dolichostenomelia), and the arm span is substantially greater than the body length. The distance from the pubis to the heel (lower segment) is increased and, compared with the distance from the crown to the pubis (upper segment), results in a diminished upper segment–lower segment ratio. Hand findings are nonspecific and include long, thin fingers (arachnodactyly) that are hyperextensible. The thumb may be adducted across the narrow palm (*Steinberg sign*). The *wrist sign*, in which the thumb and 5th finger appreciably overlap when encircling the thin wrist, is another feature.

Long, gracile ribs may contribute to abnormalities of the anterior thorax, such as sternal depression (pectus excavatum, "funnel chest") or prominence (pectus carinatum, "pigeon breast"). Scoliosis can be a problem among older children and adolescents.

Progressive *cardiovascular defects* contribute to the substantial morbidity of Marfan syndrome. Echocardiography has permitted the early diagnosis of patients with an increased risk of cardiac complications. As in adults, aortic root dilatation, with or without auscultatory evidence of aortic insufficiency, occurs in 80–100% of cases and may be congenital. In contrast to adults, frank aortic regurgitation is less common in children, perhaps because of the amount of distention required to cause aortic dysfunction. Mitral valve prolapse (MVP) occurs as frequently as aortic dilatation and tends to be progressive in nature in contrast to the more static lesion of idiopathic MVP. MVP is the most common cause of morbidity in children with Marfan syndrome and may manifest with arrhythmias, heart failure, thromboemboli, or endocarditis.

DIAGNOSIS. If the family history is negative, the diagnosis of the Marfan syndrome is based on clinical criteria (see Table 24–15). In general, sporadic or fresh mutation cases should

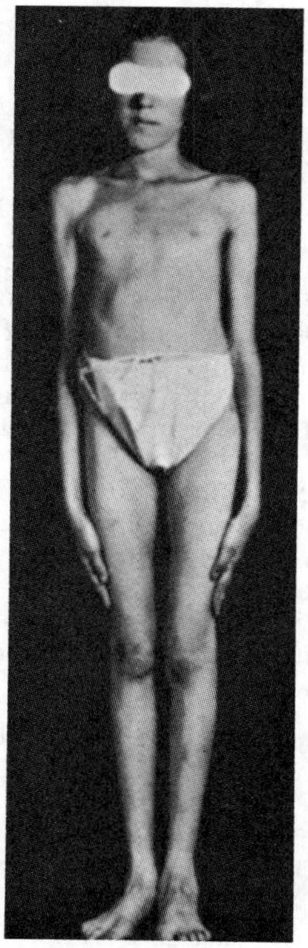

Figure 24–37. Arachnodactyly.

present with the major manifestations of this disorder, whereas in cases in which a 1st-degree relative is unequivocally affected, milder manifestations with at least one major malformation are supportive of the diagnosis. Tall stature with an abnormally low upper segment–lower segment ratio is the most consistent presenting feature. Echocardiography should demonstrate at least aortic root dilatation. Other abnormalities, such as mitral valve prolapse, mitral regurgitation, or aortic regurgitation, are supportive findings. As noted previously, a slit lamp examination is indicated in all suspected cases. The differential diagnosis is noted in Table 24–15.

TREATMENT. Therapy for Marfan syndrome focuses on prevention of complications and genetic counseling. Because of the complexity of management required by some affected individuals, periodic referral to a multidisciplinary center with experience in Marfan syndrome is advisable. For example, some centers now routinely use β-adrenergic blocking agents for possible prevention of aortic dilatation.

The pediatrician should work in concert with the pediatric subspecialists and coordinate a rational approach to expectant monitoring for potential complications. Annual evaluations for problems such as scoliosis, cardiac valvular disease, and ophthalmologic problems are imperative. Physical therapy may improve neuromuscular tone in infancy. Moderate nontraumatic physical activity should be encouraged as tolerated. However, maximal exertion should be discouraged because of the stresses that increased cardiac output places on the aorta. All affected patients should receive bacterial endocarditis prophylaxis before dental or other invasive surgical procedures. Chest pain should be considered a medical emergency and suggests acute aortic dilatation.

Optimal management of the pregnant adolescent with Marfan syndrome has not been established. However, the risk that the pregnancy will worsen cardiovascular abnormalities is of concern. Although data are lacking, it is reasonable to suggest that young women with aortic regurgitation should avoid pregnancy. Those with mild aortic dilatation should be monitored echocardiographically at regular intervals. Although β-adrenergic blockers have not been shown to be teratogenic, the prenatally exposed offspring of women with Marfan syndrome should be monitored in the neonatal period for problems such as hypotension, bradycardia, or hypoglycemia.

PROGNOSIS. Longevity with Marfan syndrome is decreased, primarily because of the increased risk of cardiovascular complications. These concerns and others can present not only medical problems but also psychologic stresses for the affected child and the parents, particularly during adolescence. Awareness of these issues and referral for support services may facilitate a positive perspective toward this condition.

GENETIC COUNSELING. The heritable nature of Marfan syndrome makes recurrence risk (genetic) counseling mandatory. Approximately 15–30% of the cases of Marfan syndrome are the first affected individuals in their families. The fathers of these sporadic cases have been on average 7–10 yr older than fathers in the general population. This paternal age effect suggests that these cases represent fresh dominant mutations with minimal recurrence risks to any future offspring of the normal parents. Children of affected individuals, however, have a 50% risk of being affected. Genetic counseling is especially important in newly diagnosed cases and in adolescence. This is best done by professionals who have expertise in the issues surrounding this chronic, debilitating disorder.

LUTHER K. ROBINSON

Arn PH, Scherer LR, Haller JA Jr, et al: Outcome of pectus excavatum in patients with Marfan syndrome and in the general population. J Pediatr 115:954, 1989.

Beighton P, dePaepe A, Danks D, et al: International nosology of heritable disorders of connective tissue, Berlin, 1986. Am J Med Genet 29:581, 1988.

Gross DM, Robinson LK, Smith LT, et al: Severe perinatal Marfan syndrome. Pediatrics 84:83, 1989.

Hollister DW, Godfrey M, Sakai LY, et al: Immunohistologic abnormalities of the microfibrillar-fiber system in the Marfan syndrome. N Engl J Med 323:152, 1990.

Kainulainen K, Pulkinen L, Savolainen A, et al: Location on chromosome 15 of the gene defect causing Marfan syndrome. N Engl J Med 323:935, 1990.

Morse RP, Rockenmacher S, Pyeritz RE, et al: Diagnosis and management of infantile Marfan syndrome. Pediatrics 86:888, 1990.

Pyeritz RE: Maternal and fetal complications of pregnancy in the Marfan syndrome. Am J Med 71:784, 1981.

Pyeritz RE, McKusick VA: The Marfan syndrome: Diagnosis and management. N Engl J Med 300:772, 1979.

Sisk HE, Zahka KG, Pyeritz RE: The Marfan syndrome in early childhood: Analysis of 15 patients diagnosed at less than 4 years of age. Am J Cardiol 52:353, 1983.

Super M: Diagnosing Marfan syndrome. Br Med J 296:1347, 1988.

Tayel S, Kurczynski TW, Levine M, et al: Marfanoid children: Etiologic heterogeneity and cardiac findings. Am J Dis Child 145:90, 1991.

Vetter U, Mayerhofer R, Lang D, et al: The Marfan syndrome—analysis of growth and cardiovascular manifestation. Eur J Pediatr 149:452, 1990.

24.58 ARTHROGRYPOSIS

Arthrogryposis multiplex congenita is a heterogeneous group of congenital disorders of unknown but probably multiple etiologies characterized by extreme stiffness and contracture of joints (usually flexion involving distal and proximal joints and the spinal column) and associated hypoplasia or absence of development of muscle, bone, and soft tissues. Although it often occurs alone, arthrogryposis may be part of a complex of multisystemic congenital anomalies or genetic and chromosomal diseases.

EPIDEMIOLOGY AND ETIOLOGY. Most cases are sporadic, occurring in about 3 of 1,000 live births, although rare cases of autosomal recessive inheritance are reported. Many of the etiologic theories postulate disorders of fetal joint mobility and include abnormalities of hormones, fetal blood supply, and mechanical restriction (e.g., bands, oligohydramnios, multiple fetuses, bicornate uterus), in utero infection, and myopathy or neuropathy.

PATHOLOGY. Thick inelastic articular capsules and atrophic muscle fibers with fibrosis and fatty infiltration are noted at autopsy. Anterior horn cell degeneration in the spinal cord has also frequently been found.

CLINICAL MANIFESTATIONS. Arthrogryposis multiplex congenita is occasionally associated with a prenatal history of reduced fetal movement, oligohydramnios, and breech presentation. It is present at birth, and, although the lesions are static, untreated deformities progress as the child grows.

The affected limbs appear cylindric with loss of the normal contours and skin creases. The skin appears thickened, and there may be dimples near joints. Structural deformities are common, including flexion contractures of knees, elbows, wrists, and other joints, dislocation of the hips and other joints, clubfoot, and scoliosis. There may be webbing across affected joints. Similar deformities occur in association with myelomeningocele, myelodysplasia, and Potter syndrome. Defects of the palate or vertebrae and absence of the sacrum and fibula may also occur. The elbows and knees may also be ankylosed in extension. Some cases of arthrogryposis are associated with diastrophic dwarfism, myotonic muscular dystrophy, various congenital myopathies, and neurogenic diseases (see Sec. 21.9). Mental retardation is relatively infrequent.

TREATMENT AND PROGNOSIS. Therapy consists of massage, passive movements, gradual correction of deformities by splints and plaster casts, and orthopedic surgery. Appropriate management plus good family support, including efforts to promote independence at an early age, result in most children functioning adequately as adults. Many remain partially dependent on others.

RICHARD E. BEHRMAN

Beckerman RC, Buchino JJ: Arthrogryposis multiplex congenita as a part of an inherited symptom complex: Two case reports and a review of the literature. Pediatrics 61:417, 1978.

Carlson WO, Speck GJ, Vicari V, et al: Arthrogryposis multiplex congenita: A long-term follow-up study. Clin Orthop 194:115, 1985.

Sarawa JM, Lernos C, Gonclaves I, et al: Arthrogryposis multiplex with renal and hepatic abnormalities in a female infant. J Pediatr 117:763, 1990.

24.59 METABOLIC BONE DISEASE

Bone is a dynamic organ capable of rapid turnover, weight bearing, and withstanding the stresses of a variety of physical activities. It is constantly being formed (modeling) and reformed (remodeling). It is the major body reservoir for calcium, phosphorus, and magnesium. Disorders that affect this organ and the process of mineralization are designated "metabolic bone diseases."

Since bone growth and turnover rates are high during childhood, many clinical features of metabolic bone diseases are more prominent in children than in adults. Recent advances in our knowledge of bone metabolism, the process of mineralization, interactions of the vitamin D–PTH–endocrine axis, and metabolism of vitamin D to active compounds have improved treatment of metabolic bone diseases.

The human skeleton consists of a protein matrix, largely comprised of a collagen-containing protein, osteoid, on which is deposited a crystalline mineral phase. Although collagen-containing osteoid comprises 90% of bone protein, other proteins are present, including osteocalcin, which contains gamma-carboxyglutamic acid. Synthesis of osteocalcin is vitamin K dependent and, in high bone turnover states, serum osteocalcin values are often elevated.

The microfibrillar matrix of osteoid permits deposition of highly organized calcium phosphate crystals, including hydroxyapatite $[C_{10}(PO_4)_6 \cdot 6H_2O]$ and octacalcium phosphate $[Ca_8(H_2PO_4)_6 \cdot 5H_2O]$, plus less oganized amorphous calcium phosphate, calcium carbonate, sodium, magnesium, and citrate. Hydroxyapatite is deep within bone matrix, whereas amorphous calcium phosphate coats the surface of newly formed or remodeled bone.

Bone growth occurs in children by the process of calcification of the cartilage cells present at the ends of bone. In accord with the prevailing extracellular fluid calcium and phosphate concentrations, mineral is deposited in those chondrocytes or cartilage cells set to undergo mineralization. The main function of the vitamin D–PTH–endocrine axis is to maintain the extracellular fluid calcium and phosphate concentrations at appropriate levels to permit mineralization.

Other hormones also appear to regulate the growth and mineralization of cartilage, including growth hormone acting through somatomedins, thyroid hormones, insulin, androgens, and estrogens during the pubertal growth spurt. By contrast, supraphysiologic concentrations of glucocorticoids impair cartilage function and bone growth.

24.60 RICKETS

See also Sec. 4.29.

Rates of bone formation are coordinated with alterations in mineral metabolism at both the intestine and kidney. Inadequate dietary intake or intestinal absorption of calcium causes a fall in serum calcium and its ionized fraction. This serves as the signal for PTH synthesis and secretion, resulting in greater bone resorption to raise serum calcium, enhanced distal tubular reabsorption of calcium, and higher rates of synthesis by the kidney of 1,25-dihydroxy vitamin D (1,25$[OH]_2$D or calcitriol), the most active metabolite of vitamin D (Fig. 24–38). Calcium homeostasis thus is controlled at the intestine, since the availability of 1,25$(OH)_2$D will ultimately determine the fraction of ingested calcium that is absorbed.

By contrast, phosphate homeostasis is regulated by the kidney, since intestinal phosphate absorption is nearly complete and since renal excretion determines the serum level. Excessive intestinal phosphate absorption causes a fall in

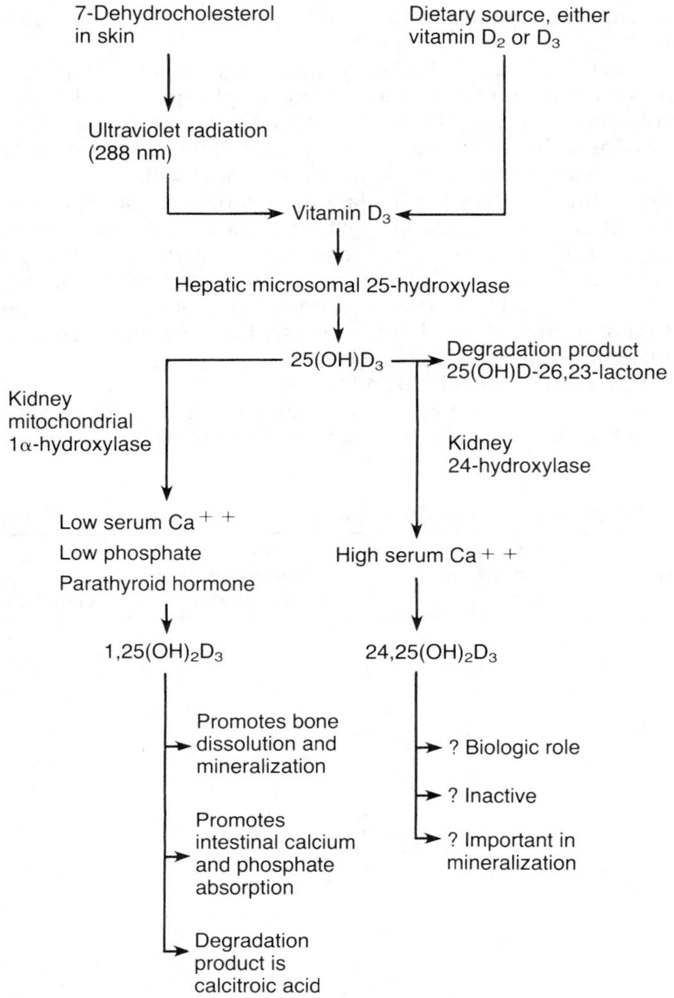

Figure 24–38. The metabolic pathway of vitamin D, indicating its conversion to the hormone $1,25(OH)_2D_3$ and to $24,25(OH)_2D_3$. Vitamin D_2 (ergosterol) of plant origin appears to undergo similar metabolic steps.

serum ionized calcium and a rise in PTH secretion, resulting in phosphaturia, thus lowering serum phosphate and permitting calcium to rise. Hypophosphatemia blocks PTH secretion and promotes renal $1,25(OH)_2D$ synthesis. This latter compound also promotes greater intestinal phosphate absorption.

An understanding of the metabolism of vitamin D is necessary to appreciate rickets (see Fig. 24–38). The skin contains 7-dehydrocholesterol, which is converted to vitamin D_3 by ultraviolet radiation; other inactive vitamin D sterols are also produced. Reduced skin exposure ultraviolet light (from smog or clothing) results in rickets (Sec. 4.29). Vitamin D_3 is then transported in the blood stream to the liver by a vitamin D binding protein (DBP); DBP binds all forms of vitamin D. The plasma concentration of free or nonbound vitamin D is much lower than the level of DBP-bound vitamin D metabolities.

Vitamin D also can enter the metabolic pathway by ingestion of dietary vitamin D_2 (ergocalciferol) or vitamin D_3 (cholecalciferol), both of which are absorbed from the intestine along with other fat-soluble vitamins because of the action of bile salts. After absorption, ingested vitamin D is transported by chylomicrons to the liver where, along with skin-derived vitamin D_3, it is converted to 25-hydroxy vitamin D (25[OH]D) by the action of an hepatic microsomal enzyme requiring oxygen, NADPH, and magnesium to hydroxylate vitamin D at the 25th carbon atom. The 25(OH)D is next transported by DBP to the kidney, where it undergoes further metabolism. 25(OH)D is the main circulating vitamin D metabolite in humans at a concentration of 20–80 ng/mL (Table 24–16). Since its synthesis is weakly regulated by feedback, its plasma level rises in summer and falls in winter. High vitamin D intake raises the plasma level of 25(OH)D to many times above normal, but the parent vitamin D itself is absorbed by adipose tissue.

In the kidney, the 25(OH)D undergoes further hydroxylation, depending on the prevailing serum concentration of calcium, phosphate, and PTH. If calcium or phosphate is reduced or PTH is elevated, the enzyme 25(OH)D-1α-hydroxylase is activated and $1,25(OH)_2D$ is formed (see Fig. 24–38). This metabolite circulates at a level that is only 0.1% of the level of 25(OH)D (see Table 24–16) and acts on the intestine to increase the active transport of calcium and stimulate phosphate absorption. Because 1α-hydroxylase is a mitochondrial enzyme that is tightly regulated by feedback, the synthesis of $1,25(OH)_2D$ declines after serum calcium or phosphate returns to normal. Excessive $1,25(OH)_2D$ is converted to an inactive metabolite. In the presence of normal or elevated serum calcium or phosphate concentrations, the renal 25(OH)D-24-hydroxylase is activated, producing 24,25-dihydroxy vitamin D ($24,25[OH]_2D$), which is a pathway for the removal of excess vitamin D, since the serum levels of $24,25(OH)_2D$ (1–5 ng/mL) become higher after ingestion of large amounts of vitamin D. Although hypervitaminosis D and production of inactive metabolites can occur after oral dosing (Sec. 4.31), extensive skin exposure to sunlight does not usually produce toxic levels of $25(OH)D_3$, suggesting natural regulation of the production of this metabolite in cutaneous tissue.

Serum $1,25(OH)_2D$ levels are higher in children than in adults, are not subject to seasonal variability, and peak in the 1st yr of life and again during the adolescent growth spurt. These values must be interpreted in light of the prevailing serum calcium, phosphate, and PTH values and also with regard to the entire vitamin D metabolite profile.

Mineral deficiency prevents the normal process of bone mineral deposition. If mineral deficiency occurs at the growth plate, growth slows and bone age is retarded—a condition called *rickets*. Poor mineralization of trabecular bone resulting in a greater proportion of unmineralized osteoid is the condition of *osteomalacia*. Rickets is found only in growing children prior to fusion of the epiphyses, whereas osteomalacia is present at all ages. All patients with rickets have osteomalacia, but not all patients with osteomalacia have rickets. These conditions should not be confused with *osteoporosis*, a condition of equal loss of bone volume and mineral, caused in childhood by glucocorticoid administration, found in Turner and Klinefelter syndromes, or as an idiopathic condition.

TABLE 24–16. Vitamin D Metabolite Values in Plasma of Normal Healthy Subjects

Metabolite	Plasma Value
Vitamin D_2	1–2 ng/mL
Vitamin D_3	1–2 ng/mL
25 $(OH)D_2$	4–10 ng/mL
25 $(OH)D_3$	12–40 ng/mL
Total 25 (OH)D	15–50 ng/mL
24, 25 $(OH)_2D$	1–4 ng/mL
1, 25 $(OH)_2D$	
—Infancy	70–100 pg/mL
—Childhood	30–50 pg/mL
—Adolescence	40–80 pg/mL
—Adulthood	20–35 pg/mL

Rickets may be classified as calcium-deficient or phosphate-deficient rickets. Because both calcium and phosphate ions comprise bone mineral, the insufficiency of either type in the extracellular fluid that bathes the mineralizing surface of bone results in rickets and osteomalacia. The two types of rickets are distinguishable by their clinical manifestations (Table 24–17).

24.61 FAMILIAL HYPOPHOSPHATEMIA

(Vitamin D Resistant Rickets, X-Linked Hypophosphatemia)

The most commonly encountered form of rickets is familial hypophosphatemia. The usual mode of inheritance is X-linked dominant, indicating that some mothers of affected children exhibit clinical evidence of disease such as bowing or short stature, whereas others manifest only fasting hypophosphatemia. Autosomal recessive and sporadic forms have also been reported.

PATHOGENESIS. Pathogenic mechanisms involve defects in the proximal tubular reabsorption of phosphate and in the conversion of 25(OH)D to $1,25(OH)_2D$. The latter defect is evidenced by low-normal serum $1,25(OH)_2D$ levels despite hypophosphatemia and by the finding that further phosphate depletion of subjects with familial hypophosphatemia does not stimulate $1,25(OH)_2D$ synthesis as it does in normal subjects. Both a renal tubular reabsorption defect and reduced $1,25(OH)_2D$ synthesis are found in an animal model of this disease. In addition, oral phosphate supplementation alone cannot completely heal bone disease; the correction of osteomalacia requires $1,25(OH)_2D$ therapy.

CLINICAL MANIFESTATIONS. Children with familial hypophosphatemia present with bowing of the lower extremities related to weight bearing at the age of walking. Tetany

TABLE 24–17. Clinical Variants of Rickets and Related Conditions

Type	Serum Calcium Level	Serum Phosphorus Level	Alkaline Phosphatase Activity	Urine Concentration of Amino Acids	Genetics
I. Calcium deficiency with secondary hyperparathyroidism (Deficiency of vitamin D; low 25 (OH)D and no stimulation of higher $1,25(OH)_2D$ values)					
1. Lack of vitamin D					
a. Lack of exposure to sunlight	N or L	L	E	E	
b. Dietary deficiency of vitamin D	N or L	L	E	E	
c. Congenital	N or L	L	E	E	
2. Malabsorption of vitamin D	N or L	L	E	E	
3. Hepatic disease	N or L	L	E	E	
4. Anticonvulsive drugs	N or L	L	E	E	
5. Renal osteodystrophy	N or L	E	E	V	
6. Vitamin D dependent type I	L	N or L	E	E	AR
II. Primary phosphate deficiency (no secondary hyperparathyroidism)					
1. Genetic primary hypophosphatemia	N	L	E	N	XD
2. Fanconi syndromes					
a. Cystinosis	N	L	E	E	AR
b. Tyrosinosis	N	L	E	E	AR
c. Lowe syndrome	N	L	E	E	XR
d. Acquired	N	L	E	E	
3. Renal tubular acidosis, type II proximal	N	L	E	N	
4. Oncogenic hypophosphatemia	N	L	E	N	
5. Phosphate deficiency or malabsorption					
a. Parenteral hyperalimentation	N	L	E	N	
b. Low phosphate intake	N	L	E	N	
III. End-organ resistance to $1,25(OH)_2D_3$					
1. Vitamin D dependent type II (several variants)	L	L or N	E	E	AR
IV. Related conditions resembling rickets					
1. Hypophosphatasia	N	N	L	Phosphoethanolamine elevated	AR
2. Metaphyseal dysostosis					
a. Jansen type	E	N	E	N	AD
b. Schmidt type	N	N	N	N	AD

N = normal; L = low; E = elevated; V = variable; X = X-linked; A = autosomal; D = dominant; R = recessive.

is not present, and the profound myopathy, rachitic rosary, and Harrison groove (pectus deformity) characteristic of calcium-deficient rickets are not evident. These children develop a waddling gait, smooth (rather than angular) bowing of the lower extremities, coxa vara, genu varus, genu valgum, and short stature. The adult height of untreated patients is 130–165 cm.

Pulp deformities and a lesion called "intraglobular dentin" are characteristic tooth abnormalities, although enamel defects are found only occasionally. By contrast, calcium-deficient rickets usually results in enamel defects. Periapical infections are found in both forms of rickets.

Roentgenographic findings include metaphyseal widening and fraying and coarse-appearing trabecular bone. Cupping of the metaphysis occurs at the proximal and distal tibia and at the distal femur, radius, and ulna.

LABORATORY FINDINGS. There is a normal or slightly reduced serum calcium level (9–9.4 mg/dL; 2.24–2.34 mM/L), a moderately reduced serum phosphate level (1.5–3 mg/dL; 0.48–0.96 mM/L), elevated alkaline phosphatase activity, and no evidence of secondary hyperparathyroidism. Urinary phosphate excretion is large, despite hypophosphatemia, indicating a defect in renal tubular phosphate reabsorption. This disorder is typical of pure phosphate-deficient rickets since aminoaciduria, glucosuria, bicarbonaturia, and kaliuria are never found. In potential obligate heterozygotes, who later develop disease, serum phosphate levels may remain normal for the first several months of life. The first laboratory abnormality is often a rise in serum alkaline phosphatase activity. The serum phosphate level probably remains normal for several months, since the glomerular filtration rate is quite low in neonates. Parathyroid hyperplasia with elevated serum PTH values is occasionally found, usually in sporadic cases.

TREATMENT. Oral phosphate supplements coupled with a vitamin D analog to offset the secondary hyperparathyroidism that may accompany an oral phosphate load is the preferred treatment. Oral phosphate is usually given every 4 hr for at least 5 times a day, since urinary excretion is constant and patients quickly become hypophosphatemic. Young children should receive 0.5–1 g/24 hr, whereas older children require 1–4 g/24 hr. Phosphate can be given as Joulie solution (dibasic sodium phosphate, 136 g/L, and phosphoric acid, 58.8 g/L), which contains 30.4 mg of phosphate/mL. Thus, a 5-mL dose given every 4 hr, 5 times daily, provides 760 mg of phosphate. Patient compliance is readily assessed because almost all of this dose is excreted in a 24-hr urine collection. The main side effect of oral phosphate therapy is diarrhea, which often improves spontaneously.

Providing a vitamin D analog is important for complete bone healing and prevention of secondary hyperparathyroidism. Classically, vitamin D_2 was used at 2,000 IU/kg/24 hr, but more recently, dihydrotachysterol at a dosage of 0.02 mg/kg/24 hr or $1,25(OH)_2D$ at 20–50 ng/kg/24 hr has been effectively used.

Familial hypophosphatemia was previously treated with 50,000–200,000 IU/24 hr (1.25–10 mg) of vitamin D_2, but this caused hypervitaminosis D with nephrocalcinosis, hypercalcemia, and permanent renal damage.

The term *vitamin D resistant rickets* was used in the past to describe rickets in which patients failed to respond to a dose of vitamin D that would cure vitamin D deficiency. If appropriate doses of vitamin D or any of its metabolites fail to heal rickets, and if serum phosphate is not reduced, metaphyseal dysplasia should be considered (Sec. 24.45).

With early diagnosis and good compliance, the bowing deformities can be minimized, and an adult height above 170 cm may be achievable. Corrective osteotomies should always be deferred until rickets appears healed roentgenographically and until the serum alkaline phosphatase level is in the normal range. Surgery prior to bone healing may be followed by redevelopment of deformity and bowing. In some patients, aggressive medical management may obviate the need for surgical intervention. Patients undergoing osteotomy should stop taking all vitamin D preparations before surgery and should not start them again until they are again ambulating to avoid immobilization hypercalcemia. Since $1,25(OH)_2D$ has such a short half-life, it can be stopped just prior to surgery, whereas vitamin D_2 should be discontinued at least 1 mo before surgery. An additional advantage of $1,25(OH)_2D$ therapy is that it augments intestinal phosphate absorption and may improve phosphate balance. However, $1,25(OH)_2D$ should not be used without concomitant oral phosphate.

Certain patients have hypophosphatemia and hyperphosphaturia but no roentgenographic evidence of rickets. This condition, inherited as an autosomal dominant disorder, has been called *hypophosphatemic bone disease*. The serum concentrations of $1,25(OH)_2D$ are normal, and the renal tubular phosphate excretion defect is not as marked as in familial hypophosphatemic rickets. Short stature is not as prominent. Oral phosphate and $1,25(OH)_2D$ have been used to treat this disorder.

24.62 VITAMIN D DEPENDENT RICKETS

(Pseudovitamin D Deficiency, Hypocalcemic Vitamin D Resistant Rickets)

Vitamin D dependent rickets appears at age 3–6 mo in children who have been receiving dosages of vitamin D (400–600 IU/24 hr) that ordinarily prevent rickets. Serum calcium and phosphate levels are low, and alkaline phosphatase activity is elevated. This condition is a calcium-deficient form of rickets because patients have secondary hyperparathyroidism, aminoaciduria, glucosuria, renal tubular bicarbonate wasting, and renal tubular acidosis. These children also develop dental enamel hypoplasia. While the rickets and biochemical features of this autosomal recessive disorder can be treated with a massive dosage of vitamin D_2 (200,000–1 million IU/24 hr), the use of relatively low-dose $1,25(OH)_2D$ at 1–2 μg/24 hr will heal this disorder. The current hypothesis to account for these findings is that the enzyme activity of 25(OH)D-1α-hydroxylase is deficient or greatly reduced. As evidence of this hypothesis, the serum levels of $1,25(OH)_2D$ are low, despite hypocalcemia, hypophosphatemia, and elevated PTH levels.

Some patients with vitamin D dependent rickets fail to reverse their rickets after treatment either with high-dose vitamin D_2 or $1,25(OH)_2D$ at 1–2 μg/24 hr. Hypocalcemia, hypophosphatemia, aminoaciduria, and rickets persist in the presence of extremely high circulating levels of $1,25(OH)_2D$, usually above 180 pg/mL. A defect in the binding of $1,25(OH)_2D$ to either cytoplasmic or nuclear receptors in skin and bone cells is the pathophysiologic mechanism in this subset of patients. An abnormal gene product is produced by the vitamin D receptor gene in these patients. A single amino acid substitution in an important DNA-binding site in the receptor causes this disorder, thus preventing the binding of $1,25(OH)_2D$ and its receptor to the nucleus. This form of the disease, which is particularly prevalent among children of 1st-cousin marriages, is termed *vitamin D dependency, type II*, or hereditary resistance to $1,25(OH)_2D$. Some patients have short stature and alopecia totalis. Rickets can sometimes be reversed by administration of 15–30 μg/24 hr of $1,25(OH)_2D$, but absent hair does not regrow.

24.63 HEPATIC RICKETS

Rickets is not uncommon in children with hepatic disorders, particularly in extrahepatic biliary atresia, where failure of bile salt secretion prevents adequate absorption of vitamin D and other fat-soluble vitamins. Rickets may also occur in neonatal hepatitis and following hepatocellular damage induced by total parenteral nutrition. Although it was initially thought that hepatic disease would impair 25-hydroxylation and thus reduce serum 25(OH)D levels, it is now believed that reduced absorption of vitamin D accounts for rickets. The usual findings of nutritional rickets are seen—reduced serum 25(OH)D values, hypocalcemia, roentgenographic evidence, and elevated serum alkaline phosphatase activity (bone and hepatic isoenzyme levels are raised). Because rickets mainly relates to vitamin D malabsorption, this form can be treated with high enough doses to overcome malabsorption. Thus, 4,000–10,000 IU of vitamin D_2 (100–250 μg), 50 μg of 25(OH)D or 0.2 μg/kg of $1,25(OH)_2D$ should be given daily, along with oral calcium. Calcium supplements are particularly indicated in infants having ascites who are receiving loop diuretics, such as furosemide, which result in hypercalciuria.

24.64 RICKETS ASSOCIATED WITH ANTICONVULSANT THERAPY

A small group of children receiving chronic anticonvulsant therapy will present with calcium-deficient rickets, despite apparently adequate vitamin D intake. This condition is more common after the combination of phenobarbital and phenytoin, but it has been associated with almost all anticonvulsant drugs. Affected patients have reduced serum levels of 25(OH)D and may have normal levels of $1,25(OH)_2D$. Because these anticonvulsants induce hepatic cytochrome P-450 hydroxylation enzyme activities, 25(OH)D is readily converted to more polar, inactive metabolites, thus accounting for lower serum 25(OH)D concentrations. However, this condition is much more complex because many patients have a low intake of dairy products, which represent the major dietary source of calcium, and very poor exposure to sunlight. Thus, the relatively normal serum $1,25(OH)_2D$ values are actually subnormal in relation to the degree of hypocalcemia, hypophosphatemia, and secondary hyperparathyroidism.

In children receiving chronic anticonvulsant therapy, the serum values of calcium, phosphate, and alkaline phosphatase activity should be evaluated periodically. This form of rickets usually can be prevented by providing an extra 500–1,000 IU of vitamin D_2 each day and by ensuring that the dietary intake of calcium is adequate.

24.65 ONCOGENOUS RICKETS

(Primary Hypophosphatemic Rickets Associated with Tumor)

Rickets associated with a tumor of mesenchymal origin that resolves upon removal of the tumor has been described in more than 60 cases. These tumors, which cause a phosphate-deficient form of rickets, are mostly benign, may become apparent only years after the development of rickets, and may be located in sites difficult to detect, such as the small bones of the hands and feet, abdominal sheath, nasal antrum, and pharynx. This syndrome is also associated with the epidermal nevus syndrome, neurofibromatosis (von Recklinghausen disease), and linear nevus syndrome.

In addition to hypophosphatemia and hyperphosphaturia, glycinemia and glycinuria are sometimes found in this form of rickets. Evidence suggests that these tumors elaborate a still-unidentified substance, which causes phosphaturia and impairs the conversion of 25(OH)D to $1,25(OH)_2D$. Serum 25(OH)D levels are normal, and serum $1,25(OH)_2D$ levels are low but rapidly rise to normal after tumor excision. This surgery also cures the bone pain and myopathy, which, if untreated, may confine the child to a wheelchair. Children with acquired or late-appearing hypophosphatemic rickets should undergo bone roentgenographic examination and/or bone scan to search for tumors. If a tumor cannot be removed or is metastatic, treatment with $1,25(OH)_2D$ and oral phosphate is often beneficial.

24.66 RICKETS ASSOCIATED WITH RENAL TUBULAR ACIDOSIS

Rickets may be present in primary renal tubular acidosis (RTA), particularly in type II or proximal RTA. Hypophosphatemia and phosphaturia are common in these syndromes, which are characterized by hyperchloremic metabolic acidosis, varying degrees of bicarbonaturia, and frequently hypercalciuria and hyperkaliuria (see Sec. 18.29). Bone demineralization without overt rickets usually is detected in type I and distal RTA. In type I there is an inability to form an adequately acid urine at all levels of serum bicarbonate; in type II, there is a lowered renal threshold for bicarbonate and impaired urinary acidification at normal levels of serum bicarbonate (see Sec.6.8). The metabolic bone disease that occurs in both types may also be characterized by bone pain, growth retardation, osteopenia, and occasionally pathologic fractures. Although acute metabolic acidosis in vitamin D deficient animals may impair the conversion of 25(OH)D to $1,25(OH)_2D$, resulting in reduced levels of this active metabolite, the circulating levels of $1,25(OH)_2D$ in patients with either type of RTA are normal. If patients with RTA have azotemia and loss of renal mass, serum $1,25(OH)_2D$ levels may be reduced.

Bone demineralization in distal RTA probably relates to dissolution of bone, since the calcium carbonate in bone may serve as a buffer against the metabolic acidosis that is due to the hydrogen ions retained by patients with RTA.

Administration of sufficient bicarbonate to reverse acidosis will stop bone dissolution and the hypercalciuria that is common in distal RTA. Proximal RTA is treated with both bicarbonate and oral phosphate supplements to heal bone disease. Doses of phosphate similar to those used in familial hypophosphatemia should be used (Sec. 24.61). Vitamin D is needed to offset the secondary hyperparathyroidism that complicates oral phosphate therapy.

24.67 HYPOPHOSPHATASIA

Hypophosphatasia is an autosomal recessive disorder that roentgenographically resembles rickets and is defined by low serum alkaline phosphatase activity. Hypophosphatasia is now recognized to be an inborn error of metabolism in which there is deficient activity of the tissue-nonspecific (liver/bone/kidney) alkaline phosphatase. Activity of the intestinal and placental enzyme is normal. There is considerable heterogeneity in the severity of the disease. Some cases appear at birth, and diagnosis has even been made in utero by roentgenographic examination of the fetus. The disease may appear in a lethal neonatal or perinatal form *(congenital lethal hypophosphatasia)*, a severe infantile form, or a milder form occurring in childhood or late adolescence *(hypophosphatasia tarda)*. The lethal form is characterized by a moth-eaten appearance at the ends of the long bones, by severe deficiency of ossification throughout the skeleton, and by marked shortening of the long bones. Patients with the mild disease may present with bowing of the legs and variable statural shortening. Since calcium accumulation by mature chondrocytes does not occur, patients may appear to have rickets, and in the neonatal and infantile form, they may have hypercalcemia.

Unusual clinical manifestations include wormian bones in the calvarium, poor calcification of the frontal, parietal, and occipital bones, and premature loss of deciduous or permanent teeth owing to hypoplasia of dental cementum. Because of the hypercalcemia in the infantile form, nephrocalcinosis is also found. In the childhood form, bone pain, frequent fractures, and milder skeletal deformities are evident, as well as premature tooth loss. The metaphyseal defect consists of irregular ossification, punched-out areas, and metaphyseal cupping.

In hypophosphatasia, large quantities of phosphoethanolamine are found in the urine because this compound cannot be degraded in the absence of adequate alkaline phosphatase activity. Plasma inorganic pyrophosphate and pyridoxal-5-phosphate are also elevated for the same reason. Although no satisfactory therapy has been found, infusion of plasma rich in alkaline phosphatase activity has been helpful in healing bone in short-term studies. The clinical course of this condition often improves spontaneously as the child matures, although early death from renal failure or flail chest leading to pneumonia may also occur in the severe infantile form of the disorder. Rare patients presenting identical clinical and roentgenographic patterns have normal serum alkaline phosphatase activities. Their disease has been labeled *pseudohypophosphatasia* and may represent the presence of a mutant alkaline phosphatase isozyme that reacts to artificial substrates in an alkaline environment (i.e., in a test tube) but not in vivo with natural substrates.

24.68 PRIMARY CHONDRODYSTROPHY
(Metaphyseal Dysplasia)

In this condition bowing of the legs, short stature, and a waddling gait appear in the absence of abnormalities of serum calcium, phosphate, alkaline phosphatase activity, or vitamin D metabolites. Metaphyseal chondrodysplasia *(Jansen type)* is typified by cupped and ragged metaphyses, which develop mottled calcification at the distal ends of bone over time. Hypercalcemia, with serum values of 13–15 mg/dL may occur. The spine may also be deformed by the irregular growth of vertebrae. The *Schmidt type* of metaphyseal chondrodysplasia is less severe, although the roentgenographic appearance of the knees and extreme bowing of the lower limbs resemble signs seen in patients with familial hypophosphatemia. The hip abnormalities are more debilitating, however. Patients with both types of metaphyseal chondrodysplasia have lifelong short stature.

Metaphyseal dysotosis, or *Pyle disease,* results from defects in endochondral bone formation and metaphyseal modeling. The long ends of bones are splayed, resulting in an "Erlenmeyer flask" defect. Short stature is not present, and serum chemical levels are normal. Leonine features develop if the facial bones are involved.

No effective forms of treatment are available for the chondrodystrophies or the dysostosis.

24.69 IDIOPATHIC HYPERCALCEMIA

Medical attention was initially drawn to hypercalcemia shortly after World War II ended, when excessive quantities of vitamin D were used to enrich food for infants in England. Although many infants were exposed to high levels of vitamin D, only a few developed hypercalcemia, failure to thrive, and decline in renal function. These infants had roentgenographic evidence of osteosclerosis and dense bones at the metaphyses. This disorder disappeared with reduction in the vitamin D content of milk. Subsequently, at least three separate forms of hypercalcemia of unknown origin have been described.

Williams syndrome, or the elfin facies syndrome, consists of a constellation of manifestations, of which hypercalcemia is an infrequent finding. The characteristic facial features include a small mandible, prominent maxilla, and upturned nose. The upper lip has a Cupid's bow curve. Small peg-like teeth with numerous caries are common. Feeding problems and failure to thrive during the 1st yr of life are usual. Mild mental retardation and an unusual "cocktail party patter" personality are typical. The types of cardiac lesions found separately or together include supravalvular aortic stenosis, peripheral pulmonary stenosis, hypoplasia of the aorta, and atrial or ventricular septal defects. In hypercalcemic patients, nephrocalcinosis and sclerotic long bones are sometimes evident.

Williams syndrome is sporadic, and some children have hypervitaminosis D without evidence of increased maternal or infantile vitamin D intake. In most cases, the circulating values for vitamin D metabolites are normal. Patients with this disorder slowly excrete an infused calcium load and have evidence for increased production of 25(OH)D from vitamin D. Impaired calcitonin secretion to an infused calcium load has also been reported. Treatment is directed at social and educational problems.

Children may also have mild *idiopathic hypercalcemia,* which is usually transient. Phenotypic features of Williams syndrome are not found. These patients have hypercalciuria and sometimes nephrocalcinosis, possibly resembling the English infants who received excessive vitamin D after World War II. However, no evidence for abnormalities in vitamin D metabolism has been found.

Familial hypocalciuric hypercalcemia is an autosomal dominant condition in which affected children have asymptomatic hypercalcemia without hypercalciuria. Pancreatitis may occur in some families and, in a few kindreds, neonates may present with life-threatening parathyroid hyperplasia. Instead of serum calcium levels of 12–15 mg/dL, typically found in the parent, these infants have levels exceeding 18 mg/dL. All these children have had mild parathyroid hyperplasia despite hypercalcemia, indicating that the parathyroid gland does not respond appropriately to the signal of hypercalcemia. Vitamin D metabolism is normal. Only the infants with serious hyperparathyroidism require treatment—an emergency parathyroidectomy. Although serum magnesium is elevated, it is not a serious concern.

24.70 HYPERPHOSPHATASIA

Excessive elevation of the bone isozyme of alkaline phosphatase in serum and significant growth failure characterize hyperphosphatasia. Osteoid proliferation in the subperiosteal portion of bone results in separation of the periosteum from the bone cortex. Bowing and thickening of the diaphyses are common, along with osteopenia. The disease usually has its onset by 2–3 yr of age, when painful deformity developing in the extremities leads to abnormal gait and sometimes fractures. Other common findings include pectus carinatum, kyphoscoliosis, and rib fraying. The skull is large and the cranium is thickened (widened diploë) and may be deformed. Roentgenographically, the bony texture is variable; dense areas (showing a teased cotton-wool appearance) are interspersed with radiolucent areas and general demineralization. Long bones appear cylindric, lose metaphyseal modeling, and contain pseudocysts showing a dense bony halo.

In this autosomal recessive disorder, serum levels of both calcium and phosphate are normal, whereas urinary leucine amino acid peptidase activity and serum acid phosphatase are increased. This disorder is often called *juvenile Paget disease* because, as in adult-onset Paget disease, calcitonin may reduce the rapid bone turnover found in this disorder; in children the disorder is more generalized and symmetric.

Transient hyperphosphatasia occurs between 2 mo and 2 yr of age, has no associated symptoms, and is usually detected during routine (screening) laboratory evaluation for some unrelated complaint. Both liver and bone isoenzyme fractions are elevated; however, there are no other manifestations of hepatic or bone dysfunction. The etiology is unknown. Resolution usually occurs within 4–6 mo.

Familial hyperphosphatemia, an autosomal dominant trait, is another benign condition that is distinguished from the transient infantile form by persistent and asymptomatic elevations of serum alkaline phosphatase levels.

RUSSELL WALLACE CHESNEY

Chesney RW: Requirements and upper limits of vitamin D intake in the term neonate, infant, and older child. J Pediatr 116:159, 1990.
Chesney RW, DeLuca HF, Gertner JM, et al: Circulating levels of vitamin D metabolites in children with the Williams syndrome. N Engl J Med 313:888, 1985.
Chesney RW: Metabolic bone diseases. Pediatrics 5:227, 1984.
Chesney RW, Kaplan BS, Phelps M, et al: Renal tubular acidosis does not alter the circulating values of calcitriol (1,25$(OH)_2$-vitamin D). J Pediatr 104:51, 1984.
Culler FL, Jones KL, Deftos LJ: Impaired calcitonin secretion in patients with Williams syndrome. J Pediatr 107:720, 1985.
Eil C, Lieberman UA, Rosen JF, et al: Cellular defect in hereditary vitamin D-dependent rickets type II: Defective nuclear uptake of 1,25-dihydroxyvitamin D in cultured skin fibroblasts. N Engl J Med 304:1588, 1981.
Finberg L: Metabolic bone disease. *In:* Gershwin ME, Robbins DL (eds): Musculoskeletal Diseases of Children. New York, Grune & Stratton, 1983, p 447.
Fraser DR: The physiological economy of vitamin D. Lancet 1:969, 1983.
Glorieux FH, Marie PJ, Pettifor JM, et al: Bone response to phosphate salts, ergocalciferol and calcitriol in hypophosphatemic vitamin D-resistant rickets. N Engl J Med 303:1023, 1980.
Harrison HE, Harrison HC: Disorders of Calcium and Phosphate Metabolism in Childhood and Adolescence. Philadelphia, WB Saunders, 1979.
Markowitz ME, Rosen JF, Smith C, et al: 1,25-Dihydroxyvitamin D_3-treated hypoparathyroidism: 35 patient years in 10 children. J Clin Endocrinol Metab 55:727, 1982.
Opshaug O, Maurseth K, Howlid H, et al: Vitamin D metabolism in hypophosphatasia: Case report. Acta Paediatr Scand 71:517, 1982.
Rosen JF, Chesney RW: Circulating calcitriol concentrations in health and disease of infancy and childhood. J Pediatr 103:1, 1983.
Scriver CR: Rickets and the pathogenesis of impaired tubular transport of phosphate and other solutes. Am J Med 57:43, 1974.
Scriver CR, Reade T, Halal F, et al: Autosomal hypophosphatemic bone disease responds to 1,25$(OH)_2D_3$. Arch Dis Child 56:203, 1981.
Whyte MP: Hypophosphatasia. *In:* Scriver CR, Beauded A, Sly WS, Valle D (eds): The Metabolic Basis of Inherited Disease. New York, McGraw-Hill, 1989, p 2843.

24.71 FANCONI SYNDROME

(Rickets Associated with Multiple Defects of the Proximal Renal Tubule; de Toni-Debré-Fanconi Syndrome)

Generalized aminoaciduria, renal glycosuria, and phosphaturia resulting in hypophosphatemia characterize Fanconi syndrome. Associated but inconstant renal tubular abnormalities include excessive bicarbonaturia leading to renal tubular acidosis, hyperkaliuria leading to hypokalemia, sodium wasting, uricosuria, proteinuria, and hyposthenuria. Clinical hallmarks are linear growth failure and rickets resistant to doses of vitamin D that are ordinarily adequate for treatment of nutritional deficiency (see Sec. 4.29).

ETIOLOGY. Fanconi syndrome occurs with genetically transmitted inborn errors of metabolism (cystinosis, fructose intolerance, galactosemia, glycogenosis, Lowe syndrome, tyrosinemia, and Wilson disease) and with some acquired diseases, including exposure to environmental toxins, for example, heavy metals (Cd, Pb, Hg) or certain drugs (outdated tetracycline, gentamicin, azathioprine). Most commonly, it is idiopathic, and its occurrence in this form may be sporadic or inherited as a mendelian dominant or recessive trait, including X-linked recessive. The following description of the primary idiopathic form is representative of the syndrome in general.

PATHOGENESIS. Studies suggest an abnormality in some final common pathway for normal membrane transport in the proximal renal tubules. There may be deficient energy production, abnormalities in membrane structure, or both, leading to impaired tubular uptake or back-leak of solutes. Also, loss of bicarbonate in the urine leads to proximal RTA (see Sec. 18.29 and 24.66). Renal potassium wasting results from excessive urinary losses of bicarbonate and glucose. Urinary sodium losses are obligatory because of the large excretion of urinary anions. Serum calcium level is normal to low; urinary calcium levels vary. A vasopressin-resistant urinary concentrating defect is often present but is unexplained. A syndrome similar to Fanconi syndrome can be produced in rodents and dogs upon administration of maleic acid, a tubular toxin, and occurs in the Basenji breed of dogs in which excessive urinary losses of amino acids, sugar, and phosphate result from decreased proximal RTA of the glomerular filtrate.

Rickets can result from the combined effects of metabolic acidosis and hypophosphatemia or from hypophosphatemia alone. Simple calcium deficiency does not appear to play a role in the bone disease. Vitamin D resistance may be due to impaired conversion of vitamin D to its biologically active metabolite, 1,25$(OH)_2D_3$, by abnormal proximal tubular cells in the presence of metabolic acidosis.

Microscopic findings are nonspecific. Renal tubules may show dilatation, variation in size and shape, swelling of epithelial cells, and atrophy. Foci of interstitial fibrosis are common. Enlarged mitochondria may be seen on electron microscopy. Typically, glomerular architecture is preserved until late in the disease.

CLINICAL MANIFESTATIONS. Primary Fanconi syndrome typically presents either in the first 6 mo of life or in the 3rd–4th decade. In infancy, vomiting, polydipsia, polyuria, and constipation occur. Episodes of weakness, fever with dehydration, and metabolic acidosis may also occur. Failure to thrive is often pronounced, especially in linear growth.

Roentgenographic signs of rickets or osteopenia may appear despite a history of adequate vitamin D intake and the absence of glomerular insufficiency, indicating a renal tubular cause.

LABORATORY DATA. Usually, a hyperchloremic metabolic acidosis is noted, with normal "anion gap" (see Sec. 6.8), hypokalemia, hypophosphatemia, and hypouricemia. Fractional excretion of phosphate is elevated. Alkaline phosphatase activity is elevated if rickets is present. Glycosuria occurs at normal serum glucose concentrations. There is generalized nonspecific aminoaciduria. Urinary pH is inappropriately elevated, with low levels of urinary ammonia and titratable acid. When the glomerular filtration rate falls late in the course of the disease, there may be a "paradoxic" improvement in the levels of serum electrolytes and an amelioration of aminoaciduria, glycosuria, and phosphaturia.

DIAGNOSIS. There is no definitive diagnostic test for idiopathic Fanconi syndrome. Aminoaciduria, diminished tubular reabsorption of phosphate, and elevated alkaline phosphatase activities accompany other forms of rickets. In a child with stunted growth and rickets refractory to ordinary doses of vitamin D the presence of renal glycosuria indicates multiple tubular dysfunction. Metabolic acidosis and hypokalemia are corroborative. Fluid deprivation to test urinary concentrating ability is risky in the face of obligatory hyposthenuria, and glucose loading may cause profound symptomatic hypokalemia by shifting potassium into cells.

TREATMENT. The clinical and biochemical expressions vary from one patient to another; accordingly, treatment is not uniform. For patients with secondary Fanconi syndrome, underlying causes should be sought. In those with primary

Fanconi syndrome, symptomatic therapy can restore mineral and electrolyte balance, prolong survival, and often permit a normal life. Rickets can be corrected and skeletal deformities prevented, but fully normal growth rates are rarely achieved.

Rickets or osteopenia responds to large doses of vitamin D. The usual starting dose is 5,000 units/24 hr, which should be increased gradually to a maximal dose of 2,000–4,000 units/kg/24 hr. Most patients require at least 25,000 units to heal rickets. Dihydrotachysterol may be substituted for vitamin D at a starting dose of 0.05–0.1 mg/24 hr (1 mg is equivalent to 120,000 units of vitamin D). In recent years, $1,25(OH)_2D_3$ has become the preferred form of vitamin D therapy because of its greater potency and shorter half-life, should hypercalcemia occur. Serum calcium levels must be followed closely (weekly at first, then monthly) to avoid hypercalcemia from vitamin D overdose. Hypophosphatemia can be treated by oral supplementation with 1–3 g of neutral phosphate/24 hr given in 4–5 equally spaced doses through the waking hours. If abdominal pain or diarrhea ensues, therapy should be discontinued temporarily and then reinstituted at a lower dose. Phosphate should not be given without concomitant vitamin D to avoid causing or aggravating hypocalcemia, and causing secondary hyperparathyroidism.

Correcting metabolic acidosis due to excessive bicarbonaturia may require large amounts of alkali. From 2 to 15 mEq/kg/24 hr of alkali may be needed, as sodium bicarbonate solution (1 mEq of base = 1 mL), *Shohl* solution (140 g of citric acid, 90 g of sodium citrate qs to 1 L with water; 1 mEq of base = 1 mL), or *Polycitra* (5 mL = 550 mg of potassium citrate, 500 mg of sodium citrate, 334 mg of citric acid; 2 mEq of base = 1 mL). Doses should be adjusted to raise serum bicarbonate only to near normal levels (18–20 mEq/L). Attempts to normalize serum bicarbonate may exaggerate urinary bicarbonate loss as a result of extracellular fluid volume expansion with excessive sodium loads. Alkali is administered 1–1½ hr after meals in 3–4 divided doses/day, and, if Polycitra is not used, extra potassium should be given at a starting dose of 2–3 mEq/kg/24 hr. Extra salt and water should be provided to counter excessive losses, especially in warm weather.

Chesney RW: Etiology and pathogenesis of the Fanconi syndrome. Miner Electrolyte Metab 4:303, 1980.

Cohn RM, Roth KS: Metabolic Disease: A Guide to Early Recognition. Philadelphia, WB Saunders, 1983, p 258.

Foreman JW, Roth KS: The Human renal Fanconi syndrome—then and now. Nephron 51:301, 1989.

24.72 CYSTINOSIS

(Lignac Syndrome; Fanconi Syndrome with Cystinosis)

Cystinosis presents the clinical and laboratory features of Fanconi syndrome with the additional distinctive finding of abnormal accumulation of cystine in various tissues (see also Sec. 8.5 and 24.71).

PATHOGENESIS. The cause is unknown. Increased cellular uptake of cystine results in accumulation in lysosomes, where it cannot be maintained in reduced form. It also appears that there is a failure in lysosomal release of this amino acid. No specific enzyme defect has yet been identified. Tissue levels of cystine do not correlate with the degree of renal tubular dysfunction; accordingly, a simple toxic effect of cystine on tubules is not the cause of Fanconi syndrome in cystinosis.

Cystine is deposited in the reticuloendothelial system, especially in spleen, liver, lymph nodes, and bone marrow, but not in muscle or brain. Deposits occur in renal tubular cells, cornea, and conjunctiva. Cystine also accumulates in peripheral blood leukocytes and fibroblasts. Early renal changes are similar to those of primary Fanconi syndrome; the characteristic "swan neck" lesion consists of atrophy and shortening of the proximal tubule just beneath the glomerulus. Birefringent cystine crystals may be seen in interstitial tissue and rarely in tubular cells; they are sometimes recognizable only on electron microscopy. With advancing renal failure, the kidneys become shrunken and contracted, with glomerular sclerosis and interstitial fibrosis.

CLINICAL MANIFESTATIONS. Cystinosis is inherited as an autosomal recessive trait. There are three clinical patterns. Patients with the *infantile or nephropathic form* present with Fanconi syndrome at 3–12 mo of age. A generalized aminoaciduria is found without predominance of cystine. The glomerular filtration rate falls progressively, and chronic renal failure develops within the 1st decade. Severe growth failure and hypothyroidism accompany this state. Distinctive clinical features include blond hair and fair complexion, owing to a defect in melanin synthesis, and photophobia secondary to deposit of cystine crystals on the conjunctivae. The *adolescent* or *intermediate form* is characterized by mild renal involvement, with onset in the 2nd decade and slow progression. Growth failure is not a feature of this form. The *adult type* of cystinosis (benign) causes no renal disease. Cystine crystals may be found in the cornea, bone marrow, and leukocytes.

LABORATORY DATA. Other than the deposition of cystine crystals, laboratory abnormalities are similar to those described for the Fanconi syndrome. Tubular proteinuria characterizes the early phase of nephropathic cystinosis, but glomerular proteinuria supervenes as renal failure ensues.

DIAGNOSIS. In the asymptomatic newborn infant from an affected family the diagnosis of cystinosis can be made by measuring the cystine content of leukocytes or fibroblasts, which will be 80–100 times normal. Later, granular and circinate irregularities in the peripheral pigmentation of the retina may be noted. Cystine crystals may be detected in the bone marrow, lymph nodes, conjunctivae, and rectal mucosa. Slit lamp examination shows crystals in the cornea. Prenatal diagnosis can be made by finding an increased concentration of cystine in amniotic fluid cells. Cystinosis must not be confused with cystinuria, which is an inborn error of specific amino acid transport, with neither cystine deposition nor Fanconi syndrome.

TREATMENT. Early on, symptomatic therapy for tubular dysfunction is similar to that for primary Fanconi syndrome. In addition, cysteamine, a sulfhydryl binder, has been shown to lower intracellular cystine in vivo and to slow the rate of progression of renal (glomerular) failure in some children. If administered early, it may attenuate but not reverse some features of the Fanconi syndrome.

For patients with end-stage renal failure, hemodialysis and renal transplantation are recommended. Hemodialysis does not lower tissue cystine levels. Children with cystinosis appear to do as well after kidney transplantation as those with other forms of chronic kidney failure, but long-term survivors may experience progressive photophobia or retinopathy. Cysteamine eye drops may be helpful. Transplantation has increased survival but has been associated with long-term extrarenal manifestations, such as swallowing dysfunction, myopathy, pancreatic endocrine and exocrine insufficiency, and various central nervous system problems (e.g., seizures, cerebral atrophy).

Broyer M, Guillot M, Gubler MC, et al: Infantile cystinosis: A reappraisal of early and late symptoms. Adv Nephrol 11:137, 1981.

Cohn RM, Roth KS: Metabolic Disease: A Guide to Early Recognition. Philadelphia, WB Saunders, 1983, p 237.

Foreman JW: Cystinosis. Sermin Nephrol 9:62, 1989.

Gahl WA: Cystinosis coming of age. Adv Pediatr 33:95, 1986.

24.73 OCULOCEREBRORENAL DYSTROPHY
(Lowe Syndrome)

This rare disorder is transmitted as an X-linked recessive trait. In addition to Fanconi syndrome, organic aciduria, decreased production of urinary ammonia, and occasionally heavy proteinuria occur. Distinctive clinical features include congenital cataracts, glaucoma, and buphthalmos that lead to severe visual impairment. Severe hypotonia and hyporeflexia appear in the 1st yr. Mental retardation is severe and often progressive. Rickets, marked osteopenia, and pathologic fracture may develop as a result of metabolic acidosis and phosphate depletion.

PATHOGENESIS. The pathogenesis is not known, but recent in vitro studies have suggested an abnormality in collagen metabolism. Pathologic studies have shown splitting of the glomerular basement membranes, with marked variation in their thickness. These changes may not be confined to the kidney.

CLINICAL FEATURES. Early in life the eye findings and mental retardation predominate; the Fanconi syndrome becomes clinically apparent later. If the patient survives childhood, the Fanconi syndrome may resolve spontaneously, only to be supplanted by chronic renal failure. There is no specific therapy. Treatment is supportive, as in primary Fanconi syndrome.

Abbassi V, Lowe CU, Calcagno PL: Oculo-cerebro-renal syndrome: A review. Am J Dis Child 15:145, 1968.

For advice and support to families with Lowe syndrome, contact the Lowe's Syndrome Association, 607 Robinson Street, West Lafayette, IN 47906.

24.74 RENAL OSTEODYSTROPHY

The term renal osteodystrophy designates the alterations in skeletal growth and remodeling that occur in children with chronic renal disease because of abnormalities in mineral and bone metabolism. These abnormalities include malabsorption of calcium, phosphate retention, hyperfunction of the parathyroid glands; cutaneous, vascular, and visceral calcifications; and impairment in the renal production of biologically active vitamin D. Renal osteodystrophy can ocur with tubular dysfunction while glomerular filtration remains intact (see Sec. 18.36, 18.37, and 24.66) but more commonly follows progressive loss of nephrons, with glomerular insufficiency and uremia.

The condition was formerly called renal (uremic) rickets or renal dwarfism because severe linear growth failure was associated with rickets-like roentgenographic changes. These findings were first thought to be due primarily to a mineralization defect resulting from vitamin D deficiency, but secondary hyperparathyroidism is an equally important contributor to the clinical and roentgenographic findings. Since the advent of pediatric dialysis and kidney transplantation, renal osteodystrophy has emerged as a major complication of chronic renal failure in childhood, along with acidosis, anemia, and caloric deficiency (Sec. 18.37).

PATHOGENESIS. Early in the course of chronic renal insufficiency (GFR 25–50 mL/min/1.73m^2) with a normal dietary intake of phosphorus, there appears to be a phosphate-mediated suppression of renal tubular synthesis of 1,25(OH)$_2$D$_3$, leading to malabsorption of calcium and phosphorus and, through unknown mechanisms, to defective mineralization of osteoid (osteomalacia). Serum calcium is maintained, and serum phosphorus may actually be normal to low as a result of raised parathyroid hormone levels (PTH), leading to increased bone resorption and increased renal phosphate excretion. Proof of this hypothesis comes from studies in which dietary phosphate restriction resulted in raised serum 1,25(OH)$_2$D$_3$ levels and improvement in secondary hyperparathyroidism. At some critical renal threshold, for example, when glomerular filtration rate falls to approximately 25–30% of normal, the phosphaturic renal response to elevated PTH is lost, and compensatory hyperparathyroidism supervenes in an attempt to restore serum calcium to normal. The consequences are roentgenographic and histologic evidence of exaggerated osteoclast-mediated resorption of bone (osteitis fibrosa). Also, endosteal fibrosis, increased bone turnover, and replacement of regularly textured lamellar bone with disorganized and structurally deficient woven bone are seen. Chronic metabolic acidosis probably contributes to the bony changes by increasing calcium resorption from bone and increasing renal excretion before severe renal failure ensues.

The pathology varies. On biopsy, trabecular bone may show predominant osteomalacia, predominant osteitis fibrosa, or, most commonly, a mixed pattern. Osteitis fibrosa predominates in dialyzed patients. A subgroup of patients has been described in whom fracturing osteomalacia and low bone turnover have resulted from accumulation of aluminum at the mineralization front. These patients have been exposed to either orally administered aluminum phosphate binders or aluminum-containing dialysis solutions.

Roentgenographic abnormalities at the epiphyseal growth plate may occasionally resemble those of nutritional rickets but are often quite distinct; histologically, they reflect osteitis fibrosa rather than rickets. The growth plate is not actually increased in longitudinal width but appears to be because of the formation of a bar of metaphyseal fibrosis with dysplastic trabeculas. The concomitant defect in mineralization leads to a failure in modeling, with persistence of cartilage, an expanded epiphyseal diameter, and frequent overriding of the lateral border of the metaphysis.

CLINICAL MANIFESTATIONS. The younger the child at onset of chronic renal failure and the longer the duration of renal failure, the greater will be the incidence and severity of osteodystrophy. In children with congenital diseases of the kidney, which predominate under the age of 5 yr, the interval between the onset of disease and end-stage renal failure is longer than it is in the glomerulonephritides, which occur later in childhood. However, in children with congenital nephropathies, bone disease is accelerated because it occurs at a time of maximal growth and bone modeling and remodeling.

The earliest sign of renal osteodystrophy is usually growth failure, to which anemia, metabolic acidosis, protein-calorie malnutrition, hormonal disorders, and trace mineral deficiencies associated with chronic renal failure may contribute. Growth failure may occur with no roentgenographic skeletal abnormalities. With advancing (untreated) disease, additional clinical manifestations appear, including muscle weakness, bone pain, bone deformities, slipped epiphyses, metaphyseal fractures, metastatic calcification, and pruritus. Genu varum, frontal bossing, and dental abnormalities are particularly evident in young children. Tetany is rare (despite hypocalcemia) because of the combined protective effects of metabolic acidosis and hyperparathyroidism.

LABORATORY DATA. There may be mild hypocalcemia, but the Ca × P product is usually elevated by increased levels of serum phosphorus. Elevated alkaline phosphatase activity reflects increased bone turnover but is not as reliable a sign in children as in adults.

In roentgenograms of the hands and wrists, subperiosteal erosions of the middle and distal phalanges may be sensitive early indicators of osteitis fibrosa. Erosions may also occur in the distal clavicle and on inner aspects of the distal femur and proximal tibia. Elevated serum levels of PTH generally give the earliest indication of bone disease and may be found when glomerular filtration rates are reduced to as little as 50–75 mL/min/1.73 m^2. The degree of elevation of PTH correlates with roentgenographic and histologic evidence of osteitis fibrosa, but the degree of histologic osteomalacia does not correlate well with chemical abnormalities in serum or with roentgenographic evidence of rickets, osteopenia, or coarsening of trabeculas.

TREATMENT. Renal osteodystrophy can usually be successfully managed by (1) controlling hyperphosphatemia, (2) supplying adequate oral calcium intake, and (3) providing extra vitamin D. Treatment should begin early because growth failure in infancy can greatly influence the attainment of ultimate stature. An unresolved question is whether therapy should be initiated before definite roentgenographic or biochemical abnormalities appear, but recent literature suggests that a raised PTH level is an indication to begin dietary phosphate restriction.

Hyperphosphatemia should be controlled with oral administration of phosphate binders if dietary restriction is not sufficient. Aluminum-containing binders should be avoided whenever possible because of the risks of aluminum intoxication. However, when there are no satisfactory alternatives, aluminum hydroxide or aluminum carbonate gel can be given at a starting dose of 20–30 mg/kg/24 hr in divided doses with meals and can be subsequently adjusted to keep the serum phosphorus between 4 and 5 mg/dL. The total dose of aluminum should not exceed 50 mg/kg/24 hr. Long-term treatment with high-dose aluminum-containing binders has been reported to cause osteomalacic osteodystrophy and a progressive, irreversible encephalopathy with dementia. Calcium supplementation in the form of calcium carbonate should be added to the diet to provide 1–1.5 g of elemental calcium per day. Calcium carbonate is preferred because, of the available calcium preparations, it contains the highest percentage of elemental calcium and it affords some degree of phosphate binding, particularly when given with meals. Strict control of acidosis should be achieved by administering sodium bicarbonate. Starting doses are usually 1–2 mEq/kg/24 hr, divided into thirds and given 1 hr after meals (see Sec. 24.71 for specific agents).

Some form of vitamin D appears necessary for successful treatment of uremic osteodystrophy. The preferred form is 1,25$(OH)_2D_3$, although the long-term advantage of this form over dihydrotachysterol (DHT) has not been demonstrated. This therapy is indicated for symptomatic bone disease with hypocalcemia, secondary hypoparathyroidism, and evidence of osteitis fibrosa on roentgenography or bone biopsy. Starting doses are 15–40 ng/kg/24 hr and should be divided and given 8–12 hr apart to reduce the risk of hypercalcemia. Stepwise adjustments in the dose and indefinite biochemical monitoring are indicated, as with DHT treatment (later). When hypercalcemia ensues, it is usually very short-lived because of the extremely short half-life of 1,25$(OH)_2D_3$.

DHT has been favored over vitamin D because it has a better ratio of therapeutic to toxic effects and because its shorter half-life will reduce complications if hypercalcemia occurs. Starting doses are 0.1–0.2 mg/24 hr, and the dosage is increased weekly or biweekly in stepwise fashion to normalize levels of serum calcium and to heal roentgenographic abnormalities. Doses can be lowered once these goals are achieved. Frequent measurements of serum calcium and phosphorus are required, weekly at first, then monthly. Evidence suggests that the "set-point" of serum calcium at which PTH is released is elevated in chronic renal failure. Thus the therapeutic goal of vitamin D therapy is to raise serum calcium to 10.5–11.0 mg/dL.

Hemodialysis or chronic peritoneal dialysis may either ameliorate or exacerbate bone disease; the effect cannot be predicted. Unrecognized or untreated hypercalcemia may accelerate renal insufficiency or foster metastatic calcification of the tympanic membranes, cornea, conjunctiva, skin, and vascular tree. When hypercalcemia is found, administration of vitamin D must be suspended until the serum calcium level is normal; therapy can then be reinstituted at a lower dose.

Autotransplantation of the parathyroid gland is preferred over parathyroidectomy in carefully selected patients with severe secondary hyperparathyroidism refractory to medical therapy. Indications include severe bone pain, mental aberrations, severe pruritus, fractures, chronic hypercalcemia, and, less commonly, metastatic calcification. In all cases marked elevation of serum PTH levels should be proved prior to surgery.

MICHAEL E. NORMAN

Foreman JW, Chan JCM: Chronic renal failure in infants and children. J Pediatr 113:793, 1988.
Malluche H, Faugere M: Renal osteodystrophy. N Engl J Med 321:317, 1989.
Norman ME: Vitamin D in bone disease. Pediatr Clin North Am 29:947, 1982.
Norman ME, Mazur AT, Borden S, et al: Early diagnosis of juvenile renal osteodystrophy. J Pediatr 97:226, 1980.
Polinsky MS, Gruskin AB: Aluminum toxicity in children with chronic renal failure. J Pediatr 105:758, 1984.
Mehls O, Salusley IB: Recent advances and controversies in childhood renal osteodystrophy. Pediatr Nephrol 1:212, 1987.

25

UNCLASSIFIED DISEASES

25.1 SUDDEN INFANT DEATH SYNDROME

DEFINITION. The sudden and unexpected death of an infant, for reasons that are unclear even after an autopsy, is the most common manner of death in the 1st year of life following the neonatal period. In the typical case this *sudden infant death syndrome (SIDS)* occurs in an apparently healthy infant of 2–3 mo of age who has been put to bed without suspicion that anything is out of the ordinary. Some time later the infant is found dead, and a conventional autopsy fails to reveal a cause of death. Although these infants appear healthy before death, detailed perinatal histories and more intensive studies of cardiorespiratory and neurologic function have produced evidence that some affected children have not been normal earlier. The needs to separate this tragic condition from child abuse and to supply stricken families with psychologic support have been highlighted mainly through the efforts of families who have had infants die in this way.

EPIDEMIOLOGY. SIDS is a worldwide phenomenon; incidence rates vary from 0.2 to 3.0/1,000 live births. Part of this variation may reflect the thoroughness with which other diagnoses are sought and the accuracy of reporting. In the United States the average incidence ranges from 1.6 to 2.3/1,000 live births, with considerable ethnic variation. The rates per 1,000 live births are 0.5 among Asians; 1.3 among whites; 1.7 among Hispanics; 2.9 among blacks (5.0 for blacks of low socioeconomic status); and 5.9 among American Indians. The incidence in American Indians may be artifactually high because detailed post mortem examination is not generally performed. Incidence peaks at 2–3 mo of age; few cases occur before 2 wk or after 6 mo of age. Males are at higher risk than females. The incidence of SIDS is higher during the colder months of the year.

Since the greatest number of deaths occur between midnight and 9:00 A.M., SIDS has been presumed to take place during sleep, but it is difficult to prove that SIDS actually occurs during sleep; the association with sleep may only reflect the larger proportion of time that infants in the susceptible age group spend sleeping. However, there may be additional vulnerability to cardiorespiratory collapse during sleep (see later).

A variety of genetic, environmental, and social factors have been associated with increased risk of SIDS, including premature births, especially with history of apnea or bronchopulmonary dysplasia; low birthweight for gestational age; cold weather; young unmarried mother; lack of prenatal care; poor socioeconomic conditions, including crowding; maternal history of smoking, anemia, or narcotic ingestion; history of a sibling with SIDS; and history of an apparent life-threatening event (ALTE), referred to in the earlier literature as a "near miss" or aborted episode of SIDS (i.e., an episode in which an infant ceases to breathe, develops cyanosis or pallor, and becomes unresponsive but is successfully resuscitated). The increased risk of SIDS in black infants does not persist when adjustments are made for family income and maternal education. The risk of SIDS varies inversely with maternal age and directly with parity. The Apgar scores of infants with SIDS average lower than those of their surviving peers. Breast-feeding is not associated with a decreased risk. The peak incidence of SIDS (2–3 mo) coincides with normally low levels of circulating immunoglobulins, but no specific pathogens have been found.

In a family having an infant with SIDS the risk for the next or a subsequent child varies from 5/1,000 to 10/1,000 or about 5 times the usual risk. Familial recurrences suggest an inborn error of metabolism. Twins or triplets are probably not at higher risk for SIDS than subsequent siblings, nor is the risk higher for monozygotic than for dizygotic twins. Evidence suggests that environmental factors (prenatal or postnatal) are important rather than genetic factors, with no evidence for mendelian inheritance of susceptibility.

PATHOLOGY. Although their significance is controversial, a wide variety of findings have been reported in infants dying of SIDS: retarded postnatal growth, increased pulmonary arterial smooth muscle, increased right ventricular muscle mass, increased extramedullary hematopoiesis, retention of brown fat, hyperplastic adrenal chromaffin tissue, brain stem gliosis, and intrathoracic petechiae. Attention has been focused particularly on the increase in smooth muscle in the larger pulmonary arteries extending to smaller blood vessels close to the alveoli. This suggests that infants with SIDS had been subjected to chronic hypoxia. The increased hypoxanthine concentrations in the vitreous humor in victims of SIDS also suggest that SIDS is preceded by a long period of respiratory failure and hypoxia. However, there is no direct evidence of this hypoxia, and the failure to find hyperplasia of the carotid bodies post mortem weighs against the presence of chronic hypoxia.

PATHOGENESIS. It seems likely that SIDS may have several etiologies. In addition, several rare conditions may masquerade as SIDS. For example, prolonged sleep apnea in infancy has been associated with a space-occupying lesion (left temporal lobe astrocytoma), with a congenital central nervous system (CNS) anomaly (absence of the corpus callosum), and with the neuromuscular dysfunction accompanying infantile botulism. Sudden death has also been caused by vascular rings, usually with antecedent evidence of upper airway obstruction. Infants with familial prolongation of the Q-T interval on an electrocardiogram (ECG) (*Romano-Ward* and *Jervell* and *Lange-Nielsen* syndromes) and inborn errors of metabolism may die suddenly. Accidental suffocation and child abuse should be considered. When such conditions as the aforementioned are excluded, patients with SIDS may share a common etiology involving an abnormality in cardiorespiratory control in which state of consciousness or CNS activity plays a modulating role. Because there is no satisfactory animal model, much of the research in this field has focused on respiratory and cardiovascular controls in groups of infants believed to be at increased risk for SIDS, including siblings of infants with SIDS and infants with an ALTE. Unfortunately, there is still uncertainty as to whether there is any relationship between ALTE and SIDS.

Respiratory Pauses. The precise role of apneic episodes or respiratory pauses in the pathogenesis of SIDS remains unclear. Prolonged apnea and cyanosis during sleep have been observed in infants who died subsequently of what was presumed to be SIDS, and upper airway obstruction, with prolonged pauses in respiration and bradycardia, has been noted in infants with an ALTE. It is uncertain, however, whether apnea of central or of obstructive origin is more important in the genesis of SIDS. Difficulties in reconciling much of the reported data stem from arbitrary definitions of apnea and from absence of standards for the normal frequency and duration of respiration pauses (Sec. 9.31). In studies of a group of normal full-term infants during the first 4 mo of life, the mean duration of respiratory pauses (defined as durations of expiratory phase greater than average by 2 standard deviations or more) was 5–7 sec, and some lasted as long as 13 sec. Pauses were longer and less frequent in quiet sleep than in rapid eye movement (REM) sleep in these infants. In infants who experienced an ALTE, the pauses were not abnormal with respect either to frequency or to duration. None of the normal or high-risk infants studied had any apneic episode longer than 13 sec during the first 4 mo of life. In a prospective study of more than 9,000 infants, Southall did not observe respiratory pauses in those who subsequently died of SIDS that were longer than those seen in the survivors. In contrast, others have noted prolonged apneic periods (15 sec or longer) in study populations that have included prematurely born infants with apnea. In addition, transient decreases of the instantaneously recorded heart rate during sleep to approximately 70/min have been noted in both normal infants and those with an ALTE without cyanosis or other evidence of cardiorespiratory embarrassment.

Brain Stem Defects and Carotid Body Defects. Some evidence suggests that infants with SIDS have an abnormality in the CNS, presumably at the level of the brain stem: abnormalities in evoked auditory brain stem potentials have been observed in some infants with an ALTE; a higher than normal resting $Pa{CO_2}$ and a blunted ventilatory response to CO_2 have been found in a group of infants with an ALTE. However, the data with respect to ventilatory responsiveness are conflicting, other studies showing that responsiveness to CO_2 in infants with an ALTE is normal or increased. The observations that there are abnormalities in brain stem reactive astrocytes and delayed disappearance of dendritic spines in infants with SIDS have led some to suggest a defect in brain stem neural circuits that control respiratory or cardiac stability. Infants with markedly decreased responses to CO_2, especially during sleep, may have other disorders, such as failure of automatic control of ventilation or Ondine curse, that should not be confused with SIDS. Although previous studies have shown controversial results regarding hyperplasia of carotid glomus cells, more recent studies have demonstrated major differences in neurotransmitter levels of SIDS carotid bodies compared with age-matched controls: both dopamine and noradrenaline are much higher in SIDS than control carotid bodies. The integrity of carotid bodies in early life is important not only for O_2 responsiveness but also for survival, as some mammals die if deprived of the carotid body in early life.

Abnormal Upper Airway Function. Upper Airway Obstruction. The young infant may be vulnerable to upper airway obstruction for anatomic and developmental reasons, including posterior displacement of the tongue and decreased airway diameter following flexion of the neck. Vulnerability to airway obstruction may be enhanced by viral respiratory illnesses. Immature or abnormal neuromuscular control of the oropharyngeal muscle may also lead to airway obstruction. Patency of the upper airway may be maintained by muscles such as the genioglossus, the activation of which is coordinated with excitation of respiratory muscles; phase shifts in the contraction of these muscles could lead to upper airway obstruction, but it is not known whether this occurs in SIDS.

Hyperreactive Airway Reflexes. The laryngeal chemoreflex system, mediated through the superior laryngeal nerve, is capable of overriding central and peripheral respiratory drive mechanisms, and a number of studies are focusing on the maturation of this system in early life. Because the introduction of some fluids into the larynx can stimulate this reflex, presumably leading to apnea, gastroesophageal reflux with aspiration might be an underlying mechanism for SIDS in some infants. With massive reflux there are clear-cut episodes of apnea and severe bradycardia. Moreover, such episodes cease when feedings are thickened and the infants are kept continuously upright. On the other hand, the normal infant demonstrates gastroesophageal reflux at least up to 2 mo of age, and it is difficult, therefore, to know to what extent apneic episodes can be attributed to mild or moderate reflux.

Cardiac Abnormalities. Although electrical instability may be present in the young heart, there is no convincing evidence to indicate that cardiac arrhythmias play a role in SIDS. Southall's prospective study did not detect a difference between the infants who died of SIDS and the normal infants with respect to cardiac rhythm.

Findings in Infants Who Later Died of SIDS. Several infants who died subsequently of SIDS have been studied before death. Shannon found that such infants have abnormal heart rate variability, and Southall observed that some of the infants who died subsequently of SIDS had a greater number of episodes of tachycardia than age-matched normal full-term infants. In response to auditory stimuli one infant has shown greater than normal lability and poorer stabilization of cardiac rate.

Findings in Infants at High Risk for SIDS. Siblings of Infants with SIDS. Although one group of infant siblings of infants with SIDS was found to have an increased incidence and longer duration of periodic breathing in sleep than a control group, another group of siblings of victims with SIDS had an increased respiratory rate and a decreased incidence of breathing pauses in sleep; these latter siblings could not be differentiated from normal infants in terms of the frequency of long pauses (more than 10 sec). Siblings of victims with SIDS also have had a faster heart rate in early infancy than control infants, with a delay in the normal decrease in heart rate with age. Finally, siblings of infants with SIDS have had longer sleep cycles during both quiet and active or REM sleep before 12 wk of age compared with normal controls, raising the possibility of a higher arousal threshold.

Infants with an ALTE. In one group of infants with ALTE, detailed neurologic examination has revealed consistent abnormalities of muscle tone, particularly shoulder hypotonia in infants under 3 mo of age. Another group of 21 infants with ALTE (found to be unresponsive, cyanotic, and apneic, and having had mouth-to-mouth resuscitation) studied during the first 4 mo of life had, in comparison with normal infants, faster heart rates, less heart rate variability (both beat-to-beat and overall variability), shorter Q-T intervals even when corrected for the increased heart rate, and normal or increased ventilatory responses to elevated concentrations of inspired CO_2. Similar groups of infants with ALTE have had an increase in the frequency and duration of respiratory pauses on exposure to gases with low oxygen tension. Although the ventilatory or arousal responses to increased CO_2 or decreased O_2 have been proposed as potentially important mechanisms in SIDS, neither discriminates between the normal and the high risk for SIDS group.

Studies of the respiratory control mechanisms of parents of victims with SIDS have given conflicting results. Earlier studies suggested a significantly lower ventilatory response to CO_2 with or without the imposition of added resistance to breathing. More recent studies demonstrated normal responses to both hypercapnia and hypoxia, leading to the conclusion that parents of victims with SIDS have normal chemosensitivity and respiratory drive.

Differences in results among investigations of infants at risk for SIDS may be owing to differences in the techniques used to measure cardiorespiratory function, in the criteria used for patient selection and the populations studied, in the methods used to stage sleep, and in the sleep states of the infants who are studied.

Abnormal Autonomic Nervous System and Chemical Mediators. The increased heart rate and decreased heart rate variability, the smaller Q-T index, and the greater ventilatory response to CO_2 found in infants who have experienced an ALTE suggest that these infants have an abnormality in the autonomic nervous system, possibly an increase in sympathetic nervous activity. Consistent with this is the finding of increased levels of dopamine in the carotid bodies of infants who have died of SIDS; dopamine could inhibit carotid discharge, especially during hypoxia. Whether the hypothetical increase in sympathoadrenal activity is secondary to hypoxia or to some other stimulus is unknown. The possible roles of such chemical mediators as catecholamines, endorphins, and serotonin in cardiorespiratory function, in the response to such stresses as hypoxia and hypercapnia, and in the maturation of these responses during sleep represent important areas of research. Short-chain opioid peptides, such as β-casomorphine, cleaved and absorbed by a permeable gastrointestinal tract epithelium, have been hypothesized to be related to SIDS, possibly in infants with abnormal or immature autonomic nervous systems.

DIAGNOSIS. Some infants at risk for SIDS may have physiologic handicaps before birth. In the neonatal period they may demonstrate low Apgar scores and abnormalities in control of respiration, heart rate, and temperature, and they may have postnatal growth retardation. ALTE remains a diagnosis that can be made only by exclusion of such conditions as seizure disorders, other neurologic abnormalities, inborn errors of metabolism, hypoglycemia, cardiac anomalies and arrhythmias, vascular anomalies (especially vascular ring), massive gastroesophageal reflux, infantile botulism, and fulminant infection.

In suspected cases investigation should include (1) blood chemistries (serum glucose, Na, K, Cl, Ca, P, Mg, and BUN); (2) pH and blood gas analysis; (3) chest roentgenogram (including magnification films of the upper airways) and upper gastrointestinal study with barium swallow; (4) a 12-lead ECG and 12- to 24-hr ECG monitoring for rhythm analysis; (5) an electroencephalogram; and (6) esophageal pH studies made concomitantly with measurements of respiration. Four- to 8-hr sleep studies may prove useful in some cases, especially when ALTEs are suspected to occur during sleep.

HOME MONITORING OF HIGH-RISK INFANTS. As technology has improved and more parents have become informed about SIDS, their desire to monitor ventilation or heart rate has increased. This monitoring requires knowledge of the normal ranges during sleep of heart rate, of heart rate variability, of respiratory rate, and of frequency and duration of respiratory pauses so that infants most likely to benefit from monitoring can be identified.

Apnea monitors based on impedance may not detect complete airway obstruction as infants continue to make respiratory movements. Since serious apnea may be missed if only thoracoabdominal movements are monitored, monitoring of heart rate should also be included. It is unknown whether measuring heart rate and heart rate variability with a high degree of precision will increase the ability to detect the infant at high risk for SIDS.

There is little objective information available on which to base a decision about whether home monitoring is necessary or desirable or how long it should go on. The abilities of members of the household to handle monitors and to make the appropriate responses to true or false alarms are critical factors in the decision. When monitoring is used for infants thought to be at special risk after a thorough evaluation, parents should receive appropriate training in cardiopulmonary resuscitation and the proper use of the monitoring equipment. There should also be documentation of the monitoring, timely re-evaluation of the patient at least by 6 mo of age, supportive counseling, and planned termination of monitoring. Some think that home monitoring programs should not be independent from research evaluating the program and its effects.

Even if it were possible to prevent SIDS in all infants at high risk, some cases would occur among those not recognized as being at risk. For this reason, and because, by definition, death comes swiftly and without forewarning, psychologic and emotional support should be provided to all members of the family in cases of SIDS and confusion with child abuse should be avoided.

ROBERT B. MELLINS
GABRIEL G. HADDAD

Grethen JK, Schulman J, Croen LA: Sudden infant death syndrome among Asians in California. J Pediatr 116:525, 1990.
Haddad GG, Bazzy AR, Chang SL, et al: Heart rate pattern during respiratory pauses in normal infants during sleep. J Develop Physiol 6:329, 1984.
Haddad GG, Donnelly DF: Chemo-baroreceptors-brain stem interactions: Critical role in early life. *In:* The Sudden Infant Death Syndrome: Cardiorespiratory Mechanisms and Interventions. New York, New York Academy of Sciences, 1988, pp 221–227.
Haddad GG, Leistner HL, Lai TL, et al: Ventilation and ventilatory pattern during sleep in aborted sudden infant death syndrome. Pediatr Res 15:879, 1981.
Harper RM, Leake B, Hoffman H, et al: Periodicity of sleep states is altered in infants at risk for the sudden infant death syndrome. Science 213:1030, 1981.
Harper RM, Leake B, Hoppenbrouwers T, et al: Polygraphic studies of normal infants and infants at risk for the sudden infant death syndrome: Heart rate and heart rate variability as a function of state. Pediatr Res 12:778, 1978.
Kinney HC, Feliano JJ: Brain stem research in sudden infant death syndrome. Pediatrician 15:240, 1988.
Kraus SF, Greenland S, Bulterys M: Risk factors for sudden death syndrome in the U.S. Collaborative Perinatal Project. J Epidemiol 18:113, 1989.
Leistner HL, Haddad GG, Epstein RA, et al: Heart rate and heart rate variability during sleep in aborted sudden infant death syndrome. J Pediatr 97:51, 1980.
Lewis NC, McBride JT, Brooks JG: Ventilatory chemosensitivity in parents of infants with sudden infant death syndrome. J Pediatr 113:307, 1988.
Meadow R: Suffocation, recurrent apnea, and sudden infant death. J Pediatr 117:351, 1990.
Naeye RL: Pulmonary arterial abnormalities in the sudden infant death syndrome. N Engl J Med 289:1167, 1973.
Perrin DG, Becher LE, Madapallimatum A, et al: Sudden infant death syndrome: Increased carotid-body dopamine and noradrenalin content. Lancet 2:535, 1984.
Peterson DR, Sabotta EE, Daling JR: Infant mortality among subsequent siblings of infants who died of sudden infant death syndrome. J Pediatr 108:911, 1986.
Rognum TO, Saugstad OD: Hypoxanthine levels in vitreous humor: Evidence of hypoxia in most infants who die of sudden infant death syndrome. Pediatrics 87:306, 1991.
Shannon DC, Kelly DH: SIDS and near-SIDS. N Engl J Med 306:959, 1022, 1982.
Southall DP, Richards JM, de Swiet D, et al: Identification of infants destined to die during infancy; evaluation of predictive importance of prolonged apnea and disorders of cardiac rhythm or conduction: First report of a multicentered prospective study into the sudden infant death syndrome. Br Med J 286:1092, 1983.
Steinschneider A: Prolonged apnea and the sudden infant death syndrome: Clinical and laboratory observations. Pediatrics 50:646, 1972.
Valdes-Dapena MA: Sudden infant death syndrome: Overview of recent research developments from a pediatric pathologist's perspective. Pediatrician 15:222, 1988.
Waggener TB, Southall DP, Scott LA: Analysis of breathing patterns in a prospective population of term infants does not predict susceptibility to sudden infant death syndrome. Pediatr Res 27:113, 1990.
Williams A, Vawter G, Reid L: Increased muscularity of the pulmonary circulation in victims of sudden infant death. Pediatrics 63:18, 1979.

25.2 AMYLOID DISEASES

DEFINITION AND CLASSIFICATION. The amyloid diseases include a number of entities of diverse etiology having in common the extracellular deposition of a proteinaceous fibrillar material that interferes with organ function.

The underlying mechanisms of local or systemic deposition may be inflammatory, hereditary, or neoplastic, and the clinical manifestations of amyloidosis depend on the site and the amount of deposited amyloid. Classification is based on the clinical features of the amyloid diseases and on the chemical characterization of the deposited fibrils.

Amyloidosis (AL) or deposition of light chain-related amyloid is the most common form in adults and either represents primary amyloid disease or associated myeloma and related plasma cell dyscrasias. It has also been identified in agammaglobulinemia. A variety of secondary forms also occur exclusively in adults (e.g., senile, hemodialysis associated). Table 25–1 indicates the spectrum of disorders that may occur in childhood. With the exception of cystic fibrosis and *familial Mediterranean fever* (FMF) (autosomal recessive), the other familial disorders appear to be autosomal dominants.

ETIOLOGY AND PATHOGENESIS. Significant insight into the complexity of these diseases has come with recognition of their heterogeneity and the elucidation of the nature of some of the amyloid fibrils. All deposited amyloid appears homogeneous and eosinophilic with conventional staining techniques, emits an apple-green fluorescence when stained with Congo red under polarized light, and by electron microscopy contains two discrete components. The major fibrillar component has a characteristic periodicity, and the minor rod-like or P component (pentamer with a hollow core) appears to be physically and chemically identical in all amyloids. The latter also circulates as a soluble serum protein whose role in tissue infiltration is not established. The deposited fibril, which has an x-ray diffusion pattern of a β-pleated sheet, is used as the basis of the chemical classification of the various disorders (e.g., AA, AL, thyroxine-binding prealbumin).

It appears that all deposited amyloid fibrils have a soluble precursor and that when there is a pathologic deposition, either the amount of precursor is increased or more of it becomes insoluble through unknown mechanisms.

Because the nature of the associated disorders varies with the amyloid protein subunits, it is necessary to consider the pathogenesis of the major types of amyloid individually. Some researchers suggest disordered functioning of the immune system in the pathogenesis of AL; others consider all types of AL as being the result primarily of the overproduction of normal or, perhaps in some cases, an unusual "amyloidogenic" protein.

In the AA type of amyloid, the AA protein appears to be derived by proteolysis from a serum AA protein (SAA), which circulates complexed to a high-density lipoprotein. It has also been found complexed to albumin. SAA behaves like an acute phase protein rising and then falling with the onset and resolution of inflammation. Its synthesis is stimulated by interleukin 1.

Even though proteolysis of the amyloid precursors seems to play a role in the deposition of the fibrils, when once formed they resist phagocytosis and proteolytic degradation. The body has few mechanisms to remove these deposits, a factor that may well account for the generally relentless progression of the diseases.

INCIDENCE. AL is a rare disease among children. Primary disease associated with myeloma or plasma cell dyscrasias has not been reported. Among the diseases giving rise to AA (secondary) AL in children are rheumatoid arthritis, regional ileitis, cystic fibrosis, and, on rare occasions, chronic suppurative disorders. Among children in the United States with juvenile rheumatoid arthritis, the frequency of AL is low; for unknown reasons it is more common in certain European countries. Regional ileitis is more frequently complicated by AL than ulcerative colitis. AL in children is rarely associated with Hodgkin disease and renal carcinoma. In young adults AL is being seen with increased frequency as a consequence of the suppurative and infectious complications of drug addiction. In developing countries endemic infectious diseases such as leprosy and malaria may give rise to secondary AL.

TABLE 25–1. Amyloid Diseases in Children and Youth

Clinical Syndrome	Fibril Precursor	Fibril	Onset (Yr)	Features
Secondary* (AA)	SSA	AA	Variable	Kidney, liver, spleen esp. Tbc, osteomyelitis
Chronic infections				
Juvenile rheumatoid disease				
Inflammatory bowel disease				
Behçet disease				
Hodgkin disease				
Substance abuse†				
Cystic fibrosis‡	SSA	AA	Variable	Pulmonary disease
Familial (AF§)				
Portuguese-Japanese (FAP type I)	TBPA(TT)	TBPA(TT)	20–40	Neuropathic (lower extremities, autonomic) cerebellar signs
Iowa (FAP type III)	Unknown	Unknown Apolipoprotein A1	20–40	Neuropathic and renal (upper and lower extremities, autonomic)
Israel (FAP type II)	Unknown	Unknown	20's	Neuropathic (upper and lower extremities, autonomic)
Familial Mediterranean fever (FMF)	SAA	AA	10–30	Inflammatory serositis, nephropathy
Derbyshire, England	Unknown	Unknown	10–30	Deafness, urticaria, fever, renal disease
Iceland	Cystatin C‖	Cystatin C	20–40	Cerebral hemorrhage

*Inflammation associated.
†Intravenous or subcutaneous foreign substances.
‡Probably secondary to a combination of chronic pulmonary infection and the basic pathophysiology of cystic fibrosis.
§Familial amyloid fibrils are identified by the notation AF with the country of origin indicated by a subscript initial.
‖Cystatin C is an abnormal lysosomal proteinase inhibitor formally known as γ-trace.
AF = amyloid fibril; FAP = familial amyloidotic polyneuropathy; SAA = serum AA; TBPA = thyroxine-binding prealbumin; TT = transthyretin.

Some of the rare familial forms of AL, especially those associated with FMF (most common among Sephardic Jews) as well as the Portuguese type, can affect children. The localized forms of AL, such as those involving the skin, are rare in children.

CLINICAL MANIFESTATIONS. The clinical features of all types of AL arise from the infiltration of tissues by amyloid deposits, with the ultimate destruction of the affected organs. Symptoms depend on the tissues involved; particularly when the liver, kidney, or heart is affected, functional impairment may lead to death. In certain localized forms of AL, for example, the cutaneous ones, the disease remains limited; otherwise it tends to be progressive, and even with control or treatment of the underlying disease significant regression is rare. An exception is FMF, the AL of which often improves with the administration of colchicine.

Secondary (AA) AL occurs with underlying disorders that are usually severe and protracted; sometimes, however, amyloid deposits appear rapidly or with mild disease. In secondary AL, deposits occur predominantly in the kidneys, spleen, liver, and adrenals and rarely involve the heart, musculoskeletal, nervous, or gastrointestinal systems. Since amyloid in the kidney is deposited primarily in the glomeruli, the major manifestations are proteinuria, hyposthenuria, and hematuria; as the disease progresses, the nephrotic syndrome and ultimately renal failure make their appearance and, if left untreated, lead to death. Renal vein thrombosis is a common complication; hypertension is rare.

Hepatic and splenic enlargements may be massive but are generally asymptomatic or give rise only to abdominal discomfort, because liver function is usually not significantly impaired. Tests of liver function may be only minimally altered, with increased hepatic alkaline phosphatase activity and Bromsulphalein retention, with or without increased transaminase activities. Intrahepatic cholestasis with elevated bilirubin concentration may occur.

Amyloid deposition is common in older patients with cystic fibrosis; deposits are found principally in the spleen, liver, and kidneys and are localized mainly in blood vessels. As the life span of these patients continues to increase, AL may become a clinical complication of this disorder.

There are many familial forms of AL, each with characteristic clinical features and often with unique geographic distribution. Because of the variety and rarity of these forms, the review by Andrade and associates should be consulted for a complete clinical description. Table 25–1 summarizes the salient features of the most common hereditary types affecting children and adolescents. Several have prominent neuropathic components in addition to marked visceral involvement.

Probably the most common and widespread of the familial forms of AL is associated with FMF in Sephardic Jews and certain other ethnic groups of the Middle East. It has also been recognized rarely in patients of Anglo-Saxon or northern European origins. FMF is a recurrent inflammatory disease of unknown etiology characterized by acute self-limited episodes (24–48 hr) of fever accompanied by abdominal, chest, or joint pains and often a transient erythematous rash. In most patients, clinical manifestations begin at 5–15 yr, but the disease may start in infancy. Acute attacks occur usually 1–2 times a month, but the frequency varies greatly and the duration of an episode may be for as long as 1 week. A variety of forms of serositis occur, but peritonitis, pleuritis, and arthritis are the most common types. AL is the most serious complication and is usually manifest as a relentless progression of renal failure and death, which may occur during childhood. The appearance of AL is not related to the frequency or severity of attacks and may precede their onset.

Independent inheritance of FMF and AL is suggested by the appearance in certain individuals and families of AL as the first or sole clinical manifestation of the syndrome.

The diagnosis of FMF is based on the typical clinical features in the proper familial setting. Laboratory findings are nonspecific. Leukocytosis and increased erythrocyte sedimentation rate and acute phase reactants occur during acute attacks. A variant of FMF has been reported in which patients have high serum IgD levels and large numbers of plasma cells with cytoplasmic IgD in the bone marrow.

The AL of FMF is unique in that its appearance can be delayed or prevented and the deposits made to regress by the administration of colchicine, 0.5 mg 1–3 times/day, a regimen that also aborts the febrile attacks. Recurrence of clinical manifestations may occur when the drug is discontinued. Since colchicine can produce chromosomal alterations and azoospermia, it should be used with caution in children and in adults in their reproductive period. To date, however, no fetal abnormalities have been attributed to the drug.

DIAGNOSIS. AL can be suspected clinically, but histologic studies are needed to establish the diagnosis. Ideally, biopsy is made of a clinically involved organ, but if biopsy of an affected organ is not advisable, rectal or gingival biopsy will yield positive results in more than 90% of cases even when the rectum or gums are not obviously clinically involved. However, a positive result on a rectal biopsy does not necessarily prove that renal or hepatic dysfunction is due to AL; the patients may have another associated disease.

In the differential diagnosis other causes of nephrotic syndrome must be ruled out when renal involvement is prominent or other causes of hepatosplenomegaly must be ruled out when there is significant liver involvement.

TREATMENT. With the exception of the AL associated with FMF, there is no effective treatment for AL because the material resists resorption. However, treatment of the underlying disease may halt progression and perhaps may also achieve some spontaneous resorption. In the AA protein type, eradication of a septic focus may be of help. Although the administration of colchicine may be effective in FMF, it has been disappointing in the treatment of the other types. Use of dimethyl sulfoxide, usually with concurrent alkylating agent therapy, has occasionally benefited these patients. The renal manifestations can be managed by dialysis and, if necessary, transplantation, which has been about as effective as in other types of renal failure. Amyloid has been found to involve transplanted kidneys after periods of 5–10 yr.

PROGNOSIS. In the absence of effective therapy the systemic forms of AL tend to be progressive and result in death in 1–5 yr, most often from renal failure or sepsis. The course can be slowed by dialysis or transplantation. The prognosis for many children with FMF treated with colchicine is good to excellent in the absence of renal disease.

RICHARD E. BEHRMAN

Andrade C, Araki S, Block WD, et al: Hereditary amyloidosis. Arthritis Rheum 13:902, 1970.

Benson MD: Hereditary amyloidosis: Disease entity and clinical model. Hosp Pract 23:165, 1988.

Breathmach SM: Amyloid and amyloidosis. Am Acad Dermatol 18:1, 1988.

Castile R, Schwachman H, Travis W, et al: Amyloidosis as a complication of cystic fibrosis. Am J Dis Child 139:728, 1985.

Cohen AS, Conners LH: The pathogenesis and biochemistry of amyloidosis. J Pathol 151:1, 1987.

Filipowicz-Sosnowski AM, Roztropowicz-Densiewicz K, Rosenthal CJ, et al: The amyloidosis of juvenile rheumatoid arthritis—comparative studies in Polish and American children. Arthritis Rheum 21:699, 1978.

Hauser WA: New frontiers in the study of amyloidosis. N Engl J Med 323:542, 1990.

Hawkins PN: Amyloidosis. Blood Rev 2:270, 1988.

Hawkins PN, Lavender JP, Myers MJ, et al: Diagnostic radionuclide imaging of amyloid. Lancet 1:1413, 1988.

Hawkins PN, Lavender JP, Pepys MB: Evaluation of systemic amyloidosis by scintigriphy with ^{123}I-labeled serum amyloid P component. N Engl J Med 323:508, 1990.

Levy M, Eliakim M: Long-term colchicine prophylaxis in familial mediterranean fever. Br Med J 2:808, 1977.
Majeed HA, Carroll JE, Khuffash FA, et al: Long-term colchicine prophylaxis in children with familial Mediterranean fever (recurrent hereditary polyserositis). J Pediatr 116:997, 1990.
McGlennen RC, Burke BA, Dehner LP: Systemic amyloidosis complicating cystic fibrosis: A retrospective pathologic study. Arch Pathol Lab Med 110:879, 1986.
Skinner M, Pinnette A, Travis WD, et al: Isolation and sequence analyses of amyloid protein AA from a patient with cystic fibrosis. J Lab Clin Med 112:413, 1988.
Van Der Meer JWM, Radl J, Meyer CJLM, et al: Hyperimmunoglobulinemia D and periodic fever: A new syndrome. Lancet 1:1087, 1984.

25.3 SARCOIDOSIS

Sarcoidosis, a chronic, multisystem, granulomatous disease of unknown etiology, occurs most frequently in young adults but can occur during childhood. The initial clinical presentation is extremely variable depending on the organ systems involved but in most pediatric cases includes weight loss, cough, fatigue, bone and joint pain, and anemia. Definitive diagnosis requires demonstration of the characteristic noncaseating, granulomatous lesions in an appropriate biopsy. The granulomas in sarcoidosis resemble those caused by microbial agents (e.g., mycobacteria and fungi) or by hypersensitivity to organic agents. These similarities have led to the speculation that microbes or organic dusts may be inciting agents. However, despite extensive studies, the etiology remains obscure.

Epidemiologic studies indicate that sarcoidosis is particularly prevalent in the southeastern United States and occurs more frequently in blacks than in whites. Familial clustering of this disease has been observed and suggests a genetic predisposition; however, the mode of inheritance is unclear.

The granulomatous lesions of sarcoidosis may occur in almost any organ of the body. Typically, the granulomas are not necrotic and contain epithelioid cells, macrophages, and giant cells in the center surrounded by a mixture of monocytes, lymphocytes, and fibroblasts. Activated lymphocytes and macrophages within the granulomas release a variety of mediators, such as interleukin 1, interleukin 2, interferon, and other cytokines, that are thought to promote and maintain granulomatous lesions. During active disease, lymphocytes in and around the granulomas are predominantly helper T lymphocytes; as the lesions resolve, the T lymphocytes decrease in number and shift to predominantly suppressor cells. These lesions usually heal with complete preservation of the parenchyma; however, in approximately 20% of the lesions, fibroblasts proliferate at the periphery of the granuloma and may produce fibrotic scar tissue.

The lung is the most frequently affected organ; pulmonary involvement is variable in its extent and characteristics. Parenchymal infiltrates, miliary nodules, and hilar and paratracheal lymphadenopathy (Fig. 25–1) occur. Pulmonary function tests primarily show restrictive changes. Peripheral lymphadenopathy, eye changes consisting of uveitis or iritis, skin lesions, and hepatic involvement occur frequently. The clinical manifestations of sarcoidosis in the older child are different from those of the very young, which consist of a maculopapular erythematous rash, uveitis, and arthritis; pulmonary changes are minimal. The arthritis, which can be confused with rheumatoid arthritis, produces large, painless, boggy synovial effusions of the tendon sheaths; there is little limitation of motion.

There are no specific diagnostic tests. An elevated erythrocyte sedimentation rate, hyperproteinemia, hypercalcemia, hypercalciuria, eosinophilia, and an elevated angiotensin-converting enzyme level are common. The Kveim test, consisting of intradermal injection of material from a sarcoid lesion and observation for the formation of a granuloma several weeks later, is used infrequently for diagnosis because of difficulty in obtaining a standardized test material and reports of varying sensitivity and specificity of the test. Biopsy of tissue from affected areas is the most valuable diagnostic measure. Significant eye disease and renal damage from hypercalciuria can occur without symptoms; therefore, all patients with sarcoidosis should be evaluated at the initial presentation and monitored at regular intervals for evidence of ocular disease and hypercalciuria.

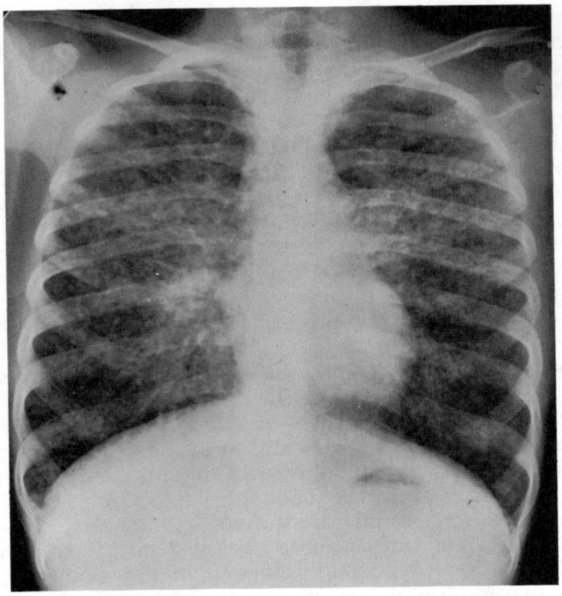

Figure 25–1. Sarcoidosis in a white 10-yr-old girl. There are widely disseminated peribronchial infiltrations, multiple small nodular densities, overaeration of the lungs, and hilar adenopathy.

Because of its protean manifestations, the differential diagnosis of sarcoidosis is extremely broad; it includes tuberculosis, the various pulmonary mycoses, lymphoma, and inflammatory ocular lesions such as phlyctenular conjunctivitis.

Treatment is symptomatic and supportive. Adrenal corticosteroids may suppress the acute manifestations, especially the inflammatory ocular lesions, progressive pulmonary disease, and the hypercalcemia/hypercalciuria. Pulmonary function tests are useful in following the progress of lung involvement, and angiotensin-converting enzyme levels have been shown to correlate with disease activity.

The prognosis and natural history of sarcoidosis in children are uncertain. Spontaneous recovery may occur after a prolonged illness of several months to several years, or the condition may be very chronic, involving progressive lung disease. Eye involvement may lead to blindness.

MARGARET W. LEIGH

Bresnitz EA, Strom BL: Epidemiology of sarcoidosis. Epidemiol Rev 5:124, 1983.
Hetherington S: Sarcoidosis in young children. Am J Dis Child 136:13, 1982.
Kendig EL: Sarcoidosis. *In:* Kendig EL, Chernick V (eds): Disorders of the Respiratory Tract in Children. 4th ed. Philadelphia, WB Saunders, 1983, p 710.
Pattishall EN, Strope GL, Denny FW: Pulmonary function in children with sarcoidosis. Am Rev Respir Dis 133:94, 1986.
Pattishall EN, Strope GL, Spinola SM, et al: Childhood sarcoidosis. J Pediatr 108:169, 1986.
Thomas PD, Hunninghake GW: Current concepts of the pathogenesis of sarcoidosis. Am Rev Respir Dis 135:747, 1987.

25.4 PROGERIA

The Hutchinson-Gilford progeria syndrome was first described in 1886. Since then there have been more than 100 patients with this condition. It has occurred on all continents and in all races of people. This condition may be an autosomal dominant trait. It has occurred in one of a twin pair and in two sets of identical twins. Paternal age is also increased significantly.

Children with progeria are usually considered to be normal in early infancy, but manifestations such as "scleroderma," midfacial cyanosis, and "sculptured nose" may suggest the existence of the syndrome at birth. Profound growth failure occurs during the 1st year of life. The characteristic facies, alopecia, loss of subcutaneous fat, abnormal posture, stiffness of joints, and bone and skin changes become apparent during the 2nd year (Fig. 25–2). Motor and mental development are normal.

Features almost *always* present when the condition has become apparent are short stature; weight distinctly low for height; failure to complete sexual maturation; diminished subcutaneous fat; head disproportionately large for face; micrognathia; prominent scalp veins; generalized alopecia; prominent eyes; "plucked-bird appearance"; delayed and abnormal dentition; pyriform thorax; short, dystrophic clavicles; "horse-riding" stance; wide-based shuffling gait; and coxa valga, thin limbs, and prominent, stiff joints.

Features *frequently* present are skin that is thin, taut, dry, wrinkled, brown-spotted in various areas, or "sclerodermatous" over the lower abdomen, proximal thighs, and buttocks; prominent superficial veins; loss of eyebrows and eyelashes; persistently patent anterior fontanel; "sculptured," beaked nasal tip; faint nasolabial cyanosis; thin lips; protruding ears; absence of ear lobes; thin, high-pitched voice; dystrophic nails; and progressive radiolucency of terminal phalanges.

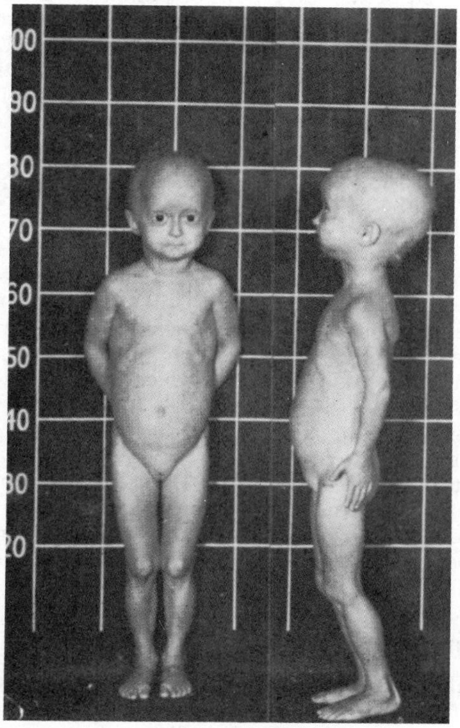

Figure 25–2. A 4.5-yr-old girl with height age of 1.75 yr and bone age of 4 yr. (From Wilkins L: Diagnosis and Treatment of Endocrine Disorders in Childhood and Adolescence, 3rd ed, 1965. Courtesy of Charles C Thomas, Publisher, Springfield, Illinois.)

Insulin resistance, abnormal collagen, increased metabolic rate, and variable abnormalities of serum lipids are found, but there are no demonstrable abnormalities of thyroid, parathyroid, pituitary, or adrenal function. Growth hormone responses are normal. Studies of cultured skin fibroblasts show reduced replicative life spans, increased fractions of heat-labile cellular enzymes, and increased tissue procoagulant activity. Increased hyaluronic acid has been noted in the urine of all patients tested.

Progeric patients ordinarily develop atherosclerosis and die of cardiac or cerebral vascular disease between 7 and 27 yr of age, with a median age of 13.4 yr at death. One patient from Japan died at the age of 40. Many features associated with normal aging such as cataracts, presbycusis, presbyopia, arcus senilis, osteoarthritis, or senile personality changes are not found.

No effective treatment for this condition exists, but physiotherapy has been effective in preventing contractures. Whether or not low doses of acetylsalicylic acid would delay vascular obstructions is not known. There are now support groups for the families of children with progeria, and a Progeria Registry now exists, which may help to better define the incidence and genetic basis of the disorder.

FRANKLIN L. DeBUSK

Brown TW: Personal communications.
DeBusk FL: The Hutchinson-Gilford progeria syndrome. J Pediatr 80:697, 1972.
Goldstein S: Studies on age-related diseases in cultured skin fibroblasts. J Invest Dermatol 73:19, 1979.

25.5 HISTIOCYTOSIS SYNDROMES IN CHILDHOOD

The childhood histiocytoses constitute a rare and diverse group of disorders. An international group, The Histiocyte Society, has proposed a system for the classification of the childhood histiocytoses that includes the syndromes grouped formerly as "histiocytosis X" (i.e., Hand-Schüller-Christian disease, eosinophilic granuloma, and Letterer-Siwe disease). These disorders are now called Langerhans cell histiocytoses (LCH) (Table 25–2). Although the diagnosis and treatment of these disorders are frequently the province of the pediatric oncologist, the majority of the LCH are not thought to be malignant. In classes I and II histiocytosis, the cellular infiltrate is thought to be the result of an uncontrolled reaction of a normal antigen-processing cell. The rarity of the histiocytoses has prevented epidemiologic studies. The only form that has a genetic component is familial erythrophagocytic lymphohistiocytosis.

Pathology. Grossly, the lesions of class I histiocytosis (LCH) are granulomatous and, when visible, they are yellow-brown. The hallmark of these lesions is the presence of Langerhans cells by light microscopy. These cells have deeply indented nuclei and low nuclear/cytoplasmic ratios as well as the characteristic, tennis racket-shaped Birbeck granules seen on electron microscopy. The lesions of LCH may consist of either pure histiocytic infiltrate or mixed histiocytic, eosinophilic lesions.

The class II histiocytoses represent the largest group of disorders and include the nonmalignant histiocytoses in which the accumulating mononuclear cell is of the phagocytic (antigen-processing) type. This contrasts with the class I diseases in which the reactive process involves the antigen-presenting or dendritic cell type. Characteristic findings on lymph node biopsy include infiltration of the node without

TABLE 25–2. Classification of Childhood Histiocytoses

Class I	Class II	Class III
	Diseases Included	
Langerhans cell histiocytosis	Infection-associated hemophagocytic syndrome (IAHS) Familial erythrophagocytic lymphohistiocytosis (FEL)	Malignant histiocytosis Acute monocytic leukemia True histiocytic lymphoma
	Cellular Characteristics of the Lesions	
Langerhans cells with Birbeck granules	Morphologically normal reactive macrophages with prominent erythrophagocytosis	Neoplastic cellular proliferation of cells with macrophages or their precursors

effacement of nodal architecture by cytologically normal-appearing activated histiocytes. Striking erythrophagocytosis (and in fact phagocytosis of all cellular blood elements) is characteristic of both *infection-associated hemophagocytic syndrome* (IAHS) and *familial erythrophagocytic lymphohistiocytosis* (FEL). Other rare class II histiocytoses may enter into the differential diagnosis of lymphadenopathy or skin lesions in which histiocytic infiltration is prominent.

CLASS I HISTIOCYTOSES

Clinical Manifestations. The LCH have an extremely variable presentation. *The skeleton* is involved in 80% of patients and may be the only affected site in the child over 5 yr of age. Lesions may be single or multiple and are seen most commonly in the skull (Fig. 25–3). They may be asymptomatic or associated with pain and local swelling. Involvement of the spine may result in collapse of the vertebral body, which can be seen roentgenographically and may result in secondary compression of the spinal cord. In flat and long bones, osteolytic lesions with sharp borders occur and there is no evidence of reactive new bone formation. These lesions will not usually have positive uptake on a ^{99}Tc diphosphonate bone scan. Lesions involving weight-bearing long bones may result in pathologic fractures. Chronically draining, infected ears are commonly associated with destruction in the mastoid area. Bony destruction of the mandible and maxilla may result in teeth that on roentgenograms appear to be floating free. With response to therapy, there may be complete healing.

Skin involvement occurs in about one half of the patients at some time during their course (usually a seborrheic dermatitis of the scalp). The lesions may spread to involve the back, palms, and soles. The exanthem may be petechial or hemorrhagic, even in the absence of thrombocytopenia.

Localized or disseminated *lymphadenopathy* is present in approximately 33% of patients. *Hepatosplenomegaly* occurs in approximately 20%. Various degrees of hepatic malfunction may occur, including jaundice and ascites.

Exophthalmos, when present, is often bilateral and is caused by retro-orbital accumulation of granulomatous tissue. *Gingival* mucous membranes may be involved with infiltrative lesions that appear superficially like candidiasis. In 10–15% of patients, *pulmonary* infiltrates are found on roentgenograms. The lesions may vary from diffuse fibrosis and disseminated nodular infiltrates to diffuse cystic changes. Rarely, pneumothorax may be a complication. If the lungs are severely involved, tachypnea and progressive respiratory failure may result.

Pituitary dysfunction or hypothalamic involvement may result in growth retardation. In addition, there may be diabetes insipidus; patients suspected of having LCH should demonstrate the ability to concentrate their urine before going to the operating room for a biopsy. Rarely, panhypopituitarism may occur. Other symptomatic involvement of the CNS is uncommon but may be serious; histiocytes can be demonstrated in the cerebrospinal fluid when neurologic disease is present.

Patients who are affected more severely may have *systemic manifestations,* including fever, weight loss, malaise, irritability, and failure to thrive. Bone marrow involvement may cause anemia and thrombocytopenia.

Diagnosis. Tissue biopsy is diagnostic. Skin lesions, when present, are the easiest site from which to obtain the diagnosis. Roentgenograms of the entire skeleton should be performed to assess the degree of bone involvement, and a computed tomography (CT) scan of the chest should be obtained to assess the pulmonary status. Liver function should be measured because hepatic infiltration may result in intrahepatic bile duct obstruction with superimposed parenchymal damage. Blood counts should be followed and bone marrow should be assessed if counts are low.

Treatment. For patients with localized bony disease, curettage may be curative, but a full evaluation of the extent of the disease should be performed. For patients with disseminated and progressive disease, treatment programs incorporate a variety of cancer chemotherapeutic agents, including prednisone, etoposide, methotrexate, cyclophosphamide, and vinblastine. Approximately 50% of patients will have some response to chemotherapy, and combination regimens have been tried. Current therapeutic investigations include administration of biologic response modifiers such as thymic factors.

Prognosis. Impaired organ function is the most important prognostic factor. Approximately 40% of patients show organ dysfunction: hematopoietic (36%), hepatic (10%), and pulmonary (5%). Patients who are over 2 yr of age and have no evidence of organ dysfunction have a good prognosis; approximately 90% of these children survive for 5 yr. Those who are less than 2 yr at diagnosis and have no organ dysfunction have an intermediate prognosis; about 65% of these children survive for 5 yr. Patients who have organ involvement, regardless of age, have the worst prognosis; approximately 45% of these children survive for 5 yr. In an evaluation of patients who had survived for 5 yr, it was found that at least one half had active disease during the 5-yr period. This disease can come and go without therapy over a period of decades. Of the long-term survivors, about one half have significant functional impairment. Diabetes insipidus, growth failure, intellectual impairment, or other neurologic deficits are the most common findings, although chronic lung disease is the most severe problem and is the cause of most of the late deaths.

CLASS II HISTIOCYTOSES

Familial Erythrophagocytic Lymphohistiocytosis (FEL). FEL is characterized by the presence of hemophagocytosis and a positive family history. This disease is rare and is almost always rapidly fatal, with an autosomal recessive pattern of inheritance. Affected children, usually under 3–4 yr at the time of diagnosis, present most often with a fever of unknown

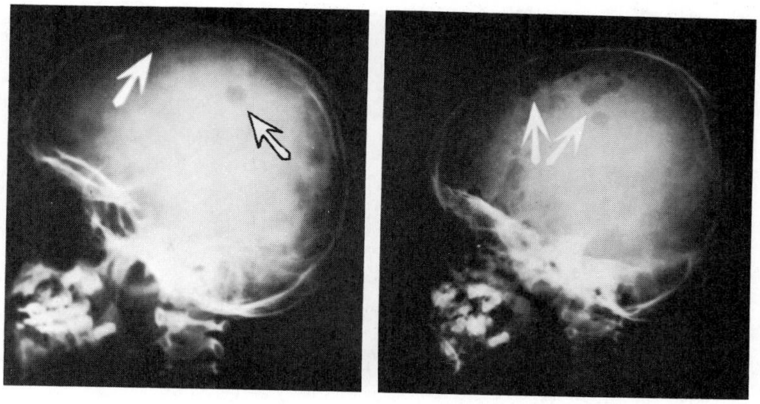

Figure 25–3. Two skull roentgenograms from patients with LCH. The patient on the left was over 2 yr of age and had involvement limited to isolated bone lesions. She had a good recovery. The patient on the right was under 2 yr of age and had extensive bone disease, febrile course, anemia, severe skin eruption, generalized adenopathy, hepatosplenomegaly, pulmonary infiltration, and a fatal outcome despite antitumor chemotherapy. These patients represent opposite ends of the clinical spectrum of LCH.

origin and weight loss. They may have hepatosplenomegaly and a maculopapular skin eruption. The CNS may be involved (e.g., aseptic meningitis).

The diagnosis of FEL rests on the identification of a lymphohistiocytic infiltrate, often with very marked erythrophagocytosis, together with an appropriate clinical and family history. The diagnosis may be made from an examination of the lymph nodes, spleen, liver, bone marrow, or lungs. Because this disease usually has a fulminant downhill course, cytotoxic chemotherapy has been employed in its treatment, but no definitive therapy has been established.

Infection-Associated Hemophagocytic Syndrome (IAHS). IAHS has been reported in association with a variety of infections including viral (EBV, CMV), bacterial, fungal, and parasitic, usually in the setting of immunodeficiency. The clinical symptoms are similar to FEL and include fever and other constitutional symptoms, liver function and coagulation abnormalities, and anemia. If the diagnosis is made in a setting of iatrogenic immunodeficiency, immunosuppressive treatment should be withdrawn and supportive care should be instituted along with specific therapy for underlying infection.

CLASS III HISTIOCYTOSES

These disorders are characterized and treated consistent with the type of malignancy that they manifest (see Chapter 17).

BRIGID LEVENTHAL

Berry DH, Gresik MV, Humphrey GB, et al: Natural history of histiocytosis X: A POG study. Med Pediatr Oncol 14:1, 1986.
Henter J, Elenden G: Familial hemophagocytic lymphohistiocytosis. Acta Paediatr 80:269, 1991.
Lahey ME: Histiocytosis X: An analysis of prognostic factors. J Pediatr 87:184, 1975.
Lichtenstein L: Histiocytosis X: Integration of eosinophilic granuloma of bone, Letterer-Siwe disease and Schüller-Christian disease as related manifestations of a single nosologic entity. Arch Pathol 56:84, 1953.
Komp DM, El Mahdi A, Starling KA, et al: Quality of survival in histiocytosis X: A Southwest Oncology Group study. Med Pediatr Oncol 8:35, 1980.
Komp DM, Herson J, Starling KA, et al: Staging system for histiocytosis X: A Southwest Oncology Group study. Cancer 47:798, 1981.
Writing group of the Histiocyte Society: Histiocytosis syndromes in childhood. Lancet 1:208, 1987.

25.6 HEMORRHAGIC SHOCK AND ENCEPHALOPATHY

This syndrome of unknown etiology is characterized by a prodromal illness of vomiting, diarrhea, listlessness, and fever, leading to profound circulatory collapse, signs of encephalopathy, acidosis, often disseminated intravascular coagulopathy, and signs of impaired hepatic and renal function. The onset of illness is sudden in previously well children usually less than 1 yr of age, but the syndrome has occurred as late as 14 yr. The prodrome usually lasts for 1–2 days, but occasionally there is no prodrome. Clinical manifestations include signs of shock, often resistant to volume correction; seizures, coma, and hypotonia followed by decerebrate posturing, spasticity, and signs of increased intracranial pressure; hyperpyrexia; watery or bloody diarrhea; petechiae and bleeding from the respiratory tract or venipuncture sites; and hepatomegaly. Laboratory studies reveal severe metabolic acidosis; markedly deranged clotting studies with subsequent thrombocytopenia and anemia; elevated blood urea, creatinine, transaminases, and bilirubin; and occasionally mild hypernatremia. Bacterial, viral, and toxicologic investigations have been negative. Decreased plasma α_1 antitrypsin and α_2 antitrypsin and increased levels of circulating proteolytic enzymes suggest a defect in protease inhibitor production or release may be involved in the pathogenesis. Mortality and central nervous system morbidity are high, despite intensive treatment of shock, elevated intracranial pressure, bleeding, and acidosis. At autopsy brains are edematous and soft to liquid in consistency, intestines have mucosal and submucosal hemorrhages and inflammatory infiltrates, and the liver has patchy swelling and degeneration of hepatocytes without fatty or other changes suggesting Reye syndrome. The differential diagnosis includes septicemia, viremia, Reye syndrome, toxic shock and other toxin-induced diseases, heat stroke, viral hemorrhage fevers, and poisonings.

RICHARD E. BEHRMAN

Levin M, Kay JDS, Gould JD, et al: Haemorrhagic shock and encephalopathy: A new syndrome with high mortality in young children. Lancet 2:64, 1983.
Levin M, Pincott JR, Hjelm M, et al: Hemorrhagic shock and encephalopathy: Clinical, pathologic, and biochemical features. J Pediatr 114:194, 1989.
Sofer S, Phillip M, Hershkowits J, et al: Hemorrhagic shock and encephalopathy syndrome. Its association with hyperthermia. AJDC 140:1252, 1986.
Whittington LK, Roscelli JD, Parry Wh: Hemorrhagic shock and encephalopathy: Further description of a new syndrome. J Pediatr 106:599, 1985.

26

ENVIRONMENTAL HEALTH HAZARDS

26.1 RADIATION INJURY

The possibility of untoward biologic effects of radiation is of special interest in pediatrics since these effects may be most serious in growing tissues. By judicious limitation of roentgenic procedures during childhood a margin of safety for unavoidable radiation exposure later in life can be preserved (Sec. 6.56).

Ionizing radiation produces injury in the same manner regardless of the type of particle or ray emitted. The variation is quantitative rather than qualitative. Absorption of energy may cause molecules in the path of the radiations to become ionized. In attaining stability these molecules may form substances that alter, temporarily or perhaps permanently, biochemical processes within the cell or its environment. These effects on cellular structures result in the deaths of persons exposed to ionizing radiation, the death of certain cancer cells treated with roentgen rays, genetic mutations, and the production of cancer as a late effect of exposures to radiation.

Susceptibility of tissues to roentgen rays is generally greater in rapidly mitosing and in undifferentiated cells. Because of an abundance of this type of tissue in the abdomen, a patient is more likely to have radiation sickness from roentgen therapy to this region than from comparable exposure elsewhere.

DOSAGE FACTORS. Radiation absorption increases with the volume of the child's body exposed, with prolongation of exposure, or with an increase in amperage or voltage. Absorption decreases in relation to the effectiveness of filters used and with an increase in distance between the patient and the roentgen tube.

Adverse acute effects of roentgen rays are diminished when the total dose is administered in several exposures separated by sufficient time for recovery from the subclinical effects of each. Repeated exposures may produce pathologic effects not manifested until years later. Some of the chemical changes produced in cells by roentgen rays are irreversible and may lie dormant until aging, infection, hormonal alterations, or further exposure to toxic agents activates them.

The infant may be more susceptible to the effects of roentgen rays than the adult. Moreover, even if there are no essential differences in susceptibility, the infant's longer life span provides more time for such changes to develop.

EARLY EFFECTS OF IRRADIATION. Exposure of the entire body to 100 roentgens usually produces illness in humans. A dose of about 400 roentgens will cause death in 50% of exposed persons. Higher doses can be tolerated if only a part of the body is exposed. Death results within hours to days when the entire body is exposed to the overwhelming dosage of an atomic bomb.

Symptoms of radiation sickness, which vary with the exposure, are malaise, fever, nausea, vomiting, and diarrhea. Leukopenia develops rapidly, and in more severe instances thrombocytopenia may appear within 1 wk. When the initial symptoms are not severe, they are followed by a temporary period of well-being. Epilation begins about 2 wk after the exposure. The leukopenia increases susceptibility to infection, and the low platelet count predisposes to hemorrhage. When autopsy does not reveal the cause of death, one can only assume that the radiation injury was responsible for lethal "cytochemical changes." If the patient survives for 6 wk, death is not likely from these effects of radiation. Bone marrow transplantation and granulocyte-macrophage colony-stimulating factors (GMCSF) may be indicated for severe pancytopenia.

Only a small percentage of deaths caused by an atomic explosion can be attributed to radiation effects alone; thermal and blast injuries account for most of them. Traumatic injuries do not heal effectively in persons with radiation sickness.

Clinical observation of the effects of radiation on children with genetic disease has led to a new understanding of molecular biology. Children with ataxia-telangiectasia are markedly predisposed to lymphoma, and when treated for it with the usual doses of radiotherapy, they sometimes suffer severe reactions (Sec. 11.19). These patients have defective repair of DNA after damage by γ-radiation, analogous to defective repair of DNA damage by ultraviolet light (UV) in xeroderma pigmentosum (Sec. 23.15). The defects in repair after γ-radiation or UV damage are enzyme mediated and nonoverlapping. Another interaction involving genetics, neoplasia, and radiosensitivity may occur in the heritable (usually bilateral) form of retinoblastoma. For example, radiogenic tumors of the orbit occur more frequently and after a shorter latent period than in patients with nonheritable cancers given similar doses of radiotherapy.

LATE EFFECTS OF IRRADIATION. Within the decade following the detonations of the atomic bombs in Japan there was a significant rise in the incidence of leukemia in proportion to exposure to the explosions. An increase in leukemia rates has been observed at doses as low as 20–49 rad among Hiroshima survivors of all ages. Children 10 yr of age at the time of the bombing were more susceptible to leukemogenesis than were older persons. When girls (younger than 10 yr of age) exposed to 50 rad or more reached the usual age for breast cancer (i.e., 35–45 yr), the frequency of this neoplasm was increased and now exceeds that for females who were older when exposed.

A committee of the National Academy of Sciences has reported that new dosimetry concerning exposures to the atomic bombs lowers the doses that produce late effects by about two thirds. The new dosimetry is based on re-evaluation of the physical effects of the bomb, such as effects on roof tiles and buttons, and revisions in mathematical modeling of the dose-response relationships (i.e., the shape of the curve).

In Great Britain and in the United States, in utero exposures to diagnostic radiation have been reported to increase the relative risk of death from cancer before 10 yr of age by about 50%. No such effect was found among children exposed in utero to the atomic bomb. However, subsequent analysis of cancer among persons exposed in utero, made when these persons were 40 yr old, suggest that adult cancers are beginning to occur excessively. Cancer involving the breast, which is the most sensitive site for radiation carcinogenesis 30 yr after exposure, had not yet occurred.

Among persons exposed in utero to radiation from the

Hiroshima atomic bomb (beginning at 10–19 rad) before the 18th wk of gestation, small head circumference occurred excessively. The effect increased in frequency and severity with increasing dose. Mental retardation occurred in those exposed to doses of 50 rad or more and affected the majority exposed in the 8th to 15th wk of gestation to 150 rad or more. Because of the catastrophic effects of the bomb, the observations at low doses may not apply directly to medical radiology. This question might be clarified by studying the head size of Soviet children exposed in utero at less than 18 wk of gestational age to radiation from the nuclear reactor accident at Chernobyl.

Complex chromosomal abnormalities were still found in the peripheral lymphocytes of atomic bomb survivors more than 35 yr after exposure, including those who were in utero, but not among persons conceived after the explosion. On the basis of animal experimentation, there is no doubt that point mutations occurred, but no effect could be demonstrated among the 75,000 first-generation offspring examined.

Small opacities of the posterior capsule of the lens have developed in 85% of those who epilated soon after the bomb explosion; the lesions are asymptomatic. Only 10 of the thousands of survivors have grade III or IV radiation-induced cataracts.

Radiation-induced premature aging has been described in animals, characterized by early senescence and death in middle age from diseases that ordinarily beset the elderly members of the species. This has not been demonstrated in humans.

Thyroid disease has occurred in children in the Marshall Islands who were exposed to fallout from nuclear weapons tests in the South Pacific in 1954. Two children, who were 1 yr old when exposed to a thyroid dose of 5,000 rad, developed severe hypofunction. Older persons developed less marked hypothyroidism, benign tumors, and, in a few instances, thyroid cancer. At Chernobyl, a goiter area, about 500 children received thyroid doses of more than 1,000 rem. Their exposures were at a lower dose and lower dose rate than those of the children of the Marshall Islands. (Fallout from the weapons tests had potent short-lived radioiodines that were not present in the plume from the reactor accident at Chernobyl.) Thyroid disorders may be prevented by ingestion of iodine after an acute exposure.

Therapeutic doses of partial-body radiation may predispose to cancer. This is indicated by reports of a greater incidence of leukemia among adults treated for ankylosing spondylitis and of thyroid tumors among persons treated in early infancy for thymic enlargement. That repeated small doses of radiation to the entire body may predispose to leukemia is indicated by the increased occurrence of this disease among radiologists in the past.

Effects of exposure of parts of the body include temporary sterility, dermatitis, bone and skin tumors, and developmental defects of teeth. Arrest in bone growth may occur in children who received cancericidal doses of roentgen rays.

Radon gas comes from radioactive decay of uranium deposits in soil and occurs more in some locales than others. Residential exposures are estimated to cause up to 13,000 deaths from lung cancer each year in the United States. Local health departments can provide information about exposures in their jurisdictions. Homes with radon levels greater than 4 pCi/L should be modified to reduce exposure, which can enhance lung cancer rates due to cigarette smoking.

There is controversy about the leukemogenic and other effects of *electromagnetic radiation*, as from transformers or electric blankets. This form of radiation is nonionizing, and the mechanism by which it might induce leukemia is not clear.

LOW-LEVEL RADIATION. Claims that low levels of radiation can induce cancer are based on data from persons in the area of fallout from nuclear weapons tests in Nevada in the 1950s. Increased mortality from leukemia has been reported in children in southwestern Utah and in military participants on maneuvers at the test site. The exposures were presumably low. Worries about low-dose exposures were amplified by the near meltdown at a nuclear power plant at Three Mile Island and at Chernobyl where "radiophobia" affects most of the population. In addition, controversial claims have been made that atomic energy workers in decades past now have increased cancer rates. The findings are not in accord with expectation based on a linear or quadratic extrapolation from effects at high or intermediate levels, as among Japanese atomic bomb survivors. The question about low-level effects is unlikely to be solved by further epidemiologic studies because the number of exposed persons needed for study far exceeds the number available. However, the Chernobyl accident, if appropriately studied, could provide important insights into this issue. Judgments will probably eventually be based on a knowledge of the fundamental biology of radiation carcinogenesis.

PREVENTIVE MEASURES. Exposures to ionizing radiation should be limited to situations in which commensurate benefits are expected. The average whole-body exposure of the general population, based on the genetically significant dose, should not exceed 100 mrem/yr, according to the National Council on Radiation Protection and Measurements.

It is thought that radiation changes within somatic cells are incompletely additive throughout life. The child of today is likely to have repeated exposures to ionizing radiation, and there is a possibility that tolerance may be dissipated. The pediatrician should limit as much as possible the exposure of patients (and self) to the emanations of roentgen ray machines and radioisotopes but should not refrain from using them for essential diagnostic and therapeutic procedures (Sec. 6.56). The patient's gonads should be shielded whenever possible.

Roentgen therapy should never be used except when the indications are unmistakable or the risk justified, as, for example, in the treatment of malignant tumors. Great care must be exercised to avoid unnecessary damage to osseous growth centers and tooth buds.

ROBERT W. MILLER

American Academy of Pediatrics, Committee on Environmental Hazards: Radon exposure: A hazard to children. Pediatrics 83:799, 1989.
Boice JD Jr, Fraumeni JF Jr (eds): Radiation Carcinogenesis: Epidemiology and Biological Significance. New York, Raven Press, 1984.
Committee on the Biological Effects of Ionizing Radiations: Health Effects of Exposure to Low Levels of Ionizing Radiation. Washington, DC, National Academy Press, 1990.
Evans HJ: Leukaemia and (preconception) radiation. Nature 345:16, 1990.
Machado SG, Land CE, McKay FW: Cancer mortality and radioactive fallout in southwestern Utah. Am J Epidemiol 125:44, 1987.
Miller RW, Boice JD Jr: Radiogenic cancer after prenatal or childhood exposure. *In*: Upton AC, Albert RE, Burns F, et al (eds): Radiation Carcinogenesis. New York, Elsevier-North Holland, 1986, p 379.
Miller RW, Brent RL: Low-dose radiation exposure (and IQ). Science 247:1166, 1990.
Miller RW, Mulvihill JJ: Small head size after atomic irradiation. Teratology 14:355, 1976.
Monson RR: Epidemiology and exposure to electromagnetic fields. Am J Epidemiol 131:774, 1990.
Neel JV, Satoh C, Gorki K, et al: Search for mutations altering protein charge and/or function in children of atomic bomb survivors: Final report. Am J Hum Genet 42:663, 1988.
Robbins J, Merino MJ, Boice JD Jr, et al: Thyroid cancer: A lethal endocrine neoplasm. Ann Intern Med (in press).
Task Group of Committee 1 of the International Commission on Radiological Protection: Developmental Effects of Irradiation on the Brain of the Embryo and Fetus. ICRP publication 49. Oxford, Pergamon Press, 1986, p 43.
Yoshimoto Y, Kato H, Schull WJ: Risk of cancer among children exposed in utero to A-bomb radiations, 1950–84. Lancet 2:665, 1988.

FOOD POISONING

The inadvertent consumption of poisonous foodstuffs is a significant cause of illness worldwide. *Salmonella* food poisoning continues to be a major problem in the United Kingdom, most recently related to contaminated eggs. In the United States, the incidence of mushroom poisoning has increased dramatically over the past decade. With the availability of rapid transportation of foodstuffs, poisoning by *Vibrio parahaemolyticus*, once limited to Japan, now occurs worldwide. Not only is the incidence of food-borne illness increasing, but also the types of poisoning have increased.

Food poisoning occurs by two mechanisms. First, contamination of usually innocuous foodstuffs by toxins or bacteria is the most common cause of poisoning; either foods may intrinsically contain toxins that manifest themselves under certain conditions (e.g., solanine poisoning and fish poisoning) or foods may become contaminated by bacterial or chemical toxins. Second, ingestion of intrinsically poisonous foodstuffs may occur; mushroom poisoning is the major example.

26.2 BACTERIAL FOOD POISONING

Salmonella Food Poisoning

Species of *Salmonella* (Sec. 12.28) account for most cases of food poisoning in the United States and the United Kingdom. In 1982, 612 of 702 outbreaks of food poisoning in the United Kingdom were attributed to *Salmonella; S. typhimurium* accounted for 44% of the cases.

EPIDEMIOLOGY. Poultry is the most frequently implicated identifiable contaminated food source. Meat products, particularly pork, are also associated with outbreaks. In rural epidemics of *Salmonella* food poisoning, unpasteurized milk is often the cause. Sporadically, contaminated chocolate bars, roast beef, and marijuana have been linked to epidemics of salmonellosis; in the latter cases, unusual strains are often involved. A number of outbreaks of *Salmonella* food poisoning have occurred in hospitals.

Because the organism is readily killed at normal cooking temperatures and by pasteurization, improper storage of precooked food and consumption of raw milk are the most common causes of *Salmonella* poisoning. Cream-filling of pastries that have been baked and are subsequently stored above 7° C may also lead to contamination.

PATHOPHYSIOLOGY. Large inocula of the organism are required to produce illness in humans. As a result, the attack rate of *Salmonella* poisoning following ingestion of contaminated food ranges from 25–65%. *Salmonella* species produce disease by invasion and infection of the gastrointestinal mucosa.

CLINICAL MANIFESTATIONS. The incubation period after ingestion of contaminated food ranges from 12–48 hr. The most common manifestation is diarrhea, which is often bloody. Vomiting and abdominal pain are less prominent clinical features. Headache, chills, and fever may also occur. These symptoms usually resolve within 48 hr. Gastrointestinal infection may disseminate in newborns, in persons with immunoincompetence, and in patients with chronic diseases. Bacteremia and meningitis may occur, and the mortality rate is about 3/1,000.

TREATMENT. Oral or parenteral correction of fluid and electrolyte losses may be required for patients with gastroenteritis. The routine use of antimicrobial therapy is not indicated, since prolongation of carriage occurs in adults and relapses occur in children.

Many isolates are resistant to ampicillin, particularly *Salmonella* acquired from animals fed tetracycline or other antimicrobial agents. Thus, cefotaxime or ceftriaxone should be included in the initial therapy for patients with bacteremia or meningitis. Uncomplicated *Salmonella* gastroenteritis should be treated in infants younger than 3 mo of age, in patients undergoing immunosuppressive therapy, and in the chronically ill.

Staphylococcal Food Poisoning

Ingestion of foodstuffs contaminated by enterotoxigenic strains of *Staphylococcus aureus* or, less commonly, coagulase-negative staphylococci is one of the major causes of epidemic food poisoning in the United States (Sec. 12.19).

EPIDEMIOLOGY. Contamination of food by *S. aureus* results from improper storage of previously cooked, proteinaceous food or from poor hygiene by food handlers. Whereas milk and milk products are the most frequently identified sources of staphylococcal poisoning, ham, salads containing potatoes or eggs, and cream-filled baked goods account for 50% of the outbreaks. Food that has been cooked but stored above 7° C for more than 4 hr is responsible for two thirds of the outbreaks. The remainder have been attributed to food handlers who were either staphylococcal carriers or who were actively infected.

Most epidemics occur wherever many persons are fed from a common source. Fifty per cent of the 131 outbreaks in the United States between 1977 and 1981 occurred in restaurants or schools, and 30% occurred at home.

From a public health standpoint, it is imperative to diagnose and confirm an outbreak of staphylococcal food poisoning. The acute onset of gastrointestinal illness in two or more persons with exposure to a common food source should raise suspicion, which may be confirmed if one of the following is documented: (1) demonstration of staphylococcal enterotoxin in food; (2) identical staphylococcal phage types isolated from food, food handler, and patient; (3) identical phage types recovered from six or more persons; or (4) presence of more than 10^5 colony-forming units of *S. aureus* per gram of food.

PATHOGENESIS. Staphylococcal gastroenteritis is caused by the ingestion of one of five immunologically distinct enterotoxins: A, B, C, D, and E. Enterotoxin A is the most frequently encountered; enterotoxins C and D are often associated with milk outbreaks, whose incidence has decreased in recent years. All of the staphylococcal enterotoxins produce an identical clinical syndrome, but the mechanisms by which they produce disease are unknown. Staphylococcal enterotoxins do not directly affect the gut or mucosal lining. Evidence suggests that the effector site for the toxin is within the autonomic nervous system.

CLINICAL MANIFESTATIONS. The incubation period between ingestion and the onset of clinical symptoms is about 4 hr (range 1–8 hr). Usually, nausea and abdominal pain precede vomiting and diarrhea. The illness is generally self-limited, resolving within 48 hr.

TREATMENT. Hospitalization for the correction of fluid and electrolyte abnormalities is rarely required. Parenteral rehydration may be required in severe cases. There is no antitoxin available, and the mortality rate is 0.03%, with most fatalities occurring in the severely debilitated.

Clostridium botulinum Food Poisoning (Botulism)

Clostridium botulinum is an unusual cause of food-borne illness in the United States. Over the past decade, approximately 40 cases per year have been reported; most have occurred in infants. (See Sec. 12.39 for clinical manifestations and treatment.)

The ingestion of preformed toxin is responsible for the clinical manifestations of botulism in adults, whereas gastrointestinal colonization with toxin-producing strains causes the illness in infants. Eight antigenically distinct but physiologically similar neurotoxins have been identified: A, B, C_1, C_2, D, E, F, and G. Botulinum toxin affects the peripheral nervous system by blocking the presynaptic release of acetylcholine. Although the exact mechanism of inhibition of release of acetylcholine is unclear, in vitro studies have shown that the toxin negatively influences Ca^{2+}-dependent acetylcholine release. Higher than physiologic concentrations of Ca^{2+} are required to counter the action of the neurotoxin.

Because the spores of *C. botulinum* are ubiquitous, contamination of foodstuffs occurs frequently. Anaerobic conditions, temperatures below 121° C, and pH above 4.5 are required for bacterial growth and toxin production. Most outbreaks of botulism are associated with improperly canned foods, particularly with foods that have been canned at home. The incidence of botulism is particularly high in Alaska, where local dishes such as fermented fish heads and seal flippers have been linked to outbreaks. In infants, honey is frequently identified as a source of poisoning.

Botulinum toxin serotypes causing infantile botulism have a distinct geographic distribution in the United States; west of the Mississippi River most sporadic cases are caused by *C. botulinum* type A, whereas eastern cases tend to involve type B. Type F has also been identified from infants with botulism.

Other Bacterial Food Poisonings

In the United Kingdom, the incidence of food poisoning caused by *C. perfringens* is second in frequency only to those caused by *Salmonella*; in the United States it is comparable with that of infections caused by *Shigella*. Meat products other than poultry are the typical sources of outbreaks. Following ingestion of contaminated foodstuffs, the organism replicates in the small intestine, producing a heat-labile enterotoxin. The toxin acts throughout the small intestine, where it impairs glucose absorption and promotes secretion of fluid (see Sec. 12.38 for clinical manifestations and treatment).

Bacillus cereus is an unusual cause of food poisoning in the United States. Outbreaks have resulted from the ingestion of contaminated Chinese food, lamb, and vegetables. Illness results either from the ingestion of preformed toxin or from gastrointestinal colonization and subsequent in vivo toxin production. The toxin activates intestinal adenyl cyclase, resulting in hyperperistalsis and secretory diarrhea. Ingestion of the preformed toxin gives rise to a clinical syndrome indistinguishable from that of staphylococcal food poisoning. Gastrointestinal colonization produces a syndrome with a longer incubation period. In both instances, the illness is self-limited and does not typically require specific therapy.

V. parahaemolyticus is also an unusual cause of food poisoning in the United States. Because this is a marine organism, ingestion of raw or improperly prepared seafood is the most common source of outbreaks. The organism produces a hemolysin, which causes gastrointestinal hypersecretion in vitro. The organism is also capable of invading the intestinal mucosa. Abdominal pain, diarrhea, vomiting, and nausea occur 4–96 hr after consumption of contaminated food. The illness is self-limited, usually resolving within 72 hr without specific therapy.

26.3 NONBACTERIAL FOOD POISONING

Mushroom Poisoning

The consumption of wild mushrooms, a favorite pastime in Europe, is becoming increasingly popular in the United States, with concomitant increases in fatal cases of mushroom poisoning.

There are four clinical syndromes and seven classes of toxins associated with wild mushroom poisoning. The clinical syndromes are divided according to the predominant system involved and the rapidity of onset of symptoms. The toxins produced by wild mushrooms are categorized as follows: cyclopeptides, monomethylhydrazine, muscarine, coprine, ibotenic acid, psilocybin, and unknown.

GASTROINTESTINAL—DELAYED ONSET. Amanita Poisoning. Poisoning from species of *Amanita* and *Galerina* account for 95% of the fatalities from mushroom intoxication, although the mortality rate for this group is 5–10%. Most species produce two classes of cyclopeptide toxins: (1) phalloidins, which are heptapeptides believed to be responsible for the early symptoms of *Amanita* poisoning; and (2) amanitotoxin, which is an octapeptide that inhibits RNA polymerase and subsequent production of messenger RNA. Cells with high turnover rates, such as those in the gastrointestinal mucosa, kidney, and liver, are the most severely affected.

Histopathologically, *Amanita* poisoning causes cellular necrosis, which may occur throughout the gastrointestinal tract, the most heavily exposed site. Acute yellow atrophy of the liver and necrosis of the proximal renal tubules are found in lethal cases.

The clinical course produced by poisoning with *Amanita* or *Galerina* species is biphasic, after an initial 6- to 12-hr latent period. Six to 24 hr following ingestion, patients develop nausea, vomiting, and severe abdominal pain. Profuse, watery diarrhea follows shortly thereafter and may last for 12–24 hr. During this time, as much as 9 L of fluid may be lost. Twenty-four to 48 hr after poisoning, jaundice, hypertransaminasemia (peaking at 72–96 hr), renal failure, and coma are noted. Death occurs 4–7 days after the ingestion. A prothrombin time less than 10% of control is a poor prognostic factor.

The treatment of *Amanita* poisoning is both supportive and specific. Fluid loss during the early course of the illness is profound, requiring aggressive therapy for correction of this loss in patients with severe diarrhea. In the late phase of the disease, management of renal and hepatic failure is also necessary.

Specific therapy for *Amanita* poisoning is designed to remove the toxin rapidly and to block binding at its target site. Because amanitotoxin may be recovered from the duodenum up to 36 hr after ingestion, aspiration of duodenal contents will significantly decrease toxin load. Forced diuresis should be avoided, since this increases renal exposure.

Although cytochrome C protects mice from lethal doses of amanitotoxin, clinical trials with this agent have failed to demonstrate any benefit. Intravenous penicillin G (250 mg/kg/24 hr) administered as a continuous infusion combined with silibinin, the water-soluble form of the flavolignone silymarin, in an intravenous dosage of 20–50 mg/kg/24 hr act synergistically to inhibit binding of both toxins and to interrupt enterohepatic recirculation of amanitotoxin. Finally, two patients with severe hepatic failure following mushroom ingestion were treated successfully by liver transplantation.

Monomethylhydrazine Intoxication. Species of *Gyromitra* contain monomethylhydrazine (CH_3NHNH_2), which inhibits central nervous system (CNS) enzymatic production of γ-aminobutyric acid (GABA). Monomethylhydrazine also oxidizes iron in hemoglobin, resulting in methemoglobinemia. Patients with *Gyromitra* poisoning develop vomiting, diarrhea, hematochezia, and abdominal pain within 6–24 hr of ingestion of the toxin. Symptoms of CNS depression and seizures develop later in the clinical course. Hemolysis and methemoglobinemia are potential life-threatening complications of monomethylhydrazine poisoning. Severe methemoglobinemia may require dialysis.

Hypovolemia from gastrointestinal fluid losses and seizures require supportive intervention. Pyridoxal phosphate, the coenzyme that catalyzes the production of GABA, can reverse the effects of monomethylhydrazine when administered in high dosages. Pyridoxine hydrochloride (25 mg/kg) is administered intravenously at a frequency dependent on clinical improvement. Parenteral administration of methylene blue is indicated if the methemoglobin concentration exceeds 30%. Blood transfusions may be required for significant hemolysis.

AUTONOMIC NERVOUS SYSTEM—RAPID ONSET. Muscarine Poisoning. Mushrooms of the genera *Inocybe* and, to a lesser degree, *Clitocybe* contain muscarine or muscarine-related compounds. These quaternary ammonium derivatives bind to postsynaptic receptors, producing an exaggerated cholinergic response.

The clinical syndrome is characterized by the following hypercholinergic response: the onset of symptoms is rapid (30 min–2 hr after consumption) and consists of diaphoresis, excessive lacrimation, salivation, miosis, urinary and fecal incontinence, and vomiting. Respiratory distress caused by bronchospasm and increased bronchopulmonary secretions is the most serious complication. The symptoms subside spontaneously within 6–24 hr.

Atropine sulfate, the specific antidote, is administered intravenously (0.1 mg/kg). This is repeated until the pulmonary symptoms resolve or the patient becomes overtly tachycardic.

Coprine Ingestion. *Coprinus atramentarius* and *Clitocybe clavipes* contain coprine. Like disulfiram (Antabuse), coprine inhibits the metabolism of acetaldehyde following ethanol ingestion. The clinical symptomatology results from accumulation of acetaldehyde.

Coprine intoxication becomes apparent after ethanol ingestion and may occur up to 5 days after consuming the mushroom. Hyperemia of the face and trunk, tingling of the hands, metallic taste, tachycardia, and vomiting occur acutely. Hypotension may result from intense peripheral vasodilatation.

The syndrome is typically self-limited and lasts only several hours. No specific antidote is available. If hypotension is severe, vascular re-expansion with isotonic parenteral solutions may be required. Small oral doses of propranolol have also been suggested.

CENTRAL NERVOUS SYSTEM—RAPID ONSET. Ibotenic Acid and Muscimol Intoxication. Although *Amanita muscaria* and *A. pantherina* may contain muscarine (see earlier), the toxins responsible for the CNS symptoms following ingestion of these mushrooms are muscimol and ibotenic acid. Muscimol, a hallucinogen, and ibotenic acid, an insecticide, have anticholinergic effects. One half to 2 hr following ingestion, ataxia, hallucinations, and euphoria occur. Nausea and vomiting may be associated. With large ingestions, coma and seizures may also develop. If large amounts of muscarine are contained in the mushroom, symptoms of cholinergic crisis may also occur.

Specific therapy must be carefully selected. If an exaggerated cholinergic response is observed, atropine should be administered. Because ingestions of *A. muscaria* are frequently associated with anticholinergic findings, the acetylcholinesterase inhibitor physostigmine is used to reverse the delirium and coma.

Indole Intoxication. Mushrooms belonging to the genus *Psilocybe* ("magic mushrooms") contain psilocybin and psilocin, two psychotropic compounds. Within 30 min after ingestion, patients develop euphoria and hallucinations, often accompanied by tachycardia and mydriasis. Fever and seizures have also been observed in children with psilocybin poisoning. These symptoms are short-lived, usually lasting 6 hr after consumption of the mushroom. Severely agitated patients may respond to diazepam.

GASTROINTESTINAL—RAPID ONSET. Many mushrooms from a variety of genera produce local gastrointestinal symptoms. The causative toxins are diverse and largely unknown.

Within an hour of ingestion, patients develop acute abdominal pain, nausea, vomiting, and diarrhea. Symptoms may last from hours to days, depending on the species.

Treatment is mainly supportive. Patients with large fluid losses may require parenteral fluid therapy. It is imperative to differentiate ingestion of mushrooms of this class from ingestions of *Amanita* and *Galerina* species containing cyclopeptide toxins (see earlier).

Solanine Poisoning

Solanine is a mixture of several related toxins found in "greened" and sprouted potatoes. Potatoes exposed to light and allowed to sprout produce a number of alkaloidal glycosides containing the cholesterol derivative solanidine. Two of these glycosides, α-solanine and α-chaconine, are found in highest concentration in the peels of greened potatoes and in the sprouts. The solanine alkaloids bind to serum cholinesterase, suggesting a possible pathophysiologic mechanism.

Clinical manifestations of solanine intoxication occur within 7–19 hr after ingestion. The most common symptoms are vomiting and diarrhea; in more severe instances of poisoning, fever, generalized abdominal pain, coma, and hypovolemic shock occur.

Treatment of solanine poisoning is largely supportive. In the most severe cases, symptoms resolve within 11 days. Atropine treatment has not been evaluated.

Seafood Poisoning

CIGUATERA FISH POISONING. Major outbreaks of ciguatera fish poisoning have been reported in Florida, Hawaii, and the Virgin Islands; however, with modern methods of transportation, the illness now occurs worldwide. Grouper is the most frequently identified source of the toxin, followed by snapper, kingfish, amberjack, dolphin, and barracuda.

The source of this poisoning is the dinoflagellate *Gambierdiscus toxicus*, a microscopic organism found in the food chain along coral reefs, which contains high concentrations of ciguatoxin and maitotoxin. After ingestion of the organism by small fish, the toxin is absorbed and concentrated in fish flesh and musculature. Larger fish consume the smaller fish, and again the toxin is absorbed from the gastrointestinal tract and concentrated in the musculature.

Ciguatoxin, a lipid with a molecular weight of approximately 1,100 daltons, increases the sodium permeability of excitable membranes. This action is inhibited by calcium and tetrodotoxin.

The onset of symptoms following ingestion of fish containing ciguatoxin is rapid, usually occurring within 2–30 hr. The illness is often biphasic. The earliest symptoms are diarrhea, vomiting, and abdominal pain; the second phase includes myalgias and circumoral or extremity dysesthesias. The dysesthesia is characterized by reversal of hot and cold sensation. Tachycardia, bradycardia, and hypertension occur infrequently.

Treatment of ciguatera fish poisoning is supportive. Gastric lavage is recommended to remove any remaining toxin. Intravenous fluids may be required for severe diarrhea, and parenteral administration of calcium can be used to treat hypotension. In a few patients with coma, mannitol has successfully reversed the neurologic manifestations of intoxication. However, further studies are needed before a blanket recommendation for mannitol therapy can be made. Most cases are self-limited; symptoms may last up to 3 wk.

SCOMBROID (PSEUDOALLERGIC) FISH POISONING. Epidemics have been associated with the ingestion of members of the Scombresocidae or Scombridae families, notably albacore, mackerel, tuna, bonita, and kingfish. Nonscombroid fish and marine mammals, such as mahi-mahi (dolphin) and bluefish, have also been linked to outbreaks of poisoning.

The "scombrotoxin," either histamine or the product of the action of the toxin on fish flesh, is responsible for the clinical syndrome. Histidine is found in high concentrations in the flesh of scombroid fish; the action of bacterial decarboxylases during putrification converts the histidine to histamine. Fish containing more than 20 mg of histamine per 100 g of flesh are toxic. In patients receiving isoniazid, a potent histaminase blocker, ingestion of fish flesh containing lower concentrations of histamine may be toxic.

The onset of clinical illness is acute and occurs within 10 min–2 hr following ingestion. The most common symptoms include diarrhea, flushing, diaphoresis, urticaria, nausea, and headache. Abdominal pain, tachycardia, oral burning, dizziness, respiratory distress, and facial swelling also occur. The illness is usually self-limited, terminating within 8–10 hr.

Treatment is mainly supportive. Gastric lavage decreases continued absorption of histamine. With severe diarrhea, fluid replacement may be necessary. Antihistamines have been variably successful. Four patients with severe toxicity treated with cimetidine (a histamine blocker) responded rapidly. Since data are limited, cimetidine or ranitidine should be reserved for severe cases.

PARALYTIC SHELLFISH POISONING. Filter-feeding mollusks, such as the black mussel and sea scallop, may become contaminated during dinoflagellate blooms, or "red tides." The dinoflagellates *Gonyaulax catenella, G. tamerensis,* and *G. grindleyi* are often responsible for these "red tides" and contain several potent neurotoxins. Saxitoxin is the most important of the neurotoxins responsible for paralytic shellfish poisoning. This toxin prevents nerve conduction by inhibiting the sodium-potassium pump. Although six other toxins have been isolated from contaminated scallops, these toxins may be bioconverted to less toxic structures.

The onset of clinical symptoms of paralytic shellfish poisoning occurs rapidly, 30 min–2 hr after ingestion. Paresthesias are the most common complaints and occur circumorally, in a stocking-glove distribution, or both. Vertigo, ataxis, and the sensation of floating occur less commonly. In severe cases, respiratory failure due to diaphragmatic paralysis may result.

There is no known antidote for paralytic shellfish poisoning. Supportive care, including mechanical ventilation, may be needed. Although the symptoms are usually self-limited and short-lived, weakness and malaise may persist for weeks following ingestion.

STEPHEN C. ARONOFF

SALMONELLA

Holmberg SD, Osterholm MT, Senger KA, et al: Drug-resistant *Salmonella* from animals fed antimicrobials. N Engl J Med 311:617, 1984.
Public Health Laboratory Service: Food poisoning and *Salmonella* surveillance in England and Wales: 1982. Br Med J 288:306, 1984.

STAPHYLOCOCCAL FOOD POISONING

Breckinridge JC, Bergdoll MS: Outbreak of food-borne gastroenteritis due to a coagulase-negative enterotoxin-producing *Staphylococcus*. N Engl J Med 284:541, 1972.
Carpenter CCJ: Mechanisms of bacterial diarrheas. Am J Med 68:313, 1980.
Holmberg SD, Blake PA: Staphylococcal food poisoning in the United States: New facts and old misconceptions. JAMA 251:457, 1984.

BOTULISM

Centers for Disease Control: Botulism in the United States, 1979. J Infect Dis 142:302, 1980.

VIBRIO PARAHAEMOLYTICUS

Rodrick GE, Hood MA, Blake NJ: Human *Vibrio* gastroenteritis. Med Clin North Am 66:665, 1982.

MUSHROOM POISONING

Editorial: Mushroom poisoning. Lancet 2:351, 1980.
Hanrahan JP, Gordon MA: Mushroom poisoning: Case reports and a review of therapy. JAMA 251:1057, 1984.
Klein AS, Hart J, Brems JJ, et al: *Amanita* poisoning: Treatment and the role of liver transplantation. Am J Med 86:187, 1989.
Litten W: The most poisonous mushrooms. Sci Am 232:90, 1975.
McCormick DJ, Avbel AJ, Biggons RB: Nonlethal mushroom poisoning. Ann Intern Med 90:332, 1979.
McDonald A: Mushrooms and madness: Hallucinogenic mushrooms and some psychopharmacological implications. Can J Psychiatry 25:586, 1980.
Mitchell DH: *Amanita* mushroom poisoning. Ann Rev Med 31:51, 1980.
Rumack BH, Spoerke DG (eds): POISINDEX System®: A Computerized Poison Information System. Denver, CO, Micromedex, Inc, Vol 68, 1991.

SOLANINE POISONING

Editorial: Potatoe poisoning. Lancet 2:681, 1979.
McMillan M, Thompson JC: An outbreak of suspected solanine poisoning in school boys: Examination of criteria of solanine poisoning. Q J Med 48:227, 1979.

CIGUATERA FISH POISONING

Lawrence DN, Enriquez MB, Lumish RM, et al: Ciguatera fish poisoning in Miami. JAMA 244:254, 1980.
Morris JG, Lewin P, Hargrett NT, et al: Clinical features of ciguatera fish poisoning. Arch Intern Med 142:1090, 1982.
Palafox NA, Jain LG, Pinano AZ, et al: Successful treatment of Ciguatera fish poisoning with intravenous mannitol. JAMA 259:2740, 1988.
Withers NW: Ciguatera fish poisoning. Ann Rev Med 33:97, 1982.

SCOMBROID FISH POISONING

Blakesley ML: Scombroid poisoning: Prompt resolution of symptoms with cimetidine. Ann Emerg Med 12:104, 1983.
Gilbert RJ, Hobbs G, Murray CK, et al: Scombrotoxic fish poisoning: Features of the first 50 incidents to be reported in Britain (1976–9). Br Med J 281:71, 1980.
Hughes JM, Potter ME: Scombroid fish poisoning: From pathogenesis to prevention. N Engl J Med 324:766, 1991.
Morrow JD, Margolies GR, Rowland J, et al: Evidence that histamine is the causative toxin of scombroid fish poisoning. N Engl J Med 324:716, 1991.

PARALYTIC SHELLFISH POISONING

Hughes JM, Merson MH: Fish and shellfish poisoning. N Engl J Med 295:1117, 1976.
Popkiss MEE, Horstman DA, Harpur D: Paralytic shellfish poisoning: A report of 17 cases in Cape Town. S Afr Med J 55:1017, 1979.
Shimizu Y, Yoshioka M: Transformation of paralytic shellfish toxins as demonstrated in scallop homogenates. Science 212:547, 1981.

CHEMICAL AND DRUG POISONING

26.4 PRINCIPLES OF MANAGEMENT

In 1987, 1,166,940 poisoning cases were reported by 63 centers that participated in the National Data Collection System of the American Association of Poison Control Centers (AAPCC). More than 90% of the cases occurred in the home. Children aged 5 yr and younger accounted for 62.2% of all cases. Accidental cases totaled 88.9%, while 5.8% were reported as suicidal. More than 90% of instances involved a single substance. Only 397 fatalities were reported: 22 in those 6 yr of age or younger.

The AAPCC data likely represent some skewing of cases away from reports of suicide with heavier emphasis on accidental cases, owing to the kinds of questions referred to a poison center. Many suicidal patients are taken directly to an emergency facility, which may or may not report to or request consultation from a poison information center. The peak age of suicide attempts for children is 13–17 yr (Sec. 3.37 and 10.3). Thus, pediatricians have to contend with two major groups of children in regard to poisoning: (1) those age 5 and younger exposed to plants, household products, medications, and so on; and (2) the adolescent exposed most frequently to medications. Once the diagnosis of poisoning or potential poisoning is entertained, the pediatrician should follow a specific management plan to ensure optimum care.

Management Plan for Poisoning and Overdose

Initial contact with a poisoned patient will usually be over the telephone. The following data should be obtained at the time of initial contact:

Phone Number. Getting the caller's telephone number is necessary in case the phone contact is accidentally broken and to permit follow-up calls.

Address. This may be crucial if emergency equipment needs to be dispatched or if the person on the phone becomes hysterical or develops lethargy, convulsions, and so on.

Evaluation of Severity. Although many callers may begin with a description of symptoms or signs such as a convulsion, it is vital to evaluate the current status of the patient in terms of immediate danger, potential danger, and no danger. Further history may be necessary to evaluate an asymptomatic patient.

Weight and Age. This permits estimation of potential toxicity.

Time of Ingestion. This permits interpretation of onset of symptoms or signs as well as evaluation of laboratory data and other prognostic information.

Past Medical History. Brief information should be elicited to determine the usual health status of the patient as a basis for interpreting signs. It will also suggest interactions of chronic medications or allergies with the current ingestion.

Type of Exposure. Product names and ingredients should be obtained from labels or from the POISINDEX System.

Amount of Exposure. How many tablets or how much fluid has been consumed should be estimated. Tablets or fluid remaining in the container should be counted or measured.

Route of Exposure. It should be determined if the exposure was by ingestion, inhalation, local application to the eyes or skin, or parenteral.

Caller's Relationship to Victim. It is important to determine if the call is from a baby-sitter, friend, relative, or stranger and who gives permission to treat the patient.

Such basic information should be a standard procedure in every office or clinic where such cases may be reported. Written records should be kept of each event. It may be acceptable practice either to see the patient or to treat and observe the patient at home, depending on the exposure and patient's condition. If treatment is at home, then follow-up calls *must* be made at approximately ½, 1, and 4 hr after exposure. Any change in the patient's condition may warrant a change in the decision to treat at home. Since as many as half the histories obtained from poisoned patients will have an error of some magnitude, the physician must be ready to change treatment or disposition decisions in light of changes in onset of symptoms or new history. Lomotil is an example of a drug for which even careful follow-up may be inadequate. Because of the idiosyncratic nature of its ingestion, *all* children consuming this drug younger than age 6 yr *must* be hospitalized and monitored for 24 hr; delayed onset of coma for 8–12 hr requires that these patients receive intensive medical observation.

INITIAL MEDICAL CARE

If after telephone consultation or direct primary evaluation the decision is made to have the patient seen by others, transportation appropriate to the patient's condition should be arranged. The site of initial medical contact should also be considered in relation to the exposure history. For example, if it is expected that respiratory support will be required, then paramedic transport to a well-equipped emergency facility is mandatory. Once the decision is made, then the receiving personnel should be notified so that proper preparation can be made, including notification of the poison center if that has not yet been done. Before transport, all product containers thought likely to be related to the exposure should be gathered up and brought with the patient. If the patient has vomited spontaneously or by induction with syrup of ipecac, this emesis should be saved and brought with the patient.

Once the patient has arrived in the appropriate medical care setting, initial attention should focus on life support, with primary emphasis on cardiorespiratory care. Shock, arrhythmias, and convulsions must be dealt with as in the case of any other critically ill patient (Sec. 6.35–6.37). There are few poisons for which there is an antidote. Except for the poisons listed below, specific treatment directed at the poison can be delayed until the physician is satisfied that the patient's condition is stable. The following poisons require simultaneous use of an antagonist and life support measures.

CARBON MONOXIDE. Oxygen (100%) should be administered as early as possible to reduce the concentration of carbon monoxide in the blood and increase oxygen transport to tissues. Symptomatic patients or those with high toxin levels may be candidates for hyperbaric oxygen therapy (see Sec. 6.35 and 14.70).

CYANIDE. Oxygen should be supplied immediately, followed by specific antidotal treatment. Although the antidote that is available in the United States is not ideal, appropriate doses should be administered to a symptomatic patient with cyanide poisoning. The antidote kit contains the following: (1) amyl nitrite inhalers, which may be broken under the patient's nose for 30 sec of each minute while the sodium nitrite solution is being readied; (2) sodium nitrite 3% solution, which should be administered at a dose of 0.33 mL/kg (10 mg/kg) to a maximum dose of 10 mL/patient with normal hemoglobin; and (3) sodium thiosulfate 25% solution, which should be administered next at a dose of 1.65 mL/kg to a maximum dose of the entire ampule. These agents produce methemoglobin, which may help remove cyanide by competition for the cytochrome. An alternative antidote, a hydroxocobalamin-thiosulfate mixture, is available outside the United States; it should be given in doses of 4–10 g. Hydroxocobalamin alone cannot be given in sufficient quantity to be effective.

OPIATES AND RELATED POISONS. Naloxone in sufficient doses is very effective in treating these poisonings. A minimum dose of 0.4 mg can be given to any patient, regardless of age or weight. If there is failure of response, up to 2.0 mg should be administered rapidly intravenously to larger children and adolescents. This may be repeated as necessary. Newborns to infants 6 mo of age should be given a dose of 10–100 μg/kg.

SUBSTANCES PRODUCING METHEMOGLOBINEMIA. Although relatively uncommon, exposure to aniline dyes, nitrobenzene, azo compounds, and nitrites may produce methemoglobinemia that is unresponsive to oxygen administration. The diagnosis is suggested by comparing a drop of the patient's blood with that of the physician. If there is at least 20% methemoglobinemia, the patient's blood will be relatively brown when dried on a sheet of filter paper; the color would be red at a lower percentage of methemoglobin. Methylene blue at a dose of 0.1–0.2 mL/kg (1–2 mg/kg) per dose of a 1% solution is therapeutic. If two doses are unsuccessful, exchange transfusion may be required.

CHOLINERGIC AGENTS. Children exposed to organophosphate insecticides and carbamates may develop salivation, lacrimation, urination, defecation, and fasciculations. Atropine at a dose of 0.05 mg/kg to a maximum initial dose of 2–5 mg should be administered while the patient is being decontaminated with soap and water. Repeated doses of atropine may be necessary if the patient is unresponsive. In severe cases or when the cholinesterase level falls to 25% of normal or lower, pralidoxime, a cholinesterase regenerator, may be indicated. The dosage is 25–50 mg/kg given over 30 min intravenously every 8–12 hr in young children, to a maximum of 1 g/dose in older children.

OTHER "ANTIDOTES." These are not generally required immediately and may be administered after the diagnosis is confirmed (e.g., ethanol for ethylene glycol or methanol poisoning or *N*-acetyl-L-cysteine for acetaminophen overdose).

PREVENTING ABSORPTION

The goal of therapy is to reduce the amount of the poison taken up by the body. In some cases, this may be preventative (e.g., a child who ingested something just prior to calling the physician may have absorbed very little). In other cases, it may be desirable to reduce further absorption (e.g., oral activated charcoal following oral or intravenous theophylline overdosage). Before using any of these techniques, their safety should be evaluated for the particular child.

EMESIS. Administration of syrup of ipecac, 15–30 mL, followed by a clear liquid such as water results in vomiting in over 95% of children younger than age 5 yr. The airway may be protected by positioning the patient on the left side with the head down (spanking position). Emesis should not be induced if the patient is comatose, is convulsing, or has ingested strong acids or bases. Treatment of hydrocarbon ingestions with emesis is controversial (Sec. 26.7). Emesis should be avoided when there is a significant risk of aspiration. Data in adolescents and adults have brought into question whether emesis affects outcome; it produces only an average of 8–30% recovery of ingested material. The initial emesis should be saved for diagnostic analysis. Apomorphine is contraindicated in children and adolescents.

LAVAGE. Gastric washout is relatively fast and about as effective as emesis. Complications in adults have included esophageal perforation. It is probably unsafe in young children in whom there may be airway obstruction and in whom cuffed endotracheal tubes cannot be used. Only in rare instances does lavage change the outcome of poisoning. If the procedure is done, warm saline should be used in young children and warm tap water in older children; a large bore tube, No. 32–36 French, should be employed to remove fragments of tablets and capsules.

CHARCOAL. The administration of a good grade of activated charcoal (*not* burned toast or universal antidote) may be the most effective and safest procedure to prevent absorption. Charcoal is capable of adsorbing almost all drugs and many other chemicals. It should be given as a water slurry with a minimum dose of 15–30 g in a child and 30–100 g in an adolescent. Repeat doses of 20 g should be administered every 2 hr until the charcoal appears in the stool. Super activated carbon is 3–5 times as adsorptive as regular charcoal and comes premixed in a liquid.

CATHARTIC. Sorbitol (maximum 1 g/kg), magnesium sulfate (maximum 250 mg/kg), sodium citrate (maximum 250 mg/kg), or phosphosoda (maximum 250 mg/kg) can be used to hasten emptying of the gastrointestinal tract once the ingested material has passed through the stomach. These agents should be used cautiously in young children. They may be useful in older children following administration of activated charcoal, especially for hydrocarbons and agents that delay bowel motility.

ENHANCING EXCRETION

FORCED DIURESIS. Forced diuresis is an overused technique for treating poisoned children. It has little general use, and its administration is even questionable in phenobarbital and salicylate ingestion, since alkalinization without diuresis may be just as effective. Acid diuresis is contraindicated for agents such as amphetamines, phencyclidine, and so on, owing to aggravation of renal problems with myoglobinuria and methemoglobinemia.

HEMODIALYSIS. Once heralded as the answer to many poisonings, hemodialysis is now used rarely and selectively. Many drugs have very large volumes of distribution so that even if there is good clearance by dialysis, total-body removal may be extremely small. For example, after a digoxin or tricyclic antidepressant overdose, only a small percentage of the drug can be removed by dialysis. The major indications for hemodialysis are severe salicylate intoxication unresponsive to standard care, poisoning with methanol and ethylene glycol with blood levels above 20 mg/dL and acidosis, and symptomatic theophylline overdoses with blood levels at 60–100 μg/dL or higher.

HEMOPERFUSION OVER ACTIVATED CHARCOAL OR RESIN. Hemoperfusion over activated charcoal or resin may be helpful in some situations when there is a small volume of distribution and the agent is well adsorbed. It may be valuable in theophylline, salicylate, and paraquat poisoning of patients who have not responded well to other forms of therapy. It is not recommended for poisonings with tricyclic antidepressants, acetaminophen, digoxin, and so on, since it does not remove substantial amounts of total-body load or change the clinical outcome.

LABORATORY EVALUATION

In some cases (e.g., poisoning with salicylates, acetaminophen, iron, methanol, and ethylene glycol), the laboratory provides data sufficient to change the treatment plan. In other instances (e.g., opiates, in which there is definitive treatment unrelated to levels, and cyanide, in which it would be too late if the physician waited for laboratory assistance), the laboratory data may be helpful but will not likely change treatment. "Drug screens" are generally not helpful. The best way to use the laboratory is to discuss the case with the technologist and provide appropriate samples and clinical data so that specific analysis can be interpreted. There is little use in doing certain portions of the screen if it is already known what the patient has consumed and that symptoms are consistent with its toxicity. If a "toxic screen" is obtained, it is important to know the specific drugs that are included in the test.

Blumer JL, Reed MD (eds): Pediatric Toxicology. Pediatr Clin North Am 33(2), 1986.
Dine MS, McGoven ME: Intentional poisoning of children: An overlooked category of child abuse. Pediatrics 70:32, 1982.
Ellenhorn MJ, Barceloux DG: Medical Toxicology: Diagnosis and Treatment in Human Poisonings. New York, Elsevier, 1988.
Goldfrank LR: Toxicologic Emergencies: A Comprehensive Handbook of Problem Solving. New York, Appleton-Century-Crofts, 1982.
Matthew H, Lawson AAH: Treatment of Common Acute Poisonings, 4th ed. New York, Churchill-Livingstone, 1979.
Rumack BH: Poisoning. In: Kempe CH, Silver HR, O'Brien D (eds): Current Pediatrics Therapy. Los Altos, CA, Lange Medical Publications, 1984.
Rumack BH, Rosen P: Emesis: Safe and effective? Ann Emerg Med 10:551, 1981.
Rumack BH, Spoerke DG (eds): POISINDEX System®: A Computerized Poison Information System. Denver, CO, Micromedex, Inc, 1989.
Veltri JC, Schmitz BF, Matyrunas N, et al: 1987 Annual Report of the American Association of Poison Control Centers National Data Collection System. Am J Emerg Med 6:479, 1988.

26.5 ACETAMINOPHEN

Acetaminophen has become the most widely used analgesic antipyretic, owing, in part, to the finding of a relationship between Reye syndrome and salicylates (Sec. 13.96). Consequently, acetaminophen is more available for accidental or intentional use by young children and adolescents in the home. There are significant differences in the degree of toxicity that may occur in children younger than age 6 yr and in the older child.

PATHOPHYSIOLOGY. Acetaminophen is primarily metabolized to the sulfate or glucuronide (94%), and the shift from sulfate to glucuronide predominance between ages 9 and 12 yr parallels the change in degree of toxicity at these ages. A small amount of acetaminophen is excreted unchanged, and the remaining approximately 4% is metabolized by cytochrome P_{450} and glutathione to the mercapturic acid conjugate. This latter pathway produces the toxicity of acetaminophen; when hepatic stores of glutathione are depleted to less than 70% of normal, the highly reactive intermediate metabolites combine with hepatic macromolecules and produce cellular damage.

Although therapeutic peak plasma levels of acetaminophen usually occur at 1–2 hr when hepatic function is normal, measurement prior to 4 hr cannot be used to determine the severity of an overdose. If there is pre-existing hepatic disease, or if the therapeutic half-life is measured after the onset of hepatotoxicity, then the half-life may be extended to 4 hr or more. Because the half-life primarily reflects the sulfate and glucuronide pathways and not the toxic metabolite, it does not relate to the degree of toxicity. The volume of distribution is approximately 1 L/kg and does not vary with the quantity of absorbed drug as does that of a salicylate.

CLINICAL AND LABORATORY MANIFESTATIONS. If untreated, patients who have overdosed pass through four stages of toxicity (Table 26–1). Without a history of ingestion or high index of suspicion the pediatrician may not diagnose the ingestion. If there is a history of acetaminophen ingestion, the plasma level should be assessed at 4 hr or more after ingestion. Interpretation of this level should be plotted on the nomogram (Fig. 26–1) to determine whether antidotal treatment is indicated. SGOT, SGPT, bilirubin, and prothrombin time should be followed daily in all patients with levels in the toxic range on the nomogram.

TREATMENT. Therapy for patients with potentially toxic plasma levels of acetaminophen as determined from the nomogram is most effective if oral *N*-acetyl-L-cysteine (Mucomyst) is administered prior to 16 hr post ingestion. It should be administered until up to 24 hr after ingestion, and the mode of administration should be as an initial loading dose of 140 mg/kg. Follow-up doses of 70 mg/kg should be given at 4-hr intervals for 17 additional doses (3 days). The drug should be diluted to a 5% concentration, which may be swallowed by the patient or instilled into the stomach or duodenum by gastric tube.

Intravenous use of this agent is possible in the United States only through investigational centers. The oral form is not an approved nonpyrogenic form. Cysteamine and methionine have been abandoned as therapies for the toxic ingestion of acetaminophen.

TABLE 26–1. Stages in the Clinical Course of Acetaminophen Toxicity

Stage	Time Following Ingestion	Characteristics
I	½–24 hr	Anorexia, nausea, vomiting, malaise, pallor, diaphoresis
II	24–48 hr	Resolution of above; upper quadrant abdominal pain and tenderness; elevated bilirubin, prothrombin time, hepatic enzymes; oliguria
III	72–96 hr	Peak liver function abnormalities; anorexia, nausea, vomiting, malaise may reappear
IV	4 days–2 wk	Resolution of hepatic dysfunction

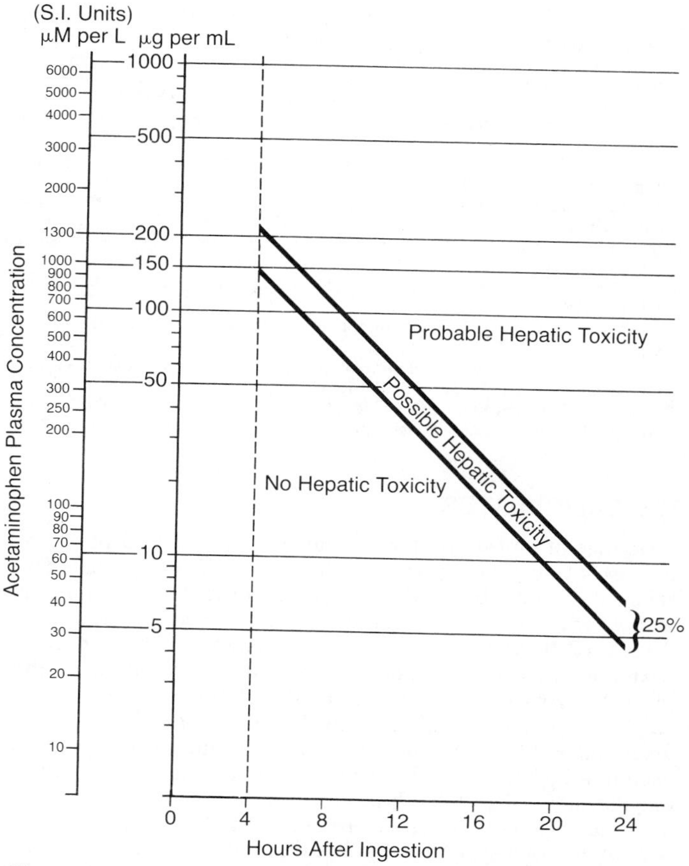

Figure 26–1. Rumack-Matthew nomogram for acetaminophen poisoning. Semilogarithmic plot of plasma acetaminophen levels versus time. *Cautions for the use of this chart:* (1) The time coordinates refer to time after *ingestion*. (2) Serum levels drawn before 4 hr may not represent peak levels. (3) The graph should be used only in relation to a single acute ingestion. (4) The lower *solid line* 25% below the standard nomogram is included to allow for possible errors in acetaminophen plasma assays and estimated time from ingestion of an overdose. (From Rumack BH, Spoerke DG [eds]: POISINDEX System: A Computerized Poison Information System. Copyright © Micromedex, Inc, Denver, CO, Vol 68, 1991. Adapted from Rumack BH, Matthew H: Acetaminophen poisoning and toxicity. Pediatrics 55:871–876, 1975. Copyright 1975. Reproduced by permission of Pediatrics.)

PROGNOSIS. Children younger than age 6 yr are unlikely to develop significant toxicity following ingestion of even relatively large doses of acetaminophen. In a large series, 55 of 417 children developed potentially toxic plasma levels following ingestion, but only 3 of the 417 developed SGOT peaks of greater than 1,000 IU/L, which is considered a toxic response. In two other series totaling 2,787 cases, no patients had toxic plasma levels and only 35 were hospitalized. Nevertheless, at this time children with a significant ingestion should have the plasma level measured and receive treatment with the antidote if the level falls within the toxic range on the nomogram. Adolescents have a higher incidence (23.2%) of toxic plasma levels following ingestion than children, and 29% of those with toxic levels are likely to develop SGOT of greater than 1,000 IU/L. Even after a serious case of hepatotoxicity, the mortality rate is well under 0.5%. Patients who recover have no sequelae when followed at 3–12 mo after the acute toxicity.

Baselt RC, Cravery RH: Deposition of Toxic Drugs and Chemicals in Man, 3rd ed. Chicago, Year Book Medical Publishers, 1989.

Lauterburg BH, Vaishnav Y, Stillwell WG, et al: The effects of age and glutathione depletion on hepatic glutathione turnover in vivo determined by acetaminophen probe analysis. J Pharmacol Exp Ther 213:54, 1980.

Linden CH, Rumack BH: Acetaminophen overdose. Emerg Clin North Am 2:103, 1984.

Mancini RE, Sonaware BR, Yaffe SJ: Developmental susceptibility to acetaminophen toxicity. Res Commun Chem Pathol Pharmacol 27:603, 1980.

Miller RP, Roberts RJ, Fisher LJ: Acetaminophen elimination kinetics in neonates, children, and adults. Clin Pharmacol Ther 19:284, 1976.

Peterson RG, Rumack BH: Age as a variable in acetaminophen overdose. Arch Intern Med 141:390, 1981.

Rumack BH: Acetaminophen overdose in young children. Am J Dis Child 138:428, 1984.

Rumack BH, Matthew H: Acetaminophen poisoning and toxicity. Pediatrics 55:871, 1975.

Rumack BH, Peterson RG: Acetaminophen overdose: Incidence, diagnosis and management in 416 patients. Pediatrics 62:898, 1978.

Rumack BH, Peterson RG, Koch GC, et al: Acetaminophen overdose: 662 cases with evaluation of oral acetylcysteine treatment. Arch Intern Med 141:380, 1981.

26.6 SALICYLATES

Incidence of ingestion of salicylates has gradually dropped as the use of acetaminophen has increased. Toxicity related to salicylates must be considered in therapeutic situations as well as when there has been an overdose. See also Sec. 6.23.

PATHOPHARMACOLOGY. Understanding the pharmocokinetics of salicylates permits a clearer evaluation of the plasma levels of salicylate and other laboratory data (Sec. 6.23). The usual half-life of salicylate is 1–2 hr. This may be extended to 25–30 hr once the urine becomes acidic and ion excretion becomes limited. The normal volume of distribution of salicylate is 0.15 L/kg, but with significant toxicity this may increase to 0.3–0.4 L/kg as protein binding is saturated and central nervous system and other distribution occurs. In cases of chronic toxicity, the metabolism of salicylates plays an insignificant role, urine excretion becomes minimal, and further doses add to the accumulated pool of drug in the patient.

Ionization of salicylate is related to the absorption and excretion of salicylate. In an alkaline state (e.g., urine of pH 7), this weak acid (pK approximately 3.0) is mostly ionized. Thus, it does not cross cell membranes very well and stays in the glomerular filtrate, permitting the drug to be excreted. As the urine pH becomes acid, less and less of the drug is ionized, reabsorption from glomerular filtrate occurs, and excretion decreases. Therapy directed at changing urine pH, therefore, affects urine excretion. In some circumstances, patients with various illnesses (e.g., juvenile rheumatoid arthritis) who are doing well on aspirin will suddenly develop problems after dietary changes. A large increase in use of orange juice, for example, will enhance excretion and reduce the plasma salicylate level, perhaps exacerbating the basic disease. Conversely, large ingestions of cranberry juice may acidify the urine, decrease excretion of salicylate, and raise plasma levels to toxic ranges.

CLINICAL MANIFESTATIONS. Young infants may have few signs of toxicity other than dehydration or hyperpnea. Temperature elevation may occur, leading to increased dosages of salicylates in a patient with salicylate toxicity. Older children demonstrate hyperpnea, vomiting, and progressive lethargy as the drug is distributed throughout the CNS. Tinnitus and sudden deafness may occur early in patients with salicylate toxicity. In adolescents, salicylate level measurement is required to distinguish hyperpnea from the "hyperventilation syndrome" (Sec. 3.32).

Although a large number of complex metabolic phenomena are involved following a salicylate ingestion, the clinically important relationships can be easily summarized:

Phase 1. Salicylates directly stimulate the respiratory center following absorption. The increased respiratory rate results in respiratory alkalosis and obligate alkaluria as a compensatory mechanism. Both K^+ and Na^+ are lost along with bicarbonate in the urine. This phase may last for as long as 12 hr after ingestion in an adolescent and may be totally missed in a young infant.

Phase 2. When sufficient K^+ has been lost to deplete the kidney of this ion, an exchange of K^+ for H^+ occurs and the urine becomes relatively acid. The hypokalemia is initially limited to renal tissue and is not reflected either in serum K^+ or on the electrocardiogram. This "paradoxical aciduria" occurs in the presence of a continued respiratory alkalosis. As this phase progresses, hypokalemia is reflected throughout the rest of the body. This phase may begin within hours after ingestion in a young child and may last as long as 12–24 hr in an adolescent.

Phase 3. Eventually dehydration, hypokalemia, and progressive accumulation of lactic acid and other metabolic acids predominate over the respiratory alkalosis. The patient's rapid breathing is in response to the acidosis rather than to primary respiratory center drive. The plasma level of salicylate is generally higher than in phase 1 or 2 because of inability to excrete salicylate in an acid urine and because of continued absorption from the intestine. Uncoupling of oxidative phosphorylation and other metabolic activity contribute a small amount to this phenomenon. The patient is acidotic, with an even more acid urine. This phase may begin 4 to 6 hr after ingestion in a young infant, or 24 hr or more after ingestion in an adolescent. This is also the presentation of chronic salicylate poisoning following repeated therapeutic dosing in the face of dehydration.

The more severe cases may develop pulmonary edema or hemorrhage, although both of these complications are rare. Hyperglycemia or hypoglycemia has also been observed. Virtually all seriously poisoned patients will be more than 5% dehydrated, usually 10% or more.

LABORATORY DATA. Following a single acute ingestion of salicylate, plasma level should be measured 6 hr or more after ingestion and plotted on the nomogram (Fig. 26–2). Levels observed before 6 hr may not reflect peak levels. The nomogram cannot be used when the drug has accumulated over several ingestions, because patients with chronic salicylate toxicity may have very low levels in relation to the severity of their illness, owing to a 3- to 4-fold increase in the volume of distribution. Levels in chronic toxicity may be in the therapeutic range of 10–20 mL/dL.

In all patients with salicylate poisoning serious enough to be hospitalized, the plasma levels should be plotted on semilog paper against time. Although the concept of half-life is not precisely correct in salicylate overdoses, calculation of this value from these plots is important. By seeing whether the apparent half-life decreases with therapy, the success of that therapy can be monitored. As long as the relative half-life is greater than 10–15 hr, treatment is not optional.

Urine pH and volume should be measured hourly in all seriously poisoned children. Plasma pH should be checked at regular intervals. K^+ and other electrolytes are critical to calculating replacement fluid therapy; serum K^+ will lag behind the K^+ status of the kidney. Prothrombin time should also be measured in all severely poisoned patients. Arterial blood gas measurements, as well as other ancillary laboratory measures required for the general support of the patient, should be performed. Hepatotoxicity from salicylate in severe, chronic cases will be demonstrated by SGOT, SGPT, bilirubin, and prothrombin abnormalities. Ferric chloride or Phenistix only indicate presence of the drug and should not be substituted for salicylate measurements. Neither of these tests will detect unhydrolized aspirin (acetylsalicylic acid) in tablets or vomitus.

TREATMENT. Dehydration and electrolyte abnormalities

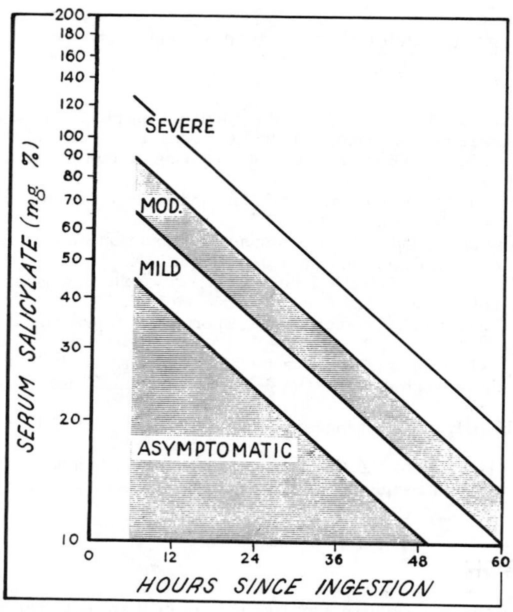

Figure 26–2. The Done nomogram for salicylate poisoning. *Cautions for the use of this chart*: (1) The patient has taken a single acute ingestion and is not suffering from chronic toxicity. (2) The blood level to be plotted on the nomogram was drawn 6 hr after *ingestion*. (3) Levels in the toxic range drawn before 6 hr should be treated. (4) If levels measured before 6 hr are in the nontoxic range, further measurements should be taken to see if the level is increasing. (From Done AK: Salicylate intoxication: Significance of measurements of salicylates in blood in cases of acute ingestion. Pediatrics 26:800–807, 1960. Copyright 1960. Reproduced by permission of Pediatrics.)

should be corrected after initiating activated charcoal, emesis, and other general acute measures (Sec. 6.16 and 26.4).

Phase 1. If dehydration and electrolyte losses have occurred for several hours, the patient may have a relative depletion of body bicarbonate, which requires treatment. Failure to administer sufficient bicarbonate, *even in the presence of an alkaline plasma,* may result in progression to phase 2. Plasma pH should be carefully monitored throughout bicarbonate infusion. Potassium should be carefully administered, even if the serum potassium is normal; urine potassium may be measured to document quantitative excretion.

Phase 2. It is critical to correct bicarbonate and potassium losses in patients in this phase. Insufficient potassium results in further depletion of body stores and continued failure to alkalinize the urine. At least 20–40 mEq/L of potassium is required.

Phase 3. Following correction of the usual severe dehydration, therapy is directed toward adding potassium and administering bicarbonate. Usually at least 40 mEq/L of potassium is required.

In all of these phases, alkalinization of the urine assists in excretion of salicylate.

Forced diuresis of 3–6 mL/kg/hr is not as important as alkalinization. Minimum fluid maintenance should result in at least 2 mL/kg/hr of urine flow. However, forced diuresis may aggravate pulmonary edema and adds little therapeutically once good alkalinization of the urine has been achieved. Acetazolamide and *tris*(hydroxymethyl)aminomethane are not recommended because of associated complications. Glucose should be administered and carefully monitored throughout the course of treatment.

Hemodialysis may be useful in severe toxicity when alkalinization has not been successful. No specific plasma levels should be used as an indication for this modality, since even very high levels of salicylate, above 100 mL/dL, have responded to alkalinization. *Peritoneal dialysis* is almost totally useless, even with addition of albumin. *Charcoal hemoperfusion* may be a useful adjunct; however, it is easier to correct fluid and electrolyte problems with hemodialysis.

Anderson RJ, Potts DE, Gabow PA, et al: Unrecognized adult salicylate intoxication. Ann Intern Med 85:745, 1976.
Done AK: Salicylate intoxication: Significance of measurements of salicylates in blood in cases of acute ingestion. Pediatrics 26:800, 1960.
Garrettson LK, Procknal JA, Levy G: Fetal acquisition and neonatal elimination of a large amount of salicylate: Study of a neonate whose mother regularly took therapeutic doses of aspirin during pregnancy. Clin Pharmacol Ther 17:98, 1975.
Gaudreault P, Temple AR, Lovejoy FH: The relative severity of acute versus chronic salicylate poisoning in children: A clinical comparison. Pediatrics 70:566, 1982.
Hill JB: Experimental salicylate poisoning: Observations on the effects of altering blood pH on tissue and plasma salicylate concentrations. Pediatrics 47:658, 1971.
Jacobsen D, Wiik-Larsen, Bredesen JE: Haemodialysis or hemoperfusion in severe salicylate poisoning. Hum Toxicol 7:161, 1988.
Levy G: Clinical pharmacokinetics of aspirin. Pediatrics 62(Suppl 5):867, 1978.
Levy G, Yaffe SJ: Relationship between dose and apparent volume of distribution of salicylate in children. Pediatrics 54:713, 1974.
Prescott LF, Balali-Mood M, Critchley JA, et al: Diuresis or urinary alkalinization for salicylate poisoning? Br Med J 285:1381, 1982.
Rumack CM, Guggenheim MA, Rumack BH, et al: Neonatal intracranial hemorrhage and maternal use of aspirin. Obstet Gynecol 58(Suppl):52, 1981.
Snodgrass W, Rumack BH, Peterson RG: Salicylate toxicity following therapeutic doses in young children. Clin Toxicol 18:247, 1981.
Temple AR: Acute and chronic effects of aspirin toxicity and their treatment. Arch Intern Med 141:364, 1981.

26.7 HYDROCARBONS

Accidental ingestion of products containing hydrocarbons involves an extremely wide array of chemical substances, and many factors are involved in determining whether a particular exposure will produce systemic or local toxicity. The following general classification of hydrocarbons relates to acute exposure and lists only representative examples.

1. High likelihood of systemic toxicity following ingestion.
   Halogenated and aliphatic hydrocarbons
   - Trichloroethane
   - Trichlorethylene
   - Carbon tetrachloride
   - Methylene chloride
   - Aromatic
   - Benzene
   - Hydrocarbons with additives
   - Heavy metals
   - Insecticides
   - Herbicides
   - Nitrobenzene
   - Aniline
2. Systemic and local toxicity unlikely.
   - Toluene
   - Xylene
   - Petroleum ether (benzine)
   - Petroleum naphtha ("lighter fluid")
   - VM & P naphtha ("paint thinner")
   - Mineral spirits (stoddard solvent, white spirit, mineral turpentine, petroleum spirits)
   - Turpentine
3. Local toxicity (e.g., aspiration) highly likely after ingestion. Systemic toxicity unlikely.
   - Mineral seal oil
   - Signal oil
   - Furniture polish mixtures
   - Gasoline

Kerosene
Charcoal lighter fluid

4. Generally nontoxic after ingestion in over 95% of cases.
   Asphalt or tar
   Lubricants (motor oil, transmission oil, cutting oil, household oil and heavy grease)
   Mineral or liquid petrolatum

PATHOPHYSIOLOGY. Once absorbed through ingestion, inhalation, or dermal routes, hydrocarbons can produce many kinds of *systemic toxicity*. The most common is CNS depression related to the anesthetic properties of certain hydrocarbons. Because most commercial products are mixtures or impure distillates, it is not possible to be precise about each product. In most cases, even following ingestion of hazardous hydrocarbons, the blood concentration may remain low enough to avoid CNS depression. Myocardial sensitization may follow ingestion of halogenated or nonhalogenated hydrocarbons. Hepatic toxicity, while usually related to carbon tetrachloride, is associated with many substances. Primary respiratory irritation with chemical pneumonitis, as well as irritation of the gastrointestinal tract, may occur. Renal and hematologic toxicity is usually related to long-term exposure. In some instances when there is high concentration of a hydrocarbon in the atmosphere, inhaling oxygen-poor air may produce anoxia or other findings not related to the toxicity of the actual hydrocarbon. Methylene chloride, found in most paint strippers, is an example of a substance that is metabolized after absorption to another substance, carbon monoxide, which produces systemic toxicity. Nitrobenzene or aniline-related compounds produce methemoglobinemia.

Local toxicity includes defatting of skin, irritation of mucous membranes, and most importantly, **aspiration pneumonitis** (see Sec. 14.60). Furniture polishes are the most common products containing mineral seal oil, the most notorious of the substances producing aspiration pneumonitis. During the act of swallowing, the very small amount of this substance that passes into the pulmonary tree is all that is required to produce significant pneumonitis. The chemical has very low viscosity and consequently is capable of spreading to involve large surface areas of the lung after only 0.1–0.2 mL is inhaled. Interstitial inflammation, hyperemia (sometimes with hemorrhage), and alveolar necrosis result.

CLINICAL MANIFESTATIONS. Aspiration pneumonia is characterized by coughing, which usually is the first clinical finding. Chest roentgenograms may be unremarkable for as long as 8–12 hr after aspiration. Most commonly, however, infiltrates will be seen by 2–3 hr after ingestion. Fever occurs later and may persist for as long as 10 days after ingestion. Accompanying leukocytosis may be misleading, since in most cases of aspiration pneumonitis, no bacteria are present in the lung. Later in the course of this illness, after resolution of most clinical findings and 2–3 wk after exposure, pneumatoceles may appear on the chest roentgenogram.

Older children, adolescents, and adults may be involved in solvent abuse. Symptoms of CNS depression, congestive heart failure, headache, vertigo, ataxis, euphoria, and renal and hepatic damage may be seen acutely. White matter changes have been reported in chronic abusers.

TREATMENT. Emesis may be useful in patients who have no other contraindication to vomiting and have consumed a hydrocarbon whose primary toxicity is systemic. When aspiration pneumonitis is likely and systemic toxicity is unlikely, emesis should not be induced. Instillation of vegetable oils or mineral oil into the stomach in an attempt to prevent absorption is contraindicated. Similarly, corticosteroids should be avoided, since they do not provide any benefit and may be harmful. Antibiotics should not be given prophylactically. Fever and leukocytosis usually result from the pyrogenic effect of the agent; bacterial pneumonia occurs in only a small percentage of cases.

Anas N, Nanasonthi V, Ginsburg CM: Criteria for hospitalizing children who have ingested products containing hydrocarbons. JAMA 246:840, 1981.
Banner W, Walson PD: Systems toxicity following gasoline aspiration. Am J Emerg Med 3:292, 1983.
Bergson PS, Hales SW, Lustganter MP: Pneumatoceles following hydrocarbon ingestion. Am J Dis Child 129:49, 1975.
Brown J, Burke B, Dajani AS: Experimental kerosene pneumonia: Evaluation of some therapeutic regimens. J Pediatr 84:396, 1984.
Dice WH, Ward G, Kelley J: Pulmonary toxicity following gastrointestinal ingestion of kerosene. Ann Emerg Med 11:138, 1982.
Kulig K, Rumack BH: Hydrocarbon ingestion. Curr Topics Emerg Med 3:1, 1981.
Rosenberg NL, Kleinschmidt-DeMaster BK, Davis KA, et al: Toluene abuse causes diffuse central nervous system white matter changes. Ann Neurol 23:611, 1988.
Rumack BH: Hydrocarbon ingestions in perspective. J Am Coll Emerg Phys 6:4, 1977.
Travner P, Harrison DJ, Bell GM: Acute renal failure due to interstitial nephritis induced by "glue-sniffing" with subsequent recovery. Scot Med J 33:2116, 1988.

26.8 IRON

Iron poisoning occurs frequently in childhood, related partially to the prevalence of iron-containing tablets in many homes and to the resemblance of many iron tablets to candy. Although iron poisoning rarely results in death, prompt action may be lifesaving. The severity of iron poisoning is related to the amount of elemental iron absorbed. Death has been reported after ingestion of as little as 650 mg of elemental iron, an amount contained in only 10 iron sulfate tablets. Absorption of 60 mg/kg is probably necessary for development of significant iron poisoning.

CLINICAL MANIFESTATIONS. The diagnosis of iron poisoning is usually made by history. Roentgenographic confirmation is often possible, because undisintegrated iron tablets are radiopaque.

Five phases may be observed with serious iron poisoning:

1. The local irritative effects of iron on the gastrointestinal mucosa have their onset 30 min–2 hr after ingestion and usually subside after 6–12 hr. They are the result of local necrosis and hemorrhage at the sites of iron contact. Nausea, vomiting, diarrhea, abdominal pain, hematemesis, and bloody diarrhea result. Severe hypotension may also occur.
2. The next phase of 2–6 hr is seen as a period of apparent recovery. The patient appears better, which may lead the physician to a false sense of security. During this time iron accumulates in mitochondria and various organs.
3. About 12 hr after ingestion the cellular damage produced by the iron produces manifestations. Hypoglycemia and a metabolic acidosis may occur, attributable to an impairment of electron transport by the damaged mitochondrial membranes. Lactic and citric acids accumulate owing to development of anaerobic metabolism and interference with the Krebs cycle.
4. After apparent recovery, 2–4 days after ingestion, severe hepatic necrosis with elevation of SGOT, SGPT, and abnormalities of bilirubin and prothrombin may occur.
5. There may be scarring and stenosis of the pyloric area 2–4 wk after ingestion as a result of the local irritative action during the first phase. This stenosis may be symptomatic and occasionally requires surgical intervention.

Not all patients demonstrate the phases in easily discernible increments. Most children with a history of ingestion develop few, if any, signs or symptoms, but they should be followed for 4–6 hr before being considered free of toxicity.

LABORATORY FINDINGS. The measurement of free iron in the serum is the best way to determine the potential for toxicity. This should be done by assessing levels of total serum iron and of total serum iron-binding capacity; if the total iron exceeds the iron-binding capacity, then free iron exists. Toxicity is unlikely unless there is at least 50 mg/kg or more of free iron. Total iron levels in excess of 350 mg/kg, regardless of iron-binding capacity, may also be toxic. In many instances, it is not possible to obtain a rapid assay. Usually, levels of serum iron greater than 300 mg/kg will be seen in patients who have diarrhea, vomiting, leukocytosis, hyperglycemia, and positive abdominal roentgenograms. Vomiting has some correlation with high toxicity, and its absence has some correlation with low toxicity.

TREATMENT. If the patient has not vomited, emesis should be induced. Lavage with a large-bore tube may be useful. Whereas 250 mg/kg oral dose of a saline cathartic may be helpful, activated charcoal is of little value. Emergency gastrotomy to remove tablets may be considered if large numbers remain in the stomach after lavage in a symptomatic patient.

Oral bicarbonate (2%) or dilute phosphosoda (1:4) forms a less soluble complex, but clinical benefits are questionable. Oral deferoxamine is expensive, may increase absorption, and is generally not used by this route in treating an acute overdose.

Supportive care for hypotension and the other severe problems associated with phases 1 and 3 should be instituted as for any other life-threatening illness (Sec. 6.34 and 26.4). If there is free serum iron of greater than 50 mg/dL, if the total iron level is greater than 350 mg/dL, or if the patient is symptomatic, then *parenteral deferoxamine* should be given. In severe cases, 10–15 mg/kg/hr for up to 24 hr may be given intravenously. For less severe cases, 90 mg/kg up to a 1 g/dose may be given intramuscularly every 8 hr for three doses. The total dose should not exceed 6.0 g intravenously or intramuscularly. Once the deferoxamine iron chelate is achieved, the complex will be excreted, imparting a reddish (vin rosé) color to the urine. Although some believe that administering deferoxamine in this way can be used to predict serum free iron by evaluating urine color, at best this gives an indication of presence but not severity. The use of chelation in renal failure requires hemodialysis to remove the complex.

Bayer MJ, Rumack BH: Poisoning and Overdose. Gaithersburg, MD, Aspen Publishers, 1983.
Boehnert M, Lacouture PG, Guttmacher A, et al: Massive iron overdose treated with high-dose deferoxamine infusion (abstr). Vet Hum Toxicol 28:291, 1985.
Czajka PA, Conrad JD, Duffy JP: Iron poisoning: An in vitro comparison of bicarbonate and phosphate lavage solutions. J Pediatr 98:491, 1981.
Fischer DS, Parkman R, Finch SC: Acute iron poisoning in children. JAMA 218:1179, 1971.
Gleason WA Jr, deMello DE, deCastro FJ, et al: Acute hepatic failure in severe iron poisoning. J Pediatr 38:140, 1979.
Helfer RE, Rodgerson DO: The effect of deferoxamine on the determination of serum iron and iron-binding capacity. J Pediatr 68:804, 1966.
Knasel AL, Collins-Barrow MD: Applicability of early indicators of iron toxicity. J Natl Med Assoc 78:1037, 1986.
Lacouture PG, Wason S, Temple AR, et al: Radiopacity of drugs and plants in vitro—limited usefulness. Vet Hum Toxicol 23:2, 1981.
Lovejoy FH: Chelation therapy in iron poisoning. J Toxicol Clin Toxicol 19:871, 1982–83.
Tarkka M, Anttila S, Sutinen S: Bronchial stenosis after aspiration of an iron tablet. Chest 93:433, 1988.

26.9 CYCLIC ANTIDEPRESSANTS

This group of drugs includes the tricyclics and a variety of associated agents primarily used as antidepressants. Table 26–2 lists these agents by structural classification as well as by relative toxicity. The mortality rate from all of these agents is estimated to be 7–12%. If exposures involving only accidental ingestion reported to poison centers in children younger than 5 yr old are considered, then the mortality rate is lower.

TABLE 26–2. Cyclic Antidepressants

Generic	Trade Name	Structural Classification	CNS Toxicity	CV Toxicity
Amitriptyline	Elavil Amitid Endep Amitril	Tricyclic	++++	++++
Amoxapine*	Ascendin	Tricyclic	++++	+
Clomipramine	INV	Tricyclic	++++	++++
Desipramine	Norpramin Pertofrane	Tricyclic	++++	++++
Doxepin	Adapin Sinequan	Tricyclic	++++	++++
Imipramine	Tofranil Presamine SK-Pramine Janimine	Tricyclic	++++	++++
Loxapine	Loxatane	Tricyclic	++++	+
Maprotiline†	Ludiomil	Tetracyclic	++++	++++
Mianserin	INV‡	Tetracyclic	?	?
Nortriptyline	Aventyl Pamelor	Tricyclic	++++	++++
Protriptyline	Vivactyl	Tricyclic	++++	++++
Trazodone	Desyrel	Miscellaneous¶	+	+
Trimipramine	Surmontil	Tricyclic	++++	++++
Viloxazine	INV§	Bicyclic	?	?
Zimelidine	INV§	Bicyclic	?	?

*Amoxapine is structurally similar to loxapine, an antipsychotic agent, and appears to have similar toxicity. Amoxapine is an active metabolite of loxapine.
†Available evidence suggests that maprotiline may have less cardiovascular toxicity when compared with the tricyclic antidepressants.
‡Investigational or newly released drug; tetracyclic antidepressant toxicity to be determined.
§Investigational or newly released drug; bicyclic antidepressant toxicity to be determined.
¶This agent has a unique dual bicyclic structure.
Combination products: Combination products containing tricyclic antidepressants include Limbitrol (amitriptyline and chlordiazepoxide); Etrafon, Perphenyline, Triavil, and Triptazine (amitriptyline and perphenazine).
From Rumack BH, Spoerke DG (eds): POISINDEX System®: A Computerized Poison Information System. Denver, CO, Micromedex, Inc, 1989, with permission of author and publisher.

PATHOPHYSIOLOGY. Cyclic antidepressants, notably the tricyclics, are structurally similar to the phenothiazines and have similar anticholinergic, adrenergic, and α-blocking properties. Following absorption, these agents are extensively bound to plasma proteins and also bind to tissue and cellular sites, including the mitochondria. The blood:tissue ratio varies from 1:10 to 1:30, which explains the ineffectiveness of forced diuresis and dialysis techniques in removal of the drug. They block the neuronal reuptake of norepinephrine, 5-hydroxytryptamine, serotonin, or dopamine. Therapeutic doses, initially, may cause drowsiness and difficulty concentrating and thinking; dulling of depressive ideation may explain the efficacy of these agents in depressive disorders. Hallucinations, excitement, and confusion have occurred in a small percentage of patients during antidepressant therapy. These agents also have a slight α-adrenergic blocking effect. Trazodone inhibits the neuronal uptake of serotonin and has antiserotonin and α-adrenergic blocking properties.

CLINICAL MANIFESTATIONS. The initial presentation is the onset of the anticholinergic syndrome including tachycardia, pupillary dilatation, dryness of mucous membranes, urinary retention, hallucinations, and flushing. Although hypertension also may initially occur, hypotension rapidly develops and is a serious sign. Convulsions, coma, and major arrhythmias ensue as tissue saturation occurs. Cardiac findings include quinidine-like effects such as slowing of myocardial conduction, multifocal premature ventricular contractions, ventricular tachycardia, flutter, and fibrillation. In addition to widening of the QRS complex, QT prolongation occurs with T wave flattening or inversion, ST segment depression, right bundle branch block, and complete heart block.

CNS toxicity includes manifestations of depression, lethargy, and hallucinations. Choreoathetosis and myoclonus have been reported and must be differentiated from generalized seizures. Coma, when it occurs, has a mean duration of 6.4 hr but may last for longer than 24 hr.

A withdrawal syndrome in neonates delivered of patients who have been taking tricyclics has occurred, with tachypnea, irritability, and restlessness lasting the 1st mo of life. Amoxapine differs from other tricyclics; there is significantly greater incidence of seizures and coma. Cardiovascular toxicity is less prominent, and seizures and coma may be associated with normal QRS complexes.

Loxapine is similar to its metabolite amoxapine in having a greater incidence of CNS toxicity and a lesser incidence of cardiovascular toxicity.

Exposure to the tetracyclics appears to be associated with a higher incidence of cardiovascular effects than does exposure to the tricyclics. Bicyclics are similar to tetracyclics but additionally appear to cause less anticholinergic toxicity. Trazodone, which has a uniquely different structure, appears to result in little CNS or cardiovascular toxicity.

Children should be observed and their electrocardiogram monitored for at least 6 hr. If any tissue manifestations (such as a QRS interval longer than 0.12 or an altered mental status) are present, then patients should be monitored for 24 hr. Catastrophic deterioration has been observed in patients who at first appear mildly, if at all, poisoned and whose condition then rapidly becomes seriously toxic. Only completely asymptomatic children should be discharged after 6 hr. Others should be admitted to intensive care units and monitored for at least 24 hr.

LABORATORY FINDINGS. Laboratory tests may be helpful in establishing the type of agent ingested. However, because these agents have extremely high volumes of distribution, blood level measurements may not be helpful in establishing severity. The observation of signs and symptoms is extremely helpful and should be relied on when laboratory test results are negative.

TREATMENT. Following general life support measures, efforts should be made to *prevent absorption*. Emesis should be avoided in children showing clinical manifestations because of the danger of aspiration from vomiting following onset of coma. Activated charcoal should be administered at a dose of 50–100 g in adolescents and 15–30 g in younger children. Repeated doses of activated charcoal should be given to all symptomatic children at a dose of 10–20 g every 2–6 hr. Obtunded patients may have this agent administered through a small-bore nasogastric tube. Multiple-dose charcoal will remove drug being re-excreted in the gastrointestinal tract. Single-dose *cathartics* such as sorbitol, magnesium, or sodium sulfate should be administered.

Although there is controversy as to which *antiarrhythmic drugs* should be given and in what order, the following is generally accepted. Sodium bicarbonate should be administered in doses sufficient to achieve a pH of 7.45–7.55. Phenytoin is indicated if conduction defects occur, such as QRS complex increased beyond 0.12 or prolonged QT interval. The dose of phenytoin is 15 mg/kg, up to 1.0 g intravenously, not to exceed a rate of 0.5 mg/kg/min. Some experts prefer prophylactic loading of phenytoin. Children with ventricular arrhythmias should have their acidosis corrected immediately with bicarbonate or mechanical hyperventilation. Phenytoin should be the first agent administered, followed by lidocaine at a loading dose of 1 mg/kg/dose and by appropriate maintenance doses thereafter. Bretylium tosylate should not be used in hypotensive patients or in those with fixed cardiac output. In adolescents, propranolol may be used at a dose of 1.0 mg intravenously every 2–5 min, until a response occurs. In younger children, the dose is 0.1 mg intravenously, until a maximum of 1.0 mg has been given. Physostigmine should be used only rarely. It is an exceptionally dangerous agent, especially if given rapidly. It is most useful in supraventricular arrhythmias. In children, 0.5 mg intravenously should be given over 2–3 min; it may be repeated 2 to 3 times.

Patients with *seizures* should be primarily treated with diazepam at a dose of up to 10 mg intravenously in an adolescent or 0.1–0.3 mg/kg, up to 10 mg, in a child. Phenytoin should then be given. Physostigmine may be used for myoclonic seizures or choreoathetosis but is not very effective for generalized seizures.

Hypotension may respond to norepinephrine but usually does not respond to dopamine. Severe hypotension is very serious and may require fluids and an intra-aortic balloon. *Hypertension* usually responds to physostigmine. Patients who have a seriously deteriorating course may have such a significant degree of tissue loading that they cannot be saved. Although hemodialysis and charcoal hemoperfusion have been attempted, these procedures are rarely helpful in such overdoses.

Albertson TE, Derlet RW, Foulke GE, et al: Superiority of activated charcoal alone compared with ipecac and activated charcoal in the treatment of acute toxic ingestions. Ann Emerg Med 18:56, 1989.

Burks JS, Walker JE, Rumack BH, et al: Tricyclic antidepressant poisoning—reversal of coma, choreoathetosis, and myoclonus by physostigmine. JAMA 230(10):1405, 1974.

Callaham M, Kassel D: Epidemiology of fatal tricyclic antidepressant ingestion: Implications for management. Ann Emerg Med 14:1, 1985.

Callaham M, Schumaker H, Pentel P: Phenytoin prophylaxis of cardiotoxicity in experimental amitriotyline poisoning. Pharmacol Exp Ther 245:216, 1988.

Ellison DW, Pentel PR: Clinical features and consequences of seizures due to cyclic antidepressant overdose. Am J Emerg Med 7:5, 1989.

Kulig K, Rumack BH, Sullivan JB, et al: Amoxapine overdose: Coma and seizures without cardiotoxic effects. JAMA 248:1092, 1982.

Lavoie RW, Gansert GG, Weiss RE: Initial ECG findings in 187 cases of cyclic antidepressant overdose (abstract). Ann Emerg Med 18:446, 1989.

Molloy DW, Penner SB, Rabson J, et al: Use of sodium bicarbonate to treat tricyclic antidepressant–induced arrhythmias in a patient with alkalosis. Can Med Assoc J 130:1457, 1984.

Rumack BH: Anticholinergic poisoning: Treatment with physostigmine. Pediatrics 52:449, 1973.

Rumack BH, Spoerke DG (eds): POISINDEX System®. A Computerized Poison Information System. Denver, CO, Micromedex, Inc, Vol 68, 1991.

Shannon MW, Merola J, Lovejoy FH Jr: Hypotension in severe tricyclic antidepressant overdose. Am J Emerg Med 6:439, 1988.

Sjöqvist F, Bergfors PG, Borga O, et al: Plasma disappearance of nortriptyline in a newborn infant following placental transfer from an intoxicated mother: Evidence of drug metabolism. J Pediatr 80:1046, 1972.

26.10 ALKALIS AND ACIDS

The incidence of severe injury from this variety of ingestions has dropped dramatically following the removal from the market of liquid corrosive drain cleaners. These agents had the tenacious capacity to coat the esophagus and produce major tissue destruction.

PATHOPHYSIOLOGY. *Alkaline agents* tend to produce liquefaction necrosis (e.g., when the strong base binds to the fats and oils in the tissue and produces a soap [saponification]). Tablets such as Clinitest tend to lodge at about the level of the aortic arch in the esophagus and produce circumferential burns. Crystalline drain cleaners may produce a small streak-like burn; they result in circumferential burns in only 15% of all cases. Solutions of greater than 4% NaOH may produce very widespread circumferential burns. Linear streak burns usually do not constrict and form obstructions, but circumferential burns are likely to develop esophageal strictures, which may become totally occlusive. Alkaline agents in the crystal form may spare the mouth and hypopharynx as they travel across these areas on the saliva. Once in the esophagus, they may then produce damage. Common household bleach (5.4% or less), while producing hyperemia, is less likely to produce burns.

Strong acid agents, such as sulfuric, nitric, or hydrochloric acid, are frequently concentrated at the pyloric end of the stomach, resulting in scarification and eventually stricture formation. They may also seriously damage the esophagus and other areas of the stomach, leading to necrosis and perforation.

Two other sources of alkaline irritation include *disc batteries* and *automatic dishwasher detergents.* Complications may occur when disc batteries lodge in the esophagus, gastrointestinal tract, nose, or ears. Localized tissue necrosis with possible tracheoesophageal fistula or burns may occur due to leaking contents. Most automatic dishwasher compounds have a pH of from 10.5 to 12.5. Actual burn development depends on several factors, including free alkalinity, composition, formulation, viscosity, and concentration.

CLINICAL MANIFESTATIONS. When burns of the esophagus or hypopharynx have occurred, swallowing is likely to be impeded, and consequently the child may drool excessively. Burns on lips and tongue may be seen. No correlation exists between oral and esophageal burns; either can exist without the other. Pain and difficulty swallowing may be encountered. Occasionally, when the diagnosis has been missed, the patient will present with esophageal strictures and vomiting.

TREATMENT (see Sec. 13.22). If the patient can swallow safely, milk or water should be administered, 1–2 cups in the first few minutes after ingestion. Following this, the child should be kept from having anything orally. Esophagoscopy should be performed between 12 and 24 hr after ingestion, to determine whether a circumferential burn exists. Performing this procedure earlier may be of less value, since the full extent of the burns may not be apparent. If there are significant burns, the patient should remain on clear liquids to avoid possible esophageal perforation. At 2–3 wk after injury, patients may develop strictures, necessitating a feeding gastrostomy. Endoscopic dilation and a colonic interposition or a gastric tube may then be necessary as a more definitive procedure.

Administering acids (such as fruit juice) to children who have consumed bases and bases to children after acid ingestion is contraindicated, since an exothermic reaction may occur and aggravate the injury. Surgical evaluation in significant cases is mandatory.

Ferguson MK, Migliore M, Staszak VM, et al: Early evaluation and therapy for caustic esophageal injury. Am J Surg 157:116, 1989.
French RJ, Tabb HG, Rutledge LJ: Esophageal stenosis produced by ingestion of bleach. South Med J 63:1140, 1970.
Gaudreault P, Parent M, McGuigan MA: Predictability of esophageal injury from signs and symptoms: A study of 378 children. Pediatrics 71:761, 1983.
Haller JA, Andrews HG, White JJ, et al: Pathophysiology and management of acute corrosive burns of the esophagus. J Pediatr Surg 6:578, 1971.
Leape LL, Ashcraft KW, Scarpelli DG, et al: Hazard to health—liquid lye. N Engl J Med 284:578, 1971.
Linden CH, Buner JM, Kulig K, et al: Acid ingestion: Toxicity following systemic absorption. Vet Hum Toxicol 25:282, 1983.
Lorette JJ Jr, Wilkinson JA: Alkaline chemical burn to the face requiring full-thickness skin grafting. Ann Emerg Med 17:739, 1988.
Maull KI, Osmand AP, Maull CD: Liquid caustic ingestions: An in vitro study of the effects of buffer, neutralization, and dilation. Ann Emerg Med 14:1160, 1985.
O'Konek S, Bierbach H, Atzpodien W: Unexpected metabolic acidosis in severe lye poisoning. Clin Toxicol 18:225, 1981.
Penner GE: Acid ingestion: Toxicology and treatment. Ann Emerg Med 9:374, 1980.
Pense SC, Wood WJ, Stempel TK, et al: Tracheoesophageal fistula secondary to muriatic acid ingestion. Burns 14:35, 1988.
Rumack BH: Soap solution contraindicated in acid ingestion (letter). J Am Coll Emerg Phys 8:124, 1979.
Rumack BH, Burrington JD: Caustic ingestions: A rational look at diluents. Clin Toxicol 11:27, 1977.
Scher LA, Maull KI: Emergency management and sequelae of acid ingestion. J Am Coll Emerg Phys 7:206, 1978.

26.11 IBUPROFEN

The anti-inflammatory agent ibuprofen, which has become available as an over-the-counter drug, is likely to be involved in progressively more accidental and intentional overdoses because of its wider distribution.

PATHOPHYSIOLOGY. Peak plasma levels occur after 1–1½ hr. The volume of distribution is 0.11–0.13 L/kg, which is similar to that seen with salicylates. Only about 10% of the drug is excreted unchanged; the rest is metabolized in the liver. About 90% of a therapeutic dose of ibuprofen is bound to protein, and its half-life is about 2 hr.

LABORATORY FINDINGS. The drug can be measured in plasma; levels of 20–30 μg/mL at 2 hr are therapeutic. Levels in the 70–100 μg/mL range 2 hr after ingestion are not associated with symptoms, but mild symptoms of gastrointestinal upset and lethargy occur at 3 hr in the range of 80–200 μg/mL (Fig. 26–3). Seriously toxic findings have been seen at a 2-hr level of 360 μg/mL, but levels as high as 704 μg/mL have been seen without toxicity.

CLINICAL MANIFESTATIONS. Gastrointestinal disorders including nausea, epigastric pain, and upper gastrointestinal tract bleeding have been reported. Renal failure and toxicity have been noted in adults and children with marked increase in serum potassium and creatinine and blood urea nitrogen levels. Hypotension has occurred but is rare. Nystagmus, diplopia, headache, tinnitus, and transient deafness have all been reported.

The most serious problems with this drug are lethargy, coma, and transient apnea. Although not reported in adults or adolescents, children 1–1½ yr of age have developed apnea following ingestion of 2.8–7.6 g. Lethargy and drowsiness are common and occur in pediatric patients following ingestion of 120–230 mg/kg. Acid-base disturbances are not common. Acidosis is seen especially in younger children. Anaphylactoid reactions have been reported with circulatory collapse, angioedema, and pruritus.

TREATMENT. Respiratory and cardiovascular support should be given immediately. Emesis, unless contraindicated by the patient's condition, may be useful. Ingested amounts of less than 100 mg/kg are not likely to produce toxicity (see Fig. 26–3); however, as in any ingestion, the history should be cautiously interpreted. Hypotension should be treated with dopamine or norepinephrine. Although the manufacturer recommends alkaline diuresis, this is unlikely to be beneficial because of 90% protein binding. Hemodialysis and charcoal hemoperfusion may be of benefit because of the small volume of distribution.

In general, good supportive care of coma or apnea until the drug is metabolized should permit resolution of the overdose in 24 hr. Children with a history of ingestion should be observed at least 6 hr to be certain that apnea and CNS depression do not occur.

Barry WS, Meinzinger MM, Howse CR: Ibuprofen overdose and exposure in utero: Results from a postmarketing voluntary reporting system. Am J Med 77:35, 1984.
Court H, Streete P, Volans GN: Acute poisoning with ibuprofen. Hum Toxicol 2:381, 1983.
Court H, Street RJ, Volans GN: Overdose with ibuprofen causing unconsciousness and hypotension. Br Med J 282:1073, 1981.
Hall AH, Rumack BH: Treatment of patients with ibuprofen overdose. Ann Emerg Med 17:185, 1988.
Hall AH, Smolinske SC, Conrad FL, et al: Ibuprofen overdose: 126 cases. Ann Emerg Med 15:1308, 1986.

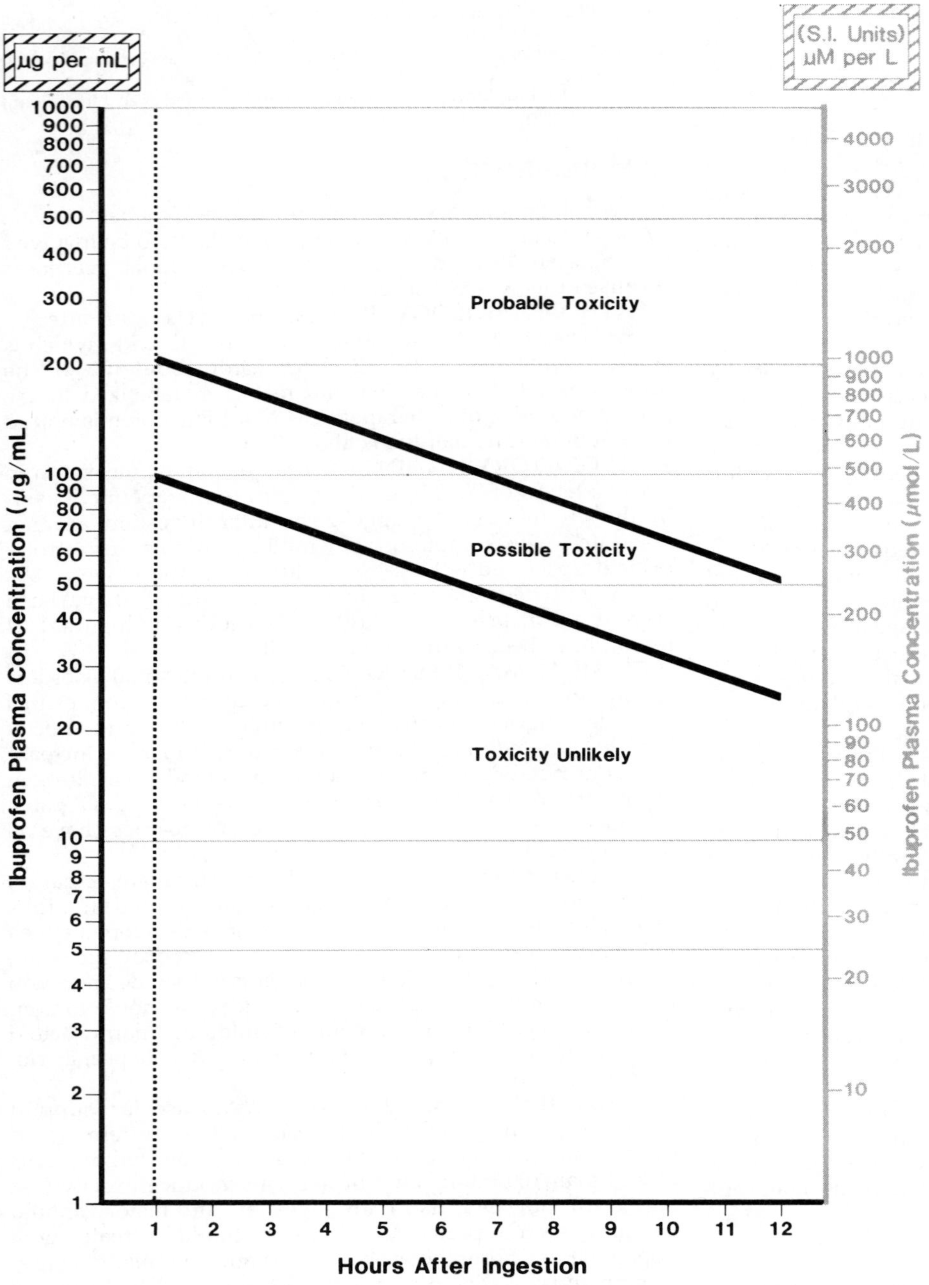

Figure 26–3. Nomogram for ibuprofen poisoning. *Cautions for the use of this chart*: (1) The time coordinates refer to time after *ingestion*. (2) Plasma levels obtained sooner than 1 hr or later than 12 hr after ingestion cannot be interpreted. (3) The nomogram may aid in predicting which initially asymptomatic or mildly symptomatic patients have the potential to develop symptoms or more severe symptomatology later. (From Hall AH, et al: Ibuprofen overdose: 126 cases. Ann Emerg Med 15:1308, 1986.)

Nomogram Prediction of Toxicity Development

	Portion of Nomogram		
	Probable Toxicity	**Possible Toxicity**	**Toxicity Unlikely**
Severe Symptoms	24%	17%	0%
Symptoms	65%	33%	24%
Asymptomatic	35%	67%	76%

Hall AH, Smolinske SC, Kulig KW, et al: Ibuprofen overdose: A prospective study. West J Med 148:653, 1988.
Hunt DP, Leigh RJ: Overdose with ibuprofen causing unconsciousness and hypotension. Br Med J 281:1458, 1980.
Joubert DW: Zomepirac overdose and review of literature on acute toxicity of nonsteroidal antiinflammatory agents. Drug Intell Clin Pharmacol 16:328, 1982.
Katona BG, Wigley FM, Walters JK, et al: Aseptic meningitis from over-the-counter ibuprofen. Lancet 1:59, 1988.
Poirier TI: Reversible renal failure associated with ibuprofen: Case report and review of the literature. Drug Intell Clin Pharmacol 18:27, 1984.
Rumack BH, Spoerke DG (eds): POISINDEX System®: A Computerized Poison Information System. Denver, CO, Micromedex, Inc, Vol 68, 1991.

26.12 PLANTS

Ingestion or exposure to plants both inside the home and outside in backyards and fields is one of the most common accidental poisoning problems. Table 26–3 lists the 20 most frequent exposures in young children. Fortunately, most plant

TABLE 26–3. Frequency of Plant Exposures by Plant Type*

Botanical Name	Common Name	Frequency
Philodendron spp	Philodendron	6,565
Dieffenbachia spp	Dumbcane	4,124
Euphorbia pulcherrima	Poinsettia	3,214
Capsicum annuum	Pepper	2,737
Crassula spp	Jade plant	2,424
Ilex spp	Holly	2,330
Brassaia & Schefflera spp	Schefflera	2,085
Spathiphyllum spp	Peace lily	1,712
Toxicodendron radicans	Poison ivy	1,662
Epipremnum aureum	Pothos, Devil's ivy	1,625
Phytolacca americana	Pokeweed, Inkberry	1,597
Saintpaulia spp	African violet	1,360
Pyracantha spp	Firethorn	1,233
Rhododendron spp	Rhododendron, Azalea	1,048
Ficus benjamina	Weeping fig tree	1,023
Solanum dulcamara	Climbing Nightshade	959
Chrysanthemum spp	Chrysanthemum	952
Chlorophytum comosum	Spider plant	920
Aloe spp	Aloe	862
Ficus elastica	Rubber plant	825

*From Litovitz TL, et al: 1990 Annual Report of The American Association of Poison Control Centers National Data Collection System. Am J Emerg Med 9(5):497, 1991.

ingestions result in little or no toxicity, and those children developing clinical manifestations usually can be dealt with symptomatically. The following are some of the common groups, their major findings, and treatment.

Arum Family

Examples are dieffenbachia, caladium, and philodendron. In this family, the entire plant contains various concentrations of calcium oxalate crystals. The most common problems occur in the oropharynx and include irritation of the lips, tongue, and mucous membrane. Intense pain and swelling may be seen. Washing of the affected area may be helpful, along with ice chips to chew and relieve pain. Corticosteroids may be helpful in very serious cases. Systemic toxicity is extremely rare.

Anticholinergic (Atropine and Related) Family

Examples are jimson weed, deadly nightshade, and potato (see also Sec. 26.3). All parts of these plants, especially the green portions, contain solanaceous (atropinic) alkaloids. Findings include tachycardia, dryness, flushing, hypertension, delirium, hallucinations, thirst, and, in some cases, coma and convulsions. If the syndrome is very severe, physostigmine may be used in doses similar to that with the cyclic antidepressants. If the findings are mild, then the patient should receive no treatment but be carefully observed.

Castor Bean and Jequirity Bean

These plants contain toxalbumins: ricin in castor bean, and abrin in jequirity bean. Severe, crampy diarrhea along with nausea, vomiting, CNS depression, shock, and convulsions may occur. Hemolytic anemia may occur with ricin, whereas renal failure is more common with abrin. There is no specific treatment. Children should be managed symptomatically, and urine flow should be monitored. Activated charcoal should be administered.

Foxglove

These plants contain the classic cardiac glycoside digitalis. Substantial similarity to overdose with any of the digitalis glycosides exists. Bradycardia with nausea and vomiting are seen as heart block gradually progresses. FAB fragments (Digibind) are effective in treatment. Potassium levels should be monitored. Treatment by phenytoin loading should be considered, as well as administration of activated charcoal to prevent further absorption.

Oleander

Oleander contains cardiac glycosides somewhat different from those of foxglove. In addition to local irritation, patients exhibit nausea, vomiting, diarrhea, and, in severe cases, A-V block, with ST segment depression and severe bradycardia. It is unknown whether FAB fragments (Digibind) will help. Potassium levels should be carefully followed. Phenytoin or atropine may be useful, as well as oral activated charcoal.

Hemlock

Poison hemlock contains the alkaloid coniine, which initially produces hyperactivity followed by CNS depression and respiratory failure. There is no specific treatment. Activated charcoal should be administered soon after ingestion, and respirations should be monitored. The intoxication is similar to that of nicotine.

Water hemlock contains the agent cicutoxin, which is likely to cause the rapid onset of hyperactivity, leading to convulsions within 30 min. Abdominal pain, emesis, and salivation are usually seen. Dilatation of the pupils is usual after onset of major signs. There is no specific treatment. Control of seizures with diazepam and administration of activated charcoal, if the patient can swallow, may be helpful. Supportive care should be provided.

BARRY H. RUMACK

Frohne D, Pfander HJ: A Color Atlas of Poisonous Plants. London, Wolfe Publishing, 1984.
Hardin JW, Arena JM: Human Poisoning from Native and Cultivated Plants. Durham, NC, Duke University Press, 1974.
Kingsbury JM: Poisonous Plants of the United States and Canada. Englewood Cliffs, NJ, Prentice-Hall, 1964.
Klein-Schwartz W, Oderda GM: Jimson weed intoxications in adolescents and young adults. Am J Dis Child 138:737, 1984.
Lampe KF, McConn MA: AMA Handbook of Poisonous and Injurious Plants. Chicago, American Medical Association, 1985.
Mitchel J, Rook A: Botanical Dermatology. Vancouver, Greengrass, 1979.
Rumack BH, Spoerke DG (eds): POISINDEX System®. A Computerized Poison Information System. Denver, CO, Micromedex, Inc, Vol 68, 1991.
Saravanapavananthan N, Ganeshamoorthy J: Yellow oleander poisoning: A study of 170 cases. Forensic Sci Int 26:247, 1988.
Veltri JC, Litovitz TL: 1983 Annual Report of the American Association of Poison Control Centers, National Data Collection System. Am J Emerg Med 1990.

MERCURY

Mercury, both inorganic and organic, causes acute and chronic poisoning. However, it is still widely used today in the household, in medicine, in agriculture, and in industry. Its effects may be either reversible or irreversible, depending on the compound and quantity of exposure. In acute poisoning, the effects of mercury exposure appear predominantly in the gastrointestinal tract and kidney, and in chronic poisoning, in the CNS and skin. Incidents of mercury poisoning of human communities have occurred in many areas of the world. Therefore, understanding the implications and mechanisms of environmental pollution by mercurial compounds has become essential for preventing and remedying contamination.

26.13 Acute and Chronic Mercury Poisoning

ETIOLOGY. Mercury vapor is highly toxic. Mercurous chloride, or calomel, is still used as an antiseptic in some skin creams. Aqueous thimerosal (Merthiolate) has been serving for years as a topical antiseptic. The mercurial diuretic chlormerodrin has been employed in the roentgenographic scanning of kidney and brain. Phenylmercuric salts are used in paints and as a fungicide for seeds. Methylmercury compounds have been used extensively as fungicides and have been the reported cause of poisonings resulting from the ingestion of bread made from wheat treated with these compounds. Mercuric salts have wide application in industries whose pollution has led to problems of environmental contamination, notably of methylmercury poisoning, which results from the ingestion of contaminated fish.

CLINICAL MANIFESTATIONS. Exposure to high concentrations of mercury vapor may cause pulmonary irritation or pneumonitis, nausea, vomiting, diarrhea, abdominal pain, and headache. Oral intake of mercury may cause stomatitis; gingivitis; esophagitis; gastroenteritis with excessive salivation; nausea, vomiting, and abdominal pain; and severe, bloody diarrhea. Patients with kidney damage develop anuria, albuminuria, and uremia and frequently die. CNS symptoms include ataxia, slurring of speech, numbness of the hands and feet, visual and hearing impairment, and delirium.

TREATMENT. Emergency treatment of acute mercury poisoning consists of (1) intravenous correction of fluid and electrolyte losses to prevent peripheral vascular collapse and (2) gastric lavage to remove the mercury in the stomach. Lavage is done first with milk and then repeated with 2–5% sodium bicarbonate.

The most effective antidote for acute mercury poisoning is BAL (British antilewisite or dimercaprol). The drug is administered intramuscularly in a 10% solution with a recommended dosage of 5 mg/kg for the first injection and 3 mg/kg every 4 hr for 2 days; this dose is then tapered to every 6 hr for 1 day, followed by administration every 12 hr for 7 days. BAL may protect against kidney damage from acute poisoning when given within 3 hr after ingestion of mercury. It may produce unpleasant side effects, such as nausea, vomiting, and fever, as the dose is increased. Penicillamine (*N*-acetyl-D,L-penicillamine) is used in patients who have adverse reactions to BAL. One method of administration is to give 100 mg/kg orally in four divided doses, to a maximum of 1,000 mg/24 hr.

Symptomatic treatment is also important. Hydroxyzine and chlorpromazine may be useful for restlessness and tolazoline for tachycardia.

Peritoneal dialysis or hemodialysis may be indicated for acute renal failure.

Chronic mercury poisoning generally results from occupational exposure in adults and is rare in children. However, both acrodynia and Minamata disease are important clinical conditions in children in which the CNS and skin are most frequently involved. The symptoms are diverse and variable, and in severe cases they are irreversible.

26.14 Acrodynia

(Pink Disease, Swift Disease, Feer Disease, Erythredema; Dermatopolyneuritis)

Acrodynia (Greek, "painful extremities"), which is principally a syndrome of chronic mercury poisoning in infants and young children, consists of many unusual symptoms that in the well-established cases are so distinctive that there is practically no differential diagnosis. In few other conditions does extreme and persistent misery play such a prominent part of the clinical picture.

ETIOLOGY. Most cases of acrodynia represent the clinical response to repeated contact with or ingestion of mercury in products such as house paints, wallpapers, teething powders, vermifuges, and diaper rinses. The interval between mercury exposure and onset of symptoms may vary from 1 wk to several months. The condition is probably the manifestation of a sensitization to mercury in the hypersensitive child.

PATHOLOGY. Pathologic findings are mainly present in the CNS. Degeneration and chromatolysis of the cerebral and cerebellar cortex are prominent.

CLINICAL MANIFESTATIONS. The natural course of acrodynia is prolonged, extending from several months to a year. There are all grades of severity. The child becomes listless, no longer interested in play, restless, and irritable. Generalized inconstant rashes, which are protean, recur from time to time. Early, the tips of the fingers, toes, and nose acquire a pinkish color, and later the hands and feet become a dusky pink, with patchy areas of ischemia and cyanotic congestion. The coloring shades off at the wrists and ankles. These changes in the extremities are the most distinctive features of the syndrome and are responsible for the term *pink disease*. Frequently the cheeks and the tip of the nose acquire a scarlet color.

As the disease becomes established, the sweat glands are enormously dilated and enlarged and perspiration is profuse. Secondary infection may lead to a severe pyoderma. There is desquamation of the soles and palms, which, although usually superficial, may be severe and recur during the course of the disease. The fingers and toes appear edematous; the swelling is due to hyperplasia and hyperkeratosis of the skin. An outstanding symptom is constant pruritus with excruciating pain in the hands and feet. Children will rub their hands together for hours, and older children will complain of a severe burning sensation.

The nails become dark and frequently drop off. Occasionally, gangrene of the toes and fingers develops and trophic ulcers may result from the constant rubbing of the hands and feet. The hair tends to fall out and is often pulled out by the child.

There is photophobia without evidence of local inflammation of the eyes. The children shield their eyes or bury their faces in their pillows. The lax ligaments and hypotonia permit the children to assume unusual positions (Fig. 26–4).

In extreme cases the teeth may be lost; necrosis of the jaw bones frequently follows. Initially, the gums appear normal except for a slightly deeper red color; later they become inflamed and swollen. Salivation then becomes pronounced, and the saliva often flows from the mouth in a constant stream. Anorexia is prominent, but because of the excessive perspiration large quantities of water are consumed. There may be diarrhea, and prolapse of the rectum is a frequent complication. The blood pressure and pulse rate may be increased significantly. Fever is usually not present unless there is some complication such as a urinary tract infection or bronchopneumonia.

Neurologic symptoms are an important part of the syndrome and include neuritis, mental apathy, and irritability. Early in the disease the tendon reflexes may be normal or increased, but later they disappear. There is not a true motor paralysis, but because of the soft, flabby musculature the child has no desire to walk and remains hypotonic, listless, and hypomotile. Severe pain prevents normal sleep. A child with acrodynia never appears happy or comfortable; the child does not play or smile but appears dejected and melancholic, a picture of abject misery.

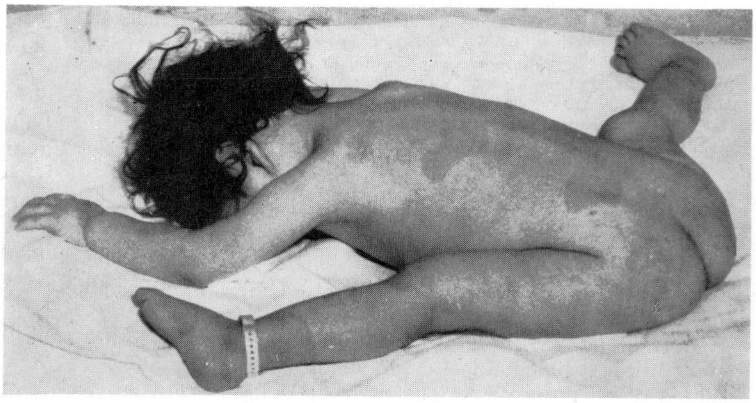

Figure 26–4. Extreme hypotonia and photophobia in an infant with acrodynia. This bizarre position may be maintained for hours.

LABORATORY DATA. There are no characteristic changes in the blood or cerebrospinal fluid. Proteinuria may occur, and a nephrotic syndrome may develop. Slit lamp examination may show a lenticular gray or red-brown reflex.

PREVENTION. The withdrawal of mercury from various household products has led to a marked decrease in the incidence of acrodynia. However, mercurial drugs should be avoided in pediatric practice whenever possible, and the physician should be alert to other sources of mercury, especially food contaminated by agricultural processes and industrial waste.

TREATMENT. The treatment of acrodynia includes (1) the removal of mercury, (2) the administration of antidotes, and (3) careful initiation of supportive measures.

BAL is an effective antidote, especially when given early in the disease. The dose and possible side effects are the same as for acute poisonings (Sec. 26.14). L-Penicillamine (*N*-acetyl-D,L-penicillamine) has been used to successfully treat acrodynia and has an advantage over BAL in that it can be given orally. The effective dose is 30 mg/kg daily in 2–3 divided doses for 4 wk or until symptoms improve. Side effects include fever, rashes, proteinuria, leukopenia, and thrombocytopenia.

Barbiturates, paraldehyde, hydroxyzine, or chlorpromazine may be used for irritability and pain. Nourishing foods containing proteins, minerals, and vitamins should be given. Frequently, nasogastric tube feeding is necessary for severe anorexia. Intravenous replacement of fluid and electrolytes may be required for dehydration. Appropriate antibiotics should be given for secondary pyogenic infections of the skin and urinary system.

26.15 Minamata Disease

Minamata disease is a form of mercury poisoning that occurred among adults and children living in towns facing Minamata Bay, Kumamoto prefecture, Japan, from 1953 to 1966. The disease has become symbolic of the catastrophic health risks of industrial pollution (Sec. 26.17).

ETIOLOGY. The causative agent of this disease is methylmercury, released as industrial waste during the manufacture of acetaldehyde and vinyl chloride and absorbed into the body by the ingestion of contaminated fish and shellfish. Congenital Minamata disease was produced by placental transfer of methylmercury to the fetus from the pregnant mother who had eaten contaminated fish. The fetus is more sensitive than the mother or the postnatal infant to toxic effects of methylmercury.

PATHOLOGY. Various degrees of regressive changes in the brain have been observed. Degeneration and loss of granular cells in the cortex of the cerebellum and central convolutions are prominent. In the congenital type more severe and widespread damage of the nerve cells in the cerebral and cerebellar cortices has been demonstrated.

CLINICAL MANIFESTATIONS. The principal symptoms in the infantile form of Minamata disease include disturbances in hand coordination, in gait, and in speech. Difficulty in masticating and swallowing and visual blurring also occur. Some patients complain of numbness and pain in the extremities, and in severe cases there are involuntary movements. Tremor, clouded consciousness, convulsions, and rigidity of the extremities are observed. Some patients have impaired hearing and constriction of the visual field. More generalized damage to the nervous system results from fetal poisoning, the principal clinical features of which include physical retardation, severe mental disturbance, delay in development, abnormal movement, or lack of smoothness in movement.

LABORATORY DATA. Mercury content in the hair of most Minamata disease patients is high, more than 20 ppm. Some patients have abnormal electroencephalograms and constricted visual fields. In the congenital form most patients have an abnormal pneumoencephalogram, cortical atrophy, and microcephalus. Chromosomal aberrations are not found.

PREVENTION. The environment should be kept free of mercury hazards. Pregnant women should be especially careful because of the high sensitivity of fetuses to mercury. The maximum safe concentration of mercury in food is 0.3 ppm of methylmercury. A level of over 40–50 ppm of mercury in the hair is considered dangerous.

TREATMENT. In the early stages, elimination of organic mercury exposure may be sufficient. Foods suspected of contamination should not be eaten. Since mercury is transmitted to infants in human milk, breast feeding should be discontinued. BAL is effective in eliminating systemic mercury, and the dosage regimen is identical to that prescribed in acrodynia and acute poisonings. The diet should contain nourishing foods rich in proteins, minerals, and vitamins. In severe cases tube feeding is necessary. Symptomatic treatment is increasingly important as time goes on. Anticonvulsive drugs are indicated for seizures. Damage is irreversible, and survivors require extensive rehabilitation, re-education, and long-term care.

TARO AKABANE

Agocs MM, Etzel RA, Parrish RG, et al: Mercury exposure from interior latex paint. N Engl J Med 323:1096, 1990.
Amin-Zaki L, Elhassani S, Majeed MA, et al: Studies of infants postnatally exposed to methylmercury. J Pediatr 85:81, 1974.
Clarkson TW: Mercury—an element of mystery. N Engl J Med 323:1137, 1990.
Harada Y, Moriyama H: Congenital Minamata disease. Bull Inst Constitut Med Kumamoto Univ 26:1, 1976.
Jaffe KM, Shurtleff DB, Robertson WO: Survival after acute mercury vapor poisoning. Am J Dis Child 137:749, 1983.

Rohyans J, Walson PD, Wood GA, et al: Mercury toxicity following merthiolate ear irrigations. J Pediatr 104:311, 1984.
Rumack BH: Acute poisoning. *In*: Gellis SS, Kagan BM (eds): Current Pediatric Therapy, 11th ed. Philadelphia, WB Saunders, 1984.
Takeuchi T: Study group of Minamata disease. *In*: Katsuma M (ed): Minamata Disease, Japan. Kumamoto University, 1966.
Warkany J, Hubbard DM: Acrodynia and mercury. J Pediatr 42:365, 1953.

26.16 INCREASED LEAD ABSORPTION AND LEAD POISONING

(Plumbism)

It is estimated that 17% of children in the United States aged 6 mo to 6 yr have blood lead (Pb) levels greater than 15 μg/dL of whole blood (0.72 μmol/L). Most children are asymptomatic, although biochemical evidence of disturbed hemosynthesis is often present. As sustained lead levels rise above 10–15 μg/dL (0.5–0.72 μmol/L), such children are at a progressively increasing risk for future neurobehavioral and cognitive deficits, which can impede progress in school. Chronically increased lead absorption is most prevalent in preschool-aged children who live in old, deteriorated dwellings. Most affected children are being identified through screening programs. Acute lead colic and lead encephalopathy, the most severe forms of this chronic disorder, are now rare. Chelation therapy substantially reduces mortality, but 50% or more of the survivors of encephalopathy treated *after* the onset of symptoms have sustained, severe, permanent brain damage. This emphasizes the importance of treating cases in the early asymptomatic phase, if the degree of residual injury is to be reduced. In many areas of the United States, lead poisoning is a reportable disease. Blood lead levels have replaced EP and FEP measurements as the primary screening test.

EXPOSURE. The lead contents of food, water, and air have decreased substantially during the past decade. The amount ingested daily in food and beverage in a 2-yr-old child is 15–20 μg. Uncontaminated drinking water contains less than 20 μg/L of lead. Air lead levels even in congested cities now average about 0.2 μg/m³. Such usual exposures are associated with an average blood lead level of 6 μg (range, 1–15 μg) and are without evident adverse effects on health. (See Table 26–4 for abbreviations used in this section.)

With the recent substantial reductions of lead in food, drinking water, and air, it is now recognized that lead in interior household dust, exterior surface soil, and old residential paints constitute the major sources of overexposure to lead in children in the United States and will continue to be the major sources for the foreseeable future. House dust in old housing may average from 600–3,000 μg Pb/g, exterior surface soil from 2,000–16,000 μg Pb/g. Multilayered chips of old lead pigment paints may contain 20,000–100,000 μg Pb/cm². Increased absorption of lead occurs among children living near lead processing smelters and among children of workers who bring leaded dust into their homes on their work clothes. Sporadic cases of clinical plumbism have been traced to other sources with very high concentrations of lead, including (1) lead shot, fishing or curtain weights, and leaded jewelry swallowed and retained in the stomach, where the lead is dissolved and absorbed; (2) juices conveyed or stored in improperly lead-glazed earthenware; (3) lead type or toys; (4) Asiatic and Mexican folk medicines and cosmetics (azarcon, greta, paylooah, surma, al kohl); (4) "soft" drinking water conveyed in lead pipes or stored in lead-lined cisterns; (6) lead-soldered vessels used in cooking; (7) fumes from burning painted wood or casings of storage batteries; and (8) dust from sanding and burning of paint containing lead. The above exposures cause *inorganic* lead poisoning. Sniffing of leaded gasoline by older children and adolescents causes *organic* lead poisoning characterized by toxic encephalopathy.

EPIDEMIOLOGY. The report of the Agency for Toxic Substances and Disease Registry (ATSDR) on the nature and extent of lead poisoning in children in the United States (July 1988) provides the most current estimates of environmental exposures to lead and its impact on preschool-aged children. The number of potentially exposed children younger than 7 yr of age living in old housing with lead paint at potentially toxic levels is about 12 million. About 5.9 million children younger than 6 yr of age live in the oldest housing with the highest lead content of paint. For the oldest housing that is also deteriorated, 1.8–2.0 million children are at elevated risk for toxic lead exposures. According to the US Census Bureau (1983), 41.8 (52%) million dwelling units were built before 1950 but are still occupied and constitute the greatest hazard. The highest surface soil levels and interior household dust levels are found in and about such housing. The hand-to-mouth route constitutes the major pathway of lead into the blood of children. Both exterior surface soil lead and interior paint contribute significantly to interior household dust. Exposure to house dust containing greater than 1,000 μg Pb/g of dust in a preschool child with hand-to-mouth activity may easily produce blood lead values in the range of 16–60 μg/dL. The more severe degrees of poisoning are generally associated with repetitive ingestion (pica) of lead paint flakes or some uncommon source (see under Exposure).

TABLE 26–4. Laboratory Test Results Usually Associated with Various Levels of Lead Absorption

	Acceptable	Increasing Risk of CNS Residua			
Blood Lead (PbB) Groups	***0***	***I***	***II***	***III***	***IV***
Indicator of internal dose (soft tissue concentrations):					
PbB (μg/dL whole blood)*†	<10	10–24	25–39	40–60	>60
Indicators of disturbed heme synthesis:					
PBGS‡			<75%	<30%	<10–15%
ALAU (mg/m²/24 hr)§	1.1 ± 0.37	1.1 ± 0.37	1.1 ± 0.37	>2	>6
EP (μg/dL whole blood)‖	≤35	≤35	35–75	76–169	≥170
FEP (μg/dL erythrocytes)¶	50 ± 20	92–197	198–444	≥445	

*Conversion factor for PbB: $\frac{\mu g/dL}{20.72} = \mu mol/L$

†Mean normal value for PbB is 6 μg/dL.

‡Results vary according to method; however, for most methods when PbB ≥ 50–60 μg, then porphobilinogen synthase (PBGS) ≤ 10–15% of normal for each method.

§Less specific screening methods give values for δ-aminolevulinic acid (ALAU) as 0.5–1.0 mg/m²/24 hr higher than values shown above. See Nordberg GF: Effects and Dose-Relationships of Toxic Metals. New York, Elsevier, 1976.

‖Note results expressed as μg erythrocyte protoporphyrin (EP)/dL whole blood as used in many screening programs.

¶Normal values based on several reports. "Free" erythrocyte protoporphyrin (FEP) values calculated from EP values on basis of 38% hematocrit. EP and FEP values are for microfluorometric extraction methods.

METABOLISM. Lead absorption from the gastrointestinal tract is affected by age, diet, and nutritional deficiencies. Although adults absorb 5–10% of dietary lead and retain little of it, young children absorb 40–50% and retain 20–25%. Spontaneous urinary excretion of lead in infants and young children normally is about 1 mg/kg/24 hr; it may increase in acute poisoning. Animal studies show that diets high in fat, and especially those low in calcium, magnesium, iron, zinc, or copper, increase the absorption of lead. Diets suboptimal in calcium and iron are prevalent among children in low income groups. The total-body lead burden is divided into two major components: bone, in which the amount increases with age and in adults has a half-life of about 20 yr, and soft tissues, in which the half-life is 20–30 days. Although most of the lead sequestered in bone is temporarily removed from the active metabolic pool, it is slowly recirculated back to the soft tissue pool and serves as a major reservoir for the maintenance of elevated blood levels long after excessive assimilation of new lead has ceased. The toxicity of lead is related to its concentration in the small mobile soft tissue pool.

PATHOPHYSIOLOGY. The principal toxic effects occur in the CNS and peripheral nervous system, in the erythroid cells in the bone marrow, and in the kidney. The developing nervous system is now recognized as the system most sensitive to the toxic effects of lead in fetuses and young children. Abnormal cardiac conduction and thyroid function have also been reported in severe cases. Lead causes partial inhibition in the synthesis of heme at several enzymatic steps (see Fig. 8–40). Ferrochelatase and porphobilinogen synthase are the enzymes most sensitive to inhibition by lead. The following combination is pathognomonic for lead poisoning: increased activity of δ-aminolevulinic acid synthase and decreased activity of porphobilinogen synthase in erythrocytes, increased δ-aminolevulinic acid in plasma and urine, normal or slightly increased urinary porphobilinogen and uroporphyrin, increased urinary coproporphyrin, and increased "free" erythrocyte protoporphyrin. Although the porphyrin found in the circulating erythrocytes in lead poisoning and in iron deficiency is zinc protoporphyrin, this metabolite is generally measured as "free" erythrocyte protoporphyrin. Compensatory erythroid hyperplasia and reticulocytosis result. Basophilic stippling is best seen in bone marrow normoblasts. There is a dose-dependent decrease in 5-pyrimidine nucleotidase activity, which underlies the basophilic stippling of erythrocytes. As the concentration of lead in blood increases above 50–60 μg/dL, hemoglobin decreases. Lead can cause a mild, well-compensated, hemolytic, normocytic anemia that can be distinguished morphologically from the hypochromic, microcytic anemia of iron deficiency. Low-level lead exposure also has subtle effects on growth rate, stature, and balance.

Severe acute lead poisoning may be responsible for the Fanconi syndrome (generalized renal aminoaciduria, mellituria, hyperphosphaturia, and hypophosphatemia) because of acute proximal renal tubular injury; the lesion is reversible. Lead nephropathy, characterized by hyperuricemia with or without gout, has been reported as a sequel of chronic plumbism in Australian children. Acute lead encephalopathy in the very young is characterized by massive cerebral edema due primarily to a generalized increase in vascular permeability. Neuronal destruction also occurs. In suckling animals, but not in mature animals, slowness in learning and behavioral changes can be induced by doses of lead insufficient to produce histopathologic changes.

CLINICAL MANIFESTATIONS. The chronic course of unrecognized lead poisoning is characterized by recurrent symptomatic episodes, which may abate spontaneously. The earliest symptoms are hyperirritability, anorexia, and decreased play activity. Sporadic vomiting, intermittent abdominal pain, and constipation are manifestations of lead colic. Colic may occur at blood levels of lead as low as 60 μg/dL, but children with levels of up to 250 μg/dL may appear clinically well. Loss of recently acquired developmental skills may occur. Anemia may be present.

The above symptoms usually, but not always, appear 4–6 wk prior to the start of acute encephalopathy, which is heralded by the sudden onset of persistent vomiting, ataxia, impairment of consciousness, coma, and seizures. In younger children massive cerebral edema is almost always present, although the classic signs of increased intracranial pressure may not be found. In older children and adolescents a toxic encephalopathy without massive cerebral edema is more likely. Subtle premonitory behavioral changes may not be appreciated.

Acute encephalopathy, in which blood lead concentration almost always exceeds 100 μg/dL and usually exceeds 150 μg/dL, is most common during the summer. The diagnosis can usually be made without lumbar puncture, which is very dangerous. If examination of the cerebrospinal fluid is considered essential for differential diagnosis, the least amount of fluid required should be obtained (several drops). In lead encephalopathy, the fluid changes consist of mild pleocytosis, mild to moderate increase in protein, and increased pressure. Observation for inappropriate secretion of antidiuretic hormone, partial heart block, and profoundly impaired renal function must be maintained in the seriously ill child. Peripheral neuropathy, manifested in adults principally by motor weakness in the distal muscles of the arms and legs, is rare in children.

CLINICAL DIAGNOSIS. Symptoms are subtle and nonspecific, and physical examination generally reveals little or nothing abnormal unless there is acute encephalopathy. Plumbism should be included in the differential diagnosis of anemia, seizure disorders, mental retardation, severe behavioral disorders, colicky abdominal pain, and the cerebral and abdominal crises of sickle cell disease. Isolated seizures and self-limited episodes of vomiting during the recent past may represent episodes of clinical plumbism, particularly if the child lives in or visits an old house, if a parent is unavailable for much of the time, and if a history of pica for any substance is obtained. Recent changes of address, recent renovations in the home, and especially time spent unsupervised or with baby-sitters and relatives should be ascertained, since persistent pica is particularly associated with such histories. This information is essential in planning the appropriate management for each patient. Emphasis must be placed on environmental sampling for sources of lead and laboratory data. Whenever an index case is found, all housemates should be examined. The possibility of uncommon sources should be ascertained (see under Exposure).

LABORATORY DIAGNOSIS. Because clinical diagnosis is exceedingly difficult in children prior to the occurrence of severe injury to the nervous system, early diagnosis depends on laboratory determinations. At least two tests are required: (1) an indicator of the internal accumulation of lead and (2) an indicator of adverse metabolic effect (see Table 26–4). Blood lead and "free" erythrocyte protoporphyrin can be determined in micro blood samples, as well as in venous blood obtained in hematology Vacutainers containing EDTA as anticoagulant. Special precautions are needed to prevent contamination of blood and urine samples by exogenous lead. Serial tests are needed to determine trends. Iron deficiency may cause "free" erythrocyte protoporphyrin to be as high as 500 μg/dL of packed red blood cells when the blood lead level is normal; higher values generally indicate lead toxicity (blood lead groups III and IV; see Table 26–4) with or without iron deficiency. In groups III and IV, toxic effects increase exponentially. In emergencies, when these tests are not immediately available and acute lead encephalopathy is a diagnostic possibility, a strongly positive qualitative urinary coproporphyrin test result, many stippled erythroblasts in bone marrow, glycosuria, and hypophosphatemia constitute presumptive evidence of plumbism. Recent experimental studies have shown in chronically lead poisoned rats that a single dose of edathamil calcium disodium (CaEDTA) is associated with an increase in brain lead; therefore, the diagnostic CaEDTA mobilization test for lead in urine is *not* recommended. Radiopaque flecks in the intestinal tract indicate recent ingestion of foreign matter containing lead. Broad bands of increased density at the metaphyses of the long bones usually represent increased storage of lead in bone, but roentgenograms of long bones may be normal or equivocal in severe acute plumbism.

Short-term responses to treatment may be monitored by changes in blood levels of lead and in δ-aminolevulinic acid levels in urine. Serial "free" erythrocyte protoporphyrin tests, which change slowly, are useful to monitor long-term responses to therapy and trends in lead absorption. Blood lead values should be obtained, since some local laws, requiring the abatement of housing hazards, are dependent on the measurement of lead in the child.

TREATMENT. The cornerstone of therapy is prompt separation of the child from the source(s) of lead, followed by timely reduction of lead hazards in the home environment. Removal of hazards is usually the local health agency's responsibility. Children and pregnant women (because of the exquisite sensitivity of the fetus to lead) should remain out of the home *day and night* until the abatement of lead paint hazards has been completed, the premises have been vacuumed with a high-efficiency particle accumulator (HEPA) vacuum, scrubbed with high-phosphate detergents 2 or 3 times, and vacuumed with a HEPA vacuum again, to remove the fine particulate lead generated by the deleading processing. The deleaded areas should then be repainted. The sanding and burning of paint with an open flame torch should be prohibited. Thereafter, wet cleaning with high phosphate detergents for dust control should be continued, particularly in old housing areas. Play in dirt areas adjacent to such housing should also be avoided. Preschool-aged children should be tested periodically according to the latest Centers for Disease Control and Early Periodic Screening, Diagnosis and Treatment guidelines, to determine trends in lead absorption.

Most children detected in current screening programs are asymptomatic and fit the requirements for groups I, II, and III (see Table 26–4). For those in group I, the above measures and improved diet should suffice, and chelation therapy is probably not advisable. Chelation therapy may be of benefit in selected cases in group II.

Chelation therapy is advised for children in groups III and IV, including the asymptomatic ones. Intramuscular therapy with CaEDTA should be limited to 5 days at a daily dose of 1,000 mg/m^2 in two divided portions, when venous blood levels are greater than 50 but less than 90–100 μg/dL whole blood. Chelation therapy prior to the onset of symptoms may lessen the risk of cerebral injury. Repeat courses of CaEDTA are often indicated in children with higher body lead burdens. Treatment with oral CaEDTA is contraindicated. CaEDTA may soon be replaced largely by meso-2,3-dimercaptosuccinic acid (DMSA) for the treatment of asymptomatic and mildly symptomatic lead toxicity. DMSA has recently been approved for treatment of lead poisoning by the Food and Drug Administration. DMSA can be given orally, has to date not been associated with serious adverse side effects, does not induce acute zinc depletion as does CaEDTA, and has been given for up to 4 wk in a few subjects without adverse side effects. In animals, DMSA is more effective than CaEDTA in reducing the lead content of brain, kidney, and blood. In those with a higher body lead burden, it is likely that multiple courses will be required. DMSA treatment protocols are now being studied.

Patients who have symptomatic plumbism (colic, seizures, acute encephalopathy) should be treated promptly with chelating agents if presumptive laboratory test results are positive. Because the onset and clinical course of encephalopathy are unpredictable, the risk of delay outweighs the risk of a few days of chelation therapy. If subsequent tests do not indicate an increased absorption of lead, treatment should be discontinued and the presumptive diagnosis reconsidered.

When acute encephalopathy is present or when blood lead levels are greater than 90–100 μg/dL whole blood, a regimen of BAL and CaEDTA is recommended; the dose for BAL is 500 mg/m^2/24 hr and for CaEDTA, 1,500 mg/m^2/24 hr. The drugs are injected simultaneously at separate intramuscular sites in six divided doses each day for 5 days, after an initial priming dose of BAL only. If repeated 5-day courses are needed, a daily dose of 1,000 mg/m^2/24 hr of CaEDTA or DMSA is safer and adequate. If the patient becomes anuric, administration of CaEDTA, but not BAL, should be temporarily withheld. CaEDTA is a nonmetabolizable drug that is excreted solely by the kidney; side effects include hypercalcemia, elevation of blood urea nitrogen levels, and renal injury. Side effects of BAL include vomiting, hypertension, and tachycardia. The side effects of each drug require careful evaluation, because some of them are also features of acute lead encephalopathy. BAL may occasionally evoke intravascular hemolysis in patients with severe glucose-6-phosphate dehydrogenase deficiency.

Fluid and electrolyte management is critical in lead encephalopathy. After an initial infusion of 10% dextrose in water (and of mannitol, if necessary to decrease intracranial pressure) to establish urine flow, continuous intravenous infusion should be restricted to basal requirements and a minimal estimate of the amounts required for correction of losses due to vomiting, dehydration, and activity associated with seizures. It is prudent to administer parenteral fluids initially in the same manner in mildly symptomatic patients and in asymptomatic ones who have very high tissue levels of lead, until the trend of the clinical course becomes clear. The use of enemas to remove lead from the lower bowel should never be permitted to delay treatment of symptomatic patients.

Seizures can be controlled initially with diazepam and thereafter with repeated doses of paraldehyde until the patients state of consciousness is significantly improved. As the dose of paraldehyde is lowered, long-term anticonvulsant therapy with phenytoin or phenobarbital is started (see Sec. 20.17–20.23). When lead poisoning results from ingestion of lead paint, effective long-term management requires the cooperative efforts of local health department personnel, the medical social worker, the psychologist or psychiatrist, and the pediatrician. Control of hand-to-mouth activity and pica is very difficult to accomplish, although behavioral modification may help.

PROGNOSIS. Sequelae are related to the degree and duration of excessive lead ingestion. Recurrence of clinical manifestations increases the chance of permanent injury. Residual brain damage may not be evident until the child reaches school age. Some survivors of encephalopathy may require residential care; sequelae include seizure disorders, impaired mentation, and attentional deficit. Seizures and altered behavior tend to abate during adolescence, but intellectual deficits persist. Blindness and hemiparesis are restricted to the most severe cases of encephalopathy.

There is general agreement that blood lead levels, if sustained during early childhood at levels greater than 10–15 μg/L (0.5–0.72 μmol/L) present an unacceptable risk for long-lasting but subtle injury to the nervous system, even if no symptoms are ever detected. In a study of over 2,000 children, a dose-response relationship was shown between the frequency of behavioral and attentional problems in school and the dentine lead content of shed deciduous teeth. Follow-up of a smaller sample of these children at 18–20 yr of age has revealed that those with the highest dentine lead content at 6–8 yr of age were 6 times more likely to have dropped out of school and 7 times more likely to have a reading disability than those with the lowest dentine lead content during the elementary school years. Some of these children had blood lead values during the preschool years averaging 35 μg/L. A new statement by the Centers for Disease Control on preventing lead poisoning in young children is anticipated in the near future since previous statements are out of date in the light of recent research.

PREVENTION. Various agencies in the United States have taken steps during the past decade to reduce air lead levels, enforce the drinking water standard for lead, and reduce the lead content of foods (particularly canned foods); lead additives in automotive fuels were virtually eliminated in 1988. The use of lead additives in residential paints was banned by the United States Consumer Product Safety Commission in 1977. However, until the large stock of older residential housing is renovated or replaced, screening programs will be needed for early detection of lead toxicity in young children.

J. JULIAN CHISOLM, JR.

Aaseth J: Recent advances in the therapy of metal poisonings with chelating agents. Hum Toxicol 2:257, 1983.

Agency for Toxic Substances and Disease Registry (ATSDR): The nature and extent of lead poisoning in children in the United States: A report to Congress. Atlanta, July 1988.

Baker EL Jr, Follard DS, Taylor TA, et al: Lead poisoning in children of lead workers: Home contamination with industrial dust. N Engl J Med 296:260, 1977.

Bellinger D, Leviton A, Waternaux C, et al: Longitudinal analyses of prenatal and postnatal lead exposure and early cognitive development. N Engl J Med 316:1037, 1987.

Bornschein RL, Succop PA, Krafft KM, et al: Exterior surface dust lead, interior house dust lead and childhood lead exposure in an urban environment. *In:* Hemphill DD (ed): Trace Substances in Environmental Health—XX. Columbia, MO, University of Missouri, 1987, p 322.

Chisolm JJ Jr: Increased lead absorption and acute lead poisoning. *In:* Gellis SS, Kagan DM (eds): Current Pediatric Therapy. Philadelphia, WB Saunders, 1986, p 667.

Chisolm JJ Jr, Barltrop D: Recognition and management of increased lead absorption. Arch Dis Child 54:249, 1979.

Clark CS, Bornschein RL, Succop PA, et al: Condition and type of housing as an indicator of potential environmental lead exposure and pediatric blood lead levels. Environ Res 38:46, 1985.

Cory-Slechta DA: Mobilization of lead over the course of DMSA chelation therapy and long-term efficacy. J Pharmacol Exp Ther 246:84, 1988.

Cory-Slechta DA, Weiss B, Cox C: Mobilization and redistribution of lead over the course of CaEDTA chelation therapy. J Pharmacol Exp Ther 243:804, 1987.

Emmerson BT: The clinical differentiation of lead gout from primary gout. Arthritis Rheum 11:623, 1968.

Fulton M, Raab G, Thomson G, et al: Influence of blood lead on the ability and attainment of children in Edinburgh. Lancet 1:1221, 1987.

Graziano JH, LoIacono NL, Meyer P: Dose-response study of oral 2,3-dimercaptosuccinic acid in children with elevated blood lead concentrations. J Pediatr 113:751, 1988.

Lourie RS, Layman EM, Millican FK: Why children eat things that are not food. Children 10:143, 1963.

Lyngbye T, Hansen GN, Trillingsgaard A, et al: Learning disabilities in children: Significance of low-level lead exposure and confounding factors. Acta Paediatr Scand 79:352, 1990.

Mahaffey KR: Nutritional factors in lead poisoning. Nutr Rev 39:353, 1981.

McMichael AJ, Baghurst PA, Wigg NR, et al: Port Pirie cohort study: Environmental exposure to lead and children's abilities at the age of 4 years. N Engl J Med 319:468, 1988.

Needleman HL, Gunnoe C, Leviton A, et al: Deficits in psychological and classroom performance of children with elevated dentine lead levels. N Engl J Med 300:689, 1979.

Nriagu JO: Lead and Lead Poisoning in Antiquity. New York, John Wiley & Sons, 1983.

Perlstein MA, Attala R: Neurologic sequelae of plumbism in children. Clin Pediatr 5:292, 1966.

Rabinowitz MD, Wetherill GW, Kopple JD: Kinetic analysis of lead metabolism in healthy humans. J Clin Invest 58:260, 1976.

Smith MA, Grant LD, Sors AI (eds): Lead Exposure and Child Development: An International Assessment. Dordrecht, Kluwer Academic Publishers, 1989.

26.17 CHEMICAL POLLUTANTS

As chemicals increasingly permeate our environment, there is a need to consider the special exposures and vulnerability of the fetus and child. Each pediatrician should be alert for evidence of new environmental effects on child health. Virtually all known human teratogens and carcinogens have been discovered by alert clinicians.

Intrauterine Effects

METHYLMERCURY. In the mid 1950s methylmercury caused the first epidemic of congenital cerebral palsy attributable to intrauterine exposures to a chemical pollutant (Sec. 26.13–26.15). It was associated with severe, sometimes fatal, neurologic disorders in the population at large and was traced to contamination of fish by waste dumped into Minamata Bay, Japan, by a factory that made vinyl plastics. Similar episodes have occurred in Alamogordo, New Mexico, and Iraq due to grain treated prior to planting with a methylmercury-containing fungicide that was mistakenly used for animal feed or baking.

POLYCHLORINATED BIPHENYLS (PCBs). In 1968, in Kyushu, Japan, there was an epidemic of chloracne, and women who were pregnant at the time gave birth to infants who were small for gestational age and had, among other findings, dark skin that cleared with time. The outbreak was traced to contamination of cooking oil by PCBs, a heat-transfer agent, through pinhole erosions in pipes during the manufacture of the oil. PCBs from factory waste have now been found in major waterways of the United States and other countries. In Taiwan an episode virtually identical to that in Kyushu occurred. Comprehensive health examinations were made of about 100 children who were conceived after their mothers were exposed to PCBs. The children, from 1 mo to 7 yr of age, had an increased frequency of defects of the skin, hair, and nails, and 11 were born with teeth. They were exposed in utero to PCBs that had been stored in their mothers' fat. Compounds similar to PCBs, *polybrominated biphenyls (PBBs),* were accidentally mixed with animal feed in Michigan and widely distributed within the state. Animals became ill and died, but no fetal effects or overt illnesses have been found in human beings.

DIOXIN. In 1976 a runaway reaction in a factory in Seveso, Italy, spewed a chemical cloud downwind over farms and homes. Many animals died, and 2 wk later about 40 exposed children developed chloracne. The chemical in the cloud was dioxin, a potent teratogen in laboratory animals. No human teratogenesis has been found among the abortuses or liveborn children of Seveso women exposed early in pregnancy. The highest exposures yet known occurred among children of Seveso, several of whom had blood levels greater than 20,000 parts per trillion 2 wk after exposure, as compared with less than 20 parts per trillion among unexposed persons. In Missouri, horse arenas and roads were sprayed with waste oil to which dioxin had been added; about 60 horses died, and foals were born malformed. Transient illness, but not chloracne, occurred in one arena owner and her two children. Further contamination from the same source was subsequently recognized in Times Beach, Missouri, and the inhabitants had to be relocated.

CIGARETTE SMOKE. On the average, the birthweight of infants whose mothers smoke heavily during pregnancy is

200 g less than normal, and perinatal morbidity is increased when medical care is inadequate (Sec. 9.7).

TRANSPLACENTAL CARCINOGENESIS. The discovery that cancer of the cervix or vagina occurs in women after intrauterine exposure to diethylstilbestrol raises the possibility that other chemicals, including pollutants, may also be transplacental carcinogens. Four children have now been reported with fetal hydantoin syndrome and neuroblastoma, suggesting that phenytoin is a transplacental carcinogen. Among other possible carcinogens is benzene, which causes leukemia after heavy occupational exposures.

Lactational Effects

Because of chemical pollution, new questions are being raised about the safety of breast feeding. PCBs, PBBs, dioxin, and certain pesticides are stored in fat and are not readily cleared from the body except in the fat of breast milk. Japanese infants whose mothers were exposed post partum to PCB-contaminated cooking oil were exposed to high levels in their mothers' milk while nursing. Elsewhere, samples of breast milk have rarely shown high levels of these chemicals. When unusual exposures occur, however, before advice on breast feeding is given, the milk should be tested (e.g., for dioxin in Seveso, for PBBs in Michigan, or for PCBs in upper New York State). No general recommendation against breast feeding should be made because of its many benefits. Cow's milk may also contain these chemicals, but tests are routinely made to determine that the milk sold commercially does not exceed limits set by federal regulation. Game fish have also been contaminated from PCB-polluted waters.

Effects of Other Exposures

ASBESTOS. Although asbestos is a naturally occurring chemical, its capacity to induce cancer is related to its physical properties. Long, thin fibers are carcinogens, whereas short, thick ones are not. The latent period from exposure until the development of mesothelioma is usually more than 30 yr. Exposure in childhood may thus induce cancer in adulthood. Asbestos dust brought home on a father's work clothes has been implicated as the cause of mesothelioma in his daughter (onset at 34 yr), as well as in his wife.

Bronchogenic carcinoma is induced by exposure to asbestos, especially among cigarette smokers; the risk is about 5 times greater than it is in cigarette smokers not exposed to asbestos and 54 times greater than in persons exposed to neither. From 1947–1973, asbestos fibers were sprayed on new schoolroom ceilings in the United States; about 10,000 schools were treated. With time and abuse, the asbestos frayed and fibers floated through the schoolrooms. In theory the exposure could increase the frequencies of mesothelioma and bronchogenic carcinoma. As yet, no increases have been observed in young adults, but sufficient time may not yet have passed to allow for both deterioration of asbestos and the latent period. Asbestos in schools is being removed, sealed with plastic, or contained by dropped ceilings. The interaction between asbestos exposure and the use of cigarettes in causing lung cancer adds to the reasons for urging young persons not to smoke.

WATER. About 200 chemicals have been found in small amounts in various water supplies. Some are known to cause human cancer after heavy occupational exposure, but the claim that regional increases in cancer mortality rates are attributable to chemicals in the water supply is not generally accepted. Fluoride, added to water or naturally occurring, is not associated with human cancer.

AIR. Major air pollutants generated by fossil fuel consumption are sulfur oxides, carbon monoxide, photochemical oxidants (especially ozone), and nitrogen oxides. The most common respiratory diseases associated with these pollutants are asthma, chronic bronchitis, and emphysema. Automotive exhausts add lead to the atmosphere and, in enclosed spaces, can cause intense pollution with carbon monoxide to which children have been especially susceptible, as in underground garages or at skating rinks where gasoline-powered vehicles were used to scrape the ice. Some industries have caused specific diseases in neighboring residential areas through air pollution with asbestos, beryllium, lead, methylmercury, or dioxin. There is an increased mortality from lung cancer among persons living in counties with arsenic-emitting smelters or petrochemical industries.

WORK CLOTHES. Illnesses in the child are at times traceable to a parent's work clothes; toxicity from lead, beryllium, and asbestos has occurred. Pediatricians, in considering the origins of noninfectious diseases, should ask about parental occupation, unusual household exposures, and neighborhood factories. A growing number of studies have found an association between childhood cancer or birth defects and exposure of the father to chemicals or radiation before conception of the child. These occurrences may be due to chance and cannot be explained by Mendelian genetics.

FOOD. In addition to the foregoing chemical pollutants that may enter the food chain, many other chemicals are intentionally added to food to improve appearance, taste, texture, or preservation. Evaluation of the safety of these chemicals is difficult because of problems in measuring exposures and in separating them from the effects of the myriad of variables that may confound interpretation of the alleged untoward effects.

Interactions

Little is known about the interactions of chemicals with one another, with physical or viral agents, or with susceptibilities. Furthermore, chemicals may be activated or inactivated by metabolic processes, thus altering their disease potential. One would expect children with heritable methemoglobin reductase deficiency to be especially susceptible to the effects of nitrates or aniline dyes. Other children from the general population may be exceptionally resistant. Some chemicals photosensitize the skin as a consequence of an interaction with a physical agent, ultraviolet light. Asbestos greatly potentiates the capacity of cigarette smoke to induce lung cancer. An interaction between old viruses and new chemicals may explain the increased frequency of diseases.

Susceptibility to chemical pollutants varies markedly from conception through adolescence. Exposures also vary as the environment changes from that within the uterus to the nursery, home, school, neighborhood, recreational area, and, occasionally, the hospital. Greater attention must be given by pediatricians to the effects of chemical pollutants, and environmental experts must become more aware of the special biology and surroundings of the fetus and child.

ROBERT W. MILLER

Arundel SE, Kinnier-Wilson LM: Parental occupations and cancer: A review of the literature. J Epidemiol Commun Health 40:30, 1986.

Chisolm JJ Jr: Fouling one's own nest. Pediatrics 62:614, 1978.

Evans HJ: Leukemia and [preconception] radiation. Nature 345:16, 1990.

Gough M: Dioxin, Agent Orange: The Facts. New York, Plenum Press, 1986.

International Programme on Chemical Safety: Environmental Health Criteria 101. Methylmercury. Geneva, WHO, 1990, p 144.

Mehta PS, Mehta AS, Mehta SJ, et al: Bhopal tragedy's health effects: A review of methylisocyanate toxicity. JAMA 264:2781, 1990.

Miller RW: Chemical and radiation hazards to children: Highlights of a meeting. J Pediatr 101:495, 1982.

Miller RW: Congenital PCB poisoning: A re-evaluation. Environ Health Perspect 60:211, 1985.
Miller RW: Frequency and environmental epidemiology of childhood cancer. *In*: Pizzo PA, Poplack D (eds): Principles and Practice of Pediatric Oncology. New York, JB Lippincott, 1989.
Mocarelli P, Pocchiari F, Nelson N: Preliminary report of 2,3,7,8-tetrachlorodibenzo-*p*-dioxin exposure to humans—Seveso, Italy. MMWR 37:733, 1988.
Mossman BT, Gee BL: Asbestos-related diseases. N Engl J Med 320:1721, 1989.
Rogan WJ, Gladen BC, Hung K-L et al: Congenital poisoning by polychlorinated biphenyls and their contaminants in Taiwan. Science 241:334, 1988.

26.18 VENOM DISEASES: POISONING BY SNAKES, LIZARDS, AND MARINE ANIMALS

The fear of venomous animals dates from antiquity, but knowledge of venomous disease remains limited. As modern transportation makes remote areas of the world more accessible, as interest in outdoor recreation activities expands, and as long as humans remain interested in domesticating wild animal species, contact with venomous animals is likely to increase.

SNAKE BITES

Of the more than 3,500 known species of snakes, only 200 that belong to four families are poisonous to humans. They have in common a modified salivary gland that secretes and stores venom and one or more maxillary fangs for conducting the venom to the victim.

The Colubridae family includes most of the world's snakes, but only the African boomslang *(Dispholidus typus)*, the vine, twig, or bird snake *(Thelotornis kirtlandi)*, and the Japanese yamakagashi *(Rhabdophis tigrinus)* have been associated with human fatalities.

The Elapidae family includes many of the world's deadliest snakes. The Afro-Asian cobras, the African mambas, the Indo-Malayan kraits, and the New World coral snakes are poisonous members of this family. The elapids are particularly numerous and diverse in Australia, where all dangerous land snakes are elapids (black tiger snake, brown snake, death adder, taipan, and copperheads).

The Hydrophidae family includes 52 different species of poisonous sea snakes that inhabit tropical waters throughout the world.

The Viperidae (true vipers) are poisonous and inhabit Europe, Africa, and Asia; the subfamily Crotalidae (pit vipers) are common in America and Southeast Asia. Many species have adapted to relatively cool climates, spending the winter in hibernation and, therefore, showing seasonal variations in growth and reproduction. Species common to North America include rattlesnakes, water moccasins, and copperheads.

EPIDEMIOLOGY. It has been estimated that 300,000 poisonous snake bites are responsible for the 30,000 to 40,000 deaths that occur throughout the world each year. The largest number of fatalities occurs in Southeast Asia; most are due to cobra bites. In the Western Hemisphere, most fatalities occur in Brazil. Approximately 45,000 persons are bitten by snakes every year in the United States, and about 20% of these are bitten by poisonous snakes; the fatalities are fewer than 20 and are usually due to bites by rattlesnakes (e.g., eastern and western diamondback rattlesnakes). Snake bites most often occur in the extremities following provocation or handling. Larger snakes are capable of injecting more venom into their victims. Snakes rarely exhaust their venom in a single bite, and the amount of venom injected is variable. Snake bites in children tend to be more serious than in adults because of the relatively large volume of venom injected into the small child.

CLINICAL MANIFESTATIONS. The venoms of most species of snakes are a complex mixture of proteins in the form of enzymes, toxins, polypeptides, and nontoxic proteins. Although the role of these various constituents is not completely understood, the activity of the venom of a particular species is usually either necrotizing or hemorrhagic as manifest by hemolysis, abnormalities in blood coagulation, alternation in vascular permeability, and circulatory collapse.

Local Effects. Bites by members of the Viperidae (true vipers) and Crotalidae (pit vipers) are characterized by the immediate appearance of localized pain and swelling extending along the entire limb and tender enlargement of regional lymph nodes. Necrosis of the skin with formation of bullae, ecchymosis, and discoloration soon follows. This is associated with local edema and the oozing of serosanguineous fluid into the bullae and subcutaneous tissue. This may be followed by extensive tissue necrosis and gangrene.

The signs and symptoms associated with bites by members of the Elapidae family vary among species. The eastern coral snake bite causes minimal pain and tissue destruction; cobra bites are characterized by severe pain with extensive necrosis and sloughing. Bites by the Hydrophidae are painless; fang marks are inconspicuous; and no local reaction is observed.

Systemic Effects. A bite by a member of the Viperidae family or subfamily Crotalidae produces predominately hemorrhagic symptoms. Hemorrhagic signs include bleeding from fang puncture sites, venipuncture sites, and into subcutaneous tissue. Epistaxis, hematuria, hemoptysis, hematemesis, and subconjunctival, retroperitoneal, and intracranial hemorrhage are often observed. Hypotension and shock are not uncommon, and myocardial toxicity may occur and may be manifest as an abnormal electrocardiogram or cardiac arrhythmia. Acute renal insufficiency may develop. Neurologic abnormalities occur and include delirium, disorientation, coma, and seizures. Death following envenomation by these reptiles is usually secondary to intracranial hemorrhage.

The venoms of other species of poisonous snakes are predominately neurotoxic, and death is secondary to respiratory paralysis. Cobra bites often produce immediate drowsiness, followed by progressive involvement of cranial nerves with resultant ptosis and ophthalmoplegia. Palatal and pharyngeal paralysis is associated with slurred speech and difficulty in handling oral secretions. Varying degrees of motor paralysis occur and is often associated with seizures and coma. The reaction to the bite of the sea snake differs from that of the cobra bite in that the aforementioned sequence is heralded by diffuse myalgia and progressive muscular weakness. The bite of the eastern coral snake initially produces paresthesia in the involved extremity, followed rapidly by involvement of the cranial nerves, respiratory insufficiency, and death.

TREATMENT. Initially, one should determine whether the attacking snake is poisonous; knowledge of the species indigenous to the geographic area is helpful. Examination of the wound may be informative, since bites by nonpoisonous species lack distinct fang punctures and do not cause local pain or swelling. There is also a lack of progressive symptomatology from nonpoisonous snake bites. Bites on the extremities and into adipose tissue are less dangerous than bites into highly vascularized area such as the face.

Local Measures. When the victim has been bitten on an extremity, a tourniquet should be placed above the bite area, tightly enough to occlude venous and lymphatic return but loosely enough to preserve distal pulses. Tourniquets are potentially dangerous and have caused gangrene, bleeding into the occluded limb, and permanent peripheral nerve injury. The involved extremity should be immobilized and, if possible, the patient should avoid exercise, including walking, thus lessening the lymphatic spread of the venom. Applying ice directly to the wound or cooling the involved extremity may be harmful and should be avoided. Incision and suction soon after the bite can remove substantial amounts of venom from the wound and should *only* be performed when transportation to a medical facility cannot be accomplished within a period of several hours. The skin should be cleansed, and a single linear incision 1 cm in length and 0.5 cm in depth should be made through each fang mark. Suction with cups provided in commercial snake bite kits or oral suction should be continued for at least 1 hr before the tourniquet is released. The risks of this procedure are considerable and include infection, particularly when nonsterile equipment or mouth suction is used, and persistent bleeding in patients with hypocoagulable blood. Amputation of the involved digit or extremity is not indicated, and every effort should be made to move the patient as quickly and as comfortably as possible to a medical facility.

The wound should be cultured, irrigated with saline, and treated with a topical antiseptic preparation. Extensive swelling that compromises the peripheral circulation is an indication for immediate fasciotomy. The administration of aspirin and/or intramuscular injections is contraindicated in patients with hypocoagulable blood. Surgical debridement of vesicles and necrotic skin can often be delayed for 1 wk.

Systemic Measures. Specific therapy with antivenom (see later) should be followed by appropriate supportive therapy, which often consists of blood transfusion for bites by snakes with a strongly hematotoxic venom. Adjustment of fluid and electrolyte balance is indicated in the presence of vomiting, renal insufficiency, and shock. Systemic complications that require therapy include paralysis, respiratory insufficiency, disseminated intravascular coagulation, and cardiac arrhythmias. Tetanus prophylaxis with toxoid or antitoxin is indicated if the child has not been adequately immunized, and parenteral therapy with a broad-spectrum penicillin is indicated to prevent secondary bacterial infection. Pain is often severe and may require narcotic administration. Nonpoisonous snake bites generally require no treatment.

Serum Therapy. Snake venom antisera or antivenoms are prepared by hyperimmunization of horses against one or more venoms. Although the chemical composition of snake venom varies from species to species, there is enough antigenic similarity between venoms of related species to produce clinically useful polyvalent antisera. Two antivenom preparations are commercially available in the United States.* Antivenom for the treatment of bites by exotic species can usually be obtained through local zoologic societies. These products can cause anaphylaxis and will cause serum sickness in 30–75% of patients, depending on the amount administered. Administration, therefore, is best performed in a hospital setting, following skin testing with the normal horse serum present in the commercial antivenom kits. Severe allergic reactions have occurred after a negative skin test, and some patients have been safely treated even after a positive test (see Sec. 11.45). Some clinicians routinely give epinephrine subcutaneously or antihistamines intravenously before infusing antivenom. After bites by unidentified snakes or snakes known not to be highly poisonous, antivenom treatment should be withheld until the development of local symptoms. Following bites by the most dangerous rattlesnakes, antivenom therapy should be administered prior to the development of signs and symptoms. Rapid spread of local swelling is considered an absolute indication for antivenom as is immediate pain or any other symptom of envenomation following bites by coral snakes.

*Wyeth Antivenin (Crotalidae) polyvalent: venom effective against rattlesnakes, water moccasins, and copperheads. Wyeth Antivenin (*Micrurus fulvius*): effective against North American coral snake venom.

GILA MONSTER

The Gila monster is the only lizard poisonous to humans. The two species (*Heloderma suspectum* and *H. horridum*) inhabit the Sahuaro desert regions of Arizona and New Mexico. Most bites occur during attempted capture or in handling captive animals. After a bite, it is often difficult to remove the lizard. There is considerable injury locally, severe pain, erythema, and edema. The venom contains a potent neurotoxin. Initial systemic features include nausea and vomiting and are followed rapidly by generalized weakness, cranial nerve paralysis, and respiratory insufficiency. Fatalities are uncommon. No antivenom is available. Treatment consists of local care of the wound and supportive therapy as described for snake bites.

VENOMOUS MARINE ANIMALS

Venomous fish include certain sharks, scorpion fish, weevers, toadfish, catfish, and stingrays. Among the venomous fish of the world, the family Scorpaenidae is considered the most dangerous in both the number and the severity of injuries produced. These fish inhabit tropical waters and are especially plentiful around coral reefs; well camouflaged with their environment, they pose a risk for scuba divers, snorkelers, swimmers, and surfers. In addition, many species, including the lionfish, are imported into this country each year by private and commercial collectors. Accordingly, aquarists are also at risk for envenomation.

CLINICAL MANIFESTATIONS. The clinical manifestations of poisoning are remarkably similar in all cases. There is immediate pain at the puncture site that spreads to involve the entire extremity. The venom produces local ischemia and circumscribed cyanosis, followed by edema and erythema that may spread to involve the entire extremity. Tissue necrosis is localized, may be extensive, and contributes to secondary bacterial infection. The wound produced by stingrays is unique in that the laceration is several centimeters deep and often contains bony and epithelial fragments of the venom apparatus. Systemic manifestations include pallor, nausea, vomiting, diaphoresis, and loss of consciousness. Convulsions, paralysis, and death have been reported.

TREATMENT. Treatment consists of the appropriate application of a tourniquet and copious irrigation of the wound to remove fragments of the venom apparatus. The only available antivenom is one for stonefish venom. Although effective for most types of Scorpaenidae, this product is only indicated for stonefish envenomations.* Many venoms are heat labile; for this reason immersion of the involved extremity in water as hot as can be tolerated is recommended. Tetanus toxoid or antitoxin should be administered except when the immune status of the patient is adequate. Broad-spectrum antibiotic therapy should be prescribed to prevent superinfection. Narcotics may be required to control pain.

COELENTERATE STINGS

The venomous coelenterates include hydroids, jellyfish, sea anemones, and coral. They are equipped with tentacles that have a venom apparatus consisting of nematocysts or nettle cells. The stings vary from a mild stinging sensation produced

*Health Services Department, Sea World in San Diego (619-222-6363), Steinbart Aquarium, San Francisco (415-221-8014), and Sea World of Ohio in Aurora (216-562-8101).

by the smaller jellyfish to an extremely painful, almost shock-like sensation produced by the most dangerous member of the phylum (Portuguese man-of-war). The local signs include erythema and urticaria. Systemic involvement may be manifested by weakness, chills, fever, nausea, and vomiting. In extreme situations, there may be respiratory failure and death.

The intensity of symptoms depends on the length of time the tentacles remain in contact with the skin; the tentacles should therefore be removed as promptly as possible. Before removal, inactivation of remaining nematocysts to prevent discharge into the victim is accomplished by irrigation with acetic acid or vinegar solutions. Rinsing with fresh water, alcoholic solutions, suntan lotion, sand, and so on is not recommended since such treatment has been associated with discharge of additional venom into the victim. Caution must be observed since some species of jellyfish have powerful nematocysts that may penetrate gloves and other clothing. Topical treatment consists of warm soaks with normal saline. Antihistamines and corticosteroids are indicated in the presence of extensive swelling and urticaria.

Prevention of stings is best accomplished by caution when swimming in tropical waters. Damaged tentacles, which often float in water following a storm, are capable of inflicting stings, as are jellyfish washed up on beaches and often presumed to be dead.

WILLIAM T. SPECK

Bucherl W: Venomous Animals and Their Venoms, vols I and II. New York, Academic Press, 1986.
Halstead BW: Poisonous and Venomous Marine Animals of the World, vols I and II. Washington, DC, US Government Printing Office, 1965 and 1967.
Kizer KW, McKinney HE, Auerbach PS: Scorpaenidae envenomation: A five-year poison center experience. JAMA 253:307, 1985.
Watt CH: Poisonous snakebite: Treatment in the United States. JAMA 240:654, 1978.

26.19 MAMMALIAN BITES

In the United States, 1–3.5 million emergency department visits occur each year as a result of mammalian bite injuries. Over 80% of these episodes are due to dog bites, 6% to cat bites, and 1–3% to human bites. Ten per cent of bite injuries require surgical closure, and 1–2% result in hospitalization.

EPIDEMIOLOGY. Most animal bites follow provocation and are to the hand. Ferrets may attack the face of infants without provocation. Closed-fist injuries (lacerations over the 3rd and 4th metacarpal following a blow to the mouth) are the most common form of human bite. Rat bites occur typically on the lower extremities.

CLINICAL MANIFESTATIONS. The diagnosis of a mammalian bite is usually straight forward and requires a compatible history and evidence of cutaneous injury. Crush injuries may accompany dog and human bites, while severe damage to facial cartilage may follow ferret bites in young infants. Cat bites are typically deep punctures, while rat and squirrel bites tend to be superficial. Bites to the hand, especially closed-fist injuries, may damage tendons, tendon compartments, deep fascia, bone, and/or joint capsules.

Infectious Complications (see Sec. 12.37 and 12.82 for discussions of tetanus and rabies). Because of the numerous bacterial species in mammalian oral cavities and on the victim's skin, contamination of bite injuries is universal; wound infections, cellulitis, and lymphangitis appearing 24–36 hr after the injury are the most common precipitating causes for hospitalization of bite injuries. Four percent of dog bites, 35% of cat bites, and almost all closed-fist injuries become infected locally. The etiologies of infections following mammalian bites are polymicrobial and consist of mixed anaerobic and aerobic bacteria. In one study, an average of three different bacterial species were isolated from infected dog bites while a mean of five different species were recovered from infected human bites. In general, anaerobic bacteria are recovered from over half of all bite victims with infected wounds. *Pasteurella multocida* is a common pathogen in infected dog and cat bites, while viridans streptococci, *Staphylococcus aureus*, and *Bacteroides* species are likely to be recovered from infected human bites. Approximately half of the bites inflicted by monkeys become infected; the bacterial etiology of these infections parallels those of human bites. Bites that occur in fresh water (e.g., domestic piranha) may become infected with *Aeromonas hydrophilia*.

Besides wound infections, osteomyelitis, septic arthritis, abscesses, and bacterial tenosynovitis uncommonly follow mammalian bites. In immunoincompetent patients, bacteremia and meningitis may follow mammalian bites; *P. multocida* meningitis and sepsis is particularly important in this patient population following dog or cat bites.

Noninfectious Complications. Significant cosmetic and functional damage may accompany severe bites. Although rare, hemorrhagic shock may occur following attacks by "pack" animals such as stray dogs. Finally, psychologic stress and subsequent fear of animals may be a consequence of animal bites.

PREVENTION. Children's interactions with pets should be closely supervised to prevent the animal from becoming provoked by the child. Dogs should not be permitted to run free. Stray animals should be reported promptly to local authorities. Ferrets should not be kept as pets in families with small children. It is illegal to keep ferrets as pets in California, Georgia, and New Hampshire.

TREATMENT. Most bite wounds can be managed in an ambulatory setting. Hospitalization is recommended for patients with (1) extensive injury that may require operative repair or grafts; (2) injury to or breach of tendon, joint capsule, bone, or facial cartilage; (3) extensive local infection; (4) infection that developed during prophylaxis; and (5) anticipated poor compliance.

Aside from tetanus and rabies prophylaxis, the preliminary care for mammalian bites requires cleansing, high-pressure irrigation, and debridement. Because of the high risk for infection, physical scrubbing rather than passive soaking with povidone-iodine solution is recommended for initial decontamination. Additional cleansing is achieved by high-pressure saline irrigation using a large syringe (or Waterpik) and a large-bore needle. Under local anesthesia, devitalized tissue is removed and the wound is explored for injury to underlying structures such as bone, joint capsules, tendons, or cartilage. For noncomplicated bites, re-irrigation is recommended following exploration.

Whether severe mammalian bites should be sutured initially is controversial. Because of the relatively low incidence of infection, clean, recent (< 8 hr old), adequately decontaminated dog bites may be closed initially using tape or suture with a low risk of subsequent infection (3%). Noninfected, fresh (< 12 hr old) mammalian bites of the hands or face may be closed primarily, if needed, but must be followed closely; sutures should be removed at the earliest sign of infection. Closed-fist injuries are particularly susceptible to infection. Other wounds that require closure should be thoroughly decontaminated, irrigated, and debrided; packed with gauze; and re-evaluated 4–7 days later for possible infection.

Aerobic and anaerobic bacterial cultures followed by antimicrobial therapy are indicated for the treatment of infected bite wounds. Since most of these infections have a polymicrobial etiology, initial therapy should be broad. For superficial infections, orally administered amoxicillin-clavulanate (Augmentin; 50 mg/kg/24 hr in three doses) is sufficiently broad and effective; erythromycin (40 mg/kg/24 hr in four doses) is an alternative in penicillin-allergic patients. Therapy may be changed after culture results are known. Severe infections require hospitalization and parenteral antimicrobial therapy. Ampicillin-sulbactam (Unasyn; 25–50 mg ampicillin/kg/dose every 6 hours) has an identical spectrum of activity to amoxicillin-clavulanate and may be used initially. Cefoxitin (30–40 mg/kg/24 hr every 6 hours) is another option. Since clindamycin (30–40 mg/kg/24 hr in four doses) is active against most anaerobes, *S. aureus*, and aerobic streptococci but not against *P. multocida*, this agent should be used initially for the treatment of infected human bites in penicillin-allergic and nonallergic patients. Because a significant minority of *P. multocida* and *Bacteroides* species isolates are resistant to oxacillin (100 mg/kg/24 hr in six doses), oxacillin plus penicillin (100,000 U/kg/24 hr in six doses) and cefoxitin alone are additional options for empiric therapy. Erythromycin or minocycline are alternatives for the penicillin-allergic patient.

Little comparative data are available addressing the efficacy of prophylactic antibiotic use. Accepted indications for prophylaxis include (1) any cat, human, or monkey bite; (2) wounds planned for delayed closure; (3) any bites of the hands or face; (4) bites that have not or cannot be adequately debrided; and (5) victims who are infants, diabetics, or immunocompromised. Oral administration of amoxicillin-clavulanate, erythromycin, or minocycline (in older patients; 4 mg/kg/24 hr in two doses) for 3 days should be adequate prophylaxis in these cases.

STEPHEN C. ARONOFF

Brook I: Microbiology of human and animal bite wounds in children. Pediatr Infect Dis J 6:29, 1987.

Feder HM, Shanley JD, Barbera JA: Review of 59 patients hospitalized with animal bites. Pediatr Infect Dis J 6:24, 1987.

Goldstein EJC, Citron DM, Wield B, et al: Bacteriology of human and animal bite wounds. J Clin Microbiol 8:667, 1978.

Paisley JW, Lauer BA: Severe facial injuries to infants due to unprovoked attacks by pet ferrets. JAMA 259:2005, 1988.

Revord ME, Goldfarb J, Shurin SB: *Aeromonas hydrophilia* wound infection in a patient with cyclic neutropenia following a piranha bite. Pediatr Infect Dis J 7:70, 1988.

Trott A: Care of mammalian bites. Pediatr Infect Dis J 6:8, 1987.

27

LABORATORY MEDICINE AND REFERENCE TABLES

27.1 LABORATORY TESTING AND REFERENCE VALUES (Table 27–2) IN INFANTS AND CHILDREN

For a number of reasons—genetic heterogeneity, biologic and environmental variability, and inhomogeneity of subclinical health status—normal values for many laboratory tests do not show a Gaussian bell-shaped curve of distribution. As a result, the population mean and standard deviation are frequently less useful than the range of normal values, generally given as the 95% normal range, that is, the range of values obtained in testing a normal population minus the lowest 2.5% and the highest 2.5%. As shown in Table 27–1, serum sodium, which is tightly controlled physiologically, has a distribution that is essentially Gaussian in a large group of children. This is indicated by the fact that the mean value ± 2 standard deviations gives a range very close to that actually observed in 95% of the children. On the other hand, serum creatine kinase, which is subject to diverse influences and is not actively controlled, does not show a Gaussian distribution, as evidenced by the lack of agreement between the range actually observed and that predicted by the mean value ± 2 standard deviations.

A refinement of referencing that is used with increasing frequency is reporting the value obtained together with the percentile of normal values into which the value obtained falls. This method is useful when one is testing for risk factors such as serum cholesterol.

A further modification that is necessary for many tests performed in infants and children is calculating the age-related adjustment of the normal range. Both age adjustment and the use of percentiles are illustrated in the normal values for serum cholesterol in Table 27–2.

A final modification needed for reporting normal ranges is referencing to the Tanner stage of sexual maturation, which is most useful in assessing pituitary and gonadal function.

ACCURACY AND PRECISION OF LABORATORY TESTS. An important consideration in interpreting the results of a laboratory test is the technical accuracy of the test. Because of improvements in methods of analysis and elimination of analytic interferences, the accuracy of most tests is limited primarily by their precision. Accuracy is a measure of the nearness of the test result to the actual value, whereas precision is a measure of the reproducibility of a result. No test can be more accurate than it is precise. Analysis of precision by repetitive measurements of a single sample gives rise to a Gaussian distribution with a meaningful mean and standard deviation. The estimate of precision generally used is the coefficient of variation (CV):

$$CV = \text{Standard deviation/mean} \times 100\ (\%)$$

The CV is not likely to be constant over the full range of values obtained in clinical testing but ordinarily is about 5% in the normal range. The CV is generally not reported but is always known by the laboratory. It is particularly important in assessing the significance of changes in laboratory results. For example, a common situation is the need to assess hepatotoxicity incurred as a result of administration of a therapeutic drug and reflected in the serum alanine aminotransferase (ALT) value. If serum ALT increases from 25 U/L to 40 U/L, is the change significant? The CV for ALT is 7%. Using the value obtained plus or minus 2 × CV to express the extremes of imprecision, it can be seen that a value of 25 is unlikely to reflect an actual concentration of greater than 29 U/L, and a value of 40 U/L is unlikely to reflect an actual concentration of less than 34 U/L. Therefore, the change in the value as obtained by testing is likely to reflect a real change in circulating ALT levels, and continued monitoring of ALT is indicated even though both values for ALT are within normal limits. "Likely" in this case is only a probability. Inherent biologic variability is such that the results of two successive tests may suggest a trend that will disappear on further testing.

The precision of a test may also be indicated by providing confidence limits for a given result. Ordinarily, 95% confidence limits are used, indicating that it is 95% certain that the value obtained lies between the two limits reported. Confidence limits are calculated using the mean and standard deviation (SD) of replicate determinations:

$$95\%\ \text{Confidence limits} = \text{mean} \pm t \times SD$$

where t is a constant derived from the number of replications. In most cases t = 2.

PREDICTIVE VALUE (PV) OF LABORATORY TESTS (see also Sec. 5.3). Predictive value theory deals with the usefulness of tests as defined by their sensitivity (ability to detect a disease) and specificity (ability to define absence of a disease).

$$\text{Sensitivity} = \text{No. positive by test/no. with disease} \times 100$$

$$\text{Specificity} = \text{No. negative by test/no. without disease} \times 100$$

TABLE 27–1. Gaussian and Non-Gaussian Laboratory Values in 458 Normal School Children Aged 7–14 Yr

	Serum Sodium (mM/L)	Serum Creatine Kinase (U/L)
Mean	141	68
SD*	1.7	34
Mean ± 2 SD	138–144	0–136
Actual 95% range	137–144	24–162

*SD = standard deviation

The PV of a positive test = true +/total + × 100, and the PV of a negative test = true −/total − × 100, where total + is the sum of true + and false +, and total − is the sum of true − and false −. The problems addressed by the theory are false-negative and false-positive tests; these are major considerations in interpreting screening tests in general and neonatal screening tests specifically.

Testing for human immunodeficiency virus (HIV) seroreactivity serves to illustrate some of these considerations. If it is assumed that approximately 1,000,000 of 200,000,000 residents of the United States are infected with HIV (prevalence = 0.5%) and that 90% of those infected show the appropriate antibodies, we can consider the usefulness of a simple test with 99% sensitivity and 99.5% specificity. If the total population of the United States were screened, it would be possible to identify most of those infected with HIV:

$$1{,}000{,}000 \times 0.9 \times 0.99 = 891{,}000\ (89.1\%)$$

There would be 109,000 false-negative test results. Even with a 99.5% specificity, the number of false-positive test results would be larger than the number of true positive results:

$$199{,}000{,}000 \times 0.005 = 995{,}000$$

There would be 198,005,000 true negative results.

$$\text{PV of positive test} = \frac{891{,}000}{891{,}000 + 995{,}000} \times 100 = 47\%$$

$$\text{PV of negative test} = \frac{198{,}005{,}000}{198{,}005{,}000 + 109{,}000} \times 100 = 99.9\%$$

Given the high cost associated with follow-up of false-positive test results, the anguish produced by a false-positive result, and the limited effectiveness of current treatment, it is easy to see why universal screening for HIV seropositivity has received a low priority.

By contrast, we can consider the screening of 100,000 individuals from groups at increased risk for HIV in whom the overall prevalence of disease is 10%, all other considerations being unchanged.

$$\text{True positive results} = 0.9 \times 0.99 \times 10{,}000 = 8{,}910$$

$$\text{False-positive results} = 0.005 \times 90{,}000 = 450$$

$$\text{False-negative results} = 10{,}000 - 8{,}910 = 1{,}090$$

$$\text{PV of positive result} = \frac{8{,}910}{8{,}910 + 450} \times 100 = 95\%$$

$$\text{PV of negative result} = \frac{89{,}550}{89{,}550 + 1090} \times 100 = 99\%$$

It is clear from these two hypothetical testing strategies that the diagnostic efficiency of testing is heavily dependent on the prevalence of the disease being tested for, even if the test is a superior one like the test for HIV antibodies.

NEONATAL SCREENING TESTS. Most neonatal screening tests are more problematic in a theoretical sense than would be the case with widespread screening for HIV. First, almost all the diseases detected in neonatal screening programs have a very low prevalence, and second, the tests are, for the most part, quantitative rather than qualitative. In general, the strategy is to use the initial screening test to separate a highly suspect group of patients from normal infants (i.e., to increase the prevalence) and then to follow this suspect group aggressively. This strategy is illustrated by a scheme used in screening newborns for congenital hypothyroidism, the prevalence of which is 25/100,000 live-born infants. The initial test performed is for thyroxine in whole blood, and infants with the lowest 10% of test results are considered suspect. If all infants with hypothyroidism were in the suspect group, the prevalence of disease in this group would be 250/100,000 infants. The original samples obtained from the suspect group are retested for thyroxine and then tested for thyroid-stimulating hormone. This second round of testing results in an even more highly suspect group comprising 0.1% of the infants screened and having a prevalence of hypothyroidism of 25,000/100,000 subjects. This final group is aggressively pursued for further testing and treatment. Even with a 1,000-fold increase in prevalence, 75% of the population aggressively tested is euthyroid. The justifications advanced for the program are that treatment is easy and effective and that the alternative, long-term custodial care, is both unsatisfactory and expensive.

TESTING IN DIFFERENTIAL DIAGNOSIS. The use of laboratory tests in differential diagnosis will satisfy predictive value theory because a correct differential diagnosis should result in a relatively high prevalence of the disease under consideration. An example of testing in differential diagnosis is the use of urinary vanillylmandelic acid (VMA) for diagnosis of neuroblastoma. Galen and Gambino pointed out that a simple spot test for VMA was not useful in general screening programs because of the low prevalence of neuroblastoma (3/100,000) and the low sensitivity of the test (69%). Even though the specificity of urinary VMA was 99.6%, testing of 100,000 children would produce 2 true positive test results, 400 false-positive results, and 1 false-negative result. The predictive value of a positive test in this setting is 0.5%, and the predictive value of a negative test is 99.99%, not much different from the assumption that neuroblastoma is not present at all. However, testing for urinary VMA in a 3-year-old child with an abdominal mass gives a useful result because the prevalence of neuroblastoma is at least 50% in 3-year-old children with abdominal masses. If 100 such children are tested and the prevalence of neuroblastoma in the group is assumed to be 50%, satisfactory predictive values are obtained:

$$\text{PV of positive test} = \frac{0.69 \times 50}{0.69 \times 50 + 0.004 \times 50} \times 100 = 99\%$$

$$\text{PV of negative test} = \frac{0.996 \times 50}{0.996 \times 50 + 0.31 \times 50} \times 100 = 76\%$$

Here a test with a low sensitivity is quite powerful in differential diagnosis because the predictive value of a positive result is almost 100% in the setting of high prevalence.

RISK FACTORS AND PREDICTIVE VALUE. When a given laboratory value within the spectrum of the reference range is considered a risk factor, it is generally true that, in the absence of clinical manifestations, the value has no predictive worth as an indicator of disease and has little value in predicting the likelihood of future disease in any individual case.

JOHN F. NICHOLSON
MICHAEL A. PESCE

Galen RS, Gambino SR: Beyond Normality. New York, Academic Press, 1975.
Novogroder M: Neonatal screening for hypothyroidism. Pediatr Clin North Am 27(4):881, 1980.

TABLE 27–2. REFERENCE RANGES FOR LABORATORY TESTS

Prefixes Denoting Decimal Factors

Prefix	*Symbol*	*Factor*
mega	M	10^6
kilo	k	10^3
hecto	h	10^2
deka	da	10^1
deci	d	10^{-1}
centi	c	10^{-2}
milli	m	10^{-3}
micro	μ	10^{-6}
nano	n	10^{-9}
pico	p	10^{-12}
femto	f	10^{-15}

To conserve space, the following common abbreviations are used.

Abbreviations

Ab	absorbance
AI	angiotensin I
AU	arbitrary unit
*c*AMP	adenosine 3′,5′-cyclic phosphate
cap	capillary
CH_{50}	dilution required to lyse 50% of indicator RBC; indicates complement activity
CHF	congestive heart failure
CKBB	brain isoenzyme of creatine kinase
CKMB	heart isoenzyme of creatine kinase
CNS	central nervous system
conc.	concentration
d	diem, day, days
F	female
g	gram
hr	hour, hours
Hb	hemoglobin
HbCO	carboxyhemoglobin
hpf	high power field
HPLC	high pressure liquid chromatography
IFA	indirect fluorescent antibody
IU	International Unit of hormone activity
L	liter
M	male
MCV	mean corpuscular value
mEq/L	milliequivalents per liter
min	minute, minutes
mm^3	cubic millimeter; equivalent to microliter (μL)
mm Hg	millimeters of mercury
mo	month, months
mol	mole
mOsm	milliosmoles
MW	relative molecular weight
nm	nanometer (wavelength)
Pa	pascals
pc	postprandial
RBC	red blood cell(s); erythrocyte(s)
RIA	radioimmunoassay
RID	radial immunodiffusion
RT	room temperature
s	second, seconds
SD	standard deviation
std.	standard
therap.	therapeutic
U	International Unit of enzyme activity
V	volume
WBC	white blood cell
WHO	World Health Organization
wk	week, weeks
yr	year, years

Symbols

>	greater than
⩾	greater than or equal to
<	less than
⩽	less than or equal to
±	plus/minus
≃	approximately equal to

Abbreviations for Specimens

S	serum
P	plasma
(H)	heparin
(LiH)	lithium heparin
(E)	EDTA
(C)	citrate
(O)	oxalate
W	whole blood
U	urine
F	feces
CSF	cerebrospinal fluid
AF	amniotic fluid

Key to Comments

30°, 37°	temperature of enzymatic analysis (centigrade)
a	atomic absorption
b	optical density
c	colorimetry
d	Ektachem, proprietary analytic system of Eastman Kodak Co.
e	enzyme-amplified immunoassay
f	values in older females higher than those in older males
g	electrophoresis
h	gas chromatography
i	radioimmunoassay
l	fluorescence-activated cell sorting
m	values obtained are significantly method-dependent
n	nephelometry
o	borate affinity chromatography
p	high pressure liquid chromatography
q	cation exchange chromatography
r	radial immunodiffusion
s	values in older males higher than those in older females
v	fluorometric method
w	ion-selective electrode
x	fluorescence polarization
z	enzymatic assay

De Schepper J, Derde MP, Goubert P, et al: Reference values for fructosamine concentrations in children's sera: Influence of protein concentration, age and sex. Clin Chem 34(12): 2444, 1988.

Dickinson JC, Hamilton PB: The free amino acids of human spinal fluid determined by ion exchange chromatography. J Neurochem 13:1179, 1966.

Endocrine Sciences, Tarzana, CA.

Gibson LE, di Sant'Agnese PA, Schwachman H: Procedure for the quantitative iontophoretic sweat test for cystic fibrosis. Rockville, MD, Cystic Fibrosis Foundation, 1985, pp 1–4.

Gillard BK, Simbala JA, Goodglick L: Reference intervals for amylase isoenzymes in serum and plasma of infants and children. Clin Chem 29(6):1119, 1983.

Hoffman G, Aramaki S, Blum-Hoffman E, et al: Quantitative analysis for organic acids in biological samples: Batch isolation followed by gas chromatographic-mass spectrometric analysis. Clin Chem 35(4):587, 1989.

Jedeikin R, Makela SK, Shennan AT, et al: Creatine kinase isoenzymes in serum from cord blood and the blood of healthy full-term infants during the first three postnatal days. Clin Chem 28(2):317, 1982.

Jung D, Lun L, Zinsmeyer J, et al: The concentration of hypoxanthine and lactate in the blood of healthy and hypoxic newborns. J Perinat Med 13:43, 1985.

Knight JA, Haymond RE: γ-glutamyltransferase and alkaline phosphatase activities compared in serum of normal children and children with liver disease. Clin Chem 27(1):48, 1981.
Landry A, Gartland GL, Abo T, et al: Enumeration of human lymphocyte subpopulations by immunofluorescence: A comparative study using automated flow microfluorometry and fluorescence microscopy. J Immunol Methods 58:337, 1983.
Lockitch G, Halstead AC, Albersheim S, et al: Age and sex specific pediatric reference intervals for biochemistry analyses as measured on the Ektachem-700 analyzer. Clin Chem 34(8):1622, 1988.
Lockitch G, Halstead AC, Quigley G, et al: Age and sex specific pediatric reference intervals: Study design and methods illustrated by measurement of serum proteins with the Behring LN nephelometer. Clin Chem 34(8):1618, 1988.
Lockitch G, Halstead AC, Wadsworth L, et al: Age and sex specific pediatric reference intervals and correlations for zinc, copper, selenium, iron, vitamins A and E, and related proteins. Clin Chem 34(8):1625, 1988.
Mayo Clinic Laboratories, Rochester, MN, 1989.
Meites S (ed): Pediatric Clinical Chemistry, Reference (Normal) Values, 3rd ed. Washington, D.C., Clinical Chemistry, 1989.
Nichols Institute Reference Laboratories, San Juan Capistrano, CA.
Pesce MA, Boudourian S: Clinical significance of plasma galactose and erythrocyte galactose-1-phosphate measurements in transferase-deficient galactosemia and in individuals with below-normal transferase activity. Clin Chem 28:301, 1982.
Pesce MA, Boudourian S, Harris RC, et al: Enzymatic micromethod for measuring galactose-1-phosphate uridylyltransferase in erythrocytes. Clin Chem 23:1711, 1977.
Pesce MA, Boudourian S, Nicholson JF: A new microfluorometric method for the measurement of galactose-1-phosphate in erythrocytes. Clin Chem Acta 118:177, 1982.
Rosenthal P, Pesce MA: Long-term monitoring of D-lactic acidosis in a child. J Pediatr Gastroenterol Nutr 4:674, 1985.
Sherry B, Jack RM, Weber A, et al: Reference interval for prealbumin for children two to 36 months old. Clin Chem 34(9):1878, 1988.
Taylor WJ, Caviness MHD: A Textbook for the Clinical Application of Therapeutic Drug Monitoring. Irving, TX, Abbott Laboratories, Diagnostic Division, 1986.
Syva Company: TDM Serum Sample Guide. Palo Alto, CA, Syva Company, 1986.
Unten SK, Hokama Y: Enzyme immunoassay for C-reactive protein analysis. J Clin Lab Anal 1:205, 1987.
Visnapu LA, Karlson LK, Dubinsky EJ, et al: Pediatric reference ranges for serum aldolase. Am J Clin Pathol 91(4):476, 1989.

TABLE 27–2. Reference Ranges for Laboratory Tests

Test	Specimen	Reference Range		Factor	Reference Range (SI)	Comments
Acetaminophen. See end of table under Drugs						
Acetone						
Semiquantitative	S, P(O)	Negative (<3 mg/dL)			Negative (<0.5 mmol/L)	
Quantitative		0.3–2.0 mg/dL		× 0.1722	0.05–0.34 mmol/L	
Semiquantitative	U	Negative			Negative	
Activated partial thromboplastin time (APTT)	P(C)	25–35 s			25–35 s (APTT)	
		Infant: <90 s			Infant: <90 s	
Adrenocorticotropic hormone (ACTH)	P(H)	Cord blood	130–160 pg/mL	× 1	130–160 μg/L	
		1–7 d postnatal	100–140 pg/mL		100–140 μg/L	
		Adult				
		0800 hr	25–100 pg/mL		25–100 μg/L	
		1800 hr	<50 pg/mL		<50 μg/L	
Alanine aminotransferase (ALT, GPT)	S	0–5 d	6–50 U/L	× 1	6–50 U/L	37° s d (Lockitch et al)
		1–19 y	5–45 U/L		5–45 U/L	
Albumin	P	Premature 1 d	1.8–3.0 g/dL	× 10	18–30 g/L	c (Meites)
		Full-term <6 d	2.5–3.4 g/dL		25–34 g/L	
		<5 yr	3.9–5.0 g/dL		39–50 g/L	
		5–19 yr	4.0–5.3 g/dL		40–53 g/L	
	U	4–16 yr	3.35–15.3 mg/24 h/1.73 m²			e (Meites)
	CSF	10–30 mg/dL			100–300 mg/L	
Aldolase	S	10–24 mo	3.4–11.8 U/L	× 1	3.4–11.8 U/L	z (Visnapu et al)
		25 mo–16 yr	1.2– 8.8 U/L		1.2– 8.8 U/L	
Aldosterone	S, P(H,E)					
		Newborn	5–60 ng/dL	× 0.0277	0.14–1.7 nmol/L	
		1 wk–1 yr	1–160 ng/dL		0.03–4.4 nmol/L	
		1–3 yr	5–60 ng/dL		0.14–1.7 nmol/L	
		3–5 yr	<5–80 ng/dL		<0.14–2.2 nmol/L	
		5–7 yr	<5–50 ng/dL		<0.14–1.4 nmol/L	
		7–11 yr	5–70 ng/dL		0.14–1.9 nmol/L	
		11–15 yr	<5–50 ng/dL		<0.14–1.4 nmol/L	
		Adult (Na diet)				
		Supine	3–10 ng/dL		0.08–0.3 nmol/L	
		Upright F	5–30 ng/dL		0.14–0.8 nmol/L	
		M	6–22 ng/dL		0.17–0.61 nmol/L	
		2–3 × higher during pregnancy				
		Adrenal vein	200–800 ng/dL		5.5–22 nmol/L	
		Low Na diet: increases 2- to 5-fold				
		Florinef suppression	<4 ng/dL		<0.1 nmol/L	
		ACTH or angiotensin stimulation, 1 hr: increases 2- to 5-fold				

TABLE 27–2. Reference Ranges for Laboratory Tests *Continued*

Test	Specimen	Reference Range			Factor	Reference Range (SI)	Comments
	U	*Total Urinary Na*	*Plasma Renin Activity*	*Urinary Aldosterone*		*Urinary aldosterone*	
		<20 mmol/d	5–24 ng AI/mL/hr	>35–80 µg/d	× 2.77	>97–220 nmol/d	
		50 mmol/d	2–7 ng AI/mL/hr	13–33 µg/d		36–91 nmol/d	
		100 mmol/d	1–5 ng AI/mL/hr	5–24 µg/d		14–66 nmol/d	
		150 mmol/d	0.5–4 ng AI/mL/hr	3–19 µg/d		8–53 nmol/d	
		200 mmol/d		1–16 µg/d		3–44 nmol/d	
		250 mmol/d		1–13 µg/d		3–36 nmol/d	
		(assuming normal serum Na, K, and extracellular volume)					
Alkaline phosphatase, leukocyte. See Neutrophil alkaline phosphate							
Alkaline phosphate, serum. See Phosphatase, alkaline							

Test	Specimen	Reference Range	Factor	Reference Range (SI)	Comments
Amino acids	CSF				q (Dickinson et al)
Taurine		6.3 ± 1.8 µmol/L	× 1	6.3 ± 1.8 µmol/L	
Aspartic acid		0.9 ± 0.5 µmol/L		0.9 ± 0.5 µmol/L	
Threonine		25.0 ± 10.0 µmol/L		25.0 ± 10.0 µmol/L	
Serine + asparagine		38.0 ± 23.0 µmol/L		38.0 ± 23.0 µmol/L	
Glutamine		509.0 ± 144.0 µmol/L		509.0 ± 144.0 µmol/L	
Proline		0.6 ± — µmol/L		0.6 ± — µmol/L	
Glutamic acid		7.0 ± 4.9 µmol/L		7.0 ± 4.9 µmol/L	
Glycine		6.6 ± 1.8 µmol/L		6.6 ± 1.8 µmol/L	
Alanine		23.0 ± 9.4 µmol/L		23.0 ± 9.4 µmol/L	
Valine		14.0 ± 5.5 µmol/L		14.0 ± 5.5 µmol/L	
Half cystine		0.2 ± — µmol/L		0.2 ± — µmol/L	
Methionine		2.6 ± 1.6 µmol/L		2.6 ± 1.6 µmol/L	
Isoleucine		4.4 ± 1.3 µmol/L		4.4 ± 1.3 µmol/L	
Leucine		11.0 ± 3.6 µmol/L		11.0 ± 3.6 µmol/L	
Tyrosine		9.1 ± 5.0 µmol/L		9.1 ± 5.0 µmol/L	
Phenylalanine		9.2 ± 5.8 µmol/L		9.2 ± 5.8 µmol/L	
Ornithine		5.7 ± 1.8 µmol/L		5.7 ± 1.8 µmol/L	
Lysine		19.0 ± 6.6 µmol/L		19.0 ± 6.6 µmol/L	
Histidine		13.0 ± 4.4 µmol/L		13.0 ± 4.4 µmol/L	
Arginine		20.0 ± 5.8 µmol/L		20.0 ± 5.8 µmol/L	

Test	Specimen	Reference Range			Factor	Reference Range (SI)	Comments
Amino acids, plasma	P(H)						q (Nichols Institute)
		0–30 d	*>1 mo–16 yr*	*> 16 yr*			
Phosphoserine		0–30	0–12	3–7 µmol/L	× 1		
Taurine		74–216	22–192	27–168 µmol/L			
Aspartic acid		0–17	5–59	0–24 µmol/L			
Hydroxyproline		20–70	0–40	0–40 µmol/L			
Threonine		114–335	73–160	79–193 µmol/L			
Serine		94–243	90–226	73–167 µmol/L			
Asparagine		20–58	28–246	14–104 µmol/L			
Glutamic acid		0–50	0–210	0–88 µmol/L			
Glutamine		538–958	52–669	415–964 µmol/L			
Proline		107–177	67–238	102–336 µmol/L			
Glycine		224–514	89–360	120–554 µmol/L			
Alanine		236–410	142–484	210–661 µmol/L			
Citrulline		8–28	1–55	12–55 µmol/L			
2-Aminobutyric acid		6–29	0–42	3–38 µmol/L			
Valine		80–246	110–271	141–317 µmol/L			
Cysteine		70–167	0–106	16–167 µmol/L			
Methionine		9–41	0–90	6–40 µmol/L			
Isoleucine		27–53	34–85	36–98 µmol/L			
Leucine		46–109	55–165	75–175 µmol/L			
Tyrosine		42–99	29–86	21–87 µmol/L			
Phenylalanine		42–110	22–98	37–88 µmol/L			
Homocystine		0–0	0–0	0–0 µmol/L			
Tryptophan		17–71	24–79	20–95 µmol/L			
Ornithine		49–151	15–143	30–106 µmol/L			
Lysine		114–269	68–266	83–238 µmol/L			
1-Methylhistidine		0–27	0–27	0–27 µmol/L			
Histidine		49–114	52–124	31–107 µmol/L			
3-Methylhistidine		0–10	0–6	0–4 µmol/L			
Arginine		22–88	6–187	36–145 µmol/L			

Table continued on following page

TABLE 27–2. Reference Ranges for Laboratory Tests *Continued*

Test	Specimen	Reference Range		Factor	Reference Range (SI)		Comments
Amino acids, urine	U						q (Nichols Institute)
		0–30 d (µmol/g creatinine)	*>1 mo (µmol/g creatinine)*		*0–30 d (mmol/mol creatinine)*	*>1 mo (mmol/mol creatinine)*	
Phosphoserine		0–53	0–35	× 0.1131	0–6.0	0–4.0	
Taurine		1521–6922	0–1450		172–783	0–164	
Phosphoethanolamine		0–23	23–203		0–2.6	2.6–23	
Aspartic acid		78–172	0–82		8.8–19.5	0–9.3	
Hydroxyproline		210–2413	0–210		23.7–273	0–23.7	
Threonine		99–509	27–265		11.2–57.6	3.1–30	
Serine		80–1096	86–566		9.1–124	9.7–64	
Asparagine		0–438	0–107		0–49.5	0–12.1	
Glutamic acid		34–363	0–80		3.8–41.1	0–9	
Glutamine		256–1096	168–849		29–124	9.7–64	
Sarcosine		93–850	93–850		10.5–96.1	10.5–96.1	
Proline		74–537	0–57		8.4–60.7	0–6.4	
Glycine		1423–7143	0–2953		161–808	0–334	
Alanine		403–715	68–534		45.6–80.9	7.7–60.4	
Citrulline		9–212	8–106		1.0–24	0.9–12	
2-Aminobutyric acid		354–1061	44–221		40–120	5–25	
Valine		18–314	7–50		2.0–35.5	0.8–5.6	
Cysteine		226–812	5–177		25.8–91.9	0.6–20	
Methionine		15–71	6–111		1.7–8	0.7–12.5	
Homocitrulline		0–266	0–266		0–30.1	0–30.1	
Cystathionine		27–111	3–23		3.1–12.5	0.3–2.6	
Isoleucine		43–179	0–65		4.9–20.2	0–7.3	
Leucine		17–72	15–57		1.9–8.1	1.7–6.5	
Tyrosine		27–97	19–145		3–11	2.2–16.4	
Phenylalanine		39–156	17–102		4.4–17.7	1.9–11.5	
β-Alanine		0–1202	0–1202		0–136	0–136	
3-Aminoisobutyric acid		0–111	0–111		0–12.5	0–12.5	
4-Aminoisobutyric acid		0–2643	0–2643		0–299	0–299	
Homocystine		0–0	0–0		0–0	0–0	
Argininosuccinic acid		0–9	0–7		0–1.0	0–0.8	
Ethanolamine		840–3492	57–308		95–395	6.5–34.8	
Tryptophan		0–106	0–106		0–12	0–12	
Hydroxylysine		0–106	0–106		0–12	0–12	
Ornithine		34–156	1–44		3.9–17.7	0.1–5.0	
Lysine		74–1282	0–548		8.4–145.0	0–62.0	
1-Methylhistidine		72–425	0–691		8.1–48.1	0–78.2	
Histidine		148–721	0–1353		16.7–81.6	0–153.0	
3-Methylhistidine		115–401	19–413		13–45.4	2.1–46.7	
Anserine		0–561	0–561		0–63.5	0–63.5	
Carnosine		0–127	0–127		0–14.4	0–14.4	
Arginine		50–73	8–32		5.6–8.3	0.9–3.6	
Aminolevulinic acid (ALA)	S	15–23 µg/dL (lower in child)		× 0.076	1.1–1.8 µmol/L		
	U	1.3–7.0 mg/24 hr		× 7.626	9.9–53.4 µmol/d		
Ammonia nitrogen	S, P(LiH)	Newborn	90–150 µgN/dL	× 0.714	64–107 µmol/L		z q
		0–2 wk	79–129 µgN/dL		56–92 µmol/L		
		>1 mo	29–70 µgN/dL		21–50 µmol/L		
		Thereafter	15–45 µgN/dL		11–32 µmol/L		
	P(LiH)	1–90 d	59–202 µgN/dL	× 0.714	42–144 µmol/L		d (Meites)
		3 mo–3 yr	48–195 µgN/dL		34–139 µmol/L		
	U		500–1,200 mgN/24 hr	0.0714	36–86 mmol/d		
Amniotic fluid analysis (Ab 450 nm)	AF		28 wk 0–0.048 A		0–0.048 A		
			40 wk 0–0.02 A		0–0.02 A		
Amphetamine. See end of table under Drugs							
Amylase	S	1–19 yr	35–127 U/L	× 1	35–127 U/L		c (Meites)
Pancreatic isoenzymes	S, P(H)	Cord blood 8 mo	0–34%	× 0.01	0–0.34 fraction of total		(Gillard et al)
		9 mo–4 yr	5–56%		0.05–0.56 fraction of total		
		5–19 yr	23–59%		0.23–0.59 fraction of total		
Androstenedione	S	M					(Endocrine Sciences)
		Tanner 1 <9.8 yr	8–50 ng/dL	× 0.03479	0.28–1.74 nmol/L		
		Tanner 2 9.8–14.5 yr	31–65 ng/dL		1.08–2.26 nmol/L		
		Tanner 3 10.7–15.4 yr	50–100 ng/dL		1.74–3.48 nmol/L		
		Tanner 4 11.8–16.2 yr	48–140 ng/dL		1.67–4.87 nmol/L		
		Tanner 5 12.8–17.3 yr	65–210 ng/dL		2.26–7.30 nmol/L		
		Adult	75–205 ng/dL		2.61–7.13 nmol/L		

TABLE 27–2. Reference Ranges for Laboratory Tests *Continued*

Test	Specimen	Reference Range	Factor	Reference Range (SI)	Comments
Androstenedione *(Continued)*		F			
		Tanner 1 <9.2 yr 8–50 ng/dL		0.28–1.74 nmol/L	
		Tanner 2 9.2–13.7 yr 42–100 ng/dL		1.46–3.48 nmol/L	
		Tanner 3 10.0–14.4 yr 80–190 ng/dL		2.78–6.61 nmol/L	
		Tanner 4 10.7–15.6 yr 77–225 ng/dL		2.68–7.83 nmol/L	
		Tanner 5 11.8–18.6 yr 80–240 ng/dL		2.78–8.35 nmol/L	
		Adult Follicular 85–275 ng/dL		2.96–9.57 nmol/L	
		Luteal 85–275 ng/dL		2.96–9.57 nmol/L	
Anion gap (Na − (Cl + CO_2))	P(H)	7–16 mmol/L		7–16 mmol/L	
Antideoxyribonuclease B titer (Anti-DNAse tit)	S	≤170 units		≤170 units	
Antidiuretic hormone (hADH, vasopressin)	P(E)	*Plasma Osmols* / *Plasma ADH*	× 1	*Plasma ADH*	
		270–280 mOsm/kg <1.5 pg/mL		<1.5 ng/L	
		280–285 mOsm/kg <2.5 pg/mL		<2.5 ng/L	
		285–290 mOsm/kg 1–5 pg/mL		1–5 ng/L	
		290–295 mOsm/kg 2–7 pg/mL		2–7 ng/L	
		295–300 mOsm/kg 4–12 pg/mL		4–12 ng/L	
Anti-streptolysin-O titer (ASO titer)	S	≤166 Todd units 170–330 Todd units in school-aged children			
α_1-Antitrypsin	S	0–5 d 143–440 mg/dL	× 0.01	1.43–4.40 g/L	n (Lockitch et al)
		1–9 yr 147–245 mg/dL		1.47–2.45 g/L	
		9–19 yr 152–317 mg/dL		1.52–3.17 g/L	
	F	<1 yr			r (Meites)
		breast milk <4.4 mg/g solid			
		formula <2.9 mg/g solid			
		6 mo–44 yr			
		cow milk, regular diet <1.7 mg/g solid			
Ascorbic acid. See Vitamin C					
Aspartate aminotransferase (AST, SGOT)	S	0–5 d 35–140 U/L	× 1	35–140 U/L	37° s (Lockitch et al)
		1–9 yr 15–55 U/L		15–55 U/L	
		10–19 yr 5–45 U/L		5–45 U/L	
Base excess	W(H)	Newborn (−10)–(−2) mmol/L		(−10)–(−2) mmol/L	
		Infant (−7)–(−1) mmol/L		(−7)–(−1) mmol/L	
		Child (−4)–(+2) mmol/L		(−4)–(+2) mmol/L	
		Thereafter (−3)–(+3) mmol/L		(−3)–(+3) mmol/L	
Bicarbonate	S, P	Arterial 21–28 mmol/L		Arterial 21–28 mmol/L	
		Venous 22–29 mmol/L		Venous 22–29 mmol/L	
Bile acids, total	S, fasting	0.3–2.3 μg/mL	× 1	0.3–2.3 mg/L	
	S, 2-hr pc	1.8–3.2 μg/mL		1.8–3.2 mg/L	
	F	120–225 mg/24 hr	× 1	120–225 mg/24 hr	
Bilirubin	S, P				
		Premature / *Full-term*		*Premature* / *Full-term*	
Total	S	Cord blood <2.0 mg/dL <2.0 mg/dL	× 17.10	<34 μmol/L <34 μmol/L	
		0–1 d <8.0 mg/dL <6.0 mg/dL		<137 μmol/L <103 μmol/L	
		1–2 d <12.0 mg/dL <8.0 mg/dl		<205 μmol/L <137 μmol/L	
		2–5 d <16.0 mg/dL <12.0 mg/dL		<274 μmol/L <205 μmol/L	
		>5 d <2.0 mg/dL 2–1.0 mg/dL		<34 μmol/L 3.4–17.1 μmol/L	
	U	Negative		Negative	
	AF	28 wk <0.075 mg/dL (or Ab450 <0.048)	× 17.10	<1.3 μmol/L (or Ab450 <0.048)	
		40 wk <0.025 mg/dL (or Ab450 <0.02)		<0.43 μmol/L (or Ab450 <0.02)	
Conjugated	S	0–0.2 mg/dL	× 17.10	0–3.4 μmol/L	
Bleeding time (BBT)					
Ivy		Normal 2–7 min Borderline 7–11 min		Normal 2–7 min Borderline 7–11 min	
Simplate (G–D)		2.75–8 min		2.75–8 min	
Blood volume	W (H)	M 52–83 mL/kg F 50–75 mL/kg	× 0.001	M 0.052–0.083 L/kg F 0.050–0.075 L/kg	
Brucellosis, agglutinins	S	≤1:8	× 1	≤1:8	

Table continued on following page

TABLE 27–2. Reference Ranges for Laboratory Tests *Continued*

Test	Specimen	Reference Range		Factor	Reference Range (SI)	Comments
C-Peptide	P	0.5–2 µg/L (fasting)		× 1	0.5–2 µg/L (fasting)	i (Nichols Institute)
C-reactive protein	S	Cord blood	52–1,330 ng/mL	× 1	52–1,330 µg/L	e (Unten et al)
		2–12 yr	67–1,800 ng/mL		67–1,800 µg/L	
CSF. See Cerebrospinal fluid						
Calcitonin	S, P(HE)	M 3–26 pg/mL		× 0.28	M 0.8–7.2 pmol/L	(Nichols Institute)
		F 2–17 pg/mL			F 0.6–4.7 pmol/L	
		Higher in newborn infants				
Calcium, ionized (Ca)	S, P(H), W(H)	Cord blood	5.0–6.0 mg/dL	× 0.25	1.25–1.50 mmol/L	
		Newborn				
		3–24 hr	4.3–5.1 mg/dL		1.07–1.27 mmol/L	
		24–48 hr	4.0–4.7 mg/dL		1.00–1.17 mmol/L	
		Thereafter	4.8–4.92 mg/dL		1.12–1.23 mmol/L	
		or	2.24–2.46 mEq/L	×0.5	1.12–1.23 mmol/L	
Calcium, total	S	Cord blood	9.0–11.5 mg/dL	× 0.25	2.25–2.88 mmol/L	
		Newborn				
		3–24 hr	9.0–10.6 mg/dL		2.3–2.65 mmol/L	
		24–48 hr	7.0–12.0 mg/dL		1.75–3.0 mmol/L	
		4–7 d	9.0–10.9 mg/dL		2.25–2.73 mmol/L	
		Child	8.8–10.8 mg/dL		2.2–2.70 mmol/L	
		Thereafter	8.4–10.2 mg/dL		2.1–2.55 mmol/L	
	U	Ca in diet				
		Ca-free	5–40 mg/24 hr	× 0.025	0.13–1.0 mmol/24 hr	
		Low to average	50–150 mg/24 hr		1.25–3.8 mmol/24 hr	
		Average (20 mmol/24 h)	100–300 mg/24 hr		2.5–7.5 mmol/24 hr	
	CSF	2.1–2.7 mEq/L or		× 0.50	1.05–1.35 mmol/L	
		4.2–5.4 mg/dL		× 0.25	1.05–1.35 mmol/L	
	F	Average 0.64 g/24 hr		× 25	16 mmol/24 hr	
Carbamazepine. See end of table under Drugs						
Carbon dioxide	W(H)	Newborn	27–40 mm Hg	× 0.1333	3.6–5.3 kPa	
		Infant	27–41 mm Hg		3.6–5.5 kPa	
Partial pressure (pCO_2)		Thereafter				
		M	35–48 mm Hg		4.7–6.4 kPa	
		F	32–45 mm Hg		4.3–6.0 kPa	
Total (tCO_2)	S, P(H)	Cord blood	14–22 mmol/L		14–22 mmol/L	
		Premature	14–27 mmol/L		14–27 mmol/L	
		Newborn	13–22 mmol/L		13–22 mmol/L	
		Infant	20–28 mmol/L		20–28 mmol/L	
		Child	20–28 mmol/L		20–28 mmol/L	
		Thereafter	23–30 mmol/L		23–30 mmol/L	
Carbon monoxide	W(E)	Nonsmokers	<2% HbCO	× 0.01	HbCO fraction <0.02	
		Smokers	<10%		<0.10	
		Lethal	>50%		>0.5	
Carboxyhemoglobin. See Carbon monoxide						
β-Carotene	S	Infant	20–70 µg/dL	× 0.0186	0.37–1.30 µmol/L	
		Child	40–130 µg/dL		0.74–2.42 µmol/L	
		Thereafter	60–200 µg/dL		1.12–3.72 µmol/L	
Catecholamines, fractionated	P(E)	Norepinephrine				
		Supine	100–400 pg/mL	× 5.911	591–2,364 pmol/L	
		Standing	300–900 pg/mL		1,773–5,320 pmol/L	
		Epinephrine				
		Supine	<70 pg/mL	× 5.458	<382 pmol/L	
		Standing	<100 pg/mL		<546 pmol/L	
		Dopamine (no postural change)	<30 pg/mL	× 6.528	<196 pmol/L	
	U	Norepinephrine				
		0–1 yr	0–10 µg/24 hr	× 5.911	0–59 nmol/24 hr	
		1–2 yr	0–17 µg/24 hr		0–100 nmol/24 hr	
		2–4 yr	4–29 µg/24 hr		24–171 nmol/24 hr	
		4–7 yr	8–45 µg/24 hr		47–266 nmol/24 hr	
		7–10 yr	13–65 µg/24 hr		77–384 nmol/24 hr	
		Thereafter	15–80 µg/24 hr		87–473 nmol/24 hr	

TABLE 27–2. Reference Ranges for Laboratory Tests *Continued*

Test	Specimen	Reference Range		Factor	Reference Range (SI)	Comments
Catecholamines, fractionated *(Continued)*		Epinephrine				
		0–1 yr	0–2.5 µg/24 hr	× 5.458	0–13.6 nmol/24 hr	
		1–2 yr	0–3.5 µg/24 hr		0–19.1 nmol/24 hr	
		2–4 yr	0–6.0 µg/24 hr		0–32.7 nmol/24 hr	
		4–7 yr	0.2–10 µg/24 hr		1.1–55 nmol/24 hr	
		7–10 yr	0.5–14 µg/24 hr		2.7–76 nmol/24 hr	
		Thereafter	0.5–20 µg/24 hr		2.7–109 nmol/24 hr	
		Fractionated Dopamine				
		0–1 yr	0–85 µg/24 hr	× 6.528	0–555 nmol/24 hr	
		1–2 yr	10–140 µg/24 hr		65–914 nmol/24 hr	
		2–4 yr	40–260 µg/24 hr		261–1,697 nmol/24 hr	
		Thereafter	65–400 µg/24 hr		424–2,611 nmol/24 hr	
Catecholamines, total	U					
Free		0–1 yr	10–15 µg/24 hr		10–15 µg/24 hr	
		1–5 yr	15–40 µg/24 hr		15–40 µg/24 hr	
		6–15 yr	20–80 µg/24 hr		20–80 µg/24 hr	
		Thereafter	30–100 µg/24 hr		30–100 µg/24 hr	
Cerebrospinal fluid						
Pressure	CSF	70–180 mm water			70–180 mm water	
Volume	CSF	Child	60–100 mL	× 0.001	0.06–0.10 L	
		Adult	100–160 mL		0.1–0.16 L	
Ceruloplasmin	S	0–5 d	5–26 mg/dL	× 10	50–260 mg/L	n f (Lockitch et al)
		1–19 yr	20–46 mg/dL		200–460 mg/L	
Chloral hydrate. See end of table under Drugs						
Chloride	S, P(H)	Cord blood	96–104 mmol/L	× 1	96–104 mmol/L	
		Newborn	97–110 mmol/L		97–110 mmol/L	
		Thereafter	98–106 mmol/L		98–106 mmol/L	
	CSF		118–132 mmol/L	× 1	118–132 mmol/L	
	U	Infant	2–10 mmol/24 hr	× 1	2–10 mmol/24 hr	
		Child	15–40 mmol/24 hr		15–40 mmol/24 hr	
		Thereafter	110–250 mmol/24 hr (varies greatly with Cl intake)		110–250 mmol/24 hr	
	Sweat	Normal	<40 mmol/L	× 1	<40 mmol/L	(Gibson et al)
		Borderline	45–60 mmol/L		45–60 mmol/L	
		Cystic fibrosis	>60 mmol/L		>60 mmol/L	
Cholesterol, total	S	1–3 yr	45–182 mg/dL	× 0.0259	1.15–4.70 mmol/L	z (Lokitch et al)
		4–6 yr	109–189 mg/dL		2.80–4.80 mmol/L	
	S	M		× 0.0259		(Mayo Clinic Laboratories)

M:

	Percentiles 5	75	95		SI 5	75	95
6–9 yr	126	172	191 mg/dL	6–9 yr	3.26	4.45	4.94 mmol/L
10–14 yr	130	179	204 mg/dL	10–14 yr	3.36	4.63	5.28 mmol/L
15–19 yr	114	167	198 mg/dl	15–19 yr	2.95	4.32	5.12 mmol/L

F:

	Percentiles 5	75	95		SI 5	75	95
6–9 yr	122	173	209 mg/dL	6–9 yr	3.16	4.47	5.41 mmol/L
10–14 yr	124	174	217 mg/dL	10–14 yr	3.21	4.50	5.61 mmol/L
15–19 yr	125	175	212 mg/dL	15–19 yr	3.23	4,53	5.48 mmol/L

Test	Specimen	Reference Range		Factor	Reference Range (SI)	Comments
Chorionic gonadotropin β-subunit (β-hCG)	S, P(E)	Child and Male, nondetectable				
		F (post-conception)				
		7–10 d	>5.0 mIU/mL	× 1.0	>5.0 IU/L	
		30 d	>100 mIU/mL		>100 IU/L	
		40 d	>2,000 mIU/mL		>2,000 IU/L	
		10 wk	50,000–100,000 mIU/mL		50,000–100,000 IU/L	
		10 wk	10,000–20,000 mIU/mL		10,000–20,000 IU/L	
		Trophoblastic disease	>100,000		>100,000 IU/L	
Clotting time, Lee-White, 37° C	W	Glass tubes	5–8 min (5–15 min at RT)		Glass tubes 5–8 min (5–15 min at RT)	
		Silicone tubes	about 30 min prolonged		Silicone tubes about 30 min prolonged	

Table continued on following page

TABLE 27–2. Reference Ranges for Laboratory Tests *Continued*

Test	Specimen	Reference Range		Factor	Reference Range (SI)	Comments
Coagulation factor assays	P(C)					
Factor I. See Fibrinogen						
Factor II		0.5–1.5 U/mL or 60–150% of normal		× 1	0.5–1.5 kU/L 60–150 AU	
Factor IV. See Calcium						
Factor V		0.5–2.0 U/mL or 60–150% of normal		× 1	0.5–2.0 kU/L 60–150 AU	
Factor VII		65–135% of normal		× 1	65–135 AU	
Factor VIII		60–145% of normal		× 1	60–145 AU	
Factor VIII antigen		50–200% of normal		× 1	50–200 AU	
Factor IX		60–140% of normal		× 1	60–140 AU	
Factor X		60–130% of normal		× 1	60–130 AU	
Factor XI		65–135% of normal		× 1	65–135 AU	
Factor XII		65–150% of normal		× 1	65–150 AU	
Factor XII (fibrin stabilizing factor, FSF)	W(C,O)	Minimal hemostatic level 0.02–0.05 U/mL or 1–2% or normal		× 1,000 × 1	20–50 U/L or 1–2 AU	
Complement components						
Total hemolytic complement activity	P(E)	75–160 U/mL >33% of plasma CH_{50}		× 1	75–160 IU/mL >0.33 of plasma CH_{50}	
Total complement decay rate (functional)	P(E)	~10–20% Deficiency >50%		× 0.01	~0.10–0.20 (fraction of decay rate) 0.50 (fraction of decay rate)	
Classic pathway components						
Clq	S	Cord blood	1.0–14.9 mg/dL	× 10	10–149 mg/L	
		1 mo	2.2–6.2 mg/dL		22–62 mg/L	
		6 mo	1.2–7.6 mg/dL		12–76 mg/L	
		Adult	5.1–7.9 mg/dL		51–79 mg/L	
Clr	S		2.5–3.8 mg/dL	× 10	25–38 mg/L	
Cls (Cl esterase)	S		2.5–3.8 mg/dL	× 10	25–38 mg/L	
C2	S	Cord blood	1.6–2.8 mg/dL	× 10	16–28 mg/L	
		1 mo	1.9–3.9 mg/dL		19–39 mg/L	
		6 mo	2.4–3.6 mg/dL		24–36 mg/L	
		Adult	1.6–4.0 mg/dL		16–40 mg/L	
C3	S	Cord blood	57–116 mg/dL	× 10	570–1,160 mg/L	n (Meites)
		1–3 mo	53–131 mg/dL		530–1,310 mg/L	
		3 mo–1 yr	62–180 mg/dL		620–1,800 mg/L	
		1–10 yr	77–195 mg/dL		770–1,950 mg/L	
		Adult	83–177 mg/dL		830–1,770 mg/L	
C4	S	Cord blood	7–23 mg/dL	× 10	70–230 mg/L	n (Meites)
		1–3 mo	7–27 mg/dL		70–270 mg/L	
		3 mo–10 yr	7–40 mg/dL		70–400 mg/L	
		Adult	15–45 mg/dL		150–450 mg/L	
C5	S	Cord blood	3.4–6.2 mg/dL	× 10	34–62 mg/L	
		1 mo	2.3–6.3 mg/dL		23–63 mg/L	
		6 mo	2.4–6.4 mg/dL		24–64 mg/L	
		Adult	3.8–9.0 mg/dL		38–90 mg/L	
C6	S	Cord blood	1.0–4.2 mg/dL	× 10	10–42 mg/L	
		1 mo	2.2–5.2 mg/dL		22–52 mg/L	
		6 mo	3.7–7.1 mg/dL		37–71 mg/L	
		Adult	4.0–7.2 mg/dL		40–72 mg/L	
C7	S		4.9–7.0 mg/dL	× 10	49–70 mg/L	
C8	S		4.3–6.3 mg/dL	× 10	43–63 mg/L	
C9	S		4.7–6.9 mg/dL	× 10	47–69 mg/L	
Alternative pathway components						
C4 binding protein	S		18.0–32.0 mg/dL	× 10	180–320 mg/L	
Factor B (C3 proactivator) RID	P(E)	Cord blood	7.8–15.8 mg/dL	× 10	78–158 mg/L	
		1 mo	6.2–28.6 mg/dL		62–286 mg/L	
		6 mo	16.9–29.3 mg/dL		169–293 mg/L	
		Adult	14.7–33.5 mg/dL		147–335 mg/L	
Nephelometry	S	Newborn	14–33 mg/dL	× 10	140–330 mg/L	
		Adult	20–45 mg/dL		200–450 mg/L	
Properdin	S	Cord blood	1.3–1.7 mg/dL	× 10	13–17 mg/L	
		1 mo	0.6–2.2 mg/dL		6–22 mg/L	
		6 mo	1.3–2.5 mg/dL		13–25 mg/L	
		Adult	2.0–3.6 mg/dL		20–36 mg/L	
Regulatory protein b1H-globulin (C3b inactivator-accelerator)	S	Cord blood	26–42 mg/dL	× 10	260–420 mg/L	
		1 mo	24–56 mg/dL		240–560 mg/L	
		6 mo	33–61 mg/dL		330–610 mg/L	
		Adult	40–72 mg/dL		400–720 mg/L	
Cl inhibitor (esterase inhibitor)	P(E)		17.4–24.0 mg/dL	× 10	174–240 mg/L	

TABLE 27–2. Reference Ranges for Laboratory Tests *Continued*

Test	Specimen	Reference Range	Factor	Reference Range (SI)	Comments
Complement components *(Continued)*					
Complement decay rate (functional)	S	<20% decay rate	× 0.01	<0.20 (fraction of decay rate)	
		Deficiency >50% decay rate		>0.50 (fraction of decay rate)	
C3b inactivator (KAF)	S	Cord blood 1.8–2.6 mg/dL	× 10	18–26 mg/L	
		1 mo 1.5–3.9 mg/dL		15–39 mg/L	
		6 mo 2.3–4.3 mg/dL		23–43 mg/L	
		Adult 2.6–5.4 mg/dL		26–54 mg/L	
S protein	S	41.8–60.0 mg/dL	× 10	418–600 mg/L	
Copper	S	0–5 d 9–46 μg/dL	× 0.157	1.4–7.2 μmol/L	fa (Lockitch et al)
		1–9 yr 80–150 μg/dL		12.6–23.6 μmol/L	
		10–14 yr 80–121 μg/dL		12.6–19.0 μmol/L	
		15–19 yr 64–160 μg/dL		11.3–25.2 μmol/L	
	U	5–18 yr 0.36–7.56 mg/mol creatinine	× 15.7	6–119 μmol/mol creatinine	
Coproporphyrin	U	34–234 μg/24 hr	× 1.5	51–351 nmol/24 hr	
	F (24-hr)	<30 μg/g dry wt	× 1.5	<45 nmol/g dry wt	
		400–1,200 μg/24 hr		600–1,800 nmol/24 hr	
Corticobinding globulin (CBG). See Transcortin					
Cortisol	S, P(H)	Newborn 1–24 μg/dL	× 27.59	28–662 nmol/L	
		Adults			
		0800 hr 5–23 μg/dL		138–635 nmol/L	
		1,600 hr 3–15 μg/dL		82–413 nmol/L	
		2,000 hr ≤50% of 0800 h	× 0.01	Fraction of 0800 hr ≤0.50	
Cortisol, free	U	Child 2–27 μg/24 hr	× 2.759	5.5–74 nmol/24 hr	
		Adolescent 5–55 μg/24 hr		14–152 nmol/24 hr	
		Adult 10–100 μg/24 hr		27–276 nmol/24 hr	
Creatine kinase	S	Cord blood 70–380 U/L	× 1	70–380 U/L	30° s (Jedeikin et al)
		5–8 hr 214–1175 U/L		214–1175 U/L	
		24–33 hr 130–1200 U/L		130–1200 U/L	
		72–100 hr 87–725 U/L		87–725 U/L	
		Adult 5–130 U/L		5–130 U/L	
Creatinine kinase isoenzymes	S	*CKMB* / *CKBB*			
		Cord blood 0.3–3.1% / 0.3–10.5%			
		5–8 hr 1.7–7.9% / 3.6–13.4%			
		24–33 hr 1.8–5.0% / 2.3–8.6%			
		72–100 hr 1.4–5.4% / 5.1–13.3%			
		Adult 0–2% / 0			
Creatinine					
Jaffe, kinetic, or enzymatic	S, P	Cord blood 0.6–1.2 mg/dL	× 88.4	53–106 μmol/L	
		Newborn 0.3–1.0 mg/dL		27–88 μmol/L	
		Infant 0.2–0.4 mg/dL		18–35 μmol/L	
		Child 0.3–0.7 mg/dL		27–62 μmol/L	
		Adolescent 0.5–1.0 mg/dL		44–88 μmol/L	
		Adult			
		M 0.6–1.2 mg/dL		53–106 μmol/L	
		F 0.5–1.1 mg/dL		44–97 μmol/L	
Jaffe, manual	S, P	0.8–1.5 mg/dL	× 88.4	70–133 μmol/L	
	AF	After 37-wk gestation >2.0 mg/dL	× 88.4	After 37-wk gestation >180 μmol/L	
Creatinine	U	Premature 8.1–15.0 mg/kg/24 hr	× 8.84	72–133 μmol/kg/24 hr	md (Meites)
		Full-term 10.4–19.7 mg/kg/24 hr		92–174 μmol/kg/24 hr	
		1.5–7 yr 10–15 mg/kg/24 hr		88–133 μmol/kg/24 hr	
		7–15 yr 5.2–41 mg/kg/24 hr		46–362 μmol/kg/24 hr	
Creatinine clearance (endogenous)	S, P, and U	Newborn 40–65 mL/min/1.73 m²			
		<40 yr			
		M 97–137 mL/min/1.73 m²			
		F 88–128 mL/min/1.73 m²			
		Decreases ~6.5 mL/min/decade			
Cyclic AMP	P(E)	M 5.6–10.9 ng/mL	× 3.04	M 17–33 nmol/L	
		F 3.6–8.9 ng/mL		F 11–27 nmol/L	
	U	<3.3 mg/24 h or	× 3040	<10,000 nmol/24 hr	
		<1.64 mg/g creatinine		<6,000 nmol cAMP/g creatinine	
Dehydroepiandrosterone	S	M			(Endocrine Sciences)
		Tanner 1 <9.8 yr 31–345 ng/dL	× 0.03467	1.07–11.96 nmol/L	
		Tanner 2 9.8–14.5 yr 110–495 ng/dL		3.81–17.16 nmol/L	
		Tanner 3 10.7–15.4 yr 170–585 ng/dL		5.89–20.28 nmol/L	
		Tanner 4 11.8–16.2 yr 160–640 ng/dL		5.55–22.19 nmol/L	
		Tanner 5 12.8–17.3 yr 250–800 ng/dL		8.67–31.21 nmol/L	
		Adult 160–800 ng/dL		5.55–27.74 nmol/L	

Table continued on following page

TABLE 27–2. Reference Ranges for Laboratory Tests *Continued*

Test	Specimen	Reference Range	Factor	Reference Range (SI)	Comments
Dehydroepiandrosterone *(Continued)*		F			
		Tanner 1 <9.2 yr 31–345 ng/dL		1.07–11.96 nmol/L	
		Tanner 2 9.2–13.7 yr 150–570 ng/dL		5.20–19.76 nmol/L	
		Tanner 3 10.0–14.4 yr 200–600 mg/dL		6.93–20.80 nmol/L	
		Tanner 4 10.7–15.6 yr 200–780 ng/dL		6.93–24.27 nmol/L	
		Tanner 5 11.8–18.6 yr 215–850 ng/dL		7.45–29.47 nmol/L	
		Adult Follicular 160–800 ng/dL		5.55–27.74 nmol/L	
		Luteal 160–800 ng/dL		5.55–27.74 nmol/L	
Dehydroepiandrosterone sulfate (DHEA-sulfate, DHEAS)		M			(Endocrine Sciences)
		Tanner 1 <9.8 yr 20–170 μg/dL	× 0.026	0.52–4.42 μmol/L	
		Tanner 2 9.8–14.5 yr 70–180 μg/dL		1.82–4.68 μmol/L	
		Tanner 3 10.7–15.4 yr 90–180 μg/dL		2.34–4.68 μmol/L	
		Tanner 4 11.8–16.2 yr 220–304 μg/dL		5.72–7.90 μmol/L	
		Tanner 5 12.8–17.3 yr 120–370 μg/dL		3.12–9.62 μmol/L	
		Adult 180–450 μg/dL		4.68–11.70 μmol/L	
		F			
		Tanner 1 <9.2 yr 40–200 μg/dL		1.04–5.20 μmol/L	
		Tanner 2 9.2–13.7 yr 81–145 μg/dL		2.11–3.77 μmol/L	
		Tanner 3 10.0–14.4 yr 129–210 μg/dL		3.35–5.46 μmol/L	
		Tanner 4 10.7–15.6 yr 170–330 μg/dL		4.42–8.58 μmol/L	
		Tanner 5 11.8–18.6 yr 117–325 μg/dL		3.04–8.45 μmol/L	
		Adult Follicular 120–315 μg/dL		3.12–8.19 μmol/L	
		Luteal 120–315 μg/dL		3.12–8.19 μmol/L	
Diazepam. See end of table under Drugs					
Differential count. See Leukocyte differential count					
Digitoxin. See end of table under Drugs					
Digoxin. See end of table under Drugs					
Dihydrotestosterone (DHT)	S	M			(Endocrine Sciences)
		Tanner 1 <9.8 yr <3 ng/dL	× 0.03443	<0.10 nmol/L	
		Tanner 2 9.8–14.5 yr 3–17 ng/dL		0.10–0.59 nmol/L	
		Tanner 3 10.7–15.4 yr 8–33 ng/dL		0.28–1.14 nmol/L	
		Tanner 4 11.8–16.2 yr 22–52 ng/dL		0.76–1.79 nmol/L	
		Tanner 5 12.8–17.3 yr 24–65 ng/dL		0.83–2.24 nmol/L	
		Adult 30–85 ng/dL		1.03–2.93 nmol/L	
		F			
		Tanner 1 <9.2 yr <3 ng/dL		<0.10 nmol/L	
		Tanner 2 9.2–13.7 yr 5–12 ng/dL		0.17–0.41 nmol/L	
		Tanner 3 10.0–14.4 yr 7–19 ng/dL		0.24–0.65 nmol/L	
		Tanner 4 10.7–15.6 yr 4–13 ng/dL		0.14–0.45 nmol/L	
		Tanner 5 11.8–18.6 yr 3–18 ng/dL		0.10–0.62 nmol/L	
		Adult Follicular 4–22 ng/dL		0.14–0.76 nmol/L	
		Luteal 4–22 ng/dL		0.14–0.76 nmol/L	
Diphenylhydantoin. See end of table under Drugs					
Disaccharide absorption test	S	Change in glucose from fasting value	× 0.055	Change in glucose from fasting value	
		Normal >30 mg/dL		Normal >1.67 mmol/L	
		Inconclusive 20–30 mg/dL		Inconclusive 1.11–1.67 mmol/L	
		Abnormal <20 mg/dL		<1.11 mmol/L	
Dithionite tube test. See Sickle cell tests					
Electrophoresis, Hemoglobin. See Hemoglobin electrophoresis					
Eosinophil count	W(E,H) capillary	50–350 cells/mm³ (μL)	× 10^6	50–350 × 10^6 cells/L	
Epinephrine. See Catecholamines, fractionated					

TABLE 27–2. Reference Ranges for Laboratory Tests *Continued*

Test	Specimen	Reference Range	Factor	Reference Range (SI)	Comments
Erythrocyte count (RBC count)	W(E)	Millions of cells/mm^3 (μL)		× 10^{12} cells/L	
		Cord blood 3.9–5.5	× 1	3.9–5.5	
		1–3 d (capillary) 4.0–6.6		4.0–6.6	
		1 wk 3.9–6.3		3.9–6.3	
		2 wk 3.6–6.2		3.6–6.2	
		1 mo 3.0–5.4		3.0–5.4	
		2 mo 2.7–4.9		2.7–4.9	
		3–6 mo 3.1–4.5		3.1–4.5	
		0.5–2 yr 3.7–5.3		3.7–5.3	
		2–6 yr 3.9–5.3		3.9–5.3	
		6–12 yr 4.0–5.2		4.0–5.2	
		12–18 yr			
		M 4.5–5.3		4.5–5.3	
		F 4.1–5.1		4.1–5.1	
		18–49 yr			
		M 4.5–5.9		4.5–5.9	
		F 4.0–5.2		4.0–5.2	
Erythrocyte Sedimentation Rate (ESR)					
Westergren, modified	W(E)	Child 0–10 mm/hr		0–10 mm/hr	
		Adult			
		M < 50 yr 0–15 mm/hr		0–15 mm/hr	
		F < 50 yr 0–20 mm/hr		0–20 mm/hr	
Wintrobe		Child 0–13 mm/hr		0–13 mm/hr	
		Adult			
		M 0–9 mm/hr		0–9 mm/hr	
		F 0–20 mm/hr		0–20 mm/hr	
ZETA		41–54%		41–54 AU	
Erythropoietin RIA	S	<5–20 mU/mL	× 1	<5–20 U/L	
Hemagglutination		25–125 mU/mL		25–125 U/L	
Bioassay		5–18 mU/mL		5–18 U/L	
Estradiol	S	M	× 36.71		(Endocrine Sciences)
		Tanner 1 <9.8 yr 0.5–1.1 ng/dL		18–40 pmol/L	
		Tanner 2 9.8–14.5 yr 0.5–1.6 ng/dL		18–59 pmol/L	
		Tanner 3 10.7–15.4 yr 0.5–2.5 ng/dL		18–92 pmol/L	
		Tanner 4 11.8–16.2 yr 1.0–3.6 ng/dL		37–132 pmol/L	
		Tanner 5 12.8–17.3 yr 1.0–3.6 ng/dL		37–132 pmol/L	
		Adult 0.8–3.6 ng/dL		29–132 pmol/L	
		F			
		Tanner 1 <9.2 yr 0.1–2.0 ng/dL		4–73 pmol/L	
		Tanner 2 9.2–13.7 yr 1.0–2.4 ng/dL		37–88 pmol/L	
		Tanner 3 10.0–14.4 yr 0.7–6.0 ng/dL		26–220 pmol/L	
		Tanner 4 10.7–15.6 yr 2.1–8.5 ng/dL		77–312 pmol/L	
		Tanner 5 11.8–18.6 yr 3.4–17 ng/dL		125–624 pmol/L	
		Adult Follicular 3–10 ng/dL		110–367 pmol/L	
		Luteal 7–30 ng/dL		257–1,100 pmol/L	
Estradiol, urinary	U	Adult M 0–6 μg/24 hr	× 3.671	Adult M 0–22 nmol/24 hr	
		Adult F		Adult F	
		Follicular 0–3 μg/24 hr		Folicular 0–11 nmol/24 hr	
		Ovulatory peak 4–14 μg/24 hr		Ovulatory peak 15–51 nmol/24 hr	
		Luteal 4–10 μg/24 hr		Luteal 15–37 nmol/24 hr	
Estriol (E3), free	S	*Wk of gestation*			
		25 3.5–10.0 μg/L	× 3.47	12.1–34.7 nmol/L	
		28 4.0–12.5 μg/L		13.9–43.4 nmol/L	
		30 4.5–14.0 μg/L		15.6–48.6 nmol/L	
		32 5.0–16.0 μg/L		17.4–55.5 nmol/L	
		34 5.5–18.5 μg/L		19.1–64.2 nmol/L	
		36 7.0–25.0 μg/L		24.3–86.8 nmol/L	
		37 8.0–28.0 μg/L		27.8–97.2 nmol/L	
		38 9.0–32.0 μg/L		31.2–111.0 nmol/L	
		39 10.0–34.0 μg/L		34.7–118.0 nmol/L	
		40–41 10.5–25.0 μg/L		36.4–86.8 nmol/L	
	AF	*Wk*			
		16–20 1.0–3.2 ng/mL (95% range)	× 3.47	3.5–11.1 nmol/L (95% range)	
		20–24 2.1–7.8 ng/mL (95% range)		7.3–27.1 nmol/L (95% range)	
		24–28 2.1–7.8 ng/mL (95% range)		7.3–27.1 nmol/L (95% range)	
		28–32 4.0–13.6 ng/mL (95% range)		13.9–47.2 nmol/L (95% range)	
		32–36 3.6–15.5 ng/mL (95% range)		12.5–53.8 nmol/L (95% range)	
		36–38 4.6–18.0 ng/mL (95% range)		16.0–62.5 nmol/L (95% range)	
		38–40 5.4–19.8 ng/mL (95% range)		18.7–68.7 nmol/L (95% range)	

Table continued on following page

TABLE 27–2. Reference Ranges for Laboratory Tests *Continued*

Test	Specimen	Reference Range		Factor	Reference Range (SI)	Comments
Estriol (E3), total	S	*Pregnancy (wk)*				
		24–28	30–170 ng/mL	× 3.47	104–590 nmol/L	
		28–32	40–220 ng/mL		140–760 nmol/L	
		32–36	60–280 ng/mL		208–970 nmol/L	
		36–40	80–350 ng/mL		280–1,210 nmol/L	
		Adult M and nonpregnant F	<2 ng/mL		<7 nmol/L	
	U	*Pregnancy (wk)*				
		30	6–18 mg/24 hr	× 3.47	21–62 μmol/24 hr	
		35	9–28 mg/24 hr		31–97 μmol/24 hr	
		40	13–42 mg/24 hr		45–146 μmol/24 hr	
		Decrease of >40% of previous value suggests fetus at risk			Fraction of previous value of <0.60 suggests fetus at risk	
Estrogens, total	S	Child	<30 pg/L	× 1	<30 ng/L	
		M	40–115 pg/L		40–115 ng/L	
		F cycle (days)				
		1–10 d	61–394 pg/L		61–394 ng/L	
		11–20 d	122–437 pg/L		122–437 ng/L	
		21–30 d	156–350 pg/L		156–350 ng/L	
		Prepubertal	≤40 pg/L		≤40 ng/L	
	U, 24 hr	Child	<10 μg/24 hr	× 1	<10 μg/24 hr	
		Adult (M)	5–25 μg/24 hr		5–25 μg/24 hr	
		F				
		Preovulation	5–25 μg/24 hr		5–25 μg/24 hr	
		Ovulation	28–100 μg/24 hr		28–100 μg/24 hr	
		Luteal peak	22–80 μg/24 hr		22–80 μg/24 hr	
		Pregnancy	<45,000 μg/24 hr		<45,000 μg/24 hr	
		Postmenopausal	<10 μg/24 hr		<10 μg/24 hr	
Ethanol. See end of table under Drugs						
Ethosuximide. See end of table under Drugs						
Fat, fecal	F (72-hr)	Infant, breast-fed	<1 g/24 hr	× 1	<1 g/24 hr	
		0–6 yr	<2 g/24 hr		<2 g/24 hr	
		Adult				
		Normal diet	<7 g/24 hr		<7 g/24 hr	
		Fat-free diet	<4 g/24 hr		<4 g/24 hr	
		Coefficient of fat absorption (%)			Absorbed fraction	
		Infant		× 0.01		
		Breast-fed	>93		>0.93	
		Formula-fed	>83		>0.83	
		>1 yr	≥95		≥0.95	
Free fatty acids	S	Premature 10–55 d	0.15–0.71 mmol/L	× 1	0.15–0.71 mmol/L	(Meites)
Ferric chloride test	U	Negative			Negative	
Ferritin	S	Newborn	25–200 ng/mL	× 1	25–200 μg/L	
		1 mo	200–600 ng/mL		200–600 μg/L	
		2–5 mo	50–200 ng/mL		50–200 μg/L	
		6 mo–15 yr	7–140 ng/mL		7–140 μg/L	
		Adult				
		M	15–200 ng/mL		15–200 μg/L	
		F	12–150 ng/mL		12–150 μg/L	
α-Fetoprotein (AFP)	S maternal		*Median*		*Median*	
		15 wk	34 ng/mL	× 1	34 μg/L	
		16 wk	38 ng/mL		38 μg/L	
		17 wk	44 ng/mL		44 μg/L	
		18 wk	49 ng/mL		49 μg/L	
		19 wk	56.5 ng/mL		56.5 μg/L	
		20 wk	66 ng/mL		66 μg/L	
	AF		*Mean*			
		15 wk	13.5 ± 3.42 μg/mL			
		16 wk	11.7 ± 3.38 μg/mL			
		17 wk	10.3 ± 3.03 μg/mL			
		18 wk	9.5 ± 3.22 μg/mL			
		19 wk	7.1 ± 2.86 μg/mL			
		20 wk	5.0 ± 2.45 μg/mL			

TABLE 27–2. Reference Ranges for Laboratory Tests *Continued*

Test	Specimen	Reference Range	Factor	Reference Range (SI)	Comments
Fibrin degradation products					
Agglutination (Thrombo-Wellco test)	W; special tube thrombin and proteolytic inhibitors	<10 μg/mL	× 1	<10 mg/L	
	U:2 mL in special tube (see above)	<0.25 μg/mL	× 1	<0.25 mg/L	
Fibrinogen	P(NaC)	Newborn 125–300 mg/dL	× 0.01	1.25–3.00 g/L	
		Adult 200–400 mg/dL		2.00–4.00 g/L	
Folate	S	Newborn 7.0–32 ng/mL	× 2.265	15.9–72.4 nmol/L	
		Thereafter 1.8–9 ng/mL		4.1–20.4 nmol/L	
	W(E)	150–450 ng/mL RBCs		340–1020 nmol/L cells	
Follicle-stimulating hormone (FSH)	S	M			(Endocrine Sciences)
		Tanner 1 <9.8 yr <1–3 mIU/mL	× 1	<1–3 U/L	
		Tanner 2 9.8–14.5 yr 2–7 mIU/mL		2–7 U/L	
		Tanner 3 10.7–15.4 yr 2–8 mIU/mL		2–8 U/L	
		Tanner 4 11.8–16.2 yr 2–8 mIU/mL		2–8 U/L	
		Tanner 5 12.8–17.3 yr 1–8 mIU/mL		1–8 U/L	
		Adult 1–8 mIU/mL		1–8 U/L	
		F			
		Tanner 1 <9.2 yr <1–5 mIU/mL		<1–5 U/L	
		Tanner 2 9.2–13.7 yr <1–6 mIU/mL		<1–6 U/L	
		Tanner 3 10.0–14.4 yr 1.5–9 mIU/mL		1.5–9 U/L	
		Tanner 4 10.7–15.6 yr 2–9 mIU/mL		2–9 U/L	
		Tanner 5 11.8–18.6 yr 1–9 mIU/mL		1–9 U/L	
		Adult Follicular 1–9 mIU/mL		1–9 U/L	
		Midcycle 4–30 mIU/mL		4–30 U/L	
		Luteal <1–7 mIU/mL		<1–7 U/L	
Fructosamine	S	0–3 yr 1.56–2.27 mmol/L	× 1	1.56–2.27 mmol/L	c (De Schepper et al)
		3–6 yr 1.73–2.34 mmol/L		1.73–2.34 mmol/L	
		6–9 yr 1.82–2.56 mmol/L		1.82–2.56 mmol/L	
		9–15 yr 2.02–2.63 mmol/L		2.02–2.63 mmol/L	
Galactose	S	Newborn 0–20 mg/dL	× 0.0555	0–1.11 mmol/L	
	P	5 mo–17 yr 0.0–0.5 mg/dL		0.0–0.03 mmol/L	z (Pesce et al)
	U	Newborn ≤60 mg/dL	× 0.0555	≤3.33 mmol/L	
		Thereafter 14 mg/24 hr	× 0.00555	<0.08 mmol/24 hr	
Galactose-l-PO_4	W(H)	5 mo–17 yr 0–44 μg/g Hgb	× 0.0038	0–0.17 μmol/g Hgb	v (Pesce et al)
Galactose-l-PO_4 uridylyltransferase	W(H)	18–26 U/g Hgb	× 1	18–26 U/g Hgb	(Pesce et al)
Gastrin	S(fasting)	Children <10–125 pg/mL	× 1	<10–125 ng/L	m (Dickinson et al)
Glucose	S	Cord blood 45–96 mg/dL	× 0.0555	2.5–5.3 mmol/L	
		Newborn			
		1 d 40–60 mg/dL		2.2–3.3 mmol/L	
		>1 d 50–90 mg/dL		2.8–5.0 mmol/L	
		Child 60–100 mg/dL		3.3–5.5 mmol/L	
		Adult 70–105 mg/dL		3.9–5.8 mmol/L	
	W, (H)	Adult 65–95 mg/dL		3.6–5.3 mmol/L	
	CSF	Adult 40–70 mg/dL		2.2–3.9 mmol/L	
Quantitative, enzymatic	U	<0.5 g/24 hr	× 5.55	<2.8 mmol/24 hr	
Qualitative	U	Negative		Negative	
Glucose, 2 hr pc	S	<120 mg/dL (For diabetes, see Glucose tolerance test, oral)	× 0.0555	<6.7 mmol/L	
Glucose-6-phosphate dehydrogenase in erythrocytes	W(E,H,C)				
Bishop, modified		Adult		Adult	
		3.4–8.0 U/g Hb	× 0.0645	0.22–0.52 mU/mll Hb	
		98.6–232 U/10^{12} RBC	× 10^{-3}	0.10–0.23 nU/10^6 RBC	
		1.16–2.72 U/mL RBC	× 1	1.16–2.72 kU/L RBC	
		Newborn: 50% higher		Newborn: 50% higher	

Table continued on following page

TABLE 27–2. Reference Ranges for Laboratory Tests *Continued*

Test	Specimen	Reference Range	Factor	Reference Range (SI)	Comments
Glucose tolerance test (GTT), oral	S	Normal Diabetic		Normal Diabetic	
Adult dose: 75 g		Fasting 70–105 mg/dL >115 mg/dL	× 0.0555	3.9–5.8 mmol/L >6.4 mmol/L	
Child dose: 1.75 g/kg of ideal		60 min 120–170 mg/dL ≥200 mg/dL		6.7–9.4 mmol/L ≥11 mmol/L	
weight up to maximum of 75 g		90 min 100–140 mg/dL ≥200 mg/dL		5.6–7.8 mmol/L ≥11 mmol/L	
		120 min 70–120 mg/dL ≥140 mg/dL		3.9–6.7 mmol/L ≥7.8 mmol/L	
γ-Glutamyltranspeptidase (GGT, GGTP)	S	Cord blood 37–193 U/L	× 1	37–193 U/L	37° s (Knight et al)
		0–1 mo 13–147 U/L		13–147 U/L	
		1–2 mo 12–123 U/L		12–123 U/L	
		2–4 mo 8–90 U/L		8–90 U/L	
		4 mo–10 yr 5–32 U/L		5–32 U/L	
		10–15 yr 5–24 U/L		5–24 U/L	
Growth hormone (hGH, somatotropin)	S, P(E,H) Fast, at rest	Cord blood 10–50 ng/mL	× 1	10–50 μg/L	
		Newborn 10–40 ng/mL		10–40 μg/L	
		Child <5 ng/mL		<5 μg/L	
		Adult			
		M <5 ng/mL		<5 μg/L	
		F <8 ng/mL		<8 μg/L	
Ham's test. See Acidified serum test					
Haptoglobin (Hp)	S				
RID		30–175 mg/dL	× 10	300–1750 mg/L	mg/L
Sephadex		40–180 mg Hb bound/dL of serum			
Nephelometry		Newborn 5–48 mg/dL	× 10	50–480 mg/L	
		Thereafter 25–175 mg/dL		250–1750 mg/L	
HDL cholesterol	S	1–13 yr 35–84 mg/dL	× 0.0259	0.9 –2.15 mmol/L	fm (Meites)
		14–19 yr 35–65 mg/dL		0.90–1.65 mmol/L	
Hematocrit (HCT, Hct)	W(E)	*Per cent Packed Red Cells (V Red Cells/V Whole Blood Cells × 100)*		*Volume Fraction (V Red Cells/ V Whole Blood)*	
Calculated from MCV and RBC (electronic displacement or laser)		1 d (capillary) 48–69%	× 0.01	0.48–0.69	
		2 d 48–75%		0.48–0.75	
		3 d 44–72%		0.44–0.72	
		2 mo 28–42%		0.28–0.42	
		6–12 yr 35–45%		0.35–0.45	
		12–18 yr			
		M 37–49%		0.37–0.49	
		F 36–46%		0.36–0.46	
		18–49 yr			
		M 41–53%		0.41–0.53	
		F 36–46%		0.36–0.46	
Hemoglobin (Hb)	W(E)	1–3 d (capillary) 14.5–22.5 g/dL	× 0.155	2.25–3.49 mmol/L	MW Hgb = 64,500
		2 mo 9.0–14.0 g/dL		1.40–2.17 mmol/L	
		6–12 yr 11.5–15.5 g/dL		1.78–2.40 mmol/L	
		12–18 yr			
		M 13.0–16.0 g/dL		2.02–2.48 mmol/L	
		F 12.0–16.0 g/dL		1.86–2.48 mmol/L	
		18–49 yr			
		M 13.5–17.5 g/dL		2.09–2.27 mmol/L	
		F 12.0–16.0 g/dL		1.86–2.48 mmol/L	
	P(H)	<10 mg/dL	× 0.155	<1.55 μmol/L	
		<3 mg/dL with butterfly set-up and 18—g needle		<0.47 μmol/L with butterfly set-up and 18-g needle	
	U	Negative		Negative	
		Per cent of Total Hemoglobin		*Fraction of Total Hemoglobin*	
Glycohemoglobin	W(H)	1–5 yr 2.1–7.7%	× 0.01	1–5 yr 0.021–0.077	
Hemoglobin A1c		5–16 yr 3.0–6.2%		5–16 yr 0.030–0.062	q (Meites)
Total glycohemoglobin	W(H)	4–16 yr 6.0–10.0%		4–16 yr 0.060–0.100	o (Meites)
Hemoglobin A	W (E,C,H)	>95%	× 0.01	Fraction of hemoglobin >0.95	
Hemoglobin A_2 (HbA_2)	W (E,O)	Adult: 1.5–3.5% (2 SD) Lower in infants <1 yr		0.015–0.035 (2 SD) mass fraction	
Hemoglobin electrophoresis	W (H,E,C)	HbA >95%	× 0.01	HbA >0.95 mass fraction	
		HbA_2 1.5–3.5%		HbA_2 0.015–.035 mass fraction	
		HbF <2%		HbF <0.02 mass fraction	

TABLE 27–2. Reference Ranges for Laboratory Tests *Continued*

Test	Specimen		Reference Range	Factor	Reference Range (SI)	Comments
Hemoglobin (Hb) *(Continued)*						
Hemoglobin F	W (E)					
Alkali denaturation		1 d	63–92 %HbF	× 0.01	0.62–0.92 mass fraction	
		5 d	65–88 %HbF		0.65–0.88 mass fraction	
		3 wk	55–85 %HbF		0.55–0.85 mass fraction	
		6–9 wk	31–75 %HbF		0.31–0.75 mass fraction	
		3–4 mo	<2–59 %HbF		<0.02–0.59 mass fraction	
		6 mo	<2–9 %HbF		<0.02–0.09 mass fraction	
		Adult	<2 %HbF		<0.02 mass fraction	
Hemoglobin H (HbH)	W (H,E,C)					
Isopropranol precipitation		No precipitation at 40 min			No precipitation at 40 min	
Homovanillic acid	U (24-hr)	0–1 yr	<32.2 mg/g creatinine	× 0.62	< 20 mmol/mol creatinine	p (Meites)
		2–4 yr	<22 mg/g creatinine		<14 mmol/mol creatinine	
		5–19 yr	<14 mg/g creatinine		<8 mmol/mol creatinine	
17-Hydroxycorticosteroids (17-OHCS)	U	0–1 yr	0.5–1.0 mg/24 hr	× 2.76	1.4–2.8 μmol/24 hr	(Conversion based on hydrocortisone MW 362)
		Child	1.0–5.6 mg/24 hr		2.8–15.5 μmol/24 hr	
		Adult				
		M	3.0–10.0 mg/24 hr		8.2–27.6 μmol/24 hr	
		F	2.0–8.0 mg/24 hr		5.5–22 μmol/24 hr	
			or 3–7 mg/g creatinine	× 3.12	or 0.9–2.5 mmol/mol creatinine	
5-Hydroxyindoleacetic acid (5-HIAA)						
Qualitative	U	Negative			Negative	
Quantitative	U	2–8 mg/24 hr		× 5.230	10.5–42 μmol/24 hr	7
17-Hydroxyprogesterone (17-OHP)	S	1 wk	60–150 ng/dL	× 0.03029	1.82–4.54 nmol/L	
		30–60 d	M: 120–200 ng/dL		3.63–6.06 nmol/L	
			F: <150 ng/dL		<4.54 nmol/L	
		M				
		Tanner 1 <9.8 yr	3–90 ng/dL		0.09–2.73 nmol/L	
		Tanner 2 9.8–14.5 yr	5–115 ng/dL		0.15–3.48 nmol/L	
		Tanner 3 10.7–15.4 yr	10–138 ng/dL		0.30–4.18 nmol/L	
		Tanner 4 11.8–16.2 yr	29–180 ng/dL		0.88–5.45 nmol/L	
		Tanner 5 12.8–17.3 yr	24–175 ng/dL		0.73–5.30 nmol/L	
		Adult	27–199 ng/dL		0.82–6.03 nmol/L	
		F				
		Tanner 1 <9.2 yr	3–82 ng/dL		0.09–2.48 nmol/L	
		Tanner 2 9.2–13.7 yr	11–98 ng/dL		0.33–2.97 nmol/L	
		Tanner 3 10.0–14.4 yr	11–155 ng/dL		0.33–4.69 nmol/L	
		Tanner 4 10.7–15.6 yr	18–230 ng/dL		0.55–6.97 nmol/L	
		Tanner 5 11.8–18.6 yr	20–265 ng/dL		0.61–8.03 nmol/L	
		Adult Follicular	15–70 ng/dL		0.45–2.12 nmol/L	
		Luteal	35–290 ng/dL		1.06–8.78 nmol/L	
Hydroxyproline free and bound	U	3 d	33–112 μmol/24 hr	× 1	33–112 μmol/24 hr	c (Meites)
		10 d	148–225 μmol/24 hr		148–225 μmol/24 hr	
		20 d	229–310 μmol/24 hr		229–310 μmol/24 hr	
Hypoxanthine	W	12–36 hr	2.7–11.2 μmol/L	× 1	2.7–11.2 μmol/L	(Jung et al)
		3 d	1.3–7.9 μmol/L		1.3–7.9 μmol/L	
		5 d	0.6–5.7 μmol/L		0.6–5.7 μmol/L	
	CSF	0–1 mo	1.8–5.5 μmol/L		1.8–5.5 μmol/L	(Meites)
Immunoglobulin A (IgA)	S	Cord blood	1.4–3.6 mg/dL	× 10	14–36 mg/L	n (Meites)
		1–3 mo	1.3–53 mg/dL		13–530 mg/L	
		4–6 mo	4.4–84 mg/dL		44–840 mg/L	
		7 mo–1 yr	11–106 mg/dL		110–1,060 mg/L	
		2–5 yr	14–159 mg/dL		140–1,590 mg/L	
		6–10 yr	33–236 mg/dL		330–2,360 mg/L	
		Adult	70–312 mg/dL		700–3,120 mg/L	
Immunoglobulin D (IgD)	S	Newborn	None detected	× 10	None detected	
		Thereafter	0–8 mg/dL		0–80 mg/L	
Immunoglobulin E (IgE)	S	M	0–230 IU/mL	× 1	0–230 kIU/L	
		F	0–170 IU/mL		0–170 kIU/L	
Immunoglobulin G (IgG)	S	Cord blood	636–1,606 mg/dL	× 0.01	6.36–16.06 g/L	n (Meites)
		1 mo	251–906 mg/dL		2.51–9.06 g/L	
		2–4 mo	176–601 mg/dL		1.76–6.01 g/L	
		5–12 mo	172–1,069 mg/dL		1.72–10.69 g/L	
		1–5 yr	345–1,236 mg/dL		3.45–12.36 g/L	
		6–10 yr	608–1,572 mg/dL		6.08–15.72 g/L	
		Adult	639–1,349 mg/dL		6.39–13.49 g/L	

Table continued on following page

TABLE 27–2. Reference Ranges for Laboratory Tests *Continued*

Test	Specimen		Reference Range	Factor	Reference Range (SI)	Comments
Immunoglobulin M (IgM)	S	Cord blood	6.3–25 mg/dL	× 10	63–250 mg/L	n (Meites)
		1 mo–4 mo	17–105 mg/dL		170–1,050 mg/L	
		5 mo–9 mo	33–126 mg/dL		330–1,260 mg/L	
		10 mo–1 yr	41–173 mg/dL		410–1,730 mg/L	
		2–8 yr	43–207 mg/dL		430–2,070 mg/L	
		9–10 yr	52–242 mg/dL		520–2,420 mg/L	
		Adult	56–352 mg/dL		560–3,520 mg/L	
Insulin (12-hr fasting)	S	Newborn	3–20 μU/mL	× 1.0	3–20 mU/L	
		Thereafter	7–24 μU/mL		7–24 mU/L	
Insulin with oral glucose tolerance test	S		Insulin			
		0 min	7–24 μU/mL	× 1	7–24 mU/L	
		30 min	25–231 μU/mL		25–231 mU/L	
		60 min	18–276 μU/mL		18–276 mU/L	
		120 min	16–166 μU/mL		16–166 mU/L	
		180 min	4–38 μU/mL		4–38 mU/L	
Iron	S	Newborn	100–250 μg/dL	× 0.179	17.90–44.75 μmol/L	
		Infant	40–100 μg/dL		7.16–17.90 μmol/L	
		Child	50–120 μg/dL		8.95–21.48 μmol/L	
		Thereafter				
		M	50–160 μg/dL		8.95–28.64 μmol/L	
		F	40–150 μg/dL		7.16–26.85 μmol/L	
		Intoxicated child	280–2,550 μg/dL		50.12–456.5 μmol/L	
		Fatally poisoned child	>1,800 μg/dL		>322.2 μmol/L	
Iron-binding capacity, total (TIBC)	S	Infant	100–400 μg/dL	× 0.179	17.90–71.60 μmol/L	
		Thereafter	250–400 μg/dL		44.75–71.60 μmol/L	
17-Ketogenic steroids (17-KGS)	U	0–1 yr	<1.0 mg/24 hr	× 3.467	<3.5 μmol/24 hr	Conversion based on dehydroepi-androsterone, MW 288
		1–10 yr	<5 mg/24 hr		<17 μmol/24 hr	
		11–14 yr	<12 mg/24 hr		<42 μmol/24 hr	
		Thereafter				
		M	5–23 mg/24 hr		17–80 μmol/24 hr	
		F	3–15 mg/24 hr		10–52 μmol/24 hr	
Ketone bodies						
Qualitative	S	Negative			Negative	
	U	Negative			Negative	
Quantitative	S	0.5–3.0 mg/dL		× 10	5–30 mg/L	
17 Ketosteroid (17-KS), total	U	14 d–2 yr	<1 mg/24 hr	× 3.467	<3.5 μmol/24 hr	Zimmerman reaction Conversion based on dehydroepi-androsterone, MW 288
		2–6 yr	<2 mg/24 hr		< 7 μmol/24 hr	
		6–10 yr	1–4 mg/24 hr		3.5–14 μmol/24 hr	
		10–12 yr	1–6 mg/24 hr		3.5–21 μmol/24 hr	
		12–14 yr	3–10 mg/24 hr		10–35 μmol/24 hr	
		14–16 yr	5–12 mg/24 hr		17–42 μmol/24 hr	
		Thereafter				
		M, 18–30 yr	9–22 mg/24 hr		31–76 μmol/24 hr	
		>30 yr	8–20 mg/24 hr		28–70 μmol/24 hr	
		F, decreases with age	6–15 mg/24 hr		21–52 μmol/24 hr Decreases with age	
LDL-Cholesterol (LDLC)	S, P(E)		M (mg/dL) / F (mg/dL)		M (mmol/L) / F (mmol/L)	
		Cord blood	10–50 / 10–50	× 0.0259	0.26–1.30 / 0.26–1.30	
		1–9 yr	60–140 / 60–150		1.55–3.63 / 1.55–3.89	
		10–19 yr	50–170 / 50–170		1.30–4.40 / 1.30–4.40	
		20–29 yr	60–175 / 60–160		1.55–4.53 / 1.55–4.14	
		30–39 yr	80–190 / 70–170		2.07–4.92 / 1.81–4.40	
		40–49 yr	90–205 / 80–190		2.33–5.31 / 2.07–4.92	
		Recommended (desirable) range for adults	<130 mg/dl		1.68–4.53 mg/dL	
Lactate						
L(+)-lactate	W(H)	Venous	0.5–2.2 mmol/L		0.5–2.2 mmol/L	
		Arterial	0.5–1.6 mmol/L		0.5–1.6 mmol/L	
		Inpatients				
		Venous	0.9–1.7 mmol/L		0.9–1.7 mmol/L	
		Arterial	<1.25 mmol/L		<1.25 mmol/L	
D(−)-lactate	P(H)	6 mo–3 yr	0.0–0.3 mmol/L	× 1	0.0–0.3 mmol/L	z (Rosenthal et al)

TABLE 27–2. Reference Ranges for Laboratory Tests *Continued*

Test	Specimen	Reference Range		Factor	Reference Range (SI)	Comments
Lactate dehydrogenase (LD)	S	<1 yr	170–580 U/L	× 1	170–580 U/L	37° m (Meites)
		1–9 yr	150–500 U/L		150–500 U/L	
		10–19 yr	120–330 U/L		120–330 U/L	
Isoenzymes	S		*Percentage of Total Activity*			(Meites)
			1–6 yr / *7–19 yr*			
		LD1	20–38 / 20–35			
		LD2	27–38 / 31–38			
		LD3	16–26 / 19–28			
		LD4	5–16 / 7–13			
		LD5	3–13 / 5–12			
Lead	W(H)	Child	<10 μg/dL	× 0.0483	<0.48 μmol/L	
		Adult	<40 μg/dL		<1.93 μmol/L	
		Acceptable for industrial exposure	<60 μg/dL		<2.90 μmol/L	
		Toxic	≥100 μg/dL		≥4.83 μmol/L	
	U (24-hr)	<80 μg/L		× 0.00483	<0.39 μmol/L	
Lecithin/sphingomyelin (L/S) ratio	AF	2.0–5.0 indicates probable fetal lung maturity (>3.0 IDM)			2.0–5.0 indicates probable fetal lung maturity	
Lecithin phosphorus	AF	>0.10 mg/dL indicates probably adequate fetal lung maturity		× 0.3229	>0.33 mmol/L indicates probably adequate fetal lung maturity	
Leukocyte count (WBC)	W(E)		× 1,000 cells/mm³ (μL)		× 10⁹ cells/L	
		Birth	9.0–30.0		9.0–30.0	
		24 hr	9.4–34.0		9.4–34.0	
		1 mo	5.0–19.5		5.0–19.5	
		1–3 yr	6.0–17.5		6.0–17.5	
		4–7 yr	5.5–15.5		5.5–15.5	
		8–13 yr	4.5–13.5		4.5–13.5	
		Adult	4.5–11.0		4.5–11.0	
Cell count	CSF	Premature	0–25 mononuclear cells/μL	× 10^6	0–25 × 10^6 cells/L	
			0–10 polymorphonuclear cells/μL		0–10 × 10^6 cells/L	
			0–1,000 RBC/μL		0–1,000 × 10^6 cells/L	
		Newborn	0–20 mononuclear cells/μL		0–20 × 10^6 cells/L	
			0–10 polymorphonuclear cells/μL		0–10 × 10^6 cells/L	
			0–800 RBC/μL		0–800 × 10^6 cells/L	
		Neonate	0–5 mononuclear cells/μL		0–5 × 10^6 cells/L	
			0–10 polymorphonuclear cells/μL		0–10 × 10^6 cells/L	
			0–50 RBC/μL		0–50 × 10^6 cells/L	
		Thereafter	0–5 mononuclear cells/μL (numbers of cells in very young infants are greater than those in the CSF of older individuals without substantial implications for growth and development in most instances)		0–5 cells/L	
Leukocyte differential	W(E)					
Myelocytes		0		× 0.01	0	
Neutrophils—"bands"		3–5%			0.03–0.05 no. fraction	
Neutrophils—"segs"		54–62%			0.54–0.62 no. fraction	
Lymphocytes		25–33%			0.25–0.33 no. fraction	
Monocytes		3–7%			0.03–0.07 no. fraction	
Eosinophils		1–3%			0.01–0.03 no. fraction	
Basophils		0–0.75%			0–0.0075 no. fraction	
Leukocyte differential		*Cells/mm³ (μL)*				
Myelocytes		0		× 1	0 × 10^6 cells/L	
Neutrophils—"bands"		150–400			150–400 × 10^6 cells/L	
Neutrophils—"segs"		3,000–5,800			3,000–5,800 × 10^6 cells/L	
Lymphocytes		1,500–3,000			1,500–3,000 × 10^6 cells/L	
Monocytes		285–500			285–500 × 10^6 cells/L	
Eosinophils		50–250			50–250 × 10^6 cells/L	
Basophils		15–50			15–50 × 10^6 cells/L	
Lymphocytes	CSF		62% ± 34%	× 0.01	0.62 ± 0.34 no. fraction	
Monocytes			36% ± 20%		0.36 ± 0.20 no fraction	
Neutrophils			2% ± 5%		0.02 ± 0.05 no. fraction	
Histiocytes			0–rare		0–rare	
Ependymal cells			0–rare		0–rare	
Eosinophils			0–rare		0–rare	
Lipase	S	1–4 yr	18–95 U/L	× 1	18–95 U/L	37° (Meites)
		5–14 yr	21–128 U/L		21–128 U/L	
		15–19 yr	28–149 U/L		28–149 U/L	

Table continued on following page

TABLE 27–2. Reference Ranges for Laboratory Tests *Continued*

Test	Specimen	Reference Range	Factor	Reference Range (SI)	Comments
Lipoprotein electrophoresis	S	Distinct β band; negligible chylomicron and pre-β bands			
Lithium. See end of table under Drugs					
Long-acting thyroid-stimulating hormone (LATS)	S	Undetectable		Undetectable	
Luteinizing hormone (LH)	S	M			(Endocrine Sciences)
		Tanner 1 <9.8 yr <1–4 mIU/mL	× 1	<1–4 U/L	
		Tanner 2 9.8–14.5 yr <1–5 mIU/mL		<1–5 U/L	
		Tanner 3 10.7–15.4 yr 2–10 mIU/mL		2–10 U/L	
		Tanner 4 11.8–16.2 yr 2–10 mIU/mL		2–10 U/L	
		Tanner 5 12.8–17.3 yr 4.5–11 mIU/mL		4.5–11 U/L	
		Adult 3–10 mIU/mL		3–10 U/L	
		F			
		Tanner 1 <9.2 yr <1–4 mIU/mL		<1–4 mIU/L	
		Tanner 2 9.2–13.7 yr <1–5 mIU/mL		<1–5 U/L	
		Tanner 3 10.0–14.4 yr <1–10 mIU/mL		<1–10 U/L	
		Tanner 4 10.7–15.6 yr 3–11 mIU/mL		3–11 U/L	
		Tanner 5 11.8–18.6 yr 2–12 mIU/mL		2–12 U/L	
		Adult Follicular 3–11 mIU/mL		3–11 U/L	
		Midcycle 18–70 mIU/mL		18–70 U/L	
		Luteal 2–11 mIU/mL		2–11 U/L	
Lymphocyte subpopulations	W(H)	*Percentage of Mononuclear Cells in Adults*		*Fraction of Mononuclear Cells in Adults*	
Total T cells (OKT3)		43–69	× 0.01	0.43–0.69	1 (Landry et al)
Helper T cells (OKT4)		26–55		0.26–0.55	
Suppressor T cells (OKT8)		9–28		0.09–0.28	
Total B cells (HB2)		5–17		0.05–0.17	
Monocytes (MMA)		8–32		0.08–0.32	
Natural killer cells (HNK)		5–20		0.05–0.20	
Lysergic acid diethylamide. See end of table under Drugs					
Magnesium	P(H)	0–6 d 1.2–2.6 mg/dL	× 0.411	0.48–1.05 mmol/L	d (Meites)
		7 d–2 yr 1.6–2.6 mg/dL		0.65–1.05 mmol/L	
		2–14 yr 1.5–2.3 mg/dL		0.60–0.95 mmol/L	
	U (24-hr)	1–6 mo			
		Breast-fed 0.04–1.55 mmol/L	× 1	0.04–1.55 mmol/L	
		Formula-fed 0.04–1.40 mmol/L		0.04–1.55 mmol/L	
Mean corpuscular hemoglobin (MCH)	W(E)	Birth 31–37 pg/cell	× 0.0155	0.48–0.57 fmol/cell	
		1–3 d (capillary) 31–37 pg/cell		0.48–0.57 fmol/cell	
		1 wk–1 mo 28–40 pg/cell		0.43–0.62 fmol/cell	
		2 mo 26–34 pg/cell		0.40–0.53 fmol/cell	
		3–6 mo 25–35 pg/cell		0.39–0.54 fmol/cell	
		0.5–2 yr 23–31 pg/cell		0.36–0.48 fmol/cell	
		2–6 yr 24–30 pg/cell		0.37–0.47 fmol/cell	
		6–12 yr 25–33 pg/cell		0.39–0.51 fmol/cell	
		12–18 yr 25–35 pg/cell		0.39–0.54 fmol/cell	
		18–49 yr 26–34 pg/cell		0.40–0.53 fmol/cell	
Mean corpuscular hemoglobin concentration (MCHC)	W(E)	*Percentage Hb/cell or g Hb/dL RBC*		*mmol Hb/L RBC*	
		Birth 30–36	× 0.155	4.65–5.58	
		1–3 d (capillary) 29–37		4.50–5.74	
		1–2 wk 28–38		4.34–5.89	
		1–2 mo 29–37		4.50–5.74	
		3 mo–2 yr 30–36		4.65–5.58	
		2–18 yr 31–37		4.81–5.74	
		>18 yr 31–37		4.81–5.74	
Mean corpuscular volume (MCV)	W(E)	1–3 d (capillary) 95–121 μm³	× 1	95–121 fL	
		0.5–2 yr 70–86 μm³		70–86 fL	
		6–12 yr 77–95 μm³		77–95 fL	
		12–18 yr			
		M 78–98 μm³		78–98 fL	
		F 78–102 μm³		78–102 fL	
		18–49 yr			
		M 80–100 μm³		80–100 fL	
		F 80–100 μm³		80–100 fL	

TABLE 27–2. Reference Ranges for Laboratory Tests *Continued*

Test	Specimen	Reference Range		Factor	Reference Range (SI)	Comments
Metanephrines, total	U (24-hr)	<1 yr	<15.9 μmol/g creatinine	× 0.1131	<1.80 mmol/mol creatinine	(Meites)
		1–2 yr	<14.8 μmol/g creatinine		<1.67 mmol/mol creatinine	
		3–4 yr	<12.8 μmol/g creatinine		<1.45 mmol/mol creatinine	
		5–8 yr	<11.7 μmol/g creatinine		<1.32 mmol/mol creatinine	
		9–13 yr	<10.5 μmol/g creatinine		<1.19 mmol/mol creatinine	
Methemoglobin (MetHb)	W(E,H,C)	0.06–0.24 g/dL or		× 155	9.3–37.2 μmol/L	
		0.78 ± 0.37% of total Hb		× 0.01	0.0078 ± 0.0037 (mass fraction)	
Methylmalonic acid	U	6–12 wk	0–57 mg/g creatinine	× 0.9579	0–55 mmol/mol creatinine	h (Meites)
Microsomal antibodies, thyroid. See Thyroid microsomal antibodies						
Mucopolysaccharides	U	<2 yr	<50 μg/g creatinine	× 0.1131	<5.7 mg/mmol creatinine	(Meites)
		2–4 yr	<25 μg/g creatinine		<2.8 mg/mmol creatinine	
		4–15 yr	<20 μg/g creatinine		<2.3 mg/mmol creatinine	
Myoglobin	S	6–85 ng/mL		× 1	6–85 pg/L	
	U	Negative			Negative	
Niacin (nicotinic acid)	U	0.3–1.5 mg/24 hr		× 8.113	2.43–12.17 μmol/24 hr	
Occult blood	F	Negative (<2 mL blood/24 hr in ~100–200 g stool)			Negative	
	U	Negative			Negative	
Organic acids	U	ADULT				(Hoffman et al)
Lactic		115–407 μM/g creatinine		× 8.8402	13–46 mmol/mol creatinine	
2-Hydroxyisobutyric		not detected			not detected	
Glycolic		159–486 μM/g creatinine			18–55 mmol/mol creatinine	
3-Hydroxybutyric		not detected–18 μM/g creatinine			not detected–2.0 mmol/mol creatinine	
3-Hydroxyisobutyric		36–168 μM/g creatinine			4.1–19 mmol/mol creatinine	
2-Hydroxyisovaleric		not detected			not detected	
3-Hydroxyisovaleric		61–221 μM/g creatinine			6.9–25 mmol/mol creatinine	
Methylmalonic		not detected			not detected	
4-Hydroxybutyric		2.7–51 μM/g creatinine			0.3–5.8 mmol/mol creatinine	
Ethylmalonic		3.5–37 μM/g creatinine			0.4–4.2 mmol/mol creatinine	
Succinic		4.4–141 μM/g creatinine			0.5–16 mmol/mol creatinine	
Fumaric		1.8–7 μM/g creatinine			0.2–0.8 mmol/mol creatinine	
Glutaric		5.3–23 μM/g creatinine			0.6–2.6 mmol/mol creatinine	
3-Methylglutaric		not detected			not detected	
Adipic		7–309 μM/g creatinine			0.8–35 mmol/mol creatinine	
Pyruvic		23–70 μM/g creatinine			2.6–7.9 mmol/mol creatinine	
Pyroglutamic		8–557 μM/g creatinine			0.9–63 μM/g creatinine	
2-Oxoisovaleric		not detected			not detected	
Acetoacetic		not detected			not detected	
Mevalonic		0.5–1.9 μM/g creatinine			0.06–0.22 mmol/mol creatinine	
2-Hydroxyglutaric		7–460 μM/g creatinine			0.8–52 mmol/mol creatinine	
3-Hydroxy-3-methylglutaric		not detected–88			not detected–10 mmol/mol creatinine	
p-Hydroxyphenylacetic		31–195 μM/g creatinine			3.5–22 mmol/mol creatinine	
2-Oxoisocaproic		not detected			not detected	
Suberic		not detected–26 μM/g creatinine			not detected–2.9 mmol/mol creatinine	
Orotic		not detected			not detected	
cis-Aconitic		24–389 μM/g creatinine			2.7–44 mmol/mol creatinine	
Homovanillic		8–49 μM/g creatinine			0.9–5.5 mmol/mol creatinine	
Azeleic		11–137 μM/g creatinine			1.3–5.5 mmol/mol creatinine	
Isocitric		318–743 μM/g creatinine			36–84 mmol/mol creatinine	
Citric		619–1998 μM/g creatinine			70–226 mmol/mol creatinine	
Sebacic		not detected			not detected	
4-Hydroxyphenyl lactic		1.8–23 μM/g creatinine			0.2–2.6 mmol/mol creatinine	
2-Oxoglutaric		35–654 μM/g creatinine			4–74 mmol/mol creatinine	
5-Hydroxyindoleacetic		not detected–64 μM/g creatinine			not detected–7.2 mmol/mol creatinine	
Succinylacetone		not detected			not detected	
Orotic acid	U	0–20.1 mg/g creatinine		× 0.7247	0–14.6 mmol/mol creatinine	cm (Meites)
Osmolality	S	Child and adult	275–295 mOsm/kg H_2O			
	U	50–1,400 mOsm/kg H_2O, depending on fluid intake. After 12 hr of fluid restriction, normal range is >850 mOsm/kg H_2O				
	U (24-hr)	300–900 mOsm/kg H_2O				

Table continued on following page

TABLE 27–2. Reference Ranges for Laboratory Tests *Continued*

Test	Specimen	Reference Range		Factor	Reference Range (SI)		Comments
Osmotic fragility test (RBC fragility) pH 7.4, 20° C	W(H)	*NaCl*	*Per cent Hemolysis*		*NaCl*	*Hemolyzed Fraction*	
		0.30 g/dL	97–100	× 0.01 (Hemolyzed fraction)	3.0 g/L	0.97–1.00	
		0.35 g/dL	90–99		3.5 g/L	0.90–0.99	
		0.40 g/dL	50–95		4.0 g/L	0.50–0.95	
		0.45 g/dL	5–45		4.5 g/L	0.05–0.45	
		0.50 g/dL	0–6		5.0 g/L	0.00–0.06	
		0.55 g/dL	0		5.5 g/L	0.00	
Sterile incubation at 37° C		*NaCl*	*Per cent Hemolysis*		*NaCl*	*Hemolyzed Fraction*	
		0.20 g/dL	95–100	× 0.01 (Hemolized fraction)	2.0 g/L	0.95–1.00	
		0.30 g/dL	85–100		3.0 g/L	0.85–1.00	
		0.35 g/dL	75–100		3.5 g/L	0.75–1.00	
		0.40 g/dL	65–100		4.0 g/L	0.65–1.00	
		0.45 g/dL	55–95		4.5 g/L	0.55–0.95	
		0.50 g/dL	40–85		5.0 g/L	0.40–0.85	
		0.55 g/dL	15–70		5.5 g/L	0.15–0.70	
		0.60 g/dL	0–40		6.0 g/L	0.00–0.40	
		0.65 g/dL	0–10		6.5 g/L	0.00–0.10	
		0.70 g/dL	0–5		7.0 g/L	0.00–0.05	
		0.85 g/dL	0		8.5 g/L	0.00	
Oxygen, partial pressure of (Po_2)	W(H), arterial	Birth	8–24 mm Hg	× 0.133	1.1–3.2 kPa		
		5–10 min	33–75 mm Hg		4.4–10.0 kPa		
		30 min	31–85 mm Hg		4.1–11.3 kPa		
		>1 hr	55–80 mm Hg		7.3–10.6 kPa		
		1 d	54–95 mm Hg		7.2–12.6 kPa		
		Thereafter (decreases with age)	83–108 mm Hg		11–14.4 kPa		
Oxygen saturation	W(H), arterial	Newborn	85–90%	× 0.01	0.85–0.90 Saturated fraction		
		Thereafter	95–99%		0.95–0.99 Saturated fraction		
Po_2. See Oxygen, partial pressure							
Po_2 at half saturation (Po_2 [0.5] or P_{50})	W(H), arterial	25–29 mm Hg		× 0.133	3.3–3.9 kPa		
Paraldehyde. See end of table under Drugs							
Parathyroid hormone	S						
C-terminal (mid-molecule)		1–16 yr	51–217 pg/mL	× 0.1053	5.4–22.8 pmol/L		m (Nichols Institute)
Intact (IRMA)		1–18 yr	1–43 pg/mL		0.1–4.5 pmol/L		
Intact N-terminal specific		2–13 yr	14–21 pg/mL		1.5–2.2 pmol/L		
Partial thromboplastin time (PTT)	W(NaC)						
Nonactivated		60–85 s (Platelin)			60–85 s		
Activated		25–35 s (differs with method)			25–35 s		
pH	W(H), arterial				*H+ Concentration*		
		Premature (48 hr)	7.35–7.50		31–44 nmol/L		
		Birth, full-term	7.11–7.36		43–77 nmol/L		
		5–10 min	7.09–7.30		50–81 nmol/L		
		30 min	7.21–7.38		41–61 nmol/L		
		>1 hr	7.26–7.49		32–54 nmol/L		
		1 d	7.29–7.45		35–51 nmol/L		
		Thereafter	7.35–7.45		35–44 nmol/L		
		Must be corrected for body temperature					
	U	Newborn/neonate	5–7		0.1–10 μmol/L		
		Thereafter (average 6)	4.5–8		0.01–32 μmol/L (average 1.0 μmol/L)		
	F		7.0–7.5		31–100 nmol/L		
Phenacetin. See end of table under Drugs							
Phenobarbital. See end of table under Drugs							
Phensuximide. See end of table under Drugs							

TABLE 27–2. Reference Ranges for Laboratory Tests *Continued*

Test	Specimen	Reference Range	Factor	Reference Range (SI)	Comments
Phenylalanine	S	Premature 2.0–7.5 mg/dL Newborn 1.2–3.4 mg/dL Thereafter 0.8–1.8 mg/dL	× 60.54	120–450 μmol/L 70–210 μmol/L 50–110 μmol/L	
	U	10 d–2 wk 1–2 mg/24 hr 3–12 yr 4–18 mg/24 hr Thereafter trace–17 mg/24 hr	× 6.054	6–12 μmol/24 hr 24–110 μmol/24 hr trace–103 μmol/24 hr	
Phenylpyruvic acid, qualitative	U	Negative by $FeCl_3$ test		Negative by $FeCl_3$ test	
Phenytoin. See end of table under Drugs					
Phosphatase, acid Prostatic (RIA)	S	<3.0 ng/mL	× 1	<3.0 μg/L	
Roy Brower and Hayden 37° C		0.11–0.60 U/L		0.11–0.60 U/L	
Phosphatase, alkaline	S	1–9 yr 145–200 U/L 10–11 yr 130–560 U/L M / F 12–13 yr 200–495 U/L 150–420 U/L 14–15 yr 130–525 U/L 70–230 U/L 16–19 yr 65–260 U/L 50–130 U/L	× 1	1–9 yr 145–420 U/L 10–11 yr 130–560 U/L M / F 12–13 yr 200–495 U/L 105–420 U/L 14–15 yr 130–525 U/L 70–230 U/L 16–19 yr 65–260 U/L 50–130 U/L	37° C md (Lockitch et al)
Phospholipids, total	S, P(E)	Newborn 75–170 mg/dL Infant 100–275 mg/dL Child 180–295 mg/dL Adult 125–275 mg/dL	× 0.01	0.75–1.70 g/L 1.00–2.75 g/L 1.80–2.95 g/L 1.25–2.75 g/L	
Phosphorus, inorganic	S, P(H)	0–5 d 4.8–8.2 mg/dL 1–3 yr 3.8–6.5 mg/dL 4–11 yr 3.7–5.6 mg/dL 12–15 yr 2.9–5.4 mg/dL 16–19 yr 2.7–4.7 mg/dL	× 0.3229	1.55–2.65 mmol/L 1.25–2.10 mmol/L 1.20–1.80 mmol/L 0.95–1.75 mmol/L 0.90–1.50 mmol/L	d (Meites)
Plasma volume	P(H)	M 25–43 mL/kg F 28–45 mL/kg	× 0.001	M 0.025–0.043 L/kg F 0.028–0.045 L/kg	
Platelet count (thrombocyte count)	W(E)	Newborn 84–478 × 10^3/mm³ (μL) (after 1 wk same as adult) Adult 150–400 × 10^3/mm³ (μL)	× 10^6	84–478 × 10^9/L 150–400 × 10^9/L	
Porphobilinogen (PBG) Quantitative Qualitative	 U U	 0–2.0 mg/24 hr Negative	 × 4.42	 0–8.8 μmol/24 hr Negative	
Potassium	S	<2 yr 3.0–6.0 mmol/L 2–12 yr 3.5–7.0 mmol/L >12 yr 3.5–5.0 mmol/L	× 1	3.0–6.0 mmol/L 3.5–7.0 mmol/L 3.5–5.0 mmol/L	w (Meites)
	p(H)	3.4–4.5 mmol/L		3.5–4.5 mmol/L	
	U (24-hr)	2.5–125 mmol/L (varies with diet)		2.5–125 mmol/L (varies with diet)	
Prealbumin (transthyretin)	P	2–6 mo 142–330 mg/L 6–12 mo 120–274 mg/L 1–3 yr 108–259 mg/L	× 1	142–330 mg/L 120–274 mg/L 108–259 mg/L	n (Sherry et al)
Pregnanetriol	U	2 wk–2 yr 0.02–0.2 mg/24 hr 2–5 yr <0.5 mg/24 hr 5–15 yr <1.5 mg/24 hr >15 yr <2.0 mg/24 hr	× 2.972	0.06–0.6 μmol/24 hr <1.5 μmol/24 hr <4.5 μmol/24 hr <5.9 μmol/24 hr	
Primidone. See end of table under Drugs					
Progesterone	S	M Tanner 1 <9.8 yr <10–33 ng/dL Tanner 2 9.8–14.5 yr <10–33 ng/dL Tanner 3 10.7–15.4 yr <10–48 ng/dL Tanner 4 11.8–16.2 yr 10–108 ng/dL Tanner 5 12.8–17.3 yr 21–82 ng/dL Adult 13–97 ng/dL	 × 0.03180	 <0.32–1.05 nmol/L <0.32–1.05 nmol/L <0.32–1.53 nmol/L 0.32–3.43 nmol/L 0.67–2.61 nmol/L 0.41–3.08 nmol/L	(Endocrine Sciences)

Table continued on following page

TABLE 27–2. Reference Ranges for Laboratory Tests *Continued*

Test	Specimen	Reference Range	Factor	Reference Range (SI)	Comments
Progesterone *(Continued)*		F			
		Tanner 1 <9.2 yr <10–33 ng/dL		<0.32–1.05 nmol/L	
		Tanner 2 9.2–13.7 yr <10–55 ng/dL		<0.32–1.75 nmol/L	
		Tanner 3 10.0–14.4 yr 10–450 ng/dL		0.32–14.31 nmol/L	
		Tanner 4 10.7–15.6 yr <10–1,300 ng/dL		<0.32–41.34 nmol/L	
		Tanner 5 11.8–18.6 yr <10–950 ng/dL		<0.32–30.21 nmol/L	
		Adult Follicular 15–70 ng/dL		0.48–2.23 nmol/L	
		Luteal 200–2,500 ng/dL		6.36–79.50 nmol/L	
Prolactin	S	M 3–18 ng/mL	× 0.0426	M 0.13–0.77 nmol/L	(Endocrine Sciences)
		F 3–24 ng/mL		F 0.13–1.02 nmol/L	
		Higher in newborn infants		Higher in newborn infants	
Propranolol. See end of table under Drugs					
Protein					
Total	S	Premature 4.3–7.6 g/dL	× 10	43–76 g/L	
		Newborn 4.6–7.4 g/dL		46–74 g/L	
		1–7 yr 6.1–7.9 g/dL	× 10	61–79 g/L	(Meites)
		8–12 yr 6.4–8.1 g/dL		64–81 g/L	
		13–19 yr 6.6–8.2 g/dL		66–82 g/L	
Electrophoresis	S				
Albumin		Premature 3.0–4.2 g/dL		30–42 g/L	
		Newborn 3.6–5.4 g/dL		36–54 g/L	
		Infant 4.0–5.0 g/dL		40–50 g/L	
		Thereafter 3.5–5.0 g/dL		35–50 g/L	
α₁-Globulin		Premature 0.1–0.5 g/dL		1–5 g/L	
		Newborn 0.1–0.3 g/dL		1–3 g/L	
		Infant 0.2–0.4 g/dL		2–4 g/L	
		Thereafter 0.2–0.3 g/dL		2–3 g/L	
α₂-Globulin		Premature 0.3–0.7 g/dL		3–7 g/L	
		Newborn 0.3–0.5 g/dL		3–5 g/L	
		Infant 0.5–0.8 g/dL		5–8 g/L	
		Thereafter 0.4–1.0 g/dL		4–10 g/L	
β-Globulin		Premature 0.3–1.2 g/dL		3–12 g/L	
		Newborn 0.2–0.6 g/dL		2–6 g/L	
		Infant 0.5–0.8 g/dL		5–8 g/L	
		Thereafter 0.5–1.1 g/dL		5–11 g/L	
γ-Globulin		Premature 0.3–1.4 g/dL		3–4 g/L	
		Newborn 0.2–1.0 g/dL		2–10 g/L	
		Infant 0.3–1.2 g/dL		3–12 g/L	
		Thereafter 0.7–1.2 g/dL (higher in blacks)		7–12 g/L (higher in blacks)	
Protein Total urinary	U (24-hr)	1–14 mg/dL		10–140 mg/L	
		50–80 mg/24 hr (at rest)		50–80 mg/24 hr	
		<250 mg/24 hr after intense exercise		<250 mg/24 hr after intense exercise	
Electrophoresis		*Average Total Protein*		*Fraction of Total Protein*	
Albumin		37.9%	× 0.01	0.379	
α₁-globulin		27.3%		0.273	
α₂-globulin		19.5%		0.195	
β-globulin		8.8%		0.088	
γ-globulin		3.3%		0.033	
Protein					
Total protein (column)	CSF	Lumbar 8–32 mg/dL	× 10	80–320 mg/L	
Turbidimetry		Lumbar			
		Premature 40–300 mg/dL		400–3,000 mg/L	
		Newborn 45–120 mg/dL		450–1,200 mg/L	
		Child 10–20 mg/dL		100–200 mg/L	
		Adolescent 15–20 mg/dL		150–200 mg/L	
		Thereafter 15–45 mg/dL		150–450 mg/L	
Electrophoresis		Prealbumin 2–7% of total	× 0.01	0.02–0.07 fraction of total	
		Albumin 56–76% of total		0.56–0.76 fraction of total	
		α₁-Globulin 2–7% of total		0.02–0.07 fraction of total	
		α₂-Globulin 4–12% of total		0.04–0.12 fraction of total	
		β-Globulin 8–18% of total		0.08–0.18 fraction of total	
		γ-Globulin 3–12% of total		0.03–0.12 fraction of total	

TABLE 27–2. Reference Ranges for Laboratory Tests *Continued*

Test	Specimen	Reference Range	Factor	Reference Range (SI)	Comments
Prothrombin time (PT)					
One-stage (quick)	W(NaC)	In general, 11–15 s (varies with type of thromboplastin) Newborn: prolonged by 2–3 s		11–15 s Newborn: prolonged by 2–3 s	
Two-stage modified (Ware and Seegers)	W(NaC)	18–22 s		18–22 s	
Quinidine. See end of table under Drugs					
RBC count. See Erythrocyte count					
RBC fragility. See Osmotic fragility					
Red cell volume	W(H)	M 20–36 mL/kg F 19–31 mL/kg	× 0.001	M 0.020–0.036 L/kg F 0.019–0.031 L/kg	
Renin (renin activity, plasma; PRA)	P(E)	0–3 yr <16.6 ng/mL/hr 3–6 yr <6.7 ng/mL/hr 6–9 yr <4.4 ng/mL/hr 9–12 yr <5.9 ng/mL/hr 12–15 yr <4.2 ng/mL/hr 15–18 yr <4.3 ng/mL/hr Normal sodium diet Supine 0.2–2.5 ng/mL/hr Upright 0.3–4.3 ng/mL/hr Low sodium diet Upright 2.9–24 ng/mL/hr	× 1	<16.6 μg/L/hr <6.7 μg/L/hr <4.4 μg/L/hr <5.9 μg/L/hr <4.2 μg/L/hr <4.3 μg/L/hr 0.2–2.5 μg/L/hr 0.3–4.3 μg/L/hr 2.9–24 μg/L/hr	
Reticulocyte count	W (E,H,O)	Adults 0.5–1.5% of erythrocytes, or 25,000–75,000/mm^3 (μL)	× 0.01 × 10^6	0.005–0.015 number fraction 25,000–75,000 × 10^6/L	
	W (capillary)	1 d 0.4–6.0% 7 d <0.1–1.3% 1–4 wk <1.0–1.2% 5–6 wk <0.1–2.4% 7–8 wk 0.1–2.9% 9–10 wk <0.1–2.6% 11–12 wk 0.1–1.3%	× 0.01	0.004–0.060 number fraction <0.001–0.013 number fraction <0.001–0.012 number fraction <0.001–0.024 number fraction 0.001–0.029 number fraction <0.001–0.026 number fraction 0.001–0.013 number fraction	
Retinol-binding protein (RBP)	S	0–5 d 0.8–4.5 mg/dL 1–9 yr 1.0–7.8 mg/dL 10–13 yr 1.3–9.9 mg/dL 14–19 yr 3.0–9.2 mg/dL	× 10	8–45 mg/L 10–78 mg/L 13–99 mg/L 30–92 mg/L	n (Lockitch et al)
Reverse triiodothyronine (rT_3)	S	1–5 yr 15–71 ng/dL 5–10 yr 17–79 ng/dL 10–15 yr 19–88 ng/dL Adults 30–80 ng/dL	× 0.0154	0.23–1.1 nmol/L 0.26–1.2 nmol/L 0.29–1.36 nmol/L 0.46–1.23 nmol/L	
Riboflavin (vitamin B_2)	U	1–3 yr 500–900 μg/g creatinine 4–6 yr 300–600 μg/g creatinine 7–9 yr 270–500 μg/g creatinine 10–15 yr 200–400 μg/g creatinine Adult 80–269 μg/g creatinine	× 0.3	150–270 μmol/mol creatinine 90–180 μmol/mol creatinine 81–150 μmol/mol creatinine 60–1200 μmol/mol creatinine 24–81 μmol/mol creatinine	
Salicylate. See end of table under Drugs					
Sediment	U				
Casts		Hyaline seen occasionally (0–1)hpf RBC Not seen WBC Not seen Tubular epithelial Not seen Transitional and squamous epithelial Not seen		Hyaline seen occasionally (0–1)/hpf RBC Not seen WBC Not seen Tubular epithelial Not seen Transitional and squamous epithelial Not seen	
Cells		RBC 0–2/hpf WBC M 0–3/hpf F and children 0–5/hpf Epithelial Few (more frequent in newborn) Bacterial, no organism/oil immersion Field unspun Spun <20 organisms/hpf		RBC 0–2/hpf WBC M 0–3/hpf F and children 0–5/hpf Epithelial Few (more frequent in newborn) Bacterial, no organism/oil immersion Field unspun Spun <20 organisms/hpf	

Table continued on following page

TABLE 27–2. Reference Ranges for Laboratory Tests *Continued*

Test	Specimen	Reference Range	Factor	Reference Range (SI)	Comments
Sedimentation rate. See Erythrocyte sedimentation rate					
Selenium	S	0–5 d 5.7–9.4 μg/dL 1–9 yr 9.6–16.1 μg/dL 10–19 yr 10.3–18.5 μg/dL	× 0.127	0.72–1.20 μmol/L 1.22–2.05 μmol/L 1.31–2.35 μmol/L	a (Lockitch et al)
Sickle cell tests					
Sodium metabisulfite	W(E,H,O)	Negative			
Dithionite test	W(E,H,O)	Negative			
Sodium	S,P(LiH, NH_4H)	Newborn 134–146 mmol/L Infant 139–146 mmol/L Child 138–145 mmol/L Thereafter 136–146 mmol/L	× 1	134–146 nmol/L 139–146 nmol/L 138–145 nmol/L 136–146 nmol/L	
	U (24-hr)	(depending on diet) 40–220		40–220 nmol/L	
	Sweat	Normal <40 mmol/L Indeterminate 45–60 mmol/L Cystic fibrosis >60 mmol/L	× 1	<40 mmol/L 45–60 mmol/L >60 mmol/L	(Gibson et al)
Somatomedin C (IGF-1)	S	*M* / *F* <3 yr 0.08–1.1 / 0.11–2.2 U/mL 3–5 yr 0.12–1.6 / 0.18–2.4 U/mL 6–10 yr 0.22–2.8 / 0.40–4.5 U/mL 11–12 yr 0.28–3.7 / 0.99–6.8 U/mL 13–14 yr 0.90–5.6 / 1.20–5.9 U/mL 15–17 yr 0.91–3.1 / 0.71–4.1 U/mL	× 1,000	*M* / *F* 80–110 / 110–220 U/L 120–1,600 / 180–2,400 U/L 220–2,800 / 400–4,500 U/L 280–3,700 / 990–6,800 U/L 900–5,600 / 1,200–5,900 U/L 911–3,100 / 710–4,100 U/L	m (Nichols Institute)
		M / *F* Tanner 1 0–2.0 / 0–3.0 U/mL Tanner 2 0.3–3.4 / 0.6–4.0 U/mL Tanner 3 0.8–4.4 / 1.1–4.3 U/mL Tanner 4 0.8–3.8 / 0.8–4.0 U/mL Tanner 5 0.7–3.5 / 0.9–4.1 U/mL		*M* / *F* 0–2,000 / 0–3,000 U/L 300–3,400 / 600–4,000 U/L 800–4,400 / 1,100–4,300 U/L 800–3,800 / 800–4,000 U/L 700–3,500 / 900–4,100 U/L	m (Nichols Institute)
Specific gravity	U	Adult 1.002–1.030 After 12-hr fluid restriction >1.025		Adult 1.002–1.030 After 12-hr fluid restriction >1.025	
	U (24-hr)	1.015–1.025			
Sucrose hemolysis and sugar-water tests for paroxysmal nocturnal hemoglobinuria (PNH)	W(C,O)	≤5% lysis 6–10% lysis, questionable	× 0.01	Lysed fraction ≤0.05 0.06–0.10 questionable	
T_3. See Triiodothyronine					
T_4. See Thyroxine					
Testosterone	S	M Tanner 1 <9.8 yr <3–10 ng/mL Tanner 2 9.8–14.5 yr 18–150 ng/mL Tanner 3 10.7–15.4 yr 100–320 ng/mL Tanner 4 11.8–16.2 yr 220–620 ng/mL Tanner 5 12.8–17.3 yr 350–970 ng/mL Adult 350–1,030 ng/mL	× 3.4672	<10–35 nmol/L 62–520 nmol/L 347–1,110 nmol/L 763–2,150 nmol/L 1,214–3,363 nmol/L 1,214–3,571 nmol/L	(Endocrine Sciences)
		F Tanner 1 <9.2 yr <3–10 ng/mL Tanner 2 9.2–13.7 yr 7–28 ng/mL Tanner 3 10.0–14.4 yr 15–35 ng/mL Tanner 4 10.7–15.6 yr 13–32 ng/mL Tanner 5 11.8–18.6 yr 20–38 ng/mL Adult 10–55 ng/mL		<10–35 nmol/L 24–97 nmol/L 52–121 nmol/L 45–111 nmol/L 69–132 nmol/L 35–191 nmol/L	
Free	*S*	*M* / *% Free* Cord blood 5–22 pg/mL 2.0–4.4% 1–15 d 1.5–31 pg/mL 0.9–1.7% 1–3 mo 3.3–18 pg/mL 0.4–0.8% 3–5 mo 0.7–14 pg/mL 0.4–1.1% 5–7 mo 0.4–4.8 pg/mL 0.4–1.0% 1–10 yr 0.15–0.6 pg/mL 0.4–0.9% Puberty not defined Adult 52–280 pg/mL 1.5–3.2%	× 3.4673	*pmol/L* / *Fraction Free* Cord blood 17–76 0.02–0.044 1–15 d 5.2–107 0.009–0.017 1–3 mo 11.4–62 0.004–0.008 3–5 mo 2.4–49 0.004–0.011 5–7 mo 1.4–16.6 0.004–0.011 1–10 yr 0.5–2.1 0.004–0.009 Puberty not defined Adult 180–971 0.015–0.032	(Endocrine Sciences)

Test	Specimen	Reference Range	Factor	Reference Range (SI)	Comments
Testosterone *(Continued)*		F			(Endocrine Sciences)
		Age / Value / % Free		Age / *pmol/L* / *Fraction Free*	
		Cord blood 4–16 pg/mL 2.0–3.9%		Cord blood 13.9–55 0.02–0.039	
		1–15 d 0.5–2.5 pg/mL 0.8–1.5%		1–15 d 1.7–8.7 0.008–0.015	
		1–3 mo 0.1–1.3 pg/mL 0.4–1.1%		1–3 mo 0.3–4.5 0.004–0.011	
		3–5 mo 0.3–1.1 pg/mL 0.5–1.0%		3–5 mo 1.1–3.8 0.005–0.01	
		5–7 mo 0.2–0.6 pg/mL 0.5–0.8%		5–7 mo 0.7–2.1 0.005–0.008	
		1–10 yr 0.15–0.6 pg/mL 0.4–0.9%		1–10 yr 0.5–2.1 0.004–0.009	
		Puberty not defined		Puberty not defined	
		Adult 1.1–6.3 pg/mL 0.5–0.8%		Adult 3.8–21.8 0.005–0.008	
Theophylline. See end of table under Drugs					
Thiamine (vitamin B_1)	S	0–2.0 μg/dL	× 37.68	0.0–75.4 nmol/L	
	U (acidified with HCl)	1–3 yr 176–200 μg/g creatinine	× 0.426	75–85 μmol/mol	
		4–6 yr 121–400 μg/g creatinine		52–170 μmol/mol	
		7–9 yr 181–350 μg/g creatinine		77–149 μmol/mol	
		10–12 yr 181–300 μg/g creatinine		77–128 μmol/mol	
		13–15 yr 151–250 μg/g creatinine		64–107 μmol/mol	
		Thereafter 66–129 μg/g creatinine		28–55 μmol/mol	
Thrombin time	W(NaC)	Control time ± 2 s when control is 9–13 s		Control time ± 2 s when control is 9–13 s	
Thromboplastin time, Activated. See Activated partial thromboplastin time (APTT)					
Thyroglobulin (Tg)	S	<50 ng/mL (higher in newborn infants)	× 1	<50 μg/L	
Thyroid microsomal antibodies	S	Nondetectable (hemagglutination) or <1:10 (Indirect Fluorescent Antibody)		Nondetectable (hemagglutination) or <1:10 (IFA)	
Thyroid thyroglobulin tanned RBC agglutination test	S	Children ≤1:4 dilution		≤1:4 dilution	
		Thereafter ≤1:10 dilution		≤1:10 dilution	
Thyroid-stimulating hormone (hTSH)	S, P(H)	Cord blood 3–12 μU/L	× 1	3–12 mU/L	
		Newborn 3–18 μU/L		3–18 mU/L	
		Thereafter 2–10 μU/L		2–10 mU/L	
Thyroid uptake of radioactive iodine	Activity over thyroid gland	2 hr <6%	× 0.01	2 hr <0.06	
		6 hr 3–20%		6 hr 0.03–0.20	
		24 hr 8–30%		24 hr 0.08–0.30	
Thyroid uptake of $^{99m}TcO_4$	Activity over thyroid gland	After 24 hr, 0.4–3.0%	× 0.01	Fractional uptake, 0.004–0.03	
Thyrotropin-releasing hormone (hTRH)	P	5–60 pg/mL	× 2.759	14–165 pmol/L	
Thyroxine-binding globulin (TBG)	S	Range		Range	
		Cord blood 1.4–9.4 mg/dL	× 10	14–94 mg/L	
		1–4 wk 1.0–9.0 mg/dL		10–90 mg/L	
		1–12 mo 2.0–7.6 mg/dL		20–76 mg/L	
		1–5 yr 2.9–5.4 mg/dL		29–54 mg/L	
		5–10 yr 2.5–5.0 mg/dL		25–50 mg/L	
		10–15 yr 2.1–4.6 mg/dL		21–46 mg/L	
		Adult 1.5–3.4 mg/dL		15–34 mg/L	
Thyroxine					
Free (FT_4)	S	0.8–2.4 ng/dL	× 12.87	10–31 pmol/L	
Total (T_4)	S	Cord blood 8–13 μg/dL	× 12.87	103–168 nmol/L	
		Newborn 11.5–24 μg/dL (lower in low birthweight infants)		148–310 nmol/L	
		Neonate 9–18 μg/dL		116–232 nmol/L	
		Infant 7–15 μg/dL		90–194 nmol/L	
		1–5 yr 7.3–15 μg/dL		94–194 nmol/L	
		5–10 yr 6.4–13.3 μg/dL		83–172 nmol/L	
		Thereafter 5–12 μg/dL		65–155 nmol/L	
		Newborn screen (filter paper) 6.2–22 μg/dL		80–284 nmol	
Tourniquet test		<5–10 petechiae in 2.5-cm circle on forearm (halfway between systolic and diastolic); pressure maintained for 5 min		<5–10 petechiae in 2.5-cm circle on forearm (halfway between systolic and diastolic); pressure maintained for 5 min	
		0–8 petechiae in 6-cm circle (50 mm Hg for 15 min)		0–8 petechiae in 6-cm circle (50 mm Hg for 15 min)	
		10–20 petechiae in 5-cm circle (80 mm Hg)		10–20 petechiae in 5-cm circle (80 mm Hg)	

Table continued on following page

TABLE 27–2. Reference Ranges for Laboratory Tests *Continued*

Test	Specimen		Reference Range	Factor	Reference Range (SI)	Comments
Transcortin	S	M	1.5–2.0 mg/dL	× 10	15–20 mg/L	
		F				
		Follicular	1.7–2.0 mg/dL		17–20 mg/L	
		Luteal	1.6–2.1 mg/dL		16–21 mg/L	
		Postmenopausal	1.7–2.5 mg/dL		17–25 mg/L	
		Pregnancy				
		21–28 wk	4.7–5.4 mg/dL		47–54 mg/L	
		33–40 wk	5.5–7.0 mg/dL		55–70 mg/L	
Transferrin (siderophilin)	S	1–3 yr	218–347 mg/dL	× 0.01	2.18–3.47 g/L	n (Lockitch et al)
		4–9 yr	208–378 mg/dL		2.08–3.78 g/L	
		10–19 yr	224–444 mg/dL		2.24–4.44 g/L	
Triglycerides	S after ≥12-hr fast		*M mg/dL*; *F mg/dL*		*M g/L*; *F g/L*	
		Cord blood	10–98; 10–98	× 0.01	0.10–0.98; 0.10–0.98	
		0–5 yr	30–86; 32–99		0.30–0.86; 0.32–0.99	
		6–11 yr	31–108; 35–114		0.31–1.08; 0.35–1.14	
		12–15 yr	36–138; 41–138		0.36–1.38; 0.41–1.38	
		16–19 yr	40–163; 40–128		0.40–1.63; 0.40–1.28	
		20–29 yr	44–185; 40–128		0.44–1.85; 0.40–1.28	
		Adults: Recommended (desirable) levels			Adults: Recommended (desirable) levels	
		M	40–160 mg/dL		0.40–1.60 g/L	
		F	35–135 mg/dL		0.35–1.35 g/L	
Triiodothyronine						
Free	S	Cord blood	20–240 pg/dL	× 0.01536	0.3–3.7 pmol/L	
		1–3 d	200–610 pg/dL		3.1–9.4 pmol/L	
		6 wk	240–560 pg/dL		3.7–8.6 pmol/L	
		Adult (20–50 yr)	230–660 pg/dL		3.5–10.0 pmol/L	
Resin uptake test (T_3RU)	S	Newborn	26–36%	× 0.01	0.26–0.36 fractional uptake	
		Thereafter	26–35%		0.26–0.35 fractional uptake	
Total	S	Cord blood	30–70 ng/dL	× 0.0154	0.46–1.08 nmol/L	
		Newborn	75–260 ng/dL		1.16–4.00 nmol/L	
		1–5 yr	100–260 ng/dL		1.54–4.00 nmol/L	
		5–10 yr	90–240 ng/dL		1.39–3.70 nmol/L	
		10–15 yr	80–210 ng/dL		1.23–3.23 nmol/L	
		Thereafter	115–190 ng/dL		1.77–2.93 nmol/L	
Tyrosine	S	Premature	7.0–24.0 mg/dL	× 0.0552	0.39–1.32 mmol/L	
		Newborn	1.6–3.7 mg/dL		0.088–0.20 mmol/L	
		Adult	0.8–1.3 mg/dL		0.044–0.07 mmol/L	
Urea nitrogen	S, P	Cord blood	21–40 mg/dL	× 0.357	7.5–14.3 mmol urea/L	
		Premature (1 wk)	3–25 mg/dL		1.1–9 mmol urea/L	
		Newborn	3–12 mg/dL		1.1–4.3 mmol urea/L	
		Infant/child	5–18 mg/dL		1.8–6.4 mmol urea/L	
		Thereafter	7–18 mg/dL		2.5–6.4 mmol urea/L	
Uric acid	S	1–5 yr	1.7–5.8 mg/dL	× 59.48	100–350 μmol/L	z (Meites)
		6–11 yr	2.2–6.6 mg/dL		130–390 μmol/L	
		12–19 yr				
		M	3.0–7.7 mg/dL		180–460 μmol/L	
		F	2.7–5.7 mg/dL		160–340 μmol/L	
Urinary sediment. See Sediment						
Urine, volume	U (24-hr)	Newborn	50–300 mL/24 hr	× 0.001	0.050–0.300 L/24 hr	
		Infant	350–550 mL/24 hr		0.350–0.550 L/24 hr	
		Child	500–1,000 mL/24 hr		0.500–1.000 L/24 hr	
		Adolescent	700–1,400 mL/24 hr		0.700–1.400 L/24 hr	
		Thereafter				
		M	800–1,800 mL/24 hr		0.800–1.800 L/24 hr	
		F	600–1,600 mL/24 hr (varies with intake and other factors)		0.600–1.600 L/24 hr	
Valporic acid. See end of table under Drugs						
Vanillylmandelic acid (VMA)	U	0–1 yr	<18.8 mg/g creatinine	× 0.5709	<11 mmol/mol creatinine	p (Meites)
		2–4 yr	<11.0 mg/g creatinine		<6 mmol/mol creatinine	
		5–19 yr	<8.0 mg/g creatinine		<5 mmol/mol creatinine	
Vitamin A (retinol)	S	1–6 yr	20–43 μg/dL	× 0.0349	0.7–1.5 μmol/L	p (Lockitch et al)
		7–12 yr	25–48 μg/dL		0.9–1.7 μmol/L	
		13–19 yr	26–72 μg/dL		0.9–2.5 μmol/L	
Vitamin B. See Thiamine						
Vitamin B_2. See Riboflavin						

TABLE 27–2. Reference Ranges for Laboratory Tests *Continued*

Test	Specimen	Reference Range		Factor	Reference Range (SI)	Comments
Vitamin B_6	P(E)	3.6–18 ng/mL		× 4.046	14.6–72.8 nmol/L	
Vitamin B_{12}	S	Newborn Thereafter	175–800 pg/mL 140–700 pg/mL	× 0.738	129–590 pmol/L 103–157 pmol/L	
Vitamin C	P(O,H,E)		0.6–2.0 mg/dL	× 56.78	34–113 μmol/L	
Vitamin D_2, 25-hydroxy	P(H)	Summer Winter	15–80 ng/mL 14–42 ng/mL	× 2.496	37–200 nmol/L 35–105 nmol/L	
Vitamin D_3, 1,25-dihydroxy (calcitriol)	S		25–45 pg/mL	× 2.4	60–108 pmol/L	
Vitamin E (tocopherol)	S	1–6 yr 7–19 yr	3.0–9.0 mg/L 4.4–10.4 mg/L	× 2.32	7–21 μmol/L 10–24 μmol/L	p (Lockitch et al)
WBC. See Leukocytes						
Xylose absorption test (0.5 g/kg in H_2O 25 g)	S	Child (1 hr) Adult (2 hr)	>20 mg/dL >25 mg/dL	× 0.0667	>1.33 mmol/L >1.67 mmol/L	
	U (5-hr)	Child 16–33% of ingested dose		× 0.01	0.16–0.33 (fraction ingested dose)	
		Adult 5-g dose 25-g dose	 >1.2 g/5 hr >4.0 g/5 hr	× 6.66	 >8.00 mmol/5 hr >26.64 mmol/5 hr	
	S	70–150 μg/dL		× 0.153	10.7–22.9 μmol/L	
Zinc	S	1–19 yr	64–118 μg/dL	× 0.1530	9.8–18.1 μmol/L	a (Lockitch et al)
	U	5–18 yr	10.1–95.9 mg/mol creatinine	× 0.0153	0.15–1.47 mmol/mol creatinine	

		Reference Range					Reference Range				
		Peak		*Trough*			*SI Peak*		*SI Trough*		
Drugs *Antibiotics*	**Specimen**	*Therapeutic (μg/mL)*	*Toxic (μg/mL)*	*Therapeutic (μg/mL)*	*Toxic (μg/mL)*	***Factor***	*Therapeutic (μmol/L)*	*Toxic (μmol/L)*	*Therapeutic (μmol/L)*	*Toxic (μmol/L)*	**Comments**
Amikacin	S	20–25	>30	1–4	>8	× 1.708	34–43	>51	1.7–6.8	>14	xe (Taylor et al)
Chloramphenicol	S	10–20	>25			× 3.095	31–62	>77			e (Taylor et al)
Gentamicin	S	6–10	>12	0.5–2.0	>2.0	× 2.064	12–21	>25	1.0–4.1	>4.1	ex (Taylor et al)
Netilmicin	S	6–10	>12	0.5–2.0	>2	× 2.103	13–21	>25	1.1–4.2	>4.2	ex (Taylor et al)
Tobramycin	S	6–10	>12	0.5–2.0	>2	× 2.139	13–21	>26	1.1–4.3	>4.3	ex (Taylor et al)
Vancomycin	S	30–40	>60	5–10	>20	× 0.303	9.1–12.1	>18.2	1.5–3.0	>6.1	ex (Sylva Co.)

Other Drugs	Specimen	Reference Range		Factor	Reference Range (SI)	Comments
Acetaminophen	S, P(H,E)	Therap. conc. Toxic conc.	10–30 μg/mL >200 μg/mL	× 6.62	66–200 μmol/L >1,300 μmol/L	xz
Amphetamine	S, P(H,E)	Therap. conc. Toxic conc.	20–30 ng/mL >200 ng/mL	× 7.396	150–220 nmol/L >1,500 nmol/L	
Amitriptyline (includes nortriptyline)	S	Therap. conc.	100–250 ng/mL	× 1	Therap. conc. 100–250 μg/L	(Sylva Co.)
Nortriptyline (only)		Therap. conc.	50–150 ng/mL	× 1	Therap. conc. 50–150 μg/L	
Caffeine	S, P	Therap. conc. for neonatal apnea	5–20 μg/mL	× 5.150	26–103 μmol/L	e (Sylva Co.)
Carbamazepine	S, P(H,E) at trough	Therap. conc. Toxic conc.	8–12 μg/mL >15 μg/mL	× 4.233	34–51 μmol/L >63 μmol/L	ex (Sylva Co.)
Chloral hydrate	S	As trichloroethanol Therap. conc. Toxic conc.	 2–12 μg/mL >20 μg/mL	× 6.694	 13–80 μmol/L >134 μmol/L	
Diazepam	S, P(H,E) at trough	Therap. conc. Toxic conc.	100–1,000 ng/mL >5,000 ng/mL	× 3.512	350–3,500 nmol/L >17,500 nmol/L	
Digitoxin	S, P(H,E) (6-hr post)	Therap. conc. Toxic conc.	20–35 ng/mL >45 ng/mL	× 1.307	26–46 nmol/L >59 nmol/L	x
Digoxin	S, P(H,E) (12-hr post)	Therap. conc. CHF Arrhythmias Toxic conc. Child Adult	 0.8–1.5 ng/mL 1.5–2.0 ng/mL >2.5 ng/mL >3.0 ng/mL	× 1.281	 –1.9 nmol/L 1.9–2.6 nmol/L >3.2 nmol/L >3.8 nmol/L	xe

Table continued on following page

TABLE 27–2. Reference Ranges for Laboratory Tests *Continued*

Test	Specimen	Reference Range		Factor	Reference Range (SI)	Comments
Diphenylhydantoin	See Phenytoin					
Doxepin (includes desmethyldoxepine)	S, P	Therap. conc.	110–250 ng/mL	× 1	Therap. conc. 110–250 μg/L	(Sylva Co.)
Ethanol	W(O),S	Toxic conc. CNS depression	50–100 mg/dL >100 mg/dL	× 0.2171	11–22 mmol/L >22 mmol/L	
Ethosuximide	S, P(H,E) at trough	Therap. conc. Toxic conc.	40–100 μg/mL >150 μg/mL	× 7.084	280–700 μmol/L >1,060 μmol/L	xe
Imipramine (includes desipramine)	S	Therap. conc.	150–250 ng/mL	× 1	150–250 μg/L	e (Sylva Co.)
Lithium	S, P(not LiH)	12 hr after dose Therap. conc. Toxic conc.	 0.6–1.2 mmol/L >2 mmol/L	× 1	Therap. conc. 0.6–1.2 mmol/L Toxic conc. >2 mmol/L	
Lysergic acid diethylamide	 P(E) U	After hallucinogenic dose 0.005–0.009 μg/mL 0.001–0.050 μg/mL		× 3089	After hallucinogenic dose 15.5–27.8 nmol/L 3.1–155 nmol/L	
Methotrexate	S, P	After high-dose therapy Toxic >5 μmol/L at 24 hr Toxic >1 μmol/L at 48 hr		× 1	After high-dose therapy Toxic >5 μmol/L at 24 hr Toxic >1 μmol/L at 48 hr	e
Paraldehyde	S, P(H,E)	Therap. conc. Sedation Anesthesia Toxic conc. Lethal conc.	 10–100 μg/mL >200 μg/mL 20–40 μg/mL >50 μg/mL	× 7.567	 75–750 μmol/L >1,500 μmol/L 150–300 μmol/L >375 μmol/L	
Phenacetin	P(E)	Therap. conc. Toxic conc.	1–20 μg/mL 50–250 μg/mL	× 5.580	5.6–110 μmol/L 280–1,400 μmol/L	
Phenobarbital	S, P(H,E) at trough	Therap. conc. Toxic conc. Slowness, ataxia, nystagmus Coma with reflexes without reflexes	15–40 μg/mL 35–80 μg/mL 65–117 μg/mL >100 μg/mL	× 4.306	65–170 μmol/L 150–345 μmol/L 280–504 μmol/L >430 μmol/L	xe
Phensuximide (both parent and *N*-desmethyl metabolite)	S, P(H,E)	Therap. conc.	40–60 μg/mL	× 5.71	228–343 μmol/L	
Phenytoin	S, P(H,E)	Therap. conc.	10–20 μg/mL	× 3.964	40–80 μmol/L	
Primidone	S, P(H,E) at trough	Therap. conc. Toxic conc. Toxic (neonatal)	5–12 μg/mL >15 μg/mL >20 μg/mL	× 4.582	23–55 μmol/L >69 μmol/L >92 μmol/L	(Taylor and Caviness)
Procainamide	S, P(H,E)	Therap conc. Toxic conc. (also consider conc. of metabolite N-acetyl-procainamide [NAPA])	4–10 μg/mL >10–12 μg/mL	× 4.25	17–42 μmol/L 42–51 μmol/L	
Propranolol	S, P(H,E) at trough	Therap. conc.	50–100 ng/mL	× 3.856	190–380 nmol/L	
Quinidine	S, P(H,E)	Therap. conc. Toxic conc.	2–5 μg/mL >6 μg/mL	× 3.083	6.2–15.5 μmol/L >18.5 μmol/L	
Salicylate	S, P(H,E) at trough	Therap. conc. Toxic conc.	15–30 mg/dL >30 mg/dL	× 0.0724	1.1–2.2 mmol/L >2.2 mmol/L	
Theophylline	S, P(H,E)	Therap. conc., bronchodilator Premature apnea Toxic conc.	10–20 μg/mL 5–10 μg/mL >20 μg/mL	× 5.550	56–110 μmol/L 28–56 μmol/L >166 μmol/L	xz
Valproic acid	S, P(H,E) at trough	Therap. conc. Toxic conc.	50–100 μg/mL >100 μg/mL	× 6.934	350–700 μmol/L >700 μmol/L	

JOHN F. NICHOLSON
MICHAEL A. PESCE

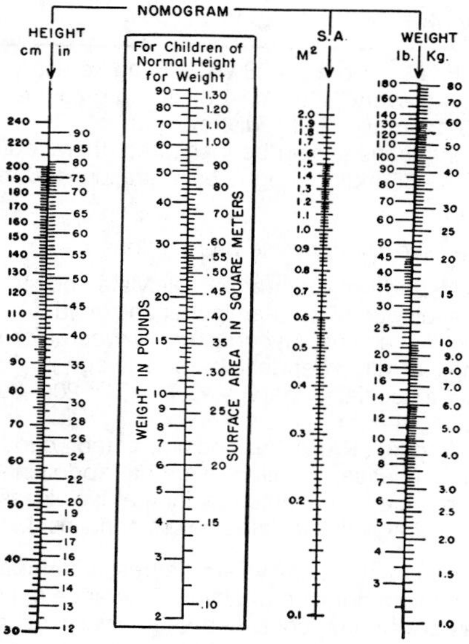

Figure 27–1. Nomogram for estimation of surface area. The surface area is indicated where a straight line that connects the height and weight levels intersects the surface area column; or the patient is roughly of average size, from the weight alone (*enclosed area*). (Nomogram modified from data of E. Boyd by C.D. West.)

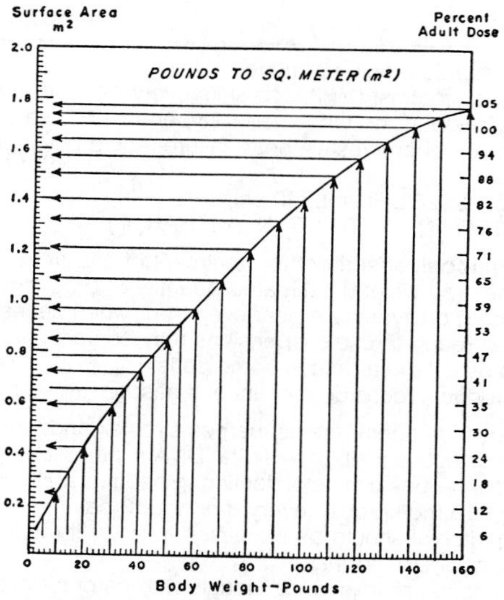

Figure 27–2. Relations between body weight in pounds, body surface area, and adult dosage. The surface area values correspond with those set forth by Crawford and associates (1950). Note that the 100% adult dose is for a patient weighing about 140 lb and having a surface area of about 1.7 m^2. (From Talbot NB, et al: Metabolic Homeostasis—A Syllabus for Those Concerned with the Care of Patients. Cambridge, Harvard University Press, 1959.)

TABLE 27–3 DRUG DOSAGES (Drugs Listed Alphabetically by Generic Name)

KEY:

NB	newborn (birth to end of 1st mo)
IN	infant (1–12 mo)
CH	child (1–12 yr)
AD	adult
caps	capsules
div	divided
D/W	dextrose in water
IM	intramuscular
inj	injection
IV	intravenous
LO	linguo-occlusal
ointm	ointment
PO	per os,oral
PR	per rectum
prn	pro re nata, when necessary
SC	subcutaneous
SL	sublingual
sol	solution
susp	suspension
tabl	tablets

†	available as generic preparation
‡	available also under other brand name(s)
g	gram
mg	milligram = 10^{-3} g
μg	microgram = 10^{-6} g (sometimes abbreviated mcg)
ng	nanogram = 10^{-9} g
kg	kilogram = 10^3 g
mL	milliliter = 10^{-3} liter ≃ cm^3 = cc (cubic centimeter)
℞	prescription

Acetaminophen, paracetamol, APAP, NAPAP
℞ antipyretic, analgesic: IN, CH = PO: 60 mg/kg/24 hr, div, every 4–6 hr, prn
†, LIQUIPRIN, TYLENOL, ‡; tabl, liquid preparations
Caution: Massive overdose may cause hepatic necrosis through formation of a toxic metabolite. Lesser overdoses frequently cause reversible jaundice (Sec. 26.5).

Acetazolamide, carbonic anhydrase inhibitor
℞ as adjunct in the treatment of convulsive disorders (ketotic effect): CH = PO: 8–30 mg/kg/24 hr, div, every 6–8 hr
†, DIAMOX; tabl

Acetylcysteine, mucolytic agent; detoxifying agent in acetaminophen overdose
℞ to loosen tenacious bronchial secretions by local application to the bronchial tree with nebulizer: 3–5 mL 20% sol diluted with equal volume of sterile water or saline, or 6–10 mL of 10% sol, every 6-8 hr; or by direct instillation: 1–2 mL of 10% or 20% sol every 1–4 hr
℞ in acetaminophen overdose: IN, CH, AD = PO: 140 mg/kg/1st dose, followed by 70 mg/kg/dose every 4 hr for a total of 72 hr
MUCOMYST; vials 10% (100 mg/mL) or 20% (200 mg/mL)

Acetylsalicylic acid, ASA
℞ antipyretic, analgesic, anti-inflammatory: IN, CH = PO: 30–65 mg/kg/24 hr, div, every 4–6 hr, prn. This dosage corresponds to 27–58 mg salicylate sodium/kg/24 hr, or 20–50 mg salicylic acid/kg/24 hr
℞ antirheumatic: CH = PO: 65–130 mg/kg/24 hr, div, every 4–6 hr
†, ASPIRIN, BUFFERIN, ‡: tabl; also contained in many combination products
Caution: Acute or chronic overdose may cause life-threatening poisoning syndrome (Sec. 6.23 and 26.6).

Table continued on following page

TABLE 27–3 Drug Dosages *Continued*

ACTH, adrenocorticotropic hormone
℞ of infantile spasms: IM: 24–40 units every 12 hr, or 2.5–4.0 units/kg every 12 hr. Observe for hypertension, use with caution in presence of congestive heart failure, acute psychosis, ocular herpes
10 units/mL, 20 units/mL, 40 units/mL vials
CORTICOTROPIN, CORTROSYN, ACTHAR; inj

Activated charcoal, adsorbent for treatment of oral drug overdose
PO: 10 times (by weight) estimated quantity of drug ingested or 0.25–1 g/kg orally; may repeat every 4 hr when necessary
Commercial ready-to-use suspensions may contain sorbitol, which induces osmotic diarrhea in some patients
Multiple products, consider continuous nasogastric administration

Acyclovir, antiviral agent against herpes simplex and varicella-zoster virus by selective inhibition of viral DNA synthesis
℞ in clinical herpes simplex infection in neonates: NB = IV (over 60 min): 10 mg/kg/dose every 8 hr, for 10 days
Dosing interval should be increased to 24 hr if renal function is less than 25% of normal
℞ in immunocompromised individuals with herpes simplex or varicella-zoster virus infection: CH = IV (over 60 min): 250 mg/m²/dose every 8 hr; AD = IV (over 60 min): 5 mg/kg/dose every 8 hr
℞ in severe first episode of herpes genitalis: CH, AD = LO: 5% ointm
ZOVIRAX; inj, ointm

Albuterol, catecholamine analog; β-adrenergic receptor agonist with preferential effect on β_2-adrenergic receptors
℞ bronchodilator: CH = PO: 0.1 mg/kg, div, every 8 hr; 6–12 yr, 2 mg 3–4 times/24 hr; nebulization 0.01–0.03 mL/kg of 5 mg/mL solution. See bronchodilator aerosols below.
VENTOLIN, PROVENTIL; tab, liquid, inhalation

Allopurinol, analogue of hypoxanthine; inhibitor of xanthine oxidase and thereby of the terminal steps of uric acid biosynthesis
℞ against hyperuricemia and urate deposition in tissues and kidneys, especially in patients receiving antineoplastic chemotherapy: CH = PO: 10 mg/kg/24 hr, div or in single daily dose. Note that allopurinol and its metabolite alloxanthine (oxypurinol) inhibit xanthine oxidase, and that reduced glomerular filtration requires lowering the dose to compensate for delayed excretion. A high urine output should be established—with a neutral or slightly alkaline urine pH—to allow for excretion of uric acid precursors.
Caution: If azathioprine or mercaptopurine, which are metabolized by xanthine oxidase, are to be given concomitantly with allopurinol, the dosage of azathioprine or mercaptopurine should be reduced substantially (to ¼–⅓ of usual dosage).
†, ZYLOPRIM; tabl

Aluminum hydroxide, antacid
℞ for treatment of peptic ulcer: CH = PO: 5–15 mL/dose every 3–6 hr, or 1 and 3 hr after meals and at bedtime
℞ for prophylaxis of gastrointestinal bleeding:
IN = PO (by nasogastric tube): 2–5 mL every 1–2 hr
CH = PO (by nasogastric tube): 5–15 mL every 1–2 hr
℞ against hyperphosphatemia: IN, CH = PO: 50–150 mg/kg/24 hr, div, every 4–6 hr
Note: May cause constipation, aluminum toxicity, phosphorus depletion. Inhibits gastric emptying. Interferes with absorption of tetracyclines
†, AMPHOJEL; susp (320 mg/5 mL), tabl (300 mg, 600 mg), gel liquid (600 mg/5 mL)

Aluminum hydroxide and **magnesium hydroxide,** antacid
Note: Magnesium-containing antacids are laxative. In renal failure, magnesium and aluminum may be retained. Interferes with absorption of tetracyclines
℞ for treatment of peptic ulcer: same as for aluminum hydroxide alone.
†, MAALOX, ‡; susp, tabl

Amikacin, sulfate, antimicrobial aminoglycoside effective primarily against gram-negative micro-organisms.
NB <7 days or <28 wk = IM, IV (over 20–30 min): 7.5 mg/kg once daily; 28–34 wk, 7.5 mg/kg every 18 hr; >34 wk, 7.5 mg/kg every 12 hr; NB >7 days <28 wk, 7.5 mg/kg every 18 hr; 28–34 wk, 7.5 mg/kg every 12 hr; >34 wk, 7.5 mg/kg every 8 hr
IN, CH = 15–20 mg/kg/24 hr, div, every 8 hr
Serum concentrations should be monitored; therapeutic peak concentration 25–35 mg/L, trough concentration <10 mg/L (see Table 27–2).

Aminophylline. See Theophylline preparations.

Aminosalicylate sodium, para-aminosalicylate sodium, PAS sodium; structural analogue of para-aminobenzoic acid with weak bacteriostatic activity against *Mycobacterium tuberculosis,* used only in combination with other antituberculous agents
℞ as adjunct to isoniazid therapy: CH = PO: 200–300 mg/kg/24 hr, div, every 4–6 hr
†, PAMISYL-Sodium, PARASAL-Sodium, ‡; tabl, caps
Note: Frequent nausea, vomiting, diarrhea, abdominal pain, and poor acceptance by patients restrict the usefulness of this substance. 1 g of aminosalicylate sodium contains 4.7 mEq Na^+.

Amobarbital, central nervous system depressant of barbiturate class with intermediate duration of action. Tolerance to its hypnotic effect may develop on continued use. Initially, hypnotic effect lasts 3–8 hr
℞ for sedation: IN, CH = PO, IM: 1–2 mg/kg/24 hr, div, every 6 hr
℞ for sleep: IN, CH = PO, IM: 2–3 mg/kg/dose, repeat prn after 12–24 hr
†, AMYTAL; tabl, elixir amobarbital sodium, †, AMYTAL sodium; inj, caps

Amoxicillin, acid-resistant ampicillin congener
IN, CH = PO: 20–40 mg/kg/24 hr, div, every 8 hr
†, AMOXIL, LAROTID; ‡, caps, oral susp, pediatric drops

Amoxicillin + clavulanic acid; combination of a β-lactam antibiotic with a β-lactamase (penicillinase) inhibitor. The addition of clavulanic acid extends the activity of amoxicillin from Group A and other streptococci, *Streptococcus pneumoniae,* many strains of *Escherichia coli* and *Proteus mirabilis*, non–β-lactamase-producing strains of staphylococci, *Neisseria gonorrhoeae,* and *Haemophilus influenzae* to include β-lactamase–producing strains of *H. influenzae, E. coli, P. mirabilis* as well as *Klebsiella pneumoniae, Staphylococcus aureus* (but not methicillin-resistant strains), *Moraxella catarrhalis, Bacteroides fragilis,* and *Legionella pneumophila. Pseudomonas aeruginosa,* many strains of *Serratia,* and *Enterobacter* are resistant.
℞ for otitis media, sinusitis, lower respiratory tract, skin, soft tissue, and urinary tract infections: CH = PO: amoxicillin 20–40 mg/kg/24 hr + clavulanic acid 5–10 mg/kg/24 hr, div, every 8 hr
Note: May cause diarrhea, abdominal pain, urticaria and other rashes, due possibly to clavulanic acid alone. Amoxicillin is available as single component.
AUGMENTIN; tabl of 2 strengths: 250 mg amoxicillin + 125 mg clavulanic acid, and 500 mg amoxicillin + 125 mg clavulanic acid; oral susp with amoxicillin 125 mg + clavulanic acid 31.25 mg/5 mL, or amoxicillin 250 mg + clavulanic acid 62.5 mg/5 mL

Amphotericin B; antifungal agent of the "polyene" type (nystatin, another example); insoluble in water, unstable below pH 4, should be given IV. Effective through binding to sterol components of the membrane of sensitive fungi, thereby altering its permeability; interference with renal function of patients seems an extension of the mode of action of this drug, demanding caution and continued monitoring during amphotericin B therapy.
Owing to potential toxicity for a variety of biologic functions, amphotericin B should be used only in progressive and potentially fatal infections with fungi sensitive to it.
Use as solution of amphotericin B at concentration of 0.1 mg/mL in 5% dextrose (all other drugs, including antimicrobial agents, and electrolytes must be kept away from the colloidal suspension of amphotericin B).
See Sec. 9.75 and 12.103 for dose and administration. Optimal dose and duration of therapy not clearly determined.
Available as lyophilized powder containing sodium deoxycholate as emulsifier. Colloidal suspension prepared by adding required volume of sterile water and shaking appropriately, subsequently diluted in 5% sterile dextrose in water to a final concentration of

TABLE 27–3 Drug Dosages *Continued*

amphotericin B of 0.1 mg/mL, for slow IV administration; FUNGIZONE intravenous; inj

Ampicillin; acid-resistant penicillin congener effective against many gram-positive and gram-negative organisms. Drug is effectively destroyed by β-lactamase.
NB <7 days <2,000 g = IV (over 15–30 min), IM: 50 mg/kg/24 hr, div, every 12 hr; >2,000 g, div, every 8 hr
NB >7 days <2,000 g = IV (over 15–30 min), IM: 100 mg/kg/24 hr, div, every 8 hr; >2,000 g, div, every 6 hr
℞ for septicemia: IV: 100–200 mg/kg/24 hr, div, every 4 hr
IN, CH = PO: 50–100 mg/kg/24 hr, div, every 4–6 hr
℞ for meningitis: IV (over 15–30 min) 200–400 mg/kg/24 hr, div, every 4 hr (usual maximum: 12 g/24 hr)
Other infections: 100–200 mg/kg/24 hr, div, every 4–6 hr
ampicillin sodium, for injection, OMNIPEN-N, PENBRITIN-S, ‡; inj
ampicillin trihydrate, †, OMNIPEN, PENBRITIN, ‡; caps, oral susp, pediatric drops

Ampicillin/sulbactam; combination of a β-lactam antibiotic with a β-lactamase (penicillinase) inhibitor. The addition of sulbactam extends the activity of ampicillin to include β-lactamase–producing strains of *H. influenzae, E. coli, P. mirabilis, K. pneumoniae, S. aureus* (but not methicillin-resistant strains), *Moraxella catarrhalis, B. fragilis,* and *Legionella pneumophila* (see Amoxicillin + clavulanic acid, above)

Atenolol; synthetic, relatively selective β_1-(cardioselective) adrenoreceptor blocking agent that possesses no membrane-stabilizing or intrinsic sympathomimetic effects. B_1-Antagonist properties are relative, and at higher doses atenolol inhibits β_2-adrenoreceptors, which are chiefly located in the bronchial and vascular musculature.
IN, CH = PO: 1.0–1.3 mg/kg/24 hr, once daily or div, every 12 hr
TENORMIN; inj, tabl

Atropine sulfate, *dl*-hyoscyamine; anticholinergic agent used mainly in premedication for anesthesia, as antiarrhythmic agent and as antispasmodic. Dosage varies according to indications and sensitivity of patients. On the average for IN, CH = SC, PO (IV): 0.01 mg/kg/dose, to be repeated prn after 2 hr until desired effect is obtained or adverse effects preclude further increase; for continued ℞: PO: 0.04 mg/kg/24 hr, div, every 6 hr, preferably with meals. Much higher doses may be necessary in the management of insecticide (acetylcholinesterase inhibitor) intoxication.
†; inj, tabl
Caution: As for belladonna, below.

Azathioprine; an imidazolyl derivative of 6-mercaptopurine and immunosuppressive antimetabolite. The drug is cleaved in the body to mercaptopurine. Both compounds are pharmacologically active.
CH = PO: 3–5 mg/kg/24 hr once daily. Maintenance dose usually 1–3 mg/kg/24 hr administered once daily.
Note: Limited experience for treatment of children with rheumatoid arthritis. The primary metabolic pathway for azathioprine is via xanthine oxidase, which is inhibited by allopurinol. Patients receiving concurrent allopurinol should have azathioprine dose reduced to approximately ⅓ to ¼ the usual dose.
IMURAN; inj, tabl

Aztreonan, monobactam antibiotic that possesses a unique monocyclic β-lactam nucleus that is effective against a wide spectrum of gram-negative aerobic pathogens.
NB <7 days old <2,000 g: 60 mg/kg/24 hr, div, every 12 hr; <7 days >2,000 g: 90 mg/kg/24 hr, div, every 8 hr; >7 days <2,000 g: 90 mg/kg/24 hr, div, every 8 hr; >2,000 g, 120 mg/kg/24 hr, every 6 hr; NB administration is IV for 15–20 min or IM
IN, CH = IV, IM: 90–120 mg/kg/24 hr, div, every 6–8 hr
AZACTAM; inj

Beclomethasone diproprionate, chlorinated synthetic corticosteroid
℞ topical treatment to the bronchial tissues in long-term, steroid-dependent asthma. Delivered from metered-dose aerosol unit, releasing approximately 50 μg beclomethasone by activation of the dispenser unit: CH (6–12 yr): 1–2 inhalations every 6–8 hr. Effect usually apparent within 1–4 wk after beginning of steroid inhalations
Caution: On transfer from systemic steroid therapy for asthma to inhalation therapy, adrenocortical competency of the patient must be watched and supported, if indicated, since inhalation therapy does not contribute to systemic corticosteroid supply.
VANCERIL inhaler

Belladonna tincture, aqueous-alcoholic extract of belladonna leaves; anticholinergic preparation; used chiefly as antispasmodic
Contains the equivalent of approximately 0.3 mg atropine sulfate/mL. Usual dose: 1 drop/4.5 kg (10 lb) body weight 15–30 min before meals, 3 times/day
Caution: Erythematous skin, persistently dilated pupils, or tachycardia are indications for discontinuing, then lowering dose. Extreme hypersensitivity may exist in patients with Down syndrome.

Bisacodyl, cathartic, structurally related to phenolphthalein
℞ laxative: PO: 0.3 mg/kg/dose, 6–8 hr before desired large bowel action. *Note:* tablets are enteric-coated and should be swallowed whole, with the added precaution of avoiding oral antacids or milk within at least 1 hr of ingestion.
DULCOLAX; tabl, suppos

Brompheniramine maleate; alkylamine; antihistamine with mild anticholinergic and mild sedative effects
℞ antiallergic effect: CH = PO: 0.5 mg/kg/24 hr, div, every 6 hr
†, DIMETANE; elixir, tabl, inj

Bronchodilator aerosols
℞ in acute asthmatic attack, provided effective inhalation is possible (e.g., in early stages of attack or with assisted ventilation [IPPB] or as continuous nebulization. Effectiveness of a delivered dose depends on microdispersion in the aerosol generated from different types of nebulizers, breathing mechanics, and patient minute ventilation. Onset of effect usually occurs within 2–5 min after inhalation of aerosol. Risk of self-overuse or overdosage in children is high with aerosol preparations, particularly in emergency situations. These limitations apply to all bronchodilator aerosols (epinephrine, racemic epinephrine, isoproterenol, metaproterenol, isoetharine, albuterol), some of which can be dispensed from "metered" nebulization nozzles, and products for use in adults. Patients and their families should be warned against over self-medication from home aerosol preparations. Nevertheless, aerosol/nebulization of selective β_2-agonist bronchodilating drugs can be a safe, highly effective means of reversing acute airways bronchoconstriction.

Bumetanide, saluretic with a duration of action of approximately 2 hr when administered IV. Bumetanide inhibits sodium reabsorption in the ascending limb of the loop of Henle ("loop diuretic"), inhibits chloride and sodium reabsorption, and interferes with concentration of urine. One milligram of bumetanide possesses a diuretic potency equivalent to approximately 40 mg of furosemide.
IN, CH = PO, IV, IM: 0.01–0.02 mg/kg/dose; if needed may be repeated at intervals of 4–8 hr
BUMEX; tabl, inj

Caffeine, CNS stimulant and vasoconstrictor of cerebral vessels
℞ against vascular headache and as an analeptic: CH = PO: 10 mg/kg/24 hr, div, prn every 4–6 hr; single dose usually 2–3 mg/kg/dose.
℞ against neonatal apnea; loading dose 10 mg/kg followed by maintenance therapy 2.5–5 mg/kg/24 hr, div, every 12–24 hr
Note: Above dosages should be doubled if citrated caffeine preparation is used. Serum concentrations may be monitored; therapeutic concentrations are 8–11 mg/L. In newborn, because caffeine elimination is markedly diminished compared with adult (including parturient women), transplacentally acquired blood concentrations of caffeine are maintained within a possibly effective range for several days after delivery. Danger of toxic manifestations owing to accumulation exists if additional caffeine is administered without appropriate dose adjustment.

Table continued on following page

TABLE 27–3 Drug Dosages *Continued*

Calcium gluconate $[CH_2OH(CHOH)_4COO]_2Ca \cdot H_2O$
1 g equivalent to 89 mg elemental calcium or to 4.46 mEq Ca^{2+}. Solution "10%" contains 100 mg/mL of calcium gluconate. This concentration equivalent to elemental calcium, 8.9 mg/mL or Ca^{2+} 0.45 mEq/mL.
℞ to compensate for manifestations of hypocalcemia (tetany, seizures, myocardial insufficiency, hypoparathyroidism). Urgency and severity of clinical situation dictate dose and route of administration: IN, CH = IV (infused slowly, with monitoring of heart for bradycardia, arrest): "10%" calcium gluconate solution: 1–2 mL/kg/dose, equivalent to Ca 0.45–0.90 mEq/kg/dose, repeat prn after 6 hr. Daily dose needed might be as high as Ca 2.7 mEq/kg/24 hr.
Caution: Do not use any calcium preparation for intramuscular injection because of risk of sterile abscess formation. Extravascular leakage may cause local necrosis.
IN, CH = PO: calcium gluconate 500 mg/kg/24 hr, equivalent to elemental calcium 45 mg/kg/24 hr or Ca^{2+} 2.3 mEq/kg/24 hr, div, every 4–8 hr
Note: Concomitant oral intake of phosphate exerts a major influence on the amount of calcium made available for absorption in the intestine.
†, powder, tabl

Calcium lactate $[CH_3CHOHCOO]_2Ca \cdot 5H_2O$
1 g of Ca lactate equivalent to 130 mg elemental calcium or to 6.49 mEq Ca^{2+}.
IN, CH = PO: 500 mg/kg/24 hr, equivalent to elemental calcium 65 mg/kg/24 hr or Ca^{2+} 3.2 mEq/kg/24 hr, div, every 4–8 hr
Note: Concomitant oral intake of phosphate exerts major influence on amount of calcium available for absorption in intestine. To ensure appropriate absorption in neonatal transient hypoparathyroidism, a calcium:phosphorus ratio of 4:1 (by weight, corresponding to 3:1 on molar basis) should be achieved in the feeding. This would require 10 g calcium lactate powder added to a daily formula containing 500 mL of whole cow's milk.
†, powder, tabl

Captopril, competitive inhibitor of angiotensin I–converting enzyme, antihypertensive agent, congestive heart failure
℞ for cardiovascular response: NB = PO: 0.1–0.4 mg/kg/dose administered every 6–24 hr; IN = PO: 0.5–0.6 mg/kg/24 hr, div, every 6–12 hr; CH = PO: 0.15 mg/kg every 4–8 hr. Dose may be slowly increased to desired effect
Note: May cause renal impairment, neutropenia, immunodeficiency, rashes, and disturbances of taste. Adjust dose with renal failure. Limited experience in children.
CAPOTEN; tabl

Carbamazepine, anticonvulsant agent; structurally related to tricyclic antidepressants
IN, CH = PO: initially 10 mg/kg/24 hr, div, every 8–12 hr; to be increased progressively, if needed, to 20 mg/kg/24 hr, div, every 12 hr or as a single daily dose, if tolerated. Usual maintenance dose range 20–30 mg/kg/24 hr
Note: Carbamazepine is a potent inducer of hepatic microsomal metabolizing enzymes that may stimulate the metabolism of numerous other drugs metabolized via the liver.
TEGRETOL; tabl, chew tabl, susp

Carbenicillin disodium; semisynthetic penicillin susceptible to destruction by penicillinase
℞ for systemic use: NB = IV (over 15–30 min), IM: initial dose 100 mg/kg, followed by maintenance therapy according to the following criteria:
≤2000 g + ≤7 days old: 225 mg/kg/24 hr, div, every 8 hr
≤2000 g + >7 days old: 400 mg/kg/24 hr, div, every 6 hr
>2000 g + ≤7 days old: 300 mg/kg/24 hr, div, every 6 hr
>2000 g + >7 days old: 400 mg/kg/24 hr, div, every 6 hr
IN, CH = IV (over 15–30 min), IM: 400–600 mg/kg/24 hr, div, every 4 hr (IV) or every 6 hr (IM). IM injection is painful. GEOPEN; inj; 1 g carbenicillin disodium contains 5.3 mEq Na^+
℞ for treatment of urinary tract infection only: CH = PO: 10–30 mg/kg/24 hr, div, every 6 hr carbenicillin indanyl sodium, GEOCILLIN; tabl

Carbinoxamine maleate, ethanolamine; antihistamine with mild anticholinergic effect and low incidence of sedation and drowsiness
℞ antiallergic effect: IN, CH = PO: 0.6 mg/kg/24 hr, div, every 6 hr
RONDEC; liquid, tabl, oral drops; component of many combination products

Cascara sagrada aromatic fluid extract; contains anthraquinones as active ingredients
℞ laxative: IN = PO: 1–2 mL/dose; CH = PO: 2–8 mL/dose

Cephalosporins, semisynthetic derivatives of 7-amino cephalosporanic acid, structurally related to penicillins
a. **First-generation cephalosporins:** active against most gram-positive cocci (excluding enterococci and methicillin-resistant *Staphylococcus aureus*), some strains of *Escherichia coli, Klebsiella pneumoniae,* and *Proteus mirabilis*
Note: First-generation drugs do not cross the blood-brain barrier and thus are ineffective for treatment of infections within the central nervous system.
Cefadroxil: relatively resistant against β-lactamases; absorption appears unaffected by food intake; minimal inhibitory concentrations for *E. coli, P. mirabilis, Klebsiella* species may be maintained in urine for about 20 hr after single dose
℞ CH = PO: 30 mg/kg/24 hr, div, every 12 hr
DURICEF, ULTRACEF; caps, powder for oral susp
Cefazolin sodium: NB = IV (over 15–30 min), IM: 40 mg/kg/24 hr, div, every 12 hr; IN, CH = IV (over 15–30 min), IM: 50–100 mg/kg/24 hr, div, every 6 hr
ANCEF, KEFZOL; inj
Cephalexin: IN, CH = PO: 25–50 mg/kg/24 hr, div, every 6 hr
KEFLEX; inj
Cephalothin: NB = IV (over 15–30 min), IM: ≤ 7 days old: 40 mg/kg/24 hr, div, every 12 hr; >7 days old: 60 mg/kg/24 hr, div, every 8 hr; IN, CH = IV: 80–160 mg/kg/24 hr, div, every 4 hr
KEFLIN; inj
Cephapirin sodium: CH = IV, IM: 40–80 mg/kg/24 hr, div, every 6 hr
CEFADYL; inj
Cephradine: CH = PO: 50–100 mg/kg/24 hr, div, every 6 hr; IV, IM: 50–100–300 mg/kg/24 hr, div, every 6 hr
ANSPOR, VELOSEF; caps, oral susp, inj
b. **Second-generation cephalosporins:** more active against gram-negative bacteria such as *Haemophilus influenzae* type b, *Neisseria gonorrhoeae,* and enteric gram-negative bacilli
Note: Some second-generation cephalosporins cross the blood-brain barrier and may be effective for treatment of bacterial meningitis. See later.
Cefaclor: effective against some β-lactamase–producing ampicillin-resistant strains of *H. influenzae*; absorption not affected by food intake.
℞ for treatment of otitis media and infections of the upper and lower respiratory tracts, urinary tract, skin, and soft tissues with susceptible organisms: IN, CH = PO: 20–40 mg/kg/24 hr, div, every 8 hr
CECLOR: powder for oral susp, caps
Cefamandole: IN, CH = IV, IM: 50–150 mg/kg/24 hr, div, every 4–6 hr
Note: May cause rash neutropenia, and cross-reaction with penicillin. Adjust dose with renal disease. Cefamandole does not effectively cross into the central nervous system and should not be used in the treatment of bacterial meningitis.
MANDOL; vials, plastic bags, inj
Cefoxitin: IN(>3 mo old), CH = IV, IM: 80–160 mg/kg/24 hr, div, every 4–6 hr
MEFOXIN; vials, infusion bottles, inj
Cefuroxime: IN (>3 month old), CH: IV, IM: 50–100 mg/kg/24 hr, div, every 6–8 hr
℞ in bacterial meningitis: IN, CH = IV: 200–240 mg/kg/24 hr, div, every 6–8 hr
ZINACEF; vials, infusion bottles, inj; tabs

TABLE 27–3 Drug Dosages *Continued*

c. **Third-generation cephalosporins:** less active against gram-positive cocci than older cephalosporins but more active against most strains of enteric gram-negative bacilli (except *Clostridium difficile*), moderately active against *Pseudomonas aeruginosa*, highly active against *H. influenzae* and *N. gonorrhoeae*.

Ceftriaxone sodium: biliary and renal excretion.

℞ misc. infection 50–75 mg/kg/12–24 hr (not to exceed 2 g) divided every 12 hr; meningitis 80–100 mg/kg/24 hr (not to exceed 4 g) divided every 12 hr.

Cefotaxime sodium: NB <7 days old IV, IM 100 mg/kg/24 hr, div, every 12 hr; >7 days old, 150 mg/kg/24 hr, div, every 8 hr; IN, CH = IV, IM: 100–200 mg/kg/24 hr, div, every 6–8 hr

℞ in bacterial meningitis: 200 mg/kg/24 hr, div, every 6 hr

Note: May cause hypersensitivity reactions in penicillin-sensitive patients. Adjust dose in patients with renal failure.

CLAFORAN; vials, inj

Ceftazidime: possesses antipseudomonal activity

NB = IV, IM: <7 days <2,000 g, 100 mg/kg/24 hr, div, every 12 hr; >2,000 g, 100 mg/kg/24 hr, div, every 8 hr; >7 days, 100–150 mg/kg/24 hr, div, every 8 hr

IN, CH = IV, IM: 100–150 mg/kg/24 hr, div, every 8 hr (meningitis, 150 mg/kg/24 hr, div, every 8 hr)

FORTAZ; TAZIDIME; inj

Ceftizoxime: not metabolized, excreted unchanged by the kidneys. Limited data on safety and effectiveness in children.

CEFIZOX; vials, inj

Moxalactam (lamoxactam): not metabolized, almost entirely excreted by kidneys; effective against *H. influenzae*

IN, CH = IV, IM: 150 mg/kg/24 hr, div, every 6–8 hr

℞ in neonatal meningitis: NB = IV: initial dose of 100 mg/kg, followed by 100 mg/kg/24 hr in NB 1–7 days old, div, every 12 hr; and 150 mg/kg/24 hr in NB 8–28 days old, div, every 8 hr

Note: Can interfere with hemostasis through three different mechanisms: hypoprothrombinemia, platelet dysfunction, or immune-mediated thrombocytopenia, resulting in bleeding. Local irritation after IM injection and phlebitis from IV administration are common.

MOXAM; vials, inj

Cefixime: orally available agent effective against many gram-positive and gram-negative organisms; possesses no antistaphylococcal or antipseudomonal activity

IN, CH = PO: 8 mg/kg/24 hr, div every 12–24 hr (max: 400 mg/24 hr)

SUPRAX; liquid, tabl

Chloral hydrate; trichloro derivative of acetaldehyde; tolerance to its hypnotic effect may develop

℞ for sedation: IN, CH = PO: 25 mg/kg/24 hr, div, every 6–8 hr

℞ for sleep: IN, CH = PO, (PR): 25–75 mg/kg/dose, (maximum total daily dose: 1.5–2.0 g/24 hr)

†, NOCTEC, SOMNOS, ‡; elixir, syrup, suppos

Chloramphenicol; derivative of dichloracetic acid combined to a structure containing a nitrobenzene ring

NB = IV (over 15–30 min), PO:

≤ 14 days old, regardless of weight: 25 mg/kg/24 hr, div, every 12 hr

15–30 days old and ≤2,000 g: 25 mg/kg/24 hr, div, every 4 hr

15–30 days old and >2,000 g: 50 mg/kg/24 hr, div, every 4 hr

IN, CH = PO: 50–100 mg/kg/24 hr, div, every 6 hr; IV (over 15–30 min): 100 mg/kg/24 hr, div, every 4 hr

Caution: Newborn infants are susceptible to development of high blood levels and gray-baby syndrome on usual doses; therefore, careful monitoring (of blood levels, if available) is mandatory. Dose-duration–related suppression of erythrocyte production is reversible; weekly hematocrit or hemoglobin and reticulocyte count are mandatory. Idiosyncratic aplastic anemia occasionally occurs without warning and may be lethal. Use only when specifically indicated. Monitor serum concentrations; in NB may be desirable to quantitate succinate concentration.

CHLOROMYCETIN; caps chloramphenicol palmitate, CHLOROMYCETIN palmitate; oral susp chloramphenicol sodium succinate, CHLOROMYCETIN sodium succinate; inj

Chloroquine, a 4-aminoquinoline antimalarial agent; drug of choice for the treatment of attacks of malaria caused by *Plasmodium vivax, P. ovale, P. malariae,* and susceptible strains of *P. falciparum*. Not advised for use in treatment of juvenile rheumatoid arthritis.

℞ oral treatment of uncomplicated attacks (excluding those caused by chloroquine-resistant *P. falciparum*):

Chloroquine diphosphate: CH = PO:

first day: 25 mg/kg/first 24 hr (equivalent to base: 15 mg/kg/first 24 hr), div in initial dose of 16.5 mg/kg (equivalent to base 10 mg/kg) and subsequent dose of 8.5 mg/kg (equivalent to base 5 mg/kg) 6 hr later;

second and third days: 8.5 mg/kg/24 hr (equivalent to base 5 mg/kg/24 hr), as single daily dose

℞ intramuscular treatment of severe illness (excluding malaria caused by chloroquine-resistant *P. falciparum*):

Chloroquine dihydrochloride: CH = IM: 6 mg/kg/dose (equivalent to base 5 mg/kg/dose), every 12 hr, until clinical response is obtained and treatment can be completed by the oral route

℞ clinical prophylaxis of malaria (prevention of clinical manifestations from infection with any of the *Plasmodium* species):

Chloroquine diphosphate: CH = PO: 8.5 mg/kg/dose (equivalent to base 5 mg/kg/dose) once every 7 days, beginning 2 wk before entering the malarious area and continuing for 8 wk after return. For eradication of *P. vivax* and *P. ovale,* treatment for 14 days with primaquine should be considered on leaving malarious area.

chloroquine diphosphate, ARALEN diphosphate, (RESOCHIN) diphosphate, tabl; chloroquine dihydrochloride, ARALEN dihydrochloride, inj; (1 mg chloroquine base is equivalent to 1.65 mg chloroquine diphosphate or 1.2 mg chloroquine dihydrochloride)

Caution: Irreversible retinal damage may occur with prolonged use; frequent ophthalmologic examination necessary to detect early changes. *Note:* Chloroquine does *not* cause hemolysis in individuals with G-6-PD deficiency

Chlorothiazide; saluretic, inhibiting sodium reabsorption and interfering with dilution of urine

IN, CH = PO: 20 mg/kg/24 hr, div, every 12 hr

†, DIURIL; tabl, oral susp

Chlorpheniramine maleate; alkylamine; antihistamine with anticholinergic and mild sedative effects

℞ antiallergic effect: CH = PO: 0.35 mg/kg/24 hr, div, every 6 hr

†, CHLORTRIMETON, ‡; tabl, syrup, inj

Chlorpromazine; phenothiazine with aliphatic side chain

℞ for sedation: CH = PO: 2 mg/kg/24 hr, div, every 4–6 hr, prn; IM, slow IV: 2 mg/kg/24 hr

†THORAZINE; suppos; chlorpromazine hydrochloride, THORAZINE hydrochloride; tabl, syrup, inj

Caution: Overdose may produce parkinsonian syndrome. Diphenhydramine may be antidotal

Chlortetracycline; see Tetracyclines

Chlorthalidone; nonthiazide saluretic with protracted duration of action

CH = PO: 1–2 mg/kg/24 hr, as single dose;

†HYGROTON; tabl

Cholestyramine, ion-exchange resin for treatment of cholestatic jaundice and hyperlipidemia

Toxicity includes constipation, vitamin A, D, and K deficiencies, and altered medication absorption.

PO: 240 mg/kg/24 hr, div, every 8–12 hr with meals

QUESTRAN, CHOLYBAR; 4-g packets, 378-g tins, 4-g cholestyramine per 9-g Questran

Cimetidine; H_2-receptor antagonist competitively inhibits secretion of gastric acid.

℞ for treatment of duodenal and gastric ulcers and for relief of symptoms caused by gastroesophageal reflux: compatible with

Table continued on following page

TABLE 27–3 Drug Dosages *Continued*

concomitant treatment with oral antacids (which should be administered at frequent intervals and in adequate doses) or other therapeutic modalities.
IN, CH = IV, PO: 20–40 mg/kg/24 hr, div, every 4–6 hr
Note: Cimetidine may compete with hepatic metabolism of other hepatically metabolized drugs. Many possible drug interactions. May cause gynecomastia, rash, and neutropenia.
TAGAMET; tabl, inj

Clindamycin; semisynthetic derivative of lincomycin
NB <7 days <2,000 g, 10 mg/kg/24 hr, div, every 12 hr; >7 days <2,000 g, 15 mg/kg/24 hr, div, every 8 hr; <7 days >2,000 g, 15 mg/kg/24 hr, div, every 8 hr; >7 days >2,000 g, 20 mg/kg/24 hr, div, every 6 hr
IN, CH: 20–45 mg/kg/24 hr, div, every 6–8 hr
Note: Therapy may be associated with the development of pseudomembranous colitis.
clindamycin hydrochloride, CLEOCIN hydrochloride; caps clindamycin palmitate hydrochloride, CLEOCIN pediatric; oral susp clindamycin phosphate, CLEOCIN phosphate; inj

Clonazepam; benzodiazepine with selective anticonvulsant effect
CH = PO: start with 0.01–0.05 mg/kg/24 hr, div, every 8 hr, and progressively increase up to 0.3 mg/kg/24 hr, div, every 8 hr, if needed.
Caution: Concomitant use of clonazepam and valproate sodium may lead to petit mal status.
CLONOPIN; tabl
Co-Trimoxazole; see Sulfonamides

Cloxacillin sodium monohydrate; penicillinase-resistant penicillin
IN, CH = PO: 50–100 mg/kg/24 hr, div, every 6 hr (expressed in terms of the base)
TEGOPEN; caps, oral susp

Codeine phosphate or sulfate; narcotic analgesic
℞ as antitussive: CH = 1–1.5 mg/kg/24 hr, div, every 4 hr, prn
℞ against moderately severe pain: CH = PO: 4 mg/kg/24 hr, div, every 4–6 hr, prn; SC: 3 mg/kg/24 hr, div, every 4–6 hr, prn
†; tabl, oral susp, inj; mostly in combination with other drugs

Colistin sodium methanesulfonate, colistimethate sodium, and colistin sulfate, polymyxin E; polypeptide antimicrobial agent with cationic detergent activity
℞ inhibition of gastrointestinal flora, justified only in selected cases (gastroenteritis with susceptible organism): IN, CH = PO (colistin sulfate): 5–15 mg/kg/24 hr, div, every 8 hr; IM, IV (by slow infusion): 3–5 mg/kg/24 hr, div, every 8 hr
Caution against pathogen overgrowth; monitor for nephrotoxicity and ototoxicity.
colistimethate sodium, COLY-MYCIN N; inj colistin sulfate, COLY-MYCIN S; oral susp

Corticosteroids
℞ physiologic replacement: *cortisone:* PO: 1 mg/kg/24 hr, div, every 8 hr; IM: 0.5 mg/kg/24 hr, every 24 hr. (*Note:* "Increased demand" under stressful situation; e.g., in children with congenital adrenogenital syndrome, receiving replacement therapy, for stressful situation in which 2 mg/kg/24 hr of cortisol may be safer)
℞ use in pharmacologic doses (leukemia, lymphoma, nephrosis, rheumatic carditis, certain types of tuberculosis, immunologic reactions, and other types of autoimmune disease): adjust dosage to the specific situation.
cortisone: PO: 10 mg/kg/24 hr, div, every 6–8 hr; IM: 3–6 mg/kg/24 hr, div, every 12 hr
prednisone: PO: 2 mg/kg/24 hr, div, every 6–8 hr (or analogue in equally effective dosage; see following table)
(For continued treatment after initial response, adjust dosage, frequency of administration, and duration of treatment according to type of disease and side effects to be avoided.)
℞ in status asthmaticus refractory to other types of treatment: methylprednisolone 2–4 mg/kg/24 hr, div, every 4–6 hr
℞ in endotoxin shock: methylprednisolone 2–4 mg/kg/24 hr, div, every 4–6 hr

Relative Potencies of Corticosteroids:

Drug	Anti-inflammatory Effect (mg)	Sodium-Retaining Effect (mg)
Hydrocortisone (cortisol)	100	100
Cortisone	80	80
Prednisolone	20	100
Prednisone	20	100
Methylprednisolone	16	0
Triamcinolone	16	0
Dexamethasone	2	0
Desoxycorticosterone	0	2

dexamethasone, DECADRON, GAMMACORTEN, ‡; tabl, elixir dexamethasone sodium phosphate, DECADRON phosphate; inj
hydrocortisone, †, CORTEF, HYDROCORTONE, ‡; tabl, oral susp hydrocortisone sodium phosphate, †, HYDROCORTONE phosphate; inj hydrocortisone sodium succinate, †, SOLU-CORTEF; inj
methylprednisolone, MEDROL; tabl methylprednisolone sodium succinate, SOLU-MEDROL; inj
prednisone, †, DELTASONE, METICORTEN, ‡; tabl
prednisolone, †, DELTA-CORTEF, METICORTELONE, ‡; tabl
triamcinolone, ARISTOCORT, KENACORT; tabl, syrup
Caution: May inhibit clinical signs of infection.

Cortisone; see Corticosteroids

Cromolyn sodium
℞ topical prophylaxis of bronchial asthma, allergic rhinitis: not useful in the treatment of acute asthmatic attack because it is not a bronchodilator. CH (≥5 yr) = inhalation of 20 mg every 6 hr; nebulize contents of one ampule (2 ml) every 6–8 hr; aerosol inhaler, 1–2 puffs 4 times daily.
AARANE, INTAL; inhalation with Spinhaler, sol, nasal spray

Cyclizine hydrochloride; antihistamine, antiemetic, and anticholinergic agent
℞ for prevention and relief of symptoms of motion sickness: CH (6–10 yr) = PO: 3 mg/kg/24 hr, div, every 8 hr. The 1st dose should be taken about 20 min before departure.
MAREZINE; tabl; cyclizine lactate for IM inj

Cyclosporine; cyclic polypeptide immunosuppressant agent produced as a metabolite from a fungus. Cyclosporine is a potent immunosuppressive drug that prolongs survival of transplants involving skin, heart, kidney, pancreas, bone marrow, and lung. The drug's mechanism of action remains to be elucidated but appears to include inhibition of T cell-dependent B cell activation, expansion of unprimed T helper and cytotoxic T cell subsets, clonal expansion of aloe-reactive cells, and induction of γ-interferon secretion.
IN, CH = PO: 14–18 mg/kg daily and tapered downward to a maintenance dose approximately 5–10 mg/kg/24 hr, div, every 12–24 hr. The oral absorption of cyclosporine is highly variable. IV (slow infusion over 2–6 hr): 2–6 mg/kg/24 hr, div, every 12–24 hr.
Note: Renal function must be monitored closely. Dosage frequently adjusted to obtain desired trough blood concentration, which is dependent upon type of assay used for cyclosporin determination (consult pharmacology/clinical pathology)
SANDIMMUNE; oral sol, inj

Cyproheptadine hydrochloride; piperidine; serotonin and histamine antagonist with mild anticholinergic and mild sedative effects
℞ antiallergic effect: CH = PO: 0.25–0.5 mg/kg/24 hr, div, every 4–6 hr
†, PERIACTIN; tabl, syrup

Dantrolene sodium; antispasmodic used in the management of chronic muscle spasticity resulting from upper motoneuron disorders (e.g., spinal cord injury, cerebral palsy, multiple sclerosis). Dantrium works directly on skeletal muscle; it disassociates

TABLE 27–3 Drug Dosages *Continued*

the excitation-contraction coupling, probably by interfering with the release of calcium from the sarcoplasmic reticulum. Common medication used in conjunction with other drugs in structured therapeutic environments. CH = PO: 1 mg/kg/24 hr, div, every 12 hr, increasing to a maximum 3 mg/kg/24 hr, div, every 6–12 hr

℞ malignant hyperthermal crisis: IV (rapid infusion): 1 mg/kg repeated immediately until signs of malignant hyperthermia resolve, up to a total dose of 10 mg/kg; maintenance 4–8 mg/kg/24 hr (IV/PO), div, every 6 hr, for 1–3 days.

Caution: Use may be associated with hepatotoxicity

DANTRIUM; caps, IV

Deferoxamine, chelating agent for treatment of iron intoxication. May cause hypotension; contraindicated in renal failure or acute anuria unless concomitant hemodialysis is used.

IV: 10–15 mg/kg/hr infusion

DESFERAL; 500 mg/vial inj

Demeclocycline; see Tetracyclines

Desmopressin acetate, synthetic analogue of vasopressin indicated as replacement therapy in the management of central diabetes insipidus. Toxicities include headache, abdominal cramping, and excessive water retention. Nasal insufflation: 5–30 μg/24 hr divided every 12–24 hr. Dose determined by patient response

DDAVP; inj; nasal insufflation

Dexamethasone; see Corticosteroids

Dextroamphetamine sulfate; noncatecholamine sympathomimetic agent

℞ in minimal brain dysfunction: drug treatment not recommended below age of 3 yr or in nonstructured therapeutic situation. CH (above 3 yr) = PO: initiate treatment with 2.5 mg/dose given at onset of daytime activities and again 4–6 hr later. If needed, increase at weekly intervals by increments of 2.5 mg/dose and adjust respective size of separate doses according to response. Daily dose should not exceed 1 mg/kg/24 hr.

℞ in narcolepsy: PO: proceed for dosage as in minimal brain dysfunction. End points: control of symptoms, maximal dose.

To avoid insomnia do not administer closer than 6 hr before bedtime. **Caution** against diversion of CNS stimulants from legitimate use in patient to misuse in adults.

†, DEXEDRINE; tabl

Caution: Severe mental depression may follow withdrawal. Overdose may produce extreme restlessness and psychotic behavior.

Dextromethorphan hydrobromide; D-isomer of a codeine analog, and probably free of addictive effects

℞ antitussive agent: IN, CH = PO: 1 mg/kg/24 hr, div, every 6–8 hr

†, ROMILAR; syrup; contained in many combination products

Diazepam; benzodiazepine with anxiolytic and muscle-relaxant effects

℞ in status epilepticus: NB, IN, CH = IV (slowly, as controlled "push" injection): 0.1–0.5 mg/kg/dose; may be repeated at 3–5 min intervals; may administer IM if IV not possible (efficacy may be diminished).

℞ for symptomatic relief of anxiety, sedation, muscle relaxation: IN, CH = PO: 0.1–0.3 mg/kg/24 hr, div, every 4–8 hr; dosage adjusted according to clinical response.

†, VALIUM; tabl, inj

Caution: Confusion and prolonged extreme drowsiness may follow overdose or concurrent ingestion of alcohol in any form.

Diazoxide, nondiuretic benzothiazide derivative with several prominent actions: (1) relaxation of smooth muscles in the peripheral arterioles after IV injection only; (2) hyperglycemic effect (beginning 1 hr after administration and lasting for approximately 8 hr) through inhibition of release of insulin; (3) retention of sodium and concomitantly of water; (4) hyperuricemic effect

℞ for emergency reduction of hypertension: CH = IV (injection within 30 sec of calculated amount of undiluted diazoxide solution into a peripheral vein): 5 mg/kg/dose, may administer as timed infusion. If 1st injection fails to elicit adequate response within 30 min, administer a 2nd complementary dose. Hypotensive effect usually lasts 2–12 hr. As soon as possible, switch to oral regimen with alternative antihypertensive medication.

℞ for hyperinsulinemic hypoglycemia: NB, IN = PO: 8–15 mg/kg/24 hr, div, every 8–12 hr; CH = PO: 3–8 mg/kg/24 hr, div, every 8–12 hr. Slow dosage titration is necessary for optimal response.

Note: Diazoxide is ineffective against hypertension due to pheochromocytoma. A concurrently administered thiazide diuretic (which characteristically exerts a diuretic response) may potentiate the antihypertensive, hyperglycemic, and hyperuricemic effects of diazoxide.

Caution: hypotensive circulatory failure (responding to catecholamine such as norepinephrine), congestive heart failure (responding to plasma volume depletion by saluretic), and hyperosmolar coma in patients with diabetes mellitus (responding to insulin) may occur.

HYPERSTAT; inj, proglycem; cap, susp

Dicloxacillin sodium monohydrate; penicillinase-resistant penicillin

IN, CH = PO: 12.5–25 mg/kg/24 hr, div, every 6 hr

DYNAPEN; caps, oral susp

Digoxin; cardiac glycoside with rapid onset of action and half-life of approximately 48 hr

℞ for digitalization: 0.5 × digitalizing dose initially, 0.25 × digitalizing dose 8 and 16 hr later.

(Digitalizing dose: NB = IV, IM: 0.010–0.030 mg/kg div in fractions, or PO: 0.040 mg/kg, div in fractions.

IN = IV, IM 0.030–0.040 mg/kg div in fractions, or PO: 0.050 mg/kg, in fractions

CH = IV, IM, PO: same doses as indicated for NB)

℞ for maintenance: begin maintenance dosage 24 hr after 1st fraction of digitalizing dose. NB = PO: 0.050–0.010 mg/kg/24 hr, div, every 12 hr. IN, CH = PO: 0.015 mg/kg/24 hr, div, every 12 hr

Note: Digitalizing and maintenance doses must be adjusted to clinical condition and response of the patient. Systemic absorption from IM administration may be erratic and unpredictable. Serum digoxin concentrations may be monitored to assist in therapy. Caution is needed in interpreting serum digoxin concentrations in patients <6 mo of age due to the presence of immunoreactive digoxin-like substances (consult pharmacology or clinical pathology textbooks).

†, LANOXIN; tabl, elixir, inj

Caution: Fatal arrhythmia may follow overdose.

Digoxin immune FAB; antigen-binding fragments (FAB) derived from specific antidigoxin antibodies in sheep used in the treatment of digoxin overdose or intoxication. Digoxin FAB antibodies bind digoxin, rendering drug unavailable to bind to their site of action. The FAB fragment-digoxin complex will accumulate in blood, may be easily quantitated, and is excreted slowly by the kidney. FAB fragment-digoxin complex is not pharmacologically active. Dose of digoxin immune FAB is dependent upon amount of digoxin reversal desired. More specific information about dose, intervals, and monitoring should be obtained from a clinical pharmacy or pharmacology service or a poison control center.

Dimenhydrinate, chlorotheophylline salt of diphenhydramine

℞ for the prevention and treatment of motion sickness: CH = PO: 5 mg/kg/24 hr, div, every 6 hr

†, DRAMAMINE; tabl, oral susp, suppos

Dimercaprol in oil; metal chelating agent used in the treatment of arsenic, gold, mercury, and lead poisoning.

℞ in the treatment of heavy metal poisoning depending upon severity of intoxication. Doses range from 12–24 mg/kg/24 hr, div, every 4 hr via IM injection.

BAL in oil; IM inj

Dioctyl sodium sulfosuccinate; wetting agent, emulsifier, demulcent

℞ as stool softener: IN, CH = PO: 5 mg/kg/24 hr, div, with meals

†, COLACE, DOXINATE, ‡; caps, oral sol, syrup

Table continued on following page

TABLE 27–3 Drug Dosages *Continued*

Diphenhydramine hydrochloride; ethanolamine; antihistamine with mild anticholinergic, sedative, antiemetic, and antitussive effects
℞ antiallergic effect; sometimes used as sedative. IN, CH = PO, IM, IV: 5 mg/kg/24 hr, div, every 6–8 hr
†, BENADRYL; caps, elixir, inj

Diphenoxylate hydrochloride + atropine sulfate; opiate analog (diphenoxylate) combined with an anticholinergic (atropine) used as short-term adjunctive therapy in the management of diarrhea. Need for routine use of this drug in infants and children is questionable.
℞ for symptomatic short-term use as an antidiarrheal: CH = PO: 0.3–0.4 mg/kg/24 hr, div, every 4–12 hr
†, LOMOTIL; tabl, liquid

Dobutamine, β-adrenergic inotropic agent used for short-term treatment of cardiac failure due to depressed cardiac contractility. Heart rate, blood pressure, and cardiac electrical activity should be monitored during infusion. Do not mix with sodium bicarbonate. IV: 0.0025–0.020 mg/kg/min constant infusion, depending on patient response.
DOBUTREX; 250-mg vials for injection

Dopamine, α- and β-adrenergic as well as dopaminergic agent (positive inotropic effect on heart)
℞ to increase cardiac output and improve organ perfusion: IV infusion (into large vein): Example: to prepare a solution containing 0.400 mg/mL, mix 100 mg dopamine HCl in 250 mL 5% D/W or appropriate electrolyte solution with pH below 7.0 (do not include bicarbonate!), and infuse at rate adjusted to response in patient, beginning with 0.002–0.005 mg/kg/min and increasing by increments of 0.005 mg/kg/min if needed up to 0.020 mg/kg/min. In case of extravasation causing peripheral ischemia, use phentolamine (REGITINE) for local infiltration.
INTROPIN; inj

Doxycycline; see Tetracyclines

Dronabinol Δ-9-tetrahydrocannabinol (Δ-9-THC) is used as adjunctive therapy in the treatment of nausea and vomiting associated with cancer chemotherapy, most often in patients who have failed to respond adequately to conventional antiemetic treatment. Dronabinol therapy may be associated with disturbing psychotomimetic reactions.
℞ CH = PO: 5 mg/m^2 beginning 1–3 hr before chemotherapy and every 2–4 hr thereafter. Dose may be increased as necessary to control emesis (usually 2.5 mg/m^2 dose).
Note: Dronabinol may have profound effects on mental status; patient should be cautioned.
MARINOL; gelatin caps

Edrophonium chloride; cholinesterase inhibitor with short duration of action
℞ for myasthenia in NB of myasthenic mother = IV (slowly) or IM: 0.2 mg/kg/dose. Symptoms should be relieved almost immediately. Continue cholinesterase-inhibiting treatment, if indicated, with pyridostigmine.
℞ for differential diagnosis of myasthenic crisis, or as adjunct treatment to carotid massage in supraventricular tachycardia: NB, IN, CH = IV: 0.05 mg/kg/dose, and watch for effect after 15–30 s, *or* IM: 0.1 mg/kg/dose, and expect effect after 2–10 min
If edrophonium test is given during "cholinergic crisis," weakness of affected muscles, including respiratory muscles, will worsen or not improve. Ventilation should be assisted, if needed, and bradycardia can be influenced by atropine. If recovery from weakness occurs, continuation of cholinesterase inhibition is indicated using inhibitors with longer duration of action, such as pyridostigmine, neostigmine, ambenonium. Their dosage must be individually titrated and adjusted.
Manifestations of overdosage with cholinesterase-inhibiting medication: increase in muscle weakness and worsening of respiratory difficulty and dysphagia after each dose of drug; fasciculations of muscles; excessive salivation, increase in bronchial secretion; vomiting, diarrhea, pallor, sweating, bradycardia.
TENSILON; inj

Caution: Administration during cholinergic crisis may cause paralysis of respiratory muscles. Use only when ventilatory assistance is available.

Ephedrine, phenylethylamine (direct and indirect sympathomimetic)
℞ for treatment of asthma in subacute stage; tolerance develops. CH = PO: 3 mg/kg/24 hr, div, every 4–6 hr. Contained in many antiasthma preparations; should be replaced with more selectively active drug
ephedrine hydrochloride; ephedrine sulfate; caps, tabl, syrup
Caution: Acute overdose may produce seizures and coma.

Epinephrine, catecholamine (α- and β-adrenergic agonist)
℞ bronchodilator (β_2 stimulatory effect), in acute asthma attack: IN, CH = SC: 0.01 mg/kg/dose, repeat prn every 20 min, 2 times
Note: With epinephrine solution 1:1000 this corresponds to 0.01 mL/kg/dose.
Caution: Cardiac arrhythmia or acute hypertension may follow overdose.

Epinephrine racemic, Inhalation treatment of acute spasmodic croup.
Inhalation: 0.25–0.5 mL of 2.25% solution diluted in 3 mL of saline given via nebulizer.
VAPONEPHRINE; Inhalation 2.25% solution

Ergotamine, adrenergic blocking agent as well as direct vasoconstrictor of vessels to the brain, and serotonin antagonist
℞ against acute attack of vascular headache (migraine): older child and adolescent = IM, SC (in acute attack): 0.25–0.50 mg/dose, in single application. Minimal effective dose should be established for each patient by titration of the amount required to control headaches in that patient. Older child and adolescent = SL, PO (at 1st symptoms of attack): 1 mg/dose; if no improvement within following 30 min, repeat same dose once.
Note: Signs of therapeutic overdosage: nausea, vomiting, diarrhea, tingling of hands and feet, weakness, muscle pain.
ergotamine tartrate: CYNERGEN; inj, tabl ergotamine tartrate + caffeine: CAFERGOT, tabl, suppos dihydroergotamine mesylate: D.H.E.45, inj

Erythromycin; macrolide antimicrobial agent
IN, CH = PO: 30–50 mg/kg/24 hr, div, every 6 hr; IV: 15–20 mg/kg/24 hr, div, every 6 hr
erythromycin, †, ILOTYCIN, ‡; tabl erythromycin estolate, ILOSONE; tabl, oral susp erythromycin ethylsuccinate, PEDIAMYCIN, EES ‡; tabl, oral susp, drops erythromycin gluceptate, ILOTYCIN gluceptate IV; inj erythromycin lactobionate, ERYTHROCIN lactobionate IV; inj erythromycin stearate, ERYTHROCIN stearate, ‡; tabl

Ethacrynic acid; saluretic, inhibiting chloride and sodium reabsorption and interfering mainly with concentration of urine
CH = PO: approximately 1 mg/kg/dose, as single daily dose. Adjust according to effect, and repeat prn on alternate days; dosage in infants and children not firmly established (PO, IV)
EDECRIN; tabl ethacrynate sodium, IV, sodium EDECRIN; inj (IV only)

Ethambutol hydrochloride; antituberculous agent used concomitantly with isoniazid
℞ in the treatment of tuberculosis as part of multiple drug regimen. Conditions for safe use in children not firmly established. In adults: 15–25 mg/kg/24 hr, as single daily dose, for course of treatment or retreatment. *Because of rare side effects of optic neuritis and decreased visual acuity,* eye examinations are indicated before inception of treatment and at monthly intervals thereafter.
MYAMBUTOL; tabl

Ethosuximide; anticonvulsant agent of the succinimide type
CH = PO: 20–30 mg/kg/24 hr, div, every 12 hr
ZARONTIN; caps, syrup

Fentanyl; Fentanyl citrate; potent narcotic analgesic, addictive. A fentanyl dose of 0.1 mg possesses an approximate equivalent analgesic activity to 10 mg of morphine or 75 mg of meperidine.

TABLE 27–3 Drug Dosages *Continued*

℞ against severe pain; NB, IN, CH = IV, IM: 0.5–5 μg/kg/dose every 1–4 hr; may be administered as a continuous intravenous infusion: 1–5 μg/kg/hr

Fluconazole; synthetic broad-spectrum *bis*-triazole antifungal drug. Selective inhibitor of fungal cytochrome P_{450} sterol C-14 α-demethylation; limited data in pediatrics available.
℞ for the treatment of fungal infections; CH = PO, IV: 3–6 mg/kg/24 hr, div, every 12–24 hr
DIFLUCAN; tabl, inj

Flucytosine; fluorinated pyrimidine antifungal agent. Mechanism of drug action remains to be elucidated but may be a result of competitive inhibition of fungal cell purine and pyrimidine metabolism, or may be due to intracellular metabolism to 5-fluorouracil. Flucytosine is used in combination with other antifungal agents.
℞ in combination with other antifungal agents: IN, CH = PO: 50–150 mg/kg/24 hr, div, every 6–8 hr.
Note: May cause bone marrow suppression.
ANCOBON: caps

Fluroquinolones; relatively new class of antimicrobial agents that inhibit the action of microbial DNA gyrase (topoisomerase 2). Drugs in this class include ciprofloxacin, enoxacin, norfloxacin, ofloxacin, and so on. Many of these drugs possess potent activity against a wide range of pathogens, including *Pseudomonas aeruginosa,* and are available for oral administration. The use of these drugs in pediatrics, primarily for the treatment of children with cystic fibrosis, has been limited owing to concern about possible fluroquinolone-induced joint damage. Toxicity studies in animals have shown destructive lesions of growing cartilage following administration of these agents. Reports of arthropathy in teenage patients with cystic fibrosis have appeared in the literature, suggesting caution in the use of this class of compounds in patients whose skeletal growth is incomplete.

Furosemide; saluretic with a duration of action of about 2 hr when given IV; inhibits chloride and sodium reabsorption and interferes with concentration of urine
IN, CH = PO: start with 2 mg/kg/dose; if needed, increase progressively to 3–6 mg/kg/dose, at intervals of 6–8 hr. IV: start with 1 mg/kg/dose; if needed, increase progressively to 6 mg/kg/dose, with an interval of at least 2 hr between doses
LASIX; tabl, oral sol, inj

Gentamicin sulfate; antimicrobial aminoglycoside
NB = IV (30–60 min), IM: <7 days <34 wk <1,500 g, 3 mg/kg every 24 hr; <34 wk >1,500 g, 2.5 mg/kg every 18 hr; >34 wk >1,500 g, 2.5 mg/kg every 12 hr; >7 days and term NB, 5 mg/kg/24 hr, div, every 12 hr.
IN, CH = IM, IV (30–60 min): 5–7.5 mg/kg/24 hr, div, every 6–8 hr
Serum concentrations should be monitored, therapeutic peak concentration 5–10 mg/L, trough <2 mg/L (see Table 27–2). Dosage and interval may require modification for treatment of patients with cystic fibrosis.
GARAMYCIN; inj
Caution: Ototoxic; nephrotoxic.

Griseofulvin; antifungal agent
℞ against deep-seated mycotic infections (skin, hair, nails) with organisms of the species *Microsporum, Trichophyton, Epidermophyton:* CH = PO (microcrystalline): 10 mg/kg/24 hr for 4–6 wk (4–6 mo for fingernails, 6–12 mo for toenails)
Note: "Ultramicrosize" form is an ultramicrocrystalline suspension for which 125 mg is biologically equivalent to 250 mg of a "microsize" preparation. The daily dose of an ultramicrosize preparation is reduced to 5 mg/kg/24 hr and offers comparable efficacy without additional advantages.
griseofulvin, microcrystalline, †, FULVICIN-U/F, GRIFULVIN V, ‡; tabl, oral susp griseofulvin, ultramicrocrystalline GRIS-PEG; tabl

Hydralazine hydrochloride; phthalazine derivative; causes relaxation of vascular smooth muscles, especially of arterioles
℞ as antihypertensive in long-term treatment: CH = PO: initially 0.75 mg/kg/24 hr, div, every 6 hr; increase progressively until desired response or daily maximum dose of 3.5 mg/kg/24 hr is reached
℞ for emergency reduction of hypertension: IV (immediate onset of action), IM (onset of action after 15–20 min): 0.15 mg/kg/dose; repeat prn every 30–90 min up to daily dose of 1.7–3.6 mg/kg/24 hr; switch to oral administration if conditions permit
Note: Hydralazine may produce sodium retention and usually increases plasma renin activity.
Caution: May induce lupus erythematosus–like syndrome; frequency related to dosage.
†, APRESOLINE, ‡; tabl, inj

Hydrochlorothiazide; saluretic, inhibiting sodium reabsorption and interfering with dilution of urine
IN, CH = PO: 2 mg/kg/24 hr, div, every 12 hr
†, ESIDRIX, HYDRODIURIL, ‡; tabl

Hydroxyzine hydrochloride; neuroleptic agent of the piperazine type, with sedative and antihistamine effects
℞ for sedation or antihistamine effect: CH = PO: 2 mg/kg/24 hr, div, every 6–8 hr, prn
ATARAX: tabl, syrup; VISTARIL IM: inj (IM) hydroxyzine pamoate, VISTARIL; caps, oral susp

Ibuprofen; nonsteroidal anti-inflammatory agent of the propionic acid class that possesses analgesic and antipyretic activities. The drug's mechanism of action remains to be described but may involve prostaglandin synthetase inhibition. Pharmacologic effect appears to be equivalent to that of equipotent doses of acetaminophen or aspirin.
℞ as antipyretic or for mild analgesia, CH = PO: 10–15 mg/kg/dose at intervals of 4–6 hr
℞ for juvenile rheumatoid arthritis, CH = PO: 30–70 mg/kg/24 hr, div, every 4–6 hr
Note: complete scope of associated adverse reactions in infants and children remains to be described. Adverse effects appear to be similar to those associated with aspirin administration including gastritis, platelet dysfunction, and possible compromise in renal function. Drug should be used cautiously in patients with renal insufficiency.
† ADVIL, MEDIPRIN, MOTRIN, NUPRIN; tabs, caps, susp

Imipramine hydrochloride; tricyclic antidepressant
℞ against enuresis, as adjunct therapy to proper medical and educational approach, after age 4 yr: CH (after age 4 yr) = PO: 25 mg/24 hr, to be given in single dose before bedtime; if response unsatisfactory, dose may be increased slowly to 100 mg/24 hr
†, TOFRANIL; tabl

Indomethacin; nonsteroidal anti-inflammatory agent used in the treatment of inflammatory disorders and for pharmacologic management of patent ductus arteriosus in premature infants.
Note: May cause GI irritation and bleeding and decreased glomerular filtration rate.
℞ as anti-inflammatory: CH = PO: 1–3 mg/kg/24 hr, div, every 6–8 hr
℞ for closure of ductus arteriosus: IN = IV: <48 hr, 0.2 mg/kg for 1 dose, then 2 doses of 0.1 mg/kg; 2–7 days of age, 3 doses of 0.2 mg/kg; >7 days of age, 0.2 mg/kg once, then 2 doses of 0.25 mg/kg
INDOCIN; PO, inj

Ipecac; emetic agent used in the adjunctive management of poisoning or intoxication. Active ingredient emetidine produces local gastric irritation and central effect, resulting in emesis, which usually occurs within 15–35 min of drug administration.
℞ to induce vomiting:
IN >8 mo of age, CH = PO: 15–30 ml/dose: if no effect occurs same dose may be repeated in 30 min
IN <8 mo of age = PO: 1 mL/kg single dose
Note: Children usually vomit 3–5 times within 1 h of receiving Ipecac. Ipecac should be available in all households with young infants and children but should not be administered except on the advice of a physician or a poison control center.

Iron preparations
℞ Daily maintenance iron requirement: elemental iron: PO: 0.5–1 mg/kg/24 hr, in single dose or divided

Table continued on following page

TABLE 27–3 Drug Dosages *Continued*

℞ In iron deficiency anemia, as elemental iron: PO: 6 mg/kg/24 hr, div, with meals

Note: Iron supply at this dosage level ought to be continued for 2–3 mo to compensate for the deficits in erythrocytes and iron stores. Only iron in the ferrous form (Fe^{2-}) is absorbed from the gastrointestinal tract. The content of elemental iron in different preparations varies. The percentage of dry weight as elemental iron of ferrous choline citrate is 20; ferrous fumarate, 33; ferrous gluconate, 12; ferrous lactate, 19; ferrous sulfate, 20; and iron-dextran complex (ferric hydroxide), 2.

℞ Dose calculation for parenteral iron administration: elemental Fe deficit = 2.5 mg/kg × deficit of hemoglobin concentration (in g/dL) in blood. (The deficit of the hemoglobin concentration is obtained as the difference between the measured and the desirable value, expressed in g/dL.) When iron has to be supplied by the parenteral route, deep IM injection is preferable to IV administration. In either case, a test dose of approximately 25 mg elemental Fe in the form of the dextran complex should precede the administration of the total dose. If the total dose is large, it should be divided in separate daily doses of which none should exceed 5 mg/kg/24 hr of elemental iron.

Note: An additional 20–30% of the calculated deficit is needed to restore the tissue iron reserves.

Caution: Acute overdose may lead to shock, CNS depression, death (Sec 26.8).

Isoniazid, INH, isonicotinic acid hydrazide; tuberculostatic agent

℞ in the treatment of active tuberculosis, in combination with other antituberculous drugs: IN, CH = PO, IM: 10–20 mg/kg/24 hr, div, every 8–12 hr; maximum daily dose: 500 mg/24 hr. AD = PO, IM: 5–10 mg/kg/24 hr, div, every 8–12 hr; maximum daily dose: 300 mg/24 hr

℞ for prophylaxis of complications in recent conversion to positive tuberculin reaction (primary tuberculosis), or after suspected exposure: IN, CH = PO: 5–10 mg/kg/24 hr, as single dose, or div, every 12 hr; maximum daily dose: 300 mg/24 hr

Note: "Slow" acetylators (homozygous) need only about 0.20–0.50 of this dose to reach therapeutically effective plasma concentrations achieved by "rapid" acetylators (homozygous and heterozygous). Higher than necessary plasma concentrations of unmetabolized isoniazid seem not to be associated with risk of isoniazid hepatotoxicity.

†, INH; tabl, syrup, inj

Caution: Formation of toxic metabolite in some patients may lead to hepatic necrosis with usual doses (rare under 20 yr of age).

Isoproterenol hydrochloride; β-adrenergic agent

℞ to overcome atrioventricular block: IV infusion: Example: to prepare a solution containing 0.004 mg/mL, mix 1 mg isoproterenol in 250 mL 5% D/W or appropriate electrolyte solution and infuse at rate adjusted to response in patient (beginning with approximately 0.0001–0.0002 mg/kg/min)

†, ISUPREL; inj

Kanamycin sulfate; antimicrobial aminoglycoside

NB = IM, IV (over 20–30 min):

≤ 2,000 g and ≤ 7 days old: 15 mg/kg/24 hr, div, every 12 hr
≤ 2,000 g and > 7 days old: 20 mg/kg/24 hr, div, every 12 hr
> 2,000 g and ≤ 7 days old: 20 mg/kg/24 hr, div, every 12 hr
> 2,000 g and > 7 days old: 30 mg/kg/24 hr, div, every 8 hr

IN, CH = IM, IV (over 20–30 min): 6–15 mg/kg/24 hr, div, every 8–12 hr. Usual duration of therapy: 7–10 days; not indicated in long-term therapy because of ototoxic hazard.

Caution: Ototoxic, nephrotoxic.

KANTREX; inj

Lidocaine hydrochloride; anesthetic agent used systemically for its antiarrhythmic effects; delayed slow diastolic depolarization, diminished automaticity. Does not affect normal conduction but seemingly improves conduction velocity in damaged areas of myocardium. In therapeutic doses does not depress myocardial contractility or atrioventricular conduction.

℞ for ventricular tachyarrhythmia; IN, CH = IV loading dose: 1 mg/kg/dose may be repeated every 5–10 min to desired effect until total dose of 5 mg/kg has been administered. Maintenance therapy administered by continuous infusion: 20–50 μg/kg/min (max: 4 mg/min)

Caution: Excessive depression of cardiac conductivity may occur; electrocardiographic (ECG) monitoring is indicated during treatment. Monitoring of serum lidocaine concentrations may also assist in therapy; seizurogenic metabolite of lidocaine may accumulate in patients with compromised renal function.

†, XYLOCAINE hydrochloride; IV, inj

Lincomycin hydrochloride; antimicrobial macrolide

CH = PO: 30–60 mg/kg/24 hr, div, every 8 hr. IM, IV (over 1–4 hr, as 10 mg/mL sol): 10–20 mg/kg/24 hr, div, every 8–12 hr

LINCOCIN; caps, syrup, inj

Loperimide; synthetic antidiarrheal agent used as short-term adjunctive therapy in the management of diarrhea. Drug slows intestinal motility thus affecting water and electrolyte movement through the bowel. Decreased peristaltic activity of the bowel results from a direct effect of loperimide on the circular and longitudinal muscles of the intestinal wall. Need for routine use of this drug in infants and children is questionable. CH = PO: 0.4–1.5 mg/kg/24 hr, div, every 6–12 hr

IMODIUM; caps, liquid

Lorazepam; benzodiazepine that possesses antianxiety and sedative effects. Most experience with use of this drug in children is limited to its use as an alternative agent in the treatment of status epilepticus.

℞ for the treatment of status epilepticus: IN, CH = IV (slowly, as controlled "push" injection): 0.05 mg/kg/dose, which may be repeated every 15–20 min for 2 doses; may administer IM if IV not possible (efficacy may be diminished)

†, ATIVAN; inj, tabs

"Lytic cocktail," mixture of narcotic analgesic, antihistamine, and phenothiazine

℞ for temporary heavy sedation: IM (deep, after mixing the 3 components in 1 syringe): meperidine (DEMEROL), 2 mg/kg/dose, plus promethazine (PHENERGAN), 1 mg/kg/dose, plus chlorpromazine (THORAZINE), 1 mg/kg/dose (maximum single dose not to exceed meperidine, 50 mg, promethazine, 25 mg, and chlorpromazine, 25 mg)

Caution: Use may be associated with prolonged sedation, seizures, severe respiratory depression, and respiratory arrest. Monitor patients closely following administration.

Magnesium hydroxide, $Mg(OH)_2$

℞ as cathartic: PO: 40 mg/kg/dose

milk of magnesia, susp, "8%" containing $Mg(OH)_2$ 80 mg/mL

Magnesium sulfate, $MgSO_4 \cdot 7H_2O$, Epsom salt; 1 g of the salt is equivalent to 98.6 mg elemental Mg or to 8.11 mEq Mg^{2-}

℞ as cathartic: PO: ($MgSO_4 \cdot 7H_2O$): 250 mg/kg/dose

℞ in hypomagnesemia: IM (in solution containing $MgSO_4 \cdot 7H_2O$ 500 mg/mL, equivalent to Mg^{2-} 4 mEq/mL, also labeled "50%"): $MgSO_4 \cdot 7H_2O$ 100 mg/kg/dose, equivalent to Mg^{2-} 0.8 mEq/kg/dose, repeat every 4–6 hr

IV (in solution containing $MgSO_4 \cdot 7H_2O$ 100 mg/mL, equivalent to Mg^{2-} 0.08 mEq/mL, also labeled "10%"): Infuse slowly $MgSO_4 \cdot 7H_2O$ up to 100 mg/kg/dose, equivalent to Mg^{2-} 0.08 mEq/kg/dose

†; crystalline salt, sterile sol for inj available as 50%, 25%, and 10%

Mannitol; osmotic diuretic

℞ test dose for oliguria: CH = IV: 0.2 g/kg/dose, injected within 3–5 min

℞ in cerebral edema: CH = IV: 1–2.5 g/kg/dose, injected as 15–25% sol over 30–60 min

†, OSMITROL, ‡; IV inj

Mebendazole; anthelmintic agent that blocks glucose uptake by the susceptible parasites and interferes with their survival

℞ against pinworms (*Enterobius vermicularis;* cure rate 90–100%): CH = PO: 100 mg/dose; as single dose; against whipworms (*Trichuris trichiura;* cure rate 61–75%), roundworms (*Ascaris lumbricoides;* cure rate 91–100%), and hookworms (*Ancylo-*

TABLE 27–3 Drug Dosages *Continued*

stoma duodenale, Necator americanus; cure rate 96%): alternative method = PO: 200 mg/24 hr, div, every 12 hr, for 3 consecutive days. If patient is not free of parasites 3 wk after treatment a 2nd course is indicated

Note: Not extensively studied in children under 2 yr of age.

VERMOX; chewable tabl

Meperidine hydrochloride; synthetic narcotic analgesic agent; addictive

℞ against severe pain: IN, CH = PO, SC, IM: 6 mg/kg/24 hr, div, prn every 4–6 hr (maximum single dose; 100 mg)

†, DEMEROL hydrochloride, ‡; tabl, elixir, inj

Caution: May produce respiratory depression, seizures, coma in some sensitive patients. Naloxone is antidote.

Metaproterenol sulfate; catecholamine analog; β-adrenergic receptor agonist with relatively selective effect on β_2-adrenergic receptors.

℞ bronchodilator: IN, CH (<6 yr of age) = PO: 1.3–2.6 mg/kg/24 hr, div, every 6–8 hr; >6 yr of age: 10–20 mg/dose administered 3–4 times daily

†, ALUPENT; METAPREL; syrup, tabl, inhalation

Methacycline; see Tetracyclines

Methenamine mandelate; urinary antibacterial agent effective in a nonspecific manner against micro-organisms by liberating formaldehyde on decomposing in urine at pH below 5.5

℞ for prevention of bacterial growth in urine, provided pH is sufficiently low: CH = PO: initially 100 mg/kg/24 hr, div, every 6 hr, followed by 50 mg/kg/24 hr, div, every 6 hr

Note: Should not be used (and is useless) when urine acidification is contraindicated or not attainable (as in infections with urea-splitting bacteria). If situation permits, acidification of urine below pH 5.5 might be implemented by adjusting acid load of intake.

†, MANDELAMINE, tabl, oral susp methenamine hippurate, HIPREX; tabl

Methicillin sodium; semisynthetic penicillinase-resistant penicillin

NB = IM, IV (over 15–30 min): according to the following criteria:

≤ 2,000 g and ≤ 14 days old: 50 mg/kg/24 hr, div, every 12 hr

≤ 2,000 g and 15–30 days old: 75 mg/kg/24 hr, div, every 8 hr

> 2,000 g and ≤ 14 days old: 75 mg/kg/24 hr, div, every 8 hr

> 2,000 g and 15–30 days old: 100 mg/kg/24 hr, div, every 6 hr

IN, CH = IV (over 15–30 min), IM: 200–400 mg/kg/24 hr, div, every 4 hr (IV) or every 6 hr (IM)

CELBENIN, STAPHCILLIN; inj

Methyldopa; antihypertensive agent, inhibitor of aromatic amino acid decarboxylase, and precursor of α-methylnorepinephrine. Probably lowers arterial blood pressure by stimulation of central inhibitory α-adrenergic receptors, false neurotransmission, or reduction of plasma renin activity

℞ as antihypertensive in long-term treatment: CH = PO: initially 10 mg/kg/24 hr, div, every 6–12 hr; decrease or increase the dose progressively at intervals of 2 days until adequate response achieved; maximum daily dosage: 65 mg/kg/24 hr

℞ for hypertensive crisis: CH = IV: 20–40 mg/kg/24 hr, div, every 6 hr

Caution: Positive direct Coombs test develops in 10–20% of patients on prolonged treatment, usually between 6 and 12 mo of continued administration. Positive indirect Coombs test, fever, and liver dysfunction occur less frequently. If evidence of hemolysis or liver dysfunction is present, methyldopa should be discontinued and not reinstituted.

ALDOMET; tabl

Methylphenidate hydrochloride; piperidine derivative structurally related to amphetamine; CNS stimulant with more prominent effects on mental than on motor activities

℞ in minimal brain dysfunction (MBD): drug treatment of MBD not recommended below the age of 3 yr or in nonstructured therapeutic situation. CH (over 3 yr) = PO: initiate treatment with 5 mg dose given at the onset of daytime activities and again 4–6 hr later; if needed, increase the dose at weekly intervals by increments of 5 mg/dose and adjust the size of the respective doses (early morning and mid-day) according to the response of the patient; daily dose usually should not exceed 2 mg/kg/24 hr. To avoid insomnia do not administer closer than 6 hr before bedtime. (For MBD, see Sec. 3.39.)

Caution: Reduction of growth rate and weight gain may accompany prolonged use. Chronic abuse can lead to tolerance.

℞ in narcolepsy: PO: proceed for dosage adjustment as in MBD, with correction of the abnormal symptomatology as the end point.

RITALIN; tabl

Metoclopramide hydrochloride; gastrointestinal prokinetic agent that increases lower esophageal sphincter pressure, rate of gastric emptying, and augments gastrointestinal peristaltic activity. Use of this drug for the treatment of symptomatic gastroesophageal reflux in infants and children remains controversial. Drug is also used for the treatment of diabetic gastroparesis and as an adjunctive measure facilitating small bowel intubation when the tube does not pass the pylorus with conventional maneuvers. High-dose metoclopramide therapy has been shown to be an effective aid in the adjunctive management of nausea and vomiting associated with cancer chemotherapy.

℞ for gastroesophageal reflux or gastrointestinal dismotility: CH = PO: 0.1 mg/kg/dose administered 4 times a day

℞ for prevention of chemotherapy-induced emesis: 2–3 mg/kg/dose administered before and after chemotherapeutic drug; timing of dose and actual regimen are dependent upon the specific chemotherapeutic agent administered.

Caution: Metoclopramide possesses dopamine receptor antagonist activity; thus, acute dystonic reactions may occur and are relatively frequent with high-dose therapy. Diphenhydramine may be used to treat metoclopramide (or phenothiazine)-induced acute dystonic reaction. It may be appropriate to co-administer diphenhydramine with high-dose metoclopramide to prevent dystonic reactions in patients receiving this therapy for nausea and vomiting associated with cancer chemotherapy.

†, REGLAN; tabs, syrup, inj

Metolazone; saluretic, inhibiting sodium reabsorption, and interfering with dilution of urine. A quinazoline diuretic with pharmacologic properties similar to those of thiazide diuretics. Dosage is titrated to effect in the management of edema as an antihypertensive agent. CH = PO: 0.2–-0.4 mg/kg/24 hr, div, every 12–24 hr

DIULO; *ZAROXOLYN;* tabs

Metoprolol tartrate; a relatively selective β_1-adrenoreceptor antagonist, used in the treatment of hypertension and other cardiovascular disorders. CH = PO: 1–5 mg/kg/24 hr, div, every 12 hr, dose adjusted to patient response.

Caution: Experience with the use of this drug in children is limited. Despite relatively selective β_1-adrenoreceptive antagonism, it should be used cautiously in patients with bronchospastic disorders.

LOPRESSOR; tabs, inj

Metronidazole hydrochloride; synthetic antibacterial agent highly active against most obligate anaerobes including *Bacteroides* species such as *B. fragilis,* and *Clostridium* and *Peptostreptococcus* species. The drug is also effective in the treatment of amebiasis, *Giardia,* and *Trichomonas.*

℞ for amebiasis: CH = PO: 35–50 mg/kg/24 hr, div, every 8 hr

℞ for the treatment of anaerobic infections: IV

NB <2,000 g, 15 mg/kg/24 hr, div, every 12 hr

NB >2,000 g, <7 days: 15 mg/kg/24 hr, div, every 8 hr

NB >2,000 g, >7 days: 30 mg/kg/24 hr, div, every 8 hr

℞ for giardiasis: CH = PO: 15 mg/kg/day, div, every 8 hr

℞ for trichomonas vaginitis: CH = PO: 15 mg/kg/24 hr, div, every 8 hr, for 7 days.

Topical therapy: Apply and rub in thin film twice daily to affected area. May be administered as vaginal suppositories.

Caution: Patient should not ingest alcohol for 24 hr after receiving a dose of this drug (disulfiram-type reaction). Drug interactions possible; may prolong anticoagulant effect of warfarin-type anticoagulants.

†, FLAGYL; tabs, inj

Table continued on following page

TABLE 27–3 Drug Dosages *Continued*

Mezlocillin sodium; semisynthetic penicillin susceptible to destruction by penicillinase.
℞ for systemic use: NB = IV (over 15–30 min), IM when IV not possible: <7 days, 150 mg/kg/24 hr, div, every 12 hr; >7 days, 225 mg/kg/24 hr, div, every 8 hr; IN, CH: 200–300 mg/kg/24 hr, div, every 4–6 hr
Note: Each gram of drug contains 1.85 mEq of sodium; IM injection is painful.
MEZLIN; inj

Miconazole; synthetic antifungal imidazole derivative effective against systemic infections with *Coccidioides immitis, Candida albicans, Cryptococcus neoformans, Paracoccidioides brasiliensis*. IV infusion alone is inadequate for the treatment of fungal meningitis and urinary bladder infection; intrathecal administration and bladder instillation must also be carried out.
℞ for treatment of proved coccidioidomycosis, candidosis, cryptococcosis, or paracoccidioidomycosis: CH = IV (after dilution with isotonic saline or 5% D/W and over 30–60 min): 20–40 mg/kg/24 hr, div, every 8 hr, until clinical and laboratory tests no longer indicate activity of fungal infection. Dose may vary with type of fungus involved.
MONISTAT IV; ampules for IV inj

Mineral oil; indigestible liquid hydrocarbon with limited absorbability; lubricant
℞ mild laxative: PO: 0.5 mL/kg/dose
†, liquid petrolatum; plain liquid or emulsion

Minocycline; see Tetracyclines

Minoxidil; direct-acting peripheral vasodilator
℞ in severely hypertensive patients who do not adequately respond to maximum therapeutic doses of a diuretic and 2 other antihypertensive agents. Usually a β-adrenergic blocking agent has to be given concomitantly to prevent tachycardia and increased myocardial workload, as well as a diuretic such as hydrochlorothiazide, chlorthalidone, or furosemide to prevent serious fluid retention. CH = PO: initial dosage 0.2 mg/kg/24 hr as single dose; thereafter dosage may be increased stepwise to 0.25–1.0 mg/kg/24 hr under careful titration of the size and frequency of administration of the doses according to the individual needs of the patient. Therapy is usually associated with extensive hirsutism.
LONITEN; tabl

Morphine sulfate; narcotic analgesic agent; addictive
℞ against severe pain: CH = SC: 0.6–1.2 mg/kg/24 hr, div, prn every 4 hr, equivalent to 0.1–0.2 mg/kg/dose, to be repeated prn every 4 hr
†; inj
Caution: Overdose produces severe respiratory depression, hypothermia, coma. Naloxone antidotal.

Mupirocin; topical antibacterial ointment that inhibits bacterial protein synthesis by reversibly binding to bacterial isoleucyl transfer-RNA synthetase. Antibacterial spectrum of activity limited to gram-positive organisms only, including methicillin-resistant and β-lactamase–producing strains of staphylococci. No drug is absorbed systemically following topical administration. Mupirocin has been used in surgical dressings, as a prophylactic agent in the care of venous catheter access sites, and in topical management of impetigo.
℞ for topical application: applied to affected skin area every 8 hr
BACTROBAN; oint

Nafcillin sodium; semisynthetic penicillinase-resistant penicillin
NB = IM, IV (over 15–30 min):
<2,000 g <7 days of age: 50 mg/kg/24 hr, div, every 12 hr
<2,000 g >7 days of age: 75 mg/kg/24 hr, div, every 8 hr
>2,000 g <7 days of age: 50 mg/kg/24 hr, div, every 8 hr
>2,000 g >7 days of age: 75 mg/kg/24 hr, div, every 6 hr
IN, CH: 150–200 mg/kg/24 hr, div, every 4–6 hr
†; UNIPEN, NAFCIL; caps, tabl, oral susp, inj

Nalidixic acid, antimicrobial agent effective against a selected group of gram-negative bacteria, apparently by inhibiting DNA synthesis
℞ for treatment of selected cases of urinary tract infection, when infective organisms can be shown to be sensitive: IN (>3 mo), CH = PO: 55 mg/kg/24 hr, div, every 6 hr, for 10–14 days
Note: If prolonged treatment is indicated, daily dose should be reduced to 33 mg/kg/24 hr, div, every 6 hr, and periodic evaluation for adverse side effects should be made. Resistance of initially sensitive micro-organisms develops in about 25% of infections and can occur within 48 hr. If resistance is suspected, a therapeutic alternative must be chosen. Action of nalidixic acid is antagonized by nitrofurantoin.
NEGGRAM; oral susp, caplets
Caution: Even therapeutic doses may cause increased intracranial pressure, toxic psychosis, seizures in some patients.

Naloxone hydrochloride; opioid antagonist; nonaddictive
℞ in respiratory depression due to opioids: NB, IN, CH = IV, IM, SC: 0.01 mg/kg/dose, to be repeated prn after 2–3 min up to 3 times. After satisfactory response the dose must be repeated every 1–2 hr, as long as opioid depression persists. May require frequent repetitive doses or administration as a continuous IV infusion, depending on the elimination characteristics of the specific opioid agonist.
NARCAN, NARCAN neonatal; inj

Naproxen; nonsteroidal anti-inflammatory agent of the arylacetic acid group that possesses antipyretic and analgesic activities. Experience with this drug in children has been mostly limited to use in the treatment of juvenile rheumatoid arthritis.
℞ for rheumatoid arthritis: CH = PO: 10 mg/kg/24 hr, div, every 12 hr
NAPROSYN, ANAPROX; tabs

Neomycin sulfate; antimicrobial aminoglycoside
℞ inhibition of gastrointestinal flora; justified only in selected cases (danger of hyperammonemia, enterocolitis with pathogenic *Escherichia coli*): IN, CH = PO: 50–100 mg/kg/24 hr, div, every 6–8 hr
Caution: Possible overgrowth of abnormal organisms.
†, MYCIFRADIN sulfate, ‡; oral susp, tabl

Netilmicin sulfate; antimicrobial aminoglycoside. NB = IM, IV (slowly over 30–60 min): <7 days of age, 5 mg/kg/24 hr, div, every 12 hr; >7 days of age, 7.5 mg/kg/24 hr, div, every 8 hr. IN, CH = IM, IV (slowly over 30–60 min): 7.5 mg/kg/24 hr, div, every 8 hr. Serum concentrations may be monitored; therapeutic peak concentration is 5–10 mg/L, trough is <2 mg/L (see Table 27–2)

Niclosamide; anthelmintic agent useful particularly against cestodes, which under the effect of the drug become susceptible to the proteolytic action of intestinal secretions
℞ against *Diphyllobothrium latum* (fish tapeworm) and *Taenia saginata* (beef tapeworm): CH = PO: 1,000 mg, as single dose; Adult = PO: 1500 mg, as single dose
℞ against *T. solium* (pork tapeworm): same dose as for fish and beef tapeworms. Since viability of ova contained in the segments is not affected by the drug and there is risk of cysticercosis with *T. solium* if ova spill out of digested segments, it is mandatory to give an adequate purge 1 hr after niclosamide administration to clear the bowel of all dead segments before they can be digested
℞ against *Hymenolepis nana* (dwarf tapeworm): CH = PO: 1,000 mg/24 hr, as single daily dose, for 5 consecutive days. Adult = PO: 1500 mg/24 hr, as single daily dose, for 5 consecutive days
Note: Niclosamide tablets must be thoroughly chewed before being swallowed or finely ground and mixed with some liquid before they are ingested to be fully effective. Niclosamide is available in the U.S.A. from the Parasitic Disease Drug Service, Bureau of Epidemiology, Centers for Disease Control, Atlanta, GA 30333.
YOMESAN; tabl

Nifedipine; calcium channel antagonist used in pediatrics as an antihypertensive agent.

TABLE 27–3 Drug Dosages *Continued*

℞ for hypertensive emergencies: CH = PO: 0.25–0.5 mg/kg/dose, administered every 6–8 hr. Contents of gelatin capsule may be placed sublingually for immediate onset of activity.
Caution: may cause severe hypotension, flushing, tachycardia, and palpitations.

Nitrofurantoin; nitrofuran-substituted hydantoin; antimicrobial agent effective against selected organisms, by interfering with enzyme systems of the microorganisms
℞ in the treatment of urinary tract infections, when infecting organisms are shown to be sensitive or likely to respond by clinical experience: IN (>3 mo), CH = PO: 5–7 mg/kg/24 hr, div, every 6 hr (with meals to minimize gastric upset), for 10–14 days. Repeated treatment courses with nitrofurantoin should be separated by "rest" periods. For long-term suppressive therapy dosage should be reduced, possibly to as low as 2 mg/kg/24 hr, div, every 6 hr
Note: Because of rapid elimination by the kidneys, bacteriostatic concentrations are achieved only in urine. Better antibacterial activity is obtained in acid urine.
Caution: Hemolysis occurs in G-6-PD–deficient individuals and in newborns because of insufficient detoxification capabilities. Nitrofurantoin should not be given to pregnant women at term or to women who breast feed.
†, FURADANTIN, MICRODANTIN, ‡; oral susp, tabl, caps

Nitroprusside; sodium nitrosylpentacyanoferrate, $Na_2Fe(CN)_5 \cdot NO \cdot 2H_2O$; vasodilator by direct action on smooth muscles of blood vessels; effect appears almost immediately and ends promptly, 1–10 min after stopping of administration of nitroprusside
℞ for emergency reduction of hypertension: IV infusion: Example: to prepare a solution of nitroprusside containing 0.1 mg/mL, dissolve 50 mg nitroprusside first in 2–3 mL 5% dextrose in water, and transfer this amount to 500 mL 5% dextrose water,* and start continuous infusion using a microdrip regulator or an infusion pump that allows precise measurement of flow; begin with infusion rate of 0.003 mg/kg/min (equivalent to 0.03 mL/kg/min of solution containing 0.1 mg/mL nitroprusside), and decrease or increase dosage according to response, for which there exists a wide dosage range (0.0005–0.008 mg/kg/min)
*Only 5% dextrose in water solution should be used to prepare nitroprusside solution, and no other drug should be added. To prevent decomposition of nitroprusside by exposure to light, protect infusion bottle and possibly tubing from light; for instance, by wrapping in aluminum foil.
Caution: Fall in arterial blood pressure is dose-dependent, with risk of hypotensive circulatory failure on overdosage if careful monitoring of blood pressure does not lead to prompt adjustment of infusion rate.
Note: In patients receiving concomitant antihypertensive medications, a smaller dosage of nitroprusside is required for comparable reduction of hypertension.
NIPRIDE; powder for preparation of solution prior to inj

Nystatin; antifungal agent; 1 mg = 2,000 units; seems to be active by altering permeability of cell membrane of yeasts
℞ for topical treatment of candidosis of the buccal cavity (thrush) and the gastrointestinal tract. Very poorly absorbed. In oral candidosis, spread nystatin suspension into recesses of mouth: NB (<2000 g) = PO: 200,000–400,000 units/24 hr, div, every 4–6 hr. NB (>2000 g), IN = PO: 400,000–800,000 units/24 hr, div, every 4–6 hr. CH = PO: 800,000–2,000,000 units/24 hr, div, every 4–6 hr
†, MYCOSTATIN, NILSTAT; oral susp, tabl

Oxacillin sodium; semisynthetic penicillinase-resistant penicillin
NB = IM, IV: <2,000 g, <7 days of age, 50 mg/kg/24 hr, div, every 12 hr; >7 days of age, 100 mg/kg/24 hr, div, every 8 hr; >2,000 g, <7 days of age, 75 mg/kg/24 hr, div, every 8 hr; >7 days of age, 150 mg/kg/24 hr, div, every 6–8 hr; IN, CH = PO, IM, IV: 50–200 mg/kg/24 hr, div, every 4–6 hr
BACTOCILL, PROSTAPHLIN; caps, oral susp, inj

Oxtriphylline; choline salt of theophylline; thus, pharmacologic action is identical to that of theophylline (see Theophylline), and 100 mg of oxtriphylline is equivalent to 64 mg of theophylline base.
CHOLEDYL, elix, tabs, SA tab

Paraldehyde; cyclic ether compound that decomposes to acetaldehyde on exposure to light and air; rapidly acting hypnotic agent
℞ in status epilepticus: CH = IM (injection remote from nerves because of risk of damage): 0.15 g/kg/dose, corresponding to 0.15 mL/kg/dose of paraldehyde solution containing 1 g/mL; occasionally 1 additional dose may be given after 30 min, prn
Note: Use glass syringe because paraldehyde reacts with plastic equipment. When given IV, injection should be slow, and paraldehyde solution should be diluted with isotonic sodium chloride solution to lessen risk of thrombophlebitis. IV use is not recommended.
℞ to calm agitation: CH = PO, IM (PR, diluted in equal amount of olive oil): 0.15 mL/kg/dose, to be repeated prn after 4–6 hr
Caution: Before use, make sure that drug is not decomposed (acetaldehyde, acetic acid).
†, PARAL; liquid for inj, oral use (risk of gastric irritation), and rectal use

Pemoline, an oxazolidone; structurally different from amphetamine and methylphenidate; CNS stimulant with minimal sympathomimetic effects
℞ in minimal brain dysfunction: drug treatment of MBD not recommended below the age of 3 yr or in nonstructured therapeutic situation: CH (so far insufficient data have been accumulated in children below the age of 6 yr to assess efficacy and safety in this age group) = PO: initiate treatment with approximately 1 mg/kg/24 hr, as single dose each morning. If needed, increase dosage at weekly intervals by increments of 0.5 mg/kg/24 hr. On this schedule of titration of dose therapeutic response may not become evident until 4th wk of continued administration. Daily dose should not exceed 3 mg/kg/24 hr
Note: Insomnia, anorexia, and weight loss have been observed. The degree of reduced growth pattern on continued treatment is not yet established. Drug treatment of MBD should be discontinued at appropriate intervals to observe behavior of the patient and assess indication for further treatment. (See Sec. 3.39.)
CYLERT; tabl

Penicillin G, benzylpenicillin; potassium penicillin G (1 mg = 1,595 units); sodium penicillin G (1 mg = 1,667 units). One million units of these salts of penicillin contains either 1.68 mEq K^+ or Na^-; in other terms, 1 g contains either 2.7 mEq K^- or 2.8 mEq Na^-.
NB = IV (over 15–30 min), IM:
<2,000 g, 50,000 units/kg/24 hr, div, every 12 hr.
℞ for meningitis: 100,000 units/kg/24 hr, div, every 12 hr
>2,000 g, 75,000 units/kg/24 hr, div, every 8 hr
℞ for meningitis: 150,000–200,000 units/kg/24 hr, div, every 8 hr
IN, CH = PO, IM, IV (15–30 min): 100,000–250,000 units/kg/24 hr, div, every 4–6 hr
℞ for meningitis: 200,000–300,000 units/kg/24 hr, div, every 4 hr
(The higher doses should be chosen for meningitis caused by group B streptococci.)
IN, CH = PO, IM, IV (over 15–30 min): 25,000–50,000 units/kg/24 hr, equivalent to 15.5–31 mg/kg/24 hr, div, every 4–6 hr; if given PO, administer penicillin G 0.5 hr before or 2 hr after the meal.
℞ in severe infections: IV: 200,000–400,000 units/kg/24 hr, equivalent to 125–250 mg/kg/24 hr, as continuous drip infusion or div, every 2–4 hr
℞ for prophylaxis of rheumatic fever: PO: 200,000 units/dose, equivalent to 125 mg/dose, twice daily, spaced from meals (see Sec 11.74)

Penicillin G benzathine, for injection: combination of 1 mole of dibenzylethylenediamine with 2 moles of penicillin G; 1 mg = 1,211 units
℞ for prophylaxis of rheumatic fever: CH = IM: 600,000–1,200,000 units, equivalent to 500–1,000 mg penicillin G, once a month
†, BICILLIN L-A, PERMAPEN, ‡; susp for inj
†, PENTIDS, PFIZERPEN G, ‡; tabl, caps, oral susp, inj (IV)

Table continued on following page

TABLE 27–3 Drug Dosages *Continued*

Penicillin G procaine, for injection; combination of penicillin G with procaine, mole for mole (1 mg = 1009 units)
NB = IM: 50,000 units/kg/24 hr, equivalent to 50 mg/kg/24 hr, in single daily dose. IN, CH = IM: 25,000–50,000 units/kg/24 hr, equivalent to 25–50 mg/kg/24 hr, in single daily dose
†, CRYSTICILLIN, DURACILLIN A.S., ‡; susp for IM inj

Penicillin V, phenoxymethyl penicillin; acid-resistant penicillin; 1 mg = 1695 units
IN, CH = PO: 25,000–50,000 units/kg/24 hr, equivalent to 15–30 mg/kg/24 hr, div, every 6–8 hr. *Note:* 400,000 units = 250 mg (approx).
†, PEN-VEE K, VEETIDS, ‡; tabl, oral susp, drops

Pentazocine hydrochloride; narcotic analgesic of the benzomorphan type; addictive
℞ against severe pain: Clinical experience in children under 12 yr of age is limited. Adult = PO: 50 mg/dose, to be repeated prn after 3–4 hr; IM, SC (pentazocine lactate); 30 mg/dose, to be repeated prn after 4 hr
FORTRAL, TALWIN; tabl (hydrochloride); inj (lactate)
Caution: As for *morphine,* above.

Pentobarbital, central nervous system depressant of barbiturate class with short duration of action; tolerance to hypnotic effect may develop on continued use; initially, hypnotic effect of 3–5 hr
℞ for sedation: IN, CH = PO, IM: 1–3 mg/kg/24 hr, div, every 6 hr
℞ for sleep: IN, CH = PO, IM: 2–6 mg/kg/dose, repeat prn after 12–24 hr
†, NEMBUTAL elixir, pentobarbital sodium, †, NEMBUTAL sodium; inj, caps, suppos

Phenobarbital, central nervous system depressant of barbiturate class with long duration of action; initially, hypnotic effect of 8–12 hr; tolerance to hypnotic effect may develop on continued use
℞ for sedation: IN, CH = PO, IM: 2–3 mg/kg/24 hr, div, every 8–12 hr
℞ for sleep: IN, CH = PO, IM: 2–3 mg/kg/dose, repeat prn after 12–24 hr
℞ as anticonvulsant for long-term therapy: IN, CH = PO: start with 1.5 mg/kg/24 hr, div, every 12 hr; increase according to tolerance and therapeutic effect to 4–6 mg/kg/24 hr, div, every 12 hr, or as single daily dose, preferably at bedtime in order to minimize daytime drowsiness from hypnotic effect (see also Sec. 20.21)
℞ as adjunct in treatment of status epilepticus: IN, CH = IV: 10–20 mg/kg loading dose by slow IV injection, followed prn after interval of 5 min by 5–10 mg/kg/dose, to be repeated at 20-min intervals until seizures are controlled or a total dose of 40 mg/kg is reached.
Caution: All barbiturates, including phenobarbital, are respiratory depressants. Serum concentrations should be monitored.
†, LUMINAL; elixir, tabl phenobarbital sodium, †, LUMINAL sodium; inj

Phenolphthalein; laxative acting primarily on the colon
CH = PO: 1 mg/kg/dose
†, tabl, oral susp; component of several preparations

Phenoxybenzamine hydrochloride; α-adrenergic receptor antagonist used primarily for the symptomatic treatment of pheochromocytoma-associated episodes of hypertension. The bioavailability of phenoxybenzamine from capsules appears to range between 20 and 30%.
℞ in the treatment of pheochromocytoma: 1–2 mg/kg/24 hr, div, every 6–12 hr, titrated to clinical effect.
DIBENZYLINE, caps

Phenylephrine hydrochloride; catecholamine with exclusively α-adrenergic action; peripheral vasoconstrictor
℞ to increase blood pressure in orthostatic hypotension, or
℞ to trigger vagal reflex in response to blood pressure increase, in the treatment of atrial tachyarrhythmia: PO: 1 mg/kg/24 hr, div, every 4 hr; SC, IM: 0.1 mg/kg/dose, repeat prn by monitoring response
Caution: With regard to hypertensive state and peripheral ischemia.
†, NEO-SYNEPHRINE hydrochloride; inj, elixir; also available as nose drops for local decongestant effect

Phenytoin, diphenylhydantoin; anticonvulsant agent; effective also in certain types of cardiac arrhythmias; antiarrhythmic effects similar to those of lidocaine: delayed slow diastolic depolarization, diminished automaticity; may facilitate conduction in damaged myocardial areas; does not depress myocardial activity
℞ as anticonvulsant for long-term therapy: IN, CH = PO: 3–8 mg/kg/24 hr, div, every 8–12 hr
℞ as adjunct in the treatment of status epilepticus: NB, IN, = IV (slow infusion under monitoring of heart rate): 15–20 mg/kg/dose (see also Sec. 20.21)
℞ as adjunct in the treatment of ventricular tachyarrhythmia: CH = IV (over 5 min): 2–4 mg/kg/dose; may be repeated prn and at beginning of maintenance therapy. Serum concentration should be monitored; therapeutic range is 10–20 mg/L (see Table 27–2).
Note: Phenytoin disposition is most often characterized by nonlinear (Michaelis-Menton) pharmacokinetics. Phenytoin is highly protein bound (>90%) and may be associated with protein binding displacement interaction; therapy is associated with unpredictable effects upon the activity of hepatic drug metabolizing enzymes. Caution should be used in generic substitution because all generic preparations may not be bioequivalent.
†, DILANTIN; oral susp phenytoin sodium, †, DILANTIN sodium; caps, inj

Piperacillin sodium; semisynthetic broad-spectrum aminobenzylpenicillin. Each gram of piperacillin contains 1.85 mEq of sodium. The drug is not absorbed when administered orally and is available only for parenteral administration.
NB = IM, IV (15–30 min): 100 mg/kg/24 hr, div, every 12 hr
IN, CH = IM, IV (15–30 min): 200–300 mg/kg/24 hr, div, every 4–6 hr in treating children with cystic fibrosis

Primaquine, 8-aminoquinoline antimalarial agent, used for prophylaxis against *Plasmodium vivax, P. ovale,* and *P. malariae* and for "radical" cure for *P. vivax* and *P. ovale*
IN, CH = PO: 0.55 mg/kg/24 hr (equivalent to 0.3 mg/kg/24 hr of base), as single daily dose, for 14 days
Note: Degree of intravascular hemolysis in individuals with G-6-PD deficiency is related to dosage and particular variant of the deficiency.
Primaquine diphosphate; tabl

Primidone; a deoxybarbiturate that is partially metabolized to phenobarbital; anticonvulsant agent
℞ for long-term therapy of selected types of convulsive disorder: CH = PO: 10 mg/kg/24 hr, div, every 8–12 hr (see also Sec. 20.21)
Note: Serum concentration monitoring should include evaluation of both PEMA and phenobarbital (see Table 27–2).
MYSOLINE; oral susp, tabl

Probenecid, competitive inhibitor of tubular secretion and reabsorption of organic acids
℞ for uricosuric action (acetylsalicylic acid antagonizes this effect), or
℞ in conjunction with penicillin G or V, or ampicillin, methicillin, oxacillin, cloxacillin, nafcillin to achieve longer persistence of therapeutic blood and tissue concentrations of the antimicrobial agent. CH = PO: initial dose of 25 mg/kg, followed by 40 mg/kg/24 hr, div, every 6 hr
BENEMID; tabl

Procainamide hydrochloride; antiarrhythmic agent with general cardiodepressant effects; diminished myocardial excitability (decreased threshold potential, prolonged refractory period), reduced conduction velocity, diminished automaticity; decreases myocardial contractility; effects similar to those of quinidine
℞ for ventricular tachyarrhythmia: IN, CH = IM: 20–30 mg/kg/24 hr, div, every 4–6 hr; IV loading dose 10–15 mg over 30 min

TABLE 27–3 Drug Dosages *Continued*

followed by continuous IV maintenance infusion of 20–80 μg/kg/min; PO: 15–50 mg/kg/24 hr, div, every 3–6 hr. Serum concentration should be monitored for both procainamide and its active metabolite *N*-acetyl procainamide (NAPA) (see Table 27–2).
†, PRONESTYL; tabl, caps, inj

Prochlorperazine; piperazine-type phenothiazine with pronounced antiemetic effect
℞ for sedation: CH (over 2 yr old) = PO: 0.4 mg/kg/24 hr, div, every 6–8 hr, prn. IM: 0.2 mg/kg/24 hr, div, every 8–12 hr, prn
†, COMPAZINE; suppos prochlorperazine edisylate, COMPAZINE edisylate; oral liquid, syrup, inj
Caution: May produce parkinsonian syndrome and acute dystonic reaction. Diphenhydramine may be antidotal. Other antiemetic agents may be more desirable for use in children.

Promethazine hydrochloride; phenothiazine with aliphatic side chain that affords antihistaminic activity.
℞ for sedation, prevention or treatment of motion sickness, and as antihistamine; CH = PO: 1 mg/kg/24 hr, divided into half dose at bedtime and quarter doses every 6 hr of the remaining daytime
†, PHENERGAN; syrup, tabl, suppos

Propantheline bromide, antispasmodic synthetic antimuscarinic agent as well as partial ganglionic blocking drug
℞ as adjunctive therapy against spasms in the gastrointestinal tract: CH = PO: 1.5 mg/kg/24 hr, div, every 6 hr, with meals, if applicable. IM: 0.8 mg/kg/24 hr, div, every 6 hr
†, PRO-BANTHINE; tabl, inj

Propoxyphene hydrochloride, and propoxyphene napsylate; opioid analgesic with less dependence liability than seen with codeine
℞ against mild to moderately severe pain: CH = PO: 2–3 mg/kg/24 hr, div, every 6 hr
propoxyphene hydrochloride, †, DARVON, ‡; caps propoxyphene napsylate, DARVON-N; oral susp, tabl

Propranolol hydrochloride; β-adrenergic blocking agent (β_1 and β_2); racemic mixture of D- and L-propranolol, of which only L form has adrenergic blocking activity
℞ against selected forms of supraventricular and ventricular tachycardia: IN, CH = IV: 0.01–0.10 mg/kg/dose, given slowly; repeat every 6–8 hr prn. PO: 0.5–4.0 mg/kg/24 hr, div, every 6–8 hr
℞ as antihypertensive in long-term therapy: CH = PO: initially 1 mg/kg/24 hr, div, every 6 hr, and progressive increase of dosage, if needed to achieve adequate response, up to 5 mg/kg/24 hr, div, every 6 hr. Combination with diuretic or hydralazine is indicated because propranolol blocks physiologic compensatory mechanisms such as adrenergic inotropic and chronotropic responses, as well as renin activity (see also Sec. 15.81).
℞ for prevention of migraine attack in severe cases and to combat the manifestations of thyrotoxicosis: propranolol requirements vary widely from patient to patient because of individual differences in severity of underlying disease, endogenous sympathetic neuronal activity, sensitivity of β-adrenergic receptors to blockade, degree of protein binding, hepatic blood flow. For comparable effect, oral dose should be 6–10 times higher than intravenous dose in spite of good absorption from the gut because of inactivation of important fraction of propranolol in liver after entrance through portal vein (i.e., first-pass effect).
Measures in case of exaggerated response: against bradycardia, atropine; if no response, isoproterenol, *cautiously;* against cardiac failure, digitalization and diuretics; against hypotension, epinephrine; against bronchospasm, isoproterenol, theophylline (aminophylline)
†, INDERAL; tabl, inj

Protamine sulfate; protamines are low-molecular weight basic proteins that bind tightly to heparin in vitro, thus neutralizing its anticoagulant effect. Protamine is used to reverse the effects of heparin. Protamine 1 mg is capable of binding to and thus neutralizing approximately 100 units of heparin. The dose of protamine to be administered is based on the expected amount of heparin remaining in the body as determined by the heparin elimination half-life ($t_{1/2}$).
Caution: Protamine dose should be calculated cautiously because excess protamine may cause anticoagulation.
PROTAMINE, inj

Pseudoephedrine hydrochloride; indirectly acting sympathomimetic
℞ as nasal decongestant by systemic route: CH = PO: 4 mg/kg/24 hr, div, every 6 hr
†, SUDAFED, ‡; syrup, caps; contained in many combination products

Pyrantel pamoate, anthelmintic agent effective by means of neuromuscular paralysis of the parasite
℞ against pinworms (*Enterobius vermicularis*), *Ascaris lumbricoides,* and hookworms (*Necator americanus, Ancylostoma duodenale*): pyrantel pamoate has not been extensively studied in infants and children below 2 yr of age, hence particular attention should be given to children of this age group during treatment of parasitic infestation with pyrantel. CH = PO: 11 mg/kg/dose, as single dose and without regard to food intake or time of day; purging not necessary prior to, during, or after therapy
Note: In pinworm infestation, in which possibility of reinfection with eggs from the host exists, a 2nd treatment 2–3 wk after the 1st might be indicated.
ANTIMINTH; oral susp

Pyridostigmine bromide, cholinesterase inhibitor
℞ for diagnosis of myasthenia gravis: see Edrophonium chloride
℞ in myasthenia gravis: NB, IN, CH = IM: 0.1 mg/kg/dose, and continue with PO medication. PO: frequency of dosage and size of dose must be adjusted individually to provide optimum compensation during cycle of daily activities; average effective dose: 7 mg/kg/24 hr, div, every 4–5 hr
℞ for reversal of nondepolarizing muscle relaxants (tubocurarine, gallamine, pancuronium): IV (preceded by IV injection of atropine to prevent excessive secretions and bradycardia): 0.15 mg/kg/dose, and watch for recovery that ought to occur after 15–30 min; assure appropriate ventilation until complete recovery
MESTINON; tabl, syrup, inj
Caution: As for Edrophonium chloride.

Pyrimethamine, inhibitor of dihydrofolate reductase, antimalarial agent; for use in treatment of toxoplasmosis (see Sec. 12.117)
℞ for clinical prophylaxis of malaria, especially effective against *Plasmodium falciparum:* IN, CH = PO: 0.5–0.75 mg/kg/dose, once every 7 days. Begin prophylaxis 2 wk before entering malarious area and continue for 8 wk after leaving. To eradicate *P. vivax* and *P. ovale* infections, treatment for 14 days with primaquine should be considered immediately on leaving malarious area while pyrimethamine prophylaxis is still in effect (see also Sec. 12.114)
Note: Hematologic abnormalities (anemia, thrombocytopenia, leukopenia) secondary to folic and folinic acid depletion can be prevented or reversed by IM administration of folinic acid (leucovorin) without affecting the efficacy of pyrimethamine.
DARAPRIM; tabl

Quinacrine hydrochloride, mepacrine hydrochloride; acridine derivative formerly used as antimalarial agent and against infestation with tapeworms, presently regarded as drug of choice against giardiasis
℞ against *Giardia lamblia (Lamblia intestinalis):* CH = PO: 6 mg/kg/24 hr, div, every 8 hr, for 5 consecutive days; maximum daily dose: 300 mg/24 hr
ATABRINE; tabl

Quinidine gluconate, quinidine sulfate, and quinidine polygalacturonate; alkaloid with general cardiodepressant effects: diminished myocardial excitability (decrease in threshold potential), reduced conduction velocity (widening of QRS complex, possibility of A-V block), increased refractory period, diminished automaticity, especially in ectopic sites; depresses myocardial contractility with risk of congestive heart failure if myocardial damage present

Table continued on following page

TABLE 27–3 Drug Dosages *Continued*

℞ against atrial tachycardia (usually after digitalization), or ventricular tachyarrhythmia: IN, CH = 2 mg/kg test dose PO, IM, (IV) to exclude idiosyncrasy. For treatment: PO (quinidine sulfate): 30 mg/kg/24 hr, div, every 4–5 hr. IV, IM (quinidine gluconate): 2–10 mg/kg/dose, prn every 3–6 hr

quinidine gluconate, QUINAGLUTE; tabl, inj quinidine sulfate, †, QUINIDEX, ‡; tabl quinidine polygalacturonate. CARDIOQUIN; tabl

Caution: Overdose may lead to cardiac arrest.

Quinolone, see Fluroquinolone.

Ranitidine hydrochloride; H_2-receptor antagonist competitively inhibits secretion of gastric acid

℞ for treatment of duodenal and gastric ulcers, for relief of symptoms caused by gastroesophageal reflux and prophylaxis against stress ulcers in critically ill children; compatible with concomitant treatment with oral antacids (which should be administered at frequent intervals and in adequate doses) or other therapeutic modalities. NB, IN, CH = IV: 1–3 mg/kg/24 hr, div, every 6–12 hr; PO: 2–6 mg/kg/24 hr, div, every 8–12 hr

Ranitidine may be administered as a continuous 24-hr infusion. Ranitidine dosage is often titrated to effect (i.e., measurement of hydrogen ion excretion (pH) of gastric aspirate).

ZANTAC; tabl, inj

Reserpine, alkaloid that depletes stores of catecholamines and serotonin in many organs, including the brain

℞ as antihypertensive in long-term treatment: CH = PO: initially 0.02 mg/kg/24 hr, as single daily dose or div, every 12 hr; for maintenance, dose usually reduced to 0.005–0.01 mg/kg/24 hr

Note: See Sec. 15.81. Reserpine may induce mental depression, nasal congestion.

†, SANDRIL, SERPASIL; tabl, elixir

Ribavirin; synthetic nucleoside antiviral drug. Ribavirin possesses antiviral inhibitory activity in vitro against respiratory syncytial virus (RSV), influenza virus, and herpes simplex virus. Various protocols exist for the use of this compound; the drug is usually reserved for use in the treatment of severe lower respiratory tract infections due to RSV. Ribavirin is administered by the aerosol route as a continuous aerosolization for 12–18 hr daily for 3–7 days. Aerosol solution is usually prepared in sterile water, without preservatives, to a final concentration of 20 mg/ml (see Sec. 12.76)

VIRAZOLE; aerosol

Rifampin; synthetic antimicrobial and antimycobacterial agent, interfering with RNA-polymerase of infecting organisms

℞ in treatment of tuberculosis, in conjunction with at least 1 other antituberculous agent (isoniazid), and

℞ in carriers of *Neisseria meningitidis* resistant to penicillin and sulfonamide; treatment course of 4 consecutive days (possibility of rapid emergence of resistance): IN, CH = PO: 10–20 mg/kg/24 hr, in single daily dose (1 hr before or 2 hr after meal); maximum daily dose: 600 mg (= adult dose)

Note: Rifampin is a potent inducer of hepatic drug metabolizing enzymes that may reduce the activity of a number of medications including anticoagulants, corticosteroids, cyclosporine, cardiac glycoside drugs, oral contraceptives, and opioid analgesics. Rifampin administration may cause the urine, feces, saliva, sputum, sweat, and tears to turn red-orange color. Permanent discoloration of soft contact lenses may occur.

RIFADIN, RIMACTANE; caps, inj

Salicylate sodium

℞ antipyretic, analgesic, anti-inflammatory: CH, Adolescents = PO: 25–50 mg/kg/24 hr, div, every 4–6 hr, prn

℞ antirheumatic: CH, Adolescents = PO: 50–100 mg/kg/24 hr, div, every 6 hr

†, tabl

Caution: See Sec. 26.6.

Scopolamine methylbromide; also methscopolamine bromide, an antimuscarinic agent and quaternary ammonium compound that essentially lacks the central nervous system actions (sedation or excitement, amnesia, euphoria, hallucinations, unexpected behavior) of scopolamine

℞ as adjunctive therapy in the treatment of spasms in the gastrointestinal and urinary tracts: CH = PO: 0.15 mg/kg/24 hr, div, every 6 hr; SC, IM: 0.01 mg/kg/dose, repeat prn every 6–8 hr

PAMINE; tabl, inj

Caution: As for Belladonna.

Secobarbital, central nervous system depressant of the barbiturate class with a short duration of action; tolerance to the hypnotic effect may develop on continued use; initially, hypnotic effect of 3–5 hr

℞ for sedation: IN, CH = PO, IM: 2–5 mg/kg/24 hr, div, every 6–8 hr

℞ for sleep: IN, CH = PO, IM: 3–6 mg/kg/dose, repeat prn after 12–24 hr

†, SECONAL elixir secobarbital sodium, †, SECONAL sodium; inj, caps, suppos

Senna syrup; contains anthraquinones, sennosides A and B, which stimulate the intramural nerve plexuses of the colon

℞ as laxative: CH = PO: 0.15 mL/kg/dose; to be repeated only once per wk, if indicated, to avoid interfering with normal bowel motility and not inducing laxative dependence

†; syrup

Simethicone; antiflatulent available as an individual agent and as an ingredient in many antacid preparations. Frequently used for symptomatic relief of the symptoms associated with excessive gas in the digestive tract (i.e., conditions such as colic, lactose intolerance, or air swallowing). Dosage is titrated to clinical effect and patient tolerance.

†, MYLICON, drops, tabs, liquid

Sodium sulfate, $Na_2SO_4 \cdot 10H_2O$, Glauber salt; 1 g of salt traps about 30 mL of water to make the solution isosmotic

℞ as salinic cathartic: CH = PO: 300 mg/kg/dose

†; crystalline substance to be dissolved in a liquid for PO administration

Spironolactone; aldosterone antagonist and potassium-sparing diuretic, which interferes with sodium reabsorption

℞ as diuretic in selected cases (with normal renal function), most effective in combination with a potassium-wasting diuretic: CH = PO: 1.5–3 mg/kg/24 hr, div, every 6–12 hr

Note: Monitoring of serum concentration of potassium, of potassium intake, and of renal function is indicated during treatment with spironolactone.

†; ALDACTONE; tabl

Streptomycin sulfate; antimicrobial aminoglycoside

Caution: Because this drug when administered in large doses and/or for long periods can damage the 8th cranial nerve in adults, children, and transplacentally in fetuses, its indications are stringently selective today.

℞ in tuberculous meningitis and progressive tuberculosis, in association with isoniazid and other anti-tuberculous medication: CH = IM: 20–40 mg/kg/24 hr, div, every 12 hr, for 2–3 mo; maximum daily dose regardless of weight: 1 g/24 hr. See Table 27–2.

†; susp, inj

Sulfonamides; analogs of para-aminobenzoic acid, interfering with the synthesis of tetrahydrofolic acid in sensitive bacteria

Sulfadiazine, sulfisoxazole, and *trisulfapyrimidines:* IN, CH = PO: initial dose 75 mg/kg/1st dose, followed by 120–150 mg/kg/24 hr, div, every 4–6 hr. IV (over 30 min), SC: 100–110 mg/kg/24 hr, div, every 4–6 hr

Sulfadiazine, †; tabl sulfadiazine sodium, †; inj sulfisoxazole, †, GANTRISIN; tabl sulfisoxazole acetyl, GANTRISIN acetyl; oral susp, syrup sulfisoxazole diolamine, GANTRISIN diolamine; inj trisulfapyrimidines (equal parts of sulfadiazine, sulfamerazine, and sulfamethazine), †, ‡; tabl, oral susp

Sulfamethoxazole: IN, CH = PO: initial dose 50–60 mg/kg/1st dose, followed by 50–60 mg/kg/24 hr, div, every 12 hr

GANTANOL; oral susp, tabl

Trimethoprim-sulfamethoxazole (combination of TMP + SMX): IN (>2 mo old), CH = PO: 6–12 mg TMP + 30–60 mg SMX/kg/24 hr, div, every 12 hr

TABLE 27–3 Drug Dosages *Continued*

℞ in severe urinary tract or *Shigella* infection: CH = PO, IV: 8–10 mg TMP + 40–60 mg SMX/kg/24 hr, div, every 6–8 hr

℞ against *Pneumocystis carinii*: CH = PO, IV: 15–20 mg TMP + 75–100 mg SMX/kg/24 hr, div, every 6–8 hr

Caution: Do not use in infants less than 2 mo old. Reduce dose in severe renal insufficiency. May cause bone marrow depression.

BACTRIM, SEPTRA; susp: 40 mg TMP + 200 mg SMX/5 mL; tabl: 80 mg TMP + 400 mg SMX/tabl or 160 mg TMP + 800 mg SMX/tabl; ampule: 80 mg TMP + 400 mg SMX/5 mL

Terbutaline sulfate, catecholamine; β-adrenergic receptor agonist with preferential effect on β_2-adrenergic receptors

℞ bronchodilator: PO: 0.10–0.15 mg/kg/24 hr, div, every 8 hr. β_2-selectivity is reduced with increasing dosage. SC: 0.005 mg/kg/dose, to be repeated prn after 20 min, once only

BRETHINE, BRICANYL; tabl, inj

Tetracyclines; a group of derivatives of polycyclic naphthacenecarboxamide

Chlortetracycline hydrochloride: CH = PO: 25–50 mg/kg/24 hr, div, every 6 hr

AUREOMYCIN; caps, inj (IV)

Demeclocycline and *demeclocycline hydrochloride:* CH = PO: 7–13 mg/kg/24 hr, div, every 6–12 hr

DECLOMYCIN; pediatric drops, syrup DECLOMYCIN hydrochloride; caps, tabl

Doxycycline monohydrate and *doxycycline hyclate:* CH = PO: 5 mg/kg/24 hr, div, every 12 hr

†, VIBRAMYCIN monohydrate; oral susp †, VIBRAMYCIN hyclate; caps, inj (IV)

Methacycline hydrochloride: CH = PO: 7–13 mg/kg/24 hr, div, every 6–12 hr

RONDOMYCIN; caps, syrup

Minocycline hydrochloride: CH = PO, IV: initial dose 4 mg/kg, followed by 4 mg/kg/24 hr, div, every 12 hr

MINOCIN, VECTRIN; caps, syrup, inj (IV)

Oxytetracycline, oxytetracycline hydrochloride, oxytetracycline calcium: same dosage as tetracycline hydrochloride, below

TERRAMYCIN; tabl, inj (IM) TERRAMYCIN hydrochloride; †, caps, inj (IV, IM) TERRAMYCIN calcium; pediatric drops, syrup

Tetracycline hydrochloride: CH = PO: 25–50 mg/kg/24 hr, div, every 8 hr; IM (often very painful): 15–25 mg/kg/24 hr, div, every 8–12 hr; IV: 10–20 mg/kg/24 hr, div, every 12 hr

†, ACHROMYCIN V, PANMYCIN, ‡; caps, inj (IV, IM); sol for IM inj contains local anesthetic. Pediatric drops, oral susp, and syrup prepared with tetracycline base

Note: Tetracyclines have limited indications in infancy and childhood because of their accumulation in bone and teeth and their potential to interfere with growth. Their use should be avoided insofar as possible until formation of dental enamel is complete in most permanent teeth (at about 8 yr), to avoid unsightly discolored, pitted teeth. Tetracyclines may cause increased intracranial pressure in infants (pseudotumor cerebri).

Theophylline; methylxanthine commonly used in acute and chronic management of reversible airways disease (asthma), and neonatal apnea, bronchopulmonary dysplasia, among others. Cellular mechanism of action originally believed to be a result of phosphodiesterase inhibition; however, pharmacologic effect is most likely a result of adenosine receptor antagonism.

℞ in neonatal apnea: IV, PO: initial loading dose 5 mg/kg followed by maintenance therapy depending upon age; preterm NB (<36 wk): 1–2 mg/kg/24 hr, div, every 8–12 hr; term infants (>36 wk): 2–4 mg/kg/24 hr, div, every 8–12 hr

℞ in status asthmaticus: initial loading dose IV: 4–7 mg/kg/dose, infused after dilution in equal volume of intravenous fluid over 20–30 min, followed by maintenance IV: 20 mg/kg/24 hr, div, every 4–6 hr, or by continuous IV drip; switch to PO maintenance as soon as possible. Daily theophylline dose adjustment necessary relative to patient age and hepatic and cardiac function.

℞ oral maintenance: PO: 20 mg/kg/24 hr, div, every 6 hr; as conditions permit, taper to lowest effective dosage, usually around 10 mg/kg/24 hr, div, every 6 hr. Time-release theophylline preparations permit extension of the dosage interval (i.e., administration every 8–12 hr).

Note the content of theophylline in the following formulations: theophylline (anhydrous), 100%; aminophylline, 85%; theophylline monoethanolamine, 75%; dihydroxypropyltheophylline, 70%; oxtriphylline, choline salt, 64%; theophylline sodium glycinate, 50%; theophylline calcium salicylate, 48%. Serum concentration should be monitored; therapeutic range for neonatal apnea, 7–13 mg/L; in the management of bronchospasm, 10–20 mg/L (see Sec. 11.41).

theophylline, †, ELIXOPHYLLIN elixir, ELIXICON oral susp, SLO-PHYLLIN caps, oral susp, SOMOPHYLLIN caps, ‡: component of many combination products aminophylline, †, SOMOPHYLLIN oral liquid, ‡; inj, oral preparations

Caution: Circulatory collapse, seizures, coma may result from acute or chronic overdose.

Thioridazine hydrochloride; phenothiazine of the piperidine type

℞ for sedation and neuroleptic effect: CH = PO: 1 mg/kg/24 hr, div, every 8 hr

MELLARIL; oral liquid, tabl

Caution: Overdose may produce parkinsonian syndrome. Diphenhydramine may be antidotal.

Ticarcillin disodium; semisynthetic penicillin susceptible to penicillinase; each gram of drug contains 5.2 mEq of sodium.

NB = IV (over 20–30 min), IM: <7 days <2,000 g, 150 mg/kg/24 hr, div, every 12 hr; >2,000 g, 225 mg/kg/24 hr, div, every 8 hr; >7 days <2,000 g, 225 mg/kg/24 hr, div, every 8 hr; >7 days >2,000 g, 300 mg/kg/24 hr, div, every 8 hr

IN, CH = IV (over 20–30 min), IM: 200–300 mg/kg/24 hr, div, every 4–6 hr. IM injection is painful.

TICAR; IV and IM inj

Ticarcillin + clavulanic acid; combination of a β-lactam antibiotic (ticarcillin) with a β-lactamase (penicillinase) inhibitor (clavulanic acid). The addition of clavulanic acid extends the activity of ticarcillin to include β-lactamase–producing strains of *Haemophilus influenzae,* and other drug-resistant pathogens. Doses administered as either IM or IV are the same as those for ticarcillin noted above.

Tobramycin sulfate: antimicrobial aminoglycoside

NB = IV (30–60 min), IM: <7 days <34 wk <1,500 g, 3 mg/kg every 24 hr; <34 wk >1,500 g, 2.5 mg/kg every 18 hr; >34 wk >1,500 g, 2.5 mg/kg every 12 hr; >7 days and term NB, 5 mg/kg/24 hr, div, every 12 hr

IN, CH = IV (30–60 min), IM: 5–7.5 mg/kg/24 hr, div, every 6–8 hr. Serum concentration should be monitored; therapeutic peak concentration 5–10 mg/L, trough <2 mg/L (see Table 27–2). Dosage and interval may require modification for the treatment of patients with cystic fibrosis.

Caution: Ototoxic; nephrotoxic.

†, NEBCIN; inj

Tolmentin sodium; nonsteroidal anti-inflammatory agent of the indole class that possesses analgesic and antipyretic activities. The drug's mechanism of action remains to be described but may involve prostaglandin synthetase inhibition. The drug is most often used in the treatment of juvenile rheumatoid arthritis.

℞ for juvenile rheumatoid arthritis: CH = PO: 15 mg/kg/24 hr

Triamterene; potassium-sparing diuretic; inhibits the reabsorption of Na^+ in exchange for K^+ and H^+; its effect is potentiated by concomitant use of diuretics that act more proximally

CH = PO: 2–4 mg/kg/24 hr, div, every 12 hr (after meals).

Note: For maintenance, dosage must be adjusted to needs of individual patient; in conjunction with other diuretics dosage usually can be decreased.

Caution: Because of the risk of hyperkalemia, serum potassium concentrations and potassium intake should be watched.

DYRENIUM; caps

Trimethadione; oxazolidinedione; anticonvulsant agent

℞ as an adjunct in the treatment of convulsive disorders: CH = PO: 20 mg/kg/24 hr, div, every 8 hr; if needed, dosage can be progressively adjusted to 40 mg/kg/24 hr, div, every 8 hr

Table continued on following page

TABLE 27–3 Drug Dosages *Continued*

Note: The methylated metabolite of trimethadione accumulates progressively in the body and is partially responsible for anticonvulsant effect.
TRIDIONE; tabl, caps, oral susp

Trimethoprim; see Sulfonamides

Tripelennamine hydrochloride: an ethylenediamine with antihistamine, mild cholinergic, and slight sedative effects
℞ antiallergic effect: CH = PO: 5 mg/kg/24 hr, div, every 6 hr
†, PYRIBENZAMINE hydrochloride; tabl tripelennamine citrate, PYRIBENZAMINE citrate; elixir

Valproic acid, valproate; carboxylic acid (dipropylacetic acid), antiepileptic agent chemically unrelated to other antiseizure medications. Mechanism of anticonvulsant activity remains unknown but may be associated with increasing brain concentrations of γ-aminobutyric acid (GABA). Valproate may be used as monotherapy in combination with other anticonvulsants in the treatment of a wide range of seizure disorders.
℞ for treatment of seizures: CH = PO: 15 mg/kg/24 hr, div, every 8–12 hr; if needed, dosage may be increased, generally on a weekly basis, in increments of 5–10 mg/kg/24 hr up to a maximum recommended dose of 30–60 mg/kg/24 hr, div, every 8–12 hr
Caution: Valproate is highly protein bound (>90%) and may be associated with drug-protein displacement interactions. Valproate may retard hepatic drug metabolizing enzymes, slowing the metabolism of, and thus leading to increases in serum concentrations of other drugs, most notably other anticonvulsant agents. Fatal hepatic dysfunction has been reported in patients receiving valproate. Patients at primary risk for this fatal drug-induced toxicity appear to be children ≤2 years of age who are receiving valproate concurrently with other anticonvulsant agents. Thus, valproate should be used with extreme caution in children under the age of 2 years. Serum concentrations may be monitored, therapeutic range 50–100 mg/L (see Sec. 20.21).
†, DEPAKENE; caps, syrup; DEPAKOTE; enteric-coated tabs

Vancomycin, complex glycopeptide that inhibits synthesis of cell wall in gram-positive bacteria and is effective against methicillin-resistant staphylococci; in oral application effective in pseudomembraneous colitis caused by toxin-producing bacteria such as *Clostridium difficile* and *Staphylococcus aureus*; excreted mainly by kidneys
NB = IV: 20–30 mg/kg/24 hr, div, every 12 hr if ≤1 wk old, every 8 hr if >1 wk old
CH = IV (<500 mg/30 min): 40 mg/kg/24 hr, div, every 6–8 hr
Note: Reduce dosage in renal insufficiency. Therapy may be associated with ototoxicity and renal impairment, skin rashes ("red-man" syndrome), and hematologic side effects. Serum concentration should be monitored, therapeutic peak concentration 30–40 mg/L, trough 5–10 mg/L (see Table 27–2).
†, VANCOCIN; inj

Verapamil; calcium channel blocker. Toxic effects include allergic reactions, urticaria, bronchospasm, hypotension, decreased cardiac output, and asystole. Cardiac monitoring should be used during administration.
IN = IV: 0.1–0.2 mg/kg infused over 2 min
CH = IV: 0.1–0.3 mg/kg infused over 2 min
Maintenance dose = 1–2 mg/kg every 8 hr
CALAN, ISOPTIN; IV 2.5 mg/mL vial inj; PO tabs: 80, 120 mg

Vidarabine, antiviral agent used for treatment of neonatal herpes simplex infections.
IN = IV: 15–30 mg/kg infused over 12 hr every 24 hr for 10 days.
Note: May rarely cause hepatic and hematologic toxicity.
VIRA-A; 200 mg/mL vial inj

MICHAEL D. REED

TABLES 27–4 to 27–8: CONVERSION TABLES

TABLE 27–4. Method for Conversion of Milligrams to Milliequivalents per Liter (or to Millimoles per Liter)

mg = milligrams   mL = milliliter
g = grams   1 mL = 1.000027 cc
dL = deciliter = 100 mL

$$\text{mEq/L (milliequivalents per liter)} = \frac{\text{mg/L}}{\text{equivalent weight}}$$

$$\text{Equivalent weight} = \frac{\text{atomic weight}}{\text{valence of element}}$$

For example: A sample of blood serum contains 10 mg of Ca in 1 dL (100 mL). The valence of Ca is 2, and the atomic weight is 40. The equivalent weight of Ca is therefore 40 ÷ 2, or 20. The milliequivalents of Ca per liter are 10 (mg/dL) × 10 (dL/L) ÷ 20, or 5 milliequivalents per liter.

$$\text{mM/L (millimoles per liter)} = \frac{\text{mg/L}}{\text{molecular weight}}$$

Vol. % (volumes per cent) = mM/L × 2.24 for a gas whose properties approach that of an ideal gas, such as oxygen or nitrogen. For carbon dioxide the factor is 2.226.

TABLE 27–5. Factors for Conversion of Concentration Expressed in Milliequivalents per Liter to Milligrams per Deciliter (100 mL), and Vice Versa, for Common Ions That Occur in Physiologic Solutions

Element or Radical	mEq/L	to mg/dL	mg/dL	to mEq/L
Sodium	1	2.30	1	0.4348
Potassium	1	3.91	1	0.2558
Calcium	1	2.005	1	0.4988
Magnesium	1	1.215	1	0.8230
Chloride	1	3.55	1	0.2817
Bicarbonate (HCO_3)	1	6.1	1	0.1639
Phosphorus valence 1	1	3.10	1	0.3226
Phosphorus valence 1.8	1	1.72	1	0.5814
Sulfur valence 2	1	1.60	1	0.625

Example: To convert milliequivalents of magnesium per liter to milligrams per deciliter (100 mL), multiply by the factor 1.215.
To convert milligrams of potassium per deciliter (100 mL) to milliequivalents per liter, multiply by the factor 0.2558.

TABLE 27–6. Milliequivalents and Milligrams of Cations and Anions Present in a Millimole of Salts Commonly Used in Physiologic Solutions

Salt	mM/L	mg/L	Cation	Anion	mEq/L	mg/L	mEq/L	mg/L
Sodium chloride (NaCl)	1	58.5	Na^+	Cl^-	1	23.0	1	35.5
Potassium chloride (KCl)	1	74.6	K^+	Cl^-	1	39.1	1	35.5
Sodium bicarbonate ($NaHCO_3$)	1	84.0	Na^+	HCO_3^-	1	23.0	1	61.0
Sodium lactate ($CH_3CHOHCOONa$)	1	112.0	Na^+	$Lactate^-$	1	23.0	1	89.0
Potassium phosphate (K_2HPO_4) dibasic	1	174.2	K^+	HPO_4^{2-}	2	78.2	1	96.0
Potassium phosphate (KH_2PO_4) monobasic	1	136.1	K^+	$H_2PO_4^-$	1	39.1	1	97.0
Calcium chloride anhydrous ($CaCl_2$)		111.0	Ca^{2+}	Cl^-	2	40.0	2	71.0
Calcium chloride dihydrate ($CaCl_2 \cdot 2H_2O$)	1	147.0	Ca^{2+}	Cl^-	2	40.0	2	71.0
Magnesium chloride anhydrous ($MgCl_2$)	1	95.2	Mg^{2+}	Cl^-	2	24.3	2	71.0
Magnesium chloride hexahydrate ($MgCl_2 \cdot 6H_2O$)	1	203.3	Mg^{2+}	Cl^-	2	24.3	2	71.0
Ammonium chloride (NH_4Cl)	1	53.5	NH_4^+	Cl^-	1	18.0	1	35.5

TABLE 27–7. Conversion of Apothecary's Measures to Metric Equivalents

1 grain = 64 mg
60 minims = 1 fl dram = 3.7 mL
1 mL = 16.23 minims

TABLE 27–8. Equivalent Temperature Readings (Celsius and Fahrenheit)*

C	F	C	F	C	F	C	F
0	32.0	37.2	99	39.2	102.6	41.2	106.2
20	68.0	37.4	99.3	39.4	102.9	41.4	106.5
30	86.0	37.6	99.7	39.6	103.3	41.6	106.9
31	87.8	37.8	100.1	39.8	103.7	41.8	107.2
32	89.6	38.0	100.4	40.0	104	42	107.6
33	91.4	38.2	100.8	40.2	104.4	43	109.4
34	93.2	38.4	101.2	40.4	104.7	44	111.2
35	95.0	38.6	101.5	40.6	105.1	100	212
36	96.8	38.8	101.8	40.8	105.4		
37	98.6	39.0	102.2	41.0	105.8		

*To convert Celsius (centigrade) readings to Fahrenheit, multiply by 1.8 and add 32. To convert Fahrenheit readings to Celsius, subtract 32 and divide by 1.8.

TABLES 27–9 TO 27–11: NUTRITIONAL VALUES

TABLE 27–9. Composition of Commonly Used Oral and Parenteral Solutions

Fluid	CHO *g/dL*	Prot* *g/dL*	Calories *per L*	Na *mEq/L*	K *mEq/L*	Cl *mEq/L*	HCO_3† *mEq/L*	Ca *mEq/L*	P‡ *mEq/L*	Mg *mEq/L*	Osm§ *mOsm/kgH_2O*
						Oral					
Apple juice¶	11.9	0.1	480	0.4	26			3	4.5		700
Coca-Cola¶	10.9		435	4.3	0.1		13.4				656
Gatorade	5.9		250	21	2.5	17			6.8		377
Ginger ale¶	9.0		360	3.5	0.1		3.6				565
Grape juice¶	16.6	0.2	672	0.4	30		32				1027
Grapefruit juice¶ (canned, sugar added)	17.8	0.6	736	0.2	35			6.5			591
Hydra-lyte	2.5		100	84	10	59	15	<1	<1		300
Lytren	7.0		280	30	25	25	36	4	5	4	267**
Milk	4.9	3.5	670	22	36	28	30	60	54		260**
Orange juice¶	10.4	0.7	444	0.2	49		50				654
Pedialyte	5.0		200	30	20	30	28	4		4	387
Pepsi-Cola	12.0		480	6.5	0.8		7.3				—
Pineapple juice (canned)¶	13.5	0.4	556	0.2	38			7.5	9		783
Prune juice¶	19	0.4	776	0.9	60			7	20		—
Root beer¶				3.5	3.9						588
Seven-Up¶	8.0		320	7.5	0.2			0.3			564
Tomato juice (canned, salted)¶	4.3		172	100	59	150	10	3	18		592

Table continued on following page

TABLE 27–9. Composition of Commonly Used Oral and Parenteral Solutions *Continued*

Fluid	CHO *g/dL*	Prot*	Calories *per L*	Na *mEq/L*	K *mEq/L*	Cl *mEq/L*	HCO_3† *mEq/L*	Ca *mEq/L*	P‡ *mEq/L*	Mg *mEq/L*	Osm§ *mOsm/kgH_2O*
						Parenteral					
CHO†† in H_2O	5–10		200–400								266–532
Isotonic saline	0–5		0–200	154		154					292–558
½ Isotonic saline	2.5–5		100–200	77		77					280–415
3% (M/2) saline				513		513					969
5% Saline				855		855					1616
2.14% Ammonium chloride						400					
M/6 Sodium lactate				167			167				
5% Sodium bicarbonate				595			595				
Lactated Ringer solution	0–5–10		0–200–400	130	4	109	28	3			261–531–801
Modified Butler 1 (a)	5		200	25	20	22	23		3	3	360
Modified Butler 2 (b)	5–10		200–400	56	25	49	26		12	5	423–719**
Talbot (c)	5		200	40	35	40	20		15		409
Ordway (d)	3.5		140	26	27	53					281**
Gastric replacement (e)	5–10		200–400	63	17	150	(contains 71 mEq/L NH_4^+)				555–812**
Intestinal replacement (f)	10		390	80	36	64	60	5		3	800**
Protein hydrolysate 5% (g)		5	850	35	19	20		5	30	2	430**
Protein hydrolysate 10% (h)		10	1700	60	31	44		10	60	4	860**
Amino-acid preparation (i)		8.5		10					20		850**
Human plasma protein fraction (j)		5		110	2	50	50				
Blood‡‡		3		95	4	50	40		2	1–2	
Dextran 10% (low mol. wt.) (k)	5		200								
Dextran 10% in saline (l)				154		154					
Dextran 6% (high mol. wt.) (m)	5–10		200–400								
Dextran 6% in saline (n)				154		154					
Mannitol 20%§§											

AVAILABLE ADDITIVES

Glucose 50%	0.5 g/mL
Sodium chloride	0.5, 1, 2.5 and 5 mEq/mL
Sodium lactate	4 and 5 mEq/mL
Sodium bicarbonate	5 (4.2%) and 9 (7.5%) mEq/mL
Potassium chloride	1, 2 and 3 mEq/mL
Potassium phosphate	3 mEq/mL
Potassium acetate	2 and 2.5 mEq/mL
Calcium gluconate 10%	9.0 mg (0.45 mEq) calcium/mL
Calcium chloride 10%	27.2 mg (1.36 mEq) calcium/mL
Ammonium chloride	4 mEq/mL
Magnesium sulfate ($MgSO_4 \cdot 7H_2O$) 50% (also 10%, 12.5% and 25% available)	4 mEq/mL

SELECTED U.S. COMMERCIAL PREPARATIONS
(possible slight variations in composition from values in Table)

(A, Abbott; C, Cutter; M, McGaw; P, Pharmacia; T, Travenol)

(a)	Ionosol MB in D5W (A); Isolyte P with 5% Dextrose (M)
(b)	Ionosol B in D5W (A); Electrolyte #2 with 10% Invert Sugar (C,M); 10% Travert in Electrolyte #2 (T)
(c)	Ionosol T in D5W (A); Isolyte M (M)
(d)	Ordway solution with 3.5% Dextrose (C)
(e)	Ionosol G in D10W (A); Isolyte G with 5% Dextrose (M)
(f)	Ionosol D with 10% Invert Sugar (A); 10% Travert with Electrolyte #1 (T)
(g)	Amigen 5% (T)
(h)	Amigen 10% (T)
(i)	Free Amine 2 (M)
(j)	Plasmatein (A); Plasmanate (C)
(k)(l)	LMD 10% (A); Dextran 40 (C,M); Rheomacrodex (P); Gentran 40 (T)
(m)(n)	Dextran 75 (A); Macrodex (P); Gentran 75 in 10% Travert (T)

*Protein or amino acid equivalent.
†Actual or potential bicarbonate, such as acetate, lactate, citrate.
‡Calculated according to valence of 1.8.
§Osmolality except for values shown,** which are osmolarity (in mOsm/L).
¶Composition varies slightly depending on source.
**See § above.
††Glucose (dextrose, fructose or invert sugar).
‡‡Red cell contents not included in calculations.
§§Also available: mannitol 5%, 10%, 15%, and 20%.
(Sources: Church CF, Church HN: Food Values of Portions Commonly Used [Bowes and Church]. 11th ed. Philadelphia, JB Lippincott, 1970; Kastrup EK, Boyd JR: Facts and Comparisons. 1978. St. Louis, Facts and Comparisons, Inc., 1978; Murray BN, Peterson LJ: Unpublished observations. Additional values in Wendland BE, Arbus GS: Can Med Assoc J 121:564, 1979.)

TABLE 27–10. Food Composition Table for Short Method of Dietary Analysis

Food and Approximate Measure	Weight g	Food Energy kcal	Protein g	Fat g	Carbohydrate g	Calcium mg	Iron mg	Vitamin A Value IU	Thiamine mg	Riboflavin mg	Niacin mg	Ascorbic Acid mg
Milk, cheese, cream; related products												
Cheese: blue, cheddar (1 cu in, 17 g), cheddar process (1 oz), Swiss (1 oz)	30	105	6	9	1	165	0.2	345	0.01	0.12	Trace	0
cottage (from skim) creamed (½ c)	115	120	16	5	3	105	0.4	190	0.04	0.28	0.1	0
Cream: half-and-half (cream and milk) (2 tbsp)	30	40	1	4	2	30	Trace	145	0.01	0.04	Trace	Trace
For light whipping add 1 pat butter												
Milk: whole (3.5% fat) (1 c)	245	160	9	9	12	285	0.1	350	0.08	0.42	0.1	2
fluid, nonfat (skim) and buttermilk (from skim)	245	90	9	Trace	13	300	Trace	—	0.10	0.44	0.2	2
milk beverage (1 c): cocoa, chocolate drink made with skim milk. For malted milk add 4 tbsp half-and-half (270 g)	245	210	8	8	26	280	0.6	300	0.09	0.43	0.3	Trace
milk desserts, custard (1 c) 248 g, ice cream (8 fl oz) 142 g		290	8	17	29	210	0.4	785	0.07	0.34	0.1	1
cornstarch pudding (248 g), ice milk (1 c) 187 g		280	9	10	40	290	0.1	390	0.08	0.41	0.3	2
White sauce, med (½ c)	130	215	5	16	12	150	0.2	610	0.06	0.22	0.3	Trace
Egg: 1 large	50	80	6	6	Trace	25	1.2	590	0.06	0.15	Trace	0
Meat, poultry, fish, shellfish, related products												
Beef, lamb, veal: lean and fat, cooked, inc. corned beef (3 oz) (all cuts)	85	245	22	16	0	10	2.9	25	0.06	0.19	4.2	0
lean only, cooked; dried beef (2 + oz) (all cuts)	65	140	20	5	0	10	2.4	10	0.05	0.16	3.4	0
Beef, relatively fat, such as steak and rib, cooked (3 oz)	85	350	18	30	0	10	2.4	60	0.05	0.14	3.5	0
Liver: beef, fried (2 oz)	55	130	15	6	3	5	5.0	30,280	0.15	2.37	9.4	15
Pork, lean and fat, cooked (3 oz) (all cuts)	85	325	20	24	0	10	2.6	0	0.62	0.20	4.2	0
lean only, cooked (2 + oz) (all cuts)	60	150	18	8	0	5	2.2	0	0.57	0.19	3.2	0
ham, light cure, lean and fat, roasted (3 oz)	85	245	18	19	0	10	2.2	0	0.40	0.16	3.1	0
Luncheon meats: bologna (2 sl), pork sausage, cooked (2 oz), frankfurter (1), bacon, broiled or fried crisp (3 sl)		185	9	16	—	5	1.3	—	0.21	0.12	1.7	0
Poultry												
chicken: flesh only, broiled (3 oz)	85	115	20	3	0	10	1.4	80	0.05	0.16	7.4	0
fried (2 + oz)	75	170	24	6	1	10	1.6	85	0.05	0.23	8.3	0
turkey, light and dark, roasted (3 oz)	85	160	27	5	0	—	1.5	—	0.03	0.15	6.5	0
Fish and shellfish												
salmon (3 oz) (canned)	85	130	17	5	0	165	0.7	60	0.03	0.16	6.8	0
fish sticks, breaded, cooked (3-4)	75	130	13	7	5	10	0.3	—	0.03	0.05	1.2	0
mackerel, halibut, cooked	85	175	19	10	0	10	0.8	515	0.08	0.15	6.8	0
bluefish, haddock, herring, perch, shad, cooked (tuna canned in oil, 20 g)	85	160	19	8	2	20	1.0	60	0.06	0.11	4.4	0
clams, canned; crab meat, canned; lobster; oyster, raw; scallop; shrimp, canned	85	75	14	1	2	65	2.5	65	0.10	0.08	1.5	0
Mature dry beans and peas, nuts, peanuts, related products												
Beans: white with pork and tomato, canned (1 c)	260	320	16	7	50	140	4.7	340	0.20	0.08	1.5	5
red (128 g), lima (96 g), cowpeas (125 g), cooked (½ c)		125	8	—	25	35	2.5	5	0.13	0.06	0.7	—
Nuts: almonds (12), cashews (8), peanuts (1 tbsp), peanut butter (1 tbsp), pecans (12), English walnuts (2 tbsp), coconut (¼ c)	15	95	3	8	4	15	0.5	5	0.05	0.04	0.9	—
Vegetables and vegetable products												
Asparagus, cooked, cut spears (⅔ c)	115	25	3	Trace	4	25	0.7	1,055	0.19	0.20	1.6	30
Beans: green (½ c) cooked 60 g; canned 120 g		15	1	Trace	3	30	0.4	340	0.04	0.06	0.3	8
Lima, immature, cooked (½ c)	80	90	6	1	16	40	2.0	225	0.14	0.08	1.0	14
Broccoli spears, cooked (⅔ c)	100	25	3	Trace	4	90	0.8	2,500	0.09	0.20	0.8	90
Brussels sprouts, cooked (⅔ c)	85	30	3	Trace	5	30	1.0	450	0.07	0.12	0.7	75
Cabbage (110 g); cauliflower, cooked (80 g); and sauerkraut, canned (150 mg) (reduced ascorbic acid value by one third for kraut) (⅔ c)		20	1	Trace	4	35	0.5	80	0.05	0.05	0.3	37
Carrots, cooked (⅔ c)	95	30	1	Trace	7	30	0.6	10,145	0.05	0.05	0.5	6
Corn, 1 ear, cooked (140 g); canned (130 g) (½ c)		75	2	Trace	18	5	0.4	315	0.06	0.06	1.1	6
Leafy greens: collards (125 g), dandelions (120 g), kale (75 g), mustard (95 g), spinach (120 g), turnip (100 g cooked, 150 g canned) (⅔ c cooked and canned) (reduce ascorbic acid one half for canned)		30	3	Trace	5	175	1.8	8,570	0.11	0.18	0.8	45

Table continued on following page

TABLE 27–10. Food Composition Table for Short Method of Dietary Analysis *Continued*

Food and Approximate Measure	Weight *g*	Food Energy *kcal*	Protein *g*	Fat *g*	Carbohydrate *g*	Calcium *mg*	Iron *mg*	Vitamin A Value *IU*	Thiamine *mg*	Riboflavin *mg*	Niacin *mg*	Ascorbic Acid *mg*
Peas, green (½ c)	80	60	4	1	10	20	1.4	430	0.22	0.09	1.8	16
Potatoes, baked, boiled (100 g), 10 pc. French fried (55 g) (for fried, add 1 tbsp cooking oil)		85	3	Trace	30	10	0.7	Trace	0.08	0.04	1.5	16
Pumpkin, canned (½ c)	115	40	1	1	9	30	0.5	7,295	0.03	0.06	0.6	6
Squash, winter, canned (½ c)	100	65	2	1	16	30	0.8	4,305	0.05	0.14	0.7	14
Sweet potato, canned (½ c)	110	120	2	—	27	25	0.8	8,500	0.05	0.05	0.7	15
Tomato, 1 raw, ⅔ c canned, ⅔ c juice	150	35	2	Trace	7	14	0.8	1,350	0.10	0.06	1.0	29
Tomato catsup (2 tbsp)	35	30	1	Trace	8	10	0.2	480	0.04	0.02	0.6	6
Other, cooked (beets, mushrooms, onions, turnips) (½ c)	95	25	1	—	5	20	0.5	15	0.02	0.10	0.7	7
Other commonly served raw, cabbage (½ c, 50 g), celery (3 sm stalks, 40 g), cucumber (¼ med, 50 g), green pepper (½, 30 g), radishes (5, 40 g)		10	Trace	Trace	2	15	0.3	100	0.03	0.03	0.2	20
carrots, raw (½ carrot)	25	10	Trace	Trace	2	10	0.2	2,750	0.02	0.02	0.2	2
lettuce leaves (2 lg)	50	10	1	Trace	2	34	0.7	950	0.03	0.04	0.2	9
Fruits and fruit products												
Cantaloupe (½ med)	385	60	1	Trace	14	25	0.8	6,540	0.08	0.06	1.2	63
Citrus and strawberries: orange (1), grapefruit (½), juice (½ c), strawberries (½ c), lemon (1), tangerine (1)		50	1	—	13	25	0.4	165	0.08	0.03	0.3	55
Yellow, fresh: apricots (3), peach (2 med); canned fruit and juice (½ c) or dried, cooked, unsweetened: apricot, peaches (½ c)		85	—	—	22	10	1.1	1,005	0.01	0.05	1.0	5
Other, dried: dates, pitted (4), figs (2), raisins (¼ c)	40	120	1	—	31	35	1.4	20	0.04	0.04	0.5	—
Other, fresh: apple (1), banana (1), figs (3), pear (1)		80	—	—	21	15	0.5	140	0.04	0.03	0.2	6
Grain products												
Enriched and whole grain: bread (1 sl, 23 g), biscuit (½), cooked cereals (½ c), prepared cereals (1 oz); Graham crackers (2 lg), macaroni, noodles, spaghetti (½ c, cooked), pancake (1, 27 g), roll (½), waffle (½, 38 g)		65	2	1	16	20	0.6	10	0.09	0.05	0.7	—
Unenriched: bread (1 sl, 23 g), cooked cereal (½ c), macaroni, noodles, spaghetti (½ c), popcorn (½ c), pretzel sticks, small (15), roll (½)		65	2	1	16	10	0.3	5	0.02	0.02	0.3	—
Desserts												
Cake, plain (1 pc), doughnut (1). For iced cake or doughnut add value for sugar (1 tbsp). For chocolate cake add chocolate (30 g)	45	145	2	5	24	30	0.4	65	0.02	0.05	0.2	—
Cookies, plain (1)	25	120	1	5	18	10	0.2	20	0.01	0.01	0.1	—
Pie crust, single crust (⅐ shell)	20	95	1	6	8	3	0.3	0	0.04	0.03	0.3	—
Flour, white, enriched (1 tbsp)	7	25	1	Trace	5	1	0.2	0	0.03	0.02	0.2	0
Fats and oils												
Butter, margarine (1 pat, ½ tbsp)	7	50	Trace	6	Trace	1	0	230	—	—	—	—
Fats and oils, cooking (1 tbsp), French dressing (2 tbsp)	14	125	0	14	0	0	0	0	0	0	0	0
Salad dressings, mayonnaise type (1 tbsp)	15	80	Trace	9	1	2	0.1	45	Trace	Trace	Trace	0
Sugars, sweets												
Candy, plain (½ oz), jam and jelly (1 tbsp), syrup (1 tbsp), gelatin dessert, plain (½ c), beverages, carbonated (1 c)		60	0	0	14	3	0.1	Trace	Trace	Trace	Trace	Trace
Chocolate fudge (1 oz), chocolate syrup (3 tbsp)		125	1	2	30	15	0.6	10	Trace	0.02	0.1	Trace
Molasses (1 tbsp), caramel (½ oz)		40	Trace	Trace	8	20	0.3	Trace	Trace	Trace	Trace	Trace
Sugar (1 tbsp)	12	45	0	0	12	0	Trace	0	0	0	0	0
Miscellaneous												
Chocolate, bitter (1 oz)	30	145	3	15	8	20	1.9	20	0.01	0.07	0.4	0
Sherbet (½ c)	96	130	1	1	30	15	Trace	55	0.01	0.03	Trace	2
Soups: bean, pea (green) (1 c)		150	7	4	22	50	1.6	495	0.09	0.06	1.0	4
noodle, beef, chicken (1 c)		65	4	2	7	10	0.7	50	0.03	0.04	0.9	Trace
clam chowder, minestrone, tomato, vegetable (1 c)		90	3	2	14	25	0.9	1,880	0.05	0.04	1.1	3

*From Wilson ED, Fisher KH, Fuqua ME: Principles of Nutrition. 2nd ed. New York, John Wiley & Sons, 1965, pp 528–33.

TABLE 27–11. Nutritive Value of Baby Foods (Per Serving)*

Food	Serving g	Energy kcal	Protein g	Fat g	Carbo-hydrate g	Sodium mg	Calcium mg	Iron mg	Vitamin A Value IU	Thiamine mg	Ribo-flavin mg	Niacin mg	Ascorbic Acid mg
Cereals													
Barley	2.4	9	0.3	0.1	1.8	1	19	1.1		0.07	0.07	0.9	0
High protein	2.4	9	0.9	0.1	1.1	1	17	1.8		0.06	0.07	0.8	0
Mixed	2.4	9	0.3	0.1	1.8	1	18	1.5		0.06	0.07	0.8	0
Oatmeal	2.4	10	0.3	0.2	1.7	1	18	1.8		0.07	0.06	0.9	0
Rice	2.4	9	0.2	0.1	1.9	1	20	1.8		0.06	0.05	0.8	0
Dinners, jar													
Beef and egg noodle	213	122	5.4	4.0	15.7	37	18	0.9	1,400	0.06	0.08	1.2	3
Chicken and noodles, jr.	213	109	4.1	3.0	16.1	36	36	0.8	1,900	0.06	0.07	1.1	3
Macroni and ham, jr.	213	127	6.8	2.9	18.0	101	159	0.8	1,100	0.12	0.21	1.7	5
Turkey and rice, jr.	213	104	3.8	2.9	15.3	33	50	0.6	2,200	0.02	0.06	0.6	3
Spaghetti, tomato, beef, jr.	213	135	5.4	2.7	21.6	42	39	1.1	1,500	0.14	0.15	2.3	5
Fruits													
Applesauce jr.	213	79	0.1	0.0	21.9	5	10	0.4	20	0.03	0.06	0.1	81
Applesauce, apricots jr.	220	104	0.5	0.5	27.3	6	13	0.6	745	0.03	0.07	0.3	39
Bananas, tapioca jr.	220	147	0.8	0.4	39.1	21	17	0.7	100	0.03	0.04	0.5	57
Peaches	220	157	1.3	0.4	41.6	10	11	0.6	400	0.03	0.07	1.4	42
Pears	213	93	0.6	0.2	24.7	4	18	0.5	70	0.03	0.06	0.4	47
Meats, poultry													
Beef	99	105	14.3	4.9	0	65	8	1.6	100	0.01	0.16	3.3	2
Chicken	99	148	14.6	9.5	0	50	54	1.0	200	0.01	0.16	3.4	2
Ham	99	123	14.9	6.6	0	66	5	1.0	30	0.14	0.19	2.8	2
Lamb	99	111	15.0	5.2	2.5	73	7	1.6	30	0.02	0.20	3.2	2
Turkey	99	128	15.2	7.0	0	72	28	1.3	600	0.02	0.25	3.4	2
Egg yolks	94	191	9.4	16.3	0.9	37	72	2.6	1,200	0.07	0.25	1.45	1
Vegetables													
Beans	206	51	2.5	0.3	11.8	3	133	2.2	900	0.04	0.21	0.7	17
Beets	128	43	1.7	0.1	9.8	106	18	0.4	40	0.01	0.06	0.2	4
Carrots	213	67	1.7	0.4	15.4	104	49	0.8	25,000	0.05	0.09	1.1	12
Mixed	213	88	3.1	0.8	17.4	77	24	0.9	9,000	0.06	0.07	1.4	5
Peas	213	113	7.0	1.1	19.0	15	34	1.9	700	0.15	0.13	2.0	9
Squash	213	51	1.8	0.4	12.0	3	50	0.7	4,000	0.02	0.14	0.8	17
Sweet potatoes	220	113	2.4	0.3	30.7	49	35	0.8	15,000	0.06	0.08	0.8	21

*Data from Pennington JAT (ed): Bowes and Church's Food Values of Portions Commonly Used, 15th ed. New York, Harper & Row, 1989.

INDEX

Note: Page numbers in *italics* refer to illustrations; page numbers followed by t refer to tables.